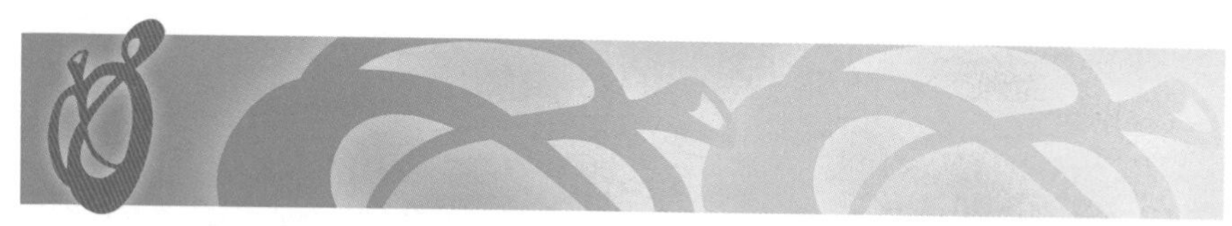

BRAUNWALD'S HEART DISEASE

A Textbook of Cardiovascular Medicine

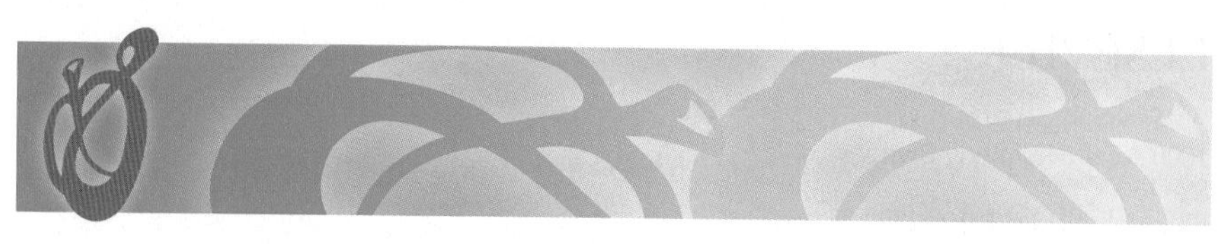

BRAUNWALD'S HEART DISEASE

A Textbook of Cardiovascular Medicine

NINTH EDITION

Edited by

Robert O. Bonow, MD
Max and Lilly Goldberg Distinguished Professor of Cardiology
Vice Chairman, Department of Medicine
Director, Center for Cardiac Innovation
Northwestern University Feinberg School of Medicine
Chicago, Illinois

Douglas L. Mann, MD
Lewin Chair and Professor of Medicine, Cell Biology, and Physiology
Chief, Division of Cardiology
Washington University School of Medicine in St. Louis
Cardiologist-in-Chief
Barnes-Jewish Hospital
Saint Louis, Missouri

Douglas P. Zipes, MD
Distinguished Professor
Professor Emeritus of Medicine, Pharmacology, and Toxicology
Director Emeritus, Division of Cardiology and the Krannert Institute of Cardiology
Indiana University School of Medicine
Indianapolis, Indiana

Peter Libby, MD
Mallinckrodt Professor of Medicine
Harvard Medical School
Chief, Cardiovascular Division
Brigham and Women's Hospital
Boston, Massachusetts

Founding Editor and Online Editor

Eugene Braunwald, MD, MD(Hon), ScD(Hon), FRCP
Distinguished Hersey Professor of Medicine
Harvard Medical School
Chairman, TIMI Study Group
Brigham and Women's Hospital
Boston, Massachusetts

ELSEVIER
SAUNDERS

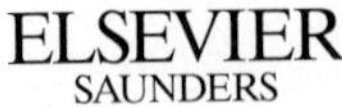

SAUNDERS

1600 John F. Kennedy Blvd.
Ste. 1800
Philadelphia, PA 19103-2899

BRAUNWALD'S HEART DISEASE: A TEXTBOOK OF CARDIOVASCULAR MEDICINE.

Single Volume: 978-1-4377-0398-6
Two-Volume Set: 978-1-4377-2708-1
International Edition: 978-0-8089-2436-4

Library of Congress Cataloging-in-Publication Data

Robert O. Bonow … [et al.].—9th ed.
p. ; cm.
Heart disease
Includes bibliographical references and index.
ISBN 978-1-4377-0398-6 (single volume : hardcover : alk. paper)—ISBN 978-1-4377-2708-1 (two-volume set : hardcover : alk. paper)—ISBN 978-0-8089-2436-4 (international ed. : hardcover : alk. paper)
1. Heart—Diseases. 2. Cardiology. I. Braunwald, Eugene, 1929- II. Bonow, Robert O. III. Title: Heart disease.
[DNLM: 1. Heart Diseases. 2. Cardiovascular Diseases. WG 210]
RC681.H36 2012
616.1'2—dc22

2010044324

Executive Publisher: Natasha Andjelkovic
Developmental Editor: Anne Snyder
Publishing Services Manager: Patricia Tannian
Team Manager: Radhika Pallamparthy
Senior Project Manager: Sarah Wunderly
Project Manager: Joanna Dhanabalan
Design Direction: Steven Stave

Printed in China

Last digit is the print number: 9 8 7 6 5 4 3 2 1

Dedication

We are proud to dedicate the ninth edition of *Braunwald's Heart Disease* to its founder, Eugene Braunwald, MD. The first edition of this work, published 30 years ago, established a standard of excellence that is rarely, if ever, achieved in publishing. Dr. Braunwald personally wrote half of the book and expertly edited the rest. He did the same for the next four editions, taking a 6-month sabbatical every 4 to 5 years to accomplish that. For the sixth edition, published in 2001, he invited two of us (PL, DPZ) to share the experience with him, increasing the editors by one (ROB) for the seventh edition. A new editor (DLM) joined for the eighth edition, and Dr. Braunwald no longer directly participated in the day-to-day editing of the print text, while still contributing some of the key chapters. However, he kept his finger on the pulse of the text and for that edition began *twice-weekly* electronic updates. Incorporating the most recent research, reviews, and opinions into the electronic text has continued through this ninth edition, making *Braunwald's Heart Disease* truly a living work and setting it apart from other texts. Dr. Braunwald, through his research, teaching, and mentorship, has shaped much of contemporary cardiovascular medicine, and it is with gratitude and admiration that we dedicate this edition of *his work* to him.

Robert O. Bonow

Douglas L. Mann

Douglas P. Zipes

Peter Libby

Acknowledgments

The editors gratefully acknowledge communication and correspondence from colleagues all over the world who have offered insightful suggestions to improve this text. We particularly wish to acknowledge the following individuals who have provided careful and studious commentary on numerous chapters: Shabnam Madadi, MD, Cardiac Imaging Center, Shahid Rajaei Heart Center, Tehran, Iran; Azin Alizadeh Asl, MD, Tabriz University of Medical Sciences and Madani Heart Hospital, Tabriz, Iran; Leili Pourafkari, MD, Razi Hospital, Tabriz, Iran; Banasiak Waldemar, MD, Centre for Heart Disease, Military Hospital, Wroclaw, Poland; Carlos Benjamín Alvarez, MD, PhD, Sacré Coeur Institute, Buenos Aires, Argentina; Elias B. Hanna, MD, Division of Cardiology, Louisiana State University, New Orleans, Louisiana.

We are also indebted to Dr. Jun-o Deguchi, Dr. Michael Markl, Dr. Vera Rigolin, and Dr. Carol Warnes for the images used on the cover.

Dr. Libby thanks Sara Karwacki for expert editorial assistance.

To:

Pat, Rob, and Sam

Laura, Stephanie, Jonathan, and Erica

Joan, Debra, Jeffrey, and David

Beryl, Oliver, and Brigitte

CONTRIBUTORS

William T. Abraham, MD
Professor of Internal Medicine, Physiology, and Cell Biology; Chair of Excellence in Cardiovascular Medicine; Director, Division of Cardiovascular Medicine; Deputy Director, The Davis Heart and Lung Research Institute, The Ohio State University, Columbus, Ohio
Devices for Monitoring and Managing Heart Failure

Michael A. Acker, MD
Professor of Surgery, University of Pennsylvania School of Medicine; Chief, Division of Cardiovascular Surgery, University of Pennsylvania Medical Center, Philadelphia, Pennsylvania
Surgical Management of Heart Failure

Michael J. Ackerman, MD, PhD
Professor of Medicine, Pediatrics, and Pharmacology; Consultant, Cardiovascular Diseases and Pediatric Cardiology; Director, Long QT Syndrome Clinic and the Windland Smith Rice Sudden Death Genomics Laboratory, Mayo Clinic, Rochester, Minnesota
Genetics of Cardiac Arrhythmias

Philip A. Ades, MD
Professor of Medicine, Division of Cardiology, Fletcher-Allen Health Care, University of Vermont College of Medicine, Burlington, Vermont
Exercise and Sports Cardiology

Elliott M. Antman, MD
Professor of Medicine, Harvard Medical School; Senior Investigator, TIMI Study Group, Brigham and Women's Hospital, Boston, Massachusetts
Design and Conduct of Clinical Trials; ST-Segment Elevation Myocardial Infarction: Pathology, Pathophysiology, and Clinical Features; ST-Segment Elevation Myocardial Infarction: Management; Guidelines: Management of Patients with ST-Segment Elevation Myocardial Infarction

Piero Anversa, MD
Professor of Anesthesia and Medicine; Director, Center for Regenerative Medicine, Brigham and Women's Hospital, Harvard Medical School, Boston, Massachusetts
Cardiovascular Regeneration and Tissue Engineering

Gary J. Balady, MD
Professor of Medicine, Boston University School of Medicine; Director, Non-Invasive Cardiovascular Laboratories, Section of Cardiology, Boston Medical Center, Boston, Massachusetts
Exercise and Sports Cardiology

Kenneth L. Baughman, MD (deceased)
Professor of Medicine, Harvard Medical School; Director, Advanced Heart Disease, Division of Cardiovascular Medicine, Brigham and Women's Hospital, Boston, Massachusetts
Myocarditis

Joshua Beckman, MD, MSc
Assistant Professor of Medicine, Harvard Medical School; Director, Cardiovascular Fellowship, Cardiovascular Division, Brigham and Women's Hospital, Boston, Massachusetts
Anesthesia and Noncardiac Surgery in Patients with Heart Disease; Guidelines: Reducing Cardiac Risk with Noncardiac Surgery

Michael A. Bettmann, MD
Professor and Vice Chair for Interventional Services, Department of Radiology, Wake Forest University Baptist Medical Center, Medical Center Boulevard, Winston-Salem, North Carolina
The Chest Radiograph in Cardiovascular Disease

Deepak L. Bhatt, MD, MPH
Associate Professor of Medicine, Harvard Medical School; Chief of Cardiology, VA Boston Healthcare System; Director, Integrated Interventional Cardiovascular Program, Brigham and Women's Hospital & VA Boston Healthcare System; Senior Investigator, TIMI Study Group, Brigham and Women's Hospital, Boston, Massachusetts
Percutaneous Coronary Intervention; Guidelines: Percutaneous Coronary Intervention; Endovascular Treatment of Noncoronary Obstructive Vascular Disease

William E. Boden, MD
Professor of Medicine and Preventive Medicine; Clinical Chief, Division of Cardiovascular Medicine, University at Buffalo Schools of Medicine & Public Health; Medical Director, Cardiovascular Services, Kaleida Health; Chief of Cardiology, Buffalo General and Millard Fillmore Hospitals, Buffalo, New York
Stable Ischemic Heart Disease; Guidelines: Chronic Stable Angina

Robert O. Bonow, MD
Max and Lilly Goldberg Distinguished Professor of Cardiology; Vice Chairman, Department of Medicine; Director, Center for Cardiovascular Innovation, Northwestern University Feinberg School of Medicine, Chicago, Illinois
Cardiac Catheterization; Nuclear Cardiology; Guidelines: Infective Endocarditis; Care of Patients with End-Stage Heart Disease; Valvular Heart Disease; Guidelines: Management of Valvular Heart Disease; Appropriate Use Criteria: Echocardiography

Eugene Braunwald, MD, MD(Hon), ScD(Hon), FRCP
Distinguished Hersey Professor of Medicine, Harvard Medical School; Founding Chairman, TIMI Study Group, Brigham and Women's Hospital, Boston, Massachusetts
Unstable Angina and Non–ST Elevation Myocardial Infarction; Guidelines: Unstable Angina and Non–ST Elevation Myocardial Infarction

Alan C. Braverman, MD
Alumni Endowed Professor in Cardiovascular Diseases; Professor of Medicine; Director, Marfan Syndrome Clinic; Director, Inpatient Cardiology Firm, Washington University School of Medicine, St. Louis, Missouri
Diseases of the Aorta

J. Douglas Bremner, MD
Professor of Psychiatry and Radiology, Department of Psychiatry and Behavioral Sciences, Emory University School of Medicine & Atlanta VAMC, Atlanta, Georgia
Psychiatric and Behavioral Aspects of Cardiovascular Disease

Hugh Calkins, MD
Nicholas J. Fortuin Professor of Cardiology; Professor of Medicine, The Johns Hopkins Medical University School of Medicine; Director of the Arrhythmia Service and Clinical Electrophysiology Laboratory, The Johns Hopkins Hospital, Baltimore, Maryland
Hypotension and Syncope

Christopher P. Cannon, MD
Associate Professor of Medicine, Harvard Medical School; Senior Investigator, TIMI Study Group, Cardiovascular Division, Brigham and Women's Hospital, Boston, Massachusetts
Approach to the Patient with Chest Pain; Unstable Angina and Non–ST Elevation Myocardial Infarction; Guidelines: Unstable Angina and Non–ST Elevation Myocardial Infarction

John M. Canty, Jr., MD
Albert and Elizabeth Rekate Professor of Medicine; Chief, Division of Cardiovascular Medicine, University at Buffalo, Buffalo, New York
Coronary Blood Flow and Myocardial Ischemia

Agustin Castellanos, MD
Professor of Medicine, University of Miami Miller School of Medicine; Director, Clinical Electrophysiology, University of Miami/Jackson Memorial Medical Center, Miami, Florida
Cardiac Arrest and Sudden Cardiac Death

Bernard R. Chaitman, MD
Professor of Medicine; Director, Cardiovascular Research, St. Louis University School of Medicine, Division of Cardiology, St. Louis, Missouri
Exercise Stress Testing; Guidelines: Exercise Stress Testing

Ming Hui Chen, MD, MMSc
Assistant Professor of Medicine, Harvard Medical School; Director, Cardiac Health for Hodgkin's Lymphoma Survivors; Associate in Cardiology, Department of Cardiology, Children's Hospital Boston, Boston, Massachusetts
The Cancer Patient and Cardiovascular Disease

Heidi M. Connolly, MD
Professor of Medicine, Mayo Clinic College of Medicine; Consultant, Division of Cardiovascular Diseases, Mayo Clinic, Rochester, Minnesota
Echocardiography

Mark A. Creager, MD
Professor of Medicine, Harvard Medical School; Director, Vascular Center, Brigham and Women's Hospital, Boston, Massachusetts
Peripheral Artery Diseases

Edécio Cunha-Neto, MD, PhD
Associate Professor of Immunology, University of São Paulo; Researcher of the Cardiac Immunology Laboratory, The Heart Institute (INCOR), University of São Paulo Medical School, São Paulo, Brazil
Chagas' Disease

Charles J. Davidson, MD
Professor of Medicine; Medical Director, Bluhm Cardiovascular Institute; Clinical Chief, Division of Cardiology, Northwestern University Feinberg School of Medicine, Chicago, Illinois
Cardiac Catheterization

Vasken Dilsizian, MD
Professor of Medicine and Diagnostic Radiology; Chief, Division of Nuclear Medicine; Director, Cardiovascular Nuclear Medicine and PET Imaging, University of Maryland School of Medicine, Baltimore, Maryland
Nuclear Cardiology

Stefanie Dimmeler, PhD
Professor and Director of the Institute of Cardiovascular Regeneration, Centre for Molecular Medicine, Goethe-University Frankfurt, Frankfurt, Germany
Emerging Therapies and Strategies in the Treatment of Heart Failure

Pamela S. Douglas, MD
Ursula Geller Professor of Research in Cardiovascular Diseases, Division of Cardiovascular Medicine, Duke University Medical Center, Durham, North Carolina
Cardiovascular Disease in Women

Andrew C. Eisenhauer, MD
Assistant Professor of Medicine, Harvard Medical School; Director, Interventional Cardiovascular Medicine Service; Associate Director, Cardiac Catheterization Laboratory, Brigham and Women's Hospital; Director, Cardiac Quality Assurance, Partners Health Care, Boston, Massachusetts
Endovascular Treatment of Noncoronary Obstructive Vascular Disease

Linda L. Emanuel, MD, PhD
Buehler Professor of Geriatric Medicine; Director, The Buehler Center on Aging, Northwestern University Feinberg School of Medicine, Chicago, Illinois
Care of Patients with End-Stage Heart Disease

Edzard Ernst, MD, PhD, FMed Sci, FRCP, FRCP(Edin)
Chair in Complementary Medicine, Peninsula Medical School, University of Exeter, Exeter, United Kingdom
Complementary and Alternative Approaches to Management of Patients with Heart Disease

James C. Fang, MD
Professor of Medicine, Division of Cardiovascular Medicine, Case Western Reserve University School of Medicine, Harrington-McLaughlin Heart and Vascular Institute, University Hospitals, Cleveland, Ohio
The History and Physical Examination: An Evidence-Based Approach

G. Michael Felker, MD, MHS
Associate Professor of Medicine, Division of Cardiology, Duke University School of Medicine, Durham, North Carolina
Diagnosis and Management of Acute Heart Failure Syndromes

Gerasimos S. Filippatos, MD
Head, Heart Failure Unit, Attikon University Hospital, Department of Cardiology, University of Athens, Athens, Greece
Diagnosis and Management of Acute Heart Failure Syndromes

Stacy D. Fisher, MD
Director of Women's and Complex Heart Disease, Department of Cardiology, University of Maryland Comprehensive Heart Center, Baltimore, Maryland
Cardiovascular Abnormalities in HIV-Infected Individuals

Lee A. Fleisher, MD
Roberts D. Dripps Professor and Chair of Anesthesiology and Critical Care; Professor of Medicine, University of Pennsylvania School of Medicine, Philadelphia, Pennsylvania
Anesthesia and Noncardiac Surgery in Patients with Heart Disease; Guidelines: Reducing Cardiac Risk with Noncardiac Surgery

Thomas Force, MD
Wilson Professor of Medicine, Thomas Jefferson University; Clinical Director, Center for Translational Medicine, Thomas Jefferson University Hospital, Philadelphia, Pennsylvania
The Cancer Patient and Cardiovascular Disease

J. Michael Gaziano, MD, MPH
Professor of Medicine, Harvard Medical School; Chief, Division of Aging, Brigham and Women's Hospital; Director, Massachusetts Veterans Epidemiology and Research Information Center (MAVERIC), VA Boston Healthcare System, Boston, Massachusetts
Global Burden of Cardiovascular Disease; Primary and Secondary Prevention of Coronary Heart Disease

Thomas A. Gaziano MD, MSc
Assistant Professor, Harvard Medical School; Associate Physician, Cardiovascular Medicine, Brigham & Women's Hospital, Boston, Massachusetts
Global Burden of Cardiovascular Disease

Jacques Genest, MD
Professor of Medicine; Scientific Director, Center for Innovative Medicine, McGill University Health Center, McGill University, Montreal, Quebec, Canada
Lipoprotein Disorders and Cardiovascular Disease

Mihai Gheorghiade, MD
Professor of Medicine and Surgery; Director, Experimental Therapeutics/Center for Cardiovascular Innovation; Northwestern University Feinberg School of Medicine, Chicago, Illinois; Co-Director, Duke Cardiovascular Center for Drug Development, Raleigh, North Carolina
Diagnosis and Management of Acute Heart Failure Syndromes

Ary L. Goldberger, MD
Professor of Medicine, Harvard Medical School & Wyss Institute for Biologically Inspired Engineering at Harvard University; Director, Margret and H.A. Rey Institute for Nonlinear Dynamics in Medicine, Beth Israel Deaconess Medical Center, Boston, Massachusetts
Electrocardiography; Guidelines: Electrocardiography

Samuel Z. Goldhaber, MD
Professor of Medicine, Harvard Medical School; Director, Venous Thromboembolism Research Group; Staff Cardiologist, Cardiovascular Medicine Division, Brigham and Women's Hospital, Boston, Massachusetts
Pulmonary Embolism

Larry B. Goldstein, MD
Professor, Department of Medicine (Neurology), Duke Stroke Center; Center for Clinical Health Policy Research, Duke University and Durham VA Medical Center, Durham, North Carolina
Prevention and Management of Stroke

Richard J. Gray, MD
Medical Director, Sutter Pacific Heart Centers, California Pacific Medical Center, San Francisco, California
Medical Management of the Patient Undergoing Cardiac Surgery

Barry Greenberg, MD
Professor of Medicine; Director, Advanced Heart Failure Treatment Program, University of California, San Diego, California
Clinical Assessment of Heart Failure

Bartley P. Griffith, MD
The Thomas E. and Alice Marie Hales Distinguished Professor/ Professor of Surgery & Chief, Division of Cardiac Surgery, Department of Surgery, Division of Cardiac Surgery, University of Maryland School of Medicine, Baltimore, Maryland
Assisted Circulation in the Treatment of Heart Failure

William J. Groh, MD, MPH
Associate Professor of Medicine, Division of Cardiology, Indiana University, Indianapolis, Indiana
Neurologic Disorders and Cardiovascular Disease

Joshua M. Hare, MD
Louis Lemberg Professor of Medicine; Professor of Biomedical Engineering; Professor of Molecular and Cellular Pharmacology; Director, Interdisciplinary Stem Cell Institute, University of Miami Miller School of Medicine, Miami, Florida
The Dilated, Restrictive, and Infiltrative Cardiomyopathies

Gerd Hasenfuss, MD
Professor and Chair, Department of Cardiology and Pneumology, Heart Center, University of Goettingen; Chair of Heart Research Center, Goettingen, Germany
Mechanisms of Cardiac Contraction and Relaxation

David L. Hayes, MD
Professor of Medicine, College of Medicine; Consultant, Division of Cardiovascular Diseases, Mayo Clinic, Rochester, Minnesota
Pacemakers and Implantable Cardioverter-Defibrillators; Guidelines: Cardiac Pacemakers and Cardioverter-Defibrillators

Maria de Lourdes Higuchi, MD
Director of Laboratory of Research on Cardiac Inflammation and Infection, Heart Institute (INCOR), University of São Paulo Medical School, São Paulo, Brazil
Chagas' Disease

L. David Hillis, MD
Professor and Chair, Internal Medicine, University of Texas Health Science Center, San Antonio, Texas
Toxins and the Heart

Farouc A. Jaffer, MD, PhD
Assistant Professor of Medicine, Cardiology Division and Cardiovascular Research Center, Department of Medicine, Massachusetts General Hospital, Harvard Medical School, Boston, Massachusetts
Molecular Imaging in Cardiovascular Disease

Mariell Jessup, MD
Professor of Medicine; Associate Chief for Clinical Affairs, Cardiovascular Division, University of Pennsylvania School of Medicine; Medical Director, Penn Heart and Vascular Center, University of Pennsylvania Health System, Philadelphia, Pennsylvania
Surgical Management of Heart Failure

Andrew M. Kahn, MD, PhD
Assistant Professor of Medicine, University of California, San Diego, California
Clinical Assessment of Heart Failure

Jan Kajstura, PhD
Associate Professor, Departments of Anesthesia and Medicine, and Cardiovascular Division, Brigham and Women's Hospital, Harvard Medical School, Boston, Massachusetts
Cardiovascular Regeneration and Tissue Engineering

Norman M. Kaplan, MD
Clinical Professor of Internal Medicine, University of Texas Southwestern Medical Center at Dallas, Dallas, Texas
Systemic Hypertension: Therapy; Guidelines: Treatment of Hypertension

Adolf W. Karchmer, MD
Professor of Medicine, Harvard Medical School; Division of Infectious Disease, Beth Israel Deaconess Medical Center, Boston, Massachusetts
Infective Endocarditis

Irwin Klein, MD
Professor of Medicine and Cell Biology; Associate Chairman, Department of Medicine, North Shore University Hospital, Manhasset, New York
Endocrine Disorders and Cardiovascular Disease

Harlan M. Krumholz, MD, SM
Harold H. Hines, Jr, Professor of Medicine and Epidemiology and Public Health; Section of Cardiovascular Medicine, Department of Medicine, Section of Health Policy and Administration, School of Public Health, Yale University School of Medicine; Center for Outcomes Research and Evaluation, Yale–New Haven Hospital, New Haven, Connecticut
Clinical Decision Making in Cardiology

Raymond Y. Kwong, MD, MPH
Assistant Professor of Medicine, Harvard Medical School; Director of Cardiac Magnetic Resonance Imaging, Cardiovascular Division, Brigham and Women's Hospital, Boston, Massachusetts
Cardiovascular Magnetic Resonance Imaging; Appropriate Use Criteria: Cardiovascular Magnetic Resonance

Philippe L. L'Allier, MD
Associate Professor of Medicine, Department of Medicine; Director, Interventional Cardiology; Desgroseillers-Bérard Chair in Interventional Cardiology, Montreal Heart Institute, University of Montreal, Montreal, Canada
Intravascular Ultrasound Imaging

Richard A. Lange, MD
Professor and Executive Vice Chairman, Medicine, University of Texas Health Science Center, San Antonio, Texas
Toxins and the Heart

Thomas H. Lee, MD
Professor of Medicine, Harvard Medical School; Network President, Partners Healthcare System, Boston, Massachusetts
Measurement and Improvement of Quality of Cardiovascular Care; Guidelines: Pregnancy and Heart Disease

Annarosa Leri, MD
Associate Professor, Departments of Anesthesia and Medicine and Cardiovascular Division, Brigham and Women's Hospital, Harvard Medical School, Boston, Massachusetts
Cardiovascular Regeneration and Tissue Engineering

Martin M. LeWinter, MD
Professor of Medicine and Molecular Physiology and Biophysics; Director, Heart Failure and Cardiomyopathy Program, University of Vermont College of Medicine; Attending Cardiologist, Fletcher Allen Health Care, Burlington, Vermont
Pericardial Diseases

Peter Libby, MD
Mallinckrodt Professor of Medicine, Harvard Medical School; Chief of Cardiovascular Medicine, Brigham and Women's Hospital, Boston, Massachusetts
Molecular Imaging in Cardiovascular Disease; The Vascular Biology of Atherosclerosis; Risk Markers for Atherothrombotic Disease; Lipoprotein Disorders and Cardiovascular Disease; Primary and Secondary Prevention of Coronary Heart Disease; Peripheral Artery Diseases

Steven E. Lipshultz, MD
George Batchelor Professor and Chairman, Department of Pediatrics; Batchelor Family Endowed Chair in Pediatric Cardiology; Professor of Epidemiology and Public Health; Professor of Medicine (Oncology); Associate Executive Dean for Child Health, Leonard M. Miller School of Medicine, University of Miami; Chief-of-Staff, Holtz Children's Hospital of the University of Miami–Jackson Memorial Medical Center; Director, Batchelor Children's Research Institute; Associate Director, Mailman Center for Child Development; Member, the Sylvester Comprehensive Cancer Center, Miami, Florida
Cardiovascular Abnormalities in HIV-Infected Individuals

Peter Liu, MD
Heart & Stroke/Polo Professor of Medicine and Physiology, Peter Munk Cardiac Centre, University Health Network, University of Toronto; Scientific Director, Institute of Circulatory and Respiratory Health, Canadian Institutes of Health Research, Toronto, Ontario, Canada
Myocarditis

Brian F. Mandell, MD, PHD
Professor and Chairman, Department of Medicine, Cleveland Clinic Foundation Lerner College of Medicine of Case Western Reserve University; Center for Vasculitis Care and Research, Department of Rheumatic and Immunologic Disease, The Cleveland Clinic, Cleveland, Ohio
Rheumatic Diseases and the Cardiovascular System

Douglas L. Mann, MD
Lewin Chair and Professor of Medicine, Cell Biology, and Physiology; Chief, Division of Cardiology, Washington University School of Medicine in St. Louis; Cardiologist-in-Chief, Barnes-Jewish Hospital, Saint Louis, Missouri
Pathophysiology of Heart Failure; Management of Heart Failure Patients with Reduced Ejection Fraction; Guidelines: Management of Heart Failure; Emerging Therapies and Strategies in the Treatment of Heart Failure

Barry J. Maron, MD
Director, Hypertrophic Cardiomyopathy Center, Minneapolis Heart Institute Foundation, Minneapolis, Minnesota
Hypertrophic Cardiomyopathy

Kenneth L. Mattox, MD
Professor and Vice Chairman, Distinguished Service Professor, Michael E. DeBakey Department of Surgery, Baylor College of Medicine, Houston, Texas
Traumatic Heart Disease

Peter A. McCullough, MD, MPH
Consultant Cardiologist, Chief Academic and Scientific Officer, St. John Providence Health System, Providence Park Heart Institute, Novi, Michigan
Interface Between Renal Disease and Cardiovascular Illness

Darren K. McGuire, MD, MHSc
Associate Professor, Internal Medicine, The University of Texas Southwestern Medical Center at Dallas, Dallas, Texas
Diabetes and the Cardiovascular System

Bruce McManus, MD, PhD
Professor of Pathology and Laboratory Medicine, Faculty of Medicine, University of British Columbia; Co-Director, Institute for Heart and Lung Health; Director, NCE CECR Centre of Excellence for Prevention of Organ Failure (PROOF Centre); Director, UBC James Hogg Research Centre, St. Paul's Hospital, University of British Columbia, Vancouver, British Columbia, Canada
Primary Tumors of the Heart

Mandeep R. Mehra, MBBS
Dr. Herbert Berger Professor of Medicine and Head of Cardiology; Assistant Dean for Clinical Services, University of Maryland School of Medicine, Baltimore, Maryland
Assisted Circulation in the Treatment of Heart Failure

John M. Miller, MD
Professor of Medicine, Krannert Institute of Cardiology, Indiana University School of Medicine; Director, Clinical Cardiac Electrophysiology, Clarian Health Partners, Indianapolis, Indiana
Diagnosis of Cardiac Arrhythmias; Guidelines: Ambulatory Electrocardiographic and Electrophysiologic Testing; Therapy for Cardiac Arrhythmias

David M. Mirvis, MD
Professor Emeritus, University of Tennessee Health Science Center, Memphis, Tennessee
Electrocardiography; Guidelines: Electrocardiography

Fred Morady, MD
McKay Professor of Cardiovascular Disease; Professor of Medicine, University of Michigan Health System, CVC Cardiovascular Medicine, Ann Arbor, Michigan
Atrial Fibrillation: Clinical Features, Mechanisms, and Management; Guidelines: Atrial Fibrillation

David A. Morrow, MD, MPH
Associate Professor of Medicine, Harvard Medical School; Senior Investigator, TIMI Study Group; Director, Samuel A. Levine Cardiac Unit, Brigham and Women's Hospital, Boston, Massachusetts
ST-Segment Elevation Myocardial Infarction: Management; Stable Ischemic Heart Disease; Guidelines: Chronic Stable Angina

Dariush Mozaffarian, MD, DrPH
Associate Professor, Division of Cardiovascular Medicine, Brigham and Women's Hospital and Harvard Medical School; Departments of Epidemiology and Nutrition, Harvard School of Public Health, Boston, Massachusetts
Nutrition and Cardiovascular Disease

Paul S. Mueller, MD, MPH
Associate Professor of Medicine, Mayo Clinic, Rochester, Minnesota
Ethics in Cardiovascular Medicine

Robert J. Myerburg, MD
Professor of Medicine and Physiology, University of Miami Miller School of Medicine, Miami, Florida
Cardiac Arrest and Sudden Cardiac Death

Elizabeth G. Nabel, MD
Professor of Medicine, Harvard Medical School; President, Brigham and Women's Hospital, Boston, Massachusetts
Principles of Cardiovascular Molecular Biology and Genetics

L. Kristin Newby, MD, MHS
Associate Professor of Medicine, Division of Cardiovascular Medicine, Duke University Medical Center, Durham, North Carolina
Cardiovascular Disease in Women

Patrick T. O'Gara, MD
Professor of Medicine, Harvard Medical School; Director, Clinical Cardiology, Cardiovascular Division, Brigham and Women's Hospital, Boston, Massachusetts
The History and Physical Examination: An Evidence-Based Approach

Jae K. Oh, MD
Professor of Medicine, Mayo Clinic College of Medicine, Consultant in Cardiovascular Diseases; Co-Director of the Echocardiography Laboratory, Mayo Clinic, Rochester, Minnesota
Echocardiography

Jeffrey Olgin, MD
Ernest Gallo-Kanu Chatterjee Distinguished Professor; Chief, Division of Cardiology; Chief, Cardiac Electrophysiology, University of California, San Francisco, California
Specific Arrhythmias: Diagnosis and Treatment

Lionel H. Opie, MD, DPhil, DSc
Professor of Medicine and Director Emeritus, Hatter Institute for Cardiovascular Research Institute, University of Cape Town, Cape Town, South Africa
Mechanisms of Cardiac Contraction and Relaxation

Catherine M. Otto, MD
Professor of Medicine, J. Ward Kennedy-Hamilton Endowed Chair in Cardiology; Director, Training Programs in Cardiovascular Disease, University of Washington School of Medicine; Associate Director, Echocardiography Laboratory; Co-Director, Adult Congenital Heart Disease Clinic, University of Washington Medical Center, Seattle, Washington
Valvular Heart Disease; Guidelines: Management of Valvular Heart Disease

Jeffrey J. Popma, MD
Associate Professor of Medicine, Harvard Medical School; Director, Interventional Cardiology Clinical Services, Beth Israel Deaconess Medical Center, Boston, Massachusetts
Coronary Arteriography; Guidelines: Coronary Arteriography; Percutaneous Coronary Intervention; Guidelines: Percutaneous Coronary Intervention

Reed E. Pyeritz, MD, PhD
Professor of Medicine and Genetics; Vice-chair for Academic Affairs, Department of Medicine, University of Pennsylvania School of Medicine, Philadelphia, Pennsylvania
Inherited Causes of Cardiovascular Disease

B. Soma Raju, MD
Professor & Head, Department of Cardiology, Hyderabad, Andhra Pradesh, India
Rheumatic Fever

José A.F. Ramires, MD, PhD
Head Professor of Cardiology and Director of Clinical Cardiology, Division of The Heart Institute (INCOR), University of São Paulo Medical School; Director of Health System and President of Professors Evaluation Committee, University of São Paulo, São Paulo, Brazil
Chagas' Disease

Margaret M. Redfield, MD
Professor of Medicine, Division of Cardiovascular Medicine, Mayo Clinic, Rochester, Minnesota
Heart Failure with Normal Ejection Fraction

Andrew N. Redington, MD
Professor and Head, Division of Cardiology, Paediatrics, Hospital for Sick Children, University of Toronto, Toronto, Canada
Congenital Heart Disease

Stuart Rich, MD
Professor of Medicine, Section of Cardiology, Center for Pulmonary Hypertension, University of Chicago, Chicago, Illinois
Pulmonary Hypertension

Paul M Ridker, MD, MPH
Eugene Braunwald Professor of Medicine, Harvard Medical School; Director, Center for Cardiovascular Disease Prevention, Brigham and Women's Hospital, Boston, Massachusetts
Risk Markers for Atherothrombotic Disease; Primary and Secondary Prevention of Coronary Heart Disease

Dan M. Roden, MD
Professor of Medicine and Pharmacology; Director, Oates Institute for Experimental Therapeutics; Assistant Vice-Chancellor for Personalized Medicine, Vanderbilt University School of Medicine, Nashville, Tennessee
Principles of Drug Therapy

Michael Rubart, MD
Assistant Professor of Pediatrics, Indiana University School of Medicine, Indianapolis, Indiana
Genesis of Cardiac Arrhythmias: Electrophysiologic Considerations

Marc S. Sabatine, MD, MPH
Associate Professor of Medicine, Harvard Medical School; Vice Chair, TIMI Study Group; Associate Physician, Division of Cardiovascular Medicine, Brigham and Women's Hospital, Boston, Massachusetts
Approach to the Patient with Chest Pain

Luis A. Sanchez, MD
Professor of Surgery and Radiology, Section of Vascular Surgery, Department of Surgery, Washington University School of Medicine, St. Louis, Missouri
Diseases of the Aorta

Janice B. Schwartz, MD
Clinical Professor of Medicine and Bioengineering and Therapeutic Sciences, University of California, San Francisco; Director, Research, Jewish Home of San Francisco, San Francisco, California
Cardiovascular Disease in the Elderly

Christine E. Seidman, MD
Thomas W. Smith Professor of Medicine and Genetics, Department of Medicine and Genetics, Brigham & Women's Hospital, Harvard Medical School, Howard Hughes Medical Institute, Boston, Massachusetts
Inherited Causes of Cardiovascular Disease

J. G. Seidman, PhD
Henrietta B. and Frederick H. Bugher Professor of Genetics, Department of Genetics, Harvard Medical School, Boston, Massachusetts
Inherited Causes of Cardiovascular Disease

Dhun H. Sethna, MD
Staff Cardiologist, Carilion Clinic, Christiansburg, Virginia
Medical Management of the Patient Undergoing Cardiac Surgery

Jeffrey F. Smallhorn, MBBS, FRACP, FRCP(C)
Professor of Pediatrics; Program Director, Pediatric Cardiology, Department of Pediatrics, University of Alberta, Edmonton, Alberta
Congenital Heart Disease

Virend K. Somers, MD, PhD
Professor of Medicine, Division of Cardiovascular Diseases, Mayo Clinic College of Medicine, Rochester, Minnesota
Sleep Apnea and Cardiovascular Disease; Cardiovascular Manifestations of Autonomic Disorders

Andrei C. Sposito
Associate Professor of Cardiology, University of Campinas; Past Director of The Heart Institute (INCOR), Brasilia, São Paulo, Brazil
Chagas' Disease

Charles D. Swerdlow, MD
Clinical Professor of Medicine, David Geffen School of Medicine at UCLA; Cedars-Sinai Heart Institute, Los Angeles, California
Pacemakers and Implantable Cardioverter-Defibrillators; Guidelines: Cardiac Pacemakers and Cardioverter-Defibrillators

Jean-Claude Tardif, MD
Professor of Medicine, University of Montreal; Director, Montreal Heart Institute Research Center; Endowed Research Chair in Atherosclerosis, Montreal Heart Institute, Université de Montréal, Montreal, Canada
Intravascular Ultrasound Imaging

Allen J. Taylor, MD
Professor of Medicine, Georgetown University; Director, Advanced Cardiovascular Imaging, Cardiology Section, Washington Hospital Center and Medstar Health Cardiovascular Research Institute, Washington, DC
Cardiac Computed Tomography; Appropriate Use Criteria: Cardiac Computed Tomography

David J. Tester, BS
Senior Research Technologist II-Supervisor, Mayo Clinic, Windland Smith Rice Sudden Death Genomics Laboratory, Rochester, Minnesota
Genetics of Cardiac Arrhythmias

Judith Therrien, MD
Associate Professor of Medicine, Department of Cardiology, McGill University, Montreal, Quebec, Canada
Congenital Heart Disease

Paul D. Thompson, MD
Professor of Medicine, University of Connecticut, Farmington, Connecticut; Director, Cardiology, Hartford Hospital, Hartford, Connecticut
Exercise-Based, Comprehensive Cardiac Rehabilitation

Robert W. Thompson, MD
Professor of Surgery, Division of General Surgery, Vascular Surgery Section, Radiology, and Cell Biology and Physiology, Washington University, St. Louis, Missouri
Diseases of the Aorta

Marc D. Tischler, MD
Associate Professor of Medicine, University of Vermont College of Medicine; Director, Cardiac Ultrasound Laboratory; Co-Director, Cardiac Magnetic Resonance Unit, Department of Internal Medicine, Burlington, Vermont
Pericardial Diseases

Peter I. Tsai, MD
Assistant Professor, Division of Cardiothoracic Surgery, Michael E. DeBakey Department of Surgery, Ben Taub General Hospital, Baylor College of Medicine, Houston, Texas
Traumatic Heart Disease

Zoltan G. Turi, MD
Professor of Medicine, Robert Wood Johnson Medical School; Director, Section of Vascular Medicine; Director, Cooper Structural Heart Disease Program, Cooper University Hospital, Camden, New Jersey
Rheumatic Fever

James E. Udelson, MD
Professor of Medicine, Department of Medicine; Chief, Division of Cardiology, The Cardiovascular Center, Tufts Medical Center and Tufts University School of Medicine, Boston, Massachusetts
Nuclear Cardiology; Appropriate Use Criteria: Nuclear Cardiology

Viola Vaccarino, MD, PhD
Professor and Chair, Department of Epidemiology, Emory University Rollins School of Public Health; Professor, Department of Medicine, Division of Cardiology, Emory University School of Medicine, Atlanta, Georgia
Psychiatric and Behavioral Aspects of Cardiovascular Disease

Ronald G. Victor, MD
Burns and Allen Professor of Medicine; Associate Director, Clinical Research; Director, Hypertension Center, The Heart Institute, Cedars-Sinai Medical Center, Los Angeles, California
Systemic Hypertension: Mechanisms and Diagnosis

Alexandra Villa-Forte, MD, MPH
Center for Vasculitis Care and Research, Department of Rheumatic and Immunologic Diseases, Cleveland Clinic, Cleveland, Ohio
Rheumatic Diseases and the Cardiovascular System

Matthew J. Wall, Jr., MD
Professor, Michael E. DeBakey Department of Surgery, Baylor College of Medicine; Deputy Chief of Surgery, Ben Taub General Hospital, Houston, Texas
Traumatic Heart Disease

Carole A. Warnes, MD, FRCP
Professor of Medicine, Mayo Clinic College of Medicine; Consultant, Division of Cardiovascular Diseases, Internal Medicine and Pediatric Cardiology, Mayo Clinic College of Medicine, Rochester, Minnesota
Pregnancy and Heart Disease; Guidelines: Pregnancy and Heart Disease

Gary D. Webb, MD
Professor, University of Cincinnati College of Medicine; Director, Cincinnati Adolescent and Adult Congenital Heart Center, Cincinnati Children's Hospital Heart Institute, Cincinnati, Ohio
Congenital Heart Disease

John G. Webb, MD
MacLeod Professor of Heart Valve Intervention, University of British Columbia; Director Cardiac Catheterization, St. Paul's Hospital, Vancouver, Canada
Percutaneous Therapies for Structural Heart Disease in Adults

Ralph Weissleder, MD, PhD
Professor, Harvard Medical School; Center for Systems Biology and Department of Radiology, Massachusetts General Hospital, Boston, Massachusetts
Molecular Imaging in Cardiovascular Disease

Jeffrey I. Weitz, MD, FRCP(C)
Professor of Medicine & Biochemistry, McMaster University; HSFO/J.F. Mustard Chair in Cardiovascular Research; Canada Research Chair (Tier 1) in Thrombosis; Executive Director, Thrombosis and Atherosclerosis Research Institute, Hamilton General Hospital Campus, Hamilton, Ontario, Canada
Hemostasis, Thrombosis, Fibrinolysis, and Cardiovascular Disease

Christopher J. White, MD
Professor of Medicine; Chairman, Department of Cardiology, Ochsner Clinic Foundation, New Orleans, Louisiana
Endovascular Treatment of Noncoronary Obstructive Vascular Disease

Stephen D. Wiviott, MD
Instructor of Medicine, Harvard Medical School; Investigator, TIMI Study Group; Associate Physician, Division of Cardiology, Brigham and Women's Hospital, Boston, Massachusetts
Guidelines: Management of Patients with ST-Segment Elevation Myocardial Infarction

Clyde W. Yancy, MD
Professor of Medicine; Chief, Division of Cardiology, Northwestern University Feinberg School of Medicine, Chicago, Illinois
Heart Disease in Varied Populations

Andreas M. Zeiher, MD
Professor of Cardiology; Chair, Department of Medicine, University of Frankfurt, Frankfurt, Germany
Emerging Therapies and Strategies in the Treatment of Heart Failure

Douglas P. Zipes, MD
Distinguished Professor; Professor Emeritus of Medicine, Pharmacology, and Toxicology; Director Emeritus, Division of Cardiology and the Krannert Institute of Cardiology, Indiana University School of Medicine, Indianapolis, Indiana
Genesis of Cardiac Arrhythmias: Electrophysiologic Considerations; Diagnosis of Cardiac Arrhythmias; Guidelines: Ambulatory Electrocardiographic and Electrophysiologic Testing; Therapy for Cardiac Arrhythmias; Pacemakers and Implantable Cardioverter-Defibrillators; Guidelines: Cardiac Pacemakers and Cardioverter-Defibrillators; Specific Arrhythmias: Diagnosis and Treatment; Atrial Fibrillation: Clinical Features, Mechanisms, and Management; Guidelines: Atrial Fibrillation; Hypotension and Syncope; Cardiovascular Disease in the Elderly; Neurologic Disorders and Cardiovascular Disease

PREFACE TO THE NINTH EDITION

Advances in cardiovascular science and practice continue at a breathtaking rate. As the knowledge base expands, it is important to adapt our learning systems to keep up with progress in our field. We are pleased to present the ninth edition of *Braunwald's Heart Disease: A Textbook of Cardiovascular Medicine* as the hub of an ongoing, advanced learning system designed to provide practitioners, physicians-in-training, and students at all levels with the tools needed to keep abreast of rapidly changing scientific foundations, clinical research results, and evidence-based medical practice.

In keeping with the tradition established by the previous editions of *Braunwald's Heart Disease*, the ninth edition covers the breadth of cardiovascular practice, highlighting new advances and their potential to transform the established paradigms of prevention, diagnosis, and treatment. We have thoroughly revised this edition to keep the content vibrant, stimulating, and up-to-date. Twenty-four of the 94 chapters are entirely new, including nine chapters that cover topics not addressed in earlier editions. We have added 46 new authors, all highly accomplished and recognized in their respective disciplines. All chapters carried over from the eighth edition have been thoroughly updated and extensively revised. This edition includes nearly 2500 figures, most of which are in full color, and 600 tables. We have continued to provide updated sections on current guidelines recommendations that complement each of the appropriate individual chapters.

A full accounting of these changes in the new edition cannot be addressed in the space of this Preface, but we are pleased to present a number of the highlights. The ninth edition includes two entirely new chapters—ethics in cardiovascular medicine by Paul Mueller and design and conduct of clinical trials by Elliot Antman—that supplement the initial section on the fundamentals of cardiovascular disease. Thomas Gaziano has joined J. Michael Gaziano in authoring the first chapter on the global burden of cardiovascular disease. With recognition of the increasing relevance of genetics, J.G. Seidman joins Reed Pyeritz and Christine Seidman in the updated chapter on inherited causes of cardiovascular disease, and David Tester and Michael Ackerman have contributed a new chapter on the genetics of cardiac arrhythmias.

Acknowledging the unremitting burden and societal impact of heart failure, the section on heart failure receives continued emphasis and has undergone extensive revision, including five new chapters. Barry Greenberg teams with Andrew Kahn in addressing the clinical approach to the patient with heart failure; Mihai Georghiade, Gerasimos Filippatos, and Michael Felker provide a fresh look at the evaluation and management of acute heart failure; Michael Acker and Mariell Jessup address advances in surgical treatment the failing heart; Mandeep Mehra and Bartley Griffith discuss the role of device therapy in assisted circulation; and William Abraham reviews the emerging role of devices for monitoring and managing heart failure.

The chapters that address cardiovascular imaging have kept abreast of all of the exciting advances in this field. Raymond Kwong and Allen Taylor have written excellent and comprehensive new chapters on cardiac magnetic resonance and cardiac computed tomography, respectively, with accompanying sections addressing the American College of Cardiology appropriate use criteria for the use of these advanced technologies. Updated ACC appropriate use criteria also follow the chapters on echocardiography and nuclear cardiology. In addition, the imaging section has been further enhanced by the inclusion of two new chapters focusing on the evolving applications of intravascular ultrasound, authored by Jean-Claude Tardif and Philippe L'Allier, and cardiovascular molecular imaging, provided by Peter Libby, Farouc Jaffer, and Ralph Weissleder.

In recognition of the growing importance of atrial fibrillation in cardiovascular practice, a new chapter devoted to the evaluation and treatment of this rhythm disturbance, authored by Fred Morady and Douglas Zipes, has been added to the section on cardiac arrhythmias. The other updated chapters in the heart rhythm section continue to inform our readers on the current state-of-the-art in this important aspect of heart disease.

Dariush Mozaffarian and Edzard Ernst have added expertly authored new chapters on nutrition and complementary medicine, respectively, to the section on preventive cardiology. In the atherosclerotic disease section, Marc Sabatine joins Chris Cannon in the revised discussion of the approach to the patient with chest pain, and William Boden joins David Morrow in a new chapter on stable ischemic heart disease. Deepak Bhatt teams with Jeffrey Popma in creating a new chapter on percutaneous coronary intervention, and he joins Andrew Eisenhauer and Christopher White in updating the discussion on endovascular treatment of noncoronary vascular disease. We welcome John Webb to our authorship team with his new chapter on catheter-based interventions in structural heart disease that includes discussion of the exciting novel catheter-based techniques for repair and replacement of cardiac valves. Our other new chapters include a fresh commentary on diseases of the aorta by Alan Braverman, Robert Thompson, and Luis Sanchez; diabetes and cardiovascular disease by Darren McGuire; hemostasis, thrombosis, and fibrinolysis by Jeffrey Weitz; and psychiatric and behavioral aspects of cardiovascular disease by Viola Vaccarino and Douglas Bremner. Finally, we are delighted that José Ramires, Andrei Sposito, Edécio Cunha-Neto, and Maria de Lourdes Higuchi have expanded our discussion of the global nature of cardiovascular disease by contributing an excellent chapter on the pathophysiology, evaluation, and treatment of Chagas' disease.

We are indebted to all of our authors for their considerable time, effort, and commitment to maintaining the high standards of *Braunwald's Heart Disease.* As excited as we are about bringing this edition of the text to fruition, we are even more energized regarding the expanding *Braunwald's Heart Disease* website. The electronic version of this work on the companion Expert Consult website includes greater content in terms of figures and tables than the print version can accommodate. Figures and tables can be downloaded directly from the website for electronic slide presentations. In addition, we have a growing portfolio of video and audio content that supplements the print content of many of our chapters. Dr. Braunwald personally updates the chapter content on a weekly basis, thus creating a truly unique living textbook with expanding content that includes the latest research, clinical trials, and expert opinion.

Moreover, the family of *Braunwald's Heart Disease* companion texts continues to expand, providing detailed expert content for the subspecialist across the broad spectrum of cardiovascular conditions. These include: *Clinical Lipidology*, edited by Christie Ballantyne; *Clinical Arrhythmology and Electrophysiology*, authored by Ziad Issa, John Miller, and Douglas Zipes; *Heart Failure*, edited by Douglas Mann; *Valvular Heart Disease*, by Catherine Otto and Robert Bonow; *Acute Coronary Syndromes*, by Pierre Théroux; *Preventive Cardiology*, by Roger Blumenthal, JoAnne Foody, and Nathan Wong; *Cardiovascular Nursing*, by Debra Moser and Barbara Riegel; *Mechanical Circulatory Support*, by Robert Kormos and Leslie Miller; *Hypertension*, by Henry Black and William Elliott; *Cardiovascular Therapeutics*, by Elliott Antman and Marc Sabatine; *Vascular Medicine*, by Marc Creager, Joshua

Beckman, and Joseph Loscalzo; and recent atlases on cardiovascular imaging such as *Cardiovascular Magnetic Resonance*, by Christopher Kramer and Gregory Hundley; *Cardiovascular Computed Tomography*, by Allen Taylor; and *Nuclear Cardiology*, by Ami Iskandrian and Ernest Garcia.

The ninth edition of *Braunwald's Heart Disease* does indeed represent the central hub of a burgeoning cardiovascular learning system that can be tailored to meet the needs of all individuals engaged in cardiovascular medicine, from the accomplished subspecialist practitioner to the beginning student of cardiology. *Braunwald's Heart Disease* aims to provide the necessary tools to navigate the ever-increasing flow of complex information seamlessly.

Robert O. Bonow

Douglas L. Mann

Douglas P. Zipes

Peter Libby

PREFACE—ADAPTED FROM THE FIRST EDITION

Cardiovascular disease is the greatest scourge affecting the industrialized nations. As with previous scourges—bubonic plague, yellow fever, and smallpox—cardiovascular disease not only strikes down a significant fraction of the population without warning but also causes prolonged suffering and disability in an even larger number. In the United States alone, despite recent encouraging declines, cardiovascular disease is still responsible for almost 1 million fatalities each year and more than half of all deaths; almost 5 million persons afflicted with cardiovascular disease are hospitalized each year. The cost of these diseases in terms of human suffering and material resources is almost incalculable. Fortunately, research focusing on the causes, diagnosis, treatment, and prevention of heart disease is moving ahead rapidly.

In order to provide a comprehensive, authoritative text in a field that has become as broad and deep as cardiovascular medicine, I chose to enlist the aid of a number of able colleagues. However, I hoped that my personal involvement in the writing of about half of the book would make it possible to minimize the fragmentation, gaps, inconsistencies, organizational difficulties, and impersonal tone that sometimes plague multiauthored texts.

Since the early part of the 20th century, clinical cardiology has had a particularly strong foundation in the basic sciences of physiology and pharmacology. More recently, the disciplines of molecular biology, genetics, developmental biology, biophysics, biochemistry, experimental pathology, and bioengineering have also begun to provide critically important information about cardiac function and malfunction. Although *Heart Disease: A Textbook of Cardiovascular Medicine* is primarily a clinical treatise and not a textbook of fundamental cardiovascular science, an effort has been made to explain, in some detail, the scientific bases of cardiovascular diseases.

Eugene Braunwald
1980

CONTENTS

PART I FUNDAMENTALS OF CARDIOVASCULAR DISEASE

PART II MOLECULAR BIOLOGY AND GENETICS

PART III EVALUATION OF THE PATIENT

Look for these other titles in the Braunwald's Heart Disease Family

Braunwald's Heart Disease Companions

PIERRE THÉROUX
Acute Coronary Syndromes

ELLIOTT M. ANTMAN & MARC S. SABATINE
Cardiovascular Therapeutics

CHRISTIE M. BALLANTYNE
Clinical Lipidology

ZIAD ISSA, JOHN M. MILLER, & DOUGLAS P. ZIPES
Clinical Arrhythmology and Electrophysiology

DOUGLAS L. MANN
Heart Failure

HENRY R. BLACK & WILLIAM J. ELLIOTT
Hypertension

ROGER S. BLUMENTHAL, JOANNE M. FOODY, & NATHAN D. WONG
Preventive Cardiology

ROBERT L. KORMOS & LESLIE W. MILLER
Mechanical Circulatory Support

CATHERINE M. OTTO & ROBERT O. BONOW
Valvular Heart Disease

MARC A. CREAGER, JOSHUA A. BECKMAN, & JOSEPH LOSCALZO
Vascular Disease

Braunwald's Heart Disease Imaging Companions

ALLEN J. TAYLOR
Atlas of Cardiac Computed Tomography

CHRISTOPHER M. KRAMER & W. GREGORY HUNDLEY
Atlas of Cardiovascular Magnetic Resonance

AMI E. ISKANDRIAN & ERNEST V. GARCIA
Atlas of Nuclear Imaging

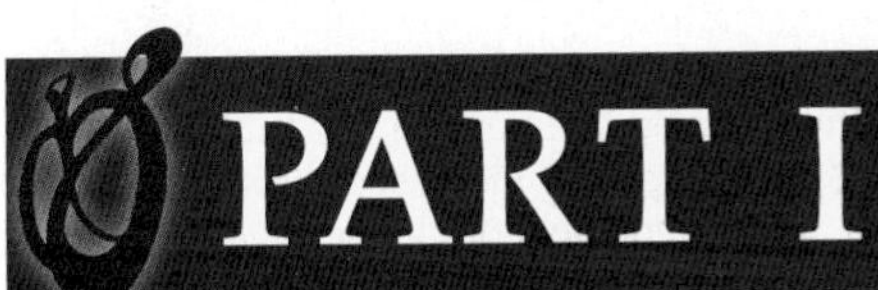

PART I

FUNDAMENTALS OF CARDIOVASCULAR DISEASE

CHAPTER 1 Global Burden of Cardiovascular Disease

Thomas A. Gaziano and J. Michael Gaziano

Over the last decade, cardiovascular disease (CVD) has become the single largest cause of death worldwide. In 2004, CVD caused an estimated 17 million deaths and led to 151 million disability-adjusted life years (DALYs) lost—about 30% of all deaths and 14% of all DALYs lost that year.[1] Like many high-income countries during the last century, low- and middle-income countries are seeing an alarming increase in the rates of CVD, and this change is accelerating. In 2001, 75% of global deaths and 82% of total DALYs lost caused by coronary heart disease (CHD) occurred in low- and middle-income countries.[2]

This chapter reviews the features of the epidemiologic transition underlying this shift in CVD morbidity and mortality and evaluates the transition in different regions of the world. A survey of the current burden of risk factors and behaviors associated with CVD and their regional variations and trends follows. The next section reviews the economic impact of CVD and the cost-effectiveness of various strategies to reduce it. The chapter ends with a discussion of the diverse challenges posed by the increasing burden of CVD for various regions of the world and potential solutions to this global problem.

Shifting Burdens

CVD now causes the most deaths in all developing regions with the exception of sub-Saharan Africa, where it leads causes of death in those older than 45 years. Between 1990 and 2001, of all deaths in low- and middle-income countries, deaths from CVD increased from 26% to 28%, a reflection of the rapid pace of the epidemiologic transition (**Fig. 1-1**). Within the six World Bank–defined low- and middle-income regions, there exist vast differences in the burden of CVD (**Fig. 1-2**), with CVD death rates as high as 58% in eastern Europe and as low as 10% in sub-Saharan Africa. These numbers compare with a CVD death rate of 38% in high-income countries.

Epidemiologic Transitions

Humans evolved under conditions of pestilence and famine and have lived with these for most of recorded history. Before 1900, infectious diseases and malnutrition constituted the most common cause of death in almost every part of the world. These conditions, along with high infant and child mortality rates, resulted in a mean life expectancy of approximately 30 years. But thanks largely to improved nutrition and public health measures, communicable diseases and malnutrition have declined and life expectancy has increased dramatically. Increased longevity and the impact of smoking, high-fat diets, and other risk factors for chronic diseases have now combined to make CVD and cancer the leading causes of death in most countries. These changes began in higher income countries, but as they gradually spread to low- and middle-income countries, CVD mortality rates have increased globally. In absolute numbers, CVD causes four to five times as many deaths in developing countries as in developed countries.

The overall increase in the global burden of CVD and the distinct patterns in the various regions result in part from the epidemiologic transition, which includes four basic stages (**Table 1-1**)[3,4]: pestilence and famine, receding pandemics, degenerative and man-made diseases, and delayed degenerative diseases. Movement through these stages has dramatically shifted the causes of death over the last two centuries, from infectious diseases and malnutrition in the first stage to CVD and cancer in the third and fourth stages. Although the transition through the age of pestilence and famine has occurred much later in the low- and middle-income countries, it has also occurred more rapidly, driven largely by the transfer of low-cost agricultural technologies and public health advances.

The first stage, pestilence and famine, is characterized by the predominance of malnutrition and infectious disease and by the infrequency of CVD as a cause of death. CVD, which accounts for

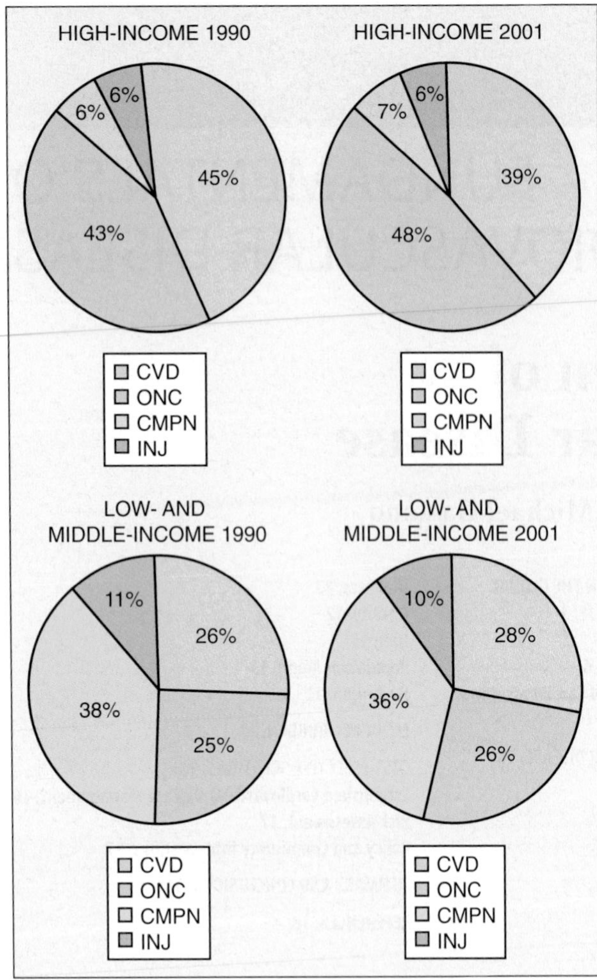

FIGURE 1-1 Changing pattern of mortality, 1990 to 2001. CMPN = communicable, maternal, perinatal, and nutritional diseases; CVD = cardiovascular disease; INJ = injury; ONC = other noncommunicable diseases. *(From Mathers CD, Lopez A, Stein D, et al: Deaths and disease burden by cause: Global burden of disease estimates for 2001 by World Bank Country Groups, 2005. Disease Control Priorities Working Paper 18 [http://www.dcp2.org/file/33/wp18.pdf].)*

less than 10% of deaths, takes the form of rheumatic heart disease and other cardiomyopathies caused by infection and malnutrition.

Per capita income and life expectancy increased during the age of receding pandemics as the emergence of public health systems, cleaner water supplies, and improved food production and distribution combined to drive down deaths from infectious disease and malnutrition. These advances, in turn, increased the productivity of the average worker, further improving the economic situation. The change most characteristic of this phase is a precipitous decline in infant and child mortality accompanied by a substantial increase in life expectancy. Rheumatic valvular disease, hypertension, and stroke cause most CVD. CHD often occurs at a lower prevalence rate compared with stroke, and CVD accounts for 10% to 35% of deaths.

During the stage of degenerative and man-made diseases, continued improvements in economic circumstances, combined with urbanization and radical changes in the nature of work-related activities, led to dramatic changes in diet, activity levels, and behaviors such as smoking. The increase in availability of foods with high saturated fat content coupled with decreased physical activity led to an increase in atherosclerosis. In this stage, CHD and stroke predominate, and between 35% and 65% of all deaths are related to CVD. Typically, the ratio of CHD to stroke is 2:1 to 3:1.

In the age of delayed degenerative diseases, CVD and cancer have remained the major causes of morbidity and mortality, with CVD accounting for 25% to 40% of all deaths. However, the age-adjusted CVD mortality rate has declined, aided by preventive strategies such as smoking cessation programs and effective blood pressure control, acute hospital management (including the use of coronary care units), and technologic advances such as invasive revascularization. Reductions in risk behaviors and factors may make even greater contributions to the decline in age-adjusted rates of death. In many cases, these result from concerted efforts by public health officials and health care communities. In other cases, secular trends play a role. For example, the widespread availability of fresh fruits and vegetables year-round in developed countries, and thus increased consumption, may have contributed to declining mean cholesterol levels before effective drug therapy was widely available. CHD, stroke, and congestive heart failure are the primary forms of CVD during this phase, with CHD remaining a significantly greater cause of death in all regions. Congestive heart failure dramatically increases as people live longer because of improved survival from myocardial infarction (MI). Japan and Portugal have been an exception to this transition, with rates of CHD never exceeding those of stroke. A further characteristic of the CVD transition in developed countries is that members of higher socioeconomic classes tend to pass through them first, whereas there is a lag for those of lower socioeconomic status.

TABLE 1-1 Four Typical Stages of the Epidemiologic Transition

STAGE	DESCRIPTION	TYPICAL PROPORTION OF DEATHS CAUSED BY CVD (%)	PREDOMINANT TYPES OF CVD
Pestilence and famine	Predominance of malnutrition and infectious diseases as causes of death; high rates of infant and child mortality; low mean life expectancy	<10	Rheumatic heart disease, cardiomyopathies caused by infection, malnutrition
Receding pandemics	Improvements in nutrition and public health leading to decrease in rates of deaths caused by malnutrition and infection; precipitous decline in infant and child mortality rates	10-35	Rheumatic valvular disease, hypertension, CHD, stroke
Degenerative and man-made diseases	Increased fat and caloric intake and decreased physical activity leading to emergence of hypertension and atherosclerosis; with increased life expectancy, mortality from chronic, noncommunicable diseases exceeds mortality from malnutrition and infectious diseases	35-65	CHD, stroke
Delayed degenerative diseases	CVDs and cancer are major causes of morbidity, mortality; better treatment and prevention efforts help avoid deaths in those with disease, delay primary events; age-adjusted CVD mortality declines; CVD affecting older and older individuals	40-50	CHD, stroke, congestive heart failure

Modified from Omran AR: The epidemiologic transition: A theory of the epidemiology of population change. Milbank Q 49:509, 1971; and Olshansky SJ, Ault AB: The fourth stage of the epidemiologic transition: The age of delayed degenerative diseases. Milbank Q 64:355, 1986.

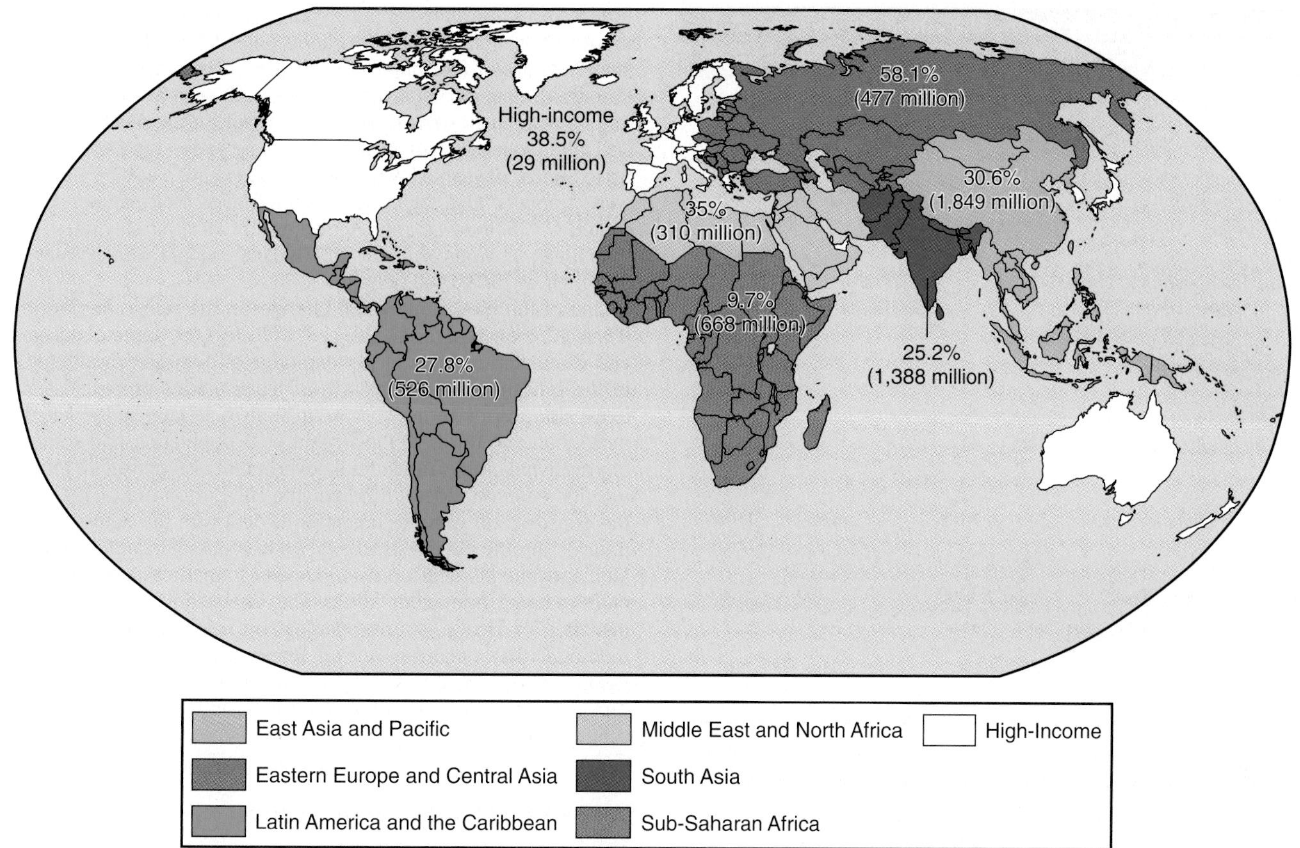

FIGURE 1-2 Cardiovascular disease deaths as a percentage of all deaths in each region and total regional population, 2001. *(Data from Mathers CD, Lopez A, Stein D, et al: Deaths and disease burden by cause: Global burden of disease estimates for 2001 by World Bank Country Groups, 2005. Disease Control Priorities Working Paper 18 [http://www.dcp2.org/file/33/wp18.pdf].)*

Is There a Fifth Phase: Age of Inactivity and Obesity?

Troubling trends in certain risk behaviors and risk factors may foreshadow a new phase of the epidemiologic transition, the age of inactivity and obesity.[5] In many parts of the industrialized world, physical activity continues to decline while total caloric intake increases at alarming rates, resulting in an epidemic of overweight and obesity. As a consequence, rates of type 2 diabetes, hypertension, and lipid abnormalities associated with obesity are rising, trends that are particularly evident in children.[6,7] These changes are occurring at a time when measurable improvements in other risk behaviors and risk factors, such as smoking, have slowed. If these trends continue, age-adjusted CVD mortality rates, which have declined over the past several decades in developed countries, could level or even increase in the coming years. This trend pertains particularly to age-adjusted stroke death rates. Also of concern, even in the developing world, is the increase in obesity. According to a recent study, one in five Chinese is overweight or obese.[8] Other new data indicate that as many as 40% of South African women may be overweight.

Epidemiologic Transition in the United States

Like other high-income countries, the United States has proceeded through four stages of the epidemiologic transition and is perhaps entering the fifth phase. Given the large amount of economic, social, demographic, and health data available (**Table 1-2**), the United States serves as a useful reference point for other countries.

Age of Pestilence and Famine (Before 1900)

The United States, like almost all other countries and regions, first experienced pestilence and famine. About half of the Pilgrims arriving in the New World in November 1620 died of infection or malnutrition by the following spring. In addition, the infectious diseases that the immigrants brought with them from Europe had a devastating impact on Native American populations. At the end of the 1800s, the U.S. economy was still largely agrarian, with more than 60% of the population living in rural settings. By 1900, life expectancy had increased to 47.8 years for men and 50.7 years for women. Infectious diseases—primarily tuberculosis, pneumonia, and diarrheal diseases—accounted for more deaths than any other cause. CVD accounted for less than 10% of all deaths. Tobacco products were beyond the economic reach of a large segment of the population.

Age of Receding Pandemics (1900-1930)

Early in the 20th century, the pace of industrialization accelerated. The population of urban areas outnumbered that of rural areas for the first time by 1920. By 1930, 56% of the population lived in or near urban centers. The shift from a rural, agriculture-based economy to an urban, industry-based economy had a number of consequences on cardiovascular risk behaviors and factors. The railway network in place at the turn of the century could move food from the farm to the city. Because the trains were not refrigerated, however, perishable foodstuffs such as fresh fruits and vegetables could not readily be transported, whereas cereal grains and livestock could. As a result, consumption of fresh fruits and vegetables declined and consumption of meat and processed grains increased. In addition, the manufacture of factory-rolled cigarettes made them more portable and more affordable for much of the population.

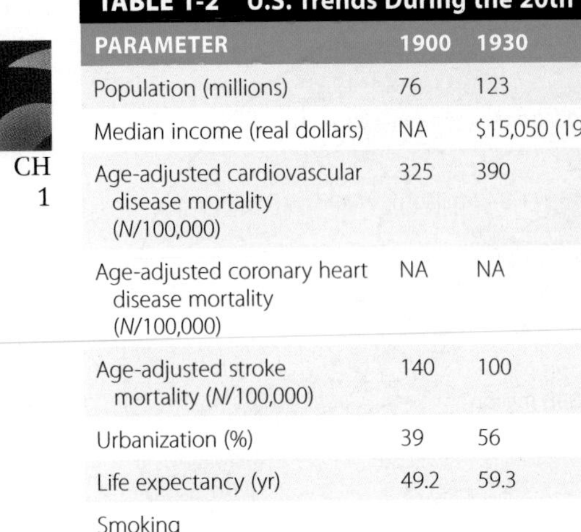

TABLE 1-2 U.S. Trends During the 20th Century

PARAMETER	1900	1930	1970	2000
Population (millions)	76	123	203	281
Median income (real dollars)	NA	$15,050 (1947)	$26,333	$29,058
Age-adjusted cardiovascular disease mortality (N/100,000)	325	390	699	341
Age-adjusted coronary heart disease mortality (N/100,000)	NA	NA	448	186
Age-adjusted stroke mortality (N/100,000)	140	100	148	57
Urbanization (%)	39	56	74	76
Life expectancy (yr)	49.2	59.3	70.8	76.9
Smoking				
Cigarettes per capita (N)	54	1,185	3,969	1,977
Smokers (%)	NA	NA	37.4	23.3
Total caloric intake (kcal)	3,500	3,300	3,200	3,800
Fat intake (% of total calories)	31.6	37.3	41.2	33
Cholesterol level (mg/dL)	NA	NA	216	204
Overweight or obese (%)	NA	NA	47.7	64.5

NA = not available.

Population: U.S. Bureau of the Census: Current Population Reports, P60-203, Measuring 50 Years of Economic Change Using the March Current Population Survey. Washington, DC, U.S. Government Printing Office, 1998; and U.S. Bureau of the Census: Money Income in the United States, 2000, P60-213. Washington, DC, U.S. Government Printing Office, 2001.

Cardiovascular disease, coronary heart disease, stroke mortality: Morbidity & Mortality: 2002 Chart Book on Cardiovascular, Lung, and Blood Diseases. Bethesda, Md, National Heart, Lung, and Blood Institute, 2002.

Urbanization: Measuring America: The Decennial Censuses, 1790 to 2000: U.S. Bureau of the Census, Washington, DC, U.S. Government Printing Office, 2002.

Life expectancy: Arias E: United States life tables, 2000. *In* National Vital Statistics Report, vol 51, no 3. Atlanta, National Center for Health Statistics, Centers for Disease Control and Prevention, 2002.

Smoking: Federal Trade Commission: Cigarette report for 2001 (http://www.ftc.gov/os/2003/06/ 2001cigreport.pdf).

Total caloric intake and fat intake: Nutrient content of the U.S. food supply, 1909-1994: A summary. Washington, DC, U.S. Department of Agriculture, 1998; and Kennedy ET, Bowman SA, Powell R: Dietary-fat intake in the U.S. population. J Am Coll Nutr 18:207, 1999.

Cholesterol level and obesity: National Center for Health Statistics: Health, United States, 2002. (http://www.cdc.gov/nchs/data/hus/hus02.pdf).

By 1900, a public health infrastructure had emerged; 40 states had health departments, and many larger towns had major public works efforts to improve water supply and sewage systems. Municipal use of chlorine to disinfect water was becoming widespread, and improvements in food handling such as pasteurization were introduced. The Flexner Report of 1910, which examined carefully the quality of medical education in the United States and Canada, was the first step toward organized quality improvement in health care personnel that, along with other public health changes, contributed to dramatic declines in infectious disease mortality rates throughout the century. These rates fell dramatically, from a crude death rate of approximately 800/100,000 people in 1900 to approximately 340/100,000 people in 1930. Life expectancy increased by 10 years between 1900 and 1930, to 57.8 years for men and 61.1 years for women. Age-adjusted CVD mortality rates, at approximately 390/100,000 people, were in the midst of their steady climb up from slightly more than 300/100,000 people in 1900. This increase was largely driven by rapidly rising CHD rates.

Age of Degenerative Man-Made Diseases (1930-1965)

By the middle of the 20th century, the United States was predominantly an industrial economy, with 64% of the population living in urban and suburban settings. With continued mechanization and urbanization, activity levels declined considerably. The prevalence of smoking, one of the major contributors to premature mortality and chronic disease, hit its zenith among adult men at 57% in 1955 and among women 10 years later at 34%.[9] Deaths from infectious diseases had fallen to fewer than 50/100,000 people/yr, and life expectancy was up to almost 70 years. However, almost 52% of men and 34% of women were smokers, and fat consumption (much of it saturated) represented 41% of total calories. Age-adjusted CHD mortality rates were at their peak, at approximately 225/100,000 people. Stroke rates were also high, at 75/100,000 people.

One of the most remarkable changes in the years after World War II was the growth of the health care industry. Only some of this growth was stimulated by rises in per capita gross domestic product (GDP). In the private sector, the growth of labor unions propelled a major expansion in private health care insurance. In fact, by the late 1950s, more than two thirds of the working U.S. population had some form of private insurance. The federal government also played an important role. Increases in federal funding (the Hill-Burton Act of 1948) led to the construction of more hospitals to deal with the acute manifestations of chronic illnesses. In 1966, two key federal insurance programs, Medicare and Medicaid, provided access to medical care for the medically indigent and older adults. The establishment of the National Institutes of Health, spurred largely by scientific achievements in medicine that occurred during World War II, not only promoted health-related research but also transformed medical education by providing financial support for the establishment of full-time medical school faculty.

Age of Delayed Degenerative Diseases (1965-2000)

A decline in age-adjusted CVD mortality rates began in the mid-1960s, and substantial reductions in age-adjusted rates of mortality from both stroke and CHD have followed since then (**Fig. 1-3**). These reductions have occurred in whites and blacks, men and women, and all age groups. Age-adjusted CHD mortality rates fell approximately 2%/yr, and stroke rates fell 3%/yr in the 1970s and 1980s. At the beginning of the 21st century, the nation was fully industrialized, with only 2% of the population involved in farming and a per capita GDP of approximately $37,800. **Table 1-3** provides an overview of CVD in 2005, the last year for which complete statistics are available.

Two significant advances have contributed to the decline in CVD mortality rates—new therapeutic approaches and prevention measures targeted at those with CVD and those potentially at risk for it.[10] Treatments once considered advanced, including the establishment of emergency medical systems, coronary care units, and widespread use of new diagnostic and therapeutic technologies such as echocardiography, cardiac catheterization, angioplasty, bypass surgery, and implantation of pacemakers and defibrillators, have now become the standard of care. Advances in drug development have also had a major beneficial impact on acute and chronic outcomes. Efforts to improve the acute management of MI have led to the application of lifesaving drugs such as beta-adrenergic blocking agents, percutaneous coronary intervention, thrombolytics, angiotensin-converting enzyme (ACE) inhibitors, and others (see Chaps. 49 and 55). The widespread use of an "old" drug, aspirin has also reduced the risk of dying of acute or secondary coronary events. Low-cost pharmacologic treatment for hypertension (see Chap. 46) and the development of highly effective cholesterol-lowering drugs such as statins have also made major contributions to primary and secondary prevention by reducing deaths from CVD (see Chaps. 47 and 49).

In concert with these advances, public health campaigns have indicated that certain behaviors increase the risk of CVD and that lifestyle modifications can reduce risk. In this regard, smoking cessation has been a model of success. In 1955, 57% of men smoked cigarettes; today, 23% of men smoke. Among women, the prevalence of smoking has fallen from a high of 34% in 1965 to 18.5% currently. Campaigns beginning in the 1970s have resulted in dramatic improvements in the detection and treatment of hypertension. This intervention likely has had an immediate and profound effect on stroke rates and a more subtle effect on CHD rates. Similar public health messages concerning saturated fat and cholesterol largely account for the decline in overall fat consumption as a percentage of total calories, from approximately 45% in 1965 to 34% in 1995, and the decline in population mean cholesterol levels, from 220 mg/dL in the early 1960s to 203 mg/dL by 2002.[11]

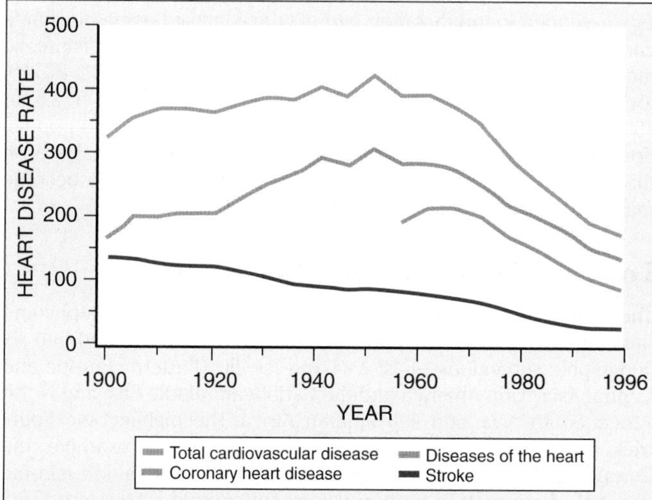

FIGURE 1-3 Increase and decline in age-adjusted heart disease rates through the epidemiological transition in the United States, 1900 to 1996. Rate is per 100,000 population, standardized to the 1940 U.S. population. Diseases are classified according to International Classification of Diseases (ICD) codes in use when the deaths were reported. ICD classification revisions occurred in 1910, 1921, 1930, 1939, 1949, 1958, 1968, and 1979. Death rates before 1933 do not include all states. Comparability ratios were applied to rates for 1970 and 1975. *(From Centers for Disease Control and Prevention (CDC): Achievements in public health, 1900-1999: Decline in deaths from heart disease and stroke—United States, 1900-1999. MMWR Morbid Mortal Wkly Rep 48:649, 1999.)*

A main characteristic of the age of delayed degenerative diseases is the steadily rising age at which a first CVD event occurs or at which people die of CVD. Despite declines in age-adjusted mortality, the aging of the population will maintain CVD as the predominant cause of morbidity and mortality. Life expectancy at birth is 74.8 years for men and 80.1 years for women, and at age 65 is 16.8 years for men and 19.8 for women. CVD still causes most morbidity and mortality, but it afflicts an older population than it did in the middle of the century.

Age of Inactivity and Obesity

Overweight and obesity have increased at an alarming pace, and only a minority of the population meets minimal physical activity recommendations, favoring the development of even more diabetes and hypertension in the future. Increases in childhood obesity and physical inactivity are leading to an upsurge in diabetes and hypertension among younger individuals.[6,7] Fortunately, recent trends in the first decade of this century suggest that there may be a tapering in the increases in obesity among adults, although the rates of obesity remain alarmingly high, at almost 34%.[12] Rates of detection and treatment of hypertension have plateaued.[13] The decline in smoking rates has leveled off, with approximately 20% of adults classified as current smokers.[14] These worrisome changes in CVD risk behaviors and factors may slow the rate of decline and could even contribute to future increases in age-adjusted rates of CVD unless they are prevented. However, continued progress in the development and application of therapeutic advances appears to have offset the effects from the changes in obesity and diabetes rates. For example, cholesterol levels continue to decline. Overall, in this decade, the age-adjusted death rate has continued to decline by about 3%/yr, from 342 to 263/100,000.

Current Worldwide Variations in the Global Burden of Cardiovascular Disease

An epidemiologic transition much like the one that occurred in the United States is occurring worldwide. However, the rate of transition

TABLE 1-3 Cardiovascular Disease in the United States, 2005

TYPE	PREVALENCE (MILLIONS)	CRUDE MORTALITY (THOUSANDS)	PERCENTAGE OF TOTAL DEATHS	RATE/100,000
Cardiovascular disease	80.0	864.5	35.3	288.8
Hypertension	73.6	57.4	2.3	18.4
Ischemic heart disease	16.8	445.7	18.2	150.4
Stroke	6.5	143.6	5.9	48.4
Congestive heart failure	5.7	292.2	1.2	19.9
Rheumatic heart disease	NA	3.4	0.14	1.1
	ANNUAL EVENTS (THOUSANDS)			
Myocardial infarction	1255			
New	785			
Recurrent	470			
Stroke	795			
New	610			
Recurrent	185			
CABG	448			
PTCA	1313			
Valve surgery*	106			

*Total costs, $403.1 billion—direct, $257.6 billion; indirect, $145.5 billion.

CABG = coronary artery bypass grafting; NA = not available; PTCA = percutaneous transluminal coronary angioplasty.

Data from American Heart Association: 2009 Heart and Stroke Statistical Update. Dallas, American Heart Association, 2009; Kung H, Hoyert DL, Xu J, Murphy SL: Deaths: Final Data for 2005. National Vital Statistics Reports; vol. 56 no. 10. Hyattsville, Md, National Center for Health Statistics, 2008; and American Heart Association. Heart Disease and Stroke Statistics—2008 Update. Dallas, American Heart Association, 2008.

varies widely, leading to large discrepancies in disease burden. After a review of high-income countries that have followed a transition similar to that in the United States, other high-income regions that have followed a somewhat different course will be described. Finally, the status of the epidemiologic transition in low- and middle-income countries, where data are more limited, will be summarized.

High-Income Countries

Approximately 940 million people (15% of the world's population) live in high-income countries, including the United States, Canada, Australia, New Zealand, Japan, and the countries of the European Union. The movement of most of these countries through the epidemiologic transition, with rising levels of risk factors and CVD death rates until the 1960s, and then declines in both over the next 40 years, is similar to what has occurred in the United States. CHD is the dominant form, with rates that tend to be twofold to fivefold higher than stroke rates. There are two notable exceptions. In Portugal, stroke rates for men and women are higher than CHD rates. The same is true in Japan, where stroke causes more fatalities than CHD. In both of these countries, however, the pattern seems to be moving toward that seen in other high-income countries, with more rapid declines in stroke than in CHD rates.

In high-income countries, despite the overall increase in CVD burden, the age-adjusted death rates for CVD are declining, predominantly driven by large stroke rate reductions. This age-adjusted decline results largely from preventive interventions that allow people to avoid disease, treatments to prevent death during an acute manifestation of disease (particularly stroke or MI), and interventions that prolong survival once CVD is manifest. Thus, the average age of death from CVD continues to climb and, as a result, affects a larger population in retirement. Almost 80% of deaths in high-income countries occur in those older than 60 years, compared with 42% in low- and middle-income countries.[2] Between 1990 and 2020, CHD deaths alone are anticipated to increase by 120% for women and 137% for men in developing countries.[15] However, distinct differences remain in the severity of the burden affecting the various populations.

The rates of CVD in Western Europe tend to be similar to those in the United States. However, the absolute rates vary threefold among the countries of Western Europe, with a clear north-south gradient of higher CHD and stroke rates in the north. The highest CVD rates in the European high-income countries (two to three times higher than the median rates) are in Finland, Ireland, and Scotland. Although still high, deaths from CHD among Finnish men of working age have decreased by almost 80% over the last 30 years, from 508 deaths/100,000 in 1967 to 126/100,000 in 2003. A program called "Success in Finland" has contributed to this decline, including a more than 40% decrease in CHD death rates in men and women between 1989 and 1999. The Scottish government is also taking measures to decrease rates, including banning smoking in all enclosed places as of spring 2006. The lowest CVD rates in Europe are in the Mediterranean countries of France, Spain, and Italy, where age-adjusted CHD rates are less than 125 and 40/100,000 for men and women, respectively.[16] Although both stroke and CHD rates are higher in northern Europe, the disparity in CHD rates is much greater. For example, CHD rates for men are 222% higher in Finland than in Spain, whereas stroke rates are only 21% higher. CVD rates in Canada, New Zealand, and Australia are similar to rates in the United States. Rapid declines in CHD and stroke rates since the early 1970s have signaled that the high-income countries were in the fourth phase of the epidemiologic transition, the age of delayed degenerative diseases. In these countries, however, the rapidly increasing rate of obesity seems to indicate that many may be entering the fifth phase. CVD death rates continue to decline, at least in part because of the technical advances in treating CVD.

JAPAN. This country is unique among high-income countries. As its rates of communicable diseases fell in the early part of the 20th century, stroke rates increased dramatically; by the middle of the century, they were the highest in the world. CHD rates, however, did not rise as sharply as in other industrialized nations and have remained lower than in any other industrialized country. Overall, CVD rates have fallen 60% since the 1960s, largely because of a decrease in age-adjusted stroke rates. Japanese men and women currently have the highest life expectancies in the world—86 years for women and 79 years for men. The difference between Japan and other industrialized countries may stem in part from genetic factors, but it is more likely that a fish- and plant-based, low-fat diet and resultant low cholesterol levels have played a more important role. As is true for so many countries, dietary habits in Japan are undergoing substantial changes. Since the late 1950s, cholesterol levels have progressively increased. A study that analyzed diet and cholesterol levels in a cohort of rural Japanese men found that their carbohydrate intake decreased significantly, from 84% in 1958 to 62% in 1999, whereas protein and fat intake increased dramatically, from 11% to 18% for protein and 5% to 20% for fat.[17] Although average cholesterol levels rose from 152.5 to 194.2 mg/dL, the incidence of coronary artery disease in this population remains low. This situation could change, however, because there seems to be a long lag phase before dietary changes become manifest as CHD events.

Low- and Middle-Income Countries

The World Bank places countries in regions based on geography and income level. Low- and middle-income countries are divided into six geographic subregions—East Asia and Pacific, (Eastern) Europe and Central Asia, Latin America and the Caribbean, Middle East and North Africa, South Asia, and sub-Saharan Africa. The high-income countries, however, are not geographically distinct. For example, the Europe and Central Asia region is made up of low- and middle-income countries from eastern Europe, whereas the wealthier western European countries are part of the high-income region, as defined by the World Bank. Significant costs and infrastructure limitations prohibit most low- and middle-income countries from having completely representative demographic surveys, vital registration systems, or disease registries; therefore, the review highlights countries with large populations and reliable data.

The six regions that constitute the low- and middle-income countries have a high degree of heterogeneity with respect to the phase of the epidemiologic transition, as illustrated by the dominant disease rates in each region (**Fig. 1-4**). The two regions where stroke still exceeds CHD as a cause of CVD death are the East Asia and Pacific and sub-Saharan Africa regions (**Fig. 1-5**). The East Asia and Pacific region appears to be following more of a Japanese-style transition, with relatively high stroke rates, whereas in Africa this may reflect their position in an earlier stage of the epidemiologic transition. Hypertensive heart disease is the largest single contributor among the remaining causes of CVD morbidity and mortality, accounting for as much as 11% in Middle East and North African countries and as little as 2% in the South Asia region.

The variability in disease prevalence in the various regions likely results from multiple factors. First, the countries are in various phases of the epidemiologic transition described earlier. Second, the regions may have cultural and/or genetic differences that lead to varying levels of CVD risk. For example, per capita consumption of dairy products (and thus consumption of saturated fat) is much higher in India than in China, although rising in both countries. Third, certain additional competing pressures exist in some regions, such as war or infectious diseases (e.g., human immunodeficiency virus/acquired immunodeficiency syndrome [HIV/AIDS]) in sub-Saharan Africa.

In many low- and middle-income countries, the age-adjusted death rates for CHD are increasing. Because CHD afflicts a younger population in developing regions, an increased number of deaths affect the working-age population. For some developing countries, the severity of the epidemiologic transition has appeared to follow a reverse social gradient, with members of lower socioeconomic groups suffering the highest rates of CHD and highest levels of various risk factors.[18] Unfortunately, reductions in risk factors do not follow the same trend. Compared with people in the upper and middle socioeconomic strata, those in the lowest stratum are less likely to acquire and apply information on risk factors and behavior modifications or to have access to advanced treatments. Consequently, CVD mortality rates decline later in those of lower socioeconomic status.

EAST ASIA AND PACIFIC

Demographic and Social Indices

The East Asia and Pacific (EAP) region is the most populated low- and middle-income region in the world, with almost 1.9 billion people. The gross national income (GNI) per capita is $1630, ranging from $2720 in Thailand to $430 in Laos.[19] In 2004, total health expenditure was 4.4% of total GDP, or $62 per capita. China is the most populated country, representing almost 70% of the region.

Life expectancy has risen quickly across the EAP region. Nowhere is this more evident than in China, which saw its life expectancy increase from 37 years in the mid-1950s to 71 years in 2000. This increase has been accompanied by a large rural to urban migration pattern, rapid urban modernization, aging of the population, decreased birth rates, major dietary changes, increased tobacco use, and a transition to work involving physical inactivity.

Burden of Disease

According to the World Health Organization (WHO) Global Burden of Disease (GBD) Project, CVD caused more than 4.4 million deaths in the EAP region in 2004, approximately 1.2 million from CHD and 2.2 million from cerebrovascular diseases.[1] The prevalence of angina and cerebrovascular diseases was 8.2 and 9.1 million people, respectively. The numbers of DALYs lost caused by CHD were 11.8 million for CHD and 24.2 million for cerebrovascular diseases. Between 1950 and 1990, the rate of CVD mortality increased threefold as a percentage of total deaths in China.

Stroke and CHD are the most prevalent forms of CVD in the EAP region. Together they account for between 60% and 77% of CVD mortality in China.[20] In contrast to North America and Europe, stroke is the leading cause of CVD in most areas of the EAP region.[21] In the country as a whole, China appears to be straddling the second and third stages of a Japanese-style epidemiologic transition. Among men aged 35 to 64 years in China, stroke death rates are 217 to 243/100,000, versus CHD death rates of 64 to 106/100,000.[20]

Even with high stroke rates, CHD is emerging as a large and growing burden in East Asia. Data from the largest death registration and classification study in China have shown that CHD accounts for 13% to 22% of overall CVD deaths and 4% to 9% of total deaths, with the higher percentages seen in urban areas. In 2004, the WHO estimated that almost 400,000 people died in China from CHD, and 652,000 cases were diagnosed.[21] The age-adjusted mortality from CHD was 80 to 128/100,000 for men and 57 to 98/100,000 for women. Higher rates were seen in urban versus rural areas (by a factor of six), higher income compared with lower income areas, and northeastern areas of China compared with southern areas.

CHD rates have grown quickly over the past two decades in China. Age-adjusted CHD mortality increased 39% in women and 41% in men aged 35 to 74 years between 1984 and 1999. Furthermore, the incidence of CHD increased by 2.7% annually in men and 1.2% annually in women. Although rates are higher, hospitalizations are somewhat low. Acute MI accounted for 4.1% of all hospital discharges in 2004 in large cities, and 2.1% of discharges in smaller cities and rural areas.[21]

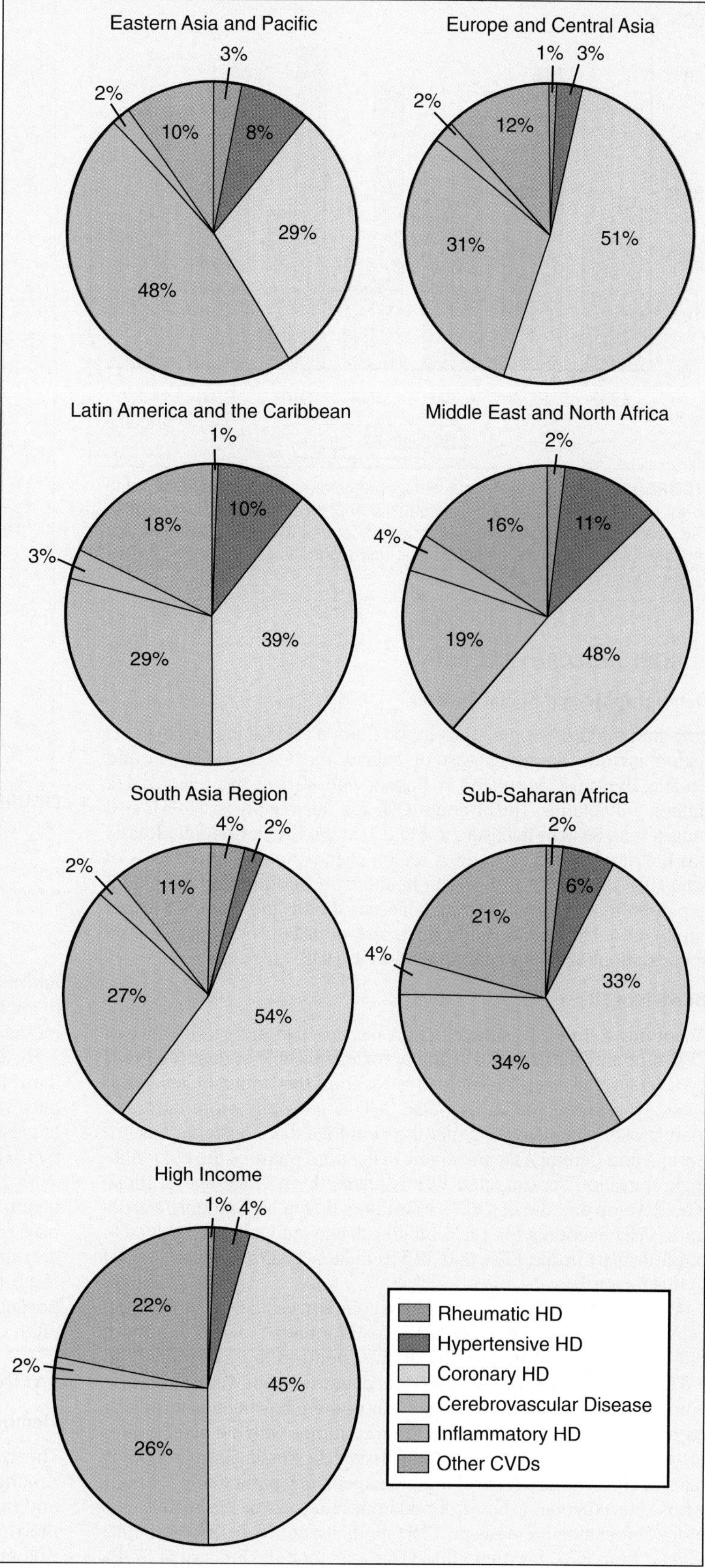

FIGURE 1-4 Cardiovascular disease deaths by specific cause by region.

The data for the burden of CHD in the Pacific Islands is much more limited. However, estimates from the WHO GBD Project suggest that Pacific Island age-standardized CHD rates exceed those in China by at least twofold to threefold; CHD age-standardized death rates range from 110/100,000 in the Federated States of Micronesia to 125/100,000 in Samoa and up to 181/100,000 in Nauru.[1]

CH 1

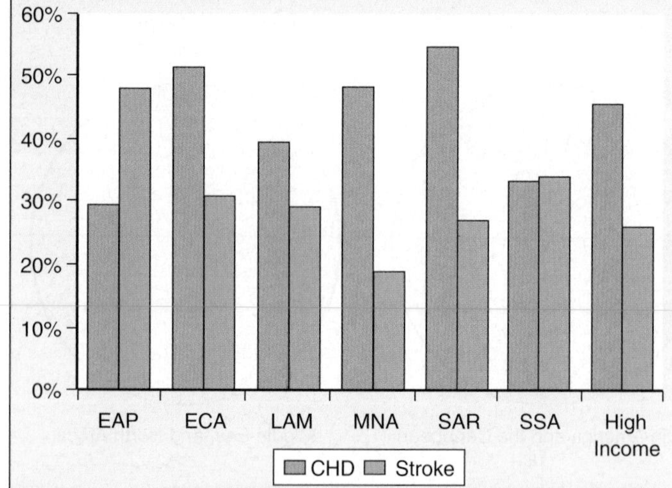

FIGURE 1-5 Comparison of percentages of cardiovascular disease mortality attributable to coronary heart disease (CHD) and stroke by developing region. EAP = East Asia and Pacific; ECA = Europe and Central Asia; LAM = Latin America and the Caribbean; MNA = Middle East and North Africa; SAR = South Asia Region; SSA = sub-Saharan Africa.

EUROPE AND CENTRAL ASIA

Demographic and Social Indices

Low- and middle-income areas in the Europe and Central Asia (ECA) region include countries east of Poland, the Czech Republic, and Croatia; the most populated is Russia, with 30% of the region's 472 million inhabitants. The average GNI for the region is $1,954; GNI ranges from $330 in Tajikistan to $11,220 in the Czech Republic. Russia has a GNI of $4,460.[19] The ECA region spends an average of 6.6% of total GDP on public and private health care, and the average health expenditure per capita is $250. Tajikistan spends the least, at $14 per capita, and Hungary spends the most, at $800 per capita. Russia spends about $245 per capita, or 6% of its GDP.[19]

Burden of Disease

According to the GBD study, the ECA has the highest regional rates of CVD mortality in the world, with approximately 60% of deaths caused by CVD. Overall rates resemble those seen in the United States in the 1960s, when CVD was at its peak. CHD is generally more common than stroke, which suggests that the countries that constitute Eastern Europe and Central Asia are largely in the third phase of the epidemiologic transition. As expected in this phase, the average age of those who develop and die of CVD is lower than that in high-income economies. CHD accounts for 1.685 million deaths annually (roughly 30% of all deaths) in the ECA, and 18.510 million DALYs are lost to CHD in this region.[2]

Although the GBD study provides a common estimate for the whole ECA region, an analysis of country-level information reveals important differences in CHD profiles among the countries in this region (**Fig. 1-6**) and compared with high-income countries from Western Europe. Since the dissolution of the Soviet Union, there has been a surprising increase in CVD rates in some of these countries, with the highest rates in Ukraine, Bulgaria, Belarus, and Russia.[22] In Russia, increased CVD rates have contributed to falling life expectancy, particularly for men, whose life expectancy has dropped from 71.6 years in 1986 to 59 years today. Percentage increases in CHD mortality between 1980 and 1992 ranged from 8.3% for men and 7.8% for women in Hungary, to 57.4% and 45.7%, respectively, in Romania.[23]

In contrast, CHD death rates have declined remarkably in ECA countries that experienced economic and market transformations in the early 1990s. In Poland, Slovenia, Hungary, the Czech Republic, and Slovakia, CHD rates declined dramatically throughout the 1990s, across both sexes, ages, and residential and educational groups.[24] In the meantime, in the former Soviet Republics (FSRs), where economic

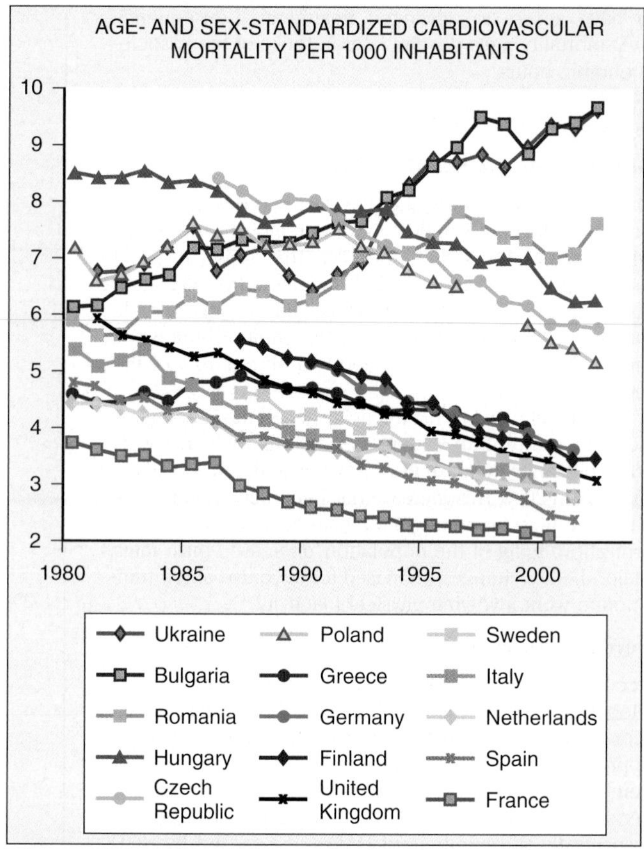

FIGURE 1-6 Trends in age- and sex-standardized cardiovascular mortality in selected European countries. *(From European Society of Cardiology: Cardiovascular Diseases in Europe: Euro Heart Survey and National Registries of Cardiovascular Diseases and Patient Management 2004 [http://www.escardio.org/guidelines-surveys/ehs/documents/ehs-cvd-report-2006.pdf].)*

and market transformations were delayed, CHD mortality continued to increase throughout the early 1990s, and has only experienced modest declines since then.

By 2002, CHD mortality in all ECA countries was still much higher than that in Western Europe or North America; however, the highest rates were seen in the FSRs, with the Russian Federation claiming the highest rates of CHD deaths in the world.[25] Importantly, deaths caused by CHD in these countries are not restricted to older adults. The GBD study has estimated that 601,000 (35.7%) of all CHD deaths in the ECA region occur in the working-age population (ages 15 to 69 years). High rates of CHD are especially troublesome in Ukraine and other FSRs in transition, where health systems are not sufficiently financed to respond to a high demand for chronic disease treatment, and out-of-pocket health care expenditures incurred by patients' households are often catastrophic.[26]

LATIN AMERICA AND THE CARIBBEAN

Demographic and Social Indices

The Latin America and Caribbean region (LAM) comprises Central America, South America, and most island nations in the Caribbean, and has a total population of about 560 million.[27] Brazil, the region's most populous country, has a third of the population, with Argentina, Colombia, Mexico, Peru, and Venezuela making up another third. The Caribbean nations, including the Dominican Republic, Jamaica, and Haiti, account for less than 10% of the population in the region. Average GNI per capita in the region is approximately $5500 dollars (purchasing power parity [PPP] $9321)[28] and all the countries spend less than 10% of their GDP on health care.[29] This level of spending translates into health care expenditures that range from $28 in Haiti to $775 in Barbados per capita.

Burden of Disease

The WHO GBD study ranked CHD as the single leading cause of mortality in the region, estimating it to be responsible for 11% of all deaths in 2004. An additional 8% can be attributed to stroke. Overall, CVD causes 28% of all deaths. Data available from the Pan American Health Organization (PAHO) also indicate that circulatory diseases accounted for 29% of all deaths in the region in 2004. In contrast, TB, malaria, HIV/AIDS, and other communicable diseases account for 10% of deaths. Unlike high-income countries, where CHD dominates among circulatory diseases, CHD and CVD are equivalent contributors to mortality, at 35% and 29%, respectively, indicating relatively higher rates of untreated hypertension in this region. No regional data on morbidity from CHD are readily available, but a household survey conducted in Brazil found that about 3.6% of the population, or around 7 million people, reported having heart disease.[30] In addition, CHD accounts for about 1% of total hospitalizations in the country. In 2002, Haiti and Guyana had the highest mortality rates for stroke (176/100,000 and 175/100,000, respectively) whereas Colombia and El Salvador had the lowest (37/100,000 and 38/100,000, respectively).[31]

An assessment of the trends in mortality caused by CHD and stroke in the Americas from 1970 to 2000 has shown a decline of about 60% for each condition in both the United States and Canada.[32] The reductions in Latin America ranged from 25% to 40% among men and 20% to 50% among women. Venezuela had the highest CVD rate in 2000 (137/100,000), whereas Brazil had the highest stroke rate (86/100,000 for men and 62/100,000 for women). The lower reductions in Latin America are attributed to rapid lifestyle changes—dietary changes, increased smoking, increased obesity, and less exercise.

With some exceptions, similar regional trends likely apply to age-adjusted CHD mortality. For example, in Brazil, age-adjusted circulatory disease mortality has declined 3.9% annually, and age-adjusted CHD mortality has declined 3.6% annually.[33] The decline, seen across all age groups and both genders, was most significant in those 44 years of age and younger. In another study analyzing trends in age-adjusted CHD mortality from 1970 to 2002, Argentina, Brazil, Chile, Colombia, and Puerto Rico all experienced declines, ranging from 2% to 68%.[32]

Over the same period, however, age-adjusted CHD mortality trended upward in Mexico, Costa Rica, and Venezuela. Together, CHD (13%), cerebrovascular disease (9.7%), and hypertensive heart disease (3.2%) accounted for almost 25% of all deaths in Mexico in 2004, and 9.9% of deaths were attributed to high blood pressure.[34] One explanation is that these countries may have been in an earlier stage of development and are likely catching up with the rest of the region. For example, in Mexico, although age-adjusted CHD mortality increased from 90% to 94% over the three-decade period, the age-adjusted mortality was 82/100,000 in men and 53/100,000 in women in 2000, falling within the overall range of 21 to 136/100,000 for the region.

MIDDLE EAST AND NORTH AFRICA

Demographic and Social Indices

The 17 countries of the Middle East and North Africa (MNA) region represent 6% of the world's population (306 million people). Egypt and Iran are the two most populous countries in the region, with Egypt having 24% of total inhabitants and Iran 22%. According to the World Bank indicators from 2005, the GNI per capita for the region is $2,198 ($6,084 PPP).[19] GNI per capita for individual countries ranges from $600 ($920 PPP) in Yemen to $30,630 ($24,010 PPP) in Kuwait. Approximately 5.6% of the total GDP for the MNA region is used for public and private health care, according to World Bank data from 2004. The average health expenditure per capita is $103. Egypt spends $64 per capita, and Iran spends $158. At $34, Yemen spends the least amount on health care per capita, and the United Arab Emirates spend the most, $711.[19]

Burden of Disease

Statistics from the 2002 WHO GBD study show that about 5% of CVD deaths in low- and middle-income countries occur in the MNA region. Over 35% of all deaths in the region are attributable to CVD. CHD, the leading cause of mortality in 2001, accounted for 16.9% of total mortality and almost half of CVD mortality. Cerebrovascular disease causes 6.8% of total deaths and 19% of CVD deaths. This translates into approximately 323,000 deaths in 2001 in the region.[2]

Mortality rates for the region have declined over time, whereas life expectancy has increased from 64.05 years in 1990 to 67.35 years in 2001. The crude death rate for the region has notably decreased. The newest data show that the crude death rate was 7.55% in 1990 and 6.15% in 2001. Also in 2001, 1.235 million deaths in the MNA region were attributable to noncommunicable diseases.[2] For CVD specifically, the number of deaths reported was 671,000. However, with the increase in life expectancy, there is an expectation that CHD will increase in the region.

Individual country surveys have shown that Iran may have a higher burden than other countries, including Saudi Arabia and Jordan. A study of a random sample of 3,723 people in Iran found that 11.3% had coronary symptoms and an additional 1.4% had had an MI. The age-adjusted prevalence was therefore 12.7%.[28] Another study, done in Saudi Arabia and involving 17,232 people from the general population, found that 5.5% were diagnosed with CHD. The data also showed that the prevalence was higher—6.2% compared with 4%—in urban versus rural areas.[35] In Jordan, a study found that a total of 5.9% out of 3,083 participants were told that they had an MI.[36] A 2001 Tunisian study of 20% of the male population found age-standardized rates of MI of only 163.8 in Tunis, 161.9 in Ariana, and 170.5/100,000 in Ben Arous.[37]

SOUTH ASIA

Demographic and Social Indices

The South Asia region (SAR), one of the world's most densely populated regions, comprises about 20% of the world's population, with a total of more than 1.4 billion residents. Home to almost 75% of the region's inhabitants, India is the largest country in the region. Average GNI per capita for the region is $692 ($3142 PPP), according to World Bank Indicators in 2005. GNI per capita ranges from $270 ($1530 PPP) in Nepal to $2560 in the Maldives. India is close to the average, with a GNI per capita of $730 ($3460 PPP). Figures from 2004 indicate that all countries spend an average of 4.6% of their total GDP, or $27 per capita, on health care. The Maldives spends the most per capita, at $208, and India spends $31, or 5% of its GDP. The lowest expenditure for health care is $14 per capita in Pakistan, Nepal, and Bhutan.[19]

Burden of Disease

In 2001, based on statistics from the GBD study, more than 25% of CVD deaths in low- and middle-income countries occurred in the SAR. Similarly, CVD accounts for more than 25% of all deaths in this region. This translated into a total of 3.4 million CVD deaths in 2001; CHD was the leading cause of mortality that year. CHD was responsible for 13.6% of total mortality, or 1.8 million deaths, and more than 50% of CVD mortality. CVD accounted for 6.8% of all deaths and 27% of CVD deaths. By comparison, communicable diseases were responsible for 43% of total mortality.[2]

Over time, regional mortality rates have declined as life expectancy has increased, from 57.2 years in 1990 to 60.7 years in 2001. The crude death rate for the region has decreased significantly; in 1990, it was 11.4% but had fallen to 9.75% in 2001.[2] However, deaths from CHD in India are increasing; from 1990 to 2000, CHD deaths rose from 1.17 million to 1.59 million. It is predicted that annual deaths from CHD will be approximately 2.03 million by 2010.[38] Similarly, overall CVD burden is expected to increase as well. In the 30-year period from 1990 to 2020, a 111% increase in CVD deaths is expected.[27]

Several studies in India and Pakistan have suggested substantial morbidity caused by CHD in this region. An estimated 31.8 million people are living with CHD in India alone,[27] a 10-fold increase over 40 years ago, which translates into an overall prevalence of about 11% in urban India and an age-adjusted prevalence of 9%, based on 2001 figures. Additional evidence suggests that women are more likely than men to have CVD in India.[39] The Initiative for Cardiovascular Health's National Cardiovascular Disease Database cited a study in India that found prevalence in men was more than 6% and in women more than

10%. More recently, a CHD study in Pakistan found a prevalence of about 6% in men and 4% in women, but active ischemia was twice as high in women. The study's authors[40] suggested that one in five adults in urban areas of Pakistan has CHD and, of these, it is estimated that only 25% are aware of their disease and are seeking medical care. Despite this, a survey of hospital data in Delhi has revealed that almost 25% of all medical admissions are because of CHD. Patients who do not seek treatment die at a rate of 7% to 8%/yr.[27]

Contrary to the epidemiologic transition in developed countries, recent evidence suggests that individuals in the SAR who have a lower socioeconomic status are developing a higher burden of CHD first. One possible explanation is that a higher proportion of the poor use tobacco products.[38]

Another demographic trend is the considerable increase in urban residents, normally associated with increased rates of CHD. Currently, about 30% of all inhabitants in the region live in an urban setting, a number that is expected to reach 43% by 2021.[41] Among urban dwellers, CHD prevalence has increased from 7% in 1980 to 9.7% in 1990 to 10.5% in 2000. CHD prevalence is increasing in urban areas as well, from 2.5% in 1980 to 4% in 1990 to 4.5% in 2000.[27] More recent data from the rural region of Andhra Pradesh in South India have suggested that the prevalence may actually be even higher in many rural regions.[42] CHD death rates were higher than 15% in this study, meaning that the rural/urban protection no longer exists—or the urban rates, if more carefully measured, could be much higher.

The rise in CHD mortality contributes to the economic burden in the Indian subcontinent. Data indicate that symptoms of CHD arise a full 10 years earlier here than in Western European and Latin American countries.[43] In India, 52% of CVD deaths occur among those younger than 70 years,[41] resulting in a considerable burden from CHD on working-age citizens.[27]

SUB-SAHARAN AFRICA

Demographic and Social Indices

Sub-Saharan Africa (SSA), as defined by the World Bank, comprises 31 island and continental nations. Approximately 782 million people lived in SSA in 2006, with Nigeria being the most populous nation (145 million) and Mauritius and Cape Verde having the smallest populations (1 million). The average annual population growth rate for 2000 to 2006 (4.7%) was almost twice the rate for 1990 to 2000 (2.5%). The average GNI per capita was $830 (U.S. dollars), on a gradient of $100 per capita in Burundi to $5570 in Botswana. Overall, the SSA region also had the lowest average life expectancy, 50 years.

Average public and private health care expenditures for the region are 6.3% of the total GDP, an average of $45 per capita according to 2004 World Bank indicators. The range of health care expenditures per capita for the region is similar to the GDP range for this region, from $3 in Burundi to $511 in Seychelles. Nigeria spends $23 per capita, or 4.6% of its total GDP.[19]

Burden of Disease

CHD was the leading cause of death in low- and middle-income countries in 2001, accounting for 11.8% (5.7 million) of all deaths, and in the SSA region, CHD accounted for 3.2% of all deaths.[2] In 2001, CVD accounted for 46% of all deaths caused by noncommunicable diseases (1,048,000) in SSA, and CHD accounted for 33% of all cardiovascular diseases (343,000). Stroke was responsible for 4.5% of the global burden of disease and 9.5% of the regional mortality in low- and middle-income countries in 2001. The burden of HIV/AIDS was 5.1% globally, with middle- and low-income countries contributing only 5.3% of mortality in the region.

Human Immunodeficiency Virus and Cardiovascular Disease

Given the large burden of disease caused by HIV/AIDS, the potential risk of CVD among those being treated with antiretroviral medications is of growing concern (see Chap. 72). HIV-positive men older than 50 years have a greater prevalence of dyslipidemia, diabetes, and peripheral artery disease (50% of cases were asymptomatic) compared with their noninfected counterparts.[44] Of note, 55% of these HIV-infected men are prior smokers, and they are also more likely to have used antihypertensive drugs, lipid-lowering agents, and antidiabetic medications. A recent study of 95 patients initiating antiretroviral drugs indicated that patients who had high baseline lipid levels showed a marked increase in lipoprotein(a).[45] Grover and colleagues[46] have conducted a randomized controlled trial comparing lipid level changes after 32 weeks of treatment with two different highly active retroviral therapy (HAART) regimens, atazanavir and nelfinavir. Levels of total cholesterol and low-density lipoprotein (LDL) increased significantly more among patients using nelfinavir (+24%, +28%) compared with those using atazanavir (+4%, +1%), increasing the 10-year risk of CHD by 50% in the former group. These data indicate that the interaction of positive HIV status, HAART therapy, and risk for CVD warrants continued attention.

Global Trends in Cardiovascular Disease

Examination of regional trends is helpful for estimating global trends in the burden of disease, particularly CVD. Because 85% of the world's population lives in low- and middle-income countries, rates in these countries largely drive global rates of CVD. Even as rates fall in high-income countries, CVD rates worldwide are accelerating because most low- and middle-income countries are entering the second and third phases of the epidemiologic transition, marked by rising CVD rates. The economic impact of chronic diseases could be dominated by CVD. Over the next decade or so, countries such as China, India, and Russia could forego between $200 and $550 billion in national income as a result of heart disease, stroke, and diabetes.[47]

In 1990, CVD accounted for 28% of the world's 50.4 million deaths and 9.7% of the 1.4 billion lost DALYs. By 2001, CVD was responsible for 29% of all deaths and 14% of the 1.5 billion lost DALYs.[44] By 2020, the world population will grow to 7.8 billion and 32% of all deaths will be caused by CVD; by 2030, when the population is expected to reach 8.2 billion, 33% of all deaths will be caused by CVD (**Table 1-4**).[22] By 2030, WHO predicts that worldwide, CVD will be responsible for 24.2 million deaths.[22] Of these, 14.9% of deaths in men and 13.1% of deaths in women will be caused by CHD, and stroke will account for 10.4% of all deaths in men and 11.8% of all deaths in women.

Risk Factors

Table 1-5 displays the population-attributable fractions (PAF) of deaths caused by CHD for leading risk factors. Elevated levels of blood pressure and cholesterol remain the leading causes of CHD; tobacco, obesity, and physical inactivity remain important contributors. Diabetes is not listed because the GBD project considers it a disease, not a risk factor. The PAFs add up to more than 100% because there is interaction among the risk factors. Unique features regarding some CHD risk factors in the developing countries are described below.

Hypertension

Elevated blood pressure is an early indicator of the epidemiologic transition. A rising mean population blood pressure is apparent as populations industrialize and move from rural to urban settings. The high rate of undetected and therefore untreated hypertension presents a major concern in developing countries; throughout Asia, this likely contributes to the high prevalence of hemorrhagic stroke.

Worldwide, approximately 62% of strokes and 49% of cases of CHD are attributable to suboptimal (>115 mm Hg systolic) blood pressure, a factor thought to account for more than 7 million deaths annually. In a recent study,[48] it was estimated that 14% of deaths and 6% of DALYs lost globally were caused by nonoptimal levels of blood pressure. Although hypertension is usually defined as a systolic blood pressure higher than 140 mm Hg, Lawes and associates[48] have found that just over 50% of the attributable CVD burden occurs in those with a systolic blood pressure less than 145 mm Hg.

TABLE 1-4 Contribution of Various Disease Categories to Global Mortality

	POPULATION (MILLIONS)	TOTAL DEATHS (MILLIONS)	TOTAL DEATHS (%) CMPN	INJURY	NON-CMPN, NON-CVD	ALL CVDS	CHD	STROKE
1990								
World	5267	50.4	34.2	10.1	27.4	28.4	12.4	8.7
High income	798	7.12	6.4	6.2	42.8	44.6	23.4	11.1
Low and middle income	4470	43.3	38.7	10.7	24.8	25.7	10.6	8.3
2001								
World	6148	56.2	32.3	9.2	29.3	29.1	12.5	9.6
High income	929	7.9	7.0	6.0	48.5	38.5	17.3	9.9
Low and middle income	5219	48.3	36.4	9.7	26.2	27.6	11.8	9.5
2020*								
World	7800	65.1				31.5	13.6	10.6
2030*								
World	8200	74.5				32.5	14.0	11.1

CMPN = communicable diseases, maternal and perinatal conditions, and nutritional deficiency.
Data for 2020 and 2030 adapted from Mackay J, Mensah G: Atlas of Heart Disease and Stroke. Geneva, World Health Organization, 2004.

TABLE 1-5 Risk Factor Population-Attributable Fractions* for Mortality from Congenital Heart Disease

WORLD BANK REGION	HIGH BLOOD PRESSURE (%)	CHOLESTEROL (%)	TOBACCO (%)	OVERWEIGHT AND OBESITY (%)	PHYSICAL INACTIVITY (%)
East Asia and Pacific	41	32	6	10	19
Europe and Central Asia	61	55	17	24	20
Latin America and Caribbean	47	49	10	23	20
Middle East and North Africa	48	47	11	22	20
South Asia Region	39	43	10	5	19
Sub-Saharan Africa	43	15	5	8	20
Low- and middle-income	47	43	11	14	20
High-income	49	52	15	19	19

*PAFs may total >100%. See text for details.
Adapted from Lopez AD, Mathers CD, Ezzati M, et al (eds): Global Burden of Disease and Risk Factors. New York, World Bank Group, 2006.

Tobacco

By many accounts, tobacco use is the most preventable cause of death in the world. Over 1.3 billion people worldwide use tobacco; more than 1 billion smoke[49] and the rest use oral or nasal tobacco. More than 80% of tobacco use occurs in low- and middle-income countries, and if current trends continue unabated, there will be more than 1 billion deaths caused by tobacco during the 21st century.[30] Smoking-related CHD deaths in the developing world totaled 360,000 in 2000, compared with 200,000 cerebrovascular deaths that year.[50]

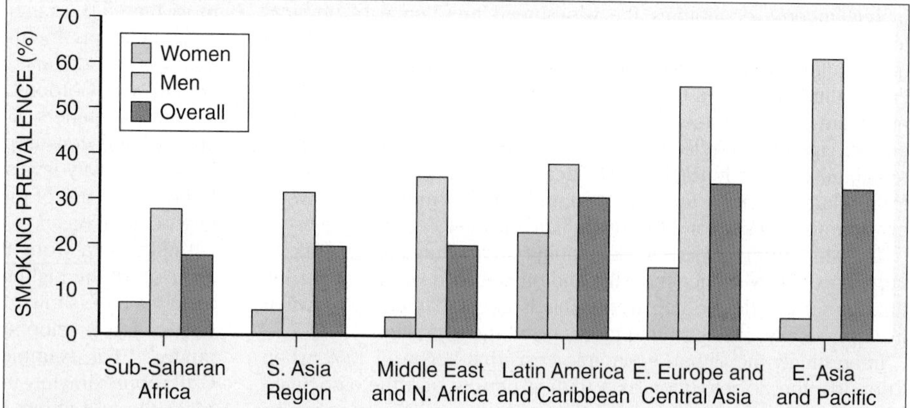

FIGURE 1-7 Smoking prevalence by sex in those 15 years of age or older (2000 estimates). *(From Jha P, Chaloupka FJ, Moore J, et al: Tobacco addiction.* In *Jamison DT, Breman JG, Measham AR, et al [eds]: Disease Control Priorities in the Developing Countries, 2nd ed. New York, Oxford University Press, 2006, pp. 869-886)*

The use of tobacco varies greatly across the world (**Fig. 1-7**). In general, more men than women smoke, and smoking is now more common in the developing world than in the developed world, where it is on the decline. Tobacco use is most common in Russia (>60% male prevalence), Indonesia (>60% male prevalence), and China (≈60% male prevalence).[49] Together, these three countries account for almost half of the world's users of tobacco. China alone has an estimated 311 million smokers.[49] Tobacco use is also prevalent in Latin America, the Pacific Islands (which have some of the highest female smoking rates in the world), and the Middle East.[49] Sub-Saharan Africa is currently a relatively low-prevalence tobacco-using area, with the exception of South Africa and parts of East Africa. Ezzati and coworkers[50] have calculated that in 2000, more than 1.62 million CVD deaths worldwide, or 11% of the total, were caused by smoking; 1.17 million were men and 670,000 occurred in the developing world. Globally, smoking-related CHD deaths totaled approximately 890,000, compared with 420,000 smoking-related cerebrovascular deaths.[50]

Other forms of tobacco use beyond cigarette smoking increase the risk for CHD. Bidis (hand-rolled cigarettes common in South Asia), kreteks (clove and tobacco cigarettes), hookah (flavored tobacco smoked through a water pipe), and smokeless tobacco are all linked to an increased risk for CHD.[30,51] The combined use of different forms of tobacco is associated with a higher risk of MI than using one type.

Second-hand smoke (SHS) also has now been well established as a cause of CHD. Using a conservative random effects model, Barnoya and Glantz[52] found that SHS is associated with a 1.31-fold increased risk of CHD (95% confidence interval [CI], 1.21 to 1.41). Their review of the biologic and epidemiologic literature on SHS concluded that the effects of chronic SHS exposure on increased CHD risk are substantial, rapid, and almost as large (80% to 90%) as those of active smoking.[52] These observations may explain the large and immediate drop seen in communities such as Helena, Montana, and in Scotland, which implemented smoke-free laws and found 20% to 40% decrease in admissions for MI, controlling for time, locality, and other variables.[53,54]

Lipids

Worldwide, high cholesterol levels cause some 56% of ischemic heart disease and 18% of strokes, amounting to 4.4 million deaths annually. Unfortunately, most developing countries have limited data on cholesterol levels, and often only total cholesterol values are collected. In high-income countries, mean population cholesterol levels are generally falling, but in low- and middle-income countries, there is wide variation in these levels. Generally, the ECA region has the highest levels, with the EAP and sub-Saharan Africa regions having the lowest levels.[55] As countries move through the epidemiologic transition, mean population plasma cholesterol levels typically rise. Changes accompanying urbanization clearly play a role, because plasma cholesterol levels tend to be higher in urban residents than in rural residents. This shift results largely from the greater consumption of dietary fats, primarily from animal products and processed vegetable oils, and from decreased physical activity.

Physical Inactivity

In high-income economies, the widespread prevalence of physical inactivity produces a high population-attributable risk (PAR) of cardiovascular consequences. The November 2007 Health and Healthcare Gallup poll found that 59% of adults say that they participate in moderate exercise three times a week, and 32% say that they participate in vigorous exercise three times a week.[55a] These numbers have remained essentially unchanged since 2001. Current guidelines call for moderate exercise for at least 30 minutes, 5 or more days a week, or vigorous exercise for 20 minutes, 3 days a week.

The shift from physically demanding, agriculture-based work to largely sedentary service industry- and office-based work is occurring throughout the developing world. This is accompanied by a switch from physically demanding to mechanized transportation.

Interestingly, the Cuban economic crisis that began in 1989, when Cuba lost the Soviet Union as a trading partner, and the associated hardship for its people improved their overall cardiovascular health. The crisis worsened for the next 5 years, and complete recovery did not take place until 2000. Sustained food rationing led to a reduction in per capita food intake, and the lack of public transportation caused by fuel shortages meant that more people were walking and riding bicycles. During the crisis period, the proportion of physically active adults increased from 30% to 67%, and a 1.5-unit shift in body mass index (BMI) distribution was observed.[56] From 1997 to 2002, deaths attributed to diabetes, CHD, and stroke decreased by 51%, 35%, and 20%, respectively.

Diabetes

Diabetes mellitus affects approximately 180 million people worldwide, and the number is expected to double by 2030.[14] Of those with diabetes, 90% have type 2 diabetes, approximately 80% of whom live in low- and middle-income countries. Future growth will be highest in developing regions such as Asia, Latin America and the Caribbean, and sub-Saharan Africa, where growth rates of diabetes are expected to be between 105% and 162%, compared with about 72% in the United States and 32% in Europe.[57,58] In addition, most cases are and will remain within the 45- to 64-year-old age group in developing countries, whereas those older than 65 years are most affected in developed countries.

Rising rates of obesity, as well as an aging and urbanized population, likely link to the diabetes epidemic. Almost 90% of type 2 diabetes cases are related to obesity, and diabetes and its related complications are the costliest consequences of obesity. Mortality from diabetes is also increasing. About 1.1 million people died of diabetes in 2005, and that number is estimated to increase by 50% in 10 years.[14]

Interestingly, Asian countries face a relatively larger burden of diabetes compared with the Europe and Central Asia or Latin America and Caribbean regions. For example, India and China have the largest numbers of diabetics—32 million and 21 million, respectively—in the world.[58] Indonesia, Pakistan, and Bangladesh are in the top 10 in terms of high absolute number of diabetics. Asian populations may have a higher risk for developing diabetes, even at a lower BMI, because of a greater tendency toward visceral obesity. In addition, this population may experience both undernutrition (during the perinatal period) and rapid weight gain (during childhood), a combination that increases the risk for insulin resistance.[59]

Obesity

Obesity is increasing throughout the world, particularly in developing countries, where the trajectories are steeper than those experienced by developed countries. According to the latest WHO data, there are approximately 1.1 billion overweight adults in the world, with 115 million of them known to be living with obesity-related problems in the developing world.[60] A 2005 compilation of population-based surveys has revised this number to about 1.3 billion and estimated that 23% of adults older than 20 years are overweight (BMI > 25) and an additional 10% are obese (BMI > 30).[61,62] In developing countries such as Egypt, Mexico, and Thailand, rates of overweight are increasing at two to five times the rate of those in the United States. In China, over an 8-year period, the prevalence of BMI greater than 25 increased by more than 50% in men and women.[61]

Explanations for this rapid trajectory are complex; they include changes in dietary patterns, physical activity, and urbanization. Popkin and Gordon-Larsen[61] have reported that use of edible oils, caloric sweeteners, and animal source foods is increasing. Annual animal food consumption tripled in China from the 1950s to 1990s. Physical activity levels are expected to decline as urbanization leads to increased use of motorized vehicles and a change to more sedentary occupations.

Unlike data from the 1980s, which showed that obesity was a problem of the higher income group in developing countries, recent analyses have shown that the poor are relatively more susceptible to obesity as a developing country's GNP approaches the middle-income range.[63,64] For example, once a country reaches $2500 per capita of GNP (approximately the median GNP for lower middle–income countries), the probability of being obese is higher among women in the lower income group than in the higher income group.

Reports have focused on two groups. Women are more affected than men, with the number of overweight women generally exceeding underweight women based on data from 36 developing countries.[65] In the same survey, the prevalence of overweight women exceeded 20% in more than 90% of surveyed countries. Even rural areas in 50% of the countries surveyed experienced these rates. Adolescents are at particular risk, with 1 in 10 children currently estimated to be overweight.[61,66] The number of overweight children is increasing in

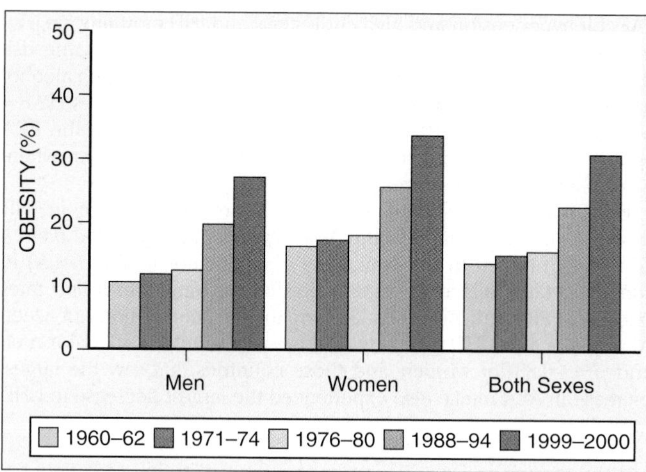

FIGURE 1-8 Trends in obesity (body mass index > 30) among Americans aged 20 to 74 years. *(From the National Health Examination Survey and the National Health and Nutrition Examination Surveys: Healthy weight, overweight, and obesity among U.S. adults [http://www.cdc.gov/nchs/data/nhanes/databriefs/adultweight.pdf].)*

countries as diverse as China, Brazil, India, Mexico, and Nigeria. Brazil saw an alarming rise, from 4% to 14% over a two-decade period.

In many high-income countries, the mean BMI is rising at an alarming rate, even as mean plasma cholesterol levels are falling and age-adjusted hypertension levels remain fairly stable during the fourth phase (the age of delayed degenerative diseases). In the United States, weight gain is occurring among all sectors of the population; however, rates are increasing faster among minorities and women. The percentage of adults classified as overweight in the United States has been stable since the 1960s, but the prevalence of obesity doubled between 1980 and 2002, rising from 15% to 30% (**Fig. 1-8**).[67,68]

Diet

As we have evolved, selective pressures have favored the ability to conserve and store fat as a defense against famine. This adaptive mechanism has become unfavorable in light of the larger portion sizes, processed foods, and sugary drinks that many people now regularly consume. From 1971 to 2000, the daily caloric intake of the typical U.S. woman rose 22%, from 1542 to 1877 kcal, and the typical U.S. man increased his intake by 7%, from 2450 to 2618 kcal.[69] As per capita income increases, so does consumption of fats and simple carbohydrates, but intake of plant-based foods decreases. A key element of this dietary change is an increase in the intake of saturated animal fats and inexpensive hydrogenated vegetable fats, which contain atherogenic trans fatty acids. New evidence suggests that the high intake of trans fats may also lead to abdominal obesity, another risk factor for CVD.

China provides a good example of such a nutritional transition—rapid shifts in diet linked to social and economic changes. The China Nationwide Health Survey[20] has found that between 1982 and 2002, calories from fat increased from 25% to 35% in urban areas and from 14% to 28% in rural areas, as calories from cereals decreased from 70% to 47%. As recently as 1980, the average BMI for Chinese adults was about 20, and fewer than 1% had a BMI of 30 or higher. From 1992 to 2002, the number of overweight adults increased by 41%, whereas the number of obese adults increased by 97%.

China and other countries in transition have the opportunity to spare their populations from the high levels of trans fats that North Americans and Europeans have consumed over the last 50 years by avoiding government policies that can contribute to the CVD burden. For example, the European Union (EU) Common Agricultural Policy (CAP) program, which subsidizes dairy and meat commodities, has increased the availability and consumption of products containing saturated fats. The CAP program has contributed to an estimated 9800 additional CHD deaths and 3000 additional stroke deaths in the EU, 50% of them premature.[70]

Another facet of the nutritional transition for countries adopting a Western diet is the introduction of soft drinks and other high-sugar beverages, which is associated with weight gain and increased risk of type 2 diabetes. A recent study of American women has shown that these beverages may be linked to CHD. Drinking full-calorie sugar-sweetened beverages on a regular basis was associated with a higher risk of CHD, even after accounting for other unhealthful lifestyle or dietary factors.[71]

Population Aging

Average life expectancy will reach 73 years by 2025, according to the WHO. This rise relates to a decline in overall infant mortality and fertility rates. Although older adults will represent a greater percentage of the developed world's population—more than 20% of the U.S. population will be older than 65 by 2025—developing regions such as Asia and Latin America will almost double their relative proportion of older adults to 10% of their populations.[72]

The time of transition to an older population is markedly shorter in developing countries. For example, whereas it took the United States and Canada more than 65 years to double their over-65 population, China will do so in 26 years, Tunisia in 24, and Brazil in 21.[73] Currently, 77% of the growth in the older population is occurring in developing regions. Such acute changes in the population structure leave less time to expand an already overburdened health infrastructure to address the chronic diseases of older adults, which prominently include cardiovascular conditions.

By Region

EAST ASIA PACIFIC. Hypertension makes up the largest PAF of disease burden for CHD in the East Asia and Pacific region, followed closely by tobacco use.[43] Slightly more recent data from China suggest a minimally lower overall prevalence of hypertension, 19%. In the Pacific region, hypertension is high and increasing over time. American Samoan men had a hypertension prevalence of 46% in 2002, compared with 40% 20 years prior.[74]

Tobacco use is a large and growing cause of CHD in East Asia. Smoking rates are extremely high in men but lower in women. In China, smoking rates are above 60% in men and below 10% in women. Tobacco use is high in many Pacific Islanders as well. Tongan men have a smoking prevalence greater than 60%, and Samoan and Tuvaluan men have rates higher than 50%.[49] More than 50% of Nauruan women smoke (higher than men), and Samoan and Tuvaluan women have smoking rates ranging from 20% to 40%.[49] The attributable burden of CHD caused by smoking mirrors these patterns.

The Asia-Pacific collaboration estimated a PAR for obesity in China of 3%, largely caused by lower estimates of overweight (15-17%) and obesity (2-3%) coming from the China National Nutrition Survey of 2002.[75] Other East Asian countries have slightly higher PARs for obesity, such as 4% in Malaysia, 6% in Thailand, and 8% in Mongolia.[75] High rates of obesity exist in the Pacific Islands.[76] Using higher Polynesian-specific standards of obesity (defined as BMI ≥ 32 as opposed to 30 in other populations),[77] McGarvey and colleagues found that 71% of American Samoan women were obese in 2002, along with 61% of men.[74] The rates of obesity more than doubled over 20 years in men, and increased by almost 50% in women.

Hyperlipidemia is generally less common in East Asia than in the Pacific Islands. Rates of hypercholesterolemia (total cholesterol ≥ 5.20 mmol/L) increased from 18% in 1982 to 31% in 1998 in adults aged 35-59.[21] Recent prevalence values for the Pacific lack precision, though studies in Samoa from the 1990s showed that the prevalence of total cholesterol ≥ 5.5 mmol/L was 36% and had almost doubled since prior measurements 10 years earlier.

Diabetes rates in East Asia are low but rising. The rate of diabetes in urban areas is 3% compared with 2% in rural areas.[21] The PAR of CHD in China is 6% in urban areas and 5% in rural areas.[21] In the

Western Pacific, where rates of diabetes are among the highest in the world,[74] CHD PAR is likely higher, though no good studies exist. The prevalence of diabetes, like obesity and hypercholesterolemia, is rapidly growing, especially in more modernized areas. In American Samoa, the adult prevalence of type 2 diabetes was 22% in men and 18% in women,[74] almost double that of men and women in independent (and less economically developed) Samoa. However, in all areas across Samoa, rates of diabetes almost doubled between 1991 and 2003.[74] The PAR for nonoptimal glucose, measured as a continuum for adults older than 30 years in the entire East Asia and Pacific regions, was estimated at 14% for men and 15% for women.[78]

EASTERN EUROPE AND CENTRAL ASIA. Of the four major modifiable risk factors for ischemic heart disease (IHD)—smoking, obesity (BMI > 30), raised blood pressure, and high cholesterol (>200 mg/dL)—many are more prevalent in the Europe and Central Asia regions than in other regions of the world. The reported prevalence of tobacco use among men is highest in Ukraine (62%); among women, the highest reported prevalence is in Serbia (27%). In those countries for which data exist, the highest prevalence of increased blood pressure is found in men in Croatia (50%) and women in Bosnia-Herzegovina (45%); the prevalence of obesity is highest among men in Croatia (22%) and women in Turkey (30%). Data on mean cholesterol levels were scarce; some survey results have suggested that mean levels in Hungary range from 172 to 205 mg/dL for males aged 14 years and older and from 170 to 213 mg/dL for women, and in Romania from 192 to 216 mg/dL for men and 189 to 217 mg/dL for women aged 30 years and older.[79]

However, these traditional risk factors for IHD do not explain all the variation in IHD mortality in the ECA region. From the mid-1980s to the mid-1990s, the WHO MONICA study attempted to develop a model to explain IHD risk across various countries based on traditional risk factors. The study found that using a risk score based on the Framingham risk factors for heart disease as a single explanatory variable for IHD incidence explained 22% of the variation in IHD risk for men and 10% for women. However, after excluding the five FSR populations that were in the study (four in Russia and one in Lithuania) from the model, the variation in IHD risk for men explained by the model increased to 31%, indicating that the traditional risk factors were not sufficient in predicting true risk of IHD in FSR populations. Vast increases in alcohol consumption and/or deaths being wrongly attributed to IHD at a time of very high total mortality were suggested as possible explanations for this discrepancy in results.[80] Another study in the Arkhangelsk region of Russia calculated a 10-year Framingham IHD risk score (also based on smoking, BMI, blood pressure, and cholesterol) for their study population of 7% to 8%, which implies an annual incidence of IHD of 7 to 8/1000 adults. However, according to official data for the region, the annual incidence of IHD at the time of the study (November 1999 to November 2000) was 16.9/1000 adults, further suggesting that these traditional risk factors do not explain all the risk for IHD in the Russian population.[81]

In 2004, the INTERHEART study identified low fruit and vegetable intake, physical inactivity, stress, and diabetes as important risk factors for IHD in addition to the traditional risk factors discussed earlier.[82] However, researchers in Croatia investigated these risk factors in a population of MI patients in southern Croatia and found that although important risk factors for MI in their population were diabetes (odds ratio [OR], 2.83; $p < 0.001$), current smoking (OR, 2.58; $p < 0.001$), abnormal ratio of apolipoprotein B to apolipoprotein A-I (apo B/apo A-1) (OR, 2.23; $p = 0.005$), abdominal obesity (OR, 1.96; $p = 0.007$), and hypertension (OR, 1.68; $p = 0.007$), physical activity and fruit and vegetable intake did not correlate significantly with MI risk. Alcohol consumption was found to be a protective factor (OR, 0.63; $p = 0.005$). The PAF of IHD mortality in ECA caused by seven of the INTERHEART risk factors was reported recently.[83] The total PAF for IHD risk factors adds up to more than 100% because risk factors overlap—that is, some cases of IHD are caused by multiple factors and are attributed to each factor. The PAF for mortality and years of life lost caused by smoking, hypertension, hypercholesterolemia, and overweight and obesity are higher in ECA than in any other region of the world. For example, the PAFs for hypertension and high cholesterol and IHD mortality are 61% and 55%, respectively, in ECA, whereas the PAF for these same risk factors is below 50% in all other regions of the world. Although alcohol intake may protect against IHD risk in high-income countries (PAF = −12%), the estimated PAF of alcohol for IHD mortality in the ECA region is 7%, second only to Latin America and the Caribbean, where alcohol intake has an estimated PAF of 8% for IHD mortality.

Researchers have sought to explain better the variation in IHD mortality in Europe and Central Asia by analyzing additional factors. One study pointed to the availability of alpha-linoleic acid (ALA) in some vegetable oils as an explanation for the variation of IHD rates between FSRs and non-FSRs; Spearman rank correlations between ALA intake and CHD mortality in this study were $\rho = -0.84$ for men and $\rho = -0.83$ for women, and those countries that saw the largest increase in ALA intake also experienced the largest decrease in CHD mortality.[84]

LATIN AMERICA. Among risk factors for IHD in the population at large, tobacco and obesity loom largest. A recent population-based study called CARMELA, carried out in seven Latin American cities (Barquisimeto, Venezuela; Bogota, Colombia; Buenos Aires, Argentina; Lima, Peru; Mexico City, Mexico; Quito, Ecuador; and Santiago, Chile) has estimated the prevalence of obesity (BMI > 30) at 23% and smoking at 30% of the population older than 25 years.[85] Obesity prevalence was highest in Mexico City and tobacco use highest in Santiago. Similarly, a population study in a Brazilian state found that 55% of those older than 20 years were obese or overweight (BMI > 25) —a dramatic increase from the previous decade, when these rates were under 32%. More than a third of the population smoked, a stable rate from the previous decade. Even in patients who have had CHD events, the relative importance of abdominal obesity as measured by waist-to-hip ratio was found to be higher, with a PAR of 48% compared with 30% for the rest of the world regions.[86] Smoking also had a slightly higher PAR, 38%, compared with 35% for the other regions.

Hypertension was diagnosed in 18% of patients in the CARMELA study, but studies by country have shown the prevalence to be higher in certain regions. For example, the prevalence was 29% in Buenos Aires and 32% in the Brazilian state of Rio Grande do Sul. Of those diagnosed with hypertension in the Brazilian study, 50% were unaware of their condition, and only 10% were being adequately treated.[87] In Costa Rica, where the public health system is thought to be accessible to 98% of the population, 25% of the population older than 20 years was noted to have hypertension.[88] Treatment was more widespread, with between 44% and 48% of the patients achieving their target.

Diabetes is an emerging epidemic for most Latin American countries, and for Mexico in particular. The prevalence of diabetes was highest in Mexico City, at 9% in the CARMELA study, compared with an average prevalence of 7% for the region. A national survey of 400 Mexican cities in 2000 estimated the prevalence at 8%.[89] Diabetes mortality increased 23% from 1998 to 2002 in Mexico, reaching 53.2 deaths/100,000 and making it the leading cause of mortality in women and the second most common cause in men. Treatment was being offered to 85% of patients, but less than 50% were achieving a target fasting glucose level lower than 140 mg/dL.

Urban diets are also propagating an alarming rise in hypercholesterolemia. In a nationwide survey of Brazilian cities performed to raise awareness about the problem, a cholesterol level higher than 200 mg/dL was present in 40% of the population and a cholesterol level higher than 240 mg/dL was present in 13%. Cholesterol levels higher than 240 mg/dL were seen in 14% of the population in the CARMELA study. In Mexico, the prevalence of hypercholesterolemia is slightly lower, at 9%, but reached a striking level (8%), even in those younger than 30 years.[89]

MIDDLE EAST AND NORTH AFRICA. Iraq, Jordan, Saudi Arabia, Syria, Kuwait, and Egypt have reported risk factors for CVD-IHD to the WHO STEPwise Surveillance study.[89a] An alarming number of people in Egypt, 76.4%, are overweight or obese. Rates for overweight and obesity are also high in Iraq and Jordan, at about 67%. Overweight and obesity are lowest in Kuwait, at 18.2%. Low intake of fresh fruits and vegetables ranges from 79% in Egypt to 95.7% in Syria. Physical inactivity (levels of activity of 10 minutes or less per day) is fairly common in the region, with a prevalence ranging from 32.9% in Syria to 56.7% in Iraq. The largest prevalence of hypertension is also found in Iraq, where about 40.4% of citizens are affected. Hypertension is least prevalent in Egypt, at 24.6%. Hypercholesterolemia rates range from 19.3% in Saudi Arabia to 42% in Kuwait. Diabetes, also a major risk factor for CHD, is most prevalent in Saudi Arabia, at 17.9%, and least prevalent in Iraq, 10.4%. Daily smoking ranges from 12.9% in Saudi Arabia to 24.7% in Syria.

Clustering of components for the metabolic syndrome appears to occur in the region. A study done in 2008 in the United Arab Emirates of 817 people showed a prevalence of 23.3% for diabetes; 20.8% had hypertension, 10.3% were smokers and, overall, 22.7% had metabolic syndrome.[90] However, rates appear to vary within regions and within countries. In one Iranian study, noted earlier, the age-adjusted rate for metabolic syndrome was 49%.[28] However, another study conducted in Iran in 2007 with a random sample of 3000 Iranians showed lower prevalence rates for similar risk factors; the prevalence of diabetes was 6.3%, smoking, 21.6%, and high blood pressure, 13.7%.[91]

The 2004 INTERHEART study found that in the Middle East and North Africa region, 47.9% had electrocardiographic changes indicative of a new MI. The PAR rates were as follows: smoking, 45.5%; self-reported hypertension, 9.2%; self-reported diabetes, 15.5%; lipids, 70.5%; and obesity, 25.9%. All nine risk factors together accounted for 95% of all causes of MI.[43]

SOUTH ASIA. Of all the low- and middle-income regions, this region has the highest prevalence of diabetes. In 2006, Goyal and Yusuf[41] estimated that the prevalence was 3.8% in rural areas and 11.8% in urban areas. Similarly, IC Health reported a prevalence of 14% in an Indian urban setting in 2000.[92] According to the INTERHEART study, 11.8% of all MIs in the South Asia region result from diabetes.[43]

Rates for hypertension are even higher. According to Goyal and Yusuf,[41] data from 2004 have shown that hypertension affects 20% to 40% of urban residents and 12% to 17% of rural residents. This is an estimated total of 118 million people in India.[41] In addition, an urban study on hypertension and socioeconomic status published in 2000 showed rates of 54% in low-income groups and 40% in high-income groups. INTERHEART found a prevalence for hypertension of 19.3% attributable to MI.[43]

Smoking rates in the region are also high, and alarmingly high in children. Goyal[41] has reported that of those between the ages of 12 and 60, 56% used tobacco in 2002. Another study showed sixth graders smoking two to three times more tobacco than eighth graders.

The IC Health report identified overweight and obesity as a growing issue in Indian populations. In northern India, prevalence measured by waist circumference soared from 33.2% to 45% in 2001 and 2003, respectively. Urban South Asia had high waist-to-hip ratios as well, increasing 16% (63% to 79%) between 2001 and 2003. There is also evidence of a positive correlation between obesity and age. In 2000, the prevalence, as measured by BMI, was 31% in those aged 20 to 40 and 38% in those older than 40 years in seven urban cities. Similarly, the prevalence from 2001 to 2003 in several areas of the region, as measured by BMI, was 31% in 20- to 69-year-olds. The rate from the same study measured by waist circumference was 32%.[93] According to INTERHEART, abdominal obesity accounts for 37.7% of MI cases.[43]

In addition to factors already mentioned, the INTERHEART study reported that there are other noteworthy risk factors attributable to MI for the South Asia region. Low intake of fruits and vegetables accounts for 18.3% of MI, lack of exercise 27.1%, and lipids 58.7%. In total, all nine risk factors explain 89.4% of all causes of MI.[43]

SUB-SAHARAN AFRICA. CVD worldwide is largely driven by modifiable risk factors, such as smoking, lack of physical activity, and diet high in fat and salt. The INTERHEART study showed that smoking, hypertension, abdominal obesity, physical activity, and a high-risk diet associated positively with risk of MI.[82] In addition, the GBD project estimated that the PAFs for individual risk factors for IHD in low- and middle-income countries in 2001 were as follows: high blood pressure, 44%; high cholesterol, 46%; overweight and obesity, 16%; low fruit and vegetable intake, 30%; physical inactivity, 21%; and smoking, 15%.[93] The upward trend in CVD in sub-Saharan Africa likely results from the increasing prevalence of some of these modifiable risk factors. Hypertension may have occurred in as many as 71% of all cases of CVD treated at an urban hospital in Zaire, and there was a positive association with higher social class.[94] Smoking in Africa has increased by 40% since the early 1980s and ranges from 28% among black men in a cohort in Durban, South Africa, to 32.5% of male civil servants in the Accra Civil Service. Steyn and colleagues[95] have found that 89.2% of the PAR for MI could be explained by smoking history (self-reported), diabetes history (self-reported), hypertension history (self-reported), abdominal obesity (waist-to-hip ratio), and ratio of apo A to apo A-I. Additionally, the authors showed that the OR and PAR for the African cohort are much higher than their counterparts elsewhere. Not controlling the impact of these modifiable risk factors through prevention will result in even greater future increases in the CVD burden in this population.[96]

In sub-Saharan Africa, the PAF for IHD mortality attributable to certain risk factors has been determined to be as follows: high blood pressure, 43% (versus 47% worldwide); low fruit and vegetable intake, identical to the rest of the world at 25%; physical inactivity, 20%; overweight and obesity, 8%, and smoking, 5%.[55]

In a review of the incidence of trends in stroke over the past 40 years, Feigin and associates[98] have shown that trends diverge between high-income and low- to middle-income countries. Specifically, they found a 42% decrease in stroke incidence in high-income countries and an increase of more than 100% in low- to middle-income countries; this was thought to be an indication of the increased rates of smoking and high blood pressure. In 2007 to 2008, stroke incidence in the latter exceeded those in the former for the first time. Death from stroke in low- to middle-income countries accounts for almost 86% of stroke deaths worldwide, with the DALYs lost in these countries being almost seven times higher than those in high-income countries.[98] The risk of coronary artery disease in black South African stroke patients may resemble that of their white counterparts, likely caused by silent MI in the black population being more common than previously thought. In a review of stroke in sub-Saharan Africa, Connor and coworkers[99] have found that the region has lower absolute numbers of incident stroke compared with high-income countries. However, the absolute numbers by themselves may not adequately convey the burden of stroke in the region. For example, compared with New Zealand, South African stroke survivors were much more likely to need help with at least one ADL (activity of daily living; 200 versus 173/100,000), which translates into substantial physical and economic challenges for families and communities of these survivors. Without adequate intervention, deaths from stroke and related heart disease are expected to increase to 5 million in 2020, from 3 million in 1998.[101] Findings in the Democratic Republic of the Congo and Nigeria underscore the need for prevention. In the Congo, a hospital-based clinical study has shown that hemorrhagic strokes are present in 52% of the study population and ischemic strokes are present in 48%; ischemic stroke was most significantly associated with mortality (hazard ratio [HR] = 4.28; $p < 0.001$).[101] In Nigeria, the dominant modifiable risk factor for stroke is hypertension, yet the lack of neurologists and lack of an agenda related to stroke are cited as elements that will fuel the increased rates of stroke, according to WHO predictions.[102]

Economic Burden

Despite some overlap, at least three approaches can measure the economic burden associated with CHD.[103] The first source of financial burden is defined by the costs incurred in the health care system itself and reported in the cost of illness studies. In these studies, the cost of CHD includes the costs of hospitalizations for angina and MI, as well as heart failure attributable to CHD. In addition, there are the costs of specific treatments or procedures related to CVD, such as thrombolytics, catheterization, and percutaneous coronary intervention. Furthermore, there are costs associated with outpatient management and

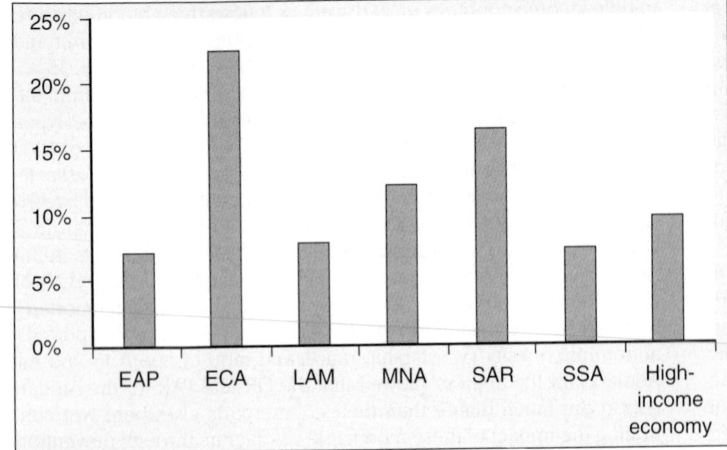

FIGURE 1-9 Percentage of health care expenditures attributed to high blood pressure. EAP = East Asia and Pacific; ECA = Europe and Central Asia; LAM = Latin America and the Caribbean; MNA = Middle East and North Africa; SAR = South Asia Region; SSA = sub-Saharan Africa.

secondary prevention, including office visits and pharmaceutical costs. In addition, nursing home, rehabilitation (inpatient and outpatient), and home nursing costs require consideration.

The second economic assessment is based on microeconomic studies that assess the household impact of catastrophic health care events such as MI. These studies look at out-of-pocket expenses incurred by the individual or family that might have other downstream economic impacts, such as loss of savings or sale of property to cover medical costs. Given that in many developing countries without an extensive insurance scheme, health care costs are almost entirely borne by individuals,[104] microeconomic studies to date have not considered CHD exclusively and have more generally looked at chronic diseases overall. Furthermore, the limited data do not confirm the causality between chronic disease and individual or household poverty.[103] However, expenditures for CHD or its addictive risk factors, such as smoking, could lead to substantial and even impoverishing costs.

The third method of determining financial burden from CHD is based on macroeconomic analyses. These assessments consider lost worker productivity or economic growth that is lost by having adults with CHD or their caregivers partially or completely out of the work force as a result of their illness. The data for the impact of chronic diseases on labor supply and productivity are more robust. An additional cost not often accounted for is the intangible loss of welfare associated with pain disability or suffering by the individual. These indirect costs are often accounted for by willingness-to-pay analyses, asking generally how much would an individual pay to avert suffering or premature death from CHD. The gains are not merely improved work performance, but also enjoying activities beyond production. Studies in the United States have suggested that as much as 1% to 3% of GDP is attributable to CVD, with almost 50% of that related to CHD.[105] In China, annual direct costs of CVD are estimated at more than $40 billion (U.S. dollars), or roughly 4% of GNI. In South Africa, 2% to 3% of the country's GNI is devoted to the direct treatment of CVD, which equates to roughly 25% of South African health care expenditures. Indirect costs have been estimated to be more than double those of direct costs. Although few cost of illness studies for CHD have been done in other regions, cost of illness studies have reported on the financial burdens attributed to risk factors for CHD. For example, the direct costs caused by diabetes in Latin American and Caribbean countries were estimated at $10 billion (U.S. dollars). Indirect costs were estimated at over $50 billion in the year 2000. Studies are limited, but suggest that obesity-related diseases are responsible for 2% to 8% of all health care expenditures in developed countries. In India and China, the costs for obesity are about 1.1% and 2.1% of GDP, respectively.

The costs attributable to nonoptimal levels of blood pressure as mediated through stroke and MI were recently evaluated for all regions of the world.[106] Globally, the health care costs of elevated blood pressure were estimated at $370 billion (U.S. dollars) for the year 2001. This amount represented approximately 10% of all global health care expenditures for that year. Regional variations do exist, with hypertension being responsible for up to 25% of health care costs in the Eastern European region (**Fig 1-9**). Over a 10-year period, blood pressure–related health care costs could equal $1 trillion (U.S. dollars) globally. Indirect health care costs attributed to blood pressure could be almost four times as much.

That a high proportion of CVD burden occurs earlier among adults of working age augments its macroeconomic impact in developing countries. Under current projections, in developing countries such as South Africa, CVD will strike 40% of adults between the ages of 35 and 64 years, compared with 10% in the United States.[15] India and China will have death rates in the same age group that are two and three times those of most developed countries. Given the large populations in these two rapidly growing economies, this trend could have profound economic effects over the next 25 years as workers in their prime succumb to CVD.

Cost-Effective Solutions

The large reductions in age-adjusted CVD mortality rates that have occurred in high-income countries result from three complementary types of interventions. One strategy targets those with acute or established CVD. A second entails risk assessment and targeting those at high risk caused by multiple risk factors for intervention before their first CVD event. The third strategy uses mass education or policy interventions directed at the entire population to reduce the overall level of risk factors. This section highlights the variety of cost-effective interventions. Much work remains undone in developing countries to determine the best strategies given limited resources, but, if implemented, these interventions could go a long way toward reducing the burden. **Table 1-6** lists the cost-effectiveness ratios for many of the high-yield interventions that could be or have been adopted in developing regions.

Established Cardiovascular Disease Management

Those at highest risk are those suffering an MI or stroke; as many as 50% die before they ever receive medical attention. For those who do make it to a hospital, standard medical therapies were examined in two cost-effectiveness analyses.[107,108]

Four incremental strategies were evaluated for the treatment of MI and compared with a strategy of no treatment as a base case for the six World Bank low- and middle-income regions. The four strategies compared were as follows: aspirin; aspirin and atenolol; aspirin, atenolol, and streptokinase; and aspirin, atenolol, and tissue plasminogen activator (t-PA). The incremental cost per quality-adjusted life-year (QALY) gained for both the aspirin and beta blocker interventions was under $25 for all six regions. Costs per QALY gained for streptokinase were between $630 and $730 across the regions. Incremental cost-effectiveness ratios for t-PA were around $16,000 per QALY gained, compared with streptokinase. Minor variations occurred among regions because of small differences in follow-up care based on regional costs.

Secondary prevention strategies are equally cost-effective in developing countries. Studies have shown that a combination of aspirin, ACE inhibitor, beta blocker, and statin for secondary prevention can lead to acceptable cost-effectiveness ratios in all developing regions.[109] Use of currently available generic agents, even in the absence of the so-called polypill, could be highly cost effective, on the order of $300 to $400/person per QALY gained.[110]

TABLE 1-6 Cost-Effectiveness for Coronary Heart Disease Interventions in Developing Regions

TREATMENT OR INTERVENTION	COST-EFFECTIVENESS RATIO (U.S. $/DALY)*
Drug Treatments	
Acute myocardial infarction	
ASA, BB	11-22
ASA, BB, SK	634-734
ASA, BB, t-PA	15,860-18,893
Secondary treatment (CHD†)	
Multidrug regimen (ASA, BB, ACEI, statin)	1,686-2,026
Coronary artery bypass grafting	24,040-72,345
Policy Interventions	
Tobacco	
Price increase of 33%	2-85
Nonpolicy interventions	33-1,432
Salt reduction†; 2-8 mm Hg reduction in BP	Cost saving—250
Fat-related interventions‡	
Reduced saturated fat intake	Cost saving—2,900
Trans fat replacement: 7% reduction in CHD	50-1,500

ACEI = angiotensin-converting enzyme inhibitor; ASA = aspirin; BB = beta-blocker; SK = streptokinase; t-PA = tissue plasminogen activator.
*Across six World Bank regions.
†Range includes different estimates of cost of interventions, as well as blood pressure reduction (<$0.50-1.00).
‡Range includes estimates of cost of interventions (<$0.50-6.00).
Adapted from Gaziano TA: Cardiovascular disease in the developing world and its cost-effective management. Circulation 112:3547, 2005; and Gaziano TA, Galea G, Reddy KS: Scaling up interventions for chronic disease prevention: The evidence. Lancet 370:1939, 2007.

Risk Assessment

Primary prevention is paramount for the large number of individuals who are at high risk for CVD. Given limited resources, finding low-cost prevention strategies is a top priority. Using prediction rules or risk scores to identify those at higher risk to target specific behavioral or drug interventions is a well-established primary prevention strategy and has proven to be cost effective in developing countries.[109,110] Most have included age, sex, hypertension, smoking status, diabetes mellitus, and lipid values, whereas others have also included family history.[111,112] Many investigators have examined whether additional laboratory-based risk factors can add to predictive discrimination of the risk factors used in the Framingham Heart Study Risk Score. The recent analyses in the Atherosclerosis Risk in Communities (ARIC) Study[113] and the Framingham Offspring Study[114,115] have suggested that little additional information is gained when other blood-based novel risk factors are added to the traditional risk factors. Although the Reynolds Risk Score[116] for women, which added family history, high-sensitivity C-reactive protein (hsCRP), and hemoglobin A1c levels, only had a marginally higher C-statistic (0.808) than the Framingham covariates (0.791), it correctly reclassified many individuals at intermediate risk (see Chap. 44). Some women deemed low risk by the Framingham Risk Score were reclassified as intermediate or high risk according to the Reynolds Risk Score and thus would have been eligible for more aggressive management. Also, some women who were initially high risk according to the Framingham score were reclassified as lower risk and thus would not have needed treatment.

More attention is now focused on developing risk scores that would be easier to use in clinical practice without the loss of predictive discrimination in resource-poor countries. In high-income countries, a prediction rule that requires a laboratory test is an inconvenience; in low-income countries, with limited testing facilities, it may be too expensive for widespread screening or preclude its use altogether. In response to this real concern, WHO recently released risk prediction charts for different regions of the world, with and without cholesterol.[117,118] A study based on the U.S. NHANES follow-up cohort has demonstrated that a non–laboratory-based risk tool that uses information obtained in a single encounter (e.g., age, systolic blood pressure, BMI, diabetes status, smoking status) can predict CVD outcomes as well as one that requires laboratory testing with a C-statistic of 0.79 for men and 0.83 for women that were no different from the Framingham-based risk tool.[119] Furthermore, the results of the goodness of fit tests suggest that the non–laboratory–based model is well calibrated across a wide range of absolute risk levels and without changes in classification of risk.

Policy and Community Interventions

Education and public policy interventions that have reduced smoking rates, lowered mean blood pressure levels, and improved lipid profiles have contributed to the reduction in CHD rates.[10] Education and policy efforts directed at tobacco consumption have contributed substantially to the reductions in CVD. In addition, salt and cholesterol reduction has been evaluated by WHO investigators as a cost-effective strategy to reduce stroke and MI in low- and middle-income countries.[120] Community interventions have reduced levels of multiple risk factors and, in some cases, CHD mortality.

TOBACCO. Tobacco control can be conceptualized in terms of strategies that reduce the supply of, or demand for, tobacco. Most public health and clinical strategies to date have focused on reducing demand through economic disincentives (taxes), health promotion (media and packaging efforts), restricted access (to advertising and tobacco), or clinical assistance for cessation. The WHO effort to expedite the creation of a global treaty against tobacco use was a key milestone. In May 2003, the WHO World Health Assembly unanimously adopted the WHO Framework Convention in Tobacco Control (FCTC), the first global tobacco treaty.[30] The FCTC had been ratified by 164 countries as of April 2009, making it one of the most widely embraced treaties in the United Nations. The FCTC has spurred efforts for tobacco control across the globe by providing rich and poor nations with a common framework of evidence-based legislation and implementation strategies known to reduce tobacco use.

In 2006, Jha and colleagues[121] presented a landmark analysis of tobacco control cost-effectiveness. They calculated the reductions in future tobacco deaths caused by a range of tax, treatment, and non-price interventions among smokers alive in 2000. They found that a 33% price increase would reduce by between 19.7 and 56.8 million (5.4% to 15.9% of total) deaths in smokers from the developing world who were alive in 2000. Calculations show that nicotine replacement therapy (NRT) could reduce the number of deaths by between 2.9 and 14.3 million (0.8% to 4.0% of total) in the 2000 cohort. A range of non-price interventions such as advertising bans, health warnings, and smoke-free laws would reduce deaths by between 5.7 and 28.6 million (1.6% to 7.9% of total) in that cohort. These reductions would translate into developing world cost-effectiveness values of between $3 and $42 dollars per QALY saved for tax increases (not including tax revenue), $55 to $761 per QALY for NRT, and $54 to $674 per QALY for non-price measures.

Of critical importance for patients who have had a coronary event, smoking cessation saves lives at a higher rate than any individual medical treatment. Mohiuddin and associates[122] have conducted a randomized controlled trial of a behavioral and medication smoking cessation program for smokers who were hospitalized with a coronary event in the critical care unit. They were able almost to triple smoking cessation rates and decrease all-cause mortality at 1 year by an absolute risk of 9% (77% reduction in relative risk). This reduction corresponded with a number needed to treat (NNT) of 11 for smoking cessation to prevent one death in the year following a major coronary cardiac event. This NNT for secondary prevention is more favorable than that for statins, beta blockers, or even aspirin.[123]

SALT AND LIPID REDUCTIONS. The cost-effectiveness analyses on salt reduction as a result of public education are favorable.[124,125] The intervention ranges from being cost saving to $200 per DALY averted. The results of a campaign for reducing saturated fat and replacing it with polyunsaturated fat is also likely to be cost effective. In the base case, a 3% decline in cholesterol and a $6 per capita education cost were assumed. This resulted in a cost as low as $1800 per DALY averted in the South Asia region and up to $4000 per DALY averted in the Middle East and North Africa region. However, if the cost for the education plan were halved, the ratio is approximately $900 per DALY and would be cost-saving if the reduction could be achieved for under $0.50 per capita, which may be possible in areas with much less expensive access to media.

COMMUNITY INTERVENTIONS. In the 1970s and 1980s, a series of population-based community intervention studies were conducted to reduce risk factors for chronic disease; these have been reviewed elsewhere.[126] They focused on changes in health behaviors or risk factors, such as tobacco use, body weight, cholesterol, and blood pressure, as well as a reduction in CVD morbidity and mortality. In general, they included a combination of community-wide actions and those focused on individuals identified as high risk.

One of the earliest and most often cited community interventions is the North Karelia project, begun in 1972 in Finland. The community-based interventions included health education, screening, hypertension control program, and treatment. Over the first 5 years of the study, reductions in risk factors and a decline in CHD mortality of 2.9%/yr versus a 1%/yr decline in the rest of Finland were noted. During the next 10 years, declines were greater in the rest of Finland. Over 25 years of follow-up, a large decline in CHD occurred in the North Karelia region (73%) and the rest of Finland (63%). Although the overall difference in the decline in CHD deaths was not significantly greater in the study area of North Karelia, the reduction in male tobacco-related cancers was significant. A similar study in the Stanford, California, area showed reductions in risk factors: cholesterol (2%), blood pressure (4%), and smoking rates (13%) when compared with sites without the intervention, but no impact on disease end-points.

Later, community interventions in high-income countries showed mixed results, with some showing improvements in risk factors beyond the secular decline that was occurring throughout most of the developed economies, and others with no additional decline. However, a meta-analysis of the randomized multiple risk factor interventions has shown net significant decreases in systolic blood pressure (4.2 mm Hg), smoking prevalence (4.2%), and cholesterol (0.14 mmol/L).[127] The declines in total and CHD mortality of 3% and 4% were not significant. The limitation to all the projects includes the challenge of detecting small changes that may be significant on a population level. It is possible that a 10% reduction in mortality could have been missed.

Several community intervention studies have been conducted in developing countries, including Mauritius and South Africa. The Mauritius project, among other interventions, resulted in a government-sponsored program that changed the prime cooking oil from a predominantly saturated fat palm oil to a soybean oil high in unsaturated fatty acids. Overall total cholesterol levels fell 14% during the 5-year study period (1987 to 1992).[128] Changes in other risk factors were mixed, with declines in blood pressure and smoking rates and increases in obesity and diabetes. The Coronary Risk Factor Study in South Africa compared a control community to two communities receiving two different levels of intensity of interventions.[129] The interventions included mass media messages, group-sponsored educational sessions, and blood pressure screening and follow-up with the health sector when appropriate. Both high- and low-intensity interventions showed improvements in blood pressure, smoking rates, and high-density lipoprotein (HDL)–to–total cholesterol ratio over the control community, but with little difference between the two intervention communities.

One other significant reduction of CHD came not through a concerted community intervention, but through changes in fiscal policy. In Poland, reductions in subsidies for animal products such as butter and lard led to a switch from saturated to polyunsaturated fats, mainly rapeseed- and soybean-based oils. A decrease in CHD mortality of greater than 25% between 1991 and 2002 could not be explained by increased fruit consumption or declines in smoking.

Summary and Conclusions

CVD remains a significant global problem. A key challenge for developing economies, unlike developed economies, is the swift pace of economic and social transformation in a postindustrial world with rapid globalization. Although CVD rates have declined in high-income countries, they are increasing in almost every other region of the world. From a worldwide perspective, the rate of change in the global burden of CVD is accelerating, reflecting the changes in low- and middle-income economies, which represent 85% of the world's population. The consequences of this preventable epidemic will be substantial on many levels—individual mortality and morbidity, family suffering, and staggering economic costs—both the direct costs of diagnosis and treatment and the indirect costs of lost productivity.

Different regions of the world face different stages of the epidemic. Currently, Eastern European countries and members of the former Soviet Republic are facing enormous burdens, with over 50% of all deaths attributed to CVD. Meanwhile, countries in sub-Saharan Africa are just beginning to see increases in these chronic illnesses while still grappling with HIV/AIDS. No single global solution to the rising burden of CVD exists, given the vast differences in social, cultural, and economic circumstances. High-income countries must minimize disparities, reverse unfavorable trends in CVD risk factors and behaviors, and deal with the increasing prevalence of CVD in an aging population. The most complex challenges face the low- and middle-income countries.

Reduction in the disease burden will require changes at the policy level and at the personal level. In the long run, the allocation of resources to lower-cost strategies will likely be more cost effective than dedicating resources to the high-cost management of CVD. From a societal perspective, efforts to strengthen tobacco control strategies, improve dietary choices, and increase physical activity will be paramount. At the personal level, risk assessment strategies and treatment modalities require simplification. Furthermore, alternative uses of allied health workers such as community health workers will need evaluation, given the reduced human resources in most developing countries. High-income countries must share the burden of research and development into every aspect of prevention and treatment with leading and emerging middle-income countries. Through further expansion of the knowledge base, particularly regarding the economic consequences of various treatment and prevention strategies, the efficient transfer of low-cost preventive and therapeutic strategies may alter the natural course of the epidemiologic transition in every part of the world, and thus reduce the excess global burden of preventable CVD.

REFERENCES

1. World Health Organization: The Global Burden of Disease: 2004 Update. Geneva, World Health Organization, 2008.
2. Lopez AD, Mathers CD, Ezzati M, et al (eds): Global Burden of Disease and Risk Factors. New York, World Bank Group, 2006, p 552.

Epidemiologic Transitions

3. Olshansky SJ, Ault AB: The fourth stage of the epidemiologic transition: The age of delayed degenerative diseases. Milbank Q 64:355, 1986.
4. Omran AR: The epidemiologic transition: A theory of the epidemiology of population change. Milbank Q 49:509, 1971.
5. Gaziano JM: Fifth phase of the epidemiologic transition: The age of obesity and inactivity. JAMA 303:275, 2010.
6. Hannon TS, Rao G, Arslanian SA: Childhood obesity and type 2 diabetes mellitus. Pediatrics 116:473, 2005.
7. Muntner P, He J, Cutler JA, et al: Trends in blood pressure among children and adolescents. JAMA 291:2107, 2004.
8. Wu Y: Overweight and obesity in China. BMJ 333:362, 2006.

Epidemiologic Transition in the United States

9. Centers for Disease Control and Prevention (CDC): State-specific prevalence of cigarette smoking and quitting among adults—United States, 2004. MMWR Morb Mortal Wkly Rep 54:1124, 2005.
10. Ford ES, Ajani UA, Croft JB, et al: Explaining the decrease in U.S. deaths from coronary disease, 1980-2000. N Engl J Med 356:2388, 2007.
11. Carroll MD, Lacher DA, Sorlie PD, et al: Trends in serum lipids and lipoproteins of adults, 1960-2002. JAMA 294:1773, 2005.
12. Flegal KM, Carroll MD, Ogden CL, Curtin LR: Prevalence and trends in obesity among US adults, 1999-2008. JAMA 303:235, 2010.
13. Chobanian AV, Bakris GL, Black HR, et al: The Seventh Report of the Joint National Committee on Prevention, Detection, Evaluation, and Treatment of High Blood Pressure: The JNC 7 report. JAMA 289:2560, 2003.
14. Centers for Disease Control and Prevention (CDC): Cigarette smoking among adults—United States, 2007. MMWR Morb Mortal Wkly Rep 57:1221, 2008.

Current Worldwide Variations in the Global Burden of CVD

15. Leeder S, Raymond S, Greenberg H, et al: A Race Against Time: The Challenge of Cardiovascular Disease in Developing Countries. New York, Columbia University Press, 2004..
16. Petersen S, Peto V, Rayner M, et al: European Cardiovascular Disease Statistics, 2005 (http://www.heartstats.org/uploads/documents%5CPDF.pdf).
17. Adachi H, Hino A: Trends in nutritional intake and serum cholesterol levels over 40 years in Tanushimaru, Japanese men. J Epidemiol 15:85, 2005
18. Reddy KS: Cardiovascular disease in non-Western countries. N Engl J Med 350:2438, 2004.
19. Bank TW (ed): World Development Indicators. Washington DC, World Bank Group, 2007, p 402.
20. Liu L: Cardiovascular diseases in China. Biochem Cell Biol 85:157, 2007.
21. Zhang XH, Lu ZL, Liu L: Coronary heart disease in China. Heart 94:1126, 2008.
22. Mackay JMG: Atlas of Heart Disease and Stroke. Geneva, World Health Organization, 2004.
23. La Vecchia C, Levi F, Lucchini F, Negri E: Trends in mortality from major diseases in Europe, 1980-1993. Eur J Epidemiol 14:1, 1998.
24. Kesteloot H, Sans S, Kromhout D: Dynamics of cardiovascular and all-cause mortality in Western and Eastern Europe between 1970 and 2000. Eur Heart J 27:107, 2006.
25. Mirzaei M, Truswell AS, Taylor R, Leeder SR: Coronary heart disease (CHD) epidemics: Not all the same. Heart 95:740, 2009.
26. Xu K, Evans DB, Kawabata K, et al: Household catastrophic health expenditure: A multicountry analysis. Lancet 362:111, 2003.
27. Gupta R: Burden of coronary heart disease in India. Ind Heart J 57:632, 2005.
28. Nabipour I, Amiri M, Imami SR, et al: The metabolic syndrome and nonfatal ischemic heart disease; a population-based study. Int J Cardiol 118:48, 2007.
29. Lim SS, Gaziano TA, Gakidou E, et al: Prevention of cardiovascular disease in high-risk individuals in low-income and middle-income countries: Health effects and costs. Lancet 370:2054, 2007.
30. Balbinotto Neto G, Silva EN: The costs of cardiovascular disease in Brazil: A brief economic comment. Arq Bras Cardiol 91:198, 2008.
31. Lavados PM, Hennis AJ, Fernandes JG, et al: Stroke epidemiology, prevention, and management strategies at a regional level: Latin America and the Caribbean. Lancet Neurol 6:362, 2007.
32. Rodríguez T, Malvezzi M, Chatenoud L, et al: Trends in mortality from coronary heart and cerebrovascular diseases in the Americas: 1970-2000. Heart 92:453, 2006.
33. Curioni C, Cunha CB, Veras RP, André C: The decline in mortality from circulatory diseases in Brazil. Rev Panam Salud Publica 25:9, 2009.
34. Stevens G, Dias RH, Thomas KJ, et al: Characterizing the epidemiological transition in Mexico: National and subnational burden of diseases, injuries, and risk factors. PLoS Med 5:e125, 2008.
35. Al-Nozha MM, Arafah MR, Al-Mazrou YY, et al: Coronary artery disease in Saudi Arabia. Saudi Med J 25:1165, 2004.
36. Nsour M, Mahfoud Z, Kanaan MN, Balbeissi A: Prevalence and predictors of nonfatal myocardial infarction in Jordan. East Mediterr Health J 14:818, 2008.
37. Ben Romdhane H, Bougatef S, Skhiri H, et al: The first Tunisian cardiovascular diseases register: Processes and results. Rev Epidemiol Sante Publique 52:558, 2004.
38. Ghaffar A, Reddy KS, Singhi M: Burden of non-communicable diseases in South Asia. BMJ 328:807, 2004.
39. Ahmad N, Bhopal R: Is coronary heart disease rising in India? A systematic review based on ECG defined coronary heart disease. Heart 91:719, 2005.
40. Jafar TH, Qadri Z, Chaturvedi N: Coronary artery disease epidemic in Pakistan: More electrocardiographic evidence of ischaemia in women than in men. Heart 94:408, 2008.
41. Goyal A, Yusuf S: The burden of cardiovascular disease in the Indian subcontinent. Indian J Med Res 124:235, 2006.
42. Joshi R, Chow CK, Raju PK, et al: Fatal and nonfatal cardiovascular disease and the use of therapies for secondary prevention in a rural region of India. Circulation 119:1950, 2009.
43. Yusuf S, Hawken S, Ounpuu S, et al: Effect of potentially modifiable risk factors associated with myocardial infarction in 52 countries (the INTERHEART study): Case-control study. Lancet 364:937, 2004.
44. Palacios R, Alonso I, Hidalgo A, et al: Peripheral arterial disease in HIV patients older than 50 years of age. AIDS Res Hum Retroviruses 24:1043, 2008.
45. Mauss S, Berger F, Schmutz G, et al: Lipoprotein(a) in patients initiating antiretroviral therapy. HIV Med 9:415, 2008.

Global Trends in Cardiovascular Disease

46. Grover SA, Coupal L, Gilmore N, Mukherjee J: Impact of dyslipidemia associated with highly active antiretroviral therapy (HAART) on cardiovascular risk and life expectancy. Am J Cardiol 95:586, 2005.
47. World Health Organization: Preventing Chronic Diseases: A Vital Investment. Geneva, World Health Organization, 2005.
48. Lawes CM, Vander Hoorn S, Rodgers A: Global burden of blood-pressure-related disease, 2001. Lancet 371:1513, 2008.
49. Shafey O, Eriksen M, Ross H, Mackay J: The Tobacco Atlas, 3rd ed. Atlanta, American Cancer Society, 2009.
50. Ezzati M, Henley SJ, Thun MJ, Lopez AD: Role of smoking in global and regional cardiovascular mortality. Circulation 112:489, 2005.
51. Teo KK, Ounpuu S, Hawken S, et al: Tobacco use and risk of myocardial infarction in 52 countries in the INTERHEART study: A case-control study. Lancet 368:647, 2006.
52. Barnoya J, Glantz SA: Cardiovascular effects of secondhand smoke: Almost as large as smoking. Circulation 111:2684, 2005.
53. Sargent RP, Shepard RM, Glantz SA: Reduced incidence of admissions for myocardial infarction associated with public smoking ban: Before and after study. BMJ 328:977, 2004.
54. Pell JP, Haw S, Cobbe S, et al: Smoke-free legislation and hospitalizations for acute coronary syndrome. N Engl J Med 359:482, 2008.
55. Ezzati M, Vander Hoorn S, Lopez AD, et al: Comparative quantification of mortality and burden of disease attributable to selected risk factors. *In* Lopez AD, Mathers CD, Ezzati E, et al (eds): Global Burden of Disease and Risk Factors. New York, Oxford University Press, 2006, pp 241-396.

55a. Few Americans Meet Exercise Targets. Gallup Poll, January 2008. (http://www.gallup.com/poll/103492/few-americans-meet-exercise-targets.aspx).

56. Franco M, Orduñez P, Caballero B, et al: Impact of energy intake, physical activity, and population-wide weight loss on cardiovascular disease and diabetes mortality in Cuba, 1980-2005. Am J Epidemiol 166:1374, 2007.
57. Hossain P, Kawar B, El Nahas M: Obesity and diabetes in the developing world—a growing challenge. N Engl J Med, 2007. 356:213, 2007.
58. Wild S, Roglic G, Green A, et al: Global prevalence of diabetes: Estimates for the year 2000 and projections for 2030. Diabetes Care 27:1047, 2004.
59. Haslam DW, James WP: Obesity. Lancet 366:1197, 2005.
60. Misr, A, Khurana L: Obesity and the metabolic syndrome in developing countries. J Clin Endocrinol Metab 93(Suppl 1):S9, 2008.
61. Popkin BM, Gordon-Larsen P: The nutrition transition: Worldwide obesity dynamics and their determinants. Int J Obes Relat Metab Disord 28(Suppl 3):S2, 2004.
62. Kelly T, Yang W, Chen CS, et al: Global burden of obesity in 2005 and projections to 2030. Int J Obes (Lond) 32:1431, 2008.
63. Raymond SU, Leeder S, Greenberg HM: Obesity and cardiovascular disease in developing countries: A growing problem and an economic threat. Curr Opin Clin Nutr Metab Care 9:111, 2006.
64. Monteiro CA, Moura EC, Conde WL, Popkin BM: Socioeconomic status and obesity in adult populations of developing countries: a review. Bull World Health Organ 82:940, 2004.
65. Mendez MA, Monteiro CA, Popkin BM: Overweight exceeds underweight among women in most developing countries. Am J Clin Nutr 81:714, 2005.
66. Poskitt EM: Countries in transition: Underweight to obesity non-stop? Ann Trop Paediatr 29:1, 2009.
67. Hedley AA, Ogden CL, Johnson CL, et al: Prevalence of overweight and obesity among US children, adolescents, and adults, 1999-2002. JAMA 291:2847, 2004.
68. Flegal KM, Carroll MD, Ogden CL, Johnson CL: Prevalence and trends in obesity among US adults, 1999-2000. JAMA 288:1723, 2002.
69. Centers for Disease Control and Prevention (CDC): Trends in intake of energy and macronutrients—United States, 1971-2000. MMWR Morb Mortal Wkly Rep 53:80, 2004.
70. Lloyd-Williams F, O'Flaherty M, Mwatsama M, et al: Estimating the cardiovascular mortality burden attributable to the European Common Agricultural Policy on dietary saturated fats. Bull World Health Organ 86:535, 2008.
71. Fung TT, Malik V, Rexrode KM, et al: Sweetened beverage consumption and risk of coronary heart disease in women. Am J Clin Nutr 89:1037, 2009.
72. UN Office of the High Representative for the Least Developed Countries: Landlocked Developing Countries and Small Island Developing States, 2009 (http://www.un.org/special-rep/ohrlls/ldc/list.htm).
73. Population Reference Bureau: Speed of population aging in selected countries, 2009 (http://www.prb.org/Home/Publications/GraphicsBank/Aging.aspx).
74. Friedman JE, Kurtis JD, McGarvey ST: The dual burden of infectious and non-communicable diseases in the Asia-Pacific region: Examples from the Philippines and the Samoan Islands. Med Health R I 90:346, 2007.
75. World Bank: Health, nutrition and population statistics, 2007 (http://go.worldbank.org/N2N84RDV00).
76. Anderson I, Crengle S, Kamaka ML, et al: Indigenous health in Australia, New Zealand, and the Pacific. Lancet 367:1775, 2006.
77. Keighley ED, McGarvey ST, Turituri P, Viali S: Farming and adiposity in Samoan adults. Am J Hum Biol 18:112, 2006.
78. Danaei G, Lawes CM, Vander Hoorn S, et al: Global and regional mortality from ischaemic heart disease and stroke attributable to higher-than-optimum blood glucose concentration: Comparative risk assessment. Lancet 368:1651, 2006.
79. World Health Organization: WHO Global InfoBase, 2008 (http://www.who.int/infobase).
80. Kuulasmaa K, Tunstall-Pedoe H, Dobson A, et al: Estimation of contribution of changes in classic risk factors to trends in coronary-event rates across the WHO MONICA Project populations. Lancet 355:675, 2000.
81. Averina M, Nilssen O, Brenn T, et al: High cardiovascular mortality in Russia cannot be explained by the classical risk factors. The Arkhangelsk Study 2000. Eur J Epidemiol 18:871, 2003.
82. Anand SS, Islam S, Rosengren A, et al: Risk factors for myocardial infarction in women and men: Insights from the INTERHEART study. Eur Heart J 29:932, 2008.
83. Carevic V, Rumboldt M, Rumboldt Z: Coronary heart disease risk factors in Croatia and worldwide: Results of the Interheart study. Acta Med Croatica 61:299, 2007.
84. Zatonski W, Campos H, Willett W: Rapid declines in coronary heart disease mortality in Eastern Europe are associated with increased consumption of oils rich in alpha-linoleic acid. Eur J Epidemiol 23:3, 2008.
85. Schargrodsky H, Hernández-Hernández R, Champagne BM, et al: CARMELA: Assessment of cardiovascular risk in seven Latin American cities. Am J Med 121:58, 2008.
86. Lanas F, Avezum A, Bautista LE, et al: Risk factors for acute myocardial infarction in Latin America: The INTERHEART Latin American study. Circulation 115:1067, 2007.
87. Gus I, Harzheim E, Zaslavsky C, et al: Prevalence, awareness, and control of systemic arterial hypertension in the state of Rio Grande do Sul. Arq Bras Cardiol 83:429, 2004.

88. Cerdas M: Epidemiology and control of hypertension and diabetes in Costa Rica. Ren Fail 28:693, 2006.
89. Garcia-Garcia G, Aviles-Gomez R, Luquin-Arellano VH, et al: Cardiovascular risk factors in the Mexican population. Ren Fail, 28:677, 2006.
89a. World Health O: The Work of WHO in the Eastern Mediterranean Region: Annual Report of the Regional Director, 2007. (http://www.emro.who.int/rd/annualreports/2007/chapter1_6.htm).
90. Baynouna LM, Revel AD, Nagelkerke NJ, et al: High prevalence of the cardiovascular risk factors in Al-Ain, United Arab Emirates. An emerging health care priority. Saudi Med J 29:1173, 2008.
91. Hatmi ZN, Tahvildari S, Gafarzadeh Motlag A, Sabouri Kashani A: Prevalence of coronary artery disease risk factors in Iran: A population based survey. BMC Cardiovasc Disord 7:32, 2007.
92. Ajay VS, Gupta R, Panniyammakkal J, et al: National Cardiovascular Disease Database, Delhi Ministry of Health and Family Welfare, Government of India. Geneva, World Health Organization, 2002.
93. Lopez AD, Mathers CD, Ezzati E, et al: Measuring the global burden of disease and risk factors, 1990-2001. *In* Lopez AD, Mathers CD, Ezzati E, et al (eds): Global Burden of Disease and Risk Factors. New York, Oxford University Press, 2006, pp 1-14.
94. Akinboboye O, Idris O, Akinkugbe O: Trends in coronary artery disease and associated risk factors in sub-Saharan Africans. J Hum Hypertens 17:381, 2003.
95. Steyn K, Sliwa K, Hawken S, et al: Risk factors associated with myocardial infarction in Africa: The INTERHEART Africa Study. Circulation 112:3554, 2005.
96. Mensah GA: Ischaemic heart disease in Africa. Heart 94:836, 2008.
97. Feigin VL, Lawes CMM, Bennett DA, Barker-Collo SL, Parag V: Worldwide stroke incidence and early case fatality reported in 56 population-based studies: a systematic review. The Lancet Neurol 8:355, 2009.
98. Mathers CD, Lopez AD, Murray CJL, et al: The burden of disease and mortality by condition: Data, methods, and results for 2001. *In* Lopez AD, Mathers CD, Ezzati E, et al (eds): Global Burden of Disease and Risk Factors. New York, Oxford University Press, 2006, pp 45-240.
99. Connor MD, Walker R, Modi G, Warlow CP: Burden of stroke in black populations in sub-Saharan Africa. Lancet Neurol 6:269, 2007.
100. Kengne AP, Anderson CS: The neglected burden of stroke in Sub-Saharan Africa. Int J Stroke 1:180, 2006.
101. Longo-Mbenza M, Tshinkwela L, Pukuta JM: Rates and predictors of stroke-associated case fatality in black Central African patients. Cardiovasc J Africa 19:72, 2008.
102. Wahab KW: The burden of stroke in Nigeria. Int J Stroke 3:290, 2008.

Economic Burden

103. Suhrcke M, Nugent RA, Stuckler D, Rocco L: Chronic Disease: An Economic Perspective. 2006 (http://www.oxha.org/ initiatives/economics/chronic-disease-an-economic-perspective).
104. Schieber GJ, Gottret P, Fleisher LK, Leive AA: Financing global health: Mission unaccomplished. Health Aff (Millwood) 26:921, 2007.
105. Thom T, Haase N, Rosamond W, et al: Heart disease and stroke statistics—2006 update: A report from the American Heart Association Statistics Committee and Stroke Statistics Subcommittee. Circulation 113:e85, 2006.
106. Gaziano TA, Bitton A, Anand S, Weinstein MC: The global cost of nonoptimal blood pressure. J Hypertens 27:1472, 2009.

Cost-Effective Solutions

107. Gaziano T, Reddy KS, Paccaud F, Horton S: Cardiovascular disease. *In* Jamison DT, Breman JG, Measham AR, et al (eds): Disease Control Priorities in Developing Countries. 2nd ed. New York, Oxford University Press, 2006, pp 645-662.
108. Gaziano TA: Cardiovascular disease in the developing world and its cost-effective management. Circulation 112:3547, 2005.
109. Gaziano TA, Steyn K, Cohen DJ, et al: Cost-effectiveness analysis of hypertension guidelines in South Africa: Absolute risk versus blood pressure level. Circulation 112:3569, 2005.
110. Gaziano TA, Opie LH, Weinstein MC: Cardiovascular disease prevention with a multidrug regimen in the developing world: A cost-effectiveness analysis. Lancet 368:679, 2006.
111. Ferrario M, Chiodini P, Chambless LE, et al: Prediction of coronary events in a low incidence population. Assessing accuracy of the CUORE Cohort Study prediction equation. Int J Epidemiol 34:413, 2005.
112. Wilson PW, D'Agostino RB, Levy D, et al: Prediction of coronary heart disease using risk factor categories. Circulation 97:1837, 1998.
113. Folsom AR, Chambless LE, Ballantyne CM, et al: An assessment of incremental coronary risk prediction using C-reactive protein and other novel risk markers: The Atherosclerosis Risk in Communities Study. Arch Intern Med 166:1368, 2006.
114. Wang TJ, Gona P, Larson MG, et al: Multiple biomarkers for the prediction of first major cardiovascular events and death. N Engl J Med 355:2631, 2006.
115. Ware JH: The limitations of risk factors as prognostic tools. N Engl J Med 355:2615, 2006.
116. Ridker PM, Buring JE, Rifai N, Cook NR: Development and validation of improved algorithms for the assessment of global cardiovascular risk in women: The Reynolds Risk Score. JAMA 297:611, 2007.
117. Lindholm LH, Mendis S: Prevention of cardiovascular disease in developing countries. Lancet 370:720, 2007.
118. Mendis S, Lindholm LH, Mancia G, et al: World Health Organization (WHO) and International Society of Hypertension (ISH) risk prediction charts: Assessment of cardiovascular risk for prevention and control of cardiovascular disease in low and middle-income countries. J Hypertens 25:1578, 2007.
119. Gaziano TA, Young CR, Fitzmaurice G, et al: Laboratory-based versus non-laboratory-based method for assessment of cardiovascular disease risk: The NHANES I Follow-up Study cohort. Lancet, 371:923, 2008.
120. Asaria P, Chisholm D, Mathers C, et al: Population-wide interventions to prevent chronic diseases. Lancet 370:2044, 2007.
121. Jha P, Chaloupka FJ, Moore J, et al: Tobacco addiction. *In* Jamison DT, Breman JG, Measham AR, et al (eds): Disease Control Priorities in Developing Countries. 2nd ed. New York, Oxford University Press, 2006, pp 869-886.
122. Mohiuddin SM, Mooss AN, Hunter CB, et al: Intensive smoking cessation intervention reduces mortality in high-risk smokers with cardiovascular disease. Chest 131:446, 2007.
123. Ong HT: Beta blockers in hypertension and cardiovascular disease. BMJ 334:946, 2007.
124. Jamison DT, Breman JG, Measham AR, et al (eds): Disease Control Priorities in the Developing Countries, 2nd ed. New York, Oxford University Press, 2006.
125. Bibbins-Domingo K, Chertow GM, Coxson PG, et al: Projected effect of dietary salt reductions on future cardiovascular disease. N Engl J Med 362:590, 2010.
126. Gaziano TA, Galea G, Reddy KS: Scaling up interventions for chronic disease prevention: The evidence. Lancet 370:1939, 2007.
127. Ebrahim S, Smith GD: Systematic review of randomised controlled trials of multiple risk factor interventions for preventing coronary heart disease. BMJ 314:1666, 1997.
128. Uusitalo U, Feskens EJ, Tuomilehto J, et al: Fall in total cholesterol concentration over five years in association with changes in fatty acid composition of cooking oil in Mauritius: cross sectional survey. BMJ (Clinical Research Ed.) 313(7064):1044-1046, 1996.
129. Steyn K, Steyn M, Swanepoel AS, et al: Twelve-year results of the Coronary Risk Factor Study (CORIS). International Journal of Epidemiology 26(5):964-971, 1997.

CHAPTER 2 Heart Disease in Varied Populations

Clyde W. Yancy

Changing Demographics of the U.S. Population

Cardiovascular disease (CVD) and stroke remain the leading causes of death and disability in the United States. These illnesses afflict the entire U.S. population. In the past, data extracted from large epidemiologic studies and major clinical trials in racially homogeneous cohorts have assessed risk and described the natural history of CVD. Earlier questions regarding the generalizability of these risks and disease traits to a more heterogeneous populace (i.e., varied populations) have been quelled by the replication of similar risk profiles and features in contemporary racially and ethnically diverse population surveys. The risk for heart disease and stroke is ubiquitous and affects all populations. Moreover, current data suggest that racial or ethnic attributes of CVD may vary significantly among populations. Given the consequences of heart disease, it is imperative that the practice of cardiovascular medicine address the nuanced risk profiles and differing presentations of disease within varied populations.

The emerging importance of these varied populations directly relates to the changing U.S. demographic. Currently, 14% of the U.S. population is black and 16% is Hispanic, and the Asian cohort is growing rapidly.[1] When added to the Native American population, the aggregate representation of these varied populations now approaches 40%, and a majority population in the United States likely will no longer exist by 2050. The population mosaic of the United States is changing, and the natural history of CVD reflects this increasing heterogeneity. Cardiovascular practitioners and scientists must be aware of the epidemiology, pathophysiology, and treatment of heart disease in varied U.S. populations (**Fig. 2-1**).

Distribution of Known Risk Factors for Heart Disease

The incidence of known risk factors for CVD is alarmingly high in varied populations (see Chaps. 44, 45, 47, and 64). The Third National Health and Nutrition Examination Survey (NHANES III) contains data on the distribution of hypertension among non-Hispanic white, non-Hispanic black, and Hispanic groups. Hypertension affects at least 33 million whites, almost 6 million blacks, and 1.3 million Hispanics. The rate of hypertension in blacks is approximately 40% (among the highest in the world); in whites, 25.6% in men and 23.8% in women; and in Hispanics, 14.6% in men and 14% in women (see Fig. 44-2). Worse disease severity accompanies a higher prevalence of hypertension in blacks. The prevalence of stage 3 hypertension [>180/110 mmHg] is 8.5% for blacks, compared with 1% for whites. The mean systolic and diastolic blood pressure (BP) for blacks is 125/75 mm Hg, compared with 122/74 mm Hg for whites. For hypertensive blacks, the difference in BP versus that for normotensive blacks is 30/20 mm Hg, whereas for hypertensive whites, the difference in BP is 23/15 mm Hg.[2]

Diabetes, a deadly risk factor for CVD, currently affects 17 million Americans. The incidence of the disease has increased 49% in the last decade, likely because of the alarming incidence of obesity. Blacks have the highest prevalence of hemoglobin A1c (HbA1c) $\geq$ 7%. In individuals 40 to 74 years of age, the prevalence of diabetes is 11.2% for whites, 18.2% for blacks, and 20.3% for Hispanics. Despite the higher incidence of diabetes in Hispanics, mortality rates from diabetes are highest in blacks—28.4/100,000 for men and 39.1/100,000 for women. This compares to 23.4/100,000 and 25.7/100,000 for white men and white women, respectively.[3] Hypertension concomitantly occurs in 75.4% of blacks with diabetes, 70.7% of Hispanics with diabetes, and 64.5% of whites with diabetes.

Insulin resistance, along with obesity, hypertension, and dyslipidemia, constitutes the metabolic syndrome, which is associated with excessive CVD. Applying the National Cholesterol Education Program Adult Treatment Panel III (NCEP ATP III) criteria to the NHANES III database, the incidence of the metabolic syndrome might exceed 30% for the U.S. population older than 20 years, but increases to more than 40% in older adults and is highest in the varied populations.[4-6] Hispanics have the highest incidence of the metabolic syndrome—31.9% overall, and 35% in Hispanic women. Despite the high incidence of insulin resistance and the metabolic syndrome, Hispanics have a lower prevalence of hypertension than blacks. When the influence of obesity, body fat distribution, and insulin concentrations is followed prospectively in whites and Hispanics, each factor independently associates with the development of hypertension—with the greatest risk in subjects with the highest body mass index (BMI; >30 kg/m^2) and the highest insulin concentration (>95 pmol/L). There appears to be no additional CVD risk for Hispanic ethnicity as compared with whites.[7]

The incidence of overweight or obesity—defined by a BMI higher than 25 kg/m^2 as overweight, higher than 30 kg/m^2 as obese, and higher than 40 kg/m^2 as morbidly obese—is alarming in the U.S. population, and the varied populations are disproportionately affected. The prevalence of overweight and obesity is likely 60% or higher in the United States, and one third of all children and adolescents are overweight or obese.[8]

The prevalence of both overweight and obesity is higher in blacks than in whites, and higher in Hispanics than in whites. The mean BMI is 29.2 kg/m^2 for blacks, 28.6 kg/m^2 for Hispanics, and 26.3 kg/m^2 for whites. Black women are on average 17 pounds heavier than white women of comparable age and socioeconomic status. Six of the 15 states with the highest prevalence of hypertension are in the southeastern United States (corresponding with the "stroke belt"), and half of all blacks live in this region. The highest prevalence of obesity, at 44%, is in black women, and in the southeastern United States, a

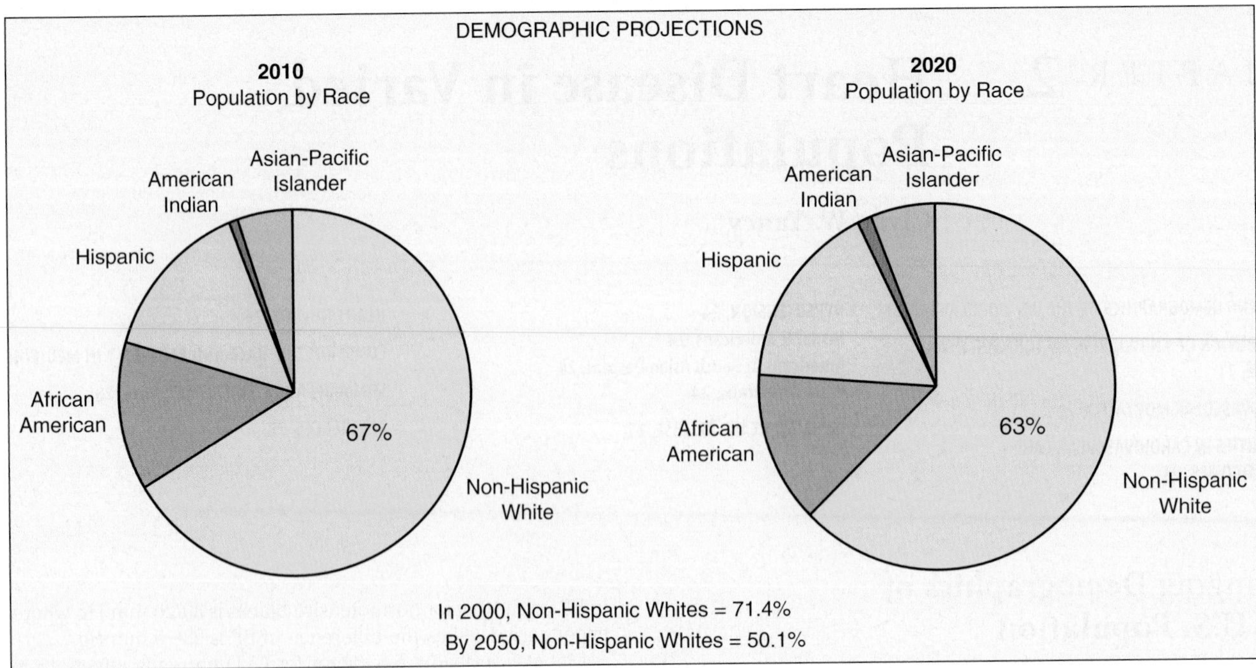

FIGURE 2-1 United States population estimates from the U.S. Census Bureau *(http://www.census.gov/population/www/projections/usinterimproj/natprojtab01a.pdf).*

striking 71% of black women are obese.[9,10] Although Asians have lesser rates of overweight and obesity, standard BMI weight class definitions may be inappropriate for this population.

The International Collaborative Study on Hypertension in Blacks (ICSHIB) has demonstrated an important interaction of BMI and hypertension across the African Diaspora. Seven populations of West African origin were identified. A striking linear relationship was noted between BMI and the percentage of the respective population with hypertension, varying from a less than 15% incidence of hypertension in Africans in Nigeria, with a mean BMI of less than 24 kg/m^2, to a hypertension incidence of almost 35% in the Chicago area, where the mean BMI was 29 kg/m^2.[11] Overall, 22% of the U.S. population, but 40% of black women, are physically inactive. Data from the Coronary Artery Risk Development in Young Adults study (CARDIA) have demonstrated that black women have a higher BMI (at least 27 kg/m^2), higher energy intake, lower levels of physical activity, and lower overall physical fitness than white women.[12] Thus, obesity and physical inactivity contribute to the development of hypertension and subsequent heart disease in blacks.

Dyslipidemia is an important modifiable risk factor for heart disease in the United States, and treatment of lipid disorders decreases the incidence of heart disease. Several reports have suggested that blacks have lower low-density lipoprotein (LDL) cholesterol concentrations and less hypercholesterolemia than whites. The CARDIA study identified the prevalence of high LDL cholesterol levels in young adults; LDL cholesterol exceeded 160 mg/dL in 10% and 5% of young black men and women, respectively, compared with 9% and 4% of young white men and women. High-density lipoprotein (HDL) cholesterol levels were higher in black men than in white men.[13] Lipoprotein(a)—Lp(a)—is a known risk factor for coronary heart disease (CHD), and levels are two- to threefold higher in blacks.

Several important dietary variations in varied populations, including increased sodium consumption, reduced potassium consumption, and decreased calcium intake, potentially associate with an increased incidence of CVD. The Treatment of Mild Hypertension Study (TOMHS) demonstrated dissimilar urinary Na^+ levels and Na^+/K^+ ratios for blacks versus whites, especially in lower socioeconomic levels. This difference relates to dietary electrolyte intake, and higher intake of dietary sodium links to the incidence of hypertension. The required daily intake of sodium is low, at 20 to 40 mmol; recently, the recommended daily allowance for sodium was set at 2300 mg for the general population but at 1500 mg (~25 mmol) for the black population.[14] Unfortunately, current sodium consumption in the United States averages 140 to 150 mmol/day (8 to 10 g/day), and is highest in blacks and Hispanics. Sodium intake relates directly to hypertension, whereas potassium intake relates inversely to hypertension. Blacks generally consume diets low in potassium; such diets are typically associated with concurrent increases in sodium intake, caloric intake, and alcohol consumption, and are common in industrialized countries. Blacks also consume diets low in calcium, and perhaps low in magnesium as well; intake of calcium and magnesium is associated with lower BP. The Dietary Approaches to Stop Hypertension (DASH) trial tested the potential benefit of a diet rich in fruits, vegetables, and low-fat dairy products, and reduced in saturated and total fats, in controls and in patients with known hypertension. The diet increased potassium intake from 1700 to 4100 mg/day, with a corresponding drop in sodium intake. The DASH diet most greatly affected those with the highest sodium intake, achieving a 12-mm Hg reduction in BP in blacks, equivalent to the results expected from pharmacologic intervention with a single drug to control BP.[15]

Studies have shown that hypovitaminosis D may be an important risk factor for heart disease. Blacks have disproportionately low levels of vitamin D, with a 10-fold greater prevalence of low vitamin D levels compared with whites. Low levels of vitamin D are related to darker skin and obesity. Hypovitaminosis D is associated with a greater incidence of heart failure, higher incidence of myocardial infarction (MI), decreased insulin sensitivity, and elevated BP.[16,17] In NHANES III, low levels of vitamin D may explain approximately half of the excess prevalence of hypertension in blacks as compared with whites.[18] Although mechanisms of disease related to low levels of vitamin D are not entirely clear, the association of proinflammatory states and increased oxidative stress are plausible considerations.

In the setting of hypertension, rates of left ventricular (LV) hypertrophy (as determined by electrocardiography) are highest in blacks—31% as compared with 10% in whites—and the pattern of hypertrophy, as determined by echocardiography, is more of the concentric type known to be associated with increased cardiovascular events.[19] These findings have been confirmed using cardiac magnetic resonance imaging. Black men and women have a two- to threefold higher incidence of LV hypertrophy compared with whites, even after controlling for body surface area, fat-free mass, height, systolic BP, and socioeconomic status.[19]

LV mass correlates with systolic BP and predicts heart disease. The CARDIA study[12] has demonstrated a higher incidence of increased LV mass in young black adults and a close relationship among obesity, systolic BP elevation, and LV mass. Smoking rates are generally higher in blacks and Hispanics, and may be increasing in teens and young adults.

Among newer risk factors for heart disease, hypertriglyceridemia and tissue plasminogen activator inhibitor-1 are less prevalent in blacks[20]; and homocysteine, C-reactive protein, and interleukin-6 are more prevalent in blacks.[21] Coronary calcium scores are highest in non-Hispanic whites and lowest in Hispanics, whereas an elevated score may be most predictive of a worse prognosis in blacks and least predictive in Asians. However, these analyses are confounded by the confluence of other risk factors for coronary artery disease (CAD).[22] Hyperuricemia and microalbuminuria may demonstrate subtle differences in these varied populations, but inadequate data points prevent definitive comment.

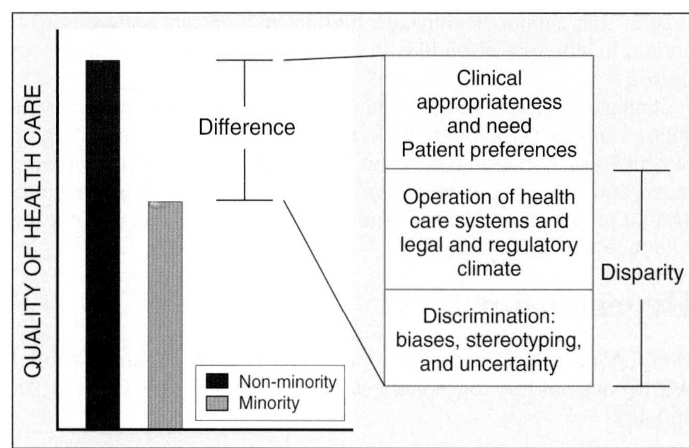

FIGURE 2-2 Identifying differences versus disparities that account for varied health care experiences as a function of race. *(From Smedley BD, Stith AY, Nelson AR [eds]: Unequal Treatment: Confronting Racial and Ethnic Disparities in Health Care. Washington, DC, National Academies Press, 2003.)*

Cardiovascular Mortality

Heart disease is the leading cause of death for all segments of the U.S. population, including the varied populations (see Chap. 1). Of these groups, blacks experience the highest rates of mortality from heart disease, and CVD causes at least 35% of the difference between blacks and whites in life-years lost. The CVD mortality rate for blacks is 1.6 times that of whites, a ratio identical to the black-to-white mortality ratio in 1950.[16] Hispanics are twice as likely as all other groups to die from diabetes, and Native Americans also die disproportionately from diabetes. The average annual death rate caused by heart disease, expressed as deaths per 100,000, is 422.8 for black men and 298.2 for black women, and 306.6 for white men and 215 for white women. For those in the 45- to 64-year age range, the rates are 188 for Native Americans, 143 for Hispanics, and 90 for Asians and Pacific Islanders. CVD is the leading cause of death in women, affecting 41% of whites, 41% of blacks, 33% of Hispanics, and 37% of Asians.

The prevalence of CHD is higher in blacks, with a prevalence of 7.1% for men and 9.0% for women, compared with 6.9% for white men and 5.4% for white women. Average annual CHD death rates are 272 and 193/100,000 for black men and women, compared with 249 and 153/100,000 for white men and women. CHD death rates in blacks are the highest in the world. Death rates from stroke are also higher in blacks; compared with whites, young black men and women have a threefold increased risk of ischemic stroke and a fourfold increased risk of stroke death. The stroke death rate is highest in the southeastern United States. The five states with the highest death rates from heart failure, and 10 of the 15 states with the highest rates of end-stage renal disease (ESRD), are also in this region.

The prevalence of CHD in Mexican Americans is 7.2% for men and 6.8% for women. The prevalence of MI in Mexican Americans is 4.1% for men and 1.9% for women, compared with 5.2% for white men and 2.0% for white women, and 4.3% for black men and 3.3% for black women. Death rates are similar for Hispanics and whites.[23]

Disparities in Cardiovascular Care and Outcomes

The foregoing information establishes important population differences regarding CVD risk and outcomes. The complete explanation for these differential outcomes is lacking, but likely reflects a complex interplay of cultural, political, physiologic, and genetic variances. Differences in health care quality metrics and outcomes contrast with disparities in racial and ethnic health care. Differences may be entirely appropriate because of the indications (or absence thereof) for care, or simply because of patient preferences for indicated interventions. Disparities in health care refers to differences in the quality of health care that are not the result of clinical needs, preferences (i.e., patient choices), or appropriateness of the intervention, and instead reflect limited access to care and health care systems, or providers who are not culturally, linguistically, or economically sensitive to all patient cohorts (**Fig. 2-2**).[24]

Minorities refuse certain procedures (e.g., coronary artery bypass grafting [CABG]) at a higher rate than other groups, but not enough to account for major differences in outcomes. Greater issues pertain at the level of the health care delivery system. Language barriers pose obstacles for many patients. Almost 14 million Americans are not proficient in English, and 1 in 5 Spanish speakers report not seeking health care because of language issues. Almost 8 million Hispanics and about 1 in 20 Native Americans do not speak English well. The language barrier in Asians varies from 1% in persons of Hawaiian origin to 15% for those of Japanese origin to 55% for persons of Cambodian origin. Lack of health insurance and geographic isolation contribute further to these disparities.

Providers may contribute to disparities in health care through subconscious stereotyping, clinical uncertainty because of cultural ignorance, and delay in referral for indicated procedures. Inexplicably, blacks are less likely to achieve lipid reduction goals, despite clear indications for therapy and evidence for statin efficacy. Physicians also give fewer referrals for cardiac catheterization to black women compared with white men or women and to black men, despite similar articulation of symptoms and reasonable indications for further evaluation.[25,26]

These patient, system, and provider issues result in a strikingly dissimilar application of indicated therapies. In a survey of 4 million patients with acute MI, as indexed in the National Hospital Discharge Survey (NHDS), black men and women underwent coronary angiography and CABG at much lower rates. A separate Medicare survey has suggested that the CABG rate is fourfold higher in whites than in blacks, even after adjusting for age and gender. An analysis of Hispanics and whites with a diagnosis of MI has revealed that Hispanics were discharged on 38% fewer medications; they also were less likely to receive percutaneous coronary interventions. Studies done at Veterans Health Administration medical centers are intriguing because these facilities theoretically have removed any access to care issues; however, referral for cardiac procedures was higher for whites than for other groups. Blacks refused invasive procedures twice as often and were much less likely to receive thrombolytic therapy or CABG. Patients with ESRD have access to Medicare funding for health care needs, which theoretically reduces disparities. A longitudinal survey of health care disparities from Medicare beneficiaries with ESRD is compelling; before developing ESRD, whites were 300% more likely to undergo cardiac catheterization, angioplasty, or CABG, after controlling for socioeconomic variables. This disparity fell to a 40% difference after the onset of ESRD and Medicare funding. These data suggest that similar health care funding may significantly diminish certain health care disparities in cardiovascular care, but differences persist.

Strategies to overcome disparate health care remain under investigation and development. Improved access to care, multilingual patient tools, community-focused efforts, enhanced cultural competence, and broader uptake of evidence-based guideline-driven strategies for all patients serve as immediate interventions that can reduce evidence of disparate care.

Hypertension

Varied populations bear a disproportionate burden of cardiovascular risk because of the consequences of hypertension (see Chaps. 1, 45, and 46).

Hispanic Americans

A paradox exists in Hispanics. Despite a higher incidence of diabetes and obesity, the prevalence of hypertension is lower than that in the general population. Hypertension among Hispanics varies by gender and by country of origin. Puerto Rican origin is associated with the highest incidence of hypertension, followed by Cuban origin and Mexican origin. Mexican Americans have the lowest rates of hypertension awareness, so BP control can be more difficult.[7] The lower incidence of hypertension in Hispanics of Mexican origin, as compared with other Hispanics, may result from a modernization phenomenon, implicating acclimatization to a North American lifestyle as a factor in the development of hypertension. In Puerto Rico, urban men with a high school education have a BP 8 mm Hg higher than less educated men. This is not the same experience seen in other North American ethnic groups, for whom education is associated with lower BP values.

Americans of South Asian Descent

Hypertension is a significant concern in the Indian subcontinent and is an important cardiovascular risk for South Asians worldwide, including Americans of South Asian ancestry. The World Health Organization has reported that Indian men 40 to 55 years of age have the highest BP among 20 developing countries (see Chap. 1). The prevalence of hypertension in South Asian countries has increased from less than 2% in 1950 to more than 20% currently. This increased risk rises further with emigration to North America, and varies directly with the degree of urbanization.[27] The Study of Health Assessment and Risk in Ethnic Groups (SHARE) carried out in Canada has reported that South Asians have the highest self-reported incidence of hypertension. Coincident with the hypertension risk is a growing risk of diabetes, dyslipidemia (perhaps related to a genetic predisposition to a low HDL level), and obesity. Tobacco consumption and per capita fat consumption are similarly increasing in South Asians. Taken together, the confluence of these risk factors contributes to the alarming rate of hypertension and to the increasing rate of symptomatic CAD.[28]

Black Americans

Hypertension in U.S. blacks represents the most prolific variance in heart disease and CVD risk factors in the varied populations; they experience perhaps the highest prevalence of hypertension in the world.[29] An estimated 5.6 million blacks have hypertension. The Hypertension and Detection Follow-up Program has found that severe hypertension (diastolic BP > 115 mm Hg) is five- to sevenfold more likely in blacks than in whites. The differential experience of hypertension is evident in childhood, with a higher recorded BP noted before 10 years of age in black versus white children. Hypertension in blacks has somewhat pathologic consequences, with a 50% higher frequency of heart failure, a four- to sixfold higher incidence of developing ESRD (see Chap. 93),[30] a 38% higher risk of stroke, and a higher risk of death from stroke (see Chap. 62).[31] Overall, mortality caused by hypertension and its consequences is four- to fivefold more likely in blacks than in whites.

Hypertensive heart disease manifests as LV hypertrophy, which is a separate risk factor for sudden death and coronary events. A substudy of the African American Study of Kidney Disease has revealed echocardiographic criteria consistent with LV hypertrophy in 67% and 74%, respectively, of African American men and women with hypertension.[32] The CARDIA study[12] has demonstrated that LV mass is higher and independently correlates with systolic BP in young black men. Increased LV mass is associated with an increased rate of death and thus contributes to the excess rate of morbidity and mortality caused by CVD in blacks. CAD is the leading putative cause of heart failure in whites, but pooled data from published clinical trials have suggested that hypertension may be the leading imputed cause of heart failure in blacks.

Variances in the pathophysiology of stroke may also exist. Blacks typically have more occlusive disease in the large- and medium-sized intracranial arteries, whereas whites typically have more occlusive disease in the extracranial arteries. The incidence of hemorrhagic stroke is also higher; similar observations have been made in the setting of ESRD. Hypertensive nephrosclerosis is the leading cause of ESRD for blacks, who also disproportionately populate the hemodialysis cohort. A nocturnal dip in BP and earlier onset of proteinuria have been noted in blacks; both of these observations are associated with a higher incidence of hypertension-induced nephrosclerosis. Several purported mechanisms may explain in part the excess burden of hypertension in blacks. Peripheral vascular resistance may be higher in some blacks with hypertension, and certain vasodilatory responses are blunted in blacks, in a manner suggesting subtle differences in nitric oxide homeostasis. Plasma renin activity and urinary kallikrein excretion are lower in age-matched black hypertensives versus white hypertensives, and insulin levels are higher in blacks. Much has been written about sodium sensitivity in blacks, including a theoretical assertion that genetic pressure during the African Diaspora (active slave trading from West Africa to North America) led to selective expression favoring genes that promote salt retention, which now predispose to hypertension. This conjecture remains unproven, yet prevalent.[33] Rates of hypertension in rural West Africa are the lowest in the world, but populations of West African origin in the Caribbean and in North America demonstrate dramatic rises in BP that may be related to increases in BMI.[34] Some blacks appear to be more sodium sensitive than others, and salt restriction leads to a greater reduction in systolic BP in blacks (~12 mm Hg) than in whites.[15,35] A genetic basis for sodium sensitivity may exist. The epithelial sodium channel (ENaC) is responsible for the final reabsorption of filtered sodium from the distal nephron and has at least eight single-nucleotide polymorphisms. One of these polymorphisms (T594M) is found only in people of West African descent, and is found four times more often in hypertensive blacks than in normotensive blacks. However, variations in a single gene do not likely account for more than 2% to 4% of the difference in hypertension among races.[36]

Cytokine polymorphisms are other attractive candidates to explain the excess risk of hypertension-related CVD in blacks. Transforming growth factor beta-1 (TGF-β1) is associated with stimulation of fibrosis, extracellular matrix turnover, glomerular hyperplasia, and left LV hypertrophy. In blacks, TGF-β1 is overexpressed, with higher circulating levels. A described polymorphism at codon 25 of the TGF-β1 gene involving the substitution of arginine for proline is associated with higher TGF-β1 levels and is seen more frequently in blacks.[37,38]

Angiotensin-converting enzyme (ACE) inhibitors and angiotensin receptor blockers (ARBs) reduce angiotensin II–mediated stimulation of TGF-β1, which may be clinically important to the treatment of hypertension in blacks. Beta-adrenergic receptor blockers (beta blockers) are reportedly less effective as monotherapy for hypertension in blacks, but data suggest visceral obesity strongly correlates with exaggerated sympathetic nervous system activity in black women.[39]

THERAPY. Therapy of hypertension in blacks should focus on BP reduction to goal to lower CVD risk (see Chap. 46). The treatment of hypertension is similar for all demographic groups, and should follow published guideline-based recommendations for optimal care.[40,41] Responsiveness to monotherapy with ACE inhibitors, ARBs, and beta blockers may be lower compared with diuretics and calcium channel blockers in blacks, but these differences are corrected when diuretics are added to neurohormonal antagonists. The African American Study of Kidney Disease and Hypertension (AASK) has prospectively addressed the impact of three antihypertensive drug classes on glomerular filtration rate (GFR) decline in hypertension. Diabetic patients were excluded. Patients with established hypertension-induced nephrosclerosis and reduced GFR (20 to 60 mL/min/1.73 m^2), a clinical composite that included a 50% reduction in GFR, ESRD, or death, were most favorably treated by an ACE inhibitor, compared with a beta blocker or calcium channel blocker. This study showed that black patients with hypertension uniformly require a multidrug regimen to achieve adequate BP control.[42,43]

The Antihypertensive and Lipid-Lowering Treatment to Prevent Heart Attack Trial (ALLHAT) was a large trial that tested the ability of a calcium channel blocker– and ACE inhibitor–based antihypertensive regimen to lower cardiovascular morbidity and mortality, compared with a diuretic-based regimen. Of the 33,357 patients in the trial, 35% (11,674) were black. All patients had hypertension and at least one additional cardiovascular risk factor. The primary outcome was an aggregate of fatal CHD or nonfatal myocardial infarction. Secondary outcomes included all-cause mortality, stroke, combined CVD (including CHD death, nonfatal myocardial infarction [MI], stroke, angina, coronary revascularization, heart failure, and peripheral vascular disease), and ESRD. There was no difference as a function of race between the treatment groups on the primary outcome. For the calcium channel blocker–based regimen as compared with the diuretic-based regimen, the incidence of heart failure (a secondary outcome) was higher, and for the ACE inhibitor–based regimen as compared with the diuretic-based regimen, BP was higher (i.e., blacks had a lower achieved BP on diuretic-based therapy); stroke and combined CVD outcomes were also higher. For the calcium channel blocker– and ACE inhibitor–based regimen, the observed differences did not yield a statistically significant difference in treatment effects by race.[44,45] Thus, the key consideration is goal BP reduction, and diuretic therapy is the preferred initial therapy for all patients with hypertension. An algorithm to guide the management of high BP in blacks is depicted in **Fig. 2-3**[46] and its features are highlighted in **Table 2-1.**

Ischemic Heart Disease

Rates of ischemic heart disease are increasing in varied populations because of concurrent and often disproportionate risk factors for CAD. Rates of CAD are increasing in Asians, Hispanics, Native Americans, and Americans of South Asian origin. The rates of CAD in these groups are approaching but do not exceed the rate seen in whites. This is not the case for blacks, however, who have the highest overall CAD mortality rate of any ethnic group in the United States and the highest prevalence of acute MI in the 35- to 54-year age range.[23]

The presentation is usually unstable angina or a non-ST elevation infarct rather than a typical ST-segment elevation event. Despite this increased incidence of disease, obstructive epicardial CAD appears less often on angiography. Not infrequently, angiographic studies show normal epicardial vessels, but autopsy studies have demonstrated a greater extent of atherosclerosis in blacks, despite a lesser degree of obstructive CAD. As noted, interventions with thrombolytic therapy, percutaneous coronary intervention, and CABG surgery are all less frequently applied.

TABLE 2-1 Management of Black Patients with Hypertension

- Increase dietary potassium intake
- Limit dietary sodium intake to <2.4 g/day
- Increase physical activity
- Weight loss
- All antihypertensive medications and combinations are effective:
  - Multiple drug combinations may be required to achieve control.
  - ACE inhibitors and beta blockers as monotherapy may be less effective, but should be used when indicated (e.g., renal disease, heart failure, post-MI).
  - Thiazide diuretics and calcium channel blockers may have greater blood pressure–lowering efficacy.
  - There is a higher incidence of angioedema when using ACE inhibitors.

From Douglas JG, Bakris GL, Epstein M, et al: Management of high blood pressure in African Americans: Consensus statement of the Hypertension in African Americans Working Group of the International Society on Hypertension in Blacks. Arch Intern Med 163:525, 2003.

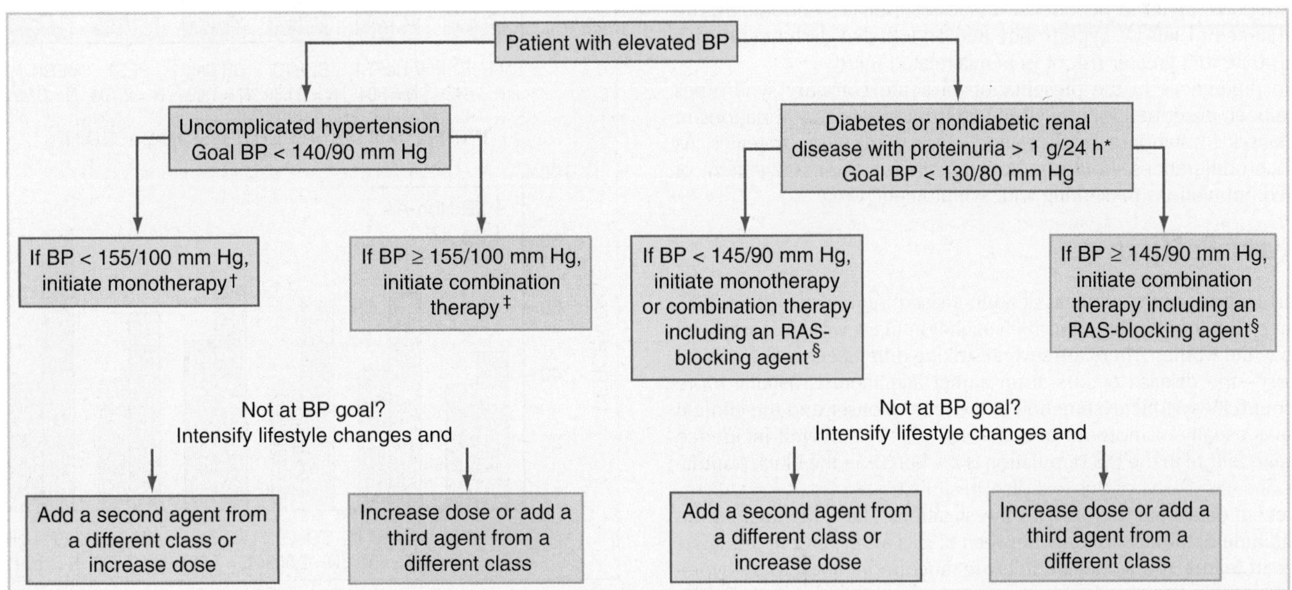

FIGURE 2-3 Hypertension treatment algorithm for blacks, from the International Society of Hypertension in Blacks (ISHIB). *Preferable BP goal for patients with renal disease with proteinuria higher than 1 g/24 hr is less than 125/75 mm Hg. †Initiate monotherapy at the recommended starting dose with an agent from any of the following classes: diuretics, beta blockers, calcium channel blockers (CCBs), ACE inhibitors, or ARBs. ‡To achieve BP goals more expeditiously, initiate low-dose combination therapy with any of the following combinations: beta blocker–diuretic, ACE inhibitor–diuretic, ACE inhibitor–CCB, or ARB–diuretic. §Consider specific clinical indications when selecting agents. RAS = renin-angiotensin system. *(From Douglas JG, Bakris GL, Epstein M, et al: Management of high blood pressure in African Americans: Consensus statement of the Hypertension in African Americans Working Group of the International Society on Hypertension in Blacks. Arch Intern Med 163:525, 2003.)*

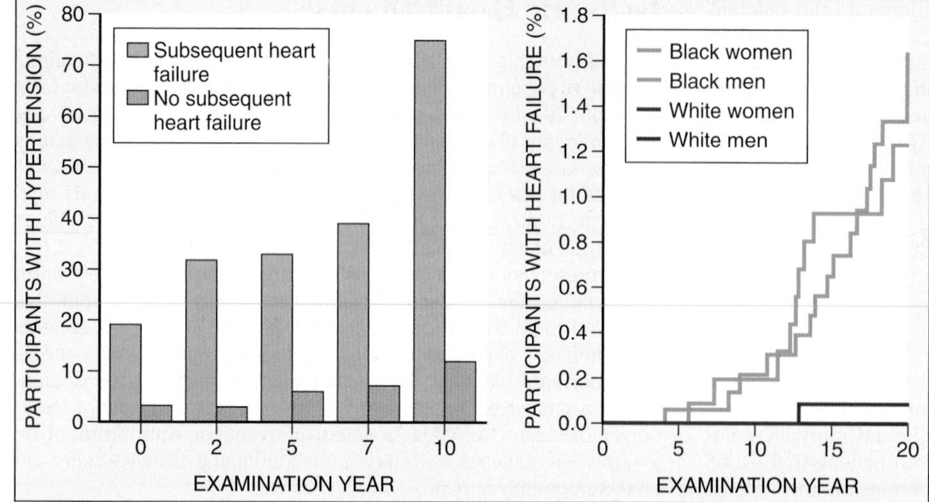

FIGURE 2-4 In the CARDIA study, note the striking association of hypertension identified as a young adult with the subsequent development of heart failure, and the significant variance in risk for the eventual development of heart failure in blacks versus whites. *(From Bibbins-Domingo K, Pletcher MJ, Lin F, et al: Racial differences in incident heart failure among young adults. N Engl J Med 360:1179, 2009.)*

The rationale for the excess prevalence of CAD in blacks less likely relates to pathophysiologic variances, as suggested in the discussion on hypertension, and more likely relates to the overabundance of cardiovascular risk factors. Obesity, LV hypertrophy, type 2 diabetes, and physical inactivity are all more common in blacks. However, total cholesterol levels may be lower in blacks and HDL levels may be higher, whereas Lp(a) levels are higher, as noted previously. Thus the relationship among total cholesterol, plaque formation, and coronary events may be weaker in blacks.[47]

The excess prevalence of LV hypertrophy likely confounds the ischemic burden in the setting of CAD, and may be related to excess mortality and sudden death (see Chap. 41). Mechanisms to support this theory remain unclear. The increase in LV mass with a disproportionately less robust vascular supply may lead to a lower threshold for arrhythmias and more damage caused by ischemic events. The potent vasoconstrictor endothelin-1 is present in higher levels in blacks. TGF-β1, which is higher in hypertensive blacks, stimulates endothelin. The confluence of left LV hypertrophy and endothelial dysfunction may contribute to a greater risk of ischemia-related injury.

No differences in the presentation of acute coronary syndromes have been described for any ethnic group, nor have any variations in responses to standard medical and revascularization strategies. As such, no differences should be contemplated in the management of varied populations presenting with symptomatic CAD.

Heart Failure

Heart failure occurs in blacks at an increased frequency, perhaps 50% higher overall, and more than 100% higher in black women compared with white women. There are several striking differences in the natural history—the disease occurs at an earlier age, there is usually more profound LV systolic dysfunction at the time of onset, and the clinical class is usually of more advanced severity.[48,49] The overall incidence of heart failure in the U.S. population is 2%, but 3% in the black population. See also Part 4 of this text, Heart Failure.

Recent data from the CARDIA investigations[50] have highlighted the magnitude of the dissimilarity between blacks and whites in the onset of heart failure. Young black adults are much more likely to be hypertensive, with a baseline incidence rate of almost 33%; more than 60% of those affected are either untreated or not treated to goal BP reductions. Even after enrollment in the CARDIA study for 10 years, the number untreated or not treated to goal remained at almost 50%, a prominent portrayal of disparate care. In this group of at-risk individuals, the subsequent development of heart failure at an early age is almost 20-fold greater than in whites (**Fig. 2-4**).[50] These findings generate a compelling public health message, and suggest the need for early detection and treatment to goal BP in young black adults as a strategy to prevent heart failure.

Not surprisingly, the leading putative cause of LV dysfunction in blacks with heart failure is hypertension. A survey of published clinical trials and registries has suggested that the incidence of hypertension as the likely cause of heart failure in this population varies from approximately 30% to almost 60% (**Fig. 2-5**). True cause and effect is lacking, because little mechanistic data support the conversion from hypertensive heart disease to systolic dysfunction. Data from spontaneously hypertensive salt-sensitive animals suggest that the conversion from left LV hypertrophy to overt heart failure (with systolic dysfunction) is associated with an increase in the progenitors of endothelin. Recent provocative theories have suggested that nitric oxide

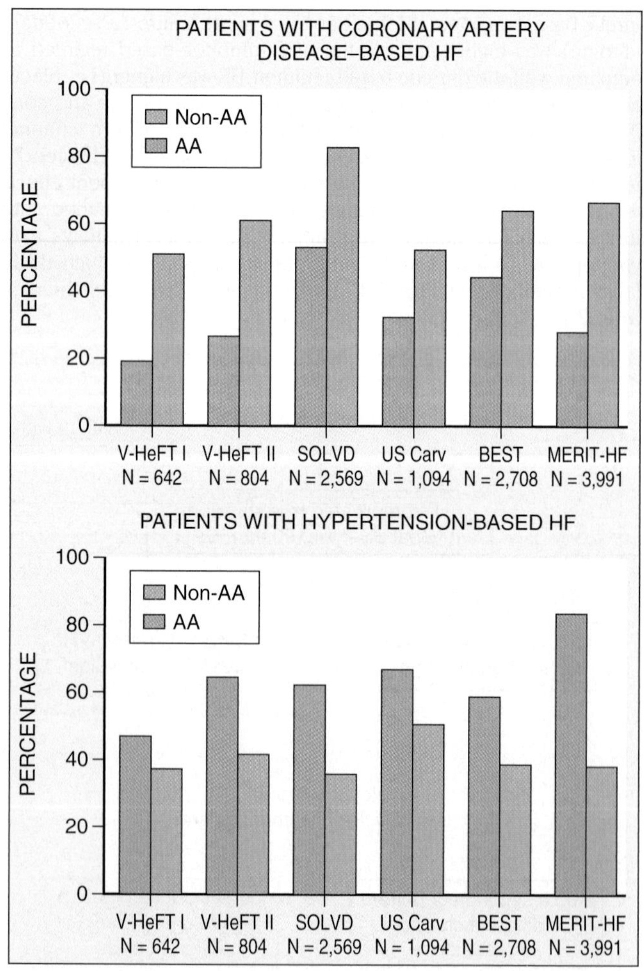

FIGURE 2-5 Multiple heart failure (HF) trials have identified a greater association of nonischemic causes for left ventricular dysfunction than ischemic causes in blacks versus whites.[1-6] AA = African American. *(Adapted from the BEST Investigators: N Engl J Med 344:1659, 2001; Packer M et al: N Engl J Med 334:1349, 1996; MERIT-HF Studay Group: Lancet 353:2001, 1999; Cohn JN et al: N Engl J Med 314:1547, 1986; Cohn JN et al: N Engl J Med 325:303, 1991; The SOLVD Investigators: N Engl J Med 325:293, 1991.)*

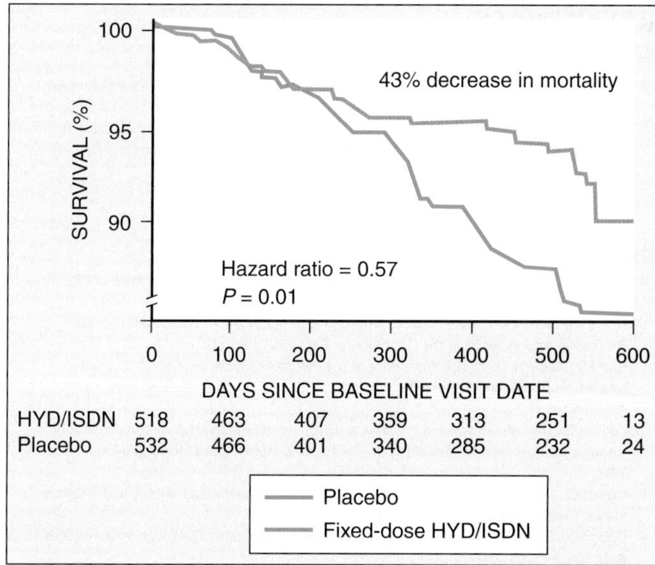

FIGURE 2-6 Primary results from the African American Heart Failure Trial, demonstrating a .40% survival advantage for blacks on isosorbide dinitrate (ISDN)–hydralazine (HYD) plus standard medical therapy, compared with placebo plus standard medical therapy. *(From Taylor AL, Zeische S, Yancy CW, et al: Combination of isosorbide dinitrate and hydralazine in blacks with heart failure. N Engl J Med 351:2049, 2004.)*

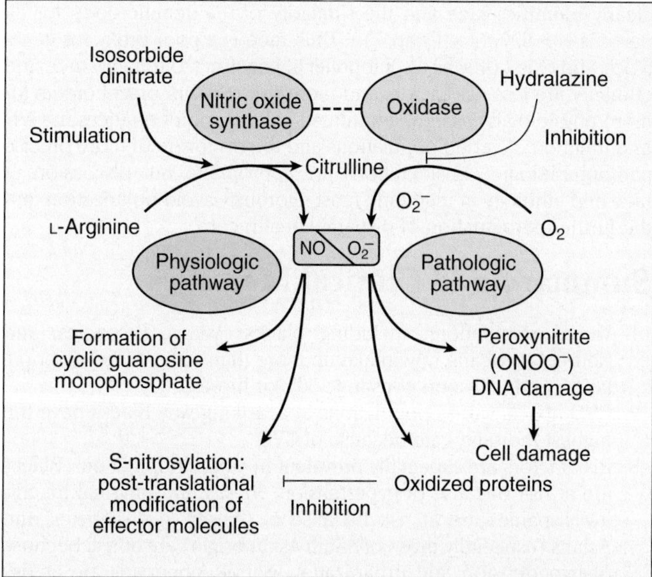

FIGURE 2-7 Nitroso-redox balance in heart failure. Exhaustion of nitric oxide synthetic capability results in excessive super oxide and reactive oxygen species production, which disrupts DNA and predisposes to vasoconstriction. Exogenous administration of nitrates plus hydralazine restores nitroso-redox balance and improves vascular homeostasis (see also Fig. 25-8). *(Adapted from Hare JM: Nitroso-redox balance in the cardiovascular system. N Engl J Med 351:2112, 2004.)*

deficiency, as seen in blacks, leads to increased calcineurin-mediated LV hypertrophy and to increased apoptotic activity mediated by *bax* and *bak*.[51] This combination of a growth stimulus and an apoptotic environment represents plausible, if not yet proven, mechanisms of LV dysfunction in the setting of hypertension alone.

The current evidence-based guideline recommendations remain the best approach to care for all those with heart failure.[52] In the 2005 American College of Cardiology (ACC)/American Heart Association (AHA) Diagnosis and Management of Chronic Heart Failure in the Adult guidelines (and in the 2009 focused update), a class I recommendation is given to the following statement: "Groups of patients including (a) high-risk ethnic minority groups (e.g., blacks), (b) groups under-represented in clinical trials, and (c) any groups believed to be underserved should, in the absence of specific evidence to direct otherwise, have clinical screening and therapy in a manner identical to that applied to the broader population (level of evidence: B)." Taken in aggregate, the data demonstrate that all approved therapeutic strategies for heart failure are effective, yield improved outcomes, and should be used in all patients.

The African American Heart Failure Trial, A-HeFT, extended the treatment options for blacks with heart failure to include combined vasodilator therapy with isosorbide dinitrate and hydralazine (**Fig. 2-6**).[53] The ACC/AHA and Heart Failure Society of America guideline statements strongly recommend the adjunctive use of combined vasodilator therapy in addition to ACE inhibitors, ARBs, and beta blockers for blacks with symptomatic heart failure (see Chap. 28).[54] The imputed but unproven mechanism of benefit targets nitric oxide deficiency and increased oxidative stress, which occur in blacks but are not unique to them (**Fig. 2-7**).[55] A prospective substudy in A-HeFT has addressed the genetic profiles of the patients and their responsiveness to combined vasodilator therapy. Preliminary data outputs implicate potentially important variances in nitric oxide synthase and aldosterone synthase.[56,57] Several other candidate polymorphisms may predict heart failure in blacks, but the usefulness of these observations must await additional prospectively acquired data from larger population cohorts (**Table 2-2**).

Confirmation of these results may allow for application of the benefits of combined vasodilator therapy to all suitable candidates, irrespective of race, and may lead to the early clinical application of pharmacogenomics, or "personalized medicine."

TABLE 2-2 Putative Genetic Markers of Cardiovascular Risk in African Americans

GENETIC POLYMORPHISM	CLINICAL IMPLICATIONS
Beta$_1$-adrenergic receptor; Gly389	Subsensitive beta$_1$ receptor; decreased affinity for agonist, less cAMP generation
Beta$_1$-adrenergic receptor; ARG389–alpha 2C Del322-325 receptor	Presence of both polymorphisms associated with increased risk for heart failure in blacks; relative risk = 10.11 when both are present
NOS 3 Glu298Glu	Subsensitive nitric oxide system; better responsiveness to ISDN/HYD
Aldosterone synthase (CYP11B2 344 TT allele)	? Excessive fibrosis; better responsiveness to ISDN/HYD
TGF-β1, codon 25	40% higher TGF-β1 levels; higher endothelin levels; more fibrosis
G protein 825-T allele	Marker of low-renin hypertension, LV hypertrophy, and stroke

cAMP = cyclic adenosine monophosphate; ISDN/HYD = isosorbide dinitrate–hydralazine.
Adapted from McNamara DM, Tam SW, Sabolinski ML, et al: Endothelial nitric oxide synthase NOS3. polymorphisms in African Americans with heart failure: Results from the A-HeFT trial. J Card Fail 15:191, 2009; and McNamara DM, Tam SW, Sabolinski ML, et al: Aldosterone synthase promoter polymorphism predicts outcome in African Americans with heart failure: Results from the A-HeFT Trial. J Am Coll Cardiol 48:1277, 2006.

Construct of Race and Ethnicity in Medicine

The inclusion of race or ethnicity in any discussion of medicine is problematic. Ethnicity can be defined, for example, as being of Hispanic descent or not. But within those of Hispanic descent, multiple populations exist, and not all observations for one Hispanic group can be extrapolated to all Hispanics. Race is best defined according to geographic origins—for which there are those of African, Asian, European, and Native American descent—but admixture is high, and race is neither scientific nor physiologic. Some have argued that continental ancestry obviates traditional racial designations. Furthermore, the Human Genome Project has failed to identify any genotype that clearly identifies race and the similarity of the genetic code for all persons is > 99% (see Chap. 7).[58] Thus, race is a poor proxy for genotypes, and exists only as a sociopolitical construct. Ultimately, race and ethnicity are less risk factors and more risk markers, placeholders for more physiologic risks. The continued elucidation of nuances in CVD as a function of varied populations and the discovery of more precise pathophysiologic considerations are appropriate, but discussion of race and ethnicity in medicine must rigorously avoid polarization and the further perpetuation of disparate health care.

Summary and Clinical Messages

1. Varied populations, including blacks, Asians, Hispanics, and Native Americans, now make up more than 30% of the U.S. population, and will soon constitute 50% or more.
2. CVD affects varied populations in a striking way. Blacks have the highest mortality rate because of CVD.
3. Risk factors are especially prevalent in varied populations. Blacks are at risk because of hypertension, obesity, and physical inactivity, Hispanics are at risk because of obesity and diabetes, and Asians (especially those of South Asian origin) are at risk because of hypertension and urbanization. Native Americans are at risk because of diabetes.
4. Disparate outcomes in CVD occur in varied populations because of discrepancies in access to care, insurance deficits, and persistent bias in health care decision making.
5. The treatment of hypertension is effective for all individuals. Decisions regarding therapy should be evidence-based and guideline-driven. Compelling other indications for aggressive therapy, such as renal insufficiency, post-MI, and heart failure, supersede considerations of race per se.
6. Blacks with hypertension have especially high risk for complications because of hypertension—especially renal disease, stroke, and heart failure—and merit aggressive treatment, including lower goal BP reductions and earlier use of combination agents or multidrug regimens.
7. Ischemic heart disease occurs at a lower frequency in Hispanics as compared with whites, at a similar frequency for Asians as compared with whites, and at a higher frequency in blacks as compared with whites, although epicardial obstructive CAD occurs less frequently. Hypertension and left ventricular hypertrophy are the leading risk factors in blacks, whereas dyslipidemia may be more of an issue in whites. Thrombolytic therapy, percutaneous coronary interventions, and CABG are carried out less frequently in blacks, especially black women, thus contributing to disparate outcomes.
8. Heart failure is notably different in blacks. The disease occurs at an earlier age, with more advanced LV dysfunction and worse clinical class severity. The incidence of heart failure is higher and morbidity is much worse in blacks; the mortality risk may be similar overall, but higher in younger patients. All patients respond similarly to neurohormonal antagonists for heart failure, and current established treatment guidelines should be followed. Combined vasodilator therapy, isosorbide dinitrate and hydralazine, is especially effective for certain patients with heart failure who are currently described as black, but likely are better characterized by pharmacogenomic and other more physiologic biomarkers.
9. A genomic basis for the differential expression of CVD in varied populations may exist, thus supplanting part of this discussion regarding race and ethnicity in medicine. The exact contribution of certain candidate single-nucleotide polymorphisms to the clinical expression of CVD remains unclear, and requires more investigation, but personalized medicine based on pharmacogenomics and pharmacokinetics is anticipated.
10. Race or ethnicity should be used with caution in medicine. Heterogeneity within races is greater than heterogeneity among races, and biologic certainty regarding race-based decisions cannot be ensured. Clinical decisions should be made on an individual basis.

REFERENCES

General

1. U.S. Census Bureau: U.S. Census Bureau News. U.S. Department of Commerce (http://www.census.gov).
2. Ostchega Y, Dillon CF, Hughes JP, et al: Trends in hypertension prevalence, awareness, treatment, and control in older U.S. adults: Data from the National Health and Nutrition Examination Survey 1988 to 2004. J Am Geriatr Soc 55:1056, 2007.
3. Mensah GA, Mokdad AH, Ford ES, et al: State of disparities in cardiovascular health in the United States. Circulation 111:1233, 2005.

Hypertension

4. Ford ES, Li C, Sattar N: Metabolic syndrome and incident diabetes: Current state of the evidence. Diabetes Care 31:1898, 2008.
5. Ford ES: Prevalence of the metabolic syndrome defined by the International Diabetes Federation among adults in the U.S. Diabetes Care 28:2745, 2005.
6. Ford ES, Giles WH, Dietz WH: Prevalence of the metabolic syndrome among US adults: Findings from the third National Health and Nutrition Examination Survey. JAMA 287: 356, 2002.
7. Centers for Disease Control and Prevention (CDC): Hypertension-related mortality among Hispanic subpopulations—United States, 1995-2002. MMWR Morb Mortal Wkly Rep 55:177, 2006.
8. Ogden CL, Carroll MD, Curtin LR, et al: Prevalence of overweight and obesity in the United States, 1999-2004. JAMA 295:1549, 2006.
9. Ogden CL: Disparities in obesity prevalence in the United States: Black women at risk. Am J Clin Nutr April;89:1001, 2009.
10. Ogden CL, Carroll MD, Curtin LR, et al: Prevalence of overweight and obesity in the United States, 1999-2004. JAMA 295:1549, 2006.
11. Bassett DR Jr, Fitzhugh EC, Crespo CJ, et al: Physical activity and ethnic differences in hypertension prevalence in the United States. Prev Med 34:179, 2002.
12. Flack JM, Ferdinand KC, Nasser SA: Epidemiology of hypertension and cardiovascular disease in African Americans. J Clin Hypertens Greenwich 51(Suppl 1):5, 2003.
13. Clark LT, Shaheen S: Dyslipidemia in racial/ethnic groups. *In* Ferdinand KC, Armani A (eds): Cardiovascular Disease in Racial and Ethnic Minorities (Contemporary Cardiology). New York, Humana, 2009, pp 119-138.
14. Food and Nutrition Board, Institute of Medicine, National Academies: Dietary reference intakes (DRIs): Recommended intakes for individuals. (http://iom.edu/en/Global/News%20Announcements/~/media/Files/Activity%20Files/Nutrition/DRIs/DRISummaryListing2.ashx).
15. Bray GA, Vollmer WM, Sacks FM, et al: A further subgroup analysis of the effects of the DASH diet and three dietary sodium levels on blood pressure: Results of the DASH-Sodium Trial. Am J Cardiol 94:222, 2004.
16. Zittermann A, Schleithoff SS, Tenderich G, et al: Low vitamin D status: A contributing factor in the pathogenesis of congestive heart failure? J Am Coll Cardiol 41:105, 2003.
17. Giovannucci E, Liu Y, Hollis BW, Rimm EB: 25-hydroxyvitamin D and risk of myocardial infarction in men: A prospective study. Arch Intern Med 168:1174, 2008.
18. Scragg R, Sowers M, Bell C: Serum 25-hydroxyvitamin D, ethnicity, and blood pressure in the Third National Health and Nutrition Examination Survey. Am J Hypertens 20:713, 2007.
19. Drazner MH, Dries DL, Peshock RM, et al: Left ventricular hypertrophy is more prevalent in blacks than whites in the general population: The Dallas Heart Study. Hypertension 46:124, 2005.
20. Lutsey PL, Cushman M, Steffen LM, et al: Plasma hemostatic factors and endothelial markers in four racial/ethnic groups: The MESA study. J Thromb Haemost 412:2629, 2006.
21. Hassan MI, Aschner Y, Manning CH, et al: Racial differences in selected cytokine allelic and genotypic frequencies among healthy, pregnant women in North Carolina. Cytokine 21:10, 2003.
22. Nasir K, Shaw LJ, Liu ST, et al: Ethnic differences in the prognostic value of coronary artery calcification for all-cause mortality. J Am Coll Cardiol 50:953, 2007.
23. Lloyd-Jones D, Adams RJ, Brown TM, et al: Heart Disease and Stroke Statistics—2010 Update. A Report from the American Heart Association (http://www.circ.ahajournals.org/cgi/content/abstract/CIRCULATIONAHA.109.192667v1).
24. Smedley BD, Stith AY, Nelson AR (eds): Unequal Treatment: Confronting Racial and Ethnic Disparities in Health Care. Washington, DC, National Academies Press, 2003.
25. Greene JD, Hamilton P, Hutchinson S, Huber J: The effect of patients' race on provider treatment choices in coronary care: A literature review for model development. Policy Polit Nurs Pract 10:40, 2009.
26. Venkat A, Hoekstra J, Lindsell C, et al: The impact of race on the acute management of chest pain. Acad Emerg Med 10:1199, 2003.
27. Reddy KS, Naik N, Prabhakaran D: Hypertension in the developing world: A consequence of progress. Curr Cardiol Rep 8:399, 2006.
28. Deedwania PC, Davidson MH, Ballantyne CM: Treating dyslipidemia in high-risk patients: Case reviews and discussion. Postgrad Med 116(Suppl):21, 2004.
29. Centers for Disease Control and Prevention (CDC): National Health and Nutrition Examination Survey NHANES 1999-2004 (http://www.cdc.gov/nchs/about/major/nhanes/nhanes99-02.htm. 10-11-2004. 10-5-2004).
30. Ruilope LM, Izzo JL: Renal risk. *In* Izzo JL, Sica D, Black H (eds): Hypertension Primer: The Essentials of High Blood Pressure: Basic Science, Population Science, and Clinical Management. 4th ed. Dallas, American Heart Association, 2008, pp 139-150.
31. Rosamond W, Flegal K, Friday G, et al: Heart disease and stroke statistics—2007 update. A report from the American Heart Association Committee and Stroke Statistics Subcommittee. Circulation 115:e69, 2007.
32. Peterson GE, de Backer T, Gabriel A, et al: Prevalence and correlates of left ventricular hypertrophy in the African American Study of Kidney Disease Cohort Study. Hypertension 50:1033, 2007.
33. Grim CE, Robinson M: Salt, slavery and survival—hypertension in the African diaspora. Epidemiology 14:120, 2003.
34. Cappuccio FP, Kerry SM, Adeyemo A, et al: Body size and blood pressure: An analysis of Africans and the African diaspora. Epidemiology 19:38, 2008.

35. Scisney-Matlock M, Bosworth HB, Giger JN, et al: Strategies for implementing and sustaining therapeutic lifestyle changes as part of hypertension management in African Americans. Postgrad Med 121:147, 2009.
36. Baker EH, Ireson NJ, Carney C, et al: Transepithelial sodium absorption is increased in people of African origin. Hypertension 38:76, 2001.
37. August P, Sharma V, Ding R, et al: Transforming growth factor beta and excess burden of renal disease. Trans Am Clin Climatol Assoc 120:61, 2009.
38. Suthanthiran M, Gerber LM, Schwartz JE, et al: Circulating transforming growth factor-beta1 levels and the risk for kidney disease in African Americans. Kidney Int 76:72, 2009..
39. Nesbitt S, Victor RG: Pathogenesis of hypertension in African Americans. Congest Heart Fail 10:24, 2004.
40. Mancia G, Grassi G: Joint National Committee VII and European Society of Hypertension/ European Society of Cardiology guidelines for evaluating and treating hypertension: A two-way road? J Am Soc Nephrol 16(Suppl 1):S74, 2005.
41. Britov AN, Bystrova MM: New guidelines of the Joint National Committee (USA) on Prevention, Diagnosis and Management of Hypertension. From JNC VI to JNC VII. Kardiologiia 43:93, 2003.
42. Onuigbo MA: RAAS blockade, renal failure, ESRD, and death among African Americans in the AASK Posttrial Cohort Study. Arch Intern Med 168:2383, 2008.
43. Norris K, Bourgoigne J, Gassman J, et al: Cardiovascular outcomes in the African American Study of Kidney Disease and Hypertension AASK. Trial. Am J Kidney Dis 48:739, 2006.
44. Wright JT Jr, Probstfield JL, Cushman WC, et al: ALLHAT findings revisited in the context of subsequent analyses, other trials, and meta-analyses. Arch Intern Med 169:832, 2009.
45. Wright JT Jr, Dunn JK, Cutler JA, et al: Outcomes in hypertensive black and nonblack patients treated with chlorthalidone, amlodipine, and lisinopril. JAMA 293:1595, 2005.
46. Douglas JG, Bakris GL, Epstein M, et al: Management of high blood pressure in African Americans: Consensus statement of the Hypertension in African Americans Working Group of the International Society on Hypertension in Blacks. Arch Intern Med 163:525, 2003.
47. Watson KE: Novel and emerging risk factors in racial/ethnic groups. *In* Ferdinand KC, Armani A (eds): Cardiovascular Disease in Racial and Ethnic Minorities (Contemporary Cardiology). New York, Humana, 2009.

Heart Failure

48. Ishizawar D, Yancy C: Racial differences in heart failure therapeutics. Heart Fail Clin 6:65, 2010.
49. Yancy CW: Heart failure in African Americans. Am J Cardiol 96:3i, 2005.
50. Bibbins-Domingo K, Pletcher MJ, Lin F, et al: Racial differences in incident heart failure among young adults. N Engl J Med 360:1179, 2009.
51. Woolert KC, Drexler H: Regulation of cardiac remodeling by nitric oxide: Focus on cardiac myocyte hypertrophy and apoptosis. *In* Jugdutt BI (ed): The Role of Nitric Oxide in Heart Failure. New York, Kluwer, 2004, pp 71-80.
52. Hunt SA, Abraham WT, Chin MH, et al: 2009 focused update incorporated into the ACC/AHA 2005 Guidelines for the Diagnosis and Management of Heart Failure in Adults: A report of the American College of Cardiology Foundation/American Heart Association Task Force on Practice Guidelines: Developed in collaboration with the International Society for Heart and Lung Transplantation. Circulation 119:e391, 2009.
53. Taylor AL, Ziesche S, Yancy CW, et al: Early and sustained benefit on event-free survival and heart failure hospitalization from fixed-dose combination of isosorbide dinitrate/hydralazine: Consistency across subgroups in the African-American Heart Failure Trial. Circulation 115:1747, 2007.
54. Heart Failure Society of America: HFSA 2006 Comprehensive Heart Failure Practice Guideline. J Card Fail 12:e1, 2006.
55. Hare JM: Nitroso-redox balance in the cardiovascular system. N Engl J Med 351:2112, 2004.
56. McNamara DM, Tam SW, Sabolinski ML, et al: Endothelial nitric oxide synthase (NOS3) polymorphisms in African Americans with heart failure: results from the A-HeFT trial. J Card Fail 15:191, 2009.
57. McNamara DM, Tam SW, Sabolinski ML, et al: Aldosterone synthase promoter polymorphism predicts outcome in African Americans with heart failure: results from the A-HeFT Trial. J Am Coll Cardiol 48:1277, 2006.
58. Serre D, Paabo S: Evidence for gradients of human genetic diversity within and among continents. Genome Res 14:1679, 2004.

CHAPTER 3 Ethics in Cardiovascular Medicine

Paul S. Mueller

Clinical ethics "provides a structured approach for identifying, analyzing, and resolving" moral problems and ethical dilemmas that arise while caring for patients.[1] Four ethics principles address most of these problems—beneficence, nonmaleficence, respect for patient autonomy, and justice.[2] Beneficence refers to the clinician's duty to promote the best interests of patients. Nonmaleficence refers to the duty to prevent or avoid doing harm to patients. Respect for patient autonomy refers to the duty to respect patients' values, goals, and rights of self-determination. Justice refers to the duty to treat patients fairly (i.e., based on medical need, not on patient characteristics such as ethnicity and gender). When caring for a patient, these principles can be at odds with each other. For example, a cardiologist's desire to promote good (e.g., prescribing a statin drug to a patient with coronary artery disease) may be at odds with a patient's autonomy (e.g., declining a statin drug to avoid side effects).

Because of the growing prevalence of patients living with heart disease, the increasingly complex nature of treatments for heart disease (e.g., devices), and the fact that heart disease remains a major cause of death, it is reasonable to expect that clinicians will care for patients who have heart disease as well as challenging medical and psychosocial problems that precipitate ethical dilemmas. Therefore, clinicians should be familiar with common clinical ethical dilemmas. In this chapter, these dilemmas and how to address them are reviewed.

Common Ethical Dilemmas in Cardiovascular Medicine

Promoting Beneficence

Beneficence requires that clinicians promote the interests of patients, which take precedence over the clinicians' self-interests. Beneficent clinicians maintain clinical competence and strive for quality, safety, and continuous improvement in clinical practice. Beneficence requires that clinicians completely and clearly share their assessments and recommendations with patients and ensure that patients understand them. Recommendations should not be presented as a menu of choices, but as a hierarchy of options based on efficacy, safety, and patients' health care–related values, preferences and goals.

Consider the case of an 84-year-old man with coronary artery disease (CAD) and metastatic prostate cancer admitted to the hospital for congestive heart failure (CHF). Echocardiography reveals markedly reduced left ventricular systolic function; he meets the criteria for an implantable cardioverter-defibrillator (ICD) for primary prevention. Although the patient has an indication for ICD implantation, he also has significant comorbid disease. In this situation, the beneficent clinician avoids making a paternalistic treatment decision and pressuring the patient to comply with the recommendation. Instead, the clinician should describe the benefits and risks of ICD implantation and therapy. If ICD implantation and therapy are expected to benefit the patient (e.g., longevity) and are consistent with the patient's values, preferences, and goals, the clinician should proceed with device implantation. If, on the other hand, ICD implantation and therapy are not expected to benefit the patient, or are inconsistent with the patient's values, preferences, and goals (e.g., avoidance of invasive procedures), they should be avoided. Notably, if the patient declines ICD implantation and therapy, he should be offered treatments that minimize symptoms and promote quality of life. Referral to a palliative medicine specialist should also be considered, especially in light of his heart disease and cancer (see Chap. 34).

Preventing and Avoiding Harm to Patients

The ethics principle of nonmaleficence is closely coupled with the principle of beneficence. Weighing the potential benefits versus the potential harms of a diagnostic or therapeutic intervention is common in clinical practice. Needless to say, clinicians should prevent or minimize harms associated with any intervention.

Most clinicians are familiar with U.S. Food and Drug Administration (FDA) black box warnings and recalls of drugs. A scenario unique to cardiology practice, however, is the implantable cardiac device advisory, also known as a recall or safety alert. The motivation for advisories is nonmaleficence. Clinicians typically learn about advisories via a letter from the device manufacturer. Many patients, however, learn about advisories from the media. Nevertheless, clinicians are responsible for addressing advisories with patients. Patients with devices that have an advisory alert might experience several harms such as device malfunction (i.e., inappropriate therapy or failure to deliver therapy), harms associated with device replacement, and psychological harm (e.g., anxiety) because of the advisory itself. Recent advisories have cited device failure risks of about 3% or less. However, the risk of complications associated with replacing an advisory device (e.g., pocket infection and death) is not trivial, up to 8%.[3] Therefore, clinicians should not categorically recommend advisory device replacement because such an approach would cause unnecessary harm.

When discussing device advisories with a patient, the clinician should explain the reasons for the advisory in clear language (checking frequently for patient understanding) and determine the patient's concerns. The clinician should base his or her recommendations on the patient's clinical status, indications for device therapy, nature of the advisory, and published guidelines.[4]

Nonmaleficence also requires that clinicians not abandon patients.[5] Consider the scenario of a multidisciplinary health care team frustrated by a 62-year-old woman with alcoholic cardiomyopathy who is frequently admitted to the hospital for volume overload because of dietary indiscretion and medication nonadherence. Despite the patient's behavior, the team is obligated to care for the patient. Furthermore, the team should attempt to discern the reasons for the patient's behavior (e.g., low literacy, lack of access to nutritious low-sodium food) and address the reasons, if possible (e.g., by scheduling a visiting nurse). Social workers and chaplains can be very helpful in these situations. The team should not summarily dismiss the patient from its care unless a suitable alternative care team is identified and the patient and alternative team agree to the transfer of care.

Finally, conflicts of interests should not compromise clinicians' nonmaleficence duties.[5] For example, a clinician's relationships with industry should not interfere with his or her clinical decision making (e.g., the clinician should choose diagnostic or therapeutic interventions based on clinical safety, benefits, and costs to the patient, not based on his or her relationships with industry). Such relationships should be fully disclosed to patients and others when appropriate.

Ensuring Informed Consent and Informed Refusal

Informed consent derives from the principle of respect for patient autonomy. For patients to be autonomous, they must be informed about their illness and diagnostic and treatment options. Therefore, clinicians have an ethical duty to inform patients about their illness and diagnostic and treatment options.

Clinicians also have a legal duty. The term *informed consent* was first used in the 1957 court case *Salgo v Stanford University*. In this case, the patient, who developed paralysis after an invasive procedure, claimed that he was not sufficiently informed of the risks associated with the procedure. The court agreed, concluding that a clinician breaches his or her duty to the patient if the clinician withholds information necessary for the patient to make an informed decision. The 1972 court case *Canterbury v Spence* established the "reasonable patient" standard—that is, clinicians should provide the information that a reasonable patient would need to know in order to make an informed decision.[6] This standard is widely used today.

The elements of informed consent include information (e.g., diagnosis, proposed intervention, risks, benefits of and alternatives to the proposed intervention), patient decision-making capacity, and patient voluntariness. A signed consent form should not be equated with informed consent. Instead, clinicians should engage patients in a meaningful conversation about their diagnoses and treatment options and these conversations should be documented. Although informed consent should be obtained for most interventions, under certain circumstances consent is presumed (e.g., emergencies) or must be obtained from a surrogate decision maker (e.g., the patient is a child or the patient lacks decision-making capacity).[6]

Many patients with decision-making capacity refuse medical interventions, including recommendations for diagnostic testing, lifestyle changes, drugs, devices, and therapeutic procedures. Clinicians should respect these decisions.[5] Although some clinicians may regard such refusals as wrong, these refusals are not necessarily irrational. Consider the case of an 82-year-old woman with symptomatic aortic stenosis who refuses aortic valve replacement (AVR). Here, the clinician should determine whether the patient is adequately informed about the risks and benefits of AVR and the risks and benefits of refusing AVR (informed refusal). If the patient is fully informed and remains steadfast in her refusal, the clinician should respect the patient's decision, not abandon her, and formulate an alternative plan of care. Adequate documentation of the patient's informed refusal of AVR in her medical record is essential.

Handling Medical Errors

Unfortunately, errors (unintended acts or omissions that harm or have the potential to harm patients) occur. Consider the case of a 59-year-old man who presents with angina, undergoes coronary angiography, and experiences anaphylaxis. The medical record documents an allergy to contrast dye. Not surprisingly, the cardiologist caring for the patient may experience negative emotions when he or she realizes that an error has been made. Nevertheless, he or she is ethically obligated to disclose the error to the patient.[5]

The ethical rationale for disclosing errors to patients is strong. First, clinicians should act in the best interests of the patient. Nondisclosure does not serve the patient and damages trust because many patients eventually learn of errors. Instead, clinicians should disclose errors and their clinical implications to patients. Patients who have experienced errors should not be abandoned. Second, respect for patient autonomy requires that clinicians disclose errors to patients to allow for informed decision-making. In the case example, the patient has the right to know about the error so that he can act on it according to his health care–related values, preferences, and goals. Third, justice requires that patients be given what is due to them, including information about their medical condition and compensation if appropriate (e.g., for injury). Finally, clinicians should participate in efforts to prevent errors.

Most patients want to know about errors, even minor ones. Also, there are benefits to disclosing errors. For patients, disclosing errors informs them, resolves uncertainty, and promotes trust. For clinicians, disclosing errors may reduce stress, foster patient forgiveness, promote trust, and reduce litigation. Nevertheless, clinicians may feel uncomfortable disclosing errors to patients. The following steps can lessen this burden[7]:

1. Disclosure should be done in private; the patient's loved ones and essential members of the health care team should be present. Interruptions should be avoided.
2. Before disclosing the error, the clinician should discern the patient's perception of the problem. For example, the cardiologist in the case example might ask, "Do you know why you got so ill after the angiogram?" Such questions allow for correction of misinformation.
3. When disclosing the error, the clinician should speak clearly and check for comprehension (e.g., "May I clarify anything?").
4. After disclosing the error, the clinician should sincerely apologize and inform the patient that the clinician and organization will act to prevent future errors. The clinician should avoid attributing blame to others (e.g., "The nurse must have forgotten to tell me about your allergy.").
5. The clinician should acknowledge the patient's response to the disclosure by using empathic statements (e.g., "I can see that you are upset by this news.").
6. The clinician should describe a treatment and follow-up plan.
7. The clinician should document the discussion in writing.

Addressing Refusals of and Requests for Withdrawal of Life-Sustaining Treatments

Respect for patient autonomy is the ethics principle that underlies a patient's right to refuse or request the withdrawal of medical treatments. A patient also has the right to refuse previously consented treatments if their health care–related values, preferences, and goals have changed. Regardless of the clinician's intent, beginning or continuing a treatment that a patient has refused may be viewed from a legal standpoint as battery.[5]

Dying patients identify strengthening relationships with loved ones, addressing pain and other symptoms, and avoiding prolongation of the dying process as features of quality end-of-life care. Dying patients (or their surrogates) may refuse or request the withdrawal of life-sustaining treatments (e.g., mechanical ventilation, hemodialysis, artificially administered hydration and nutrition, device therapies) that are perceived by the patients (or surrogates) as burdensome. Withdrawal of life-sustaining treatments from dying patients who no longer want the treatment is widely practiced.[5,6]

Several U.S. court decisions have clarified patients' rights to refuse or request the withdrawal of life-sustaining treatments. In the 1976 *Quinlan* case, the New Jersey Supreme Court declared that the right to privacy includes the right to refuse unwanted medical treatments, including life-sustaining treatments.[6] In the 1990 *Cruzan* case, the U.S. Supreme Court affirmed that competent persons have the right to refuse unwanted medical treatments and that this right applies to incompetent persons through previously expressed wishes (e.g., advance directive [AD]; see later) and surrogate decision-makers. However, for situations involving patients who lack decision-making capacity and do not have ADs, the court deferred to the states on how surrogates should exercise patients' rights to refuse medical treatments.

Carrying out a patient's request to refuse or withdraw a life-sustaining treatment is not the same as physician-assisted suicide (PAS) or euthanasia. In PAS, the patient intentionally terminates his or her life using a means provided by a clinician (e.g., prescription of a potentially lethal drug). In euthanasia, the clinician intentionally terminates the patient's life. In PAS and euthanasia, a new pathology is introduced (e.g., drug), the intent of which is the patient's death. In contrast, when a patient dies after a treatment is refused or withdrawn, the cause of death is the underlying disease. The intent is avoidance of, or freedom from, treatments in which the perceived burdens outweigh the perceived benefits.[5,6] For example, consider the case of an 81-year-old man who has ischemic cardiomyopathy and an ICD and is also dying of lung cancer. The patient requests withdrawal of ICD support; he understands the implications of his request. In this situation, the patient's cardiologist should grant the patient's request. Withdrawing ICD support is painless and may prevent unwanted and uncomfortable shocks during the last days of the patient's life. When death occurs, the patient's underlying disease, not withdrawal of ICD support, is the cause of death.

Clinicians caring for patients who refuse or request the withdrawal of life-sustaining treatments should be certain the patients have decision-making capacity and are informed of the consequences of and alternatives to carrying out their request. Indeed, many patients lack decision-making capacity when decisions to withhold or withdraw life-sustaining treatments are made. Also, life-sustaining treatments are more likely to be withheld from patients who lack capacity than those who have capacity.[6] These observations emphasize the importance of proactively discussing and documenting patients' end-of-life values, preferences, and goals, and identifying a surrogate when they have decision-making capacity. Cardiologists and other clinicians who care for patients with heart disease should also engage in these discussions with patients, especially after milestone cardiac events have occurred, such as myocardial infarction, hospitalization for CHF, or implantation of a device.

At times, clinicians may conscientiously object to patients' requests to withhold or withdraw life-sustaining treatment. Nevertheless, clinicians must acknowledge patients' authority over their bodies and their right to refuse unwanted interventions. If, after careful exploration of a patient's values, preferences, and goals and the alternatives to withholding or withdrawing the treatment, the patient's decision remains unchanged, and carrying out the request violates the clinician's conscience, the clinician should transfer the patient's care to a colleague.[5]

Fostering Advance Care Planning

Respect for patient autonomy is the ethics principle that underlies advance care planning. Advance care planning is a process in which patients, working with their clinicians and loved ones, articulate their values, preferences, and goals regarding future health care decisions (e.g., life-sustaining treatments at the end of life) (see Chap. 34).

One form of advance care planning is the do not resuscitate (DNR) order. In general, cardiopulmonary resuscitation (CPR) is the default standard of care for cardiac arrest unless a DNR order has been written for the patient. A DNR order is unusual in that it requires a patient's consent to prevent a procedure (CPR) from being carried out. Notably, in a study involving more than 430,000 hospitalized older adults who underwent in-hospital CPR between 1992 and 2005, the survival to hospital dismissal was only 18%; among those hospitalized for myocardial infarction and CHF, the survival to hospital dismissal was 20%.[8]

A number of factors are associated with having a DNR order—advanced age, female gender, white race, reduced cognition, and diagnosis, especially cancer.[9] Despite similar prognoses, however, patients with coronary artery disease and severe CHF are less likely to have DNR orders than patients with lung cancer. The reasons for these observations are unclear, but may reflect perceptions among clinicians and patients that effective therapies are almost always available for CHF but not for other diseases, resulting in fewer DNR orders for patients with CHF. Also, patients with CHF and their clinicians may perceive the value of CPR and the length and quality of life after CPR differently than patients with other diseases and their clinicians.[10]

Although most patients hospitalized with severe CHF prefer to be resuscitated, many do not.[11] Few patients with CHF discuss resuscitation preferences with their clinicians.[12] Furthermore, clinicians are not always accurate in predicting the CPR preferences of patients with CHF. Nevertheless, as patients with severe CHF become more symptomatic and disabled, they are less likely to prefer being resuscitated. DNR orders tend to be written a few days before death, suggesting that the DNR order is more a marker for impending death than the result of a planned decision.[9] Nevertheless, patients who are informed about CPR (e.g., how it is done and outcomes) are more likely to forego CPR. These observations suggest that clinicians should engage patients more actively in discussions about CPR, the outcomes of CPR, and DNR orders. In fact, the Joint Commission requires that health care institutions have formal procedures for DNR orders.[13]

Advance care planning also includes completion of an advance directive. ADs are health care instructions used when a patient lacks decision-making capacity. The AD should be regarded as an extension of the autonomous patient. Common types of ADs are the health care power of attorney, in which a patient designates another person for making future health care decisions, the living will, in which a patient lists preferences about future treatments, and the combined AD, which has features of both a health care power of attorney and a living will.[14] Professional organizations such as the American Medical Association[15] and American College of Physicians[5] have endorsed wider use of ADs. Most patients and the general public also endorse the use of ADs. Finally, the Patient Self-Determination Act (PSDA) requires health care institutions that participate in Medicare and Medicaid programs to ask patients whether they have an AD, inform patients of their right to complete an AD, and incorporate patient ADs into the medical record. All 50 states and the District of Columbia have laws for complying with the PSDA.[6]

However, even though adult patients have favorable views of ADs, fewer than 25% have ADs.[14] Similarly, most cardiac care unit patients do not have ADs and do not recall discussing end-of-life care with their clinicians.[12] Regarding patients with implantable cardiac devices, few discuss management of their devices with their clinicians at the end of life (e.g., device deactivation).[16] Evidence suggests that although many patients with ICDs have ADs, few, if any, of their ADs address the device.[17] Unfortunately, some patients who have ICDs experience painful and multiple shocks during the dying process.[18,19] However, patients who have ICDs and have engaged in advance care planning are less likely to experience shocks at the end of life.

These observations suggest that clinicians who care for patients with heart disease should promote advance care planning. Given the prevalence of heart disease and the fact that heart disease is a major cause of death, cardiologists and other clinicians who care for patients with heart disease are uniquely positioned, like oncologists who care for patients with cancer, to engage these patients in advance care planning. Many patients with heart disease have experienced a milestone event, such as myocardial infarction, CHF, or implantation of a device, that might prompt them to contemplate end-of-life matters. They should be encouraged to discuss their end-of-life values, preferences, and goals with their loved ones and to complete an AD. Patients who have implantable cardiac devices should be encouraged to incorporate their preferences about end-of-life management of their devices into their AD.

Ensuring Appropriate Surrogate Decision Making

Patients who lack decision-making capacity are incapable of being autonomous. For these patients, clinicians must rely on surrogate decision-makers to make decisions for patients. If the patient's AD names a surrogate, this choice should be honored. If the patient does not have an AD, the ideal surrogate is one who best understands the patient's health care values, preferences, and goals. Many states, however, specify by law a hierarchy of surrogates (e.g., spouse, followed by adult child) in the absence of an AD.

Notably, some states do not specify a hierarchy and the surrogate is identified by the patient's loved ones, clinicians, and other interested persons.[5]

The ethical principle of respect for patient autonomy requires that a surrogate follow instructions in the patient's AD, if one exists. In the absence of an AD, a surrogate should use "substituted judgment" (i.e., base their decision on the patient's previously stated values, preferences, and goals, as closely as possible to those the patient would make if capable). To achieve substituted judgment, a useful question to ask the surrogate is, "If (your loved one) could wake up for 15 minutes and understand his or her condition fully, and then had to return to it, what would he or she tell you to do?"[20] Nevertheless, surrogates may not know the patient's health care–related values, preferences, and goals. In these situations, the surrogate should use the "best interest" standard (i.e., make a decision that is in the best interests of the patient).[6]

Addressing Requests for Interventions

Many patients (or their surrogates) make requests for specific diagnostic and therapeutic interventions. Many requests are reasonable and within standards of care; clinicians generally should grant these requests. However, clinicians are not obligated to grant requests for interventions that are ineffective or violate their consciences.[5,6]

Patients may also request interventions of questionable efficacy that support uncontroversial ends.[6,21] Consider the case of a 56-year-old man who requests screening for CAD with computed tomography. His best friend has just experienced a myocardial infarction and he has thought about screening CT ever since seeing a billboard advertisement for it. The requested intervention (CT screening for CAD) is of questionable efficacy, yet supports an uncontroversial end (e.g., patient health). Such requests reflect the gap between clinical evidence and practice. In addition, patients' health care–related values, goals, and experiences often prompt these requests. Rather than simply granting such requests, clinicians should determine the patients' values, goals, and experiences that underlie them, inform patients of the benefits and risks of the requested interventions, and formulate mutually agreed on plans with patients.

Patients may also request effective interventions that support controversial ends.[6,21] Consider the case of an 80-year-old woman who has been in the cardiac care unit for more than 1 month and is dependent on a mechanical ventilator for respiratory failure; she lacks decision-making capacity. Believing the prospects that the patient will be weaned from the ventilator and experience a meaningful recovery are slim, the clinician recommends withdrawal of mechanical ventilation and initiation of palliative care. The patient's husband, however, believes that the ventilator is doing exactly what it is intended to do—keep his wife alive. He requests that mechanical ventilation continue indefinitely and claims that his request is consistent with his wife's previously expressed wishes. Such requests reflect a gap between a patient's and clinician's values regarding a desired end. In the case example, the patient's husband requests that mechanical ventilation continue, which is effective in treating the patient's respiratory failure. On the other hand, the clinician believes that the patient will not recover and therefore regards continuing mechanical ventilation as futile.

Futility, however, is hard to define.[15] Qualitative or quantitative futility assessments are value-laden—that is, what a clinician regards as futile may be acceptable to the patient (or surrogate). When responding to requests for effective interventions that support controversial ends, the clinician should avoid summarily declaring the intervention as futile. Instead, the clinician should seek to understand the patient's health care–related values, preferences, and goals and the motive underlying the request. In general, if the requested intervention supports the patient's values, preferences, and goals, the request should be granted. If not, the clinician should clearly and empathetically explain why the intervention is not appropriate. Overall, the clinician's aim should be to formulate and implement a mutually agreed on plan with the patient. For situations in which uncertainty remains, ethics consultation can be very useful (see later). If implementation of the intervention violates the clinician's conscience, the clinician should arrange for the transfer of the patient's care to a colleague or, if necessary, another institution.[5,6]

Maintaining Patient Confidentiality

The ethics principle of respect for patient autonomy requires that clinicians maintain patient confidentiality. Clinicians need access to patients' medical information, ask sensitive questions (e.g., about sexual history), and conduct thorough physical examinations to assess and treat patients properly. Patients should trust that their personal and medical information will be kept confidential. For millennia and across diverse geographic regions, codes of ethics have declared the clinician's duty to maintain patient confidentiality.[5,15] Similarly, there are legal duties to maintain patient confidentiality.

At times, however, clinicians are ethically and legally obligated to breach patient confidentiality. For example, most jurisdictions have laws for mandatory reporting of infectious diseases. Here, the clinician's duty to protect the public's health overrides the duty to maintain patient confidentiality. Consider the case of a 28-year-old man who presents with recurrent syncope, with the last episode resulting in a car accident. Evaluation reveals recurrent polymorphic ventricular tachycardia in the setting of long-QT syndrome. His cardiologist recommends medications and ICD implantation. Preferring natural therapies to allopathic treatment, he declines. The cardiologist wonders whether the patient should be allowed to drive. Although the patient has the right to refuse recommended treatment, the patient also poses a risk to himself and others if he drives, and should be advised not to drive. If the patient refuses and therefore poses a risk to others, the clinician is justified in breaching confidentiality by reporting the patient to the relevant civil authorities. Needless to say, these situations can be difficult for clinicians. However, valuable assistance can be obtained from colleagues such as social workers and health care institution–based attorneys.

Bedside Allocation of Health Care Resources

The ethics principle of justice requires that clinicians treat patients fairly.[2] Injustice occurs when health care–related decisions are based on patient-specific factors such as gender, ethnicity, and religion, not on medical need.[5,15]

Consider the case of an 83-year-old African American woman who presents with angina. Coronary angiography reveals a 90% stenosis of the left main coronary artery and a 90% stenosis of the right coronary artery. Believing that he is being a good steward of scarce health care resources, the patient's cardiologist offers the patient medical management rather than coronary artery bypass grafting (CABG). However, the cardiologist's rationale for withholding surgery from the patient is wrong for several reasons. First, if the standard of care for the patient's coronary artery disease is CABG and relevant contraindications do not exist, the patient should be offered surgery. Second, the cardiologist may be the patient's only advocate and therefore should act to promote the patient's interests. Third, the patient may actually decline surgery and not offering surgery to her deprives the patient of the opportunity to decline it. Finally, withholding surgery from the patient falsely presumes that the cost savings will be applied to health care needs elsewhere.

Notably, in cardiology practice, evidence suggests a tendency for health care resources to be allocated according to race and gender. For example, African American and other minority patients are less likely to receive coronary angiography, coronary angioplasty, and CABG than white patients (see Chap. 1).[22] ICD implantation and therapy are less likely to be provided to women and ethnic or racial minority patients than white men.[23] The ethics principle of justice requires that clinicians avoid these allocation inequities and work to eliminate them.

Approaching Ethical Dilemmas in Clinical Practice

A useful approach to clinical ethical dilemmas begins with a careful review of the medical indications, patient preferences, quality of life, and contextual features of the case. Medical indications include identifying the patient's medical problems, treatments, and clinician's and patient's goals of treatment. Reviewing patient preferences is self-explanatory; however, it also includes identifying the appropriate surrogate if the patient lacks decision-making capacity. Quality of life includes determining the prospects of restoring the patient—with or without treatment—to normal life, deficits that the patient will experience if treatment is successful, and clinician's and patient's definitions of quality of life. Contextual features include family, religious, financial, legal, and other issues that might affect decision making. This approach does not suggest or specify a hierarchy of ethical priority. Instead, it allows for proper exposition and analysis of the ethically relevant facts (i.e., the facts related to the four ethics principles) of the case. It also usually defines the ethical problem of the case and suggests a solution.[1]

Nevertheless, cardiologists and other clinicians who care for patients with heart disease may encounter daunting ethical dilemmas that are difficult to resolve. In these situations, ethics consultation can be very helpful. In fact, the Joint Commission requires health care institutions to have processes for addressing ethical concerns that arise while caring for patients.[13] Clinicians should be familiar with these processes at their institutions.

REFERENCES

1. Jonsen AR, Siegler M, Winslade WJ: Clinical Ethics: A Practical Approach to Ethical Decisions in Clinical Medicine. 5th ed. New York, McGraw-Hill, 2002.
2. Beauchamp TL, Childress JF: Principles of Biomedical Ethics. 6th ed. New York, Oxford University Press, 2008.
3. Gould PA, Krahn AD: Complications associated with implantable cardioverter-defibrillator replacement in response to device advisories. JAMA 295:1907, 2006.
4. Carlson MD, Wilkoff BL, Maisel WL, et al: Recommendations from the Heart Rhythm Society Task Force on Device Performance Policies and Guidelines Endorsed by the American College of Cardiology Foundation (ACCF) and the American Heart Association (AHA) and the International Coalition of Pacing and Electrophysiology Organizations (COPE). Heart Rhythm 3: 1250, 2006.
5. Snyder L, Leffler C; for the Ethics and Human Rights Committee, American College of Physicians. Ethics manual: fifth edition. Ann Intern Med 142:560, 2005.
6. Mueller PS, Hook CC, Fleming KC: Ethical issues in geriatrics: a guide for clinicians. Mayo Clin Proc 79:554, 2004.
7. Murphy JG, McEvoy MT: Revealing medical errors to your patients. Chest 133:1064, 2008.
8. Ehlenbach WJ, Barnato AE, Curtis JR, et al: Epidemiologic study of in-hospital cardiopulmonary resuscitation in the elderly. New Engl J Med 361:22, 2009.
9. Loertscher LL, Reed DA, Bannon MP, Mueller PS: Cardiopulmonary resuscitation and do-not-resuscitate orders: a guide for clinicians. Am J Med 123:4, 2010.
10. Wachter RM, Luce JM, Hearst N, Lo B: Decisions about resuscitation: inequities among patients with different diseases but similar prognoses. Ann Intern Med 111:525, 1989.
11. Formiga F, Chivite D, Ortega C, et al: End-of-life preferences in elderly patients admitted for heart failure. QJM 97:803, 2004.
12. Kirkpatrick JN, Kim AY: Ethical issues in heart failure: overview of an emerging need. Perspect Biol Med 49:1, 2006.
13. The Joint Commission: Organizational Ethics Issues, 2010 (http://www.jcrinc.com/Organizational-Ethics-Statements/Ethics-Committee/Organizational-Ethics-Issues).
14. Nishimura A, Mueller PS, Evenson LK, et al: Patients who complete advance directives and what they prefer. Mayo Clin Proc 82:1480, 2007.
15. American Medical Association Council on Ethical and Judicial Affairs: Code of Medical Ethics of the American Medical Association: Current Opinions and Annotations, 2008-2009 ed. Chicago, AMA Press, 2008.
16. Goldstein NE, Mehta D, Siddiqui S, et al: "That's like an act of suicide" patients' attitudes toward deactivation of implantable defibrillators. J Gen Intern Med 23(Suppl 1):7, 2008.
17. Berger JT, Gorski M, Cohen T: Advance health planning and treatment preferences among recipients of implantable cardioverter defibrillators: an exploratory study. J Clin Ethics 17:72, 2006.
18. Goldstein NE, Lampert R, Bradley E, et al: Management of implantable cardioverter defibrillators in end-of-life care. Ann Intern Med 141:835, 2004.
19. Lewis WR, Luebke DL, Johnson NJ, et al: Withdrawing implantable defibrillator shock therapy in terminally ill patients. Am J Med 119:892, 2006.
20. Quill TE: Terri Schiavo—a tragedy compounded. N Engl J Med 352:1630, 2005.
21. Weijer C, Singer PA, Dickens BM, Workman S: Bioethics for clinicians: 16. Dealing with demands for inappropriate treatment. CMAJ 159:817, 1998.
22. Kressin NR, Petersen LA: Racial differences in the use of invasive cardiovascular procedures: review of the literature and prescription for future research. Ann Intern Med 135:352, 2001.
23. Redberg RF: Disparities in use of implantable cardioverter-defibrillators: moving beyond process measures to outcomes data. JAMA 298:1564, 2007.

CHAPTER 4 Clinical Decision Making in Cardiology

Harlan M. Krumholz

Clinical decision making is central to all patient care activities and involves making a diagnosis and selecting actions from among alternatives. Clinicians are continually faced with decisions, some that are made deliberately and others urgently. Some decisions can be made in full partnership with patients; others must be made on behalf of patients. In most cases, these decisions must be made under conditions of uncertainty. All these decisions have consequences and some will ultimately determine the likelihood that a patient will survive illness and recover without disability.

Clinical decision making is growing increasingly complex as the array of diagnostic and therapeutic options expands rapidly. The number of journals and published articles is burgeoning, challenging physicians to keep pace with advances in medical knowledge. Moreover, the relevance of systematic reviews quickly becomes dated.[1] In addition, the cost of care is escalating, which creates pressure to consider value when selecting among clinical strategies. The time available to make decisions is often brief, particularly with the shortening of the average patient visit.

The goal of this chapter is to highlight key issues in clinical decision making in cardiology. The true breadth of the science of clinical decision making is enormous, spanning the disciplines of statistics, sociology, psychology, economics, and political science, among others. Moreover, there are many issues to consider, including hypothesis generation and refinement, use and interpretation of diagnostic tests, causal reasoning, diagnostic verification, therapeutic decision making, and cognitive tools and pitfalls.[2] Despite the breadth of this topic, clinicians should be familiar with a key set of concepts that can enhance their decision-making skills and ensure that the best interest of each patient is promoted.

Diagnostic Decision Making

Making the correct diagnosis is critical to the proper care of patients. Diagnoses can classify a patient by underlying pathophysiology, prognosis, and response to therapy. Delays in diagnosis, or an incorrect diagnosis, can have marked adverse consequences for patients.

There are many conceptual models that underlie the approach of clinicians in various circumstances. Deductive inference starts with a hypothesis that can be tested. Observations and test results can be assessed for their consistency with the hypothesis. Knowledge progresses according to the acceptance, rejection, and refinement of hypotheses. Inductive inference starts with empiric observations, which leads to the development of an applicable hypothesis. Medical diagnosis is most often based on inductive inference, asking the question: "Given the patient's condition, what is the likelihood of different diseases?"

There are many types of diagnostic reasoning that clinicians use. In his classic article, Kassirer considered three major types—probabilistic, causal and deterministic.[3] The probabilistic approach relies on estimates of the likelihood of various conditions and outcomes and is usually based on clinical evidence. Causal (physiologic) reasoning is rooted in an extrapolation of an understanding of mechanism from basic science (anatomic, physiologic, biochemical). Deterministic (rule-based) reasoning is usually in the form of unambiguous rules that are followed to expedite decision making. These strategies can be complementary.

Diagnostic Testing

Practitioners use diagnostic tests to reduce uncertainty about the presence of disease, and good decision making requires a thorough understanding of the strengths and limitations of each diagnostic test. A diagnostic test can be based on information from the history, physical examination, laboratory test, or any other source. This information is used to increase or decrease the probability of a given diagnosis.

Test characteristics convey information about the performance of a test and can be expressed in terms of sensitivity, specificity, likelihood ratio, and positive and negative predictive values. For clinicians to be able to incorporate diagnostic test results into clinical decision making, they should be familiar with the following definitions.

SENSITIVITY AND SPECIFICITY (see Chaps. 14 and 17). These can be defined as follows:

- Sensitivity: Among those with disease, the proportion with a positive test (true positive)
- Specificity: Among those without disease, the proportion with a negative test (true negative)

Knowledge of these test characteristics can assist in the interpretation of results and their implications for the patient. High-sensitivity tests have low false-negative rates. A test with a high sensitivity will be positive in almost all individuals with the condition being tested. Thus, a negative test with high sensitivity makes the diagnosis highly unlikely, essentially ruling out the condition. Conversely, a test with high specificity will have a low false-positive rate. A test with a high specificity will be negative in almost all individuals without the condition being tested. Thus, a positive test with high specificity makes the diagnosis highly likely.

The test characteristics, however, are not always an intrinsic characteristic of the test. The skill with which someone performs the test will affect its sensitivity and specificity. Inexperienced or inexpert physicians or technicians may produce findings that have considerably lower sensitivity and specificity than is possible under the best conditions.

In addition, some tests will vary in sensitivity and specificity with each patient. In the case of echocardiography, the sensitivity and specificity of the test for a specific finding such as a vegetation will vary based on the patient's ability to be imaged (see Chap. 15). Echocardiography will have a lower sensitivity and specificity in individuals who cannot be imaged well compared with patients whose body habitus can yield outstanding images. In contrast, computed tomography (CT) images (see Chap. 19) tend not to vary by patient and have a more consistent sensitivity and specificity. In considering the characteristics of a test that varies by patient, it is important to take into account the circumstances of each clinical situation.

Studies that define the sensitivity and specificity of a specific test may also be flawed, and clinicians should be alert to problems with these estimates. In high-quality studies, the diagnostic test should be compared with a gold standard that is measured independently. Stable estimates of test characteristics require large study populations. The study of test characteristics may be too small to define the performance of the tests with precision. An analysis of published studies of diagnostic accuracy has found that only 5% reported a priori sample size calculations.[4]

Several types of bias may also threaten the validity of studies of diagnostic tests. Studies of tests in populations that do not resemble those seen in clinical practice (spectrum bias) may artificially inflate estimates of test performance. Partial verification bias may occur if the gold standard is applied differentially to individuals based on the results of the test evaluated in that particular study. Some studies have even used the test being evaluated as part of the definition of the reference standard (incorporation bias). These biases should be considered in assessing the quality of published estimates of sensitivity and specificity and their relevance to practice.

PREDICTIVE VALUES

- Positive predictive value (PPV): Among those with a positive test, the proportion that has the disease

$$PPV = sens \times prev/[sens \times prev + (1 - spec) \times (1 - prev)]$$

- Negative predictive value (NPV): among those with a negative test, the proportion that does not have the disease

$$NPV = spec \times (1 - prev)/[(1 - spec) \times prev + spec \times (1 - prev)]$$

Predictive values are more clinically informative than sensitivity and specificity (see Chaps. 14 and 17). This value conveys information about how the test result translates into the likelihood that the patient has the disease. The key insight about predictive values is that unlike sensitivity and specificity, they are highly dependent on disease prevalence. If the prevalence is low, a positive highly specific test will still not yield a high likelihood of disease (i.e., the test has a low positive predictive value, despite the exemplary test characteristic). The implication is that even with a test with high specificity, the screening of a low-risk population will still yield many false-positives.

EXAMPLE. A young woman comes to your office with a result of a positive exercise stress test caused by electrocardiographic changes, despite good exercise tolerance. She has no traditional risk factors for coronary artery disease, including family history, and wonders whether this is likely an indication that she has heart disease. If her risk of disease were to be 1 in 1 million and the stress test were to have a sensitivity and specificity of 75%, you could calculate that for every 4 million women in her risk group, 4 would have disease and 3 would have a positive test. Of the almost 4 million without disease, 1 million would have a positive test. Therefore, for every 1 million positive tests, only about 3 would represent a true positive. Even if the screening test had a sensitivity and specificity of 99%, then for every 10 million women screened, 10 would have disease and 9 of them would have a positive test. Of the approximately 10 million without disease, 100,000 would have a positive test. Thus, for every approximate 100,000 positive tests, only 9 would represent a true positive.

BAYES' THEOREM. Bayes' theorem relates the change in probability given new information. The posterior, or post-test, probability is a function of the prior, or pretest probability (or disease prevalence) and the likelihood ratio. This theorem provides a way to revise estimates based on new information. In essence, it relates a conditional probability, the probability of A given B. The conceptual issue is that it formalizes the incorporation of prior information into the interpretation of new information.

LIKELIHOOD RATIO

- Likelihood ratio (LR): The ratio of the probability of a certain test result in people who have the disease to the probability in people who do not have the disease

$$LR+ = sens/(1 - spec)$$

$$LR- = (1 - sens)/spec$$

The LR, which is an expression of diagnostic accuracy, can range from 0 to infinity. The post-test odds that a patient has the disease can be calculated with the LR: pretest odds × LR. An LR value of 1.0 does not modify the post-test probability, thus indicating a test that provides no useful information. If the LR is much greater than 1, it is providing substantial information. The effect of the LR on pretest probabilities is not linear. Nomograms facilitate the conversion of pretest to post-test probabilities.

The likelihood ratio may indicate whether the test is useful, but if the prevalence is low, the test may still not be a good indicator of disease. An important implication of testing patients with very low or high pretest probabilities of disease is that test results may be more likely to mislead than enlighten. False-positives and false-negatives should be expected in these situations.

DEFINING ABNORMAL. Another important issue in the use of diagnostic tests is the definition of normal. By convention, test results are often characterized in a binary fashion (normal-abnormal), which is a translation from a continuous result. Expert decision makers appreciate that thresholds are often arbitrary and have no special meaning. In some cases, thresholds are based on a Gaussian distribution of results in a nondiseased population and defines abnormal as more than 2 standard deviations from the mean. Alternatively, the threshold may be designated based on a range beyond which disease becomes more probable. In other cases, it could be that the cut point is based on information about the range in which treatment is effective. In any case, clinicians should appreciate that not all abnormal designations are equivalent and a value that barely crosses the threshold may carry different information than one that is far across the threshold. Clinicians lose information and potentially undermine decisions when they focus on tests as binary instead of continuous outcomes.

The value of a test in discriminating disease in a population is often characterized by its performance across a range of thresholds for defining disease, producing what is described as a receiver operator characteristic (ROC) curve. These curves were developed in the 1950s in studies differentiating signal to noise. The area under the ROC curve is a measure of the discrimination of a test, where an area under the ROC curve with a value of 0.5 identifies a test with no diagnostic value, and 1.0 provides perfect discrimination. These curves are not only used to determine the overall discrimination of a test across a spectrum of test values, but often to determine the optimal cutoff for what constitutes an abnormal value, balancing the best combination of sensitivity and specificity.

TEST ORDERING. Decisions about test ordering are often difficult, because too few studies have compared alternative testing strategies for patients with a given set of signs and symptoms. A test can reduce uncertainty about a diagnosis and risk, but the key question is whether patients undergoing the test have better outcomes than those who are not tested.

The construct of number needed to treat can also apply to screening tests.[5] The number needed to screen, which is defined as the number of people who need to be screened over a defined period to prevent an adverse event, takes into account the number of people tested to identify those with a specific condition that may be amenable to a specific treatment strategy. The metric can convey how many must be tested for one individual to experience a benefit.

EXAMPLE. A middle-aged man with hyperlipidemia is about to be started on statin therapy. You remember a recent article that identified a single-nucleotide polymorphism (SNP) that predicts the risk of myopathy and can identify individuals with a risk of almost 20% (see Chap. 10). Then you realize that in the published study, of more than 8000 patients taking a statin, only about 10 cases of myopathy, which were reversible, were attributable to this SNP. The benefit is very modest (a reversible adverse event) and the number screened is high, raising questions about the usefulness of using this test in practice.[6]

In deciding about whether to recommend diagnostic tests, clinicians should envision the actions that would occur based on the results. If findings would not change clinical strategies in ways likely to improve outcomes or reduce future testing, the test should probably not be ordered.[7] Ultimately, we need more evidence that addresses how particular testing strategies relate to patient outcomes.

Decisions about testing need to consider the risks of the test itself (e.g., radiation exposure or invasive instrumentation) as well as the downstream risks and benefits of the procedures and tests that may occur as a result of a positive test. For example, radiation exposure as a result of testing can be substantial.[8] Moreover, even if a test does not have intrinsic risk, it may lead to more interventions and eventually result in net harm and wasteful use of scarce resources. At every step of deciding about diagnostic testing, the clinician should be sure how a test result will be used and how it will promote the best interests of the patient.

Therapeutic Decision Making

Decisions about therapy involve weighing risks and benefits to determine the best course of action, and understanding the goals of the patient. The key questions for clinical decision makers are whether an intervention can improve the quantity and/or quality of the patient's life, and how the risks, benefits, and requirements align with the patient's preferences. Moreover, the benefit is often best understood in a probabilistic framework, because most interventions do not provide direct benefit for each person who is treated.

Clinicians should be aware of the strength of the evidence in support of therapeutic decisions. The strongest evidence derives from well-conducted randomized trials (see Chap. 6). Observational studies and case series can provide useful information, but are usually less definitive. Regardless of design, clinicians should not assume that all published studies, including randomized trials, are of high quality. Criteria for assessing studies are available, although a description is beyond the scope of this chapter.

Clinical practice guidelines from the American College of Cardiology (ACC) and the American Heart Association (AHA) grade their recommendations with information about the strength and type of evidence. Level of evidence A is associated with evidence derived from multiple randomized trials or meta-analyses. Level of evidence B is based on a single trial or nonrandomized trials. Level of evidence C is based solely on the consensus opinion of experts, case studies or standard of care, which may be derived primarily from causal reasoning. The recommendations are also organized into class I (strongly recommended), II (some uncertainty, with IIa favoring treatment more strongly than IIb), and III (not recommended).

Unfortunately, even if high-quality studies are available, precise estimates of risks and benefits are not often available for individual patients. Although the internal validity of a study may be strong, the external validity, or generalizability, may be less clear because patients in routine practice often do not resemble those enrolled in trials. The extrapolation of the trial results may be difficult. Moreover, clinicians must reconcile average results from large numbers of patients to the decision about an individual patient who will experience the consequence of the decision only once.

Decision Analysis. Decision analysis in medicine was developed to assist in making decisions. This approach seeks to make explicit the assumptions that underlie recommendations, and is commonly applied in therapeutic decisions. The method takes into account the probabilities of different outcomes and the value (or usefulness) of various outcomes from the patient's perspective. When repeating the analysis, with varying assumptions about probabilities and usefulness, this approach can reveal how sensitive the decision is to particular factors and under what conditions a specific strategy is favored. A decision analysis cannot mandate a choice. It is a tool intended to assist in illuminating the trade-offs inherent in a decision occurring under conditions of uncertainty. What can be most beneficial about this approach is the need to state explicitly all the assumptions that are relevant to the decision-making process.

EXAMPLE. The decision about whether to administer fibrinolytic therapy to patients who are 80 years of age and older was controversial when the therapy was first introduced. Some clinicians had concerns that the bleeding risk might offset the benefit of restoring blood flow in the coronary artery. A decision analysis modeled the decision, incorporating estimates of the risks and benefits of therapy.[9] In addition, the analysis evaluated the decision across a range of estimates for risk and benefit. The study demonstrated that across a broad range of estimates of risks and benefits, the decision to treat was, on average, favored. The analysis provided the insight that even a small relative reduction in risk produces a substantial absolute reduction in the number of deaths, which overshadowed the risk of bleeding. Using the best estimates for benefit, the decision favored treatment until the risk of hemorrhagic stroke rose to above 4%.

Evaluating the Evidence

The interpretation of evidence has many subtleties. Several topics bear particular emphasis, because they are commonly the source of misunderstanding and can compromise the quality of decisions.

***P* Values.** Statistical issues play a key role in therapeutic decision making. The *P* value, in particular, has taken on great weight in clinical studies. This value represents the probability that the result observed, or a more extreme one, could have occurred under the null hypothesis. The null hypothesis generally proposes that there is no effect, and the *P* value represents the probability that the observation occurred by chance in the absence of an effect of the factor studied. If the null hypothesis is rejected, then the alternative hypothesis is usually favored, suggesting the presence of an effect. The *P* value conveys the probability of the data given that the null hypothesis is true, but not the probability that the null hypothesis is true given the data. The *P* value is not a measure of the probability that the null hypothesis is false. In fact, under the right conditions, the probability that the null hypothesis is false may be low, even with a P value < 0.05. There are other views about how to approach statistical inference. Bayesian statisticians reject *P* values in favor of the approach of using data to update their estimates of a certain parameter. There is growing support for the Bayesian approach, but hypothesis testing continues to dominate.

Because the *P* value is so commonly used in clinical research, clinicians need to be aware of several key issues. First, the threshold of 0.05 for statistical significance is arbitrary. A *P* value of 0.04 implies that the data could occur 4% of the time if the null hypothesis is true and a *P* value of 0.06 suggests that the data would occur 6% of the time. Is the difference between 6% and 4% enough to reject the null hypothesis in one case and accept it in another? Clinicians should understand that *P* values are continuous values and are one piece of information among many. Second, *P* values do not inform clinical importance. A large study sample can produce a small *P* value, despite a clinically inconsequential difference between groups. Clinicians need to examine the size of the effects in addition to the statistical tests of whether the results could have occurred by chance. Statistics cannot supplant clinical judgment.

Expressions of Risk and Benefit. Clinical decisions involve the balancing of benefit and risk. The expression of benefit and risk can influence decisions. Clinicians need to have an understanding of these expressions, because they are the foundation for making decisions from clinical evidence.

The relative benefit (or risk) of an intervention is often expressed as a relative risk or odds ratio. Risk is the probability of an event and odds is the probability that an event will occur against the probability that it will not occur. A probability of 25% (1 in 4) represents odds of 1:3 or 1/3. The relative risk ratio of an event conveys the relative probability that an event will occur when two groups are compared. The odds ratio expresses the odds of the event in one group compared with another.

Despite its widespread use, the odds ratio is less helpful than relative risk in clinical decision making. The expressions are similar when baseline event rates are low (<5%), but deviate with higher risk and larger treatment effects.[10] The odds ratio can express associations but, unlike the risk ratio, it cannot express the relative size of the treatment effect; if clinicians assume it to be equivalent to risk, it may lead to overestimates of the treatment effect when the outcome is common. The odds ratio is often used in clinical research because of its mathematic properties and is good for identifying associations in certain situations, but clinicians need to know its limitations for estimates of treatment effect.

The relative benefit of any intervention may vary depending on patient characteristics, which are often explored in subgroup analyses. For example, fibrinolytic therapy was effective in the treatment of suspected acute myocardial infarction (AMI) and subgroup analyses revealed the benefit to be substantial in patients with ST-elevation but not in those without it (see Chap. 55).[11] The challenge is that subgroup analyses introduce the possibility that associations have occurred only by chance. In the Second International Study of Infarct Survival (ISIS-2), the authors provided perspective on subgroup analyses by demonstrating that patients born under the astrological signs of Gemini or Libra were significantly less likely to benefit from fibrinolytic therapy.[11a] Thus, subgroup analysis is capable of producing important insights, but must be interpreted with caution. A weakness of relative benefit estimates is that they do not convey information about what is achieved for patients at varying levels of risk. A small relative reduction in risk may be meaningful for a high-risk patient, whereas a large relative reduction may be inconsequential for a very low-risk patient. Absolute risk reduction, the difference between two rates, varies with the risk of an individual patient. For example, a risk ratio of 2.0 does not distinguish between baseline risks of 80% and 30% and between 0.08%, and 0.03%. In one case the absolute difference is 50% (5,000/10,000) and in the other it is 0.05% (5/10,000). In one case, 1 person out of 2 is benefited and in the other, 1 out of 2,000 is benefited. Unfortunately absolute benefit is not emphasized adequately in many articles.[12]

Number needed to treat (NNT), which can be calculated as the inverse of the absolute risk reduction, represents the number of people who need to be treated to prevent an adverse event. NNTs are a useful approach to express risk and benefit that incorporates the patient's baseline risk and a convenient way to express a trial result. For decision making with an individual patient, the baseline risk, which cannot be assumed to be the same as that of people in a trial, will strongly influence the estimate. Therefore, the NNT from the trial may need to be modified for an individual patient.

EXAMPLE. Physicians and their patients are often in a position to decide about whether aspirin should be used for primary prevention of cardiovascular disease (see Chap. 49). To make the example easier, let us assume that the patient is male and a physician, the group for which there is the most data. Some of the best information about this topic is from the Physicians' Health Study (PHS) Research Group, which enrolled 22,071 doctors in a randomized, double-blind, placebo-controlled trial of the effect of 325 mg of aspirin every other day (versus placebo) on cardiovascular risk.[13] The study was terminated early because the findings strongly favored aspirin. The investigators reported a 44% reduction in the risk of an AMI. The relative reduction sounds impressive, but the absolute reduction in risk is less compelling. The overall risk of an AMI in this population was low, 440/100,000/year in the placebo group. Thus, a 44% reduction in a low-risk population only averted about 186 events/100,000 treated (in the trial, 100 AMIs [93% nonfatal] were averted with 54,560 person-years of treatment). In other words, about 540 physicians needed to take aspirin every other day for 1 year for one person to avoid an AMI. The other 539 did not experience a benefit. On the other hand, there was a strong trend toward a doubling of the admittedly small risk of incurring a hemorrhagic stroke (relative risk, 2.14; 95% confidence interval, 0.96 to 4.77; $P = 0.06$). Overall, there were 11 extra hemorrhagic strokes. For every 9 AMIs that were avoided, there was one additional hemorrhagic stroke. The overall risk of stroke was slightly but nonsignificantly elevated in the aspirin group (relative risk, 1.22; 95% confidence interval, 0.93 to 1.60; $P = 0.15$), which also represented 11 extra strokes. The risk of death was not significantly different in the two groups (relative risk, 0.96; 95% confidence interval, 0.80 to 1.14; $P = 0.64$). The expression of the result as an absolute risk reduction provides a perspective for the individual patient that is easier to understand than the relative reduction in risk. The main point is that the reporting of a large relative reduction in risk provides only part of the relevant information to make this decision, and that presentation can affect the decision.

The evidence that 540 physicians need to take aspirin every other day for 1 year for one person to benefit, with a cost of an additional stroke for every 9 AMIs averted, is hard to translate into action without incorporating preferences. Some patients may find that result favorable and others may not. Also, people can be overwhelmed by too much information, and information on risk may be difficult to understand.

The findings from this study were reinforced in a meta-analysis of all the primary prevention trials. The very small absolute benefit, even in the higher risk primary prevention groups, might lead many patients to decide not to take aspirin in this setting.[14]

RISK STRATIFICATION. Risk stratification is often used to estimate patient risk and assist in decision making. This approach generally uses the results of statistical models that have identified prognostic factors and incorporated them into a tool that could assist clinicians. In recent years, many tools have been developed to assist in the rapid assessment of patients. For example, the Thrombolysis in Myocardial Infarction (TIMI) risk score for unstable angina non–ST-segment elevation MI uses seven readily available variables to predict the risk of death and ischemic events (see Chap. 56).[15] The number of risk factors produced a range of risk from 5% (0/1 risk factors) to 41% (6/7 risk factors).

In evaluating risk stratification studies, it is important to consider whether the score or approach has been validated in populations similar to the patients to whom it is applied in practice. The predictors should have been collected independently of knowledge of the outcome. The outcome and time frame should be appropriate for clinical decisions. The value of the stratification should also be clear. Improving precision in risk estimates without consequence is like ordering tests that have no implications for treatment. On the other hand, risk stratification can assist in the calculation of absolute benefit and put the balance of risks and benefits of an intervention in proper perspective.

RISK-TREATMENT PARADOX. Several studies have shown a risk-treatment paradox in which the higher risk patients are least likely to receive interventions that are expected to provide a benefit.[16,17] This pattern is paradoxical because the high-risk patients would be expected to have the most to gain from an intervention that reduces risk, assuming that the relative reduction in risk is constant across groups defined by their baseline risk. The source of the paradox is not known, although some have suggested that it is related to an aversion to the treatment of patients with a limited functional status.[18] Another possibility is that concerns about the harm associated with an intervention are increased in the highest risk patients.

OUTCOMES AND TIMING. Additional considerations in assessing the potential effect of interventions are the outcome that is evaluated and the time period assessed. Articles about patients with cardiovascular disease often focus on cardiovascular events, including cardiovascular death, but patients would be expected to have more interest in all-cause mortality. If averting cardiovascular death merely leads to death from other causes, then there is little value to the patient. This issue is particularly important for older patients with other conditions, often called competing risks.[19] Moreover, even a short-term advantage in mortality, conferred for example by bypass surgery, may not be valued by the patient if other conditions and complications diminish the quality of that time. Quality of life and health status are commonly neglected in clinical studies, but are very important to patients. Thus, narrowly focusing on specific outcomes may obscure important insights about an intervention. The challenge is that evaluating many outcomes in a trial can increase the likelihood of false-positive findings. Another important issue with outcomes is that intermediate or surrogate outcomes, such as change in ejection fraction, do not always correspond to outcomes such as survival.

OUTCOME TYPES. In evaluating evidence, clinicians should be particularly attuned to the outcomes that are assessed. Ideally, interventions are assessed for their effect on a patient's quality or quantity of life. Many studies use surrogate outcomes, measures that are more distantly related to the patient's experience but are expected to be related to the likelihood that a patient's quality or quantity of life will be affected.[19a] These surrogate outcomes often reflect information about a patient's biology and, in epidemiologic studies, have prognostic value. However, it is not possible to know that an intervention that modifies a surrogate outcome has the expected effect on patients. There are many examples in medicine of changes in surrogate measures that did not translate into benefits for patients. Clinicians evaluating the medical literature should know whether the outcome reflects the patient's experience.

EXAMPLE. Low-density lipoprotein (LDL) levels are understood to reflect an individual's atherogenic milieu and are predictive of future cardiovascular outcomes (see Chap. 47). Moreover, some interventions that lower LDL levels reduce patient risk. Studies of interventions often have this laboratory measure as their outcome. Drugs can even be approved solely on their ability to modify LDL levels. However, knowledge that an intervention reduces LDL levels cannot be assumed to predict the patient's experience. Torcetrapib, a cholesteryl ester transfer protein (CETP) inhibitor, is very effective in reducing LDL levels (as well as increasing high-density lipoprotein [HDL] levels) and was predicted to reduce cardiovascular risk markedly. However, the trial results have shown that the subjects in the torcetrapib group have a higher mortality, even though they also have marked reductions in LDL and increases in HDL.[20]

EFFICACY AND EFFECTIVENESS. Efficacy is what is achieved by interventions under ideal circumstances, such as in the setting of a clinical trial. In contrast, effectiveness describes the effect in actual practice. There are many reasons why actual practice is different from the trial environment. Patients may differ in their biologic response or their adherence to intervention protocols and may be treated by less skilled individuals who have less infrastructure support. Therapeutic decisions are often based on the assumption that the efficacy and effectiveness of interventions are identical, which is not always the case.

COMPLETENESS OF EVIDENCE. In evaluating the evidence, there is one additional consideration for clinicians. The medical literature is skewed by publication bias. Such selective publication can distort the evidence available in the medical literature, compromising systematic reviews and meta-analyses, impairing evidence-based clinical practice, and undermining guideline recommendations. Studies have suggested that less than half of the trials registered in ClinicalTrials.gov, the Internet-based registry of clinical trials managed by the U.S. National Library of Medicine, had been published.[21] Many trials that are published lack complete safety data.[22] Data that are not published can have important public health implications, as was demonstrated in the case of rofecoxib (Vioxx).[23] Clinicians are handicapped by not knowing what is not in the literature, and should at least be aware that information on the safety and effectiveness profile of interventions may not be complete. This unfortunate fact heightens the uncertainty around treatment decisions.

ACCURACY OF TEST RESULTS. An important aspect of clinical decision making is the validity of the primary information on which the decisions are based. Clinicians need to ensure that the evidence is coherent and consistent. Does the evidence, in its totality, make sense? Clinicians must be prepared to review the primary data, particularly when information is inconsistent. Errors can occur in analyzing, interpreting, or reporting results. Excellent clinicians recognize the possibility that the information with which they are provided is not correct.

Cognitive Errors

Even with good information, cognitive errors can undermine clinical decisions.[24] Some examples of these errors are described below.

HEURISTICS OR RULES OF THUMB. Clinicians tend to rely on heuristics, or rules of thumb, to assess probabilities and support complex cognitive tasks required for decision making. These heuristics can be useful because they allow shortcuts in reasoning, but are also vulnerable to important errors and can undermine decisions.

Many medical heuristics are familiar. The principle of Occam's razor suggests that a clinician should choose the simplest explanation for a set of observations. Sutton's law, named for a bank robber who explained why he robbed banks by stating "because that's where the money is," encourages clinicians to focus their attention where they will obtain the greatest yield.

Heuristics can be useful but may contribute to errors. The following limited set provides some examples of the heuristics that may be helpful in some settings but can cause cognitive errors in others.

The availability heuristic leads clinicians to estimate probability by how readily they can remember examples. Clinicians may estimate the probability of a disease because of its ease of recall. Thus, a more recent experience with a certain illness may make someone believe that it is more common than it is. A patient who has suffered a rare adverse event with a medication could lead a clinician to avoid that treatment.

The anchoring heuristic leads people to stay with their initial impressions. This heuristic can be misleading if clinicians do not refine initial impressions. A form of this heuristic, called premature closure, can lead clinicians to stop pursuing alternative explanations prematurely.

FRAMING EFFECTS. Like their patients, clinicians are sensitive to the framing of information. That is, the same truth is acted on differently depending on how the information is presented. Clinicians (and patients) need to recognize their sensitivity to the framing of the data. Clinicians are more likely to use a new therapy when presented with the relative reduction in risk rather than the absolute reduction.[25] When presented with trial results, physicians rated treatment effectiveness higher when presented with relative risk reductions compared with absolute risk reductions.[26] Physicians can address this error by reframing decisions and being aware of the effect of the presentation of the data on perceptions of benefit.

BLIND OBEDIENCE. The unwavering acceptance of the diagnosis of an authority (test or person) can lead to ignoring information that is clearly discordant. Wise clinicians have the courage to question authority when the information does not provide a clear answer. The persistence of good decision makers and their refusal to follow the crowd blindly often leads to important insights. The best interests of the patient should guide clinicians and give them the strength to question authority respectfully, when appropriate.

Shared Decision Making

Clinical decisions are not the sole domain of physicians. The principle of autonomy maintains that patients retain control over their bodies and must consent to undergo interventions, except in rare circumstances (see Chap. 3). Informed consent is the cornerstone of this concept. Unfortunately, there is little consensus about how best to involve patients actively in decision making. Nevertheless, given the need to align goals of therapy with the patient's preferences and values, it is important to engage them, if possible. This approach is most appropriate for major decisions, those with intermediate or low certainty, and those that are not emergent.

There are many aspects of communicating risks and benefits. First, this information takes many forms. The dimensions of risk and benefit include their identity, permanence, timing, probability, and value to an individual patient.[27] All should be considered in decision making. Unfortunately, there is relatively little evidence to guide physicians about how best to convey risks to patients.[28]

It is known that patients do not always understand benefit and risk well. For example, in a study of patients who had given consent for elective percutaneous coronary intervention, an intervention that does not improve survival or prevent AMI in this context (see Chap. 57), 75% thought it would prevent an AMI and 71% thought that it would improve survival.[29] Moreover, only 46% could identify at least one possible complication. Among this group, 67% stated that they should be involved at least equally with the physician in making decisions. Others have also found that patients often have unrealistic expectations of benefit.[30] These deficiencies in patient understanding need to be addressed for shared decision making to occur.

The manner in which information is presented may influence patients. Like physicians, patients are also susceptible to framing effects.[31] Patients tend to be more likely to choose a therapy that is presented as having an advantage over an alternative in relative rather than absolute terms. The relative effect is almost always much greater than the absolute change. Patients may also be influenced by the order in which information is provided.

Some techniques have been proposed to help clinicians convey risk.[32] First, clinicians should avoid descriptive terms only because they may not have a consistent meaning to patients. Terms such as *low risk* may be difficult for people to interpret. If clinicians express risk as ratios, they should use a consistent denominator (e.g., 40 of 1000 and 5 of 1000 instead of 1 in 25 and 1 in 200). Clinicians should offer a number of perspectives, revealing multiple ways of thinking about risk. Use absolute numbers, not relative risks. It is helpful to use visual aids, if possible, because poor numeracy or literacy skills may be a barrier for many patients. Many patients do not understand risk communication formats.[33] In addition, clinicians should recognize that information and data are not the same, and it is incumbent on the clinician to communicate health information that is meaningful to the patient.

Shared decision making can be understood as having five phases: assess, advise, agree, assist, and arrange. First, the clinician must assess the patient. Then, the clinician should advise the patient of the options, with their benefits and risks. Next, the clinician and patient should agree on a plan that is aligned with the patient's preferences and values. The clinician should then assist the patient in implementing the plan. Finally, the patient and clinician arrange follow-up.

ADOPTION OF INNOVATION. In the course of clinical decision making, physicians are continually exposed to new information and innovation. Decisions must be made about whether to adopt new practices. The Diffusion of Innovations models, promoted by Everett Rogers, describes an S-shaped curve whereby some people adopt early and others later, with most adopting after an initial delay.[34] In medicine, this type of diffusion is commonly observed.

A cumulative meta-analysis has shown that evidence often becomes conclusive much longer before it is incorporated into authoritative texts and review articles.[35] On the other hand, the experience with spironolactone has shown that even when new therapies are adopted, they may be applied to populations that were excluded from the trials because of concerns about risks (see Chap. 28).[36] The appreciation of the need to improve the appropriate incorporation of new knowledge into clinical practice has spurred efforts to improve quality of care.

The best way to determine whether evidence is sufficiently strong to support practice change is by referring to Clinical Practice Guidelines, Appropriate Use Criteria, and Performance Measures that are published by the ACC and the AHA.[37-40] Guidelines grade and synthesize the current evidence and provide recommendations about practice. Other trustworthy recommendations on specific topics are available from the U.S. Preventive Services Task Force and the Cochrane Collaboration. Performance measures are distinct from guidelines in that they identify key processes of care that are considered essential for high-quality care.[41]

Decision-Making Support

Good clinical decision making can only occur in the context of good systems. The information on which the decision is based should be reliable. System errors, including problems with policies and procedures, inefficient processes, and communication obstacles, commonly contribute to mistakes in decision making.[42] Lack of decision support can lead to oversight. Lack of systems to diagnose and learn from decision-making errors will increase the likelihood that they will occur again. There is a need to regard good decision making as a team effort and not as an individual skill.

Conclusion

Clinical decision making is the cornerstone of good clinical care. Physicians must not only have knowledge of the field, but be prepared to use it in ways that optimize the care and outcomes of patients. Good judgment requires an ability to interpret evidence, weigh risks and benefits, and understand and promote the preferences and values of patients.

Classic Reading List

Eddy D: Clinical Decision Making: From Theory to Practice: A Collection of Essays From the Journal of the American Medical Association. Sudbury, Mass, Jones & Bartlett, 1996.

Guyatt GH, Rennie D, Meade M, Cook D (eds): Users' Guides to the Medical Literature: A Manual for Evidence-Based Clinical Practice. 2nd ed. New York, McGraw-Hill, 2008.

Laupacis A, Sackett DL, Roberts RS: An assessment of clinically useful measures of the consequences of treatment. N Engl J Med 318:1728, 1988.

Rembold CM: Number needed to screen: Development of a statistic for disease screening. BMJ 317:307, 1998.

Tversky A, Kahneman D: Judgment under uncertainty: Heuristics and biases. Science 185:1124, 1974.

REFERENCES

Clinical Decision Making

1. Shojania KG, Sampson M, Ansari MT, et al: How quickly do systematic reviews go out of date? A survival analysis. Ann Intern Med 147:224, 2007.
2. Kassirer JP, Kopelman RI: Learning Clinical Reasoning. Baltimore, Williams & Wilkins, 1991.

Diagnostic Decision Making and Testing

3. Kassirer JP: Diagnostic reasoning. Ann Intern Med 110:893, 1989.
4. Bachmann LM, Puhan MA, ter Riet G, Bossuyt PM: Sample sizes of studies on diagnostic accuracy: Literature survey. BMJ 332:1127, 2006.

4a. Froelicher VF, Lehmann KG, Thomas R, et al: The electrocardiographic exercise test in a population with reduced workup bias: diagnostic performance, computerized interpretation, and multivariable prediction. Ann Intern Med 128:965, 1998.

4b. Punglia RS, D'Amico AV, Catalona WJ, et al: Effect of verification bias on screening for prostate cancer by measurement of prostate-specific antigen. N Engl J Med 349:335, 2003.

5. Rembold CM: Number needed to screen: Development of a statistic for disease screening. BMJ 317:3072, 1998.
6. SEARCH Collaborative Group: SLCO1B1 variants and statin-induced myopathy—a genomewide study. N Engl J Med 359:789, 2008.
7. Chen J, Krumholz HM: How useful is computed tomography for screening for coronary artery disease? Screening for coronary artery disease with electron-beam computed tomography is not useful. Circulation 113:125, 2006.
8. Fazel R, Krumholz HM, Wang Y, et al: Exposure to low-dose ionizing radiation from medical imaging procedures. N Engl J Med 361:849, 2009.

Therapeutic Decision Making

9. Krumholz HM, Pasternak RC, Weinstein MC, et al: Cost effectiveness of thrombolytic therapy with streptokinase in elderly patients with suspected acute myocardial infarction. N Engl J Med 327:7, 1992.
10. Schwartz LM, Woloshin S, Welch HG: Misunderstandings about the effects of race and sex on physicians' referrals for cardiac catheterization. N Engl J Med 341:279, 1999.
11. Fibrinolytic Therapy Trialists' (FTT) Collaborative Group: Indications for fibrinolytic therapy in suspected acute myocardial infarction: Collaborative overview of early mortality and major morbidity results from all randomised trials of more than 1000 patients. Lancet 343:311, 1994.

11a. ISIS-2 (Second International Study of Infarct Survival) Collaborative Group: Randomised trial of intravenous streptokinase, oral aspirin, both, or neither among 17 187 cases of suspected acute myocardial infarction: ISIS-2. Lancet 332:349, 1988.

12. Schwartz LM, Woloshin S, Dvorin EL, Welch HG: Ratio measures in leading medical journals: Structured review of accessibility of underlying absolute risks. BMJ 333:1248, 2006.
13. Steering Committee of the Physicians' Health Study Research Group: Final report on the aspirin component of the ongoing Physicians' Health Study. N Engl J Med 321:129, 1989.
14. Antithrombotic Trialists' (ATT) Collaboration: Aspirin in the primary and secondary prevention of vascular disease: Collaborative meta-analysis of individual participant data from randomised trials. Lancet 373:1849, 2009.
15. Antman EM, Cohen M, Bernink PJ, et al: The TIMI risk score for unstable angina/non-ST elevation MI: A method for prognostication and therapeutic decision making. JAMA 284:835, 2000.
16. Ko DT, Mamdani M, Alter DA: Lipid-lowering therapy with statins in high-risk elderly patients: The treatment-risk paradox. JAMA 291:1864, 2004.
17. Lee DS, Tu JV, Juurlink DN, et al: Risk-treatment mismatch in the pharmacotherapy of heart failure. JAMA 294:1240, 2005.
18. McAlister FA, Oreopoulos A, Norris CM, et al: Exploring the treatment-risk paradox in coronary disease. Arch Intern Med 167:1019, 2007.
19. Welch HG, Albertsen PC, Nease RF, et al: Estimating treatment benefits for the elderly: The effect of competing risks. Ann Intern Med 124:577, 1996.

19a. Krumholz HM, Lee TH: Redefining quality—implications of recent clinical trials. N Engl J Med 358:2537, 2008.

20. Barter PJ, Caulfield M, Eriksson M, et al: Effects of torcetrapib in patients at high risk for coronary events. N Engl J Med 357:2109, 2007.
21. Ross JS, Mulvey GK, Hines EM, et al: Trial publication after registration in ClinicalTrials.Gov: A cross-sectional analysis. PLoS Med 6:e1000144, 2009.
22. Ioannidis JP, Lau J: Completeness of safety reporting in randomized trials: An evaluation of 7 medical areas. JAMA 285:437, 2001.
23. Ross JS, Madigan D, Hill KP, et al: Pooled analysis of rofecoxib placebo-controlled clinical trial data: lessons for postmarket pharmaceutical safety surveillance. Arch Intern Med 169:1976, 2009.

Accuracy of Test Results: Cognitive Errors

24. Scott IA: Errors in clinical reasoning: causes and remedial strategies. BMJ 338:b1860, 2009.
25. Forrow L, Taylor WC, Arnold RM: Absolutely relative: How research results are summarized can affect treatment decisions. Am J Med 92:121, 1992.
26. Naylor CD, Chen E, Strauss B: Measured enthusiasm: Does the method of reporting trial results alter perceptions of therapeutic effectiveness? Ann Intern Med 117:916, 1992.

Shared Decision Making

27. Bogardus ST Jr, Holmboe E, Jekel JF: Perils, pitfalls, and possibilities in talking about medical risk. JAMA 281:1037, 1999.
28. Epstein RM, Alper BS, Quill TE: Communicating evidence for participatory decision making. JAMA 291:2359, 2004.
29. Holmboe ES, Fiellin DA, Cusanelli E, et al: Perceptions of benefit and risk of patients undergoing first-time elective percutaneous coronary revascularization. J Gen Intern Med 15:632, 2000.
30. Whittle J, Conigliaro J, Good CB, et al: Understanding of the benefits of coronary revascularization procedures among patients who are offered such procedures. Am Heart J 154:662, 2007.
31. Malenka DJ, Baron JA, Johansen S, et al: The framing effect of relative and absolute risk. J Gen Intern Med 8:543, 1993.
32. Paling J: Strategies to help patients understand risks. BMJ 327:745, 2003.
33. Sheridan SL, Pignone MP, Lewis CL: A randomized comparison of patients' understanding of number needed to treat and other common risk reduction formats. J Gen Intern Med 18:884, 2003.

Adoption of Innovation

34. Rogers EM: A prospective and retrospective look at the diffusion model. J Health Commun 9:13, 2004.
35. Antman EM, Lau J, Kupelnick B, et al: A comparison of results of meta-analyses of randomized control trials and recommendations of clinical experts. Treatments for myocardial infarction. JAMA 268:240, 1992.
36. Masoudi FA, Gross CP, Wang Y, et al: Adoption of spironolactone therapy for older patients with heart failure and left ventricular systolic dysfunction in the United States, 1998-2001. Circulation 112:39, 2005.
37. Antman EM, Hand M, Armstrong PW, et al: 2007 Focused update of the ACC/AHA 2004 guidelines for the management of patients with ST-elevation myocardial infarction: A report of the American College of Cardiology/American Heart Association Task Force on Practice Guidelines: Developed in collaboration with the Canadian Cardiovascular Society endorsed by the American Academy of Family Physicians: 2007 Writing Group to Review New Evidence and Update the ACC/AHA 2004 Guidelines for the Management of Patients With ST-Elevation Myocardial Infarction, Writing on Behalf of the 2004 Writing Committee. Circulation 117:296, 2008.

38. Hendel RC, Berman DS, Di Carli MF, et al: ACCF/ASNC/ACR/AHA/ASE/SCCT/SCMR/SNM 2009 appropriate use criteria for cardiac radionuclide imaging: A report of the American College of Cardiology Foundation Appropriate Use Criteria Task Force, the American Society of Nuclear Cardiology, the American College of Radiology, the American Heart Association, the American Society of Echocardiography, the Society of Cardiovascular Computed Tomography, the Society for Cardiovascular Magnetic Resonance, and the Society of Nuclear Medicine. Endorsed by the American College of Emergency Physicians. J Am Coll Cardiol 53:2201, 2009.
39. Krumholz HM, Anderson JL, Bachelder BL, et al: ACC/AHA 2008 performance measures for adults with ST-elevation and non-ST-elevation myocardial infarction: a report of the American College of Cardiology/American Heart Association Task Force on Performance Measures (Writing Committee to Develop Performance Measures for ST-Elevation and Non-ST-Elevation Myocardial Infarction) developed in collaboration with the American Academy of Family Physicians and American College of Emergency Physicians endorsed by the American Association of Cardiovascular and Pulmonary Rehabilitation, Society for Cardiovascular Angiography and Interventions, and Society of Hospital Medicine. J Am Coll Cardiol 52:2046, 2008.
40. Patel MR, Dehmer GJ, Hirshfeld JW, et al: ACCF/SCAI/STS/AATS/AHA/ASNC 2009 appropriateness criteria for coronary revascularization: a report by the American College of Cardiology Foundation Appropriateness Criteria Task Force, Society for Cardiovascular Angiography and Interventions, Society of Thoracic Surgeons, American Association for Thoracic Surgery, American Heart Association, and the American Society of Nuclear Cardiology endorsed by the American Society of Echocardiography, the Heart Failure Society of America, and the Society of Cardiovascular Computed Tomography. J Am Coll Cardiol 53:530, 2009.
41. Spertus JA, Eagle KA, Krumholz HM, et al: American College of Cardiology and American Heart Association methodology for the selection and creation of performance measures for quantifying the quality of cardiovascular care. Circulation 111:1703, 2005.

Decision-Making Support

42. Graber ML, Franklin N, Gordon R: Diagnostic error in internal medicine. Arch Intern Med 165:1493, 2005.

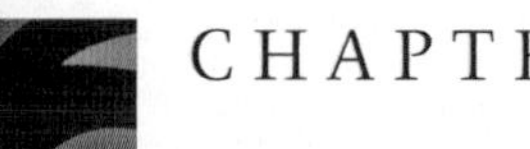

CHAPTER 5 Measurement and Improvement of Quality of Cardiovascular Care

Thomas H. Lee

In recent years, measurement and improvement of quality has become an important focus for cardiovascular leaders and researchers because of a combination of factors, including advances in measurement of quality and changes in the health care environment. This trend has been made possible by clinical research that has helped define evidence-based medicine for common cardiovascular syndromes (i.e., knowledge of which interventions improve patient outcomes). This growing body of knowledge has made possible the development of guidelines more comprehensive and explicit than those for any other specialty of medicine. The availability of these guidelines has in turn enabled the development of measures to assess the reliability with which the guidelines' recommendations are implemented.

Interest in report cards on quality has been intensified by concerns about quality, safety, and costs of care.[1] Data on gaps in quality and on costs are now publicly reported for hospitals and physicians,[2] and the prominence of these data has grown with the advent of new insurance products, in which providers receive bonuses for higher measured quality (pay for performance)[3,4] or larger percentages of health care costs are borne by patients. Data on provider costs and quality are frequently provided to patients in these consumer-directed health plans so that in theory, they might choose providers of superior efficiency and quality.[5]

Measurement of quality of cardiovascular care had been building momentum, even before these recent trends in the health care marketplace, and numerous U.S. agencies have been actively involved in the development of measures and dissemination of data for several years (**Table 5-1**). Statewide report cards on cardiac surgery and percutaneous coronary interventions for hospitals and individual physicians have been introduced in some states.[6] The National Committee for Quality Assurance (NCQA) has developed measures of quality for managed care organizations known as the health plan employer and data set (HEDIS).[7] Measures for cardiovascular quality of care delivered by hospitals have been introduced by the Joint Commission,[8] and data on the volume of cardiovascular procedures have been disseminated via organizations such as the Leapfrog Group.[9] Data on rates of readmission to hospitals are being reported publicly by the U.S. Department of Health and Human Services.[10] This phenomenon has not been limited to the United States; detailed data on cardiovascular and other outcomes are available via the Internet for hospitals in the United Kingdom[11] and other countries.

Guidelines and Quality Measures

Amid calls for caution and expression of concern, health care professionals have responded with a variety of initiatives aimed at improving care. The most prominent of these responses in cardiovascular medicine has been the development of guidelines, particularly those from the American College of Cardiology (ACC) and the American Heart Association (AHA). Guidelines are written to describe a consensus on the diagnostic or therapeutic interventions appropriate for most patients in most cases. Guidelines are written with the expectation that individual physicians will use discretion in the treatment of individual patients and *not* follow the guidelines in certain cases.

These guidelines often provide the basis for measures of quality.[12] In contrast to guidelines, quality metrics often reflect rules or standards of care that should be followed for almost all patients. When the clinician believes that the rule is not appropriate for a patient, the reasons should be documented. When such standards are not met, the implication is that an error has occurred (e.g., failure to recommend aspirin for patients with acute myocardial infarction).

A subset of quality metrics can be considered for performance measurement for the purposes of public reporting, external comparisons, and pay for performance reimbursement systems.[12] Because the stakes are high in these settings, performance measures tend to be written to define the minimum standards of adequate care, as opposed to the targets that might define excellent care. For example, a 2004 report from the National Cholesterol Education Program supported a low-density lipoprotein (LDL) cholesterol goal of less than 70 mg/dL for high-risk patients,[13] which represented a modification of 2002 guidelines that recommended a target cholesterol level below 100 mg/dL for this population (see Chap. 49). In contrast, a higher LDL cholesterol target has been used by NCQA for its HEDIS measure for cholesterol management in high-risk patients. Until 2006, the HEDIS measure required managed care organizations to report the percentage of such patients who achieved an LDL level below 130 mg/dL. The NCQA rationale was that although experts agreed that a level below 100 mg/dL reflects excellent care, the strength of evidence was such that physicians should be faulted only if they allowed patients with coronary disease to have a level above 130 mg/dL. In 2006, the HEDIS LDL target was changed to 100 mg/dL, which remains higher than the goal supported in current guidelines.

The practical implication of this relationship between performance measures and guidelines in cardiovascular medicine is that performance measures are usually closely linked to class I indications from the ACC/AHA guidelines (i.e., conditions for which there is evidence or general agreement that a given procedure or treatment is useful and effective). Failure to perform interventions that are less strongly supported by evidence is too often a matter of judgment to use as a quality measure.

The ACC and AHA have articulated basic principles for selecting and creating performance measures.[14] These principles define a first phase in which measurement sets are constructed, followed by a second phase in which measure feasibility is assessed, and a third in which performance is measured (**Table 5-2**). The types of pitfalls that might compromise the usefulness or validity of measures as they are developed or applied are explored in detail. Using these principles, AHA/ACC workgroups have developed performance measures for patients with acute myocardial infarction, heart failure, and nonvalvular atrial fibrillation or atrial flutter (**Tables 5-3, 5-4, 5-5, and 5-6**).[15-17] The appendices of references 15, 16, and 17 include detailed specifications for the collection of data for these measures.

TABLE 5-1 Key Organizations Involved in Measurement of Quality of Cardiovascular Care

ORGANIZATION	MAJOR ACTIVITY	FOCUS	WEBSITE
American College of Cardiology (ACC)	Guidelines Applied in Practice (GAP); ACC/AHA Task Force on Performance Measures	Health care providers	www.acc.org
American Heart Association (AHA)	Get with the Guidelines; ACC/AHA Task Force on Performance Measures	Health care providers	www.americanheart.org
American Medical Association (AMA)	Physician Consortium for Quality Improvement	Physicians	www.ama-assn.org
Centers for Medicare and Medicaid Services (CMS)	Hospital Quality Initiative	Physicians and hospitals	www.cms.org
The Joint Commission (formerly JCAHO)	ORYX Initiatives	Accreditation of hospitals	www.jointcommission.org
Leapfrog Group	Publication of volume data for cardiac procedures at hospitals	Hospitals	www.leapfroggroup.org
National Committee for Quality Assurance (NCQA)	Health Plan Employer and Data Set (HEDIS); Heart Stroke Provider Recognition Program	Accreditation of health plans; physician provider recognition programs	www.ncqa.org
National Quality Forum (NQF)	Hospital Performance Measures Project	Hospitals	www.qualityforum.org

TABLE 5-2 Summary of Performance Measurement Development Strategy*

PHASE	TASKS
I. Constructing measurement sets	Defining the target population Identifying dimensions of care that should be quantified (e.g., problem diagnosis, patient education, treatment, patient self-management) Synthesizing and reviewing the literature Defining and operationalizing potential measures Selecting measures for inclusion in the performance measures set
II. Determining measure feasibility	Definition of sample (e.g., document sources of case identification and attrition; develop an algorithm to assign patients to providers) Feasibility of measures—report validity, reliability, and completeness of collected data
III. Measuring performance	Determining reporting unit (i.e., level at which information will be reported) Determining number and range of measures Evaluating performance

*Recommended by American College of Cardiology/American Heart Association.

Modified from Spertus JA, Eagle KA, Krumholz HM, et al: American College of Cardiology and American Heart Association Methodology for the Selection and Creation of Performance Measures for Quantifying the Quality of Cardiovascular Care. Circulation 111:1703, 2005.

TABLE 5-3 American College of Cardiology/American Heart Association Inpatient Heart Failure Performance Measures

PERFORMANCE MEASURE	DESCRIPTION
Evaluation of left ventricular systolic (LVS) function	Heart failure (HF) patients with documentation in hospital record that LVS function was assessed before arrival, during hospitalization, or is planned after discharge
ACE inhibitor (ACEI) or angiotensin receptor blocker (ARB) for LV systolic dysfunction (LVSD)	HF patients with LVSD and without both ACEI and ARB contraindications who are prescribed an ACEI or ARB at discharge
Anticoagulant at discharge for HF patients with atrial fibrillation (AF)	HF patients with chronic or recurrent AF and without warfarin contraindications who are prescribed warfarin at discharge
Discharge instructions	HF patients discharged home with written instructions and educational material addressing all the following: activity level, diet, discharge medications, follow-up appointment, weight monitoring, and what to do if symptoms worsen
Adult smoking cessation advice/counseling	HF patients with history of smoking cigarettes who are given smoking cessation advice or counseling during hospital stay

Modified from Bonow RO, Bennett S, Casey DE, et al: ACC/AHA clinical performance measures for adults with chronic heart failure: A report of the American College of Cardiology/American Heart Association Task Force on Performance Measures (Writing Committee to Develop Heart Failure Clinical Performance Measures): Endorsed by the Heart Failure Society of America. Circulation 112:1853, 2005.

METHODOLOGIC ISSUES

Many of the methodologic issues that affect clinical research influence the measurement of cardiovascular quality, with two major additional themes. First, the performance data for individual physicians and hospitals may be made public in some cases; as a general rule, the more widely data are disseminated, the greater the demand for methodologic rigor. Second, the collection and analysis of data for quality measurement is rarely funded as well as in clinical trials. Thus, the desire for methodologic rigor must be weighed against the cost of collecting and analyzing the data.

Claims Data

The least expensive type of information used for quality measurement is claims data, which are collected for the purposes of mediating payment, not promoting quality of care. Thus, there is little or no quality control for claims data regarding issues such as the accuracy of diagnoses. These data have the advantage of being readily available for large populations, but error rates in diagnoses are high, and information that is not required for payment is unavailable (e.g., whether heart failure is caused by systolic or diastolic dysfunction, or whether blood pressure levels were controlled).

Retrospective Chart Review

This method can be used to collect more accurate clinical data, but such reviews are expensive and are complicated by the existence of multiple medical records for most patients. Patients generally have separate

TABLE 5-4 American College of Cardiology/American Heart Association Outpatient Performance Measures for Heart Failure

PERFORMANCE MEASURE	DESCRIPTION
Initial laboratory tests	Initial laboratory evaluation of patients with newly diagnosed heart failure (HF)—complete blood cell count; blood urea nitrogen, blood glucose, serum electrolyte, serum creatinine, thyroid-stimulating hormone levels
Left ventricular systolic (LVS) assessment	HF patients with documentation that LVS has been assessed
Weight measurement	Measurement of patient's weight at each outpatient visit to assess change in volume status
Blood pressure measurement	Measurement of patient's blood pressure at each outpatient visit
Assessment of clinical symptoms of volume overload	Assessment of clinical symptoms of volume overload at each outpatient visit (e.g., dyspnea, fatigue, orthopnea)
Assessment of clinical signs of volume overload	Completion of a physical examination pertaining to volume status assessment in patients diagnosed with HF at each HF visit (e.g., peripheral edema, rales, hepatomegaly, ascites, jugular venous pressure, S_3 or S_4 gallop)
Assessment of activity level	Evaluation of impact of HF on activity level at each outpatient visit using standardized scale or assessment tool
Patient education	Percentage of patients who were provided with patient education on disease management and health behavior changes during one or more visits within period of assessment
Beta blocker therapy	Prescription of beta blockers in patients with HF and LVS dysfunction (LVSD)
ACE inhibitor (ACEI) or angiotensin receptor blocker (ARB) therapy for patients with HF who have LVSD	Prescription of ACEI or ARB for management of outpatient HF patients with LVSD
Warfarin therapy for patients with atrial fibrillation (AF)	Use of warfarin in patients with both HF and AF

Modified from Bonow RO, Bennett S, Casey DE, et al: ACC/AHA clinical performance measures for adults with chronic heart failure: A report of the American College of Cardiology/American Heart Association Task Force on Performance Measures (Writing Committee to Develop Heart Failure Clinical Performance Measures): Endorsed by the Heart Failure Society of America. Circulation 112:1853, 2005.

records at each hospital to which they have been admitted, as well as at the office of their primary care physician and the specialists from whom they have received care. None of these records is complete unless all these health care providers are part of an integrated delivery system with a single electronic medical record. Even when all records are available for review, data collection from paper records is limited by the completeness, accuracy, and legibility of record keeping.

The increasing use of electronic medical records potentially will assist the use of measures based on clinical data instead of administrative data.[18] However, significant barriers include the difficulty of integration of data from medical records used by different providers in the absence of a single national patient identification number, and the failure of many physicians to use key-coded fields of the electronic record (e.g., problem lists and medication lists) reliably.

Prospective Data Collection

Collection of key data for quality measurement is becoming an increasingly common and important tactic for quality improvement. Standard data forms for patients undergoing cardiac surgery or percutaneous coronary intervention (PCI) are now used at many medical centers. At

TABLE 5-5 American College of Cardiology/American Heart Association ST-Segment Elevation and Non–ST-Segment Elevation Myocardial Infarction Performance Measures

PERFORMANCE	DESCRIPTION
Aspirin at arrival	Acute myocardial infarction (AMI) patients without aspirin contraindications who received aspirin within 24 hours before or after hospital arrival
Aspirin prescribed at discharge	AMI patients without aspirin contraindications who are prescribed aspirin at hospital discharge
Beta blocker at arrival	AMI patients without beta blocker contraindications who received a beta blocker within 24 hours after hospital arrival
Beta blocker prescribed at discharge	AMI patients without beta blocker contraindications who are prescribed a beta blocker at hospital discharge
Low-density lipoprotein (LDL) cholesterol assessment	AMI patients with documentation of LDL cholesterol level in the hospital record (or documentation that testing was done during the hospital stay or is planned for after discharge
Lipid-lowering therapy at discharge	AMI patients with elevated LD cholesterol (≥100 mg/dL) who are prescribed a lipid-lowering medication at hospital discharge
ACEI or ARB for left ventricular systolic dysfunction (LVSD) at discharge	AMI patients with LVSD and without both ACEI and ARB contraindications who are prescribed an ACEI or ARB at hospital discharge
Time to fibrinolytic therapy	Median time from arrival to administration of fibrinolytic therapy in patients with ST-segment elevation or left bundle branch block (LBBB) on the electrocardiogram (ECG) performed closest to hospital arrival time; AMI patients receiving fibrinolytic therapy during the hospital stay and having time from hospital arrival to fibrinolysis ≤ 30 min
Time to percutaneous coronary intervention (PCI)	Median time from arrival to PCI in patients with ST-segment elevation or left bundle branch block (LBBB) on ECG performed closest to hospital arrival time; AMI patients receiving PCI during hospital stay and having time from hospital arrival to PCI ≤ 90 min
Reperfusion therapy	AMI patients with ST-segment elevation on ECG performed closest to arrival who receive fibrinolytic therapy or primary PCI
Adult smoking cessation advice and counseling	AMI patients with a history of smoking cigarettes who are given smoking cessation advice or counseling during hospital stay

Modified from Krumholz HM, Anderson JL, Brooks NH, et al: ACC/AHA clinical performance measures for adults with ST-elevation and non-ST-elevation myocardial infarction: A report of the ACC/AHA Task Force on Performance Measures (ST-Elevation and Non-ST-Elevation Myocardial Infarction Performance Measures Writing Committee). Circulation 113:732, 2006.

some institutions, the data collected via these protocols are used for institutional data bases or for regional collaborations.[19-21] Many hospitals now report data on specific cardiovascular patient populations to national data bases such as the Society of Thoracic Surgery or the American College of Cardiology's National Cardiovascular Data Registry. Participation in such data bases allows comparison of institutional performance to regional and national benchmarks.

TABLE 5-6 American College of Cardiology/American Heart Association Performance Measures for Patients with Atrial Fibrillation or Atrial Flutter

PERFORMANCE MEASURE	DESCRIPTION
Assessment of thromboembolic risk factors	Nonvalvular atrial fibrillation patients for whom assessment of thromboembolic risk factors is documented
Chronic anticoagulation therapy	Prescription of warfarin for all patients with any high-risk factor or more than one moderate-risk factor
Monthly international normalized ratio (INR) assessment	Frequency of monitoring of INR

Modified from Estes NAM 3rd, Halperin JL, Calkins H, et al: ACC/AHA/Physician Consortium 2008 clinical performance measures for adults with nonvalvular atrial fibrillation or atrial flutter: A report of the American College of Cardiology/American Heart Association Task Force on Performance Measures and the Physician Consortium for Performance Improvement (Writing Committee to Develop Performance Measures for Atrial Fibrillation). Circulation 117:1101, 2008.

Collection of Patient Outcome Data

Collection of patient outcome data (e.g., 1-year mortality or functional status) is expensive and difficult. Administrative sources such as the National Death Index can provide information on whether individual patients have died in the United States; analogous resources are available in many other countries. However, obtaining information on the cause of death or on the status of patients who have not died requires interviews or surveys. Even when such data are available, the results should be adjusted for clinical and socioeconomic factors that are likely to influence the results. Therefore, many quality measures focus on processes such as the use of medications (e.g., beta blockers after acute myocardial infarction) or tests (e.g., measurement of LDL cholesterol) that are expected to lead to better outcomes.

Collection of Patient Experience Data

Surveys are widely used to collect information on patients' experiences and satisfaction with the care provided by hospitals and individual physicians. Patient satisfaction tends to be higher in patients who are older, have better physical function, and are not depressed. Research in patients with acute myocardial infarction indicates that patient satisfaction does not correlate well with other measures of quality of care, including survival.[22]

Definition of Quality

A variety of definitions of quality have been proposed, reflecting the complexity of the health care system and its heterogeneous stakeholders. An increasingly popular operational definition of quality is based on error reduction and the recognition that there are three major types of errors in health care—errors of underuse, overuse, and misuse. Underuse is the failure to provide a medical intervention when it is likely to produce a favorable outcome for a patient, such as the failure to prescribe an angiotensin-converting enzyme inhibitor for a patient with left ventricular dysfunction. Overuse occurs when an intervention becomes common practice, even though its benefits do not justify the potential harm or costs, such as performance of exercise testing in asymptomatic patients with a low risk for cardiovascular disease. Misuse occurs when a preventable complication eliminates the benefit of an intervention. An example is continued administration of a statin to a patient with muscle tenderness and weakness, suggesting possible myopathy.

The relationship between guidelines and these three types of errors is close and complex. In ACC/AHA guidelines, class I indications sometimes define rules that, if not applied for an appropriate patient, would suggest an error of underuse. Class III indications define potential errors of overuse. The ACC/AHA guidelines tend to focus on two aspects of quality:

- Complying with evidence-based medicine (i.e., doing the right thing for the patient)
- Procedural quality (i.e., performing interventions correctly)

Failure to comply with evidence-based medicine may constitute an error of underuse (e.g., failure to use a beta blocker after acute myocardial infarction) or of overuse (e.g., performance of coronary angiography in a patient without clinical evidence of coronary artery disease). Failure to perform an intervention correctly can constitute an error of misuse (e.g., continued administration of a statin in a patient with symptoms of myopathy).

Outcomes (e.g., mortality, complication rates) are the measure of performance of greatest interest to patients and clinicians, but adjusting for the effects of comorbid medical conditions, severity of the underlying disease, and socioeconomic status is a formidable challenge. This challenge is particularly great when analyses are restricted to administrative claims data. Nevertheless, severity adjustment models for hospital 30-day mortality using Medicare claims data for patients with heart failure and acute myocardial infarction have reported performance approaching that of clinical data extracted from medical record reviews.[23,24] These models have been endorsed by the National Quality Forum and are believed to have performance sufficient for use for public reporting. However, it should be noted that similar models are necessary for other outcomes for non-Medicare patients and for other diagnoses.

A surrogate marker for quality that is used by the public and by professional organizations is procedure volume. The relationship between volume and patient outcomes has been demonstrated in numerous studies focusing on hospitals and physicians.[25,26] These relationships are complex; for some procedures, outcomes are associated with the volume for the hospital, whereas for other procedures, outcomes are associated with the volume for the individual physician. The ACC/AHA guidelines acknowledge research on the relationship between volume and outcome in guidelines, such as those for the use of PCI for patients with acute myocardial infarction.[27] These guidelines recommend that elective PCI should be performed by experienced operators (at least 75 procedures/year) at high-volume facilities (at least 400 procedures/year). Analysis of data for all 34 nonfederal hospitals in New York State and for all 264 percutaneous coronary intervention operators indicate that these thresholds distinguish good from poor outcome rates.[26]

Dynamic Nature of Quality of Cardiovascular Care

Although gaps in quality continue to exist for patients with cardiovascular disease of all races and both genders, there has been a steady trend toward improvement. For example, the HEDIS measure for percentage of patients with acute myocardial infarction who receive a prescription for beta blockers within 7 days of hospital discharge was retired in 2007 because there was uniformly excellent performance among U.S. health plans (**Fig. 5-1**).[28] The key steps in such progress include rigorous research, followed by development of consensus guidelines and then performance measures for health plans, hospitals, and physicians. These performance measures are used for benchmarking, internal quality improvement programs, public reporting, and pay for performance contracts. In this context, hospitals and physicians are quick to share best practices and implement systems that improve the reliability of care. However, it should not be assumed that improvement in the reliability of performance of key processes of care automatically leads to improvement in patient outcomes,[29-31] just as it should not be assumed that hospitals ranked as leading cardiovascular centers under public reporting systems have better outcomes than hospitals with lower rankings.[32]

Hospitals

For hospitals in the United States, measures of cardiovascular care mandated by the Joint Commission have recently become important foci for quality improvement. These measures are part of a program

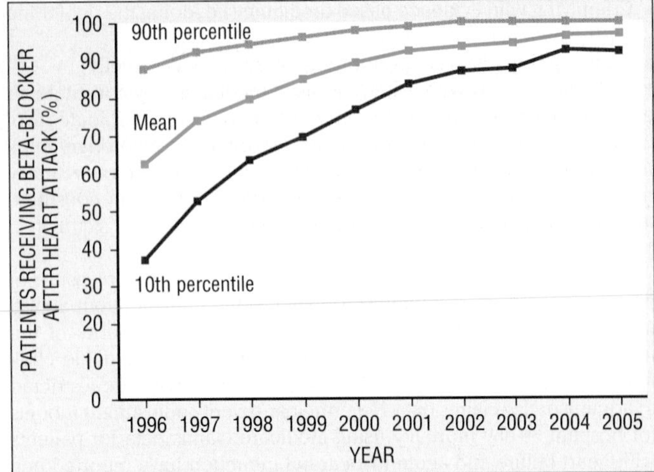

FIGURE 5-1 Use of beta blocker treatment after myocardial infarction, 1996-2005. *(From Lee TH: Eulogy for a quality measure. N Engl J Med. 357:1175, 2007.)*

called the ORYX Initiative, which integrates outcomes and other performance measurement data into the accreditation process for hospitals. Two of the core foci of the ORYX initiative are acute myocardial infarction and heart failure. Comparisons of hospitals on these measures can be made on the Joint Commission website.[8] Despite broad acceptance of these measures, researchers have found wide variability in adherence to guideline-recommended treatments and corresponding differences in patient outcomes (**Figs. 5-2 and 5-3**).

An issue of considerable controversy is the appropriateness of using mortality and other quality data to compare and rank institutions in public reporting forums. Critics of the use of mortality data note the limitations of risk adjustment and the inability of any single measure, including mortality, to capture quality of care.[33] Safety, for example, is just one dimension of quality, and it is sometimes in conflict with the goal of achieving optimal long-term patient outcomes. Thus, a procedural mortality rate of zero should not be regarded as a reflection of ideal care.[34]

Physicians

Cardiovascular surgeons and cardiologists who perform PCI are evaluated on their actual outcomes data via public report cards in some states. In these reports, analyses attempt to adjust for the risk of complications and for emergency procedures, allowing calculation of a risk-adjusted mortality rate for individual physicians and hospitals. Thus far, limited data suggest that the public does not use such data extensively,[5] although the public disclosure of performance data is believed to be a powerful driver for individual institutions to improve their care.

Nonprocedural care by physicians is often assessed by HEDIS measures developed by the NCQA (**Table 5-7**).[7] These measures were developed for the evaluation of health insurance plans, and therefore most rely on analyses of medical and pharmacy claims data. In recent years, however, there has been a shift toward measures that are less focused on measuring processes and are more closely tied to patient outcome. Therefore, measures that require review of medical records for some data have been introduced (e.g., blood pressure and LDL cholesterol levels).

NCQA also administers a program called the Heart/Stroke Recognition Program in collaboration with the AHA and the American Stroke Association. This program is designed to identify physicians who are providing excellent care to patients who have cardiovascular disease or a history of stroke. In this voluntary program, physicians seeking recognition must audit a sample of their office records and report on their rates of success in meeting specific performance measures (**Table 5-8**). A similar physician recognition program for diabetes care has been administered by NCQA for several years, and some employers now pay a bonus to physicians who meet the standards of these two programs.

Considerable controversy exists around measurement and public reporting of efficiency of the care delivered by physicians and other providers.[35,36] Interest in efficiency measurement has become intense because of rising health care costs, but the data and analytic tools available for efficiency measurement are primitive at best, particularly for the care delivered by individual physicians. Key questions that remain unresolved include whether physician efficiency should be evaluated globally (i.e., for a wide range of diagnoses) or narrowly (for specific conditions), whether analyses should be performed for individual physicians or groups, and which uses of these data are appropriate.

Improvement Strategies

The ACC, AHA, and a wide range of other organizations are attempting to develop and disseminate tools for improvement in the reliability of delivery of evidence-based cardiovascular care. The AHA's Get With the Guidelines program has enrolled more than 2 million patients with myocardial infarction, heart failure, or stroke from more than 1400 hospitals nationwide. The ACC's Guidelines Applied in Practice Initiative has used tactics known as continuous quality improvement (CQI) to help physicians and hospitals improve compliance with guidelines. These CQI tools are based on principles adapted from industrial manufacturers and seek to improve quality and efficiency through repetitive cycles of process and outcomes measurement, design, and implementation of interventions to improve the processes of care and remeasurement to assess the impact of interventions. Regional and national collaboratives have been organized to promote comparisons of performance and sharing of best practices.[20,21]

Research that has evaluated the impact of CQI programs on the quality of cardiovascular care has yielded mixed but encouraging results. Factors associated with effective improvement initiatives include the following: hospital commitment to an explicit goal motivated by internal and external pressures; senior management support; innovative protocols; flexibility in refining standardized protocols; uncompromising individual clinical leaders; collaborative teams; data feedback to monitor progress and identify problems and successes; and an organizational culture that fosters resilience to challenges.[37]

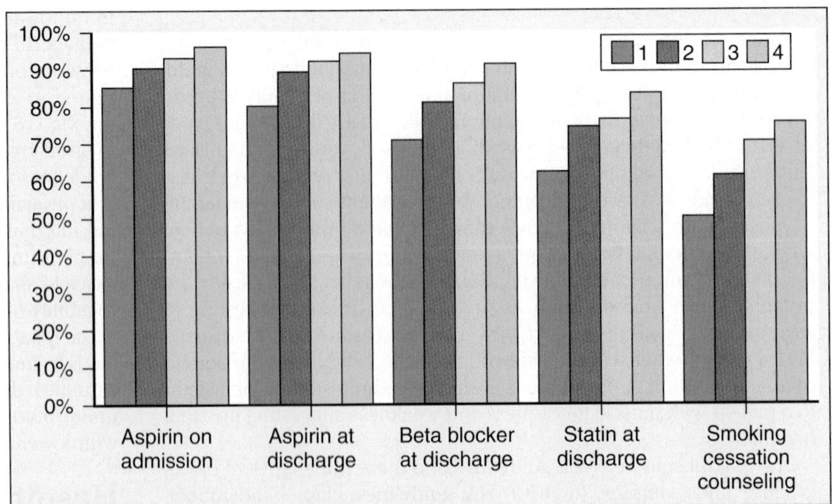

FIGURE 5-2 Compliance by quartile with guidelines for acute myocardial infarction. Bars show percentage compliance for quartiles of hospitals grouped by performance. *(From Peterson ED, Roe MT, Mulgund J, et al: Association between hospital process performance and outcomes among patients with acute coronary syndromes. JAMA 295:1912, 2006.)*

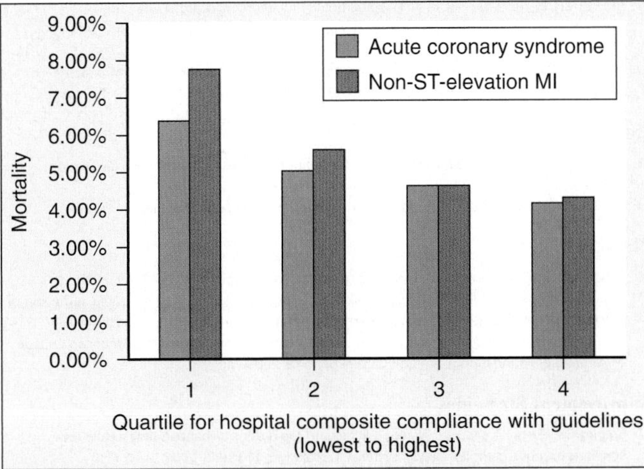

FIGURE 5-3 In-hospital mortality for patients with acute coronary syndrome and non-ST-elevation myocardial infarction correlated with hospital compliance with guidelines. Bars show percentage compliance for quartiles of hospitals grouped by performance. *(From Peterson ED, Roe MT, Mulgund J, et al: Association between hospital process performance and outcomes among patients with acute coronary syndromes. JAMA 295:1912, 2006.)*

TABLE 5-7 Cardiovascular HEDIS Measures

MEASURE	DESCRIPTION	MEAN PERFORMANCE (%)*
Persistence of beta blocker treatment after a heart attack	Percentage of patients >18 yr old who were hospitalized and discharged alive during measurement year with diagnosis of AMI and who received persistent beta blocker treatment for 6 mo after discharge	71.9
Controlling high blood pressure	Percentage of patients 45-85 yr old with diagnosis of hypertension and whose blood pressure was adequately controlled (<140/90 mm Hg) during measurement year	62.2
Cholesterol screening and management	Percentage of patients 18-75 yr old who had evidence of an acute cardiovascular event (hospitalization for AMI, coronary artery bypass grafting, or percutaneous transluminal coronary angioplasty) and whose low-density lipoprotein cholesterol was screened and controlled to <100 mg/dL in year following event	58.7

*Data are for commercial population for 2007.
From National Committee for Quality Assurance (NCQA): The State of Health Care Quality 2008 (http://www.ncqa.org/Portals/0/Newsroom/SOHC/SOHC_08.pdf).

TABLE 5-8 Measures of the Heart/Stroke Provider Recognition Program of the National Committee for Quality Assurance

Proportion of patients with blood pressure < 140/90 mm Hg
Lipid testing
Proportion of patients with low-density lipoprotein cholesterol < 100 mg/dL
Use of aspirin or other antithrombotics
Smoking status and cessation advice

From National Committee for Quality Assurance (NCQA): Heart/stroke recognition program. (www.ncqa.org/tabloid/140/Default.aspx).

Computerized physician order entry systems are being implemented at many academic medical centers in the United States, as well as a smaller number of community hospitals. These systems have been shown to improve compliance with guidelines to as high as 100% for selected quality measures for acute myocardial infarction and congestive heart failure.[38] Other research has shown that administrative and leadership cultures oriented toward quality improvement appear to be important predictors of success in reducing door to balloon times for patients with acute myocardial infarction who undergo PCI.[37]

Future Perspectives

Public reporting on the quality and efficiency of cardiac care is likely to become increasingly common in the years ahead because of changes in the U.S. and other health care systems, as well as the availability of new and larger data bases of administrative and clinical information. Reporting has thus far been focused on health plans and hospitals but can be expected to focus on groups and even individual physicians. Cardiovascular disease will be among the most prominent areas for such reporting because of the relative wealth of scientific knowledge and guidelines on cardiovascular conditions, as well as the high prevalence and costs of these conditions.

REFERENCES

1. Lee TH, Mongan JJ: Chaos and Organization in Health Care. Cambridge, Mass, MIT Press, 2009.
2. Lee TH, Meyer GS, Brennan TA: A middle ground on public accountability. N Engl J Med 350:2409, 2004.
3. Epstein AM, Lee TH, Hamel MB: Paying physicians for high-quality care. N Engl J Med 350:406, 2004.
4. Bufalino V, Peterson ED, Burke GL, et al: Payment for quality: Guiding principles and recommendations. Principles and recommendations from the American Heart Association's Reimbursement, Coverage, and Access Policy Development Workgroup. Circulation 113:1151, 2006.
5. Lee TH, Zapert K: Do high-deductible health plans threaten quality of care? N Engl J Med 353:1202, 2005.
6. Jha AK, Epstein AM: The predictive accuracy of the New York State coronary artery bypass surgery report-card system. Health Aff (Millwood) 25:844, 2006.
7. National Committee for Quality Assurance (NCQA): HEDIS 2010 measures (http://www.ncqa.org/tabloid/170/Default.aspx).
8. The Joint Commission: Performance measurement initiatives. (http://www.jointcommission.org/PerformanceMeasurement/PerformanceMeasurement).
9. Leapfrog Group: (http://www.leapfroggroup.org).
10. U.S. Department of Health and Human Services: Hospital Compare, 2010 (http://www.Hospitalcompare.hss.gov).
11. Dr Foster Intelligence: Dr Foster Quality Accounts (http://www.drfosterhealth.co.uk/quality-accounts).

Guidelines and Performance Measures

12. Bonow RO, Masoudi FA, Rumsfeld JS, et al: ACC/AHA classification of care metrics: Performance measures and quality metrics: A report of the American College of Cardiology/American Heart Association Task Force on Performance Measures. Circulation 118:2662, 2008.
13. Grundy SM, Cleeman JI, Merz NB, et al: Implications of recent clinical trials for the National Cholesterol Education Program Adult Treatment Panel III Guidelines. Circulation 110:227, 2004.
14. Spertus JA, Bonow RO, Chan P, et al: ACC/AHA 2010 methodology for the selection and creation of performance measures for quantifying the quality of cardiovascular care update: A report of the American College of Cardiology/American Heart Association Task Force on Performance Measures. J Am Coll Cardiol 56:1767, 2010.
15. Krumholz HM, Anderson JL, Bachelder BL, et al: ACC/AHA 2008 performance measures for adults with ST-elevation and non-ST-elevation myocardial infarction: A report of the ACC/AHA Task Force on Performance Measures (Writing Committee to Develop ST-Elevation and Non-ST-Elevation Myocardial Infarction). Circulation 118:2596, 2008.
16. Bonow RO, Bennett S, Casey DE Jr, et al: A report of the American College of Cardiology/American Heart Association Task Force on Performance Measures (Writing Committee to Develop Heart Failure Clinical Performance Measures): Endorsed by the Heart Failure Society of America. Circulation 112:1853, 2005.
17. Estes NAM 3rd, Halperin JL, Calkins H, et al: ACC/AHA/Physician Consortium 2008 clinical performance measures for adults with nonvalvular atrial fibrillation or atrial flutter: A report of the American College of Cardiology/American Heart Association Task Force on Performance Measures and the Physician Consortium for Performance Improvement (Writing Committee to Develop Performance Measures for Atrial Fibrillation). Circulation 117:1101, 2008.
18. Persell SD, Wright JM, Thompson JA, et al: Assessing the validity of national quality measures for coronary artery disease using an electronic health record. Arch Intern Med 116:2272, 2006.
19. Moscucci M, Rogers EK, Montoye C, et al: Association of a continuous quality improvement initiative with practice and outcome variations of contemporary percutaneous coronary interventions. Circulation 113:814, 2006.
20. Brush JE, Rensing E, Song F, et al: A statewide collaborative initiative to improve the quality of care for patients with acute myocardial infarction and heart failure. Circulation 119:1609, 2009.
21. Krumholz HM, Bradley EH, Nallamouthu BK, et al: A campaign to improve the timeliness of primary percutaneous coronary intervention: Door-to-Balloon: An Alliance for Quality. JACC Cardiovasc Interv 1:97, 2008.

22. Lee DS, Tu JV, Chong A, et al: Patient satisfaction and its relationship with quality and outcomes of care after acute myocardial infarction. Circulation 118;1938, 2008.

Definition of Quality

23. Krumholz HA, Wang Y, Mattera JA, et al: An administrative claims model suitable for profiling hospital performance based on 30-day mortality rates among patients with acute myocardial infarction. Circulation 113:1683, 2006.
24. Krumholz HA, Wang Y, Mattera JA, et al: An administrative claims model suitable for profiling hospital performance based on 30-day mortality rates among patients with heart failure. Circulation 113:1693, 2006.
25. Kuntz RE, Normand S-LT: Measuring percutaneous coronary intervention quality by simple case volume. Circulation 112:1088, 2005.
26. Hannan EL, Wu C, Walford G, et al: Volume-outcome relationships for percutaneous coronary interventions in the stent era. Circulation 112:1171, 2005.
27. Smith SC Jr, Feldman TE, Hirshfeld JW Jr, et al: ACC/AHA/SCAI 2005 guideline update for percutaneous coronary intervention: A report of the American College of Cardiology/American Heart Association Task Force on Practice Guidelines. ACC/AHA/SCAI Writing Committee to Update the 2001 Guidelines. Circulation 113:e1, 2006.

Dynamic Nature of Quality of Cardiovascular Care

28. Lee TH: Eulogy for a quality measure. N Engl J Med 357:1175, 2007.
29. Fonarow GC, Abraham WT, Albert NM, et al: Association between performance measures and clinical outcomes for patients hospitalized with heart failure. JAMA. 297:61, 2007.
30. Peterson ED, Roe MT, Mulgund J, et al: Association between hospital process performance and outcomes among patients with acute coronary syndromes. JAMA 295:1912, 2006.
31. Bradley EH, Herrin J, Elbel B, et al: Hospital quality for acute myocardial infarction: Correlation among process measures and relationship with short-term mortality. JAMA 296:72, 2006.
32. Wang OJ, Wang Y, Lichtman JH, et al: "America's Best Hospitals" in the treatment of acute myocardial infarction. Arch Intern Med 167:1342, 2007.

Hospitals

33. Shahian DM, Normand S-LT: Comparison of "risk-adjusted" hospital outcomes. Circulation 117:1955, 2008.
34. Lee TH, Torchiana DF, Lock JE: Is zero the ideal death rate? N Engl J Med 357:111, 2007.

Physicians

35. Milstein A, Lee TH: Comparing physicians on efficiency. N Engl J Med 357:2649, 2007.
36. Krumholz HM, Keenan PS, Brush JE Jr, et al: Standards for measures used for public reporting of efficiency in health care: A scientific statement from the American Heart Association Interdisciplinary Council on Quality of Care and Outcomes research and the American College of Cardiology Foundation. J Am Coll Cardiol 52:1518, 2008.

Improvement Strategies

37. Bradley EH, Curry LA, Webster TR, et al: Achieving rapid door-to-balloon times: How top hospitals improve complex clinical systems. Circulation. 113:1048, 2006.
38. Butler J, Speroff T, Arbogast PG, et al: Improved compliance with quality measures at hospital discharge with a computerized physician order entry system. Am Heart J 151:643, 2006.

CHAPTER 6 Design and Conduct of Clinical Trials

Elliott M. Antman

Despite many decades of advances in diagnosis and management, cardiovascular disease (CVD) remains the leading cause of death in the United States and other high-income countries, as well as many developing countries.[1] Interventions to treat CVD are therefore a major focus of contemporary clinical research. Therapeutic recommendations in cardiovascular medicine are no longer based on nonquantitative pathophysiologic reasoning but instead are evidence-based. Rigorously performed trials are required before regulatory approval and clinical acceptance of new treatments (drugs, devices, and biologics). Thus, the design, conduct, analysis, interpretation, and presentation of clinical trials are a central feature of the professional life of the contemporary cardiovascular specialist.[2,3] Case-control studies and registry observations are integral to epidemiologic and outcomes research, are not strictly clinical trials, and will not be discussed in this chapter.[4]

Constructing the Research Question

Before embarking on a clinical trial, investigators should review the FINER criteria for a good research question (**Table 6-1**), the phases of evaluation of new therapies (**Table 6-2**), and familiarize themselves with the processes of designing and implementing a research project, as well as drawing conclusions from the findings (see Fig. 6e-1 on website).[2,3,5-8] A clinical trial may be designed to test for superiority of the investigational treatment over control but also may be designed to show therapeutic similarity between the investigational and control treatments (noninferiority design) (**Fig. 6-1**; **Table 6-3**).

In a noninferiority trial, investigators specify a noninferiority criterion (M) and consider the investigational treatment to be therapeutically similar to control (standard) therapy if, with a high degree of confidence, the true difference in treatment effects is less than M (see Fig. 6-1).[9] Specification of the noninferiority margin M involves considerable discussion between the investigators (advocating for clinical perception of minimally important difference) and regulatory authorities (advocating for assurance that the investigational treatment maintains a reasonable fraction of the efficacy of the standard treatment based on prior trials). The investigational therapy may satisfy the definition of noninferiority but may or may not also show superiority compared with control therapy.[10] Thus, superiority can be considered a special case of noninferiority, where the entire confidence interval for the difference in treatments (investigational-to-control ratio) falls in favor of the investigational treatment (see Fig. 6-1). Investigators can stipulate that a trial is being designed to test both noninferiority and superiority (see Table 6-3). For a trial that is configured only as a noninferiority trial, it is acceptable to test for superiority conditional on having demonstrated noninferiority. Because of the subjective nature of the choice of M, the reverse is not true—trials configured for superiority cannot later test for noninferiority unless the margin M was prespecified.

Regardless of the design of the trial, it is essential that investigators provide a statement of the hypothesis being examined, using a format that permits biostatistical assessment of the results (see Fig. 6-e1 on website). Typically, a null hypothesis (H_O) is specified (e.g., no difference exists between the treatments being studied) and the trial is designed to provide evidence leading to rejection of H_O in favor of an alternative hypothesis (H_A; a difference exists between treatments).[2,5] To determine whether H_O may be rejected, investigators specify type I (α) and type II (β) errors referred to as the false-positive and false-negative rates, respectively. Conventionally, α is set at 5%, indicating a willingness to accept a 5% probability that a significant difference will occur by chance when there is no true difference in efficacy. Regulatory authorities may on occasion demand a more stringent level of α—for example when a single large trial is being proposed rather than two smaller trials—to gain approval of a new treatment. The value of β represents the probability that a specific difference in treatment efficacy might be missed and the investigators incorrectly fail to reject H_O when there is a true difference in efficacy. The power of the trial is given by the quantity ($1-\beta$) and is selected by the investigators (typically, between 80% and 90%). Using the quantities α, β, and the estimated event rates in the control group, the sample size of the trial can be calculated using standardized formulas for comparison of dichotomous outcomes or for a comparison of the rate of development of events over a follow-up period (time to failure). Table 6-3 summarizes the major features and concepts for superiority and noninferiority trials designed to change the standard of care for patients with a cardiovascular condition.

TABLE 6-1 FINER Criteria for a Good Research Question

Feasible
Interesting
Novel
Ethical
Relevant

From Hulley SB, Cummings SF, Browner WS, et al: Designing Clinical Research, 3rd ed. Philadelphia, Lippincott Williams & Wilkins, 2007.

TABLE 6-2 Phases of Evaluations of New Therapies

PHASE	FEATURES	PURPOSE
I	First administration of new treatment	Safety—is further investigation warranted?
II	Early trial in patients	Efficacy—dose ranging, AEs, pathophysiologic insights
III	Large scale comparison vs standard treatment	Registration pathway—definitive evaluation
IV	Monitoring in clinical practice	Postmarketing surveillance

Modified from Meinert C: Clinical trials. Design, conduct, and analysis. New York, Oxford University Press, 1986; and Stanley K: Design of randomized controlled trials. Circulation115:1164, 2007.

TABLE 6-3 Trial Designs to Replace Standard of Care

PARAMETER	SUPERIORITY	NONINFERIORITY OBJECTIVE 1	NONINFERIORITY OBJECTIVE 2
Goal	Test beats control	Test beats placebo	Test as good as standard
H_O H_A	$P_{test} = P_{control}$ $P_{test} < P_{control}$	Assessment of test made against putative placebo	$P_{test} \geq P_{standard} + M$ $P_{test} < P_{standard} + M$
Source of data	Trial	Historical data	Trial
Type I error	Set by regulatory authorities, typically 0.05	Set by regulatory authorities, typically 0.05	Set by regulatory authorities, typically 0.05
Type II error (power)	Set by investigator	N/A	Set by investigator
Major threats to validity	Assay sensitivity; bias	Assay constancy	Assay sensitivity; bias
Inferential reasoning from trial	Results in study cohort yield estimate of $P_{test} - P_{control}$ in population of patients with same clinical characteristics and disease state	Combining results from the trial ($P_{test} - P_{standard}$) and historical data ($P_{standard} - P_{placebo}$) yields estimate of ($P_{test} - P_{placebo}$) in population of patients with same clinical characteristics and disease state	Results in study cohort yield estimate of $P_{test} - P_{standard}$ in population of patients with same clinical characteristics and disease state
Generalizability to universe of *all* patients with the disease state	Related to enrollment criteria; the more restrictive they are, the less generalizable are the results to the entire universe of patients with the disease state	Enrollment criteria of prior trials and medical practice concurrent with those trials determines generalizability of estimate of $P_{standard} - P_{placebo}$ to contemporary practice	Related to enrollment criteria; the more restrictive they are, the less generalizable are the results to the entire universe of patients with the disease state

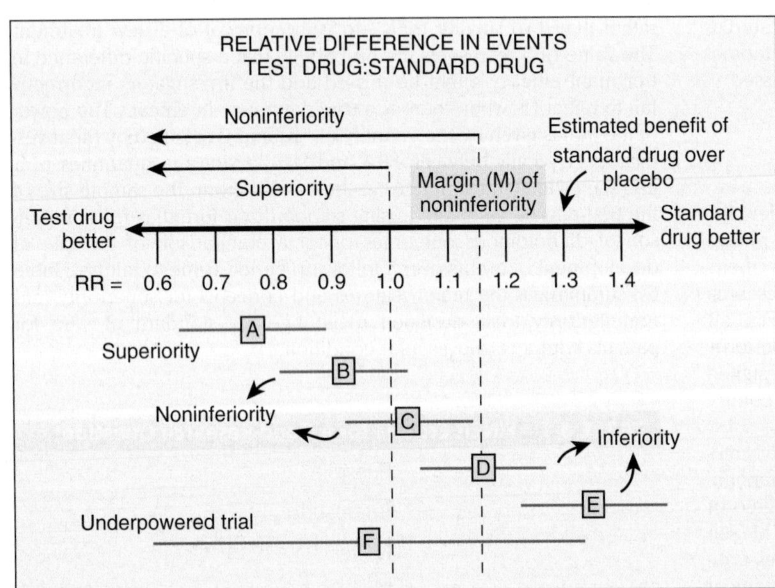

FIGURE 6-1 Example of design and interpretation of noninferiority trials. The margin (M) for noninferiority is prespecified based on prior trials comparing the standard drug with placebo. Examples of hypothetical trials A to F are shown, of which some (trials B and C) satisfy the definition of noninferiority. Trial A not only satisfies the criteria for noninferiority but because the confidence interval is entirely to the left of a relative risk of 1.0, the trial also shows superiority of the test drug compared with the standard drug.

Clinical Trial Design

Controlled Trials

The randomized controlled trial (RCT) is considered the gold standard for the evaluation of new treatments (**Fig. 6-2**). The allocation of subjects to control and test treatments is not determined or even influenced by the investigator but is based on an impartial scheme (usually a computer algorithm). Randomization reduces the likelihood of patient selection bias in allocation of treatment, enhances the likelihood that any baseline differences between groups are random so that comparable groups of subjects can be compared, and validates the use of common statistical tests.[2] Randomization may be fixed over the course of the trial or may be adaptive, based on the distribution of treatment assignments in the trial to a given point, baseline characteristics, or observed outcomes (see Fig. 6-2).[11] Fixed randomization schemes are more common and are specified further according to the allocation ratio (equal or unequal assignment to study groups), stratification levels, and block size (i.e., constraining the randomization of patients to ensure a balanced number of assignments to the study groups, especially if stratification [e.g., based on enrollment characteristics] is used in the trial). During the course of a trial, investigators may find it necessary to modify one or more treatments in response to evolving data (internal or external to the trial) or a recommendation from the trial's Data Safety Monitoring Board (DSMB) (adaptive design, as indicated in Fig. 6-2). The most desirable situation is for the control group to be studied contemporaneously and to be a collection of subjects distinct from the treatment group. Other trial formats that have been used in cardiovascular investigations include nonrandomized concurrent and historic controls (**Figs. 6-3A and B**), crossover designs (**Fig. 6-3C**), withdrawal trials (**Fig. 6-3D**), and group or cluster allocations (groups of subjects or investigative sites are assigned as a block to test or control). Depending on the clinical circumstances, the control agent may be placebo or an active treatment (standard of care).[2]

Other Forms of Controlled Studies

Trials in which the investigator selects the subjects to be allocated to the control and treatment groups are nonrandomized, concurrent control studies (see Fig. 6-3A). In this type of trial design, clinicians do not leave the allocation of treatment in each patient to chance and there is no need for patients to accept the concept of randomization. It is, however, difficult for investigators to match subjects in the test and control groups for all relevant baseline characteristics, introducing the possibility of selection bias that could influence the conclusions of the trial.

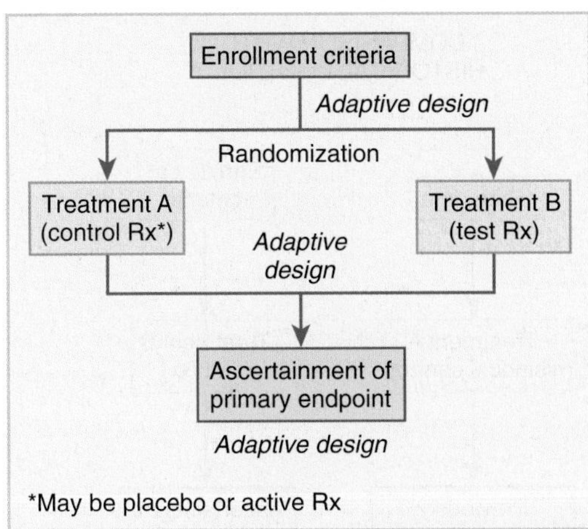

FIGURE 6-2 Basic structure of a randomized control trial (RCT). The investigators specify the enrollment criteria for the study population. Allocation to the treatment groups occurs through a randomization scheme, subjects are followed, and the primary endpoint is ascertained. The design of the RCT may be adapted at several levels as the investigators respond to evolving aggregate data, prior to unblinding, and advice from the Data Safety Monitoring Board.

Clinical trials that use historical controls compare a test intervention with data obtained earlier in a nonconcurrent, nonrandomized control group (see Fig. 6-3B). Potential sources for historical controls include previously published trials in cardiovascular medicine and electronic databases of clinic populations or registries. The use of historical controls allows investigators to offer the treatments(s) being investigated to all subjects enrolled in the trial. The major drawbacks are bias in the selection of the control population and failure of the historical controls to reflect accurately the contemporary picture of the disease under study.

The crossover design is a special case of the RCT in that each subject serves as his or her own control (see Fig. 6-3C). The appeal of this design is the ability to use the same subject for both test and control groups, thereby diminishing the influence of interindividual variability and allowing a smaller sample size. However, important limitations to crossover design are the assumptions that the effects of the treatment assigned during the first period have no residual effect on the treatment assigned during the second period, and that the patient's condition does not change during the periods being compared.

In a fixed sample size design, the trialists specify the necessary sample size before patient recruitment, whereas in an open or closed sequential design, subjects are enrolled only if the evolving test-control difference from previous subjects remains within prespecified boundaries.[11] Trials with a fixed design can be configured to continue until the requisite number of endpoints is reached (event driven), thus ensuring that enough endpoints will occur to provide intended power to evaluate the null and alternative hypotheses. When both the patient and investigator are aware of the treatment assignment, the trial is said to be unblinded. Single-blind trials mask the treatment from the patient but permit it to be known by the investigator, double-blind trials mask the treatment assignment from both the patient and investigator,[2] and triple-blind trials also mask the actual treatment assignment from the DSMB and provide data only in the form of group A and group B.

Withdrawal Studies

A withdrawal study evaluates the patient's response to discontinuation of treatment or reduction in the intensity of treatment for a cardiovascular condition (see Fig. 6-3D). Because patients previously experiencing incapacitating side effects would have been taken off the test intervention, they are not available for withdrawal. This bias toward selection of patients who tolerate a test intervention can overestimate benefit and underestimate toxicity associated with the treatment. Also, changes in the natural history of the disease in a given patient may influence the response to withdrawal of therapy.

Factorial Design

In a factorial design, multiple treatments can be compared with control within a single trial through independent randomizations (**Fig. 6-4**). Because CVD patients typically receive multiple therapies, the factorial design is more reflective of actual clinical practice than trials in which only a single intervention is randomized. Multiple comparisons can be efficiently performed in a single large factorial design trial that is smaller than the sum of two independent clinical trials. Each intervention should be evaluated individually against control and the possibility of interaction between the factors should be evaluated, because the validity of comparisons within each factor depends on the absence of interaction. Factorial designs may not be appropriate if there is an a priori reason to anticipate interactions (e.g., resulting from related mechanisms of action; see Fig. 6-4).

Selection of Endpoint of Clinical Trial

Evaluation of new treatments in the face of rising costs and reduced mortality rates for cardiovascular illnesses has resulted in two major approaches to the selection of endpoints. The first is to use a composite endpoint with a perceived logical grouping of events believed to be similarly affected by the treatments being studied.[2] During the course of a trial but prior to unblinding, investigators may assess the aggregate (all treatment groups combined) event rate for the primary endpoint to ascertain whether the initial estimates of the event rate in the control arm and anticipated treatment effect of the intervention were reasonable.[11] A low aggregate event rate may reflect inaccuracies in the control rate or treatment effect; investigators may respond by modifying the sample size or expanding the definition of the primary endpoint (another example of adaptive design; see Fig. 6-2).

Some investigators use a phrase such as MACE (***m***ajor ***a***dverse ***c***ardiac ***e***vents) to refer to the composite endpoint that they selected, but readers need to evaluate the methods sections in clinical trial reports rigorously because such phrases may be used differently across trial groups. Interpretation of composite endpoints is challenging when the various component elements show different quantitative or qualitative responses to a new treatment. For example, the new treatment may reduce a nonfatal element such as hospitalization for heart failure but may increase total mortality.

The balance of benefit and risk associated with a new treatment may be described using terms such as *net clinical benefit*, *net clinical outcome*, or *NACE* (***n***et ***a***dverse ***c***ardiac ***e***vents). Such terms typically combine elements of efficacy and safety (e.g., cardiovascular death, nonfatal myocardial infarction [MI], nonfatal stroke, nonfatal major bleed) and provide clinicians with a summary statement about what to expect from a new treatment. Although this is appealing, controversy remains because of a lack of agreement on weighting schemes to interpret composite endpoints, especially when nonfatal safety elements (e.g., bleeding) are combined with efficacy elements (e.g., prevention of MI).

Another approach is to use a surrogate endpoint as a substitute for measuring more traditional clinical outcomes. Surrogate endpoints are attractive to investigators because they are often measured on an interval (continuous) scale and can lead to trials with a smaller sample size. However, the field of cardiology is replete with examples of the trials configured around surrogate endpoints that not only failed to demonstrate benefit, but actually uncovered harm (e.g., increased mortality) associated with a new treatment. Surrogate endpoints are useful if they lie in the causal pathway of a disease and if interventions that affect them are reliably associated with changes in clinical outcomes. **Figure 6-5** illustrates a range of settings in which surrogate endpoints failed to serve as useful substitutes for measuring hard clinical events in cardiovascular trials.

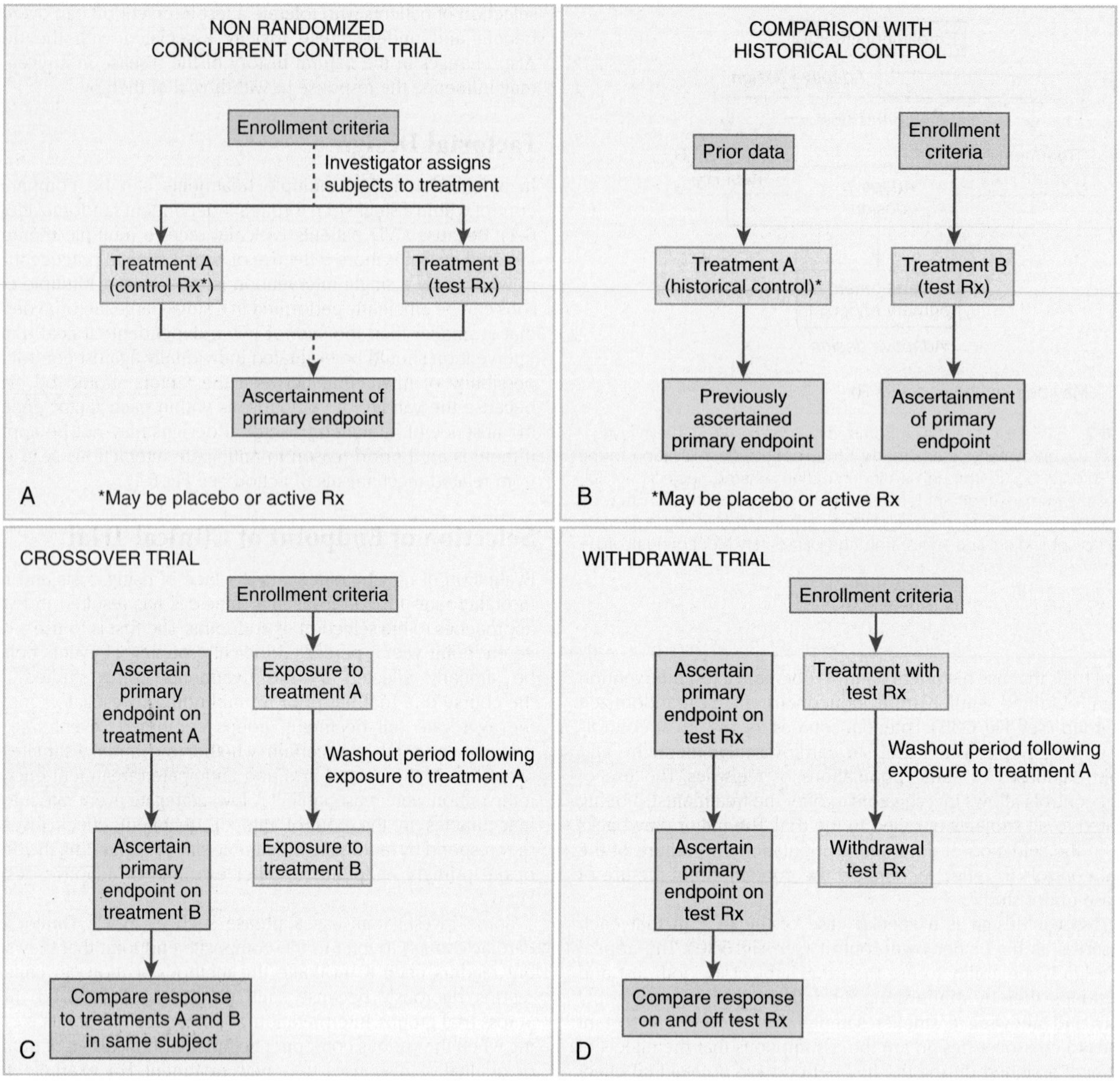

NON RANDOMIZED CONCURRENT CONTROL TRIAL

Enrollment criteria

Investigator assigns subjects to treatment

Treatment A (control Rx*)

Treatment B (test Rx)

Ascertainment of primary endpoint

A *May be placebo or active Rx

COMPARISON WITH HISTORICAL CONTROL

Prior data

Enrollment criteria

Treatment A (historical control)*

Treatment B (test Rx)

Previously ascertained primary endpoint

Ascertainment of primary endpoint

B *May be placebo or active Rx

CROSSOVER TRIAL

Enrollment criteria

Exposure to treatment A

Ascertain primary endpoint on treatment A

Washout period following exposure to treatment A

Exposure to treatment B

Ascertain primary endpoint on treatment B

Compare response to treatments A and B in same subject

C

WITHDRAWAL TRIAL

Enrollment criteria

Treatment with test Rx

Ascertain primary endpoint on test Rx

Washout period following exposure to treatment A

Withdrawal test Rx

Ascertain primary endpoint on test Rx

Compare response on and off test Rx

D

FIGURE 6-3 Other forms of controlled studies. **A,** Features of nonrandomized concurrent control trial. **B,** Design features of a trial using an historical control group. **C,** Design features of a crossover trial. (For an example of this type of trial to evaluate an intervention for angina pectoris, refer to Cole PL, Beamer AD, McGowan N, et al: Efficacy and safety of perhexiline maleate in refractory angina. A double-blind placebo-controlled clinical trial of a novel antianginal agent. Circulation 81:1260, 1990.) **D,** Design features of a withdrawal trial. *(For an example of the use of this type of trial to evaluate the use of digoxin in patients with chronic heart failure, refer to Packer M, Gheorghiade M, Young JB, et al: Withdrawal of digoxin from patients with chronic heart failure treated with angiotensin-converting-enzyme inhibitors. RADIANCE Study. N Engl J Med 329:1, 1993.)*

Key Issues

During the Course of the Trial

Contemporary trials require surveillance of multiple issues on a regular basis (see Fig. 6-e2 on the website). The determination as to whether an event (efficacy, safety) has occurred is the responsibility of a clinical events committee (CEC). Members of a CEC typically are experts in the field, are blinded to the treatment assignment, and adjudicate events according to a charter established and agreed to prior to initiation of enrollment. Because it would not be possible for investigators to maintain equipoise as the events in a trial begin to accumulate, the DSMB assesses the data at prespecified intervals to ascertain whether the accumulating evidence strongly suggests an advantage of one treatment (see Fig. 6-e2 on the website).[2,12]

Stopping boundaries to guide the DSMB are usually agreed on prior to the initiation of enrollment. Such stopping boundaries need to take into account the uncertainty of the evidence at iterative interim looks at the data and the play of chance, which may produce a situation in which one treatment appears to be favorable. During these interim looks at the data, members of the DSMB inspect the differences between treatment groups expressed as a standardized normal statistic (Z_i). Usually, Z_i plots depict evidence of superiority of the test treatment in the upward (positive) direction and inferiority of the test treatment in the downward direction. Stopping boundaries may be symmetric (**Fig. 6-6**) or asymmetric. Investigators and DSMB members may agree to use an asymmetric stopping boundary scheme that requires less compelling evidence to cross a lower bound for inferiority of a new treatment when an acceptable standard treatment is clinically available and the new treatment is associated with safety concerns (e.g., intracranial hemorrhage during the evaluation of a new fibrinolytic).[12] The DSMB may also be called on to determine whether a particular dose group should be discontinued (adaptive design) and whether the trial is futile (e.g., that conditional on the data accumulated at the *-ith* look, there is only a 10% chance that H_0 would be rejected at the end of the trial).

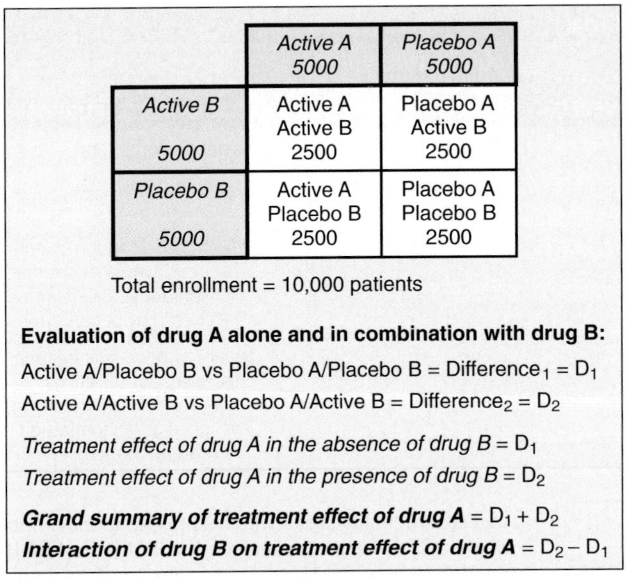

	Active A 5000	*Placebo A* 5000
Active B 5000	Active A Active B 2500	Placebo A Active B 2500
Placebo B 5000	Active A Placebo B 2500	Placebo A Placebo B 2500

Total enrollment = 10,000 patients

Evaluation of drug A alone and in combination with drug B:

Active A/Placebo B vs Placebo A/Placebo B = Difference$_1$ = D$_1$

Active A/Active B vs Placebo A/Active B = Difference$_2$ = D$_2$

Treatment effect of drug A in the absence of drug B = D$_1$

Treatment effect of drug A in the presence of drug B = D$_2$

Grand summary of treatment effect of drug A = D$_1$ + D$_2$

Interaction of drug B on treatment effect of drug A = D$_2$ – D$_1$

FIGURE 6-4 Factorial design of clinical trial. In this example, 10,000 patients are randomized to receive or not receive two interventions (drug A and drug B). Each patient will fall into one of the following four categories: Active A/Active B, Placebo A/Active B, Active A/Placebo B, Placebo A/Placebo B. *Bottom*, Differences in event rates for the comparisons permit an assessment of the treatment effect of drug A in the presence and absence of drug B. See text for further discussion. *(From Antman E: Medical therapy for acute coronary syndromes: An overview. In Califf R, Braunwald E [eds]: Acute Myocardial Infarction and Other Acute Ischemic Syndromes. Philadelphia, Current Medicine, 1996, pp 10.1-10.25.)*

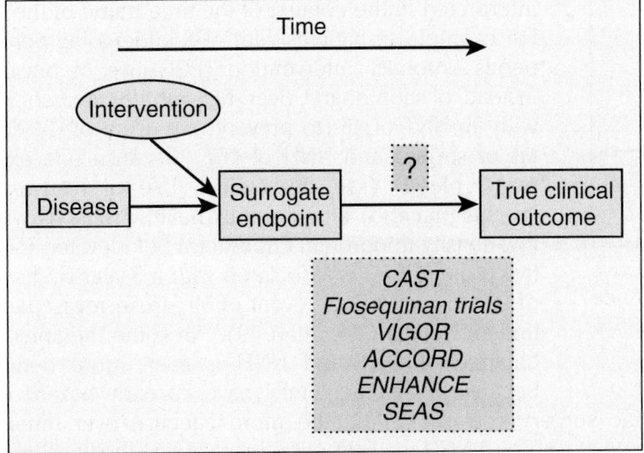

FIGURE 6-5 Surrogate endpoints. Selection of a surrogate endpoint in a clinical trial provides reliable information for clinicians if the surrogate endpoint is in the causal pathway of the disease with respect to clinical outcomes and the intervention acts on the surrogate endpoint so as to truly affect clinical outcome. Some examples of trials of cardiovascular medicine for which this paradigm failed include the following: CAST (Cardiac Arrhythmia Suppressor Trial), studies of flosequinan; VIGOR (Vioxx GI Outcomes Research); ACCORD (Action to Control Cardiovascular Risk in Diabetes); ENHANCE (Ezetimibe and Simvastatin in Hypercholesterolemia Enhances Atherosclerosis Regression); and SEAS (Simvastatin and Ezetimibe in Aortic Stenosis). *(Modified from Fleming TR, DeMets DL: Surrogate end points in clinical trials: Are we being misled? Ann Intern Med 125:605, 1996.)*

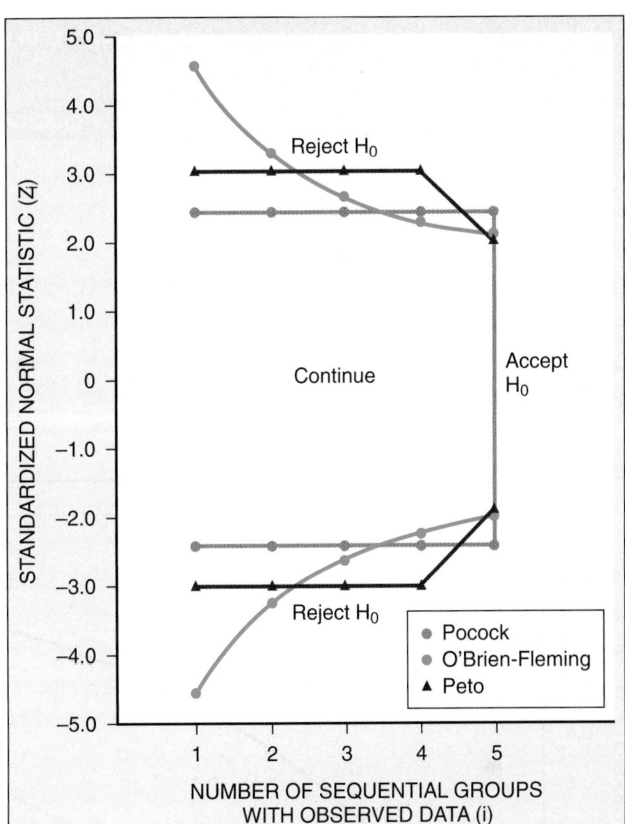

FIGURE 6-6 Sequential stopping boundaries used in monitoring a clinical trial. Shown are three sequential stopping boundaries for the standardized normal statistic (Z_i) for up to five sequential groups (of patients enrolled in the trial by the *-ith* analysis), with a final two-sided significance level of 0.05. *(From Friedman LM, Furberg CD, DeMets DL: Fundamentals of Clinical Trials, 4th ed. New York, Springer Verlag, 1998.)*

During the Analytic Phase of the Trial

Prior to unblinding the results of the trial (i.e., revealing patient outcomes by treatment group to the investigators), investigators should have finalized a statistical analysis plan (SAP). Key features of the SAP include a definition of the cohorts of trial subjects to be analyzed (**Table 6-4**), the statistical test(s) to be used to analyze the primary endpoint (e.g., for comparison of proportions or time to event), conventions for handling missing data, time windows for analyzing data (e.g., randomization through common study end date), and subgroups of interest (see Fig. 6-e2 on the website).[3,7] Depending on the exact definitions used for the analytic cohorts (see Table 6-4), the denominators may vary; this may lead to slight variations in the estimates of event rates and treatment effects. Ideally, the main results of the trial will be similar in the intention to treatment and per protocol cohorts. If they are not, an explanation should be sought from additional analyses of the data.

Not all patients will respond to a given treatment in a clinical trial to the same extent. The role of pharmacogenomics in determining the response to therapeutic agents is discussed in Chap. 10. Given that not all patients will respond to a given treatment, it is of clinical interest to inspect the data stratified by subgroups of interest.[13] Although such an approach may initially seem appealing, a number of considerations limit the investigator's ability to draw conclusions from subgroup analyses. Typically, subgroups involve univariate analyses of the data (e.g., men versus women) but the clinical picture is more complex, such that an individual patient will belong to multiple subgroups. Responses in subgroups should be evaluated by an interaction test, which determines whether the relative efficacy of treatments differs among the subgroups being examined. A quantitative interaction is said to be present when the treatment effect varies in magnitude but not in direction across subgroups.[13] A qualitative interaction is said to be present when the direction of the treatment effect varies among the subgroups.[13] Note that a qualitative interaction must also be a quantitative interaction. Importantly, the multiplicity of subgroup analyses inflates the false-positive rate (**Fig. 6-7**).[13] Rather than relying on a *P* value for a subgroup response, investigators and readers should focus on a graphic display of subgroup data depicting the point estimates and confidence intervals for the treatment effect. Such an

TABLE 6-4 Examples of Definitions of Analytic Cohorts in a Clinical Trial

ANALYTIC COHORT	REFERENCE DATE	EXCLUDE IF PROTOCOL VIOLATIONS DISCOVERED	REQUIRE THAT SUBJECT RECEIVED AT LEAST ONE DOSE OF STUDY DRUG	TREATMENT ASSIGNMENT FOR ANALYTIC PURPOSES
Intention to treat	Randomization	No	No	As per randomization
Modified intention to treat	May start at initial dose of study drug	No (may vary)	May introduce this requirement	As per randomization
Per protocol	Initial dose of study drug	Yes	Yes	Usually as per randomization, but sensitivity analyses that account for actual treatment received may be performed
Safety	Usually at time of initial dose of study drug	No	Yes	Usually as per actual treatment received, but sensitivity analyses that use treatment assigned at randomization may be performed

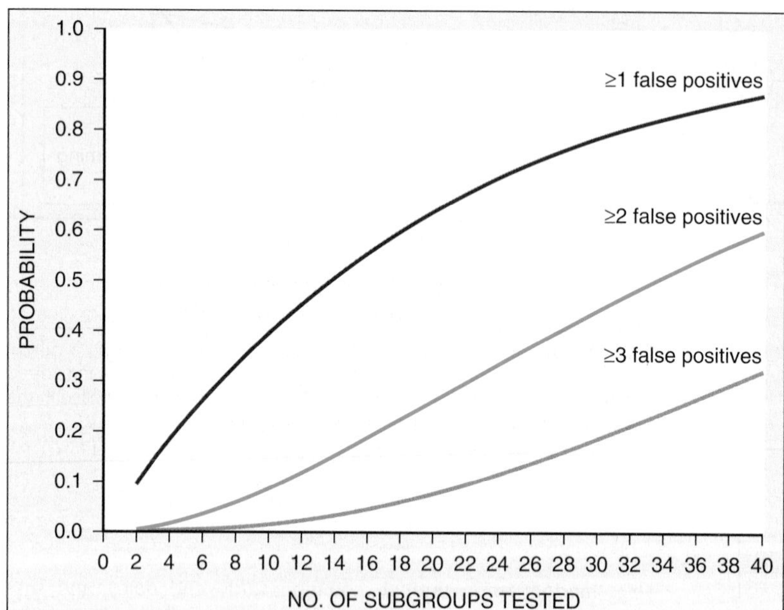

FIGURE 6-7 Probability that multiple subgroup analyses will yield at least one (red line), two (blue line), or three (yellow line) false-positive results. *(From Lagakos SW: The challenge of subgroup analyses—reporting without distorting. N Engl J Med 354:1667, 2006.)*

approach provides a summary of the range of plausible treatment effects observed in a trial.[13]

Measures and Detection of Treatment Effect

Events in a clinical trial may be measured on a nominal (dichotomous), categorical, or interval (continuous) scale.[14] Clinical trials reports should use descriptive statistics, graphic displays, and estimates of the precision of the observations appropriate for the scale of measurement being used in the trial.[14,15] A common assessment in a cardiovascular trial is comparison of the proportion of patients experiencing a dichotomous event (e.g., dead versus alive) during the follow-up period of the trial.[5] When the outcome is an undesirable cardiovascular response and the data are arranged as investigational group compared with control group, a relative risk (RR) or odds ratio (OR) of less than 1 indicates benefit of the investigational treatment (see Fig. 6-1).

Interpretation of the treatment effect should take into account the absolute risk of the outcomes. The absolute risk difference (ARD) is the difference in events in the treatment group and the control group, and is particularly useful when expressed as the number of patients that must be treated ($N = 1/\text{ARD}$), or number needed to treat (NNT), to observe the beneficial effect in one patient. Similarly, the absolute risk increase (ARI) in adverse events with the investigational treatment can be converted into the number needed to harm (NNH). By comparing the NNT and NNH for a given treatment, clinicians can assess the risk-benefit balance and also benchmark the treatment effects of the new therapy against other treatments used in contemporary cardiovascular practice. Another useful metric is to express the outcome for every 1000 patients treated.

The number needed to treat (or harm) should be interpreted in the context of the time frame of the trial. For example, in patients with ACS undergoing percutaneous coronary intervention (PCI), use of prasugrel instead of clopidogrel over 14.5 months is associated with an NNT of 46 (to prevent one event of CV death, MI, or stroke) and NNH of 167 (to cause one excess major bleed) (see Chap. 55).[16] Use of rosuvastatin (versus placebo) in apparently healthy persons with a low-density lipoprotein cholesterol but elevated C-reactive protein level is associated with a 5-year NNT value of 20 (to prevent one event of MI, stroke, revascularization, or death) (see Chap. 49).[17] In some therapies, the balance of NNT and NNH is even more complex because a treatment may have an early hazard (e.g., cardiac surgery versus PCI) but be more effective over time; the balance of NNT and NNH may also vary according to the baseline risk at the time of randomization.[18]

The interplay of variables set by investigators during the design of a clinical trial, the characteristics of the patients studied, and the features of the treatment being investigated influence the relative difference in events in the treatment groups (see Fig. 6-e3 on website).[19] The interface of the patient and the treatment may change over the course of exposure to the treatment (e.g., lower risk of events over time as the patient moves from the acute to chronic phases of a disease) and background therapy may also change during the course of the trial (e.g., treatments added or removed or doses modified). While these considerations can influence the likelihood of a "positive" trial, they also impact on the ability to detect a signal of harm (see Fig. 6-e4 on website).

Future Perspectives

Trialists, peer-reviewers, and journal editors now have checklists and templates that codify the reporting of clinical trials (see Table 6-e1 on website). Clinicians can refer to guides for reading and interpreting clinical trials (see Table 6-e2 on website).[3] These advances, however, only deal with clinical trials that reach the point where they are reported in a publicly available format. Considerable concern has been expressed in the past that some clinical trials, especially those with negative results, were never reported. The introduction of a requirement to register clinical trials on a web-based repository (e.g., www.clinicaltrials.gov) was an important step forward, but specific details are typically limited on such postings.[20] Contemporary requirements that clinical trials post a final study report within a reasonable period after study completion (1 year) will assist those investigators planning future trials, clinicians seeking the latest information about treatments, and writing committees for guidelines documents who need up-to-date and complete data to formulate recommendations.[21]

As part of its road map to transform clinical research, the National Institutes of Health launched the Clinical and Translational Science Award (CTSA) program in 2006. Clinical trials play an integral role in contemporary CTSA efforts because they intersect at the level of translation of basic science to human studies, usually in health volunteers (T1), translation of new knowledge in patients with disease (T2), translation of discoveries into the care of patients (T3), and translation to improve global health (T4).[22,23] An exciting new dimension to the continuum of CTSA-related investigation is community-based participatory research (CBPR).[24] The advent of CBPR promises to break down barriers between trialists and the community that they wish to serve by engaging community representatives in the planning of clinical trials. Investigators will need to build on the rigor and lessons learned from traditional clinical trials as CBPR projects are formulated and implemented.

REFERENCES

Constructing the Question and Clinical Trial Design

1. Lloyd-Jones D, Adams RJ, Brown TM, et al: Heart disease and stroke statistics—2010 update. A report from the American Heart Association. Circulation 121:e46, 2010.
2. Stanley K: Design of randomized controlled trials. Circulation 115:1164, 2007.
3. Stanley K: Evaluation of randomized controlled trials. Circulation 115:1819, 2007.
4. Krumholz HM: Outcomes research: Generating evidence for best practice and policies. Circulation 118:309, 2008.
5. Gauvreau K: Hypothesis testing: proportions. Circulation 114:1545, 2006.
6. Davis RB, Mukamal KJ: Hypothesis testing: Means. Circulation 114:1078, 2006.
7. Rao SR, Schoenfeld DA: Survival methods. Circulation 115:109, 2007.
8. Oakes D, Peterson DR: Survival methods: Additional topics. Circulation 117:2949, 2008.
9. Kaul S, Diamond GA: Making sense of non-inferiority: A clinical and statistical perspective on its application to cardiovascular clinical trials. Prog Cardiovasc Dis 49:284, 2007.
10. Connolly SJ, Ezekowitz MD, Yusuf S, et al: Dabigatran versus warfarin in patients with atrial fibrillation. N Engl J Med 361:1139, 2009.
11. Mehta C, Gao P, Bhatt DL, et al: Optimizing trial design: Sequential, adaptive, and enrichment strategies. Circulation 119:597, 2009.
12. Slutsky AS, Lavery JV: Data safety and monitoring boards. N Engl J Med 350:1143, 2004.

Key Issues During the Trial and Measurement of the Treatment Effect

13. Lagakos SW: The challenge of subgroup analyses—reporting without distorting. N Engl J Med 354:1667, 2006.
14. Larson MG: Descriptive statistics and graphical displays. Circulation 114:76, 2006.
15. Sullivan LM: Estimation from samples. Circulation 114:445, 2006.
16. Wiviott SD, Braunwald E, McCabe CH, et al: Prasugrel versus clopidogrel in patients with acute coronary syndromes. N Engl J Med 357:2001, 2007.
17. Ridker PM, MacFadyen JG, Fonseca FAH, et al: Number needed to treat with rosuvastatin to prevent first cardiovascular events and death among men and women with low low-density lipoprotein cholesterol and elevated high-sensitivity C-reactive protein: Justification for the use of statins in Prevention: An Intervention Trial Evaluating Rosuvastatin (JUPITER). Circ Cardiovasc Qual Outcomes 2:616, 2009.
18. Serruys PW, Morice MC, Kappetein AP, et al: Percutaneous coronary intervention versus coronary-artery bypass grafting for severe coronary artery disease. N Engl J Med 360:961, 2009.
19. Antman EM, DeMets D, Loscalzo J: Cyclooxygenase inhibition and cardiovascular risk. Circulation 112:759, 2005.
20. De Angelis C, Drazen JM, Frizelle FA: Clinical trial registration: A statement from the International Committee of Medical Journal Editors. N Engl J Med 351:1250, 2004.
21. Tse T, Williams RJ, Zarin DA: Reporting "basic results" in ClinicalTrials.gov. Chest 136:295, 2009.
22. Westfall JM, Mold J, Fagnan L: Practice-based research—"Blue Highways" on the NIH roadmap. JAMA 297:403, 2007.
23. Szilagyi PG: Translational research and pediatrics. Academic Pediatrics 9:71, 2009.
24. Horowitz CR, Robinson M, Seifer S: Community-based participatory research from the margin to the mainstream: Are researchers prepared? Circulation 119:2633, 2009.

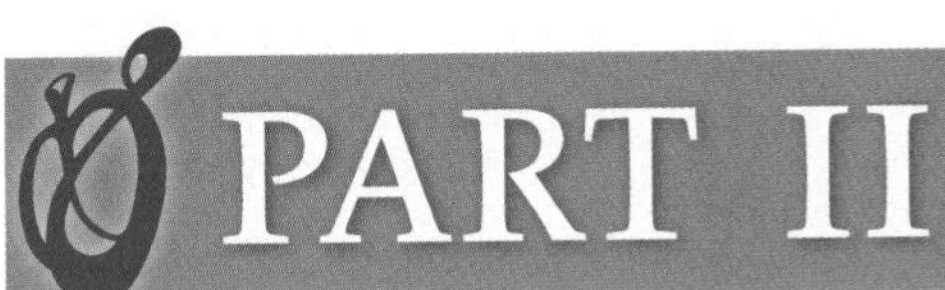

PART II

MOLECULAR BIOLOGY AND GENETICS

CHAPTER 7 Principles of Cardiovascular Molecular Biology and Genetics

Elizabeth G. Nabel

Molecular biology and genetics furnish the scientific underpinnings of cardiovascular medicine. Recent discoveries of the genetic bases and molecular pathways of cardiovascular disease have been extraordinary. We are learning about the pathophysiology of rare single-gene disorders as well as common, multigene diseases. New approaches, such as genome-wide association studies and large-scale DNA sequencing, have led to new gene discoveries that generate new hypotheses to be tested using molecular and cellular approaches.

This chapter highlights the basic principles of molecular biology and genetics. It is designed as a brief review and reference source, intended to prepare the reader for discussions of specific cardiovascular applications in other chapters in this text and in the contemporary literature. References are provided for general coverage of a topic.

Principles of Cell Biology and the Cell Cycle

All living organisms are composed of cells, and all cells arise from preexisting cells.[1,2] Cells are organized into compartments. Prokaryotes, such as bacteria, contain a single cell compartment bounded by a membrane or membranes. Eukaryotes, such as mammals, segregate genetic material into a nucleus that contains the genetic material, surrounded by a cytoplasm, bounded in turn by the plasma membrane that marks the periphery of the cell. The cytoplasm contains other discrete compartments, also bounded by membranes. Understanding the execution of genetic instructions in a cell requires consideration of the nature of the various compartments and how they function to create regions with different properties.

The mammalian cell is a highly compartmentalized structure (**Fig. 7-1**). The outer membrane, called the plasma membrane, is a lipid bilayer intended to exclude an aqueous environment, such as extracellular fluid. The plasma membrane is studded with a class of transmembrane proteins called receptors. A receptor has a binding site that recognizes some ligand on the exterior side of the membrane. Binding of the ligand usually triggers a change in the protein, which is transmitted to the cytoplasmic face by a conformational change in the receptor protein, or as movement of the whole protein into the interior. These events, in turn, trigger other changes within the cell and thus provide a means for responding to the environment. This type of relationship is called signal transduction.

The cytoplasm contains networks of membranes. Membrane sheets make up the endoplasmic reticulum (ER) and the Golgi apparatus. ER consists of a continuous sheet of highly folded membranes extending from the outer nuclear membrane, and can be divided into two types, which are part of the same membrane sheet. Rough ER has ribosomes, the small particles concerned with the synthesis of proteins, on its surface, whereas smooth ER does not. The Golgi apparatus consists of stacks of separate cisternae. Proteins that have been modified in the ER enter the Golgi apparatus, undergo further modifications, and then exit. The ER and Golgi apparatus sort proteins according to destination, using signals inherent in the protein sequence. This process of directing proteins to their final destination is called protein sorting or trafficking. Mitochondria are specialized organelles in the cytoplasm that generate energy stored in the form of adenosine triphosphate from the oxidation of carbon-containing compounds such as sugars or fats. Lysosomes are membrane-bound bodies that contain hydrolytic enzymes, which further process proteins and other macromolecules within the cell. Cell shape is determined by the cytoskeleton, which contains networks of protein fibers extending across and around the cell. The three classes of fibers are actin filaments, microtubules, and intermediate filaments.

The most important feature of the nucleus is genetic material. The nucleus has a granular microscopic appearance because of chromatin. Between cell divisions, chromatin forms a single dense mass. When a cell divides, its chromatin can be seen to consist of a discrete number of stringlike structures, called chromosomes. A common feature of cells, except those that have reached a final, specialized state of development (terminal differentiation), is their ability to divide. Many structural changes occur within a cell during division. Membranes and the cytoskeleton undergo extensive reorganization. The cell is organized by a new structure, called the spindle, which allows the distribution of chromosomes to daughter cells. These changes halt many of the former activities of the cell—gene expression, protein synthesis and secretion, and cell motility.

The cell cycle—the period between the release of a newly formed cell as a progeny of a division and its own division into two daughter cells—consists of two parts. Interphase, a relatively long period,

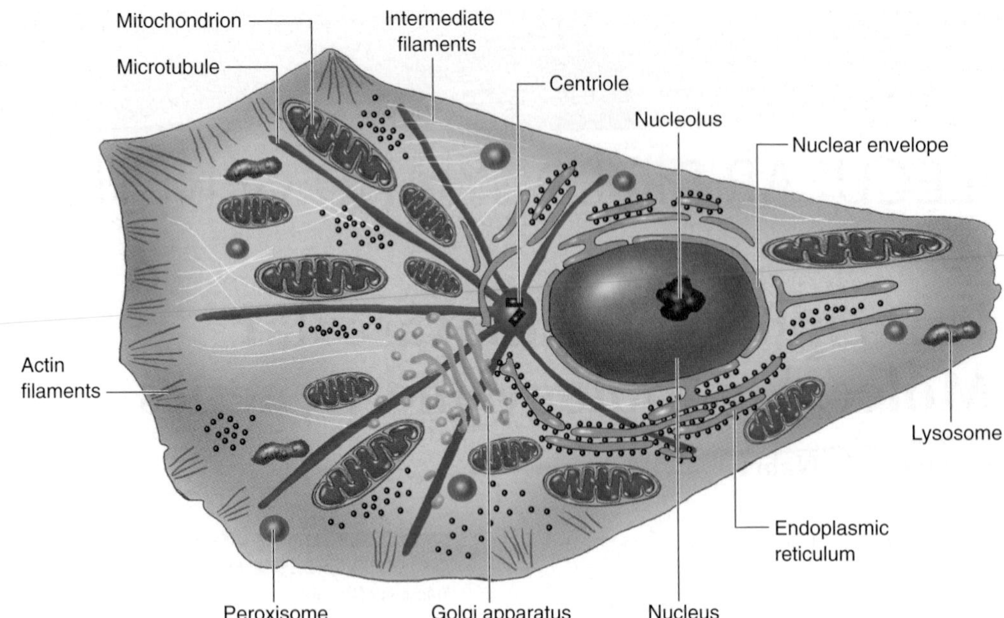

FIGURE 7-1 Schematic illustration of the structure of a mammalian cell, demonstrating structures common to most cells.

represents the time during which the cell engages in its synthetic activities and reproduces its subcellular components. During interphase, the cell has a discrete nuclear compartment, containing a compact mass of chromatin. During mitosis, a relatively short period of time, the actual division into two daughter cells occurs. The spindle replaces the internal organization of the cell and individual chromosomes become apparent. The products of the mitotic divisions that generate the organism are called the somatic cells. During embryonic development, many of the somatic cells proceed through the cell cycle. In the adult organism, many cells are terminally differentiated and no longer divide. They remain in a stationary phase in which there is no DNA synthesis, equivalent to a perpetual interphase.

Mitosis recapitulates the chromosome constitution of the cell. Each daughter cell starts its life with two copies of each chromosome. These copies are called homologues. The total number of chromosomes is called the diploid set and has 2n members (see Chap. 8). During interphase, a growing cell duplicates its chromosomal material. At the beginning of mitosis, each chromosome appears to split longitudinally to generate two copies, called sister chromatids. The cell now contains 4n chromosomes, organized as 2n pairs of sister chromatids. Mitosis consists of four phases—prophase, metaphase, anaphase, and telophase—ending in cytokinesis, in which the cell divides and each daughter cell has the same complete set of chromosomes, one member of each pair derived from each parent (**Fig. 7-2**). Each phase consists of distinct movements of the centromere, the central constriction region of the chromosome. These movements are essential to separation of the pairs of chromosomes into each daughter cell and completion of cell division.

Just before mitosis, double-stranded chromosomal breaks or other DNA damage is repaired by a series of cell cycle checkpoints. Under normal conditions, cellular DNA is repaired and the cell completes mitosis. Cells in which DNA is not repaired undergo apoptosis, or programmed cell death.[3] This mechanism allows the perpetuation of cell division in which chromosomal DNA is intact. Carcinogenesis can result when cell division escapes checkpoint control, and cells with double-stranded DNA break or other forms of damaged DNA divide uncontrollably.

The essential proteins in cell cycle checkpoint control are cyclins and cyclin-dependent kinases (CDKs; **Fig. 7-3**). CDKs are holoenzyme complexes that contain cyclin regulatory subunits and CDK catalytic subunits. Four distinct phases of the cell cycle are regulated by cyclin-CDK complexes—gap 1 or G1 phase, DNA replication or S phase, gap 2 or G2 phase, and mitosis or M phase. Restriction point control in the G1 phase is mediated by two CDKs, the cyclin D– and cyclin E–dependent kinases. The D-type cyclins (D1, D2, and D3) interact in combination with two catalytic partners, CDK4 and CDK6, early in G_1 to yield at least six holoenzymes expressed in tissue-specific patterns. Cyclin E enters into a complex with its catalytic partner CDK2 and collaborates with the cyclin D–dependent kinases to complete phosphorylation of the retinoblastoma tumor suppressor protein (Rb) late in G1, which results in transit through the G1-S checkpoint into S phase.

Endogenous inhibitors of the cyclins-CDKs, termed the *cyclin-dependent kinase inhibitors*, or CKIs, are expressed throughout G1 to inhibit phosphorylation and activation of cyclin-CDK complexes, resulting in G1 arrest. The CKIs function to prevent transition through the G1 checkpoint and inhibit mitosis, leading to growth arrest of cells. CKIs are classified into two families on the basis of their structures and CDK targets. The CIP/KIP proteins are broadly acting inhibitors that alter the activities of cyclin D–, cyclin E–, and cyclin A–dependent kinases. This family includes p21(Cip1), p27(Kip1), and p57(Kip2). All three contain characteristic motifs in their amino-terminal regions that bind cyclin and CDK substrates. p21(Cip1) functions as a downstream effector of the transcription factor and tumor suppressor gene, p53, to cause DNA damage repair and/or promote apoptosis.

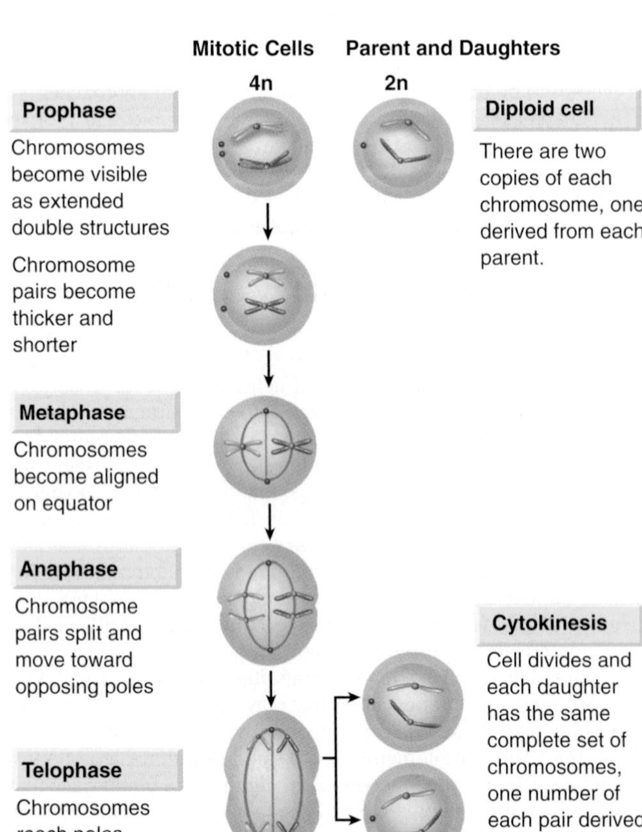

FIGURE 7-2 The process of mitosis in a mammalian cell, in which the genetic material is duplicated and distributed during cell division.

p27(Kip1) is a potent inhibitor of cell proliferation in normal and diseased tissues and is a critical mediator in tissue injury, inflammation, and wound repair. The INK4 (inhibitor of CDK4) family of proteins consists of INK4A (p16), INK4B (p15), INK4C (p18), and INK4D (p19). These CKIs contain multiple ankyrin repeats, bind only to CDK4 and CDK6 and not to other CDKs, and specifically inhibit the catalytic subunits of CDK4 and CDK6. The INK4 proteins are important regulators of tumor growth, but their role in cardiovascular disease is less well defined.

Injury to the heart or blood vessels leads to a remodeling process that is adaptive under normal conditions or maladaptive in conditions of disease pathophysiology (see Chaps. 25 and 43). In response to physiologic stimuli, vascular smooth-muscle cells (VSMCs) within the media proliferate and migrate into the intima to form a multilayered vascular wound, or neointima. Normally, this is a self-limited process that results in a well-healed vascular wound and preservation of luminal blood flow. In certain vascular diseases, however, VSMC proliferation becomes excessive, leading to a pathologic lesion in the blood vessel, which in turn produces clinical symptoms. These diseases often involve systemic or local inflammation, which exacerbates the VSMC proliferative response. The CIP/KIP CKIs are important regulators of tissue remodeling in the vasculature.[4] p27(Kip1) is constitutively expressed in VSMCs and endothelial cells of arteries and is downregulated after vascular injury or exposure of VSMCs and endothelial cells to mitogens. After a proliferative burst, VSMCs synthesize and secrete extracellular matrix molecules, which signal to VSMCs and endothelial cells, leading to induction of p27(Kip1) and p21(Cip1) and suppression of cyclin E-CDK2. Expression of the CIP/KIP CKIs leads to cell cycle arrest and inhibition of cell division.[5] p27(Kip1) is also an important regulator of tissue inflammation through its effects on T-lymphocyte proliferation. In the vasculature, p27(Kip1) mediates vascular repair through its regulation of proliferation, inflammation, and bone marrow progenitor cells. Genetic deletion of p27(Kip1) in mice results in a benign hyperplasia of epithelial and mesodermal cells in multiple organs, including the heart and vasculature.

p21(Cip1) is required for growth and differentiation in the heart, bone, skin, and kidney, and it confers susceptibility to apoptosis.[6] This CKI functions in a p53-dependent and p53-independent manner. In the heart, p21(Cip1) is expressed independently of p53 in cardiac myocytes; overexpression of p21(Cip1) within myocytes leads to hypertrophy.

Most human cancer cells sustain mutations that alter the functions of p53 or Rb by direct mutation of gene sequences or by targeting genes that act epistatically to prevent their normal function. Rb limits cell proliferation by preventing entry into the S phase. The mechanism is blockage of E2F transcription factors from activating genes required for DNA replication and nucleotide metabolism. p53 is mutated in more than 50% of human cancers. The protein accumulates in response to cellular stress from DNA damage, hypoxia, and oncogene activation. p53 initiates a transcriptional program that triggers cell cycle arrest or apoptosis. When activated by p53, p21(Cip1) induces apoptosis in tumor and other cells.

The cell cycle functions as the major regulator of cell division. DNA replication and cytokinesis depend on normal functioning of the cell cycle. The cyclins, CDKs, and CKIs are important mediators of carcinogenesis, tissue inflammation, and wound repair.

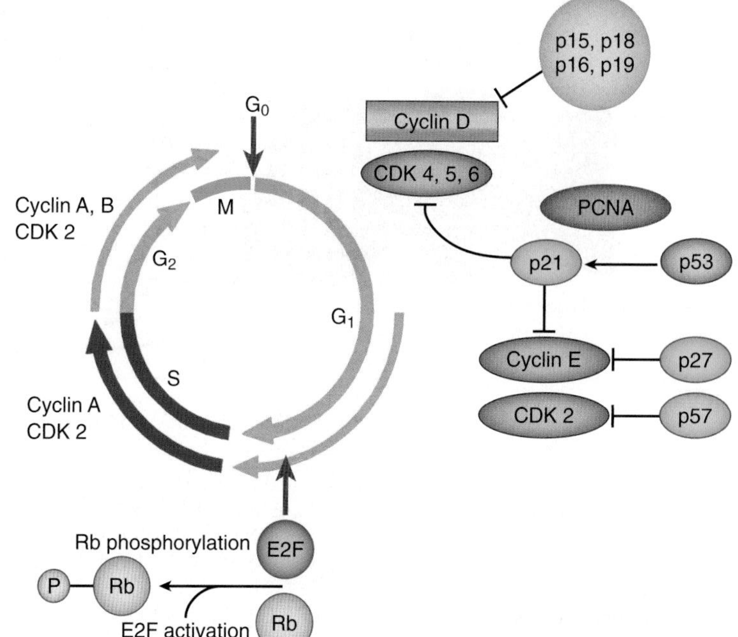

FIGURE 7-3 The mammalian cell cycle. The cyclins, cyclin-dependent kinases, and cyclin-dependent kinase inhibitors active in each phase are shown.

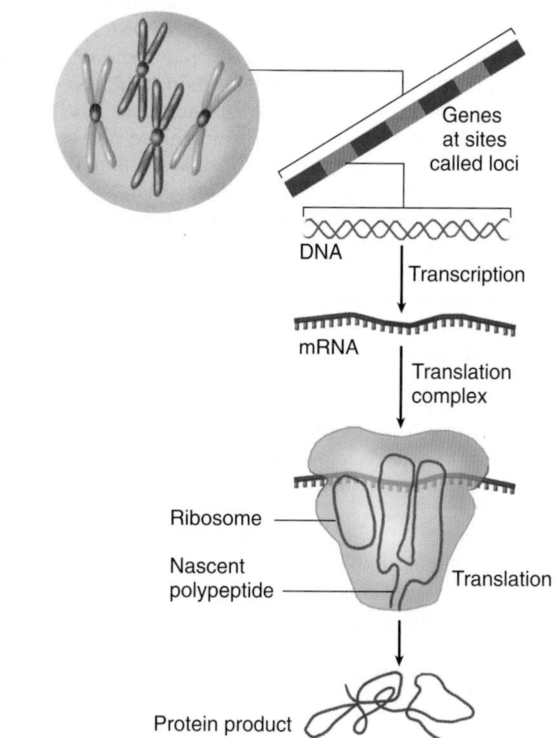

FIGURE 7-4 Depiction of the storage of genetic information in homologous chromosomes, which contain genes made up of DNA. Genetic expression involves transcription of DNA into RNA, which is translated on a ribosome into protein.

The Genetic Code: DNA, RNA, and Protein

DNA

DNA's double helical structure is deceptively simple, yet the rules encoded in this structure specify the form and function of all cells within an organism (**Fig. 7-4**). DNA consists of two long strands of polydeoxyribonucleotides that twist around each other clockwise to form an unbroken double helix. Alternating deoxyribose phosphate groups form the backbone of the helix, with the phosphate group making a 5′-3′ phosphodiester bond between the fifth carbon of one pentose ring and the third carbon of the next pentose ring (**Fig. 7-5**). Nucleic acid bases attached to the sugar groups of each strand face each other within the helix, perpendicular to the strand axis. The order of the nucleic acids specifies the eventual sequence of the protein product of the gene. There are four bases, the purines adenine and guanine (A and G) and the pyrimidines cytosine and thymine (C and T). During assembly of the double helix, a purine can pair only with a pyrimidine, and a pyrimidine with a purine. Each base pair (bp) forms one of the rungs in the twisted ladder of the DNA molecule, which can be millions of bases long. The two strands of DNA, which are held together by hydrogen bonds between complementary base pairs, have opposite chemical polarities. One strand is oriented in a 5′ to 3′ direction, whereas the other is in a 3′ to 5′ direction. Enzymes that recognize specific DNA sequences also recognize the polarity of

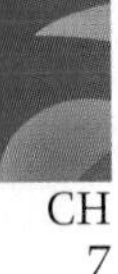

CH 7

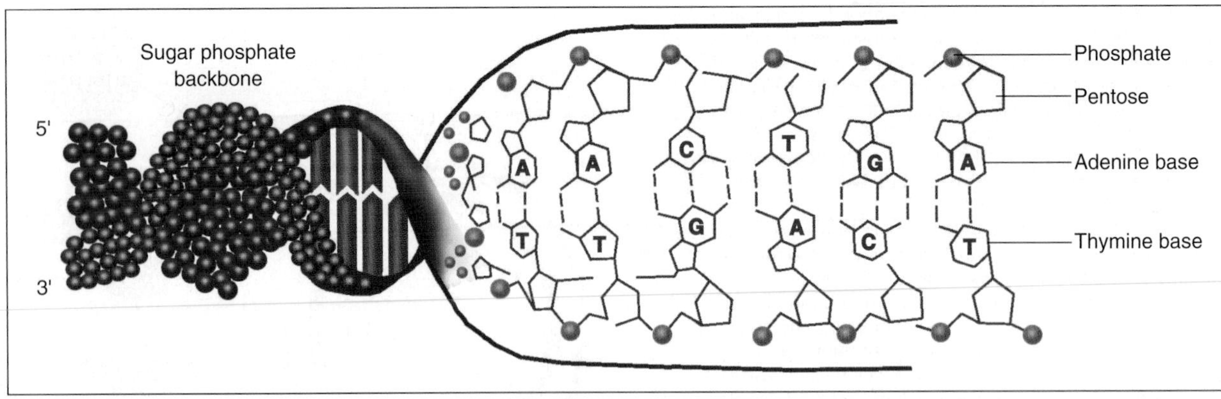

FIGURE 7-5 Schematic representation of the DNA double helix. The specificity of genetic information is carried in the four bases—guanine, adenine, thymine, and cytosine—that extend inward from a sugar phosphate backbone and form pairs with complementary bases on the opposing strand.

the strand. An enzyme "reads" the nucleotide sequences on the two strands in opposite directions. Because the structure of the helical backbone is invariant, enzymes responsible for DNA copying, cleavage, and repairing strand breaks can act anywhere along the length of the DNA strand.

An important consequence of the A-T and G-C pairing is that the sequence of nucleotides on one strand of the double helix determines the sequence on the complementary strand. This base pairing rule is critical for the storage, retrieval, and transfer of genetic material, whether it be for duplication of DNA into a daughter cell, repair of a damaged DNA strand, or reading as a template for RNA transcription.

Chromosomes are long double helical strands of DNA tightly coiled into compacted, discrete lengths by nuclear proteins. Each chromosome varies in length and base pair composition. In human cells, the nucleus contains 23 different pairs of chromosomes, each with a specific length and base pair sequence. The combined DNA sequences (approximately 3×10^9) on all the chromosomes within a cell comprise the genome.[7,8] The information carried in the genome is identical in all cells of an organism and varies little among members of a species. Indeed, the genome of humans is approximately 99% identical among individuals.[9]

During cell division, enzymes called polymerases unwind the DNA helix in each chromosome and copy each of the two strands separately along their entire length. Each daughter cell inherits a DNA molecule containing one old and one new strand. Each of these strands can in turn generate a new strand that faithfully reproduces the original template. This fidelity of DNA replication is essential for accurate transfer of genetic information. Errors in this process are a common source of gene mutations, which are inherited in successive rounds of cell division.

A gene is a section of base sequences used as a template for the copying process of transcription, and therefore is the fundamental unit of inherited DNA information. Genes comprise only a small fraction of the DNA carried on a chromosome. Only 1% to 2% of its bases encode proteins, and the full complement of protein-coding sequences still remains to be established. The human genome contains an estimated 30,000 distinct genes.[7,8] The protein coding information contained within a single gene is not continuous, but instead is encoded in multiple discontinuous packets called exons. Between these exons are variably sized stretches of DNA called introns. The function of these introns is not known. They probably contain the bulk of the regulatory information controlling the expression of the approximately 30,000 protein-coding genes, and other functional elements such as non–protein-coding genes and the sequence determinants of chromosome dynamics. Even less is known about the function of the roughly half of the genome consisting of highly repetitive sequences or of the remaining noncoding, nonrepetitive DNA.

RNA

Transcription, the first step in the expression of genetic information, serves to carry the genetic information out of the nucleus and into the cytoplasm, where the synthesis of proteins occurs. In this process, transcription of DNA to RNA requires the assembly of a template called messenger RNA (mRNA) in the nucleus (**Fig. 7-6**). A specialized enzyme called RNA polymerase copies one of the two DNA strands (the antisense strand), creating a complementary stretch of sequence that is an exact copy of the sense strand. RNA structure differs slightly from that of DNA. One of the RNA bases, uracil, replaces the DNA base thymine, and the RNA sugar phosphate component ribose replaces DNA deoxyribose. Ribose renders the RNA molecule much more susceptible to degradation than the more stable deoxyribose, which allows RNA to respond more rapidly to shifts in cellular signaling and move quickly to the cytoplasm for protein production.

From Genes to Proteins

The complex and highly regulated process of converting a gene to a protein involves two major steps, transcription of the DNA by RNA in the nucleus and translation of RNA into protein in the cytoplasm. Transcription begins in the nucleus by copying the DNA sequence of the gene into mRNA (see Fig. 7-6). The single-stranded RNA is modified at both ends. At the 5′ end, a nucleotide structure called a cap is added to increase translation efficiency by allowing ribosomes to bind to RNA. At the 3′ end, a nucleotide recognizes an A/T-rich sequence in a noncoding region and trims the transcript downstream by about 20 bp. An enzyme that adds a stretch of adenosine to form a polyA tail, which stabilizes the transcript, modifies the newly cleaved 3′ end. The transcript then undergoes splicing to remove intronic sequences. This is a highly regulated process, because unspliced transcripts are highly unstable and are cleared rapidly from the cell. Splicing is an important control point in gene expression; it must be absolutely precise, because the deletion or addition of a single nucleotide at the splice junction would throw the subsequent three-base codon translation of the RNA out of frame. The full significance of RNA splicing is not completely understood, but it must represent a critical point in the regulation of gene expression because of the large expanses of intron sequences and the inability of transcripts to leave the nucleus until their introns are removed.

Once in the cytoplasm, mRNA provides a template for translation or protein synthesis. Translation occurs on a macromolecular complex, like an assembly line, composed of ribosomes. The ribosomes read and translate the nucleotide sequence in mRNA into an amino acid sequence; that is, the four-base mRNA code is translated into the 20–amino acid alphabet of proteins. This genetic code is remarkably simple and has been conserved in most organisms. Every three RNA nucleotides encode for a single amino acid; the codon therefore is a triplet of bases. Permutations of the four RNA nucleotides result in 64 different triplets ($4 \times 4 \times 4$), so that any of the 20 amino acids can be specified by more than one codon. One of the triplets, AUG, specifies methionine, the amino acid that starts each protein. Three other triplets, UAA, UGA, and UAG, program the ribosome to end translation and are therefore called stop codons.

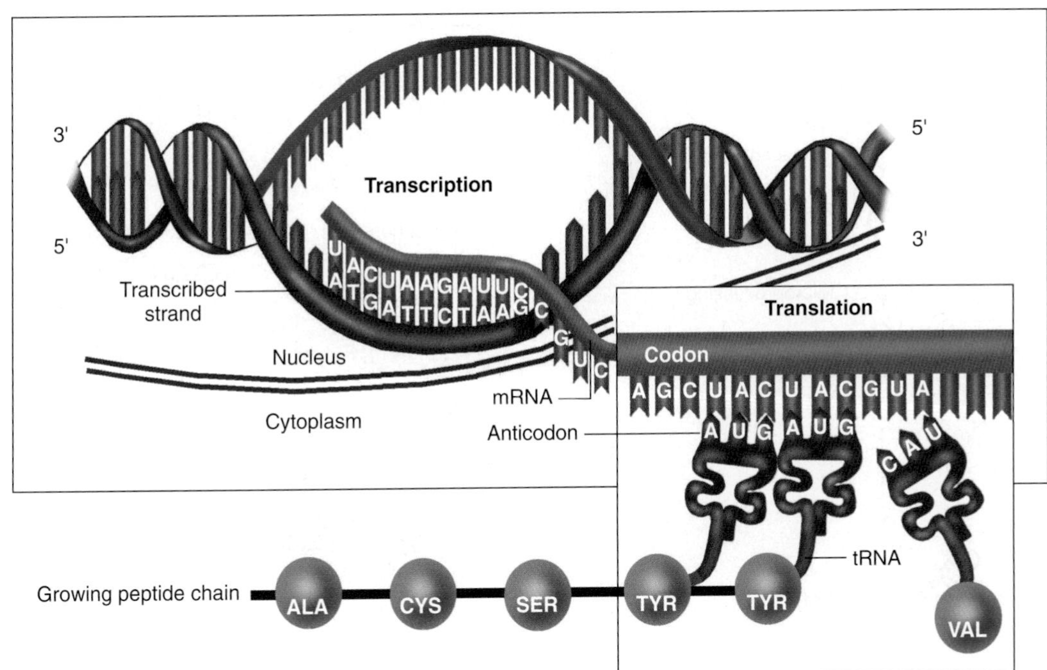

FIGURE 7-6 The flow of genetic information. Transcription in the nucleus creates a complementary ribonucleic acid copy from one of the DNA strands in the double helix. mRNA is transported into the cytoplasm, where it is translated into protein.

The conversion of a codon into an amino acid requires an adapter molecule, called transfer RNA (tRNA), to decode mRNA. Each tRNA uses a unique three-base sequence or anticodon to line up with the complementary codon in mRNA (see Fig. 7-6). Ribosomal enzymes link adjoining amino acids, which frees them from the tRNA adapters and adds them to the growing amino acid chain. The order of the amino acids is specified by the order of the codons on the corresponding mRNA template. Translation then completes the transfer of information from DNA in the nucleus to a unique protein structure.

Because the genetic code is preserved across species, human genetic sequences can be transferred into bacteria, yeast, or insect cells, where the sequences will be replicated and decoded into RNA and protein. This principle constitutes the basis of recombinant DNA technology, which is used to produce recombinant proteins for research and therapeutic purposes (e.g., tissue plasminogen activator).

The process of gene expression requires controlled and precise regulation at multiple steps. Only a small number of genes are expressed within a cell at a given time. One set of genes is constitutively expressed in most cells, referred to colloquially as housekeeping genes. These genes are necessary for cell replication, energy generation, and survival functions. A second set of genes is expressed in a lineage-specific manner (i.e., within certain cells); they are required for cell-specific functions such as contractility. The precise regulation of lineage-specific genes determines the unique identity and function of a particular cell. Another set of genes is induced in response to environmental stimuli. These are required to produce the complex and dynamic patterns of gene expression, which allow an organism to respond to internal and external signals.

Recently, post-transcriptional regulation by small noncoding RNAs, such as microRNAs (miRNAs), has emerged as a central regulator of many cardiovascular processes. miRNAs are a large class of evolutionarily conserved, small, noncoding RNAs, typically 20 to 26 nucleotides in length, that primarily function post-transcriptionally by interacting with the 3′ untranslated region (UTR) of specific target mRNAs in a sequence-specific manner.[10] The first animal miRNA was described in 1993 as a regulator of developmental timing in *Caenorhabditis elegans* (a roundworm). Recognition that miRNAs are widespread in all eukaryotes, including vertebrates, did not occur until 10 years later. More than 650 miRNAs are encoded in the human genome, and each is thought to target more than 100 mRNAs, resulting in mRNA degradation or translational inhibition. Interactions between miRNAs and mRNAs are thought to require sequence homology in the 5′ region of the miRNA, but significant variance in the degree of complementation in the remaining sequences allows a single miRNA to target a wide range of mRNAs, often regulating multiple genes within a common pathway. As a result, more than one third of mRNAs in the mammalian genome are thought to be regulated by one or more miRNAs. miRNAs regulate gene expression at the post-translational level by mRNA degradation, translation repression, or miRNA-mediated mRNA decay (**Fig. 7-7**). The transcription of miRNA genes is mediated by RNA polymerase II (pol II). Inside the nucleus, the pre-miRNA has a stem loop structure that is cleaved by the ribonuclease endonuclease Drosha, leaving a cleaved pre-miRNA that is exported from the nucleus. In the cytoplasm, the ribonuclease endonuclease Dicer further cleaves the pre-miRNA into a mature double-stranded miRNA, which is incorporated into the RNA-induced silencing complex (RISC), allowing preferential strand separation of the mature miRNA to repress mRNA translation or destabilize mRNA transcripts through cleavage or deadenylation.

Despite advances in miRNA discovery, the role of miRNAs in physiologic and pathophysiologic processes is just emerging. miRNAs play diverse roles in fundamental biologic processes, such as lineage development, cell proliferation, differentiation, apoptosis, stress response, and tumorigenesis. For example, identification of miRNAs expressing specific cardiac cell types has led to the discovery of important regulatory roles for these small RNAs during cardiomyocyte differentiation, cell cycle, and stages of cardiac hypertrophy in the adult, suggesting that miRNAs may be almost as important as transcription factors in regulating gene expression.[11] A similar story is developing for miRNA regulation of smooth-muscle cell fate and plasticity.[12]

Principles and Techniques of Molecular Biology

Recombinant DNA technologies developed in the 1970s as a response to the need for sufficient quantities of DNA for biochemical analysis. The method refers to the clipping of a segment out of surrounding DNA using sequence-specific endonucleases known as restriction

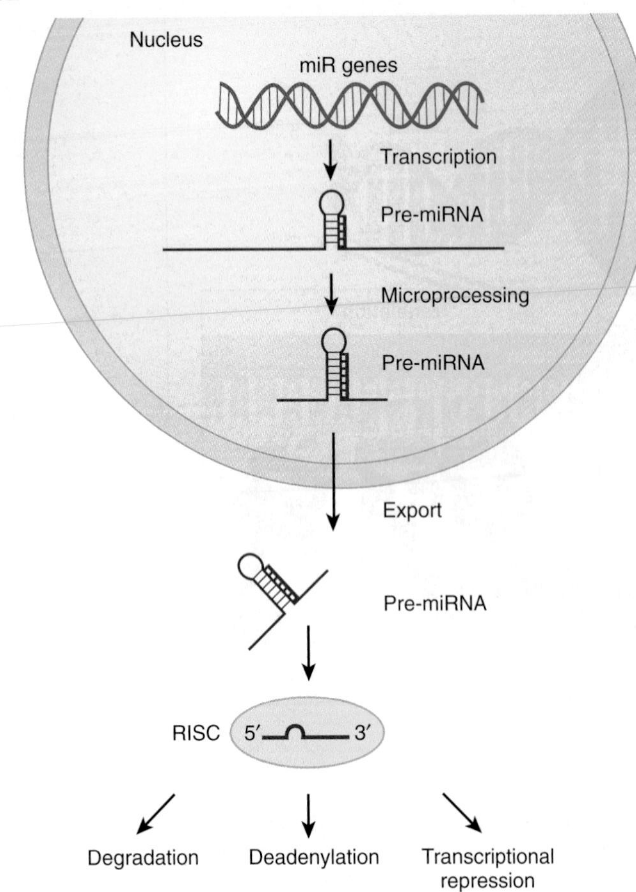

FIGURE 7-7 miRNA biogenesis and function. The process of miRNA within the nucleus and cytoplasm is shown (see text for details).

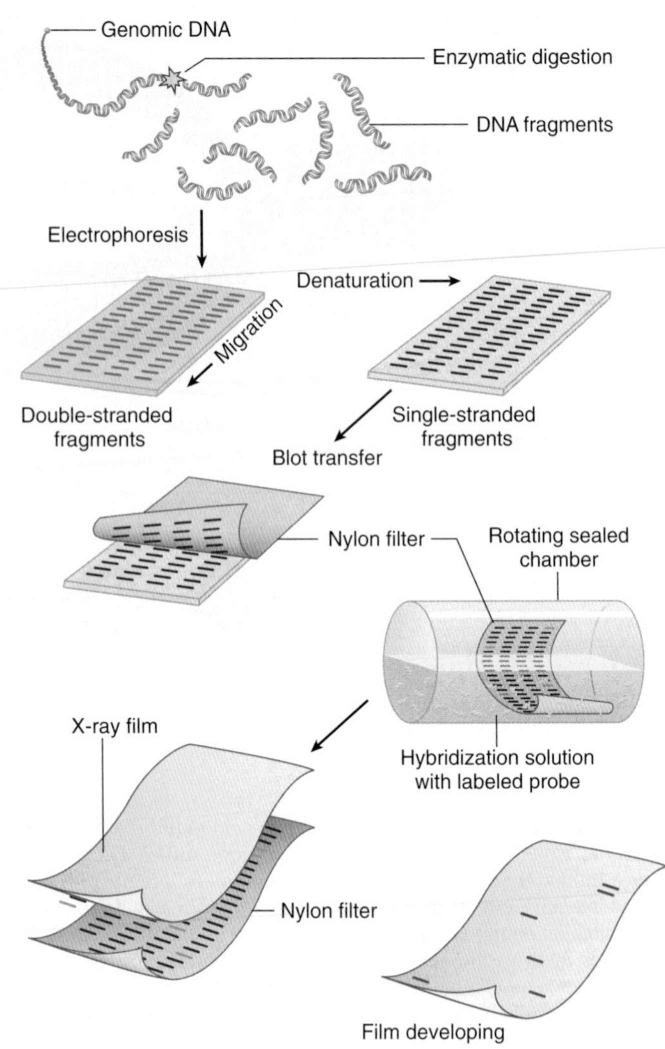

FIGURE 7-8 The process of Southern blotting to identify genomic DNA is shown.

enzymes. The segment can then be inserted at will into a vector that permits copying it millions of times (see later). The success of recombinant DNA techniques has fueled most of the advances in molecular biology over the past 40 years. These approaches are used routinely for the analysis of gene structure, expression, and organization, regulatory pathways whereby cells control gene expression, and discovery of novel genes and therapeutics. As a consequence, these advances have changed the face of medical research. For example, recombinant DNA technologies mass produce therapeutic proteins, such as recombinant tissue plasminogen activator. The techniques of molecular biology, like the structure of DNA itself, are surprisingly simple. The basic approaches are described here; see in-depth reviews for a primer on how to perform these techniques.[13]

Cloning DNA

Molecular cloning provides a means to produce millions of copies of a DNA sequence or gene within bacterial cells. A DNA fragment is first inserted into a cloning vector. The most commonly used vectors are small, circular DNA molecules called plasmids or bacterial viruses called phages. The vectors also contain genetic information that allows the bacterial cell to replicate the DNA sequence. After insertion of a DNA sequence, the plasmid or phage vector is introduced into a bacterial cell. The growing bacterial culture replicates the vector containing the DNA sequence in hundreds of copies per cell, yielding multiple identical clones of the original DNA sequence. The vectors are then harvested from the bacterial culture using the same restriction enzymes used to insert the DNA sequence into the vector.

The molecular biologist uses restriction endonucleases derived from bacteria as molecular scissors that cut DNA motifs at predictable sequences. Each restriction enzyme recognizes a specific nucleotide sequence. These recognition sites occur randomly along the DNA of any organism and consist of a short symmetric sequence motif called a palindrome, which is repeated in opposing orientation on both strands of the double-helix DNA. For example, the enzyme EcoRI from the bacteria *Escherichia coli* recognizes and cuts the sequence GAATTC in double-strand DNA at GA and AG junctions. Most restriction enzymes cleave their palindromic sequence asymmetrically, leaving a single-stranded overhang on each end of the cut. These "sticky" ends have unique and complementary sequences that can be used to connect a fragment of human DNA with complementary ends of DNA from another source. An enzymatic reaction connects the continuous double-stranded DNA to form a smooth splice. These principles are used to construct various DNA rearrangements for multiple purposes such as gene cloning, generating knockout mice, or constructing recombinant DNA therapies.

Blotting Techniques

Blotting is a tool that permits identification of DNA, RNA, or protein by its molecular size. Analysis of DNA is referred to as a Southern blot, RNA identification is a Northern blot, and protein isolation is a Western blot. The principles of blotting techniques are straightforward.[10] A mixture of molecules to be analyzed is subjected to gel electrophoresis, which separates different species according to size and/or electrical charge (**Fig. 7-8**). An agarose gel is used, in which the molecules are loaded into wells at one end. The gel is submerged into a buffer and subjected to an electrical current. The molecules migrate across the electrical field. Because DNA and RNA are acids that carry a negative charge, they migrate toward the positive pole of the gel. The agarose matrix hinders the migration of larger molecules so that the molecules also separate by size. When the electrophoresis is completed, the gel is removed from the buffer, and a nylon filter and dry absorbent material are placed on top. The buffer from the gel is blotted into the absorbent material, carrying with it the separated molecules, which remain on the nylon filter. The filter is treated to fix the molecules on its surface permanently, creating a mirror image of the original gel. The filter is then bathed with a tagged molecule (the probe) that recognizes (hybridizes to) the molecule of interest and washed to remove the unbound probe. For Southern (DNA) and Northern (RNA) blots, the probe is a small fragment of nucleic acid that carries a complementary sequence to the molecule being investigated. The nucleic acid is tagged with a radioactive element detectable by exposure to x-ray film or other techniques. The position of the hybridized probe, which appears as a band, provides an estimate of the size of DNA or RNA segment. By running parallel lanes of molecular markers of known size, the precise size of the DNA or RNA element is determined. For protein identification (Western blot), the probe consists of a tagged antibody that recognizes the target protein, and size markers are run to identify protein size.

Blotting techniques are also used for other purposes, including mapping the position of restriction sites in a specific gene following restriction enzyme digestion, and in cytogenetic analysis to compare restriction sites in genomic DNA from test and reference samples.

Polymerase Chain Reaction

The polymerase chain reaction (PCR) is an amplification procedure that takes place in a test tube (**Fig. 7-9**). The segment of DNA or RNA to be amplified is combined in a test tube with two short oligonucleotide primers (chemically synthesized single-stranded DNA fragments). The primers initiate the amplification, which then proceeds in a series of cycles in which the original DNA, called the template, is separated into single strands. The separation of the strands allows the primers to bind or anneal to the respective complementary sequences at each end of the single strands. A heat-stable DNA polymerase enzyme adds nucleotide bases at the ends of each primer, reading across the single DNA strand and generating a complementary copy. By the time the polymerase has reached the end of the single strand, a new double-stranded sequence has been generated. The cycle begins again, heating and separating the double strand, followed by the generation of a new strand by the primer and polymerase. Each round of PCR amplification doubles the number of DNA templates. Creating millions of copies of a DNA segment is possible in several hours by PCR, even when the starting material is a single copy of DNA. The entire amplification is carried out in a sealed test tube or well in a specially designed machine that can be programmed to heat and cool the sample automatically. PCR has now become a commonplace tool to generate a sufficient quantity of identical genetic material for analysis.

Principles of Molecular Genetics

Genotype and the Identification of Disease-Causing Genes

The discovery of the structure and function of DNA in 1953 laid the foundation for molecular genetics.[14] Sequencing of the human genome added to this tool kit.[7,8] Physicians and scientists have molecular genetics tools with which they can pursue diagnoses and treatments. Three concepts are important: genotype, genomics, and proteomics. Genotype is the composite of DNA sequences within an individual's set of genes, or the complete sequence of an individual's DNA on all 23 pairs of chromosomes. Genomics is the expression of gene sequences as RNA; its focus is on which genes are expressed. Proteomics is the study of proteins expressed within a cell or organism, and seeks to understand the networks of protein-protein interactions.

Historically, the field of genetics focused on monogenic disorders—that is, diseases caused by a single-gene deletion or mutation (see Chap. 8). With the newer tools of genomics and proteomics, attention has turned to the evaluation of genetic susceptibility to complex disease traits, such as coronary artery disease and diabetes. Understanding the genetic basis of complex diseases requires knowledge of gene sequences, proteins encoded by the genes, and functions of the proteins. However, it is becoming increasingly clear that complex cardiovascular problems will not be resolved solely by deriving the nucleotide sequence of the human genome or by unraveling the approximately 30,000 loci that encode the corresponding proteins or

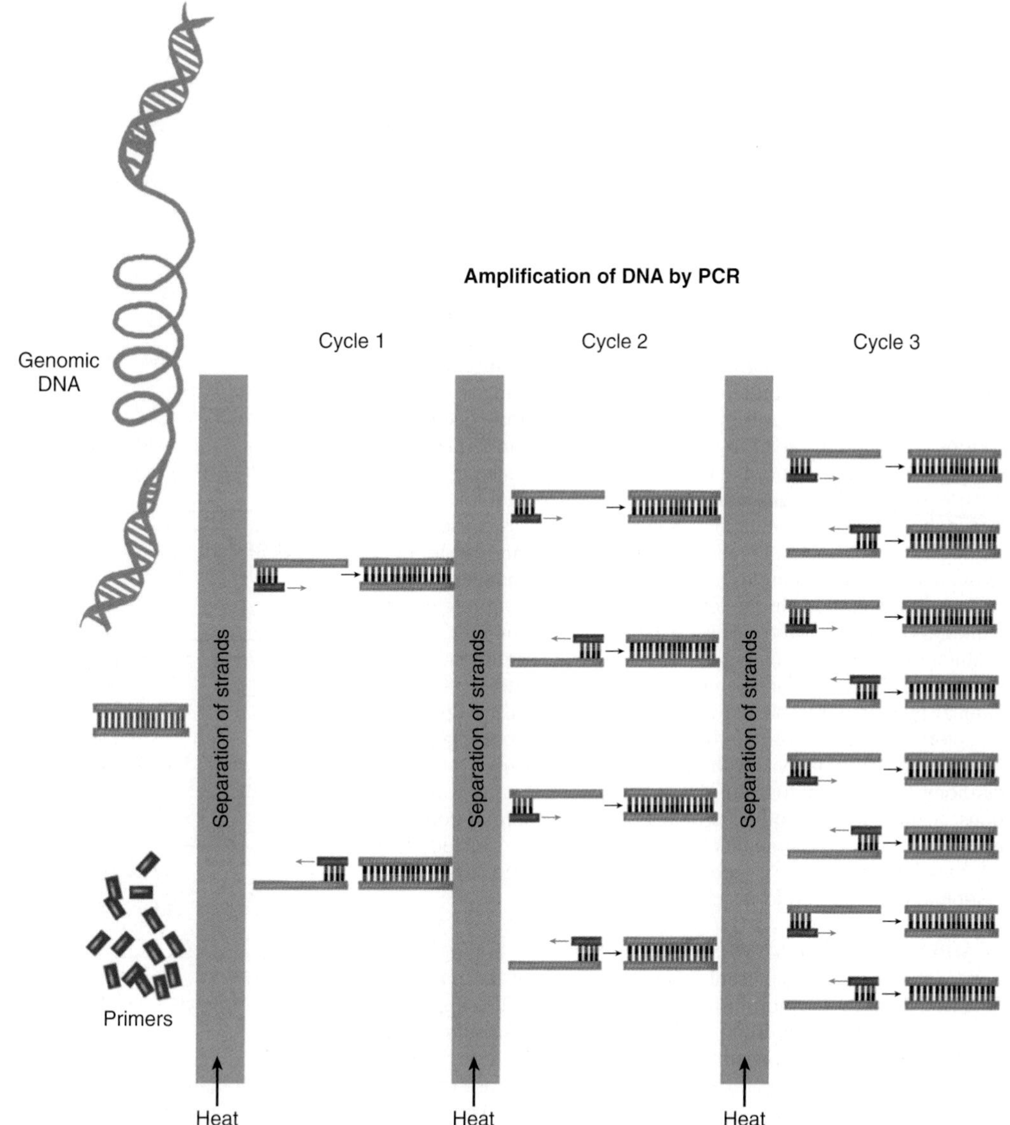

FIGURE 7-9 DNA amplification with the polymerase chain reaction (PCR). Synthetic primers corresponding to the 5′ and 3′ ends of the DNA sequence are chemically synthesized. The double-stranded DNA is melted by heating to 92°C, followed by cooling to 72°C to anneal the primers. A heat-stable DNA polymerase amplifies each strand of the target sequence, producing two copies of the DNA sequence. The process is repeated multiple times to achieve amplification of the target sequence.

regulate other genes. Considerable work is required to define the molecular mechanisms precisely whereby changes in an individual gene or set of genes specifies or confers risk for a specific disease.

MONOGENIC DISORDERS. Medical genetics has classically focused on single-gene or monogenic diseases, in which the cause is traced to a missing or mutated gene. An excellent resource is Online Mendelian Inheritance in Man (OMIM), which contains information on all known mendelian disorders and over 12,000 genes.[15] Monogenic disorders (see Chap. 8) are rare and typically are inherited in a mendelian or autosomal manner. Interestingly, our understanding of the mechanism whereby single genes cause disease, even though these mechanisms are uncommon, has led to an understanding of the pathogenesis of more common cardiovascular diseases.

The role of genetic factors in cardiovascular disease is reviewed in more detail elsewhere (see Chap. 8). Briefly, each gene exists in two copies, known as alleles. An individual is homozygous at a given locus if the two alleles are identical, or heterozygous if the alleles are different. A genotype comprises an individual's set of alleles and constitutes the genetic factors that create a phenotype. A phenotype is the visible or measurable properties resulting from a genotype, such as coronary artery disease or obesity. Phenotype can also be defined as the effect of gene action, whether caused by a single gene or the entire genotype.

Differences in nucleotide sequences, either between two individuals or among all individuals within a population, constitute genetic variation. Differences that arise in nucleotide sequences and lead to a structural change in the proteins they encode are called mutations. A mutation is defined as occurring in less than 1% of a given population. Examples of mutations include missense, nonsense, frame shift, deletion, and insertion (**Fig. 7-10**). Missense mutations result from substitutions of one or more nucleotides in such a way as to change the primary sequence of the encoded protein. They alter the function of the protein by changing its primary structure. A nonsense mutation introduces a premature stop codon into a gene, resulting in a truncated gene product that can display alterations in function and be unstable. Insertions or deletions of nucleotides add or subtract amino acids from the resulting proteins, if the nucleotide changes lead to an addition or deletion of a triplet. Frame shift mutations occur when codons of a gene are read in the wrong reading frame. These mutations typically cause abnormal protein structure because of the introduction of out-of-frame termination codons, which lead to premature termination of proteins. Mutations in introns and exons cause splicing errors that also lead to alterations in protein structure or premature termination. Finally, mutations in the promoters or enhancers of genes can lead to alterations in the levels of expression of a protein or the temporal or spatial patterns of gene expression of a protein.

Mutations in single genes lead to monogenic cardiovascular diseases (see Chap. 8). For example, although the primary defect in familial hypercholesterolemia is a deficit of low-density lipoprotein receptors (LDLRs), more than 600 mutations in the LDLR gene have been identified in patients with this disorder.[16] Similarly, hypertrophic cardiomyopathy, an autosomal dominant disease, is caused by mutations in the genes encoding proteins of the myocardial contractile apparatus.[17] Other monogenic cardiovascular disorders include familial long-QT syndrome,[18] venous thrombosis caused by factor V Leiden,[19] and inherited forms of hypertension.[20]

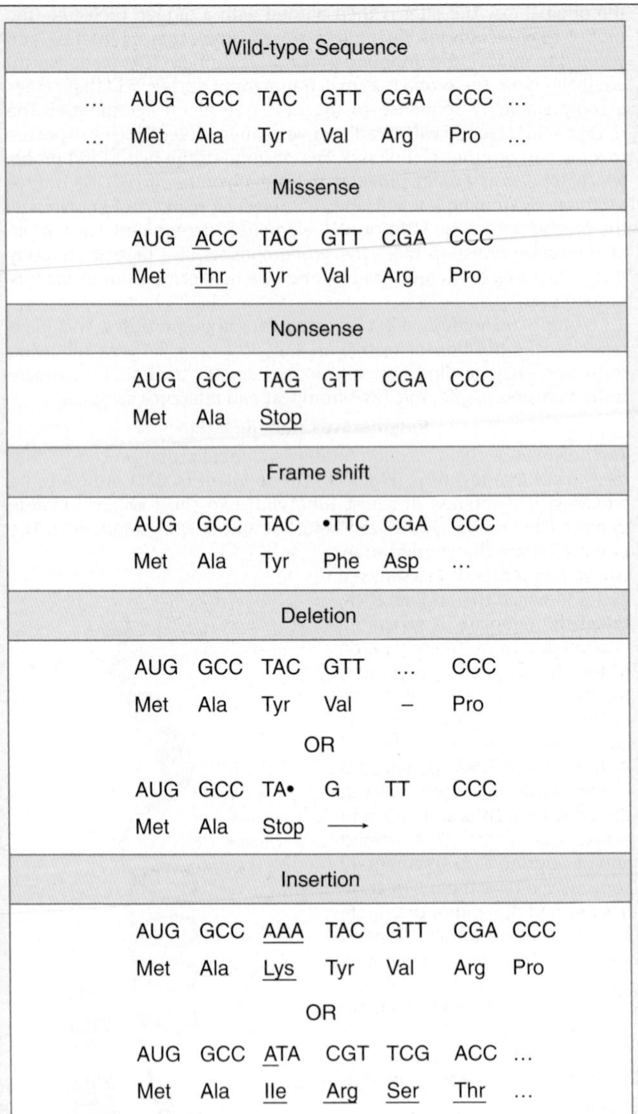

FIGURE 7-10 Different types of mutations that alter the structure and expression of human genes.

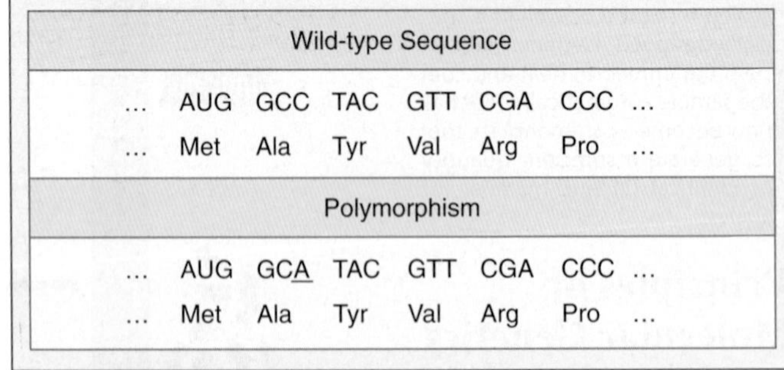

FIGURE 7-11 A polymorphism is a nucleotide substitution that does not alter the primary amino acid structure of the resulting protein.

COMPLEX TRAIT ANALYSIS. Polymorphisms are common variations, defined as being present in more than 1% of the population. Single-nucleotide polymorphisms (SNPs) are nucleotide substitutions that do not alter protein structure (**Fig. 7-11**). SNPs are useful markers to map genes to chromosomal loci. An SNP may be a marker of disease susceptibility (i.e., it can associate with a disease caused by a direct effect of the SNP on the disease or linkage with a nearby susceptibility locus). Putative and confirmed SNPs are accessible through the dbSNP, a public database maintained by the National Center for Biotechnology Information.[21]

A haplotype is a set of SNPs grouped in a contiguous genetic region and inherited en bloc in a given population. Haplotypes may have a true association with a disease or may only appear to be associated because of confounding factors. If an SNP is associated with a disease, it is likely that the SNP is inherited as part of a haplotype in which other SNPs are also statistically associated with the disease. This nonrandom association of alleles is called linkage disequilibrium. Linkage disequilibrium exists when alleles at two distinct locations in the genome are inherited together more frequently than expected.

Because an SNP may be a marker rather than a cause of disease, proof of causality requires demonstration of altered gene function.

An international effort has identified all SNPs on all 22 somatic chromosomes in 300 individuals from diverse backgrounds in Asia, Africa, Europe, and the Americas. This project, called the Haplotype Map, or HapMap, was initiated to construct a genome-wide map of SNP clusters on the basis of DNA samples from different human populations, and it was completed in 2005.[9] The HapMap provides an SNP road map for performing linkage analysis, association studies, and evaluation of SNP partners for contribution to a disease. SNPs, then, provide insight into the genetic basis for disease for several reasons—direct causal agents of altered gene function, markers of disease, regardless of causality, and genome-wide markers for genetic studies, because of their presence at high density throughout the genome.

LINKAGE ANALYSIS AND ASSOCIATION STUDIES. Two types of genetic studies examine inheritance—linkage analysis and association studies. Linkage studies are performed in families to study coinheritance of two traits passed down from parent to child. SNP analyses are used because these markers can reveal coinheritance of two traits or alleles in close proximity to each other on a chromosomal locus. The genes encoding the two traits typically reside in close proximity, and hence the alleles are linked. Linkage is determined by an LOD score, the logarithm of the odds that markers are linked at a particular distance, divided by the odds that they are linked at 50% coinheritance (not linked at all). Linkage analysis is commonly used to identify and study mendelian traits. Allele-sharing methods are also used to compare similarity of alleles in closely affected individuals, such as sibling pairs.

Population-based association studies are useful for investigations of common disorders without clear mendelian inheritance. Association studies often use a case-control approach in which experimental and reference groups are compared. Careful consideration of the most appropriate control population is necessary to draw valid conclusions and infer gene function from these studies. Case-control studies should be sufficiently powered with a large enough sample size to achieve statistical significance. In this approach, known SNPs in candidate genes are investigated using the alleles of a given SNP as variables, which are then associated with the presence or absence of disease or a particular outcome. If SNPs in a candidate gene are not known, the gene is directly sequenced in a subset of the study and in control populations to determine which SNPs are differentially represented in the two populations. Confirmation of SNPs is then performed in the remainder of the population using PCR-based techniques. Validation requires testing the association in an independent cohort. A limitation of the association approach is the bias inherent in selection of candidate genes. Only those genes known or of interest are often chosen for investigation. In contrast, identification of genes by positional cloning has frequently led to unanticipated discoveries.

GENOME-WIDE ASSOCIATION STUDIES. A genome-wide association approach is a study that surveys most of the genome for causal genetic variants.[22] Because no assumptions are made about the genomic location of the causal variants, the approach exploits the strength of association studies without having to guess the identity of the causal genes. Genome-wide association studies (GWAS) represent an unbiased yet comprehensive approach, even in the absence of convincing evidence regarding the function or location of causal genes.[23-25]

Genome-wide scans of SNPs are performed on high-throughput platforms and simultaneously assay hundreds of thousands or even millions of SNPs. By taking advantage of the physical distribution of SNPs throughout the genome, chromosomal regions between SNPs can be associated with a disease using statistical methods. Using this approach, investigators have discovered novel SNPs within or in close proximity to genes that cause or are associated with diseases, often complex cardiovascular diseases.[26-29] Often, these SNP discoveries have led to the generation of hypotheses regarding disease causation that require replication, validation, and follow-up functional studies. Data from GWAS funded by the National Institutes of Health are available in a public database called dbGaP (database genotype and phenotype), maintained by the National Center for Biotechnology Information.[30,31] Investigators will use GWAS combined with large-scale DNA sequencing to study genetic susceptibility to complex cardiovascular diseases, genetic modifiers of diseases, and gene-environment interactions.

Genomics

Genomics is the study of gene function through the parallel measurements of genomes, most commonly using the techniques of microarrays and serial analysis of gene expression (SAGE). Microarray usage in drug discovery is expanding, and its applications include basic research and target discovery, biomarker determination, pharmacology, toxicogenomics, target selectivity, development of prognostic tests, and disease subclass determination.

The basic technique involves extraction of RNA from biologic samples in normal or test states (**Fig. 7-12**).[32] The RNA is copied while incorporating fluorescent nucleotides or a tag that is later stained with fluorescence. The labeled RNA is then hybridized to a microarray, the excess is washed off, and the microarray is scanned under laser light. The end result is 4000 to 5000 measurements of gene expression per biologic sample. Because a complete experiment might involve hundreds of microarrays, the resultant RNA expression data sets can vary greatly in size.

cDNA MICROARRAYS. cDNA (complementary DNA) microarrays are created from probe cDNA libraries (500 to 5000 bases) by spotting a cDNA corresponding to an individual gene or probe at a precise location on a microscope slide. Each microarray measures two samples and provides a relative measurement level for each RNA molecule. Target RNAs labeled with a fluorescent dye are hybridized to the cDNA microarray surface, along with a control sample. The two RNA samples compete for binding to each probe. RNA that matches the cDNA sequence hybridizes to the cDNA spot on the microscope slide. The fluorescent labels are laser activated, and the signal intensities from fluorescent probes binding cDNA spots are compared. The comparison reflects the ratios of RNA abundance for each expressed gene. Normalization strategies that allow for the standardization of interarray comparisons are applied, followed by analytic methods (see earlier).

OLIGONUCLEOTIDE ARRAYS. Oligonucleotide arrays are created by the attachment of synthetic nucleotide probes (12- to 80-mer oligonucleotides) representative of unique portions of genes to an array surface. cDNA is synthesized from the experimental mRNA sample, followed by an in vitro transcription step to create biotin-labeled cRNA, which hybridizes to the microarray target. The microarray is treated with a fluorescent dye tagged to avidin (a protein that binds tightly to biotin) and subjected to laser activation. With oligonucleotide arrays, each microarray

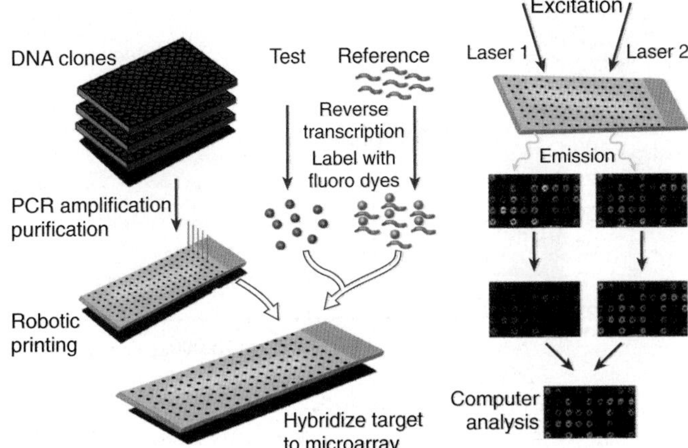

FIGURE 7-12 Detection of differential expression of mRNA from cells or tissues using gene expression profiling. After mRNA is isolated from cells or tissues, it is analyzed by hybridization to fluorescent-labeled cDNA clones imprinted onto a microscope slide. The fluorescent labels are laser-activated, and the signal intensities from fluorescent probes binding cDNA spots are compared.

measures a single sample and provides an absolute measurement level of each RNA molecule. Signal intensities are measured as a reflection of expression level for each gene.

SAGE. SAGE is a technique for characterization of gene expression based on direct sequencing of transcripts. Its major strength is determination and analysis of transcripts when the sequence is unknown. SAGE requires approximately 10-fold larger quantities of mRNA for analysis and hence is much more labor intensive than some array platforms, even with automated sequencers, because the simplest two-sample comparison requires sequencing of approximately 1.5×10^6 bases. This factor alone poses difficulties when RNA abundance is low, whereas a major advantage is its higher sensitivity for changes in expression level.

After acquisition of data by image processing, data are analyzed in three steps—normalization, filtering, and computation. Normalization accounts for technical factors, such as array manufacturing, differences in dye incorporation, and irregularities in probe distribution during hybridization, and is performed to allow meaningful comparisons among individual arrays. Filtering of data refers to the selection of those data likely to represent significant findings. Typical criteria for filtering include assessment of signal quality and the degree of change in gene expression level. Differential gene expression in microarray analysis is often defined by a 1.5- to 2-fold difference in relative gene expression level.

Determination of similarity and dissimilarity is a critical component of data analysis. Two general approaches are used, supervised and unsupervised. Supervised methods are used for finding genes with expression levels that are significantly different among groups of samples and finding genes that accurately predict a characteristic of the sample. Two commonly used supervised techniques include nearest neighbors and support vector machines. Users of unsupervised methods try to find internal structure or relationships in a data set instead of trying to determine how best to predict a correct answer. Four commonly used unsupervised techniques include hierarchical clustering, self-organizing maps, relevance networks, and principal component analysis. These computational approaches are then followed by a statistical analysis. Microarray data require validation by independent testing of RNA expression levels using quantitative reverse transcription PCR or conventional Northern blotting techniques.

Proteomics

Proteomics is the study of proteins expressed by the genome.[33] Genomics and proteomics should be viewed as complementary components of the genetic spectrum, beginning with DNA and ending with modified proteins. Proteins are the final product of the human genome and ultimately define human biology. Proteins are responsible for biologic form and function. Scientists have estimated that there are six to seven times as many proteins as genes (~200,000) in humans because of splicing, exchange of structural cassettes among genes during transcription, and post-translational modifications. The field of proteomics seeks to understand the complex interactions of all proteins expressed in a tissue or organism under normal or perturbed conditions.

There are five basic elements to any proteomic analysis—sample acquisition, protein extraction, protein separation, protein sequence determination, and sequence comparison to reference data bases for protein identification. Sample acquisition is straightforward and involves obtaining a tissue biopsy or fluid sample from an individual (under informed consent). Protein extraction is generally performed by chemical methods, generally with methanol, to remove all DNA, RNA, carbohydrates, and lipids. Extracted proteins must be separated for identification, and this step has traditionally been performed by two-dimensional gel electrophoresis. In the first dimension, proteins are separated by mass; in the second dimension, they are separated by isoelectric point or net charge. Because most spots on a two-dimensional gel contain multiple protein constituents, alternate methods for separating and identifying proteins, including liquid chromatography, have evolved. Liquid chromatography uses solid- and liquid-phase media to separate proteins according to biochemical properties, including molecular mass, isoelectric point, and hydrophobicity. These liquid chromatography separations can be performed in series to improve resolution. Other types of chromatographic columns can be used to improve sensitivity and specificity, such as affinity chromatography, in which a column contains antibodies specific to certain functions to achieve the desired separation. Following separation, the protein is identified, generally using some form of mass spectrometry (**Fig. 7-13**). Mass spectrometry converts proteins or peptides to charged species that can be separated on the basis of their mass-to-charge ratio. Several mass spectrometry ionization methods are in use, including electrospray ionization and matrix-assisted laser desorption ionization (MALDI). Peptide sequences identified with these methods must next be analyzed by comparison with known data base sequences to determine the unequivocal identity of the protein.

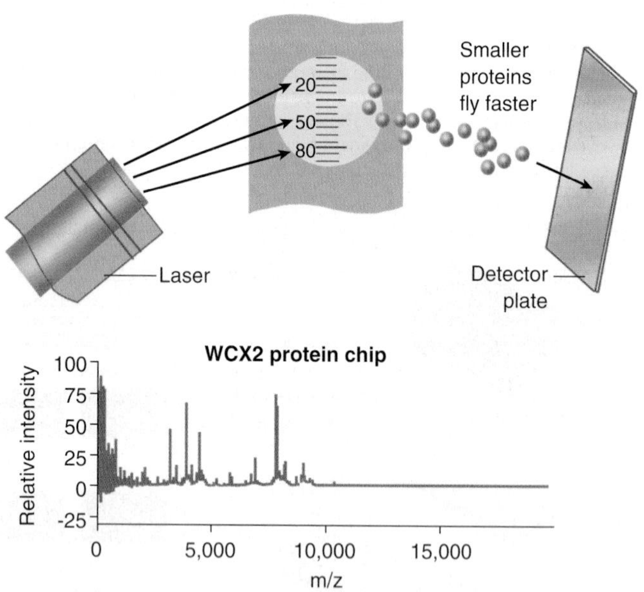

FIGURE 7-13 Mass spectrometry to identify separated proteins. A sample of serum or plasma is applied to the surface of a protein-binding chip, and the chip is irradiated with a laser from which bound proteins are launched as ions. A time of flight to detection by an electrode is a measure of the mass-to-charge ratio (m/z) of the ion. The center panel represents the detector plate, where ions separate by time of flight, biochemical property, and size. The numbers represent protein size (in kDa).

Once proteins in a given proteome have been identified, their relative abundance levels are determined to compare relative abundance of proteins in a normal or diseased state. Finally, a thorough analysis of a proteome should include some measure of function, whether in cultured cells or in animal models. This approach is similar to functional genomic analysis, in which it is critical to gauge the importance of a gene or mutation through determination of gene function.

Proteomic analysis is currently limited by sensitivity, specificity, and throughput. However, this field and its methodologies are developing rapidly. The application of proteomics to cardiovascular disease holds great promise for understanding the function of the cardiovascular system in all its complexity.

Genetic Modification of Mice to Study Human Cardiovascular Disease

The techniques for generating genetically modified mice have had a tremendous impact on cardiovascular research. The mouse is a small animal with a short gestation period (21 days). However, there is remarkable conservation of the molecular pathways that control cardiovascular development and function between mice and humans. Similar genes and signaling pathways regulate the development of the heart and vasculature in both species. With completion of the sequencing of the mouse and human genomes, comparative genetics is now possible. Thus, genetically modified mice have become an essential animal model to study cardiovascular genetics, developmental biology, and physiology. Limitations of mouse models to study human cardiovascular disease are evident, but because of the simplicity of genetic manipulation in the mouse, it has become a standard starting place for hypothesis testing before evaluation in a larger animal. This section briefly describes the principles of four approaches to genetic modification in the mouse—transgenics, gene deletion or knockout, conditional knockout, and studies of mouse physiology.

Transgenic Mice

Creation of a transgenic mouse involves four steps: cloning of the gene of interest; fusion of the gene to transcriptional regulatory sequences that program its expression in all tissues of the mouse or in specific tissues; injection of the purified transgene into the male pronucleus of a fertilized one-cell mouse embryo; and reimplantation of the injected embryo into a foster mother. The injected transgene randomly integrates into a chromosome of the fertilized embryo, resulting in a founder mouse that expresses the injected transgene and passes the transgene to 50% of its progeny. Comparative studies can then be performed between the transgenic mouse and a nontransgenic littermate mouse as a control. Similar techniques have been used to create transgenic rabbits, rats, and pigs.

Refinements of these techniques have assisted more sophisticated transgenic models. Cell-specific promoters program transgene expression exclusively in cardiomyocytes, endothelial cells, and vascular smooth-muscle cells, creating a transgenic mouse with restricted expression in the cardiovascular system. Although overexpression of a transgene results in a gain of function, it is also possible to eliminate the function of a single gene by overexpressing a dominant negative mutant of that gene, the encoded protein of which interferes with the function of the wild-type protein. Expression of a transgene can also be turned on or off by administration of a simple drug such as tetracycline using a tet operon system. These mice allow precisely timed transgene expression as well as a comparison in the same animal of the phenotypes of transgene on and off states.

Gene Inactivation or Knockout Approaches

Gene deletion is a complementary approach to transgenesis for studying the role of a specific gene in mouse development and physiology (**Fig. 7-14**). In gene deletion studies, the expression of one or more genes is knocked out to produce a loss-of-function mutant mouse. The knockout approach involves the following: construction of a targeting vector containing the gene of interest with a deletion or nonsense mutation; transfection of a pluripotent mouse embryonic stem cell with the targeting vector; homologous recombination between the targeting construct and one copy of the endogenous gene, producing an embryonic stem cell with a homozygous deletion of the gene of interest; injection of the mutant embryonic stem cell into a fertilized mouse blastocyst; and implantation of the blastocyst into a foster mother. The resulting mouse pup is a chimera in which all tissues, including the gonads, are derived in part from the mutant embryonic stem cells and in part from the wild-type cells of the injected blastocysts. This chimeric animal is bred to a wild-type animal, and fertilization of a wild-type egg with a mutant sperm from the chimera produces a heterozygous knockout mouse in which one copy of the gene of interest in all cells is mutant and the other copy is wild type. Heterozygous animals are then bred with each other to produce homozygous knockouts that have deletions of the gene of interest in all cells. The absence of the gene in the knockout animal produces a specific phenotype that reveals the direct function of the gene in development and normal and perturbed physiology. Creation of a knockout mouse is technically more challenging than transgenesis and often takes 9 to 12 months to complete.

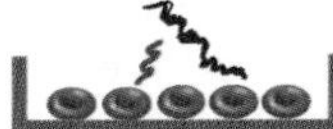

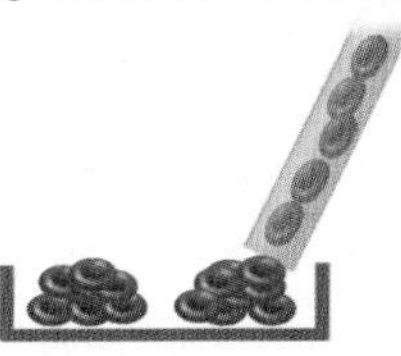

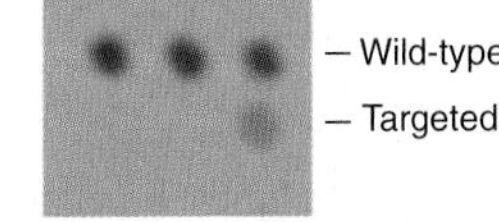

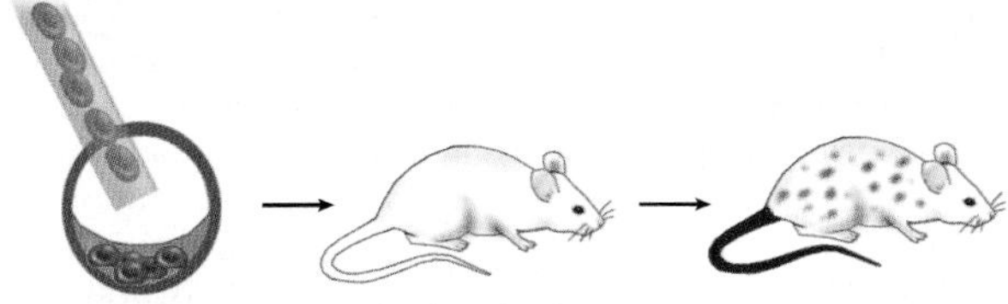

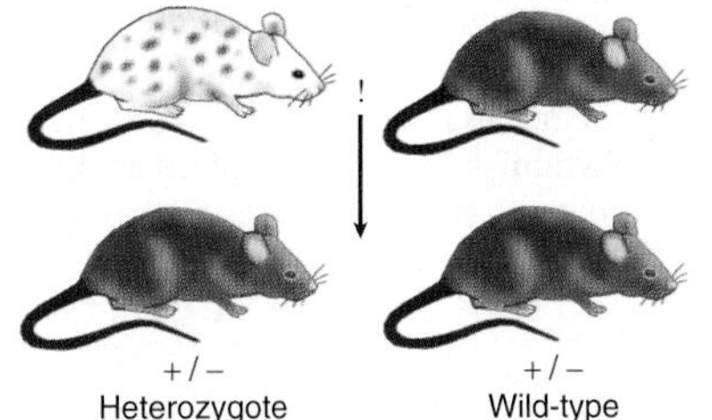

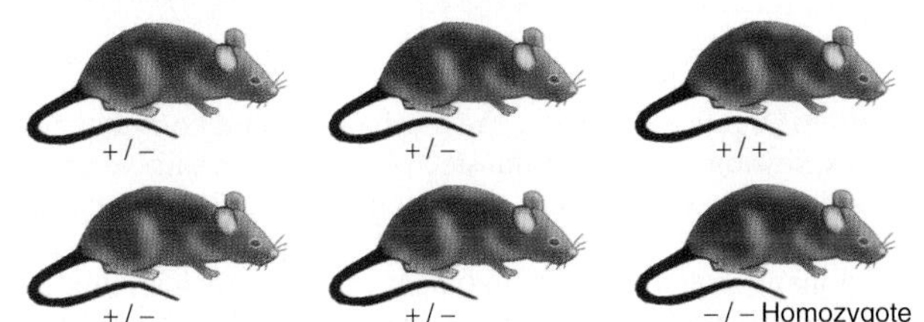

FIGURE 7-14 Scheme for generating heterozygous and homozygous gene knockout mice by homologous recombination in mouse embryonic stem cells. ES cell = embryonic stem cell.

Conditional Knockout Mice

Inactivation of important genes commonly results in early embryonic lethal phenotypes that are difficult to analyze and understand. As a result, methods have been developed to delete genes in a tissue-specific fashion and to inactivate genes at different times in development. In addition, it is often of interest to produce specific mutations of genes rather than eliminate their expression completely. Homologous recombination is also used to introduce specific mutations into wild-type genes; the difference in technique is that these "knock-ins" use a targeting construct containing a mutant gene rather than a gene deletion. Other homologous recombination approaches permit introduction of a distinct or unrelated gene into a foreign genetic locus to regulate the new gene under the control of the promoter of the targeted locus.

Another approach to tissue-specific gene deletion is use of a bacterial phage recombination system called Cre-lox. A P1 bacteriophage encodes an enzyme called Cre that catalyzes recombination of DNA between two specific sequences (called loxP sites) that signal recombination. This system has been adapted in mice by producing a targeting construct in which the gene of interest is flanked by loxP sites (a floxed allele). Mice homozygous for the floxed allele are bred with transgenic mice that express the Cre recombinase in a tissue-specific manner (e.g., endothelial cells, vascular smooth-muscle cells, cardiomyocytes). The resulting mice have a deletion of the gene of interest only in the tissue expressing the Cre recombinase. By placing the Cre transgene under the control of a tetracycline-responsive promoter, gene deletion is programmed only following tetracycline feeding.

Studies of Mouse Physiology

Realizing the potential of mouse genetics requires technologies that can characterize the phenotype of mutant mice. The mouse is technically challenging because the heart and blood vessels are small in size and the resting heartbeat is more than 500 beats/min. Miniaturized instrumentation and microsurgical techniques have helped solve these problems. With these techniques, it is possible to take physiologic measurements in anesthetized and intubated mice, including aortic blood pressures, left ventricular pressure tracings, and cardiac hemodynamics before and after infusion of pharmacologic agents, such as dobutamine or isoproterenol. Noninvasive imaging of the heart and vasculature has improved substantially, and two-dimensional echocardiography is routine in fetal and adult mice. Magnetic resonance imaging renders clear images of cardiac structure and function. These noninvasive techniques are used to measure end-systolic and end-diastolic left ventricular dimensions, left ventricular wall thickness and mass, and shortening fraction. Myocardial infarctions produced by coronary artery ligation, wire injuries to vessels that simulate angioplasty, and aortic banding to induce left ventricular hypertrophy are commonly performed in gene-modified mice. Exercise testing, 24-hour electrocardiographic recordings on conscious mice using implanted transducers, and electrophysiologic studies to detect inducible cardiac arrhythmias are also standard techniques. With the availability of techniques to study cardiovascular physiology, genetically modified mice now provide an accurate and convenient way to evaluate the function of specific genes in cardiovascular disease.

Gene Transfer

Gene transfer is the introduction and expression of recombinant genes in mammalian cells. Gene transfer aims to introduce recombinant genes into target cells to study the mechanisms and consequences of gene expression. Genes are transfected into cells using vectors. The recombinant gene undergoes transcription into RNA and translation into protein by host enzymes, culminating in the expression of the recombinant protein. The recombinant protein remains intracellular or is secreted into the extracellular space or circulation. Gene expression is transient or stable, depending on whether integration into chromosomes occurs. The efficiency of DNA uptake and gene expression, often referred to as transfection efficiency, depends on many factors, including delivery of DNA to the cell, uptake of DNA into the cytoplasm, degradation of DNA in endosomes, release of DNA from endosomes into the cytoplasm, transport to the nucleus, and persistence in the nucleus.

In vivo gene transfer is performed by cell-mediated or direct gene transfer methods. Cell-mediated or ex vivo gene transfer involves removing autologous cells from the host and transfecting the cells with the vector in vitro. Genetically modified cells are reintroduced into the host by infusion or injection. Ex vivo gene transfer permits the introduction of recombinant genetic material into a specific cell—for example, endothelial or smooth-muscle cells—and analysis of recombinant gene expression within that cell type.

In vivo gene transfer uses the direct introduction of recombinant genes into target cells and tissues. Targeted gene transfer in the vasculature has been performed with cell-specific promoters to achieve gene expression within endothelial cells or smooth-muscle cells. Both ex vivo and in vivo gene transfer approaches have been used in the development of animal models of vascular disease and in clinical trials of gene transfer to the cardiovascular system.

Vectors

Transfection of appropriate target cells represents the critical first step in gene transfer. As a result, development of gene transfer methods has represented a significant area of research in the field. Viral and nonviral vectors have been used in vascular gene transfer studies. A common feature of these methods is the efficient delivery of genes into cells. Vectors differ, however, in their processing of foreign DNA and the frequency of integration into chromosomal DNA. In the case of retroviral and lentiviral vectors, the transferred sequences are integrated in a stable fashion into the chromosomal DNA of the target cell. Other methods of gene transfer result primarily in the introduction of foreign DNA into target cell nuclei in an unintegrated form. These methods result in high, but transient, gene expression. The vectors include adenovirus, adeno-associated virus, and cationic liposomes.

RETROVIRUSES. Retroviruses were the first vectors used in gene transfer studies, dating back to the 1980s. Initial interest in retroviruses as vectors arose from the observation that these vectors stably transduce almost 100% of proliferating target cells in culture. Retroviral vectors have been used in cardiovascular gene transfer studies, primarily in ex vivo studies, but their use has been limited by low transfection efficiencies.

LENTIVIRUSES. Lentiviruses are a subclass of retroviruses that have been adapted as gene transfer vectors. They are an attractive vector because in contrast to retroviruses, lentiviruses integrate into the genome of nondividing cells. The lentiviral genome enters a cell as RNA, is reverse-transcribed to DNA, and DNA integrates into the host genome at a random position using a viral integrase enzyme. This provirus is propagated into host daughter cells during host cell division. Lentiviral vectors have a lower tendency to integrate in sites that lead to mutagenesis than retroviruses, but the clinical experience with lentiviral vectors is still limited. Lentiviral vectors are produced using a packaging cell line, similar to retroviruses. Packaging plasmids encode the virion proteins, such as the capsid and the reverse transcriptase, while a second plasmid carries the gene of interest to be delivered by the vector.

ADENOVIRUS. Adenovirus types 2 and 5 are the two serotypes used as vectors in cardiovascular gene transfer. The adenovirus genome is linear double-stranded DNA, approximately 36 kb in length and divided into 100 map units, each of which is 360 bp in length. The DNA contains short inverted terminal repeats (ITRs) at the end of the genome that are required for viral DNA replication. The gene products are organized into early (E1 to E4) and late (L1 to L5) regions on the basis of expression before or after initiation of DNA replication. Adenoviruses have a lytic life cycle characterized by attachment to an adenoviral glycoprotein receptor on mammalian cells and entry into cells by receptor-mediated endocytosis. Adenoviral capsid proteins protect adenoviruses from lysosomal degradation and viral DNA translocates to the nucleus. Expression of viral genes depends on cellular transcription factors and expression of the adenoviral E1 region, which encodes a transactivator of viral gene expression. During lytic infection, the viral genome replicates to several thousand copies per cell. The viral genome associates with core proteins and is packaged into capsids by self-assembling of major capsid proteins.

The adenovirus genome is rendered replication-deficient to generate a vector. Vectors are constructed by homologous recombination in a cell line known as 293 cells by cotransfection of (1) a bacterial plasmid containing the cDNA of interest and a small region of adenoviral genome deleted from the E1A and E1B regions (these regions regulate adenoviral transcription and are required for viral replication), and (2) an incomplete adenoviral genome. Homologous recombination between the two DNAs generates a recombinant genome in which the foreign gene replaces the E1 region. Viral stock is further propagated in 293 cells to a high titer, generally 10^9 to 10^{10} plaque-forming units (pfu)/mL.

Adenoviral vectors have several additional advantages, including efficient infection of mammalian cells and expression in nondividing cells in vitro and in vivo. These vectors are relatively stable and can be grown and concentrated to a high titer. Extrachromosomal replication of the vector greatly reduces the chance of mutation by random integration and dysregulation of host cellular genes. However, a number of shortcomings limit their use as gene transfer vectors. Gene expression in vascular and myocardial cells following adenoviral infection is short-lived, persisting only for several weeks. Host immune response to adenoviral proteins presents a major limitation to their in vivo use.

Adeno-Associated Virus. Adeno-associated virus (AAV) is a defective human parvovirus that has attractive features as a gene transfer vector. This viral vector is prepared at high titers, is not normally pathogenic in humans, and infects many cell types in vitro. The AAV genome is a single-stranded, linear, 5-kb DNA molecule. The wild-type AAV integrates in a site-specific fashion into a single 7-kb region on human chromosome 19. The AAV genome is flanked by 145 bp-inverted terminal repeats containing the sequences required for packaging, DNA replication, and integration. The coding region contains two open reading frames, which are deleted and replaced with one or more cDNAs plus transcriptional regulatory units during vector construction. AAV vectors accept transgene cassettes of only 4 to 5 kb; this limits the types of transgenes that can be used. Propagation of AAV vectors requires complex packaging, including AAV Rep and Cap proteins and five adenoviral proteins (E1A, E1B, E2A, E4, and VA). These complex packaging requirements have precluded construction of a helper cell line for AAV. Currently, vectors are constructed by cotransfection of cells with the AAV vector and a nonpackageable plasmid containing the AAV Rep and Cap proteins. This is followed by infection of the transfected cells with wild-type or mutant helper adenovirus. AAV is separated from contaminating adenovirus by heat treatment and equilibrium density gradation centrifugation. Protocols for constructing AAV vectors are described elsewhere.

The AAV vectors infect multiple cell types in vitro, but their usefulness in vivo is uncertain. Further limitations include a lack of packaging cell lines and a requirement for coinfection with adenovirus, making it difficult to prepare large quantities of pure AAV vectors. Deletion of viral genes during vector construction limits the ability of these vectors to integrate in a site-specific manner but does raise the possibility of insertional mutagenesis.

Cationic Liposomes. Cationic lipids are preparations of positively charged lipids that spontaneously complex with negatively charged DNA to form DNA-lipid conjugates. The lipid component assists delivery of DNA to cells by fusion with plasmid membrane or with endosomal membranes after endocytosis. Following release from endosomes, plasmid DNA is maintained in an extrachromosomal form. Cationic liposomes have been used in arterial gene transfer studies in many animal models, including rats, rabbits, dogs, and pigs. Advantages of cationic liposomes include a favorable safety profile, lack of viral coding sequences, and no cDNA size constraints. They have produced minimal biochemical, hemodynamic, or cardiac toxicity in animals or humans. These vectors have straightforward preparation for experimental and clinical use. The limitations include a low transfection efficiency and short-term gene expression.

Polymers. Nucleic acids and drugs have been applied to polymer gels coated onto stents or balloons and directly applied to arteries. Many early polymers were associated with intense inflammatory reactions. Newer formulations have been successfully used in the development of drug-eluting stents.

Future Directions

Molecular and cellular biology represent the foundation of cardiovascular research. These approaches have advanced our understanding of the pathogenesis of cardiovascular diseases, led to the development of useful animal models, and provided the basic principles for molecular therapies. Cardiovascular research has embraced molecular genetics as the arena in which major advances are occurring. The mechanisms whereby single genes cause cardiovascular disease are now understood, and these mechanisms have provided insight into the pathophysiology of complex cardiovascular disorders. Future directions will focus on several areas. The first is new gene and protein discoveries made in the fields of genomics and proteomics. These discoveries will generate hypotheses about disease pathophysiology that will require functional analysis in cellular and animal models. Genotyping and DNA sequencing will be standard components of clinical trials, and discoveries will only be as good as the characterization of clinical phenotypes by thoughtful, observant physicians who detect unusual patterns of disease in their patients. Second, translational research will be increasingly important as gene and protein discoveries lead to new biomarkers, diagnostic tools, and molecular therapies. Third, stem cell advances will affect clinical medicine, but it is not yet known how and to what extent. Physicians, scientists, and clinical investigators are essential to realizing the promise of molecular genetics and applying research advances to the care of cardiovascular patients.

REFERENCES

Cell Biology and Signaling

1. Alberts B, Johnson A, Lewis J, et al: Molecular Biology of the Cell. New York, Taylor & Francis, 2007.
2. Lewin B: Genes IX. Boston, Jones and Bartlett, 2008.
3. Edinger AL, Thompson CB: Death by design: Apoptosis, necrosis and autophagy. Curr Opin Cell Biol 16:663, 2004.
4. Boehm M, Olive M, True AL, et al: Bone marrow-derived immune cells regulate vascular disease through a p27Kip1-dependent mechanism. J Clin Invest 114:419, 2004.
5. Langenickel TH, Olive M, Boehm M, et al: KIS protects against adverse vascular remodeling by opposing stathmin-mediated vascular SMC migration in mice. J Clin Invest 118:3848, 2008.
6. Olive M, Mellad JA, Beltran LE, et al: p21Cip1 modulates arterial wound repair through the stromal cell-derived factor-1/CXCR4 axis in mice. J Clin Invest 118:2050, 2008.

Molecular Basis of Genetics

7. Lander ES, Linton LM, Birren B, et al: Initial sequencing and analysis of the human genome. Nature 409:860, 2001.
8. Venter JC, Adams MD, Myers EW, et al: The sequence of the human genome. Science 291:1304, 2001.
9. International HapMap Consortium: A second-generation human haplotype map of over 3.1 million SNPs. Nature 449:851, 2007.
10. Zhao Y, Srivastava D: A developmental view of microRNA function. Trends Biochem Sci 32:189, 2007.
11. Cordes KR, Srivastava D: MicroRNA regulation of cardiovascular development. Circ Res 104:724, 2009.
12. Cordes KR, Sheehy NT, White MP, et al: miR-145 and miR-143 regulate smooth muscle cell fate and plasticity. Nature 460:705, 2009.
13. Sambrook J, Russell DW: Molecular Cloning: A Laboratory Manual. Cold Spring Harbor, NY, Cold Spring Harbor Laboratory, 2001.
14. Watson JD, Crick FHC: Molecular structure of nucleic acids: A structure for deoxyribose nucleic acid. Nature 171:737, 1953.
15. National Center for Biotechnology Information: OMIM: Online Mendelian Inheritance in Man (http://www.ncbi.nlm.nih.gov/omim).
16. Cohen JC, Boerwinkle E, Mosley TH, et al: Sequence variations in PCSK9, low LDL, and protection against coronary heart disease. N Engl J Med 354:1264, 2006.
17. Morita H, Rehm HL, Menesses A, et al: Shared genetic causes of cardiac hypertrophy in children and adults. N Engl J Med 358:1899, 2008.
18. Sanguinetti MC, Tristani-Firouzi M: hERG potassium channels and cardiac arrhythmia. Nature 440:463, 2006.
19. Watkins H, Farrall M: Genetic susceptibility to coronary artery disease: From promise to progress. Nat Rev Genet 7:163, 2006.
20. Newton-Cheh C, Johnson T, Gateva V, et al: Genome-wide association study identifies eight loci associated with blood pressure. Nat Genet 2009 May 10. [Epub ahead of print] PMID:19430483.
21. National Center for Biotechnology Information: Single Nucleotide Polymorphism (dbSNP) (http://www.ncbi.nlm.nih.gov/SNP).
22. Hirschhorn JN, Daly MJ: Genome-wide association studies for common disease and complex traits. Nat Rev Genet 6:95, 2005.
23. McCarthy MI, Abecasis GR, Cardon LR, et al: Genome-wide association studies for complex traits: Consensus, uncertainty and challenges. Nat Rev Genet 9:356, 2008.
24. Zeggini E, Ioannidis JPA: Meta-analysis in genome-wide association studies. Pharmacogenomics 10:191, 2009.
25. Hardy J, Singleton A: Genomewide association studies and human disease. N Engl J Med 360:1759, 2009.
26. Wellcome Trust Case Control Consortium: Genome-wide association study of 14,000 cases of seven common diseases and 3,000 shared controls. Nature 447:661, 2007.
27. Manolio TA, Brooks LD, Collins FS: A HapMap harvest of insights into the genetics of common disease. J Clin Invest 118:1590, 2008.
28. Ding K, Kullo I: Genome-wide association studies for atherosclerotic vascular disease and its risk factors. Circ Cardiovasc Genet 2:63, 2009
29. Frayling TM, Timpson NJ, Weedon MN, et al: A common variant in the FTO gene is associated with body mass index and predisposes to childhood and adult obesity. Science 316:889, 2007.
30. National Center for Biotechnology Information: Database Genotypes and Phenotypes (dbGaP) (http://www.ncbi.nlm.nih.gov/sites/entrez?Db=gap).
31. Mailman MD, Feolo M, Jin Y, et al: The NCBI dbGaP database of genotypes and phenotypes. Nat Genet 39:1181, 2007.
32. Butte A: The use and analysis of microarray DNA. Nat Rev Drug Disc 1:951, 2002.
33. Gstaiger M, Aebersold R: Applying mass spectrometry-based proteomics to genetics, genomics and network biology. Nat Rev Genet 10:617, 2009.

CHAPTER 8 Inherited Causes of Cardiovascular Disease

J.G. Seidman, Reed E. Pyeritz, and Christine E. Seidman

Application of human genomic technologies to the study of myocardial diseases has revealed a considerable role for genetics in cardiac pathologies. Over the past 20 years, scores of genes and thousands of mutations have been discovered to cause inherited and sporadic cardiomyopathies, arrhythmias, and congenital malformations. In addition to delineating the fundamental cause for these disorders, molecular information provides insights into pathophysiology and a rational approach for improved classification. Clinical application of genetic discoveries has facilitated accurate diagnosis and enabled the preclinical recognition of individuals at risk for disease development. Genetic understanding has also enabled analyses of the relevance of precise molecular causes and their effect on the natural history and clinical expression of disease. The prospect that genetic insights will fuel development of highly specific, novel therapeutics that can diminish, delay, or even prevent the emergence of disease in individuals with gene mutations is of great importance.

The opportunities for harnessing genetic insights to improve medical diagnosis and affect management and therapy rationalize the establishment of clinical molecular diagnostic laboratories. Although more widely used in other medical fields, molecular genetics has equally great potential to advance cardiovascular medicine. This chapter discusses the genetic basis of specific myocardial diseases, emphasizing contributions to adult cardiology, and outlines future expectations for this emerging field. Familiarity with basic human genetic concepts[1] is assumed (see Chap. 7).

Genetic Causes of Cardiomyopathy

Hypertrophic cardiomyopathy (HCM), dilated cardiomyopathy (DCM), and arrhythmogenic right ventricular dysplasia (ARVD) were previously denoted as idiopathic and are now recognized as single-gene disorders. In familial cardiomyopathies, gene mutations are inherited as autosomal dominant traits (see Chaps. 68 and 69). De novo mutations in these same genes will produce sporadic cases of cardiomyopathy. Disease penetrance (the likelihood of clinical manifestations in gene carriers) for HCM, DCM, and ARVD is extremely high, and for HCM it approaches 100%. However, clinical severity can vary, even among affected family members with an identical mutation. Modifying factors that may contribute to differences in the expression of these cardiomyopathies include background genes and lifestyle. Genomic mutations that cause HCM, DCM, and ARVD are present at conception, yet the emergence of overt pathology usually takes years or even decades.

An intriguing observation emerging from the discovery of genetic causes for cardiomyopathies is that different mutations in some genes cause either HCM or DCM. Despite this overlap, individual mutations in these genes typically produce only one pathologic condition, HCM or DCM. The current repertoire of ARVD genes indicates a completely distinct genetic substrate (see Chap. 9). Most cardiomyopathy gene mutations alter structural proteins with highly specialized functions in contraction, force transmission, or cell-to-cell communication. The following sections examine molecular causes of these myocardial disorders and define the clinical relevance of genetic causes to diagnosis and management.

Gene Mutations Causing Cardiac Hypertrophy

Unexplained left ventricular hypertrophy (LVH) occurs in approximately 1 of 500 individuals.[2] LVH that occurs without underlying hypertension or valvular heart disease, or has another cause, often prompts the diagnosis of HCM (see Chap. 69). The discovery of human mutations that cause LVH indicates that there are two major genetic subtypes, HCM and metabolic cardiomyopathies. In addition to distinct molecular causes, the marked differences in histopathology, disease mechanisms, and clinical manifestations[3] provide considerable rationale for this subdivision (**Table 8-1**). Mutations in genes encoding the contractile proteins of the sarcomere are the most common cause of HCM. Mutations in genes encoding proteins with functions in general myocyte biology cause metabolic cardiomyopathies. Approximately 70% of patients with unexplained LVH and a family history of cardiomyopathy have sarcomere protein gene mutations (see Table 8-1). Metabolic gene mutations occur in approximately 10% of patients with unexplained LVH. Mutations in unidentified genes are presumed to account for the remaining cases.

SARCOMERE PROTEIN GENE MUTATIONS. HCM is caused by mutations in genes that encode the protein constituents of the cardiac sarcomere.[4] These mutations are transmitted as an autosomal dominant trait, conveying a 50% risk to each offspring of affected individuals. More than 900 mutations have been described (see http://cardiogenomics.med.harvard.edu),[5] and they are often unique to individual families. More than half of all HCM mutations occur in genes that encode thick-filament components of the sarcomere, either the beta-cardiac myosin heavy chain (βMHC; *MYH7*) or cardiac myosin binding protein C (*MYBPC3*). Most other HCM mutations occur in the other thick-filament proteins— regulatory myosin light chain (*MYL2*), essential myosin light chain (*MYL3*), or titin (*TTN*) or in thin-filament proteins—cardiac troponin I (*TNNI3*), cardiac troponin T (*TNNT2*), alpha-tropomyosin (*TPM1*), or actin (*ACTC*). Rare HCM mutations have been reported in genes that encode Z-disc proteins (myozenin-2 [MYOZ2], telethonin [TCAP], muscle LIM protein [CSRP]), which connect sarcomere units together.

Most HCM mutations produce dominant-negative polypeptides that are incorporated into cardiac myofilaments, and thereby produce defective sarcomeres. Two recent studies have suggested that *MYBPC3* mutations lead to reduced amounts of mature protein and thereby reduce sarcomere function.[6,7] In most cases, however, incorporation of mutant proteins into the sarcomere perturbs normal biophysical functions and produces enhanced contraction, but markedly impaired relaxation.[8,9] The impact of different mutations on sarcomere function may correlate with some differences in clinical expression, including the age at onset of hypertrophy, natural history, and arrhythmias that are associated with sudden death.

TABLE 8-1 Cardiac Hypertrophy Disease Genes

LOCUS	SYMBOL	NAME	FUNCTION	DISEASE
1q32	*TNNT2*	Cardiac troponin T	Sarcomere	HCM
2q31	*TTN*	Titin	Sarcomere	HCM
3p21	*MYL3*	Essential myosin light chain	Sarcomere	HCM
3p21-p14	*TNNC1*	Cardiac troponin C	Sarcomere	HCM
11p11.2	*MYBPC3*	Cardiac myosin binding protein C	Sarcomere	HCM
12q23-q24	*MYL2*	Regulatory myosin light chain	Sarcomere	HCM
14q12	*MYH7*	Beta-myosin heavy chain	Sarcomere	HCM
14q12	*MYH6*	Alpha-myosin heavy chain	Sarcomere	HCM
15q14	*ACTC*	Cardiac actin	Sarcomere	HCM
15q22	*TPM1*	Alpha-tropomyosin	Sarcomere	HCM
19p13.2	*TNNI3*	Cardiac troponin I	Sarcomere	HCM
7q36	*PRKAG2*	Protein kinase, AMP-activated, noncatalytic, $gamma_2$	Metabolism	PRKAG2 cardiomyopathy
Xq22	*GLA*	Alpha-galactosidase A	Lysosome, metabolism	Fabry disease
Xq24	*LAMP2*	Lysosome-associated membrane protein B	Lysosome, metabolism	Danon disease

AMP = adenosine monophosphate.

First-degree family members of HCM patients have a 50% risk of inheriting the mutation and developing disease, because the lifelong penetrance of HCM mutations is more than 95%. Because HCM mutations cause latent or subtle disease in childhood and adolescence, at-risk individuals require longitudinal clinical assessment of disease status,[10] unless their status is defined by gene-based diagnosis. The advent of Clinical Laboratory Improvement Amendment (CLIA)-approved gene-based HCM diagnosis provides efficient and accurate mutation status in individuals of any age (see www.genetests.org). Gene-based diagnosis typically reveals a single mutation in HCM patients, although two disease-causing mutations in the same or a different sarcomere protein gene are sometimes found in those with particularly severe disease. Genetic diagnosis of family members focuses clinical follow-up only on mutation carriers and alleviates the need for cardiac studies in individuals free of mutations.[11]

Thick-Filament Proteins

Missense mutations in βMHC (encoded by *MYH7* on chromosome 14) are prevalent causes of HCM and account for approximately 25% to 40% of cases.[5,12] Abundantly expressed in the adult heart, βMHC accounts for 70% of total ventricular myosin. A 200,000 kDa protein, βMHC contains a carboxyl terminal rod, a hinge region, and an amino terminal globular head that interacts with actin to produce force. HCM mutations occur throughout the head domain and hinge region, and are uncommon in the rod.

Clinical presentation of HCM caused by βMHC mutations is often apparent by late adolescence, and affected individuals typically develop substantial hypertrophy. Although the clinical course associated with βMHC and other sarcomere protein gene mutations is heterogeneous, *MYH7* mutations that substantially alter protein structure and function cause more severe disease. Increased risk for sudden death (Arg403Gln) and the development of end-stage heart failure (Arg719Trp) characterize several βMHC defects, and rare individuals with homozygous *MYH7* mutations[13] are at very high risk for these adverse outcomes. However, determinants of disease expression and prognosis are likely multifactorial and involve gene-gene and gene-environment interactions.[14]

Cardiac myosin binding protein C (MyBPC), a 137-kDa protein encoded by *MYBPC3* on chromosome 11, provides structural support to the sarcomere by binding myosin heavy chain and titin (see later), and modulates myosin ATPase activity and cardiac contractility in response to adrenergic stimulation.[15] Missense, splice-site, and deletion-insertion mutations in MyBPC collectively account for approximately 40% of cases of HCM.[5,12] Individuals with MyBPC mutations can have delayed clinically expression of LVH until age 50 years or older. Consistent with this observation, symptoms from HCM caused by *MYBPC3* mutations are often less severe than those produced by *MYH7* mutations. The milder phenotypes of *MYBPC3* mutations have enabled some defects to escape evolutionary selection, and founder MyBPC mutations are observed in populations from the Netherlands[16] and among 4% of individuals of southeast Indian ancestry.[17] Even these mutations are not entirely benign, however, because with recent increases in human longevity, mutation carriers demonstrate substantially increased risks (eightfold) for heart failure.

Mutations in the giant 34350 amino acid (3000kDa) titin molecule, encoded by the *TTN* gene on chromosome 2, can cause HCM.[18] Spanning the sarcomere from the Z-disc to the M-line, titin probably assembles contractile filaments and provides elasticity through serial springlike elements. The considerable costs associated with genetic analyses of this huge gene have impeded comprehensive analyses in the HCM population. The few *TTN* mutations reported in HCM have produced phenotypes indistinguishable from other sarcomere gene mutations.[19]

The regulatory (encoded by *MYL2*) and essential (encoded by *MYL3*) myosin light chains belong to the EF hand superfamily of proteins with a helix-loop-helix motif that help determine the speed and force of actomyosin sliding by interacting with the head-rod junction of myosin heavy chains.[18] Mutations in myosin light chains are rarely genetic causes of HCM, accounting for less than 5% of cases. One essential myosin light chain mutation (Met149Val) is associated with a distinctive HCM morphology—midcavitary hypertrophy—associated with hemodynamic obstruction. Essential myosin light chain mutations may distort the stretch-activated response, an intrinsic property of muscle resulting in oscillatory power and regional contraction properties of the heart that are particularly important for papillary muscle functions.

Thin-Filament Proteins

Approximately 5% of HCM is thought to be attributable to cardiac troponin T (cTnT) mutations.[5,12] Encoded by *TNNT2* on chromosome 1, cTnT is a 36- to 39-kDa amino acid peptide that links the troponin complex to alpha-tropomyosin and functions as a key regulator of contractile function. Several distinct isoforms are expressed in cardiac tissue via alternative splicing of 16 exons. Historically, the clinical phenotype of cTnT mutations has been characterized as modest hypertrophy,[12] but with increased risk of sudden death. Other cTnT mutations are associated with better long-term survival. Rare homozygous cTnT mutations have been identified in consanguineous families. Doubling the dose of mutant cTnT peptide has markedly increased sudden death in children with homozygous mutations.[9]

Cardiac troponin I (cTnI) missense mutations cause about 3% of HCM cases.[18,20] The cardiac-specific isoform of troponin I (encoded by *TNNI3* on chromosome 19) is a 27- to 31-kDa protein that functions as the inhibitory subunit of the troponin complex, reducing actin-myosin interaction. Initial clinical findings reported with cTnI defects have suggested a greater predisposition for apical hypertrophy than occurs with other HCM genes. However, morphologic manifestations associated with larger numbers of *TNNI3* mutations indicate a range of morphologic phenotypes, although restrictive physiology may be particularly common.

Mutations in alpha-cardiac actin rarely cause HCM. Encoded by the *ACTC* gene on chromosome 15, alpha-cardiac actin is a 41-kDa protein. Human mutations are clustered in proximity to the myosin-binding site and may alter protein folding. The clinical phenotype of *ACTC* mutation is mild with respect to degree of hypertrophy and incidence of sudden death. Most *ACTC* mutations, like other HCM genes, produce all types of hypertrophic morphologies, but the Glu-101Lys missense mutation identified in multiple affected families uniformly causes apical hypertrophy.[21] Although the mechanisms for selective apical remodeling are unknown, *ACTC* Glu101Lys, like essential myosin light chain mutations, may particularly affect stretch activation responses.

Mutations in alpha-tropomyosin, which is encoded by *TPM1* on chromosome 15, account for less than 5% of HCM in most populations.[5,12] However, these defects are prevalent in Finland, because of a founding mutation.[22] Clinical phenotypes of HCM caused by *TPM1* mutations include variable degrees of hypertrophy and relatively good survival. Although alpha-tropomyosin protein is expressed in fast skeletal and cardiac muscle, HCM mutations produce disease that is restricted to the heart. The absence of skeletal myopathy may reflect the fact that HCM mutations often occur in a domain of alpha-tropomyosin that interacts with the cardiac-specific isoform of cTnT. Alterations in calcium sensitivity may also affect the tissue specificity of *TPM1* mutations.

DISEASE MECHANISM AND EMERGING THERAPEUTIC STRATEGIES. Insights into the pathogenetic mechanisms of βMHC mutations have come from the study of animal models engineered to carry human HCM mutations.[23] Mice and rabbits with HCM mutations recapitulate the clinical features of human disease with cardiac hypertrophy, myocyte disarray, and diastolic dysfunction. Investigations of the biophysical properties of a mouse carrying HCM mutation Arg-403Gln have demonstrated unexpected enhanced myosin functions, including actin-activated ATPase activity, force generation, and velocity of actin translocation along myosin. Analyses of HCM mutation cTnT Phe110 have also shown increased calcium sensitivity of force generation and increased ATPase activity.[24] Together these data imply that changes in sarcomere contractile force due to HCM mutations stimulate hypertrophic remodeling. These studies also highlight increased energy requirements by mutant sarcomeres that increase oxidative stress in HCM myocytes. Treatment of HCM animals with *N*-acetylcysteine to increase thiol pools protecting against oxidative stress have salutary effects on myocardial fibrosis. Animal studies also indicate the important role of intracellular calcium in linking alterations of muscle contraction with myocyte growth. Changes in calcium cycling by mutant sarcomeres occur early and in advance of histopathology as a result of diminished levels of calcium transport proteins such as calsequestrin and ryanodine receptors, with ultimate depletion of sarcoplasmic reticulum Ca^{2+} levels.[25,26] Treatment of HCM mice with diltiazem blunts this effect and restores normal calcium cycling between the sarcoplasmic reticulum and cytoplasm, thereby interrupting the signals leading to hypertrophic remodeling. These animal studies have prompted ongoing clinical trials (see http://clinicaltrials.gov) involving diltiazem treatment of genotype-positive individuals who have no clinical signs of HCM. Translation of mechanistic insights derived from HCM models to human clinical trials is expected.

Gene Mutations Causing Metabolic Cardiomyopathy

LVH can result from mutations in genes encoding metabolic proteins.[27,28] Patients with metabolic cardiomyopathy are often misdiagnosed with HCM because of the cardiac morphology and contractile parameters, when assessed by echocardiography or magnetic resonance imaging. In contrast, cardiac histopathology readily distinguishes these cardiomyopathies. The prominent myocyte and myofibrillar disarray that characterizes HCM is absent from metabolic cardiomyopathies, which show myocyte-filled vacuoles that contain lipid (*GLA* mutations), glycogen (*PRKAG2* mutations), or lysosomal remnants (*LAMP2* mutations).[28] The clinical course of metabolic cardiomyopathies is different from that of HCM, and two gene causes (*LAMP2* and *GLA*) are encoded on chromosome X, resulting in a different pattern of inheritance than that of HCM. Gene-based diagnosis is available in CLIA-approved molecular laboratories, enabling accurate diagnosis of metabolic cardiomyopathies.

CARDIAC FABRY DISEASE. Mutation of the lysosomal hydrolase alpha-galactosidase A protein, encoded by *GLA* on chromosome X, causes Fabry disease. Although systemic manifestations—including nephropathy, sensorineural deafness, skin lesions, and autonomic dysfunction—occur with Fabry disease, cardiac manifestations predominate in some patients.[29] Symptoms include angina, exercise intolerance, and palpitations, and diagnostic studies show concentric cardiac hypertrophy and progressive electrophysiologic deficits. The shortened duration of the PR interval may indicate the severity of cardiac disease. Missense and splice-site *GLA* mutations reduce enzymatic activity and increase cardiac globotriaosylceramide levels. Diagnosis should prompt enzyme replacement therapy with recombinant alpha-galactosidase A administration, which reduces cardiac hypertrophy and normalizes cardiac electrophysiology.

CARDIAC DANON DISEASE. Mutation in the X-linked lysosome-associated membrane protein-2 (*LAMP2*) causes Danon disease, a multisystem disorder involving the nervous system, liver, and skeletal and heart muscle, or predominantly marked LVH occurring with subclinical systemic disease.[28,30] *LAMP2* mutations are clinically distinguished from HCM by male predominance and early disease onset, typically in childhood. The electrocardiogram shows strikingly increased voltage with ventricular preexcitation, and echocardiograms demonstrate massive concentric hypertrophy. *LAMP2* cardiomyopathy is associated with frequent ventricular arrhythmias that can become refractory to medical management. Cardiac dysfunction is progressive and may prompt consideration of transplantation, albeit with thorough consideration of systemic involvement. Arrhythmias and heart failure account for the shortened life expectancy in most patients. Affected males often die during the second decade of life; survival in females is better, but may be complicated by heart failure.

Disease Mechanism

LAMP2 mutations produce a functionally null allele and resultant accumulation of autophagic vacuoles in the tissues of affected males.[30,31] Female carriers have half-normal *LAMP2* levels and do not exhibit systemic disease, although some increase in adult-onset heart failure has been reported. Rarely, massive cardiac hypertrophy occurs in females with *LAMP2* mutation, presumably because of the unfortunate inactivation of the normal X chromosome, with resultant *LAMP2* deficiency. The mechanisms whereby deficiency in lysosomal proteins causes hypertrophy and electrophysiologic dysfunction are incompletely understood, but the profound consequences of these mutations indicate critical roles for lysosomes in the heart.

GLYCOGEN STORAGE CARDIOMYOPATHY. Genetic studies of families and sporadic cases of unexplained LVH with conduction abnormalities (e.g., ventricular preexcitation [Wolff-Parkinson-White syndrome], progressive atrioventricular block, atrial fibrillation) have led to the identification of a glycogen storage cardiomyopathy caused by mutations in the gamma$_2$ regulatory subunit (*PRKAG2*) of adenosine monophosphate-activated protein kinase (AMPK).[27] Histologic examination demonstrates hypertrophied myocytes containing vacuoles filled with glycogen and glycogen-protein complexes (amylopectin). In addition to cardiac hypertrophy, ventricular preexcitation typically occurs early and causes symptoms. Progressive conduction disease occurs with increasing age, necessitating permanent pacemaker implantation in 30% of affected individuals. Conduction system disease helps discriminate *PRKAG2* cardiomyopathy from HCM caused by sarcomere protein gene mutations. Severe clinical outcomes occur in some patients with *PRKAG2* mutations, including neonatal cardiac progression to end-stage heart failure or transplantation and sudden cardiac death.[32]

Disease Mechanism

PRKAG2 mutations result in constitutive activation of AMPK activity, leading to glycogen accumulation.[27,32] Because the gamma$_2$ subunit is expressed solely in the heart, *PRKAG2* mutations cause only a glycogen cardiomyopathy, without the systemic manifestations found in *GAA* and *LAMP2* mutations. AMPK is an energy sensor activated under conditions of energy depletion and alters substrate uptake, activation of glucose transport, stimulation of beta oxidation of fatty acids, inactivation of cholesterol synthesis, inhibition of creatine kinase, and transcriptional regulation of several genes. The target proteins altered by constitutive activation of AMPK from *PRKAG2* mutations resulting in glycogen accumulation are unknown. Arrhythmias associated with glycogen storage cardiomyopathy are caused, at least in part, by glycogen-filled myocytes that disrupt the annulus fibrosis, which provides an anatomic insulator to prevent ventricular preexcitation.[33]

Gene Mutations Causing Dilated Cardiomyopathy

Idiopathic DCM occurs in approximately 1 in 2500 individuals (see Chap. 68).[34] Approximately half of patients who undergo evaluations for DCM retain the idiopathic designation, and clinical studies of first-degree relatives have shown that 30% to 50% of cases are familial, implying a genetic cause. Most DCM mutations are transmitted as autosomal dominant traits, but other modes of transmission (e.g., recessive, X-linked, or matrilineal) also occur.[35]

By convention, DCM genes are categorized according to whether conduction system disease or extracardiac manifestations accompany DCM (**Table 8-2**). Additional phenotypes can emerge with time or be subclinical and unappreciated unless they are thoroughly investigated. Human DCM mutations occur in genes encoding proteins that participate in a wide range of myocyte functions, including contractile force generation and transmission, metabolism, calcium homeostasis, RNA splicing, and transcriptional regulation.[2,35] Many DCM genes have

TABLE 8-2 Dilated Cardiomyopathy Disease Genes and Loci

LOCUS	SYMBOL	NAME	ADDITIONAL PHENOTYPE	DISEASE
1q32	*TNNT2*	Cardiac troponin T	None	DCM
1q42-q43	*ACTN2*	Alpha-actinin		
2q31	*TTN*	Titin	None	DCM
6q12-q16	*CMD1K*	Unknown	None	DCM
6q22.1	*PLN*	Phospholamban	None	DCM
9q13-q22	*CMD1B*	Unknown	None	DCM
9q22-q31	Unknown	Unknown	None	DCM
10 q 22.2-q23.3	*LDBD2*	Cipher ZASP	Left ventricular noncompaction	DCM
10q22.3-q23.2	*LDB3*	LIM domain-binding protein 3		DCM
11p11.2	*MYBPC3*	Cardiac myosin binding protein C	None	DCM
11p15.1	*CLP (CSRP3)*	Cardiac muscle LIM protein	None	DCM
12p12.1	*ABCC9*	ATP-sensitive K channel	None	DCM
14q12	*MYH7*	Beta-myosin heavy chain	None	DCM
15q14	*ACTC*	Cardiac actin	None	DCM
15q22	*TPM1*	Alpha-tropomyosin	None	DCM
16p11	*CTF1*	Cardiotrophin 1	None	DCM
1p1-q21	*LMNA*	Lamin A/C	Conduction disease, skeletal myopathy	DCM
2q14-q22	*CMD1H*	Unknown	Conduction disease	DCM
2q35	*DES*	Desmin	Skeletal myopathy	DCM
3p22-p25	Unknown	Unknown	Conduction disease	DCM
5q33	*SGCD*	Delta-sarcoglycan	Skeletal myopathy	MD
6q23-q24	*EYA4*	Eyes absent 4	Skeletal myopathy, sensorineural hearing loss	DCM with hearing loss
10q22-q23	*MVCL*	Metavinculin	Mitral valve prolapse	DCM
17q12	*TCAP*	Telethonin	Limb-girdle muscular dystrophy	
19q13.2	Unknown	Unknown	Conduction disease	DCM
Xp21.2	*DMD*	Dystrophin	Skeletal myopathy	DMD
Xq28	*TAZ*	Tafazzin	Skeletal myopathy	Barth syndrome
Xq28	*EMD*	Emerin	Skeletal myopathy	Emerin muscular dystrophy

ATP = adenosine triphosphate.

been analyzed in CLIA-approved laboratories (see www.genetests.org and www.hpcgg.org/LMM), but because the compendium of DCM genes remains incomplete, these analyses are informative in fewer than 50% of idiopathic DCM cases. When a pathogenic DCM mutation is found, the genotype and risk for DCM development in relatives can be ascertained. Studies of families with DCM mutations show incomplete penetrance, and infrequently an adult mutation carrier does not develop DCM.

ISOLATED DILATED CARDIOMYOPATHY. Gene mutations affecting sarcomere proteins, calcium-handling proteins, and other unidentified molecules cause DCM unaccompanied by extracardiac manifestations or conduction system diseases. Sarcomere mutations are most common,[36] and mutations have been identified in genes that encode actin (*ACTC*), beta-cardiac myosin heavy chain (*MYH7*), cardiac troponin I (*TNNI3*), cardiac troponin T (*TNNT2*), alpha-tropomyosin (*TPM1*), titin (*TTN*), and cardiac troponin C (*TNNC1*). DCM mutations in sarcomere protein genes, like HCM, show autosomal dominant inheritance. Clinical manifestations occur earlier than with other DCM genes, and childhood presentation with rapid progression to heart failure has been recognized. In contrast, adults with DCM caused by sarcomere mutations can show only mild functional deficits and NYHA Class I or II symptoms.

MUTATIONS IN SARCOMERE PROTEIN GENES. The histopathology of DCM caused by sarcomere mutations is notably different from that of HCM.[36,37] Degenerating myocytes and increased interstitial fibrosis occur without myocyte disarray, which serves to discriminate between primary DCM and the end-stage, burnt-out phase of HCM. The DCM mutations found in sarcomere protein genes are indistinguishable from those causing HCM. Most DCM mutations produce missense amino acids or small deletions, and mutant peptides are incorporated into the sarcomere. The location of a sarcomere gene mutation does not predict whether it will cause HCM or DCM (**Fig. 8-1**). Although the proximity of HCM and DCM mutations is remarkable, only one cardiac remodeling phenotype occurs from a particular mutation.

Human DCM mutations also occur in the giant muscle protein titin, which interacts with sarcomeres.[35,37] DCM mutations are often localized in the cardiac-specific N2B domain that interacts with I-bands, the extensible thin filaments flanking Z-discs, and may cause deficits in force transmission. At the Z-disc, titin interacts with alpha-actinin, telethonin (encoded by *TCAP*), muscle LIM protein (encoded by *CLP*) and cipher ZASP (encoded by *LBD3*).[35,36] Mutations in these Z-disc interacting proteins reportedly cause DCM, but disease penetrance is incomplete. In addition to DCM, patients have elevated serum levels of muscle creatine phosphokinase (CPK), suggestive of a subclinical skeletal myopathy. Mutations in Z-disc proteins may render the titin–Z-disc complex unstable, and impair normal detection and modulation of mechanical stresses in the heart.

MUTATIONS AFFECTING CALCIUM REGULATION. Dominant mutations in phospholamban (*PLN*) cause DCM by altering Ca^{2+} handling.[35] Affected patients develop fulminant DCM and heart failure and require cardiac transplantation early in middle age. Phospholamban is the reversible inhibitor of the cardiac sarcoendoplasmic reticulum $Ca2^{+}$-ATPase (SERCA) that regulates basal cardiac contractility. Phospholamban inhibition of SERCA is released following phosphorylation via beta-adrenergic stimulation of the heart. Dominant DCM mutations in the *PLN* mutation can prevent phosphorylation or cause superinhibition of SERCA; either change results in chronic delay in Ca^{2+} reuptake after sarcomere contraction.

Human DCM mutations in the regulatory SUR2A subunit (encoded by *ABCC9*) of KATP (ATP-sensitive potassium channels) may impair the ability of the heart to decode metabolic signals during stress adaptation.[38] KATP channels are multimeric proteins containing an inwardly rectifying potassium channel pore (Kir6.2), a regulatory SUR2A subunit, and an ATPase-harboring ATP-binding cassette protein. DCM mutations render KATP channels insensitive to ADP-induced conformation changes, which alter channel opening and closure. Mice engineered to lack cardiac KATP channels are susceptible to calcium overload, and develop the pathophysiology of human KATP mutations, DCM, and arrhythmias.

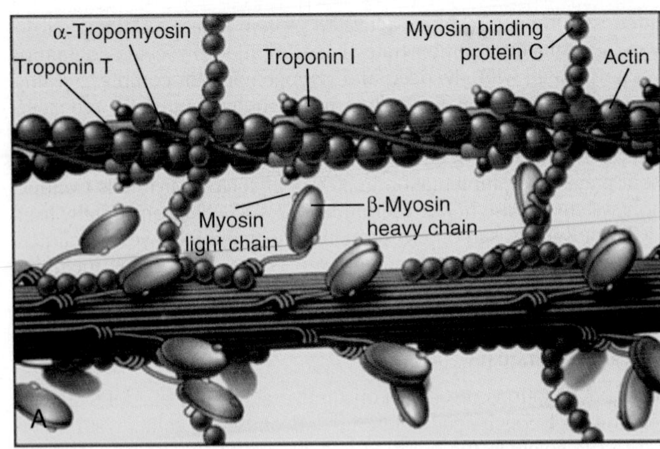

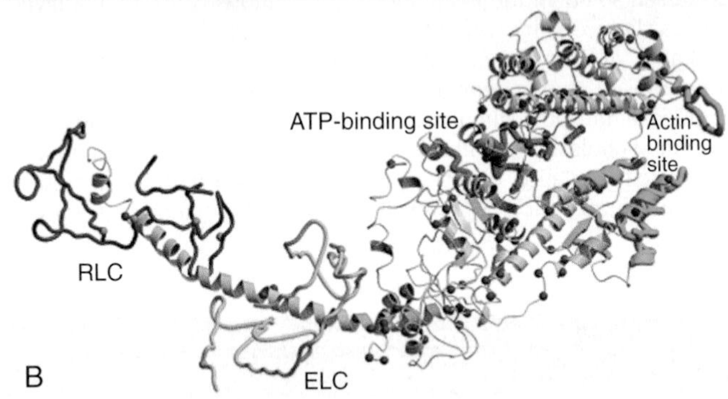

FIGURE 8-1 **A,** Major protein components of the sarcomere that are mutated in human hypertrophic cardiomyopathy (HCM) and dilated cardiomyopathy (DCM). HCM and DCM caused by sarcomere proteins mutations are not accompanied by extracardiac clinical findings. Mutations in the thick-filament proteins, myosin binding protein C, and beta-myosin heavy chain are the most common causes for HCM. **B,** Computer reconstruction of the three-dimensional crystal structure of myosin head (silver)[71] and essential (yellow) and regulatory light chains (purple). Myosin protein residues that bind actin (green) and adenosine triphosphate (tan) are indicated. Human mutations that cause HCM (blue spheres) and DCM (red spheres) are distributed throughout these proteins. Note the close proximity of the HCM and DCM mutations.

Disease Mechanism

Reduced fractional shortening or ejection fraction is a diagnostic clinical feature of dilated cardiomyopathy. These measures are consistent with impaired contractile function. Biophysical analyses of mutant proteins and animal models have been used to explore the mechanisms whereby sarcomere mutations cause DCM. Impaired contractile force is the consequence of DCM mutations affecting both thick- and thin-filament proteins. Depressed contractility, the net result of DCM mutations in sarcomere proteins, is a fundamentally opposite effect to that produced by HCM mutations. Studies of isolated sarcomeres and proteins from multiple DCM models have confirmed the hypothesis that DCM-causing mutations directly or indirectly affect force production or force transmission.[8] Pathways activated by altered myocyte force or aberrant calcium cycling, which lead to myocardial remodeling in DCM, are unknown.

MUTATIONS WITH CONDUCTION SYSTEM DISEASE. DCM with associated conduction system disease can reflect mutation in at least three distinct loci (see Table 8-2). The disease gene at only one chromosome locus (1q12) has been identified to date, lamin A/C (*LMNA*). Dominant mutations in the nuclear envelope protein lamin A/C most commonly cause DCM that occurs with progressive conduction system abnormalities (**Fig. 8-2**).[39] Disease onset usually occurs in

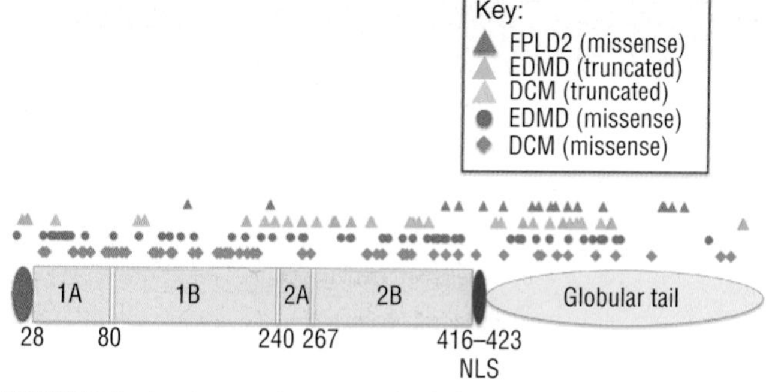

FIGURE 8-2 Lamin mutations cause familial partial lipodystrophy, Dunigan type (FPLD2); Emery-Dreifuss muscular dystrophy (EDMD); and dilated cardiomyopathy (DCM). Symbols indicate the location of mutations in lamin (residues 1-416, rod region; residues 1-28, head; residues 28-66, coil 1A; residues 78-227, coil 1B; residues 240-253, coil 2A; residues 267-408, coil 2B; residues 416-423, nuclear localization signal [nls]; residues 423-666, globular tail). All FPLD2 mutations are missense mutations (purple triangles), most of which occur in the globular tail region. Some DCM mutations (green triangles) and some EDMD mutations (blue triangles) cause truncations, while other DCM mutations (blue squares) and EDMD mutations (red circles) are missense mutations. The pattern of lamin mutations that cause DCM and EDMD suggests that lamin haploinsufficiency can cause either DCM or EDMD, depending on genetic or environmental modifiers.

the third to fourth decade of life. Electrophysiologic dysfunction usually precedes systolic dysfunction by many years, but because arrhythmias are often silent, conduction system disease may be undetected until heart failure symptoms prompt evaluation. The increased incidence of sudden death associated with *LMNA* mutations necessitates careful surveillance and appropriate intervention. Progressive cardiac dysfunction occurs despite progressive pacemaker implantation, indicating that *LMNA* mutations cause primary defects in all myocytes.

Ubiquitously expressed in all cells, lamin A/C participates in nuclear dissociation and reassembly during mitosis (see Chap. 9), but its function in terminally differentiated myocytes is unclear.[38] Analyses of myocytes and fibroblasts from mice deficient in lamin A/C have demonstrated deformities of the nucleus and the desmin cytoskeletal network, impaired mechanotransduction, diminished viability during periods of mechanical strain, and impaired activation of transcriptional programs in response to mechanical strain. Similar deformities of the nuclear architecture appear in skin fibroblasts of patients with *LMNA* mutations. Such mutations may impair normal adaptive mechanisms to mechanical strain; this is an appealing mechanism, but it fails to account for early-onset and progressive electrophysiologic abnormalities.

The shared muscle and cardiac phenotypes in patients with lamin or emerin mutations (*EMD,* encoded by *EMD* on chromosome Xq28) likely relate to their common functions in supporting nuclear membrane integrity. Long-term survival in some patients with DCM *LMNA* mutations is associated with late-onset skeletal myopathy.

Disease Mechanism

The mechanism whereby lamin A/C mutations cause myocyte death is largely unknown. Because lamin A/C null mutations (i.e., haploinsufficiency) cause disease, we know that a 50% reduction in the amount of lamin A/C is sufficient to cause disease. Presumably, myocyte death leads to reduced contractile function and cardiac dilation. Conduction system cell death, although probably unrelated to the ventricular dysfunction, adds to the complexities of treating this disease.

MUTATIONS WITH EXTRACARDIAC MANIFESTATIONS. A variety of extracardiac manifestations can accompany DCM, but skeletal myopathy is the most common, presumably because many molecules are common to all striated muscle cells. Extracardiac phenotypes can precede or follow the onset of DCM.

Mutations in genes encoding protein components of the dystrophin-associated sarcoglycan complex, a protein scaffold that connects the nucleus to the extracellular matrix through the sarcolemma in all muscle cells,[40] cause DCM and skeletal myopathy. Because the dystrophin gene (*DMD*) is encoded at chromosome Xq33, males are more susceptible to disease, although females can develop DCM later in life.[41] Unlike Duchenne muscular dystrophy mutations that alter amino acid sequences, DCM mutations in *DMD* can occur in regulatory sequences and lead to more prominent involvement of the heart. Cardiac disease also predominates in some mutations in muscle delta-sarcoglycan (*SGCD*, encoded at chromosome 5q33), but mutations in *SGCD* and *DMD* usually also cause subclinical skeletal myopathy.

Diverse extracardiac manifestations accompany DCM as part of Barth syndrome.[42] Clinical features include early onset of heart failure in young boys, skeletal myopathy, neutropenia, and growth retardation. Mutations in tafazzin (*TAZ,* encoded on chromosome X), a molecule with putative enzyme functions involved in cardiolipin metabolism, cause Barth syndrome. Levels of the mitochondrial phospholipid cardiolipin are reduced, which may alter mitochondrial structure and disrupt the function of respiratory chain proteins.

EYA4, a transcriptional coactivator that may function as a nuclear phosphatase, causes DCM and sensorineural hearing loss.[35] Human mutations abolish *EYA4-SIX* protein interactions essential for translocation of the transcription coactivator into the nucleus. Genes regulated by *EYA4* are unknown.

Disease Mechanism

Studies of gene mutations causing DCM with extracardiac manifestations have demonstrated that the encoded proteins are expressed in both tissues; cardiac disease is independent and does not arise secondary to dysfunction of another organ system. Mutations causing DCM with skeletal muscle disease (e.g., *DMD, SGCD*) disrupt processes shared between myocytes. Mutations causing DCM and dysfunction of organ systems with vastly different functions (e.g., *EYA4, TAZ*) may alter distinct cellular functions in affected organ systems. Although studies have not identified a uniform myocyte pathway or function that is perturbed by DCM mutations, most gene mutations cause early myocyte death and increased extracellular matrix remodeling, processes that lead to systolic dysfunction and cardiac dilation.

MITOCHONDRIAL MUTATIONS CAUSING DILATED CARDIOMYOPATHY. Mutations in genes that direct synthesis of ATP by oxidative phosphorylation can cause pleiomorphic diseases, frequently including DCM.[43,44] Proteins involved in oxidative phosphorylation are primarily encoded in the nuclear genome, but 13 are encoded in the mitochondrial genome. Unlike nuclear gene defects, mitochondrial mutations are inherited through the maternal lineage. Because the mitochondrial chromosome is present in multiple copies and mutations are often heteroplasmic, not all copies are affected. These issues, coupled with the variable energy needs of different tissues, account for the considerable clinical diversity of mitochondrial gene mutations. Whereas most mitochondrial defects cause cardiomyopathy in the context of pleiomorphic syndromes such as Kearns-Sayre syndrome, ocular myopathy, MELAS (***m***itochondrial ***e***ncephalomyopathy with ***l***actic ***a***cidosis, and ***s***trokelike episodes), and MERRF (***m***yoclonus ***e***pilepsy with ***r***agged ***r***ed ***f***ibers), particular mitochondrial mutations may produce predominant or exclusive cardiac disease. In addition, an association between heteroplasmic mitochondrial mutations and DCM has been recognized. Deficits in energy may be a shared mechanism whereby mutations in mitochondrial genes and tafazzin cause DCM.

Gene Mutations Causing Arrhythmogenic Right Ventricular Dysplasia

ARVD,[45] a cardiomyopathy characterized by fibrofatty degeneration of the myocardium with progressive dysfunction, electrical instability, and sudden death (see Chap. 68), occurs in approximately 1 in 5000 people in the United States (see Chap. 9). Male sex may be associated

TABLE 8-3 Arrhythmogenic Right Ventricular Cardiomyopathy Disease Genes and Loci

LOCUS	SYMBOL	NAME	ADDITIONAL PHENOTYPE
1q42-q43	*RyR2*	Ryanodine receptor	Catecholaminergic polymorphic ventricular tachycardia
2q32.1-q32.3	—	—	Left ventricular involvement
3p23	—	Unknown	—
6p24	*DSP*	Desmoplakin	—
10p12-p14	—	Unknown	Early onset, high penetrance
10q22	—	Unknown	Myofibrillar myopathy
12p11	*PKP2*	Plakophilin-2	—
14q12-q22	—	Unknown	—
14q23-q24	—	Unknown	—
17q21	*JUP*	Junctional plakoglobin	Naxos, Carvajal syndromes (recessive)
18q12	*DSG2*	Desmoglein-2	—
18q12.1	*DSC2*	Desmocollin-2	—

with higher disease penetrance.[46] ARVD occurs as an isolated cardiomyopathy or in the context of two related disorders, Naxos or Carvajal syndrome, which prominently manifest in skin (palmar-plantar keratosis), hair (woolly), and either predominantly the right ventricle (Naxos) or left ventricle (Carvajal). The higher prevalence of ARVD in some countries, particularly Italy, is not accounted for by founder mutations and may reflect surveillance and/or clinical awareness.

Recessive mutations in plakoglobin (*JUP*) cause Naxos and Carvajal syndromes. Cardiac disease in these disorders is comparable to that found in ARVD.[45] Dominant mutations in five genes cause isolated ARVD; the genes at other loci identified through linkage studies are unknown. Mutations occur in desmoplakin (*DSP*), plakophilin-2 (*PKP2*), desmoglein-2 (*DSG2*), and desmocollin-2 (*DSC2*), each of which encodes a protein component of desmosomes - highly organized cell membrane structures that maintain structural and functional contacts between adjacent cells (**Table 8-3**). Less common mutations occur in the cardiac ryanodine receptor (*RyR2*). Whether distinct mutations in these genes are associated with clinical expression is unknown.

Disease Mechanism

Experimental models of ARVD indicate that mutations may render desmosomes inappropriately sensitive to mechanical stresses, resulting in myocyte death. In addition, analyses of signal transduction processes induced by mutant desmosome proteins can lead to reprogrammed myocyte cell biology so that these cells adopt a fibrofatty lineage, therein accounting for ARVD histopathology.[47]

Genetic Causes of Congenital Heart Malformations

Heart malformations are among the most common human congenital defects, occurring in 5 to 7/1000 live births (see Chap. 65).[48] Higher rates (10%) are observed in stillbirths and in children with another congenital anomaly, particularly when cytogenetic abnormalities are evident. With major advances in corrective surgery, survival and reproductive fitness of patients with congenital heart disease have improved. This has aided in the discovery of dominant gene mutations that cause congenital heart defects. Epidemiologic data also indicate that recessive mutations cause heart malformations, because the incidence of these structural defects is increased in children from consanguineous matings.

Most congenital heart disease cases appear as sporadic occurrences. Uncovering the roles of genetics in isolated cases is an active research endeavor. Sporadic cases can reflect de novo dominant mutations, recessive mutations, or complex genetics (e.g., sequence variations in multiple genes that collectively increase risk for aberrant heart development). The recent advent of technologies used to assess genome-wide variation in populations (see Chap. 7) provides new opportunities to identify those common sequence variations responsible for congenital heart malformations.

Gene mutations causing congenital heart malformations typically alter transcription factors (*GATA4, TBX1, TBX5, NKX2-5,* and *ZIC3*) or signaling proteins (*JAG1, KRAS, NOTCH1, PTPN11*) that direct and integrate temporal-spatial interactions of cells and tissues during cardiac development (**Table 8-4**). Unlike gene mutations causing adult-onset disease (e.g., cardiomyopathies), remarkably few structural protein genes (e.g., *CRELD1, ELN, MYH6*) are implicated in congenital heart malformations. Congenital heart disease mutations alter gene dosage, most often producing haploinsufficiency or loss of one functional copy (or allele) of the encoded molecule, which implies that expression levels of these molecules are critical for normal cardiac morphogenesis.

Congenital heart disease gene mutations vary in expressivity. Some mutation carriers may exhibit one preponderant malformation, and others may have anatomically distinct malformations. Whether the diversity of malformations triggered by one mutation reflects background genes, fetal environment, or epigenetic factors is unknown. In addition to congenital structural heart defects, mutations in some disease genes (e.g., *NKX2-5*) produce additional phenotypes that take years to emerge, implying the need for longitudinal clinical evaluations.

Mendelian forms of congenital heart disease can be classified into three broad categories—isolated cardiovascular malformations, pleiotropic syndromes that frequently include congenital cardiovascular defects, and syndromes that only occasionally affect the cardiovascular system. Common examples of these first two categories, more likely to be seen by adult cardiologists, are considered here. A more complete presentation of additional disorders and syndromes is discussed in Online Mendelian Inheritance in Man.[49]

Isolated Congenital Heart Disease

ATRIAL AND VENTRICULAR SEPTAL DEFECTS. Familial aggregation of isolated atrial and ventricular defects can arise from autosomal dominant mutations in a variety of cardiac transcription factor genes. Detailed evaluations are important to assess the involvement of the cardiac conduction system and other organ systems. For example, coexistence of upper limb malformations, even in a first-degree relative, should prompt consideration of hand-heart syndromes (e.g., Holt-Oram syndrome).

TABLE 8-4 Gene Mutations and Loci in Congenital Heart Disease

LOCUS	GENE	FUNCTION	MALFORMATIONS
1p31-p21	Unknown	—	AVCD
1q42	*LEFTY A*	Left-right axis	Heterotaxy
3p22	*CFC1*	Nodal-related signaling	Heterotaxy
3p25.3	*CRELD1*	Cell adhesion	ASD, VSD, AVC, heterotaxy
4p16	*EVC, EVC1*	Unknown	ASD, primum, Ellis-van Creveld
5p	*DNAH5*	Dynein, microtubule motor	Heterotaxy, Kartagener syndrome
5p	Unknown	—	ASD, aneurysm
5q	*NKX2-5*	Transcription	VSD, TOF, conduction system
7p21	*DNAH11*	Dynein, microtubule motor	Heterotaxy, Kartagener syndrome
7q21	*SEMA3E*	Semaphorin, neural guidance	TOF, PDA, AVC, CHARGE syndrome
7q11.2	*ELN*	Vascular integrity	SVAS, PA stenosis
8q12	*CHD7*	Chromodomain helicase	TOF, PDA, AVC, CHARGE syndrome
8p23.1-p22	*GATA4*	Transcription	ASD
9p21	*DNAI1*	Dynein, microtubule motor	Heterotaxy, Kartagener syndrome
9q34.3	*NOTCH1*	Signaling	Bicuspid aortic valve
11p15.4	Unknown	—	MVP
12p12.1	*KRAS*	Signaling	PS, ASD, VSD, PDA, Noonan syndrome
12q24.1	*PTPN11*	Signaling	PS, ASD, VSD, PDA, Noonan syndrome
12q24.1	*TBX5*	Transcription	ASD, VSD, TOF, conduction system, Holt-Oram syndrome
12q24	Unknown	—	PDA
20q13	*SALL4*	Transcription	VSD, TOF, TA, Okihiro syndrome
20p12	*JAG1*	Signaling	PS, VSD, TOF, Alagille syndrome
14q12	*MYH6*	Alpha-myosin	ASD
16p11.2	Unknown	—	MVP
22q 11.2	*TBX1*	Transcription	TOF, TGA, DORV, DiGeorge syndrome
Xq26.2	*ZIC3*	—	Heterotaxy
Xq28	Unknown	—	MVP

ASD = atrial septal defect; AVC = atrioventricular conduction; AVCD = atrioventricular conduction disturbance; DORV = double outlet right ventricle; MVP = mitral valve prolapse; PA = pulmonary artery; PDA = patent ductus arteriosus; PS = pulmonic stenosis; SVAS = supraventricular arterial stenosis; TA = tricuspid atresia; TOF = tetralogy of Fallot; TGA = transposition of the great arteries; VSD = ventricular septal defect.

Isolated hereditary defects in atrial septation are usually ostium secundum defects. Affected family members may have other structural defects, including atrial septal aneurysms, ventricular septal defects (VSDs), and atrioventricular canal or aortic or pulmonary valve disease. Spontaneous closure of septation defects caused by gene mutation is uncommon; these defects usually require surgical correction.

Dominant mutations in *GATA4*, *MYH6*, *NKX2-5*, and an unidentified gene on chromosome 5p cause isolated familial atrial septal defects.[50] Loss of one gene copy (hemizygosity) of *GATA4* may also cause heart malformations in patients with chromosome 8p23 interstitial deletions. *GATA4* is a member of a zinc finger transcription factor gene family, which recognizes a consensus sequence motif in target gene promoters.[51] Although *GATA4* is also expressed in developing gut epithelium and gonads, the effects of human mutations appear limited to the heart.

Dominant mutations in *NKX2-5* (encoded on chromosome 5q34) cause inherited septation defects associated with postnatal onset of electrophysiologic disease (**Fig. 8-3**).[50,51a,52] *NKX2-5* is a member of the NK gene family of transcription factors that contains a homeobox sequence motif and is the mammalian homologue of the *Drosophila tinman* gene (so-named because deletions abrogate development of the dorsal vessel, the insect's heart equivalent). Heart malformations

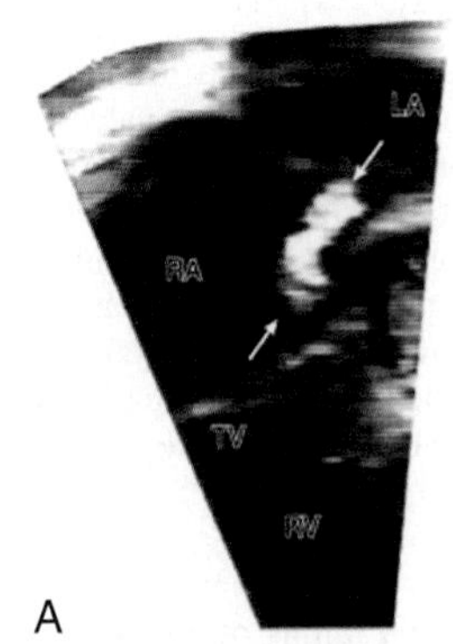

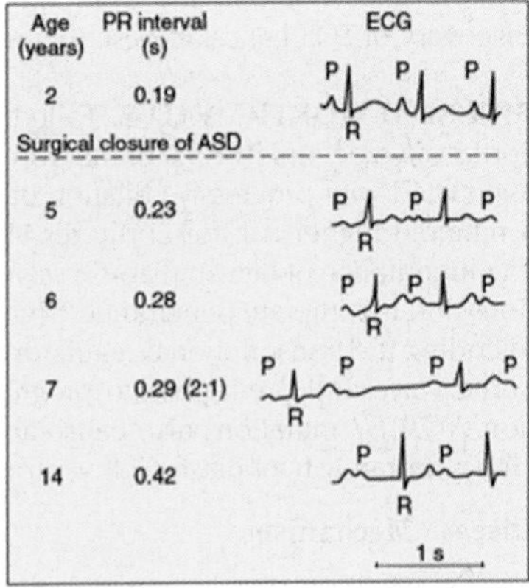

FIGURE 8-3 Clinical manifestations of *NKX2-5* mutations. **A,** Doppler echocardiography detects atrial septal defect (ASD). **B,** The electrocardiogram (ECG) shows progressive atrioventricular delay through 6 years of age. By 7 years of age, 2:1 atrioventricular block is evident. A pacemaker was implanted at 14 years of age. LA = left atrium; RA = right atrium; RV = right ventricle; TV = tricuspid valve. *(From Schott JJ, Benson DW, Basson CT, et al: Congenital heart disease caused by mutations in the transcription factor NKX2-5. Science 281:108, 1998.)*

arising from *NKX2-5* mutations vary more than those caused by *GATA4* mutations and include secundum- or cribriform-type atrial septal defects (ASDs), VSDs (muscular type), tetralogy of Fallot (TOF), and double-orifice mitral valve. Adult-onset LVH caused by *NKX2-5* does not always involve demonstrable structural malformations.[50]

CH 8

NKX2-5 mutation produces electrophysiologic defects, including progressive atrioventricular conduction delay with Wenckebach-type second-degree heart block, sick sinus, and atrial fibrillation. In some individuals, electrophysiologic manifestations occur without structural heart defects. Atrioventricular conduction delays evolve insidiously and necessitate permanent pacemaker implantation, even decades after diagnosis of the structural malformation (see Fig. 8-3B), necessitating longitudinal evaluations of affected individuals. Electrocardiographic abnormalities in a patient with apparently sporadic ASD should prompt a detailed family history and evaluation of close relatives.

Disease Mechanism

NKX2.5 and *GATA4* encode interacting transcription factors that bind DNA. Analyses of human mutations indicate that *GATA4* and *NKX2.5* mutations disrupt interactions with cognate DNA sequences and reduce transcriptional activation of target genes. *NKX2.5* specifies cardiac progenitor cells from mesoderm tissue in mammalian and lower species.[51] *GATA4* regulates genes critical for myocardial differentiation and function, including troponin C, alpha-cardiac myosin heavy chain, and brain natriuretic peptide. Complete ablation of *NKX2.5* or *GATA4* in experimental models results in failed cardiac development, and thus is lethal.

TETRALOGY OF FALLOT. TOF, the most prevalent form of cyanotic heart disease, comprises a malpositioned aorta that overrides both ventricles, ventricular septal defect, pulmonary stenosis, and right ventricular hypertrophy (see Chap. 65). TOF occurs in 1 of 3000 live births and accounts for 10% of all major congenital heart disease.[53] With contemporary corrective surgery strategies, early lethality from TOF is rare, but long-term sequelae, including arrhythmia and ventricular dysfunction, can persist.

TOF occurs in isolation or as a component of multisystem disorders such as DiGeorge syndrome or Alagille syndrome. Microscopic deletions of chromosome 22q11.2 cause DiGeorge syndrome, accounting for 15% of TOF cases. Trisomy 21 (Down syndrome) accounts for 7% of TOF cases.[54,55]

Mutations in cardiac transcription factor genes (*NKX2.5*, *TBX1*, *GATA4*) cause isolated TOF and other malformations. TOF also occurs in the context of Alagille syndrome, caused by mutation in the transmembrane receptor *NOTCH2* or its ligand *JAG1*, and in the Holt-Oram syndrome, caused by mutation in *TBX5*. Microscopic deletions or insertions at chromosome 1q21.1 are found in 1% of nonsyndromic sporadic cases of TOF, and less commonly at 3p25.1 and 7p21.3.[56] Discovery of TOF genes at these loci is an active area of research.

BICUSPID AORTIC VALVE. Failed development of a trileaflet aortic valve occurs in 1.5% of the population. Bicuspid aortic valve is associated with progressive dilation of the proximal aorta and carries a ninefold higher risk for aortic dissection (see Chaps. 60 and 66).[57] The inheritance of bicuspid aortic valve accompanies dominant mutations and incomplete penetrance.[58] Inactivating mutations in the gene encoding the transcriptional regulator *NOTCH1* rarely cause bicuspid aortic valve and predispose to progressive postnatal valve calcification. *NOTCH1* mutations also cause aortic stenosis and aortic insufficiency or, rarely, hypoplastic left ventricle or TOF.

Disease Mechanism

NOTCH receptors and ligands constitute a gene family of transmembrane receptors with diverse roles in signaling cellular differentiation and cell fate. Activation of NOTCH receptors stimulates proteolytic cleavage and release of domains that translocate to the nucleus and participate in transcriptional activation.

MITRAL VALVE PROLAPSE. Mitral valve prolapse (MVP) is a prevalent abnormality that can arise alone (see Chap. 66) or in the context of heritable connective tissue disorders (e.g., Marfan syndrome; see Chap. 60). MVP is associated with myxomatous degeneration or a thickening, enlargement, and redundancy of the leaflets and chordae involved in changes in collagen distribution. Familial MVP can show distinctive billowing of the mitral leaflets or excessive systolic mitral annular expansion. Isolated familial MVP exhibits age- and sex-dependent expression,[59] with autosomal dominant inheritance. MVP maps to four genetic loci. One disease gene is filamin A (*FMNA*), encoded on Xq28.[60-63] *FMNA* mutations inactivate the gene and result in minimal valvular defects in women, but cause significant degeneration of all cardiac valves in men.[63]

Inherited Syndromes with Major Cardiovascular Malformations (see Chap. 65)

HOLT-ORAM SYNDROME. Dysplasia of the upper limbs and cardiac septal defects characterize this prototypic hand-heart disorder.[64] Arm deformities are usually bilateral but often asymmetric in severity, and range from subtle abnormalities of the radius and thumb (distally placed and triphalangeal) to phocomelia. Hypoplasia of the clavicles or shoulders may be present. Heart malformations occur in 85% of patients with Holt-Oram syndrome and include secundum ASDs, VSDs, patent ductus arteriosus (PDA), and a wide spectrum of complex heart and vascular malformations. Patients can develop electrophysiologic deficits beyond the atrioventricular node; conduction system disturbances can occur in the absence of structural heart disease. Patients with apparently sporadic atrial septal defects should be carefully examined for subtle limb malformations, because detection of Holt-Oram syndrome substantially increases the recurrence risk for offspring from 3% (empirical recurrence risk of an isolated septal defect) to 50%.

Holt-Oram syndrome results from mutations in *TBX5*, a member of the T-box transcription factor gene family,[64] which shares conserved DNA-binding sequences, denoted as the T-box. Mutations typically inactivate one gene copy and reduce physiologic levels by half, but clinical expression varies considerably among family members. Parental manifestations do not reliably predict the severity of malformations in offspring.

Disease Mechanism

The transcription factors TBX5, GATA4, and NKX2.5 interact with one another and regulate expression of genes required for cardiac septation. TBX5 and NKX2.5 interact to regulate expression of ID2 and other downstream genes required for the normal morphology and function of the atrioventricular and bundle branch conduction systems.[65] TBX5 presumably also regulates the expression of genes expressed in the developing forelimb, accounting for the skeletal abnormalities observed in Holt-Oram syndrome.

NOONAN SYNDROME. This autosomal dominant cardiofacial syndrome occurs with a prevalence of 1 in 1000 to 2500 live births.[49] The pleiotropic features of Noonan syndrome include facial dysmorphism (hypertelorism, ptosis), short stature, pectus deformity, cubitus valgus, neck webbing, congenital lymphedema, and congenital heart defects (in 80% of patients). Additional manifestations include mental retardation, hematopoietic abnormalities that can evolve into leukemia, and cryptorchidism. Lymphatic dysplasia of the lower limbs is common but causes clinical difficulties in less than 20% of cases. Chylothorax and a protein-losing enteropathy represent the severe end of the spectrum.

Valvular pulmonic stenosis is the most common congenital heart defect and is found in 40% of patients with Noonan syndrome. Valve cusps are thickened and dysplastic, even in the absence of hemodynamic compromise. Pulmonary artery hypoplasia or infundibular subvalvular remodeling can occur and result in a cardiomyopathy that is hypertrophic, often asymmetric, and predominant in either ventricle. ASD occurs in about one third of patients with Noonan syndrome, usually in association with pulmonic stenosis. VSD and PDA each occur in about 10% of cases. Congenital anomalies of coronary arteries arise occasionally and unexpectedly during evaluation of more obvious defects.

Mutations in eight genes—*PTPN11*, *SOS1*, *RAF1*, *KRAS*, *BRAF*, *MEK1*, *MEK2*, and *HRAS*[66]—cause about 75% of Noonan syndrome cases. These genes encode proteins that participate in the Ras/Raf/MEK/ERK signal transduction pathway. Mutations in *PTPN11*, which encodes SHP-2, a tyrosine phosphatase with a Src homology 2 (SH2) domain, occur in approximately 50% of patients with Noonan syndrome.

Disease Mechanism

Noonan syndrome mutations activate components of the Ras/Raf pathway. Binding of guanosine diphosphate (GDP) and guanosine triphosphate (GTP) by RAS proteins regulates intracellular signals that control cell proliferation, differentiation, and survival.

DIGEORGE SYNDROME. DiGeorge syndrome (DGS; also known as velocardiofacial syndrome [VCFS], and chromosome 22q11.2 deletion syndrome), is an autosomal dominant disorder characterized by outflow tract defects of the heart, hypocalcemia arising from parathyroid hypoplasia, thymic hypoplasia and, frequently, neurologic abnormalities.[67] Clinical manifestations can be subtle, accounting for incomplete disease penetrance. DiGeorge syndrome is caused by a microdeletion on chromosome 22q11, which is inherited or arises de novo in approximately 1 of 2000 to 4000 live births. Microdeletions arise from homologous recombination between flanking sequences on 22q11, excising approximately 3 million base pairs encompassing the *TBX1* gene, which accounts for most phenotypes associated with DiGeorge syndrome.

Disease Mechanism

Disturbance of cervical neural crest migration into the derivatives of the pharyngeal arches and pouches account for the phenotypes found in patients with DiGeorge syndrome. TBX1 is required for appropriate neural crest migration, but the target gene(s) regulated by this transcription factor, which account for the diverse phenotypes found in DiGeorge syndrome, are unknown.

TRISOMY 21 (DOWN SYNDROME). With an occurrence of 1 in 600 births, trisomy 21 is the most common defect of human chromosome dosage.[68] Clinical features include characteristic abnormal facies, mental retardation, conductive hearing loss, and major congenital heart malformations (in 40% to 50% of cases). Patients have increased risk for hematologic malignancy disease (10- to 20-fold above normal) and progressive dementia of the Alzheimer type at a younger than expected age (fifth decade). Premature aging of the vasculature also occurs.

Atrioventricular canal defects are the prototypic cardiac anomaly of Down syndrome, causing pulmonary hypertension from increased blood flow. Other complex cardiac malformations, with the exception of transposition of the great arteries, occur in one third of patients. Older patients develop MVP at a higher frequency than age- and sex-matched control subjects, and adult patients are predisposed to fenestrations in the aortic and pulmonary valve cusps.

In most patients, the three copies of chromosome 21 reflect maternal errors in meiosis, events that increase exponentially with maternal age. Risk for trisomy 21 rises steeply after age 35, and reaches 4% in women older than 45 years. Critical regions within chromosome 21 for Down syndrome phenotypes have been identified, and they contain genes that may be implicated in trisomy 21 heart disease. The genes responsible for the cardiac abnormalities associated with this condition, however, have not been identified.

TURNER SYNDROME. About 1 in 2500 females has Turner syndrome.[69] Classic morphologic features include short stature, webbed neck, and bowed arms, but clinical findings are variable and often mild. Diagnosis sometimes occurs only during evaluation for short stature or amenorrhea.

Approximately 20% to 50% of patients with Turner syndrome have heart defects.[61] Aortic coarctation (postductal type) occurs in 50% to 70% of patients with heart disease. Other malformations occur alone or in combination with coarctation, including bicuspid aortic valve, dilation of the ascending aorta, hypoplastic left heart, and partial anomalous pulmonary venous drainage without an accompanying ASD. Cardiac conduction system abnormalities, including repolarization abnormalities and QT prolongation, can occur. Hypertension is common, even without coarctation or following repair, and may reflect a high frequency of renal anomalies in patients with Turner syndrome. Blood pressure elevation is strongly associated with dilation of the ascending aorta, so aggressive treatment is warranted. Treatment of children with human growth hormone to increase mature height has no apparent deleterious effect on cardiac performance.[70]

Turner syndrome is caused by complete or partial absence of the X chromosome, resulting in a 45,X karyotype. Mosaicism can also result in Turner syndrome with 46,XX or 46,XY karyotypes; these patients are less likely to have cardiovascular defects.

Future Perspectives

Mendelian disorders affecting the heart commonly cause cardiovascular disease. Most cardiomyopathy disease genes encode structural proteins involved in critical contractile processes. Mutant structural proteins incorporated into functional complexes cause disease by their disruptive effects.

In contrast, congenital heart disease mutations affect transcription factors and signaling molecules that regulate cardiac development. These gene mutations usually reduce the levels of the encoded protein by half, implying that normal cardiac embryogenesis requires physiologic doses of these genes. Congenital heart disease gene mutations have a wide range of clinical expression. Increasingly available clinical gene-based diagnoses of cardiomyopathy and congenital heart disease can provide early accurate diagnosis and evaluation of risk assessment in family members.

Therapies for cardiomyopathy and congenital heart disease remain limited. With gene discoveries and the development of animal models for these conditions, ongoing discoveries of pathways affected by mutant genes will increase and fuel the development of targeted therapies. Given the long latency of many cardiovascular genetic diseases, this knowledge can advance opportunities for intervention and disease prevention.

REFERENCES

1. Lewis R: Human Genetics: Concepts and Applications. New York, Harper and Row, 2008.
2. Morita H, Seidman J, Seidman CE: Genetic causes of human heart failure. J Clin Invest 115:518, 2005.
3. Alcalai R, Seidman JG, Seidman CE: Genetic basis of hypertrophic cardiomyopathy: From bench to the clinics. J Cardiovasc Electrophysiol 19:104, 2008.
4. Ahmad F, Seidman JG, Seidman CE: The genetic basis for cardiac remodeling. Annu Rev Genomics Hum Genet 6:185, 2005.
5. Morita H, DePalma SR, Arad M, et al: Molecular epidemiology of hypertrophic cardiomyopathy. Cold Spring Harb Symp Quant Biol 67:383, 2002.
6. Michels M, Lamers JM, Winegrad S, et al: Cardiac myosin-binding protein C mutations and hypertrophic cardiomyopathy: Haploinsufficiency, deranged phosphorylation, and cardiomyocyte dysfunction. Circulation 119:1473, 2009.
7. Marston S, Copeland O, Jacques A, et al: Evidence from human myectomy samples that MYBPC3 mutations cause hypertrophic cardiomyopathy through haploinsufficiency. Circ Res 105:219, 2009.
8. Debold EP, Schmitt JP, Patlak JB, et al: Hypertrophic and dilated cardiomyopathy mutations differentially affect the molecular force generation of mouse alpha-cardiac myosin in the laser trap assay. Am J Physiol Heart Circ Physiol 293:H284, 2007.
9. Ho CY, Lever HM, DeSanctis R, et al: Homozygous mutation in cardiac troponin T: Implications for hypertrophic cardiomyopathy. Circulation 102:1950, 2000.
10. Maron BJ, Maron MS, Wigle ED, Braunwald E: The 50-year history, controversy, and clinical implications of left ventricular outflow tract obstruction in hypertrophic cardiomyopathy: From idiopathic hypertrophic subaortic stenosis to hypertrophic cardiomyopathy. J Am Coll Cardiol 54:191, 2009.
11. Hershberger RE, Cowan J, Morales A, Siegfried JD: Progress with genetic cardiomyopathies: Screening, counseling, and testing in dilated, hypertrophic, and arrhythmogenic right ventricular dysplasia/cardiomyopathy. Circ Heart Fail 2:253, 2009.
12. Richard P, Charron P, Carrier L, et al: Hypertrophic cardiomyopathy: Distribution of disease genes, spectrum of mutations, and implications for a molecular diagnosis strategy. Circulation 107:2227, 2003.
13. Nishi H, Kimura A, Harada H, et al: Possible gene dose effect of a mutant cardiac beta-myosin heavy chain gene on the clinical expression of familial hypertrophic cardiomyopathy. Biochem Biophys Res Commun 200:549, 1994.

14. Bos JM, Towbin JA, Ackerman MJ: Diagnostic, prognostic, and therapeutic implications of genetic testing for hypertrophic cardiomyopathy. J Am Coll Cardiol 54:201, 2009.
15. Carrier L: Cardiac myosin-binding protein C in the heart. Arch Mal Coeur Vaiss 100:238, 2007.
16. Alders M, Jongbloed R, Deelen W, et al: The 2373insG mutation in the MYBPC3 gene is a founder mutation, which accounts for nearly one-fourth of the HCM cases in the Netherlands. Eur Heart J 24:1848, 2003.
17. Dhandapany PS, Sadayappan S, Xue Y, et al: A common MYBPC3 (cardiac myosin binding protein C) variant associated with cardiomyopathies in South Asia. Nat Genet 41:187, 2009.
18. Morimoto S: Sarcomeric proteins and inherited cardiomyopathies. Cardiovasc Res 77:659, 2008.
19. Bos JM, Poley RN, Ny M, et al: Genotype-phenotype relationships involving hypertrophic cardiomyopathy-associated mutations in titin, muscle LIM protein, and telethonin. Mol Genet Metab 88:78, 2006.
20. Mogensen J, Murphy RT, Kubo T, et al: Frequency and clinical expression of cardiac troponin I mutations in 748 consecutive families with hypertrophic cardiomyopathy. J Am Coll Cardiol 44:2315, 2004.
21. Arad M, Penas-Lado M, Monserrat L, et al: Gene mutations in apical hypertrophic cardiomyopathy. Circulation 112:2805, 2005.
22. Jääskeläinen P, Miettinen R, Kärkkäinen P, et al: Genetics of hypertrophic cardiomyopathy in eastern Finland: Few founder mutations with benign or intermediary phenotypes. Ann Med 36:23, 2004.
23. Tsoutsman T, Lam L, Semsarian C: Genes, calcium and modifying factors in hypertrophic cardiomyopathy. Clin Exp Pharmacol Physiol 33:139, 2006.
24. Chang AN, Harada K, Ackerman MJ, Potter JD: Functional consequences of hypertrophic and dilated cardiomyopathy-causing mutations in alpha-tropomyosin. J Biol Chem 280:34343, 2005.
25. Semsarian C, Ahmad I, Giewat M, et al: The L-type calcium channel inhibitor diltiazem prevents cardiomyopathy in a mouse model. J Clin Invest 109:1013, 2002.
26. Tardiff JC: Sarcomeric proteins and familial hypertrophic cardiomyopathy: Linking mutations in structural proteins to complex cardiovascular phenotypes. Heart Fail Rev 10:237, 2005.
27. Arad M, Seidman CE, Seidman JG: AMP-activated protein kinase in the heart: Role during health and disease. Circ Res 100:474, 2007.
28. Arad M, Maron BJ, Gorham JM, et al: Glycogen storage diseases presenting as hypertrophic cardiomyopathy. N Engl J Med 352:362, 2005.
29. Clarke JT: Narrative review: Fabry disease. Ann Intern Med 146:425, 2007.
30. Yang Z, Vattam: Danon disease as a cause of autophagic vacuolar myopathy. Congenit Heart Dis 2:404, 2007.
31. Eskelinen EL: Roles of LAMP-1 and LAMP-2 in lysosome biogenesis and autophagy. Mol Aspects Med 27:495, 2006.
32. Burwinkel B, Scott JW, Bührer C, et al: Fatal congenital heart glycogenosis caused by a recurrent activating R531Q mutation in the gamma 2-subunit of AMP-activated protein kinase (PRKAG2), not by phosphorylase kinase deficiency. Am J Hum Genet 76:1034, 2005.
33. Arad M, Moskowitz IP, Patel VV, et al: Transgenic mice overexpressing mutant PRKAG2 define the cause of Wolff-Parkinson-White syndrome in glycogen storage cardiomyopathy. Circulation 107:2850, 2003.
34. Maron BJ, Towbin JA, Thiene G, et al: Contemporary definitions and classification of the cardiomyopathies: An American Heart Association Scientific Statement from the Council on Clinical Cardiology, Heart Failure and Transplantation Committee; Quality of Care and Outcomes Research and Functional Genomics and Translational Biology Interdisciplinary Working Groups; and Council on Epidemiology and Prevention. Circulation 113:1807, 2006.
35. Kimura A: Molecular etiology and pathogenesis of hereditary cardiomyopathy. Circ J 72(Suppl A):A38, 2008.
36. Chang AN, Potter JD: Sarcomeric protein mutations in dilated cardiomyopathy. Heart Fail Rev 10:225, 2005.
37. LeWinter MM, VanBuren P: Sarcomeric proteins in hypertrophied and failing myocardium: An overview. Heart Fail Rev 10:173, 2005.
38. Kane GC, Liu XK, Yamada S, et al: Cardiac KATP channels in health and disease. J Mol Cell Cardiol 38:937, 2005.
39. Malhotra R, Mason PK: Lamin A/C deficiency as a cause of familial dilated cardiomyopathy. Curr Opin Cardiol 24:203, 2009.
40. Heydemann A, McNally EM: Consequences of disrupting the dystrophin-sarcoglycan complex in cardiac and skeletal myopathy. Trends Cardiovasc Med 17:55, 2007.
41. Kaspar RW, Allen HD, Montanaro F: Current understanding and management of dilated cardiomyopathy in Duchenne and Becker muscular dystrophy. J Am Acad Nurse Pract 21:241, 2009.
42. Sparagna GC, Lesnefsky EJ: Cardiolipin remodeling in the heart. J Cardiovasc Pharmacol 53:290, 2009.
43. Blum A: Heart failure—new insights. Isr Med Assoc J 11:105, 2009.
44. Ingwall JS: Energy metabolism in heart failure and remodelling. Cardiovasc Res 81:412, 2009.
45. Basso C, Corrado D, Marcus FI, et al: Arrhythmogenic right ventricular cardiomyopathy. Lancet 373:1289, 2009.
46. Corrado D, Thiene G: Arrhythmogenic right ventricular cardiomyopathy/dysplasia: Clinical impact of molecular genetic studies. Circulation 113:1634, 2006.
47. Lombardi R, Dong J, Rodriguez G, et al: Genetic fate mapping identifies second heart field progenitor cells as a source of adipocytes in arrhythmogenic right ventricular cardiomyopathy. Circ Res 104:1076, 2009.
48. Lloyd-Jones D, Adams R, Carnethon M, et al: Heart disease and stroke statistics—2009 update: A report from the American Heart Association Statistics Committee and Stroke Statistics Subcommittee. Circulation 119:480, 2009.
49. National Center for Biotechnology Information: OMIM: Online Mendelian Inheritance in Man (http://www.ncbi.nlm.nih.gov/omim).
50. Maslen CL: Molecular genetics of atrioventricular septal defects. Curr Opin Cardiol 19:205, 2004.
51. Joziasse IC, van de Smagt JJ, Smith K, et al: Genes in congenital heart disease: Atrioventricular valve formation. Basic Res Cardiol 103:216, 2008.
51a. Schott JJ, Benson DW, Basson CT, et al: Congenital heart disease caused by mutations in the transcription factor NKX2-5. Science 281:108, 1998.
52. Bajolle F, Zaffran S, Bonnet D: Genetics and embryological mechanisms of congenital heart diseases. Arch Cardiovasc Dis 102:59, 2009.
53. Ferencz C, Rubin JD, McCarter RJ, et al: Congenital heart disease: Prevalence at livebirth. The Baltimore-Washington Infant Study. Am J Epidemiol 121:31, 1985.
54. Marelli AJ, Mackie AS, Ionescu-Ittu R, et al: Congenital heart disease in the general population: Changing prevalence and age distribution. Circulation 115:163, 2007.
55. Yagi H, Furutani Y, Hamada H, et al: Role of TBX1 in human del22q11.2 syndrome. Lancet 362:1366, 2003.
56. Greenway SC, Pereira AC, Lin JC, et al: De novo copy number variants identify new genes and loci in isolated sporadic tetralogy of Fallot. Nat Genet 41:931, 2009.
57. Tadros TM, Klein MD, Shapira OM: Ascending aortic dilatation associated with bicuspid aortic valve: Pathophysiology, molecular biology, and clinical implications. Circulation 119:880, 2009.
58. McBride KL, Pignatelli R, Lewin M, et al: Inheritance analysis of congenital left ventricular outflow tract obstruction malformations: Segregation, multiplex relative risk, and heritability. Am J Med Genet A 134:180, 2005.
59. Horne BD, Camp NJ, Muhlestein JB, Cannon-Albright LA: Evidence for a heritable component in death resulting from aortic and mitral valve diseases. Circulation 110:3143, 2004.
60. Donaldson MD, Gault EJ, Tan KW, Dunger DB: Optimising management in Turner syndrome: From infancy to adult transfer. Arch Dis Child 91:513, 2006.
61. Doswell BH, Visootsak J, Brady AN, Graham JM Jr: Turner syndrome: An update and review for the primary pediatrician. Clin Pediatr (Phila) 45:301, 2006.
62. Vergara P, Digilio MC, De Zorzi A, et al: Genetic heterogeneity and phenotypic anomalies in children with atrioventricular canal defect and tetralogy of Fallot. Clin Dysmorphol 15:65, 2006.
63. Kyndt F, Gueffet JP, Probst V, et al: Mutations in the gene encoding filamin A as a cause for familial cardiac valvular dystrophy. Circulation 115:40, 2007.
64. Hatcher CJ, McDermott DA: Using the TBX5 transcription factor to grow and sculpt the heart. Am J Med Genet A 140:1414, 2006.
65. Moskowitz IP, Kim JB, Moore ML, et al: A molecular pathway including Id2, Tbx5, and Nkx2-5 required for cardiac conduction system development. Cell 129:1365, 2007.
66. Tidyman WE, Rauen KA: The RASopathies: Developmental syndromes of Ras/MAPK pathway dysregulation. Curr Opin Genet Dev 19:230, 2009.
67. Emanuel BS: Molecular mechanisms and diagnosis of chromosome 22q11.2 rearrangements. Dev Disabil Res Rev 14:11, 2008.
68. Antonarakis SE, Lyle R, Dermitzakis ET, et al: Chromosome 21 and down syndrome: From genomics to pathophysiology. Nat Rev Genet 5:725, 2004.
69. Bondy CA: Turner syndrome 2008. Horm Res 71(Suppl 1):52, 2009.
70. Rosenfeld RG: The future of research into growth hormone responsiveness. Horm Res 71(Suppl 2):71, 2009.
71. Rayment I, Rypniewski WR, Schmidt-Bäse K, et al: Three-dimensional structure of myosin subfragment-1: a molecular motor. Science 261:50, 1993.

CHAPTER 9 Genetics of Cardiac Arrhythmias

David J. Tester and Michael J. Ackerman

Cardiac arrhythmia encompasses a large and heterogeneous group of electrical abnormalities of the heart, with or without underlying structural heart disease. Cardiac arrhythmias can be innocuous, can predispose to the development of potentially lethal stroke or embolus, or can present emergently with a life-threatening condition that may result in sudden cardiac death (SCD), one of the most common causes of death in the developed countries. In the United States for example, an estimated 300,000 to 400,000 individuals die suddenly each year, with the vast majority involving older adults; 80% are caused by ventricular fibrillation (VF) in the context of ischemic heart disease. In comparison, SCD in the young is relatively uncommon, with an incidence between 1.3 and 8.5/100,000 patient-years.[1] However, tragically, thousands of otherwise healthy individuals younger than 20 years die suddenly each year without warning. Most SCD in the young can be attributed to structural cardiovascular anomalies identifiable at autopsy; however, as much as 30% of sudden death in the young remains unexplained following a complete autopsy and medicolegal investigation (see Chap. 41).

Potentially lethal and inheritable arrhythmia syndromes under the umbrella of the cardiac channelopathies, including congenital long-QT syndrome (LQTS), Brugada syndrome (BrS), catecholaminergic polymorphic ventricular tachycardia (CPVT), and related disorders, involve electrical disturbances with the propensity to produce fatal arrhythmias in the setting of a structurally normal heart. These often unassuming electrical abnormalities can cause the heart of an unsuspecting individual to develop a potentially lethal arrhythmia, leading to the sudden and early demise of someone who is otherwise healthy.[1] It is now recognized that almost one third of autopsy-negative sudden unexplained deaths in the young[2] and approximately 10% of sudden infant death syndrome (SIDS) are caused by pathogenic mechanisms involving these genetically inherited cardiac channelopathies.[3,4]

Through molecular advances in the field of cardiovascular genetics, the underlying genetic bases responsible for many inherited cardiac arrhythmia syndromes have come to light, and for others their underlying genetic substrates are on the cusp of discovery. Over the past decade, a particular set of themes, including extreme genetic heterogeneity, reduced or incomplete penetrance, and variable expressivity have proven to be commonplace among the cardiac channelopathies. However, for some disorders, important genotype-phenotype correlates have been recognized that have a diagnostic, prognostic, and therapeutic impact.

Given the potentially devastating impact of these genetic disorders on families and their communities, we will provide the clinical description, genetic basis, and genotype-phenotype correlates associated with these inherited arrhythmia syndromes. Specifically, in this chapter, we will discuss the cardiac channelopathies, focusing first on the subset of QT-opathies—LQTS, Andersen-Tawil syndrome (ATS), Timothy syndrome (TS), short-QT syndrome (SQTS), drug-induced torsades de pointes (TdP)—and then on the other channelopathies—BrS, idiopathic ventricular fibrillation (IVF), progressive cardiac conduction defect (PCCD), sick sinus syndrome (SSS), CPVT, ankyrin-B syndrome, and familial atrial fibrillation (AF).

QT-opathies

Long-QT Syndrome

CLINICAL DESCRIPTION AND MANIFESTATIONS. Congenital LQTS comprises a distinct group of cardiac channelopathies characterized by delayed repolarization of the myocardium, QT prolongation (QTc > 480 msec as the 50th percentile among LQTS cohorts), and increased risk for syncope, seizures, and SCD in the setting of a structurally normal heart and otherwise healthy individual. The incidence of LQTS may exceed 1/2500 persons.[5,6] Individuals with LQTS may or may not manifest QT prolongation on a resting 12-lead surface electrocardiogram (ECG). This repolarization abnormality is almost always without consequence; however, rarely, triggers such as exertion, swimming, emotion, auditory stimuli (e.g., alarm clock), or the postpartum period can cause the heart to become electrically unstable and develop potentially life-threatening and sometimes lethal arrhythmia of TdP (see Chap. 39) Although the cardiac rhythm most often spontaneously returns to normal, resulting in only an episode of syncope, 5% of untreated and unsuspecting LQTS individuals succumb to a fatal arrhythmia as their sentinel event. However, it is estimated that almost 50% of individuals experiencing SCD stemming from this very treatable arrhythmogenic disorder may have exhibited prior warning signs (e.g., exertional syncope, family history of premature sudden death) that went unrecognized. LQTS may explain approximately 20% of autopsy-negative sudden unexplained deaths in the young and 10% of SIDS cases.[2,3]

GENETIC BASIS FOR LONG-QT SYNDROME. LQTS is a genetically heterogeneous disorder largely inherited in an autosomal dominant pattern, previously known as Romano-Ward syndrome.[6] Rarely, LQTS is inherited as the recessive trait first described by Jervell and Lange-Nielsen and is characterized by a severe cardiac phenotype and sensorineural hearing loss. Spontaneous and sporadic germline mutations can account for almost 5% to 10% of LQTS. Hundreds of mutations have now been identified in 12 LQTS susceptibility genes, with two of the first three canonical LQTS susceptibility genes discovered in 1995. Approximately 75% of patients with a clinically robust diagnosis of LQTS host either loss or gain of function mutations in one of these three major LQTS genes (**Table 9-1**)—*KCNQ1*-encoded I_{Ks} (Kv7.1) potassium channel (LQT1, ~35%, loss of function), *KCNH2*-encoded I_{Kr} (Kv11.1) potassium channel (LQT2, ~30%, loss of function), *SCN5A*-encoded I_{Na} (Nav1.5) sodium channel (LQT3, ~10%, gain of function)—that are responsible for the orchestration of the cardiac action potential[7,8] (**Fig. 9-1**). Approximately 5% to 10% of patients have multiple mutations in these genes and patients with multiple mutation LQTS present at a younger age and with greater expressivity[7] (see Chap. 7).

The nine minor LQTS susceptibility genes encode for either key cardiac *ch*annel *i*nteracting *p*roteins (ChIPs), which generally regulate the native ion channel current, or for structural membrane scaffolding proteins, which function in proper localization of channels to the plasma membrane and collectively explain perhaps 5% of LQTS. The vast majority of mutations are coding region single-nucleotide substitutions or small insertions or deletions resulting in nonsynonymous missense (amino acid substitution for another amino acid), nonsense (amino acid

TABLE 9-1 Summary of Heritable Arrhythmia Syndrome Susceptibility Genes

GENE	LOCUS	PROTEIN
Long-QT Syndrome		
Major LQTS Genes		
KCNQ1 (LQT1)	11p15.5	I_{Ks} potassium channel alpha subunit (KvQT1, Kv7.1)
KCNH2 (LQT2)	7q35-36	I_{Kr} potassium channel alpha subunit (HERG, Kv11.1)
SCN5A (LQT3)	3p21-p24	Cardiac sodium channel alpha subunit (NaV1.5)
Minor LQTS Genes (listed alphabetically)		
AKAP9	7q21-q22	Yotiao
ANKB	4q25-q27	Ankyrin-B
CACNA1C	12p13.3	Voltage-gated L-type calcium channel (CaV1.2)
CAV3	3p25	Caveolin-3
KCNE1	21q22.1	Potassium channel beta subunit (MinK)
KCNE2	21q22.1	Potassium channel beta subunit (MiRP1)
KCNJ2	17q23	I_{K1} potassium channel (Kir2.1)
SCN4B	11q23.3	Sodium channel beta$_4$ subunit
SNTA1	20q11.2	Syntrophin-alpha 1
Andersen-Tawil Syndrome		
KCNJ2 (ATS1)	17q23	I_{K1} potassium channel (Kir2.1)
Timothy Syndrome		
CACNA1C	2p13.3	Voltage-gated L-type calcium channel (CaV1.2)
Short-QT Syndrome		
KCNH2 (SQT1)	7q35-36	I_{Kr} potassium channel alpha subunit (HERG, Kv11.1)
KCNQ1 (SQT2)	11p15.5	I_{Ks} potassium channel alpha subunit (KvLQT1, Kv7.1)
KCNJ2 (SQT3)	17q23	I_{K1} potassium channel (Kir2.1)
CACNA1C (SQT4)	2p13.3	Voltage-gated L-type calcium channel (CaV1.2)
CACNB2 (SQT5)	10p12	Voltage-gated L-type calcium channel beta$_2$ subunit
Brugada Syndrome		
SCN5A (BrS1)	3p21-p24	Cardiac sodium channel alpha subunit (NaV1.5)
GPD1L	3p22.3	Glycerol-3-phosphate dehydrogenase 1–like
CACNA1C	2p13.3	Voltage-gated L-type calcium channel (CaV1.2)
CACNB2	10p12	Voltage-gated L-type calcium channel beta$_2$ subunit
SCN1B	19q13	Sodium channel beta$_1$ subunit
KCNE3	11q13.4	Potassium channel beta subunit (MiRP2)
Idiopathic Ventricular Fibrillation		
SCN5A	3p21-p24	Cardiac sodium channel alpha subunit (NaV1.5)
ANKB	4q25-q27	Ankyrin-B
RYR2	1q42.1-q43	Ryanodine receptor 2
DPP6	7q36	Dipeptidyl peptidase-6
SCN3B	11q23	Sodium channel beta$_3$ subunit
Progressive Cardiac Conduction Defect		
SCN5A	3p21-p24	Cardiac sodium channel alpha subunit (NaV1.5)
Sick Sinus Syndrome		
SCN5A	3p21-p24	Cardiac sodium channel alpha subunit (NaV1.5)
HCN4	15q24-q25	Hyperpolarization-activated cyclic nucleotide-gated channel 4
ANKB	4q25-q27	Ankyrin-B
Catecholaminergic Polymorphic Ventricular Tachycardia		
RYR2 (CPVT1)	1q42.1-q43	Ryanodine receptor 2
CASQ2 (CPVT2)	1p13.3	Calsequestrin 2
Ankyrin-B Syndrome		
ANK2	4q25-q27	Ankyrin-B
Familial Atrial Fibrillation		
KCNQ1	11p15.5	I_{Ks} potassium channel alpha subunit (KvLQT1, Kv7.1)
KCNJ2	17q23	I_{K1} potassium channel (Kir2.1)
KCNA5	12p13	I_{Kur} potassium channel (Kv1.5)
SCN5A	3p21-p24	Cardiac sodium channel alpha subunit (NaV1.5)
NPPA	1p36	Atrial natriuretic peptide precursor A
NUP155	5p13	Nucleoporin, 155 kDa
GJA5	1q21	Connexin 40

substitution for a termination codon), splice site alterations (resulting in exon skipping or intron inclusion), or frameshift mutations (altered normal amino acid coding resulting in an early termination).[7-9] Recently, a few large gene rearrangements involving hundreds to thousands of nucleotides resulting in single or multiple whole exon deletions or duplications have been described.[10,11] Importantly, there is no quintessential mutational hot spot within these genes, because the vast majority of unrelated families have their own unique private mutation. In 2010, it is important to note that almost 20% to 25% of clinically definitive cases of LQTS remain genetically elusive.

In contrast to rare, pathogenic, LQTS-associated channel mutations present in less than 0.04% (1/2500) of persons and in 75% of clinically robust LQTS patients, comprehensive genetic testing of *KCNQ1*, *KCNH2*, and *SCN5A* of more than 1300 ostensibly healthy volunteers has revealed that approximately 4% of whites and up to 8% of nonwhites host rare, nonsynonymous genetic variants (allelic frequency < 0.5%) in these specific cardiac channel genes.[12] A total of 79 distinct channel variants were detected in these healthy subjects, including 14 variants in *KCNQ1*, 28 in *KCNH2*, and 37 in *SCN5A*. Currently, over 1500 genetic tests are clinically available diagnostic tests for numerous disorders, including clinical genetic testing for the cardiac channelopathies. However, this background noise rate of genetic variation is known for only a handful of diseases as compared with the major LQTS susceptibility genes. This has enabled a case-control mutational analysis of the properties and localization of case-associated mutations compared with the compendium of presumably innocuous variants. The probabilistic rather than binary nature of genetic testing is depicted in **Fig. 9-2**, which shows that rare mutations other than missense mutations (approximately 20% of the LQTS spectrum of mutations) are high-probability LQTS-associated mutations, whereas the probability of pathogenicity for the most common mutation type, missense mutations (i.e. single amino acid substitutions), is strongly location-dependent. For example, missense mutations localizing to the transmembrane-spanning pore domains of the LQT1- and LQT2-associated potassium channels are high-probability disease

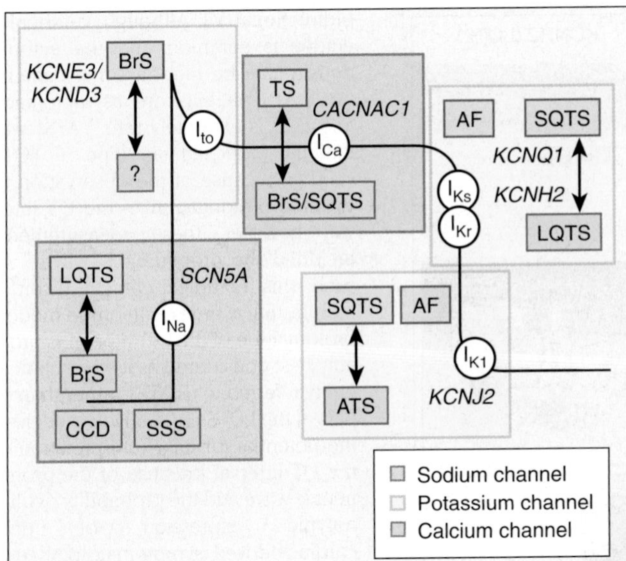

FIGURE 9-1 Cardiac action potential disorders. Illustrated are the key ion currents (white circles) along the ventricular cardiocyte's action potential that are associated with potentially lethal cardiac arrhythmia disorders. Disorders resulting in gain of function mutations are shown in green rectangles and those with loss of function mutations are shown in blue rectangles. For example, whereas gain of function mutations in the *SCN5A*-encoding cardiac sodium channel responsible for I_{Na} lead to LQTS, loss of function SCN5A mutations result in BrS, CCD, and SSS.

mutations, whereas a similarly rare missense mutation that localizes to the domain I-II linker of the Nav1.5 sodium channel is indeterminate, a variant of uncertain significance (VUS). Without cosegregation or functional data, such a mutation has a point estimate for probability of pathogenicity of less than 50%.

In addition to this background frequency (4% to 8%) of rare variants in health, 15 unique common polymorphisms (allelic frequency > 0.5%) have been identified in the four potassium channel subunit genes (*KCNQ1*, *KCNH2*, *KCNE1*, and *KCNE2*) and eight common polymorphisms have been identified in the sodium channel gene (*SCN5A*). Many of these rare and common polymorphisms represent innocent bystanders; however, a layer of complexity is added to the genetics of these channelopathies and the management of patients when otherwise apparently innocuous variants can modify disease. For example, the most common sodium channel variant, H558R, with a minor allelic frequency of approximately 29% in African Americans, 20% in whites, 23% in Hispanics, and 9% in Asians, can provide a modifying effect on the disease state through intragenic complementation (the interaction of two mutations within the same gene that produce a novel functional effect) of other SCN5A mutations.[13] Several studies have indicated that some of these common polymorphisms may be clinically informative and relevant to the identification of those at risk for cardiac arrhythmias, particularly in the setting of TdP-inducing drugs or other environmental factors (see later).

GENOTYPE-PHENOTYPE CORRELATES. Specific genotype-phenotype associations in LQTS have emerged, suggesting relatively gene-specific triggers, electrocardiographic patterns, and response to therapy (**Fig. 9-3**).[14] Swimming and exertion-induced cardiac events are strongly associated with mutations in *KCNQ1* (LQT1), whereas auditory triggers and events occurring during the postpartum period most often occur in patients with LQT2. Although exertional or emotional stress-induced events are most common in LQT1, events occurring during periods of sleep or rest are most common in LQT3. Characteristic gene-suggestive electrocardiographic patterns have been described earlier. LQT1 is associated with a broad-based T wave, LQT2 with a low-amplitude notched or biphasic T wave, and LQT3 with a long isoelectric segment followed by a narrow-based T wave.

However, exceptions to these relatively gene-specific T wave patterns exist and due caution must be exercised with making a pregenetic test prediction of the particular LQTS subtype involved, because the most common clinical mimicker of the LQT3-appearing ECG is seen in patients with LQT1. It is important to keep this in mind because the underlying genetic basis heavily influences the response to standard LQTS pharmacotherapy (beta blockers). Beta blockers are extremely protective in LQT1 patients, moderately protective in LQT2, and may not be sufficiently protective for those with LQT3.[15,16] Consequently, targeting the pathologic, LQT3-associated late sodium current with agents such as mexiletine, flecainide, or ranolazine may represent a gene-specific therapeutic option for LQT3.[17,18] Attenuation in repolarization with clinically apparent shortening in the QTc has been demonstrated with such a strategy, although there is no evidence-based demonstration of survival benefit thus far. Realistically however, at least a 30-year study may be needed for the latter.

In addition, intragenotype risk stratification has been realized for the two most common subtypes of LQTS based on mutation type, mutation location, and cellular function.[19-24] Patients with LQT1 with Kv7.1 missense mutations localizing to the transmembrane-spanning domains clinically have a twofold greater risk of a LQT1-triggered cardiac event than LQT1 patients with mutations localizing to the C-terminal region. Trumping location, patients with mutations resulting in a greater degree of Kv7.1 loss of function at the cellular in vitro level (i.e. dominant negative) have a twofold greater clinical risk

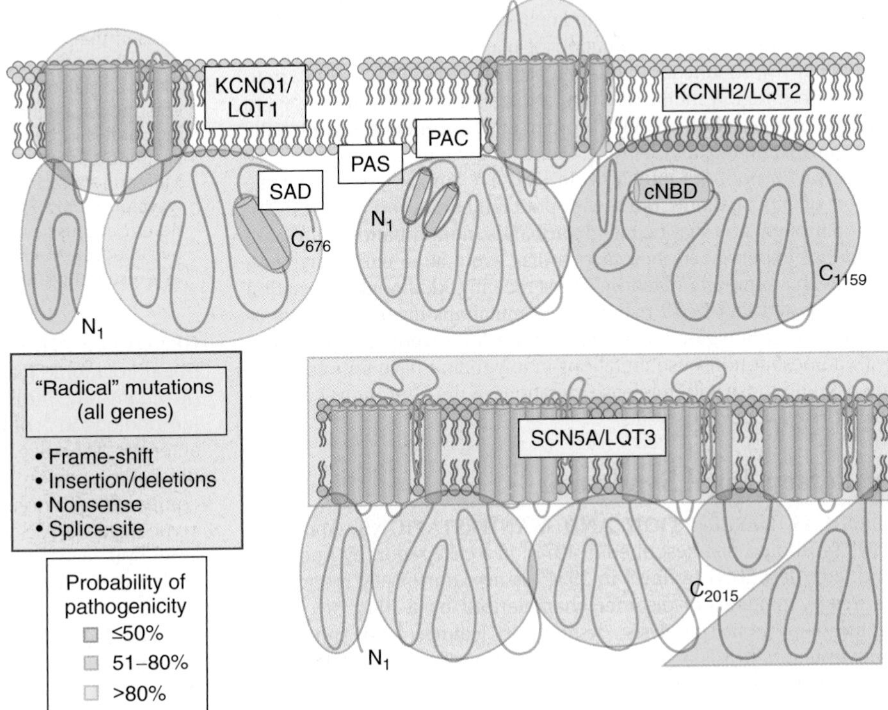

FIGURE 9-2 Probabilistic nature of LQTS genetic testing. Depicted are the three major ion channels causative for LQTS, with areas of probability of pathogenicity shown for mutations localizing to these respective areas. Whereas "radical" mutations have a >90% probability of being a true pathogenic mutation, the level of probability for missense mutations varies, depending on their location for each channel protein. Missense mutations residing in red shaded areas have a high probability (>80%) of being pathogenic, those in blue are possibly (51-80%) pathogenic, and those in yellow shaded areas truly represent variants of uncertain significance (VUS; $P = 0.5$) clinically. SAD = subunits assembly domain; PAS = Per-Arnt-Sim domain; PAC = PAS-associated C-terminal domain; cNBD = cyclic nucleotide binding domain.

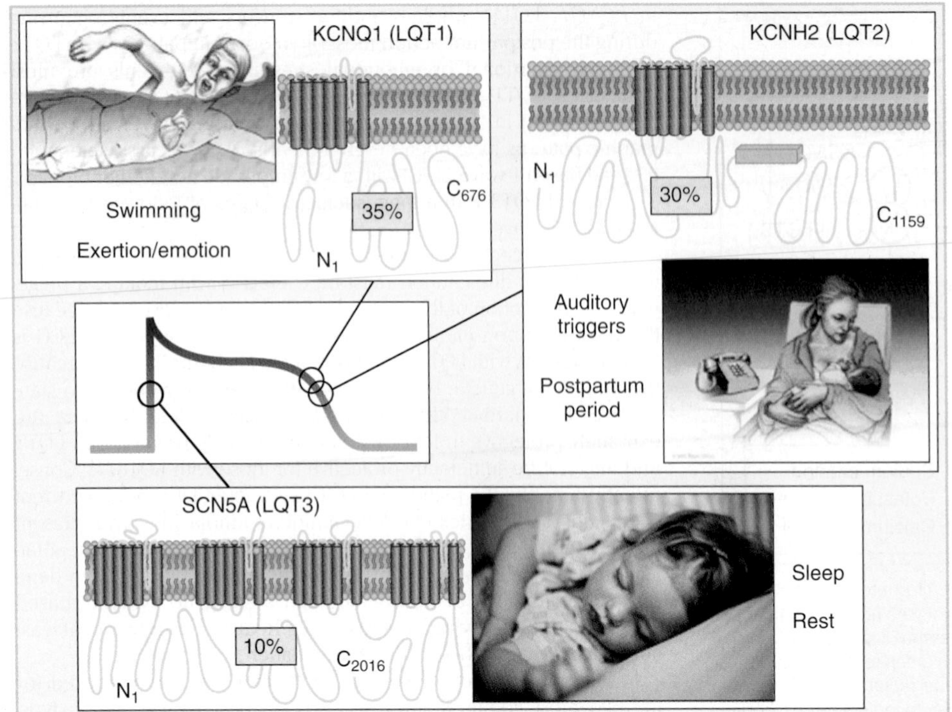

FIGURE 9-3 Genotype-phenotype correlations in long-QT syndrome. Of clinically strong LQTS cases, 75% are caused by mutations in three genes (35% *KCNQ1*, 30% *KCNH2*, and 10% in *SCN5A*) encoding for ion channels that are critically responsible for the orchestration of the cardiac action potential. Genotype-phenotype correlations have been observed, including the following: swimming, exertion, emotion, and LQT1; auditory triggers, postpartum period, and LQT2; and sleep, rest, and LQT3.

than those mutations that damage the biology of the Kv7.1 channel less severely (haploinsufficiency). Adding to the traditional clinical risk factors, molecular location and cellular function are independent risk factors used for the evaluation of patients with LQTS.[22] Akin to molecular risk stratification in LQT1, patients with LQT2 secondary to Kv11.1 pore region mutations have a longer QTc and a more severe clinical manifestation of the disorder, and experience significantly more arrhythmia-related cardiac events at a younger age than LQT2 patients with nonpore mutations in Kv11.1.[19] Similarly, in a Japanese cohort of LQT2 patients, those with pore mutations had a longer QTc and, although not significant in probands, nonprobands with pore mutations experienced their first cardiac event at an earlier age than those with a nonpore mutation.[23] Most recently, additional information has suggested that LQT2 patients with mutations involving the transmembrane pore region have the greatest risk for cardiac events, those with frameshift nonsense mutations in any region have an intermediate risk, and those with missense mutations in the C-terminus have the lowest risk for cardiac events.[24]

Andersen-Tawil Syndrome

CLINICAL DESCRIPTION AND MANIFESTATIONS. Andersen-Tawil syndrome, first described in 1971[25] in a case report by Andersen and later described by Tawil in 1994[26] is now universally recognized as a rare, multisystem disorder characterized by a triad of clinical features—periodic paralysis, dysmorphic features, and ventricular arrhythmias.[27] ATS is a heterogenous disorder that is sporadically or autosomal dominant–derived and has a high degree of variable phenotypic expression and incomplete penetrance, with as much as 20% of mutation-positive carriers being nonpenetrant. The mean age of onset for periodic paralysis has been reported to be 5 years (range, 8 months to 15 years) and slightly older, 13 years (range, ~4 to 25 years) for cardiac symptoms.

Electrocardiographic abnormalities of ATS may include pronounced QTc prolongation, prominent U waves, and ventricular ectopy, including polymorphic ventricular tachycardia (VT), bigeminy, and bidirectional VT. Although ventricular ectopy is common and the ectopic density can be high in some patients, most ATS patients are asymptomatic and SCD is extremely rare.[28] ATS1 was initially proposed as type 7 LQTS (LQT7) because of the observation of extreme prolongation of the QT interval; however, these measurements included the prominent U wave.[29] As such, this complex clinical disorder, manifesting at times with only a modest prolongation of the QT interval, is probably best considered as its own clinical entity, referred to as ATS1 rather than as part of the LQTS regime. However, given the potential for false interpretation of the QT interval because of the prominent U wave and the probability of phenotypic expression of only cardiac-derived symptomatology (e.g., syncope, palpitations, ventricular rhythm disturbances), a considerable number of ATS patients are conceivably misdiagnosed with classic LQTS. Similarly, the presence of bidirectional VT, an accepted hallmark feature of CPVT (see later) often leads to a misdiagnosis of ATS as the potentially lethal disorder CPVT. Correctly distinguishing between ATS and CPVT is critical, because the treatment strategies are different.[30]

GENETIC BASIS FOR ANDERSEN-TAWIL SYNDROME. To date, over 30 unique mutations in *KCNJ2* have been described as causative for ATS1. Mutations in *KCNJ2* account for approximately two thirds of ATS, but the molecular basis of the residual third of ATS cases remains genetically and mechanistically elusive. Localized to chromosome 17q23, *KCNJ2* encodes for Kir2.1, a small potassium channel alpha subunit expressed in brain, skeletal muscle, and heart, that is critically responsible for the inward rectifying cardiac I_{K1} current (see Table 9-1 and Fig. 9-1). In the heart, I_{K1} plays an important role in setting the heart's resting membrane potential, buffering extracellular potassium, and modulating the action potential waveform. Most *KCNJ2* mutations described in ATS are missense mutations that cause a loss of function of I_{K1}, either through a dominant negative effect on the Kir2.1 subunit assembly or through haploinsufficiency as a result of protein trafficking defects.[31]

GENOTYPE-PHENOTYPE CORRELATES. Genotype-specific electrocardiographic features of ATS are beginning to emerge. In a study by Zhang and colleagues examining the electrocardiographic T-U morphology, 91% of *KCNJ2* mutation-positive ATS1 patients had characteristic T-U wave patterns (including prolonged terminal T wave downslope, a wide T-U junction, and biphasic and enlarged U waves) compared with none of the 61 unaffected family members or 29 genotype-negative ATS patients.[29] Also, whereas the U-wave is markedly abnormal in ATS1, it is typically normal in LQTS. Thus, this *KCNJ2* gene-specific electrocardiographic feature of T-U morphology can be useful in differentiating ATS1 patients from *KCNJ2* mutation-negative ATS and LQT1, LQT2, and LQT3 patients, and may facilitate a cost-effective approach toward genetic testing of the appropriate disorder.

Timothy Syndrome

CLINICAL DESCRIPTION AND MANIFESTATIONS. In 1992 and 1995, cases of a novel arrhythmia syndrome associated with congenital heart disease and syndactyly were described. A decade later, in 2004, Splawski and associates[32] identified the molecular basis for this novel, rare, multisystem, highly lethal arrhythmia disorder and termed it *Timothy syndrome* (TS) after Katherine Timothy, the study coordinator who meticulously phenotyped these cases. All 17 children in this study had extreme QT prolongation and simple syndactyly (webbing of the toes and fingers). Most had life-threatening arrhythmias, including 2:1 atrioventricular block, TdP, and VF, and 10 of 17 (59%) children died at a mean age of 2.5 years. Additional common features included dysmorphic facial features, congenital heart disease, immune deficiency, and developmental delay.

Genetic Basis for Timothy Syndrome. Remarkably, in all unrelated patients for whom DNA was available, Splawski and coworkers[32] identified the same recurrent sporadic de novo missense mutation, *G406R*, in the alternatively spliced exon 8A of the *CACNA1C*-encoded cardiac L-type calcium channel ($Ca_v1.2$), which is important for excitation-contraction coupling in the heart and, like the cardiac sodium channel *SCN5A*, mediates an inward depolarizing current in cardiomyocytes (see Table 9-1 and Fig. 9-1). Through the mechanism of alternative splicing, the human L-type Ca channel consists of two mutually exclusive isoforms, one containing exon 8A and the other with exon 8. A year later, in 2005, Splawski and colleagues[33] described two cases of atypical TS (TS2) with similar features of TS yet without syndactyly. As with other TS cases, these two atypical cases were identified as having sporadic de novo *CACNA1C* mutations not in exon 8A, but rather in exon 8. One case hosted a mutation analogous to the classic TS mutation, *G406R*, whereas the other case hosted a *G402R* missense mutation. Unlike other channelopathies, in which there are no mutational hot spots, these three missense mutations (two in exon 8, *G402R* and *G406R* and one in exon 8A, *G406R*) account for all TS cases analyzed to date and confer gain of function to the L-type Ca channels through impaired channel inactivation.

Short-QT Syndrome

CLINICAL DESCRIPTION AND MANIFESTATIONS. SQTS, first described in 2000 by Gussak and associates,[34] is associated with a short QT interval (usually ≤320 msec) on a 12-lead ECG, paroxysmal atrial fibrillation, syncope, and an increased risk for SCD. Giustetto and coworkers[35] have analyzed the clinical presentation of 29 patients with SQTS, the largest cohort studied to date, and found that 62% of the patients were symptomatic, with cardiac arrest being the most common symptom (31% of patients) and frequently the first manifestation of the disorder. A history of syncope was found in 25% of patients, and almost 30% had a family history of SCD. Symptoms including syncope or cardiac arrest most often occurred during periods of rest or sleep. Almost one third presented with AF. SCD was observed during infancy, suggesting the potential role for SQTS as a pathogenic basis in some cases of SIDS.[36,37]

Genetic Basis for Short-QT Syndrome. SQTS is most often inherited in an autosomal dominant manner; however, some de novo sporadic cases have been described. To date, mutations in five genes (see Table 9-1) have been implicated in the pathogenesis of SQTS, including gain of function mutations in the potassium channel–encoding genes *KCNH2* (SQT1), *KCNQ1* (SQT2), and *KCNJ2* (SQT3) and loss of function mutations in *CACNA1C* (SQT4) and *CACNB2b* (SQT5), encoding for L-type calcium channel alpha and beta subunits, respectively (see Table 9-1 and Fig. 9-1).[36,38] However, despite the identification of these five SQTS susceptibility genes, it remains unknown as to what proportion of SQTS is expected to be genotype-positive for types 1 to 5 and what proportion awaits genetic elucidation.

GENOTYPE-PHENOTYPE CORRELATES IN SHORT-QT SYNDROME. Although there are insufficient data to define genotype-phenotype correlations in SQTS clearly, because probably less than 50 cases have been described in the literature to date, gene-specific electrocardiographic patterns are beginning to emerge. The typical pattern consists of a QT interval of ≤320 msec (QTc ≤ 340 msec) and tall, peaked T waves in the precordial leads with either no or a short ST segment present. The T waves tend to be symmetric in SQT1 but asymmetric in SQT types 2 to 4. In SQT2, inverted T waves can be observed. In SQT5, a BrS–like ST elevation in the right precordial lead may be observed.[36]

Drug-Induced Torsades de Pointes

CLINICAL DESCRIPTION AND MANIFESTATIONS. Drug-induced QT prolongation and/or drug-induced TdP is a constant concern for physicians prescribing certain drugs that can produce such unwanted and potentially life-threatening side-effects (see Chaps. 10 and 37). The estimated incidence of antiarrhythmic drug-induced TdP has ranged from 1% to 8%, depending on the drug and dose.[39] Drug-induced TdP and subsequent sudden death are rare events, but the list of potential QT liability or torsadogenic drugs is extensive. It includes not only antiarrhythmic drugs such as quinidine, sotalol, and dofetilide, but also many noncardiac medications such as antipsychotics, methadone, antimicrobials, antihistamines, and the gastrointestinal stimulant cisapride (see www.qtdrugs.org for a comprehensive list).[40]

I_{Kr} CHANNEL BLOCKERS AND THE REPOLARIZATION RESERVE. In addition to their intended function and intended target of action, the vast majority of medications with a potential unwanted TdP-predisposing side effect are I_{Kr} channel blockers, also referred to as HERG channel blockers. In effect, QT-prolonging drugs create an LQT2-like phenotype through reduced repolarization efficiency and subsequent lengthening of the cardiac action potential.[41] However, I_{Kr} drug blockade alone does not appear sufficient to provide the potentially lethal TdP substrate. One particular hypothesis notes that cardiac repolarization relies on the interaction of several ion currents that provide some level of redundancy to protect against extreme QT prolongation by QT liability drugs.[39] This so-called repolarization reserve may be reduced through anomalies in the repolarization machinery, namely as a result of common or rare genetic variants in critical ion channels that produce a subclinical loss of the repolarizing currents I_{Ks} and I_{Kr}. Recent studies have revealed that 10% to 15% of patients with drug-induced TdP host rare ion channel mutations. A recent smaller study has found potential LQTS susceptibility mutations in 40% of cases of seemingly isolated, drug-induced LQTS.[42] Furthermore, functional characterization of those mutations suggested that these mutations are somewhat weaker than the loss of function mutations associated with classic, autosomal dominant LQTS, furthering the multihit hypothesis that underlies reduced repolarization reserve.

Common Ion Channel Polymorphisms. Among the common polymorphisms of the *KCNH2*-encoding I_{Kr} potassium channel (see Chap. 10), the K897T and R1047L polymorphisms have received the most attention. Paavonen and colleagues[43] have observed that T897-KCNH2 channels exhibit slower activation kinetics with a higher degree of inactivation, an alteration expected to decrease channel function and perhaps alter drug sensitivity, because several commonly used drugs inhibiting I_{Kr} channel function bind preferentially to the inactivated state of the channel. These data suggest that T897 channels may genetically reduce repolarization reserve, and facilitate a proarrhythmic response that may be enhanced in the setting of I_{Kr} channel–blocking drugs, compared with wild-type K897 channels. K897T appears to affect the QTc response to ibutilide in a gender-specific manner. In a study by Sun and associates,[44] among 105 AF patients treated with dofetilide, R1047L was overrepresented among those patients who developed drug-induced TdP compared with patients who were free of TdP. In addition to these common potassium channel alpha subunit polymorphisms, three common polymorphisms (D85N-KCNE1, T8A-KCNE2, and Q9E-KCNE2) involving auxiliary beta subunits have been implicated in drug-induced arrhythmia susceptibility.[40]

In addition to genetic variants in major repolarizing channels, variants of the major depolarizing channel Nav1.5 may provide a substrate for a proarrhythmic response in the setting of I_{Kr} channel–blocking drugs or in patients with other risk factors for drug-induced TdP. The most prominent channel polymorphism to confer arrhythmia susceptibility in an ethnic-specific manner is S1103Y-SCN5A, originally annotated as the Y1102 variant. This polymorphism, seen in 13% of African Americans, but not observed in any white or Asian controls (>1000 subjects), was overrepresented in arrhythmia cases (56.5%) compared with controls (13%) involving African Americans (odds ratio, 8.7).[39,40] S1103Y has very subtle alterations in channel kinetics in heterologous expression studies when studied under basal conditions. However, functional and modeling studies have supported the potential for QT prolongation, reactivation of calcium channels, early afterdepolarizations, and arrhythmias, particularly in the setting of concomitant exposure to I_{Kr} channel–blocking drugs.

Additionally, genetic variation or individual differences in drug elimination or metabolism may contribute to individual risk for drug induced-TdP. For example, patients with genetically mediated reduction in CYP3A enzymatic activity could be vulnerable to drug-induced TdP in the setting of I_{Kr} channel blockers that depend on the cytochrome P-450 enzyme CYP3A for metabolism.[13,40]

Other Channelopathies

Brugada Syndrome

CLINICAL DESCRIPTION AND MANIFESTATIONS. Brugada syndrome is a heritable arrhythmia syndrome that is characterized by an electrocardiographic pattern consisting of coved-type ST-segment elevation (2 mm) followed by a negative T wave in the right precordial leads, V_1 through V_3 (often referred to as type 1 Brugada electrocardiographic pattern), and an increased risk for sudden death resulting from episodes of polymorphic ventricular tachyarrhythmias.[45,46] The penetrance and expressivity of the disorder are highly variable, ranging from lifelong asymptomatic individuals to SCD during the first year of life. BrS is generally considered a disorder involving young men, perhaps greatest among Southeast Asian men, with arrhythmogenic manifestation first occurring at an average age of 40 years and with sudden death typically occurring during sleep.[47,48] Sudden unexplained nocturnal death (SUND) in young men is endemic to Southeast Asia and is now considered phenotypically, genetically, and functionally the same disorder as BrS. However, BrS has been demonstrated in children and infants. In a 2007 population study of 30 children (younger than 16 years) affected by BrS from 26 families, fever represented the most common precipitating factor for arrhythmic cardiac events, including syncope and SCD.[49]

GENETIC BASIS OF BRUGADA SYNDROME. BrS is inherited as an autosomal dominant trait; however, over 50% of BrS cases may be sporadic. Approximately 20% to 30% of BrS cases stem from loss of function mutations in the *SCN5A*-encoded cardiac sodium channel (see Table 9-1 and Fig. 9-1) and is classified as BrS type 1 (BrS1). In 2009, an international compendium of *SCN5A* mutations in patients referred for BrS genetic testing reported almost 300 distinct mutations in 438 of 2111 (21%) unrelated patients, and the mutation detection yield ranged from 11% to 28% across nine centers.[50] The yield of mutation detection may be significantly higher among familial forms than in sporadic cases. Schulze-Bahr and coworkers[13] have identified *SCN5A* mutations in 38% of their familial BrS cases compared with none in 27 sporadic cases ($P = 0.001$). Most of the mutations were missense (66%), followed by frameshift (13%), nonsense, (11%), splice-site (7%), and in-frame deletions or insertion (3%) mutations. Approximately 3% of the genotype-positive patients hosted multiple putative pathogenic *SCN5A* mutations and, like the genotype-phenotype observations in LQTS,[7] patients hosting multiple *SCN5A* mutations tend to be younger at diagnosis (29.7 ± 16 years) than those having a single mutation (39.2 ± 14.4 years). Again, like LQTS, there is no particular mutational hot spot because almost 80% of the BrS-related *SCN5A* mutations occur as "private" single-family mutations (**Fig. 9-4**). However, almost 10% of the 438 unrelated, *SCN5A* mutation–positive patients hosted one of four mutations: *E1784K* (14 patients), *F861WfsX90* (11 patients), *D356N* (8 patients), and *G1408R* (7 patients). Interestingly, the most commonly occurring BrS1 mutation, *E1784K*, has also been reported as the most commonly seen LQT3-associated *SCN5A* mutation, illustrating how the same DNA alteration in a given gene can lead to two distinct cardiac arrhythmia syndromes, most likely as a result of other environmental or genetic modifying factors. *E1784K* represents the quintessential example of a cardiac sodium channel mutation with the capacity to provide for a mixed clinical phenotype of LQT3, BrS, and conduction disorders.[51]

In addition to pathogenic mutations in *SCN5A*, common polymorphisms may have a modifying effect on the disorder. Bezzina and colleagues[52] have described an Asian-specific haplotype of six *SCN5A* promoter polymorphisms in near-complete linkage disequilibrium that occurred with an allelic frequency of 22% and was comparatively absent in whites and blacks. These promoter region polymorphisms may modulate the variability in cardiac conduction and partially contribute to the observed higher prevalence of BrS in the Asian population. Brugada and associates[46] have provided data supporting the common polymorphism H558R as a modulator of the BrS phenotype, for which the minor allele R558 provided a less severe clinical course in their 75 genotyped Brugada patients. Patients homozygous for H558 had longer QRS complex duration in lead II, higher J-point elevation in lead V_2, and higher aVR sign, and trended toward more symptoms than H558R or R558 homozygotes.

In addition to primary mutations of the sodium channel, mutations in genes that modulate the sodium channel function are proposed to cause BrS (see Table 9-1). Recently, mutations in the glycerol-3-phosphate dehydrogenase 1–like protein encoded by *GPD1L* were found to affect trafficking of the sodium channel to the plasma membrane, thus reducing overall sodium current giving rise to the BrS phenotype.[53] However, mutations involving the L-type calcium channel alpha and beta subunits encoded by the *CACNA1C* and *CACNB2b* genes, respectively, were implicated in approximately 10% of BrS cases, with concomitant short QT intervals.[54] Other minor causes of BrS include mutations in the sodium channel $beta_1$ subunit encoded by *SCN1B* and in a putative beta subunit of the transient outward potassium channel (I_{to}) encoded by *KCNE3*.[55,56] Mechanistically, either decreases in the inward sodium or calcium currents or increases in the outward Kv4.3 potassium current produce the BrS phenotype through perturbations of the respective channel alpha subunits or channel interacting proteins (see Fig. 9-1).[47] However, the genetic cause of more than two thirds of clinically diagnosed BrS cases remains elusive, suggesting a high degree of genetic heterogeneity for this disorder.

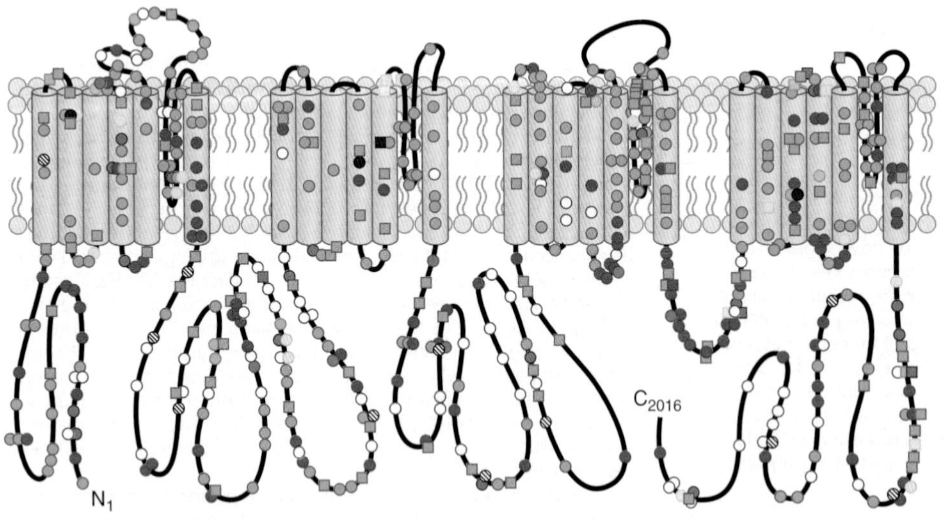

FIGURE 9-4 Sodium channelopathies. Depicted is the linear topology of the 2016–amino acid–containing cardiac sodium channel isoform with mutation location and their associated disorders. Circles denote missense mutations and squares represent radical mutations including frameshift insertion or deletion, in-frame insertion or deletion, nonsense, and splice-site mutations.

GENOTYPE-PHENOTYPE CORRELATES IN BRUGADA SYNDROME. Because most BrS cases are genetically undefined, genotype-phenotype correlations in BrS have not been analyzed to the same degree as in LQTS. Perhaps the two most robust observations involve longer His-ventricular (HV) intervals in patients with BrS1 and, within the subset of BrS1, patients with nonsense, frameshift, premature truncation causing mutations exhibit a more severe phenotype.[57] Unlike LQTS genetic testing, in which the triad of diagnostic, prognostic, and therapeutic impact has been fulfilled, Brugada syndrome genetic testing is currently limited by its lower yield (25% for BrS versus 75% for LQTS) and relative absence of a therapeutic contribution from knowing the genotype.

Idiopathic Ventricular Fibrillation

CLINICAL DESCRIPTION AND MANIFESTATIONS. VF is a major cause of SCD and ultimately is the final common arrhythmic pathway for all the aforementioned channelopathies. In the absence of identifying structural or genetic abnormalities to explain the VF or the out-of-hospital cardiac arrest, the VF is termed *idiopathic ventricular fibrillation* (IVF). In essence, like SIDS, IVF is a diagnosis of exclusion and can stem from several underlying mechanisms. IVF may account for as much as 10% of sudden deaths, especially in the young. About 30% of IVF-labeled individuals will have recurrent episodes of VF. In 20%, there is a family history of SD or IVF, suggesting a hereditary component in some cases.[58] Unfortunately, most IVF cases are often only recognized after their first out-of-hospital cardiac arrest. Haissaguerre and colleagues[59] have noted that J point elevation (1 mm above baseline) on inferolateral electrocardiographic leads (so-called early repolarization, which is generally considered benign) was significantly overrepresented (31%) and was greater in magnitude in 206 subjects who experienced cardiac arrest caused by IVF compared with 412 (5%; $P < 0.001$) age-, gender-, race-, and level of physical activity–matched controls. Those patients with early repolarization were more often males and had a personal history of syncope or cardiac arrest during sleep than those without early repolarization.[59] Similarly, Rosso and associates[60] have noted an overrepresentation of J point elevation in their 45 IVF patients compared with controls (45% versus 13%; $P = 0.001$), with the same observation of male predominance in those with early repolarization. Obviously, the vexing clinical conundrum with respect to this inferolateral early repolarization syndrome is this background rate of a similarly appearing early repolarization pattern seen in 5% to 10% of healthy controls.

GENETIC BASIS FOR IDIOPATHIC VENTRICULAR FIBRILLATION. IVF has been thought to be clinically, genetically, and mechanistically most closely linked with BrS. As many as 20% of IVF cases have been diagnosed subsequently with BrS, depending on the diagnostic criteria used.[37] Like BrS, loss of function SCN5A mutations have been identified in cases of IVF where there are no electrocardiographic stigmata at rest or with provocation for BrS. However, some case reports of IVF have identified mutations in other arrhythmia susceptibility genes, such as *ANKB*, which encodes for ankyrin-B, and *RYR2*, which encodes for the cardiac ryanodine receptor. These particular IVF cases ultimately represented atypical presentations of LQTS or CPVT. For most IVF cases, their genetic mechanism remains undefined.

However, three new IVF susceptibility genes have been recently elucidated. First, Haissaguerre and coworkers[59] have reported finding a rare, functionally uncharacterized, missense mutation in the *KCNJ8*-encoding pore-forming subunit Kir6.1 of the ATP-sensitive potassium channel in a 14-year-old girl with IVF. Second, Alders and colleagues[58] have embarked on a genome-wide, haplotype-sharing analysis involving three distantly related IVF pedigrees and identified a haplotype on chromosome 7q36 that was conserved among all affected individuals and in 7 of 42 independent IVF patients, suggesting a risk locus for IVF. This chromosome segment contains part of the *DPP6* gene which encodes for dipeptidyl peptidase-6, a putative component of the transient outward current (I_{to}; Kv4.3) in the heart. Furthermore, the investigators showed a 20-fold increase in *DPP6* messenger RNA (mRNA) expression in the myocardium of haplotype carriers compared with controls, suggesting that *DPP6* may be a candidate gene for IVF. However, to date, no IVF-associated coding region mutations have been identified in *DPP6*. Third, Valdivia and coworkers[61] have identified a mutation in the *SCN3B*-encoded sodium channel NaV beta$_3$ subunit that precipitates intracellular retention of NaV1.5, functionally mimicking a trafficking defective SCN5A loss of function, in a 20-year-old man with IVF.

Progressive Cardiac Conduction Defect

CLINICAL DESCRIPTION AND MANIFESTATIONS. Cardiac conduction disease (CCD) causes a potentially life-threatening alteration in normal impulse propagation through the cardiac conduction system. CCD can be a result of a number of physiologic mechanisms ranging from acquired to congenital and with or without structural heart disease. PCCD, also known as Lev-Lenègre disease, is one of the most common cardiac conduction disturbances in the absence of structural heart disease. It is characterized by progressive (age-related) alteration of impulse propagation through the His-Purkinje system, with right or left bundle branch block and widening of the QRS complex, leading to complete atrioventricular (AV) block, syncope, and occasionally sudden death.[48]

GENETIC BASIS FOR PROGRESSIVE CARDIAC CONDUCTION DEFECTS. In 1999, Schott and colleagues[62] further expanded the spectrum of loss of function SCN5A disease with the inclusion of familial PCCD. They identified a splice-site *SCN5A* mutation (c.3963+2T > C) associated with an autosomal dominant inheritance pattern in a large French family. Since then, investigators have identified over 30 PCCD-associated mutations in *SCN5A* (see Fig. 9-4). These mutations present with a loss of function phenotype through reduced current density and enhanced slow inactivation of the channel. As with most loss of function SCN5A diseases, the phenotypic expression of PCCD can be complex and is often present with a concomitant BrS or BrS-like phenotype. In fact, Probst and associates[49] have shown that PCCD is the prevailing phenotype in BrS-associated *SCN5A* mutation carriers, where the penetrance of conduction defects was 76%.

In 2009, Meregalli and associates demonstrated that *SCN5A* mutation type can have a profound effect on the severity of PCCD and BrS.[57] Studying 147 individuals hosting one of 32 different *SCN5A* mutations, they found that patients with a premature truncation mutation (M_T—nonsense or frameshift) or a severe loss of function missense mutation ($M_{inactive}$; >90% reduction in peak I_{Na}) had a significantly longer PR interval compared with patients with missense mutations having less impairment to the sodium current (M_{active}; 90% reduction). Furthermore, patients with a truncation mutation had significantly more episodes of syncope than those with an active mutation (M_{active}). These data suggest that those mutations with a more deleterious loss of sodium current produce a more severe phenotype of syncope and conduction defect, providing the first evidence for intragenotype risk stratification associated with SCN5A loss of function disease.

When CCD is associated with a concomitant phenotype of LQTS, the QRS is usually narrow and the conduction defect is commonly intermittent 2:1 AV block. Patients with LQT2, TS1, or ATS1 may also have dysfunctional AV conduction.

Sick Sinus Syndrome

CLINICAL DESCRIPTION AND MANIFESTATIONS. Sinus node dysfunction (SND) or SSS, manifesting as inappropriate sinus bradycardia, sinus arrest, atrial standstill, tachycardia-bradycardia syndrome, or chronotropic incompetence, is the primary cause leading up to pacemaker implantation and has been attributed to the dysfunction of the sinoatrial (SA) node[31,48] (see Chap. 39). SSS commonly occurs in older adults (1 in 600 cardiac patients older than 65 years) with acquired cardiac conditions, including cardiomyopathy, congestive heart failure, ischemic heart disease, or metabolic disease. However, in a significant number of patients, there are no identifiable cardiac anomalies or cardiac conditions underlying sinus node dysfunction (idiopathic SND), which can occur at any age, including in utero. Additionally, familial forms of idiopathic SND consistent with autosomal dominant inheritance with reduced penetrance and recessive forms with complete penetrance have been reported.

GENETIC BASIS OF SICK SINUS SYNDROME. Mutational analysis of small cohorts and case reports of patients with idiopathic SSS have so far implicated three genes—*SCN5A*, *HCN4*, and *ANKB* (see Table 9-1). To date,

15 SSS-associated mutations have been reported in *SCN5A*.[48,63] The mutations produced nonfunctional sodium channels through loss of expression or channels with mild to severe loss of function through an altered biophysical mechanism of the channel. In 2003, based on prior observations of arrhythmias and conduction disturbances, Benson and coworkers[64] examined *SCN5A* as a candidate gene for congenital SSS in 10 pediatric patients from seven families who were diagnosed during their first decade of life and identified compound heterozygote mutations (*T220I* + *R1623X, P1298L* + *G1408R*, and *delF1617* + *R1632H*) in five individuals from three of the seven families, implicating *SCN5A* in autosomal recessive SSS. Not surprisingly, many of the *SCN5A*-positive patients displayed a mixed phenotype consisting of SSS, BrS, and/or CCD (see Fig. 9-4). The expressivity of the mixed phenotype can be highly variable within affected families. In 2007, the case of a 12-year-old boy with SSS, CCD, and recurrent VT was presented. The patient was identified with an *L1821fsX10* frameshift mutation that displayed a unique channel phenotype of 90% reduced current density (consistent with BrS-SSS-CCD), yet an increase in late sodium current relative to the peak current (consistent with LQT3) for those channels expressed. As illustrated by this family, in which the mutation was present in six asymptomatic family members but two displayed only mild ECG phenotypes, this disorder is often associated with incomplete or low penetrance.

Two loss of function mutations in the hyperpolarization-activated cyclic nucleotide-gated channel 4 gene, *HCN4*, have been identified in two cases of idiopathic SND. The *HCN4* gene encodes the so-called I_f or pacemaker current and plays a key role in automaticity of the sinus node. In one study, a heterozygous single-nucleotide deletion (c.1631delC) creating a frameshift mutation (*P544fsX30*) with early truncation of the protein was identified in an idiopathic SND patient; in a second study, another patient with idiopathic SND had a missense mutation (*D553N*) that resulted in abnormal trafficking of the pacemaker channel.[65] Interestingly, although the frameshift mutation identified in a 66-year-old woman produced a mild phenotype associated with sinus rhythm during exercise, the *D553N* missense mutation identified in a 43-year-old woman was associated with severe bradycardia, recurrent syncope, QT prolongation, and polymorphic VT with TdP, suggesting the potential for lethality in *HCN4*-mediated disease. Whether the preliminary 10% to 15% yield for defective *HCN4*-encoded pacemaker channels in idiopathic SND, derived from the two small cohorts, is durable will require further studies involving much larger cohorts.

In 2008, Le Scouarnec and colleagues[66] reported the genetic and molecular mechanisms involving *ANK2* (also known as *ANKB*)-encoded ankyrin-B in two large families with high penetrance and severe SND. Ankyrin-B is essential for normal membrane organization of the ion channels and transporters in the cardiocytes in the SA node and is required for proper physiologic cardiac pacing. Dysfunction of ankyrin-B–based trafficking pathway causes abnormal electrical activity in the SA node and SND. Like the sodium channel, variants in *ANK2* cause a variety of cardiac dysfunctions (see later).

Catecholaminergic Polymorphic Ventricular Tachycardia

CLINICAL DESCRIPTION AND MANIFESTATIONS. CPVT is a heritable arrhythmia syndrome that classically manifests with exercise-induced syncope or sudden death, is predominantly expressed in the young, and closely mimics the phenotypic byline of LQT1 but appears to be far more lethal.[67,68] Like LQT1, swimming is a potentially lethal arrhythmia-precipitating trigger in CPVT. Both LQT1 and CPVT have been shown to underlie several cases of unexplained drowning or near-drowning in young healthy swimmers. However, CPVT is associated with a completely normal resting ECG (perhaps bradycardia and U waves) and is electrocardiographically suspected following exercise or catecholamine stress testing that demonstrates significant ventricular ectopy with the hallmark feature of bidirectional VT.

Clinically, a presentation of exercise-induced syncope and a QTc shorter than 460 msec should always prompt first consideration of and need to rule out CPVT, rather than so-called concealed or normal QT interval LQT1. Furthermore, exercise-induced premature ventricular complexes in bigeminy is far more likely than the more specific but less sensitive finding of bidirectional VT.[69] CPVT is generally associated with a structurally normal heart. Once thought to manifest only during childhood, more recent studies have suggested that the age of first presentation can vary from infancy to 40 years. The lethality of CPVT is illustrated by mortality rates of 30% to 50% by age 35 years and the presence of a positive family history of young (younger than 40 years) SCD for more than one third of CPVT patients and in as many as 60% of families hosting *RyR2* mutations.[67] Moreover, approximately 15% of autopsy-negative sudden unexplained death in the young and some cases of SIDS have been attributed to CPVT.[1,70]

GENETIC BASIS OF CATECHOLAMINERGIC POLYMORPHIC VENTRICULAR TACHYCARDIA. Perturbations in key components of intracellular calcium–induced calcium release from the sarcoplasmic reticulum serve as the pathogenic basis for CPVT (see Chap. 35). Inherited in an autosomal dominant fashion, mutations in the *RYR2*-encoded cardiac ryanodine receptor–calcium release channel represent the most common genetic subtype of CPVT (CPVT1), accounting for 60% of clinically strong cases of CPVT (**Fig. 9-5**; see Table 9-1). Gain of function mutations in RyR2 lead to leaky calcium release channels and excessive calcium release, particularly during sympathetic stimulation, which can precipitate calcium overload, delayed depolarizations (DADs), and ventricular arrhythmias.[67] Again, most unrelated CPVT families are identified with their own unique *RYR2* mutation and approximately 5% of unrelated mutation-positive patients host multiple putative pathogenic mutations.[71]

RYR2 is one of the largest genes in the human genome, with 105 exons that transcribe or translate one of the largest cardiac ion channel proteins, comprising 4967 amino acid residues. Although there does not appear to be any specific mutation hot spots, there are three regional hot spots or domains where unique mutations reside (see Fig. 9-5). This observation has lent itself toward targeted genetic testing of *RYR2* (~61 exons) rather than a comprehensive 105-exon scan. More than 90% of RYR2 mutations discovered to date represent missense mutations; however, perhaps as many as 5% of unrelated CPVT patients host large gene rearrangements consistent with large whole-exon deletions, akin to what has been observed in LQTS.[71]

Strikingly, almost one third of possible atypical LQTS cases (QTc < 480 msec) with exertion-induced syncope have also been identified as *RYR2* mutation–positive.[71] It has been reported that almost 30% of patients with CPVT have been misdiagnosed as having LQTS with normal QT intervals or concealed LQTS, indicating the critical importance of properly distinguishing between CPVT and LQTS at the clinical level, because risk assessments and treatment strategies of these unique disorders may vary. Similarly, some patients diagnosed with CPVT, based on the presence of bidirectional VT on exercise, have been identified as carriers of *KCNJ2* mutations that are associated with the rarely lethal ATS.[30] The misdiagnosis of ATS as the potentially lethal disorder CPVT may lead to a more aggressive prophylactic therapy (i.e., implantable cardioverter-defibrillator) than necessary. A rare subtype of autosomal recessive CPVT involves mutations in *CASQ2*-encoded calsequestrin (CPVT2).[67]

Ankyrin-B Syndrome

The *ANK2* gene encodes ankyrin-B protein, a member of a large family of proteins that anchor various integral membrane proteins to the spectrin-based cytoskeleton. Specifically, ankyrin-B is involved in anchoring the Na^+,K^+-ATPase, Na^+/Ca^{2+} exchanger, and InsP3 receptor to specialized microdomains in the cardiomyocyte transverse tubules.[72] Loss of function mutations of *ANK2* were shown originally to cause a dominantly inherited cardiac arrhythmia with an increased risk for SCD associated with a prolonged QT interval; subsequently, the label type 4 long-QT syndrome (LQT4) was assigned to this *ANK2* pedigree. Since then, this disorder has been more correctly renamed SSS with bradycardia, or the ankyrin-B syndrome.[72]

In 2003, Mohler and associates[73] described the first human *ANK2* mutation (*E1425G*) identified in a large multigenerational French kindred presenting with atypical LQTS and displaying a phenotype of prolonged QT interval, severe sinus bradycardia, polyphasic T waves, and AF. Following this sentinel discovery, significant loss of function ankyrin-B variants of differing degrees of functionality have now been identified in patients with various arrhythmia phenotypes, including bradycardia, SND, delayed cardiac conduction block, IVF, AF, drug-induced LQTS, exercise-induced VT, and CPVT. In addition, 2% to 4% of ostensibly healthy white controls and 8% to 10% of black controls (including the most common black-specific variant, *L1622I*) also host rare variants in *ANK2*, underscoring the challenge in distinguishing pathogenic mutations that truly mediate an ankyrin-B syndrome from rare *ANK2* variants of uncertain signficance.[72] Individuals hosting *ANK2* variants displaying a more severe loss of function in vitro tend to have a more severe cardiac phenotype and may be at an increased risk for SCD.

Familial Atrial Fibrillation

CLINICAL DESCRIPTION AND MANIFESTATIONS. AF is the most common cardiac arrhythmia, with a prevalence of about 1% in the general population and 6% in people older than 65 years.[74] AF is usually associated with underlying cardiac pathology, including cardiomyopathy, valvular disease, hypertension, and atherosclerotic cardiovascular disease, and is responsible for more than one third of cardioembolic episodes. However, AF can present even at an early age without any identifiable cardiac anomalies and is termed *lone AF*, accounting for 2% to 16% of all AF cases. Furthermore, approximately one third of lone AF patients have a family history of AF, suggesting a familial form of the disease (see Chap. 40).[75]

GENETIC BASIS FOR FAMILIAL ATRIAL FIBRILLATION. Although most familial forms of AF remain genetically elusive, over the past decade several genetic loci and causative genes have been described and recently reviewed.[74,75] In 1996, Brugada and colleagues[76] identified three families with autosomal dominant AF. The age of onset ranged from in utero to 45 years. Genetic linkage analysis of these families revealed a novel locus for AF on chromosome 10 (10q22). In 2003, a second locus at 6q14-16, again associated with autosomal dominant inheritance, was identified.[77] To date, the underlying causative genes for both loci remain unknown.

However, in 2003, an AF-associated locus on chromosome 11 in a large four-generation family and subsequent identification of an SQTS-like gain of function mutation, *S140G-KCNQ1*, in Kv11.1 (I_{Ks}) was identified, thus providing for the first time a causal link between a cardiac potassium ion channel mutation and familial AF. Interestingly, a second de novo mutation involving codon 141 of *KCNQ1* was identified in a patient with a severe form of AF and SQTS presenting in utero.[74] An R27C mutation in *KCNE2*, which encodes for a KCNQ1-interacting protein, was discovered[78] in two AF families and produced an I_{Ks} gain of function phenotype when coexpressed with wild-type *KCNQ1*. In 2005, a V93I mutation in *KCNJ2* in 1 of 30 unrelated Chinese AF families was identified. Whereas loss of function *KCNJ2* mutations yield ATS1, the AF-associated V93I mutation conferred gain of function biophysical properties to the Kir2.1 channels. Finally, in 2006, a loss of function mutation in the *KCNA5* gene responsible for the Kv1.5 potassium channel I_{Kur} in a family with AF was discovered.

In addition to these potassium channels, Nav1.5 has been implicated in lone and familial AF. AF is a fairly common arrhythmia among patients with loss of function SCN5A-opathies; in particular, up to 15% to 20% of BrS patients develop AF.[64] In 2008, a novel SCN5A mutation (*M1875T*) in a family characterized with juvenile onset of atrial arrhythmias that progressed to AF in the absence of structural heart disease or ventricular arrhythmias was described.[79] Functional studies of this mutant channel produced an increased peak current density and a depolarizing shift of activation (gain of function). Additionally, Darbar and coworkers[80] have identified SCN5A channel mutations in approximately 3% of AF cases (see Fig. 9-4).

Lastly, non-ion channel genes have been implicated in familial and lone AF.[74] In 2008, Hodgson-Zingman and colleagues identified a frameshift mutation in the *NPPA* gene in a large family with AF. *NPPA* encodes for the atrial natriuretic peptide, which modulates ionic currents in myocardial cells and may shorten atrial conduction time. The clinical phenotype of neonatal onset of AF, with an autosomal recessive inheritance pattern, was recently linked to a mutation in *NUP155*, which encodes for a member of the nucleoporins family of proteins. In 2006, Gollob and associates[81] identified four heterozygote *GJA5* missense mutations in 4 of 15 patients with early-onset idiopathic AF. Most interestingly, three of the four mutations were shown to be in cardiac tissue only (somatic) and not germline in origin. *GJA5* encodes for the cardiac gap junction protein connexin 40 that is selectively expressed in atrial myocytes and mediates the finely orchestrated electrical activation of the atria.

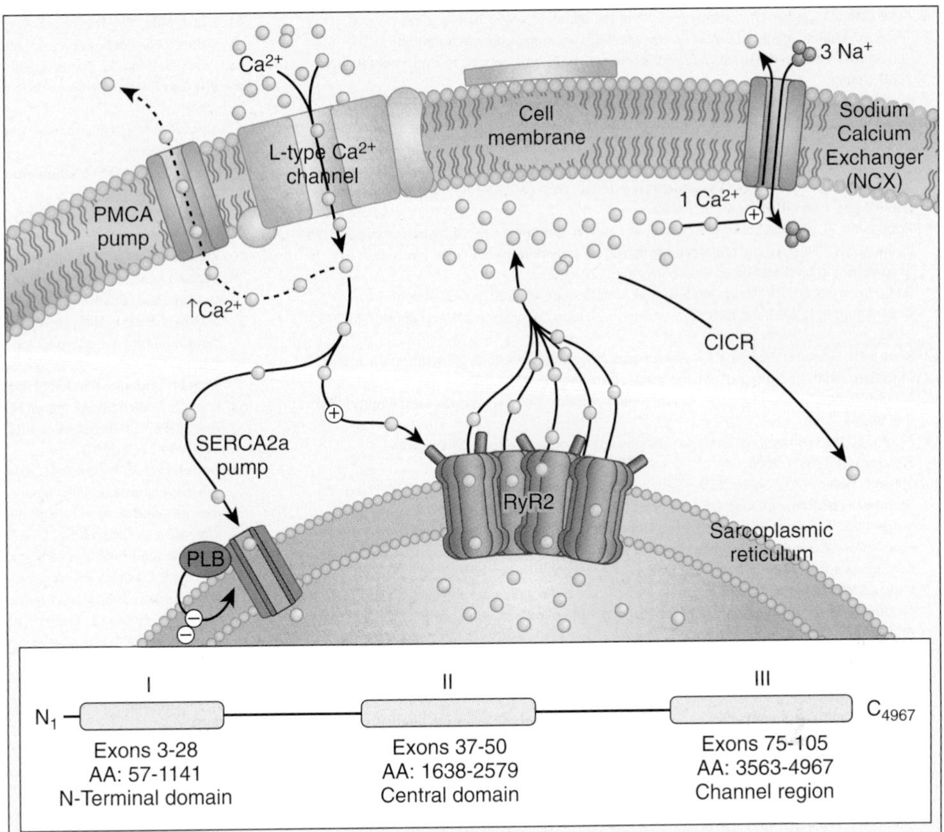

FIGURE 9-5 Catecholaminergic polymorphic ventricular tachycardia, a disorder of intracellular calcium handling. Perturbations in key components of the calcium-induced calcium release (CICR) mechanism responsible for cardiac excitation-contraction coupling is the pathogenic basis for CPVT. At the center of this mechanism is the *RYR2*-encoded cardiac ryanodine receptor calcium release channel located in the sarcoplasmic reticulum membrane. Mutations in *RyR2* are clustered and distributed in three hot spot regions of this 4967–amino acid (AA) protein—domain I or N-terminal domain (AA 57-1141), domain II or central domain (AA 1638-2579), and domain III or channel region (AA 3563-4967). PLB = phospholamban; PMCA = plasma membrane Ca^{2+}-ATPase; SERCA2a = sarcoplasmic reticulum Ca^{2+}-ATPase.

Conclusions

The relatively new discipline of the heritable arrhythmia syndromes and cardiac channelopathies has exploded over the past decade. The pathogenic insights into the molecular underpinnings for almost all these syndromes have progressed throughout the evolution of discovery, translation, and incorporation into clinical practice. This bench to bedside maturation now requires the learned interpretation of the genetic tests available for these syndromes, with a clear understanding of the diagnostic, prognostic, and therapeutic implications associated with genetic testing for these channelopathies.

REFERENCES

1. Tester DJ, Ackerman MJ: The role of molecular autopsy in unexplained sudden cardiac death. Curr Opin Cardiol 21:166, 2006.
2. Tester DJ, Ackerman MJ: Postmortem long QT syndrome genetic testing for sudden unexplained death in the young. J Am Coll Cardiol 49:240, 2007.
3. Arnestad M, Crotti L, Rognum TO, et al: Prevalence of long-QT syndrome gene variants in sudden infant death syndrome. Circulation 115:361, 2007.
4. Van Norstrand DW, Ackerman MJ: Sudden infant death syndrome: Do ion channels play a role? Heart Rhythm 6:272, 2009.
5. Schwartz PJ, Stramba-Badiale M, Crotti L, et al: Prevalence of the congenital long-QT syndrome. Circulation 120:1761, 2009.

6. Ackerman MJ: Cardiac channelopathies: It's in the genes. Nat Med 10:463, 2004.
7. Tester DJ, Will ML, Haglund CM, et al: Compendium of cardiac channel mutations in 541 consecutive unrelated patients referred for long QT syndrome genetic testing. Heart Rhythm 2:507, 2005.
8. Napolitano C, Priori SG, Schwartz PJ, et al: Genetic testing in the long QT syndrome: Development and validation of an efficient approach to genotyping in clinical practice. JAMA 294:2975, 2005.
9. Kapplinger JD, Tester DJ, Salisbury BA, et al: Spectrum and prevalence of mutations from the first 2,500 consecutive unrelated patients referred for the FAMILION (R) long QT syndrome genetic test. Heart Rhythm 6:1297, 2009.
10. Koopmann TT, Alders M, Jongbloed RJ, et al: Long QT syndrome caused by a large duplication in the KCNH2 (HERG) gene undetectable by current polymerase chain reaction-based exon-scanning methodologies. Heart Rhythm 3:52, 2006.
11. Eddy C-A, MacCormick JM, Chung S-K, et al: Identification of large gene deletions and duplications in KCNQ1 and KCNH2 in patients with long QT syndrome. Heart Rhythm 5:1275, 2008.
12. Kapa S TD, Salisbury BA, Wilde AA, Ackerman MJ: Distinguishing long QT syndrome-causing mutations from "background" genetic noise. Heart Rhythm 5:S76, 2008.
13. Schulze-Bahr E: Susceptibility genes and modifiers for cardiac arrhythmias. Prog Biophys Mol Biol 98:289, 2008.
14. Ackerman MJ: Genotype-phenotype relationships in congenital long QT syndrome. J Electrocardiol 38:64, 2005.
15. Villain E, Denjoy I, Lupoglazoff JM, et al: Low incidence of cardiac events with B-blocking therapy in children with long QT syndrome. Eur Heart J 25:1405, 2004.
16. Vincent GM, Schwartz PJ, Denjoy I, et al: High efficacy of beta-blockers in long-QT syndrome type 1: Contribution of noncompliance and QT-prolonging drugs to the occurrence of beta-blocker treatment "failures." Circulation 119:215, 2009.
17. Moss AJ, Windle JR, Hall WJ, et al: Safety and efficacy of flecainide in subjects with Long QT-3 syndrome (DeltaKPQ mutation): a randomized, double-blind, placebo-controlled clinical trial. Ann Noninv Electrocardiol 10:59, 2005.
18. Moss AJ, Zareba W, Schwarz KQ, et al: Ranolazine shortens repolarization in patients with sustained inward sodium current due to type-3 long-QT syndrome. J Cardiovasc Electrophysiol 19:1289, 2008.
19. Moss AJ, Zareba W, Kaufman ES, et al: Increased risk of arrhythmic events in long-QT syndrome with mutations in the pore region of the human ether-a-go-go-related gene potassium channel. Circulation 105:794, 2002.
20. Jons C, Moss AJ, Lopes CM, et al: Mutations in conserved amino acids in the KCNQ1 channel and risk of cardiac events in type-1 long-QT syndrome. J Cardiovasc Electrophysiol 20:859, 2009.
21. Shimizu W, Horie M, Ohno S, et al: Mutation site-specific differences in arrhythmic risk and sensitivity to sympathetic stimulation in the LQT1 form of congenital long QT syndrome: Multicenter study in Japan. J Am Coll Cardiol 44:117, 2004.
22. Moss AJ, Shimizu W, Wilde AAM, et al: Clinical aspects of type-1 long-QT syndrome by location, coding type, and biophysical function of mutations involving the KCNQ1 gene. Circulation 115:2481, 2007.
23. Nagaoka I, Shimizu W, Itoh H, et al: Mutation site dependent variability of cardiac events in Japanese LQT2 form of congenital long-QT syndrome. Circulation Jl 72:694, 2008.
24. Shimizu W, Moss A, Wilde A, et al: Genotype-phenotype aspects of type-2 long-QT syndrome. J Am Coll Cardiol 54:2063, 2009.
25. Andersen ED, Krasilnikoff PA, Overvad H: Intermittent muscular weakness, extrasystoles, and multiple developmental anomalies. A new syndrome? Acta Paediatrica Scandinavica 60:559, 1971.
26. Tawil R, Ptacek LJ, Pavlakis SG, et al: Andersen's syndrome: potassium-sensitive periodic paralysis, ventricular ectopy, and dysmorphic features. Ann Neurol 35:326, 1994.
27. Yoon G, Oberoi S, Tristani-Firouzi M, et al: Andersen-Tawil syndrome: Prospective cohort analysis and expansion of the phenotype. Am J Med Genet A 140:312, 2006.
28. Peters S, Schulze-Bahr E, Etheridge SP, et al: Sudden cardiac death in Andersen-Tawil syndrome. Europace 9:162, 2007.
29. Zhang L, Benson DW, Tristani-Firouzi M, et al: Electrocardiographic features in Andersen-Tawil syndrome patients with KCNJ2 mutations: Characteristic T-U-wave patterns predict the KCNJ2 genotype. Circulation 111:2720, 2005.
30. Tester DJ, Arya P, Will M, et al: Genotypic heterogeneity and phenotypic mimicry among unrelated patients referred for catecholaminergic polymorphic ventricular tachycardia genetic testing. Heart Rhythm 3:800, 2006.
31. Wilde AAM, Bezzina CR: Genetics of cardiac arrhythmias. Heart 91:1352, 2005.
32. Splawski I, Timothy KW, Sharpe LM, et al: Cav1.2 calcium channel dysfunction causes a multisystem disorder including arrhythmia and autism. Cell 119:19, 2004.
33. Splawski I, Timothy KW, Decher N, et al: Severe arrhythmia disorder caused by cardiac L-type calcium channel mutations. Proc Natl Acad Sci U S A 102:8089, 2005.
34. Zareba W, Cygankiewicz I: Long QT syndrome and short QT syndrome. Prog Cardiovasc Dis 51:264, 2008.
35. Giustetto C, Di Monte F, Wolpert C, et al: Short QT syndrome: Clinical findings and diagnostic-therapeutic implications. E Heart Jl 27:2440, 2006.
36. Zareba W, Cygankiewicz I: Long QT syndrome and short QT syndrome. Progress in Cardiovascular Diseases 51:264, 2008.
37. Sarkozy A, Brugada P: Sudden cardiac death: What is inside our genes? Can J Cardiol 21:1099, 2005.
38. Brugada R, Hong K, Dumaine R, et al: Sudden death associated with short-QT syndrome linked mutations in HERG. Circulation 109:30, 2004.
39. Roden DM: Long QT syndrome: Reduced repolarization reserve and the genetic link. J Intern Med 259:59, 2006.
40. Fitzgerald PT, Ackerman MJ: Drug-induced torsades de pointes: The evolving role of pharmacogenetics. Heart Rhythm 2:S30, 2005.
41. Modell SM, Lehmann MH: The long QT syndrome family of cardiac ion channelopathies: A HuGE review. Genet Med 8:143, 2006.
42. Itoh H, Sakaguchi T, Ding W-G, et al: Latent genetic backgrounds and molecular pathogenesis in drug-induced long-QT syndrome. Circ Arrhythm Electrophysiol 2:511, 2009.
43. Paavonen KJ, Chapman H, Laitenen PJ, et al: Functional characterization of the common amino acid 897 polymorphism of the cardiac potassium channel KCNH2 (HERG). Cardiovasc Res 59:603, 2003.
44. Sun Z, Milos PM, Thompson JF, et al: Role of KCNH2 polymorphism (R1047L) in dofetilide-induced *Torsades de Pointes*. J Mol Cell Cardiol 37:1031, 2004.
45. Chen PS, Priori SG: The Brugada syndrome. J Am Coll Cardiol 51:1176-1180, 2008.
46. Brugada P, Benito B, Brugada R, et al: Brugada syndrome: Update 2009. Hellenic J Cardiol 50:352, 2009.
47. Shimizu W: Clinical impact of genetic studies in lethal inherited cardiac arrhythmias. Circ J 72:1926, 2008.
48. Ruan Y, Liu N, Priori SG: Sodium channel mutations and arrhythmias. Nat Rev Cardiol 6:337, 2009.
49. Probst V, Denjoy I, Meregalli PG, et al: Clinical aspects and prognosis of Brugada syndrome in children. Circulation 115:2042, 2007.
50. Kapplinger J, Tester D, Alders M, et al: An international compendium of mutations in the *SCN5A*-encoded cardiac sodium channel in patients referred for Brugada syndrome genetic testing. Heart Rhythm 7:33, 2010.
51. Makita N, Behr E, Shimizu W, et al: The E1784K mutation in SCN5A is associated with mixed clinical phenotype of type 3 long QT syndrome. J Clin Invest 118:2219, 2008.
52. Bezzina CR, Shimizu W, Yang P, et al: Common sodium channel promoter haplotype in asian subjects underlies variability in cardiac conduction. Circulation 113:338, 2006.
53. London B, Michalec M, Mehdi H, et al: Mutation in glycerol-3-phosphate dehydrogenase 1 like gene (GPD1-L) decreases cardiac Na^+ current and causes inherited arrhythmias. Circulation 116:2260-2268, 2007.
54. Antzelevitch C, Pollevick GD, Cordeiro JM, et al: Loss of function mutations in the cardiac calcium channel underlie a new clinical entity characterized by ST-segment elevation, short QT intervals, and sudden cardiac death. Circulation 115:442, 2007.
55. Watanabe H, Koopmann TT, Le SS, et al: Sodium channel β1 subunit mutations associated with Brugada syndrome and cardiac conduction disease in humans. J Clin Invest 118:2260, 2008.
56. Delpon E, Cordeiro JM, Nunez L, et al: Functional effects of KCNE3 mutation and its role in the development of Brugada syndrome. Circ Arrhythm Electrophysiol 1:209, 2008.
57. Meregalli PG, Tan HL, Probst V, et al: Type of SCN5A mutation determines clinical severity and degree of conduction slowing in loss of function sodium channelopathies. Heart Rhythm 6:341, 2009.
58. Alders M, Koopmann TT, Christiaans I, et al: Haplotype-sharing analysis implicates chromosome 7q36 harboring DPP6 in familial idiopathic ventricular fibrillation. Am J Hum Genet 84:468, 2009.
59. Haissaguerre M, Chatel S, Sacher F, et al: Ventricular fibrillation with prominent early repolarization associated with a rare variant of KCNJ8/KATP channel. J Cardiovasc Electrophysiol 20:93, 2009.
60. Rosso R, Kogan E, Belhassen B, et al: J-point elevation in survivors of primary ventricular fibrillation and matched control subjects: Incidence and clinical significance. J Am Coll Cardiol 52:1231, 2008.
61. Valdivia C, Mederios-Domingo A, Ye B, et al: Idiopathic ventricular fibrillation associated with loss of function of the *SCN3B*-encoded sodium channel β3 subunit. Cardiovasc Res 2010 (in press).
62. Schott JJ, Alshinawi C, Kyndt F, et al: Cardiac conduction defects associate with mutations in SCN5A. Nat Genet 23:20, 1999.
63. Lei M, Huang CLH, Zhang Y: Genetic Na^+ channelopathies and sinus node dysfunction. Prog Biophys Mol Biol 98:171, 2008.
64. Benson DW, Wang DW, Dyment M, et al: Congenital sick sinus syndrome caused by recessive mutations in the cardiac sodium channel gene (*SCN5A*). J Clin Invest 112:1019, 2003.
65. Ueda K, Nakamura K, Hayashi T, et al: Functional characterization of a trafficking-defective HCN4 mutation, D553N, associated with cardiac arrhythmia. J Biol Chem 279:27194, 2004.
66. Le Scouarnec S, Bhasin N, Vieyres C, et al: Dysfunction in ankyrin-B–dependent ion channel and transporter targeting causes human sinus node disease. Proc Natl Acad Sci U S A 105:15617-15622, 2008.
67. Liu N, Ruan Y, Priori SG: Catecholaminergic polymorphic ventricular tachycardia. Prog Cardiovasc Dis 51:23, 2008.
68. Tester DJ, Kopplin LJ, Will ML, et al: Spectrum and prevalence of cardiac ryanodine receptor (RyR2) mutations in a cohort of unrelated patients referred explicitly for long QT syndrome genetic testing. Heart Rhythm 2:1099, 2005.
69. Horner JM, Ackerman MJ: Ventricular ectopy during treadmill exercise stress testing in the evaluation of long QT syndrome. Heart Rhythm 5:1690, 2008.
70. Tester DJ, Dura M, Carturan E, et al: A mechanism for sudden infant death syndrome (SIDS): Stress-induced leak via ryanodine receptors. Heart Rhythm 4:7339, 2007.
71. Medeiros-Domingo A, Bhuiyan Z, Tester D, et al: The RYR2-encoded ryanodine receptor/calcium release channel in patients diagnosed previously with either catecholaminergic polymorphic ventricular tachycardia or genotype negative, exercise-induced long QT syndrome: A comprehensive open reading frame mutational analysis. J Am Coll Cardiol 54:2065, 2009.
72. Mohler PJ, Le Scouarnec S, Denjoy I, et al: Defining the cellular phenotype of "ankyrin-B syndrome" variants: Human ANK2 variants associated with clinical phenotypes display a spectrum of activities in cardiomyocytes. Circulation 115:432, 2007.
73. Mohler PJ, Healy JA, Xue H, et al: Ankyrin-B syndrome: Enhanced cardiac function balanced by risk of cardiac death and premature senescence. PLoS ONE 2:e1051, 2007.
74. Campuzano O, Brugada R: Genetics of familial atrial fibrillation. Europace 11:1267, 2009.
75. Darbar D: Genetics of atrial fibrillation: Rare mutations, common polymorphisms, and clinical relevance. Heart Rhythm 5:483, 2008.
76. Brugada R, Tapscott T, Czernuszewicz GZ, et al: Identification of a genetic locus for familial atrial fibrillation. New Engl J Med 336:905, 1997.
77. Ellinor PT, Shin JT, Moore RK, et al: Locus for atrial fibrillation maps to chromosome 6q14-16. Circulation 107:2880, 2003.
78. Olson TM, Alekseev AE, Liu XK, et al: Kv1.5 channelopathy due to KCNA5 loss-of-function mutation causes human atrial fibrillation. Human Molecular Genetics 15:2185, 2006.
79. Makiyama T, Akao M, Shizuta S, et al: A novel SCN5A gain-of-function mutation M1875T associated with familial atrial fibrillation. J Am Coll Cardiol 52:1326, 2008.
80. Darbar D, Kannankeril PJ, Donahue BS, et al: Cardiac sodium channel (SCN5A) variants associated with atrial fibrillation. Circulation 117:1927, 2008.
81. Gollob MH, Jones DL, Krahn AD, et al: Somatic mutations in the connexin 40 gene (GJA5) in atrial fibrillation. New Engl J Med 354:2677, 2006.

CHAPTER 10 Principles of Drug Therapy

Dan M. Roden

Importance of Correct Drug Use

In 2007, Americans spent $289 billion on pharmaceuticals.[1] Adverse drug reactions are estimated to be the fourth to sixth most common cause of death in the United States, costing $19 to $27 billion annually, and accounting directly for 3% to 6% of all hospital admissions.[2] The prevalence of heart disease and the increasing use of not only acute interventional therapies but also long-term preventive therapies translate into a dominant role of cardiovascular drugs in these costs, a projected $52.3 billion in 2009, almost 20% of all drug costs according to the American Heart Association. Moreover, with increasing success not only in heart disease but also in other therapeutic areas, cardiovascular physicians are increasingly encountering patients receiving multiple medications for noncardiovascular indications. The goal of this chapter is to outline principles of drug action and interaction that allow the safest and most effective therapy for an individual patient.

Key Decision in Drug Therapy: Risk Versus Benefit

The fundamental assumption underlying administration of any drug is that the real or expected benefit exceeds the anticipated risk. The benefits of drug therapy are initially defined in small clinical trials, perhaps involving several thousand patients, before a drug's marketing and approval. Ultimately, the efficacy and safety profile of any drug are determined after the compound has been marketed and used widely in hundreds of thousands of patients.

When a drug is administered for the acute correction of a life-threatening condition, the benefits are often self-evident; insulin for diabetic ketoacidosis, nitroprusside for hypertensive encephalopathy, or lidocaine for ventricular tachycardia are examples. Extrapolation of such immediately obvious benefits to other clinical situations may not be warranted, however.

The efficacy of lidocaine to terminate ventricular tachycardia led to its widespread use as a prophylactic agent in cases of acute myocardial infarction until it was recognized that in this setting, the drug does not alter mortality. The outcome of the Cardiac Arrhythmia Suppression Trial (CAST) highlights the difficulties in extrapolating from an incomplete understanding of physiology to chronic drug therapy. CAST tested the hypothesis that suppression of ventricular ectopic activity, a recognized risk factor for sudden death after myocardial infarction, would reduce mortality; this notion was highly ingrained in cardiovascular practice in the 1970s and 1980s. In CAST, sodium channel–blocking antiarrhythmics did suppress ventricular ectopic beats but also unexpectedly increased mortality threefold. Similarly, the development of a first-generation cholesterol ester transport protein (CETP) inhibitor achieved the goal of elevating high-density lipoprotein (HDL) and lowering low-density lipoprotein (LDL) cholesterol levels, but mortality was increased.[3] Thus, the use of arrhythmia suppression or of HDL elevation as a surrogate marker did not achieve the desired drug action, reduction in mortality, likely because the underlying pathophysiology or full range of drug actions was incompletely understood.

Similarly, drugs with positive inotropic activity increase cardiac output in patients with heart failure, but also increase in mortality, likely because of drug-induced arrhythmias. Nevertheless, clinical trials with these agents suggest symptom relief. Thus, the prescriber and patient may elect therapy with positive inotropic drugs because of this benefit while recognizing the risk. This illustrates the continuing personal relationship between the prescriber and patient and emphasizes the need for a clear understanding of the expected benefit of therapy, disease pathophysiology, and response to drug therapy in the drug development and prescribing processes.

Variability in Drug Action

Despite increasing understanding of the mechanisms of drug action, efficacy is far from uniform for any drug and dose. Drugs interact with specific molecular targets to effect changes in whole-organ and whole-body function. The targets with which drugs interact to produce beneficial effects may or may not be the same as those with which drugs interact to produce adverse effects. Drug targets may be in the circulation, at the cell surface, or within cells. Many newer drugs have been developed to interact with a desired drug target specifically; examples of such targets are 3-hydroxy-3-methyl-glutaryl-CoA (HMG-CoA) reductase, angiotensin-converting enzyme (ACE), G protein–coupled receptors (e.g., alpha, beta, angiotensin II, histamine), and platelet IIb/IIIa receptors. On the other hand, many drugs widely used in cardiovascular therapeutics were developed when the technology to identify specific molecular targets simply was not available; digoxin, amiodarone, and aspirin are examples. Some, like amiodarone, have many drug targets. In other cases, however, even older drugs turn out to have rather specific molecular targets. The actions of digitalis glycosides are mediated primarily by the inhibition of Na^+,K^+-ATPase. Aspirin permanently acetylates a specific serine residue on the cyclooxygenase (COX) enzyme, an effect that is thought to mediate its analgesic effects and its gastrointestinal (GI) toxicity.

The risks of drug therapy may be a direct extension of the pharmacologic actions for which the drug is actually being prescribed. Excessive hypotension in a patient taking an antihypertensive agent or bleeding in a patient taking a platelet IIb/IIIa receptor antagonist are examples. In other cases, adverse effects develop as a consequence of pharmacologic actions that were not appreciated during a drug's initial development and use in patients. Rhabdomyolysis with HMG-CoA reductase inhibitors (statins), angioedema during ACE inhibitor therapy, torsades de pointes during treatment with noncardiovascular drugs such as thioridazine or pentamidine, or atrial fibrillation with bisphosphonates[4] are examples. Importantly, these rarer but serious effects generally become evident only after a drug has been marketed and extensively used. Even rare adverse effects can alter the overall perception of risk versus benefit and can prompt removal of the drug from the market, particularly if alternate therapies thought to be safer are available. For example, withdrawal of the first insulin sensitizer, troglitazone, after recognition of

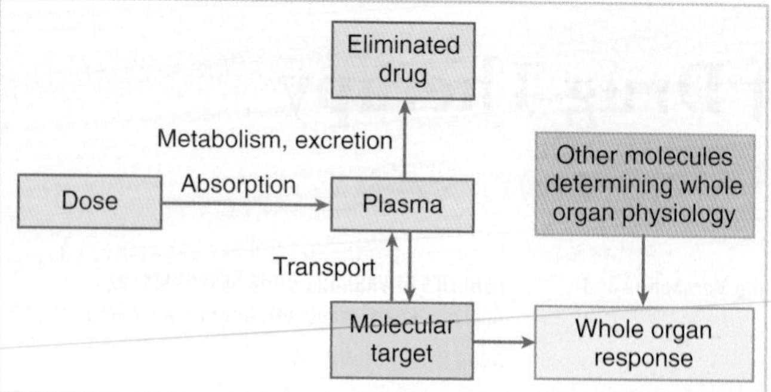

FIGURE 10-1 A model for understanding variability in drug action. When a dose of a drug is administered, the processes of absorption, metabolism, excretion, and transport determine its access to specific molecular targets that mediate beneficial and toxic effects. The interaction between a drug and its molecular target then produces changes in molecular, cellular, whole-organ, and ultimately whole-patient physiology. This molecular interaction does not occur in a vacuum, but rather in a complex biologic milieu modulated by multiple factors, some of which are disturbed to cause disease. DNA variants in the genes responsible for the processes of drug disposition (green), the molecular target (blue), or the molecules determining the biologic context in which the drug-target interaction occurs (brown) all can contribute to variability in drug action.

hepatotoxicity was further spurred by the availability of other new drugs in this class.

The recognition of multiple COX isoforms led to the development of specific COX-2 inhibitors to retain aspirin's analgesic effects but reduce GI side effects. However, one of these, rofecoxib, was withdrawn because of an apparent increase in cardiovascular mortality. The events surrounding the withdrawal of rofecoxib have important implications for drug development and utilization. First, specificity achieved by targeting a single molecular entity may not necessarily reduce adverse effects; one possibility is that by inhibiting COX-2, the drug removes a vascular protective effect of prostacyclin. Second, drug side effects may include not only readily identifiable events such as rhabdomyolysis or torsades de pointes, but also an increase that may be difficult to detect in events such as myocardial infarction that are common in the general population.[5]

MECHANISMS UNDERLYING VARIABLE DRUG ACTIONS. Two major processes determine how the interaction between a drug and its target molecule can generate variable drug actions in a patient (**Fig. 10-1**). The first, pharmacokinetics, describes drug delivery to and removal from the target molecule and includes the processes of absorption, distribution, metabolism, and excretion. These are collectively termed *drug disposition*. Robust mathematical techniques, applicable across drugs and drug classes, to analyze variability in drug disposition have been developed and result in a series of principles that can be used to adjust drug dosages to enhance the likelihood of a beneficial effect and minimize toxicity.

The second process, pharmacodynamics, describes how the interaction between a drug and its target generates downstream molecular, cellular, whole-organ, and whole-body effects. Pharmacodynamic sources of variability in drug action arise from the specifics of the target molecule and the biologic context in which the drug-target interaction occurs; thus, methods for analysis of pharmacodynamics tend to be drug or drug class specific.

This contemporary view of drug actions identifies a series of molecules that mediate drug actions in patients—drug-metabolizing enzymes, drug transport molecules, drug targets, and molecules modulating the biology in which the drug-target interaction occurs. *Pharmacogenetics* is the term used to describe the concept that individual variants in the genes controlling these processes contribute to variable drug actions. The way in which variability across multiple genes, up to whole genomes, explains differences in drug response among individuals and populations is termed *pharmacogenomics*.[6-8]

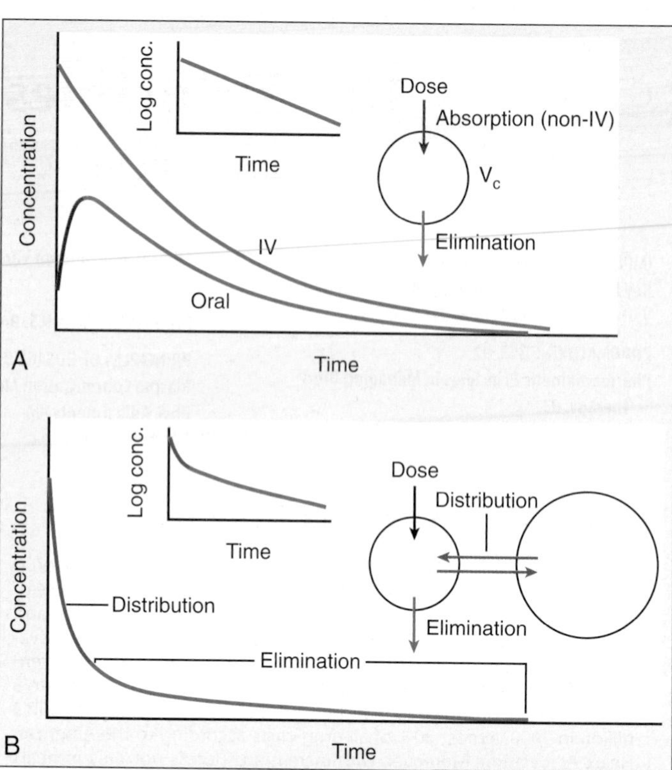

FIGURE 10-2 Models of plasma concentrations as a function of time after a single dose of a drug. **A,** The simplest situation is one in which a drug is administered as a rapid intravenous bolus into a volume (V_c), where it is instantaneously and uniformly distributed. Elimination then takes place from this volume. In this case, drug elimination is monoexponential; that is, a plot of the logarithm of concentration versus time is linear (inset). When the same dose of drug is administered orally, a distinct absorption phase is required before drug entry into V_c. Most absorption (shown here in red) is completed before elimination (shown in green), although the processes overlap. In this example, the amount of drug delivered by the oral route is less than that delivered by the intravenous route, assessed by the total areas under the two curves, indicating reduced bioavailability. **B,** In this example, drug is delivered to the central volume, from which it is not only eliminated but also undergoes distribution to the peripheral sites. This distribution process (blue) is more rapid than elimination, resulting in a distinct biexponential disappearance curve (inset).

Pharmacokinetics

Administration of an intravenous drug bolus results in maximal drug concentrations at the end of the bolus and then a decline in plasma drug concentrations over time (**Fig. 10-2A**). The simplest case is one in which this decline occurs monoexponentially over time. A useful parameter to describe this decline is the half-life ($t_{1/2}$), the time in which 50% of the drug is eliminated; for example, after two half-lives, 75% of the drug has been eliminated, after three half-lives, 87.5%. A monoexponential process can be considered almost complete in four or five half-lives.

In some cases, the decline of drug concentrations following administration of an intravenous bolus dose is multiexponential. The most common explanation is that drug is not only eliminated (represented by the terminal portion of the time-concentration plot) but also undergoes more rapid distribution to peripheral tissues. Just as elimination may be usefully described by a half-life, distribution half-lives can also be derived from curves such as those shown in Fig. 10-2B.

The plasma concentration measured immediately after a bolus dose can be used to derive a volume into which the drug is distributed. When the decline of plasma concentrations is multiexponential, multiple distribution compartments can be defined; these volumes of distribution can be useful in considering dose adjustments in cases of disease but rarely correspond exactly to any physical volume, such as plasma or total body water. With drugs that are highly tissue bound (e.g., some antidepressants), the volume of distribution can exceed total body volume by orders of magnitude.

Drugs are often administered by nonintravenous routes, such as oral, sublingual, transcutaneous, or intramuscular. With such routes of

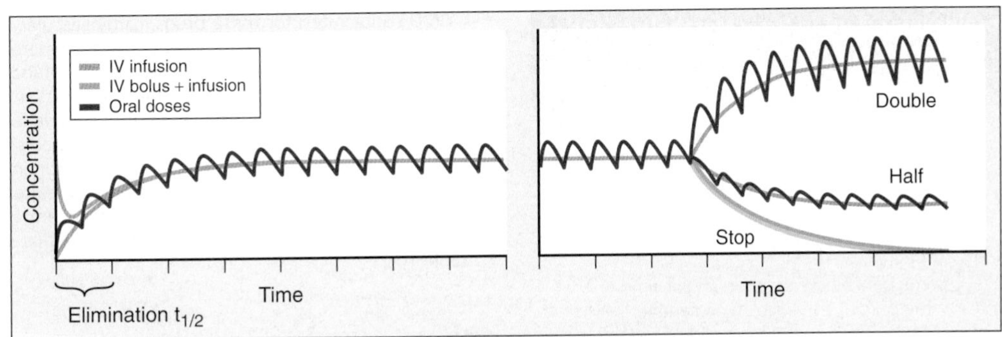

FIGURE 10-3 Time course of drug concentrations when treatment is started or dose changed. **Left,** The hash lines on the abscissa indicate one elimination half-life ($t_{1/2}$). With a constant rate intravenous infusion (gold), plasma concentrations accumulate to steady state in four or five elimination half-lives. When a loading bolus is administered with the maintenance infusion (blue), plasma concentrations are transiently higher but may dip, as shown here, before achieving the same steady state. When the same drug is administered by the oral route, the time course of drug accumulation is identical (red); in this case the drug was administered at intervals of 50% of a $t_{1/2}$. Steady-state plasma concentrations during oral therapy fluctuate around the mean determined by intravenous therapy. **Right,** This plot shows that when dosages are doubled, or halved, or the drug is stopped during steady-state administration, the time required to achieve the new steady state is 4 to 5 × $t_{1/2}$, and is independent of the route of administration.

administration, there are two differences from the intravenous route (see Fig. 10-2A). First, concentrations in plasma demonstrate a distinct rising phase as the drug slowly enters plasma. Second, the total amount of drug that actually enters the systemic circulation may be less than that achieved by the intravenous route. The relative amount of drug entering by any route, compared with the same dose administered intravenously, is termed *bioavailability*. Bioavailability may be reduced because drug undergoes metabolism before entering the circulation or because drug is simply not absorbed from its site of administration.

Drug elimination occurs by metabolism followed by the excretion of metabolites and unmetabolized parent drug, generally by the biliary tract or kidneys. The term *clearance* is the most useful way of quantifying drug elimination. Clearance can be viewed as a volume that is cleared of drug in any given period. Clearance may be organ specific (e.g., renal clearance, hepatic clearance) or whole-body clearance.

Pharmacokinetic Principles in Managing Drug Therapy

Bioavailability. Some drugs undergo such extensive presystemic metabolism that the amount of drug required to achieve a therapeutic effect is much greater (and often more variable) than that required for the same drug administered intravenously. Thus, small doses of intravenous propranolol (5 mg) may achieve heart rate slowing equivalent to that observed with much larger oral doses (80 to 120 mg). Propranolol is actually well absorbed but undergoes extensive metabolism in the intestine and liver before entering the systemic circulation. Another example is amiodarone; its physicochemical characteristics make it only 30% to 50% bioavailable when administered orally. Thus, an intravenous infusion of 0.5 mg/min (720 mg/day) is equivalent to 1.5 to 2 g/day orally.

Distribution. Rapid distribution can alter the way in which intravenous drug therapy should be initiated. When lidocaine is administered intravenously, it displays a prominent and rapid distribution phase ($t_{1/2}$ = 8 minutes) before slower elimination ($t_{1/2}$ = 120 minutes). As a consequence, an antiarrhythmic effect of lidocaine may be transiently achieved but rapidly lost following a single bolus, not as a result of elimination but of rapid distribution. Administration of larger bolus doses to circumvent this problem results in dose-related toxicity, often seizures. Hence, administration of a lidocaine loading dose of 3 to 4 mg/kg should occur over 10 to 20 minutes as a series of intravenous boluses (e.g., 50 to 100 mg every 5 to 10 minutes) or an intravenous infusion (e.g., 20 mg/min over 10 to 20 minutes).

Time Course of Drug Effects. With repeated doses, drug levels accumulate to a steady state, the condition under which the rate of drug administration is equal to the rate of drug elimination in any given period. As illustrated in **Fig. 10-3**, the elimination half-life describes not only the disappearance of a drug but also the time course of drug accumulation to steady state. It is important to distinguish between steady-state plasma concentrations, achieved in four to five elimination half-lives, and steady-state drug effects, which may take longer to achieve. For some drugs, clinical effects develop immediately on access to the molecular target—nitrates for angina, nitroprusside to lower blood pressure, and sympathomimetics to treat shock are examples. In other situations, drug effects follow plasma concentrations, but with a lag, and several explanations are possible. First, an active metabolite may need to be generated to achieve drug effects. Second, time may be required for translation of the drug effect at the molecular site to a physiologic endpoint; inhibition of synthesis of vitamin K–dependent clotting factors by warfarin ultimately leads to a desired elevation of the international normalized ratio, but the development of this desired effect occurs only as levels of clotting factors fall. Third, penetration of a drug into intracellular or other tissue sites of action may be required before development of drug effect. One mechanism underlying such penetration is the variable function of specific drug uptake and efflux transport proteins that control intracellular drug concentrations. Variable tissue penetration is widely invoked to explain the lag time between administration of amiodarone and the development of its effects, although the precise details underlying this phenomenon remain elusive.

Metabolism and Excretion. Drug metabolism most often occurs in the liver, although extrahepatic metabolism (in the circulation, intestine, lungs, and kidneys) is increasingly well defined. Phase I drug metabolism generally involves oxidation of the drug by specific drug-oxidizing enzymes, a process that renders the drug more water soluble (and hence more likely to undergo renal excretion). Additionally, drugs or their metabolites often undergo conjugation with specific chemical groups (phase II) to enhance water solubility; these conjugation reactions are catalyzed by specific transferases.

The most common enzyme systems mediating phase I drug metabolism are those of the cytochrome P-450 superfamily, termed *CYPs*. Multiple CYPs are expressed in human liver and other tissues. A major source of variability in drug action is variability in CYP activity, caused by variability in CYP expression and/or genetic variants that alter CYP activity. The most abundant CYP in human liver and intestine is CYP3A4 and a closely related isoform, CYP3A5. These CYPs metabolize up to 50% of clinically used drugs. CYP3A activity varies widely among individuals, for reasons that are not entirely clear. One mechanism underlying this variability is the presence of a polymorphism in this CYP3A5 gene that reduces its activity. **Table 10-1** lists CYPs and other drug-metabolizing enzymes important in cardiovascular therapy. Reduction in clearance, by disease, drug interactions, or genetic factors, will increase drug concentrations and hence drug effects. An exception is drugs whose effects are mediated by the generation of active metabolites. In this case, inhibition of drug metabolism may lead to accumulation of the parent drug but loss of therapeutic efficacy (see later).

Excretion of drugs or their metabolites, generally into the urine or bile, is accomplished by glomerular filtration or specific drug transport molecules, whose level of expression and genetic variation are only now being explored.[9] One widely-studied transporter is P-glycoprotein, the product of expression of the *MDR1* (or *ABCB1*) gene. Originally identified as a factor mediating multiple drug resistance in patients with cancer, P-glycoprotein expression is now well recognized in normal enterocytes, hepatocytes, renal tubular cells, the endothelium of the capillaries forming the blood-brain barrier, and the testes. In each of these sites, P-glycoprotein expression is restricted to the apical aspect of polarized cells, where it acts to enhance drug efflux. In the intestine, P-glycoprotein pumps substrates back into the lumen, thereby limiting bioavailability. In the liver and kidney, it promotes drug excretion into bile or urine. In central nervous system capillary endothelium, P-glycoprotein–mediated

TABLE 10-1 Proteins Important in Drug Metabolism and Elimination

PROTEIN*	SUBSTRATES
CYP3A4, CYP3A5	Erythromycin, clarithromycin; quinidine, mexiletine; many benzodiazepines; cyclosporine, tacrolimus; many antiretrovirals; HMG-CoA reductase inhibitors (atorvastatin, simvastatin, lovastatin; not pravastatin); many calcium channel blockers
CYP2D6†	Some beta blockers—propranolol, timolol, metoprolol, carvedilol; propafenone; desipramine and other tricyclics; codeine‡; debrisoquine; dextromethorphan
CYP2C9†	Warfarin, phenytoin, tolbutamide, losartan‡
CYP2C19†	Omeprazole, clopidogrel,‡ mephenytoin
P-glycoprotein	Digoxin
N-acetyltransferase†	Procainamide, hydralazine, isoniazid
Thiopurine methyl-transferase†	6-Mercaptopurine, azathioprine
Pseudocholinesterase†	Succinylcholine
UDP-glucuronosyl-transferase†	Irinotecan‡

*Full CYP listing available at http://medicine.iupui.edu/flockhart.
†Clinically important genetic variants described; see text.
‡Prodrug bioactivated by drug metabolism.

efflux is an important mechanism limiting drug access to the brain. Drug transporters play a role not only in drug elimination but also in drug uptake into many cells, including hepatocytes and enterocytes. Variable function of drug transporters has been implicated in the differing clinical effects of many cardiovascular drugs, including digoxin, verapamil, spironolactone, quinidine, ibutilide, and simvastatin.

Clinical Relevance of Variable Drug Metabolism and Elimination

When a drug is metabolized and eliminated by multiple pathways, absence of one of these, because of genetic variants, drug interactions, or dysfunction of excretory organs, generally does not affect drug concentrations or actions. By contrast, if a single pathway plays a critical role, the drug is more likely to exhibit marked variability in plasma concentration and thus action, a situation that has been termed *high-risk pharmacokinetics*.[10]

One scenario is a drug that is bioactivated—that is, metabolized to active and potent metabolites that mediate drug action. Decreased function of such a pathway reduces or eliminates drug effect. Bioactivation of clopidogrel by CYP2C19 is an example; individuals with reduced CYP2C19 activity (caused by genetic variants or possibly by interacting drugs; **Table 10-2** and see Table 10-1) have an increased incidence of cardiovascular events following stent placement.[11-13] Similarly, the widely used analgesic codeine undergoes CYP2D6-mediated bioactivation to an active metabolite, morphine, and patients with reduced CYP2D6 activity display reduced analgesia. A small group of individuals with multiple functional copies of CYP2D6, and hence increased enzymatic activity, has been identified; in this group, codeine may produce nausea and euphoria, presumably because of rapid morphine generation. A third example is the angiotensin receptor blocker losartan, which is bioactivated by CYP2C9; reduced antihypertensive effect is a risk with common genetic variants that reduce CYP2C9 activity or with coadministration of CYP2C9 inhibitors, such as phenytoin.

A second high-risk pharmacokinetic scenario is a drug eliminated by only a single pathway. In this case, there is a risk that absence of activity of that pathway will lead to marked accumulation of drug in plasma, failure to form downstream metabolites, and a consequent risk of drug toxicity caused by high drug concentrations. A simple example is the dependence of sotalol or dofetilide elimination on renal function; failure to decrease the dosage in a patient with renal dysfunction leads to accumulation of these drugs in plasma and an increased risk for drug-induced QT prolongation and torsades de pointes.

Similarly, administration of CYP2D6-metabolized beta blockers, including metoprolol and carvedilol, to patients with defective enzyme activity may produce exaggerated heart rate slowing. The weak beta-blocking actions of the antiarrhythmic propafenone are also increased in patients with reduced CYP2D6 activity. Some antidepressants are CYP2D6 substrates; for these drugs, cardiovascular adverse effects are more common in CYP2D6 poor metabolizers, whereas therapeutic efficacy is more difficult to achieve in ultrarapid metabolizers.

The concept of high-risk pharmacokinetics extends from drug metabolism to transporter-mediated drug elimination. The most widely recognized example is digoxin, which is eliminated primarily by P-glycoprotein–mediated efflux into bile and urine. Administration of a wide range of structurally and mechanistically unrelated drugs has been empirically recognized to increase digoxin concentrations; the common mechanism is inhibition of P-glycoprotein–mediated elimination (see Table 10-2).

Pharmacodynamics

Drugs can exert variable effects, even in the absence of pharmacokinetic variability. As indicated in Figure 10-1, this can arise as a function of variability in the molecular targets with which drugs interact to achieve their beneficial and adverse effects, as well as variability in the broader biologic context within which the drug-target interaction takes place. Variability in the number or function of a drug's target molecules can arise because of genetic factors (see later) or because disease alters the number of target molecules or their state (e.g., changes in the extent of phosphorylation). Examples of variability in the biologic context are high dietary salt, which can inhibit the antihypertensive action of beta blockers, or hypokalemia, which increases the risk for drug-induced QT prolongation. In addition, disease itself modulates drug response, as indicated in the following cases: the effect of lytic therapy in a patient with no clot is manifestly different from that in a patient with acute coronary thrombosis; the arrhythmogenic effects of digitalis depend on serum potassium levels; and the vasodilating effects of nitrates, beneficial in patients with coronary disease with angina, can be catastrophic in patients with aortic stenosis.

Principles of Dosage Optimization

The goals of drug therapy should be defined before the initiation of drug treatment. These may include acute correction of serious pathophysiology, acute or chronic symptom relief, or changes in surrogate endpoints (e.g., blood pressure, serum cholesterol, international normalized ratio) that have been linked to beneficial outcomes in target patient populations. The lessons of CAST and of positive inotropic drugs should make prescribers skeptical about such surrogate-guided therapy in the absence of controlled clinical trials.

When the goal of drug therapy is to correct a disturbance in physiology acutely, the drug should be administered intravenously in doses designed to achieve a therapeutic effect rapidly. This approach is best justified when benefits clearly outweigh risks. As discussed earlier for lidocaine, large intravenous drug boluses carry with them a risk of enhancing drug-related toxicity; therefore, even with the most urgent of medical indications, this approach is rarely appropriate. An exception is adenosine, which must be administered as a rapid bolus because it undergoes extensive and rapid elimination from plasma by uptake into almost all cells. As a consequence, a slow bolus or infusion rarely achieves sufficiently high concentrations at the desired site of action (the coronary artery perfusing the atrioventricular node) to terminate arrhythmias. Similarly, the time course of anesthesia depends on anesthetic drug delivery to and removal from sites in the central nervous system.

The time required to achieve steady-state plasma concentrations is determined by the elimination half-life (see earlier). The administration of a loading dose may shorten this time, but only if the kinetics of distribution and elimination are known a priori in an individual subject and the correct loading regimen is chosen. Otherwise, overshoot or undershoot during the loading phase may occur (see Fig. 10-3). Thus, the initiation of drug therapy by a loading strategy should be used only when the indication is acute.

Two dose-response curves describe the relationship between drug dose and the expected cumulative incidence of a beneficial effect or an adverse effect (**Fig. 10-4**). The distance along the X axis describing

TABLE 10-2 Drug Interactions: Mechanisms and Examples

MECHANISM	DRUG	INTERACTING DRUG(S)	EFFECT
Decreased bioavailability	Digoxin	Antacids	Decreased digoxin effect because of decreased absorption
Increased bioavailability	Digoxin	Antibiotics	By eliminating gut flora that metabolize digoxin, some antibiotics may increase digoxin bioavailability. (NOTE: Some antibiotics also interfere with P-glycoprotein. expressed in the intestine and elsewhere, another effect that can elevate digoxin concentration.)
Induction of hepatic metabolism	**CYP3A substrates** Quinidine Mexiletine Verapamil Cyclosporine	Phenytoin Rifampin Barbiturates St. John's wort	Loss of drug effect because of increased metabolism
Inhibition of hepatic metabolism	**CYP2C9 substrates** Warfarin Losartan	Amiodarone Phenytoin	Decreased warfarin requirement Diminished conversion of losartan to its active metabolite, with decreased antihypertensive control
	CYP3A substrates Quinidine Cyclosporine HMG-CoA reductase inhibitors: lovastatin, simvastatin, atorvastatin (not pravastatin) Cisapride, terfenadine, astemizole*	Ketoconazole Itraconazole Erythromycin Clarithromycin Some calcium blockers Some HIV protease inhibitors (especially ritanovir)	Increased risk for drug toxicity
	CYP2D6 substrates Beta blockers (see Table 10-1), propafenone Desipramine Codeine	Quinidine (even ultralow dose) Fluoxetine, paroxetine	Increased beta blockade Increased beta blockade, increased adverse effects Decreased analgesia (caused by failure of biotransformation to the active metabolite morphine)
	CYP2C19 Clopidogrel	Omeprazole, possibly other proton pump inhibitors	Decreased clopidogrel efficacy reported
Inhibition of drug transport	**P-glycoprotein transport** Digoxin	Amiodarone, quinidine, verapamil, cyclosporine, itraconazole, erythromycin	Digoxin toxicity
	Renal tubular transport Dofetilide	Verapamil	Slightly increased plasma concentration and QT effect
	Monoamine transport Guanadrel	Tricyclic antidepressants	Blunted antihypertensive effects
Pharmacodynamic interactions	Aspirin	Warfarin	Increased therapeutic antithrombotic effect; increased risk of bleeding
	NSAIDs	Warfarin	Increased risk of GI bleeding
	Antihypertensive drugs	NSAIDs	Loss of blood pressure lowering
	QT-prolonging antiarrhythmics	Diuretics	Increased torsades de pointes risk caused by diuretic-induced hypokalemia
	Supplemental potassium	ACE inhibitors	Hyperkalemia
	Sildenafil	Nitrates	Increased and persistent vasodilation; risk of myocardial ischemia

NSAIDs = nonsteroidal antiinflammatory drugs.
*Withdrawn because of severe toxicity due to drug interactions.

the difference between these curves, often termed the *therapeutic ratio* (or *index* or *window*), provides an index of the likelihood that a chronic dosing regimen that provides benefits without adverse effects can be identified. Drugs with especially wide therapeutic indices can often be administered at infrequent intervals, even if they are rapidly eliminated (see Fig. 10-4, A and C).

When expected adverse effects are serious, the most appropriate treatment strategy is to start at low doses and reevaluate the necessity for increasing drug dosages once steady-state drug effects have been achieved. This approach has the advantage of minimizing the risk of dose-related adverse effects but carries with it a need to titrate doses to efficacy. Only when stable drug effects are achieved should increasing drug dosage to achieve the desired therapeutic effect be considered. An example is sotalol; because the risk of torsades de pointes increases with drug dosage, the starting dose should be low.

In other cases, anticipated toxicity is relatively mild and manageable. It may then be acceptable to start at dosages higher than the minimum required to achieve a therapeutic effect, accepting a greater than minimal risk of adverse effects; some antihypertensives can be administered in this fashion. However, the principle of using the lowest dose possible to minimize toxicity, particularly toxicity that is unpredictable and unrelated to recognized pharmacologic actions, should be the rule.

Occasionally, dose escalation into the high therapeutic range results in no beneficial drug effect and no side effects. In this circumstance, the prescriber should be alert to the possibility of drug

CH 10

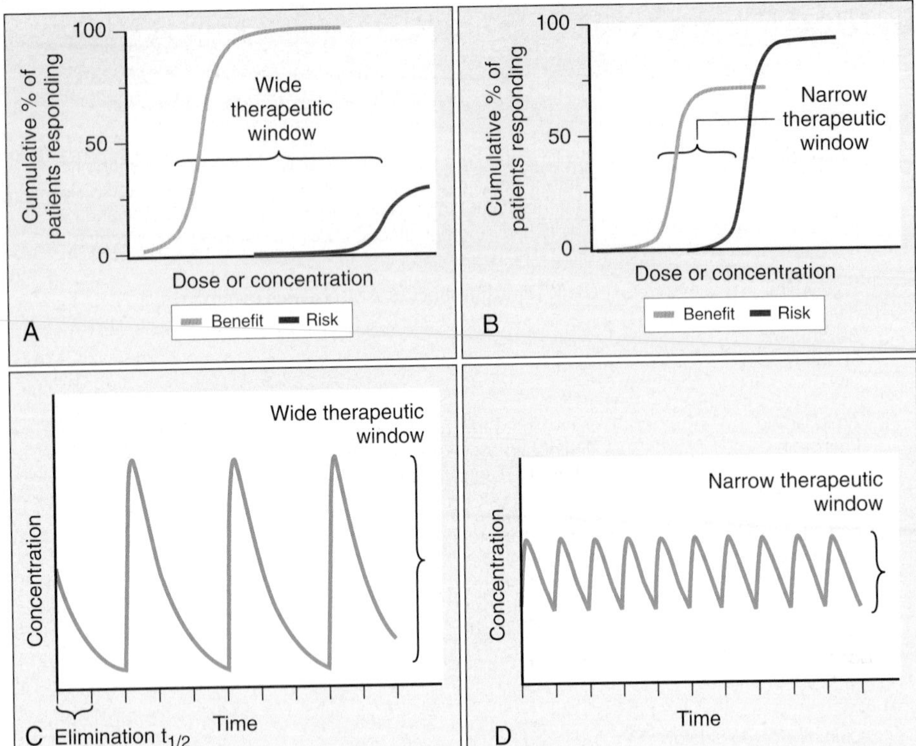

FIGURE 10-4 The concept of a therapeutic ratio. **A, B,** Two dose- (or concentration-) response curves. The blue lines describe the relationship between dose and cumulative incidence of beneficial effects, and the magenta line depicts the relationship between dose and dose-related adverse effects (risk). A drug with a wide therapeutic ratio displays separation between the two curves, a high degree of efficacy, and low degree of dose-related toxicity **(A)**. Under these conditions, a wide therapeutic ratio can be defined. In **B,** conversely, the curves describing cumulative efficacy and cumulative incidence of adverse effects are positioned near each other, the incidence of adverse effects is higher, and the expected beneficial response is lower. These characteristics define a narrow therapeutic ratio. **C, D,** Steady-state plasma concentrations with oral drug administration as a function of time with wide (left) and narrow (right) therapeutic ratios. The hash marks on the abscissae indicate one elimination half-life. **C,** When the therapeutic window is wide, drug administration every three elimination half-lives can produce plasma concentrations that are maintained above the minimum for efficacy and below the maximum beyond which toxicity is anticipated. **D,** The opposite situation is illustrated. To maintain plasma concentrations within the narrow therapeutic range, the drug must be administered more frequently.

interactions at the pharmacokinetic or pharmacodynamic level. Depending on the nature of the anticipated toxicity, dose escalation beyond the usual therapeutic range may occasionally be acceptable, but only if anticipated toxicity is not serious and is readily manageable.

Plasma Concentration Monitoring

For some drugs, curves such as those shown in Figures 10-4A and B relating drug concentration to cumulative incidence of beneficial and adverse effects can be generated. With such drugs, monitoring plasma drug concentrations to ensure that they remain within a desired therapeutic range (i.e., above a minimum required for efficacy and below a maximum likely to produce adverse effects) may be a useful adjunct to therapy. Monitoring drug concentrations may also be useful to ensure compliance and to detect pharmacokinetically based drug interactions that underlie unanticipated efficacy and/or toxicity at usual dosages. Samples for measurement of plasma concentrations should generally be obtained just before the next dose, at steady state. These trough concentrations provide an index of the minimum plasma concentration expected during a dosing interval.

On the other hand, patient monitoring, whether by plasma concentration or other physiologic indices, to detect incipient toxicity is best accomplished at the time of anticipated peak drug concentrations. Thus, patient surveillance for QT prolongation during therapy with sotalol or dofetilide is best accomplished 1 to 2 hours after the administration of a dose of drug at a steady state.

A lag between the time courses of drug in plasma and drug effects may exist (see earlier). In addition, monitoring plasma drug concentrations relies on the assumption that the concentration measured is in equilibrium with that at the target molecular site. Importantly, it is only the fraction of drug not bound to plasma proteins that is available to achieve such equilibration. Variability in the extent of protein binding can therefore affect the free fraction and anticipated drug effect, even in the presence of apparently therapeutic total plasma drug concentrations. Basic drugs such as lidocaine and quinidine are not only bound to albumin but also bind extensively to $alpha_1$ acid glycoprotein, an acute-phase reactant whose concentrations are increased in a variety of stress situations, including acute myocardial infarction. Because of this increased protein binding, drug effects may be blunted, despite achieving therapeutic total drug concentrations in these situations.

Dose Adjustments

Polypharmacy is common in patients with varying degrees of specific organ dysfunction. Although treatment with an individual agent may be justified, the practitioner should also recognize the risk of unanticipated drug effects, particularly drug toxicity, during therapy with multiple drugs.

The presence of renal disease mandates dose reductions for drugs eliminated primarily by renal excretion, including digoxin, dofetilide, procainamide, and sotalol. A requirement for dose adjustment in cases of mild renal dysfunction is dictated by available clinical data and the likelihood of serious toxicity if drug accumulates in plasma because of impaired elimination. Renal failure reduces the protein binding of some drugs (e.g., phenytoin); in this case, a total drug concentration value in the therapeutic range may actually represent a toxic value of unbound drug.

Advanced liver disease is characterized by decreased hepatic drug metabolism and portocaval shunts that decrease clearance, particularly first-pass clearance. Moreover, such patients frequently have other profound disturbances of homeostasis, such as coagulopathy, severe ascites, and altered mental status. These pathophysiologic features of advanced liver disease can profoundly affect not only the dose of a drug required to achieve a potentially therapeutic effect but also the perception of risks and benefits, thereby altering the prescriber's assessment of the actual need for therapy.

Heart disease similarly carries with it a number of disturbances of drug elimination and drug sensitivity that may alter the therapeutic doses or the practitioner's perception of the desirability of therapy on the basis of evaluation of risks and benefits. Patients with left ventricular hypertrophy often have baseline QT prolongation, and thus risks of QT-prolonging antiarrhythmics may increase; most guidelines suggest avoiding QT-prolonging antiarrhythmics in such patients (see Chaps. 37 and 39; see also www.azcert.org).

In heart failure (see Chap. 28), hepatic congestion can lead to decreased clearance and thus an increased risk for toxicity with usual doses of certain drugs, including some sedatives, lidocaine, and beta blockers. On the other hand, gut congestion can lead to decreased absorption of orally administered drugs and decreased effects. In addition, patients with heart failure may demonstrate reduced renal perfusion and require dose adjustments on this basis. Heart failure is also characterized by a redistribution of regional blood flow, which can lead to reduced volume of distribution and enhanced risk for drug toxicity. Lidocaine is probably the best-studied example; loading doses of lidocaine should be reduced in patients with heart failure because of altered distribution, whereas maintenance doses should be reduced in heart failure and liver disease because of altered clearance.

Age is also a major factor in determining drug doses, as well as sensitivity to drug effects. Doses in children are generally administered on a milligram per kilogram body weight basis, although firm data to guide therapy are often not available. Variable postnatal maturation of drug disposition systems may present a special problem in the neonate. Older persons often have reduced creatinine clearance, even with a normal serum creatinine level, and dosages of renally excreted drugs should be adjusted accordingly (see Chap. 80). Systolic dysfunction with hepatic congestion is more common in older adults, and vascular disease and dementia are common, which can lead to increased postural hypotension and risk of falling. Therapies such as sedatives, tricyclic antidepressants, or anticoagulants should be initiated only when the practitioner is convinced that the benefits of such therapies outweigh this increased risk.

Genetics of Variable Drug Responses

Figure 10-1 highlights candidate pathways in which DNA variants may influence drug responses—those encoding drug metabolism and transport, drug targets, and biologic context and disease. Examples are presented here.

There are common polymorphisms in CYP2D6, CYP2C9, and CYP2C19 that influence the metabolism of widely-used cardiovascular drugs (see Table 10-1). Those who are homozygous for loss of function variants (poor metabolizers [PMs]) are at greatest risk for aberrant drug responses. However, for drugs with very narrow therapeutic margins (e.g., warfarin, clopidogrel), even heterozygotes may display unusual drug sensitivity. Although PMs make up a minority of subjects in most populations, many drugs in common use can inhibit these enzymes (see Table 10-2), and thereby "phenocopy" the PM trait. Omeprazole, and possibly other proton pump inhibitors, block CYP2C19 and have been associated with an increase in cardiovascular events during clopidogrel therapy.[10,14] Similarly, specific inhibitors of CYP2D6 and CYP2C9 can phenocopy the PM trait when coadministered with substrate drugs.

A variant in *SLCO1B1*, a gene encoding a drug uptake transporter in liver, has been associated with a markedly increased risk for simvastatin-induced myopathy.[15] This variant has also been associated with variability in the extent to which statins lower LDL cholesterol levels.

The heart rate slowing and blood pressure effects with beta blockers and beta agonists have been associated with polymorphisms in the drug targets, the $beta_1$ and $beta_2$ receptors. Variability in warfarin dose requirements has been clearly associated with variants in both *CYP2C9*, which mediates elimination of the active enantiomer of the drug, and *VKORC1*, part of the vitamin K complex that is the drug target.[16] The effect of hormone replacement therapy on HDL cholesterol has been linked to a polymorphism in the estrogen receptor.

An example of a variant modulating biologic context in which the drug acts is susceptibility to stroke in patients receiving diuretics; this has been linked to a polymorphism in the alpha-adducing gene whose product plays a role in renal tubular sodium transport. Torsades de pointes during QT-prolonging antiarrhythmic therapy has been linked to polymorphisms not only in the ion channel that is the drug target but to many other ion channel genes. In addition, this adverse effect sometimes occurs in patients with clinically latent congenital long-QT syndrome, emphasizing the interrelationship among disease, genetic background, and drug therapy (see Chaps. 9 and 39).[17] Drugs can also bring out latent Brugada syndrome (see www.brugadadrugs.org).

An example of a tumor genotype determining response to therapy is the anticancer drug trastuzumab, which is effective only in cancers that do not express the Her2/neu receptor . Because the drug also potentiates anthracycline-related cardiotoxicity, toxic therapy can be avoided in patients who are receptor negative (see Chap. 73).

Very common polymorphisms in genes regulating cardiovascular function have been associated with many cardiovascular phenotypes, including variable drug responses. One of the best-studied human polymorphisms is the insertion-deletion (I-D) variant in the ACE gene that determines ACE activity. DD individuals, homozygous for the D allele, have higher plasma ACE activity and thus are assumed to have higher concentrations of the pressor peptide angiotensin II than individuals with the II genotype. Many associations have been reported between the DD genotype and worse outcomes in cardiovascular disease. However, a very large study (almost 38,000 patients) found no effect of this polymorphism on a range of outcomes such as myocardial infarction or death in patients treated for hypertension with ACE inhibitors.[18] Whether this reflects a true nonassociation or whether the ACE I-D polymorphism may predict outcomes in more precisely defined patient subsets remains to be seen. More generally, it is important to recognize that genomic science is in its infancy, and thus reported associations—especially in small populations—require independent confirmation and assessment of clinical importance and cost-effectiveness before they can or should enter clinical practice.

Technologies to screen hundreds of thousands of polymorphisms in large populations are now routine research tools that can identify genes contributing to variability in physiology, disease susceptibility, or variable drug responses. Examples are baseline QT interval, risk of obesity, diabetes, atrial fibrillation, and premature myocardial infarction, and responses to drugs such as HMG-CoA reductase inhibitors or inhaled $beta_2$ agonists (see Chap. 7).[19-23]

Applying Pharmacogenetic Information to Practice

This discussion highlights the tantalizing prospect that some variability in responses to drugs, including the development of some severe adverse drug reactions, could be reduced by the incorporation of pharmacogenetic information into practice. In 2007, the U.S. Food and Drug Administration began systematically including pharmacogenetic information in drug labels.[24] There are substantial barriers to this vision, however, including cost, varying levels of evidence supporting a role for genetics, and implementation (e.g., how fast and accurately a genetic test result can be delivered).

One scenario in which pharmacogenetic testing would be appealing is a drug with these characteristics: (1) carries a risk of a severe adverse reaction; (2) confers a truly important clinical benefit; (3) has no alternate therapies; and (4) involves a genetic test to discriminate those individuals at risk from those not at risk, preferably in a randomized clinical trial. Preprescription genotyping to prevent serious skin rash with the antiretroviral agent abacavir is now routine practice because it meets these criteria.[25] In cardiovascular medicine, clinical trials of a prospective, genotype-guided approach to warfarin therapy started in late 2009.[26] As methods to generate whole human genome sequences very rapidly become perfected, the day may come when this information becomes part of every patient's electronic health record, and variants known to affect drug response, such as those in drug-metabolizing enzymes, will be routinely accessed and used to modify dosing on a patient by patient basis.

Drug Interactions

Table 10-2 summarizes mechanisms that may underlie important drug interactions. Drug interactions may be based on altered pharmacokinetics (absorption, distribution, metabolism, and excretion). In addition, drugs can interact at the pharmacodynamic level. A trivial example is the coadministration of two antihypertensive drugs, leading to excessive hypotension. Similarly, coadministration of aspirin and warfarin leads to an increased risk for bleeding, although benefits of the combination can also be demonstrated.

The most important principle in approaching a patient receiving polypharmacy is to recognize the high potential for drug interactions.

A complete medication history should be obtained from each patient at regular intervals; patients will often omit topical medications such as eye drops, health food supplements, and medications prescribed by other practitioners unless specifically prompted. Each of these, however, carries a risk of important systemic drug actions and interactions. Even high dosages of grapefruit juice, which contains CYP3A and P-glycoprotein inhibitors, can affect drug responses. Beta blocker eye drops can produce systemic beta blockade, particularly with CYP2D6 substrates (e.g., timolol) in patients with defective CYP2D6 activity. St. John's wort induces CYP3A and P-glycoprotein activity (like phenytoin and other drugs) and thus can markedly lower plasma concentrations of drugs such as cyclosporine and oral contraceptives. As with many other interactions, this may not be a special problem as long as both drugs are continued. However, if a patient stabilized on cyclosporine stops taking St. John's wort, plasma concentrations of the drug can rise dramatically and toxicity can ensue. Similarly, initiation of St. John's wort may lead to markedly lowered cyclosporine concentrations and a risk of organ rejection. A number of other natural supplements have been associated with serious drug toxicity and have been withdrawn from the market; phenylpropanolamine-associated stroke is an example.

Prospects for the Future

The past 25 years have seen dramatic advances in the treatment of heart disease, in no small part because of the development of highly effective and well-tolerated drug therapies such as HMG-CoA reductase inhibitors, ACE inhibitors, and beta blockers. These developments, along with improved nonpharmacologic approaches, have led to dramatically enhanced survival of patients with advanced heart disease. Thus, polypharmacy in an aging and chronically ill population is becoming increasingly common. In this milieu, drug effects become increasingly variable, reflecting interactions among drugs, underlying disease and disease mechanisms, and genetic backgrounds.

An increasing understanding of the genetic basis of variable drug actions includes the promise of reducing such variability. However, the logistics of implementing such a strategy and the costs of individualizing therapy on the basis of genetics are major outstanding issues. An alternate view is that effective therapies are available and have not been adequately delivered to populations that would benefit. These two perspectives are not mutually exclusive. With such increasing complexity, the relationship between the prescriber and patient remains the centerpiece of modern therapeutics. Each initiation of drug therapy represents a new clinical experiment. Prescribers must always be vigilant regarding the possibility of unusual drug effects, which could provide clues about unanticipated and important mechanisms of beneficial and adverse drug effects.

REFERENCES

Importance of Correct Drug Use

1. Hartman M, Martin A, McDonnell P, et al: National health spending in 2007: Slower drug spending contributes to lowest rate of overall growth since 1998. Health Aff 28:246, 2009.
2. Moore TJ, Cohen MR, Furberg CD: Serious adverse drug events reported to the Food and Drug Administration, 1998-2005. Arch Intern Med 167:1752, 2007.
3. Barter PJ, Caulfield M, Eriksson M, et al: Effects of torcetrapib in patients at high risk for coronary events. N Engl J Med 357:2109, 2007.
4. Black DM, Delmas PD, Eastell R, et al: Once-yearly zoledronic acid for treatment of postmenopausal osteoporosis. N Engl J Med 356:1809, 2007.
5. Brownstein JS, Sordo M, Kohane IS, et al: The tell-tale heart: Population-based surveillance reveals an association of rofecoxib and celecoxib with myocardial infarction. PLoS ONE 2:e840, 2007.
6. Giacomini KM, Brett CM, Altman RB, et al: The pharmacogenetics research network: From SNP discovery to clinical drug response. Clin Pharmacol Ther 81:328, 2007.
7. Roden DM, Altman RB, Benowitz NL, et al: Pharmacogenomics: Challenges and opportunities. Ann Intern Med 145:749, 2006.
8. Weinshilboum RM, Wang L: Pharmacogenetics and pharmacogenomics: Development, science, and translation. Annu Rev Genomics Hum Genet 7:223, 2006.

Pharmacokinetics

9. Kim RB: Transporters and drug discovery: Why, when, and how. Mol Pharm 3:26, 2006.
10. Roden DM, Stein CM: Clopidogrel and the concept of high-risk pharmacokinetics. Circulation 119:2127, 2009.
11. Collet JP, Hulot JS, Pena A, et al: Cytochrome P450 2C19 polymorphism in young patients treated with clopidogrel after myocardial infarction: A cohort study. Lancet 373:309, 2009.
12. Mega JL, Close SL, Wiviott SD, et al: Cytochrome P-450 polymorphisms and response to clopidogrel. N Engl J Med 360:354, 2009.
13. Simon T, Verstuyft C, Mary-Krause M, et al: Genetic determinants of response to clopidogrel and cardiovascular events. N Engl J Med 360:363, 2009.

Genetics of Variable Drug Responses

14. Ho PM, Maddox TM, Wang L, et al: Risk of adverse outcomes associated with concomitant use of clopidogrel and proton pump inhibitors following acute coronary syndrome. JAMA 301:937, 2009.
15. Link E, Parish S, Armitage J, et al: SLCO1B1 variants and statin-induced myopathy—a genomewide study. N Engl J Med 359:789, 2008.
16. International Warfarin Pharmacogenetics Consortium: Estimation of the warfarin dose with clinical and pharmacogenetic data. N Engl J Med 360:753, 2009.
17. Roden DM, Viswanathan PC: Genetics of acquired long QT syndrome. J Clin Invest 115:2025, 2005.
18. Arnett DK, Davis BR, Ford CE, et al: Pharmacogenetic association of the angiotensin-converting enzyme insertion/deletion polymorphism on blood pressure and cardiovascular risk in relation to antihypertensive treatment: The Genetics of Hypertension-Associated Treatment (GenHAT) study. Circulation 111:3374, 2005.
19. Newton-Cheh C, Eijgelsheim M, Rice KM, et al: Common variants at ten loci influence QT interval duration in the QTGEN Study. Nat Genet 41:399, 2009.
20. Manolio TA, Brooks LD, Collins FS: A HapMap harvest of insights into the genetics of common disease. J Clin Invest 118:1590, 2008.
21. McPherson R, Pertsemlidis A, Kavaslar N, et al: A common allele on chromosome 9 associated with coronary heart disease. Science 316:1488, 2007.
22. Helgadottir A, Thorleifsson G, Manolescu A, et al: A common variant on chromosome 9p21 affects the risk of myocardial infarction. Science 316:1491, 2007.
23. Gudbjartsson DF, Arnar DO, Helgadottir A, et al: Variants conferring risk of atrial fibrillation on chromosome 4q25. Nature 448:353, 2007.
24. Woodcock J, Lesko LJ: Pharmacogenetics–tailoring treatment for the outliers. N Engl J Med 360:811, 2009.
25. Mallal S, Phillips E, Carosi G, et al: HLA-B*5701 screening for hypersensitivity to abacavir. N Engl J Med 358:568, 2008.
26. Shurin SB, Nabel EG: Pharmacogenomics—ready for prime time? N Engl J Med 358:1061, 2008.

CHAPTER 11 Cardiovascular Regeneration and Tissue Engineering

Piero Anversa, Jan Kajstura, and Annarosa Leri

The traditional view that the reparative ability of the heart is limited by the inability of terminally differentiated cardiomyocytes to undergo cell division after the first weeks of life has been challenged by recent studies suggesting that the heart is capable of limited self-regeneration. Current evidence suggests that there are at least four potential sources of cells that can account for new cardiomyocytes after birth[1]: adult cardiomyocytes (mononucleated) may reenter the cell cycle and divide[2]; bone marrow–derived cardiac stem or progenitor cells that possess the capacity to differentiate into cardiomyocytes may populate the heart after injury[3]; cells that are derived from the embryonic epicardium may give rise to cardiomyocytes; and niches of cardiac stem or cardiac progenitor cells (CPCs) may give rise to cardiomyocytes. In the following chapter, we will focus on the emerging role of CPCs and exogenous progenitor cells in myocardial homeostasis and tissue repair. Recent developments in tissue engineering will also be reviewed briefly. The clinical application of stem cell biology is discussed in Chap. 33.

Cardiac Stem Cells

The observation that niches of primitive cells reside in the adult hearts of small and large mammals, including humans, and that these primitive cells possess the ability to form cardiomyocytes, endothelial cells (ECs), and smooth muscle cells (SMCs) that can organize into coronary vessels, has provided new insights into the mechanisms of myocardial homeostasis and myocardial tissue repair. Thus far, several different classes of CPCs have been characterized in the embryonic, fetal, postnatal, and adult heart based on cell surface markers (**Fig. 11-1**),[1] although it should be recognized that a definitive marker for CPCs has not yet been identified. Several different populations have been identified and characterized, including c-Kit$^+$ cells, Sca-1$^+$ cells, side population cells, and cells expressing the protein Islet-1. Some side population cells express Kit and/or Sca-1 and, similar to Kit$^+$ CPCs and Sca-1$^+$ CPCs, side population cells can generate cardiomyocytes in vitro and in vivo. In addition to Kit$^+$ CPCs, Sca-1$^+$ CPCs, and side population cells, a fourth population of CPCs expresses the transcription factor Islet-1. Experiments using lineage tracing have shown that Islet-1–expressing cells can differentiate into endothelial, endocardial, smooth muscle, conduction system, right ventricular, and atrial myogenic lineages during the development of the embryonic heart. Islet-1–expressing cells are also present in the adult mammalian heart but are limited to the right atrium, are found in smaller numbers than in embryonic hearts, and have no known physiologic role.

Recently, epicardium-derived progenitor cells have been described that show angiogenic potential. Whether c-Kit$^+$, Sca-1$^+$, and cardiac SP cells comprise three different cell populations has also not been entirely resolved. However, the observation that these different undifferentiated cells share common characteristics and can differentiate into myocytes, ECs, and SMCs suggests that they arise from a general CPC compartment. Cardiac stem cells have also been obtained by growing self-adherent clusters (termed *cardiospheres*) from subcultures of murine or human biopsy specimens. Other laboratories have generated cardiac SP cell–derived cardiospheres by adapting a method used for creating a neurosphere and have claimed that cardiac neural crest cells contribute to cardiac SP cells. Cardiosphere-derived cardiac stem cells as well as c-Kit$^+$ cardiac stem cells are capable of long-term self-renewal and can differentiate into the major specialized cell types of the heart: myocytes and vascular cells (i.e., cells with endothelial or smooth muscle markers). Thus far, the origin and mechanisms maintaining the cardiac stem cell pool are unclear. Two recent studies have suggested that c-Kit$^+$ and cardiac SP cells may derive from the bone marrow, but these studies cannot entirely exclude the hypothesis that specific subpopulations of cardiac stem cells originate from distinct sources and may represent remnants from embryonic development in selected niches within the heart.

The current focus in the field of stem cell biology is to gain a better understanding of the growth and differentiation potential of different classes of CPCs. Understanding CPC function is critical for the implementation of CPCs in the treatment of the chronically decompensated human heart (see Chap. 33). There is emerging evidence that the heart has the capacity to undergo limited self-regeneration, at least in part, through the activation of endogenous stem cell compartments.[3] Regeneration conforms to a hierarchical archetype in which slowly dividing stem cells give rise to proliferating, lineage-restricted progenitor-precursor cells, which then become highly dividing amplifying cells that eventually reach terminal differentiation and growth arrest (**Fig. 11-2**). Stem cells have a high propensity for cell division, which is maintained throughout the lifespan of the organ and organism. In contrast, the less primitive, transient amplifying cells represent a group of dividing cells that have a limited capacity for proliferation. Amplifying cells divide and concurrently differentiate and, when complete differentiation is reached, the ability to replicate is permanently lost. Taken together, these observations suggest that multipotent resident CPCs contribute to the homeostatic maintenance of myocytes, ECs, SMCs, and fibroblasts in the heart. The discovery that activated CPCs translocate to areas of cardiac injury, where they grow and differentiate, suggests that myocardial regeneration is feasible.

The observation that the adult atrial and ventricular myocardium contains a pool of CPCs, which are self-renewing, clonogenic, and multipotent in vitro and can regenerate cardiomyocytes and coronary vessels in vivo, has raised the possibility that these cells can repair injured hearts. In theory, CPCs could be isolated from myocardial biopsy samples and, following their expansion in vitro, could be implanted within regions of myocardial damage, where they could reconstitute the lost myocardium. Alternatively, portions of infarcted or injured myocardium can be restored by cytokine activation of resident CPCs, which migrate to the site of injury and subsequently form myocytes and vascular structures[4]; this would allow necrotic or scarred tissue to be replaced by new, mechanically effective myocardium (**Fig. 11-3**). These two forms of therapy are not mutually exclusive and, in fact, complement each other. In a heart severely depleted of its CPC compartment, the identification and expansion of the remaining functionally competent CPCs may be the preferable option,

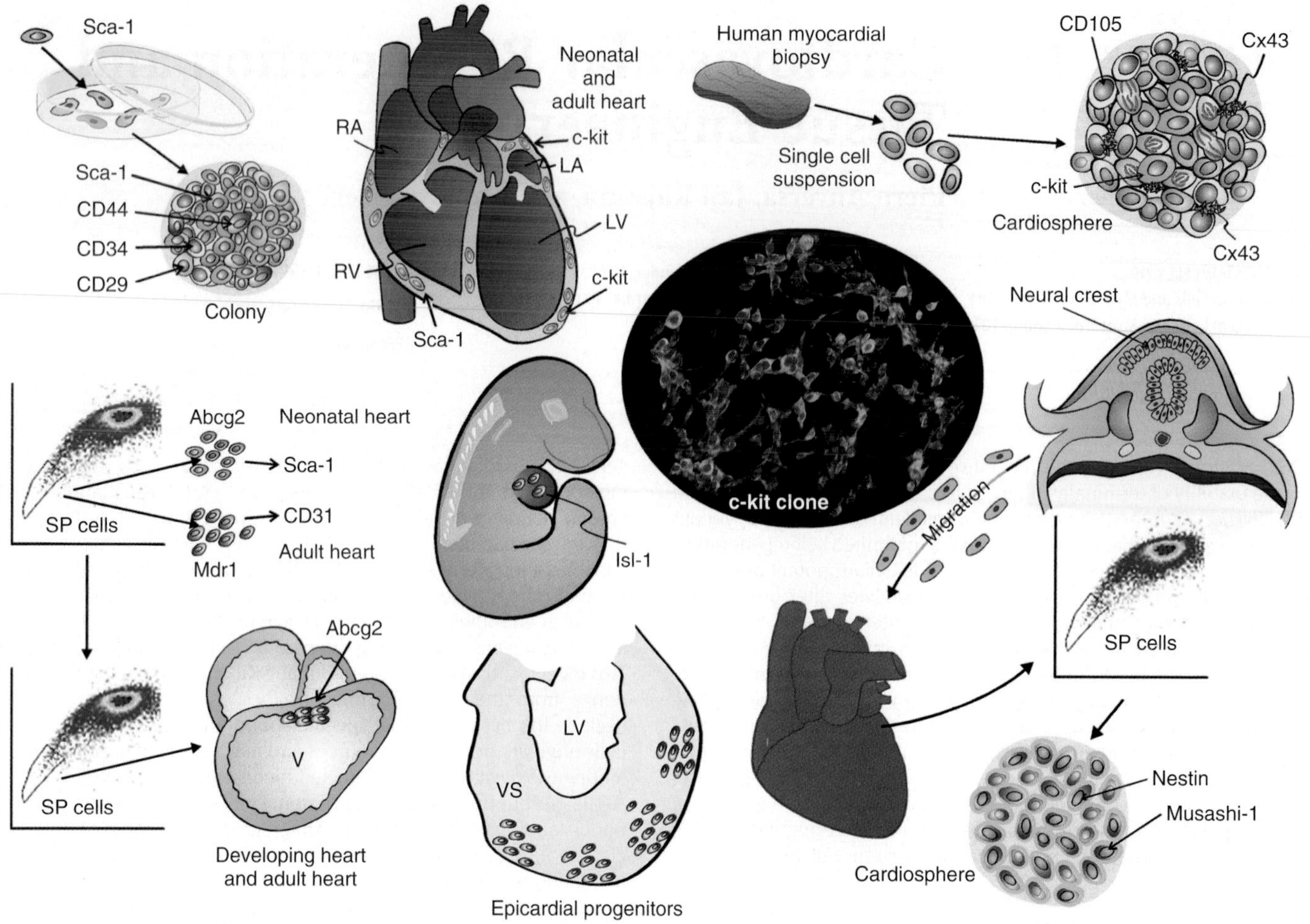

FIGURE 11-1 Cardiac progenitor cell classes. This scheme illustrates the CPC classes described so far: c-kit[7,8] *(Beltrami A, Barlucchi L, Torella D, et al: Cell 114:763, 2003)*, Sca-1 *(Oh H, Bradfute SB, Gallardo TD, et al: Proc Natl Acad Sci U S A 100:12313, 2003; Rosenblatt-Velin N, Lepore MG, Cartoni C, et al: J Clin Invest 115:1724, 2005; Oyama T, Nagai T, Wada H, et al: J Cell Biol 176:329, 2007)*, Isl-1 *(Laugwitz KL, Moretti A, Lam J, et al: Nature 433:647, 2005)*, and Musashi-1 *(Tomita Y, Matsumura K, Wakamatsu Y, et al: J Cell Biol 170:1135, 2005)*, positive cells, side population *(Martin CM, Meeson AP, Robertson SM, et al: Dev Biol 265:262, 2004; Pfister O, Mouquet F, Jain M, et al: Circ Res 97:52, 2005)*, cardiospheres *(Smith RR, Barile L, Cho HC, et al: Circulation 115:896, 2007)*, epicardial progenitors *(Limana F, Zacheo A, Mocini D, et al: Circ Res 101:1255, 2007; Cai CL, Martin JC, Sunet Y, et al: Nature 454:104, 2008; Zhou B, Ma Q, Rajagopal S, et al: Nature 454:109, 2008)*. LA = left atrium; LV = left ventricle; RA = right atrium; RV = right ventricle. *(Reproduced with permission from Leri A: Circulation 120:2515, 2009.)*

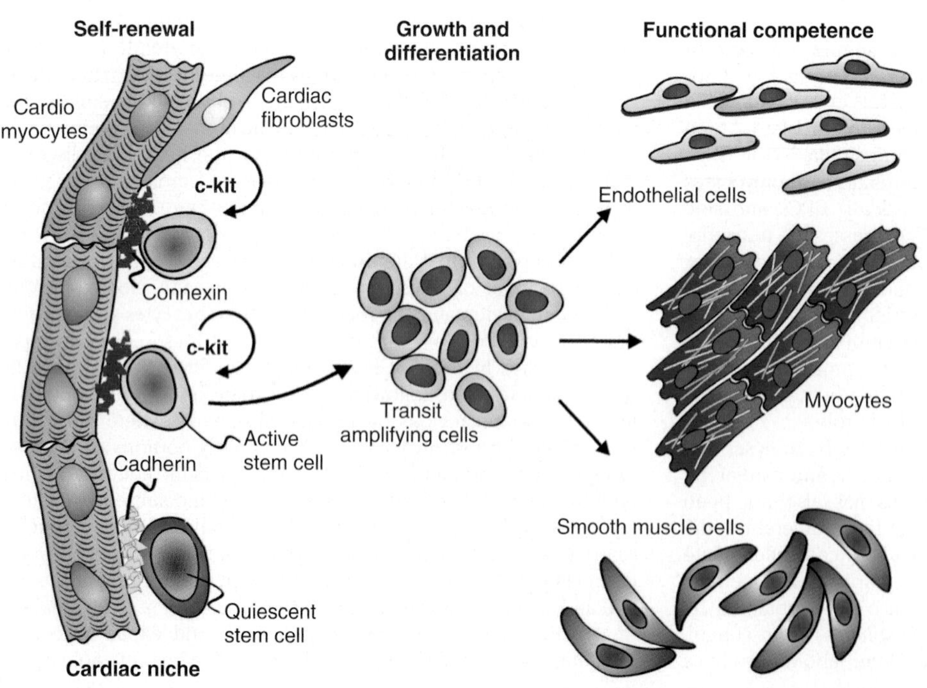

FIGURE 11-2 Hierarchy of CPC growth and differentiation. Cardiac niches contain quiescent stem cells that undergo asymmetric division, forming a daughter CPC (self-renewal) and a daughter-committed cell. Following activation, daughter-committed cells leave the niche area and give rise to rapidly proliferating transit-amplifying cells (growth and differentiation), which progress into fully mature myocytes, SMCs, and ECs (functional competence). CPCs in the niches are connected structurally and functionally to the supporting cells by gap and adherens junctions made by connexins and cadherins, respectively. Myocytes and fibroblasts act as supporting cells.

whereas in the presence of a relatively intact CPC pool, the administration of cytokines may be as effective as direct cell implantation.

Cardiac Stem Cells and Myocardial Repair

Experimental efforts with different classes of CPC have yielded consistent results with respect to myocardial regeneration.[1,3] In most cases, different degrees of myocardial regeneration, characterized by a combination of cardiomyocytes and coronary vessels, have been documented to occur in conjunction with improved cardiac function. Although these experimental findings have been encouraging, they have not yet achieved the objective of restoring the structural and functional integrity of the pathologically remodeled heart. In this regard, several important questions remain unanswered. At present, the classes of CPCs that are available for myocardial regeneration appear to lack the inherent ability to mature into adult cardiomyocytes or to form the vascular framework typical of the fully differentiated myocardium. Although only a small fraction of the CPC populations approaches the adult phenotype, these cells are electrically excitable and exhibit calcium transients that are characteristic of functionally competent myocytes that can contribute to improved ventricular performance (**Fig. 11-4**). Similarly, the capillary density of the newly formed tissue is significantly smaller than that of the mature organ, whereas the number of resistance arterioles markedly exceeds control values. Moreover, it is also not known whether the limited capillary growth is dictated by the size of the new cardiomyocytes, which are in close proximity to the formed capillaries, or by a defect in vasculogenesis at the capillary level. The need to define the developmental origin and molecular control of progenitor cell growth and differentiation in the embryonic, fetal, and early postnatal heart of transgenic mice is important for the identification of resident CPCs, as well as their potential role in the adult organ.[5,6] The early preclinical work with CPCs has led to interest in using these cells in clinical studies.[7-9]

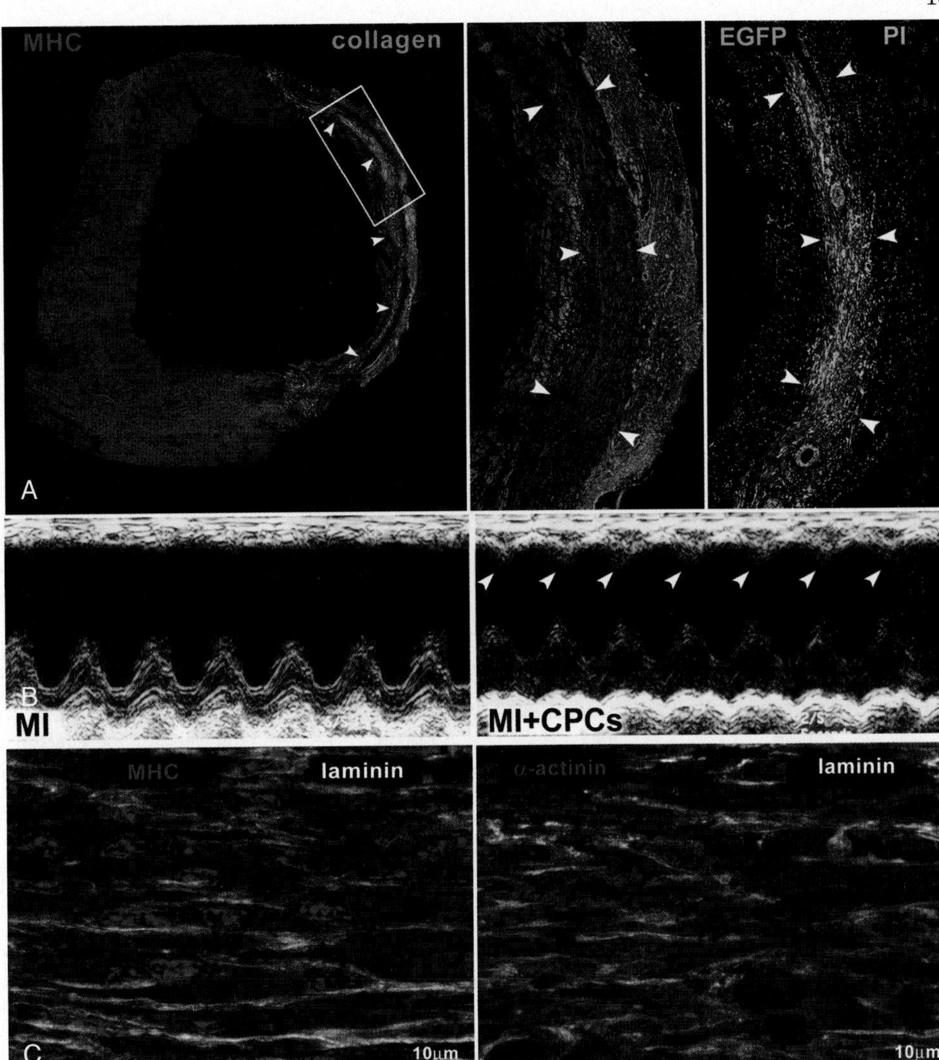

FIGURE 11-3 CPCs and myocardial regeneration. **A,** Enhanced green fluorescent protein (EGFP)–labeled CPCs were injected in the border zone of healed infarcts. Twenty days later, a band of regenerated myocytes developed within the scarred tissue. The area included in the rectangle is shown at higher magnification in the adjacent panels. Newly formed myocytes expressed myosin heavy chain (MHC, red; arrowheads) and EGFP (green) collagen (blue), propidium iodide (PI), (white). **B,** M-mode echocardiography. Note the reappearance of contraction (arrowheads) in infarcted hearts treated with CPCs (MI + CPCs). **C,** New myocytes generated by CPCs express MHC (red) and alpha-cardiac actinin (red). Laminin (white) defines the boundary of regenerated myocytes. *(From Rota M, Padin-Iruegas ME, Misao Y, et al: Local activation or implantation of cardiac progenitor cells rescues scarred infarcted myocardium improving cardiac function. Circ Res 103:107, 2008.)*

Cardiac Stem Cells and Myocardial Aging

As noted in Chap. 28, the prevalence of heart failure (HF) increases dramatically with aging.[10] The traditional view of aging is that the heart is a postmitotic organ characterized by a predetermined number of myocytes that are established at birth, and that are largely preserved throughout life until the death of the organism.[11] According to this, the generation of new myocytes only occurs in the fetal heart, and postnatal cardiac growth and organ hypertrophy in the adult only occur through myocyte enlargement. Based on this paradigm, the development of heart disease in older subjects has been considered to arise secondary to the loss of myocytes, which results from ischemic injury, hypertension, diabetes, and other disorders that foster cell death.

In recent years, our understanding of the biology of the adult and senescent heart in animals and humans has changed dramatically.[3,12] The recognition that CPCs reside in the heart and are capable of generating different cardiac cell lineages has provided the missing link between the identification of small dividing myocytes and the uncertainty concerning the origin of these repopulating cells. These studies have argued against the idea that all cardiomyocytes have the same age and that their age corresponds to the age of the organ and organism (see Fig. 11-e1 on website). These studies have further suggested that the turnover and growth of coronary vascular SMCs and ECs may be regulated by the commitment and differentiation of CPCs to a greater extent than the ability of these mature cells to reenter the cell cycle and divide. A recent study[13] took advantage of the incorporation of carbon-14, which was released during above-ground nuclear bomb tests, into genomic DNA of human cardiomyocytes to calculate rates of turnover in cardiac myocytes. Levels of carbon-14 in the atmosphere rose sharply as a result of nuclear testing and dropped precipitously once the Limited Nuclear Test Ban Treaty was signed in 1963. As a result, cells that were "born" during times of high carbon-14 levels were able to be dated precisely because subjects living during this period incorporated carbon-14 into the DNA of newly generated cardiomyocytes. This study showed that cardiomyocytes renew throughout life and that at age 25 years, 1% of myocytes turn over annually, whereas the turnover rate decreases to 0.45% at the age of 75. During an average lifespan, fewer than 50% of cardiomyocytes are renewed.

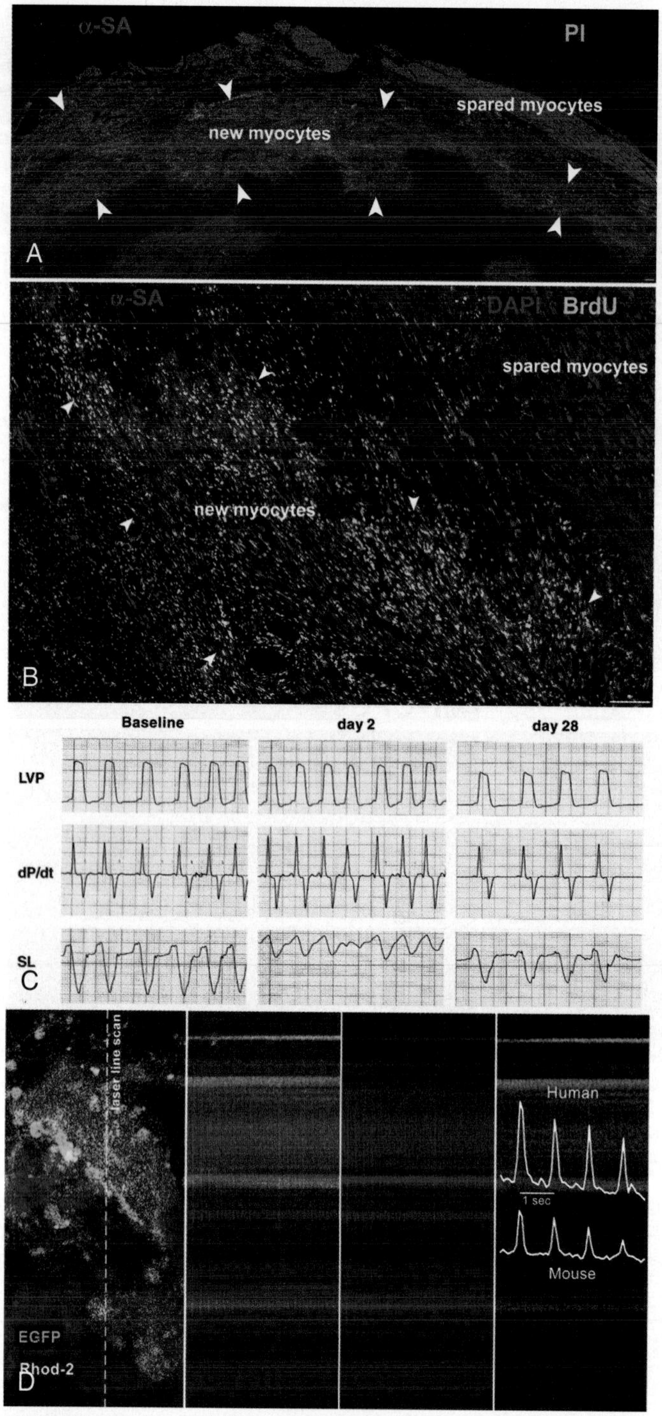

CH 11

FIGURE 11-4 Myocardial regeneration. **A-C,** IGF-1 and hepatocyte growth factor (HGF) were injected intramyocardially to activate resident CPCs acutely after infarction in dogs. **A,** Newly formed myocytes (alpha-sarcomeric actin [α-SA], red) are clustered together (arrowheads; PI, propidium iodide, green). **B,** Bright blue fluorescence in nuclei of regenerated myocytes corresponds to BrdU labeling. **C,** Myocardial contraction was measured by sonomicrometer crystals. Left panels, Baseline conditions before coronary artery occlusion. Central panels, Recordings at 2 days after infarction. Right panels, Recordings at 28 days after infarction. The loss of function and paradoxical motion at 2 days (bottom center) is followed by significant recovery of contraction at 28 days (bottom right). **D,** Human CPCs (hCPCs) labeled by EGFP were injected in the border zone of an acutely infarcted immunodeficient mouse. Two weeks later, calcium transient in EGFP-positive human myocytes (green) and EGFP-negative mouse myocytes were recorded by two-photon microscopy and laser line scan imaging (calcium indicator Rhod-2, red). The synchronicity in calcium tracings between these myocyte populations documents their functional integration. LVP = left ventricular pressure; SL = segment length. *(**A-C,** From Linke A, Müller P, Nurzynska D, et al: Stem cells in the dog heart are self-renewing, clonogenic, and multipotent and regenerate infarcted myocardium, improving cardiac function. Proc Natl Acad Sci U S A 102:89661, 2005; **D,** From Bearzi C, Rota M, Hosoda T, et al: Human cardiac stem cells. Proc Natl Acad Sci U S A 104:14068, 2007.)*

The critical question that needs to be addressed is whether the senescent heart develops, at least in part, because of the effects of aging on the number and/or function of progenitor cells. Both CPCs and myocytes in humans and animals undergo replicative senescence with severe telomere shortening, which fosters irreversible growth arrest and activation of cell death.[14] As senescent CPCs and poorly contracting hypertrophied myocytes accumulate, the pool of functionally competent CPCs is reduced and cardiac decompensation supervenes, leading to a senescent cardiac phenotype.[15,16] If aging does adversely affect the CPC compartment, exhausting its growth reserve, the possibility to implement cell therapy to overcome the myopathy would not be feasible, and alternative approaches will have to be developed. However, observations in humans and animals suggest that this is not the case, and that a small pool of CPCs expresses telomerase and possesses relatively long telomeres, suggesting that regeneration of cardiomyocytes and coronary vessels may be accomplished in the older heart. Activation of resident CPCs dramatically changes the structure and function of the senescent rat heart[16] and prolongs the lifespan in an animal model (**Fig. 11-5**). Whether the older human heart retains a restricted pool of relatively young CPCs that may be locally activated or expanded in vitro for subsequent delivery to the myocardium rescuing the aging myopathy remains an important unanswered question.

Cardiac Stem Cells and Gender

Epidemiologic studies have shown that women are less susceptible to cardiovascular disease, maintain preserved left ventricular function more effectively, and have a longer life expectancy than men.[10] These genetically determined differences delay the onset of the aging myopathy in women.[15,17] Myocyte death and myocyte formation are well balanced for a long time in the female heart, but not in the male heart (see Fig. 11-e2 on website). These factors have profound consequences with regard to the anatomy, structural composition, and performance of the heart. Alterations in cell turnover occur early in life in males, leading to the accumulation of older cells. Loss of CPCs, cellular aging, and a shift in the pattern of cell death from apoptosis to necrosis become apparent prematurely in the male myocardium, whereas the senescent heart phenotype develops only later in life in women. Cell necrosis alters the orderly organization of myocardial structure by promoting inflammation, fibroblast activation, and collagen deposition, dramatically affecting the growth reserve of the heart.

Studies have suggested that estrogen plays an important role in reducing the risks for cardiovascular diseases. Estrogen induces transcription of the catalytic subunit of the telomerase protein (TERT), because an estrogen response element is present in the TERT promoter.[18] Downstream effector pathways of the estrogen-estrogen receptor system involve the activation of the phosphatidylinositol 3-kinase (PI3K)/Akt cascade, which exerts multiple beneficial effects on cardiac function and biology. In human cells, estrogen activates PI3K/Akt signaling,[19] which in turn potentiates human telomerase activity through TERT phosphorylation.[18] Estrogens phosphorylate insulin-like growth factor 1 (IGF-1) receptors,[20] mimicking the effects of IGF-1, which is a powerful inducer of CPC division and survival.[4,16] The protein kinase Akt, a distal effector of IGF-1 activation, regulates a broad range of physiologic responses, including metabolism, gene transcription, and cell viability. Women possess higher levels of nuclear localized phospho-Akt in the myocardium[21] relative to comparably aged men (see Fig. 11-e3 on website). The female heart preserves its myocyte compartment up to approximately 90 years of age whereas the male heart loses 64×10^6 myocytes/year during adulthood and senescence.[17] Similarly, myocyte death occurs in heart failure but differs significantly in women and men.[22] The reduced incidence of myocyte death in women is apparent in spite of a longer duration of the heart failure. Familial hypertrophic cardiomyopathies are more detrimental in men than in women,[23] and the female heart remodels less in aortic stenosis. Thus, the female heart withstands cardiac injury better than the male heart. Whether this gender difference is dictated by a defective stem cell compartment that conditions senescence and death of cardiac cells at a significantly younger age in men than in women has not been established. If the female heart were to acquire a more robust cardiac stem cell compartment than the male heart, local factors within the female myocardium might have to be present to protect the CPC pool size during the process of aging in life.[24,25] Although cardiac myocytes can synthesize estrogen, it is not known whether CPCs can synthesize estrogen.[26] Estrogen protects the heart from myocyte apoptosis, fibroblast activation, and remodeling after infarction.[27] The formation of estrogen locally may enhance telomerase function in cardiac cells and phosphorylation of IGF-1 receptors in CPCs and myocytes, stimulating their growth, survival, and differentiation. Further details about gender-related differences in cardiac regeneration can be found in the online supplement on the website.

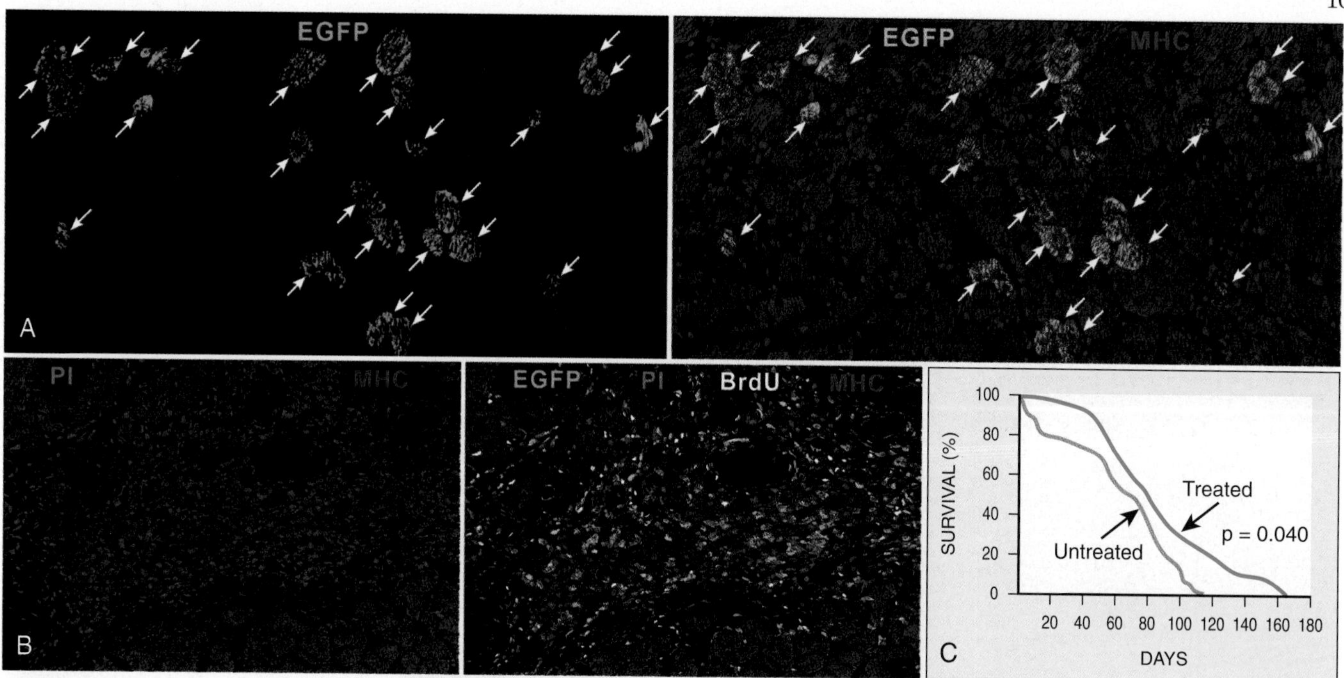

FIGURE 11-5 CPCs and the senescent heart. **A, B,** CPCs within atrial and apical niches of the rat heart were infected with a retrovirus carrying EGFP. IGF-1 and increasing concentrations of HGF were injected intramyocardially to induce the migration of CPCs from their sites of storage to areas of injury in the midregion of the left ventricle. Forty-five days later, newly formed EGFP-positive (green) cardiomyocytes (MHC, red; arrows) were scattered throughout the left ventricle in a 28- to 29-month-old rat **(A)**. A large area of myocardial damage **(B)** was replaced by BrdU-positive (white) regenerated myocytes in the heart of a rat ~29 months of age. **C,** Mortality in untreated (yellow line) and treated (blue line) animals at 27 months. Growth factor administration increased life expectancy at 27 months by 44%, from 57 to 82 days. *(From Gonzalez A, Rota M, Nurzynska D, et al: Activation of cardiac progenitor cells reverses the failing heart senescent phenotype and prolongs lifespan. Circ Res 102:597, 2008.)*

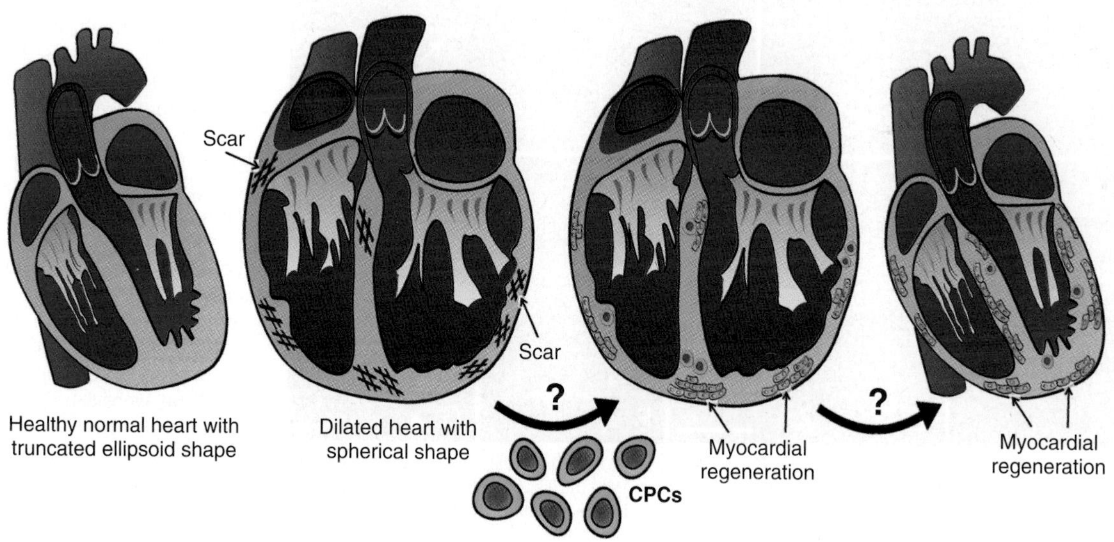

FIGURE 11-6 Ventricular remodeling and heart failure. Ventricular remodeling is coupled with progressive chamber dilation and thinning of the walls. The heart loses its truncated ellipsoid shape and assumes a more spherical configuration. Myocardial regeneration may reverse this process, transforming a dilated failing heart into a normal, functionally competent organ.

Cardiac Stem Cells and Myocardial Diseases

The prevalence of chronic HF has increased dramatically in recent years (see Chap. 28).[10] One potential role for cardiac stem cells in the advanced stages of heart failure would be to modulate endogenous CPCs to regenerate cardiac muscle and/or to create new blood vessel formation.[28] In theory, this would allow the chronically dilated failing heart to "reverse remodel" into a smaller, more elliptically shaped ventricle that is mechanically more efficient (**Fig. 11-6**). However, the observation that the failing heart has a limited capacity to regenerate itself has raised a number of important questions vis-à-vis cardiac stem cells. Although alterations in coronary perfusion, endothelial function, and myocyte mechanics have and will continue to represent the primary goal of the management of HF patients, the answers to these

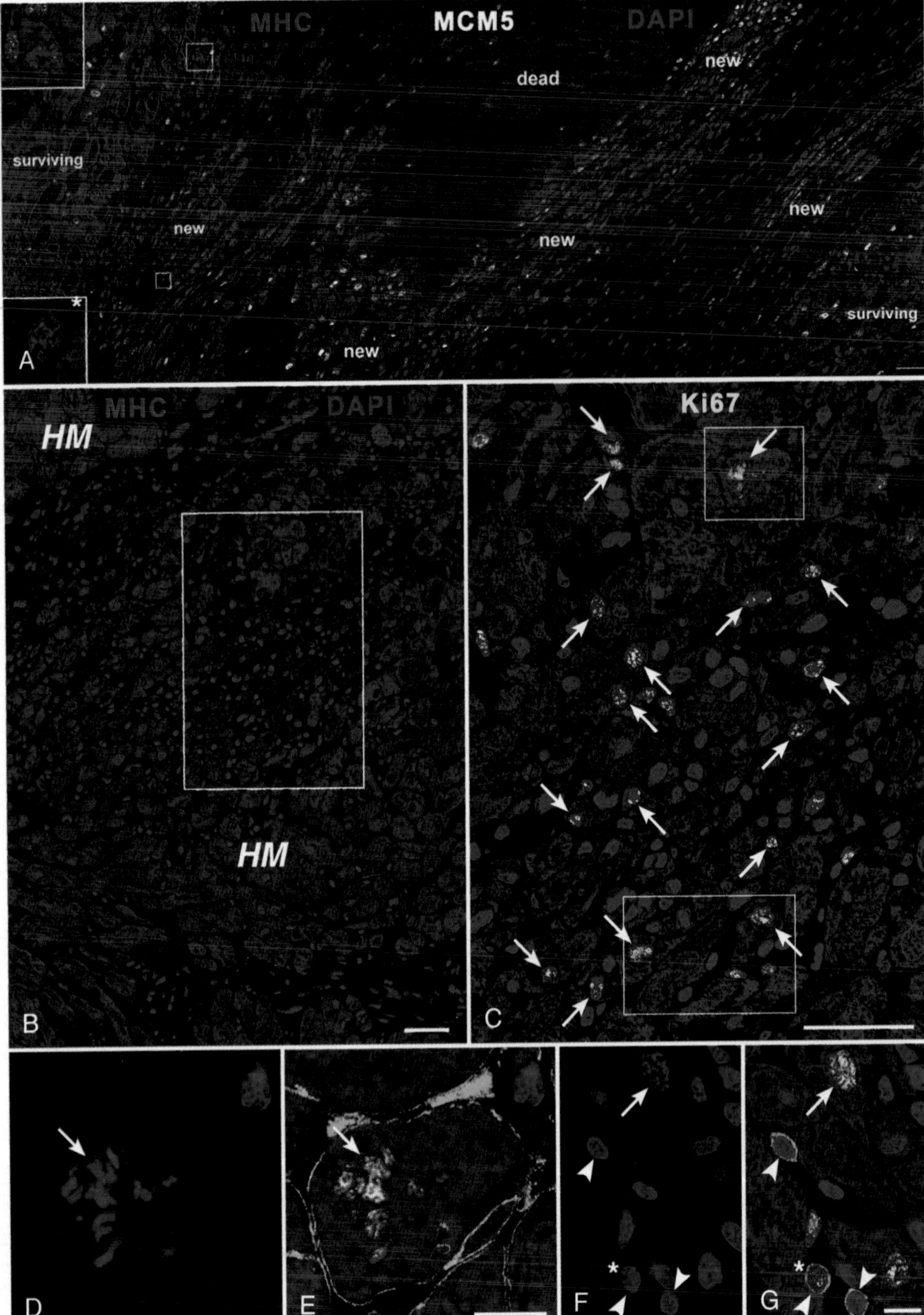

FIGURE 11-7 Myocardial regeneration in the human heart. **A,** Clusters of highly proliferating regenerated cardiomyocytes within the infarcted tissue. Myocytes are labeled by cardiac MHC (red) and nuclei by DAPI (blue). Most of these cells are positive for the cell cycle protein MCM5 (white). Two dividing small myocytes are shown in the insets**. B-G,** Intense myocardial growth in the hypertrophied heart of patients with chronic aortic stenosis. **B,** The rectangle delimits a low-power field containing a cluster of small poorly differentiated myocytes within the hypertrophied myocardium (HM). **C,** The area in the rectangle is illustrated at higher magnification; Ki67 (yellow) labels a large number of myocyte nuclei (arrows). **D-G,** The two small rectangles delimit areas shown at higher magnification. A mitotic nucleus with metaphase chromosomes (**D and E;** arrows) is positive for Ki67 (**E,** yellow) and the boundary of the cell is defined by laminin (**E,** green). Another mitotic nucleus (**F,** arrow) is labeled by Ki67 (**G,** yellow; arrow). c-Kit-positive CPCs (**G,** green; arrowheads) are near the mitotic myocyte. One shows Ki67 (**G,** yellow; asterisk). *(From Urbanek K, Quaini F, Tasca G, et al: Intense myocyte formation from cardiac stem cells in human cardiac hypertrophy. Proc Natl Acad Sci U S A 100:10440, 2003.)*

questions could lead to the development of new therapeutic strategies to treat the failing heart. Progress in this field will require new information about the optimization of cell type and cell preparation, as well as optimization of cell delivery modalities (see Chap. 33).

In contrast to myocardial regeneration in HF, multipotent CPCs undergo lineage commitment and form cardiac structures de novo following acute myocardial infarction.[29] However, the magnitude of the infarct may exceed the response of CPCs and tissue reconstitution such that cardiogenic shock supervenes. In spite of this negative outcome, the presence of small foci of spontaneous myocardial regeneration derived from the activation of endogenous progenitor cells has provided strong evidence in favor of the possibility that the infarcted tissue can be replaced partly by new cardiomyocytes and coronary vessels. Large clusters of newly formed cardiomyocytes have also been identified in human chronic aortic stenosis[30] (**Fig. 11-7**). However, the mechanism whereby new myocardium can be formed in a region with little or no blood supply and the unfavorable environment of the infarct is unclear. Opening of collateral vessels may provide enough oxygen for cell growth and function and explain the presence of viable CPCs within the infarct. Similarly, oxygen diffusion from the blood in the left ventricular chamber to the endomyocardium may preserve progenitor cells in the ischemic region. Alternatively, CPCs may migrate from the surviving myocardium to the infarct and differentiate into myocytes and coronary vasculature.

Although the CPC pool is enhanced acutely after infarction in humans, this compensatory growth response is attenuated in chronic HF, in which telomerase activity is decreased and CPC division is impaired by telomeric shortening, leading to irreversible growth arrest. Moreover, CPC apoptosis is increased, resulting in a decline of the number of functionally-competent CPCs. The duration of the cardiac disease, coupled with the compensatory long-term replicative growth of CPCs, may lead to telomere attrition, activation of the p53 and $p16^{INK4a}$ pathways and, ultimately, to the senescent cell phenotype (see Fig. 11-e4 on website). Therefore, the formation of myocytes and coronary vessels cannot counteract the chronic loss of parenchymal cells and vascular structures, suggesting that the negative balance between myocardial regeneration and death results in progressive ventricular dilation and deterioration of ventricular performance. Similar findings have been obtained in prolonged pressure overload hypertrophy[30] and in the decompensated aging myopathy.[15] Nevertheless, the recognition that the human heart possesses a stem cell compartment that, although compromised, is still present in end-stage failure points to a potentially important role of CPCs in cardiac repair in the failing heart. The residual functional CPCs may be isolated from myocardial biopsy samples and, following their growth in vitro, the expanded CPCs can be administrated back to the same patient. This therapeutic approach would offer the same advantages of autologous

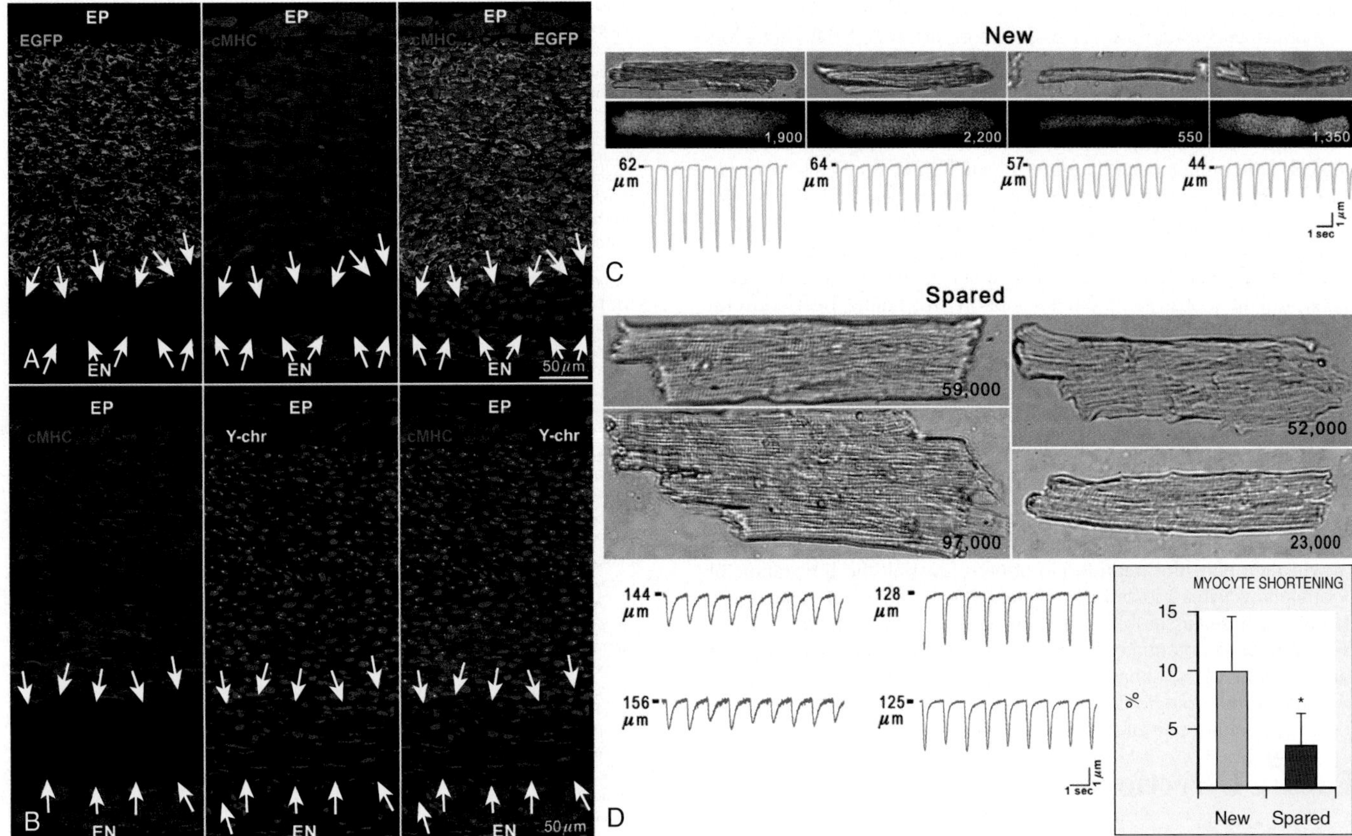

FIGURE 11-8 Bone marrow cells (BMCs) regenerate infarcted myocardium. **A, B,** Male BMCs from beta-actin EGFP mice injected in the border zone of acutely infarcted female hearts promoted myocardial regeneration. EGFP expression **(A)** and Y chromosome (**B,** Y-chr) localization in newly formed myocytes demonstrate that these cells originated from the delivered BMCs. **A,** EGFP (green), newly formed myocytes (MHC, red), and their merge. **B,** Regenerated myocytes (MHC, red), distribution of Y-chr (white dots), and their merge (arrows, nonregenerated infarct). **C,** BMCs from transgenic mice in which EGFP was under the control of the alpha-MHC promoter. At 30 days, newly formed EGFP-positive myocytes were electrically excitable. **D,** Spared myocytes had depressed fractional shortening. Values are mean ± SD. $P < 0.05$ versus new myocytes. EN = endocardium; EP = epicardium. *(From Rota M, Kajstura J, Hosoda T, et al: Bone marrow cells adopt the cardiomyogenic fate in vivo. Proc Natl Acad Sci U S A 104:17783, 2007.)*

cell transplantation. Preclinical studies have been completed and two phase I clinical trials, testing the safety of CPCs and cardiospheres, are in progress (see http://clinicaltrials.gov; Identifier: NCT00474461 and NCT00893360).

Exogenous Stem Cells

Exogenous progenitor stem cells comprise at least two different groups of cells, bone marrow–derived stem cells and a circulating pool of stem or progenitor cells, which at least in part are derived from the bone marrow. Bone marrow–derived stem cells are the best studied cells thus far, and have been used in most of the clinical trials in acute and chronic myocardial infarction and/or idiopathic dilated cardiomyopathy (see Chap. 33).[31-37] Bone marrow contains a complex assortment of progenitor cells, including hematopoietic stem cells (HSCs), the so-called side population cells (SP cells, defined by the expression of the Abcg2 transporter and allowing export of Hoechst dye), mesenchymal stem cells (MSCs) or stromal cells, and multipotential adult progenitor cells (MAPCs), a subset of MSCs. Bone marrow–derived endothelial progenitor cells (EPCs), mononuclear cells (MCs), CD34-positive cells, and MSCs have been tested in small and large animal models of cardiac injury, and have been used in a variety of clinical trials (see Chap. 33).[38-41] In general, these interventions have had a positive impact on outcomes in clinical trials, supporting the feasibility and safety of this therapeutic approach. However, the mechanism for the beneficial effects of HSCs is not at all clear, and the point of hypothesis that HSCs can regenerate infarcted myocardial tissue has been and continues to be controversial.[1,28,42] Several laboratories have shown experimentally that c-Kit–positive HSCs, EPCs, MCs, CD34-positive cells, and MSCs are capable of generating cardiomyocytes and coronary vessels after acute infarction. In most cases, a significant recovery of ventricular function has been reported, along with the formation of new vascular and nonvascular structures. Thus far, c-Kit–positive HSCs have produced the most striking experimental results[43-45] with respect to cardiac repair and restoration of ventricular performance (**Fig. 11-8**). Because of several technical issues, including the lack of a human grade monoclonal c-Kit antibody, this class of stem cells has not been used in clinical trials. The number of differentiated and functionally integrated myocytes derived from transplanted stem cells that has been observed in some studies is too small to explain the observed improvements in cardiac function, and several other mechanisms have been proposed for the beneficial effects of stem cells. One such suggestion is that improved cardiac function might be driven by paracrine mechanisms that lead to enhanced neovascularization, improved scar formation, and/or cytoprotection. In this regard, it should be noted that CPCs should be more effective than stem or progenitor cells from other organs, including the bone marrow and/or adipose tissue, in terms of regenerating new myocardium, insofar as CPCs are programmed to create heart muscle and, on activation, can rapidly generate parenchymal cells and coronary vessels. Further details about exogenous progenitor cells and cardiac regeneration can be found in the online supplement on the website.

Tissue Engineering

Regeneration of the infarcted heart, whether promoted by HSCs or CPCs, has only partly reconstituted necrotic myocardium. Moreover,

CH 11

the structural organization of the newly formed tissue resembles fetal-neonatal myocardium, with areas of more advanced differentiation. Furthermore, the newly generated myocardium lacks the complex architecture of cardiomyocyte bundles within the ventricular wall. These limitations may be overcome by the use of bioengineered scaffolds that can drive an orderly growth of myocytes and coronary vessels.[46] In contrast to cell therapy, in which individual cells integrate into the scar tissue, tissue engineering in its pure sense aims at providing tissue grafts. Larger constructs of heart muscle can be generated by using heart cell populations to form engineered heart tissue. So far, it has been challenging to generate tissue in vitro with contractile force and at a size sufficient to support the failing heart. Several culture conditions have been used in combination with cell mixtures (e.g., neonatal cardiomyocytes, fibroblasts, skeletal myoblasts, adult and embryonic stem cells) for creating myocardial tissue in vitro. Implantation of engineered rat heart tissue from neonatal rat cardiomyocyte in rats after myocardial infarction improved the contractile function and was shown to be electrically coupled to the native myocardium. Recently, self-assembling peptide hydrogels consisting of individual interwoven nanofibers that can be engineered to deliver specific proteins to the myocardium have been modified to tether growth factors to the peptide nanofibers, favoring the integration of neonatal myocytes and/or CPCs implanted with the tethered peptide.[47] In this study, self-assembling peptide nanofibers with tethered IGF-1 were shown to potentiate the action and differentiation of delivered and resident CPCs, enhancing cardiac repair after infarction. Thus, bioengineered biologic devices and CPCs may have to be combined for a successful repair of the injured heart.

Future Directions

In this chapter, we have reviewed the literature that supports the concept that the heart has an endogenous repair system that arises, at least in part, secondary to CPCs and circulating progenitor cells. Nonetheless, several fundamental areas of stem cell research have to be addressed for this field to move forward. One important question involves the determination of whether distinct classes of human stem cells influence the efficacy of cardiac repair. Another important question is whether the expression of a single stem cell antigen or a combination of epitopes in CPCs is linked to the formation of a preferential cardiac cell progeny. Similarly, the impact of age, gender, and type and duration of the heart failure on stem cell proliferation and lineage commitment needs to be better understood. Additionally, there is little understanding concerning the difference in the regeneration potential of primitive and partly committed CPCs. Furthermore, an apparent dichotomy exists between our incomplete knowledge of basic mechanisms that regulate stem cell growth, differentiation, and death and the number of patients who have been treated with cells of bone marrow origin. It is hoped that ongoing clinical trials (see Chap. 33) will address this important question.

REFERENCES

Cardiac Stem Cells

1. Anversa P, Leri A, Rota M, et al: Concise review: Stem cells, myocardial regeneration, and methodological artifacts. Stem Cells 25:589, 2007.
2. Bersell K, Arab S, Haring B, Kühn B: Neuregulin1/ErbB4 signaling induces cardiomyocyte proliferation and repair of heart injury. Cell 138:257, 2009.
3. Anversa P, Kajstura J, Leri A, Bolli R: Life and death of cardiac stem cells: A paradigm shift in cardiac biology. Circulation 113:1451, 2006.
4. Rota M, Padin-Iruegas ME, Misao Y, et al: Local activation or implantation of cardiac progenitor cells rescues scarred infarcted myocardium improving cardiac function. Circ Res 103:107, 2008.
5. Chien KR, Domian IJ, Parker KK: Cardiogenesis and the complex biology of regenerative cardiovascular medicine. Science 322:1494, 2008.
6. Parmacek MS, Epstein JA: Cardiomyocyte renewal. N Engl J Med 361:86, 2009.
7. Smith RR, Barile L, Cho HC, et al: Regenerative potential of cardiosphere-derived cells expanded from percutaneous endomyocardial biopsy specimens. Circulation 115:896, 2007.
8. Bearzi C, Rota M, Hosoda T, et al: Human cardiac stem cells. Proc Natl Acad Sci U S A 104:14068, 2007.
9. Bearzi C, Leri A, Lo Monaco F, et al: Identification of a coronary vascular progenitor cell in the human heart. Proc Natl Acad Sci U S A 106:15885, 2009.
10. Lloyd-Jones D, Adams R, Carnethon M, et al: Heart disease and stroke statistics—2009 update: A report from the American Heart Association Statistics Committee and Stroke Statistics Subcommittee. Circulation 119:e21, 2009.
11. Rubart M, Field LJ: Cardiac regeneration: Repopulating the heart. Annu Rev Physiol 68:29, 2006.
12. Anversa P, Rota M, Urbanek K, et al: Myocardial aging—a stem cell problem. Basic Res Cardiol 100:482, 2005.
13. Bergmann O, Bhardwaj RD, Bernard S, et al: Evidence for cardiomyocyte renewal in humans. Science 324:98, 2009.
14. Collado M, Blasco MA, Serrano M: Cellular senescence in cancer and aging. Cell 130:223, 2007.
15. Chimenti C, Kajstura J, Torella D, et al: Senescence and death of primitive cells and myocytes lead to premature cardiac aging and heart failure. Circ Res 93:604, 2003.
16. Gonzalez A, Rota M, Nurzynska D, et al: Activation of cardiac progenitor cells reverses the failing heart senescent phenotype and prolongs lifespan. Circ Res 102:597, 2008.
17. Olivetti G, Giordano G, Corradi D, et al: Gender differences and aging: effects on the human heart. J Am Coll Cardiol 26:1068, 1995.
18. Kimura A, Ohmichi M, Kawagoe J, et al: Induction of hTERT expression and phosphorylation by estrogen via Akt cascade in human ovarian cancer cell lines. Oncogene 23:4505, 2004.
19. Simoncini T, Hafezi-Moghadam A, Brazil DP, et al: Interaction of oestrogen receptor with the regulatory subunit of phosphatidylinositol-3-OH kinase. Nature 407:538, 2000.
20. Santen RJ, Fan P, Zhang Z, et al: Estrogen signals via an extra-nuclear pathway involving IGF-1R and EGFR in tamoxifen-sensitive and -resistant breast cancer cells. Steroids 74:586, 2009.
21. Camper-Kirby D, Welch S, Walker A, et al: Myocardial Akt activation and gender: Increased nuclear activity in females versus males. Circ Res 88:1020, 2001.
22. Guerra S, Leri A, Wang X, et al: Myocyte death in the failing human heart is gender dependent. Circ Res 85:856, 1999.
23. Stefanelli CB, Rosenthal A, Borisov AB, et al: Novel troponin T mutation in familial dilated cardiomyopathy with gender-dependent severity. Mol Genet Metab 83:188, 2004.
24. Ordovas JM: Gender, a significant factor in the cross talk between genes, environment, and health. Gend Med S111, 2007.
25. Kudlow BA, Kennedy BK, Monnat RJ Jr: Werner and Hutchinson-Gilford progeria syndromes: mechanistic basis of human progeroid diseases. Nat Rev Mol Cell Biol 8:394-404, 2007.
26. Grohé C, Kahlert S, Löbbert K, Vetter H: Expression of oestrogen receptor alpha and beta in rat heart: Role of local oestrogen synthesis. J Endocrinol 156:R1, 1998.
27. Donaldson C, Eder S, Baker C, et al: Estrogen attenuates left ventricular and cardiomyocyte hypertrophy by an estrogen receptor-dependent pathway that increases calcineurin degradation. Circ Res 104:265, 2009.
28. Leri A, Kajstura J, Anversa P: Cardiac stem cells and mechanisms of myocardial regeneration. Physiol Rev 85:1373, 2005.
29. Urbanek K, Torella D, Sheikh F, et al: Myocardial regeneration by activation of multipotent cardiac stem cells in ischemic heart failure. Proc Natl Acad Sci U S A 102:8692, 2005.
30. Urbanek K, Quaini F, Tasca G, et al: Intense myocyte formation from cardiac stem cells in human cardiac hypertrophy. Proc Natl Acad Sci U S A 100:10440, 2003.

Exogenous Stem Cells and Tissue Engineering

31. Wollert KC, Meyer GP, Lotz J, et al: Intracoronary autologous bone-marrow cell transfer after myocardial infarction: the BOOST randomised controlled clinical trial. Lancet 364:141, 2004.
32. Assmus B, Honold J, Schächinger V, et al: Transcoronary transplantation of progenitor cells after myocardial infarction. N Engl J Med 355:1222, 2006.
33. Schächinger V, Erbs S, Elsässer A, et al; REPAIR-AMI Investigators: Intracoronary bone marrow-derived progenitor cells in acute myocardial infarction. N Engl J Med 355:1210, 2006.
34. Lunde K, Solheim S, Aakhus S, et al: Intracoronary injection of mononuclear bone marrow cells in acute myocardial infarction. N Engl J Med 355:1199, 2006.
35. Meyer GP, Wollert KC, Lotz J, et al: Intracoronary bone marrow cell transfer after myocardial infarction: Eighteen months' follow-up data from the randomized, controlled BOOST (BOne marrOw transfer to enhance ST-elevation infarct regeneration) trial. Circulation 113:1287, 2006.
36. Yousef M, Schannwell CM, Köstering M, et al: The BALANCE Study: Clinical benefit and long-term outcome after intracoronary autologous bone marrow cell transplantation in patients with acute myocardial infarction. J Am Coll Cardiol 53:2262, 2009.
37. Fischer-Rasokat U, Assmus B, Seeger FH, et al: A pilot trial to assess potential effects of selective intracoronary bone marrow-derived progenitor cell infusion in patients with non-ischemic dilated cardiomyopathy: Final 1-year results of the TOPCARE-DCM trial. Circ Heart Fail 118:1425, 2009.
38. Perin EC, Dohmann HF, Borojevic R, et al: Improved exercise capacity and ischemia 6 and 12 months after transendocardial injection of autologous bone marrow mononuclear cells for ischemic cardiomyopathy. Circulation 110:II213, 2004.
39. Amado LC, Schuleri KH, Saliaris AP, et al: Multimodality noninvasive imaging demonstrates in vivo cardiac regeneration after mesenchymal stem cell therapy. J Am Coll Cardiol 48:2116, 2006.
40. Kawamoto A, Iwasaki H, Kusano K, et al: CD34-positive cells exhibit increased potency and safety for therapeutic neovascularization after myocardial infarction compared with total mononuclear cells. Circulation 114:2163, 2006.
41. Losordo DW, Schatz RA, White CJ, et al: Intramyocardial transplantation of autologous CD34+ stem cells for intractable angina: A phase I/IIa double-blind, randomized controlled trial. Circulation 115:3165, 2007.
42. Laflamme MA, Murry CE: Regenerating the heart. Nat Biotechnol 23:845, 2005.
43. Orlic D, Kajstura J, Chimenti S, et al: Bone marrow cells regenerate infarcted myocardium. Nature 410:701, 2001.
44. Kajstura J, Rota M, Whang B, et al: Bone marrow cells differentiate in cardiac cell lineages after infarction independently of cell fusion. Circ Res 96:127, 2005.
45. Rota M, Kajstura J, Hosoda T, et al: Bone marrow cells adopt the cardiomyogenic fate in vivo. Proc Natl Acad Sci U S A 104:17783, 2007.
46. Segers VF, Lee RT: Stem-cell therapy for cardiac disease. Nature 451:937, 2008.
47. Padin-Iruegas ME, Misao Y, Davis ME, et al: Cardiac progenitor cells and biotinylated insulin-like growth factor-1 nanofibers improve endogenous and exogenous myocardial regeneration after infarction. Circulation 120:876, 2009.

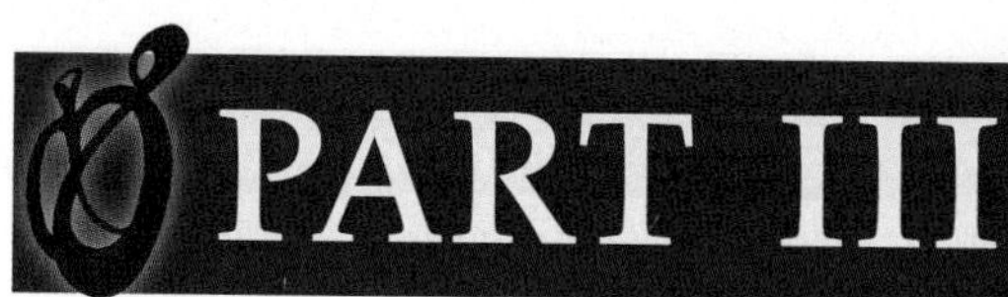

PART III

EVALUATION OF THE PATIENT

CHAPTER 12 The History and Physical Examination: An Evidence-Based Approach

James C. Fang and Patrick T. O'Gara

The approach to the patient with known or suspected cardiovascular disease begins with a directed history and targeted physical examination, the scope of which depends on the clinical context at the time of presentation. Elective ambulatory encounters allow comparatively more time for the development of a comprehensive assessment, whereas emergency department visits and urgent bedside consultations require a more focused strategy. The elicitation of the history should not be delegated to a trainee or other health care provider. The history often provides clues linking seemingly disparate aspects of the patient's presentation. It helps to assess the patient's personal attitudes—his or her intelligence, comprehension, acceptance, denial, motivation, fear, and prejudices. Insight of this nature allows a more informed approach to shared treatment decisions. The interview can reveal genetic influences and the impact of other medical conditions on the manifesting illness. Although time constraints challenge careful history taking,[1] concerns regarding health care costs, driven in part by premature medical imaging, may reverse this trend.

Declining physical examination skills have raised great concerns. Only a minority of internal medicine and family practice residents recognize classic cardiac findings. Performance does not predictably improve with experience.[2] Lessened bedside skills have increased the unnecessary use of noninvasive imaging.

The use of handheld cardiac ultrasound devices may characterize chamber size, ventricular function, and valve performance more reliably than the physical examination.[3,4] Nevertheless, the history and physical examination remain desirable and cost-effective. Educational efforts, including repetition, patient-centered teaching conferences, and visual display feedback of auscultatory and Doppler echocardiographic findings, should help improve competence.[5-7]

The evidence base that justifies correlations between the history and physical examination and cardiovascular disease has been established most rigorously for heart failure, valvular heart disease, and coronary artery disease. Vital signs, pulmonary congestion, and mitral regurgitation (MR) contribute importantly to bedside assessment in the patient with an acute coronary syndrome (ACS).[8,9] The physical examination informs clinical decision making in real time and should guide therapy before biomarker results are available. Accurate auscultation provides important insight into many valvular and congenital heart lesions.[10] This chapter aims to review the fundamentals of the cardiovascular history and physical examination in light of the evidence base from correlative studies. See earlier editions of this text for further detail.

History

The major symptoms associated with cardiac disease include chest discomfort, dyspnea, fatigue, edema, palpitations, and syncope. Cough, hemoptysis, and cyanosis are additional examples. Claudication, limb pain, edema, and skin discoloration can indicate a vascular disorder. The differential diagnosis of chest discomfort can be narrowed by careful attention to its location, radiation, triggers, mode of onset, duration, alleviating factors, and associated symptoms (see Chap. 53).

Angina pectoris must be distinguished from the pain associated with pulmonary embolism, pericarditis, aortic dissection, esophageal reflux, and costochondritis. Although a history of chest discomfort alone does not suffice to render a diagnosis of ACS, several aspects of the presenting symptom increase or decrease the likelihood of ACS. For example, pain that is sharp (likelihood ratio [LR], 0.3; 95% confidence interval [CI], 0.2 to 0.5), pleuritic (LR, 0.2; 95% CI, 0.1 to 0.3), positional (LR, 0.3; 95% CI, 0.2 to 0.5), or reproducible with palpation (LR, 0.3; 95% CI, 0.2 to 0.4) is usually noncardiac, whereas discomfort that radiates to both arms or shoulders (LR, 4.1; 95% CI, 2.5 to 6.5) or is precipitated by exertion (LR, 2.4; 95% CI, 1.5 to 3.8) increases the likelihood of ACS.[11] Less classic symptoms (anginal equivalents) such as indigestion, belching, and dyspnea should also command the clinician's attention when other features of the presentation suggest ACS, even in the absence of chest discomfort. Less typical presentations are more common in women, older patients, and patients with diabetes. Dyspnea may occur with exertion, recumbency (orthopnea), or even with standing (platypnea). Paroxysmal nocturnal dyspnea of cardiac origin usually occurs 2 to 4 hours after the onset of sleep, compels the patient to sit upright or stand, and subsides gradually over several minutes. The patient's partner should be questioned about any signs of sleep-disordered breathing, such as loud snoring and/or periods of apnea. Pulmonary embolism often causes dyspnea of sudden onset. Patients may use a variety of terms to describe their awareness of the heartbeat (palpitations), such as *flutters*, *skips*, or *pounding*. The likelihood of a cardiac arrhythmia is modestly increased with a known history of cardiac disease (LR, 2.03; 95% CI, 1.33 to 3.11) and decreased when symptoms resolve within 5 minutes (LR, 0.38; 95% CI, 0.22 to 0.63) or in the presence of panic disorder (LR, 0.26; 95% CI, 0.07 to 1.01).[12] A report of a regular, rapid-pounding sensation in the neck (LR, 1.77; 95% CI, 25 to 1251) or visible neck pulsations associated with

TABLE 12-1 Comparison of Three Methods of Assessing Cardiovascular Disability

CLASS	NYHA FUNCTIONAL CLASSIFICATION	CCS FUNCTIONAL CLASSIFICATION	SPECIFIC ACTIVITY SCALE
I	Patients with cardiac disease but without resulting limitations of physical activity. Ordinary physical activity does not cause undue fatigue, palpitation, dyspnea, or anginal pain.	Ordinary physical activity, such as walking and climbing stairs, does not cause angina. Angina occurs with strenuous or rapid or prolonged exertion at work or recreation.	Patients can perform to completion any activity requiring >7 metabolic equivalents (METs; e.g., can carry 24 lb up eight steps; carry objects that weigh 80 lb; do outdoor work [shovel snow, spade soil]; do recreational activities [skiing, basketball, squash, handball, jog/walk 5 mph]).
II	Patients with cardiac disease resulting in slight limitation of physical activity. They are comfortable at rest. Ordinary physical activity results in fatigue, palpitation, dyspnea, or angina pain.	Slight limitation of ordinary activity. Walking or climbing stairs rapidly, walking uphill, walking or stair climbing after meals, in cold, in wind, or when under emotional stress, or only during the few hours after awakening. Walking more than two blocks on the level and climbing more than one flight of ordinary stairs at a normal pace and in normal conditions.	Patients can perform to completion any activity requiring >5 METs (e.g., have sexual intercourse without stopping, garden, rake, weed, roller skate, dance fox trot, walk at 4 mph on level ground), but cannot and do not perform to completion activities requiring ≥7 METs.
III	Patients with cardiac disease resulting in marked limitation of physical activity. They are comfortable at rest. Less than ordinary physical activity causes fatigue, palpitation, dyspnea, or anginal pain.	Marked limitation of ordinary physical activity. Walking one to two blocks on the level and climbing more than one flight in normal conditions.	Patients can perform to completion any activity requiring >2 METs (e.g., shower without stopping, strip and make bed, clean windows, walk 2.5 mph, bowl, play golf, dress without stopping), but cannot and do not perform to completion any activities requiring ≥5 METs.
IV	Patients with cardiac disease resulting in inability to carry on any physical activity without discomfort. Symptoms of cardiac insufficiency or of the anginal syndrome may be present even at rest. If any physical activity is undertaken, discomfort is increased.	Inability to carry on any physical activity without discomfort—anginal syndrome may be present at rest.	Patients cannot or do not perform to completion activities requiring ≥2 METs. Cannot carry out activities listed above (Specific Activity Scale, Class III).

From Goldman L, Hashimoto B, Cook EF, Loscalzo A: Comparative reproducibility and validity of systems for assessing cardiovascular functional class: advantages of a new specific activity scale. Circulation 64:1227, 1981.

palpitations (LR, 2.68; 95% CI, 1.25 to 5.78) increases the likelihood that atrioventricular nodal reentrant tachycardia (AVNRT) is the responsible arrhythmia. The absence of a regular, rapid-pounding sensation in the neck makes detecting AVNRT much less likely (LR, 0.07; 95% CI, 0.03 to 0.19).[12] Cardiac syncope occurs suddenly and restoration of consciousness occurs quickly. Patients with neurocardiogenic syncope may have an early warning (nausea, yawning), appear ashen and diaphoretic, and revive more slowly, albeit without signs of seizure or a prolonged postictal state. The complete history requires information pertaining to traditional cardiovascular risk factors, a general medical history, occupation, social habits, medications, drug allergies or intolerance, family history, and systems review.

It is extremely important to obtain a semiquantitative assessment of symptom severity and to document any change over time. The New York Heart Association (NYHA) and Canadian Cardiovascular Society (CCS) functional classification systems have served for decades and remain useful for patient care and clinical research, despite their inherent limitations (**Table 12-1**).[13,14]

Physical Examination

The physical examination can help determine the cause of a given symptom, assess disease severity and progression, and evaluate the impact of specific therapies.

General Appearance

The examination begins with an appreciation of the general appearance of the patient, including his or her age, posture, demeanor, and general health status. Is the patient in pain, resting quietly, or visibly diaphoretic with a foreboding sense of doom? Diaphoresis is not volitional and implies serious disease. Does the patient choose to avoid certain positions to reduce or eliminate pain? The pain of acute pericarditis, for example, is often minimized by sitting up, leaning forward, and breathing shallowly. The respiratory pattern is also important. Pursing of the lips, a breathy quality to the voice, and an increased anteroposterior chest diameter would favor a pulmonary rather than cardiovascular cause of dyspnea. Pallor suggests that anemia may contribute to exercise intolerance or dyspnea. Certain congenital syndromes may be apparent from the patient's general appearance (see Chaps. 8 and 65). Emaciation suggests chronic heart failure or another systemic disorder (e.g., malignancy, infection). The vital signs, including height, weight, temperature, pulse rate, blood pressure (both arms), respiratory rate, and peripheral oxygen saturation, can guide diagnosis and management. The height and weight permit the calculation of body mass index (BMI) and body surface area (BSA). Waist circumference (measured at the iliac crest) and waist-to-hip ratio (using the widest circumference around the buttocks) assess central obesity and are predictors of long-term cardiovascular risk.[15,16] In patients with palpitations, a resting heart rate less than 60 beats/min may indicate a clinically significant arrhythmia (LR, 3.00; 95% CI, 1.27 to 7.08).[12] Mental status should be assessed. The observation of respiration during sleep may reveal signs of disordered breathing (e.g., Cheyne-Stokes respiration, obstructive sleep apnea).

SKIN. Central cyanosis is present with significant right-to-left shunting at the level of the heart or lungs, which allows deoxygenated blood to reach the systemic circulation. It is also a feature of hereditary methemoglobinemia. Peripheral or acrocyanosis of the fingers, toes, nose, and ears reflects reduced blood flow because of small vessel constriction seen in severe heart failure, shock, or peripheral vascular disease. Differential cyanosis affecting the lower but not the upper extremities occurs with a patent ductus arteriosus (PDA) and pulmonary artery (PA) hypertension with right-to-left shunting at the great vessel level. Hereditary telangiectases on the lips, tongue, and mucous membranes (Osler-Weber-Rendu syndrome) resemble spider nevi and, when in the lungs, can cause right-to-left shunting and central cyanosis. Scleroderma can also cause telangiectasias. Tanned or bronze discoloration of the skin in unexposed areas can suggest iron overload and hemochromatosis. Jaundice, often first evident in the sclerae, has a broad differential diagnosis. Ecchymoses are often present with warfarin, aspirin, and/or thienopyridine use, whereas petechiae are a feature of thrombocytopenia, and purpuric skin lesions can be seen with endocarditis and other causes of leukocytoclastic vasculitis. Various lipid disorders can manifest with xanthomas, subcutaneously, along tendon sheaths, or over the extensor surfaces of the extremities. Xanthoma within the palmar creases is specific for type III hyperlipoproteinemia (pre-beta, intermediate density). The leathery, cobblestone, plucked-chicken appearance of the skin in the axilla and skin folds of a young person is highly characteristic for pseudoxanthoma elasticum, a disease with multiple cardiovascular manifestations, including premature atherosclerosis.[17] Extensive lentiginoses (freckle-like brown macules and café-au-lait spots over the trunk and neck) may be part of developmental delay cardiovascular syndromes (e.g., LEOPARD, LAMB, Carney) with multiple atrial myxomas, atrial septal defect (ASD), hypertrophic cardiomyopathy, and valvular stenoses (see Chap. 8). In a patient with heart failure or syncope, cardiovascular sarcoid should be suspected by the presence of lupus pernio, erythema nodosum, or granuloma annulare.

HEAD AND NECK. The dentition should always be assessed as a source of infection and an index of general health and hygiene. A high-arched palate suggests Marfan syndrome and other connective tissue disease syndromes. A large protruding tongue with parotid enlargement may suggest amyloidosis. A bifid uvula has been described in patients with Loeys-Dietz syndrome. Orange tonsils are characteristic of Tangier disease. Ptosis and ophthalmoplegia suggest muscular dystrophies, and congenital heart disease is often accompanied by hypertelorism, low-set ears, micrognathia, and a webbed neck, as with Noonan, Turner, and Down syndromes. Proptosis, lid lag, and stare denote Graves' hyperthyroidism. Blue sclerae, mitral or aortic regurgitation (AR), and a history of recurrent nontraumatic skeletal fractures are observed in patients with osteogenesis imperfecta. Premature arcus senilis may be associated with hyperlipidemia.

The funduscopic examination is underused in the evaluation of patients with hypertension, atherosclerosis, diabetes, endocarditis, neurologic symptoms, or known carotid or aortic arch disease. Lacrimal hyperplasia sometimes occurs in sarcoidosis. The mitral facies of rheumatic mitral stenosis (pink, purplish patches with telangiectasias over the malar eminences) can also accompany other disorders associated with pulmonary hypertension and reduced cardiac output. Palpation of the thyroid gland assesses its size, symmetry, and consistency.

EXTREMITIES. The temperature of the extremities, presence of clubbing, arachnodactyly, and nail findings can be quickly surmised, often while talking to the patient. Clubbing implies the presence of central shunting (**Fig. 12-1**). The unapposable "fingerized" thumb occurs in Holt-Oram syndrome. Arachnodactyly characterizes the Marfan syndrome. Janeway lesions (nontender, slightly raised hemorrhages on the palms and soles), Osler's nodes (tender, raised nodules on the pads of the fingers or toes), and splinter hemorrhages (linear petechiae in the middle of the nail bed) may occur in endocarditis.

Lower extremity or presacral edema with elevated jugular venous pressure occurs in many volume-overloaded states, including heart failure. A normal jugular venous pressure with additional signs of venous disease, such as extensive varicosities, medial ulcers, or brownish pigmentation from hemosiderin deposition, suggests chronic venous insufficiency. Edema also can complicate dihydropyridine calcium channel blocker therapy. Anasarca is rare in heart failure unless long-standing, untreated, and accompanied by hypoalbuminemia. Asymmetrical swelling can reflect local or unilateral venous thrombosis, lymphatic obstruction, or the sequelae of previous vein graft harvesting. Homan's

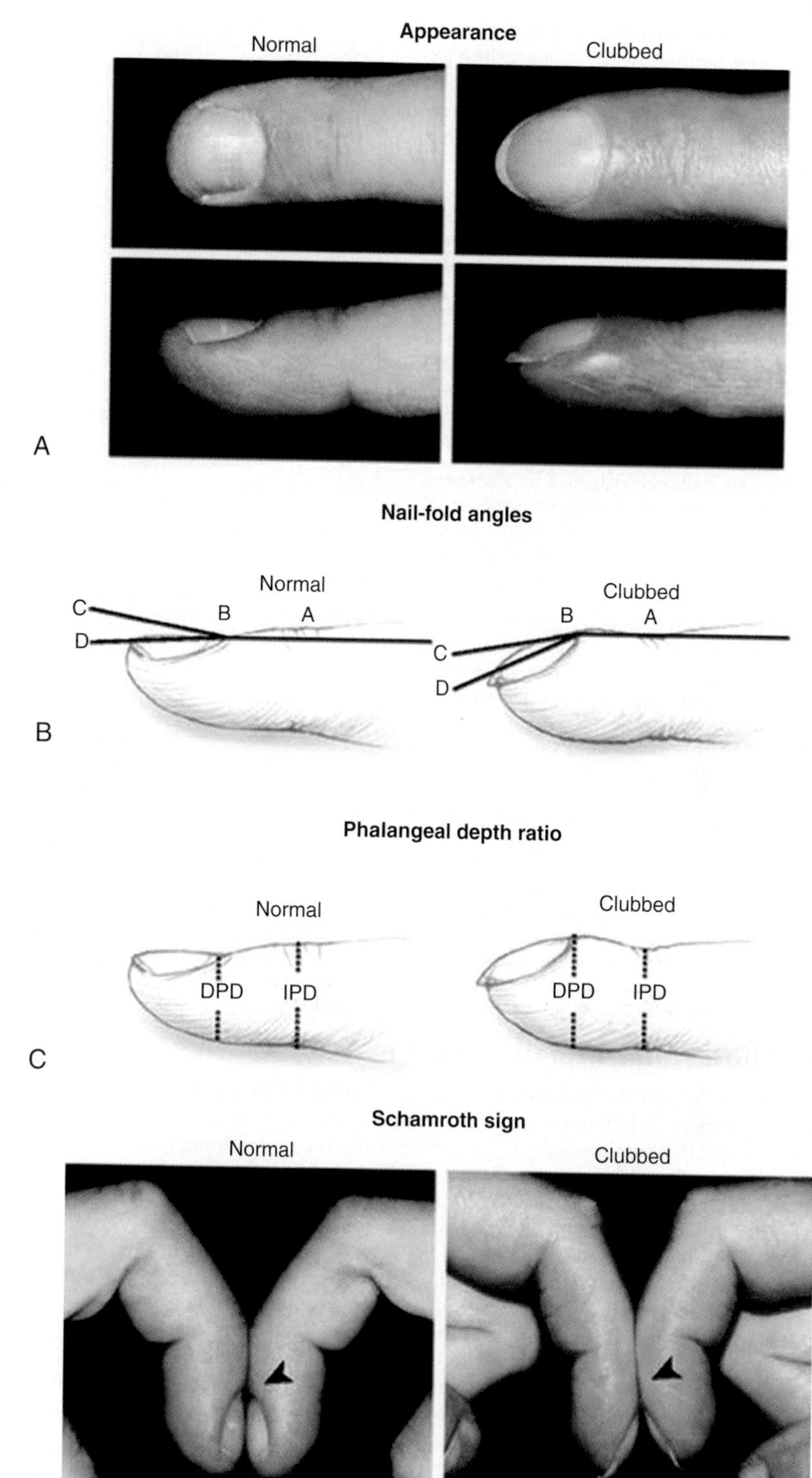

FIGURE 12-1 **A,** Normal finger viewed from above and in profile, and the changes occurring in established clubbing, viewed from above and in profile. **B,** The finger on the left demonstrates normal profile (ABC) and normal hyponychial (ABD) nail fold angles of 169 and 183 degrees, respectively. The clubbed finger on the right shows increased profile and hyponychial nail fold angles of 191 and 203 degrees, respectively. **C,** Distal phalangeal finger depth (DPD)–interphalangeal finger depth (IPD) represents the phalangeal depth ratio. In normal fingers, the IPD is greater than the DPD. In clubbing, this relationship is reversed. **D,** Schamroth sign. In the absence of clubbing, nail to nail opposition of the index fingers creates a diamond-shaped window (arrowhead). In clubbed fingers, the loss of the profile angle caused by the increase in tissue at the nail bed causes obliteration of this space (arrowhead). *(From Myers KA, Farquhar DR: Does this patient have clubbing? JAMA 286:341, 2001.)*

sign (calf pain on forceful dorsiflexion of the foot) is neither specific nor sensitive for deep venous thrombosis. Muscular atrophy and absent hair in an extremity should suggest chronic arterial insufficiency or a neuromuscular disorder.

Chest and Abdomen. Cutaneous venous collaterals over the anterior chest suggest obstruction of the superior vena cava or subclavian vein, especially in the presence of indwelling catheters or leads. Asymmetric breast enlargement unilateral to an implanted device may also be present. Thoracic cage abnormalities, such as pectus carinatum (pigeon chest) or pectus excavatum (funnel chest), may accompany connective tissue disorders; the barrel chest of emphysema or advanced kyphoscoliosis may be associated with cor pulmonale. The severe kyphosis of ankylosing spondylitis should prompt careful auscultation for AR. The straight back syndrome (loss of normal kyphosis of the thoracic spine) can accompany mitral valve prolapse (MVP). Cyanotic congenital heart disease may result in asymmetry of the chest wall, with the left hemithorax displaced anteriorly. A thrill may be present over well-developed intercostal artery collaterals in patients with aortic coarctation.

The cardiac impulse may be prominent in the epigastrium in patients with emphysema or substantial obesity. The liver is often enlarged and tender in heart failure; systolic hepatic pulsations signify severe tricuspid regurgitation (TR). Patients with infective endocarditis may have splenomegaly. Ascites can occur with advanced and chronic right heart failure or constrictive pericarditis. The aorta may normally be palpated between the epigastrium and umbilicus in thin patients and children. The sensitivity of palpation for the detection of abdominal aortic aneurysm (AAA) disease increases as a function of aneurysm diameter and varies according to body size. Palpation alone cannot establish this diagnosis in most patients. Arterial bruits in the abdomen should be noted.

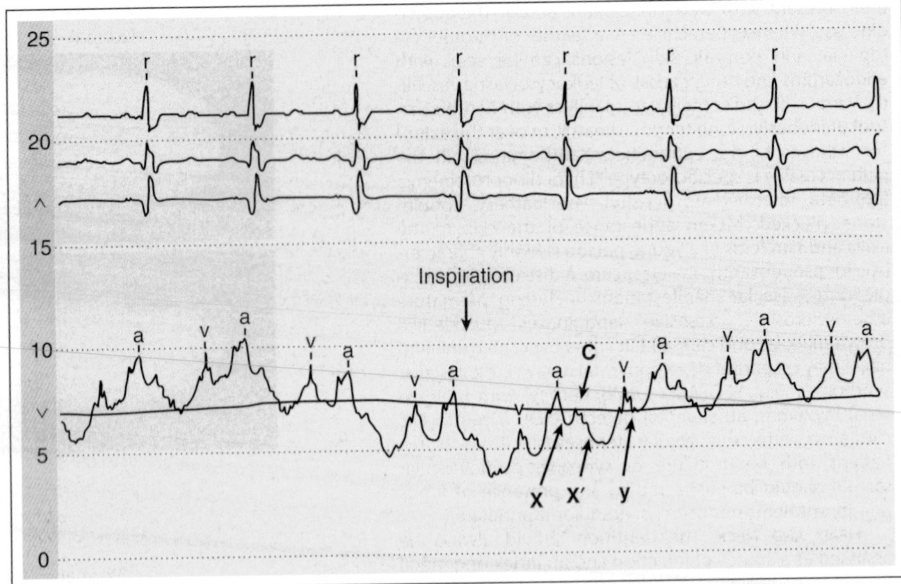

FIGURE 12-2 The normal jugular venous waveform recorded at cardiac catheterization. Note the inspiratory fall in pressure and the dominant *X/X′* descent.

TABLE 12-2 Distinguishing Jugular Venous Pulse from Carotid Pulse

FEATURE	INTERNAL JUGULAR VEIN	CAROTID ARTERY
Appearance of pulse	Undulating two troughs and two peaks for every cardiac cycle (biphasic)	Single brisk upstroke (monophasic)
Response to inspiration	Height of column falls and troughs become more prominent	No respiratory change to contour
Palpability	Generally not palpable (except in severe TR)	Palpable
Effect of pressure	Can be obliterated with gentle pressure at base of vein/clavicle	Cannot be obliterated

Cardiovascular Examination

Jugular Venous Pressure and Waveform. The jugular venous pressure aids in the estimation of volume status at the bedside. The external (EJV) or internal (IJV) jugular vein may be used, although the IJV is preferred because the EJV is valved and is not directly in line with the superior vena cava (SVC) and right atrium (RA). The EJV is easier to visualize when distended, and its appearance has been used to discriminate between a low and high central venous pressure (CVP) when tested in a group of attending physicians, residents, and medical students.[18] An elevated left EJV pressure may also signify a persistent left-sided SVC or compression of the innominate vein from an intrathoracic structure such as a tortuous or aneurysmal aorta. If an elevated venous pressure is suspected but venous pulsations cannot be appreciated, the patient should be asked to sit with the feet dangling over the side of the bed. The pooling of blood in the lower extremities with this maneuver may reveal venous pulsations. SVC syndrome should be suspected if the venous pressure is elevated, pulsations are still not discernible, and the head and neck appear dusky or cyanotic. In the hypotensive patient in whom hypovolemia is suspected, the patient may need to be lowered to a supine position to gauge the waveform in the right supraclavicular fossa.

The venous waveform can sometimes be difficult to distinguish from the carotid artery pulse. The venous waveform has several characteristic features (**Fig. 12-2** and **Table 12-2**) and its individual components can usually be identified. The *a* and *v* waves, and *x* and *y* descents, are defined by their temporal relation to electrocardiographic events and heart sounds (S_1, S_2). The estimated height of the venous pressure indicates the central venous, or RA, pressure. Although observers vary widely in the estimation of the CVP, knowledge that the pressure is elevated, and not its specific value, can still inform diagnosis and management.

The venous pressure is measured as the vertical distance between the top of the venous pulsation and the sternal inflection point, where the manubrium meets the sternum (angle of Louis). A distance of more than 3 cm is considered abnormal, but the distance between the angle of Louis and mid-RA can vary considerably, especially in obese patients.[19]

In 160 consecutive patients receiving chest computed tomography (CT) scans, this distance ranged considerably according to body position. At 45 degrees, values ranged widely among patients, from 6 to 15 cm, and correlated independently with smoking status, age, and anteroposterior chest dimension.[18] In general, use of the sternal angle as a reference leads to systematic underestimation of venous pressure. Other body surface reference sites have been proposed. A point 5 cm below the fourth or fifth intercostal space at the left sternal border on the anterior chest wall may be the most accurate. Practically, however, the use of even relatively simple landmarks has proven difficult, and critical care nurses vary by several centimeters in trying to locate an external reference point to measure the CVP. Venous pulsations above the clavicle are clearly abnormal, because the distance from the right atrium is at least 10 cm. The correlation of the bedside assessment of CVP with direct measurements is only fair. Measurements made at the bedside, which are in units of centimeters of blood or water, should be converted to millimeters of mercury (1.36 cm H_2O = 1.0 mm Hg) for comparison with hemodynamic measurements.

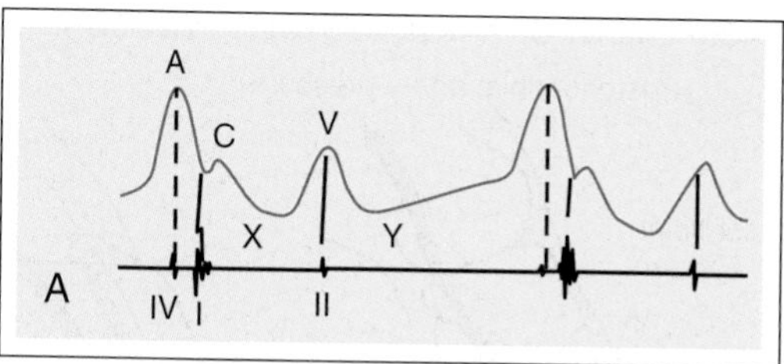

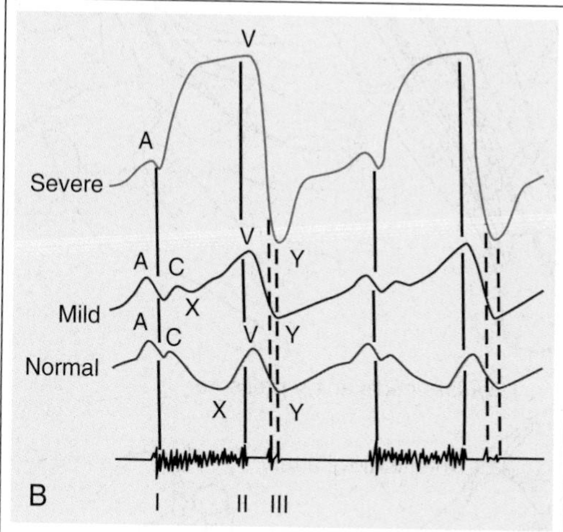

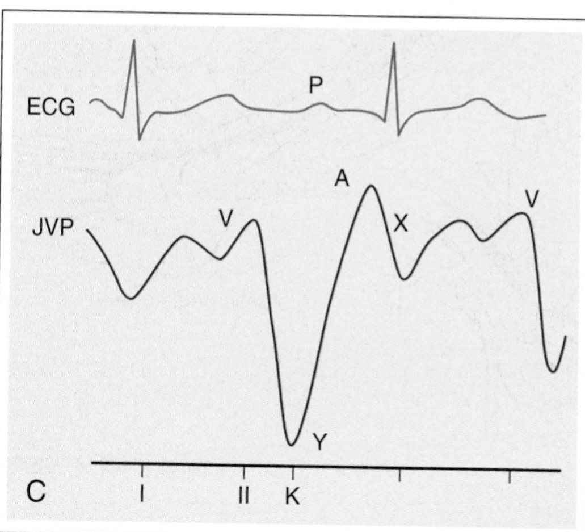

FIGURE 12-3 Abnormal jugular venous waveforms. **A,** Large *a* waves associated with reduced RV compliance or elevated RV end-diastolic pressure. The phonocardiographic tracing (below) shows timing of the corresponding right-sided S_4. **B,** Normal jugular venous waveform (bottom), mild TR (middle), and severe TR (top), with corresponding phonocardiogram. With severe TR, there is "ventricularization" of the jugular venous waveform, with a prominent *V* wave and rapid *Y* descent. The *X* descent is absent. **C,** Jugular venous waveform in constrictive pericarditis with a prominent *Y* descent. Note the timing of the pericardial knock (K) relative to S_2. The abrupt rise in pressure after the nadir of the *Y* descent is caused by the rapid rise in venous pressure with ventricular filling. JVP = jugular venous pulse. *(From Abrams J: Synopsis of Cardiac Physical Diagnosis. 2nd ed. Boston, Butterworth Heinemann, 2001, pp 25-35.)*

The venous waveforms include several distinct peaks (*a*, *c*, and *v*; see Fig. 12-2). The *a* wave reflects RA presystolic contraction, occurs just after the electrocardiographic P wave, and precedes the first heart sound (S_1). A prominent *a* wave indicates reduced right ventricular (RV) compliance. A cannon *a* wave occurs with A-V dissociation and RA contraction against a closed tricuspid valve (TV; **Fig. 12-3**). The presence of cannon *a* waves in a patient with wide complex tachycardia identifies the rhythm as ventricular in origin. The *a* wave is absent with AF. The *x* descent reflects the fall in RA pressure after the *a* wave peak. The *c* wave interrupts this descent as ventricular systole pushes the closed TV into the RA. In the neck, the carotid pulse may also contribute to the *c* wave. The *x′* descent follows because of atrial diastolic suction created by ventricular systole pulling the TV downward. In normal individuals, the *x′* descent is the predominant waveform in the jugular venous pulse. The *v* wave represents atrial filling, occurs at the end of ventricular systole, and follows just after S_2. Its height is determined by RA compliance and by the volume of blood returning to the RA, either antegrade from the vena cavae and/or retrograde through an incompetent TV. The *v* wave is smaller than the *a* wave because of the normally compliant RA. In patients with ASD, the *a* and *v* waves may be of equal height; in TR, the *v* wave is accentuated. With TR, the *v* wave will merge with the *c* wave because retrograde flow and antegrade right atrial filling occur simultaneously (see Fig. 12-3). The *y* descent follows the *v* wave peak and reflects the fall in RA pressure after TV opening. Resistance to ventricular filling in early diastole blunts the *y* descent, as is the case with pericardial tamponade or tricuspid stenosis (TS). The *y* descent will be steep when ventricular diastolic filling occurs early and rapidly, as with pericardial constriction or isolated severe TR. The normal venous pressure should fall by at least 3 mm Hg with inspiration. A rise in venous pressure (or its failure to decrease) with inspiration (the Kussmaul sign) is associated with constrictive pericarditis and also with restrictive cardiomyopathy, pulmonary embolism, RV infarction, and advanced systolic heart failure. A Kussmaul sign occurs with right-sided volume overload and reduced right ventricular compliance. Normally, the inspiratory increase in right-sided venous return is accommodated by increased right ventricular ejection, facilitated by an increase in the capacitance of the pulmonary vascular bed. In states of RV diastolic dysfunction and volume overload, the right ventricle cannot accommodate the enhanced volume and the pressure rises.

The abdominojugular reflux or passive leg elevation can elicit venous hypertension. The abdominojugular reflux requires firm and consistent pressure over the upper abdomen, preferably the right upper quadrant, for at least 10 seconds. A sustained rise of more than 3 cm in the venous pressure for at least 15 seconds after resumption of spontaneous respiration is a positive response. The patient should be coached to refrain from holding his or her breath or performing a Valsalva-like maneuver that could falsely elevate the venous pressure. The abdominojugular reflux is useful in predicting heart failure and a PA wedge pressure higher than 15 mm Hg.[20]

TABLE 12-3 Important Aspects of Blood Pressure Measurement

- Patient seated comfortably, back supported, bared upper arm, legs uncrossed
- Arm should be at heart level
- Cuff length/width should be 80%/40% of arm circumference
- Cuff should be deflated at <3 mm Hg/sec
- Column or dial should be read to nearest 2 mm Hg
- First audible Korotkoff sound is systolic pressure; last sound, diastolic pressure
- No talking between subject and observer

MEASURING THE BLOOD PRESSURE. Auscultatory measurement of blood pressure (see Chap. 45 for further details) yields lower systolic and higher diastolic values than direct intra-arterial recording.[21] Nurse-recorded blood pressure is usually closer to the patient's average daytime blood pressure. Blood pressure should be measured with the patient seated using an appropriately sized cuff (**Table 12-3**). A common source of error in clinical practice is the use of an inappropriately small cuff, which results in overestimation of the true blood pressure and has particular relevance for obese patients.

On occasion, the Korotkoff sounds may disappear soon after the first sound, only to recur later before finally disappearing as phase 5. This auscultatory gap is more likely to occur in older hypertensive patients with target end-organ damage. The systolic pressure should be recorded at the first Korotkoff sound and not when the sound reappears. This finding should be distinguished from pulsus paradoxus (see later). Korotkoff sounds may be heard all the way down to 0 mm Hg with the cuff completely deflated in children, in pregnant patients, in patients with chronic severe AR or in the presence of a large arteriovenous (AV) fistula. In these cases, both the phase 4 and 5 pressures should be noted.

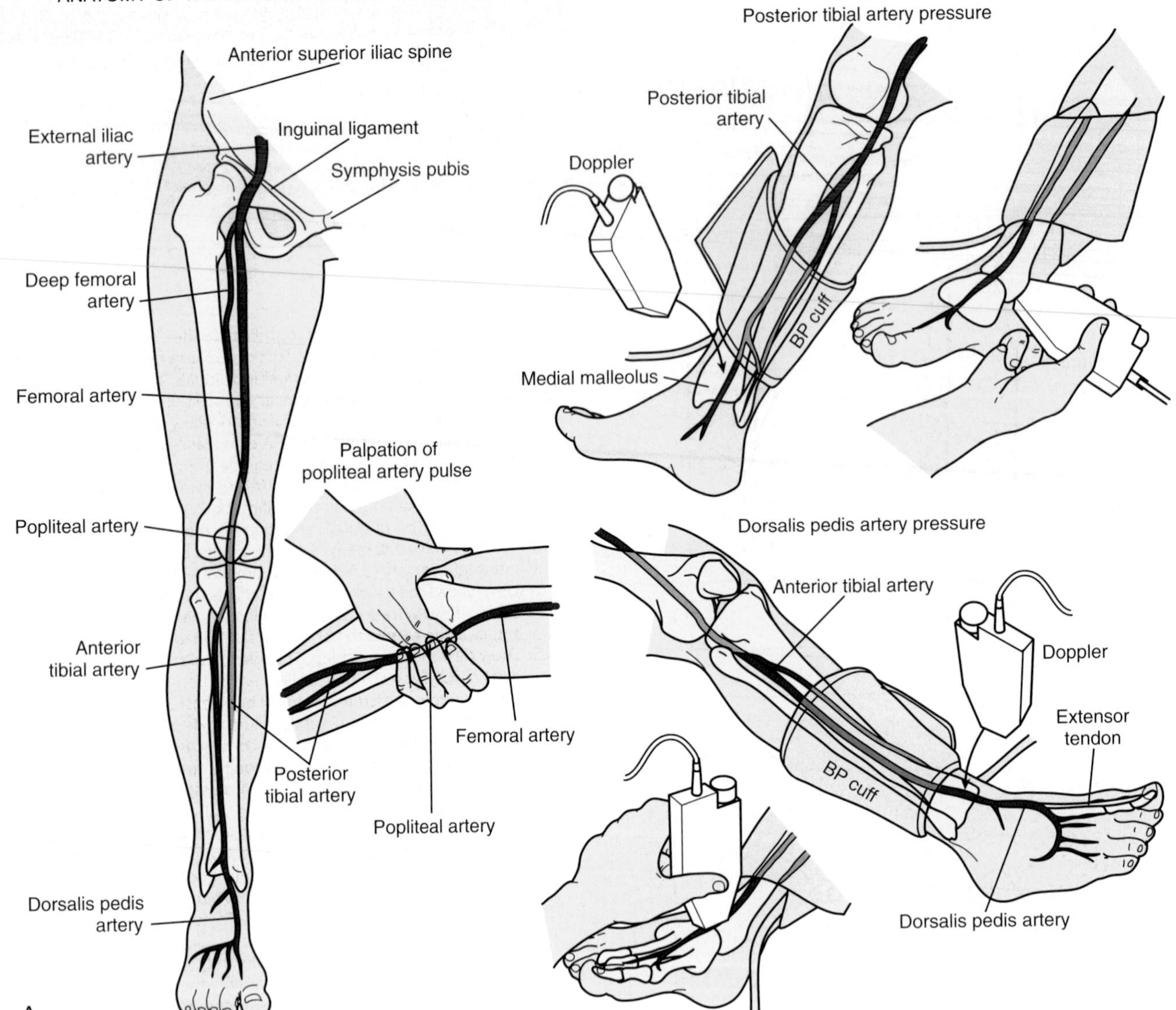

FIGURE 12-4 Measurement of the lower extremity blood pressures. *(From Khan NA, Rahim SA, Anand SS, et al: Does the clinical examination predict lower extremity peripheral arterial disease? JAMA 295:536, 2006.)*

Blood pressure should be measured in both arms either in rapid succession or simultaneously; normally the measurements should differ by less than 10 mm Hg, independent of handedness. As many as 20% of normal subjects, however, have a more than 10-mm Hg arm blood pressure differential in the absence of symptoms or other examination findings, an observation of uncertain relevance.[22] A blood pressure differential of more than 10 mm Hg can be associated with subclavian artery disease (atherosclerotic or inflammatory), supravalvular aortic stenosis, aortic coarctation, or dissection. Systolic leg pressures may exceed arm pressures by as much as 20 mm Hg; greater leg-arm pressure differences are seen in patients with severe AR (Hill sign) and patients with extensive and calcified lower extremity peripheral arterial disease (PAD). Leg blood pressure should be measured using large thigh cuffs with auscultation at the popliteal artery or using a standard large arm cuff on the calf with simultaneous auscultation at the posterior tibial artery (**Fig. 12-4**; see also Fig. 61-4). Measurement of lower extremity blood pressures forms the basis of the ankle-brachial index (ABI), a powerful predictor of cardiovascular mortality (see Chap. 61).

Consideration should be given to ambulatory blood pressure monitoring when uncertainty exists about the significance of recordings obtained in the clinic. This approach is especially useful for the patient with suspected white coat hypertension (see Chap. 45).[23] Masked hypertension (caused by severe PAD) should be suspected when normal or even low blood pressures are recorded and evidence of hypertensive end-organ damage is present.

Orthostatic hypotension (a fall in blood pressure of more than 20 mm Hg systolic and/or more than 10 mm Hg diastolic in response to moving from a supine to a standing position within 3 minutes) may be accompanied by a lack of compensatory tachycardia, a response suggestive of autonomic insufficiency, as can be seen in patients with diabetes or Parkinson's disease. The heart rate–blood pressure response to standing is also influenced by age, hydration, medications, food, conditioning, and ambient temperature and humidity.

An increase in pulse pressure can represent increased vascular stiffness, usually because of aging or arteriosclerosis. Aortic stiffness is increased in patients with Marfan syndrome and other connective tissue disorders and may contribute to a propensity for dissection. The single best measure of vascular stiffness is unknown.[24] Peripheral indices may not correlate well with central aortic stiffness, which is a primary determinant of ventricular-vascular coupling. One measure, the augmentation index, is the percentage increase in systolic pressure created by the premature return of the reflected wave during late systole. Such measurements can be obtained using peripheral tonometry and translated into central stiffness indices using mathematical transfer functions, but are not routinely available in practice.

ASSESSING THE PULSES. The carotid artery pulse wave occurs within 40 milliseconds of the ascending aortic pulse and reflects aortic valve and ascending aortic function. The aortic pulse is best appreciated in the epigastrium (abdominal aorta). The peripheral arterial pulses should be assessed (see Chap. 61). The temporal arteries can be easily palpated and aid in the diagnosis of temporal arteritis or polymyalgia rheumatica. One of the two pedal pulses may not be palpable in a normal subject because of unusual anatomy (posterior tibial, <5%; dorsal pedis, <10%), but each pair should be symmetric. True congenital absence of a pulse is rare (<2%) and, in most cases, pulses can be obtained with a handheld Doppler device when not palpable.[25] Concomitant palpation of the brachial or radial pulse with the femoral pulse should routinely be performed; a femoral delay in a patient with hypertension may indicate aortic coarctation.

The contour of the pulses depends on the stroke volume, ejection velocity, vascular capacity and compliance, and systemic resistance. The palpable pulse reflects the merging of both the antegrade pulsatile flow of blood and reflection of the propagated pulse returning from the peripheral arteries. The arterial pulse upstroke increases with distance from the heart. Normally, the incident (or percussion wave) begins with systolic ejection (just after S_1) and is the predominant monophasic pulse appreciated at the bedside (**Fig. 12-5**). The incisura or dicrotic notch signifies aortic valve closure. A bounding pulse may occur in hyperkinetic states such as fever, anemia, and thyrotoxicosis, or in pathologic states such as severe bradycardia, AR, or arteriovenous fistula. A bifid pulse is created by two distinct pressure peaks. This phenomenon may occur with fever or after exercise in a normal individual and is consistent with increased vascular compliance. With chronic severe AR, a large stroke volume ejected rapidly into a noncompliant arterial tree (as with hypertension or aging) produces a reflected wave of sufficient amplitude to be palpated during systole. Hypertrophic obstructive cardiomyopathy (HOCM) can rarely produce a bifid systolic pulse with percussion and tidal (or reflected) waves (see Fig. 12-5).

A more than 10 mm Hg fall in systolic pressure with inspiration (pulsus paradoxus) is considered pathologic and a sign of pericardial or pulmonary disease, and can also occur in obesity and pregnancy without clinical disease.[26] Pulsus paradoxus is measured by noting the difference between the systolic pressure at which the Korotkoff sounds are first heard (during expiration) and the systolic pressure at which the Korotkoff sounds are heard with each beat, independent of respiratory phase. Between these two pressures, the sounds are heard only intermittently (during expiration). The cuff pressure must be decreased slowly to appreciate the finding. Tachycardia, AF, and tachypnea make its assessment difficult. Pulsus paradoxus may be palpable when the pressure difference exceeds 15 to 20 mm Hg (see Chap. 75).[27] Pulsus paradoxus is not specific for pericardial tamponade and can accompany massive pulmonary embolus, hemorrhagic shock, severe obstructive lung disease, or tension pneumothorax.

Pulsus alternans is defined by the beat-to-beat variability of the pulse amplitude (**Fig. 12-6**). It is present when only every other phase 1 Korotkoff sound is audible as the cuff pressure is slowly lowered, in a patient with a regular heart rhythm, independent of the respiratory cycle. Pulsus alternans is generally seen in severe heart failure and is exaggerated in severe AR, hypertension, and hypovolemic states. It is attributed to cyclic changes in intracellular calcium levels and action potential duration. Association with electrocardiographic T wave alternans appears to increase arrhythmic risk.[28]

Severe aortic stenosis (AS) may be suggested by a weak and delayed pulse (pulsus parvus et tardus) and best appreciated by careful palpation of the carotid arteries (see Fig. 12-5 and Chap. 66). The delay is assessed during simultaneous auscultation of the heart sounds; the carotid upstroke should be coincident with S_1. This finding is less accurate in older hypertensive patients with reduced vascular compliance and stiffer carotid arteries. An abrupt carotid upstroke with rapid fall-off characterizes the pulse of AR (Corrigan or water hammer pulse). The carotid upstroke is also rapid in

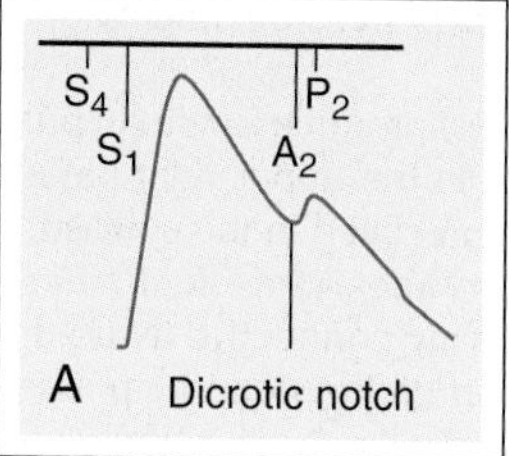

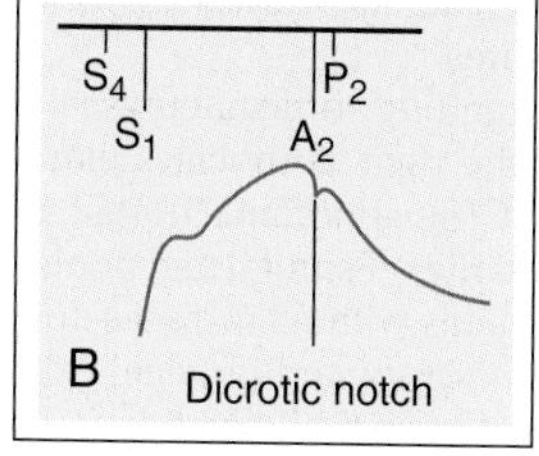

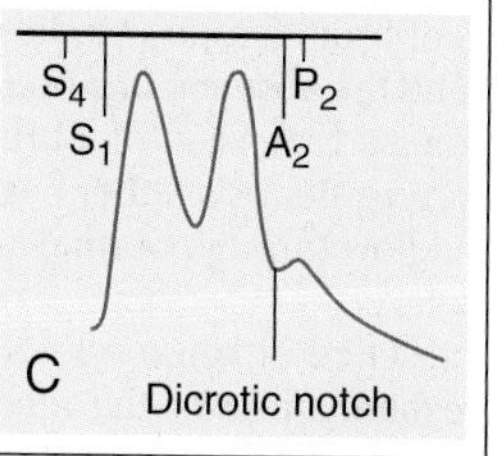

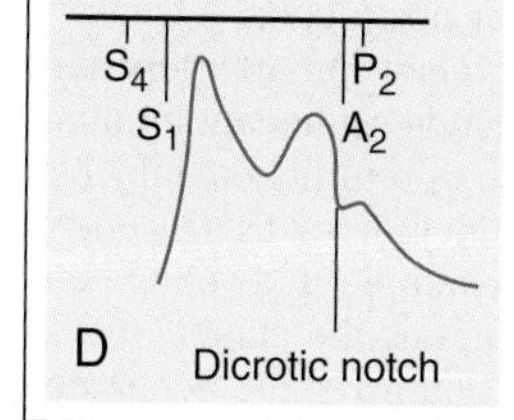

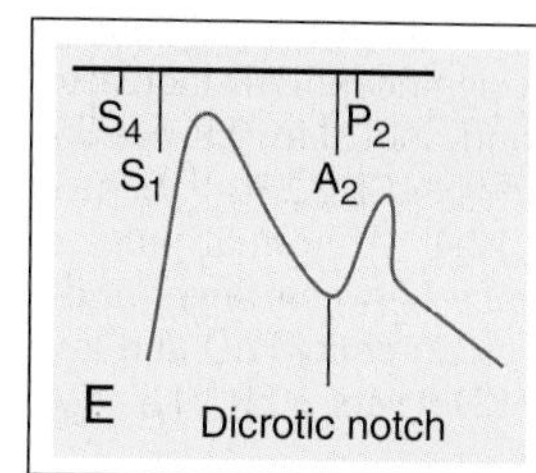

FIGURE 12-5 Carotid pulse waveforms and heart sounds. **A,** Normal. **B,** AS—anacrotic pulse with slow upstroke and peak near S_2. **C,** Severe AR—bifid pulse with two systolic peaks. **D,** HOCM—bifid pulse with two systolic peaks. The second peak (tidal or reflected wave) is of lower amplitude than the initial percussion wave. **E,** Bifid pulse with systolic and diastolic peaks as may occur with sepsis or intra-aortic balloon counterpulsation. A_2 = aortic component of S_2; P_2 = pulmonic component of S_2; S_1 = first heart sound; S_2 = second heart sound; S_4 = fourth heart sound. *(From Chatterjee K: Bedside evaluation of the heart: The physical examination. In Chatterjee K, Parmley W [eds]: Cardiology: An Illustrated Text/Reference. Philadelphia, JB Lippincott, 1991, pp 3.11-3.51; and Braunwald E: The clinical examination. In Braunwald E, Goldman L [eds]: Primary Cardiology. 2nd ed. Philadelphia, Elsevier, 2003, p 36.)*

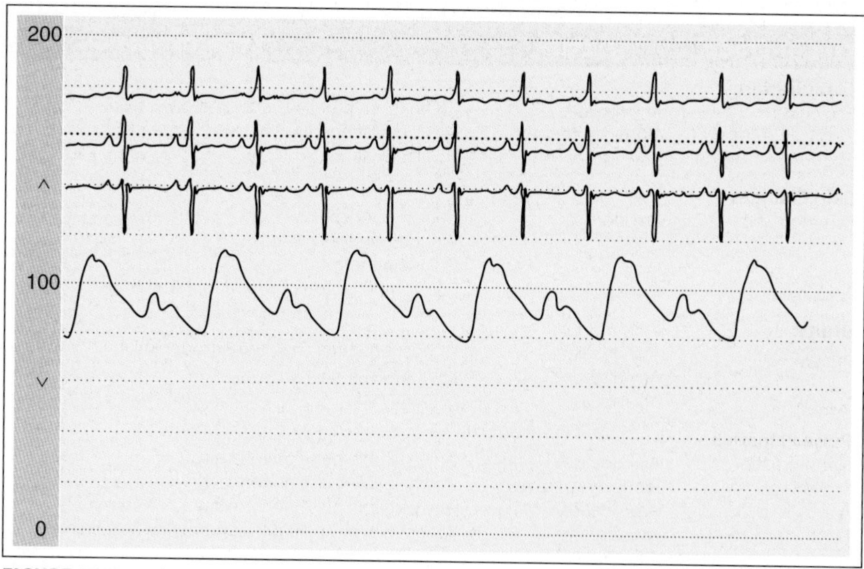

FIGURE 12-6 Pulsus alternans in a patient with severe left ventricular systolic dysfunction. The systolic pressure varies from beat to beat independently of the respiratory cycle. The rhythm is sinus throughout.

older patients with isolated systolic hypertension and wide pulse pressures.

Ascending aortic aneurysms may rarely produce a systolic pulsation near the right sternoclavicular joint or in the upper right parasternal region. The abdominal aorta can be appreciated in the epigastric area (see earlier). Femoral and popliteal artery aneurysms should be sought in patients with AAA disease or underlying connective tissue disease.

The history and physical examination findings can help assess the level of arterial obstruction in lower extremity claudication (see Chap. 61). Auscultation for aortic and femoral artery bruits should be routine. The correlation between the presence of a bruit and the degree of vascular obstruction is weak.[29] A cervical bruit is a poor indicator of the degree of carotid artery narrowing, and the absence of a bruit does not exclude significant luminal compromise. Extension of a bruit into diastole or a thrill generally indicates severe stenosis. Other causes of a bruit include AV fistulas and enhanced flow through normal arteries as, for example, in a young patient with fever.

Integrating the clinical history and presence of atherosclerotic risk factors improves the accuracy of the examination for the identification of lower extremity PAD.[25] In an asymptomatic patient, the presence of a femoral bruit (LR, 4.8; 95% CI, 2.4 to 9.5) or any abnormality of the pulse (LR, 3.1; 95% CI, 3.1 to 6.6) increases the likelihood of PAD. The likelihood of significant PAD increases when there are lower extremity symptoms and cool skin (LR, 5.9; 95% CI, 4.1 to 8.6), pulse abnormalities (LR, 4.7; 95% CI, 2.2 to 9.9), or any bruit (LR, 5.6; 95% CI, 4.7 to 6.7; **Table 12-4**). Abnormal pulse oximetry, defined by a more than 2% difference between finger and toe oxygen saturation, can also indicate lower extremity PAD and is comparable to the ABI (LR, 30; 95% CI, 7.6 to 121.0 versus LR, 24.8; 95% CI, 6.2 to 99.8).[30]

INSPECTION AND PALPATION OF THE HEART. The apical heartbeat may be visible in thin-chested adults. The left anterior chest wall may heave in patients with enlarged and hyperdynamic left ventricles. Right upper parasternal and sternoclavicular pulsations suggest ascending aortic aneurysm disease. A left parasternal heave indicates RV pressure or volume overload. A pulsation in the third intercostal space to the left of the sternum can indicate PA hypertension. In very thin, tall patients, or in patients with emphysema and flattened diaphragms, the RV impulse may be visible in the epigastrium and should be distinguished from a pulsatile liver edge.

Palpation of the heart should begin with the patient in the supine position at 30 degrees. If the heart is not palpable in this position, the patient should be examined in the left lateral decubitus position with the left arm above the head or in the seated position, leaning forward. The point of maximal impulse is normally over the left ventricular apex in the midclavicular line at the fifth intercostal space. It is smaller than 2 cm in diameter, and moves quickly away from the fingers. It is best felt at end-expiration, when the heart is closest to the chest wall. The normal impulse may not be palpable in obese or muscular patients or in those with thoracic cage deformities.

Left ventricular (LV) cavity enlargement displaces the apex beat leftward and downward. A sustained apex beat is a sign of LV pressure overload (AS, hypertension). A palpable, presystolic impulse corresponds to a fourth heart sound (S_4) and reflects the atrial contribution to ventricular diastolic filling of a noncompliant LV. A prominent, rapid, early filling wave in patients with advanced systolic heart failure may result in a palpable third heart sound (S_3), which may be present when the gallop itself is not audible. A large ventricular aneurysm may yield a palpable and visible ectopic impulse discrete from the apex beat. HOCM rarely may cause a triple-cadence apex beat, with contributions from a palpable S_4 and the two components of the systolic pulse.

A parasternal lift occurs with RV pressure or volume overload. Signs of TR (jugular venous *cv* waves) and/or PA hypertension (loud, single, or palpable P_2) should be sought. An enlarged RV impulse can extend across the precordium and obscure left-sided findings. Rarely, patients with severe MR will have a prominent left parasternal impulse because of systolic expansion of the left atrium (LA) and forward displacement of the heart. The parasternal movement of an enlarged LA will begin and end after the LV apex beat; RV and LV impulses, on the other hand, occur simultaneously. Lateral retraction of the chest wall may also be present with isolated RV enlargement because of posterior displacement of the systolic LV impulse. Systolic and diastolic thrills signify turbulent, high-velocity blood flow, and help localize the origins of heart murmurs.

AUSCULTATION OF THE HEART

Heart Sounds

FIRST HEART SOUND (S_1). The normal first heart sound (S_1) comprises mitral (M_1) and tricuspid (T_1) valve closure. The two components are usually best heard at the lower left sternal border in younger subjects. Normal splitting of S_1 is accentuated with complete right bundle branch block. The intensity of S_1 depends on both the distance

TABLE 12-4 Likelihood Ratios for Various Symptoms or Signs of Peripheral Arterial Disease*

TYPE OF STUDY	SEVERITY	SYMPTOM OR SIGN	Likelihood Ratio (95% CI) POSITIVE	NEGATIVE
Claudication				
Screening	Any disease	"Definite" or "probable" claudication	3.30 (2.30-4.80)†	
	Moderate to severe	No claudication		0.57 (0.43-0.76)
	Any disease	No claudication		0.89 (0.78-1.00)
Skin Changes				
Symptomatic	Any disease	Cooler to touch	5.90 (4.10-8.60)	0.92 (0.89-0.95)
		Wounds or sores	5.90 (2.60-13.40)	0.98 (0.97-1.00)
		Discoloration	2.80 (2.40-3.30)	0.74 (0.69-0.79)
Screening	Moderate to severe	Hair, temperature, color, or atrophic change	1.50 (1.20-1.70)†	0.81 (0.72-0.92)†
Bruits				
Symptomatic	Any disease	At least one bruit (iliac, femoral, popliteal)	5.60 (4.70-6.70)†	0.39 (0.34-0.45)†
	Any disease	Femoral bruit	5.70 (4.70-7.00)	0.74 (0.70-0.78)
Screening	Any disease	Femoral bruit	4.80 (2.40-9.50)	0.83 (0.73-0.95)
Pulse Palpation				
Symptomatic	Any disease	Any palpable pulse abnormality	4.70 (2.20-9.90)	0.38 (0.23-0.64)
Screening	Moderate to severe	Any palpable pulse abnormality	3.00 (2.30-3.90)	0.44 (0.30-0.66)
	Any disease	Any palpable pulse abnormality	3.10 (1.40-6.60)	0.48 (0.22-1.04)
	Any disease	Absence of any palpable abnormality (in a lipid research clinic study)		0.27 (0.16-0.44)
	Any disease	Absence of any palpable abnormality (in high prevalence of diabetes)		0.87 (0.79-0.97)

*Stratified by symptomatic or screening studies.

†Results statistically homogeneous (all $P > 0.20$). Moderate to severe peripheral arterial disease defined by ankle-brachial index < 0.50.

Modified from Khan NA, Rahim SA, Anand SS, et al: Does the clinical examination predict lower extremity peripheral arterial disease? JAMA 295:536, 2006.

over which the anterior leaflet of the mitral valve must travel after onset of systole and its mobility. S_1 intensity increases in the early stages of rheumatic mitral stenosis when the valve leaflets are still pliable, in hyperkinetic states, and with short PR intervals (<160 milliseconds). S_1 becomes softer in the late stages of mitral stenosis, when the leaflets are rigid and calcified, with contractile dysfunction, beta-adrenergic receptor blockers, and long PR intervals (>200 milliseconds). Other factors that can decrease the intensity of the heart sounds and murmurs include mechanical ventilation, obstructive lung disease, obesity, pendulous breasts, pneumothorax, or pericardial effusion.

SECOND HEART SOUND (S_2). The second heart sound (S_2) comprises aortic (A_2) and pulmonic (P_2) valve closure. With normal, or physiologic, splitting, the A_2-P_2 interval increases during inspiration and narrows with expiration. The individual components are best heard at the second left interspace in the supine position. The A_2-P_2 interval widens with complete right bundle branch block because of delayed pulmonic valve closure, and with severe MR because of premature aortic valve closure, although the normal respiratory variation persists in both conditions. Unusually narrow but physiologic splitting of S_2, with an increase in the intensity of P_2 relative to A_2, indicates PA hypertension. With fixed splitting, the A_2-P_2 interval is wide and remains unchanged during the respiratory cycle, and indicates ostium secundum ASD. Reversed, or paradoxical, splitting occurs as a consequence of a pathologic delay in aortic valve closure, as may occur with complete left bundle branch block, RV apical pacing, severe AS, HOCM, and myocardial ischemia. A_2 is normally louder than P_2 and can be heard at most sites across the precordium. When both components can be heard at the lower left sternal border or apex, or when P_2 can be palpated at the second left interspace, pulmonary hypertension is present. The intensity of A_2 and P_2 decreases with aortic and pulmonic stenosis, respectively. A single S_2 may result.

SYSTOLIC SOUNDS. An ejection sound is a high-pitched, early systolic sound that coincides in timing to the upstroke of the carotid pulse and is usually associated with congenital bicuspid aortic or pulmonic valve disease, or in some patients with aortic or pulmonic root dilation and normal semilunar valves. The ejection sound accompanying pulmonic valve disease decreases in intensity with inspiration—the only right-sided cardiac event to behave in this manner. Ejection sounds disappear as the culprit valve loses its pliability over time. Contrary to expectation, these sounds are often better heard at the lower left sternal border than at the base of the heart. Nonejection clicks, which occur after the upstroke of the carotid pulse, are related to MVP. A systolic murmur may or may not follow the click. With standing, ventricular preload decreases and the click and murmur move closer to S_1. With squatting, ventricular preload increases, the prolapsing mitral valve tenses later in systole, and the click and murmur move away from S_1 (**Fig. 12-7**).

DIASTOLIC SOUNDS. The high-pitched OS of mitral stenosis occurs a short distance after S_2; the A_2-OS interval is inversely proportional to the LA-LV diastolic pressure gradient. The intensity of both the S_1 and OS decreases with progressive calcification and rigidity of the anterior mitral leaflet. A pericardial knock (PK) is a high-pitched early diastolic sound, which corresponds in timing to the abrupt cessation of ventricular expansion after atrioventricular valve opening and with the prominent *y* descent seen in the jugular venous waveform in patients with constrictive pericarditis.[31,32] A tumor plop is rarely heard with atrial myxoma; it is a low-pitched sound that may be appreciated only in certain positions and arises from the diastolic prolapse of the tumor across the mitral valve. A diastolic murmur may be present, although most myxomas cause no sound. A third heart sound (S_3) occurs during the rapid filling phase of ventricular diastole. An S_3 may be normal in children, adolescents, and young adults, but indicates systolic heart failure in older adults and carries important prognostic weight (see later). A left-sided S_3 is a low-pitched sound best heard over the LV apex in the left lateral decubitus position, whereas a right-sided S_3 is usually heard at the lower left sternal border or in the subxiphoid position with the patient supine and may become louder with inspiration. A fourth heart sound (S_4) occurs during the atrial filling phase of ventricular diastole and is thought to indicate presystolic ventricular expansion. An S_4 is especially common in patients with an accentuated atrial contribution to ventricular filling (e.g., left ventricular hypertrophy).

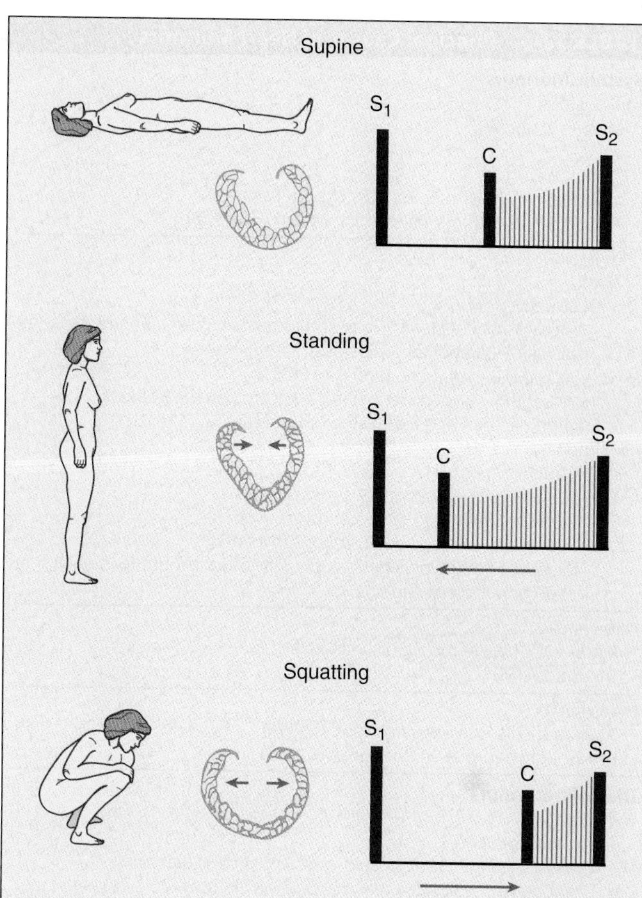

FIGURE 12-7 Behavior of the nonejection click (C) and systolic murmur of mitral valve prolapse. With standing, venous return decreases, the heart becomes smaller, and prolapse occurs earlier in systole. The click and murmur move closer to S_1. With squatting, venous return increases, causing an increase in left ventricular chamber size. The click and murmur occur later in systole and move away from S_1. *(From Shaver JA, Leonard JJ, Leon DF: Examination of the Heart. Part IV: Auscultation of the Heart. Dallas, American Heart Association, 1990, p 13.)*

Cardiac Murmurs (See **Table 12-5** and **Figure 12-8**, see Fig. 12-7 and Chap. 66).

Heart murmurs result from audible vibrations caused by increased turbulence and are defined by their timing within the cardiac cycle. Not all murmurs indicate valvular or structural heart disease. The accurate identification of a functional (benign) systolic murmur can obviate the need for echocardiography in many healthy subjects. The magnitude, dynamic variability, and duration of the pressure difference between two cardiac chambers, or between the ventricles and their respective great arteries, dictate the duration, frequency, configuration, and intensity of the murmur. Intensity is graded on a scale of 1 to 6; a palpable thrill is present with murmurs of grade 4 intensity or higher. Other important attributes that aid in identification include location, radiation, and response to bedside maneuvers, including quiet respiration.

SYSTOLIC MURMURS. Systolic murmurs are early, midsystolic, late, or holosystolic in timing. Acute severe MR results in a decrescendo early systolic murmur because of collapse of the LV-LA pressure gradient during systole, due to the steep rise in pressure within the noncompliant left atrium (**Fig. 12-9**). Severe MR associated with posterior mitral leaflet prolapse or flail radiates anteriorly and to the base; MR caused by anterior leaflet involvement radiates posteriorly and to the axilla. With acute TR in patients with normal PA pressures, an early systolic murmur, which increases in intensity with inspiration, may be audible at the lower left sternal border, and regurgitant *cv* waves may be visible in the jugular venous pulse. Midsystolic murmurs begin after S_1 and end before S_2; they are usually crescendo-decrescendo in configuration. Aortic stenosis or sclerosis causes most midsystolic murmurs in adults. Accurate characterization of the severity of the valve lesion

TABLE 12-5 Principal Causes of Heart Murmurs

Systolic Murmurs

- Early systolic
  - Mitral—acute MR
  - VSD
    - Muscular
    - Nonrestrictive with pulmonary hypertension
  - Tricuspid—TR with normal pulmonary artery pressure
- Midsystolic
  - Aortic
    - Obstructive
      - Supravalvular—supravalvular aortic stenosis, coarctation of the aorta
      - Valvular—AS and aortic sclerosis
      - Subvalvular—discrete, tunnel, or HOCM
    - Increased flow, hyperkinetic states, AR, complete heart block
    - Dilation of ascending aorta, atheroma, aortitis
  - Pulmonary
    - Obstructive
      - Supravalvular—pulmonary artery stenosis
      - Valvular—pulmonic valve stenosis
      - Subvalvular—infundibular stenosis (dynamic)
      - Increased flow, hyperkinetic states, left-to-right shunt (e.g., ASD)
    - Dilation of pulmonary artery
- Late systolic
  - Mitral—MVP, acute myocardial ischemia
  - Tricuspid—TVP
- Holosystolic
  - Atrioventricular valve regurgitation (MR, TR)
  - Left-to-right shunt at ventricular level (VSD)

Diastolic Murmurs

- Early diastolic
  - Aortic regurgitation
    - Valvular—congenital (bicuspid valve), rheumatic deformity, endocarditis, prolapse, trauma, postvalvulotomy
    - Dilation of valve annulus—aortic dissection, annuloaortic ectasia, cystic medial degeneration, hypertension, ankylosing spondylitis
    - Widening of commissures—syphilis
  - Pulmonic regurgitation
    - Valvular—postvalvulotomy, endocarditis, rheumatic fever, carcinoid
    - Dilation of valve annulus—pulmonary hypertension; Marfan syndrome
    - Congenital— isolated or associated with tetralogy of Fallot, VSD, pulmonic stenosis
- Mid-diastolic
  - Mitral
    - Mitral stenosis
    - Carey Coombs murmur (mid-diastolic apical murmur in acute rheumatic fever)
    - Increased flow across nonstenotic mitral valve (e.g., MR, VSD, PDA, high-output states, complete heart block)
  - Tricuspid
    - Tricuspid stenosis
    - Increased flow across nonstenotic tricuspid valve (e.g., TR, ASD, and anomalous pulmonary venous return)
  - Left and right atrial tumors (myxoma)
  - Severe or eccentric AR (Austin Flint murmur)
- Late diastolic
  - Presystolic accentuation of mitral stenosis murmur
  - Austin Flint murmur of severe or eccentric AR

Continuous Murmurs

- PDA
- Coronary AV fistula
- Ruptured sinus of Valsalva aneurysm
- Aortic septal defect
- Cervical venous hum
- Anomalous left coronary artery
- Proximal coronary artery stenosis
- Mammary souffle of pregnancy
- Pulmonary artery branch stenosis
- Bronchial collateral circulation
- Small (restrictive) ASD with MS
- Intercostal AV fistula

From Braunwald E, Perloff JK: *In* Zipes DP, Libby P, Bonow RO, Braunwald E (eds): Braunwald's heart disease: A Textbook of Cardiovascular Medicine. 7th ed. Philadelphia, Elsevier, 2005, pp 77-106; and Norton PJ, O'Rourke RA: Approach to the patient with a heart murmur. *In* Braunwald E, Goldman L (eds): Primary Cardiology. 2nd ed. Philadelphia, Elsevier, 2003, pp 151-168.

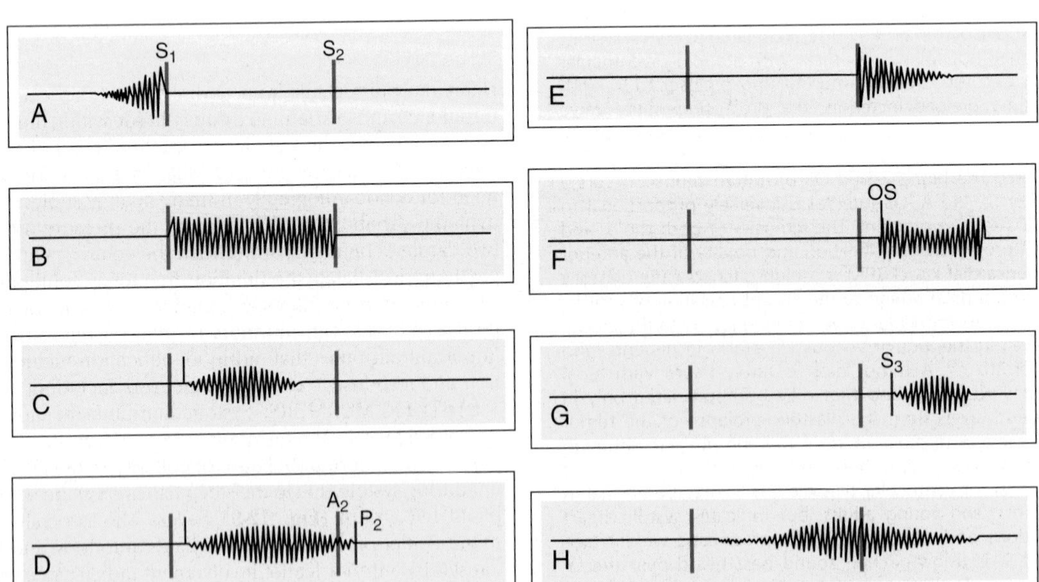

FIGURE 12-8 Diagram of principal heart murmurs. **A,** Presystolic accentuation of the murmur of MS with sinus rhythm. **B,** Holosystolic murmur of chronic, severe MR or TR, or VSD without severe pulmonary hypertension. **C,** Ejection sound and crescendo-decrescendo murmur of bicuspid AS. **D,** Ejection sound and crescendo-decrescendo murmur that extends to P_2 in bicuspid PS. **E,** Early decrescendo diastolic murmur of AR or PR. **F,** Opening snap and mid-diastolic rumble of MS. **G,** Diastolic filling sound (S_3) and mid-diastolic murmur associated with severe MR, TR, or ASD with significant left-to-right shunt. **H,** Continuous murmur of PDA that envelops S_2. OS = opening snap. *(Modified from Wood P: Diseases of the Heart and Circulation. Philadelphia, Lippincott, 1968; and O'Rourke RA, Braunwald E: Physical examination of the cardiovascular system. In Kasper D, Braunwald E, Fauci A, et al [eds]: Harrison's Principles of Internal Medicine. 16th ed. New York, McGraw-Hill, 2005, p 1309.)*

at the bedside depends on cardiac output, stiffness of the carotid arteries, and associated findings. Other causes of a midsystolic heart murmur include HOCM, pulmonic stenosis (PS), and increased pulmonary blood flow in patients with a large ASD and left-to-right shunt. An isolated grade 1 or 2 midsystolic murmur in the absence of symptoms or other signs of heart disease is a benign finding that does not warrant further evaluation, including echocardiography.[33] A grade 1 or 2 midsystolic murmur can often be heard at the left sternal border with pregnancy, hyperthyroidism, or anemia. Healthy children and adolescents can also commonly have such murmurs. A late apical systolic murmur usually indicates MVP; one or more nonejection clicks may be present. A similar murmur may be heard transiently during an episode of acute myocardial ischemia. In this setting, the MR is caused by apical tethering and malcoaptation of the leaflets in response to structural and functional changes of the ventricle and mitral annulus. The intensity of the murmur will vary with LV afterload. Holosystolic murmurs, which are plateau in configuration, derive from the continuous and wide pressure gradient between two cardiac chambers—the left ventricle and LA with chronic MR, the right ventricle and RA with chronic TR, and the left ventricle and right ventricle with a membranous ventricular septal defect (VSD) without pulmonary hypertension. MR is best heard over the cardiac apex, TR at the lower left sternal border, and a VSD at the mid-left sternal border where a thrill is palpable in most patients. Although there are several causes of primary TR, it most commonly occurs secondary to PA hypertension, right ventricular enlargement, annular dilation, papillary muscle displacement, and failure of tricuspid leaflet coaptation.

DIASTOLIC MURMURS. Diastolic murmurs invariably signify cardiac disease. Chronic AR causes a high-pitched, decrescendo, early to mid-diastolic murmur. With primary aortic valve disease, the murmur is best heard along the left sternal border, whereas with root enlargement and secondary AR, the murmur tends to radiate along the right sternal border. A midsystolic murmur caused by augmented and accelerated forward flow is also present with moderate to severe AR, and need not signify valve or outflow tract obstruction. The diastolic murmur is both softer and of shorter duration in acute AR because of the rapid rise in LV diastolic pressure and the diminution of the aortic–LV diastolic pressure gradient. Additional features of acute AR include tachycardia, a soft S_1, and the absence of peripheral findings of significant diastolic run-off. The murmur of pulmonic regurgitation (PR) is heard along the left sternal border and is most often caused by annular enlargement from chronic PA hypertension (Graham Steell murmur). Signs of RV pressure overload are present. PR can also occur with a congenitally deformed valve and is invariably present after repair of tetralogy of Fallot. In these settings, the murmur is relatively softer and lower pitched. The severity of PR after surgical repair can be underappreciated. Mitral stenosis is the classic cause of a mid- to late diastolic murmur (see Fig. 66-20). Mitral stenosis may also be "silent"—for example, in patients with low cardiac output or large body habitus. The murmur is best heard over the apex in the left lateral decubitus position, is low-pitched (rumbling), and introduced by an OS in the early stages of the disease. Presystolic accentuation (an increase in the intensity of the murmur in late diastole following atrial contraction) occurs in patients in sinus rhythm. Left-sided events usually obscure findings in patients with rheumatic TS. Functional mitral stenosis or TS refers to mid-diastolic murmurs created by increased, accelerated transvalvular flow, without valvular obstruction, in the setting of severe MR, severe TR, or ASD with a large left-to-right shunt. The low-pitched mid- to late apical diastolic murmur sometimes associated with AR (Austin Flint murmur) can be distinguished from mitral stenosis on the basis of its response to vasodilators and the presence of associated findings. Less common causes of a mid-diastolic murmur include atrial myxoma, complete heart block, and acute rheumatic mitral valvulitis (Carey Coombs murmur).

CONTINUOUS MURMURS. A continuous murmur implies a pressure gradient between two chambers or vessels during both systole and diastole. These murmurs begin in systole, peak near S_2, and then continue into diastole. They can be difficult to distinguish from systolic and diastolic murmurs in patients with mixed aortic or pulmonic valve disease. Examples include the murmurs associated with PDA, ruptured sinus of Valsalva aneurysm, and coronary, great vessel, or hemodialysis AV fistulas. The cervical venous hum and mammary souffle of pregnancy are two benign variants.

DYNAMIC AUSCULTATION. Simple bedside maneuvers can help identify heart murmurs and characterize their significance (**Table 12-6**). Right-sided events, except for the pulmonic ejection sound, increase with inspiration and decrease with expiration; left-sided events behave oppositely (100% sensitivity, 88% specificity). The intensity of the murmurs associated with MR, VSD, and AR will increase in response to maneuvers that increase LV afterload (handgrip, vasopressors) and decrease after exposure to vasodilating agents (amyl nitrite). Squatting abruptly increases ventricular preload and afterload, whereas rapid standing suddenly decreases preload. In patients with MVP, the click and murmur will move away from S_1 with squatting because of the delay in onset of leaflet prolapse at higher ventricular volumes. With rapid standing, the click and murmur move closer to S_1, because prolapse occurs earlier in systole at a smaller chamber dimension. The murmur of HOCM behaves in a directionally similar manner, becoming softer and shorter with squatting (95%

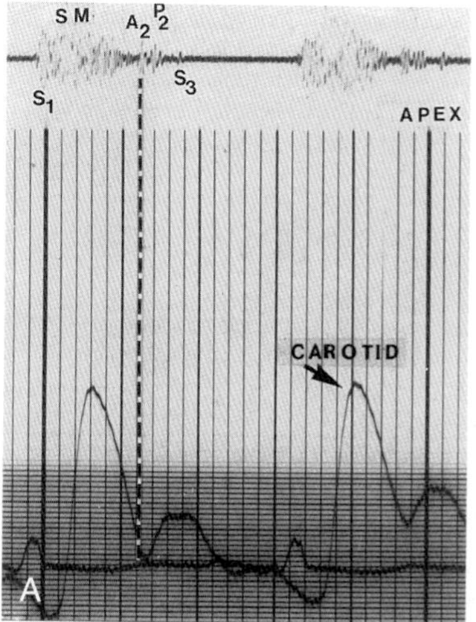

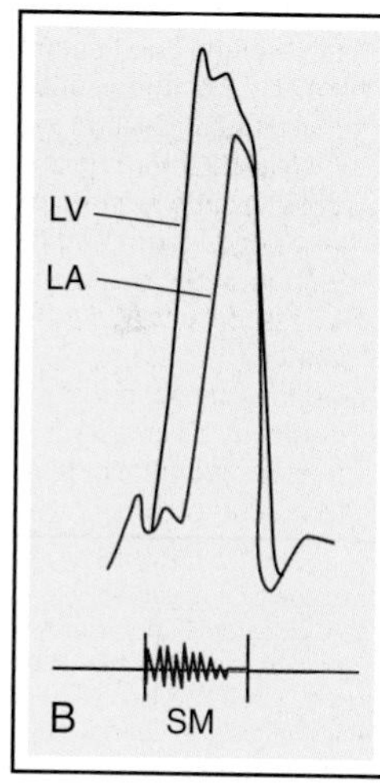

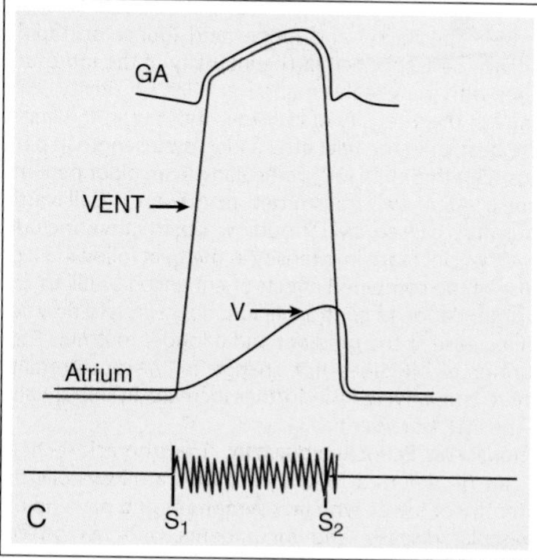

FIGURE 12-9 **A,** Phonocardiogram (top) of a patient with acute severe mitral regurgitation showing a decrescendo early systolic murmur and diastolic filling sound (S_3). **B,** LV and LA pressure waveforms demonstrating the abrupt rise in LA pressure and attenuation of the LV-LA pressure gradient, resulting in the duration and configuration of the murmur. **C,** Phonocardiogram depicting great artery (GA), ventricular (VENT), and atrial pressures with resultant phonocardiogram in chronic MR or TR. Note the holosystolic timing and plateau configuration of the murmur, both of which derive from the large ventricular-atrial pressure gradient throughout systole. SM = systolic murmur; V = *v* wave. *(From Braunwald E, Perloff JK: Physical examination of the heart and circulation. In Zipes D, Libby P, Bonow RO, Braunwald E [eds]: Braunwald's Heart Disease. A Textbook of Cardiovascular Medicine. 7th ed. Philadelphia, Elsevier, 2005, p 97.)*

CH 12

TABLE 12-6 Interventions for Altering Intensity of Cardiac Murmurs

Respiration: Right-sided murmurs generally increase with inspiration. Left-sided murmurs usually are louder during expiration.
Valsalva maneuver: Most murmurs decrease in length and intensity. Two exceptions are the systolic murmur of HOCM, which usually becomes much louder, and that of MVP, which becomes longer and often louder. After release of the Valsalva maneuver, right-sided murmurs tend to return to baseline intensity earlier than left-sided murmurs.
Exercise: Murmurs caused by blood flow across normal or obstructed valves (e.g., PS and MS) become louder with both isotonic and isometric (handgrip) exercise. Murmurs of MR, VSD, and AR also increase with handgrip exercise.
Positional changes: With standing, most murmurs diminish; two exceptions are the murmur of HOCM, which becomes louder, and that of MVP, which lengthens and often is intensified. With squatting, most murmurs become louder, but those of HOCM and MVP usually soften and may disappear. Passive leg raising usually produces the same results as squatting.
Postventricular premature beat or AF: Murmurs originating at normal or stenotic semilunar valves increase in intensity during the cardiac cycle after a ventricular premature beat or in the beat after a long cycle length in AF. By contrast, systolic murmurs caused by AV valve regurgitation do not change, diminish (papillary muscle dysfunction), or become shorter after a premature beat (MVP).
Pharmacologic interventions: During the initial relative hypotension after amyl nitrite inhalation, murmurs of MR, VSD, and AR decrease in intensity, whereas the murmur of AS increases in intensity because of increased stroke volume. During the later tachycardia phase, murmurs of MS and right-sided lesions also become louder. This intervention may help distinguish the murmur of the Austin Flint phenomenon from that of MS. The response in MVP often is biphasic (softer and then louder than control).
Transient arterial occlusion: Transient external compression of both brachial arteries by bilateral cuff inflation to 20 mm Hg greater than peak systolic pressure augments the murmurs of MR, VSD, and AR, but not murmurs from other causes.

From Bonow RO, Carabello BA, Chatterjee K, et al: ACC/AHA 2006 guidelines for the management of patients with valvular heart disease: A report of the American College of Cardiology/American Heart Association Task Force on Practice Guidelines (Writing Committee to Revise the 1998 Guidelines for the Management of Patients with Valvular Heart Disease) developed in collaboration with the Society of Cardiovascular Anesthesiologists endorsed by the Society for Cardiovascular Angiography and Interventions and the Society of Thoracic Surgeons. J Am Coll Cardiol 48:e18, 2006.

sensitivity, 85% specificity) and longer and louder on rapid standing (95% sensitivity, 84% specificity). The intensity of the murmur of HOCM also increases with the Valsalva maneuver (65% sensitivity, 95% specificity). A change in the intensity of a systolic murmur in the first beat after a premature beat, or in the beat after a long cycle length in patients with AF, suggests AS rather than MR, particularly in an older patient in whom the murmur of AS is well transmitted to the apex (Gallavardin effect). Systolic murmurs caused by LV outflow obstruction, including those caused by AS, will increase in intensity in the beat following a premature beat because of the combined effects of enhanced LV filling and postextrasystolic potentiation of contractile function. Forward flow accelerates, causing an increase in the gradient and a louder murmur. The intensity of the murmur of MR does not change in the postpremature beat, because there is relatively little further increase in mitral valve flow or change in the LV-LA gradient.

INDICATIONS FOR ECHOCARDIOGRAPHY. Transthoracic echocardiography (TTE) can be deferred for patients with a midsystolic murmur of grade 2 intensity or lower, who lack symptoms and have no other signs of cardiovascular disease, and for patients with benign continuous murmurs (**Fig. 12-10**).[33] Other patients should undergo echocardiographic study to characterize cardiac structure and function and to estimate PA pressures.

Integrated Evidence-Based Approach

Heart Failure (see Chap. 26)

HISTORY. Both exertional and resting symptoms should be explored. Common symptoms include dyspnea, fatigue, exercise limitation, orthopnea, and edema. In a review of 22 studies of adult patients presenting to an emergency room with dyspnea, the probability of heart failure was best predicted by a past history of heart failure (LR, 5.8; 95% CI, 4.1 to 8.0), paroxysmal nocturnal dyspnea (PND) (LR, 2.6; 95% CI, 1.5 to 4.5), a third heart sound (LR, 11; 95% CI, 4.9 to 25.0), or atrial fibrillation (LR, 3.8; 95% CI, 1.7 to 8.8).[34] An initial clinical impression of heart failure by the physician was one of the stronger clinical predictors of this diagnosis (LR, 4.4; 95% CI, 1.8 to 10.0). With the exception of PND, these same features were also predictive of heart failure when there was concomitant pulmonary disease.[34]

Severe and sudden-onset dyspnea indicates acute pulmonary edema, typically precipitated by ischemia, arrhythmia, sudden left-sided valvular regurgitation, and/or accelerated hypertension. It is important to exclude other causes, such as pulmonary embolism and pneumothorax. The extent of limitation should also be defined because functional capacity, as assessed by NYHA class, strongly and independently predicts mortality for patients with heart failure. Self-reported functional capacity and objectively measured cardiovascular performance can differ substantially. Symptoms that occur at rest may have greater predictive value for the diagnosis of heart failure compared with exertional symptoms. Orthopnea is not specific for heart failure and can occur in patients with severe ascites or emphysema. Trepopnea, which is dyspnea or discomfort in the lateral decubitus position, may also be present. Patients with heart failure prefer sleeping on their right side, and trepopnea likely accounts for the predominance of right-sided pleural effusions in this population. Paroxysmal nocturnal dyspnea is also common in heart failure. Cheyne-Stokes respirations occur when awake. The prevalence of central sleep apnea or Cheyne-Stokes respirations ranges from 20% to 62% in various heart failure studies[35] and portends an increased mortality risk. Lower extremity edema is usually pitting and becomes more prominent as the day progresses for the ambulatory patient. Clinically evident edema likely indicates a volume excess of at least 3 to 4 kg. In patients with advanced right heart failure, uncomfortable hepatomegaly and ascites may predominate. Patients with chronic heart failure often lack pulmonary rales or lower extremity edema.[36] In 50 patients referred for heart transplantation, the combination of rales, edema, and an elevated jugular venous pressure were absent in 18 of 43 subjects with a measured PA wedge pressure higher than 22 mm Hg; this combination of findings, however, had a sensitivity of 58% and a specificity of 100% for the diagnosis of heart failure.[37]

Few studies have explored the predictive values of various symptoms of heart failure. Symptoms often correlate poorly with objective evidence of cardiac dysfunction at rest. The available literature is also limited by small sample sizes, lack of proper controls, retrospective designs, variable interviewers and definitions, and referral bias. In a systematic review, orthopnea only modestly predicted increased filling pressures. Dyspnea and edema were similarly useful but were most predictive when combined with physical examination findings (S_3, tachycardia, elevated jugular venous pressure, low pulse pressure, rales, abdominojugular reflux). When combined with other findings, a total of three or more symptoms or signs predicted a more than 90% likelihood of increased filling pressures if severe LV dysfunction was not known. In contrast, if one or no findings or symptoms were present, there was less than a 10% likelihood of increased filling pressures. Several studies have used this approach for the diagnosis of heart failure.[38] The most commonly used system, the Framingham criteria, has only modest specificity (63%) and sensitivity (63%) when an ejection fraction (EF) less than 0.40 is used to define heart failure.[39]

The distinction between systolic and nonsystolic heart failure can be made at the bedside with modest accuracy. Systolic function is also more likely to be preserved when patients are female or older, and have an increased body mass index, but such findings lack adequate specificity and sensitivity to guide therapy.[40,41] Furthermore, diastolic dysfunction is not mutually exclusive of systolic dysfunction.

PHYSICAL EXAMINATION. The assessment of volume status is critical. Most patients with heart failure who require hospital admission will do so because of volume overload,[42] and failure to relieve it has negative prognostic impact. Four signs are commonly used to predict elevated filling pressures: jugular venous distention–abdominojugular reflux, presence of an S_3 and/or S_4, rales, and pedal edema. In general, diagnostic accuracy is improved by using a combination of findings rather than relying on isolated clinical findings that have limited predictive value.[38]

Some clinicians advocate a clinical assessment of the heart failure patient along two basic hemodynamic axes—volume status (dry or wet) and perfusion status (warm or cold)—which may be useful in guiding therapy.[43] There also appears to be prognostic usefulness of this approach, particularly when assessing patients at discharge following admission for heart failure. For example, advanced heart failure patients discharged with a wet or cold profile experience worse outcomes (HR, 1.5; 95% CI,1.1 to 12.1; $P = 0.017$) in comparison with those discharged warm and dry (HR, 0.9; 95% CI, 0.7 to 2.1; $P = 0.5$).[44] Specialized cardiology training may be required to achieve this level of diagnostic precision from the physical examination. For example, emergency department physicians' interobserver agreement in identifying these hemodynamic profiles was poor (k-statistic, 0.28; 95% CI, 0.01 to 0.51).[45]

Jugular Venous Pressure. The jugular venous pressure provides the readiest bedside assessment of LV filling pressure. In the Evaluation Study of Congestive Heart Failure and Pulmonary Artery Catheterization Effectiveness (ESCAPE) trial, 82% of patients (149 of 181) who had an estimated RA pressure higher than 8 mm Hg (10.5 cm H_2O) had a measured RA pressure higher than 8 mm Hg. Conversely, the same investigators were able to predict the 9 of the 11 patients with an RA pressure lower than 8 mm Hg.[44] Although the jugular venous pressure estimates RV filling pressure, it has a predictable relationship with PA wedge pressure. In 1000 consecutive patients with advanced heart failure undergoing right heart catheterization, Drazner and colleagues[46] have found that the RA pressure reliably predicts the PA wedge pressure (r = 0.64); the positive predictive value of an RA pressure higher than 10 mm Hg for a PA wedge pressure higher than 22 mm Hg was 88%. In addition, the PA systolic pressure could be estimated as twice the wedge pressure (r = 0.79). In the ESCAPE trial, an estimated RA pressure higher than 12 mm Hg and two-pillow orthopnea were the only bedside parameters (including gastrointestinal distress, fatigue, dyspnea, rales, ascites, edema, and hepatomegaly) that provided incremental value in predicting a PA wedge pressure higher than 22 mm Hg and compared favorably with brain natriuretic peptide levels.[44]

An elevated venous pressure has prognostic significance. Drazner and associates[47] have demonstrated that the presence of jugular venous distention at the time of enrollment in a large clinical heart failure trial (11% of the Studies of Left Ventricular Dysfunction [SOLVD] treatment study participants), after adjusting for other markers of disease severity, predicts heart failure hospitalizations (relative risk [RR], 1.32; 95% CI, 1.08 to 1.62), death from pump failure (RR, 1.37; 95% CI, 1.07 to 1.75), and death plus heart failure hospitalization (RR, 1.30; 95% CI, 1.11 to 1.53; **Fig. 12-11**). They extended these observations to asymptomatic individuals enrolled in the SOLVD prevention study, in which jugular venous distention was less common (1.7% of study population).[48] These findings are especially noteworthy in that the presence of jugular venous distention was reported in a "yes" or "no" format by the multiple investigators who participated in the trial. In patients presenting with dyspnea, the abdominojugular reflux is useful in predicting heart failure (LR, 6.0; 95% CI, 0.8 to 51), and suggests a PA wedge pressure higher than 15 mm Hg (LR, 6.7; 95% CI, 3.3 to 13.4).[20] The presence of jugular venous distention, either at rest or inducible, had the best combination of sensitivity (81%), specificity (80%), and predictive accuracy (81%) for elevation of the PA wedge pressure (>18 mm Hg).

THIRD AND FOURTH HEART SOUNDS. The third heart sound (S_3) predicts ejection fraction (EF) poorly because it reflects primarily diastolic rather than systolic performance. In patients with heart failure, an S_3 is equally prevalent in those with or without LV systolic dysfunction (EF cut point, 0.50).[49] The most rigorous contemporary assessment of the S_3 was conducted by Marcus and coworkers in 100 patients with various cardiovascular conditions undergoing elective cardiac catheterization.[50,51] Cardiology fellows ($n = 18$; k-statistic, 0.37; $P < 0.001$) and faculty ($n = 26$, k-statistic, 0.29; $P = 0.003$) performed better than residents ($n = 102$; no significant agreement) in the identification of a phonocardiographically confirmed S_3. Furthermore, an S_3 heard by a cardiology fellow or faculty physician predicted an increase in both LV end-diastolic pressure (LVEDP) (>15 mm Hg) and B-type natriuretic peptide (>100 pg/mL), and depressed ventricular systolic function (EF < 0.50), although sensitivities were low (32% to 52%; **Fig. 12-12**). An S_4 had comparable sensitivity (40% to 46%), but inferior specificity (72% to 80% for an S_4 versus 87% to 92% for an S_3; **Table 12-7**). In several earlier studies of heart failure patients referred for transplantation, a third heart sound was frequently heard but poorly predicted elevated filling pressures.[37] The prevalence of an S_3 in a less ill cohort with systolic dysfunction (SOLVD prevention study) was 5.1%.[48] The lack of an auscultatory S_3 cannot exclude a diagnosis of heart failure, but its presence reliably indicates ventricular dysfunction.

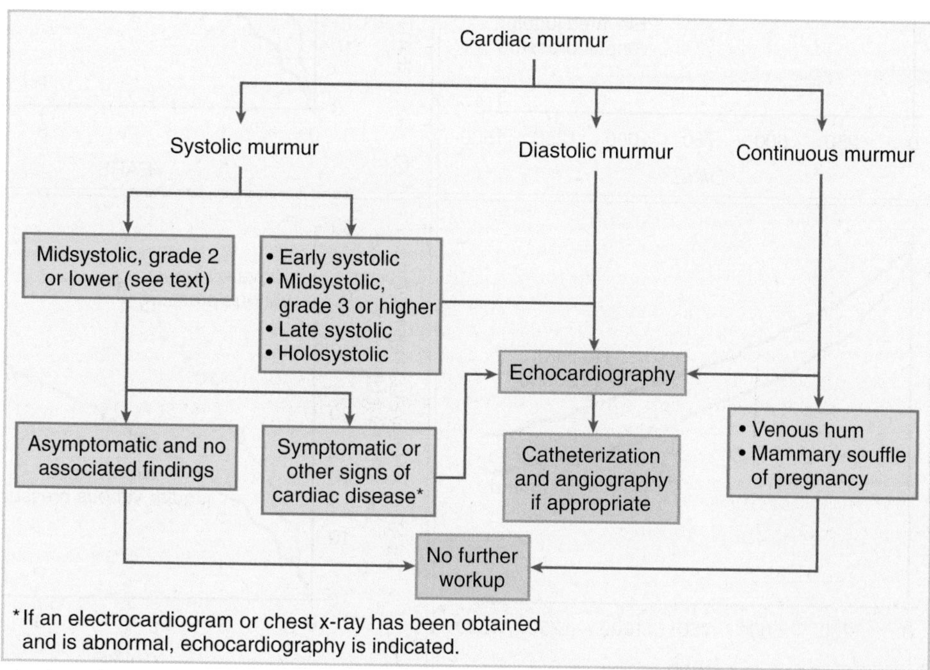

FIGURE 12-10 Strategy for the evaluation of heart murmurs. *(From Roldan CA, Shively BK, Crawford MH: Value of the cardiovascular physical examination for detecting valvular heart disease in asymptomatic subjects. Am J Cardiol 77:1327, 1996; and Bonow RO, Carabello BA, Chatterjee K, et al: ACC/AHA 2006 guidelines for the management of patients with valvular heart disease: A report of the American College of Cardiology/American Heart Association Task Force on Practice Guidelines (Writing Committee to Revise the 1998 Guidelines for the Management of Patients with Valvular Heart Disease) developed in collaboration with the Society of Cardiovascular Anesthesiologists: Endorsed by the Society for Cardiovascular Angiography and Interventions and the Society of Thoracic Surgeons. J Am Coll Cardiol 48:e1, 2006.)*

The prognostic value of an S_3 in chronic heart failure was established by the studies of Drazner and colleagues using the SOLVD treatment and prevention studies.[46-48] The investigators found that an S_3 predicted cardiovascular morbidity and mortality (see Fig. 12-11). The relative risk for heart failure hospitalization and death in patients with an S_3 in the prevention and treatment cohorts was of comparable magnitude. These observations remained significant after adjustment for markers of disease severity and were even more powerful when combined with the presence of an elevated jugular venous pressure. An S_3 also portends a higher risk of adverse outcomes in other settings, such as myocardial infarction (MI) and noncardiac surgery.

RALES AND EDEMA. In three older studies of chronic heart failure patients, approximately 75% to 80% of participants lacked rales despite elevated PA wedge pressures, presumably because of enhanced lymphatic drainage.[37] The chest radiograph similarly lacked sensitivity for increased filling pressures in these studies. Therefore, in patients with chronic LV systolic dysfunction, the absence of rales cannot exclude increased left heart filling pressures. Pedal edema is neither sensitive nor specific for the diagnosis of heart failure and has low predictive value as an isolated variable.

VALSALVA MANEUVER. The blood pressure response to the Valsalva maneuver can be measured invasively with an intra-arterial line, or noninvasively using a blood pressure cuff or commercially available devices. The Valsalva maneuver has four phases, and a normal response is sinusoidal in appearance (**Fig. 12-13**). In a normal response, Korotkoff sounds are audible only during phases I and IV, because the systolic pressure normally rises at the onset and release of the strain phase. There are two recognized abnormal responses to the Valsalva maneuver in heart failure: absence of the phase IV overshoot, and the square-wave response (**Fig. 12-14**). The absent overshoot pattern indicates decreased systolic function; the square-wave response indicates elevated filling pressures and appears to be independent of EF.[52] The responses can be quantified using the pulse amplitude ratio. This ratio compares the minimum pulse pressure at the end of the strain phase with the maximum pulse pressure at the onset of the strain phase; a higher ratio is consistent with a square-wave response.

OTHER FINDINGS. In the absence of hypertension, the pulse pressure is determined by the stroke volume and vascular stiffness and can be used to assess cardiac output. In a chronic heart failure cohort (EF, 0.18 ± 0.06), the proportional pulse pressure ([systolic − diastolic]/systolic) correlated well with cardiac index ($r = 0.82$; $P < 0.001$), stroke volume index ($r = 0.78$; $P < 0.001$), and the inverse of systemic vascular resistance ($r = 0.65$; $P < 0.001$). Using a proportional pulse pressure of 25%, the cardiac index could be predicted: if the value was lower than 25%, the cardiac index was less than 2.2 liters/min/m^2 in 91% of patients; if the value was higher than 25%, the cardiac index was higher than 2.2 liters/min/m^2 in 83% of patients.[37] However, the best assessment for systemic perfusion and cardiac index appears to be the overall clinical impression—the so-called "cold profile". Specialized heart failure clinicians' gestalt performed better than proportional pulse pressure, systolic blood pressure, cool extremities, or fatigue in predicting an invasively measured cardiac index lower than 2.3 liters/min/m^2.[44] This prediction rule has not been reported in other patient

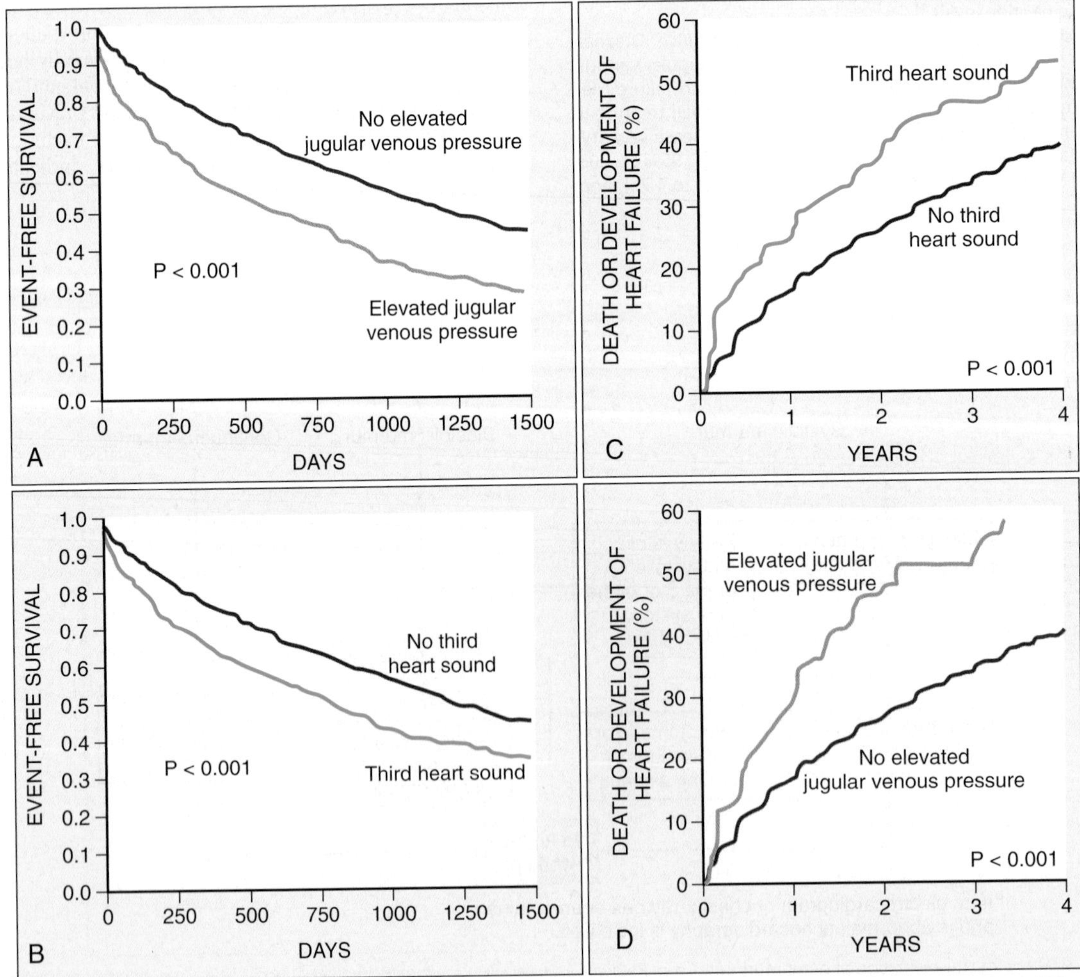

FIGURE 12-11 Kaplan-Meier plots demonstrating the prognostic value of an elevated jugular venous pressure and S_3 in symptomatic (**A** and **B**) and asymptomatic (**C** and **D**) heart failure patients with systolic dysfunction. (***A, B,*** *From Drazner MH, Rame JE, Stevenson LW, Dries DL: Prognostic importance of elevated jugular venous pressure and a third heart sound in patients with heart failure. N Engl J Med 345:574, 2001;* ***C, D*** *from Drazner MH, Rame JE, Dries DL: Third heart sound and elevated jugular venous pressure as markers of the subsequent development of heart failure in patients with asymptomatic left ventricular dysfunction. Am J Med 114:431, 2003.*)

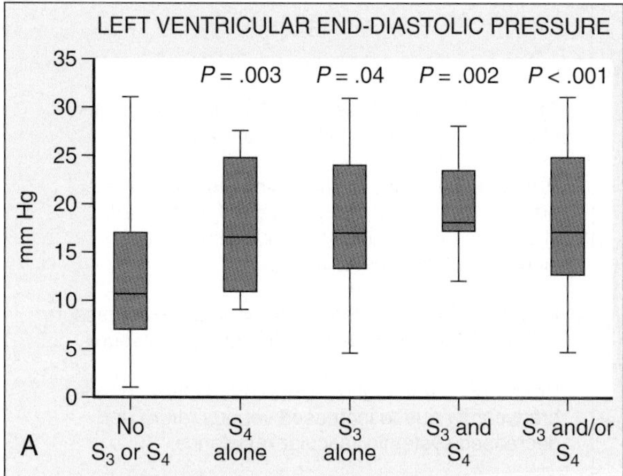

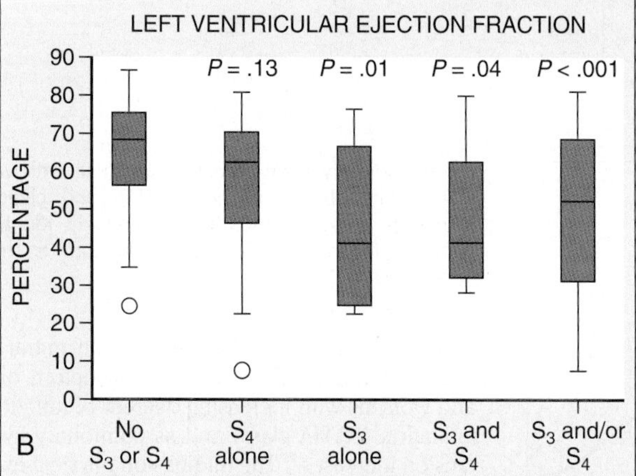

FIGURE 12-12 Median LVEDP **(A)** and LVEF **(B)** for patients based on phonocardiographic presence of a third and/or fourth heart sound. Median, interquartile ranges, error bars, and outlier values (circles) are shown; *P* values are compared with first column. *(From Marcus GM, Gerber IL, McKeown BH, et al: Association between phonocardiographic third and fourth heart sounds and objective measures of left ventricular function. JAMA 293:2238, 2005.)*

groups, in larger cohorts, or in more contemporary studies. An increase in the intensity of the pulmonic component of the second heart sound (P_2) is strongly suggestive of PA hypertension. If P_2 can be heard at the apex, the PA systolic pressure is likely to be more than 50 mm Hg. Pleural effusions are also common in heart failure and are typically right-sided, presumably because of a preference for the right lateral decubitus position during sleep in heart failure patients. Dullness to percussion is the simplest finding to elicit when identifying a pleural effusion and is superior (LR, 8.7; 95% CI, 2.2 to 33.8) to auscultatory percussion, decreased breath sounds, asymmetrical chest expansion, increased vocal resonance, crackles, or pleural friction rubs. In contrast, absence of reduced tactile vocal fremitus makes a pleural effusion less likely (negative LR, 0.21; 95% CI, 0.12 to 0.37).[53]

Valvular Heart Disease (see Chap. 66)

A careful history and physical examination can reveal much information regarding lesion severity, natural history, indications for surgery, and outcomes in patients with valvular heart disease. LV dysfunction from coronary artery disease is a common confounder. Nevertheless, the history in any patient with known or suspected valvular heart disease should rely on the use of a functional classification scheme (see Table 12-1). Currently, onset of even mild functional limitation is an indication for mechanical correction of the responsible valve lesion.[33] Valvular heart disease is most often first suspected because of a heart murmur. Cardiologists can detect systolic heart murmurs with fair reliability (kappa, 0.30 to 0.48) and can usually rule in or rule out AS, HOCM, MR, MVP, TR, and functional murmurs.[54]

However, diagnostic inaccuracies exist, and some have advocated the routine use of handheld ultrasound devices to improve detection rates.[55] Kobal and associates have compared the test characteristics of physical examination by board-certified cardiologists with handheld ultrasound performed by trained medical students.[3] Cardiologists' and students' sensitivities for the recognition of valve lesions that cause a systolic murmur were 62% and 93%, respectively. Sensitivities were 16% for cardiologists and 75% for students in the detection of lesions responsible for a diastolic murmur. In this study, overall sensitivity for cardiologists in the detection of valvular heart disease was 50% versus 89% for the students using cardiac ultrasound ($P < 0.001$).[3] Spencer and coworkers had previously reported that cardiologists missed 59% of the cardiovascular findings on physical examination.[56] Only 2 of 10 subjects with valvular heart disease detected by transesophageal echocardiography (TEE), but not by physical examination, had a clinically important valve lesion. In addition, dynamic auscultation was able to distinguish functional from pathologic murmurs with a specificity of 98% and a positive predictive value of 92%.

TABLE 12-7 Test Characteristics of Computerized Heart Sounds Detection*

SOUND	LVEDP > 15 MM HG (%)	LVEF < 50% (%)	BNP > 100 PG/ML (%)
S_3			
Sensitivity	41 (26-58)	52 (31-73)	32 (20-46)
Specificity	92 (80-98)	87 (76-94)	92 (78-98)
Positive predictive value	81 (58-95)	57 (34-78)	85 (62-97)
Negative predictive value	65 (53-76)	84 (73-92)	48 (36-60)
Accuracy	69 (58-78)	78 (68-86)	56 (45-67)
S_4			
Sensitivity	46 (31-63)	43 (23-66)	40 (26-54)
Specificity	80 (66-90)	72 (59-82)	78 (61-90)
Positive predictive value	66 (46-82)	34 (18-54)	72 (52-87)
Negative predictive value	64 (51-76)	79 (66-88)	47 (34-60)
Accuracy	64 (54-74)	64 (54-74)	55 (44-66)
S_3 and/or S_4			
Sensitivity	68 (52-82)	74 (52-90)	57 (42-70)
Specificity	73 (59-85)	64 (52-76)	72 (55-86)
Positive predictive value	68 (52-82)	42 (26-58)	75 (59-87)
Negative predictive value	73 (59-85)	88 (75-95)	53 (38-67)
Accuracy	71 (61-80)	67 (56-76)	63 (52-73)

*Data are presented as percentage (95% CI).

Modified from Marcus GM, Gerber IL, McKeown BH, et al: Association between phonocardiographic third and fourth heart sounds and objective measures of left ventricular function. JAMA 293:2238, 2005.)

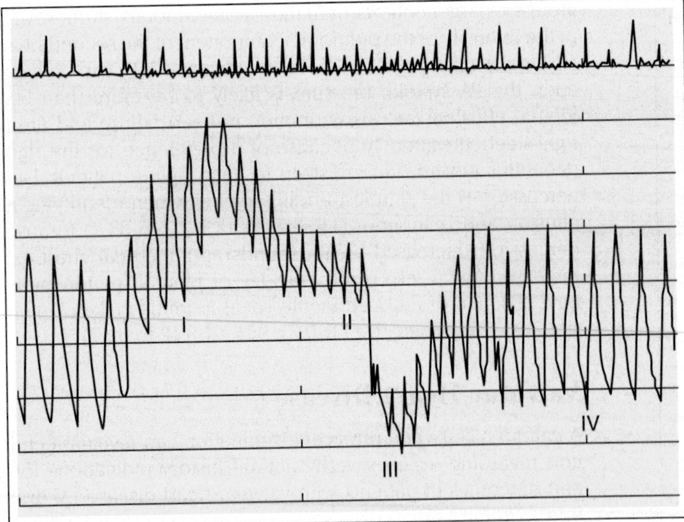

Phase I: Increase in systolic pressure with initial strain due to increase in intrathoracic pressure

Phase II: Decrease in stroke volume and pulse pressure and reflex tachycardia with continued strain due to decrease in venous return and increase in vascular resistance

Phase III: Brief, sudden decrease in systolic pressure due to sudden decrease in intrathoracic pressure

Phase IV: Overshoot of systolic pressure and reflex bradycardia due to increased venous return and decreased systemic vascular resistance

FIGURE 12-13 Normal Valsalva response. *(From Nishimura RA, Tajik AJ: The Valsalva maneuver—3 centuries later. Mayo Clin Proc 79:577, 2004.)*

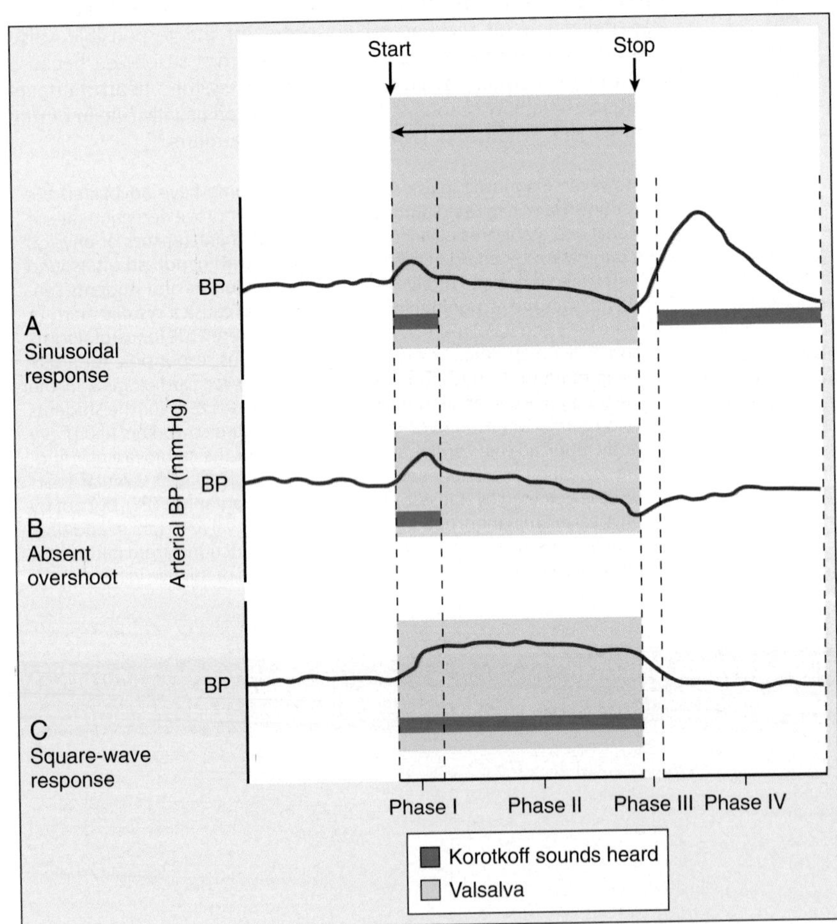

FIGURE 12-14 Abnormal Valsalva responses assessed using the pattern of Korotkoff sounds. **A,** Normal sinusoidal response with sounds intermittent during strain and release. **B,** Briefly audible sounds during initial strain phase suggest only impaired systolic function in the absence of fluid overload. **C,** Persistence of Korotkoff sounds throughout strain phase suggests elevated left ventricular filling pressures. BP = blood pressure. *(From Shamsham F, Mitchell J: Essentials of the diagnosis of heart failure. Am Fam Physician 61:1319, 2000.)*

A study of young military recruits yielded similar findings.[57] Physical examination performed by cardiology fellows or faculty could detect a pathologic murmur with 100% sensitivity, 67% specificity, 30% positive predictive value, and 100% negative predictive value, using TTE as the reference standard. Thus, a careful and complete cardiac examination can first identify asymptomatic individuals with valvular heart disease for whom TTE and clinical follow-up are indicated. It can similarly identify patients for whom further evaluation is not necessary.

MITRAL STENOSIS. In patients with mitral stenosis, survival declines following symptom onset and worsens with increasing degrees of functional limitation (NYHA class) and as pulmonary hypertension increases.[33] The findings on physical examination will vary with the chronicity of the disease, heart rate, rhythm, and cardiac output. It can be difficult to estimate the severity of the valve lesion in older patients with less pliable valves, rapid AF, or low cardiac output. Severe mitral stenosis is suggested by the following: (1) a long or holodiastolic murmur, indicating a persistent LA-left ventricle gradient; (2) a short A_2-OS interval, consistent with greater degrees of LA pressure elevation; (3) a loud P_2 (or single S_2) and/or a right ventricular lift, suggestive of pulmonary hypertension; and (4) elevated jugular venous pressure with *cv* waves, hepatomegaly, and lower extremity edema, all signs of right heart failure. Neither the intensity of the diastolic murmur nor the presence of presystolic accentuation in patients with sinus rhythm accurately reflects lesion severity.

MITRAL REGURGITATION. The symptoms associated with MR depend on its severity and time course of development. The acute severe MR that occurs with papillary muscle rupture or endocarditis usually results in sudden and profound dyspnea from pulmonary edema. Examination findings may be misleading because the LV impulse is usually neither enlarged nor displaced, and the systolic murmur is early in timing and decrescendo in configuration (see Fig. 12-9). The murmur may be loudest at the lower left sternal border or in the axilla rather than at the apex. A new systolic murmur early following MI may not be audible in a ventilated or obese patient; hence, vigilance for MR requires a high clinical index of suspicion.

Chronic severe MR is suggested by the following: (1) an enlarged, displaced, but dynamic LV apex beat; (2) an apical systolic thrill (murmur intensity grade 4 or higher); (3) a mid-diastolic filling complex comprising an S_3 and a short, low-pitched murmur, indicative of accelerated and enhanced diastolic mitral inflow; (4) wide but physiologic splitting of S_2 because of early aortic valve closure; and (5) a loud P_2 or right ventricle lift. The examiner should strive to distinguish MR from other causes of a systolic heart murmur, based on location, radiation, timing, configuration, response to bedside maneuvers, and behavior following a premature beat (see earlier). The findings in patients with MVP can vary daily, depending on left ventricular loading conditions. The combination of a nonejection click and mid-to late systolic murmur predicts MVP best, as confirmed by TTE criteria (LR, 2.43).

AORTIC STENOSIS. A slowly rising carotid upstroke (pulsus tardus), reduced carotid pulse amplitude (pulsus parvus), reduced intensity of A_2, and mid-to-late peaking of the systolic murmur help gauge the severity of AS. The intensity of the murmur depends on cardiac output and body size (peak momentum transfer)[58] and does not reliably indicate stenosis severity.

Munt and coworkers have reported that no single physical examination finding has both a high sensitivity and high specificity for the diagnosis of severe AS (valve area < 1.0 cm^2).[59] Univariate predictors of outcome (death, aortic valve replacement) included carotid upstroke delay and amplitude, systolic murmur grade and peak, and a single S_2. However, on multivariate Cox regression analysis, only carotid upstroke amplitude predicted outcome.[59] Clinical experience has established the difficulty of assessing carotid upstroke characteristics in older patients, in patients with hypertension, and in low output states. It is also challenging to distinguish the murmur of significant AS from that caused by mild or even moderate degrees of AS. Aortic sclerosis is defined by focal calcification and thickening of the leaflets without restriction of motion and a peak transaortic velocity of less than 2.5 milliseconds. The murmur can be of grade 2 or 3 intensity, but peaks in midsystole. The carotid upstroke should be normal and A_2 should be preserved, and the electrocardiogram (ECG) should lack evidence of left ventricular hypertrophy. TTE is often necessary to clarify this distinction, especially in older patients with hypertension. The findings will affect decisions regarding the frequency of clinical and TTE follow-up. Signal analysis of digitally captured cardiovascular sounds using spectral display can distinguish the murmur of aortic sclerosis from that caused by hemodynamically significant AS.[10] The differential diagnosis of a systolic murmur related to LV outflow obstruction includes valvular AS, HOCM, discrete membranous subaortic stenosis (DMSS), and supravalvular aortic stenosis (SVAS). The presence of an ejection sound indicates a valvular cause. HOCM can be distinguished on the basis of the response of the murmur to the Valsalva maneuver and standing or squatting. Patients with DMSS will commonly have a diastolic murmur indicative of AR, but not an ejection sound, whereas in patients with SVAS, the right arm blood pressure is more than 10 mm Hg higher than the left arm blood pressure.

AORTIC REGURGITATION. Patients with acute severe AR present with pulmonary edema and symptoms and signs of low forward cardiac output. Tachycardia is invariably present; systolic blood pressure is not elevated, and the pulse pressure is not widened. S_1 is soft because of premature closure of the mitral valve. As noted, both the intensity and duration of the diastolic murmur are attenuated by the rapid rise in LV diastolic pressure and diminution of the aortic–LV diastolic pressure gradient. Interestingly, in patients with acute type A aortic dissection, the presence of a diastolic murmur (heard in almost 30% of cases) does little to change the pretest probability of dissection (LR, 1.4; 95% CI, 1.0 to 2.0).[60,61] Acute severe AR is poorly tolerated and mandates surgical correction. Typical symptoms associated with chronic severe AR include dyspnea, fatigue, chest discomfort, and palpitations. As is the case for chronic MR, mild or moderate degrees of chronic AR are well tolerated and insufficient to cause symptoms, absent other cardiovascular abnormalities. The typical decrescendo diastolic blowing murmur suggests chronic AR. A midsystolic murmur indicative of augmented LV outflow is invariably heard at the base. Aortic valve stenosis may coexist. The absence of the diastolic murmur significantly reduces the likelihood of moderate or greater AR (LR, 0.1) and of mild or greater AR (LR, 0.2 to 0.3). The presence of a typical diastolic murmur increases the likelihood of moderate or greater AR (LR, 4.0 to 8.3) and of mild or greater AR (LR, 8.8 to 32.0).[60]

In addition, in patients with chronic AR, the intensity of the murmur correlates with the severity of the lesion. A grade 3 diastolic murmur has an LR of 4.5 (95% CI, 1.6 to 14.0) for distinguishing severe AR from mild or moderate AR.[60] Data regarding the significance of an Austin Flint murmur (low-pitched, mid-to-late apical diastolic murmur) are conflicting. Little evidence supports the historical claims of the importance of almost all the eponymous peripheral signs of chronic AR, of which there are at least 12.[62] The Hill sign (brachial-popliteal systolic blood pressure gradient > 20 mm Hg) may be the single exception (sensitivity, 89% for moderate to severe AR), although its supporting evidence base is also weak.[62]

TRICUSPID VALVE DISEASE. The symptoms and signs of TS are usually obscured by left-sided valve lesions. An elevated jugular venous pressure with a delayed *y* descent, abdominal ascites, and edema suggest severe TS. The auscultatory findings are difficult to appreciate but mimic those of mitral stenosis and may increase during inspiration. TR may be primary in origin (Ebstein anomaly, prolapse, endocarditis, carcinoid syndrome), but occurs more often as a secondary complication of PA hypertension, RV enlargement, and annular dilation. The symptoms of TR resemble those of TS. Severe TR is manifested by elevated jugular venous pressure with prominent *cv* waves, a parasternal lift, pulsatile liver, ascites, and edema. The intensity of the holosystolic murmur of TR increases with inspiration (Carvallo sign). Murmur intensity does not accurately reflect the severity of the valve lesion.

PULMONIC VALVE DISEASE. PS may cause exertional fatigue, dyspnea, lightheadedness, and chest discomfort (right ventricular angina). Syncope denotes severe obstruction. The midsystolic murmur of PS is best heard at the second left interspace. With severe PS, the interval between S_1 and the pulmonic ejection sound narrows, the murmur peaks in late systole and may extend beyond A_2, and P_2 becomes inaudible. Signs of significant RV pressure overload include a prominent jugular venous *a* wave and a parasternal lift. Pulmonic regurgitation (PR) occurs most commonly as a secondary manifestation of significant PA hypertension and annular dilation, but it may also reflect a primary valve disorder (e.g., congenital bicuspid valve) or develop as a complication of RV outflow tract surgery (e.g., for tetralogy of Fallot). The diastolic murmur of secondary PR (Graham Steell murmur) can be distinguished from that caused by AR on the basis of its increase in intensity with inspiration, its later onset (after A_2 and with P_2), and its slightly lower pitch. When a typical murmur is audible, the likelihood of PR increases (LR, 17), but the absence of a murmur does not exclude PR (LR, 0.9).[60] With severe PA hypertension and PR, P_2 is usually palpable and there are signs of RV pressure and volume overload (e.g., parasternal lift, prominent jugular venous *a* wave).

PROSTHETIC HEART VALVES (see Fig. 66-44). The differential diagnosis of recurrent functional limitation following valve replacement surgery includes prosthetic valve dysfunction, arrhythmia, and impairment of ventricular performance. Prosthetic valve dysfunction can occur as a result of thrombosis, pannus ingrowth, infection, and structural deterioration. Symptoms mimic those observed with native valve disease and may occur acutely or develop gradually over time. The first clue that prosthetic valve dysfunction may be present is often a change in the quality of the heart sounds or the appearance of a new murmur. The heart sounds with a bioprosthetic valve resemble those generated by native valves. A bioprosthesis in the mitral position is usually associated with a midsystolic murmur (from turbulence created by systolic flow across the valve struts as they project into the LV outflow tract) and a soft, mid-diastolic murmur that occurs with normal LV filling. The diastolic murmur is usually heard only in the left lateral decubitus position at the apex. A high-pitched or holosystolic apical murmur signifies paravalvular or bioprosthetic regurgitation that requires TEE verification and careful follow-up. Depending on the magnitude of the regurgitant volume, a diastolic murmur may be audible. Clinical deterioration can occur rapidly after the first expression of bioprosthetic failure.

A bioprosthesis in the aortic position is invariably associated with a grade 2 or 3 midsystolic murmur at the base. A diastolic murmur of AR is abnormal under any circumstance and merits additional investigation. Bioprosthetic stenosis from pannus ingrowth in the mitral or aortic position is relatively uncommon. A decrease in the intensity of the opening or closing sounds of a mechanical prosthesis, depending on its type, is a worrisome finding. A high-pitched apical systolic murmur in patients with a mechanical mitral prosthesis, or a decrescendo diastolic murmur in patients with a mechanical aortic prosthesis, indicates paravalvular regurgitation or prosthetic dysfunction. Patients with prosthetic valve thrombosis may present with signs of shock, muffled heart sounds, and soft murmurs.

Pericardial Disease (see Chap. 75)

PERICARDITIS. The typical pain of acute pericarditis starts abruptly, is sharp, and varies with position. It can radiate to the trapezius ridge. Associated fever or history of a recent viral illness may provide additional clues. A pericardial friction rub is almost 100% specific for the diagnosis, although its sensitivity is not as high, because the rub may wax and wane over the course of an acute illness, or may be difficult to elicit. This leathery or scratchy, typically two- or three-component sound may also be monophasic. It is usually necessary to auscultate the heart in several positions. The ECG may provide additional clues related to ST-segment elevations and PR-segment depression. A transthoracic echocardiogram is routinely obtained to assess the volume and appearance of any effusion and whether there are early signs of hemodynamic compromise.

PERICARDIAL TAMPONADE. Pericardial tamponade occurs when intrapericardial pressure equals or exceeds right atrial pressure. In the subacute and chronic settings, the most common symptom is dyspnea (sensitivity, 87% to 88%).[63] Typical findings on examination include tachycardia, pulsus paradoxus, elevated jugular venous pressure, and tachypnea (sensitivities, 76% to 82%).[63] Hypotension (sensitivity, 26%) and muffled heart sounds (sensitivity, 28%) are relatively insensitive indicators of tamponade. A pulsus paradoxus more than 12 mm Hg in a patient with a large pericardial effusion predicts tamponade with a sensitivity of 98%, a specificity of 83%, and a positive LR of 5.9 (95% CI, 2.4 to 14). A pulsus paradoxus more than 10 mm Hg predicts tamponade with a positive LR of 3.3 (95% CI, 1.8 to 6.3). A pulsus paradoxus less than 10 mm Hg significantly lowers the likelihood that tamponade is present (negative LR, 0.03; 95% CI, 0.01 to 0.24).[63] Echocardiography must still be performed in all patients with suspected pericardial tamponade.

CONSTRICTIVE PERICARDITIS. Constrictive pericarditis is an uncommon clinical entity that occurs in the setting of previous chest radiation, cardiac or mediastinal surgery, chronic tuberculosis, or malignancy. Dyspnea, fatigue, weight gain, abdominal bloating, and leg swelling dominate the presentation, yet a high index of suspicion is warranted. The diagnosis is most often first suspected after inspection of the jugular venous pressure and waveforms, with elevation and inscription of the classic M or W contour caused by prominent *x* and *y* descents and a Kussmaul sign. Evidence of pleural effusions (right > left) and ascites can often be found. Rarely, a pericardial knock is audible. Distinction from restrictive cardiomyopathy is often not possible on the basis of the history and physical examination alone.

Future Perspectives

The history and physical examination will not lose their important roles in the assessment of the patient with known or suspected cardiovascular disease. Increasing concerns regarding the escalating costs of medical care, driven in large part by expenses related to imaging, may reinforce the value of these time-honored traditions. However, they will become more relevant only in relation to their proven value to provide incremental information regarding diagnosis, prognosis, and response to therapy. Additional studies are needed to establish the accuracy and performance characteristics of the history and examination, with the same rigor applied to other diagnostic testing. For example, a prospective study to assess the comparative effectiveness of the physical examination versus routine surveillance echocardiography in the longitudinal follow-up of stable patients with prosthetic heart valves would help to determine the incremental benefit of imaging for clinical decision making in this setting. Recognition of the need to reestablish the mentored patient evaluation as a dedicated component of clinician training programs, along with mechanisms to allow practice, repetition, and feedback, are essential. The routine incorporation of handheld Doppler echocardiography and/or spectral display of the heart sounds may improve learner performance and bedside accuracy.

ACKNOWLEDGMENT

The authors wish to acknowledge the previous contributions of Drs. Eugene Braunwald, Joseph Perloff, Robert O'Rourke, and James A. Shaver, which have laid the foundation for this chapter.

REFERENCES

General Physical Examination

1. Laukkanen A, Ikaheimo M, Luukinen H: Practices of clinical examination of heart failure patients in primary health care. Cent Eur J Public Health 14:86, 2006.
2. Vukanovic-Criley JM, Criley S, Warde CM, et al: Competency in cardiac examination skills in medical students, trainees, physicians, and faculty: A multicenter study. Arch Intern Med 166:610, 2006.
3. Kobal SL, Trento L, Baharami S, et al: Comparison of effectiveness of hand-carried ultrasound to bedside cardiovascular physical examination. Am J Cardiol 96:1002, 2005.
4. Decara JM, Kirkpatrick JN, Spencer KT, et al: Use of hand-carried ultrasound devices to augment the accuracy of medical students' bedside cardiac diagnoses. J Am Soc Echocardiogr 18:2573, 2005.
5. Hoyte H, Jensen T, Gjesdal K: Cardiac auscultation training of medical students: A comparison of electronic sensor-based and acoustic stethoscopes. BMC Med Educ 5:14, 2005.
6. Barrett MJ, Lacey CS, Sekara AE, et al: Mastering cardiac murmurs: The power of repetition. Chest 126:470, 2004.
7. March SK, Bedynek JL Jr, Chizner MA: Teaching cardiac auscultation: Effectiveness of a patient-centered teaching conference on improving cardiac auscultatory skills. Mayo Clin Proc 80:1443, 2005.
8. Wiviott SD, Morrow DA, Frederick PD, et al: Performance of the thrombolysis in myocardial infarction risk index in the National Registry of Myocardial Infarction-3 and -4: A simple index that predicts mortality in ST-segment elevation myocardial infarction. J Am Coll Cardiol 44:783, 2004.
9. Wiviott SD, Morrow DA, Frederick PD, et al: Application of the thrombolysis in myocardial infarction risk index in non-ST-segment elevation myocardial infarction: Evaluation of patients in the National Registry of Myocardial Infarction. J Am Coll Cardiol 47:1553, 2006.
10. Tavel ME: Cardiac auscultation: A glorious past—and it does have a future! Circulation 113:1255, 2006.
11. Swap CJ, Nagurney JT: Value and limitations of chest pain history in the evaluation of patients with suspected acute coronary syndromes. JAMA 294:2623, 2005.
12. Thavendiranathan P, Bagai A, Khoo C, et al: Does this patient with palpitations have a cardiac arrhythmia? JAMA 302:2135, 2009.
13. The Criteria Committee of the New York Heart Association: Nomenclature and Criteria for Diagnosis. 9th ed. Boston, Little Brown, 1994.
14. Campeau L: Grading of angina pectoris. Circulation 54:522, 1975.
15. de Koning L, Merchant AT, Pogue J, Anand SS: Waist circumference and waist to hip ratio as predictors of cardiovascular events: Meta-regression analysis of prospective studies. Eur Heart J 28:850-856, 2007.
16. Redberg RF, Benjamin EJ, Bittner V, et al: ACCF/AHA 2009 performance measures for primary prevention of cardiovascular disease in adults: A report of the American College of Cardiology Foundation/American Heart Association task force on performance measures (writing committee to develop performance measures for primary prevention of cardiovascular disease): Developed in collaboration with the American Academy of Family Physicians; American Association of Cardiovascular and Pulmonary Rehabilitation; and Preventive Cardiovascular Nurses Association: endorsed by the American College of Preventive Medicine, American College of Sports Medicine, and Society for Women's Health Research. Circulation 120:1296, 2009.
17. von Beckerath O, Gaa J, von Mohrenfels CW, von Beckerath N: Intermittent claudication in a 28-year-old man with pseudoxanthoma elasticum. Circulation 118:102, 2008.

Assessment of Venous Pressure

18. Seth R, Magner P, Matziner F, vanWalraven C: How far is the sternal angle from the mid-right atrium? J Gen Intern Med 17:852, 2002.
19. Ramana RK, Senegala T, Lichtenberg R: A new angle on the Angle of Louis. Congest Heart Fail 12:196, 2006.
20. Wiese J: The abdominojugular reflux sign. Am J Med 109:59, 2000.

Assessment of Arterial Pulses and Blood Pressure

21. Pickering TG, Hall JE, Appel LJ, et al: Recommendations for blood pressure measurement in humans and experimental animals: Part 1: Blood pressure measurement in humans: A statement for professionals from the Subcommittee of Professional and Public Education of the American Heart Association Council on High Blood Pressure Research. Hypertension 45:142, 2005.
22. Lane D, Beevers M, Barnes N, et al: Inter-arm differences in blood pressure: When are they clinically significant? J Hypertens 20:1089, 2002.
23. Ogedegbe G, Pickering TG, Clemow L, et al: The misdiagnosis of hypertension: The role of patient anxiety. Arch Intern Med 168:2459, 2008.
24. Williams B, Lacy PS, Thom SM, et al: Differential impact of blood pressure-lowering drugs on central aortic pressure and clinical outcomes: Principal results of the Conduit Artery Function Evaluation (CAFE) study. Circulation 113:1213, 2006.
25. Khan NA, Rahim SA, Anand SS, et al: Does the clinical examination predict lower extremity peripheral arterial disease? JAMA 295:536, 2006.

26. Lee JC, Atwood JE, Lee HJ, et al: Association of pulsus paradoxus with obesity in normal volunteers. J Am Coll Cardiol 47:1907, 2006.
27. Sagrista-Sauleda J, Angel J, Sambola A, et al: Low-pressure cardiac tamponade: Clinical and hemodynamic profile. Circulation 114:945, 2006.
28. Weiss JN, Karma A, Shiferaw Y, et al: From pulsus to pulseless: The saga of cardiac alternans. Circ Res 98:1244, 2006.
29. Magyar MT, Nam EM, Csiba L, et al: Carotid artery auscultation—anachronism or useful screening procedure? Neurol Res 24:705, 2002.
30. Parameswaran GI, Brand K, Dolan J: Pulse oximetry as a potential screening tool for lower extremity arterial disease in asymptomatic patients with diabetes mellitus. Arch Intern Med 165: 442, 2005.
31. Michaels AD, Viswanathan MN, Jordan MV, Chatterjee K: Computerized acoustic cardiographic insights into the pericardial knock in constrictive pericarditis. Clin Cardiol 30:450, 2007.
32. Sharif D, Radzievsky A, Rosenschein U: Recurrent pericardial constriction: Vibrations of the knock, the calcific shield, and the evoked constrictive physiology. Circulation 118:1685, 2008.
33. Bonow RO, Carabello BA, Chatterjee K, et al: ACC/AHA 2006 guidelines for the management of patients with valvular heart disease: A report of the American College of Cardiology/American Heart Association Task Force on Practice Guidelines (Writing Committee to Revise the 1998 Guidelines for the Management of Patients with Valvular Heart Disease) developed in collaboration with the Society of Cardiovascular Anesthesiologists endorsed by the Society for Cardiovascular Angiography and Interventions and the Society of Thoracic Surgeons. J Am Coll Cardiol 48:e1, 2006.

Assessment of Heart Failure

34. Wang CS, Fitzgerald JM, Schulzer M, et al: Does this dyspneic patient in the emergency department have congestive heart failure? JAMA 294:1944, 2005.
35. Givertz MM, Fang JC: Diastolic heart failure. *In* Baughman KL, Baumgartner WA (eds): Treatment of Advanced Heart Disease. New York, Taylor and Francis, 2006, pp 227-246.
36. Hunt SA, Abraham WT, Chin MH, et al: ACC/AHA 2005 Guideline Update for the Diagnosis and Management of Chronic Heart Failure in the Adult: A report of the American College of Cardiology/American Heart Association Task Force on Practice Guidelines (Writing Committee to Update the 2001 Guidelines for the Evaluation and Management of Heart Failure): Developed in collaboration with the American College of Chest Physicians and the International Society for Heart and Lung Transplantation: Endorsed by the Heart Rhythm Society. Circulation 112:e154, 2005.
37. Stevenson LW, Perloff JK: The limited reliability of physical signs for estimating hemodynamics in chronic heart failure. JAMA 261:884, 1989.
38. Rohde LE, Beck-da-Silva L, Goldraich L, et al: Reliability and prognostic value of traditional signs and symptoms in outpatients with congestive heart failure. Can J Cardiol 20:697, 2004.
39. Marantz PR, Tobin JN, Wassertheil-Smoller S, et al: The relationship between left ventricular systolic function and congestive heart failure diagnosed by clinical criteria. Circulation 77:607, 1988.
40. Thomas JT, Kelly RF, Thomas SJ, et al: Utility of history, physical examination, electrocardiogram, and chest radiograph for differentiating normal from decreased systolic function in patients with heart failure. Am J Med 112:437, 2002.
41. Smith GL, Masoudi FA, Vaccarino V, et al: Outcomes in heart failure patients with preserved ejection fraction: Mortality, readmission, and functional decline. J Am Coll Cardiol 41:1510, 2003.
42. Fonarow GC, Adams KF Jr, Abraham WT, et al: Risk stratification for in-hospital mortality in acutely decompensated heart failure: Classification and regression tree analysis. JAMA 293:572, 2005.
43. Nohria A, Tsang SW, Fang JC, et al: Clinical assessment identifies hemodynamic profiles that predict outcomes in patients admitted with heart failure. J Am Coll Cardiol 41:1797, 2003.
44. Drazner MH, Hellkamp AS, Leier CV, et al: Value of clinician assessment of hemodynamics in advanced heart failure: The ESCAPE trial. Circ Heart Fail 1:170, 2008.
45. Chaudhry A, Singer AJ, Chohan J, et al: Inter-rater reliability of hemodynamic profiling of patients with heart failure in the ED. Am J Emerg Med 26:196, 2008.
46. Drazner MH, Hamilton MA, Fonarow G, et al: Relationship between right and left-sided filling pressures in 1000 patients with advanced heart failure. J Heart Lung Transplant 18:1126, 1999.
47. Drazner MH, Rame JE, Stevenson LW, Dries DL: Prognostic importance of elevated jugular venous pressure and a third heart sound in patients with heart failure. N Engl J Med 345:574, 2001.
48. Drazner MH, Rame JE, Dries DL: Third heart sound and elevated jugular venous pressure as markers of the subsequent development of heart failure in patients with asymptomatic left ventricular dysfunction. Am J Med 114:431, 2003.
49. Malki Q, Sharma ND, Afzal A, et al: Clinical presentation, hospital length of stay, and readmission rate in patients with heart failure with preserved and decreased left ventricular systolic function. Clin Cardiol 25:149, 2002.
50. Marcus GM, Gerber IL, McKeown BH, et al: Association between phonocardiographic third and fourth heart sounds and objective measures of left ventricular function. JAMA 293:2238, 2005.
51. Marcus GM, Vessey J, Jordan MV, et al: Relationship between accurate auscultation of a clinically useful third heart sound and level of experience. Arch Intern Med 166:617, 2006.
52. Felker GM, Cuculich PS, Gheorghiade M: The Valsalva maneuver: A bedside "biomarker" for heart failure. Am J Med 119:117, 2006.
53. Wong CL, Holroyd-Leduc J, Strauss SE: Does this patient have a pleural effusion. JAMA 301:309, 2009.

Assessment of Valvular Heart Disease

54. Attenhofer Jost CH, Turina J, Mayer K, et al: Echocardiography in the evaluation of systolic murmurs of unknown cause. Am J Med 108:614, 2000.
55. Vourvouri EC, Poldermans D, Deckers JW, et al: Evaluation of a hand-carried cardiac ultrasound device in an outpatient cardiology clinic. Heart 91:171, 2005.
56. Spencer KT, Anderson AS, Bharqava A, et al: Physician-performed point-of-care echocardiography using a laptop platform compared with physical examination in the cardiovascular patient. J Am Coll Cardiol 37:2013, 2001.
57. Shry EA, Smithers MA, Mascette AM: Auscultation versus echocardiography in a healthy population with precordial murmur. Am J Cardiol 87:1428, 2001.
58. Kuperstein R, Feinberg MS, Eldar M, Schwammenthal E: Physical determinants of systolic murmur intensity in aortic stenosis. Am J Cardiol 95:774, 2005.
59. Munt B, Legget ME, Kraft CD, et al: Physical examination in valvular aortic stenosis: Correlation with stenosis severity and prediction of clinical outcome. Am Heart J 137:298, 1999.
60. Choudhry NK, Etchells EE: The rational clinical examination. Does this patient have aortic regurgitation? JAMA 281:2231, 1999.
61. Klompas M: Does this patient have an acute thoracic aortic dissection? JAMA 287:2262, 2002.
62. Babu AN, Kymes SM, Carpenter Fryer SM: Eponyms and the diagnosis of aortic regurgitation: What says the evidence? Ann Intern Med 138:736, 2003.

Pericardial Tamponade

63. Roy CL, Minor MA, Brookhart MA, Choudry NK: Does this patient with a pericardial effusion have cardiac tamponade? JAMA 297:1810, 2007.

CHAPTER 13 Electrocardiography

David M. Mirvis and Ary L. Goldberger

The technology and the clinical usefulness of the electrocardiogram (ECG) have continuously advanced over the past two centuries.[1,2] Early demonstrations of the heart's electrical activity during the last half of the 19th century were closely followed by direct recordings of cardiac potentials by Waller in 1887. Invention of the string galvanometer by Einthoven in 1901 provided a direct method for registering electrical activity of the heart. By 1910, use of the string galvanometer had emerged from the research laboratory into the clinic. Subsequently, the ECG became the first and most common bioelectric signal to be computer-processed and the most commonly used cardiac diagnostic test.

Recent advances have extended the importance of the ECG. It is a vital test for determining the presence and severity of acute myocardial ischemia, localizing sites of origin and pathways of tachyarrhythmias, assessing therapeutic options for patients with heart failure, and identifying and evaluating patients with genetic diseases who are prone to arrhythmias. Achievements in physiology and technology, as discussed later in this chapter, have expanded the possibilities of extracting more information about the heart's electrical activity from the ECG that will extend these clinical applications further.

It is the goal of this chapter to review the physiologic bases for electrocardiographic patterns in health and in disease, outline the criteria for the most common electrocardiographic diagnoses in adults, describe critical aspects of the clinical application of the ECG, and suggest future opportunities for the clinical practice of electrocardiography.

FUNDAMENTAL PRINCIPLES

The ECG is the final outcome of a complex series of physiologic and technologic processes. First, transmembrane ionic currents are generated by ion fluxes across cell membranes and between adjacent cells. These currents are synchronized by cardiac activation and recovery sequences to generate a cardiac electrical field in and around the heart that varies with time during the cardiac cycle. This electrical field passes through numerous other structures, including the lungs, blood, and skeletal muscle, that perturb the cardiac electrical field.

The currents reaching the skin are then detected by electrodes placed in specific locations on the extremities and torso that are configured to produce leads. The outputs of these leads are amplified, filtered, and displayed by a variety of devices to produce an electrocardiographic recording. In computerized systems, these signals are digitized, stored, and processed by pattern recognition software. Diagnostic criteria are then applied, either manually or with the aid of a computer, to produce an interpretation.

Genesis of Cardiac Electrical Fields

IONIC CURRENTS AND CARDIAC ELECTRICAL FIELD GENERATION DURING ACTIVATION. Transmembrane ionic currents (see Chap. 35) are ultimately responsible for the potentials that are recorded as an ECG. Current may be modeled as being carried by positively charged or negatively charged ions. A positive current moving in one direction is equivalent to a negative current of equal strength moving in the opposite direction. Through a purely arbitrary choice, electrophysiological currents are considered to be the movement of positive charge.

The process of generating the cardiac electrical field during activation is illustrated in **Figure 13-1**. A single cardiac fiber, 20 mm in length, is activated by a stimulus applied to its left-most margin (see Fig. 13-1A). Transmembrane potentials (V_m) are recorded as the difference between intracellular and extracellular potentials (Φ_i and Φ_e, respectively). Figure 13-1B plots V_m along the length of the fiber at the instant (t_0) at which activation has reached the point designated as X_0. As each site is activated, it undergoes depolarization, and the polarity of the transmembrane potential converts from negative to positive, as represented in the typical cardiac action potential. Thus, sites to the left of the point X_0 that have already undergone excitation have positive transmembrane potentials (i.e., the inside of the cell is positive relative to the outside of the cell), whereas those to the right of X_0 that remain in a resting state have negative transmembrane potentials. Near the site undergoing activation (site X_0), the potentials reverse polarity over a short distance.

Figure 13-1C displays the direction and magnitude of transmembrane currents (I_m) along the fiber at the instant (t_0) at which excitation has reached site X_0. Current flow is inwardly directed in fiber regions that have just undergone activation (i.e., to the left of point X_0) and outwardly directed in neighboring zones still at rest (i.e., to the right of X_0). Sites of outward current flow are current sources and those with inward current flow are current sinks. As depicted in the figure, current flow is most intense in each direction near the site of activation, X_0.

Because the border between inwardly and outwardly directed currents is relatively sharp, these currents may be visualized as if they were limited to the sites of maximal current flow, as depicted in Figure 13-1D, and separated by a distance, d, that is usually 1.0 mm or less. As activation proceeds along the fiber, the source-sink pair moves to the right at the speed of propagation in the fiber.

THE CARDIAC DIPOLE. Two point sources of equal strength but of opposite polarity located very near each other, such as the current source and current sink illustrated in Figure 13-1D, can be represented as a current dipole. Thus, activation of a fiber can be modeled as a current dipole that moves in the direction of activation.

Such a dipole is fully characterized by three parameters—strength or dipole moment, location, and orientation. In this case, the location of the dipole is the site undergoing activation (point X_0), and its orientation is in the direction of activation (i.e., from left to right along the fiber in Fig. 13-1). Dipole moment is proportional to the rate of change of intracellular potential—that is, action potential shape.

A current dipole produces a characteristic potential field with positive potentials projected ahead of it and negative potentials projected behind it. The actual potential recorded at any site within this field is directly proportional to the dipole moment, inversely proportional to the square of the distance from the dipole to the recording site, and directly proportional to the cosine of the angle between the axis of the dipole and a line drawn from the dipole to the recording site.

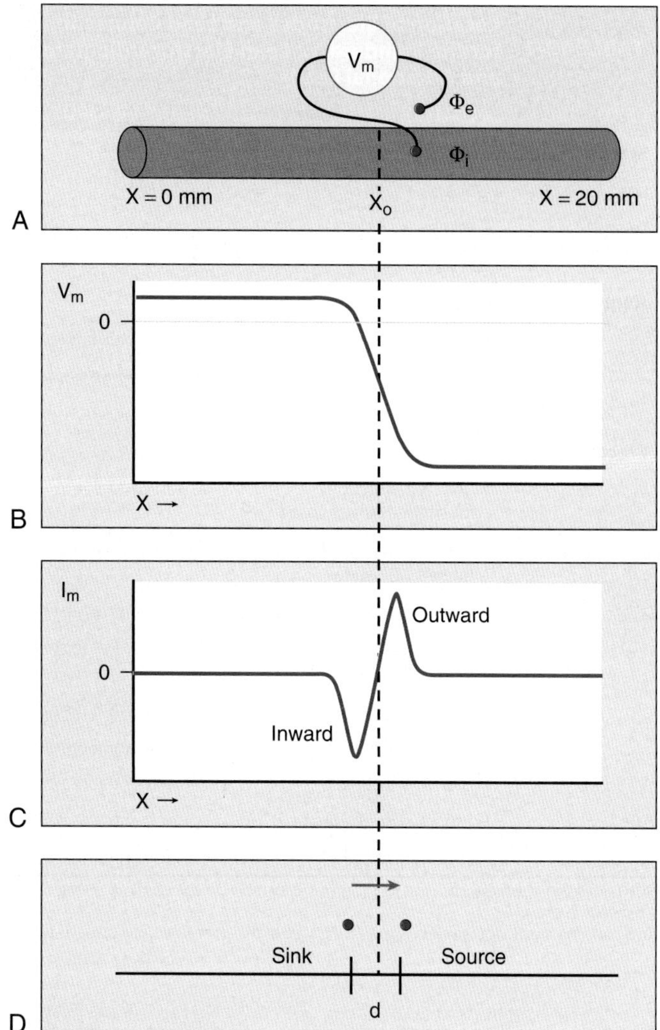

FIGURE 13-1 Example of potentials and currents generated by the activation of a single (e.g., ventricular) cardiac fiber. **A,** Intracellular (Φ_i) and extracellular (Φ_e) potentials are recorded with a voltmeter (V_m) from a fiber 20 mm in length. The fiber is stimulated at site X = 0 mm, and propagation proceeds from left to right. **B,** Plot of transmembrane potential (V_m) at the instant in time at which activation reaches point X_0 as a function of the length of the fiber. Positive potentials are recorded from activated tissue to the left of site X_0, and negative ones are registered from not yet excited areas to the right of site X_0. **C,** Membrane current (I_m) flows along the length of the fiber at time t_0. The outward current is the depolarizing current that propagates ahead of activation site X_0, whereas an inward one flows behind site X_0. **D,** Representation of the sites of peak inward and outward current flow as two point sources, a sink (at the site of peak inward current flow) and a source (at the site of peak outward current flow) separated by distance d. The dipole produced by the source-sink pair is represented by the arrow. *(Modified from Barr RC: Genesis of the electrocardiogram. In MacFarlane PW, Lawrie TDV [eds]: Comprehensive Electrocardiography. New York, Pergamon Press, 1989.)*

Cardiac Wave Fronts. This example from one cardiac fiber can be generalized to the more realistic case in which multiple adjacent fibers are activated in synchrony. Activation of each fiber creates a dipole oriented in the direction of activation to produce an activation front. All the individual dipoles in this wave front can be represented by a single dipole with a strength and orientation equal to the (vector) sum of all the simultaneously active component dipoles. Thus, an activation front propagating through the heart can be represented by a single dipole that projects positive potentials ahead of it and negative potentials behind it.

This relationship among the direction of movement of an activation wave front, the orientation of the current dipole, and the polarity of potentials is critical in electrocardiography. An electrode senses positive potentials when an activation front is moving toward it and negative potentials when the activation front is moving away from it.

Solid Angle Theorem. One important and common method of estimating the potentials projected to some point away from an activation front is an application of the solid angle theorem. A solid angle is a geometric measure of the size of a region when viewed from a distant site. It equals the area on the surface of a sphere of unit radius constructed around an electrode that is cut by lines drawn from the recording electrode to all points around the boundary of the region of interest. This region may be a wave front, zone of infarction, or any other region in the heart.

The solid angle theorem states that the potential recorded by a remote electrode (Φ) is defined by the following equation:

$$\Phi = (\Omega/4\pi)(V_{m2} - V_{m1})K$$

where Ω is the solid angle, $V_{m2} - V_{m1}$ is the potential difference across the boundary under study, and K is a constant reflecting differences in conductivity.

This equation suggests that the recorded potential equals the product of two factors. First, the solid angle reflects spatial parameters, such as the size of the boundary of the region under study and the distance from the electrode to that boundary. The potential will increase as the boundary size increases and as the distance to the electrode decreases. A second set of parameters includes nonspatial factors, such as the potential difference across the surface (i.e., $V_{m2} - V_{m1}$) and intracellular and extracellular conductivity (i.e., K). Nonspatial effects include, as one example, myocardial ischemia which changes transmembrane action potential shapes and alters conductivity.

The dipole model, although useful in describing cardiac fields and understanding clinical electrocardiography, has significant theoretical limitations. These limits result primarily from the inability of a single dipole to represent more than one wave front that is propagating through the heart at any one instant accurately. As will be discussed, during much of the time of ventricular excitation, more than one wave front is present. Other approaches, such as the direct estimation of epicardial potentials from body surface recordings,[3] represent other important, albeit more complex, approaches.

Cardiac Electrical Field Generation During Ventricular Recovery. The cardiac electrical field during recovery (phases 1 through 3 of the action potential) is generated by forces analogous to those described during activation. However, recovery differs in several important ways from activation. First, intercellular potential differences and, hence, the directions of current flow during recovery are the opposite of those described for activation. As a cell undergoes recovery, its intracellular potential becomes progressively more negative. For two adjacent cells, the intracellular potential of the cell whose recovery has progressed further is more negative than that of the adjacent, less recovered cell. Intracellular currents then flow from the less recovered toward the more recovered cell. An equivalent dipole can then be constructed for recovery, just as for activation. Its orientation points from less to more recovered cells—that is, the opposite to that of a dipole during activation.

The moment, or strength, of the recovery dipole also differs from that of the activation dipole. As noted, the strength of the activation dipole is proportional to the rate of change in transmembrane potential. Rates of change in potential during the recovery phases of the action potential are considerably slower than during activation, so that the dipole moment at any one instant during recovery is less than during activation.

A third difference between activation and recovery is the rate of movement of the activation and recovery dipoles. Activation is rapid (as fast as 1 msec in duration) and occurs over only a small distance along the fiber. Recovery, in contrast, lasts 100 msec or longer and occurs simultaneously over extensive portions of the fiber.

These features result in characteristic electrocardiographic differences between activation and recovery patterns. All other factors being equal (an assumption that is often not true, as described later), electrocardiographic waveforms generated during recovery of a linear fiber with uniform recovery properties may be expected to be of opposite polarity, lower amplitude, and longer duration than those generated by activation. As will be described, these features are explicitly demonstrated in the clinical ECG.

Role of Transmission Factors. These activation and recovery fields exist within a complex three-dimensional physical environment (the volume conductor) that modifies the cardiac electrical field in significant ways. The contents of the volume conductor are called transmission factors to emphasize their effects on transmission of the cardiac electrical field throughout the body. They may be grouped into four broad categories—cellular factors, cardiac factors, extracardiac factors, and physical factors.

Cellular factors determine the intensity of current fluxes that result from local transmembrane potential gradients. These include intracellular and extracellular resistances and the concentrations of relevant ions, especially the sodium ion. Lower ion concentrations, for example, reduce the intensity of current flow and reduce extracellular potentials.

Cardiac factors affect the relationship of one cardiac cell to another. The following are two major factors: (1) anisotropy, the property of cardiac tissue that results in greater current flow and more rapid propagation along the length of a fiber than across its width; and (2) the presence of connective tissue between cardiac fibers that disrupts effective electrical coupling of adjacent fibers. Recording electrodes oriented along the long axis of a cardiac fiber register higher potentials than electrodes oriented perpendicular to the long axis. Waveforms recorded from fibers with little or no intervening connective tissue are narrow in width and smooth in contour, whereas those recorded from tissues with abnormal fibrosis are prolonged, with prominent notching.

Extracardiac factors encompass all the tissues and structures that lie between the activation region and the body surface, including the ventricular walls, intracardiac blood, lungs, skeletal muscle, subcutaneous fat, and skin. These tissues alter the cardiac field because of differences in the electrical resistivity of adjacent tissues—that is, the presence of electrical inhomogeneities within the torso. For example, intracardiac blood has much lower resistivity (162 Ω cm) than the lungs (2150 Ω cm). When the cardiac field encounters the boundary between two tissues with differing resistivity, the field is altered. Differences in torso inhomogeneities can have significant effects on ECG potentials, especially when the differences are exaggerated as in patients with congestive heart failure.[4]

Other transmission factors reflect basic laws of physics. Changes in the distance between the heart and recording electrode reduce potential magnitudes in proportion to the square of the distance. A related factor is the eccentricity of the heart within the chest. The right ventricle and anteroseptal aspect of the left ventricle are located closer to the anterior chest wall than other parts of the left ventricle and atria. Therefore, electrocardiographic potentials will be higher on the anterior than on the posterior chest, and waveforms projected from the anterior left ventricle to the chest wall will be greater than those generated by posterior regions.

An additional physical factor affecting the recording of cardiac signals is cancellation. This results when two or more wave fronts that are simultaneously active during activation or repolarization have different orientations. The vectorial components of the wave fronts that are oriented in opposite directions cancel each other when viewed from remote electrode positions. The magnitude of this effect is substantial. During both the QRS and ST-T waves, as much as 90% of cardiac activity is obscured by cancellation.

As a result of all these factors, body surface potentials have an amplitude of only 1% of the amplitude of transmembrane potentials, are smoothed in detail so that surface potentials have only a general spatial relationship to the underlying cardiac events, preferentially reflect electrical activity in some cardiac regions over others, and reflect only limited amounts of total cardiac electrical activity.

Recording Electrodes and Leads

Potentials generated by the cardiac electrical generator and modified by transmission factors are sensed by electrodes placed on the torso that are configured to form various types of leads.

ELECTRODE CHARACTERISTICS. Electrocardiographic potentials are affected by the properties of the dermal and epidermal layers of the skin, the electrolytic paste applied to the skin, the electrode itself, and the mechanical contact between the electrode and skin. The net effect is equivalent to a complex electrical circuit that includes resistances, capacitances, and voltages produced by these different components and the interfaces between them.

ELECTROCARDIOGRAPHIC LEAD SYSTEMS. Electrodes are connected to form leads. The electrocardiographic leads are bipolar leads that record the potential difference between two electrodes. One electrode is designated as the positive input. The potential at the other, or negative, electrode is subtracted from the potential at the positive electrode to yield the bipolar potential. The actual potential at either electrode is not known, and only the difference between them is recorded.

In some cases, as described later, multiple electrodes are electrically connected together to represent the negative member of the bipolar pair. This electrode network or compound electrode is referred to as a reference electrode. The lead then records the potential difference between a single electrode serving as the positive input, the exploring electrode, and the potential in the reference electrode.

TABLE 13-1 Location of Electrodes and Lead Connections for the Standard 12-Lead Electrocardiogram and Additional Leads

LEAD TYPE	POSITIVE INPUT	NEGATIVE INPUT
Standard Limb Leads		
Lead I	Left arm	Right arm
Lead II	Left leg	Right arm
Lead III	Left leg	Left arm
Augmented Limb Leads		
aVR	Right arm	Left arm plus left leg
aVL	Left arm	Right arm plus left leg
aVF	Left leg	Left arm plus right arm
Precordial Leads*		
V_1	Right sternal margin, fourth intercostal space	Wilson central terminal
V_2	Left sternal margin, fourth intercostal space	Wilson central terminal
V_3	Midway between V_2 and V_4	Wilson central terminal
V_4	Left midclavicular line, 5th intercostal space	Wilson central terminal
V_5	Left anterior axillary line†	Wilson central terminal
V_6	Left midaxillary line†	Wilson central terminal
V_7	Posterior axillary line†	Wilson central terminal
V_8	Posterior scapular line†	Wilson central terminal
V_9	Left border of spine†	Wilson central terminal

*The right-sided precordial leads V_3R to V_6R are taken in mirror image positions on the right side of the chest.

†The exploring electrodes for leads V_5 to V_9 are placed at the same horizontal plane as the electrode for V_4.

The standard clinical ECG includes recordings from 12 leads. These 12 leads include three standard limb leads (leads I, II, and III), six precordial leads (leads V_1 through V_6), and three augmented limb leads (leads aVR, aVL, and aVF). Definitions of the positive and negative inputs for each lead are listed in **Table 13-1**.

STANDARD LIMB LEADS. The standard limb leads record the potential differences between two limbs, as detailed in Table 13-1 and illustrated in **Figure 13-2** (top panel). Lead I represents the potential difference between the left arm (positive electrode) and right arm (negative electrode), lead II displays the potential difference between the left leg (positive electrode) and right arm (negative electrode), and lead III represents the potential difference between the left leg (positive electrode) and left arm (negative electrode). The electrode on the right leg serves as an electronic reference that reduces noise and is not included in these lead configurations.

The electrical connections for these leads are such that the leads form a triangle, known as the Einthoven triangle. In it, the potential in lead II equals the sum of potentials sensed in leads I and III, as shown by this equation:

$$\mathrm{I} + \mathrm{III} = \mathrm{II}$$

This relationship is known as Einthoven's law or Einthoven's equation.

PRECORDIAL LEADS AND THE WILSON CENTRAL TERMINAL. The precordial leads register the potential at each of the six designated torso sites (see Fig. 13-2, bottom, left panel) in relation to a reference potential.* To do so, an

*The precordial electrodes and the augmented limb leads (see later) are often referred to as "unipolar" leads. Unipolar leads register the potential at one site in relation to an absolute zero potential. Referring to these leads as unipolar leads is based on the notion that the reference electrode—that is, the Wilson central terminal or the combination of two limb electrodes—represents a true zero potential. The choice of using the term *bipolar* for these leads reflects the recognition that the reference electrode is not at zero potential but yields the average of the potentials sensed at the sites of the electrodes making up the compound electrode.[2]

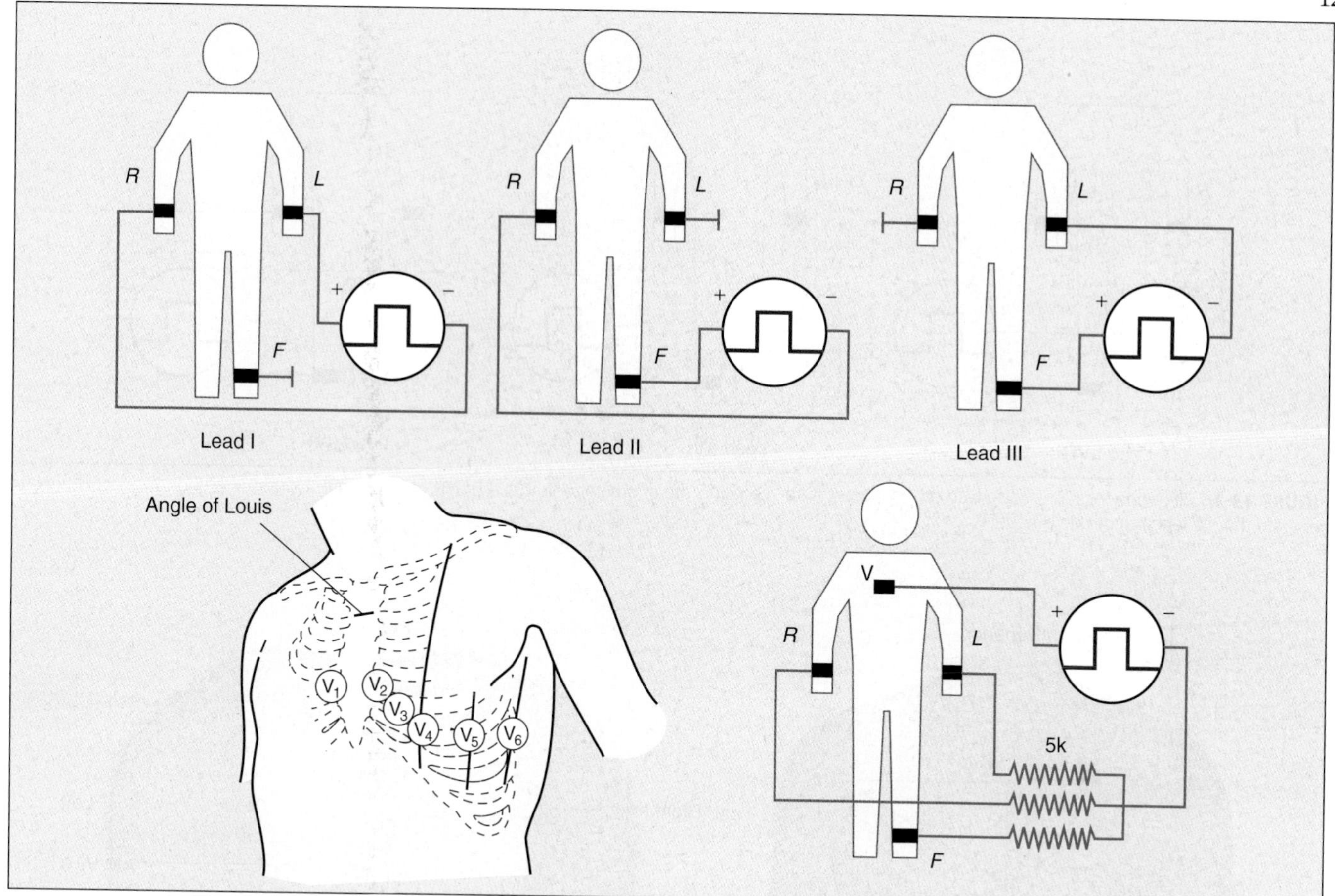

FIGURE 13-2 Top, Electrode connections for recording the standard limb leads I, II, and III. R, L, and F indicate locations of electrodes on the right arm, left arm, and left foot, respectively. **Bottom,** Electrode locations and electrical connections for recording a precordial lead. **Left,** The positions of the exploring electrode (V) for the six precordial leads. **Right,** Connections to form the Wilson central terminal for recording a precordial (V) lead. *(From Goldberger AL: Clinical Electrocardiography: A Simplified Approach. 7th ed. St. Louis, CV Mosby, 2006.)*

exploring electrode is placed on each precordial site and connected to the positive input of the recording system (see Fig. 13-2, bottom, right panel).

The negative, or reference, input is composed of a compound electrode known as the Wilson central terminal. This terminal is formed by combining the output of the left arm (LA), right arm (RA), and left leg (LL) electrodes through 5000-Ω resistances (see Fig. 13-2, bottom, right panel). The potential in each V lead can be expressed as

$$V_i = E_i - WCT$$

where

$$WCT = (LA + LL + RA)/3,$$

and V_i is the potential recorded in precordial lead i, E_i is the voltage sensed at the exploring electrode for lead V_i, and WCT is the potential in the composite Wilson central terminal. Thus, the potential in the Wilson central terminal is the average of the potentials in the three limb leads.

The potential recorded by the Wilson central terminal remains relatively constant during the cardiac cycle, so that the output of a precordial lead is determined predominantly by time-dependent changes in the potential at the precordial site.[2,5] The waveforms registered by these leads preferentially reflect potentials generated in cardiac regions near the electrode, as well as those generated by all cardiac sources active at any instant during the cardiac cycle.

Augmented Limb Leads. The three augmented limb leads are designated aVR, aVL, and aVF. The exploring electrode (**Fig. 13-3**) that forms the positive input is the right arm electrode for lead aVR, the left arm electrode for lead aVL, and the left leg electrode for aVF. The reference potential for the augmented limb leads is formed by connecting the two limb electrodes that are not used as the exploring electrode. For lead aVL, for example, the exploring electrode is on the left arm and the reference electrode is the combined output of the electrodes on the right arm and the left foot. Thus,

$$aVR = RA - (LA + LL)/2$$

$$aVL = LA - (RA + LL)/2$$

and

$$aVF = LL - (RA + LA)/2$$

This modified reference system was designed to produce a larger amplitude signal than if the full Wilson central terminal were used as the reference electrode. When the Wilson central terminal was used, the output was small, in part because the same electrode potential was included in both the exploring and the reference potential input. Eliminating this duplication results in a theoretical increase in amplitude of 50%.

The 12 leads are commonly divided into subgroups corresponding to the cardiac regions to which they are thought to be most sensitive. Various definitions of these groupings have been offered in the literature—for example, anterior lead groups have been defined as including V_2 through V_4 or only V_2 and V_3, and leads I and aVL have been described as being lateral or anterobasal.[5] These designations are nonspecific and the recommendation of expert committees has been not to use them in electrocardiographic interpretation, except in the case of localizing myocardial infarction.[6] We recommend that the conventional names of the leads be used to describe the distribution of electrocardiographic findings.

Other Lead Systems. Other lead systems have been developed to detect diagnostically important information not recorded by the standard 12-lead ECG and to increase the efficiency of recording, transmitting, and storing an ECG. Expanded lead systems include the recording of additional right precordial leads to assess right ventricular abnormalities, such as right ventricular infarction in patients with evidence of inferior infarction,[6] and left posterior leads (see Table 13-1) to help detect acute posterolateral infarctions.

Electrode arrays of 80 or more electrodes deployed on the anterior and posterior torso can be used to display body surface potentials as

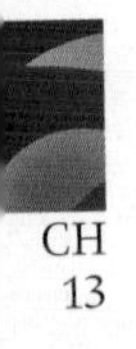

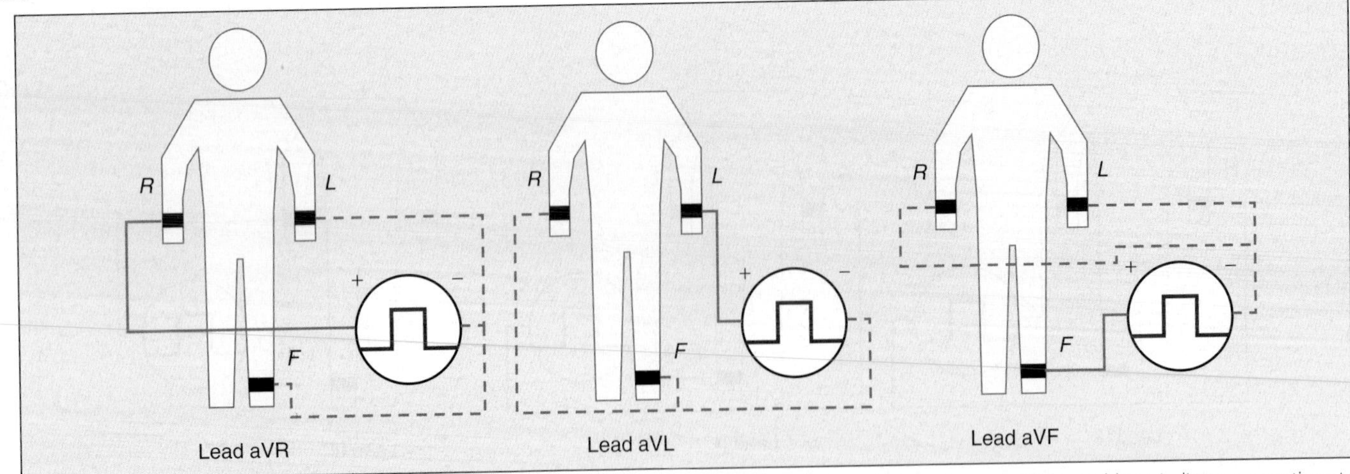

FIGURE 13-3 Electrode locations and electrical connections for recording the augmented limb leads aVR, aVL, and aVF. Dotted lines indicate connections to generate the reference electrode potential.

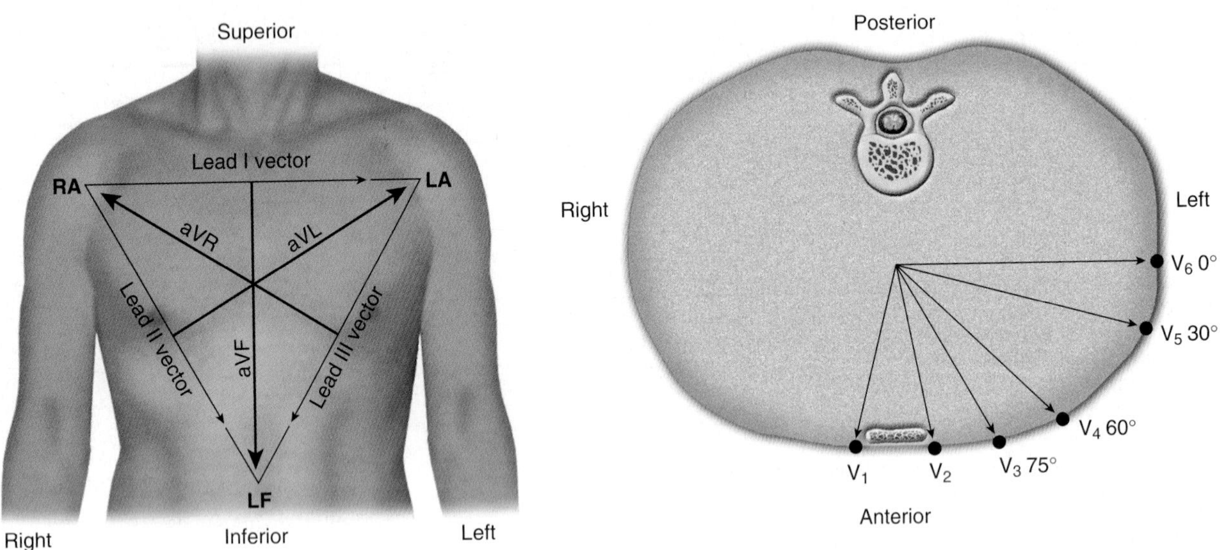

FIGURE 13-4 Lead vectors for the three standard limb leads, the three augmented limb leads (**left**), and the six unipolar precordial leads (**right**).

body surface isopotential maps. These maps portray cardiac potentials at all torso sites at any one instant in time. They thus depict the spatial distribution of cardiac activity, whereas the standard scalar ECG depicts the potential at one site over time. Maps also capture information projected to all regions of the torso, improving the accuracy of, for example, detecting ST-segment elevation acute myocardial infarction.[7]

Other arrays have sought to reduce the number of electrodes to reduce the time and mechanical complexity of a full recording, especially during emergency situations. For example, a full 12-lead ECG can be reconstructed, with high accuracy, from lead sets requiring only five electrodes.[8] Modified lead systems are also used in ambulatory ECG recording, exercise stress testing, and bedside cardiac monitoring, as described in other chapters, to simplify application and reduce motion artifact during exercise. The waveforms they produce are significantly different than those recorded from the standard electrocardiographic sites, including diagnostically important changes in waveform intervals and amplitudes.[9]

Other lead systems that have had clinical usefulness include those designed to record a vectorcardiogram (VCG). The VCG depicts the orientation and strength of a single cardiac dipole or vector that best represents overall cardiac activity at each instant during the cardiac cycle. Lead systems for recording the VCG record the three orthogonal or mutually perpendicular components of the dipole moment—the horizontal (*x*), frontal (*y*), and sagittal or anteroposterior (*z*) axes. Clinical use of the VCG has waned in recent years but, as described later, vectorial principles remain important for understanding the origins of electrocardiographic waveforms.

Lead Vectors and Heart Vectors. A lead can be represented as a vector referred to as the lead vector. For simple two-electrode leads, such as leads I, II, and III, the lead vectors are directed from the negative electrode toward the positive one (**Fig. 13-4**). For the augmented limb and precordial leads, the origin of the lead vectors lies at the midpoint of the axis connecting the electrodes that make up the compound electrode. That is, for lead aVL, the vector points from the midpoint of the axis connecting the right arm and left leg electrodes toward the left arm (see Fig. 13-4, left). For each precordial lead, the lead vector points from the center of the triangle formed by the three standard limb leads to the precordial electrode site (see Fig. 13-4, right).

As described earlier, instantaneous cardiac activity can also be approximated as a single vector (the heart vector) or dipole representing the vector sum of the various active wave fronts. Its location, orientation, and intensity vary from instant to instant as cardiac activation proceeds.

The amplitude of the potentials sensed in a lead equals the length of the projection of the heart vector on the lead vector, multiplied by the length of the lead vector:

$$V_L = (H)(\cos\tau)(L)$$

where L and H are the length of the lead and heart vectors, respectively, and τ is the angle between the two vectors, as illustrated in **Figure 13-5**.

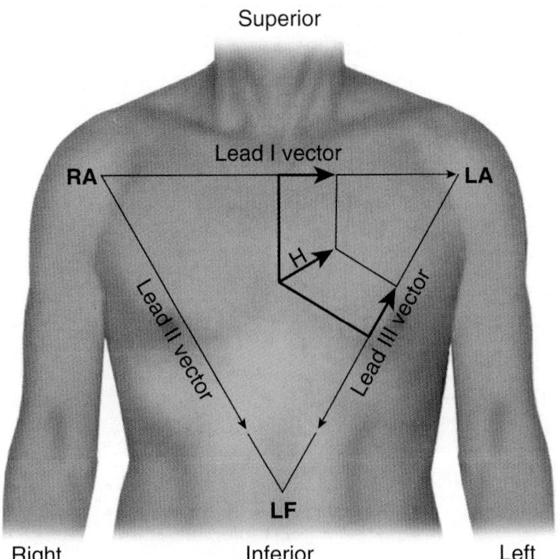

FIGURE 13-5 The heart vector H and its projections on the lead axes of leads I and III. Voltages recorded in lead I will be positive and potentials in lead III will be negative.

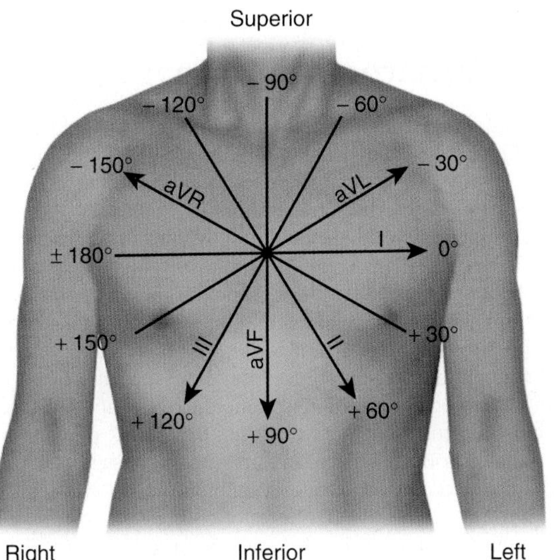

FIGURE 13-6 The hexaxial reference system constructed from the lead axes of the six frontal plane leads. The lead axes of the six frontal plane leads have been rearranged so that their centers overlay one another. These axes divide the plane into 12 segments, each subtending 30 degrees. Positive ends of each axis are labeled with the name of the lead.

Thus, if the projection of the heart vector on the lead vector points toward the positive pole of the lead axis, the lead will record a positive potential. If the projection is directed away from the positive pole of the lead axis, the potential will be negative. If the projection is perpendicular to the lead axis, the lead will record zero potential.

HEXAXIAL REFERENCE FRAME AND ELECTRICAL AXIS. The lead axes of the six frontal plane leads can be superimposed to produce the hexaxial reference system. As depicted in **Figure 13-6**, the six lead axes divide the frontal plane into 12 segments, each subtending 30 degrees.

These concepts allow calculation of the mean electrical axis of the heart. The orientation of the mean electrical axis represents the direction of activation in an "average" cardiac fiber. This direction is determined by the properties of the cardiac conduction system and activation properties of the myocardium. Differences in the relation of cardiac to torso anatomy contribute relatively little to shifts in the axis.[10]

The process for computing the mean electrical axis during ventricular activation in the frontal plane is illustrated in **Figure 13-7**. First, the mean force during activation is represented by the area under the QRS waveform, measured as millivolt-milliseconds. Areas above the baseline are assigned a positive polarity and those below the baseline have a negative polarity. The overall area equals the sum of the positive and the negative areas.

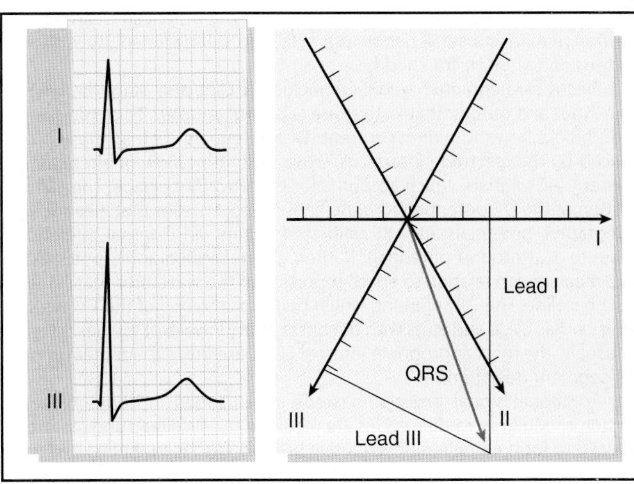

FIGURE 13-7 Calculation of the mean electrical axis during the QRS complex from the areas under the QRS complex in leads I and III. Magnitudes of the areas of the two leads are plotted as vectors on the appropriate lead axes, and the mean QRS axis is the sum of these two vectors. *(From Mirvis DM: Electrocardiography: A Physiologic Approach. St. Louis, Mosby-Year Book, 1993.)*

Second, the area in each lead (typically two are chosen) is represented as a vector oriented along the appropriate lead axis in the hexaxial reference system (see Fig. 13-6), and the mean electrical axis equals the resultant or vector sum of the two vectors. An axis directed toward the positive end of the lead axis of lead I—that is, oriented directly away from the right arm and toward the left arm—is designated as an axis of 0 degrees. Axes oriented in a clockwise direction from this zero level are assigned positive values and those oriented in a counterclockwise direction are assigned negative values.

The mean electrical axis during ventricular activation in the horizontal plane can be computed in an analogous manner by using the areas under and lead axes of the six precordial leads (see Fig. 13-4, right). A horizontal plane axis located along the lead axis of lead V_6 is assigned a value of 0 degrees, and those directed more anteriorly have positive values.

This process can be applied to compute the mean electrical axis for other phases of cardiac activity. Thus, the mean force during atrial activation is represented by the areas under the P wave, and the mean force during ventricular recovery is represented by the areas under the ST-T wave.

Electrocardiographic Processing and Display Systems

Electrocardiographic waveforms are also influenced by the characteristics of the electronic systems used to digitize, amplify, and filter the sensed signals. In computerized systems, analog signals are converted to a digital form at rates of 1000/sec (Hz) to as high as 15,000 Hz.[2] Too low a sampling rate will miss brief signals such as notches in QRS complexes or pacemaker spikes, and will reduce the accuracy of waveform morphologies. Too fast a sampling rate may introduce artifacts, including high-frequency noise, and requires extensive digital storage capacity. In general, the sampling rate should be at least twice the frequency of the highest frequencies of interest in the signal being recorded (up to approximately 500 Hz in adults[2]).

The standard amplifier gain for routine electrocardiography is 1000. Lower (e.g., 500 or half-standard) or higher (e.g., 2000 or double standard) gains may be used to compensate for unusually large or small signals, respectively.

Electrocardiographic amplifiers respond differently to the range of signal frequencies included in an electrophysiologic signal system, and they include filters to reduce the amplitude of specific frequency ranges of the signal intentionally. Low-pass filters reduce the distortions caused by high-frequency interference from, for example, muscle tremor and external electrical devices. High-pass filters reduce the effects of body motion or respiration.

The bandwidth of an amplifier defines the frequency range over which the amplifier accurately amplifies the input signals and is determined by specific characteristics of the amplifier and any added filters. Waveform components with frequencies outside the bandwidth of the amplifier will be artifactually reduced or increased in amplitude. For routine electrocardiography, the standards of the American Heart Association require an overall bandwidth of 0.05 to 150 Hz for adults, with an extension to 250 Hz for children.[2]

Electrocardiographic amplifiers include a capacitor stage between the input and output; that is, they are capacitor coupled. This configuration blocks unwanted direct current (DC) potentials, such as those produced by the electrode interfaces, while permitting flow of alternating current (AC) signals, which accounts for the waveform shape. The elimination of the DC potential from the final product means that electrocardiographic potentials are not calibrated against an external reference level (e.g., a ground potential). Rather, electrocardiographic potentials are measured in relation to another portion of the waveform that serves as a baseline. The T-P segment, which begins at the end of the T wave of one cardiac cycle and ends with the onset of the P wave of the next cycle, is usually the most appropriate internal ECG baseline (e.g., for measuring ST-segment deviation).

Additional signal processing steps are included in computerized systems.[2] Multiple cardiac cycles are recorded for each lead and are processed to form a single representative beat for each lead that is used for interpretation. This step reduces the effects of beat-to-beat variation in the waveforms.

The representative beats from all leads may then be electronically overlaid on each other to produce a single, global pattern. Electrocardiographic intervals are then measured from this single pattern. This approach has the advantage of identifying the earliest onset and latest ending of an electrocardiographic interval in all leads. The beginning or end of a waveform may appear to be isoelectric in a given lead if the electrical forces at that time are perpendicular to the lead axis. The forces will, however, be detected in other leads, so that a more accurate measurement may be made than if determined only from a recording from a single lead.

Cardiac potentials are most commonly displayed as the classic scalar ECG. Scalar recordings depict the potentials recorded from each lead as a function of time. For standard electrocardiography, amplitudes are displayed on a scale of 1 mV- to 10-mm on the vertical axis and time as 400 msec/cm on the horizontal scale. Leads are generally displayed in three groups, the three standard limb leads followed by the three augmented limb leads followed by the six precordial leads.

Alternative display formats have been proposed in which the six limb leads are displayed in the sequence of the frontal plane reference frame (see Fig. 13-6). In addition, the polarity of lead aVR is reversed.[11] That is, waveforms are displayed in this order: lead aVL, lead I, lead aVR (reversed in polarity), lead II, lead aVF, and lead III. Proposed advantages of this system include facilitating estimation of the electrical axis by presenting the leads in the order in which they appear on the frontal plane reference frame and emphasizing the relevance of abnormalities in lead aVR by reversing its polarity. This approach has also been extended to display the inverted form of all 12 leads, producing a 24-lead ECG in which waveforms are shown at 30-degree increments in the frontal plane and as if recorded on the back and right torso in the horizontal plane.[12]

Interpreting the Electrocardiogram

The recorded or displayed electrocardiographic tracings are, finally, compared with various diagnostic criteria to identify specific abnormalities. In some cases, the electrocardiographic criteria are derived from physiologic constructs and are the sole basis for a diagnosis with no anatomic or physiologic correlation. For example, the electrocardiographic criteria for intraventricular conduction defects (see later) are diagnostic without reference to an anatomic standard.

For other electrocardiographic diagnoses, the criteria are based on statistical correlations between anatomic or physiologic findings and electrocardiographic measurements in large populations. For example, the electrocardiographic diagnostic criteria for ventricular hypertrophy depend on correlations between various electrocardiographic patterns and anatomic measures of chamber size in large populations. As a result, many different sets of criteria have been proposed for common abnormalities (e.g., left ventricular hypertrophy). The various criteria have different predictive accuracies that are empirically determined, so that the final electrocardiographic diagnosis is not absolute but represents a statistical probability that the abnormality exists based on the presence (positive predictive accuracy) or absence (negative predictive accuracy) of a specific set of electrocardiographic findings.

Another issue related to electrocardiographic interpretation is the variability in the terminology used to describe waveform patterns. Often, several different diagnostic statements, which may contain vague terminology, may be used to describe identical or similar findings. A lexicon of preferred diagnostic statements has recently been proposed to reduce these problems.[13]

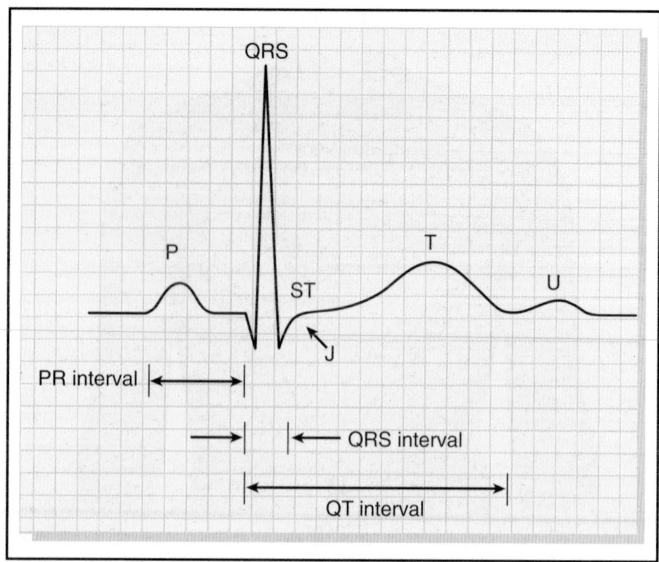

FIGURE 13-8 The waves and intervals of a normal electrocardiogram. *(From Goldberger AL: Clinical Electrocardiography: A Simplified Approach. 7th ed. St. Louis, CV Mosby, 2006.)*

Normal Electrocardiogram

The waveforms and intervals that make up the standard ECG are displayed in **Figure 13-8**, and a normal 12-lead ECG is shown in **Figure 13-9**. The P wave is generated by activation of the atria, the PR segment represents the duration of atrioventricular (AV) conduction, the QRS complex is produced by the activation of the two ventricles, and the ST-T wave reflects ventricular recovery (see Chap. 35).

Table 13-2 lists normal values for the various intervals and waveforms of the ECG. The range of normal values of these measurements reflects the substantial interindividual variability related to, among other factors, differences in age, gender, body habitus, heart orientation, and physiology. In addition, significant differences in electrocardiographic patterns may occur within the same person in ECGs recorded days, hours, or even minutes apart. These intraindividual variations may be caused by technical issues (e.g., changes in electrode position) or the biologic effects of changes in posture, temperature, or eating, and may be sufficiently large to alter diagnostic evidence for conditions such as chamber hypertrophy.[14]

The values shown in Table 13-2 have been typically used in clinical electrocardiography. Other normal ranges for various measures, as will be described in the sections that follow, have been suggested. These proposals are based on changes in the demographics of the population as well as differences in recording methods, especially the use of digital signals and computerized analysis systems, which have occurred over the past decades. Computerization of electrocardiographic interpretation facilitates the identification and use of different criteria for various population subgroups based on, for example, age, gender, and race, that were not previously feasible. For example, the substantial differences in the duration of the normal PR interval between genders and among different age groups[15] suggest that a single range of normal values for all subjects may be inappropriate and could lead to over- or underdiagnosis of clinically important conditions.

Atrial Activation and the P Wave

ATRIAL ACTIVATION. Atrial activation begins with impulse generation in the atrial pacemaker complex in or near the sinoatrial (SA) node. Once the impulse leaves this pacemaker site, atrial activation begins in one or, in many cases, simultaneously in several areas of the right atrium.[16] Propagation then proceeds rapidly along the crista terminalis and moves anteriorly toward the lower portion of the right atrium.

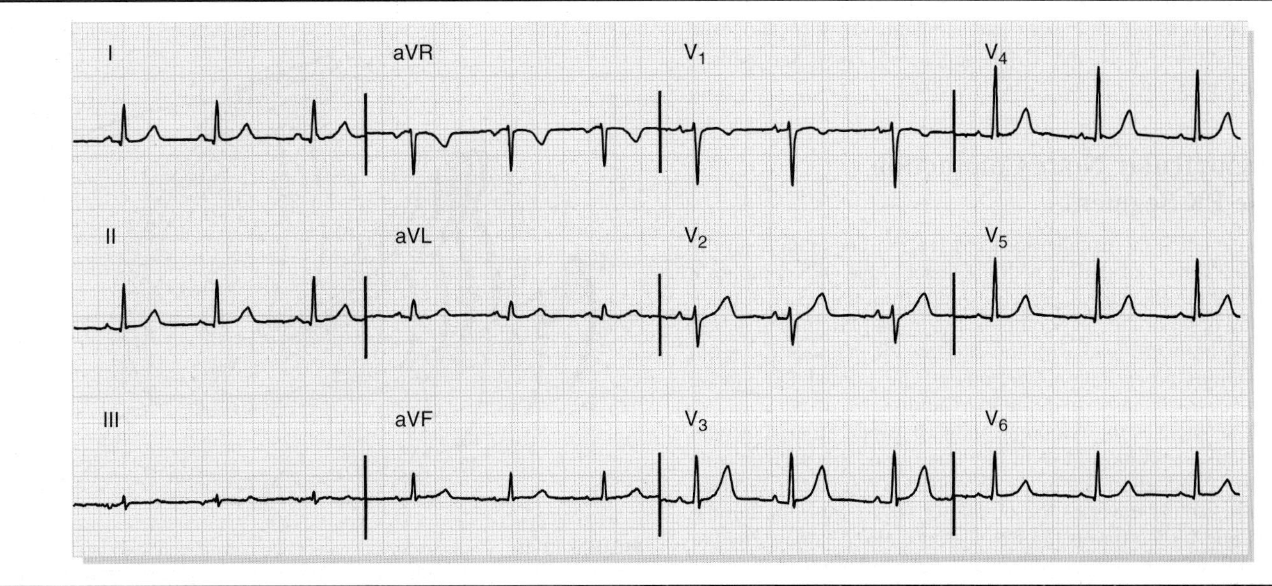

FIGURE 13-9 Normal electrocardiogram recorded from a 48-year-old woman. The vertical lines of the grid represent time, with lines spaced at 40-msec intervals. Horizontal lines represent voltage amplitude, with lines spaced at 0.1-mV intervals. Every fifth line in each direction is typically darkened. The heart rate is approximately 72 beats/min, the PR interval, QRS, and QT_c durations measure about 140, 84, and 400 msec, respectively, and the mean QRS axis is approximately +35 degrees.

TABLE 13-2 Normal Values for Durations of Electrocardiographic Waves and Intervals in Adults

WAVE OR INTERVAL	DURATION (MSEC)
P wave duration	<120
PR interval	<200
QRS duration	<110-120*
QT interval (corrected)	≤440-450*

*See text for further discussion.

Interatrial spread is more complex. In most people, the left atrium is activated first by propagation across Bachmann's bundle, which extends from the anterior right atrium, above the fossa ovalis to the left atrium, near the right upper pulmonary vein. Other routes of interatrial spread include paths within the fossa ovalis or near the coronary sinus either alone or, more commonly, in combination with conduction in Bachmann's bundle.[16,17]

At the same time, activation spreads through the interatrial septum, beginning high on the right side and moving around the fossa ovalis to reach the top of the interventricular septum. The last area to be activated is over the inferolateral aspect of the left atrium.

Thus, right atrial activation begins before activation of the left atrium, left atrial activation continues after the end of right atrial activation, and both atria undergo activation during much of the middle of the overall atrial activation period.

NORMAL P WAVE. These patterns of atrial activation produce the normal P wave. Activation beginning high in the right atrium and proceeding simultaneously leftward toward the left atrium and inferiorly toward the AV node corresponds to a mean frontal plane P wave axis of approximately 60 degrees. Based on this orientation of the heart vector, normal atrial activation projects positive or upright P waves in leads II and usually in leads I, aVL, and aVF. The pattern in leads aVL and III may be upright or downward, depending on the exact orientation of the mean axis.

P wave patterns in the precordial leads correspond to the direction of atrial activation wave fronts in the horizontal plane. Atrial activation early in the P wave is over the right atrium and is oriented primarily anteriorly; later, it shifts posteriorly as activation proceeds over the left atrium. Thus, the P wave in the right precordial leads (V_1 and, occasionally, V_2) is upright or, often, biphasic, with an initial positive deflection followed by a later negative one. In the more lateral leads, the P wave is upright and reflects continual right to left spread of the activation fronts. Variations in this pattern may reflect differences in pathways of interatrial conduction.[17]

The upper limit for a normal P wave duration is conventionally set at 120 msec as measured in the lead with the widest P wave. The amplitude in the limb leads is normally less than 0.25 mV and the terminal negative deflection in the right precordial leads is normally less than 0.1 mV in depth.

ATRIAL REPOLARIZATION. The potentials generated by atrial repolarization are not usually seen on the surface ECG because of their low amplitude (usually less than 100 μV) and because they are superimposed on the much higher amplitude QRS complex. They may be observed as a low-amplitude wave with a polarity opposite that of the P wave (the T_a wave) during atrioventricular block and may have special significance in influencing ST-segment patterns during exercise testing. Deviation of the PR segment is, as described later, also an important marker of acute pericarditis and, less commonly, of atrial infarction.

HEART RATE VARIABILITY. Ongoing attention continues to be directed to the analysis of beat-to-beat changes in heart rate and related dynamics, termed *heart rate variability* (HRV), to gain insight into neuroautonomic control mechanisms (see Chaps. 36 and 94) and their perturbations with aging, disease, and drug effects. For example, relatively high-frequency (0.15 to 0.5 Hz) fluctuations mediated by the vagus nerve traffic occur phasically, with heart rate increasing during inspiration and decreasing during expiration. Attenuation of this respiratory sinus arrhythmia, and related short-term heart rate variability, is a consistent marker of physiologic aging and also occurs with diabetes mellitus, congestive heart failure, and a wide range of other cardiac and noncardiac conditions that alter autonomic tone. Relatively lower frequency (0.05 to 0.15 Hz) physiologic oscillations in heart rate are associated with baroreflex activation and appear to be jointly regulated by sympathetic and parasympathetic interactions. Various complementary signal processing techniques are being developed to analyze heart rate variability and its interactions with other physiologic signals.[18] These methods include time domain statistics, frequency domain techniques based on spectral methods (Fourier and other wave decomposition), and newer computational tools derived from nonlinear dynamics and complex systems.[19] Free, open source methods to measure heart rate variability are available at the National Institutes of Health (NIH)–sponsored PhysioNet website (http://www.physionet.org/tutorials/hrv-toolkit).

Atrioventricular Node Conduction and the PR Segment

The PR segment is the usually isoelectric region beginning with the end of the P wave and ending with the onset of the QRS complex. It forms part of the PR interval, which extends from the onset of the P wave to the onset of the QRS complex. The overall PR interval is best determined from the lead with the shortest PR intervals (to avoid missing various preexcitation syndromes). The normal PR interval measures 120 to 200 msec in duration in adults.

The PR segment is the temporal bridge between atrial activation and ventricular activation. Most of the time during this segment represents slow conduction within the AV node. On exiting the AV node, the impulse rapidly traverses the bundle of His to enter the bundle branches, and it then travels through the specialized intraventricular conduction paths to activate ventricular myocardium. The segment ends when enough ventricular myocardium has been activated to initiate the recording of the QRS complex.

The PR segment appears isoelectric because the potentials generated by the conduction system structures are too small to produce detectable voltages on the body surface at the normal amplifier gains used in clinical electrocardiography. Signals from elements of the conduction system can be recorded from intracardiac recording electrodes placed against the base of the interventricular septum near the bundle of His (see Chap. 35).

Ventricular Activation and the QRS Complex

Normal ventricular activation is a complex process that is dependent on interactions between the physiology and anatomy of the specialized ventricular conducting system and the ventricular myocardium.

VENTRICULAR ACTIVATION. Ventricular activation is the product of two temporally overlapping events, endocardial activation and transmural activation.[20] Endocardial activation is guided by the anatomic distribution and physiology of the His-Purkinje system. The broadly dispersed ramifications of this treelike (fractal) system and the rapid conduction within it result in the near-simultaneous activation of multiple endocardial sites and the depolarization of most of the endocardial surfaces of both ventricles within several msec.

The sequence of ventricular endocardial activation is depicted in **Figure 13-10**. Earliest activity begins in three sites: (1) the anterior paraseptal wall of the left ventricle; (2) the posterior paraseptal wall of the left ventricle; and (3) the center of the left side of the septum. These loci generally correspond to the sites of insertion of the branches of the left bundle branch. Septal activation begins on the left side and spreads across the septum from left to right and from apex to base. Wave fronts sweep from these initial sites of activation in anterior and inferior and then superior directions to activate the anterior and lateral walls of the left ventricle. The posterobasal areas of the left ventricle are the last to be activated.

Excitation of the right ventricle begins near the insertion point of the right bundle branch, close to the base of the anterior papillary muscle, and spreads to the free wall. The final areas to be activated are the pulmonary conus and the posterobasal areas. Thus, in both ventricles, the overall endocardial excitation pattern begins on septal surfaces and sweeps down toward the apex and around the free walls to the posterior and basal regions in an apex to base direction.

The activation fronts then move from endocardium to epicardium. Excitation of the endocardium begins at sites of Purkinje–ventricular muscle junctions and proceeds by muscle cell to muscle cell conduction in an oblique direction toward the epicardium.

NORMAL QRS COMPLEX. The sequence of endocardial and transmural activation results in the characteristic waveforms of the QRS complex.

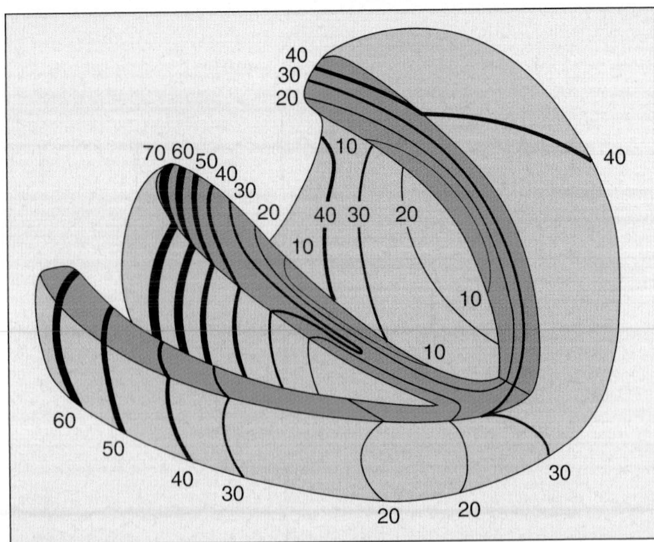

FIGURE 13-10 Activation sequence of the normal right and left ventricles. Portions of the left and right ventricles have been removed so that the endocardial surfaces of the ventricles and the interventricular septum can be seen. Isochrone lines connect sites that are activated at equal instants after the earliest evidence of ventricular activation. *(From Durrer D: Electrical aspects of human cardiac activity: A clinical-physiological approach to excitation and stimulation. Cardiovasc Res 2:1, 1968.)*

Terminology for the QRS Complex

QRS patterns are described by the sequence of waves constituting the complex. An initial negative deflection is called the Q wave, the first positive wave is the R wave, and the first negative wave after a positive wave is the S wave. A second upright wave following an S wave is an R′ wave. Tall waves are denoted by upper case letters and smaller ones by lower case letters. A monophasic negative complex is referred to as a QS complex. Thus, for example, the overall QRS complex may be described as qRS if it consists of an initial small negative wave (the q wave) followed by a tall upright one (the R wave) and a deep negative one (an S wave). In an RSr′ complex, initial R and S waves are followed by a small positive wave (the r′ wave). In each case, the deflection must cross the baseline to be designated a discrete wave; changes in waveform direction that do not cross the baseline result in notches.

Early QRS Patterns. The complex pattern of activation described earlier can be simplified into two vectors, the first representing septal activation and the second representing left ventricular free wall activation (**Fig. 13-11**). Initial activation of the interventricular septum corresponds to a vector oriented from left to right in the frontal plane and anteriorly in the horizontal plane, corresponding to the anatomic position of the septum within the chest. This vector produces an initial positive wave in leads with axes directed to the right (lead aVR) or anteriorly (lead V_1). Leads with axes directed to the left (leads I, aVL, V_5, and V_6) will register initial negative waves (septal q waves). These initial forces are normally of low amplitude and are brief (less than 30 msec). The absence of these septal q waves, with QS complexes in the right precordial leads or as initial R waves in leads I and V_{5-6}, is usually a normal variant and not associated with any cardiac disease.[21]

Mid and Late QRS Patterns. Subsequent parts of the QRS complex reflect activation of the free walls of the left and right ventricles. Because right ventricular muscle mass is considerably smaller than that of the left ventricle, it contributes little to normal QRS complexes recorded in the standard ECG. Thus, the normal QRS can be considered to represent only septal and left ventricular activity, with relatively little meaningful oversimplification.

The complex interrelationships among cardiac position, conduction system function, and ventricular geometry[22] result in a wide range of normal QRS patterns in the six limb leads. The QRS pattern in leads II, III, and aVF may be predominantly upright with qR complexes or these leads may show rS or RS patterns. Lead I may record an isoelectric RS pattern or a predominantly upright qR pattern.

The wide range of QRS patterns, especially in the inferior leads, can be interpreted by referring to the hexaxial reference system in Figure 13-6. The normal mean QRS axis in adults lies between −30 degrees and +90 degrees. If the mean axis is near 90 degrees, the QRS complex in leads II, III, and aVF will be predominantly upright, with qR complexes; lead I will record an isoelectric RS pattern because the heart vector lies perpendicular to the lead axis. If the mean axis is nearer 0 degrees, the patterns will be reversed; leads I and aVL will register a predominantly upright qR pattern, and leads II, III, and aVF will show rS or RS patterns.

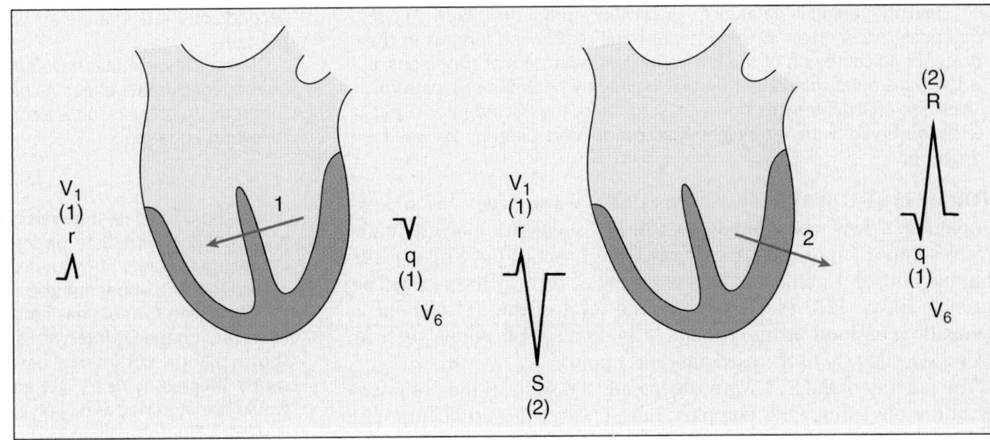

FIGURE 13-11 Schematic representation of ventricular depolarization as two sequential vectors representing septal **(left)** and left ventricular free wall **(right)** activation. QRS waveforms generated by each stage of activation in leads V_1 and V_6 are shown.

Mean QRS axes more positive than +90 degrees (usually with an rS pattern in lead I) represent right axis deviation (RAD), with axes between +90 and +120 degrees referred to as moderate RAD and axes between +120 and +180 degrees referred to as marked RAD. Axes more negative than −30 degrees (with an rS pattern in lead II) represent left axis deviation (LAD), with axes between −30 and −45 degrees called moderate LAD and those between −45 and −90 degrees called marked LAD. Mean QRS axes of approximately −80 to −90 degrees are sometimes referred to as superior axis deviation, and have been reported in cases of severe chronic obstructive lung disease.

Mean axes lying between −90 degrees and −180 degrees (or, equivalently, between +180 degrees and +270 degrees) are referred to as extreme axis deviations or, alternatively, as right superior axis deviations. The term *indeterminate axis* is applied when all six extremity leads show biphasic (QR or RS) patterns, indicating a mean axis that is perpendicular to the frontal plane. This finding can occur as a normal variant or may be seen in a variety of pathologic conditions.

Normal QRS patterns in the precordial leads follow an orderly progression from right (V_1) to left (V_6). In leads V_1 and V_2, left ventricular free wall activation generates S waves following the initial r waves generated by septal activation (an rS pattern). These S waves are produced by the spread of activation in the free wall to the left and posteriorly, with generation of a heart vector directed away from the axes of these leads.

Patterns in the midprecordial leads V_3 and V_4 reflect the activation front in the ventricular free wall, first approaching the exploring electrode, and followed by its moving leftward and posteriorly to more remote regions of the left ventricle and away from the exploring electrode. In leads V_3 and V_4, this generates an R or r wave as it moves toward the electrode, followed by an S wave as it moves away from the electrode to produce rS or RS complexes. As the exploring electrode moves laterally to the left, the R wave becomes more dominant and the S wave becomes smaller (or is totally lost) because of the greater time period during which the activation front moves toward the positive end of the electrode. In the leftmost leads (i.e., leads V_5 and V_6), the pattern also includes the septal q wave to produce a qRs or qR pattern.

Thus, in the precordial leads, the QRS complex is usually characterized by a consistent progression from an rS complex in the right precordial leads to a qR pattern in the left precordial leads. The site during this transition at which the pattern changes from an rS to an Rs configuration—the lead in which an isoelectric RS pattern is present—is known as the transition zone and normally occurs in leads V_3 or V_4. An example of a normal precordial QRS pattern is shown in Figure 13-9. An altered location of the transition zone may occur for a variety of reasons; transition zones that are shifted to the right to lead V_2 are early transitions, and those that are shifted leftward to V_5 or V_6 are delayed transitions.[2]

Normal variabilities in QRS amplitudes, axes, and duration QRS are related to demographic and physiologic factors. QRS amplitudes are greater in men than in women, with higher amplitudes in African Americans than in those of other races. In addition, the location of the mitral papillary muscles in relation to the septum affects duration and frontal plane axis,[22] and left ventricular mass (within the normal range) affects both QRS amplitude and duration.[23]

QRS Duration. The upper normal value for QRS duration is traditionally reported as less than 120 msec (and often as less than 110 msec) measured in the lead with the widest QRS duration. Women, on average, have somewhat shorter QRS durations than men (by ≈5 to 8 msec).

The Intrinsicoid Deflection. An additional feature of the QRS complex is the intrinsicoid deflection. An electrode overlying the ventricular free wall will record a rising R wave as transmural activation proceeds toward it. Once the activation front reaches the epicardium, the full thickness of the wall under the electrode will be in an active state. At that moment, the electrode will register negative potentials as activation proceeds in remote cardiac areas. The sudden reversal of potential, with a sharp downslope, is the intrinsicoid deflection and approximates the timing of activation of the epicardium under the electrode. The term *ventricular activation time* (VAT) is sometimes used with reference to the surface ECG.

Ventricular Recovery and the ST-T Wave

Sequence of Ventricular Recovery. The ST-T wave of the electrocardiogram reflects activity during the plateau phase (the ST segment) and the later repolarization phases (the T wave) of the cardiac action potential.

Ventricular repolarization, like activation, occurs in a characteristic geometric pattern. Differences in recovery timing occur both across the ventricular wall and between regions of the left ventricle.[24] Transmural differences in recovery times are the net result of two effects, differences in action potential duration across the ventricular wall and the relatively slow spread of activation across the wall. As activation moves from endocardium to epicardium, sites further away from the endocardium are activated later in time. However, action potential durations are longest near the endocardium and shortest near the epicardium. Differences in action potential duration are greater than differences in activation times, so that recovery is completed near the epicardium before it is completed near the endocardium. For example, one endocardial site may be excited 10 msec earlier than the overlying epicardium (i.e., transmural activation may require 10 msec), and the action potential duration at the endocardium may be 22 msec longer than on the epicardium. As a result, recovery will be completed 12 msec earlier in the epicardium than in the endocardium.

The resulting recovery dipole will then be directed away from sites of less recovery (the endocardium) toward sites of greater recovery (near the epicardium). The orientation of this dipole is in the same direction as transmural activation dipoles, as described earlier. The result, in normal persons, is relatively concordant QRS and ST-T wave vectorial patterns.

The identification of midwall cells (M cells; see Chap. 35) has suggested that the origins of the ST-T wave may be more complex. These cells have action potentials that are longer than those of endocardial or epicardial cells.[24] The ST-T wave begins when epicardial cells begin to recover ahead of both M and endocardial cells, with current flowing from midmyocardial and endocardial regions toward the epicardium. The result is the rising phase of the T wave. These currents reach maximal intensity when the epicardium is fully repolarized at the peak of the T wave. As endocardial regions begin to repolarize, a second set of currents flowing from M cells to endocardial cells is generated. This current, flowing in the opposite direction to the first, initiates the descending limb of the T wave. These relationships suggest that the interval between the peak and the end of the T wave (the T_p-T_e interval) may be a measure of transmural dispersion of recovery properties and may be related to arrhythmogenesis.

Similarly, regional differences in recovery properties exist. Action potentials are shortest in the anterior-basal region and longest in the posterior-apical region of the left ventricle. Under normal conditions, it is the transmural gradients that predominantly determine ST patterns. These regional differences, however, account for the discordant ST-T patterns observed with intraventricular conduction defects, as will be described.

NORMAL ST-T WAVE. The normal ST-T wave begins as a low-amplitude, slowly changing wave (the ST segment) that gradually evolves into a larger wave, the T wave. The onset of the ST-T wave is the junction, or J point, and it is normally at or near the isoelectric baseline of the ECG (see Fig. 13-9). The level of the ST segment is generally measured at the J point or, in some applications such as exercise testing, 40 or 80 msec after the J point.

The polarity of the ST-T wave is generally the same as the net polarity of the preceding QRS complex. Thus, T waves are usually upright in leads I, II, aVL, and aVF and the lateral precordial leads. They are negative in lead aVR and variable in leads III, V_1, and V_2.

The amplitude of the normal J point and ST segment varies with race, gender, and age.[15] It is typically highest in lead V_2 and it is higher in young men than in young women and higher in African Americans than in whites. Recent recommendations for the upper limits of normal J point elevation in leads V_2 and V_3 are 0.2 mV for men older than 40 years, 0.25 mV for men younger than 40 years, and 0.15 mV for women. In other leads, the recommended upper limit is 0.1 mV.[25]

J WAVE. A J wave is a dome or hump-shaped wave that appears at the end of the QRS complex. It may be prominent as a normal variant (see later) and in certain pathologic conditions, such as systemic hypothermia (where it is sometimes referred to as an Osborn wave) and the Brugada pattern (see Chaps. 9 and 39). Its origin has been related to a prominent notch (phase 1) of the action potentials on the epicardium but not on the endocardium.[24]

U WAVE. The T wave may be followed by an additional low-amplitude wave known as the U wave. This wave, usually less than 0.1 mV in amplitude, normally has the same polarity as the preceding T wave. It is largest in the leads V_1 and V_2, and it is most often seen at slow heart rates. Its electrophysiologic basis is uncertain; it may be caused by the late repolarization of the Purkinje fibers, by the long action potential of midmyocardial M cells, or by delayed repolarization in areas of the ventricle that undergo late mechanical relaxation.[24]

QT INTERVAL. The QT interval extends from the onset of the QRS complex to the end of the T wave. Thus, it includes the total duration of ventricular activation and recovery and, in a general sense, corresponds to the duration of the ventricular action potential. Accurately measuring the QT interval is challenging for several reasons, including identifying the beginning of the QRS complex and end of the T wave, determining which lead(s) to use, and adjusting the measured interval for rate, QRS duration, and gender.[25]

Because the onset of the QRS and the end of the T wave do not occur simultaneously in every lead, the QT interval duration will vary from lead to lead by as much as 50 to 65 msec. When the interval is to be measured from a single lead, the lead in which the interval is the longest, most commonly lead V_2 or V_3, and in which a prominent U wave is absent should be used. In automated electrocardiographic systems, the interval is typically measured from a composite of all leads, with the interval beginning with the earliest onset of the QRS in any lead and ending with the latest end of the T wave in any lead.

The duration of the QT interval varies widely in the general population. This is a result of the substantial variation in measurements between repeated recordings in the same person (explaining as much as one third of the variation), as well as interindividual variations in various biologic, pharmacologic, metabolic, and genetic factors.[14,26] The normal QT interval decreases as heart rate increases, as does the duration of the normal ventricular action potential duration and refractoriness. Thus, the normal range for the QT interval is rate-dependent. This variability is related in part to genotypic differences affecting heart rate as well as the structure and function of repolarization channels.[14] Rate adaptation occurs in two phases, with a rapid phase that changes the QT interval within 30 seconds of a rate change and a slower one that responds over several minutes.

Numerous formulas have been proposed to correct the measured QT interval for this rate effect. A commonly used formula was developed by Bazett in 1920. The result is a corrected QT interval, or QT_c, defined by the following equation:

$$QT_c = QT/\sqrt{RR}$$

where the QT and RR intervals are measured in seconds. The normal QT_c is generally accepted to be less than or equal to 440* and is slightly longer, on average, in women younger than 40 years. Others have suggested that the upper limit be set at 450 or even 460.

The Bazett formula has limited accuracy in predicting the effects of heart rate on the QT interval. Large data base studies have, for example, shown that the QTc interval based on the Bazett formula remains significantly affected by heart rate and that as many as 30% of normal ECGs would be diagnosed as having a prolonged QT interval when this formula is used.[27] The formula, in general, overcorrects the QT interval at high heart rates and undercorrects at low rates.

Many other formulas and methods for correcting the QT interval for the effects of heart rate, including linear, logarithmic, hyperbolic, and exponential functions, have been developed and tested. Each has a different normal range. A joint committee of the American Heart Association and the American College of Cardiology has recently recommended using a linear regression function.[25] Several linear models have been proposed; one formula that has been shown to be relatively insensitive to heart rate[27] is

$$QT_c = QT + 1.75\,(HR - 60)$$

where HR is the heart rate and the intervals are measured in milliseconds.

QT Dispersion. As noted, the QT interval varies from lead to lead. In normal persons, the QT interval varies by up to 65 msec between leads, and is typically longest in leads V_2 and V_3. This range of intervals, referred to as QT dispersion, has been related to electrical instability and the risk of ventricular arrhythmogenesis, as described further below, although its practical clinical usefulness remains limited.[25]

QRST Angle. The concordance between the orientation of the normal QRS complex and the normal ST-T wave described earlier can be expressed vectorially. An angle can be visualized in three-dimensional space between the vector representing the mean QRS force and the vector representing the mean ST-T force. This angle is the spatial QRST angle. The angle between the two vectors in the frontal plane represents a reasonable simplification and is normally less than 60 degrees and usually less than 30 degrees. Abnormalities of the QRST angle reflect abnormal relationships between the properties of activation and recovery.

Ventricular Gradient. If the two vectors representing mean activation and mean recovery forces are added, a third vector known as the ventricular gradient is created. This vector represents the net area under the QRST complex. The concept of the ventricular gradient was originally developed to assess the variability that exists in regional repolarization properties; the greater these differences, the larger will be the ventricular gradient. In addition, because changes in activation patterns produced, for example, by bundle branch block cause corresponding changes in recovery patterns (see later), no change in the ventricular gradient typically results. The ventricular gradient should thus allow a measure of regional recovery properties that is independent of the activation pattern. This measurement has possible relevance to the genesis of reentrant arrhythmias that may be caused, in part, by abnormal regional variations in refractory periods.

Normal Variants

These descriptions of the waveforms of the normal ECG represent patterns most often observed in normal adults. Numerous variations occur in subjects without heart disease. These variations are important to recognize because they may be mistaken for significant

*The QT_c is traditionally reported in units of seconds or msec. However, the units of the QTc will vary with the formula used for the rate correction. Based on the Bazett formula, for example, it is a ratio of seconds to the square root of seconds, which is equivalent to the square root of seconds. If the denominator of the Bazett formula is considered as unitless, then the QT_c by this formula will have traditional units of seconds or msec.

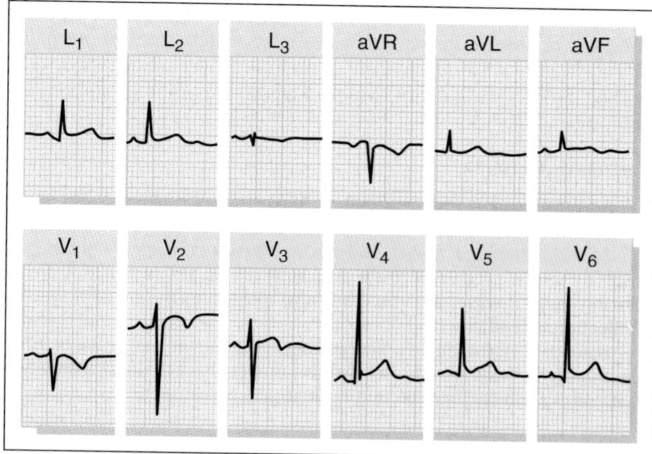

FIGURE 13-12 Normal tracing with a juvenile T wave inversion pattern in leads V_1, V_2, and V_3, as well as early repolarization pattern manifested by ST-segment elevation in leads I, II, aVF, V_4, V_5, and V_6. *(Courtesy of Dr. C. Fisch.)*

abnormalities and lead to an erroneous and potentially harmful diagnosis of heart disease.

T waves can be inverted in the right precordial leads in normal persons (**Fig. 13-12**). T waves are commonly inverted in all precordial leads at birth but usually become upright as time passes. A persistent juvenile pattern with inverted T waves in leads to the left of V_1 occurs in 1% to 3% of adults and is more common in women than in men and more common in African Americans than in other racial or ethnic groups.

The ST segment can be significantly elevated in normal persons, especially in the right and midprecordial leads (**Fig. 13-13**). The elevation begins from an elevated J point and is commonly associated with notching of the downstroke of the QRS complex.[28] This occurs in 2% to 5% of the population and is most prevalent in young adults, especially in African American men and those who are athletically active.

The pattern is commonly referred to as early repolarization. The pathogenesis may relate to specific ion channel changes during early portions of repolarization, to regional variations in repolarization time or, alternatively, to deeper than normal penetration of Purkinje fibers so that transmural activation time is shortened.[28,29] Although typically found as a benign condition, especially in young adults and athletes, recent studies have suggested an unexpected association with ventricular tachyarrhythmias and sudden cardiac arrest with ventricular fibrillation.[30,31] However, the implications of this reported association remain uncertain.

Abnormal Electrocardiogram*

Atrial Abnormalities

Various pathophysiologic events alter the normal sequence of atrial activation to produce abnormal P wave patterns. Three general categories of P wave changes are described here—abnormal patterns of activation, left atrial abnormalities, and right atrial abnormalities.

ABNORMAL ATRIAL ACTIVATION AND CONDUCTION. Small shifts in the site of initial activation within the SA node or away from the SA node to other ectopic sites within the atria can lead to major changes in the pattern of atrial activation and, hence, in the morphology of P waves. These shifts can occur as escape rhythms if the normal SA nodal pacemaker fails or as accelerated ectopic rhythms if the automaticity of an ectopic site is enhanced (see Chap. 39).

P wave patterns can suggest the site of impulse formation and the path of subsequent activation based on simple vectorial principles. For example, a negative P wave in lead I suggests that the origin of activation is in the left atrium. Inverted P waves in the inferior leads generally correspond to a posterior atrial site. However, the correlations of P wave patterns with location of origin are highly variable. Because of this, these electrocardiographic patterns may, as a group, be best referred to as ectopic atrial rhythms.

Conduction delays within the atria alter the duration and pattern of P waves.[17,32] When conduction from the right to the left atrium within Bachmann's bundle is delayed, P wave duration is prolonged beyond 120 msec and P waves appear to have two humps in lead II (often referred to as P mitrale; see Chap. 66). With more advanced block or when interatrial conduction is predominantly through the coronary sinus, the sinus node impulses reach the left atrium only after passing inferiorly to near the AV junction and then superiorly through the left atrium. In this case, P waves are wide and biphasic (an initial positive wave followed by a negative deflection) in the inferior leads.

LEFT ATRIAL ABNORMALITY. Anatomic or functional abnormalities of the left atrium that alter the P waves in the clinical ECG include atrial dilation, atrial muscular hypertrophy, elevated intra-atrial pressures, and delayed conduction. Because these abnormalities commonly coexist and can produce the same electrocardiographic effects, the resulting electrocardiographic patterns may best be referred to as left atrial abnormality (LAA) rather than in terms suggesting a particular pathologic basis.[33]

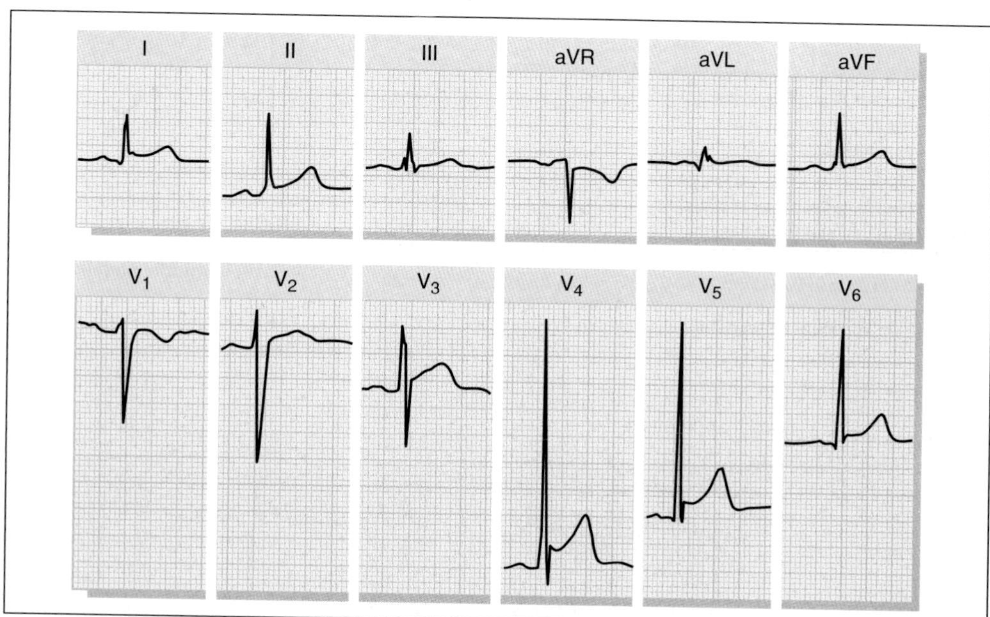

FIGURE 13-13 Normal variant pattern with the "early repolarization" variant of ST-segment elevation. The ST-segment elevation is most marked in the midprecordial lead V_4. Reciprocal ST-segment depression and PR-segment depression are absent (except in lead aVR), findings that may be helpful in the differential diagnosis of ischemia and pericarditis, respectively. Note also that lead II has a baseline recording shift. *(From Goldberger AL: Myocardial Infarction: Electrocardiographic Differential Diagnosis. 4th ed. St. Louis, Mosby-Year Book, 1991.)*

*All the diagnostic criteria that will be presented here apply only to adults.

Diagnostic Criteria

The most commonly used criteria for diagnosing left atrial abnormality are listed in **Table 13-3** and illustrated in **Figures 13-14 and 13-15**.

MECHANISMS FOR ELECTROCARDIOGRAPHIC ABNORMALITIES. Increases in left atrial mass or chamber size cause increases in P wave amplitudes and durations. Because the left atrium is generally activated relatively late during P wave inscription, the changes produce prolonged P wave durations and increased P terminal forces in the right precordial leads.

DIAGNOSTIC ACCURACY. Comparisons of the various electrocardiographic abnormalities to echocardiographic criteria for left atrial enlargement have demonstrated the limited sensitivity and high specificity for standard electrocardiographic criteria. Based on two-dimensional echocardiographic standards, the classic P wave patterns of LAA have sensitivities of only 12% to 70% and specificities of over 90% for detecting enlarged left atria.[34] In general, the low overall predictive accuracy of these criteria render them of limited clinical value for assessing atrial size.

CLINICAL SIGNIFICANCE. The electrocardiographic findings of left atrial abnormality are associated with more severe left ventricular dysfunction in patients with ischemic heart disease (see Chap. 54) and with more severe valve damage in patients with mitral or aortic valve disease (see Chap. 66). Patients with left atrial abnormalities also have a higher than normal incidence of paroxysmal atrial tachyarrhythmias, including atrial fibrillation.[35]

RIGHT ATRIAL ABNORMALITY. The electrocardiographic features of right atrial abnormality are illustrated in Figures 13-14 and 13-15. They include abnormally high P wave amplitudes in the limb and right precordial leads. As in the case of left atrial abnormality, the term *right atrial abnormality* is preferred over other terms, such as right atrial enlargement, which suggest a particular underlying pathophysiology.

Diagnostic Criteria

Criteria commonly used to diagnose right atrial abnormality are listed in Table 13-3.

MECHANISMS FOR ELECTROCARDIOGRAPHIC ABNORMALITIES. Greater right atrial mass generates greater electrical force early during atrial activation, producing taller P waves in limb leads and increasing the initial P wave deflection in lead V_1.

DIAGNOSTIC ACCURACY. Imaging studies have shown that the electrocardiographic findings of right atrial abnormality have limited sensitivity but high specificity for detecting right atrial enlargement.[34]

TABLE 13-3 Common Diagnostic Criteria for Left and Right Atrial Abnormalities

LEFT ATRIAL ABNORMALITY	RIGHT ATRIAL ABNORMALITY*
Prolonged P wave duration > 120 msec in lead II	Peaked P waves with amplitudes in lead II > 0.25 mV (P pulmonale)
Prominent notching of P wave, usually most obvious in lead II, with interval between notches of 0.40 msec (P mitrale)	Prominent initial positivity in lead V_1 or V_2 > 0.15 mV
Ratio between the duration of the P wave in lead II and duration of the PR segment > 1.6	Increased area under initial positive portion of the P wave in lead V_1 to > 0.06 mm-sec
Increased duration and depth of terminal- negative portion of P wave in lead V_1 (P terminal force) so that area subtended by it > 0.04 mm-sec	Rightward shift of mean P wave axis to more than +75 degrees
Leftward shift of mean P wave axis to between −30 and −45 degrees	

*In addition to criteria based on P wave morphologies, right atrial abnormalities are suggested by QRS changes, including (1) Q waves (especially qR patterns) in the right precordial leads without evidence of myocardial infarction and (2) low-amplitude (<600 μV) QRS complexes in lead V_1 with a threefold or greater increase in lead V_2.

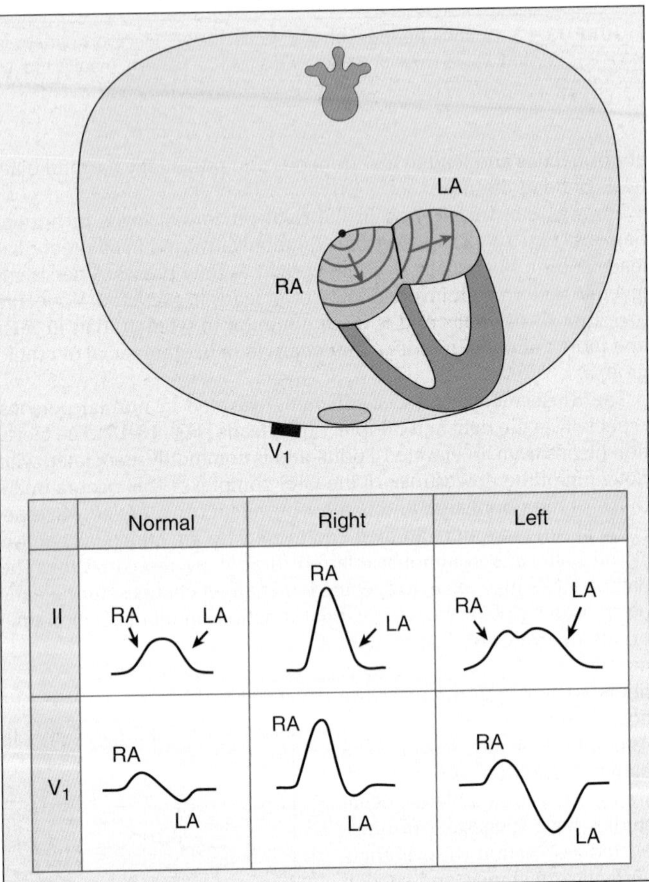

FIGURE 13-14 Schematic representation of atrial depolarization (diagram) and P wave patterns associated with normal atrial activation **(left panel)** and with right **(middle panel)** and left **(right panel)** atrial abnormalities. *(Modified from Park MK, Guntheroth WG: How to Read Pediatric ECGs. 3rd ed. St. Louis, Mosby-Year Book, 1993.)*

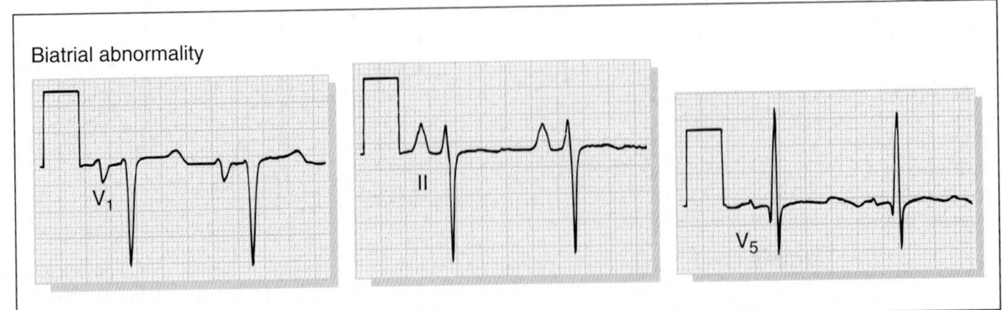

FIGURE 13-15 Biatrial abnormality, with tall P waves in lead II (right atrial abnormality) and an abnormally large terminal negative component of the P wave in lead V_1 (left atrial abnormality). The P wave is also notched in lead V_5.

CLINICAL SIGNIFICANCE. Patients with chronic obstructive pulmonary disease and this electrocardiographic pattern (often referred to as P pulmonale) have more severe pulmonary dysfunction and significantly reduced survival than do others (see Chap. 78). However, comparison of electrocardiographic and hemodynamic parameters has not demonstrated a close correlation of P wave patterns and right atrial hypertension.

OTHER ATRIAL ABNORMALITIES. Patients with abnormalities in both atria—that is, biatrial abnormality—can have electrocardiographic patterns reflecting each defect. Suggestive findings include large biphasic P waves in lead V_1 and tall and broad P waves in leads II, III, and aVF (see Fig. 13-15). P wave and PR segment changes can also be seen in patients with atrial infarction or pericarditis, as described later in this chapter.

Ventricular Hypertrophy

LEFT VENTRICULAR HYPERTROPHY. Left ventricular hypertrophy (LVH) produces changes in the QRS complex, the ST segment, and the T wave. The most characteristic finding is increased amplitude of the QRS complex. R waves in leads facing the left ventricle (i.e., leads I, aVL, V_5, and V_6) are taller than normal, and S waves in leads overlying the right ventricle (i.e., V_1 and V_2) are deeper than normal. These changes are illustrated in **Figure 13-16**.

ST-T wave patterns vary widely in patients with LVH. The ST segment may be normal or elevated in leads with tall R waves. In many patients, however, the ST segment is depressed and followed by an inverted T wave (**Fig. 13-17**). In most cases, the ST segment slopes downward from a depressed J point and the T wave is asymmetrically inverted. These LVH-related repolarization changes usually occur in patients with QRS changes but may appear alone. Particularly prominent inverted T waves, so-called giant negative T waves, are characteristic of hypertrophic cardiomyopathy with predominant apical thickening (Yamaguchi syndrome; see Fig. 13-46).

Other QRS changes seen in cases of LVH include widening of the QRS complex beyond 110 msec, a delay in the intrinsicoid deflection, and notching of the QRS complex. Additional electrocardiographic abnormalities may include prolongation of the QT interval and evidence of left atrial abnormality.

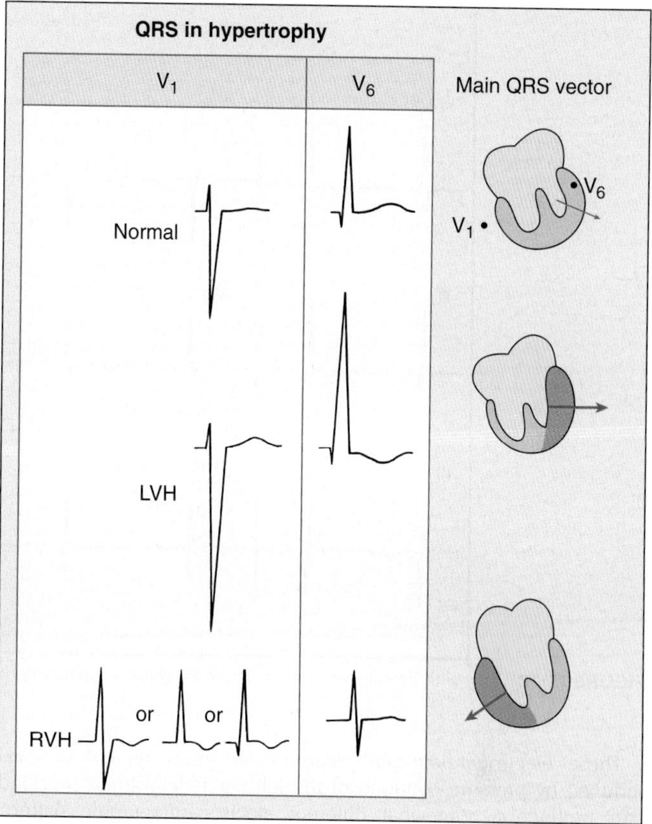

FIGURE 13-16 LVH increases the amplitude of electrical forces directed to the left and posteriorly. In addition, repolarization abnormalities can cause ST-segment depression and T wave inversion in leads with a prominent R wave (formerly referred to as a strain pattern). RVH can shift the QRS vector to the right; this effect is usually associated with an R, RS, or qR complex in lead V_1, especially when caused by severe pressure overload. T wave inversions may be present in the right precordial leads. *(From Goldberger AL: Clinical Electrocardiography: A Simplified Approach. 7th ed. St. Louis, CV Mosby, 2006.)*

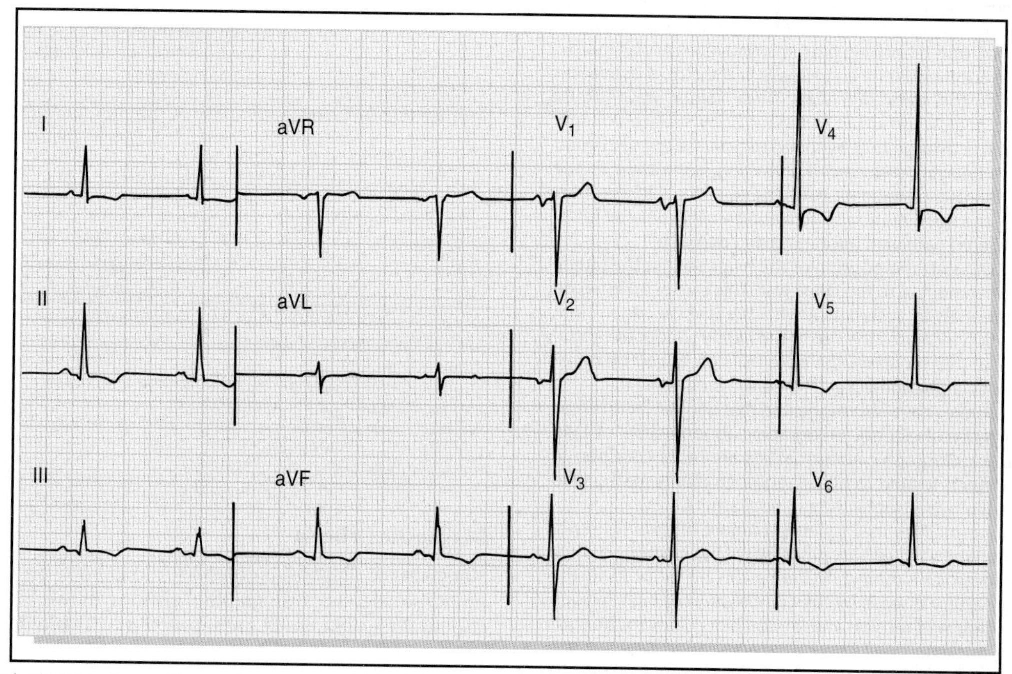

FIGURE 13-17 Marked LVH pattern with prominent precordial lead QRS voltages. ST depression and T wave inversion can be seen with severe LVH in leads with a predominant R wave (compare with Fig. 13-18). Left atrial abnormality is also present.

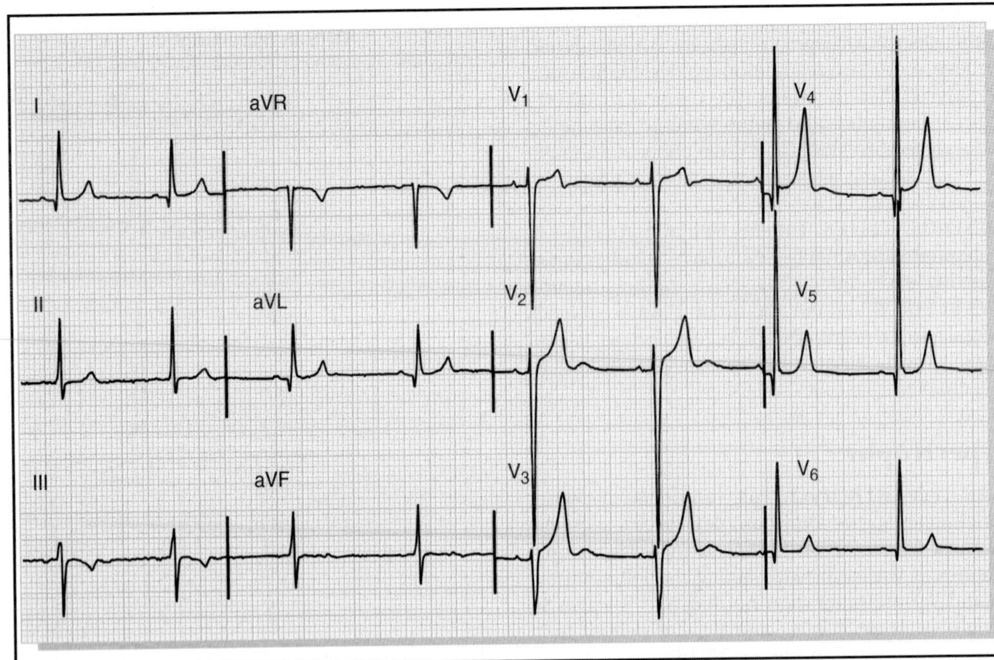

FIGURE 13-18 LVH with prominent positive anterior T waves from a patient with severe aortic regurgitation. The serum potassium level was normal.

These electrocardiographic features are most typical of LVH induced by pressure overload of the left ventricle. Volume overload can produce a somewhat different electrocardiographic pattern, including tall, upright T waves, and sometimes narrow (less than 25 msec) but deep (0.2 mV or greater) Q waves in leads facing the left side of the septum or the left ventricular free wall (**Fig. 13-18**). These distinctions have limited value in diagnosing hemodynamic conditions and their use in electrocardiographic diagnoses has been discouraged.[33]

MECHANISMS FOR ELECTROCARDIOGRAPHIC ABNORMALITIES. Electrocardiographic changes of LVH result from abnormalities at the cellular, tissue, and volume conductor levels. These abnormalities may be compounded by changes caused by concomitant clinical conditions, such as myocardial ischemia.

At the cellular level, hypertrophy is associated with a form of electrical remodeling that alters action potential shape and duration.[36] These include heterogeneous changes in the function and distribution of ion channels, myocyte size and branching patterns, and intercellular matrix.

These effects are augmented by an increase in the size of activation fronts moving across the thickened wall. These larger wave fronts subtend larger solid angles and result in higher body surface voltage. Prolonged transmural activation time required to activate the thickened wall, combined with delayed endocardial activation, contribute to the high voltage as well as QRS prolongation. Notching of the QRS complex can be produced by the fractionation of activation wave fronts by intramural scarring associated with wall thickening and damage.

In addition, LVH can shift the position of the heart so that the lateral free wall lies closer than normal to the chest wall. This causes an increase in body surface potentials in accordance with the inverse square law. Also, ventricular dilation increases the size of the highly conductive intraventricular blood pool that increases the potentials produced by transmural activation fronts, a phenomenon termed the *Brody effect.*

Recent genome studies have also suggested that genetic factors may influence the emergence of electrocardiographic abnormalities of LVH. For example, electrocardiographic abnormalities are more common in carriers of genetic defects related to hypertrophic cardiomyopathy who do not have ventricular hypertrophy than in noncarriers.[37]

ST-T segment abnormalities may reflect a primary disorder of repolarization that accompanies the cellular processes of hypertrophy or they may reflect subendocardial ischemia. Ischemia can be induced in the absence of coronary artery disease by the combination of high oxygen demand caused by high wall tension and limited blood flow to the subendocardium of the thickened wall. There is no association between the ST segment shifts and hemodynamic work, so the term *strain* used to describe these changes is best avoided and the term *secondary ST-T wave abnormalities* should be used.[33]

TABLE 13-4 Common Diagnostic Criteria for Left Ventricular Hypertrophy

MEASUREMENT	CRITERIA
Sokolow-Lyon voltages	$SV_1 + RV_5 > 3.5$ mV RaVL > 1.1 mV
Romhilt-Estes point score system*	Any limb lead R wave or S wave > 2.0 mV (3 points) *or* SV_1 or $SV_2 \geq 3.0$ mV (3 points) *or* RV_5 to $RV_6 \geq 3.0$ mV (3 points) ST-T wave abnormality, no digitalis therapy (3 points) ST-T wave abnormality, digitalis therapy (1 point) Left atrial abnormality (3 points) Left axis deviation ≥ −30 degrees (2 points) QRS duration ≥ 90 msec (1 point) Intrinsicoid deflection in V_5 or $V_6 \geq 50$ msec (1 point)
Cornell voltage criteria	SV_3 + RaVL ≥ 2.8 mV (for men) SV_3 + RaVL >2.0 mV (for women)
Cornell regression equation	Risk of LVH = $1/(1+ e^{-exp})$†
Cornell voltage duration measurement	QRS duration × Cornell voltage > 2,436 mm-sec‡ QRS duration × sum of voltages in all leads > 1,742 mm-sec

Voltages are in mV, QRS is QRS duration in msec, PTF is the area under the P terminal force in lead V_1 (in mm-sec), and gender = 1 for men and 2 for women. LVH is diagnosed present if exp < −1.55.

*Probable left ventricular hypertrophy is diagnosed if 4 points are present and definite left ventricular hypertrophy is diagnosed if 5 or more points are present.

†For subjects in sinus rhythm, exp = 4.558 − 0.092 (SV_3 + RaVL) − 0.306 TV_1 − 0.212 QRS − 0.278 $PTFV_1$ − 0.559 (gender).

‡For women, add 8 mm.

Diagnostic Criteria

Many sets of diagnostic criteria for LVH have been developed based on these electrocardiographic abnormalities. Several of the more commonly used criteria are presented in **Table 13-4**.*

*A comprehensive list of criteria has been presented by Hancock and colleagues.[33]

Most methods assess the presence or absence of LVH as a binary function, indicating that either LVH does or does not exist based on an empirically determined set of criteria. For example, the Sokolow-Lyon and Cornell voltage criteria require that voltages in specific leads exceed certain values. The Romhilt-Estes point score system assigns point values to amplitude and other criteria, including QRS axis and P wave patterns; definite LVH is diagnosed if 5 points are computed, and probable LVH is diagnosed if 4 points are computed. The Cornell voltage-duration method includes measurement of QRS duration as well as amplitudes.

Other methods seek to quantify left ventricular mass as a continuum. Diagnosis of LVH can then be based on a computed mass that exceeds an independently determined threshold. One set of criteria applying this approach is the Cornell regression equation shown in Table 13-4.

Diagnostic Accuracy. The relative diagnostic accuracy of these methods has been tested using autopsy, radiographic, echocardiographic and, most recently, magnetic resonance imaging measurements of left ventricular size as standards. Results are highly variable, varying with the specific electrocardiographic criteria that are tested, the imaging method that is relied on to determine anatomic measurements, and the population that is studied. For example, sensitivities are substantially lower when tested in the general population than in a high-risk population, such as hypertensive patients.[38] Accuracy also varies with gender (with women having lower voltages than men), with race (with African Americans having higher voltages than other racial groups), and with body habitus (with obesity reducing electrocardiographic voltages).

In general, these studies have reported low sensitivity and high specificity. Sensitivities vary from approximately 10% in the general population to approximately 50% in cohorts with hypertension who are at greater risk of having LVH.[38] A recent review of 21 studies has reported that the median sensitivity for six commonly used electrocardiographic criteria varies from 10.5% to 21% and the median specificity varies from 89% to 99%.[39] Accuracies tend to be higher for the Cornell voltage, voltage-duration, and regression methods than for others.

Thus, all methods are limited as screening tests in which high sensitivity (few false-negatives) is critical but have good reliability as diagnostic tests when few false-positives are desired. As a result, in the general population, a negative ECG has a minimal effect on the pretest likelihood of LVH, whereas a positive ECG would substantially increase the likelihood.[39] Because of the variability in the accuracy of the criteria from one trial to another, no one criterion can be established as the preferred method.[33] Using multiple criteria may increase the accuracy of electrocardiographic screening.

Repolarization abnormalities associated with QRS findings increase the correlation with anatomic LVH. ST and T wave abnormalities are associated with a threefold greater prevalence of anatomic LVH in patients without coronary artery disease.

Confounding Electrocardiographic Abnormalities. Concomitant electrocardiographic abnormalities may interfere with the diagnosis of LVH and reduce the accuracy of standard electrocardiographic criteria. Intraventricular conduction defects may affect the accuracy of electrocardiographic criteria for LVH. In left anterior fascicular block, the larger R waves in leads I and aVL and smaller R waves but deeper S waves in leads V_5 and V_6 make criteria relying on R wave amplitude less valuable.

Left bundle branch block (LBBB) makes the diagnosis of LVH difficult because of the extensive reordering of left ventricular activation (see later). In addition, the high prevalence of LVH in patients with LBBB makes assessment of the accuracy of criteria difficult. Some have concluded that the diagnosis should not be attempted in this setting, whereas others think that the diagnosis can be made. Left atrial abnormalities and QRS durations longer than 155 msec, as well as precordial lead voltage criteria, have relatively high specificity for LVH in the presence of LBBB.

The delay in right ventricular activation that occurs with right bundle branch block (see later) increases the cancellation of left ventricular forces during the middle of the QRS complex.[40] This reduces the amplitude of the S wave in the right precordial leads and of the R waves in the left precordial leads, and thus reduces the accuracy of electrocardiographic criteria for LVH. Diagnostic criteria for LVH in patients with conduction defects have been suggested.[33]

Clinical Significance

An accurate electrocardiographic diagnosis of LVH is important to detect hypertrophy, assess prognosis, and monitor progression or regression of hypertrophy during treatment. Although imaging methods may provide a more direct assessment of structural LVH, the ECG remains critical in clinical settings because of its simplicity and limited expense, and because electrocardiographic findings may provide independent, clinically important information concerning, for example, prognosis.

The presence of electrocardiographic criteria for LVH identifies a subset of the general population and of those with hypertension with a significantly increased risk for cardiovascular morbidity and mortality. Among patients with hypertension, the LIFE study[41] has reported that declines in electrocardiographic measures such as the Cornell and Sokolow-Lyon voltages during antihypertensive therapy correlate with a decrease in left ventricular mass and with lower likelihoods of cardiovascular mortality and morbidity independently of the extent of blood pressure lowering. A 1-SD decrease in the Cornell product was associated with a 22% decrease in cardiovascular deaths.

Patients with repolarization abnormalities have, on average, more severe degrees of LVH and more commonly have symptoms of left ventricular dysfunction, in addition to a greater risk of future cardiovascular events. In the LIFE study cited earlier, hypertensive patients with LVH-related ST-T wave abnormalities were 1.8 times as likely to develop congestive heart failure and 2.8 times as likely to experience heart failure–related death than patients without such ST-T wave changes.[41]

RIGHT VENTRICULAR HYPERTROPHY. The electrocardiographic effects of right ventricular hypertrophy (RVH) differ in fundamental ways from those of LVH (see Chap. 78). The right ventricle is considerably smaller than the left ventricle and produces electrical forces that are largely cancelled by those generated by the larger left ventricle. Thus, for RVH to be manifested on the ECG, it must be severe enough to overcome the masking effects of the larger left ventricular forces. In addition, increasing dominance of the right ventricle changes the ECG in fundamental ways, whereas an enlarged left ventricle produces predominantly quantitative changes in underlying normal waveforms.

The electrocardiographic changes associated with moderate to severe concentric hypertrophy of the right ventricle include abnormal, tall R waves in anteriorly and rightward-directed leads (leads aVR, V_1, and V_2), and deep S waves and abnormally small r waves in leftward-directed leads (I, aVL, and lateral precordial leads; **Fig. 13-19**). These changes result in a reversal of normal R wave progression in the precordial leads, a shift in the frontal plane QRS axis to the right, and the presence of S waves in leads I, II, and III ($S_1S_2S_3$ pattern).

Less severe hypertrophy, especially when limited to the outflow tract of the right ventricle that is activated late during the QRS complex, produces less marked changes. Electrocardiographic abnormalities may be limited to an rSr′ pattern in V_1 and persistence of s (or S) waves in the left precordial leads. This pattern is typical of right ventricular volume overload such as that produced by an atrial septal defect.

Diagnostic Criteria

These electrocardiographic abnormalities form the basis for the diagnostic criteria for RVH. The most commonly relied on criteria for the ECG diagnosis of RVH are listed in **Table 13-5**. The diagnostic accuracies of these criteria remain unclear. Although the older literature has suggested very high specificities for many of the listed criteria, these estimates were often based on small and highly selective populations. The sensitivities and specificities in the general population remain to be accurately determined.

Mechanisms for Electrocardiographic Abnormalities. These electrocardiographic patterns result from three effects of RVH:

1. Current fluxes between hypertrophied cells are stronger than normal and produce higher than normal voltage on the body surface.
2. Activation fronts moving through the enlarged right ventricle are larger than normal and produce higher surface potentials, as predicted by the solid angle theorem.
3. The activation time of the right ventricle is prolonged.

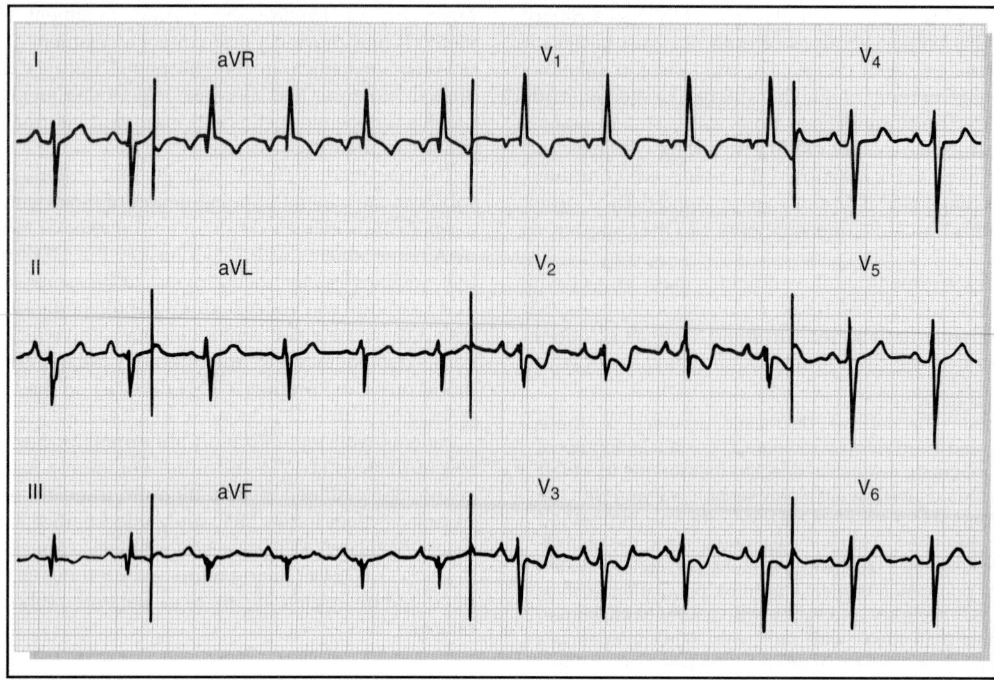

FIGURE 13-19 RVH pattern most consistent with severe pressure overload. Note the combination of findings, including (1) a tall R wave in V_1 (as part of the qR complex), (2) right axis deviation, (3) T wave inversion in V_1 through V_3, (4) delayed precordial transition zone (rS in V_6), and (5) right atrial abnormality. An S_1Q_3 pattern is also present and can occur with acute or chronic right ventricular overload syndromes.

TABLE 13-5 Common Diagnostic Criteria for Right Ventricular Hypertrophy

R in $V_1 \geq 0.7$ mV
QR in V_1
R/S in $V_1 > 1$ with $R > 0.5$ mV
R/S in V_5 or $V_6 < 1$
S in V_5 or $V_6 > 0.7$ mV
R in V_5 or $V_6 \geq 0.4$ mV with S in $V_1 \leq 0.2$ mV
Right axis deviation (>90 degrees)
S_1Q_3 pattern
$S_1S_2S_3$ pattern
P pulmonale

From Murphy ML, Thenabadu PN, de Soyza N, et al: Reevaluation of electrocardiographic criteria for left, right and combined cardiac ventricular hypertrophy. Am J Cardiol 53:1140, 1984.

Right ventricular activation now ends after the completion of left ventricular activation so that its effects are no longer canceled by the more powerful forces of the left ventricle and become manifest in the ECG. Because the right ventricle is located anteriorly as well as to the right of the left ventricle, the effects produce increased potentials in leads directed anteriorly and to the right, especially late during the QRS complex.

Chronic Obstructive Pulmonary Disease

Chronic obstructive pulmonary disease (see Chap. 78) can induce electrocardiographic changes by producing RVH, changing the position of the heart within the chest, and hyperinflating the lungs (**Fig. 13-20**). QRS changes caused by the insulating and positional changes produced by hyperinflation of the lungs include reduced amplitude of the QRS complex, right axis deviation in the frontal plane, and delayed transition in the precordial leads, probably reflecting a vertical and caudal shift in heart position caused by hyperinflation and a flattened diaphragm. Evidence of true RVH includes the following: (1) right axis deviation more positive than 110 degrees; (2) deep S waves in the lateral precordial leads; and (3) an $S_1Q_3T_3$ pattern, with an S wave in lead I (as an RS or rS complex), an abnormal Q wave in lead III, and an inverted T wave in the inferior leads.

The electrocardiographic evidence of RVH has limited value in assessing the severity of pulmonary hypertension or lung disease. QRS changes do not generally appear until ventilatory function is significantly depressed, with the earliest change commonly being a rightward shift in the mean QRS axis, and the correlation with ventilatory function or hemodynamics is poor. The presence of right atrial abnormality, an $S_1S_2S_3$ pattern, or both is associated with reduced survival.

Pulmonary Embolism

Acute right ventricular pressure overload such as that produced by pulmonary embolism can produce characteristic electrocardiographic patterns (**Fig. 13-21**; see Chap. 77). These include the following: (1) a QR or qR pattern in the right ventricular leads; (2) an $S_1Q_3T_3$ pattern with an S wave in lead I and new or increased Q waves in lead III and sometimes aVF, with T wave inversions in those leads; (3) ST-segment deviation and T wave inversions in leads V_1 to V_3; and (4) incomplete or complete right bundle branch block (RBBB). Sinus tachycardia is usually present. Occasionally, with massive pulmonary obstruction, a right ventricular current of injury pattern is seen, with ST elevations in the right midprecordial leads.

Electrocardiographic findings of acute right ventricular overload in patients with pulmonary embolism correspond to obstruction of much of the pulmonary arterial bed and significant pulmonary hypertension. However, even with major pulmonary artery obstruction, the ECG is notoriously deceptive and may show little more than minor or nonspecific waveform changes, or it may even be normal. The classic $S_1Q_3T_3$ pattern occurs in only about 10% of cases of acute pulmonary embolism (see Chap. 77). Furthermore, the specificity of this finding is limited, because it can occur with other causes of pulmonary hypertension. An analysis of the ECGs of patients with right ventricular dilation caused by acute pulmonary embolism has reported positive predictive accuracies of 23% to 69%.[42]

BIVENTRICULAR HYPERTROPHY. Hypertrophy of both ventricles produces complex electrocardiographic patterns. In contrast to biatrial enlargement, the result is not the simple sum of the two sets of abnormalities. The effects of enlargement of one chamber may cancel the effects of enlargement of the other. The greater left

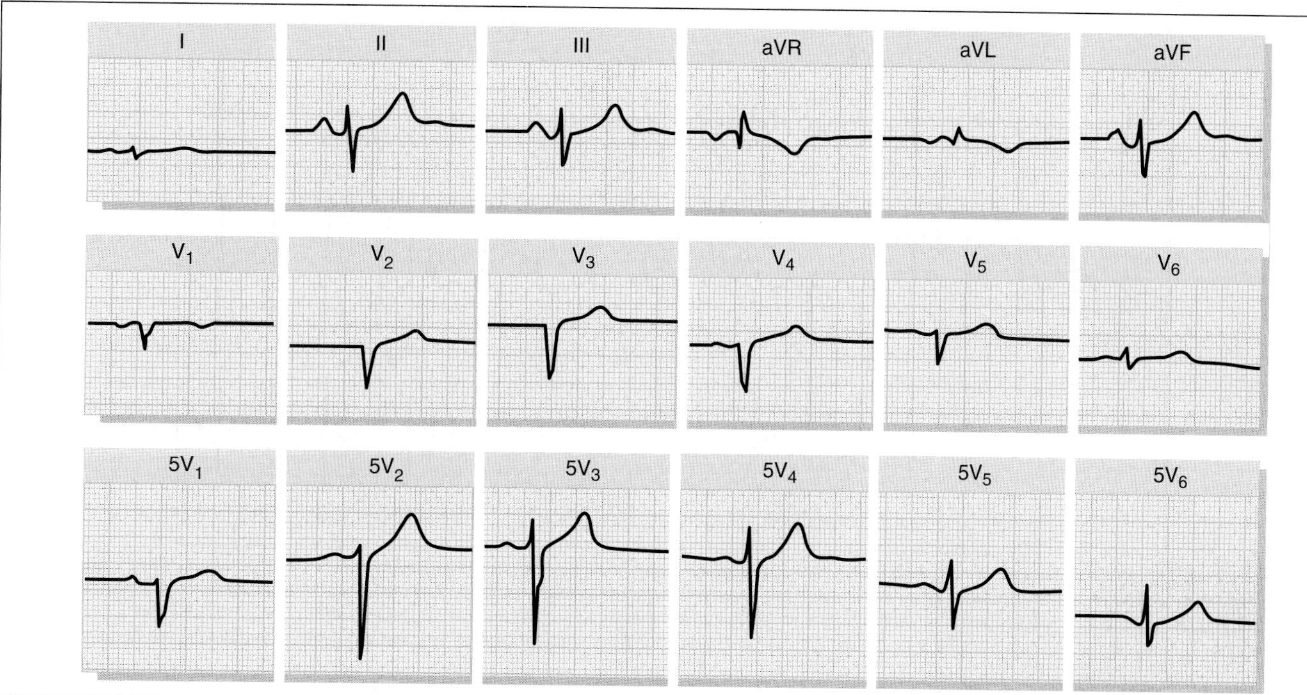

FIGURE 13-20 Pulmonary emphysema simulating anterior infarction in a 58-year-old man with no clinical evidence of coronary disease. Note the relative normalization of R wave progression with placement of the chest leads an interspace below their usual position (e.g., $5V_1$, $5V_2$). *(From Chou TC: Pseudo-infarction (noninfarction Q waves).* In *Fisch C [ed]: Complex Electrocardiography. Vol 1. Philadelphia, FA Davis, 1973.)*

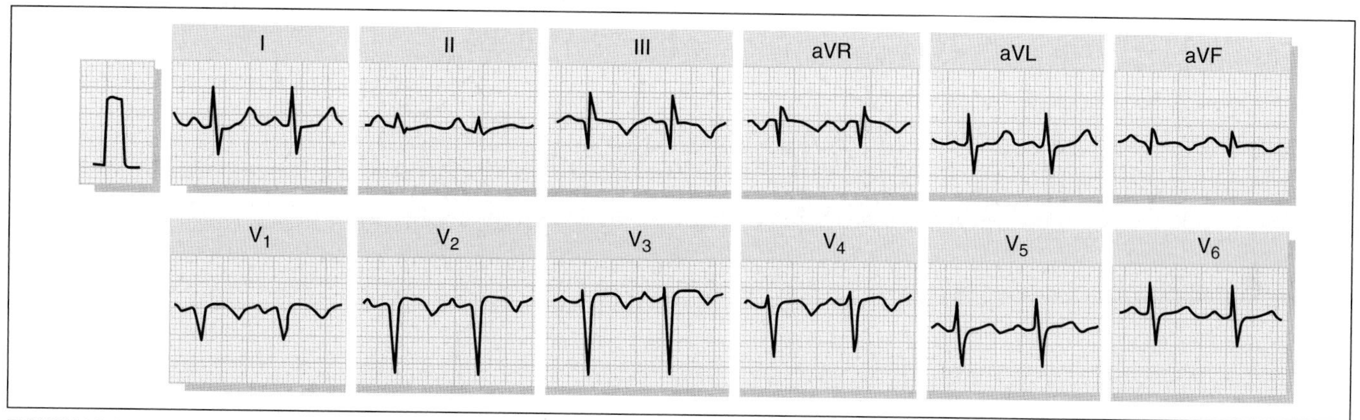

FIGURE 13-21 Acute cor pulmonale secondary to pulmonary embolism simulating inferior and anterior infarction. This tracing exemplifies the classic pseudoinfarct patterns sometimes seen: an $S_1Q_3T_3$, a QR in V_1 with poor R wave progression in the right precordial leads (clockwise rotation), and right precordial to midprecordial T wave inversion (V_1 to V_4). Sinus tachycardia is also present. The S_1Q_3 pattern is usually associated with a QR or QS complex, but not an rS, in aVR. Furthermore, acute cor pulmonale per se does not cause prominent Q waves in II (only in III and aVF). *(From Goldberger AL: Myocardial Infarction: Electrocardiographic Differential Diagnosis. 4th ed. St. Louis, Mosby-Year Book, 1991.)*

ventricular forces generated in LVH increase the degree of RVH needed to overcome the dominance of the left ventricle, and the anterior forces produced by RVH may cancel or be canceled by enhanced posterior forces generated by LVH.

Because of these factors, specific electrocardiographic criteria for RVH or LVH are seldom observed with biventricular enlargement. Rather, electrocardiographic patterns are usually a modification of the features of LVH, such as the following: (1) tall R waves in the right and left precordial leads; (2) vertical heart position or right axis deviation in the presence of criteria for LVH; (3) deep S waves in the left precordial leads in the presence of electrocardiographic criteria for LVH; or (4) a shift in the precordial transition zone to the left in the presence of LVH. The presence of prominent left atrial abnormality or atrial fibrillation with evidence of right ventricular or biventricular enlargement (especially LVH with a vertical or rightward QRS axis) should suggest chronic rheumatic valvular disease (**Fig. 13-22**; see Chap. 66).

Intraventricular Conduction Delays

Delays in intraventricular conduction of cardiac impulses may result from abnormalities in the His-Purkinje system or in ventricular muscle, and may be caused by structural changes or by the functional properties of the cardiac conduction system.[43] Although the conduction abnormalities to be described will be referred to in specific anatomic terms (e.g., right bundle branch block), the electrocardiographic changes may be caused by abnormalities in various sites within the ventricles. Hence, the anatomic references are not intended to localize sites of impaired function precisely.

FASCICULAR BLOCK. Under normal conditions, activation of the left ventricle begins almost simultaneously at the insertion points of the fascicles of the left bundle branch. Absolute or relative delays in conduction in a fascicle, fascicular block, results in an abnormal

CH 13

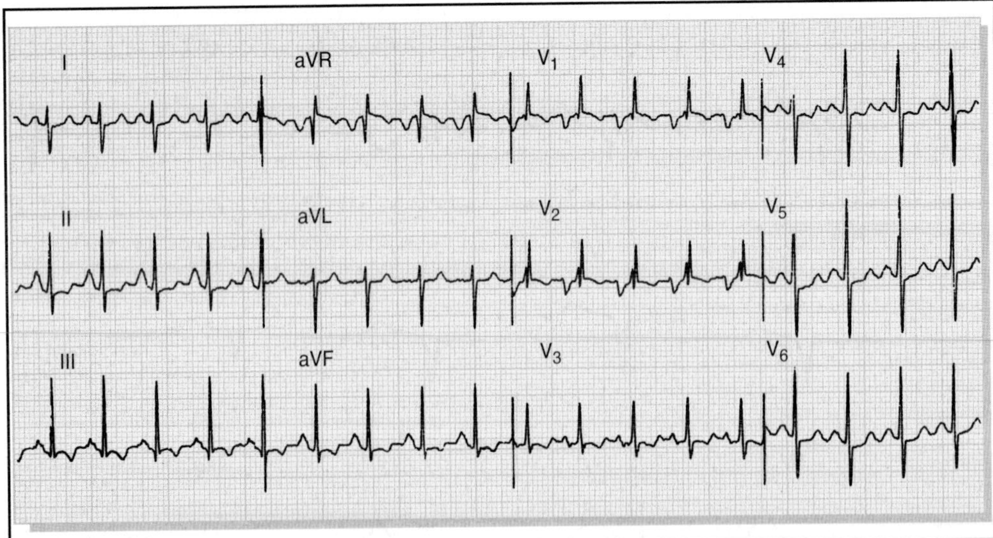

FIGURE 13-22 ECG from a 45-year-old woman with severe mitral stenosis showing multiple abnormalities. The rhythm is sinus tachycardia. Right axis deviation and a tall R wave in lead V_1 are consistent with right ventricular hypertrophy. The very prominent biphasic P wave in lead V_1 indicates left atrial abnormality and enlargement. The tall P waves in lead II suggest concomitant right abnormality. Nonspecific ST-T changes and incomplete right bundle branch block are also present. The combination of right ventricular hypertrophy and marked left or biatrial abnormality is highly suggestive of mitral stenosis. *(From Goldberger AL: Clinical Electrocardiography: A Simplified Approach. 7th ed. St. Louis, CV Mosby, 2006.)*

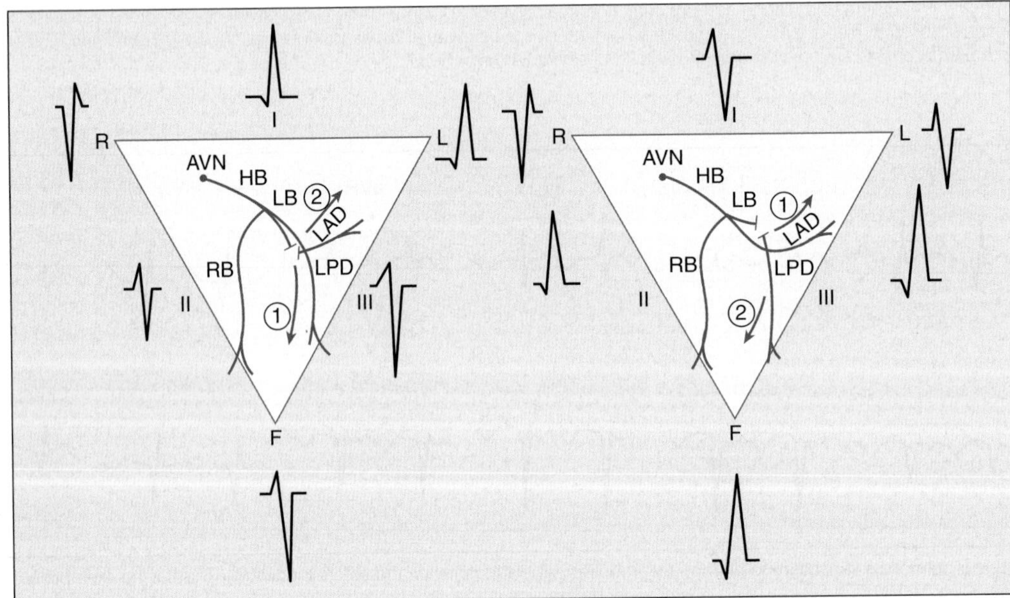

FIGURE 13-23 Diagrammatic representation of fascicular blocks in the left ventricle. **Left,** Interruption of the left anterior fascicle or division (LAD) results in an initial inferior (1) followed by a dominant superior (2) direction of activation. **Right,** Interruption of the left posterior fascicle or division (LPD) results in an initial superior (1) followed by a dominant inferior (2) direction of activation. AVN = atrioventricular node; HB = His bundle; LB = left bundle; RB = right bundle. *(Courtesy of Dr. C. Fisch.)*

sequence of early left ventricular activation that, in turn, leads to characteristic electrocardiographic patterns. Even modest delays in conduction through the affected structure may be enough to alter ventricular activation patterns sufficiently to produce characteristic electrocardiographic patterns; a complete block of conduction is not required.

Left Anterior Fascicular Block. The electrocardiographic features of left anterior fascicular block (LAFB) are listed in **Table 13-6** and illustrated in **Figure 13-23**. The most characteristic finding is marked left axis deviation.

The left anterior fascicle normally activates the anterosuperior portion of the left ventricle early during the QRS complex. With LAFB, this region is activated later than normal, resulting in unbalanced inferior and posterior forces early during ventricular activation (initiated by the left posterior fascicle) and unopposed anterosuperior forces later during the QRS complex (the region activated late).

TABLE 13-6 Common Diagnostic Criteria for Unifascicular Blocks

Left Anterior Fascicular Block
Frontal plane mean QRS axis = −45 to −90 degrees
qR pattern in lead aVL
QRS duration < 120 msec
Time to peak R wave in aVL ≥ 45 msec
Left Posterior Fascicular Block
Frontal plane mean QRS axis = +90 to +180 degrees
rS pattern in leads I and aVL with qR patterns in leads III and aVF
QRS duration < 120 msec
Exclusion of other factors causing right axis deviation (e.g., right ventricular overload patterns, lateral infarction)

These changes are manifest on the ECG as a leftward shift of the mean frontal plane QRS axis. The characteristic pattern in the inferior leads includes initial r waves (caused by early unopposed activation of the inferoposterior left ventricle) followed by deep S waves (caused by late unopposed activation of the anterosuperior left ventricle; left axis deviation with rS patterns). The left-looking leads (e.g., leads I and aVL) show a qR pattern.

However, LAFB is not synonymous with left axis deviation. Axis shifts to between 30 and 45 degrees commonly reflect other conditions, such as LVH, without conduction system damage, and such patterns are best referred to as (moderate) left axis deviation rather than LAFB.

LAFB can also produce prominent changes in the precordial leads. Leads V_4 through V_6 commonly show deep S waves (a delayed transition) produced by the late activation of the anterosuperior left ventricle. The overall QRS duration is not prolonged; fascicular block alters the sequence but not the overall duration of left ventricular activation.

Damage to the left anterior fascicle is a very common occurrence because of the delicate nature of the structure. Left anterior fascicular block is common in persons without overt cardiac disease, as well as in persons with a wide range of conditions. In patients with coronary artery disease, the presence of LAFB may be associated with an increased risk of cardiac death.[44] Commonly associated conditions include myocardial infarction, especially occlusion of the left anterior descending coronary artery, LVH, hypertrophic and dilated cardiomyopathy, and various cardiac degenerative diseases. The development of LAFB with rS complexes in leads II, III, and aVF can mask the Q waves of an inferior myocardial infarction.

Left Posterior Fascicular Block. Conduction delay in the left posterior fascicle is considerably less common than delay in the anterior fascicle because of its thicker structure and more protected location near the left ventricular inflow tract. Conduction delay results in early unopposed activation of the anterosuperior left ventricular free wall, followed by late activation of the inferoposterior aspect of the left ventricle—that is, the reverse of the pattern observed with LAFB.

The electrocardiographic features of left posterior fascicular block (LPFB; see Table 13-6 and Fig. 13-23), reflect this altered activation pattern. Right axis deviation, with rS patterns in leads I and aVL as well as qR complexes in the inferior leads, is the result of early unopposed activation forces from the anterosuperior aspect of the left ventricle (activated early via the left anterior fascicle and producing the initial q and r waves) and of late unopposed forces from the inferoposterior free wall (activated late via the left posterior fascicle and generating the late S and R waves). As in the case of LAFB, the overall activation time of the ventricles is not prolonged, and the QRS duration remains normal.

LPFB can occur in patients with almost any cardiac disease but is unusual in otherwise healthy persons. Other conditions that augment or appear to augment the rightward electrical forces in the frontal plane, such as right ventricular overload syndromes and extensive lateral infarction, can produce similar electrocardiographic patterns and must be excluded before a diagnosis of LPFB can be made.

Other Forms of Fascicular Block. Electrocardiographic patterns that suggest left septal fascicular block have also been described. The most common electrocardiographic finding attributed to this form of block is the absence of septal q waves. It has been recommended that this term not be used because clear diagnostic criteria have not been developed.[43]

TABLE 13-7 Common Diagnostic Criteria for Bundle Branch Blocks

Complete Left Bundle Branch Block
QRS duration ≥ 120 msec
Broad, notched, or slurred R waves in leads I, aVL, V_5 and V_6
Small or absent initial r waves in right precordial leads (V_1 and V_2) followed by deep S waves
Absent septal q waves in leads I, V_5, and V_6
Prolonged time to peak R wave (>60 msec) in V_5 and V_6
Complete Right Bundle Branch Block
QRS duration ≥ 120 msec
rsr′, rsR′,, or rSR′, patterns in leads V_1 and V_2
S waves in leads I and V_6 ≥ 40 msec wide
Normal time to peak R wave in leads V_5 and V_6 but >50 msec in V_1

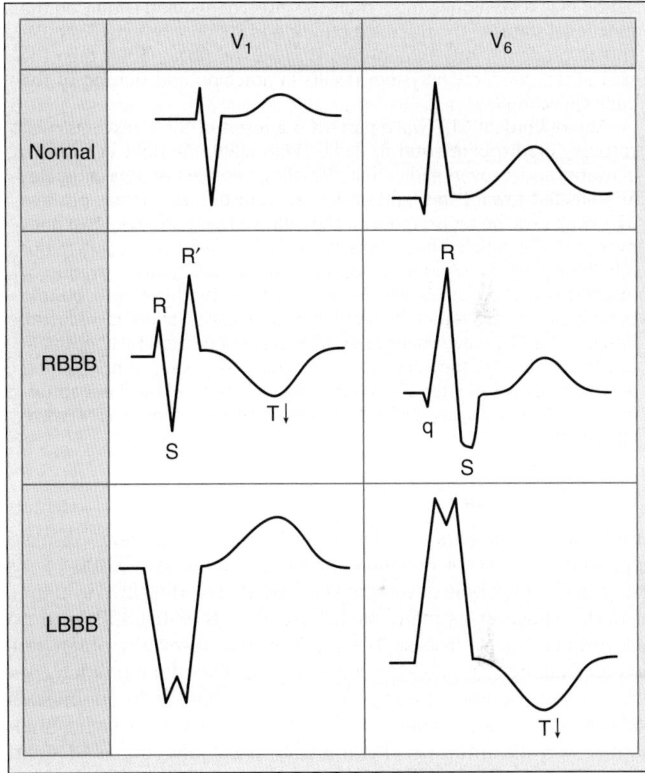

FIGURE 13-24 Comparison of typical QRS-T patterns in RBBB and LBBB with the normal pattern in leads V_1 and V_6. Note the secondary T wave inversions (arrows) in leads with an rSR′ complex with RBBB and in leads with a wide R wave with LBBB. *(From Goldberger AL: Clinical Electrocardiography: A Simplified Approach. 6th ed., St. Louis, CV Mosby, 1999.)*

LEFT BUNDLE BRANCH BLOCK. LBBB results from conduction delay or block in any of several sites in the intraventricular conduction system, including the main left bundle branch, each of the two fascicles, the distal conduction system of the left ventricle or, less commonly, the fibers of the bundle of His that become the main left bundle branch. The result is extensive reorganization of the activation and recovery patterns of the left ventricle that produces extensive changes in the QRS complex and ST-T wave.

ECG Abnormalities

LBBB produces a prolonged QRS duration, abnormal QRS patterns, and ST-T wave abnormalities (**Fig. 13-24**). Commonly accepted diagnostic criteria for LBBB are listed in **Table 13-7**. Basic requirements include a prolonged QRS duration to 120 msec or more, broad and commonly notched R waves in leads I and aVL and the left precordial leads, narrow r waves followed by deep S waves in the right precordial leads, and absent septal q waves. R waves are typically tall and S waves are deep. The mean QRS axis with LBBB is highly variable; it can be normal, deviated to the left or, rarely, deviated to the right. In addition to these features, some require a prolonged time to the peak of the R wave (> 60 msec) in the left precordial leads to diagnose LBBB.[43]

ST-T wave changes are prominent with LBBB. In most cases, the ST segment and T wave are discordant with the QRS complex. That is, the ST segment is depressed and the T wave is inverted in leads with positive QRS waves (e.g., leads I, aVL, V_5, and V_6), and the ST segment is elevated and the T wave is upright in leads with negative QRS complexes (e.g., leads V_1 and V_2).

An incomplete form of LBBB may result from lesser degrees of conduction delay in the left bundle branch system. Electrocardiographic features include the following: (1) modest prolongation of the QRS complex (between 100 and 119 msec); (2) loss of septal q waves; (3) slurring and notching of the upstroke of tall R waves; and (4) delay in the time to the peak of the R wave in left precordial leads. The pattern commonly is similar to that of LVH.

Mechanisms for the Electrocardiographic Abnormalities. The electrocardiographic abnormalities of LBBB result from an almost completely reorganized pattern of left ventricular activation.[45] The site and timing of septal activation vary, suggesting differences in the pathophysiology of LBBB. Initial septal activation typically occurs on the right (rather than on the left) septal surface. This leads to right to left (rather than left to right) activation of the septum, resulting in the absence of normal septal q waves in the ECG. In some cases, earliest left septal activation occurs high along the septum, remote from the left side conduction system, suggesting transseptal activation. In other cases, earliest left septal activation occurs in the midseptal region in or just anterior to the left posterior fascicle, suggesting activation by slow conduction within the left bundle system rather than by transseptal spread. Other patients with LBBB have near-normal left septal activation time, indicating a more peripheral site of block.

After septal activation, activation of the left ventricular free wall is also varied. The spread of activation may be disrupted by regions of block, which may, for example, require the activation of the anterior left ventricule by fronts moving though the inferior or apical portions of the left ventricle. These blocks may be fixed, caused by scarring, or may be transient, related to functional derangements in conduction. Overall activation may then require more than 180 msec, depending largely on the functional status of the distal left bundle and Purkinje systems. Irregular spread predominantly through working muscle fibers rather than the specialized conduction system results in notching and slurring of the wide QRS complex.

The discordant ST-T wave pattern is a result of the transventricular recovery gradients referred to earlier. With LBBB, the right ventricle is activated and recovers earlier than the left, so recovery vectors or dipoles are directed toward the right and away from the left. Hence, positive ST-T waves will be registered over the right ventricle and negative ones over the left ventricle. These transventricular gradients play only a minor role during normal conduction because the simultaneous activation of multiple regions cancels the forces that they produce; with bundle branch block, activation is sequential and cancellation is reduced. Because the ST-T wave changes with LBBB are generated by abnormalities in conduction, they are called secondary ST-T wave abnormalities; as will be discussed later, ST-T wave changes produced by direct abnormalities of the recovery process are referred to as primary ST- T wave abnormalities.

Clinical Significance

LBBB usually appears in patients with underlying heart disease; approximately 30% of patients with heart failure have LBBB.[46,47] As many as 70% of people developing LBBB had preceding ECG evidence of LVH.[46] However, as many as 12% of patients with LBBB have no demonstrable heart disease. The prevalence and severity of left ventricular dysfunction increase progressively as QRS duration increases.

LBBB has significant prognostic implications. Even in persons without overt heart disease, LBBB is associated with a higher than normal risk of cardiovascular mortality from infarction and heart failure. The risk of heart failure increases progressively as QRS duration increases.[48] LBBB is associated with substantially higher than expected risks of high-grade atrioventricular block and cardiac death, mostly because of sudden death outside the hospital setting. Among patients with coronary artery disease, the presence of LBBB correlates with more extensive disease, more severe left ventricular dysfunction, and reduced survival rates.

Patients with associated left or, rarely, right axis deviation have more severe clinical manifestations. Left axis deviation is associated with more severe conduction system disease that includes the fascicles and the main left bundle, whereas right axis deviation suggests dilated cardiomyopathy with biventricular enlargement.

The abnormal ventricular activation pattern of LBBB itself induces hemodynamic changes that are superimposed on the abnormalities caused by the underlying heart disease. These include premature movement of the septum into the left ventricle that is followed by delayed contraction of the posterior and lateral walls of the left ventricle.[49] As a result, when the lateral wall does contract, blood pushes the compliant septum toward the right ventricular cavity rather than out the aortic valve, reducing the ejection fraction and efficiency. Severe left ventricular dyssynergy, with a delay of more than 60 msec between septal and lateral wall contraction, is found in 60% of patients with QRS durations of 120 to 150 msec and in 70% of those with QRS durations over 150 msec (see Chaps. 28 and 38).

A major impact of LBBB lies in obscuring or simulating other electrocardiographic patterns. The diagnosis of LVH is complicated by the increased QRS amplitude and axis shifts intrinsic to LBBB; in addition, the very high prevalence of anatomic LVH in combination with LBBB makes defining criteria with high specificity difficult. The diagnosis of myocardial infarction may be obscured; as will be described, the emergence of abnormal Q waves with infarction is dependent on a normal initial sequence of ventricular activation, which is absent with LBBB. In addition, electrocardiographic patterns of LBBB, including low R wave amplitude in the midprecordial leads and ST-T wave changes, can simulate anterior infarct patterns.

RIGHT BUNDLE BRANCH BLOCK. Right bundle branch block is a result of conduction delay in any portion of the right-sided intraventricular conduction system. The delay can occur in the main right bundle branch itself, in the bundle of His, or in the distal right ventricular conduction system. The latter is the common cause of RBBB after a right ventriculotomy is performed, for example, to correct the tetralogy of Fallot.

Electrocardiographic Abnormalities

Major features of RBBB are illustrated in Figure 13-24 and commonly used diagnostic criteria are listed in Table 13-7. As with LBBB, the QRS complex duration exceeds 120 msec. The right precordial leads show prominent and notched R waves with rsr′, rsR′, or rSR′ patterns, whereas leads I and aVL and the left precordial leads demonstrate wide S waves that are longer in duration than the preceding R wave. The ST-T waves are, as in LBBB, discordant with the QRS complex, so T waves are inverted in the right precordial leads (and other leads with a terminal R′ wave) and upright in the left precordial leads and in leads I and aVL.

The mean QRS axis is not altered by RBBB. Axis shifts can occur, however, as a result of the simultaneous occurrence of fascicular block along with RBBB (see later). This combination of RBBB with LAFB (producing left axis deviation) or LPFB (producing right axis deviation) is termed *bifascicular block*.

Features indicative of incomplete RBBB, produced by lesser delays in conduction in the right bundle branch system, are commonly seen. This finding is most frequently characterized by an rSr′ pattern in lead V_1 with a QRS duration between 100 and 120 msec. Although these electrocardiographic changes of incomplete RBBB are commonly attributed to conduction defects, they can reflect RVH (especially with a rightward QRS axis) without intrinsic dysfunction of the conduction system. An rSr′ morphology in lead V_1 (and sometimes V_2) with a narrow QRS duration (≤ 100 msec) is a common physiologic or positional variant.

Mechanism for Electrocardiographic Abnormalities. With delay or block in the proximal right bundle branch system, activation of the right side of the septum is initiated only after slow transseptal spread of activation from the left septal surface.[49] The right ventricular anterior free wall is then excited slowly, followed by activation of the lateral right ventricular wall and, finally, the right ventricular outflow tract.

The result is delayed and slow activation of the right ventricle. Much or all of the right ventricle undergoes activation after depolarization of the left ventricle has been completed. This reduces the cancellation of right ventricular activation forces by the more powerful left ventricular activation forces. The late and unopposed emergence of right ventricular forces produces increased anterior and rightward voltage in the later half of the ECG, as well as a prolonged QRS complex. Discordant ST-T wave patterns are generated by the same mechanisms as for LBBB; with RBBB, recovery forces are directed toward the earlier activated left ventricle and away from the right.

A substantial proportion of patients with RBBB have abnormalities of left ventricular activation that are similar to those in patients with LBBB.[49] This suggests that many patients with RBBB have a diffuse, biventricular conduction system disease.

Clinical Significance

RBBB is a common finding in the general population, and many persons with RBBB have no clinical evidence of structural heart disease. The high prevalence of RBBB corresponds to the relative fragility of the right bundle branch, as suggested by the development of RBBB after the minor trauma produced by right ventricular catheterization.

In some reports, RBBB is an independent predictor of cardiovascular mortality. The new onset of RBBB predicts a higher rate of coronary artery disease, congestive heart failure, and cardiovascular mortality. When cardiac disease is present, the coexistence of RBBB suggests advanced disease with, for example, more extensive multivessel disease and reduced long-term survival in patients with ischemic heart disease. An entity known as the Brugada syndrome[50] has been described, in which an RBBB-like pattern with persistent ST-segment elevation in the right precordial leads is associated with susceptibility to ventricular tachyarrhythmias and sudden cardiac death (see Chaps. 9 and 39).

RBBB interferes with other electrocardiographic diagnoses, although to a lesser extent than LBBB. The diagnosis of RVH is more difficult to make with RBBB because of the accentuated positive potentials in lead V_1. RVH is suggested, although with limited accuracy, by the presence of an R wave in lead V_1 that exceeds 1.5 mV and a rightward shift of the mean QRS axis. The usual criteria for LVH can be applied but have lower sensitivities than with normal conduction. The combination of left atrial abnormality or left axis deviation with RBBB also suggests underlying LVH.

Multifascicular Blocks. The term *multifascicular block* refers to conduction delay or block in more than one of the structural components of the specialized conduction system—that is, the left bundle branch, the left anterior and posterior fascicles of the left bundle branch, and the right bundle branch. Conduction delay in any two fascicles is termed *bifascicular block,* and delay in all three fascicles is termed *trifascicular block*. The term *bilateral bundle branch block* has been used to refer to concomitant conduction abnormalities in both the left and right bundle branch systems.

Bifascicular block can have several forms: (1) RBBB with LAFB, characterized by the electrocardiographic pattern of RBBB plus left axis deviation beyond −45 degrees (**Fig. 13-25**); (2) RBBB with LPFB, with an electrocardiographic pattern of RBBB and a mean QRS axis deviation to the right of +120 degrees (**Fig. 13-26**); or (3) LBBB alone that may be caused by delay in both the anterior and posterior fascicles. This form of LBBB represents one of the inadequacies of current electrocardiographic terminology and the simplification inherent in the trifascicular schema of the conduction system.[43] The electrophysiologic consequences of these abnormalities are discussed in Chaps. 35 and 38.

Trifascicular block involves conduction delay in the right bundle branch plus delay in the main left bundle branch or in both the left anterior and the left posterior fascicles. The resulting electrocardiographic pattern is dependent on the relative degree of delay in the affected structures and on the shortest conduction time from the atria to the ventricles through any one part of the conducting system. Ventricular activation begins at the site of insertion of the branch with the fastest conduction time and spreads from there to the remainder of the ventricles. For example, if conduction in the right and left bundle branches exists and the delay in the right bundle branch is shorter than the delay in the left bundle branch, activation will begin in the right ventricle and the QRS pattern will resemble that of LBBB. If the delay were longer in the right bundle branch than in the left bundle branch, the electrocardiographic pattern would be that of RBBB. The fascicle with the longest delay can vary with, for example, the heart rate and lead to changing or alternating conduction patterns (**Fig. 13-27**).

What distinguishes electrocardiographic patterns of trifascicular block from those of bifascicular block is an increase in the overall conduction time from the AV node to the ventricles. In bifascicular block, conduction time through the unaffected fascicle (and hence, overall conduction time) is normal in the absence of concomitant AV nodal conduction delay. In trifascicular block, however, the delay in conduction through even the least affected fascicle is abnormal and results in relative prolongation of the overall conduction time from the AV node to the ventricular myocardium. (Note that only delay, not block, of conduction is required. If block were present in all fascicles, conduction would fail and complete heart block would result. This situation is perhaps best illustrated by cases of alternating bundle branch block (see Fig. 13-27); if the block were total in one bundle branch, development of block in the other would produce complete AV block rather than a change in bundle branch block patterns.) Thus, a diagnosis of trifascicular block requires an electrocardiographic pattern of bifascicular block plus evidence of prolonged conduction below the AV node.

This delay in conduction is most specifically observed as a prolongation of the His-ventricular (HV) time in intracardiac recordings. On the surface ECG, the delay in conduction delay may be manifest as a prolonged PR interval. However, the PR interval includes conduction time in the AV node as well as in the intraventricular conduction system. Prolonged intraventricular conduction may be insufficient to extend the PR interval beyond normal limits, whereas a prolonged PR interval can reflect delay in the AV node rather than in all three intraventricular fascicles.

Thus, it should be noted that the finding of a prolonged PR interval in the presence of an electrocardiographic pattern consistent with

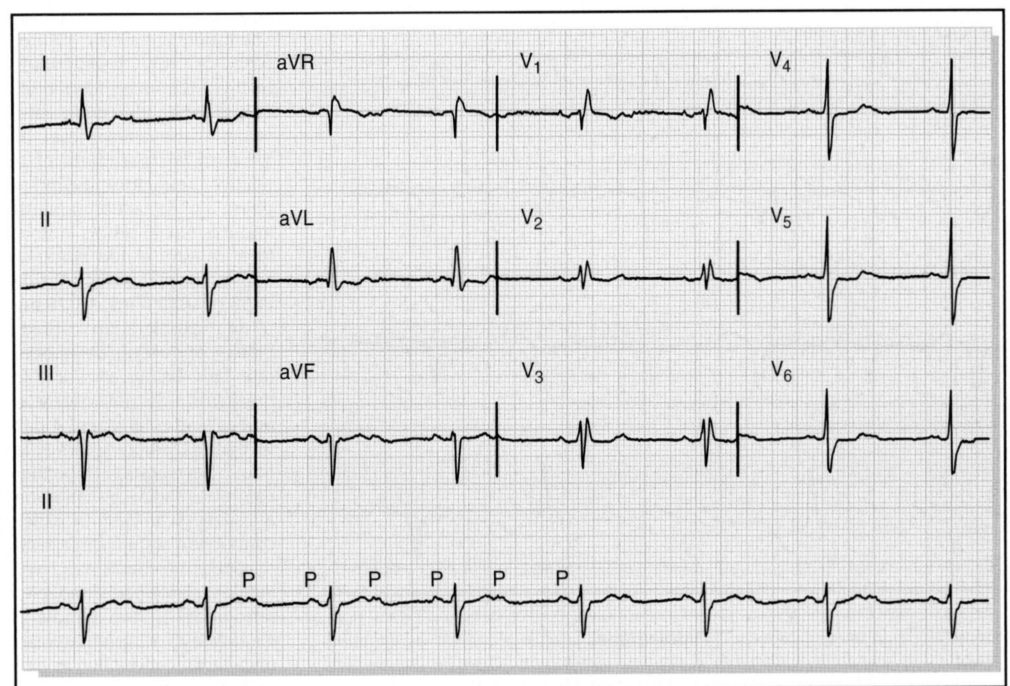

FIGURE 13-25 Sinus rhythm at 95 beats/min with 2:1 AV block. Conducted ventricular beats show a pattern consistent with bifascicular block with delay or block in the right bundle and left anterior fascicle. The patient underwent pacemaker implantation for presumed infrahisian block.

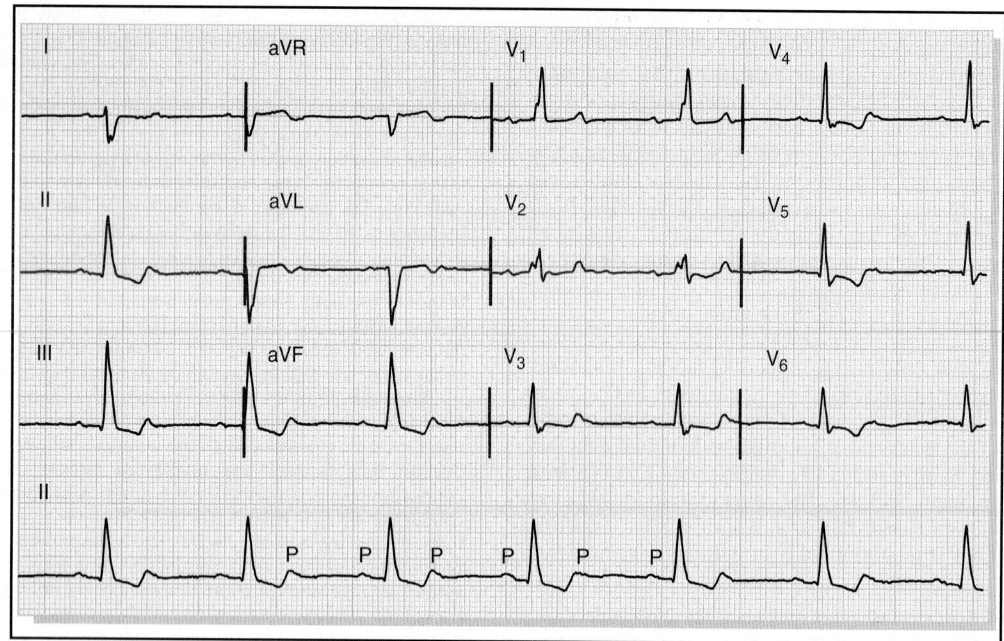

FIGURE 13-26 Sinus rhythm with a 2:1 atrioventricular block. QRS morphology in the conducted beats is consistent with bifascicular block with delay or block in the right bundle and left posterior fascicle. Subsequently, complete heart block was also noted. The patient underwent pacemaker implantation for presumed infrahisian block.

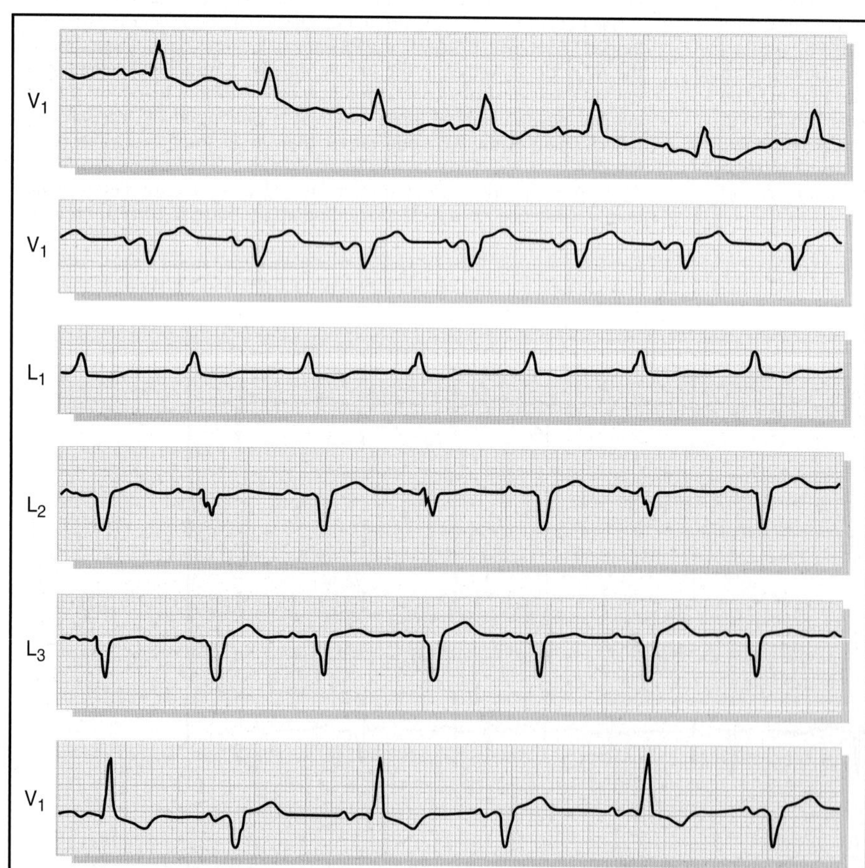

FIGURE 13-27 Multifascicular block manifested by alternating bundle branch blocks and PR intervals. **Top panel,** Lead V_1 RBBB with a PR interval of 280 msec. **Middle panel,** Lead V_1 LBBB with a PR interval of 180 msec. **Lower panel,** RBBB alternating with LBBB, along with alternation of the PR interval. The electrocardiographic records shown in leads I, II, and III (L1 to L3) exhibit left anterior fascicular block. An alternating bundle branch block of this type is consistent with trifascicular conduction delay. *(From Fisch C: Electrocardiography of Arrhythmias. Philadelphia, Lea & Febiger, 1990.)*

bifascicular block is not diagnostic of trifascicular block, whereas the presence of a normal PR interval does not exclude this finding.

The major clinical implication of a multifascicular block is its relation to advanced conduction system disease. It may be a marker for severe myocardial disease and may identify patients at risk for heart block (see Figs. 13-25 and 13-26), as discussed in Chaps. 35, 38, and 39.

Rate-Dependent Conduction Block (Aberration). Intraventricular conduction delays can result from the effects of changes in the heart rate, as well as from fixed pathologic lesions in the conduction system. Rate-dependent block or aberration (see Chap. 39) can occur at relatively high or low heart rates. In acceleration (tachycardia)-dependent block, conduction delay occurs when the heart rate exceeds a critical value. At the cellular level, this aberration is the result of encroachment of the impulse on the relative refractory period (sometime during phase 3 of the action potential) of the preceding impulse, which results in slower conduction. This form of rate-related block is relatively common and can have the electrocardiographic pattern of RBBB or LBBB (**Figs. 13-28 and 13-29**).

In deceleration (bradycardia)-dependent block, conduction delay occurs when the heart rate falls below a critical level. Although the mechanism is not clearly established, it may reflect abnormal phase 4 depolarization of cells so that activation occurs at lower resting potentials. Deceleration-dependent block is less common than acceleration-dependent block and is usually seen only in patients with significant conduction system disease (**Fig. 13-30**).

Other mechanisms of ventricular aberration include concealed conduction (anterograde or retrograde) in the bundle branches (see Figs. 13-28 and 13-29), premature excitation, depressed myocardial conduction as a result of drug effects or hyperkalemia (see Fig. 13-49, top), and the effect of changing cycle length on refractoriness (the Ashman phenomenon; see Chaps. 29

and 32). The duration of the refractory period is a function of the immediately preceding cycle length: the longer the preceding cycle, the longer the subsequent refractory period. Therefore, abrupt prolongation of the immediately preceding cycle can result in aberration as part of a long cycle–short cycle sequence. These so-called Ashman beats usually have an RBBB morphology (see Fig. 13-28).

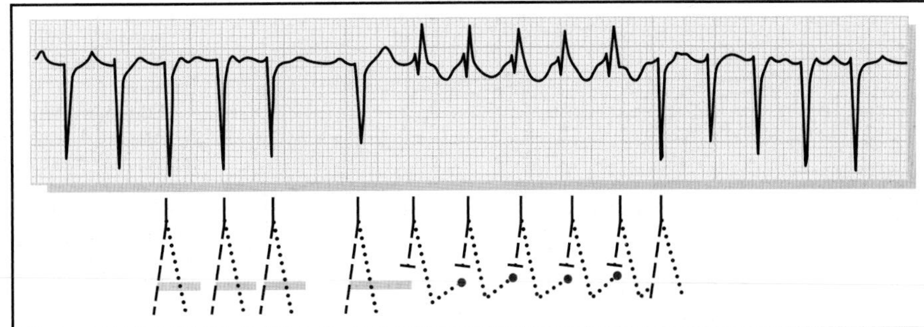

FIGURE 13-28 Atrial tachycardia with a Wenckebach (type I) second-degree AV block, ventricular aberration resulting from the Ashman phenomenon, and probably concealed transseptal conduction. The long pause of the atrial tachycardia is followed by five QRS complexes with RBBB morphology. The RBBB of the first QRS reflects the Ashman phenomenon. The aberration is perpetuated by concealed transseptal activation from the left bundle (LB) into the right bundle (RB) with block of anterograde conduction of the subsequent sinus impulse in the RB. Foreshortening of the R-R cycle, a manifestation of the Wenckebach structure, disturbs the relationship between transseptal and anterograde sinus conduction, and RB conduction is normalized. In the ladder diagram below the tracing, the **solid lines** represent the His bundle, the **dashes** represent the RB, the **dots** represent the LB, and the **solid horizontal bars** denote the refractory period. P waves and the AV node are not identified in the diagram. *(Courtesy of Dr. C. Fisch.)*

OTHER FORMS OF CONDUCTION ABNORMALITIES

NOTCHING. The presence of multiple deflections within the QRS complex (e.g., rSr, Rsr′, rSR′ or multiple r′ patterns) or the presence of high-frequency notches within the R and S wave without overall prolongation of the QRS complex may also reflect forms of intraventricular conduction defects, especially in patients with known coronary artery disease. These findings have reported sensitivities and specificities of over 85% for the presence of myocardial scars or ventricular aneurysms, but more definitive studies are needed.[51]

PERI-INFARCTION BLOCK. This term refers to conduction delay in the region of a myocardial infarction. It is manifest in electrocardiographic leads with pathologic Q waves when the terminal portion of the QRS complex is wide and directed opposite to the Q wave, such as a QR complex in leads III and aVF. A related abnormality is peri-ischemic block, manifested by a reversible widening of the QRS complex in electrocardiographic leads with ST-segment elevation caused by acute injury.[43]

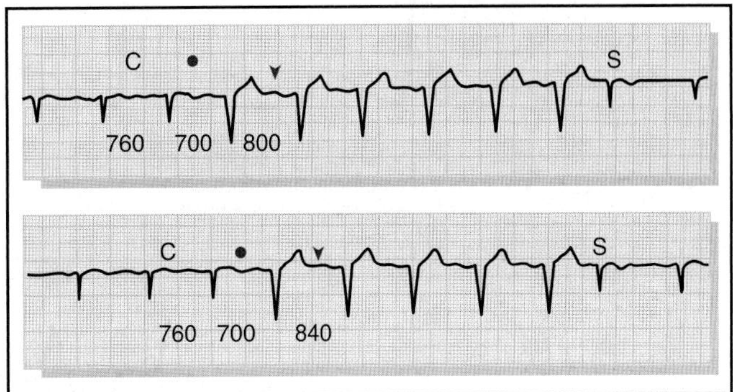

FIGURE 13-29 Acceleration-dependent QRS aberration with the paradox of persistence at a longer cycle and normalization at a shorter cycle than what initiated the aberration. The duration of the basic cycle (C) is 760 msec. LBBB appears at a cycle length of 700 msec **(dot)** and is perpetuated at cycle lengths **(arrowheads)** of 800 and 840 msec; conduction normalizes after a cycle length of 600 msec. Perpetuation of LBBB at a cycle length of 800 and 840 msec is probably caused by transseptal concealment, similar to that described in Figure 13-31. Unexpected normalization of the QRS (S) following the atrial premature contraction is probably caused by equalization of conduction in the two bundles; however, supernormal conduction in the left bundle cannot be excluded. *(From Fisch C, Zipes DP, McHenry PL: Rate dependent aberrancy. Circulation 48:714, 1973.)*

Myocardial Ischemia and Infarction

The ECG remains a key test for the diagnosis of acute and chronic coronary syndromes.[52-56] The findings vary considerably, depending importantly on four major factors: (1) the duration of the ischemic process (acute versus evolving/chronic); (2) its extent (transmural versus nontransmural); (3) its topography (anterior versus inferior-posterior-lateral or right ventricular); and (4) the presence of other underlying abnormalities (e.g., LBBB, Wolff-Parkinson-White syndrome, or pacemaker patterns) that can mask or alter the classic patterns.

A key clinical distinction is between ST-segment elevation myocardial infarction (or ischemia; STEMI) and non-STEMI because of the therapeutic implications. Emergency coronary reperfusion therapy has only proven to be consistently efficacious in the former syndrome.

REPOLARIZATION (ST-T WAVE) ABNORMALITIES. The earliest and most consistent electrocardiographic finding during acute severe ischemia is deviation of the ST segment as a result of a current of injury mechanism[6] (see Chap. 54). Under normal conditions, the ST segment is usually nearly isoelectric because almost all healthy myocardial cells attain approximately the same potential during the initial to middle phases of repolarization, corresponding to the plateau phase of the ventricular action potential.

Ischemia, however, has complex time-dependent effects on the electrical properties of myocardial cells. Severe acute ischemia can reduce the resting membrane potential, shorten the duration of the action potential in the ischemic area, and decrease the rate of rise and amplitude of phase 0 (**Fig. 13-31**). These changes cause a voltage gradient between normal and ischemic zones that leads to current flow between these regions. Resulting currents of injury are represented on the surface ECG by deviation of the ST segment.

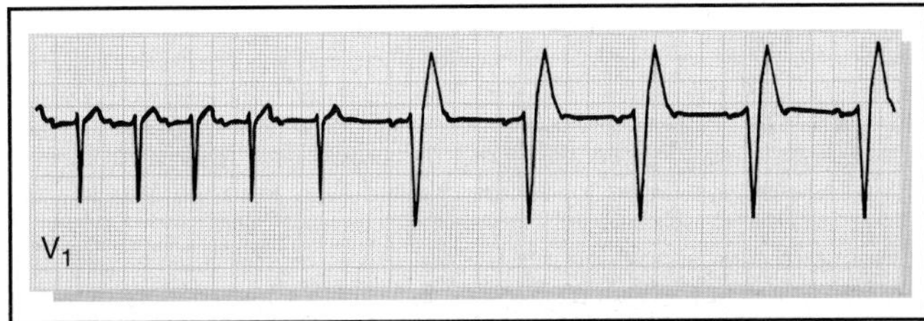

FIGURE 13-30 Deceleration-dependent aberration. The basic rhythm is sinus with a Wenckebach (type I) AV block. With 1:1 AV conduction, the QRS complexes are normal in duration; with a 2:1 AV block or after the longer pause of a Wenckebach sequence, LBBB appears. Slow diastolic depolarization (phase 4) of the transmembrane action potential during the prolonged cycle is implicated as the cause of the LBBB. *(Courtesy of Dr. C. Fisch.)*

Both "diastolic" and "systolic" injury currents have been proposed to explain ischemic ST-segment elevations (**Fig. 13-32**).[57] According to the diastolic current of injury hypothesis, ischemic ST-segment elevation is attributable to negative (downward) displacement of the electrical diastolic baseline (the TQ segment of the ECG). Ischemic cells remain relatively depolarized during phase 4 of the ventricular action potential (i.e., lower membrane resting potential; see Fig. 13-31) and depolarized muscle carries a negative extracellular charge relative to repolarized muscle. Therefore, during electrical diastole, current (the diastolic current of injury) will flow between the partly or completely depolarized ischemic myocardium and the neighboring, normally repolarized, uninjured myocardium. The injury current vector will be directed away from the more negative ischemic zone toward the more positive normal myocardium. As a result, leads overlying the ischemic zone will record a

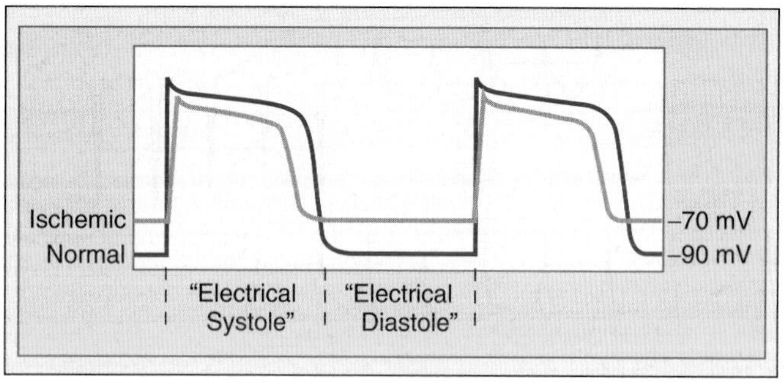

FIGURE 13-31 Acute ischemia may alter ventricular action potentials by inducing lower resting membrane potential, decreased amplitude and velocity of phase 0, and an abbreviated action potential duration (pathologic early repolarization). These electrophysiologic effects create a voltage gradient between ischemic and normal cells during different phases of the cardiac electrical cycle. The resulting currents of injury are reflected on the surface ECG by deviation of the ST segment (see Fig. 13-32).

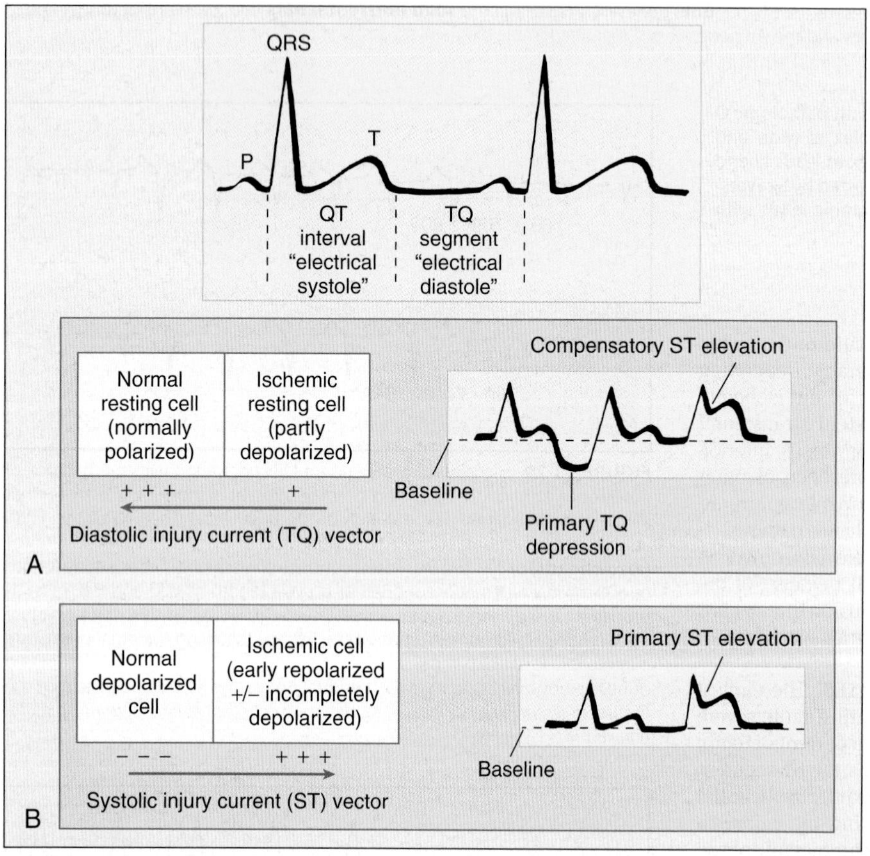

FIGURE 13-32 Pathophysiology of ischemic ST elevation. Two basic mechanisms have been advanced to explain the elevation seen with acute myocardial injury. **A,** Diastolic current of injury. In this case (first QRS-T complex), the ST vector will be directed away from the relatively negative, partly depolarized, ischemic region during electrical diastole (TQ interval), and the result will be primary TQ depression. Conventional alternating-current ECGs compensate for the baseline shift, and an apparent ST-segment elevation (second QRS-T complex) results. **B,** Systolic current of injury. In this case, the ischemic zone will be relatively positive during electrical systole because the cells are repolarized early and the amplitude and upstroke velocity of their action potentials may be decreased. This injury current vector will be oriented toward the electropositive zone, and the result will be primary ST-segment elevation. *(Modified from Goldberger AL: Myocardial Infarction: Electrocardiographic Differential Diagnosis. 4th ed. St. Louis, Mosby-Year Book, 1991.)*

negative deflection during electrical diastole and produce depression of the TQ segment.

TQ-segment depression, in turn, appears as ST-segment elevation because the electrocardiographic recorders in clinical practice use AC-coupled amplifiers that automatically compensate for any negative shift in the TQ segment. As a result of this electronic compensation, the ST segment will be proportionately elevated. Therefore, according to the diastolic current of injury theory, ST-segment elevation represents an apparent shift. The true shift, observable only with DC-coupled electrocardiographic amplifiers, is the negative displacement of the TQ baseline.

Current evidence suggests that ischemic ST-segment elevations (and hyperacute T waves) are also related to systolic injury currents. Three factors may make acutely ischemic myocardial cells relatively positive in comparison to normal cells with respect to their extracellular charge during electrical systole (QT interval): (1) pathologic early repolarization (shortened action potential duration); (2) decreased action potential upstroke velocity; and (3) decreased action potential amplitude (see Fig. 13-34). The presence of one or more of these effects will establish a voltage gradient between normal and ischemic zones during the QT interval such that the current of injury vector will be directed toward the ischemic region. This systolic current of injury mechanism will result in primary ST-segment elevation, sometimes with tall, positive (hyperacute) T waves.

When acute ischemia is transmural (whether caused by diastolic or systolic injury currents, or both), the overall ST vector is usually shifted in the direction of the outer (epicardial) layers, and ST-segment elevation and sometimes tall, positive (hyperacute) T waves are produced over the ischemic zone (**Fig. 13-33**). Reciprocal ST depression can appear in leads reflecting the contralateral surface of the heart. Occasionally, the reciprocal changes can be more apparent than the primary ST-segment elevations. When ischemia is confined primarily to the subendocardium, the overall ST vector typically shifts toward the inner ventricular layer and the ventricular cavity such that the overlying (e.g., anterior precordial) leads show ST-segment depression, with ST-segment elevation in lead aVR (see Fig. 13-33). This subendocardial ischemia pattern is the typical finding during spontaneous episodes of angina pectoris or during symptomatic or asymptomatic (silent) ischemia induced by exercise or pharmacologic stress tests (see Chaps. 14 and 57).

Multiple factors can affect the amplitude of acute ischemic ST deviations. Profound ST-segment elevation or depression in multiple leads usually indicates very severe ischemia. Conversely, prompt resolution of ST-segment elevation following thrombolytic therapy or percutaneous coronary interventions[54,58] is a specific marker of successful reperfusion. These relationships are not universal, however, because severe ischemia or even infarction can occur with slight or absent ST-T changes. Furthermore, a relative increase in T wave amplitude (hyperacute T waves) can accompany or precede the ST-segment elevations as part of the injury current pattern attributable to ischemia with or without infarction (**Fig. 13-34**).

QRS CHANGES. With actual infarction, depolarization (QRS) changes often accompany repolarization (ST-T) abnormalities (**Fig. 13-35**). Necrosis of sufficient myocardial tissue can lead to decreased R wave amplitude or Q waves in the anterior, lateral, or inferior leads as a result of loss of electromotive forces in the infarcted area. Local conduction delays caused by acute ischemia can also contribute to Q wave pathogenesis in selected cases. Abnormal Q waves were once considered markers of transmural myocardial infarction, whereas subendocardial (nontransmural) infarcts were thought not to produce Q waves. However, careful experimental and clinical electrocardiographic-pathologic correlative studies have indicated that transmural infarcts can occur without Q waves and that subendocardial infarcts can be associated with Q waves.[55,59] Accordingly, infarcts are better classified electrocardiographically as Q wave or non–Q-wave rather than as transmural or nontransmural, based on the ECG. The findings may be somewhat different with posterior or lateral infarction (**Fig. 13-36**). Loss of depolarization forces in these regions can reciprocally *increase* R wave amplitude in lead V_1 and sometimes V_2, rarely without causing diagnostic Q waves in any of the conventional leads. The differential diagnosis of prominent right precordial R waves is presented in **Table 13-8**.

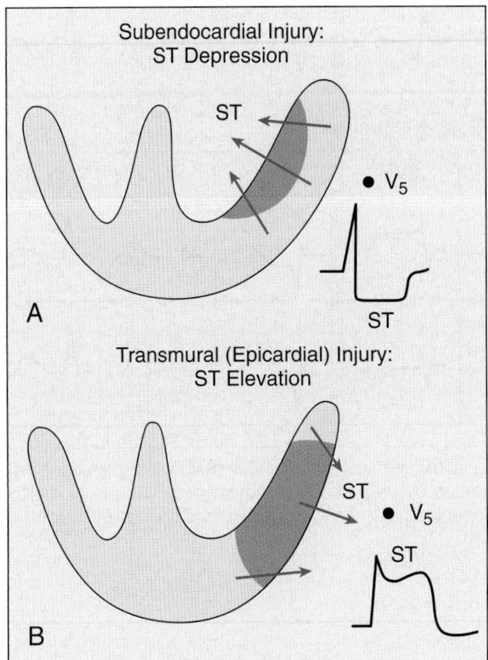

FIGURE 13-33 Current of injury patterns with acute ischemia. **A,** With predominant subendocardial ischemia, the resultant ST vector is directed toward the inner layer of the affected ventricle and the ventricular cavity. Overlying leads therefore record ST depression. **B,** With ischemia involving the outer ventricular layer (transmural or epicardial injury), the ST vector is directed outward. Overlying leads record ST-segment elevation. Reciprocal ST-segment depression can appear in contralateral leads.

EVOLUTION OF ELECTROCARDIOGRAPHIC CHANGES. Ischemic ST-segment elevation and hyperacute T wave changes may occur as the earliest sign of acute infarction (STEMI) and are typically followed within a period ranging from hours to days by evolving T wave inversion and sometimes Q waves in the same lead distribution (see Fig. 13-35 and Chap. 54). T wave inversion from evolving or chronic ischemia correlates with increased ventricular action potential duration, and these ischemic changes are often associated with QT prolongation. The T wave inversions can resolve after days or weeks, or persist indefinitely. The extent of the infarct may be an important determinant of T wave evolution. In one series,[60] T waves that were persistently negative for more than 1 year in leads with Q waves were associated with a transmural infarction with fibrosis of the entire wall; in contrast, T waves that were positive in leads with Q waves correlated with nontransmural infarction, with viable myocardium within the wall.

TABLE 13-8 Differential Diagnosis of Tall R Waves in Leads V1 and V2

Physiologic and Positional Factors

Misplacement of chest leads
Normal variants
Displacement of heart toward right side of chest (dextroversion), congenital or acquired

Myocardial Injury

Lateral or "true posterior" myocardial infarction (see Fig. 13-39)
Duchenne muscular dystrophy (see Chap. 92)

Ventricular Enlargement

Right ventricular hypertrophy (usually with right axis deviation)
Hypertrophic cardiomyopathy

Altered Ventricular Depolarization

Right ventricular conduction abnormalities
Wolff-Parkinson-White patterns (caused by posterior or lateral wall preexcitation)

Modified from Goldberger AL: Clinical Electrocardiography: A Simplified Approach. 7th ed. St. Louis, CV Mosby, 2006.

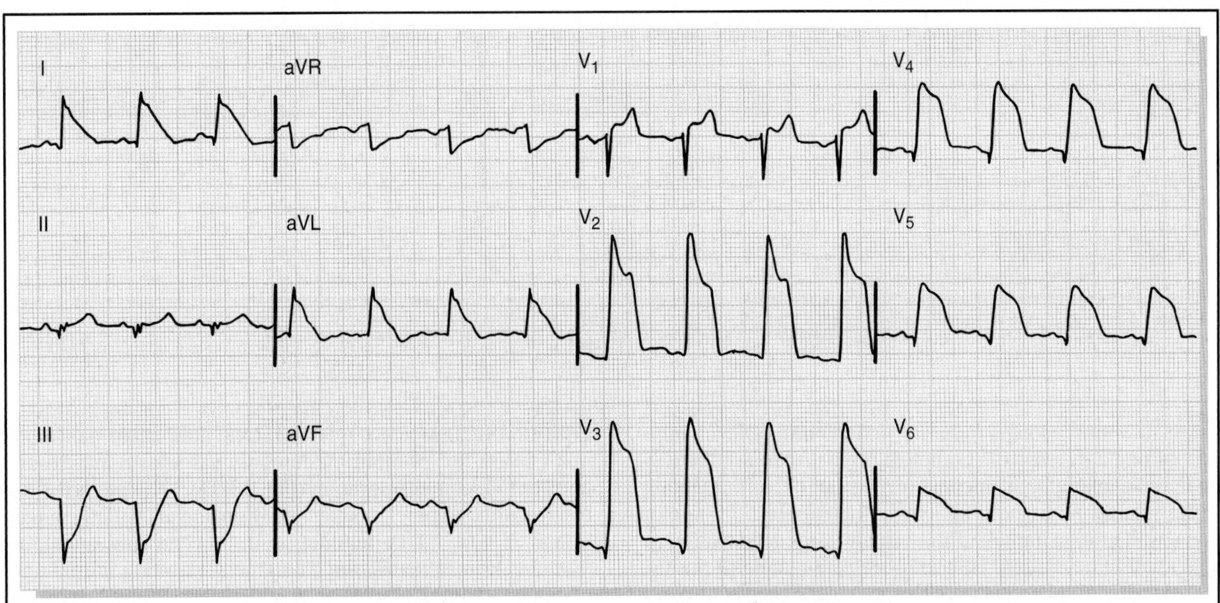

FIGURE 13-34 Hyperacute phase of extensive anterolateral myocardial infarction. Marked ST-segment elevation melding with prominent T waves is present across the precordium, as well as in leads I and aVL. ST-segment depression, consistent with a reciprocal change, is seen in leads III and aVF. Q waves are present in leads V_3 through V_6. Marked ST-segment elevations with tall T waves caused by severe ischemia are sometimes referred to as a monophasic current of injury pattern. A paradoxical increase in R wave amplitude (V_2 and V_3) may accompany this pattern. This tracing also shows left axis deviation with small or absent inferior R waves, which raises the possibility of a prior inferior infarct.

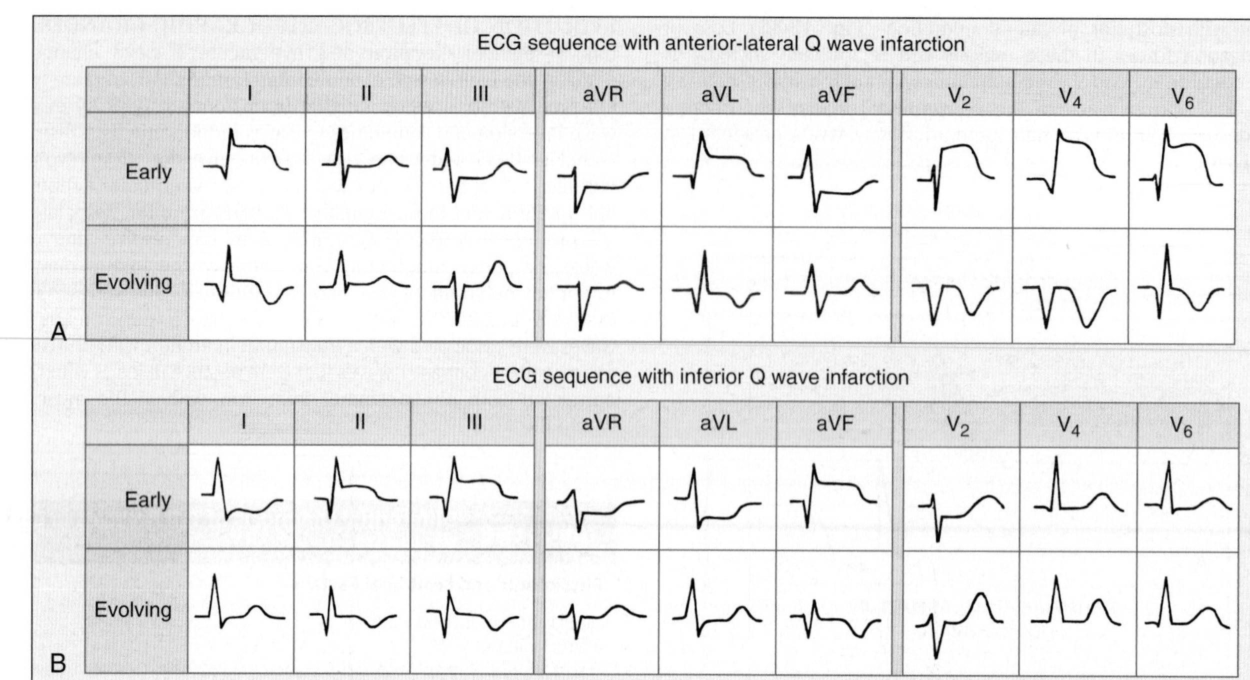

FIGURE 13-35 Sequence of depolarization and repolarization changes with acute anterior-lateral **(A)** and acute inferior wall **(B)** Q wave infarctions. With anterior-lateral infarcts, ST-segment elevation in leads I, aVL, and the precordial leads can be accompanied by reciprocal ST-segment depression in leads II, III, and aVF. Conversely, acute inferior (or posterior) infarcts can be associated with reciprocal ST-segment depression in leads V_1 to V_3. *(Modified from Goldberger AL: Clinical Electrocardiography: A Simplified Approach. 6th ed. St. Louis, CV Mosby, 1999.)*

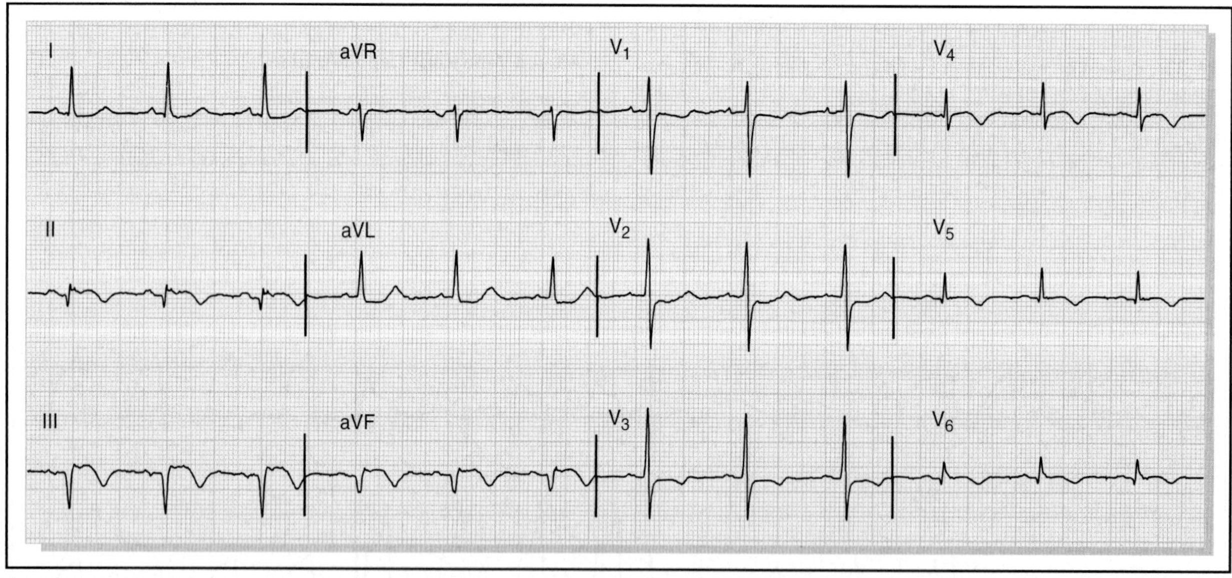

FIGURE 13-36 Evolving inferoposterolateral infarction. Note the prominent Q waves in II, III, and aVF, along with ST-segment elevation and T wave inversion in these leads, as well as V_3 through V_6. ST depression in I, aVL, V_1, and V_2 is consistent with a reciprocal change. Relatively tall R waves are also present in V_1 and V_2.

In the days to weeks or longer following infarction, the QRS changes can persist or begin to resolve.[61] Complete normalization of the ECG following Q wave infarction is uncommon but can occur, particularly with smaller infarcts and when the left ventricular ejection fraction and regional wall motion improve. This is usually associated with spontaneous recanalization or good collateral circulation and is a positive prognostic sign. In contrast, persistent Q waves and ST-segment elevation several weeks or more after an infarct correlate strongly with a severe underlying wall motion disorder (akinetic or dyskinetic zone), although not necessarily a frank ventricular aneurysm. The presence of an rSR(′) or similar complex in the midleft chest leads or lead I is another reported marker of ventricular aneurysm.

OTHER ISCHEMIC ST-T PATTERNS. Reversible transmural ischemia caused, for example, by coronary vasospasm may result in very transient ST-segment elevation (**Fig. 13-37**).[55] This pattern is the classic electrocardiographic marker of Prinzmetal variant angina (see Chaps. 56 and 57). Depending on the severity and duration of such noninfarction ischemia, the ST-segment elevation can either resolve completely within minutes or be followed by T wave inversion that can persist for hours or even days. Some patients with ischemic chest pain have deep coronary T wave inversion in multiple precordial leads (e.g., V_1 through V_4), with or without cardiac enzyme level elevations. This finding is typically caused by severe ischemia associated with a high-grade stenosis in the proximal left anterior descending (LAD)

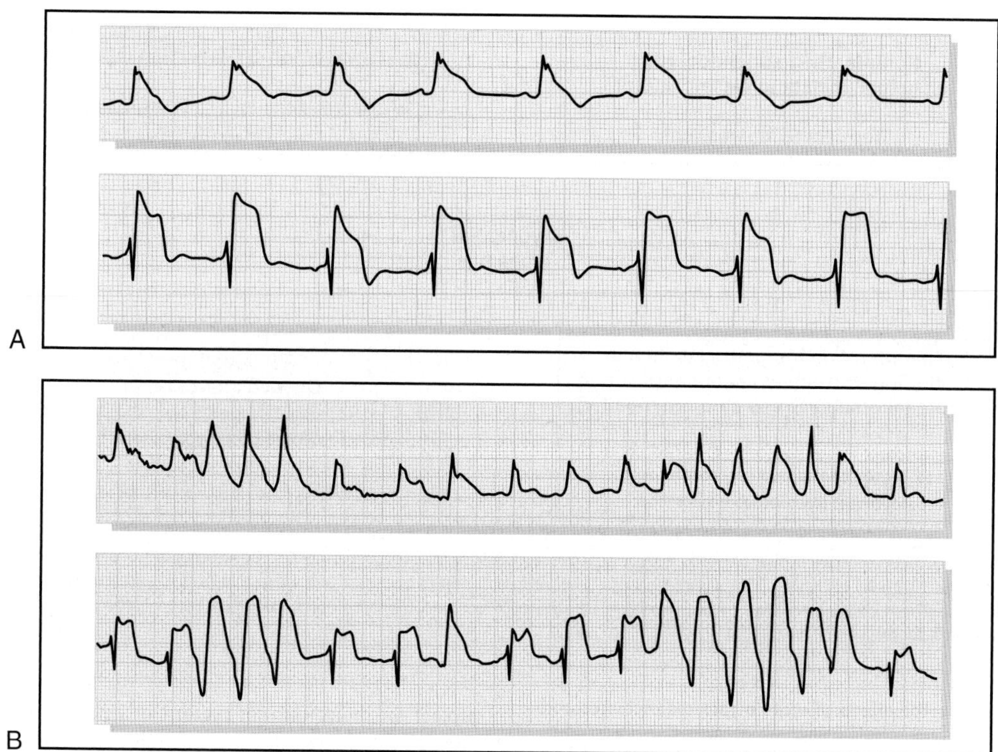

FIGURE 13-37 **A,** Prinzmetal angina with ST segment and T wave alternans. **B,** ST segment and T wave alternans associated with nonsustained ventricular tachycardia. *(Courtesy of Dr. C. Fisch.)*

coronary artery system (referred to as the LAD-T wave pattern or Wellens T waves). The T wave inversion can actually be preceded by a transient ST-segment elevation that resolves by the time the patient arrives at the hospital. These T wave inversions, in the setting of unstable angina, can correlate with segmental hypokinesis of the anterior wall and suggest a myocardial stunning syndrome. The natural history of this syndrome is unfavorable, with a high incidence of recurrent angina and myocardial infarction. On the other hand, patients whose baseline ECG already shows abnormal T wave inversion can experience paradoxical T wave normalization (pseudonormalization) during episodes of acute transmural ischemia (**Fig. 13-38**). The four major classes of acute electrocardiographic–coronary artery syndromes in which myocardial ischemia leads to different electrocardiographic findings are summarized in **Figure 13-39**.

Ischemic U Wave Changes

Alterations in U wave amplitude or polarity have been reported with acute ischemia or infarction.[62] For example, exercise-induced transient inversion of precordial U waves has been correlated with severe stenosis of the left anterior descending coronary artery. Rarely, U wave inversion can be the earliest electrocardiographic sign of acute coronary syndromes.

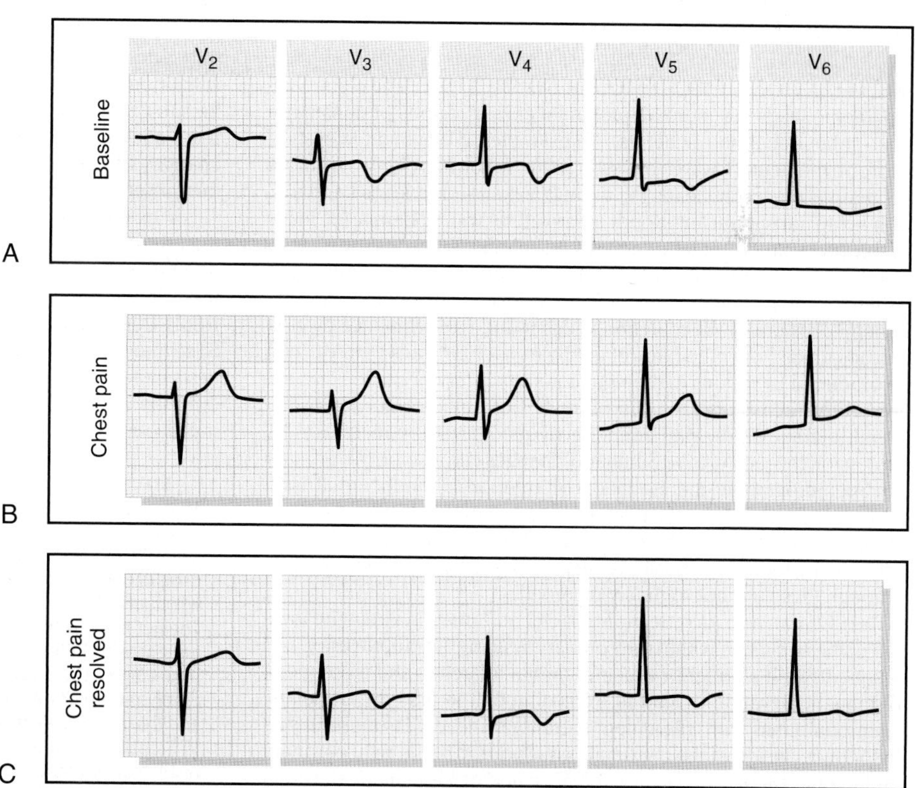

FIGURE 13-38 Pseudo (paradoxical) T wave normalization. **A,** Baseline ECG of a patient with coronary artery disease shows ischemic T wave inversion. **B,** T wave "normalization" during an episode of ischemic chest pain. **C,** Following resolution of the chest pain, the T waves have reverted to their baseline appearance. *(From Goldberger AL: Myocardial Infarction: Electrocardiographic Differential Diagnosis. 4th ed. St. Louis, Mosby-Year Book, 1991.)*

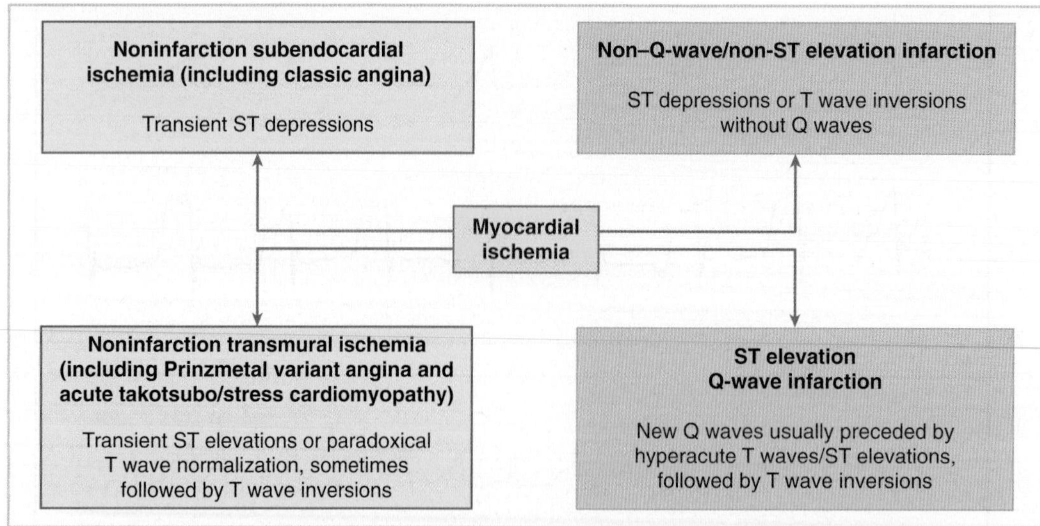

FIGURE 13-39 Variability of electrocardiographic patterns with acute myocardial ischemia. The ECG may also be normal or nonspecifically abnormal. Furthermore, these categorizations are not mutually exclusive. For example, a non–Q-wave infarct can evolve into a Q wave infarct, ST-segment elevation can be followed by a non–Q-wave infarct or ST-segment depression, and T wave inversion can be followed by a Q wave infarct. *(Modified from Goldberger AL: Myocardial Infarction: Electrocardiographic Differential Diagnosis. 4th ed. St. Louis, Mosby-Year Book, 1991.)*

QT INTERVAL DISPERSION. The effects of acute myocardial ischemia and infarction on the disparity among QT intervals in various electrocardiographic leads, referred to as QT dispersion, have generated interest. The greater the difference between maximum and minimum QT intervals—that is, increased QT dispersion—the greater the variability in myocardial repolarization. An increased index has been proposed as a marker of arrhythmia risk after myocardial infarction and as a marker of acute ischemia with atrial pacing. The practical usefulness of QT dispersion measurements in patients with coronary syndromes appears limited, despite initial enthusiasm[63-65] (see Chaps. 35 and 36).

LOCALIZATION OF ISCHEMIA OR INFARCTION. The electrocardiographic leads are more helpful in localizing regions of transmural than subendocardial ischemia. As examples, ST-segment elevation and/or hyperacute T waves are seen in the following: (1) two or more contiguous precordial leads (V_1 through V_6) and/or in leads I and aVL with acute transmural anterior or anterolateral wall ischemia; (2) leads V_1 to V_3 with anteroseptal or apical[66] ischemia; (3) leads V_4 to V_6 with apical or lateral ischemia; (4) leads II, III, and aVF with inferior wall ischemia; and (5) right-sided precordial leads with right ventricular ischemia. Posterior wall infarction, which induces ST-segment elevation in leads placed over the back of the heart, such as leads V_7 to V_9,[5] can be produced by lesions in the right coronary artery or the left circumflex artery. Such blockages can produce both inferior and posterior-lateral injuries, which may be indirectly recognized by reciprocal ST depression in leads V_1 to V_3. Similar ST changes can also be the primary electrocardiographic manifestation of anterior subendocardial ischemia. Posterolateral or inferolateral wall infarction with reciprocal changes can sometimes be differentiated from primary anterior wall ischemia by the presence of ST-segment elevations in posterior leads, although these are not routinely recorded.

The ECG can also provide more specific information about the location of the occlusion within the coronary system (the culprit lesion).[6,56] In patients with an inferior wall myocardial infarction, the presence of ST-segment elevation in lead III exceeding that in lead II, particularly when combined with ST-segment elevation in lead V_1, is a useful predictor of occlusion in the proximal to midportion of the right coronary artery (**Fig. 13-40**). In contrast, the presence of ST-segment elevation in lead II equal to or exceeding that in lead III, especially in concert with ST-segment depression in leads V_1 to V_3 or ST-segment elevation in leads I and aVL, suggests occlusion of the left circumflex coronary artery or a distal occlusion of a dominant right coronary artery. Right-sided ST-segment elevation is indicative of acute right ventricular injury and usually indicates occlusion of the proximal right coronary artery. Of note is the finding that acute right ventricular infarction can project an injury current pattern in leads V_1 through V_3 or even V_4, thereby simulating anterior infarction. In other cases, simultaneous ST-segment elevation in V_1 (V_2R) and ST-segment depression in V_2 (V_1R) can occur (see Fig. 13-40). Lead aVR may provide important clues to artery occlusion in myocardial infarction (MI). Left main (or severe multivessel) disease should be considered when leads aVR and V_1 show ST-segment elevation, especially in concert with diffuse prominent ST depression in other leads.

These and other criteria proposed for localization of the site of coronary occlusion based on the initial ECG[56,67-70] still require additional validation in larger populations. Current and future criteria will always be subject to limitations and exceptions based on variations in coronary anatomy, the dynamic nature of acute electrocardiographic changes, the presence of multivessel involvement, collateral flow, and the presence of ventricular conduction delays.

For example, in some cases, ischemia can affect more than one region of the myocardium (e.g., inferolateral; see Fig. 13-35). Not uncommonly, the ECG will show the characteristic findings of involvement in each region. Sometimes, however, partial normalization can result from cancellation of opposing vectorial forces. Inferior lead ST-segment elevation accompanying acute anterior wall infarction suggests either occlusion of a left anterior descending artery that extends onto the inferior wall of the left ventricle (the wrap-around vessel) or multivessel disease with jeopardized collaterals.

ELECTROCARDIOGRAPHIC DIAGNOSIS OF BUNDLE BRANCH BLOCKS AND MYOCARDIAL INFARCTION. The diagnosis of MI is often more difficult in cases in which the baseline ECG shows a bundle branch block pattern, or a bundle branch block develops as a complication of the infarct. The diagnosis of Q wave infarction is not usually impeded by the presence of RBBB, which affects primarily the terminal phase of ventricular depolarization. The net effect is that the criteria for the diagnosis of a Q wave infarct in a patient with RBBB are the same as in patients with normal conduction (**Fig. 13-41**). The diagnosis of infarction in the presence of LBBB is considerably more complicated and confusing, because LBBB alters the early and the late phases of ventricular depolarization and produces secondary ST-T changes. These changes may mask and/or mimic MI findings. As a result, considerable attention has been directed to the problem of diagnosing acute and chronic MI in patients with LBBB[71] (**Fig. 13-42**).

Infarction of the left ventricular free (or lateral) wall ordinarily results in abnormal Q waves in the midprecordial to lateral precordial leads (and selected limb leads). However, the initial septal depolarization forces with LBBB are directed from right to left. These leftward forces produce an initial R wave in the midprecordial to lateral precordial leads, usually masking the loss of electrical potential (Q waves) caused by the infarction. Therefore, acute or chronic left ventricular free wall infarction by

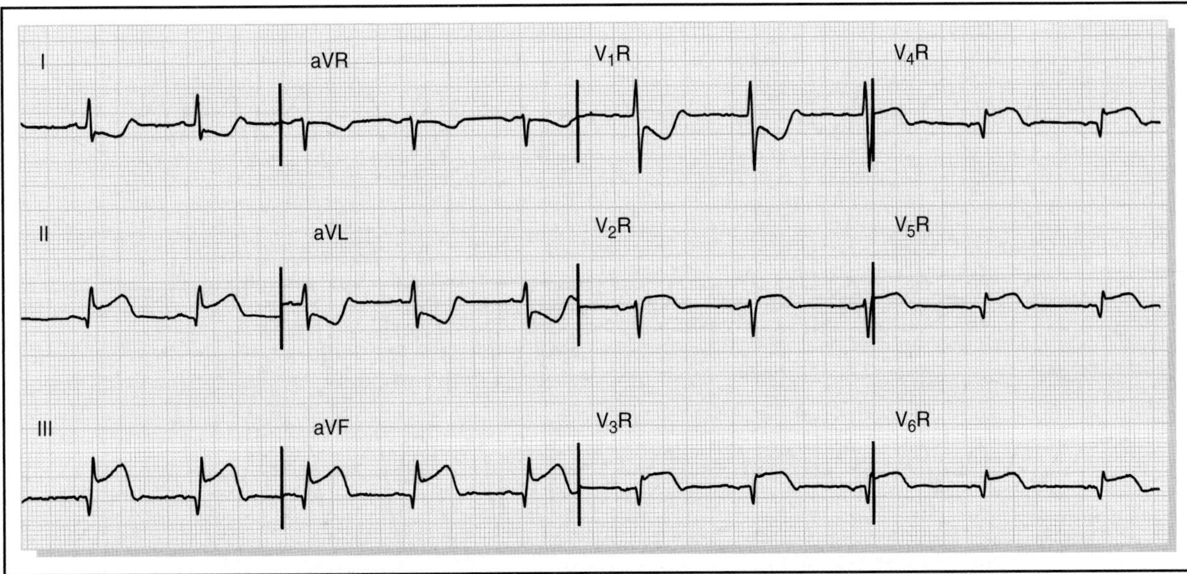

FIGURE 13-40 Acute right ventricular infarction with acute inferior wall infarction. Note the ST-segment elevation in the right precordial leads, as well as in leads II, III, and aVF, with reciprocal changes in leads I and aVL. ST-segment elevation in lead III greater than in lead II and right precordial ST-segment elevation are consistent with proximal to middle occlusion of the right coronary artery. The combination of ST-segment elevation in conventional lead V_1 (V_3R here) and ST-segment depression in lead V_2 (lead V_1R here) has also been reported with acute right ventricular ischemia or infarction.

itself will not usually produce diagnostic Q waves in the presence of LBBB. Acute or chronic infarction involving both the free wall and septum (or the septum itself) may produce abnormal Q waves (usually as part of QR-type complexes) in leads V_4 to V_6. These initial Q waves probably reflect posterior and superior forces from the spared basal portion of the septum (**Fig. 13-43**). Thus, a wide Q wave (40 msec) in one or more of these leads is a reliable sign of underlying infarction. The sequence of repolarization is also altered in LBBB, with the ST-segment and T wave vectors being directed opposite the QRS complex. These changes can mask or simulate the ST segment changes of actual ischemia.

The following points summarize the ECG signs of myocardial infarction in LBBB:

1. ST-segment elevation with tall, positive T waves is frequently seen in the right precordial leads with uncomplicated LBBB. Secondary T wave inversions are characteristically seen in the lateral precordial leads. However, the appearance of ST-segment elevations in the lateral leads or ST-segment depressions or deep T wave inversions in leads V_1 to V_3 strongly suggests underlying ischemia. More marked ST-segment elevations (>0.5 mV) in leads with QS or rS waves may also be caused by acute ischemia, but false-positive findings occur, especially with large-amplitude negative QRS complexes.[6]
2. The presence of QR complexes in leads I, V_5, or V_6 or in II, III, and aVF with LBBB strongly suggests underlying infarction.
3. Chronic infarction is also suggested by notching of the ascending part of a wide S wave in the midprecordial leads (Cabrera sign) or the ascending limb of a wide R wave in lead I, aVL, V_5, or V_6 (Chapman sign).

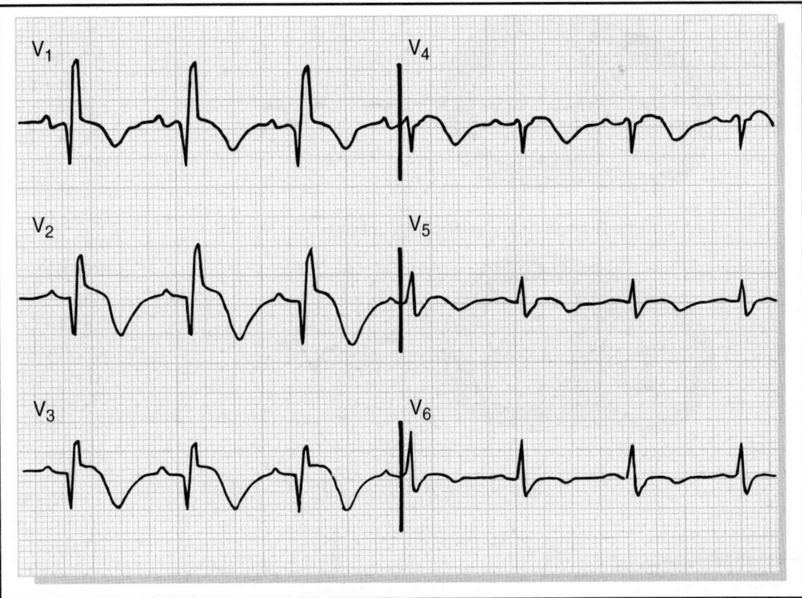

FIGURE 13-41 RBB with acute anterior infarction. Loss of anterior depolarization forces results in QR-type complexes in the right precordial to midprecordial leads, with ST-segment elevations and evolving T wave inversions (V_1 through V_6).

Similar principles can apply to the diagnosis of acute and chronic infarction in the presence of right ventricular pacing. Comparison between an ECG exhibiting the LBBB prior to the infarction and the present ECG is often helpful to show these changes.

The diagnosis of concomitant LAFB and inferior wall infarction can also pose challenges. This combination can result in loss of the small r waves in the inferior leads, so that leads II, III, and aVF show QS, not rS, complexes. LAFB, however, will occasionally hide the diagnosis of inferior wall infarction. The inferior orientation of the initial QRS forces caused by the fascicular block can mask inferior Q waves, with resultant rS complexes in leads II, III, and aVF. In other cases, the combination of LAFB and inferior wall infarction will produce qrS complexes in the inferior limb leads, with the initial q wave the result of the infarct and the minuscule r wave the result of the fascicular block.

ATRIAL INFARCTION. A number of ECG clues to the diagnosis of atrial infarction have been suggested, including localized deviations of the PR segment (e.g., PR elevation in lead V_5 or V_6 or the inferior leads,[72,73] changes in P wave morphology, and atrial arrhythmias). The sensitivity and specificity of these signs are limited, however. Diffuse PR-segment changes (PR elevation in aVR with depression in the inferolateral leads) with acute ventricular infarction usually indicate concomitant pericarditis (see later).

ELECTROCARDIOGRAPHIC DIFFERENTIAL DIAGNOSIS OF ISCHEMIA AND INFARCTION. The ECG has important limitations in sensitivity and specificity in the diagnosis of coronary syndromes.[55]

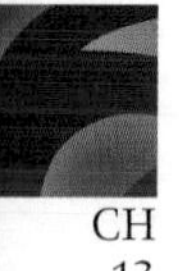

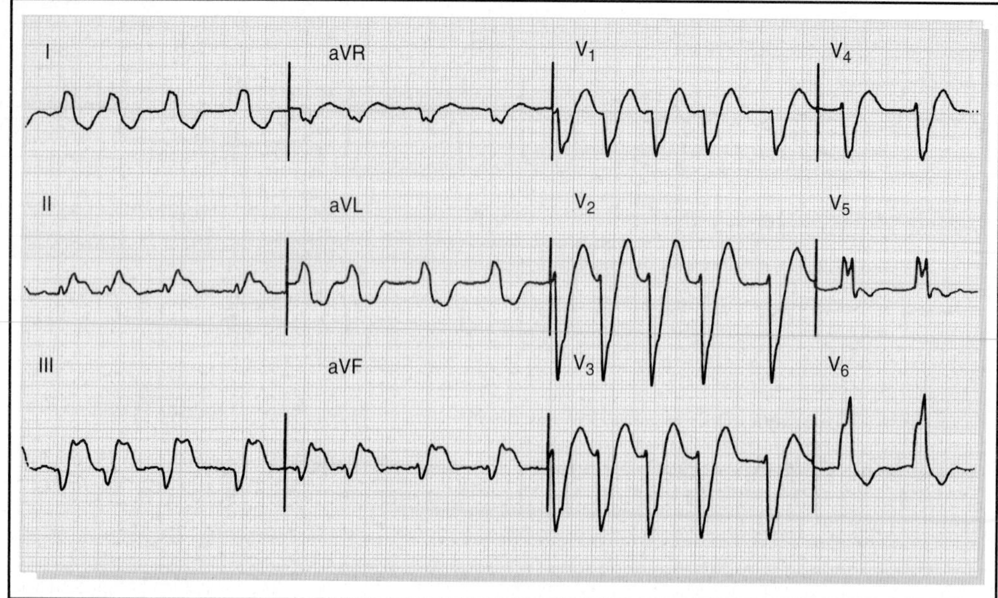

FIGURE 13-42 Complete LBBB with acute inferior myocardial infarction. Note the prominent ST-segment elevation in leads II, III, and aVF, with reciprocal ST-segment depression in leads I and aVL superimposed on secondary ST-T changes. The underlying rhythm is atrial fibrillation.

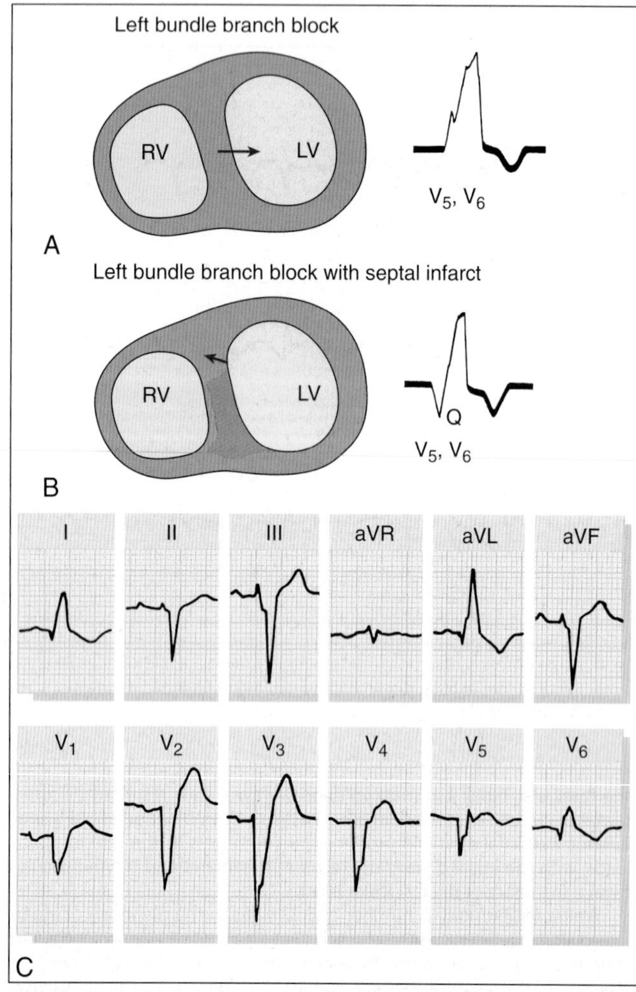

FIGURE 13-43 **A,** With uncomplicated LBBB, early septal forces are directed to the left. Therefore, no Q waves will be seen in V_5 and V_6 (right panel). **B,** With LBBB complicated by anteroseptal infarction, early septal forces can be directed posteriorly and rightward (left panel). Therefore, prominent Q waves may appear in leads V_5 and V_6 as a paradoxical marker of septal infarction (right panel). **C,** Anterior wall infarction (involving septum) with LBBB. Note the presence of QR complexes in leads I, aVL, V_5, and V_6. (***A** and **B** modified from Dunn MI, Lipman BS: Lipman-Massie Clinical Electrocardiography. 8th ed. Chicago, Year Book, 1989.*)

An initially normal ECG does not exclude ischemia or even acute infarction.[74] If the initial ECG is not diagnostic, but the patient remains symptomatic and there is high clinical suspicion for acute ischemia, it is recommended that the ECG be repeated at 5- to 10-minute intervals.[54] However, a normal ECG throughout the course of an alleged acute infarct is distinctly uncommon. As a result, prolonged chest pain without diagnostic electrocardiographic changes on repeat ECGs should always prompt a careful search for noncoronary causes of chest pain (see Chap. 53). Pathologic Q waves can be absent, even in patients with depressed left ventricular function caused by severe coronary disease and a previous infarct. As noted, the diagnosis of acute or chronic infarction can be completely masked by ventricular conduction disturbances, especially those resulting from LBBB, as well as ventricular pacing and Wolff-Parkinson-White preexcitation. On the other hand, diagnostic confusion can arise because Q waves, ST-segment elevation, ST-segment depression, tall positive T waves, and deep T wave inversion can be seen in a wide variety of noncoronary settings.

NONINFARCTION Q WAVES. Q waves simulating coronary artery disease can be related to one (or a combination) of the following four factors[55] (**Table 13-9**): (1) physiologic or positional variants; (2) altered ventricular conduction; (3) ventricular enlargement; and (4) myocardial damage or replacement. Depending on the electrical axis, prominent Q waves (as part of QS- or QR-type complexes) can also appear in the limb leads (aVL with a vertical axis and III and aVF with a horizontal axis). A QS complex can appear in lead V_1 as a normal variant, but rarely in leads V_1 and V_2. Prominent Q waves can be associated with a variety of other positional factors that alter the orientation of the heart vis-à-vis a given lead axis. Poor R wave progression, sometimes with actual QS waves, can be caused solely by improper placement of chest electrodes above their usual position. In cases of dextrocardia, provided that no underlying structural abnormalities are present, normal R wave progression can be restored by recording leads V_2 to V_6 on the right side of the chest (with lead V_1 placed in the V_2 position) A rightward mediastinal shift in the left pneumothorax can contribute to the apparent loss of left precordial R waves. Other positional factors associated with slow R wave progression include pectus excavatum and congenitally corrected transposition of the great vessels.

An intrinsic change in the sequence of ventricular depolarization can lead to pathologic, noninfarct Q waves. The two most important conduction disturbances associated with pseudoinfarct Q waves are LBBB and the Wolff-Parkinson-White (WPW) preexcitation patterns. With LBBB, QS complexes can appear in the right precordial to midprecordial leads and, occasionally, in one or more of leads II, III, and aVF. Depending on the location of the bypass tract, WPW preexcitation can mimic anteroseptal,

TABLE 13-9 Differential Diagnosis of Noninfarction Q Waves (with Selected Examples)

Physiological or Positional Factors
Normal variant "septal" Q waves
Normal variant Q waves in V_1-V_2, III, and aVF
Left pneumothorax or dextrocardia—loss of lateral R wave progression
Myocardial Injury or Infiltration
Acute processes—myocardial ischemia without infarction, myocarditis, hyperkalemia (rare cause of transient Q waves)
Chronic myocardial processes—idiopathic cardiomyopathies, myocarditis, amyloid, tumor, sarcoid
Ventricular Hypertrophy or Enlargement
Left ventricular (slow R wave progression)*
Right ventricular (reversed R wave progression† or poor R wave progression, particularly with chronic obstructive lung disease)
Hypertrophic cardiomyopathy (can simulate anterior, inferior, posterior, or lateral infarcts; see Fig. 13-47)
Conduction Abnormalities
Left bundle branch block (slow R wave progression*)
Wolff-Parkinson-White patterns

*Small or absent R waves in the right precordial to midprecordial leads.
†Progressive decrease in R wave amplitude from V_1 to the midlateral precordial leads.
Modified from Goldberger AL: Clinical Electrocardiography: A Simplified Approach. 7th ed. St. Louis, CV Mosby, 2006.

lateral, or inferior-posterior infarction. LAFB is often cited as a cause of anteroseptal infarct patterns; however, LAFB usually has only minor effects on the QRS complex in horizontal plane leads. Probably the most common findings are relatively prominent S waves in leads V_5 and V_6. Slow R wave progression is not a consistent feature of LAFB, although minuscule q waves in leads V_1 to V_3 have been reported in this setting. These small q waves can become more apparent if the leads are recorded one interspace above their usual position and disappear in leads that are one interspace below their usual position. As a general clinical rule, however, prominent Q waves (as part of QS or QR complexes) in the right precordial to midprecordial leads should not be attributed to LAFB alone.

Slow ("Poor") R Wave Progression

In contrast, slow R wave progression, a nonspecific finding, is commonly observed with LVH and with acute or chronic right ventricular overload. Q waves in such settings can reflect a variety of mechanisms, including a change in the balance of early ventricular depolarization forces and altered cardiac geometry and position. A marked loss of R wave voltage, sometimes with frank Q waves from lead V_1 to the lateral chest leads, can be seen with chronic obstructive pulmonary disease (see Fig. 13-20). The presence of low limb voltage and signs of right atrial abnormality (P pulmonale) can serve as additional diagnostic clues. This loss of R wave progression may, in part, reflect right ventricular dilation. Furthermore, downward displacement of the heart in an emphysematous chest can play a major role in the genesis of poor R wave progression in this syndrome. Partial or complete normalization of R wave progression can be achieved in these cases simply by recording the chest leads an interspace lower than usual (see Fig. 13-20).

Other Pseudoinfarct Patterns in Ventricular Overload. A variety of pseudoinfarct patterns can occur with acute cor pulmonale caused by pulmonary embolism (see Chap. 77). Acute right ventricular overload in this setting can cause slow R wave progression and sometimes right precordial to midprecordial T wave inversion (formerly referred to as right ventricular strain), mimicking anterior ischemia or infarction. The classic $S_1Q_3T_3$ pattern can occur but is neither sensitive nor specific. A prominent Q wave (usually as part of a QR complex) can also occur in lead aVF along with this pattern (see Fig. 13-21). However, acute right overload by itself does not cause a pathologic Q wave in lead II. Right heart overload, acute or chronic, may also be associated with a QR complex in lead V_1 and simulate anteroseptal infarction.

Pseudoinfarct patterns are an important finding in patients with hypertrophic cardiomyopathy, and the ECG can simulate anterior, inferior, posterior, or lateral infarction. The pathogenesis of depolarization abnormalities in this cardiomyopathy is not certain. Prominent inferolateral Q waves (leads II, III, aVF, and V_4 to V_6) and tall, right precordial R waves are probably related to increased depolarization forces generated by the markedly hypertrophied septum (**Fig. 13-44**). Abnormal septal depolarization can also contribute to bizarre QRS complexes.

Q Wave Pathogenesis with Myocardial Damage. Loss of electromotive force associated with myocardial necrosis contributes to R wave loss and Q wave formation in MI cases. This mechanism of Q wave pathogenesis, however, is not specific for coronary artery disease with infarction. Any process, acute or chronic, that causes sufficient loss of regional electromotive potential can result in Q waves. For example, replacement of myocardial tissue by electrically inert material such as amyloid or tumor can cause noninfarction Q waves (see Chap. 74). A variety of dilated cardiomyopathies associated with extensive myocardial fibrosis can be characterized by pseudoinfarct patterns. Ventricular hypertrophy can also contribute to Q wave pathogenesis in this setting. Finally, Q waves caused by myocardial injury, whether ischemic or nonischemic in origin, can appear transiently and do not necessarily signify irreversible heart muscle damage. Severe ischemia can cause regional loss of electromotive potential without actual cell death (electrical stunning phenomenon). Transient conduction disturbances can also cause alterations in ventricular activation and result in noninfarctional Q waves. In some cases, transient Q waves may represent unmasking of a prior Q wave infarct. New but transient Q waves have been described in patients with severe hypotension from a variety of causes, as well as with tachyarrhythmias, myocarditis, Prinzmetal angina, protracted hypoglycemia, phosphorus poisoning, and hyperkalemia.

Fragmented QRS

Because Q waves are not always present and can regress or even disappear over time, alternative electrocardiographic markers of prior infarction are being evaluated, including a fragmented QRS complex

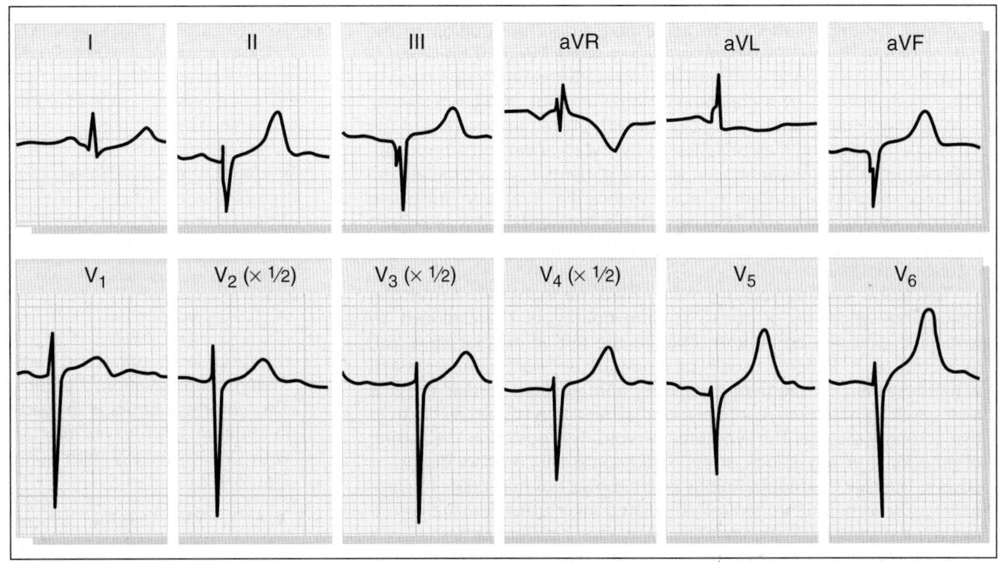

FIGURE 13-44 Hypertrophic cardiomyopathy simulating inferolateral infarction. This 11-year-old girl had a family history of hypertrophic cardiomyopathy. Note the W-shaped QS waves and the qrS complexes in the inferior and lateral precordial leads. *(From Goldberger AL: Myocardial Infarction: Electrocardiographic Differential Diagnosis. 4th ed. St. Louis, Mosby-Year Book, 1991.)*

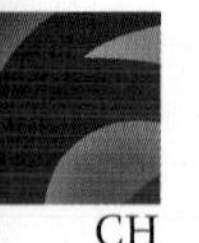

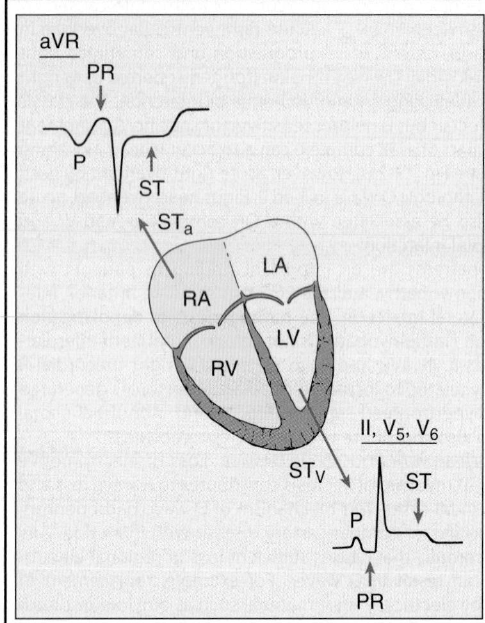

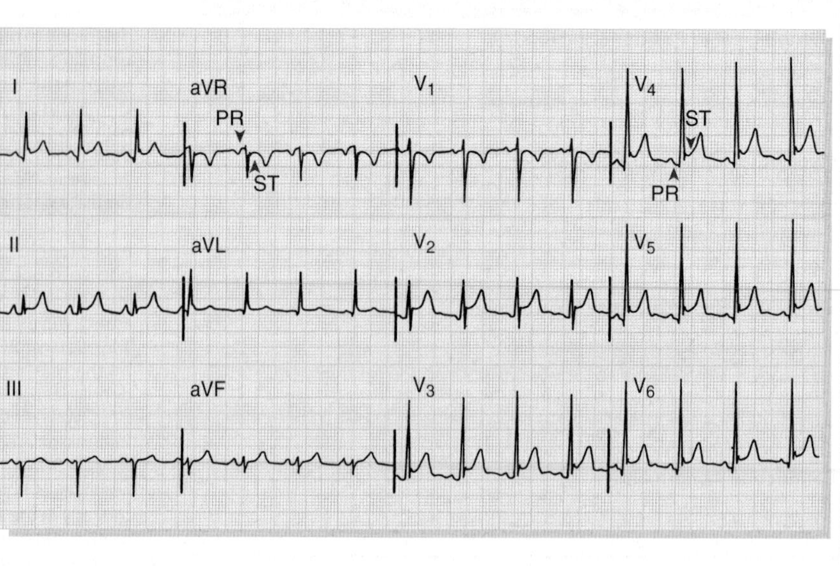

FIGURE 13-45 Acute pericarditis is often characterized by two apparent injury currents, one atrial and the other ventricular. The atrial injury current vector (ST_a) is usually directed upward and to the right and produces PR-segment elevation in aVR with reciprocal PR depression in II, V_5, and V_6. The ventricular injury current (ST_V) is directed downward and to the left, associated with ST-segment elevation in leads II, V_5, and V_6. This characteristic PR-ST segment discordance is illustrated in the bottommost tracing. Note the diffuse distribution of ST-segment elevation in acute pericarditis (e.g., I, II, and V_2 through V_6, with reciprocal changes in aVR and perhaps minimally in V_1). *(From Goldberger AL: Myocardial Infarction: Electrocardiographic Differential Diagnosis. 4th ed. St. Louis, Mosby-Year Book, 1991.)*

(fQRS).[51] Further investigations in a wide range of populations are required to confirm preliminary findings and to develop consistent replicable definitions of QRS fragmentation. The possibly related patterns of peri-infarction block and QRS notching with MI have been discussed earlier.

ST-T Changes Simulating Ischemia. The differential diagnosis of STEMI (or ischemia)[52,55,75] caused by obstructive coronary disease subtends a wide variety of diagnoses, including acute pericarditis (see Chap. 75; **Fig. 13-45** and Fig. 75-2), acute myocarditis (see Chap. 70), normal variants, including classic early repolarization patterns (see Fig. 13-13), takotsubo (stress) cardiomyopathy,[76] Brugada patterns[50] (see Chap. 39), and a number of other conditions listed in **Table 13-10**. Acute pericarditis, in contrast to acute myocardial infarction, typically induces diffuse ST-segment elevation, usually in most of the chest leads and also in leads I, aVL, II, and aVF. Reciprocal ST-segment depression is seen in lead aVR. An important clue to acute pericarditis, in addition to the diffuse nature of the ST-segment elevation, is the frequent presence of PR-segment elevation in aVR, with reciprocal PR segment depression in other leads, caused by a concomitant atrial current of injury (see Fig. 13-45). Abnormal Q waves do not occur with acute pericarditis and the ST-segment elevation may be followed by T wave inversion after a variable period. Acute myocarditis can, in some patients, exactly simulate the electrocardiographic pattern of acute myocardial infarction, including ST-segment elevation and Q waves. These myocarditic pseudoinfarct findings can be associated with a rapidly progressive course and increased mortality.

Takotsubo cardiomyopathy, also called transient left ventricular ballooning syndrome or stress cardiomyopathy, is characterized by reversible wall motion abnormalities of the left ventricular apex and midventricle.[76,77] Patients, usually postmenopausal women, may present with chest pain, ST-segment elevations, and elevated cardiac enzyme levels, exactly mimicking acute myocardial infarction caused by obstructive coronary disease. The syndrome is typically reported in the setting of emotional or physiologic stress. Fixed epicardial coronary disease is absent. The exact pathophysiology is not known but may relate to coronary vasospasm or neurogenically mediated myocardial damage, resulting in a transmural (ST-segment elevation) injury current pattern.

A variety of factors such as digitalis, ventricular hypertrophy, hypokalemia, and hyperventilation can cause ST-segment depression mimicking subendocardial ischemia. Similarly, tall positive T waves do not invariably represent hyperacute ischemic changes but can reflect normal variants, hyperkalemia, cerebrovascular injury, and left ventricular volume loads resulting from mitral or aortic regurgitation, among other causes. ST-segment elevation, J point elevations, and tall positive T waves are also common findings in leads V_1 and V_2 with LBBB or LVH patterns. In addition, tall T waves may be seen occasionally in the left chest leads with LVH, especially with volume (diastolic) overload syndromes (see Fig. 13-18).

TABLE 13-10 Differential Diagnosis of ST-Segment Elevation

Myocardial ischemia or infarction
Noninfarction, transmural ischemia (e.g., Prinzmetal angina pattern, takotsubo syndrome; see Fig. 13-40)
Acute myocardial infarction (see Fig. 13-37)
Post myocardial infarction (ventricular aneurysm pattern)
Acute pericarditis (see Fig. 13-48)
Normal variants (including the classic early repolarization pattern; see Fig. 13-16)
LVH, LBBB (V_1-V_2 or V_3 only)
Other (rarer)
Acute pulmonary embolism (right midchest leads)
Hypothermia (J wave, Osborn wave; see Fig. 13-53)
Myocardial injury
Myocarditis (may resemble myocardial infarction or pericarditis)
Tumor invading the left ventricle
Hypothermia (J wave, Osborn wave) (see Fig. 9-53)
DC cardioversion (just following)
Intracranial hemorrhage
Hyperkalemia*
Brugada pattern (RBBB-like pattern and ST-segment elevations in right precordial leads)*
Type 1C antiarrhythmic drugs*
Hypercalcemia*

*Usually most apparent in V_1 to V_2.

Modified from Goldberger AL: Clinical Electrocardiography: A Simplified Approach. 7th ed. St. Louis, CV Mosby, 2006.

T WAVE INVERSION. When caused by physiologic variants, T wave inversion is sometimes mistaken for ischemia. T waves in the right precordial leads can be slightly inverted, particularly in leads V_1 and V_2. Some adults show persistence of the juvenile T wave pattern (see Fig. 13-12), with more prominent T wave inversion in right precordial to midprecordial leads showing an rS or RS morphology. Such patterns, especially associated with LBBB-type premature ventricular beats or relevant family history, also raise strong consideration of arrhythmogenic right ventricular cardiomyopathy (dysplasia).[29,78] The other major normal variant that can be associated with notable T wave inversion is the early repolarization pattern (see Fig. 13-13). Some subjects, especially athletes, with this variant have prominent, biphasic T wave inversion in association with the ST-segment elevation. This pattern, which may simulate the initial stages of an evolving infarct, is most prevalent in young black men and athletes. These functional ST-T changes are probably the result of regional disparities in repolarization and can be normalized by exercise.

Primary and Secondary T Wave Inversions

A variety of pathologic factors can alter repolarization and cause prominent T wave inversion (**Fig. 13-46**). As noted earlier, T wave alterations are usefully classified as primary or secondary. Primary T wave changes are caused by alterations in the duration or morphology of ventricular action potentials in the absence of changes in the activation sequence. Examples include ischemia, drug effects, and metabolic factors. Prominent primary T wave inversion (or in some cases, tall positive T waves) is also a well-described feature of the ECG in cerebrovascular accidents, particularly with subarachnoid hemorrhage. The so-called cerebrovascular accident (CVA) T wave pattern is characteristically seen in multiple leads, with a widely splayed appearance usually associated with marked QT prolongation (see Figs. 13-46 and 92-18). Some studies have implicated structural damage (myocytolysis) in the hearts of patients with such T wave changes, probably induced by excessive sympathetic stimulation mediated via the hypothalamus. A role for concomitant vagal activation in the pathogenesis of such T wave changes, which are usually associated with bradycardia, has also been postulated. Similar T wave changes have been reported after truncal vagotomy, radical neck dissection, and bilateral carotid endarterectomy. In addition, the massive diffuse T wave inversion seen in some patients after Stokes-Adams syncope may be related to a similar neurogenic mechanism. Patients with subarachnoid hemorrhage can also show transient ST elevation, as well as arrhythmias, including torsades de pointes. Ventricular dysfunction can even occur.

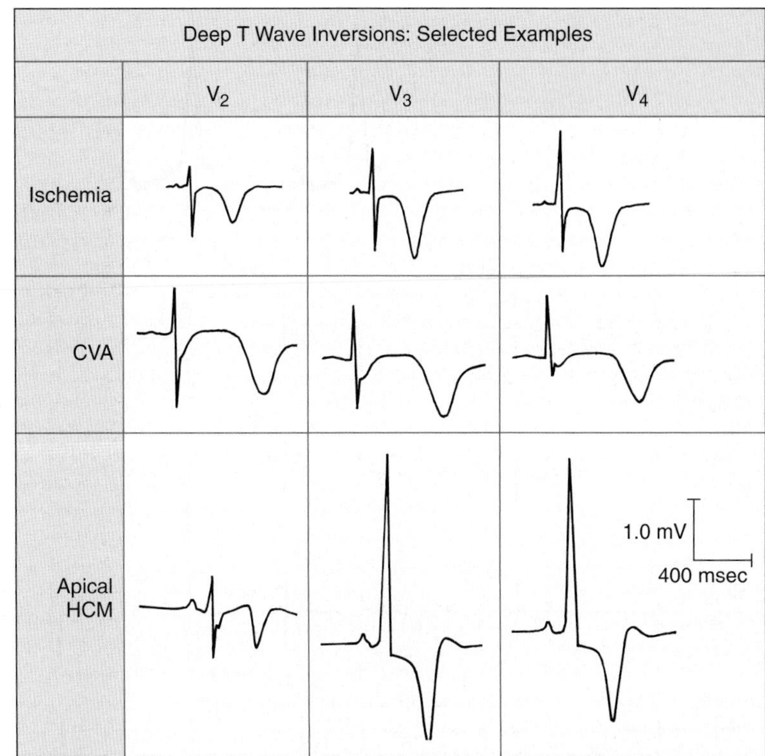

FIGURE 13-46 Deep T wave inversion can have various causes. Note the marked QT prolongation in conjunction with the cerebrovascular accident (CVA) T wave pattern caused here by subarachnoid hemorrhage. Apical hypertrophic cardiomyopathy (HCM) is another cause of deep T wave inversion that can be mistaken for coronary disease. *(From Goldberger AL: Deep T wave inversions. ACC Curr J Rev 5:28, 1996.)*

In contrast to these primary T wave abnormalities, secondary T wave changes are caused by altered ventricular activation, without changes in action potential characteristics. Examples include bundle branch block, Wolff-Parkinson-White preexcitation, and ventricular ectopic or paced beats. In addition, altered ventricular activation (associated with QRS interval prolongation) can induce persistent T wave changes that appear after normal ventricular depolarization has resumed. The term *cardiac memory T wave changes* has been used in this context to describe repolarization changes subsequent to depolarization changes caused by ventricular pacing, intermittent LBBB, intermittent Wolff-Parkinson-White preexcitation, and other alterations of ventricular activation[79] (see Chaps. 36 and 39). Finally, the term *idiopathic global T wave inversion* has been applied in cases in which no identifiable cause for often marked diffuse repolarization abnormalities can be found. An unexplained female preponderance has been reported.

Drug Effects

Numerous drugs can affect the ECG, often in association with nonspecific ST-T alterations.[52,53,80] More marked changes, as well as AV and intraventricular conduction disturbances, can occur with selected agents. The proarrhythmic effects of antiarrhythmic medications are described in Chaps. 10 and 37.

The digitalis effect[80] refers to the relatively distinctive "scooped" appearance of the ST-T complex and shortening of the QT interval, which correlates with abbreviation of the ventricular action potential duration (**Fig. 13-47**). Digitalis-related ST-T changes can be accentuated by an increased heart rate during exercise and result in false-positive stress test results (see Chap. 14). Digitalis effect can occur with therapeutic or toxic doses of the drug. The term *digitalis toxicity* refers specifically to systemic effects (nausea and anorexia, among other effects) or conduction disturbances and arrhythmias caused by drug excess or increased sensitivity.

The electrocardiographic effects and toxicities of other cardioactive agents can be anticipated, in part, from ion channel effects (see Chap. 35). Inactivation of sodium channels by class 1 agents (e.g., quinidine, procainamide, disopyramide, flecainide) can cause QRS prolongation. Classes 1A and 3 agents (e.g., amiodarone, dronedarone, dofetilide, ibutilide, sotalol) can induce an acquired long QT(U) syndrome (see Chap. 37). Psychotropic drugs (e.g., tricyclic antidepressants and phenothiazines), which have class 1A-like properties, can also lead to QRS and QT(U) prolongation. Toxicity can produce asystole or torsades de pointes. Right axis shift of the terminal 40 msec frontal plane QRS axis may be a helpful additional marker of tricyclic antidepressant overdose. QT prolongation has been reported with methadone, as discussed below in the section on ECG Guidelines. Cocaine (see Chap. 73) can cause a variety of ECG changes including those of STEMI, as well as life-threatening arrhythmias.

Electrolyte and Metabolic Abnormalities

In addition to the structural and functional cardiac conditions already discussed, numerous systemic metabolic aberrations affect the ECG, including electrolyte abnormalities and acid-base disorders, as well as systemic hypothermia.[52,53]

CALCIUM. Hypercalcemia and hypocalcemia predominantly alter the action potential duration. An increased extracellular calcium concentration shortens the ventricular action potential duration by shortening phase 2 of the action potential. In contrast, hypocalcemia prolongs phase 2 of the action potential. These cellular changes correlate with abbreviation and prolongation of the QT interval (ST segment portion) with hypercalcemia and hypocalcemia, respectively (**Fig. 13-48**). Severe hypercalcemia (e.g., serum Ca^{2+} >15 mg/dL) can also be associated with decreased T wave amplitude, sometimes with T wave notching or inversion. Hypercalcemia sometimes produces a high takeoff of the ST segment in leads V_1 and V_2 and can thus simulate acute ischemia (see Table 13-10).

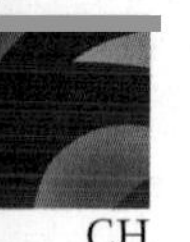

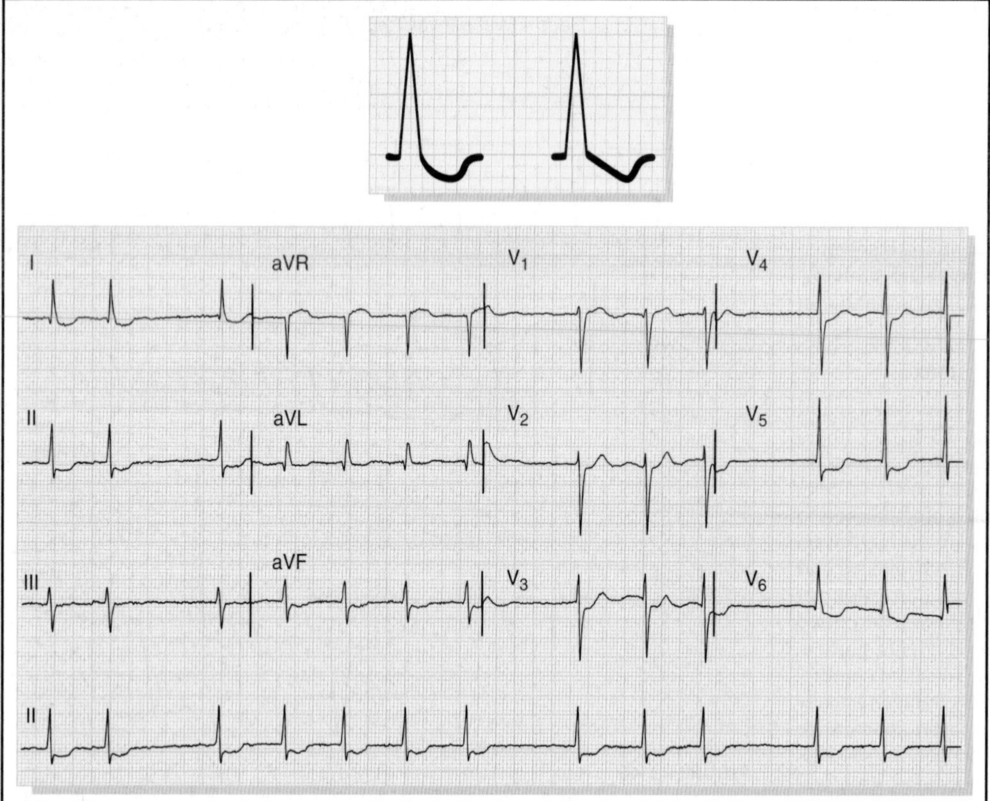

FIGURE 13-47 Top panel, Digitalis effect. Digitalis glycosides characteristically produce shortening of the QT interval with a scooped or downsloping ST-T complex. **Bottom panels,** Digitalis effect in combination with digitalis toxicity. The underlying rhythm is atrial fibrillation. A group beating pattern of QRS complexes with shortening of the R-R intervals is consistent with nonparoxysmal junctional tachycardia with exit (AV Wenckebach) block. ST-segment depression and scooping (lead V_6) are consistent with the digitalis effect, although ischemia or LVH cannot be excluded. Findings are strongly suggestive of digitalis excess; the serum digoxin level was higher than 3 ng/mL. The digitalis effect does not necessarily imply digitalis toxicity, however. *(**Top panel** from Goldberger AL: Clinical Electrocardiography: A Simplified Approach. 6th ed. St. Louis, CV Mosby, 1999.)*

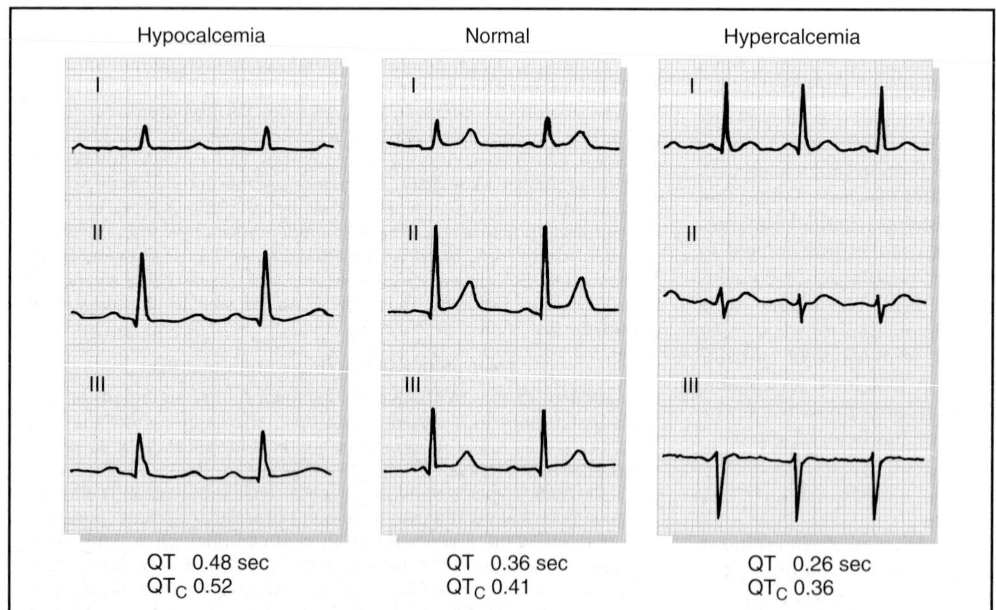

FIGURE 13-48 Prolongation of the QT interval (ST segment portion) is typical of hypocalcemia. Hypercalcemia may cause abbreviation of the ST segment and shortening of the QT interval. *(From Goldberger AL: Clinical Electrocardiography: A Simplified Approach. 6th ed. St. Louis, CV Mosby, 1999.)*

Potassium. Hyperkalemia is associated with a distinctive sequence of ECG changes (**Fig. 13-49A**). The earliest effect is usually narrowing and peaking (*tenting*) of the T wave. The QT interval is shortened at this stage, associated with decreased action potential duration. Progressive extracellular hyperkalemia reduces atrial and ventricular resting membrane potentials, thereby inactivating sodium channels, which decreases V_{max} and conduction velocity. The QRS begins to widen and P wave amplitude decreases. PR interval prolongation can occur, followed sometimes by second- or third-degree AV block. Complete loss of P waves may be associated with a junctional escape rhythm or so-called *sinoventricular* rhythm. In the latter instance, sinus rhythm persists with conduction between the SA and AV nodes and occurs without producing an overt P wave. Moderate to severe hyperkalemia occasionally induces ST elevations in the right precordial leads (V_1 and V_2) and simulates an ischemic current of injury or Brugada-type patterns.[50] However, even severe hyperkalemia can be associated with atypical or nondiagnostic ECG findings. Very marked hyperkalemia leads to eventual asystole, sometimes preceded by a slow undulatory ("sine-wave") ventricular flutter-like pattern. The electrocardiographic triad of (1) peaked T waves (from hyperkalemia), (2) QT prolongation (from hypocalcemia), and (3) LVH (from hypertension) is strongly suggestive of chronic renal failure (see Chap. 93).

Electrophysiologic changes associated with hypokalemia, in contrast, include hyperpolarization of myocardial cell membranes and increased action potential duration. The major electrocardiographic manifestations are ST depression with flattened T waves and increased U wave prominence (see Fig. 13-49B). The U waves can exceed the amplitude of T waves. Clinically, distinguishing T waves from U waves can be difficult or impossible from the surface ECG. Indeed, apparent U waves in hypokalemia and other pathologic settings may actually be part of T waves whose morphology is altered by the effects of voltage gradients between M, or midmyocardial, cells, and adjacent myocardial layers.[81] The prolongation of repolarization with hypokalemia, as part of an acquired long QT(U) syndrome, predisposes to torsades de pointes. Hypokalemia also predisposes to tachyarrhythmias from digitalis.

Magnesium. Specific electrocardiographic effects of mild to moderate isolated abnormalities in magnesium ion concentration are not well characterized. Severe hypermagnesemia can cause AV and intraventricular conduction disturbances that may culminate in complete heart block and cardiac arrest (Mg^{2+} > 15 mEq/L). Hypomagnesemia is usually associated with hypocalcemia or hypokalemia. Hypomagnesemia can potentiate certain digitalis toxic arrhythmias. The role of magnesium deficiency in the pathogenesis and treatment of the acquired long QT(U) syndrome with torsades de pointes is discussed in Chaps. 9 and 39.

OTHER FACTORS. Isolated hypernatremia or hyponatremia does not produce consistent effects on the ECG. Acidemia and alkalemia are often associated with hyperkalemia and hypokalemia, respectively. Systemic hypothermia may be associated with the appearance of a distinctive convex elevation at the junction (J point) of the ST segment and QRS complex (J wave or Osborn wave; **Fig. 13-50**). The cellular mechanism of this type of pathologic J wave appears to be related to an epicardial-endocardial voltage gradient associated with the localized appearance of a prominent epicardial action potential notch.

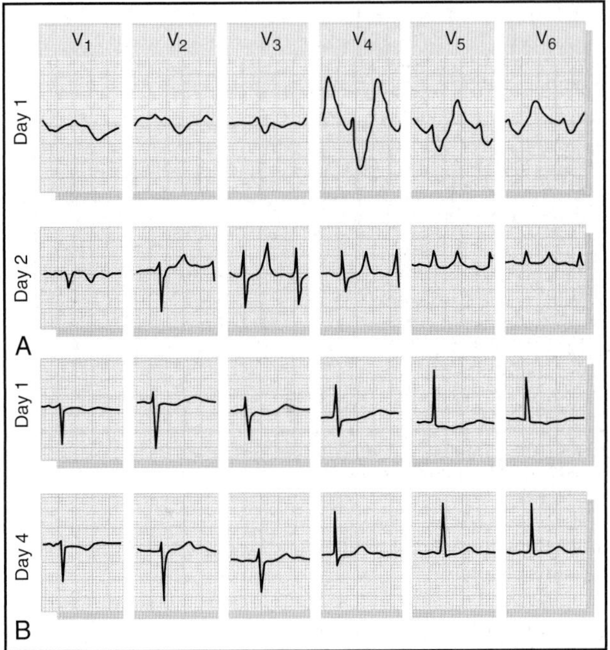

FIGURE 13-49 Electrocardiographic changes in hyperkalemia **(A)** and hypokalemia **(B)**. **A,** On day 1, at a K^+ level of 8.6 mEq/liter, the P wave is no longer recognizable and the QRS complex is diffusely prolonged. Initial and terminal QRS delays are characteristic of K^+-induced intraventricular conduction slowing and are best illustrated in leads V_2 and V_6. On day 2, at a K^+ level of 5.8 mEq/liter, the P wave is recognizable, with a PR interval of 0.24 second; the duration of the QRS complex is approximately 0.10 second, and the T waves are characteristically "tented." **B,** On day 1, at a K^+ level of 1.5 mEq/liter, the T and U waves are merged. The U wave is prominent and the QU interval is prolonged. On day 4, at a K^+ level of 3.7 mEq/liter, the tracing is normal. *(Courtesy of Dr. C. Fisch.)*

Nonspecific QRS and ST-T Changes

Low QRS voltage is said to be present when the total amplitude of the QRS complexes in each of the six extremity leads is 0.5 mV or less or 1.0 mV or less in leads V_1 through V_6. Low QRS voltage can relate to a variety of mechanisms, including increased insulation of the heart by air (chronic obstructive pulmonary disease) or adipose tissue (obesity); replacement of myocardium, for example, by fibrous tissue (ischemic or nonischemic cardiomyopathy), amyloid, or tumor; or to short-circuiting (shunting) effects resulting from low resistance of the fluids (especially with pericardial or pleural effusions, or anasarca). The combination of relatively low limb voltage (QRS voltage < 0.8 mV in each of the limb leads), relatively prominent QRS voltage in the chest leads (SV_1 or SV_2 + RV_5 or RV_6 > 3.5 mV), and slow R wave progression (R wave less than the S wave amplitude in V_1 through V_4) has been reported as a relatively specific but not sensitive sign of dilated-type cardiomyopathies (referred to as the ECG–congestive heart failure triad).[52]

Many factors in addition to ischemia (e.g., postural changes, meals, drugs, hypertrophy, electrolyte and metabolic disorders, central nervous system lesions, infections, pulmonary diseases) can affect the ECG. Ventricular repolarization is particularly sensitive to these effects, which can lead to a variety of nonspecific ST-T changes. The term is usually applied to slight ST depression or T wave inversion or to T wave flattening without evident cause. Care must be taken not to overinterpret such changes, especially in subjects with a low prior probability of heart disease. At the same time, subtle repolarization abnormalities can be markers of coronary or hypertensive heart disease or other types of structural heart disease; these probably account for the association of relatively minor but persistent nonspecific ST-T changes with increased cardiovascular mortality in middle-aged men and women.[82]

Alternans Patterns

The term *alternans* applies to conditions characterized by the sudden appearance of a periodic beat-to-beat change in some aspect of cardiac electrical or mechanical behavior. These abrupt (period-doubling) changes (AAAA > ABAB pattern) are reminiscent of a generic class of patterns observed in perturbed nonlinear control systems. Many different examples of electrical alternans have been described clinically[83,84]; a number of others have been reported in the laboratory. Most familiar is total electrical alternans with sinus tachycardia, a specific but not highly sensitive marker of pericardial effusion with tamponade physiology (**Fig. 13-51**; see Chap. 75). This finding is associated with an abrupt transition from a 1 : 1 to a 2 : 1 pattern in the "to-fro" swinging motion of the heart in the effusion (see Fig. 15-72). Other alternans patterns have primary electrical rather than mechanical causes. ST-T alternans has long

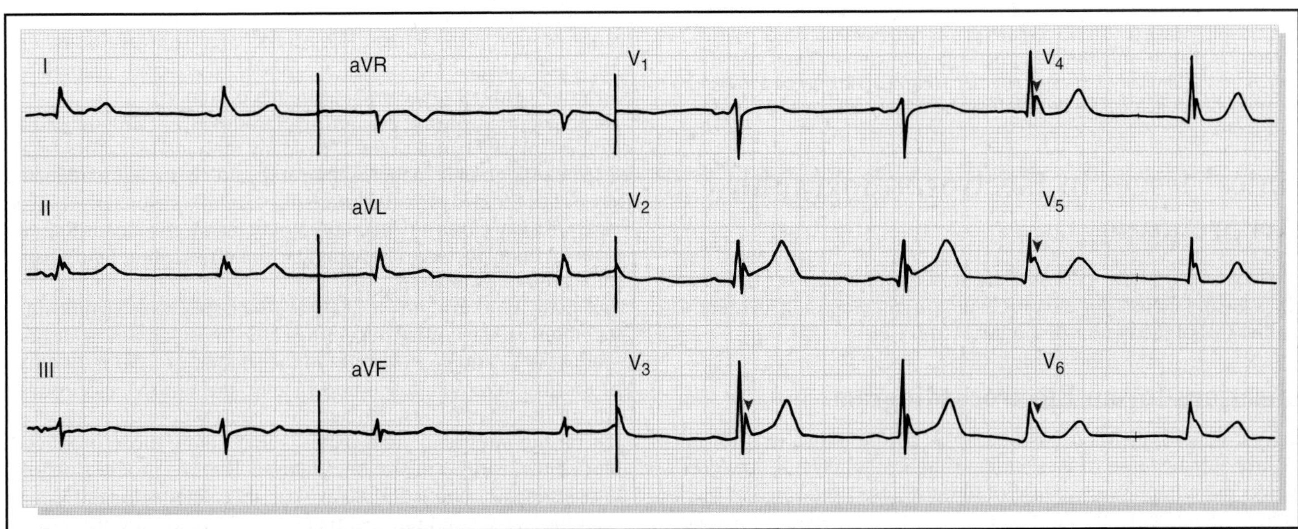

FIGURE 13-50 Systemic hypothermia. The arrowheads (leads V_3 through V_6) point to the characteristic convex J waves, termed *Osborn waves*. Prominent sinus bradycardia is also present. *(From Goldberger AL: Clinical Electrocardiography: A Simplified Approach. 6th ed. St. Louis, CV Mosby, 1999.)*

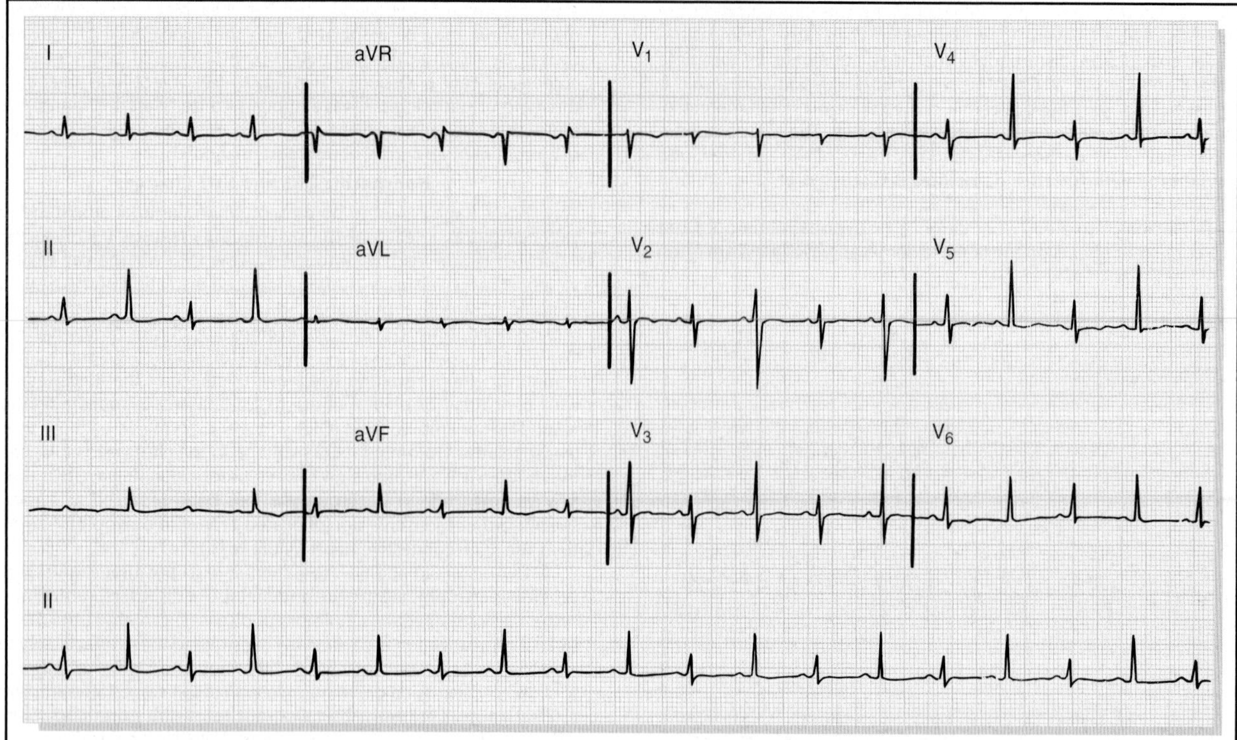

FIGURE 13-51 Total electrical alternans (P-QRS-T) caused by pericardial effusion with tamponade. This finding, particularly in concert with sinus tachycardia and relatively low voltage, is a highly specific, although not sensitive, marker of cardiac tamponade.

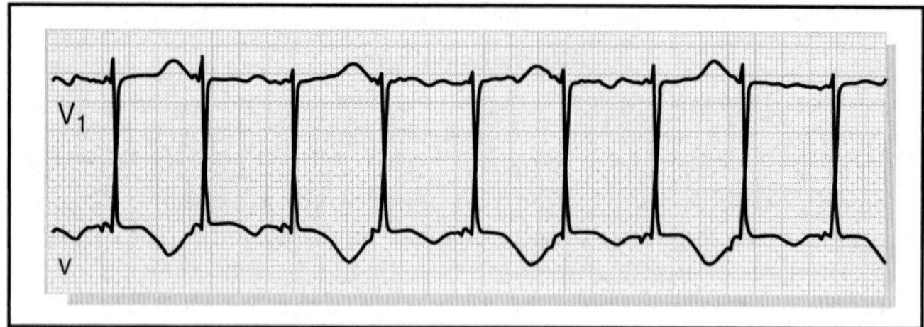

FIGURE 13-52 The QT(U) interval is prolonged (approximately 600 msec) with TU wave alternans. The tracing was recorded in a patient with chronic renal disease shortly following dialysis. This type of repolarization alternans may be a precursor to torsades de pointes. *(Courtesy of Dr. C. Fisch.)*

been recognized as a marker of electrical instability in cases of acute ischemia, where it may precede ventricular tachyarrhythmia (see Fig. 13-37). Considerable interest continues to be directed at the detection of microvolt T wave (or ST-T) alternans as a noninvasive marker of the risk of ventricular tachyarrhythmias in patients with chronic heart disease. (see Chap. 36). Similarly, T-U wave alternans (**Fig. 13-52**) may be a marker of imminent risk of torsades de pointes in hereditary or acquired long-QT syndromes.

Clinical Issues in Electrocardiographic Interpretation

The effectiveness of the ECG as a diagnostic tool depends on factors such as the indications for the procedure, proper recording technique, and the skills of the reader of the ECG.

Indications for an Electrocardiogram

Relatively limited attention has been paid to the indications for an ECG, probably because of its seeming simplicity, safety, and low cost. However, the cumulative expense of low-cost tests performed at high volume is significant, and the potential risk to the patient of missed or false diagnoses of cardiac disease can be substantial. Recommendations for performing ECGs have been proposed by various organizations; these are described and discussed in the section at the end of this chapter.

Whereas most reviews tend to focus on preventing overuse, the ECG may be underused in other important clinical situations. For example, over one third of patients evaluated for angina pectoris in outpatient settings do not have an ECG recorded[85] and only one fourth of patients with ST-segment elevation myocardial infarction transported to emergency rooms have a prehospital ECG, with resulting delays in revascularization procedures.[86]

Technical Errors and Artifacts

Technical errors can lead to clinically significant diagnostic mistakes. Artifacts that may interfere with interpretation can come from movement of the patient or electrodes, electrical disturbances related to current leakage and grounding failure, and external sources such as electrical stimulators or cauteries.[87] Electrical artifacts can simulate life-threatening arrhythmias (**Fig. 13-53**), and excessive body motion can cause excessive baseline wander that could simulate an ST-segment shift of myocardial ischemia or injury.

Misplacement of one or more electrodes is a common cause for errors in interpretation of the ECG. Many limb lead switches produce electrocardiographic patterns that can aid in their identification.[88] Reversal of the two arm electrodes, for example, results in an inverted P and QRS waveforms in lead I but not in lead V_6, two leads that would normally be expected to have similar polarities. Other lead misplacements are not as obvious.

As many as one third of ECGs are recorded with significant misplacement of precordial electrodes. The most common errors are placing the V_1 and V_2 electrodes in the second or third rather than in the fourth intercostal space and placing the V_4 to V_6 electrodes too high on the lateral chest. Placing the right precordial electrodes too high on the chest can yield patterns that mimic those produced by anterior myocardial infarction (delayed R wave progression) or an intraventricular conduction delay (e.g., rSr′ patterns in lead V_1).

Another very common technical error is recording the ECG with nonstandard high- and low-pass filter settings.[89] Increasing the low-frequency cutoff to reduce baseline wander and respiratory effects

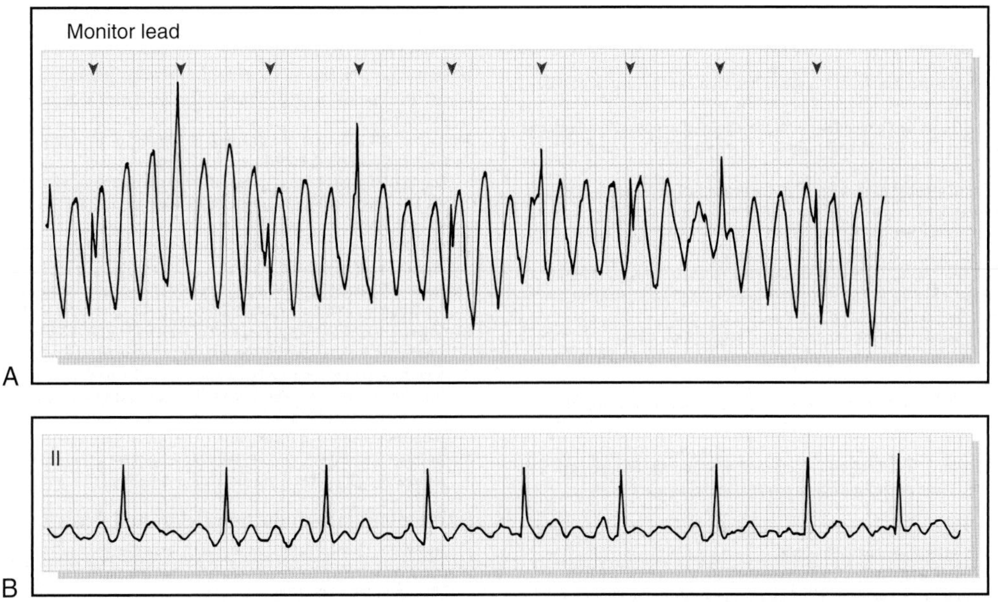

FIGURE 13-53 Artifacts simulating serious arrhythmias. **A,** Motion artifact mimicking ventricular tachyarrhythmia. Partly obscured normal QRS complexes (arrowheads) can be seen with a heart rate of ≈100 beats/min. **B,** Parkinsonian tremor causing baseline oscillations mimicking atrial fibrillation. The regularity of QRS complexes may provide a clue to this artifact.

can produce a range of artifactual ST segment abnormalities. Lowering the high-frequency cutoff to reduce motion and tremor artifacts reduces R wave amplitudes and Q wave measurements and decreases the accuracy of diagnoses of hypertrophy and infarction.[2] Low-pass filtering may also alter electrocardiographic features such as J waves in early repolarization.[90]

Other technical issues reflect characteristics of computerized systems. Clinically relevant differences in measurements may be reported by systems of different manufacturers and by different software versions from the same manufacturer.[91] Other differences result from the differences in the signals used for computerized interpretation and for graphic display. For example, intervals measured by eye may be significantly shorter than those reported by software because the software determines the interval from an overlay of patterns from all leads, whereas manual methods typically rely on the analysis of the waveform from a single lead. Differences in intervals, such as the duration of the Q wave or the QRS complex, may exceed 5 msec, sufficient to alter the diagnosis of conduction defects and infarction.

Reading Competency

Developing and maintaining competency in interpretation of the ECG is critical to successful clinical practice. The Accreditation Council for Graduate Medical Education and the American College of Cardiology recommend supervised and documented interpretation of a minimum of 3500 ECGs covering a broad spectrum of diagnoses and clinical settings over a 3-year training period.[92]

Errors in interpreting ECGs are common and may be increasing in frequency. Studies assessing the accuracy of routine interpretations have demonstrated significant numbers of errors that can lead to clinical mismanagement, including failure to detect and triage patients with acute myocardial ischemia and other life-threatening situations appropriately. In one recent study of patients with acute myocardial infarction who were eligible for but who did not receive revascularization, an interpretation not correctly identifying ST segment elevation was the cause of not undergoing revascularization in 34%.[93]

A final issue concerns overreliance on computerized interpretations. Although computerized diagnostic algorithms have become more accurate and serve as important adjuncts to the clinical interpretation of ECGs, measurements and diagnoses are not currently sufficiently accurate to be relied on in critical clinical environments without expert review. Overall error rates in interpreting abnormal ECGS may be as high as 16%,[94] with error rates exceeding 50% for rhythm abnormalities.[95]

Various tools are available to assess and improve proficiency. The Adult Clinical Cardiology Self-Assessment Program (ACCSAP) contains a self-assessment examination in electrocardiography and is useful for identifying knowledge levels of proficiency and areas of specific weakness.[92] A number of websites feature ECGs for self-assessment and clinical instruction. ECG Wave-Maven (http://ecg.bidmc.harvard.edu) provides free access to more than 400 case studies of ECGs, with answers and multimedia adjuncts.

Future Perspectives

Clinical electrocardiography represents a mature and canonical cardiovascular technology based on extensive electrophysiologic and clinical correlates that have been elaborated over more than a century of study. Advances in other fields have challenged the use of the ECG.[2] For example, imaging techniques provide a more direct assessment of cardiac structural abnormalities than the ECG. Thus, it is important to assess the role of the ECG in adding value within the overall spectrum of cardiac diagnostic tests.[2]

Recent advances in biomedical engineering and technology, clinical therapeutics, and basic science suggest that important new clinically relevant information may be derived from the ECG. Methods to estimate direct cardiac potentials from surface recordings will permit a more direct understanding of the abnormal physiology underlying electrocardiographic patterns, and extracting "hidden information" in the ECG using advanced mathematics techniques will expand its clinical usefulness. Full application of the capabilities of computerized systems will permit the development of more accurate diagnostic criteria based on population subsets and clinical covariates. Continued research correlating electrocardiographic patterns with genomic and biomarker patterns will promote greater understanding of the variation in electrocardiographic patterns seen in common disorders. Also, the development of new treatments will likely expand the role of the ECG as urgent revascularization and cardiac resynchronization have done in the recent past. The historic richness of the surface ECG as a source of basic physiologic and clinical information continues to support the expectation of future unanticipated areas for exploration and discovery.

REFERENCES

Fundamental Principles

1. Wellens HJJ, Gorgels AP: The electrocardiogram 102 years after Einthoven. Circulation 109:652, 2004.
2. Kligfield P, Gettes L, Bailey JJ, et al: Recommendations for the standardization and interpretation of the electrocardiogram. Part I: The electrocardiogram and its standardization. J Am Coll Cardiol 49:1109, 2007.
3. MacLeod R, Kornreich F, van Oosterom A, et al: Report of the first virtual visualization of the reconstructed electrocardiographic display symposium. J Electrocardiol 38:385, 2005.
4. Madias J: The resting electrocardiogram in the management of patients with congestive heart failure: Established applications and new insights. PACE 30:123, 2007.
5. Bacharova L, Selvester RH, Engblom H, Wagner GS: Where is the central terminal located? In search of understanding the use of the Wilson central terminal for production of 9 of the 12 electrocardiogram leads. J Electrocardiol 38:119, 2005.
6. Wagner G, Macfarlane P, Wellens H, et al: AHA/ACC/HRS Recommendations for the Standardization and Interpretation of the Electrocardiogram. Part VI: Acute Myocardial Ischemia. J Am Coll Cardiol 53:1003, 2009.
7. Owens C, McClelland A, Walsh S, et al: Comparison of value of leads from body surface maps to 12-lead electrocardiogram for diagnosis of acute myocardial infarction. Am J Cardiol 102:257, 2008.
8. Sejersten M, Wagner GS, Pahlm O, et al: Detection of acute ischemia from the EASI-derived electrocardiogram and the 12-lead electrocardiogram acquired in clinical practice. J Electrocardiol 40:120, 2007.
9. Farrell RM, Syed A, Syed A, Gutterman DD: Effects of limb electrode placement on the 12- and 16- lead electrocardiogram. J Electrocardiol 41:536, 2008.
10. Engblom H, Foster JE, Martin TN, et al: The relationship between electrical axis by 12-lead electrocardiogram and anatomical axis of the heart by cardiac magnetic resonance imaging in healthy subjects. Am Heart J 150:507, 2005.
11. Sgarbossa EB, Barold SS, Pinski SL, et al: Twelve-lead electrocardiogram: The advantages of an orderly frontal display including lead aVR. J Electrocardiol 37:141, 2004.
12. Perron A, Lim T, Pahlm-Webb, et al: Maximal increase in sensitivity with minimum loss of specificity for diagnosis of acute coronary occlusion achieved by sequentially adding leads from the 24-lead electrocardiogram to the orderly sequenced 12-lead electrocardiogram. J Electrocardiol 40:463, 2007.
13. Mason JW, Hancock EW, Gettes LS, et al: Recommendations for the standardization and interpretation of the electrocardiogram. Part II: Electrocardiography diagnostic statement list. J Am Coll Cardiol 49:1128, 2007.

Normal Electrocardiogram

14. Schijvenaars BJA, van Herpen G, Kors JA: Intraindividual variability in electrocardiograms. J Electrocardiol 41:190, 2008.
15. Mason JW, Ramseth DJ, Chanter DO, et al: Electrocardiographic reference ranges derived from 79,743 ambulatory subjects. J Electrocardiol 40:228, 2007.
16. Lemery R, Birnie D, Tang ASL, et al: Normal atrial activation and voltage during sinus rhythm in the human heart. J Cardiovasc Electrophysiol 18:402, 2007.
17. Holmqvist F, Husser D, Tapanainen JM, et al: Interatrial conduction can be accurately determined using standard 12-lead electrocardiography: Validation of P-wave morphology using electroanatomic mapping in man. Heart Rhythm 5:413, 2008.
18. Thomas RJ, Mietus JE, Peng C-K, et al: Differentiating obstructive from central and complex sleep apnea using an automated electrocardiogram-based method. Sleep 30:1756, 2007.
19. Cerutti S, Hoyer D, Voss A: Multiscale, multiorgan and multivariate complexity analyses of cardiovascular regulation. Philos Transact A Math Phys Eng Sci 367:1337, 2009.
20. Ramanathan C, Jia P, Ghanem R, et al: Activation and repolarization of the normal human heart under complete physiological condition. Proc Nat Acad Sci U S A 103:6309, 2006.
21. MacAlpin RN: Clinical significance of QS complexes in V_1 and V_2 without other electrocardiographic abnormality. Ann Noninvasive Electrocardiol 9:39, 2004.
22. Hakacova N, Robinson AMC, Olson CW, et al: The relationship between mitral papillary muscle positions and characteristics of the QRS complex. J Electrocardiol 41:487, 2008.
23. Carlsson MB, Tragardh E, Engblom H, et al: Left ventricular mass by 12-lead electrocardiogram in healthy subjects: Comparison to cardiac magnetic resonance imaging. J Electrocardiol 39:67, 2006.
24. Antzelevitch C: Cellular basis for the repolarization waves of the ECG. Ann N Y Acad Sci 1080:268, 2006.
25. Rautaharju PM, Surawicz B, Gettes LS, et al: Recommendations for the standardization and interpretation of the electrocardiogram. Part IV: The ST segment, T and U waves. J Am Coll Cardiol 53:982, 2009.
26. Sohaib AMA, Papacosta O, Morris RW, et al: Length of the QT interval: Determinants and prognostic implications in a population-based prospective study. J Electrocardiol 41:704, 2008.
27. Luo S, Michler K, Johnston P, Macfarlane PW: A comparison of commonly used QT correction formulae: The effect of heart rate on the QTc of normal ECGs. J Electrocardiol 37(Suppl):81, 2004.
28. Boineau JP: The early repolarization variant—an electrocardiographic enigma with both QRS and J-STT anomalies. J Electrocardiol 40:3e1, 2007.
29. Wellens HJ: Early repolarization revisited. N Engl J Med 358:19, 2008.
30. Haissaguerre M, Derval N, Sacher F, et al: Sudden cardiac death associated with early repolarization. N Engl J Med 358:2016, 2008.
31. Rosso R, Kogan E, Belhassen B, et al: J-point elevation in survivors of primary ventricular fibrillation and matched control subjects. J Am Coll Cardiol 52:1231, 2008.

Atrial Abnormalities; Ventricular Hypertrophy and Enlargement

32. Ariyarajah V, Assad N, Tandar A, Spodick DH: Interatrial block. Pandemic prevalence, significance and diagnosis. Chest 128:970, 2005.
33. Hancock EW, Deal B, Mirvis DM, et al: Recommendations for the standardization and interpretation of the electrocardiogram. Part V: ECG changes associated with cardiac chamber hypertrophy. J Am Coll Cardiol 53:982, 2009.
34. Lee KW, Appleton CP, Lester SJ, et al: Relation of electrocardiographic criteria for left atrial enlargement to two-dimensional echocardiographic left atrial volume measurements. Am J Cardiol 99:113, 2007.
35. de Bacquer D, Willekins J, De Backer G: Long-term prognostic value of P-wave characteristics for the development of atrial fibrillation in subjects aged 55 to 74 years at baseline. Am J Cardiol 100:850, 2007.
36. Bacharova L: Electrical and structural remodeling in left ventricular hypertrophy. Ann Noninvas Elecrophysiol 12:260, 2007.
37. Konno T, Shimizu M, Ino H, et al: Differences in diagnostic value of four electrocardiographic voltage criteria for hypertrophic cardiomyopathy in a genotyped population. Am J Cardiol 96:1308, 2005.
38. Ang DSC, Lang CC: The prognostic value of the ECG in hypertension: Where are we now? J Human Hypertens 22:460, 2008.
39. Pewsner D, Juni P, Egger M, et al: Accuracy of electrocardiography in diagnosis of left ventricular hypertrophy in arterial hypertension: Systematic review. Brit Med J 335:711, 2007.
40. Chan PG, Logue M, Kligfield P: Effect of right bundle branch block on electrocardiographic amplitudes, including combined voltage criteria used for the detection of left ventricular hypertrophy. Ann Noninvas Electrophysiol 11:230, 2006.
41. Okin PM, Devereux RB, Nieminen MS, et al: Electrocardiographic strain pattern and prediction of new onset congestive heart failure in hypertensive patients: The Losartan Intervention for Endpoint Reduction in Hypertension (LIFE) study. Circulation 113:67, 2006.
42. Sukhija R, Aronow WS, Kakar P: Electrocardiographic abnormalities in patients with right ventricular dilatation due to acute pulmonary embolism. Cardiology 105:57, 2006.

Intraventricular Conduction Delays and Preexcitation

43. Surawicz B, Childers R, Deal BJ, Gettes LS, et al: Recommendations for the standardization and interpretation of the electrocardiogram. Part III: Intraventricular conduction disturbances. Circulation 119:e235, 2009.
44. Biagini E, Elhendy A, Schinkel AF, et al: Prognostic significance of left anterior hemiblock in patients with suspected coronary artery disease. J Am Coll Cardiol 45:858, 2005.
45. Varma N, Jia P, Rudy Y: Electrocardiographic imaging of patients with heart failure with left bundle branch block and response to cardiac resynchronization therapy. J Electrocardiol 40:S174, 2007.
46. Imanishi R, Seto S, Ichimaru S, et al: Prognostic significance of incident complete left bundle branch block observed over a 40-year period. Am J Cardiol 98:644, 2006.
47. Kashani A, Barold S: Significance of QRS complex duration in patients with heart failure. J Am Coll Cardiol 46:2183, 2005.
48. Dhingra R, Pencina MJ, Wang TJ, et al: Electrocardiographic QRS duration and the risk of congestive heart failure. Hypertension 47:861, 2006.
49. Fantoni C, Kawabata M, Massaro R, et al: Right and left ventricular activation sequence in patients with heart failure and right bundle branch block. J Cardiovasc Electrophysiol 16:112, 2005.
50. Antzelevitch C, Brugada P, Borggrefe M, et al: Brugada syndrome: Report of the second consensus conference. Heart Rhythm 2:429, 2005.
51. Das MK, Khan B, Jacob S, et al: Significance of a fragmented QRS complex versus a Q wave in patients with coronary artery disease. Circulation 113:2495, 2006.

Myocardial Ischemia and Infarction

52. Goldberger AL: Clinical Electrocardiography: A Simplified Approach. 7th Edition. St. Louis, Mosby/Elsevier, 2006.
53. Surawicz B, Knilans T: Chou's Electrocardiography in Clinical Practice: Adult and Pediatric. 6th ed. Philadelphia, WB Saunders, 2008.
54. Antman EM, Anbe DT, Armstrong PW, et al: ACC/AHA guidelines for the management of patients with ST-elevation myocardial infarction. A report of the ACC/AHA Task Force on Practice Guidelines J Am Coll Cardiol 44:E1, 2004.
55. Goldberger AL: Myocardial Infarction: Electrocardiographic Differential Diagnosis. 4th ed. St. Louis, Mosby-Year Book, 1991.
56. Zimetbaum PJ, Josephson ME: Use of the electrocardiogram in acute myocardial infarction. N Engl J Med 348:933, 2003.
57. Kleber AG: ST-segment elevation in the electrocardiogram: A sign of myocardial ischemia. Cardiovasc Res 45:111, 2000.
58. Brodie BR, Stuckey TD, Hansen C, et al: Relation between electrocardiographic ST-segment resolution and early and late outcomes after primary percutaneous coronary intervention for acute myocardial infarction. Am J Cardiol 95:343, 2005.
59. Moon JC, De Arenaza DP, Elkington AG, et al: The pathologic basis of Q-wave and non-Q-wave myocardial infarction: A cardiovascular magnetic resonance study. J Am Coll Cardiol 44:554, 2004.
60. Bosimini E, Giannuzzi P, Temporelli PL, et al: Electrocardiographic evolutionary changes and left ventricular remodeling after acute myocardial infarction: Results of the GISSI-3 Echo substudy. J Am Coll Cardiol 35:127, 2000.
61. Voon WC, Chen YW, Hsu CC, et al: Q-wave regression after acute myocardial infarction assessed by Tl-201 myocardial perfusion SPECT. J Nucl Cardiol 11:165, 2004.
62. Correale E, Battista R, Ricciardiello V, et al: The negative U wave: A pathogenetic enigma but a useful, often overlooked bedside diagnostic and prognostic clue in ischemic heart disease. Clin Cardiol 27:674, 2004.
63. Chen A, Kusumoto FM: QT dispersion: Much ado about something? Chest 125:1974, 2004.
64. Rautaharju PM: Why did QT dispersion die? Card Electrophysiol Rev 6:295, 2002.
65. Kligfield P, Okin PM, Lee KW, et al: Significance of QT dispersion. Am J Cardiol 91:1291, 2003.
66. Bogaty P, Boyer L, Rousseau L, Arsenault M: Is anteroseptal myocardial infarction an appropriate term? Am J Med 113:37, 2002.
67. Yamaji H, Iwasaki K, Kusachi S, et al: Prediction of acute left main coronary artery obstruction by 12-lead electrocardiography. ST segment elevation in lead aVR with less ST segment elevation in lead V1. J Am Coll Cardiol 38:1348, 2001.
68. Nikus KC, Sclarovsky S: ST-segment elevation in lead aVR as a sign of left main disease—perpetuating an error? Am J Cardiol 94:542, 2004.
69. Kurum T, Birsin A, Ozbay G, et al: Differentiating the infarct-related artery on initial electrocardiogram in single or multi-vessel disease in acute inferior myocardial infarction and

evaluating involvement of vessels using correspondence analysis. Angiology 56:385, 2005.
70. Wang SS, Paynter L, Kelly RV, et al: Electrocardiographic determination of culprit lesion site in patients with acute coronary events. J Electrocardiol 42:46, 2009.
71. Tabas JA, Rodriguez RM, Seligman HK, Goldschlager NF: Electrocardiographic criteria for detecting acute myocardial infarction in patients with left bundle branch block: A meta-analysis. Ann Emerg Med 523:29, 2008.
72. Jim MH, Miu R, Siu CW: PR-segment elevation in inferior leads: An atypical electrocardiographic sign of atrial infarction. J Invasive Cardiol 16:219, 2004.
73. Neven K, Crijns H, Gorgels A: Atrial infarction: A neglected electrocardiographic sign with important clinical implications. J Cardiovasc Electrophysiol 14:306, 2003.
74. Welch RD, Zalenski RJ, Frederick PD, et al: Prognostic value of a normal or nonspecific initial electrocardiogram in acute myocardial infarction. JAMA 286:1977, 2001.
75. Wang K, Asinger RW, Marriott HJ: ST-segment elevation in conditions other than acute myocardial infarction. N Engl J Med 349:2128, 2003.
76. Sharkey SW, Windenberg DC, Lesser JR, et al: Natural history and expansive clinical profile of stress (tako-tsubo) cardiomyopathy. J Am Coll Cardiol 55:333, 2010.
77. Prasad A, Lerman A, Rihal CS: Apical ballooning syndrome (Tako-Tsubo or stress cardiomyopathy): A mimic of acute myocardial infarction. Am Heart J 155:408, 2008.
78. Bauce B, Frigo G, Marcus F, et al: Comparison of clinical features of arrhythmogenic right ventricular cardiomyopathy in men versus women. Am J Cardiol 102:1252, 2008.
79. Shvilkin A, Bojovic B, Vajdic B, et al: Vectorcardiographic determinants of cardiac memory during normal ventricular activation and continuous ventricular pacing. Heart Rhythm 6:943, 2009.

Drug Effects; Electrolyte and Metabolic Abnormalities; Nonspecific QRS and ST-T Abnormalities; Alternans Patterns

80. Sundqvist K, Jogestrand T, Nowak J: The effect of digoxin on the electrocardiogram of healthy middle-aged and elderly patients at rest and during exercise: A comparison with the ECG reaction induced by myocardial ischemia. J Electrocardiol 35:213, 2002.
81. Antzelevitch C, Shimizu W, Yan GX, et al: The M cell: Its contribution to the ECG and to normal and abnormal electrical function of the heart. J Cardiovasc Electrophysiol 10:1124, 1999.
82. Greenland P, Xie X, Liu K, et al: Impact of minor electrocardiographic ST-segment and/or T-wave abnormalities on cardiovascular mortality during long-term follow-up. Am J Cardiol 91:1068, 2003.
83. Maury P, Racka F, Piot C, Davy JM: QRS and cycle length alternans during paroxysmal supraventricular tachycardia: What is the mechanism? J Cardiovasc Electrophysiol 13:92, 2002.
84. Chow T, Kereiakes DJ, Onufer J, et al: Does microvolt T-wave alternans testing predict ventricular tachyarrhythmias in patients with ischemic cardiomyopathy and prophylactic defibrillators? The MASTER (Microvolt T Wave Alternans Testing for Risk Stratification of Post-Myocardial Infarction Patients) trial. J Am Coll Cardiol 53:1245, 2009.

Clinical Issues in Electrocardiographic Interpretation

85. Li J, Reaven NL, Funk SE, et al: Frequency of electrocardiographic recordings in patients presenting with angina pectoris (from the Investigation of National Coronary Disease Identification). Am J Cardiol 103:312, 2009.
86. Diercks DB, Kontos MC, Chan AY, et al: Utilization and impact of pre-hospital electrocardiograms for patients with acute ST-segment elevation myocardial infarction. J Am Coll Cardiol 53:161, 2009.
87. Patel, SI, Souter MJ: Equipment-related electrocardiographic artifacts. Anesthesiology 108:38, 2000.
88. Rowlands DJ: Inadvertent interchange of electrocardiogram limb lead connections: Analysis of predicted consequences. J Electrocardiol 41:84, 2008.
89. Kligfield P, Okin PM: Prevalence and clinical implications of improper filter settings in routine electrocardiography. Am J Cardiol 99:711, 2007.
90. Garcia-Niebla J, Serra-Autonell G: Effect of inadequate low-pass filter application. J Electrocardiol 42:303, 2009.
91. Kligfield P, Hancock EW, Helfenbein ED, et al: Relation of QT interval measurements to evolving automated algorithms from different manufacturers of electrocardiographs. Am J Cardiol 98:88, 2006.
92. Myerburg RJ, Chaitman BR, Ewy GA, Lauer MS: Task Force 2: Training in electrocardiography, ambulatory electrocardiography, and exercise testing. J Am Coll Cardiol 51:348, 2008.
93. Tricomi AJ, Magid DJ, Rumsfeld JS, et al: Missed opportunities for reperfusion therapy for ST-segment elevation myocardial infarction: Results of the Emergency Room Quality in Myocardial Infarction (EDQMI) study. Am Heart J 155:47, 2008.
94. Guglin ME, Thatai D: Common errors in computer electrocardiogram interpretation. Int J Cardiol 106:232, 2006.
95. Shah AP, Rubin SA: Errors in computerized electrocardiogram interpretation of cardiac rhythm. J Electrocardiol 40:385-390, 2007.

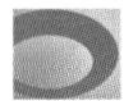

GUIDELINES

DAVID M. MIRVIS AND ARY L. GOLDBERGER

Electrocardiography

Guidelines for the performance of electrocardiograms have evolved little in recent years. The most widely cited guidelines were published by the American College of Cardiology and American Heart Association (ACC/AHA) in 1992[1] and are summarized in Tables 13G-1 through 13G-3. Other professional groups have also published guidelines for use in specific populations and clinical settings (see later).

The ACC/AHA guidelines[1] use the convention of classifying indications according to one of three classes. Class I indications are conditions for which it is generally agreed that ECGs are useful. Class II indications are conditions for which opinions differ with respect to the usefulness of ECGs. Class III indications are conditions for which it is generally agreed that ECGs have little or no usefulness.

Indications for the ECG can be considered for several different subpopulations—those with known heart disease (**Table 13G-1**), those with suspected heart disease or at high risk for heart disease (**Table 13G-2**), and those without evidence of heart disease (**Table 13G-3**). In addition, more specific recommendations have been proposed for the use of the ECG in special groups, including preoperative patients, persons with dangerous occupations, athletes, and those taking medications associated with electrophysiologic effects.

PATIENTS WITH KNOWN CARDIOVASCULAR DISEASE

The guidelines[1] support the use of ECGs in the baseline evaluation of all patients with known cardiovascular disease, when important clinical changes occur, for following the course of disease, and for the evaluation of response to therapies likely to produce electrocardiographic changes (see Table 13G-1). Thus, in patients with known cardiac disease, ECGs are warranted as part of a baseline examination, after initiating therapy known to produce electrocardiographic changes that correlate with therapeutic responses, progression of disease, or adverse effects, for intermittent follow-up after changes in signs or symptoms such as syncope, chest pain, and extreme fatigue or relevant laboratory findings, and after significant intervals (usually 1 year or longer) in the absence of clinical changes. Follow-up ECGs are not considered appropriate for patients with mild chronic cardiovascular conditions that are not considered likely to progress (e.g., mild mitral valve prolapse). ECGs at each visit are considered inappropriate for patients with stable heart disease who are seen frequently (e.g., within 4 months) and have no evidence of clinical change.

PATIENTS SUSPECTED OF HAVING CARDIOVASCULAR DISEASE

In patients suspected of having cardiac disease or at high risk for cardiac disease, an ECG is appropriate as part of an initial evaluation in the presence of signs or symptoms suggesting cardiac disease, in patients with important risk factors such as cigarette abuse, diabetes mellitus, peripheral vascular disease, or a family history of cardiac disease, during therapy with cardioactive medications, and during follow-up if clinical events develop or at prolonged intervals if clinically stable (see Table 13G-2). In the follow-up of patients at increased risk for heart disease, ECGs every 1 to 5 years are considered appropriate, but routine screening ECGs more frequently than yearly are not supported for patients who remain clinically stable.

PATIENTS WITHOUT KNOWN OR SUSPECTED CARDIOVASCULAR DISEASE

The various guidelines differ in their recommendations for the use of ECGs to screen for cardiovascular disease in healthy people. In the ACC/AHA guidelines, ECGs are considered appropriate screening tests in patients without apparent or suspected heart disease who are 40 years of age or older (see Table 13G-3). Earlier guidelines from the AHA recommended that ECGs be obtained at ages 20, 40, and 60 years. In contrast, the U.S. Preventive Services Task Force (USPSTF) and the task force assembled by the Canadian government did not find evidence to support the use of screening ECG.

The ACC/AHA guidelines also recommend ECGs for patients for whom drugs with a high incidence of cardiovascular effects (e.g., chemotherapy) or for whom exercise testing is planned, and for people of any age in occupations with high cardiovascular demands or whose cardiovascular status might affect the safety of other people (e.g., airline pilots).

In populations without known disease or significant risk factors, it has become common practice to include an ECG as part of routine health examinations and on any admission to a hospital. These ECGs are assumed

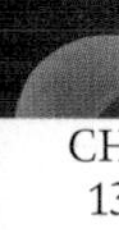

CH 13

TABLE 13G-1 ACC/AHA Guidelines for Electrocardiography in Patients with Known Cardiovascular Disease or Dysfunction

INDICATION	CLASS I (INDICATED)	CLASS II (EQUIVOCAL)	CLASS III (NOT INDICATED)
Baseline or initial evaluation	All patients	None	None
Response to therapy	Patients in whom prescribed therapy is known to produce changes in the ECG that correlate with therapeutic responses or progression of disease Patients in whom prescribed therapy may produce adverse effects that may be predicted from or detected by changes in the ECG	None	Patients receiving pharmacologic or nonpharmacologic therapy not known to produce changes in the ECG or to affect conditions that may be associated with such changes
Follow-up	Patients with a change in symptoms, signs, or relevant laboratory findings Patients with an implanted pacemaker or antitachycardia device Patients with symptoms such as the following, even in the absence of new symptoms or signs, after an interval of time appropriate for the condition or disease: syncope and near-syncope, unexplained change in the usual pattern of angina pectoris, and who have no new chest pain or worsening dyspnea Extreme and unexplained fatigue, weakness and prostration; palpitations, new signs of congestive heart failure; new organic murmur or pericardial friction rub; new findings suggesting pulmonary hypertension; accelerating or poorly controlled systemic arterial hypertension; evidence of a recent cerebrovascular accident; unexplained fever in patients with known valvular disease; new onset of cardiac arrhythmia or inappropriate heart rate; chronic known congenital or acquired cardiovascular disease	None	Adult patients whose cardiovascular condition is usually benign and unlikely to progress (e.g., patients with asymptomatic mild mitral valve prolapse, mild hypertension, or premature contractions in absence of organic heart disease) Adult patients with chronic stable heart disease seen at frequent intervals (e.g., 4 months) and unexplained findings
Before surgery	All patients with known cardiovascular disease or dysfunction, except as noted under Class II	Patients with hemodynamically insignificant congenital or acquired heart disease, mild systemic hypertension, or infrequent premature complexes in absence of organic heart disease	None

TABLE 13G-2 ACC/AHA Guidelines for Electrocardiography in Patients Suspected of Having or at Increased Risk for Cardiovascular Disease or Dysfunction

SETTING	CLASS I (APPROPRIATE)	CLASS II (EQUIVOCAL)	CLASS III (INAPPROPRIATE)
Baseline or initial evaluation	All patients suspected of having or being at increased risk for cardiovascular disease Patients who may have used cocaine, amphetamines, or other illicit drugs known to have cardiac effects Patients who may have received an overdose of a drug known to have cardiac effects	None	None
Response to therapy	To assess therapy with cardioactive drugs in patients with suspected cardiac disease To assess response to administration of any agent known to result in cardiac abnormalities or abnormalities on the ECG (e.g., antineoplastic drugs, lithium, antidepressant agents)	To assess response to administration of any agent known to alter serum electrolyte concentration	To assess response to administration of agents known not to influence cardiac structure or function
Follow-up once	Presence of any change in clinical status or laboratory findings suggesting interval development of cardiac disease or dysfunction Periodic follow-up of patients (e.g., every 1 to 5 yr) known to be at increased risk for cardiac disease Follow-up of patients after resolution of chest pain	None	Follow-up ECGs more often than yearly not indicated for patients who remain clinically stable, not at increased risk for development of cardiac disease, and not demonstrated to have cardiac disease with previous studies
Before surgery	As part of preoperative evaluation of any patient with suspected, or at increased risk of developing, cardiac disease or dysfunction	None	None

to be of value in detecting unknown abnormalities, serving as a baseline against which to compare later tracings, and assessing the future risk of cardiovascular events.

There is little evidence to support these practices, and the recommendations for routine clinical screening by numerous organizations, including the USPSTF,[2] do not include an ECG. It is clear, as described in earlier sections of this chapter, that many commonly encountered electrocardiographic abnormalities in clinically normal people raise the risk of various forms of cardiac morbidity and mortality. Although the proportion of persons subjected to routine screening ECGs who have these abnormalities may be substantial, the overall sensitivity and specificity of the ECG for identifying individual patients who will have future events and the number of therapeutic or diagnostic changes provoked by routine electrocardiographic findings are too low to warrant universal screening.

TABLE 13G-3 **ACC/AHA Guidelines for Electrocardiography in Patients with No Apparent or Suspected Heart Disease or Dysfunction**

SETTING	CLASS I (APPROPRIATE)	CLASS II (EQUIVOCAL)	CLASS III (INAPPROPRIATE)
Baseline or initial evaluation	Persons aged 40 yr or older undergoing physical examination Before administration of pharmacologic agents known to have high incidence of cardiovascular effects (e.g., antineoplastic agents) Before exercise stress testing People of any age in special occupations that require very high cardiovascular performance (e.g., fire fighters, police officers) or whose cardiovascular performance is linked to public safety (e.g., pilots, air traffic controllers, critical process operators, bus or truck drivers, railroad engineers)	To evaluate competitive athletes	Routine screening or baseline ECG in asymptomatic persons <40 yr with no risk factors
Response to therapy	To evaluate patients in whom prescribed therapy (e.g., doxorubicin) is known to produce cardiovascular effects	None	To assess treatment known not to produce any cardiovascular effects
Follow-up	To evaluate asymptomatic persons >40 yr of age	None	To evaluate asymptomatic adults who have had no interval change in symptoms, signs, or risk factors and who have had a normal ECG within recent past
Before surgery	Patients >40 yr of age Patients being evaluated as donor for heart transplantation or as recipient of noncardiopulmonary transplant	Patients 30-40 yr of age	Patients <30 yr with no risk factors for coronary artery disease

The consequences of high rates of false-positive results, including unnecessary diagnostic testing, overtreatment, and labeling, especially in populations with a low prevalence of disease, may outweigh the benefits of screening

SPECIAL POPULATIONS

Persons with Dangerous Occupations

Recommendations for screening of persons with dangerous jobs or jobs that place others at risk—for example, airline pilots and bus drivers—are also controversial. Although no specific data defining the value of routine screening are available, some groups, including the USPSTF, recognize the potential for benefit in relation to the possible risk to others.[2]

Preoperative Evaluation

The routine recording of the ECG before noncardiac surgery in patients without other indications, although a common practice, has also been challenged. Routine electrocardiographic recording may be recommended for patients with one or more risk factors undergoing vascular surgery and for patients with known peripheral or cerebrovascular disease undergoing intermediate-risk procedures. It may be reasonable in patients without risk factors undergoing vascular procedures or with risk factors who are undergoing intermediate-risk procedures.[3]

However, routine preoperative or postoperative ECGs are not recommended for asymptomatic persons undergoing low-risk procedures.[3,4] Although electrocardiographic abnormalities are common in these patients, the findings do not have predictive value for postoperative cardiac events beyond that established by routine clinical examinations. In these cases, use of the ECG may be based on clinical judgment rather than on rigid protocol requirements.

Screening of Athletes

The routine screening of competitive athletes by electrocardiography remains unsettled.[5,6] Proposals to include the ECG are based on its high sensitivity in detecting the most common underlying causes of athlete deaths such as hypertrophic cardiomyopathy and the long-QT interval syndromes. It is thus proposed that prospective identification of these abnormalities can reduce the occurrence of sudden death by facilitating the disqualification of high-risk affected persons.

Evidence of the success of this approach has been reported, and both the European Society of Cardiology and the International Olympic Committee recommend including the ECG as part of pre-participation medical review.[5] In contrast, the AHA does not recommend routine electrocardiographic screening,[6] largely because of the cost, the lack of an organized system to achieve the goal, and the risks of false-positive recordings. Rather, they recommend a more complete examination if suggestive abnormalities are found in the personal and family history or on physical examination.

Cardioactive Drug Administration

The role of the ECG as a baseline and in the follow-up of patients taking drugs with potential cardioactive effects, especially QT(U) interval prolongation, remains poorly defined and, in some cases, controversial. One example is the suggestion by an expert panel on electrocardiographic screening in methadone treatment to "obtain a pretreatment electrocardiogram for all patients to measure the QTc interval and a follow-up electrocardiogram within 30 days and annually. Additional electrocardiography is recommended if the methadone dosage exceeds 100 mg/day or if patients have unexplained syncope or seizures."[7] This proposal, which has provoked considerable debate and discussion, has not been formally endorsed by national cardiology societies.

REFERENCES

1. Schlant RC, Adolph RJ, DiMarco JP, et al: Guidelines for electrocardiography. A report of the ACC/AHA Task Force on Assessment of Diagnostic and Therapeutic Cardiovascular Procedures (Committee on Electrocardiography). J Am Coll Cardiol 19:473, 1992.
2. Agency for Health Care Research and Quality: Guide to Clinical Preventive Services, 2008 (http://www.ahrq.gov).
3. Goldberger AL, O'Konski M: Utility of the routine electrocardiogram before surgery and on general hospital admission. Critical review and new guidelines. Ann Intern Med 105:552, 1986.
4. Fleisher LA, Beckman JA, Brown KA, et al: ACC/AHA 2007 Guidelines on Perioperative Cardiovascular Evaluation and Care for Noncardiac Surgery. J Am Coll Cardiol 50:1707, 2007.
5. Corrado D, Pelliccia A, Bjornstad HH, et al: Cardiovascular pre-participation screening of young competitive athletes for prevention of sudden death. Eur Heart J 26:516, 2005.
6. Maron BJ, Thompson PD, Ackerman MJ, et al: Recommendations and considerations related to preparticipation screening for cardiovascular abnormalities in competitive athletes. Circulation 115:1643, 2007.
7. Krantz MJ, Martin J, Stimmel B, et al: QTc interval screening in methadone treatment. Ann Intern Med 150:387, 2009.

CHAPTER 14 Exercise Stress Testing

Bernard R. Chaitman

Exercise is a common physiologic stress used to elicit cardiovascular abnormalities not present at rest and to determine the adequacy of cardiac function.[1-14] Exercise electrocardiography is one of the most frequent noninvasive modalities used to assess patients with suspected or proven cardiovascular disease. The test is mainly used to estimate prognosis and determine functional capacity, the likelihood and extent of coronary artery disease (CAD), and the effects of therapy. Hemodynamic and electrocardiographic measurements, combined with ancillary techniques such as metabolic gas analysis or cardiac imaging (see Chaps. 15 and 17) enhance the information content of exercise testing in selected patients.

Exercise Physiology

Anticipation of dynamic exercise results in an acceleration of ventricular rate caused by vagal withdrawal, increase in alveolar ventilation, and increased venous return, primarily as a result of sympathetic venoconstriction.[12] In normal persons, the net effect is to increase resting cardiac output before the start of exercise. The magnitude of hemodynamic response during exercise depends on the severity of the exercise and the amount of muscle mass involved. In the early phases of exercise in the upright position, cardiac output is increased by an augmentation in stroke volume mediated through the use of the Frank-Starling mechanism and heart rate; the increase in cardiac output in the later phases of exercise is primarily caused by a sympathetic-mediated increase in ventricular rate. At fixed submaximal workloads below anaerobic threshold, steady-state conditions are usually reached after the second minute of exercise, following which heart rate, cardiac output, blood pressure, and pulmonary ventilation are maintained at reasonably constant levels. During strenuous exertion, sympathetic discharge is maximal and parasympathetic stimulation is withdrawn, resulting in vasoconstriction of most circulatory body systems, except for that in exercising muscle and in the cerebral and coronary circulations. Venous and arterial norepinephrine release from sympathetic postganglionic nerve endings, as well as plasma renin levels, are increased; the catecholamine release enhances ventricular contractility. As exercise progresses, skeletal muscle blood flow is increased, oxygen extraction increases by as much as threefold, total calculated peripheral resistance decreases, and systolic blood pressure, mean arterial pressure, and pulse pressure usually increase. Diastolic blood pressure does not change significantly. The pulmonary vascular bed can accommodate as much as a sixfold increase in cardiac output with only modest increases in pulmonary artery pressure, pulmonary capillary wedge pressure, and right atrial pressure; in normal individuals, this is not a limiting determinant of peak exercise capacity.

Cardiac output increases by four- to sixfold above basal levels during strenuous exertion in the upright position, depending on genetic endowment and level of training.[12,13] The maximum heart rate and cardiac output are decreased in older persons, partly because of decreased beta-adrenergic responsivity.[15,16] Maximum heart rate (HR) can be estimated from the following formula:

$$HR = 220 - \text{age (in years)}$$

with a standard deviation of 10 to 12 beats/min. This formula tends to overestimate maximum heart rate in a female population. The formula HR = 206 − 0.88 (age in years) provides a more accurate estimate of maximum heart rate in women.[16a] The age-predicted maximum heart rate is a useful measurement for safety reasons. However, the wide standard deviation in the various regression equations used and the impact of drug therapy limit the usefulness of this parameter in estimating the exact age-predicted maximum for an individual patient.[8]

In the postexercise phase, hemodynamics return to baseline within minutes of termination of exercise. Vagal reactivation is an important cardiac deceleration mechanism after exercise and is accelerated in well-trained athletes but blunted in patients with chronic heart failure (see later, "Nonelectrocardiographic Observations"). Intense physical work or significant cardiorespiratory impairment may interfere with achievement of a steady state, and an oxygen deficit occurs during exercise. The total oxygen uptake in excess of the resting oxygen uptake during the recovery period is the oxygen debt.[4,5]

Patient's Position

At rest, the cardiac output and stroke volume are higher when the person is in a supine position than when in an upright position. With exercise, in normal supine persons, the elevation of cardiac output results almost entirely from an increase in heart rate, with little augmentation of stroke volume. In the upright posture, the increase in cardiac output in normal individuals results from a combination of elevations in stroke volume and heart rate. A change from supine to upright posture causes a decrease in venous return, left ventricular end-diastolic volume and pressure, stroke volume, and cardiac index. Renin and norepinephrine levels are increased. End-systolic volume and ejection fraction are not significantly changed. In normal individuals, end-systolic volume decreases and ejection fraction increases to a similar extent from rest to exercise in the supine and upright positions. The magnitude and direction of change in end-diastolic volume from rest to maximum exercise in both positions are small and may vary according to the patient population studied. The net effect on exercise performance is an approximate 10% increase in exercise time, cardiac index, heart rate, and rate pressure product at peak exercise in the upright as compared with the supine position.

Cardiopulmonary Exercise Testing

Cardiopulmonary exercise testing involves measurements of respiratory oxygen uptake ($\dot{V}O_2$), carbon dioxide production ($\dot{V}CO_2$), and ventilatory parameters during a symptom-limited exercise test. The patient usually wears a nose clip and breathes through a nonrebreathing valve that separates expired air from room air. During testing, it is important that there be no air leaks in the system. Important measurements of expired

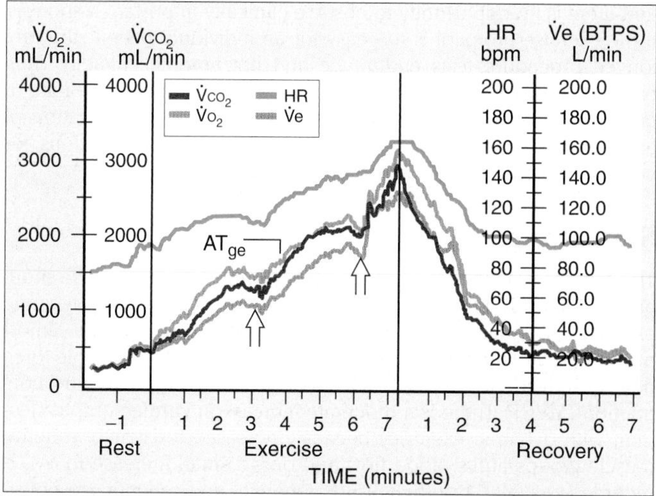

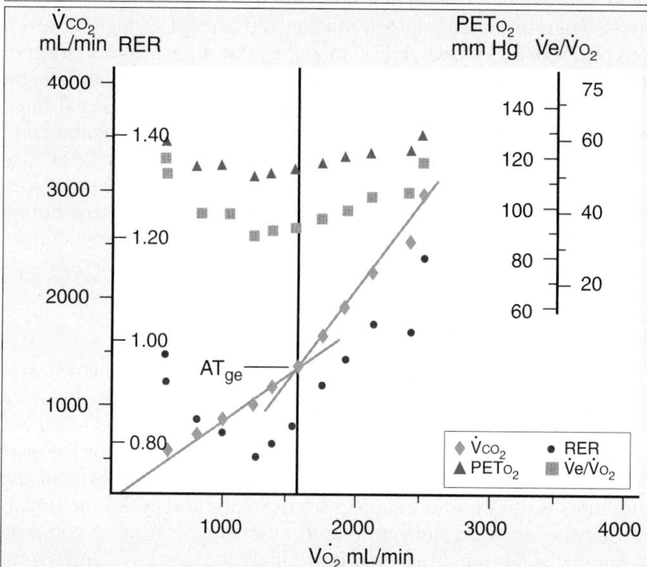

FIGURE 14-1 Cardiopulmonary exercise test in a healthy 53-year-old man using the Bruce protocol. The progressive linear increase in work output, HR, and oxygen consumption ($\dot{V}O_2$) is noted, with steady-state conditions reached after 2 minutes in each of the first two stages **(top)**. Open arrows indicate the beginning of each new 3-minute stage. The subject completed 7 minutes and 10 seconds of exercise, and peak $\dot{V}O_2$ was 3.08 liters/min. The anaerobic threshold (AT$_{ge}$), determined by the V slope method, is the point at which the slope of the relative rate of increase in $\dot{V}CO_2$ relative to $\dot{V}O_2$ changes; it occurred at a $\dot{V}O_2$ of 1.5 liters/min, or 49% of peak $\dot{V}O_2$, within predicted values for a normal sedentary population **(bottom)**. The AT$_{ge}$ determined by the point at which the $\dot{V}O_2$ and $\dot{V}CO_2$ slopes intersect (1.8 liters/min; **top**) is slightly greater than the AT$_{ge}$ determined by the V slope method **(bottom)**. The V slope method usually provides a more reproducible estimate of AT$_{ge}$. bpm = beats/min; PETO_2 = end-tidal pressure of oxygen; RER = respiratory exchange ratio; $\dot{V}e/\dot{V}O_2$ = ratio of ventilation to oxygen uptake.

gas are PO_2, PCO_2, and air flow. Ventilatory measurements include respiratory rate, tidal volume, and minute ventilation ($\dot{V}e$). PO_2 and PCO_2 are sampled breath by breath or by the use of a mixing chamber. The $\dot{V}O_2$ and $\dot{V}CO_2$ can be computed from ventilatory volumes and differences between inspired and expired gases.[4,5] Under steady-state conditions, $\dot{V}O_2$ and $\dot{V}CO_2$ measured at the mouth are equivalent to total-body oxygen consumption and carbon dioxide production. The relationship among work output, oxygen consumption, heart rate, and cardiac output during exercise is linear (**Fig. 14-1**). The slope of the $\dot{V}O_2$–work relationship is a measure of the biochemical efficiency of exercise.

The maximum oxygen consumption represents the largest amount of oxygen a person can use while performing dynamic exercise involving a large part of total muscle mass. It is determined by the equation:

TABLE 14-1 Cardiopulmonary Exercise Test Parameters Used to Differentiate Cardiac and Pulmonary Causes of Exertional Dyspnea

PARAMETER	CARDIAC	PULMONARY
Peak $\dot{V}O_2$	Reduced	Reduced
V_T	May be reduced	May be reduced
$\dot{V}$emax	≤80% of MVV	>80% of MVV*
SpO_2	>90% throughout exercise	May drop to <90%*
CO	May be reduced	Normal
Preexercise PFT	Normal	May have obstructive or restrictive pattern*
FEV_1 postexercise	No change from preexercise	≥15% decrease from preexercise†
PEF postexercise	No change from preexercise	≥15% decrease from preexercise†

*These responses should not be considered the gold standard for defining a pulmonary limitation to exercise. Rather, a $\dot{V}$emax > 80% of MVV, a drop in Spo2, and/or abnormal resting PFT values indicate a pulmonary limitation that must be supported by additional testing (e.g., rule out cardiac shunts, coexisting cardiac and pulmonary disease).
†Compatible with exercise-induced bronchospasm.
MVV = maximal voluntary ventilation; PEF = peak expiratory flow; PFT = pulmonary function test.
From Arena R, Myers J, Williams MA, et al: Assessment of functional capacity in clinical and research settings. A Scientific Statement from the American Heart Association Committee on Exercise, Rehabilitation, and Prevention of the Council on Clinical Cardiology and the Council on Cardiovascular Nursing. Circulation 116:329, 2007.

$$\dot{V}O_2\text{max} = \text{cardiac output (heart rate} \times \text{stroke volume)} \times \text{maximal arteriovenous oxygen difference}$$

This represents the largest amount of oxygen a person can use while performing dynamic exercise involving a large part of total muscle mass. The $\dot{V}O_2$max decreases with age, typically by an average of 10%/decade in nonathletic subjects with an increased rate of decline in older subjects, is usually lower in women than in men, and can vary among individuals as a result of genetic factors.[4,5,10,13,14] $\dot{V}O_2$max is diminished by the degree of cardiovascular impairment and by physical inactivity. In untrained persons, the arterial-mixed venous oxygen difference at peak exercise is relatively constant (14 to 17 vol-%), and $\dot{V}O_2$max is an approximation of maximum cardiac output. Measured $\dot{V}O_2$max can be compared with predicted values from empirically derived formulas based on age, gender, weight, and height.[3] Most clinical studies that use exercise as a stress to assess cardiac reserve report the peak $\dot{V}O_2$ (the highest $\dot{V}O_2$ attained during graded exercise testing) rather than $\dot{V}O_2$max. Peak exercise capacity is decreased when the ratio of measured to predicted $\dot{V}O_2$max is less than 85% to 90%. Estimating peak $\dot{V}O_2$ from work rate or treadmill time in individual patients may lead to misinterpretation of data if exercise equipment is not correctly calibrated, if the patient holds on to the front handrails, or if the patient fails to achieve steady state, is obese, or has peripheral vascular disease, pulmonary vascular disease, or cardiac impairment. In some patients with cardiovascular or pulmonary disease, $\dot{V}O_2$ does not increase linearly as work rate is increased, and may be overestimated. The measurements obtained with cardiopulmonary exercise testing are useful for understanding an individual patient's response to exercise and can be useful in the diagnostic evaluation of a patient with unexplained dyspnea or exercise impairment, or in quantifying the degree of disability (**Table 14-1**).[6,8]

Oximetry, performed noninvasively, can be used to monitor arterial oxygen saturation, provided that a good signal pulse is obtained; the value normally does not decrease by more than 5% during exercise. In general, pulse oximeters are useful in monitoring trending phenomena, but may not be reliable in determining absolute magnitude of change. A significant desaturation should be confirmed with arterial blood gases.

ANAEROBIC THRESHOLD. Anaerobic threshold is a theoretical point during dynamic exercise when muscle tissue switches over to anaerobic metabolism as an additional energy source. All tissues do not shift simultaneously, and there is a brief interval during which exercise muscle tissue shifts from predominantly aerobic to anaerobic metabolism.[4,5] Lactic acid begins to accumulate when a healthy untrained subject reaches about 50% to 60% of the maximal capacity for aerobic metabolism. The increase in lactic acid becomes greater as exercise becomes more intense, resulting in metabolic acidosis. As lactate is formed, it is buffered in the serum by the bicarbonate system, resulting in increased carbon dioxide excretion, which causes reflex hyperventilation. The gas exchange anaerobic threshold is the point at which $\dot{V}e$ increases disproportionately relative to $\dot{V}O_2$ and work; it usually occurs at 40% to 60% of $\dot{V}O_2$ max in normal untrained individuals, with a wide range of normal values between 35% and 80%. Below the anaerobic threshold, carbon dioxide production is proportional to oxygen consumption. Above the anaerobic threshold, carbon dioxide is produced in excess of oxygen consumption. The anaerobic threshold determination is influenced by age, modality (e.g., arm versus leg, ergometer versus treadmill), and exercise protocol. There are several methods to determine anaerobic threshold, including the following: (1) the V slope method, the point at which the rate of increase in $\dot{V}CO_2$ relative to $\dot{V}O_2$ increases (see Fig. 14-1); (2) the point at which the $\dot{V}O_2$ and $\dot{V}CO_2$ slopes intersect; and (3) the point at which there is a systemic increase in $\dot{V}e/\dot{V}O_2$ without a concomitant increase in $\dot{V}e/\dot{V}CO_2$ (see Fig. 14-1). The anaerobic threshold is a useful parameter because work below this level encompasses most activities of daily living. Values below 40% of predicted $\dot{V}O_2$ may indicate significant cardiovascular disease, pulmonary disease, limited oxygen delivery to the tissues, or mitochondrial abnormalities. An increase in anaerobic threshold with training can enhance an individual's capacity to perform sustained submaximal activities, with consequent improvement in quality of life and daily living. Changes in anaerobic threshold and peak $\dot{V}O_2$ with repeat testing can be used to assess disease progression, response to medical therapy, and improvement in cardiovascular fitness with training.

Ventilatory Parameters. In addition to peak $\dot{V}O_2$, minute ventilation and its relation to $\dot{V}CO_2$ and oxygen consumption are useful indices of cardiac and pulmonary function.[4,5] Exercise-induced changes in tidal minute $\dot{V}e$ and breathing pattern (tidal volume, VT, and inspiratory frequency) are measured, along with assessment of ventilatory reserve. The ventilatory reserve determination corresponds to how closely the peak minute ventilation achieved (ventilatory demand) during exercise, $\dot{V}e$max, approaches maximum ventilatory capacity. Oxygen pulse, defined as the amount of oxygen consumed per heartbeat, may decrease during exercise in patients with exercise-induced myocardial ischemia but usually remains normal in patients with pulmonary disease. Responses such as the VT, $\dot{V}e/\dot{V}CO_2$ slope, $\dot{V}e/\dot{V}CO_2$ at peak exercise, oscillatory ventilation, oxygen uptake on kinetics, rate of recovery of $\dot{V}O_2$, and oxygen uptake efficiency slope are being used with greater frequency to classify functional limitations and risk-stratify cardiac patients.

The respiratory exchange ratio represents the amount of carbon dioxide produced divided by the amount of oxygen consumed. The respiratory exchange ratio ranges from 0.7 to 0.85 at rest and is partly dependent on the predominant fuel used for cellular metabolism (e.g., the respiratory exchange ratio for predominant carbohydrate use is 1.0, whereas the respiratory exchange ratio for predominant fatty acid use is 0.7). At high exercise levels, carbon dioxide production exceeds $\dot{V}O_2$, and a respiratory exchange ratio greater than 1.1 often indicates that the subject has performed at maximal effort.

Metabolic Equivalent. In current use, the term *metabolic equivalent* (MET) refers to a unit of oxygen uptake in a sitting, resting person; 1 MET is equivalent to 3.5 mL O_2/kg/min of body weight. Measured $\dot{V}O_2$ in mL O_2/kg/min divided by 3.5 mL O_2/kg/min determines the number of METs associated with activity. Work activities can be calculated in multiples of METs; this measurement is useful to determine exercise prescriptions, assess disability, and standardize the reporting of submaximal and peak exercise workloads when different protocols are used. An exercise workload of 3 to 5 METs is consistent with activities such as raking leaves, light carpentry, golf, and walking at 3 to 4 mph. Workloads of 5 to 7 METs are consistent with exterior carpentry, singles tennis, and light backpacking. Workloads in excess of 9 METs are compatible with heavy labor, handball, squash, and running at 6 to 7 mph.

Exercise Protocols

The main types of exercise are isotonic or dynamic exercise, isometric or static exercise, and resistive (combined isometric and isotonic) exercise. Dynamic protocols are most frequently used to assess cardiovascular reserve, and those suitable for clinical testing should include a low-intensity warm-up phase. In general, approximately 8 to 12 minutes of continuous progressive exercise, during which the myocardial oxygen demand is elevated to the patient's maximal level, is optimal for diagnostic and prognostic purposes.[8] The protocol should include a suitable recovery or cool-down period. If the protocol is too strenuous for an individual patient, the test must be terminated early, and there is no opportunity to observe clinically important responses. If the exercise protocol is too easy for an individual patient, the prolonged procedure tests endurance and not aerobic capacity. Thus, exercise protocols should be individualized to accommodate a patient's limitations. Protocols may be set up at a fixed duration of exercise for a certain intensity to meet minimal qualifications for certain industrial tasks or sports programs.

Static Exercise

This form of isometric exercise generates force with little muscle shortening and produces a greater blood pressure response than dynamic exercise.[11] The increase in heart rate and blood pressure are almost proportional to the force exerted relative to the greatest possible force that an individual can evoke (percentage maximum voluntary contraction [MVC]). There is a moderate increase in cardiac output (less than with dynamic exercise) because increased resistance in active muscle groups limits blood flow, and only a small increase in $\dot{V}O_2$ is recorded, usually insufficient to generate an ischemic response. Stroke volume remains largely unchanged, except at high levels of tension (>50% MVC), wherein it may decrease. In a common form of static exercise, the patient's maximal force on a hand dynamometer is recorded. The patient then sustains 20% to 30% of maximal force for 3 to 5 minutes while the electrocardiogram (ECG) is obtained and blood pressure recorded. When heavy dynamic resistance exercise such as lifting weights is performed (resistive exercise), the cardiovascular response is a combination of the responses that occur during both dynamic aerobic exercise and isometric exercise, reflecting a combined volume and pressure load.

Dynamic Exercise

ARM ERGOMETRY. Arm crank ergometry protocols involve arm cranking at incremental workloads of 10 to 20 watts (W) for 2- or 3-minute stages. The heart rate and blood pressure responses to a given workload of arm exercise usually are greater than those for leg exercise. A bicycle ergometer with the axle placed at the level of the shoulders is used, and the subject sits or stands and cycles the pedals so that the arms are fully extended alternately. The most common frequency is 50 rpm. In normal individuals, maximal $\dot{V}O_2$ and $\dot{V}e$ for arm cycling approximate 50% to 70% of the same measures as leg cycling. Peak $\dot{V}O_2$ and peak heart rate are approximately 70% of the measures during leg testing.

BICYCLE ERGOMETRY. Bicycle protocols involve incremental workloads calibrated in W or kilopond-meters per minute (kpm)[17]; 1 W is equivalent to approximately 6 kpm. Because exercise on a cycle ergometer is not weight bearing, kilopond-meters per minute or watts can be converted to oxygen uptake in milliliters per minute. In mechanically braked bicycles, work is determined by force and distance and requires a constant pedaling rate of 60 to 80 rpm, according to the patient's preference. Electronically braked bicycles provide a constant workload despite changes in pedaling rate and are less dependent on a patient's cooperation. They are more costly than a mechanically braked bicycle but are preferred for diagnostic and prognostic assessment. Most protocols start with a power output of 10 or 25 W/min (150 kpm), usually followed by increases of 25 W every 2 or 3 minutes until endpoints are reached. Younger subjects can start at 50 W, with increases in 50-W increments every 2 minutes. A ramp protocol differs from the staged protocols in that the patient starts at 3 minutes of unloaded pedaling at a cycle speed of 60 rpm. Work rate is increased by a uniform amount each minute, ranging from 5- to 30-W increments, depending on a patient's expected performance. Exercise is terminated if the patient is unable to maintain a cycling frequency above 40 rpm. In the cardiac catheterization laboratory, hemodynamic measurements can be made during supine bicycle ergometry at rest and at one or two submaximal workloads. The bicycle ergometer is associated with a lower maximal $\dot{V}O_2$ and anaerobic threshold than the treadmill; maximal heart rate, maximal $\dot{V}e$, and maximal lactate values are often similar. The relationship between peak $\dot{V}O_2$ on cycle

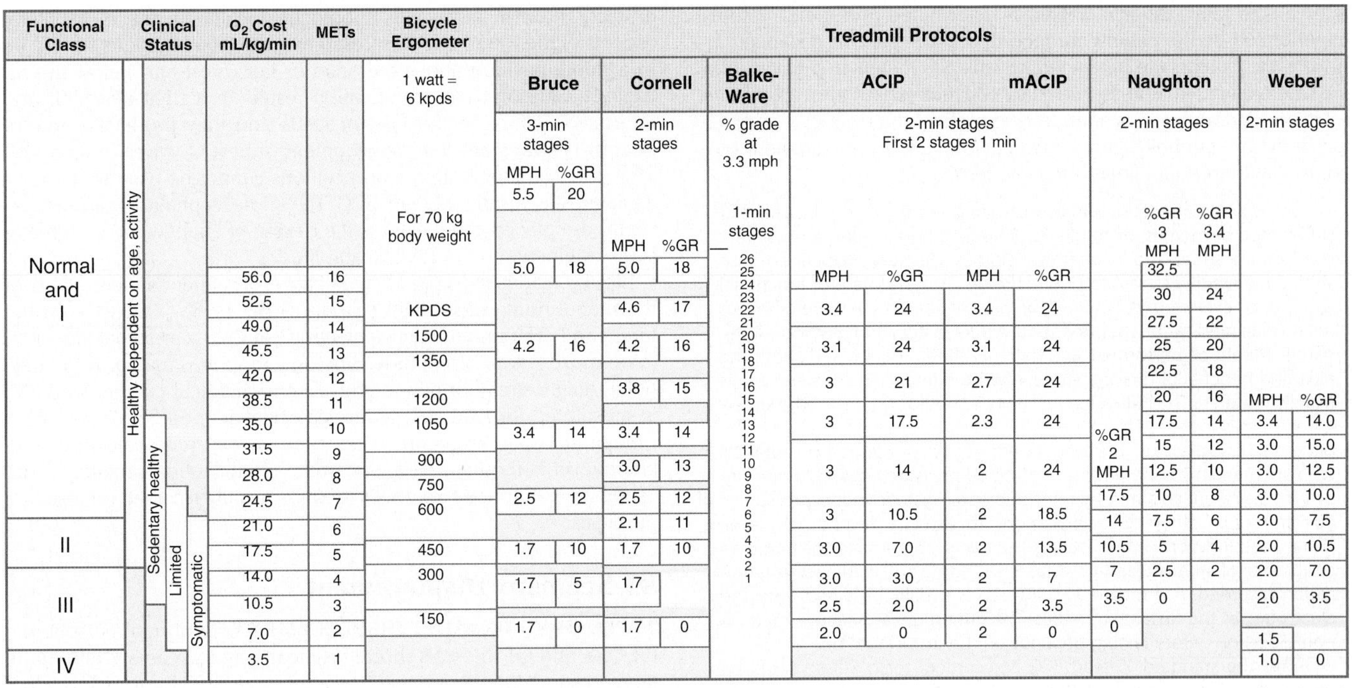

Functional Class	Clinical Status	O_2 Cost mL/kg/min	METs	Bicycle Ergometer	Treadmill Protocols: Bruce		Cornell		Balke-Ware	ACIP		mACIP		Naughton			Weber	
				1 watt = 6 kpds; For 70 kg body weight	3-min stages		2-min stages		% grade at 3.3 mph; 1-min stages	2-min stages; First 2 stages 1 min				2-min stages			2-min stages	
				KPDS	MPH	%GR	MPH	%GR		MPH	%GR	MPH	%GR	%GR 2 MPH	%GR 3 MPH	%GR 3.4 MPH	MPH	%GR
					5.5	20												
Normal and I	Healthy dependent on age, activity	56.0	16		5.0	18	5.0	18	26 25 24						32.5			
		52.5	15				4.6	17	23 22	3.4	24	3.4	24		30	24		
		49.0	14	1500					21 20						27.5	22		
		45.5	13	1350	4.2	16	4.2	16	19 18	3.1	24	3.1	24		25	20		
		42.0	12				3.8	15	17 16	3	21	2.7	24		22.5	18		
		38.5	11	1200					15 14						20	16		
	Sedentary healthy	35.0	10	1050	3.4	14	3.4	14	13 12	3	17.5	2.3	24		17.5	14	3.4	14.0
		31.5	9	900			3.0	13	11 10						15	12	3.0	15.0
		28.0	8	750					9 8	3	14	2	24		12.5	10	3.0	12.5
	Limited	24.5	7	600	2.5	12	2.5	12	7 6	3	10.5	2	18.5	17.5	10	8	3.0	10.0
II	Symptomatic	21.0	6				2.1	11	5 4					14	7.5	6	3.0	7.5
		17.5	5	450	1.7	10	1.7	10	3 2	3.0	7.0	2	13.5	10.5	5	4	2.0	10.5
III		14.0	4	300	1.7	5	1.7		1	3.0	3.0	2	7	7	2.5	2	2.0	7.0
		10.5	3							2.5	2.0	2	3.5	3.5	0		2.0	3.5
		7.0	2	150	1.7	0	1.7	0		2.0	0	2	0	0			1.5	
IV		3.5	1														1.0	0

FIGURE 14-2 Estimated oxygen cost of bicycle ergometer and selected treadmill protocols. The standard Bruce protocol starts at 1.7 mph and 10% grade (5 METs), with a larger increment between stages than protocols such as the Naughton, ACIP, and Weber, which start at less than 2 METs at 2 mph and increase by 1- to 1.5-MET increments between stages. The Bruce protocol can be modified by two 3-minute warm-up stages at 1.7 mph and 0% grade and 1.7 mph and 5% grade. mACIP = modified ACIP. *(Modified from Fletcher GF, Balady G, Amsterdam EA, et al: Exercise Standards for Testing and Training. A statement for health care professionals from the American Heart Association. Circulation 104:1694, 2001.)*

ergometry and treadmill is consistent, even though peak $\dot{V}O_2$ is generally less with cycle ergometry. One formula to harmonize the discrepancy in peak $\dot{V}O_2$ is as follows:

$$\text{Treadmill METs} = 0.98\,(\text{cycle ergometry METs}) + 1.85$$

Multiplication of the value obtained from this equation by 3.5 produces a treadmill peak $\dot{V}O_2$ value in mL O_2/kg/min.[10]

TREADMILL PROTOCOL. The treadmill protocol should be consistent with the patient's physical capacity and the purpose of the test. In healthy individuals, the standard Bruce protocol is popular, and a large diagnostic and prognostic data base has been published using this protocol.[1,2,7,8] The Bruce multistage maximal treadmill protocol has 3-minute periods to allow achievement of a steady state before workload is increased (**Fig. 14-2**; see Fig. 14-1). In older individuals or those whose exercise capacity is limited by cardiac disease, the protocol can be modified by two 3-minute warm-up stages at 1.7 mph and 0% grade and 1.7 mph and 5% grade. A limitation of the Bruce protocol is the relatively large increase in $\dot{V}O_2$ between stages and the additional energy cost of running as compared with walking at stages in excess of Bruce's stage III. The Naughton and Weber protocols use 1- to 2-minute stages with 1-MET increments between stages; these protocols may be more suitable for patients with limited exercise tolerance, such as patients with compensated congestive heart failure. The Asymptomatic Cardiac Ischemia Pilot (ACIP) trial and modified ACIP (mACIP) protocols use 2-minute stages, with 1.5-MET increments between stages after two 1-minute warm-up stages with 1-MET increments. The ACIP protocols were developed to test patients with established CAD and result in a linear increase in heart rate and $\dot{V}O_2$, distributing the time to occurrence of ST-segment depression over a wider range of heart rate and exercise time than protocols with more abrupt increments in workload between stages. The mACIP protocol produces a similar aerobic demand as the standard ACIP protocol for each minute of exercise and is well suited for short or older individuals who cannot keep up with a walking speed of 3 mph (see Fig. 14-2).

Ramp protocols start the patient at a relatively slow treadmill speed, which is gradually increased until the patient has a good stride. The ramp angle of incline is progressively increased at fixed intervals (e.g., 10 to 60 seconds), starting at zero grade, with the increase in grade calculated on the basis of the patient's estimated functional capacity so that the protocol will be complete at approximately 8 to 12 minutes.[8] If the test duration is too short (e.g., <6 minutes), ramp protocols using modest increases in workload may still demonstrate a nonlinear relationship between $\dot{V}O_2$ and work rate. In a ramp protocol, the rate of work increase is continuous and steady-state conditions are not reached. A limitation of ramp protocols is the need to estimate functional capacity from an activity scale; underestimation or overestimation of functional capacity occasionally results in an endurance test or premature cessation. One formula for estimating $\dot{V}O_2$ from treadmill speed and grade is as follows:

$$\dot{V}O_2\left(\text{mL } O_2 \times \text{kg}^{-1} \times \text{min}^{-1}\right) = (\text{mph} \times 2.68) \times [0.1 + (\text{grade} \times 1.8)] + 3.5$$

where grade is expressed as a fraction (e.g., 5% grade = 0.05). $\dot{V}O_2$ can be converted to METS by dividing by 3.5. The peak $\dot{V}O_2$ is usually the same regardless of treadmill protocol used; the difference is the rate of time at which the peak $\dot{V}O_2$ is achieved.

It is important to encourage patients not to grasp the handrails of the treadmill during exercise, particularly the front handrails. Functional capacity can be overestimated by as much as 20% in tests in which handrail support is permitted, and $\dot{V}O_2$ is decreased. Because the degree of handrail support is difficult to quantify from one test to another, more consistent results can be obtained during serial testing when handrail support is not permitted.

WALK TEST. A 6-minute walk test or a long-distance corridor walk test can be used to provide an estimate of functional capacity in patients who cannot perform bicycle or treadmill exercise, such as older patients or those with heart failure, claudication, or orthopedic limitations.[18] During a 6-minute walk test, patients are instructed to walk down a 100-foot corridor at their own pace, attempting to cover as much ground as possible in 6 minutes. At the end of the 6-minute interval, the total distance walked is determined and the symptoms experienced by the patient are recorded. During a long-distance corridor walk, patients are instructed to walk 400 meters in a hallway on a 20 meter/segment course for 10 laps (40 meters/lap) after a 2-minute warm-up. Performance of walk tests as a clinical measure of ambulatory function requires highly skilled personnel following a rigid protocol to elicit reproducible and reliable results.

Techniques. Patients should be instructed not to eat, drink alcohol or caffeinated beverages, or smoke for 3 hours before testing and to wear comfortable shoes and loose-fitting clothes. Unusual physical exertion should be avoided before testing. If the test is performed for functional capacity or exercise prescription, the patient should continue on his or her routine medications as prescribed. A brief history and physical examination should be performed, and patients should be advised about the risks and benefits of the procedure. A written informed consent form is usually required. The indication for the test should be known. The supervising physician should be made aware of any recent deterioration in the patient's clinical status. The test should not be performed on subjects who are markedly hypertensive (e.g., blood pressure > 220/120 mm Hg) or who have unexplained hypotension (e.g., systolic blood pressure < 80 mm Hg) or other contraindications to exercise testing (see later, "Safety and Risks of Exercise Testing"). In many laboratories, the presence or absence of atherosclerotic risk factors is noted and cardioactive medication recorded. A standard 12-lead ECG is usually obtained, with the electrodes at the distal extremities. The timing of cardioactive medication ingestion before testing depends on the test indication.

After the standard 12-lead ECG is recorded, torso ECGs should be obtained with the patient in the supine position and in the sitting or standing position. Postural changes can elicit labile ST-T wave abnormalities. Hyperventilation is not recommended before exercise. If a false-positive test result is suspected, hyperventilation should be performed after the test, and the hyperventilation tracing compared with the maximal ST-segment abnormalities observed. The ECG should be obtained and blood pressure recorded in both positions, and patients should be instructed on how to perform the test.

Adequate skin preparation is essential for high-quality recordings, and the superficial layer of skin needs to be removed to augment signal-to-noise ratio. The areas of electrode application are rubbed with an alcohol-saturated pad to remove oil and rubbed with free sandpaper or a rough material to reduce skin resistance to 5000 Ω or less. Silver chloride electrodes with a fluid column to avoid direct metal to skin contact produce high-quality tracings; these electrodes have the lowest offset voltage. The electrode fluid column can dry out over time and should be verified prior to application. This can be a cause of poor-quality tracings.

Cables connecting the electrodes and recorders should be light, flexible, and properly shielded. In a small minority of patients, a fishnet jersey may be required over the electrodes and cables to reduce motion artifact. The electrode-skin interface can be verified by tapping on the electrode and examining the monitor or by measuring skin impedance. Excessive noise indicates that the electrode needs to be replaced; replacement before the test rather than during exercise can save time. The electrocardiographic signal can be digitized systematically at the patient's end of the cable by some systems, reducing power line artifact. Cables, adapters, and the junction box have a finite life span and require periodic replacement to obtain the highest quality tracings. Exercise equipment should be calibrated regularly. Room temperature should be between 64° and 72°F (18° and 22°C) and humidity less than 60%.

Treadmill walking should be demonstrated to the patient. The heart rate, blood pressure, and ECG should be recorded at the end of each stage of exercise, immediately before and immediately after stopping exercise, at the onset of an ischemic response, and for each minute for at least 5 to 10 minutes in the recovery phase. A minimum of three leads should be displayed continuously on the monitor during the test. There is some controversy about optimal patient position in the recovery phase. In the sitting position, less space is required for a stretcher, and patients are more comfortable immediately after exertion. The supine position increases end-diastolic volume and has the potential to augment ST-segment changes.[8]

Electrocardiographic Measurements

Lead Systems

The Mason-Likar modification of the standard 12-lead ECG requires that the extremity electrodes be moved to the torso to reduce motion artifact. The arm electrodes should be located in the most lateral aspects of the infraclavicular fossae, and the leg electrodes should be in a stable position above the anterior iliac crest and below the rib cage. The Mason-Likar modification results in a right axis shift and increased voltage in the inferior leads and may produce a loss of inferior Q waves and the development of new Q waves in lead aVL. Thus, the body torso limb lead positions cannot be used to interpret a diagnostic resting 12-lead ECG. The more cephalad the leg electrodes are placed, the greater is the degree of change and the greater is the augmentation of R wave amplitude.

Bipolar lead groups place the negative, or reference, electrode over the manubrium (CM_5), right scapula (CB_5), or RV_5 (CC_5), or on the forehead (CH_5), and the active electrode at V_5 or a proximate location to optimize R wave amplitude. Bipolar lead groups may provide additional diagnostic information and, in some medical centers, lead CM_5 is substituted for lead aVR in the Mason-Likar–modified lead system. Bipolar leads are frequently used when only a limited electrocardiographic set is required (e.g., in cardiac rehabilitation programs). The use of more elaborate lead set systems is usually reserved for research purposes.

ST-Segment Displacement

TYPES OF ST-SEGMENT DISPLACEMENT. In normal persons, the PR, QRS, and QT intervals shorten as heart rate increases. P amplitude increases, and the PR segment becomes progressively more downsloping in the inferior leads. J point, or junctional, depression is a normal finding during exercise (**Fig. 14-3**). In patients with myocardial ischemia, however, the ST segment usually becomes more horizontal (flattens) as the severity of the ischemic response worsens. With progressive exercise, the depth of ST-segment depression may increase, involving more electrocardiographic leads, and the patient may develop angina. In the immediate postrecovery phase, the ST-segment displacement may persist, with downsloping ST segments and T wave inversion, gradually returning to baseline after 5 to 10 minutes (**Figs. 14-4 and 14-5**). Ischemic ST-segment displacement may be seen only during exercise, emphasizing the importance of adequate skin preparation and electrode placement to capture high-quality recordings during maximum exertion (**Fig. 14-6**). In about 10% of patients, the ischemic response may appear only in the recovery phase. This is a relevant finding, and the prevalence of reversible perfusion defects by single-photon emission computed tomography criteria (see Chap. 17) is comparable to those observed when the ischemic ST-segment response occurs during and after exercise. Patients should not leave the exercise laboratory area until the postexercise ECG has returned to baseline. **Figure 14-7** illustrates eight different electrocardiographic patterns seen during exercise testing.

MEASUREMENT OF ST-SEGMENT DISPLACEMENT. For purposes of interpretation, the PQ junction is usually chosen as the isoelectric point. The TP segment represents a true isoelectric point but is an impractical choice for most routine clinical measurements. The development of 0.10 mV (1 mm) or more of J point depression measured from the PQ junction, with a relatively flat ST-segment slope (e.g., <0.7 to 1 mV/sec), depressed 0.10 mV or more 80 ms after the J point (ST80) in three consecutive beats, with a stable baseline, is considered to be an abnormal response (**Fig. 14-8**). In general, the ST60 measurement should be used at heart rates higher than 130/min. The ST segment at rest may occasionally be depressed. When this occurs, the J point and ST60 or ST80 measurements should be depressed an additional 0.10 mV or more to be considered abnormal. In most laboratories, the exercise ECG is printed out in a 3 × 4 format, or 2.5 sec/three-lead group. To maximize the opportunity of meeting the above criteria, some laboratories have adopted a strategy of recording a full 10 seconds of electrocardiographic data with leads II, aVF, and V_5 when the tracing starts to show abnormal beats below the ischemic threshold. This 10-second tracing increases the likelihood of capturing consecutive abnormal beats with a stable baseline.

When the degree of resting ST-segment depression is 0.1 mV or greater, the exercise ECG becomes less specific, and myocardial

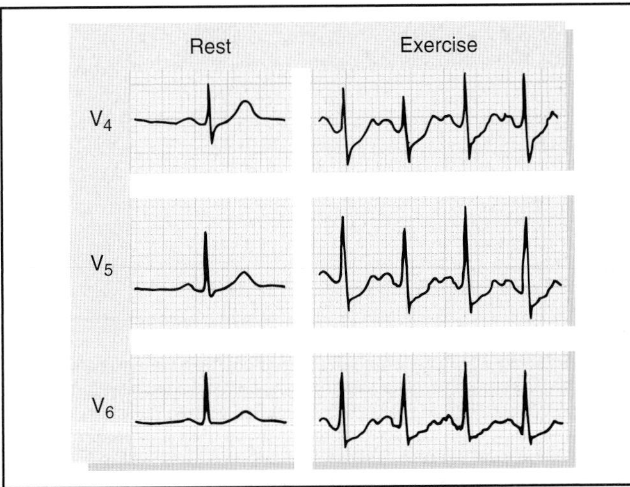

FIGURE 14-3 J point depression of 2 to 3 mm in leads V_4 to V_6, with rapid upsloping ST segments depressed approximately 1 mm 80 milliseconds after the J point. The ST-segment slope in leads V_4 and V_5 is 3.0 mV/sec. This response should not be considered abnormal.

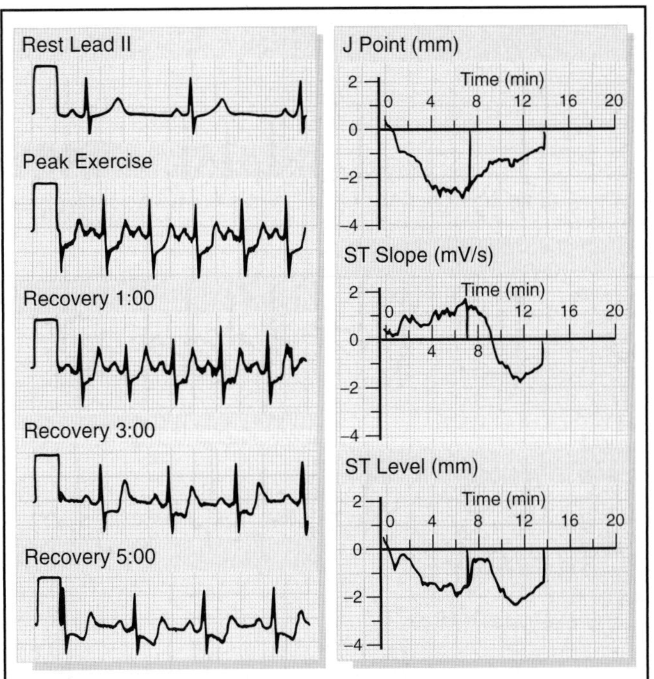

FIGURE 14-5 Bruce protocol. In this type of ischemic pattern, the J point at peak exertion is depressed 2.5 mm, the ST-segment slope is 1.5 mV/sec, and the ST-segment level is depressed 1.6 mm at 80 milliseconds after the J point. This "slow upsloping" ST segment at peak exercise indicates an ischemic pattern in patients with a high pretest prevalence of coronary disease. A typical ischemic pattern is seen at 3 minutes of the recovery phase when the ST segment is horizontal and 5 minutes after exertion when the ST segment is downsloping. **Right panels,** Exercise is discontinued at the vertical line at 7.5 minutes.

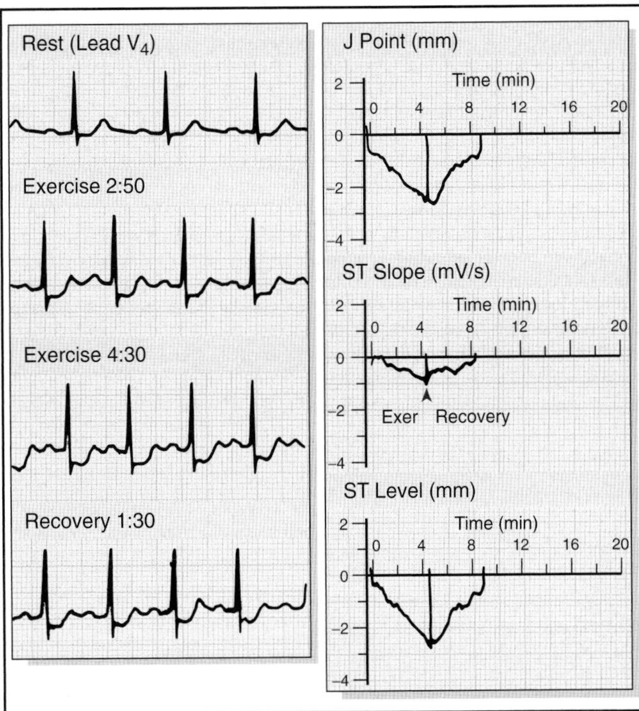

FIGURE 14-4 Bruce protocol. In lead V_4, the exercise electrocardiographic result is abnormal early in the test, reaching 0.3 mV (3 mm) of horizontal ST-segment depression at the end of exercise. The ischemic changes persist for at least 1.5 minutes into the recovery phase. **Right panel,** Continuous plot of the J point, ST slope, and ST-segment displacement at 80 milliseconds after the J point (ST level) during exercise and in the recovery phase. Exercise ends at the vertical line at 4.5 minutes (red arrow). The computer trends permit a more precise identification of initial onset and offset of ischemic ST segment depression. This type of electrocardiographic pattern, with early onset of ischemic ST-segment depression, reaching more than 3 mm of horizontal ST-segment displacement and persisting several minutes into the recovery phase, is consistent with a severe ischemic response.

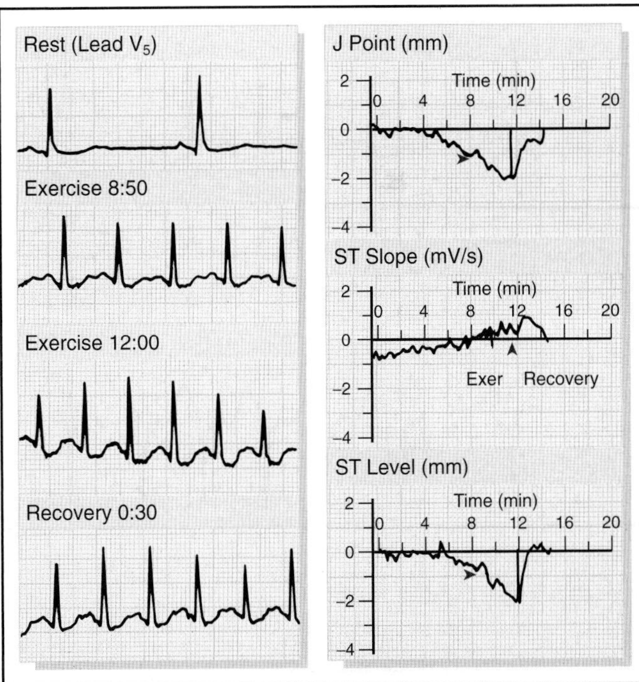

FIGURE 14-6 Bruce protocol. The exercise electrocardiographic result is not yet abnormal at 8:50 minutes but becomes abnormal at 9:30 minutes (horizontal arrowheads, **right panel**) of a 12-minute exercise test and resolves in the immediate recovery phase. This electrocardiographic pattern, in which the ST segment becomes abnormal only at high exercise workloads and returns to baseline in the immediate recovery phase, may indicate a false-positive result in an asymptomatic individual without atherosclerotic risk factors. Exercise myocardial perfusion imaging would provide more diagnostic and prognostic information if this were an older person with several atherosclerotic risk factors. Vertical arrowhead indicates termination of exercise.

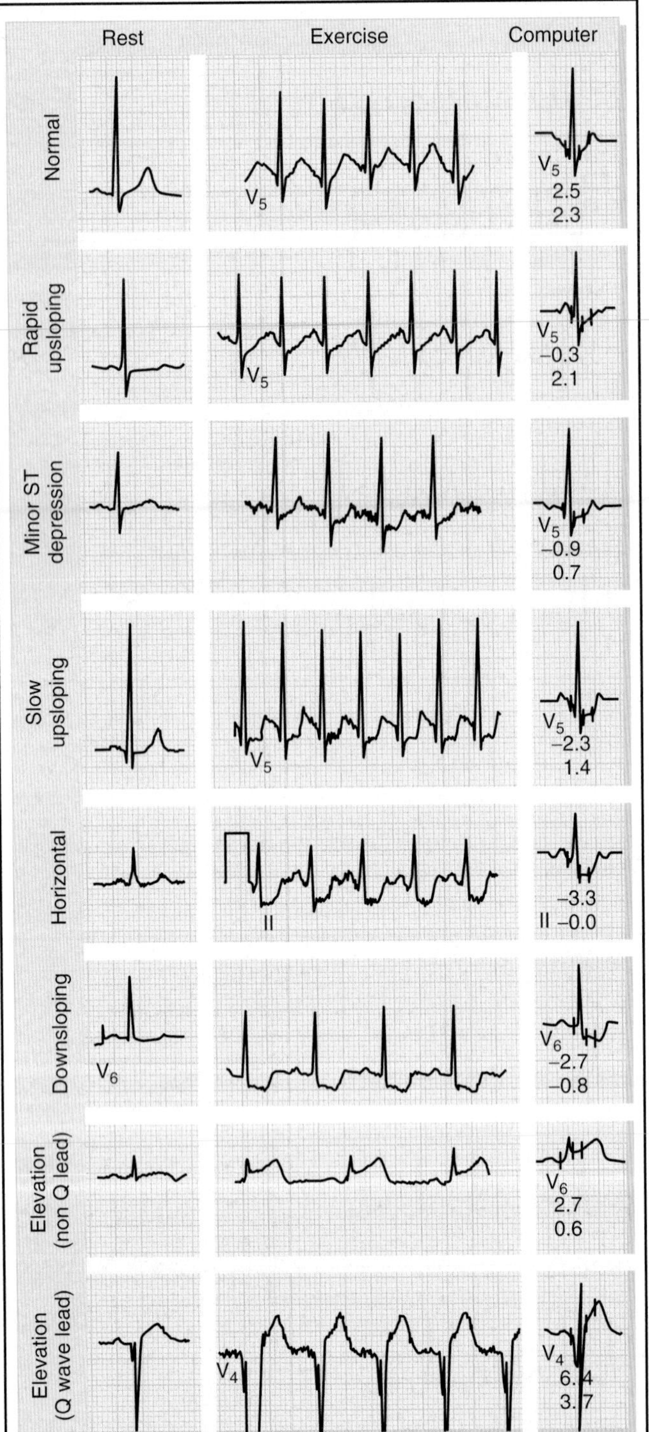

FIGURE 14-7 Eight typical exercise electrocardiographic patterns at rest and at peak exertion. The computer-processed incrementally averaged beat corresponds with the raw data taken at the same time point during exercise and is illustrated in the last column. The patterns represent worsening electrocardiographic responses during exercise. In the column of computer-averaged beats, ST80 displacement (top number) indicates the magnitude of ST-segment displacement 80 milliseconds after the J point relative to the PQ junction or E point. ST-segment slope measurement (bottom number) indicates the ST-segment slope at a fixed time point after the J point to the ST80 measurement. At least three noncomputer average complexes with a stable baseline should meet criteria for abnormality before the exercise electrocardiographic result can be considered abnormal (see Fig. 14-9). The normal and rapid upsloping ST-segment responses are normal responses to exercise. J point depression with rapid upsloping ST segments is a common response in an older, apparently healthy person. Minor ST-segment depression can occur occasionally at submaximal workloads in patients with coronary disease; in this figure, the ST segment is depressed 0.09 mV (0.9 mm) 80 milliseconds after the J point. The slow upsloping ST-segment pattern often demonstrates an ischemic response in patients with known coronary disease or those with a high pretest clinical risk of coronary disease. Criteria for slow upsloping ST-segment depression include J point and ST80 depression of 0.15 mV or more and ST-segment slope of more than 1.0 mV/sec. Classic criteria for myocardial ischemia include horizontal ST-segment depression observed when both the J point and ST80 depression are 0.1 mV or more and the ST-segment slope is within the range of 1.0 mV/sec. Downsloping ST segment depression occurs when the J point and ST80 depression are 0.1 mV and the ST segment slope is −1.0 mV/sec. ST-segment elevation in a non–Q-wave noninfarct lead occurs when the J point and ST60 are 1.0 mV or higher and represents a severe ischemic response. ST-segment elevation in an infarct territory (Q wave lead) indicates a severe wall motion abnormality and, in most cases, is not considered an ischemic response. *(From Chaitman BR: Exercise electrocardiographic stress testing. In Beller GA [ed]: Chronic Ischemic Heart Disease. In Braunwald E [series ed]: Atlas of Heart Diseases. Vol 5. Chronic Ischemic Heart Disease. Philadelphia, Current Medicine, 1995, pp 2.1-2.30.)*

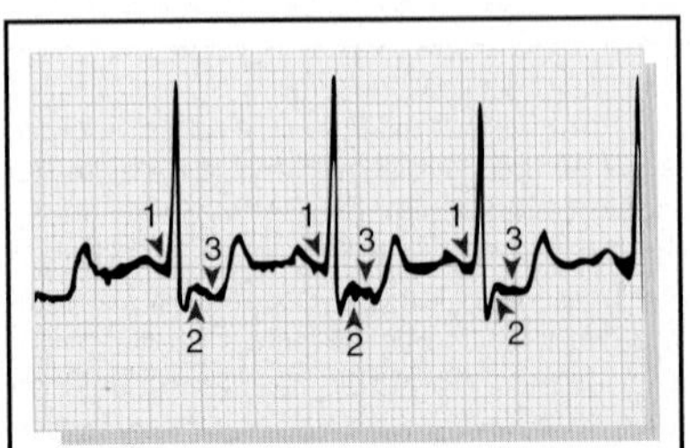

FIGURE 14-8 Magnified ischemic exercise-induced electrocardiographic pattern. Three consecutive complexes with a relatively stable baseline are selected. The PQ junction (1) and J point (2) are determined; the ST80 (3) is determined 80 milliseconds after the J point. In this example, average J point displacement is 0.2 mV (2 mm) and ST80 is 0.24 mV (24 mm). The average slope measurement from the J point to ST80 is −1.1 mV/sec.

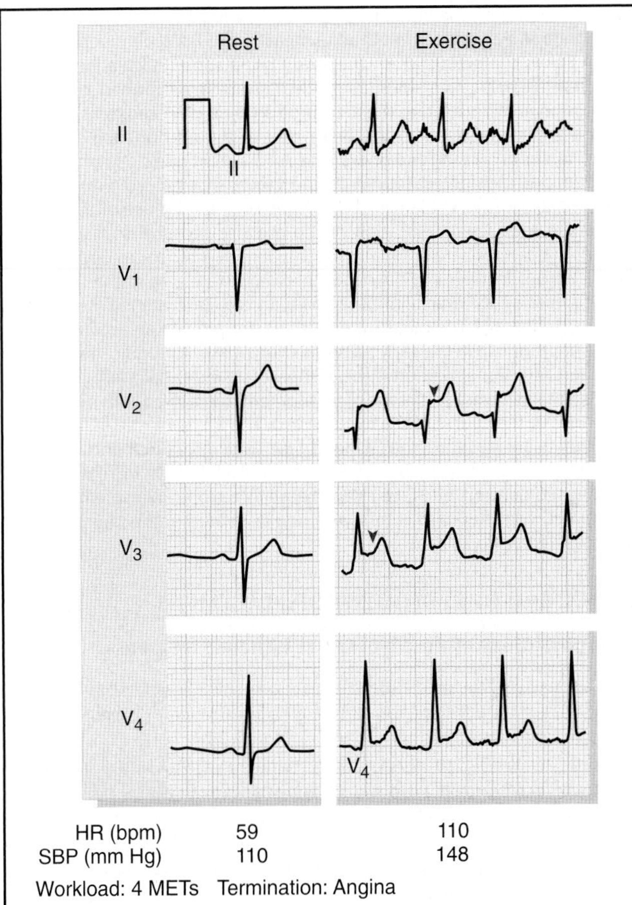

FIGURE 14-9 A 48-year-old man with several atherosclerotic risk factors and a normal resting electrocardiographic result developed marked ST-segment elevation (4 mm [arrows]) in leads V_2 and V_3, with lesser degrees of ST-segment elevation in leads V_1 and V_4 and J point depression with upsloping ST segments in lead II, associated with angina. This type of electrocardiographic pattern is usually associated with a full-thickness, reversible myocardial perfusion defect in the corresponding left ventricular myocardial segments and high-grade intraluminal narrowing at coronary angiography. Rarely, coronary vasospasm produces this result in the absence of significant intraluminal atherosclerotic narrowing. SBP = systolic blood pressure. *(From Chaitman BR: Exercise electrocardiographic stress testing. In Beller GA [ed]: Chronic Ischemic Heart Disease. In Braunwald E [series ed]: Atlas of Heart Diseases. Vol 5. Chronic Ischemic Heart Disease. Philadelphia, Current Medicine, 1995, pp 2.1-2.30.)*

imaging modalities should be considered.[2] In patients with early repolarization and resting ST-segment elevation, return to the PQ junction is normal. Therefore, the magnitude of exercise-induced ST-segment depression in a patient with early repolarization should be determined from the PQ junction and not from the elevated position of the J point before exercise. Exercise-induced ST-segment depression does not localize the site of myocardial ischemia, nor does it indicate which coronary artery is involved. Exercise-induced ST-segment elevation is relatively specific for the territory of myocardial ischemia and the coronary artery involved (**Fig. 14-9**).

UPSLOPING ST SEGMENTS. Junctional or J point depression is a normal finding during maximal exercise, and a rapid upsloping ST segment (more than 1 mV/sec) depressed less than 0.15 mV (1.5 mm) after the J point should be considered to be normal (see Fig. 14-3). Occasionally, however, the ST segment is depressed 0.15 mV (1.5 mm) or more at 80 milliseconds after the J point. This type of slow upsloping ST segment may be the only electrocardiographic finding in patients with well-defined obstructive CAD and may depend on the lead set used (see Figs. 14-5 and 14-7). In patient subsets with a high CAD prevalence, a slow upsloping ST segment depressed 0.15 mV or more at 80 milliseconds after the J point should be considered abnormal. The importance of this finding in asymptomatic individuals or those with a low CAD prevalence is less certain. Increasing the degree of ST-segment depression at 80 milliseconds after the J point to 0.2 mV (2.0 mm) or more in patients with a slow upsloping ST segment increases specificity but decreases sensitivity.[1,7,8]

ST-SEGMENT ELEVATION. Exercise-induced ST-segment elevation may occur in an infarct territory where Q waves are present or in a noninfarct territory. The development of 0.10 mV (1 mm) or more of J point elevation, persistently elevated higher than 0.10 mV at 60 milliseconds after the J point in three consecutive beats with a stable baseline, is considered an abnormal response (see Fig. 14-7). This finding occurs more frequently in patients with anterior myocardial infarctions tested early after the index event and decreases in frequency by 6 weeks. As a group, postinfarct patients with exercise-induced ST-segment elevation have a lower ejection fraction than those without, greater severity of resting wall motion abnormalities, and worse prognosis. Exercise-induced ST-segment elevation in leads with abnormal Q waves is not a marker of more extensive CAD and rarely indicates myocardial ischemia. Exercise-induced ST-segment elevation may occasionally occur in a patient who has regenerated embryonic R waves after an acute myocardial infarction; the clinical significance of this finding is similar to that observed when Q waves are present.

When ST-segment elevation develops during exercise in a non–Q-wave lead in a patient without a previous myocardial infarction, the finding should be considered as likely evidence of transmural myocardial ischemia caused by coronary vasospasm or a high-grade coronary narrowing (Fig. 14-9). This finding is relatively uncommon, occurring in approximately 1% of patients with obstructive CAD. The electrocardiographic site of ST-segment elevation is relatively specific for the coronary artery involved, and myocardial perfusion scintigraphy usually reveals a defect in the territory involved.

T WAVE CHANGES. The morphology of the T wave is influenced by body position, respiration, hyperventilation, drug therapy, and myocardial ischemia or necrosis. In patient populations with a low CAD prevalence, pseudonormalization of T waves (inverted at rest and becoming upright with exercise) is a nondiagnostic finding (**Fig. 14-10**). In rare cases, this finding may be a marker for myocardial ischemia in a patient with documented CAD, although it would need to be substantiated by an ancillary technique, such as the concomitant finding of a reversible myocardial perfusion defect.

OTHER ELECTROCARDIOGRAPHIC MARKERS. Changes in R wave amplitude during exercise are relatively nonspecific and are related to the level of exercise performed. When the R wave amplitude meets voltage criteria for left ventricular hypertrophy, the ST-segment response cannot be used reliably to diagnose CAD, even in the absence of a left ventricular strain pattern. Loss of R wave amplitude, commonly seen after myocardial infarction, reduces the sensitivity of the ST-segment response in that lead to diagnose obstructive CAD. Adjustment of the extent of ST-segment depression by R wave height in individual leads has not been consistently shown to improve the diagnostic value of the exercise ECG for CAD. U wave inversion can occasionally be seen in the precordial leads at heart rates of 120 beats/min. Although this finding is relatively specific for CAD, it is relatively insensitive.

COMPUTER-ASSISTED ANALYSIS. The use of computers has facilitated the routine analysis of and measurements required from the exercise ECG and can be performed online as well as offline. When the raw electrocardiographic data are of high quality, the computer can filter and average or select median complexes from which the degree of J point displacement, ST-segment slope, and ST-segment displacement 60 to 80 milliseconds (ST60 to ST80) after the J point can be measured.[8] The selection of ST60 or ST80 depends on the heart rate response. At ventricular rates higher than 130 beats/min, the ST80 measurement may fall on the upslope of the T wave, and the ST60 measurement should be used instead. In some computerized systems, the PQ junction or isoelectric interval is detected by scanning before the R wave for the 10-millisecond

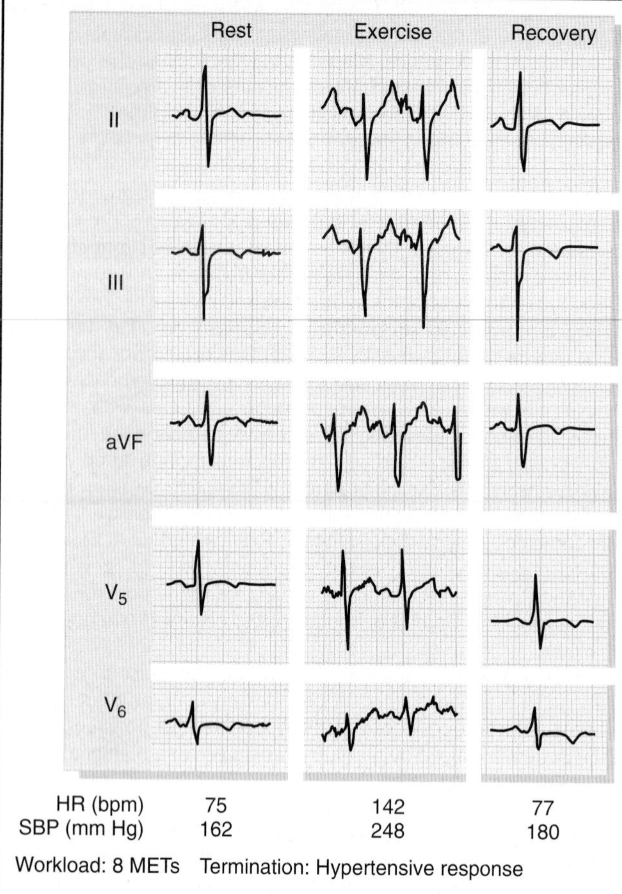

FIGURE 14-10 Pseudonormalization of T waves in a 49-year-old man referred for exercise testing. The patient had previously been seen for typical angina. The resting ECG in this patient with CAD shows inferior and anterolateral T wave inversion, an adverse long-term prognosticator. The patient exercised to 8 METs, reaching a peak heart rate of 142 beats/min and a peak systolic blood pressure of 248 mm Hg. At that point, the test was stopped because of hypertension. During exercise, pseudonormalization of T waves occurs, and it returns to baseline (inverted T wave) in the postexercise phase. The patient denied chest discomfort, and no arrhythmia or ST-segment displacement was noted. Transient conversion of a negative T wave at rest to a positive T wave during exercise is a nonspecific finding in patients without prior myocardial infarction and does not enhance the diagnostic or prognostic content of the test; however, the ability to exercise to 8 METs without ischemic changes in the ST segment places this patient into a subset of lower risk. SBP = systolic blood pressure. *(From Chaitman BR: Exercise electrocardiographic stress testing. In Beller GA [ed]: Chronic Ischemic Heart Disease. In Braunwald E [series ed]: Atlas of Heart Diseases. Vol 5. Chronic Ischemic Heart Disease. Philadelphia, Current Medicine, 1995, pp 2.1-2.30.)*

interval with the least slope. J point, ST slope, and ST levels are determined (see Figs. 14-4, 14-5, and 14-6); the ST integral can be calculated from the area below the isoelectric line from the J point to ST60 or ST80. Computerized treatment of electrocardiographic complexes permits reduction of motion and myographic artifacts. However, the averaged or median beats may occasionally be erroneous because of electrocardiographic signal distortion caused by noise, baseline wander, or changes in conduction, and identification of the PQ junction and ST segment onset can be imperfect. Therefore, it is crucial to ensure that the computer-determined averages or median complexes reflect the raw electrocardiographic data; physicians should program the computer to print out raw data during exercise and inspect the raw data to be certain that the QRS template is accurately reproduced, and that the placement of the fiducial points is correctly placed at the PQ junction and J point before accepting the automatic measurements.

ST/Heart Rate Slope Measurements. Heart rate adjustment of ST-segment depression appears to improve the sensitivity of the exercise test, particularly the prediction of multivessel CAD.[19] The ST/heart rate slope depends on the type of exercise performed, number and location of monitoring electrodes, method of measuring ST-segment depression, and clinical characteristics of the study population. Calculation of the maximal ST/heart rate slope in mV/beats/min is performed by linear regression analysis relating the measured amount of ST-segment depression in individual leads to the heart rate at the end of each stage of exercise, starting at the end of exercise. An ST/heart rate slope of 2.4 mV/beats/min is considered abnormal, and values that exceed 6 mV/beats/min are suggestive evidence of three-vessel CAD. The use of this measurement requires modification of the exercise protocol so that increments in heart rate are gradual, as in the Cornell protocol, as opposed to more abrupt increases in heart rate between stages, as in the Bruce or Ellestad protocols, which limit the ability to calculate valid ST/heart rate slopes statistically. The measurement does not provide an accurate estimate of prognosis in the early postinfarction phase. A modification of the ST/heart rate slope method is the ST/heart rate index calculation, which represents the average change of ST-segment depression with heart rate throughout the course of the exercise test. The ST/heart rate index measurements are less than the ST/heart rate slope measurements, and an ST/heart rate index of 1.6 is defined as abnormal. A slight increase in the prognostic content of ST segment/heart rate slope measurements as compared with standard criteria was demonstrated in the Multiple Risk Factor Interventional Trial.[1,8]

MECHANISM OF ST-SEGMENT DISPLACEMENT

Pathophysiology of the Myocardial Ischemic Response

Myocardial oxygen consumption ($M\dot{O}_2$) is determined by heart rate, systolic blood pressure, left ventricular end-diastolic volume, wall thickness, and contractility (see Chaps. 24 and 52).[1,2,7,8,12] The rate-pressure or double product (heart rate × systolic blood pressure) increases progressively with increasing work and can be used to estimate the myocardial perfusion requirement in normal persons and in many patients with CAD. The heart is an aerobic organ with little capacity to generate energy through anaerobic metabolism. Oxygen extraction in the coronary circulation is almost maximal at rest. The only significant mechanism available to the heart to increase oxygen consumption is to increase perfusion, and there is a direct linear relationship between $M\dot{O}_2$ and coronary blood flow in normal individuals. The principal mechanism for increasing coronary blood flow during exercise is to decrease resistance at the coronary arteriolar level. In patients with progressive atherosclerotic narrowing of the epicardial vessels, an ischemic threshold occurs, and exercise beyond this threshold can produce abnormalities in diastolic and systolic ventricular function, electrocardiographic changes, and chest pain. The subendocardium is more susceptible to myocardial ischemia than the subepicardium because of increased wall tension, causing a relative increase in myocardial oxygen demand in the subendocardium. Dynamic changes in coronary artery tone at the site of an atherosclerotic plaque may result in diminished coronary flow during static or dynamic exercise instead of the expected increase that normally occurs from coronary vasodilation in a normal vessel; that is, perfusion pressure distal to the stenotic plaque actually falls, as during exercise, resulting in reduced subendocardial blood flow. Thus, regional left ventricular myocardial ischemia may result not only from an increase in myocardial oxygen demand during exercise but also from a limitation of coronary flow as a result of coronary vasoconstriction, or inability of vessels to vasodilate sufficiently as a result of diffuse atherosclerosis and abnormal endothelial function at or near the site of an obstructive atherosclerotic plaque.

Some patients with chronic angina have a warm-up phenomenon that can be demonstrated using sequential exercise testing.[20] Under these conditions, the time to angina and ischemic ST-segment depression can be prolonged and can occur at a higher rate-pressure product on the second of two exercise tests performed within 10 to 30 minutes of each other. Improvement in performance on the second test is related to the magnitude of myocardial ischemia produced on the first test and usually myocardial ischemia of more than moderate intensity is required to produce the warm-up response.

In normal persons, the action potential duration of the endocardial region is longer than that of the epicardial region, and ventricular repolarization is from epicardium to endocardium. The action potential duration is shortened in the presence of myocardial ischemia and electrical gradients are created, resulting in ST-segment depression or elevation, depending on the surface electrocardiographic leads. At the molecular level, activation of sarcolemmal ATP-sensitive potassium (K_{ATP}) channels by ischemic ATP depletion may play a role. Transgenic mice with homozygous knockout of the *Kir6.2* channel gene, which encodes the pore-forming subunit of cardiac surface K_{ATP} channels, lack the ability to generate an ST-segment elevation response to acute coronary occlusion.[21] Increased myocardial oxygen demand associated with a failure to increase or with an actual decrease in regional coronary blood flow usually causes ST-segment depression; ST-segment elevation may occasionally occur in patients with more severe coronary flow reduction.

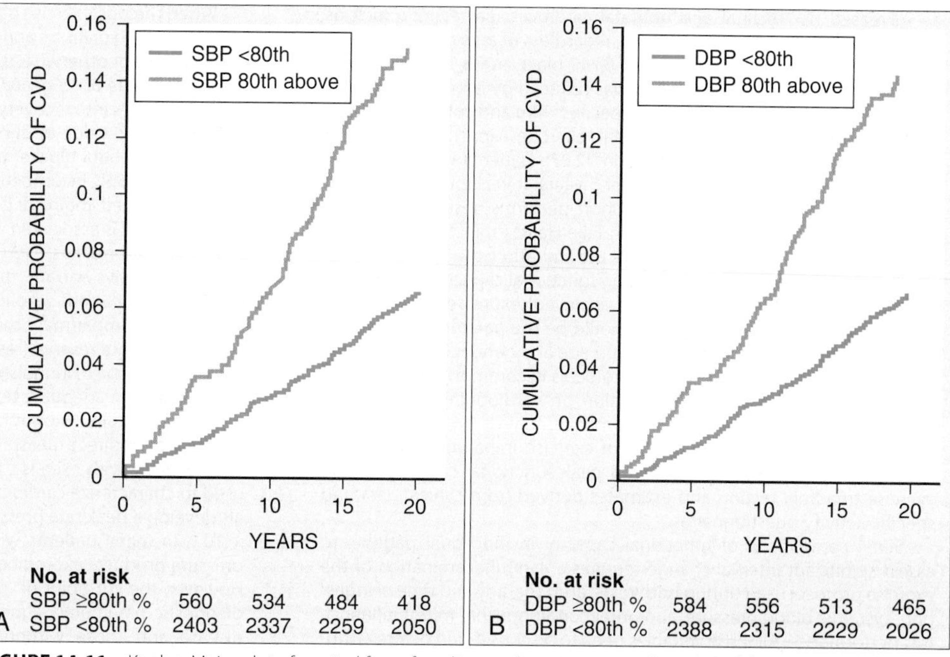

FIGURE 14-11 Kaplan-Meier plot of survival free of cardiovascular events according to the presence of systolic blood pressure (SBP; **A**) and diastolic blood pressure (DBP; **B**) in excess of gender-specific 80 percentile obtained at the midpoint of the second stage of exercise using the standard Bruce protocol in 3045 study participants followed for 20 years. CVD = cardiovascular disease. *(From Lewis GD, Gona P, Larson MG, et al: Exercise blood pressure and the risk of incident cardiovascular disease (from the Framingham Heart Study). Am J Cardiol 101:1614, 2008.)*

NONELECTROCARDIOGRAPHIC OBSERVATIONS

The ECG is only one part of the exercise response, and symptoms, abnormal hemodynamics or heart rate response, and reduced functional capacity are even more important than ST-segment shifts in determining long-term prognosis.

Blood Pressure. The normal exercise response is to increase systolic blood pressure progressively with increasing workloads to a peak response ranging from 160 to 200 mm Hg, with the higher range of the scale in older patients with less compliant vascular systems.[1,7,8] As a group, black patients tend to have a higher systolic blood pressure response than white patients. At high exercise workloads, it is sometimes difficult to obtain a precise determination of systolic blood pressure by auscultation. In normal persons, the diastolic blood pressure does not usually change significantly. Failure to increase systolic blood pressure beyond 120 mm Hg, a sustained decrease greater than 10 mm Hg repeatable within 15 seconds, or a fall in systolic blood pressure below standing resting values during progressive exercise, when the blood pressure has otherwise been increasing appropriately, is abnormal and reflects inadequate elevation of cardiac output because of left ventricular systolic pump dysfunction or an excessive reduction in systemic vascular resistance. Exertional hypotension ranges from 3% to 9% in symptomatic patients and is higher in patients with three-vessel or left main CAD. Conditions other than myocardial ischemia that have been associated with a failure to increase or with an actual decrease in systolic blood pressure during progressive exercise are cardiomyopathy, cardiac arrhythmias, vasovagal reactions, left ventricular outflow tract obstruction, ingestion of antihypertensive drugs, hypovolemia, and prolonged vigorous exercise.

It is important to distinguish between a decline in blood pressure in the postexercise phase and a decrease in or failure to increase systolic blood pressure during progressive exercise. The incidence of postexertional hypotension in asymptomatic subjects was 1.9% in 781 asymptomatic volunteers in the Baltimore Longitudinal Study on Aging, with a 3.1% incidence noted in subjects younger than 55 years and a 0.3% incidence in patients older than 55 years.[22] In this series, most hypotensive episodes were symptomatic, and only two patients had hypotension associated with bradycardia and vagal symptoms. Although ST-segment abnormalities suggestive of ischemia occurred in one third of the patients with hypotension, none of the patients had a cardiac event during 4 years of follow-up. Rarely, in young patients, vasovagal syncope can occur in the immediate postexercise phase, progressing through sinus bradycardia to several seconds of asystole and hypotension before reverting to sinus rhythm. An exaggerated blood pressure increase with exercise is associated with an increased risk of future hypertension, greater prevalence of left ventricular hypertrophy, and an augmented rise of angiotensin II during the test, in otherwise normotensive individuals.[23-25] In the Framingham Heart Study, an exaggerated blood pressure response to submaximal exercise in middle-aged adults was associated with significant increased incidence of cardiovascular events over a 20-year follow-up (**Fig. 14-11**). This type of response in patients with a high prevalence of CAD is associated with more extensive CAD and more extensive myocardial perfusion defects. Occasionally, a marked hypertensive response may cause new exercise-induced wall motion abnormalities in the absence of CAD.

Maximal Work Capacity. This variable is one of the most important prognostic measurements obtained from an exercise test (**Fig. 14-12**).[1,2,7,8,10,26-30] Maximal work capacity in normal individuals is influenced by familiarization with the exercise test equipment, level of training, and environmental conditions at the time of testing. In patients with known or suspected CAD, a limited exercise capacity is associated with

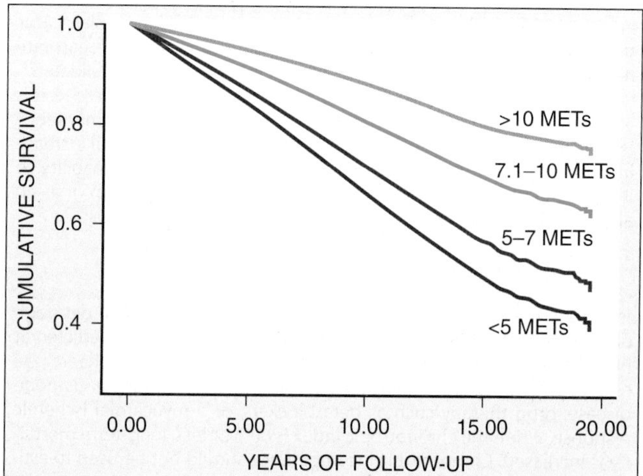

FIGURE 14-12 Cumulative 20-year survival rates in 6749 black and 8911 white male U.S. veterans with and without cardiovascular disease. Survival is significantly reduced with each decrement in peak aerobic capacity. The relationship was similar for those with and without cardiovascular disease and for blacks and whites. *(From Kokkinos P, Myers J, Kokkinos JP, et al: Exercise capacity and mortality in black and white men. Circulation 117:614, 2008.)*

an increased risk of fatal and nonfatal cardiovascular events, such as acute coronary syndromes and stroke, regardless of age, gender, race, or abdominal adiposity. In one series of 6,749 black and 8,911 white male veterans, the adjusted risk of death was reduced by approximately13% for each 1-MET increase in exercise capacity.[26] Kim and colleagues[31] have validated the prognostic value of peak exercise capacity using seven age- and gender-based nomograms in 22,275 patients without known heart disease followed for a median of 5 years. It was found that that a model based on a Veterans Affairs cohort performs best in men and a model based on the St. James Women Take Heart Project performs best in women. In general, the more severe the limitation, the worse the CAD extent and prognosis. When estimating functional capacity, the amount of work performed (or exercise stage achieved) expressed in METs, not the number of minutes of exercise, should be the parameter measured. Estimates of peak functional capacity for age and gender have been well established for most of the exercise protocols in common use, subject to the limitations described in the section on cardiopulmonary testing. Comparison of an individual's performance against normal standards provides an estimate of the degree of exercise impairment. There is a rough correlation between observed peak functional capacity during exercise treadmill testing and estimates derived from clinical data and specific activity questionnaires.

Serial comparison of functional capacity in individual patients to assess significant interval change requires a careful examination of the exercise protocol used during both tests, drug therapy and time of ingestion, systemic blood pressure, and other conditions that might influence test performance. All these variables need to be considered before attributing changes in functional capacity to progression of CAD or worsening of left ventricular function. Major reductions in exercise capacity usually indicate significant worsening of cardiovascular status; modest changes may not.

Submaximal Exercise. The interpretation of exercise test results for diagnostic and prognostic purposes requires consideration of maximal work capacity. When a patient is unable to complete moderate levels of exercise or reach at least 85% to 90% of age-predicted maximum, the level of exercise performed may be inadequate to test cardiac reserve. Thus, ischemic electrocardiographic, scintigraphic, or ventriculographic abnormalities may not be evoked and the test may be nondiagnostic. Nondiagnostic test results are more common in patients with peripheral vascular disease, orthopedic limitation, or neurologic impairment and in patients with poor motivation. Pharmacologic stress imaging studies should be considered in this setting.[1,2]

Heart Rate Response. The sinus rate increases progressively with exercise, mediated in part through sympathetic and parasympathetic innervation of the sinoatrial node and circulating catecholamines. In some patients who may be anxious about the exercise test, there may be an initial overreaction of heart rate and systolic blood pressure at the beginning of exercise, with stabilization after approximately 30 to 60 seconds. An inappropriate increase in heart rate at low exercise workloads may also occur in patients who are in atrial fibrillation, physically deconditioned, hypovolemic, or anemic, or who have marginal left ventricular function. The prognostic importance of an early abnormal acceleration of heart rate during low-level exercise is controversial.[32] This parameter should not be used to estimate prognosis because heart rate reserve and heart rate recovery have been more extensively validated.[1]

When the heart rate fails to increase appropriately with exercise, it is associated with an adverse prognosis.[1,33-35] Chronotropic incompetence is determined by decreased heart rate sensitivity to the normal increase in sympathetic tone during exercise and is defined as the inability to increase heart rate to at least 85% of age-predicted maximum or as an abnormal heart rate reserve. HR reserve is calculated as follows:

$$\%\ \text{HR reserve}_{\text{used}} = (\text{HR}_{\text{peak}} - \text{HR}_{\text{rest}})/(220 - \text{age} - \text{HR}_{\text{rest}})$$

The term *chronotropic index* refers to a heart rate increment per stage of exercise that is below normal or a peak heart rate below predicted at maximal workloads. It reflects an inability to use up all the heart rate reserve. This finding may indicate autonomic dysfunction, sinus node disease, drug therapy such as beta blockers, or a myocardial ischemic response. When the chronotropic index is 80% or less, long-term mortality is increased. Chronotropic incompetence should not be used to estimate prognosis in patients on beta blocker therapy.

Heart Rate Recovery. Abnormal heart rate recovery (HRR) refers to a relatively slow deceleration of heart rate following exercise cessation. This type of response reflects decreased vagal tone and is associated with increased mortality.[8,34,36-38]

$$\text{HRR} = \text{HR}_{\text{peak}} - \text{HR}_{\text{1 minute later}}$$

When the postexercise phase includes an upright cool-down, a value of 12 beats/min or less is abnormal. For patients undergoing stress echocardiography or otherwise assuming a supine position immediately after exercise, a value of 18 beats/min or less is abnormal. When HRR is measured 2 minutes into recovery, a value of 22 beats/min or less is abnormal. The prognostic value of abnormal HRR is independent of the exercise level attained, beta blocker usage, severity of CAD, left ventricular function, chronotropic incompetence, Duke treadmill score, and presence of exercise-induced angina or ischemic electrocardiographic abnormalities. Abnormal HRR is associated with increased abnormal and high-risk myocardial perfusion scans, even in patients without exercise test results that would normally warrant further testing.[37] A submaximal heart rate response in a patient who is poorly motivated to complete the test or has a physical impairment that limits ability to perform sufficient exercise to test heart rate reserve (resulting in a nondiagnostic test, as described earlier) should be distinguished from a patient with chronotropic incompetence and an adequate test for prognostic estimates.

Rate-Pressure Product. The heart rate–systolic blood pressure product, an indirect measure of myocardial oxygen demand, increases progressively with exercise, and the peak rate-pressure product can be used to characterize cardiovascular performance. Most normal individuals develop a peak rate pressure product of 20 to 35 mm Hg $\times$ beats/min $\times\ 10^{-3}$. In many patients with significant ischemic heart disease, rate-pressure products exceeding 25 mm Hg $\times$ beats/min $\times\ 10^{-3}$ are unusual. However, the cut point of 25 mm Hg $\times$ beats/min $\times\ 10^{-3}$ is not a useful diagnostic parameter; significant overlap exists between patients with disease and those without disease. Furthermore, cardioactive drug therapy significantly influences this measurement.

Chest Discomfort. Characterization of chest discomfort during exercise can be a useful diagnostic finding, particularly when the symptom complex is compatible with typical angina pectoris. In some patients, the exercise level during the test may exceed that which the patient exhibits in daily activities. Exercise-induced chest discomfort usually occurs after the onset of ischemic ST-segment abnormalities and may be associated with diastolic hypertension. In some patients, however, chest discomfort may be the only signal that obstructive CAD is present. In patients with chronic stable angina, exercise-induced chest discomfort occurs less frequently than ischemic ST-segment depression. The severity of myocardial ischemia in a patient with exercise-induced angina and a normal ECG can often be assessed using a myocardial imaging technique.[1,2] The new development of an S_3, holosystolic apical murmur, or basilar rales in the early recovery phase of exercise enhances the diagnostic accuracy of the test.

Exercise Test Indications

The most frequent indications for exercise testing are to aid in establishing the diagnosis of CAD, determining functional capacity, and estimating prognosis. The indications continue to evolve, with some that are uniformly accepted and others that are more controversial. The American Heart Association and American College of Cardiology Exercise Task Force have determined several categories of test indications drawn from a large body of published literature on exercise testing[1] (see later, "Guidelines"). Exercise testing should not be used to screen very low-risk asymptomatic individuals because the test has limited diagnostic and prognostic value in this situation, and the resultant undesirable consequences of a false-positive exercise test result might include unnecessary follow-up, additional procedures, anxiety, and exercise restrictions.[7,8]

Diagnostic Use of Exercise Testing

Appreciation of the noninvasive test literature to diagnose CAD requires an understanding of standard terminology such as *sensitivity*, *specificity*, and *test accuracy* (**Table 14-2**).[1,2,7,8] In patients selected for coronary angiography, the sensitivity of the exercise ECG in patients with CAD is approximately 68% and specificity is 77%. In patients with single-vessel disease, the sensitivity ranges from 25% to 71%, with exercise-induced ST displacement most frequent in patients with left anterior descending CAD, followed by those with right CAD and those with isolated left circumflex CAD. In patients with multivessel CAD, sensitivity is approximately 81% and specificity is 66%. The sensitivity and specificity for left main or three-vessel CAD are approximately 86% and 53%, respectively. The exercise ECG tends to be less sensitive

TABLE 14-2 Terms Useful for Evaluation of Test Results

TERM	DEFINITION
True positive (TP)	Abnormal test result in individual with disease
False positive (FP)	Abnormal test result in individual without disease
True negative (TN)	Normal test result in individual without disease
False negative (FN)	Normal test result in individual with disease
Sensitivity	Percentage of patients with CAD who have an abnormal result = TP/(TP + FN)
Specificity	Percentage of patients without CAD who have a normal result = TN/(TN + FP)
Predictive value of a positive test	Percentage of patients with an abnormal result who have CAD = TP/(TP + FP)
Predictive value of a negative test	Percentage of patients with a normal result who do not have CAD = TN/(TN + FN)
Test accuracy	Percentage of true test results = (TP + TN)/total number tests performed
Likelihood ratio	Odds of a test result being true abnormal test result: sensitivity/(1 − specificity); normal test result: specificity/(1 − sensitivity)
Relative risk	Disease rate in persons with a positive test result/ disease rate in persons with a negative test result

TABLE 14-3 Noncoronary Causes of ST-Segment Depression

Anemia
Cardiomyopathy
Digitalis use
Glucose load
Hyperventilation
Hypokalemia
Intraventricular conduction disturbance
Left ventricular hypertrophy
Mitral valve prolapse
Preexcitation syndrome
Severe aortic stenosis
Severe hypertension
Severe hypoxia
Severe volume overload (aortic, mitral regurgitation)
Sudden excessive exercise
Supraventricular tachyarrhythmias

in patients with extensive anterior wall myocardial infarction and when a limited exercise electrocardiographic lead set is used. Approximately 75% to 80% of the diagnostic information on exercise-induced ST-segment depression in patients with a normal resting ECG is contained in leads V_4 to V_6. The exercise ECG is less specific when patients in whom false-positive results are more common are included, such as those with valvular heart disease, left ventricular hypertrophy, marked resting ST segment depression, or digitalis therapy. **Table 14-3** lists the more common causes of noncoronary exercise–induced ST-segment depression.

Selective referral of patients with a positive test result for further study decreases the rate of detection of true-negative test results and increases the rate of detection of false-positive results, thus increasing sensitivity and decreasing specificity.[1,2,7] Froelicher and Myers,[8] in a study of 814 consecutive patients who presented with angina pectoris and agreed to undergo both exercise testing and coronary angiography, have reported an exercise electrocardiographic sensitivity of 45% and specificity of 85% for obstructive CAD using visual analysis in this population, with reduced workup bias. Computerized ST-segment measurements were similar to visual ST-segment measurements in this study. A false-positive result is more common when only the inferior lead group (leads I, III, aVF) is abnormal at high exercise workloads.

The magnitude of coronary atherosclerosis is often underestimated in a luminal angiogram when intravascular ultrasonographic studies are performed (see Chap. 22), and may be extensive even if the most severe luminal narrowing appears less than 50%. A mildly abnormal coronary angiogram does not eliminate the possibility that a patient's symptoms may be ischemic in origin.

BAYES' THEOREM. The depth of exercise-induced ST-segment depression and the extent of the myocardial ischemic response can be thought of as continuous variables. Cut points such as 1 mm of horizontal or downsloping ST-segment depression as compared with baseline cannot completely distinguish patients with disease from those without disease, and the requirement of more severe degrees of ST-segment depression to improve specificity will decrease sensitivity. Sensitivity and specificity are inversely related, and false-negative and false-positive results are to be expected when electrocardiographic or angiographic cut points are selected to optimize the diagnostic accuracy of the test.

The use of Bayes' theorem incorporates the pretest risk of disease and the sensitivity and specificity of the test (likelihood ratio) to calculate the post-test probability of CAD. The patient's clinical information and exercise test results are used to make a final estimate about the probability of CAD. Atypical or probable angina in a 50-year-old man or a 60-year-old woman is associated with an approximately 50% probability for CAD before exercise testing is performed. The diagnostic power of the exercise test is maximal when the pretest probability of CAD is intermediate (30% to 70%).

MULTIVARIATE ANALYSIS. Multivariate analysis of noninvasive exercise tests to estimate post-test risk also can provide important diagnostic information. Multivariate analysis offers the potential advantage that it does not require that the tests be independent of each other or that sensitivity and specificity remain constant over a wide range of disease prevalence rates (see later, "Exercise Testing in Determining Prognosis"). However, the multivariate technique critically depends on how patients are selected to establish the reference data base.[39] Both bayesian and multivariate approaches are commonly used to provide diagnostic and prognostic estimates of patients with CAD. For example, Morise and colleagues[40] have developed and validated a pretest scoring technique from multivariate models that incorporates age, gender and estrogen status, angina symptoms, obesity, and atherosclerotic risk factors to provide a robust pretest diagnostic and prognostic estimate of death or myocardial infarction that can be applied to estimate post-test risk of events based on the results of exercise or pharmacologic stress testing using bayesian principles.

SEVERITY OF ELECTROCARDIOGRAPHIC ISCHEMIC RESPONSE. The exercise electrocardiographic result is more likely to be abnormal in patients with more severe coronary arterial obstruction, with more extensive CAD, and after more strenuous levels of exercise. Early onset of angina, ischemic ST-segment depression, and fall in blood pressure at low exercise workloads are the most important exercise parameters associated with an adverse prognosis and multivessel CAD.[1,2,7,8] Additional adverse markers include profound ST-segment displacement, ischemic changes in five or more electrocardiographic leads, and persistence of the changes late in the recovery phase of exercise (**Table 14-4**).

Exercise Testing in Determining Prognosis

Exercise testing provides not only diagnostic information but also, more importantly, prognostic data.[1,2,7,8] The value of exercise testing to estimate prognosis must be considered in light of what is already known about a patient's risk status.[26-30,39,41-52] Left ventricular dysfunction, CAD extent, electrical instability, and noncoronary comorbid conditions must be taken into consideration when estimating long-term outcome.

TABLE 14-4 Exercise Parameters Associated with Adverse Prognosis and Multivessel Coronary Artery Disease

Duration of symptom-limiting exercise < 5 METs
Failure to increase systolic blood pressure ≥ 120 mm Hg, or a sustained decrease ≥ 10 mm Hg, or below rest levels, during progressive exercise
ST-segment depression ≥ 2 mm, downsloping ST segment, starting at <5 METs, involving ≥5 leads, persisting ≥5 min into recovery
Exercise-induced ST-segment elevation (aVR excluded)
Angina pectoris at low exercise workloads
Reproducible sustained (>30 sec) or symptomatic ventricular tachycardia

ASYMPTOMATIC POPULATION. The prevalence of an abnormal exercise electrocardiographic result in middle-aged asymptomatic men ranges from 5% to 12%. The risk of developing a cardiac event such as angina, myocardial infarction, or death in men is approximately nine times greater when the test result is abnormal than normal although, over 5 years of follow-up, generally one in four men will suffer a cardiac event, and this will most likely be angina. The data illustrate the difficulty in identifying asymptomatic subjects destined to develop abrupt changes in plaque morphology based on an abnormal exercise ECG in an individual with occult chronic ischemic heart disease. The future risk of cardiac events is greatest if the test result is strongly positive or if an asymptomatic subject has multiple atherosclerotic risk factors that predispose to accelerated atherosclerosis. Target extracardiac end-organ damage, such as peripheral vascular disease, proteinuria, or stroke, further escalates the risk in accordance with bayesian principles. Selection of asymptomatic subjects for an exercise test should be based on the atherosclerotic risk profile that can be used to provide a global risk estimate of the likelihood of death, myocardial infarction, or stroke. Appropriate asymptomatic subjects for exercise testing would be those with an estimated annual risk greater than 1% or 2%/year. In asymptomatic middle-aged or older men with several atherosclerotic risk factors, a markedly abnormal exercise response is associated with a significantly increased risk of subsequent cardiac events, particularly when there is additional supporting evidence for underlying CAD (e.g., abnormal imaging findings). Serial change of a negative exercise ECG result to a positive one in an asymptomatic person carries the same prognostic importance as an initially abnormal test result. However, the finding that an asymptomatic individual with an initially abnormal test result has significant worsening of electrocardiographic abnormalities at lower exercise workloads may indicate significant CAD progression; this warrants a more aggressive diagnostic workup. The prevalence of an abnormal exercise ECG result in middle-aged asymptomatic women ranges from 20% to 30%.[1,2,7,8] In general, the prognostic value of an ST-segment shift in women is less than in men (see later, "Specific Clinical Applications: Women").

SYMPTOMATIC PATIENTS. Exercise testing should be performed (unless this is not feasible or unless there are contraindications) before coronary angiography in patients with chronic ischemic heart disease. This should be done because the prognostic functional, hemodynamic, and ischemic threshold information contained in the test complements the anatomic information and can be used to help formulate a decision on the potential benefit of performing a coronary revascularization procedure during the catheterization if the sole procedure indication is to prevent future cardiac events (see Chap. 57). Unfortunately, stress testing is underused in this clinical setting; in a series of 23,887 Medicare fee-for-service beneficiaries older than 65 years undergoing elective percutaneous coronary intervention (PCI), only 44.5% had a stress test within 90 days of the procedure.[44] Patients who have excellent exercise tolerance (e.g., more than 10 METs) and satisfactory management of their global atherosclerotic risk usually have an excellent prognosis, regardless of the anatomic extent of CAD.[1,2,7,8,41] The test provides an estimate of the functional significance of angiographically documented coronary artery stenoses. The impact of exercise testing in patients with proven or suspected CAD was studied by Weiner and associates[2] in 4083 medically treated patients in the CASS study. A high-risk patient subset was identified (12% of the population), with an annual mortality rate of 5% when exercise workload was less than Bruce stage I (less than 4 METs) and the exercise ECG exhibited 0.1-mV (1-mm) ST-segment depression or higher. A low-risk patient subset (34% of the population) who could exercise into Bruce stage III or higher and who had a normal exercise electrocardiographic result had an annual mortality rate of less than 1% over 4 years of follow-up. Similar electrocardiographic and workload parameters were useful in risk-stratifying patients with three-vessel CAD likely to benefit from coronary bypass grafting.

Mark and coworkers[2] have developed a treadmill score based on 2842 consecutive patients with chest pain in the Duke data bank; these patients underwent treadmill testing using the Bruce protocol and cardiac catheterization.[1] Patients with left bundle branch block (LBBB) or those with exercise-induced ST elevation in a Q wave lead were excluded. The treadmill (TM) score is calculated as follows:

$$\text{TM score} = \text{exercise time} - (5 \times \text{ST-segment deviation}) - (4 \times \text{TM angina index})$$

Angina index was assigned a value of 0 if angina was absent, 1 if typical angina occurred during exercise, and 2 if angina was why the patient stopped exercising. Exercise-induced ST-segment deviation was defined as the largest net ST-segment displacement in any lead. The 13% of patients with a TM score of −11 or less had a 5-year survival rate of 72% as compared with a 97% survival rate among the 34% of patients at low risk with a TM score of +5 or higher. The score added independent prognostic information to that provided by clinical data, coronary anatomy, and left ventricular ejection fraction. The Duke TM score is not as effective in estimating risk in subjects 75 years of age or older (see later, "Older Patients").[45] Lauer and colleagues[41] have developed a more comprehensive multivariate model that includes age, gender, smoking history, hypertension, diabetes or typical angina, and exercise findings of functional capacity, ST-segment changes, symptoms, heart rate recovery, and frequent ventricular ectopy postexercise in 33,268 patients referred for suspected CAD who were followed a median of 6.2 years and validated the model in 5,821 patients (**Fig. 14-13**). In this study, both the Duke and Lauer scores classified patients into lower and higher risk patients subsets. However, the Lauer nomogram had better performance characteristics (discrimination and calibration) in predicting 3-year event rates as well as in the validation set. The Duke score tended to overestimate the intermediate- and high-risk categories; 64% of patients placed in this category by the Duke score were reclassified correctly as lower risk (0% to 3% mortality over 3 years). Exercise scoring systems can be used to identify prognostically intermediate- to high-risk patients in whom coronary angiography would be indicated to define coronary anatomy. However, the decision to perform coronary revascularization should take into consideration the fact that in patients with less extensive CAD (e.g., one to two vessels narrowed and well-preserved left ventricular function), a similar degree of exercise-induced myocardial ischemia does not carry the same significant increased risk of cardiac events as in patients with more extensive disease (e.g., three vessels narrowed or impaired left ventricular function). When estimating prognosis in individual patients from the population-based data collected over approximately the last three decades, consideration should be given to the fact that actual survival rates currently are likely to be greater because of more aggressive treatment of atherosclerotic risk factors and the use of noninvasive testing to identify the highest risk subjects who would benefit from coronary revascularization.

SILENT MYOCARDIAL ISCHEMIA. In patients with documented CAD, the presence of exercise-induced ischemic ST-segment depression confers an increased risk of subsequent cardiac events, regardless of whether angina occurs during the test. The magnitude of the prognostic gradient in patients with an abnormal exercise electrocardiographic result with or without angina varies considerably in the published literature, most likely a feature of patient selection. In the CASS data bank, 7-year survival in patients with silent (see Chap. 57)

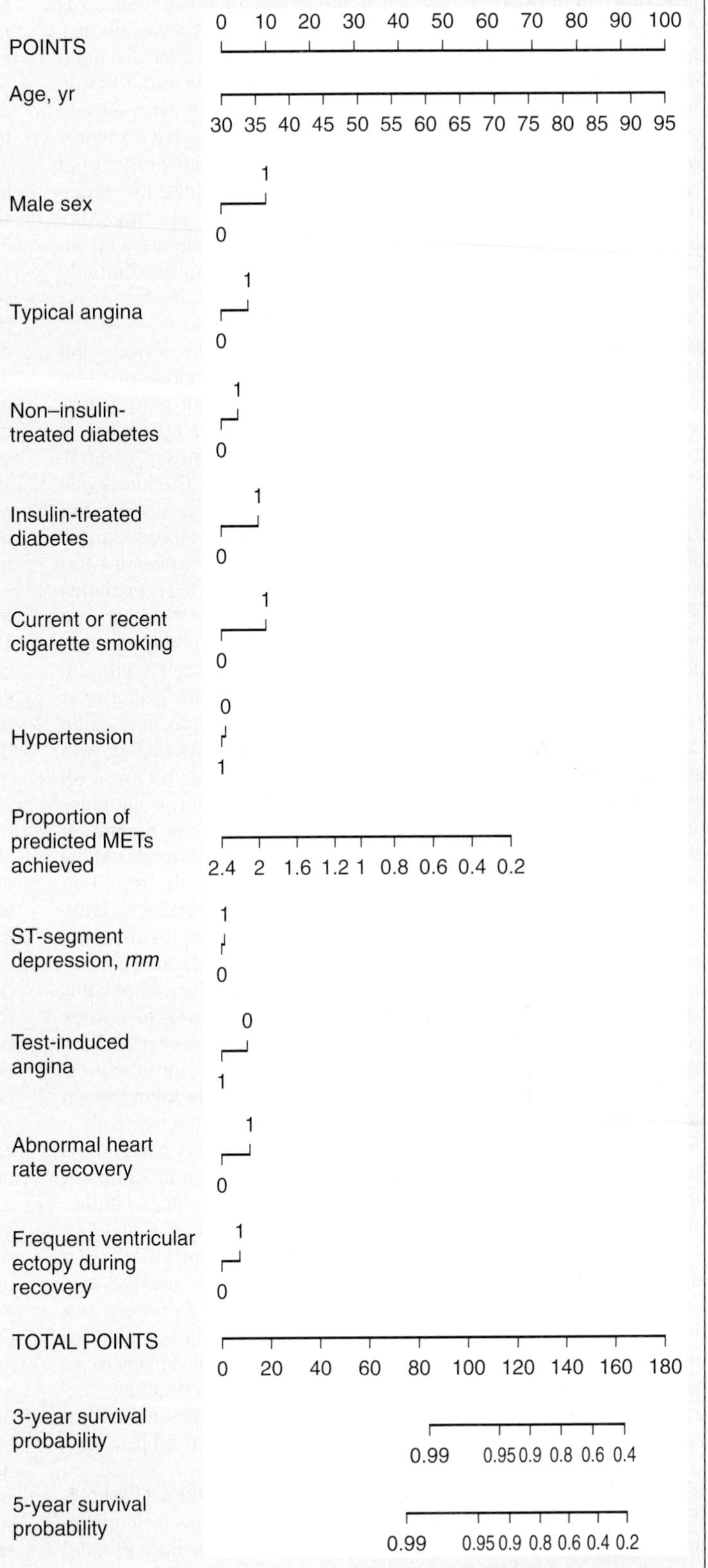

FIGURE 14-13 Nomogram of multivariable proportional hazards prediction model of total mortality derived from 33,268 patients and validated in 5,821 subjects. To determine risk, draw a vertical line from each risk marker to the top line, labeled "POINTS," to calculate points for each risk marker. The sum of all the points is then marked on the line labeled "TOTAL POINTS." Drop vertical lines from there to yield the 3- and 5-year survival probabilities. For binary variables, 1 means "yes" and 0 means "no." *(From Lauer MS, Pothier CE, Magid DJ, et al: An externally validated model for predicting long-term survival after exercise treadmill testing in patients with suspected coronary artery disease and a normal electrocardiogram. Ann Intern Med 147:821, 2007.)*

or symptomatic exercise-induced myocardial ischemia was similar in patients stratified by coronary anatomy and left ventricular function, with the worst survival in patients with the most extensive CAD.

ACUTE CORONARY SYNDROMES. The prognostic risk assessment after an acute coronary syndrome (see Chaps. 55 and 56) should incorporate findings from the history, physical examination, resting 12-lead ECG, and level of serum markers to optimize mortality and morbidity estimates and to categorize patients into low-, intermediate-, and high-risk groups.[46,47] Exercise testing should be considered in the outpatient evaluation of low-risk patients with unstable angina (biomarker negative) who are free of active ischemic signs (e.g., electrocardiographic changes) or symptoms for a minimum of 8 to 12 hours, and in hospitalized low- to intermediate-risk ambulatory patients who are free of angina or heart failure symptoms for at least 48 hours. In many intermediate- or high-risk patients, coronary angiography will have been performed during the acute phase of the illness; CAD extent, left ventricular function, and degree of coronary revascularization, if performed, should then be incorporated to determine the need and potential incremental value of the exercise test data to determine overall predischarge prognostic risk estimates. Patients who cannot perform or complete an exercise test for clinical reasons have a worse prognosis than those who can complete the protocol. Low functional capacity or abnormal hemodynamic responses to exercise are generally more predictive of an adverse prognosis than electrocardiographic measures of exercise-induced ischemia in patients with an acute coronary syndrome who have undergone partial or complete revascularization.

MYOCARDIAL INFARCTION. Exercise testing after myocardial infarction (both non–ST-segment and ST-segment elevation) is useful to determine the following: (1) functional capacity for activity prescription after hospital discharge; (2) assessment of adequacy of medical therapy and need to use supplemental diagnostic or treatment options; and (3) assessment of prognosis.[1,2,7,8,46-50] The incidence of fatal or nonfatal cardiac events associated with exercise testing after myocardial infarction is low and is slightly greater for symptom-limited protocols compared with submaximal tests. A low-level exercise test (achievement of 5 to 6 METs, or 70% to 80% of age-predicted maximum) is frequently performed before hospital discharge to establish the hemodynamic response and functional capacity. The ability to complete 5 to 6 METs of exercise or 70% to 80% of age-predicted maximum in the absence of an abnormal ECG or blood pressure response is associated with a 1-year mortality rate of 1% to 2% and may help guide the timing of early hospital discharge. Parameters associated with increased risk include inability to perform or complete the low-level predischarge exercise test, poor exercise capacity, inability to increase or a decrease in exercise systolic blood pressure, and angina or exercise-induced ST-segment depression at low workloads. Many postinfarct patients referred for exercise testing have been prescribed beta-adrenergic blocking agents and angiotensin-converting enzyme inhibitors. Although beta-adrenergic blocking drugs may attenuate the ischemic response, they do not interfere with poor functional capacity as a marker of adverse prognosis and should be continued in patients referred for testing. The relative prognostic value of a 3- to 6-week postdischarge exercise test is minimal once clinical variables and the results of the low-level predischarge test are taken into consideration. For this reason, the timing of the exercise test after the infarct event favors predischarge exercise testing to allow implementation of a definitive treatment plan in patients in whom coronary anatomy is known, as well as risk stratification of patients in whom coronary anatomy has not yet been determined. In many medical centers, predischarge exercise testing is performed within 3 to 4 days in uncomplicated patients after acute myocardial infarction (e.g. absence of recurrent chest pain, heart failure, renal insufficiency, hemodynamic instability, or cardiac arrhythmia). A 3- to 6-week test may be useful for clearing patients to return to work in occupations involving physical labor in whom the MET expenditure is likely to be higher than that on a predischarge test. In patients with baseline electrocardiographic abnormalities that compromise interpretation, myocardial imaging should be added to standard exercise testing.

RISK STRATIFICATION IN THE EMERGENCY DEPARTMENT. Patients who present to the emergency department are a heterogeneous population, with a large range of pretest risk for CAD. Clinical algorithms can identify lower risk persons who can safely be risk-stratified further using exercise testing.[51-54] In one series of 1000 symptomatic low-risk patients with chest pain, possibly of cardiac origin, who presented to the emergency department, Amsterdam and associates[52] have reported a positive, negative, and nondiagnostic exercise test result in 13%, 64%, and 23%, respectively. There were no adverse effects of exercise testing. Khare and coworkers[53] have studied a slightly lower risk population of 1194 patients admitted to a chest pain unit using exercise (81% of the subjects) with or without imaging and reported positive, negative, and indeterminate results in 5%, 91% and 4% of patients, respectively. Of patients with a positive noninvasive test result who underwent cardiac catheterization, only 27% had significant obstructive CAD. There is an increasing use of multidetector cardiac computed tomography (MDCT) in the emergency department setting to screen for high-risk coronary pathology as an alternative approach to exercise or pharmacologic stress testing (see Chap. 19). However, additional research is required to determine the cost-effectiveness and usefulness of this strategy and whether MDCT might be more optimally used as a complementary approach for patients who have an abnormal or indeterminate exercise and/or pharmacologic test result.

The accuracy of exercise testing in the emergency department setting follows bayesian principles, with the greatest diagnostic and prognostic estimates in intermediate-risk clinical patient subsets. Exercise testing in the emergency department should not be performed in the following situations: (1) new or evolving electrocardiographic abnormalities are noted on the rest tracing; (2) the levels of cardiac enzymes are abnormal; (3) the patient cannot adequately perform exercise; (4) the patient reports worsening or persistent chest pain symptoms; or (5) clinical risk profiling indicates that imminent coronary angiography is likely. Several series of clinically low-risk subjects have reported 6-month cardiac event rates lower than 1% with a normal exercise test result.

PREOPERATIVE RISK STRATIFICATION BEFORE NONCARDIAC SURGERY. Exercise electrocardiography before elective noncardiac surgery provides an objective measurement of functional capacity and the potential to identify the likelihood of perioperative myocardial ischemia in patients with a low ischemic threshold (see Chap. 85).[55] In patients with intermittent claudication and no prior history of cardiac disease, approximately 20% to 25% will have an abnormal exercise electrocardiographic result. In patients with a prior history of myocardial infarction or an abnormal resting ECG, 35% to 50% will have an abnormal exercise electrocardiographic result. Exercise testing may be useful in the evaluation of asymptomatic patients with peripheral arterial disease (see Chap. 61) and ankle brachial index readings lower than 0.90.[56] The risks of perioperative cardiac events and adverse long-term outcome are significantly increased in patients with abnormal exercise electrocardiographic results at low workloads. Coronary angiography with revascularization, when feasible, should be considered in such patients before noncardiac operative interventions that are considered high risk, such as aortic and other major vascular surgery and anticipated prolonged procedures associated with large fluid shifts or blood loss. Cardiopulmonary exercise testing may be used to risk-stratify patients prior to lung resection or organ transplantation.[57,58] In one series of 134 patients with end-stage liver disease referred for transplantation, a low preoperative peak $\dot{V}O_2$ during exercise was associated with significant reduced 1-year survival, longer duration of hospitalization, and greater need for postoperative oxygen support.[57]

CONGESTIVE HEART FAILURE. Cardiac and peripheral compensatory mechanisms are activated in patients with chronic congestive heart failure to restore impaired left ventricular performance partially or completely (see Chaps. 25 and 28). Abnormal baroreflex function and increased norepinephrine spillover, sympathetic discharge, downregulation of beta-adrenergic receptors, depletion of myocardial sympathetic stores, and increased peripheral and central chemosensitivity with abnormally increased ventilatory response to exercise characterize the disease process resulting in the cardiopulmonary response to exercise.[59-68] There is a wide range of exercise capacity in patients who have a markedly reduced ejection fraction, with some patients having near-normal peak exercise capacity. The magnitude of exercise capacity impairment is a function of the relative inability to augment stroke volume and abnormalities in skeletal muscle metabolism, which may be the predominant cause of functional limitation in a significant proportion of patients with heart failure. Fatigue may be related to altered skeletal muscle metabolism secondary to chronic physical deconditioning, impaired perfusion, and chronic anemia. Symptoms in patients with congestive heart failure are related to an excessive increase in blood lactate level during low exercise levels, reduction in quantity of oxygen consumed at peak exertion, and disproportionate increase in ventilation at submaximal and peak workloads. The increased ventilatory requirement assessed by the hyperventilatory response to exercise and increase in pulmonary dead space leads to rapid shallow breathing during exercise. Exercise oscillatory ventilation (EOV), characterized by the regular alteration of tidal volume with a crescendo-decrescendo pattern without interposed apnea, occurs in 12% to 30% of ambulatory heart failure patients managed at tertiary referral centers, is more common in patients with more advanced disease, and may be associated with an increased risk of sudden cardiac death (**Fig. 14-14**). EOV can be defined as an oscillatory pattern at rest that persists for 60% or more of the exercise test at an amplitude 15% or more of the average resting value. Dyspnea and fatigue are the usual reasons for exercise termination. Arterial desaturation does not usually occur unless there is associated pulmonary disease.

Peak $\dot{V}O_2$ measurements, defined as the highest $\dot{V}O_2$ values observed during the last 20 to 30 seconds of maximum exertion, in patients with compensated congestive heart failure are useful for risk-stratifying patients who have achieved anaerobic threshold to determine the subsequent incidence of cardiac events (**Fig. 14-15**).[1,8] The

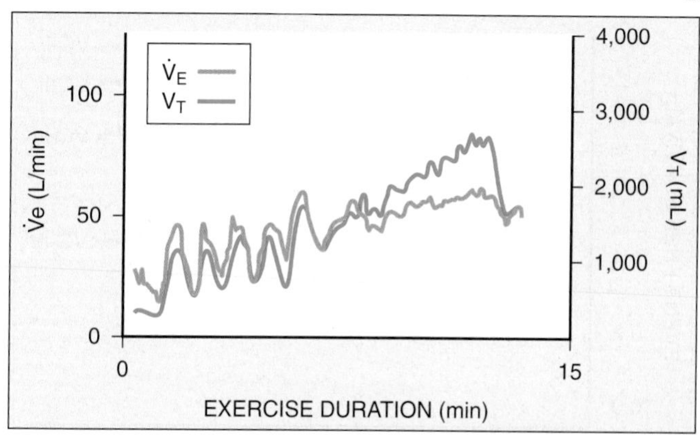

FIGURE 14-14 Oscillation of $\dot{V}e$ during exercise in a patient with chronic, stable New York Heart Association Class III heart failure. Ventilatory oscillation resolved during the final phase of exercise. Oscillation of $\dot{V}_T$ is also shown; in this patient, the magnitude of breath to breath $\dot{V}_T$ oscillation varied by more than 250% during a single oscillatory cycle. *(From Olson LJ, Arruda-Olson AM, Somers VK, et al: Exercise oscillatory ventilation. Instability of breathing control associated with advanced heart failure. Chest 133:474, 2008.)*

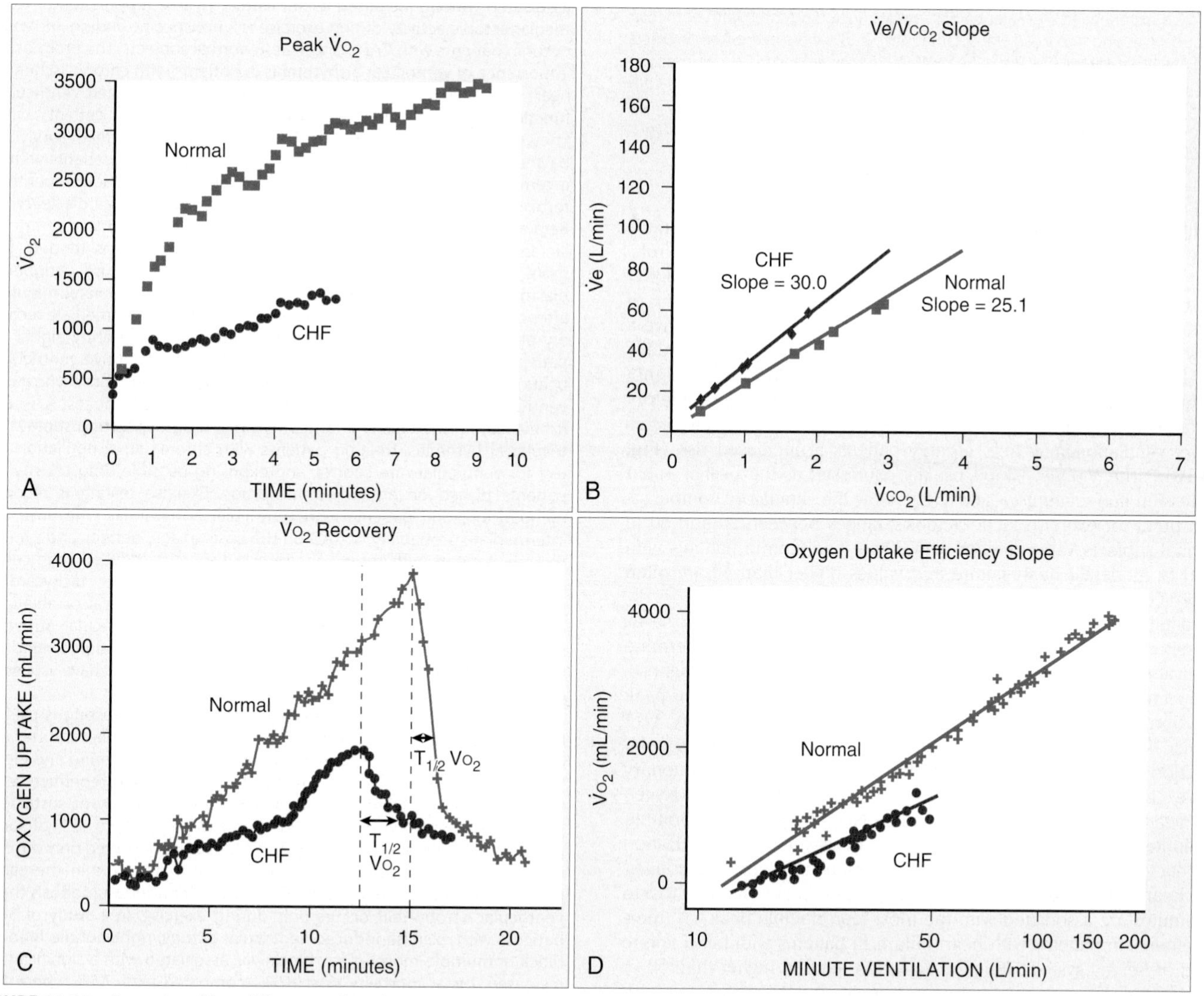

FIGURE 14-15 Examples of four different cardiopulmonary exercise test methods used to estimate prognosis in patients with cardiovascular disease. **A,** The peak $\dot{V}O_2$ responses are taken from a normal subject and a typical patient with chronic heart failure (CHF) of the same age. **B,** The $\dot{V}e/\dot{V}CO_2$ slope is derived from the regression line between $\dot{V}e$ and $\dot{V}CO_2$, excluding points beyond the ventilatory threshold. **C,** $\dot{V}O_2$ in recovery shows a more graded recovery response in the heart failure patient (i.e., longer recovery time), despite the lower exercise capacity. $T_{1/2}$ represents the time required for a 50% fall from the peak $\dot{V}O_2$ value. **D,** The oxygen uptake efficiency slope is derived by plotting $\dot{V}O_2$ against the log of $\dot{V}e$; a steeper slope reflects a lower $\dot{V}e$ for any given $\dot{V}O_2$—that is, more efficient ventilation. CHF = congestive heart failure. *(From Myers J: Applications of cardiopulmonary exercise testing in the management of a cardiovascular and pulmonary disease. Int J Sports Med 26:S49, 2005.)*

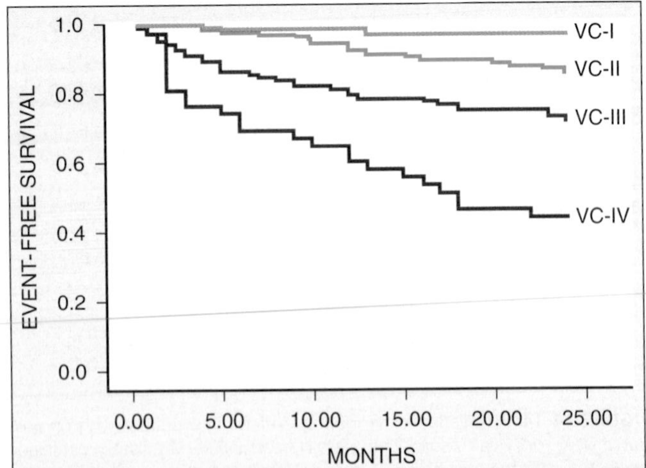

FIGURE 14-16 Kaplan-Meier analysis for 2-year major cardiac-related events. Subjects meeting criteria for VC-1 ($\dot{V}e/\dot{V}CO_2$ slope ≤ 29.9; $N = 144$) experienced four cardiac events (including two heart transplantations); 97.2% were event-free. Subjects meeting VC-II criteria ($\dot{V}e/\dot{V}CO_2$ slope, 30-35.9; $N = 149$) experienced 22 major cardiac events (including three left ventricular assist devices); 85.2% were event-free. Subjects meeting VC-III criteria ($\dot{V}e/\dot{V}CO_2$ slope 36-44.9; $N = 112$) experienced 31 major cardiac events (including three left ventricular assist devices and two heart transplantations); 72.3% were event-free. Subjects who met VC-IV criteria ($\dot{V}e/\dot{V}CO_2$ slope ≥ 45; $N = 43$) experienced 24 major cardiac events (including two left ventricular assist devices and five heart transplantations); 44.2% were event-free ($p < 0.001$). *(From Arena R, Myers J, Abella J, et al: Development of a ventilatory classification system in patients with heart failure. Circulation 115:2410, 2007.)*

ability to achieve a peak $\dot{V}O_2$ higher than 18 mL O_2/kg/min and anaerobic threshold higher than 14 mL O_2/kg/min is associated with a relatively good long-term prognosis and maximal cardiac output higher than 8 liters/min/m^2. Patients who are unable to achieve a peak $\dot{V}O_2$ of 10 mL O_2/kg/min and anaerobic threshold of 8 mL O_2/kg/min have a poor prognosis, and their maximal exercise cardiac output is usually less than 4 liters/min/m^2. When the peak $\dot{V}O_2$ ranges from 10 to 18 mL/kg/min, the prognostic risk is moderate; in this setting, ventilatory parameters such as a $\dot{V}e/\dot{V}CO_2$ slope higher than 35 or exercise oscillatory ventilation may help identify patients at increased risk (**Fig. 14-16**).[68] The $\dot{V}e/\dot{V}CO_2$ slope, usually expressed as the best-fit linear regression line relating $\dot{V}e$ and $\dot{V}CO_2$ below the ventilatory compensation point for exercise lactic acidosis, ranges between 20 and 30 in normal subjects. Values higher than 30 are common in patients with mild to moderate heart failure and values higher than 40 are often observed in those with more severe heart failure.

Patients with heart failure should be encouraged to exercise as closely as possible to a respiratory exchange ratio of 1.15 to determine motivation and ensure that the peak $\dot{V}O_2$ measurement is prognostically reliable. Failure of $\dot{V}O_2$ to decrease within 30 seconds after peak exertion, and accumulation of a large oxygen debt (recovery $\dot{V}O_2$/work), is associated with more severe reductions in left ventricular ejection fraction and moderate to severe impairment of pulmonary gas exchange. Inability to increase oxygen pulse (milliliters of oxygen per beat) is related to a lack of or a minimal increase of stroke volume. A blunted heart rate response caused by postsynaptic desensitization of beta-adrenergic receptors is not uncommon in patients with congestive heart failure. Exercise protocols that limit exercise duration to 5 to 7 minutes are associated with the most reproducible peak $\dot{V}O_2$ measurements in patients with heart failure. In patients with heart failure with preserved systolic function (ejection fraction higher than 50%), impaired exercise ventilation appears to be a more robust predictor of mortality and subsequent hospitalization than peak $\dot{V}O_2$. The interpretation of cardiopulmonary exercise test results in patients with heart failure can occasionally be difficult, because some patients hyperventilate during exercise, producing falsely low peak oxygen consumption, and it can be difficult to distinguish patients who are deconditioned from those who have impaired exercise performance and low peak $\dot{V}O_2$ caused by cardiac pathology. Randomized controlled trials of long-term moderate exercise training in patients with chronic heart failure have reported a 15% to 20% improvement in peak $\dot{V}O_2$ and prolonged onset of anaerobic metabolism. Thus, clinical decisions such as listing a patient for cardiac transplantation based on peak $\dot{V}O_2$ measurements need to take into consideration interval training effects, as well as changes in pharmacologic therapy, such as beta blockers. Walk tests can also be used to evaluate functional capacity and estimate prognosis in patients unable to exercise on a bicycle ergometer or treadmill. However, in patients with moderate to severe heart failure, peak $\dot{V}O_2$ measurements are more reliable than the walk test for clinical decisions.

Cardiac Arrhythmias and Conduction Disturbances

The genesis of cardiac arrhythmias includes reentry, triggered activity, and enhanced automaticity (see Chap. 35). Increased catecholamine levels during exercise accelerate impulse conduction velocity, shorten the myocardial refractory period, increase the amplitude of afterpotentials, and increase the slope of phase 4 spontaneous depolarization of the action potential. Other potentiators of cardiac rhythm disturbance include metabolic acidosis and exercise-induced myocardial ischemia. Ventricular premature complexes occur frequently during exercise testing and increase with age.[69] Repetitive forms occur in 0% to 5% of asymptomatic subjects without suspected cardiac disease and are not associated with an increased risk of cardiac death. Suppression of ventricular ectopic activity during exercise is a nonspecific finding and may occur in patients with CAD, as well as in normal subjects. The prognostic importance of ventricular arrhythmias in patients with chronic ischemic heart disease after adjustment for baseline, clinical, and left ventricular function characteristics is low. Approximately 20% of patients with known heart disease and 50% to 75% of sudden cardiac death survivors have repetitive ventricular beats induced by exercise. In patients with a recent myocardial infarction, the presence of exercise-induced repetitive forms is associated with an increased risk of subsequent cardiac events. Beta-adrenergic blocking drugs may suppress exercise-induced ventricular arrhythmias. Exercise-induced ventricular arrhythmias tend to be more frequent in the recovery phase of exercise because peripheral plasma norepinephrine levels continue to increase for several minutes after cessation of exercise, and vagal tone is high in the immediate recovery phase. Five-year all-cause mortality rates are significantly higher in patients who have frequent ventricular ectopy or repetitive ventricular beats in the recovery phase of exercise as compared with those who have ventricular arrhythmias that occur only during exercise. The test is useful for evaluating the effects of antiarrhythmic drugs, detecting supraventricular arrhythmias, treating patients with chronic atrial fibrillation to test for ventricular rate control, and exposing possible drug toxicity in patients placed on antiarrhythmic drugs. Exercise testing is recommended for adult patients with ventricular arrhythmias who have an intermediate probability of CAD on the basis of age, gender, and symptoms, in patients with known or suspected exercise-induced ventricular arrhythmias, including catecholaminergic ventricular tachycardia, regardless of age, and in evaluating response to medical or ablation therapy in patients with known exercise-induced ventricular arrhythmias. Exercise testing may occasionally be useful to evaluate middle-aged or older patients without evidence of CAD who have isolated premature ventricular complexes.

Evaluation of Ventricular Arrhythmias. Exercise testing is useful for the assessment of patients with ventricular arrhythmias and has an important adjunctive role, along with ambulatory monitoring and electrophysiologic studies.[1,2,7,8,69-71] Exercise testing provokes repetitive ventricular premature beats in most patients with a history of sustained ventricular tachyarrhythmia and, in approximately 10% to 15% of such patients, spontaneously occurring arrhythmias are observed only during exercise testing. Frequent ventricular ectopy that occurs in the early postexercise phase is associated with a worse long-term prognosis than ventricular ectopy that occurs only during exercise. In a study of 585 patients with exercise-induced ventricular ectopy, right bundle branch block or multiple-morphology block was associated with a significantly increased 2-year mortality rate (6.9%) compared with 2.5% when the morphology was an LBBB configuration or 1.8% in 2340 age-, gender-, and risk factor–matched control patients without ventricular ectopy.[71] In patients with adrenergic-dependent rhythm disturbances (including monomorphic ventricular tachycardia and polymorphic ventricular tachycardia related to long-QT syndromes), ambulatory electrocardiography or event monitoring may fail to capture the arrhythmia, particularly if the patient is relatively sedentary.

Supraventricular Arrhythmias. Supraventricular premature beats induced by exercise are observed in 4% to 10% of normal persons and in up to 40% of patients with underlying heart disease. Sustained supraventricular tachyarrhythmias occur in only 1% to 2% of patients, although the frequency may be as high as 10% to 15% in patients referred for management of episodic supraventricular arrhythmias. The presence of supraventricular arrhythmias is not diagnostic for ischemic heart disease, nor do they predict adverse long-term cardiovascular outcomes.

Atrial Fibrillation. Patients with chronic atrial fibrillation (see Chap. 40) tend to have a rapid ventricular response in the initial stages of exercise, and 60% to 70% of the total change in heart rate usually occurs within the first few minutes of exercise. The effect of digitalis preparations and beta-adrenergic and selected calcium antagonists, such as diltiazem, on attenuating this rapid increase in heart rate for individual patients can be measured using exercise testing. Pharmacologic control of the ventricular rate does not necessarily result in a significant increase in exercise capacity, which in many patients is related to the underlying cardiac disease process and not to adequacy of control of the ventricular rate.

Sinus Node Dysfunction. In general, patients with sinus node dysfunction have a lower heart rate at submaximal and maximal workloads compared with control subjects. However, as many as 40% to 50% of patients will have a normal exercise heart rate response.

Atrioventricular Block. Exercise testing may help determine the need for atrioventricular (AV) sequential pacing in selected patients. In patients with congenital AV block, exercise-induced heart rates are low and some patients develop symptomatic rapid junctional rhythms that can be suppressed with DDD devices (see Chap. 38). In patients with acquired conduction disease, exercise can occasionally elicit advanced AV block.

Left Bundle Branch Block. Exercise-induced ST segment depression is found in most patients with LBBB and cannot be used as a diagnostic or prognostic indicator, regardless of the degree of ST-segment abnormality. In patients who are referred to a tertiary center and in whom exercise testing is carried out, the new development of exercise-induced transient left hemiblock was found to be 0.3% and the new development of LBBB was 0.4%, with a slightly greater incidence in older patients. The relative risk of death or other major cardiac events in patients with exercise-induced LBBB is increased approximately threefold over the risk in patients without this abnormality. In one series, permanent LBBB was reported in approximately 50% of patients who developed transient LBBB during exercise and who were monitored for an average of 6.6 years.[8] High-grade AV block did not develop in any of the patients in this 15-patient series. The development of ischemic ST-segment depression before the LBBB pattern appears or in the recovery phase after the LBBB has resolved does not attenuate the diagnostic yield of the ST segment shift. The ventricular rates at which the LBBB appears and disappears can be significantly different (**Fig. 14-17**).

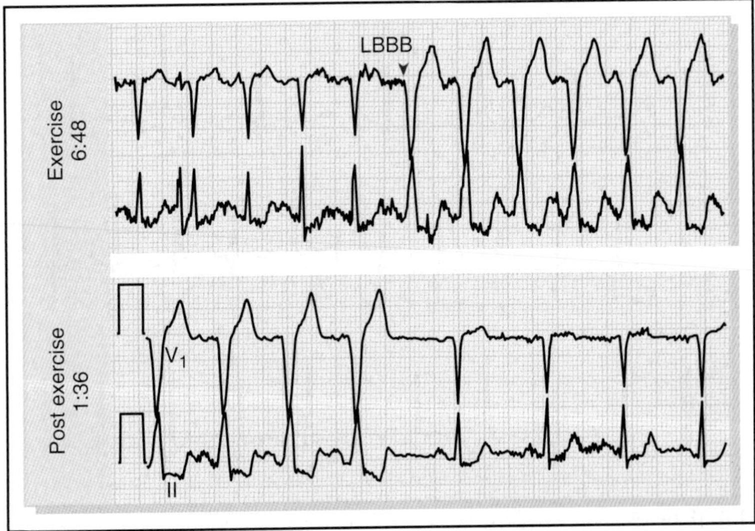

FIGURE 14-17 A 58-year-old hypertensive diabetic man with prior history of cigarette smoking was referred for evaluation of dyspnea and early fatigability during exercise. At 6:48 minutes into the test, the patient developed a rate-related LBBB at a heart rate of 133 beats/min, which persisted during exercise and resolved at 1:36 minutes into the postexercise phase. The abnormal 2.5- to 3-mm downsloping ST-segment depression in lead II during the LBBB is nondiagnostic for CAD because of the conduction disturbance. The test was stopped because of dyspnea at a peak heart rate of 138 beats/min (85% of predicted) and estimated workload of 6 METs. Peak blood pressure at the end of exercise was 174/94 mm Hg. Time to onset and offset of LBBB occurred at different ventricular rates related to fatigue in the left bundle, a common finding.

Right Bundle Branch Block. The resting ECG in patients with right bundle branch block (RBBB) is frequently associated with T wave and ST-segment changes in the early anterior precordial leads (V_1 to V_3). Exercise-induced ST-segment depression in leads V_1 to V_4 is a common finding in patients with RBBB and is nondiagnostic (**Fig. 14-18**). The new development of exercise-induced ST-segment depression in leads V_5 and V_6 or leads 2 and aVF, reduced exercise capacity, and inability to increase systolic blood pressure adequately are useful for detecting patients who have CAD and a high clinical pretest risk of disease. The presence of RBBB decreases the sensitivity of the test. The new development of exercise-induced RBBB is relatively uncommon, occurring in approximately 0.1% of test results.

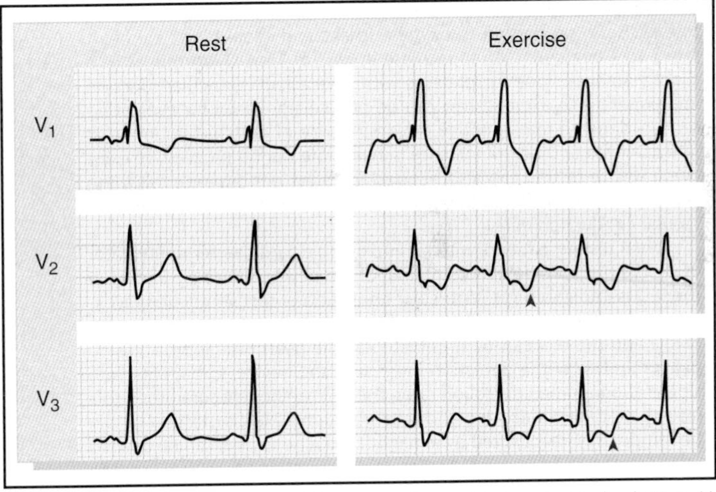

FIGURE 14-18 Exercise-induced ST-segment depression is noted in leads V_2 to V_3 (arrowheads) in this patient with a resting RBBB pattern. Exercise-induced horizontal or downsloping ST-segment responses in the early anterior precordial leads (V_1 through V_4) are common in patients with RBBB and are secondary to the conduction disturbance. The presence of this finding in leads V_1 through V_4 is not diagnostic of obstructive coronary disease; however, if ischemic changes are seen in lead II or aVF, or in leads V_5 or V_6, the specificity for coronary disease is improved.

Preexcitation Syndrome. The presence of Wolff-Parkinson-White syndrome invalidates the use of ST-segment analysis as a diagnostic method for detecting CAD in preexcited as well as normally conducted beats; false-positive ischemic changes are frequently registered (**Fig. 14-19**). In patients with persistent preexcitation, exercise may normalize the QRS complex, with disappearance of the delta wave in 20% to 50% of cases, depending on the series studied. Abrupt disappearance of the delta wave is presumptive evidence of a longer anterograde effective refractory period of the accessory pathway. Progressive disappearance of the delta wave is less reassuring and occurs when the improvement in AV node conduction is greater than in the accessory pathway; this finding does not preclude a possible significant or even critical shortening of the anterograde effective refractory period in the accessory pathway under the influence of sympathetic stimulation. Exercise-induced disappearance of the delta wave is more frequent with left-sided than right-sided accessory pathway positions. Although tachyarrhythmias appearing during an exercise test in patients with Wolff-Parkinson-White syndrome are rare, they provide an opportunity to evaluate AV conduction velocity when they do occur. The presence of Wolff-Parkinson-White syndrome does not cause a limitation of physical work capacity.

CH 14

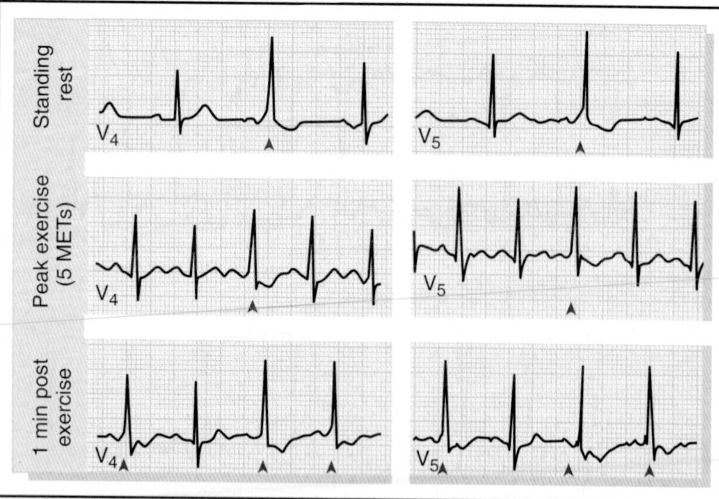

FIGURE 14-19 A 61-year-old man with atypical angina and a hiatal hernia was referred for diagnostic exercise testing. The test was stopped because of dyspnea. The standing resting ECG shows an intermittent Wolff-Parkinson-White pattern (arrowheads). In the nonpreexcited beats, ST-segment depression does not occur at peak exercise or in the postexercise phase. However, in the preexcited beats (arrowheads), an additional 1.3 mm of downsloping ST-segment depression is noted as compared with baseline during and after exertion.

Cardiac Pacemakers and Implantable Cardioverter-Defibrillator Devices. The exercise protocol used to assess chronotropic responsiveness in patients before and after cardiac pacemaker insertion should adjust for the fact that many patients with such devices are older persons and may not tolerate high exercise workloads or abrupt and relatively large increments in work between stages of exercise.[72,73] An optimal physiologic cardiac pacemaker should normalize the heart rate response to exercise in proportion to oxygen uptake and should increase heart rate 2 to 4 beats/min for an increase in $\dot{V}O_2$ of 1 mL O_2/kg/min, with a slightly steeper slope for patients with severe left ventricular function impairment. The exercise test can be particularly useful for evaluating sensor-triggered rate-adaptive pacing in terms of both maximum heart rate achieved and rate of increase in heart rate during progressive exercise. Exercise testing can also be used to assess performance following cardiac resynchronization therapy in patients with heart failure and ventricular conduction delay.

When testing patients with an implantable cardioverter-defibrillator (ICD), the program detection interval of the device should be known. If the ICD is implanted for ventricular fibrillation or fast ventricular tachycardia, the rate will normally exceed that attainable during sinus tachycardia and the test can be terminated as the heart rate approaches 10 beats/min below the detection interval of the device. In patients with slower programmed detection rates, the ICD can be reprogrammed to a faster rate to avoid accidental discharge during exercise testing or can be temporarily deactivated by a magnet. Exercise testing can be used to test the efficacy of tachycardic detection algorithms that apply criteria such as suddenness of onset and R-R variability.

Specific Clinical Applications

INFLUENCE OF DRUGS AND OTHER FACTORS. Patients with CAD demonstrate individual variability in time to onset of exercise-induced angina, time to onset of exercise-induced ischemic ST-segment depression of 0.1 mV or higher, and cardiovascular efficiency during exercise testing.[7,8] The average individual variability in time to onset of exercise-induced myocardial ischemia or peak anaerobic capacity approximates as much as 20% in placebo-controlled trials of antianginal drugs. Average increases in exercise duration approach 40 to 60 seconds after 2 to 4 weeks and as long as 90 seconds after 12 weeks of placebo therapy.[74] Variability can be reduced by the patient's familiarization with the exercise protocol and equipment, controlling for antianginal drug therapy at the time of testing, and stable test performance conditions. When two or three exercise tests are conducted within weeks of each other, the greatest increase in exercise time usually occurs between the first test and the second test. The mechanisms of the attenuation response with reexercise may be the results of ischemic preconditioning, familiarization with the exercise protocol, and improved musculoskeletal efficiency, but do not appear to be dependent on exercise protocol intensity or downregulation of myocardial contractility induced by the initial ischemic stimulus. In cold-sensitive individuals, exercise testing in a cooler environment results in onset of ischemic ST-segment depression earlier than under normal temperature-controlled conditions. Conditions that increase carbon monoxide levels, such as chronic cigarette smoking, lower the ischemic response threshold.

Digitalis glycosides can produce exertional ST-segment depression, even if the effect is not evident on the resting ECG, and can accentuate ischemic exercise-induced ST-segment changes, particularly in older individuals. Absence of ST-segment deviation during an exercise test in a patient receiving a cardiac glycoside is considered a valid negative response. Hypokalemia in patients on long-term diuretic therapy can be associated with exercise-induced ST-segment depression. In a double-blind randomized study of 40 patients with chronic stable angina on background antianginal drug therapy and preserved left ventricular function (75% with prior history of hypertension), 3 weeks of therapy with hydrochlorothiazide and amiloride increased placebo-corrected treadmill exercise time by 44 seconds and reduced the extent of exercise-induced ST-segment depression.[75] Anti-ischemic drug therapy with nitrates, beta-blocking drugs, or calcium channel blocking drugs prolongs the time to onset of ischemic ST-segment depression, increases exercise tolerance and, in a small minority of patients (10% to 15%), may normalize the exercise electrocardiographic response in patients with documented CAD.[7,8] The time and dose of drug ingestion may affect exercise performance. In some laboratories, cardioactive drug therapy is withheld for three to five half-lives and digitalis for 1 to 2 weeks before diagnostic testing, but this is impractical in many cases. In 336 patients with stable angina, documented CAD, preserved rest left ventricular function, and absence of uncontrolled hypertension, high-dose angiotensin-converting enzyme inhibition failed to change the time to exercise-induced angina or ischemic ST-segment depression or improve peak exercise capacity after 16 weeks of therapy compared with placebo.[76]

WOMEN. The diagnostic accuracy of exercise-induced ST-segment depression for obstructive CAD is lower in women than in men. Populations of young and middle-aged women have less extensive CAD than men, resulting in a lower sensitivity to detect CAD using noninvasive tests such as exercise testing in this age group. Women tend to have a greater release of catecholamines during exercise, which could potentiate coronary vasoconstriction and augment the incidence of abnormal exercise electrocardiographic results, as well as a lower prevalence of CAD compared with men, and false-positive results have been reported to be more common during menses or preovulation and in postmenopausal women on isolated estrogen replacement therapy.[77] The initial evaluation of women with suspected CAD and a normal resting ECG with adequate exercise capability should be an exercise electrocardiographic treadmill study. The exercise electrocardiographic data should be integrated with peak exercise capacity achieved, heart rate, and blood pressure changes to optimize prognostic accuracy.[77-81] In asymptomatic women, a low exercise capacity, low heart rate recovery, and failure to reach target heart rate are more important predictors of outcome than exercise-induced ECG changes (**Fig. 14-20**). Morise and colleagues[81] have reported mortality rates ranging from 0.2% for a low-risk score to 7% for a high-risk score based on five clinical and three exercise test variables after an average 2.6-year follow-up in 442 symptomatic women referred for their first exercise test. In symptomatic women with an intermediate to high likelihood of CAD, imaging procedures should be considered as the initial test when the resting ECG is abnormal or exercise capacity is questionable.

HYPERTENSION. Exercise testing has been used in an attempt to identify patients who have an abnormal blood pressure response and are destined subsequently to develop hypertension.[23-25] In

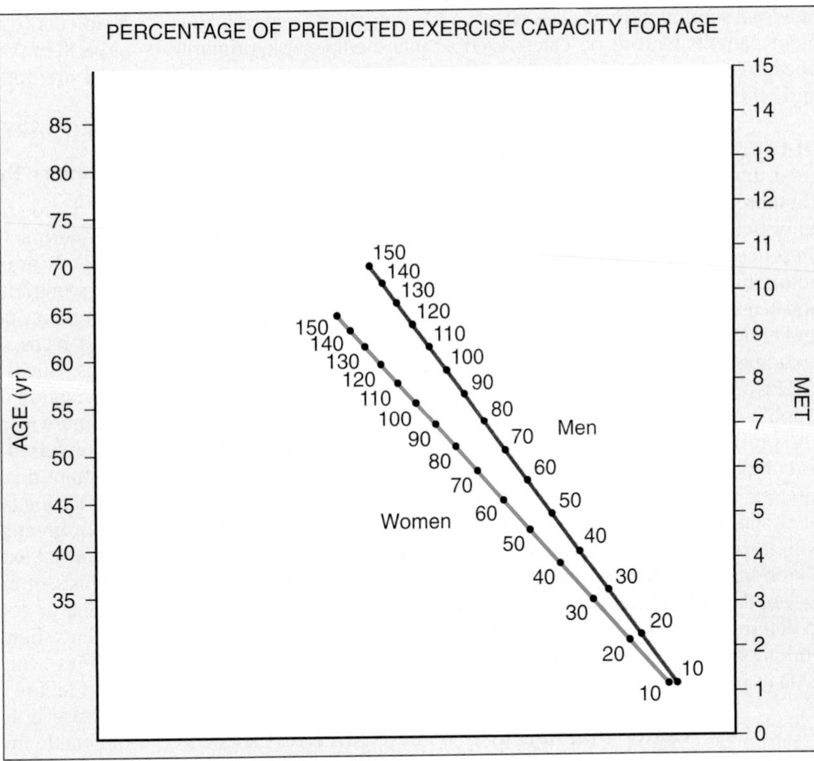

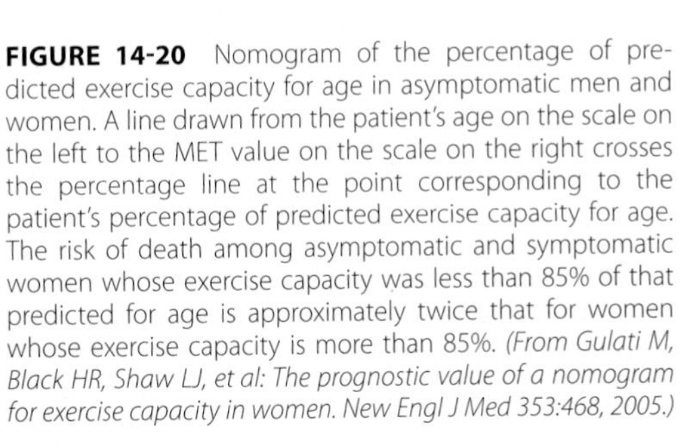

FIGURE 14-20 Nomogram of the percentage of predicted exercise capacity for age in asymptomatic men and women. A line drawn from the patient's age on the scale on the left to the MET value on the scale on the right crosses the percentage line at the point corresponding to the patient's percentage of predicted exercise capacity for age. The risk of death among asymptomatic and symptomatic women whose exercise capacity was less than 85% of that predicted for age is approximately twice that for women whose exercise capacity is more than 85%. *(From Gulati M, Black HR, Shaw LJ, et al: The prognostic value of a nomogram for exercise capacity in women. New Engl J Med 353:468, 2005.)*

asymptomatic normotensive individuals, an exaggerated exercise systolic and diastolic blood pressure response during exercise, an exaggerated peak systolic blood pressure response to 214 mm Hg or higher, or an elevated systolic or diastolic blood pressure at the third minute of recovery is associated with significant increased long-term risk of hypertension (**Fig. 14-21**).[82] Severe systemic hypertension may interfere with subendocardial perfusion and cause exercise-induced ST-segment depression in the absence of atherosclerosis, even when the resting ECG does not show significant ST or T wave changes. Beta- and calcium channel blocking drugs decrease submaximal and peak systolic blood pressure in many hypertensive patients. Exercise tolerance is decreased in patients with poor blood pressure control. In a cross-sectional study of 2545 treated hypertensive Italian patients with preserved left ventricular function (ejection fraction > 45%) and average age of 70 years, diastolic dysfunction was found in 26% to 46% of subjects, a finding associated with decreased exercise capacity in other reports.[83,84]

OLDER PATIENTS. Maximal aerobic capacity $\dot{V}O_2$max declines 5% to 10% per decade in sedentary men and women, with an approximately 50% reduction in exercise capacity between the ages of 30 and 80 years, accelerating in the later decades of life.[1,2,14] The exercise protocol in older patients should be selected according to estimated aerobic capacity. In patients with limited exercise tolerance, the test should be started at the slowest speed, with a 0% grade, and adjusted according to the patient's ability. Older patients may need to grasp the handrails for support. The frequency of abnormal exercise electrocardiographic patterns is higher in older than in younger individuals, and the risk of cardiac events is significantly increased because of a concomitant increase in the prevalence of more extensive CAD.[13,85]

The greater test sensitivity of the exercise ECG in older subjects is accompanied by a slight reduction in specificity. Cardiac arrhythmias, chronotropic incompetence, and hypertensive responses are more common in older individuals. The value of exercise testing to estimate prognosis in older subjects was evaluated in 3107 patients from Olmstead County, of whom 512 were 65 years of age or older. Workload expressed in METs was the only variable associated with all-cause mortality in subjects 65 years of age or older, whereas workload and exercise-induced angina were predictive of cardiac death or nonfatal myocardial infarction.[86] In subjects 75 years of age or older, the Duke

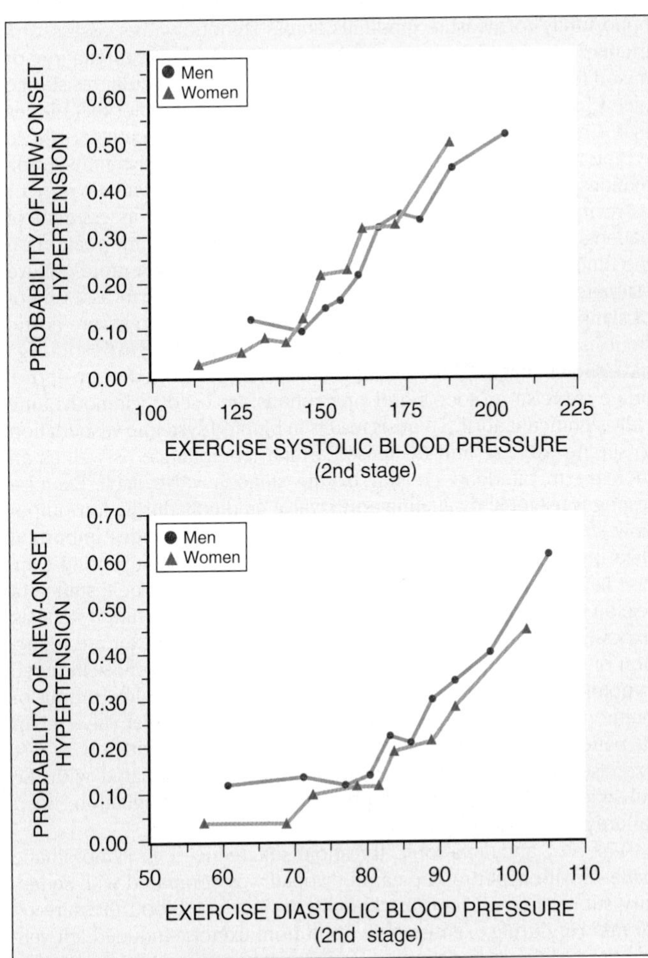

FIGURE 14-21 Probability of developing systemic hypertension within 8 years after exercise testing as a function of exercise-induced systolic **(top panel)** and diastolic **(bottom panel)** blood pressure responses in men and women. Crude probabilities of developing hypertension are displayed for mean systolic or diastolic blood pressure values for each exercise response during the second stage of treadmill testing. *(From Singh JP, Larson MG, Manolio TA, et al: Blood pressure response during treadmill testing is a risk factor for new onset hypertension. The Framingham Heart Study. Circulation 99:1831, 1999.)*

treadmill scoring system is less effective for estimating prognosis. Most older patients tend to be categorized as intermediate risk, primarily because they cannot exercise long enough to be classified as low risk, and other scoring systems should be considered.[39]

DIABETES MELLITUS. Coronary atherosclerosis and peripheral vascular disease are significantly increased in adult diabetic patients as compared with nondiabetic patients (see Chap. 64); the likelihood of atherosclerosis correlates closely with the duration of diabetes and the presence of microvascular disease, peripheral vascular disease, and autonomic neuropathy.[87,88] In patients with autonomic dysfunction and sensory neuropathy, the perception of angina may be diminished, and abnormal rest and exercise-induced heart rate (e.g., chronotropic incompetence) and blood pressure responses are common.[89] Once CAD is established, the incidence of exercise-induced electrocardiographic changes is similar to the incidence in nondiabetic persons. The probability of an adverse cardiac outcome in a diabetic person as compared with a nondiabetic person for a similar abnormal exercise test result is likely to be increased because of the increased risk of dyslipidemia, impaired fibrinolysis, and hypertension associated with the diabetic process. Patients with diabetes who wish to enroll in a moderate- to high-intensity exercise program are considered to have a class IIa indication for exercise testing.[1] Further research is required to determine optimal noninvasive test procedures for diagnosing early endothelial dysfunction and the presence and extent of obstructive CAD in patients with diabetes.

VALVULAR HEART DISEASE AND HYPERTROPHIC CARDIOMYOPATHY. The hemodynamics of exercise provide an excellent opportunity to measure gradients across stenotic valves, assess ventricular function in patients with primary valvular regurgitation or mixed lesions, and assess pulmonary and systemic vascular resistance (see Chap. 66).[90-92] The use of echocardiographic Doppler techniques (see Chap. 15) is particularly valuable for evaluating patients whose symptoms are out of proportion to the degree of hemodynamic abnormalities observed at rest and assessing the results of valvulotomy or valve replacement. Clinical and exercise noninvasive assessment of patients with valvular heart disease can provide useful information on the timing of operative intervention and help achieve a more precise estimate of a patient's degree of incapacitation than can assessment of symptoms alone. Studies of adults with moderate to severe aortic stenosis (e.g., valve area, 0.5 to 1.5 cm^2; mean gradients, 18 to 64 mm Hg) have shown that exercise testing can be safely performed when appropriate exercise protocols and precautions are used.[90] Hemodynamically significant aortic stenosis results in blunted systemic vasodilation to supine exercise and decreased arterial compliance, as well as an increase in afterload created by the stenotic valve itself. Exercise testing is useful in evaluating aortic valve gradients during low-output flow states and, with Doppler echocardiography, provides important data on left ventricular functional reserve. Hypotension during exercise in asymptomatic patients with aortic stenosis may be a sufficient reason to consider valve replacement.[90] In patients with mitral stenosis, excessive heart rate response to relatively low levels of exercise, reduction of cardiac output with exercise (manifested by exercise-induced hypotension), and chest pain (ischemia secondary to low output or pulmonary hypertension) are indicators that favor earlier valve repair. In patients with mitral valve prolapse without regurgitation at rest, exercise-induced mitral regurgitation has been associated with the subsequent development of progressive mitral regurgitation, heart failure symptoms, or syncope.

Peak $\dot{V}O_2$ and anaerobic threshold are reduced in symptomatic patients with hypertrophic cardiomyopathy as compared with sedentary subjects (see Chap. 69). Inability to increase blood pressure by 20 mm Hg during exercise may result from exercise-induced left ventricular systolic dysfunction and is associated with an adverse prognosis. Abnormal blood pressure responses in patients with hypertrophic cardiomyopathy may normalize after transcoronary alcohol septal ablation, associated with only a slight increase in exercise time. Exercise testing is relatively safe in patients with hypertrophic cardiomyopathy and resting or inducible gradients.[93] Patients with high resting gradients (e.g., more than 4 meters/sec), New York Heart Association class III or IV symptoms, and a history of important ventricular arrhythmias are not generally tested.

CORONARY REVASCULARIZATION

Coronary Bypass Grafting

The degree of improvement in exercise-induced myocardial ischemia and aerobic capacity after coronary bypass grafting (see Chap. 57) depends in part on the degree of revascularization achieved and on left ventricular function. Exercise-induced ischemic ST-segment depression may persist when incomplete or, rarely, even when complete revascularization is achieved, albeit at higher exercise workloads. Stress imaging studies are likely to provide more useful information regarding the site and extent of myocardial ischemia after coronary revascularization procedures than the exercise ECG, and are the preferred modality when noninvasive testing is performed for management decisions. The diagnostic and prognostic usefulness of exercise testing late after coronary revascularization (e.g., 5 to 10 years) is much greater than early (less than 1 year) testing, because a late abnormal exercise response is more likely to indicate graft occlusion, stenosis, or progression of CAD, particularly in the presence of typical angina or conditions of accelerated atherosclerosis, such as diabetes mellitus, hemodialysis, or immunosuppressive therapy.[94] In selected patients with severe left ventricular dysfunction and symptomatic heart failure, coronary bypass surgery is associated with a significant increase in exercise capacity when a large amount of dysfunctional but viable myocardium (e.g., more than 25% of left ventricular mass) is revascularized.

Percutaneous Coronary Intervention

The risk of restenosis after PCI is time-dependent; stent restenosis usually occurs within the first 12 months after PCI, and is significantly reduced (less than 10%) with the use of drug-eluting stents (see Chap. 58). In the early post-PCI phase (less than 1 month), an abnormal exercise electrocardiographic result may be secondary to a suboptimal result, impaired coronary vascular reserve in a successfully dilated vessel, or incomplete revascularization.[95] Thus, exercise electrocardiography has a low diagnostic accuracy to detect restenosis or an incomplete dilation in the periprocedural phase. The optimal time to perform an exercise test after PCI depends in part on the success of the procedure and the degree of revascularization obtained. In an otherwise asymptomatic patient, a 6- to 12-month postprocedure test allows sufficient time to document restenosis should it occur and allows the dilated vessel an opportunity to heal. Serial conversion of an initially normal exercise test result after PCI to an abnormal result in the initial 6 months after the procedure, particularly when it occurs at a lower exercise workload, is usually associated with restenosis. The use of exercise myocardial imaging in selected patients enhances the diagnostic content of the test and can help localize the territory of myocardial ischemia and guide indications for repeat coronary angiography in patients who have undergone multivessel or multilesion PCI.

Clinical stent thrombosis or access site complications were not increased in one randomized trial of exercise testing performed early after coronary stenting.[96]

CARDIAC TRANSPLANTATION AND LEFT VENTRICULAR ASSIST DEVICES. Cardiopulmonary exercise testing is useful for selecting patients with end-stage heart failure for cardiac transplantation and for evaluating left ventricular assist devices (LVADs; see Chap. 32).[97-101] In a multicenter series of 67 subjects with various LVAD implants, peak $\dot{V}O_2$ increased from 13.7 mL O_2/kg/min after 30 days to 18.9 mL O_2/kg/min after 120 days, despite no change in peak LVAD flow and a progressive reduction on rest left ventricular ejection fraction.[97] A peak $\dot{V}O_2$ of less than 10 mL O_2/kg/min is associated with a poor short-term outcome.[59] The use of percentage of predicted $\dot{V}O_2$, which adjusts an individual patient's peak $\dot{V}O_2$ for age, gender, and weight rather than weight alone, and assessment of $Ve/\dot{V}CO_2$ slope measurements have been shown to enhance prognostic estimates further in patients with a low peak exercise $\dot{V}O_2$. In patients with initial poor exercise capacity awaiting heart transplantation, the ability to increase peak oxygen uptake with increased peak oxygen pulse identifies a relatively lower risk group in whom cardiac transplantation could be deferred if the patient's clinical status is stable.

Exercise performance in transplant recipients is influenced by the fact that the donor heart is surgically denervated without efferent parasympathetic or sympathetic innervation, and by the occurrence of rejection and scar formation, systemic and pulmonary vascular resistance, level of training, and development of coronary atherosclerosis in the graft. Exercise hyperpnea in some patients may be related to persistent increased peripheral chemoreceptor sensitivity. Maximal oxygen uptake and work capacity are reduced after cardiac transplantation compared with measures in age-matched control subjects, but usually are markedly improved compared with preoperative findings.[100] Abnormalities of the ventricular rate response include a resting tachycardia caused by parasympathetic denervation, a slow heart rate response during mild to moderate exercise, a more rapid response during more strenuous exercise, and a more prolonged time for the ventricular rate to return to baseline during recovery. The transplanted heart relies heavily on the Frank-Starling mechanism to increase cardiac output during mild to moderate exercise. Systemic vascular resistance may be increased because of cyclosporine therapy. Sympathetic reinnervation of the sinus node may occur after cardiac transplantation and may partially restore a normal heart rate response to exercise, but in most patients will not return exercise capacity to normal. The exercise ECG is relatively insensitive for detecting coronary artery vasculopathy after cardiac transplantation. However, the new development of an abnormal exercise electrocardiographic result several years after cardiac transplantation may indicate focal intraluminal narrowing.

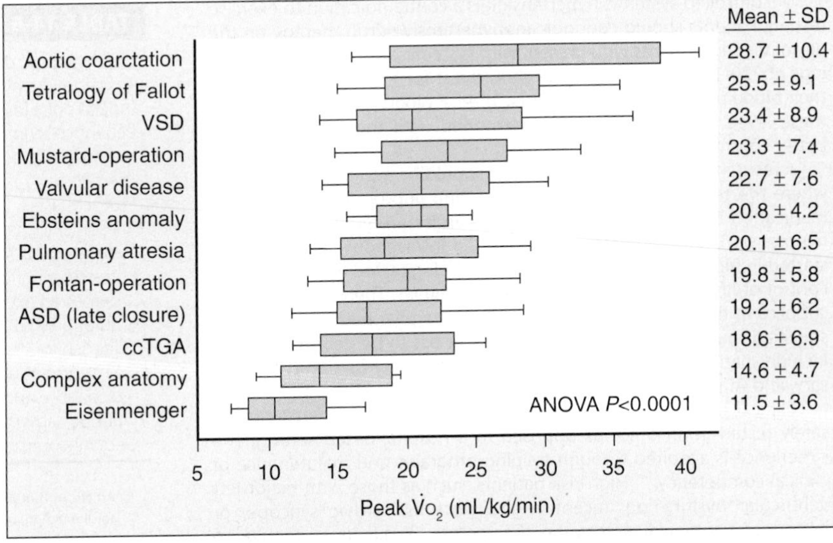

FIGURE 14-22 Distribution of peak $\dot{V}O_2$ measurements in different diagnostic categories of a consecutive series of patients with adult congenital heart disease ($N = 335$) who underwent cardiopulmonary exercise testing. Peak $\dot{V}O_2$ measurements were predictive of death and repeat hospital admissions over a median follow-up of 304 (range, 17-580) days. Cardiopulmonary exercise capacity (peak $\dot{V}O_2$) was significantly worse in patients with cyanotic lesions, pulmonary hypertension, and complex pathology. ANOVA = analysis of variance between groups; ASD = atrial septal defect; ccTGA = congenitally corrected transposition of the great vessels; VSD = ventricular septal defect. *(From Diller GP, Dimopoulos K, Okonko D, et al: Exercise intolerance in adult congenital heart disease: comparative severity, correlates, and prognostic implication. Circulation 112:828, 2005.)*

ADULT CONGENITAL HEART DISEASE AND PULMONARY HYPERTENSION. Exercise capacity is usually decreased in adults with congenital heart disease, even in the absence of symptoms (see Chaps. 65 and 78).[102,103] Chronotropic response to exercise, pulmonary arterial hypertension, impaired pulmonary function, and underlying cardiac anatomy are important determinants of peak exercise capacity. Low peak $\dot{V}O_2$ measurements are associated with increased hospital admissions and survival (**Fig. 14-22**). Patients with simple noncyanotic lesions, with biventricular hearts without pulmonary arterial hypertension, have a significantly greater exercise capacity and better prognosis than patients with complex or cyanotic lesions and pulmonary arterial hypertension. Exercise testing with Doppler echocardiography may be useful in assessing dynamic changes in pulmonary vascular compliance. In a study of 191 patients with idiopathic and familial pulmonary artery hypertension, exercise-induced hypertensive tricuspid regurgitation velocities were observed in 32% of 291 relatives compared with 10% of age-matched controls.[104]

TABLE 14-5 Absolute Contraindications to Exercise Testing
Acute myocardial infarction (<2 days)
High-risk unstable angina
Decompensated heart failure
Uncontrolled cardiac arrhythmias with symptoms or hemodynamic compromise
Advanced atrioventricular block
Acute myocarditis or pericarditis
Severe symptomatic aortic stenosis
Severe hypertrophic obstructive cardiomyopathy
Uncontrolled hypertension
Acute systemic illness (pulmonary embolism, aortic dissection)

SAFETY AND RISKS OF EXERCISE TESTING

Exercise testing has an excellent safety record.[105] The risk is determined by the clinical characteristics of the patient referred for the procedure. In nonselected patient populations, the mortality is less than 0.01% and morbidity is less than 0.05%. The risk is greater when the test is performed soon after an acute ischemic event. In a survey of 151,941 tests conducted within 4 weeks of an acute myocardial infarction, mortality was 0.03%, and 0.09% of patients tested either had a nonfatal reinfarction or were resuscitated from cardiac arrest.[106] The relative risk of a major complication is about twice as great when a symptom-limited protocol is used as compared with a low-level protocol. Nevertheless, in the early postinfarction phase, the risk of a fatal complication during symptom-limited testing is only 0.03%. The risk is less for low-risk patients who are seen in the emergency department and who undergo exercise testing for risk stratification. Exercise testing can be safely performed in patients with compensated congestive heart failure, with no major complications reported in 1,286 tests in which a bicycle ergometer was used.[107] The risk of exercise testing in patients referred for life-threatening ventricular arrhythmias was examined by Young and associates[108] in a series of 263 patients who underwent 1,377 tests; 2.2% developed sustained ventricular tachyarrhythmias that required cardioversion, cardiopulmonary resuscitation, or antiarrhythmic drugs to restore sinus rhythm. The ventricular arrhythmias were more frequent in tests performed on patients who were receiving antiarrhythmic drug therapy as compared with the baseline drug-free state. In contrast to the high risk in the aforementioned patient subsets, the risk of complications in asymptomatic subjects is extremely low, with no fatalities reported in several series.[1,7,8]

The risk of incurring a major complication during exercise testing can be reduced by performing a careful history and physical examination before the test and observing patients closely during exercise with monitoring of the ECG, arterial pressure, and symptoms. The standard 12-lead ECG should be verified before the test for any acute or recent changes. The contraindications to exercise testing are well defined (**Table 14-5**). Patients with critical obstruction to left ventricular outflow are at increased risk of cardiac events during exercise. In selected patients, low-level exercise can be useful in determining the severity of the left ventricular outflow tract obstruction. The cool-down period should be prolonged to at least 2 minutes in patients with left ventricular outflow tract obstruction or stenotic valves to avoid sudden pressure-volume shifts, which occur in the immediate postexercise phase.

Uncontrolled systemic hypertension is a contraindication to exercise testing. Patients should continue antihypertensive drug therapy on the day of testing. Patients who present with systemic arterial pressure readings of 220/120 mm Hg or higher should rest for 15 to 20 minutes, and their blood pressure should be remeasured. If blood pressure remains at these levels, the test should be postponed until the hypertension is better controlled.

A resuscitation cart and defibrillator should be available in the room where the test procedure is carried out, and appropriate cardioactive medication should be available to treat cardiac arrhythmias, AV block, hypotension, and persistent chest pain. An intravenous line should be started in high-risk patients, such as those being tested for adequacy of control of life-threatening ventricular arrhythmias. The equipment and supplies in the cart should be checked on a regular basis. A previously specified routine for cardiac emergencies needs to be determined; this includes patient transfer and admission to a coronary care unit, if necessary, and ACLS certification for personnel performing the test.

Clinical judgment is required to determine which patients can be safely tested in an office as opposed to a hospital-based setting. The experience is acquired through training programs and maintenance of clinical competency.[109] High-risk patients, such as those with major left ventricular dysfunction, recent angina pectoris, cardiac syncope, or important ventricular ectopy on the pretest examination, should be tested in the hospital. Low-risk patients, such as asymptomatic individuals and those with a low pretest risk of disease, can be tested by specially trained nurses or physician assistants who have received advanced cardiac life support certification, with a physician in close proximity.

Termination of Exercise

The use of standard test indications to terminate an exercise test reduces risk (see Table 14G-2). Termination of exercise should be determined in part by the patient's recent activity level. The rate of perceived patient exertion can be estimated by the Borg scale. The scale is linear, with values of 9 for very light, 11 for fairly light, 13 for somewhat hard, 15 for hard, 17 for very hard, and 19 for very, very hard. Borg readings of 14 to 16 approximate anaerobic threshold, and readings of 18 or higher approximate a patient's maximum exercise capacity. It is helpful to grade exercise-induced chest discomfort on a 1 to 4 scale, with 1 indicating the initial onset of chest discomfort and 4 the most severe chest pain the patient has ever experienced. The exercise technician should note the onset of grade 1 chest discomfort on the work sheet, and the test should be stopped when the patient reports grade 3 chest pain. In the absence of symptoms, it is prudent to stop exercise when a patient demonstrates 0.3 mV (3 mm) or higher of ischemic ST segment depression or 0.1 mV (1 mm) or higher of ST-segment elevation in a noninfarct lead without an abnormal Q wave. Significant worsening of ambient ventricular ectopy during exercise or the unsuspected appearance of ventricular tachycardia is an indication to terminate exercise. A progressive, reproducible decrease in systolic blood pressure of 10 mm Hg or more may indicate transient left ventricular dysfunction or an inappropriate decrease in systemic vascular resistance, and is an indication to terminate exercise. The test should be stopped if the arterial blood pressure is 250 to 270/120 to 130 mm Hg or higher. Ataxia can indicate cerebral hypoxia.

The exercise test report should contain basic demographic data, the indication for testing, a brief description of the patient's profile, and exercise test results (**Table 14-6**).

TABLE 14-6 Exercise Test Report Information

Demographic data: Name, patient identifier, date of birth and age, gender, weight, height, test date
Indication(s) for test
Patient descriptors: Atherosclerotic risk profile, drug usage, resting electrocardiographic findings
Exercise test results
Protocol used
Reason(s) for stopping exercise
Hemodynamic data: Resting and peak heart rate, resting and peak blood pressure, percentage of maximum achieved heart rate, maximum rate of perceived exertion (Borg scale), peak workload, peak METs, total exercise duration in minutes
Evidence for myocardial ischemia: Time to onset and offset of ischemic ST-segment deviation or angina, maximum depth of ST-segment deviation, number of abnormal exercise electrocardiographic leads, abnormal systemic blood pressure responses
General comments

REFERENCES

1. Gibbons RJ, Balady GJ, Bricker JT, et al: ACC/AHA 2002 guideline update for exercise testing. Summary article: A report of the ACC/AHA Task Force on Practice Guidelines (Committee to Update the 1997 Exercise Testing Guidelines). J Am Coll Cardiol 40:1531, 2002.
2. Gibbons RJ, Abrams J, Chatterjee K, et al: ACC/AHA 2002 Guideline update for the management of patients with chronic stable angina. A Report of the American College of Cardiology/American Heart Association Task Force on Practice Guidelines (Committee to Update the 1999 Guidelines for the Management of Patients with Chronic Stable Angina) (http://www.acc.org/qualityandscience/clinical/guidelines/stable/stable_clean.pdf).
3. Thompson WR, Gordon NF, Pescatello LS: ACSM's Guidelines for Exercise Testing and Prescription. 8th ed. Philadelphia, Lippincott Williams & Wilkins, 2010.
4. Wasserman K, Hansen JE, Sue DY, et al: Principles of Exercise Testing and Interpretation. Including Pathophysiology and Clinical Applications. 4th ed. Philadelphia, Lippincott Williams & Wilkins, 2005.
5. American Thoracic Society/American College of Chest Physicians: Statement on cardiopulmonary exercise testing. Am J Respir Crit Care Med 167:211, 2003.

Exercise Physiology

6. Skinner JS: Exercise Testing and Exercise Prescription for Special Cases: Theoretical Basis and Clinical Application. 3rd ed. Philadelphia, Lippincott Williams & Wilkins, 2005.
7. Ellestad MH: Stress Testing: Principles and Practice. 5th ed. New York, Oxford University Press, 2003.
8. Froelicher VF, Myers J: Exercise and the Heart. 5th ed. Philadelphia, WB Saunders, 2006.
9. Paridon SM, Alpert BS, Boas SR, et al: Clinical stress testing in the pediatric age group: A statement from the American Heart Association Council on Cardiovascular Disease in the Young, Committee on Atherosclerosis, Hypertension, and Obesity in Youth. Circulation 113:1905, 2006.
10. Arena R, Myers J, Williams MA, et al: Assessment of functional capacity in clinical and research settings. A Scientific Statement from the American Heart Association Committee on Exercise, Rehabilitation, and Prevention of the Council on Clinical Cardiology and the Council on Cardiovascular Nursing. Circulation 116:329, 2007.
11. Williams MA, Haskell WL, Ades P, et al: Resistance exercise in individuals with and without cardiovascular disease: 2007 update. A Scientific Statement from the American Heart Association Council on Clinical Cardiology and Council on Nutrition, Physical Activity, and Metabolism. Circulation 116:572, 2007.
12. Hall JE: Guyton and Hall Textbook of Medical Physiology. 12th ed. Philadelphia, Saunders, 2010.
13. Ingelsson E, Larson MG, Vasan RS, et al: Heritability, linkage, and genetic associations of exercise treadmill test responses. Circulation 115:2917, 2007.
14. Fleg JL, Morrell CH, Bos AG, et al: Accelerated longitudinal decline of aerobic capacity in healthy older adults. Circulation 112:674, 2005.
15. Tanaka H, Monahan KD, Seals DR: Age-predicted maximal heart rate revisited. J Am Coll Cardiol 37:153, 2001.
16. Correia LCL, Lakatta EG, O'Connor FC, et al: Attenuated cardiovascular reserve during prolonged submaximal cycle exercise in healthy older subjects. J Am Coll Cardiol 40:1290, 2002.

16a. Gulati M, Shaw LJ, Thisted RA, et al: Heart rate response to exercise stress testing in asymptomatic women: The St. James Women Take Heart Project. Circulation 122:130, 2010.

17. Maeder M, Wolber T, Atefy R, et al: Impact of the exercise mode on exercise capacity. Bicycle testing revisited. Chest 128:2804, 2005.
18. Newman AB, Simonsick EM, Naydeck BL, et al: Association of long distance corridor walk performance with mortality, cardiovascular disease, mobility limitation and disability. JAMA 295:2018, 2006.

Electrocardiographic Measures

19. Okin PM, Prineas RJ, Grandits G, et al: Heart rate adjustment of exercise-induced ST segment depression identifies men who benefit from a risk factor reduction program. Circulation 96:2899, 1997.
20. Bogaty P, Poirier P, Boyer L, et al: What induces the warm-up ischemia/angina phenomenon: Exercise or myocardial ischemia? Circulation 107:1858, 2003.
21. Li RA, Leppo M, Miki T, et al: Molecular basis of electrocardiographic ST-segment elevation. Circ Res 87:837, 2000.

Nonelectrocardiographic Observations

22. Fleg JL, Lakatta EG: Prevalence and significance of postexercise hypotension in apparently healthy subjects. Am J Cardiol 57:1380, 1986.
23. Miyai N, Arita M, Miyashita K, et al: Blood pressure response to heart rate during exercise test and risk of future hypertension. Hypertension 39:761, 2002.
24. Shim CY, Ha JW, Park S, et al: Exaggerated blood pressure response to exercise is associated with augmented rise of angiotensin II during exercise. J Am Coll Cardiol 52:287, 2008.
25. Lewis GD, Gona P, Larson MG, et al: Exercise blood pressure and the risk of incident cardiovascular disease (from the Framingham Heart Study). Am J Cardiol 101:1614, 2008.
26. Kokkinos P, Myers J, Kokkinos JP, et al: Exercise capacity and mortality in black and white men. Circulation 117:614, 2008.
27. Hooker SP, Sui X, Colabianchi N, et al: Cardiorespiratory fitness as a predictor of fatal and nonfatal stroke in asymptomatic women and men. Stroke 39:2950, 2008.
28. Kodama S, Saito K, Tanaka S, et al: Cardiorespiratory fitness as a quantitative predictor of all-cause mortality and cardiovascular events in healthy men and women. A meta-analysis. JAMA 301:2024, 2009.

29. Peterson PN, Magid DJ, Ross C, et al: Association of exercise capacity on treadmill with future cardiac events in patients referred for exercise testing. Arch Intern Med 168:174, 2008.
30. Gulati M, Pandey DK, Arnsdorf MF, et al: Exercise capacity and the risk of death in women. The St. James Women Take Heart Project. Circulation 108:1554, 2003.
31. Kim ESH, Ischwaran H, Blackstone E, Lauer MS: External prognostic validations and comparisons of age- and gender- adjusted exercise capacity predictions. J Am Coll Cardiol 50:1867, 2007.
32. Chaitman BR: Should early acceleration of heart rate during exercise be used to risk stratify patients with suspected or established coronary artery disease? Circulation 115:430, 2007.
33. Jouven X, Empana JP, Schwartz PJ, et al: Heart-rate profile during exercise as a predictor of sudden death. N Engl J Med 352:1951, 2005.
34. Adabag AS, Grandits GA, Prineas RJ, et al: Relation of the heart rate parameters during exercise test to sudden death and all-cause mortality in asymptomatic men. Am J Cardiol 101:1437, 2008.
35. Girotra S, Keelan M, Weinstein AR, et al: Relation of heart rate response to exercise with prognosis and atherosclerotic progression after coronary artery bypass grafting. Am J Cardiol 103:1386, 2009.
36. Chaitman BR: Abnormal heart rate responses to exercise predict increased long-term mortality regardless of coronary disease extent. The question is why? J Am Coll Cardiol 42:2049, 2003.
37. Gera N, Taillon LA, Ward RP: Usefulness of abnormal heart rate recovery on exercise stress testing to predict high-risk findings on single-photon emission computed tomography myocardial perfusion imaging in men. Am J Cardiol 103:611, 2009.
38. Morise AP: Heart rate recovery: Predictor of risk today and target of therapy tomorrow? Circulation 110:2778, 2004.

Diagnostic and Prognostic Applications

39. Morise AP, Jalisi F: Evaluation of pretest and exercise test scores to assess all-cause mortality in unselected patients presenting for exercise testing with symptoms of suspected coronary artery disease. J Am Coll Cardiol 42:842, 2003.
40. Morise A, Evans M, Jalisi F, et al: A pretest prognostic score to assess patients undergoing exercise or pharmacological stress testing. Heart 93:200, 2007.
41. Lauer MS, Pothier CE, Magid DJ, et al: An externally validated model for predicting long-term survival after exercise treadmill testing in patients with suspected coronary artery disease and a normal electrocardiogram. Ann Intern Med 147:821, 2007.
42. Myers J, Prakash M, Froelicher V, et al: Exercise capacity and mortality among men referred for exercise testing. N Engl J Med 346:793, 2002.
43. Gehi AK, Ali S, Na B, et al: Inducible ischemia and the risk of recurrent cardiovascular events in outpatients with stable coronary heart disease. The Heart and Soul Study. Arch Intern Med 168:1423, 2008.
44. Lin GA, Dudley RA, Lucas FL, et al: Frequency of stress testing to document ischemia prior to elective percutaneous coronary intervention. JAMA 300:1765, 2008.
45. Lai S, Kaykha A, Yamazaki T, et al: Treadmill scores in elderly men. J Am Coll Cardiol 43:606, 2004.
46. Anderson JL, Adams CD, Antman EM, et al: ACC/AHA 2007 Guidelines for the management of patients with unstable angina/non-ST-elevation myocardial infarction. J Am Coll Cardiol 50:e1, 2007.
47. Antman EM, Hand M, Armstrong, et al: 2007 Focused update of the ACC/AHA 2004 guidelines for the management of patients with ST-elevation myocardial infarction. A Report of the American College of Cardiology/American Heart Association Task Force on Practice Guidelines. J Am Coll Cardiol 51:210, 2008.
48. Dutcher JR, Kahn J, Grines C, Franklin B: Comparison of left ventricular ejection fraction and exercise capacity as predictors of two- and five-year mortality following acute myocardial infarction. Am J Cardiol 99:436, 2007.
49. De Luca G, Suryapranata H, van't Hof AWJ, et al: Prognostic assessment of patients with acute myocardial infarction treated with primary angioplasty. Implications for early discharge. Circulation 109:2737, 2004.
50. Fernandez-Avilés F, Alonso JJ, Castro-Beiras A, et al: Routine invasive strategy within 24 hours of thrombolysis versus ischaemia-guided conservative approach for acute myocardial infarction with ST-segment elevation (GRACIA-1): A randomised controlled trial. Lancet 364:1045, 2004.
51. Stein RA, Chaitman BR, Balady GJ, et al: Safety and utility of exercise testing in emergency room chest pain centers: An advisory from the Committee on Exercise, Rehabilitation and Prevention, Council on Clinical Cardiology, American Heart Association. Circulation 102:1463, 2000.
52. Amsterdam EA, Kirk JD, Diercks DB, et al: Immediate exercise testing to evaluate low-risk patients presenting to the emergency department with chest pain. J Am Coll Cardiol 40:251, 2002.
53. Khare RK, Powell ES, Venkatesh AK, Courtney DM: Diagnostic uncertainty and costs associated with current emergency department evaluation of low risk chest pain. Crit Pathw Cardiol 7:191, 2008.
54. Jeetley P, Burden L, Stoykova B, Senior R: Clinical and economic impact of stress echocardiography compared with exercise electrocardiography in patients with suspected acute coronary syndrome but negative troponin: A prospective randomized controlled study. Eur Heart J 28:204, 2007.
55. Fleisher LA, Beckman JA, Brown KA, et al: ACC/AHA 2007 Guidelines on perioperative cardiovascular evaluation and care for noncardiac surgery: Executive summary. A report of the American College of Cardiology/American Heart Association Task Force on Practice Guidelines (Writing Committee to Revise the 2002 Guidelines on Perioperative Cardiovascular Evaluation for Noncardiac Surgery). Circulation 116:1971, 2007.
56. McDermott MM, Guralnik JM, Ferrucci L, et al: Asymptomatic peripheral arterial disease is associated with more adverse lower extremity characteristics than intermittent claudication. Circulation 117:2484, 2008.
57. Dharancy S, Lemyze M, Boleslawski E, et al: Impact of impaired aerobic capacity on liver transplant candidates. Transplantation 86:1077, 2008.
58. Benzo R, Kelley GA, Recchi L, et al: Complications of lung resection and exercise capacity: A meta-analysis. Respir Med 101:1790, 2007.
59. Hunt SA, Abraham WT, Chin MH, et al: 2009 Focused update incorporated into the ACC/AHA 2005 guidelines for the diagnosis and management of heart failure in adults. A report of the American College of Cardiology Foundation/American Heart Association Task Force on Practice Guidelines. J Am Coll Cardiol 53:e1, 2009.
60. Chase P, Arena R, Myers J, et al: Relation of the prognostic value of ventilatory efficiency to body mass index in patients with heart failure. Am J Cardiol 101:348, 2008.
61. Borlaug BA, Melenovsky V, Russel SD, et al: Impaired chronotropic and vasodilator reserves limit exercise capacity in patients with heart failure and a preserved ejection fraction. Circulation 114:2138, 2006.
62. Myers J, Arena R, Dewey R, et al: A multivariate scoring system for predicting risk in heart failure. Am Heart J 156:1177, 2008.
63. Hsich E, Gorodeski EZ, Starling RC, et al: Importance of treadmill exercise time as an initial prognostic screening tool in patients with systolic left ventricular dysfunction. Circulation 119:3189, 2009.
64. Corrà U, Mezzani A, Giordano A, et al: Exercise haemodynamic variables rather than ventilatory efficiency indexes contribute to risk assessment in chronic heart failure patients treated with carvedilol. Eur Heart J 30:3000, 2009.
65. Guazzi M, Myers J, Arena R: Cardiopulmonary exercise testing in the clinical and prognostic assessment of diastolic heart failure. J Am Coll Cardiol 46:1883, 2005.
66. Guazzi M, Raimondo R, Vicenzi M, et al: Exercise oscillatory ventilation may predict sudden cardiac death in heart failure patients. J Am Coll Cardiol 50:299, 2007.
67. Olson LJ, Arruda-Olson AM, Somers VK, et al: Exercise oscillatory ventilation. Instability of breathing control associated with advanced heart failure. Chest 133:474, 2008.
68. Arena R, Myers J, Abella J, et al: Development of a ventilatory classification system in patients with heart failure. Circulation 115:2410, 2007.
69. Zipes DP, Camm AJ, Borggrefe M, et al: ACC/AHA/ESC 2006 guidelines for the management of patients with ventricular arrhythmias and the prevention of sudden cardiac death. A report of the American College of Cardiology/ American Heart Association Task Force and the European Society of Cardiology Committee for Practice Guidelines (Writing Committee to Develop Guidelines for Management of Patients With Ventricular Arrhythmias and the Prevention of Sudden Cardiac Death). J Am Coll Cardiol 48:e247, 2006.
70. Haugaa KH, Leren IS, Berge KE, et al: High prevalence of exercise-induced arrhythmias in catecholaminergic polymorphic ventricular tachycardia mutation-positive family members diagnosed by cascade genetic screening. Europace 12:417, 2010.
71. Eckart RE, Field ME, Hruczkowski TW, et al: Association of electrocardiographic morphology of exercise-induced ventricular arrhythmia with mortality. Ann Intern Med 149:451, 2008.
72. Melzer C, Korber T, Theres H, et al: How can the rate-adaptive atrioventricular delay be programmed in atrioventricular block pacing? Europace 9:319, 2007.
73. Salukhe TV, Dimopoulos K, Sutton R, et al: Instantaneous effects of resynchronization therapy on exercise performance in heart failure patients: The mechanistic role and predictive power of total isovolumic time. Heart 94:59, 2008.

Specific Clinical Applications

74. Chaitman BR: Efficacy and safety of a metabolic modulator drug in chronic angina: Review of evidence from clinical trials. J Cardiovasc Pharmacol Therapeut 9:S47, 2004.
75. Finimundi HC, Caramori PA, Parker JD: Effect of diuretic therapy on exercise capacity in patients with chronic angina and preserved left ventricular function. J Cardiovasc Pharmacol 49:275, 2007.
76. Pepine CJ, Rouleau JL, Annis K, et al: Effects of angiotensin-converting enzyme inhibition on transient ischemia. The Quinapril Anti-Ischemia and Symptoms of Angina Reduction (QUASAR) Trial. J Am Coll Cardiol 42:2049, 2003.
77. Mieres JH, Shaw LJ, Arai A, et al: Role of noninvasive testing in the clinical evaluation of women with suspected coronary artery disease. Consensus Statement from the Cardiac Imaging Committee, Council on Clinical Cardiology, and the Cardiovascular Imaging and Intervention Committee, Council on Cardiovascular Radiology and Intervention, American Heart Association. Circulation 111:682, 2005.
78. Gulati M, Black HR, Shaw LJ, et al: The prognostic value of a nomogram for exercise capacity in women. N Engl J Med 353:468, 2005.
79. Mora S, Redberg RF, Cui Y, et al: Ability of exercise testing to predict cardiovascular and all-cause death in asymptomatic women. A 20-year follow-up of the Lipid Research Clinics Prevalence Study. JAMA 290:1600, 2003.
80. Kavanagh T, Mertens DJ, Hamm LF, et al: Peak oxygen intake and cardiac mortality in women referred for cardiac rehabilitation. J Am Coll Cardiol 42:2139, 2003.
81. Morise AP, Lauer MS, Froelicher VF: Development and validation of a simple exercise test score for use in women with symptoms of suspected coronary artery disease. Am Heart J 144:818, 2002.
82. Singh JP, Larson MG, Manolio TA, et al: Blood pressure response during treadmill testing as a risk factor for new-onset hypertension. The Framingham Study. Circulation 99:1831, 1999.
83. Zanchetti A, Cuspidi C, Comarella L, et al: Left ventricular diastolic dysfunction in elderly hypertensives: results of the APROS-diadys study. J Hypertens 25:2158, 2007.
84. Grewal J, McCully RB, Kane GC, et al: Left ventricular function and exercise capacity. JAMA 301:286, 2009.
85. Jeger RV, Zellweger MJ, Kaiser C, et al: Prognostic value of stress testing in patients over 75 years of age with chronic angina. Chest 125:1124, 2004.
86. Goraya TY, Jacobsen SJ, Pellikka PA, et al: Prognostic value of treadmill exercise testing in elderly persons. Ann Intern Med 132:862, 2000.
87. Albers AR, Krichavsky MZ, Balady GJ: Stress testing in patients with diabetes mellitus. Diagnostic and prognostic value. Circulation 113:583, 2006.
88. Lyerly GW, Sui X, Church TS, et al: Maximal exercise electrocardiography responses and coronary heart disease mortality among men and diabetes mellitus. Circulation 117:2734, 2008.
89. Ho PM, Maddox TM, Ross C, et al: Impaired chronotropic response to exercise stress testing in patients with diabetes predicts future cardiovascular events. Diabetes Care 31:1531, 2008.
90. Bonow RO, Carabello BA, Chatterjee K, et al: 2008 Focused update incorporated into the ACC/AHA 2006 guidelines for the management of patients with vascular heart disease. A Report of the American College of Cardiology/ American Heart Association Task Force on Practice

Guidelines (Writing Committee to Revise the 1998 Guidelines for the Management of Patients With Valvular Heart Disease). J Am Coll Cardiol 52:e1, 2008.

91. Picano E, Pibarot P, Lancellotti P, et al: The emerging role of exercise testing and stress echocardiography in valvular heart disease. J Am Coll Cardiol 54:2251, 2009.
92. Laskey WK, Kussmaul WG, Noordergraaf A: Systemic arterial response to exercise in patients with aortic valve stenosis. Circulation 119:996, 2009.
93. Gimeno JR, Tome-Esteban M, Lofiego C, et al: Exercise-induced ventricular arrhythmias and risk of sudden cardiac death in patients with hypertrophic cardiomyopathy. Eur Heart J 30:2599, 2009.
94. Krone RJ, Hardison RM, Chaitman BR, et al: Risk stratification after successful coronary revascularization: The lack of a role for routine exercise testing. J Am Coll Cardiol 38:136, 2001.
95. Smith SC, Feldman T, Hirshfeld JW, et al: ACC/AHA/SCAI 2005 Guideline update for percutaneous coronary intervention. A report of the American College of Cardiology/American Heart Association Task Force on Practice Guidelines (ACC/AHA/SCAI Writing Committee to Update the 2001 Guidelines for Percutaneous Coronary Intervention). J Am Coll Cardiol 47:e1, 2006.
96. Roffi M, Wenaweser P, Windecker S, et al: Early exercise after coronary stenting is safe. J Am Coll Cardiol 42:1569, 2003.
97. Maybaum S, Mancini D, Xydas S, et al: Cardiac improvement during mechanical circulatory support. A prospective multicenter study of the LVAD Working Group. Circulation 115:2497, 2007.
98. Haft J, Armstrong W, Dyke DB, et al: Hemodynamic and exercise performance with pulsatile and continuous-flow left ventricular assist devices. Circulation 116:I-8, 2007.
99. Kavanagh T, Mertens DJ, Shephard RJ: Long-term cardiorespiratory results of exercise training following cardiac transplantation. Am J Cardiol 91:190, 2003.
100. Myers J, Geiran O, Simonsen S, et al: Clinical and exercise test determinants of survival after cardiac transplantation. Chest 124:2000, 2003.
101. Ciarka A, Cuylits N, Vachiery JL, et al: Increased peripheral chemoreceptors sensitivity and exercise ventilation in heart transplant recipients. Circulation 113:252, 2006.
102. Diller GP, Dimopoulos K, Okonko D, et al: Exercise intolerance in adult congenital heart disease. Comparative severity, correlates, and prognostic implication. Circulation 112:828, 2005.
103. Glaser S, Opitz CF, Bauer U, et al: Assessment of symptoms and exercise capacity in cyanotic patients with congenital heart disease. Chest 125:368, 2004.

Safety and Risks of Exercise Testing

104. Grunig E, Weissmann S, Ehlken N, et al: Stress Doppler echocardiography in relatives of patients with idiopathic and familial pulmonary arterial hypertension. Results of a multicenter European analysis of pulmonary artery pressure response to exercise and hypoxia. Circulation 119:1747, 2009.
105. Myers J, Arena R, Franklin B, et al: Recommendations for clinical exercise laboratories: A scientific statement from the American Heart Association. Circulation 119:3144, 2009.
106. Hamm LF, Crow RS, Stull GA, Hannan P: Safety and characteristics of exercise testing early after acute myocardial infarction. Am J Cardiol 63:1193, 1989.
107. Tristani FE, Hughes CV, Archibald DG, et al: Safety of graded symptom-limited exercise testing in patients with congestive heart failure. Circulation 76:VI-54, 1987.
108. Young DZ, Lampert S, Graboys TB, Lown B: Safety of maximal exercise testing in patients at high risk for ventricular arrhythmia. Circulation 70:184, 1984.
109. Myerburg RJ, Chaitman BR, Ewy GA, Lauer MS: Task Force 2: Training in electrocardiography, ambulatory electrocardiography, and exercise testing. J Am Coll Cardiol 51:348, 2008.

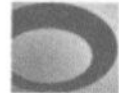

GUIDELINES

BERNARD R. CHAITMAN

Exercise Stress Testing

Several sets of guidelines for the performance of exercise testing have been published by the American Heart Association and by committees commissioned jointly by the American College of Cardiology and the American Heart Association (ACC/AHA). The use of exercise testing is addressed in guidelines for specific clinical syndromes, including chronic stable angina,[1] acute coronary syndromes,[2,3] coronary revascularization,[4-6] congestive heart failure,[7,8] perioperative cardiac evaluation,[9] valvular heart disease,[10] congenital heart disease[11] and pulmonary hypertension,[12] cardiac arrhythmias[13,14] and syncope,[15] and the use of exercise as a stressor for cardiac imaging studies.[16,17]

CLINICAL PRACTICE GUIDELINES

The purpose of developing clinical practice guidelines (CPGs) by the ACC/AHA, summarized by Antman and Peterson,[18] is to summarize the evidence on randomized controlled trials and, if unavailable, other forms of trials, meta-analyses, and registry data to provide evidence-based standards of care. Appropriate use criteria (AUC) were subsequently developed in response to potential overuse or misuse of advanced technologies and to determine whether a particular approach to care is reasonable in a given clinical scenario. The AUC do not have the same rigorous evidence-based standard because randomized controlled or other trial data may not have been done in the various clinical scenarios presented. The CPG itself may not always have the strongest scientific evidence on which to base its recommendations; for example, of 16 ACC/AHA CPG recommendations, a median of 11% were classified as level of evidence A, whereas 48% were level of evidence C.[19] Therefore, clinicians must always use excellent clinical judgment armed with information contained in guidelines such as CPGs or AUC for guiding individual patient care.

The CPGs generally consist of four levels of recommendations based on the level of benefit to risk. Thus, in a Class I recommendation, the benefit greatly outweighs the risk, whereas in a Class III recommendation, the risk is greater than or the same as the benefit. For Class IIa and IIb recommendations, the benefit is greater than the risk and greater than or the same as the risk, respectively. The three levels of evidence to support the recommendations outlined range from A to C. Level A evidence includes multiple population risk strata evaluated and general consistency of direction and magnitude of effect, whereas level C evidence contains very limited (one or two) population risk strata evaluated, and level B is intermediate levels of evidence.

EXERCISE TEST PERFORMANCE AND TRAINING

Absolute and relative contraindications to exercise testing are illustrated in the ACC/AHA exercise test guidelines published in 2002 (**Table 14G-1**)

TABLE 14G-1 ACC/AHA Guidelines: Absolute and Relative Contraindications to Exercise Testing

Absolute
Recent significant change in the rest electrocardiogram (ECG) suggestive of significant ischemia or other acute cardiac event
Acute systemic infection accompanied by fever, body aches, or lymphadenopathy
Acute myocardial infarction (within 2 days)
High-risk unstable angina
Uncontrolled cardiac arrhythmias causing symptoms or hemodynamic compromise
Symptomatic severe aortic stenosis
Uncontrolled symptomatic heart failure
Acute pulmonary embolus or pulmonary infarction
Acute myocarditis or pericarditis
Acute aortic dissection

Relative*
Left main coronary stenosis
Moderate stenotic valvular heart disease
Electrolyte abnormalities
Severe arterial hypertension (suggested definition: systolic blood pressure > 200 mm Hg and/or diastolic blood pressure > 110 mm Hg)
Tachyarrhythmias or bradyarrhythmias
Hypertrophic cardiomyopathy and other forms of outflow tract obstruction
Mental or physical impairment leading to inability to exercise adequately
High-degree atrioventricular block
Neuromuscular, musculoskeletal, or rheumatoid disorders known to be exacerbated by exercise
Ventricular aneurysm
Uncontrolled endocrine disorder (e.g., diabetes, thyroid)
Chronic infectious diseases (mononucleosis, hepatitis, AIDS)

*Relative contraindications can be superseded if benefits outweigh risks of exercise. In some cases, the patients can be exercised with caution and/or using low-level exercise endpoints, particularly if they are asymptomatic at rest

From Gibbons RJ, Balady GJ, Bricker JT, et al: ACC/AHA 2002 guideline update for exercise testing: Summary article. A report of the ACC/AHA Task Force on Practice Guidelines (Committee to Update the 1997 Exercise Testing Guidelines). Circulation 106:1883, 2002 and adapted by the ACSM (Thompson WR, Gordon NF, Pescatello LS: ACSM's Guidelines for Exercise Testing and Prescription. 8th ed. Philadelphia, Lippincott Williams & Wilkins, 2010.)

and updated by the American College of Sports Medicine in 2009.[20] Indications for termination of exercise testing are summarized in **Table 14G-2**. Relative indications for termination of testing or contraindications to testing can be superseded when the clinician considers that the benefit exceeds the risks. Exercise testing should be performed under the supervision of a physician, who should be in the vicinity and immediately available during all exercise tests. A properly trained nonphysician (i.e., nurse, physician assistant, or exercise physiologist or specialist) can perform the direct supervision for healthy younger persons and those with stable chest pain syndromes. An ACC/AHA Clinical Competence Statement on exercise testing published in 2008[20,21] recommends that cardiology trainees be exposed to at least 2 months, or the equivalent, of active participation in a fully equipped exercise testing laboratory, and should perform a minimum of 200 exercise tests reviewed by faculty. More advanced levels of training (an additional 100 tests) are required for competence in advanced forms of exercise testing; these include arrhythmia evaluation, ventilatory gas studies, pulmonary function testing as part of cardiopulmonary stress testing, stress echocardiographic techniques, and nuclear cardiology. The statement also lists specific skills needed for test supervision and interpretation, and recommends that medical centers have a program of quality assurance to ensure systematic review and critique of a significant sample of exercise tests.

CLINICAL INDICATIONS FOR EXERCISE TESTING

Diagnosis of Obstructive Coronary Artery Disease

When the clinical question is whether obstructive coronary artery disease (CAD) is present or absent in a patient (i.e., diagnosis), the ACC/AHA guidelines consider exercise testing to be most appropriate for patients with an "intermediate" pretest probability of CAD, such as patients with atypical or probable angina or younger patients with typical angina. Definitions of pretest risk status according to age, gender, and symptoms are summarized in **Table 14G-3**. Patients with a low pretest probability of CAD are less likely to have their management altered by exercise testing; therefore, exercise testing is not strongly supported by these guidelines in these populations (**Table 14G-4**). Exercise electrocardiography alone is

TABLE 14G-2 ACC/AHA Guidelines: Indications for Terminating Exercise Testing

Absolute

- Drop in systolic blood pressure >10 mm Hg from baseline blood pressure despite an increase in workload, when accompanied by other evidence of ischemia
- Moderate to severe angina (defined as three of four on exercise angina scale)
- Increasing nervous system symptoms (e.g., ataxia, dizziness, near-syncope)
- Signs of poor perfusion (cyanosis or pallor)
- Technical difficulties in monitoring electrocardiogram (ECG) or systolic blood pressure
- Subject's desire to stop
- Sustained ventricular tachycardia
- ST elevation (≥1.0 mm) in leads without diagnostic Q waves (other than V_1 or aVR)

Relative

- Drop in systolic blood pressure >10 mm Hg from baseline blood pressure despite an increase in workload, in the absence of other evidence of ischemia
- ST or QRS changes, such as excessive ST-segment depression (>2 mm of horizontal or downsloping ST segment depression) or marked axis shift
- Arrhythmias other than sustained ventricular tachycardia, including multifocal PVCs, triplets of PVCs, supraventricular tachycardia, heart block, or bradyarrhythmias
- Fatigue, shortness of breath, wheezing, leg cramps, or claudication
- Development of bundle-branch block or IVCD that cannot be distinguished from ventricular tachycardia
- Increasing chest pain
- Hypertensive response (suggested definition: systolic blood pressure > 250 mm Hg and/or a diastolic blood pressure > 115 mm Hg)

IVCD = intraventricular conduction delay; PVCs = premature ventricular contractions.
From Gibbons RJ, Balady GJ, Bricker JT, et al: ACC/AHA 2002 guideline update for exercise testing: Summary article. A report of the ACC/AHA Task Force on Practice Guidelines (Committee to Update the 1997 Exercise Testing Guidelines). Circulation 106:1883, 2002.

TABLE 14G-4 ACC/AHA Guidelines for Exercise Testing to Diagnose Obstructive Coronary Artery Disease

CLASS	INDICATION
I	Adult patients (including those with complete right bundle branch block or less than 1 mm of resting ST-segment depression) with an intermediate pretest probability of CAD on the basis of gender, age, and symptoms (specific exceptions are noted under Classes II and III, below)
IIa	Patients with vasospastic angina
IIb	1. Patients with a high pretest probability of CAD by age, symptoms, and gender 2. Patients with a low pretest probability of CAD by age, symptoms, and gender 3. Patients with less than 1 mm of baseline ST-segment depression and taking digoxin 4. Patients with electrocardiographic criteria for left ventricular hypertrophy and less than 1 mm of baseline ST-segment depression
III	1. Patients with the following baseline ECG abnormalities: • Preexcitation (Wolff-Parkinson-White) syndrome • Electronically paced ventricular rhythm • More than 1 mm of resting ST-segment depression • Complete left bundle branch block 2. Patients with a documented myocardial infarction or prior coronary angiography demonstrating significant disease who have an established diagnosis of CAD; however, ischemia and risk can be determined by testing.

From Gibbons RJ, Balady GJ, Bricker JT, et al: ACC/AHA 2002 guideline update for exercise testing: Summary article. A report of the ACC/AHA Task Force on Practice Guidelines (Committee to Update the 1997 Exercise Testing Guidelines). Circulation 106:1883, 2002.

TABLE 14G-3 Pretest Probability of Coronary Artery Disease by Age, Gender, and Symptoms

AGE (yr)	GENDER	TYPICAL OR DEFINITE ANGINA PECTORIS	ATYPICAL OR PROBABLE ANGINA PECTORIS	NONANGINAL CHEST PAIN	ASYMPTOMATIC
30-39	Men	Intermediate	Intermediate	Low	Very low
	Women	Intermediate	Very low	Very low	Very low
40-49	Men	High	Intermediate	Intermediate	Low
	Women	Intermediate	Low	Very low	Very low
50-59	Men	High	Intermediate	Intermediate	Low
	Women	Intermediate	Intermediate	Low	Very low
60-69	Men	High	Intermediate	Intermediate	Low
	Women	High	Intermediate	Intermediate	Low

From Gibbons RJ, Balady GJ, Bricker JT, et al: ACC/AHA 2002 guideline update for exercise testing: Summary article. A report of the ACC/AHA Task Force on Practice Guidelines (Committee to Update the 1997 Exercise Testing Guidelines). Circulation 106:1883, 2002.

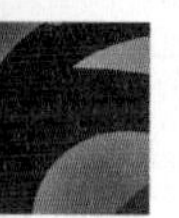

TABLE 14G-5 ACC/AHA Guidelines: Risk Assessment and Prognosis in Patients with Symptoms or Prior History of Coronary Artery Disease

CLASS	INDICATION
I	1. Patients undergoing initial evaluation with suspected or known CAD, including those with complete right bundle (indicated) branch block or less than 1 mm of resting ST-segment depression (specific exceptions noted below in class IIb) 2. Patients with suspected or known CAD, previously evaluated, now presenting with significant change in clinical status 3. Low-risk unstable angina patients 8 to 12 hr after presentation who have been free of active ischemic or heart failure symptoms 4. Intermediate-risk unstable angina patients 2 to 3 days after presentation who have been free of active ischemic or heart failure symptoms
IIa	Intermediate-risk unstable angina patients who have initial cardiac markers that are normal, a repeat ECG without significant change, and cardiac markers 6 to 12 hr after onset of symptoms that are normal and no other evidence of ischemia during observation
IIb	1. Patients with the following resting electrocardiographic abnormalities: • Preexcitation (Wolff-Parkinson-White) syndrome • Electronically paced ventricular rhythm • 1 mm or more of resting ST-segment depression • Complete left bundle branch block or any interventricular conduction defect with QRS duration > 120 msec 2. Patients with stable clinical course who undergo periodic monitoring to guide treatment
III	1. Patients with severe comorbidity likely to limit life expectancy and/or candidacy for revascularization 2. High-risk unstable angina patients

From Gibbons RJ, Balady GJ, Bricker JT, et al: ACC/AHA 2002 guideline update for exercise testing: Summary article. A report of the ACC/AHA Task Force on Practice Guidelines (Committee to Update the 1997 Exercise Testing Guidelines). Circulation 106:1883, 2002.

TABLE 14G-6 Risk Stratification Before Discharge: Class I Recommendations

1. Noninvasive stress testing is recommended for low-risk patients (see Table 14G-7) who have been free of ischemia at rest or with low-level activity and of HF for a minimum of 12 to 24 hr (level of evidence: C).
2. Noninvasive stress testing is recommended for patients at intermediate risk (see Table 14G-7) who have been free of ischemia at rest or with low-level activity and of HF for a minimum of 12 to 24 hr (level of evidence: C).
3. Choice of stress test is based on the resting ECG, ability to perform exercise, local expertise, and technologies available. Treadmill exercise is useful for patients able to exercise in whom the ECG is free of baseline ST-segment abnormalities, bundle branch block, left ventricular (LV) hypertrophy, intraventricular conduction defect, paced rhythm, preexcitation, and digoxin effect (level of evidence: C).
4. An imaging modality should be added in patients with resting ST-segment depression (≥0.10 mV), LV hypertrophy, bundle branch block, intraventricular conduction defect, preexcitation, or digoxin who are able to exercise. In patients undergoing a low-level exercise test, an imaging modality can add sensitivity (level of evidence: B).
5. Pharmacologic stress testing with imaging is recommended when physical limitations (e.g., arthritis, amputation, severe peripheral vascular disease, severe chronic obstructive pulmonary disease, or general debility) preclude adequate exercise stress (level of evidence: B).
6. Prompt angiography without noninvasive risk stratification should be performed for failure of stabilization with intensive medical treatment (level of evidence: B).
7. A noninvasive test (echocardiography or radionuclide angiography) is recommended to evaluate LV function in patients with definite ACS who are not scheduled for coronary angiography and left ventriculography (level of evidence: B).

From Anderson JL, Adams CD, Antman EM, et al: ACC/AHA 2007 Guidelines for the management of patients with unstable angina/non ST-elevation myocardial infarction: A report of the American College of Cardiology/American Heart Association Task Force on Practice Guidelines (Writing Committee to Revise the 2002 Guidelines for the Management of Patients With Unstable Angina/Non ST-Elevation Myocardial Infarction) Developed in Collaboration with the American College of Emergency Physicians, the Society for Cardiovascular Angiography and Interventions, and the Society of Thoracic Surgeons Endorsed by the American Association of Cardiovascular and Pulmonary Rehabilitation and the Society for Academic Emergency Medicine. J Am Coll Cardiol 50:e1, 2007.

considered inappropriate as an initial diagnostic test if the patient has an electrocardiographic pattern likely to lead to a nondiagnostic tracing and in which concomitant imaging studies would provide more useful information.[16,17].

Risk Assessment and Prognosis in Patients with Coronary Disease

The ACC/AHA guidelines emphasize that exercise testing should be used to improve risk stratification as part of a process that begins with the assessment of routinely available data from the clinical examination and other laboratory tests.[1-3,9] The decision of whether to order an exercise test should reflect the probability that test results might alter management, and the interpretation of the results should be considered in the context of the patient's overall clinical status.

The recommendations endorse the routine use of exercise testing for risk stratification of patients with suspected or known CAD (**Table 14G-5**) who are clinically stable or after a change in clinical status. The guidelines emphasize the importance of considering multiple types of data from the exercise test (e.g., exercise duration) and encourage the use of scoring tools to integrate the multivariable data into a risk prediction tool. Risk stratification procedures before noncardiac operations follow the same general principles (**Fig. 14G-1**).

For low-risk patients with unstable angina in the emergency room, the guidelines support exercise testing early after presentation in patients if they have been free of active ischemic or heart failure symptoms for 8 to 12 hours.[2,20] A longer delay (2 to 3 days) is recommended for patients with an intermediate risk of complications, although the guidelines indicate that there is good supportive evidence for earlier exercise testing as part of chest pain management protocols for stable patients from this population if there is no evidence of active ischemia (Class I indication). The guidelines discourage exercise testing for patients in whom the procedure would be dangerous (e.g., high-risk unstable angina patients), unlikely to add accurate information (e.g., patients with certain resting electrocardiographic abnormalities), or unlikely to change management (e.g., patients with stable clinical courses or who were poor candidates for revascularization; see Table 14G-5).

After Acute Myocardial Infarction

Recommendations for the use of exercise testing after acute myocardial infarction (**Table 14G-6**) reflect an overall strategy for risk stratification and management described in the ACC/AHA guidelines on acute myocardial infarction.[2,3] In this approach high-risk patients should undergo invasive evaluation to determine whether he or she is a candidate for coronary revascularization procedures. For patients at lower risk for complications (low prognostic GRACE or TIMI risk score), exercise testing (in patients suitable for the procedure) is recommended to identify prognostic high-risk patients. **Table 14G-7** illustrates risk gradients based on noninvasive test results. An intermediate- to high-risk result would normally lead to cardiac catheterization in a patient initially managed with a conservative or selective invasive approach. ACC/AHA/SCAI/ASNC guideline[5] and appropriateness[6] criteria provide three levels of evidence for coronary revascularization in various patient subsets. When the initial exercise test result is negative, a second symptom-limited exercise test can be repeated at 3 to 6 weeks for patients undergoing vigorous activity during leisure time activities or at work, or exercise training as part of cardiac rehabilitation.

Special Populations

The ACC/AHA guidelines discourage routine exercise testing for asymptomatic persons without known CAD and conclude that only weak evidence is available to support its appropriateness for asymptomatic patients with multiple risk factors or patients about to embark on an exercise

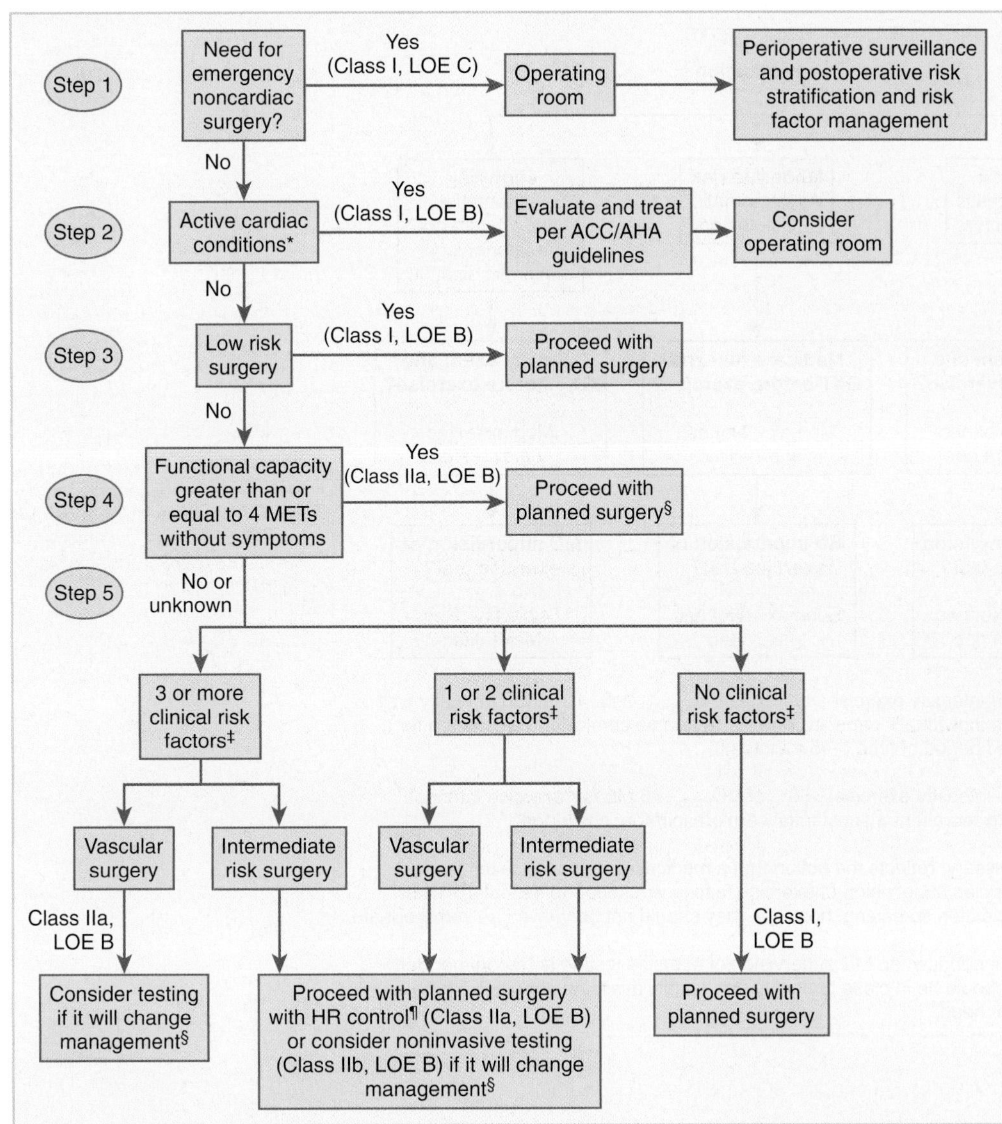

FIGURE 14G-1 Strategies for exercise test evaluation before noncardiac operative procedures. *Active cardiac conditions = acute coronary syndrome (ACS), decompensated heart failure (HF), serious arrhythmias, severe valvular disease; ‡clinical risk factors = history of ischemic heart disease, compensated or prior heart failure, history of cerebrovascular accident (CVA), diabetes mellitus, renal insufficiency (Cr > 2 mg/dL); §noninvasive testing may be considered before surgery in specific patients with risk factors if it will change management; ¶consider perioperative beta blockade for populations in which this has been shown to reduce cardiac morbidity/mortality. LOE = level of evidence; MET = metabolic equivalent. [§,¶] *(From Fleisher LA, Beckman JA, Brown KA, et al: ACC/AHA 2007 guidelines on perioperative cardiovascular evaluation and care for noncardiac surgery: Executive summary. A report of the American College of Cardiology/American Heart Association Task Force on Practice Guidelines (Writing Committee to Revise the 2002 Guidelines on Perioperative Cardiovascular Evaluation for Noncardiac Surgery). Circulation 116:1971, 2007.)*

program. The guidelines are more supportive of exercise testing of patients with diabetes who are about to start vigorous exercise programs because of the high risk for atherosclerotic disease in this population. **Figure 14G-2**, from the American College of Sports Medicine, provides guidance on exercise testing for asymptomatic subjects and direct physician supervision requirements.

Exercise testing is useful for assessing functional capacity in patients with valvular heart disease, particularly patients with regurgitant lesions[10] (**Table 14G-8**). The guidelines note that exercise testing is usually not needed for symptomatic patients with stenotic valvular heart disease, and that severe aortic stenosis is classically considered to be a contraindication to exercise testing. However, the guidelines acknowledge that there are subsets of asymptomatic patients with stenotic valvular lesions in whom exercise testing may help assess functional capacity, such as determination of whether they are actually asymptomatic.

The ACC/AHA heart failure guidelines support the use of exercise testing with imaging, where appropriate (**Table 14G-9**), and cardiopulmonary exercise testing for the evaluation of patients for cardiac transplantation or concomitant pulmonary disease in whom the cause of dyspnea is unclear.[7,8] A peak $\dot{V}O_2$ <10 mL/kg/min with achievement of anaerobic metabolism in a patient is an absolute indication for cardiac transplantation in suitable patients, whereas a peak [$\dot{V}O_2$ between 11 and 14 mL/kg/min or 55% of predicted and major daily limitation is a relative indication. When the peak $\dot{V}O_2$ exceeds 15 mL/kg/min, there is insufficient indication for transplantation without other indications.

The guidelines endorse exercise testing for patients with heart rhythm disorders when the test is intended to diagnose exercise-induced arrhythmias or evaluate therapy (e.g., settings for rate-adaptive pacemakers, or impact of therapy for patients with exercise-induced arrhythmias).[13-15] However, there is little support for exercise testing for heart rhythm abnormalities that in isolation are not associated with a higher risk of cardiovascular complications, such as isolated ventricular or atrial premature beats (**Table 14G-10**).

Exercise testing is useful for the evaluation of unoperated patients with congenital heart disease to establish an objective measurement of functional capacity, to aid in the assessment of the functional significance of what appears to be an intermediate-severity left-sided obstructive lesion such as stenotic valve or subvalvular narrowing, in the follow-up of operated or nonoperated patients with coarctation of the aorta, to determine the potential of serious exercise-induced cardiac arrhythmias, and in the

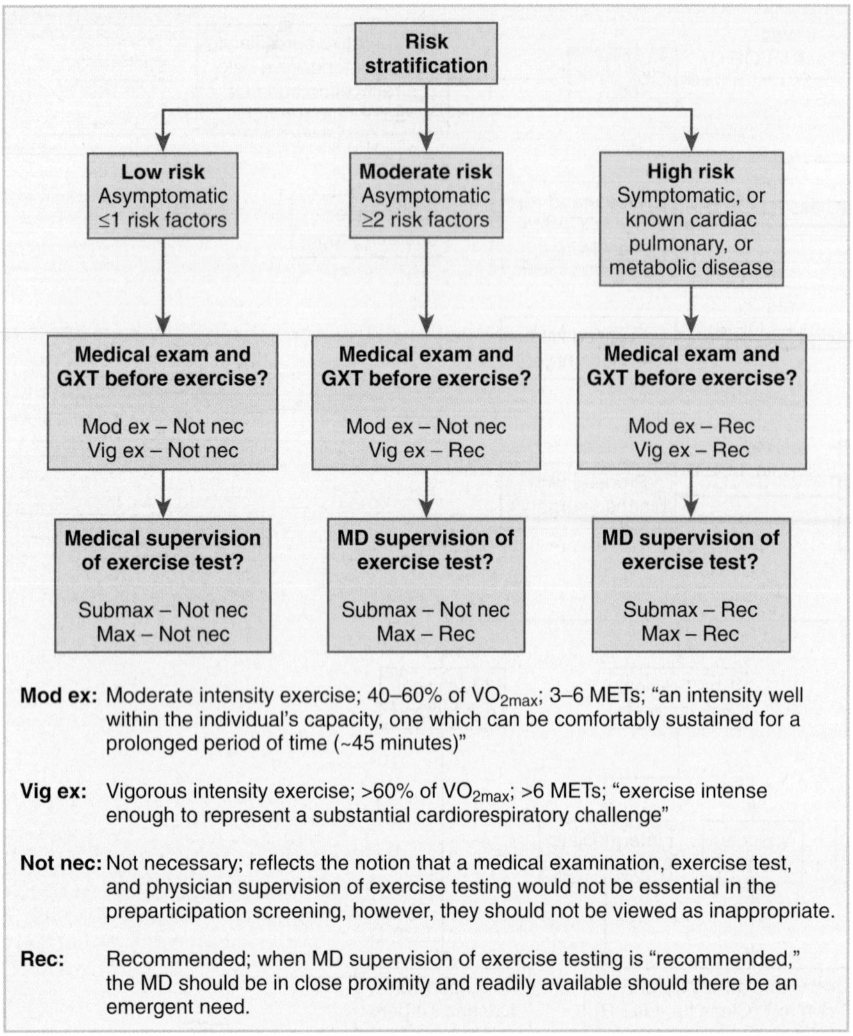

FIGURE 14G-2 Exercise testing and testing supervision recommendations based on risk stratification. GXT = graded exercise test. *(From Thompson WR, Gordon NF, Pescatello LS: ACSM's Guidelines for Exercise Testing and Prescription. 8th ed. Philadelphia, Lippincott Williams & Wilkins, 2010.)*

TABLE 14G-7 **Noninvasive Risk Stratification**

High Risk (Greater than 3% Annual Mortality Rate)
Severe resting LV dysfunction (LV ejection fraction [EF] < 0.35)
High-risk treadmill score (score of −11 or lower)
Severe exercise LV dysfunction (exercise LVEF < 0.35)
Stress-induced large perfusion defect (particularly if anterior)
Stress-induced multiple perfusion defects of moderate size
Large, fixed perfusion defect with LV dilation or increased lung uptake (thallium-201)
Stress-induced moderate perfusion defect with LV dilation or increased lung uptake (thallium-201)
Echocardiographic wall motion abnormality (involving more than two segments) developing at a low dose of dobutamine (10 μg/kg/min or less) or at a low heart rate (less than 120 beats/min)
Stress echocardiographic evidence of extensive ischemia
Intermediate Risk (1% to 3% Annual Mortality Rate)
Mild to moderate resting LV dysfunction (LVEF = 0.35-0.49)
Intermediate-risk treadmill score (−11 to 5)
Stress-induced moderate perfusion defect without LV dilation or increased lung intake (thallium-201)
Limited stress echocardiographic ischemia with a wall motion abnormality only at higher doses of dobutamine involving ≤two segments
Low Risk (Less than 1% Annual Mortality Rate)
Low-risk treadmill score (score of 5 or higher)
Normal or small myocardial perfusion defect at rest or with stress*
Normal stress echocardiographic wall motion or no change of limited resting wall motion abnormalities during stress*

*Although the published data are limited, patients with these findings will probably not be at low risk in the presence of either a high-risk treadmill score or severe resting LV dysfunction (LVEF < 0.35).

From Gibbons RJ, Abrams J, Chatterjee K, et al: ACC/AHA 2002 guideline update for the management of patients with chronic stable angina: A report of the American College of Cardiology/American Heart Association Task Force on Practice Guidelines (Committee to Update the 1999 Guidelines for the Management of Patients with Chronic Stable Angina) (http://www.acc.org/qualityandscience/clinical/guidelines/stable/stable_clean.pdf).

TABLE 14G-8 ACC/AHA Guidelines for Exercise Testing in Patients with Valvular Heart Disease

Class IIa

1. Exercise stress testing for chronic aortic regurgitation (AR) is reasonable for assessment of functional capacity and symptomatic response in patients with a history of equivocal symptoms (level of evidence: B).
2. Exercise stress testing for patients with chronic AR is reasonable for the evaluation of symptoms and functional capacity before participation in athletic activities (level of evidence: C).
3. Graded exercise testing is a reasonable diagnostic evaluation in the adolescent or young adult with aortic stenosis (AS) who has a Doppler mean gradient > 30 mm Hg or a peak velocity > 3.5 m/sec (peak gradient > 50 mm Hg) if the patient is interested in athletic participation, or if the clinical findings and Doppler findings are disparate (level of evidence: C)
4. Exercise testing is reasonable for the initial evaluation of adolescent and young adult patients with tricuspid regurgitation (TR), and serially every 1 to 3 yr (level of evidence: C).

Class IIb

1. Exercise stress testing in patients with radionuclide angiography may be considered for assessment of LV function in asymptomatic or symptomatic patients with chronic AR (level of evidence: B).
2. Exercise testing in asymptomatic patients with AS may be considered to elicit exercise-induced symptoms and abnormal blood pressure responses (level of evidence: B).

Class III

1. Exercise testing should not be performed in symptomatic patients with AS (level of evidence: B).

From Bonow RO, Carabello BA, Chatterjee K, et al: 2008 Focused update incorporated into the ACC/AHA 2006 guidelines for the management of patients with vascular heart disease. A Report of the American College of Cardiology/American Heart Association Task Force on Practice Guidelines (Writing Committee to Revise the 1998 Guidelines for the Management of Patients With Valvular Heart Disease). J Am Coll Cardiol 52:e1, 2008.

TABLE 14G-9 ACC/AHA Guidelines for Exercise Testing in Patients with Compensated Heart Failure (HF)

Class IIa

1. Noninvasive imaging to detect myocardial ischemia and viability is reasonable in patients presenting with HF who have known coronary artery disease and no angina, unless the patient is not eligible for revascularization of any type (level of evidence: B).
2. Maximal exercise testing with or without measurement of respiratory gas exchange and/or blood oxygen saturation is reasonable in patients presenting with HF to help determine whether HF is the cause of exercise limitation when the contribution of HF is uncertain (level of evidence: C).
3. Maximal exercise testing with measurement of respiratory gas exchange is reasonable to identify high-risk patients presenting with HF who are candidates for cardiac transplantation or other advanced treatment (level of evidence: B).

From Hunt SA, Abraham WT, Chin MH, et al: ACC/AHA 2005 guideline update for the diagnosis and management of chronic heart failure in the adult—summary article. A report of the American College of Cardiology/American Heart Association Task Force on Practice Guidelines (Writing Committee to Update the 2001 Guidelines for the Evaluation and Management of Heart Failure). J Am Coll Cardiol 46:1116, 2005.

TABLE 14G-10 Recommendations for Exercise Testing in Patients with Heart Rhythm Disorders

Class I

1. Exercise testing is recommended for adult patients with ventricular arrhythmias who have an intermediate or greater probability of having coronary heart disease (CHD) by age, gender, and symptoms to provoke ischemic changes or ventricular arrhythmias (level of evidence: B).*
2. Exercise testing, regardless of age, is useful for patients with known or suspected exercise-induced ventricular arrhythmias, including catecholaminergic ventricular tachycardia (VT), to provoke the arrhythmia, achieve a diagnosis, and determine the patient's response to tachycardia (level of evidence: B).

Class IIa

1. Exercise testing can be useful for evaluating response to medical or ablation therapy in patients with known exercise-induced ventricular arrhythmias (level of evidence: B).

Class IIb

1. Exercise testing may be useful in patients with ventricular arrhythmias and a low probability of CHD by age, gender, and symptoms (level of evidence: C).*
2. Exercise testing may be useful in the investigation of isolated premature ventricular complexes (PVCs) in middle-aged or older patients without other evidence of CHD (level of evidence: C).

Class III

1. See Table 1 in the ACC/AHA 2002 guideline update for exercise testing[†] for contraindications (level of evidence: B).

*See Table 4 in the ACC/AHA 2002 guideline update for exercise testing (†Gibbons RJ, Balady GJ, Bricker JT, et al: ACC/AHA 2002 guideline update for exercise testing: Summary article. A report of the ACC/AHA Task Force on Practice Guidelines [Committee to Update the 1997 Exercise Testing Guidelines]. Circulation 106:1883, 2002) for further explanation of CHD probability.

From Zipes DP, Camm AJ, Borggrefe M, et al: ACC/AHA/ESC 2006 guidelines for the management of patients with ventricular arrhythmias and the prevention of sudden cardiac death. A report of the American College of Cardiology/American Heart Association Task Force and the European Society of Cardiology Committee for Practice Guidelines (Writing Committee to Develop Guidelines for Management of Patients With Ventricular Arrhythmias and the Prevention of Sudden Cardiac Death). J Am Coll Cardiol 48:e247, 2006.

functional assessment of dyspnea in patients with CAD—pulmonary artery hypertension (**Table 14G-11**).[11,12] In idiopathic pulmonary hypertension, exercise testing using a 6-minute walk test or cardiopulmonary testing is often part of the routine diagnostic evaluation, and can be used to assess the adequacy of pulmonary vascular reserve during a right heart catheterization with direct measurement of pulmonary artery pressures. Treatment decisions are not usually made solely on the basis of exercise echocardiography-determined pulmonary hypertension.[12]

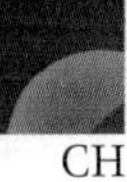

CH 14

TABLE 14G-11 ACC/AHA Guidelines for Exercise Testing in Patients with Unoperated Congenital Heart Disease and for Patients with Primary Pulmonary Hypertension

Atrial Septal Defect

Class IIa

Maximal exercise testing can be useful to document exercise capacity in patients with symptoms that are discrepant with clinical findings or to document changes in oxygen saturation in patients with mild or moderate pulmonary artery hypertension (PAH) (level of evidence: C).

Class III

Maximal exercise testing is not recommended in atrial septal defect (ASD) with severe PAH (level of evidence: B).

Aortic Stenosis

Class IIa

1. In asymptomatic young adults younger than 30 years, exercise stress testing is reasonable to determine exercise capability, symptoms, and blood pressure response (level of evidence: C).
2. Exercise stress testing is reasonable for patients with a mean Doppler gradient > 30 mm Hg or peak Doppler gradient > 50 mm Hg if the patient is interested in athletic participation or if clinical findings differ from noninvasive measurements (level of evidence: C).
3. Exercise stress testing is reasonable for the evaluation of an asymptomatic young adult with a mean Doppler gradient > 40 mm Hg or a peak Doppler gradient > 64 mm Hg or when the patient anticipates athletic participation or pregnancy (level of evidence: C).
4. Exercise stress testing can be useful to evaluate blood pressure response or elicit exercise-induced symptoms in asymptomatic older adults with AS (level of evidence: B).

Class III

1. Exercise stress testing should not be performed in symptomatic patients with AS or those with repolarization abnormality on the ECG or systolic dysfunction on the echocardiogram (level of evidence: C).

Subaortic Stenosis

Class IIa

1. Stress testing to determine exercise capability, symptoms, electrocardiographic changes or arrhythmias, or increase in LV outflow tract (LVOT) gradient is reasonable in the presence of otherwise equivocal indications for intervention (level of evidence: C).
2. Exercise testing, dobutamine stress testing, positron emission tomography, or stress sestamibi with adenosine studies can be useful to evaluate the adequacy of myocardial perfusion (level of evidence: C).

Coarctation of the Aorta

Class IIb

1. Routine exercise testing may be performed at intervals determined by consultation with the regional adult congenital heart disease (ACHD) center (level of evidence: C).

Pulmonary Arterial Hypertension

Class II

1. It is reasonable to include a 6-minute walk test or similar nonmaximal cardiopulmonary exercise test as part of the functional assessment of patients with CAD-PAH (level of evidence: C).

From Warnes CA, Williams RG, Bashore TM, et al: ACC/AHA 2008 guidelines for the management of adults with congenital heart disease: A report of the American College of Cardiology/American Heart Association Task Force on Practice Guidelines (Writing Committee to Develop Guidelines for the Management of Adults With Congenital Heart Disease). J Am Coll Cardiol 52:e143, 2008; and McLaughlin VV, Archer SL, Badesch DB, et al: ACCF/AHA 2009 expert consensus document on pulmonary hypertension. A report of the American College of Cardiology Foundation Task Force on Expert Consensus Documents and the American Heart Association. J Am Coll Cardiol 53:1573, 2009.

REFERENCES

1. Gibbons RJ, Abrams J, Chatterjee K, et al: ACC/AHA 2002 guideline update for the management of patients with chronic stable angina: A report of the American College of Cardiology/American Heart Association Task Force on Practice Guidelines (Committee to Update the 1999 Guidelines for the Management of Patients with Chronic Stable Angina) (http://www.acc.org/qualityandscience/clinical/guidelines/stable/stable_clean.pdf).
2. Anderson JL, Adams CD, Antman EM, et al: ACC/AHA 2007 guidelines for the management of patients with unstable angina/non ST-elevation myocardial infarction: A report of the American College of Cardiology/American Heart Association Task Force on Practice Guidelines (Writing Committee to Revise the 2002 Guidelines for the Management of Patients With Unstable Angina/Non ST-Elevation Myocardial Infarction) Developed in Collaboration with the American College of Emergency Physicians, the Society for Cardiovascular Angiography and Interventions, and the Society of Thoracic Surgeons Endorsed by the American Association of Cardiovascular and Pulmonary Rehabilitation and the Society for Academic Emergency Medicine. J Am Coll Cardiol 50:e1, 2007.
3. Antman EM, Hand M, Armstrong, et al: 2007 focused update of the ACC/AHA 2004 guidelines for the management of patients with ST-elevation myocardial infarction. A report of the American College of Cardiology/American Heart Association Task Force on Practice Guidelines. J Am Coll Cardiol 51:210, 2008.
4. Smith SC, Feldman T, Hirshfeld JW, et al: ACC/AHA/SCAI 2005 guideline update for percutaneous coronary intervention. A report of the American College of Cardiology/American Heart Association Task Force on Practice Guidelines (ACC/AHA/SCAI Writing Committee to Update the 2001 Guidelines for Percutaneous Coronary Intervention). J Am Coll Cardiol 47:e1, 2006.
5. Hirsch AT, Haskal ZJ, Hertzer NR, et al: ACC/AHA 2005 guidelines for the management of patients with peripheral arterial disease (lower extremity, renal, mesenteric, and abdominal aortic): A collaborative report from the American Association for Vascular Surgery/Society for Vascular Surgery, Society for Cardiovascular Angiography and Interventions, Society for Vascular Medicine and Biology, Society of Interventional Radiology, and the ACC/AHA Task Force on Practice Guidelines (Writing Committee to Develop Guidelines for the Management of Patients With Peripheral Arterial Disease) (http://www.acc.org/clinical/guidelines/pad/index.pdf).
6. Patel MR, Dehmer GJ, Hirshfeld JW, et al: ACCF/SCAI/STS/AATS/AHA/ASNC 2009 appropriateness criteria for coronary revascularization. A report of the American College of Cardiology Foundation Appropriateness Criteria Task Force, Society for Cardiovascular Angiography and Interventions, Society of Thoracic Surgeons, American Association for Thoracic Surgery, American Heart Association, and the American Society of Nuclear Cardiology. J Am Coll Cardiol 53:530, 2009.
7. Hunt SA, Abraham WT, Chin MH, et al: ACC/AHA 2005 guideline update for the diagnosis and management of chronic heart failure in the adult—summary article. A report of the American College of Cardiology/American Heart Association Task Force on Practice Guidelines (Writing Committee to Update the 2001 Guidelines for the Evaluation and Management of Heart Failure). J Am Coll Cardiol 46:1116, 2005.

8. Hunt SA, Abraham WT, Chin MH, et al: 2009 focused update incorporated into the ACC/AHA 2005 guidelines for the diagnosis and management of heart failure in adults. A report of the American College of Cardiology Foundation/American Heart Association Task Force on Practice Guidelines. J Am Coll Cardiol 53:e1, 2009.
9. Fleisher LA, Beckman JA, Brown KA, et al: ACC/AHA 2007 guidelines on perioperative cardiovascular evaluation and care for noncardiac surgery: Executive summary. A report of the American College of Cardiology/American Heart Association Task Force on Practice Guidelines (Writing Committee to Revise the 2002 Guidelines on Perioperative Cardiovascular Evaluation for Noncardiac Surgery). Circulation 116:1971, 2007.
10. Bonow RO, Carabello BA, Chatterjee K, et al: 2008 focused update incorporated into the ACC/AHA 2006 guidelines for the management of patients with vascular heart disease. A Report of the American College of Cardiology/American Heart Association Task Force on Practice Guidelines (Writing Committee to Revise the 1998 Guidelines for the Management of Patients With Valvular Heart Disease). J Am Coll Cardiol 52:e1, 2008.
11. Warnes CA, Williams RG, Bashore TM, et al: ACC/AHA 2008 guidelines for the management of adults with congenital heart disease: A report of the American College of Cardiology/American Heart Association Task Force on Practice Guidelines (Writing Committee to Develop Guidelines for the Management of Adults With Congenital Heart Disease). J Am Coll Cardiol 52:e143, 2008.
12. McLaughlin VV, Archer SL, Badesch DB, et al: ACCF/AHA 2009 expert consensus document on pulmonary hypertension. A report of the American College of Cardiology Foundation Task Force on Expert Consensus Documents and the American Heart Association. J Am Coll Cardiol 53:1573, 2009.
13. Zipes DP, Camm AJ, Borggrefe M, et al: ACC/AHA/ESC 2006 guidelines for the management of patients with ventricular arrhythmias and the prevention of sudden cardiac death. A report of the American College of Cardiology/American Heart Association Task Force and the European Society of Cardiology Committee for Practice Guidelines (Writing Committee to Develop Guidelines for Management of Patients With Ventricular Arrhythmias and the Prevention of Sudden Cardiac Death). J Am Coll Cardiol 48:e247, 2006.
14. Goldberger JJ, Cain ME, Hohnloser SH, et al: American Heart Association/American College of Cardiology Foundation/Heart Rhythm Society scientific statement on noninvasive risk stratification techniques for identifying patients at risk for sudden cardiac death: A scientific statement from the American Heart Association Council on Clinical Cardiology Committee on Electrocardiography and Arrhythmias and Council on Epidemiology and Prevention. J Am Coll Cardiol 52:1179, 2008.
15. Strickberger SA, Benson W, Biaggioni I, et al: AHA/ACCF Scientific Statement on the Evaluation of Syncope. From the American Heart Association Councils on Clinical Cardiology, Cardiovascular Nursing, Cardiovascular Disease in the Young, and Stroke, and the Quality of Care and Outcomes Research Interdisciplinary Working Group; and the American College of Cardiology Foundation in Collaboration with the Heart Rhythm Society. J Am Coll Cardiol 47:473, 2006.
16. Brindis RG, Douglas PS, Hendel RC, et al: ACCF/ASNC Appropriateness criteria for single-photon emission computed tomography myocardial perfusion imaging (SPECT MPI). A report of the American College of Cardiology Foundation Quality Strategic Directions Committee Appropriateness Criteria Working Group and the American Society of Nuclear Cardiology. J Am Coll Cardiol 46:1587, 2005.
17. Douglas PS, Khandheria B, Stainback RF, et al: ACCF/ASE/ACEP/AHA/ASNC/SCAI/SCCT/SCMR 2008 appropriateness criteria for stress echocardiography. A report of the American College of Cardiology Foundation Appropriateness Criteria Task Force, American Society of Echocardiography, American College of Emergency Physicians, American Heart Association, American Society of Nuclear Cardiology, Society for Cardiovascular Angiography and Interventions, Society of Cardiovascular Computed Tomography, and Society for Cardiovascular Magnetic Resonance. J Am Coll Cardiol 51:1127, 2008.
18. Antman EM, Peterson ED: Tools for guiding clinical practice from the American Heart Association and the American College of Cardiology. What are they and how should clinicians use them? Circulation 119:1180, 2009.
19. Tricoci P, Allen JM, Kramer JM, et al: Scientific evidence underlying the ACC/AHA clinical practice guidelines. JAMA 301:831, 2009.
20. Thompson WR, Gordon NF, Pescatello LS: ACSM's Guidelines for Exercise Testing and Prescription. 8th ed. Philadelphia, Lippincott Williams & Wilkins, 2010.
21. Myerburg RJ, Chaitman BR, Ewy GA, Lauer MS: Task Force 2: Training in electrocardiography, ambulatory electrocardiography, and exercise testing. J Am Coll Cardiol 51:349, 2008.

CHAPTER 15 Echocardiography

Heidi M. Connolly and Jae K. Oh

Even with advances in other cardiovascular imaging modalities, such as cardiac magnetic resonance imaging (CMR) and computed tomography (CT), echocardiography remains the most frequently used and usually the initial imaging test to evaluate all cardiovascular diseases related to a structural, functional, or hemodynamic abnormality of the heart or great vessels. Echocardiography uses ultrasound beams reflected by cardiovascular structures to produce characteristic lines or shapes caused by normal or altered cardiac anatomy in one, two, or three dimensions by M (motion)–mode, two-dimensional, or three-dimensional echocardiography, respectively. Doppler examination and color flow imaging provide reliable assessment of cardiac hemodynamics and blood flow.[1] The creation of contrast agents that pass through the pulmonary circulation after intravenous administration has improved delineation of structures on the left side of the heart and made real-time myocardial perfusion imaging a clinical reality.[2] Transesophageal echocardiography (TEE) has markedly improved resolution of echocardiographic images, including real-time three-dimensional images, and tissue Doppler imaging and strain imaging have enhanced the ability to assess systolic and diastolic function.[3]

Reliable noninvasive hemodynamic evaluation and confident delineation of cardiovascular structures by echocardiography have dramatically reduced the clinical necessity for hemodynamic cardiac catheterization. Increasingly, patients undergo valvular or congenital heart surgery on the basis of an echocardiographic diagnosis (see Chaps. 65 and 66). Echocardiographic units are also being miniaturized to become an extension of a clinician's physical examination.[4] In our opinion, the appreciation of cardiac anatomy and hemodynamics by bedside echocardiography makes a physician's clinical evaluation, including physical examination, more relevant to the care of patients. For all physicians who care for patients with a cardiovascular problem, it is essential to know how echocardiographic images are obtained, what type of information echocardiography can provide, and how it should be used for management.

M-Mode, Two-Dimensional, and Three-Dimensional Transthoracic Echocardiography

An echocardiographic examination currently begins with real-time two-dimensional echocardiography, which produces high-resolution tomographic images of cardiac structures and their movements. These images are usually obtained from four standard transducer locations—parasternal, apical, subcostal, and suprasternal (**Fig. 15-1A**)—by manual rotation and angulation of the transducer (Fig. 15-1B,C). Qualitative and quantitative measurements of cardiac dimensions, area, and volume are derived from two-dimensional images or M-mode recordings derived from two-dimensional images.[5] Also, two-dimensional echocardiography provides the framework for Doppler examination and color flow imaging. Newer matrix transducers with more than 3000 elements allow three-dimensional or multidimensional images of the heart (**Figs. 15-2 to 15-5**). Customized as well as preformatted images (equivalent to two-dimensional views) can be obtained or derived from a full-volume three-dimensional

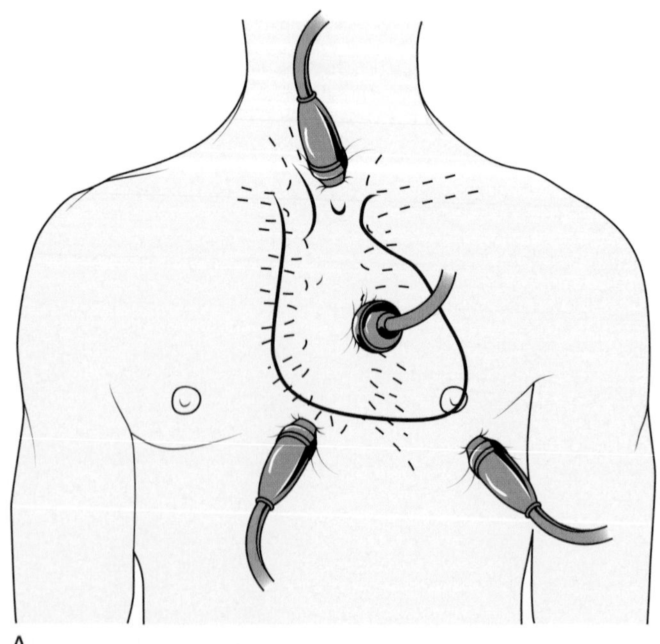

FIGURE 15-1 A, Four standard transducer positions—parasternal, apical, subcostal, and suprasternal—used to visualize the heart and great vessels. *(Modified from Bansal RC, Tajik AJ, Seward JB, Offord KP: Feasibility of detailed two-dimensional echocardiographic examination in adults: Prospective study of 200 patients. Mayo Clin Proc 55:291, 1980. Used with permission of Mayo Foundation for Medical Education and Research.)*

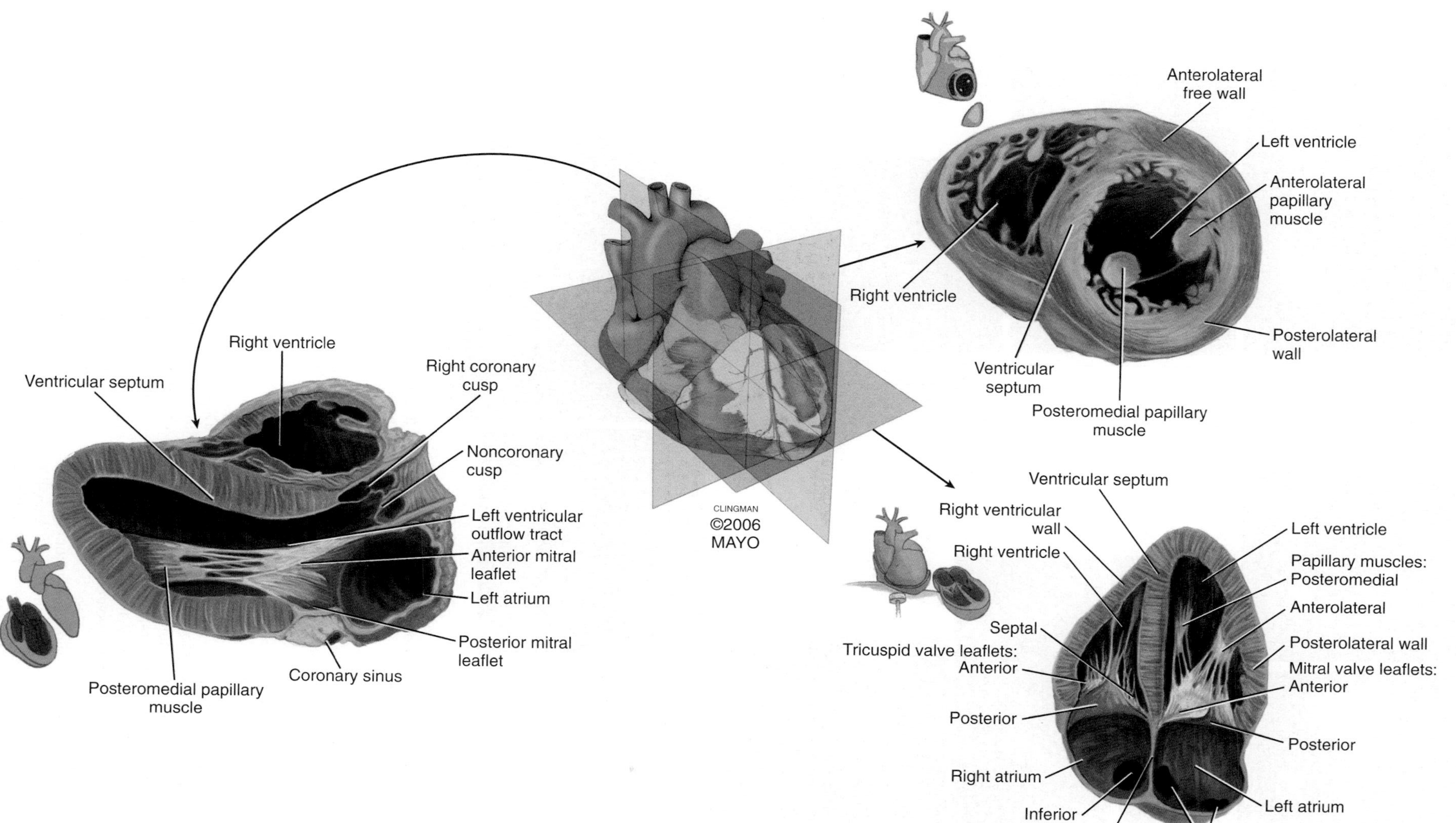

FIGURE 15-1, cont'd **B,** Diagram of cardiac structures from standard tomographic planes: parasternal long-axis view **(left),** parasternal short-axis view **(upper right),** and apical four-chamber view **(lower right).**

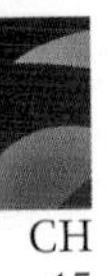

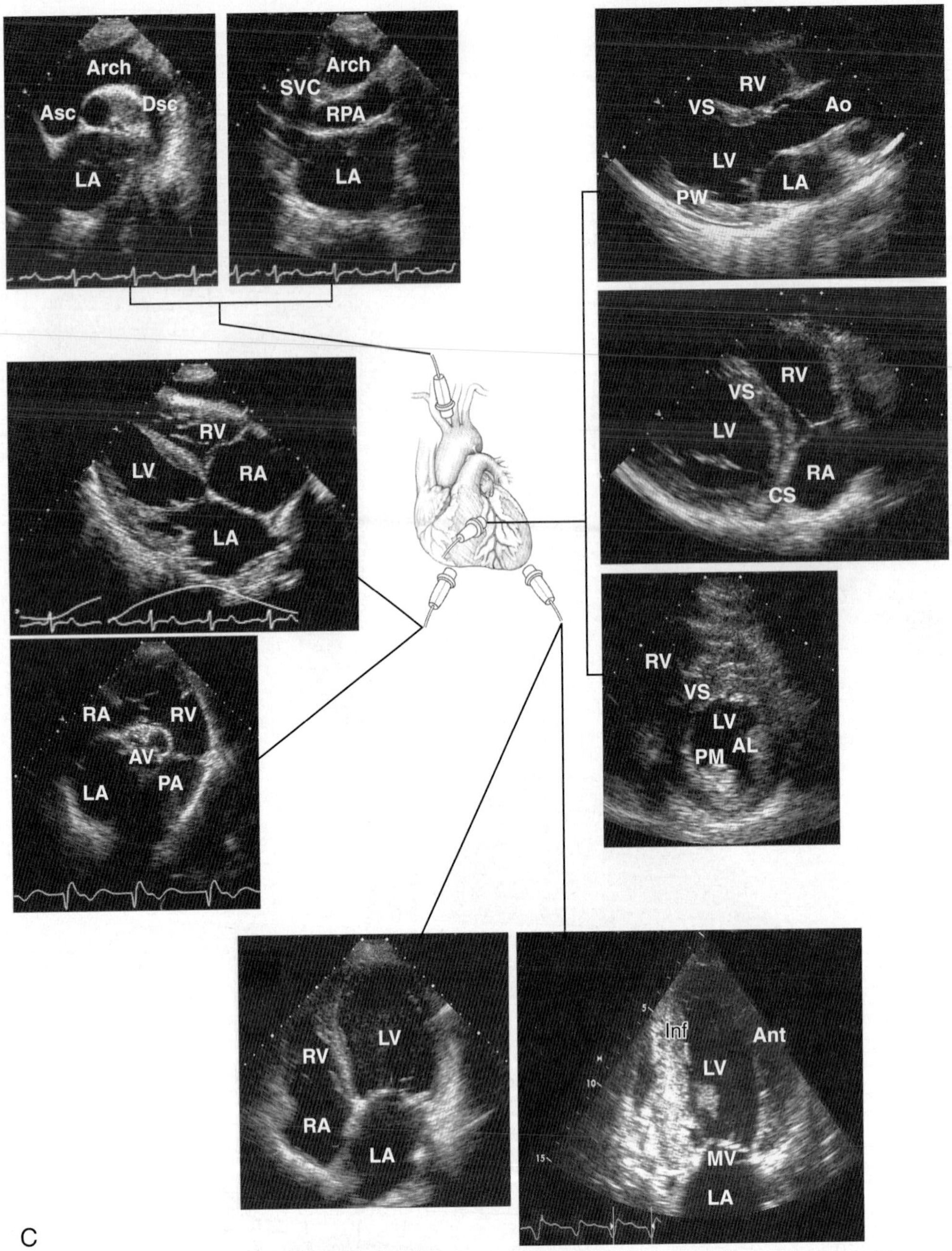

FIGURE 15-1, cont'd **C,** Still frame two-dimensional echocardiographic images from various tomographic views: parasternal long-axis view **(right upper),** parasternal right ventricular inflow view **(right middle),** parasternal short-axis view **(right lower),** apical four-chamber view **(left bottom),** apical two-chamber view **(right bottom),** subcostal four-chamber and short-axis views **(left middle and lower),** and suprasternal long- and short-axis views **(left upper).** These images are similar to the appearance of the diagram in **B.** AL = anterolateral; Ao = aorta; Asc = ascending aorta; AV = aortic valve; CS = coronary sinus; Dsc = descending aorta; LA = left atrium; MV = mitral valve; PA = pulmonary artery; PM = papillary muscle; PW = posterior wall; RA = right atrium; RPA = right pulmonary artery; RV = right ventricle; SVC = superior vena cava; VS = ventricular septum. *(Modified from Tajik AJ, Seward JB, Hagler DJ, et al: Two-dimensional real-time ultrasonic imaging of the heart and great vessels: Technique, image orientation, structure identification, and validation. Mayo Clin Proc 53:271, 1978. Used with permission of Mayo Foundation for Medical Education and Research.)*

echocardiographic image. This shortens the examination time and minimizes variation in acquisition of cardiovascular images. With advances and clinical experience in three-dimensional and multidimensional echocardiographic imaging, visualization and quantitation of cardiovascular structure, function, and hemodynamics will improve. It may be feasible in the near future for an echocardiogram to begin with three-dimensional images.

An M-mode recording is derived from two-dimensional tomographic images and graphically represents the motion of cardiac structures. It is used primarily to measure cardiac chamber size and timing of cardiac events and to display subtle abnormalities of cardiac motion. Thus, it is important to recognize the characteristic M-mode features to understand the pathophysiologic mechanisms of cardiovascular disorders.

Measurement of cardiac dimensions from M-mode echocardiography has been standardized (**Fig. 15-6**). For these measurements, an M-mode cursor is drawn as a straight line from the transducer position in any direction in the sector to record the movement of the cardiac structure of interest. However, this traditional M-mode method may overestimate the dimensions of the structure if the direction of the ultrasound beam is oblique to that structure. Anatomic M-mode allows the M-mode cursor to be positioned in any direction from anywhere in the heart; this allows a more reliable recording of cardiac structures. **Figure 15-7** demonstrates the dynamic changes of cardiac structures documented with M-mode, two-dimensional, and three-dimensional echocardiography.

TRANSESOPHAGEAL ECHOCARDIOGRAPHY

With the proximity of the major cardiovascular structures (heart, aorta, and pulmonary arteries) to the esophagus, TEE provides excellent evaluation of cardiovascular anatomy, function, hemodynamics, and blood flow.

TEE is now considered essential in the evaluation of mitral valve lesions, the left atrium or its appendage, an intracardiac mass, an atrial septal defect, endocarditis and its complications, and thoracic aortic lesions such as aortic dissection (see Chaps. 60, 65, 66, 67, and 74). Patients with atrial fibrillation (AF) undergo direct-current cardioversion without chronic anticoagulation if TEE does not show intracardiac thrombus (see Chap. 40), and with ablation procedures, AF has become one of the most common reasons for referral for TEE.[6,7] Another routine clinical use of TEE is in the operating room to assess the result of various valvular and repair procedures. Since its clinical introduction more than 20 years ago, TEE has been a low-risk procedure, with a complication rate less than 0.1% when transthoracic echocardiography (TTE) is not diagnostic.[8]

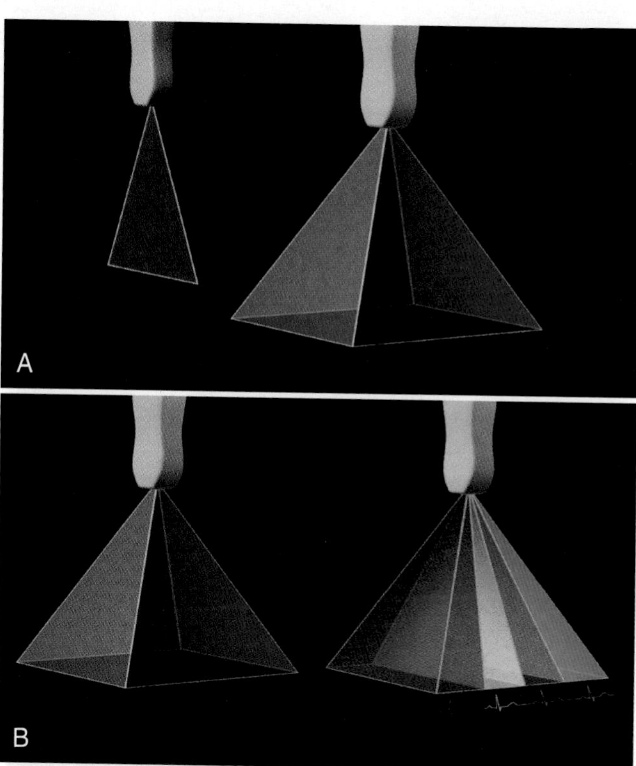

FIGURE 15-2 **A,** Schematic diagram of two-dimensional tomographic image acquisition **(left)** and three-dimensional full-volume acquisition **(right).** **B,** Three-dimensional full-volume images are usually patched together from four pyramidal volumes. *(Courtesy of Joe Maalouf, MD.)*

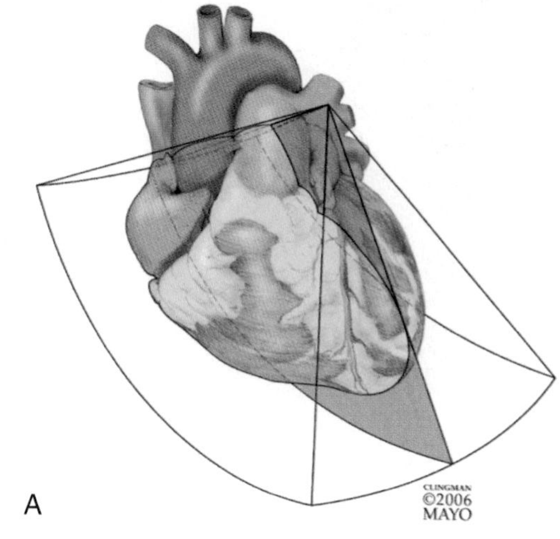

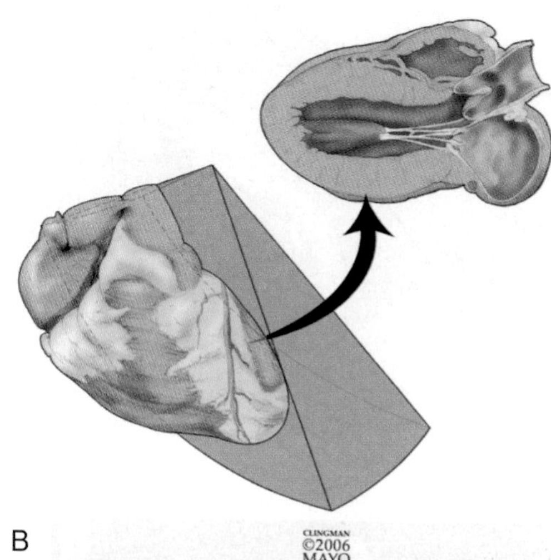

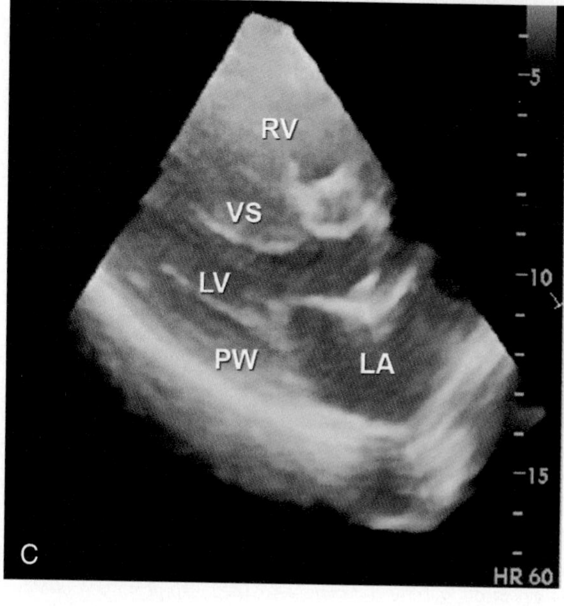

FIGURE 15-3 **A,** Parasternal long-axis view of three-dimensional echocardiography pyramidal imaging. **Shaded area,** Center of pyramidal image along parasternal long-axis view. **B,** Removal of half the pyramidal image from left side of the heart produces a three-dimensional image of the parasternal long-axis view. **C,** Still frame of real-time three-dimensional imaging along parasternal long-axis view. The image can be rotated and tilted freely. This image was rotated clockwise to show better the mitral inflow area and left ventricular outflow tract area. LA = left atrium; LV = left ventricle; PW = posterior wall; RV = right ventricle; VS = ventricular septum. *(Modified from Oh JK, Seward JB, Tajik AJ: The Echo Manual. 3rd ed. Philadelphia, Lippincott Williams & Wilkins, 2006. Used with permission of Mayo Foundation for Medical Education and Research.)*

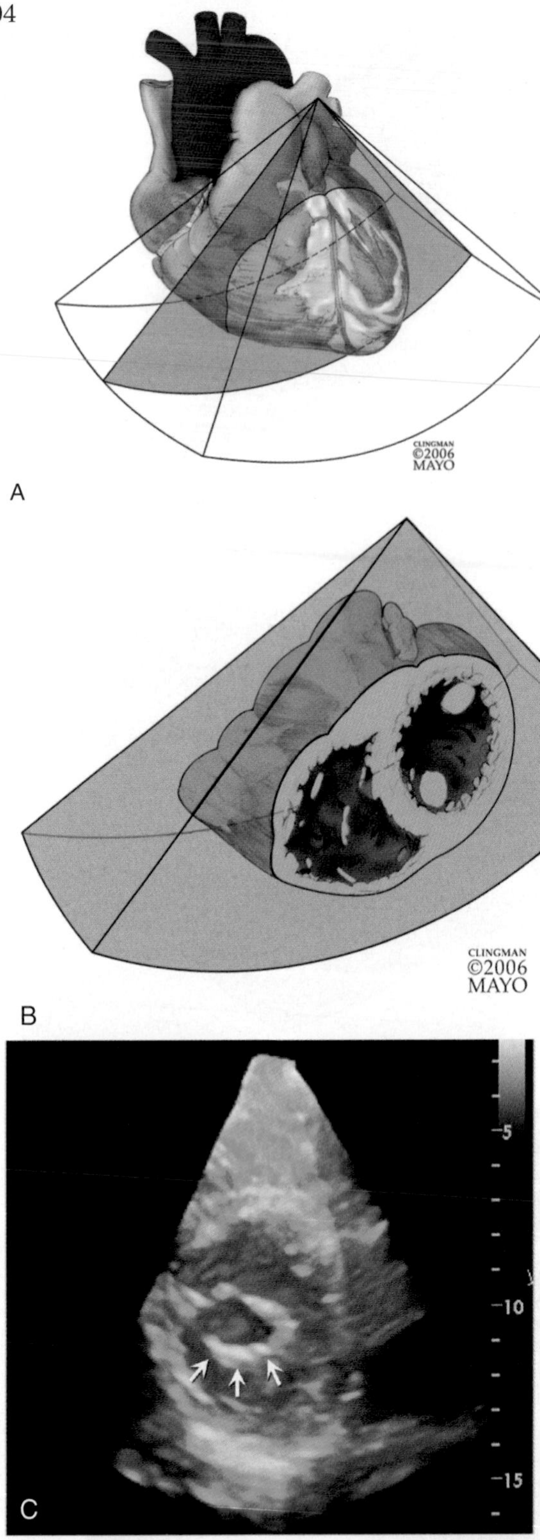

FIGURE 15-4 **A,** Three-dimensional pyramidal imaging along parasternal short-axis view. **Shaded area,** Midportion of the pyramid. **B,** Diagram of the view from the apex after half the pyramid was cropped away. **C,** Three-dimensional echocardiographic image along parasternal short-axis view from patient with mitral stenosis. Note fish-mouth appearance of mitral valve orifice (arrows). *(Modified from Oh JK, Seward JB, Tajik AJ: The Echo Manual. 3rd ed. Philadelphia, Lippincott Williams & Wilkins, 2006. Used with permission of Mayo Foundation for Medical Education and Research.)*

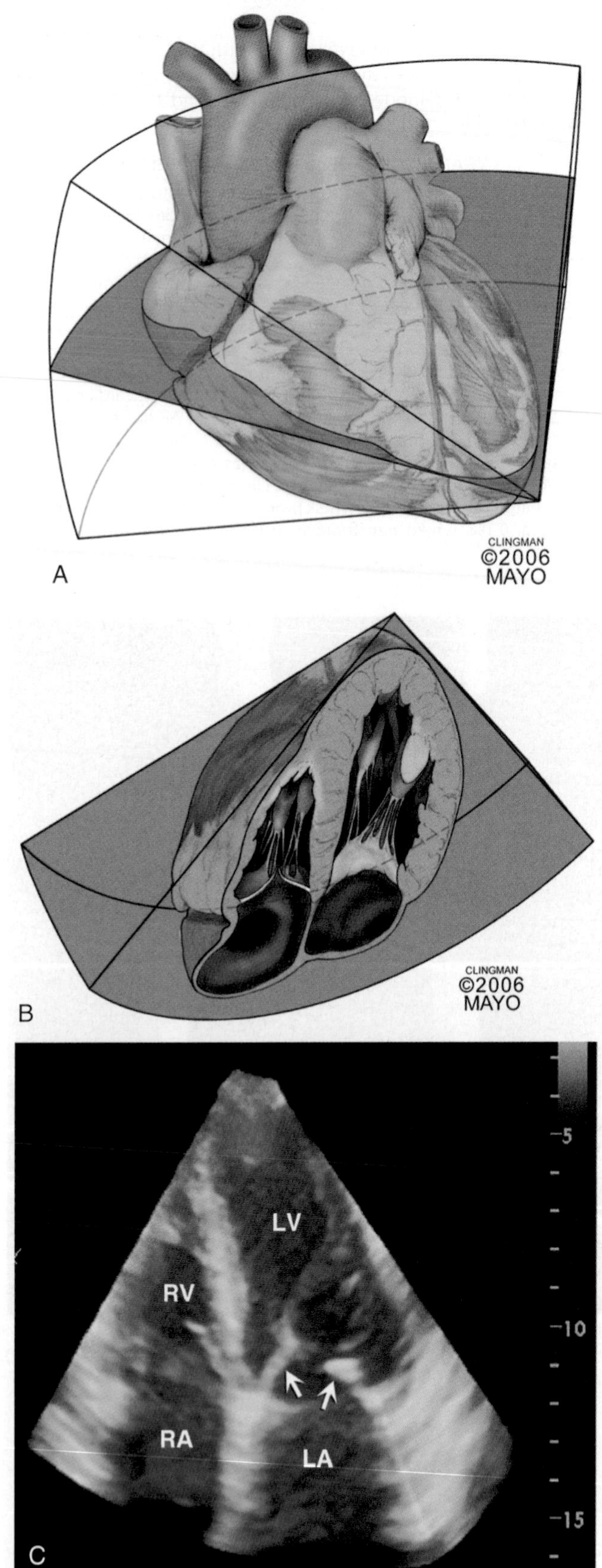

FIGURE 15-5 **A,** Three-dimensional pyramidal image of apical four-chamber view. **Shaded area,** Midportion of the pyramid. **B,** Cropping of the top half of the pyramid shows the four chambers clearly, with much better definition of the spatial relationships of various cardiac structures. **C,** Still frame of real-time three-dimensional imaging of apical four-chamber view from patient with mitral stenosis. The thickened and restricted motion of the mitral valve (arrows) is well shown. LA = left atrium; LV = left ventricle; RA = right atrium; RV = right ventricle. *(Modified from Oh JK, Seward JB, Tajik AJ: The Echo Manual. 3rd ed. Philadelphia, Lippincott Williams & Wilkins, 2006. Used with permission of Mayo Foundation for Medical Education and Research.)*

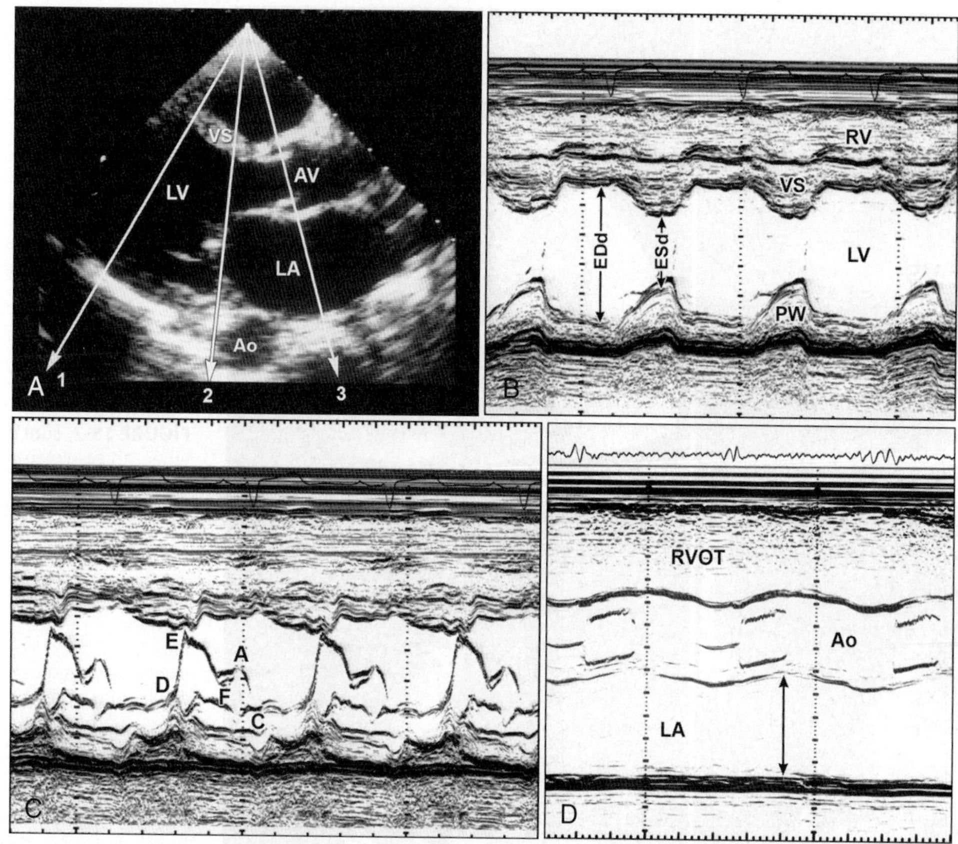

FIGURE 15-6 **A,** An M-mode cursor is placed along different levels (1, ventricular; 2, mitral valve; 3, aortic valve level) of the heart, with parasternal long-axis two-dimensional echocardiographic guidance. **B,** EDd and ESd are end-diastolic and end-systolic dimensions, respectively, of the left ventricle (LV). **C,** M-mode echocardiogram of the anterior mitral leaflet. A = peak of late opening with atrial systole; C = closure of mitral valve; D = end systole before mitral valve opening; E = peak of early opening; F = mid-diastolic closure. **D,** Level of aortic valve. Double-headed arrow indicates the dimension of the left atrium (LA) at end systole. Ao = aorta; AV = aortic valve; PW = posterior wall; RV = right ventricle; RVOT = right ventricular outflow tract; VS = ventricular septum. *(From Oh JK, Seward JB, Tajik AJ: The Echo Manual. 3rd ed. Philadelphia, Lippincott Williams & Wilkins, 2006. Used with permission of Mayo Foundation for Medical Education and Research.)*

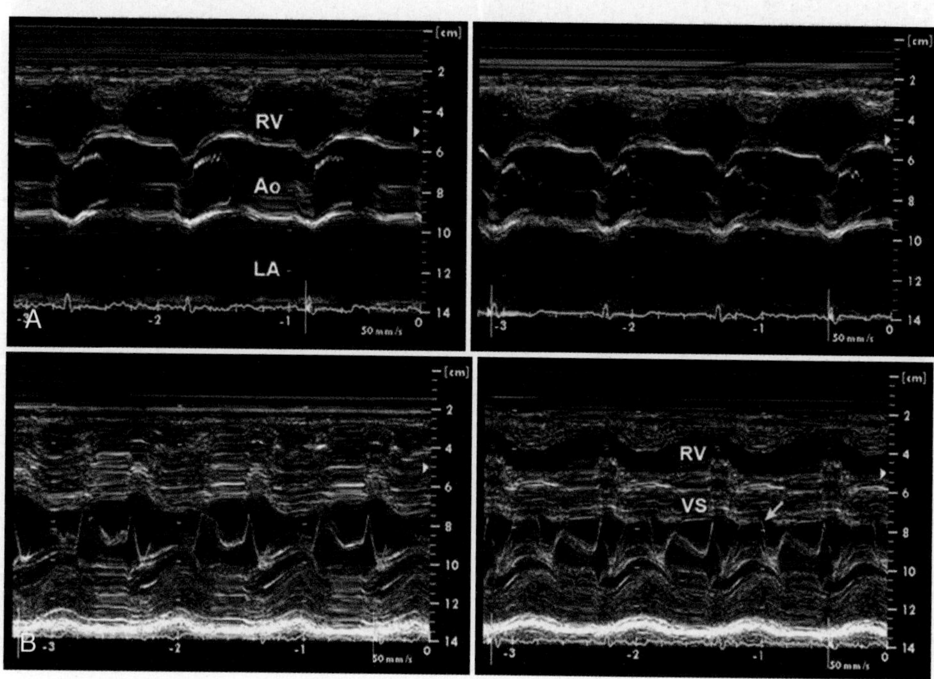

FIGURE 15-7 **A,** M-mode echocardiogram of aortic valve of 58-year-old man with heart failure and dysproteinemia. **Left,** Baseline M-mode echocardiogram shows normal aortic valve opening. **Right,** With Valsalva maneuver, patient developed loud murmur and midsystolic closure of aortic valve. **B, Left,** M-mode echocardiogram of mitral valve at baseline. **Right,** With Valsalva maneuver, patient developed systolic anterior motion of mitral valve (arrow) from dynamic left ventricular outflow tract (LVOT) obstruction.

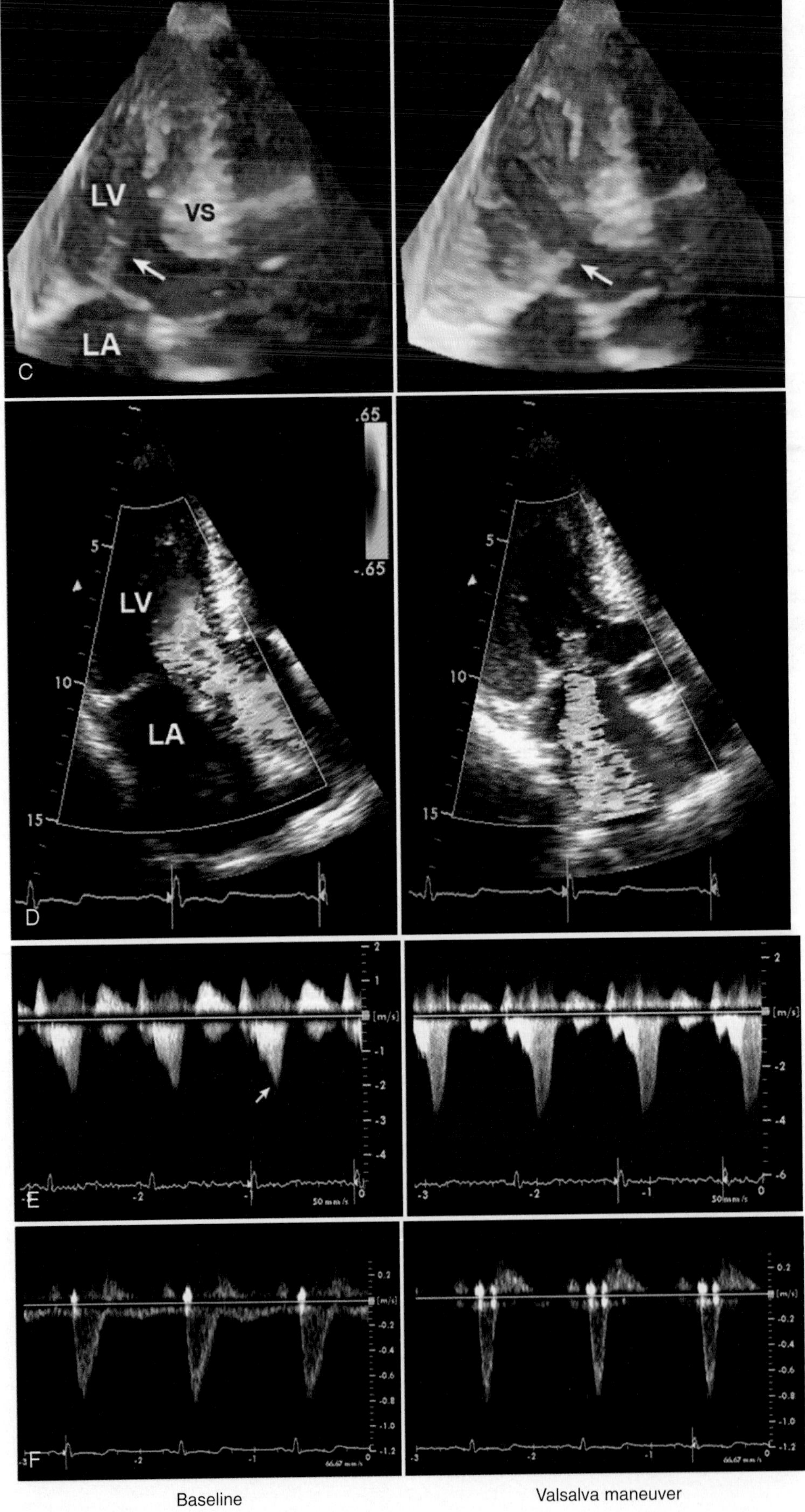

FIGURE 15-7, cont'd **C,** Still frames of real-time three-dimensional echocardiograms from patient in **A** at baseline **(left)** and with Valsalva maneuver **(right).** Note mild systolic anterior motion (arrow on left) at baseline without pronounced LVOT obstruction. With Valsalva maneuver, systolic anterior motion is more pronounced, obstructing LVOT (arrow on right). Ventricular septum (VS) is thick. This patient has systemic amyloidosis with cardiac involvement. A subset of patients with cardiac amyloidosis present with dynamic LVOT obstruction (as in this case), which is sometimes misdiagnosed as hypertrophic obstructive cardiomyopathy. **D,** Systolic frame of two-dimensional and color flow imaging of same patient. **Left,** At baseline, there is no mitral regurgitation. **Right,** With Valsalva maneuver, marked mitral regurgitation develops, with a typical lateral direction of mitral regurgitation caused by systolic anterior motion, as in hypertrophic cardiomyopathy. **E,** Recordings of continuous-wave Doppler examination across the LVOT from apical transducer position at baseline **(left)** and with Valsalva maneuver **(right)** show dagger-shaped systolic velocities below the baseline, characteristic of dynamic LVOT gradient or obstruction. The peak velocity is 4 m/sec with Valsalva maneuver, which equals a gradient of 64 mm Hg. **F,** Recordings of pulsed-wave Doppler examination from suprasternal notch transducer position with sample volume in a proximal descending thoracic aorta at baseline **(left)** and with Valsalva maneuver **(right)** show marked reduction in flow duration and midsystolic flow reversal with Valsalva maneuver. Ao = aorta; LA = left atrium; LV = left ventricle; RV = right ventricle.

The TEE probe is equipped with a multiplane transducer that rotates in a 180-degree arc, which produces a continuum of transverse and longitudinal image planes. These TEE images are identified by an icon that indicates the degree of transducer rotation (**Fig. 15-8**). The transverse plane, in the short axis of the body, is designated 0 degrees, and the longitudinal plane, in the long axis of the body, is designated 90 degrees. Normally, from the midesophagus (35 to 40 cm from the teeth), the short axis of the heart is imaged at 45 to 60 degrees of rotation and the long axis at 120 to 135 degrees.

TEE tomographic views can be displayed similarly to those of TTE with the electronic transducer at the bottom or, for the opposite orientation, at the top of the screen (**Fig. 15-9**). With the addition of a three-dimensional transducer to the TEE probe, this method provides exceptional real-time three-dimensional images that have been especially valuable in surgical patients.[9]

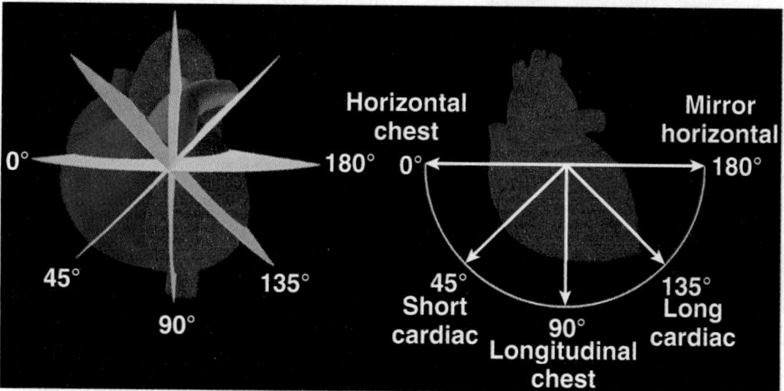

FIGURE 15-8 For transesophageal echocardiography, array rotations of selected degrees (0, 45, 90, 135, and 180) permit a logical sequence of standard transducer orientations and resultant images. Such a display helps the examiner acquire the desired views: 0-degree transverse orientation, which is horizontal to the chest at the midesophageal level; 45-degree short-axis orientation to the base of the heart from the midesophagus; 90-degree longitudinal orientation, which is in the sagittal plane of the body; 135-degree long-axis orientation to the heart from the midesophagus; and 180-degree rotation, which produces a mirror-image transverse plane. *(Modified from Seward JB, Khandheria BK, Freeman WK, et al: Multiplane transesophageal echocardiography: Image orientation, examination technique, anatomic correlations, and clinical applications. Mayo Clin Proc 68:523, 1993. Used with permission of Mayo Foundation for Medical Education and Research.)*

Primary Views

Four primary TEE views are obtained by rotating the transducer array from 0 to 140 degrees (see Fig. 15-9): (1) 0 degrees (transverse plane); the four-chamber view or an oblique view of the basal structures is obtained from this position; (2) 45- to 60-degree short-axis view of the aortic valve; this image is similar to the transthoracic parasternal short-axis view at the level of the aortic valve; (3) 65- to 100-degree longitudinal transducer orientation; this produces images oblique to the long axis of the heart; and (4) 125 to 140 degrees, the true long axis of the left atrium and the left ventricular outflow tract (LVOT); this is analogous to the transthoracic parasternal long-axis view.

Secondary Longitudinal Views

With the transducer array at 75 to 90 degrees, the plane is sagittal to the body and oblique to the long axis of the heart. Sequential leftward (counterclockwise) and rightward (clockwise) rotations of the probe shaft develop a series of longitudinal TEE views,[1] including the following: (1) counterclockwise rotation of the probe, producing a two-chamber view; (2) slight clockwise rotation of the scope from the neutral position, producing a long-axis view of the right ventricular outflow tract (RVOT); (3) further rightward rotation, producing a long-axis view of the proximal ascending aorta; and (4) still further rightward clockwise rotation, producing a long-axis view of the venae cavae and atrial septum.

Transgastric Views

The short-axis view of the left ventricle and right ventricle is obtained with the transducer tip in the stomach (about 40 to 45 cm from the incisors) and the transducer array at 0 degrees. Anteflexion of the transducer tip optimizes the basal short-axis view of the ventricles, and retroflexion of the tip results in a more apical short-axis view. The longitudinal two-chamber view of the left ventricle is obtained with the transducer array at 75 to 90 degrees, and clockwise rotation shows both right ventricular (RV) inflow and outflow areas. The LVOT and aortic valve can be imaged with the array at 110 to 135 degrees.

Views of the Aorta, Pulmonary Artery, and Pulmonary Veins

The ascending aorta is clearly visualized from the 120- to 135-degree transducer position. The arch and descending aorta are imaged by directing the transducer to face posteriorly (see Diseases of the Aorta). Aortic aneurysm, aortic dissection, and atheromatous plaques are reliably detected with TEE. The main, right, and proximal portion of the left pulmonary arteries are visualized from the 0-degree transverse transducer position if the probe is pulled slightly higher from the left atrial (LA) view. Pulmonary veins are becoming important structures to be imaged, with increasing catheter-based or surgical procedures involving the structure. From the 45- to 60-degree short-axis view of the aortic

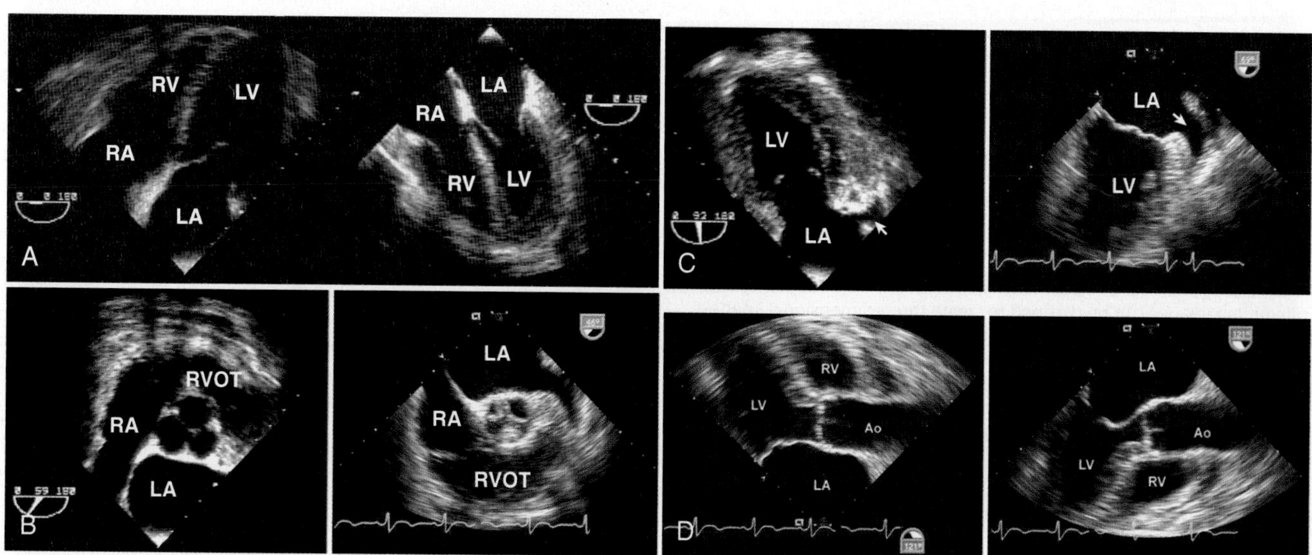

FIGURE 15-9 **A,** Four-chamber view (0 degrees with retroflexion of the transducer tip). Two different image orientations on the screen are shown: apex-up **(left)** and apex-down **(right)** views. **B,** Short-axis view (45 to 60 degrees) of the aortic valve in two different image displays. **Left,** Image display of left atrium (LA) at the bottom and right ventricular outflow tract (RVOT) at the top, similar to transthoracic parasternal short-axis view. **Right,** Image display of LA at the top and RVOT at the bottom. **C, Left** and **right,** Two-chamber view (65 to 100 degrees with leftward rotation of the transesophageal echocardiographic shaft). Arrow indicates the LA appendage in two different image displays. **D, Left** and **right,** Long-axis view (125 to 140 degrees) of the left ventricle (LV). Ao = aorta; RA = right atrium; RV = right ventricle. *(Modified from Oh JK, Seward JB, Tajik AJ: The Echo Manual. 3rd ed. Philadelphia, Lippincott Williams & Wilkins, 2006. Used with permission of Mayo Foundation for Medical Education and Research.)*

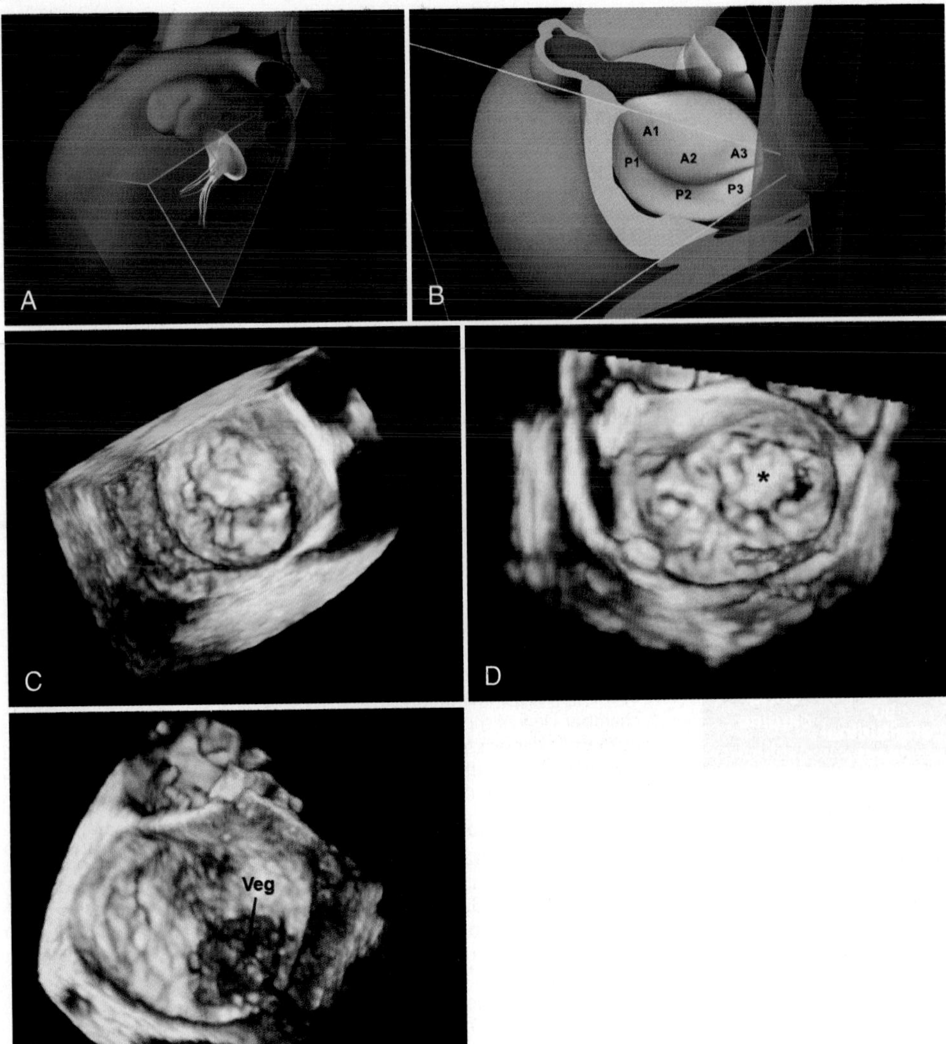

FIGURE 15-10 **A,** Schematic diagram of three-dimensional TEE visualizing the mitral valve. **B,** Schematic left atrial view of the mitral valve from three-dimensional TEE. Anterior (A) and posterior (P) leaflets and their scallops are numbered. **C,** Still frame of three-dimensional TEE image of normal mitral valve viewed from left atrium. **D,** Still frame image of myomatous mitral valve with prolapse (asterisk) of P3 scallop from left atrial perspective. **E,** Three-dimensional TEE image of mitral valve vegetation (Veg) attached to P2 and P3 regions.

valve, the probe is rotated clockwise to image the right pulmonary veins as a Y structure. Left pulmonary veins are best visualized by rotating the probe counterclockwise from the 120- to 130-degree long-axis view of the aorta. Pulmonary veins are also visualized from the 0-degree transverse view of the left atrium.

Real-Time Three-Dimensional Views

A full-volume or preset three-dimensional image can be obtained by TEE. Full-volume images can be cropped to create three-dimensional images of the desired structures online or offline. Because evaluation of the mitral valve structure is one of the more frequent uses of TEE, visualization of the mitral valve and its surrounding structures is preprogrammed in a certain ultrasound unit so that they are automatically visualized by pushing a three-dimensional live-imaging knob after imaging boundaries are provided (**Fig. 15-10**).

Doppler Echocardiography and Color Flow Imaging

Doppler Echocardiography

Doppler echocardiography measures blood flow velocities on the basis of the Doppler effect, which was described by Christian Doppler in 1842. When an ultrasound beam with known frequency (*fo*) is transmitted to the heart, it is reflected by red blood cells. The frequency of the reflected ultrasound waves (*fr*) increases when the red blood cells are moving toward the source of ultrasound and decreases when the red blood cells are moving away. The difference in frequency between transmitted sound and reflected sound is the frequency shift or Doppler shift: ($\Delta f = fr - fo$). The Doppler shift is related to the transmitted frequency (*fo*), the velocity of the moving target (υ), and the angle (θ) between the ultrasound beam and the direction of the moving target, as expressed in the Doppler equation (**Fig. 15-11**):

$$\Delta f = 2\, fo \times \upsilon \times \cos\theta / c$$

Once Δf is calculated, the velocity of red blood cells can be calculated as follows:

$$\upsilon = \Delta f \times c / 2\, fo$$

where c is the speed of sound in blood (1540 m/sec). If the ultrasound beam is not parallel with the direction of blood flow, angle θ is greater than 0 degrees. As angle θ increases, the corresponding cosine value becomes progressively less than 1, which results in underestimation of the Doppler shift (Δf) and hence peak velocity. Blood flow velocities measured with Doppler echocardiography are used to derive various hemodynamic data.

There are two forms of Doppler echocardiography: the pulsed-wave form and the continuous-wave form (**Fig. 15-12**; see also Fig. 15-7). Pulsed-wave Doppler is location specific. A single crystal sends a short burst of ultrasound at a pulse repetition frequency and receives sound beams reflected from moving red blood cells from a specified location that is determined by placement of a "sample volume." Thus, the maximal frequency shift that pulsed-wave Doppler can measure is half the pulse repetition frequency, called the Nyquist frequency. If the frequency shift is higher than the Nyquist frequency, aliasing occurs; that is, the frequency shift or the corresponding velocity higher than the Nyquist frequency is cut off at the Nyquist frequency or velocity, and the remaining frequency shift is recorded on the top or bottom of the opposite side of baseline. In continuous-wave Doppler, the transducer sends ultrasound waves and receives the reflected ultrasound waves continuously with the use of two separate crystals. Therefore, the maximal frequency shift and velocity recorded with continuous-wave Doppler are not limited by the pulse repetition frequency or Nyquist phenomenon. Unlike pulsed-wave Doppler, continuous-wave Doppler measures all frequency shifts (i.e., velocities) along its beam path; hence, it is used to detect and to record the highest flow velocity available.

Color Flow Imaging or Color Doppler

Color flow imaging, or color Doppler, is a form of pulsed-wave Doppler that displays blood flow or myocardial velocities in various colors (usually red, blue, and green) or their combinations, depending on the velocity, direction, and turbulence. At each sampling site, the frequency shift is measured, converted to a digital format, automatically correlated (autocorrelation) with a preset color scheme, and displayed as color flow superimposed on two-dimensional imaging (**Fig. 15-13**). For intracavitary flow, blood flow directed toward the transducer has a positive frequency shift and is color coded in shades of red. Blood flow directed away from the transducer has a negative frequency shift and is color coded in shades of blue. The lighter shades within each primary color are assigned to higher velocities within the Nyquist limit. When flow velocity is higher than the Nyquist frequency limit, color aliasing occurs and is depicted as a color reversal. Turbulence reflects the degree of the variance from the mean velocity of a region and is coded usually in a shade of green. Therefore, abnormal blood flow is easily recognized by combinations of multiple colors according to the directions, velocities, and degrees of turbulence. The width and size of abnormal intracavitary blood flows are used to evaluate the degree of valvular regurgitation or cardiac shunt.

Almost all structural and hemodynamic abnormalities of the heart produce a disturbance in blood flow and hence abnormality in color flow imaging. An exception is wide-open flow or regurgitation with laminar flow. Color Doppler is used also for determination of diastolic function and timing of intracardiac events (see Evaluation of Systolic and Diastolic Function). Figure 15-7 demonstrates dynamic changes of valvular regurgitation and hemodynamics recorded with Doppler

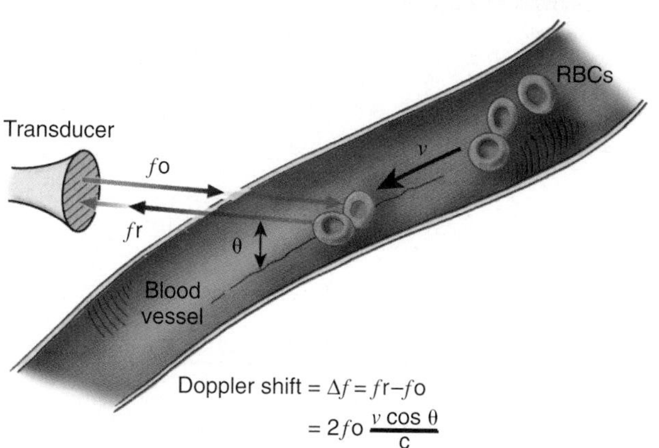

FIGURE 15-11 Diagram of the Doppler effect (see text for explanation). RBCs = red blood cells. *(From Oh JK, Seward JB, Tajik AJ: The Echo Manual. 3rd ed. Philadelphia, Lippincott Williams & Wilkins, 2006. Used with permission of Mayo Foundation for Medical Education and Research.)*

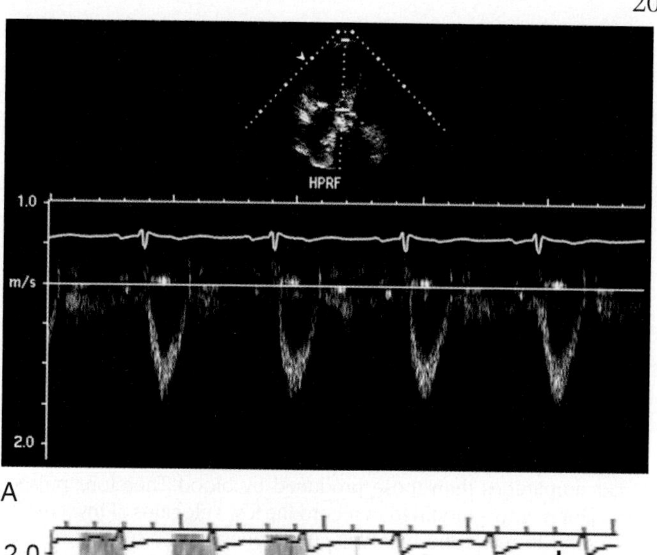

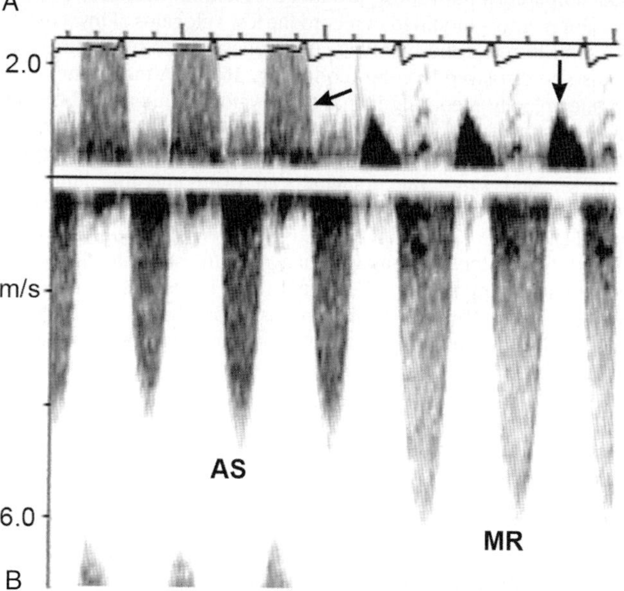

FIGURE 15-12 **A,** Pulsed-wave Doppler records flow velocity from a specific location. The sample volume was in the left ventricular outflow tract, and its velocity was 1.5 m/sec. **B,** Continuous-wave Doppler records all velocities along the path of the ultrasound beam. Therefore, a slight angulation of the transducer may record entirely different velocities. This continuous-wave recording was obtained from the apical window with a pencil probe in a patient with severe aortic stenosis (AS) and moderate mitral regurgitation (MR). A slight change in the direction of the continuous-wave Doppler probe recorded both AS and MR signals as well as aortic regurgitation (left arrow) and mitral inflow (down arrow) during diastole. Note that the duration and peak velocity of AS are shorter and lower, respectively, than those of MR. *(**B** modified from Oh JK, Seward JB, Tajik AJ: The Echo Manual. 3rd ed. Philadelphia, Lippincott Williams & Wilkins, 2006. Used with permission of Mayo Foundation for Medical Education and Research.)*

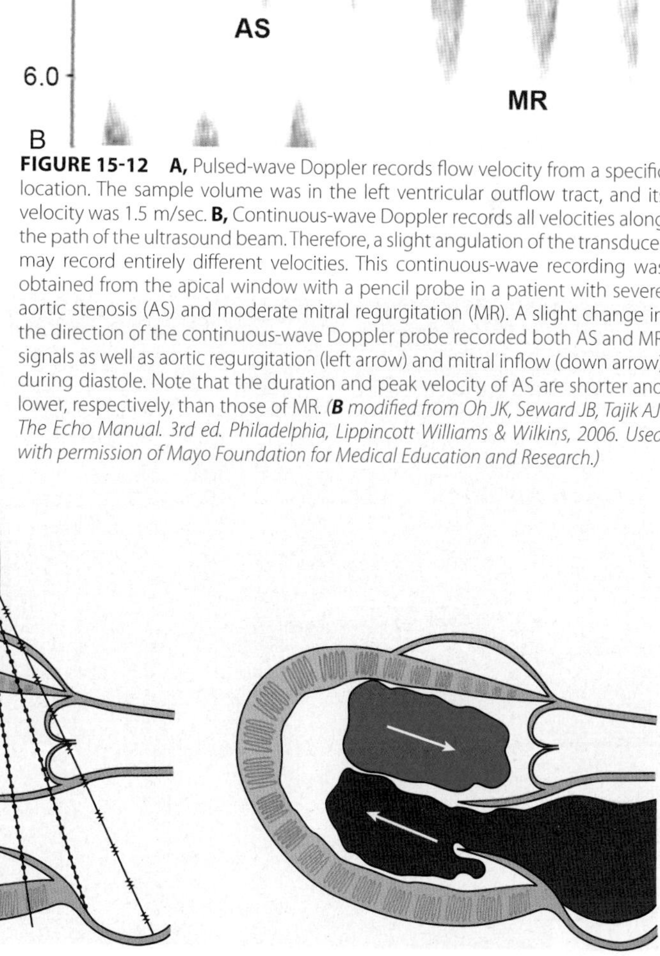

FIGURE 15-13 Drawing illustrating how color flow imaging is performed and displayed. The dots indicate multiple sampling sites (gates). The frequency shift measured at each gate is correlated automatically (autocorrelation) and converted to a preset color scheme (red for flow toward and blue for flow away from the transducer). *(Modified from Oh JK, Seward JB, Tajik AJ: The Echo Manual. 3rd ed. Philadelphia, Lippincott Williams & Wilkins, 2006. Used with permission of Mayo Foundation for Medical Education and Research.)*

echocardiography and color flow imaging. Another important use of color display in echocardiography is parametric imaging, reflecting a predetermined characteristic of blood flow, or tissue Doppler velocities, including the timing of peak velocities. M-mode of color flow imaging is helpful in determination of the timing of cardiac or flow events and assessment of diastolic function or flow propagation velocity.

Tissue Doppler and Strain Imaging

Tissue Doppler imaging (TDI) records the motion of tissue or other structures with a velocity or frequency shift much lower than that of blood flow. Doppler echocardiography for blood flow measures the velocities of red blood cells (velocity usually higher than 20 cm/sec and up to 800 cm/sec in the case of valvular disease). However, the velocities of myocardial tissue are much lower (<30 cm/sec) but with larger amplitudes than those produced by blood. Therefore, pulsed-wave Doppler was modified to record the low velocities of myocardial tissue and to reject the high velocities generated by blood flow. TDI can also be displayed in color mode (**Fig. 15-14**). A major limitation of tissue velocity recording is that tissue velocities measured by TDI may overestimate or underestimate the active component or function of the tissue because of translational motion or tethering, respectively. Strain (ε) and strain rate imaging can overcome this limitation by measuring the actual extent of stretching or contraction (see Fig. 15-14).[10]

Strain (ε) is the percentage change in muscle length during myocardial contraction and relaxation and is expressed as a percentage. By convention, shortening is represented by negative values and lengthening by positive values for both strain and strain rate.

$$\varepsilon = \Delta L/L_0 = (L_1 - L_0)/L_0 = (V_a \times t - V_b \times t)/L_0 = (V_a - V_b) \times t/L_0$$

where L_0 is the original length, L_1 is final length, ΔL is change in length, $V_a - V_b$ is the instantaneous velocity difference at points a and b, and t is time interval.

Strain rate is the rate of instantaneous change in strain calculated as the difference between two velocities normalized to the distance (d) between them and expressed as s^{-1} (see Fig. 15-e1 on website).

$$\text{Strain rate} = (V_a - V_b)/d$$

Therefore, strain (ε) is the sum of the instantaneous strain rate values over a time interval of deformation.

Tissue tracking or displacement is the integral of tissue velocity over a given time. It represents the distance a region of interest moves relative to its original location.

Tissue Doppler velocities, strain rate, displacement, and systolic strain of individual segments from healthy individuals are shown in **Tables 15-1 to 15-3**.

Speckle tracking is a method that uses two-dimensional images to quantify myocardial motion in various planes.[11] Reflection, scattering, and interference of the ultrasound beam in the myocardial tissue produce formation of speckles. Myocardial regions with unique speckle patterns in the gray-scale two-dimensional image can be tracked frame to frame throughout the cardiac cycle. Speckle tracking is another method for measurement of strain by use of angle-independent two-dimensional images instead of the angle-dependent tissue Doppler method described earlier. Hence, the speckle tracking method can provide circumferential and radial strain as well as longitudinal strain (**Fig. 15-15**).

TABLE 15-1 Velocity of Individual Segments Determined with Tissue Doppler Echocardiography

	Segment			
MEASURE	SEPTUM	LATERAL	INFERIOR	ANTERIOR
S wave, cm/sec				
Basal	5.97 ± 1.14	6.26 ± 2.44	6.52 ± 1.31	6.44 ± 2.32
Mid	6.29 ± 1.89	4.48 ± 0.92	5.21 ± 2.79	5.1 ± 1.16
Apical	4.42 ± 2.3	4.81 ± 1.97	2.97 ± 1.14	3.8 ± 2.66
E wave, cm/sec				
Basal	7.91 ± 2.16	8.54 ± 2.77	9.01 ± 2.44	8.09 ± 2.48
Mid	8.39 ± 2.5	6.85 ± 1.86	6.82 ± 3.16	7.22 ± 2.04
Apical	6.03 ± 2.95	6.74 ± 2.58	4.76 ± 1.94	4.52 ± 2.95
A wave, cm/sec				
Basal	5.99 ± 1.73	3.77 ± 1.95	5.84 ± 2.06	3.86 ± 1.75
Mid	4.87 ± 2.14	4.9 ± 1.72	2.62 ± 1.84	4.78 ± 1.7
Apical	2.69 ± 1.93	3.77 ± 2.1	3.08 ± 1.54	1.69 ± 1.45

A = late diastolic velocity; E = early diastolic velocity; S = systolic velocity.

Modified from Sun JP, Popovic ZB, Greenberg NL, et al: Noninvasive quantification of regional myocardial function using Doppler-derived velocity, displacement, strain rate, and strain in healthy volunteers: Effects of aging. J Am Soc Echocardiogr 17:132, 2004.

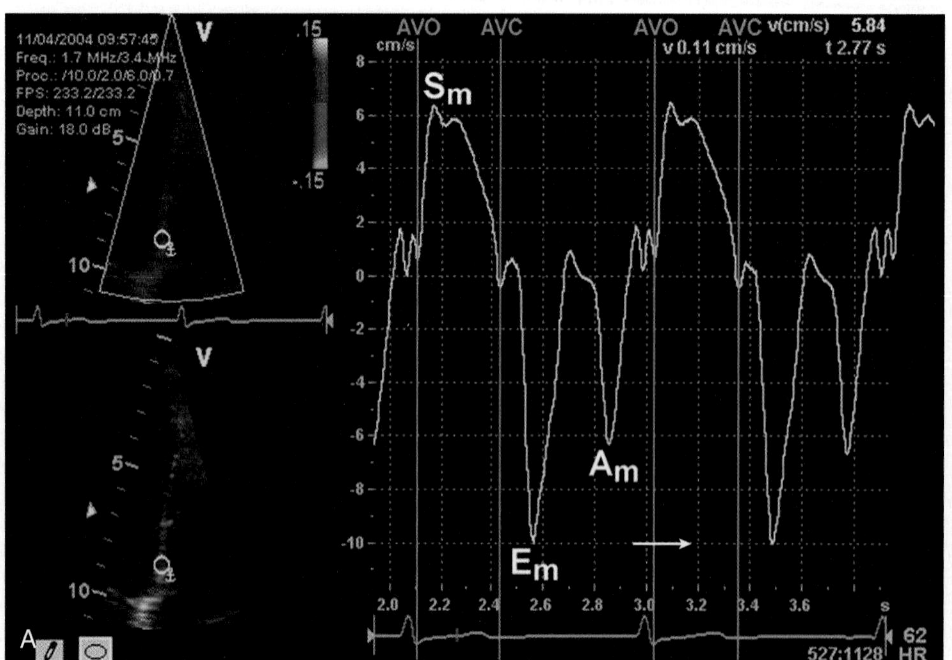

FIGURE 15-14 A, Recording of tissue velocity. The sample volume was placed at the basal portion of the inferior septum. Peak systolic velocity (S_m) was slightly more than 6 cm/sec, early diastolic velocity (E_m) was 10 cm/sec, and late diastolic velocity (A_m) was 6 cm/sec.

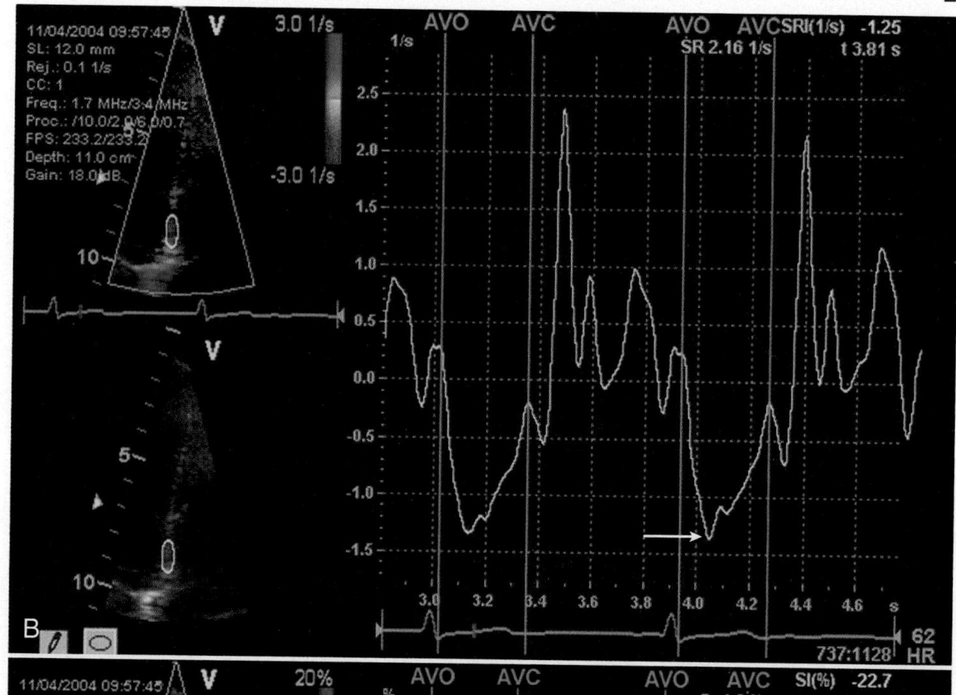

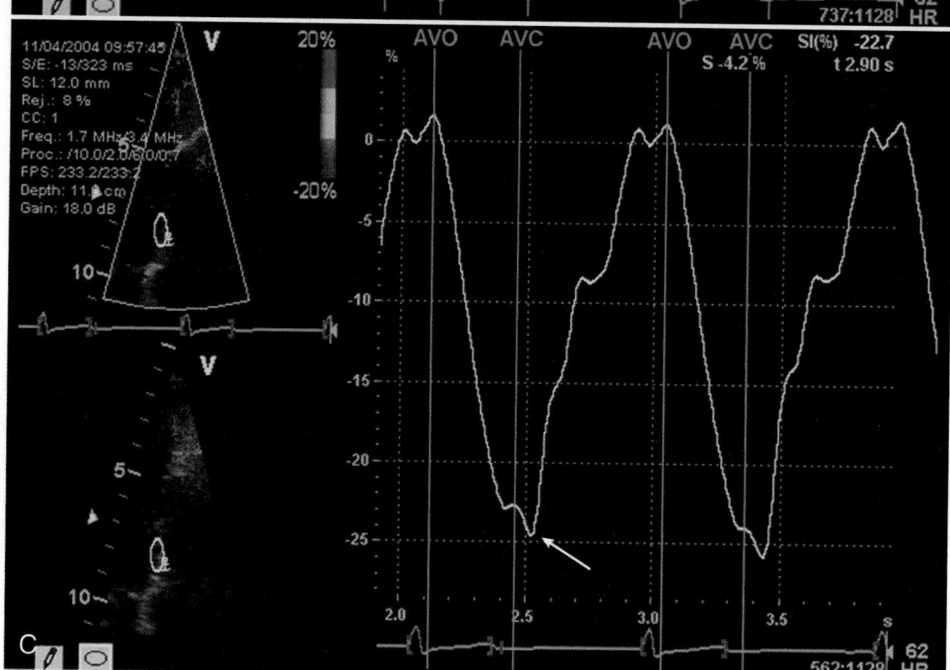

FIGURE 15-14, cont'd B, Recording of strain rate, which represents the rate of deformation; the peak negative strain rate (arrow) was −1.3/sec. **C,** Strain recording, which is the integration of the strain rates; the negative peak strain (arrow) occurred slightly after aortic valve closure (AVC). The normal strain value is usually more than −15%. AVO = aortic valve opening. *(Modified from Oh JK, Seward JB, Tajik AJ: The Echo Manual. 3rd ed. Philadelphia, Lippincott Williams & Wilkins, 2006. Used with permission of Mayo Foundation for Medical Education and Research.)*

TABLE 15-2 Strain Rate of Individual Segments

	Segment			
MEASURE	SEPTUM	LATERAL	INFERIOR	ANTERIOR
Peak systolic wave, s^{-1}				
Basal	0.99 ± 0.49	1.5 ± 0.74	0.88 ± 0.39	1.64 ± 0.9
Mid	1.25 ± 0.73	1.29 ± 0.58	0.95 ± 0.54	0.98 ± 0.68
Apical	1.15 ± 0.5	1.09 ± 0.59	1.38 ± 0.45	1.05 ± 0.63
Early diastolic wave, s^{-1}				
Basal	1.95 ± 0.89	1.92 ± 1.11	1.85 ± 0.89	2.03 ± 0.99
Mid	1.94 ± 0.97	1.71 ± 0.66	1.92 ± 1.2	1.7 ± 0.82
Apical	1.91 ± 0.66	1.81 ± 0.87	2.29 ± 0.88	1.76 ± 0.98
Late diastolic wave, s^{-1}				
Basal	1.54 ± 0.93	0.93 ± 0.59	1.18 ± 0.78	1.49 ± 0.96
Mid	1.29 ± 0.86	1.48 ± 0.77	0.78 ± 0.62	1.04 ± 0.57
Apical	0.95 ± 0.54	1.07 ± 0.68	1.68 ± 0.76	0.68 ± 0.65

Modified from Sun JP, Popovic ZB, Greenberg NL, et al: Noninvasive quantification of regional myocardial function using Doppler-derived velocity, displacement, strain rate, and strain in healthy volunteers: Effects of aging. J Am Soc Echocardiogr 17:132, 2004.

TABLE 15-3 Displacement and Systolic Strain of Individual Segments

	Segment			
MEASURE	SEPTUM	LATERAL	INFERIOR	ANTERIOR
Displacement, cm				
Basal	1.2 ± 0.19	0.93 ± 0.22	1.33 ± 0.22	1.05 ± 0.27
Mid	1.13 ± 0.27	0.91 ± 0.18	0.62 ± 0.22	1.04 ± 0.19
Apical	0.65 ± 0.24	0.82 ± 0.27	0.55 ± 0.18	0.41 ± 0.25
Systolic strain, %				
Basal	17.5 ± 5.32	18.22 ± 6.79	14.97 ± 5.74	22.19 ± 7.75
Mid	18.27 ± 6.93	18.83 ± 5.29	14.2 ± 5.14	17.95 ± 5.53
Apical	19.31 ± 6.07	17.56 ± 5.85	23.6 ± 5.17	13.17 ± 5.83

Modified from Sun JP, Popovic ZB, Greenberg NL, et al: Noninvasive quantification of regional myocardial function using Doppler-derived velocity, displacement, strain rate, and strain in healthy volunteers: Effects of aging. J Am Soc Echocardiogr 17:132, 2004.

CH 15

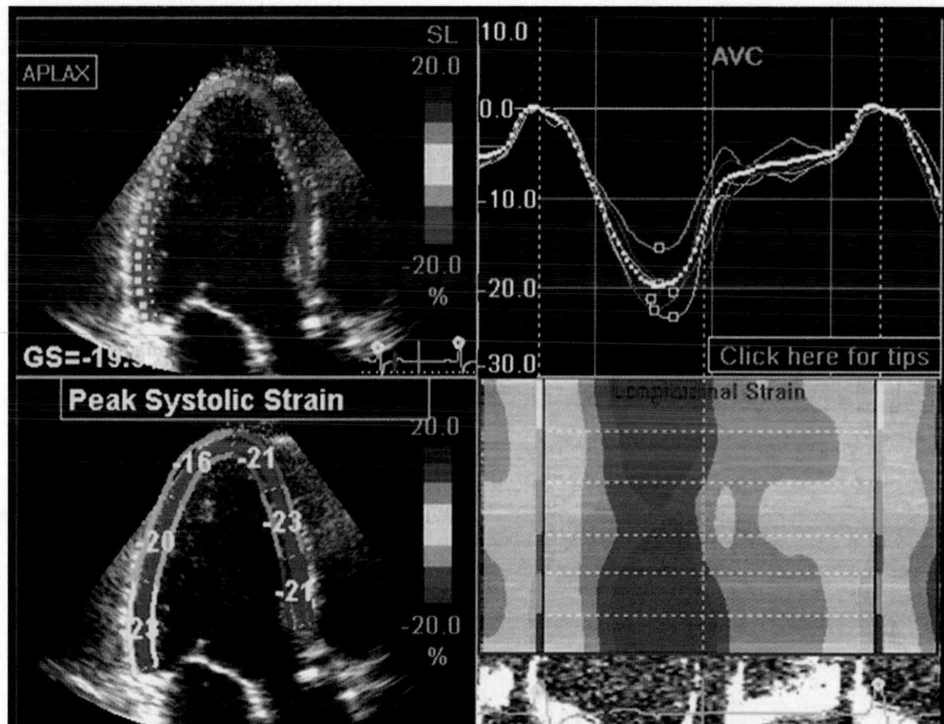

FIGURE 15-15 Speckle tracking strain imaging from apical long-axis (APLAX) view showing global longitudinal strain (GS) of −19.9%. Regional peak systolic strain is also shown in the left bottom panel. Strain curves from different LV regions are also shown in the upper right panel along with the cardiac event of aortic valve closure (AVC). The bottom right panel portrays longitudinal strain from six LV segments in a flat panel color format. The basal inferolateral segment is represented at the top and the basal anteroseptum at the bottom of the display. The horizontal axis represents time and the vertical axis represents the six LV segments.

Strain imaging also allows left ventricular (LV) rotational motion, often referred to as torsion or twist, to be assessed (**Fig. 15-16**). The spiral shape of LV myocardial fibers results in a complex three-dimensional torsion mechanism for systolic contraction and untwisting for diastolic relaxation.[12] The degree of torsion or twisting appears to be related to aging and diastolic function as well as systolic contraction. The LV myocardium consists of two layers; the subendocardial layer wraps around the LV cavity in a right-handed helical direction, and the subepicardial layer wraps around in a left-handed helical direction. Viewed from the LV apex, the apex rotates counterclockwise and the base rotates clockwise during systole.[13] As the two ends of the LV twist in opposite directions, the myocardium between the two thickens and shortens longitudinally.

The clinical applications of TDI and strain imaging are increasing and provide incremental diagnostic and prognostic value over standard two-dimensional and blood pool Doppler echocardiography. They have been used successfully in assessing regional and global systolic and diastolic function. Myocardial strain becomes abnormal during the early stage of myocardial ischemia as well as in myopathies and appears to be more sensitive for identification of ischemic segments during stress echocardiography.[14-19] TDI has been used most commonly to evaluate diastolic function and to estimate diastolic filling pressures.[20,21] Both strain imaging and TDI allow reliable determination of cardiac timing intervals, which is useful in assessing cardiac function[22] and LV intraventricular mechanical dyssynchrony.[23-26]

Contrast Echocardiography

Contrast echocardiography represents two distinct echocardiographic modalities, one using agitated saline (10 mL of saline is squirted back and forth between two syringes at least five times) to identify a right-to-left intracardiac shunt and to improve the Doppler signal from the right heart, and the other using gas-filled microbubbles that can pass through the pulmonary circulation to improve the definition of the LV endocardial border and to assess myocardial perfusion.[27] Although the issue of using gas-filled microbubbles in critically ill patients was raised by a black box warning, a subsequent multicenter retrospective analysis of 78,383 contrast doses, including more than 10,000 doses given to critically ill patients, showed no death and probable severe reaction in 8 patients (0.01%), all of whom were outpatients.[28] The safety of contrast echocardiography was validated by other studies.[29] The U.S. Food and Drug Administration subsequently revised the labeling for ultrasound contrast agents. Contraindications to the administration of a contrast agent include patients with known or suspected right-to-left, bidirectional, or transient right-to-left cardiac shunts and those with hypersensitivity to perflutren. Monitoring of vital signs, electrocardiogram, and cutaneous oxygen saturation during and for at least 30 minutes after administration of contrast agents is recommended in patients with pulmonary hypertension or unstable cardiopulmonary conditions.

Evaluation of Intra-atrial Shunts

Evaluation of an intra-atrial shunt through a patent foramen ovale (PFO) is the most frequent use of contrast echocardiography with agitated saline. Normally, when agitated saline is injected intravenously, the right atrium and right ventricle become opacified by the contrast effect of the agitated saline, and the left side of the heart remains contrast free. If there is an intra-atrial shunt through a PFO or atrial septal defect (see Chap. 65), the agitated saline appears in the left atrium immediately after the right atrium becomes opacified by bubbles from agitated saline (**Fig. 15-17**). If a patient has an intrapulmonary shunt, the bubbles do not appear in the left atrium until several cardiac cycles after they are seen in the right atrium. Another indication for agitated saline is to evaluate persistent left superior vena cava, which drains into the coronary sinus. In this case, injection of agitated saline into a left arm vein produces opacification of the enlarged coronary sinus in the left atrioventricular groove.

Left Ventricular Endocardial Border Enhancement and Assessment of Myocardial Perfusion

For left-sided heart chambers to be opacified by a contrast agent, microbubbles need to be small and stable enough to pass through the pulmonary circulation. Microbubbles 4 to 5 µm in diameter are sufficiently small to pass through the microcirculation. When exposed to ultrasound signals, they undergo volumetric oscillations.[27] Oscillations of the microbubbles create acoustic signals responsible for opacification of cardiac chambers and other areas that have blood flow. Microbubbles (usually perfluorocarbons or sulfur hexafluoride) are packaged within a stable shell made of lipid, polymer, galactose, surfactant, albumin, or some combination of these.[27] Ultrasound generates positive and negative (sinusoidal) pressures, and the ultrasound acoustic energy causes the microbubbles to compress and to expand in a nonlinear fashion if the acoustic pressure is at least as high as the resonant frequency of the microbubbles. Harmonic signals are generated by this nonlinear property of microbubbles when they are contacted by ultrasound energy. When ultrasound energy is transmitted with a high frequency (fundamental frequency) to the microbubbles, the returning signals have a second harmonic frequency, 2 *fo* (a frequency twice that of the fundamental frequency), as well as the fundamental frequency, *fo*. Therefore, modification of the imaging device to receive the signals with the second

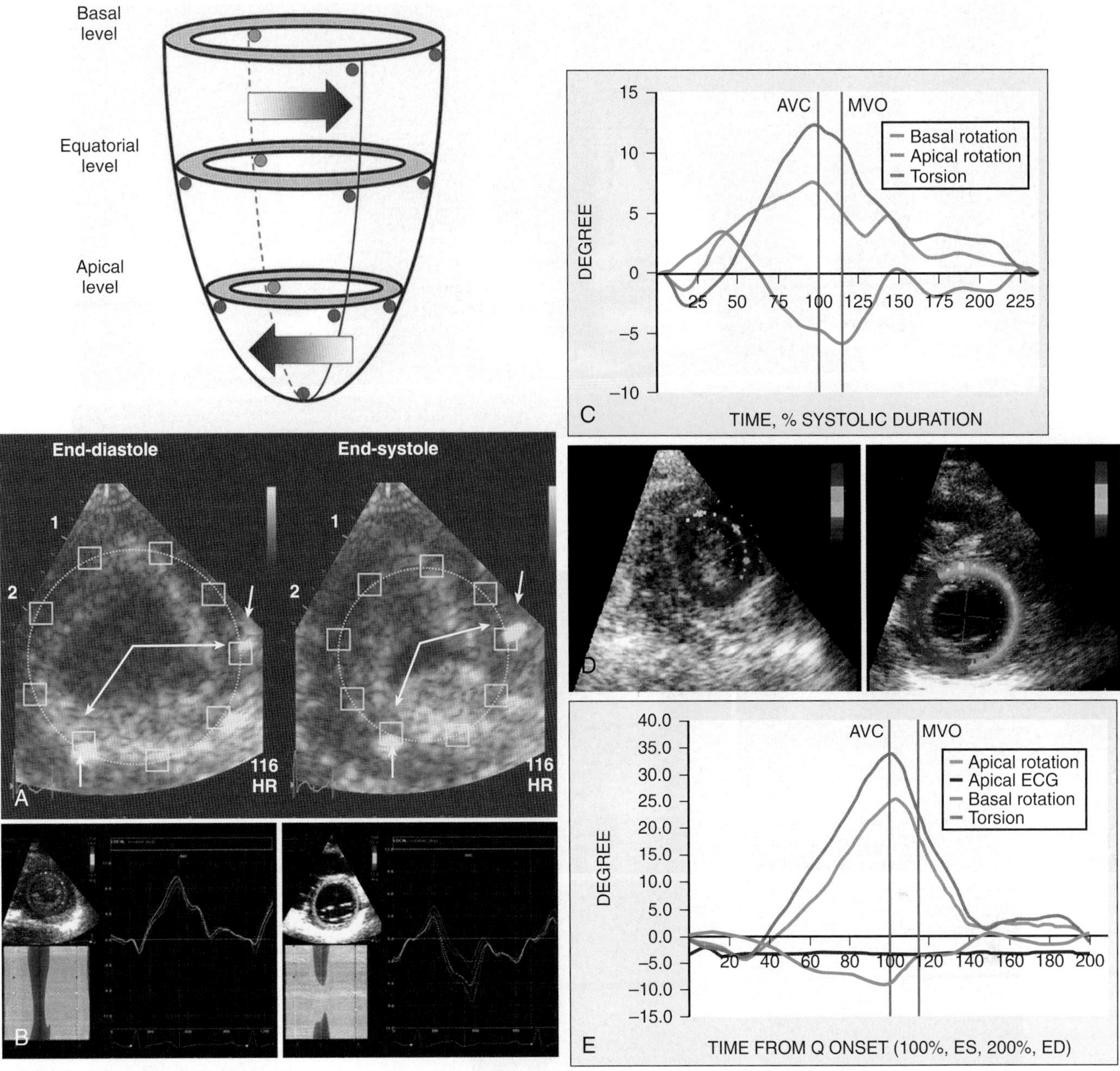

FIGURE 15-16 **A, Top,** Viewed from the apex, the apical rotation is counterclockwise (top arrow) and basal rotation is clockwise (bottom arrow). **Bottom,** Speckle tracking regions of interest are denoted by white boxes in the echocardiographic image of the animal model. Rotational changes are noted by the arrows during end-diastole and end-systole frames. **B,** Cardiac rotation in a normal person. The extent of rotation is colorized in these speckle tracking images. **Left,** Apical short-axis view with counterclockwise rotation colored blue. Maximal rotation occurred at end systole, shown as the graph above the baseline. The extent of rotation of multiple segments is shown in different colors. The rectangle below the speckle image shows colorized rotation of different segments during one cardiac cycle, which is a color M-mode image of left ventricular apical rotation. **Right,** The basal segment of the left ventricle, with clockwise rotation by color and graph. Because rotation is clockwise, the graph is recorded below the baseline. **C,** The mean apical rotation (7 degrees counterclockwise) and basal rotation (5 degrees clockwise) at the time of aortic valve closing (AVC) are shown. They resulted in a net torsion of 12 degrees. Untwisting of the torsion starts the myocardial relaxation process. MVO = mitral valve opening. **D, Left,** Apical short-axis view with speckle imaging showing exaggerated counterclockwise rotation in a patient with abnormal myocardial relaxation. **Right,** Basal short-axis view showing clockwise rotation. **E,** Quantification of the extent of the rotation and resulting torsion is shown in this graph from the same patient as in **D.** Apical counterclockwise rotation is 25 degrees (above the baseline), and the peak basal rotation is clockwise (below the baseline) 9 degrees. Both apical and basal rotation is greater than that of a normal subject. Therefore, torsion is higher than in a normal subject at 34 degrees. ED = end diastole; ES = end systole. *(**A** modified from Helle-Valle T, Crosby J, Edvardsen T, et al: New noninvasive method for assessment of left ventricular rotation: Speckle tracking echocardiography. Circulation 112:3149, 2005. Used with permission. **B-E** courtesy of C. Miyazaki, MD.)*

harmonic frequency (second harmonic imaging) enhances the detection of microbubbles. Myocardial tissue also produces a second harmonic frequency, but weaker than the nonlinearly behaving microbubbles. Therefore, tissue second harmonic imaging also improves the image quality of myocardial structures without microbubbles being in the cardiac chambers. Second harmonic imaging signals increase with higher ultrasound power, and by higher positive and negative pressures, they deform the microbubbles to the point of destruction. The ultrasound acoustic power is expressed as the mechanical index, which is calculated as follows:

$$\text{Mechanical index} = \text{acoustic power}/\sqrt{fo}$$

A mechanical index higher than 0.7 is associated with bubble destruction. Several techniques enhance second harmonic signals from microbubbles (see Fig. 15-e2 on website). The pulse-inversion method sends out two ultrasound pulses of inverted (or out of) phase to myocardial

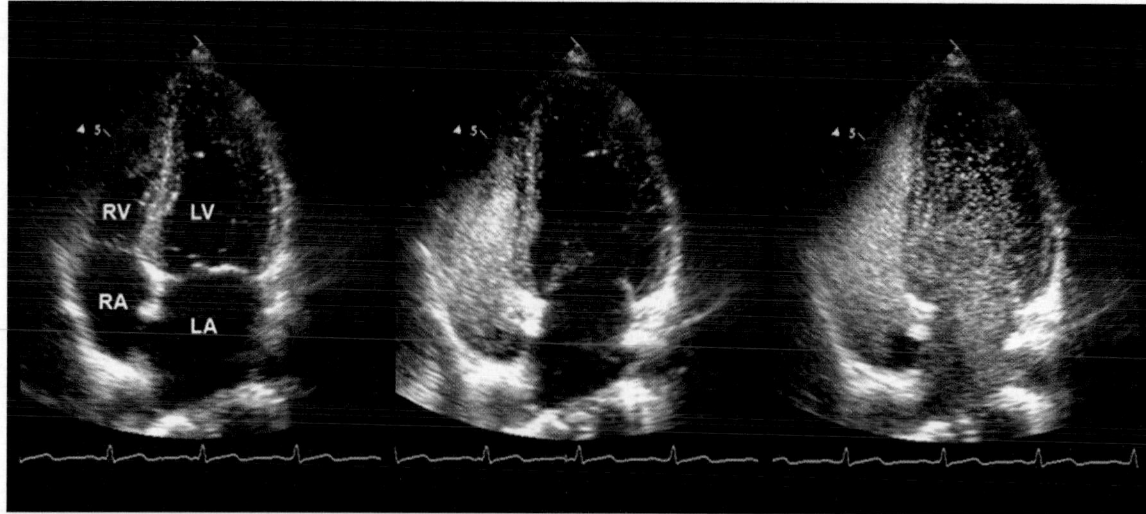

FIGURE 15-17 Apical four-chamber view demonstrating positive contrast study for right-to-left shunt through patent foramen ovale. **Left,** Before intravenous administration of agitated saline. **Center,** Opacification of right atrium by agitated saline. **Right,** Immediately after right atrial opacification, left atrium is also opacified because of a large right-to-left shunt through a patent foramen ovale.

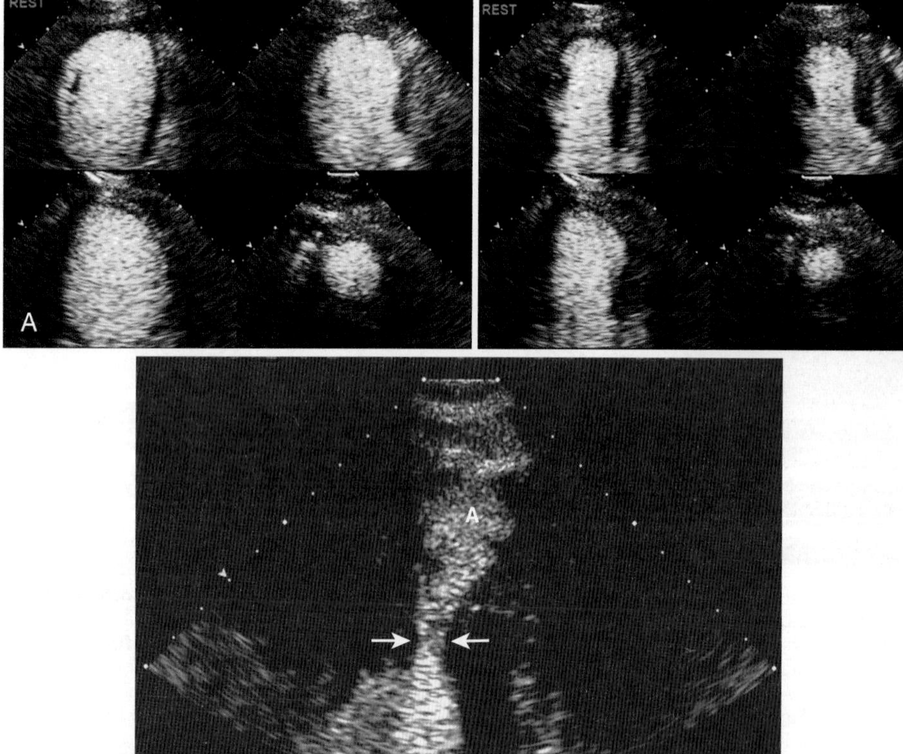

FIGURE 15-18 **A,** Harmonic imaging from apical views of the left ventricle during diastole **(left)** and systole **(right)** with intravenous myocardial contrast agent. The mechanical index was set at 0.4 to minimize destruction of microbubbles. The definition of the left ventricular endocardial border is very clear with injection of contrast agent. **B,** Apical view showing a midcavity obstruction (arrows) that was not visualized clearly with two-dimensional echocardiography without contrast injection. An apical pouch (A) is clearly seen. *(Modified from Oh JK, Seward JB, Tajik AJ: The Echo Manual. 3rd ed. Philadelphia, Lippincott Williams & Wilkins, 2006. Used with permission of Mayo Foundation for Medical Education and Research.)*

tissue and microbubbles. With its linear property, myocardial tissue produces two ultrasound signals of inverted phase at the fundamental frequency that are canceled by each other, but with their nonlinear property, microbubbles produce residual signals from two nonlinearly reflected signals. An alternative method is pulse modulation, which sends out two successive pulses, one signal with half the amplitude of the other signal. The returning signal of half-amplitude is doubled and subtracted from the other full signal. From myocardial tissue with a linear property, both signals are canceled; but from microbubbles with a nonlinear property, some signals remain to be imaged.

Because a high mechanical index may destroy the microbubbles, especially at the apex, low mechanical index (0.4 to 0.5) harmonic imaging is used to enhance the LV endocardial border definition between the blood pool and adjacent tissue or even mass. It is also important to use a sufficient amount of contrast agent to opacify the entire cavity.

LV opacification (LVO) obtained with microbubbles improves the definition of the LV border (**Fig. 15-18A**). This provides better quantitation of LV volume by the Simpson method. The correlation between LV volume measured with CMR and that measured with echocardiography is better with the use of LVO. Regional wall motion analysis can also be better with LVO. This is especially helpful during stress echocardiography. In critically ill patients in an intensive care unit, LVO is frequently necessary to assist in the echocardiographic evaluation of LV contractility and LV ejection fraction (LVEF). Also, LVO is helpful in the evaluation of intracardiac thrombus or mass and pseudoaneurysm. The presence or absence of vascularity of an intracardiac or paracardiac mass demonstrated with contrast echocardiographic pixel intensity measurements has been found to be useful in distinguishing between thrombus and tumor (see Chap. 74).[30] Another diagnostically important use of LVO is the assessment of apical or midcavity hypertrophic cardiomyopathy (HCM; see Chap. 69), which is often missed or mistaken for a dyskinetic apical segment because the epicardial motion of the hypertrophic apex appears to bulge outward unless the apical endocardium is clearly visualized, which is possible with the use of a contrast agent (Fig. 15-18B).

After microbubbles are destroyed by a high mechanical index (>1.5) of ultrasound, myocardium with normal perfusion is replenished by microbubbles within five to seven cardiac cycles (or 5 seconds), imaged

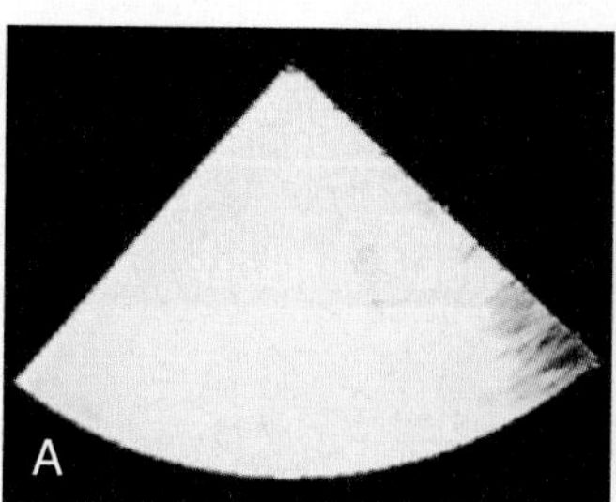

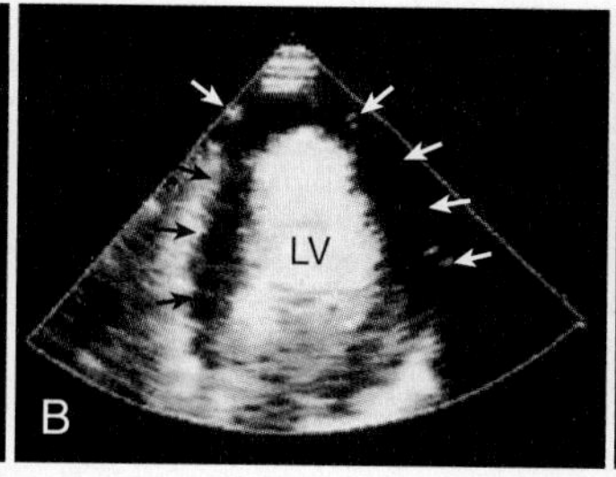

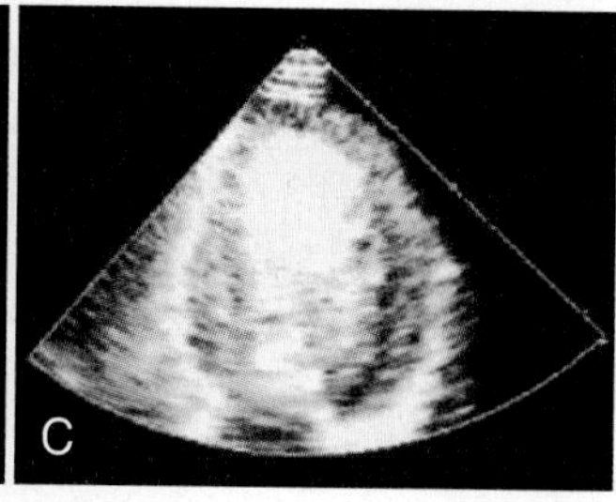

FIGURE 15-19 The process of performing real-time myocardial perfusion imaging. **A,** A high mechanical index of 1.7 is applied to the heart, destroying all microbubbles in the myocardium. **B,** Immediately after the destruction, no microbubbles are present (black areas indicated by arrows). LV = left ventricle. **C,** Myocardium with normal perfusion is replenished with the microbubbles within five to seven cardiac cycles. *(Modified from Oh JK, Seward JB, Tajik AJ: The Echo Manual. 3rd ed. Philadelphia, Lippincott Williams & Wilkins, 2006. Used with permission of Mayo Foundation for Medical Education and Research. Courtesy of Namsik Chung, MD.)*

TABLE 15-4 Reference Limits and Partition Values of Left Ventricular Size*

	Women				*Men*			
		ABNORMAL				ABNORMAL		
MEASURE	REFERENCE RANGE	*MILDLY*	*MODERATELY*	*SEVERELY*	REFERENCE RANGE	*MILDLY*	*MODERATELY*	*SEVERELY*
LV dimension								
Diastolic diameter	3.9-5.3	5.4-5.7	5.8-6.1	≥6.2	4.2-5.9	6.0-6.3	6.4-6.8	≥6.9
Diastolic diameter/BSA, cm/m^2	2.4-3.2	3.3-3.4	3.5-3.7	≥3.8	2.2-3.1	3.2-3.4	3.5-3.6	≥3.7
Diastolic diameter/height, cm/m	2.5-3.2	3.3-3.4	3.5-3.6	≥3.7	2.4-3.3	3.4-3.5	3.6-3.7	≥3.8
LV volume								
Diastolic volume, mL	56-104	105-117	118-130	≥131	67-155	156-178	179-201	≥202
Diastolic volume/BSA, mL/m^2	**35-75**	**76-86**	**87-96**	**≥97**	**35-75**	**76-86**	**87-96**	**≥97**
Systolic volume, mL	19-49	50-59	60-69	≥70	22-58	59-70	71-82	≥83
Systolic volume/BSA, mL/m^2	**12-30**	**31-36**	**37-42**	**≥43**	**12-30**	**31-36**	**37-42**	**≥43**

*Boldface measures and volumes: recommended and best validated.
BSA = body surface area.
Modified from Lang RM, Bierig M, Devereux RB, et al: Recommendations for chamber quantification: A report from the American Society of Echocardiography's Guidelines and Standards Committee and the Chamber Quantification Writing Group, developed in conjunction with the European Association of Echocardiography, a branch of the European Society of Cardiology. J Am Soc Echocardiogr 18:1440, 2005. Used with permission.

as opacified myocardium (**Fig. 15-19**); however, myocardium with no or less than normal replenishment of microbubbles because of the lack of or decreased perfusion appears dark or patchy. The destruction and replenishment of microbubbles can be imaged in real time, providing a visual assessment of myocardial contractility as well as myocardial perfusion (see Fig. 15-e3 on the website).[27] A myocardial perfusion defect may be more sensitive for the detection of myocardial ischemia than regional wall motion analysis in patients with chest pain syndrome.[31] Myocardial contrast perfusion imaging stress testing uses either dobutamine or a vasodilator such as dipyridamole or adenosine. Perfusion defects detected on myocardial contrast perfusion echocardiography with a vasodilator correlate well with perfusion defects seen on an exercise or dobutamine stress test, and perfusion defects demonstrated with myocardial contrast echocardiography correlate well with those seen on nuclear imaging (see Chap. 17). No difference in sensitivity has been found between myocardial contrast echocardiography and single-photon emission computed tomography (SPECT) for the detection of coronary artery disease (84% versus 82%, respectively).[32]

Theoretically, myocardial risk area, final infarct size, and amount of myocardial salvage by acute reperfusion therapy (a thrombolytic agent or percutaneous coronary intervention; see Chap. 55) can be measured with serial myocardial contrast perfusion echocardiography. In patients with acute myocardial infarction (MI), the evaluation of myocardial viability soon after acute reperfusion therapy is possible with a myocardial contrast perfusion study.[33,34] After TIMI 3 coronary flow has been established with acute reperfusion therapy, almost one third of the patients may not recover myocardial function because of the no-reflow phenomenon. TIMI 3 flow indicates the patency of the epicardial coronary artery but does not always indicate normal microvascular circulation. Myocardial perfusion imaging is a better way to assess the coronary microcirculation. We have performed contrast echocardiography with an intravenous contrast agent in patients who had revascularization (thrombolysis, percutaneous coronary intervention, or both) after acute MI. Normal perfusion predicted functional recovery with greatest accuracy in myocardial segments supplied by the left anterior descending coronary artery.

Myocardial contrast perfusion echocardiography has been an essential tool for alcohol ablation of the septal coronary artery in patients with obstructive HCM (see Chap. 69).[35] Because the myocardial distribution of the septal perforator artery varies, knowledge about the amount of myocardium that would be damaged by the injection of alcohol into a septal perforator is critical before the procedure is performed.

Chamber Quantitation

The American Society of Echocardiography (ASE) has published recommendations for chamber quantification with M-mode and two-dimensional echocardiography.[5] It is critical that a method for chamber quantification be standardized because cardiac function is determined from the size of the chambers, which also frequently guides the strategy for management of the patient. It is recommended that the same range of normal values for chamber dimensions and volumes be used for both TEE and TTE (**Tables 15-4 to 15-9**).[5]

Left Ventricular Dimensions

Usually, LV dimensions are measured from two-dimensional guided M-mode echocardiograms of the left ventricle at the level of mitral leaflet tips or the papillary muscle by the parasternal view (**Fig. 15-20**). If no extensive regional wall motion abnormalities are present, the LV dimensions measured at the mid-ventricular level can be used to calculate global LVEF (see Evaluation of Systolic and Diastolic Function). The thicknesses of the ventricular posterior wall and the ventricular septum (from the leading edge to the trailing edge) are measured from the same M-mode echocardiogram. These values are used to calculate LV mass. The long-axis and short-axis dimensions of the ventricle can also be obtained directly from systolic and diastolic frames of the two-dimensional parasternal long-axis view and apical view (**Fig. 15-21**). The LV end-diastolic and end-systolic dimensions are measured at the level of the tips of the mitral leaflets as the largest and the smallest LV dimensions, respectively.

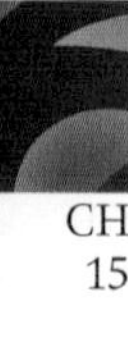

TABLE 15-5 Reference Limits and Values and Partition Values of Left Ventricular Function*

MEASURE	*Women* REFERENCE RANGE	ABNORMAL *MILDLY*	*MODERATELY*	*SEVERELY*	*Men* REFERENCE RANGE	ABNORMAL *MILDLY*	*MODERATELY*	*SEVERELY*
Linear method								
Endocardial fraction shortening, %	27-45	22-26	17-21	≤16	25-43	20-24	15-19	≤14
Midwall fractional shortening, %	15-23	13-14	11-21	≤10	14-22	12-13	10-11	≤9
Two-dimensional method								
Ejection fraction, %	**≥55**	**45-54**	**30-44**	**<30**	**≥55**	**45-54**	**30-44**	**<30**

*Boldface measures and values: recommended and best validated.

Modified from Lang RM, Bierig M, Devereux RB, et al: Recommendations for chamber quantification: A report from the American Society of Echocardiography's Guidelines and Standards Committee and the Chamber Quantification Writing Group, developed in conjunction with the European Association of Echocardiography, a branch of the European Society of Cardiology. J Am Soc Echocardiogr 18:1440, 2005.

TABLE 15-6 Reference Limits and Partition Values of Left Ventricular Mass and Geometry*

MEASURE	*Women* REFERENCE RANGE	ABNORMAL *MILDLY*	*MODERATELY*	*SEVERELY*	*Men* REFERENCE RANGE	ABNORMAL *MILDLY*	*MODERATELY*	*SEVERELY*
Linear method								
LV mass, g	67-162	163-186	187-210	≥211	88-224	225-258	259-292	≥293
LV mass/BSA, g/m²	**43-95**	**96-108**	**109-121**	**≥122**	**49-115**	**116-131**	**132-148**	**≥149**
LV mass/height, g/m	41-99	100-115	116-128	≥129	52-126	127-144	145-162	≥163
LV mass/height, g/m	18-44	45-51	52-58	≥59	20-48	49-55	56-63	≥64
Relative wall thickness, cm	0.22-0.42	0.43-0.47	0.48-0.52	≥0.53	0.24-0.42	0.43-0.46	0.47-0.51	≥0.52
Septal thickness, cm	**0.6-0.9**	**1.0-1.2**	**1.3-1.5**	**≥1.6**	**0.6-1.0**	**1.1-1.3**	**1.4-1.6**	**≥1.7**
Posterior wall thickness, cm	**0.6-0.9**	**1.0-1.2**	**1.3-1.5**	**≥1.6**	**0.6-1.0**	**1.1-1.3**	**1.4-1.6**	**≥1.7**
Two-dimensional method								
LV mass, g	66-150	151-171	172-182	≥183	96-200	201-227	228-254	≥255
LV mass/BSA, g/m²	**44-88**	**89-100**	**101-112**	**≥113**	**50-102**	**103-116**	**117-130**	**≥131**

*Boldface measures and values: recommended and best validated.

BSA = body surface area.

From Lang RM, Bierig M, Devereux RB, et al: Recommendations for chamber quantification: A report from the American Society of Echocardiography's Guidelines and Standards Committee and the Chamber Quantification Writing Group, developed in conjunction with the European Association of Echocardiography, a branch of the European Society of Cardiology. J Am Soc Echocardiogr 18:1440, 2005.

TABLE 15-7 Reference Limits and Partition Values of Right Ventricular and Pulmonary Artery Size

DIMENSION	REFERENCE RANGE	*Abnormal* MILDLY	MODERATELY	SEVERELY
RV dimension				
Basal RV diameter, cm	2.0-2.8	2.9-3.3	3.4-3.8	≥3.9
Mid RV diameter, cm	2.7-3.3	3.4-3.7	3.8-4.1	≥4.2
Base to apex length, cm	7.1-7.9	8.0-8.5	8.6-9.1	≥9.2
RVOT diameter				
Above aortic valve, cm	2.5-2.9	3.0-3.2	3.3-3.5	≥3.6
Above pulmonic valve, cm	1.7-2.3	2.4-2.7	2.8-3.1	≥3.2
Pulmonary artery diameter				
Below pulmonic valve, cm	1.5-2.1	2.2-2.5	2.6-2.9	≥3.0

Modified from Lang RM, Bierig M, Devereux RB, et al: Recommendations for chamber quantification: A report from the American Society of Echocardiography's Guidelines and Standards Committee and the Chamber Quantification Writing Group, developed in conjunction with the European Association of Echocardiography, a branch of the European Society of Cardiology. J Am Soc Echocardiogr 18:1440, 2005.

TABLE 15-8 Reference Limits and Partition Values of Right Ventricular Size and Function as Measured in the Apical Four-Chamber View

MEASURE	REFERENCE RANGE	*Abnormal* MILDLY	MODERATELY	SEVERELY
RV diastolic area, cm²	11-28	29-32	33-37	≥38
RV systolic area, cm²	7.5-16	17-19	20-22	≥23
RV fractional area change, %	32-60	25-31	18-24	≤17

Modified from Lang RM, Bierig M, Devereux RB, et al: Recommendations for chamber quantification: A report from the American Society of Echocardiography's Guidelines and Standards Committee and the Chamber Quantification Writing Group, developed in conjunction with the European Association of Echocardiography, a branch of the European Society of Cardiology. J Am Soc Echocardiogr 18:1440, 2005.

TABLE 15-9 Reference Limits and Partition Values for Atrial Dimensions and Volumes*

	Women				Men			
		ABNORMAL				ABNORMAL		
MEASURE	REFERENCE RANGE	*MILDLY*	*MODERATELY*	*SEVERELY*	REFERENCE RANGE	*MILDLY*	*MODERATELY*	*SEVERELY*
Atrial dimension								
LA diameter, cm	2.7-3.8	3.9-4.2	4.3-4.6	≥4.7	3.0-4.0	4.1-4.6	4.7-5.2	≥5.2
LA diameter/BSA, cm/m^2	1.5-2.3	2.4-2.6	2.7-2.9	≥3.0	1.5-2.3	2.4-2.6	2.7-2.9	≥3.0
RA minor axis dimension, cm	2.9-4.5	4.6-4.9	5.0-5.4	≥5.5	2.9-4.5	4.6-4.9	5.0-5.4	≥5.5
RA minor axis dimension/BSA, cm/m^2	1.7-2.5	2.6-2.8	2.9-3.1	≥3.2	1.7-2.5	2.6-2.8	2.9-3.1	≥3.2
Atrial area								
LA area, cm^2	<20	20-30	30-40	>40	<20	20-30	31-40	>40
Atrial volumes								
LA volume, mL	22-52	53-62	63-72	≥73	18-58	59-68	69-78	≥79
LA volume/BSA, mL/m^2	**22±6**	**29-33**	**34-39**	**≥40**	**22±6**	**29-33**	**34-39**	**≥40**

*Boldface measure and values: recommended and best validated.

BSA = body surface area.

Modified from Lang RM, Bierig M, Devereux RB, et al: Recommendations for chamber quantification: A report from the American Society of Echocardiography's Guidelines and Standards Committee and the Chamber Quantification Writing Group, developed in conjunction with the European Association of Echocardiography, a branch of the European Society of Cardiology. J Am Soc Echocardiogr 18:1440, 2005.

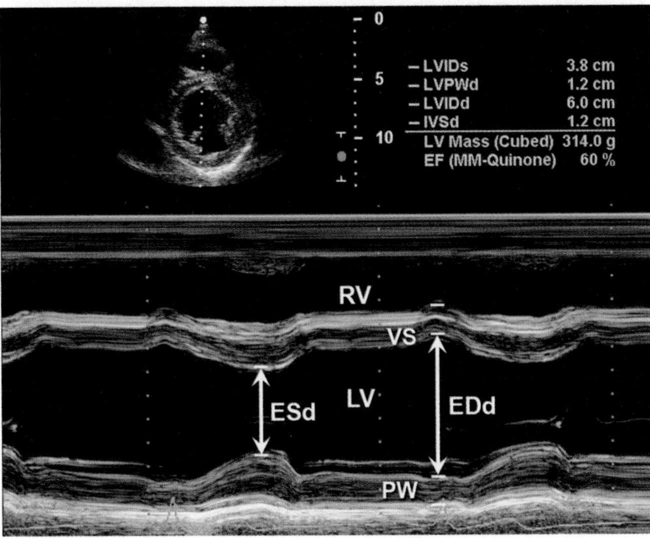

FIGURE 15-20 Two-dimensional guided M-mode echocardiogram of left ventricle (LV) at the papillary muscle level. The LV end-diastolic internal dimension (EDd) measured at the onset of QRS is 60 mm, and the LV end-systolic internal dimension (ESd) is 38 mm. Therefore,

$$\text{LV ejection fraction (LVEF)} = \frac{60^2 - 38^2}{60^2} \times 100 = 60\% \text{ (uncorrected)}$$

If apical contractility is normal:

$$\begin{aligned}\text{Corrected LVEF} &= 60\% + [(100-60)\times 15\%] \\ &= 60\% + 6\% \\ &= 66\%\end{aligned}$$

LV mass is also calculated from LV dimensions, posterior wall (PW) thickness, and ventricular septal thickness. RV = right ventricle. *(Modified from Oh JK, Seward JB, Tajik AJ: The Echo Manual. 3rd ed. Philadelphia, Lippincott Williams & Wilkins, 2006. Used with permission of Mayo Foundation for Medical Education and Research.)*

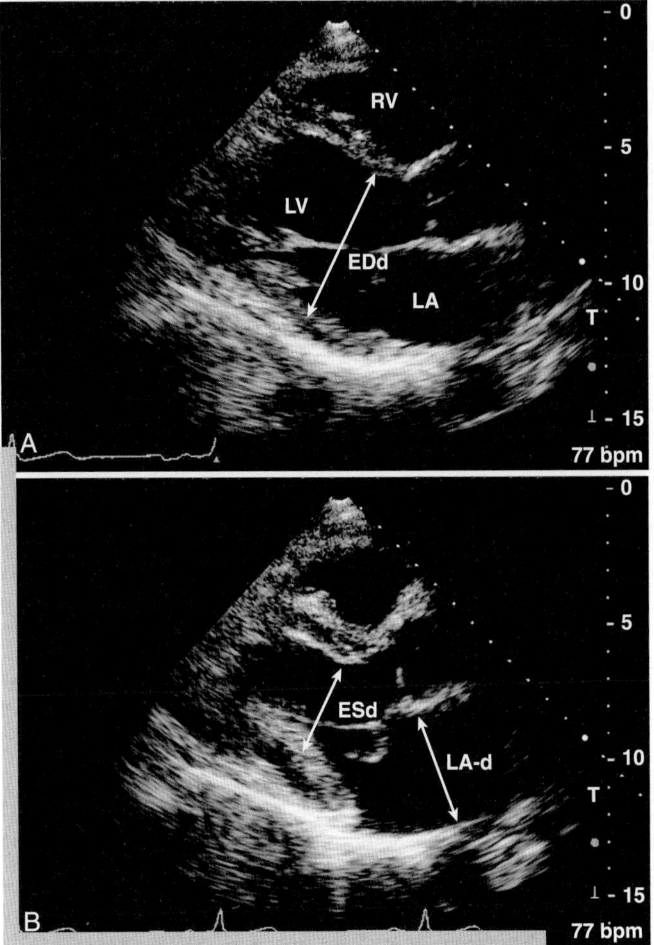

FIGURE 15-21 Measurement of LV diastolic dimensions **(A)** and systolic dimensions **(B)** from two-dimensional echocardiography. LV end-diastolic dimension (EDd) and end-systolic dimension (ESd) are measured at the level of the mitral leaflet tips (at one-third the distance along the length of the long axis) from the parasternal long-axis view. The left atrial dimension (LA-d) is measured at end systole, when it is largest. *(Modified from Oh JK, Seward JB, Tajik AJ: The Echo Manual. 3rd ed. Philadelphia, Lippincott Williams & Wilkins, 2006. Used with permission of Mayo Foundation for Medical Education and Research.)*

Right Ventricular Dimensions

Detection of RV dilation may be the first clue to RV pressure or volume overload. Chronic RV pressure overload is accompanied by an increase in RV wall thickness in addition to dilation, whereas in RV dysplasia, the RV wall is thin (see Chap. 68). The thickness of the RV wall is normally less than 5 mm and is measured best from the subcostal view at the peak of the R wave.[5] The size of the right ventricle is measured best from the apical four-chamber view. An example of

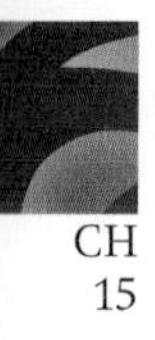

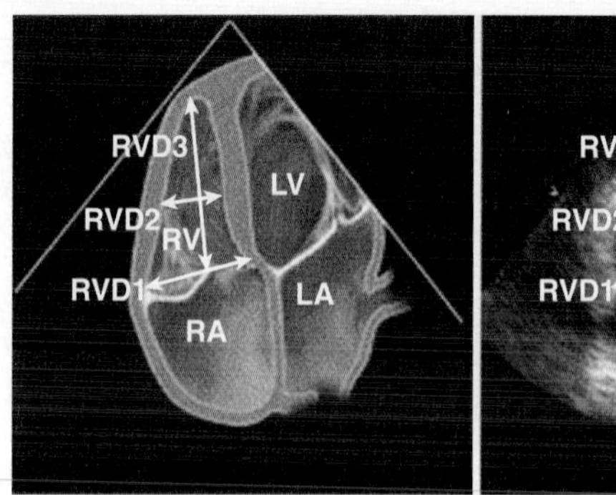

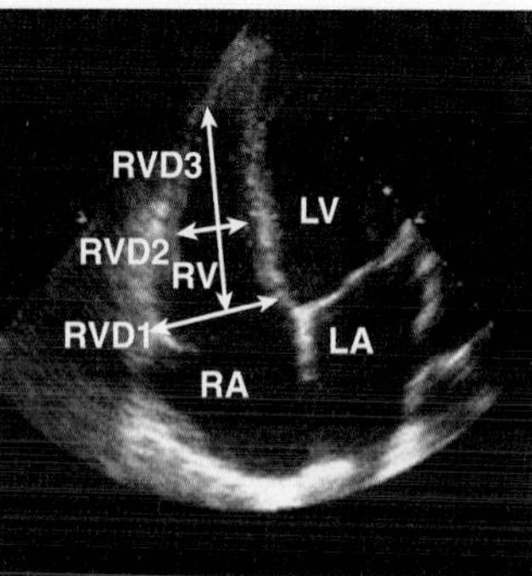

FIGURE 15-22 Measurements of right ventricular long-axis and short-axis dimensions (RVD1-RVD3) from apical four-chamber view. LA = left atrium; LV = left ventricle; RA = right atrium; RV = right ventricle. *(Modified from Lang RM, Bierig M, Devereux RB, et al: Recommendations for chamber quantification: A report from the American Society of Echocardiography's Guidelines and Standards Committee and the Chamber Quantification Writing Group, developed in conjunction with the European Association of Echocardiography, a branch of the European Society of Cardiology. J Am Soc Echocardiogr 18:1440, 2005. Used with permission.)*

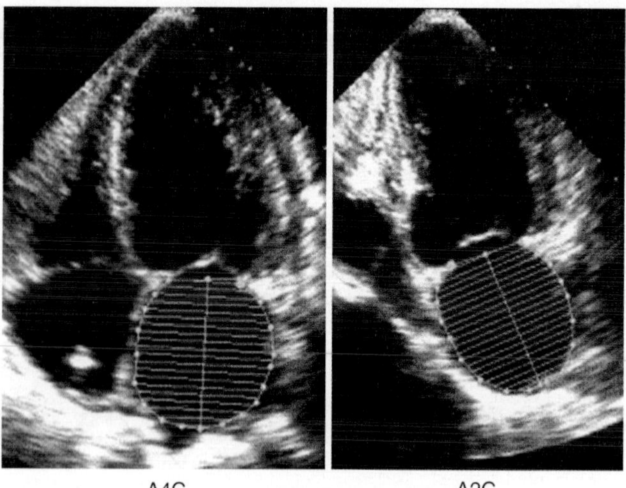

FIGURE 15-23 Left atrial volume measurement by biplane area-length method requires measurements of left atrial area from two orthogonal or apical views. A2C = apical two-chamber view; A4C = apical four-chamber view. *(Modified from Lang RM, Bierig M, Devereux RB, et al: Recommendations for chamber quantification: A report from the American Society of Echocardiography's Guidelines and Standards Committee and the Chamber Quantification Writing Group, developed in conjunction with the European Association of Echocardiography, a branch of the European Society of Cardiology. J Am Soc Echocardiogr 18:1440, 2005. Used with permission.)*

measuring the RV short axis and long axis is shown in **Figure 15-22**. The dimension of the LVOT is measured from the parasternal long-axis view, and the dimension of the RVOT is measured from the parasternal short-axis view.

Left Atrial Size and Volume

Traditionally, LA dimension is determined from the parasternal long-axis view at end systole. However, the size of the left atrium may be underestimated from the parasternal view because the chamber may enlarge longitudinally. Therefore, LA size should also be measured from apical views (from the tip of the mitral valve to the posterior wall of the left atrium). However, LA volume is a better measure of LA size and provides better prognostic value. Four different methods are available for determination of LA volume: prolate ellipse, biplane area-length, biplane Simpson, and three-dimensional echocardiography.

The prolate ellipse method requires measurement of LA dimensions from the parasternal long-axis view (D1) and apical four-chamber view (D2 and D3), from which LA volume is calculated as D1 × D2 × D3 × 0.523. The biplane area-length method requires measurements of LA area from two orthogonal apical views (A1 and A2) and LA length (L), from which LA volume is calculated as (0.85 × A1 × A2)/L (**Fig. 15-23**). When LA length is measured from two apical views, the shorter value is used to calculate LA volume. LA volume measured by the prolate ellipse method is usually 5 to 10 mL smaller than that measured by the biplane area-length method. Although LA volume can be measured by the biplane Simpson or three-dimensional volumetric method, the biplane area-length method is currently the one recommended by the ASE.[5] The influence of body surface area on LA volume is corrected by dividing LA volume by body surface area to calculate LA volume index. The normal value for all age groups for the LA volume index is 22 ± 6 mL/m^2. LA volume was measured in 230 healthy individuals (mean age, 76 years) from the Cardiovascular Health Study by the ellipsoid measurement method. The 95th percentile absolute value was 46.7 mL in women and 58.2 mL in men.[36] In healthy elderly subjects, indices of LA size correlated not with age or height but with weight and measures of body build. LA size or volume is an important determinant of LA pressure, diastolic function, and prognosis.[37]

Left Ventricular Mass

Two methods are available for calculation of LV mass from two-dimensional echocardiography: the biplane area-length method and the truncated ellipsoid method. In both methods, the LV wall volume is derived by subtracting intracavitary (endocardial) LV volume from the entire (epicardial) LV volume, including LV walls and ventricular septum. Myocardial mass is equal to the product of the volume and the specific gravity of the myocardium, 1.04 g/mL. LV mass can also be estimated from measurements of LV dimension and wall thicknesses on two-dimensional or M-mode echocardiograms. Without measurement of the major axis of the left ventricle, LV mass is obtained from the LV short-axis dimension and a simple geometric cube formula. The following equation provides a reasonable determination of LV mass in grams:

$$1.04\left[(\mathrm{LVID}+\mathrm{PWT}+\mathrm{IVST})^3-\mathrm{LVID}^3\right]\times 0.8+0.6$$

where LVID is the internal dimension, PWT is posterior wall thickness, IVST is interventricular septal thickness, 1.04 equals the specific gravity of the myocardium, and 0.8 is the correction factor. All measurements are made at end diastole (at onset of the R wave) in centimeters.

Harmonic real-time three-dimensional imaging has the potential to be the most accurate echocardiographic measure for LV volume and mass. From a pyramidal volume data set, three-dimensional echocardiography allows offline selection of anatomically correct apical views without foreshortening. Tracing of endocardial and epicardial boundaries of anatomically correct, nonforeshortened apical views provides more accurate quantification of LV volume and mass. Compared with CMR, Mor-Avi and colleagues[38] showed that interobserver variability was 37% ± 19% of measured LV mass by two-dimensional echocardiography and 7% ± 10% by real-time three-dimensional echocardiography. Intraobserver variability was 19% ± 10% and 8% ± 5%, respectively.

Left Ventricular Volume

With two-dimensional echocardiography, LV volume is calculated best by the modified Simpson method or disc summation method (**Fig. 15-24**). The apical long axis is divided by the number of cylinders created within the left ventricle, and the resulting distance (long-axis dimension/number of cylinders) becomes the height of each cylinder. Therefore, long-axis dimensions from two apical views should be similar to match the locations of each cylinder from two orthogonal views. In subjects with uniform contractility, the LV volume

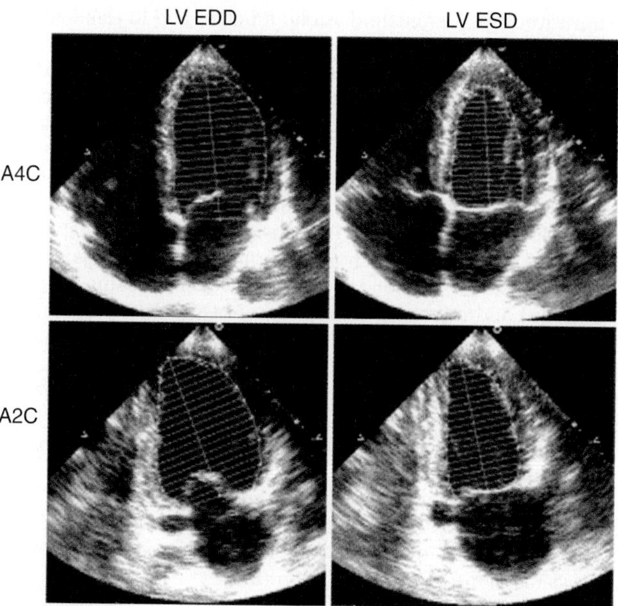

FIGURE 15-24 LV volume measurement by the biplane Simpson method requires two orthogonal apical views. The left ventricle is divided into 20 cylinders or discs, and their volumes are calculated and added to provide LV volume at end diastole (LV EDD) and end systole (LV ESD). A2C = apical two-chamber view; A4C = apical four-chamber view. *(Modified from Lang RM, Bierig M, Devereux RB, et al: Recommendations for chamber quantification: A report from the American Society of Echocardiography's Guidelines and Standards Committee and the Chamber Quantification Writing Group, developed in conjunction with the European Association of Echocardiography, a branch of the European Society of Cardiology. J Am Soc Echocardiogr 18:1440, 2005. Used with permission.)*

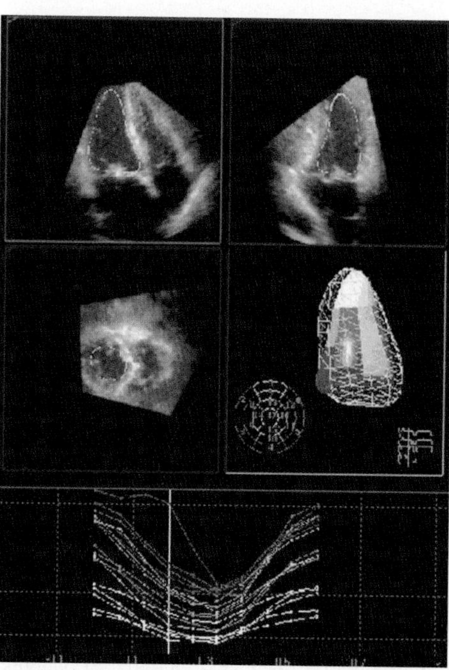

FIGURE 15-25 The LV volume cast (lower right) was created from three-dimensional echocardiography imaging. Regional LV volume changes are shown in the plot at the bottom. The color of each line corresponds to the segment of the same color in the LV cast. *(Modified from Oh JK, Seward JB, Tajik AJ: The Echo Manual. 3rd ed. Philadelphia, Lippincott Williams & Wilkins, 2006. Used with permission of Mayo Foundation for Medical Education and Research.)*

measured by single-plane disc summation is very close to that measured by the biplane Simpson method, which is preferred for LV volume measurements in patients with regional wall motion abnormalities. Reliable visualization of the LV endocardial blood-tissue border is a key for making reliable LV volume measurements with echocardiography. Contrast echocardiography and harmonic imaging have improved definition of the endocardial border.

Studies indicate that LV volume measurement is more reliable and accurate with real-time three-dimensional echocardiography; this may well become the standard mode of measuring LV volume and LVEF in the future.[39] Comparison of real-time three-dimensional echocardiography measurements of LV parameters with M-mode and two-dimensional echocardiographic and CMR measurements showed that LV volume was underestimated by two-dimensional echocardiography but much improved by real-time three-dimensional echocardiography, with standard error estimates of 17 and 16 mL for end-diastolic volume and end-systolic volume, respectively. However, the LVEF obtained with CMR was similar to that obtained with two-dimensional and real-time three-dimensional echocardiography. With three-dimensional echocardiography, a real-time LV cast can be created (**Fig. 15-25**) and regional volume changes can be displayed, which is useful for determination of LV dyssynchrony.

Evaluation of Systolic and Diastolic Function

Systolic Functional Parameters

Echocardiography can measure several parameters as an expression of systolic function of the heart. These parameters are LVEF, fractional shortening, stroke volume and cardiac index, systolic tissue velocity of the mitral annulus and myocardium, strain, and regional wall motion analysis.

LEFT VENTRICULAR EJECTION FRACTION. The most well accepted expression of global LV function is LVEF. Although LVEF has many limitations, including load dependency, it is a strong predictor of clinical outcome in almost all major cardiac conditions, and it is used to select optimal management strategies. In clinical practice, LVEF is frequently determined by visual assessment of two-dimensional echocardiographic images of the left ventricle. This assessment is reasonably reliable when it is performed by an experienced echocardiographer but varies widely among readers. Therefore, LVEF should be measured more objectively whenever possible, using volumetric measurements as described by the following equation:

$$\text{LVEF} = (\text{LVEDV} - \text{LVESV})/\text{LVEDV}$$

where LVEDV and LVESV are LV end-diastolic volume and end-systolic volume, respectively.

LVEF can also be calculated from LV dimensions measured with M-mode or two-dimensional echocardiography. M-mode or two-dimensional echocardiographic measurement of LV dimensions from the mid-ventricular level (see Fig. 15-20) is used to calculate LVEF as follows:

$$\text{LVEF} = \left(\text{LVEDD}^2 - \text{LVESD}^2\right)/\text{LVEDD}^2$$

where LVEDD and LVESD are end-diastolic dimension and end-systolic dimension, respectively. This equation is actually the percentage change in LV area, or fractional shortening of the LV short axis, which equals LVEF if the apical long-axis dimension remains the same from diastolic phase to systolic contraction. Because the apical long axis normally shortens 10% to 15% with systole, an apical correction factor is added on the basis of the contractility of the apex: 5% to 7% for normal to hyperdynamic apical contraction, 3% for hypokinetic contraction, and 0% for akinetic apex.

Because three-dimensional echocardiography can provide LV end-diastolic and end-systolic volumes closer to those measured by CMR, it will become the standard method to calculate LVEF. It can also provide regional LV volume as well as the timing of the smallest volume of each region, which may be helpful in assessing the synchronicity of LV regional contraction.

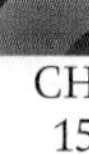

FRACTIONAL SHORTENING. Fractional shortening (FS) is a percentage change in LV dimensions with each LV contraction:

$$FS = (LVEDD - LVESD)/LVEDD$$

This systolic function parameter is now rarely used for diagnosis or clinical decision making.

STROKE VOLUME. Stroke volume (SV) can be measured as the difference between LVEDV and LVESV obtained by the Simpson method or three-dimensional echocardiography, as described. The difference should be equal to systolic volume across the LVOT if there is no valvular regurgitation. If there is mitral regurgitation (MR), regurgitant volume needs to be subtracted to obtain SV across LVOT. LVOT SV can also be obtained by the product of LVOT area and LVOT time-velocity integral (see Hemodynamic Assessment).

SYSTOLIC VELOCITY OF MYOCARDIAL TISSUE OR MITRAL ANNULUS. The systolic component of the mitral annulus measured by TDI correlates well with LVEF and has been shown to be a good predictor of clinical outcome in various cardiovascular disorders.[19]

Assessment of Diastolic Function

Assessment of diastolic function should be an integral part of an evaluation of cardiac function because about 50% of patients with heart failure have preserved LVEF (see Chap. 30). Assessment of diastolic function requires an understanding of diastology and various means to evaluate diastolic function. Currently, echocardiography is the best noninvasive way to evaluate diastolic function and to estimate filling pressures. M-mode, two-dimensional, and Doppler (blood flow, tissue, and color) echocardiography are all helpful in evaluating diastolic function. Recently, the ASE and the European Association of Echocardiography (EAE) published a guideline for assessment of diastolic function by echocardiography.[40] The following steps will ensure comprehensive assessment of diastolic function and the identification of heart failure related to diastolic dysfunction:

1. Look for M-mode and two-dimensional echocardiographic evidence of diastolic dysfunction. Abnormal myocardial relaxation, an integral part of diastolic dysfunction, decreases the slope (in M-mode) and mitral annulus motion of early diastolic filling and increases LA size. LV wall thicknesses are usually but not necessarily increased.
2. Mitral inflow velocities reflect the transmitral pressure gradient, which is usually characteristic of various stages of diastolic dysfunction. Assessment of ventricular compliance is possible from the configuration (velocities and flow duration) of mitral inflow velocities. Pulmonary vein flow velocities are also helpful.
3. Myocardial relaxation by TDI can be evaluated. Mitral annulus velocity (e′) during early diastole correlates reasonably well with the status of myocardial relaxation (tau).
4. Mitral inflow velocities (E and A), e′, mitral inflow propagation velocity, and their combination can estimate LV diastolic filling pressure at rest and with exercise.
5. These steps allow diagnosis of diastolic heart failure and separation of myocardial diastolic heart failure from pericardial diastolic heart failure (see Pericardial Diseases).

LV diastolic filling consists of a series of events that are affected by numerous factors, including myocardial relaxation, compliance, cardiac rhythm, and pericardial compliance (see Chap. 24). Normal diastolic function ensures adequate filling of the ventricles during rest and exercise without an abnormal increase in diastolic pressure or pulmonary venous congestion. The initial diastolic event is myocardial relaxation,[41] an active energy-dependent process that causes LV pressure to decrease rapidly after the end of contraction. When LV pressure falls below LA pressure, the mitral valve opens, and rapid early diastolic filling begins. Under normal circumstances, a major determinant of the driving force of early diastolic filling is the elastic recoil caused by normal relaxation of the left ventricle. Normally, 75% to 80% of LV filling occurs during this phase. During early diastolic filling, LV pressure continues to decrease until completion of myocardial relaxation (normally about 100 milliseconds) before rising after reaching minimal pressure; this loss of positive driving force results in the deceleration of mitral inflow. Later, atrial contraction produces a positive transmitral pressure gradient and inflow, accounting for 20% to 25% of LV filling in normal subjects. The proportion of LV filling during the early and late diastolic phases depends on elastic recoil (suction), rate of myocardial relaxation, chamber compliance, LA pressure, and heart rate. The LV filling pattern is the result of the transmitral pressure gradient produced by these various factors (**Fig. 15-26**).

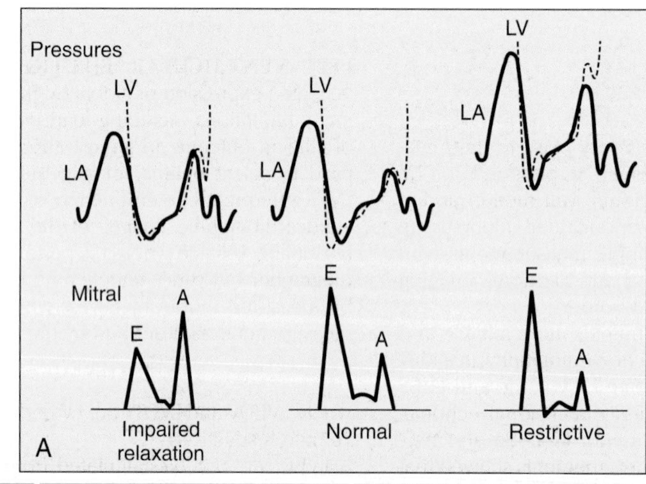

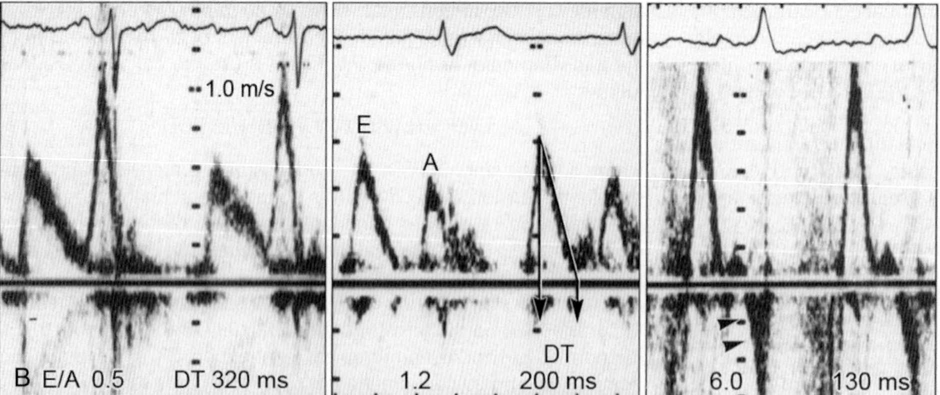

FIGURE 15-26 **A,** Left ventricular (LV) and left atrial (LA) pressure relationship and corresponding mitral inflow velocities in three different diastolic filling patterns: impaired relaxation, normal, and restrictive. **B,** Actual Doppler recordings of mitral inflow velocities, representing impaired relaxation **(left),** normal **(center),** and restrictive filling **(right)** patterns. Arrowheads indicate diastolic mitral regurgitation. A = late diastolic filling; DT = deceleration time; E = early diastolic filling. *(Modified from Oh JK, Seward JB, Tajik AJ: The Echo Manual. 3rd ed. Philadelphia, Lippincott Williams & Wilkins, 2006. Used with permission of Mayo Foundation for Medical Education and Research.)*

The transmitral pressure gradient or the relationship between LA and LV pressures is accurately reflected by mitral inflow Doppler velocities.[20] Diastolic filling is usually classified initially on the basis of the peak mitral flow velocity of the early rapid filling wave (E), peak velocity of the late filling wave caused by atrial contraction (A), E/A ratio, and deceleration time (DT), which is the time interval for the peak E velocity to reach zero baseline (see Fig. 15-26).

With myocardial relaxation, the LV cavity elongates, expands laterally, and rotates. The longitudinal motion of the mitral annulus has been shown to correlate with the rate of myocardial relaxation. The velocity of the mitral annulus can be recorded by TDI, which has become an essential part of evaluation of diastolic function by echocardiography.[42] Radial and circumferential function can also be assessed with speckle tracking strain imaging.[43]

Comprehensive assessment of diastolic filling and estimation of filling pressures by echocardiography require TDI, pulmonary vein Doppler, hepatic vein Doppler, and color M-mode of mitral inflow for propagation velocity—sometimes with an alteration in a loading condition (**Fig. 15-27**). The Valsalva maneuver is used most frequently to decrease venous return by increasing intrathoracic pressure.[44]

Grading of Diastolic Dysfunction (or Diastolic Filling Pattern)

The grading of the diastolic filling pattern (or diastolic dysfunction) is based on several parameters (see Fig. 15-27).[20,40] In most (if not all) cardiac diseases, the initial diastolic abnormality is impaired relaxation. With further progression of disease and a mild to moderate increase in LA pressure, the mitral inflow velocity pattern appears similar to a normal filling pattern (pseudonormalized). With further decrease in LV compliance and increase in LA pressure, diastolic filling becomes restrictive. Most patients with restrictive filling are symptomatic and have a poor prognosis unless the restrictive filling can be reversed by treatment. However, restrictive filling may be irreversible and represent the end stage of diastolic heart failure. Therefore, diastolic dysfunction can be graded according to the diastolic filling pattern.[40]

Grade 1 (mild dysfunction): impaired relaxation with normal filling pressure

Grade 2 (moderate dysfunction): pseudonormalized mitral inflow pattern

Grade 3 (severe reversible dysfunction): reversible restrictive (high filling pressure)

Grade 4 (severe irreversible dysfunction): irreversible restrictive (high filling pressure)

A grade 1 diastolic filling pattern usually implies a normal filling pressure despite a background of impaired myocardial relaxation. However, in patients with a marked relaxation abnormality, as in HCM, the filling pressure can still be elevated with grade 1 mitral inflow velocity pattern (E/A ratio <1.0 and DT >240 milliseconds). Because the reversibility of restrictive filling usually cannot be assessed at one clinical setting, grade 4 dysfunction was not used in the ASE and EAE recommendation.[40]

Normal Diastolic Filling Pattern

In normal young subjects, LV elastic recoil is vigorous because of normal myocardial relaxation; therefore, most filling is completed during early diastole. Thus, the E/A ratio is usually 1.5 or higher, DT is 160 to 240 milliseconds (septal), e′ is 10 cm/sec or higher, E/e′ is less than 8, and Vp is 50 cm/sec or higher. **Figure 15-28** shows mitral inflow, TDI, and color M-mode flow propagation in a young normal subject. This vigorous relaxation in normal subjects can also be seen as active motion of the mitral annulus away from the apex during early diastole in parasternal long-axis and apical four-chamber views.

With normal myocardial relaxation, the longitudinal mitral annulus diastolic velocity pattern mirrors that of normal mitral inflow: early diastolic velocity (e′) is higher than late diastolic velocity (a′). Lateral annulus velocity is always higher (normal, >15 cm/sec) than septal e′. Thus, e′

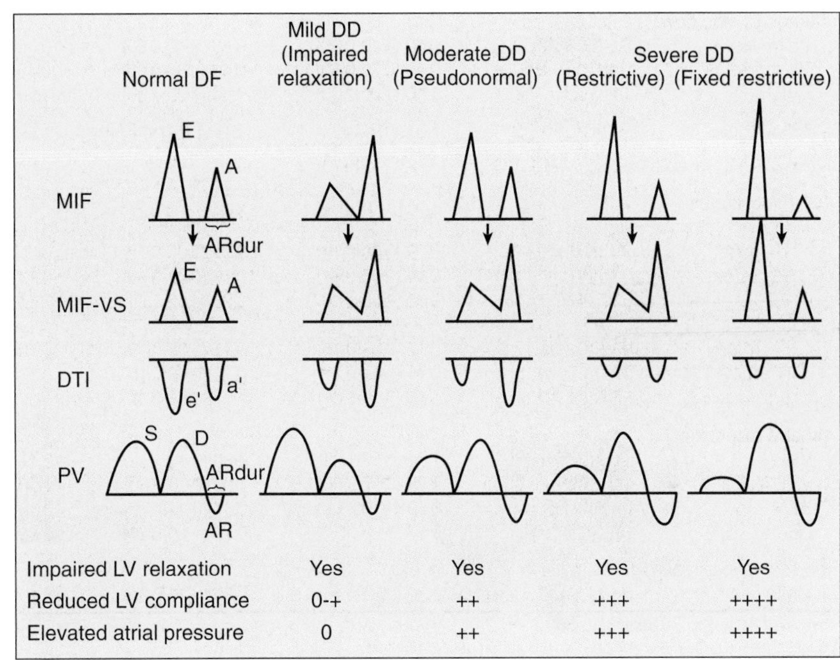

FIGURE 15-27 Diagram of various Doppler parameters for normal diastolic function (DF) and several stages of diastolic dysfunction (DD). A = late diastolic mitral inflow velocity; a′ = late diastolic mitral annulus velocity; AR = PV atrial reversal; D = diastolic forward PV velocity; DTI = Doppler tissue imaging; E = early diastolic mitral inflow velocity; e′ = early diastolic mitral annulus velocity; MIF = mitral inflow; PV = pulmonary vein; S = systolic forward PV velocity; VS = Valsalva. *(Modified from Redfield MM, Jacobsen SJ, Burnett JC Jr, et al: Burden of systolic and diastolic ventricular dysfunction in the community: Appreciating the scope of the heart failure epidemic. JAMA 289:194, 2003.)*

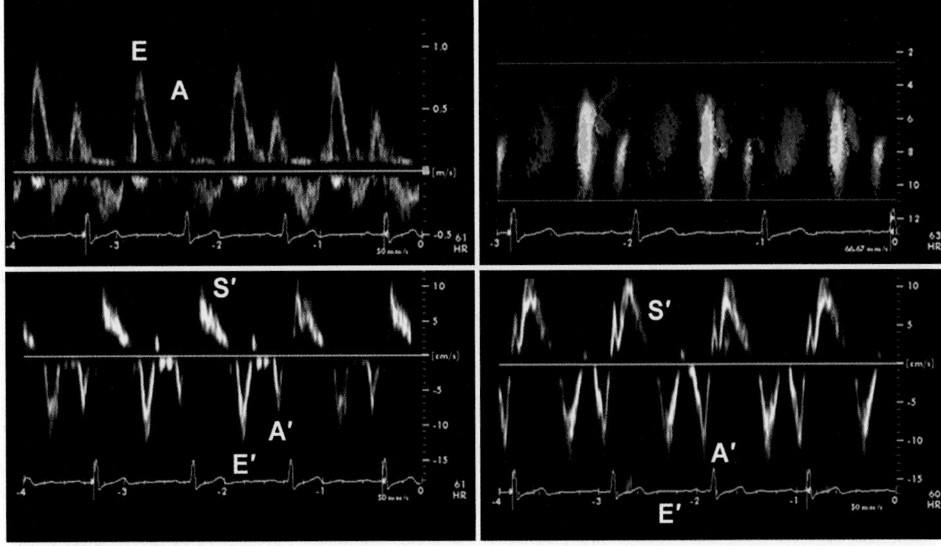

FIGURE 15-28 Mitral inflow, color M-mode, and tissue velocity of mitral annulus from a normal subject. Systolic velocity of the mitral annulus (S′) is normally greater than 7 cm/sec. Early diastolic velocity (E′) of the mitral annulus is higher from the lateral annulus **(right lower)** than from the septal annulus **(left lower).** Color M-mode shows a rapid flow, with propagation velocity >50 cm/sec. A = late diastolic filling; A′ = late diastolic velocity; E = early diastolic filling.

TABLE 15-10 Reference Ranges for Diastolic Function Parameters by Age*

PARAMETER	Age Groups (yr) 45-49	50-54	55-59	60-64	65-69	≥70
Mitral inflow						
E, m/sec	0.7 (0.5-0.9)	0.6 (0.5-0.9)	0.7 (0.5-0.9)	0.7 (0.5-0.9)	0.6 (0.4-0.8)	0.6 (0.4-1.0)
A, m/sec	0.5 (0.3-0.7)	0.5 (0.4-0.8)	0.6 (0.4-0.9)	0.6 (0.4-0.9)	0.7 (0.4-1.0)	0.8 (0.5-1.1)
E/A	1.3 (1.0-2.0)	1.2 (0.8-2.0)	1.2 (0.7-1.8)	1.0 (0.7-1.6)	1.00 (0.6-1.50)	0.8 (0.6-1.3)
E/(A-E at A)	1.50 (1.0-2.67)	1.40 (1.0-2.33)	1.29 (0.83-2.25)	1.20 (0.83-2.0)	1.00 (0.75-1.67)	1.00 (0.67-1.60)
DT, msec	208 (180-258)	217 (178-266)	210 (183-187)	222 (180-282)	227 (188-298)	242 (188-320)
A_{dur}, msec	140 (122-170)	147 (130-172)	147 (127-173)	147 (129-172)	150 (122-180)	150 (128-183)
Pulmonary vein flow						
P_S, m/sec	0.60 (0.40-0.80)	0.60 (0.40-0.80)	0.60 (0.40-0.80)	0.60 (0.40-0.80)	0.60 (0.50-0.80)	0.60 (0.40-0.80)
P_D, m/sec	0.40 (0.30-0.60)	0.40 (0.30-0.60)	0.40 (0.30-0.60)	0.40 (0.30-0.60)	0.40 (0.30-0.60)	0.40 (0.30-0.60)
P_S/P_D	1.25 (0.86-2.00)	1.40 (1.00-2.00)	1.40 (1.00-2.00)	1.50 (1.00-2.25)	1.60 (1.00-2.50)	1.67 (1.00-2.50)
$PVAR_{dur}$, msec	118 (100-140)	122 (103-142)	123 (105-157)	123 (103-160)	127 (110-152)	130 (112-170)
$PVAR_{dur} - A_{dur}$, msec	−25.0 (−53.3-0)	−25.0 (−51.7-0)	−21.6 (−50.0-11.7)	−23.3 (−51.7-13.4)	−21.7 (−55.0-12.5)	−22.3 (−51.7-31.6)
TDI, mitral annulus						
Septal						
E'_S, m/sec	0.10 (0.07-0.14)	0.09 (0.06-0.14)	0.09 (0.05-0.12)	0.09 (0.06-0.13)	0.08 (0.05-0.11)	0.07 (0.05-0.11)
A'_S, m/sec	0.10 (0.07-0.14)	0.10 (0.08-0.14)	0.11 (0.08-0.15)	0.11 (0.09-0.15)	0.11 (0.09-0.15)	0.11 (0.09-0.15)
E/E'_S	6.67 (4.62-11.25)	7.00 (4.55-11.67)	7.78 (4.62-13.33)	7.64 (5.0-12.0)	8.57 (5.45-13.33)	8.57 (4.55-16.67)
Lateral						
E'_L, m/sec	0.13 (0.09-0.17)	0.12 (0.08-0.16)	0.11 (0.07-0.15)	0.10 (0.07-0.15)	0.09 (0.07-0.12)	0.08 (0.05-0.11)
A'_L, m/sec	0.11 (0.07-0.16)	0.11 (0.07-0.15)	0.11 (0.08-0.16)	0.12 (0.08-0.17)	0.12 (0.09-0.16)	0.12 (0.08-0.18)
E/E'_L	5.38 (3.75-7.78)	5.45 (3.75-8.89)	6.0 (3.85-10.0)	6.67 (4.62-8.89)	7.0 (4.17-11.25)	7.78 (5.0-14.0)
Valsalva maneuver						
VS E/A	1.00 (0.60-1.33)	1.00 (0.57-1.33)	0.80 (0.44-1.25)	0.71 (0.43-1.20)	0.60 (0.40-1.00)	0.57 (0.30-1.00)
VS E/(A-E at A)	1.33 (0.80-2.50)	1.25 (0.67-3.00)	1.00 (0.60-2.50)	1.00 (0.50-2.00)	0.75 (0.50-1.67)	0.71 (0.33-1.50)
ΔE/A	0.37 (0-1.0)	0.40 (−0.05-1.0)	0.37 (0-1.0)	0.36 (−0.04-0.80)	0.31 (0-0.64)	0.29 (−0.04-0.70)
ΔE/(A-E at A)	0.0 (−1.3-1.0)	0.07 (−1.33-0.75)	0.17 (−1.0-0.77)	0.13 (−0.83-0.75)	0.17 (−0.58-0.57)	0.17 (−0.75-0.63)
Index of myocardial performance						
LIMP	0.30 (0.10-0.50)	0.30 (0.20-0.60)	0.30 (0.20-0.60)	0.40 (0.20-0.60)	0.40 (0.20-0.60)	0.40 (0.20-0.60)

*Data are median (5th and 95th percentiles).

A = late diastolic mitral flow velocity; A_{dur} = duration of late mitral flow; A'_L = lateral mitral annulus velocity with atrial contraction; A'_S = late diastolic lateral annular velocity; DT = deceleration time of early diastolic mitral flow; E = early diastolic mitral flow velocity; E'_L = early diastolic lateral annular velocity; E'_S = early diastolic septal annular velocity; ΔE/A = change in E/A with Valsalva; ΔE/A-E = change in E/A-E at A with Valsalva; LIMP = left ventricular index of myocardial performance; P_D = pulmonary vein diastolic flow velocity; P_S = pulmonary vein systolic flow velocity; $PVAR_{dur}$ = duration of pulmonary vein atrial flow reversal; TDI = tissue Doppler imaging; VS = peak Valsalva.

Modified from Munagala VK, Jacobsen SJ, Mahoney DW, et al: Association of newer diastolic function parameters with age in healthy subjects: A population-based study. J Am Soc Echocardiogr 16:1049, 2003.

increases with exercise in healthy subjects so that E/e′ is similar at rest and with exercise (usually <8).[45] With aging (see Chap. 80), there is a gradual decrease in the rate of myocardial relaxation as well as in elastic recoil, resulting in slower decline of LV pressure, and filling becomes slower, producing a diastolic function pattern similar to grade 1 dysfunction. At roughly the age of 65 years, E velocity approaches A velocity, and in persons older than 70 years, the E/A ratio is usually less than 1.0. The reversal of e′/a′ occurs about 10 to 15 years earlier than that of E/A. Pulmonary venous flow velocities show similar changes with aging; diastolic forward flow velocity decreases as more filling of the left ventricle occurs at atrial contraction and systolic forward flow velocity becomes more prominent. Measurements of diastolic function in 1012 subjects without a history of cardiovascular disease or abnormal two-dimensional echocardiograms showed that all diastolic function parameters are associated with age (**Table 15-10**).

Grade 1 Diastolic Dysfunction or Mild Diastolic Dysfunction

An early abnormality of diastolic filling is abnormal myocardial relaxation. Typical cardiac conditions that produce abnormal relaxation are LV hypertrophy, HCM, and myocardial ischemia or infarction as well as aging. During this stage of diastolic dysfunction, an adequate diastolic filling period is critical to maintain normal filling without increasing filling pressure. As long as LA pressure remains normal, the pressure crossover between the left ventricle and left atrium occurs late, and the early transmitral pressure gradient is decreased. Consequently, the isovolumic relaxation time (IVRT) is prolonged. Mitral E velocity is decreased and A velocity is increased, producing an E/A ratio of less than 1, with prolonged DT. Pulmonary vein diastolic forward flow velocity parallels mitral E velocity and is also decreased with compensatory increased flow in systole. The duration and velocity of pulmonary vein atrial flow reversal are usually normal, but they may be increased if atrial compliance decreases or LV end-diastolic pressure (LVEDP) is high. The e′ and mitral flow propagation velocity are reduced, usually less than 7 cm/sec (at the septal annulus) and less than 50 cm/sec, respectively. In most patients with the described mitral inflow velocity pattern, diastolic filling pressure is not increased and the E/e′ ratio is 8 or higher. In a subgroup of patients, E/e′ ratio is higher than 15, with an E/A ratio less than 1. This pattern has been designated grade 1a diastolic dysfunction to emphasize that filling pressure is increased while there is a typical grade 1 mitral inflow velocity pattern.

Grade 2 Diastolic Dysfunction or Moderate Diastolic Dysfunction

This stage is also referred to as the pseudonormalized mitral flow filling pattern, and it represents a moderate stage of diastolic dysfunction.[20] As diastolic function worsens, the mitral inflow pattern goes through a phase resembling a normal diastolic filling pattern, that is, an E/A ratio of 1 to 1.5 and normal DT (160 to 240 milliseconds). This is the result of a moderately increased LA pressure superimposed on delayed myocardial relaxation. There are several means to differentiate the pseudonormal pattern from a true normal pattern in patients with grade 2 dysfunction:

1. The e′ is usually less than 7 because myocardial relaxation is impaired.
2. Frequently, there is mid-diastolic flow because of marked impairment of myocardial relaxation (see Fig. 15-e4 on website).[46,47]
3. A decrease in preload, by having the patient sit or perform the Valsalva maneuver, may be able to unmask the underlying impaired relaxation of the left ventricle, decreasing the E/A ratio by more than 0.5. If the A velocity increases with the Valsalva maneuver, it is a positive sign.
4. Normal-appearing mitral inflow may occur in the setting of systolic dysfunction or increased wall thickness because impaired relaxation

is expected as the baseline diastolic function without increased filling pressure in those situations, and a normal E/A ratio suggests that increased LA pressure is masking the abnormal relaxation.

5. Mitral A duration is shortened in the absence of a short PR interval and prolonged pulmonary vein atrial flow reversal exceeding mitral A duration.
6. Decreased rate of flow propagation (<45 cm/sec) by color M-mode of mitral inflow occurs. This is less reliable in patients with normal LV cavity size.

Grade 3-4 Diastolic Dysfunction or Severe Diastolic Dysfunction

Severe diastolic dysfunction is also termed restrictive filling or restrictive physiology and can be present in any cardiac abnormality or in a combination of abnormalities that produce decreased LV compliance and markedly increased LA pressure. Examples include decompensated congestive systolic heart failure, advanced restrictive cardiomyopathy, severe coronary artery disease, acute severe aortic regurgitation (AR), and constrictive pericarditis. Early rapid diastolic filling into a less compliant left ventricle causes a rapid increase in early LV diastolic pressure, with rapid equalization of LV and LA pressures producing a shortened DT. Atrial contraction increases LA pressure, but A velocity and duration are shortened because LV pressure increases even more rapidly. When LV diastolic pressure is markedly increased, there may be diastolic MR during mid-diastole or with atrial relaxation. Therefore, restrictive filling with severe diastolic dysfunction is characterized by increased E velocity, decreased A velocity (markedly less than E) with an E/A ratio higher than 2, and shortened DT (<160 milliseconds) and IVRT (<70 milliseconds). Systolic forward flow velocity in the pulmonary vein is decreased because of increased LA pressure and decreased LA compliance (**Fig. 15-29**).

Because myocardial relaxation is impaired in patients with a restrictive filling pattern, mitral annulus velocity (Ea) is reduced (<7 cm/sec). The E/e′ ratio is usually higher than 15. Flow propagation velocity may not be reduced in restrictive filling when the LV cavity is small and systolic function is well preserved. The Valsalva maneuver may reverse the restrictive filling pattern to a grade 1 to 2 pattern, indicating the reversibility of high filling pressure (grade 3 diastolic filling). However, even if the restrictive filling pattern does not change with the Valsalva maneuver, reversibility cannot be excluded because the Valsalva maneuver may not be adequate or filling pressure is too high to be altered by the Valsalva maneuver.

Evaluation of Cardiac Function by Cardiac Time Intervals

Cardiac time intervals provide valuable mechanistic and diagnostic insight into systolic and diastolic function of the heart. In the 1960s, the duration of isovolumic contraction time (IVCT) and the preejection period (PEP) was studied extensively as a measure of cardiac systolic function, and LV ejection time (LVET) was used as a measure of LV SV. Although myocardial dysfunction prolongs PEP and shortens LVET, these intervals are also influenced by many hemodynamic and electrical variables. Weissler and colleagues derived an index (PEP/LVET) called systolic time interval, which was less heart rate dependent as a measure of LV systolic function. Because IVRT is also affected by LV function, Mancini and colleagues incorporated IVRT into an index called the isovolumic index, derived as (IVCT + IVRT)/LVET. The sum of IVCT and IVRT was measured by subtracting LVET from the peak of the R wave on the electrocardiogram to the onset of mitral valve opening. The isovolumic index was considered more sensitive for cardiac dysfunction than the systolic time interval because it contains IVRT as well as IVCT. However, the interval from the R wave peak to the onset of mitral valve opening contains an interval of electromechanical delay, which can be pronounced in patients with left bundle branch block. With the advent of Doppler echocardiography, it has become easier to determine cardiac time intervals more reliably. Tei and colleagues proposed an index of myocardial performance with Doppler echocardiography (IMP or Tei index) that is independent of the electromechanical delay, (IVCT + IVRT)/LVET, and can be used to identify the exact onset of isovolumic contraction.[48]

The time intervals necessary for calculation of IMP are easily obtained with Doppler echocardiography and TDI[22] as well as with M-mode echocardiography.[49] The normal value is 0.39 ± 0.05, and its mean value is 0.59 ± 0.10 in those with dilated cardiomyopathy. The IMP was evaluated for the right ventricle, especially in patients with pulmonary hypertension. When myocardial relaxation is normal, the opening of the mitral valve is initiated by rapid suction of the left ventricle; hence, the onset of mitral valve opening is close to the onset of early diastolic movement (or velocity) of the mitral annulus.[15,21] However, if myocardial relaxation is delayed, the mitral valve opens by high LA pressure. Therefore, the onset of diastolic motion of the mitral annulus follows the onset of mitral inflow. The time interval has been correlated with the degree of impairment in myocardial relaxation and LV filling pressure. With worsening of diastolic function, the time interval lengthens.

Clinical Applications of Diastolic Function Assessment

Assessment of diastolic function echocardiographically has the following clinical applications and should be an integral part of an echocardiography examination.

1. Estimation of filling pressures at rest and with exercise. In patients with reduced LV systolic function (LVEF <35%), mitral inflow E/A ratio of 1.5 or higher and DT of 140 milliseconds or higher indicate increased filling pressures. However, these parameters do not have a good correlation with filling pressure in patients with normal LVEF

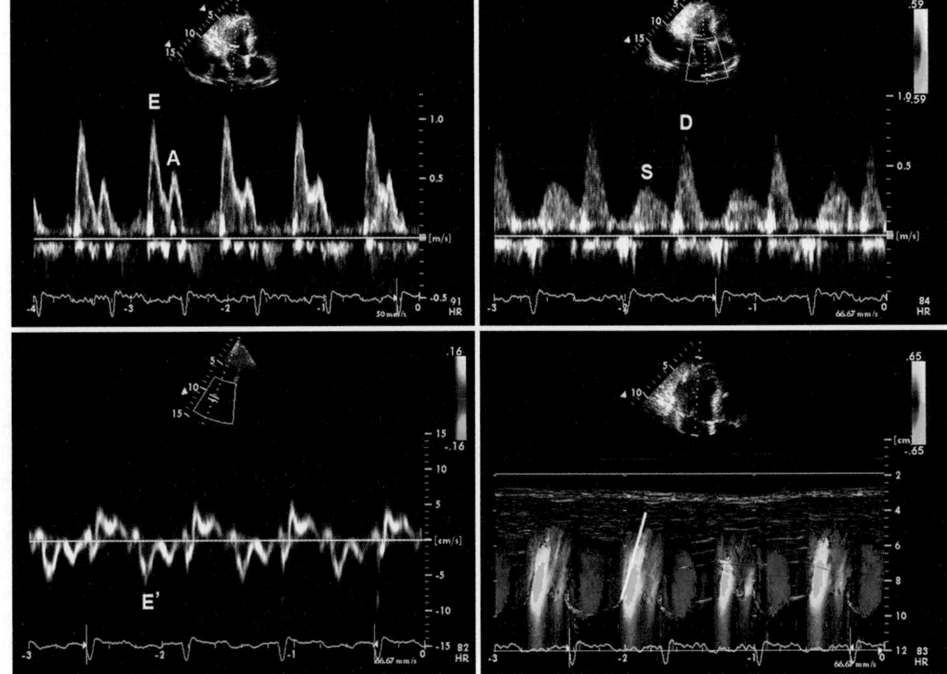

FIGURE 15-29 Mitral inflow **(upper left)**, pulmonary vein velocity **(upper right)**, septal mitral annular tissue Doppler **(lower left)**, and color M-mode **(lower right)** from a patient with restrictive diastolic dysfunction.

and diastolic heart failure. For all degrees of LVEF, E/e′ is the best parameter to estimate filling pressure; pulmonary capillary wedge pressure (PCWP) is 20 mm Hg or more if E/e′ is 15 or higher, and PCWP is normal if E/e′ is less than 8.[20,40] When E/e′ is 8 or higher but less than 15, pulmonary vein flow duration and the Valsalva maneuver can help estimate PCWP. In an important subset of patients with diastolic dysfunction, PCWP is normal at rest but increases only with exertion, causing exertional dyspnea. It is feasible and reliable to estimate PCWP with exercise by recording mitral inflow and annulus velocity.[46,50] In a normal population with normal diastolic function, filling pressure rarely increases with exercise. Diastolic dysfunction (or impaired myocardial relaxation) is usually a prerequisite for development of exercise-induced high filling pressure. These patients increase cardiac output at the expense of increased filling pressure. In this situation, mitral E velocity increases while annulus Ea velocity does not increase as much or at all, resulting in an increase in E/e′ ratio. E/e′ correlates well with simultaneously measured PCWP with exercise as well as during resting stage, and a ratio higher than 15 indicates PCWP greater than 20 mm Hg with exercise (see Fig. 15-e5 on website).[50]

2. Diagnosis of diastolic heart failure, cardiomyopathies, and constrictive pericarditis. Knowledge of the diastolic filling pattern and filling pressures allows the detection of cardiac diseases that are frequently missed or not suspected clinically, especially when the LVEF is normal. Patients with diastolic heart failure and normal LVEF have a large LA volume and evidence of impaired relaxation as well as increased filling pressure. There are several reports that TDI of myocardial relaxation can diagnose various forms of cardiomyopathy (HCM, Fabry disease, and amyloidosis) even before frank phenotypic manifestation.[51-53] The detection of constrictive pericarditis has been made much easier with the use of echocardiographic diastolic parameters and TDI (see Pericardial Diseases).[54,55]
3. Prognosis. Diastolic echocardiographic parameters, E, E/A, DT, E/e′, and LA volume, have been found to be powerful prognostic indicators for various conditions.[56-59] Even in asymptomatic patients, the presence of diastolic dysfunction portends a poor clinical outcome.

Although diastolic filling is affected by various factors, the direction of its change or progression is predictable in patients with known heart disease. Therefore, assessment of the diastolic filling pattern allows LV filling pressures and LV compliance and relaxation to be estimated and understood so that optimal treatment strategies can be offered to symptomatic patients with diastolic dysfunction.

Echocardiography in Heart Failure (see Chaps. 26 and 28)

Echocardiography is the single most useful test in the evaluation of patients with heart failure and may establish the underlying cause so that an optimal management strategy can be implemented. When a cardiac structural abnormality or systolic dysfunction is responsible for heart failure, it is usually obvious on two-dimensional echocardiography. In systolic heart failure, however, echocardiography has many roles beyond the recognition of decreased LVEF because dilation of the left ventricle alters intracardiac geometry and hemodynamics.[60] Echocardiography is also helpful in selected patients in monitoring responses to various therapies.[61-63]

LV volume is one of the most important prognostic indicators in patients with ischemic or dilated cardiomyopathy. With LV remodeling and progressive dilation of the heart, the left ventricle becomes more spherical and the mitral annulus is dilated, with apical displacement of the mitral leaflets causing functional mitral valve regurgitation (see Chap. 66). Among various echocardiographic parameters, LVEDV, DT of mitral E velocity (which is a surrogate for PCWP), and severity of MR are the strongest predictors of survival for patients with an LVEF of 35% or less.[60] In heart failure trials, echocardiography is a valuable tool for measuring or assessing LV dimensions, volumes, sphericity index, severity of MR, diastolic filling parameters, and pulmonary artery systolic pressure.

Echocardiography has been used to assess the success of biventricular pacing by documenting reverse LV remodeling and reduction in MR (see Chap. 29). Another potential role of echocardiography in biventricular pacing is to identify the patients who will benefit from the therapy because 30% to 50% of patients who receive biventricular pacing may not have improvement. Initially, time intervals measured by TDI[64-66] were used to determine indexes of mechanical dyssynchrony to identify a positive responder. However, the PROSPECT trial demonstrated that no echocardiographic parameter, including TDI-derived timing intervals, could predict positive or negative responders reliably.[67] Therefore, no patient should be denied cardiac resynchronization therapy on the basis of any echocardiography-derived dyssynchrony parameters.[68]

In the large subset of patients with heart failure and normal LVEF (see Chap. 30), assessment of LV diastolic function is useful in evaluating the severity of disease and in risk assessment.

If mitral inflow velocity clearly demonstrates a restrictive filling pattern or high filling pressure at the resting stage, the diagnosis of heart failure or constrictive pericarditis is usually secure. TDI of the septal mitral annulus is helpful in differentiating pseudonormal from true normal mitral inflow velocities and differentiating constrictive pericarditis from myocardial diseases. When plasma levels of brain natriuretic peptide (BNP) and the mitral E/e′ ratio were correlated with PCWP, the correlation was better for the mitral E/e′ ratio than for BNP.[69] Another important clinical consideration is assessment of exercise-induced increases in filling pressures responsible for symptoms of shortness of breath with exertion. Therefore, filling pressure needs to be assessed with exercise as well as at rest.

Coronary Artery Disease

Evaluation of coronary artery disease is the most common use of echocardiography. Broad applications include the diagnosis of coronary artery disease with resting or stress echocardiography, detection of complications of acute MI, assessment of myocardial viability, and risk stratification.

From the parasternal, apical, and sometimes subcostal imaging windows, two-dimensional echocardiography can visualize all LV wall segments. For purposes of regional wall motion analysis, the ASE has recommended a 16-segment model or, optionally, a 17-segment model with an addition of the apical cap (**Fig. 15-30**). The following numerical score is assigned to each wall segment on the basis of its contractile function as assessed visually: 1 = normal (>40% thickening with systole); 2 = hypokinesis (10% to 40% thickening); 3 = severe hypokinesis to akinesis (<10% thickening); 4 = dyskinesis; and 5 = aneurysm. On the basis of this wall motion analysis scheme, a wall motion score index (WMSI) is calculated to semiquantitate the extent of regional wall motion abnormalities:

$$\text{WMSI} = \frac{\text{Sum of wall motion scores}}{\text{Number of segments visualized}}$$

A normal left ventricle has a WMSI of 1, and the index increases as wall motion abnormalities become more severe. When two-dimensional echocardiography was performed simultaneously with sestamibi SPECT in patients with acute ST-segment MI (STEMI), the overall correlation between the WMSI and the perfusion defect was good. Patients with a WMSI higher than 1.7 had a perfusion defect greater than 20%. The correlation was better for patients with an anterior wall MI than for those with an inferior or lateral wall MI with a smaller infarct size. A small area of subendocardial ischemia may not demonstrate wall motion abnormality, but contrast echocardiography can demonstrate a rim of subendocardial perfusion defect.

Echocardiography is helpful in the evaluation of chest pain, especially during active chest pain. The absence of LV wall motion abnormalities during chest pain usually but not always excludes myocardial ischemia or infarction, and the presence of regional wall motion abnormalities has a high sensitivity for detection of myocardial ischemia or infarction, although it is not specific. Myocardial contrast perfusion imaging provides incremental diagnostic value for patients with chest pain, with excellent concordance with gated SPECT (77% to 84%).[31] However, routine use of echocardiography in this setting requires availability of appropriately trained personnel to perform echocardiography and to interpret its findings.

Wall motion analysis can also be performed more objectively and conveniently by speckle tracking strain imaging. Moreover, Ishii and colleagues[70] elegantly demonstrated that diastolic relaxation of the ischemic myocardial segment remains abnormal long after resolution of the regional wall motion abnormality, and the diastolic relaxation abnormality can be detected by strain imaging.

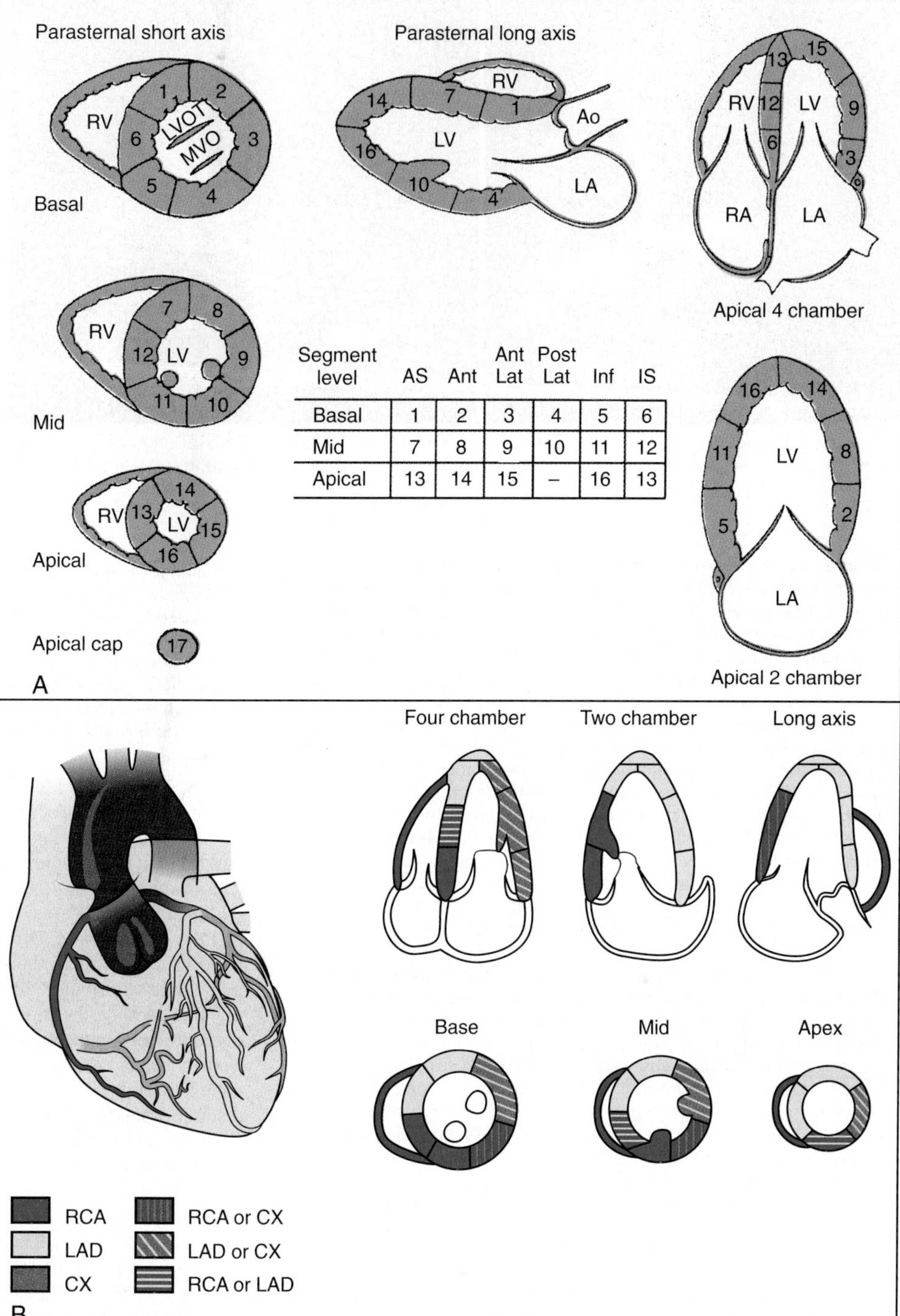

Segment level	AS	Ant	Ant Lat	Post Lat	Inf	IS
Basal	1	2	3	4	5	6
Mid	7	8	9	10	11	12
Apical	13	14	15	–	16	13

FIGURE 15-30 **A,** Diagrammatic cross sections of the left ventricle to show 17 segments for wall motion analysis. Ant = anterior; Ant Lat = anterolateral; AS = anteroseptal; Inf = inferior; IS = inferoseptal; Post Lat = posterolateral wall. **B,** Left ventricular segments from three apical views and mid-parasternal short-axis view with the corresponding coronary artery distribution. CX = circumflex artery; LAD = left anterior descending artery; RCA = right coronary artery. *(**A** modified from Oh JK, Seward JB, Tajik AJ: The Echo Manual. 3rd ed. Philadelphia, Lippincott Williams & Wilkins, 2006. Used with permission of Mayo Foundation for Medical Education and Research. **B** modified from Lang RM, Bierig M, Devereux RB, et al: Recommendations for chamber quantification: A report from the American Society of Echocardiography's Guidelines and Standards Committee and the Chamber Quantification Writing Group, developed in conjunction with the European Association of Echocardiography, a branch of the European Society of Cardiology. J Am Soc Echocardiogr 18:1440, 2005. Used with permission.)*

Echocardiography in Patients with Acute Myocardial Infarction

(see Chaps. 55 and 56)

In patients with acute MI, echocardiography has several important roles: (1) diagnosis and exclusion of acute MI in patients with prolonged chest pain and nondiagnostic electrocardiographic findings; (2) estimation of the amount of myocardium at risk and final infarct size after reperfusion therapy; (3) evaluation of patients with unstable hemodynamic findings and detection of infarct complications; (4) evaluation of myocardial viability; and (5) risk stratification.

Two-dimensional echocardiographic imaging is useful in assessing reperfused myocardial segments or infarct expansion in patients with STEMI. Persistent akinesis does not always indicate failed reperfusion. When the myocardium remains akinetic while being viable, low-dose dobutamine, contrast, or strain imaging echocardiography may be helpful to demonstrate its viability (see Chaps. 52 and 57).[71] Regional strain or strain rate can be used as a marker of acute ischemia.[72]

DETECTION OF MECHANICAL COMPLICATIONS OF ACUTE MYOCARDIAL INFARCTION. Because complications of MI can be life-threatening, reliable and timely identification of infarct-related complications is critical for optimal management. Two-dimensional and Doppler echocardiography with color flow imaging should be the first imaging modality to evaluate a clinical situation with a suspected mechanical complication or a patient with unstable hemodynamics. In addition to patients in whom precordial echocardiography is not possible for various reasons, TEE can obtain diagnostic images under the most difficult clinical situations, including in the critical care unit, in intubated patients and postoperative patients, and even during cardiopulmonary resuscitation.[73] The presence of normal systolic function in a critically ill or hemodynamically unstable patient should lead immediately to the suspicion of a mechanical complication.

NEW SYSTOLIC MURMUR: VENTRICULAR SEPTAL RUPTURE, PAPILLARY MUSCLE RUPTURE, AND ACUTE OUTFLOW OBSTRUCTION. The differential

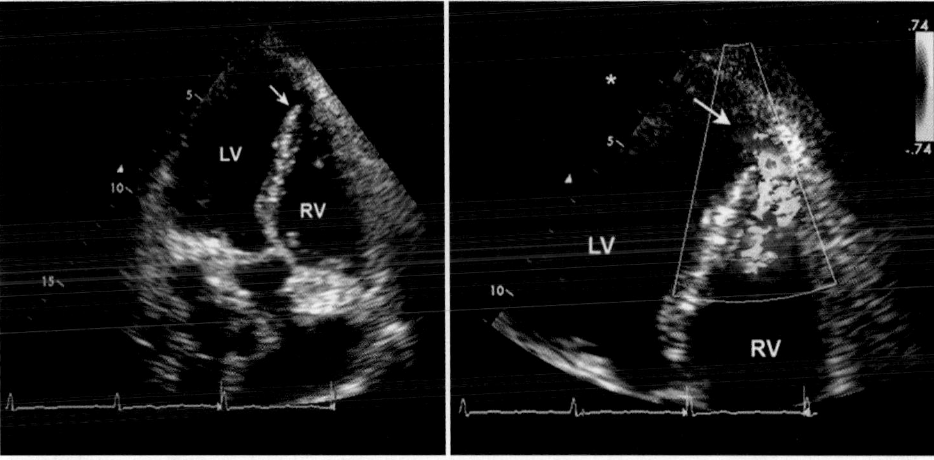

FIGURE 15-31 Left, Transthoracic apical long-axis view showing a large apical ventricular septal defect (arrow). **Right,** Color flow imaging showing a shunt from the left to right ventricle through the ventricular septal defect. LV = left ventricle; RV = right ventricle.

diagnosis of a new systolic murmur in patients with acute MI includes infarct-related ventricular septal rupture, papillary muscle dysfunction or rupture, pericardial rub, and acute LVOT obstruction. After physical examination, echocardiography is the next logical noninvasive diagnostic procedure for all patients with a new murmur, especially those who are hemodynamically unstable. Infarct-related ventricular septal defect is diagnosed by demonstration of a disrupted ventricular septum with a left-to-right shunt. The defect is always located in the region of the thinned myocardium with dyskinetic motion. The diagnosis usually can be established with a two-dimensional TTE examination (**Fig. 15-31**; see Fig. 55-35). TEE may be necessary in the small subgroup of patients with a suboptimal precordial study (see Fig. 15-e6 on website). Peak flow velocity across the rupture measured with continuous-wave Doppler imaging can estimate RV systolic pressure. When the rupture is located at the inferoseptum, the right ventricle is usually involved by the MI, which portends a poor prognosis. An inferoseptal ventricular rupture can have a serpiginous septal tear, and an anteroapical ventricular septal rupture may extend to an LV free wall rupture.

Acute MR is another important cause of systolic murmur, related to LV global or regional remodeling, papillary muscle dysfunction, papillary muscle rupture (partial or complete), and acute systolic anterior motion (SAM) of the mitral valve. For optimal management, it is important to recognize the underlying cause of ischemic MR because papillary muscle rupture mandates urgent mitral valve replacement or repair,[74] but MR caused by papillary muscle dysfunction or annulus dilation may improve with afterload reduction or coronary revascularization or both (see Chaps. 57 and 66). MR caused by acute SAM is managed by fluid, a beta blocker, or occasionally a pure alpha agonist.

Hemodynamically, papillary muscle rupture is the most serious complication involving the mitral valve. The patients usually have a small infarct in the distribution of the right coronary or circumflex coronary artery. Because the posteromedial papillary muscle is supplied by a single coronary artery (compared with the dual supply of the anterolateral papillary muscle), rupture of the posteromedial papillary muscle is more frequent. Echocardiography is the best way to diagnose papillary muscle dysfunction and rupture (see Figs. 15-e7 and 15-e8 on website). Papillary muscle rupture can be partial (incomplete) or complete. Because patients with severe MR usually present with hemodynamic decompensation, TEE may be necessary to establish clearly the diagnosis and to assess the severity of MR.

A less known but clinically important entity resulting in new systolic murmur and an unstable hemodynamic condition is acute dynamic LVOT obstruction, which is related to the compensatory hyperdynamic motion of the posterior and inferolateral walls, resulting in SAM of the mitral leaflet, which causes MR, as well as the obstruction. It is more common after anterior wall MI in elderly women who have basal septal hypertrophy caused by hypertension. It also has been noted in one third of patients with apical ballooning syndrome (see Chaps. 68 and 73).[75] Patients with acute LVOT obstruction can develop severely unstable hemodynamics, including shock and pulmonary edema. The most appropriate therapies are fluids, beta blockers, alpha agonists, avoidance of vasodilators, and inotropes. This condition is not uncommon during the postoperative period in patients who receive inotropic support.

FREE WALL RUPTURE AND PSEUDOANEURYSM. In patients with cardiac free wall rupture, two-dimensional TTE may not be able to show the site of rupture but may only demonstrate a pericardial effusion with or without Doppler characteristics of pericardial tamponade. The presence of pericardial effusion alone is not sufficient for diagnosis of a free wall rupture because pericardial effusion is common after acute MI. Contrast echocardiography or color flow imaging may help in identifying the rupture site. Negative echocardiographic findings should not exclude myocardial rupture if clinical suspicion is high. In this case, another imaging technique such as CMR should be considered. In some cases, a pseudoaneurysm forms after a free wall rupture is contained within a limited portion of the pericardial space (most frequently in the posterior wall, followed by the lateral and apical walls). A pseudoaneurysm is traditionally characterized by a small neck communication between the left ventricle and aneurysmal cavity (the ratio of the diameter of entry and the maximal diameter of the pseudoaneurysm is <0.5). However, it may have a wide neck communication[25] (see Fig. 15-e9 on website). There is always to-and-fro blood flow through the rupture site that can be documented with Doppler and color flow imaging. On occasion, a free wall rupture does not extend through the entire thickness of the wall and is contained by the epicardial layer (subepicardial aneurysm; see Fig. 15-e10 on website).

TRUE LEFT VENTRICULAR ANEURYSM AND THROMBUS. Compared with a pseudoaneurysm, a true aneurysm contains all layers of the myocardium and is characterized by myocardial thinning and bulging motion during systole. True aneurysm formation is related to transmural MI and is found most frequently at the apex, followed by the inferobasal area. A ventricular aneurysm is the consequence of infarct expansion, which indicates a poor prognosis. Ventricular aneurysms frequently harbor a thrombus and can be the focus of malignant ventricular arrhythmias. Two-dimensional echocardiography has become the most practical and reliable imaging modality for detection of LV thrombus. It is important to differentiate thrombus from chordae or artifacts frequently seen at the apex. Characteristically, a thrombus has a nonhomogeneous echo density with a margin distinct from the underlying wall, which is akinetic to dyskinetic. Contrast echocardiography is also helpful in distinguishing LV thrombus from other structures.[30]

EVALUATION OF LEFT VENTRICULAR REMODELING AND ISCHEMIC MITRAL REGURGITATION (see Chap. 57). LV remodeling represents progressive LV dilation and systolic dysfunction after acute MI. As the left ventricle dilates and develops a more spherical shape, LVEF decreases, and mitral leaflets are pulled more apically, allowing an increasing amount of MR, all of which result in worsening of heart failure and increased risk of death. Echocardiography is essential in identifying these patients and assisting clinical trials in LV remodeling by providing detailed information about LV size, LV volume, regional wall motion analysis, myocardial viability, LV filling pressures, severity of MR, and pulmonary artery systolic pressure.

Ischemic MR refers to chronic MR caused by LV remodeling due to coronary artery disease (see Chaps. 57 and 66). In patients with LV systolic dysfunction, acute pulmonary edema has been associated with the dynamic changes in ischemic MR and the resulting increase in pulmonary vascular pressure.[76] As in the acute phase of MI, chronic ischemic MR has been found to be an important prognostic indicator,[77] and even a mild degree of MR has been associated with increased mortality.[78] Whether reduction of MR by surgery or a percutaneous device procedure improves quality of life or survival has not been determined by a clinical trial.[79]

RIGHT VENTRICULAR INFARCTION. Mortality from a hemodynamically serious RV infarction is as high as that related to shock from LV infarction (see Chap. 54). RV infarction is characterized by a dilated and hypokinetic to akinetic right ventricle. The apical portion of the right ventricle may be spared because it is supplied by the left anterior descending coronary artery, whereas the basal to mid RV free walls are more commonly affected. The right atrium is also dilated, and tricuspid regurgitation (TR) develops as a result of tricuspid annulus dilation. Because RV systolic pressure is not increased, peak TR velocity is low, usually less than 2 m/sec. TDI of the tricuspid valve annulus may be helpful in identifying depressed RV function in patients with inferior wall MI. In patients with a PFO, an RV infarct creates an optimal clinical setting for a severe right-to-left shunt because of abnormal RV compliance and markedly increased right atrial (RA) pressure. This diagnosis can be confirmed with contrast echocardiography (peripheral venous injection of agitated saline) or color flow imaging. This situation is best assessed with TEE (see Fig. 15-e11 on website).

APICAL BALLOONING SYNDROME OR TAKOTSUBO CARDIOMYOPATHY. A subgroup of patients with acute MI have no coronary artery stenosis on angiography. These patients may have typical ST-segment elevation as well as elevation of troponin or creatine kinase with muscle subfraction (CK-MB). Echocardiography shows typical regional wall motion abnormalities, and these patients can also develop complications similar to those of patients with coronary artery disease. Clinical situations in which this scenario is found include coronary spasm, subarachnoid hemorrhage, pheochromocytoma, electroconvulsive treatment, and apical ballooning syndrome or takotsubo cardiomyopathy (see Chaps. 68 and 73).[74,79,80] Usually, the apical segment is involved more frequently, and acute LVOT obstruction has also occurred in this setting.

Echocardiography is extremely helpful in this syndrome for monitoring the functional and hemodynamic responses to treatment. A variant mid-ventricular form of this syndrome has been described in which apical and basal segments are spared. Only the midportion of the left ventricle was found to be akinetic on left ventriculography and echocardiography.[81] When apical ballooning was compared with STEMI by echocardiography, the extent of wall motion abnormalities was greater in patients with apical ballooning, but the diastolic filling pattern was better, indicating less transmural involvement in apical ballooning.[82] Contrast echocardiography shows relatively normal perfusion in apical ballooning, indicating that wall motion abnormalities in apical ballooning are more demand related (such as increased catecholamine level) than supply related (**Fig. 15-32**).

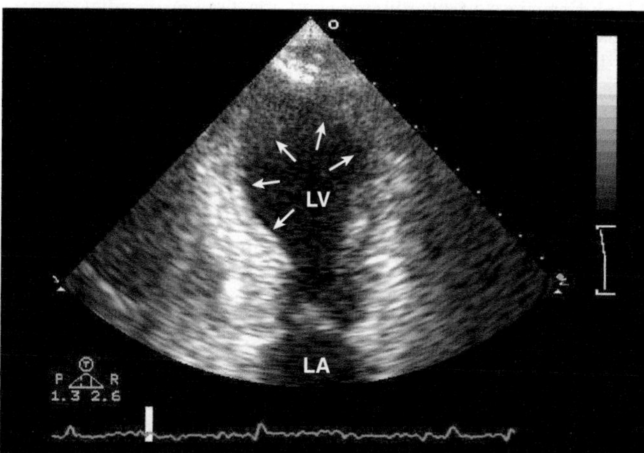

FIGURE 15-32 Apical two-chamber view demonstrates a dilated apical segment or ballooning (arrows) in a 55-year-old woman with stress-induced apical ballooning syndrome. LA = left atrium; LV = left ventricle. *(Modified from Oh JK, Seward JB, Tajik AJ: The Echo Manual. 3rd ed. Philadelphia, Lippincott Williams & Wilkins, 2006. Used with permission of Mayo Foundation for Medical Education and Research.)*

RISK STRATIFICATION BY ECHOCARDIOGRAPHY IN PATIENTS WITH ACUTE MYOCARDIAL INFARCTION. The most powerful prognostic indicators after MI are the degree of LV systolic dysfunction, LV volume, LV sphericity, extent of coronary artery disease, MR, diastolic function, and presence of heart failure[77,83,84] (see Chap. 54). Therefore, it is reasonable to predict that patients with a high WMSI have a greater chance for subsequent development of cardiac events. Most patients with Killip class II-IV heart failure after acute MI have a WMSI of 1.7 or higher. In addition to the WMSI, restrictive Doppler filling variables derived from mitral inflow velocities correlate well with the incidence of postinfarction heart failure and LV filling pressures.[60] The E/e′ ratio, a reliable parameter to estimate PCWP, was found to be a strong predictor for long-term outcome after acute MI.[62] LA volume, a surrogate for chronic diastolic dysfunction and chronic elevation of LA pressure, was also a strong predictor of outcome.[60] Stress echocardiography is sensitive in detecting residual ischemia, myocardial viability, and multivessel disease soon after MI. Often, however, patients are unable to exercise adequately soon after an acute MI, and the myocardium may remain akinetic for a period of days to weeks after successful reperfusion of the occluded coronary artery. Demonstration of viability by augmentation of contractility (with dobutamine echocardiography) or demonstration of perfusion (with contrast echocardiography) predicts functional recovery.

Stress Echocardiography

Stress echocardiography is an excellent method for comparing wall motion (regional contractility), myocardial perfusion, pressure gradient, pulmonary pressure, valvular regurgitation, or filling pressures before and after a stress to identify pathologic conditions that are not apparent at rest. Stress echocardiography requires a comparison of echocardiographic data obtained at the time of or after stress with baseline resting data, and it is essential to review resting and stress images side-by-side using digital acquisition and display.[85,86] By allowing several successive cardiac cycles to be captured and stored in memory, digitized echocardiography enhances the capability of acquiring satisfactory comparative images after exercise.

Stress echocardiography is performed with exercise or the administration of a pharmacologic agent.[1] The exercise protocol includes a treadmill exercise test, with immediate postexercise echocardiographic images, or upright or supine bicycle exercise with echocardiographic images obtained at peak exercise. Because exercise-induced regional wall motion abnormalities due to ischemia usually last for a few minutes after the termination of exercise, images taken immediately after exercise can be compared with the baseline pre-exercise images to detect exercise-induced regional wall motion abnormalities. The typical exercise echocardiography protocol is shown in **Figure 15-33**. Some centers favor a supine bicycle exercise protocol, as images can be obtained at peak exercise. Supine bicycle exercise is a preferred form of stress test for evaluation of exercise-induced hemodynamics in patients with valvular heart disease or diastolic dysfunction.

When a patient cannot exercise, stress is induced pharmacologically with dobutamine, dipyridamole, or adenosine. Dobutamine is the agent used most commonly in stress echocardiography (see Fig. 15-33). Contrast myocardial perfusion echocardiography can be used to identify ischemic myocardium. To induce a perfusion defect, adenosine or dipyridamole is most frequently used. These vasodilating agents create a "coronary steal" so that myocardial segments subtended by a stenotic coronary artery show a decrease in myocardial perfusion (see Chaps. 17 and 52).

At our institution, the patient's medications usually are not discontinued before stress echocardiography; more than one third of our patients are taking a beta blocker at the time of stress echocardiography. Atropine is used in 59% of dobutamine stress tests to augment heart rate. Stress echocardiography is safe, with no procedural mortality noted after more than 50,000 studies. Ventricular tachycardia occurred in 1.4% of exercise echocardiographic studies and in 4% of dobutamine stress echocardiographic studies. Ventricular fibrillation occurred in three patients (one with exercise and two with

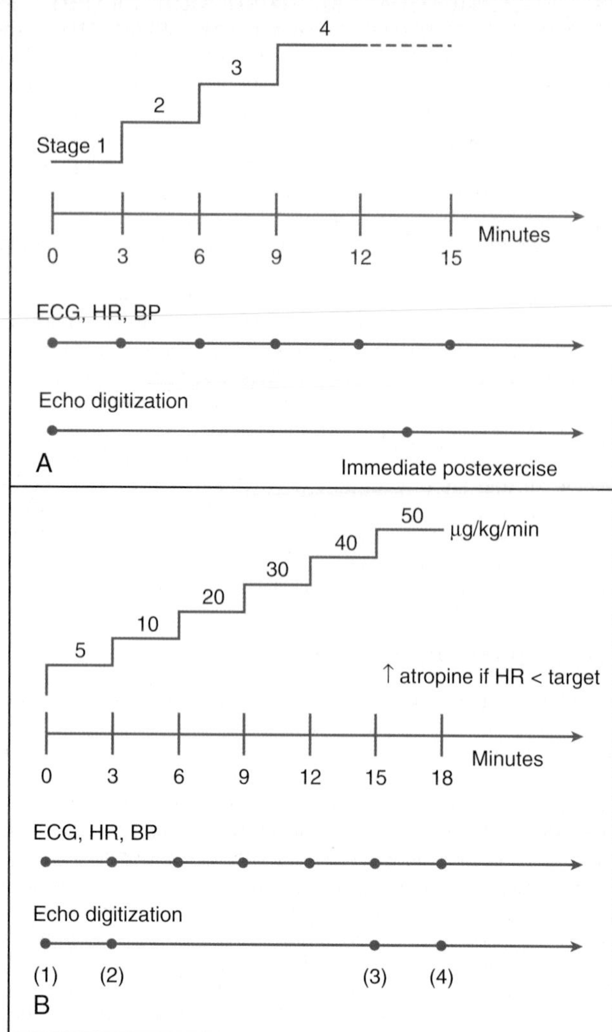

FIGURE 15-33 **A,** Typical exercise protocol. **B,** Protocol for pharmacologic dobutamine stress test. BP = blood pressure; ECG = electrocardiography; HR = heart rate. *(Modified from Oh JK, Seward JB, Tajik AJ: The Echo Manual. 3rd ed. Philadelphia, Lippincott Williams & Wilkins, 2006. Used with permission of Mayo Foundation for Medical Education and Research.)*

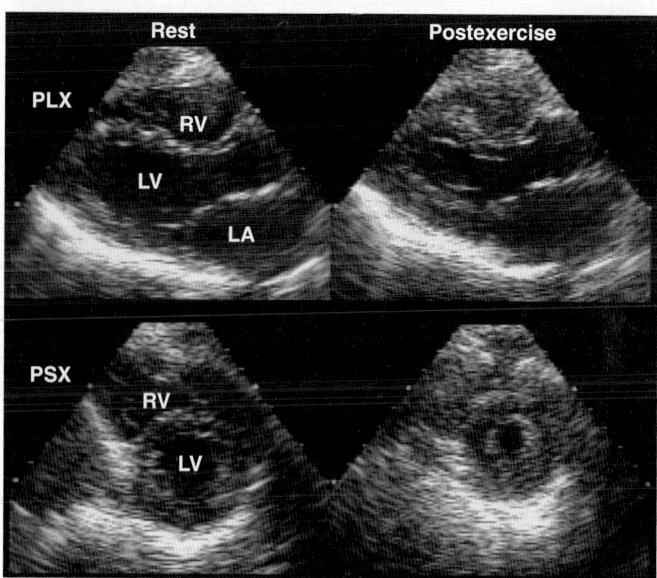

FIGURE 15-34 Still frame of end-systolic parasternal long-axis (PLX) and short-axis (PSX) views of normal exercise echocardiogram as shown in a quad-screen format. The LV cavity is smaller and the walls are hyperdynamic in the postexercise period. LA = left atrium; LV = left ventricle; RV = right ventricle. *(Modified from Oh JK, Seward JB, Tajik AJ: The Echo Manual. 3rd ed. Philadelphia, Lippincott Williams & Wilkins, 2006. Used with permission of Mayo Foundation for Medical Education and Research.)*

dobutamine). Supraventricular tachycardia and AF are more common. Stress echocardiography is safe enough that it can be supervised directly by specially trained registered nurses.[87]

DIAGNOSTIC CRITERIA FOR STRESS ECHOCARDIOGRAPHY. Normally with exercise, dobutamine, or pacing, LV wall motion becomes hyperdynamic (**Fig. 15-34**). Worsening of wall motion abnormalities or the development of new abnormalities is the hallmark of stress-induced myocardial ischemia (**Fig. 15-35**). The lack of hyperdynamic motion may indicate ischemia, but it is less specific. When the stress level is inadequate or the patient is taking a beta blocker, however, the entire LV segment may contract normally without hyperdynamic motion. Not infrequently, an akinetic myocardial segment becomes dyskinetic during stress echocardiography, but this change was not found to have any diagnostic or prognostic implication.[88]

Other adjunctive diagnostic criteria for an abnormal stress echocardiogram include LV cavity dilation and a decrease in global systolic function. These adjunctive diagnostic criteria are more specific for detection of severe coronary artery disease. Also, the response to dobutamine is different from that due to exercise. Even in patients with severe coronary artery disease, including left main coronary artery disease, the LV cavity may not dilate and global systolic function may improve with dobutamine infusion despite new wall motion abnormalities due to severe ischemia.

The use of TDI or strain imaging may be more sensitive for identification of ischemic segments.[89] Time from the QRS to the onset of regional relaxation has been found to be a good indication of ischemia. Myocardial ischemia delays the onset and the rate of regional myocardial relaxation, and the delay in relaxation can be quantified with TDI and strain rate imaging. Normally, the time from the QRS to the onset of regional myocardial relaxation is 350 to 400 milliseconds, and the interval decreases by a mean of 34% ± 10% in normal myocardial segments with high-dose dobutamine, but the reduction in the interval is less (mean, 12% ± 18%) in ischemic segments. Speckle strain imaging can be used to demonstrate delayed regional relaxation when myocardial ischemia occurs. This phenomenon has been termed diastolic stunning because the abnormality lasts longer than wall motion abnormality.[70]

Ideally, both myocardial contractility and perfusion data are available during stress echocardiography by real-time myocardial contrast perfusion imaging. A myocardial perfusion defect is usually observed as a dark area devoid of microbubbles in the subendocardium or the entire transmural myocardium area. Wall motion analysis is enhanced by LVO with use of contrast microbubbles. Currently, contrast is used for LVO in 25% of exercise studies and 50% of dobutamine echocardiography examinations in our laboratory. Biplane and three-dimensional imaging may shorten the acquisition period of postexercise or peak-exercise images. This will improve the sensitivity of stress echocardiography as well as minimize the technical strains imposed occasionally on sonographers or echocardiographers in obtaining challenging images.

DIAGNOSTIC ACCURACY. The sensitivity and specificity of stress echocardiography, with the use of wall motion criteria, are comparable to those of stress thallium or sestamibi SPECT (see Chap. 17).[85,86] In a large comparison study (112 patients), the overall sensitivity and specificity of exercise echocardiography were 85% and 88%, respectively, compared with 85% and 81% for exercise thallium imaging. The sensitivity of exercise echocardiography and exercise thallium imaging for coronary artery disease in patients with single-, double-, or triple-vessel involvement was also similar (58%, 86%, and 94% versus 61%, 86%, and 94%, respectively). However, according to our experience, the sensitivity of exercise echocardiography for prediction of multivessel disease is about 70%. When a

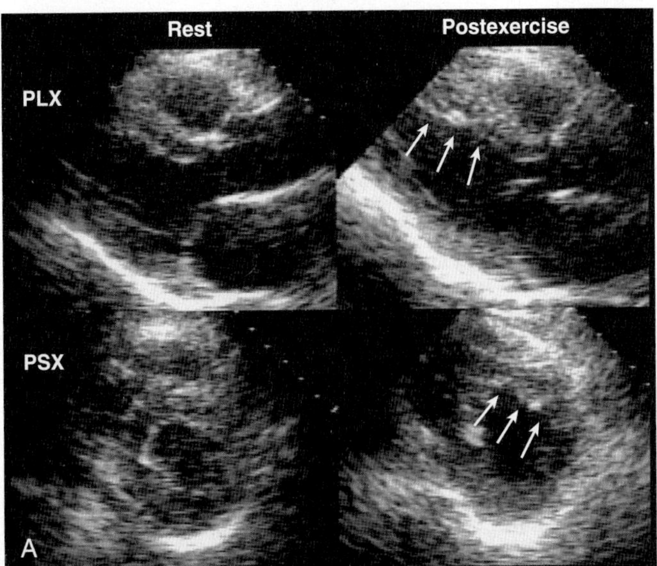

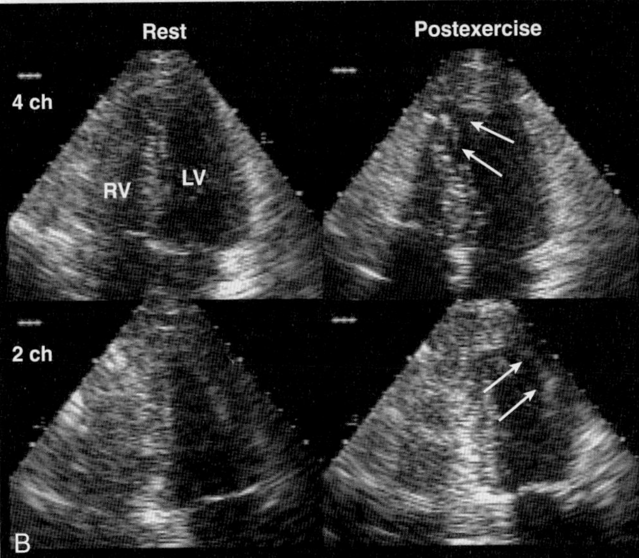

FIGURE 15-35 **A,** Still frame of end-systolic parasternal long-axis (PLX) and short-axis (PSX) views of an exercise echocardiogram positive for stress-induced myocardial ischemia. The anteroseptum and anterior wall became severely hypokinetic (arrows) with exercise. **B,** Still frame of end-systolic apical views of positive exercise echocardiogram. The apical septum and anteroapex became akinetic to dyskinetic (arrows). 2 ch = two-chamber view; 4 ch = four-chamber view; LV = left ventricle; RV = right ventricle. *(Modified from Oh JK, Seward JB, Tajik AJ: The Echo Manual. 3rd ed. Philadelphia, Lippincott Williams & Wilkins, 2006. Used with permission of Mayo Foundation for Medical Education and Research.)*

diagnostic test is used routinely, the diagnostic accuracy depends on the population of patients, the expertise of the interpreter, and the quality of the image. Patients with seemingly normal wall motion but abnormal myocardial perfusion have been observed. Some stress-induced wall motion abnormalities resolve quickly before being documented by post-stress images. Another possibility is that our visual interpretation of regional wall motion analysis is not always accurate. The ultimate technical goal of stress echocardiography for the evaluation of myocardial ischemia is to be able to assess regional contractility and myocardial perfusion at the same time. With further clinical experience, TDI, strain rate imaging, or diastolic stunning imaging by speckle strain may be able to improve the accuracy of stress echocardiography.

Stress Echocardiography as a Prognostic Indicator. The likelihood of a cardiac event (cardiac death, nonfatal infarct, or coronary revascularization) after normal stress echocardiography is extremely low. Among 1325 patients with normal findings on exercise echocardiography at Mayo Clinic, the event rate during 3 years of follow-up was less than 3%. The cardiac event rate per person-years of follow-up was 0.9%. Multivariate predictors of subsequent cardiac events were angina during a treadmill exercise test, low workload (<7 metabolic equivalents [METs] for men and <5 METs for women), LV hypertrophy, and advancing age. Therefore, an interpretation of a normal exercise echocardiogram should consider the patient's symptoms and workload.

When the outcomes of 1874 patients who had good exercise capacity (≥5 METs for women and ≥7 METs for men) but an abnormal exercise echocardiogram were analyzed, the overall cardiac death or nonfatal MI rate was 2% per person-year follow-up.[87] Diabetes mellitus, history of MI, and increase or no change in LV end-systolic size in response to exercise predicted a higher rate of a cardiac event, with risk ratio of 1.9, 2.4, and 1.6, respectively. When exercise capacity is reduced at the time of exercise echocardiography, an abnormal study is also a predictor for a cardiac event, with a worse outcome for patients with a decreased LVEF and an increase or no change in LV size with exercise. Even within a group of patients with a high pretest probability of coronary artery disease, those with a normal exercise echocardiogram had a lower event rate than those with an abnormal exercise echocardiogram (2% versus 17% at 1 year and 4% versus 25% at 3 years).[90] The prognostic value of exercise echocardiography has been confirmed in other studies. Independent predictors of cardiac events are the WMSI with exercise, ST-segment depression of 1 mm or more, and treadmill time. The prognostic value of exercise echocardiography is comparable in women and men.

A common indication for dobutamine stress echocardiography is preoperative cardiac evaluation (see Chap. 85). In 530 patients undergoing nonvascular surgery at Mayo Clinic, dobutamine stress echocardiography was a reliable predictor of postoperative events such as cardiac death and nonfatal MI. An ischemic threshold of less than 60% of age-predicted maximal heart rate identified a high-risk group (8% of patients), with 43% sustaining a postoperative event compared with 0% and 9% of patients with no ischemia or an ischemic threshold of 60% or higher, respectively.

Assessment of Myocardial Viability

In general, a myocardial segment of normal or near-normal thickness (≥6 mm) is considered viable, whereas a thinned and echodense (fibrotic) segment is considered scarred. More frequently than not, however, it is difficult to differentiate viable from nonviable myocardium by assessment of LV wall thickness alone.

It has been shown in animals that adrenergic stimulation improves contractility of a chronically ischemic or postischemic myocardium with regional wall motion abnormalities, but it does not improve contractility in infarcted myocardium. Several human studies have demonstrated that a low dose of dobutamine (5 to 20 μg/kg per minute) induces contractility in viable myocardium, whether stunned or hibernating. Dobutamine-responsive wall motion improvement predicts subsequent improvement in regional LV wall thickening after coronary revascularization (see Chaps. 52 and 57).

At least in hibernating myocardium, a biphasic response best predicts recovery of myocardial function after revascularization. During infusion of a low dose of dobutamine, coronary blood flow increases and recruitment of contractile reserve improves the wall motion of the dysfunctional myocardium. As the dobutamine dose is increased, coronary blood flow does not increase further and myocardial ischemia occurs because of stenosis of the coronary artery supplying the region, resulting in worsening of wall motion compared with the previous lower dose of dobutamine. Most of the initial improvement in wall motion takes place with a low dose of dobutamine, between 10 and 20 μg/kg per minute, and worsening occurs at a higher dose, 30 to 40 μg/kg per minute, or with atropine.

Dobutamine is not as sensitive as thallium uptake or positron emission tomography (PET) for detection of myocardial viability (see Chap. 17). However, recovery of contractility of akinetic myocardium after revascularization is better predicted by contractile reserve demonstrated by dobutamine stress echocardiography than by SPECT or PET. Assessment of myocardial perfusion with the use of contrast echocardiography is another way to demonstrate potential myocardial viability. Microbubble opacification of the myocardium indicates integrity of the microvascular circulation, but the presence of microvascular integrity may not necessarily indicate the presence of sufficient myocardium to restore myocardial contractility. Therefore, it appears that myocardial contrast echocardiography, like thallium perfusion imaging, is sensitive but less specific than dobutamine echocardiography in predicting functional recovery after revascularization. Several studies, including a multicenter dobutamine viability registry, demonstrated that the outcome of patients with severe LV dysfunction and myocardial viability shown by dobutamine is better when they undergo revascularization.

Postsystolic shortening is an important feature of ischemic myocardium. When postsystolic shortening is associated with systolic hypokinesis or akinesis, it indicates actively contracting and potentially viable myocardium. Strain imaging may be useful in assessing myocardial viability by quantifying postsystolic shortening, but these methods require further clinical investigation.

Diastolic Stress Test

Another important condition that needs further evaluation is exercise-induced increase in filling pressures. The mitral annulus Ea velocity, which reflects the status of mitral relaxation, actually increases with exercise or increased preload when myocardial relaxation is normal, but Ea velocity is not augmented as much with higher transmitral pressure gradients or with exercise when relaxation is impaired. Therefore, in normal subjects, mitral inflow E velocity and mitral annulus Ea velocity increase proportionately (roughly 25%) so that the E/e′ ratio remains less than 15 (mean, 6.6) at both the resting stage and with exercise.[53] DT decreases an average of 16 milliseconds (from 192 to 176 milliseconds). However, in patients with diastolic dysfunction and exertional dyspnea, E velocity increases with exercise, but Ea velocity remains less or increases less with exercise. Therefore, the E/e′ ratio increases with exercise compared with the resting stage in patients with diastolic dysfunction.

In patients with diastolic dysfunction, the magnitude of the E/e′ ratio response to exercise varies, with three possible patterns.[54] The first pattern is an E/e′ ratio higher than 15 (increased filling pressure) at rest, and the ratio remains elevated with exercise. The second pattern represents relatively normal filling pressure and impaired myocardial relaxation pattern on mitral inflow velocity at rest, which changes to a restrictive filling pattern with an E/e′ ratio higher than 15 with exercise. The third pattern is normal filling pressure and an E/e′ ratio less than 15 at rest and with exercise. Patients with increased filling pressure with exercise, whether or not filling pressure is normal at rest (the first and second groups), have shorter exercise duration than patients (the third group) with normal filling pressure at rest and with exercise. Simultaneous cardiac catheterization and Doppler echocardiography have been performed in patients who were undergoing exercise testing in the cardiac catheterization laboratory for evaluation of exertional dyspnea. In this population of patients, the E/e′ ratio correlated well with PCWP, not only at the resting stage but also with exercise; specifically, an E/e′ ratio higher than 15 during exercise is associated with PCWP greater than 20 mm Hg.[91] Burgess and colleagues[50] have shown a similarly good correlation between the E/e′ ratio and PCWP at rest and with exercise (see Fig. 15-e5 on website). The results of diastolic stress testing have been well correlated with exercise duration.[92]

Hemodynamic Assessment

During the past 20 years, echocardiography has gradually replaced cardiac catheterization for most hemodynamic assessments in most clinical practices. Currently at our institution, for example, less than 5% of patients undergo hemodynamic cardiac catheterization before aortic valve replacement for aortic stenosis (AS). Even the most demanding hemodynamic assessment, such as evaluation of constrictive pericarditis, is performed reliably by echocardiography, and cardiac catheterization is performed in fewer than half the patients undergoing pericardiectomy. In some situations, Doppler hemodynamic assessment is more accurate than invasive hemodynamic measurement, with the best example being the transmitral pressure gradient. Therefore, it is mandatory that all physicians who care for patients with cardiac disease be familiar with how echocardiography provides cardiac hemodynamic measurements.

Transvalvular Gradients

Doppler echocardiography records blood flow velocities (in meters per second [m/sec]), and Doppler velocities are converted to pressure gradients (in millimeters of mercury [mm Hg]) according to the simplified Bernoulli equation (**Fig. 15-36**):

$$\text{Pressure gradient}(\Delta P) = 4 \times (v_2)^2 \text{ or } (2\,v_2)^2$$

When maximal Doppler velocity is converted to pressure gradient by the simplified Bernoulli equation, it represents the maximal instantaneous gradient. Mean gradient is an average of pressure gradients during the entire flow period. Maximal instantaneous or mean gradient obtained with Doppler echocardiography has been shown to correlate well with corresponding gradients simultaneously measured by cardiac catheterization (see Chap. 20). In some clinical situations, the Doppler-derived pressure gradient is more reliable than the catheter-derived gradient because the transmitral (normal, stenotic, native, or prosthetic valve) pressure gradient may be overestimated by cardiac catheterization if PCWP is used (instead of direct LA pressure) to calculate the pressure gradient.

Intracardiac Pressures

PULMONARY ARTERY PRESSURES. Flow velocities recorded with Doppler echocardiography are used to determine various intracardiac pressures. TR velocity reflects the systolic pressure difference between the right ventricle and the right atrium (see Fig. 15-36). Therefore, RV systolic pressure can be obtained by adding the estimated RA pressure to the TR velocity$^2 \times 4$. If there is no RVOT obstruction, pulmonary artery systolic pressure is equal to the calculated RV systolic pressure. Similarly, pulmonary regurgitation velocity represents the diastolic pressure difference between the pulmonary artery and the right ventricle. Hence, pulmonary artery end-diastolic pressure can be obtained by adding RV end-diastolic pressure (which is equal to RA pressure) to (pulmonary regurgitation end-diastolic velocity)$^2 \times 4$. The pulmonary artery mean pressure correlates well with the early diastolic pressure difference between the pulmonary artery and right ventricle, hence, (pulmonary regurgitation peak velocity)$^2 \times 4$.

LEFT VENTRICULAR END-DIASTOLIC PRESSURE. AR velocity reflects the diastolic pressure difference between the aorta and the left ventricle. Hence,

$$\text{LVEDP} = \text{DBP} - (\text{AR EDV})^2 \times 4$$

where DBP is the diastolic blood pressure and EDV is end-diastolic velocity. LV end-diastolic pressure and LA pressure can also be estimated by various diastolic filling variables from mitral inflow, pulmonary venous flow velocities, TDI, and color M-mode of mitral inflow[20] (see Assessment of Diastolic Function).

Stroke Volume and Cardiac Output

According to the hydraulic orifice formula, flow (rate) across a fixed orifice is equal to the product of the cross-sectional area (CSA) of the orifice and flow velocity:

$$\text{Flow rate} = \text{CSA} \times \text{flow velocity}$$

This formula is used in all hemodynamic calculations of flow, SV, and orifice area by Doppler echocardiography.

Because flow velocity varies during ejection in a pulsatile system, individual velocities of the Doppler spectrum need to be summed (i.e., integrated) to measure the total volume of flow during a given ejection period. The sum of velocities is called the time-velocity integral (TVI). It is equal to the area enclosed by the baseline and Doppler spectrum. After the TVI is determined, SV is calculated by multiplying TVI by CSA:

$$\text{SV} = \text{CSA} \times \text{TVI}$$

The location most frequently used to determine SV is the LVOT. **Figure 15-37** shows how to calculate SV from the LVOT. Flow across the other cardiac orifices can be calculated by use of the same formula. The CSA of orifices in the heart is usually assumed to be a circle, and it is determined by measuring the orifice diameter (D):

$$\text{CSA} = (D/2)^2 \times \pi = D^2 \times 0.785$$

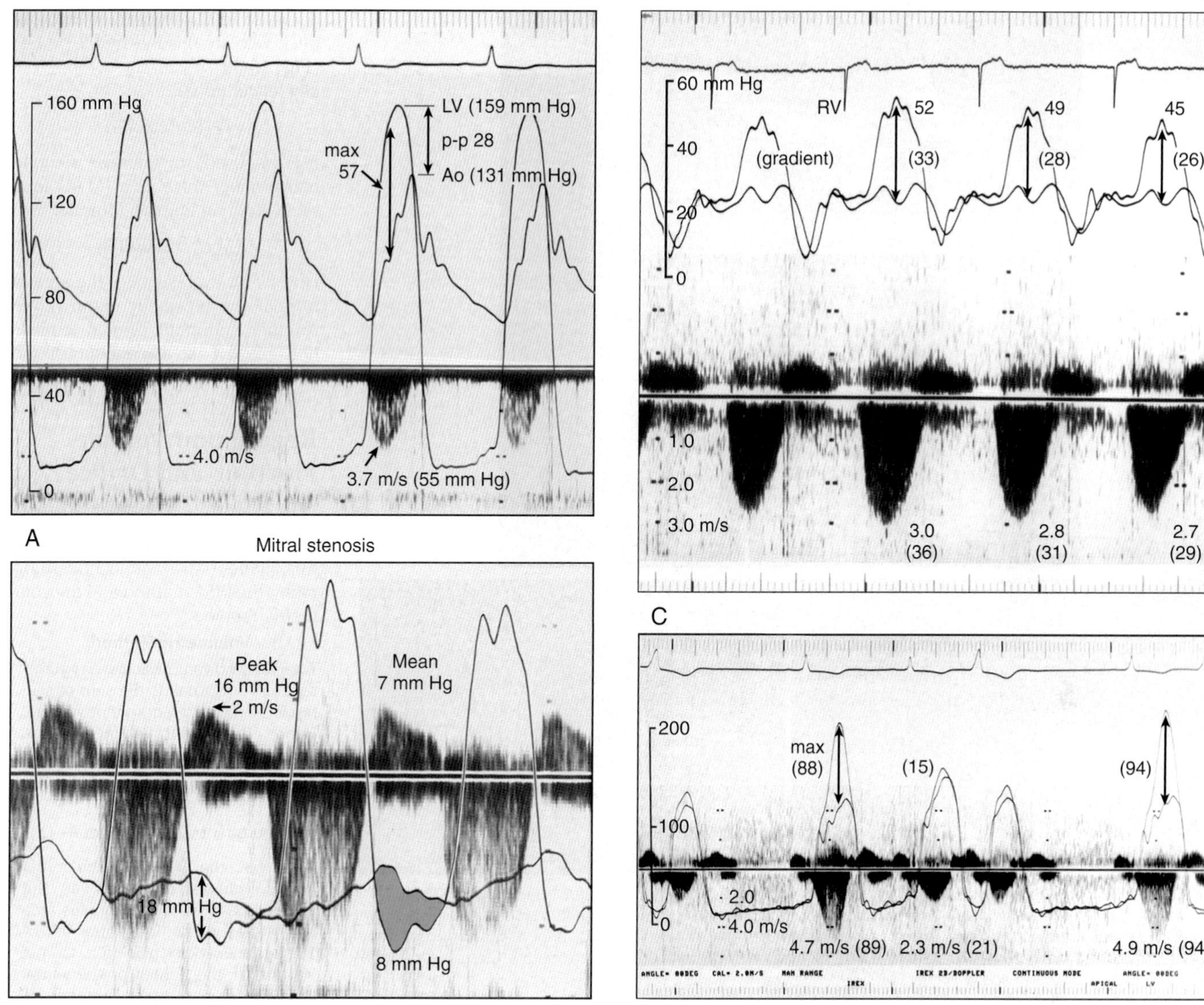

FIGURE 15-36 **A,** Simultaneous Doppler and cardiac pressure recordings show an excellent correlation between Doppler-derived and catheter-derived pressure gradients in aortic stenosis. Peak Doppler velocity (3.7 m/sec) from the third cardiac cycle is converted to a maximal instantaneous gradient (max) of 55 mm Hg, which corresponds well to the maximal gradient determined by catheter (57 mm Hg) but not to the peak-to-peak (p-p) gradient of 28 mm Hg. Ao = aorta; LV = left ventricle. **B,** Simultaneous left ventricular and left atrial pressure measurements and Doppler velocity recording of the mitral valve in mitral stenosis. Peak instantaneous and mean gradients correlate well. **C,** Simultaneous right ventricular (RV) and right atrial pressure tracings and tricuspid regurgitation velocity recording by continuous-wave Doppler echocardiography. Pressure gradients (36, 31, and 29 mm Hg) derived from the peak Doppler velocities of the second, third, and fourth beats (3.0, 2.8, and 2.7 m/sec, respectively) are close to the catheter-derived RV and right atrial gradients (arrows, 33, 28, and 26 mm Hg). **D,** Simultaneous continuous-wave Doppler and cardiac catheterization study. LV apex and outflow pressures are recorded to determine the severity of outflow obstruction. Doppler velocities are converted to pressure gradients with the simplified Bernoulli equation and correlate well with maximal (max) catheter-derived gradients. The resting gradient is 15 to 20 mm Hg, and it is markedly accentuated in the postextrasystolic contractions (second and fifth beats), with resultant gradients derived by catheter of 88 and 94 mm Hg and by Doppler of 89 and 94 mm Hg, respectively. Note that the LV pressure tracing has a late-peaking appearance corresponding to the late-peaking Doppler profile. *(**A** modified from Currie PJ, Seward JB, Reeder GS, et al: Continuous wave Doppler echocardiographic assessment of severity of calcific aortic stenosis: A simultaneous Doppler-catheter correlative study in 100 adult patients. Circulation 71:1162, 1985. Used with permission. **B-D** modified from Oh JK, Seward JB, Tajik AJ: The Echo Manual. 3rd ed. Philadelphia, Lippincott Williams & Wilkins, 2006. Used with permission of Mayo Foundation for Medical Education and Research.)*

Hence,

$$SV = D^2 \times 0.785 \times TVI$$

Cardiac output is obtained by multiplying SV by heart rate, and cardiac index is obtained by dividing cardiac output by body surface area.

Continuity Equation (see Chap. 66)

Flow rate or SV passing through a stenotic or regurgitant orifice is the same as the product of proximal (or upstream) flow rate or SV across a known area and velocity (or TVI). Because flow rate (or volume) is the product of the area and velocity (or TVI) of flow:

$$A_1 \times TVI_1 = A_2 \times TVI_2$$

where A_1 is a known area at a location proximal to the unknown area, A_2. This is the continuity equation (**Fig. 15-38**), which is used to calculate the area of a stenotic[93] or regurgitant valve. By use of the continuity equation, a stenotic or regurgitant orifice area is calculated from the following equation:

$$A_2 = A_1 \times TVI_1 / TVI_2$$

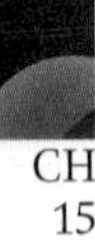

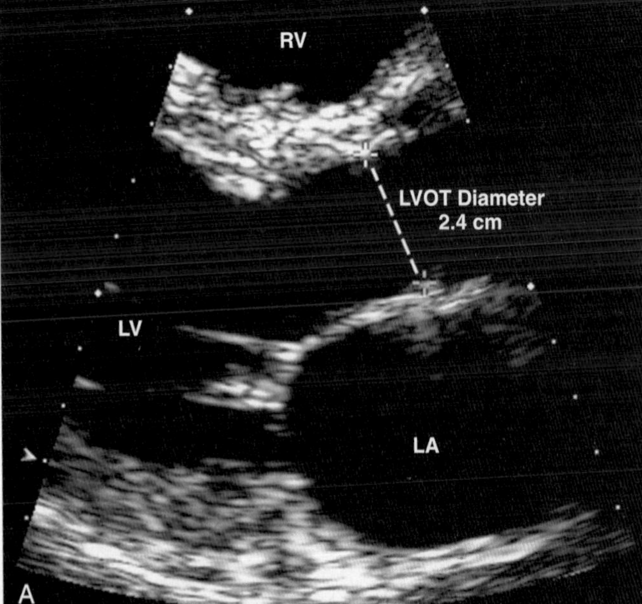

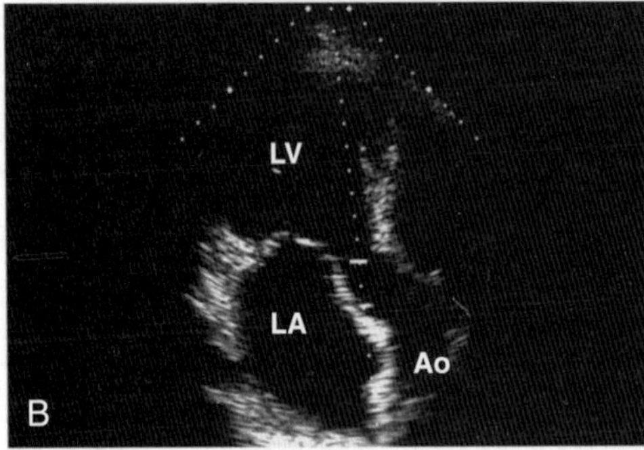

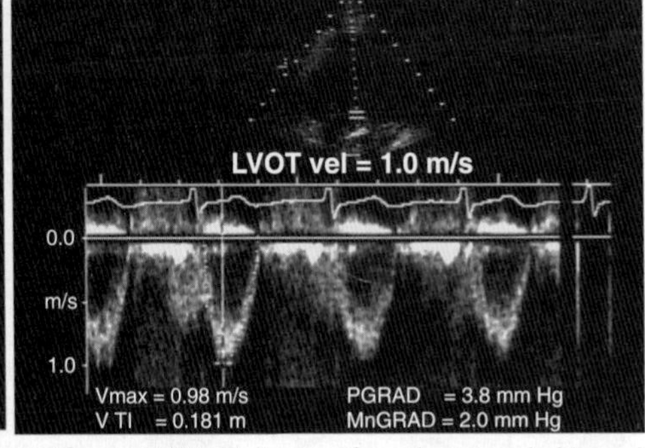

FIGURE 15-37 **A,** Step 1, Measurement of left ventricular outflow tract (LVOT) diameter from the expanded (zoom) parasternal long-axis view. The diameter is measured at the level of the aortic annulus during systole. The line is drawn from where the anterior aortic cusp meets the ventricular septum to where the posterior aortic cusp meets the anterior mitral leaflet and perpendicular to the anterior aortic wall. Distance (D) = 2.4 cm. Step 2, Calculation of LVOT area. Assuming a circular shape of LVOT,

$$\text{LVOT area } (cm^2) = \left(\frac{D}{2}\right)^2 \times \pi = D^2 \times 0.785$$

LVOT area = 4.5 cm^2 when D = 2.4 cm. LA = left atrium; LV = left ventricle; RV = right ventricle. **B, Left,** Step 3, Measurement of LVOT velocity (vel) and time-velocity integral (TVI = V TI) from the apical long-axis view. A pulsed-wave sample volume is placed at the center of the aortic annulus or 2 to 5 mm proximal to it. **Right,** TVI (cm) is the area under the velocity curve and is equal to the sum of velocities (cm/sec) during the ejection time (s). TVI was measured to be 18 cm. Step 4, Calculation of stroke volume (SV) across the LVOT.

$$\begin{aligned} \text{SV (mL)} &= \text{area}(cm^2) \times \text{TVI} \\ &= D^2 \times 0.785 \times \text{TVI} \\ &= 4.5\,cm^2 \times 18\,cm = 81\,mL \end{aligned}$$

Ao = aorta; MnGRAD = mean gradient; PGRAD = peak gradient. *(Modified from Oh JK, Seward JB, Tajik AJ: The Echo Manual. 3rd ed. Philadelphia, Lippincott Williams & Wilkins, 2006. Used with permission of Mayo Foundation for Medical Education and Research.)*

In AS, SV across the aortic valve area (A_2) is the same as SV across the LVOT (A_1). In MR, the flow rate across the regurgitant mitral valve orifice (A_2) is the same as that of a proximal isovelocity surface area known as PISA (A_1). The ratio of the areas is inversely proportional to their TVI ratio:

$$A_2/A_1 = TVI_1/TVI_2$$

Pressure Half-time

Pressure half-time (PHT) is the time for the peak pressure gradient to reach its half level and is the same as the time for peak velocity to decrease to a velocity equal to the peak velocity divided by √2 (= 1.4) (**Fig. 15-39**). It is always proportionally related to DT:

$$PHT = 0.29 \times DT$$

PHT is used to estimate stenotic native mitral valve area (MVA) indirectly from an empiric formula:

$$MVA = 220/PHT$$

However, it overestimates the area of normal and prosthetic mitral valves. Another important clinical application of PHT is assessment of the severity of AR.

Regurgitant Volume, Fraction, and Orifice Area (see Chap. 66)

Regurgitant volume can be estimated two different ways with echocardiography: the PISA method and the volumetric method.[94]

Volumetric Method

Total forward volume across a regurgitant valve (Q total) is the sum of systemic SV (Q_s) and regurgitant volume. Hence, regurgitant volume can be obtained by calculating the difference between the total forward SV and systemic SV (**Fig. 15-40**):

$$\text{Regurgitant volume} = \text{Q total} - Q_s$$

In MR, the Q total is the mitral inflow volume, calculated as the product of mitral valve annulus area and mitral inflow TVI. Mitral inflow TVI is obtained by placing a sample volume at the center of the mitral annulus during diastole. Systemic SV (Q_s) is obtained from multiplying the LVOT area by LVOT TVI. Mitral valve regurgitant volume is calculated by subtracting the LVOT SV from the mitral inflow volume. This calculation is not accurate (i.e., regurgitant volume is underestimated) if AR is pronounced. In AR, the aortic valve regurgitant volume is obtained by subtracting the mitral inflow SV (Q_s) from the LVOT forward SV (Q total).

The regurgitant fraction is the percentage of regurgitant volume compared with the total forward flow across the regurgitant valve:

$$\text{Regurgitant fraction} = (\text{regurgitant volume}/\text{Q total}) \times 100\%$$

PISA Method

The regurgitant orifice area can be estimated by the concept of PISA. As blood converges toward the regurgitant orifice, blood flow velocity increases, with the formation of multiple isovelocity shells of hemispheric shape. The flow rate at the surface of a hemispheric shell with a given flow velocity should be equal to the flow rate across the regurgitant orifice (conservation of flow or modified form of the continuity equation). By adjustment of the Nyquist limit of the color flow map, the flow velocity at a hemispheric surface proximal to the regurgitant orifice can be determined. In TTE, regurgitant flow travels away from the apical transducer position and toward the MR orifice. Hence, the blood flow converging toward the mitral regurgitant orifice in the left ventricle is color coded

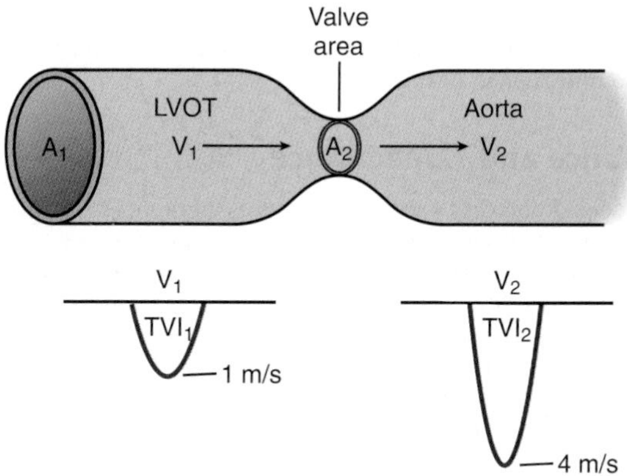

FIGURE 15-38 Diagram illustrating the continuity equation. Area$_1$ (A_1) is the known cross-sectional area. Area$_2$ (A_2) is the unknown cross-sectional area to be calculated:

$$SV_2 = SV_1$$

$$A_2 \times TVI_2 = A_1 \times TVI_1$$

LVOT = left ventricular outflow tract; SV = stroke volume; TVI = time-velocity integral. *(Modified from Oh JK, Seward JB, Tajik AJ: The Echo Manual. 3rd ed. Philadelphia, Lippincott Williams & Wilkins, 2006. Used with permission of Mayo Foundation for Medical Education and Research.)*

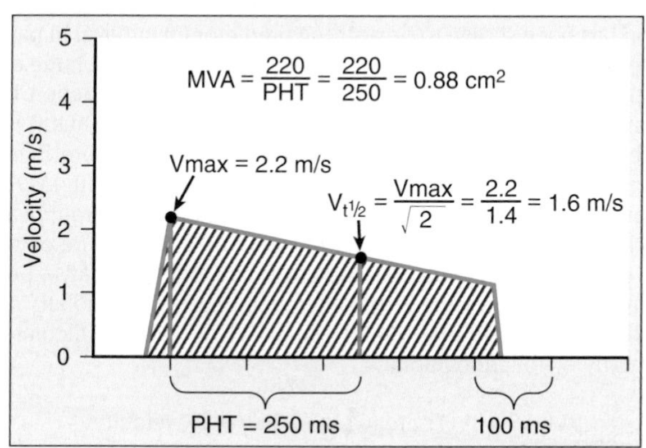

FIGURE 15-39 Diagram illustrating the calculation of pressure half-time (PHT). PHT is the time interval required for maximal pressure gradient (Pmax) to reach its half level $P_{1/2}$). Hence,

$$P_{t1/2} = 1/2\,Pmax$$

$$4 \times (V_{t1/2})^2 = 1/2(4 \times Vmax^2)$$

In this example, Vmax = 2.2 m/sec; hence, = 2.2/1.4 = 1.6 m/sec. The time interval from Vmax (2.2 m/sec) to $V_{t1/2}$ (1.6 m/sec) is PHT (= 250 milliseconds). In patients with native mitral valvular stenosis, mitral valve area (MVA) is estimated by dividing the constant, 220, by PHT. Vmax = maximal velocity; $V_{t1/2}$ = velocity at PHT. *(Modified from Oh JK, Seward JB, Tajik AJ: The Echo Manual. 3rd ed. Philadelphia, Lippincott Williams & Wilkins, 2006. Used with permission of Mayo Foundation for Medical Education and Research.)*

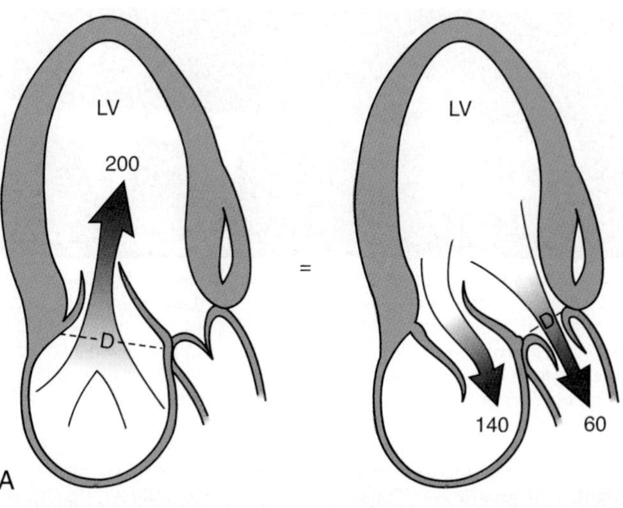

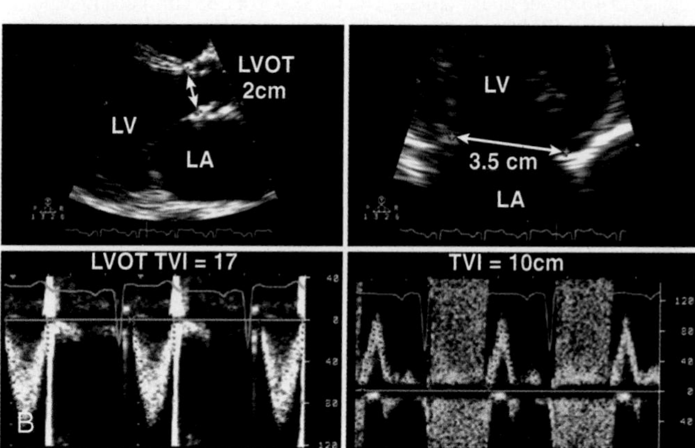

FIGURE 15-40 **A,** Estimation of regurgitant volume and regurgitant fraction using mitral regurgitation as an example. Assume that regurgitation is present only in the mitral valve. Therefore, diastolic forward flow across the mitral valve (200 mL, left) is the sum of systolic flow across the LVOT (60 mL) and mitral regurgitant volume (140 mL); what goes into the left ventricle (LV) during diastole (mitral inflow) must come out of the LV during systole (LVOT flow + mitral regurgitant flow). The diagram shows a flail posterior mitral leaflet. Mitral inflow volume is the product of mitral annulus area and mitral flow TVI (flow = area × TVI). For this volumetric calculation, the sample volume is placed at the level of the mitral annulus:

$$\text{Mitral regurgitant volume} = \text{mitral inflow} - \text{LVOT flow}$$
$$= (D^2 \times 0.785 \times TVI)\,MV - (D^2 \times 0.785 \times TVI)\,LVOT$$

D = diameter. **B,** A representative case for calculation of mitral regurgitation volume by the volumetric method. LVOT stroke volume is $(2)^2 \times 0.785 \times 17$ = 53 mL, and mitral inflow volume is $(3.5)^2 \times 0.785 \times 10$ = 96 mL. The difference, 96 mL − 53 mL = 43 mL, is the mitral regurgitation volume. LA = left atrium. *(**A** modified from Oh JK, Seward JB, Tajik AJ: The Echo Manual. 3rd ed. Philadelphia, Lippincott Williams & Wilkins, 2006. Used with permission of Mayo Foundation for Medical Education and Research.)*

blue until the velocity reaches the negative aliasing velocity of the selected color flow map, at which time the flow is color coded light orange-red. If the negative aliasing velocity is decreased, the transition from blue to red-orange occurs farther from the regurgitant orifice, providing a larger hemispheric shell radius (r) (**Fig. 15-41**). An opposite color scheme occurs if TEE is used for quantification of MR by the PISA method. After a hemisphere of blood flow with known velocity (equal to negative aliasing velocity if TTE is used or positive aliasing velocity if TEE is used) is identified, the rate of flow through a hemispheric shell is equal to the area of the hemisphere multiplied by the flow velocity (which is the aliasing velocity). The area of hemisphere is calculated as $2\pi r^2$. Hence,

$$\text{Flow rate} = 6.28\,r^2 \times \text{aliasing velocity}$$

This flow rate across PISA is equal to the flow rate across the effective regurgitant orifice (ERO):

$$\text{Flow rate} = \text{ERO} \times \text{regurgitant velocity}$$

Therefore, ERO can be obtained by dividing the flow rate by peak MR velocity across the regurgitant orifice:

$$\text{ERO} = \text{Flow rate/peak MR velocity}$$

Regurgitant volume is equal to regurgitant orifice area multiplied by the MR TVI:

$$\text{Regurgitant volume} = \text{ERO} \times \text{MR TVI}$$
$$= [6.28\,r^2 \times \text{aliasing velocity/MR velocity}] \times \text{MR TVI}$$

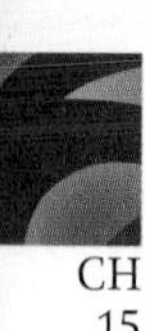

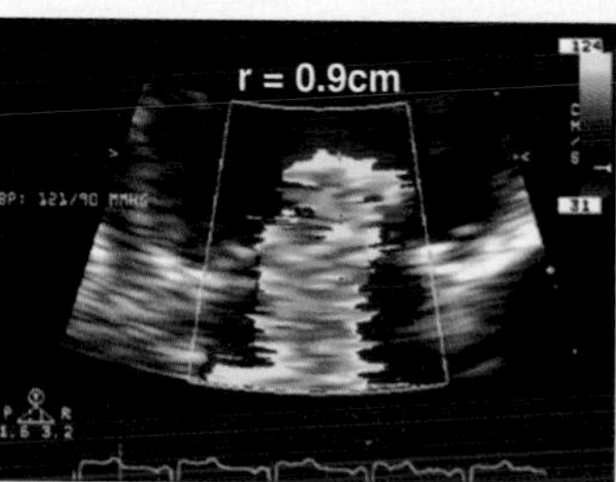

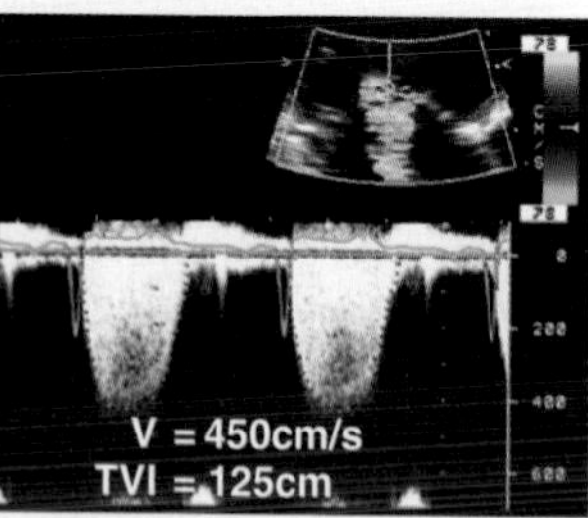

FIGURE 15-41 Calculation of mitral regurgitation orifice and volume by the proximal isovelocity surface area (PISA) method. **Left,** Mitral valve area is zoomed and color flow map baseline is shifted downward to make negative aliasing velocity of 31 cm/sec. This is the velocity of the PISA where the color changes from blue to yellow proximal to the mitral regurgitation orifice. The radius of PISA is measured from the regurgitation orifice to the surface of PISA, which is 0.9 cm. From these values, flow rate at PISA is calculated as follows: 6.28 × $(0.9)^2$ × 31 = 158 cm/sec. To obtain effective regurgitant orifice (ERO), the flow rate is divided by the peak mitral regurgitation velocity shown on the right. **Right,** Continuous-wave Doppler signal of mitral regurgitation shows the peak velocity of 4.5 m/sec or 450 cm/sec. ERO = 158/450 = 0.35 cm^2. Because volume is the product of ERO and time-velocity integral (TVI) of mitral regurgitation, mitral regurgitant volume = 0.35 × 125 = 44 mL. These values are consistent with moderate degree of mitral regurgitation.

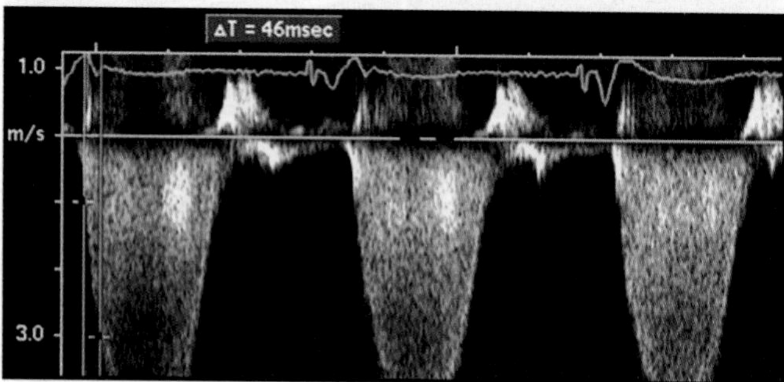

FIGURE 15-42 Continuous-wave Doppler recording of mitral regurgitation. Time interval (ΔT) from 1 m/sec to 3 m/sec of the velocity is 46 milliseconds. Therefore, dP/dt = 32/0.046 = 696 mm Hg/sec.

The PISA method has several limitations, and its accuracy is based on reliable measurement of the PISA radius, which should be at midsystole. It is more accurate for a central MR jet. It is also important to have a correct aliasing velocity to produce a hemispheric PISA.

The concept of PISA can be applied for calculation of the area of a stenotic orifice (see Fig. 15-e12 on website). This method has been validated for MVA in patients with mitral stenosis (MS); however, it should be considered that PISA proximal to a stenotic mitral orifice may not be a complete hemisphere but rather a portion of a hemisphere because of the geometry of mitral leaflets on the atrial side. Therefore, an angle correction factor may be necessary (but not in all cases):

$$\text{MVA} = [6.28\,r^2 \times \text{aliasing velocity}/\text{peak MS velocity}] \times \alpha/180\ \text{degrees}$$

where α is the angle between two mitral leaflets on the atrial side.

Rate of Left Ventricular Pressure Change During Isovolumic Contraction

The dP/dt is another index of LV contractility. During isovolumic contraction, there is no notable change in LA pressure. Therefore, MR velocity changes during this period reflect dP/dt. Usually, the interval between 1 m/sec and 3 m/sec on the MR velocity spectrum is measured (**Fig. 15-42**). For the Bernoulli equation, the pressure change from 1 m/sec to 3 m/sec is 32 mm Hg:

$$(4\times 3^2 - 4\times 1^2)$$

The dP/dt (in mm Hg/sec) is calculated from the following formula:

$$\text{dP/dt} = 32\ \text{mm Hg/sec}$$

Several studies have demonstrated a good correlation between the noninvasive Doppler-derived and catheter-derived dP/dt. Normal dP/dt is 1200 mm Hg/sec or higher.

Resistance and Capacitance

Resistance is defined as a ratio of pressure (gradient) to flow. Because Doppler echocardiography is able to determine pressure (gradient) and flow, various resistances can be calculated noninvasively with two-dimensional and Doppler echocardiographic measurements. Systemic vascular resistance (SVR) by echocardiography is determined as MR velocity/LVOT TVI. It correlates well with catheter-derived SVR (where SVR = [mean aortic pressure – RA pressure]/cardiac output). An MR velocity/LVOT TVI ratio higher than 0.27 has been shown to have a 70% sensitivity and a 77% specificity for identification of SVR greater than 14 Wood units.[95]

Pulmonary vascular resistance (PVR) is an important parameter to guide the management of patients with cardiopulmonary diseases (see Chap. 78). Because TR velocity provides pulmonary systolic pressure and TVI of the RVOT provides pulmonary flow, the TR velocity/RVOT TVI ratio has been correlated with invasively determined PVR. The following regression formula was found to be reliable in estimating PVR by TR velocity/RVOT TVI:

$$\text{PVR} = (\text{TR velocity}/\text{RVOT TVI})\times 10 + 0.16$$

Pulmonary vascular capacitance (PVCAP) is a measure of the workload on the right ventricle, and PVCAP derived by right-heart catheterization has been shown to be a strong predictor for survival in patients with pulmonary hypertension. PVCAP measures how much the aggregate pulmonary artery tree will dilate with each RV contraction. It can be calculated from measures of pulse pressure and SV. Thus, it is calculated by dividing SV by pulmonary artery pulse pressure. Echocardiography can determine SV by multiplying LVOT area with LVOT TVI. The pulmonary artery systolic pressure can be obtained from peak TR velocity, and the pulmonary artery diastolic pressure can be obtained from pulmonary regurgitation end-diastolic velocity. Because pulmonary artery pulse pressure is the difference between pulmonary artery systolic pressure and diastolic pressure, PVCAP can be calculated as follows by echocardiography[95]:

$$\text{PVCAP} = \text{LVOT area} \times \text{LVOT TVI}/4(\text{TR velocity}^2 - \text{pulmonary regurgitation velocity}^2)$$

Valvular Heart Disease (see Chap. 66)

Echocardiography provides a comprehensive and reliable hemodynamic assessment of patients with valvular heart disease, including determination of pressure gradients, stenotic and regurgitant valve orifice area, regurgitant volume, and pulmonary artery pressures. TEE complements TTE by allowing improved delineation of valvular morphology, and three-dimensional echocardiography provides better delineation of valvular structures. On the basis of a comprehensive echocardiography examination, which outlines structure, function, and hemodynamic information, physicians can decide optimal treatment strategy, including the timing of surgical intervention for patients with valvular heart disease.

Aortic Stenosis

The aortic valve is reliably visualized with two-dimensional echocardiography, which differentiates noncalcific (doming of aortic cusps in bicuspid aortic valve) from calcific AS. The two-dimensional TTE parasternal short-axis view at the level of the aortic valve is used to visualize the number of aortic cusps. Additional delineation of cusp anatomy can be obtained by TEE and three-dimensional echocardiography (**Fig. 15-43**). Important ancillary information in patients with AS readily obtained with echocardiography includes the degree of valvular calcification, aortic annulus and supravalvular ascending aorta size, degree of LV hypertrophy, and the presence and degree of subvalvular obstruction and aortic valve regurgitation.

The echocardiographic assessment of AS severity relies on acquiring the following hemodynamic Doppler parameters: peak aortic valve velocity (v), mean pressure gradient (**Fig. 15-44**), aortic valve area (AVA), and ratio of the LVOT to the aortic valve velocity or TVI. As the severity of AS increases, the valve area becomes smaller and flow velocity and pressure gradients increase. The modified Bernoulli equation is used to reliably measure the pressure gradient across the aortic valve:

$$\text{Pressure gradient} = 4 \times v^2 \text{ or } (2 \times v)^2$$

There may be a small difference between aortic valve pressure gradients obtained by Doppler and catheter methods because of the pressure recovery phenomenon. The pressure gradient depends on SV; thus, the AVA is a better measure to determine the severity of AS, especially when SV and cardiac output are decreased. AVA is calculated from the continuity equation (see Hemodynamic Assessment; see also Fig. 15-e13 on website):

$$\text{AVA} = (\text{LVOT area} \times \text{LVOT TVI})/\text{AV TVI}$$

LVOT area, LVOT TVI, and aortic valve TVI (AV TVI) are reliably measured with two-dimensional and Doppler echocardiography. All available transducer positions should be used to record the highest velocity from the aortic valve. When there is marked calcification of the aortic valve and annulus, it may be difficult to measure LVOT diameter and area. The continuity equation can be rearranged as follows:

$$\text{AVA}/\text{LVOT area} = \text{LVOT TVI}/\text{AV TVI}$$

The LVOT TVI and AV TVI ratio is inversely proportional to AVA and LVOT area ratio. Hence, LVOT TVI/AV TVI of 0.25 indicates that AVA is 25% of the LVOT area. Because the LVOT area is usually 3 to 3.5 cm^2, a ratio of less than 0.25 indicates AVA of 0.8 cm^2 or less, consistent with severe AS.

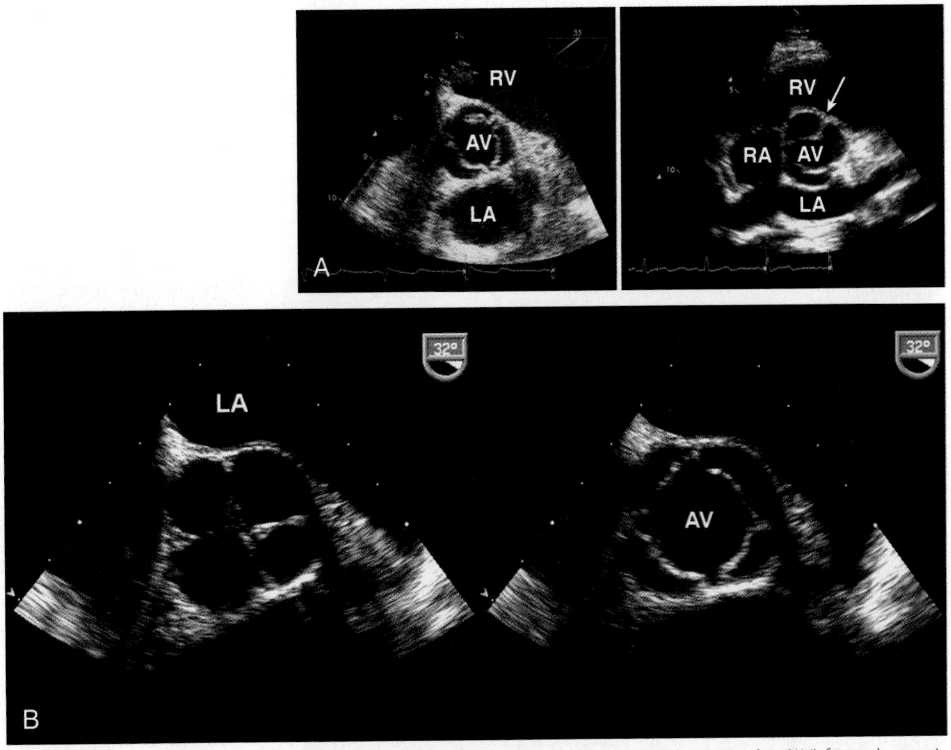

FIGURE 15-43 A, Left, Transesophageal echocardiographic image of tricuspid aortic valve (AV) from short-axis view. **Right,** Transthoracic image of a typical bicuspid aortic valve with fusion of the right and left cusps forming a raphe (arrow) and commissures at the 4- and 9-o'clock positions. LA = left atrium; RA = right atrium; RV = right ventricle. **B,** Transesophageal images of quadricuspid aortic valve in diastole **(left)** and systole **(right)**.

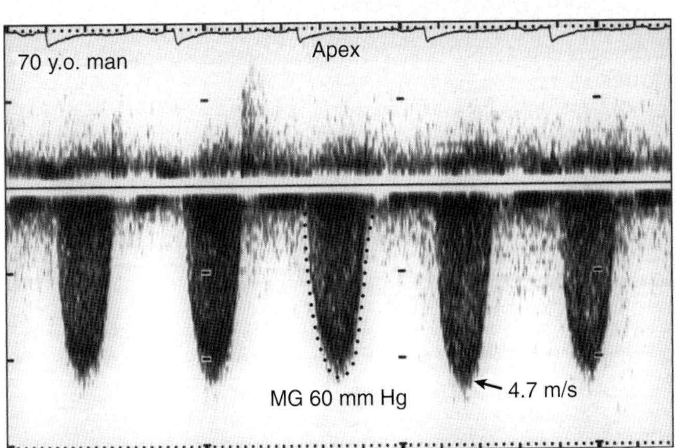

FIGURE 15-44 Continuous-wave Doppler spectra from 70-year-old man with severe aortic stenosis. The velocity was obtained from the apical window. The peak velocity is 4.7 m/sec, and the mean pressure gradient (MG) is 60 mm Hg. *(Modified from Oh JK, Seward JB, Tajik AJ: The Echo Manual. 3rd ed. Philadelphia, Lippincott Williams & Wilkins, 2006. Used with permission of Mayo Foundation for Medical Education and Research.)*

SEVERE AORTIC STENOSIS BY ECHOCARDIOGRAPHY. AS is usually severe when patients with normal LV systolic function and cardiac output demonstrate the following echocardiographic Doppler hemodynamics:

- peak aortic valve velocity of 4.5 m/sec or more;
- mean pressure gradient of 50 mm Hg or more;
- LVOT/AV TVI of 0.25 or less; or
- AVA of 0.75 cm^2 or less.

American College of Cardiology/American Heart Association (ACC/AHA) Guidelines recommendations (see Chap. 66) selected a lower degree of stenosis with which to consider aortic valve replacement in patients with symptoms, LV dysfunction, or need for coronary artery bypass graft surgery.[96] These criteria include a peak velocity of greater than 4.0 m/sec, a mean pressure gradient greater than 40 mm Hg, and an AVA less than 1.0 cm^2. The peak velocity threshold of 4 m/sec was selected because of natural history data[97] indicating a high likelihood of symptoms or other indications for surgery at this degree of stenosis (see Chap. 66).

The Doppler-derived aortic pressure gradient is generally higher and the Doppler-derived AVA is smaller than the catheter-derived aortic pressure gradient and AVA. Thus, the ACC/AHA recommendation[96] that an AVA of 1 cm^2 or less is severe AS overestimates the severity of AS when the AVA is calculated with two-dimensional Doppler echocardiography.

Determination of aortic valve hemodynamics depends on LV systolic function and cardiac output. The peak aortic velocity and mean aortic pressure gradient may be less than 4.5 m/sec and less than 50 mm Hg, respectively, in patients with severe AS when LV function and SV decrease. Conversely, AS may not be severe even when the peak velocity is 4.5 m/sec or higher and the mean gradient is 50 mm Hg or higher when cardiac output is increased, as in AR or anemia. In these situations, the LVOT/AV TVI (or velocity) ratio and AVA are more helpful in determining the severity of AS because of proportional change in velocities.

SEVERE AORTIC STENOSIS WITH LOW AORTIC PRESSURE GRADIENT. In patients with LV systolic dysfunction and reduced cardiac output, a small calculated AVA may represent true anatomically severe AS or a moderately stenotic aortic valve that may not open fully because of low SV. AS is likely to be severe if the AVA by the continuity equation is 0.75 cm^2 or less and the LVOT/AV TVI (or velocity) ratio is 0.25 or less. A dobutamine infusion is often used to increase SV and may be helpful in differentiating morphologically severe AS from pseudosevere AS. In true anatomically severe AS, the AVA remains less than 1 cm^2 and the mean gradient increases proportional to an increase in SV with dobutamine infusion (**Fig. 15-45**). Dobutamine infusion in patients with low-gradient AS also assesses contractile reserve, defined as an increase in SV of greater than 20% with dobutamine.[98,99]

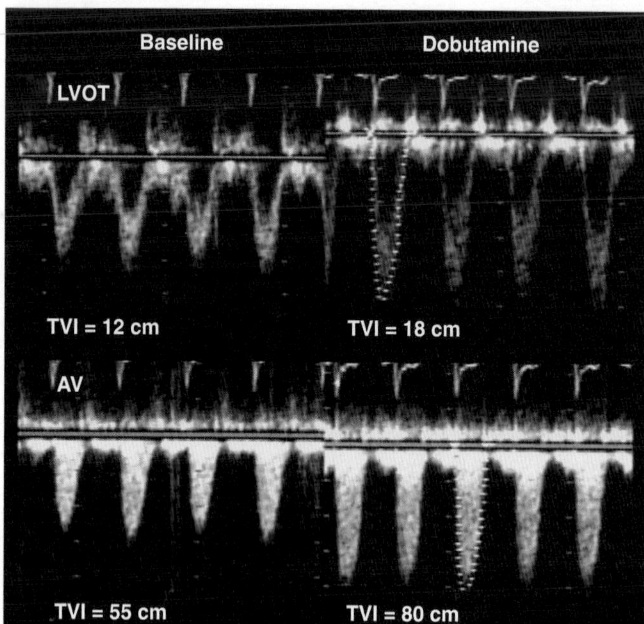

FIGURE 15-45 Example of dobutamine Doppler hemodynamic measurement in a patient with severe aortic stenosis and a low gradient. At baseline, LVOT TVI was low (12 cm), indicating a low stroke volume, and aortic valve (AV) peak velocity was 3 m/sec, with TVI of 55 cm. TVI ratio between LVOT and AV was 0.22. With infusion of dobutamine (up to 20 μg/kg/min), LVOT TVI increased to 18 cm, which is a 50% increase in stroke volume, and AV TVI increased a similar degree to 80 cm. TVI ratio was 0.23, similar to the baseline ratio. This result indicates that the aortic valve is truly stenotic, with a low gradient. The patient successfully underwent aortic valve replacement. LVOT = left ventricular outflow tract; TVI = time-velocity integral. *(Modified from Oh JK, Seward JB, Tajik AJ: The Echo Manual. 3rd ed. Philadelphia, Lippincott Williams & Wilkins, 2006. Used with permission of Mayo Foundation for Medical Education and Research.)*

Mitral Stenosis

The typical M-mode and two-dimensional echocardiographic features of rheumatic MS are shown in **Figure 15-46** (see also Fig. 66-19). The parasternal short-axis view is used to measure MVA by planimetry. Three-dimensional echocardiography may provide a better determination of the stenotic MVA (see Fig. 15-4C) in patients with calcified valves or prior commissurotomy.

Mitral balloon valvuloplasty is a successful form of intervention for many patients with MS (see Chap. 66). An echocardiographic score based on valve thickness, calcification, mobility, and subvalvular thickening can be used to predict the outcome of the procedure (**Table 15-11**). Patients with an echocardiographic score of 8 or less generally have a more favorable result from mitral balloon valvuloplasty than do those with a score higher than 8. Commissural calcification or fusion is an additional important determinant of outcome after percutaneous valvuloplasty or valvotomy.

Calculation of the MVA is the most reliable means of determining the severity of MS. Several methods in addition to planimetry of the mitral valve are available. The comprehensive echocardiographic Doppler evaluation of MS should include determination of

1. peak mitral diastolic velocity by continuous-wave Doppler echocardiography;
2. mean pressure gradient and TVI by tracing mitral velocity (**Fig. 15-47**);
3. MVA by the PHT method: MVA = 220/PHT;
4. MVA by the continuity equation and by the PISA method (see Fig. 15-e12 on website); and
5. direct measurement of MVA by two-dimensional or three-dimensional echocardiography (if the image quality is good).

The PHT method is easiest to use but is less reliable immediately after balloon valvuloplasty or in patients with severe AR or high filling pressure. This method underestimates the severity of MS in these situations because PHT becomes shortened. The continuity equation cannot be used if there is severe AR or MR. The PISA method is not affected by other valvular lesions. Thus, severe MS by echocardiography is defined as follows:

- Resting mean pressure gradient is 10 mm Hg or higher.
- MVA is 1 cm^2 or less.
- PHT is 220 milliseconds or longer.

It may be helpful to perform a Doppler hemodynamic assessment during bicycle exercise, after treadmill exercise, or during dobutamine infusion for symptomatic patients who do not clearly show severe MS. A marked increase in the transmitral gradient, LA pressure, and pulmonary artery pressure occurs with the exercise-related increase in cardiac output and heart rate. A mean gradient greater than 15 mm Hg

TABLE 15-11 Echocardiographic Score Used to Predict Outcome of Mitral Balloon Valvuloplasty*

GRADE	MOBILITY	SUBVALVULAR THICKENING	THICKENING	CALCIFICATION
1	Highly mobile valve with only leaflet tips restricted	Minimal thickening just below the mitral leaflets	Leaflets nearly normal in thickness (4-5 mm)	A single area of increased echo brightness
2	Leaflet mid and base portions have normal mobility	Thickening of chordal structures extending up to one third of the chordal length	Mid leaflets normal, considerable thickening of margins (5-8 mm)	Scattered areas of brightness confined to leaflet margins
3	Valve continues to move forward in diastole, mainly from the base	Thickening extending to the distal third of the chords	Thickening extending through the entire leaflet (5-8 mm)	Brightness extending into the midportion of the leaflets
4	No or minimal forward movement of the leaflets in diastole	Extensive thickening and shortening of all chordal structures extending down to the papillary muscles	Considerable thickening of all leaflet tissue (>8-10 mm)	Extensive brightness throughout much of the leaflet tissue

*The total echocardiographic score was derived from an analysis of mitral leaflet mobility, valvular and subvalvular thickening, and calcification, which were graded from 0 (normal) to 4 according to the above criteria. This gave a total score of 0 to 16.

Modified from Oh JK, Seward JB, Tajik AJ: The Echo Manual. 3rd ed. Philadelphia, Lippincott Williams & Wilkins, 2006. Used with permission of Mayo Foundation for Medical Education and Research.

with exercise is considered severe MS. A dobutamine-induced mean mitral pressure gradient of 18 mm Hg or higher predicted clinical events with 90% accuracy.[91]

TEE is used for patients with MS primarily to exclude LA or LA appendage thrombus after an embolic event or before mitral balloon valvuloplasty. On occasion, TEE or three-dimensional TEE or intracardiac echocardiography is performed during mitral balloon valvuloplasty to guide transseptal puncture or the position of the balloon.

Tricuspid Stenosis

Tricuspid valve morphology is assessed with two-dimensional echocardiography. The severity of tricuspid stenosis is determined by Doppler echocardiography, similar to the method described for MS. Tricuspid stenosis is considered severe when the mean gradient is 7 mm Hg or higher and the PHT is 190 milliseconds or higher (constant of 190 milliseconds was proposed for the PHT method).

Aortic Regurgitation

Structural abnormalities causing AR are usually detected on two-dimensional echocardiography. In patients with chronic severe aortic valve regurgitation, the left ventricle is dilated and pulsation of the aorta is evident.

Methods of assessing AR using echocardiographic Doppler include the following:

1. The aortic regurgitant jet area is assessed from the parasternal short-axis view relative to the short-axis area of the LVOT at the level of the aortic annulus (**Fig. 15-48**). The width of the regurgitant jet at its origin relative to the dimension of the LVOT is also a good predictor of the severity of AR (see Fig. 15-48; see also Fig. 66-11).
2. PHT measures the continuous-wave Doppler signal, which corresponds to the pressure difference between the aorta and the left ventricle (**Fig. 15-49A**). The PHT of AR becomes markedly shorter with severe AR because of a rapid increase in LV diastolic pressure and decrease in aortic pressure. However, this velocity may also be shortened by increased LV diastolic pressure from other causes.
3. Holodiastolic retrograde flow can be demonstrated in the descending thoracic aorta (Fig. 15-49B) and in the abdominal aorta in severe aortic valve regurgitation.
4. In case of acute severe AR, LV diastolic pressure increases rapidly, resulting in a restrictive diastolic filling pattern in mitral inflow.
5. Regurgitant volume and orifice area can be quantified with the volumetric or PISA method.
6. The vena contracta is the smallest neck of the color flow region at the level of the aortic valve, immediately below the flow convergence region (see Fig. 15-48). The vena contracta is usually measured from the parasternal long-axis view, and a vena contracta larger than 6 mm is specific for severe AR.

Thus, severe AR is evident by echocardiography on the basis of the following criteria:

- Regurgitant jet width/LVOT diameter ratio of 60% or higher
- Vena contracta larger than 6 mm

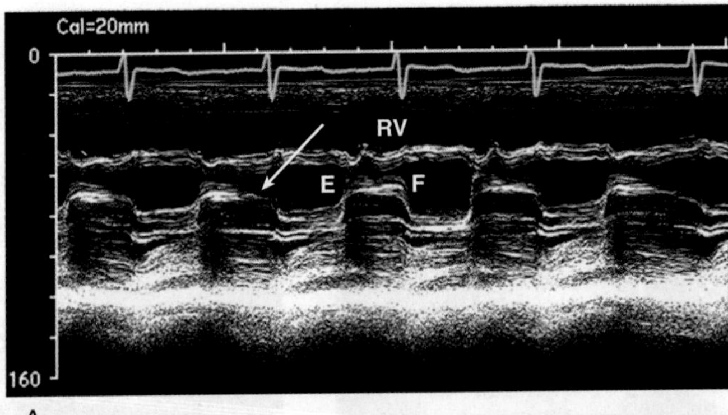

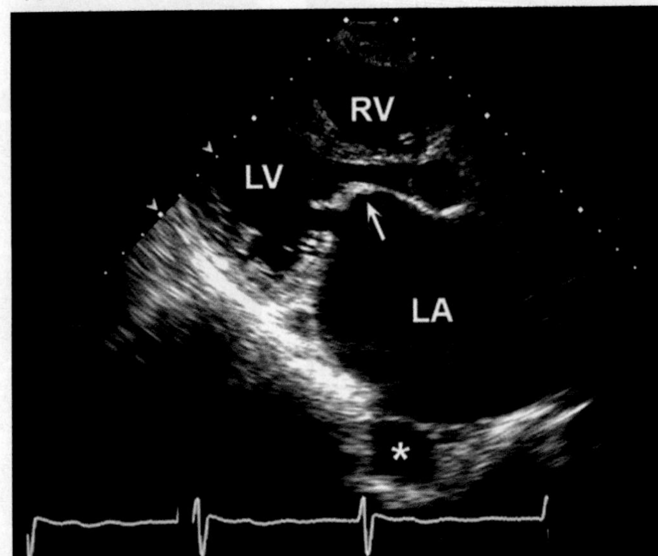

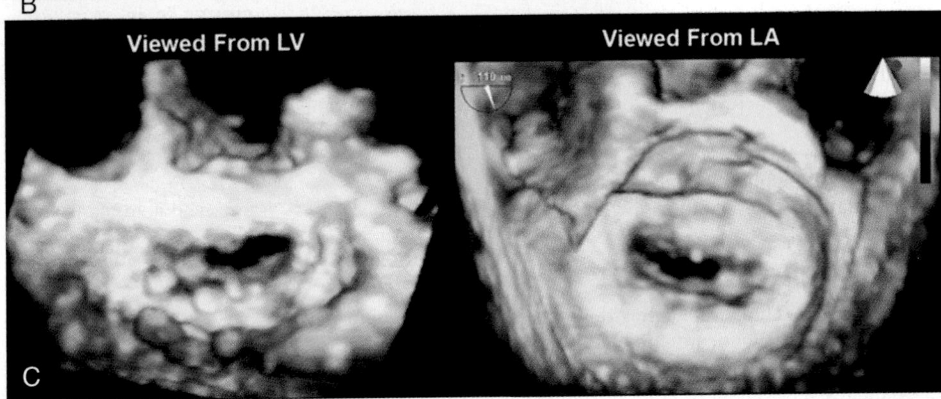

FIGURE 15-46 **A,** M-mode echocardiogram of a patient with mitral stenosis. Note the abnormal motion of the anterior mitral valve leaflet as demonstrated by the E-F slope (arrow). **B,** Two-dimensional echocardiogram of parasternal long-axis view during diastole of a patient with mitral stenosis. The mitral valve leaflets are thickened and have the typical hockey-stick appearance (arrow). Left atrium (LA) is enlarged. Asterisk indicates descending thoracic aorta; LV = left ventricle; RV = right ventricle. **C,** Three-dimensional transesophageal echocardiogram of a patient with mitral stenosis viewed from the left ventricle **(left)** and left atrium **(right)**.

CH 15

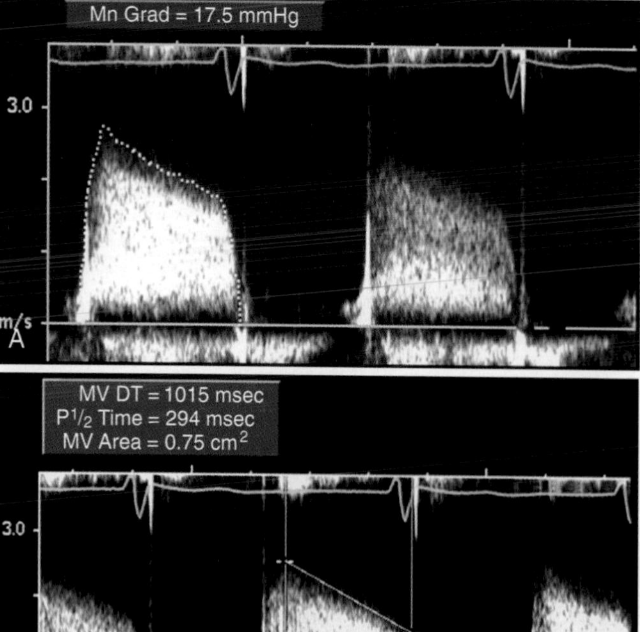

FIGURE 15-47 **A,** Continuous-wave Doppler velocity measurement from the apex in a patient with mitral stenosis. The mean gradient (Mn Grad) is 17.5 mm Hg. **B,** Pressure half-time ($P_{½}$) is drawn from peak velocity and is 294 milliseconds. Mitral valve (MV) area is calculated as 220/294 = 0.75 cm^2. DT indicates deceleration time.

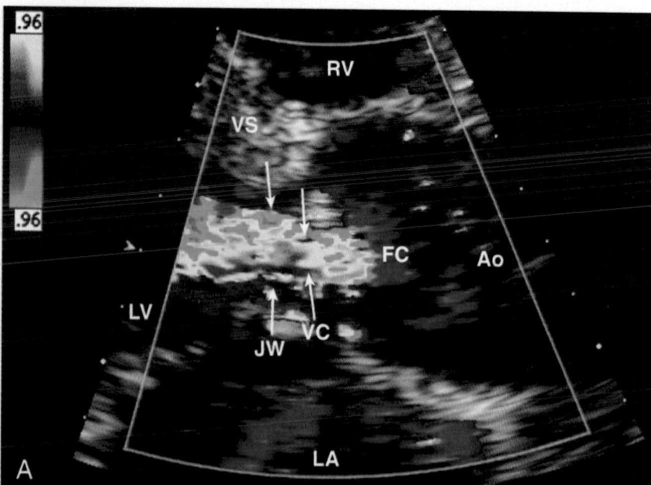

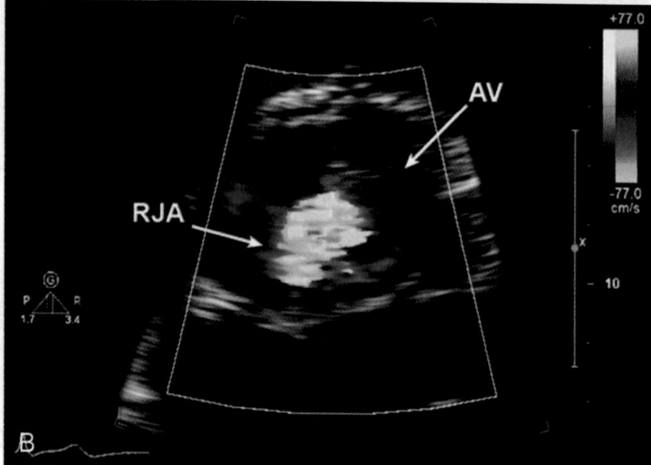

FIGURE 15-48 **A,** Color flow imaging to estimate severity of aortic regurgitation. Parasternal long-axis view showing aortic regurgitation by color flow imaging. LV outflow height and jet width (JW) are determined from the parasternal long-axis view. Vena contracta (VC) is the smallest region below the aortic valve and flow convergence (FC). The jet spreads out into the LV outflow tract. Aortic JW is about two thirds of the LV outflow tract diameter, consistent with severe aortic regurgitation. Ao = aorta; LA = left atrium; LV = left ventricle; RV = right ventricle; VS = ventricular septum. **B,** Regurgitant jet area (RJA) is measured from the parasternal short-axis view at the aortic valve (AV) level. *(**A** modified from Oh JK, Seward JB, Tajik AJ: The Echo Manual. 3rd ed. Philadelphia, Lippincott Williams & Wilkins, 2006. Used with permission of Mayo Foundation for Medical Education and Research.)*

- Regurgitant jet area/LVOT area ratio of 60% or higher
- Aortic regurgitation PHT of 250 milliseconds or less
- Restrictive mitral flow pattern (usually in acute setting)
- Holodiastolic flow reversal in the descending thoracic or abdominal aorta
- ERO of 0.30 cm^2 or larger
- Regurgitant volume of 60 mL or more
- Regurgitant fraction of 50% or higher

Mitral Regurgitation

Comprehensive echocardiography identifies the underlying cause of MR (see Chap. 66). Echocardiographic Doppler methods of assessing MR include the following.

1. Qualitative assessment by color flow imaging. The area of the regurgitant jet relative to the size of the left atrium has been shown to correlate well with regurgitant severity determined with angiography when the jet is not eccentric (see Fig. 15-e14 on website; see also Fig. 66-31). However, color flow imaging of valvular regurgitation depends on technical machine settings, loading conditions, and jet geometry. A flow jet directed against the atrial wall appears smaller than a free jet of the same regurgitant volume (Coanda effect).
2. Anterograde flow (mitral inflow) velocity increases with severe regurgitation.
3. The continuous-wave Doppler spectrum may have a characteristic configuration (due to the V wave) with increased intensity and reduced systolic velocity as the increase in LA pressure reduces the transmitral systolic gradient (see Fig. 15-e15 on website).
4. In severe MR, there may be systolic flow reversal in the pulmonary vein (see Fig. 15-e16 on website).
5. The vena contracta is the narrowest portion of the MR jet downstream from the orifice (**Fig. 15-50**). It represents the physiologic or effective orifice area of the regurgitant jet as opposed to the actual anatomic orifice area, can be measured by two-dimensional or three-dimensional echocardiography, and correlates well with other quantitative measures of MR severity.[100]
6. Regurgitant volume, fraction, and orifice area can be calculated with the volumetric or PISA method to assess the severity of MR (**Fig. 15-51**; see also Fig. 66-31). The determination of regurgitation severity should incorporate LV volume, which should increase with severe degrees of chronic AR or MR. A normal LV volume is not consistent with severe chronic AR or MR.

Severe MR is evident by echocardiography on the basis of the following criteria:

- Two-dimensional echocardiographic evidence of disruption of the mitral valve apparatus (papillary muscle rupture, flail mitral leaflet) or incomplete coaptation
- ERO of 0.40 cm^2 or larger
- MR volume of 60 mL or more
- Regurgitation fraction of 50% or more
- Vena contracta width 7 mm or more

- MR color flow jet reaching the posterior wall of the left atrium (with a high aliasing velocity of the color map)
- Pulmonary vein systolic flow reversals

MR can be dynamic, related to afterload and ischemia. On occasion, assessment of clinically important MR requires change in loading conditions or exercise. For example, the severity of MR in the operating room is usually less than that of the preoperative evaluation, and MR may need to be assessed after an increase in afterload with an isoproterenol infusion. In patients with ischemia, MR, and LV dysfunction, the ERO and MR volume may increase with exercise.[100] In patients with exercise-induced SAM of the mitral valve, MR may be evident only with exercise, with Valsalva maneuver, or in a standing position.

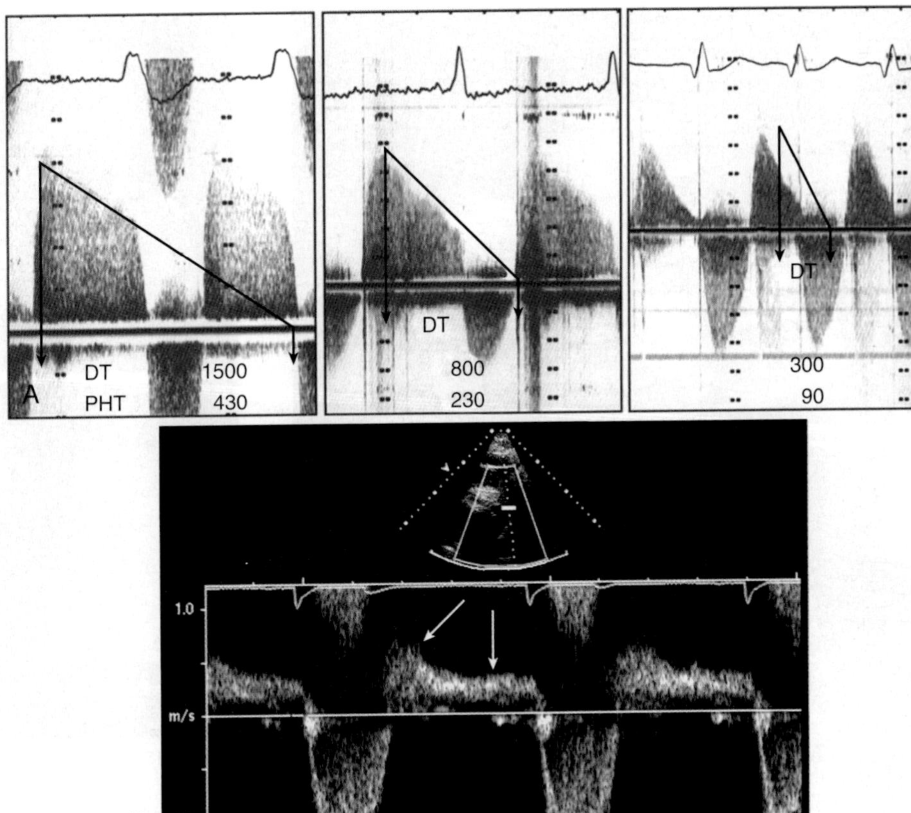

FIGURE 15-49 **A,** Continuous-wave Doppler spectra of aortic regurgitation from three patients illustrating decreased deceleration time (DT) and pressure half-time (PHT) with more severe aortic regurgitation. **Left,** Mild regurgitation, with a PHT of 430 milliseconds; **right,** severe regurgitation, with a PHT of 90 milliseconds; and **middle,** moderately severe regurgitation. **B,** Holodiastolic reversal flow (arrows) in the descending aorta indicates severe aortic regurgitation. Similar diastolic reversal can be seen in a descending thoracic aneurysm or shunt into the aorta during diastole (as in Blalock-Taussig shunt). The sample volume is usually located just distal to the takeoff of the left subclavian artery. *(Modified from Oh JK, Seward JB, Tajik AJ: The Echo Manual. 3rd ed. Philadelphia, Lippincott Williams & Wilkins, 2006. Used with permission of Mayo Foundation for Medical Education and Research.)*

MITRAL VALVE PROLAPSE. The echocardiographic diagnosis of mitral valve prolapse is primarily based on the parasternal long-axis view (see Chap. 66). Mitral valve prolapse is defined as systolic displacement (>2 mm) of one or both mitral leaflets into the left atrium, below the plane of the mitral annulus (**Fig. 15-52**; see also Fig. 66-37). The mitral leaflets are often thickened (>5 mm) or myxomatous. If a strict definition is used, the prevalence of mitral valve prolapse is 1.7% to 2.4%. The calculation of MR volume is more accurate than a visual assessment of its severity in mitral valve prolapse because the duration of MR is shorter starting from midsystole (see Fig. 15-52).

FUNCTIONAL MITRAL REGURGITATION. Functional MR is regurgitation caused by regional or global LV remodeling in ischemic or dilated cardiomyopathy without structural valve abnormalities (see Chap. 66). The functional MR jet is usually central in origin but can be eccentric, and color flow imaging tends to overestimate its severity. After 5 years, total mortality and cardiac mortality for patients with at least moderate (ERO ≥20 mm^2 and regurgitant volume ≥30 mL) ischemic MR (62% ± 5% and 50% ± 6%, respectively) were higher than for those without ischemic MR (39% ± 6% and 30% ± 5%, respectively). Severe functional MR is defined as an ERO of 20 mm^2 or higher. The major determinant of the ERO is mitral deformation (i.e., systolic mitral valvular tenting area; **Fig. 15-53**). The tenting area is determined by apical and posterior displacement of the papillary muscles and by the WMSI of the segments supporting the papillary muscles. A tenting area measuring 6 cm^2 or more usually indicates grade 3 or higher MR.

TRANSESOPHAGEAL ECHOCARDIOGRAPHY. TEE visualizes the mitral valve apparatus clearly, including identification of the flail mitral leaflet scallops (**Fig. 15-54**), and can be used in conjunction with TTE to determine the cause and severity of MR. TEE often provides invaluable clinical and anatomic information in the setting of severe acute MR and is routinely used in the operating room to assess the mitral valve before and after operative intervention. The addition of real-time three-dimensional TEE provides further anatomic information in patients undergoing mitral valve surgery for MR.[92]

Tricuspid Regurgitation

A mild degree of TR is common, and its velocity is routinely used to estimate RV systolic pressure. However, more than moderate TR has been found to adversely affect survival.[101]

Echocardiographic methods used to assess the severity of TR are similar to those used to assess MR and include the following (see Fig. 15-e17 on website):

1. assessment of regurgitant jet area with color flow imaging;
2. identification of late-peaking systolic flow reversal in the hepatic veins (**Fig. 15-55**) (this should not be confused with early-peaking systolic flow reversals caused by RV dysfunction or increased RA pressure);
3. demonstration of continuous-wave Doppler signal with increased forward flow velocity, relatively decreased TR velocity, and concave late systolic configuration of TR due to a large RA V wave (**Fig. 15-56**);
4. use of the vena contracta width to quantify the severity of TR (see Fig. 66-41); and
5. calculation of the ERO and regurgitant volume with the PISA method, as for the mitral valve.

Severe TR is defined by echocardiography on the basis of the following criteria:

- Color flow regurgitant jet area of 30% or more of RA area
- Annulus dilation (≥4 cm) or inadequate cusp coaptation
- Late systolic concave configuration of the continuous-wave signal
- Late systolic flow reversals in the hepatic vein
- ERO of 0.4 cm^2 or larger
- Regurgitant volume of 45 mL or more
- Width of vena contracta of 6.5 mm or more

Pulmonary Stenosis and Regurgitation

Pulmonary stenosis is usually an isolated congenital cardiac lesion but may be part of a more complex congenital cardiac disorder. The morphologic features of each of these lesions are easily identified on two-dimensional and Doppler echocardiography.

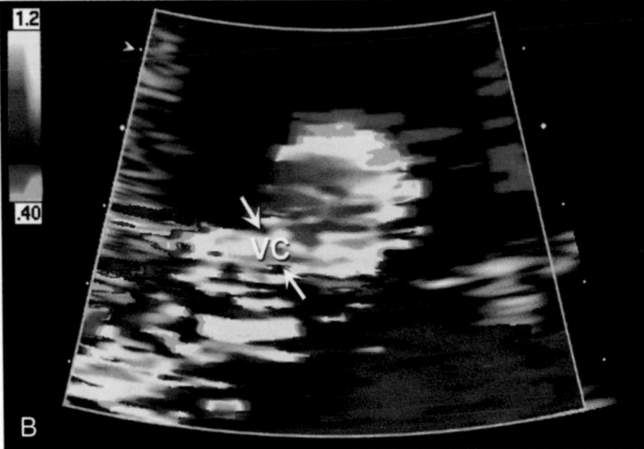

FIGURE 15-50 Measurement of the vena contracta (VC between arrows) in two different patients: **A,** with a central mitral regurgitation jet; and **B,** with an eccentric mitral regurgitation jet (note change in color flow baseline). LA = left atrium; LV = left ventricle. *(Modified from Oh JK, Seward JB, Tajik AJ: The Echo Manual. 3rd ed. Philadelphia, Lippincott Williams & Wilkins, 2006. Used with permission of Mayo Foundation for Medical Education and Research.)*

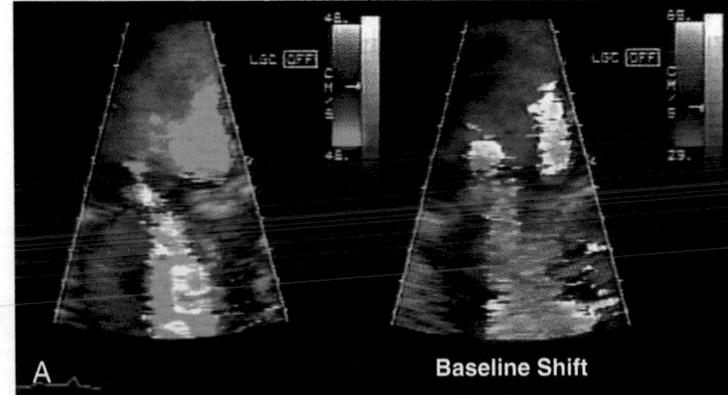

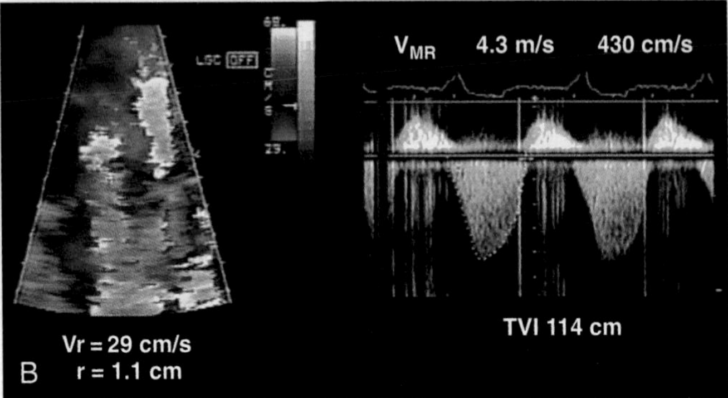

FIGURE 15-51 **A,** Apical four-chamber view and color flow imaging of mitral regurgitation, with mitral regurgitation jet zoomed. **Left,** Aliasing velocity is 46 cm/sec in either direction. The baseline for the color flow map has not been shifted. **Right**, Color flow map baseline is shifted downward so that negative aliasing velocity was reduced from 46 cm/sec to 29 cm/sec. The downward baseline shift makes the change of color flow farther from the mitral regurgitant orifice because blood flow converging toward the mitral regurgitant orifice has a lower velocity farther away from the regurgitant orifice. Therefore, a downward baseline shift makes the radius of the identified proximal isovelocity surface area (PISA) larger. **B,** The measured radius (r) was 1.1 cm, with an aliasing velocity (Vr) of 29 cm/sec. Mitral regurgitation velocity (V_{MR}) was obtained with continuous-wave Doppler from the apex, and the peak velocity was 4.3 m/sec (430 cm/sec), with a time-velocity integral (TVI) of 114 cm. From the data of PISA radius, color flow map aliasing velocity, mitral regurgitation peak velocity, and mitral regurgitation TVI, the mitral regurgitation effective regurgitant orifice and regurgitant volume can be calculated. *(Modified from Oh JK, Seward JB, Tajik AJ: The Echo Manual. 3rd ed. Philadelphia, Lippincott Williams & Wilkins, 2006. Used with permission of Mayo Foundation for Medical Education and Research.)*

Evaluation of the pulmonary valve is usually possible with two-dimensional echocardiography. Mild degrees of pulmonary regurgitation have been reported in 40% to 78% of patients with normal pulmonary valves and no structural heart disease. Identification of valve anatomy, including bicuspid valve, prolapse, dysplasia, and absence of the pulmonary valve, may help define the mechanism of regurgitation (see Fig. 15-e18A on website). Color Doppler imaging shows a diastolic jet in the RVOT, beginning at the region of the pulmonary valve (see Fig. 15-e18B on website). Planimetered jet areas, indexed for body surface area, have been shown to correlate well with the severity of pulmonary regurgitation determined angiographically. The continuous-wave Doppler profile demonstrates rapid deceleration of the regurgitation jet to baseline (**Fig. 15-57**; see also Fig. 66-42). The vena contracta width may be used to evaluate the severity of pulmonary regurgitation with color Doppler imaging; however, this technique has not been validated for the pulmonary valve.[102]

Prosthetic Valve Evaluation (see Chap. 66)

The echocardiographic evaluation of prosthetic valves requires a thorough knowledge of the normal structure and hemodynamic profiles as well as the surgical techniques used for different prostheses. Identification of prosthetic valve structural abnormalities requires an understanding of the echocardiographic characteristics, including reflectance of the prosthetic material, attenuation of the ultrasound beam, and ultrasound reverberations from the prosthesis. All these factors may cause difficulties in echocardiographic interpretation. Structural abnormalities of a prosthesis, such as dehiscence, vegetation, thrombus, and tissue prosthesis degeneration, can be assessed with two-dimensional TTE, complemented by TEE when needed because of the challenges in visualizing structures around and behind the cardiac prosthesis.

Doppler echocardiography is used to determine pressure gradients across prosthetic valves with the modified Bernoulli equation. Invasive dual-catheter pressure measurements made simultaneously across various prosthetic valves (**Fig. 15-58**) have demonstrated an excellent correlation with Doppler-derived gradients. However, because of the pressure recovery phenomenon, it has been shown in vitro that the aortic prosthetic gradients determined with Doppler velocities are overestimated compared with catheter-derived gradients. In pressure recovery, part of the kinetic energy, which is lost during flow passage through a small orifice, is recovered. Therefore, this pressure recovery results in a higher absolute pressure in the ascending aorta away from the stenotic aortic valve, accounting for the pressure gradient's being lower than the Doppler-derived pressure

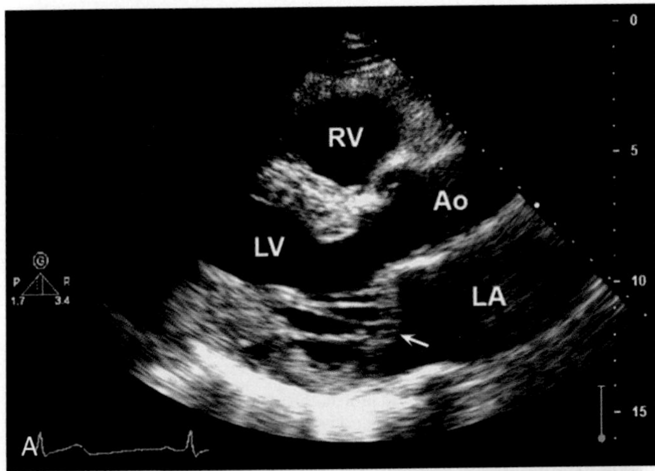

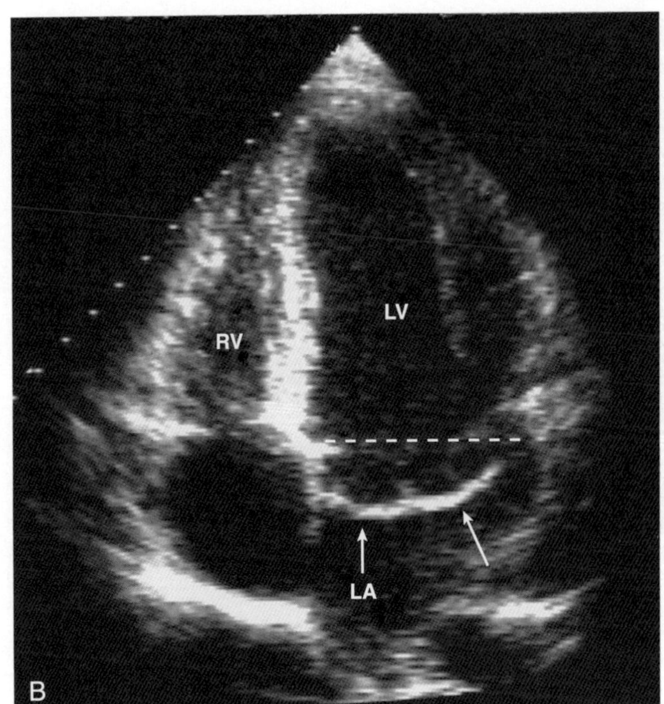

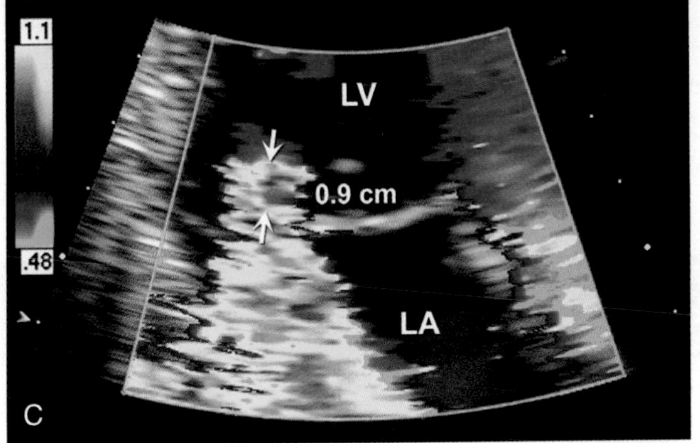

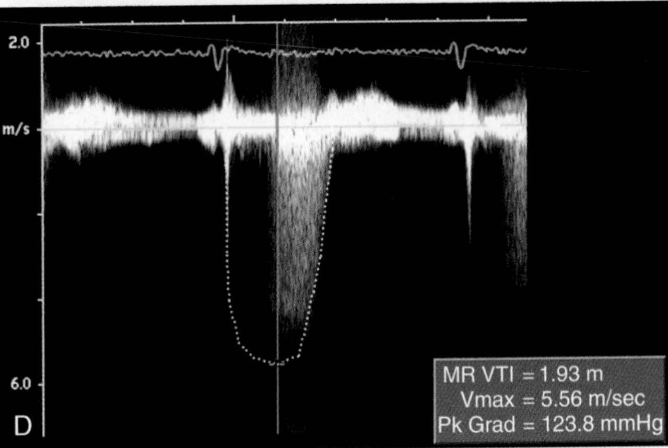

FIGURE 15-52 Mitral valve prolapse. **A,** From the parasternal long-axis view, there is systolic displacement of the anterior mitral leaflet (arrow) into the left atrium (LA) beyond the plane of the mitral annulus. Ao = aorta; LV = left ventricle; RV = right ventricle. **B,** Apical four-chamber view showing prolapse of both mitral leaflets (arrows). The dotted line indicates the plane of the mitral annulus. In general, the apical view should not be used to make the diagnosis of mitral valve prolapse. **C,** Quantification of mitral regurgitation (MR) in mitral valve prolapse. Proximal isovelocity surface area (PISA) of MR caused by mitral valve prolapse with color flow aliasing velocity of 48 cm/sec. PISA radius is 0.9 cm (arrows), which usually indicates severe MR. **D,** Continuous-wave Doppler recording of MR velocity shows mid to late systolic MR. Peak MR velocity is 556 cm/sec; hence:

$$\text{Effective regurgitant orifice (ERO)} = 6.28 \times (0.9)^2 \times 48/556 = 0.44\ \text{cm}^2$$

This finding is consistent with severe MR. MR time-velocity integral (TVI) is 193 cm if the entire systolic interval is included, which provides the following calculation of MR volume:

$$\text{MR volume} = \text{ERO} \times \text{TVI} = 0.44 \times 193 = 85\ \text{mL}$$

MR volume also indicates severe MR. However, the actual TVI is about half because MR starts at midsystole, which estimates MR volume to be about 40 mL (more consistent with moderate MR). *(**B-D** modified from Oh JK, Seward JB, Tajik AJ: The Echo Manual. 3rd ed. Philadelphia, Lippincott Williams & Wilkins, 2006. Used with permission of Mayo Foundation for Medical Education and Research.)*

gradient, which measures the highest value. Pressure recovery is less when the aorta is dilated. The discrepancy is minor in a large mechanical prosthesis and in tissue prostheses.

The prosthetic valve is inherently stenotic, and normal prosthetic flow velocity varies on the basis of the type and size of the prosthesis and its location and cardiac output. Normal Doppler values for each type of aortic, mitral, tricuspid, and pulmonary prosthesis in a large number of patients have been reported (**Tables 15-12 to 15-15**). It is important to know the normal values for each prosthesis and to have an early postoperative baseline Doppler study that can be used as an individual reference baseline for comparison with later studies. Increased flow velocities across a prosthetic valve may be caused by regurgitation from increased flow across the prosthesis or obstruction, indicating a smaller orifice.

Thrombus is the most common cause of mitral mechanical prosthesis obstruction (**Fig. 15-59**), whereas pannus formation is usually the cause of aortic mechanical prosthesis obstruction. The reduced motion of the

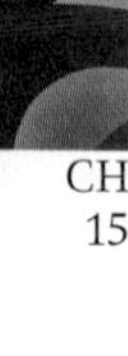

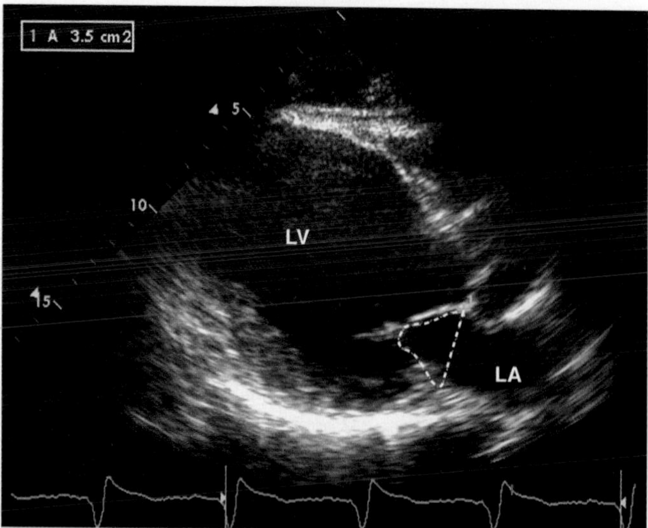

FIGURE 15-53 Parasternal long-axis view of dilated cardiomyopathy. Mitral tenting (dotted area) is caused by the markedly dilated left ventricular (LV) cavity. The tenting area is 3.5 cm^2. LA = left atrium.

disc, ball, or leaflets in an obstructed prosthetic valve may be difficult to visualize and to quantify with TTE, whereas normal and abnormal prosthetic valve motion may be visualized with TEE (see Fig. 15-e19 on website). Doppler echocardiography is the most accurate method to detect and to quantify the degree of prosthetic obstruction; however, increased flow velocities may be related to a high-output state or severe prosthetic regurgitation and should be excluded. The maximal and mean pressure gradients and the effective valve area can be calculated by the same formulas and equations described for the native valve (see Fig. 15-e20 on website). In patients with an obstructed mitral or tricuspid valve prosthesis, flow velocities increase and the PHT is prolonged. When the velocity across the mitral or tricuspid prosthesis is increased because of severe regurgitation, the PHT is normal or shortened and LVOT velocity is decreased because forward flow is decreased.

The increase in flow velocity across the obstructed aortic prosthesis is not accompanied by increased LVOT velocity, but it is with severe regurgitation. The LVOT and aortic prosthesis velocity or TVI ratio is helpful in differentiating increased flow velocity across an aortic prosthesis due to a prosthetic obstruction (ratio, ≥0.20) from increased velocity due to regurgitation (normal ratio, ≥0.3).

The PHT constant, 220, was derived for native mitral valve stenosis and not for calculation of the effective orifice area of a mitral prosthesis. Thus, the PHT method overestimates the area of a mitral prosthesis. The continuity equation is the preferred method for estimation of the functional orifice area of prosthetic aortic and mitral valves when there is no pronounced AR or MR.

TABLE 15-12 Hemodynamic Profiles of 609 Normal Aortic Valve Prostheses

TYPE OF PROSTHESIS	NO. OF PROSTHESES	PEAK VELOCITY (M/SEC)	MEAN GRADIENT (MM HG)	LVOT TVI/AV TVI
Heterograft	214	2.4 ± 0.5	13.3 ± 6.1	0.44 ± 0.21
Ball cage	160	3.2 ± 0.6	23.0 ± 8.8	0.32 ± 0.09
Björk-Shiley	141	2.5 ± 0.6	13.9 ± 7.0	0.40 ± 0.10
St. Jude Medical	44	2.5 ± 0.6	14.4 ± 7.7	0.41 ± 0.12
Homograft	30	1.9 ± 0.4	7.7 ± 2.7	0.56 ± 0.10
Medtronic-Hall	20	2.4 ± 0.2	13.6 ± 3.3	0.39 ± 0.09
Total	609	2.6 ± 0.7	15.8 ± 8.3	0.40 ± 0.16

AV = aortic valve; LVOT = left ventricular outflow tract; TVI = time-velocity integral.
Modified from Miller F Jr, Callahan J, Taylor C, et al: Normal aortic valve prosthesis hemodynamics: 609 prospective Doppler examinations [abstract]. Circulation 80(Suppl 2):II-169, 1989.

TABLE 15-13 Doppler Hemodynamic Profiles of 456 Normal Mitral Valve Prostheses

TYPE OF PROSTHESIS	NO. OF PROSTHESES	PEAK VELOCITY (M/SEC)	MEAN GRADIENT (MM HG)	EFFECTIVE AREA (CM^2)
Heterograft	150	1.6 ± 0.3	4.1 ± 1.5	2.3 ± 0.7
Ball cage	161	1.8 ± 0.3	4.9 ± 1.8	2.4 ± 0.7
Björk-Shiley	79	1.7 ± 0.3	4.1 ± 1.6	2.6 ± 0.6
St. Jude Medical	66	1.6 ± 0.4	4.0 ± 1.8	3.0 ± 0.8

Modified from Lengyel M, Miller F Jr, Taylor C, et al: Doppler hemodynamic profiles in 456 clinically and echo-normal mitral valve prostheses [abstract]. Circulation 82(Suppl 3):III-43, 1990.

TABLE 15-14 Doppler Hemodynamic Profiles of Normal Tricuspid Valve Prostheses

TYPE OF PROSTHESIS	NO. OF PROSTHESES	PEAK VELOCITY (M/SEC)	MEAN GRADIENT (MM HG)	PRESSURE HALF-TIME (M/SEC)
Heterograft	41	1.3 ± 0.2	3.2 ± 1.1	146 ± 39
Ball cage	33	1.3 ± 0.2	3.1 ± 0.8	144 ± 46
St. Jude Medical	7	1.2 ± 0.3	2.7 ± 1.1	108 ± 32
Björk-Shiley	1	1.3	2.2	144
Total	82	1.3 ± 0.2	3.1 ± 1.0	142 ± 42

Modified from Connolly HM, Miller FA Jr, Taylor CL, et al: Doppler hemodynamic profiles of eighty-six normal tricuspid valve prostheses [abstract]. J Am Coll Cardiol 17:69A, 1991.

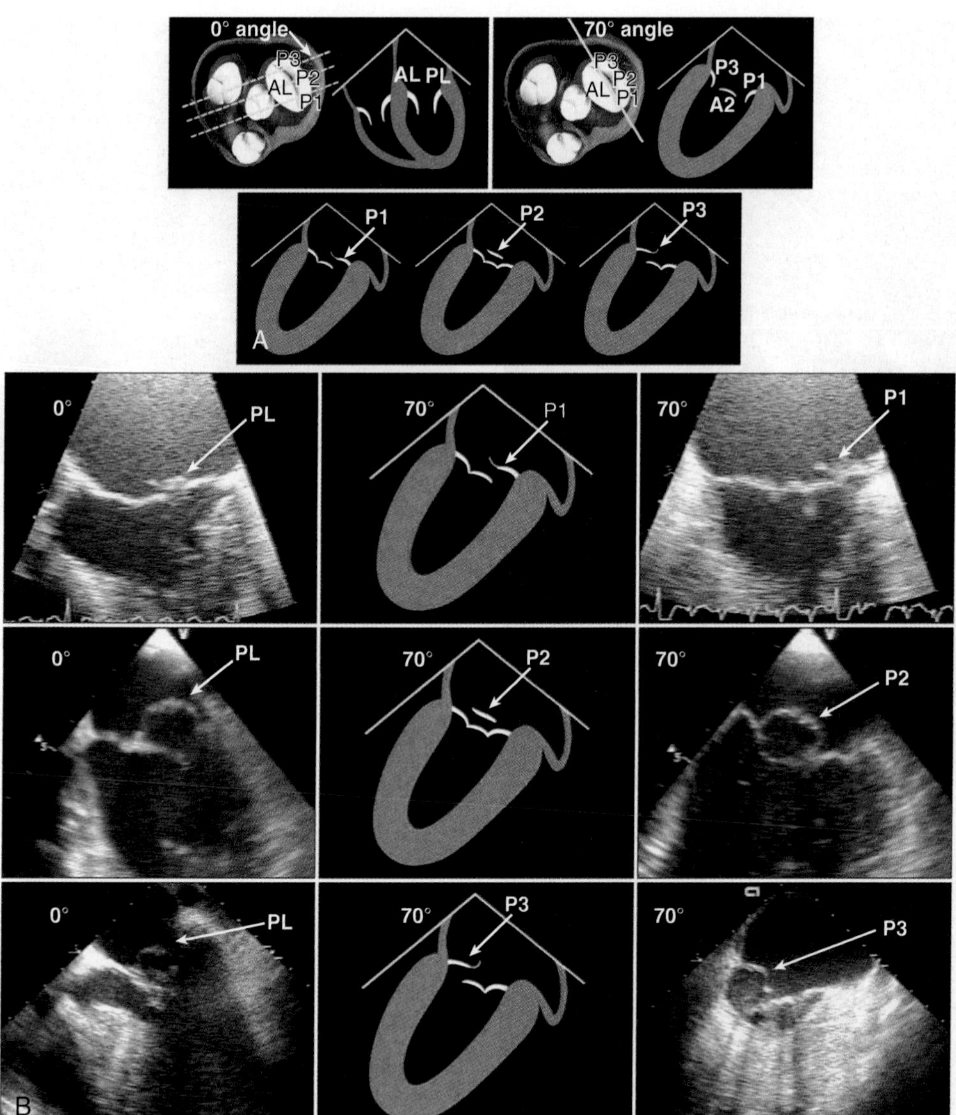

FIGURE 15-54 **A,** Transesophageal echocardiographic identification of mitral valve scallops. **Upper left,** First view at 0 degrees to determine if anterior (A) or posterior (P). AL = anterior leaflet; PL = posterior leaflet. **Upper right,** Next, the probe is rotated to about 70 degrees, cutting across the valve medial to lateral to identify the individual scallops. P3 = medial posterior scallop; P2 = middle scallop; P1 = lateral scallop; A2 = middle portion of the anterior leaflet. P2 is across from A2 and seen when flail. **Lower panels,** Examples of the three posterior leaflet flail views. **B,** Examples of flail mitral valve scallops. **Left column,** Transesophageal images at 0 degrees. The scallop location cannot be adequately assessed at 0 degrees. **Middle column,** Drawings of the lateral (P1), middle (P2), and medial (P3) flail scallops. **Right column,** The corresponding transesophageal echocardiographic images at 70 degrees. *(Modified from Oh JK, Seward JB, Tajik AJ: The Echo Manual. 3rd ed. Philadelphia, Lippincott Williams & Wilkins, 2006. Used with permission of Mayo Foundation for Medical Education and Research.)*

TABLE 15-15 Doppler Echocardiographic Data for Pulmonary Prostheses

TYPE OF PROSTHESIS	NO. OF PROSTHESES	SIZE (MM)	PEAK VELOCITY(M/SEC)	MEAN GRADIENT(MM HG)	TRIVIAL/MILD REGURGITATION (N)
Carpentier-Edwards	24	26.5 ± 1.8	2.4 ± 0.5	12.1 ± 5.3	7
Pulmonary homograft	17	24.2 ± 1.8	1.8 ± 0.6*	8.4 ± 4.8	15
Aortic homograft	3	22.3 ± 1.2	2.5 ± 0.4	14.4 ± 3.4	3
Hancock	3	26.0 ± 3.0	2.4 ± 0.5	14.0 ± 5.7	1
Ionescu-Shiley	2	25.0 ± 0.0	2.4 ± 0.4	12.5 ± 3.5	2
St. Jude Medical	1	25	2.6	12.0	1
Björk-Shiley	1	25	2.0	7.0	1

*Compared with all heterografts combined ($P = 0.002$).

Modified from Novaro GM, Connolly HM, Miller FA Jr: Doppler hemodynamics of 51 clinically and echocardiographically normal pulmonary valve prostheses. Mayo Clin Proc 76:155, 2001. Used with permission of Mayo Foundation for Medical Education and Research.

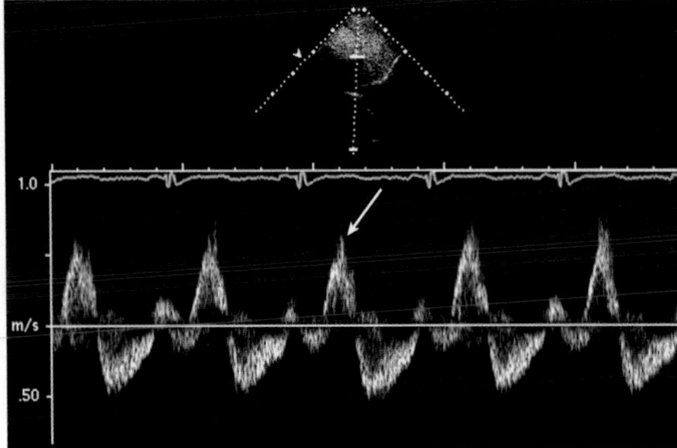

FIGURE 15-55 Tricuspid regurgitation. Pulsed-wave Doppler recording showing late systolic flow reversal (arrow) in the hepatic vein. *(Modified from Oh JK, Seward JB, Tajik AJ: The Echo Manual. 3rd ed. Philadelphia, Lippincott Williams & Wilkins, 2006. Used with permission of Mayo Foundation for Medical Education and Research.)*

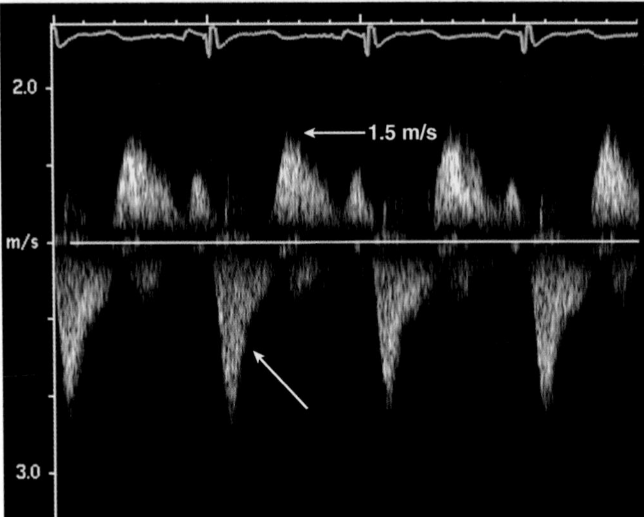

FIGURE 15-56 Continuous-wave Doppler recording of tricuspid flow in a patient with severe tricuspid regurgitation. Because of the large amount of tricuspid regurgitation, there is an indentation (arrow) in tricuspid regurgitation velocity spectrum during mid-late systole (i.e., V wave). Diastolic velocity is also increased (1.5 m/sec) from increased flow across the tricuspid valve. *(Modified from Oh JK, Seward JB, Tajik AJ: The Echo Manual. 3rd ed. Philadelphia, Lippincott Williams & Wilkins, 2006. Used with permission of Mayo Foundation for Medical Education and Research.)*

A small amount of leakage volume regurgitation is detected in about 30% of normal mechanical prostheses examined with TTE and in up to 44% and 95% of aortic and mitral prostheses, respectively, examined with TEE. The size and type of mechanical prosthesis also have an effect on the degree of regurgitation. Pathologic prosthetic valve regurgitation can be distinguished from normal regurgitation by examining the morphology of the valve and the number and location of regurgitant jets.

Color flow imaging is the principal technique used to detect prosthetic valvular regurgitation. Semiquantification of prosthetic valvular and perivalvular regurgitation is possible by use of the same criteria as for native valvular regurgitation. TEE is often necessary when mitral or tricuspid prostheses are assessed for regurgitation because of the inability to visualize the atria adequately, which is related to attenuation of the ultrasound beam. Aortic prosthetic regurgitation often requires combined TTE and TEE assessments to determine location and severity. Transverse imaging of the prosthesis sewing ring and transgastric imaging may help delineate periprosthetic AR. Periprosthetic regurgitation can be readily identified by two-dimensional and three-dimensional TTE and TEE and can be treated percutaneously under echocardiographic monitoring.[103]

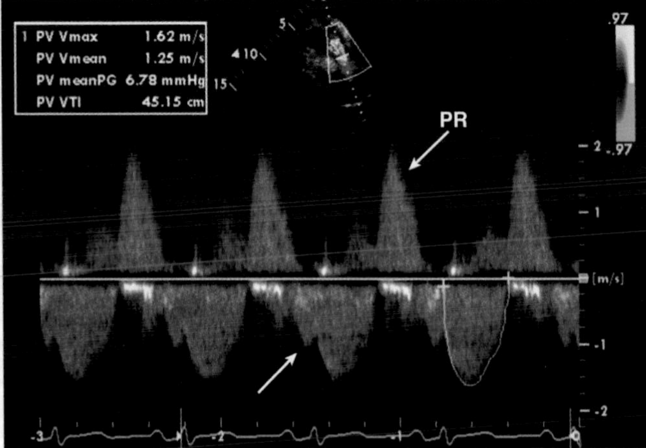

FIGURE 15-57 Continuous-wave Doppler signal showing a pulmonary regurgitant (PR) signal with a short deceleration time because of rapid equalization (downward arrow) of the right ventricular and pulmonary artery diastolic pressures before the onset of QRS. There is also diastolic flow (upward arrow) across the pulmonary valve (PV) caused by a rapid increase in right ventricular diastolic pressure. PG = pressure gradient; Vmax = maximum velocity; Vmean = mean velocity; VTI = velocity-time integral.

TEE and three-dimensional TTE and TEE complement the echocardiographic assessment of patients with prosthetic valves and are commonly used in conjunction with comprehensive hemodynamic assessment by TTE to assess patients with possible endocarditis, abscess, dehiscence, and intracardiac masses or thrombi. With TEE, filamentous prosthetic valve strands related to fibroblasts and collagen are often noted, but their role in cardioembolic events is uncertain.

Prosthesis-Patient Mismatch

A subset of patients with prosthetic aortic valves have a prosthesis that is too small in relation to body size, resulting in an increased transvalvular gradient and cardiovascular disability (see Chap. 66). Subsequent studies have defined prosthesis-patient mismatch as follows:

Mild: indexed effective orifice area >0.85 cm^2/m^2
Moderate: effective orifice area >0.65 cm^2/m^2 and ≤0.85 cm^2/m^2
Severe: effective orifice area of 0.65 cm^2/m^2 or less

More than a moderate degree of prosthesis-patient mismatch is associated with increased early mortality and increased late mortality in patients younger than 70 years or with a body mass index less than 30 kg/m^2 or an LVEF less than 50%.[104]

Infective Endocarditis

The diagnosis of infective endocarditis is frequently suggested on the basis of echocardiography, which is the diagnostic procedure of choice for detection of valvular vegetations (see Chap. 67). Identification of a vegetation is one of two major diagnostic criteria for infective endocarditis.

The echocardiographic features typical of infective endocarditis are an oscillating intracardiac mass on a valve or supporting structure or in the path of a regurgitation jet or on a device, abscesses, new partial dehiscence of a prosthetic valve, and new valvular regurgitation. The initial attachment site of a vegetation is usually on the ventricular surface of the semilunar valves and on the atrial surface of the atrioventricular valves (**Fig. 15-60**). Vegetations frequently show high-frequency flutter or oscillations and can be linear, round, irregular, or shaggy.[105]

The sensitivity for detection of vegetation is 65% to 80% with two-dimensional TTE and 95% with TEE but depends on vegetation size, location, and echocardiographic window. The yield of TTE is poor in patients with prosthetic valve endocarditis, but the sensitivity for TEE is 90%. A baseline TTE examination is often recommended for patients with suspected endocarditis (see Chap. 67). Serial studies are dictated by the patient's clinical and hemodynamic status. Right-sided valvular vegetations are often larger than left-sided ones, and TEE rarely improves the diagnostic accuracy of TTE in detecting vegetations (see Fig. 15-e21 on website). After successful medical treatment of endocarditis, vegetations frequently persist but are not associated with late complications.

By identifying and characterizing vegetations, echocardiography is useful in predicting complications related to endocarditis (**Fig. 15-61**), including embolization, destruction of valvular or intracardiac structures, abscess, and hemodynamic deterioration (**Table 15-16**). In left-sided valve endocarditis, mobility, extent, consistency, and size of the vegetation affect the frequency of complications. More than 50% of patients developed at least one complication when vegetations were larger than 10 mm. Tricuspid valve endocarditis causes pulmonary embolism in 69% of cases.

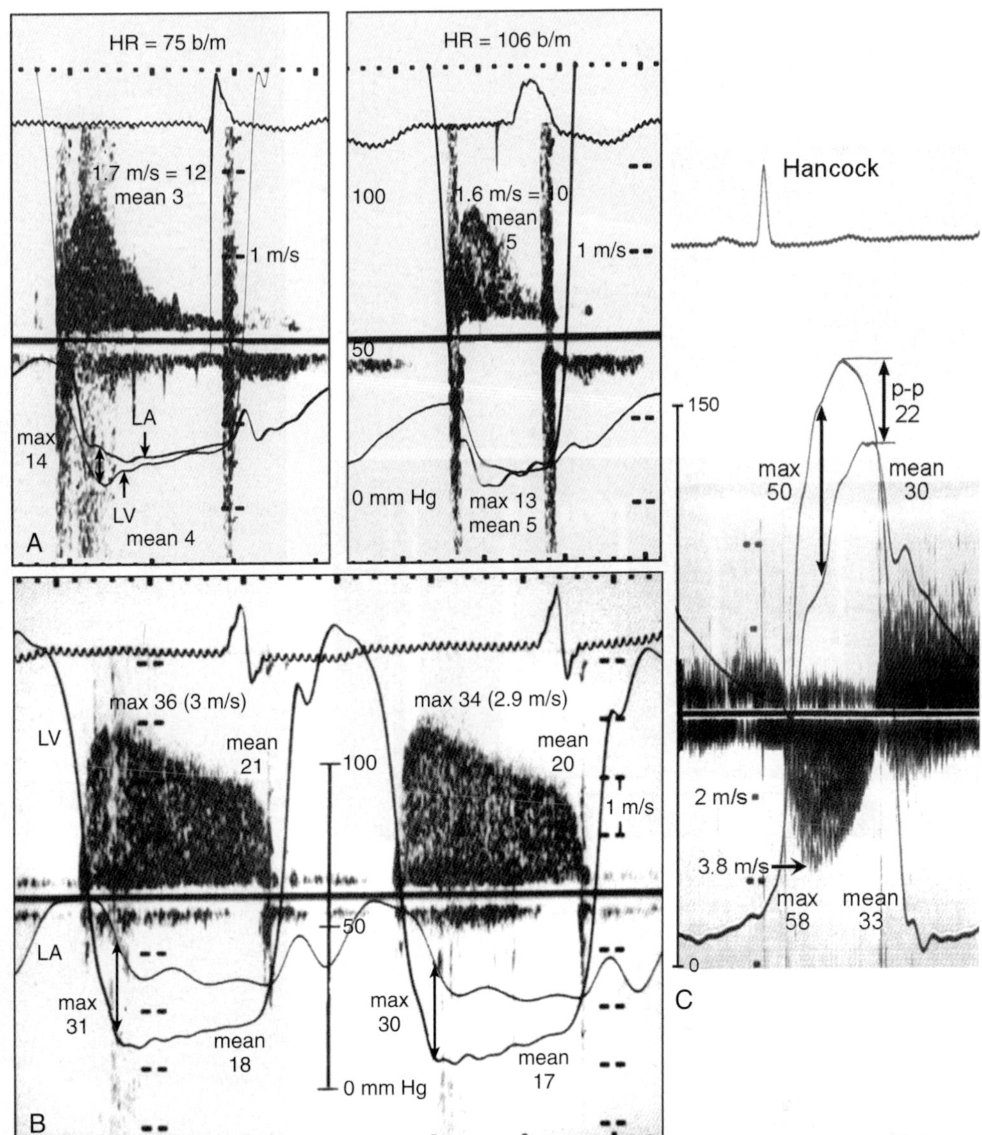

FIGURE 15-58 **A,** Simultaneous Doppler and catheterization study of a normal mechanical mitral prosthesis. The correlation between the two techniques at different heart rates (HR) is good. b/m = beats per minute; LA = left atrium; LV = left ventricle. **B,** Simultaneous continuous-wave Doppler and catheter pressure measurements in a patient with an obstructed Hancock mitral prosthesis. The maximal (36 versus 31 mm Hg) and mean (21 versus 18 mm Hg by Doppler and catheter, respectively) gradients derived from these two techniques correlate well. **C,** Simultaneous Doppler and catheterization study in a patient with a Hancock aortic prosthesis. The correlation between Doppler-derived and catheter-derived maximal (58 versus 50 mm Hg) and mean (33 versus 30 mm Hg) pressure gradients is good. A good correlation was also noted for the mechanical aortic prosthesis. Note that the peak-to-peak (p-p) gradient, which is a nonphysiologic assessment, underestimates the severity of obstruction (p-p gradient, 22 mm Hg; catheter-derived mean gradient, 30 mm Hg). (***A** modified from Oh JK, Seward JB, Tajik AJ: The Echo Manual. 3rd ed. Philadelphia, Lippincott Williams & Wilkins, 2006. Used with permission of Mayo Foundation for Medical Education and Research. **B** and **C** modified from Burstow D, Nishimura R, Bailey K, et al: Continuous wave Doppler echocardiographic measurement of prosthetic valve gradients: A simultaneous Doppler-catheter correlative study. Circulation 80:504, 1989. Used with permission.)*

Transesophageal Echocardiography in Endocarditis

The sensitivity of TEE for detection of vegetations or complications of endocarditis is higher than that of TTE. Thus, TEE should be performed in all patients who have nondiagnostic TTE findings, persistent fever, persistent positive blood cultures, or heart failure without a demonstrable cause (see Chap. 67). TEE is the diagnostic procedure of choice for exclusion of vegetation and for detection of complications of infective endocarditis. In patients with aortic valve endocarditis, TEE more frequently than TTE demonstrates anatomic complications such as involvement of subaortic structures, mitral-aortic intervalvular fibrosa aneurysm (see Fig. 15-61), perforation with communication into the left atrium, aortic annular abscess, or perforation of the mitral leaflet. In pediatric patients, TTE has a higher sensitivity for detection of vegetation, and TEE may be used less frequently.

Nonbacterial Thrombotic Endocarditis

Patients with nonbacterial thrombotic endocarditis often present with cerebral embolic events. Thus, echocardiography is performed to identify a potential cardiac source. The mitral valve is usually involved (**Fig. 15-62**), causing regurgitation. The aortic valve is involved less frequently.

Cardiomyopathies

Dilated Cardiomyopathy (see Chap. 68)

In dilated cardiomyopathy, the LV cavity is enlarged and global systolic function is decreased (**Fig. 15-63**).[106,107] End-diastolic and end-systolic dimensions and volumes are increased, and systolic function is decreased. With gradual dilation, the LV cavity becomes more spherical, with a sphericity index (short-axis dimension/long-axis dimension) nearing the value of 1 (normally, ≥1.5). LV mass is uniformly increased (eccentric hypertrophy), and wall thickness is typically within normal limits. Ventricular contractility usually is globally reduced, but regional wall motion abnormalities can be present. Similar echocardiographic findings occur in patients with cardiomyopathy related to ischemia, myocarditis, alcohol abuse, hemochromatosis, sarcoidosis, acute catecholamine crisis, acquired immunodeficiency syndrome, severe sepsis, or doxorubicin (Adriamycin) toxicity and in peripartum cardiomyopathy.

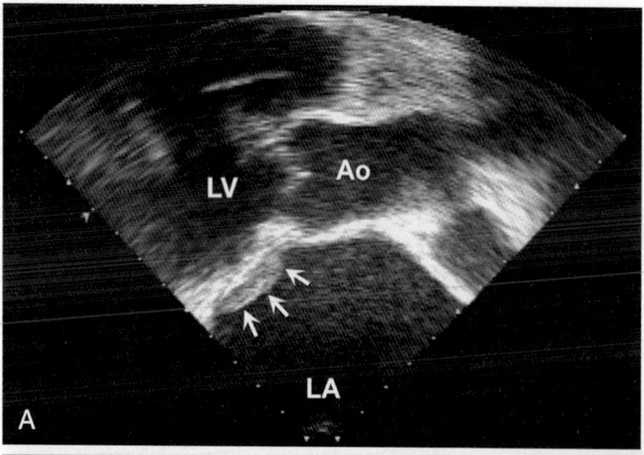

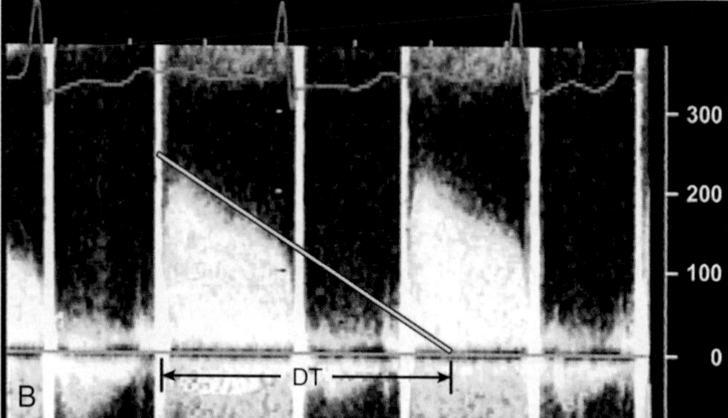

FIGURE 15-59 A, Transesophageal echocardiographic examination showing a large thrombus (arrows) attached to the atrial surface of a mitral mechanical prosthesis, causing an obstruction. Ao = aorta; LA = left atrium; LV = left ventricle. **B,** Continuous-wave Doppler recording across the obstructive mitral prosthesis. Peak mitral prosthesis velocity is higher than 2 m/sec, and pressure half-time and deceleration time (DT) are prolonged. *(Modified from Oh JK, Seward JB, Tajik AJ: The Echo Manual. 3rd ed. Philadelphia, Lippincott Williams & Wilkins, 2006. Used with permission of Mayo Foundation for Medical Education and Research.)*

Secondary features may be identified by echocardiography in patients with dilated cardiomyopathy. These include dilated mitral annulus with incomplete mitral leaflet coaptation causing functional MR, evidence of low cardiac output (decreased excursion of mitral leaflets), enlarged atrial cavities, RV enlargement, and occasionally apical mural thrombus. Intraventricular mechanical dyssynchrony caused by left or right bundle branch block is common and contributes to further cardiac dysfunction.[108] In view of the incidence (20% to 50%) of familial dilated cardiomyopathy, echocardiographic screening of immediate family members is recommended.[109]

Doppler echocardiography is useful to determine hemodynamics in patients with dilated cardiomyopathy. Important hemodynamic data routinely obtained include cardiac output and LV filling pressures and diastolic function by mitral inflow filling patterns, TDI, and color M-mode (see Fig. 15-e22 on website). Both mitral annulus systolic (S′) and early diastolic (E′) velocities are reduced in dilated cardiomyopathy.[15]

Diastolic function analysis correlates well with PCWP and has incremental prognostic power over what LVEF can provide in dilated cardiomyopathy.[110] Patients who are compensated with near-normal SV and cardiac output have an impaired relaxation pattern (grade 1 diastolic dysfunction; **Fig. 15-64A**). Patients who are decompensated have decreased SV and a restrictive diastolic filling pattern (Fig. 15-64B) because of decreased compliance and increased LV filling pressures. Patients with reversible restrictive filling have a high probability of improvement with medical therapy and excellent survival. The persistence of the restrictive filling pattern after therapy is associated with high mortality and transplantation rates.

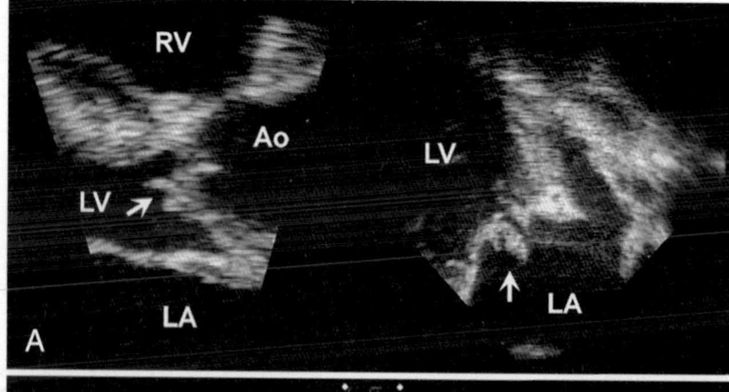

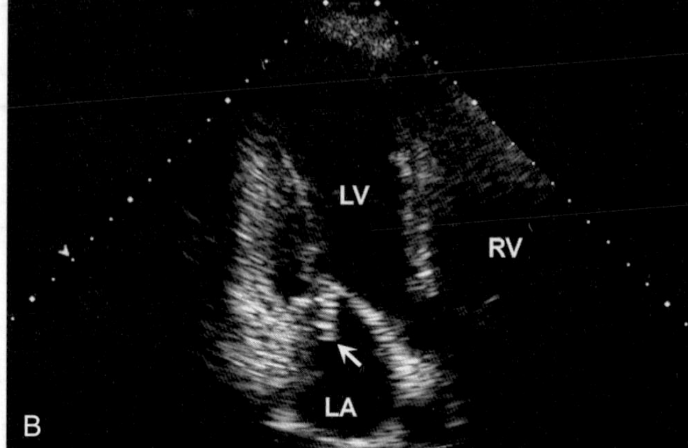

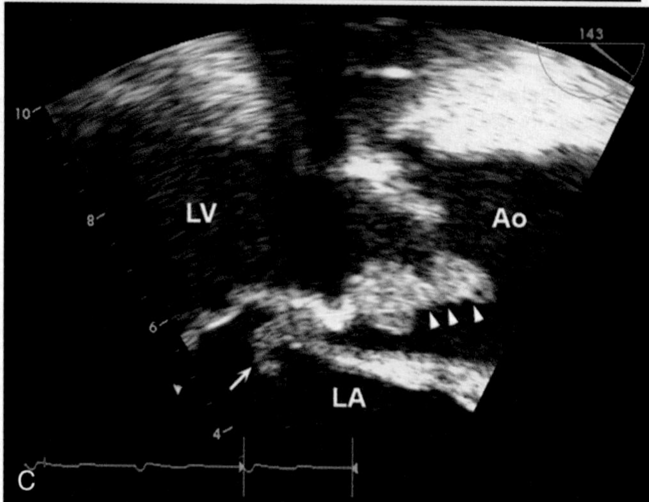

FIGURE 15-60 A, Transesophageal echocardiograms of aortic valve **(left)** and mitral valve **(right)** showing the typical attachment site for vegetation. The initial attachment site to the aortic valve is usually on the ventricular surface (left arrow). For the mitral and tricuspid valves, it is on the atrial side (right arrow). It results from the high-velocity blood jet from the high-pressure chamber to the low-pressure chamber. When the regurgitation jet is eccentric, as in mitral valve prolapse, satellite vegetation lesions can develop along the direction of the mitral regurgitation jet. **B,** Transthoracic apical view showing a mobile mass attached to the atrial surface (arrow) of the mitral valve. **C,** Vegetation (arrowheads) attached to the aortic bioprosthesis comes through (arrow) the intervalvular fibrosa into the left atrium (LA). Ao = aorta; LV = left ventricle; RV = right ventricle. *(**A** and **B** modified from Oh JK, Seward JB, Tajik AJ: The Echo Manual. 3rd ed. Philadelphia, Lippincott Williams & Wilkins, 2006. Used with permission of Mayo Foundation for Medical Education and Research.)*

Doppler-derived pulmonary artery pressure measurement also has prognostic importance in dilated cardiomyopathy. Patients with a TR velocity of 3 m/sec or higher have a higher mortality rate, a higher incidence of heart failure, a restrictive diastolic filling pattern, and more frequent hospitalizations than those with a velocity less than 3 m/sec. Therefore, a restrictive diastolic filling pattern and a high TR

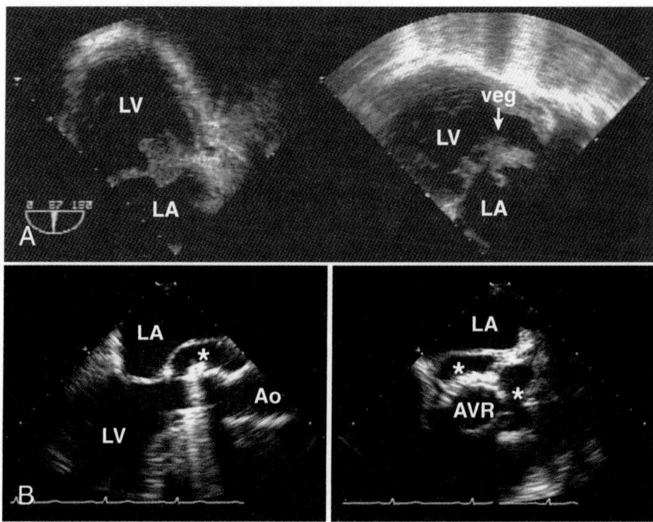

FIGURE 15-61 A, Transesophageal echocardiogram of a patient with *Staphylococcus aureus* endocarditis. Vegetation (veg) is attached to the mitral valve, specifically the anterior leaflet of the mitral valve. As a complication, the anterior leaflet of the mitral valve with vegetation had a dehiscence from the mitral annulus, causing severe mitral valve regurgitation. Pulmonary edema and a loud murmur developed suddenly during the treatment of endocarditis, and echocardiography showed the dehiscence as a complication of endocarditis. **B,** Transesophageal long-axis **(left)** and short-axis **(right)** views showing an abscess cavity (asterisk) at the aortic and mitral valve intervalvular fibrosa in a patient with prosthetic aortic valve endocarditis. The increased echodensity in the region posterior to the aortic valve is consistent with an infectious process. Ao = aorta; AVR = aortic valve prosthesis; LA = left atrium; LV = left ventricle. *(**A** modified from Oh JK, Seward JB, Tajik AJ: The Echo Manual. 3rd ed. Philadelphia, Lippincott Williams & Wilkins, 2006. Used with permission of Mayo Foundation for Medical Education and Research.)*

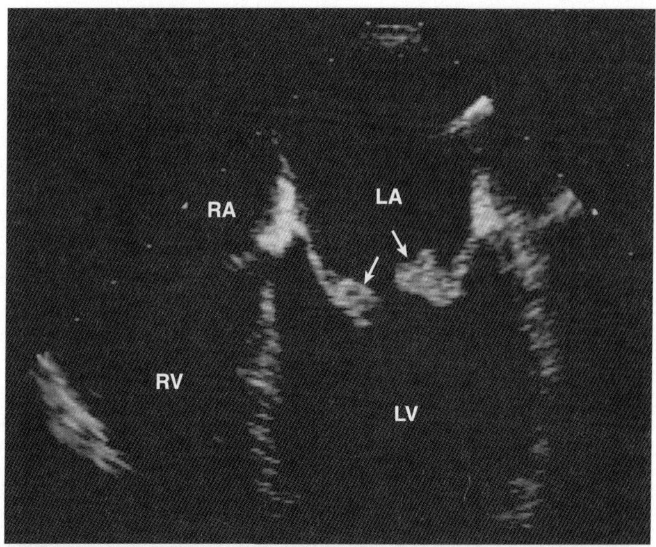

FIGURE 15-62 Transesophageal echocardiographic view of round masses attached to the tip of the mitral leaflet (arrows) of a patient with systemic lupus erythematosus and no clinical evidence of bacterial endocarditis. Diastolic frame of the horizontal transesophageal echocardiographic view of the mitral valve shows large verrucous vegetations (arrows). LA = left atrium; LV = left ventricle; RA = right atrium; RV = right ventricle. *(Modified from Oh JK, Seward JB, Tajik AJ: The Echo Manual. 3rd ed. Philadelphia, Lippincott Williams & Wilkins, 2006. Used with permission of Mayo Foundation for Medical Education and Research.)*

TABLE 15-16 Complications of Endocarditis

Structural
Cusp or leaflet rupture/flail
Perforation
Abscess
Aneurysm
Fistula
Dehiscence of prosthetic valve
Pericardial effusion (more frequent with abscess)
Hemodynamic compromise
Valvular regurgitation
Acute mitral regurgitation
Acute aortic regurgitation
Premature mitral valve closure
Restrictive mitral inflow pattern
Valvular stenosis
Shunt
Congestive heart failure
Embolization
Systemic
Cerebral
Pulmonary

Modified from Oh JK, Seward JB, Tajik AJ: The Echo Manual. 3rd ed. Philadelphia, Lippincott Williams & Wilkins, 2006. Used with permission of Mayo Foundation for Medical Education and Research.

velocity identify patients who are at increased risk for death and heart failure. MR is common in dilated cardiomyopathy and is related to the LV remodeling process (see Fig. 15-53; see Chap. 66). Treatment directed toward reverse remodeling improves MR as well as LV systolic function.

ECHOCARDIOGRAPHY IN MANAGEMENT OF DILATED CARDIOMYOPATHY. TDI and other modified techniques are used to quantify the degree of intraventricular dyssynchrony (Fig. 15-64C). However, marked differences between techniques are found for the presence of mechanical dyssynchrony, making interchangeability of these techniques uncertain. Assessment of mechanical dyssynchrony by real-time three-dimensional echocardiography might be an appropriate alternative to TDI for accurate prediction of response to cardiac resynchronization therapy (see Chap. 29).[111]

Deciding which echocardiographic parameters are most helpful in predicting a positive response to cardiac resynchronization requires further clinical experience.[1]

Hypertrophic Cardiomyopathy (see Chap. 69)

Two-dimensional echocardiography is the diagnostic method of choice for evaluation of patients with HCM (**Fig. 15-65**; see Fig. 69-1). Although asymmetric septal hypertrophy is the most common morphologic pattern, HCM can present with concentric, apical, or free wall LV hypertrophy.[112] Patients with obstructive HCM have a variable degree of MR. Obstruction in HCM is often dynamic and varies with the loading conditions, LV size, and contractility. Three-dimensional echocardiography may provide additional anatomic delineation (see Fig. 15-e23 on website). Diffuse hypertrophy of the ventricular septum and anterolateral free wall is the most common type of HCM in the West (70% to 75%), followed by basal septal hypertrophy (10% to 15%), concentric hypertrophy (5%), apical hypertrophy (<5%), and hypertrophy of the lateral wall (1% to 2%). The magnitude of hypertrophy is related to the risk of sudden death (see Chap. 69).[112]

The degree of LVOT obstruction is readily assessed with continuous-wave Doppler echocardiography, often best assessed at the right parasternal window. The continuous-wave Doppler spectrum has a characteristic late-peaking dagger-shaped appearance (**Fig. 15-66**).

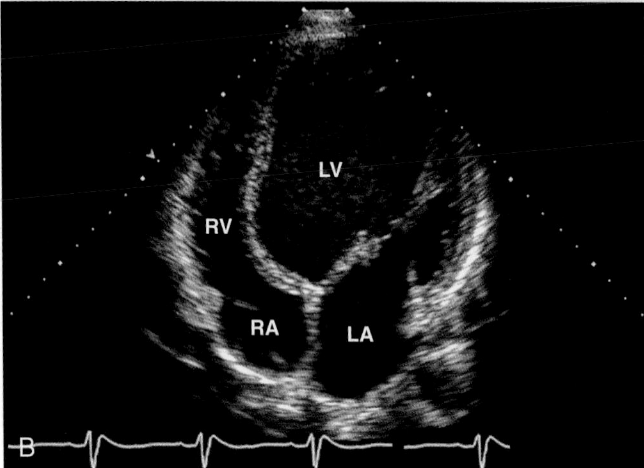

FIGURE 15-63 A, Two-dimensional echocardiography-guided M-mode echocardiogram in dilated cardiomyopathy. End-diastolic dimension (EDD = 86 mm) and end-systolic dimension (ESD = 76 mm) were markedly dilated. Contractility is globally reduced, although it is better in the posterior wall (PW) than in the ventricular septum (VS). According to the simplified Quinones method, left ventricular ejection fraction (EF) is calculated as follows:

$$EF = \frac{86^2 - 76^2}{86^2} \times 100 = 22\%$$

B, End-diastolic frame of apical four-chamber view in dilated cardiomyopathy (from the same patient as in **A**). The left ventricle (LV) is markedly dilated, and systolic function is reduced in real time. This is typical end-stage dilated cardiomyopathy, with a more spherical shape caused by more dilation of the short axis (86 mm) than of the long axis (100 mm). LA = left atrium; RA = right atrium; RV = right ventricle. *(Modified from Oh JK, Seward JB, Tajik AJ: The Echo Manual. 3rd ed. Philadelphia, Lippincott Williams & Wilkins, 2006. Used with permission of Mayo Foundation for Medical Education and Research.)*

With the simplified Bernoulli equation, the peak velocity can be converted to the peak pressure gradient across the LVOT. The correlation between Doppler-derived and catheter-derived pressure gradients is good. The dynamic nature of LVOT obstruction can be documented with continuous-wave Doppler imaging during the Valsalva maneuver, positional change (from supine to standing), or amyl nitrite inhalation (see Fig. 15-66).[1] MR frequently accompanies the obstructive form of HCM and is related to SAM of the mitral valve.

Diastolic Filling Pattern and Tissue Doppler Imaging. Markedly impaired myocardial relaxation is the predominant diastolic abnormality in HCM. Atrial contraction makes an important contribution to LV filling, and when atrial contraction is compromised because of tachycardia or AF, cardiac output decreases and pulmonary venous congestion occurs. As compliance decreases and LA pressure increases, early filling gradually increases and DT decreases. There is no significant correlation between DT and LV filling pressures in patients with HCM because DT is markedly prolonged at baseline and the same degree of increase in LA pressure does not produce similar shortening of the DT as would be expected in other disorders. Mitral annulus velocity, Ea, reflects the status of myocardial relaxation and is reduced in most patients with HCM (see Fig. 15-65B). Ea is decreased in patients with preclinical disease who have a genotype positive for HCM.[1] Strain of the myocardium is also altered in HCM (see Fig. 15-65C).

Dynamic Left Ventricular Outflow Tract Obstruction in Other Diseases. Not all dynamic LVOT obstruction is caused by HCM. Hyperdynamic LV systolic function, caused by medication or other factors, can cause dynamic LVOT obstruction hemodynamically indistinguishable from HCM in patients with basal septal hypertrophy. Elderly patients with hypertension treated with vasodilators, diuretics, or digoxin may develop dynamic obstruction and associated symptoms of dyspnea, chest pain, or hypotension exacerbated by treatment. This disorder has been called hypertensive HCM, but it is clearly different from true HCM. Dynamic LVOT obstruction is also commonly noted in the postoperative period when intravascular volume is depleted and inotropic agents are being administered. Patients with AS or mitral valve prolapse are especially vulnerable to LVOT obstruction after aortic valve replacement or mitral valve repair, respectively. Acute LVOT obstruction can occur after acute anterior-apical MI, and some patients with apical ballooning have dynamic LVOT obstruction caused by SAM and associated MR. Discrete subaortic stenosis can mimic hypertrophic obstructive cardiomyopathy (see Chap. 65); however, a continuous-wave Doppler recording of subaortic stenosis does not demonstrate a dynamic late-peaking profile but resembles that of valvular AS. Dynamic LVOT obstruction may also be an initial presentation of cardiac amyloidosis.

APICAL HYPERTROPHIC CARDIOMYOPATHY. Apical HCM may be missed by parasternal two-dimensional echocardiography because the hypertrophy is usually confined to the cardiac apex (**Fig. 15-67**; see Fig. 69-1D). Apical HCM is best visualized from apical short-axis and four-chamber views with good endocardial definition; echocardiography of patients with this condition shows thickened apical walls and obliteration of the apical cavity during systole. Because of massive apical hypertrophy, epicardial motion may suggest a dyskinetic apex. Apical hypertrophy should be differentiated from obliteration of the apical cavity caused by hypereosinophilic syndrome or abnormal apical trabeculation in noncompaction. Intravenous administration of a contrast agent is extremely helpful in delineating the small apical cavity with a configuration of the "ace of spades," typical of apical HCM (see Fig. 15-e24 on website).[113] CMR is an excellent diagnostic technique used to confirm the diagnosis of apical HCM (see Chap. 18).

MANAGEMENT OF HYPERTROPHIC OBSTRUCTIVE CARDIOMYOPATHY. By outlining the extent and location of hypertrophy, echocardiography can help guide intervention. Surgical myectomy remains the gold standard for relief of LVOT obstruction. It is the preferred method of management in the setting of diffuse septal hypertrophy or anomalous papillary muscle contributing to obstruction and in patients who have another indication for cardiac surgery.[114] Alcohol septal ablation is an effective method to reduce LVOT obstruction in selected patients. Because the myocardial area supplied by the septal perforator varies, it is critical to visualize the area to be infarcted by septal ablation before the procedure. Myocardial contrast echocardiography is well suited for this purpose (see Fig. 15-e25 on website).[52]

Other Conditions Mimicking Hypertrophic Cardiomyopathy. Although echocardiography is the diagnostic procedure of choice in HCM, many other disorders have similar echocardiographic features, including chronic hypertension, RV hypertrophy, cardiac amyloidosis (see Fig. 15-7), athlete's heart, pheochromocytoma, long-term hemodialysis, Fabry disease, and Friedreich ataxia. Therefore, the echocardiographic finding of increased LV wall thickness and dynamic LVOT obstruction should be interpreted in its clinical context. Apical hypertrophy should be differentiated from apical cavity obliteration caused by hypereosinophilic syndrome or noncompaction. Contrast and three-dimensional echocardiography is helpful in differentiating apical HCM from other entities.[115]

Athlete's Heart Versus Hypertrophic Cardiomyopathy. LV hypertrophy occurs after years of intense athletic training, and the two-dimensional echocardiographic findings of athlete's heart are similar to those of HCM (see Chap. 69). The following characteristics of athlete's heart can differentiate it from HCM:

- Symmetric hypertrophy
- Hypertrophy is rarely greater than 17 mm.
- LV cavity dimension is increased, whereas it is decreased in HCM.

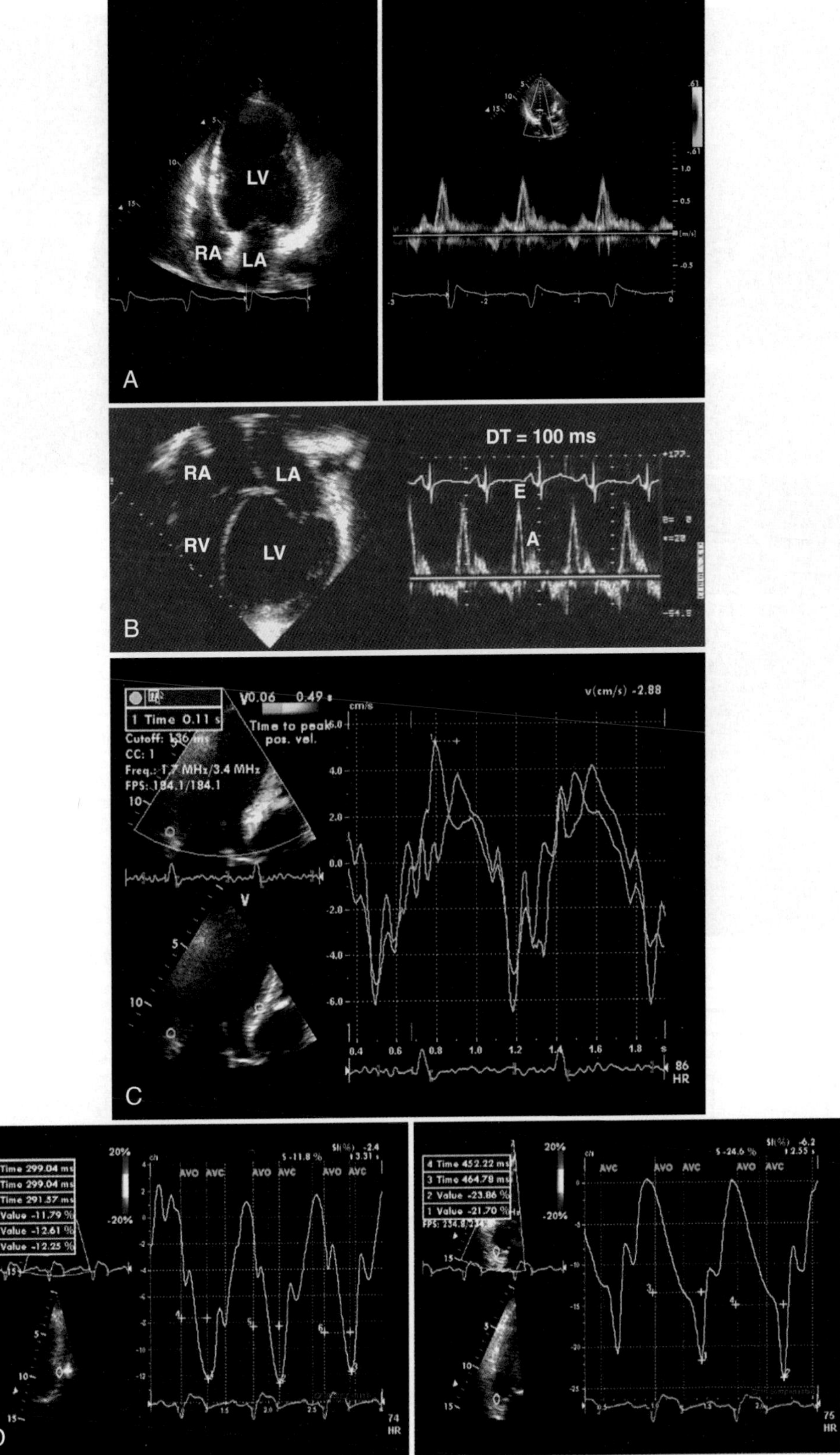

FIGURE 15-64 A, Apical four-chamber view **(left)** and pulsed-wave Doppler velocity recording of mitral valve inflow **(right)** in a patient with dilated ischemic cardiomyopathy showing a relaxation abnormality pattern with increased A velocity. Patients with this type of diastolic filling pattern usually have minimal to mild symptoms, despite severe LV systolic dysfunction. **B,** In this patient with dilated cardiomyopathy, the MV inflow velocity pattern shows restrictive physiology, with a markedly decreased A velocity and an increased E/A ratio. Deceleration time (DT) of mitral E velocity is shortened. Patients with this type of diastolic filling have increased filling pressure and symptomatic congestive heart failure. **C,** Tissue Doppler velocity recordings from the basal septal (yellow) and basal lateral (blue) walls. Septal peak velocity occurs first, then lateral peak velocity. The timing difference (+----+) is 110 milliseconds, indicating dyssynchronous contraction. **D,** Intraventricular dyssynchrony can be measured with strain imaging, which we prefer. **Left,** Strain recording from the basal septal wall. The time from the onset of QRS to peak negative strain (when the maximum contraction occurs) is measured from three cardiac cycles. The time intervals measured for the three cycles are 299, 299, and 291 milliseconds. **Right,** Strain recording from the basal lateral wall. The peak strain occurs after aortic valve closure (AVC), which is termed postsystolic shortening. The time interval measured from the onset of QRS to peak negative is 452 and 464 milliseconds, much later than that of the septal wall. The timing difference between the septal and lateral segments is more than 150 milliseconds, indicating marked dyssynchrony. AVO = aortic valve opening; LA = left atrium; LV = left ventricle; RA = right atrium; RV = right ventricle. *(**B** modified from Oh JK, Seward JB, Tajik AJ: The Echo Manual. 3rd ed. Philadelphia, Lippincott Williams & Wilkins, 2006. Used with permission of Mayo Foundation for Medical Education and Research.)*

- Diastolic function is normal (Ea >7 cm/sec).
- Tissue Doppler velocities and strain values are normal.

Restrictive Cardiomyopathy (see Chap. 68)

Early in the disease, LV systolic function is usually preserved, but diastolic function is abnormal, which causes increased atrial pressures and marked biatrial enlargement. The characteristic features of primary restrictive cardiomyopathy on two-dimensional echocardiography include normal ventricular cavity size, normal wall thicknesses, and usually preserved global systolic function, with biatrial enlargement (**Fig. 15-68**). Restrictive cardiomyopathy is accompanied by restrictive diastolic filling, but this is a nonspecific finding. The typical LV diastolic pressure tracing in restrictive

CH 15

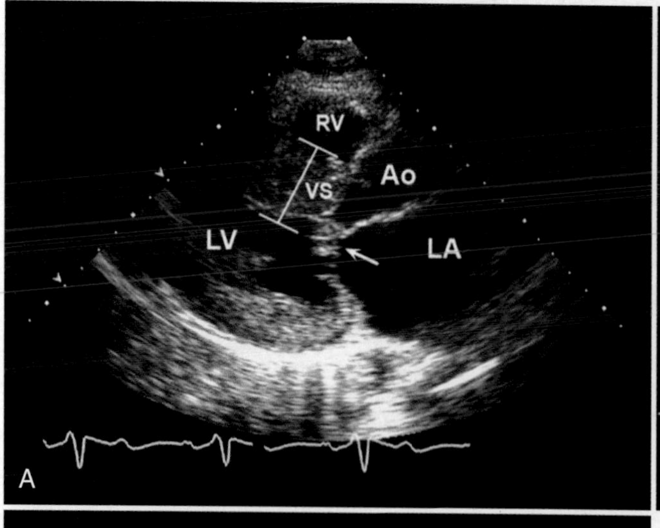

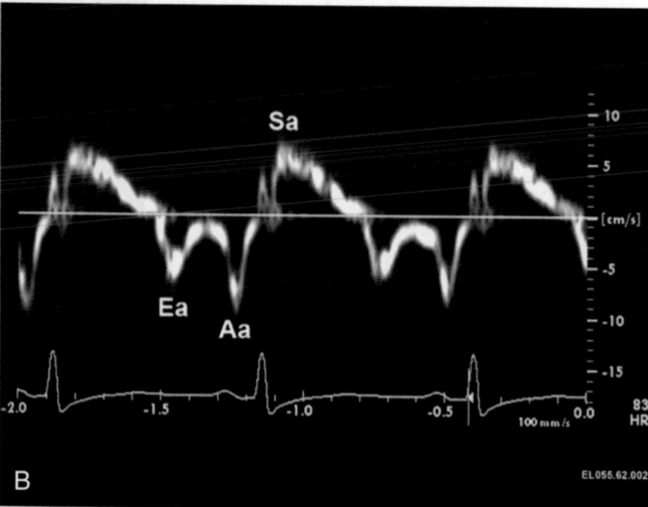

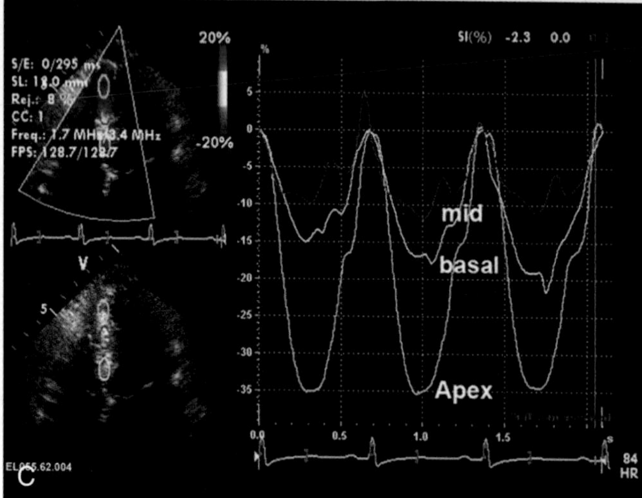

FIGURE 15-65 **A,** Two-dimensional echocardiogram of hypertrophic obstructive cardiomyopathy (systolic frame). The ventricular septum (VS) is markedly thickened (25 mm) and has an abnormal myocardial texture. Systolic anterior motion of the anterior mitral leaflet is shown, contributing to the obstruction of the left ventricular outflow tract (arrow). Ao = aorta; LA = left atrium; LV = left ventricle; RV = right ventricle. **B,** Septal mitral annulus velocity recording by tissue Doppler imaging in a 28-year-old asymptomatic patient with family history of hypertrophic cardiomyopathy. Early diastolic velocity (Ea) is reduced to 6 cm/sec. Sa indicates systolic and Aa indicates late diastolic tissue Doppler velocities. **C,** Strain from midseptum (red curve with peak negative strain of 10%) is markedly reduced and apical strain (blue curve with 35%) is increased.

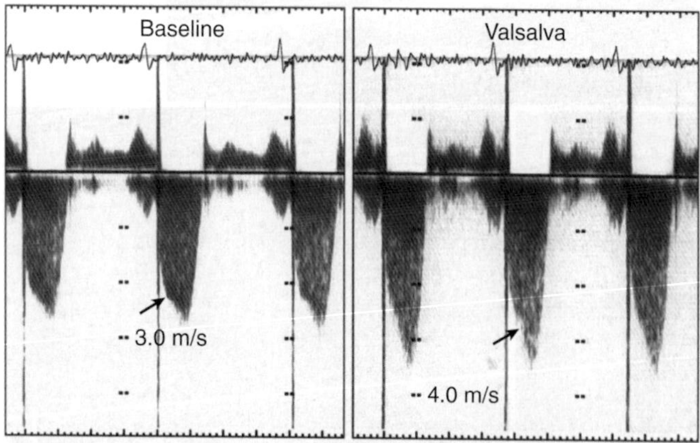

FIGURE 15-66 Continuous-wave Doppler spectra obtained from the apex showing dynamic LVOT obstruction in hypertrophic cardiomyopathy. Note the typical late-peaking configuration resembling a dagger or ski slope (arrow). The baseline **(left)** velocity is 2.8 m/sec, corresponding to the peak LVOT gradient of 31 mm Hg (= 4 × 2.8^2). With the Valsalva maneuver **(right)**, the velocity increased to 3.5 m/sec, corresponding to the gradient of 50 mm Hg. *(Modified from Oh JK, Seward JB, Tajik AJ: The Echo Manual. 3rd ed. Philadelphia, Lippincott Williams & Wilkins, 2006. Used with permission of Mayo Foundation for Medical Education and Research.)*

cardiomyopathy is the dip and plateau or square root configuration, which corresponds to shortened DT of the mitral inflow E velocity. The increase in LA pressure causes (1) the mitral valve to open at a higher pressure, resulting in a decrease in IVRT; (2) an increased transmitral pressure gradient with associated increased mitral E velocity; and (3) a decrease in pulmonary venous flow velocity during systole and an increase during diastole (**Fig. 15-69**). With high LVEDP, the atrial contribution to ventricular filling is minimal, and A velocity is usually decreased (see Fig. 15-69), causing the E/A ratio to increase markedly (>2). In contrast to constrictive pericarditis, hepatic vein diastolic flow reversal is greater during inspiration (**Fig. 15-70**). Myocardial relaxation is universally impaired so that mitral annulus E′ velocity obtained from the septal annulus is usually less than 7 cm/sec.[116]

Arrhythmogenic Right Ventricular Dysplasia/Cardiomyopathy (see Chap. 68)

The Multidisciplinary Study of Right Ventricular Dysplasia group has reported two-dimensional echocardiographic findings of arrhythmogenic RV dysplasia from 29 patients.[117] The systolic and diastolic RVOT and RV inflow tract dimensions are increased, with diastolic RVOT enlargement being most common (RVOT diameter was >25 mm in all patients). An RVOT dimension greater than 30 mm from the parasternal long-axis view had the highest sensitivity (89%) and specificity (86%) for the diagnosis of arrhythmogenic RV dysplasia. RV function

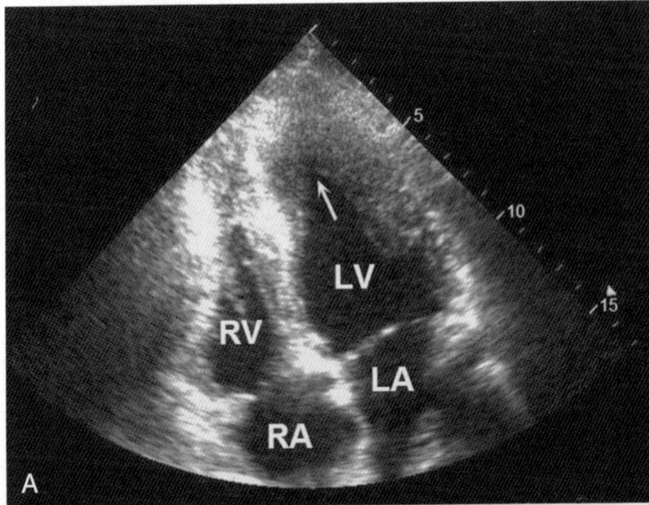

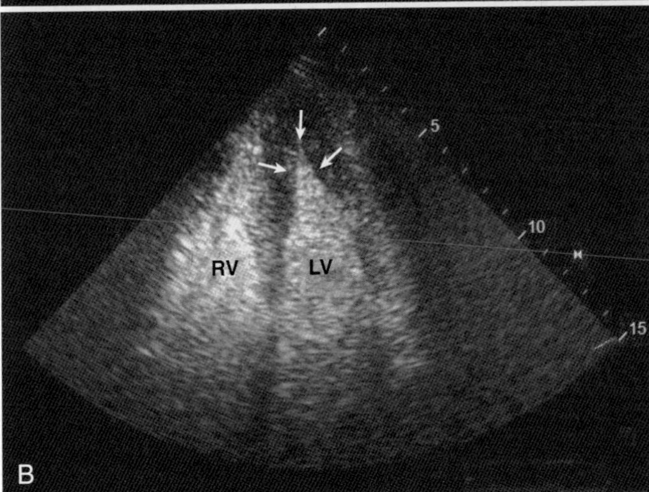

FIGURE 15-67 **A,** Two-dimensional apical four-chamber view during diastole in a patient with apical hypertrophic cardiomyopathy. The apical wall thickness during diastole is markedly increased (arrow), and the apical cavity is nearly obliterated except for a small slit during diastole. **B,** Two-dimensional apical four-chamber view with contrast shows apical hypertrophy and obliteration of the apical cavity (arrows). LA = left atrium; LV = left ventricle; RA = right atrium; RV = right ventricle.

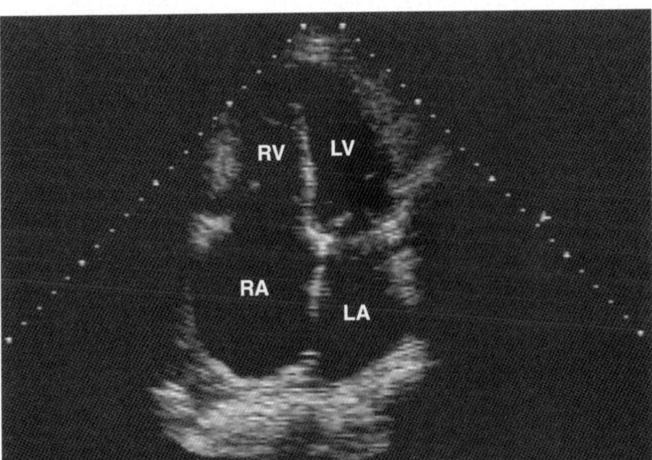

FIGURE 15-68 Apical four-chamber view of typical restrictive cardiomyopathy with normal LV cavity size, normal systolic function, and marked biatrial enlargement. LA = left atrium; LV = left ventricle; RA = right atrium; RV = right ventricle. *(Modified from Oh JK, Seward JB, Tajik AJ: The Echo Manual. 3rd ed. Philadelphia, Lippincott Williams & Wilkins, 2006. Used with permission of Mayo Foundation for Medical Education and Research.)*

was abnormal in 62%, and RV regional wall motion abnormalities were frequent, most commonly affecting the apex and anterior wall. RV trabecular derangements, hyperreflective moderator band, and sacculations were present in 54%, 34%, and 17%, respectively (see Fig. 15-e26 on website). In some patients, LV dilation and dysfunction also occur. The TR velocity is usually less than 2 m/sec, suggesting an RV systolic pressure in the low-normal range. Contrast echocardiography is useful in delineating RV morphology and contractility. CMR or CT for fat in the RV myocardium has been helpful in some patients (see Fig. 18-11).[118]

Noncompaction Cardiomyopathy (Isolated Ventricular Noncompaction)

Isolated ventricular noncompaction occurs from embryonic arrest of compaction, previously described as persistent intramyocardial sinusoids. It is characterized by segmental thickening of the LV wall consisting of a compacted epicardial layer and a thickened endocardial layer with marked trabeculations and deep intertrabecular recesses (**Fig. 15-71**; see Figs. 18-16 and 26-4). Complications related to noncompaction cardiomyopathy include heart failure (53%), thromboembolic events (24%), ventricular tachycardia (41%), and sudden death.

The following echocardiographic criteria for ventricular noncompaction have been reported:

- The absence of any coexisting cardiac anomalies
- The characteristic appearance of numerous, excessively prominent trabeculations and deep intertrabecular recesses
- Intertrabecular spaces filled by direct blood flow from the ventricular cavity, as visualized on color flow imaging
- An end-systolic ratio of noncompacted to compacted layers higher than 2

The ratio of noncompacted to compacted layers can be determined better with contrast enhancement (see Fig. 15-71). Predominant areas of the trabeculations in isolated ventricular noncompaction are midlateral, midinferior, and apical segments.[119]

Pericardial Diseases (see Chap. 75)

Detection of pericardial effusion was one of the first clinical applications of echocardiography, and echocardiography continues to be invaluable in the evaluation and management of various pericardial diseases. Pericardial effusion, tamponade, pericardial cyst, and absence of pericardium are readily recognized on two-dimensional echocardiography. The unique echocardiographic features of constrictive pericarditis and the use of TDI have added reliability and confidence to the noninvasive diagnosis of constrictive pericarditis and its differentiation from restrictive myocardial disease. Pericardiocentesis can be performed safely under the guidance of two-dimensional echocardiography.

Congenitally Absent Pericardium

Congenital absence of the pericardium demonstrates typical two-dimensional echocardiographic features. These include the appearance of RV cavity enlargement from the standard parasternal windows, mimicking the RV volume overload pattern on echocardiography (see Fig. 15-e27 on website; this finding is caused by shifting of the entire cardiac structure to the left); the displacement of the apical imaging window into the axilla (with the patient on the left side); and the appearance of compressed atria. Cardiac motion, especially the posterior wall of the left ventricle, is exaggerated. The diagnosis can be confirmed with CT or CMR (see Chaps. 18 and 19).[120]

Pericardial Cyst

A pericardial cyst is a benign fluid-filled abnormality of the pericardium that is usually detected as a mass lesion on chest radiography or as a cystic echo-free structure on two-dimensional echocardiography. Pericardial cysts are usually located on the right side (see Fig. 15-e28 on website), but they also are found in the left costophrenic angle, hilum, and superior mediastinum. They should be differentiated from tumors, cardiac chamber enlargement, and diaphragmatic hernia.

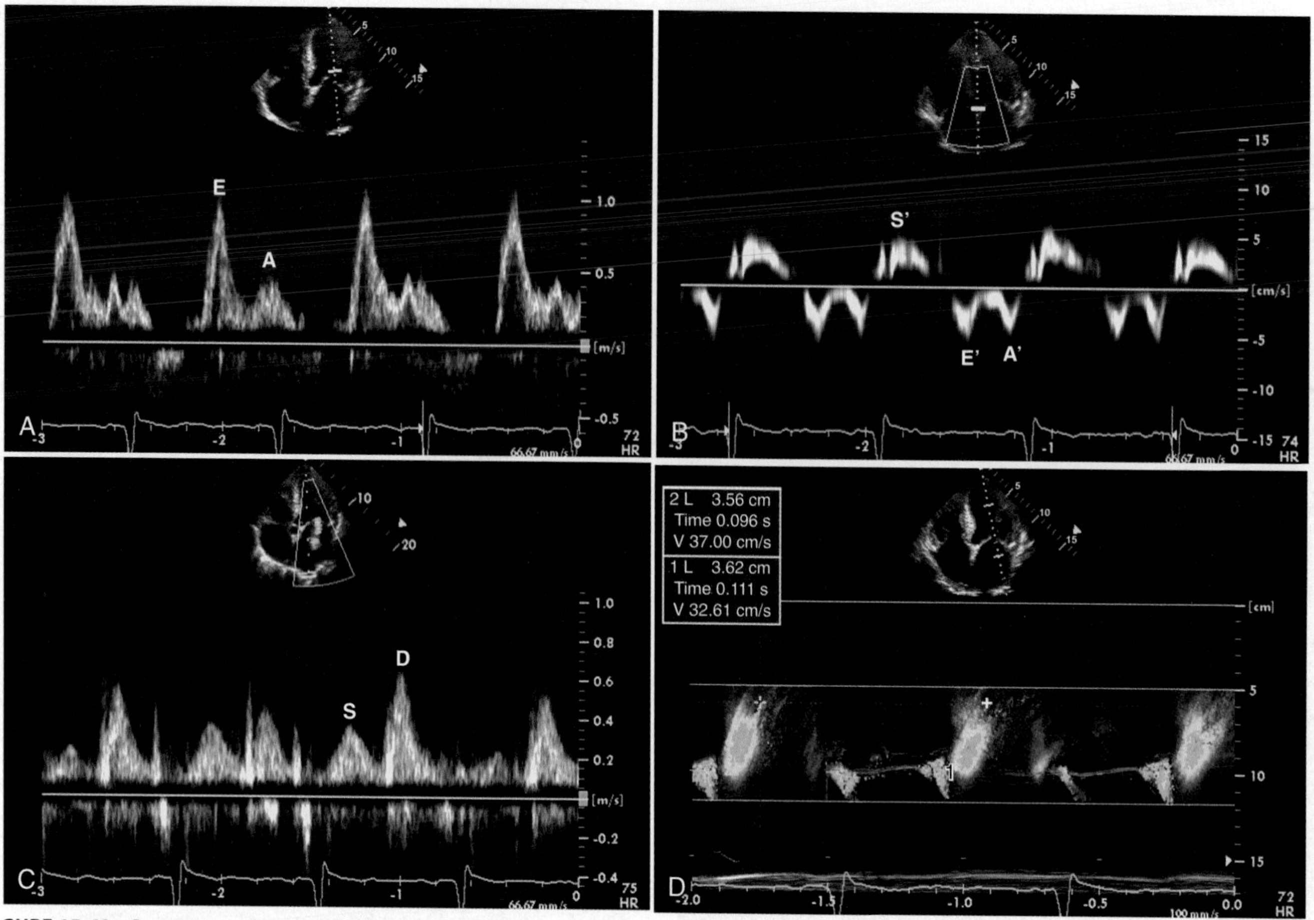

FIGURE 15-69 Restrictive cardiomyopathy. **A,** Mitral inflow. E/A ratio is higher than 2, and deceleration time is short. **B,** Tissue Doppler septal mitral annulus. E′ is decreased because of abnormal relaxation; S′ is also decreased. **C,** Pulmonary vein systolic velocity (S) is reduced and diastolic velocity (D) deceleration time is shortened. **D,** Color M-mode of mitral inflow velocity. Mitral inflow color propagation velocity (V) is reduced to 32 to 37 cm/sec. A = late diastolic mitral flow velocity; A′ = late diastolic mitral annulus velocity; E = early diastolic mitral flow velocity; E′ = early diastolic mitral annulus velocity; S′ = systolic velocity of mitral annulus.

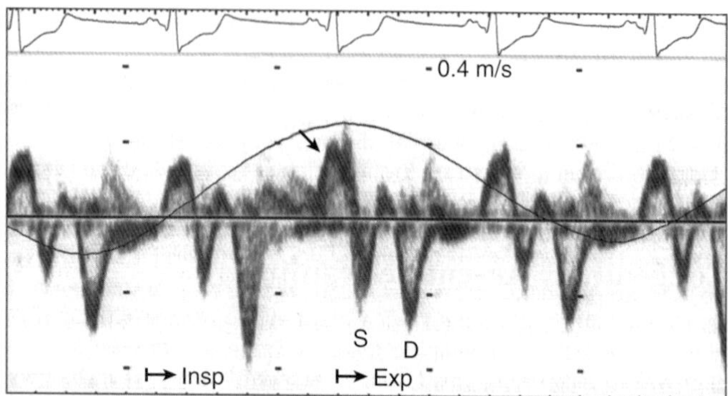

FIGURE 15-70 Hepatic vein pulsed-wave Doppler recording together with respirometer recording from a patient with restrictive physiology. Note the higher diastolic velocity (D) than systolic velocity (S) and greater reversal of diastolic flow during inspiration (Insp, arrow). Exp = expiration. *(Modified from Oh JK, Seward JB, Tajik AJ: The Echo Manual. 3rd ed. Philadelphia, Lippincott Williams & Wilkins, 2006. Used with permission of Mayo Foundation for Medical Education and Research.)*

Pericardial cysts also have a characteristic appearance on CT and CMR (see Fig. 15-e29B on website).

Pericardial Effusion and Tamponade

Pericardial effusion is detected as an echo-free space. In a large pericardial effusion, the heart may have a "swinging" motion in the pericardial cavity that causes the typical electrocardiographic manifestation of cardiac tamponade, electrical alternans (**Fig. 15-72**; see Fig. 75-7). M-mode and two-dimensional echocardiographic features caused by the characteristic hemodynamics of tamponade include (1) early diastolic collapse of the right ventricle and late diastolic RA inversion (see Figs. 75-8 and 75-9) related to increase of the intrapericardial pressure above the intracardiac pressures (diastolic collapse of the right side of the heart may not occur if right-sided heart pressure is elevated); (2) abnormal ventricular septal motion related to respiratory variation in ventricular filling; (3) respiratory variation in ventricle chamber size; and (4) plethora of the inferior vena cava with blunted respiratory changes. Clotted blood, or hemopericardium, may be seen in the pericardial sac of patients with myocardial rupture or proximal aortic dissection (see Fig. 15-e29 on website). Pneumopericardium, or air in the pericardial sac as a result of esophageal perforation, causes inadequate TTE and TEE imaging because ultrasound does not penetrate air well.

Pericardial and pleural effusions may be difficult to differentiate from each other. In the parasternal long-axis view, pericardial effusion is located anterior to the descending thoracic aorta, whereas a pleural effusion is posterior to the aorta (see Fig. 15-e30 on website). The presence of only an anterior echo-free space suggests an epicardial fat pad rather than pericardial effusion; a pericardial effusion is usually circumferential.

Doppler echocardiographic features of pericardial tamponade are more sensitive than the two-dimensional echocardiographic features. The Doppler findings of cardiac tamponade are based on the characteristic respiratory variations in intrathoracic and intracardiac hemodynamics (see Chap. 75).[1] Normally, intrapericardial pressure (hence, LA and LV diastolic pressures) and intrathoracic pressure (hence, PCWP) decrease the same degree during inspiration, but in cardiac

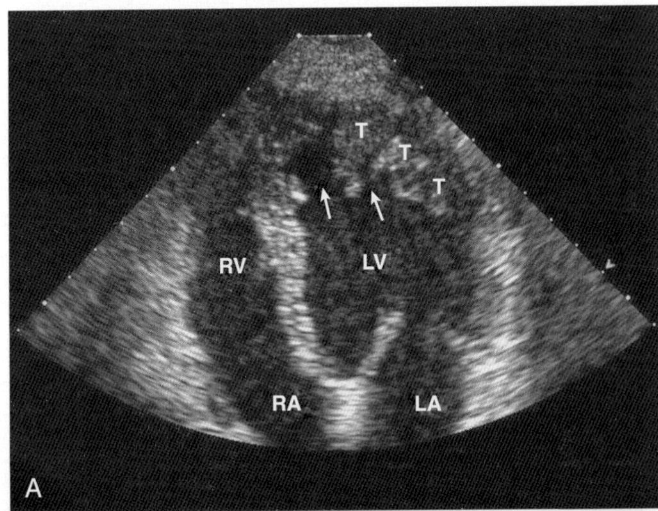

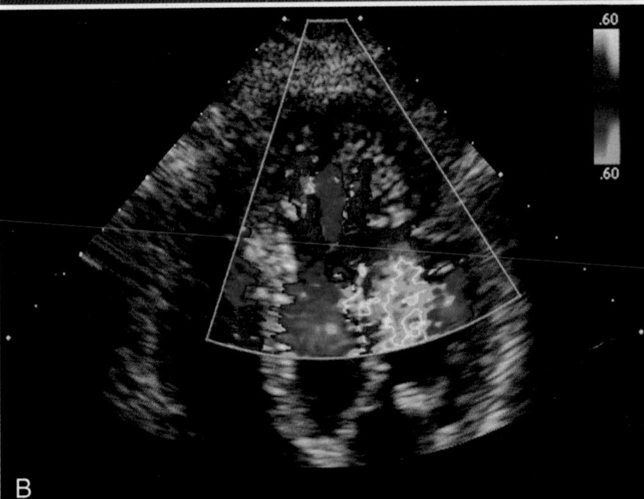

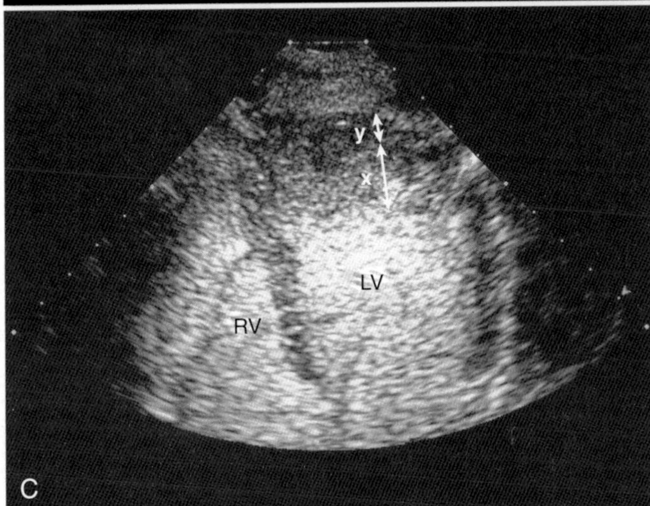

FIGURE 15-71 **A,** Apical four-chamber two-dimensional echocardiographic view showing characteristic increase in trabeculations (T) and deep recesses (arrows) in noncompaction cardiomyopathy. LA = left atrium; LV = left ventricle; RA = right atrium; RV = right ventricle. **B,** Color flow imaging showing flow into the intratrabecular recesses. **C,** Contrast administration shows trabeculations at the apex; the appearance is different from that of apical hypertrophic cardiomyopathy. With contrast enhancement, the ratio of noncompacted layer (x) to compacted layer (y) can be calculated. In this patient, x = 1.8 cm, y = 0.8 cm, with x/y = 2.3. *(Modified from Oh JK, Seward JB, Tajik AJ: The Echo Manual. 3rd ed. Philadelphia, Lippincott Williams & Wilkins, 2006. Used with permission of Mayo Foundation for Medical Education and Research.)*

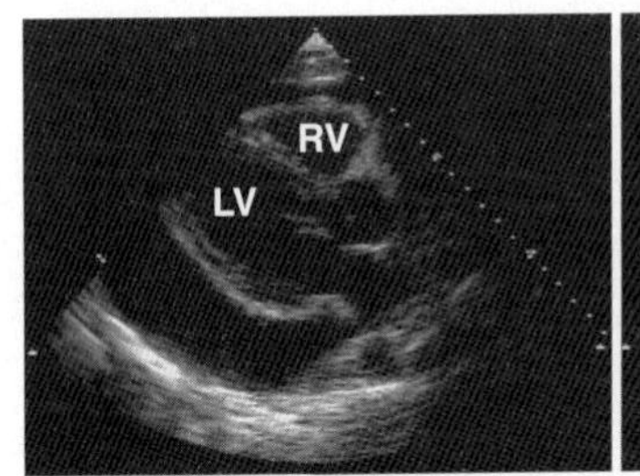

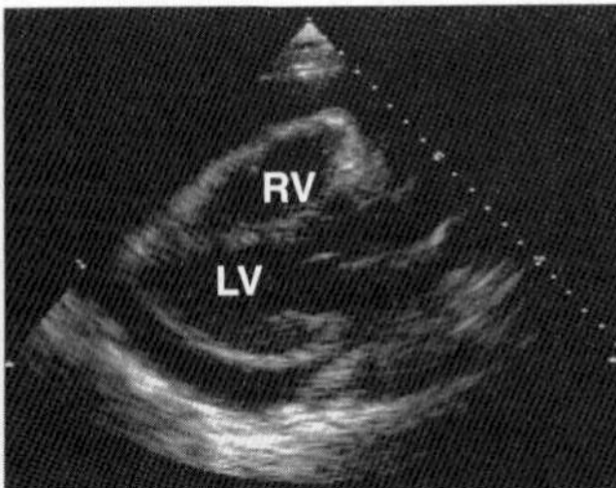

FIGURE 15-72 With a large amount of pericardial effusion, the heart has a swinging motion, which is an ominous sign of cardiac tamponade. When the LV cavity is close to the surface **(left)**, the QRS voltage increases on the electrocardiogram, but it decreases when the LV swings away from the surface **(right)**, producing electrical alternans. LV = left ventricle; RV = right ventricle. *(Modified from Oh JK, Seward JB, Tajik AJ: The Echo Manual. 3rd ed. Philadelphia, Lippincott Williams & Wilkins, 2006. Used with permission of Mayo Foundation for Medical Education and Research.)*

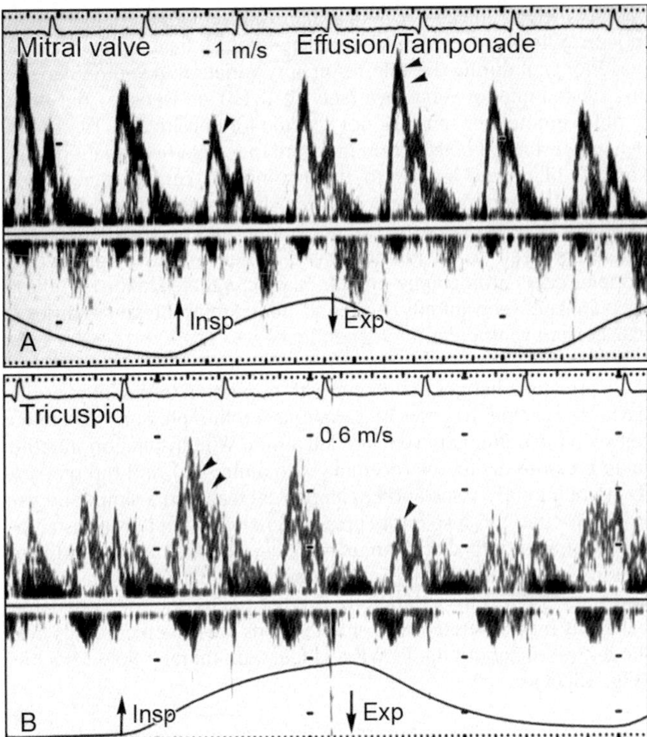

FIGURE 15-73 Typical pulsed-wave Doppler pattern of tamponade recorded with a nasal respirometer. **A,** Mitral inflow velocity decreases (single arrowhead) after inspiration (Insp) and increases (double arrowheads) after expiration (Exp). **B,** Tricuspid inflow velocity has the opposite changes. E velocity increases (double arrowheads) after inspiration and decreases (single arrowhead) after expiration. *(Modified from Oh JK, Hatle LK, Mulvagh SL, Tajik AJ: Transient constrictive pericarditis: Diagnosis by two-dimensional Doppler echocardiography. Mayo Clin Proc 68:1158, 1993. Used with permission of Mayo Foundation for Medical Education and Research.)*

tamponade, intrapericardial (and intracardiac) pressure falls substantially less than intrathoracic pressure. Therefore, the LV filling pressure gradient from PCWP to LV diastolic pressure decreases with inspiration. Consequently, mitral E velocity is reduced with inspiration. LV filling and mitral E velocity increase with expiration. In cardiac tamponade, the degree of ventricular filling depends on the other ventricle because of the relatively fixed combined cardiac volume (ventricular interdependence); thus, reciprocal changes occur in the right-sided heart chambers (**Fig. 15-73**). Increased venous return to the right-sided heart chambers with inspiration also contributes to the increased ventricular interdependence. The respiratory flow velocity changes

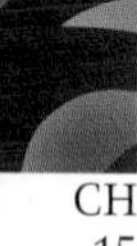

across the mitral and tricuspid valves are also reflected in the pulmonary and hepatic venous flow velocities, respectively: inspiratory decrease and expiratory increase in pulmonary vein diastolic forward flow and expiratory decrease in hepatic vein forward flow and increase in expiratory reversal flow.[1] In contrast, hepatic vein flow reversal occurs during inspiration in restrictive cardiomyopathy. Two-dimensional echocardiography can guide pericardiocentesis by locating the optimal site of puncture and by monitoring the results of the pericardiocentesis (see Chap. 75).

Constrictive Pericarditis

The pericardium is usually thickened in patients with constrictive pericarditis but may be normal in up to 20% of cases. Invasive hemodynamic features described initially (equalization of diastolic pressures) are similar to those of restrictive cardiomyopathy and other myocardial diseases. Improved understanding of the mechanism of constrictive pericarditis has allowed development of specific echocardiographic Doppler diagnostic criteria for constriction.[121] The M-mode and two-dimensional echocardiographic features of constrictive pericarditis include thickened pericardium, abnormal ventricular septal motion reflecting ventricular interdependence, flattening of the LV posterior wall during diastole, respiratory variation in ventricular size, and dilated inferior vena cava (see Fig. 15-e31 on website), but these findings are neither sensitive nor specific for constriction. The hemodynamic events of constriction in regard to respiratory variation in LV and RV filling are similar to the findings in cardiac tamponade, although the underlying pathologic mechanism is different. To establish the diagnosis of constrictive pericarditis, two hemodynamic characteristics need to be demonstrated either with two-dimensional Doppler echocardiography or with cardiac catheterization: (1) disassociation between intrathoracic and intracardiac pressures and (2) exaggerated ventricular interdependence.[1]

A thickened pericardium prevents full transmission of the intrathoracic pressure changes that occur with respiration to the intracardiac cavities, creating respiratory variations in the pressure difference between the pulmonary vein and left atrium. With inspiration, intrathoracic pressure decreases (normally 3 to 5 mm Hg), and the pressure in the pulmonary veins and capillaries decreases to a similar degree. In constriction, this inspiratory pressure change is not fully transmitted to the intrapericardial and intracardiac cavities. As a result, the driving pressure gradient for LV filling decreases immediately after inspiration and increases with expiration. This characteristic hemodynamic pattern is best illustrated with simultaneous pressure recordings from the left ventricle and the PCWP together with mitral inflow velocities (**Fig. 15-74**).[1]

Within the noncompliant, adherent pericardium, the combined ventricular volume is relatively fixed; thus, the diastolic filling of each ventricular chamber relies on the other, accounting for reciprocal respiratory changes in the filling of the ventricles in constrictive pericarditis (see Chap. 75). With inspiration, LV filling decreases and the ventricular septum shifts to the left, which allows increased RV filling. Consequently, tricuspid inflow E velocity and hepatic vein diastolic forward flow velocity increase. With expiration, LV filling increases, causing the ventricular septum to shift to the right, which limits RV filling. Tricuspid inflow decreases and hepatic vein diastolic forward flow decreases, with notable flow reversals during diastole. When the Doppler features for constrictive pericarditis were described initially, respiratory variation of 25% or more in the mitral inflow E velocity and increased hepatic vein diastolic flow reversal with expiration were proposed as diagnostic criteria for constrictive pericarditis (**Fig. 15-75**). However, it is now recognized that up to 50% of patients with constrictive pericarditis have less than 25% respiratory variation in mitral E velocity.[116] Because LA pressure is markedly elevated, the respiratory variation in mitral E velocity becomes more blunted. Therefore, the lack of respiratory variation in mitral inflow velocities should not exclude the diagnosis of constrictive pericarditis. Hepatic vein flow reversal at the beginning of expiration continues to be a reliable diagnostic feature, even in AF (**Fig. 15-76**; see Fig. 75-10). Mitral annulus velocity recorded with TDI has become a valuable Doppler parameter in establishing the diagnosis of constriction[116] and in differentiating it from myocardial disease or restrictive cardiomyopathy (**Fig. 15-77**). Myocardial relaxation is relatively well preserved in constriction unless the myocardium is also involved, as in radiation heart injury. The longitudinal motion, hence mitral septal annulus velocity, is well preserved in constriction (Ea >7 cm/sec) and increases further as the constriction becomes worse with higher filling pressure, paradoxical to its change in myocardial disease. This phenomenon has been termed annulus paradoxus.[1] Normally, the lateral mitral annulus velocity is higher than the medial mitral annulus velocity. In constrictive pericarditis, the lateral annulus is adherent to the constricted pericardium; thus, it is frequently lower than the medial annulus.

Acute dilation of the heart, pulmonary embolism, RV infarct, pleural effusion, and chronic obstructive lung disease can produce respiratory Doppler changes similar to constrictive pericarditis, and most can be differentiated on the basis of clinical features. In addition, patients with chronic obstructive lung disease may have symptoms of right-sided heart failure similar to constrictive pericarditis and may be difficult to differentiate from those who have constrictive pericarditis. Respiratory variation in ventricular filling in chronic obstructive lung disease is related to increased respiratory effort causing marked reduction in intrathoracic pressure with inspiration. This is also manifested

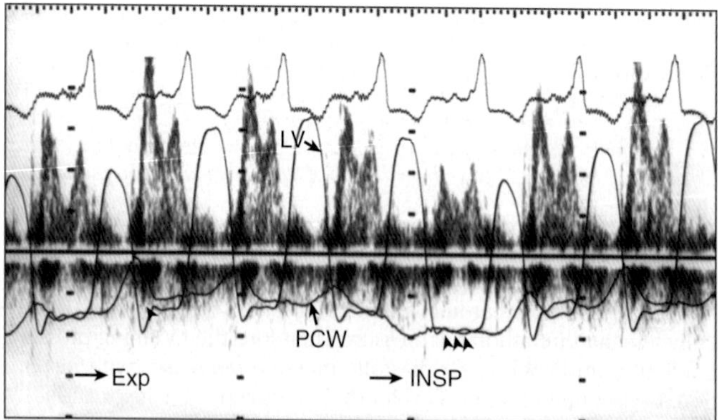

FIGURE 15-74 Constrictive perieardritis. Diagrams of left ventricular (LV) and pulmonary capillary wedge (PCW) pressure tracings to demonstrate dissociation between intrathoracic (or PCW) and intracardiac (or LV) pressure change with respiration (see text). Exp = expiration (single arrowhead); INSP = inspiration (triple arrowheads). *(Modified from Oh JK, Seward JB, Tajik AJ: The Echo Manual. 3rd ed. Philadelphia, Lippincott Williams & Wilkins, 2006. Used with permission of Mayo Foundation for Medical Education and Research.)*

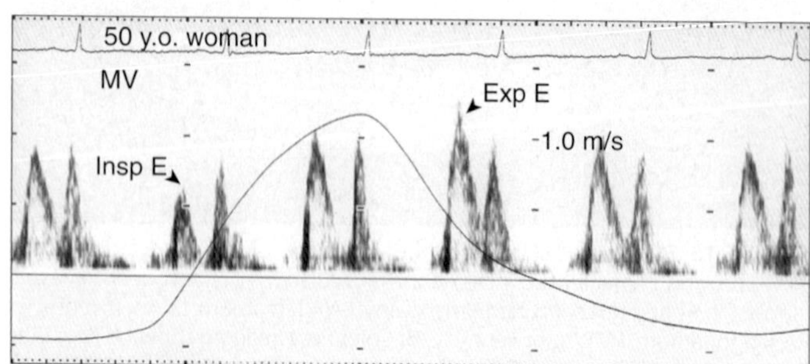

FIGURE 15-75 Typical mitral inflow pulsed-wave Doppler recordings in constrictive pericarditis along with simultaneous recording of respiration (onset of inspiration at upward deflection and onset of expiration at downward deflection). The first mitral inflow is at the onset of inspiration, and the fourth mitral inflow is soon after the onset of expiration. Mitral inflow E velocity is decreased with inspiration (first and sixth beats). MV = mitral valve. *(Modified from Oh JK, Seward JB, Tajik AJ: The Echo Manual. 3rd ed. Philadelphia, Lippincott Williams & Wilkins, 2006. Used with permission of Mayo Foundation for Medical Education and Research.)*

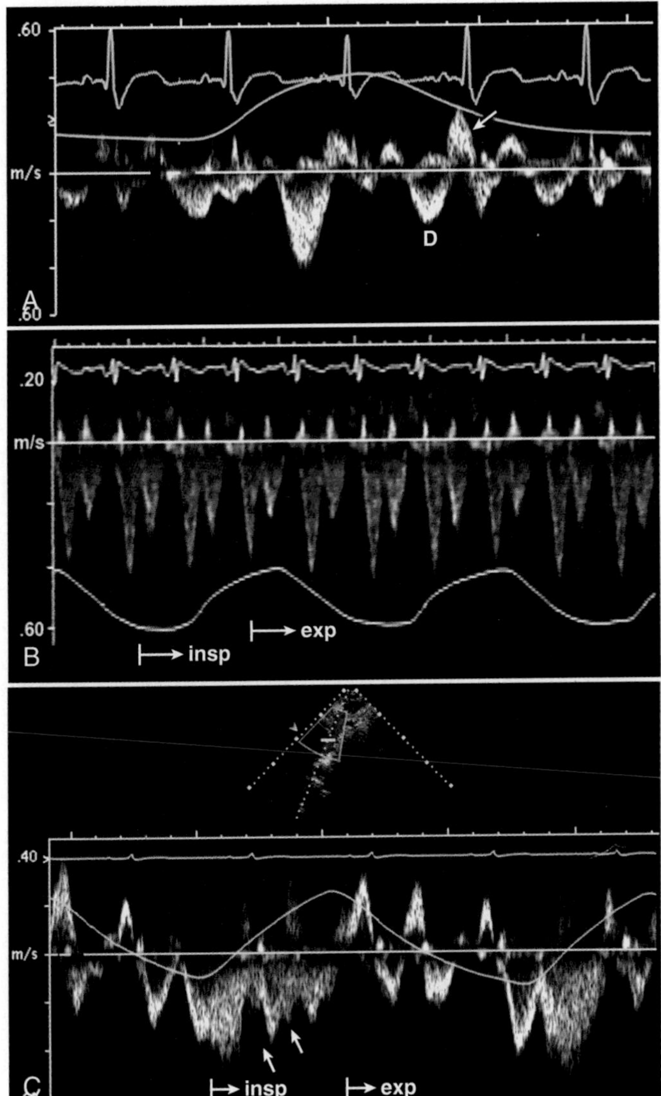

FIGURE 15-76 **A,** Pulsed-wave Doppler recording from the hepatic vein of a patient with advanced constrictive pericarditis. The hepatic vein has flow reversal after the onset of expiration (arrow), with decreased forward flow during diastole (D) compared with the flow velocities on inspiration. **B,** Superior vena cava velocity in constriction. There is no notable difference in systolic velocity with respiration. **C,** Superior vena cava velocity in chronic obstructive lung disease. There is marked increase in flow velocities (arrows) with inspiration (insp), then decrease with expiration (exp).

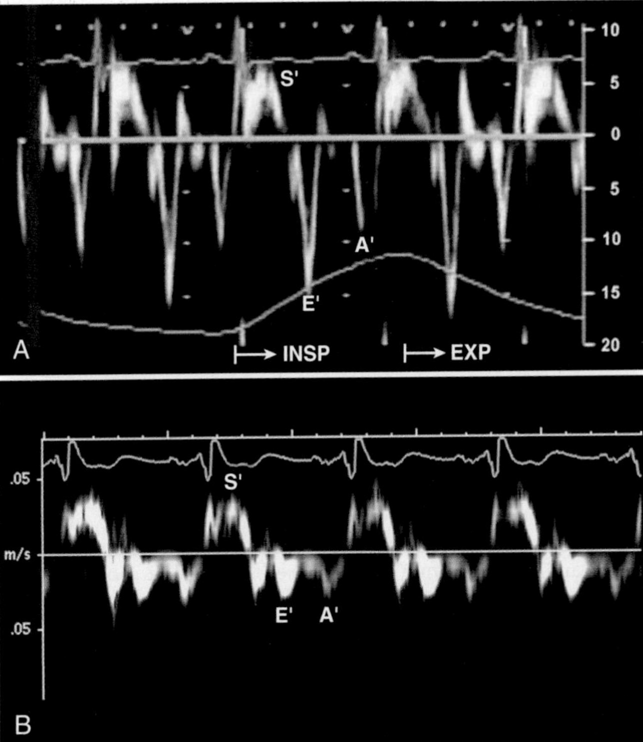

FIGURE 15-77 Tissue Doppler imaging of the septal mitral annulus in constriction **(A)** and restriction **(B)**. **A,** Early diastolic septal mitral annulus velocity (E′) is 12 cm/sec, indicating relatively normal or even greater than normal longitudinal motion of the mitral annulus. In patients with heart failure and increased jugular venous pressure, E′ velocity of 8 cm/sec or more should be equated with constrictive pericarditis until proven otherwise. **B,** E′ is markedly decreased in this patient with myocardial disease and heart failure. Decreased E′ correlates with abnormality in myocardial relaxation, which is reduced in almost all forms of cardiomyopathies. A′ = late diastolic septal mitral annulus velocity; EXP = expiration; INSP = inspiration; S′ = longitudinal systolic velocity. *(Modified from Oh JK, Seward JB, Tajik AJ: The Echo Manual. 3rd ed. Philadelphia, Lippincott Williams & Wilkins, 2006. Used with permission of Mayo Foundation for Medical Education and Research.)*

as a marked increase in forward flow velocity in the superior vena cava that is not present in patients with constrictive pericarditis (see Fig. 15-76).

AF makes the interpretation of respiratory variation in Doppler velocities difficult. Patients with constrictive pericarditis and AF still have typical two-dimensional echocardiographic features and require longer observation of Doppler velocities to detect velocity variation with respiration, regardless of underlying cardiac cycle length. Hepatic vein diastolic flow reversal with expiration is an important Doppler finding that suggests constrictive pericarditis, even when mitral inflow velocity pattern is not diagnostic.[1] On occasion, a temporary pacemaker is used to regularize the patient's rhythm in an attempt to evaluate the respiratory variation of Doppler velocities. Strain imaging may be able to add more diagnostic features useful in distinguishing pericardial from myocardial diastolic heart failure. Preliminary data suggest normal strain of the ventricular septum in constriction but decreased strain in myocardial diseases, especially at the basal septum.

Doppler echocardiographic features of constrictive pericarditis are summarized by the following:

1. restrictive mitral inflow velocity pattern with or without respiratory variation;
2. increased hepatic vein diastolic flow reversals with expiration;
3. mitral annulus septal Ea greater than 7 cm/sec;
4. less than 20 cm/sec respiratory variation in superior vena cava systolic velocity; and
5. normal strain imaging of the ventricular septum.

A subset of patients with constrictive pericarditis present with pericardial effusion. Patients usually present with clinical or hemodynamic evidence of increased filling pressures caused by a pericardial effusion, tamponade, or both.[55,122] However, constrictive hemodynamics persist even after removal or resolution of pericardial effusion and after intrapericardial pressure has normalized. This condition is called effusive-constrictive pericarditis (see Chap. 75). Most of these patients have inflammation of the pericardium that causes constriction; the constrictive hemodynamics resolve spontaneously or after treatment with anti-inflammatory agents. The condition has been termed transient constrictive pericarditis.[123] On occasion, the underlying constrictive pericarditis requires pericardiectomy.

Transient Constrictive Pericarditis

About 7% to 10% of patients with acute pericarditis have a transient constrictive phase. These patients usually have a moderate amount of pericardial fluid, and as the pericardial effusion disappears, the pericardium remains inflamed, thickened, and noncompliant, resulting in constrictive hemodynamics. The patient presents with features of chronic constrictive pericarditis, including dyspnea, peripheral edema, increased

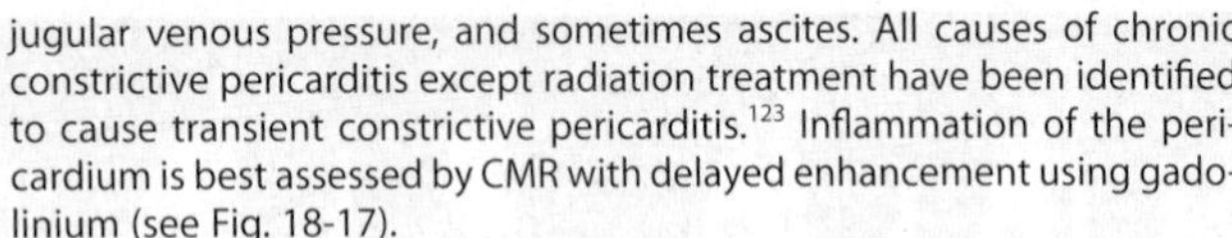

jugular venous pressure, and sometimes ascites. All causes of chronic constrictive pericarditis except radiation treatment have been identified to cause transient constrictive pericarditis.[123] Inflammation of the pericardium is best assessed by CMR with delayed enhancement using gadolinium (see Fig. 18-17).

Transesophageal Echocardiography in Pericardial Diseases

If TTE does not provide adequate imaging of the pericardium and hemodynamic assessment of ventricular filling, TEE should be considered. A loculated pericardial effusion may be difficult to detect on TTE, and TEE has been especially helpful postoperatively in patients with loculated hemopericardium as a cause of tamponade. TEE also provides useful pulmonary venous flow pulsed-wave Doppler velocities with simultaneous respirometer recording, which may be helpful in the evaluation of constrictive pericarditis. Furthermore, TEE is helpful in measuring the thickness of the pericardium.

Cardiac Diseases Caused by Systemic Illness

Multiple systemic disorders, genetic diseases, chemicals, acute illnesses such as sepsis, and medications can cause morphologic, functional, and hemodynamic abnormalities of the heart. Table 15-e1, on the website, lists various cardiac manifestations of systemic illnesses frequently seen in the echocardiography laboratory.

Amyloidosis (see Chap. 68)

Myocardial infiltration is primarily interstitial in amyloidosis, and an increase in myocardial wall thickness without dilation of the LV cavity is the predominant morphologic feature. However, normal wall thickness does not exclude the diagnosis. Amyloid deposits can affect most cardiac structures, such as the valves, thus causing multivalvular regurgitation. Amyloid deposition in the myocardium causes a characteristic sparkling appearance on two-dimensional echocardiography (**Fig. 15-78**). Importantly, the sparkling appearance alone is not diagnostic of cardiac amyloidosis; it occurs commonly with harmonic imaging or in other conditions such as hypertensive disease (especially in patients with renal failure), glycogen storage disease, and HCM.

During an early stage of cardiac amyloidosis, systolic function can be hyperdynamic, and SAM of the mitral valve with intracavitary obstruction may be present, similar to HCM. The initial diastolic abnormality in cardiac amyloidosis is abnormal relaxation (grade 1 diastolic dysfunction) resulting from increased ventricular wall thickness. As amyloid infiltration progresses, systolic function gradually deteriorates and the diastolic filling pattern becomes restrictive (grade 3-4 diastolic dysfunction), decreasing LV compliance and increasing LA pressure. Diastolic function is an important prognostic variable in cardiac amyloidosis (**Fig. 15-79**; see Fig. 26-31). The shorter the DT, the poorer the prognosis; the average survival for patients with a DT of 150 milliseconds or lower is less than 1 year, compared with 3 years if DT is higher than 150 milliseconds. TDI demonstrates decreased systolic and early diastolic velocities of the mitral annulus (usually <6 cm/sec) in cardiac amyloidosis (Fig. 15-79C). Color M-mode imaging of mitral inflow may not show delayed propagation despite marked abnormality in myocardial relaxation because of the small LV cavity. However, the longitudinal myocardial velocity gradient ([myocardial velocity at the base – myocardial velocity at mid left ventricle]/[distance between two sample sites]) appears to identify patients with heart failure.[124]

Recent data suggest increased risk of intracardiac thrombus detected by TEE in patients with amyloidosis.[125]

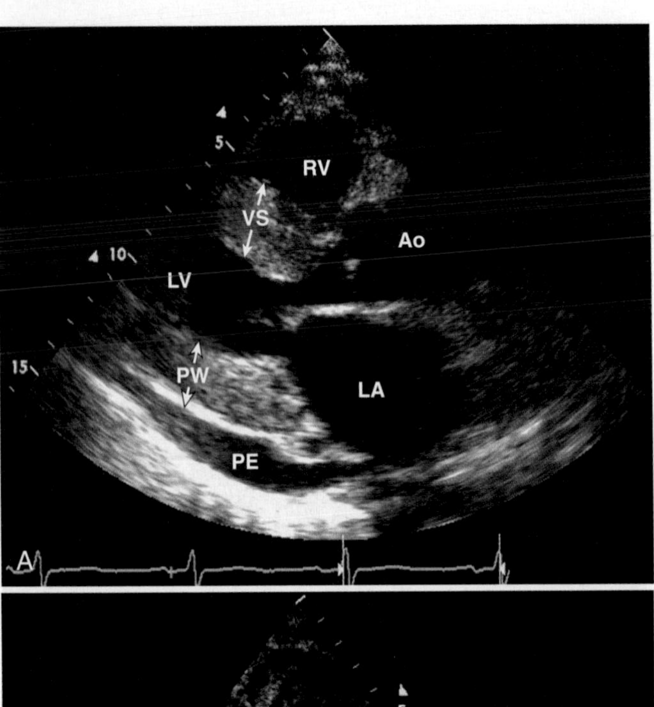

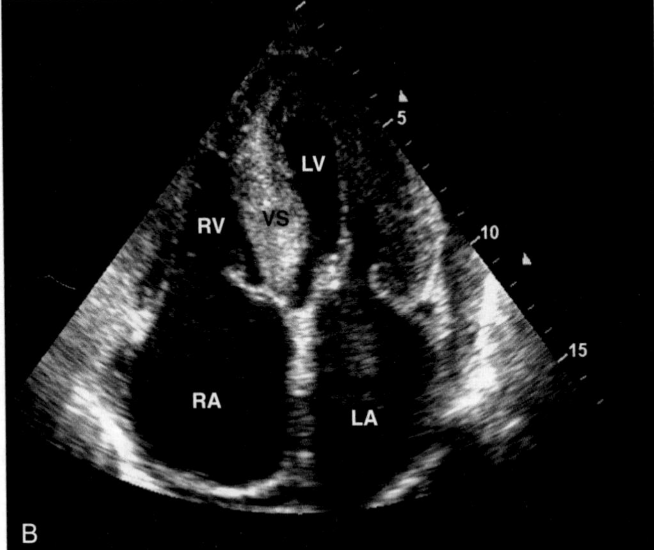

FIGURE 15-78 **A,** Parasternal long-axis view showing typical findings in cardiac amyloidosis: concentric increase in LV wall thickness, sparkling granular appearance of the myocardium, and thickened valve leaflets. Arrows indicate 23-mm-thick ventricular septum (VS) and 19-mm-thick posterior wall (PW). There is a small pericardial effusion (PE). **B,** Apical four-chamber view showing marked increase in VS wall thickness and marked dilation of both atria. Ao = aorta; LA = left atrium; LV = left ventricle; RA = right atrium; RV = right ventricle. *(Modified from Oh JK, Seward JB, Tajik AJ: The Echo Manual. 3rd ed. Philadelphia, Lippincott Williams & Wilkins, 2006. Used with permission of Mayo Foundation for Medical Education and Research.)*

Carcinoid Disease (see Chaps. 66 and 68)

Cardiac involvement in carcinoid tumors predominantly affects the endocardium and valves on the right side of the heart because the tumor substances are inactivated by the lung.[126] Left-sided valve disease is noted in 7% of cases and is usually related to a PFO, which allows the tumor substances to pass from the right atrium to the left atrium, or less commonly to high circulating levels of serotonin or to pulmonary metastasis. The characteristic tricuspid and pulmonary valve thickening causes restricted motion of the valves and secondary severe tricuspid valve regurgitation (see Figs. 15-e17 and 15-e18 on website; see Fig. 66-39), minimal tricuspid stenosis, and various degrees of pulmonic stenosis and regurgitation.

Characteristic two-dimensional echocardiographic features demonstrate tricuspid valve thickening and retraction, with limited mobility. Coaptation is incomplete, resulting in severe TR that produces an RV volume overload pattern. The pulmonary valve thickening and retraction result in mixed pulmonic stenosis and regurgitation; the pulmonary valve is characteristically difficult to image with TTE (see Fig. 15-57); however, Doppler and color flow imaging readily outlines hemodynamic features. Doppler recordings from the tricuspid and pulmonic valves demonstrate severe valve regurgitation and rapid rise in RV diastolic pressure. Liver metastasis and hepatic vein Doppler systolic flow reversal from severe TR are important features noted on

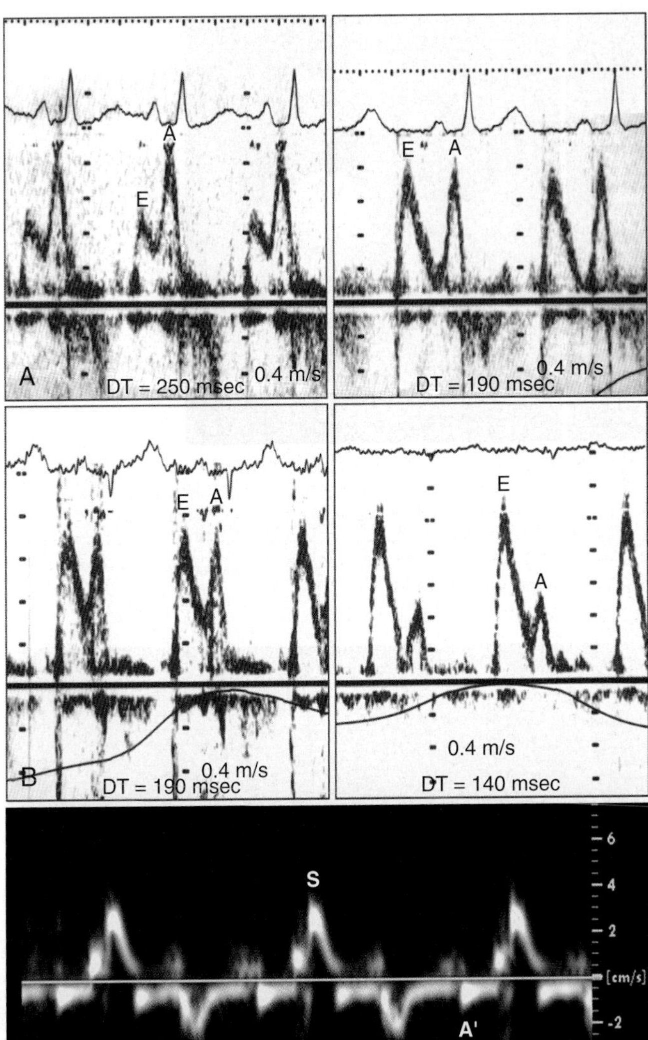

FIGURE 15-79 Serial mitral inflow Doppler velocities from two patients with cardiac amyloidosis. **A,** The initial Doppler study **(left)** showed a relaxation abnormality, with decreased E, increased A, and prolonged deceleration time (DT). Six months later **(right)**, it had become pseudonormalized, with progressive cardiac amyloidosis. **B,** In another patient, the initial study **(left)** showed a DT of 190 milliseconds, with normal E and A. Seven months later **(right)**, the mitral inflow became typical of a restrictive pattern (increased E, decreased A, and decreased DT), indicating that the initial Doppler pattern was of pseudonormalized inflow. **C,** Tissue Doppler imaging of mitral annulus in a patient with cardiac amyloidosis. Longitudinal systolic (S) and diastolic (E′ and A′) velocities are decreased: S′ = 3.4 m/sec, E′ = 2.5 cm/sec, and A′ = 1 cm/sec. *(**A** and **B** modified from Klein AL, Hatle LK, Taliercio CP, et al: Serial Doppler echocardiographic follow-up of left ventricular diastolic function in cardiac amyloidosis. J Am Coll Cardiol 16:1135, 1990. Used with permission. **C** modified from Oh JK, Seward JB, Tajik AJ: The Echo Manual. 3rd ed. Philadelphia, Lippincott Williams & Wilkins, 2006. Used with permission of Mayo Foundation for Medical Education and Research.)*

subcostal imaging. Carcinoid also may produce a metastatic tumor embedded in the myocardium (see Fig. 15-e32 on website).

The two-dimensional echocardiographic features of carcinoid heart disease are distinctive and readily distinguishable from other lesions producing right-sided heart failure. Rarely, cardiac valvular lesions resembling carcinoid involvement may develop with excessive use of appetite suppressants, ergot, or pergolide (see later).

Drug-Induced Cardiac Diseases

Drugs have been identified as responsible agents for myocardial, valvular, and pericardial abnormalities. The chemotherapy agent doxorubicin (Adriamycin) causes LV dilation and systolic dysfunction that usually occurs after a dose of more than 450 g/m^2 and may not be reversible (see Chaps. 73 and 90). Cardiac toxicity is dose related and potentiated by concurrent or previous radiotherapy. Daunorubicin (>600 mg/m^2) and cyclophosphamide (>6.2 g/m^2) cause a similar cardiomyopathy. Pericardial effusion or tamponade may also develop after cyclophosphamide treatment.

Cardiac valves may be affected by drug toxicity. Ergot alkaloids, appetite suppressants (see Fig. 15-e33 on website), and pergolide may produce valvular lesions similar to those of rheumatic or carcinoid valve disease.[127] The two-dimensional echocardiographic findings are similar to those of rheumatic valve disease, but microscopic examination shows fibrous plaque stuck on relatively normal valve tissue.

Hypereosinophilic Syndrome (see Chap. 68)

Cardiac involvement in hypereosinophilic syndrome involves thrombotic-fibrotic obliteration of the ventricular apices and endocardial thickening of the inflow areas. The majority of patients (>50%) with hypereosinophilia have characteristic echocardiographic findings, including limited motion of the posterior mitral leaflet resulting in MR, thickening of the inferobasal LV wall, endocardial thrombotic-fibrotic lesion, and biventricular apical obliteration by thrombus. Myocardial contrast imaging confirms apical thrombus (**Fig. 15-80**). Ventricular compliance is reduced, and ventricular diastolic filling is limited by apical cavity obliteration and eosinophilic endocardial involvement.

Renal Failure (see Chap. 93)

The predominant echocardiographic finding in patients with chronic renal failure is increased LV wall thickness related to LV hypertrophy from hypertension. The myocardial texture with LV hypertrophy appears similar to that of cardiac amyloidosis, but these two conditions can be distinguished by the QRS voltage on the electrocardiogram. In the early stage of chronic renal failure, systolic function is normal, but diastolic function is not because of decreased myocardial relaxation. As the disease progresses, LV systolic dysfunction occurs with decreased compliance of the myocardium, LV filling pressure increases, and the diastolic filling pattern becomes pseudonormalized or even restrictive. Small pericardial effusions are common, especially in patients undergoing chronic hemodialysis. Valvular sclerosis and mitral annulus and leaflet calcification are also common in chronic renal failure.

Sarcoidosis (see Chap. 68)

The two-dimensional echocardiographic features of myocardial involvement with sarcoidosis occur in less than 20% of sarcoid patients and include a dilated left ventricle with regional wall motion abnormalities, especially at the mid and basal levels of the left ventricle. Characteristically, the wall motion abnormalities do not correspond to a defined coronary distribution.

Sepsis

LV dilation and decreased LVEF are common in patients with sepsis and septic shock.[128] Echocardiography frequently shows a dilated left ventricle and decreased LVEF. Stroke volume may be maintained (normal LVOT TVI and velocity) or reduced. In patients who survive sepsis, LV dilation and systolic dysfunction are reversible. Certain infections result in characteristic cardiac and echocardiographic abnormalities: pericarditis in viral, bacterial, or tuberculosis infection; intracardiac mass in echinococcosis or tuberculosis; and ventricular aneurysm in Chagas disease.

Systemic Lupus Erythematosus (see Chap. 89)

Pericarditis is the most common cardiac manifestation and is found in more than two thirds of patients. Thus, one of the diagnostic criteria for systemic lupus erythematosus is the detection of pericardial effusion. The myocardium may be involved by vasculitis, resulting in myocarditis, but extensive LV diastolic dysfunction is rare. Another characteristic cardiac lesion is that of Libman-Sacks endocarditis (see Fig. 15-62).

Diseases of the Aorta (see Chap. 60)

Aortic Aneurysm

In general, aortic dilation is easily detected with TTE and TEE. When the ascending aneurysm reaches a diameter of more than 5 cm, there is increased risk of rupture, and replacement is generally indicated.[129,130] Smaller aneurysms require serial follow-up studies to measure the aorta at specific locations. Aortic root dilation, AR (**Fig. 15-81**), and

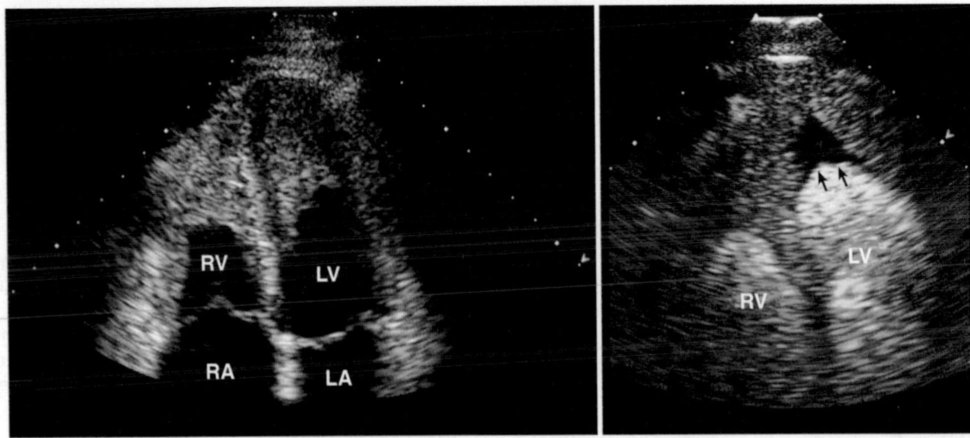

FIGURE 15-80 Apical four-chamber views in a patient with hypereosinophilic syndrome showing apical (both LV and RV) obliteration caused by deposits of thrombus and eosinophils. **Left,** Obliterative thrombus material is shown only in the apex of the left ventricle. This condition should be differentiated from apical hypertrophic cardiomyopathy, in which the apical cavity is obliterated by hypertrophied myocardium but still with a slitlike cavity inside the hyperdynamic myocardium. **Right,** Myocardial contrast shows black wedge-shaped thrombus (arrows) in the LV apex, which has good perfusion. It is very different from apical hypertrophic cardiomyopathy. LA = left atrium; LV = left ventricle; RA = right atrium; RV = right ventricle. *(Modified from Oh JK, Seward JB, Tajik AJ: The Echo Manual. 3rd ed. Philadelphia, Lippincott Williams & Wilkins, 2006. Used with permission of Mayo Foundation for Medical Education and Research.)*

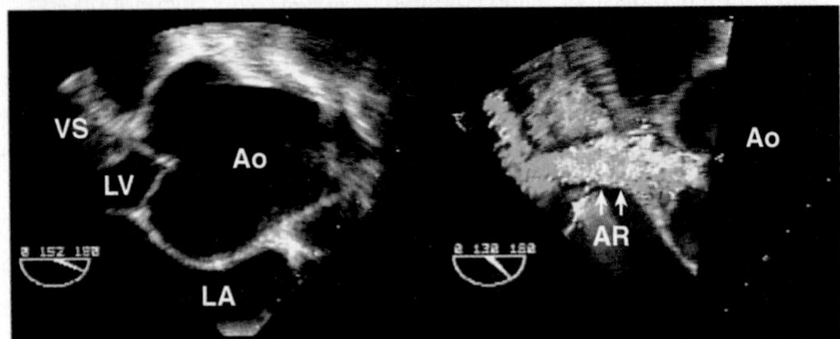

FIGURE 15-81 Multiplane transesophageal view of the aorta in a patient with Marfan syndrome. **Left,** Long-axis view of the aorta (Ao) with a transducer at 130 to 150 degrees showing the dilated sinus of Valsalva. **Right,** Color flow imaging of severe aortic regurgitation (AR, arrows). LA = left atrium; LV = left ventricle; VS = ventricular septum. *(Modified from Oh JK, Seward JB, Tajik AJ: The Echo Manual. 3rd ed. Philadelphia, Lippincott Williams & Wilkins, 2006. Used with permission of Mayo Foundation for Medical Education and Research.)*

aortic dissection are the most common cardiovascular findings in patients with Marfan syndrome and the ones of most concern.

Bicuspid Aortic Valve and Aortopathy (see Chaps. 60 and 66)

More than 50% of young patients with normally functioning bicuspid aortic valve disease have echocardiographic evidence of aortic root dilation. Aortic dilation should be monitored carefully with echocardiography.[131,132] The region of maximal dilation usually involves the mid ascending aorta (see Fig. 15-e34 on website) but may also involve the aortic sinuses. Comprehensive evaluation and monitoring with TTE is feasible in most patients. If these images are limited, alternative imaging should include TEE, CT, or CMR (see Chaps. 18 and 19). Aortic root replacement is recommended for patients with a bicuspid aortic valve whose aortic root size measures 5 cm or larger.[96]

Aneurysm of the Sinus of Valsalva

The localized absence of the media in the aortic wall results in aneurysm of the sinus of Valsalva (**Fig. 15-82**).[133] The parasternal and apical long-axis views are helpful in distinguishing this from an aneurysm of a membranous ventricular septum. A sinus of Valsalva aneurysm is located on the aortic side of the aortic valve, whereas an aneurysm of the membranous septum is located on the ventricular side of the aortic valve. These aneurysms can be distinguished confidently with comprehensive TTE and TEE examinations.

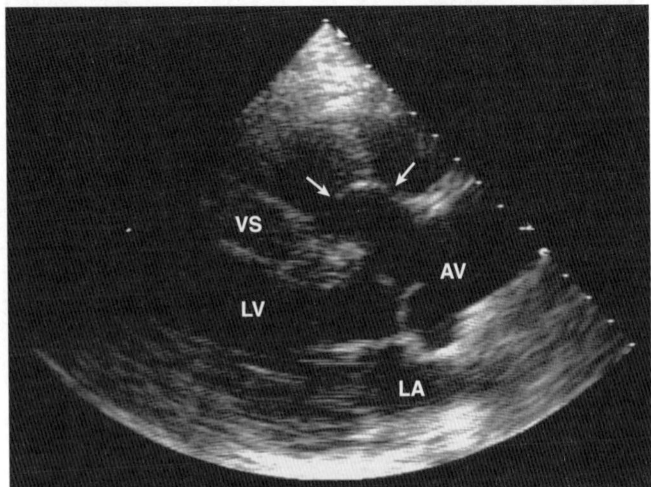

FIGURE 15-82 Transthoracic parasternal long-axis view of aneurysm (arrows) of the sinus of Valsalva. AV = aortic valve; LA = left atrium; LV = left ventricle; VS = ventricular septum. *(Modified from Meier JH, Seward JB, Miller FA Jr, et al: Aneurysms in the left ventricular outflow tract: Clinical presentation, causes, and echocardiographic features. J Am Soc Echocardiogr 11:729, 1998.)*

Atherosclerosis and Aortic Debris

On a routine TEE examination, atherosclerotic plaques and debris are common findings in elderly patients. Aortic plaques usually are irregularly shaped and frequently mobile (**Fig. 15-83**). The incidental detection of plaques in the aortic arch or proximal descending aorta is not associated with future vascular events.[134]

Aortic Dissection, Intramural Hematoma, and Aortic Ulcer (see Chap. 69)

Although most patients with aortic dissection have a dilated aorta on two-dimensional echocardiography, an intimal flap is often difficult to see on TTE (**Fig. 15-84**). Another limitation of TTE is the inability to visualize the descending thoracic aorta. Therefore, TTE is a rapid screening tool for aortic dissection, but negative findings or a suboptimal examination requires further diagnostic evaluation.

A good initial imaging modality for visualization of proximal aortic dissection is TEE. With TEE, the entire thoracic aorta can be visualized because of the intimate anatomic relation between the esophagus and

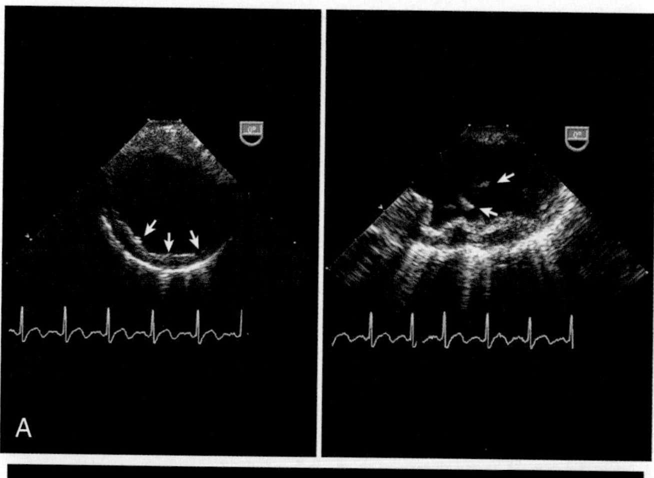

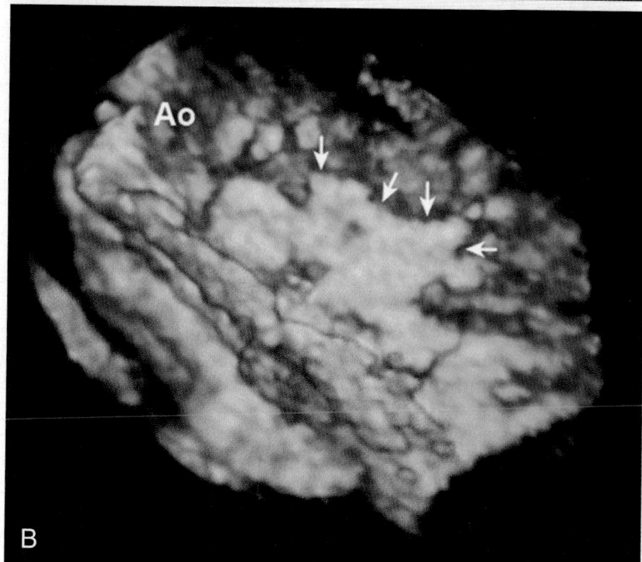

FIGURE 15-83 **A,** Transesophageal short-axis image of aortic debris in the descending thoracic aorta (**left,** arrows) and arch **(right)** with mobile irregular masses (in real time, arrows). This appearance is typical of an atherosclerotic plaque in the aorta. **B,** Aortic debris in the descending thoracic aorta (arrows) visualized by three-dimensional transesophageal echocardiographic imaging.

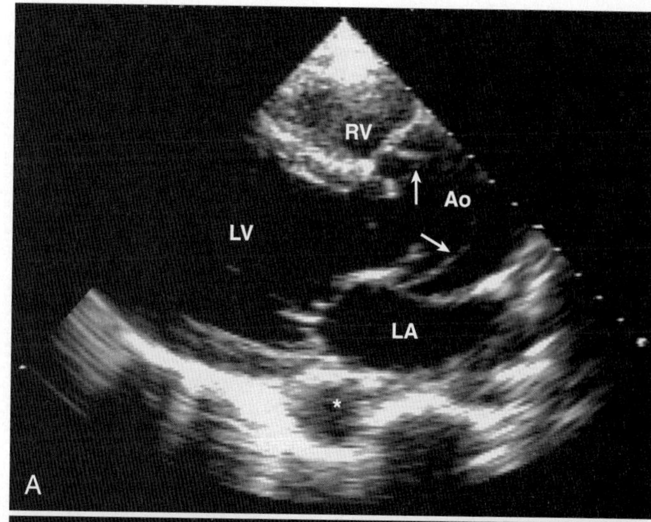

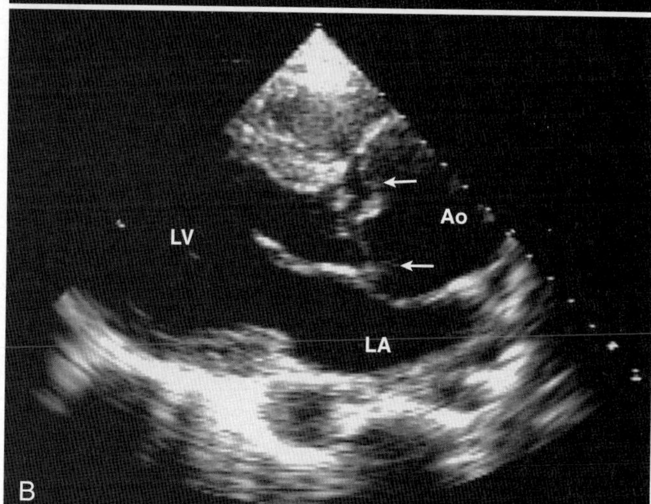

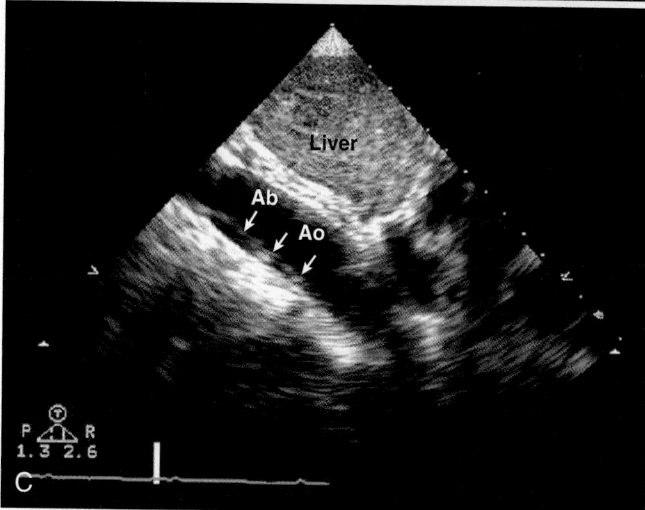

FIGURE 15-84 **A,** Transthoracic parasternal long-axis view showing a dilated ascending aorta and an undulating intimal flap in proximal aortic dissection. Systolic frame shows an intimal flap (arrows) in the aorta (Ao), which is dilated. The asterisk indicates the descending thoracic aorta, which is not dilated. **B,** Diastolic frame shows movement of the flap (arrows) toward the aortic valve. **C,** Abdominal aorta (Ab Ao) from the subcostal view also shows an intimal flap (arrows). LA = left atrium; LV = left ventricle; RV = right ventricle. *(Modified from Oh JK, Seward JB, Tajik AJ: The Echo Manual. 3rd ed. Philadelphia, Lippincott Williams & Wilkins, 2006. Used with permission of Mayo Foundation for Medical Education and Research.)*

thoracic aorta. In a horizontal transesophageal view, the distal portion of the ascending aorta and the proximal portion of the transverse aorta may not be well visualized because of the interposed trachea. However, this blind area on the horizontal plane can be visualized with the longitudinal view. With a clearer and more complete view of the entire aorta, TEE has changed the role of echocardiography in the diagnosis and management of aortic dissection (see Fig. 15-e35 on website; see Figs. 60-12 and 60-16).[1] The International Registry of Acute Aortic Dissection (IRAD) has reported imaging modalities used for diagnosis of aortic dissection. From an initial 13 international medical centers, 628 patients with acute aortic dissection were reviewed.[135] CT and TEE were the most common initial imaging tests for the diagnosis of aortic dissection.

The multicenter European Cooperative Study Group of Echocardiography was the first to demonstrate that TEE is equal to or even superior to CT and aortography for the diagnosis of aortic dissection (sensitivity, 99%). Subsequent studies validated the highly accurate diagnostic capability of TEE in aortic dissection. As TEE became more widespread in clinical use, its diagnostic sensitivity became slightly less. TEE or CT with contrast agent is the initial diagnostic procedure of choice for suspected aortic dissection. Although the diagnostic accuracy of CMR was reported by a small number of studies to be excellent, its clinical role is limited by the longer examination time, the difficulties with monitoring of patients during the procedure, and

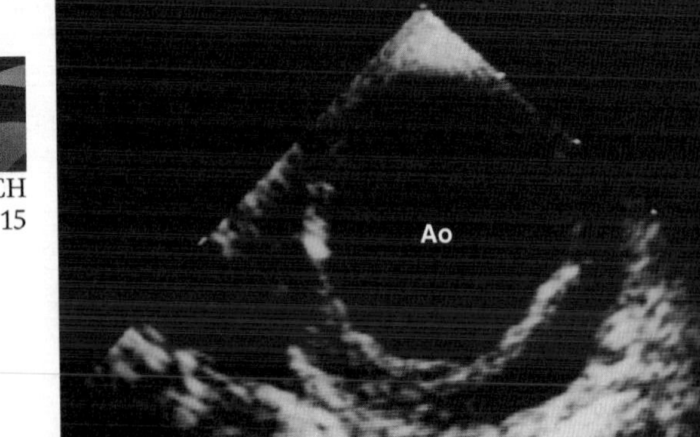

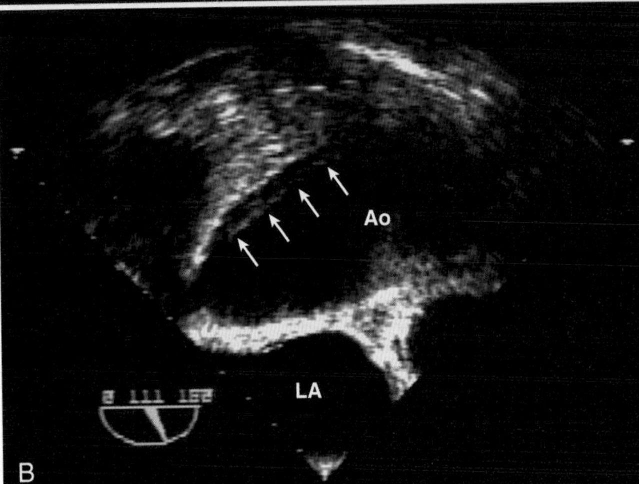

FIGURE 15-85 A, Transverse transesophageal view of the descending thoracic aorta (Ao) showing an intramural hematoma in a patient with hypertension and severe back pain. The soft tissue mass with a smooth surface appears different from aortic debris. During the next 6 months, the intramural hematoma disappeared while the patient was taking antihypertensive medications, including a beta blocker. **B,** Long-axis transesophageal view showing intramural hematoma in the ascending aorta (arrows). LA = left atrium. *(Modified from Oh JK, Seward JB, Tajik AJ: The Echo Manual. 3rd ed. Philadelphia, Lippincott Williams & Wilkins, 2006. Used with permission of Mayo Foundation for Medical Education and Research.)*

the remote location of the imaging facility from the emergency department.

Intramural hematoma is a precursor of aortic dissection. It is often associated with hypertension and advanced age. From 15% to 20% of patients with aortic dissection may present with intramural hematoma. It has been found to progress to aortic dissection or rupture in up to 45%.[136] Intramural hematoma has been reported to regress completely in 34% of patients, to progress to aortic dissection in 12%, to involve aneurysm in 20%, and to evolve to pseudoaneurysm in 24%. Intramural hematoma, best visualized on TEE, appears as increased echodensity along the wall of the aorta, corresponding to thrombus formation between the intima and the adventitia (**Fig. 15-85**; see Fig. 60-23). This should be differentiated from atheromatous plaque in the aorta, or aortitis. Intramural hematoma is also easily identified on CT and CMR (see Figs. 19-23B and 60-24), whereas aortography is the least valuable diagnostic modality.

Penetrating atherosclerotic aortic ulcer may result in intramural hematoma, aortic dissection, or aortic rupture and should be suspected in a hypertensive patient presenting with chest or back pain similar to that of aortic dissection. The ulcer is usually located in the descending aorta. With TEE, the penetrating aortic ulcer has a craterlike or focal outpouching appearance in an atherosclerotic aortic wall.

Aortitis (see Chaps. 60 and 89)

Aortitis is an inflammation of the aortic wall caused by infection (syphilitic or mycotic), giant cell arteritis, Takayasu disease, ankylosing spondylitis, rheumatoid arthritis, or relapsing polychondritis. Aortic involvement is usually an expression of the systemic nature of the underlying disease. Aortic wall thickness is increased, making it difficult to differentiate the TEE findings from those of intramural hematoma (see Fig. 15-e36 on website). Thoracic or abdominal aortic narrowing with obstruction may occur in patients with Takayasu disease. Syphilitic aortitis is uncommon but characteristically affects the ascending aorta.

Ankylosing spondylitis is characterized by aortic root thickening and dilation. Aortic regurgitation with dilation of the aorta is also seen in patients with Reiter syndrome, psoriatic arthritis, and Behçet syndrome.[137]

Cardiac Tumors and Masses (see Chap. 74)

The size, shape, location, mobility, and attachment site of a cardiac mass as well as the clinical presentation usually help in diagnostic differentiation. Accurate diagnosis is crucial, and misinterpretation may result in incorrect management, including an unnecessary surgical procedure.

Myxoma

The majority of myxomas occur in the left atrium, with attachment to the atrial septum (83% to 88%), but they have been identified in all other chambers and also attached to cardiac valves. Myxomas usually have a typical echocardiographic appearance characterized by a gelatinous and friable mass and occasionally central necrosis (**Fig. 15-86**; see also Fig. 74-1). Up to 7% of myxoma cases are familial, with the most notable condition being Carney syndrome, an autosomal dominant complex of cutaneous findings (including lentigines, ephelides, and blue nevi), cardiac myxomas (classically occurring before 40 years of age, with an atypical location, and often multiple), and endocrine abnormalities. This syndrome is caused by a gene defect on the long arm of chromosome 17. Although sporadic atrial myxomas usually are highly amenable to curative surgical resection, familial lesions frequently recur, often at locations distant from the initial site of resection. Complications associated with myxoma include embolic events occurring primarily with small myxomas, obstruction to inflow or outflow, systemic illness, and rarely metastases.

Fibroma

Fibromas are usually located in the LV free wall, in the ventricular septum, or at the apex. A fibroma is well demarcated from the surrounding myocardium by multiple calcifications (**Fig. 15-87**). Fibromas can grow into the LV cavity and interfere with ventricular filling or cause malignant arrhythmias. Also, fibromas can cause congestive heart failure. When it is located at the apex, a fibroma may be misinterpreted by other imaging modalities as apical HCM.

Papillary Fibroelastoma

Papillary fibroelastoma, or papilloma, is a benign intracardiac tumor with a characteristic appearance on echocardiograms. It is usually small (average size, <15 mm) and has a characteristic stippled edge, with a shimmering appearance at the tumor-blood interface. There are fingerlike projections consistent with the fronds that are described pathologically as a "sea anemone." The most frequent location is the aortic valve on either the aortic or ventricular surface (**Fig. 15-88**), followed by either the atrial or ventricular surface of the mitral valve.[138] Papillomas can be found in any chamber or on any surface and are usually single, but multiple tumors occur in approximately 10% of patients.

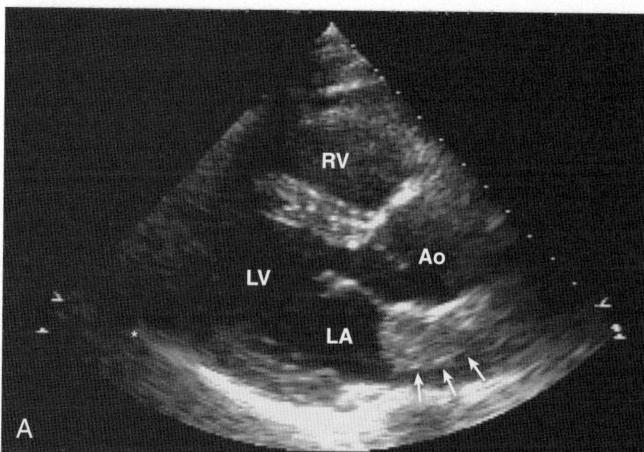

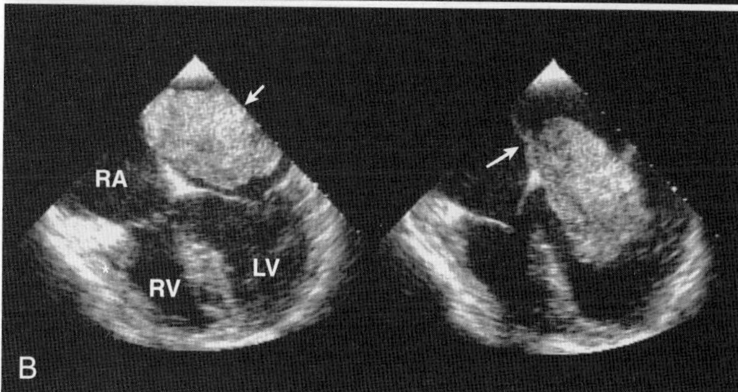

FIGURE 15-86 **A,** Left atrial myxoma (arrows) recorded from the parasternal long-axis position. The myxoma appears attached to the posterior wall of the aorta (Ao), although its attachment site is actually atrial septum. **B,** Systolic **(left)** and diastolic **(right)** frames of transesophageal view of a large left atrial myxoma (left arrow) attached to the atrial septum (right arrow). LA = left atrium; LV = left ventricle; RA = right atrium; RV = right ventricle. *(Modified from Oh JK, Seward JB, Tajik AJ: The Echo Manual. 3rd ed. Philadelphia, Lippincott Williams & Wilkins, 2006. Used with permission of Mayo Foundation for Medical Education and Research.)*

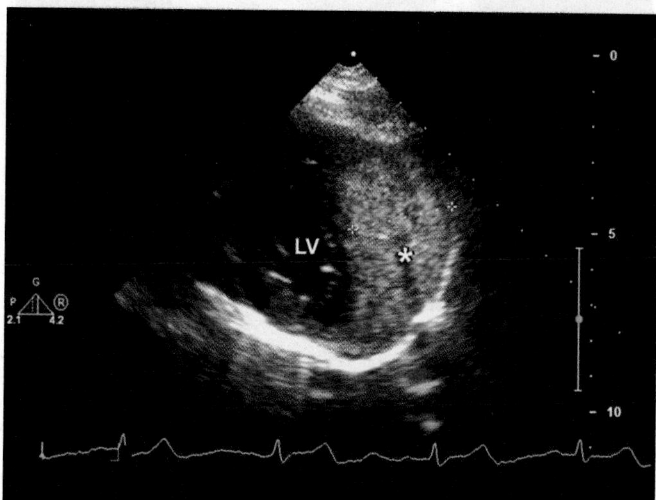

FIGURE 15-87 Parasternal short-axis view of a left ventricular (LV) fibroma (asterisk). It is large and well circumscribed in the posterior free wall. It may cause ventricular arrhythmia but does not produce any hemodynamic abnormality. Surgical removal was successful despite tumor size.

Malignant Tumors of the Heart

Angiosarcoma usually occurs in the right atrium and is commonly associated with pericardial effusion. Rhabdomyosarcoma and fibrosarcoma can occur anywhere in the heart. Synovial sarcoma is rare and usually occurs in the right atrium.

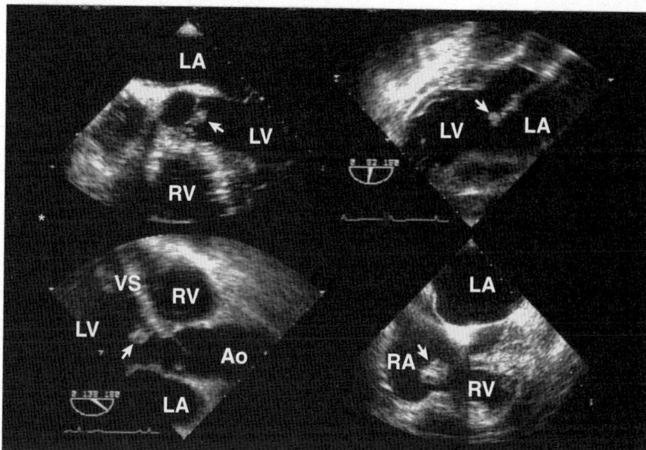

FIGURE 15-88 Transesophageal echocardiographic examples of aortic valve **(upper left)**, mitral valve **(upper right)**, left ventricular outflow tract **(lower left)**, and tricuspid valve **(lower right)** papillary fibroelastomas (arrows). These tumors were not detected with transthoracic echocardiography. Ao = aorta; LA = left atrium; LV = left ventricle; RA = right atrium; RV = right ventricle; VS = ventricular septum. *(Modified from Oh JK, Seward JB, Tajik AJ: The Echo Manual. 3rd ed. Philadelphia, Lippincott Williams & Wilkins, 2006. Used with permission of Mayo Foundation for Medical Education and Research.)*

Metastatic malignant tumors are more common than primary tumors to the heart (see Chap. 74). Most frequently, they are from the lung, breast, kidney, liver, lymphoma, melanoma (see Fig. 18-18), and osteogenic sarcoma. Whenever an RA mass is detected, the inferior vena cava should be carefully scanned because hypernephroma, hepatoma, and intravenous leiomyomatosis from the uterus tend to metastasize to the inferior vena cava and right atrium (**Fig. 15-89**).

Other Masses

Lipomatous atrial septal hypertrophy can be misinterpreted as a cardiac tumor (**Fig. 15-90**; see also Fig. 74-3). The right atrium often harbors structures that appear as a mass on two-dimensional echocardiography; these include the eustachian valve, pacemaker wire or central-line catheter infection, cyst, and thrombus. Infection and abscess in the heart can present as a mass. Echinococcal cyst, tuberculoma, or vegetations attached to the ventricular free wall or intracardiac catheter are also examples. RA thrombi may be mobile, have a characteristic snakelike appearance, and usually are associated with pulmonary embolism (see Fig. 15-e37 on website). On occasion, an RA thrombus is identified passing through a PFO, and this may cause a paradoxical embolus. A similar mobile RA structure may be seen in patients with intravenous leiomyomatosis.

TEE should be used when thrombus is suspected in the left atrium or LA appendage (**Fig. 15-91**). Ventricular thrombus is differentiated from a tumor because the thrombus is associated with abnormal regional wall motion, except apical thrombus noted in hypereosinophilic syndrome and, occasionally, in lymphoma. Contrast echocardiography can be helpful in differentiating an apical mass or thrombus. Thrombus is visualized as a dark structure on contrast echocardiography because it is not vascular. Similar findings are obtained with contrast-enhanced CMR (see Fig. 18-22).

Additional anatomic information can be obtained by three-dimensional echocardiography in patients with cardiac masses.[139]

Echocardiography in Atrial Fibrillation

(see Chap. 40)

Echocardiography has an important role in the evaluation of patients with AF and in making management decisions. During the initial evaluation, TTE is usually performed to screen for occult cardiovascular disease that may precipitate AF, and it provides information that alters the approach to therapy. Information acquired with TTE can assist with the decision about anticoagulation in patients with AF.

Prospective data from large population-based studies have established a relationship between LA diameter and the risk

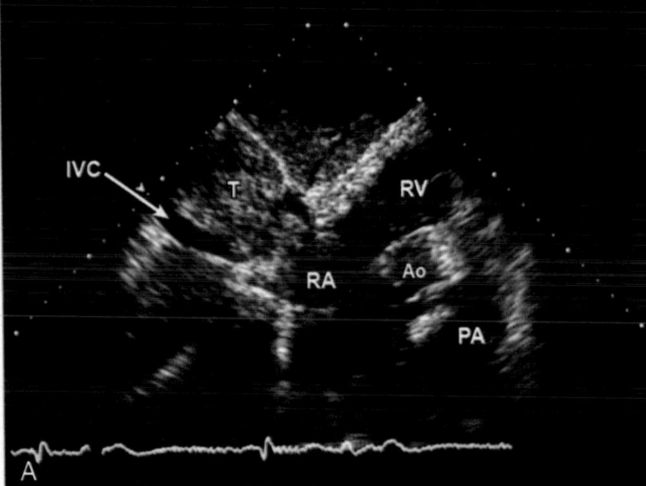

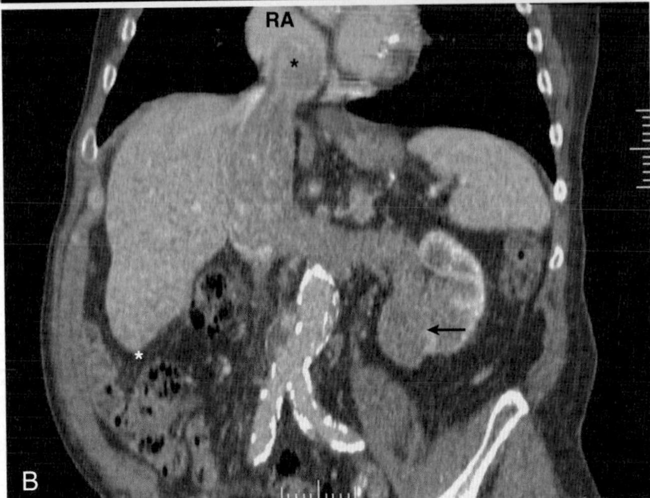

FIGURE 15-89 **A,** Subcostal transthoracic image of a tumor (T) in the inferior vena cava (IVC) extending to the level of the right atrium (RA). Ao = aorta; PA = pulmonary artery; RV = right ventricle. **B,** Computed tomography confirmed that the mass arises from the kidney (arrow) and extends from the renal vein into the inferior vena cava and presents as a mass in the right atrium (asterisk). The tumor is a hypernephroma. The patient underwent nephrectomy and removal of the mass from the inferior vena cava and right atrium.

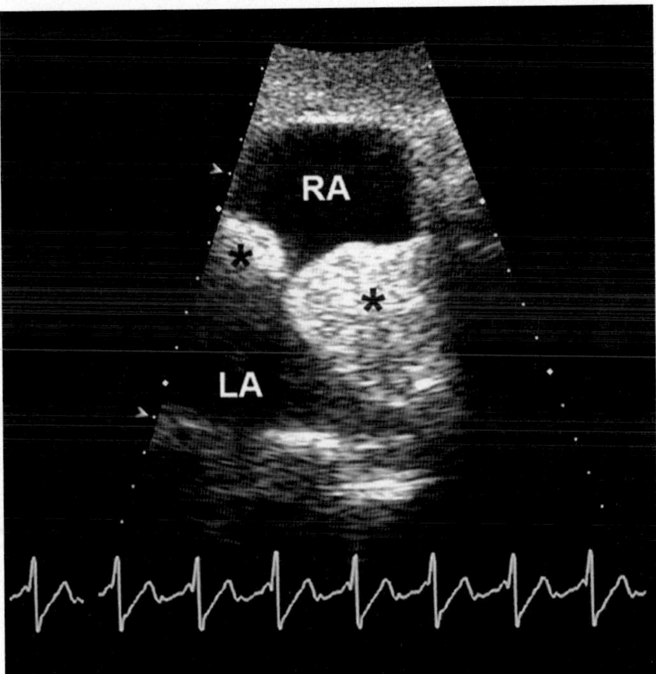

FIGURE 15-90 Subcostal long-axis view showing lipomatous hypertrophy (asterisks) involving the atrial septum. This is occasionally misinterpreted as a tumor or indeterminate mass. The characteristic features include sparing of the fossa ovalis membrane, resulting in a so-called dumbbell appearance. LA = left atrium; RA = right atrium.

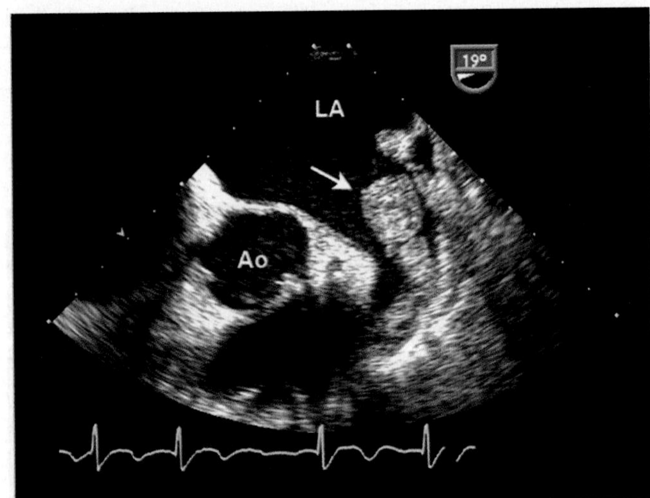

FIGURE 15-91 Transverse transesophageal view of the left atrium (LA) and its appendage with thrombus (arrow) in a patient with atrial fibrillation. Ao = aorta.

for development of AF. Recently, it was reported that LA volume is a superior measure to LA diameter for prediction of outcomes, including AF,[140] and provided prognostic information that was incremental to clinical risk factors.

TEE is frequently performed in patients with AF (see Chap. 40). The primary purpose of TEE is to detect LA appendage thrombi (see Fig. 15-91) and to identify patients at increased risk for cardiogenic embolism. Patients at moderate risk for both stroke and hemorrhagic complications with anticoagulation may benefit from risk stratification with TEE. Compared with TTE, TEE provides a superior assessment of the LA appendage in most patients. The LA appendage is a multilobed muscular extension of the left atrium, and meticulous imaging in several planes is essential because of the complexity of the structure and its anatomic variability. Common artifacts include prominent trabeculations, duplication artifacts, and adipose tissue within the transverse sinus. It is also important to image the RA appendage in patients with AF.

In sinus rhythm, the LA appendage is protected from thrombus formation by high-velocity blood flow. Function of the LA appendage can be assessed with pulsed-wave Doppler interrogation of the chamber (see Fig. 15-e38 on website) during TEE. In patients in sinus rhythm, the appendage contracts once per cardiac cycle, and flow velocities have a biphasic pattern, with peak velocities generally exceeding 40 cm/sec. Patients with AF have lower flow velocities. An LA appendage peak flow velocity less than 20 cm/sec is independently associated with increased risk of thromboembolic events.

Spontaneous echo contrast is commonly identified with TEE in patients with AF. The smokelike echo reflections are likely produced by backscatter from red blood cell aggregates at low flow rates, and they are a marker of stasis and a prothrombotic environment. Variables that have been associated with the presence of spontaneous echo contrast include age, fibrinogen levels, hematocrit, LA appendage velocity, and atherosclerotic aortic plaque. In retrospective studies, dense spontaneous echo contrast has been associated with increased thromboembolic risk.

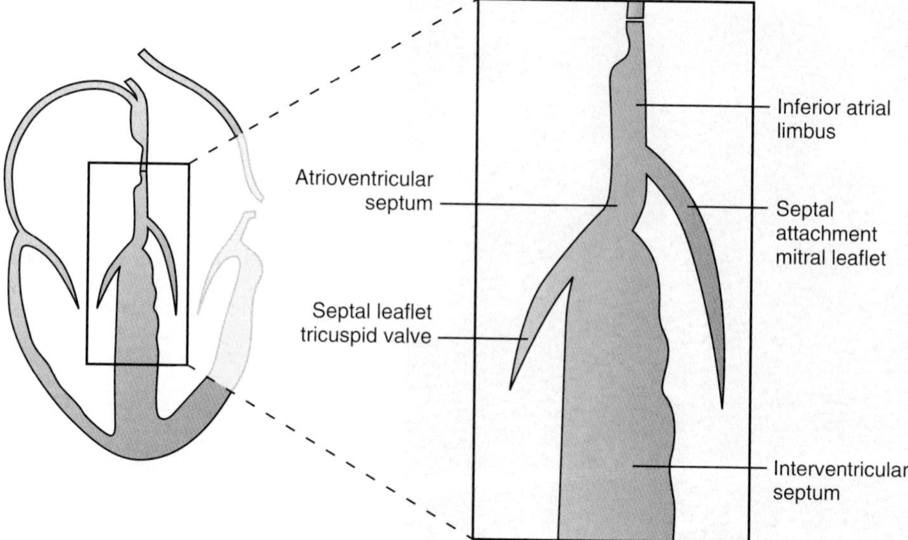

FIGURE 15-92 Diagram of the internal cardiac crux: the joining of the inflow atrial and ventricular septa and respective leaflets of the mitral and tricuspid valves form a crosslike configuration within the heart. This view is predictably obtained with an apical four-chamber view. The normal internal cardiac crux (i.e., cross) is characterized by a lower insertion of the septal leaflet of the morphologic tricuspid valve. In fact, this characteristic relationship of crux attachment of the atrioventricular valves can predict the morphology of these valves (i.e., tricuspid and mitral) and ventricular morphology. This also allows potential communication between left ventricle and right atrium through the atrioventricular septum. The morphologic tricuspid valve is always committed to the morphologic right ventricle and the mitral valve to the morphologic left ventricle. Note that with partial (i.e., primum atrial septal defect) and complete (primum atrial septal defect and inflow ventricular septal defect) congenital canal defects, the mitral valve is characteristically displaced downward. This downward displacement with loss of the atrioventricular septum (i.e., potential communication from the left ventricle directly into the right atrium) results in a deficiency of the mitral leaflet (i.e., a cleft). A large number of congenital anomalies are characterized by diagnostic alterations of the internal cardiac crux.

Transesophageal Echocardiography–Guided Cardioversion

A strategy of TEE to exclude LA thrombus, followed immediately by cardioversion, has been shown to be an efficient means of restoring sinus rhythm without requiring long-term precardioversion anticoagulation (see Chap. 40). Although TEE-guided cardioversion has been found to be a safe alternative to the standard approach of 3 to 4 weeks of anticoagulation followed by cardioversion, it has not been shown to result in a higher success rate for either initial conversion to sinus rhythm or maintenance of sinus rhythm at 1 year. The risk of stroke might be reduced by incorporating TEE into the treatment algorithm, compared with standard anticoagulation management. Preliminary data suggest that combined two-dimensional and three-dimensional TTE has comparable accuracy to TEE in evaluating the left atrium and LA appendage for thrombus.[141]

The TEE study ACUTE, a multicenter prospective randomized study, showed that TEE-guided cardioversion is a safe alternative to conventional anticoagulant therapy in patients with AF. However, controversy persists about whether TEE-guided therapy is superior to the conventional strategy, and there is concern that accelerated cardioversion might be harmful, with increased mortality. With use of either strategy, extremely low stroke rates make it difficult to justify extending the TEE-guided strategy to all patients with planned cardioversion. In the majority of patients with AF, long-term anticoagulant therapy may be recommended, regardless of rhythm status. Still, TEE-guided cardioversion should be strongly considered in certain subgroups of patients with AF, including those with hemodynamic compromise caused by poor rate control, those with persistent symptoms, and those at high risk of hemorrhage with outpatient anticoagulation therapy, keeping in mind that postcardioversion anticoagulation is still necessary.

Congenital Heart Disease (see Chap. 65)

Echocardiography has markedly changed the evaluation, diagnosis, and management of patients with congenital heart disease. A complete echocardiographic examination can establish management, reduce the need for confirmatory cardiac catheterization, and provide serial evaluation of residua and sequelae of congenital heart disease.

Systematic Tomographic Approach to Imaging in Congenital Heart Disease

In the evaluation of patients who have congenital heart defects, the echocardiographic examination must not only quantify function but also define any anatomic and physiologic deviations from normal that may be present. The systematic approach can be applied to all cardiac anomalies and conforms to the recommendations of the ASE and the Society of Pediatric Echocardiography.

For a congenital TTE examination, it is easiest to begin with examination of the upper abdomen to establish the position of the viscera and heart. The location of the heart and the base to apex orientation are established to determine levocardia (cardiac apex in the left side of the chest), mesocardia (cardiac apex in the midline), or dextrocardia (cardiac apex in the right side of the chest). In imaging of congenital anomalies, apex-down is used because it orients cardiac structures in a manner most closely resembling classic anatomic dissections and surgical approaches to the heart. Thus, four-chamber views orient the heart as though looking at the patient from the front.

The internal cardiac crux is an important echocardiographic landmark used in the evaluation of many common and complex congenital cardiac anomalies (**Fig. 15-92**). In the four-chamber plane, the components of the internal crux include the atrial septum, ventricular septum, and septal portions of the mitral and tricuspid valves. The tricuspid valve originates from the crest of the ventricular septum, whereas the septal portion of the mitral valve inserts at a higher level off the lower atrial septum. The portion of the ventricular septum between the two valves represents the atrioventricular septum (i.e., a potential communication between the left ventricle and right atrium). The anatomy of the internal cardiac crux can be used to diagnose both ventricular and atrioventricular valve morphology and abnormalities. The higher inserting morphologic mitral valve is predictably committed to the morphologic left ventricle, and the lower inserting morphologic tricuspid valve to the morphologic right ventricle. The anatomy of the crux is best imaged from a precordial apical, subcostal, or transesophageal four-chamber view. Many complex anomalies of the heart are diagnosed most confidently by their alteration of the crux anatomy, such as Ebstein anomaly, congenitally corrected transposition, double-inlet ventricle, and others (**Fig. 15-93**).

TRANSESOPHAGEAL ECHOCARDIOGRAPHY. Because of the superb visualization of cardiovascular structures, TEE is increasingly being used in the diagnosis of congenital heart disease. TEE is particularly useful in the operating room or during interventional procedures. However, intracardiac echocardiographic imaging is increasingly used for monitoring during percutaneous procedures.

FETAL CONGENITAL HEART DISEASE. High-resolution echocardiography can now be used to confidently diagnose congenital heart disease in a fetus. Fetal echocardiography is used most effectively to anticipate fetal or neonatal problems, to allow prenatal counseling, and to plan pregnancy, delivery, neonatal care, and treatment strategies.

Atrial Septal Defect

A complete TTE examination can detect most secundum atrial septal defects (**Fig. 15-94**) and primum defects or partial atrioventricular canal (**Fig. 15-95**), but sinus venosus defect (**Fig. 15-96**) is visualized in only about 70% of patients. However, TEE is exquisitely sensitive for the identification of all types of atrial septal defect, including coronary sinus atrial septal defect (see Fig. 15-e39 on the Web site), as well as associated anomalous pulmonary venous connections.

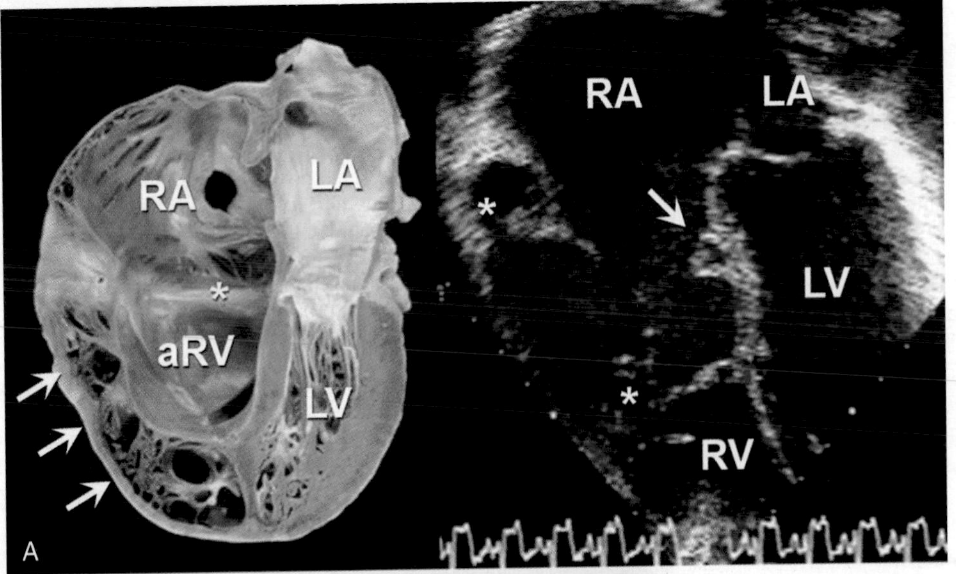

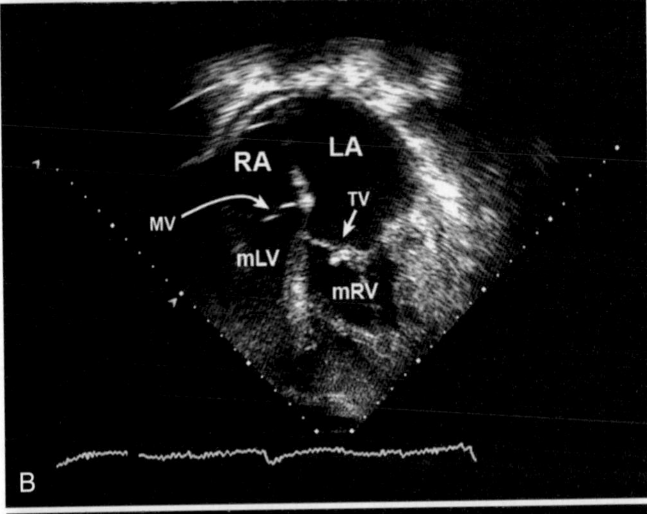

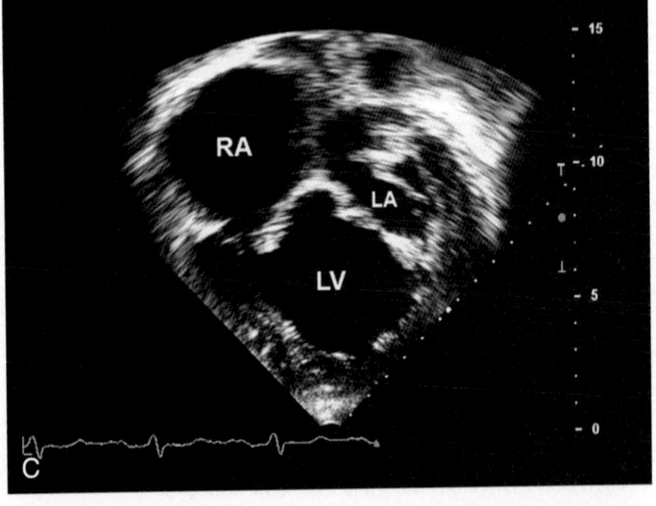

FIGURE 15-93 **A,** Ebstein anomaly. **Left,** Pathology specimen shows enlargement of the right atrium (RA) and right ventricle (RV) with a large atrialized portion of the right ventricle (aRV). The anterior tricuspid valve leaflets are tethered to the lateral wall of the RV (arrows). The left atrium (LA) and left ventricle (LV) are small. The asterisk indicates the anatomic tricuspid annulus. **Right,** Apical four-chamber view. The septal leaflet of the tricuspid valve (arrow) inserts lower than the septal attachment of the mitral valve. The portion of the RV below the tricuspid valve annulus and the downwardly displaced septal tricuspid valve leaflet (arrow) is an atrialized RV. The anterior leaflet is inserted directly into the papillary muscle (asterisk), which impairs mobility. Note that the heart cavities on the right side (RA and RV) become enlarged because of associated tricuspid regurgitation and an atrial septal defect that is usually present (not shown in this example). **B,** Congenitally corrected transposition of the great arteries. The RA communicates with a right-sided morphologically left ventricle (mLV), which connects to the pulmonary artery. The LA communicates with a left-sided morphologically right ventricle (mRV), which connects to the aorta. Four-chamber echocardiogram showing the reversed relationship of the cardiac crux (i.e., the right-sided mitral valve [MV] inserts higher than the left-sided tricuspid valve [TV]). The mLV is to the left below the RA and the mRV is below the LA. The RV is trabeculated. **C,** Double-inlet LV. Systole. The left-sided and right-sided atrioventricular valves are committed to the LV. Both atrioventricular valves can be committed to a single ventricular chamber. This is referred to as double-inlet ventricle. (***A*** *modified from Oh JK, Seward JB, Tajik AJ: The Echo Manual. 3rd ed. Philadelphia, Lippincott Williams & Wilkins, 2006. Used with permission of Mayo Foundation for Medical Education and Research.)*

Each form of atrial septal defect is normally associated with a left-to-right shunt, which eventually results in RA and RV volume overload. It is not necessary or recommended to quantify shunt volume by Doppler measurements. These assessments are often inaccurate because of the number of component measurements involved in the calculation of multiple stroke volumes. The TTE finding of an atrial septal defect with associated right-sided heart enlargement is enough to warrant closure of the defect in the absence of pulmonary hypertension. Pulmonary hypertension of a magnitude that would preclude surgical or device closure is rare and can be recognized on two-dimensional and Doppler echocardiography. Confirmation of fixed pulmonary hypertension requires cardiac catheterization and hemodynamic assessment. Routine cardiac catheterization is not required to establish the diagnosis of atrial septal defect.

Ventricular Septal Defect

There are four major categories of ventricular septal defect (see Fig. 65-8). The most common type in adults is the membranous type (**Fig. 15-97**). These are located at the junction of the muscular, atrioventricular, and outlet portions of the septum. They are adjacent to the aortic and tricuspid valves, which may eventually cause aortic or tricuspid valve regurgitation; thus, prolonged echocardiographic surveillance is recommended.

The most common ventricular septal defect in children is the muscular type (**Fig. 15-98**). They are most often located in the apical two thirds of the ventricular septum. Remote from any cardiac valve, they are not associated with progressive valve dysfunction. Most of these defects are small and close spontaneously early in life. A large muscular ventricular septal defect can cause a large left-to-right shunt, with eventual pulmonary hypertension.

The third most frequent type of ventricular septal defect is the one seen with complete atrioventricular septal defects (see Figs. 65-6 and

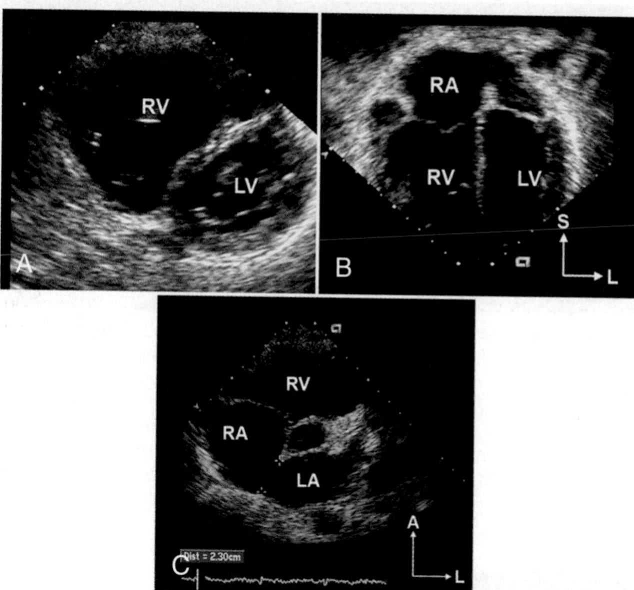

FIGURE 15-94 Two-dimensional echocardiographic features of atrial septal defect. **A,** Short-axis imaging shows RV enlargement from RV volume overload. **B,** Apical four-chamber image shows RA and RV enlargement and dropout in the atrial septum from the secundum atrial septal defect. **C,** Basal short-axis view of RA and RV enlargement and the secundum atrial septal defect (2.3 cm). A = anterior orientation; LA = left atrium; L = left orientation; LV = left ventricle; RA = right atrium; RV = right ventricle; S = superior orientation. *(Modified from Oh JK, Seward JB, Tajik AJ: The Echo Manual. 3rd ed. Philadelphia, Lippincott Williams & Wilkins, 2006. Used with permission of Mayo Foundation for Medical Education and Research.)*

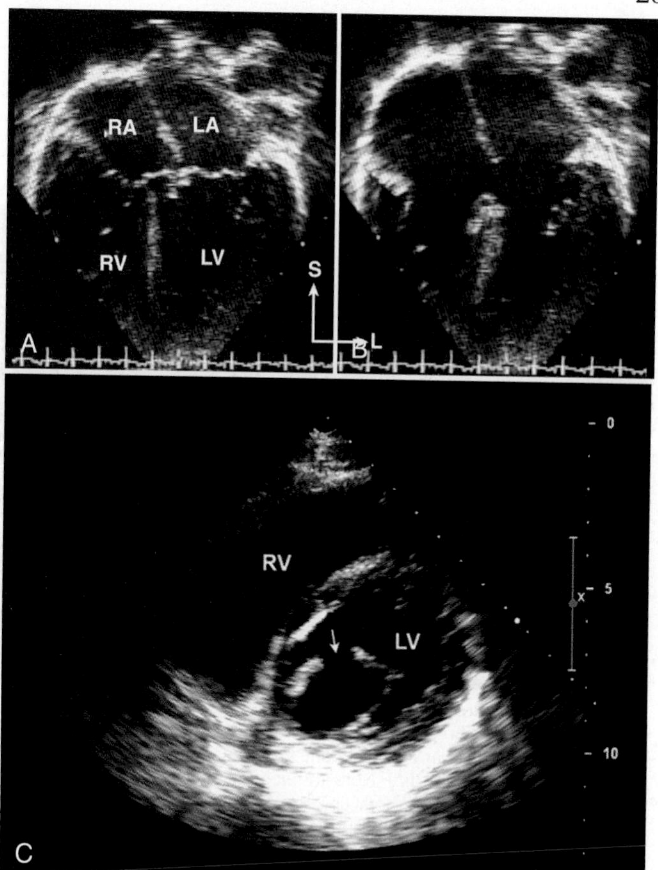

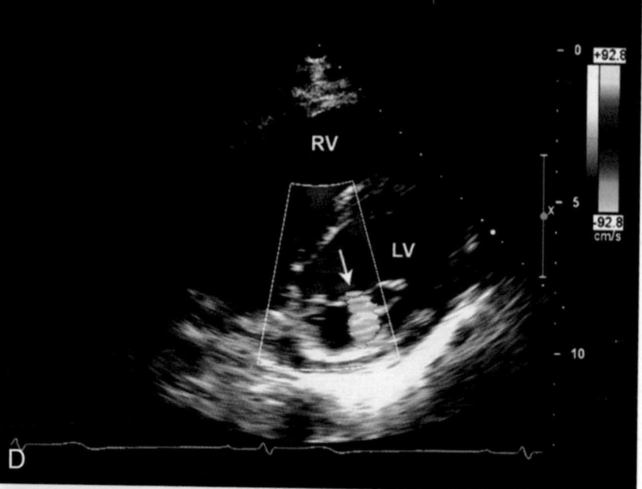

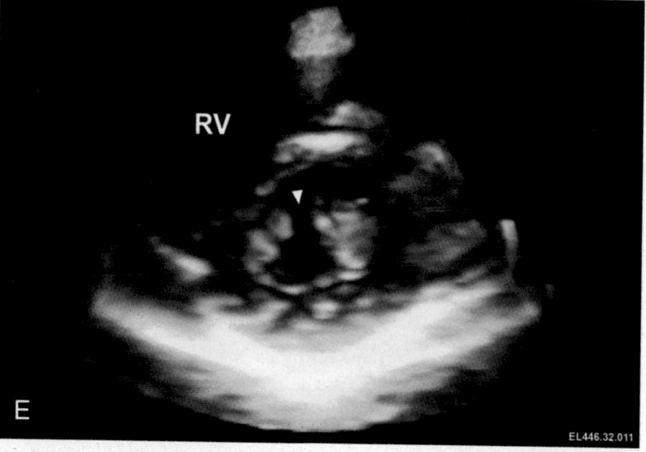

FIGURE 15-95 Primum atrial septal defect is characterized by a defect in the lower atrial septum and downward displacement of the atrioventricular valves, as seen with apical four-chamber imaging during systole **(A)** and diastole **(B)**. **C,** Short-axis two-dimensional imaging shows a mitral valve cleft (arrow). **D,** Color flow imaging shows mitral regurgitation through the cleft. **E,** The cleft (arrowhead) is visualized by three-dimensional transthoracic imaging. LA = left atrium; L = left orientation; LV = left ventricle; RA = right atrium; RV = right ventricle; S = superior orientation. *(Modified from Oh JK, Seward JB, Tajik AJ: The Echo Manual. 3rd ed. Philadelphia, Lippincott Williams & Wilkins, 2006. Used with permission of Mayo Foundation for Medical Education and Research.)*

65-7). This type usually occurs as part of a complete atrioventricular canal defect, but it may occasionally be seen in isolation.

The supracristal, or subarterial, ventricular septal defect is rare. It is located in the outlet septum, immediately adjacent to both the aortic and pulmonary valve annulus at the base of the heart. As a result, the right aortic cusp may be unsupported and prolapse into the ventricular septal defect (see Fig. 15-e40 on website). Aortic cusp prolapse restricts the functional size of the defect but distorts the aortic valve and is associated with aortic valve regurgitation. Elective repair of this ventricular septal defect is usually recommended to prevent progressive aortic cusp prolapse and regurgitation.

A comprehensive TTE examination can identify a ventricular septal defect in more than 90% of cases. Continuous-wave Doppler echocardiography can measure the blood flow velocity and gradient across the defect. A large ventricular septal defect has a smaller pressure difference between the ventricles; conversely, a small defect has a large gradient (i.e., velocity). Rarely, TEE is used to improve imaging in patients with a known or suspected ventricular septal defect.

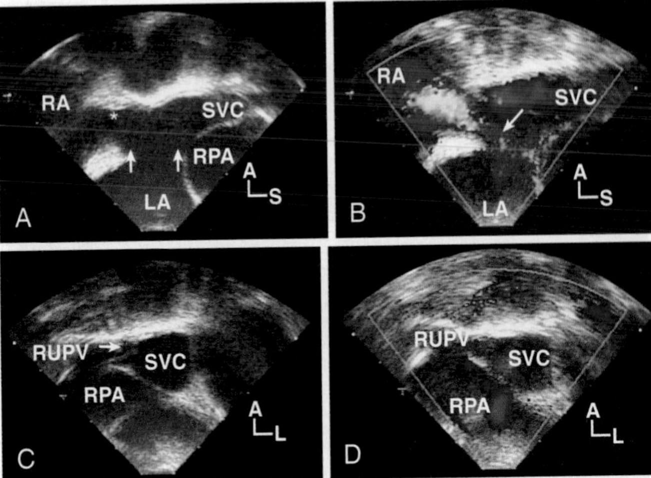

FIGURE 15-96 Sinus venosus atrial septal defect (ASD). **A,** Long-axis transesophageal examination aligned with the superior vena cava (SVC). Note the large atrial septal defect (arrows) just beneath the SVC, where this vessel enters (asterisk) the right atrium (RA). Note the volume-enlarged right pulmonary artery (RPA) and that no atrial septal tissues are attached to the wall adjacent to the RPA (absence of the superior limbus of the atrial septum). These features are pathognomonic of sinus venosus ASD. Note the intact membranous portion of the fossa ovalis. **B,** Color flow Doppler shows left-to-right shunt flow across the sinus venosus ASD. Also visualized is blood entering the SVC from the anomalously connecting right pulmonary vein *(arrow)*. **C,** Transesophageal short-axis view at the level of the RPA, which is displayed in its long axis. Normally, SVC is circular, but in this example, it has a teardrop shape because an anomalous connecting pulmonary vein (RUPV, *arrow*) enters the lateral wall of the SVC. **D,** On color flow Doppler study, note blood flow from the anomalously connecting RUPV into the SVC. A sinus venosus ASD is commonly associated with anomalous connection of the right middle and upper pulmonary veins, which enter either the RA or SVC. A = anterior orientation; L = left orientation; LA = left atrium; S = superior orientation. *(Modified from Oh JK, Seward JB, Tajik AJ: The Echo Manual. 3rd ed. Philadelphia, Lippincott Williams & Wilkins, 2006. Used with permission of Mayo Foundation for Medical Education and Research.)*

Patent Ductus Arteriosus

Echocardiographic diagnosis of patent ductus arteriosus is based on demonstration of a persistent anatomic connection and flow between the descending thoracic aorta and the pulmonary artery (**Fig. 15-99**). The best imaging views include the high left parasternal long-axis scan of the RVOT and main pulmonary artery and the suprasternal view. A

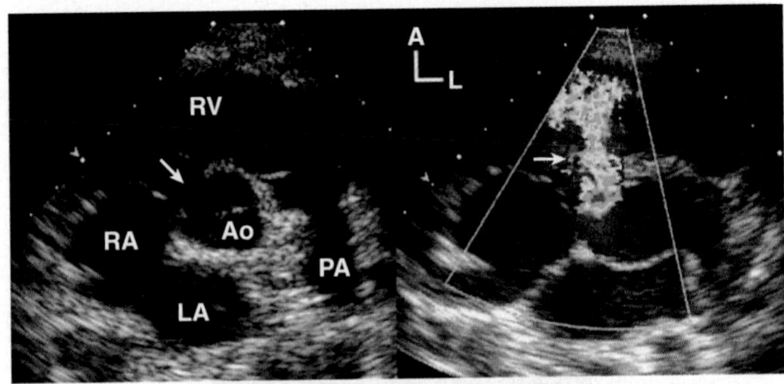

FIGURE 15-97 Membranous ventricular septal defect (VSD). **Left,** Parasternal short-axis view. The ventricular septal defect *(arrow)* is located on the medial aspect of the left ventricle outflow. **Right,** Color flow imaging shows left-to-right shunt from across the membranous VSD *(arrow)*. A = anterior orientation; Ao = aorta; L = left orientation; LA = left atrium; PA = pulmonary artery; RA = right atrium; RV = right ventricle. *(Modified from Oh JK, Seward JB, Tajik AJ: The Echo Manual. 3rd ed. Philadelphia, Lippincott Williams & Wilkins, 2006. Used with permission of Mayo Foundation for Medical Education and Research.)*

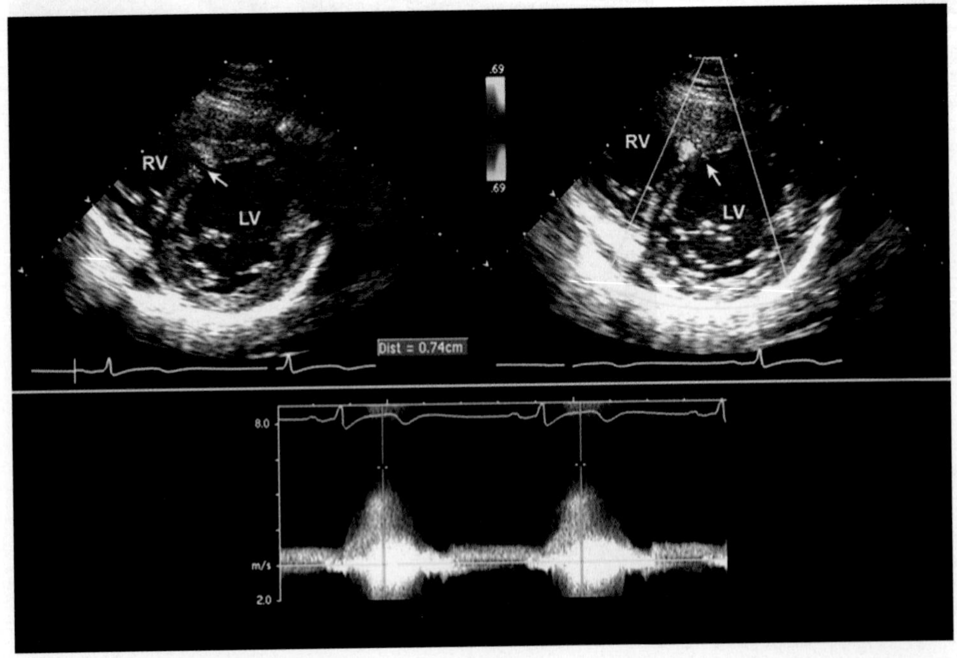

FIGURE 15-98 Muscular ventricular septal defect (VSD). **Top left,** Parasternal short-axis image demonstrating VSD (arrow). LV = left ventricle; RV = right ventricle. **Top right,** Short-axis imaging with color flow Doppler of a muscular VSD *(arrow)* shows flow from LV to RV. **Bottom,** Continuous-wave Doppler signal from the VSD demonstrates left-to-right high-velocity flow.

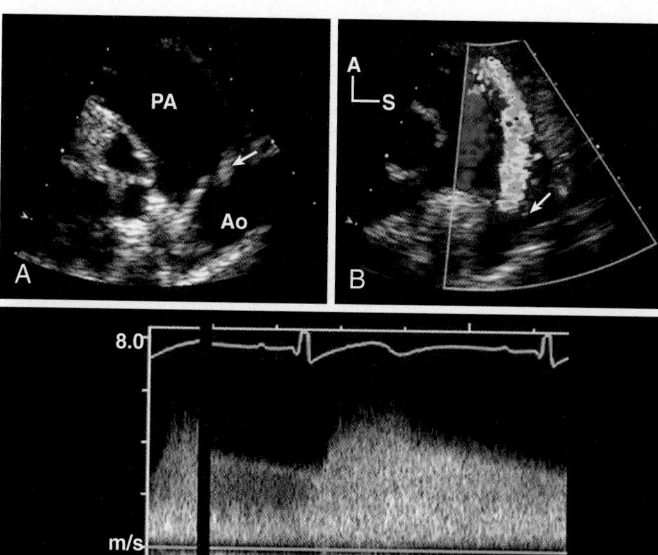

FIGURE 15-99 Patent ductus arteriosus. **A,** Parasternal short-axis image shows communication (arrow) between the aorta (Ao) and pulmonary artery (PA) by two-dimensional echocardiography, which is confirmed on color flow imaging **(B). C,** Continuous-wave Doppler signal shows high systolic velocity and persistent flow through diastole. A = anterior orientation; S = superior orientation. *(Modified from Oh JK, Seward JB, Tajik AJ: The Echo Manual. 3rd ed. Philadelphia, Lippincott Williams & Wilkins, 2006. Used with permission of Mayo Foundation for Medical Education and Research.)*

patent ductus arteriosus associated with pulmonary hypertension may be difficult to visualize with TTE or TEE because of equalization of pressures between the two vessels. High Doppler velocities across the patent ductus suggest low pulmonary artery pressure.

Coarctation of the Aorta

Aortic coarctation (see Chaps. 60 and 65) can be seen just distal to the left subclavian artery in the region opposite the origin or remnant of the ductus arteriosus, so-called juxtaductal coarctation. Coarctation of the aorta occurs in 6% to 8% of patients with congenital heart disease. With TTE, the area of aortic narrowing can often be seen from the suprasternal or high left parasternal transducer position; however, continuous-wave Doppler echocardiography is the best method to quantify the magnitude of obstruction. Doppler recordings of hemodynamically significant coarctation are characterized by an increased flow velocity in the descending thoracic aorta that extends into diastole. The systolic gradient in severe coarctation may underestimate the severity of obstruction when there is an extensive collateral network. Thus, ancillary data are obtained; in severe coarctation, a pulsed-wave examination of the abdominal aorta shows distorted flow velocity, with decreased systolic amplitude, and persistent flow in diastole (see Fig. 15-e41 on website). Abnormal abdominal flow is helpful in recognizing (re)coarctation in adults. In older patients and any patient with a repaired coarctation, CMR or CT (see Chaps. 18 and 19) has replaced angiography for definitive diagnosis and overall vascular assessment of coarctation or recoarctation (see Fig. 82-4).

REFERENCES

Transthoracic, Transesophageal, and Doppler Echocardiography

1. Oh JK, Seward JB, Tajik AJ: The Echo Manual. 3rd ed. Philadelphia, Lippincott Williams & Wilkins, 2006.
2. Mulvagh SL, Rakowski H, Vannan MA, et al: American Society of Echocardiography consensus statement on the clinical applications of ultrasonic contrast agents in echocardiography. J Am Soc Echocardiogr 21:1179, 2008.
3. Amundsen BH, Helle-Valle T, Edvardsen T, et al: Noninvasive myocardial strain measurement by speckle tracking echocardiography: Validation against sonomicrometry and tagged magnetic resonance imaging. J Am Coll Cardiol 47:789, 2006.
4. Goonewardena SN, Gemignani A, Ronan A, et al: Comparison of hand-carried ultrasound assessment of the inferior vena cava and N-terminal pro-brain natriuretic peptide for predicting readmission after hospitalization for acute decompensated heart failure. Am J Coll Cardiol Img 1:595, 2008.
5. Lang RM, Bierig M, Devereux RB, et al: Recommendations for chamber quantification: A report from the American Society of Echocardiography's Guidelines and Standards Committee and the Chamber Quantification Writing Group, developed in conjunction with the European Association of Echocardiography, a branch of the European Society of Cardiology. J Am Soc Echocardiogr 18:1440, 2005.
6. Douglas PS, Khandheria B, Stainback RF, et al: ACCF/ASE/ACEP/ASNC/SCAI/SCCT/SCMR 2007 appropriateness criteria for transthoracic and transesophageal echocardiography: A report of the American College of Cardiology Foundation Quality Strategic Directions Committee Appropriateness Criteria Working Group, American Society of Echocardiography, American College of Emergency Physicians, American Society of Nuclear Cardiology, Society for Cardiovascular Angiography and Interventions, Society of Cardiovascular Computed Tomography, and the Society for Cardiovascular Magnetic Resonance endorsed by the American College of Chest Physicians and the Society of Critical Care Medicine. J Am Coll Cardiol 50:187, 2007.
7. Shah SJ, Bardo DM, Sugeng L, et al: Real-time three-dimensional transesophageal echocardiography of the left atrial appendage: Initial experience in the clinical setting. J Am Soc Echocardiogr 21:1362, 2008.
8. Min JK, Spencer KT, Furlong KT, et al: Clinical features of complications from transesophageal echocardiography: A single-center case series of 10,000 consecutive examinations. J Am Soc Echocardiogr 18:925, 2005.
9. Grewal J, Mankad S, Freeman WK, et al: Real-time three-dimensional transesophageal echocardiography in the intraoperative assessment of mitral valve disease. J Am Soc Echocardiogr 22:34, 2009.
10. Sutherland GR, Di Salvo G, Claus P, et al: Strain and strain rate imaging: A new clinical approach to quantifying regional myocardial function. J Am Soc Echocardiogr 17:788, 2004.
11. Helle-Valle T, Crosby J, Edvardsen T, et al: New noninvasive method for assessment of left ventricular rotation: Speckle tracking echocardiography. Circulation 112:3149, 2005.
12. Notomi Y, Martin-Miklovic MG, Oryszak SJ, et al: Enhanced ventricular untwisting during exercise: A mechanistic manifestation of elastic recoil described by Doppler tissue imaging. Circulation 113:2524, 2006.
13. Sengupta PP, Khandheria BK, Korinek J, et al: Apex-to-base dispersion in regional timing of left ventricular shortening and lengthening. J Am Coll Cardiol 47:163, 2006.
14. Marwick TH: Measurement of strain and strain rate by echocardiography: Ready for prime time? J Am Coll Cardiol 47:1313, 2006.
15. Tanaka H, Kawai H, Tatsumi K, et al: Improved regional myocardial diastolic function assessed by strain rate imaging in patients with coronary artery disease undergoing percutaneous coronary intervention. J Am Soc Echocardiogr 19:756, 2006.
16. Bjork Ingul C, Rozis E, Slordahl SA, Marwick TH: Incremental value of strain rate imaging to wall motion analysis for prediction of outcome in patients undergoing dobutamine stress echocardiography. Circulation 115:1252, 2007.
17. Bellavia D, Abraham TP, Pellikka PA, et al: Detection of left ventricular systolic dysfunction in cardiac amyloidosis with strain rate echocardiography. J Am Soc Echocardiogr 20:1194, 2007.
18. Serri K, Reant P, Lafitte M, et al: Global and regional myocardial function quantification by two-dimensional strain: Application in hypertrophic cardiomyopathy. J Am Coll Cardiol 47:1175, 2006.
19. Yu CM, Sanderson JE, Marwick TH, Oh JK: Tissue Doppler imaging a new prognosticator for cardiovascular diseases. J Am Coll Cardiol 49:1903, 2007.
20. Oh JK, Hatle L, Tajik AJ, Little WC: Diastolic heart failure can be diagnosed by comprehensive two-dimensional and Doppler echocardiography. J Am Coll Cardiol 47:500, 2006.
21. Little WC, Oh JK: Echocardiographic evaluation of diastolic function can be used to guide clinical care. Circulation 120:802, 2009.
22. Kjaergaard J, Hassager C, Oh JK, et al: Measurement of cardiac time intervals by Doppler tissue M-mode imaging of the anterior mitral leaflet. J Am Soc Echocardiogr 18:1058, 2005.
23. Yu CM, Zhang Q, Fung JW, et al: A novel tool to assess systolic asynchrony and identify responders of cardiac resynchronization therapy by tissue synchronization imaging. J Am Coll Cardiol 45:677, 2005.
24. Gorcsan J 3rd, Abraham T, Agler DA, et al: Echocardiography for cardiac resynchronization therapy: Recommendations for performance and reporting—a report from the American Society of Echocardiography Dyssynchrony Writing Group endorsed by the Heart Rhythm Society. J Am Soc Echocardiogr 21:191, 2008.
25. Mele D, Pasanisi G, Capasso F, et al: Left intraventricular myocardial deformation dyssynchrony identifies responders to cardiac resynchronization therapy in patients with heart failure. Eur Heart J 27:1070, 2006.
26. Miyazaki C, Powell BD, Bruce CJ, et al: Comparison of echocardiographic dyssynchrony assessment by tissue velocity and strain imaging in subjects with or without systolic dysfunction and with or without left bundle-branch block. Circulation 117:2617, 2008.

Contrast Echocardiography

27. Kurt M, Shaikh KA, Peterson L, et al: Impact of contrast echocardiography on evaluation of ventricular function and clinical management in a large prospective cohort. J Am Coll Cardiol 53:802, 2009.
28. Wei K, Mulvagh SL, Carson L, et al: The safety of deFinity and Optison for ultrasound image enhancement: A retrospective analysis of 78,383 administered contrast doses. J Am Soc Echocardiogr 21:1202, 2008.
29. Dolan MS, Gala SS, Dodla S, et al: Safety and efficacy of commercially available ultrasound contrast agents for rest and stress echocardiography a multicenter experience. J Am Coll Cardiol 53:32, 2009.
30. Kirkpatrick JN, Wong T, Bednarz JE, et al: Differential diagnosis of cardiac masses using contrast echocardiographic perfusion imaging. J Am Coll Cardiol 43:1412, 2004.
31. Kaul S, Senior R, Firschke C, et al: Incremental value of cardiac imaging in patients presenting to the emergency department with chest pain and without ST-segment elevation: A multicenter study. Am Heart J 148:129, 2004.

32. Jeetley P, Hickman M, Kamp O, et al: Myocardial contrast echocardiography for the detection of coronary artery stenosis: A prospective multicenter study in comparison with single-photon emission computed tomography. J Am Coll Cardiol 47:141, 2006.
33. Kaul S, Ito H: Microvasculature in acute myocardial ischemia: Part II: Evolving concepts in pathophysiology, diagnosis, and treatment. Circulation 109:310, 2004.
34. Ujino K, Hillis GS, Mulvagh SL, et al: Usefulness of real-time intravenous myocardial contrast echocardiography in predicting left ventricular dilation after successfully reperfused acute myocardial infarction. Am J Cardiol 96:17, 2005.
35. Holmes DR Jr, Valeti US, Nishimura RA: Alcohol septal ablation for hypertrophic cardiomyopathy: Indications and technique. Catheter Cardiovasc Interv 66:375, 2005.

Cardiac Chamber Size and Function

36. Aurigemma GP, Gottdiener JS, Arnold AM, et al: Left atrial volume and geometry in healthy aging: The Cardiovascular Health Study. Circ Cardiovasc Imaging 2:282, 2009.
37. Abhayaratna WP, Seward JB, Appleton CP, et al: Left atrial size: Physiologic determinants and clinical applications. J Am Coll Cardiol 47:2357, 2006.
38. Mor-Avi V, Sugeng L, Weinert L, et al: Fast measurement of left ventricular mass with real-time three-dimensional echocardiography: Comparison with magnetic resonance imaging. Circulation 110:1814, 2004.
39. Mor-Avi V, Jenkins C, Kuhl HP, et al: Real-time 3-dimensional echocardiographic quantification of left ventricular volumes: Multicenter study for validation with magnetic resonance imaging and investigation of sources of error. Am J Coll Cardiol Img 1:413, 2008.
40. Nagueh SF, Appleton CP, Gillebert TC, et al: Recommendations for the evaluation of left ventricular diastolic function by echocardiography. J Am Soc Echocardiogr 22:107, 2009.
41. Zile MR, Baicu CF, Gaasch WH: Diastolic heart failure: Abnormalities in active relaxation and passive stiffness of the left ventricle. N Engl J Med 350:1953, 2004.
42. Kasner M, Westermann D, Steendijk P, et al: Utility of Doppler echocardiography and tissue Doppler imaging in the estimation of diastolic function in heart failure with normal ejection fraction: A comparative Doppler-conductance catheterization study. Circulation 116:637, 2007.
43. Knebel F, Schattke S, Bondke H, et al: Evaluation of longitudinal and radial two-dimensional strain imaging versus Doppler tissue echocardiography in predicting long-term response to cardiac resynchronization therapy. J Am Soc Echocardiogr 20:335, 2007.
44. Nishimura RA, Tajik AJ: The Valsalva maneuver—3 centuries later. Mayo Clin Proc 79:577, 2004.
45. Ha JW, Oh JK, Pellikka PA, et al: Diastolic stress echocardiography: A novel noninvasive diagnostic test for diastolic dysfunction using supine bicycle exercise Doppler echocardiography. J Am Soc Echocardiogr 18:63, 2005.
46. Ha JW, Oh JK, Redfield MM, et al: Triphasic mitral inflow velocity with middiastolic filling: Clinical implications and associated echocardiographic findings. J Am Soc Echocardiogr 17:428, 2004.
47. Lam CS, Han L, Ha JW, et al: The mitral L wave: A marker of pseudonormal filling and predictor of heart failure in patients with left ventricular hypertrophy. J Am Soc Echocardiogr 18:336, 2005.
48. Spencer KT, Kirkpatrick JN, Mor-Avi V, et al: Age dependency of the Tei index of myocardial performance. J Am Soc Echocardiogr 17:350, 2004.
49. Tham EB, Silverman NH: Measurement of the Tei index: A comparison of M-mode and pulse Doppler methods. J Am Soc Echocardiogr 17:1259, 2004.
50. Burgess MI, Jenkins C, Sharman JE, Marwick TH: Diastolic stress echocardiography: Hemodynamic validation and clinical significance of estimation of ventricular filling pressure with exercise. J Am Coll Cardiol 47:1891, 2006.
51. Galderisi M: Diastolic dysfunction and diabetic cardiomyopathy: Evaluation by Doppler echocardiography. J Am Coll Cardiol 48:1548, 2006.
52. Jassal DS, Neilan TG, Fifer MA, et al: Sustained improvement in left ventricular diastolic function after alcohol septal ablation for hypertrophic obstructive cardiomyopathy. Eur Heart J 27:1805, 2006.
53. Fukuta H, Little WC: Elevated left ventricular filling pressure after maximal exercise predicts increased plasma B-type natriuretic peptide levels in patients with impaired relaxation pattern of diastolic filling. J Am Soc Echocardiogr 20:832, 2007.
54. Choi EY, Ha JW, Kim JM, et al: Incremental value of combining systolic mitral annular velocity and time difference between mitral inflow and diastolic mitral annular velocity to early diastolic annular velocity for differentiating constrictive pericarditis from restrictive cardiomyopathy. J Am Soc Echocardiogr 20:738, 2007.
55. Sohn DW, Kim YJ, Kim HS, et al: Unique features of early diastolic mitral annulus velocity in constrictive pericarditis. J Am Soc Echocardiogr 17:222, 2004.
56. Moller JE, Pellikka PA, Hillis GS, Oh JK: Prognostic importance of diastolic function and filling pressure in patients with acute myocardial infarction. Circulation 114:438, 2006.
57. Tsang TS, Barnes ME, Gersh BJ, et al: Risks for atrial fibrillation and congestive heart failure in patients ≥65 years of age with abnormal left ventricular diastolic relaxation. Am J Cardiol 93:54, 2004.
58. Temporelli PL, Giannuzzi P, Nicolosi GL, et al; GISSI-3 Echo Substudy Investigators: Doppler-derived mitral deceleration time as a strong prognostic marker of left ventricular remodeling and survival after acute myocardial infarction: Results of the GISSI-3 echo substudy. J Am Coll Cardiol 43:1646, 2004.
59. Hillis GS, Moller JE, Pellikka PA, et al: Noninvasive estimation of left ventricular filling pressure by E/e′ is a powerful predictor of survival after acute myocardial infarction. J Am Coll Cardiol 43:360, 2004.

Heart Failure

60. Grayburn PA, Appleton CP, DeMaria AN, et al; BEST Trial Echocardiographic Substudy Investigators: Echocardiographic predictors of morbidity and mortality in patients with advanced heart failure: The Beta-blocker Evaluation of Survival Trial (BEST). J Am Coll Cardiol 45:1064, 2005.
61. Jones RH, Velazquez EJ, Michler RE, et al; STICH Hypothesis 2 Investigators: Coronary bypass surgery with or without surgical ventricular reconstruction. N Engl J Med 360:1705, 2009.
62. Anand IS, Carson P, Galle E, et al: Cardiac resynchronization therapy reduces the risk of hospitalizations in patients with advanced heart failure: Results from the Comparison of Medical Therapy, Pacing and Defibrillation in Heart Failure (COMPANION) trial. Circulation 119:969, 2009.
63. Cleland J, Freemantle N, Ghio S, et al: Predicting the long-term effects of cardiac resynchronization therapy on mortality from baseline variables and the early response a report from the CARE-HF (Cardiac Resynchronization in Heart Failure) Trial. J Am Coll Cardiol 52:438, 2008.
64. Bax JJ, Bleeker GB, Marwick TH, et al: Left ventricular dyssynchrony predicts response and prognosis after cardiac resynchronization therapy. J Am Coll Cardiol 44:1834, 2004.
65. Yu CM, Fung JW, Zhang Q, et al: Tissue Doppler imaging is superior to strain rate imaging and postsystolic shortening on the prediction of reverse remodeling in both ischemic and nonischemic heart failure after cardiac resynchronization therapy. Circulation 110:66, 2004.
66. Miyazaki C, Lin G, Powell BD, et al: Strain dyssynchrony index correlates with improvement in left ventricular volume after cardiac resynchronization therapy better than tissue velocity dyssynchrony indexes. Circ Cardiovasc Imaging 1:14, 2008.
67. Chung ES, Leon AR, Tavazzi L, et al: Results of the Predictors of Response to CRT (PROSPECT) trial. Circulation 117:2608, 2008.
68. Sonne C, Sugeng L, Takeuchi M, et al: Real-time 3-dimensional echocardiographic assessment of left ventricular dyssynchrony: Pitfalls in patients with dilated cardiomyopathy. Am J Coll Cardiol Img 2:802, 2009.
69. Dokainish H, Zoghbi WA, Lakkis NM, et al: Optimal noninvasive assessment of left ventricular filling pressures: A comparison of tissue Doppler echocardiography and B-type natriuretic peptide in patients with pulmonary artery catheters. Circulation 109:2432, 2004.

Coronary Artery Disease

70. Ishii K, Imai M, Suyama T, et al: Exercise-induced post-ischemic left ventricular delayed relaxation or diastolic stunning: Is it a reliable marker in detecting coronary artery disease? J Am Coll Cardiol 53:698, 2009.
71. Park SM, Miyazaki C, Prasad A, et al: Feasibility of prediction of myocardial viability with Doppler tissue imaging following percutaneous coronary intervention for ST elevation anterior myocardial infarction. J Am Soc Echocardiogr 22:183, 2009.
72. Lyseggen E, Rabben SI, Skulstad H, et al: Myocardial acceleration during isovolumic contraction: Relationship to contractility. Circulation 111:1362, 2005.
73. Vignon P: Hemodynamic assessment of critically ill patients using echocardiography Doppler. Curr Opin Crit Care 11:227, 2005.
74. Russo A, Suri RM, Grigioni F, et al: Clinical outcome after surgical correction of mitral regurgitation due to papillary muscle rupture. Circulation 118:1528, 2008.
75. Bybee KA, Kara T, Prasad A, et al: Systematic review: Transient left ventricular apical ballooning: A syndrome that mimics ST-segment elevation myocardial infarction. Ann Intern Med 141:858, 2004.
76. Pierard LA, Lancellotti P: The role of ischemic mitral regurgitation in the pathogenesis of acute pulmonary edema. N Engl J Med 351:1627, 2004.
77. Bursi F, Enriquez-Sarano M, Jacobsen SJ, Roger VL: Mitral regurgitation after myocardial infarction: A review. Am J Med 119:103, 2006.
78. Bursi F, Enriquez-Sarano M, Nkomo VT, et al: Heart failure and death after myocardial infarction in the community: The emerging role of mitral regurgitation. Circulation 111:295, 2005.
79. Wu AH, Aaronson KD, Bolling SF, et al: Impact of mitral valve annuloplasty on mortality risk in patients with mitral regurgitation and left ventricular systolic dysfunction. J Am Coll Cardiol 45:381, 2005.
80. Lee VH, Abdelmoneim SS, Daugherty WP, et al: Myocardial contrast echocardiography in subarachnoid hemorrhage–induced cardiac dysfunction: Case report. Neurosurgery 62:E261, 2008.
81. Hurst RT, Askew JW, Reuss CS, et al: Transient midventricular ballooning syndrome: A new variant. J Am Coll Cardiol 48:579, 2006.
82. Park SM, Prasad A, Rihal C, et al: Left ventricular systolic and diastolic function in patients with apical ballooning syndrome compared with patients with acute anterior ST-segment elevation myocardial infarction: A functional paradox. Mayo Clin Proc 84:514, 2009.
83. Wong SP, French JK, Lydon AM, et al: Relation of left ventricular sphericity to 10-year survival after acute myocardial infarction. Am J Cardiol 94:1270, 2004.
84. Vartdal T, Brunvand H, Pettersen E, et al: Early prediction of infarct size by strain Doppler echocardiography after coronary reperfusion. J Am Coll Cardiol 49:1715, 2007.
85. Pellikka PA: Stress echocardiography for the diagnosis of coronary artery disease: Progress towards quantification. Curr Opin Cardiol 20:395, 2005.
86. Armstrong WF, Zoghbi WA: Stress echocardiography: Current methodology and clinical applications. J Am Coll Cardiol 45:1739, 2005.
87. Kane GC, Hepinstall MJ, Kidd GM, et al: Safety of stress echocardiography supervised by registered nurses: Results of a 2-year audit of 15,404 patients. J Am Soc Echocardiogr 21:337, 2008.
88. Hillis GS, Oh JK, Mahoney DW, et al: Akinesia becoming dyskinesia after exercise testing: Prevalence and relationship to clinical outcome. J Am Coll Cardiol 43:599, 2004.
89. Hanekom L, Jenkins C, Jeffries L, et al: Incremental value of strain rate analysis as an adjunct to wall-motion scoring for assessment of myocardial viability by dobutamine echocardiography: A follow-up study after revascularization. Circulation 112:3892, 2005.
90. Elhendy A, Mahoney DW, Burger KN, et al: Prognostic value of exercise echocardiography in patients with classic angina pectoris. Am J Cardiol 94:559, 2004.
91. Talreja DR, Nishimura RA, Oh JK: Estimation of left ventricular filling pressure with exercise by Doppler echocardiography in patients with normal systolic function: A simultaneous echocardiographic-cardiac catheterization study. J Am Soc Echocardiogr 20:477, 2007.
92. Grewal J, McCully RB, Kane GC, et al: Left ventricular function and exercise capacity. JAMA 301:286, 2009.

Valvular Heart Disease and Endocarditis

93. Otto CM: Valvular aortic stenosis: Disease severity and timing of intervention. J Am Coll Cardiol 47:2141, 2006.
94. Enriquez-Sarano M, Avierinos JF, Messika-Zeitoun D, et al: Quantitative determinants of the outcome of asymptomatic mitral regurgitation. N Engl J Med 352:875, 2005.
95. Abbas AE, Fortuin FD, Patel B, et al: Noninvasive measurement of systemic vascular resistance using Doppler echocardiography. J Am Soc Echocardiogr 17:834, 2004.

96. Bonow RO, Carabello BA, Kanu C, et al: ACC/AHA 2006 guidelines for the management of patients with valvular heart disease: A report of the American College of Cardiology/American Heart Association Task Force on Practice Guidelines (writing committee to revise the 1998 Guidelines for the Management of Patients With Valvular Heart Disease): Developed in collaboration with the Society of Cardiovascular Anesthesiologists: Endorsed by the Society for Cardiovascular Angiography and Interventions and the Society of Thoracic Surgeons. Circulation 114:e84, 2006.
97. Pellikka PA, Sarano ME, Nishimura RA, et al: Outcome of 622 adults with asymptomatic, hemodynamically significant aortic stenosis during prolonged follow-up. Circulation 111:3290, 2005.
98. Levy F, Laurent M, Monin JL, et al: Aortic valve replacement for low-flow/low-gradient aortic stenosis operative risk stratification and long-term outcome: A European multicenter study. J Am Coll Cardiol 51:1466, 2008.
99. Tribouilloy C, Levy F, Rusinaru D, et al: Outcome after aortic valve replacement for low-flow/low-gradient aortic stenosis without contractile reserve on dobutamine stress echocardiography. J Am Coll Cardiol 53:1865, 2009.
100. Little SH, Pirat B, Kumar R, et al: Three-dimensional color Doppler echocardiography for direct measurement of vena contracta area in mitral regurgitation: In vitro validation and clinical experience. Am J Coll Cardiol Img 1:695, 2008.
101. Nath J, Foster E, Heidenreich PA: Impact of tricuspid regurgitation on long-term survival. J Am Coll Cardiol 43:405, 2004.
102. Bruce CJ, Connolly HM: Right-sided valve disease deserves a little more respect. Circulation 119:2726, 2009.
103. Sorajja P, Cabalka AK, Hagler DJ, et al: Successful percutaneous repair of perivalvular prosthetic regurgitation. Catheter Cardiovasc Interv 70:815, 2007.
104. Mohty D, Dumesnil JG, Echahidi N, et al: Impact of prosthesis-patient mismatch on long-term survival after aortic valve replacement: Influence of age, obesity, and left ventricular dysfunction. J Am Coll Cardiol 53:39, 2009.
105. Baddour LM, Wilson WR, Bayer AS, et al: Infective endocarditis: Diagnosis, antimicrobial therapy, and management of complications: A statement for healthcare professionals from the Committee on Rheumatic Fever, Endocarditis, and Kawasaki Disease, Council on Cardiovascular Disease in the Young, and the Councils on Clinical Cardiology, Stroke, and Cardiovascular Surgery and Anesthesia, American Heart Association: Endorsed by the Infectious Diseases Society of America [erratum in Circulation 112:2373, 2005. Circulation 115:e408, 2007. Circulation 116:e547, 2007. Circulation 118:e49, 2008]. Circulation 111:E394, 2005.

Cardiomyopathies

106. Maron BJ, Towbin JA, Thiene G, et al: Contemporary definitions and classification of the cardiomyopathies: An American Heart Association Scientific Statement from the Council on Clinical Cardiology, Heart Failure and Transplantation Committee; Quality of Care and Outcomes Research and Functional Genomics and Translational Biology Interdisciplinary Working Groups; and Council on Epidemiology and Prevention. Circulation 113:1807, 2006.
107. Elliott P, Andersson B, Arbustini E, et al: Classification of the cardiomyopathies: A position statement from the European Society Of Cardiology Working Group on Myocardial and Pericardial Diseases. Eur Heart J 29:270, 2008.
108. Leclercq C, Hare JM: Ventricular resynchronization: Current state of the art. Circulation 109:296, 2004.
109. Burkett EL, Hershberger RE: Clinical and genetic issues in familial dilated cardiomyopathy. J Am Coll Cardiol 45:969, 2005.
110. Troughton RW, Prior DL, Pereira JJ, et al: Plasma B-type natriuretic peptide levels in systolic heart failure: Importance of left ventricular diastolic function and right ventricular systolic function. J Am Coll Cardiol 43:416, 2004.
111. Kleijn SA, van Dijk J, de Cock CC, et al: Assessment of intraventricular mechanical dyssynchrony and prediction of response to cardiac resynchronization therapy: Comparison between tissue Doppler imaging and real-time three-dimensional echocardiography. J Am Soc Echocardiogr 22:1047, 2009.
112. Nishimura RA, Holmes DR Jr: Clinical practice: Hypertrophic obstructive cardiomyopathy [erratum in N Engl J Med 351:1038, 2004]. N Engl J Med 350:1320, 2004.
113. Moukarbel GV, Alam SE, Abchee AB: Contrast-enhanced echocardiography for the diagnosis of apical hypertrophic cardiomyopathy. Echocardiography 22:831, 2005.
114. Ommen SR, Maron BJ, Olivotto I, et al: Long-term effects of surgical septal myectomy on survival in patients with obstructive hypertrophic cardiomyopathy. J Am Coll Cardiol 46:470, 2005.
115. Frans EE, Nanda NC, Patel V, et al: Live three-dimensional transthoracic contrast echocardiographic assessment of apical hypertrophic cardiomyopathy. Echocardiography 22:686, 2005.
116. Ha JW, Ommen SR, Tajik AJ, et al: Differentiation of constrictive pericarditis from restrictive cardiomyopathy using mitral annular velocity by tissue Doppler echocardiography. Am J Cardiol 94:316, 2004.
117. Yoerger DM, Marcus F, Sherrill D, et al; Multidisciplinary Study of Right Ventricular Dysplasia Investigators: Echocardiographic findings in patients meeting task force criteria for arrhythmogenic right ventricular dysplasia: New insights from the multidisciplinary study of right ventricular dysplasia. J Am Coll Cardiol 45:860, 2005.
118. Hulot JS, Jouven X, Empana JP, et al: Natural history and risk stratification of arrhythmogenic right ventricular dysplasia/cardiomyopathy. Circulation 110:1879, 2004.
119. de Groot-de Laat LE, Krenning BJ, ten Cate FJ, Roelandt JR: Usefulness of contrast echocardiography for diagnosis of left ventricular noncompaction. Am J Cardiol 95:1131, 2005.

Pericardial Disease

120. Abbas AE, Appleton CP, Liu PT, Sweeney JP: Congenital absence of the pericardium: Case presentation and review of literature. Int J Cardiol 98:21, 2005.
121. Ha JW, Oh JK, Ommen SR, et al: Diagnostic value of mitral annular velocity for constrictive pericarditis in the absence of respiratory variation in mitral inflow velocity. J Am Soc Echocardiogr 15:1468, 2002.
122. Sagrista-Sauleda J, Angel J, Sanchez A, et al: Effusive-constrictive pericarditis. N Engl J Med 350:469, 2004.
123. Haley JH, Tajik AJ, Danielson GK, et al: Transient constrictive pericarditis: Causes and natural history. J Am Coll Cardiol 43:271, 2004.

Systemic Diseases Affecting the Heart

124. Koyama J, Davidoff R, Falk RH: Longitudinal myocardial velocity gradient derived from pulsed Doppler tissue imaging in AL amyloidosis: A sensitive indicator of systolic and diastolic dysfunction. J Am Soc Echocardiogr 17:36, 2004.
125. Feng D, Syed IS, Martinez M, et al: Intracardiac thrombosis and anticoagulation therapy in cardiac amyloidosis. Circulation 119:2490, 2009.
126. Moller JE, Pellikka PA, Bernheim AM, et al: Prognosis of carcinoid heart disease: Analysis of 200 cases over two decades. Circulation 112:3320, 2005.
127. Pritchett AM, Morrison JF, Edwards WD, et al: Valvular heart disease in patients taking pergolide. Mayo Clin Proc 77:1280, 2002.
128. Lancel S, Joulin O, Favory R, et al: Ventricular myocyte caspases are directly responsible for endotoxin-induced cardiac dysfunction. Circulation 111:2596, 2005.

Diseases of the Aorta

129. Milewicz DM, Dietz HC, Miller DC: Treatment of aortic disease in patients with Marfan syndrome. Circulation 111:e150, 2005.
130. Elefteriades JA: Natural history of thoracic aortic aneurysms: Indications for surgery, and surgical versus nonsurgical risks. Ann Thorac Surg 74:S1877, 2002.
131. Veldtman GR, Connolly HM, Orszulak TA, et al: Fate of bicuspid aortic valves in patients undergoing aortic root repair or replacement for aortic root enlargement. Mayo Clin Proc 81:322, 2006.
132. Michelena HI, Desjardins VA, Avierinos JF, et al: Natural history of asymptomatic patients with normally functioning or minimally dysfunctional bicuspid aortic valve in the community. Circulation 117:2776, 2008.
133. Banerjee S, Jagasia DH: Unruptured sinus of Valsalva aneurysm in an asymptomatic patient. J Am Soc Echocardiogr 15:668, 2002.
134. Russo C, Jin Z, Rundek T, et al: Atherosclerotic disease of the proximal aorta and the risk of vascular events in a population-based cohort: The Aortic Plaques and Risk of Ischemic Stroke (APRIS) study. Stroke 40:2313, 2009.
135. Moore AG, Eagle KA, Bruckman D, et al: Choice of computed tomography, transesophageal echocardiography, magnetic resonance imaging, and aortography in acute aortic dissection: International Registry of Acute Aortic Dissection (IRAD). Am J Cardiol 89:1235, 2002.
136. Ramanath VS, Oh JK, Sundt TM 3rd, Eagle KA: Acute aortic syndromes and thoracic aortic aneurysm. Mayo Clin Proc 84:465, 2009.
137. Tsui KL, Lee KW, Chan WK, et al: Behçet's aortitis and aortic regurgitation: A report of two cases. J Am Soc Echocardiogr 17:83, 2004.

Cardiac Tumors

138. Ngaage DL, Mullany CJ, Daly RC, et al: Surgical treatment of cardiac papillary fibroelastoma: A single center experience with eighty-eight patients. Ann Thorac Surg 80:1712, 2005.
139. Suwanjutah T, Singh H, Plaisance BR, et al: Live/real time three-dimensional transthoracic echocardiographic findings in primary left atrial leiomyosarcoma. Echocardiography 25:337, 2008.

Atrial Fibrillation

140. Tsang TS, Abhayaratna WP, Barnes ME, et al: Prediction of cardiovascular outcomes with left atrial size: Is volume superior to area or diameter? J Am Coll Cardiol 47:1018, 2006.
141. Karakus G, Kodali V, Inamdar V, et al: Comparative assessment of left atrial appendage by transesophageal and combined two- and three-dimensional transthoracic echocardiography. Echocardiography 25:918, 2008.

APPROPRIATE USE CRITERIA ROBERT O. BONOW

Echocardiography

During the past decade and a half, there has been an explosive growth in the use of cardiac imaging, particularly in the applications of echocardiography, Doppler echocardiography, and stress echocardiography.[1] The American College of Cardiology/American Heart Association (ACC/AHA) guidelines for the use of echocardiography were last updated in 2003.[2] Whether cardiac imaging, and in particular echocardiography, leads to enhanced quality of care and improved patient outcomes is unclear. It is difficult to tie an imaging test to patient outcomes, as any impact of diagnostic testing on patient-related outcomes is ultimately tied to downstream management strategies that the diagnostic tests may or may not set in motion. There have also been no prospective randomized trials designed to demonstrate the efficacy of imaging in achieving optimal patient outcomes. Thus, there is no firm foundation on which to develop evidence-based guidelines.

Against this background, the ACC has moved from the development of practice guidelines in cardiovascular imaging to the development of appropriate use criteria (AUC).[3,4] Partnering with a number of subspecialty societies, the ACC has spearheaded the delivery of AUC for imaging, which are designed to define the appropriate test for the appropriate indication in the appropriate patient. The first such criteria were developed for SPECT myocardial perfusion imaging, followed shortly thereafter with AUC for cardiac magnetic resonance (CMR), cardiac computed tomography (CT), echocardiography, and stress echocardiography. In subsequent chapters, the AUC are described for nuclear cardiology (see Chap. 17), CMR (see Chap. 18), and cardiac CT (see Chap. 19). The process used for development of appropriateness criteria is only partially evidence based and is heavily weighted by expert consensus.

The AUC for echocardiography are based on a number of common clinical scenarios in which imaging is often employed. These scenarios are then rated by a panel with a broad array of expertise (i.e., not just imaging experts) to evaluate the "appropriateness" of echocardiography in each situation, using the following definition: "An appropriate imaging study is one in which the expected incremental information, combined with clinical judgment, exceeds the expected negative consequences by a sufficiently wide margin for a specific indication that the procedure is generally considered acceptable care and a reasonable approach for the indication."[5] Rating scores are made on a scale of 1 to 9, in which a score of 9 indicates a highly appropriate use of testing. Using an iterative modified Delphi exercise process, with predefined rules, a final rating score is established for each indication and grouped as A, score 7-9, indicating an appropriate test for the specific indication (the test **is** generally acceptable and **is** a reasonable approach for the indication); U, score 4-6, indicating uncertainty for the specific indication (the test **may** be generally acceptable and **may** be a reasonable approach for the indication); and I, score 1-3, indicating an inappropriate test for that indication (the test **is not** generally acceptable and **is not** a reasonable approach for the indication).[5]

The AUC for echocardiography were first published in 2007,[6] followed by AUC for stress echocardiography in 2008.[7] The echocardiography AUC were updated in 2010.[8] These criteria are summarized in Table 15G-1.

TABLE 15G-1 Echocardiography Appropriate Use: Transthoracic, Transesophageal, and Stress

	INDICATION	APPROPRIATENESS SCORE (1-9)
	TTE for General Evaluation of Cardiac Structure and Function	
	Suspected Cardiac Etiology—General	
1.	Symptoms or conditions potentially related to suspected cardiac etiology including but not limited to chest pain, shortness of breath, TIA, stroke, or peripheral embolic event	A (9)
2.	Prior testing that is concerning for heart disease or structural abnormality including but not limited to chest x-ray, baseline scout images for stress echocardiogram, ECG, or cardiac biomarkers	A (9)
	Arrhythmias	
3.	Infrequent APCs or VPCs or palpitations without other evidence of heart disease	I (2)
4.	Frequent VPCs or exercise-induced VPCs	A (8)
5.	Sustained or nonsustained atrial fibrillation, SVT or VT	A (9)
6.	Asymptomatic isolated sinus bradycardia	I (2)
	Lightheadedness/Pre-Syncope/Syncope	
7.	Clinical symptoms or signs consistent with a cardiac diagnosis known to cause lightheadedness/pre-syncope/syncope (including but not limited to aortic stenosis, hypertrophic cardiomyopathy or heart failure)	A (9)
8.	Lightheadedness/presyncope/syncope when there is very low clinical suspicion for cardiovascular disease	I (3)
9.	Syncope when there are no other symptoms or signs of cardiovascular disease	A (7)
	Evaluation of Ventricular Function	
10.	Initial evaluation of ventricular function (e.g., screening) with no symptoms or signs of cardiovascular disease	I (2)
11.	Routine reevaluation of ventricular function with known coronary artery disease and no change in clinical status or cardiac exam	I (3)
12.	Evaluation of left ventricular function with prior ventricular function evaluation showing normal function (such as prior echocardiogram, left ventriculogram, CT, SPECT, cardiac MRI) in patients in whom there has been no change in clinical status or cardiac exam	I (1)
	Perioperative Evaluation	
13.	Routine perioperative evaluation of ventricular function with no symptoms or signs of cardiovascular disease	I (2)
14.	Routine perioperative evaluation of cardiac structure and function prior to non-cardiac solid organ transplant	U (6)
	Pulmonary Hypertension	
15.	Evaluation of suspected pulmonary hypertension including evaluation of right ventricular function and estimated pulmonary artery pressure	A (9)
16.	Routine (< 1 year) reevaluation of known pulmonary hypertension without change in clinical status or cardiac exam	I (3)
17.	Routine (≥ 1 year) reevaluation of known pulmonary hypertension without change in clinical status or cardiac exam	A (7)
18.	Reevaluation of known pulmonary hypertension if change in clinical status or cardiac exam or to guide therapy	A (9)

TABLE 15G-1 **Echocardiography Appropriate Use: Transthoracic, Transesophageal, and Stress—cont'd**

	INDICATION	APPROPRIATENESS SCORE (1-9)
	TTE for Cardiovascular Evaluation in an Acute Setting	
	Hypotension or Hemodynamic Instability	
19.	Hypotension or hemodynamic instability of uncertain or suspected cardiac etiology	A (9)
20.	Assessment/monitoring of volume status in a critically ill patient	U (5)
	Myocardial Ischemia/Infarction	
21.	Acute chest pain with suspected myocardial infarction and nondiagnostic ECG when a resting echocardiogram can be performed during pain	A (9)
22.	Evaluation of a patient without chest pain but with other features of an ischemic equivalent or laboratory markers indicative of ongoing myocardial infarction	A (8)
23.	Suspected complication of myocardial ischemia/infarction, including but not limited to acute mitral regurgitation, ventricular septal defect, free-wall rupture/tamponade, shock, right ventricular involvement, heart failure, or thrombus	A (9)
	Evaluation of Ventricular Function after Acute Coronary Syndrome (ACS)	
24.	Initial evaluation of ventricular function following ACS	A (9)
25.	Reevaluation of ventricular function following ACS during recovery phase when results will guide therapy	A (9)
	Respiratory Failure	
26.	Respiratory failure or hypoxemia of uncertain etiology	A (8)
27.	Respiratory failure or hypoxemia when a non-cardiac etiology of respiratory failure has been established	U (5)
	Pulmonary Embolism	
28.	Suspected pulmonary embolism in order to establish diagnosis	I (2)
29.	Known acute pulmonary embolism to guide therapy (e.g., thrombectomy and thrombolytics)	A (8)
30.	Routine reevaluation of prior pulmonary embolism with normal right ventricular function and pulmonary artery systolic pressure	I (1)
31.	Reevaluation of known pulmonary embolism after thrombolysis or thrombectomy for assessment of change in right ventricular function and/or pulmonary artery pressure	A (7)
	Cardiac Trauma	
32.	Severe deceleration injury or chest trauma when valve injury, pericardial effusion or cardiac injury are possible or suspected	A (9)
33.	Routine evaluation in the setting of mild chest trauma with no ECG changes or biomarker elevation	I (2)
	TTE for Evaluation of Valvular Function	
	Murmur or Click	
34.	Initial evaluation when there is a reasonable suspicion of valvular or structural heart disease	A (9)
35.	Initial evaluation when there is a very low suspicion of valvular or structural heart disease	I (2)
36.	Reevaluation in a patient without valvular disease on prior echocardiogram and no change in clinical status or cardiac exam	I (1)
37.	Reevaluation of known valvular heart disease with a change in clinical status or cardiac exam or to guide therapy	A (9)
	Native Valvular Stenosis	
38.	Routine (< 3 year) reevaluation of mild valvular stenosis without change in clinical status or cardiac exam	I (3)
39.	Routine (≥ 3 year) reevaluation of mild valvular stenosis without change in clinical status or cardiac exam	A (7)
40.	Routine (< 1 year) reevaluation of moderate or severe valvular stenosis without change in clinical status or cardiac exam	I (3)
41.	Routine (≥ 1 year) reevaluation of moderate or severe valvular stenosis without change in clinical status or cardiac exam	A (8)
	Native Valvular Regurgitation	
42.	Routine reevaluation of trace valvular regurgitation	I (1)
43.	Routine (< 3 years) reevaluation of mild valvular regurgitation without change in clinical status or cardiac exam	I (1)
44.	Routine (≥ 3 years) reevaluation of mild valvular regurgitation without change in clinical status or cardiac exam	U (4)
45.	Routine (< 1 year) reevaluation of moderate or severe valvular regurgitation without change in clinical status or cardiac exam	U (6)
46.	Routine (≥ 1 year) reevaluation of moderate or severe valvular regurgitation without change in clinical status or cardiac exam	A (8)
	Prosthetic Valve	
47.	Initial postoperative evaluation of prosthetic valve for establishment of baseline	A (9)
48.	Routine (< 3 years) reevaluation of prosthetic valve if no known or suspected valve dysfunction	I (3)
49.	Routine (≥ 3 years) reevaluation of prosthetic valve if no known or suspected valve dysfunction	A (7)
50.	Evaluation of prosthetic valve with suspected dysfunction or a change in clinical status or cardiac exam	A (9)
51.	Reevaluation of known prosthetic valve dysfunction when it would change management or guide therapy	A (9)
	Infective Endocarditis (Native or Prosthetic Valves)	
52.	Initial evaluation of suspected infective endocarditis with positive blood cultures or a new murmur	A (9)
53.	Transient fever without evidence of bacteremia or new murmur	I (2)
54.	Transient bacteremia with a pathogen not typically associated with infective endocarditis and/or documented non-endovascular source of infection	I (3)
55.	Reevaluation of infective endocarditis at high risk for progression or complication or with a change in clinical status or cardiac exam	A (9)
56.	Routine reevaluation of uncomplicated infective endocarditis when no change in management is contemplated	I (2)
	TTE for Evaluation of Intracardiac and Extracardiac Structures and Chambers	
57.	Suspected cardiac mass	A (9)
58.	Suspected cardiovascular source of embolus	A (9)
59.	Suspected pericardial conditions	A (9)

Continued

TABLE 15G-1 **Echocardiography Appropriate Use: Transthoracic, Transesophageal, and Stress—cont'd**

	INDICATION	APPROPRIATENESS SCORE (1-9)
60.	Routine reevaluation of known small pericardial effusion with no change in clinical status	I (2)
61.	Reevaluation of known pericardial effusion to guide management or therapy	A (8)
62.	Guidance of percutaneous noncoronary cardiac procedures including but not limited to pericardiocentesis, septal ablation or RV biopsy	A (9)
	TTE for Evaluation of Aortic Disease	
63.	Evaluation of the ascending aorta in the setting of a known or suspected connective tissue disease or genetic condition that predisposes to aortic aneurysm or dissection (e.g., Marfan syndrome)	A (9)
64.	Reevaluation of known ascending aortic dilation or history of aortic dissection to establish a baseline rate of expansion or when the rate of expansion is excessive	A (9)
65.	Reevaluation of known ascending aortic dilation or history of aortic dissection with a change in clinical status or cardiac exam or when findings may alter management or therapy	A (9)
66.	Reevaluation of known ascending aortic dilation or history of aortic dissection without a change in clinical status or cardiac exam when findings would not change management or therapy	I (3)
	TTE for Evaluation of Hypertension, Heart Failure, or Cardiomyopathy	
Hypertension		
67.	Initial evaluation of suspected hypertensive heart disease	A (8)
68.	Routine evaluation of systemic hypertension without suspected hypertensive heart disease	I (3)
69.	Reevaluation of known hypertensive heart disease without a change in clinical status or cardiac exam	U (4)
Heart Failure		
70.	Initial evaluation of known or suspected heart failure (systolic or diastolic) based on symptoms, signs or abnormal test results	A (9)
71.	Reevaluation of known heart failure (systolic or diastolic) with a change in clinical status or cardiac exam without a clear precipitating change in medication or diet	A (8)
72.	Reevaluation of known heart failure (systolic or diastolic) with a change in clinical status or cardiac exam with a clear precipitating change in medication or diet	U (4)
73.	Reevaluation of known heart failure (systolic or diastolic) to guide therapy	A (9)
74.	Routine (< 1 year) reevaluation of heart failure (systolic or diastolic) when there is no change in clinical status or cardiac exam	I (2)
75.	Routine (≥ 1 year) reevaluation of heart failure (systolic or diastolic) when there is no change in clinical status or cardiac exam	U (6)
Device Evaluation (including pacemaker, ICD or CRT)		
76.	Initial evaluation or reevaluation after revascularization and/or optimal medical therapy to determine candidacy for device therapy and/or to determine optimal choice of device	A (9)
77.	Initial evaluation for cardiac resynchronization therapy (CRT) device optimization after implantation	U (6)
78.	Known implanted pacing device with symptoms possibly due to device complication or suboptimal pacing device settings	A (8)
79.	Routine (< 1 year) reevaluation of implanted device without change in clinical status or cardiac exam	I (1)
80.	Routine (≥ 1 year) reevaluation of implanted device without change in clinical status or cardiac exam	I (3)
Ventricular Assist Devices and Cardiac Transplantation		
81.	To determine candidacy for ventricular assist device	A (9)
82.	Optimization of ventricular assist device settings	A (7)
83.	Reevaluation of signs/symptoms suggestive of ventricular assist device-related complications	A (9)
84.	Monitoring for rejection in a cardiac transplant recipient	A (7)
85.	Cardiac structure and function evaluation in a potential heart donor	A (9)
Cardiomyopathies		
86.	Initial evaluation of known or suspected cardiomyopathy (e.g., restrictive, infiltrative, dilated, hypertrophic or genetic cardiomyopathy)	A (9)
87.	Reevaluation of known cardiomyopathy with a change in clinical status or cardiac exam or to guide therapy	A (9)
88.	Routine (< 1 year) reevaluation of known cardiomyopathy without change in clinical status or cardiac exam	I (2)
89.	Routine (≥ 1 year) reevaluation of known cardiomyopathy without change in clinical status or cardiac exam	U (5)
90.	Screening evaluation for structure and function in first-degree relatives of a patient with inherited cardiomyopathy	A (9)
91.	Baseline and serial reevaluations in patients undergoing therapy with cardiotoxic agents	A (9)
	TTE for Adult Congenital Heart Disease	
92.	Initial evaluation of known or suspected adult congenital heart disease	A (9)
93.	Known adult congenital heart disease with a change in clinical status or cardiac exam	A (9)
94.	Reevaluation to guide therapy in known adult congenital heart disease	A (9)
95.	Routine (< 2 years) reevaluation of adult congenital heart disease following complete repair -without residual structural or hemodynamic abnormality -without a change in clinical status or cardiac exam	I (3)
96.	Routine (≥ 2 years) reevaluation of adult congenital heart disease following complete repair -without residual structural or hemodynamic abnormality -without a change in clinical status or cardiac exam	U (6)
97.	Routine (< 1 year) reevaluation of congenital heart disease following incomplete or palliative repair -with residual structural or hemodynamic abnormality -without a change in clinical status or cardiac exam	U (5)
98.	Routine (≥ 1 year) reevaluation of congenital heart disease following incomplete or palliative repair -with residual structural or hemodynamic abnormality -without a change in clinical status or cardiac exam	A (8)

TABLE 15G-1 Echocardiography Appropriate Use: Transthoracic, Transesophageal, and Stress—cont'd

INDICATION	APPROPRIATENESS SCORE (1-9)
Transesophageal Echocardiography	
TEE as Initial or Supplemental Test—General Uses	
99. Use of TEE when there is a high likelihood of a non-diagnostic TTE due to patient characteristics or inadequate visualization of relevant structures	A (8)
100. Routine use of TEE when a diagnostic TTE is reasonably anticipated to resolve all diagnostic and management concerns	I (1)
101. Reevaluation of prior TEE finding for interval change (e.g., resolution of thrombus after anticoagulation, resolution of vegetation after antibiotic therapy) when a change in therapy is anticipated	A (8)
102. Reevaluation of prior TEE finding for interval change (e.g., resolution of thrombus after anticoagulation, resolution of vegetation after antibiotic therapy) when no change in therapy is anticipated	I (2)
103. Guidance during percutaneous noncoronary cardiac interventions including but not limited to closure device placement, radiofrequency ablation, and percutaneous valve procedures	A (9)
104. Suspected acute aortic pathology including but not limited to dissection/transsection	A (9)
105. Routine assessment of pulmonary veins in an asymptomatic patient status post pulmonary vein isolation	I (3)
TEE as Initial or Supplemental Test—Valvular Disease	
106. Evaluation of valvular structure and function to assess suitability for, and assist in planning of, an intervention	A (9)
107. To diagnose/manage infective endocarditis with a low pretest probability (e.g., transient fever, known alternative source of infection or negative blood cultures/atypical pathogen for endocarditis)	I (3)
108. To diagnose/manage infective endocarditis with a moderate or high pretest probability (e.g., staph bacteremia, fungemia, prosthetic heart valve, or intracardiac device)	A (9)
TEE as Initial or Supplemental Test—Embolic Event	
109. Evaluation for cardiovascular source of embolus with no identified non-cardiac source	A (7)
110. Evaluation for cardiovascular source of embolus with a previously identified non-cardiac source	U (5)
111. Evaluation for cardiovascular source of embolus with a known cardiac source in which a TEE would not change management	I (1)
TEE as Initial Test—Atrial Fibrillation/Flutter	
112. Evaluation to facilitate clinical decision-making with regards to anticoagulation, cardioversion and/or radiofrequency ablation	A (9)
113. Evaluation when a decision has been made to anticoagulate and not to perform cardioversion	I (2)
Stress Echocardiography for Detection of CAD/Risk Assessment: Symptomatic or Ischemic Equivalent	
Evaluation of Ischemic Equivalent (Non-Acute)	
114. Low pre-test probability of CAD ECG interpretable AND able to exercise	I (3)
115. Low pre-test probability of CAD ECG uninterpretable OR unable to exercise	A (7)
116. Intermediate pre-test probability of CAD ECG interpretable AND able to exercise	A (7)
117. Intermediate pre-test probability of CAD ECG uninterpretable OR unable to exercise	A (9)
118. High pre-test probability of CAD Regardless of ECG interpretability and ability to exercise	A (7)
Acute Chest Pain	
119. Possible ACS ECG: no ischemic changes or uninterpretable ECG Low-risk TIMI score Negative troponin levels	A (7)
120. Possible ACS ECG: no ischemic changes or uninterpretable ECG Low-risk TIMI score Peak troponin: borderline, equivocal, minimally elevated	A (7)
121. Possible ACS ECG: no ischemic changes or uninterpretable ECG High-risk TIMI score Negative troponin levels	A (7)
122. Possible ACS ECG: no ischemic changes or uninterpretable ECG High-risk TIMI score Peak troponin: borderline, equivocal, minimally elevated	A (7)
123. Definite ACS	I (1)
Stress Echocardiography for Detection of CAD/Risk Assessment: Asymptomatic (Without Ischemic Equivalent)	
General Patient Populations	
124. Low global CHD risk	U (1)
125. Intermediate global CHD risk ECG interpretable	I (2)
126. Intermediate global CHD risk ECG uninterpretable	U (5)
127. High global CHD risk	U (5)

Continued

TABLE 15G-1 Echocardiography Appropriate Use: Transthoracic, Transesophageal, and Stress—cont'd

INDICATION	APPROPRIATENESS SCORE (1-9)
Stress Echocardiography for Detection of CAD/Risk Assessment: Asymptomatic (Without Ischemic Equivalent) in Patient Populations With Defined Comorbidities	
New-Onset or Newly Diagnosed Heart Failure or LV Systolic Dysfunction	
128. No prior CAD evaluation AND no planned coronary angiography	A (7)
Arrhythmias	
129. Sustained VT	A (7)
130. Frequent PVCs, exercise induced VT, or nonsustained VT	A (7)
131. Infrequent PVCs	I (3)
132. Atrial fibrillation or other SVT	U (6)
Syncope	
133. Low global CHD risk	I (3)
134. Intermediate or high global CHD risk	A (7)
Elevated Troponin	
135. Troponin elevation without symptoms or additional evidence of ACS	A (7)
Stress Echocardiography Following Prior Test Results	
Asymptomatic: Prior Evidence of Subclinical Disease	
136. Coronary calcium Agatston score < 100	I (2)
137. Low to intermediate global CHD risk Coronary calcium Agatston score between 100-400	U (5)
138. High global CHD risk Coronary calcium Agatston score between 100-400	U (6)
139. Coronary calcium Agatston score > 400	A (7)
140. Abnormal carotid intimal medial thickness (IMT ≥ 0.9 mm and/or the presence of plaque encroaching into the arterial lumen)	U (5)
Coronary Angiography (Invasive or Noninvasive)	
141. Coronary artery stenosis of unclear significance	A (8)
Asymptomatic OR Stable Symptoms, Normal Prior Stress Imaging Study	
142. Low global CHD risk Last stress imaging study < 2 years ago	I (1)
143. Low global CHD risk Last stress imaging study ≥ 2 years ago	I (2)
144. Intermediate to high global CHD risk Last stress imaging study < 2 years ago	I (2)
145. Intermediate to high global CHD risk Last stress imaging study ≥ 2 years ago	U (4)
Asymptomatic OR Stable Symptoms With Abnormal Coronary Angiography OR Abnormal Prior Stress Study, No Prior Revascularization	
146. Known CAD on coronary angiography OR prior abnormal stress imaging study Last stress imaging study < 2 years ago	I (3)
147. Known CAD on coronary angiography OR prior abnormal stress imaging study Last stress imaging study ≥ 2 years ago	U (5)
Treadmill ECG Stress Test	
148. Low risk treadmill score (e.g., Duke)	I (1)
149. Intermediate risk treadmill score (e.g., Duke)	A (7)
150. High risk treadmill score (e.g., Duke)	A (7)
New, Worsening, or Unresolved Symptoms	
151. Abnormal coronary angiography OR abnormal prior stress imaging study	A (7)
152. Normal coronary angiography OR normal prior stress imaging study	U (6)
Prior Noninvasive evaluation	
153. Equivocal, borderline, or discordant stress testing where obstructive CAD remains a concern	A (8)
Stress Echocardiography for Risk Assessment: Perioperative Evaluation for Noncardiac Surgery without Active Cardiac Conditions	
Low-Risk Surgery	
154. Perioperative evaluation for risk assessment	I (1)
Intermediate-Risk Surgery	
155. Moderate to good functional capacity (≥ 4 METs)	I (3)
156. No clinical risk factors	I (2)
157. ≥ 1 clinical risk factor Poor or unknown functional capacity (< 4 METs)	U (6)
158. Asymptomatic < 1 year post normal catheterization, noninvasive test, or previous revascularization	I (1)

TABLE 15G-1 **Echocardiography Appropriate Use: Transthoracic, Transesophageal, and Stress—cont'd**

INDICATION	APPROPRIATENESS SCORE (1-9)
Vascular Surgery	
159. Moderate to good functional capacity (≥ 4 METs)	I (3)
160. No clinical risk factors	I (2)
161. ≥1 clinical risk factor Poor or unknown functional capacity (< 4 METs)	A (7)
162. Asymptomatic < 1 year post normal catheterization, noninvasive test, or previous revascularization	I (2)
Stress Echocardiography for Risk Assessment: Within 3 Months of an Acute Coronary Syndrome	
STEMI	
163. Primary PCI with complete revascularization No recurrent symptoms	I (2)
164. Hemodynamically stable, no recurrent chest pain symptoms or no signs of HF To evaluate for inducible ischemia No prior coronary angiography since the index event	A (7)
165. Hemodynamically unstable, signs of cardiogenic shock, or mechanical complications	I (1)
UA/NSTEMI	
166. Hemodynamically stable, no recurrent chest pain symptoms or no signs of HF To evaluate for inducible ischemia No prior coronary angiography since the index event	A (8)
ACS—Asymptomatic Post-Revascularization (PCI or CABG)	
167. Prior to hospital discharge	I (1)
Cardiac Rehabilitation	
168. Prior to initiation of cardiac rehabilitation (as a stand-alone indication)	I (3)
Stress Echocardiography for Risk Assessment: Post-Revascularization (PCI or CABG)	
Symptomatic	
169. Ischemic equivalent	A (8)
Asymptomatic	
170. Incomplete revascularization Additional revascularization feasible	A (7)
171. < 5 years after CABG	I (2)
172. ≥ 5 years after CABG	U (6)
173. < 2 years after PCI	I (2)
174. ≥ 2 years after PCI	U (5)
Cardiac Rehabilitation	
175. Prior to initiation of cardiac rehabilitation (as a stand-alone indication)	I (3)
Stress Echocardiography for Assessment of Viability/Ischemia	
Ischemic Cardiomyopathy/Assessment of Viability	
176. Known moderate or severe LV dysfunction Patient eligible for revascularization Use of dobutamine only	A (8)
Stress Echocardiography for Hemodynamics (Includes Doppler During Stress)	
Chronic Valvular Disease—Asymptomatic	
177. Mild mitral stenosis	I (2)
178. Moderate mitral stenosis	U (5)
179. Severe mitral stenosis	A (7)
180. Mild aortic stenosis	I (3)
181. Moderate aortic stenosis	U (6)
182. Severe aortic stenosis	U (5)
183. Mild mitral regurgitation	I (2)
184. Moderate mitral regurgitation	U (5)
185. Severe mitral regurgitation LV size and function not meeting surgical criteria	A (7)
186. Mild aortic regurgitation	I (2)
187. Moderate aortic regurgitation	U (5)
188. Severe aortic regurgitation LV size and function not meeting surgical criteria	A (7)
Chronic Valvular Disease—Symptomatic	
189. Mild mitral stenosis	U (5)
190. Moderate mitral stenosis	A (7)
191. Severe mitral stenosis	I (3)
192. Severe aortic stenosis	I (1)
193. Evaluation of equivocal aortic stenosis Evidence of low cardiac output or LV systolic dysfunction ("low gradient AS") Use of dobutamine only	A (8)

Continued

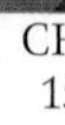

CH 15

TABLE 15G-1 Echocardiography Appropriate Use: Transthoracic, Transesophageal, and Stress—cont'd

	INDICATION	APPROPRIATENESS SCORE (1-9)
194.	Mild mitral regurgitation	U (4)
195.	Moderate mitral regurgitation	A (7)
196.	Severe mitral regurgitation Severe LV enlargement or LV systolic dysfunction	I (3)
Acute Valvular disease		
197.	Acute moderate or severe mitral or aortic regurgitation	I (3)
Pulmonary Hypertension		
198.	Suspected pulmonary hypertension Normal or indeterminate resting echo study	U (5)
199.	Routine evaluation of patients with known resting pulmonary hypertension	I (3)
200.	Reevaluation of patient with exercise induced pulmonary hypertension to evaluate response to therapy	U (5)
Contrast Use in TTE/TEE or Stress Echocardiography		
201.	Routine use of contrast All left ventricular segments visualized on noncontrast images	I (1)
202.	Selective use of contrast ≥2 contiguous left ventricular segments are NOT seen on noncontrast images	A (8)

Abbreviations: ACS = acute coronary syndrome; APC = atrial premature contraction; CABG = coronary artery bypass graft surgery; CAD = coronary artery disease; CHD = coronary heart disease; HF = heart failure; LV = left ventricular; NSTEMI = non ST-segment myocardial infarction; PCI = percutaneous coronary intervention; STEMI = ST-segment myocardial infarction; SVT = supraventricular tachycardia; TEE = transesophageal echocardiography; TTE = transthoracic echocardiography; TIA = transient ischemic attack; UA = unstable angina; VPC = ventricular premature contraction; VT = ventricular tachycardia

REFERENCES

1. Pearlman AS, Ryan T, Picard MH, Douglas P: Evolving trends in the use of echocardiography: A study of Medicare beneficiaries. J Am Coll Cardiol 49:2283, 2007.
2. Cheitlin MD, Armstrong WF, Aurigemma GP, et al: ACC/AHA/ASE 2003 guideline update for the clinical application of echocardiography: A report of the American College of Cardiology/American Heart Association Task Force on Practice Guidelines (ACC/AHA/ASE Committee to Update the 1997 Guidelines for the Clinical Application of Echocardiography). J Am Coll Cardiol 42:954, 2003.
3. Douglas PS, Wolk MJ, Brindis R, Hendel RC: Appropriateness criteria: Breaking new ground. J Am Coll Cardiol 46:2143, 2005.
4. Patel MR, Spertus JA, Brindis RG, et al: ACCF proposed method for evaluating the appropriateness of cardiovascular imaging. J Am Coll Cardiol 46:1606, 2005.
5. Brindis RG, Douglas PS, Hendel RC, et al: ACCF/ASNC appropriateness criteria for single-photon emission computed tomography myocardial perfusion imaging (SPECT MPI). A report of the American College of Cardiology Foundation Quality Strategic Directions Committee Appropriateness Criteria Working Group and the American Society of Nuclear Cardiology Endorsed by the American Heart Association. J Am Coll Cardiol 46:1587, 2005.
6. Douglas PS, Khandheria B, Stainback RF, Weissman NJ: ACCF/ASE/ACEP/ASNC/SCAI/SCCT/SCMR 2007 appropriateness criteria for transthoracic and transesophageal echocardiography. A report of the American College of Cardiology Foundation Quality Strategic Directions Committee Appropriateness Criteria Working Group, American Society of Echocardiography, American College of Emergency Physicians, American Society of Nuclear Cardiology, Society for Cardiovascular Angiography and Interventions, Society of Cardiovascular Computed Tomography, and the Society for Cardiovascular Magnetic Resonance endorsed by the American College of Chest Physicians and the Society of Critical Care Medicine. J Am Coll Cardiol 50:187, 2007.
7. Douglas PS, Khandheria B, Stainback RF, Weissman NJ: ACCF/ASE/ACEP/AHA/ASNC/SCAI/SCCT/SCMR 2008 appropriateness criteria for stress echocardiography. A Report of the American College of Cardiology Foundation Appropriateness Criteria Task Force, American Society of Echocardiography, American College of Emergency Physicians, American Heart Association, American Society of Nuclear Cardiology, Society for Cardiovascular Angiography and Interventions, Society of Cardiovascular Computed Tomography, and Society for Cardiovascular Magnetic Resonance. Endorsed by the Heart Rhythm Society and the Society of Critical Care Medicine. J Am Coll Cardiol 51:1127, 2008.
8. Douglas PS, Garcia MJ, Haines DE, et al: ACCF/ASE/ACCP/AHA/ASNC/HFSA/HRS/SCAI/SCCM/SCCT/SCMR 2010 Appropriate use criteria for echocardiography. J Am Coll Cardiol 2010. In press.

CHAPTER 16 The Chest Radiograph in Cardiovascular Disease

Michael A. Bettmann

The chest radiograph was one of the first clinical examinations to use the then-new technology of diagnostic radiography.[1] It remains the most common x-ray examination and one of the most difficult examinations to interpret. With careful evaluation, it yields a large amount of anatomic and physiologic information, but it is difficult and sometimes even impossible to extract the information that it contains. The major variables that determine what can be learned from the chest x-ray include the technical factors (milliamperage [mA], kilovoltage [kV], exposure duration) used in obtaining the radiographs, patient specific factors (e.g., body habitus, age, physiologic status, ability to stand and to take and hold a deep breath), and the training, experience, and focus of the interpreter. The aims of this chapter are to review how chest radiographs are obtained, present a basic approach to their interpretation, and discuss and illustrate common and characteristic findings relevant to cardiovascular disease in adults.

Technical Considerations

The usual chest radiograph consists of a frontal and a lateral view. The frontal view is a posteroanterior (PA) view, with the patient standing with the chest toward the recording medium and the back to the x-ray tube. The lateral is also taken with the patient standing, with the left side toward the film. For both, the x-ray tube is positioned at a distance of 6 feet from the film. This is termed a *6-foot SID* (source-image distance). The rationale for these conventions is based on physics; x-rays are created by inducing a high current across a diode, thereby generating electrons aimed at a metal target, the anode. When the electrons reach the target, x-ray photons are produced. This anode is made of special metals, rotates at a high speed, and is housed in an oil-filled container, all to preserve the target and ensure that the production of the photons is uniform and of high quality, without damage to the anode. The anode has an angled edge, so that the x-rays emerge at essentially a right angle to the incoming electron beam. The x-rays are allowed to emerge from the tube housing only through a small opening, the focal spot. The smaller the focal spot, the higher the energy required to deliver a given number of photons. Also, the smaller the focal spot, the narrower the x-ray beam (i.e., the closer to a point source), leading to improved imaging geometry. The ability of the x-rays to penetrate structures is determined by the combination of the kilovoltage, milliamperage, and time used to produce them. These factors are also the major (but not sole) determinants of the radiation exposure that the patient receives.[2,3]

In theory, x-rays emerge from the x-ray tube as a point source, remain parallel, and do not diverge from each other, and consequently there is no geometric distortion of structures as they pass through the body and are recorded on film. In reality, however, the x-rays form a cone-shaped beam. They diverge from the focal spot and become less parallel as the distance from the focal spot increases. When the incident x-rays interact with film or other recording medium, there is geometric distortion as a function of the distance from the midline of the x-ray beam and the distance of the structures from the film. If one imagines a wide-diameter structure, such as the thorax, that is perpendicular to the center of the x-ray beam, the farther from the tube an object is, the more parallel are the x-rays that penetrate it (**Figs. 16-1 and 16-2**). Conversely, the closer the object and film are to the x-ray tube, the more the incident x-rays must diverge to cover the edges of the object. Thus, the farther an object is from the source, the less geometric distortion is encountered. The greater the distance from the source, however, the more energy that must be applied to penetrate the object to be imaged and to expose the x-ray recording medium. That is, in simple terms, resolution is improved by increasing the SID but tube energy and therefore exposure to the patient must also be increased as the SID increases. To balance these opposing concerns, a standard convention has been developed; routine standing chest radiographs are obtained with an SID of 6 feet.

X-rays are blocked from the film or other recording medium to varying degrees by various structures, leading to shades of gray that allow discrimination between the heart, which is fluid-filled and relatively impervious to x-rays, and the air-filled lung parenchyma, which blocks few x-rays. The exposure that the patient receives is a function of the strength and duration of the current applied to the x-ray tube (or, more precisely and accurately, of the number, strength and duration of the x-ray photons produced—the mA, kV, and milliseconds), size of the focal spot, distance from the tube to the patient, and degree to which the x-rays are blocked and scattered within the patient. Most patient exposure is not a result of the x-rays that penetrate, but rather those that interact with tissues and are slowed and changed, and in the process deposit residual energy in tissue. This process is what is broadly referred to as scatter. As the amount of tissue that attenuates photons increases, the amount of energy deposition within the patient will increase. Patients who are very thin will require an inherently lower x-ray dose to achieve diagnostically satisfactory deposition of x-ray photons on an imaging medium, and will have less energy deposition within the body. In patients who are obese, a higher x-ray dose will be necessary to penetrate the patient and produce a diagnostic exposure. The increased soft tissue in these patients also causes more dispersion of the x-ray beam and results in a higher dose. Scatter leads not only to deposition of energy in the patient, but also deposits energy on surrounding structures. This includes personnel, if they are close to the patient (as with fluoroscopy), and the recording medium. That is, the film or other digital plate is altered not only by incident x-rays to produce an image (i.e., signal). It is also altered by scatter, which does not reflect anatomic structures but will detract from the resolution of these structures (i.e., noise). The more scatter deposited on the recording medium, the more the image quality is denigrated and the worse the resolution—signal-to-noise ratio is decreased. This is why the resolution of chest radiographs is worse in larger than in thinner patients when all other factors remain constant.

There are several additional practical considerations that relate to the physics of chest radiographs. The standard chest radiograph is obtained with deep inspiration and the patient facing the film. If patients are unable to stand, chest radiographs are generally obtained with the patient's chest toward the tube and the back toward the film, the anteroposterior (AP) position. With the standard PA view, the heart appears smaller and its size and contour are more accurately depicted than on an AP view, because the SID is larger and the heart is closer to the recording medium. With AP views, as with portable films, there is resultant greater divergence of x-rays because the heart lies relatively anteriorly (and so is farther from the film) and the SID is short. Similarly, on a standard lateral film, the right ribs appear larger than the left (see Fig. 16-2B). In both cases, this effect occurs because a structure is farther from the film. As a result, there is increased divergence of the x-rays from the midline point source and relative magnification. The side of an effusion, therefore, can generally be delineated on a lateral radiograph by determining whether the effusion is associated with the side with the ribs that appear larger or those that appear smaller (see Fig. 16-2B).

There are several inherent practical limitations to portable chest radiographs. Most are obtained with patients positioned supine or semisupine. The degree of inspiration is therefore likely to be substantially less than with an erect film, making the heart appear relatively larger and providing less optimal visualization of the lungs, because they are not optimally expanded. Furthermore, portable radiographs are invariably taken as AP views and the SID is less than 6 feet, of necessity, because of the nature of the portable x-ray machine and also because of the usual position of the patient, sitting or lying in a bed. Most portable x-ray units do not have generators sufficiently strong to be able to produce x-rays that will penetrate a patient adequately and expose the film from 6 feet. Space constraints and the patient's position are additional hurdles. Also, because exposure time must usually be longer than with fixed units, cardiac and respiratory motion are more likely to interfere and edge definition is compromised. For all these reasons, the inherent resolution is poorer with portable radiographs, making them less accurate and useful. Also because of the lower available energy with portable x-ray units and the longer exposure time necessary to compensate, radiation exposure to the patient is greater than with a standard PA film. Portable films are most useful for answering relatively simple mechanical questions, such as whether the pacemaker or automated implantable cardioverter-defibrillator (ICD) is properly positioned (**Fig. 16-3**), whether the endotracheal tube is in the correct location, and whether the mediastinum is midline.[2,4] They are generally not good at providing physiologic or complex anatomic information.

It is important to recognize that there are questions that cannot be answered accurately from a portable chest x-ray film. If the film is obtained with the patient in a less than upright position, it is impossible to exclude even a sizable pneumothorax or pleural effusion. Because of the patient's position, shorter SID, and limited tube output, it is impossible to evaluate heart size and contour or status of pulmonary vascularity. It may be possible to say whether there is acute pulmonary edema, but it is not possible to judge whether there is cardiomegaly, mild to moderate congestive heart failure, or presence or absence of a small infiltrate. Although portable chest studies may be convenient and provide some information, they should be performed only in limited situations, when clearly needed to answer specific questions.

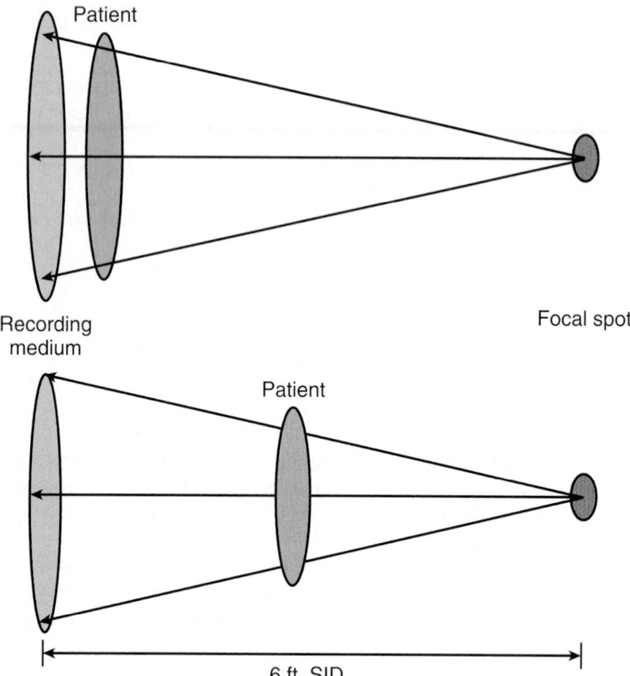

FIGURE 16-1 Position of the patient in relation to the SID between x-ray source (focal spot) and recording medium. The closer the patient is to the source, the greater the x-ray divergence and the resulting geometric distortion.

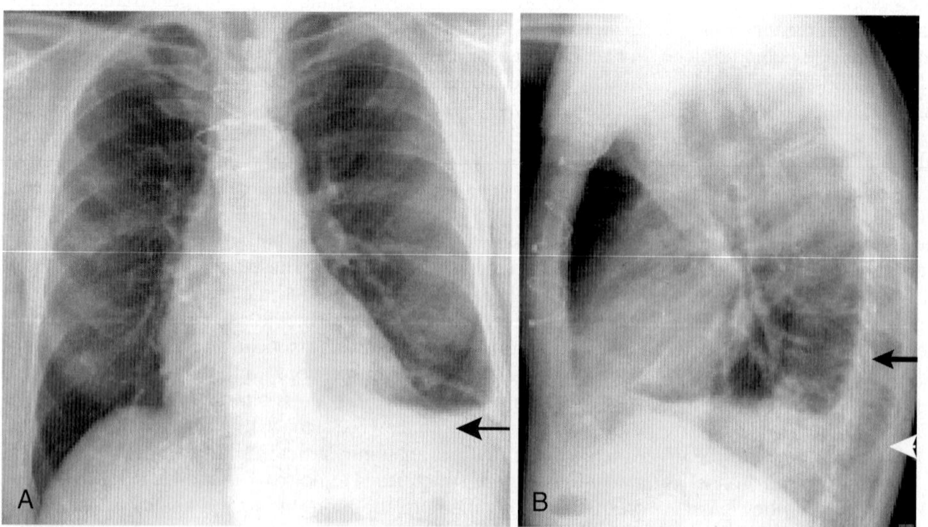

FIGURE 16-2 Standard upright chest radiographs of a 74-year-old man who has undergone aortic valve replacement. **A,** PA view shows median sternotomy wires, a left pleural effusion (arrow), and normal pulmonary vascular pattern. **B,** Lateral view. Note that the right ribs (small arrow) are magnified compared with the left (large arrow), and the effusion can be localized to the left. Also, note that the gastric air bubble is displaced inferiorly (PA view) and anteroinferiorly (lateral view), indicating an enlarged left ventricle.

Image Recording and Radiation Exposure

Until the turn of the last century, all chest radiographs were recorded on high-resolution x-ray film. With optimal technique and a cooperative patient who can hold a deep inspiration, the result is a study that clearly and accurately depicts very small structures, such as the contour of small pulmonary arteries. With x-ray film, the incident x-rays (and scattered photons) alter silver iodide crystals in an emulsion. When the film is developed, these alterations produce an image reflecting the extent to which x-rays have interacted with specific areas of the film. There is inherently very high resolution of structures because of the small size of the silver iodide crystals and their sensitivity to incident x-ray photons. This has changed as the digital age has come to imaging. With the advent of digital radiography (DR), a filmless form of radiography, chest radiographs are increasingly stored on digital media. There are two principal ways to do this. The first, less expensive approach has been called computed radiography (CR). It is essentially a digital conversion of conventionally obtained chest radiographs. For this procedure, x-rays are recorded on a reusable imaging screen, much like a fluoroscopic screen but with the ability to provide better resolution, and the image is converted to a digital format in which it is postprocessed, reviewed, and stored. The second method, DR, is the direct recording of images by digital means, without analog-to-digital conversion. There is an inherent difference with the elimination of added noise and lost information that occurs with this conversion. True DR can be accomplished in many ways. The most common is flat plate technology for reasons of resolution, usefulness and, in the long term, cost. It involves the use of an image-sensing plate that directly converts the incident photons into a digital signal rather than producing a transient conversion as with an image intensifier, reusable CR plate, or alteration of a silver iodide crystal in a film emulsion. DR is truly "filmless"; CR can be either, and the classic chest radiograph relies on film that is exposed and developed.[5-13]

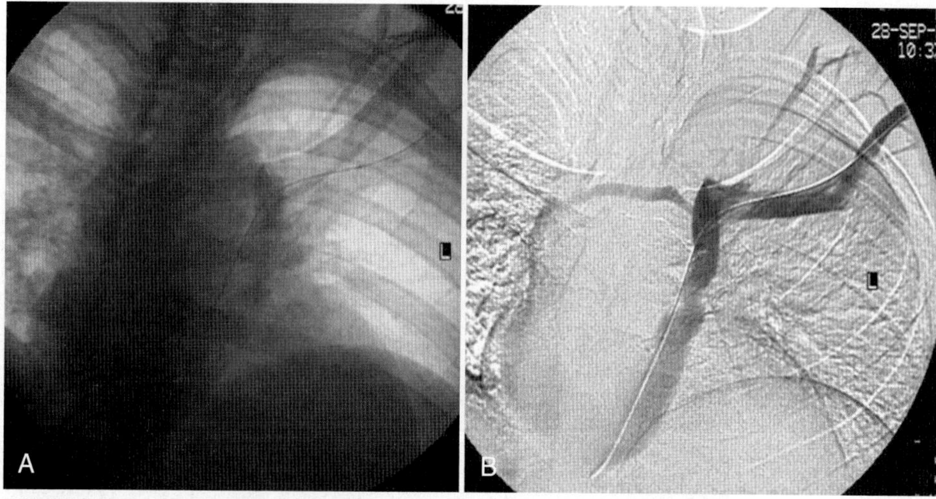

FIGURE 16-3 **A,** Portable chest x-ray demonstrating location of a guidewire (used for placement of a peripherally inserted central catheter) in a left-sided SVC. **B,** Venogram confirms variant left SVC and absent left innominate vein.

Resolution with DR may be marginally decreased because the pixel size is larger than that of the silver iodide crystals in the emulsion on x-ray film, although this is a function of the specific system used and of the exposure factors.[3,6,13] If there is a decrease, it is generally below the ability of the eye to detect and does not lessen the diagnostic usefulness of the images.[5,9] Currently, when replacement of equipment is justified, DR equipment is installed. Both DR and CR have significant advantages for several reasons. First, with the widespread adoption of picture archiving and communication systems (PACS), films that are obtained digitally or are directly converted to digital format are immediately available for review at any location where there is a PACS-enabled workstation. This adds speed and availability and obviates the problem of lost films—all films are digitally archived—and the need to go to a remote location to review a film.[14,15] The dose to an individual patient may or may not be lower as a function of patient factors and the specific imaging system.[10,11] The overall exposure to patients, however, is decreased because the need to repeat films because of inadequate positioning or exposure is substantially eliminated. That is, DR provides the ability to manipulate the image after it is obtained; the relative density (window and level), magnification, and even area included can be altered without reexposing the patient. This adds substantial information to the examination (**Fig. 16-4**). Storage of conventional x-ray films is relatively straightforward, although it is time- and space-intensive. Storage of digital images, although initially more complex, eliminates many of the major problems encountered with storage of standard x-ray films. Most PACS, rather than using stand-alone systems, now use large-volume local storage devices combined with the Internet for gaining access to images, further simplifying their availability. Integration with hospital-wide information systems allows improved access and use compared to what was available even a decade ago.[16]

The radiation exposure to the patient should always be kept in mind when any x-ray study is ordered or performed. The complexity of diagnostic radiation in the general population limits obtaining clear answers. However, a real concern is that ionizing radiation at cumulative diagnostic doses may be teratogenic and may, over decades, cause cancers. The radiation necessary for PA and lateral chest films is usually minimal in terms of radiation effects, in both the dose of a single study (generally <1 mSv) and the cumulative dose of repeated chest x-rays. In pregnant women and children, radiation exposure is always a concern because of the long latency period for radiation-induced cancer.[2] Concerns have been raised that exposure of the population has increased over the last few decades, largely because of the use of high-tech imaging such as computed tomography (CT), radionuclide studies, and cardiac interventional procedures.[17,18] The contribution from conventional imaging procedures, such as chest x-rays, is small, but the precise relationships between individual exposures and cumulative effect are not known. Despite this, and despite the lack of clarity of the relationship between diagnostic level radiation and cancer, it is always wise to limit the amount of radiation as much as possible. Consequently, each chest film should be ordered with care. Whether the dose is actually decreased with digital imaging remains an open question, because digital systems continue to evolve rapidly.

Normal Chest Radiograph

Interpreting standard PA and lateral chest radiographs is a daunting task. The amount of information present is huge, and there are countless relevant variables. It is imperative to have a systematic and standardized approach, based first on an assessment of anatomy, then of physiology, and finally of pathology. Any approach must be based on an understanding of what is normal[19,20] and must include an evaluation of the soft tissues, bones and joints, pleura, lungs and major airways, pulmonary vascularity, mediastinum and its contents, and heart and its chambers specifically, as well as the areas seen below the diaphragm and above the thorax. In the standard PA chest study, the overall heart diameter is normally less than half the transverse diameter of the thorax (**Fig. 16-5**). The heart overlies the thoracic spine, roughly 75% to the left of the spine and 25% to the right. The mediastinum is narrow superiorly, and normally the descending aorta can be defined from the arch to the dome of the diaphragm, on the left. The pulmonary hila are seen below the aortic arch, slightly higher on the left than the right. On the lateral film (**Fig. 16-6**), the left main pulmonary artery can be seen coursing superiorly and posteriorly compared with the right. On both frontal and lateral views, the ascending aorta (aortic root) is normally obscured by the main pulmonary artery and both atria. The location of the pulmonary outflow tract is usually clear on the lateral film.

Cardiac Chambers and Aorta. On the normal chest film, it is not usually possible to define individual cardiac chambers. It is imperative, however, to know their normal position and to examine the film to determine whether the size and location of each chamber and the great vessels are within the normal range. On the PA view, the right contour of the mediastinum contains the right atrium and the ascending aorta and superior vena cava (SVC). If the azygous vein is enlarged, secondary to right heart failure or SVC obstruction (**Fig. 16-7**), it may also be visible. The right ventricle, as is clear from cross-sectional imaging (**Fig. 16-8**), is located partially overlying the left ventricle on both frontal and lateral views.[21] The left atrium is located just inferior to the left pulmonary hilum. In normal individuals, there is a concavity at this level, which is the location of the left atrial appendage. The atrium constitutes the upper portion of the posterior contour of the heart on the lateral film but

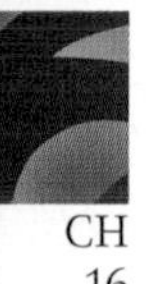

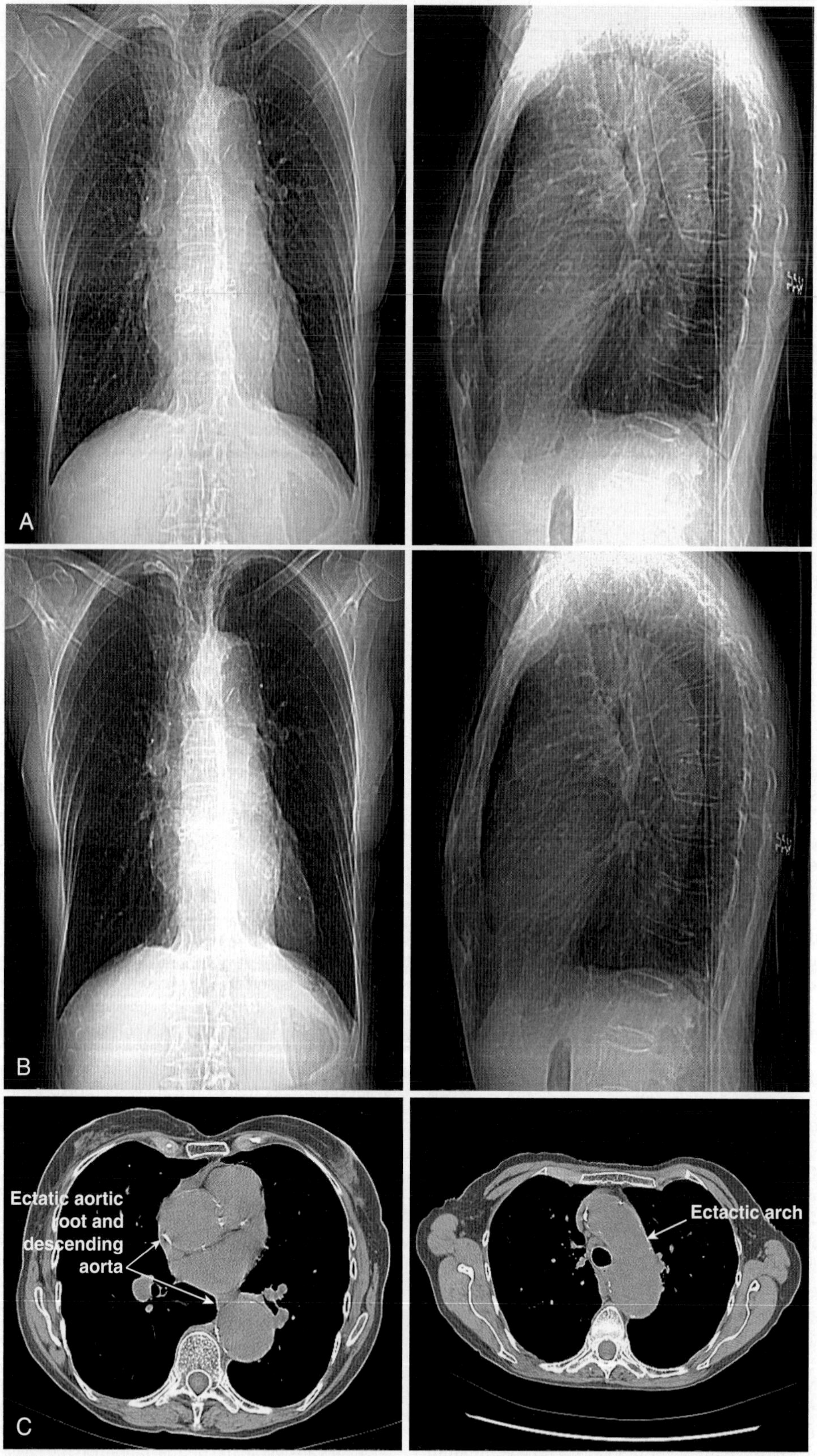

FIGURE 16-4 **A, B,** PA and lateral digital chest x-rays, with different windows and leveling. **A,** With pulmonary window and level, the lung fields, including the pulmonary vasculature, are well visualized but the mediastinal structures are not well defined. Note also flattening of the diaphragms and increased lung lucency, indicative of chronic obstructive pulmonary disease. **B,** Rewindowed, the mediastinal structures are now well seen, showing a dilated, calcified aortic root and descending thoracic aorta. Pulmonary vascularity cannot be defined in these images. **C,** CT scan at the level of the aortic root and arch confirms marked ectasia of the entire thoracic aorta.

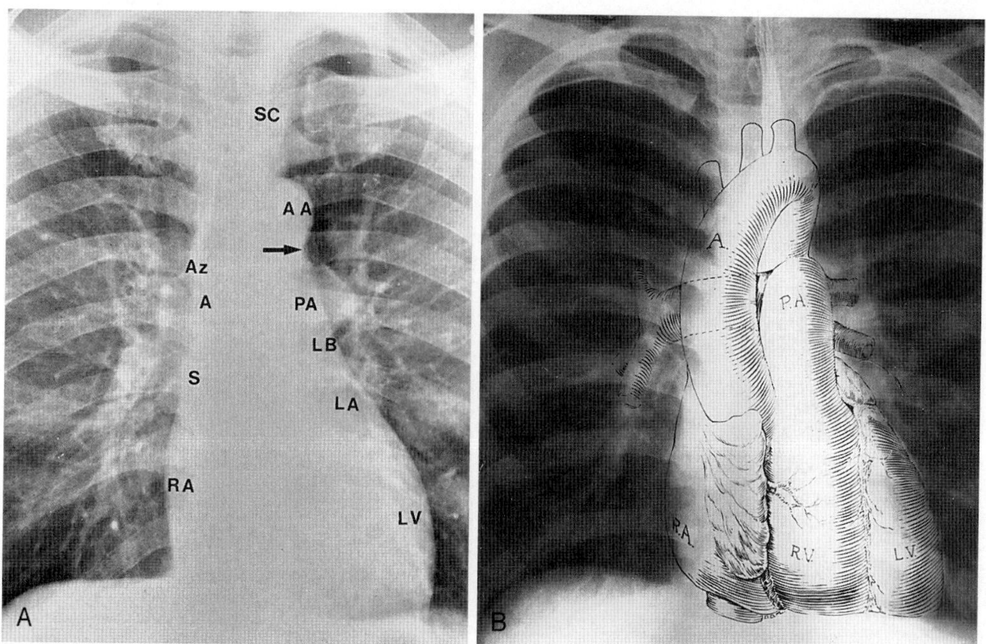

FIGURE 16-5 Frontal projection of the heart and great vessels. **A,** Left and right heart borders in the frontal projection. **B,** A line drawing in the frontal projection demonstrates the relationship of the cardiac valves, rings, and sulci to the mediastinal borders. A = ascending aorta; AA = aortic arch; Az = azygous vein; LA = left atrial appendage; LB = left lower border of pulmonary artery; LV = left ventricle; PA = main pulmonary artery; RA = right atrium; S = superior vena cava; SC = subclavian artery.

cannot normally be differentiated from the left ventricle. The left ventricle constitutes the prominent, rounded apex of the heart on the frontal view and the sloping inferior portion of the mediastinum on the lateral view (see Figs. 16-5 and 16-6).

The apex is often not clearly delineated for a reason related to x-ray attenuation. The heart is distinguishable from the lungs because it contains water density blood rather than air. Because blood attenuates x-rays to a greater extent than air, the heart appears relatively white (although less so than calcium-containing bones) and the lungs relatively black (less so than the edges of the film, where there is only air and no interposed tissue). A fat pad of varying thickness surrounds the apex of the heart (**Figs. 16-9 and 16-10**). Fat has a density greater than that of air and marginally less than that of blood. As it covers the ventricular apex, the fat pad is relatively thick and dense. As it thins out toward the left lateral chest wall, it is progressively less dense; hence, the hazy, poorly marginated appearance of the apex. Similarly, a fat pad may be seen on the lateral chest film as a wedge-shaped density overlying the anterior aspect of the left ventricle (see Figs. 16-9 and 16-10). The pericardial sac cannot normally be defined (**Fig. 16-11**). The borders of the cardiac silhouette are normally moderately but not completely sharp in contour. Even though the exposure time for a chest x-ray is very short (less than 100 milliseconds), there is usually sufficient cardiac motion to cause minor haziness of the silhouette. If a portion of the heart border does not move, as in the case of a left ventricular aneurysm, the border may be unusually sharp (**Fig. 16-12**). The aortic arch, however, is usually visible, as the aorta courses posteriorly and is surrounded by air. Most of the descending aorta is also visible. The position and the size of each can be easily evaluated (see Figs. 16-4 and 16-9) using the frontal and lateral views.

Lungs and Pulmonary Vasculature. Lung size varies as a function of inspiratory effort, age, body habitus, water content, and intrinsic pathologic processes. For example, because lung distensibility decreases with age, the lungs normally appear subtly but progressively smaller as patients age, even with maximal inspiratory effort. As lung size decreases, the heart appears relatively slightly larger, although in adults the heart does not exceed half the transverse diameter of the chest in a good-quality PA film unless there is true cardiomegaly. Also, with increasing left ventricular dysfunction, interstitial fluid in the lungs increases and lung compliance, and therefore expansion as seen on a chest x-ray, decreases. With the presence of chronic obstructive pulmonary disease, with or without bullae, the lungs appear larger and blacker, the diaphragms may appear flattened, and the relative heart size, even in the presence of heart failure, decreases. The heart often appears small or normal in size, even in the presence of cardiac dysfunction (see Fig. 16-4A). It is also important to keep in mind that evident enlargement of the cardiac silhouette on the chest film may be caused by enlargement of the heart overall, dilation of one or more chambers, or pericardial fluid (see Fig. 16-8).

In normal subjects, pulmonary vascularity has a predictable pattern.[22] Pulmonary arteries are usually easily visible centrally in the hila and progressively less so more peripherally. Centrally, the main right and left pulmonary arteries are difficult to quantify unless they are grossly enlarged, because they lie within the mediastinum (see Figs. 16-5 and 16-6). If the lung is thought of in three zones, the major arteries are central; the clearly distinguishable midsized pulmonary arteries (third and fourth order branches) are in the middle zone, and the small arteries and arterioles that are normally below the limit of resolution are in the outer zone. The visible small and midsized arteries (midzone) have sharp, clearly definable margins. As noted, this is because of the sharp border between water density and air density structures. In the standard, standing frontal (PA) chest film, the arteries in the lower zone are larger than those in the upper zone, at an equal distance from the hila. This is because of the effect of gravity on the normal, low-pressure lung circulation. That is, gravity leads to slightly greater intravascular volume at the lung bases than in the upper zones. This effect of gravity on the distribution of normal intravascular lung volume is reflected in a normal perfusion lung scan. Because the radionuclide is generally administered with the patient supine, there is a greater concentration posteriorly than anteriorly, as confirmed in the count rates. If the patient is sitting or standing when the radionuclide is injected, the count rate is greater at the lung base than at the apices.

The angles that the lungs make with the diaphragm are normally sharp and can be delineated bilaterally on frontal and lateral views, because the pleura is usually tightly applied to (not separated from) the ribs. The contour that the inferior vena cava (IVC) makes with the heart is clearly seen on the lateral film (see Fig. 16-2B). Its relationship to the rest of the cardiac silhouette varies markedly, depending on minor degrees of rotation of the patient; that is, the IVC lies on the right of the mediastinum and posterior to the contour of the heart. This contour is made up of the left atrium and ventricle, which lie toward the left side of the thorax. If the patient is placed laterally, with the left side against the film, the right is relatively slightly magnified compared with the left (see Figs. 16-2B and 16-8). If the patient rotates minimally anterior or posterior to true lateral, the relationship between the IVC and left-sided contours changes substantially. This anatomic relationship is important to understand, because in the past a formula was used (the Riegler sign) to determine left ventricular enlargement as a function of its relationship

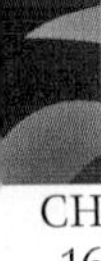

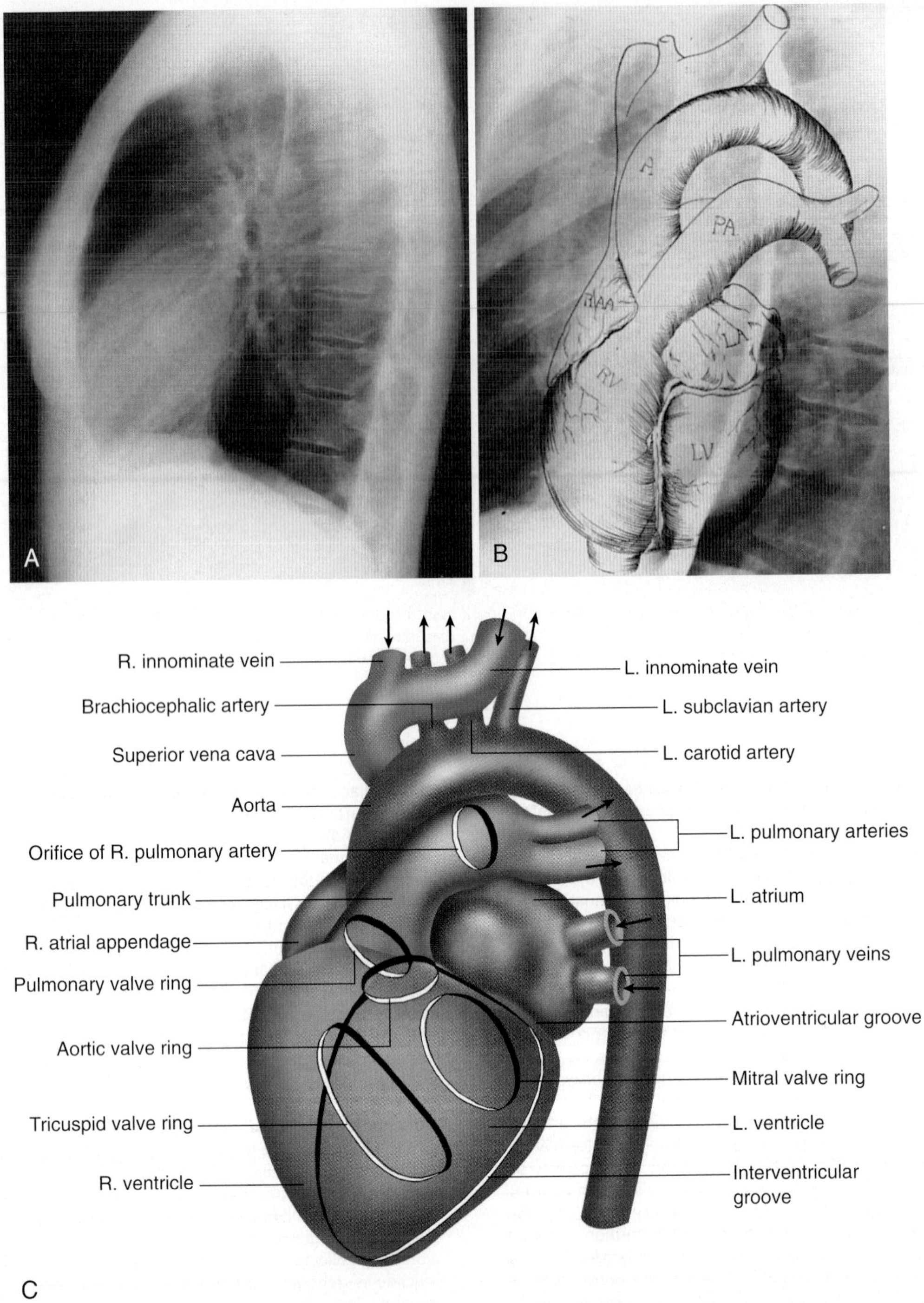

FIGURE 16-6 **A,** Lateral chest radiograph. **B,** Superimposed anatomic drawing of the cardiac chambers and great vessels. **C,** Diagram of the lateral projection of the heart showing the position of the cardiac chambers, valve rings, and sulci. Arrows indicate direction of blood flow.

to the IVC.[23] This sign, although sometimes still used, is not accurate and should not be relied on.[24,25]

Normal Variations. Anatomic variables and aging present challenges in the evaluation of chest radiographs, in addition to those posed by decreased lung compliance. The aorta and great vessels normally dilate and become more tortuous and prominent with increasing age, leading to widening of the superior mediastinum. As noted, the heart appears larger because of decreasing lung compliance although, unless there is true cardiac disease, its diameter remains less than half the transverse diameter of the chest on a PA view. There are additional important anatomic considerations. Patients who are obese are likely to have a degree of inhibition of maximal lung expansion that may make a normal heart appear slightly larger. Patients with pectus excavatum have a narrowed AP diameter of the chest, increasing the transverse diameter. Consequently, the heart may appear enlarged on the frontal view, explained by the narrow AP diameter seen on the lateral view. There may also be lack of definition of the right heart border on the frontal view because of compression by the sternum (**Fig. 16-13**). Marked kyphosis, as may occur with osteoporotic collapse of vertebral bodies or scoliosis, can also cause the heart or mediastinum to look abnormal. It is thus important to evaluate the spine and other bony structures systematically when looking at a chest radiograph. Delineation of all anatomic abnormalities is beyond the scope of this chapter. For an in-depth discussion, *Fraser and Pare's Diagnosis of Diseases of the Chest*[26] remains a useful reference.

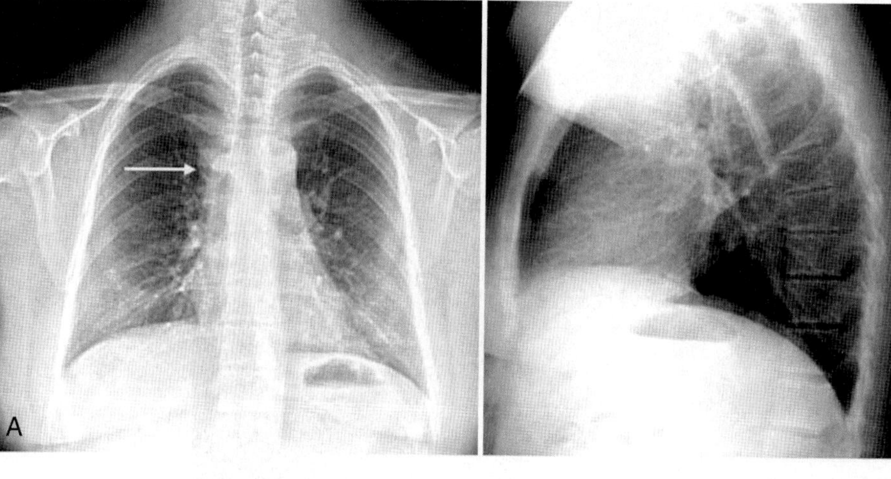
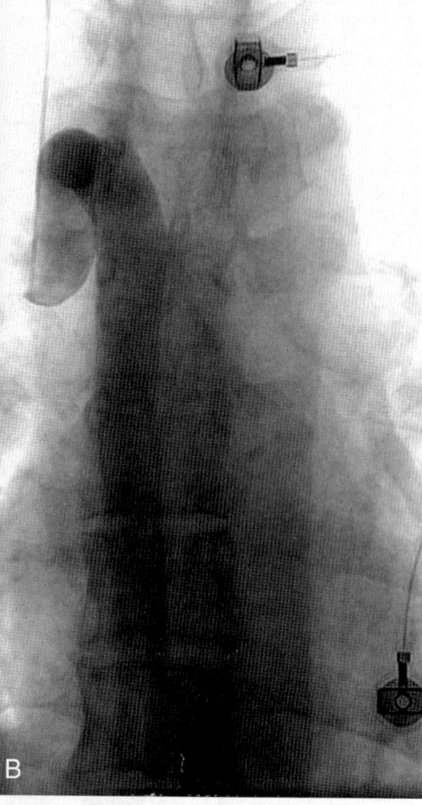

FIGURE 16-7 Radiographs of a 39-year-old renal transplant patient. **A,** Normal PA and lateral images, except for prominence in the azygous vein region (arrow). **B,** Right innominate venogram demonstrates occluded superior vena cava and markedly enlarged azygous vein, draining below the diaphragm.

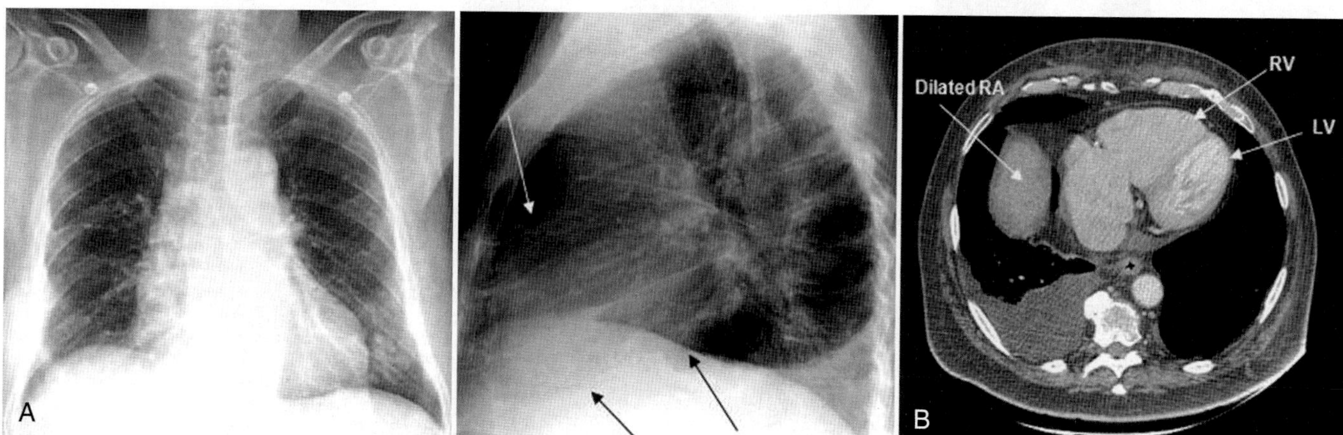

FIGURE 16-8 **A,** Radiographs of an older man with biventricular hypertrophy (note boot-shaped heart on PA view, arrows on lateral view), marked pulmonary vascular redistribution (note haziness and loss of definition of margins of pulmonary vessels throughout), and right pleural effusion. **B,** CT scan confirms biventricular hypertrophy, with right ventricle (RV) larger than left ventricle (LV), right atrial (RA) enlargement, and right pleural effusion.

Evaluating the Chest Radiograph in Heart Disease

There is no single best way to read a chest film. A systematic approach to the evaluation of a chest radiograph is imperative to distinguish normal from abnormal and to define the underlying pathology and pathophysiology. Each person must develop his or her own system. The first step is to define which type of film is being evaluated—PA and lateral, PA alone, or AP view (either portable or one obtained in the AP view because the patient is unable to stand). The next step is to determine whether prior films are available for comparison.[27] Many abnormalities are put into appropriate perspective by determining whether they are new. Common examples are a prominent aortic arch, visible major fissure related to prior inflammatory process, or widened superior mediastinum related to aortic ectasia (see Fig. 16-4), substernal thyroid, or enlarged azygous vein (see Fig. 16-7).

Any system should incorporate a routine that includes a deliberate attempt to look at areas that are easily ignored. These include the thoracic spine, neck (for masses and tracheal position), costophrenic angles, lung apices, retrocardiac space, and retrosternal space. Looking at these areas enables definition of mediastinal position and cardiac and aortic situs and the presence of pleural effusions, scarring, or diaphragmatic elevation. It is logical to evaluate the lung fields next. This should involve a careful search for infiltrates or masses, even when the primary concern is cardiovascular abnormalities. The

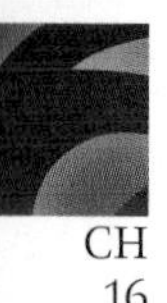

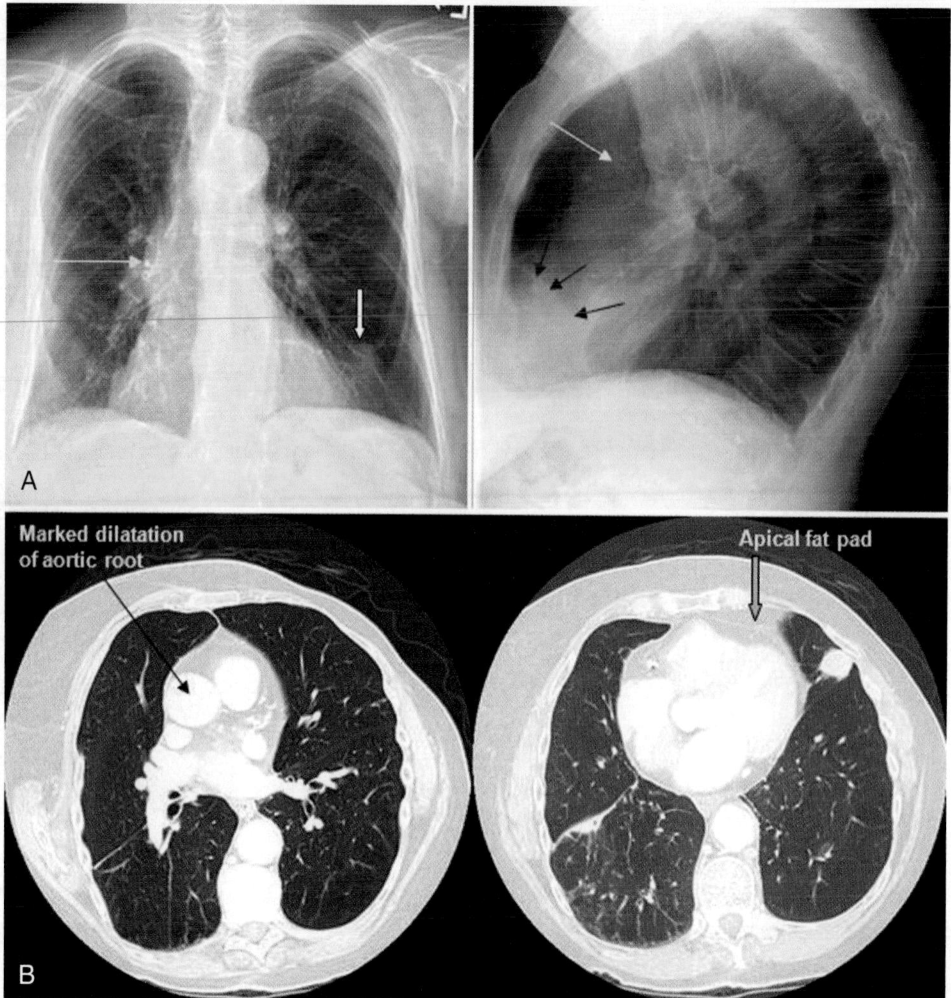

FIGURE 16-9 **A,** PA and lateral chest radiographs showing marked aortic root dilation (yellow arrows), mass versus artifact in lingula in frontal (PA) view (white arrow), with slight haziness of cardiac apex. There is a prominent apical fat pad on lateral view (short arrows). **B,** CT scan shows marked dilatation of aortic root (arrow), mass in lingula that is poorly seen on radiographs, and prominent apical fat pad (thick arrow).

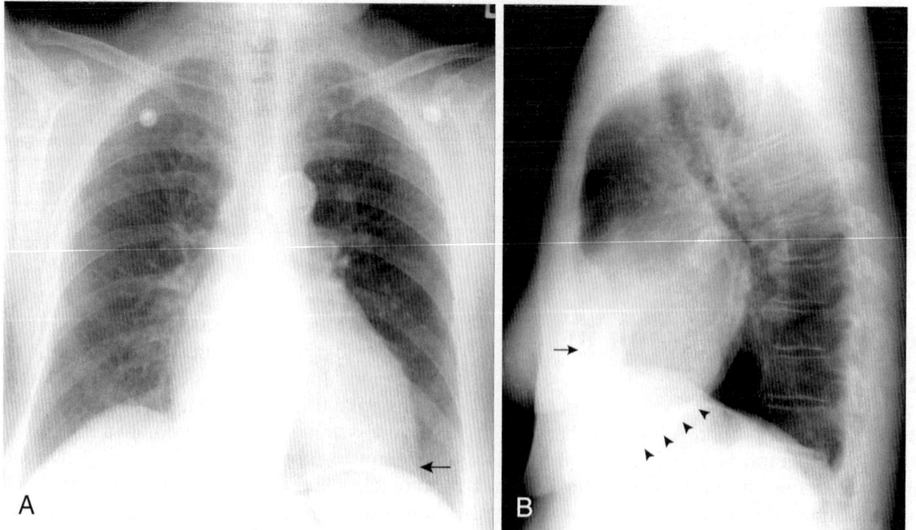

FIGURE 16-10 Chest radiographs of a 70-year-old woman with rheumatic heart disease and combined aortic stenosis and mitral stenosis. Her pulmonary capillary wedge pressure is 30 mm Hg. **A,** PA view. There is evidence of chronically elevated pulmonary venous pressures with moderate (not marked) pulmonary vascular redistribution. There is moderate left ventricular enlargement and prominence of the left atrial appendage. **B,** Lateral view. Note enlargement of the left ventricle, extending below the diaphragm and compressing the gastric bubble (arrowheads). Also note the apical fat pad, seen as the hazy density on the frontal view (**A,** arrow), and the anterior, retrosternal, well-delineated, wedge-shaped density on the lateral view (**B,** arrow).

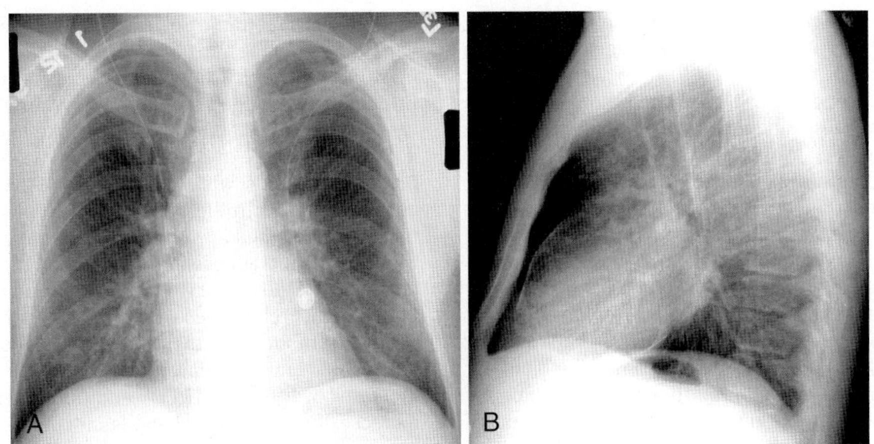

FIGURE 16-11 Chest radiographs of a 45-year-old man with calcific pericarditis. **A,** PA view is essentially normal. **B,** Lateral view demonstrates thin, irregular calcification of pericardium around the left ventricular contour.

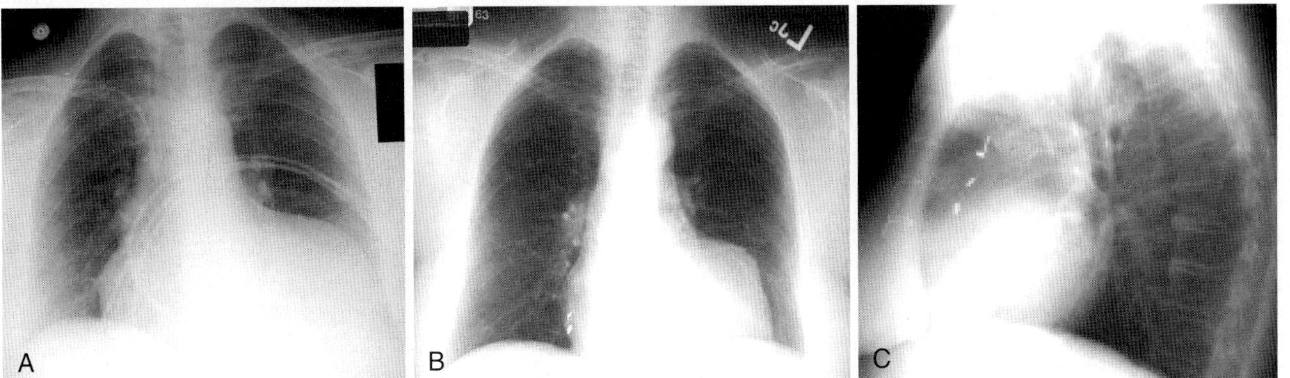

FIGURE 16-12 Chest radiographs of a 53-year-old woman with coronary artery disease and heart failure following a large anterolateral myocardial infarction. **A,** Frontal portable view suggests cardiomegaly and heart failure. Sharp horizontal contour of the left ventricle is suggestive of anterior wall aneurysm. **B, C,** PA and lateral views after revascularization and aneurysmectomy demonstrate persistence of an abnormal contour of the left ventricle, consistent with recurrent aneurysm, and clips on side branches of the saphenous vein graft to right coronary artery.

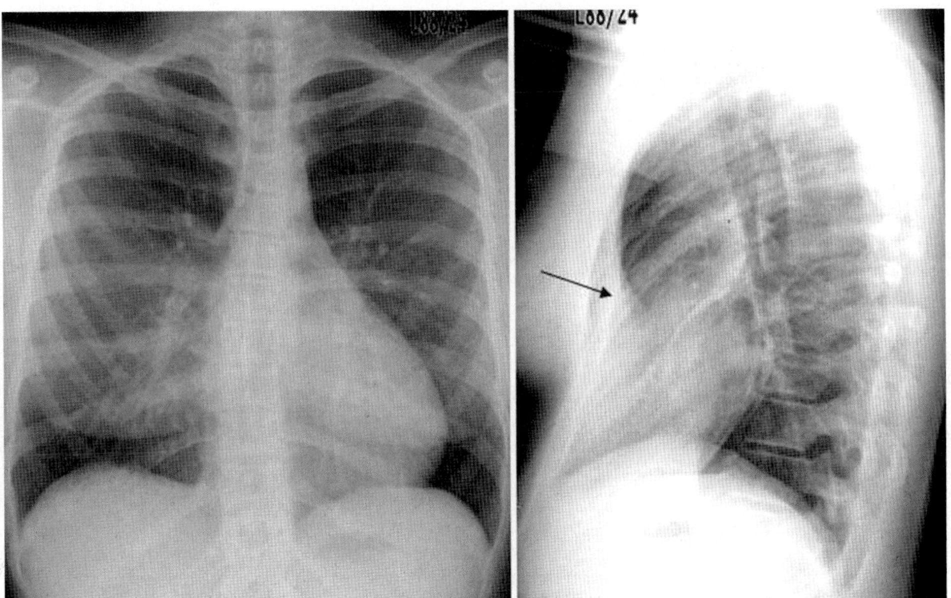

FIGURE 16-13 Routine chest radiographs of a healthy 37-year-old woman. Note hazy right mediastinal silhouette on frontal view, caused not by cardiac or pulmonary abnormalities but by pectus excavatum, as seen on lateral view. Note also the normal pulmonary vascular pattern.

logic is that many people with coronary artery disease have a history of tobacco abuse and are thus at increased risk for lung malignancies (see Fig. 16-9).

Cardiovascular disease states cause various and complex changes in the appearance of the chest radiograph. The overall size of the cardiac silhouette (see Fig. 16-8), its position (see Fig. 16-13), and the location of the ascending and descending aorta must be specifically evaluated. Dextrocardia and a right descending aorta are rare, particularly in adults, but are easy to check for and are important to recognize because of their association with congenital cardiac and abdominal situs abnormalities. It is also important to look at the site and position of the stomach. This information can be used to differentiate between a high diaphragm and a pleural effusion (see Fig. 16-2). Cardiomegaly, accurately judged by the heart diameter exceeding half the diameter of the thorax on a PA film, is a common but nonspecific finding.[28-32] It is probably most often seen as a result of ischemic cardiomyopathy following one or more myocardial infarctions (see Figs. 16-8 and 16-12).

Lungs and Pulmonary Vasculature

Evaluation of the pulmonary vascular pattern is difficult and imprecise but very important. As noted, the pattern varies with the patient's position (erect versus supine) and is altered substantially by underlying pulmonary disease. It is best to define pulmonary vascularity by looking at the middle zone of the lungs (i.e., the third of the lungs between the hilar region and peripheral region laterally) and comparing a region in the upper portion of the lungs with a region in the lower portion, at equal distances from the hilum.[22] Vessels should be larger in the lower lung but sharply marginated in the upper and lower zones. In normal individuals, the vessels taper and bifurcate and are difficult to define in the outer third of the lung. They normally become too small to be seen near the pleura (see Figs. 16-7 and 16-13).

Two distinct patterns of abnormality are recognizable. When pulmonary arterial flow is increased, as in patients with a high-output state (e.g., pregnancy, severe anemia as in sickle cell disease, hyperthyroidism) or left-to-right shunt, the pulmonary vessels are seen more prominently than usual in the periphery of the lung (**Fig. 16-14**). They are uniformly enlarged and can be traced almost to the pleura, but their margins remain clear. In contrast, in patients with elevated pulmonary venous pressure, the vessel borders become hazy, the lower zone vessels constrict and the upper zone vessels enlarge, and vessels become visible farther toward the pleura, in the outer third of the lungs (**Fig. 16-15**; see also Fig. 16-8). With increasing left ventricular end-diastolic pressure (LVEDP) or left atrial pressure, interstitial edema increases and ultimately pulmonary edema occurs (**Fig. 16-16**). There is usually a reasonably good correlation between the pulmonary vascular pattern and pulmonary capillary wedge pressure (PCWP). At a PCWP of less than 8 mm Hg, the vascular pattern is normal. As the PCWP increases to 10 to 12 mm Hg, the lower zone vessels appear equal in diameter to or smaller than the upper zone vessels. At pressures of 12 to 18 mm Hg, the vessel borders become progressively hazier because of increasing extravasation of fluid into the interstitium. This effect is sometimes evident as Kerley B lines, which are horizontal, pleural-based, peripheral linear densities. As the PCWP increases above 18 to 20 mm Hg, pulmonary edema occurs, with interstitial fluid present in sufficient amounts to cause a perihilar bat wing appearance (see Fig. 16-16).

Again, these typical appearances may be altered for various reasons. In patients with extensive pulmonary fibrosis or multiple bullae, the vascular pattern is abnormal at baseline and, as the PCWP increases, it does not change in predictable ways as definable on a chest radiograph. In patients with chronic congestive heart failure, there are chronic changes in the pulmonary vascular pattern that do not correlate with the changes that occur in patients with normal left ventricular pressure at baseline.[22,33] For example, a patient with a chronic elevation of LVEDP to 25 to 30 mm Hg resulting from ischemic myopathy or some other cause may have a normal pulmonary vascular pattern or moderate rather than marked redistribution (see Figs. 16-8 and 16-10, and compare with Fig. 16-16). In general, heart size increases over time as LVEDP and pulmonary vascular redistribution increase. If pulmonary edema is independent of left ventricular dysfunction, however, as may occur at a high altitude or following cerebral trauma, the heart size may remain normal. A more frequently encountered disparity is that in the setting of an acute, large transmural myocardial infarction, the heart is usually minimally or mildly enlarged, despite marked increase in LVEDP (see Fig. 16-16). Despite these limitations, it is important to evaluate the pulmonary vascular pattern routinely because it can provide a great deal of information.

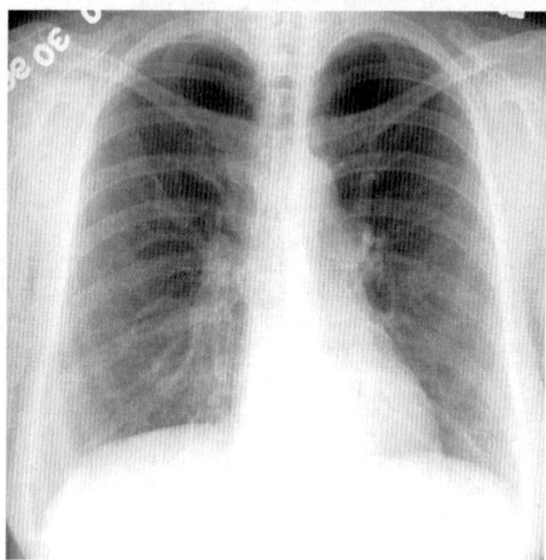

FIGURE 16-14 Chest radiograph of a 47-year-old asymptomatic woman with a small atrial septal defect. The PA view shows a normal cardiac contour, with mild pulmonary vascular plethora at the periphery of the lung fields.

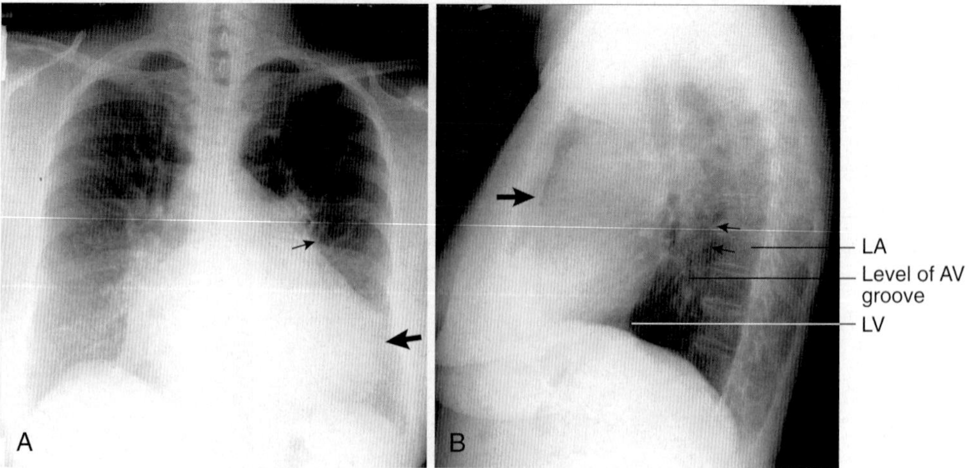

FIGURE 16-15 Chest radiographs of a 59-year-old woman with a history of rheumatic heart disease and mitral stenosis. **A,** PA view demonstrates enlarged cardiac silhouette, with suggestion of a double density seen through the heart (left atrial enlargement), prominent convexity of the left atrial appendage (small arrow), and slightly elevated cardiac apex (large arrow), suggestive of right ventricular (rather than left ventricular) enlargement. There is significant elevation of the pulmonary venous pressures. **B,** The lateral view confirms marked right ventricular (arrow) and left atrial (small arrows) enlargement. Note filling in of the retrosternal airspace. LA = left atrium; LV = left ventricle.

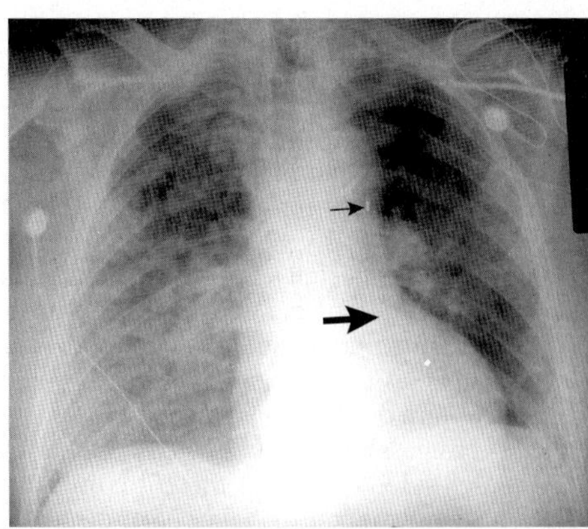

FIGURE 16-16 Patient with acute pulmonary edema. Note engorged hila bilaterally, with typical pattern of pulmonary edema on the right. Also note intra-aortic counterpulsation balloon with radiopaque tip at the top of the descending aorta (small arrow) and the balloon expanded in the aorta below it (large arrow).

Cardiac Chambers and Great Vessels

After assessing overall heart size and pulmonary vascular pattern—as a reflection, in general, of left heart physiologic status—the individual chambers should be examined. As noted, it is not possible to define individual chambers in a normal chest radiograph clearly (see Figs. 16-5 and 16-6) and, when the cardiac silhouette is enlarged, it is most often related to biventricular failure and individual chamber enlargement is not visible. In acquired valvular disease and in many types of congenital heart disease, however, individual chamber enlargement is present and crucial to plain film (and often clinical) diagnosis.[19,28,33] This information is now readily available with other more expensive imaging modalities—echocardiography, cardiac magnetic resonance imaging (CMRI), and cardiac CT (see Chaps. 15, 18, and 19).[34] Plain films have several advantages: (1) they allow fairly straightforward assessment of current status and changes over time; (2) they are routinely and readily available; (3) they are inexpensive; (4) they carry a low radiation dose.[35-39]

RIGHT ATRIUM. Right atrial enlargement is essentially never isolated except in the presence of congenital tricuspid atresia or Ebstein anomaly. Both are rarely encountered, even in the pediatric age group. The right atrium may dilate in the presence of pulmonary hypertension or tricuspid regurgitation, but right ventricular dilation usually predominates and prevents definition of the atrium. The right atrial contour blends with that of the SVC, right main pulmonary artery, and right ventricle. In adults, therefore, it is almost impossible to define, and it is pointless to try (see Fig. 16-8).

RIGHT VENTRICLE. The classic signs of right ventricular enlargement are a boot-shaped heart and filling in of the retrosternal airspace.[21] The former is caused by transverse displacement of the apex of the right ventricle as it dilates (**Fig. 16-17**; see also Fig. 16-15). In adults, it is rare for the right ventricle to dilate without left ventricular dilation, so this boot shape is not often obvious. It is most commonly seen as an isolated finding in congenital heart disease, typically in tetralogy of Fallot. As the right ventricle dilates, it expands superiorly as well as laterally and posteriorly, explaining the well-marginated increase in density in the retrosternal airspace (**Fig. 16-18**). The classic teaching is that in a lateral chest radiograph in normal patients, the soft tissue density is confined to less than one third of the distance from the suprasternal notch to the tip of the xyphoid. If the soft tissue fills in by more than one third, in the absence of other explanations, it is a reliable indication of right ventricular enlargement. There are, however, other causes of increased soft tissue density in this region that are usually readily definable and generally easy to distinguish from right ventricular enlargement. Common causes include retrosternal adenopathy, midmediastinal mass (e.g., lymphoma or thymoma), marked dilation of the main pulmonary artery (**Fig. 16-19**), and marked aortic root dilation (see Figs. 16-4 and 16-9). The most common cause of increased retrosternal soft tissue, however, is prior median sternotomy, with resultant scarring and haziness of this region (see Fig. 16-12C). Right ventricular enlargement is most often seen in mitral valve disease, secondary to pulmonary hypertension (see Figs. 16-14, 16-17, and 16-18). Less commonly, it is the result of primary pulmonary hypertension or chronic pulmonary emboli.

LEFT ATRIUM. Several classic signs define left atrial enlargement.[19,39] The first is dilation of the left atrial appendage, seen as a focal convexity where there is normally a concavity between the left main pulmonary artery and left border of the left ventricle on the frontal view (see Fig. 16-18A). Second, because of its location, as the left atrium enlarges, it elevates the left main stem bronchus. In so doing, it widens the angle

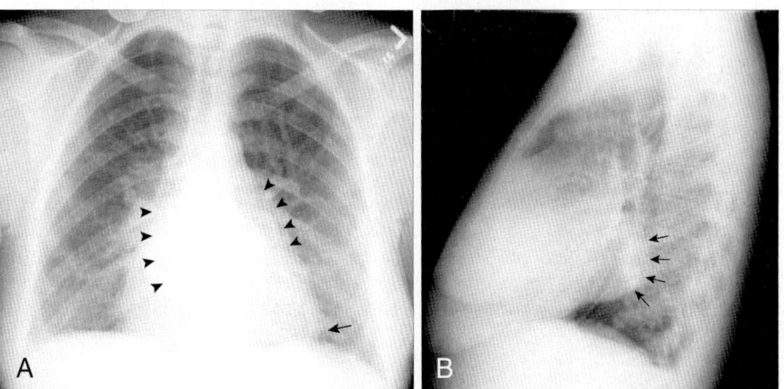

FIGURE 16-17 Chest radiographs of a 60-year-old woman with severe mitral stenosis **A,** PA view shows enlargement of the left atrium (arrowheads), prominence of the hilar vessels, and pulmonary vascular redistribution. Transverse angle of the apex suggests right ventricular (RV) enlargement (arrow). **B,** Lateral view confirms RV enlargement with filling in of the retrosternal air space. Note also marked left atrial enlargement (arrows).

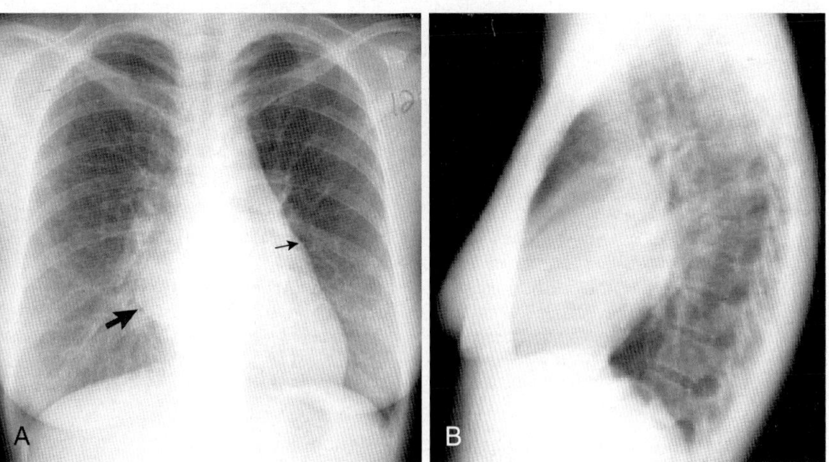

FIGURE 16-18 Chest radiographs of a 39-year-old Asian woman with rheumatic mitral stenosis. **A,** Frontal view shows normal heart size, mild vascular redistribution, and marked focal enlargement of the left atrium (small arrow), which extends to the right of the midline (large arrow). There is elevation of the left main stem bronchus. **B,** Lateral view shows dilated right ventricle, with filling in of the retrosternal airspace. The left ventricle is normal in size and contour.

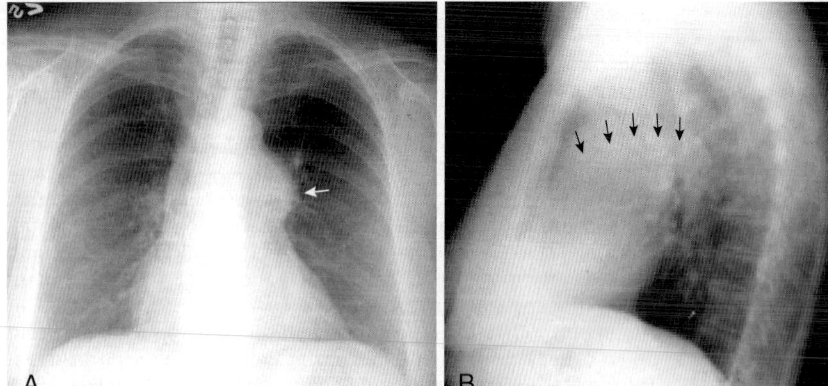

FIGURE 16-19 Chest radiographs of a 56-year-old asymptomatic woman with incidentally discovered pulmonic stenosis. **A,** PA view shows marked enlargement of the main pulmonary trunk extending into the left main pulmonary artery (arrow). **B,** Lateral view confirms prominence of the pulmonary outflow tract and main and left pulmonary arteries (arrows).

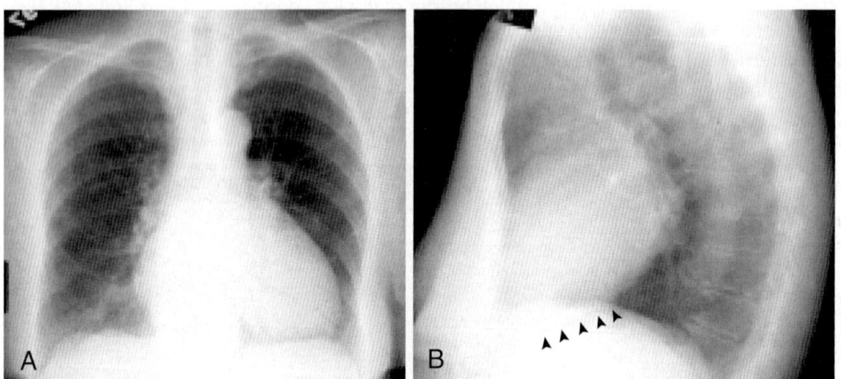

FIGURE 16-20 Chest films of a 78-year-old woman with pure mitral regurgitation and atrial fibrillation. **A,** PA view shows enlargement of the left atrium and left ventricle with mild pulmonary vascular redistribution. **B,** Lateral view confirms these findings. Arrowheads indicate prominent left ventricular contour.

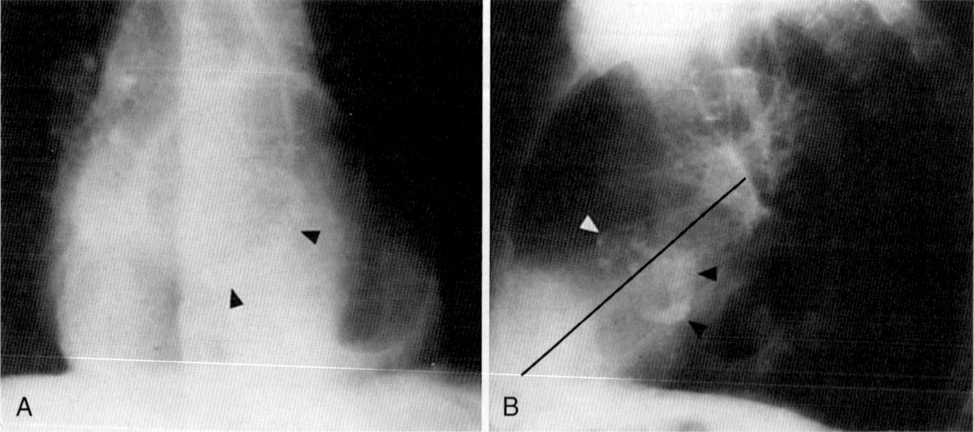

FIGURE 16-21 Mitral annulus calcification in posteroanterior **(A)** and lateral **(B)** projections. This calcification (black arrowheads) lies below the line drawn from the left main bronchus to the anterior costophrenic sulcus, which localizes it to the mitral valve. The calcified aortic valve in this patient lies more anteriorly and above this line (white arrowhead).

of the carina.[40] Third, as the left atrium enlarges posteriorly, it may cause focal bowing of the middle to low thoracic aorta toward the left (see Fig. 16-18A). This bowing is distinguishable from the tortuosity seen with progressive atherosclerosis, which involves the descending thoracic aorta in its upper portion or diffusely. Fourth, with marked left atrial enlargement, a double density can be seen on the frontal view because the left atrium projects laterally toward the right and posteriorly, and the discrete outline of the blood-filled left atrium is surrounded by air-filled lung (see Figs. 16-17 and 16-18). Finally, on the lateral film, left atrial enlargement appears as a focal, posteriorly directed bulge (see Figs. 16-15B and 16-17B).

Definable left atrial enlargement is the hallmark of mitral valve disease, and isolated left atrial enlargement in adults is most often seen in mitral stenosis (see Chap. 66). In mitral stenosis, the left atrium dilates progressively over time (because of progressive pressure increase in this low pressure left-sided chamber), there is consequent progressive evidence of pulmonary vascular redistribution, often with Kerley B lines, and there is ultimately dilation and enlargement of the right ventricle. The left ventricle, however, remains normal in size (see Figs. 16-15, 16-17, and 16-18). In contrast, in mitral regurgitation, with increased volume in the left atrium and ventricle, both dilate over time (**Fig. 16-20**). The pattern of pulmonary vascular redistribution is more variable in mitral regurgitation than in mitral stenosis, as is right ventricular dilation. It is also important to note mitral annulus calcification (see Chap. 80); this is a common finding but does not have a strong association with valvular dysfunction. It does, however, have an association with premature coronary artery disease (**Fig. 16-21**).[41]

LEFT VENTRICLE. Left ventricular enlargement is characterized by a prominent, downwardly directed contour of the apex, as distinguished from the transverse displacement seen with right ventricular enlargement. On the PA film, the overall cardiac contour is also usually enlarged, although this is a nonspecific finding. It is also important to evaluate the left ventricle on the lateral film. Here it is seen as a posterior bulge, below the level of the mitral annulus (**Fig. 16-22**). It may also be seen inferiorly, pushing the gastric bubble (see Figs. 16-8A and 16-10B). Such left ventricular enlargement is an illustration of findings that lie outside the usual confines of the chest and another example of the value of looking at the entire chest radiograph.

Focal left ventricular enlargement in adults is most commonly seen in the presence of aortic insufficiency (with aortic root dilation; see Fig. 16-22) or mitral regurgitation (with left atrial dilation; see Fig. 16-20). In contrast, because aortic stenosis is characterized by left ventricular hypertrophy rather than dilation, the left ventricle is dilated on the chest film only when aortic stenosis is accompanied by left ventricular failure.[23-25,33,42]

PULMONARY ARTERIES. The main pulmonary artery can appear abnormal in many clinical settings. In the presence of pulmonic stenosis, the main pulmonary artery and left pulmonary artery dilate (see Fig. 16-19). This dilation is thought to be caused by the jet effect on the vessel wall of the blood flow through the stenotic valve, coupled with the anatomy. That is, the main pulmonary artery continues straight into the left main pulmonary artery but the right comes off at a fairly sharp angle and is not generally affected by the jet from the stenotic valve. This enlargement can be seen with a prominent left hilum on the frontal view and a prominent pulmonary outflow tract on the lateral view. It is important to remember that the pulmonic valve lies more superiorly in the outflow tract and more anteriorly than the aorta valve (see Fig. 16-6).

AORTA. The most commonly seen abnormality of the aorta is dilation, and the way the aorta dilates is a function of the underlying pathology (see Chap. 60). It is often possible to define the pathology by a combination of the pattern of dilation and associated cardiac abnormalities.[43] On the frontal chest radiograph, aortic dilation appears as a prominence to the right of the middle mediastinum (see Fig. 16-22). There is also a prominence in the anterior mediastinum on the lateral view, behind and superior to the pulmonary outflow tract (**Fig. 16-23**; see also Figs. 16-4 and 16-9). Dilation of the aortic root is seen in the presence of aortic valve disease (both stenosis and regurgitation) but more frequently has other causes, such as long-term, poorly controlled systemic hypertension or generalized atherosclerosis with ectasia.

In aortic valve stenosis (see Chap. 66), there is usually focal dilation of the aortic root, often subtle and often without left ventricular enlargement (see Fig. 16-23). It is important to look for this, because there are often no other signs on the chest radiograph, even in the presence of a very small valve area.[42] The left ventricle generally hypertrophies in response to increased resistance to outflow, rather than dilating as it does in response to the increased volume of flow that occurs with aortic insufficiency. The wall thickening with hypertrophy is seen with echocardiography, CT, or CMRI, but the ventricle may appear entirely normal on the chest radiograph, despite tight aortic valve stenosis. Aortic valve calcification is pathognomonic of significant aortic valve disease (see Figs. 16-21 and 16-23), but is usually difficult to see on a chest radiograph because of the overlying soft tissue densities and the minimal blurring caused by cardiac motion. If calcification is present, it is much more easily seen with fluoroscopy or CT (see Fig. 19-21). Despite the decreased resolution of fluoroscopy compared with standard chest radiography, real-time visualization facilitates definition of calcification because it eliminates blurring caused by motion.[44-46]

It is important to remember that there is a subset of patients with aortic stenosis who present with left ventricular decompensation. In these patients, there is left ventricular and aortic root enlargement. To distinguish this from aortic regurgitation, it is important to look carefully for aortic valve calcification. It is not possible on a chest radiograph to establish definitively whether aortic stenosis is caused by rheumatic disease, a bicuspid valve, or degenerative changes. It can be helpful, however, to remember that rheumatic disease essentially always involves the mitral valve (see Chaps. 66 and 88), and the absence of signs of mitral stenosis generally indicates that the cause is not rheumatic.

In aortic regurgitation, aortic involvement is usually more diffuse than in aortic stenosis and is more easily seen (see Chap. 66). In pure aortic regurgitation, the left atrium is not typically enlarged. Over time, however, dilation of the mitral annulus may occur secondary to left ventricular dilation, with resultant mitral regurgitation and left atrial dilation. Although aortic regurgitation most often occurs secondary to congenital defects, degenerative valve disease, or rheumatic heart disease (with associated mitral valve disease), it may also be caused by diseases of the aortic root, including cystic medial necrosis, with or without Marfan syndrome. In cystic medial necrosis, the involvement

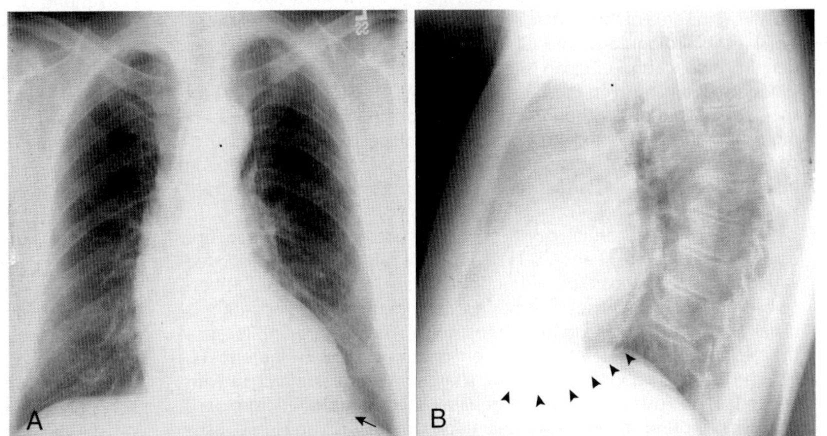

FIGURE 16-22 Chest radiographs of a 63-year-old man with chronic aortic regurgitation. **A,** PA view shows downward displacement of the apex (arrow), suggestive of left ventricular enlargement. There is prominence and enlargement of the ascending aorta, creating a convex right border of the mediastinum. **B,** Lateral view shows prominent left ventricular enlargement (arrowheads). The aortic root is markedly enlarged in the retrosternal airspace but is separate from the sternum (in contrast to findings in right ventricular enlargement; see Fig. 16-17B).

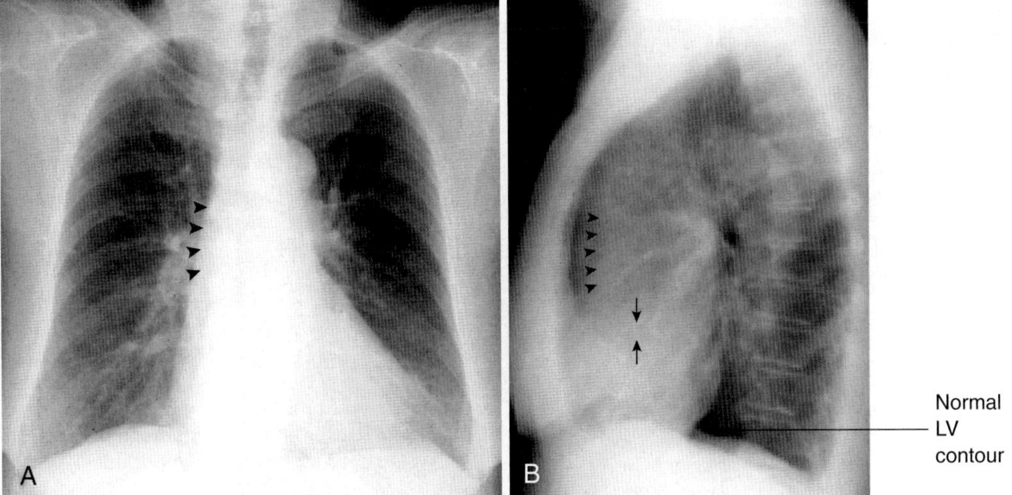

FIGURE 16-23 Chest radiographs of a 65-year-old woman with severe aortic stenosis. **A,** Frontal view shows a prominent aortic root, to the right of the midline (arrowheads). Note absence of cardiomegaly and presence of normal pulmonary vascular pattern. **B,** Lateral view demonstrates calcification of the aortic valve leaflets (arrows), suggestive of a bicuspid valve. There is a prominent, mildly dilated aortic root (arrowheads).

is diffuse and there is generally dilation of the aorta from the level of the valve at least through the arch, with a gradual transition to normal diameter (see Chap. 60). Aortic regurgitation may be caused by dilation of the valve or by aortic dissection into the valve ring. In tertiary syphilis, now rarely seen, the characteristic finding is marked dilation of the aorta from the root to the arch, with abrupt return to normal diameter at this level. Other aortic abnormalities, such as acute or chronic dissection and traumatic rupture or pseudoaneurysm, generally require a cross-sectional imaging modality for clear delineation. In the setting of suspected acute trauma to the chest or mediastinum, obtaining a chest radiograph may unnecessarily delay appropriate diagnosis and intervention, as in the case of suspected aortic rupture. The findings on the chest films are generally nonspecific and indirect, such as mediastinal widening, blood at the left apex, a large left pleural effusion (presumably blood), deviation of the trachea to the right, or rib fractures. Multislice or even helical CT can provide a rapid and accurate answer (see Chap. 19).

Pleura and Pericardium

The pleura and pericardium also require systematic evaluation. The pericardium is rarely distinctly definable on plain films of the chest.[47] There are two situations, however, in which it can be seen; in the presence of a large pericardial effusion, the visceral and parietal pericardium separate. Because there is a fat pad associated with each, it is sometimes possible to make out two parallel lucent lines (i.e., fat) on the lateral film, usually in the area of the cardiac apex, with density (fluid) between them. CMRI, echocardiography, and CT, however, are all far more reliable for defining a pericardial effusion (see Chap. 75). Nonetheless, if the cardiac silhouette is enlarged on the chest radiograph, it is important to look for specific explanations. Although cardiac dilation and valvular disease are more common causes, the presence of an unsuspected effusion is worth considering. Typically, the cardiac silhouette has a water bottle shape in the presence of a pericardial effusion, but this shape is not in itself diagnostic.

Pleural and pericardial calcification can occur, but are often not obvious (see Figs. 16-11 and 75-11). Pericardial calcification is associated with a history of pericarditis. Although there are multiple causes, tuberculosis and various viruses are the most common. Such calcification is usually thin and linear and follows the contour of the pericardium. Because the calcification is thin, it is often seen only on one view, as in Figure 16-11. Myocardial calcification secondary to a large myocardial infarction with transmural necrosis is rare but can generally be distinguished from pericardial calcification. It tends to appear thicker, more focal, and less consistent with the outer contour of the heart. Pleural calcification is easily distinguishable from pericardial calcification and is essentially pathognomonic for asbestos exposure. It is associated with a high risk of malignant mesothelioma but is not diagnostic of this type of tumor.

Additional Specific Considerations

A catalogue of all the findings associated with cardiac disease is beyond the scope of this chapter, but several additional specific entities and situations are worth considering because they are common or characteristic of certain disease states. As noted, the most common explanation for cardiomegaly and pulmonary vascular redistribution is ischemic heart disease.[20,23,24] In most patients with an acute myocardial infarction, the cardiac silhouette is not enlarged but there is pulmonary vascular redistribution, consistent with an acute increase in LVEDP. This condition is most easily defined when the chest radiograph is compared with a prior or subsequent one. After infarction, a variety of alterations can occur. Left ventricular aneurysms, either true (generally in the distribution of the left anterior descending artery; see Fig. 16-12) or false (i.e., pseudoaneurysms, usually involving the base or posterior wall) are uncommon.[48,49] Although their locations differ, their appearances are similar; there is focal prominence (of the anterolateral cardiac contour with true aneurysms), there may be linear myocardial calcification, and the cardiac margin is unusually sharp, because the area of the aneurysm does not have normal cardiac motion. Again, this is best seen in comparison with prior chest radiographs.

It is impossible to define a postinfarction ventricular septal defect on the chest radiograph because the findings are nonspecific cardiac dilation and evidence of left ventricular or biventricular failure. After percutaneous repair, however, the septal repair device can often be identified.[50]

IMPLANTABLE DEVICES AND OTHER POSTSURGICAL FINDINGS

A final important and broad area concerns the chest radiograph following surgery or other procedures. In these situations, it is crucial to recognize devices that have been implanted and changes that may occur. Among the most common are various valve prostheses,[51] pacemakers[52] and ICDs (**Fig. 16-24**), intra-aortic counterpulsation balloons (see Fig. 16-16), and ventricular assist devices (see Fig. 32-4). There are also clear changes that occur after surgery, such as the presence of clips on the side branches of saphenous veins used for coronary artery bypass grafting (see Fig. 16-12) and retrosternal blurring and effusions (see Fig. 16-2).[53] Some of these findings may be temporary, such as lines and tubes associated with surgery and effusions. Pacemakers and ICDs present specific questions (see Chap. 38). The first is whether the leads are intact[54,55] and the second is the position of the tips (see Figs. 38-32 and 38-33). Although course and tip position are generally confirmed fluoroscopically at the time of placement, malposition can occur. If there are two leads, the tips should generally be in the anterolateral wall of the right atrium and apex of the right ventricle. If the leads are not positioned in this way, the reasons should be carefully determined. That is, are they positioned because of error or anatomic variants (e.g., a persistent left SVC that empties into the coronary sinus and then the right atrium; **Fig. 16-25**)[56] or because the lead belongs in the coronary sinus (**Fig. 16-26**)? Additionally, the position of the wires and of valve prostheses can help in the definition of specific chamber enlargement (**Fig. 16-27**; see also Fig. 16-24).

Conclusion

Chest radiographs provide a wealth of physiologic and anatomic information. As such, they play a central role in the evaluation and management of patients with a wide variety of cardiovascular and other disorders. The radiation dose inherent in obtaining x-rays should always be considered. Portable chest films should be used as infrequently as possible because the information they provide is limited and may even be misleading (e.g., in defining cardiomegaly or in ruling out a pneumothorax or effusion). Standard 6-foot frontal and lateral chest x-rays, on the other hand, are almost always of value. Whether recorded conventionally or digitally, if they are evaluated carefully using a systematic approach and, whenever possible, compared with prior chest radiographs, it is hard to overstate their importance.

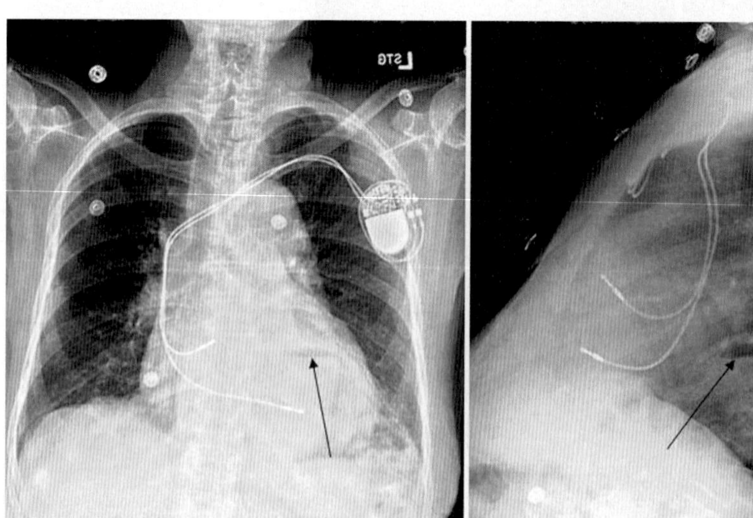

FIGURE 16-24 Radiographs of an older man with heart failure, biventricular dilation, large hiatus hernia (arrows; note air-fluid level), and pacemaker leads in the right atrium and right ventricle.

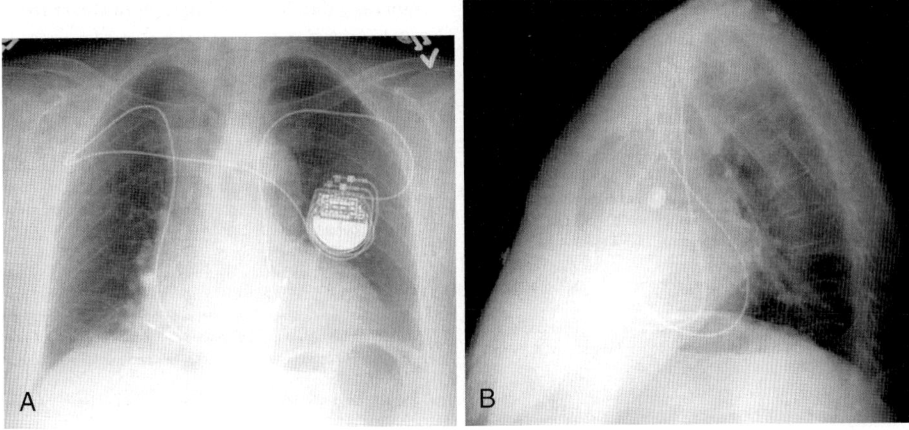

FIGURE 16-25 Chest radiographs of a 62-year-old woman with two pacemakers, with left-sided pacemaker implanted because of failure of the right. As seen on frontal **(A)** and lateral **(B)** views, the right-sided wire traverses the right superior vena cava and right atrium, and its tip lies superiorly and anteriorly in the pulmonary outflow tract. The left-sided wire traverses a persistent left superior vena cava (a normal anatomic variant) and the coronary sinus and its tip, the lower of the two, is in the right atrium.

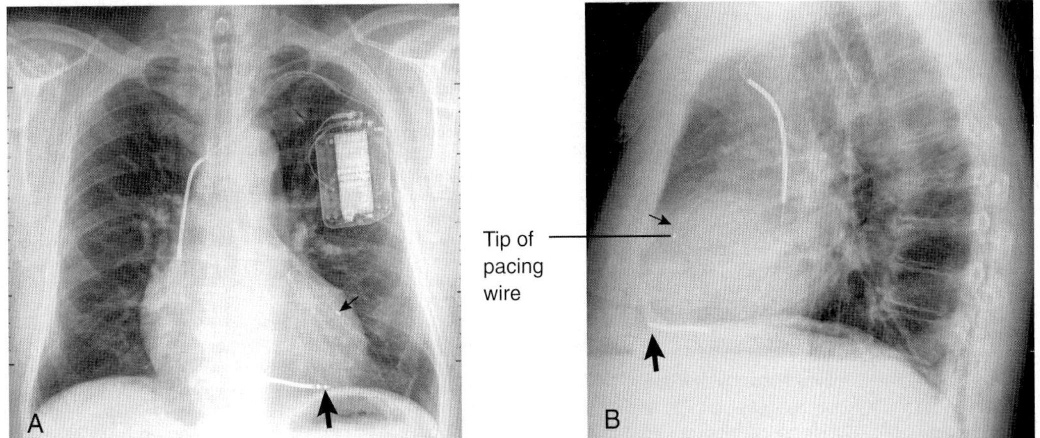

FIGURE 16-26 **A, B,** Chest radiographs of a 78-year-old man after aortic valve replacement. Note wire position (small arrow), through the coronary sinus into the great coronary vein (running parallel to the left anterior descending coronary artery), and biventricular enlargement. Also note position of the separate ICD tip in the right ventricular apex (large arrow).

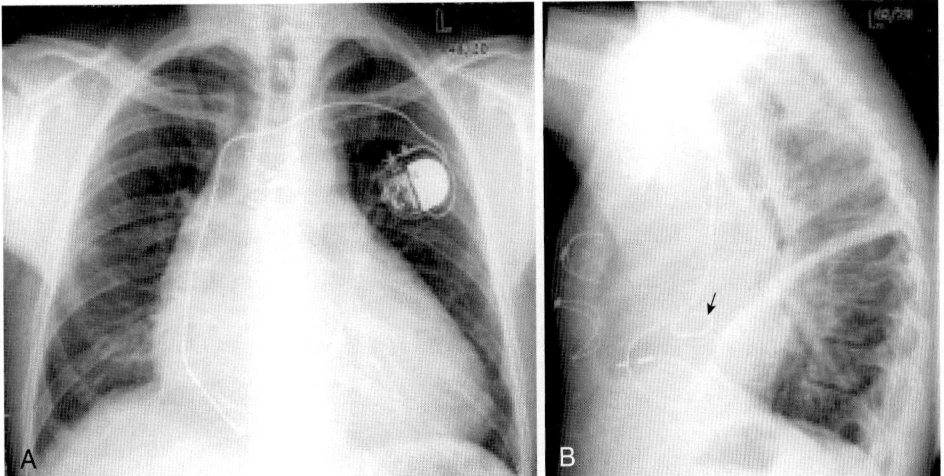

FIGURE 16-27 Chest radiographs of a 28-year-old man who has undergone aortic valve replacement with a porcine bioprosthesis. **A,** PA view. There is marked left ventricular (LV) enlargement with downwardly displaced apex. Note the pacemaker wire with its tip in the right ventricular (RV) apex. **B,** Lateral view confirms primary LV dilation, shows position of the aortic valve, and also shows the tip of the pacing wire in the RV apex. This confirms LV versus RV dilation.

REFERENCES

1. Williams FH: A method for more fully determining the outline of the heart by means of a fluoroscope together with other uses of the instrument in medicine. Boston Med Surg J 135:335, 1896.

Technical Considerations

2. Hintenlang KM, Williams JL, Hintenlang DE: A survey of radiation dose associated with pediatric plain-film chest X-ray examinations. Pediatr Radiol 32:771, 2002.
3. Volk M, Hamer OW, Feuerbach S, Strotzer M: Dose reduction in skeletal and chest radiography using a large-area flat-panel detector based on amorphous silicon and thallium-doped cesium iodide: Technical background, basic image quality parameters, and review of the literature. Eur Radiol 14:827, 2004.
4. Krivopal M, Shlobin OA, Schwartzstein RM: Utility of daily routine portable chest radiographs in mechanically ventilated patients in the medical ICU. Chest 123:1607, 2003.
5. Rong XJ, Shaw CC, Liu X, et al: Comparison of an amorphous silicon/cesium iodide flat-panel digital chest radiography system with screen/film and computed radiography systems: A contrast-detail phantom study. Med Phys 28:2328, 2000.
6. Garmer M, Hennigs SP, Jäger HJ, et al: Digital radiography versus conventional radiography in chest imaging: Diagnostic performance of a large area flat-panel detector in a clinical CT-controlled study. Am J Roentgenol 174:75, 2000.
7. Chotas HG, Dobbins JT, Ravin CE: Principles of digital radiography with large-area electronically readable detectors: A review of the basics. Radiology 210:595, 1999.
8. Bacher K, Smeets P, Bonnarens K, et al: Dose reduction in patients undergoing chest imaging: Digital amorphous silicon flat-panel detector radiography versus conventional film-screen radiography and phosphor-based computed radiography. AJR Am J Roentgenol 181:923, 2003.
9. Konen E, Greenberg I, Rozenman J: Visibility of normal thoracic anatomic landmarks on storage phosphor digital radiography versus conventional radiography. Isr Med Assoc J 7:495, 2005.
10. Pascoal A, Lawinski CP, Mackenzie A, et al: Chest radiography: A comparison of image quality and effective dose using four digital systems. Radiat Prot Dosimetry 114:273, 2005.
11. Eisenhuber E, Stadler A, Prokop M, et al: Detection of monitoring materials on bedside chest radiographs with the most recent generation of storage phosphor plates: Dose increase does not improve detection performance. Radiology 227:216, 2003.
12. Prato A, Ropolo R, Fava C: Digital chest radiography system with amorphous selenium flat-panel detectors: Qualitative and dosimetric comparison with a dedicated film-screen system. Radiol Med (Torino) 110:561, 2005.
13. Kroft LJ, Veldkamp WJ, Mertens BJ, et al: Comparison of eight different digital chest radiography systems: variation in detection of simulated chest disease. AJR Am J Roentgenol 185:339, 2005.
14. Ganten M, Radeleff B, Kampschulte A, et al: Comparing image quality of flat-panel chest radiography with storage phosphor radiography and film-screen radiography AJR Am J Roentgenol 181:171, 2003.
15. Weatherburn GC, Ridout D, Strickland NH, et al: A comparison of conventional film, CR hard copy and PACS soft copy images of the chest: Analyses of ROC curves and inter-observer agreement. Eur J Radiol 47:206, 2003.
16. Honeyman-Buck J: PACS adoption. Semin Roentgenol 38:256, 2003.
17. Correia MJ, Hellies A, Andreassi MG, et al: Lack of radiological awareness among physicians working in a tertiary-care cardiological centre. Int J Cardiol 103:307, 2005.
18. Fazel R, Krumholz HM, Wang SMY, et al: Exposure to low-dose ionizing radiation from medical imaging procedures. N Engl J Med 361:849, 2009.

Normal Chest Radiograph

19. Baron MG: The cardiac silhouette. J Thorac Imaging 15:230, 2000.
20. Ohye RG, Kulik TA: Images in cardiovascular medicine. Normal chest x-ray. Circulation 105:2455, 2002.
21. Boxt LM: Radiology of the right ventricle. Radiol Clin North Am 37:379, 1999.
22. Sharma S, Bhargave A, Krishnakumar R, et al: Can pulmonary venous hypertension be graded by the chest radiograph? Clin Radiol 53:899, 1998.
23. Hoffman RB, Rigler LG: Evaluation of left ventricular enlargement in the lateral projection of the chest. Radiology 85:93, 1965.
24. Freeman V, Mutatiri C, Pretorius M, et al: Evaluation of left ventricular enlargement in the lateral position of the chest using the Hoffman and Rigler sign. Cardiovasc J S Afr 14:134, 2003.
25. Jung G, Landwehr P, Schanzenbächer G, et al: [Value of thoracic radiography in the assessment of cardiac size. A comparison with left ventricular cardiography.] Rofo 162:368, 1995.
26. Fraser RS, Muller NL, Colman N, et al (eds): Fraser and Pare's Diagnosis of Diseases of the Chest. 4th ed. Philadelphia, WB Saunders, 1999.

Evaluating the Chest Radiograph in Heart Disease

27. Berbaum KS, Smith WL: Use of reports of previous radiologic studies. Acad Radiol 5:111, 1998.
28. Satou GM, Lacro RV, Chung T, et al: Heart size on chest x-ray as a predictor of cardiac enlargement by echocardiography in children. Pediatr Cardiol 22:218, 2001.
29. Thomas JT, Kelly RF, Thomas SJ, et al: Utility of history, physical examination, electrocardiogram, and chest radiograph for differentiating normal from decreased systolic function in patients with heart failure. Am J Med 112:437, 2002.
30. Ernst ER, Shub C, Bailey KR, et al: Radiographic measurements of cardiac size as predictors of outcome in patients with dilated cardiomyopathy. J Card Fail 7:13, 2001.
31. Petrie MC: It cannot be cardiac failure because the heart is not enlarged on the chest X-ray. Eur J Heart Fail 5:117, 2003.
32. Perez AA, Ribeiro AL, Barros MV, et al: Value of the radiological study of the thorax for diagnosing left ventricular dysfunction in Chagas' disease. Arq Bras Cardiol 80:208, 2003.
33. Hoilund-Carlsen PF, Gadsboll N, Hein E, et al: Assessment of left ventricular systolic function by the chest x-ray: comparison with radionuclide ventriculography. J Card Fail. 11:299, 2005.
34. Schmermund A, Rensing BJ, Sheedy PF, et al: Reproducibility of right and left ventricular volume measurements by electron-beam CT in patients with congestive heart failure. Int J Card Imaging 14:201, 1998.
35. Ferri C, Emdin M, Nielsen H, et al: Assessment of heart involvement. Clin Exp Rheumatol 21:S24, 2003.
36. Rothrock SG, Green SM, Costanzo KA, et al: High yield criteria for obtaining non-trauma chest radiography in the adult emergency department population. J Emerg Med 23:117, 2002.
37. Oeppen RS, Fairhurst JJ, Argent JD: Diagnostic value of the chest radiograph in asymptomatic neonates with a cardiac murmur. Clin Radiol 57:736, 2002.
38. Gardiner S: Are routine chest x ray and ECG examinations helpful in the evaluation of asymptomatic heart murmurs? Arch Dis Child 88:638, 2003.
39. Laya BF, Goske MJ, Morrison S, et al: The accuracy of chest radiographs in the detection of congenital heart disease and in the diagnosis of specific congenital cardiac lesions. Pediatr Radiol 36:677, 2006.
40. Murray JG, Brown AL, Anagnostou EA, et al: Widening of the tracheal bifurcation on chest radiographs: Value as a sign of left atrial enlargement. AJR Am J Roentgenol 164:1089, 1995.
41. Atar S, Jeon DS, Luo H, et al: Mitral annular calcification: A marker of severe coronary artery disease in patients under 65 years old. Heart 89:161, 2003.
42. Rodan BA, Chen JT, Halber MD, et al: Chest roentgenographic evaluation of the severity of aortic stenosis. Invest Radiol 17:453, 1982.
43. Yamamoto H, Shavelle D, Takasu J, et al: Valvular and thoracic aortic calcium as a marker of the extent and severity of angiographic coronary artery disease. Am Heart J 146:153, 2003.
44. Cook C, Styles C, Hopkins R: Calcification on the chest X-ray: A pictorial review. Hosp Med 62:210, 2001.
45. Li J, Galvin HK, Johnson SC, et al: Aortic calcification on plain chest radiography increases risk for coronary artery disease. Chest 121:1468, 2002.
46. Kiryu S, Raptopoulos V, Baptista J, et al: Increased prevalence of coronary artery calcification in patients with suspected pulmonary embolism. Acad Radiol 10:840, 2003.
47. Wang ZJ, Reddy GP, Gotway MB, et al: CT and MR imaging of pericardial disease. Radiographics 23:S167, 2003.
48. Kao CL, Chang JP: Left ventricular pseudoaneurysm secondary to left ventricular apical venting. Tex Heart Inst J 30:162, 2003.
49. Brown SL, Gropler RJ, Harris KM: Distinguishing left ventricular aneurysm from pseudoaneurysm. A review of the literature. Chest 111:1403, 1997.
50. Kim JH, Siegel MJ, Goldstein JA, et al: Radiologic findings of 2 commonly used cardiac septal occluders with clinical correlation. J Thorac Imaging 18:183, 2003.
51. Bordlee RP: Cardiac valve reconstruction and replacement: A brief review. Radiographics 12:659, 1992.
52. Bejvan SM, Ephron JH, Takasugi JE, et al: Imaging of cardiac pacemakers. AJR Am J Roentgenol 169:1371, 1997.
53. Kurihara Y, Yakushiji YK, Nakajima Y, et al: The vertical displacement sign: A technique for differentiating between left and right ribs on the lateral chest radiograph. Clin Radiol 54:367, 1999.
54. Morishima I, Sone T, Tsuboi H, et al: Follow-up X rays play a key role in detecting implantable cardioverter defibrillator lead fracture: A case of incessant inappropriate shocks due to lead fracture. Pacing Clin Electrophysiol 26:911, 2003.
55. Drucker EA, Brooks R, Garan H, et al: Malfunction of implantable cardioverter defibrillators placed by a nonthoracotomy approach: Frequency of malfunction and value of chest radiography in determining cause. AJR Am J Roentgenol 165:275, 1995.
56. Schummer W, Schummer C, Frober R: Persistent left superior vena cava and central venous catheter position: Clinical impact illustrated by four cases. Surg Radiol Anat 25:315, 2003.

CHAPTER 17 Nuclear Cardiology

James E. Udelson, Vasken Dilsizian, and Robert O. Bonow

The era of noninvasive radionuclide cardiac imaging in humans began in the early 1970s with the first reports of noninvasive evaluation of resting myocardial blood flow. Since that time, there have been major advances in the technical ability to image cardiac physiology and pathophysiology, including that of myocardial blood flow, myocardial metabolism, and ventricular function. Just as important has been a major growth in the understanding of how to apply the image information to care of patients and the effect of that information on clinical decision making. Ultimately, the role of information derived from any imaging procedure is to enhance the clinician's decision-making process to improve symptoms or clinical outcomes or both.

Technical Aspects of Image Acquisition, Display, and Interpretation

Single-Photon Emission Computed Tomography Imaging of Perfusion and Function

The most commonly performed imaging procedure in nuclear cardiology is single-photon emission computed tomography (SPECT) imaging of myocardial perfusion. After injection of the chosen radiotracer, the isotope is extracted from the blood by viable myocytes and retained within the myocyte for some time. Photons are emitted from the myocardium in proportion to the magnitude of tracer uptake, in turn related to perfusion. The standard camera used in nuclear cardiology studies, a gamma camera, captures the gamma ray photons and converts the information into digital data representing the magnitude of uptake and the location of the emission. The photoemissions collide along their flight path with a detector crystal. There, the gamma photons are absorbed and converted into visible light events (a scintillation event). Emitted gamma rays are selected for capture and quantitation by a collimator attached to the face of the camera-detector system. Most often, parallel hole collimators are used so that only photon emissions coursing perpendicular to the camera head and parallel to the collimation holes are accepted (**Fig. 17-1**). This arrangement allows better appropriate localization of the source of the emitted gamma rays. Photomultiplier tubes, the final major component in the gamma camera, sense the light-scintillation events and convert the events into an electrical signal to be further processed (see Fig. 17-1). The final result of SPECT imaging is the creation of multiple tomograms, or slices, of the organ of interest, composing a digital display representing radiotracer distribution throughout the organ.[1] With SPECT myocardial perfusion imaging (MPI), the display represents the distribution of perfusion throughout the myocardium.

SPECT IMAGE ACQUISITION. To construct the three-dimensional model of the heart from which tomograms are created, the myocardial perfusion data must be sampled from multiple angles over 180 or 360 degrees around the patient. Multiple images, each comprising 20 to 25 seconds of emission data, are collected. Each one of the separate "projection" images constitutes a two-dimensional snapshot of myocardial perfusion from the angle at which the projection was acquired. Then, the imaging information from each of the angles is backprojected onto an imaging matrix, creating a reconstruction of the organ of interest. The reader is referred to detailed reviews for more extensive information on the technical aspects of SPECT imaging and image reconstruction.[1]

SPECT IMAGE DISPLAY. From the three-dimensional reconstruction of the heart, computer processing techniques are used to identify the long axis of the left ventricle, and standardized tomographic images in three standard planes are derived. Short-axis images, representing donut-like slices of the heart cut perpendicular to the long axis of the heart, are displayed beginning toward the apex and moving toward the base. This tomographic orientation is similar to the short-axis view in two-dimensional echocardiography, although it is shifted counterclockwise (**Fig. 17-2A**). Tomographic slices cut parallel to the long axis of the heart and also parallel to the long axis of the body are termed vertical long-axis tomograms (Fig. 17-2B), and slices also cut parallel to the long axis of the heart but perpendicular to the vertical long-axis slices are known as horizontal long-axis tomograms (Fig. 17-2C). From all of these tomographic planes, the entire three-dimensional myocardium is sampled and displayed, minimizing overlap of structures.

Basics of Quality Control. The quality of SPECT MPI and the "accuracy" of the representation of regional myocardial perfusion are dependent on multiple quality control issues. These issues include the stability of the tracer distribution in the organ of interest during the acquisition interval, the absence of motion of the patient or organ of interest or both during the acquisition, and the absence of overlying structures that would attenuate the photon emissions from one region relative to another region across the different projection images. Those issues are related to the patient and the organ being imaged, and other quality control issues involve the camera and detector system, including the uniformity of photon detection efficiency across the camera face as well as the stability of the camera across the entire orbit of acquisition.[2]

It is important in interpreting SPECT images to be aware of possible sources of image artifacts. Discrete motion of the patient (and thus motion of the heart outside its original field) causes an abnormality in the final images that may be corrected with motion correction software. Imaging artifacts commonly occur because of the effects of overlying structures that attenuate photon emissions. These include breast attenuation in women and attenuation of the inferobasal wall related to the

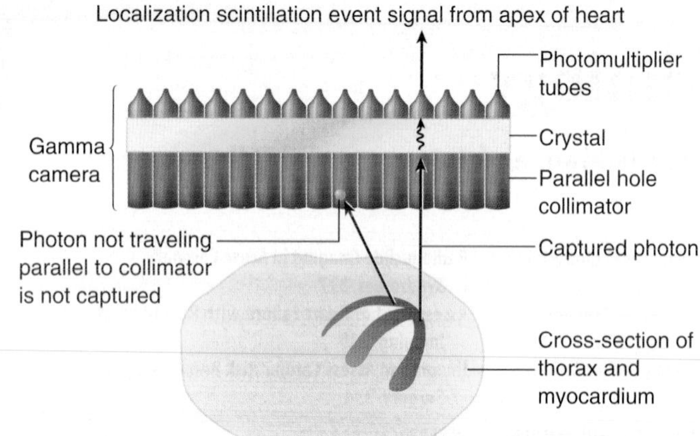

FIGURE 17-1 Capture of emitted photons by a gamma camera. Emissions are captured by a parallel hole collimator, allowing photons to interact with a detector crystal, and are recorded as scintillation events. The event is localized on the basis of where the photon interacts with the crystal.

diaphragm, most commonly seen in men. Strategies to overcome quality problems such as attenuation are described subsequently.

New Technology: High-Speed SPECT Imaging. High-speed SPECT technology introduces a new design of SPECT in terms of both photon acquisition and reconstruction algorithm. This approach uses a series of small, pixilated solid-state detector columns with cadmium zinc telluride or CsI(Tl) crystals, which provide considerably more information for each detected gamma ray. In addition, the design of the solid-state detector with wide-angle tungsten collimators combined with a novel image reconstruction algorithm provides true three-dimensional, patient-specific images localized to the heart.[3] Compared with the conventional SPECT cameras, the high-speed SPECT systems can provide up to eight-fold increase in count rates, thereby reducing imaging times significantly from 14 to 15 minutes with a conventional Anger camera to 5 to 6 minutes with the newer solid-state cameras while achieving a twofold increase in spatial resolution from 9 to 11 mm for Anger cameras to 4.3 to 4.9 mm for cadmium zinc telluride cameras. Reduced imaging times should translate to improved comfort of the patient and fewer motion artifacts. An additional advantage of high-speed SPECT imaging is the potential for administration of lower doses of radiopharmaceuticals without sacrificing image resolution and quality, thereby reducing radiation dose to patients. The reduced imaging time in concert with reduced radiopharmaceutical doses may be cost-effective, with implications for future appropriateness of SPECT imaging.[4]

SPECT PERFUSION TRACERS AND PROTOCOLS

Thallium-201

Thallium-201 (^{201}Tl) was introduced in the 1970s and propelled the clinical application of MPI as an adjunct to exercise treadmill testing. ^{201}Tl is a monovalent cation with biologic properties similar to those of potassium. As potassium is the major intracellular cation in muscle and is virtually absent in scar tissue, ^{201}Tl is a well-suited radionuclide for differentiation of normal and ischemic myocardium from scarred myocardium.[5] ^{201}Tl emits 80 keV of photon energy and has a physical half-life of 73 hours. The initial myocardial uptake early after intravenous injection of thallium is proportional to regional blood flow. First-pass extraction fraction (the proportion of tracer extracted from the blood as it passes through the myocardium) is high, in the range of 85%. It is transported across the myocyte cell membrane by the Na^+,K^+–adenosine triphosphatase (ATPase) transport system and by facilitative diffusion. Peak myocardial concentration of thallium occurs within 5 minutes of injection, with rapid clearance from the intravascular compartment. Although the initial uptake and distribution of thallium are primarily a function of blood flow, the subsequent redistribution of thallium, which begins within 10 to 15 minutes after injection, is unrelated to flow but is related to the rate of thallium clearance from myocardium, linked to the concentration gradient between myocytes and the blood levels of thallium (**Fig. 17-3A**). Thallium clearance is more rapid from normal myocardium with high thallium activity compared with myocardium with reduced thallium activity (ischemic myocardium), a process termed differential washout (Fig. 17-3B).

Thallium studies can be divided into protocols in which ^{201}Tl is administered during stress or at rest.[5] After stress, the reversal of a thallium defect from the initial peak stress to delayed 3- to 4-hour or 24-hour redistribution images is a marker of reversibly ischemic, viable myocardium. When thallium is injected at rest, the extent of thallium defect reversibility from the initial rest images to delayed redistribution images (at 3 to 4 hours) reflects viable myocardium with resting hypoperfusion. When scarred myocardium is present, the initial rest or stress thallium defect persists over time, termed an irreversible or fixed defect. However, in some patients with coronary artery disease (CAD), the initial uptake of thallium during stress may be severely decreased, and tracer accumulation from the recirculating thallium in the blood during the redistribution phase may be slow or even absent because of rapid decline of thallium levels in the blood. The result is that some severely ischemic but viable regions may show no redistribution on either early (3- to 4-hour) or late (24-hour) imaging, even if viable myocardium is present. Viable myocardium in this situation can be revealed by raising blood levels of thallium by reinjection of a small dose (1 mCi) of thallium at rest. Thus, in some patients, thallium reinjection is necessary to identify viable myocardium when there are irreversible defects on stress-redistribution images.

Technetium Tc 99m–Labeled Tracers

Technetium Tc 99m–labeled myocardial perfusion tracers were introduced in the clinical arena in the 1990s.[6] ^{99m}Tc emits 140 keV of photon energy and has a physical half-life of 6 hours. Despite the excellent myocardial extraction and flow kinetic properties of thallium, its energy spectrum of 80 keV is suboptimal for conventional gamma cameras (ideal photopeak in the 140-keV range). In addition, thallium's long physical half-life (73 hours) limits the amount of thallium that may be administered to stay within acceptable radiation exposure parameters. Thus, ^{99m}Tc-labeled tracers improve on these two limitations of thallium. Although three ^{99m}Tc-labeled tracers (sestamibi, teboroxime, and tetrofosmin) have received U.S. Food and Drug Administration (FDA) approval for detection of CAD, only sestamibi and tetrofosmin are available for clinical use at present.

Sestamibi and tetrofosmin are lipid-soluble cationic compounds with first-pass extraction fraction in the range of 60%. Myocardial uptake and clearance kinetics of both tracers are similar. They cross sarcolemmal and mitochondrial membranes of myocytes by passive distribution, driven by the transmembrane electrochemical gradient, and they are retained within the mitochondria.[5] There is minimal redistribution of these tracers compared with thallium. Thus, myocardial perfusion studies with ^{99m}Tc-labeled tracers require two separate injections, one at peak stress and the second at rest.

There are three basic protocols[4] with ^{99m}Tc-labeled tracers: (1) a single-day study, in which myocardial blood flow is interrogated at rest and at peak stress, or in the reverse order, as long as the first injected dose is low (8 to 10 mCi) and the second injected dose is high (22 to 30 mCi); (2) a 2-day study (commonly performed in patients with large body habitus), in which higher doses of the tracer are injected (20 to 30 mCi) both at rest and at peak stress to optimize myocardial count rate; and (3) a dual-isotope technique, which combines injection of thallium at rest followed by injection of a ^{99m}Tc tracer at peak stress. The last approach takes advantage of the favorable properties of each of the two tracers, including high-quality gated SPECT images from ^{99m}Tc and the potential of acquiring redistribution images from thallium (either at 4 hours before the stress study or at 24 hours after the ^{99m}Tc activity has decayed). A comparison of the properties of the available isotopes for perfusion imaging is shown in **Table 17-1**.

SPECT Image Interpretation and Reporting

SPECT myocardial perfusion images may be evaluated visually. The interpreter describes the perfusion pattern findings on stress and then visually interprets whether defects observed on the stress images are or are not reversible. Because the imaging data are digital, computer-aided quantitative analysis may also be used. Validated software programs for

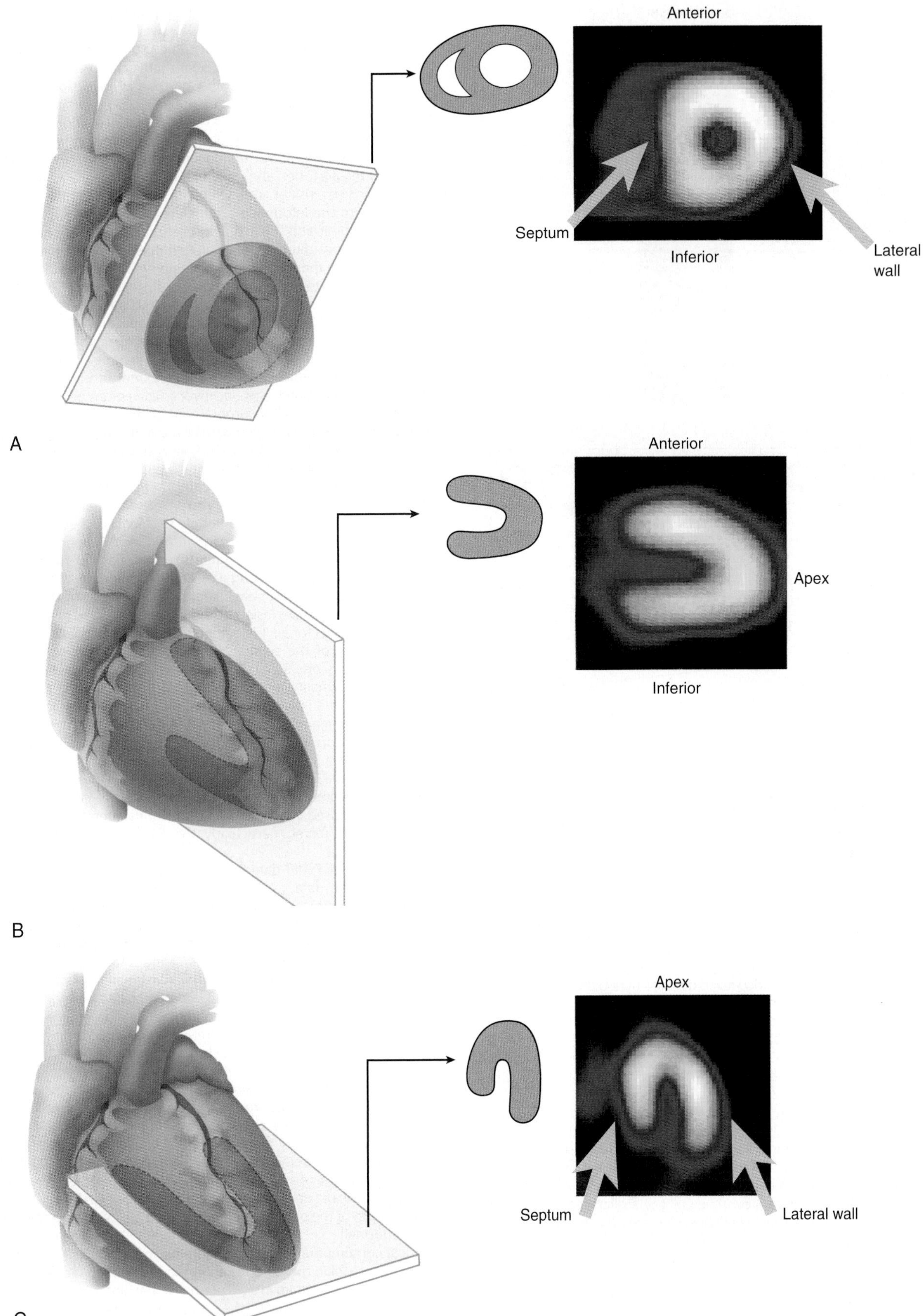

FIGURE 17-2 Standard SPECT imaging display. **A,** The short-axis images represent a portion of the anterior, lateral, inferior, and septal walls. **B,** Vertical long-axis images represent the anterior wall, apex, and inferior wall. **C,** Horizontal long-axis images represent the septum, apex, and lateral walls.

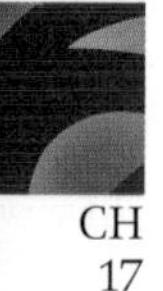

CH 17

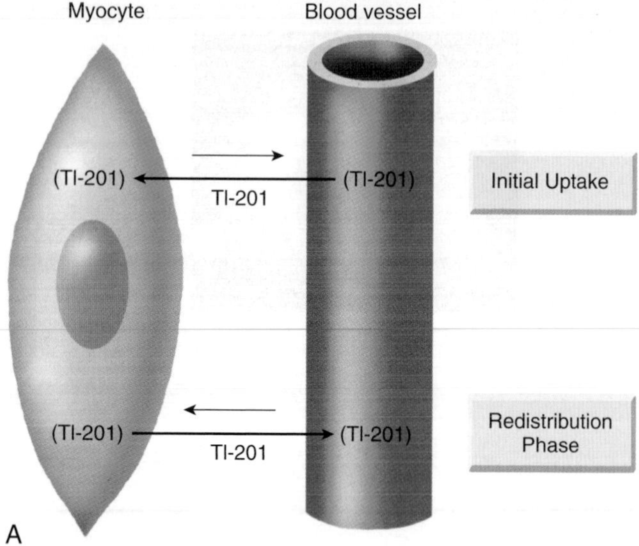

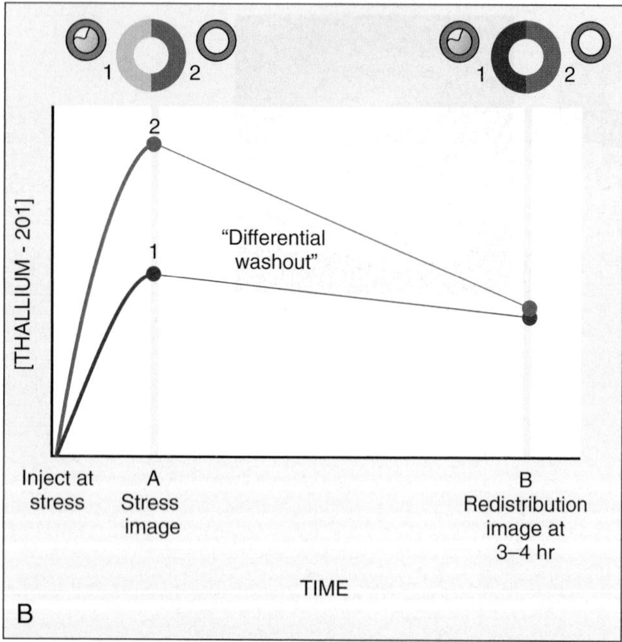

FIGURE 17-3 Thallium-201 redistribution. **A,** After initial uptake into the myocyte, an equilibrium is created between the intracellular and extracellular concentrations of thallium. After blood levels diminish during the redistribution phase, the equilibrium favors egress of thallium out of the myocyte. **B,** On the basis of that equilibrium, thallium concentration diminishes over time in zones of normal uptake while diminishing more slowly in zones with less initial thallium uptake, that is, those with diminished flow reserve or ischemia. In this example, segment 1 of the myocardial schematic is supplied by an artery with an 80% stenosis and segment 2 is supplied by a normal artery. During peak stress, normal blood flow reserve is present in segment 2; blunted flow reserve, based on the presence of stenosis, is present in segment 1, and there is less initial thallium uptake into segment 1 (time point A). Thallium washout is more rapid from the territory with initially normal uptake and slower from the ischemic zone, creating the phenomenon of differential washout. When redistribution imaging is done 3 to 4 hours later (time point B), thallium concentrations are equal in segments 1 and 2. Thus, a reversible stress defect is seen in segment 1, based on the redistribution properties and differential washout. *(Modified from Dilsizian V: SPECT and PET techniques. In Dilsizian V, Narula J [eds]: Atlas of Nuclear Cardiology. Braunwald E [series ed]. Philadelphia, Current Medicine, 2003, pp 19-46.)*

semiquantitative or fully automated quantitative analysis of SPECT myocardial perfusion images are now widely available.

General Principles of Interpretation and Reporting. For any type of image interpretation, visual or quantitative, the key elements to be reported include the presence and location of perfusion defects and whether defects on stress images are reversible on the rest images (implying stress-induced ischemia) or whether stress perfusion defects are irreversible or fixed (often implying myocardial infarction [MI]). Moreover, substantial literature has documented that the extent and the severity of the perfusion abnormality are independently associated with clinical outcomes (risk of adverse events over time) and thus contribute importantly to the information on risk stratification to be conveyed to the ordering clinician.[6] The extent of perfusion abnormality refers to the amount of myocardium or vascular territory that is abnormal, and the severity refers to the magnitude of reduction in tracer uptake in abnormal zone relative to normal. Examples of stress and rest SPECT myocardial perfusion abnormalities of varying extents and severities are shown in **Figures 17-4, 17-5,** and **17-6**. These concepts imply that it is not sufficient to describe a stress perfusion imaging test as simply "abnormal." Rather, a clinically relevant interpretation will include a description of the magnitude of abnormality as well as the extent of ischemia, extent of infarct, and localization to specific myocardial regions or vascular territories. The final report will incorporate all of the clinical data, the stress testing result, and the imaging data to provide comprehensive information to the referring clinician, in a timely and clinically meaningful way.

To minimize subjectivity in image interpretation, semiquantitative visual analysis or fully quantitative computer analysis may be applied to MPI data.[7] With semiquantitative visual analysis, a score is assigned to represent perfusion for each of multiple segments of the myocardium. A segmentation model has been standardized for this approach by dividing the myocardium into 17 segments[8] on the basis of three short-axis slices and a representative long-axis slice to depict the apex (**Fig. 17-7**). Perfusion is graded within each segment on a scale of 0 to 4, with 0 representing normal perfusion and 4 representing a very severe perfusion defect. Scores for all 17 segments are added to create a "summed" score. The sum of the segmental scores from the stress images (the summed stress score, SSS) represents the extent and severity of stress perfusion abnormality, the magnitude of perfusion defects related to both ischemia and infarction. The sum of the 17 segmental scores from the rest images (the summed rest score, SRS) represents the extent of infarction. The summed difference score (SDS) is derived by subtracting the SRS from the SSS and represents the extent and severity of stress-induced ischemia. The segmental scores can be assigned subjectively by the image interpreter or automatically by widely available software programs. As discussed subsequently, a substantial literature has validated these summed scores, particularly the SSS, as predictors of natural history outcomes.

Because SPECT MPI data are a digital representation of radiotracer distribution, the data can also be analyzed quantitatively. The most common technique involves creation of a circumferential profile of relative tracer activity around the tomogram of interest, such as a short-axis tomogram. With this technique, each short-axis tomogram is sampled at every 3 to 6 degrees for 360 degrees, along a ray extending from the center of the image (**Fig. 17-8A**). The maximum counts at a picture element (pixel) along the ray, usually occurring in the midportion of the myocardium, are recorded for each angle. The data may be plotted to create a profile of the perfusion pattern of that tomogram relative to the most "normal" area of uptake, which is assigned a value of 100% uptake (Fig. 17-8B). Circumferential profiles for an individual patient can be compared directly with a composite profile representing normal perfusion. The normal perfusion data are created from studies performed in normal subjects with a very low clinical probability of CAD or in those with known normal coronary arteries (Fig. 17-8B). A quantitative extent of abnormality can be derived for each tomogram of the individual patient (the total amount of myocardium that falls below the lower limit of normal) as well as a derivation of the severity of the perfusion abnormality (the depth of the patient's perfusion abnormality relative to the lower limit of normal).

Most contemporary computer systems and analysis programs create bull's-eye or polar maps representing perfusion of the entire three-dimensional myocardium in a two-dimensional plot (Fig. 17-8C,D). Quantitative data may be derived on the extent of global perfusion abnormality, the abnormality within vascular territories, and the extent of reversible and fixed defects (Fig. 17-8D). These are often displayed as blackout maps, in which any pixel values falling below a set number of standard deviations below the normal limits is assigned the color black, and the extent of that abnormality is expressed as a percentage of the presumed vascular territory and as a percentage of the left ventricle.

Advantages and Disadvantages of Visual and Quantitative Analysis

The accuracy of visual analysis is based on many factors, which include the experience and training of the reader as well as the quality of the imaging study. Well-trained readers will incorporate information from the raw data (such as the presence of apparent breast attenuation or an elevated diaphragm potentially attenuating the inferior wall) and adjust their threshold for interpreting an abnormality to optimize accuracy. Visual analysis is inherently subjective, however, and thus subject to variability, both between readers and within an individual reader. The quantitative programs and comparisons to normal data bases can perform with little or no human interaction. Thus, the results are highly reproducible. This approach attempts to account for potential artifacts such as breast or diaphragm attenuation by the comparison of patient image data to image data from normal, gender-matched subjects (in which, for example, the lower limit of normal for the anterolateral wall of a woman would be lower than that of a man because of the presence of breast tissue). Nonetheless, artifacts that are not accounted for by the normal data comparison, such as those introduced by motion or other suboptimal quality issues that the trained reader may recognize as likely artifactual, may often be called abnormal by quantitation. Thus, in practice, many readers will interpret MPI studies by visual analysis as well as by incorporating the quantitative data to arrive at a final conclusion. The more objective and reproducible nature of the quantitative analysis is a strength with regard to its use in clinical trials that interrogate the effect of therapies on serial changes in myocardial perfusion.

Incorporating Bayesian Principles into Image Interpretation

Although it is possible to interpret MPI data in isolation and report only on what the images demonstrate, a more accepted interpretive methodologic principle is that the final interpretation should take into account the entirety of the data at hand. Hence, the image data build

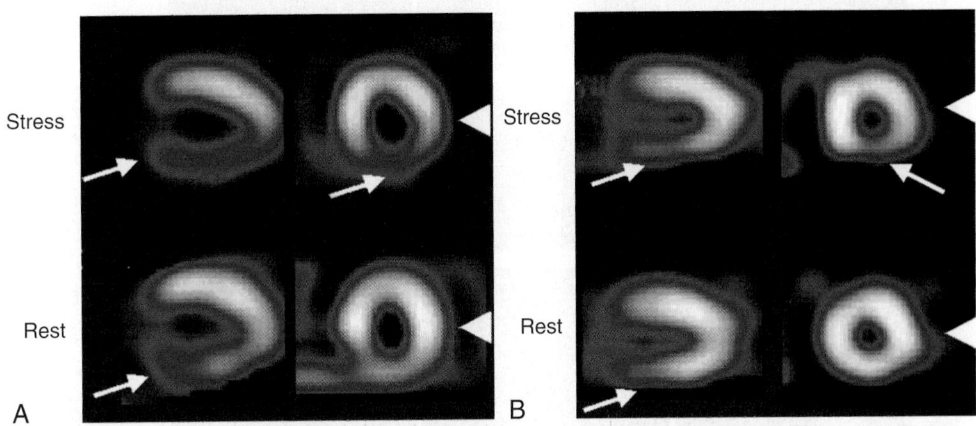

FIGURE 17-4 Abnormal SPECT images of different extent and severity. **A,** A large, moderately severe, reversible inferior wall defect (arrows) reflecting a moderately severe flow reserve abnormality. **B,** A milder reversible inferior wall defect (arrows) reflecting a less severe stenosis or a severe stenosis with well-developed collaterals minimizing the defect severity. In both patients, there is also a mild lateral wall reversible defect (arrowheads). Note how the lateral wall brightens relative to the septum on the rest images compared with the stress images.

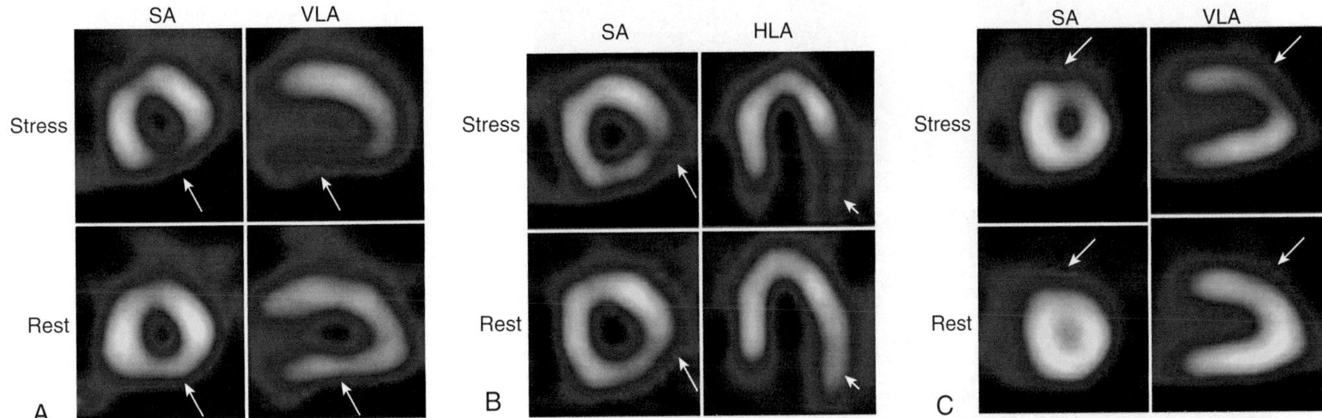

FIGURE 17-5 Examples of single vascular territory reversible defects. **A,** A reversible inferior wall defect (arrows) in the short-axis (SA) and vertical long-axis (VLA) views, consistent with inducible ischemia in the right coronary artery territory. **B,** A reversible lateral wall defect (arrows) in the SA and horizontal long-axis (HLA) views (arrowheads), consistent with inducible ischemia in the left circumflex coronary artery territory. **C,** A reversible anterior wall defect (arrows) in the SA and VLA views, consistent with inducible ischemia in the left anterior descending coronary artery territory.

TABLE 17-1 Properties of SPECT Tracers

TRACER FRACTION	PHYSICAL HALF-LIFE	UPTAKE	MYOCARDIAL CLEARANCE	DIFFERENTIAL WASHOUT	MAXIMUM EXTRACTION
Thallium-201	73 hours	Active	~50% at 6 hours	Yes	~0.70
^{99m}Tc-sestamibi	6 hours	Passive	Minimal	Minimal	0.39
^{99m}Tc-tetrafosmin	6 hours	Passive	Minimal	Minimal	0.24
^{99m}Tc-teboroxime	6 hours	Passive	~50% at 10 minutes	Yes	0.72

From Gerson MC, McGoron A, Roszell N, et al: Myocardial perfusion imaging: Radiopharmaceuticals and tracer kinetics. *In* Gerson MC (ed): Cardiac Nuclear Medicine. New York, McGraw Hill, 1997, pp 3-27.

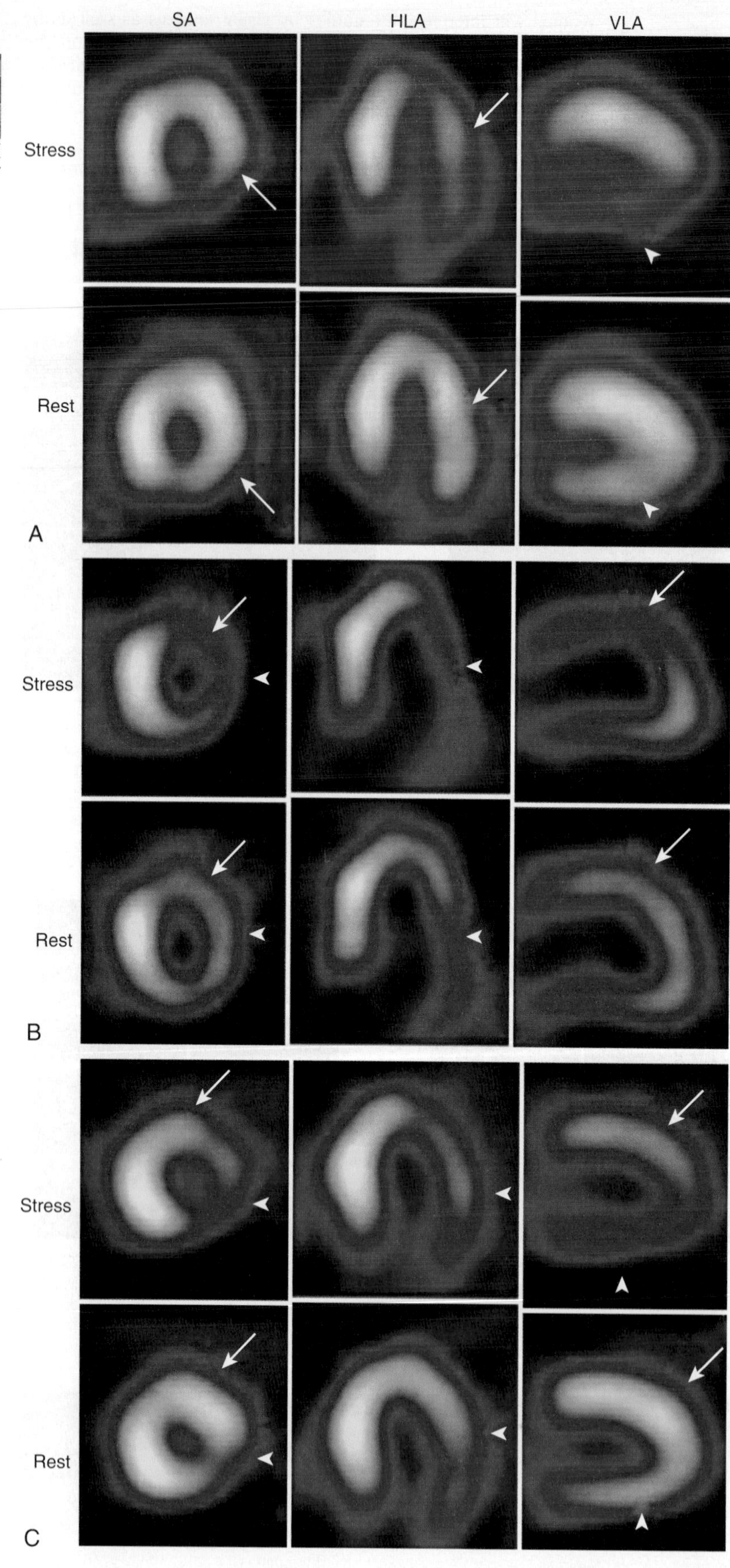

FIGURE 17-6 Examples of reversible defects in more than one vascular territory. **A,** A reversible lateral wall defect (arrows) in the short-axis (SA) and horizontal long-axis (HLA) views, consistent with inducible ischemia in left circumflex (LCX) coronary artery territory, and a reversible inferior wall defect (arrowheads) in the vertical long-axis (VLA) view, consistent with inducible ischemia in the right coronary artery (RCA) territory. **B,** A reversible anterior wall defect (arrows) in the SA and VLA views, consistent with inducible ischemia in the left anterior descending (LAD) coronary artery territory, and a reversible lateral wall defect (arrowheads) in the SA and HLA views, consistent with inducible ischemia in LCX territory. **C,** An example of perfusion abnormalities in all three major vascular territories: a reversible anterior wall defect (arrows) in the SA and VLA views, consistent with inducible ischemia in the LAD territory; a reversible lateral wall defect (arrowheads) in the SA and HLA views, consistent with inducible ischemia in the LCX territory; and a reversible inferior wall defect (arrowheads) in the VLA view, consistent with inducible ischemia in the RCA territory.

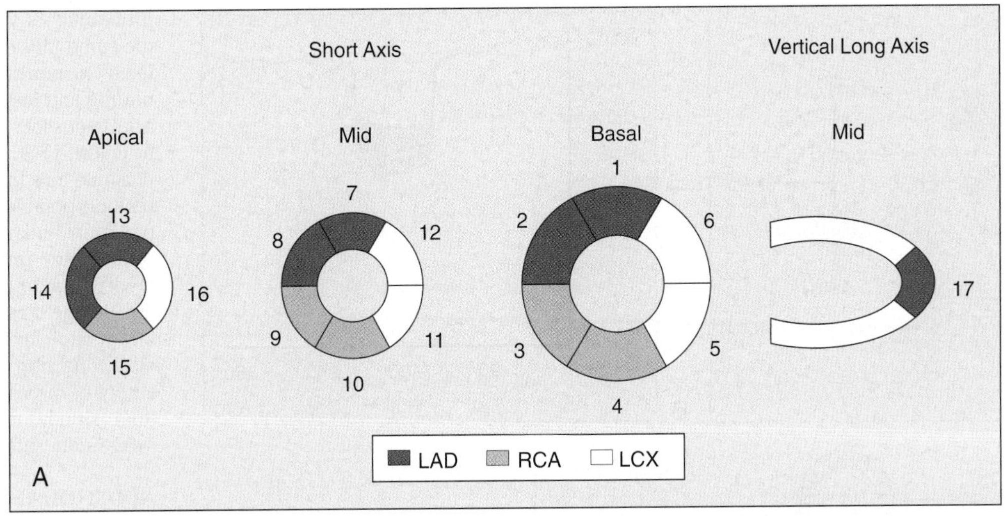

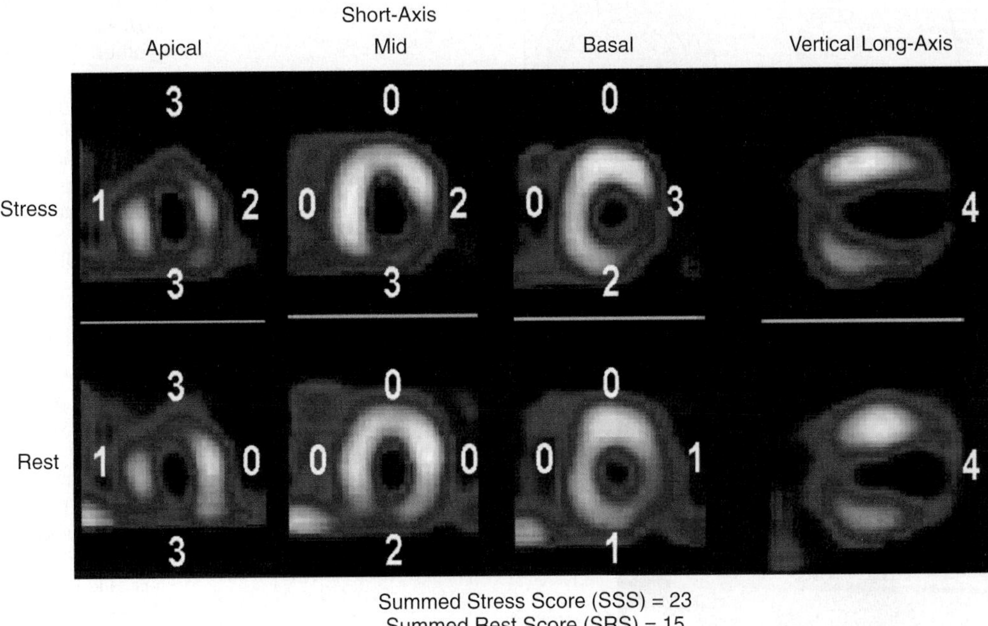

FIGURE 17-7 **A,** Standard segmental myocardial display for semiquantitative visual analysis in a 17-segment model, with corresponding vascular territory schematic. **B,** Segmental scoring of a patient whose stress and rest SPECT perfusion images show a severe apical fixed defect (in the vertical long axis), extending into the inferoapical and anteroapical walls (in the apical short axis), with evidence of reversible defects in the inferior and lateral walls (in the mid and basal short axis). The summed stress score (SSS = 23) represents extensive perfusion abnormality at stress (reflecting ischemia and infarct); the summed rest score (SRS = 15) represents the extent of infarct; and the summed difference score (SDS = SSS – SRS = 8) represents the extent of ischemia. LAD = left anterior descending (artery); LCX = left circumflex (coronary artery); RCA = right coronary artery.

on the already known clinical and stress test data, and the clinician should take all of this information into account when interpreting MPI data. An understanding of Bayesian probability principles is useful in this regard. Bayes' theorem posits that the post-test probability of disease (or risk of an event after a test) is influenced not only by the sensitivity and specificity of the test but also importantly by the pretest probability of disease (see Chap. 14). This principle is illustrated in **Figure 17-9**. For a given positive test result, the post-test probability of disease may be distinctly lower in a patient with a very low pretest probability of disease compared with a different patient with a much higher pretest probability (Fig. 17-9A). In practice, MPI results are not simply positive or negative; rather, positive (i.e., abnormal) tests can range from borderline abnormal (uncertainty whether the abnormality may be an artifact or a mild perfusion defect) to strongly abnormal (i.e., extensive and severe defects, highly likely to be real and unlikely to represent artifact). Thus, the "test positive" curve in Figure 17-9A can be thought of as a family of positivity curves, with distinct implications for post-test likelihood of disease (Fig. 17-9B).

The implication for image interpretation incorporating these concepts can be illustrated by considering a mildly positive MPI study demonstrating a small mild reversible inferobasal defect. Whereas it is possible that this defect represents a small area of inferior inducible ischemia, it is also possible that the image may reflect diaphragm attenuation of the inferobasal wall predominantly affecting the stress image. The influence of the pretest probability data (i.e., pre-MPI) is illustrated in Figure 17-9C. For a young patient with nonanginal chest pain, the pretest probability of CAD is low. If the patient undergoes an exercise treadmill test (ETT) (see Chap. 14) as the stress portion of the MPI test and exercises to a good workload with no symptoms and no electrocardiographic change, the post-ETT probability is even lower. The post-ETT probability then becomes the pre-MPI probability, as seen in Figure 17-9D. A positive test, especially a mildly positive

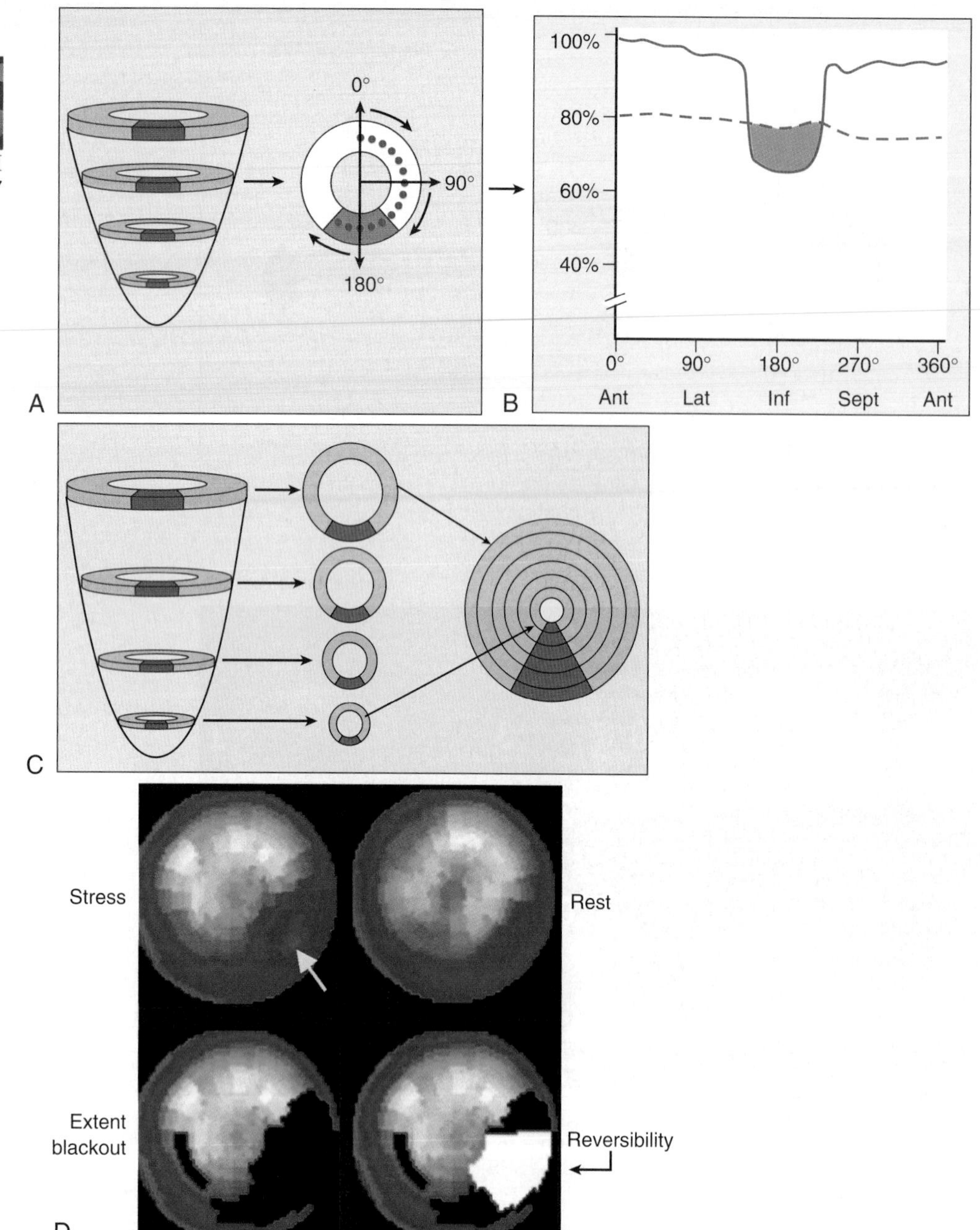

FIGURE 17-8 Quantitative analysis of SPECT imaging. **A,** Circumferential profile analysis of tracer uptake along rays emanating from the center of the short-axis tomogram. From this procedure, a circumferential profile of tracer uptake around the myocardium is developed for each short-axis tomogram. In this example, there is a perfusion defect in the inferior wall (darker purple area). **B,** The data are plotted relative to location around the myocardium (*x*-axis) and "normalized" to the point of peak uptake, which is assigned a value of 100% (*y*-axis). The patient's data (solid line) are compared with lower limits of normal (dashed line) derived from a group of subjects without coronary artery disease of the same gender. From this comparison, the quantitative extent and severity of the perfusion abnormality can be derived (red area). **C,** Data from all of the individual short-axis tomograms can be combined to create a bull's-eye polar plot, representing a two-dimensional compilation of all of the three-dimensional short-axis perfusion data. The extent of the inferior wall perfusion defect (gray area on individual profiles and polar plot) is seen on the two-dimensional map. **D,** Example of a bull's-eye polar plot for a patient with a reversible defect of the inferolateral wall (yellow arrow on the stress bull's-eye plot, upper left). The blackout area (on the extent blackout plot, lower left) represents the myocardium that falls below the lower limits of normal; in the reversibility plot (lower right), the white area represents the extent of that abnormality that is reversible (ischemic) on rest imaging. *(Images courtesy of Ernest Garcia, PhD.)*

test, is still associated with a relative low post-test probability of CAD. If it is reported as positive, there is actually a greater chance that such a result represents a false-positive as opposed to a true-positive result. In contrast, for an older patient being evaluated for anginal chest pain symptoms, who reproduces those symptoms on the treadmill with positive electrocardiographic changes, the pre-MPI probability is very high, and thus the same MPI results are far more likely to represent a true-positive finding and less likely to represent a false-positive study, as illustrated in Figure 17-9C,D. These examples illustrate how the clinical data may be incorporated into the MPI interpretation and also how Bayesian probability principles may be incorporated sequentially so that the image reader is conveying information to the referring clinician reflecting the post-test probability of disease (and risk), rather than simply reporting what the image data show in isolation.

ADDITIONAL IMPORTANT SIGNS IN SPECT IMAGING ANALYSIS BEYOND MYOCARDIAL PERFUSION. There are other abnormal findings that provide additional information beyond that provided by the perfusion pattern alone, including lung uptake of tracer (particularly ^{201}Tl) and transient ischemic dilation of the left ventricle.

Lung Uptake

In some patients, substantial tracer uptake is apparent throughout the lung fields after stress that is not present at rest (**Fig. 17-10A**). Patients with lung uptake often have severe multivessel disease, elevation of pulmonary capillary wedge pressure during exercise, and decreases in ejection fraction (EF) during exercise, all implying extensive myocardial ischemia.[5] It is likely that ischemia-induced elevation in left atrial and pulmonary pressures slows pulmonary transit of the tracer, allowing more time for extraction or transudation into the interstitial spaces of the lung, accounting for this imaging sign.

Lung uptake of ^{201}Tl has been more extensively validated than lung uptake of the ^{99m}Tc tracers sestamibi and tetrofosmin. There is minimal splanchnic or background activity after thallium stress injection, allowing image acquisition earlier after stress. In addition, the redistribution properties of thallium mandate that imaging begin relatively early after stress, and thus lung uptake may be more apparent.

With the ^{99m}Tc perfusion tracers, liver uptake is more prominent than that of the heart immediately after injection; thus, image acquisition should begin 15 to 30 minutes after exercise stress injection and 30 to 60 minutes after pharmacologic stress.[5] Thus, lung uptake, even if it had been present early after stress, may be missed with ^{99m}Tc tracers because of the more delayed onset of imaging compared with thallium.

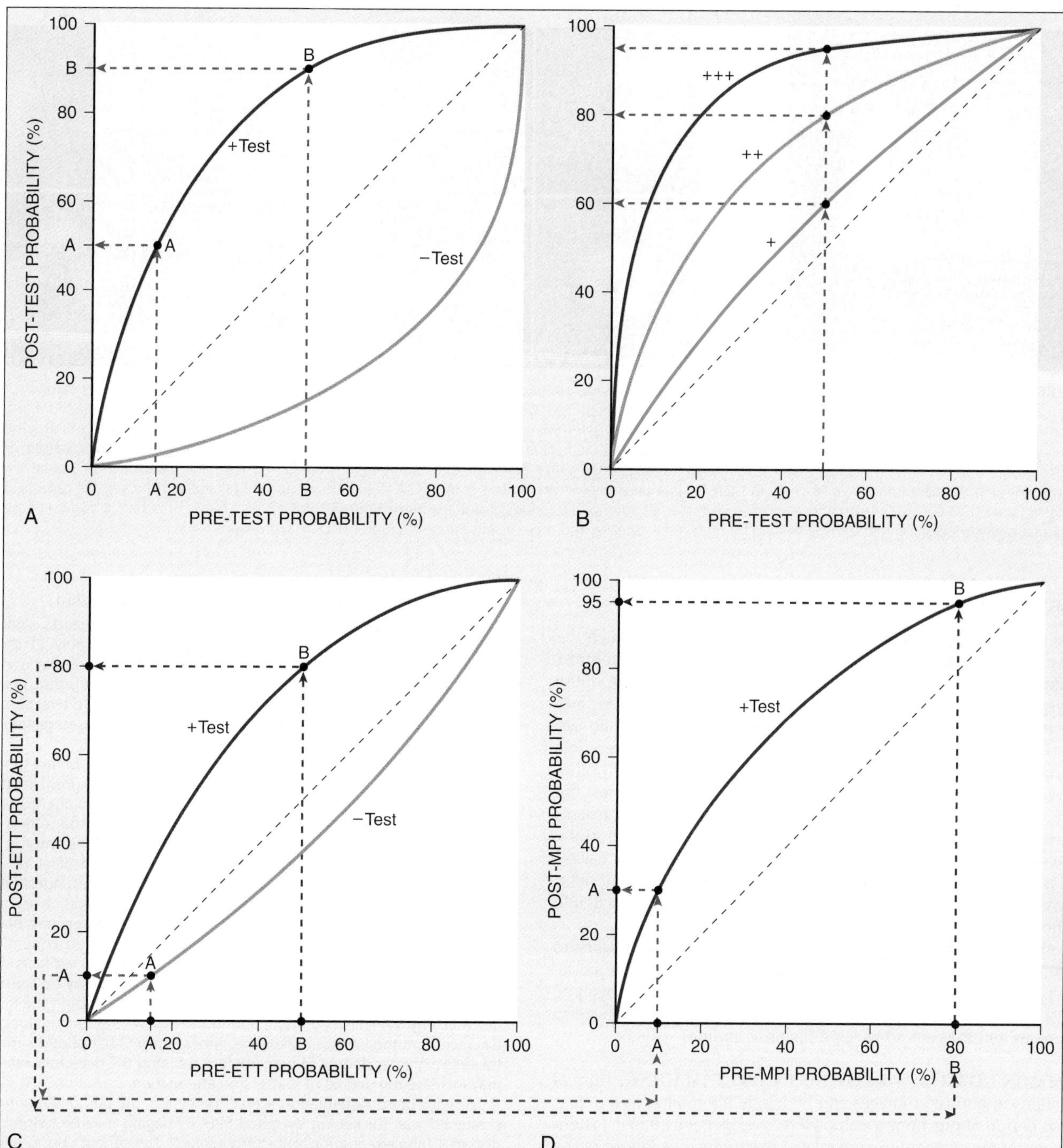

FIGURE 17-9 The influence of the pretest probability on post-test interpretation and application of Bayes' theorem. **A,** For a patient with a low pretest probability of disease (point A at 15% on the *x*-axis) with a positive test result, the post-test probability of disease (point A at 50% on the *y*-axis) is lower compared with a different patient with a higher pretest probability with the same positive test result (point B at 50% pretest probability on the *x*-axis, 90% post-test probability on the *y*-axis). In **B,** the "test positive" curve can be thought of as a family of curves influenced by how strongly positive the images might be. For a given pretest probability, the post-test probability becomes progressively higher as the image becomes more strongly abnormal. For a borderline abnormal study (+ curve), the post-test probability may be only slightly higher then the pretest value. For a strongly positive study (+++ curve), the post-test probability is very high no matter what the pretest probability. **C, D,** Sequential application of Bayes' theorem. For a young patient with nonanginal chest pain, the pretest probability of CAD is low (~15%, point A on *x*-axis of **C**). If the patient undergoes an exercise treadmill test (ETT) and exercises to a good workload with no symptoms and no electrocardiographic change, the post-ETT probability is even lower (10% on *y*-axis in **C**). The post-ETT probability then becomes the pre-MPI probability, as seen in **D** (point A on *x*-axis). A "positive" MPI test is still associated with a relative low post-test probability of CAD (point A at 30% probability on *y*-axis). If reported as positive, there is actually a greater chance that such a result represents a false-positive result (70%) as opposed to a true-positive result (30%). For an older patient with chest pain (higher pretest probability, point B on *x*-axis of **C**), who reproduces those symptoms on the treadmill with positive electrocardiographic changes, the post-ETT probability rises (point B on *y*-axis of **C**), and that becomes the high pre-MPI probability (point B on *x*-axis of **D**). Thus, the same MPI results are far more likely to represent a true-positive finding (point B on *y*-axis of **D**, 95%) and less likely to represent a false-positive study (5%).

CH 17

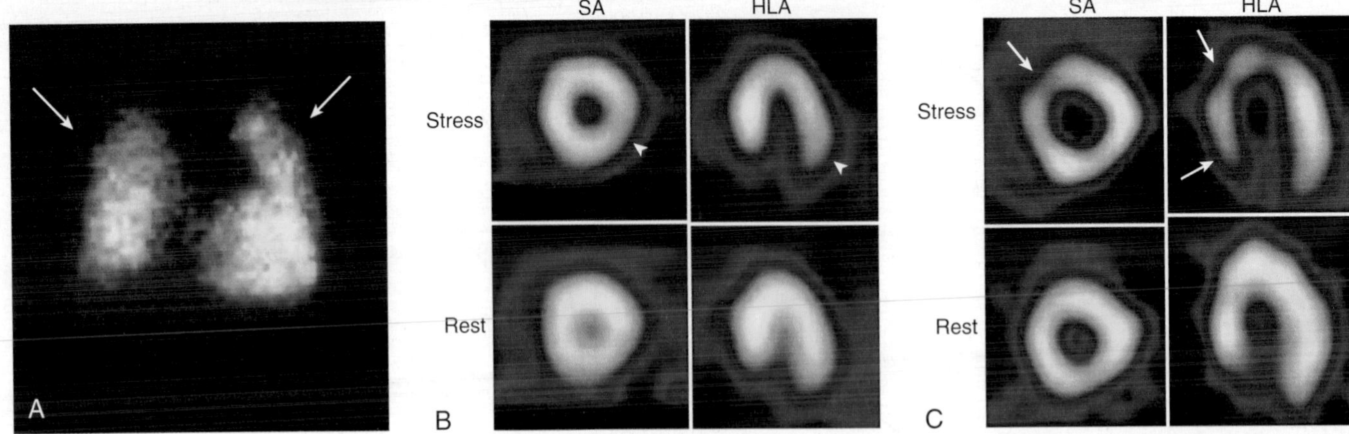

FIGURE 17-10 A, Increased lung uptake of thallium-201 (arrows), imaged in the anterior projection. Lung uptake such as this is associated with extensive CAD and an adverse prognosis. **B, C,** Transient ischemic dilation as a sign of extensive CAD. In these examples, the perfusion pattern suggests single-vessel disease, but the presence of transient ischemic cavity dilation is suggestive of more extensive and higher risk disease. In **B,** there is a reversible lateral wall defect (arrowheads) in the short-axis (SA) and horizontal long-axis (HLA) views, consistent with inducible ischemia in left circumflex coronary artery territory; the perfusion pattern of the other territories appears normal at stress and rest. However, the apparently larger left ventricular cavity at stress compared with rest in both the SA and HLA views is consistent with transient ischemic dilation. In **C,** there is an anteroseptal reversible defect in the SA view (arrows) and septal and apical reversible defects in the HLA view (arrows), all consistent with important disease in the left anterior descending coronary artery. However, there is also transient ischemic dilation of the left ventricular cavity, suggesting that there is likely to be multivessel disease, and these results suggest a high-risk clinical scenario.

Transient Ischemic Dilation of the Left Ventricle

Transient ischemic dilation refers to an imaging pattern in which the left ventricle or left ventricular (LV) cavity appears larger on the stress images than at rest (Fig. 17-10B,C).[9] For patients in whom the entire left ventricle appears larger during stress, the pathophysiology is probably related to extensive ischemia and prolonged postischemic systolic dysfunction, resulting in a dilated, dysfunctional left ventricle during the stress acquisition relative to the rest acquisition. In other patients, the epicardial silhouette appears similar at stress and rest, but there is apparent dilation of the LV cavity. This probably represents diffuse subendocardial ischemia (relatively less tracer uptake in the subendocardium, creating the appearance of an enlarged LV cavity) and is also associated with severe and extensive CAD. Contemporary processing systems can automatically quantify transient ischemic dilation.

Both lung uptake and transient ischemic dilation provide clues to more extensive CAD than may have been suspected from the perfusion pattern alone. Both signs have been associated with angiographically extensive and severe CAD and with unfavorable long-term outcomes and thus are considered high-risk findings.

COMMON NORMAL VARIATIONS IN SPECT IMAGING. Normal variations in perfusion images can be falsely interpreted as a defect. These perturbations from a completely homogeneous tracer pattern throughout the myocardium are related to structural variations of the myocardium as well as to technical factors associated with image acquisition.

One example is the "dropout" of the upper septum because of merging of the muscular septum with the membranous septum (**Fig. 17-11A**). Apical thinning is another variation of normal that can be mistaken for a perfusion defect (Fig. 17-11B). The apex is anatomically thinner than other myocardial regions, creating this appearance. In normal SPECT images, the lateral wall may often appear brighter than the contralateral septum (Fig. 17-11C). This is not due to a difference in lateral versus septal wall myocardial blood flow. Rather, during a SPECT acquisition, the camera is physically closer to the lateral myocardial wall (in proximity to the lateral chest wall) than to the septum, thus subject to less soft tissue attenuation and associated with more efficient count capture. A careful review of a series of normal volunteers or subjects with a low probability of CAD with one's own equipment is an important step in minimizing the influence of these normal variations on the sensitivity and specificity for detection of CAD.

Technical Artifacts Affecting Image Interpretation

BREAST ATTENUATION. In patients with large or dense breasts, significant attenuation may create artifacts varying considerably in their appearance and location (**Fig. 17-12**). A review of the cine display of the raw projection images may reveal the presence of potential breast attenuation.[6] Gender-matched quantitative data bases have had a favorable although modest impact on this issue, as such data bases generally consist of subjects who are of average body and breast size.

Several approaches toward minimizing the impact of breast tissue have been taken to improve specificity (lowering the false-positive rate) in women. Most well documented is the use of ^{99m}Tc-based agents with SPECT imaging with electrocardiography (ECG) gating. In the setting of a mildly to moderately severe fixed defect, most often of the anterior or anterolateral wall, that may represent breast attenuation artifact versus nontransmural MI, the presence of preserved wall motion suggests the absence of infarct and supports the interpretation of attenuation artifact (see Fig. 17-12). Specificity for ruling out CAD in women has been improved significantly with this technique,[6] as discussed subsequently.

INFERIOR WALL ATTENUATION. Inferior wall attenuation artifacts are commonly encountered in SPECT imaging. This artifact may be caused by extracardiac structures, such as the diaphragm overlapping the inferior wall (**Fig. 17-13**). In addition, during a SPECT acquisition, the longer distance from the inferior wall to the camera means that photons must traverse a greater degree of tissue before reaching the detectors, which may increase the degree of scatter and attenuation.

As with breast attenuation artifact detection, the demonstration of preserved wall thickening by gated SPECT imaging may be helpful in distinguishing attenuation artifact from infarct. The patient's positioning may also minimize the degree of attenuation. When patients are imaged in the prone position,[2,6] the inferior wall is shifted away from the diaphragm and thus less subject to attenuation (see Fig. 17-13).

ARTIFACTS RELATED TO EXTRACARDIAC TRACER UPTAKE. Tracer in extracardiac structures can cause artifacts in SPECT images. When such a structure is near the heart, increased counts may reach the detector. This may falsely elevate the number of counts the system assigns to the nearby cardiac wall, so that the cardiac region is displayed as falsely "hotter." A second possibility occurs when a nearby hot extracardiac structure causes a "ramp filter" or "negative lobe" artifact.[2] This artifact is due to a hot extracardiac structure "stealing" counts from the heart during the calculation of the summed SPECT images. The adjacent myocardium appears falsely "cool." If substantial extracardiac uptake is noted, image acquisition may be repeated after waiting a longer time before imaging. Having the patient drink cold water may enhance clearance of tracer from visceral organs, particularly the bowel.

ATTENUATION CORRECTION METHODS. Attenuation of photons refers to undetected events in the heart due to interaction of photons with the intervening soft tissue, breast, or diaphragm. Attenuation of photons can produce artifactual defects in both positron emission tomography (PET) and SPECT cardiac imaging that mimic true myocardial perfusion defects and thus reduce specificity (increase false-positive findings). The 511-keV photons emitted by positron-emitting radiotracers in PET imaging are attenuated less per centimeter of soft tissue than are the lower energy 80- to 140-keV photons typically emitted by SPECT radiotracers. In SPECT imaging, a single photon needs to travel from the heart to the camera; in PET imaging, two coincident photons (i.e., emitted simultaneously) need to travel across the entire body to reach their respective detectors (see Positron Emission Tomography). Whereas the total attenuation may actually be greater for PET than for SPECT, an important distinction in the case of PET is that the attenuation is the same along a projection line (the path the pair of photons traverse) independent of how deep in the body the annihilation took place. Thus, in PET, only the total attenuation through the whole body along a specific direction must be known. On the other hand, in SPECT, the exact depth along a projection line where the radioactive decay took place is necessary to correct for attenuation. Thus, attenuation correction for SPECT is theoretically more challenging. In recent years, several approaches to correct for attenuation in both PET and SPECT imaging have emerged, with the goal of "correcting" attenuation artifacts to minimize false-positive defects and to improve specificity.

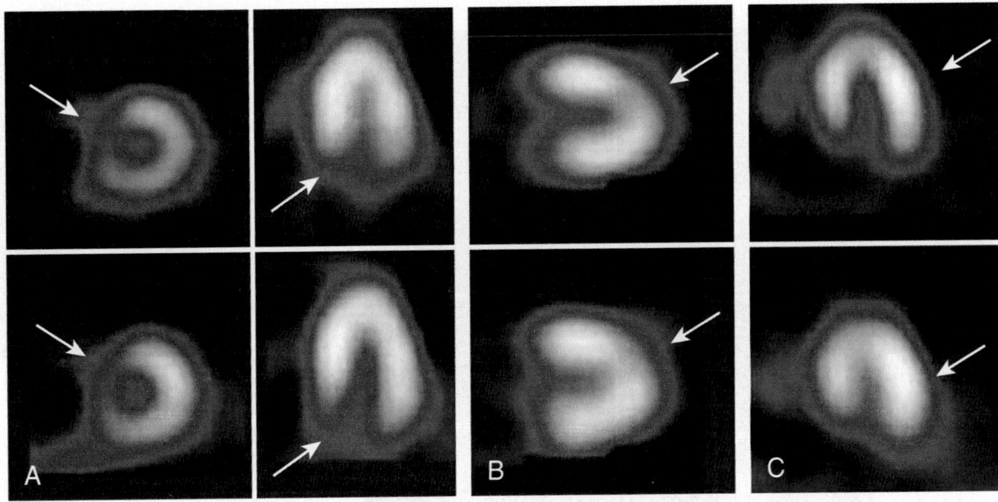

FIGURE 17-11 Normal variations in SPECT perfusion imaging. **A,** Normal "dropout" of the basal septum (arrows), which would be seen in the most basal short-axis tomograms (left) and the basal septal portion in the horizontal long-axis view (right). **B,** Normal apical thinning (arrows). **C,** The lateral wall is often slightly "hotter" than the septum, another normal variation.

PET Attenuation Correction

To measure the attenuation correction factor, a rod that rotates about the patient is filled with a relatively long-lived positron emitter, germanium-68, or a single-photon emitter, cesium-137. The rod is first made to rotate at a fixed speed in the gantry, and total coincident counts are measured without the patient (the blank scan) and repeated with the patient (the transmission scan). The ratio of coincident counts of blank scan and transmission scan yields the array of attenuation correction factors needed to correct each projection line. Once each projection line has been corrected for attenuation (and scatter), the emission data may be reconstructed into an attenuation-corrected emission image for clinical interpretation. As long as the patient does not move during the scanning procedure, cardiac PET images will be free from attenuation artifacts.

SPECT Attenuation Correction

Approaches similar to PET attenuation correction have been attempted to correct attenuation artifacts in SPECT, but these have not been widely adopted because the problem of attenuation correction is fundamentally more challenging in SPECT than in PET. There are a number of commercially available SPECT gamma cameras that have the ability to acquire transmission data and to perform attenuation correction. Several published studies suggest that incorporating attenuation correction into SPECT interpretation may increase the specificity of CAD diagnosis. However, the increased cost of SPECT attenuation correction systems and the additional time required to quality control, acquire, and process studies are factors that have slowed the widespread deployment of this technology.

TYPES OF SPECT ATTENUATION CORRECTION. Accurate attenuation correction with SPECT requires both emission and transmission acquisitions from a single study, and there are a number of potential approaches to accomplish this. The first is a sequential attenuation correction, which can be done with the emission acquisition (the clinical imaging data) after the transmission scan. However, registration between the two acquisitions can be challenging. A second approach is "interleaved" attenuation correction, in which emission and transmission scans are acquired sequentially, at each stop. Whereas this reduces the emission-transmission misalignment, the acquisition time is significantly longer. The third approach is simultaneous attenuation correction, which reduces the length of the study as well as emission-transmission misalignment. When a two-headed (90-degree) or three-headed gamma camera is used, one of the heads can be dedicated to acquire the transmission data and the other head (or two) to acquire the emission data. However, crosstalk by scattered photons between the emission and transmission photons unavoidably degrades the acquired data. For three-headed SPECT cameras, a line source can be added at one of the gaps between the three camera heads. In this approach, the opposing camera head with a fan beam collimator is then used to detect the transmitted photons. Because the fan beam collimator focuses down to a line in about 50 cm, it is possible that a portion of the patient's body will not intersect the fan beam and thus be out of the camera's field of view. This can lead to loss of data, termed truncation artifacts, in reconstruction of the attenuation image. Although a number of schemes have been proposed to account for the truncation artifact, none has proved to be clinically robust. Clinical validation has been performed for several but not all of the commercially available systems described. Despite these technical challenges, the application of attenuation correction in multicenter clinical trials, with different hardware and software approaches, has been shown to add to the diagnostic accuracy of stress myocardial perfusion SPECT, predominantly by improving specificity (**Fig. 17-14**). As a result, the American Society of Nuclear Cardiology (ASNC) and the Society of Nuclear Medicine have published a joint statement with the recommendation that the weight of current evidence is in favor of applying attenuation correction in addition to ECG gating with SPECT MPI to optimize diagnostic accuracy.[10] This recommendation, however, presumes that personnel highly knowledgeable about the technique and its stringent quality control apply the attenuation correction methodology.

Combined PET-CT and SPECT-CT Scanners

Scanners that combine PET or SPECT technology with radiographic computed tomography (CT) provide a tool for obtaining complementary anatomic and functional information in a single imaging session. CT angiography provides information on the presence and extent of luminal narrowing of epicardial coronary arteries with high sensitivity and specificity (see Chap. 19), whereas PET and SPECT provide information on the downstream functional consequences of anatomic lesions. Cardiac CT angiography is suited to determine whether an "obstructive" coronary artery stenosis is present, although the ability to accurately determine stenosis severity is limited with current-generation CT angiography

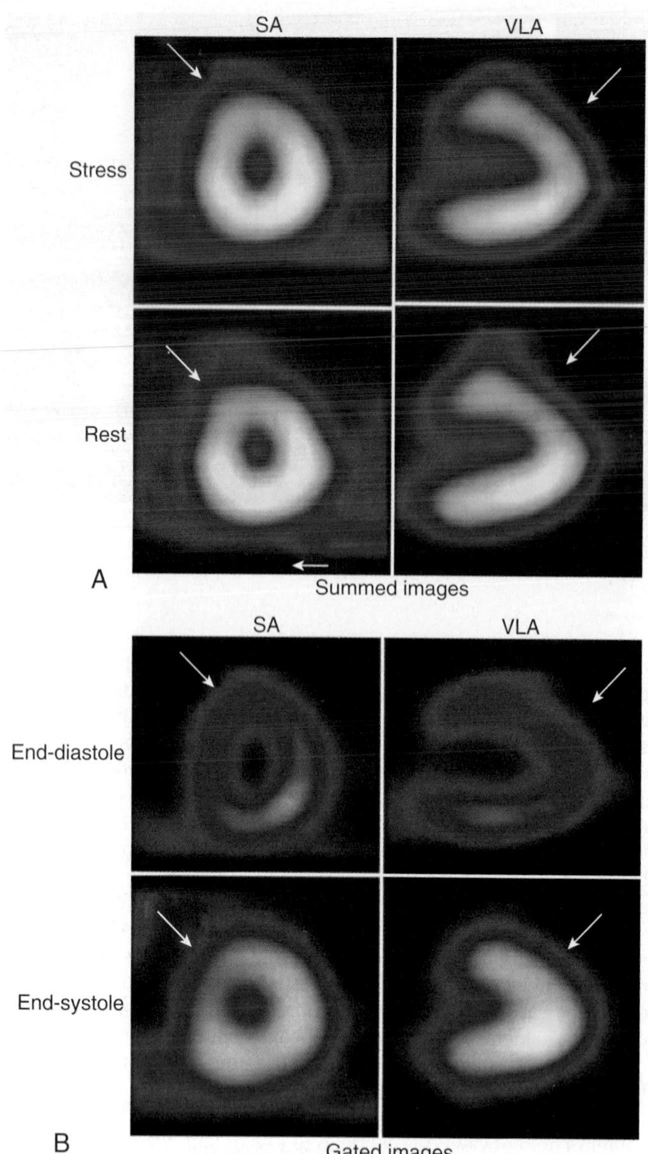

FIGURE 17-12 Differential diagnosis of a mild fixed defect by incorporation of gated functional images. **A,** The summed images demonstrate a mild fixed anterior and anteroseptal defect in the short-axis (SA) and vertical long-axis (VLA) views (arrows). There was a suggestion of breast shadowing on review of the raw cine images (not shown). Thus, this defect may represent either a nontransmural anterior infarct or an artifact consistent with breast attenuation. In this situation, the gated SPECT functional images are helpful in making this distinction. **B,** In the gated images, the same SA and VLA views are shown but frozen in end diastole and end systole. In both views, wall thickening from end diastole to end systole (arrows) appears normal. This is most consistent with an attenuation artifact, as an infarct would be expected to result in abnormal wall thickening.

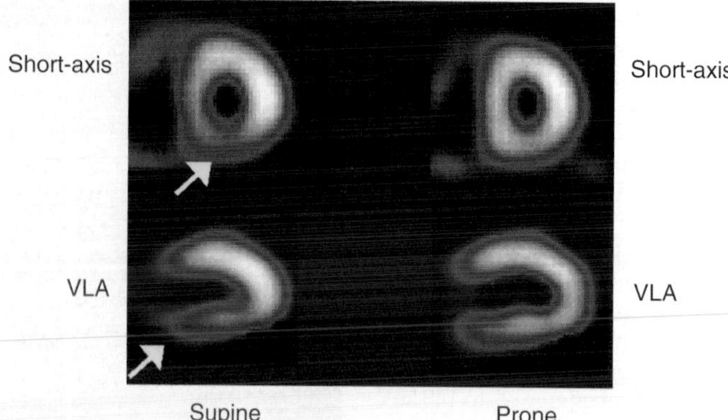

FIGURE 17-13 **Left,** Attenuation of the inferior basal wall (arrows) possibly related to attenuation by overlying left hemidiaphragm. Most commonly, this appears as a tapering of the inferior wall seen best on the vertical long-axis (VLA) image. **Right,** One solution to the problem of inferior wall attenuation is reimaging of the patient in the prone position. In this position, the inferior wall is pulled somewhat away from the diaphragm. In this example, the inferior wall appears more normal in the prone acquisition, suggesting that the apparent reduction in counts in the usual supine acquisition represented attenuation artifact.

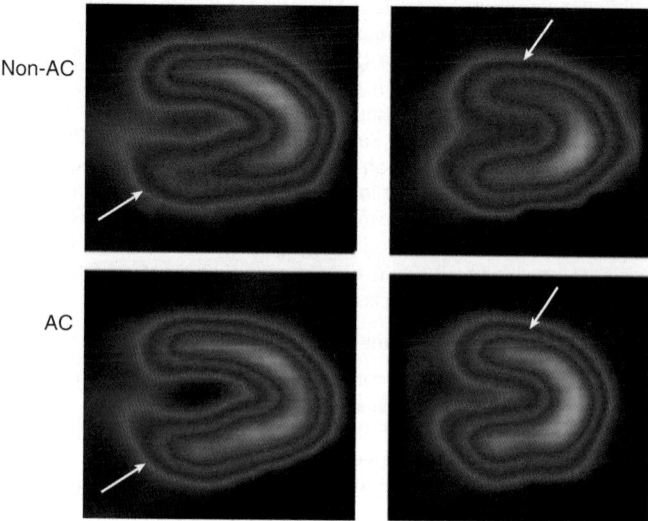

FIGURE 17-14 Impact of attenuation correction (AC). In the non-AC images (top row), there are examples of an inferior defect (left column) and an anterior defect (right column), which may represent diaphragmatic and breast attenuation, respectively, or may represent a true perfusion abnormality. With the application of AC (bottom row), both images become normal, suggesting that the abnormalities in the non-AC images were highly likely to represent artifact. *(Courtesy of Ernest Garcia, PhD.)*

systems. PET and SPECT, on the other hand, are more suited to determine if such a stenosis is physiologically significant regarding limitation of flow reserve. With the advent of hybrid PET-CT or SPECT-CT systems, such complementary information of anatomy and physiology can be realized immediately, at the same imaging session. The combination of these anatomic and functional modalities is particularly relevant in patients who have an intermediate finding on either SPECT-PET or CT angiography. The advantage of the combined scanner is that the corresponding images are spatially aligned and can be acquired during a single imaging session (**Fig. 17-15**).

CT Attenuation Correction for PET and SPECT. A subsidiary benefit of hybrid PET-CT and SPECT-CT imaging systems is in the potential to use the CT image to compute the attenuation map for the MPI data. This approach has allowed the replacement of germanium-68 or cesium-137 transmission scans with faster CT scans, reducing the overall duration of the PET procedure. One potential problem of using fast CT scans for attenuation correction, however, is the motion of the organs during respiration. The CT scanner "freezes" the heart, lungs, and liver at one point in the respiratory cycle, whereas the PET emission data are averaged over many respiratory cycles. Methods using respiratory gating to correct this problem are currently under investigation.

At present, the decision of whether a particular patient is a candidate for PET alone, CT angiography alone, or hybrid PET-CT depends on multiple factors. The age of the patient, underlying irregular heart rhythm, known coronary artery calcification or metallic implants, renal insufficiency, lung disease, or allergy to contrast medium will exclude a significant percentage of patients from being candidates for CT angiography. Given that PET can be performed in the majority of these patients, and the fact that revascularization improves survival over medical therapy only in patients with a moderate to severe degree of inducible ischemia, most patients will not require simultaneous assessment of coronary artery anatomy and myocardial perfusion with hybrid PET-CT. The incremental radiation dose from performing two diagnostic studies should also be taken into consideration.

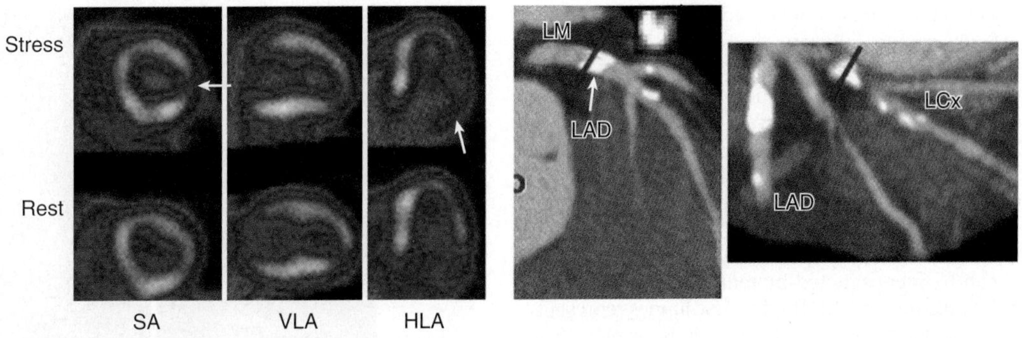

FIGURE 17-15 Combined PET images of stress and rest perfusion **(left)** and cardiac CT angiography and calcium imaging **(right).** The PET images demonstrate a lateral wall reversible defect consistent with ischemia (arrows in the short-axis [SA] and horizontal long-axis [HLA] images). However, the CT images demonstrate more extensive calcification and stenosis of the left main (LM), left anterior descending (LAD), and left circumflex (LCx) vessels. The combined information suggests that although the physiologic ischemia predominantly involves the lateral wall–LCx territory, more extensive CAD is present. VLA = vertical long axis.

Patients with low-risk stress ECG or nuclear myocardial perfusion scans show no survival advantage from revascularization over medical therapy, regardless of the angiographic extent of coronary artery stenosis (see Chap. 57). On the other hand, among younger patients with strong family history or multiple risk factors for CAD, CT angiography may not only exclude significant coronary artery luminal narrowing but also detect early atherosclerosis by quantifying the extent of calcified plaques (see Chap. 19). The latter may have important implications for aggressive risk factor modification and medical therapy. As such, hybrid PET-CT should be limited to only a small subset of patients, in whom the knowledge of both coronary anatomy and physiology would be anticipated to have an impact on clinical management (e.g., anomalous coronary anatomy or myocardial bridging and chest pain).

All other applications, such as detection of endothelial dysfunction or microvascular disease and identification of soft plaques, remain experimental at this time with limited clinical data to support widespread clinical application. In the future, with the potential development of new radiotracers that target coronary artery plaque, hybrid PET-CT images that incorporate plaque anatomy with molecular imaging may provide valuable insights into differentiation of "vulnerable" from "nonvulnerable" plaque, which may be used to portend and potentially to prevent acute MIs.

GATED SPECT DISPLAY, INTERPRETATION, AND QUANTITATION. An important advance in the use and application of SPECT MPI has been the incorporation of ECG-gated SPECT perfusion imaging for simultaneous assessment of LV function and perfusion. Before the use of gated SPECT, comprehensive information on both perfusion and function required separate testing modalities, such as SPECT MPI and separate radionuclide ventriculography (RVG) or echocardiography.

Electrocardiographically Gated Radionuclide Techniques to Assess the Physiology of Ventricular Function

To assess parameters of cardiac function with echocardiography, LV endocardial borders are drawn over several beats to derive parameters such as EF. With contrast left ventriculography, endocardial borders are drawn for either one beat or an average of several beats to calculate EF. In contrast, the commonly used radionuclide techniques to assess ventricular function create one cardiac cycle for analysis that represents an average of several hundred beats acquired during a period of 8 to 15 minutes, by use of a technique known as ECG gating (**Fig. 17-16**).

During an ECG-gated image acquisition, the patient's electrocardiogram is monitored simultaneously with the image. As the peak of an R wave is detected, the "gate" opens and a set number of milliseconds of imaging information is stored in a "frame." For a typical gated SPECT acquisition, each R-R interval is divided into eight frames. For example, if the patient's resting heart rate is 60 beats/min (1000 milliseconds per beat), an eight-frame acquisition across the cardiac cycle comprises 125 milliseconds per frame. After the first 125

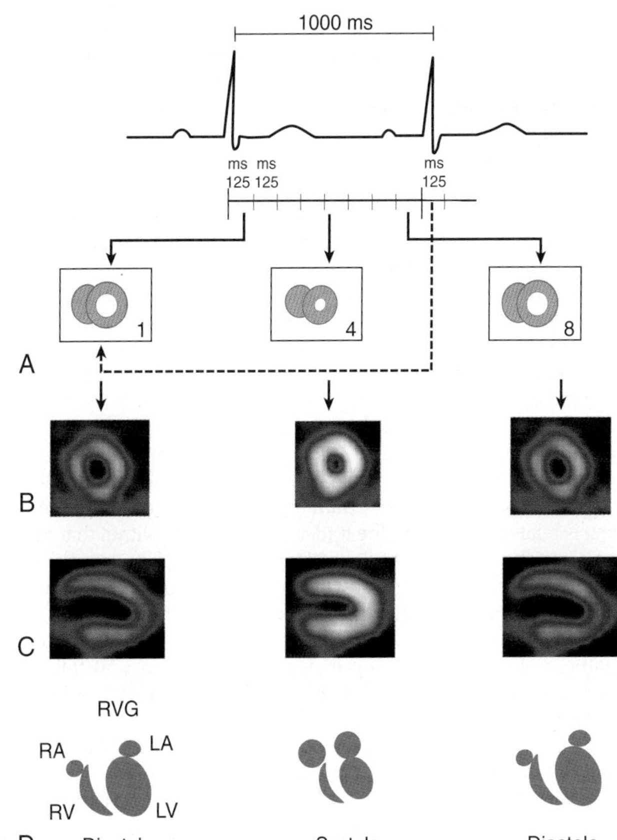

FIGURE 17-16 Basis for the technique of ECG gating. **A,** The scintigraphic acquisition data are collected in conjunction with the electrocardiogram. The R-R interval is divided into a prespecified number of frames (in this example eight frames). At a heart rate of 60 beats/min (1000 msec/beat), each of the eight frames would comprise 125 milliseconds. For the first 125 milliseconds after the peak of the initial R wave, all imaging data are recorded in frame 1; the second 125 milliseconds are recorded in frame 2 and so on until the peak of the next R wave is detected, and this is repeated for each beat in the acquisition. Frame 1 thus represents the end-diastolic events, and one of the frames in the middle of the acquisition (frame 4 in this example) represents end-systolic events. **B,** Examples of gated SPECT perfusion imaging. Short-axis images are seen at end diastole and at end systole. **C,** Similar timing with images displayed from the vertical long-axis orientation. Visually, wall thickening and brightening are seen across the course of systole. These events represent regional wall thickening and changes in global function across the cardiac cycle. **D,** ECG-gated equilibrium radionuclide ventriculographic (RVG) schematic images are shown at diastole and at end systole. LA = left atrium; LV = left ventricle; RA = right atrium; RV = right ventricle. *(Modified from Germano G, Berman DS: Acquisition and processing for gated SPECT: Technical aspects. In Germano G, Berman DS [eds]: Clinical gated cardiac SPECT. Armonk, NY, Futura, 1999, pp 93-114.)*

milliseconds of imaging data have been recorded in frame 1, the gate closes and then instantly reopens, allowing the second 125 milliseconds of information to be recorded in frame 2 (Fig. 17-16A). This sequence continues through the prespecified number of frames throughout the cardiac cycle. When the R wave of the next beat is detected by the ECG-gated system, the sequence is repeated for each beat that occurs throughout the image acquisition.

The number of counts recorded during any individual cardiac cycle is insufficient to create an interpretable image. When several hundred beats have been recorded, an average cardiac cycle representing all the recorded beats can be reconstructed by redisplaying the frames sequentially in a cine or movie format.[11] The first few frames represent systolic events, and the latter frames represent diastolic events (Fig. 17-16A).

High-quality ECG-gated images require that included cardiac cycles have reasonably homogeneous beat lengths. This is usually accomplished by beat-length windowing, whereby the computer acquisition system is programmed to accept beats into the acquisition of only certain cycle lengths. Typically, cycles with the beat length represented by the average heart rate of the patient (1000 milliseconds in the preceding example), along with cycles fluctuating up to 10% to 15% around the average beat length, are allowed into the acquisition. Cardiac cycles with cycle lengths above or below that limit are rejected. For example, the short cardiac cycle from the R wave of a normal beat to the R wave of a premature ventricular contraction (PVC) would not be allowed into the acquisition, nor would the long cycle representing the post-PVC pause. This makes physiologic sense; the short pre-PVC beat and the more prolonged post-PVC beat have distinctly different systolic and diastolic characteristics than the beats during normal sinus rhythm.

ECG-GATED SPECT IMAGING. The clinical technique most commonly used to assess ventricular function is ECG-gated SPECT imaging.[2] Normal regional systolic function is depicted as brightening of the wall during systole (Fig. 17-16B). The wall appears to thicken, and there is apparent endocardial excursion. Assessment of regional LV function by gated SPECT imaging is based on an effect known in imaging physics as the partial volume effect, sometimes referred to as the recovery coefficient effect. When objects being imaged fall below a certain thickness threshold, count (or photon) recovery from the object is related not only to the tracer concentration within that object but also to the thickness of the object.[11] For SPECT imaging, usually all myocardial wall thicknesses fall below that threshold. Although tracer concentration within the myocardium is constant during a gated SPECT image acquisition, the recovery of counts (and thus the brightness of the object being imaged) is related to wall thickness. Hence, during systolic wall thickening, it appears that the LV wall becomes brighter and thicker, even though the isotope concentration per gram of myocardial tissue is actually unchanged. This principle forms the basis for gated SPECT imaging.

Regional myocardial function is usually assessed visually, in a manner similar to the analysis performed in echocardiography. Regions that brighten normally have normal regional systolic performance, and those with diminished but apparent brightening are labeled hypokinetic. Regions with slight brightening are interpreted as severely hypokinetic, and regions with no apparent brightening as akinetic (**Fig. 17-17**). Regional function can also be analyzed by quantitative techniques and displayed in a polar map format.

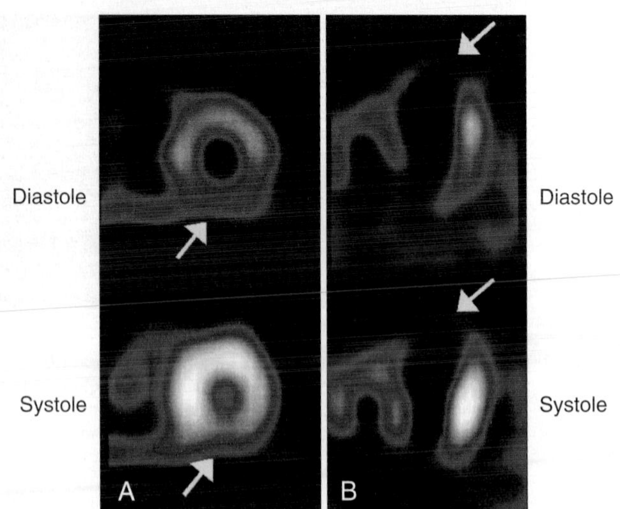

FIGURE 17-17 Examples of regional dysfunction detected by ECG-gated SPECT perfusion imaging. **A,** The severely hypokinetic inferior region appears to brighten less (arrows) than the other regions from diastole to systole. The lateral wall also brightens less than the normal septum and thus would be interpreted as hypokinetic. **B,** The akinetic apex in the horizontal long axis (arrows) appears to have no change from diastole to systole, in contrast to the normally thickening (brightening) lateral wall.

Quantitative Analysis of Global Left Ventricular Function by Gated SPECT Imaging

All contemporary camera-computer systems have software capable of quantitative analysis of global LV function. These computer-based methodologies are fully automated and thus highly reproducible. The most common method involves automated interrogation of the apparent epicardial and endocardial borders of all of the tomograms in all three orthogonal planes (**Fig. 17-18A**). These multiple two-dimensional contours are then reconstructed to create a surface-rendered three-dimensional display representing global LV function across a typical cardiac cycle (Fig. 17-18B) that can be viewed from any direction by simple maneuvering of the computer display screen or cursor.[11] The three-dimensional display is accompanied by automated calculation of EF and LV volumes.

EF measurements from automated analysis of ECG-gated SPECT MPI have been extensively validated against other quantitative techniques assessing LV function, such as equilibrium RVG, angiographic contrast left ventriculography, and cardiac magnetic resonance (CMR) imaging (see Chaps. 18 and 20).[11] Across a wide range of LV function, and even in the setting of severe perfusion defects, ECG-gated SPECT imaging provides robust, reproducible estimates of LVEF.

The incorporation of ECG-gated SPECT imaging into a SPECT acquisition is now routine in MPI and is recommended as standard by contemporary guidelines.[2] As discussed subsequently, the addition of LV function data to the perfusion information provides incremental and independent prognostic information in addition to its practical importance in management decisions. Gated SPECT imaging has also been an important advance in helping to differentiate attenuation artifacts from infarct, as regions with persistent low counts that show normal motion and thickening represent soft tissue artifacts rather than scar (see Fig. 17-12). Thus, gated SPECT has improved the specificity of perfusion imaging for ruling out of CAD, particularly in women.[6]

Planar Myocardial Perfusion Imaging

Before the widespread application of tomographic (SPECT) perfusion imaging techniques, planar imaging was the standard acquisition and display methodology. In planar imaging, three separate two-dimensional images are obtained with the gamma camera after radiotracer injection and uptake into the myocardium.[2] The three standard views are an anterior, a left anterior oblique, and a more lateral view (see Fig. 17-e1 on website).

With planar imaging, the imaging views are standard and prespecified, and the reader must account for the different orientations of the heart in assigning regional abnormalities. In contrast, because the tomographic SPECT slices are constructed along orthogonal planes that are perpendicular and parallel to an assigned long axis, SPECT images are oriented in a uniform manner for display and interpretation without influence by the individual patient's cardiac orientation.

An advantage of planar imaging over SPECT imaging is its simplicity. Each of the three views can be acquired during 5 to 8 minutes with patients lying on a table with their arms by their side. Planar imaging is less affected by patient motion than is SPECT imaging.

With planar imaging, there is no extensive image processing as with SPECT, and thus there are fewer sources of potential error and artifact. However, given the two-dimensional nature of planar imaging, in each of the standard views there is substantial overlap of myocardial regions and less ability to differentiate smaller and particularly milder perfusion abnormalities. The more standard orientation of SPECT imaging lends itself to easier understanding of the localization of perfusion abnormalities.

The original data on the sensitivity and specificity of perfusion imaging for CAD, as well as the prognostic value of perfusion imaging, were developed with planar imaging and later revalidated with SPECT imaging. In contemporary practice, planar imaging may be used for patients who do not tolerate the position that must be maintained during a SPECT acquisition, those who have difficulty coping with the larger SPECT camera being so close to the body, or those with large body habitus that surpasses the weight and size limits of SPECT systems.[6]

Quantitative analytical techniques such as the circumferential profile technique were originally developed by use of planar perfusion imaging. A substantial literature has documented that when quantitative analysis is applied to planar perfusion imaging, there is an improvement in the sensitivity to detect multivessel CAD.

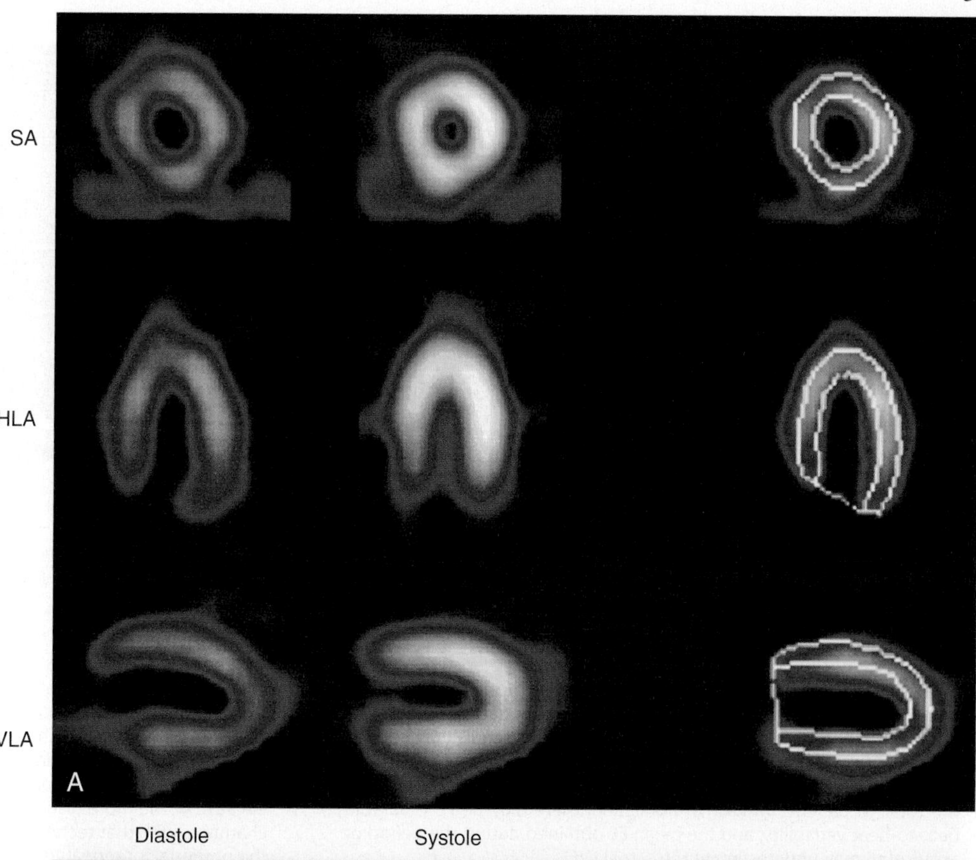

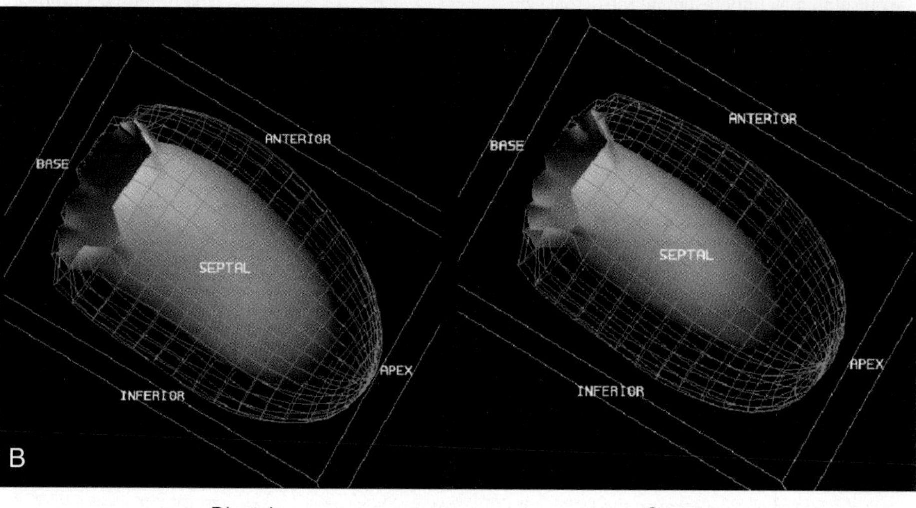

FIGURE 17-18 A, ECG-gated SPECT perfusion images in short axis (SA), vertical long axis (VLA), and horizontal long axis (HLA), shown frozen at diastole (left column) and at end systole (middle column). Endocardial and epicardial borders are shown on the diastolic frames as automatically assigned by the software analysis program (right column). **B,** From the contours that are created from all of the two-dimensional tomograms, a three-dimensionally surface-rendered image of the left ventricle can be created and displayed in multiple orientations, here frozen at end diastole (left) and end systole (right). The green "mesh" represents the epicardium, and the gray surface represents the endocardium. Ejection fraction is quantitated from the volume change. During image interpretation, gated SPECT images are displayed in the cine format as an endless loop movie rather than as the still frames depicted here.

Radionuclide Ventriculography or Angiography

RVG, also know as radionuclide angiography or blood pool imaging, may be performed by first-pass or by equilibrium gated techniques.[12] The equilibrium technique is often referred to as multiple gated acquisition (MUGA) scanning. Although the two techniques use distinct tracers and data recording, they provide similar results for global EF and chamber volumes. Both techniques provide a highly reproducible means to quantify global LV and right ventricular (RV) EF.

Equilibrium Radionuclide Angiography or Ventriculography (Gated Blood Pool Imaging). In equilibrium RVG studies, data are recorded in a computer system synchronized with the R wave of the patient's electrocardiogram, similar to ECG-gated SPECT (see Fig. 17-16). For labeling of the blood pool, ^{99m}Tc is bound to red blood cells or albumin. Image contrast is usually better with ^{99m}Tc-labeled red blood cells, but ^{99m}Tc-labeled albumin is preferable in patients in whom red blood cell labeling may be difficult. Labeling of red blood cells with ^{99m}Tc pertechnetate requires a reducing agent, stannous pyrophosphate, which is administered 15 to 30 minutes before pertechnetate injection.

Image Acquisition. Although relatively few counts are recorded during a single ECG-gated cardiac cycle, the summation of counts from 800 to 1000 cardiac cycles produces an average cardiac cycle with high resolution. Images of the heart are usually acquired in three standard projections: anterior, "best septal" left anterior oblique (best separation of the left and right ventricles), and left lateral (or left posterior oblique). The minimum framing rate for a resting RVG study is 16 frames/cycle (about 50 msec/frame).[12] For quantitative assessment of diastolic indices and regional EF, the framing rate should be increased to 32 frames/cycle (about 25 msec/frame). For adequate counting statistics, images are

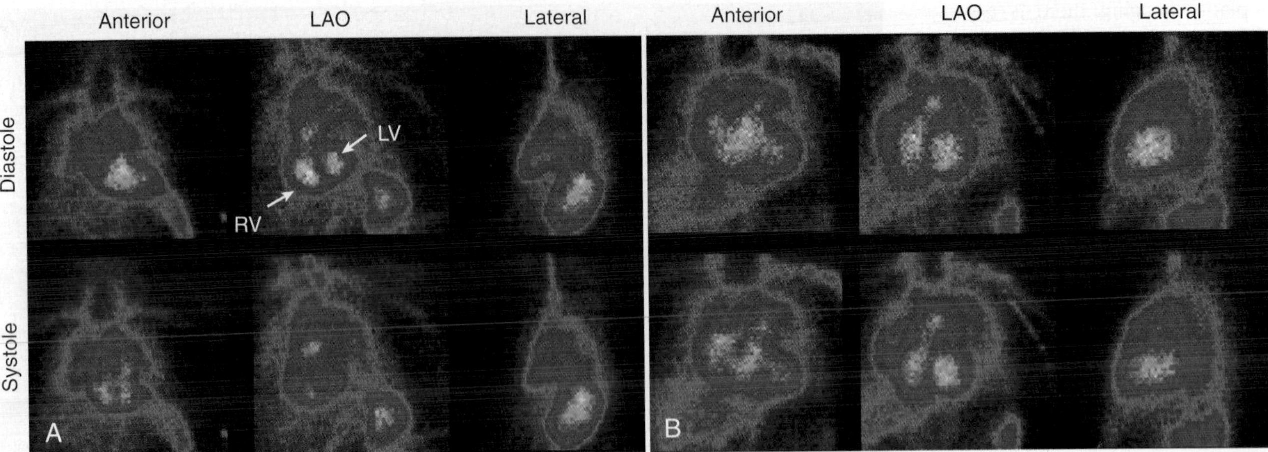

FIGURE 17-19 Equilibrium radionuclide ventriculography. The isotope (^{99m}Tc) is labeled to red blood cells, and hence the images represent the blood "pools" in the left ventricle (LV), the right ventricle (RV), the other cardiac chambers, and the great vessels as well as the spleen. Typically, three views are obtained, as shown. **A,** Normal LV function, with end-diastolic images in the top row and end-systolic images in the bottom row. LV and RV volumes diminish from diastole to systole. **B,** Images obtained in a patient with LV dysfunction. There is significant LV and RV dilation at both end diastole (top) and end systole (bottom) and severely diminished LV systolic function (i.e., much less volume change from end diastole to end systole compared with the study in **A**). LAO = left anterior oblique projection.

acquired for a preset count of at least 250,000 per frame or count density of 300 counts per pixel, which corresponds to an acquisition time of 5 to 10 minutes per projection. For exercise studies, adequate counts can be obtained in the best septal view with a 2-minute acquisition using a high-sensitivity collimator. Arrhythmias such as multiple PVCs can adversely affect the study if these beats account for more than 10% of the total. In patients with atrial fibrillation, there may be considerable beat-to-beat variability, and the mean EF obtained during the period of acquisition may underestimate the actual LVEF.[12]

Image Display and Analysis. Qualitative inspection of equilibrium studies as an endless cinematic loop of the cardiac cycle (see Fig. 17-16D) allows assessment of (1) size of heart chambers and great vessels; (2) regional wall motion; (3) global function (qualitative assessment) (**Fig. 17-19A,B**); (4) ventricular wall thickness, pericardial effusion, pericardial fat pad, or paracardiac mass; and (5) extracardiac uptake (such as splenomegaly). Quantification of systolic and diastolic indices and volumes is derived from the ventricular time-activity curve,[12] which is analogous to the angiographic time-volume curve (see Fig. 17-e2 on website). In addition to the time-activity curve, functional images, such as amplitude and phase images, can be produced that have been useful in characterizing regional asynergy and asynchrony.

First-Pass Radionuclide Angiography or Ventriculography. In first-pass RVG studies, the bolus of radioactivity passes initially through the right chambers of the heart, then through the lungs, and finally through the left-sided chambers of the heart. Radiopharmaceuticals used for this purpose must produce adequate counts in a short time at an acceptably low radiation dose to the patient.[12] Although both ^{99m}Tc-diethylenetriaminepentaacetic acid (DTPA) and ^{99m}Tc pertechnetate have short intravascular residence time, ^{99m}Tc-DTPA is the recommended radionuclide of choice because the DTPA salt enhances renal excretion.

Image Acquisition. Images are acquired very rapidly as the tracer passes through the heart chambers. Separation of the right and left ventricles is achieved because of the temporal separation of the bolus. Image quality is related to the injection technique, which should be rapid (during 2 to 3 seconds) to achieve an uninterrupted bolus (see Fig. 17-e3 on website). Images are acquired in the supine position after the rapid injection of 25 mCi of tracer through an 18-gauge or larger intravenous catheter placed in the medial antecubital or external jugular vein. The shallow (20- to 30-degree) right anterior oblique projection is used to optimize separation of the atria and great vessels from the ventricles and to view the ventricles parallel to their long axes. Although the right anterior oblique view maximizes overlap of the right and left ventricles, this is not a problem in most patients because the timing of tracer appearance reliably identifies each chamber sequentially. A 1-mCi tracer dose may be used to ensure proper positioning so that the right and left ventricles are in the field of view.

Image Analysis. To identify the RV and LV phases, regions of interest are drawn around the right and left ventricles at end diastole.[12] Time-activity curves are generated, and cycles around and including the peak time-activity curve are used to calculate EFs. In general, two to five cardiac cycles are summed for the RV phase, and five to seven cycles are summed for the LV phase. From these data, quantitative analysis of LVEF and RVEF is performed.

Comparison of Equilibrium and First-Pass Techniques. Advantages of the first-pass technique are the high target-to-background ratio, more distinct temporal separation of the cardiac chambers, and rapidity of imaging. RVEF may be more readily assessed by the first-pass technique because of the more distinct separation of this structure from the other chambers with that technique. Advantages of equilibrium technique are the potential for repeated assessment of cardiac function during rapidly varying physiologic conditions, high count density, and acquisition of images in multiple projections. In contemporary practice, the equilibrium technique is performed far more commonly.[2,6]

Positron Emission Tomography

Because of the quantitative capabilities of PET, measurement of myocardial perfusion and metabolism can be obtained with PET in absolute quantitative terms, a potential advantage compared with SPECT imaging. The radiotracers used in PET are labeled with positron-emitting isotopes that have chemical and physical properties identical to those of naturally occurring elements, such as carbon, oxygen, nitrogen, and fluorine. Incorporation of such elements allows interrogation of physiologically relevant processes in normal and diseased states.[5] Although most positron-emitting radiotracers are cyclotron produced with short half-lives, the development of generator-produced positron-emitting isotopes, such as rubidium-82 (^{82}Rb), makes it feasible for laboratories to perform cardiac PET studies without an on-site cyclotron.

Clinically available cardiac PET radiotracers fall within two broad categories, those that evaluate myocardial perfusion and those that evaluate myocardial metabolism (**Table 17-2**).[6] The perfusion tracers ^{82}Rb and [^{13}N]ammonia and the myocardial metabolic tracer 2-[^{18}F] fluoro-2-deoxyglucose (FDG) have received U.S. FDA approval.

IMAGE ACQUISITION. PET employs camera systems designed to optimize the detection of positron-emitting radioisotopes. The process by which a positron-emitting radionuclide attempts to stabilize over time is termed beta decay, which occurs when the nucleus of an atom emits a positron, a positively charged beta particle (**Fig. 17-20**). After a high-energy positron is emitted from a nucleus, it travels a few millimeters in tissue and ultimately collides with an electron (a negatively charged beta particle). This collision results in complete annihilation of both the positron and the electron, with conversion to energy in the form of electromagnetic radiation composed of two high-energy gamma rays, each with 511-keV energy. The discharged gamma rays travel in perfectly opposite directions (180 degrees from each other). PET detectors can be programmed to register only events with temporal coincidence of photons that strike at directly opposing detectors. The outcome of such selective coincidence detection is an improvement in spatial and temporal resolution of PET compared with SPECT imaging.[13] Unlike the procedure in SPECT, in which an extrinsic collimator is used to limit the direction at which photons enter the detector, the coincidence detection with PET provides "intrinsic" collimation and improves the sensitivity of the camera.

In addition, an important distinction between PET and SPECT is in the ease of labeling primary substrates for energy metabolism and membrane receptor subtypes in the heart, allowing the interrogation of such physiologic pathways in vivo. Moreover, dynamic mode PET scanning permits potential analysis of the change in tracer content in a specific region of interest in the heart with time, allowing potential interrogation of the rate of change of a physiologic process.

IMAGE ANALYSIS. Emission data are displayed as tomograms in the horizontal and vertical long-axis and short-axis views, similar to SPECT display.[13] If the data are acquired in dynamic mode, with appropriate mathematical modeling, myocardial perfusion and metabolic data can be displayed in absolute terms: in milliliters per gram per minute for blood flow and moles per gram per minute for metabolism.

TABLE 17-2 Properties of Selected Positron Emission Tomography Tracers

TRACER	PRODUCED	HALF-LIFE	COMPOUND
Perfusion			
Oxygen-15	Cyclotron	2.1 minutes	H_2O
Nitrogen-13	Cyclotron	10 minutes	NH_3
Rubidium-82	Generator	76 seconds	RbCl
Metabolism			
Carbon-11	Cyclotron	20.4 minutes	Acetate, palmitate
Fluorine-18	Cyclotron	110 minutes	Deoxyglucose

Modified from Bergmann SR: Positron emission tomography of the heart. *In* Gerson MC (ed): Cardiac Nuclear Medicine. New York, McGraw-Hill, 1997, pp 267-300.

PET PERFUSION TRACERS. PET perfusion tracers can be divided into two types: (1) freely diffusible tracers, which accumulate and wash out from myocardial tissue as a function of blood flow; and (2) nondiffusible tracers, characterized by retention in myocardial tissue as a function of blood flow.[5] The rapid physiologic washout of the freely diffusible tracers, such as [^{15}O]water, makes it possible to repeat studies in rapid sequence. The images of the distribution of such tracers are usually not visually meaningful; mathematical modeling is done to arrive at flow values at each pixel. An advantage of freely diffusible tracers is that they do not depend on a metabolic trapping mechanism that might change as a function of a changing metabolic environment.

The nondiffusible flow tracers are easier to image as the tracer is retained in myocardium for a reasonable length of time. ^{82}Rb and [^{13}N] ammonia fall into this second category of flow tracers, the more microsphere-like flow tracers. ^{82}Rb is a cation, with biologic properties similar to those of potassium and thallium, and uptake across the sarcolemmal membrane reflects active transport by the Na^+,K^+-ATPase pump. In experimental studies, its extraction fraction does not change significantly over a wide range of metabolic conditions. However, the very short half-life of 75 seconds for ^{82}Rb means that any trapped ^{82}Rb quickly disappears from the myocardium by physical decay. Despite its short half-life, ^{82}Rb is easily obtained as it is generator produced, and it can be used clinically without the need for an on-site cyclotron.

[^{13}N]Ammonia is an extractable perfusion tracer, with a physical half-life of 10 minutes. Its transport across cell membranes may occur by passive diffusion or by the active Na-K transport mechanism. Retention of [^{13}N]ammonia in the myocyte involves metabolic trapping. As with ^{82}Rb, myocardial uptake of ammonia reflects absolute blood flows up to 2 to 3 mL/g/min and plateaus at more hyperemic flows. The use of this tracer to assess myocardial blood flow has been extensively validated in both experimental and clinical studies.[13]

PET Perfusion Tracers: Research Directions

Recently, ^{18}F-labeled fluorobenzyl triphenyl phosphonium, originally developed for measurement of the mitochondrial membrane

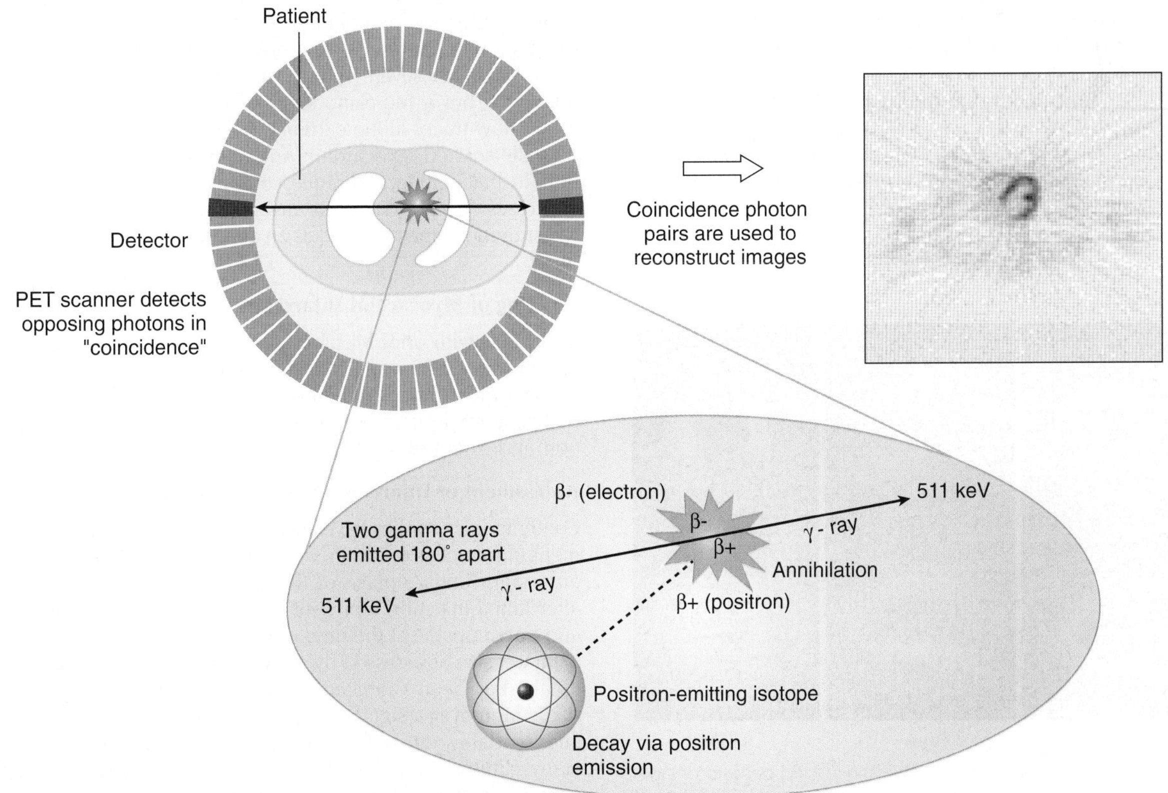

FIGURE 17-20 Schematic of positron and electron beta particle emission, with detection by a coincidence camera, as the basis of PET imaging.

potential, was introduced for MPI with PET.[14] The currently available PET myocardial perfusion tracers, ^{82}Rb chloride and [^{13}N]ammonia, have short physical half-lives and require either an on-site cyclotron or generator, thereby limiting their widespread clinical application. The longer half-life of ^{18}F (110 minutes) allows the possibility of distribution as a single-dose unit on a daily basis, which may facilitate the clinical application of myocardial perfusion PET imaging. Moreover, the longer half-life of ^{18}F would allow assessment of perfusion during treadmill exercise, rather than with vasodilator stress alone, as is currently the case with ^{82}Rb PET.

CLINICAL APPLICATION OF PET PERFUSION IMAGING. ^{82}Rb and [^{13}N]ammonia are the two PET tracers that have received U.S. FDA approval for clinical application to assess myocardial perfusion. Advantages of PET perfusion imaging over SPECT include higher spatial resolution, improved attenuation and scatter correction, and potential for quantifying regional blood flow. As a result, a number of clinical studies with either ^{82}Rb or [^{13}N]ammonia PET have shown an improvement in either the sensitivity or specificity (as high as 95%) for detection of CAD compared with SPECT (**Fig. 17-21**). However, the widespread use of PET myocardial perfusion studies in the clinical setting has been hampered by the requirement of an on-site cyclotron for [^{13}N]ammonia and the high cost of monthly generator replacement for ^{82}Rb. Moreover, the relatively short half-lives of both ^{82}Rb and [^{13}N]ammonia limit the utility of PET perfusion studies to patients undergoing pharmacologic stress only. As the exercise component of MPI studies has independent prognostic and diagnostic value, this represents an important limitation. On the other hand, the potential for quantifying myocardial blood flow and blood flow reserve in absolute terms is highly desirable, with potential clinical applications. For example, patients with multivessel CAD may have uniform decrease in flow reserve, and the relative perfusion data from SPECT may fail to detect this "balanced" ischemia. At the other extreme, detection of mild abnormalities in myocardial blood flow reserve with PET provides the potential for early identification of CAD characterized by endothelial dysfunction in asymptomatic patients with elevated cholesterol, smoking, hypertension, and insulin resistance. Studies have also shown that abnormal blood flow reserve by PET may be predictive of future cardiovascular outcome among patients with cardiomyopathies in the absence of CAD,[15] such as patients with idiopathic dilated cardiomyopathy[16] and hypertrophic cardiomyopathy[17] (see Chaps. 68 and 69).

RADIATION EXPOSURE ISSUES

Clinical decision making for the use of low-level ionizing radiation to obtain diagnostic nuclear cardiac studies must adhere to appropriate use criteria and encompass the broad range of the risk-benefit ratio, with the guiding principle to minimize exposure while obtaining the necessary high-quality diagnostic information. The prediction of risk of subsequent malignant transformation for an individual undergoing a medical diagnostic test, or procedure, employing ionizing radiation is a complex exercise with many uncertainties. Concerns about the late carcinogenic effects of exposure to low levels (i.e., <100 mSv) of ionizing radiation stem from extrapolation of exposure-outcome data in survivors of atomic bomb explosions. However, there is uncertainty about the dose-response relationship in the lower range of exposure, making assessment of the incremental risk to subjects complex, as well as of tissue-specific reparative responses that may also be manifested at lower levels of exposure.[18] Nonetheless, exposure of the patient to ionizing radiation should be at the minimum dose consistent with obtaining a diagnostic examination. Each patient procedure is unique, and the methodology to achieve minimum exposure while maintaining diagnostic accuracy needs to be viewed in this light to ensure optimal patient care.

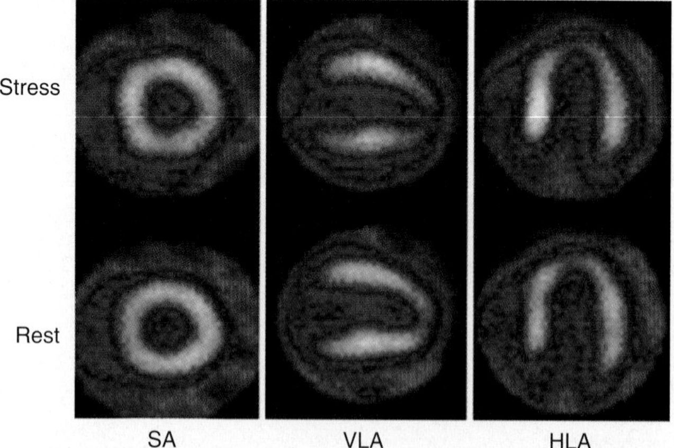

FIGURE 17-21 Example of high-quality stress and rest PET perfusion images, using ^{82}Rb as the perfusion tracer in the short axis (SA), vertical long axis (VLA), and horizontal long axis (HLA).

Assessment of the Physiology and Pathophysiology of Myocardial Blood Flow, Myocardial Metabolism, and Ventricular Function

Assessment of Myocardial Blood Flow by Radionuclide Imaging

RESTING MYOCARDIAL BLOOD FLOW. Myocardial blood flow at rest is tightly regulated to provide nutritive perfusion to viable, contractile myocytes (see Chap. 52). Although SPECT tracers to image myocardial blood flow are commonly referred to as perfusion tracers, they require viable myocyte cell membranes for uptake and retention.[5] Thus, the uptake and retention of these tracers do reflect regional flow differences, but myocyte cell membrane integrity is also a prerequisite. Although visualization of myocardial regions suggests the presence of working, viable cell membranes, lack of visualization of myocardium does not necessarily indicate the absence of viable cells. Decreased regional myocardial tracer uptake at rest could reflect either lack of cell membrane integrity in an area of infarcted myocardium or reduced blood flow secondary to hibernating but viable myocardium. A severe reduction in tracer activity usually signifies infarction, but a more moderate reduction in regional activity of a blood flow tracer alone cannot always differentiate hibernating from partially scarred myocardium in patients with ischemic LV dysfunction. In that setting, techniques that assess intact cellular metabolic processes (e.g., FDG) or the myocardial potassium space (e.g., ^{201}Tl redistribution) may be used as an adjunct to resting myocardial blood flow.[5]

Imaging of Myocardial Infarction

In patients with prior MI, blood flow to the infarcted region is usually diminished, often severely, and there are few viable myocytes within the scarred territory.[6] Thus, severely reduced uptake of a radionuclide perfusion tracer in a resting study is a good marker of presence, location, and extent of MI (**Fig. 17-22**).

Assessment of Infarct Size

Contemporary studies have used ^{99m}Tc-sestamibi to provide an assessment of infarct size.[19] As there is minimal clearance from the myocardium after initial uptake of this tracer, images acquired even hours after initial injection represent a "snapshot" of blood flow conditions and tracer uptake at the time of injection.

Infarct size as assessed by quantitative analysis of resting sestamibi uptake has been validated against many other measures of infarct size.[19] Moreover, a significant association between SPECT infarct size and mortality during long-term follow-up has been demonstrated. Many clinical trials now use "final infarct size" by sestamibi SPECT imaging as an early post-MI surrogate endpoint to assess new agents to reduce infarct size.

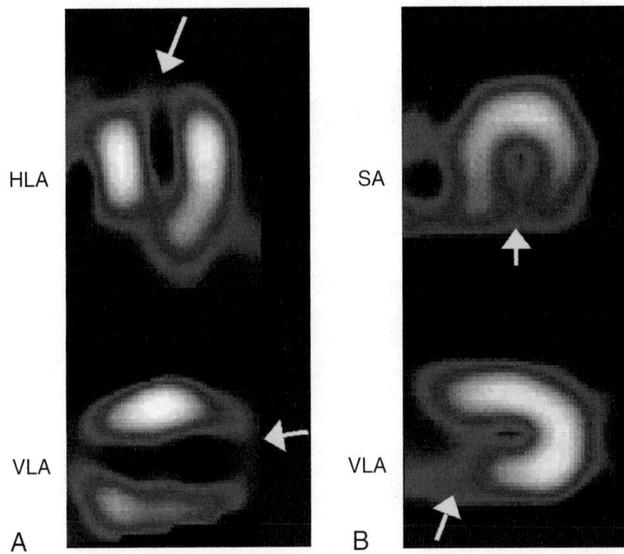

FIGURE 17-22 SPECT perfusion images demonstrating myocardial infarction in different locations. **A,** An apical infarction (arrow) in the horizontal long-axis (HLA) and vertical long-axis (VLA) views. **B,** An inferior infarction in the short-axis (SA) and VLA views. In both studies, the severity of the defect suggests minimal myocyte viability within those territories.

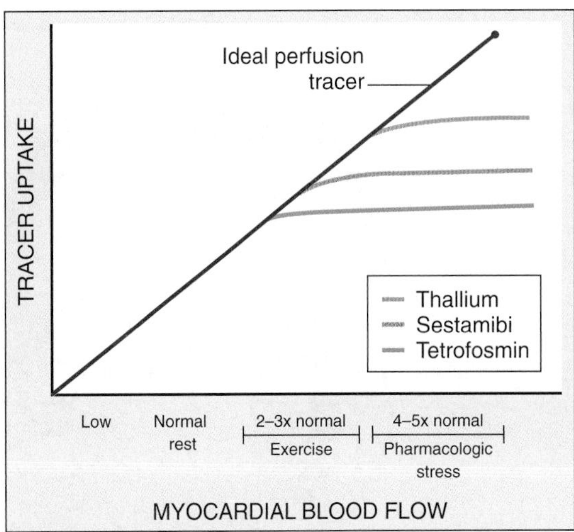

FIGURE 17-23 The relation between myocardial blood flow and perfusion tracer uptake. The ideal perfusion tracer would track myocardial blood flow across the entire range of physiologically relevant flows (red line). However, the available perfusion tracers "roll off" at higher levels of flow. The different tracers reach a plateau at different levels of myocardial blood flow, as demonstrated in this schematic example based on multiple studies in animal models.

When a tracer such as sestamibi is injected during acute infarction in the setting of an occluded infarct-related artery before reperfusion therapy, the resulting defect, even when it is imaged hours later after successful reperfusion, represents the area-at-risk of the occluded artery.[19] A second injection of sestamibi at rest with subsequent imaging can be done at a later time during the post-MI course and represents final infarct size. The change in defect size between the initial image acquired in the acute stage and the later image represents the magnitude of salvaged myocardium from reperfusion. Hence, SPECT imaging at rest in the early postinfarction period can provide important information about final infarct size and infarct zone viability.

ASSESSMENT OF MYOCARDIAL PERFUSION DURING STRESS. Coronary blood flow must respond rapidly to changing metabolic conditions and oxygen demand to meet the nutrient needs of myocytes being called on to contract more quickly and with more force. Oxygen extraction by the myocardium is nearly maximum at rest; thus, any increase in oxygen demand can be met only through increasing coronary blood flow to deliver more oxygen per unit time (see Chap. 52). The major determinants of coronary blood flow include the perfusion pressure at the head of the system (principally aortic diastolic pressure) and the downstream resistance, residing predominantly in the coronary arteriolar bed. Because aortic diastolic pressure during exercise varies little from the resting value, the major mechanism responsible for increasing coronary blood flow during stress involves a reduction in coronary vascular resistance. During exercise stress, coronary blood flow can increase approximately two to three times above resting levels. During pharmacologic stress to minimize coronary arteriolar resistance, with intravenous coronary arteriolar vasodilator agents such as dipyridamole and adenosine (discussed later), coronary blood flow can increase up to four to five times above resting levels. The magnitude of blood flow increase secondary to any stress relative to resting flow values is termed coronary blood flow reserve.[20]

Perfusion Tracers and Coronary Blood Flow Reserve

The ideal perfusion tracer should track myocardial blood flow across the entire physiologically relevant range of blood flow achievable in animal models and in humans (**Fig. 17-23**). It should be extracted rapidly (from the blood into the myocyte), as the hemodynamic conditions during peak stress are not maintained for long periods. The ideal tracer should also be extracted as completely as possible out of the bloodstream, and it should be retained in myocardium for a sufficient period to be imaged. Moreover, perturbations in metabolic conditions, such as ischemia or commonly used cardioactive drugs, should neither influence nor interfere with uptake so that the resulting regional tracer concentrations primarily reflect myocardial perfusion.[5]

Despite its excellent first-pass myocardial extraction (85%), the energy spectrum of thallium is lower (69 to 80 keV) than optimum for current gamma cameras. The 140-keV energy spectrum of ^{99m}Tc perfusion tracers results in less scatter and soft tissue attenuation, with improved spatial resolution compared with thallium.[5] However, the first-pass myocardial extraction of both sestamibi and tetrofosmin is only in the 60% range with nonlinear extraction at high flows. Thus, none of the clinically available SPECT perfusion tracers have all of the properties of an ideal perfusion tracer (see Fig. 17-23). Nonetheless, regional differences in myocardial tracer uptake during exercise or pharmacologic stress have provided important diagnostic as well as prognostic information.[6]

The PET perfusion tracer [^{13}N]ammonia displays an extraction fraction exceeding 90%; ^{82}Rb has a lower extraction fraction and reaches a plateau more rapidly at hyperemic range of flow. In the clinical setting, the evaluation of regional myocardial blood flow and flow reserve with [^{13}N]ammonia and ^{82}Rb has been validated for detection and localization of CAD.[5] As noted previously, most PET studies evaluating coronary flow reserve use pharmacologic rather than exercise stress.

Effect of a Coronary Stenosis on Coronary Blood Flow Reserve (see Chap. 52)

In animal models in which discrete coronary stenoses of varying degrees are induced, resting coronary blood flow is maintained by autoregulatory dilation of the downstream arteriolar resistance vessels until a stenosis between 80% and 90% diameter is reached (**Fig. 17-24**). As stenosis severity increases further, the arteriolar vasodilatory capacity to maintain resting flow is exhausted, at which point resting coronary blood flow diminishes.

In contrast, maximum coronary blood flow reserve begins to decrease when the upstream coronary stenosis reaches 50% diameter (see Fig. 52-13). There are three levels of resistance that influence coronary blood flow: that provided by the large conductance epicardial vessels (R1), the coronary arteriolar resistance (R2), and the resistance in the subendocardium by wall tension from the ventricular chamber

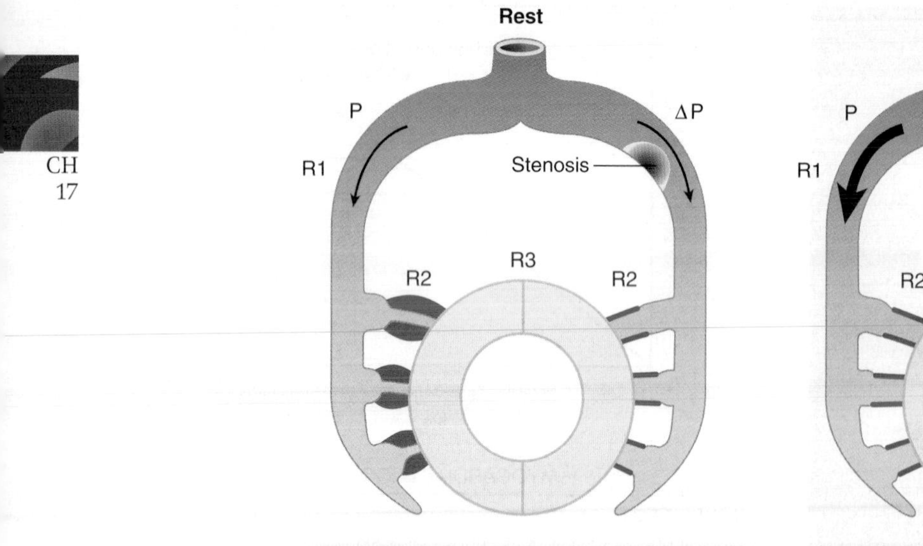

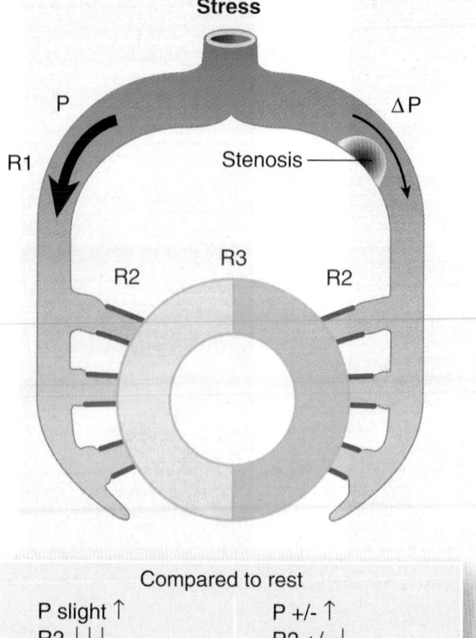

FIGURE 17-24 Effect of coronary resistance on coronary blood flow reserve. **A,** At rest, flow is driven by the pressure head (P) at the proximal end of the system. R1 refers to resistance offered by the large epicardial conductance vessels. R2 represents the coronary arteriolar resistance, which predominantly regulates coronary blood flow. R3 represents the resistance provided by wall tension in the subendocardium. At rest in the normal vessel (left vessel), some vasoconstrictor resistance is present. In the setting of an epicardial coronary stenosis (right vessel), blood flow at rest can be maintained, as coronary resistance can be lowered downstream (R2 decreased) by autoregulatory dilation of the arterioles. Thus, with lower resistance, resting flow may be maintained despite the lower pressure head at the distal end of the stenosis. A perfusion tracer would show homogeneous uptake at rest. **B,** With a demand stress or with the administration of a coronary arteriolar vasodilator such as dipyridamole or adenosine, perfusion increases substantially in the area supplied by the normal epicardial artery (left vessel) as resistance (R2) becomes minimal. However, there is blunted flow reserve in the area supplied by the stenosis (right vessel) because most vasodilator reserve at the R2 level has been used to maintain resting flow. Thus, heterogeneity of flow is established (based on the presence of the upstream stenosis) and can be imaged with a perfusion tracer as a defect in the territory supplied by the stenotic vessel. *(Modified from Follansbee WP: Alternatives to leg exercise in the evaluation of patients with coronary artery disease: Functional and pharmacologic stress modalities. In Gerson MC [ed]: Cardiac Nuclear Medicine. New York, McGraw-Hill, 1997, pp 193-236.)*

(R3) (see Fig. 17-24; see also Fig. 52-5). Under normal conditions, most of the resistance at rest is provided by R2, and most of the increase in coronary flow during heightened demand occurs through reduction of resistance at this level, potentially increasing flow as much as four times as demand increases. Normal epicardial vessels dilate slightly (R1 decreases slightly) in response to increased coronary flow as a consequence of normal endothelial cell function. Depending on the type of exercise that is performed, the R3 component may remain unchanged or may increase, with an increase in chamber radius and wall tension. Achieving maximal flow is predominantly dependent on the vasodilatory capacity of the downstream resistance vessels.[20] With a coronary stenosis, in which some vasodilatory reserve has been used to maintain resting flow, less vasodilatory reserve is available to minimize resistance during stress. Thus, in a vessel with a moderate stenosis, coronary blood flow reserve is blunted and detectable by a perfusion tracer (see Fig. 17-24).

In contrast to animal models, human CAD is more complex. Stenoses may not be discrete, the length and complexity of the stenosis may affect the coronary reserve, and impaired endothelial function plays a role (see Chap. 52).[21] In subjects with preserved endothelial function, the increased coronary flow during stress leads to coronary arterial and arteriolar vasodilation, contributing to maximal coronary flow reserve. Endothelial function is often abnormal with early atherosclerosis, or risk factors for atherosclerosis, contributing to the blunting of coronary flow reserve. The development of collaterals to the distal perfusion bed of a myocardial territory with a severe upstream coronary stenosis also influences blood flow at rest and during stress.[22]

With SPECT imaging, relative regional differences of tracer uptake can be detected and quantified (**Fig. 17-25**), whereas with PET imaging, absolute regional coronary blood flow at rest and during stress (in milliliters per gram per minute) potentially can be quantified.[5,13]

Detection of Stress-Induced Ischemia Versus Infarction with Myocardial Perfusion Imaging

In standard practice, stress and rest myocardial perfusion images are compared to determine the presence, extent, and severity of stress-induced perfusion defects and to determine whether such defects represent regions of myocardial ischemia or infarction.[2,6] Regions with stress-induced perfusion abnormalities, which have normal perfusion at rest, are termed reversible perfusion defects and represent viable regions with blunted coronary blood flow reserve (**Fig. 17-26A**; see Figs. 17-4 through 17-7 and 17-10). Strictly speaking, SPECT MPI demonstrates stress-induced reversible abnormalities in perfusion reserve, although these findings are often referred to as ischemia. Regional myocardial tissue ischemia per se is not being demonstrated, although it is indeed often present, based on a mismatch between oxygen supply and demand. Perfusion abnormalities at stress that are irreversible, or fixed, as seen on resting images (unchanged from stress to rest) most often represent infarction, particularly if the defect is severe (Fig. 17-26B; see Fig. 17-7). When both viable myocardium and scarred myocardium are present, thallium redistribution or technetium 99m tracer reversibility is incomplete, giving the appearance of partial reversibility on the delayed thallium or rest technetium 99m images.

EXERCISE STRESS TO INDUCE CORONARY HYPEREMIA. SPECT MPI is commonly performed with exercise stress to induce coronary hyperemia, particularly suitable for patients with exertional

FIGURE 17-25 Illustration of coronary blood flow reserve abnormalities, the concomitant perfusion tracer concentration differences, and the resulting tomographic images. **Left,** The myocardial blood flow profiles at rest and stress of two myocardial regions are shown, with region S (septum) supplied by a normal epicardial artery and region L (lateral wall) supplied by an artery with a significant epicardial coronary stenosis. Blood flow at stress is diminished in region L compared with S. **Right,** The perfusion tracer uptake profile is demonstrated with myocardial blood flow on the *y*-axis. Tracer uptake is diminished in region L relative to S during stress. In the resulting perfusion images, a relative "defect" of tracer uptake is seen in the lateral wall compared with the septum, whereas both regions demonstrate similar tracer uptake at rest. The lateral wall thus demonstrates a reversible perfusion defect, reflecting the blunted coronary blood flow reserve and indirectly reflecting the presence of the coronary stenosis.

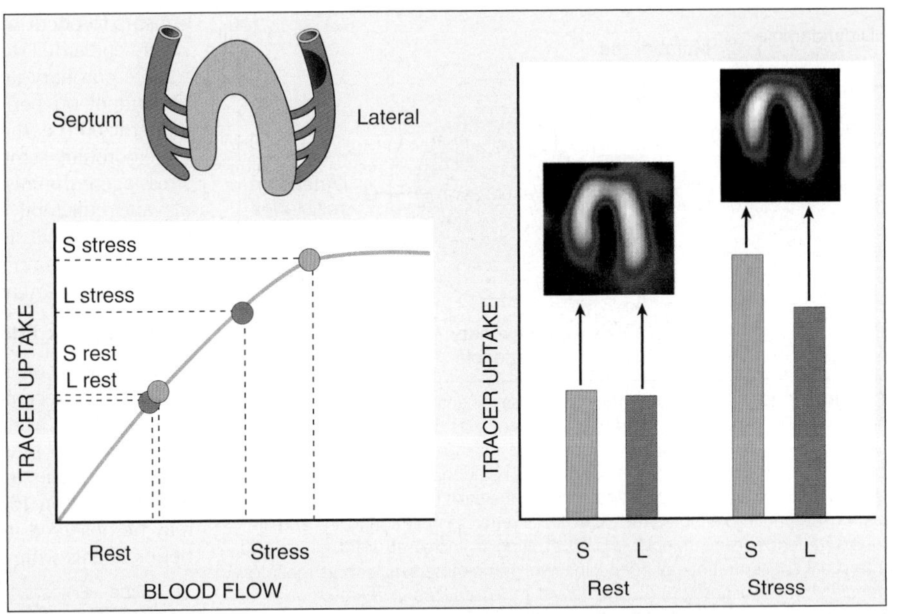

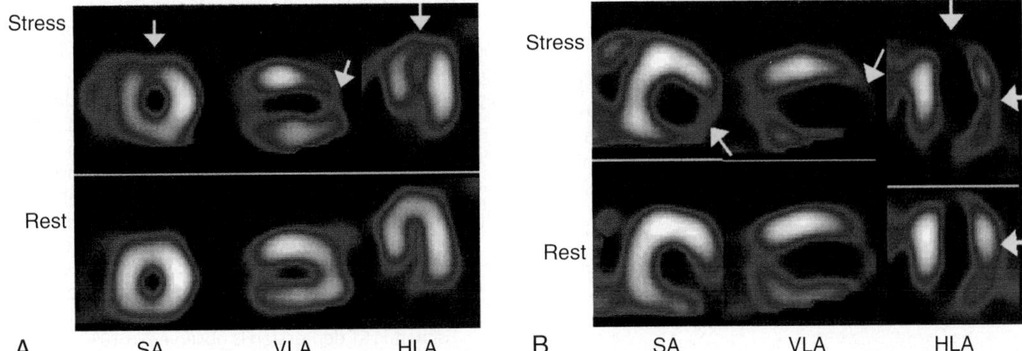

FIGURE 17-26 **A,** Example of SPECT anterior and apical reversible perfusion defects (arrows), representing inducible regional myocardial ischemia in the short axis (SA), vertical long axis (VLA), and horizontal long axis (HLA). **B,** Example of irreversible or fixed defects of the inferolateral wall in the SA and of the apex in the VLA images (arrows), representing predominant myocardial infarction. There is also evidence of a reversible lateral wall defect (arrows) in the HLA image representing lateral wall ischemia.

symptoms, as this provides the opportunity to link the symptoms induced during exercise to the location, extent, and severity of abnormal perfusion patterns.[6] Moreover, performing exercise stress in conjunction with MPI allows the opportunity to incorporate additional information on functional capacity, stress-induced electrocardiographic changes or arrhythmias, and use of heart rate reserve and heart rate recovery in the assessment of CAD probability or prognosis (see Chap. 14).[23]

PHARMACOLOGIC STRESS TO INDUCE CORONARY HYPEREMIA. Exercise stress is the preferred modality to induce coronary hyperemia as it allows a correlation between exertional symptoms and the perfusion pattern and provides information on exercise duration, workload achieved, and presence and extent of ischemic electrocardiographic changes, all of which provide important diagnostic and prognostic information.[6] However, a substantial proportion of patients are incapable of attaining a sufficient level of exercise. Patients with exertional symptoms may not exercise adequately to reproduce these symptoms, and patients may not achieve more than 85% of the maximum predicted heart rate for age (see Chap. 14), considered the optimal level of exertion to achieve coronary hyperemic responses.[6,23] As the population ages and comorbid disease states such as peripheral vascular disease and diabetes increase, the proportion of patients referred for stress testing who are unable to achieve adequate levels of exercise will increase.

In such patients, pharmacologic stress testing can be used to induce coronary hyperemia. The most widely used agents for pharmacologic stress testing can be divided into those that act as coronary arteriolar vasodilators (adenosine, dipyridamole, and regadenoson) and adrenergic agents such as dobutamine.[2,6]

Mechanism of Coronary Arteriolar Vasodilator Pharmacologic Stress

Stimulation of adenosine A_{2a} receptors on the smooth muscle cells leads to enhanced production of adenylate cyclase, increased intracellular cyclic adenosine monophosphate, and other effects that produce vasorelaxation. With maximal arteriolar vasodilation (maximal decrease in coronary resistance), coronary blood flow increases.

Adenosine is a powerful, endogenous molecule that acts as a regulator of blood flow in many organ beds, including the coronary circulation (see Chap. 52). It has many other effects mediated by different receptor subtypes (**Fig. 17-27**). Adenosine A_1 receptors are present in the sinus node and atrioventricular (AV) node and mediate diminished heart rate and AV nodal conduction. Adenosine A_{2b} receptors are present in bronchioles and the peripheral vasculature, and stimulation may result in bronchial constriction and peripheral vasodilation.

Initial studies of adenosine demonstrated that a dose of 140 μg/kg/min induced maximal coronary hyperemia, with no further increase

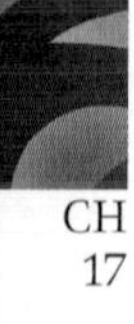

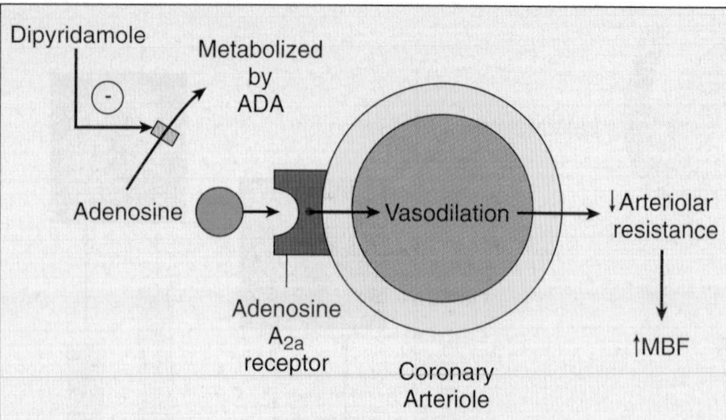

FIGURE 17-27 Schematic of the mechanism of action of dipyridamole and adenosine. Exogenously administered adenosine acts directly on its receptor to result in coronary arteriolar vasodilation and thus an increase in myocardial blood flow (MBF) as resistance is minimized. The adenosine A_{2a} receptor mediates coronary arteriolar vasodilation, which is the basis for pharmacologic stress testing. Dipyridamole blocks the intracellular retransport of adenosine and also inhibits adenosine deaminase (ADA), resulting in increased intracellular and interstitial concentrations of adenosine, which then interacts with its receptor. *(Modified from Follansbee WP: Alternatives to leg exercise in the evaluation of patients with coronary artery disease: Functional and pharmacologic stress modalities. In Gerson MC [ed]: Cardiac Nuclear Medicine. New York, McGraw-Hill, 1997, pp 193-236.)*

in maximum coronary blood flow at higher doses.[24] After the onset of intravenous adenosine infusion, maximum coronary flow occurs at an average of 84 seconds with a range of up to 125 seconds. Dipyridamole blocks the intracellular retransport of adenosine and inhibits adenosine deaminase, responsible for the intracellular breakdown of adenosine.[24] Thus, dipyridamole acts as an indirect coronary arteriolar vasodilator, increasing intracellular and interstitial concentrations of adenosine (see Fig. 17-27). The newer agent regadenoson is similar to adenosine in that it directly interacts with the adenosine A_{2a} receptor.[25]

Heterogeneity of Coronary Hyperemia with Pharmacologic Stress

With the administration of dipyridamole or adenosine, the resistance vessels in the area subtended by a normal epicardial vessel dilate, diminishing coronary resistance and resulting in an increment in coronary blood flow four to five times above normal. Coronary resistance in a bed supplied by a stenotic epicardial vessel is diminished at rest (i.e., coronary vasodilator reserve has been used), and only minor or no further reductions can take place. Thus, myocardial blood flow in that territory does not change or may even decrease slightly because of the peripheral vasodilation and drop in diastolic blood pressure characteristic of pharmacologic stress. The net result of these changes is heterogeneity in myocardial blood flow (increased in the normal territory and relatively unchanged in the territory supplied by the stenotic epicardial vessel). Perfusion tracer administration in this setting demonstrates a defect in the area supplied by the stenotic vessel (see Fig. 17-24).[24]

During exercise stress, the increase in myocardial oxygen demand and limitation of oxygen supply create a supply-demand mismatch often resulting in cellular ischemia. With pharmacologic stress, the perfusion defect may represent merely the heterogeneity in coronary flow reserve. "Demand" may change little during pharmacologic stress; there is often a reduction in blood pressure accompanied by a reflex although modest increase in heart rate, so that double product, reflecting oxygen demand, changes little during the vasodilator "stress." Thus, a supply-demand mismatch may not occur and cellular ischemia may not be present despite vasodilator-induced perfusion defects.[24]

Under certain conditions, true myocardial ischemia may indeed be present, related to development of a coronary steal. This phenomenon appears to occur when the myocardial perfusion bed supplied by a severe epicardial stenosis is also dependent on collateral vessels from remote coronary arteries. Blood flow through coronary collaterals is dependent on perfusion pressure, particularly if the collaterals are jeopardized (i.e., their parent blood vessel is compromised by a moderate coronary stenosis). In this setting, administration of a vasodilator stress agent diminishes the perfusion pressure supplying the collaterals, and collateral flow diminishes. Flow to the bed supplied by a severe epicardial stenosis may then decrease compared with resting flow, and the diminished supply may create supply-demand mismatch and true myocardial ischemia, with ECG ST segment depression.

Hemodynamic Effects of Vasodilator Pharmacologic Stress

Administration of dipyridamole, adenosine, and regadenoson results in adenosine receptor–mediated systemic as well as coronary vasodilation, with an average reduction of 8 to 10 mm Hg in systolic and diastolic blood pressure, often accompanied by a reflex increase in heart rate.[24] The magnitude of the heart rate increase is variable, usually between 10 and 20 beats/min. A blunted heart rate response may be observed in patients who are taking beta blockers or in diabetic patients with underlying autonomic insufficiency.

Side Effects Associated with Vasodilator Pharmacologic Stress. The side effects associated with pharmacologic vasodilator stress are the result of stimulation of the adenosine A_1, A_{2b}, and A_3 receptors and are common.[24-26] After dipyridamole stress, approximately 50% of patients experience some side effect. In a large registry study, more than 80% of patients undergoing adenosine stress experienced untoward side effects, most commonly flushing, chest pain, or shortness of breath.[2,24,26]

As a result of adenosine's effect on the conduction system, AV block may develop during adenosine administration. Approximately 10% of patients manifest first-degree AV block, with 5% developing either second- or third-degree AV block. AV block is more common in patients who are studied while they are taking beta blockers or heart rate–lowering calcium channel blockers. Patients with baseline evidence of second- or third-degree AV block in the absence of a pacemaker should not receive adenosine. However, patients with first-degree AV block or left bundle branch block (LBBB) appear to tolerate adenosine infusion well, without an exacerbation of conduction abnormalities.[2,6]

Ischemic ST depression is observed in 10% to 15% of patients undergoing pharmacologic vasodilator stress, probably representing the physiologic consequence of induction of a coronary steal and regional myocardial ischemia. Such patients often have extensive and severe perfusion defects on imaging and more often have collateralized multivessel disease on angiography.

Chest pain, even typical angina pectoris, develops commonly during pharmacologic vasodilator stress testing. Although it may reflect regional myocardial ischemia based on a coronary steal, chest pain may also occur in patients with no ischemic electrocardiographic changes and with normal perfusion studies because of involvement of adenosine A_1 receptors in the nociceptive pathway influencing the sensation of chest pain.[24,26] Thus, chest pain by itself is a nonspecific finding during vasodilator pharmacologic stress.

In early reports of dipyridamole testing, infrequent but severe episodes of bronchospasm occurred, possibly related to a nonspecific adenosine receptor–mediated mechanism. Thus, patients with a significant history of reactive airways disease should not undergo vasodilator stress testing.[2,6] However, patients with obstructive lung disease without a reactive airways component generally tolerate the procedure well.

New vasodilator pharmacologic stress agents have been under development that are more specific agonists at the adenosine A_{2a} receptor. Early studies suggested that the results of imaging are similar to the effects of adenosine, although side effects are fewer and less severe, consistent with greater A_{2a} receptor specificity.[25,26] One of these agents, regadenoson, is approved by the U.S. FDA for use in pharmacologic stress testing for MPI. Pivotal trials suggested imaging performance similar to that of adenosine. Some but not all side effects are slightly diminished compared with adenosine, but the overall side effect profile does not appear to be very clearly different from that of adenosine. It is administered as a bolus, however, which is more convenient than with the other vasodilator stress agents in use.[25]

Reversal of the Effects of Vasodilator Pharmacologic Stress. Methylxanthine compounds such as theophylline and caffeine act as competitive antagonists of adenosine at the receptor level, and infusion of intravenous aminophylline antagonizes the effects of the vasodilator stress agents.[2,6] As adenosine has a very short half-life (~20 to 30 seconds), administration of aminophylline is rarely required during adenosine testing; simply stopping the infusion results in cessation of symptoms within 20 to 30 seconds. After intravenous dipyridamole, infusion of aminophylline at approximately 1 to 2 mg/kg, given during 30 seconds, reverses side effects (as well as the coronary vasodilator effects), usually within 1 to 2 minutes. As the coronary vasodilator effects are reversed as well, reversal of the dipyridamole effect should be delayed until at least 1 to 2 minutes after radionuclide administration if it is clinically safe; otherwise, the true stress perfusion pattern may not be manifested. In general, side effects from vasodilator pharmacologic stress, although common, may be tolerated for this time. However, with more severe side effects, such as severe shortness of breath or bronchospasm, or with more dramatic ST-segment abnormalities, reversal of the dipyridamole effect more quickly is prudent. As caffeine is a methylxanthine compound and antagonizes the effect of adenosine at its receptor, it is critical that patients be instructed to withhold caffeine, ideally for 24 hours before vasodilator pharmacologic stress testing.

In some patients, myocardial ischemia provoked during vasodilator stress testing triggers a cascade of events that maintains ischemia even after reversal of the vasodilator effect with aminophylline. The sensation of chest pain may drive a heightened sympathetic response, with an elevation of heart rate and blood pressure. In that setting, when aminophylline has been given to reverse the effects of the vasodilator, it is safe to administer sublingual nitroglycerin or other measures to relieve myocardial ischemia. It is not safe to give sublingual nitroglycerin before aminophylline to treat signs of myocardial ischemia. Because systemic vasodilation is present during vasodilator stress testing, administration of nitroglycerin before aminophylline may result in substantial systemic hypotension.

In contemporary practice, a small number of patients may be encountered who are taking oral dipyridamole preparations for their antiplatelet effects. As dipyridamole is an adenosine deaminase inhibitor and prevents the usual rapid breakdown of adenosine, infusion of intravenous adenosine in patients receiving oral dipyridamole may be accompanied by a far more prolonged adenosine effect than usual. Thus, for adenosine testing, oral dipyridamole compounds must be stopped at an appropriate time before testing. Oral dipyridamole as background therapy does not complicate the performance of intravenous dipyridamole testing.

Protocols for Pharmacologic Stress Testing

The accepted protocols for performing vasodilator pharmacologic stress testing are listed in **Table 17-3**.[2,6] Since the original descriptions of these protocols, iterations have been studied, with the goal of shortening the test procedure or minimizing side effects, or both,[27] by shortening the duration of the adenosine infusion or adding low-level exercise.

Handgrip exercise may be used to raise peripheral blood pressure and thus coronary perfusion pressure. Reports are mixed on whether image quality is improved. This approach may be useful in patients with borderline low blood pressure before the test to avoid significant hypotension.

Low-level treadmill exercise has been increasingly applied in combination with vasodilator stress testing. Although no clear advantage in diagnostic performance has been demonstrated, a reduction in side effects of pharmacologic stress testing has been consistently demonstrated, as well as a reduction in extracardiac tracer uptake that improves image quality.[27]

Initial reports of intravenous adenosine testing described a protocol in which the dose was progressively increased. More commonly, adenosine is given now as an infusion starting with the maximum dose. This allows a shortened total infusion period of 4 minutes rather than 6 minutes, with radionuclide injected at 3 minutes into the 4-minute infusion. Published data suggest that diagnostic sensitivity is maintained while the overall time of testing is decreased.[24]

TABLE 17-3 Pharmacologic Stress Protocols

	DOSE	DURATION	ISOTOPE INJECTION
Dipyridamole	142 μg/kg/min	4 minutes by hand infusion or pump	3 minutes after completion of infusion
Adenosine	140 μg/kg/min	6-minute infusion by pump	At 3 minutes into infusion
Regadenoson	0.4 mg (5 mL) rapid IV injection, followed by 5 mL saline flush	Bolus	10-20 seconds after the saline flush

DIFFERENCES BETWEEN VASODILATOR AND EXERCISE STRESS. The perfusion images obtained by use of vasodilator pharmacologic stress are generally concordant with those obtained with maximal exercise stress in the same patient, but there are several important differences. Higher levels of coronary flow are achieved during vasodilator pharmacologic stress compared with exercise, possibly because of the increased resistance to flow with exercise caused by higher subendocardial pressures. Although theoretically this should result in increased sensitivity for detection of CAD with pharmacologic stress, that has not been clearly demonstrated. The failure to demonstrate increased sensitivity may be due to the inability of the radionuclide tracers to reflect myocardial blood flow adequately at the highest levels of flow (see Fig. 17-23).[5]

Vasodilator pharmacologic stress is less "physiologic" than exercise, and symptoms during testing (or lack thereof) cannot be as clearly linked to the perfusion pattern. Optimal diagnostic performance of MPI during exercise is often dependent on the patient's achieving a maximal level of stress, which does not always occur. In contrast, vasodilator pharmacologic stress affords generally predictable coronary flow responses.[5,24]

Anti-ischemic medications may significantly affect the results of MPI during exercise.[6] Reports have now suggested that the extent and severity of myocardial perfusion defects may also be affected in an important way by background medication during pharmacologic stress.[28,29] Thus, antianginal medications should be withheld if possible before the study.

DOBUTAMINE STRESS TO INDUCE CORONARY HYPEREMIA. In some patients, vasodilator pharmacologic stress is contraindicated because of reactive bronchospastic airways disease or background methylxanthines. In such situations, intravenous dobutamine hydrochloride may be used to induce coronary hyperemia.[2,6] Dobutamine has a relatively rapid onset of action, with a half-life of approximately 2 minutes. This agent is given starting at a dose of 5 μg/kg/min and increased in a stepwise fashion by 5 μg/kg/min every 3 minutes, to a maximum dose of 40 μg/kg/min (see Fig. 15-33B). Dobutamine is a broad adrenergic receptor agonist, at varying doses stimulating the $beta_1$, $beta_2$, and $alpha_1$ receptors. At relatively low doses, the predominant effect is an increase in contractility through adrenergic receptors. As the dose is increased beyond 10 μg/kg/min, heart rate rises steadily, and the increase in oxygen demand stimulates an increase in myocardial blood flow.

The hemodynamic response to dobutamine generally involves a modest increase in systolic blood pressure with a modest decrease in diastolic blood pressure through doses up to 20 μg/kg/min, with only small further changes after that point. As the increase in myocardial blood flow is dependent on the increase in oxygen demand, optimal sensitivity for MPI based on optimizing heterogeneity of flow is dependent on achieving an adequate heart rate response, often requiring a high dose of dobutamine.

The increment in myocardial blood flow during maximal doses of dobutamine appears to be less than that achieved during vasodilator pharmacologic stress, and hence the degree of heterogeneity of coronary flow with a coronary stenosis is also less. Thus, vasodilator stress is the preferred pharmacologic modality for MPI in patients who cannot exercise adequately. Dobutamine stress is reserved for cases in which vasodilator stress is contraindicated or cannot be performed because of background medications.[2,6]

Side effects of dobutamine are frequent and can be bothersome.[2] The most common side effects include palpitations and chest pain, and arrhythmias including PVCs and nonsustained ventricular tachycardia may be encountered. Hypotension occurs in approximately 10% of patients, possibly as a result of myocardial mechanoreceptor stimulation during increased contractility with resulting withdrawal of peripheral constrictor tone. Hypotension during dobutamine stress does not have the same prognostic implications as exercise-induced hypotension. Because of the relatively short half-life, side effects generally resolve within a few minutes of stopping of the infusion and can be aborted more quickly with intravenous beta blockade.[2,6]

Assessment of Myocardial Cellular Metabolism and Physiology by Radionuclide Imaging

MYOCARDIAL ISCHEMIA AND VIABILITY

Programmed Cell Survival

Imbalance between oxygen supply and demand results in myocardial ischemia. If the imbalance is transient (i.e., triggered by exertion), it represents reversible ischemia. However, if supply-demand imbalance is prolonged, high-energy phosphates are depleted, and regional contractile function progressively deteriorates. If the supply-demand balance is sufficiently prolonged, cell membrane rupture with cell death follows.

The myocardium has several mechanisms of acute and chronic adaptation to a temporary or sustained reduction in coronary blood flow (**Fig. 17-28**), known as stunning, hibernation, and ischemic preconditioning (see Chap. 52). These responses to ischemia preserve sufficient energy to protect the structural and functional integrity of the cardiac myocyte. In contrast to programmed cell death, or apoptosis, the term *programmed cell survival* has been used to describe the commonality between myocardial stunning, hibernation, and ischemic preconditioning despite their distinct pathophysiology.[30]

Stunned and Hibernating Myocardium

In stunned and hibernating myocardium, myocardial function is depressed at rest but myocytes remain viable. Although LV dysfunction may be reversible in both stunning and hibernation, these states differ in the relationship between myocardial perfusion and function. Stunned myocardium is most commonly observed after a transient period of ischemia followed by reperfusion (depressed function at rest but preserved perfusion). The ischemic episodes can be single or multiple, brief or prolonged, but never severe enough to result in injury. Hibernating myocardium refers to adaptive responses of the myocardium to repetitive episodes of ischemia resulting in myocardial hypoperfusion at rest[31] (depressed function and perfusion at rest). Clinically, it is likely that the adaptive responses of hibernation and stunning coexist (see Chap. 52).

Myocardial Viability

Requirements for cellular viability include (1) sufficient myocardial blood flow, (2) cell membrane integrity, and (3) preserved metabolic activity. Myocardial blood flow has to be adequate to deliver substrate to the myocyte for metabolic processes and to remove the end products of metabolism. If blood flow is severely reduced, metabolites accumulate, causing inhibition of the enzymes of the metabolic pathway, depletion of high-energy phosphates, cell membrane disruption, and cell death. Thus, with severe reduction in blood flow, perfusion tracers alone provide information about myocardial viability.[6] However, in regions in which the reduction in blood flow is less severe, perfusion information alone may be an insufficient signal to identify clinically relevant viability, and additional data, such as metabolic indices, would be important.[6]

Because cell membrane integrity, another requisite for cell survival, is dependent on preserved intracellular metabolic activity to generate high-energy phosphates, tracers that reflect cation flux (^{201}Tl), electrochemical gradients (sestamibi or tetrofosmin), or metabolic processes (FDG) provide insight into myocardial viability (**Fig. 17-29**).[5,30]

MAJOR MYOCARDIAL FUELS AND ENERGETICS IN NORMAL AND ISCHEMIC MYOCARDIUM. High-energy phosphates, such as adenosine triphosphate (ATP), provide the fuel that powers the myocyte contractile proteins (see Chap. 24). ATP is generated in the myocardium by two different but integrated metabolic processes: oxidative phosphorylation and glycolysis.[13] Fatty acids, glucose, and lactate are the major sources of energy in the heart, and depending on the arterial concentration of each and the physiologic condition, any one of these three can be the principal substrate (Fig. 17-29B). Increased uptake and use of one substrate leads to a decreased contribution by the others.

In the fasting state, long-chain free fatty acids are the preferred source of energy in the heart, with glucose accounting for only 15% to 20% of the total energy supply. When the oxygen supply is normal, high levels of ATP and tissue citrate formed by breakdown of fatty acids suppress the oxidation of glucose. When the oxygen supply is decreased, ATP and citrate levels fall, and the rate of glycolysis is accelerated. Anaerobic glycolysis can be maintained only if lactate and hydrogen ion (the byproducts of glycolysis) are removed and do not accumulate. In the setting of severe hypoperfusion, these end products of the glycolytic pathway accumulate, causing inhibition of the glycolytic enzymes and depletion of high-energy phosphates, resulting in cell membrane disruption and cell death.[30] Thus, even to maintain anaerobic glycolysis, minimally sufficient blood flow is necessary.

IMAGING OF ALTERATIONS IN MYOCARDIAL METABOLISM

Imaging of Fatty Acid Metabolism

[^{11}C]PALMITATE. Because fatty acids are the primary source of myocardial energy production in the fasting state, early PET studies focused on characterizing the kinetics of long-chain fatty acids, such as [^{11}C]palmitate.[32] Measurement by dynamic PET imaging allows determination of tracer inflow (by regional perfusion), peak accumulation, and release within a region of interest. Once the tracer is in the cell, it either (1) enters the endogenous lipid pool or (2) moves to the mitochondria, where rapid degradation by beta-oxidation results in the generation of carbon dioxide. Depending on demand, about 80% of extracted [^{11}C]palmitate is activated for transport from the lipid pool into the mitochondria for breakdown by beta-oxidation. Because of its complicated kinetic modeling and numerous confounding effects, [^{11}C]palmitate imaging has not gained wide clinical acceptance.

[^{123}I]BMIPP. Fatty acid imaging with radioiodine-labeled fatty acid analogues, such as iodine-123–labeled beta-methyliodopentadecanoic acid (BMIPP) with SPECT, is an investigational area for the assessment of ischemic memory.[33] After an ischemic episode, fatty acid metabolism may be suppressed for a prolonged time, and BMIPP imaging can demonstrate a regional metabolic defect even if perfusion has returned to normal. This metabolic signal of recent ischemia has been termed ischemic memory and may be clinically useful, for example, in patients who report to an emergency department with chest pain that resolved hours earlier. Although BMIPP is approved for clinical use in Japan, it has not yet received approval by the U.S. FDA.

Imaging of Glucose Metabolism

Whereas fatty acids are the primary source of fuel in the fasting state, increased arterial glucose concentration in the fed state results in an increase in insulin levels, stimulating glucose metabolism while inhibiting lipolysis.[5,13] The result is a switch in myocardial metabolism from predominantly fatty acid use to glucose use.

The principle of using a metabolic tracer that tracks glycolysis is based on the concept that glucose use may be preserved or increased relative to flow in hypoperfused but viable (hibernating) myocardium, termed metabolism-perfusion mismatch.[5,13,34] Myocardial glucose use is absent in scarred or fibrotic tissue, represented by metabolism-perfusion match (**Fig. 17-30**). Although the amount of energy produced by glycolysis may be adequate to maintain myocyte viability and to preserve the electrochemical gradient across the cell membrane, it may not be sufficient to sustain contractile function.[30,55]

2-[^{18}F]FLUORO-2-DEOXYGLUCOSE. FDG is a glucose analogue used to image myocardial glucose use with PET.[5,13,30] After injection of 5 to 10 mCi, FDG rapidly exchanges across the capillary and cellular membranes. It is phosphorylated by hexokinase to FDG-6-phosphate (see Fig. 17-29B) and not metabolized further or used in glycogen synthesis. Because the dephosphorylation rate of FDG is slow, it becomes trapped in the myocardium, permitting PET or SPECT imaging of regional glucose use. FDG uptake may be increased in hibernating but viable myocardium, and FDG uptake in asynergic myocardial regions with reduced blood flow at rest has become a scintigraphic marker of hibernation.

Diagnostic quality of FDG imaging is critically dependent on hormonal milieu and substrate availability. Most clinical FDG studies are performed after 50 to 75 g of glucose loading in the form of oral dextrose approximately 1 to 2 hours before the FDG injection to increase glucose metabolism, to increase FDG uptake, and to improve image quality.[5,13]

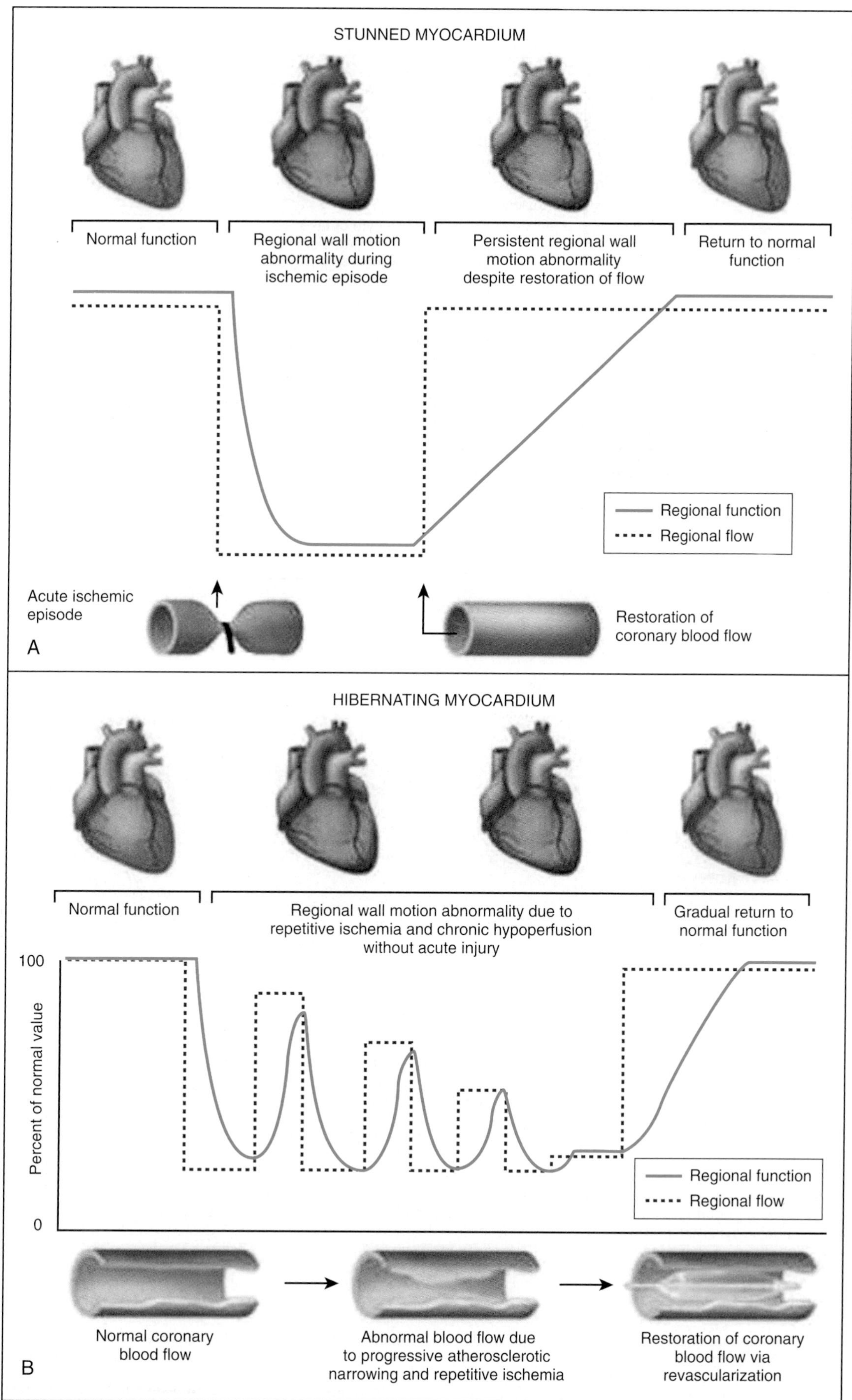

FIGURE 17-28 Pathophysiology of stunning and hibernation, representing different mechanisms of acute and chronic reversible left ventricular dysfunction. *(Modified from Dilsizian V: Myocardial viability: Reversible left ventricular dysfunction. In Dilsizian V, Narula J, Braunwald E [eds]: Atlas of Nuclear Cardiology. Philadelphia, Current Medicine, 2006.)*

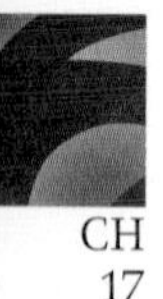

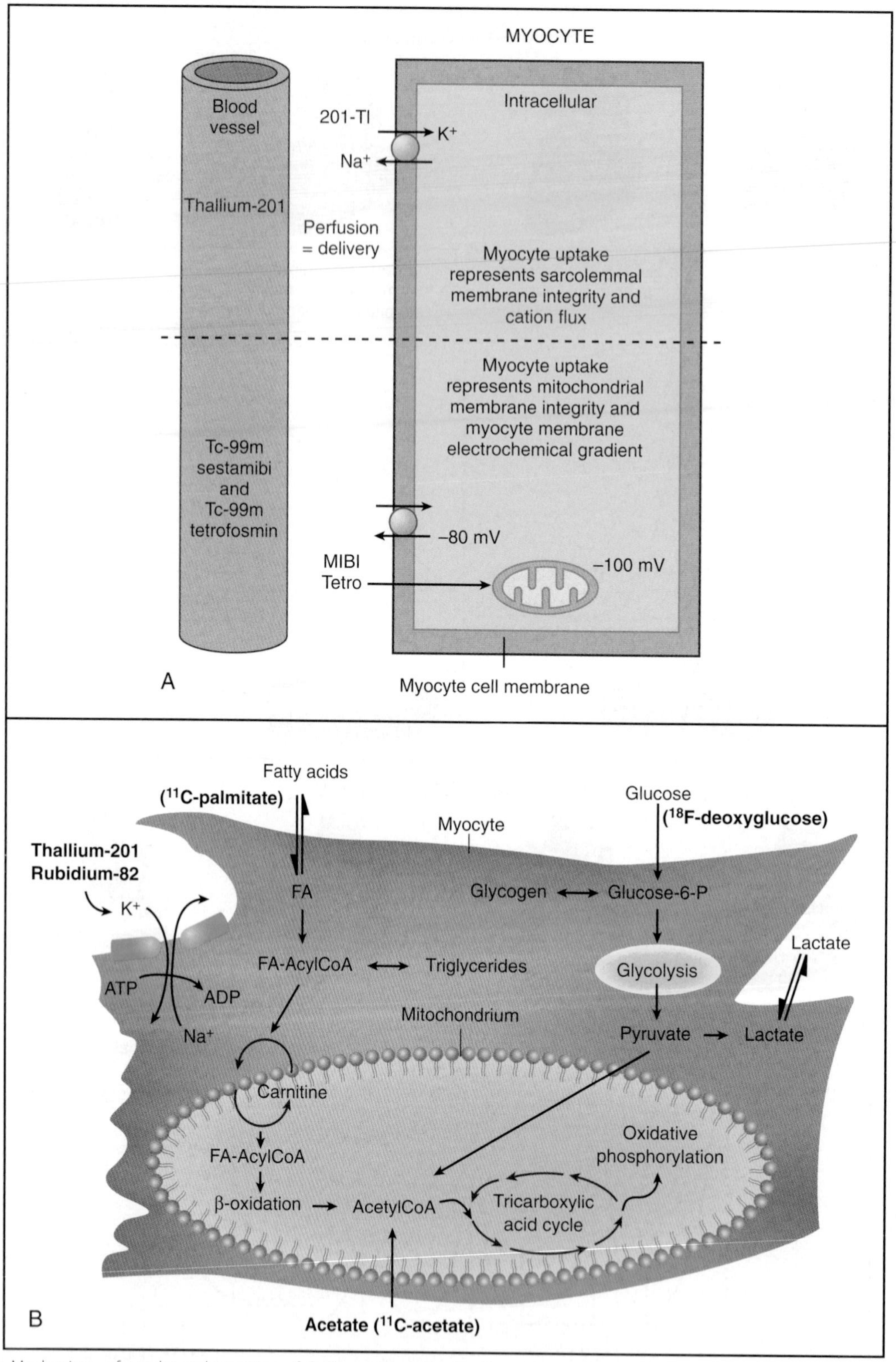

FIGURE 17-29 **A,** Mechanisms of uptake and retention of thallium-201 and technetium-99m perfusion tracers. **B,** Mechanism of uptake and retention of PET agents tracing perfusion (rubidium-82) and oxidative and anaerobic metabolism (^{11}C-acetate, ^{11}C-palmitate, and ^{18}F-deoxyglucose). ADP = adenosine diphosphate; ATP = adenosine triphosphate; CoA = coenzyme A; FA = fatty acid. *(Modified from Dilsizian V: SPECT and PET techniques. In Dilsizian V, Narula J, Braunwald E [eds]: Atlas of Nuclear Cardiology. Philadelphia, Current Medicine, 2006.)*

Although 90% of FDG images are of diagnostic quality in nondiabetic patients, the quality of FDG images after glucose loading alone is less certain in patients with clinical or subclinical diabetes, as the increase in plasma insulin levels may be attenuated, tissue lipolysis may not be inhibited, and free fatty acid levels may remain high. Standardization schemes to optimize FDG image quality in diabetic patients include[5,13] (1) intravenous insulin injections after glucose loading, (2) hyperinsulinemic-euglycemic clamping, and (3) use of nicotinic acid derivative.

Imaging of Oxidative Metabolism and Mitochondrial Function

[^{11}C]Acetate. All oxidative fuels are metabolized in the tricarboxylic acid cycle after conversion to acetyl coenzyme A. [^{11}C]Acetate is avidly extracted by the myocardium and metabolized predominantly by conversion to [^{11}C] acetyl coenzyme A in the cytosol and oxidation by the tricarboxylic acid cycle in the mitochondria to [^{11}C]carbon dioxide and water. Hence, the rapid myocardial turnover and clearance of [^{11}C]acetate in the form of [^{11}C] carbon dioxide may reflect myocardial oxidative metabolism and provide insight into mitochondrial function. In patients with recent MI and chronic stable angina, clearance rates of [^{11}C]acetate predict myocardial viability and functional recovery after revascularization. Despite encouraging data in the literature, [^{11}C]acetate remains an investigational tracer.

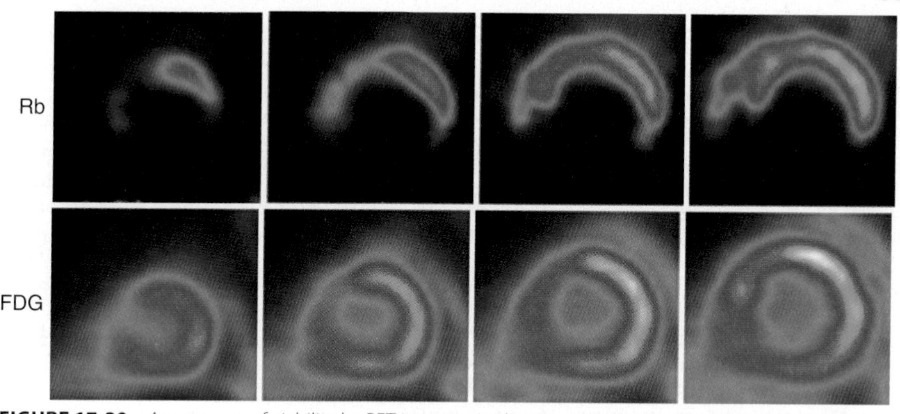

FIGURE 17-30 Assessment of viability by PET imaging. In the top row, rubidium-82 (Rb) is used as a tracer of myocardial blood flow at rest in these short-axis images starting toward the apex (left) and moving toward the base of the heart (right). Myocardial perfusion is markedly decreased in the apical, inferior, inferolateral, and septal regions. In the bottom row, 18F-fluorodeoxyglucose (FDG) is used as a tracer of myocardial glucose metabolism. FDG uptake is enhanced relative to blood flow, demonstrating a pattern of perfusion-metabolism mismatch in most abnormally perfused myocardial regions, indicative of viable or hibernating myocardium. An exception is the anteroseptal resion, which demonstrates a matched perfusion-metabolism pattern, indicative of non-viable or scarred myocardium. *(From Taegtmeyer H, Dilsizian V: Imaging myocardial metabolism and ischemic memory. Nat Clin Pract Cardiovasc Med 5[Suppl 2]:S42, 2008.)*

Assessment of Ventricular Function by Radionuclide Imaging

ASSESSING THE PHYSIOLOGY OF VENTRICULAR FUNCTION. The EF as an index of global systolic LV performance is influenced by many factors, including the intrinsic state of contractility, preload, and afterload as well as neurohormonal and inotropic influences (see Chap. 24). Despite its load dependence, EF has proved clinically useful as a marker of ventricular performance. In the aftermath of acute MI, the postinfarction EF is among the most powerful indices predictive of subsequent mortality.[6,35] The radionuclide techniques used to image ventricular function, RVG and gated SPECT imaging, have provided substantial insight into the physiology of LV function and the response to disease states.

Assessing the Left Ventricular Response to Exercise

Equilibrium gated RVG and first-pass RVG are among the few noninvasive imaging techniques that can evaluate ventricular performance during exercise.[12] Most often, this is accomplished by imaging of the patient during bicycle exercise, supine or semisupine for equilibrium RVG and upright for first-pass RVG. EF measurements during exertion can then be compared with the resting EF.[12]

This technique has been used to study the response of LV function and volumes to exercise. For example, in younger normal subjects, the normal increase in EF and cardiac output is accomplished by decreasing end-systolic volume. In contrast, among older normal subjects, the increase in EF and cardiac output during exercise is accomplished by increasing end-diastolic volume (using preload reserve). In healthy subjects, the normal EF response to exercise is an increase of more than five EF units. The underlying physiology of this increase changes as normal subjects age.[12]

The relative ease with which the EF response to exercise may be studied by RVG techniques led to many reports in the late 1970s and throughout the 1980s. However, evaluation of LV function during exercise by RVG has now been largely replaced by exercise echocardiography (see Chap. 15).

Evaluation of Left Ventricular Volumes

With the RVG technique, the counts detected from the LV region of interest are proportional to ventricular volume. The proportional relation can be estimated from a blood sample of known volume, in which the quantitative relationship between counts and volume can be determined after correction for attenuation.[2,6,12]

The major advantage of the RVG technique for evaluation of ventricular volumes (and function) over contrast ventriculographic and echocardiographic methods is that the radionuclide techniques do not require assumptions about ventricular geometry. With use of RVG techniques, volumes are calculated from count rates over a region of interest involving the left or right ventricle, or both, and are based on photon emissions from the region of interest.[12] Thus, the radionuclide techniques are not dependent on any assumption of ventricular geometry and are suitable for the study of ventricular volumes when ventricular geometry is abnormal.

Serial studies of LV volumes have been useful in evaluating the process of LV remodeling after MI and in chronic heart failure,[36] in which there is a progressive increase in LV volume in the absence of neurohormonal blockade. Serial RVG studies have shown that the effect of angiotensin-converting enzyme (ACE) inhibition is an early reduction in LV volume, which is maintained during follow-up.[36]

LV volumes may also be calculated by gated SPECT perfusion imaging, and volumetric data have been validated against other quantitative techniques.[37] At this time, there is less experience with gated SPECT perfusion imaging for serial evaluation of LV volumes compared with equilibrium RVG volumetric techniques. Nonetheless, the ability to evaluate simultaneously LV function, perfusion, and volumes demonstrates the clinical versatility of gated SPECT MPI.

Serial Evaluation of Left Ventricular Function

The quantitative nature of radionuclide analysis of ventricular function and the high reproducibility of the measurement make ECG-gated RVG or ECG-gated SPECT imaging well suited for serial follow-up of changes in LV systolic performance. There are many clinical situations in which serial changes in LV function are clinically relevant, such as in patients with heart failure,[38] those observed with valvular heart disease,[39,40] and those being treated with cardiotoxic chemotherapy.[41] Serial RVG studies demonstrating diminution in EF suggesting the early onset of myocardial dysfunction can herald the onset of a higher risk clinical course directing clinical management decisions.

The accuracy and reproducibility of the RVG technique for assessment of LV function make this technique particularly suitable for serial follow-up assessment of patients with regurgitant valvular heart disease. As an example, studies using RVG have shown that patients being observed with asymptomatic chronic severe aortic regurgitation who demonstrate the onset of LV dysfunction, even when they remain asymptomatic, are at higher risk for adverse clinical outcomes than are those with preserved LV performance.[39,40] On the basis of such RVG data, the onset of LV dysfunction in an asymptomatic patient with aortic regurgitation is an indication for surgery. Similarly, serial RVG follow-up of patients undergoing cardiotoxic chemotherapy[41] has demonstrated that a decline in EF as detected by RVG of 10% to a final level less than 50% indicates high risk for the development of subsequent heart failure.

Evaluation of Diastolic Function with Radionuclide Techniques

Although the most important quantitative variable derived from RVG evaluation of LV function in the majority of cardiac diseases is the EF, numerous other quantitative variables, including indices describing LV diastolic performance, may also be derived.

Left Ventricular Diastolic Filling. Radionuclide assessment of LV filling properties is based on analysis of the LV time-activity curve, usually obtained by equilibrium RVG techniques,[2] which represents relative volume changes throughout the cardiac cycle (see Fig. 17-e4 on website). With appropriate data acquisition methods and attention to technical considerations, several parameters of diastolic function may be computed from the time-activity curve, including the peak rate of rapid diastolic filling, the time to peak filling rate, and the relative contributions of the rapid filling period and of atrial systole to total LV stroke volume. Several studies have shown good correlation between various radionuclide and Doppler echocardiographic measures of filling, as both techniques assess physiologic events during the filling period.[2,6]

Evaluation of Diastolic Filling by Equilibrium Radionuclide Ventriculography Techniques in Disease States

Hypertrophic Cardiomyopathy. Abnormal diastolic properties of the hypertrophied ventricle are a characteristic feature of hypertrophic cardiomyopathy (HCM), contributing notably to clinical manifestations.[42] Studies using RVG evaluation of diastolic filling have demonstrated that the rate and extent of rapid filling are reduced in HCM, that the time to peak filling rate is prolonged, and that the contribution of atrial systole to total LV stroke volume is increased.[42]

Heart Failure. Radionuclide studies have provided evidence of an abnormal end-diastolic volume response to exercise in patients with heart failure and preserved systolic performance, supporting the concept of diastolic dysfunction as an underlying cause of symptoms. Patients with heart failure but preserved systolic performance do not increase end-diastolic volume during exercise, associated with a substantial increase in wedge pressure (see Fig. 17-e5 on website). In contrast, normal subjects demonstrate an increase in end-diastolic volume associated with no change in wedge pressure, recruiting preload despite no change in left atrial driving pressure. Patients with heart failure and normal systolic performance require higher filling pressures to maintain stroke volume, at the cost of an increased pulmonary wedge pressure, resulting in shortness of breath. Thus, abnormal diastolic performance, manifested by an impaired ability to recruit end-diastolic volume (preload reserve), as demonstrated by equilibrium RVG techniques, results in physiologic abnormalities leading to heart failure in these patients with normal systolic function.

Disease Detection, Risk Stratification, and Clinical Decision Making

Stable Chest Pain Syndromes

APPLICATION OF RADIONUCLIDE IMAGING: ANSWERING THE CLINICAL QUESTIONS. For patients with stable symptoms of suspected CAD who are referred for noninvasive testing, the two major goals of testing are (1) determination of whether CAD is present or absent (the diagnostic construct) and (2) determination of the longer term prognosis or risk of an adverse outcome over time (the prognostic construct). These goals of testing are linked to the two main treatment goals for patients with suspected or known CAD: (1) amelioration of symptoms in everyday life and (2) improvement in natural history.

Establishment of the presence or absence of CAD is an important goal of testing. The performance characteristics of radionuclide imaging for this purpose are often based on an angiographic definition of stenosis ≥50% or 70% stenosis in an individual epicardial vessel. This definition of CAD is in part based on seminal studies in animal models showing that a 50% stenosis begins to blunt coronary flow reserve (see Fig. 52-13). However, over time, a view has emerged that CAD is a more complex process than can be simply defined dichotomously by a 50% or even a 70% luminal stenosis. Throughout the progression of plaque growth, there is a risk of transformation from a stable plaque to an unstable plaque, with the potential for an acute coronary syndrome (ACS) that abruptly alters the natural history of the patient (see Chaps. 43 and 54).[43] Plaque encroachment of the lumen occurs later in the process but has a potentially important impact on the patient's everyday quality of life by causing symptoms related to exertional ischemia.

Patient-Related Outcomes as a "Gold Standard"

The evolution of preventive therapies (see Chap. 49), such as 3-hydroxy-3-methylglutaryl coenzyme A reductase inhibitors (statins), to reduce cardiovascular risk has focused attention on the ability of global risk scores or noninvasive testing to assess risk of future events to best target strategies to reduce risk.[44,45] Thus, from the perspective of improving natural history, knowledge of whether a stenosis greater than 50% is present in a patient with stable anginal symptoms becomes less important than knowledge of the patient's risk of a cardiovascular event (i.e., cardiac death or nonfatal MI). After initial investigations of the performance of radionuclide imaging to detect or to rule out CAD (sensitivity and specificity), the trajectory of the literature has been toward gaining more understanding of how noninvasive imaging results assess prognosis and stratify the risk of future cardiac events.[6] This has occurred in parallel with similar directions in primary prevention efforts, such as the use of a Framingham Risk Score, with a goal of lifestyle and treatment interventions to lower that risk.[44] In much the same way, risk stratification and assessment of prognosis by noninvasive imaging will inform clinical management decisions geared toward reducing risk of MI and cardiac death and optimizing the selection of patients for revascularization and medical therapies.

RISK STRATIFICATION IN STABLE CHEST PAIN SYNDROMES

Definitions for Understanding the Literature

For prognostic assessment, an important goal is to detect patients at risk for "hard" cardiac events. This definition includes nonfatal MI as well as cardiac death or all-cause mortality, irreversible events important to prevent.[46] "Soft" cardiac events include revascularization and hospital admission for unstable angina or heart failure. Such events occur more often than the hard cardiac events and thus contribute to a larger number of endpoints for data analysis. However, these events are not as important in terms of natural history and may be driven by subjective changes in symptoms and, in the case of revascularization, by the results of the imaging tests themselves.

Risk categories as described in the American College of Cardiology/American Heart Association (ACC/AHA) stable angina guidelines include (1) low risk, defined as a less than 1% per year risk of hard cardiac events; (2) intermediate risk, defined as a 1% to 3% per year risk; and (3) high risk, defined as a greater than 3% per year risk.[47] These definitions are conceptually linked to implied treatment strategies. Patients with greater than 3% per year risk would be most likely to benefit from a revascularization strategy, whereas those at low risk would be least likely to benefit from revascularization, in terms of natural history, and thus could be treated medically, with treatment directed against symptoms as well as risk factor modification.

The Relation Between the Extent of Perfusion Defect and Natural History Outcomes

Seminal studies in the 1980s demonstrated that the extent of perfusion abnormality by stress MPI has an important relationship with the subsequent likelihood of an adverse natural history outcome (cardiac death or nonfatal MI). Among patients presenting with chest pain and suspected CAD (without any prior known CAD history, such as MI or revascularization), the risk of cardiac death or MI increased as the number of reversible perfusion defects (i.e., the extent of inducible ischemia) increased (**Fig. 17-31**).

This concept has been confirmed many times by investigators around the world. Moreover, this robust concept not only applies to exercise stress MPI but also extends across the spectrum of procedural variation in nuclear cardiology, including different stressors (vasodilator pharmacologic stress, dobutamine stress), isotopes (^{201}Tl and ^{99m}Tc agents), and imaging protocols (including dual-isotope imaging).[6] An example of data on risk stratification implying therapeutic management strategies is demonstrated by the images shown in Figure 17-31A,B. In two older men with typical exertional angina, it would be predicted that the probability of CAD is very high, according to established guidelines. However, what is not established from that clinical information is the natural history risk. These examples demonstrate that patients presenting with similar symptoms might be identified as having distinct natural histories on the basis of perfusion imaging data, with distinct implications for subsequent management.

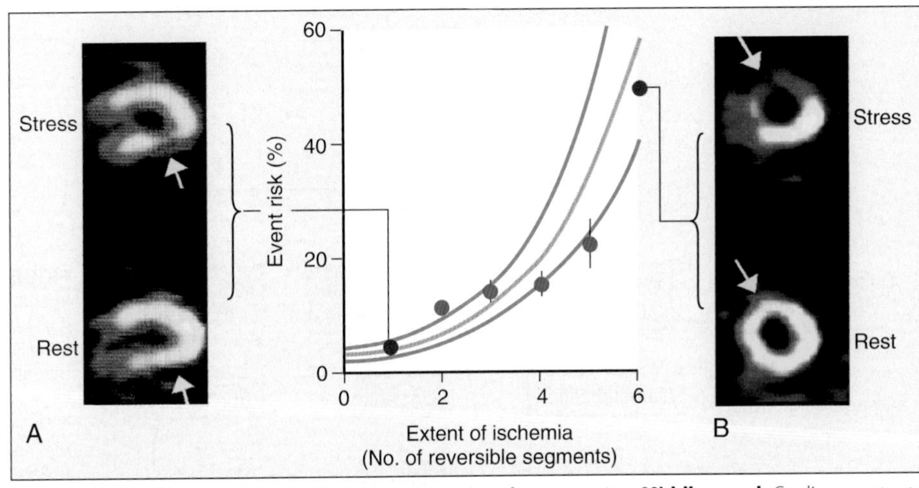

FIGURE 17-31 Prognostic implications of myocardial perfusion imaging. **Middle panel,** Cardiac event rate (risk of cardiac death or MI) during long-term follow-up plotted as a function of the extent of inducible ischemia (the number of reversible perfusion defects). There is an exponential relationship between the extent of ischemia and the risk of a cardiac event. The brown line represents modeling of data points; magenta lines represent confidence limits. *(Modified from Ladenheim ML, Pollock BH, Rozanski A, et al: Extent and severity of myocardial hypoperfusion as predictors of prognosis in patients with suspected coronary artery disease. J Am Coll Cardiol 7:464, 1986.)* **A, B,** SPECT perfusion images in two patients with stable anginal symptoms. **A,** Small area of inferoapical ischemia (arrows). When this extent of ischemia is plotted on the graph (line to red circle), the patient is placed in a low-risk category. **B,** In contrast, the large, severe area of anterior and septal ischemia in this patient places him in a high-risk group (line to red circle).

The Incremental Value of Perfusion Imaging

The term *incremental value* implies that perfusion imaging data provide information on natural history risk and outcomes that are additive to (incremental to) information from more available or less expensive tests, such as clinical data and stress ECG findings.

Stress MPI data have been shown to have incremental prognostic value when added to prognostic stress ECG instruments such as the Duke Treadmill Score, a well-validated instrument incorporating symptoms, treadmill performance, and stress ECG findings to predict natural history outcomes (see Chap. 14). In a group of 2200 patients with suspected CAD referred for nuclear testing, the Duke Treadmill Score was used to place patients in subgroups according to the risk of a hard event (**Fig. 17-32**). When information from stress MPI studies was incorporated, incremental value to predict outcome was demonstrated within each of the three Duke Treadmill Score risk categories.

The importance of this information in driving management decisions for patients can be illustrated by considering how clinicians would manage patients given certain amounts of information. Given the Duke Treadmill Score information alone, the management of low-risk patients would probably be conservative and the management of high-risk patients would be likely to involve revascularization. The optimal management of intermediate-risk patients is unclear, but many would probably be referred for catheterization. However, almost 70% of the patients in the intermediate Duke Treadmill Score category had a normal stress perfusion study (Fig. 17-32A), associated with a very low risk natural history, implying that conservative management would be a safe and effective strategy.

Another method used to demonstrate the incremental value of MPI data over clinical, stress, and even angiographic data involves the creation of a multivariable model to measure the strength of association of individual factors with the natural history outcomes.[48] This is often illustrated by assessing the incremental chi-square value measuring the strength of the association of the factor with subsequent cardiac death and nonfatal MI (Fig. 17-32B).

Identification of Treatment Benefit After Risk Stratification

Although numerous studies intimate that the extent and severity of perfusion abnormality are related to subsequent natural history risk, few studies have documented reduction in that risk associated with a particular therapy. Current information suggests that more extensive ischemia determined by MPI identifies patients in whom revascularization may lead to an improvement in outcome. In a group of more than 10,000 patients with suspected CAD studied by stress MPI, the extent of ischemic myocardium predicted reduction in the risk of death with revascularization compared with medical therapy (**Fig. 17-33**), beginning at just over 10% of ischemic myocardium.[49] As the percentage of ischemic myocardium increased, the magnitude of benefit of revascularization increased as well. Thus, MPI data can predict the magnitude of a potential treatment benefit from revascularization, helping to guide management decisions.

Prognostic Value of Normal Myocardial Perfusion Imaging

A consistent finding in studies assessing prognosis has been the benign outcome associated with a normal stress MPI study. As summarized in the ACC/AHA/ASNC Radionuclide Imaging Guidelines,[6] data on outcomes associated with a normal stress SPECT MPI study now involve almost 21,000 patients. In patients with a normal study, the hard event rate (i.e., rate of cardiac death or nonfatal MI) occurring during an average follow-up of 2 years is 0.7% per year. This concept applies across a broad spectrum of isotopes, protocols, and stressors.[6,50] The prediction of low-risk outcome after a normal MPI study extends approximately 2 years after testing (i.e., the "warranty period").[51] Patients who at baseline represent higher risk subsets (i.e., those with diabetes) have a slightly higher risk of an adverse outcome after a normal stress MPI study,[52] consistent with Bayes' theorem; that is, given a certain MPI finding, the post-test probability (outcome risk) is related in part to the pretest risk.

Even when angiographic CAD is present with a stable symptom complex, a normal stress MPI study is associated with a low-risk outcome (~0.9% per year).[6] The mechanism for a normal MPI study despite established CAD has not been conclusively demonstrated but may involve preserved endothelial function, allowing appropriate flow-mediated vasodilation during stress, reducing the impact of an angiographic stenosis on downstream myocardial perfusion. If this is true, such preserved endothelial function may identify a patient less susceptible to plaque fissuring or rupture and more likely to have a stable clinical course.

Dynamic Assessment of Prognosis by Serial Scintigraphic Studies: A New Paradigm?

Although there is an important correlation between the extent of ischemia and subsequent outcome, the specificity of such determinations is low. That is, among patients with high-risk scintigraphic signs, only a minority suffer an important cardiac event during follow-up, and the majority of "high-risk" patients remain event free. As most of these high-risk patients undergo catheterization and intervention, many patients who will not have an event are receiving interventions to prevent these events in the minority. Clinicians accept this tradeoff, but evolving data suggest that the response of scintigraphic ischemia to medical therapy may allow more precise estimates of prognosis.

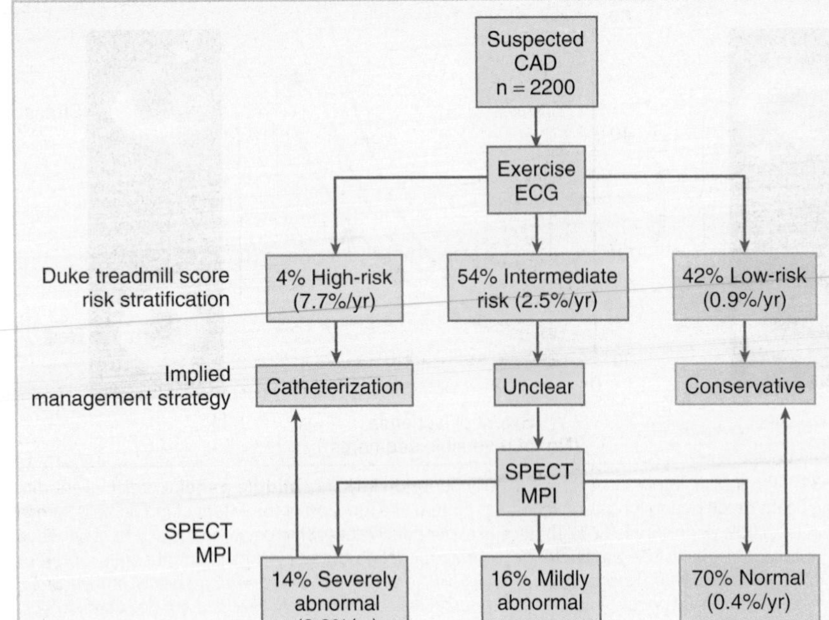

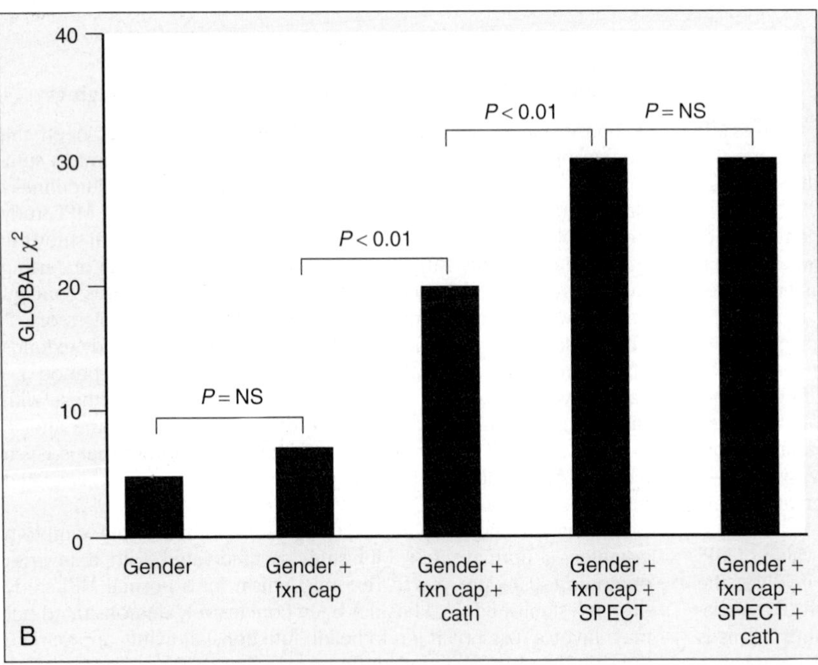

FIGURE 17-32 Incremental value of SPECT perfusion imaging. **A,** Comparison with the Duke Treadmill Score (DTS). A large group of patients with suspected CAD was initially risk stratified by the well-validated DTS. Figures in parentheses are the observed annual event rates. The majority of the population is classified as intermediate risk by DTS, and management strategy is not clear. High-risk patients may be managed aggressively, and low-risk patients may be managed conservatively. Among patients originally categorized as intermediate risk by the DTS, almost 70% had a normal SPECT perfusion study, associated with a very low event rate. After SPECT MPI, more patients are classified at the "extremes" of risk (low or high), where management is more clearly implied by the risk prediction. Thus, the imaging data allowed further stratification and had incremental value over the DTS information. **B,** The incremental value of imaging data may be expressed as the incremental chi-square value, a statistical measure of the strength of the association of clinical, demographic, stress, or imaging factors to risk stratification. Among patients with known CAD who had undergone catheterization (cath), clinical information is added on the *x*-axis, with the global chi-square value associated with the information depicted on the *y*-axis. The larger the chi-square value, the stronger the relation between the combination of factors on the *x*-axis and the natural history outcome of cardiac death or myocardial infarction. Even when anatomic information is available, the physiologic information provided by SPECT MPI adds significantly to risk prediction ability. fxn cap = functional capacity. *(**A** modified from Hachamovitch R, Berman DS, Kiat H, et al: Exercise myocardial perfusion SPECT in patients without known coronary artery disease: Incremental prognostic value and use in risk stratification. Circulation 93:905, 1996. **B** modified from Beller GA: First Annual Mario S. Verani, MD, Memorial Lecture: Clinical value of myocardial perfusion imaging in coronary artery disease. J Nucl Cardiol 10:529, 2003.)*

Among post-MI patients with strongly positive adenosine SPECT perfusion imaging studies randomized to aggressive medical therapy or to revascularization, the extent of ischemia was similarly reduced with medical therapy compared with percutaneous coronary intervention (PCI) on a follow-up SPECT perfusion study performed 6 weeks later.[28] In the Clinical Outcomes Utilizing Revascularization and Aggressive Drug Evaluation (COURAGE) trial, patients with stable CAD who were randomized to PCI in addition to optimal medical therapy had a greater reduction in scintigraphic ischemia compared with those patients randomized to optimal medical therapy alone.[53] Whether patients receiving optimal medical therapy with residual ischemia on serial testing benefit from more aggressive interventional therapy is a concept for future study. Until such data are available, the benefit of serial testing to assess for the presence of residual ischemia is uncertain.

Studies using either PET or SPECT assessment of perfusion have concordantly demonstrated improvement in stress perfusion after statin therapy (see Fig. 17-e6 on website).[54] As such therapy is unlikely to affect significantly the degree of luminal encroachment by a plaque, the data suggest that improvement in perfusion may be a result of statin-mediated improvement in endothelial function. Favorable changes in perfusion may identify cohorts of patients gaining most benefit from statin therapy in terms of vascular stability, a concept that requires longer term follow-up of such patients.

DETECTING THE PRESENCE AND EXTENT OF CORONARY ARTERY DISEASE. Noninvasive testing in patients with suspected CAD is commonly performed to determine the presence or absence of angiographic CAD. In this paradigm, angiography is the gold standard to define the presence or absence of CAD, and performance of the noninvasive test is measured by its sensitivity (percentage of true-positive test results among those with CAD as defined by angiography) as well as by its specificity (percentage of true-negative test results among those without CAD).[6,55] Published values of sensitivity to detect CAD and specificity to rule out CAD vary widely.[6] There are many factors influencing these performance characteristics that should be understood for imaging data to be incorporated appropriately into clinical decision making. These include either methodologic or physiologic factors.

Methodologic Influences on Sensitivity and Specificity

Referral Bias. The apparent accuracy of any noninvasive test to detect CAD depends on the indications for coronary angiography.

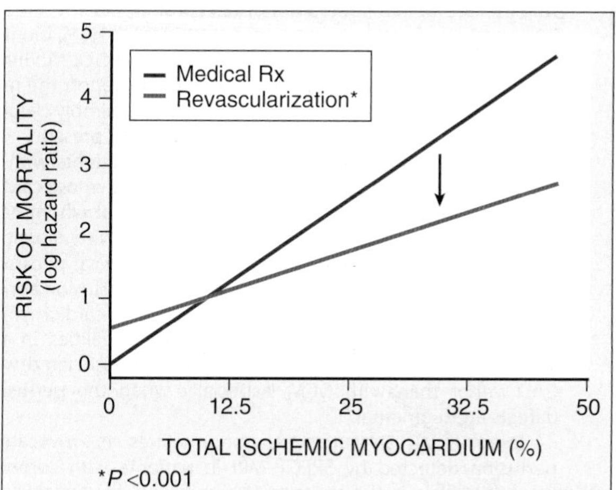

FIGURE 17-33 Predicting the magnitude of treatment benefit by revascularization. Risk of death is plotted as a function of the percentage of ischemic myocardium by SPECT perfusion imaging. The lines represent patients treated with medical therapy (medical Rx, magenta) or revascularization (blue). When the magnitude of ischemia exceeds approximately 12%, there is a potential survival benefit with revascularization. *(Modified from Hachamovitch R, Hayes SW, Friedman JD, et al: Comparison of the short-term survival benefit associated with revascularization compared with medical therapy in patients with no prior coronary artery disease undergoing stress myocardial perfusion single photon emission computed tomography. Circulation 107:2900, 2003.)*

Accuracy of a new diagnostic test is usually determined initially in patients who are undergoing coronary angiography. As the test becomes implemented in routine diagnostic strategies, its results determine which patients are to be referred for coronary angiography (**Fig. 17-34**). For example, patients with abnormal MPI are more likely to undergo coronary angiography than those with normal MPI. This results in a phenomenon termed post-test referral bias, in which the specificity of a diagnostic test declines over time as it is accepted into clinical practice and plays a gatekeeper role in determining which patients undergo angiography.[6] In its extreme form, in which only patients with an abnormal test are referred for angiography (as in Fig. 17-34), post-test referral bias drives the specificity to zero (all patients with normal coronary arteriograms have false-positive MPI results and there are no true-negatives). The same phenomenon artificially increases the sensitivity of the test and in its extreme drives the sensitivity to 100% (all patients with abnormal coronary arteriograms have true-positive MPI, with no false-negatives). This concept holds not only for MPI but also for any diagnostic test that might determine the indications for angiography.

The concept of "normalcy rate" has been developed in an attempt to compensate for this referral bias.[6] Normalcy is calculated in the same manner as specificity but includes only the imaging test results of patients with a clinically low or very low pretest likelihood of CAD, whether or not they are referred for cardiac catheterization. Normalcy rates tend to be greater than specificity.

Angiography as the Gold Standard. In humans, coronary atherosclerosis is a complex disease most often involving the coronary arteries diffusely and not merely focally. Moreover, whether a given discrete stenosis, imaged at rest during coronary angiography, results in a perfusion abnormality during stress is dependent on a number of factors besides the percentage degree of stenosis. These factors include the dilatory or constrictor response of the vessel during stress (mediated by endothelial function) and the presence or absence of collaterals.[55] For example, a vessel with 70% stenosis but with preserved endothelial function and a well-developed collateral supply may not be associated with an abnormality on stress MPI. In a diagnostic construct, such a result would be categorized as a false-negative finding, reducing MPI sensitivity. However, the MPI data may be providing the correct physiologic information about the functional significance of the angiographic finding, demonstrating that collateral flow during exercise or normal endothelial function or both are associated with preserved coronary blood flow reserve despite the coronary stenosis. This example illustrates the limitation of using angiography as a gold standard in evaluation of a physiologic modality.

Many published studies define CAD as ≥50% stenosis, whereas others use a threshold of ≥70% stenosis.[2,6] Use of the former would decrease sensitivity (as some 50% to 70% stenoses are not hemodynamically

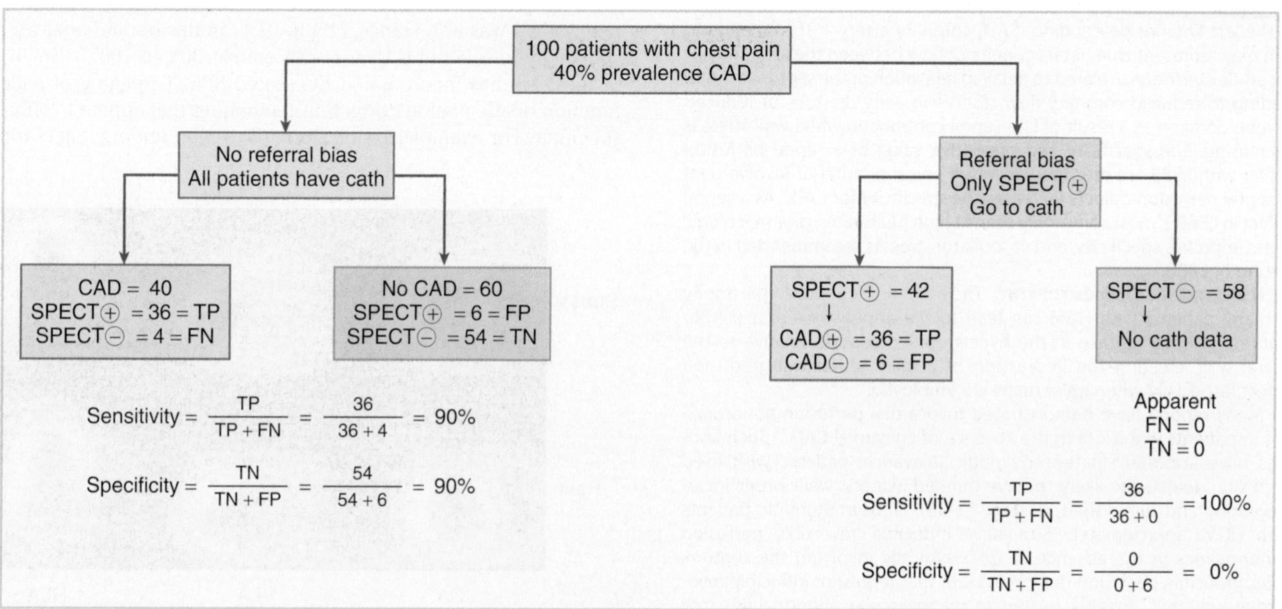

FIGURE 17-34 The effect of referral bias on specificity calculation. If the test being evaluated is used as the "gatekeeper" to coronary angiography, many patients who are true-negatives (i.e., have a normal test and do not have coronary disease) will not undergo angiography and thus will not be included in the specificity calculations (right). This has an effect of artificially reducing the apparent specificity of the noninvasive test in question. CAD = coronary artery disease; FN = false-negative; FP = false-positive; TN = true-negative; TP = true-positive. *(Modified from Rozanski A, Diamond GA, Berman D, et al: The declining specificity of exercise radionuclide ventriculography. N Engl J Med 309:518, 1983.)*

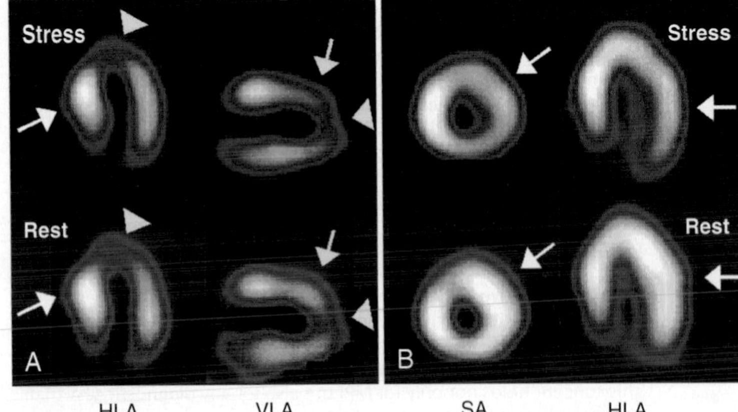

FIGURE 17-35 SPECT perfusion imaging in hypertrophic cardiomyopathy in young asymptomatic patients with normal coronary arteries. **A,** Fixed perfusion defect of the apex consistent with infarction, indicated by yellow arrowheads in the horizontal (HLA) and vertical (VLA) long-axis images, with a reversible defect of the anterior wall (yellow arrows in the VLA images). The hypertrophied septum is evident (white arrows in the HLA images). **B,** Extensive inducible silent ischemia in the anterior, lateral, and inferior walls (white arrows). Transient ischemic cavity dilation is also present, possibly related to subendocardial ischemia. *(Figures based on data from O'Gara PT, Bonow RO, Maron BJ, et al: Myocardial perfusion abnormalities in patients with hypertrophic cardiomyopathy: Assessment with thallium-201 emission computed tomography. Circulation 76:1214, 1987; and Udelson JE, Bonow RO, O'Gara PT, et al: Verapamil prevents silent myocardial perfusion abnormalities during exercise in asymptomatic patients with hypertrophic cardiomyopathy. Circulation 79:1052, 1989.)*

significant) and increase specificity. In contrast, use of the latter threshold would increase sensitivity, as more such stenoses are likely to be associated with perfusion abnormality, but decrease specificity, as any positive scan result with 50% to 70% stenosis would be considered false-positive.

Physiologic Influences on Sensitivity and Specificity

A number of disease processes involving the coronary vasculature or the myocardium may result in abnormalities in myocardial perfusion in the absence of a discrete coronary stenosis. In a diagnostic construct for CAD, such abnormalities would be labeled false-positive, reducing specificity (i.e., the test result is positive in the absence of epicardial CAD). However, MPI may actually be providing correct information about perfusion physiology.

Left Bundle Branch Block. Isolated reversible perfusion defects of the septum in patients with LBBB may be seen in the absence of stenosis of the left anterior descending (LAD) coronary artery.[2,6] This phenomenon may represent true heterogeneity of flow between the LAD and left circumflex territories, related to delayed relaxation of the septum in LBBB leading to reduced coronary flow reserve in early diastole, or reduced oxygen demand as a result of late septal contraction when wall stress is decreasing. The specificity and predictive value of a septal perfusion defect with LBBB are thus low. However, apical or anterior involvement in septal perfusion defects increases the specificity for CAD.[6] As a septal defect in LBBB is most commonly seen at high heart rates, pharmacologic stress improves specificity, and vasodilator stress is recommended in the setting of LBBB.[6]

Hypertrophic Cardiomyopathy. The asymmetric septal hypertrophy in many patients with HCM can lead to the appearance of a greater amount of tracer uptake in the hypertrophied septum relative to the lateral wall, creating the impression of a mild lateral wall perfusion defect, especially when polar maps are employed.

Many reports have demonstrated myocardial perfusion abnormalities in patients with HCM in the absence of epicardial CAD.[17] Such findings have important pathophysiologic relevance: patients with fixed perfusion defects are likely to have thinned akinetic walls on echocardiography and diminished EF (**Fig. 17-35**). Of asymptomatic patients with HCM, approximately 50% have inducible, reversible perfusion abnormalities in the absence of CAD, typically involving the septum. Thus, inducible perfusion defects in HCM that represent inducible myocardial ischemia, possibly related to microvascular abnormalities (see Chap. 69), have low specificity for CAD in patients with HCM. The blunted coronary flow reserve in patients with HCM is associated with a more unfavorable natural history.[17]

Left Ventricular Hypertrophy. As with the experience in HCM, inducible perfusion abnormalities may develop in patients with pressure overload LV hypertrophy (LVH) related to either hypertension or aortic stenosis.[6] In the absence of CAD, it is presumed that these abnormalities represent regional myocardial ischemia based on abnormal microcirculation and limited vasodilator reserve in patients with LVH. However, studies in patients with LVH by ECG criteria have generally demonstrated an accuracy of MPI for detection of CAD that is comparable to that in patients without LVH.[10] On the basis of such data, MPI is a Class I indication for CAD detection when LVH is present on ECG according to ACC/AHA guidelines.[6] SPECT imaging data in patients with LVH also have a risk stratification value similar to that in patients without LVH.[56]

Dilated Cardiomyopathy. Abnormalities in myocardial perfusion are common in patients with dilated cardiomyopathy (DCM) despite normal epicardial coronary arteries.[6] Several studies have demonstrated abnormal coronary flow reserve in these patients (see Chap. 68), and as with data in HCM, blunted flow reserve identifies a cohort of patients with DCM with a more unfavorable natural history.[16] Such data support the relevance of the perfusion abnormalities rather than simply classifying them as false-positive if epicardial CAD is not present.

An important diagnostic consideration in patients with LV systolic dysfunction involves distinguishing those whose cardiomyopathy may be primarily due to CAD (many of whom have potentially reversible LV dysfunction) from those with idiopathic DCM. Although many patients with DCM may have perfusion abnormalities detected on MPI, the absence of perfusion abnormalities virtually excludes CAD as the cause of the cardiomyopathy (**Fig. 17-36**).[57] Extensive perfusion abnormalities in the setting of LV dysfunction are virtually always associated with CAD rather than with DCM, especially when the perfusion defects are segmental.

Endothelial Dysfunction. Abnormalities in myocardial perfusion detected by SPECT MPI in patients with coronary endothelial dysfunction, in the absence of "significant" epicardial vessel stenosis, have been demonstrated. That these perfusion findings represent true abnormalities in coronary flow reserve is supported by studies showing improvement in perfusion on follow-up MPI after treatment with medical therapies directed at improving endothelial function.[58] Further support for this concept comes from CMR studies demonstrating blunted subendocardial coronary flow reserve in patients with angina and normal coronary arteries (see Chap. 18).[59]

SENSITIVITY AND SPECIFICITY OF MYOCARDIAL PERFUSION IMAGING. The 2003 ACC/AHA/ASNC Radionuclide Imaging Guidelines summarize sensitivity and specificity data from 33 studies involving 4480 patients undergoing exercise SPECT imaging.[6] Sensitivity to detect CAD was 87% (range, 71% to 97%) in this pooled analysis, and specificity to rule out CAD was 73% (range, 36% to 100%). Few if any of these studies incorporated ECG-gated SPECT imaging of regional function or attenuation correction, techniques that appear to enhance specificity. For example, in one study of women undergoing coronary

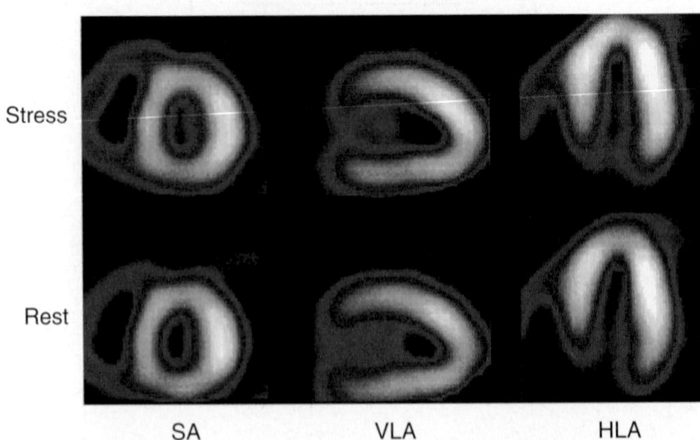

FIGURE 17-36 SPECT perfusion images at stress and rest from a patient with heart failure. The images depict a dilated left ventricle but with normal perfusion patterns, suggesting a low likelihood that coronary artery disease is the cause of heart failure. HLA = horizontal long axis; SA = short axis; VLA = vertical long axis.

angiography, specificity was improved from 76% to 96% when gated SPECT ^{99m}Tc-sestamibi imaging was used compared with nongated SPECT ^{201}Tl.[6]

Influence of Perfusion Tracer on Detection of Coronary Artery Disease

Despite the expectation of improved diagnostic accuracy with use of ^{99m}Tc-based agents, on the basis of more favorable attributes as a radioisotope for gamma camera imaging compared with ^{201}Tl, studies comparing the widely used agents have not shown significant improvement in sensitivity or specificity. An exception is the demonstration of improved specificity in women with the use of ^{99m}Tc-sestamibi compared with thallium, as noted earlier. Thus, the choice of radiotracer for MPI does not notably affect the discrimination between the presence and absence of CAD. Published studies often involve subjects who may not fully represent those who are most challenging to image. It would be expected that the ^{99m}Tc-based agents, with their greater photon energy, would offer improved performance in obese patients and those with large breasts as well as allow the option of higher quality gated images.

Influence of Automated Quantitation of Myocardial Perfusion Images in Detection of Coronary Artery Disease

There may be significant intraobserver and interobserver variability in the visual analysis of myocardial perfusion images. Several methods of quantitative analysis of MPI have been developed[1,6] to reduce the variability in reading by "objectifying" image analysis, by comparing regional uptake values with a normal data base.

Automated quantitative analysis systems are incorporated into most SPECT camera-computer equipment. Some of the most common are Emory Toolbox,[1] Cedars QPS,[60] and 4D-MSPECT (**Fig. 17-37**).[1] Although published data do not clearly demonstrate improved sensitivity or specificity of these programs over visual analysis for CAD detection, such data arise from expert centers, often where the quantitative software was developed, and the visual analysis data are derived from experienced readers in laboratories with excellent quality control.

In practice, the use of contemporary quantitative programs can improve image acquisition quality as well as interpretation. Some programs incorporate motion-sensing algorithms that interrogate the raw data and alert the technologist that motion correction may be needed.

PHARMACOLOGIC STRESS TESTING FOR DETECTION OF CORONARY ARTERY DISEASE. Reports examining the sensitivity and specificity of vasodilator pharmacologic stress combined with MPI for the detection of CAD have achieved results similar to those reported with exercise stress. A pooled analysis from the 2003 ACC/AHA/ASNC Radionuclide Imaging Guidelines involving 2465 catheterized patients in 17 studies[6] demonstrated sensitivity of 89% and specificity of 75%, similar to values from exercise SPECT MPI studies.

The more powerful hyperemic stress response achieved with vasodilator stress compared with exercise might be expected to result in improved sensitivity to detect CAD, particularly more moderate stenoses. This has not been demonstrated, possibly because of the "roll-off" property of the common perfusion tracers, caused by diffusion limitation at hyperemic blood flow levels (see Fig. 17-23).[5] Thus, the more favorable hyperemic stress achieved with pharmacologic stress is offset by the lack of linear tracer uptake in the areas with the highest flow.

The diagnostic ability of dobutamine stress imaging appears to be generally similar to that of other pharmacologic and exercise stress modalities for the detection of CAD.[6] However, because maximal coronary flow reserve is not achieved as often as with vasodilator pharmacologic stress and side effects are substantial, dobutamine is recommended only when adenosine, dipyridamole, or regadenoson is contraindicated, such as in a patient with important reactive airways disease.

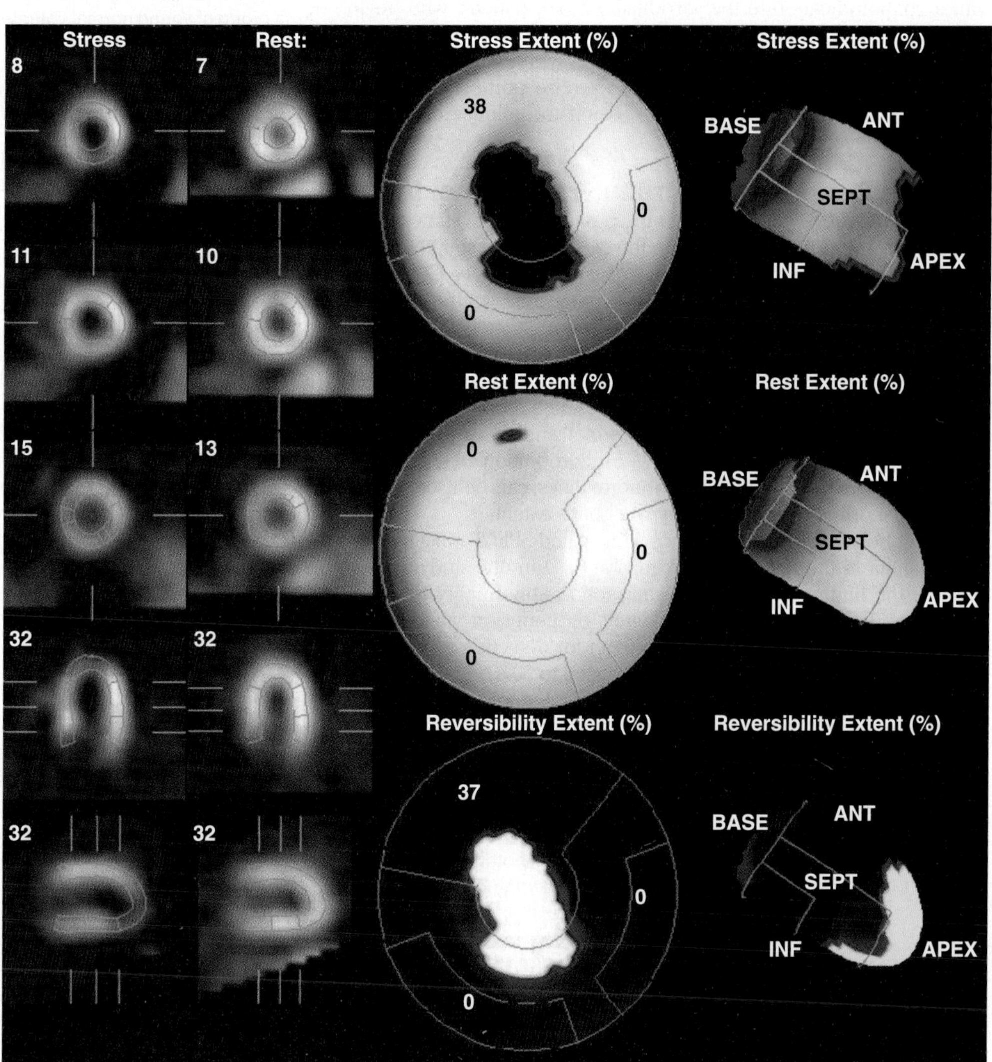

FIGURE 17-37 Automated quantitative analysis software. Selected short- and long-axis tomograms from stress and rest studies (two left columns) are automatically segmented and scored. Bull's-eye plots are created (third column) representing the stress (top) and rest (middle) data and demonstrate a large apical reversible defect. The bottom bull's-eye plot displays the extent of ischemic myocardium (white area), which measures 23% of the total myocardium. The bull's-eye information is also displayed in a three-dimensional format (right column, top, middle, and bottom, respectively). *(Images courtesy of Guido Germano, PhD.)*

EFFECT OF SUBMAXIMAL EXERCISE PERFORMANCE ON CORONARY ARTERY DISEASE DETECTION. The sensitivity of MPI to detect CAD is optimized by achieving the highest possible level of oxygen demand to stimulate the greatest increment in coronary flow reserve. In exercise ECG testing, sensitivity to detect CAD falls significantly if greater than 85% of maximum predicted heart rate for age is not achieved (see Chap. 14).[61] Because perfusion heterogeneity usually develops at a lower degree of supply-demand mismatch than electrocardiographic changes, the sensitivity of MPI to detect CAD is maintained at somewhat lower workloads. In one study, patients with CAD were stressed with MPI at a maximal workload and then again at a less than maximal workload.[2,6] There was no difference in sensitivity between the maximal and the submaximal tests. However, the extent and severity of reversible perfusion defects are diminished at submaximal compared with maximal workloads, which may affect the prognostic value of the test.

Thus, the selection of a stress protocol can be summarized as follows[2,6]: exercise is the preferred stressor, as it allows the optimal potential association of symptoms with perfusion abnormalities. The use of exercise also allows incorporation of validated stress test criteria such as the Duke Treadmill Score, heart rate reserve, or heart rate recovery with the MPI data.[23] For patients who cannot exercise adequately, vasodilator stress with adenosine, dipyridamole, or regadenoson is the procedure of choice; dobutamine is used for patients with a contraindication to the vasodilators.[2,6] For patients who begin exercise but do not reach 85% of maximum predicted heart rate for age or who do not reach an appropriate symptomatic endpoint, isotope injection can be withheld, the exercise portion of the test terminated, and vasodilator stress performed to optimize diagnostic and risk stratification information.

DETECTING AND DEFINING THE EXTENT OF CORONARY ARTERY DISEASE. In formulating a management strategy for patients, it is important to determine the extent of disease rather than just the presence or absence of disease. The term *extensive CAD* refers to angiographic patterns of CAD that have prognostic significance and suggest treatment benefit from revascularization, such as left main or severe three-vessel CAD involving the proximal LAD artery.

SPECT MPI is limited by the relative nature of the perfusion information; if all areas are hypoperfused in the presence of three-vessel CAD, the least hypoperfused area appears normal and the true extent of CAD may be underestimated. However, incorporation of other findings, including regional functional abnormalities, can be used to estimate more correctly the probability of disease extent.

Wall motion abnormalities on poststress gated SPECT imaging may be of benefit in the detection of extensive CAD. In one study,[62] incorporating the finding of poststress wall motion abnormality on gated SPECT imaging along with the degree of perfusion abnormality allowed improved sensitivity (85% to 91%) for detection of proximal 90% LAD lesions or multivessel disease related to 90% or greater proximal lesions. Similar findings have been reported to improve detection of three-vessel CAD.[63] Numerous reports suggest that the presence of transient ischemic dilation raises the probability of multivessel CAD for any given extent of perfusion abnormality.[2,6]

Findings unrelated to imaging are also useful in enhancing the diagnosis of left main or three-vessel CAD. The development of greater than 2 mm of ST depression or hypotension on ECG treadmill testing increases the likelihood of left main or three-vessel CAD.[61]

DETECTION OF CORONARY ARTERY DISEASE IN WOMEN. The detection of CAD by exercise ECG testing is problematic in women (see Chap. 81).[47,61] The use of ^{201}Tl for detection of CAD in women is limited by problems associated with breast attenuation. The use of ^{99m}Tc-labeled tracers should improve specificity as there is slightly less tissue attenuation, as demonstrated in a study comparing ^{201}Tl SPECT with ^{99m}Tc-sestamibi gated SPECT for the detection of angiographic CAD.[6] With the incorporation of gated SPECT sestamibi imaging, a specificity of 92% was achieved in one study compared with 67% with ^{201}Tl (see Fig. 17-12).

DETECTION OF CORONARY ARTERY DISEASE IN VALVULAR HEART DISEASE. Several studies have evaluated the use of MPI in the assessment of the possible copresence of CAD in patients with valvular heart disease; most of the published studies involved patients with aortic stenosis. Sensitivity of MPI has ranged from 61% to 100%, with specificity of 64% to 77%.[6] Although it is potentially useful in selected cases to assist in symptom evaluation, these performance characteristics are not sufficient to preclude the use of coronary angiography to define the presence of CAD in patients being considered for surgery (see Chap. 66).[40]

RADIONUCLIDE VENTRICULOGRAPHY FOR DETECTION OF CORONARY ARTERY DISEASE. Early reports of exercise RVG to detect CAD included predominantly patients with extensive CAD, resulting in high sensitivity. As the test was more widely applied to populations with less extensive disease, sensitivity values were lower. However, although the EF response to exercise may be a relatively insensitive marker of CAD, it is a powerful prognostic marker.[6]

As the LVEF response to exercise may be normal in many patients with less extensive CAD, a regional wall motion abnormality during exercise may be more sensitive for identification of CAD. RVG data during exercise are usually acquired in only one view, the left anterior oblique "best septal" view.[12] Thus, the view of the inferior wall is limited, and regional wall motion abnormalities are insensitive for disease of the right coronary artery.

The normal range for an exercise EF response was initially defined by a group of young normal volunteers, a population that differs from those with chest pain and normal coronary arteriograms. Post-test referral bias has also been invoked to explain the decline in specificity in exercise RVG. However, as with a normal MPI study, a preserved ventricular response to exercise is associated with a good prognosis,[12] despite the presence of CAD.

In contrast to studies of MPI demonstrating little change in the ability to detect CAD at slightly submaximal workloads, the sensitivity for detection of CAD by exercise RVG is impaired at submaximal workloads.[12] A similar problem would be expected with stress echocardiographic studies of inducible regional wall motion abnormalities.

Although exercise RVG is rarely used in contemporary practice, the EF response to exercise or the absolute value of the exercise EF is a powerful prognostic indicator in suspected or known CAD, and these data have informed the contemporary use of poststress ECG-gated SPECT imaging as well as stress echocardiography (see Chap. 15).

IMAGING IN PATIENTS WITH ESTABLISHED CORONARY ARTERY DISEASE. There are several potential roles for SPECT MPI in patients who are known to have established CAD. Clinical questions may remain after angiography regarding the "physiologic significance" of stenoses. The results of stress-rest SPECT MPI correlate generally with invasive measures of coronary flow reserve. Moreover, improvement of SPECT evidence of ischemia has been commonly documented after successful PCI, suggesting that SPECT MPI can identify the "culprit" ischemic lesion.[6]

Imaging After Coronary Artery Bypass Surgery

Studies of patients who develop recurrent symptoms after coronary artery bypass graft (CABG) surgery have demonstrated that SPECT MPI can accurately detect the presence and location of graft stenoses, even if the symptoms are atypical for ischemia.

A number of studies have concordantly demonstrated the risk stratification value of SPECT MPI in patients after CABG, especially late after CABG, even if symptoms are not present.[6] The extent of perfusion abnormality is related to the subsequent risk of cardiac death and nonfatal MI, and SPECT information has incremental predictive value over clinical and stress data. As the outcome risk is generally low in the early years after CABG, routine assessment for the presence and extent of ischemia in an asymptomatic patient is not recommended by current guidelines. Nonetheless, in a study of almost 900 asymptomatic patients studied with SPECT MPI after CABG,[6] perfusion defects were common and were associated with significantly increased relative risk of death or major events (as was impaired exercise capacity), even when controlling for time after CABG. In symptomatic post-CABG patients, such information can guide the need for catheterization and intervention. In asymptomatic patients, in whom aggressive secondary prevention strategies should be in place, the implications for clinical decision making are less clear. In this situation, the extent of SPECT abnormality is important, as a more extensive perfusion abnormality is associated with a progressively higher risk of subsequent cardiac death or MI[64] and at some threshold may justify an invasive approach.

Imaging After Percutaneous Coronary Intervention

Exercise MPI is superior in detecting the presence and location of restenosis after PCI compared with exercise ECG, and current guidelines recommend stress imaging in symptomatic post-PCI patients.[6] The extent of SPECT MPI abnormality in patients studied after PCI is correlated with the subsequent risk of cardiac death or MI on long-term follow-up, even late after PCI, and this appears to hold true in patients even in the absence of symptoms.[65] Thus, although routine assessment of asymptomatic patients after PCI with SPECT MPI is not currently recommended, important information may be gleaned by imaging of symptomatic patients to guide decisions for reintervention and in selected high-risk asymptomatic patients late after PCI to assess subsequent risk.[6]

Reports have suggested that very early after PCI, SPECT MPI may demonstrate a mild reversible defect in the territory of the treated vessel (although less severe than before PCI).[6] This may be due to delayed return of full coronary flow reserve after PCI, thus representing a true physiologic phenomenon.

Left Ventricular Function During Exercise in Patients with Known Coronary Artery Disease

The EF response to exercise (as determined by exercise RVG) can be considered a reflection of the impact of regional ischemia on global LV performance. Even among patients with three-vessel disease by angiography, the EF response to exercise may be maintained. This finding may be due to the possibility that only small areas of the left ventricle become ischemic if some of the stenoses are not physiologically significant or if distal vessels are well collateralized. Patients with three-vessel disease who have an abnormal exercise EF response are at high risk for adverse events during follow-up and thus are more likely to benefit from revascularization.[6] In contrast, patients who manifest a more normal EF response to exercise have a more favorable natural history and thus are less likely to benefit from revascularization in terms of natural history.

Detection of Preclinical Coronary Artery Disease and Risk Stratification in Asymptomatic Subjects

As sudden cardiac death is too often the first manifestation of CAD, there is interest in screening populations for CAD or for CAD risk. On the basis of Bayesian principles, the low prevalence of CAD in the general asymptomatic population results in low predictive value of a positive test, although negative predictive value is high. Current guidelines do not recommend routine stress MPI in asymptomatic populations.[6]

There may be circumstances, however, in which the baseline risk of a specific asymptomatic population may warrant testing with MPI. In a study of asymptomatic siblings of patients with known CAD, an abnormal SPECT MPI was associated with a fivefold increase in risk for cardiac events, with higher relative risk if both stress MPI and ECG were abnormal.[66] A key question in considering the use of testing such as SPECT MPI in asymptomatic populations is how the information will be used to manage or to reduce risk. Current guidelines suggest aggressive risk factor reduction in those at high clinical risk for the development of vascular disease.[67] Whether further intensification of risk factor reduction in the setting of an abnormal imaging test, or diminished aggressiveness of risk factor reduction in the setting of a normal MPI study, results in improved outcomes is unproved and worthy of study.

Patients with diabetes are at significant risk for CAD development and cardiac events. An emerging body of literature suggests that a substantial proportion of asymptomatic diabetic patients have abnormal SPECT MPI studies and that such patients may be at even higher risk for events over time. Studies have suggested that 20% to 40% of asymptomatic diabetic patients have abnormal SPECT MPI studies, often with evidence of inducible, silent ischemia.[68,69] SPECT MPI has substantial risk stratification value in patients with diabetes, with risk being higher for any given perfusion abnormality than in nondiabetic patients. A randomized trial of screening asymptomatic diabetic patients with stress SPECT MPI versus not screening showed no differences in outcomes during long-term follow-up, with event rates low in both groups.[70] Thus, guidelines at present do not suggest routine screening of asymptomatic diabetic patients with stress SPECT MPI.

Myocardial Perfusion Imaging After CT Coronary Calcium Imaging or CT Angiography

With the growing availability and use of noninvasive CT cardiac imaging (see Chap. 19), clinicians are now commonly faced with a patient with substantial coronary artery calcium (CAC), raising the possibility of multivessel CAD, or with apparent moderate or even severe stenoses seen on CT coronary angiography, raising questions about physiologic significance and risk stratification.

SPECT MPI and Coronary Calcium Imaging. Although extensive CAC and a high coronary calcium score are indicative of atherosclerosis, studies to date have suggested that even extensive CAC is associated with important myocardial perfusion abnormalities only in a minority of patients. In one study of more than 1000 patients (approximately 50% of whom were asymptomatic), among those with the highest coronary calcium scores (>400), only approximately 10% had abnormal perfusion on stress SPECT MPI, and only 5% had "high-risk" SPECT MPI perfusion patterns,[71] suggesting potential benefit from revascularization (see Fig. 17-e7A on website). Thus, the presence of even extensive CAC on CT imaging, although well validated to represent atherosclerosis deserving of aggressive risk factor modification, does not always represent obstructive stenoses resulting in stress-induced perfusion abnormalities. On the basis of this concept, stress SPECT MPI is an appropriate test to perform to evaluate the need for and potential benefit of catheterization and potential revascularization after CT imaging demonstration of CAC.[72]

Refining Risk Stratification by Incorporating Both CT Calcium Imaging and SPECT MPI. Substantial literature now documents that patients with CAC, especially if it is extensive, are at higher risk of cardiac events over time compared with those with no CAC. Yet among those with extensive calcification, many will have normal stress perfusion on MPI, a finding that extensive published data suggest is associated with low risk. How can these seemingly contradictory bodies of literature be reconciled? It is important to understand that "high risk" is a relative term, that is, patients with extensive CAC are at higher risk than those without CAC; but among those with extensive CAC, most will still not have events. For example, in the Multi-Ethnic Study of Atherosclerosis (MESA), there was a clear gradient of risk as CAC scores increased, but the absolute risk of events was low (roughly 1% per year even among those with high calcium scores).[73] Investigators have suggested that the implications of combining data from CT assessment of CAC and information from SPECT MPI may be to allow a refinement of risk stratification.[74] Conceptually, those patients with no CAC and normal SPECT MPI should have the lowest risk, and those patients with both evidence of CAC and abnormal SPECT MPI the highest risk. Patients with either CAC or abnormal SPECT MPI should have intermediate risk. Thus, information from the two testing modalities may be complementary in the sense of the ability to refine risk predictions about outcomes and potentially tailoring the aggressiveness of secondary prevention. Studies are ongoing in this regard.

SPECT MPI and CT Angiography. With the growing availability and technical evolution of multidetector CT angiography (see Chap. 19), clinicians may now be faced with new questions about the physiologic significance of noninvasively detected coronary stenoses. Whereas current CT angiography data demonstrate high sensitivity and moderate specificity to detect or to rule out obstructive stenoses, the spatial resolution is still not of a caliber such that accurate determination of the severity of an individual stenosis is consistently reliable or quantifiable. Moreover, in a coronary segment that is heavily calcified, stenoses are particularly difficult to detect, to rule out, or to quantitate. SPECT MPI can assess the physiologic significance of a stenosis during stress and potentially link the perfusion abnormality to the patient's symptoms. In one study representative of the literature to date,[75] many stenoses considered obstructive (i.e., >50% stenosis) by CT angiography were associated with normal stress SPECT MPI (see Fig. 17-e7B on website). These important data give pause to the concept of moving directly to invasive angiography (and potential PCI) after CT angiography and suggest that assessment of the physiologic significance of CT angiography–defined stenoses may be important for clinical decision making.

Radionuclide Imaging in Acute Coronary Syndromes

APPLICATION OF RADIONUCLIDE IMAGING: ANSWERING THE CLINICAL QUESTIONS. For patients with suspected ACS, radionuclide imaging techniques can both play a diagnostic role (Is the clinical syndrome due to ischemia and CAD?) and provide prognostic information. Among patients who present with an ACS and ST-segment depression or elevation, the typical role for imaging is in the stabilized patient to provide risk stratification information to drive management strategies aimed at improving natural history.

SUSPECTED ACUTE CORONARY SYNDROMES IN THE EMERGENCY DEPARTMENT. Many patients presenting to emergency departments with symptoms suggestive of ACS but with nondiagnostic initial ECG and biomarker findings are admitted to an observation unit for serial biomarker studies and possible stress testing. ^{99m}Tc-based perfusion agents may be administered to a patient in the emergency department at rest, with images acquired 45 to 60 minutes later,[76] and as there is minimal redistribution, images reflect myocardial blood flow at the time of injection.

In this setting, negative predictive value for ruling out MI is high in all observational series.[76] Patients with positive MPI have a higher risk of cardiac events during the index hospitalization as well as during follow-up (**Fig. 17-38**). Thus, rest SPECT MPI can provide information to assist triage decisions (admit or not admit) in the emergency department.

One study[76] reported that SPECT sestamibi imaging performed in the emergency department was 92% sensitive for detection of acute MI, whereas initial troponin I values in samples drawn at the same time had a sensitivity of only 39%. The maximum troponin I during the first 24 hours had a sensitivity similar to that of rest sestamibi imaging but at a distinctly later time point. Thus, acute MPI has the potential to identify ACS earlier than biomarkers. SPECT perfusion imaging data have been shown to provide incremental risk stratification value over clinical data for prediction of unfavorable cardiac events.[10] One small randomized study[77] of 46 emergency department patients with ongoing chest pain and a nondiagnostic ECG reported that an MPI-guided strategy incurred lower costs and resulted in shorter lengths of stay.

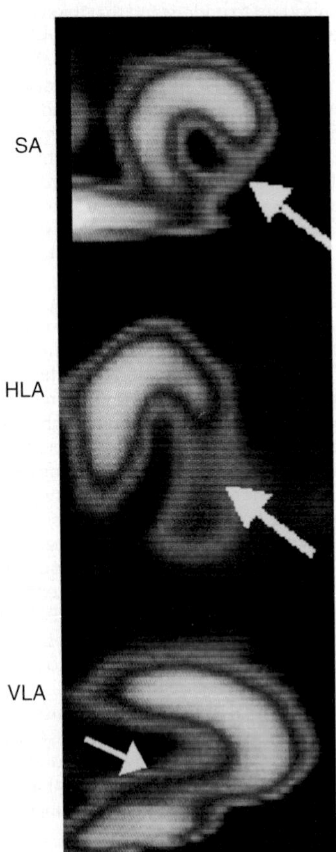

FIGURE 17-38 Example of resting SPECT images in a patient evaluated in the emergency department with chest pain and nondiagnostic initial electrocardiographic findings. A severe inferolateral resting perfusion defect (arrows) suggests resting ischemia or infarction in that territory. Subsequent emergent angiography demonstrated an occluded left circumflex artery. HLA = horizontal long axis; SA = short axis; VLA = vertical long axis.

The Emergency Room Assessment of Sestamibi for Evaluation (ERASE) of chest pain trial[78] of 2475 patients with symptoms suggestive of ACS reported a significant 20% relative reduction in unnecessary admissions of patients ultimately found not to have ACS for those randomly assigned to incorporation of MPI into the emergency department evaluation strategy. The imaging data were among the most powerful factors associated with the decision to discharge the patient appropriately from the emergency department.

Thus, evidence from controlled, randomized trials suggests that incorporation of SPECT MPI in the evaluation of emergency department patients with suspected ACS but no definitive electrocardiographic changes can improve triage decisions. The ACC/AHA/ASNC Radionuclide Imaging Guidelines classify MPI in this setting as a Class I, Level A indication.[6]

NON–ST-SEGMENT ELEVATION MYOCARDIAL INFARCTION AND UNSTABLE ANGINA. Guidelines suggest that patients with high-risk clinical characteristics in the setting of unstable angina should undergo direct catheterization.[46] Contemporary clinical trials suggest that patients with positive biomarkers, or those with a high-risk Thrombolysis in Myocardial Infarction (TIMI) score, benefit in terms of outcomes from an "invasive" strategy.[79] For patients with intermediate or low clinical risk (i.e., with "medically stabilized" unstable angina), stress MPI has been shown to have substantial risk stratification value.[6] Patients without ischemia or infarction, especially in the presence of preserved LV function, have a low-risk outcome, suggesting that such patients can be managed conservatively without catheterization (**Fig. 17-39**), whereas patients with significant inducible ischemia are at high risk and thus are selected for intervention (see Fig. 17-39). Guidelines[6] classify the use of stress MPI for detection of residual ischemia as a Class I indication.

Although the results of randomized clinical trials such as Treat Angina with Aggrastat and determine Cost of Therapy with an Invasive or Conservative Strategy (TACTICS)–TIMI 18 and others suggest slight superiority of an invasive approach in patients with unstable angina or non–ST-segment elevation MI, subgroup analyses suggest that an important proportion of patients may be well managed by the conservative strategy of risk stratification by MPI followed by more selective catheterization and intervention. Moreover, a recent large randomized trial of patients with ACS and positive troponin T found no difference in outcomes between an invasive strategy and a selectively invasive strategy in which patients were examined for the presence of ischemia before selection for catheterization while receiving contemporary aggressive medical therapy.[80] In TACTICS–TIMI 18, the troponin-positive subgroup, constituting 60% of the total population, had a larger reduction in death or MI with the early invasive strategy, whereas there was no difference in outcomes in those patients with negative troponins.[79] Therefore, TACTICS type patients without elevation of troponin or high TIMI risk score[81] may be optimally managed by a more conservative approach with risk stratification by use of imaging techniques.

ST-SEGMENT ELEVATION MYOCARDIAL INFARCTION. Clinical variables such as recurrent ischemia, heart failure, and nonacute arrhythmias during hospitalization for acute ST-segment elevation MI (STEMI) identify a subgroup of patients at high risk in whom early catheterization and intervention are indicated.[82] However, patients surviving the initial acute period may have a relatively stable course, and current guidelines suggest that noninvasive risk stratification before hospital discharge is appropriate.[6,82]

Assessment of Inducible Ischemia after Acute Myocardial Infarction

Three major determinants of natural history risk after an acute MI include residual resting LV function; the extent of ischemic, jeopardized myocardium; and the susceptibility to ventricular arrhythmias. Gated SPECT MPI, on the basis of the comprehensive ability to provide much of this information, has the potential to be the single most important test in the stable patient after STEMI.

In one of the earliest studies to examine the relation of MPI data to outcomes in stable patients after MI, ^{201}Tl scintigraphic data contained the most robust information on stratifying post-MI risk. A "low-risk" ^{201}Tl image (no reversible defects and no lung uptake) was associated with a low-risk natural history outcome after MI.[48]

An important proportion of patients after uncomplicated MI are not able to exercise, even to a submaximal workload. With use of pharmacologic stress MPI in the post-MI setting, the presence of reversible defects has been reported as the only significant predictor of cardiac events on multivariable analysis,[48] whereas the absence of reversible defects identified a low-risk cohort.

Studies in the reperfusion era have reported generally similar results about the relation of stress-induced ischemia to post-MI outcomes. In a study of 134 consecutive patients within 14 days of an uncomplicated MI, the extent of ischemia on SPECT MPI was the only significant correlate of a future cardiac event on Cox regression analysis (see Fig. 17-e8 on website). The extent of SPECT ischemia remained a strong correlate of a cardiac event in those who received thrombolytic therapy. The quantitated extent of ischemia on adenosine SPECT MPI has also been shown to be an important predictor of cardiac events in post-MI risk stratification. Post-MI patients with extensive inducible ischemia are at high risk for future cardiac events, and interventional management is likely to result in improved outcome.

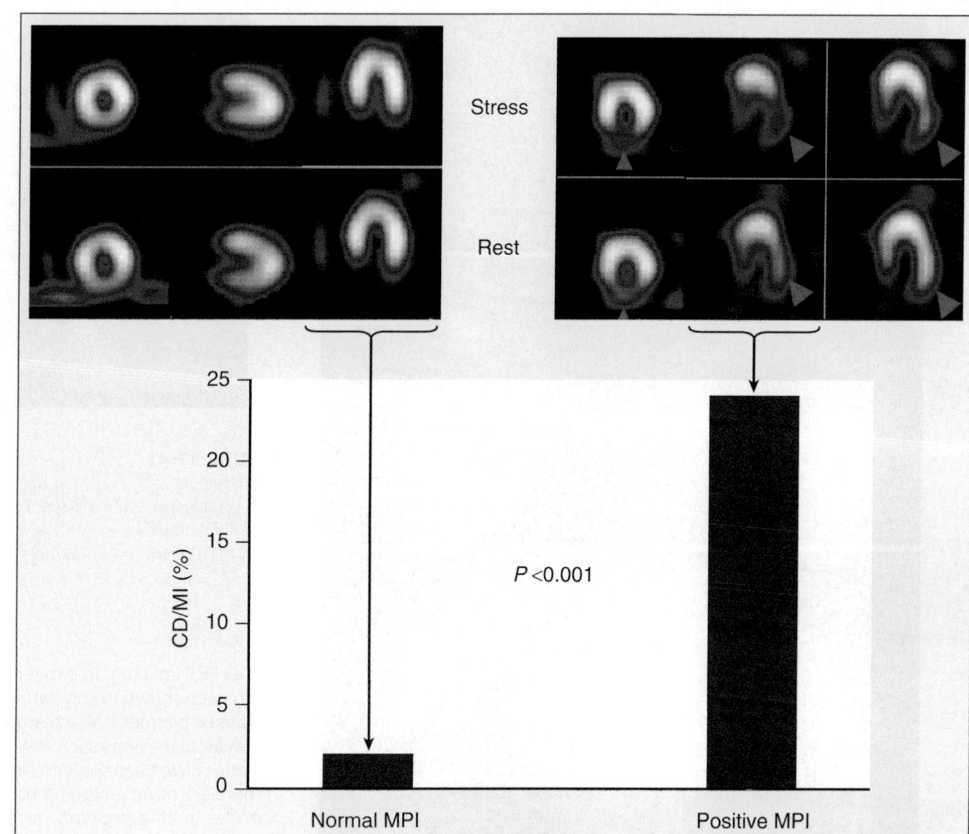

FIGURE 17-39 SPECT perfusion imaging in patients after medical stabilization of unstable angina. **Upper left,** Normal study, associated with a low risk of cardiac events during follow-up, suggesting that such a patient can be managed conservatively without catheterization but with aggressive secondary preventive strategies. The bottom graph is a summary of predictive values of SPECT imaging in the aftermath of unstable angina from multiple studies. Similar to the concepts in populations with stable chest pain, abnormal perfusion imaging after unstable angina is associated with a substantial increase in the risk of cardiac death or myocardial infarction (CD/MI) during follow-up. **Upper right,** An example of a high-risk stress-rest SPECT MPI study in the aftermath of unstable angina. Despite the stabilization of symptoms, extensive reversible perfusion abnormalities in the inferior and lateral walls suggest high risk of cardiac death or myocardial infarction, or both, during follow-up. Thus, this patient would be managed more aggressively with catheterization and intervention. *(Modified in part from Brown KA: Management of unstable angina: The role on noninvasive risk stratification. J Nucl Cardiol 4:S164, 1997.)*

Very Early Post–Myocardial Infarction Risk Stratification

Because pharmacologic vasodilator stressors induce coronary hyperemia with only minimal increments in oxygen demand, it may potentially be performed safely even very early after MI. This concept was examined in a study of 451 patients randomly assigned to a standard post-MI evaluation strategy or to a strategy incorporating dipyridamole SPECT MPI 2 to 3 days after uncomplicated MI. The testing was safe, and MPI supplied better risk stratification data predicting outcomes than the submaximal stress MPI data.[24] Thus, pharmacologic stress can safely allow management decisions to be made earlier in the post-MI course.

Studies Examining Both Perfusion Imaging and Left Ventricular Function After Acute Myocardial Infarction

As post-MI EF falls, there is a progressive increase in mortality risk. The availability of gated SPECT imaging to evaluate myocardial perfusion and LV function simultaneously raises an important question about the incremental information provided by combining the analysis of perfusion and function information within one test.

One study comprehensively evaluated LV function and adenosine SPECT MPI in patients in relation to long-term cardiac events. Both the extent of perfusion defect and LVEF provided superior risk categorization compared with either variable alone. These data strongly suggest that perfusion abnormalities and LVEF after MI have complementary roles, and their measurement together powerfully categorizes patients' risk in the post-MI setting (see Fig. 17-e8 on website).

RADIONUCLIDE IMAGING FOR ACUTE CORONARY SYNDROMES: RESEARCH DIRECTIONS

Imaging of Ischemic Memory

A possible future approach to risk stratification in patients with suspected ACS involves the imaging of fatty acid metabolism. As noted earlier, after a regional ischemic insult, abnormalities in fatty acid metabolism may persist long after perfusion has returned to normal, a finding termed ischemic memory. Imaging of fatty acid metabolism may therefore allow assessment of recent ischemia. Uptake of the radiolabeled fatty acid analogue BMIPP has been imaged with SPECT 1 to 5 days after presentation in patients with suspected ACS. In an early study, the BMIPP images showed greater sensitivity than did rest MPI in identifying the presence and site of the culprit coronary stenosis (**Fig. 17-40**).[83] Recent multicenter data have shown that SPECT imaging of fatty acid metabolism in patients presenting to emergency departments with suspected ACS adds incremental value to initial clinical information for assessment of the presence or absence of an

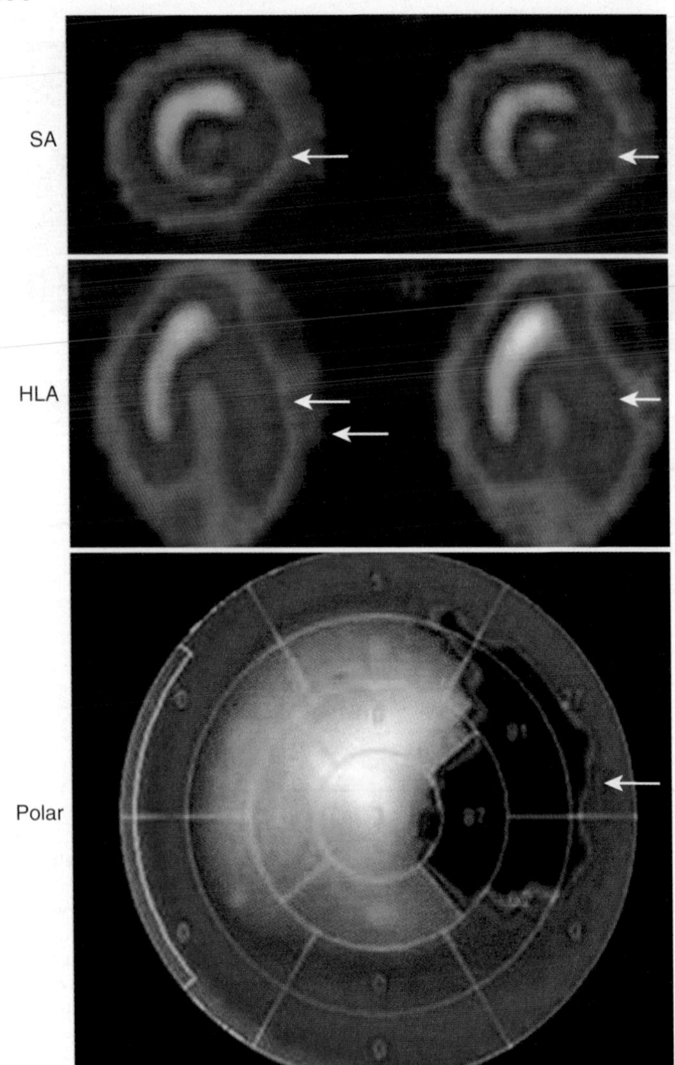

FIGURE 17-40 Iodine-123–labeled beta-methyliodopentadecanoic acid (BMIPP) imaging of ischemic memory in a patient presenting to an emergency department with a suspected acute coronary syndrome. In the top row, short-axis (SA) tomograms demonstrate a significant lateral wall defect (arrows), suggesting prolonged postischemic suppression of fatty acid metabolism, referred to as ischemic memory. Horizontal long-axis (HLA) images also demonstrate the defect (arrows), as does the polar map (bottom row). Subsequent angiography demonstrated a severe stenosis of the left circumflex coronary artery. *(Modified from Kontos MC, Dilsizian V, Weiland F, et al: Iodofiltic acid I 123 [BMIPP] fatty acid imaging improves initial diagnosis in emergency department patients with suspected acute coronary syndromes: A multicenter trial. J Am Coll Cardiol 256:290, 2010.)*

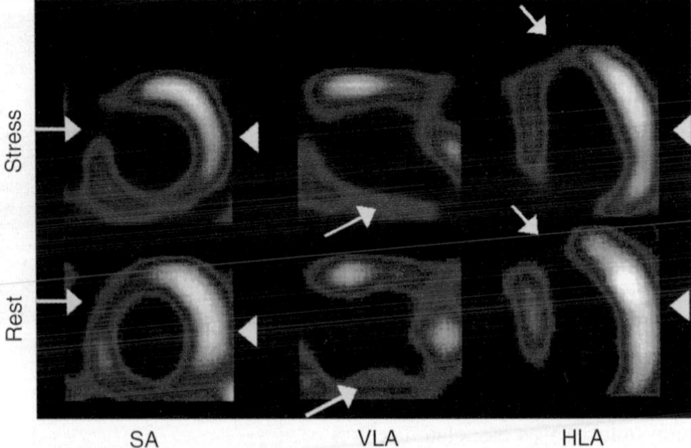

FIGURE 17-41 SPECT perfusion imaging demonstrating extensive severe fixed defects of the septum, apex, and inferior wall (arrows) suggestive of extensive prior myocardial infarction as well as extensive inducible ischemia of the lateral wall (arrowheads). This strongly suggests that coronary artery disease is the cause of the heart failure syndrome in this patient. HLA = horizontal long axis; SA = short axis; VLA = vertical long axis.

ACS.[84] Future studies will determine whether such techniques can help guide management decisions.

Imaging of Potentially Unstable Atherosclerotic Plaques and Platelet Activation. The emphasis of current cardiovascular imaging modalities is on the anatomic detection of coronary artery luminal narrowing. However, in the clinical setting, vulnerable plaques that are not flow limiting may account for the majority of cardiovascular events. Vulnerable atherosclerotic plaques typically have a necrotic lipid core with a thin fibrous cap and large amount of macrophages. When such vulnerable plaques rupture, they cause MI, sudden death, or stroke. Thus, the biologic composition and inflammatory state of an atherosclerotic plaque, rather than its degree of stenosis or size, may be the major determinants for acute clinical events.[85] Hence, the pursuit for development of noninvasive imaging techniques that target vulnerable plaques is a laudable goal.

Studies have demonstrated the clinical feasibility of direct visualization and characterization of coronary and carotid artery plaques with FDG PET imaging. In experimental studies, the intensity of FDG uptake has been shown to correlate with macrophage density and inflammatory state of plaques.[86] Vascular plaque FDG uptake has been linked to cardiovascular events such as MI and stroke.[87] Anti-inflammatory drugs and statins have been shown to attenuate FDG uptake in plaques.[88,89] Whereas there are other emerging tracers that target specific pathways and molecules in atherosclerotic lesions, such as apoptosis, $\alpha_v\beta_3$ integrins, and matrix metalloproteinase, they remain predominantly in the experimental phase. Combined functional and structural whole-body imaging will likely afford the best potential for visualization of coronary atherosclerosis and plaque inflammation.[90] However, the limitations of the partial volume effect of small plaques, low target-to-background ratio of radiopharmaceuticals, and cardiac motion make direct visualization of atherosclerotic plaques in coronary arteries with the current hybrid PET-CT technology challenging.[85]

Plaque rupture exposes the lipid core to platelet activation. ^{125}I-labeled low-density lipoprotein has been used to image atherosclerotic disease in carotid arteries. A radionuclide target for macrophages, ^{131}I-labeled monocyte chemoattractant protein 1, has been shown to accumulate in lipid-rich, macrophage-rich regions in animal models of atherosclerosis.[91] Whether these favorable results in animals can be translated to the clinical setting of patients with potentially unstable atherosclerosis is a subject of ongoing study.

Assessment of Heart Failure with Radionuclide Imaging

IS CORONARY ARTERY DISEASE THE CAUSE OF HEART FAILURE? Determination of whether LV dysfunction is due predominantly to the consequences of CAD or to one of the many other causes included in "nonischemic" cardiomyopathy is a critical early step in the management of patients with heart failure. Because CAD is the most common cause of heart failure in developed countries,[92] noninvasive assessment of myocardial ischemia and viability would identify the subgroup of patients with heart failure who have a potentially reversible degree of LV dysfunction and may benefit from revascularization. Therapeutic interventions that improve dysfunctional but viable myocardium may significantly affect global LVEF, LV remodeling, and survival. The identification of CAD in patients with heart failure also has implications in secondary prevention strategies, as recurrent MI is a common mechanism of death in patients with heart failure.

A normal stress MPI scan in a patient with heart failure and LV dysfunction is highly predictive for the absence of CAD. Studies of MPI for detection of CAD in patients with LV dysfunction have shown high sensitivity but modest specificity (**Fig. 17-41**; see Fig. 17-36).[57] The modest specificity of MPI to rule out CAD is explained in part by pathologic and CMR studies[93] demonstrating that patients with nonischemic cardiomyopathy may have patchy or larger confluent territories of fibrosis or scarring (see Chap. 18), manifested as fixed defects on SPECT MPI. Invasive studies as well as PET imaging have demonstrated attenuated coronary blood flow at rest and during hyperemic stress in nonischemic cardiomyopathy,[16,94] which could be manifested as reversible defects.

Although the presence of any perfusion abnormality is not specific for ruling out CAD, the pattern of perfusion abnormality may assist in the differentiation between CAD and nonischemic etiology of heart failure. More extensive or more severe perfusion defects, or both, are more likely to represent CAD, whereas smaller and milder defects are more likely in patients with nonischemic cardiomyopathy.[6,57]

ASSESSMENT OF MYOCARDIAL VIABILITY AND THE POTENTIAL BENEFIT OF REVASCULARIZATION. The goal of assessing viability is to optimize selection of patients with heart failure whose symptoms and natural history may improve after revascularization. Data suggest that hibernation and stress-induced ischemia are common in patients with stable heart failure, even in the absence of angina.[95] In a clinical trial of stable community-based patients with heart failure, of whom only a minority had angina, hibernation or stress-induced ischemia or both were demonstrated by SPECT imaging in approximately 70% of patients, suggesting that an important subpopulation of patients with heart failure may benefit from a noninvasive search for viability and ischemia.

Studies have demonstrated that the potential for improved heart failure symptoms after revascularization correlates with the magnitude of the PET mismatch pattern (i.e., enhanced FDG uptake relative to perfusion).[6] In a meta-analysis of outcome studies after viability imaging, patients with evidence of preserved myocardial viability[96] who underwent revascularization had a substantial reduction in the risk of cardiac death during long-term follow-up (**Fig. 17-42**). Revascularization conferred no natural history advantage in patients without substantial myocardial viability. These data suggest that noninvasive imaging of viability and ischemia can play an important role in selecting patients for revascularization, with the expectation of improving symptoms and natural history.

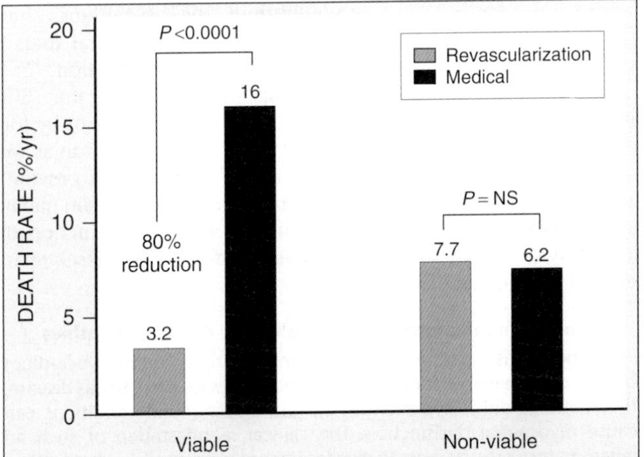

FIGURE 17-42 Meta-analysis demonstrating outcome of patients with ischemic left ventricular dysfunction after viability testing. Among patients determined to have predominantly viable myocardium, treatment with medical therapy is associated with a 16% annual risk of cardiac death. Similar patients treated with revascularization have only a 3.2% annual risk of cardiac death, representing an 80% reduction in risk with revascularization. In contrast, patients with predominantly nonviable myocardium have no difference in outcome whether they are treated with medical therapy or revascularization. These data suggest that noninvasive interrogation of myocardial viability can identify treatment strategies associated with more favorable long-term outcomes. *(Modified from Allman K, Shaw L, Hachamovitch R, Udelson JE: Myocardial viability testing and impact of revascularization on prognosis in patients with coronary artery disease and left ventricular dysfunction: A meta-analysis. J Am Coll Cardiol 39:1151, 2002.)*

Principles of Assessing Myocardial Viability by Radionuclide Techniques

The radionuclide tracers and techniques most often used to assess viability have been evaluated for their relation to preserved tissue viability directly by correlation of tracer uptake with histologically confirmed extent of tissue viability.[97] Quantitative analysis of tracer uptake correlates directly with the magnitude of preservation of tissue viability, and tracer uptake represents a continuous variable; that is, the magnitude of tracer uptake directly reflects the magnitude of preserved tissue viability.[97,98] For a dysfunctional segment or territory, the probability of functional recovery after revascularization is related to the magnitude of tracer uptake, representing the degree of preserved myocardial viability (extent of hibernation or stunning) within that territory. A dysfunctional territory with normal or only mildly reduced tracer uptake thus has a high likelihood of improved function after revascularization. In contrast, a territory with a severe reduction in tracer uptake would represent predominant infarction, and the likelihood of improved function after revascularization would be low (**Fig. 17-43**). The magnitude of potential improvement of global LV function after revascularization is in turn determined by the extent of viable dysfunctional myocardium.

Imaging Protocols for Assessment of Myocardial Viability

THALLIUM-201. The presence of ^{201}Tl after redistribution implies preserved myocyte cellular viability. However, as the absence of ^{201}Tl uptake on the redistribution images is not a sufficient sign of the absence of regional viability, iterations of the standard ^{201}Tl protocol have been investigated[5] to optimize the assessment of regional viability (**Fig. 17-44**). After ^{201}Tl reinjection, approximately 50% of regions with fixed defects on stress-redistribution imaging show significant enhancement of ^{201}Tl uptake, predictive of improvement in regional LV function.[98a] The presence of a severe ^{201}Tl defect after reinjection identifies areas with a very low probability of improvement in function.

Late redistribution imaging, 24 to 48 hours after the initial stress ^{201}Tl injection, allows more time for redistribution to occur and has good positive predictive value for improvement in function. Even with late redistribution imaging, the negative predictive value is suboptimal, as redistribution does not occur in some patients even after a prolonged time, and in addition, image quality may be poor.[5,6] In such patients, ^{201}Tl reinjection after late redistribution imaging may provide further insight into defect reversibility and hence viability.

With rest-redistribution ^{201}Tl imaging, images are obtained 15 to 20 minutes after tracer injection at rest, reflecting resting regional blood flow, and images obtained 3 to 4 hours after redistribution reflect preserved viability. The finding of a reversible resting defect may identify areas of myocardial hibernation (see Fig. 17-44). This finding appears to be an insensitive although specific sign of potential improvement in regional function.[6]

TECHNETIUM 99m SESTAMIBI AND TETROFOSMIN. Studies have demonstrated that the performance of these agents for prediction of improvement in regional function after revascularization is similar to that of ^{201}Tl.[6] Administration of nitrates to improve resting blood flow before injection of sestamibi appears to improve slightly the ability of these tracers to detect myocardial viability.[5,6]

POSITRON EMISSION TOMOGRAPHY. The extent of the PET mismatch pattern (enhanced FDG uptake relative to blood flow; see Fig. 17-30) correlates with improvement in LV function after revascularization as well as with the clinical course, magnitude of improvement in heart failure symptoms, and survival after revascularization.[5,6,13] Patients with heart failure and an extensive PET match pattern (diminished blood flow and severe reduction in FDG uptake), representing predominant infarction, are unlikely to benefit clinically from revascularization.

COMPARISON OF IMAGING TECHNIQUES FOR VIABILITY ASSESSMENT. On the basis of a meta-analysis evaluating the ability of the various radionuclide techniques to predict improvements in regional function, all the radionuclide techniques (as well as low-dose dobutamine echocardiography) perform in a relatively similar manner regarding positive and negative predictive values for

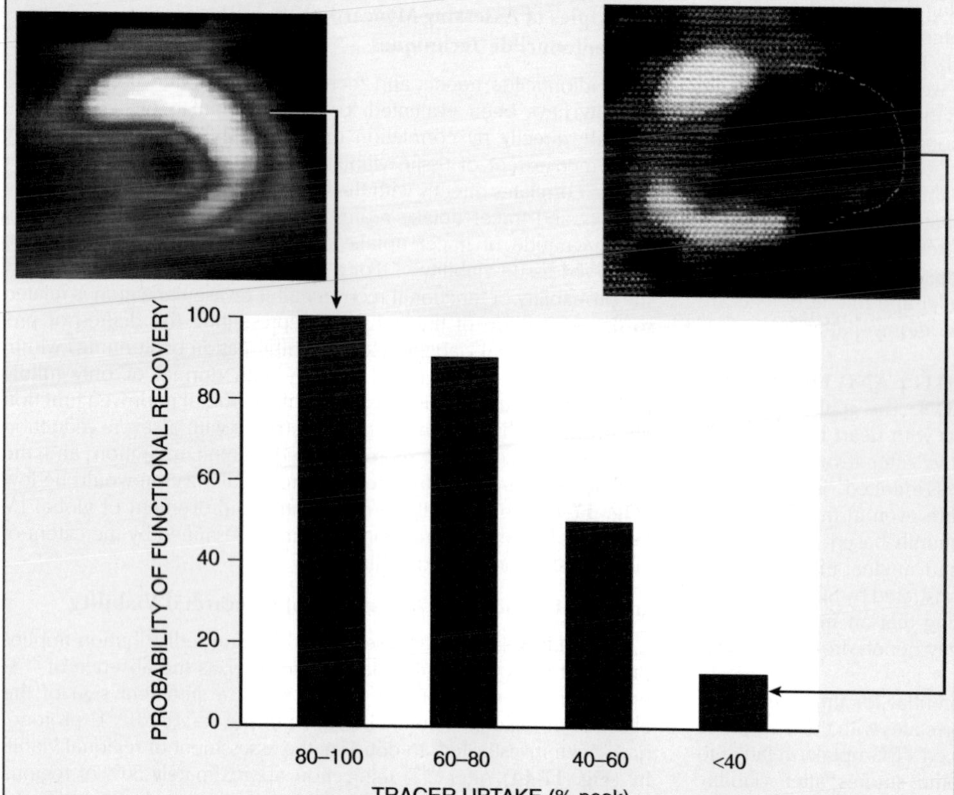

FIGURE 17-43 Relation between tracer uptake in a dysfunctional territory and the subsequent probability of functional recovery after revascularization. The probability of improved regional left ventricular function after revascularization is significantly related to the quantitative degree of tracer uptake. **Upper right,** A patient with a large, severe defect in the anterior and apical walls. The severity of the defect suggests that significant functional recovery would not be expected with revascularization. **Upper left,** Extensive myocardial viability in a patient with left ventricular dysfunction (ejection fraction 30%) and severe three-vessel coronary disease. There is substantial tracer uptake throughout the anterior wall and apex (arrow), territories with significant regional dysfunction. The retained degree of tracer uptake suggests extensive myocardial (myocyte) viability and high probability of functional recovery after revascularization. *(Modified from Bonow RO: Assessment of myocardial viability with thallium-201. In Zaret BL, Beller GA [eds]: Nuclear Cardiology: State of the Art and Future Directions. St. Louis, Mosby, 1999, pp 503-512; and Udelson JE: Assessment of myocardial viability with technetium-99m–labeled agents. In Zaret BL, Beller GA [eds]: Nuclear Cardiology: State of the Art and Future Directions. St. Louis, Mosby, 1999, pp 513-533.)*

improvements in regional function.[97] SPECT techniques appear to be slightly more sensitive, dobutamine echocardiography appears to be slightly more specific, and PET techniques appear to have better accuracy. A randomized trial of patients with moderate LV dysfunction being considered for revascularization randomly allocated to have viability information supplied by either PET imaging or SPECT stress-rest sestamibi imaging found no difference in outcomes during long-term follow-up.[99] As noted previously, a meta-analysis of observational outcome studies related to myocardial viability demonstrated no difference among the techniques commonly used to assess viability (PET versus SPECT versus dobutamine echocardiography) with regard to reduction of mortality after revascularization (see Fig. 17-42).[96]

Selection of Patients with Heart Failure for Viability Assessment

Guidelines suggest that patients with heart failure and active angina benefit in terms of natural history from revascularization and thus should be referred directly for angiography.[100] In some situations, subsequent noninvasive definition of regional viability and ischemia may be important to plan the revascularization strategy when the anatomy is known.

For patients with heart failure and no angina, recommendations are less clear. Studies suggest that ischemia and viability may be present in a significant proportion of such patients, who have potential benefit from revascularization[95]; and for most patients with heart failure, a search for underlying ischemia and viability would be an appropriate clinical strategy at some point in their evaluation. If substantial ischemia or viability of dysfunctional territories is found in the setting of vessels technically amenable to revascularization, the literature would suggest a clinical benefit from revascularization.[6] In the absence of substantial ischemia or viability, such a benefit is less likely. The imaging data can be used in decision making to help balance the risks and benefits of revascularization in a patient with heart failure and LV dysfunction by supplying information on potential benefit of a revascularization strategy.

ASSESSMENT OF LEFT VENTRICULAR FUNCTION IN HEART FAILURE. For patients with the clinical syndrome of heart failure, the distinction between those patients with preserved and those with impaired systolic function has important clinical relevance. Clinical trials evaluating the use of such therapies as ACE inhibitors, angiotensin receptor blockers, and beta blockers have focused on the subpopulation of heart failure patients with impaired systolic function.[100] Thus, accurate determination of LV function in a patient with heart failure defines the evidence-based therapeutic approach that should be undertaken.

On the basis of the quantitative and reproducible nature of the EF results, equilibrium RVG techniques have been used in large clinical trials to identify systolic dysfunction.[6,100] In contemporary practice, the ECG-gated SPECT technique is often used for determination of systolic function. The simultaneous assessment of LV systolic function as well as stress and rest perfusion by gated SPECT imaging can provide a range of information relevant to the care and clinical decision making for patients with heart failure, including the state of LV function, the probability of CAD as the cause of heart failure, and the presence and extent of viability and ischemia.

Imaging in Inflammatory and Infiltrative Cardiomyopathies

MYOCARDITIS (see Chap. 70). Inflammatory injury to the myocardium by infective agents, postinfective immune processes (i.e., Chagas disease, rheumatic carditis), hypersensitivity, and autoimmune conditions can cause myocardial dysfunction. The clinical manifestation of such an inflammatory process is acute myocarditis and cardiac allograft rejection. As myocyte necrosis is an obligatory component of myocarditis (cellular infiltrates, predominantly lymphocytes and macrophages, clustered around necrotic myocytes), ^{111}In-labeled antimyosin antibody, which specifically targets myosin heavy chain, has been used for the detection of necrosis associated with myocarditis and heart transplant rejection. In patients with biopsy-positive myocarditis, the sensitivity of an antimyosin scan is approximately 95%, with a negative predictive value of approximately 95%. However, the specificity and positive predictive value of antimyosin imaging are modest, in the 50% range.[101] In cardiac allograft recipients, there is a general relationship between the severity of transplant rejection by biopsy and the magnitude of antimyosin uptake by scintigraphy. However, the highly variable antimyosin uptake across the severity range of rejection, as well as lack of general availability, precludes antimyosin imaging as a sufficiently reliable noninvasive test for detection of transplant rejection.[102] Observational studies with myocardial perfusion, gated blood pool, and ^{123}I-metaiodobenzylguanidine (MIBG) imaging have reported regional perfusion defects, wall motion abnormalities, and sympathetic denervation in patients who present with myocarditis, in the absence of significant CAD.[6]

Sarcoid Heart Disease (see Chap. 68). Cardiac involvement occurs in about 20% of patients with sarcoidosis. In patients presenting with advanced AV block, myocardial perfusion SPECT or gallium-67 imaging (a nonspecific indicator of inflammation) along with CMR or CT can localize myocardial involvement of sarcoidosis.[6] Focal fibromuscular dysplasia found in the small coronary arteries may provide an explanation for focal ischemic injuries and reversible defects described on myocardial perfusion SPECT. Perfusion defects involving the left ventricle have been associated with AV block and heart failure, and defects involving the right ventricle on SPECT have been associated with ventricular tachycardia of RV origin.[103]

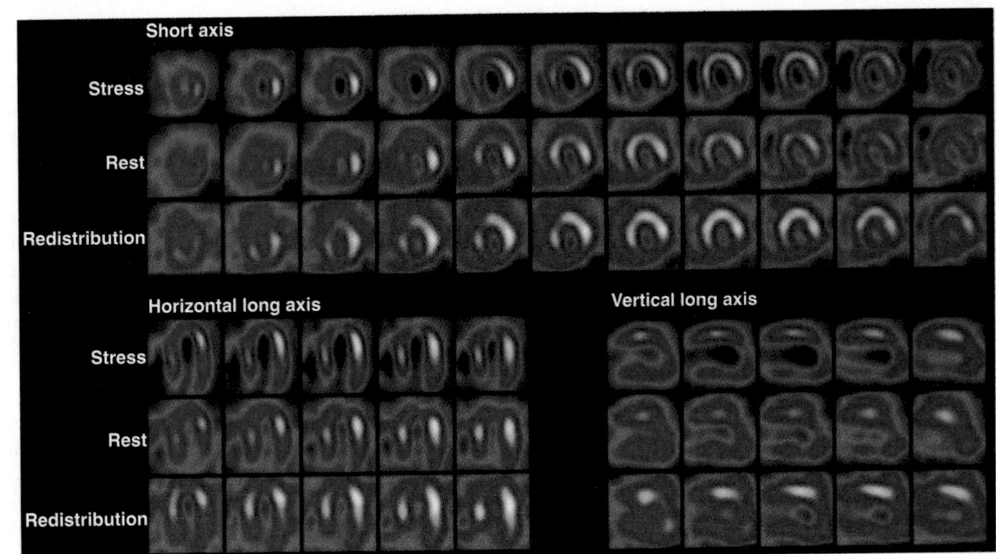

FIGURE 17-44 Rest-redistribution thallium imaging performed as part of a dual-isotope technetium-thallium stress imaging protocol in a 55-year-old patient with severe heart failure and left ventricular dysfunction (ejection fraction 30%). The initial thallium images at rest demonstrate several areas of reduced resting blood flow involving the septum, anteroapical wall, and inferior wall. Thallium redistribution imaging 4 hours later demonstrates substantial redistribution of thallium in the septal, anteroapical, and inferior regions of the left ventricle, indicating myocardial viability, with only the basal portion of the inferolateral wall representing irreversibly damaged myocardium. After the thallium redistribution image acquisition, stress imaging with ^{99m}Tc-sestamibi demonstrates inducible ischemia in the septum and anterior wall. However, without the redistribution images, routine stress-rest imaging would have given misleading information about viability because of the apparently irreversible defects in the inferior and anteroapical walls. *(From Holly TA, Bonow RO: Assessment of myocardial viability with thallium-201 and technetium-based agents. In Zaret BL, Beller GA [eds]: Nuclear Cardiology: State of the Art and Future Directions. 4th ed. Philadelphia, Mosby Elsevier, 2010, pp 594-607.)*

FDG PET imaging (with or without anatomic colocalization with CT or CMR) has gained interest recently for diagnosis and potential follow-up of cardiac sarcoidosis.[104] Because inflammatory cells, such as macrophages, contain increased membrane glucose transporters and significantly high hexose monophosphate shunt pathway activity, FDG can accumulate within areas of granulomatous inflammation and cannot diffuse out or be metabolized further. As a granuloma matures, the number of macrophages and inflammatory cells decreases, with subsequent fibrous replacement. Whereas CMR typically displays myocardial enhancement with delayed gadolinium washout in regions of myocyte replacement fibrosis (see Chap. 18), the CMR signal alone may not be able to differentiate areas of acute from chronic or mixed cardiac sarcoidosis.[105] On the other hand, FDG PET imaging in concert with either CMR or CT may be optimal for monitoring of the efficacy of therapy directed at the active inflammation in cardiac sarcoidosis and for detection of recurrence.

Cardiac Amyloidosis (see Chap. 68). Cardiac amyloidosis involves the deposition of light-chain amino acids into the myofibrils, which leads to impaired relaxation. Patients with amyloidosis may demonstrate abnormally prolonged LV diastolic filling and an increased atrial contribution to the total diastolic filling. ^{99m}Tc-pyrophosphate scintigraphy may be useful to identify patients with cardiac amyloidosis, demonstrating diffuse uptake throughout the myocardium.[6] ^{123}I-MIBG imaging has shown marked cardiac sympathetic denervation, providing insight into the pathogenesis of cardiac conduction disturbances in amyloidosis.[106]

RADIONUCLIDE IMAGING IN HEART FAILURE AND LEFT VENTRICULAR DYSFUNCTION: RESEARCH DIRECTIONS

Assessment of Cardiac Sympathetic Innervation

An emerging area of risk stratification involves the use of ^{123}I-MIBG imaging of cardiac sympathetic innervation. In the post-MI setting, the territory of abnormal MIBG uptake (corresponding to sympathetic denervation) often exceeds the final infarct size, and such patients are at higher risk for subsequent ventricular arrhythmias.[57,107] In recent multicenter prospective phase 3 studies of over 900 patients with heart failure and systolic dysfunction, 2-year event-free survival was significantly higher in patients with more preserved MIBG uptake compared with patients who showed evidence of more advanced functional denervation on MIBG imaging.[107a] Should these findings prove prognostic for specific outcomes in patients with LV dysfunction, as suggested by earlier studies, MIBG imaging may have a role in optimizing selection of post-MI or heart failure patients who may (or may not) benefit from a defibrillator.[107]

Imaging of Apoptosis

Another potential approach to evaluation of patients with LV dysfunction after MI is the visualization of apoptosis, or programmed cell death, in humans by use of ^{99m}Tc-labeled annexin V, which localizes to apoptotic cells.[108] In one study, positive uptake of this agent was seen in six of seven post-MI patients, localized to areas of resting perfusion defects.[109] This agent may herald the onset of the ability to track this process noninvasively in syndromes such as heart failure and to study approaches to attenuate the unfavorable pathophysiology of apoptosis.

Radionuclide Imaging of Cell- or Gene-Based Regenerative Therapy

Local targeted gene delivery or implantation of autologous skeletal myoblasts, bone marrow stromal cells, or hematopoietic stem cells may functionally revitalize scarred, noncontractile myocardial regions. Noninvasive assessment of the fate of myogenic cell grafts and therapeutic genes in vivo may provide insight into the mechanism by which they improve cardiac function or prevent remodeling. In animal studies, transplanted cardiomyoblasts expressing a PET reporter gene have been imaged longitudinally to gain insight into the pattern of cell survival.[110] With use of cardiac micro-PET imaging, detailed tomographic locations of transplanted cells were obtained (**Fig. 17-45**). This may become an important method to study regenerative therapies in human studies.

Imaging of the Tissue Angiotensin-Converting Enzyme Receptor System

Radionuclide imaging has been used in experimental systems to study the tissue ACE receptor system directly. By use of the radiotracer [^{18}F] fluorobenzyl-lisinopril, observations have shown a relationship

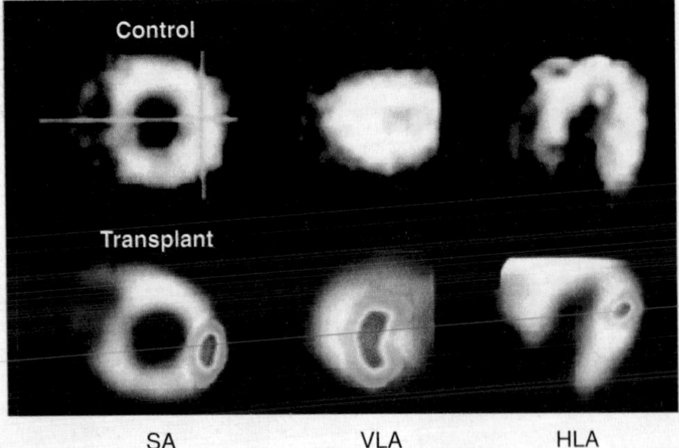

FIGURE 17-45 Cardiac micro-PET images in the short-axis (SA), vertical long-axis (VLA), and horizontal long-axis (HLA) views of a rat heart transplanted with cardiomyoblasts expressing a PET reporter gene. The gray-white uptake represents homogeneous perfusion by [^{13}N]ammonia, and the color uptake in the lateral wall represents the viable transplanted cardiomyoblasts studied in vivo **(bottom row)**. There is no uptake in the control heart, with normal perfusion **(top row)**. *(Modified from Wu JC, Chen IY, Sundaresan G, et al: Molecular imaging of cardiac cell transplantation in living animals using optical bioluminescence and positron emission tomography. Circulation 108:1302, 2003.)*

between ACE and collagen replacement, as ACE was absent in the collagen-stained areas and was increased in the juxtaposed areas of replacement fibrosis.[111] These data suggest that increased ACE may be a stimulus for collagen replacement and remodeling. In the future, noninvasive imaging with PET in patients with heart failure may allow monitoring of changes in ACE patterns in vivo, possibly reflecting progression of disease and the effect of therapies before collagen replacement ensues.

Imaging to Assess Cardiac Risk Before Noncardiac Surgery (see Chap. 85)

The clinical role of MPI for evaluation of patients before elective noncardiac surgery has grown, as CAD represents an important perioperative and long-term risk in such patients. The ischemic burden from the stress of surgery and postoperative recovery can result in MI or cardiovascular death. Prospective identification of such patients has important prognostic and preventive implications.

Initial cardiac assessment of patients undergoing noncardiac surgery should be based on (1) the prevalence of CAD in a given surgical population, (2) the type of the surgical procedure and the institutional event rate, (3) the cardiac history and risk factors, and (4) the functional capacity.[112] Surgical procedures can be classified as high-risk procedures (cardiac risk greater than 5%), such as major vascular surgery. If the institutional event rate for an elective operation is less than 2% to 3%, most screening studies are inefficient with regard to lowering of the cardiac event rate in the perioperative period.

Clinical parameters of increased risk include advanced age (older than 70 years), diabetes, history of angina or recent ACS, heart failure, and ventricular arrhythmias. Patients with known prior CAD may be considered to have a low perioperative cardiac risk on the basis of their functional capacity and symptoms. Asymptomatic patients with known CAD who have had revascularization within the past 5 years generally require no further evaluation.[112] Patients with intermediate risk on the basis of clinical predictors, functional capacity, and type of surgery are optimal candidates for further stratification by imaging procedures.

Studies of MPI using pharmacologic stress have uniformly shown that a normal MPI study predicts a low likelihood (~1%) for perioperative or longer term postoperative cardiac events.[112] Reversible perfusion defects predict an increased risk of cardiac events, and the magnitude of risk is related to the extent of ischemia. Although fixed perfusion defects (infarct) portend a lower risk than ischemia for perioperative cardiac events, the risk is higher than that with a normal scan, and patients with infarct or LV dysfunction are at higher long-term risk for death or heart failure.[112]

In clinical practice, most patients in whom extensive ischemia is demonstrated preoperatively undergo catheterization with expectation of revascularization. Clinical trial evidence supporting this point provides conflicting evidence,[113,114] and the threshold of ischemia extent above which revascularization might reduce short- or long-term cardiac risk is not known. In the contemporary era of PCI, the potential need for prolonged antiplatelet therapy after stenting must also be factored into the benefit-risk ratio in considering whether to pursue stress testing and potential catheterization.

REFERENCES

Technical Aspects of Image Acquisition, Display, and Interpretation

1. Garcia EV, Galt JR, Faber TL, Chen J: Principles of nuclear cardiology imaging. *In* Dilsizian V, Narula J, Braunwald E (eds): Atlas of Nuclear Cardiology. 3rd ed. Philadelphia, Current Medicine, 2009, pp 1-36.
2. Nichols KJ, Bacharach SL, Bergmann SR, et al; Quality Assurance Committee of the American Society of Nuclear Cardiology: Imaging guidelines for nuclear cardiology procedures: Instrumentation quality assurance and performance. J Nucl Cardiol 14:e61, 2007.
3. Erlandsson K, Kacperski K, van Gramberg D, Hutton BF: Performance evaluation of D-SPECT: A novel SPECT system for nuclear cardiology. Phys Med Biol 54:2635, 2009.
4. Bonow RO: High-speed myocardial perfusion imaging: Dawn of a new era in nuclear cardiology? J Am Coll Cardiol Img 1:164, 2008.
5. Dilsizian V: SPECT and PET perfusion imaging: Tracers and techniques. *In* Dilsizian V, Narula J, Braunwald E (eds): Atlas of Nuclear Cardiology. 3rd ed. Philadelphia, Current Medicine, 2009, pp 37-60.
6. Ficaro EP, Hansen CL; American Society of Nuclear Cardiology: Imaging Guidelines for Nuclear Cardiology Procedures. Available at: http://www.asnc.org/imageuploads/ImagingGuidelinesComplete070709.pdf. Accessed April 13, 2010.
7. Berman DS, Hachamovitch R, Germano G: Risk stratification and patient management. *In* Dilsizian V, Narula J, Braunwald E (eds): Atlas of Nuclear Cardiology. 3rd ed. Philadelphia, Current Medicine, 2009, pp 141-168.
8. Cerqueira MD, Weissman NJ, Dilsizian V, et al: Standardized myocardial segmentation and nomenclature for tomographic imaging of the heart: A statement for healthcare professionals from the cardiac imaging committee of the council on clinical cardiology of the American Heart Association. Circulation 105:539, 2002.
9. McLaughlin MG, Danias PG: Transient ischemic dilation: A powerful diagnostic and prognostic finding of stress myocardial perfusion imaging. J Nucl Cardiol 9:663, 2002.
10. Hendel RC, Corbett JR, Cullom SJ, et al: The value and practice of attenuation correction for myocardial perfusion SPECT imaging: A joint position statement from the American Society of Nuclear Cardiology and the Society of Nuclear Medicine. J Nucl Cardiol 9:135, 2002.
11. Germano G, Berman DS: Acquisition and processing for gated SPECT: Technical aspects. *In* Germano G, Berman DS (eds): Clinical Gated Cardiac SPECT. Armonk, NY, Blackwell Futura, 2006, pp 93-114.
12. Botvinick E: Assessment of cardiac function: First-pass, equilibrium blood pool, and gated myocardial SPECT. *In* Dilsizian V, Narula J, Braunwald E (eds): Atlas of Nuclear Cardiology. 3rd ed. Philadelphia, Current Medicine, 2009, pp 109-141.
13. Dilsizian V, Bacharach SL, Beanlands SR, et al: PET myocardial perfusion and metabolism clinical imaging. J Nucl Cardiol 16:651; 2009.
14. Madar I, Ravert HT, Du Y, et al: Characterization of uptake of the new PET imaging compound ^{18}F-fluorobenzyl triphenyl phosphonium in dog myocardium. J Nucl Med 47:1359, 2006.
15. Yoshinaga K, Chow BJ, William K, et al: What is the prognostic value of myocardial perfusion imaging using rubidium-82 positron emission tomography? J Am Coll Cardiol 48:1029, 2006.
16. Neglia D, Michelassi C, Trivieri MG, et al: Prognostic role of myocardial blood flow impairment in idiopathic left ventricular dysfunction. Circulation 105:186, 2002.
17. Cecchi F, Olivotto I, Gistri R, et al: Coronary microvascular dysfunction and prognosis in hypertrophic cardiomyopathy. N Engl J Med 349:1027, 2003.
18. Laskey WK, Feinendegen LE, Neumann RD, Dilsizian V: Low-level ionizing radiation from non-invasive cardiac imaging: Can we extrapolate estimated risks from epidemiologic data to the clinical setting? J Am Coll Cardiol Img 3:517, 2010.

Assessment of the Physiology and Pathophysiology of Myocardial Blood Flow, Myocardial Metabolism, and Ventricular Function

19. Gibbons RJ, Miller TD, Christian TF: Infarct size measured by single photon emission computed tomographic imaging with ^{99m}Tc-sestamibi: A measure of the efficacy of therapy in acute myocardial infarction. Circulation 101:101, 2000.
20. Kern MJ, Meier B: Evaluation of the culprit plaque and the physiological significance of coronary atherosclerotic narrowings. Circulation 103:3142, 2001.
21. Gould KL, Nakagawa Y, Nakagawa K, et al: Frequency and clinical implications of fluid dynamically significant diffuse coronary artery disease manifest as graded, longitudinal, base-to-apex myocardial perfusion abnormalities by noninvasive positron emission tomography. Circulation 101:1931, 2000.
22. He Z, Mahmarian JJ, Verani MS: Myocardial perfusion in patients with total occlusion of a single coronary artery with and without collateral circulation. J Nucl Cardiol 8:452, 2001.
23. Mark DB, Lauer MS: Exercise capacity: The prognostic variable that doesn't get enough respect. Circulation 108:1534, 2003.
24. Miller DD: Pharmacologic stressors in coronary artery disease. *In* Dilsizian V, Narula J, Braunwald E (eds): Atlas of Nuclear Cardiology. 3rd ed. Philadelphia, Current Medicine, 2009, pp 61-78.

25. Iskandrian AE, Bateman TM, Belardinelli L, et al: Adenosine versus regadenoson comparative evaluation in myocardial perfusion imaging: Results of the ADVANCE phase 3 multicenter international trial. J Nucl Cardiol 14:645, 2007.
26. Udelson JE, Heller GV, Wackers FJ, et al: A randomized, controlled dose-ranging study of the selective adenosine A_{2A} receptor agonist binodenoson for pharmacologic stress as an adjunct to myocardial perfusion imaging. Circulation 109:457, 2004.
27. Thomas GS, Prill NV, Majmundar H, et al: Treadmill exercise during adenosine infusion is safe, results in fewer adverse reactions, and improves myocardial perfusion imaging quality. J Nucl Cardiol 7:439, 2000.
28. Mahmarian JJ, Dakik HA, Filipchuk NG, et al: An initial strategy of intensive medical therapy is comparable to that of coronary revascularization for suppression of scintigraphic ischemia in high-risk but stable survivors of acute myocardial infarction. J Am Coll Cardiol 48:2458, 2006.
29. Taillefer R, Ahlberg AW, Masood Y, et al: Acute beta-blockade reduces the extent and severity of myocardial perfusion defects with dipyridamole Tc-99m sestamibi SPECT imaging. J Am Coll Cardiol 42:1475, 2003.
30. Taegtmeyer H: Modulation of responses to myocardial ischemia: Metabolic features of myocardial stunning, hibernation, and ischemic preconditioning. *In* Dilsizian V (ed): Myocardial Viability: A Clinical and Scientific Treatise. Armonk, NY, Futura, 2000, pp 25-36.
31. Selvanayagam JB, Jerosch-Herold M, Porto I, et al: Resting myocardial blood flow is impaired in hibernating myocardium: A magnetic resonance study of quantitative perfusion assessment. Circulation 112:3289, 2005.
32. Feinendegen LE: Myocardial imaging of lipid metabolism with labeled fatty acids. *In* Dilsizian V (ed): Myocardial Viability: A Clinical and Scientific Treatise. Armonk, NY, Futura, 2000, pp 349-389.
33. Dilsizian V, Bateman TM, Bergmann SR, et al: Metabolic imaging with ß-methyl-p-[^{123}I]-iodophenyl-pentadecanoic acid identifies ischemic memory after demand ischemia. Circulation 112:2169, 2005.
34. Dilsizian V, Bacharach SL, Maung KM, Smith MF: Fluorine-18-deoxyglucose SPECT and coincidence imaging for myocardial viability: Clinical and technological issues. J Nucl Cardiol 8:75, 2001.
35. Jafary F, Udelson JE: Assessment of myocardial perfusion and left ventricular function in acute coronary syndromes: Implications for gated SPECT imaging. *In* Germano G, Berman DS (eds): Clinical Gated Cardiac SPECT. Armonk, NY, Blackwell Futura, 2006, pp 259-306.
36. Anand IS, Florea VG, Solomon SD, et al: Noninvasive assessment of left ventricular remodeling: Concepts, techniques, and implications for clinical trials. J Card Fail 8:S452, 2002.
37. Germano G, Berman DS: Quantitative gated perfusion SPECT. *In* Germano G, Berman DS (eds): Clinical Gated Cardiac SPECT. Armonk, NY, Blackwell-Futura Publishing, 2006, pp 115-146.
38. Metra M, Giubbini R, Nodari S, et al: Differential effects of ß-blockers in patients with heart failure: A prospective, randomized, double-blind comparison of the long-term effects of metoprolol versus carvedilol. Circulation 102:546, 2000.
39. Borer JS, Bonow RO: Contemporary approach to aortic and mitral regurgitation. Circulation 108:2432, 2003.
40. Bonow RO, Carabello BA, Chatterjee K, et al: 2008 focused update incorporated into the ACC/AHA 2006 guidelines for the management of patients with valvular heart disease: A report of the American College of Cardiology/American Heart Association Task Force on Practice Guidelines (Writing Committee to Develop Guidelines for the Management of Patients With Valvular Heart Disease). J Am Coll Cardiol 52:e1, 2008.
41. Imitani I, Jain D, Joska TM, et al: Doxorubicin cardiotoxicity: Prevention of congestive heart failure with serial cardiac function monitoring with equilibrium radionuclide angiocardiography in the current era. J Nucl Cardiol 10:132, 2003.
42. Maron BJ: Hypertrophic cardiomyopathy: A systematic review. JAMA 287:1308, 2002.

Disease Detection, Risk Stratification, and Clinical Decision Making

43. Libby P, Ridker PM, Maseri A: Inflammation and atherosclerosis. Circulation 105:1135, 2002.
44. Third Report of the National Cholesterol Education Program (NCEP) Expert Panel on Detection, Evaluation, and Treatment of High Blood Cholesterol in Adults (Adult Treatment Panel III) Final Report. Circulation 106:3143, 2002.
45. Fletcher GF, Balady GJ, Vogel RA: Preventive cardiology: How can we do better? 33rd Bethesda Conference. J Am Coll Cardiol 40:579, 2002.
46. Anderson JL, Adams CD, Antman EM, et al: ACC/AHA 2007 guidelines for the management of patients with unstable angina/non–ST-elevation myocardial infarction: A report of the American College of Cardiology/American Heart Association Task Force on Practice Guidelines (Writing Committee to Revise the 2002 Guidelines for the Management of Patients With Unstable Angina/Non–ST-Elevation Myocardial Infarction): Developed in collaboration with the American College of Emergency Physicians, American College of Physicians, Society for Academic Emergency Medicine, Society for Cardiovascular Angiography and Interventions, and Society of Thoracic Surgeons. J Am Coll Cardiol 50:e1, 2007.
47. Gibbons RJ, Abrams J, Chatterjee K, et al: ACC/AHA 2002 guideline update for the management of patients with chronic stable angina—summary article: A report of the American College of Cardiology/American Heart Association Task Force on Practice Guidelines (Committee on the Management of Patients with Chronic Stable Angina). Circulation 107:149, 2003.
48. Beller GA: First Annual Mario S. Verani, MD, Memorial Lecture: Clinical value of myocardial perfusion imaging in coronary artery disease. J Nucl Cardiol 10:529, 2003.
49. Hachamovitch R, Hayes SW, Friedman JD, et al: Comparison of the short-term survival benefit associated with revascularization compared with medical therapy in patients with no prior coronary artery disease undergoing stress myocardial perfusion single photon emission computed tomography. Circulation 107:2900, 2003.
50. Shaw LJ, Hendel R, Borges-Neto S, et al: Prognostic value of normal exercise and adenosine ^{99m}Tc-tetrofosmin SPECT imaging: Results from the multicenter registry of 4,728 patients. J Nucl Med 44:134, 2003.
51. Hachamovitch R, Hayes S, Friedman JD, et al: Determinants of risk and its temporal variation in patients with normal stress myocardial perfusion scans. What is the warranty period of a normal scan? J Am Coll Cardiol 41:1329, 2003.
52. Giri S, Shaw LJ, Murthy DR, et al: Impact of diabetes on the risk stratification using stress single-photon emission computed tomography myocardial perfusion imaging in patients with symptoms suggestive of coronary artery disease. Circulation 105:32, 2002.
53. Shaw LJ, Berman DS, Maron DJ, et al: Optimal medical therapy with or without percutaneous coronary intervention to reduce ischemic burden: Results from the Clinical Outcomes Utilizing Revascularization and Aggressive Drug Evaluation (COURAGE) trial nuclear substudy. Circulation 117:1283, 2008.
54. Schwartz RG, Pearson TA, Kalaria VG, et al: Prospective serial evaluation of myocardial perfusion and lipids during the first six months of pravastatin therapy: Coronary artery disease regression single photon emission computed tomography monitoring trial. J Am Coll Cardiol 42:600, 2003.
55. Beller GA, Zaret BL: Contributions of nuclear cardiology to diagnosis and prognosis of patients with coronary artery disease. Circulation 101:1465, 2000.
56. Amanullah AM, Berman DS, Kang X, et al: Enhanced prognostic stratification of patients with left ventricular hypertrophy with the use of single-photon emission computed tomography. Am Heart J 140:3456, 2000.
57. Udelson JE, Shafer CD, Carrio I: Radionuclide imaging in heart failure: Assessing etiology and outcomes and implications for management. J Nucl Cardiol 9:S40, 2002.
58. Masoli O, Perez Baliño N, Sabaté D, et al: Effect of endothelial dysfunction on regional perfusion in myocardial territories supplied by normal and diseased vessels in patients with coronary artery disease. J Nucl Cardiol 7:199, 2000.
59. Panting JR, Gatehouse PD, Yang GZ, et al: Abnormal subendocardial perfusion in cardiac syndrome X detected by cardiovascular magnetic resonance imaging. N Engl J Med 346:1948, 2002.
60. Germano G, Berman DS: Quantitative gated SPECT. J Nucl Med 42:528, 2001.
61. Gibbons RJ, Balady GJ, Timothy B, et al: ACC/AHA 2002 guideline update for exercise testing: Summary article. A report of the American College of Cardiology/American Heart Association Task Force on Practice Guidelines (Committee to Update the 1997 Exercise Testing Guidelines). J Am Coll Cardiol 40:1531, 2002.
62. Sharir T, Bacher-Stier C, Dhar S, et al: Identification of severe and extensive coronary artery disease by postexercise regional wall motion abnormalities in Tc-99m sestamibi gated single-photon emission computed tomography. Am J Cardiol 86:1171, 2000.
63. Lima RSL, Watson, DD, Goode AR, et al: Incremental value of combined perfusion and function over perfusion alone by gated SPECT myocardial perfusion imaging for detection of severe three-vessel coronary artery disease. J Am Coll Cardiol 42:64, 2003.
64. Zellweger M, Lewin H, Shenghan L, et al: When to stress patients after coronary artery bypass surgery? Risk stratification in patients early and late post-CABG using stress myocardial perfusion SPECT: Implications of appropriate clinical strategies. J Am Coll Cardiol 37:144, 2001.
65. Acampa W, Petretta M, Florimonte L, et al: Prognostic value of exercise cardiac tomography performed late after percutaneous coronary intervention in symptomatic and symptom-free patients. Am J Cardiol 9:259, 2003.
66. Blumenthal RS, Becker DM, Yanek LR, et al: Comparison of coronary calcium and stress myocardial perfusion imaging in apparently healthy siblings of individuals with premature coronary artery disease. Am J Cardiol 97:328, 2006.
67. Smith SC, Greenland P, Grundy SM: Prevention Conference V: Beyond secondary prevention: Identifying the high-risk patient for primary prevention: Executive summary. Circulation 101:111, 2000.
68. Wackers FJ, Young LH, Inzucchi SE, et al; Detection of Ischemia in Asymptomatic Diabetics Investigators: Detection of silent myocardial ischemia in asymptomatic diabetic subjects: The DIAD study. Diabetes Care 27:1954, 2004.
69. De Lorenzo A, Lima RS, Siqueira-Filho AG, Pantoja MR: Prevalence and prognostic value of perfusion defects detected by stress technetium-99m sestamibi myocardial perfusion single-photon emission computed tomography in asymptomatic patients with diabetes mellitus and no known coronary artery disease. Am J Cardiol 90:827, 2002.
70. Young LH, Wackers FJ, Chyun DA, et al: Cardiac outcomes after screening for asymptomatic coronary artery disease in patients with type 2 diabetes: The DIAD study: A randomized controlled trial. JAMA 301:1547, 2009.
71. Berman DS, Wong ND, Gransar H, et al: Relationship between stress-induced myocardial ischemia and atherosclerosis measured by coronary calcium tomography. J Am Coll Cardiol 44:923, 2004.
72. Brindis RG, Douglas PS, Hendel RC, et al: ACCF/ASNC appropriateness criteria for single-photon emission computed tomography myocardial perfusion imaging (SPECT MPI): A report of the American College of Cardiology Foundation Quality Strategic Directions Committee Appropriateness Criteria Working Group and the American Society of Nuclear Cardiology endorsed by the American Heart Association. J Am Coll Cardiol 46:1587, 2005.
73. Detrano RC, Guerci AD, Carr JJ, et al: Coronary calcium as a predictor of coronary events in four racial or ethnic groups. N Engl J Med 358:1336, 2008.
74. Berman DS, Hachamovitch R, Shaw LJ, et al: Roles of nuclear cardiology, cardiac computed tomography, and cardiac magnetic resonance: Noninvasive risk stratification and a conceptual framework for the selection of noninvasive imaging tests in patients with known or suspected coronary artery disease. J Nucl Med 47:1107, 2006.
75. Schuijf JD, Wijns W, Jukema JW, et al: Relationship between noninvasive coronary angiography with multi-slice computed tomography and myocardial perfusion imaging. J Am Coll Cardiol 48:2508, 2006.
76. Wackers FJ, Brown KA, Heller GV, et al: American Society of Nuclear Cardiology position statement on radionuclide imaging in patients with suspected acute ischemic syndromes in the emergency department or chest pain center. J Nucl Cardiol 9:246, 2002.
77. Stowers SA, Eisenstein EL, Wackers FJ, et al: An economic analysis of an aggressive diagnostic strategy with single photon emission computed tomography myocardial perfusion imaging and early exercise stress testing in emergency department patients who present with chest pain but nondiagnostic electrocardiograms: Results from a randomized trial. Ann Emerg Med 35:17, 2000.
78. Udelson JE, Beshansky JR, Ballin DS, et al: Myocardial perfusion imaging for evaluation and triage of patients with suspected acute cardiac ischemia: A randomized controlled trial. JAMA 288:2693, 2002.
79. Cannon CP, Weintraub WS, Demopoulos LA, et al: Comparison of early invasive and conservative strategies in patients with unstable coronary syndromes treated with the glycoprotein IIb/IIIa inhibitor tirofiban. N Engl J Med 344:1879, 2001.
80. de Winter RJ, Windhausen F, Cornel JH, et al: Early invasive versus selectively invasive management for acute coronary syndromes. N Engl J Med 353:1095, 2005.

81. Antman EM, Cohen M, Bernink PJ, et al: The TIMI risk score for unstable angina/non–ST elevation MI: A method for prognostication and therapeutic decision making. JAMA 284:835, 2000.
82. Antman EM, Anbe DT, Armstrong PW, et al: ACC/AHA guidelines for the management of patients with ST-elevation myocardial infarction—executive summary: A report of the American College of Cardiology/American Heart Association Task Force on practice guidelines (writing committee to revise the 1999 guidelines for the management of patients with acute myocardial infarction). J Am Coll Cardiol 44:671, 2004.
83. Kawai Y, Tsukamoto E, Nozaki Y, et al: Significance of reduced uptake of iodinated fatty acid analogues for the evaluation of patients with acute chest pain. J Am Coll Cardiol 38:1888, 2001.
84. Kontos MC, Dilsizian V, Weiland F, et al: Iodofiltic acid I 123 (BMIPP) fatty acid imaging improves initial diagnosis in emergency department patients with suspected acute coronary syndromes: A multicenter trial. J Am Coll Cardiol 56:290, 2010.
85. Chen W, Dilsizian V: ^{18}F-Fluorodeoxyglucose PET imaging of coronary atherosclerosis and plaque inflammation. Curr Cardiol Rep 12:179, 2010.
86. Ogawa M, Ishino S, Mukai T, et al: ^{18}F-FDG accumulation in atherosclerotic plaques: Immunohistochemical and PET imaging study. J Nucl Med 45:1245, 2004.
87. Rudd JH, Warburton EA, Fryer TD, et al: Imaging atherosclerotic plaque inflammation with [^{18}F]-fluorodeoxyglucose positron emission tomography. Circulation 105:2708, 2002.
88. Ogawa M, Magata Y, Kato T, et al: Application of ^{18}F-FDG PET for monitoring the therapeutic effect of antiinflammatory drugs on stabilization of vulnerable atherosclerotic plaques. J Nucl Med 47:1845, 2006.
89. Tahara N, Kai H, Ishibashi M, et al: Simvastatin attenuates plaque inflammation: Evaluation by fluorodeoxyglucose positron emission tomography. J Am Coll Cardiol 48:1825, 2006.
90. Dilsizian V, Narula J: Putting the face to a name: Concurrent assessment of vascular morphology and biology. J Am Coll Cardiol Img 2:1243, 2009.
91. Jaffer F, Narula J: Molecular imaging of atherosclerosis: A biologic roadmap. *In* Dilsizian V, Narula J, Braunwald E (eds): Atlas of Nuclear Cardiology. 3rd Ed. Philadelphia, Current Medicine, 2009, pp 257-278.
92. Gheorghiade M, Sopko, G, De Luca L, et al: Navigating the crossroads of coronary artery disease and heart failure. Circulation 114:1202, 2006.
93. McCrohon JA, Moon JCC, Prasad SK, et al: Differentiation of heart failure related to dilated cardiomyopathy and coronary artery disease using gadolinium-enhanced cardiovascular magnetic resonance. Circulation 108:54, 2003.
94. Bennett SK, Smith MF, Gottlieb SS, et al: Effect of metoprolol on absolute myocardial blood flow in patients with heart failure secondary to ischemic or non-ischemic cardiomyopathy. Am J Cardiol 89:1431, 2002.
95. Cleland JG, Pennell DJ, Ray SG, et al: Myocardial viability as a determinant of the ejection fraction response to carvedilol in patients with heart failure (CHRISTMAS trial): Randomised controlled trial. Lancet 362:14, 2003.
96. Allman K, Shaw L, Hachamovitch R, Udelson JE: Myocardial viability testing and impact of revascularization on prognosis in patients with coronary artery disease and left ventricular dysfunction: A meta-analysis. J Am Coll Cardiol 39:1151, 2002.
97. Bax JJ, Poldermans D, Elhendy A, et al: Assessment of myocardial viability by nuclear imaging techniques. Curr Cardiol Rep 7:124, 2005.
98. Bonow RO: Myocardial viability and prognosis in patients with ischemic left ventricular dysfunction. J Am Coll Cardiol 39:1159, 2002.
98a. Udelson JE, Bonow RO, Dilsizian V: The historical and conceptual evolution of radionuclide assessment of myocardial viability. J Nucl Cardiol 11:318, 2004.
99. Siebelink HM, Blanksma P, Crijns H, et al: No difference in cardiac event-free survival between positron emission tomography and single-photon emission computed tomography–guided patient management. J Am Coll Cardiol 37:81, 2001.
100. Hunt SA, Abraham WT, Chin MH, et al: 2009 focused update incorporated into the ACC/AHA 2005 guidelines for the diagnosis and management of heart failure in adults: A report of the American College of Cardiology Foundation/American Heart Association Task Force on Practice Guidelines. J Am Coll Cardiol 53:e1, 2009.
101. Margazi ZJ, Anastasiou-Nana MI, Terrovitis J, et al: Indium-111 monoclonal antimyosin cardiac scintigraphy in suspected acute myocarditis: Evolution and diagnostic impact. Int J Cardiol 90:239, 2003.
102. Puig M, Ballester M, Matias-Guiu X, et al: Burden of myocardial damage in cardiac allograft rejection: Scintigraphic evidence of myocardial injury and histologic evidence of myocyte necrosis and apoptosis. J Nucl Cardiol 7:132, 2000.
103. Eguchi M, Tsuchihashi K, Hotta D, et al: Technetium-99m sestamibi/tetrofosmin myocardial perfusion scanning in cardiac and noncardiac sarcoidosis. Cardiology 94:193, 2000.
104. Ishimaru S, Tsujino I, Takei T, et al: Focal uptake of ^{18}F-fluoro-2-deoxyglucose positron emission tomography images indicates cardiac involvement of sarcoidosis. Eur Heart J 26:1538, 2005.
105. Patel MR, Cawley PJ, Heitner JF, et al: Detection of myocardial damage in patients with sarcoidosis. Circulation.120:1969, 2009.
106. Hongo M, Urushibata K, Kai R, et al: Iodine-123 metaiodobenzylguanidine scintigraphic analysis of myocardial sympathetic innervation in patients with AL (primary) amyloidosis. Am Heart J 144:122, 2002.
107. Carrió I, Cowie MR, Yamazaki J, et al: Cardiac sympathetic imaging with mIBG in heart failure. J Am Coll Cardiol Img 3:92, 2010.
107a. Jacobson AF, Senior R, Cerqueira MD, et al: Mycocardial iodine-123 meta-iodobenzylguanidine imaging and cardiac events in heart failure: Results of the prospective ADMIRE-HF (AdreView Myocardial Imaging for Risk Evaluation in Heart Failure) study. J Am Coll Cardiol 55:2222, 2010.
108. Narula J, Kietselaer B, Hofstra L: Role of molecular imaging in defining and denying death. J Nucl Cardiol 11:349, 2004.
109. Hofstra L, Liem IH, Dumont EA, et al: Visualization of cell death in vivo in patients with acute myocardial infarction. Lancet 356:209, 2000.
110. Wu JC, Chen IY, Sundaresan G, et al: Molecular imaging of cardiac cell transplantation in living animals using optical bioluminescence and positron emission tomography. Circulation 108:1302, 2003.
111. Dilsizian V, Eckelman WC, Loredo ML, et al: Evidence for tissue angiotensin converting enzyme in explanted hearts of ischemic cardiomyopathy patients using targeted radiotracer technique. J Nucl Med 48:1, 2007.
112. Fleisher LA, Beckman JA, Brown KA, et al: ACC/AHA 2007 guidelines on perioperative cardiovascular evaluation and care for noncardiac surgery: A report of the American College of Cardiology/American Heart Association Task Force on Practice Guidelines (Writing Committee to Revise the 2002 Guidelines on Perioperative Cardiovascular Evaluation for Noncardiac Surgery). J Am Coll Cardiol 50:e159, 2007.
113. Landesberg G, Mosseri M, Wolf YG, et al: Preoperative thallium scanning, selective coronary revascularization and long-term survival after major vascular surgery. Circulation 108:177, 2003.
114. McFalls EO, Ward HB, Moritz TE, et al: Coronary-artery revascularization before elective major vascular surgery. N Engl J Med 351:2795, 2004.

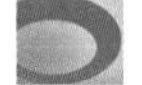

APPROPRIATE USE CRITERIA JAMES E. UDELSON

Nuclear Cardiology

The American College of Cardiology Foundation, the American Society of Nuclear Cardiology, and other organizations recently published appropriate use criteria for radionuclide imaging as a guide for clinicians to the appropriateness of ordering an imaging procedure in various clinical scenarios. The initial criteria for radionuclide imaging were published in 2005[1] and updated in 2009.[2] These criteria are meant to complement and to incorporate "disease-based" guideline recommendations as much as possible while acknowledging that many clinical scenarios faced by clinicians do not fit neatly into the evidence base from the published literature on which more formal guidelines are built. This approach has become the primary mechanism for rating procedures and tests such as radionuclide imaging and echocardiography while guidelines continue to be developed for clinical disease states and syndromes.

After development of the clinical indications to be rated, a panel with a broad array of expertise (i.e., not just imaging experts) rates the "appropriateness" of radionuclide imaging in each scenario, using the following definition: "An appropriate imaging study is one in which the expected incremental information, combined with clinical judgment, exceeds the expected negative consequences by a sufficiently wide margin for a specific indication that the procedure is generally considered acceptable care and a reasonable approach for the indication."[1] Rating scores are made on a scale of 1 to 9, in which a score of 9 indicates a highly appropriate use of testing. Using an iterative modified Delphi exercise process, with predefined rules, a final rating score is established for each indication and grouped as A, score 7-9, an appropriate test for the specific indication (the test **is** generally acceptable and **is** a reasonable approach for the indication); U, score 4-6, uncertain for the specific indication (the test **may** be generally acceptable and **may** be a reasonable approach for the indication); and I, score 1-3, an inappropriate test for that indication (the test **is not** generally acceptable and **is not** a reasonable approach for the indication) (**Table 17G-1**).[1]

As an example, for stable outpatients with chest pain syndromes, patients with an intermediate or high pretest likelihood of coronary artery disease are thought to be appropriate for nuclear imaging along with stress testing, whereas those with a low pretest likelihood who can exercise are not. Patients within 1 year of successful percutaneous coronary intervention (PCI) who had symptoms before PCI and remain asymptomatic after PCI are thought to be inappropriate candidates for single-photon emission computed tomography (i.e., routine "surveillance" stress imaging). It is likely that payers will use these criteria as a basis for reimbursement decisions at some point in the future.

TABLE 17G-1 Appropriate Use Criteria for Nuclear Cardiology

Detection of CAD: Symptomatic	
INDICATION	**APPROPRIATE USE SCORE (1-9)**
Evaluation of Ischemic Equivalent (Non-Acute)	
1. • Low pretest probability of CAD • ECG interpretable *and* able to exercise	I (3)
2. • Low pretest probability of CAD • ECG uninterpretable *or* unable to exercise	A (7)
3. • Intermediate pretest probability of CAD • ECG interpretable *and* able to exercise	A (7)
4. • Intermediate pretest probability of CAD • ECG uninterpretable *or* unable to exercise	A (9)
5. • High pretest probability of CAD • Regardless of ECG interpretability and ability to exercise	A (8)
Acute Chest Pain	
6. • Possible ACS • ECG—no ischemic changes or with LBBB or electronically ventricular paced rhythm • Low-risk TIMI score • Peak troponin: borderline, equivocal, minimally elevated	A (8)
7. • Possible ACS • ECG—no ischemic changes or with LBBB or electronically ventricular paced rhythm • High-risk TIMI score • Peak troponin: borderline, equivocal, minimally elevated	A (7)
8. • Possible ACS • ECG—no ischemic changes or with LBBB or electronically ventricular paced rhythm • Low-risk TIMI score • Negative peak troponin levels	A (8)
9. • Possible ACS • ECG—no ischemic changes or with LBBB or electronically ventricular paced rhythm • High-risk TIMI score • Negative peak troponin levels	A (8)
10. • Definite ACS	I (1)
Acute Chest Pain (Rest Imaging Only)	
11. • Possible ACS • ECG—no ischemic changes or with LBBB or electronically ventricular paced rhythm • Initial troponin negative • Recent or ongoing chest pain	A (7)
Detection of CAD/Risk Assessment Without Ischemic Equivalent	
INDICATION	**APPROPRIATE USE SCORE (1-9)**
Asymptomatic	
12. • Low CHD risk (ATP III risk criteria)	I (1)
13. • Intermediate CHD risk (ATP III risk criteria) • ECG interpretable	I (3)
14. • Intermediate CHD risk (ATP III risk criteria) • ECG uninterpretable	U (5)
15. • High CHD risk (ATP III risk criteria)	A (7)
New-Onset or Newly Diagnosed Heart Failure with LV Systolic Dysfunction Without Ischemic Equivalent	
16. • No prior CAD evaluation *and* no coronary angiography	A (8)
New-Onset Atrial Fibrillation	
17. • Part of evaluation when etiology unclear	U (6)
Ventricular Tachycardia	
18. • Low CHD risk (ATP III risk criteria)	A (7)
19. • Intermediate or high CHD risk (ATP III risk criteria)	A (8)
Syncope	
20. • Low CHD risk (ATP III risk criteria)	I (3)
21. • Intermediate or high CHD risk (ATP III risk criteria)	A (7)
Elevated Troponin	
22. • Troponin elevation without additional evidence of ACS	A (7)

CH 17

TABLE 17G-1 Appropriate Use Criteria for Nuclear Cardiology—cont'd

	INDICATION	APPROPRIATE USE SCORE (1-9)
	Risk Assessment with Prior Test Results and/or Known Chronic Stable CAD	
	Asymptomatic *or* Stable Symptoms	
	Normal Prior Stress Imaging Study	
23.	• Low CHD risk (ATP III risk criteria) • Last stress imaging study done less than 2 years ago	I (1)
24.	• Intermediate to high CHD risk (ATP III risk criteria) • Last stress imaging study done less than 2 years ago	I (3)
25.	• Low CHD risk (ATP III risk criteria) • Last stress imaging study done ≥2 years ago	I (3)
26.	• Intermediate to high CHD risk (ATP III risk criteria) • Last stress imaging study done ≥2 years ago	U (6)
	Asymptomatic *or* Stable Symptoms	
	Abnormal Coronary Angiography or Abnormal Prior Stress Imaging Study, No Prior Revascularization	
27.	• Known CAD on coronary angiography *or* prior abnormal stress imaging study • Last stress imaging study done less than 2 years ago	I (3)
28.	• Known CAD on coronary angiography *or* prior abnormal stress imaging study • Last stress imaging study done ≥2 years ago	U (5)
	Prior Noninvasive Evaluation	
29.	• Equivocal, borderline, or discordant stress testing where obstructive CAD remains a concern	A (8)
	New or Worsening Symptoms	
30.	• Abnormal coronary angiography *or* abnormal prior stress imaging study	A (9)
31.	• Normal coronary angiography *or* normal prior stress imaging study	U (6)
	Coronary Angiography (Invasive or Noninvasive)	
32.	• Coronary stenosis or anatomic abnormality of uncertain significance	A (9)
	Asymptomatic	
	Prior Coronary Calcium Agatston Score	
33.	• Agatston score less than 100	I (2)
34.	• Low to intermediate CHD risk • Agatston score between 100 and 400	U (5)
35.	• High CHD risk • Agatston score between 100 and 400	A (7)
36.	• Agatston score greater than 400	A (7)
	Duke Treadmill Score	
37.	• Low-risk Duke treadmill score	I (2)
38.	• Intermediate-risk Duke treadmill score	A (7)
39.	• High-risk Duke treadmill score	A (8)
	Risk Assessment: Preoperative Evaluation for Noncardiac Surgery Without Active Cardiac Conditions	
	INDICATION	APPROPRIATE USE SCORE (1-9)
	Low-Risk Surgery	
40.	• Preoperative evaluation for noncardiac surgery risk assessment	I (1)
	Intermediate-Risk Surgery	
41.	• Moderate to good functional capacity (≥4 METs)	I (3)
42.	• No clinical risk factors	I (2)
43.	• ≥1 clinical risk factor • Poor or unknown functional capacity (<4 METs)	A (7)
44.	• Asymptomatic up to 1 year post–normal catheterization, noninvasive test, or previous revascularization	I (2)
	Vascular Surgery	
45.	• Moderate to good functional capacity (≥4 METs)	I (3)
46.	• No clinical risk factors	I (2)
47.	• ≥1 clinical risk factor • Poor or unknown functional capacity (<4 METs)	A (8)
48.	• Asymptomatic up to 1 year post–normal catheterization, noninvasive test, or previous revascularization	I (2)
	Risk Assessment: Within 3 Months of an Acute Coronary Syndrome	
	INDICATION	APPROPRIATE USE SCORE (1-9)
	STEMI	
49.	• Primary PCI with complete revascularization • No recurrent symptoms	I (2)
50.	• Hemodynamically stable, no recurrent chest pain symptoms or no signs of HF • To evaluate for inducible ischemia • No prior coronary angiography	A (8)
51.	• Hemodynamically unstable, signs of cardiogenic shock, or mechanical complications	I (1)

TABLE 17G-1 Appropriate Use Criteria for Nuclear Cardiology—cont'd

	INDICATION	APPROPRIATE USE SCORE (1-9)
	Risk Assessment: Within 3 Months of an Acute Coronary Syndrome	
	UA/NSTEMI	
52.	• Hemodynamically stable, no recurrent chest pain symptoms or no signs of HF • To evaluate for inducible ischemia • No prior coronary angiography	A (9)
	ACS—Asymptomatic Post-Revascularization (PCI or CABG)	
53.	• Evaluation prior to hospital discharge	I (1)
	Cardiac Rehabilitation	
54.	• Prior to initiation of cardiac rehabilitation (as a stand-alone indication)	I (3)
	Risk Assessment: Post-Revascularization (Percutaneous Coronary Intervention or Coronary Artery Bypass Graft)	
	Symptomatic	
55.	• Evaluation of ischemic equivalent	A (8)
	Asymptomatic	
56.	• Incomplete revascularization • Additional revascularization feasible	A (7)
57.	• <5 years after CABG	U (5)
58.	• ≥5 years after CABG	A (7)
59.	• <2 years after PCI	I (3)
60.	• ≥2 years after PCI	U (6)
	Cardiac Rehabilitation	
61.	• Prior to initiation of cardiac rehabilitation (as a stand-alone indication)	I (3)
	Assessment of Viability/Ischemia	
	Ischemic Cardiomyopathy/Assessment of Viability	
62.	• Known severe LV dysfunction • Patient eligible for revascularization	A (9)
	Evaluation of Ventricular Function	
	Evaluation of LV Function	
63.	• Assessment of LV function with radionuclide angiography (ERNA or FP RNA) • In absence of recent reliable diagnostic information regarding ventricular function obtained with another imaging modality	A (8)
64.	• Routine use of rest/stress ECG gating with SPECT or PET MPI	A (9)
65.	• Routine use of stress FP RNA in conjunction with rest/stress gated SPECT MPI	I (3)
66.	• Selective use of stress FP RNA in conjunction with rest/stress gated SPECT MPI • Borderline, mild, or moderate stenoses in 3 vessels *or* moderate or equivocal left main stenosis in left dominant system	U (6)
	Use of Potentially Cardiotoxic Therapy (e.g., Doxorubicin)	
67.	• Serial assessment of LV function with radionuclide angiography (ERNA or FP RNA) • Baseline and serial measures after key therapeutic milestones or evidence of toxicity	A (9)

ACS = acute coronary syndrome; CABG = coronary artery bypass grafting surgery; CAD = coronary artery disease; CHD = coronary heart disease; ECG = electrocardiogram; ERNA = equilibrium radionuclide angiography; FP = first pass; HF = heart failure; LBBB = left bundle branch block; LV = left ventricular; MET = estimated metabolic equivalents of exercise; MPI = myocardial perfusion imaging; PCI = percutaneous coronary intervention; PET = positron emission tomography; RNA = radionuclide angiography; SPECT = single-photon emission computed tomography; STEMI = ST elevation myocardial infarction; UA/NSTEMI = unstable angina (UA) and non–ST elevation myocardial infarction (NSTEMI).

From Hendel RC, Berman DS, Di Carli MF, et al: ACCF/ASNC/ACR/AHA/ASE/SCCT/SCMR/SNM 2009 appropriate use criteria for cardiac radionuclide imaging: a report of the American College of Cardiology Foundation Appropriate Use Criteria Task Force, the American Society of Nuclear Cardiology, the American College of Radiology, the American Heart Association, the American Society of Echocardiography, the Society of Cardiovascular Computed Tomography, the Society for Cardiovascular Magnetic Resonance, and the Society of Nuclear Medicine. J Am Coll Cardiol 3:2201, 2009.

REFERENCES

1. Brindis RG, Douglas PS, Hendel RC, et al: ACCF/ASNC appropriateness criteria for single-photon emission computed tomography myocardial perfusion imaging (SPECT MPI). A report of the American College of Cardiology Foundation Quality Strategic Directions Committee Appropriateness Criteria Working Group and the American Society of Nuclear Cardiology Endorsed by the American Heart Association. J Am Coll Cardiol 46:1587, 2005.
2. Hendel RC, Berman DS, Di Carli MF, et al: ACCF/ASNC/ACR/AHA/ASE/SCCT/SCMR/SNM 2009 appropriate use criteria for cardiac radionuclide imaging: A report of the American College of Cardiology Foundation Appropriate Use Criteria Task Force, the American Society of Nuclear Cardiology, the American College of Radiology, the American Heart Association, the American Society of Echocardiography, the Society of Cardiovascular Computed Tomography, the Society for Cardiovascular Magnetic Resonance, and the Society of Nuclear Medicine. J Am Coll Cardiol 3:2201, 2009.

CHAPTER 18 Cardiovascular Magnetic Resonance Imaging

Raymond Y. Kwong

Over the past decade, cardiac magnetic resonance (CMR) has developed into a routine clinical imaging tool. With excellent spatial and temporal resolution, unrestricted tomographic fields, and no exposure to ionizing radiation, CMR offers detailed morphologic and functional characterization for most types of heart disease. In this chapter, the current evidence supporting the use of CMR in the diagnosis and risk stratification of patients with heart disease will be reviewed and the future directions of this technology will be discussed.

Basic Principles of Magnetic Resonance Imaging

Magnetic Field and Gradient Coil System

Magnetic resonance imaging (MRI) is based on the imaging of water (and fat, to a lesser extent) because of its abundance in the body. The hydrogen nuclei (spins) within water or fat possess magnetic moment. When a patient is placed inside the CMR scanner within a static magnetic field (B_0), spins are either aligned with or opposite the main direction of B_0. The summation of the net spins forms a magnetization vector that aligns along the longitudinal axis (*z* axis) of the magnet at static state before the deposition of any radiofrequency pulse (**Fig. 18-1**). The main B_0 field is created so that it has the same strength along each of the three orthogonal directions (known as *x*, *y*, and *z*) inside the CMR bore; thus, it is a homogeneous magnetic field. The homogeneous B_0 is fine-tuned by the computer-controlled adjustments of currents in small coils mounted within the magnet, a process known as active shimming. Apart from lining up with B_0, spins also precess (wobble about the axis of the B_0 field) at a frequency ω_0, known as the Larmor frequency, proportional to B_0 as described by the following equation:

$$\omega_0 = \gamma B_0$$

where γ is the gyromagnetic ratio (a constant for hydrogen for a given field strength). To introduce a system of spatial address of the Larmor frequency, three orthogonal sets of gradient coils are placed so that a slight linear alteration in the strength of B_0 can be created in each of the *x*, *y*, and *z* directions. As a result, magnetic spins precess at frequencies according to their locations along each of the three orthogonal axes and they can be excited selectively by specific radiofrequency pulses.

Generation of Magnetic Resonance Signal, Signal Contrast, and Image Formation

Magnetic resonance is a form of energy exchange between spins and a radiofrequency (RF) pulse that can only occur at a specific frequency. To create an image, an RF pulse with a frequency matched to the Larmor frequency of the magnetic spins will excite magnetic spins of interests to a higher energy state, which leads to a tipping down of the net magnetization vector from the *z* axis onto the *x-y* plane. There is, therefore, an increase of the transverse component (onto the *x-y* plane) and a decrease of the longitudinal component (*z* axis) of the net magnetization vector. The extent to which the magnetization vector is tipped away from the direction of B_0 (*z* axis) defines the flip angle, reflects the amount of energy deposition in tissue, and is a function of the strength and duration of the RF pulse. A set of phased array surface coils in front and behind the patient's chest is used to receive the magnetic resonance signal generated. For the purpose of imaging thin cross sections through the body, an RF pulse should only "excite" spins in that cross section and have no effect elsewhere. This can be achieved by applying a magnetic field gradient perpendicular to a prescribed slice plane; the magnetic gradient causes a spread of Larmor frequencies, and the resonance condition for the RF excitation is only met by a thin cross section whose width is determined by the frequency bandwidth of the RF pulse.

The absorbed electromagnetic energy by the spins will be released by two coexisting mechanisms termed *longitudinal magnetization recovery* and *transverse magnetization decay*. Longitudinal magnetization recovery corresponds to the exponential rate of recovery of the longitudinal component (*z* direction) of the net magnetization vector, characterized by the time constant T1, which is defined as the time to recover 63% of the original longitudinal magnetization vector. T1 is a physical characteristic of the tissue of interest, but is also affected by the field strength of the scanner, with values progressively longer at higher field strengths (in Tesla). The variation of T1 between tissue types allows one to generate images that reflect these differences. A T1-weighted scan will keep the time between delivery of two successive flip angles (repetition time) short, thus maximizing the sensitivity to differentiating tissues by the displayed signal intensity as a result of difference in their T1 values. The transverse magnetization decay results from interaction between neighboring spins (spin-spin interaction) leading to exponential loss of the transverse component of the net magnetization vector, defined by the time constant T2. T2 is also a tissue-specific parameter and is defined as the time to lose 63% of

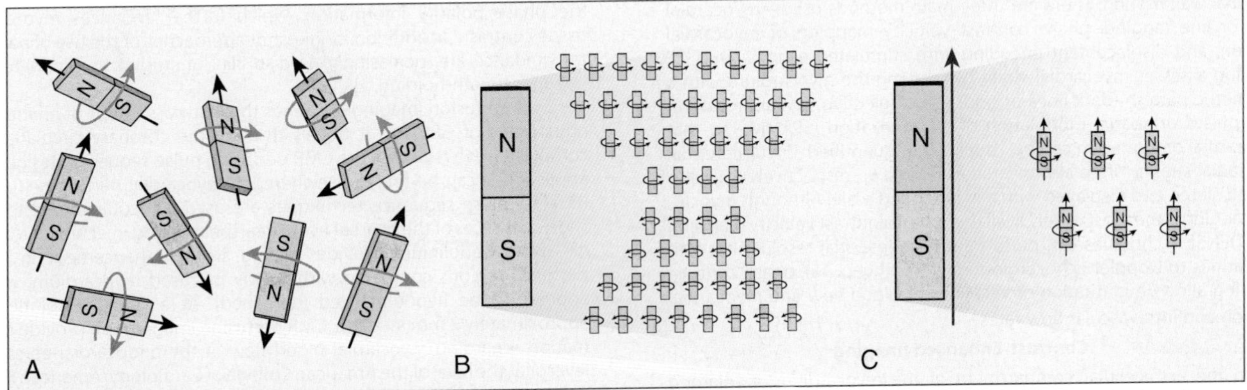

FIGURE 18-1 **A,** Spins are randomly oriented in the absence of an external magnetic field. **B,** In the presence of an external magnetic field, B_0, the spins align parallel or antiparallel to it. **C,** The difference between the parallel minus the antiparallel spins represents the spins that will create a detectable magnetic resonance signal. *(Modified from Aletras AH: Basic MRI physics. In Kwong RY (ed): Cardiovascular Magnetic Resonance Imaging. Totowa, NJ, Humana Press, 2008, pp 1-32.)*

the transverse magnetization. Unlike T1, T2 values are unrelated to the field strength of the scanner. To distinguish different tissues, contrast must be obtained, which is the difference in the magnetic resonance signals of two structures of interest. These depend on the T1, T2, and proton density of the tissues and sequence parameters. With the application of magnetic field gradients in any of the three orthogonal directions, the magnetic resonance signal can carry spatial localization information, produced by encoding steps known as slice select, phase encoding, and frequency encoding. All relevant information of the magnetic resonance signal is stored in a data matrix called the k-space, which will undergo two-dimensional inverse Fourier transformation to form an image. The choice of signal contrast weighting of the imaging method is partly dictated by the physiologic characteristics of the tissue being studied. For qualitative interpretation, signal enhancement (from T1 effects) is in general preferred over darkening (T2*) effects (see later); thus, most pulse sequences used in CMR are relative T1-weighted signal-enhancing techniques. In addition, T1-weighted pulse sequences are less prone to artifacts from adjacent air in the lungs or from cardiac motion.

Contrast Agents

For practical purposes, gadolinium-based contrast agents (GBCAs) are the only contrast materials used in clinical MRI today. After intravenous injection, a GBCA typically takes 15 to 30 seconds for a first pass through the cardiac chambers and blood vessels (first-pass phase) before it diffuses into the extracellular space. At approximately 10 to 15 minutes after injection, a transient plateau of GBCA concentration (equilibrium between contrast washing in to the extracellular space and washing out to the blood pool) is reached. Myocardial perfusion CMR and most types of magnetic resonance angiography (MRA) are performed during the first-pass phase, whereas late gadolinium enhancement (LGE) images are obtained during the equilibrium phase. There are several commercially available GBCAs in the United States, but their use in CMR is considered off-label. Mild allergic reactions from GBCA occur in 0.01% to 0.07% of patients but severe or anaphylactic reactions are rare. All GBCAs are chelated to make the compounds nontoxic and to allow renal excretion. Exposure to the nonchelated component of GBCA (Gd^{3+}) has been reported to trigger nephrogenic systemic fibrosis (NSF), which is characterized by an interstitial inflammatory reaction that leads to severe skin induration, contracture of the extremities, fibrosis of internal organs, and even death. Risk factors for developing NSF include a high-dose (>0.1 mmol/kg) of GBCA in the setting of renal insufficiency (estimated glomerular filtration rate [eGFR] < 30 mL/min/1.73 m^2), need for hemodialysis, severe renal insufficiency (eGFR < 15 mL/min/1.73 m^2), acute renal failure, presence of concurrent proinflammatory processes, and use of the specific GBCA gadodiamide (Omniscan, General Electric Healthcare), A recent review from high-volume MRI centers has shown that NSF is rare. Wertman and colleagues[1] have reviewed records over 7 years at four major U.S. tertiary care centers and reported an NSF incidence of 0.002% to 0.3%, depending on the agent used. Prince and associates[2] have reported an overall incidence of 0.02% in 83,121 patients exposed to GBCA over 10 years when routine screening for renal function was not performed. Most MRI facilities have been screening for high-risk patients in the past few years, and the reported incidence of NSF has been near zero.

TECHNICAL ASPECTS OF CARDIAC MAGNETIC RESONANCE PULSE SEQUENCES

CMR uses a range of strategies to overcome technical difficulties caused by cardiac motion, respiratory motion, and blood flow. Collection of data synchronized to the cardiac cycle (gating) is required, and thus careful placement of electrodes to obtain a reliable electrocardiographic signal is crucial. Fortunately, advances in gating technology have allowed reliable cardiac gating in almost all patients in 1.5-T and even 3-T scanners. Cardiac gating can be prospective (triggering by an electrocardiographic waveform followed by a fixed period of acquisition during all cardiac cycles) or retrospective (continuous data acquisition with subsequent reconstruction based on electrocardiographic timing). For cine imaging, retrospective gating is preferred because it covers the entire cardiac cycle and does not have the flash artifact—sudden brightness of images in the cine loop from partial recovery of longitudinal magnetization—seen in prospective gating. To reduce blurring from cardiac motion, many CMR techniques fractionate the data for an image to be acquired only within a narrow window of the cardiac cycle (segmented approach). On the other hand, other techniques can rapidly acquire data of an entire image all within a cardiac cycle (single-shot approach), thus eliminating the need for breath-holding but at the expense of lower spatial resolution and increased blurriness. Respiratory motion is contained in most situations currently by using a 5- to 15-second breath-hold if compatible with the patient's clinical conditions. Otherwise, navigator-based techniques (tracking of diaphragmatic motion to achieve combined electrocardiographic and diaphragmatic motion gating) and respiratory motion averaging are alternative strategies to suppress respiratory motion. Finally, real-time imaging involves rapid and continuous acquisition of single-shot images that overcomes respiratory and cardiac motion, but at the expense of reduced temporal and spatial resolutions.

Table 18-e1 (see website) provides a summary of the most common clinical CMR pulse sequence techniques at our center. Variations in these parameters exist among centers. CMR uses bright blood cine imaging or dark blood fast spin-echo (FSE) imaging to assess cardiac morphology and structure. Cine CMR has become the imaging reference standard for quantifying ventricular volumes, mass, and regional and global contractile function because of its lack of need for geometric assumption. Among the various cine CMR techniques, cine steady state with free precession (SSFP) is the current technique of choice for its highest image quality. It can acquire a cine movie at a high temporal resolution of 30 to 45 milliseconds during a breath-hold of less than 10 seconds, so that the whole heart in motion is captured in less than 5 minutes. T1-weighted dark blood FSE has high spatial resolution and is often used for the morphology of cardiac chambers, vascular structures, pericardium, and imaging of fat. CMR techniques have been developed to quantify intramyocardial motion to overcome the interobserver variation of visualizing regional wall motion. There are three main methods used—myocardial grid or line tagging, phase contrast velocity mapping of myocardial motion, and displacement encoding with stimulated echoes (DENSE). Tagging assesses myocardial strain by marking the myocardium with a geometric pattern (dark lines or grid) using selective spatial presaturation pulses or spatial modulation of magnetization (SPAMM), so that myocardial deformation can be visualized or quantified. Circumferential and radial strains (often abbreviated as E_{cc} and E_{rr}, respectively) can also be calculated and displayed with a color-coded scale. Although myocardial tagging is the most widely available, phase contrast velocity mapping and DENSE techniques can perform at higher spatial resolutions. With similarities to Doppler echocardiography (see Chap. 15), phase contrast imaging allows quantitation of velocities of blood flow and myocardial motion and intravascular flow rates.

Contrast-Enhanced Imaging

When the extracellular compartment of the myocardium is enlarged because of infarction, infiltration, or replacement fibrosis, influx and retention of the GBCA can be seen by T1-weighted imaging such as LGE. LGE is best detected 10 to 15 minutes after an intravenous injection of GBCA (0.1 to 0.2 mmol/kg)—hence the term *late gadolinium enhancement*. **Figure 18-2** illustrates this technique with LGE imaging of a patient with an anterior myocardial infarction (MI). Further details regarding the features of this pulse sequence are shown in Table 18-e1 (see website). Currently, both two-dimensional and three-dimensional techniques are available; each has its respective merits. A recent technique termed *phase-sensitive inversion recovery* (PSIR) reference imaging incorporates the phase polarity information, which further enhances myocardial tissue contrast.[3] In addition, single-shot approaches or the use of navigator guidance are increasingly used in clinical studies to eliminate the need for breath-holding.[4,5]

CMR perfusion imaging examines the first-pass transit of an intravenous bolus of GBCA as it travels through the coronary circulation. A comprehensive review of the CMR perfusion pulse sequence design and applications can be found elsewhere.[6] In myocardial perfusion studies, ultrafast pulse sequence techniques are used to acquire three to five short-axis slices of the heart at every heartbeat during injection of a bolus of GBCA. Gadolinium provides strong signal enhancement in well-perfused regions compared with poorly perfused myocardium, which appears to be hypoenhanced (darkened). At a spatial resolution of approximately 2 mm in-plane, CMR perfusion imaging can provide information regarding myocardial blood flow at the endocardial-epicardial level or at the level of the American College of Cardiology/American Heart Association (ACC/AHA) 17-segment model. Newer methods, such as SSFP and 3-T perfusion imaging, which provide a substantially higher signal-noise-ratio, are promising to improve image quality further.[7] T2-weighted imaging detects myocardial edema as a result of ischemic injury or inflammation. The edematous region obtained by T2-weighted imaging has been shown to have high correlation to the area at risk after an acute MI (see Fig. 58-4).[8] T2-weighted imaging complements LGE in determining the chronicity of MI and allowing for sizing of salvageable myocardium after emergent revascularization. The pulse sequence options, including the widely used black blood short inversion time inversion recovery (STIR) FSE and newer SSFP methods, and their merits are listed in Table 18-e1 (see website).[9,10]

T2* is a transverse relaxation parameter sensitive to tissue iron content. T2* imaging has been extensively validated at 1.5 T against tissue iron levels with excellent interstudy reproducibility over time and across different MRI platforms.[11,12] A T2* shorter than 20 milliseconds (normal myocardium, ~40 to 50 milliseconds) is diagnostic of myocardial iron overload and a T2* shorter than 10 milliseconds is evidence of severe iron overload.[13,14] Despite challenges from small luminal sizes, vessel tortuosity, and cardiac and respiratory motions, technical advances in coronary MRA imaging have resulted in high success rates in experienced centers[15-17] (**Fig. 18-3**). Currently, the common technique acquires a three-dimensional heart volume using navigator guidance

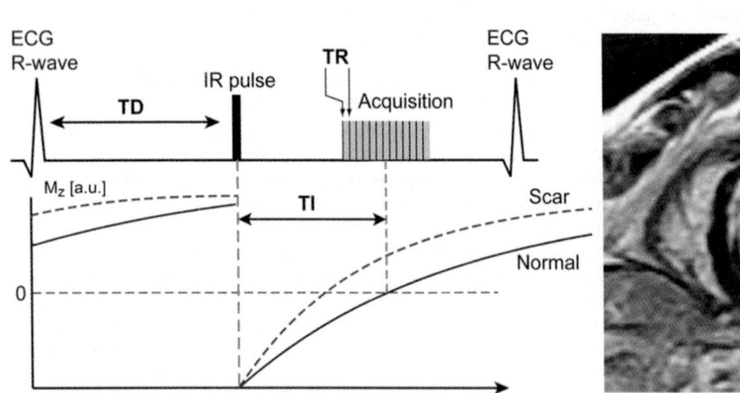

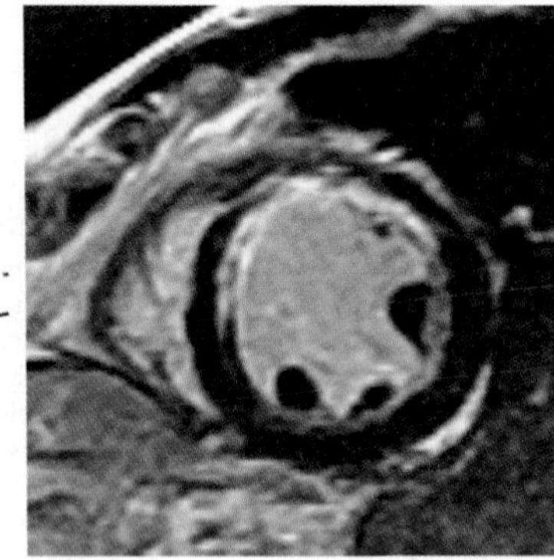

FIGURE 18-2 T1-weighted inversion recovery fast gradient echo imaging for LGE. The technique uses the difference in T1 between infarcted (T1 shortened by accumulation of gadolinium) and normal myocardium. Imaging data acquisition is set to occur at the appropriate inversion time when normal myocardium is nulled (dark) and during mid-late diastole to minimize motion blurring. The image shows differentiation of a bright infarcted anterior wall, intermediate-intensity blood pool, and dark normal myocardium.

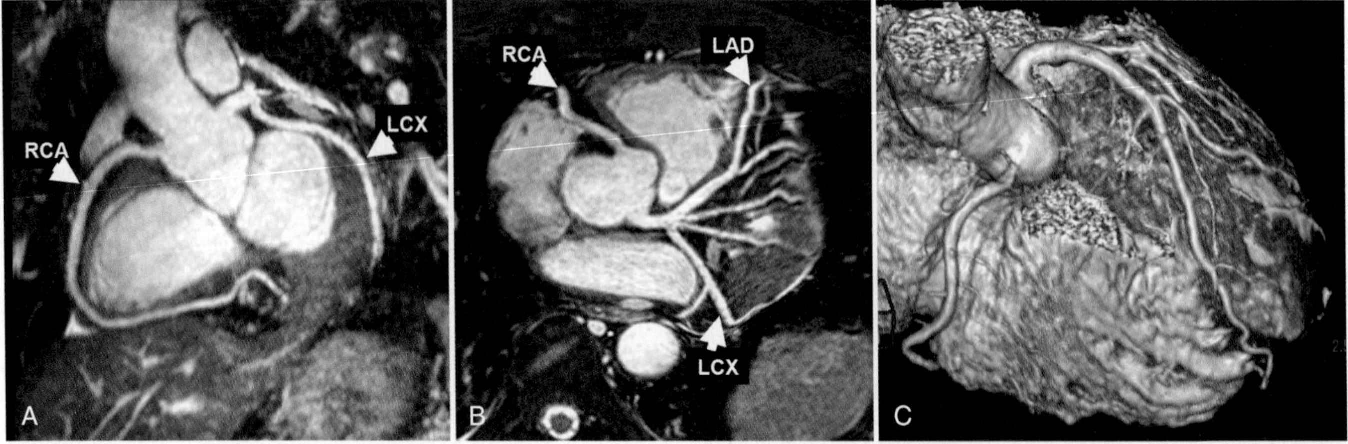

FIGURE 18-3 Free-breathing, navigator echo-gated whole-heart coronary MRA acquired with an SSFP sequence (balanced turbo field echo) with fat saturation and T2 preparation in a subject with normal coronary arteries. **A,** Left anterior oblique whole-heart coronary MRA reformatted with curved multiplanar reformatting clearly depicts the right coronary artery (RCA) and left circumflex (LCX) arteries. **B,** Oblique axial whole-heart coronary MRA reformatted with curved multiplanar reformatting visualizes the left main coronary artery, left anterior descending (LAD) artery, proximal RCA, and LCX artery. **C,** Volume-rendered image of whole-heart coronary MRA is useful for three-dimensional anatomic recognition of the coronary arteries. *(From Sakuma H, Ichikawa Y, Suzawa N, et al: Assessment of coronary arteries with total study time of less than 30 minutes by using whole-heart coronary MR angiography. Radiology 237:316, 2005.)*

at a spatial resolution (0.8 × 0.8 mm at a slice thickness of 1 mm) that is only slightly lower than computed tomography (CT; see Chap. 19). A recent consensus statement from the AHA has assigned a level of evidence of IIa for evidence supporting the use of coronary MRA in assessing coronary anomalies.[15]

Many parallel imaging techniques are routinely used to speed up CMR (k-space) data acquisition while cardiac and respiratory motions are controlled for image quality. These techniques combine information obtained separately from each element of the surface receiver coil to reduce the sampling of k-space data for faster image acquisition. Incorporating parallel imaging into pulse sequences can lead to reduced acquisition time, shorter patient breath-holds, improved temporal resolution, and/or elimination of certain artifacts. The main disadvantage of all parallel imaging techniques is a reduction in signal-to-noise ratio as a result of undersampling of the k-space lines.

Patient Safety

Most clinical (1.5-T) CMR scanners are superconducting systems in which the magnetic field created by the superconductive coil cannot be turned off. In rare emergency situations, the only way to remove the magnetic field quickly is by rapidly boiling off the cooling liquid helium as gas to the outside environment (quenching) through evacuation pipes. Every caution must be practiced to avoid an emergency quench because it carries the risk of burns or asphyxia to individuals inside the MRI scanner room, and restoration of the magnetic field is costly. A short list of common medical devices that are contraindications to the use of CMR include cochlear implants, neurostimulators, hydrocephalus shunts, metal-containing ocular implants, pacing wires, Swan-Ganz catheters, and metallic cerebral aneurysm clips. Sternal wires, mechanical heart valves and annuloplasty rings, coronary stents, nonmetallic catheters, and orthopedic or dental implants can be safely scanned at 1.5 T and even 3 T (updated safety information for medical devices can be found at www.mrisafety.com). Patient claustrophobia can almost always be managed with oral sedation or by performing the study in a short-bore scanner with an expanded diameter.

Performing Cardiac Magnetic Resonance in Patient with a Permanent Pacemaker or Defibrillator

The risks of performing MRI in the presence of a pacemaker or automated implantable cardioverter-defibrillator (ICD) include the generation of an electrical current from the metallic hardware (especially if wire loops exist), device movement induced by the magnetic field, inappropriate discharging and sensing, and heating as a result of the antenna effect.[18] A temporary pacemaker is currently an absolute contraindication to CMR, although clinical trials of pacemakers with new designs of pacing wires are underway. A number of experienced centers have reported safety in performing CMR at 1.5 T in patients with a permanent pacemaker. Roguin and coworkers[19] have reported safe and successful MRI examinations in 99% of patients using an algorithm involving careful selection and programming of the pacemaker and limiting the RF energy absorbed by the patient to less than 2.0 W/kg by any pulse sequence. A similar strategy was reported to be safe by the same group, which allowed non–pacemaker-dependent patients with ICDs implanted after 2000 to undergo CMR.[20] Collectively, evidence from combined reports of more than 250 patients in the medical literature with pacemaker models from the year 2000 or later appears to suggest that CMR at 1.5 T or less can be safely performed in a controlled setting.

Clinical Applications

The next sections of this chapter discuss clinical aspects of CMR imaging. Table 18-e2 (see website) provides a summary of the CMR protocols by study indications at our center. A detailed description of CMR protocols endorsed by the Society of Cardiovascular Magnetic Resonance (SCMR) is available at www.scmr.org.[21] In addition, the SCMR has established reporting guidelines to provide a framework for enhancing communication with referring physicians.[22]

Assessment of Coronary Artery Disease

Multicomponent CMR imaging is capable of characterizing various pathophysiologic states described within the spectrum of coronary artery disease (CAD). Current CMR protocols for CAD integrate cine SSFP, T2-weighted edema imaging, myocardial perfusion at rest and stress, and LGE imaging of myocardial scar, thus providing a comprehensive evaluation of myocardial anatomy and physiology. Coronary MRA is also performed as a part of the CMR examination in more experienced centers. Tables 18-e2 and 18-e3 (see website) summarize the CMR protocols used in our center and the typical CMR findings of CAD.

IMAGING OF MYOCARDIAL INFARCTION. LGE imaging is currently the most accurate and precise noninvasive method to quantify infarct size and morphology in patients (see Figs. 58-14 and 56-5).[23] There are easy-to-use commercial software programs and more sophisticated validated computer algorithms available for in vivo quantitation of infarct size by LGE.[24] At the clinical level, infarct size or infarct transmurality by LGE imaging correlates with markers of infarct size such as serum creatine kinase level, time to treatment, and incomplete electrocardiographic ST-segment resolution.[17] The robustness of the LGE imaging across MRI vendors was demonstrated by a recent double-blind, multicenter, randomized trial of 566 patients who underwent LGE imaging for MI.[25] LGE identified infarct location accurately and detected acute and chronic infarcts with a sensitivity of 99% and 94%, respectively. When LGE imaging is performed early (within the first 5 minutes) after contrast injection, regions of microvascular obstruction (no-reflow) can be seen as a dense hypoenhanced area within the core of a bright region of infarction (**Fig. 18-4**). This noninvasive method for quantifying microvascular obstruction has been validated against angiographic parameters of microcirculatory flow such as thrombolysis in myocardial infarction (TIMI) frame counts, intracoronary Doppler flow, and myocardial Blush score.[19] A recent study has demonstrated detection of myocardial hemorrhage as a result of reperfusion injury.[26]

With an in-plane spatial resolution of 1.5 to 2 mm and a high contrast-to-noise ratio, LGE imaging can recognize subendocardial MI undetected by single-photon emission computed tomography (SPECT) or positron emission tomography (PET). This high sensitivity of LGE in detecting MI has been shown to detect down to a few grams of infarcted tissue in the target myocardial region of distal embolization during percutaneous coronary intervention in patients with CAD.[27] There is growing evidence that these technical advantages of CMR translate to useful patient prognostic information. In a study of 195 patients referred for assessment of CAD but without a history of MI, LGE consistent with an unrecognized MI was an independent and strong predictor of cardiac death after adjustment to common clinical variables. Even infarct size in the smallest tertile was associated with a more than sevenfold unadjusted hazard of adverse events.[28]

Patients with diabetes are a particular subgroup with a high likelihood of unrecognized previous coronary events (see Chap. 64). In a study of 187 diabetics undergoing CMR for assessment of CAD, patients without clinical or electrocardiographic evidence of MI experienced a 3.6-fold elevated hazard of death if LGE consistent with MI was detected, with a Kaplan-Meier distribution for cardiac death similar to that of diabetic patients known to have had a clinical MI[29] (**Fig. 18-5**).

Other studies support the prognostic value of LGE in patients with clinically recognized MI. A recent study of 857 patients by Cheong and colleagues[30] has reported that LGE scar transmurality index is a strong independent predictor of death or cardiac transplantation at a median follow-up of 4.4 years; this provides complementary prognostic information to the left ventricular (LV) ejection fraction (**Fig. 18-6**). The same investigators also reported that LGE provides similar prognostic information in a subgroup of 349 patients with CAD and severe LV dysfunction.[31] Several pilot studies have demonstrated that tissue inhomogeneity quantified in LGE images may identify arrhythmogenic

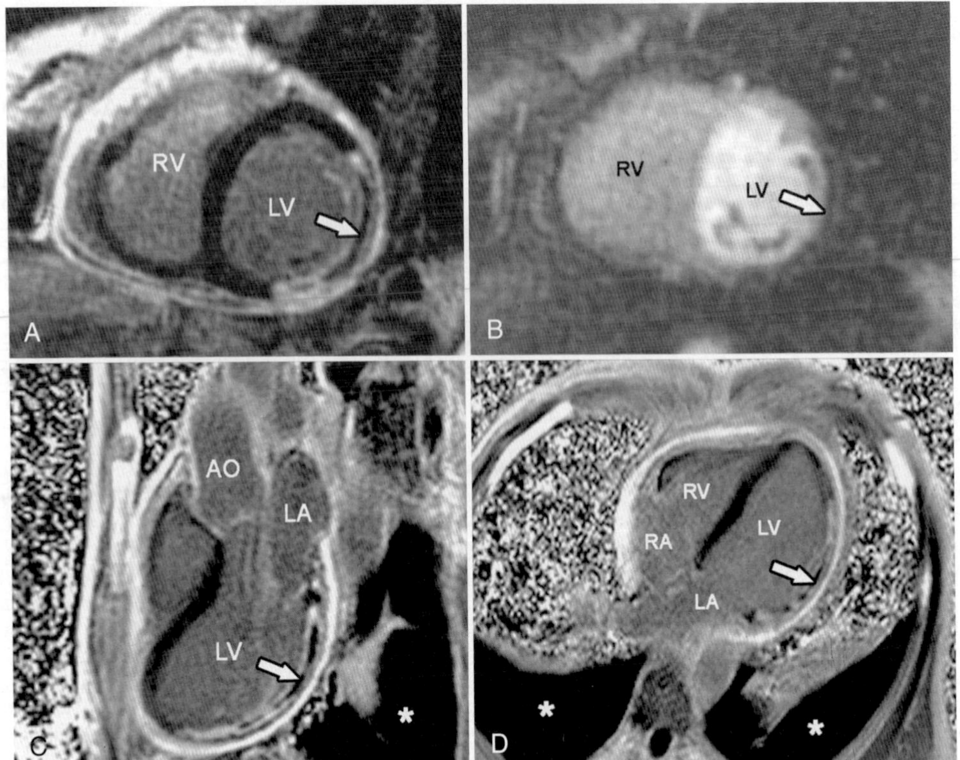

FIGURE 18-4 A 52-year-old man with history of a prior inferior MI 1 week ago was referred for assessment of myocardial viability. **A,** Short-axis LGE images reveal a transmural MI involving the lateral LV wall associated with a large and dense area of microvascular obstruction (arrow). **B,** Despite successful epicardial revascularization of the infarct-related coronary artery, first-pass myocardial perfusion imaging demonstrates a dense perfusion defect indicative of no-reflow (arrow) matching in location with the infarct. **C, D,** Long-axis LGE images confirm the extensive area of microvascular obstruction involving a large extent of the lateral LV wall. Of note, there was concurrent intense pericardial inflammation and bilateral pleural effusion (asterisk). Ao = aorta; LA = left atrium; RA = right atrium; RV = right ventricle.

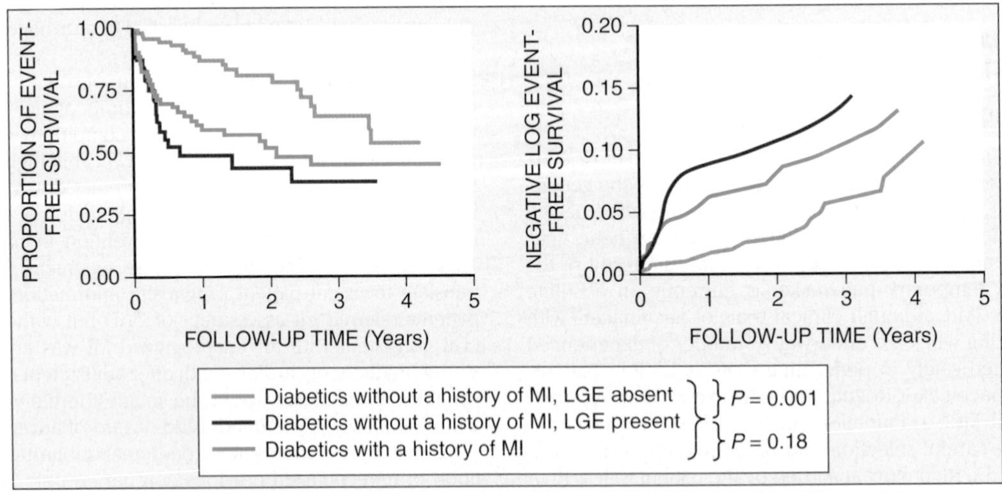

FIGURE 18-5 Kaplan-Meier event-free survival curves **(left panel)** and cumulative rate of adverse cardiac events **(right panel)** for patients with diabetes. Patients without a history of MI who had no evidence of infarction by LGE imaging (yellow curve) experienced a relatively benign clinical course, compared with worse event-free survival in patients with a known history of MI (blue curve) and patients without a history of MI who had evidence of unrecognized MI by LGE imaging (red curve). *(From Kwong RY, Sattar H, Wu H, et al: Incidence and prognostic implication of unrecognized myocardial scar characterized by cardiac magnetic resonance in diabetic patients without clinical evidence of myocardial infarction. Circulation 118:1011, 2008.)*

substrates that develop as a result of MI. Schmidt and associates[32] have reported a method for quantifying the heterogeneous peri-infarct zone, which demonstrated a strong association with inducible monomorphic ventricular tachycardia during electrophysiologic studies. Roes and coworkers,[33] using slightly different quantitative criteria, have reported that the peri-infarct zone is the strongest predictor of spontaneous ventricular arrhythmias that required appropriate ICD therapy in 91 patients with previous MI in whom ICDs were implanted for clinical indications. These findings are concordant with the observed increased in patient mortality associated with larger peri-infarct zones in a cohort of 144 post-MI patients reported by Yan and colleagues[34] (**Fig. 18-7**). Before this promising novel application can become a routine means of stratifying patients according to arrhythmic risks, future studies need to establish standardized criteria for quantifying the peri-infarct zone and demonstrate robustness in its association with serious arrhythmic events.

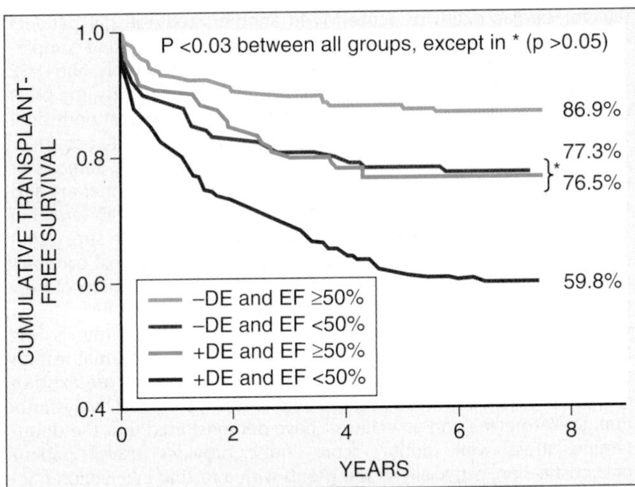

FIGURE 18-6 Transplant-free survival in a cohort of 857 patients referred for CMR assessment of coronary artery disease. Patients are stratified by left ventricular ejection fraction (EF) and the presence (+) or absence (–) of delayed contrast enhancement (DE). *(From Cheong BYC, Muthupillai R, Wilson JM, et al: Prognostic significance of delayed-enhancement magnetic resonance imaging. Circulation 120:2069, 2009.)*

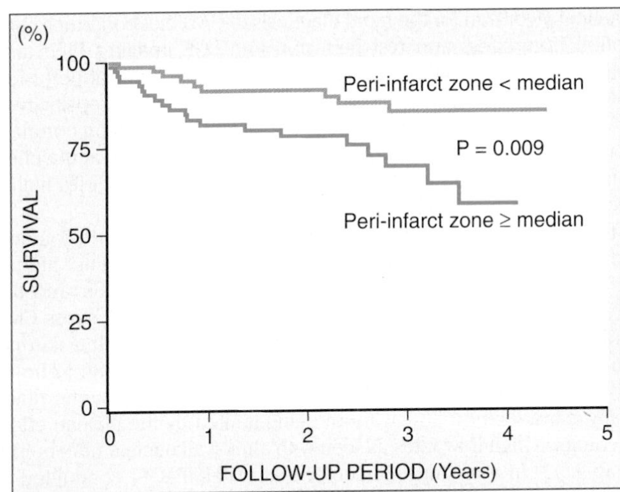

FIGURE 18-7 Kaplan-Meier survival curves for all-cause mortality, stratified by median size of the peri-infarct zone. *(From Yan AT, Shayne AJ, Brown KA, et al: Characterization of the peri-infarct zone by contrast-enhanced cardiac magnetic resonance imaging is a powerful predictor of post-myocardial infarction mortality. Circulation 114:32, 2006.)*

Assessment of Myocardial Viability and Benefit from Coronary Revascularization. Several pitfalls are often encountered in the imaging of myocardial viability. A fundamental concept defines myocardial viability as preservation of cellular function without any irreversible cellular damage. Although assessment of histologic viability could not be reliably achieved clinically, indirect markers of cellular function have been used as surrogates of myocardial viability and have created problems in comparing the usefulness of various noninvasive modalities. Recovery of regional and/or global LV systolic function after coronary revascularization is the most common clinical standard of myocardial viability, but this surrogate provides limited information about patient morbidity and mortality. Targeting different cellular processes of the hibernating myocardium, imaging modalities can yield discordant results at different stages or severity of chronic hypoperfusion, causing inconsistencies when the usefulness of these imaging modalities are compared. Consider the following two examples: (1) early development of ischemia in myocardium subtended by a critical coronary stenosis during low-dose dobutamine challenge (see Chap. 15); and (2) lack of contractile reserve when chronic and severe hypoperfusion has led to disassembly of cellular contractile filaments and myocyte dedifferentiation (see Chap. 52), despite maintenance of basic cellular metabolism and cell membrane integrity. In both these examples, the absence of contractile reserve would suggest a lack of viability. Other techniques, such as PET, which detects myocardial metabolism (see Chap. 17), or LGE imaging by CMR, which detects altered tissue relaxation characteristics of irreversibly injured myocardium, may identify these segments as viable in either example. However, recovery of contractile function, which may occur in the first example, is unlikely in the second.

End-diastolic wall thickness alone has limited accuracy in predicting the recovery of segmental function because it may include irreversibly damaged subendocardial myocardium and a thinned epicardial rim of viable myocardium, which may not be sufficient to result in improved function after successful coronary revascularization. In addition, during acute ischemia, local edema and cellular infiltrates may increase regional wall thickness. Augmentation of regional function in response to low-dose (5 to 10 μg/kg/min) dobutamine administration has been well validated in identifying segmental viability by cine CMR. Early cine CMR studies showed that contractile reserve, defined as an increase in systolic wall thickening of 2 mm, has excellent specificity and sensitivity in predicting segmental contractile recovery after revascularization (sensitivity, 89%; specificity, 94%).

In a landmark paper by Kim and associates,[35] the transmural extent of myocardial scar detected by LGE imaging was shown to predict a progressive stepwise decrease in the likelihood of function recovery accurately, despite successful coronary revascularization. This prediction of segmental functional recovery was especially strong in segments with resting akinesia or dyskinesia. For example, 88% of segments with less than 25% transmural extent of LGE improved contractile function, whereas only 4% of segments with more than 50% transmural extent of LGE improved function after revascularization. Compared with dobutamine cine CMR, LGE is easy to perform and interpret, and a 50% transmurality cutoff is sensitive in predicting segmental contractile recovery. On the other hand, the high specificity of low-dose dobutamine cine CMR provides a physiologic assessment of the midmyocardial and subepicardial contractile reserve, particularly in segments with subendocardial infarction involving less than 50% of the transmural extent. Some controversy exists as to whether dobutamine cine CMR provides additional information beyond LGE characterization of infarct transmurality in this setting. Among a few other single-center studies, Wellnhofer and coworkers[36] assessed 29 patients before and 3 months after coronary revascularization with both low-dose dobutamine cine imaging and LGE imaging, and reported better prediction of segmental contractile recovery by dobutamine cine imaging. Although local expertise and difference in opinion will continue to direct regional practice, at our center it appears that LGE imaging alone suffices to answer most questions about assessing myocardial viability. However, low-dose dobutamine cine CMR can be complementary in assessing myocardial viability early after acute MI when tissue edema is prominent or when there is a need to assess the benefit of bypass surgery in patients at high preoperative risk.

Detecting Acute Coronary Syndromes and Differentiating From Noncoronary Causes. Early studies performed in the emergency department setting indicated high sensitivity and specificity of CMR in detecting acute coronary syndromes and in risk-stratifying patients presenting with acute chest pain.[37,38] Abdel-Aty and colleagues[39] have studied 73 post-MI patients and found that qualitative assessment of T2-weighted imaging and LGE yielded a 96% specificity in differentiating acute from chronic MI. Cury and associates[40] have assessed patients presenting with acute chest pain with negative electrocardiographic findings and cardiac enzyme levels. They reported that adding T2-weighted imaging and LV wall thickness to cine and LGE imaging increases the specificity from 84% to 96% without any loss of sensitivity, thus enhancing the diagnostic certainty for acute coronary syndrome, especially in patients with prior MI. Furthermore, in patients presenting with acute chest pain, several single-center studies have reported strong diagnostic usefulness of CMR in differentiating acute coronary syndrome from noncoronary causes of chest pain.[41-43]

DETECTING AND QUANTIFYING MYOCARDIAL ISCHEMIA

Myocardial Perfusion Imaging

Numerous single-center studies and a recent multicenter study have shown that qualitative assessment of vasodilator stress CMR myocardial perfusion is rapid and accurate in detecting CAD. Improved standardization of perfusion data acquisition and analysis across CMR centers and scanner manufacturers have been developed in the past few years. Klem and coworkers[44] have proposed and validated a

practical algorithm for the rapid diagnosis of CAD that combines information from stress and rest perfusion and LGE imaging. Plein and colleagues[45] demonstrated that combined interpretation of perfusion, coronary MRA, LGE, and cine CMR reaches an excellent sensitivity of 96% while maintaining a high specificity of 83% in detecting coronary stenosis in a prospective study of patients presenting with acute chest pain. The combined multicomponent CMR approach provides higher accuracy than any single CMR component alone.

There are several technical advantages of CMR stress perfusion over radionuclide perfusion imaging. CMR perfusion imaging is not limited by attenuation artifacts, has no need for ionizing radiation, and has three- to fourfold higher spatial resolution than SPECT. A stress CMR study that includes stress and rest perfusion imaging, cine cardiac function, and viability takes 35 to 45 minutes (compared with >2 hours for SPECT). CMR perfusion also can characterize the dynamic range of myocardial blood flow without being limited by the plateau effect of counts at high flow rates, as seen with almost all nuclear tracers (see Chap. 17).[46] In a recent multicenter trial (MR-IMPACT) conducted in 18 experienced centers that enrolled 241 patients who underwent coronary angiography,[46a] CMR perfusion performed better than SPECT in detecting coronary stenosis (area under the curve, 86% versus 67%; $P = 0.01$), especially in the group of patients with multivessel stenosis (area under curve by CMR, 89% versus 70%, $P = 0.006$). This supports the notion that the higher spatial resolution obtained when characterizing subendocardial perfusion deficits by CMR may improve the detection of diffuse coronary disease as suggested by preclinical studies. CMR myocardial perfusion can also be analyzed by quantitative methods using the signal intensity versus time curves derived from LV myocardial segments. Accounting for arterial input function at different hemodynamic states and using a low dose of contrast injection—to maintain a linear relationship between contrast concentration and measured signal intensity—are prerequisites in quantitative methods. Common semiquantitative parameters include signal upslope (rate of rise of the ascending curve), upslope integral (area under the upslope), and contrast enhancement ratio (ratio of peak to baseline signal intensity; **Fig. 18-8**). Fully quantitative analysis of CMR perfusion yields absolute myocardial blood flow (in milliliters per minute per gram of tissue) using deconvolution methods and modeled compartmental analysis. The advantages of quantitative analyses include minimization of reader's bias and generation of color-coded maps of perfusion reserve (ratio of stress over rest myocardial blood flow), which may serve not only to improve the diagnosis of CAD but may test the efficacy of novel therapies.

Dobutamine Stress Cardiac Magnetic Resonance

Dobutamine stress CMR has been shown in several studies to have high sensitivities of 83% to 86% and specificities of 83% to 86% in detecting CAD and to be superior to dobutamine stress echocardiography when echocardiographic windows are inadequate, despite the use of second harmonic imaging. Such favorable results were consistent and maintained despite the presence of underlying resting wall motion abnormalities.[47] The addition of dobutamine stress myocardial perfusion imaging and myocardial tagging can serve as adjuncts to cine CMR for detecting myocardial ischemia.[48] Preliminary results of accelerated real-time cine CMR imaging, which eliminates the need for breath-holding or ECG gating during dobutamine stress, have been encouraging. Treadmill exercise CMR is currently investigational but has been shown to be feasible in highly experienced centers.

Prognostic Value. A growing number of studies have demonstrated strong prognostic values of stress CMR. Ingkanisorn and associates[37] have used adenosine stress CMR perfusion to assess 135 patients evaluated in the emergency department setting with chest pain but without electrocardiographic or serologic evidence of MI. At study follow-up, 20 patients developed clinical events (new diagnosis of significant coronary stenosis or adverse cardiac events). Stress CMR perfusion imaging was the strongest component of the CMR examination, with a sensitivity of 100% and specificity of 93% for clinical events at 1 year. Combining data from the components of a CMR study appears to provide complementary prognostic information. In a study of 513 patients, Jahnke and coworkers[49] have reported that a CMR study with normal dobutamine stress cine and normal adenosine perfusion carries a 99.2% negative 3-year event rate for cardiac death or acute MI. In another study of 254 patients referred for stress CMR, Steel and colleagues[50] found robust and complementary prognostic information of stress CMR perfusion and LGE imaging in predicting cardiac death or acute MI. In that study, the presence of LGE, despite the absence of ischemia by stress or rest perfusion, was associated with an 11-fold increase in the hazard of cardiac death or acute MI. In a pilot study of 81 patients with angiographic stenosis of intermediate severity (50% to 75%) treated with medical therapy and followed for an average of 30 months, CMR perfusion was abnormal in all 9 patients who developed adverse events.[51] Dobutamine stress CMR provides accurate patient prognostication beyond traditional coronary risk factors in patients referred for stress testing for evaluation of new symptoms or risk assessment before noncardiac surgery. In patients with normal dobutamine stress CMR, the cardiac event rate is less than 1% over the next 2 to 3 years in the presence of normal resting LV ejection fraction[49] and is only 2% in the presence of pre-existing global LV dysfunction. In a study of 200 patients with global LV dysfunction, Dall'Armellina and associates[52] have demonstrated that the dobutamine stress wall motion score index provides useful patient prognostication, especially in the group with a resting LV ejection fraction between 40% and 55%, with a more than threefold elevated hazard of experiencing hard cardiac events in those with abnormal dobutamine responses. The same investigators also reported that dobutamine stress CMR provides prognostic information regarding cardiac death or MI in women.[53]

IMAGING OF ATHEROSCLEROTIC PLAQUES. Plaque structure and activity are important factors that lead to plaque vulnerability. MRI of the carotid artery and descending aorta remains the most comprehensive noninvasive method to characterize plaque structure and activity. The carotid bifurcation is relatively immobile, large, and superficial to the skin surface, and it shows the full spectrum of atherosclerotic lesion types. Yuan and Kerwin[54] have proposed a standardized protocol that consists of two contrast-weighted imaging sequences to identify carotid plaque fibrous cap, hemorrhage, calcifications, and loose matrix. In addition, gadolinium-enhanced T1-weighted imaging helps discriminate fibrous cap from necrotic or lipid core. Carotid plaque activity such as neovascularization can be assessed by contrast-enhanced dynamic MRI that measures the transfer constant between blood and the extracellular space, with preliminary evidence of prognostic implications.[55,56] Ultrasmall superparamagnetic particles of iron oxide (USPIO) have been shown to target macrophage activity at high affinity based on histologic and electron microscopic analyses of atherosclerotic plaques. By causing signal darkening from the T2* susceptibility effect, USPIO-based CMR imaging of macrophages in carotid plaques can be performed with an optimal time window at 24 to 36 hours after USPIO injection.[57] MRI of aortic plaques is limited by signal-noise ratio in achieving submillimeter spatial resolution and blood flow artifacts. Technical improvements in aortic plaque imaging using intravascular magnetic resonance coils have been reported.[58] CMR provides accurate quantitation of aortic plaque size and composition, which complements three-dimensional MRA assessment of the thoracic aorta. Common to all imaging modalities, imaging of the coronary plaque is challenged by cardiac and respiratory motion and small vessel size, but future technical improvement using exogenous targeted contrast agents, intravascular coils, and high-field CMR may offer promise. Specifically, the fibrin-binding contrast agent EP-2104R (EPIX Pharmaceuticals, Cambridge, Mass) has been shown to allow CMR imaging of coronary thrombosis.[59] This molecule-targeting approach is advantageous because the demands for high spatial resolution and motion suppression may be less stringent.

Assessment of Cardiomyopathies

A summary of CMR protocols useful for evaluating patients with various cardiomyopathies is shown in Table 18-e2 (see website). Echocardiography will likely remain the first test for patient evaluation because of its ease of use and widespread availability (see Chap. 15). However, with its multifaceted approach within a study, CMR is considered by many experienced centers to be the best noninvasive diagnostic test for assessing the etiology in patients with a newly diagnosed

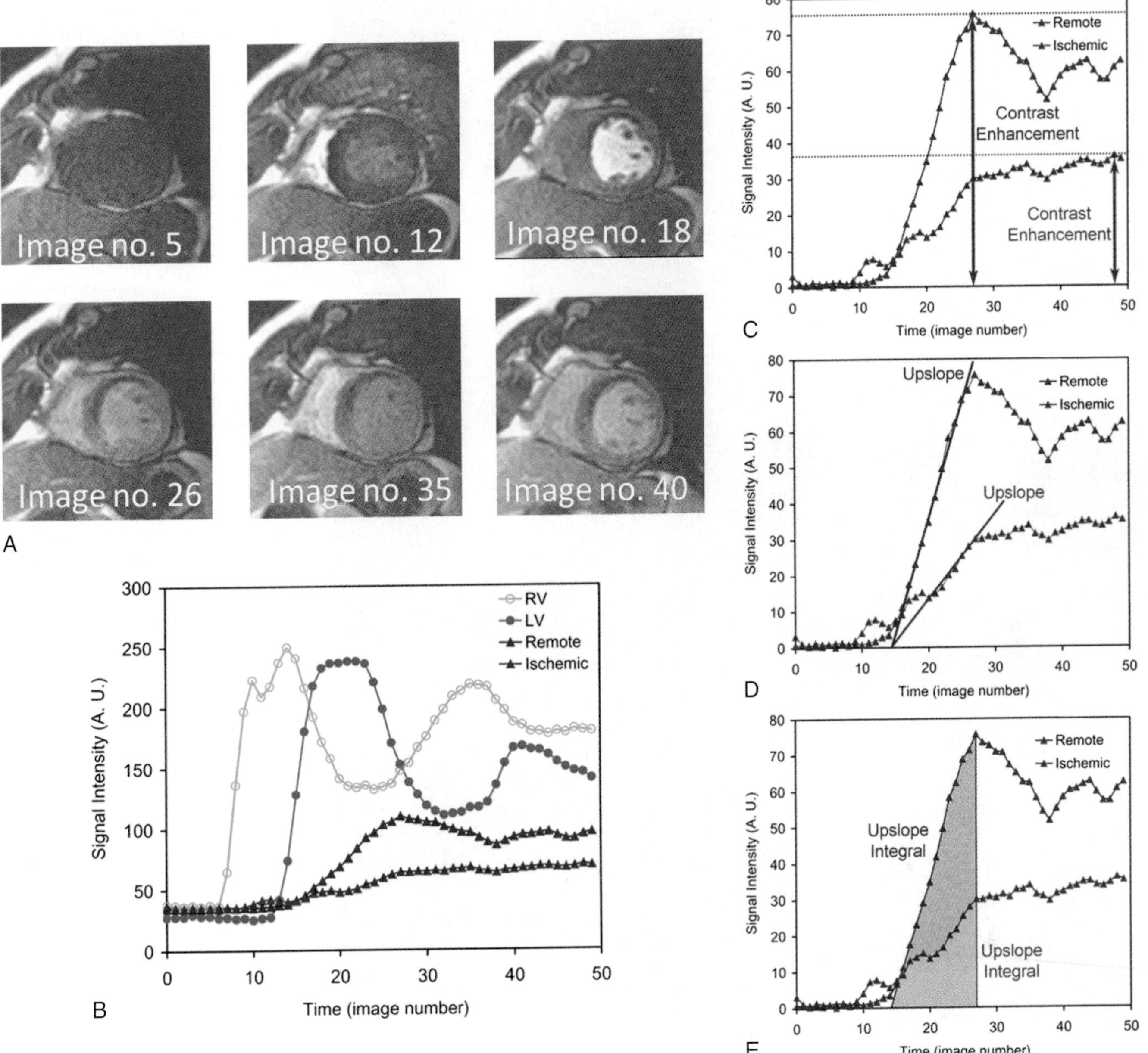

FIGURE 18-8 **A,** Qualitative interpretation of a first-pass myocardial perfusion study as a bolus of gadolinium contrast transits through the heart. Note that an anterior subendocardial perfusion defect appears starting at image 18 and persists at peak contrast enhancement (image 26) and later. **B,** Time intensity curves measured from a first-pass CMR perfusion study. The open green circles were measured in the RV cavity. The dark green circles were measured in the LV cavity. The blue triangles were measured in a sector representing normal vasodilated myocardium, and the red triangles came from a region of the myocardium with severely reduced perfusion (anterior subendocardium in this case). **C, D, E,** Methods for semiquantitative analysis of perfusion. Common semiquantitative parameters for measuring myocardial perfusion include peak contrast enhancement **(C)**, upslopes of the time-intensity curves **(D)**, and upslope integrals **(E)**. *(Courtesy of Dr. Andrew Arai, National Heart, Lung, and Blood Institute, National Institutes of Health, Bethesda, Md.)*

cardiomyopathy (**Fig. 18-9**). Table 18-e3 (see website) summarizes the CMR features—using rest and stress myocardial perfusion, regional function, LGE, and T2-weighted imaging by CMR—for differentiating myocardial viability, ischemia, infarction, and noncoronary causes of cardiomyopathy. When the LGE pattern is used to rule in nonischemic cardiomyopathy, it is important to recognize that infarction can appear nonsubendocardial at the edge of the infarction, or may be a result of microvascular obstruction or endocardial thrombus (both appear dark on LGE imaging), thus mimicking a nonischemic pattern of LGE. Comparing the LGE image against cine gradient echo or perfusion images in matching location or by using a long inversion time (600 milliseconds or longer) can help determine the presence of microvascular obstruction or thrombus.[60] Tissue tagging may help resolve any suspected regional wall motion abnormality at rest or stress or when myocardial adhesion from pericardial diseases becomes part of the issue under consideration.

HYPERTROPHIC CARDIOMYOPATHY. CMR cine imaging of LV structure and function and tissue characterization are useful for distinguishing between physiologic and pathologic forms of LV hypertrophy (LVH; see Chap. 69). Olivotto and colleagues[61] have reported that substantial overlap in LV mass index values exists among patients with hypertrophic cardiomyopathy (HCM) and normal control subjects from the Framingham Heart Study, in which at least 20% of HCM patients had a normal LV mass index. Whereas a dichotomous LV mass index cutoff value cannot be used as a diagnostic criterion for HCM,

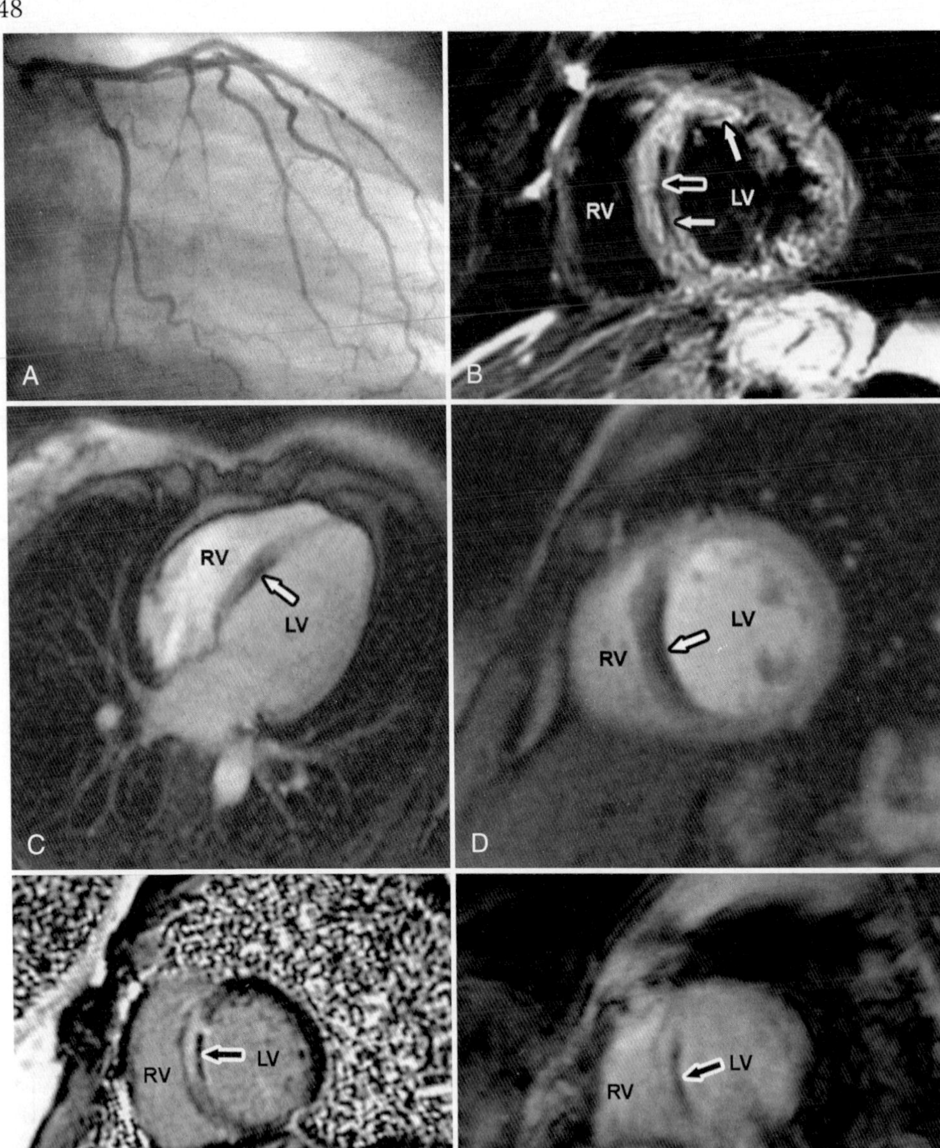

FIGURE 18-9 A 42-year-old woman was admitted with several days of chest pain and found to have transient ST-segment elevation and abnormal serum troponin levels. **A,** Whereas urgent coronary angiography did not reveal any significant coronary stenosis, multimodality CMR provided information that indicated an acute coronary event. **B,** T2-weighted fast spin-echo imaging demonstrated an area of high signal intensity consistent with transmural myocardial edema (area at risk) in the anteroseptal wall (arrows). Although there was no significant epicardial coronary stenosis, evidence of tissue no-reflow was seen in the subendocardium of the anteroseptal wall within the area at risk (black arrow). **C,** On first-pass myocardial perfusion imaging, the no-reflow zone is seen as a dense perfusion defect (**C** and **D**, arrows), and as a dark region within the gadolinium-enhanced area of infarction on late gadolinium enhancement imaging (**E**, arrow). **F,** In addition, very low signal intensity was seen in this region by T2* imaging, raising the suspicion of coexisting intramyocardial hemorrhage (arrow).

Petersen and associates[62] have observed that an end-diastolic wall thickness–to–cavity volume ratio less than 0.15 mm/mL/m^2 and lack of LGE of the ventricular myocardium can provide accurate differentiation between physiologic and pathologic LVH. Limited echocardiographic windows lead to obliquity and errors in geometric measurements. Rickers[63] has reported that CMR detects hypertrophic segments in 6% of patients in whom it was undetected by two-dimensional echocardiography. In addition, echocardiography underestimated the magnitude of hypertrophy determined by CMR in the basal anterolateral wall by 20% and the presence of extreme hypertrophy (>30-mm wall thickness) by 10%. Both findings have important prognostic implications. For apical hypertrophic cardiomyopathy, CMR can detect hypertrophied segments of the LV apex not easily identifiable by echocardiography. CMR should also be performed when discrepancy between electrocardiographic and echocardiographic evidence of hypertrophy exists. In HCM patients with severe septal hypertrophy and symptomatic dynamic LV outflow tract obstruction, CMR has advantages over echocardiography in assessing the reduction of septal thickness from surgical myectomy or alcohol septal ablation, which has implications regarding patient symptoms and outcome.[64]

LV mass index varies widely with maximal LV wall thickness because of heterogeneity of the HCM phenotype but has important prognostic implications. A markedly elevated LV mass index (men > 91 g/m^2; women > 69 g/m^2) was sensitive (100%), whereas maximal wall thickness of more than 30 mm was specific (91%) for cardiac deaths.[61] Other potential markers of adverse prognosis include right ventricular (RV) hypertrophy or myocardial edema by T2-weighted imaging.[65] Typical patterns of findings in HCM characterized by a multicomponent CMR examination are listed in Table 18-e3 (see website) and illustrated in the case example in **Figure 18-10**. This approach may offer not only accurate HCM diagnosis but also novel understanding of myocardial pathophysiology. Petersen and colleagues[66] have found that blunted endocardial myocardial blood flow and myocardial fibrosis are both related to the degree of hypertrophy, raising the intriguing possibility that microvascular dysfunction plays an important role in the development of hypertrophy and myocardial fibrosis as a substrate to sudden cardiac death. Long-term prognostic evidence using contrast-enhancing techniques by CMR is currently lacking in HCM patients, but LGE has been associated with ventricular arrhythmias[67] and progressive ventricular dilation. By its concurrent assessment of altered physiology secondary to coronary microvascular dysfunction, fibrosis, and hypertrophy, CMR will advance the understanding of myocardial substrates and triggers relevant to sudden cardiac death and guidance of ICD therapy in HCM patients.

ARRHYTHMOGENIC RIGHT VENTRICULAR CARDIOMYOPATHY. Arrhythmogenic RV cardiomyopathy (ARVC; see Chap. 68) distinguishes itself from other cardiomyopathies by a predisposition to ventricular arrhythmias that precede overt morphologic abnormalities and even histologic substrate and by diverse phenotypic manifestations, despite success in isolating the causative desmosomal mutations. CMR offers advantages over echocardiography and RV angiography by its quantitative and volumetric assessment of cardiac function and its characterization of myocardial fibrofatty tissue (see Fig. 68-14). Recent

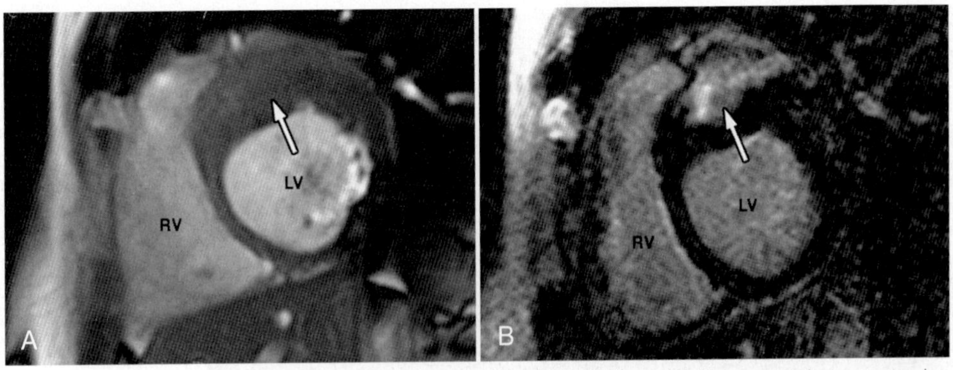

FIGURE 18-10 **A,** Patient with hypertrophic cardiomyopathy with severe panseptal hypertrophy (arrow). **B,** The septum demonstrates dense LGE (arrow) consistent with fibrosis.

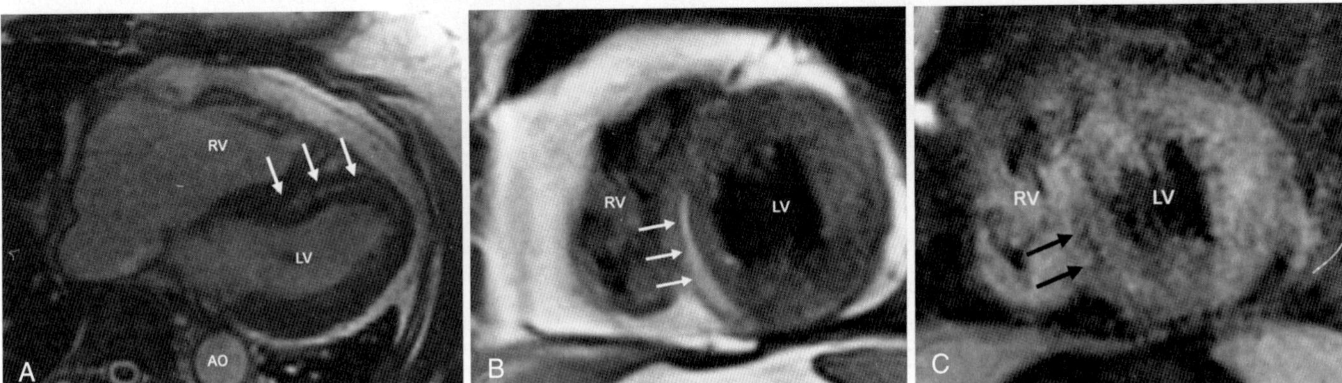

FIGURE 18-11 A 56-year-old woman presenting with recurrent presyncope was found to have nonsustained ventricular tachycardia on Holter monitoring and was referred for CMR assessment. Echocardiography was normal. **A,** Long-axis cine CMR showed an area of high signal (arrows) within the mid to distal interventricular septal wall, representing suspected fatty infiltration. The RV is normal in size, function, and morphology. **B,** Midventricular short-axis T1-weighted FSE CMR confirms a layer of fatty infiltration (arrows) in the matching inferoseptal walls of the LV. **C,** The same short-axis location acquired with a T1-weighted FSE sequence with fat saturation revealed a specific and clear nulling of a layer of fatty infiltration (black arrows).

evidence has indicated that early and predominant LV disease exists in variant groups (**Fig. 18-11**).[68] Such enthusiasm for CMR for assessing ARVC was somewhat curbed by a lack of standardized imaging protocols in the past and inherent subjectivity in interpreting myocardial fat and wall motion abnormality of the thin-walled crescent-shaped right ventricle.[69] Recent efforts toward the standardization of CMR protocols have affirmed the value of CMR as an integral component in the workup of ARVC.[70] Quantitative RV measurements by CMR are accurate and reproducible. Fat-suppressed LGE imaging of the RV myocardium using a short inversion time (<150 milliseconds) has shown high correlation with endomyocardial biopsy and inducibility of ventricular arrhythmias.[71] Fat infiltration of the RV wall as an isolated finding is of limited specificity for diagnosing ARVC. Sen-Chowdhry and associates[72] have studied 232 patients with suspected to have ARVC using clinical evaluation, genetic analysis, and a dedicated CMR protocol; 134 patients fulfilled the extended diagnostic criteria of ARVC. CMR had a sensitivity of 96% and a specificity of 78% in detecting ARVC. The authors suggested that CMR has the potential to detect patients with early disease not characterized by the task force guideline. Future studies will need to determine the diagnostic and prognostic role of CMR relative to clinical evaluation, genetic analyses, and the new immunohistochemical analysis of plakoglobin signals.[73] Jain and coworkers[74] have provided a current and detailed review of the role of CMR concurrent to the recent expansion of the genetic understanding of ARVC.

MYOCARDITIS. CMR targets three aspects of tissue abnormality in myocarditis—myocardial edema by T2-weighted imaging, regional hyperemia and capillary leak by early gadolinium enhancement ratio (EGE_r), and myocardial necrosis or fibrosis by LGE imaging. Table 18-e1 (see website) summarizes the diagnostic criteria of these techniques for acute myocarditis (see Chap. 70). Further details of these diagnostic criteria can be found in a recent expert consensus.[75] A case example of acute myocarditis is illustrated in **Figure 18-12** (see Fig. 70-5). From pooled data of single-center studies, T2-weighted imaging, EGE_r, and LGE have individual sensitivities and specificities of 70% and 71%, 74% and 83%, and 59% and 86%, respectively. An expert panel has suggested that two or more of the three tissue-based criteria provide modest sensitivity (67%) but high specificity (91%) for the diagnosis of myocarditis.[75] In cases with high index of clinical suspicion but negative CMR tissue findings, a repeat study in a few weeks may be necessary for diagnosis because inflammation may be focal and difficult to detect in the first few days of disease. Early evidence has indicated that a persistence of LGE 4 weeks after symptom onset is predictive of adverse functional and clinical outcomes.[76]

CARDIAC SARCOIDOSIS. CMR techniques and corresponding findings in cardiac sarcoidosis are listed in Tables 18-e2 and 18-e3 (see website), and a case example is shown in **Figure 18-13** (see Chap. 68). The CMR techniques described may enhance disease detection through the successive histologic stages of disease: tissue edema, noncaseating granulomatous infiltration, and patchy myocardial fibrosis. Disease activity may explain any discordance between T2-weighted and LGE findings. In 81 patients with extracardiac sarcoidosis, Patel and colleagues[77] have found that LGE imaging identifies abnormalities consistent with cardiac sarcoidosis in 26% of patients compared with 12% by the modified Japanese Ministry of Health guidelines. LGE-positive patients had a ninefold increase in the hazard of death or major dysrhythmic events requiring intervention. CMR can also be used to guide sampling during endomyocardial biopsy and thus

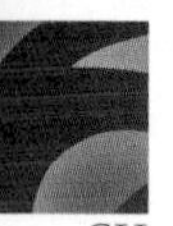

CH 18

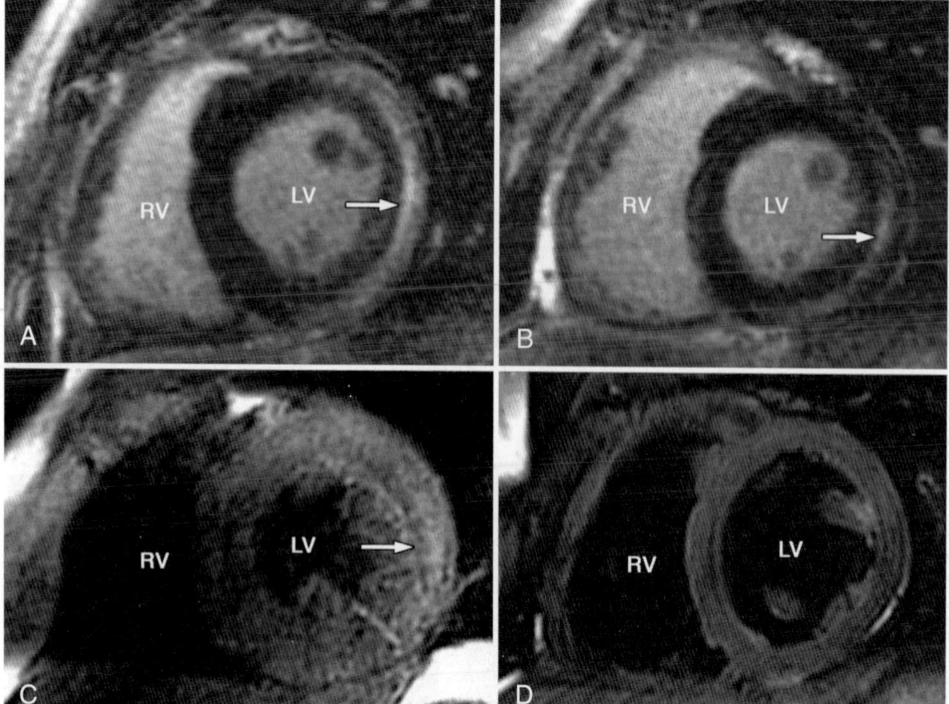

FIGURE 18-12 A 17-year-old college student presented with sudden onset of chest pain and ST-segment elevation in the anterior and anterolateral leads. Urgent coronary angiography revealed no significant coronary arterial stenosis but his serum troponin T level was markedly elevated to 100 times the upper limit of normal within the first 24 hours of presentation, and there was a large region of anterior and anterolateral hypokinesis. CMR performed during the first 48 hours of presentation showed extensive evidence of myocardial inflammation by LGE imaging involving the epicardial aspect of the anterior and anterolateral walls **(A)**, which were matched by a high signal intensity region on T2-weighted FSE edema imaging **(C)**, consistent with acute viral myocarditis. Parvovirus serology was elevated fivefold. Three months later, regional function completely resolved. There was evidence of a residual epicardial scar by LGE imaging **(B)** but with no evidence of persistent inflammation on T2-weighted edema imaging **(D)**.

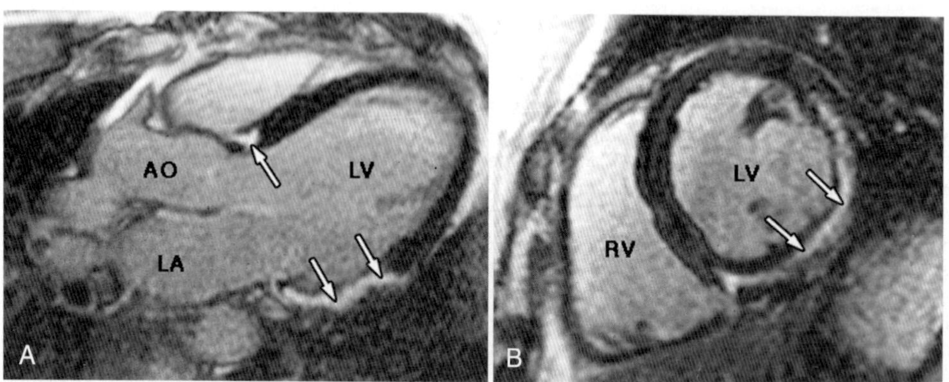

FIGURE 18-13 A 47-year-old man with no prior medical history presented with dizziness and a junctional rhythm with frequent premature ventricular contractions on a resting electrocardiogram. CMR revealed mildly reduced LV systolic function with akinesis of the basal and midinferior and inferolateral walls. LGE images (**A,** long axis; **B,** short axis) demonstrate midmyocardial and epicardial LGE (arrows). In **A,** apart from the inferolateral midwall enhancement (bottom arrows), there was a second focus of LGE seen in the basal septum (top arrow). This pattern of midmyocardial and epicardial LGE is consistent with an infiltrative process, such as sarcoidosis. AO = aorta; LA = left atrium; RV = right ventricle.

increase tissue yield. Despite being reproducible and accurate in reflecting sarcoid progression,[78] CMR is often currently limited as a monitoring tool for disease progression by a patient's need for an ICD.

CARDIAC AMYLOIDOSIS. The characteristic features of CMR techniques in cardiac amyloidosis are summarized in Table 18-e3 (see website and Chap. 68). Maceira and associates[79] were the first to report a global subendocardial LGE pattern and an inverse relationship between endocardial T1 and systemic and myocardial amyloid load. LGE was confirmed to be related to amyloid interstitial expansion in one autopsy case. Furthermore, a transmural T1 gradient across the myocardium minutes after GBCA injection was predictive of cardiac death.[80] A case example is presented in **Figure 18-14**.

IDIOPATHIC DILATED CARDIOMYOPATHY. Major advantages of CMR in evaluating suspected idiopathic dilated cardiomyopathy (IDCM) include ruling out ischemic cardiomyopathy, characterizing the pattern of myocardial scar, which has diagnostic and prognostic implications, and monitoring treatment response and disease progression by quantitation of LV structure and function (see Fig. 68-2). In prior studies involving patients with LV dysfunction,[81] LGE was observed in all patients with coronary stenosis, indicating that an ischemic cause of LV dysfunction is unlikely in the absence of LGE. In patients with cardiomyopathy but without angiographic coronary stenosis, 28% had patchy or linear midwall LGE, most often in the basal septum. This LGE pattern consistent with midwall fibrosis has been associated with adverse cardiac events, including sudden death independent of LV structure and function.[82] This finding is consistent with the postulation that LGE imaging can identify arrhythmogenic substrate. Nazarian and colleagues[83] have found that LGE involving 26% to 75% of wall thickness is predictive of the inducibility of ventricular tachycardia, independent of LV ejection fraction.

Iron Overload Cardiomyopathy. Iron overload cardiomyopathy is most often the result of repeated blood transfusions, such as in patients with thalassemia major, but can be caused by hereditary hemochromatosis, a genetic disorder caused by mutations of *HFE* or the transferrin receptor gene (see Chap. 68). In patients with transfusion-dependent thalassemia major, premature cardiac death as a result of myocardial iron toxicity occurs in 50% of patients. Serum ferritin and hepatic iron levels do not reflect cardiac iron overload caused by different transport mechanism from the heart, and chelation therapy readily removes iron from the liver. Global LV systolic function is usually preserved, especially in anemic thalassemic patients, until severe cardiac toxicity occurs, thus providing little if any guidance to chelation therapy, which can potentially reverse this cardiomyopathy. The CMR T2* technique for quantifying myocardial iron is summarized in Table 18-e1 (see website). CMR assessment of myocardial iron overload using T2* quantitation has been responsible for improved delivery of iron chelation therapy[84] by enabling the development of better chelating agents or treatment intensification. The T2* technique has also been associated with a 70% reduction of iron overload–related mortality in patients with thalassemia major since 2000; further evidence of the prognostic benefit of T2* was demonstrated in a recent study[85] of 652 thalassemic patients. Patients with a myocardial T2* shorter than 10 milliseconds had a relative risk of 160 in developing heart failure within 1 year (relative risk further increased to 270 if myocardial T2* was <6 milliseconds; **Fig. 18-15**).

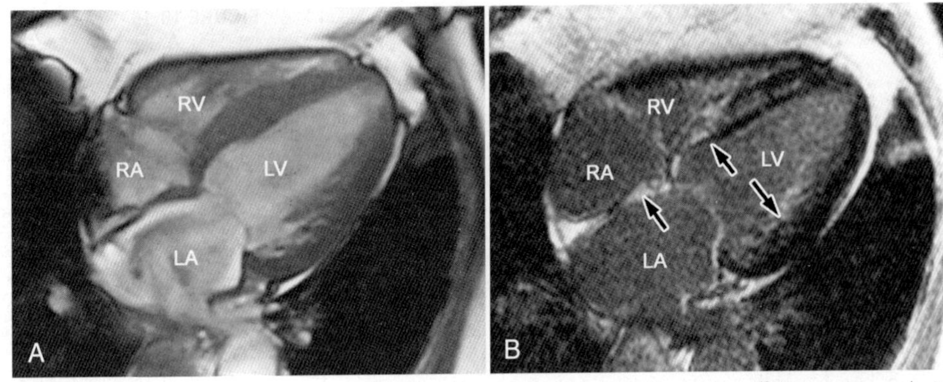

FIGURE 18-14 A 78-year-old man with a history of hypertension and chronic renal insufficiency presented with progressive dyspnea on exertion. **A,** CMR reveals left ventricular hypertrophy with severe biventricular systolic dysfunction (four-chamber long-axis cine systolic image). **B,** Matching LGE imaging shows rapid washout of the contrast agent from the blood pool with diffuse intramyocardial LGE of the septum, subendocardial LGE of the inferior wall, and diffuse atrial LGE (black arrows). This pattern is consistent with amyloidosis.

OTHER CARDIOMYOPATHIES

CHAGAS DISEASE. Chagas disease is a myocarditis caused by infection from the protozoan *Trypanosoma cruzi* endemic in Central and South America (see Chap. 71), but rare cases have been reported in North America. Although most patients have a self-limiting course once immunity develops within 10 weeks, about 30% of untreated cases will have persistent parasitemia and a latent infection that manifest 10 to 20 years later as a severe dilated cardiomyopathy often associated with ventricular arrhythmias. Once heart failure develops, the 5-year cardiac mortality rate is 50%, and sudden cardiac death is common. Rochitte and associates[86] have described the typical findings by CMR (see Table 18-e3 on website) and provided evidence supporting the role of CMR in diagnosing and monitoring patients infected with this disease during the latent period.

NONCOMPACTION. LV noncompaction is a cardiomyopathy characterized by failure of compaction of the trabecular layer (see Table 18-e3 on website and **Fig. 18-16**; see also Fig. 26-4), with a familial pattern reported in approximately 40% of patients. In a cohort-control study, Petersen and coworkers[87] have reported that a diastolic noncompacted-to-compacted thickness ratio more than 2.3 measured in a long axis is 86% sensitive and 99% specific for diagnosing this condition.

TAKOTSUBO CARDIOMYOPATHY. Transient LV apical ballooning syndrome (or takotsubo cardiomyopathy) is characterized by a transient contractile dysfunction of the LV apex, currently proposed to be caused by high catecholamine levels caused by severe emotional or physical stress (see Chap. 68). CMR can be useful for differentiating apical ballooning syndrome from an acute coronary event (see Table 18-e3 on website and Fig. 68-5.).[88] LGE in this setting represents a disproportionate expansion of extracellular matrix with increased collagen I deposition on immunohistochemical tissue staining.[89]

ENDOMYOCARDIAL DISEASE. Endomyocardial disease is a restrictive cardiomyopathy that consists of two variants, endomyocardial fibrosis and Löffler endocarditis. Both are considered the result of direct toxic effects of eosinophils on the myocardium. Hypereosinophilia, regardless of its cause, has been suggested to lead to cardiomyopathy in three stages—necrosis, thrombosis, and fibrosis—although definitive proof in humans is lacking. Hypereosinophilia is the hallmark of Löffler endocarditis whereas it is variable in endomyocardial fibrosis, which has characteristic features on CMR (see Table 18-e3 on website).

Diastolic Dysfunction

Diastolic function of the left ventricle represents a complex interplay of conditions, including myocardial relaxation, passive ventricular elastic recoil, and pericardial constraints (see Chaps. 24 and 30). Similar to other modalities, CMR quantitation of diastolic filling rates and time to peak filling are influenced by the cardiac chronotropic state and left atrial pressure. Phase contrast velocity imaging has been shown to measure mitral inflow and pulmonary venous velocities accurately (validating against Doppler echocardiography; see Chap. 15) over a practical scan time of several minutes.[90] With the advantage of unrestricted scan planes, Paelinck and coworkers[91] have found that early mitral inflow velocity (E) normalized to in vivo mitral septal tissue velocity (Ea) measured using phase contrast CMR provides strong correlation and good agreement with mean pulmonary capillary wedge pressure measured by invasive cardiac catheterization (correlation coefficient = 0.8). CMR-specific tissue grid tagging can determine the rotational and translational motions of the LV myocardium by characterizing the clockwise and anticlockwise rotation at the base and apex during systole, respectively. With adequate temporal resolution (less than 35 milliseconds), quantitation of grid distortion permits direct assessment of diastolic intramyocardial deformation measured in strain and strain rates.

Pericardial Disease

At our center, a typical CMR assessment includes cine SSFP imaging, T1- and T2-weighted double-inversion black blood fast spin-echo (FSE; half-Fourier acquisition single-shot turbo spin-echo [HASTE]), and LGE imaging of the whole heart to assess for pericardial changes (see Chap. 75). Real-time cine SSFP and phase contrast flow across the tricuspid valve are often added to the examination to enhance the detection of cardiac constriction. First-pass perfusion and pre- and postcontrast T1-weighted techniques (gradient or spin-echo) may also be necessary to determine the vascularity of a pericardial mass (e.g., differentiate tumor from thrombus). Cine myocardial tagged (dark lines or grids) imaging may be useful to identify any perimyocardial adhesion by demonstrating reduced myocardial strain. Single-shot and real-time methods increase the diagnostic yield of the study in patients with irregular heart rhythms, such as atrial fibrillation. A description of our CMR protocol is given in Table 18-e2 (see website). On T1-weighted FSE imaging, a thickness of up to 3 mm is accepted as normal, accounting for the effects from partial volume averaging, cardiac motion, inclusion of pericardial fluid, and chemical shift artifact. Pericardial sinuses are often mistaken for pathology. The transverse sinus, which lies dorsal to the ascending aorta, and the superior pericardial recess (a curvilinear space to the right of the ascending aorta) may be mistaken for an aortic dissection or a mediastinal mass. The oblique sinus behind the left atrium may be misinterpreted as an esophageal lesion or bronchogenic cyst. Enhancement of the thickened pericardium after the administration of a GBCA suggests active inflammation or pericardial fibrosis (**Fig. 18-17**). CMR is the current test of choice for differentiating constrictive pericarditis from restrictive cardiomyopathy, not only by assessing pericardial thickness but also signs of constrictive physiology. Cardiac CT can demonstrate pericardial calcifications (see Chap. 19) but is inferior to CMR because of a lack of assessment of constrictive physiology and hemodynamics and limited tissue characterization.

Pericardial cysts usually have thin smooth walls without internal septa. Their homogeneous transudative contents appear dark on T1-weighted images and bright on T2-weighted images, with no enhancement from GBCA. Proteinaceous cysts appear very bright on T1-weighted images. Pericardial metastases are far more common (from lung, breast, and lymphomas) than primary pericardial tumors (see Chap. 74). Malignant invasion of the pericardium often shows focal obliteration of the pericardial line and pericardial effusion. Most neoplasms appear dark or gray on noncontrast T1-weighted images, except metastatic melanoma because of its paramagnetic metals bound by melanin (**Fig. 18-18**). Partial absence of the pericardium is

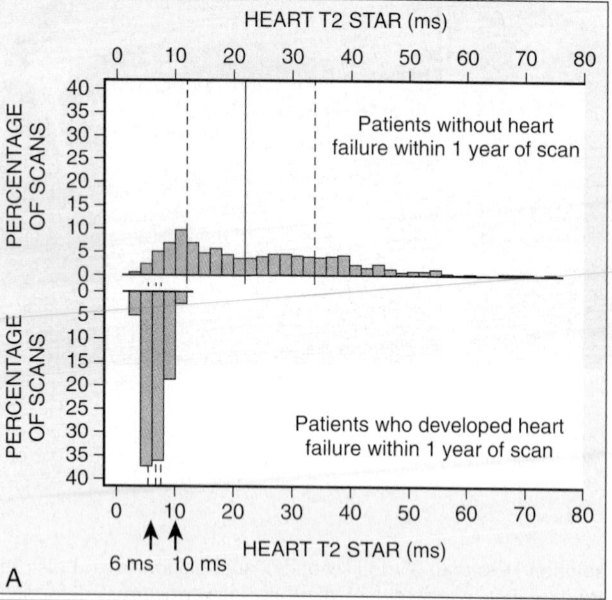

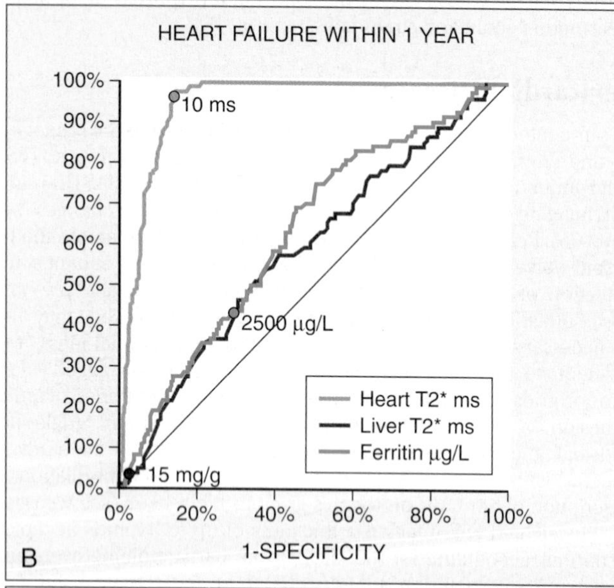

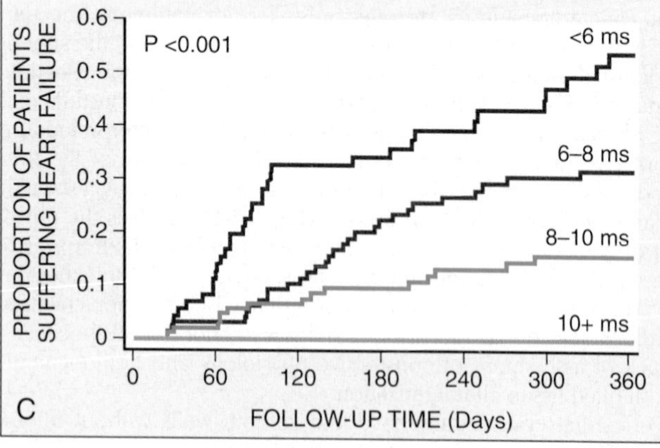

FIGURE 18-15 Outcome of patients with thalassemia major based on CMR imaging. **A,** Frequency distribution of cardiac T2* values in 80 patients who developed heart failure within 1 year of CMR (bottom) versus 572 patients who did not develop heart failure (top). Note the segregation of cardiac T2* in the patients who subsequently developed heart failure into the lowest values; 98% of patients who developed heart failure had a cardiac T2* shorter than 10 milliseconds. The solid vertical black line is the median; dashed black lines are the upper and lower quartiles. **B,** Receiver-operating characteristic curve for the prediction of heart failure within 1 year of CMR. The diagonal line shows the performance of a nondiagnostic test. Although the liver T2* and serum ferritin levels are weakly predictive, the cardiac T2* is greatly superior to both of these conventional measures ($P < 0.001$). The points marked on each line indicate a threshold of 10 milliseconds for cardiac T2*, 0.96 milliseconds for liver T2* (equivalent to 15 mg/kg dry weight), and 2500 μg/L for the serum ferritin level. **C,** Kaplan-Meier curves showing the development of heart failure over 1 year according to baseline cardiac T2* values >10, 8-10, 6-8, and <6 milliseconds ($P < 0.001$). *(From Kirk P, Roughton JB, Porter JM, et al: Cardiac T2* magnetic resonance for prediction of cardiac complications in thalassemia major. Circulation 120:1961, 2009.)*

usually left-sided and can be associated with atrial septal defect, malformation of the great vessels, patent ductus arteriosus, and defects of the sternum. Rare strangulation of the left atrium through herniation through the pericardial defect is possible. Absence of pericardium is suspected when lung tissue is seen interposed between the aorta and pulmonary artery or between the heart and diaphragm.

Adult Congenital Heart Disease

CMR can provide important diagnostic information beyond echocardiography for the assessment of congenital heart disease (see Chap. 65) based on the following factors: no need for ionizing radiation, three-dimensional tomographic imaging of thoracic structures and anatomy (compared with echocardiographic windows, which are more limited by body growth), and correlation of complex anatomy with blood flow and physiology. This section will focus on CMR assessment of common adult congenital heart diseases.

ATRIAL AND VENTRICULAR SEPTAL DEFECTS. CMR provides a noninvasive alternative to transesophageal echocardiography and even to diagnostic catheterization for assessing patients presenting with right-sided volume overload from a suspected left-to-right shunt. In this situation, a single CMR study can detect the presence of an atrial septal defect (ASD), assess suitability for transcatheter ASD closure (see Chap. 59), quantify right heart size and function by cine SSFP, determine pulmonary-to-systemic shunt ratio (Q_p/Q_s) using velocity-encoded phase contrast, and identify any coexisting anomalous pulmonary venous return using three-dimensional contrast-enhanced MRA. Phase contrast imaging positioned in a plane parallel to the atrial septum and set at a low velocity range (100 cm/sec) can visualize the ASD directly with good correlation with defect size measured invasively.[92] Phase contrast imaging of tricuspid regurgitation can estimate the pulmonary arterial systolic pressure. Because most closure devices are MRI-compatible, CMR can be used to evaluate residual shunts and proper device deployment. Patients with a ventricular septal defect (VSD) can be assessed using similar CMR techniques. In addition, LGE imaging may help determine whether a VSD has developed as a complication of MI.

ANOMALOUS PULMONARY VENOUS CONNECTION. Using a large field of view, three-dimensional MRA can capture abnormal intrathoracic structures and vascular dynamics in anomalous pulmonary venous return. Near-isotropic in-plane resolution can be achieved allowing reformatting in any plane to detect anomalous venous structures as small as 1 mm (**Fig. 18-19**). The magnitude of any left-to-right shunt can be assessed by direct blood flow measurements in the anomalous pulmonary vein or by the Q_p/Q_s ratio (see earlier), which is in general more accurate than invasive oximetry measurements caused by the errors from mixed venous return in the right atrium.

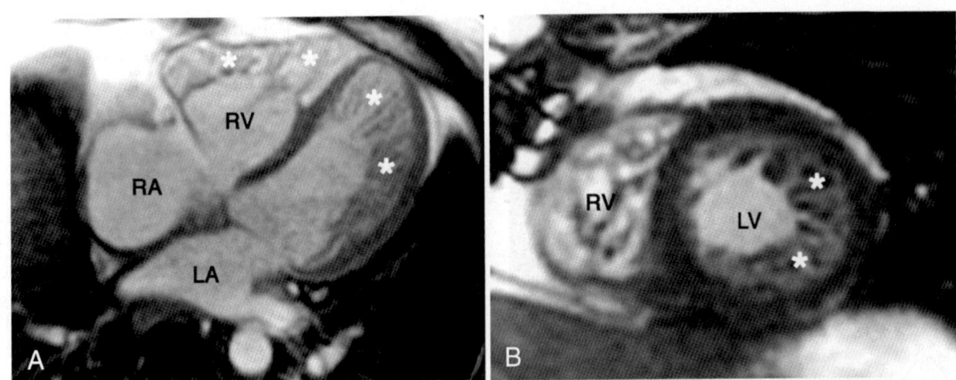

FIGURE 18-16 A 64-year-old man developed decompensated heart failure in the setting of atrial flutter. CMR revealed normal LV size and mild systolic dysfunction (ejection fraction 53%). CMR (**A,** long axis; **B,** short axis) also showed an extensive spongelike appearance of the LV and RV myocardium involving the anterior, lateral, and apical walls (asterisks), consistent with LV noncompaction. The ratio between the noncompacted and compacted myocardium is 9 for the apex and 3 for the lateral wall, values that meet diagnostic criteria for noncompaction.

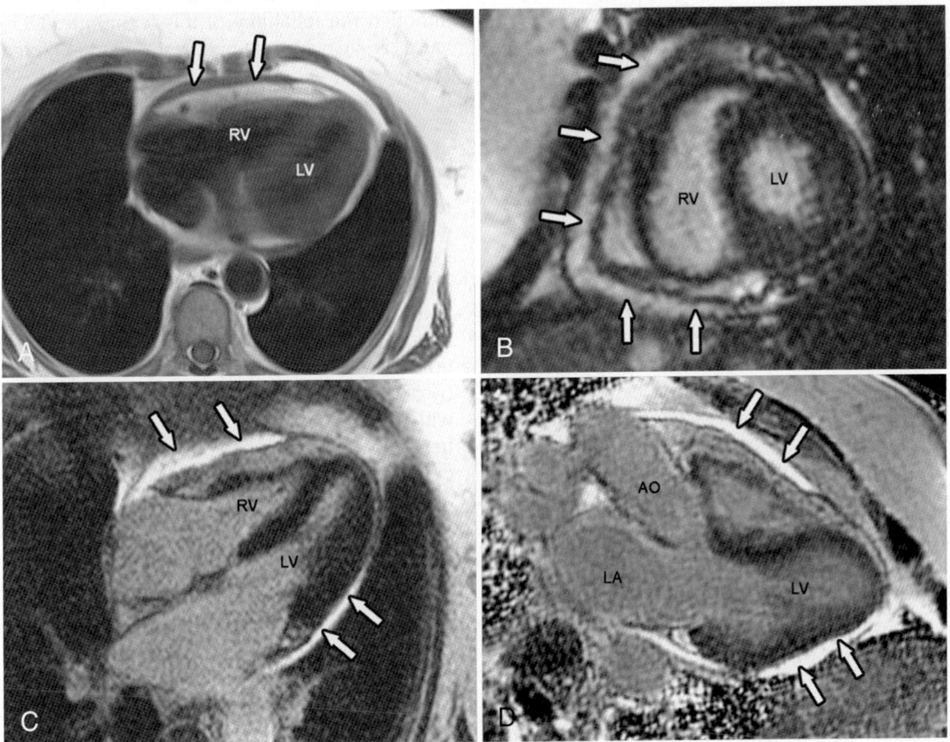

FIGURE 18-17 A 67-year-old man presented with shortness of breath and atypical chest pain. **A,** Double inversion recovery fast spin-echo imaging reveals markedly and diffusely thickened pericardium (arrows). **B, C,** The ventricles are small, whereas the atria are dilated, suggestive of constrictive physiology. With gadolinium contrast, the pericardium demonstrates marked LGE indicative of active and intense pericardial inflammation (**B-D,** arrows).

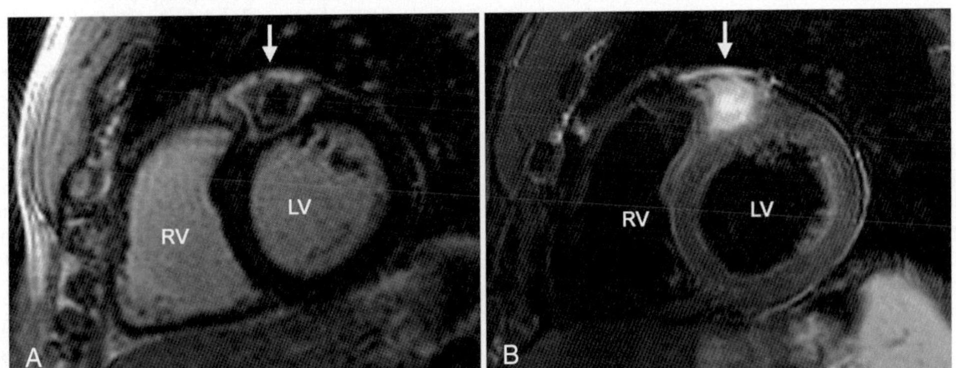

FIGURE 18-18 A 56-year-old man with a history of melanoma with pulmonary metastases presented with a suspicious lesion on a chest CT scan. CMR revealed a 2.4- × 2.2-cm mass in the basal anterior wall of the LV, which was hyperintense on T2-weighted images **(B)**, with peripheral late LGE suggestive of tumor necrosis **(A)**. These findings are consistent with a focal metastasis of the melanoma to the left ventricle.

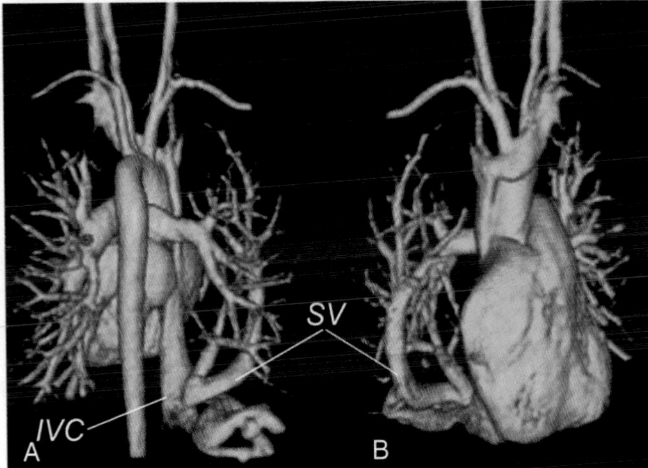

FIGURE 18-19 Posterior **(A)** and anterior **(B)** projections of a volume-rendered gadolinium-enhanced three-dimensional magnetic resonance angiogram in a 33-year-old woman with scimitar syndrome. The pulmonary venous return from the right lung drains into the inferior vena cava (IVC) through two veins that form the shape of a Turkish sword, called the scimitar vein (SV). Mesocardia is noted on the anterior projection **(B)**. Because the hemodynamic burden from the left-to-right shunt was relatively small (pulmonary-to-systemic flow ratio measured by phase contrast cine CMR of 1.3), mild right ventricular dilation (end-diastolic volume index, 124 mL/m^2; upper limit of normal, 103 mL/m^2), normal systolic function, and normal pulmonary artery pressure, no further therapy was recommended. *(Courtesy of Dr. Tal Geva, Boston Children's Hospital, Boston.)*

COARCTATION OF THE AORTA. Gadolinium-enhanced three-dimensional MRA is sufficient for defining the site of aortic narrowing in most cases (see Figs. 65-33 and 82-4). Cine SSFP, in a long-axis candy cane view, can further delineate the aortic anatomy, degree of obstruction, and aortic valvular dysfunction (caused by a coexisting bicuspid aortic valve). Cine SSFP, in a short-axis stack of the heart, can evaluate LV size, mass, and function, thus assessing the impact of chronic hypertension from aortic coarctation (see Chap. 60). Black blood FSE is useful to evaluate the entire aorta, particularly because it is less affected by metallic artifacts from an implanted endovascular stent than gradient echo techniques. Phase contrast imaging can characterize the descending-to-ascending aorta flow ratio, estimate the pressure gradient across the coarctation, and determine the degree of collateral formation.

CONOTRUNCAL ANOMALIES. Tetralogy of Fallot (TOF) is an increasingly common referral to CMR in young adults. In patients being considered for surgical repair of TOF, key elements in CMR include depiction of all sources of pulmonary blood flow (including pulmonary arterial, aortopulmonary collateral, and ductus-arterial sources) in the presence of RV outflow obstruction, quantitation of the severity of infundibular or pulmonary stenosis, assessment of RV function, and ruling out a coexisting anomalous coronary artery. In patients who have undergone surgery for TOF, CMR attempts to quantify determinants of long-term status, including formation of RV outflow aneurysms, pulmonary regurgitation fraction (especially in patients who underwent patching of the pulmonary valve with postoperative pulmonary regurgitation), biventricular size and global function, and any residual shunt.[93] Recently, LGE imaging has been proposed for detection of myocardial fibrosis that has been associated with ventricular dysfunction, exercise intolerance, and arrhythmia.[94] The principal physiologic abnormality in D-loop transposition of the great arteries (TGA, with D-loop TGA being the most common type) is profound hypoxemia caused by a ventriculoarterial discordant connection, where systemic venous blood flows to the aorta and oxygenated pulmonary venous blood returns to the lung (see Chap. 65). Survival is dependent on systemic-pulmonary circulatory mixing via a ductus arteriosus, ASD, or VSD. The arterial switch operation is now the most common corrective surgery but many adult patients have undergone an atrial switch procedure (Senning or Mustard). CMR is useful for monitoring these patients after surgical correction by assessing ventricular size and function, flow across the postoperative LV and RV outflow tracts, aortopulmonary collaterals, and other anomalies, such as coarctation of the interrupted aortic arch and pulmonary stenosis.

Valvular Heart Disease

With the capability to assess cardiac structure and function, valvular and great vessel flow hemodynamics, and three-dimensional angiography, CMR can provide complementary information to the echocardiographic evaluation of valvular heart disease (see Chap. 66). Compared with echocardiography, CMR is three-dimensional and does not involve geometric assumption of cardiac shape; thus, it is more sensitive in detecting any change in ventricular sizes, function, and myocardial mass. CMR overcomes the problem of acoustic windows in echocardiography. For aortic stenosis, arbitrary scan plane selection by CMR can visualize and allow direct planimetry of the aortic valve orifice at high spatial resolution. The results of direct planimetry of the aortic valve correlate highly with measures of aortic valve area by transthoracic and transesophageal echocardiography (see Chap. 15), although the reliability of this technique decreases when the aortic valve is heavily calcified, with markedly reduced leaflet motion. Because phase contrast CMR imaging has lower temporal resolution than echocardiography, it may underestimate the peak velocity of blood flow across a highly stenotic aortic valve compared with continuous wave Doppler. A novel application of CMR in identifying vortical blood flow in the main pulmonary artery has been shown to estimate mean pulmonary arterial pressures and differentiate patients with pulmonary hypertension.[95] The CMR approach to a patient with aortic regurgitation is shown in **Figure 18-20**. Major limitations that challenge CMR assessment of valve disease are related to irregular heart rhythms, especially atrial fibrillation or frequent ventricular premature contractions. Acquiring phase contrast flow quantitation multiple times and averaging the results may alleviate the error introduced by arrhythmias to some extent, but the results should be interpreted with caution. Most recently, three-dimensional volumetric phase contrast imaging has been developed, which allows visualization of vascular vector flow patterns of large vessels with a novel potential for assessing vascular wall shear stress or ventricular cavitary flow dynamics (**Fig. 18-21**).[96] This three-dimensional vector flow may allow advancement in the understanding between valvular dysfunction and the progression of the resultant ventricular dysfunction.

Cardiac Thrombi and Masses

Differential diagnoses of an intracardiac mass mainly include thrombus, tumor, or vegetation. LGE imaging can detect thrombus with a higher sensitivity than echocardiography by depicting high contrast between the dark thrombus and its adjacent structures and by imaging in three dimensions. Mural thrombus does not enhance on first-pass perfusion and often has a characteristic etched appearance (black border surrounding a bright center) on LGE imaging, thus providing higher diagnostic specificity than anatomic information alone[97] (**Fig. 18-22**). Weinsaft and colleagues[60] have demonstrated that setting the inversion time of LGE imaging to 600 milliseconds, which allows recovery of signal in tissues except thrombus, which stays dark, provides a sensitive method for detection of mural thrombus. Microvascular obstruction from MI can be confused with mural thrombus, but it is usually confined within the infarcted myocardium characterized by LGE. Common benign cardiac tumors include atrial myxoma, rhabdomyoma, fibroma, and endocardial fibroelastoma (see Chap. 74). Atrial myxomas are often seen as a round or multilobar mass in the left atrium (75%), right atrium (20%), or ventricles or mixed chambers (5%). It typically has inhomogeneous brightness in the center on cine SSFP imaging because of its gelatinous content and may have a pedunculated attachment to the fossa ovalis. Most malignant cardiac tumors are metastatic and are 20 times more common than primary cardiac malignancies; these include cardiac involvement from direct invasion (lung and breast), lymphatic spread (lymphomas and melanomas), and hematogenous spread (renal cell carcinoma). Cardiac involvement of renal cell carcinoma occurs more often by contiguous spread via the inferior vena cava into the right-sided chambers. Primary cardiac malignancies occur more often in children or young adults; these include angiosarcoma (see Fig. 74-4), fibrosarcoma, rhabdomyosarcoma, and liposarcoma.

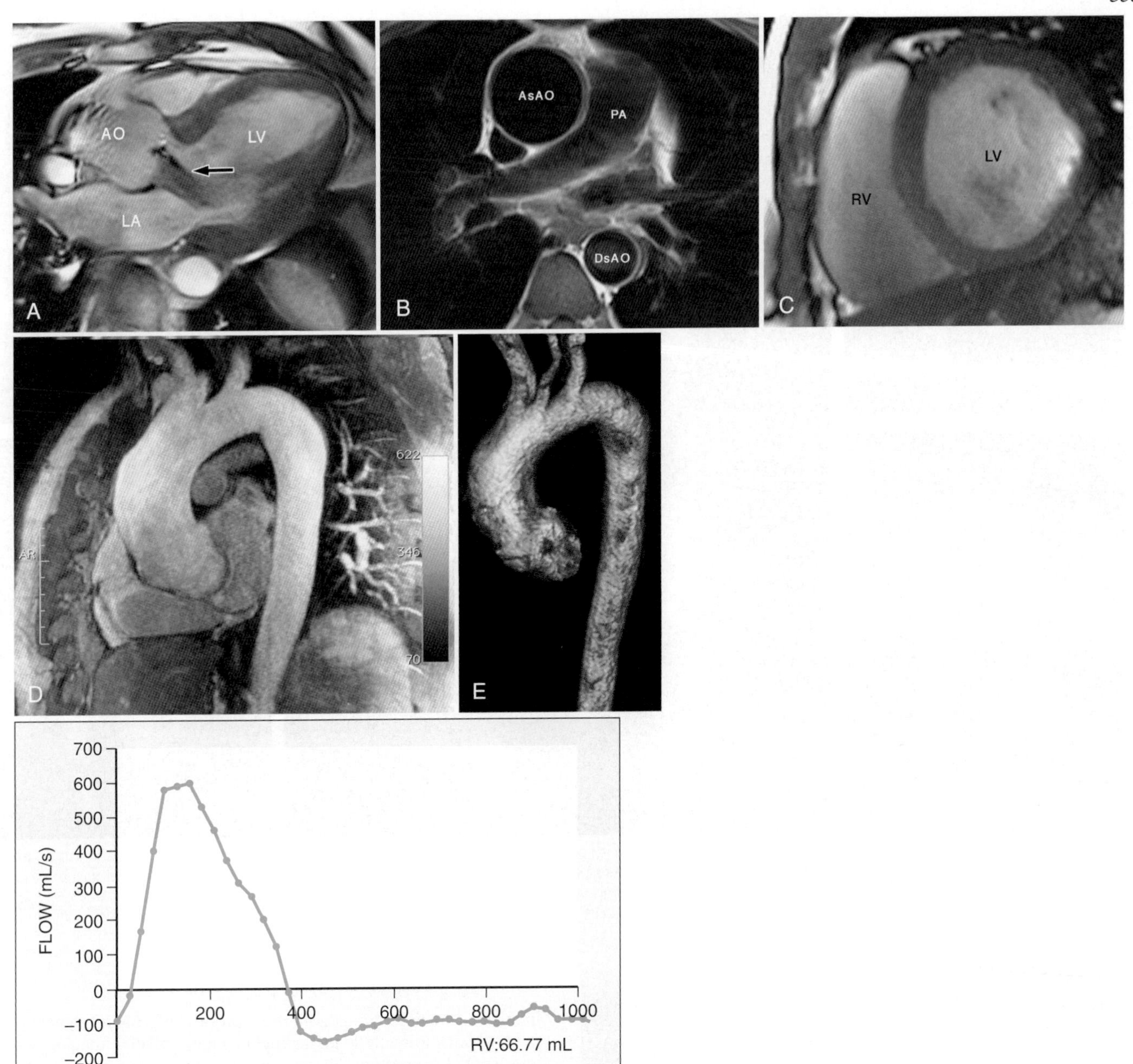

FIGURE 18-20 CMR image of a 67-year-old man with ascending aortic dilation and aortic regurgitation. **A,** Three-chamber cine SSFP showing a dilated LV with an aortic regurgitant jet (black arrow). **B,** Axial T1-weighted double-inversion recovery FSE image demonstrating dilation of the ascending aorta (AsAO). **C,** Short-axis cine CMR demonstrates dilation of the left ventricle. **D,** Maximum intensity projection (MIP) images of gadolinium-enhanced MRA. **E,** Three-dimensional volume reconstruction of gadolinium-enhanced MRA. Note that the AsAO is dilated compared with the descending aorta (DsAO). **F,** Graph of aortic valve flow from phase contrast imaging demonstrates reversal of flow in diastole, consistent with aortic regurgitation, and a calculated regurgitant volume of 66.8 mL. AO = aorta; PA = pulmonary artery; RV = right ventricle.

Novel Cardiac Magnetic Resonance Imaging Techniques

Magnetic Resonance Spectroscopy

Magnetic resonance spectroscopy (MRS) provides information regarding cellular metabolism. Free energy in adenosine triphosphate (ATP) is produced and stored primarily in mitochondria and carried to sites of energy consumption (e.g., myofibrils or ion channels) as phosphocreatine (PCr) through diffusion. Phosphorus-31 MRS assesses energy metabolism and thus the integrity of myocardial cellular functions by quantifying the concentrations and ratios of PCr and ATP. MRS is currently limited by the low signal-to-noise ratio because of the low concentration of the high-energy phosphate molecules, resulting in a limited sensitivity in detecting viable myocardium and coverage beyond the anterior LV myocardium. However, proton (^{1}H) MRS has up to a 20-fold improved sensitivity over ^{31}P MRS and thus can quantify phosphorylated and unphosphorylated creatine in any part of the LV myocardium.[98] Using ^{1}H MRS, a recent study has found that lipid overstorage in human myocytes develops in diabetics in the absence of systolic dysfunction, which may have mechanistic implications for the development of diabetic cardiomyopathy.[99]

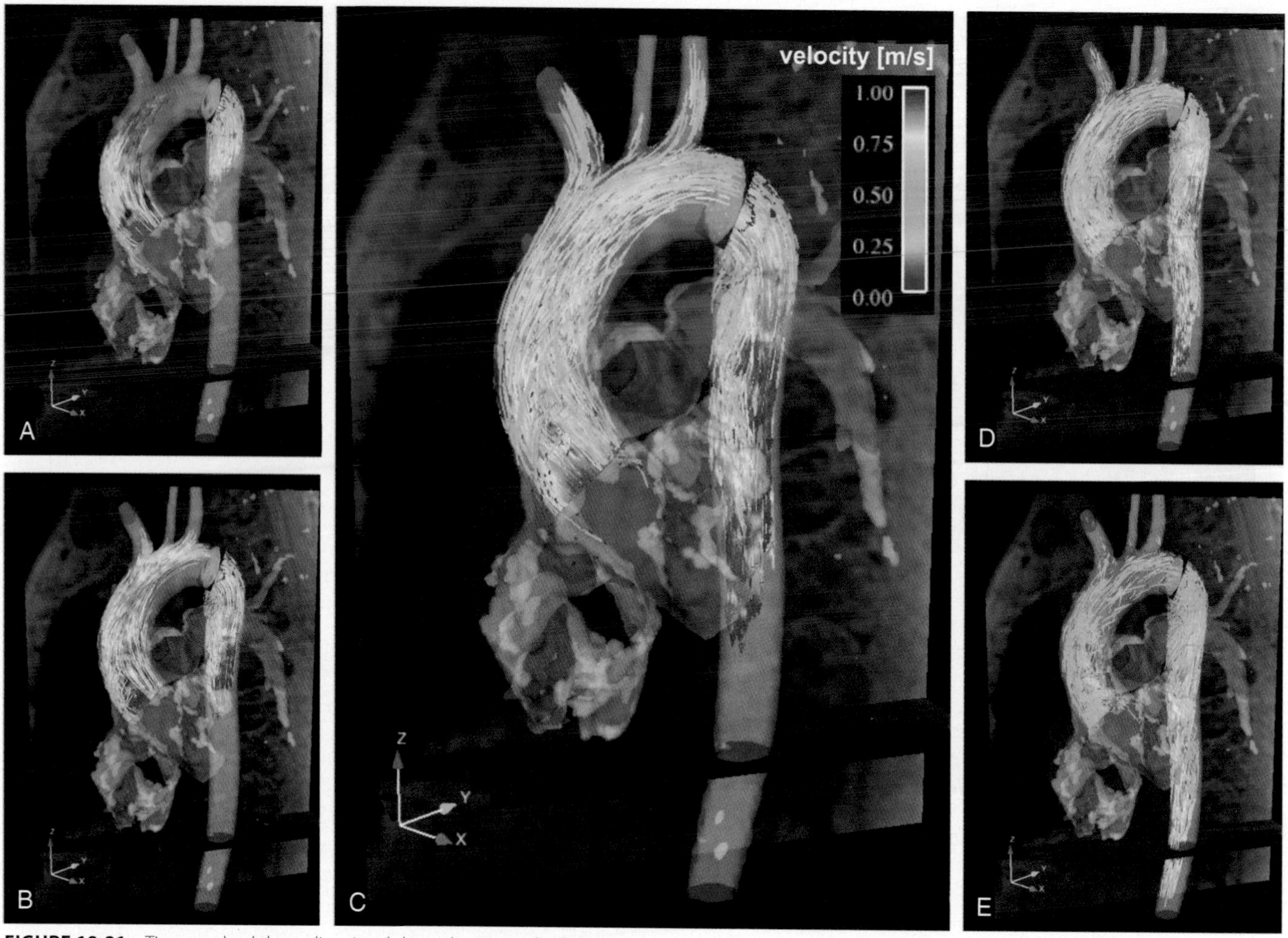

FIGURE 18-21 Time-resolved three-directional three-dimensional velocity-encoded phase contrast MRI of aortic flow. **A-E,** Blood flow visualization using phase contrast angiography (gray shaded isosurface) in combination with time-resolved three-dimensional particle traces in the thoracic aorta depicting the temporal evolution of three-dimensional blood flow in five sequential phases during ventricular systole and early diastole. The individual lines represent traces along the time-resolved velocity vector field and are color-coded according to velocity magnitude in meters per second. *(Courtesy of Dr. Michael Markl, University Hospital, Freiburg, Germany.)*

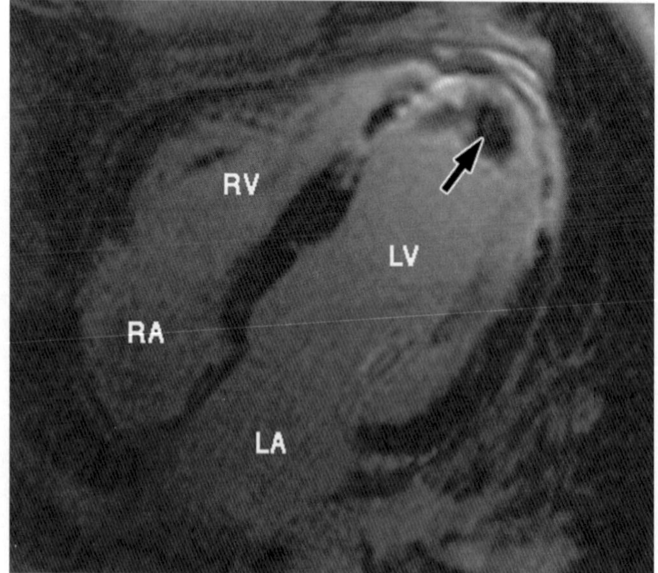

FIGURE 18-22 Characteristic etched appearance of thrombus seen on post-contrast LGE image.

Cardiac Magnetic Resonance at 3 T

Increasing the field strength offers the promise of a higher signal-noise-ratio, which indirectly leads to higher image quality, imaging speed, and spatial resolution. T1 of myocardium is lengthened at 3 T and therefore can lead to a higher contrast against blood pool or gadolinium-enhanced regions, because myocardium appears darker as a result of slower T1 signal recovery. This can also reduce the amount of contrast needed to achieve the same level of diagnostic quality in contrast-enhanced techniques. At a diagnostic level, pulse sequences such as myocardial perfusion imaging and LGE imaging are readily improved from the higher signal-to-noise ratio. In the 3-T environment, the benefit of parallel imaging can be used in more applications, thus enhancing sequence efficiency with an acceptable loss of signal-to-noise ratio. Because resonance frequencies of spins in water and fat are more widely separated at 3 T, fat suppression can be more precise, leading to better image quality. T2 and T2* are both shorter, and thus hyposignal structures such as blood clots are more easily seen as dark structures at 3 T. The elevated signal-noise-ratio also allows novel applications that are limited by low signal at 1.5 T, such as blood oxygen level deoxygenation (BOLD) perfusion and MRS. However, several technical problems exist for CMR at 3 T. RF energy deposition (as measured by specific absorption rate [SAR]) is elevated at 3 T, which can lead to patient or device heating. This can be solved by separating high SAR sequences by breath-holds so that heat dissipation occurs between successive data acquisition. Chemical shift artifacts from adjacent fat and off-resonance artifacts from through-plane blood flow, in addition to SAR limitation, can create severe artifacts in cine SSFP imaging at 3 T. This problem may be alleviated with resonance frequency tuning techniques.

Molecular Cardiac Magnetic Resonance Imaging

Molecular CMR imaging is currently experimental, but imaging molecular targets can theoretically improve the following: (1) specific disease diagnosis; (2) preclinical or early disease detection and monitoring; (3) treatment response from novel therapies; and (4) patient prognostication.[100] Gadolinium chelates combined with a fibrin-specific peptide ligand have been demonstrated to detect thrombi implanted into the left atrium or pulmonary artery and in vivo coronary thrombus within thrombogenic stents.[101,102] Nanoparticles targeting the adhesion molecule $\alpha_v\beta_3$-integrin have been used successfully for imaging angiogenesis in experimental atherosclerosis. Ultrasmall USPIO particles accumulate in macrophages in inflamed carotid plaques and have been visualized as dark regions 24 hours after USPIO injection.[57] Other examples include CMR tracking of intramyocardial transplanted mesenchymal stem cells in an experimental model of MI.[103] Newer magnetic nanoparticles such as cross-linked iron oxide may improve efficiency in labeling stem cells, with reduced immunogenicity and toxicity.

Future Perspectives

Technologic advances of CMR in the coming years will likely focus on improving the study throughput, protocol consistency, and patient tolerability to CMR examinations. Faster data collection achieved by combining efficient parallel imaging algorithms and improved surface coil elements may reduce or eliminate the need for patient breath-holding and reduce CMR scan time. With more efficient data collection methods, time-resolved techniques such as cine imaging may be replaced by real-time imaging. Three-dimensional pulse sequence techniques or performing CMR at 3 T can offset the reduction in the signal-to-noise ratio caused by data undersampling by parallel imaging. It is therefore conceivable that combinations of these methods will replace the current standard two-dimensional methods. Semiautomated cardiac localization and scanning algorithms will be developed to reduce the time required for training physicians and technologists. New contrast agents hold promise for improving the assessment of myocardial or vascular physiology. For example, a novel contrast agent with perfusion-dependent reversible binding to myocardial collagen might substantially improve the quality of CMR myocardial perfusion imaging and enable the option of performing exercise stress testing before CMR imaging.[104] Blood pool contrast agents may improve the delineation of coronary stenosis by whole-heart coronary MRA and assessment of myocardial perfusion.[105,106] Although further development is needed in interventional instrumentation and MRI hardware, CMR-guided interventions, especially for electrophysiologic applications, hold promise for improving ablative procedures. Clinical trials involving patients with pacemakers will establish criteria for selected patients to undergo CMR safely.

CMR will likely expand its role in clinical decision making and discovery of new cardiac therapies. The former is supported by the multifaceted approach of CMR in combining information regarding cardiac structure and novel physiology, a growing understanding of CMR technology and its acceptance in the clinical cardiology community, and an increasing awareness of the risk of medical radiation exposure. The latter is evidenced by the high reproducibility of quantitative CMR in reducing study sample sizes and costs required for testing new therapies in clinical trials. Ongoing studies that investigate any cost-benefit improvement by CMR will further define the future directions of CMR as a diagnostic tool.

REFERENCES

Basic Principles and Technical Aspects

1. Wertman R, Altun E, Martin DR, et al: Risk of nephrogenic systemic fibrosis: Evaluation of gadolinium chelate contrast agents at four American universities. Radiology 248:799, 2008.
2. Prince MR, Zhang H, Morris M, et al: Incidence of nephrogenic systemic fibrosis at two large medical centers. Radiology 248:807, 2008.
3. Kellman P, Arai AE, McVeigh ER, Aletras AH: Phase-sensitive inversion recovery for detecting myocardial infarction using gadolinium-delayed hyperenhancement. Magn Reson Med 47:372, 2002.
4. Sievers B, Elliott MD, Hurwitz LM, et al: Rapid detection of myocardial infarction by subsecond, free-breathing delayed contrast-enhancement cardiovascular magnetic resonance. Circulation 115:236, 2007.
5. Peters DC, Wylie JV, Hauser TH, et al: Detection of pulmonary vein and left atrial scar after catheter ablation with three-dimensional navigator-gated delayed enhancement MR imaging: Initial experience. Radiology 243:690, 2007.
6. Gerber BL, Raman SV, Nayak K, et al: Myocardial first-pass perfusion cardiovascular magnetic resonance: History, theory, and current state of the art. J Cardiovasc Magn Reson 10:18, 2008.
7. Cheng AS, Pegg TJ, Karamitsos TD, et al: Cardiovascular magnetic resonance perfusion imaging at 3-tesla for the detection of coronary artery disease: a comparison with 1.5-tesla. J Am Coll Cardiol 49:244, 2007.
8. Aletras A: Retrospective determination of the area at risk for reperfused acute myocardial infarction with T2-weighted cardiac magnetic resonance imaging: Histopathological and displacement encoding with stimulated echoes (DENSE) functional validations. Circulation 113:1865, 2006.
9. Kellman P, Aletras AH, Mancini C, et al: T2-prepared SSFP improves diagnostic confidence in edema imaging in acute myocardial infarction compared to turbo spin echo. Magn Reson Med 57:89, 2007.
10. Aletras AH, Kellman P, Derbyshire JA, Arai AE: ACUT2E TSE-SSFP: A hybrid method for T2-weighted imaging of edema in the heart. Magn Reson Med 59:229, 2008.
11. Wood JC, Otto-Duessel M, Aguilar M, et al: Cardiac iron determines cardiac T2*, T2, and T1 in the gerbil model of iron cardiomyopathy. Circulation 112:535, 2005.
12. Tanner MA, He T, Westwood MA, et al: Multi-center validation of the transferability of the magnetic resonance T2* technique for the quantification of tissue iron. Haematologica 91:1388, 2006.
13. Pennell D: MRI and iron-overload cardiomyopathy in thalassaemia. Circulation 113:f43, 2006.
14. Pennell DJ: T2* magnetic resonance and myocardial iron in thalassemia. Ann N Y Acad Sci 1054:373, 2005.
15. Bluemke DA, Achenbach S, Budoff M, et al: Noninvasive coronary artery imaging: Magnetic resonance angiography and multidetector computed tomography angiography: A scientific statement from the American Heart Association Committee on Cardiovascular Imaging and Intervention of the Council on Cardiovascular Radiology and Intervention, and the Councils on Clinical Cardiology and Cardiovascular Disease in the Young. Circulation 118:586, 2008.
16. Manning WJ, Nezafat R, Appelbaum E, et al: Coronary magnetic resonance imaging. Magn Reson Imaging Clin N Am 15:609, 2007.
17. Yang Q, Li K, Liu X, et al: Contrast-enhanced whole-heart coronary magnetic resonance angiography at 3.0-T: A comparative study with X-ray angiography in a single center. J Am Coll Cardiol 54:69, 2009.

Patient Safety

18. Nazarian S, Halperin H: How to perform magnetic resonance imaging on patients with implantable cardiac arrhythmia devices. Heart Rhythm 6:138, 2009.
19. Roguin A, Schwitter J, Vahlhaus C, et al: Magnetic resonance imaging in individuals with cardiovascular implantable electronic devices. Europace 10:336, 2008.
20. Nazarian S, Roguin A, Zviman MM, et al: Clinical utility and safety of a protocol for noncardiac and cardiac magnetic resonance imaging of patients with permanent pacemakers and implantable-cardioverter defibrillators at 1.5 tesla. Circulation 114:1277, 2006.

Standards

21. Kramer CM, Barkhausen J, Flamm SD, et al: Standardized cardiovascular magnetic resonance imaging (CMR) protocols, society for cardiovascular magnetic resonance: Board of trustees task force on standardized protocols. J Cardiovasc Magn Reson 10:35, 2008.
22. Hundley WG, Bluemke D, Bogaert JG, et al: Society for Cardiovascular Magnetic Resonance guidelines for reporting cardiovascular magnetic resonance examinations. J Cardiovasc Magn Reson 11:5, 2009.

Coronary Artery Disease

23. Kim RJ, Shah DJ: Fundamental concepts in myocardial viability assessment revisited: When knowing how much is "alive" is not enough. Heart 90:137, 2004.
24. Hsu LY, Natanzon A, Kellman P, et al: Quantitative myocardial infarction on delayed enhancement MRI. Part I: Animal validation of an automated feature analysis and combined thresholding infarct sizing algorithm. J Magn Reson Imaging 23:298, 2006.
25. Kim RJ, Albert TS, Wible JH, et al: Performance of delayed-enhancement magnetic resonance imaging with gadoversetamide contrast for the detection and assessment of myocardial infarction: An international, multicenter, double-blinded, randomized trial. Circulation 117:629, 2008.
26. Ganame J, Messalli G, Dymarkowski S, et al: Impact of myocardial haemorrhage on left ventricular function and remodelling in patients with reperfused acute myocardial infarction. Eur Heart J 30:1440, 2009.
27. Ricciardi MJ, Wu E, Davidson CJ, et al: Visualization of discrete microinfarction after percutaneous coronary intervention associated with mild creatine kinase-MB elevation. Circulation 103:2780, 2001.
28. Kwong RY, Chan AK, Brown KA, et al: Impact of unrecognized myocardial scar detected by cardiac magnetic resonance imaging on event-free survival in patients presenting with signs or symptoms of coronary artery disease. Circulation 113:2733, 2006.
29. Kwong RY, Sattar H, Wu H, et al: Incidence and prognostic implication of unrecognized myocardial scar characterized by cardiac magnetic resonance in diabetic patients without clinical evidence of myocardial infarction. Circulation 118:1011, 2008.
30. Cheong BY, Muthupillai R, Wilson JM, et al: Prognostic significance of delayed-enhancement magnetic resonance imaging: Survival of 857 patients with and without left ventricular dysfunction. Circulation 120:2069, 2009.

31. Kwon DH, Halley CM, Carrigan TP, et al: Extent of left ventricular scar predicts outcomes in ischemic cardiomyopathy patients with significantly reduced systolic function: A delayed hyperenhancement cardiac magnetic resonance study. J Am Coll Cardiol Img 2:34, 2009.
32. Schmidt A, Azevedo CF, Cheng A, et al: Infarct tissue heterogeneity by magnetic resonance imaging identifies enhanced cardiac arrhythmia susceptibility in patients with left ventricular dysfunction. Circulation 115:2006, 2007.
33. Roes SD, Borleffs CJ, van der Geest RJ, et al: Infarct tissue heterogeneity assessed with contrast-enhanced MRI predicts spontaneous ventricular arrhythmia in patients with ischemic cardiomyopathy and implantable cardioverter-defibrillator. Circ Cardiovasc Imaging 2:183, 2009.
34. Yan AT, Shayne AJ, Brown KA, et al: Characterization of the peri-infarct zone by contrast-enhanced cardiac magnetic resonance imaging is a powerful predictor of post-myocardial infarction mortality. Circulation 114:32, 2006.
35. Kim RJ, Wu E, Rafael A, et al: The use of contrast-enhanced magnetic resonance imaging to identify reversible myocardial dysfunction. N Engl J Med 343:1445, 2000.
36. Wellnhofer E, Olariu A, Klein C, et al: Magnetic resonance low-dose dobutamine test is superior to SCAR quantification for the prediction of functional recovery. Circulation 109:2172, 2004.
37. Ingkanisorn WP, Kwong RY, Bohme NS, et al: Prognosis of negative adenosine stress magnetic resonance in patients presenting to an emergency department with chest pain. J Am Coll Cardiol 47:1427, 2006.
38. Lockie T, Nagel E, Redwood S, Plein S: Use of cardiovascular magnetic resonance imaging in acute coronary syndromes. Circulation 119:1671, 2009.
39. Abdel-Aty H, Zagrosek A, Schulz-Menger J, et al: Delayed enhancement and T2-weighted cardiovascular magnetic resonance imaging differentiate acute from chronic myocardial infarction. Circulation 109:2411, 2004.
40. Cury RC, Shash K, Nagurney JT, et al: Cardiac magnetic resonance with T2-weighted imaging improves detection of patients with acute coronary syndrome in the emergency department. Circulation 118:837, 2008.
41. Codreanu A, Djaballah W, Angioi M, et al: Detection of myocarditis by contrast-enhanced MRI in patients presenting with acute coronary syndrome but no coronary stenosis. J Magn Reson Imaging 25:957, 2007.
42. Assomull RG, Lyne JC, Keenan N, et al: The role of cardiovascular magnetic resonance in patients presenting with chest pain, raised troponin, and unobstructed coronary arteries. Eur Heart J 28:1242, 2007.
43. Laissy JP, Hyafil F, Feldman LJ, et al: Differentiating acute myocardial infarction from myocarditis: Diagnostic value of early- and delayed-perfusion cardiac MR imaging. Radiology 237:75, 2005.
44. Klem I, Heitner JF, Shah DJ, et al: Improved detection of coronary artery disease by stress perfusion cardiovascular magnetic resonance with the use of delayed enhancement infarction imaging. J Am Coll Cardiol 47:1630, 2006.
45. Plein S, Ridgway JP, Jones TR, et al: Coronary artery disease: Assessment with a comprehensive MR imaging protocol—initial results. Radiology 225:300, 2002.
46. Lee DC, Simonetti OP, Harris KR, et al: Magnetic resonance versus radionuclide pharmacological stress perfusion imaging for flow-limiting stenoses of varying severity. Circulation 110:58, 2004.
46a. Schwitter J, Wacker CM, van Rossum AC, et al: MR-IMPACT: comparison of perfusion-cardiac magnetic resonance with single-photon emission tomography for the detection of coronary artery disease in a multicentre, multivendor, randomized trial. Eur Heart J 29:480, 2009.
47. Wahl A, Paetsch I, Roethemeyer S, et al: High-dose dobutamine-atropine stress cardiovascular MR imaging after coronary revascularization in patients with wall motion abnormalities at rest. Radiology 233:210, 2004.
48. Gebker R, Jahnke C, Manka R, et al: Additional value of myocardial perfusion imaging during dobutamine stress magnetic resonance for the assessment of coronary artery disease. Circ Cardiovasc Imaging 1:122, 2008.
49. Jahnke C, Nagel E, Gebker R, et al: Prognostic value of cardiac magnetic resonance stress tests: Adenosine stress perfusion and dobutamine stress wall motion imaging. Circulation 115:1769, 2007.
50. Steel K, Broderick R, Gandla V, et al: Complementary prognostic values of stress myocardial perfusion and late gadolinium enhancement imaging by cardiac magnetic resonance in patients with known or suspected coronary artery disease. Circulation 120:1390, 2009.
51. Doesch C, Seeger A, Doering J, et al: Risk stratification by adenosine stress cardiac magnetic resonance in patients with coronary artery stenoses of intermediate angiographic severity. J Am Coll Cardiol Img 2:424, 2009.
52. Dall'Armellina E, Morgan TM, Mandapaka S, et al: Prediction of cardiac events in patients with reduced left ventricular ejection fraction with dobutamine cardiovascular magnetic resonance assessment of wall motion score index. J Am Coll Cardiol 52:279, 2008.
53. Wallace EL, Morgan TM, Walsh TF, et al: Dobutamine cardiac magnetic resonance results predict cardiac prognosis in women with known or suspected ischemic heart disease. J Am Coll Cardiol Img 2:299, 2008.
54. Yuan C, Kerwin WS: MRI of atherosclerosis. J Magn Reson Imaging 19:710, 2004.
55. Kerwin WS, O'Brien KD, Ferguson MS, et al: Inflammation in carotid atherosclerotic plaque: A dynamic contrast-enhanced MR imaging study. Radiology 241:459, 2006.
56. Yuan C, Kerwin WS, Yarnykh VL, et al: MRI of atherosclerosis in clinical trials. NMR Biomed 19:636, 2006.
57. Trivedi RA, Mallawarachi C, U-King-Im JM, et al: Identifying inflamed carotid plaques using in vivo USPIO-enhanced MR imaging to label plaque macrophages. Arterioscler Thromb Vasc Biol 26:1601, 2006.
58. Larose E, Yeghiazarians Y, Libby P, et al: Characterization of human atherosclerotic plaques by intravascular magnetic resonance imaging. Circulation 112:2324, 2005.
59. Botnar RM, Perez AS, Witte S, et al: In vivo molecular imaging of acute and subacute thrombosis using a fibrin-binding magnetic resonance imaging contrast agent. Circulation 109:2023, 2004.

Cardiomyopathies

60. Weinsaft JW, Kim HW, Shah DJ, et al: Detection of left ventricular thrombus by delayed-enhancement cardiovascular magnetic resonance prevalence and markers in patients with systolic dysfunction. J Am Coll Cardiol 52:148, 2008.
61. Olivotto I, Maron MS, Autore C, et al: Assessment and significance of left ventricular mass by cardiovascular magnetic resonance in hypertrophic cardiomyopathy. J Am Coll Cardiol 52:559, 2008.
62. Petersen SE, Selvanayagam JB, Francis JM, et al: Differentiation of athlete's heart from pathological forms of cardiac hypertrophy by means of geometric indices derived from cardiovascular magnetic resonance. J Cardiovasc Magn Reson 7:551, 2005.
63. Rickers C: Utility of cardiac magnetic resonance imaging in the diagnosis of hypertrophic cardiomyopathy. Circulation 112:855, 2005.
64. Valeti U, Nishimura R, Holmes D, et al: Comparison of surgical septal myectomy and alcohol septal ablation with cardiac magnetic resonance imaging in patients with hypertrophic obstructive cardiomyopathy. J Am Coll Cardiol 49:350, 2007.
65. Abdel-Aty H, Cocker M, Strohm O, et al: Abnormalities in T2-weighted cardiovascular magnetic resonance images of hypertrophic cardiomyopathy: Regional distribution and relation to late gadolinium enhancement and severity of hypertrophy. J Magn Reson Imaging 28:242, 2008.
66. Petersen SE, Jerosch-Herold M, Hudsmith LE, et al: Evidence for microvascular dysfunction in hypertrophic cardiomyopathy: New insights from multiparametric magnetic resonance imaging. Circulation 115:2418, 2007.
67. Adabag AS, Maron BJ, Appelbaum E, et al: Occurrence and frequency of arrhythmias in hypertrophic cardiomyopathy in relation to delayed enhancement on cardiovascular magnetic resonance. J Am Coll Cardiol 51:1369, 2008.
68. Sen-Chowdhry S, Syrris P, Ward D, et al: Clinical and genetic characterization of families with arrhythmogenic right ventricular dysplasia/cardiomyopathy provides novel insights into patterns of disease expression. Circulation 115:1710, 2007.
69. Sen-Chowdhry S, McKenna WJ: The utility of magnetic resonance imaging in the evaluation of arrhythmogenic right ventricular cardiomyopathy. Curr Opin Cardiol 23:38, 2008.
70. Tandri H, Castillo E, Ferrari VA, et al: Magnetic resonance imaging of arrhythmogenic right ventricular dysplasia: Sensitivity, specificity, and observer variability of fat detection versus functional analysis of the right ventricle. J Am Coll Cardiol 48:2277, 2006.
71. Tandri H, Saranathan M, Rodriguez ER, et al: Noninvasive detection of myocardial fibrosis in arrhythmogenic right ventricular cardiomyopathy using delayed-enhancement magnetic resonance imaging. J Am Coll Cardiol 45:98, 2005.
72. Sen-Chowdhry S, Prasad SK, Syrris P, et al: Cardiovascular magnetic resonance in arrhythmogenic right ventricular cardiomyopathy revisited: Comparison with task force criteria and genotype. J Am Coll Cardiol 48:2132, 2006.
73. Asimaki A, Tandri H, Huang H, et al: A new diagnostic test for arrhythmogenic right ventricular cardiomyopathy. N Engl J Med 360:1075, 2009.
74. Jain A, Tandri H, Calkins H, Bluemke DA: Role of cardiovascular magnetic resonance imaging in arrhythmogenic right ventricular dysplasia. J Cardiovasc Magn Reson 10:32, 2008.
75. Friedrich MG, Sechtem U, Schulz-Menger J, et al: Cardiovascular magnetic resonance in myocarditis: A JACC White Paper. J Am Coll Cardiol 53:1475, 2009.
76. Wagner A, Schulz-Menger J, Dietz R, Friedrich MG: Long-term follow-up of patients paragraph sign with acute myocarditis by magnetic paragraph sign resonance imaging. MAGMA 16:17, 2003.
77. Patel MR, Cawley PJ, Heitner JF, et al: Detection of myocardial damage in patients with sarcoidosis. Circulation 120:1969, 2009.
78. Vignaux O, Dhote R, Duboc D, et al: Clinical significance of myocardial magnetic resonance abnormalities in patients with sarcoidosis: A 1-year follow-up study. Chest 122:1895, 2002.
79. Maceira AM, Joshi J, Prasad SK, et al: Cardiovascular magnetic resonance in cardiac amyloidosis. Circulation 111:186, 2005.
80. Maceira AM, Prasad SK, Hawkins PN, et al: Cardiovascular magnetic resonance and prognosis in cardiac amyloidosis. J Cardiovasc Magn Reson 10:54, 2008.
81. Senthilkumar A, Majmudar MD, Shenoy C, et al: Identifying the etiology: A systematic approach using delayed-enhancement cardiovascular magnetic resonance. Heart Fail Clin 5:349, 2009.
82. Assomull RG, Prasad SK, Lyne J, et al: Cardiovascular magnetic resonance, fibrosis, and prognosis in dilated cardiomyopathy. J Am Coll Cardiol 48:1977, 2006.
83. Nazarian S, Bluemke DA, Lardo AC, et al: Magnetic resonance assessment of the substrate for inducible ventricular tachycardia in nonischemic cardiomyopathy. Circulation 112:2821, 2005.
84. Tanner MA, Galanello R, Dessi C, et al: A randomized, placebo-controlled, double-blind trial of the effect of combined therapy with deferoxamine and deferiprone on myocardial iron in thalassemia major using cardiovascular magnetic resonance. Circulation 115:1876, 2007.
85. Modell B, Khan M, Darlison M, et al: Improved survival of thalassaemia major in the UK and relation to T2* cardiovascular magnetic resonance. J Cardiovasc Magn Reson 10:42, 2008.
86. Rochitte CE, Oliveira PF, Andrade JM, et al: Myocardial delayed enhancement by magnetic resonance imaging in patients with Chagas' disease: A marker of disease severity. J Am Coll Cardiol 46:1553, 2005.
87. Petersen SE, Selvanayagam JB, Wiesmann F, et al: Left ventricular non-compaction: insights from cardiovascular magnetic resonance imaging. J Am Coll Cardiol 46:101, 2005.
88. Wittstein IS, Thiemann DR, Lima JA, et al: Neurohumoral features of myocardial stunning due to sudden emotional stress. N Engl J Med 352:539, 2005.
89. Rolf A, Nef HM, Mollmann H, et al: Immunohistological basis of the late gadolinium enhancement phenomenon in tako-tsubo cardiomyopathy. Eur Heart J 30:1635, 2009.

Other Clinical Applications

90. Rathi VK, Doyle M, Yamrozik J, et al: Routine evaluation of left ventricular diastolic function by cardiovascular magnetic resonance: A practical approach. J Cardiovasc Magn Reson 10:36, 2008.
91. Paelinck BP, de Roos A, Bax JJ, et al: Feasibility of tissue magnetic resonance imaging: A pilot study in comparison with tissue Doppler imaging and invasive measurement. J Am Coll Cardiol 45:1109, 2005.
92. Durongpisitkul K, Tang NL, Soongswang J, et al: Predictors of successful transcatheter closure of atrial septal defect by cardiac magnetic resonance imaging. Pediatr Cardiol 25:124, 2004.
93. Knauth AL, Gauvreau K, Powell AJ, et al: Ventricular size and function assessed by cardiac MRI predict major adverse clinical outcomes late after tetralogy of Fallot repair. Heart 94:211, 2008.
94. Wald RM, Haber I, Wald R, et al: Effects of regional dysfunction and late gadolinium enhancement on global right ventricular function and exercise capacity in patients with repaired tetralogy of Fallot. Circulation 119:1370, 2009.

95. Reiter G, Reiter U, Kovacs G, et al: Magnetic resonance-derived 3-dimensional blood flow patterns in the main pulmonary artery as a marker of pulmonary hypertension and a measure of elevated mean pulmonary arterial pressure. Circ Cardiovasc Imaging 1:23, 2008.
96. Frydrychowicz A, Stalder AF, Russe MF, et al: Three-dimensional analysis of segmental wall shear stress in the aorta by flow-sensitive four-dimensional-MRI. J Magn Reson Imaging 30:77, 2009.
97. Grizzard JD: Magnetic resonance imaging of pericardial disease and intracardiac thrombus. Heart Fail Clin 5:401, 2009.

Novel Techniques

98. Horn M: Cardiac magnetic resonance spectroscopy: A window for studying physiology. Methods Mol Med 224:225, 2006.
99. McGavock JM, Lingvay I, Zib I, et al: Cardiac steatosis in diabetes mellitus: A 1H-magnetic resonance spectroscopy study. Circulation 116:1170, 2007.
100. Jaffer FA, Weissleder R: Seeing within: Molecular imaging of the cardiovascular system. Circ Res 94:433, 2004.
101. Spuentrup E, Buecker A, Katoh M, et al: Molecular magnetic resonance imaging of coronary thrombosis and pulmonary emboli with a novel fibrin-targeted contrast agent. Circulation 111:1377, 2005.
102. Botnar RM, Buecker A, Wiethoff AJ, et al: In vivo magnetic resonance imaging of coronary thrombosis using a fibrin-binding molecular magnetic resonance contrast agent. Circulation 110:1463, 2004.
103. Kraitchman DL, Gilson WD, Lorenz CH: Stem cell therapy: MRI guidance and monitoring. J Magn Reson Imaging 27:299, 2008.
104. Spuentrup E, Ruhl KM, Botnar RM, et al: Molecular magnetic resonance imaging of myocardial perfusion with EP-3600, a collagen-specific contrast agent: Initial feasibility study in a swine model. Circulation 119:1768, 2009.
105. Tang L, Merkle N, Schar M, et al: Volume-targeted and whole-heart coronary magnetic resonance angiography using an intravascular contrast agent. J Magn Reson Imaging 30:1191, 2009.
106. Paetsch I, Huber ME, Bornstedt A, et al: Improved three-dimensional free-breathing coronary magnetic resonance angiography using gadocoletic acid (B-22956) for intravascular contrast enhancement. J Magn Reson Imaging 20:288, 2004.

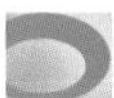

APPROPRIATE USE CRITERIA

RAYMOND Y. KWONG

Cardiovascular Magnetic Resonance

The explosive growth in cardiovascular imaging has sometimes outpaced the evidence on which the use of new technologies should be based. In an effort to guide rational use of these technologies, eight scientific organizations—American College of Cardiology Foundation, American College of Radiology, Society of Cardiovascular Computed Tomography, Society for Cardiovascular Magnetic Resonance, American Society of Nuclear Cardiology, North American Society for Cardiac Imaging, Society for Cardiovascular Angiography and Interventions, and Society of Interventional Radiology—have embarked on a process to determine the appropriateness of selected indications for cardiovascular imaging procedures.

Panelists rated 33 indications for cardiovascular magnetic resonance (CMR) imaging as appropriate (7 to 9 points), uncertain (4 to 6 points), and inappropriate (1 to 3 points), based on the following definition of appropriateness[1]:

An appropriate imaging study is one in which the expected incremental information, combined with clinical judgment, exceeds the expected negative consequences by a sufficiently wide margin for a specific indication that the procedure is generally considered acceptable care and a reasonable approach for the indication. (Negative consequences include the risks of the procedure [i.e., radiation or contrast exposure] and the downstream impact of poor test performance such as delay in diagnosis [false negatives] or inappropriate diagnosis [false positives].)

Of the 33 CMR indications, 17 were deemed appropriate, 7 were uncertain, and 9 were rated as inappropriate (**Table 18G-1**).

The panel stressed that appropriate use criteria are not substitutes for sound clinical judgment and practice experience. Medical reasons may preclude applying the appropriate use criteria to specific patients, and clinician judgment should be used at all times in applying the criteria. For example, the rating of an indication as inappropriate should not dissuade a provider from performing CMR imaging when patient- and condition-specific data support that decision, and not performing a study rated as appropriate may be the correct decision in light of unique patient, clinical, and other relevant information.

TABLE 18G-1 Joint Professional Society* Evaluation of Appropriate Indications for Cardiac Magnetic Resonance

INDICATION	APPROPRIATENESS (MEDIAN SCORE)
Detection of CAD: Symptomatic	
Evaluation of Chest Pain Syndrome (Use of Vasodilator Perfusion CMR or Dobutamine Stress Function CMR)	
Intermediate pretest probability of CAD ECG uninterpretable *or* unable to exercise	A (7)
High pretest probability of CAD	U (5)
Intermediate pretest probability of CAD ECG interpretable *and* able to exercise	U (4)
Low pretest probability of CAD ECG interpretable *and* able to exercise	I (2)
Evaluation of Chest Pain Syndrome (Use of MR Coronary Angiography)	
Intermediate pretest probability of CAD ECG interpretable *and* able to exercise	I (2)
Intermediate pretest probability of CAD ECG uninterpretable *or* unable to exercise	I (2)
High pretest probability of CAD	I (1)
Evaluation of Intracardiac Structures (Use of MR Coronary Angiography)	
Evaluation of suspected coronary anomalies	A (8)
Acute Chest Pain (Use of Vasodilator Perfusion CMR or Dobutamine Stress Function CMR)	
Intermediate pretest probability of CAD No changes on the ECG and serial cardiac enzymes negative	U (6)
High pretest probability of CAD ECG—ST-segment elevation and/or positive cardiac enzymes	I (1)

Continued

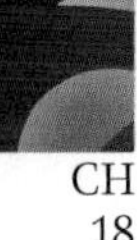

TABLE 18G-1 Joint Professional Society* Evaluation of Appropriate Indications for Cardiac Magnetic Resonance—cont'd

INDICATION	APPROPRIATENESS (MEDIAN SCORE)
Risk Assessment with Prior Test Results (Use of Vasodilator Perfusion CMR or Dobutamine Stress Function CMR)	
Coronary angiography (catheterization or CT) Stenosis of unclear significance	A (7)
Equivocal stress test (exercise, stress SPECT, or stress echo) Intermediate CHD risk (Framingham)	U (6)
Normal prior stress test (exercise, nuclear, echo, MRI) High CHD risk (Framingham) Within 1 year of prior stress test	I (2)
Risk Assessment: Preoperative Evaluation for Noncardiac Surgery	
Low-Risk Surgery (Use of Vasodilator Perfusion CMR or Dobutamine Stress Function CMR)	
Intermediate perioperative risk predictor	I (2)
Intermediate- or High-Risk Surgery (Use of Vasodilator Perfusion CMR or Dobutamine Stress Function CMR)	
Intermediate perioperative risk predictor	U (6)
Detection of CAD: Postrevascularization (PCI or CABG)	
Evaluation of Chest Pain Syndrome (Use of MR Coronary Angiography)	
Evaluation of bypass grafts History of percutaneous revascularization with stents	I (2) I (1)
Structure and Function	
Evaluation of Ventricular and Valvular Function[†]	
Assessment of complex congenital heart disease, including anomalies of coronary circulation, great vessels, and cardiac chambers and valves Procedures may include LV-RV mass and volumes, MR angiography, quantification of valvular disease, and contrast enhancement	A (9)
Evaluation for arrhythmogenic right ventricular cardiomyopathy (ARVC) Patients presenting with syncope or ventricular arrhythmia	A (9)
Evaluation of LV function following myocardial infarction *or* in heart failure patients Patients with technically limited images from echocardiogram	A (8)
Quantification of LV function Discordant information that is clinically significant from prior tests	A (8)
Evaluation of specific cardiomyopathies (infiltrative [amyloid, sarcoid], HCM, or caused by cardiotoxic therapies) Use of delayed enhancement	A (8)
Characterization of native and prosthetic cardiac valves, including planimetry of stenotic disease and quantification of regurgitant disease Patients with technically limited images from echocardiogram or TEE	A (8)
Evaluation of myocarditis or myocardial infarction with normal coronary arteries Positive cardiac enzymes without obstructive atherosclerosis on angiography	A (8)
Evaluation of LV function following myocardial infarction *or* in heart failure patients	U (6)
Evaluation of Intra- and Extracardiac Structures	
Evaluation of cardiac mass (suspected tumor or thrombus) Use of contrast for perfusion and enhancement	A (9)
Evaluation of pericardial conditions (pericardial mass, constrictive pericarditis)	A (8)
Evaluation for aortic dissection	A (8)
Evaluation of pulmonary veins prior to radiofrequency ablation for atrial fibrillation Left atrial and pulmonary venous anatomy, including dimensions of veins for mapping purposes	A (8)
Detection of Myocardial Scar and Viability	
Evaluation of Myocardial Scar (Use of Late Gadolinium Enhancement)	
To determine viability prior to revascularization Viability assessment by SPECT or dobutamine echo has provided "equivocal" or "indeterminate" results	A (9)
To determine viability prior to revascularization To establish likelihood of recovery of function with revascularization (PCI or CABG) or medical therapy	A (9)
To determine the location and extent of myocardial necrosis, including no-reflow regions Post–acute myocardial infarction	A (7)
To detect post-PCI myocardial necrosis	U (4)

*American College of Cardiology Foundation, American College of Radiology, Society of Cardiovascular Computed Tomography, Society for Cardiovascular Magnetic Resonance, American Society of Nuclear Cardiology, North American Society for Cardiac Imaging, Society for Cardiovascular Angiography and Interventions, and Society of Interventional Radiology.

†Procedures may include LV and RV mass and volumes, MR angiography, quantification of valvular disease, and delayed contrast enhancement.

CABG = coronary artery bypass grafting; CAD = coronary artery disease; CHD = congenital heart disease; CMR = cardiovascular magnetic resonance; CT = computed tomography; ECG = electrocardiogram; HCM = hypertrophic cardiomyopathy; LV = left ventricular; MRI = magnetic resonance imaging; PCI = percutaneous coronary intervention; RV = right ventricular; SPECT = single-photon emission computed tomography; TEE = transesophageal echocardiography.

Since the 2006 publication of the CMR appropriate use criteria, new published data and changes in regulation and practice may influence the current appropriate use of a few specific indications. In 2008, new Current Procedural Terminology (CPT) billing codes[2] were created that cover assessment of blood flow and velocity quantitation by phase contrast CMR imaging. There has also been a growing body of literature indicating the strong potential usefulness for CMR in assessing acute chest pain by imaging physiologic changes at the myocardial level. This has direct relevance to the indication of "Acute Chest Pain (Use of Vasodilator Perfusion CMR or Dobutamine Stress Function CMR, Intermediate pretest probability of CAD, No changes on the ECG and serial cardiac enzymes negative," which may warrant a higher appropriate indication than its current "unknown" (U[6]). (See Table 18G-1.)

REFERENCE

1. Hendel RC, Patel MR, Kramer CM, et al: ACCF/ACR/SCCT/SCMR/ASNC/NASCI/SCAI/SIR 2006 appropriateness criteria for cardiac computed tomography and cardiac magnetic resonance imaging: A report of the American College of Cardiology Foundation Quality Strategic Directions Committee Appropriateness Criteria Working Group, American College of Radiology, Society of Cardiovascular Computed Tomography, Society for Cardiovascular Magnetic Resonance, American Society of Nuclear Cardiology, North American Society for Cardiac Imaging, Society for Cardiovascular Angiography and Interventions, and Society of Interventional Radiology. J Am Coll Cardiol 48:1475, 2006.
2. Centers for Medicare and Medicaid Services (http://www.CMS.gov/Transmittals/downloads/R107ncd.pdf).

CHAPTER 19 Cardiac Computed Tomography

Allen J. Taylor

Progress in the technical developments of cardiovascular computed tomography (CT) during the past decade now enables rapid and accurate imaging of the cardiovascular system, including coronary arteries, coronary arterial wall, cardiac valves, myocardium, and associated structures. The basic principle of CT technology is the use of ionizing radiation within a gantry rotating around the patient in which x-rays are detected on a detector array (**Fig. 19-1**) and converted through reconstruction algorithms to images. It is these images, acquired at high spatial and temporal resolution, that have enabled cardiovascular medicine to enter the CT imaging era.

The most notable technical advance is progressive increase in the number of detector rows (or slices). Each row is a narrow channel, approximately 0.625 mm in width, through which x-rays are detected on scintillation crystals. The number of detector rows aligned in an array has increased from a single detector to 4, 16, and 64 (present standard technology) and now on to "wide" detectors of 256 to 320 rows. The increase in the number of rows leads to wider coverage (more of the heart viewed simultaneously, e.g., 64 rows of 0.625-mm width produces approximately 4 cm of coverage; **Table 19-1**), leading to shorter scan acquisition times and consequently reduced radiation exposure and contrast requirements. Spatial resolution within the imaging plane (the *x-y* axis) is broadly determined by the detector width and the ability to create volumes of image data (voxels) of equal size on all sides, or isotropism. The other major constraint for cardiac imaging is temporal resolution to obtain motion-free cardiac images. This requires fast gantry rotation (maximum gantry rotation times are approximately 270 to 330 msec) and image acquisition or reconstruction during periods of limited cardiac motion (end systole to mid-late diastole). At present, CT spatial resolution through reconstruction of overlapping data sets is approximately 0.5 mm^3, and temporal resolution is approximately 83 to 165 msec through the use of half-scan reconstruction techniques. Further refinements in spatial resolution are possible through the use of narrower detector widths (below 0.625 mm; high-definition CT) but require special computer reconstruction algorithms because of the reduced signal-to-noise ratios. Improvements in temporal resolution have been obtained through novel scanner designs (e.g., dual-source CT, or simultaneous imaging with two source-detector arrays leading to temporal resolutions of 83 msec through quarter-scan reconstruction), but physical forces from the weight of the rotating gantry will make further improvements difficult. Whereas the temporal and spatial resolution of cardiac CT is presently beneath that of invasive coronary angiography, it is sufficient for highly accurate diagnostic imaging.

Scan Modes

There are two basic scan modes in cardiac CT, helical and axial scanning (**Fig. 19-2**).[1] Helical scanning involves continuous radiation exposure and table movement (the patient is moved through the rotating x-ray beam), during which the detector arrays receive projection data from multiple contiguous slices of the patient. This relies on collection of a redundant or overlapping data set so that complete image data can be reconstructed after CT data acquisition (retrospective reconstruction). The reconstruction of CT data to images relies on aligning the data to the electrocardiogram and selectively including only CT data from the desired time point of the electrocardiogram (typically when cardiac motion is at a minimum and thus in a consistent position within the chest). In contrast, axial imaging involves sequential scanner "snapshots," in between which the x-ray tube is turned off and the table is moved to a different position for the next image to be acquired. The CT data are then reconstructed in a series of slices akin to slices of a loaf of bread. The major relative merit of helical CT acquisition is the ability to reconstruct data throughout the cardiac cycle, enabling great flexibility for cine evaluation of ventricular function and data editing in the event of cardiac arrhythmias. The major relative merit of axial CT acquisition is the on-off nature of x-ray exposure, leading to marked (80%) reductions in x-ray exposure but with limitations in data reconstruction, including the inability to evaluate ventricular function. Both modes produce images of similar spatial and temporal resolution and therefore provide the same diagnostic image quality. After data acquisition, images are reconstructed within the desired field of view (cardiac structures), including thin slices (for coronary arteries and evaluation of finer cardiac details), data at different time points of the cardiac cycle (to provide flexibility for resolution of motion artifacts), and thicker slices for evaluation of cardiac chambers and noncardiac anatomy. Reconstructions may be performed by selected reconstruction kernels, which are mathematical algorithms for blending of data from adjacent voxels, resulting in images with either sharp or smooth detail (**Fig. 19-3**).

RADIATION EXPOSURE

Radiation dosing is measured by the CT dose index (CTDI) and dose-length product (mGy × cm). Effective radiation (sieverts) exposure entails the application of a constant determined by the relative radiation sensitivity of the tissue. The weighting factor for the chest is 0.14. Radiation exposure must be kept to the minimum achievable that retains diagnostic image quality. Factors determining radiation exposure (**Table 19-2**) include the volume of tissue scanned (scan length in the *z* axis of the patient), the scanner settings including the tube current (mA) and tube voltage output (peak tube voltage or kVp), and the amount of overlap in the data acquired (pitch). Scanner programming, including helical or axial scanning, is also important. Helical scanning optimally includes the use of upward modulation of the tube current (**Fig. 19-4**) during desired imaging periods (e.g., mid-late diastole) and downward modulation of the tube current during periods of cardiac motion (e.g., systole and early diastole). The use of tube current modulation can spare 25% to 40% of radiation dosage.[2] Radiation exposure increases directly with tube current and according to the square of peak tube voltage. Therefore, reduced tube voltage is especially important to limit radiation exposure. Presently, 120 kVp is a standard setting, but patients beneath 180 pounds can often be successfully imaged at 100 kVp, leading to a 40% radiation sparing without any degradation in image quality.[3] Axial scan protocols

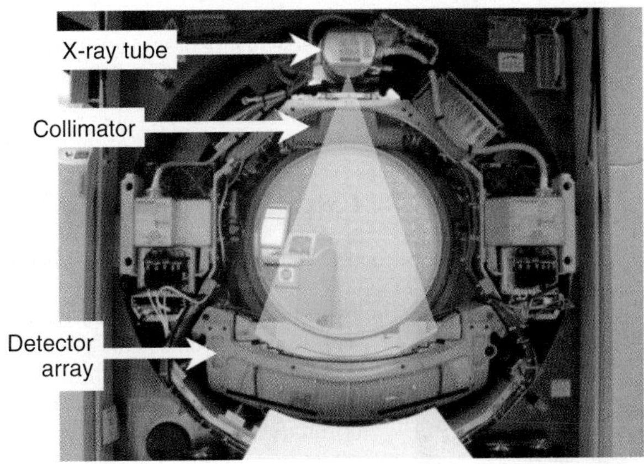

FIGURE 19-1 View within the rotating multidetector CT gantry. Key elements include the x-ray tube or source, a collimator to align the x-ray beam, and the detector array consisting of narrow channels for detection of x-ray photons. The number of detector channels determines the nomenclature (e.g., 64-row multidetector CT). The maximum number of detectors within a commercially available multidetector CT scanner is 320.

at 100 kVp can be performed at effective radiation doses of below 4 mSv, an amount equivalent to 1 year of normal background radiation. Because of evolving knowledge and technical capabilities, there is a large degree of regional variation in radiation exposure. A new mode of imaging involving helical acquisition with high pitch (no overlap) has been developed.[4,5] Preliminary data indicate the potential for very low radiation exposure of <1 to 2 mSv, but more data on image quality and diagnostic accuracy are needed.

PREPARATION OF THE PATIENT AND SCANNING SEQUENCE

The absolute requirements for patients to undergo contrast-enhanced cardiac CT angiography include the ability to receive intravenous contrast material and the ability to cooperate with breathing instructions and to hold the breath for approximately 10 to 20 seconds. Relative contraindications include high or irregular heart rates (particularly atrial fibrillation), morbid obesity, and severe coronary calcium. Each of these conditions can degrade scan quality or interpretability. Instructions to the patient include pretest, on-site, and post-test considerations (**Table 19-3**). Most centers control heart rate with beta blockers administered either orally (e.g., metoprolol 25 to 100 mg orally 1 hour before the scan) or intravenously (e.g., metoprolol 5 mg intravenously in repeated doses) to achieve a resting heart rate below 65 beats/min. Some scanners with faster gantry rotations or dual-source configurations can obtain diagnostic image quality at higher heart rates; but in general, scan quality is lower at higher heart rates.[6] Nitroglycerin (400 to 800 μg sublingually) is typically administered just before CT angiography to increase coronary artery diameter and to improve the signal-to-noise ratio.

The intravenous administration of a contrast agent is required for the performance of cardiac CT angiography. The principle is to achieve a plateau of contrast concentration in the coronary arteries that is sustained through the image acquisition. A standard three-phase injection protocol includes undiluted contrast 40 to 60 mL at a rate of approximately 5 mL/sec through an antecubital 18- to 20-gauge intravenous line, followed by a smaller volume of dilute contrast (50:50 contrast/saline for a total of 10 to 20 mL), then a bolus of saline (40 mL). The intent is to maximize contrast enhancement of the left side of the heart and arterial structures, with mild contrast enhancement of the right side of the heart and pulmonary artery. Excessive right-sided contrast enhancement can interfere with evaluation of the right coronary artery and is unnecessary for most scan indications (unless right-sided heart enhancement is judged necessary for the particular clinical indication) (**Fig. 19-5**). Timing of the scan in relationship to the contrast bolus is commonly performed by the triggered bolus method, in which contrast attenuation in the pulmonary artery or aorta is monitored, followed by automated scan initiation once an adequate CT attenuation value (110 to 180 HU) is achieved. An alternative method is to tailor scan timing on the basis of a contrast test bolus to determine the time to peak contrast attenuation, with subsequent scan programming based on the individual patient's transit time (which can vary from patient to patient according to volume status, cardiac output, and ventricular and valvular function). After peak contrast opacification, an additional delay including a patient breath-hold is programmed to last typically 6 to 10 seconds to permit even contrast opacification of the coronary circulation and stabilization of heart rate. Scan time is determined by the scanner, acquisition mode, heart rate, and scan length; for 64-row multidetector CT, it is

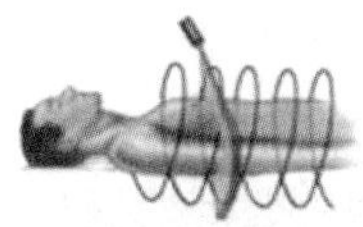
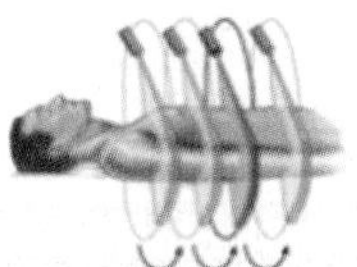

Scan mode	Helical	Axial
Synonyms	Spiral, retrospectively-gated	Triggered, step and shoot
Basic principle	X-ray tube continuously "on" with patient moved through the beam	X-ray tube on and off triggered by the ECG, with no scanning between steps as the patient is moved through the scan range
CT data acquired	Systole and diastole	Set phase (diastole, or systole) with some phase tolerance (temporal padding)
X-ray sparing maneuvers	ECG-based tube current modulation, limited scan length, use of 100 kVp in smaller patients	Limited scan length, use of 100 kVp in smaller patients
Advantages	Enables flexible reconstruction in the event of arrhythmias or artifacts; evaluation of cine images for systolic and diastolic frames (ejection fraction)	Low radiation dose, no loss in image quality for purpose of coronary or structural diagnosis
Disadvantage	Higher radiation dose	Loss of ventricular function evalution

FIGURE 19-2 Comparison of helical and axial CT scan acquisition.

TABLE 19-1 Evolution of Common Multidetector Computed Tomography Technical Parameters

	4-ROW	16-ROW	64-ROW	320-ROW
Temporal resolution (half-scan reconstruction)	250 msec	210 msec	165 msec	175 msec
Spatial resolution	1.25 mm	1 mm	0.4 mm	0.4 mm
Volume coverage	0.5-3 cm	1-2 cm	2-4 cm	15 cm
Breath-hold	30-40 sec	20 sec	10 sec	2 sec

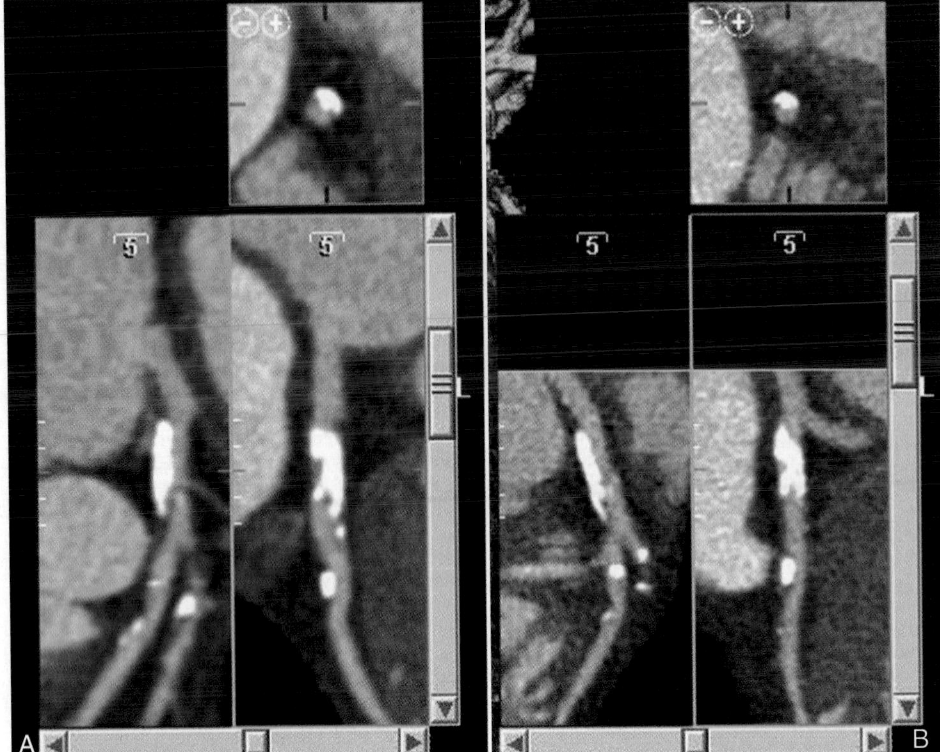

FIGURE 19-3 Reconstruction of CT data by two different reconstruction kernels. In **A,** a soft or smoothing reconstruction kernel is used. In comparison, the sharp kernel in **B** produces a grainier image. The sharp kernel results in an image with more edge definition between structures of high and low attenuation, such as coronary calcium.

typically approximately 6 seconds. A typical sequence of scan acquisition and postprocessing algorithm are shown in **Tables 19-4 and 19-5**.

Cardiac Computed Tomography Anatomy

Thin-slice cardiac CT reconstructions with isotropic voxels can be displayed in any imaging plane with minimal or no image distortion. Cardiac chambers, coronary vessels, great vessels, and other surrounding cardiac and mediastinal structures can be imaged in a multiplanar fashion (**Fig. 19-6**). Images can be displayed in orthogonal planes (axial, coronal, sagittal) or nonstandard planes (oblique planar reformats; **Fig. 19-7**). Images are evaluated in both thin- and thick-slice projections, most commonly with use of a maximal intensity projection in which the pixel within the slab volume with the highest Hounsfield number is viewed. Maximum intensity projections provide the ability to view more structures within a single planar view but can obscure details, particularly when high-density structures (such as coronary artery calcium) are present. Optimal accuracy entails the use of an interactive evaluation technique in which optimal imaging planes are selected by the interpreter.[7] Curved structures can be viewed in planar oblique multiplanar reformats through the use of curved multiplanar reformations (see Fig. 19-7) constructed with the use of centerline techniques. Volume rendered reconstructions are useful for revealing general structural relationships but not for viewing details of the coronary anatomy. In addition to image planes for

TABLE 19-2 Methods to Limit Radiation Exposure

Methods to Limit Radiation Exposure
Select appropriate patients for imaging
Limit scan length to cardiac structures
Tailor scanner settings
Tube current, mA (weight based)
Tube output, kVp (100 kVp for patients <80 kg)
Acquisition parameters
Scanning method
Axial scans: use when ventricular functional information is not needed
Helical scans: use tube current modulation

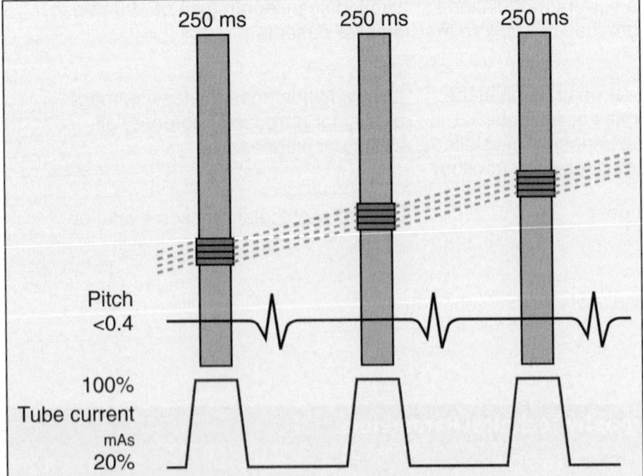

FIGURE 19-4 Helical CT acquisition with dose modulation in which the timing of increased tube current from 20% to 100% of maximum output is synchronized with the electrocardiogram (diastole). This limits the period of exposure to maximum tube current (250 msec) and results in lower radiation exposure to the patient without loss of image quality for diastolic image reconstruction.

TABLE 19-3 Patient Instructions and Preparation for Cardiac Computed Tomography

Pretest	No food 3 hours before the examination No caffeine 12 hours before the examination Drink water Take all regular medications Take premedications for contrast allergy as needed Take premedications for renal protection as needed Serum creatinine by institutional protocol (diabetics, age >60 yr, known chronic kidney disease)
On-site preparation	Intravenous line: 18- or 20-gauge, antecubital site Pulse, blood pressure, ECG monitor Beta blocker (IV or PO) (metoprolol) 25-100 mg metoprolol PO 1 hour before scan 5 mg metoprolol IV bolus Positioning Breath-hold training: observe heart rate response Nitroglycerin: 400-800 μg sublingual
Post-test	Liberal oral fluids Hold metformin 48-72 hours after administration of contrast agent

coronary artery evaluation, which can be categorized by coronary segmentation models (**Fig. 19-8**), analysis of cardiac chambers is performed with standard short-axis, horizontal long-axis, and vertical long-axis projections (**Fig. 19-9**). A complete evaluation includes the inspection of the images for noncardiac disease in the lungs, mediastinum, and great vessels.

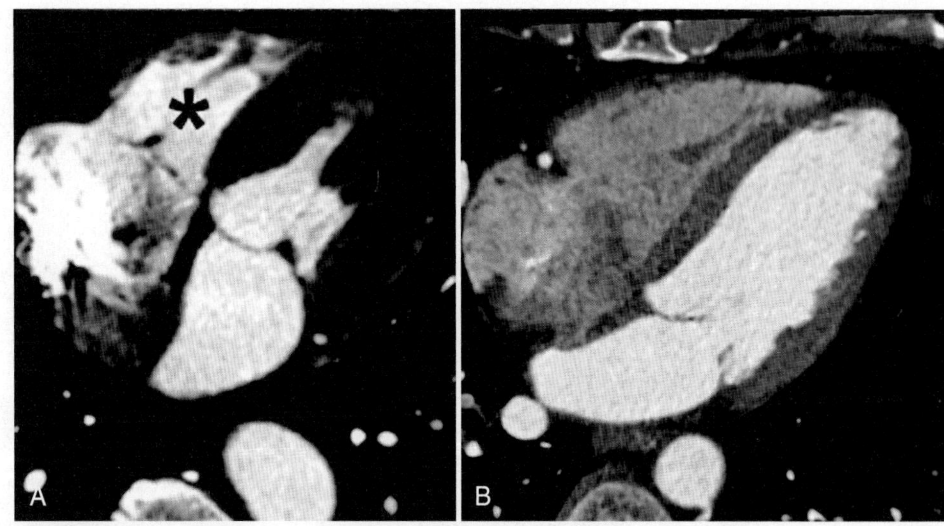

FIGURE 19-5 Timing of radiocontrast media within the right side of the heart. In **A,** timing was early as contrast medium was still contained within the right atrium and right ventricle (asterisk). This may be desirable if delineation of right-sided cardiac structures is necessary; but in general, most cardiac CT is timed after contrast material has passed through the right side of the heart, leading to a levophase image as shown in **B.**

Clinical Indications

Clinical indications for cardiovascular CT encompass a broad range of potential anatomic imaging targets and clinical scenarios. These can be broadly divided into seven categories: detection of coronary artery disease in symptomatic patients without known heart disease, coronary artery disease risk assessment in asymptomatic individuals, coronary artery disease detection in other cardiac conditions, use of CT angiography after other test results, use after revascularization, evaluation of cardiac structure and function, and evaluation of intracardiac and extracardiac structures. In general, cardiac CT is considered most appropriate in settings in which there is a generally low or intermediate pretest likelihood of coronary artery disease and in which the test results would lead to improved management of the patient. Because the technical development of cardiac CT has been rapid during the past 5 to 8 years, there are few clinical trials guiding optimal use of cardiac CT. Instead, appropriate use of cardiac CT is largely guided by expert opinion through appropriate use criteria. Multisociety appropriate use criteria were originally drafted in 2006[8] and revised in 2010[9] within a modified approach to the Rand methodology. Use of cardiac CT is judged to be appropriate when the expected incremental information, combined with clinical judgment, exceeds the expected negative consequences by a sufficiently wide margin for a specific indication that the procedure is generally considered acceptable care and a reasonable approach for the indication. Appropriate cardiac CT indications described within the 2010 update are discussed in detail at the end of this chapter. Clinical trials are needed both to compare the clinical performance of cardiac CT relative to other techniques and to demonstrate its overall effect on net health outcomes. Contraindications to cardiac CT include pregnancy, known history of anaphylactic contrast reactions, clinical instability, and renal insufficiency. Relative issues that deserve consideration of the risk and benefit of the procedure include difficulty with the breath-hold, obesity, maintaining body position, contraindications to beta blockers or nitroglycerin, and high heart rates and arrhythmias.

TABLE 19-4 Typical Cardiac Computed Tomography Scan Sequence

Scout film	Determine cardiac location
Set scan range	Limit scan range to cardiac and other relevant structures of interest
Calcium scan	If indicated Use calcium scan to refine CT angiography scan range
Nitroglycerin administration	400-800 μg sublingual
Contrast test bolus or bolus tracking	Injection of contrast agent to determine transit time or track bolus until scan is initiated with achievement of attenuation threshold
Breath-hold initiated	Permits contrast opacification to become uniform and heart rate to stabilize Prolonged scan delays may lead to increased coronary venous opacification
CT angiogram	
Image reconstruction and postprocessing/analysis	

TABLE 19-5 Typical Reconstruction Parameters for Cardiac Computed Tomography

Coronary anatomy	Half-scan reconstruction Field of view 200-250 mm Slice thickness 0.5-0.6 mm Slice increment 50% Reconstruction phases: diastole 70%-80% of the RR interval most common; end systole (40% phase) if high heart rates/helical acquisition Semi-sharp reconstruction kernel
Coronary calcium	Field of view 200-250 mm Slice thickness 2.5-3.0 mm
Ventricular function	Field of view 200-250 mm Slice thickness 2.5 mm Reconstruction phases: 0%-90% in 5%-10% increments
Noncardiac evaluation	Full field of view Slice thickness 5 mm

Coronary Artery Calcium Scanning

Coronary calcium testing is used in asymptomatic patients to refine their clinically predicted risk of incident coronary heart disease (CHD) beyond that predicted by standard cardiac risk factors. Coronary artery calcium is typically present in direct proportion to the overall extent of atherosclerosis, although typically only a minority (approximately 20%) of plaque is calcified. Arterial calcification is an active process involving the deposition of hydroxyapatite most typically in areas of prior arterial disruption or plaque rupture. Although most data regarding coronary calcium were derived by use of electron beam CT, multidetector CT has supplanted electron beam scanning. Coronary calcium is detected by a standardized protocol that should result in acceptably low levels of radiation exposure (1 to 2 mSv) and potentially lower levels with the evolution of lower 100-kVp imaging protocols.[10] CT quantification methods primarily involve the measurement

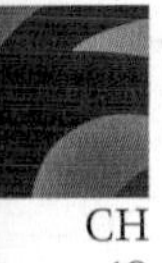

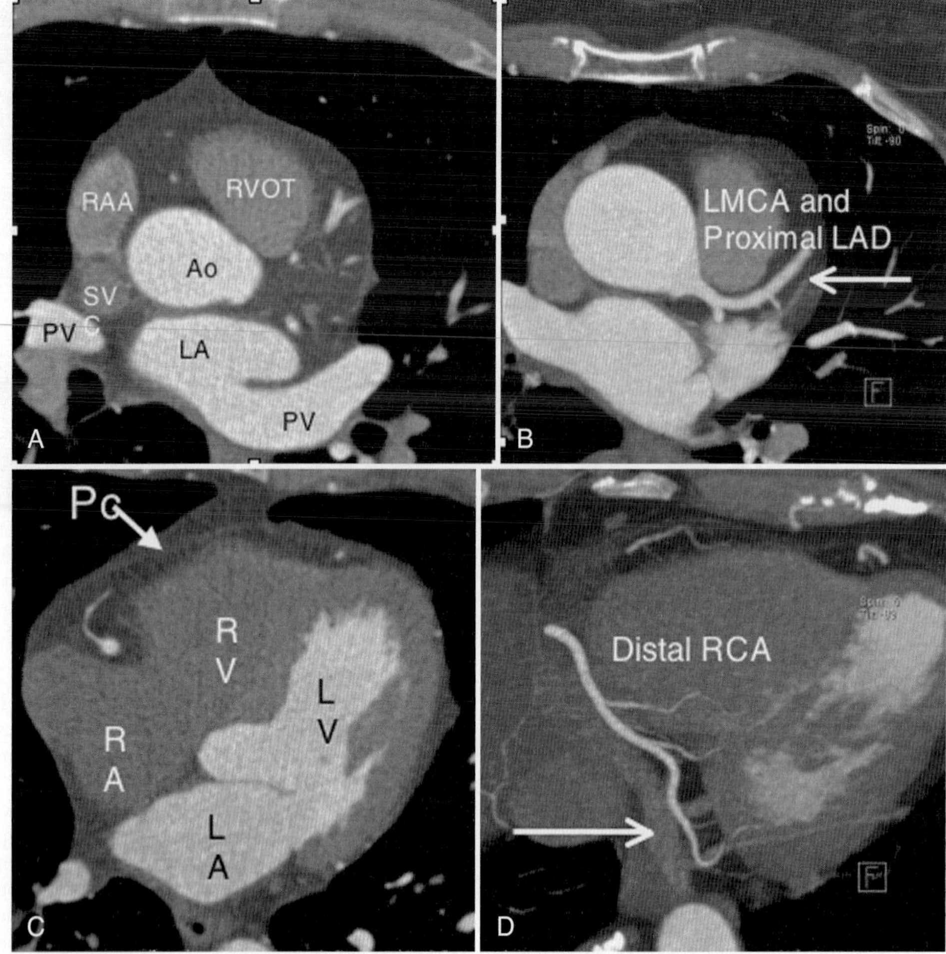

FIGURE 19-6 Overview of cardiac CT cross-sectional anatomy from axial images. **A,** Thin-slice axial projection at the level of the superior vena cava (SVC) and right ventricular outflow tract (RVOT) showing relationships of the structures at the base of the heart. Ao = aorta; LV= left ventricle; PV = pulmonary vein; RAA = right atrial appendage. **B,** Thick-slice axial maximum intensity projection showing the origin of the left main coronary artery (LMCA) and the left anterior descending (LAD) coronary artery (arrow). **C,** Midlevel four-chamber ventricular view showing the right atrium (RA), right ventricle (RV), left atrium (LA), and left ventricle (LV) and the normal pericardium (Pc). **D,** Thick-slice maximum intensity projection showing the distal right coronary artery (RCA) and the nearby coronary sinus (arrow).

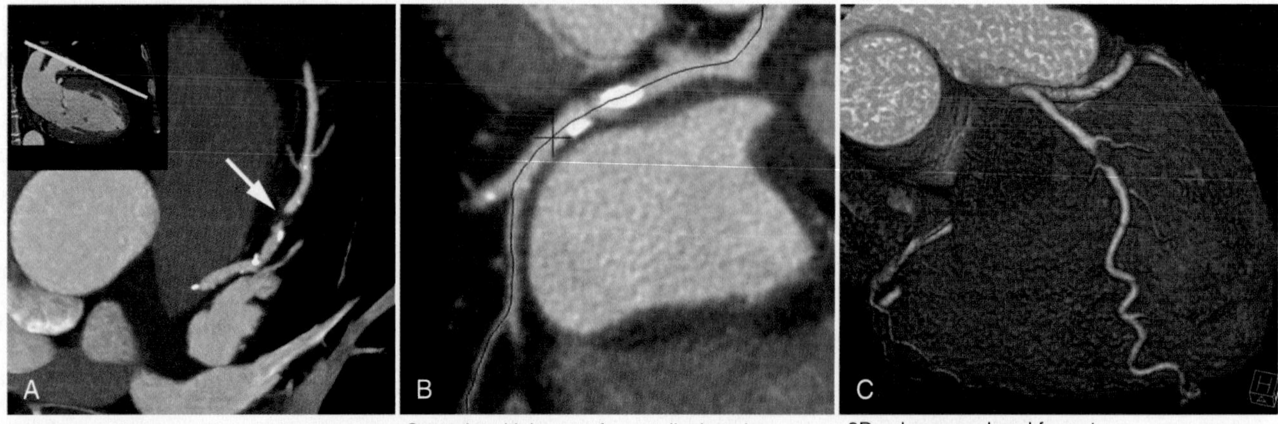

FIGURE 19-7 Three common display modes for cardiac CT. **A,** Oblique-angle multiplanar reformat displayed as a thick-slice maximum intensity projection useful for alignment of the image plane to cardiac structures. **B,** Centerline curved multiplanar reformat displayed as a thick-slice maximum intensity projection useful for display of curved structures in a two-dimensional image plane. **C,** A three-dimensional volume rendered format useful for general anatomic overview.

of the area and density of all foci of calcification (defined by a Hounsfield unit threshold of 130 units; **Fig. 19-10**). The sum of the area and density weightings across the coronary arteries is the unitless calcium score originally defined by Agatston and colleagues. Other quantification methods are available, including a calcium volume determination and mass score. Although specific advantages may include increased reproducibility of these techniques, the clinical data available for coronary calcium quantification are derived by the area-density scoring method and are the clinical standard. Calcium score reproducibility is modest, with interscan variability of 10% to 20%, being more reproducible at low heart rates and for higher calcium scores.

Coronary calcium presence and extent are dependent on age, gender, ethnicity, and standard cardiac risk factors. Calcium scores are higher for age and gender among whites (**Fig. 19-11**). It is well established that the detection of coronary calcium indicates an increased risk of incident CHD above that predicted by standard risk factors, from 2-fold for scores of up to 100 and increasing to 11-fold for scores above 1000.[11] Similar findings are shown for gender and ethnicity from the Multi-Ethnic Study of Atherosclerosis (see Fig. 19-11)[12] and among both young (aged 40 to 50 years)[13] and older[14] populations of patients. Middle-aged women with any detectable coronary artery calcium experience a CHD event risk that exceeds 2%/year.[15] Recent data indicate that the spatial distribution of coronary calcium may provide further risk stratification beyond the total calcium score. A coronary calcium coverage score was devised from the Multi-Ethnic Study of Atherosclerosis and showed greater predictive accuracy than the area-density scoring system for future CHD events.[16] This finding is in line with other observations that multivessel coronary calcium,[17] the number of calcified lesions,[18] and diffuse spotty pattern (small foci <3 mm)[19] are associated with a higher clinical risk (**Fig. 19-12**). Conversely, data from 13 studies involving 75,000 patients during 4 years show that a calcium score of 0 is associated with a very high event-free probability (99.9% per year).[20]

Based on the consistency of studies showing independent prediction of CHD risk, appropriate use criteria support the use of coronary calcium scanning as a risk stratification tool when an initial evaluation of clinical risk with risk prediction tools indicates an intermediate level of CHD risk (10% to 20% during 10 years) or in the setting of low-risk patients with a family history of premature CHD. Areas of uncertainty include patients with low to intermediate risk (6% to 10% risk), particularly among women and younger men in whom relative risk and lifetime CHD risk may be unacceptably increased. Both the National

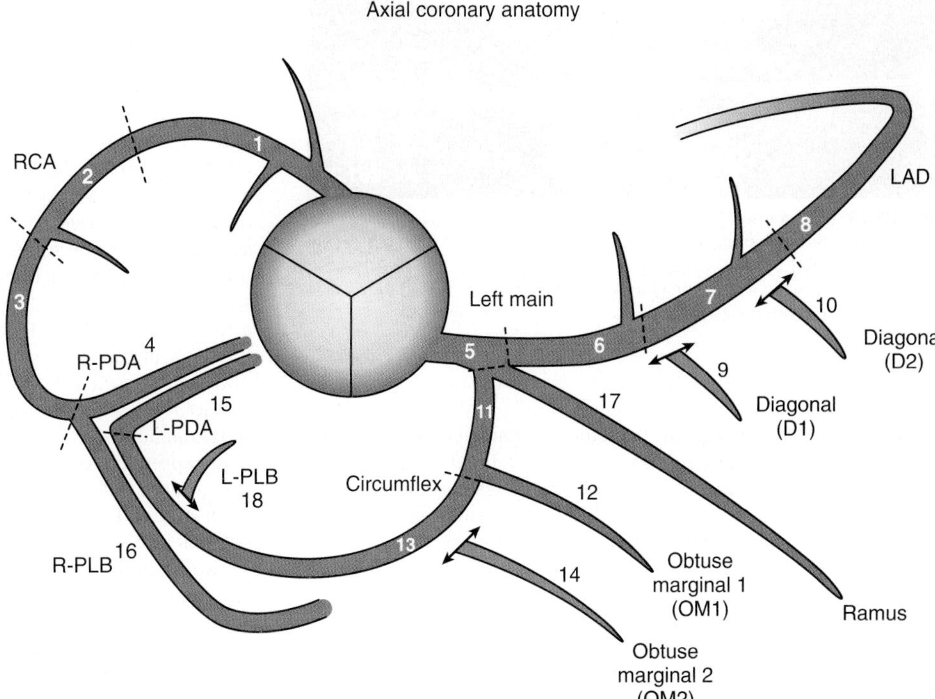

FIGURE 19-8 Axial coronary anatomic model of the coronary segments described on cardiac CT.

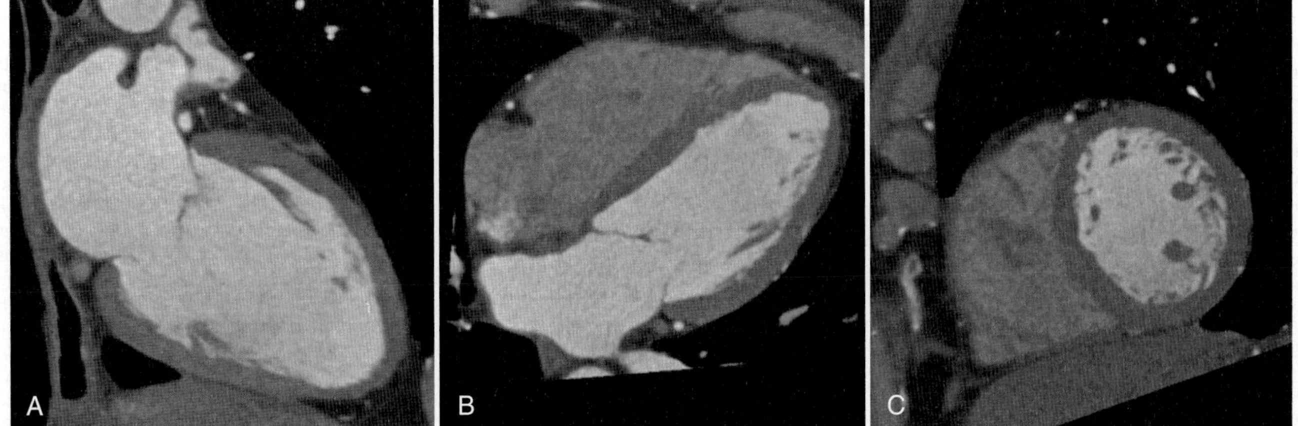

FIGURE 19-9 Standard cardiac chamber axes on cardiac CT including two-chamber **(A)**, four-chamber **(B)**, and short-axis **(C)** views. Timing of contrast in this study shows a typical levophase (right side of the heart is underfilled with contrast material) in diastole (mitral valve is in the open position).

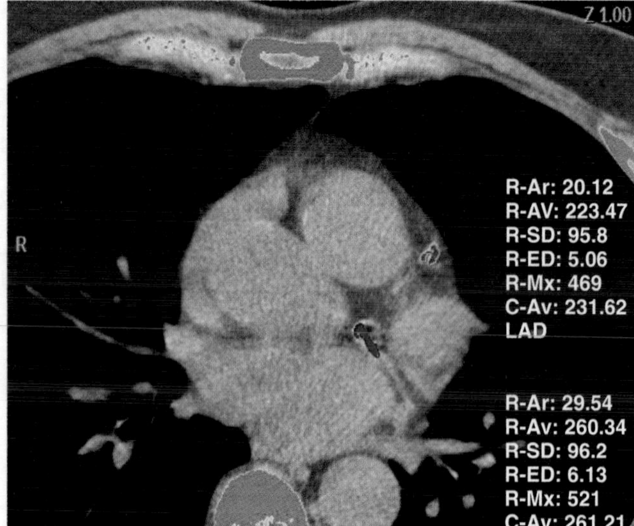

FIGURE 19-10 Example of coronary artery calcium scoring in which calcified foci are identified within the left anterior descending (orange) and left circumflex (pink outlined in blue) coronary arteries. The region's area (R-Ar) and its average density in Hounsfield units (R-Av) are displayed and used in the area-density calcium scoring calculation.

Cholesterol Education Program[21] and the Clinical Expert Consensus of the American College of Cardiology[11] indicated that the performance of coronary calcium scanning is a reasonable testing option among such patients on the basis of the possibility that such patients might be reclassified to a higher risk status by high coronary artery calcium score and subsequent patient management may be modified. At present, however, there are no data demonstrating that a strategy of coronary calcium screening improves cardiovascular outcomes. However, community-based screening cohorts[22,23] have shown up to threefold greater use of aspirin, statin cholesterol medications, and other cardiovascular risk reduction interventions in the setting of coronary calcium. Beyond recommendations for the provision of and adherence to risk-reducing therapies, an abnormal coronary calcium scan in an asymptomatic patient can be associated with an increased likelihood of silent ischemia by stress myocardial perfusion imaging (see Chap. 17),[24,25] and the absence of myocardial ischemia may moderate the risk associated with a very high calcium score.[26] However, such testing is not recommended without specific clinical trial evidence showing benefit for the patient from such an approach.

The use of serial testing to define progression of coronary calcium has been suggested as a method of further defining evolving CHD risk. Once it is present, coronary calcium tends to progress at a rate of approximately 20%/year.[27] Middle-aged individuals with a calcium score of 0 have an approximately 5%/year conversion rate from a zero to non-zero score.[28] Although observational data from referred populations suggest that individuals with clinically significant coronary calcium progression (>15%/year) may have substantially higher clinical event risk for a given calcium score,[29,30] data show that risk-reducing interventions do not retard coronary calcium progression, indicating that calcium progression is a complex phenomenon likely to involve a mixture of both plaque healing and plaque progression.[31] Because of concerns about radiation exposure, intertest variability, and undefined management implications, present guidelines do not support the performance of serial calcium testing.[11]

Coronary Computed Tomography Angiography

The primary clinical application of cardiac CT is the performance of noninvasive coronary CT angiography among patients with symptoms suggestive of myocardial ischemia. Meta-analysis of primarily single-center studies of symptomatic patients (prevalence of coronary artery disease 64%) shows that the overall accuracy of 64-row CT angiography included a sensitivity of 87% to 99% and specificity of 93% to 96%.[32] Accurate performance of cardiac CT requires proper attention to technical methods and preparation of the patient. However, even under optimal conditions, some coronary segments (~4%) will be uninterpretable because of patient or technical factors. Several recent multicenter trials support the high sensitivity of coronary CT angiography (**Table 19-6**)[33-35]; however, specificity will be reduced, particularly among patients with severe coronary artery calcification (which can render CT angiography uninterpretable, particularly at calcium scores above 400 to 1000) or obesity (due to excess image noise). Most CT angiography accuracy studies are limited by selection of patients optimized for cardiac CT, and the analysis typically involves only the more proximal coronary segments down to approximately 1.5 mm in size.

The accuracy of cardiac CT angiography must also be considered in the context of the method of stenosis evaluation. The existing literature has primarily evaluated stenosis presence along the lines of a 50% binary cut point. Qualitative grading schemes have been proposed in which normal is distinguished from arteries with evident plaque with <25% (minimal), 25% to 49% (mild), 50% to 69% (moderate), and ≥70% (severe) stenosis (**Fig. 19-13**).[36] Compared with grading by quantitative invasive coronary angiography, CT angiographic stenosis severity tends to be somewhat worse and with only a modest correlation (r = 0.5-0.6), but it correlates very well with intravascular ultrasound, probably as a consequence of better visualization of the arterial wall.[37] Similar to results with invasive coronary angiography, the determination of an anatomic stenosis is only modestly predictive of inducible ischemia. A 50% or greater stenosis on cardiac CT has a 30% to 50% likelihood of demonstrable ischemia on myocardial perfusion imaging (see Chap. 17),[38,39] underscoring the need for a multimodality approach to imaging to guide subsequent treatment of patients.

Given the high negative predictive value of cardiac CT, the test has been studied as a method to exclude coronary artery disease among patients presenting with acute chest pain. A randomized clinical trial showed that the use of cardiac CT among patients presenting to the emergency department with chest pain with a normal electrocardiogram and initial cardiac biomarkers led to more rapid discharge and cost savings compared with a conventional serial biomarker evaluation.[40] A majority of patients have normal CT angiograms and can be safely discharged, whereas approximately 20% to 50% may have some plaque identified and require further evaluation.[41]

Detection of Noncalcified Plaque

Beyond detection of coronary stenosis or coronary artery calcification, noncalcified plaque detection is an appealing but unvalidated approach to the risk assessment. Defined as any coronary arterial wall lesion with an x-ray attenuation detectably below the iodine contrast medium but higher than surrounding tissue, such plaque is difficult to quantify, with limited accuracy and reproducibility. Detection requires maximal spatial and temporal resolution and minimized image noise through higher radiation exposures. Compared with intravascular ultrasound, the correlation coefficient for plaque volumes is approximately 0.69, with a sensitivity of approximately 80%.[42] In general, noncalcified plaque severity tends to be underestimated, particularly for small plaques. Among asymptomatic patients, noncalcified plaque frequently is found along with coronary artery calcium, but it is found in only 5% to 10% of patients as the sole finding.[42,43] For this reason, screening CT angiography is not advocated in asymptomatic patients for the purpose of detecting noncalcified plaque.

Among symptomatic patients, noncalcified plaque tends to be a common finding. On the basis of correlations with intravascular ultrasound, plaques with low attenuation values (15 to 50 HU) tend to be morphologically classified as lipid rich, and those with attenuation values of approximately 100 HU tend to be fibrous plaques. This finding has generated interest in noninvasive plaque characterization and quantification as a method to detect patients with greater vulnerability for subsequent acute coronary syndromes. Plaque features proposed to be associated with greater risk for plaque rupture or acute coronary syndromes include low-attenuation plaque (plaque <30 HU), outward arterial remodeling (artery diameter ratio of the involved segment to a proximal reference of 1.1 or greater), and a spotty pattern (<3 mm in size) of calcification.[19] In particular, both low-attenuation plaque and outward arterial remodeling (Fig. 19-13B) have been associated with increased risk (HR, 23) of acute coronary events.[44] Problems with this assessment include the infrequent nature of these findings and substantial overlap and the impact of scan technique on attenuation values. More validation work is needed to further elucidate the prognostic value of plaque characterization. However, comparable to findings with invasive coronary angiography, a threefold worse cardiovascular prognosis has been found in the setting of a greater number of coronary vessels and of coronary artery segments involved with plaque.[45] Emerging methods of high-definition CT with spatial resolution of approximately 0.3 mm may overcome some of the limitations of noncalcified plaque underdetection (**Fig. 19-14**).

The Post-Revascularization Patient

In general, patients with known coronary artery disease are presently not the optimal candidates for noninvasive angiography because of the high pretest likelihood of coronary atherosclerosis. However, evaluation of coronary bypass graft patency is highly accurate, with sensitivities and specificities of nearly 100%[46] because of the large size and limited mobility of these structures (**Fig. 19-15**). However, a notable limitation to the technique among post–coronary bypass patients is the evaluation of native coronary artery disease, in which metallic clips and severe coronary calcium lead to reduced sensitivity and specificity with a high rate of unassessable coronary segments. Before reoperative coronary surgery, cardiac CT can be used to define the relationship of sternal wires to cardiac and graft structures for the purpose of planning surgical reentry techniques. High-risk findings include cardiac structures adjacent to or adherent to the sternum and coronary bypass grafts that cross into the midline (**Fig. 19-16**).[47]

Image artifact from metallic stents limits the application in patients with prior coronary stent procedures, such that small stents are difficult to evaluate and prone to noninterpretability. However, moderate to high accuracy, approximately 90%,[48] can be obtained in stents 3 mm or greater in diameter, with some dependency on stent design after optimization of reconstruction techniques (sharp kernel) and display characteristics (wide display window) (**Fig. 19-17**). Quantitative assessment of within-stent contrast density may assist in the diagnosis. A contrast density ratio of 0.81 between the stent (proximal, mid, and distal) and aorta showed a sensitivity of 90.9% and a specificity of 95.2% for in-stent stenosis for stents down to 2.5 mm in size.[49] New techniques applying high-definition CT with thinner detector arrays and iterative reconstruction techniques and using quantitative attenuation mapping may enable more accurate detection of in-stent restenosis.[50]

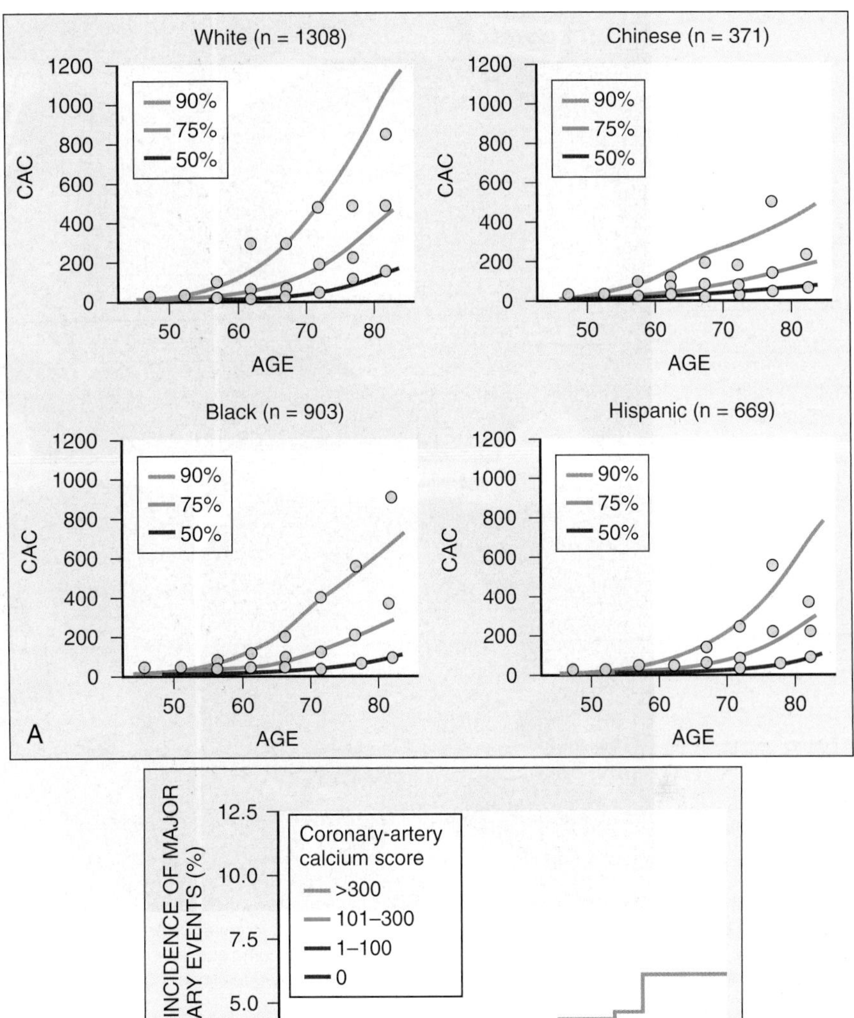

FIGURE 19-11 Data from the Multi-Ethnic Study of Atherosclerosis regarding the distribution of coronary artery calcium (CAC) scores among men relative to age and ethnicity **(A)** and major cardiovascular outcomes **(B)** observed in the study in association with higher thresholds of coronary calcium scores. *(From McClelland RL, Chung H, Detrano R, et al: Distribution of coronary artery calcium by race, gender, and age: Results from the Multi-Ethnic Study of Atherosclerosis [MESA]. Circulation 113:30, 2006; and Detrano R, Guerci AD, Carr J, et al: Coronary calcium as a predictor of coronary events in four racial or ethnic groups. N Engl J Med 358:1336, 2008.)*

Scan Artifacts

Despite optimal selection and preparation of patients, scan artifacts can occur (**Fig. 19-18**). High heart rate (>65 beats/min for single-source scanners) can lead to coronary motion artifact, particularly within the mid right coronary artery (**Fig. 19-19**). In some instances, end-systolic phases (versus diastolic phases) can resolve this issue. Newer scanners with improved temporal resolution or orthogonal x-ray sources (dual-source CT) can achieve adequate image quality at higher heart rates. Misalignment of axial image slices arises from positional changes of the heart due to motion of the patient (particularly respiratory motion), ectopic heartbeats, or abrupt changes in heart rate during scanning. Helical scan data sets generally permit editing electrocardiographic tags to delete data from ectopic beats during the scan reconstruction. Highly attenuating objects (metallic objects, coronary calcium) can produce an artifact called beam hardening, created by alteration in the energy spectrum of the x-ray beam. This artifact can particularly hamper coronary interpretation of plaques with highly dense calcified atherosclerosis. Last, images with poor signal-to-noise ratio can be the result of underpenetration due to either scan acquisition parameters or the patient's body size. Thicker slice reconstructions can improve the signal-to-noise ratio but at the expense of spatial resolution.

Ventricular and Valvular Morphology and Function

Helical scan acquisitions, with or without tube current modulation, provide the ability to reconstruct cardiac CT data from both systolic

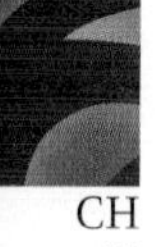

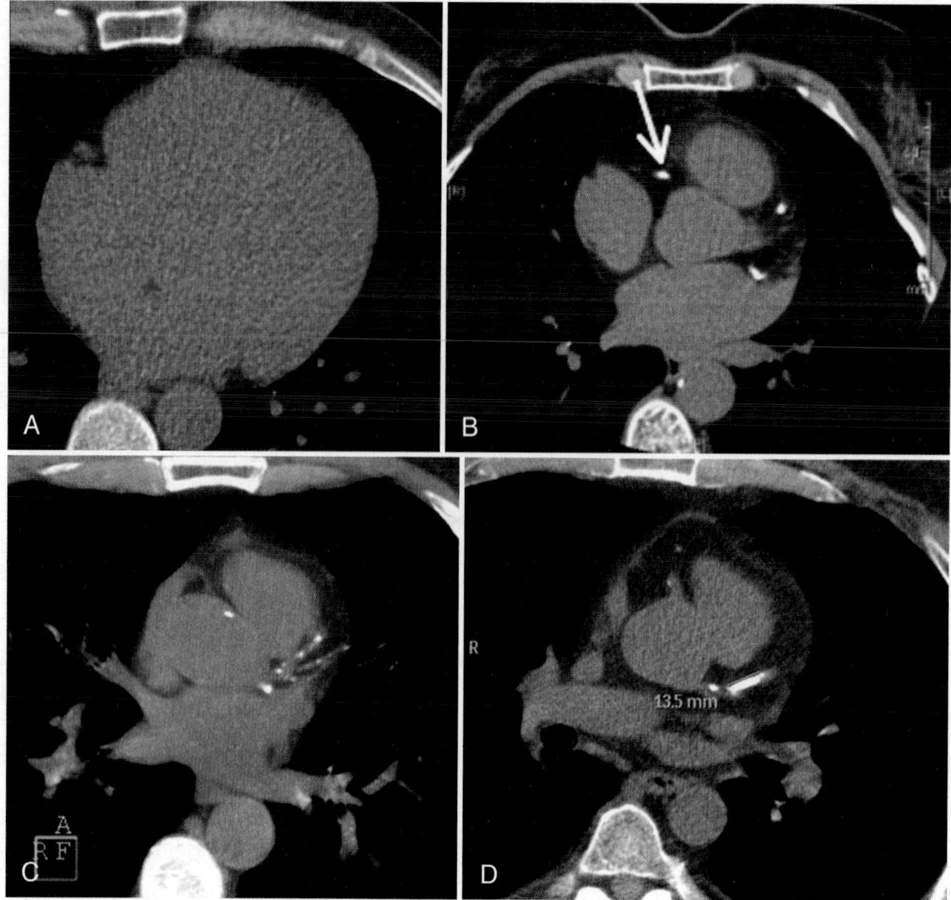

FIGURE 19-12 Distributions of coronary calcium. **A,** No detectable coronary calcium. **B,** Coronary calcium in all three epicardial coronary arteries including (clockwise) the right coronary artery (arrow) and the left anterior descending and left circumflex coronary arteries. **C,** A "spotty" or diffuse pattern of coronary calcium with multiple small (<3 mm) foci of coronary calcium. **D,** A large calcified lesion in the left anterior descending coronary artery.

TABLE 19-6 Multicenter Trials Assessing the Diagnostic Accuracy of Cardiac CT Angiography for Detection of Coronary Artery Stenosis

	N	PREVALENCE OF CAD (%)	SENSITIVITY (%)	SPECIFICITY (%)	POSITIVE PREDICTIVE VALVE (%)	NEGATIVE PREDICTIVE VALUE (%)
Budoff et al: ACCURACY	230	25	95	83	64	99
Meijboom et al	360	68	94	83	48	99
Miller et al: CORE 64	291	56	85	90	91	83

CAD = coronary artery disease.

Data from Budoff MJ, Dowe D, Jollis JG, et al: Diagnostic performance of 64-multidetector row coronary computed tomographic angiography for evaluation of coronary artery stenosis in individuals without known coronary artery disease: Results from the prospective multicenter ACCURACY (Assessment by Coronary Computed Tomographic Angiography of Individuals Undergoing Invasive Coronary Angiography) Trial. J Am Coll Cardiol 52:1724, 2008; Meijboom WB, Meijs MFL, Schuijf JD, et al: Diagnostic accuracy of 64-slice computed tomography coronary angiography: A prospective, multicenter, multivendor study. J Am Coll Cardiol 52:2135, 2008; Miller JM, Rochitte CE, Dewey M, et al: Diagnostic performance of coronary angiography by 64-row CT. N Engl J Med 359:2324, 2008.

and diastolic cardiac phases, enabling evaluation of ventricular systolic function. Such data can be displayed in cine-loop format for estimation of ejection fraction and regional wall motion or can be evaluated by quantitative segmentation software for volumetric analysis (**Fig. 19-20**). Reconstruction parameters permit thicker slice reconstructions (2 to 3 mm) with enough spatial resolution for adequate structural detail. By use of such methods, determination of left[51] and right ventricular[52,53] ejection fraction and volumes is highly accurate (±2%) compared with other methods such as cardiovascular magnetic resonance imaging (see Chap. 18). Myocardial morphology can also be reliably assessed for findings of prior myocardial infarction such as wall thinning, calcification, or fatty myocardial replacement (indicated by negative HU densities within the myocardium). Atrial morphology and volume can also be assessed. Clot in the left atrial appendage can be identified with high negative predictive value, although delayed mixing in the setting of poor flow may result in a diagnosis of pseudothrombus.

Anatomic evaluation of cardiac valves and their motion, both native[54] and prosthetic valves,[55] is also feasible (**Fig. 19-21**). Aortic stenosis can be characterized in terms of the extent of valvular calcification and by planimetry (see Chap. 66).[56] Aortic valvular calcification is directly related to valve area and can be quantitated by area-density methods.[57] Valve area planimetry is closely related to other invasive and noninvasive determinations in aortic stenosis. In aortic regurgitation, malcoaptation of the valve leaflets >0.75 cm^2 is associated with severe aortic regurgitation (**Fig. 19-22**).[58] Prosthetic

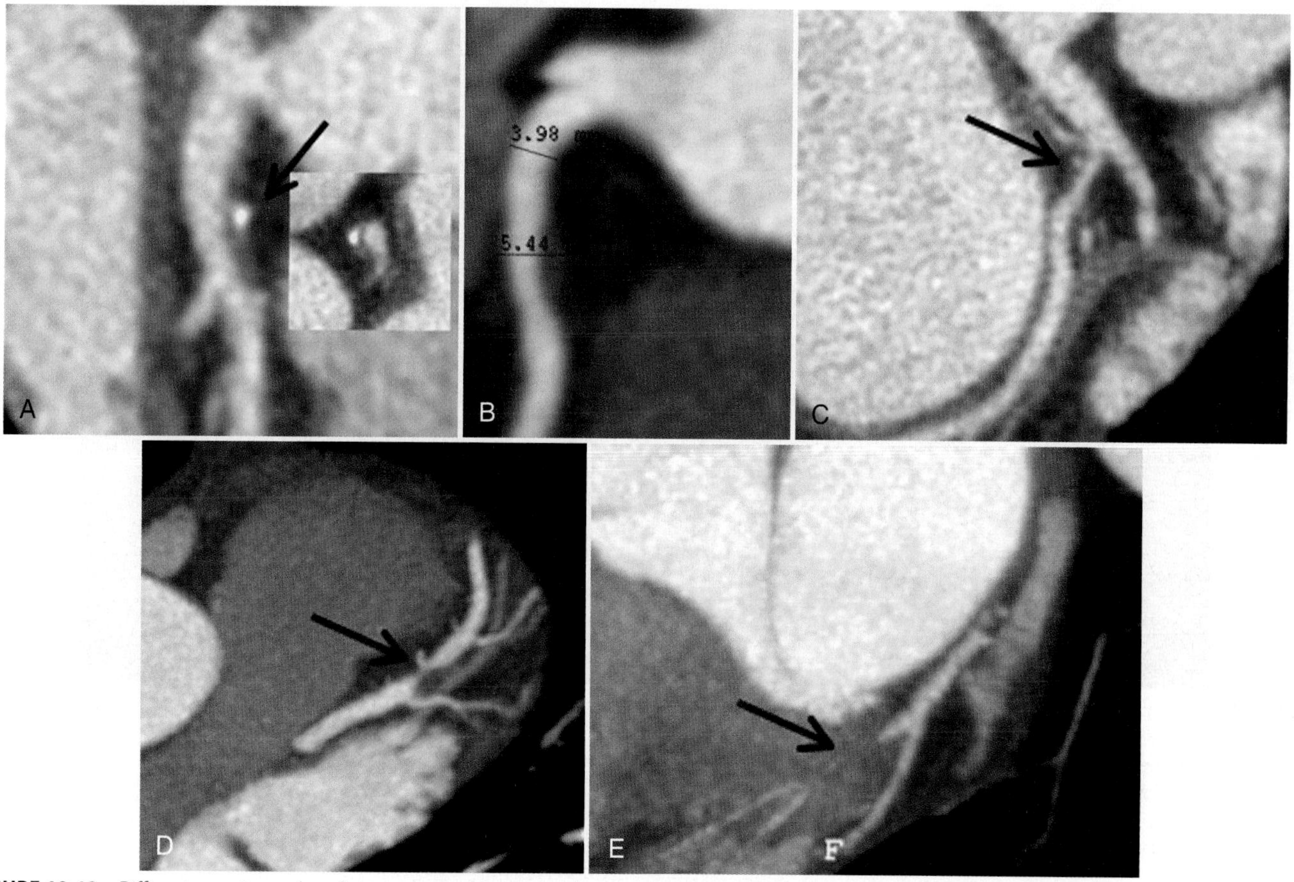

FIGURE 19-13 Different severity grades of coronary artery lesions as depicted on cardiac CT. **A,** Large mixed plaque without significant stenosis in the proximal left anterior descending coronary artery (curved multiplanar reformat) with outward arterial remodeling (arrow) as shown in the cross-sectional image **(inset)**. **B,** Large noncalcified plaque with outward arterial remodeling in the right coronary artery with mild luminal stenosis (<25%). **C,** Moderate stenosis (50%) in the proximal left circumflex coronary artery with a mixed plaque. **D,** High-grade (>70%) stenosis of the mid left anterior descending coronary artery with a noncalcified plaque. **E,** Total occlusion of the distal left circumflex coronary artery.

Standard 0.625 mm detector width | High-definition 0.312 mm detector width

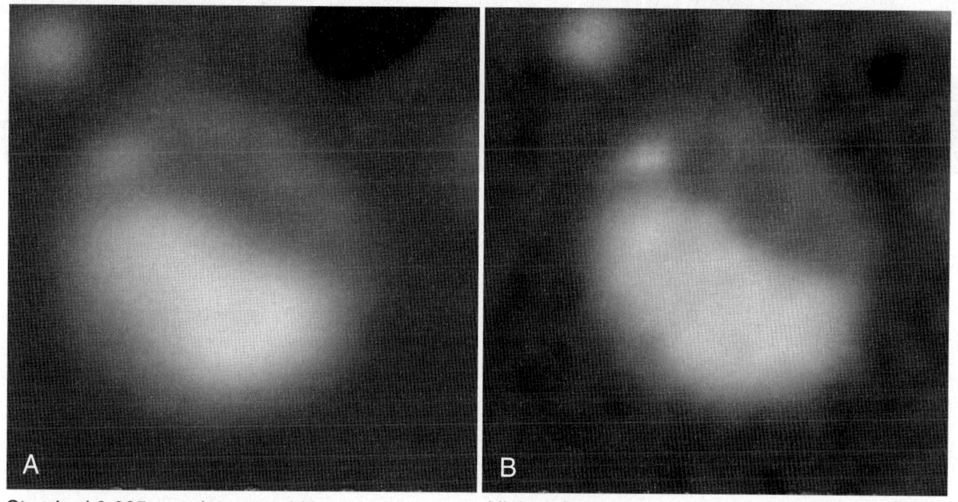

FIGURE 19-14 Thin cross section of coronary artery plaque seen with standard-definition CT (detector width 0.625 mm) and high-definition CT (detector width 0.312 mm). High-definition CT may enable more accurate detection of plaque and grading of coronary stenosis and is presently investigational.

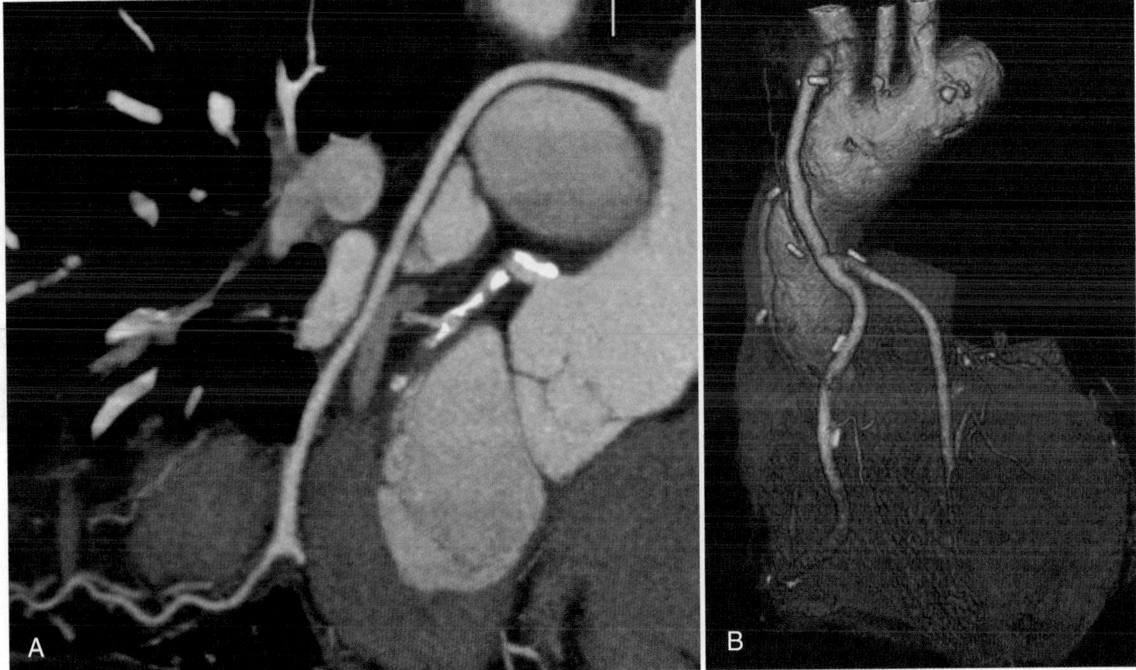

FIGURE 19-15 Cardiac CT provides high accuracy for evaluation of coronary bypass grafts because of their large size, often limited extent of calcified atherosclerosis, and limited mobility as shown in the oblique multiplanar reformat **(A)** and three-dimensional volume rendered reformat **(B)**. *(Images courtesy of Dr. Stephan Achenbach, Erlangen, Germany.)*

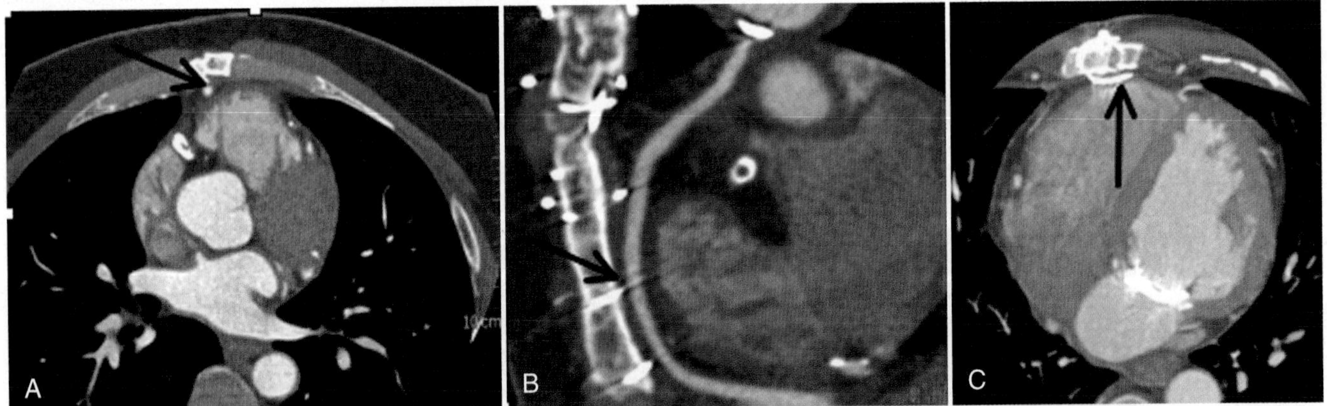

FIGURE 19-16 High-risk substernal reoperative anatomy in a patient with prior coronary bypass surgery including a coronary bypass graft immediately beneath the sternum shown in axial **(A)** and sagittal **(B)** images. In **C,** the right ventricle is immediately adjacent and adherent to the sternal wire.

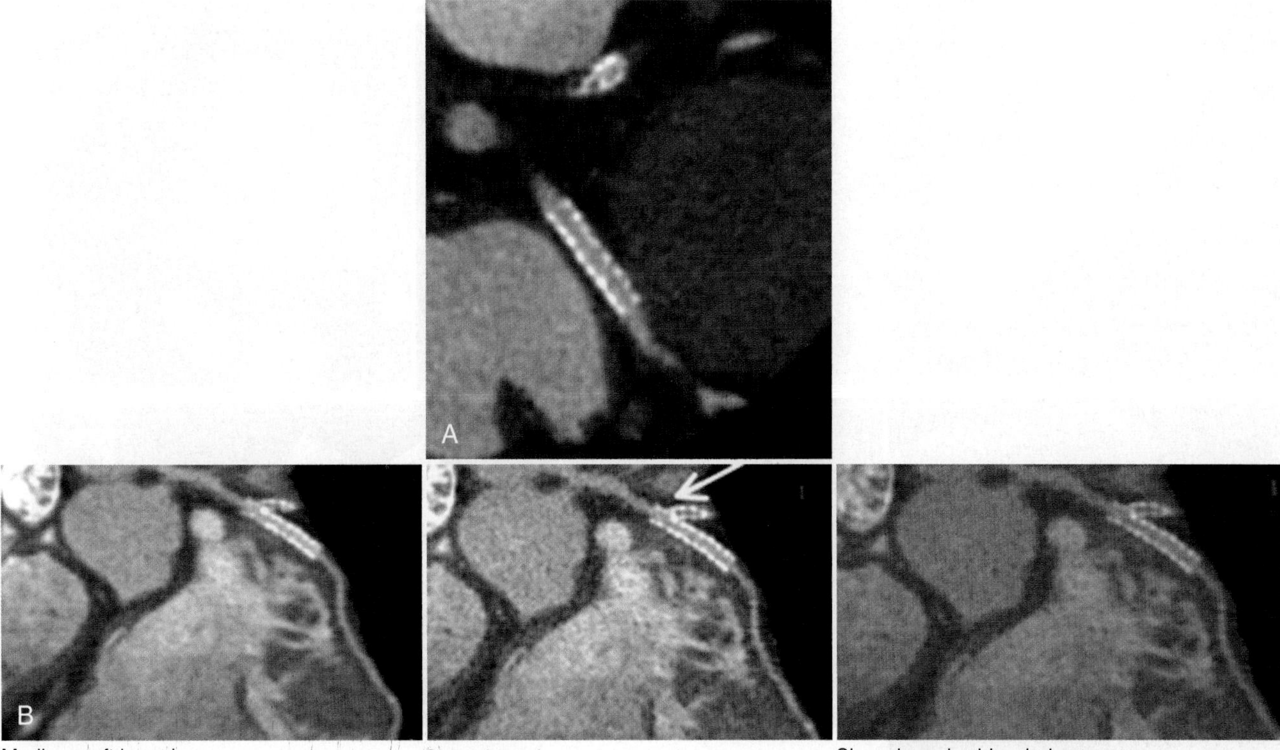

FIGURE 19-17 Stent imaging with cardiac CT. **A,** A large stent is seen with uniform contrast attenuation in the lumen, indicating patency. **B,** A small stent is seen in the left anterior descending artery with another stent in the proximal diagonal branch. Reconstruction is shown for three display settings: a medium-soft kernel, a sharp kernel, and a sharp kernel reconstruction displayed with a wide window width. Visualization of in-stent restenosis in the diagonal branch is optimized with a sharp kernel, wide window display width approach. *(Images courtesy of Dr. John Lesser, Minneapolis Heart Institute.)*

valve malfunction, including size mismatch, tissue ingrowth, and valve thrombosis, can be identified.[55,59] A weakness of cardiac CT valvular evaluations is the lack of physiologic valve flow evaluation.

Cardiac CT depicts the structural characteristics of congenital heart disease (see Chap. 65) and coronary artery anomalies, particularly as an alternative to cardiovascular magnetic resonance imaging in the setting of implanted pacemakers. However, concern about radiation exposure in young individuals requires strict attention to scan acquisition parameters, including the use of 80-kVp imaging to limit radiation exposure.

Acute Aortic Syndromes and Pulmonary Embolism

Multidetector CT provides accurate diagnosis of other serious causes of acute chest pain or ischemic equivalent symptoms to include acute aortic syndromes (aortic dissection, **Fig. 19-23A**; aortic intramural hematoma, Fig. 19-23B) and pulmonary embolism (Fig. 19-23C). Helical CT has a sensitivity of 100% and a specificity of 98% for the diagnosis of aortic dissection among individuals with low pretest likelihood (see Chap. 60).[60] Similarly, accuracy for the diagnosis of pulmonary embolism with multidetector CT is high, with a negative predictive value of 99% among patients with low to moderate pretest likelihood (see Chap. 77),[61] although accuracy for the detection of subsegmental pulmonary emboli may be limited. In spite of the accuracy of dedicated multidetector CT for these conditions and the general recommendation that such noncardiac incidental abnormalities should be detected on cardiac CT, the routine adaptation of cardiac CT protocols (such as in the triple rule-out protocol) for optimal detection of such noncoronary diagnoses is complicated and presently not recommended. Longer scan range will increase radiation exposure, requiring emphasis on radiation reduction techniques, and heighten potential for incidental scan findings. In general, thin-slice collimation, needed for coronary evaluations, is not needed for aortic or pulmonary artery evaluations, but electrocardiographic gating is necessary to avoid aortic motion artifact mimicking aortic dissection. The volume of contrast material and timing are crucial to provide optimal contrast enhancement of the pulmonary, coronary, and aortic vasculature. Last, differing pretest probabilities for aortic or pulmonary artery disease will affect the negative and positive predictive values in that sensitivity and specificity of the technique are imperfect.

EMERGING APPLICATIONS

Detection of myocardial scar and viability is a relevant measurement among patients with known cardiovascular disease. Cardiac CT may detect regions of myocardial hypoattenuation on first-pass imaging and, particularly with myocardial thickness <5 mm, suggests prior myocardial infarction and nonviable myocardium (**Fig. 19-24**). Such first-pass defects typically have a level of myocardial attenuation <50% of the surrounding myocardium and may even be <0% in the setting of fibrofatty myocyte replacement from chronic myocardial infarction, although this finding can also be present in normal individuals.[62] Infarct size on cardiac CT correlates closely with that obtained on cardiovascular magnetic resonance imaging (see Chap. 18), with slight underestimation of infarct size on first-pass imaging and comparable infarct sizing based on late enhancement imaging.[63] Late myocardial enhancement imaging involves specific cardiac CT acquisition with both the infusion of additional contrast medium and a delay of approximately 10 minutes. The kinetics of iodinated contrast material is similar to that of gadolinium, with accumulation within the interstitial space of myocardial fibrosis. Under delayed imaging, contrast preferentially accumulates within areas of scarring and can be detected on delayed imaging[64] (**Fig. 19-25**). This imaging can be accomplished with lower radiation exposure than in first-pass cardiac CT by imaging with wider collimation, axial scanning, and lower tube output and tube voltage. However optimal imaging protocols are not yet determined. Display characteristics favoring the detection of myocardial scar include the use of a narrow window width (200) and lower display center (100) and use of minimum intensity projection. Delayed enhancement on cardiac CT indicates regions of myocardium with reduced likelihood of functional recovery and patients whose ejection fraction will remain lower after myocardial infarction, particularly when a transmural pattern of delayed enhancement is present.[65]

On the basis of the relationship between myocardial flow reserve and arterial stenosis, first-pass CT stress perfusion imaging is being developed. Initial data indicate a per-vessel sensitivity of 96%, specificity of 73%, and negative predictive value of 98% for the detection of stenosis

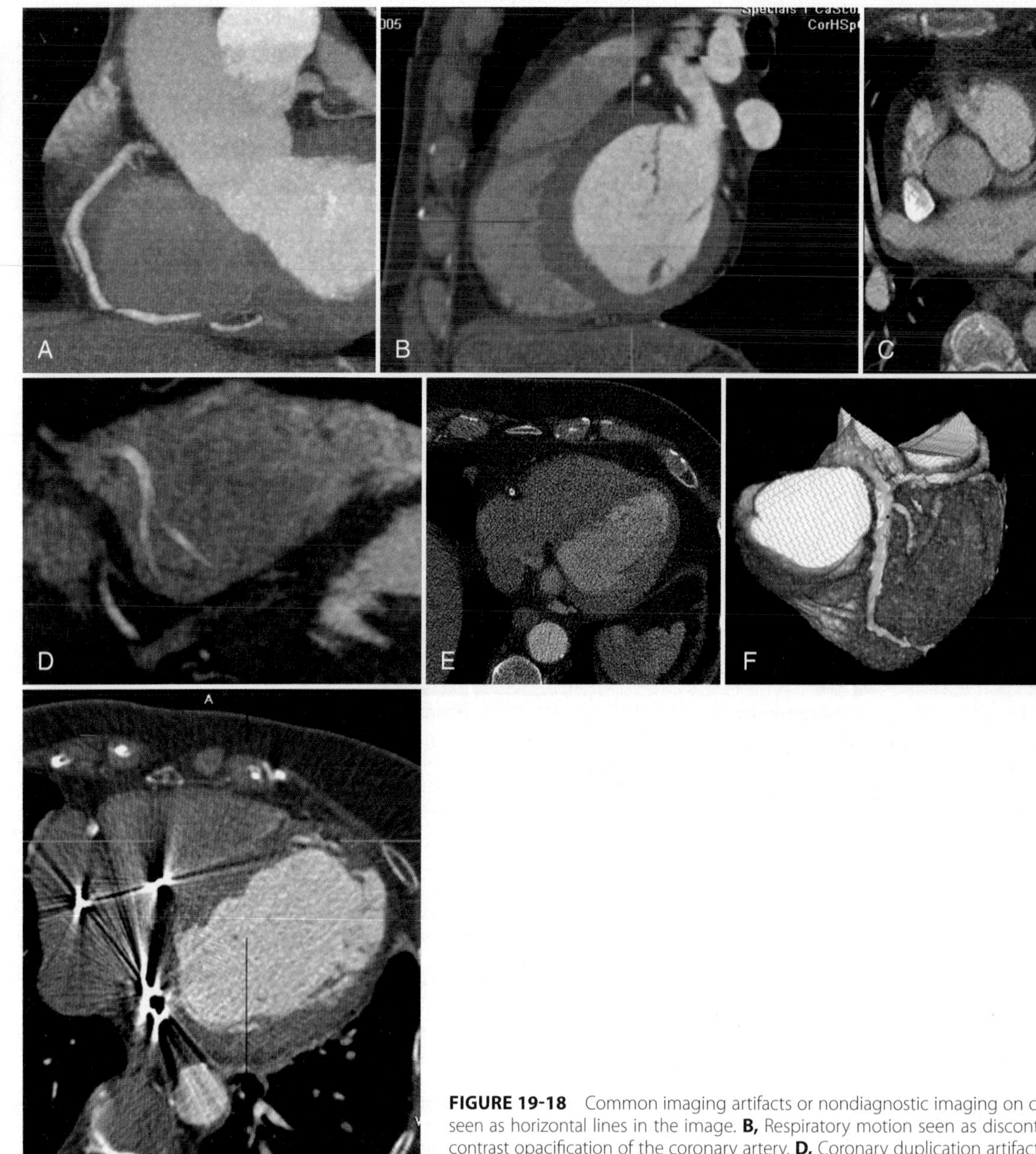

FIGURE 19-18 Common imaging artifacts or nondiagnostic imaging on cardiac CT. **A,** Registration error seen as horizontal lines in the image. **B,** Respiratory motion seen as discontinuity of the sternum. **C,** Poor contrast opacification of the coronary artery. **D,** Coronary duplication artifact from an ectopic beat. **E,** Poor signal-to-noise ratio (grainy image) due to obesity. **F,** Severe coronary calcification. **G,** Streak artifact from an implantable biventricular pacemaker. *(Images courtesy of Dr. John Lesser, Minneapolis Heart Institute.)*

of 70% or greater, with radiation exposure comparable to that of stress radionuclide imaging.[66]

Incidental Scan Findings

Incidental scan findings during cardiac CT span a broad spectrum of noncardiac vascular structures (aorta, pulmonary artery, and pulmonary veins) and the lungs, mediastinum, musculoskeletal and soft tissue structures, and gastrointestinal tract. In a series of subjects studied with multidetector CT, incidental scan findings were common (40% to 50%). Although the majority of patients do not require further evaluation, a minority (5% to 10%) will require second imaging tests or clinical follow-up. Guidelines for follow-up of pulmonary nodules include no follow-up for small (<4 mm) nodules (**Table 19-7**), although larger nodules require further evaluation.[67] Despite the absence of data showing an overall improvement in outcomes or management, present practice requires the evaluation of incidental scan findings with full field of view reconstructions by cardiovascular imagers with expertise in evaluation of other thoracic disease.[68] More data on the clinical impact and overall effect on net health outcomes from incidental findings are needed.

Training and Certification

Cardiac CT represents a new imaging modality for many cardiovascular specialists. Competency[69] and training[68] standards for cardiac CT have been published for cardiovascular specialists and broadly require a knowledge base in CT methods and case experience from 150 cardiac CT angiography cases, which can be obtained from both live (50 cases) and workstation review experience. Board certification is governed by the Certification Board of Cardiovascular Computed Tomography[70] and CT laboratory accreditation by the Intersocietal Commission for the Accreditation of Computed Tomography Laboratories or the American College of Radiology.

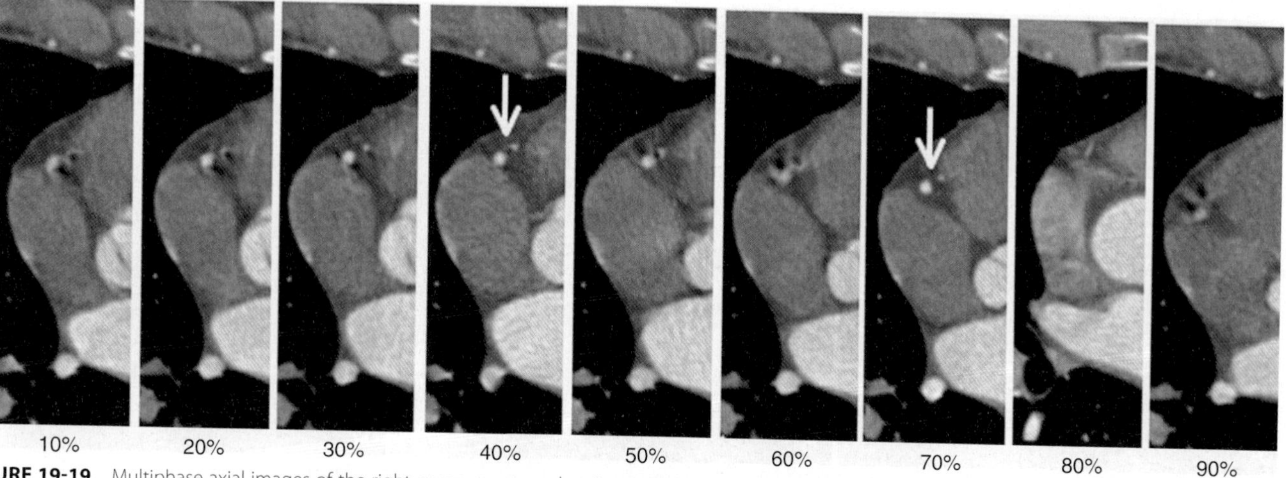

FIGURE 19-19 Multiphase axial images of the right coronary artery showing motion artifact throughout the cardiac cycle including systole (0% to 40% phases) and diastole (50% to 90%). The most motion-free images of the right coronary artery are at 40% (end systole) and 70% (mid diastole) when cardiac motion is minimized.

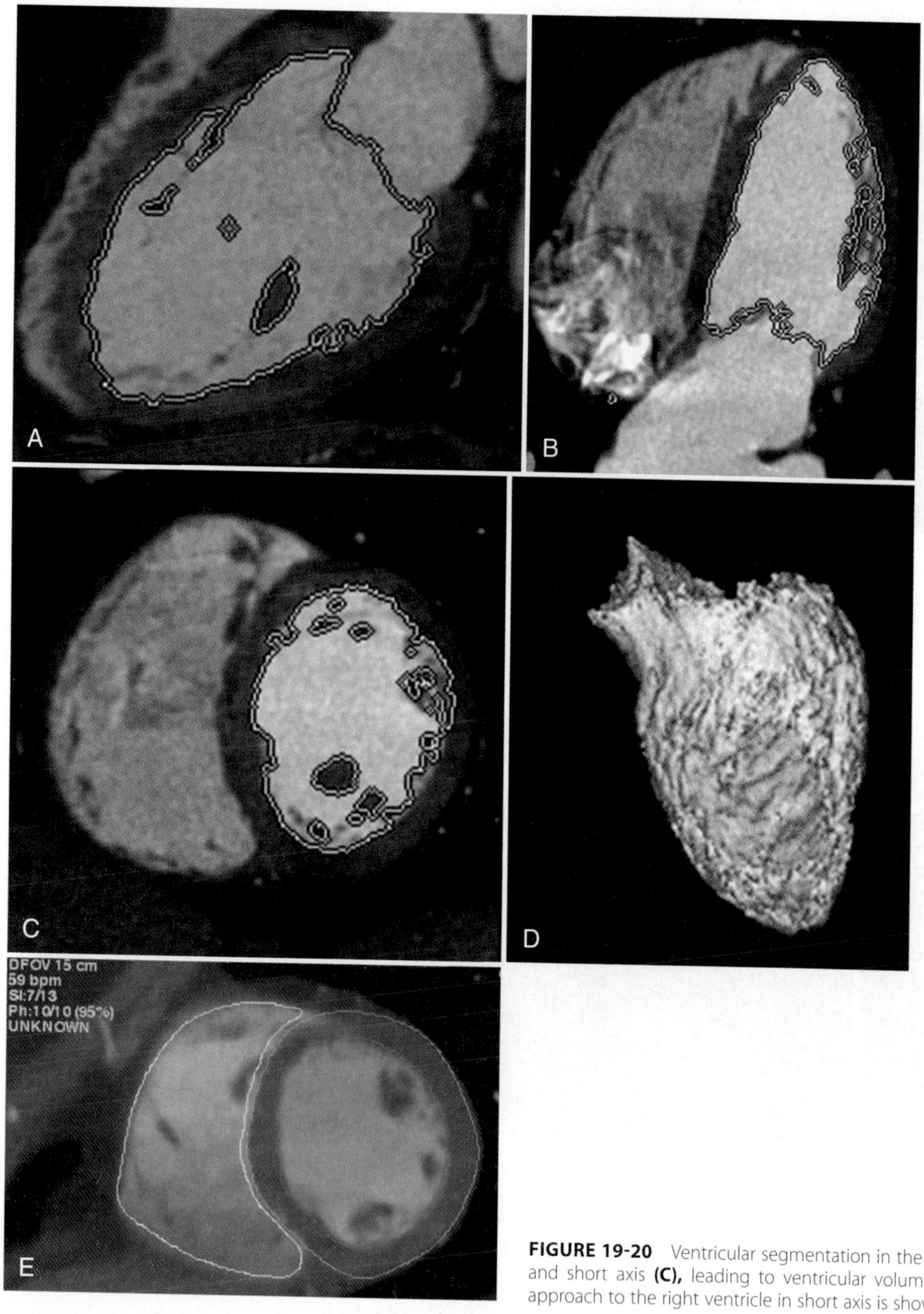

FIGURE 19-20 Ventricular segmentation in the vertical long axis **(A)**, horizontal long axis **(B)**, and short axis **(C),** leading to ventricular volume determination **(D)**. A similar segmentation approach to the right ventricle in short axis is shown in **E**.

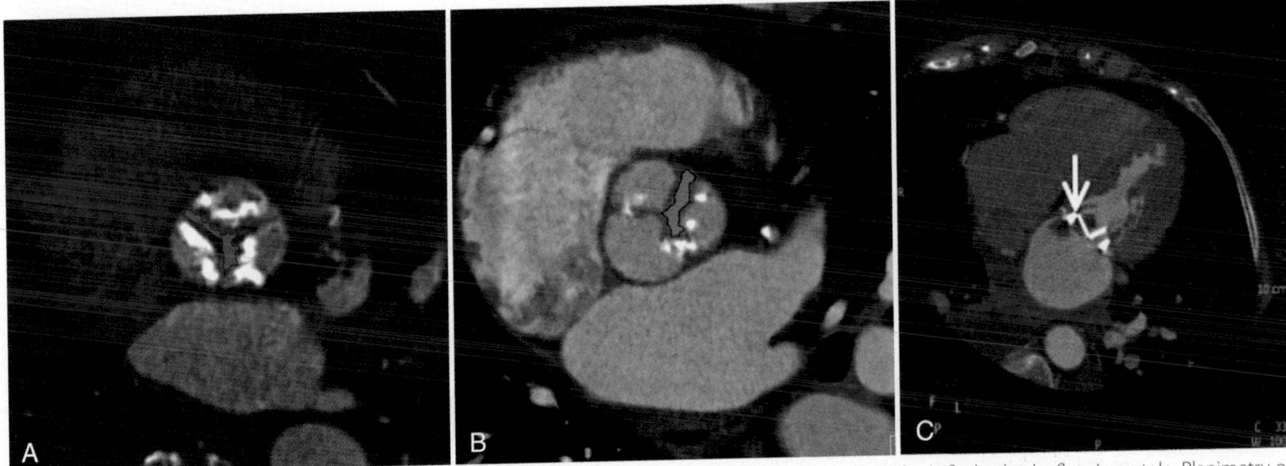

FIGURE 19-21 Valvular heart disease on cardiac CT. **A,** Aortic stenosis is characterized by restricted motion of calcified valve leaflets in systole. Planimetry of the aortic valve area showed severe aortic stenosis, with an area of 1 cm². **B,** Malcoaptation of the aortic valve leaflets in diastole with an area of 0.8 cm² consistent with severe aortic regurgitation. **C,** Bileaflet prosthetic mitral valve with a stuck leaflet from subacute valve thrombosis (arrow).

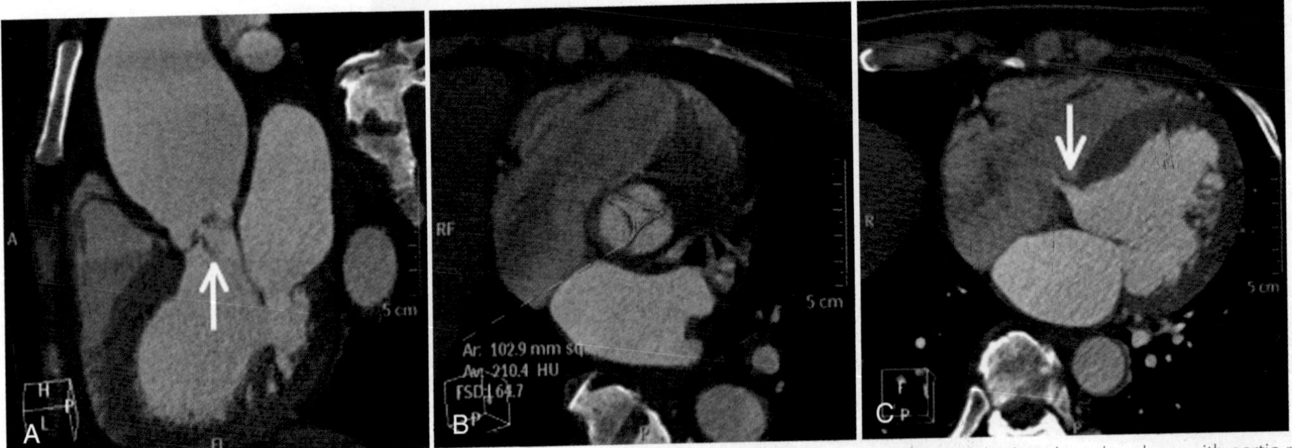

FIGURE 19-22 Aortic valve endocarditis with Gerbode defect. The aortic valve shows a low-attenuation object attached to the valve along with aortic root enlargement **(A)** and severe aortic regurgitation with malcoaptation of the valve leaflets in diastole **(B)**. A ventriculoatrial septal defect (Gerbode defect) as a complication of carditis is seen in **C** (arrow).

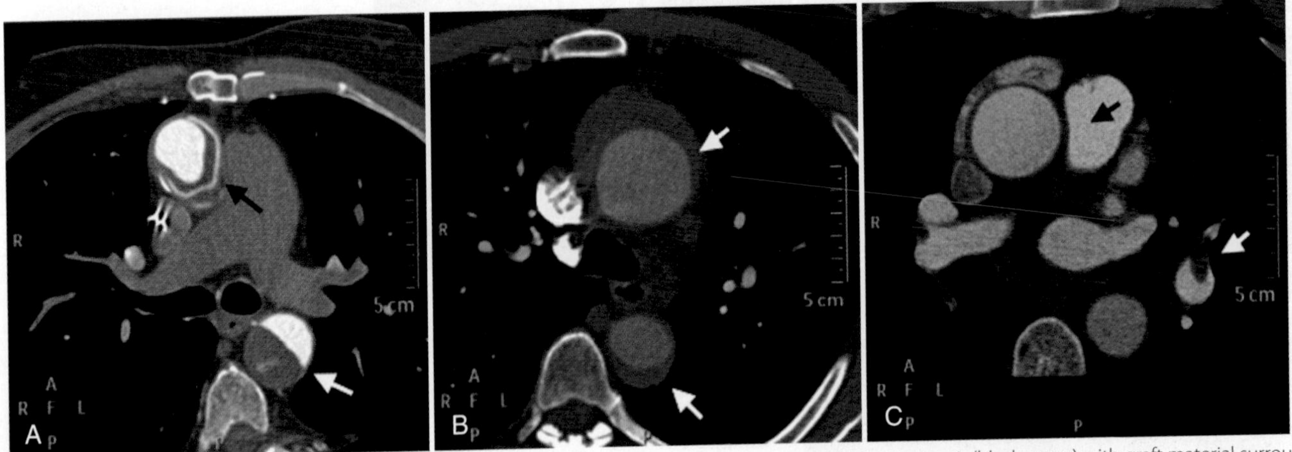

FIGURE 19-23 **A,** Descending aortic dissection (white arrow) in a patient with prior ascending aortic dissection repair (black arrow) with graft material surrounding the aortic root. First-pass contrast attenuation is seen in the true lumen of the descending aorta. **B,** Aortic intramural hematoma shown as low-attenuation material in the wall of the ascending and descending aorta (arrows). **C,** Pulmonary embolism (white arrow) in the left lower pulmonary artery seen as an area of hypoattenuation (clot). Multiple, bilateral pulmonary emboli were present, leading to delayed transit of contrast medium shown as greater contrast attenuation in the pulmonary artery (black arrow) and aorta.

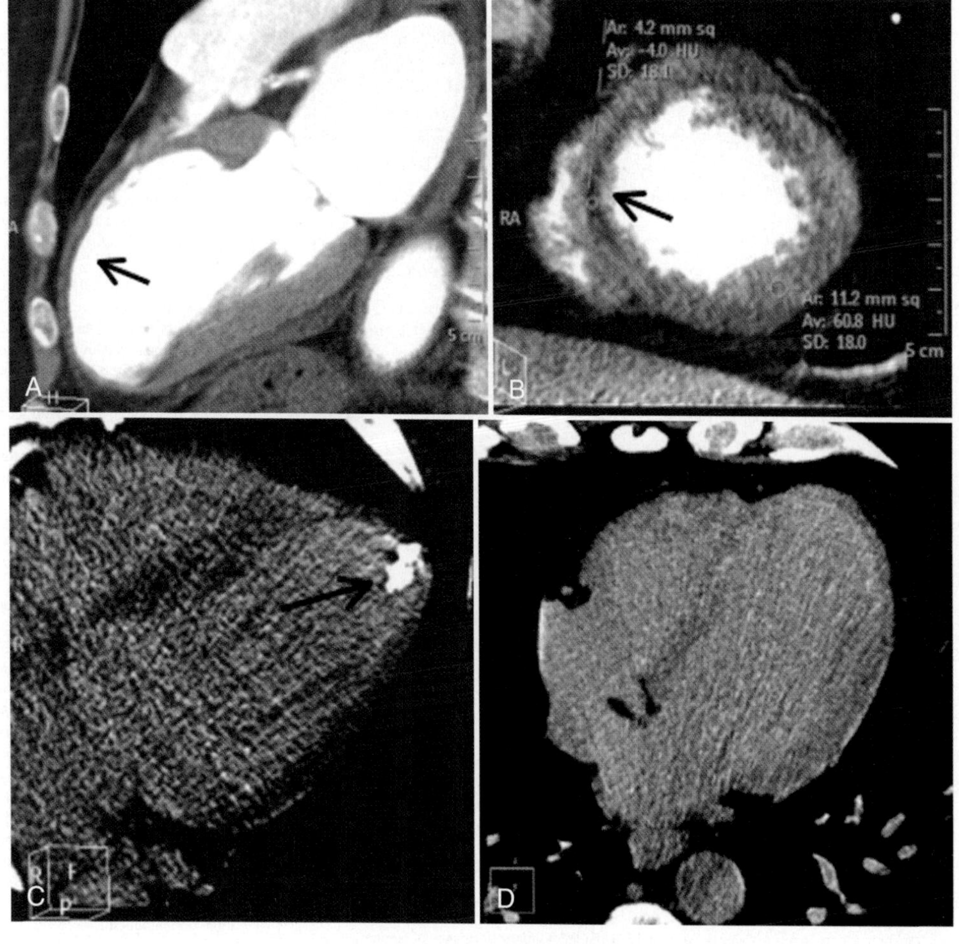

FIGURE 19-24 The spectrum of chronic myocardial infarction as seen on cardiac CT. **A,** Thinned myocardium after anteroseptal myocardial infarction (arrow). **B,** Hypoattenuation (<0 HU) of the ventricular septum indicative of chronic myocardial infarction and fibrofatty change (arrow). **C,** Calcification of the left ventricular apex (arrow). **D,** Delayed enhancement imaging (10 minutes) showing late enhancement of the anteroapex indicative of chronic scarring and nonviable myocardium.

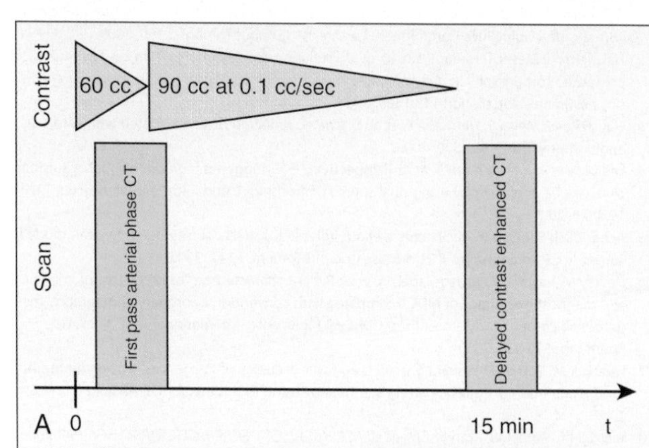

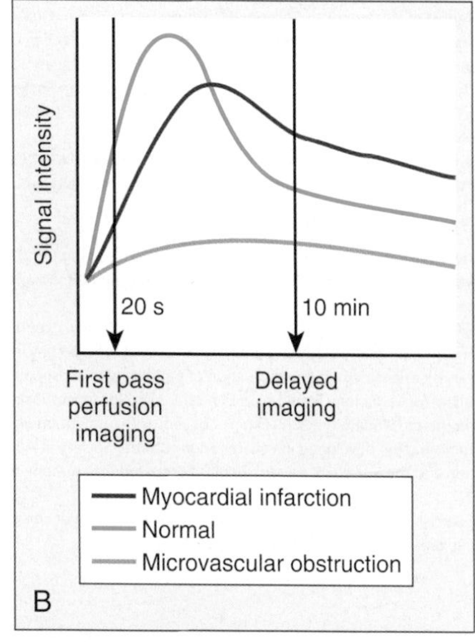

FIGURE 19-25 **A,** Cardiac CT protocol for delayed enhancement imaging with additional intravenous administration of contrast medium and delayed scanning typically performed 10 to 15 minutes after first-pass scanning. **B,** The contrast kinetics of myocardial infarction shows gradual increase in signal intensity in regions of myocardial infarction from delayed accumulation of contrast material in fibrotic regions.

TABLE 19-7 Recommendations for Follow-up and Management of Nodules <8 mm Detected Incidentally at Nonscreening Computed Tomography

NODULE SIZE (MM)*	LOW-RISK PATIENT†	HIGH-RISK PATIENT‡
≤4	No follow-up needed§	Follow-up CT at 12 months; if unchanged, no further follow-up¶
>4-6	Follow-up CT at 12 months; if unchanged, no further follow-up¶	Initial follow-up CT at 6-12 months, then at 18-24 months if no change¶
>6-8	Initial follow-up CT at 6-12 months, then at 18-24 months if no change	Initial follow-up CT at 3-6 months, then at 9-12 and 24 months if no change
>8	Follow-up CT at around 3, 9, and 24 months; dynamic contrast-enhanced CT, positron emission tomography, and/or biopsy	Same as for low-risk patient

Note: Newly detected indeterminate nodule in persons 35 years of age or older.
*Average of length and width.
†Minimal or absent history of smoking and of other known risk factors.
‡History of smoking or of other known risk factors.
§The risk of malignancy in this category (<1%) is substantially less than that in a baseline CT scan of an asymptomatic smoker.
¶Nonsolid (ground-glass) or partly solid nodules may require longer follow-up to exclude indolent adenocarcinoma.

REFERENCES

1. Abbara S, Arbab-Zadeh A, Callister TQ, et al: SCCT guidelines for performance of coronary computed tomographic angiography: A report of the Society of Cardiovascular Computed Tomography Guidelines Committee. J Cardiovasc Comput Tomogr 3:190, 2009.
2. Hausleiter J, Meyer T, Hadamitzky M, et al: Radiation dose estimates from cardiac multislice computed tomography in daily practice: Impact of different scanning protocols on effective dose estimates. Circulation 113:1305, 2006.
3. Hausleiter J, Meyer T, Hermann F, et al: Estimated radiation dose associated with cardiac CT angiography. JAMA 301:500, 2009.
4. Lell M, Marwan M, Schepis T, et al: Prospectively ECG-triggered high-pitch spiral acquisition for coronary CT angiography using dual source CT: Technique and initial experience. Eur Radiol 19:2576, 2009.
5. Achenbach S, Marwan M, Schepis T, et al: High-pitch spiral acquisition: A new scan mode for coronary CT angiography. J Cardiovasc Comput Tomogr 3:117, 2009.
6. Dewey M, Vavere AL, Arbab-Zadeh A, et al: Patient characteristics as predictors of image quality and diagnostic accuracy of MDCT compared with conventional coronary angiography for detecting coronary artery stenoses: CORE-64 Multicenter International Trial. AJR Am J Roentgenol 194:93, 2010.
7. Ferencik M, Ropers D, Abbara S, et al: Diagnostic accuracy of image postprocessing methods for the detection of coronary artery stenoses by using multidetector CT. Radiology 243:696, 2007.
8. Hendel RC, Patel MR, Kramer CM, et al: ACCF/ACR/SCCT/SCMR/ASNC/NASCI/SCAI/SIR 2006 appropriateness criteria for cardiac computed tomography and cardiac magnetic resonance imaging: A report of the American College of Cardiology Foundation Quality Strategic Directions Committee Appropriateness Criteria Working Group, American College of Radiology, Society of Cardiovascular Computed Tomography, Society for Cardiovascular Magnetic Resonance, American Society of Nuclear Cardiology, North American Society for Cardiac Imaging, Society for Cardiovascular Angiography and Interventions, and Society of Interventional Radiology. J Am Coll Cardiol 48:1475, 2006.
9. Taylor AJ, Cerqueira M, Hodgson J, et al: ACCF/SCCT/ACR/AHA/ASE/ASNC/SCMR 2010 appropriate use criteria for cardiac computed tomography. J Am Coll Cardiol 56:1864, 2010.

Coronary Artery Calcium Scanning

10. Nakazato R, Dey D, Gutstein A, et al: Coronary artery calcium scoring using a reduced tube voltage and radiation dose protocol with dual-source computed tomography. J Cardiovasc Comput Tomogr 3:394, 2009.
11. Greenland P, Bonow RO, Brundage BH, et al: ACCF/AHA 2007 clinical expert consensus document on coronary artery calcium scoring by computed tomography in global cardiovascular risk assessment and in evaluation of patients with chest pain: A report of the American College of Cardiology Foundation Clinical Expert Consensus Task Force (ACCF/AHA Writing Committee to Update the 2000 Expert Consensus Document on Electron Beam Computed Tomography) developed in collaboration with the Society of Atherosclerosis Imaging and Prevention and the Society of Cardiovascular Computed Tomography. J Am Coll Cardiol 49:378, 2007.
12. Detrano R, Guerci AD, Carr JJ, et al: Coronary calcium as a predictor of coronary events in four racial or ethnic groups. N Engl J Med 358:1336, 2008.
13. Taylor AJ, Bindeman J, Feuerstein I, et al: Coronary calcium independently predicts incident premature coronary heart disease over measured cardiovascular risk factors: Mean three-year outcomes in the Prospective Army Coronary Calcium (PACC) project. J Am Coll Cardiol 46:807, 2005.
14. Vliegenthart R, Oudkerk M, Hofman A, et al: Coronary calcification improves cardiovascular risk prediction in the elderly. Circulation 112:572, 2005.
15. Lakoski SG, Greenland P, Wong ND, et al: Coronary artery calcium scores and risk for cardiovascular events in women classified as "low risk" based on Framingham risk score: The multi-ethnic study of atherosclerosis (MESA). Arch Intern Med 167:2437, 2007.
16. Brown ER, Kronmal RA, Bluemke DA, et al: Coronary calcium coverage score: Determination, correlates, and predictive accuracy in the Multi-Ethnic Study of Atherosclerosis. Radiology 247:669, 2008.
17. Budoff MJ, Shaw LJ, Liu ST, et al: Long-term prognosis associated with coronary calcification: Observations from a registry of 25,253 patients. J Am Coll Cardiol 49:1860, 2007.
18. Williams M, Shaw LJ, Raggi P, et al: Prognostic value of number and site of calcified coronary lesions compared with the total score. J Am Coll Cardiol Img 1:61, 2008.
19. Motoyama S, Kondo T, Sarai M, et al: Multislice computed tomographic characteristics of coronary lesions in acute coronary syndromes. J Am Coll Cardiol 50:319, 2007.
20. Sarwar A, Shaw LJ, Shapiro MD, et al: Diagnostic and prognostic value of absence of coronary artery calcification. J Am Coll Cardiol Img 2:675, 2009.
21. Executive Summary of The Third Report of The National Cholesterol Education Program (NCEP) Expert Panel on Detection, Evaluation, And Treatment of High Blood Cholesterol In Adults (Adult Treatment Panel III). JAMA 285:2486, 2001.
22. Nasir K, McClelland RL, Blumenthal RS, et al: Coronary artery calcium in relation to initiation and continuation of cardiovascular preventive medications: The Multi-Ethnic Study of Atherosclerosis (MESA). Circ Cardiovasc Qual Outcomes 3:228, 2010.
23. Taylor AJ, Bindeman J, Feuerstein I, et al: Community-based provision of statin and aspirin after the detection of coronary artery calcium within a community-based screening cohort. J Am Coll Cardiol 51:1337, 2008.
24. Anand DV, Lim E, Raval U, et al: Prevalence of silent myocardial ischemia in asymptomatic individuals with subclinical atherosclerosis detected by electron beam tomography. J Nucl Cardiol 11:450, 2004.
25. He ZX, Hedrick TD, Pratt CM, et al: Severity of coronary artery calcification by electron beam computed tomography predicts silent myocardial ischemia. Circulation 101:244, 2000.
26. Rozanski A, Gransar H, Wong ND, et al: Clinical outcomes after both coronary calcium scanning and exercise myocardial perfusion scintigraphy. J Am Coll Cardiol 49:1352, 2007.
27. Taylor AJ, Bindeman J, Le TP, et al: Progression of calcified coronary atherosclerosis: Relationship to coronary risk factors and carotid intima-media thickness. Atherosclerosis 197:339, 2008.
28. Kronmal RA, McClelland RL, Detrano R, et al: Risk factors for the progression of coronary artery calcification in asymptomatic subjects: Results from the Multi-Ethnic Study of Atherosclerosis (MESA). Circulation 115:2722, 2007.
29. Raggi P, Callister TQ, Shaw LJ: Progression of coronary artery calcium and risk of first myocardial infarction in patients receiving cholesterol-lowering therapy. Arterioscler Thromb Vasc Biol 24:1272, 2004.
30. Raggi P, Cooil B, Ratti C, et al: Progression of coronary artery calcium and occurrence of myocardial infarction in patients with and without diabetes mellitus. Hypertension 46:238, 2005.
31. Burke AP, Taylor A, Farb A, et al: Coronary calcification: Insights from sudden coronary death victims. Z Kardiol 89(Suppl 2):49, 2000.

Coronary CT Angiography

32. Mowatt G, Cook JA, Hillis GS, et al: 64-Slice computed tomography angiography in the diagnosis and assessment of coronary artery disease: Systematic review and meta-analysis. Heart 94:1386, 2008.
33. Miller JM, Rochitte CE, Dewey M, et al: Diagnostic performance of coronary angiography by 64-row CT. N Engl J Med 359:2324, 2008.
34. Budoff MJ, Dowe D, Jollis JG, et al: Diagnostic performance of 64-multidetector row coronary computed tomographic angiography for evaluation of coronary artery stenosis in individuals without known coronary artery disease: Results from the prospective multicenter ACCURACY (Assessment by Coronary Computed Tomographic Angiography of Individuals Undergoing Invasive Coronary Angiography) trial. J Am Coll Cardiol 52:1724, 2008.
35. Meijboom WB, Meijs MF, Schuijf JD, et al: Diagnostic accuracy of 64-slice computed tomography coronary angiography: A prospective, multicenter, multivendor study. J Am Coll Cardiol 52:2135, 2008.
36. Raff GL, Abidov A, Achenbach S, et al: SCCT guidelines for the interpretation and reporting of coronary computed tomographic angiography. J Cardiovasc Comput Tomogr 3:122, 2009.
37. Okabe T, Weigold WG, Mintz GS, et al: Comparison of intravascular ultrasound to contrast-enhanced 64-slice computed tomography to assess the significance of angiographically ambiguous coronary narrowings. Am J Cardiol 102:994, 2008.
38. Tamarappoo BK, Gutstein A, Cheng VY, et al: Assessment of the relationship between stenosis severity and distribution of coronary artery stenoses on multislice computed tomographic angiography and myocardial ischemia detected by single photon emission computed tomography. J Nucl Cardiol 17:791, 2010.
39. Di Carli MF, Dorbala S, Curillova Z, et al: Relationship between CT coronary angiography and stress perfusion imaging in patients with suspected ischemic heart disease assessed by integrated PET-CT imaging. J Nucl Cardiol 14:799, 2007.
40. Goldstein JA, Gallagher MJ, O'Neill WW, et al: A randomized controlled trial of multi-slice coronary computed tomography for evaluation of acute chest pain. J Am Coll Cardiol 49:863, 2007.
41. Hoffmann U, Nagurney JT, Moselewski F, et al: Coronary multidetector computed tomography in the assessment of patients with acute chest pain. Circulation 114:2251, 2006.
42. Leber AW, Becker A, Knez A, et al: Accuracy of 64-slice computed tomography to classify and quantify plaque volumes in the proximal coronary system: A comparative study using intravascular ultrasound. J Am Coll Cardiol 47:672, 2006.
43. Hausleiter J, Meyer T, Hadamitzky M, et al: Prevalence of noncalcified coronary plaques by 64-slice computed tomography in patients with an intermediate risk for significant coronary artery disease. J Am Coll Cardiol 48:312, 2006.

44. Motoyama S, Sarai M, Harigaya H et al: Computed tomographic angiography characteristics of atherosclerotic plaques subsequently resulting in acute coronary syndrome. J Am Coll Cardiol 54:49, 2009.
45. Min JK, Shaw LJ, Devereux RB, et al: Prognostic value of multidetector coronary computed tomographic angiography for prediction of all-cause mortality. J Am Coll Cardiol 50:1161, 2007.
46. Hamon M, Lepage O, Malagutti P, et al: Diagnostic performance of 16- and 64-section spiral CT for coronary artery bypass graft assessment: Meta-analysis. Radiology 247:679, 2008.
47. Maluenda G, Goldstein MA, Lemesle G, et al: Perioperative outcomes in reoperative cardiac surgery guided by cardiac multidetector computed tomographic angiography. Am Heart J 159:301, 2010.
48. Sun Z, Almutairi AM: Diagnostic accuracy of 64 multislice CT angiography in the assessment of coronary in-stent restenosis: A meta-analysis. Eur J Radiol 73:266, 2010.
49. Abdelkarim MJ, Ahmadi N, Gopal A, et al: Noninvasive quantitative evaluation of coronary artery stent patency using 64-row multidetector computed tomography. J Cardiovasc Comput Tomogr 4:29, 2010.
50. Min JK, Swaminathan RV, Vass M, et al: High-definition multidetector computed tomography for evaluation of coronary artery stents: Comparison to standard-definition 64-detector row computed tomography. J Cardiovasc Comput Tomogr 3:246, 2009.

Valvular and Congenital Heart Disease, Acute Aortic Syndromes, and Pulmonary Embolism

51. van der Vleuten PA, Willems TP, Gotte MJ, et al: Quantification of global left ventricular function: Comparison of multidetector computed tomography and magnetic resonance imaging. A meta-analysis and review of the current literature. Acta Radiol 47:1049, 2006.
52. Guo YK, Gao HL, Zhang XC, et al: Accuracy and reproducibility of assessing right ventricular function with 64-section multi-detector row CT: Comparison with magnetic resonance imaging. Int J Cardiol 2008 Nov 22. [Epub ahead of print.]
53. Plumhans C, Muhlenbruch G, Rapaee A, et al: Assessment of global right ventricular function on 64-MDCT compared with MRI. AJR Am J Roentgenol 190:1358, 2008.
54. LaBounty TM, Glasofer S, Devereux RB, et al: Comparison of cardiac computed tomographic angiography to transesophageal echocardiography for evaluation of patients with native valvular heart disease. Am J Cardiol 104:1421, 2009.
55. LaBounty TM, Agarwal PP, Chughtai A, et al: Evaluation of mechanical heart valve size and function with ECG-gated 64-MDCT. AJR Am J Roentgenol 193:W389, 2009.
56. LaBounty TM, Sundaram B, Agarwal P, et al: Aortic valve area on 64-MDCT correlates with transesophageal echocardiography in aortic stenosis. AJR Am J Roentgenol 191:1652, 2008.
57. Shavelle DM, Budoff MJ, Buljubasic N, et al: Usefulness of aortic valve calcium scores by electron beam computed tomography as a marker for aortic stenosis. Am J Cardiol 92:349, 2003.
58. Feuchtner GM, Dichtl W, Muller S, et al: 64-MDCT for diagnosis of aortic regurgitation in patients referred to CT coronary angiography. AJR Am J Roentgenol 191:W1, 2008.
59. LaBounty TM, Agarwal PP, Chughtai A, et al: Hemodynamic and functional assessment of mechanical aortic valves using combined echocardiography and multidetector computed tomography. J Cardiovasc Comput Tomogr 3:161, 2009.
60. Shiga T, Wajima Z, Apfel CC, et al: Diagnostic accuracy of transesophageal echocardiography, helical computed tomography, and magnetic resonance imaging for suspected thoracic aortic dissection: Systematic review and meta-analysis. Arch Intern Med 166:1350, 2006.
61. Quiroz R, Kucher N, Zou KH, et al: Clinical validity of a negative computed tomography scan in patients with suspected pulmonary embolism: A systematic review. JAMA 293:2012, 2005.

Emerging Applications

62. Raney AR, Saremi F, Kenchaiah S, et al: Multidetector computed tomography shows intramyocardial fat deposition. J Cardiovasc Comput Tomogr 2:152, 2008.
63. Nieman K, Shapiro MD, Ferencik M, et al: Reperfused myocardial infarction: Contrast-enhanced 64-section CT in comparison to MR imaging. Radiology 247:49, 2008.
64. Lardo AC, Cordeiro MA, Silva C, et al: Contrast-enhanced multidetector computed tomography viability imaging after myocardial infarction: Characterization of myocyte death, microvascular obstruction, and chronic scar. Circulation 113:394, 2006.
65. Sato A, Hiroe M, Nozato T, et al: Early validation study of 64-slice multidetector computed tomography for the assessment of myocardial viability and the prediction of left ventricular remodelling after acute myocardial infarction. Eur Heart J 29:490, 2008.
66. Blankstein R, Shturman LD, Rogers IS, et al: Adenosine-induced stress myocardial perfusion imaging using dual-source cardiac computed tomography. J Am Coll Cardiol 54:1072, 2009.
67. MacMahon H, Austin JH, Gamsu G, et al: Guidelines for management of small pulmonary nodules detected on CT scans: A statement from the Fleischner Society. Radiology 237:395, 2005.
68. Budoff MJ, Achenbach S, Berman DS, et al: Task force 13: Training in advanced cardiovascular imaging (computed tomography) endorsed by the American Society of Nuclear Cardiology, Society of Atherosclerosis Imaging and Prevention, Society for Cardiovascular Angiography and Interventions, and Society of Cardiovascular Computed Tomography. J Am Coll Cardiol 51:409, 2008.
69. Budoff MJ, Cohen MC, Garcia MJ, et al: ACCF/AHA clinical competence statement on cardiac imaging with computed tomography and magnetic resonance: A report of the American College of Cardiology Foundation/American Heart Association/American College of Physicians Task Force on Clinical Competence and Training. J Am Coll Cardiol 46:383, 2005.
70. Min JK, Abbara S, Berman DS, et al: Blueprint of the certification examination in cardiovascular computed tomography. J Cardiovasc Comput Tomogr 2:263, 2008.

APPROPRIATE USE CRITERIA Allen J. Taylor

Cardiac Computed Tomography

Appropriate use criteria (AUC) for cardiac computed tomography (CT) were first developed in 2006[1] by the American College of Cardiology in a joint society effort. Rapid evolution in CT technology and the data on its clinical application have emerged since then, leading to an update in the AUC in 2010 (**Table 19G-1**).[2] The criteria are developed by a regimented process from the modified Delphi exercise of the Rand methodology. They adhere to the conceptual application of pretest risk or probability determination before diagnostic testing. An appropriate imaging test is defined as one in which the expected incremental information, combined with clinical judgment, exceeds the expected negative consequences by a sufficiently wide margin for a specific indication that the procedure is generally considered acceptable care and a reasonable approach for the indication. Negative consequences include the risks of the procedure (radiation or contrast exposure) and the downstream impact of poor test performance, such as delay in diagnosis (false-negatives) or inappropriate diagnosis (false-positives). Cardiac CT is performed in accordance with best practice standards as delineated in the imaging guidelines of the Society of Cardiovascular Computed Tomography[3,4] by competent and appropriately credentialed physicians. This includes the optimization of the scan protocol to limit radiation exposure. In addition, the criteria assume technical factors, including the following:

1. Cardiac CT imaging equipment is available that has the minimal technical capabilities required for the indication. Typical technical parameters for studies performed on multidetector-row scanners include CT equipment enabling 64 or more slices, sub-millimeter spatial resolution, and gantry rotation time no greater than 420 msec. Appropriate computer software must be available for image analysis.
2. Patients are optimally suited for cardiac CT under the following conditions:
   - Regular heart rate and rhythm including a heart rate at a level commensurate with the temporal resolution of the available scanner
   - Body mass index below 40 kg/m^2
   - Normal renal function
3. For CT angiography, patient requirements may include the ability to hold still and to follow breathing instructions, to tolerate beta blockers, to tolerate sublingual nitroglycerin, and to lift both arms above the shoulders.
4. All indications for cardiac CT were considered with the following important assumptions:
   - All indications should first be evaluated on the basis of the available medical literature.
   - In many cases, studies published in the medical literature are reflections of the capabilities and limitations of the test but provide minimal information about the role of the test in clinical decision making.
   - AUC development requires determination of a reasonable course of action for clinical decision making based on a risk-to-benefit trade-off as determined by individual patient indications.
5. For all stress imaging referenced in the indications, the mode of stress testing was assumed to be exercise for patients able to exercise. For patients unable to exercise, pharmacologic stress testing was assumed to be used.

These criteria were developed with the intent that they be considered both in the delivery of and in the policy positions for these services, including reimbursement. In contrast, services performed for inappropriate indications are likely to require additional documentation to justify reimbursement because of the unique circumstances or the clinical profile that must exist in such a patient. Uncertain ratings are those for which expert opinion or the available data vary or are rapidly evolving. These criteria are intended to provide a practical guide and perspective to clinicians and patients in considering cardiac CT imaging and to promote more appropriate test use, including avoidance of underuse or overuse.

TABLE 19G-1 **Appropriateness Criteria for Cardiac Computed Tomography**

Detection of CAD in Symptomatic Patients Without Known Heart Disease		
	PRETEST PROBABILITY OF CAD	**APPROPRIATE USE SCORE**
Non-Acute Symptoms Possibly Representing an Ischemic Equivalent		
1. ECG interpretable and able to exercise	Low	U
2. ECG interpretable and able to exercise	Intermediate	A
3. ECG interpretable and able to exercise	High	I
4. ECG uninterpretable or unable to exercise	Low	A
5. ECG uninterpretable or unable to exercise	Intermediate	A
6. ECG uninterpretable or unable to exercise	High	U
Acute Symptoms with Suspicion of Acute Coronary Syndrome (Urgent Presentation)		
7. Normal ECG and cardiac biomarkers	Low	A
8. Normal ECG and cardiac biomarkers	Intermediate	A
9. Normal ECG and cardiac biomarkers	High	U
10. ECG uninterpretable	Low	A
11. ECG uninterpretable	Intermediate	A
12. ECG uninterpretable	High	U
13. Nondiagnostic electrocardiogram or equivocal cardiac biomarkers	Low	A
14. Nondiagnostic electrocardiogram or equivocal cardiac biomarkers	Intermediate	A
15. Nondiagnostic electrocardiogram or equivocal cardiac biomarkers	High	U
16. Persistent ECG ST-segment elevation following exclusion of myocardial infarction		U
17. Definite myocardial infarction		I
18. Acute chest pain of uncertain cause (differential diagnosis includes pulmonary embolism, aortic dissection, and acute coronary syndrome [triple rule-out])		U
Detection of CAD/Risk Assessment in Asymptomatic Individuals Without Known Coronary Artery Disease		
	GLOBAL CHD RISK ESTIMATE	**APPROPRIATE USE SCORE**
19. Noncontrast CT for coronary calcium score	Low risk with a family history of premature CHD	A
20. Noncontrast CT—coronary calcium score	Low	I
21. Noncontrast CT—coronary calcium score	Intermediate	A
22. Noncontrast CT—coronary calcium score	High	U
23. Repeated noncontrast CT for coronary calcium score with a zero calcium score >5 years ago		U
24. Repeated noncontrast CT for coronary calcium score with a positive calcium score >2 years ago		I
25. Coronary CT angiography	Low	I
26. Coronary CT angiography	Intermediate	I
27. Coronary CT angiography	High	U
28. CT angiography for routine evaluation of coronary arteries following heart transplantation		U
Detection of CAD in Other Clinical Scenarios		
	PRETEST PROBABILITY OF CAD	**APPROPRIATE USE SCORE**
New-Onset or Newly Diagnosed Clinical Heart Failure and No Prior CAD		
29. Reduced left ventricular ejection fraction	Low	A
30. Reduced left ventricular ejection fraction	Intermediate	A
31. Reduced left ventricular ejection fraction	High	U
32. Normal left ventricular ejection fraction	Low	U
33. Normal left ventricular ejection fraction	Intermediate	U
34. Normal left ventricular ejection fraction	High	U
Preoperative Coronary Assessment Prior to Non-Coronary Cardiac Surgery		
35. Coronary evaluation before non-coronary cardiac surgery	Low	U
36. Coronary evaluation before non-coronary cardiac surgery	Intermediate	A
37. Coronary evaluation before non-coronary cardiac surgery	High	I
Arrhythmias— Etiology Unclear After Initial Evaluation		
38. New-onset atrial fibrillation (atrial fibrillation is underlying rhythm during imaging)		I
39. Nonsustained ventricular tachycardia		U
40. Syncope		U
Elevated Troponin of Uncertain Clinical Significance		
41. Elevated troponin without additional evidence of acute coronary syndrome or symptoms of suggestive of CAD		U
Use of CT Angiography in the Setting of Prior Test Results		
		APPROPRIATE USE SCORE
ECG Exercise Testing		
42. Exercise testing and Duke Treadmill Score, low-risk findings		I
43. Exercise testing and Duke Treadmill Score, intermediate-risk findings		A
44. Exercise testing and Duke Treadmill Score, high-risk findings		I
45. Normal exercise test with continued symptoms		A

TABLE 19G-1 Appropriateness Criteria for Cardiac Computed Tomography—cont'd

Use of CT Angiography in the Setting of Prior Test Results	APPROPRIATE USE SCORE
Stress Imaging Procedures	
46. Discordant ECG exercise and imaging results	A
47. Stress imaging results: equivocal	A
48. Stress imaging results: mild ischemia	U
49. Stress imaging results: moderate or severe ischemia	I
Diagnostic Impact of Coronary Calcium on the Decision to Perform Contrast CT Angiography in Symptomatic Patients	
50. Coronary calcium score <100	A
51. Coronary calcium score 100-400	A
52. Coronary calcium score 401-1000	U
53. Coronary calcium score >1000	U
Periodic Repeated Testing, Asymptomatic *or* Stable Symptoms with Prior Stress Imaging or Coronary Angiography	
54. No known CAD with last study done <2 years ago	I
55. No known CAD with last study done ≥2 years ago	I
56. Known CAD with last study done <2 years ago	I
57. Known CAD with last study done ≥2 years ago	I
Evaluation of New or Worsening Symptoms in the Setting of Past Stress Imaging Study	
58. Previous stress imaging study normal	A
59. Previous stress imaging study abnormal	U
Risk Assessment Preoperative Evaluation of Non-Cardiac Surgery Without Active Cardiac Conditions	
Low-Risk Surgery	
60. Preoperative evaluation for non-cardiac surgery risk assessment, irrespective of functional capacity	I
Intermediate-Risk Surgery	
61. Functional capacity ≥4 METs	I
62. No clinical risk predictors	I
63. Functional capacity <4 METs with one or more clinical risk predictors	U
64. Asymptomatic less than 1 year following a normal coronary angiogram, stress test, or coronary revascularization procedure	I
Vascular Surgery	
65. Functional capacity ≥4 METs	I
66. No clinical risk predictors	I
67. Functional capacity <4 METs with one or more clinical risk predictors	U
68. Asymptomatic less than 1 year following a normal coronary angiogram, stress test, or coronary revascularization procedure	I
Risk Assessment Post-Revascularization (PCI or CABG)	
Symptomatic (Ischemic Equivalent)	
69. Evaluation of graft patency after coronary bypass surgery	A
70. Prior coronary stent with stent diameter <3 mm or not known	I
71. Prior coronary stent with stent diameter ≥3 mm	U
Asymptomatic	
72. Prior coronary bypass surgery, <5 years ago	I
73. Prior coronary bypass surgery, ≥5 years ago	U
74. Prior coronary stent with stent diameter <3 mm or not known Less than 2 years after PCI	I
75. Prior coronary stent with stent diameter <3 mm or not known Greater than or equal to 2 years after PCI	I
76. Prior coronary stent with stent diameter ≥3 mm Less than 2 years after PCI	I
77. Prior coronary stent with stent diameter ≥3 mm Greater than or equal to 2 years after PCI	U
78. Prior left main coronary stent with stent diameter ≥3 mm	A
Evaluation of Cardiac Structure and Function	
Adult Congenital Heart Disease	
79. Assessment of anomalies of coronary arterial and other thoracic arteriovenous vessels	A
80. Assessment of complex adult congenital heart disease	A
Evaluation of Ventricular Morphology and Systolic Function	
81. Initial evaluation of left ventricular function following acute myocardial infarction or in heart failure patients	I
82. Evaluation of left ventricular function following acute myocardial infarction or in heart failure patients with inadequate images from other noninvasive methods	A
83. Quantitative evaluation of right ventricular function	A
84. Assessment of right ventricular morphology in suspected arrhythmogenic right ventricular dysplasia	A
85. Assessment of myocardial viability prior to myocardial revascularization for ischemic left ventricular systolic dysfunction when other imaging modalities are inadequate or contraindicated	U

Continued

CH 19

TABLE 19G-1 Appropriateness Criteria for Cardiac Computed Tomography—cont'd

Evaluation of Cardiac Structure and Function	APPROPRIATE USE SCORE
Evaluation of Intracardiac and Extracardiac Structures	
86. Characterization of native cardiac valves in individuals with suspected clinically significant valvular dysfunction when images from other noninvasive methods are inadequate	A
87. Characterization of prosthetic cardiac valves in individuals with suspected clinically significant valvular dysfunction when images from other noninvasive methods are inadequate	A
88. Initial evaluation of cardiac mass (suspected tumor or thrombus)	I
89. Evaluation of cardiac mass (suspected tumor or thrombus) with inadequate images from other noninvasive methods	A
90. Evaluation of pericardial anatomy	A
91. Evaluation of pulmonary vein anatomy prior to radiofrequency ablation for atrial fibrillation	A
92. Noninvasive coronary vein mapping prior to placement of biventricular pacemaker	A
93. Localization of coronary bypass grafts and other retrosternal anatomy prior to reoperative chest or cardiac surgery	A

CABG = coronary artery bypass grafting surgery; CAD = coronary artery disease; CHD = coronary heart disease; ECG = electrocardiogram; METs = estimated metabolic equivalents of exercise; PCI = percutaneous coronary intervention.

From Taylor AJ, Cerqueira M, Hodgson J, et al: ACCF/SCCT/ACR/AHA/ASE/ASNC/SCMR 2010 appropriate use criteria for cardiac computed tomography. J Am Coll Cardiol 2010 Oct 25. [Epub ahead of print. doi:10.1016/j.jacc2010.07.005].

- A total of 31 indications were carried forward from the 2006 document, including prior ratings of appropriate (10), uncertain (10), or inappropriate (11). Among these, 8 shifted up one category from either uncertain to appropriate or from inappropriate to uncertain. The other 23 indications had unchanged appropriateness ratings.
- One area of expansion compared with the 2006 criteria involves symptomatic patients without known heart disease. Cardiac CT is thought to be appropriate primarily for situations involving a low or intermediate pretest probability of obstructive coronary artery disease (CAD). Scenarios involving patients with a high probability of CAD are rated as uncertain with the exception of a patient with an interpretable electrocardiogram who is able to exercise and for definite myocardial infarction.
- Non–contrast-enhanced CT calcium scoring is judged appropriate for patients at intermediate coronary heart disease (CHD) risk and for the specific subset of low-risk patients in whom a family history of premature CHD is present. Intermediate risk is defined as a 10-year risk of between 10% and 20%, although individual patient exceptions to a broadened intermediate risk range of 6% to 20% are recognized for certain patient subsets with generally low absolute risk but high relative risk (younger men and women). Screening of asymptomatic patients by coronary CT angiography is considered inappropriate, as is repeated coronary calcium testing. Repeated CT angiography in asymptomatic patients or patients with stable symptoms with prior test results is broadly considered inappropriate.
- Within heart failure, CT angiography is appropriate with reduced left ventricular ejection fraction with low or intermediate pretest CAD probability.
- As part of the preoperative evaluation, CT angiography is viewed as a potential option among patients undergoing heart surgery for noncoronary indications (e.g., valve replacement surgery or atrial septal defect closure) when the pretest CAD risk is either intermediate (appropriate) or low (uncertain). In comparison, there are no appropriate indications for coronary CT angiography as part of the preoperative evaluation for noncardiac surgery.
- The evaluation of coronary stents is considered as a function of patient symptom status, time from revascularization, and stent size. Only with larger stents (≥3 mm in diameter) after long time periods (≥2 years) is stent imaging considered uncertain, and only with left main stents is imaging of stents considered appropriate.
- A strength of cardiac CT imaging is the evaluation of cardiac structure and function. Appropriate indications include coronary anomalies, congenital heart disease, evaluation of right ventricular function, evaluation of left ventricular ejection fraction when images from other techniques are inadequate, and evaluation of prosthetic heart valves. New to this document is the use of cardiac CT for evaluation of myocardial viability when other modalities are inadequate or contraindicated (uncertain) and in suspected arrhythmogenic right ventricular dysplasia (appropriate).
- The use of cardiac CT is appropriate before electrophysiologic procedures for anatomic mapping or before repeated sternotomy in reoperative cardiac surgery.

REFERENCES

1. Hendel RC, Patel MR, Kramer CM, et al: ACCF/ACR/SCCT/SCMR/ASNC/NASCI/SCAI/SIR 2006 appropriateness criteria for cardiac computed tomography and cardiac magnetic resonance imaging: A report of the American College of Cardiology Foundation Quality Strategic Directions Committee Appropriateness Criteria Working Group, American College of Radiology, Society of Cardiovascular Computed Tomography, Society for Cardiovascular Magnetic Resonance, American Society of Nuclear Cardiology, North American Society for Cardiac Imaging, Society for Cardiovascular Angiography and Interventions, and Society of Interventional Radiology. J Am Coll Cardiol 48:1475, 2006.
2. Taylor AJ, Cerqueira M, Hodgson J, et al: ACCF/SCCT/ACR/AHA/ASE/ASNC/SCMR 2010 appropriate use criteria for cardiac computed tomography. J Am Coll Cardiol 56:1864, 2010.
3. Abbara S, Arbab-Zadeh A, Callister TQ, et al: SCCT guidelines for performance of coronary computed tomographic angiography: A report of the Society of Cardiovascular Computed Tomography Guidelines Committee. J Cardiovasc Comput Tomogr 3:190, 2009.
4. Raff GL, Abidov A, Achenbach S, et al: SCCT guidelines for the interpretation and reporting of coronary computed tomographic angiography. J Cardiovasc Comput Tomogr 3:122, 2009.

CHAPTER 20 Cardiac Catheterization

Charles J. Davidson and Robert O. Bonow

Indications for Diagnostic Cardiac Catheterization

As with any procedure, the decision to recommend cardiac catheterization is based on an appropriate risk/benefit ratio. In general, diagnostic cardiac catheterization is recommended whenever it is clinically important to define the presence or severity of a suspected cardiac lesion that cannot be evaluated adequately by noninvasive techniques. Because the risk of a major complication from cardiac catheterization is less than 1% with mortality of less than 0.08%, there are few patients who cannot be studied safely in an active laboratory. Intracardiac pressure measurements and coronary arteriography are procedures that can be performed with reproducible accuracy best by invasive catheterization. Noninvasive estimation of intracardiac pressures can be obtained with echocardiography (see Chap. 15). Coronary computed tomography (CT) angiography can also be used for assessment of coronary anatomy (see Chap. 19) and provides complementary information of plaque distribution and composition. However, current limitations of spatial resolution, heart rate variability, patient cooperation, and radiation dosing limit the ability of CT to replace cardiac catheterization.

To understand the various indications for diagnostic cardiac catheterization, integration of knowledge from multiple American College of Cardiology/American Heart Association (ACC/AHA) guidelines is necessary. The diagnostic coronary angiography guidelines[1] have been updated by other groups that have addressed specific cardiac catheterization indications, including the guidelines for management of patients with valvular heart disease,[2] chronic heart failure,[3] ST elevation myocardial infarction,[4] percutaneous coronary intervention[5] and coronary artery bypass surgery,[6] unstable angina or non–ST elevation myocardial infarction,[7] and congenital heart disease.[8]

Indications for cardiac catheterization include divergent populations. At one extreme, many critically ill and hemodynamically unstable patients are evaluated during acute coronary syndromes, severe heart failure, or cardiogenic shock. At the other end of the spectrum, many procedures are performed in an outpatient setting. These settings include hospitals with or without cardiac surgical capability and freestanding or mobile laboratories.[8]

Cardiac catheterization should be considered a diagnostic test used in combination with complementary noninvasive tests. For example, cardiac catheterization in patients with valvular or congenital heart disease is best performed with full prior knowledge of noninvasive imaging and functional information. This allows catheterization to be directed and simplified without obtaining redundant anatomic information that is reliably available through echocardiography, cardiac magnetic resonance (see Chap. 18), or CT.

Identification of coronary artery disease and assessment of its extent and severity are the most common indications for cardiac catheterization in adults. The information obtained is crucial to optimize the selection of mechanical or medical therapy. In addition, dynamic coronary vascular lesions, such as spasm, myocardial bridging, and plaque rupture with thrombosis, can be identified. The consequences of coronary heart disease, such as ischemic mitral regurgitation and left ventricular (LV) dysfunction, can be defined. During percutaneous catheter intervention for acute coronary syndromes, patients are studied during evolving acute myocardial infarction, with unstable angina, or in the early period after acute myocardial injury. The optimal timing for catheterization and revascularization has been described in various guidelines[2-8] (see Chaps. 21, 55, 57, and 58).

In patients with myocardial disease and LV dysfunction, cardiac catheterization provides critical information. It can evaluate whether coronary artery disease is the cause of symptoms and quantify LV function, right-heart pressures, and cardiac outputs. In patients with angina and impaired LV function, noninvasive testing is of limited value and clinicians should proceed directly to coronary angiography.[3] Cardiac catheterization also permits quantification of the severity of both diastolic and systolic dysfunction, differentiation of myocardial restriction from pericardial constriction, assessment of the extent of valvular regurgitation, and assessment of the cardiovascular response to acute pharmacologic intervention.

In patients with valvular heart disease, cardiac catheterization provides data both confirmatory of and complementary to noninvasive echocardiography, cardiac magnetic resonance, and nuclear studies (see Chap. 66). Cardiac catheterization can define the severity of valvular stenosis or regurgitation, particularly when noninvasive studies are inconclusive or the results are disparate to clinical findings. Knowledge of coronary artery anatomy is critical in most adults older than 35 years when valve surgery is planned.[2] However, catheterization may be unnecessary in some preoperative situations, such as for patients with an atrial myxoma or young patients (<35 years) with endocarditis or acute valvular regurgitation. The identification of anomalies, the quantification of the hemodynamic consequences of the valvular lesions (such as pulmonary hypertension), and the acute hemodynamic response to pharmacologic therapy can provide useful preoperative information that helps define the operative risk and response to surgery and permits a more directed surgical approach.[2]

The current role of cardiac catheterization in certain congenital disease states has been addressed in guidelines for adults with congenital heart disease (see Chap. 65). Echocardiography with Doppler study and cardiac magnetic resonance often provide adequate information. Because gross cardiac anatomy can generally be well defined by these methods, catheterization is required only if certain hemodynamic information (e.g., quantification of shunt size,

TABLE 20-1 Relative Contraindications to Diagnostic Cardiac Catheterization

Acute gastrointestinal bleeding
Severe hypokalemia
Uncorrected digitalis toxicity
Anticoagulation with international normalized ratio >1.8 or severe coagulopathy
Previous anaphylactoid reaction to contrast media
Acute stroke
Acute renal failure or severe chronic non–dialysis-dependent kidney disease
Unexplained fever or untreated active infection
Severe anemia
Uncooperative patient

pulmonary vascular resistance, and reversibility of pulmonary arterial hypertension with a vasodilator) is important in determining the indications for surgical procedures or if percutaneous interventional methods are being used.

There is no true absolute contraindication to cardiac catheterization other than refusal of the competent patient. The procedure can be successfully performed even in the most critically ill patient with a relatively low risk. The relative contradictions to cardiac catheterization are summarized in **Table 20-1**.

Technical Aspects of Cardiac Catheterization

Catheterization Laboratory Facilities

Cardiac catheterization facilities have several venues, including traditional hospital-based laboratories with in-house cardiothoracic surgical programs, hospital-based laboratories without on-site surgical programs, freestanding laboratories, and mobile laboratories. At present, about 75% of cardiac catheterization laboratories have on-site surgical backup. The goal of the freestanding and mobile cardiac catheterization facilities is to reduce cost while offering services in a convenient location for low-risk patients. The safety of mobile catheterization in properly selected low-risk patients has been well established and appears comparable to other settings.

As a result of the documented safety and cost-effectiveness of diagnostic cardiac catheterization in the outpatient setting, there has been increasing use of this approach. About 50% of hospital-based practices are currently performed as outpatient procedures. In general, patients who require preprocedural hospitalization for diagnostic catheterization are uncommon. These include patients with severe congestive heart failure and patients with congestive heart failure renal insufficiency requiring prehydration. The need for hospitalization to change from warfarin to heparin has been replaced by use of low-molecular-weight heparin as an outpatient bridge for anticoagulation.[2]

Noninvasive testing can identify patients who would be more appropriately evaluated in a setting where cardiac surgery is available. This includes severe ischemia discovered during stress testing, ischemia at rest, known or highly suspected severe left main or proximal three-vessel disease, critical aortic stenosis, and severe comorbid disease. Most patients can be discharged on the same day within 2 to 6 hours after the procedure.

The most common reason for postprocedural hospitalization is hematoma formation necessitating additional bed rest and observation. Also, diagnosis from the procedure may require hospitalization, including the findings of severe left main or three-vessel disease. Other considerations for postprocedure hospitalization include uncompensated heart failure, unstable ischemic symptoms, severe aortic stenosis with LV dysfunction, renal insufficiency requiring further hydration, and need for continuous anticoagulation.[7]

PERSONNEL. Personnel in the catheterization laboratory include the medical director, physicians, nurses, cardiovascular fellows, physician extenders including nurse practitioners and physician assistants, and radiologic technologists. All members should be trained in cardiopulmonary resuscitation and preferably in advanced cardiac life support. For full-service laboratories, it is highly desirable for facilities to be associated with a cardiothoracic surgical program. High-risk diagnostic studies and all elective percutaneous interventions should be performed in laboratories with on-site surgical facilities.[5]

LABORATORY CASELOAD. For proficiency to be maintained, laboratories for adult studies should perform a minimum of 300 procedures per year. According to the Accreditation Council for Graduate Medical Education guidelines for diagnostic catheterization, physicians in training must spend a total of 8 months and perform more than 300 cases, including more than 200 as a primary operator, to be credentialed for level II diagnostic cardiac catheterization procedures in practice.[9] However, the minimum caseload for established physicians in practice has not been established.[10] Regular evaluation with quality indicator assessment of laboratory, physician, nurse, and technologist performance and outcomes is mandatory. The laboratory director should possess at least 5 years of catheterization experience. In a laboratory performing percutaneous coronary intervention, the director should be board certified in interventional cardiology. The director is responsible for credentialing of physicians; for review of laboratory, physician, and ancillary personnel performance; and for provision of necessary training. Other responsibilities involve establishing and maintaining quality control of staff and equipment, patient outcome monitoring, and budget oversight.

EQUIPMENT. Necessary equipment for cardiac catheterization includes the radiographic system and physiologic data monitoring, including recording and acquisition instrumentation, sterile supplies, and an emergency cart. Also necessary is support equipment consisting of a power injector, image processing with digital archiving, viewing stations, and a uniform method of report generation.

Radiographic Equipment

High-resolution x-ray imaging is required for optimal performance of catheterization procedures. The necessary equipment includes a generator, x-ray tube, image intensifier or flat panel detector, expansive modulation, video image capture, imaged display, and either digital archiving or a cine camera (see Fig. 21-5).[11] Presently, x-ray systems use a flat panel detector rather than an image intensifier and therefore do not use video cameras. The flat panel detector produces a direct digital video signal from the original visible light fluorescence without the intermediate visible light stage.

Digital acquisition and archiving permits immediate on-line review, quantitative computer analysis, image manipulation capabilities, road maps, and flicker-free images at low frame rates, thus minimizing exposure. Transfer of images between cardiac catheterization laboratories, hospitals, and physician offices can be accomplished with use of a common network. The development of Digital Imaging and Communication (DICOM) standards for cardiac angiography has allowed compatibility among different vendor systems. Increased computer storage capabilities have allowed storage with immediate access to thousands of archived cases.

Physiologic Monitors

Continuous monitoring of blood pressure and the electrocardiogram (ECG) is required during cardiac catheterization. Systemic, pulmonary, and intracardiac pressures are generally recorded by use of fluid-filled catheters connected to strain-gauge pressure transducers and then transmitted to a monitor. Equipment for determination of thermodilution and Fick cardiac output and blood gas determination as well as a standard 12-lead ECG machine is necessary.

RADIATION SAFETY. Radiation effects can be classified as either deterministic effects or stochastic effects. Both have a delay between radiation and effect. The delay may be hours to years. Deterministic effects are dose related in that below a certain dose, there is no effect. However, when a threshold is exceeded, the severity increases with dose. Examples of deterministic effects include skin erythema, desquamation, cataracts, hair loss, and skin necrosis. Skin injury is the most common deterministic effect from radiation. Early transient erythema can develop within hours, but most skin injuries do not appear for 2 to 3 weeks after exposure. The main guiding principle of x-ray exposure is ALARA (as low as reasonably achievable). This implies that no level of radiation is completely safe to patients or providers. The dose-area product (DAP) is the absorbed dose to air (air kerma) multiplied by the x-ray beam cross-sectional area at the point of measurement. It is an approximation of the total x-ray energy delivered to the patient and is a measure of the patient's risk of stochastic effect.[11]

Another measure of skin dose is the interventional reference point (IRP). This is located 15 cm from the isocenter of the x-ray tube and is an estimation of the skin entrance point of the beam.

Stochastic effects are related to probability and not proportional to dose, although the likelihood of an effect is related to dose. Examples of this effect include neoplasms and genetic defects. The estimated dose range for cardiac catheterization is 1 to 10 millisievert (mSv), which is the equivalent of 2 to 3 years of natural background radiation.[11] The typical dose is 3 to 5 mSv.

The basic principles of minimizing radiation exposure include minimizing fluoroscopic beam time for fluoroscopy, using beam collimation, positioning the x-ray source and image reception optimally, using the least magnification possible, changing the radiographic projection in long procedures to minimize entrance port skin exposure, recording the estimated patient dose, and selecting equipment with dose reduction features including low fluoroscopy mode.

For laboratory personnel, the most important factors are maximizing distance from the source of x-rays and using appropriate shielding, including lead aprons, thyroid collars, lead eyeglasses, and movable leaded barriers. Severely angulated views, particularly the left anterior oblique view, substantially increase the radiation exposure of the operators.

A method for measuring radiation exposure for personnel is required. It is recommended that two film badges be worn, one on the outside of the apron at the neck and another under the apron at the waist. The latter monitors the effectiveness of the lead apron. The maximum allowable whole-body radiation dose per year for those working with radiation is 5 roentgen-equivalents-man (rem = 50 mSv) or a maximum of 50 rem in a lifetime.[7]

Catheterization Laboratory Protocol

Preparation of the Patient for Cardiac Catheterization. Before arrival in the catheterization laboratory, the cardiologist responsible for the procedure should explain the procedure fully, including the risks and benefits, and answer questions from the patient and family. Precatheterization evaluation includes obtaining the patient's history, physical examination, and ECG. Routine laboratory studies include complete blood count with platelets, serum electrolyte determinations with creatinine and glucose concentrations, prothrombin time with international normalized ratio (INR), and partial thromboplastin time (in patients receiving heparin). Important components of the history that need to be addressed include diabetes mellitus (insulin or non–insulin requiring), kidney disease, anticoagulation status, and peripheral arterial disease as well as previous contrast media or latex allergy. Full knowledge of any prior procedures, including cardiac catheterizations, percutaneous coronary interventions, peripheral arterial interventions or surgery, and cardiac surgery, is necessary.

Patients should be fasting at least 6 hours, and an intravenous line should be established. Oral or intravenous sedation is usually administered (e.g., benzodiazepine). Pulse oximetry should be used to monitor respiratory status. Some laboratories premedicate patients with antihistamines such as diphenhydramine (25 mg intravenous push) for its anti-allergic properties and to assist in sedation. Oral anticoagulants should be discontinued and the INR should be less than 1.8 to avoid increased risk of bleeding. Aspirin or other oral antiplatelet agents are continued before the procedure. Patients with diabetes receiving metformin should have the medication discontinued the morning of the procedure and not restarted until renal function is stable at least 48 hours after the procedure.[12] All patients should receive hydration before and after the procedure. The amount of hydration is dependent on the ventricular function and baseline fluid status. However, if tolerated, a total of 1 liter of normal saline administered between initiation and completion of the procedure is recommended. Another hydration regimen that has been shown to be effective in preventing contrast nephropathy in patients with chronic kidney disease is the use of sodium bicarbonate at 3 mL/kg/km for 1 hour before the procedure and 1 mL/kg/km for 6 hours after.[13]

Those with a prior history of contrast medium allergy need prophylaxis before the procedure.[14] A recommended regimen is administration of either prednisone (60 mg by mouth) or hydrocortisone (100 mg by intravenous push) given 12 hours and immediately before the procedure. Cimetidine (300 mg), a nonselective histamine antagonist, and diphenhydramine (25 to 50 mg) may also be given by intravenous push. A common misconception is that a history of shellfish allergy predisposes the patient to contrast media reactions. The iodine in shellfish is not the allergen. Rather, tropomyosin appears to be the allergen.

Catheterization Protocol. Each physician should develop a routine for performing diagnostic catheterization to ensure efficient acquisition of all pertinent data. The particular technical approach and necessary procedures should be established individually for each patient so that the specific clinical questions can be addressed. In general, hemodynamic measurements and cardiac output determination should be made before angiography to reflect basal conditions most accurately and to guide angiography. However, in a high-risk case, the approach is to gather the most important diagnostic information first because of the possibility of an adverse event.

Right-heart catheterization should not be performed in all patients undergoing routine coronary angiography. Despite limited risks, right-heart catheterization, including screening oximetric analysis, measurement of pressures, and determination of cardiac output, has a low yield in patients with suspected coronary artery disease without other known cardiac disease. Right-heart catheterization is indicated when a patient has LV dysfunction, congestive heart failure, complicated acute myocardial infarction, valvular heart disease, suspected pulmonary hypertension, congenital disease, intracardiac shunts, or pericardial disease.

Although the use of a temporary pacemaker is not indicated for routine cardiac catheterization, operators should understand the techniques for proper insertion and use when it is needed. Even in patients with isolated left bundle branch block, right-heart catheterization can generally be safely performed with balloon flotation catheters without causing additional conduction disturbance. An example of a balloon flotation catheter (Swan-Ganz) is shown in **Figure 20-1**.

Catheters and Associated Equipment. Catheters used for cardiac catheterization are available in various lengths, sizes, and configurations. Typical catheter lengths vary between 50 and 125 cm; 100 cm is the length most commonly used for adult left-heart catheterization by the femoral approach. The outer diameter of the catheter is specified by French units, where one French unit (F) = 0.33 mm. The inner diameter of the catheter is smaller than the outside diameter because of the thickness of the catheter material. Guidewires used during the procedure must be small enough to pass through the inner diameters of both the introducer needle and the catheter. Guidewires are described by their length in centimeters, diameter in inches, and tip conformation. A commonly used wire is a 150-cm, 0.035-inch J-tip wire. The introducer sheaths are specified by the French number of the largest catheter that passes

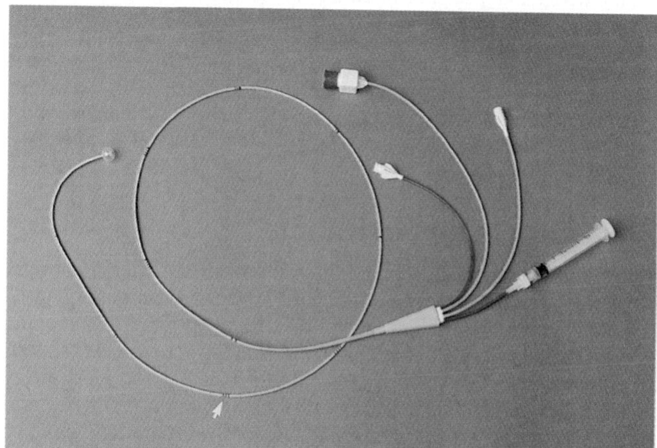

FIGURE 20-1 Typical Swan-Ganz catheter. Proximal ports, left to right, are proximal injection hub, thermistor connector, distal lumen hub, and balloon inflation valve with syringe. The distal end of the catheter has a balloon and a distal end hole. The proximal injectate port exits at 30 cm from the distal lumen (arrow). The thermistor lies just proximal to the balloon.

CH 20

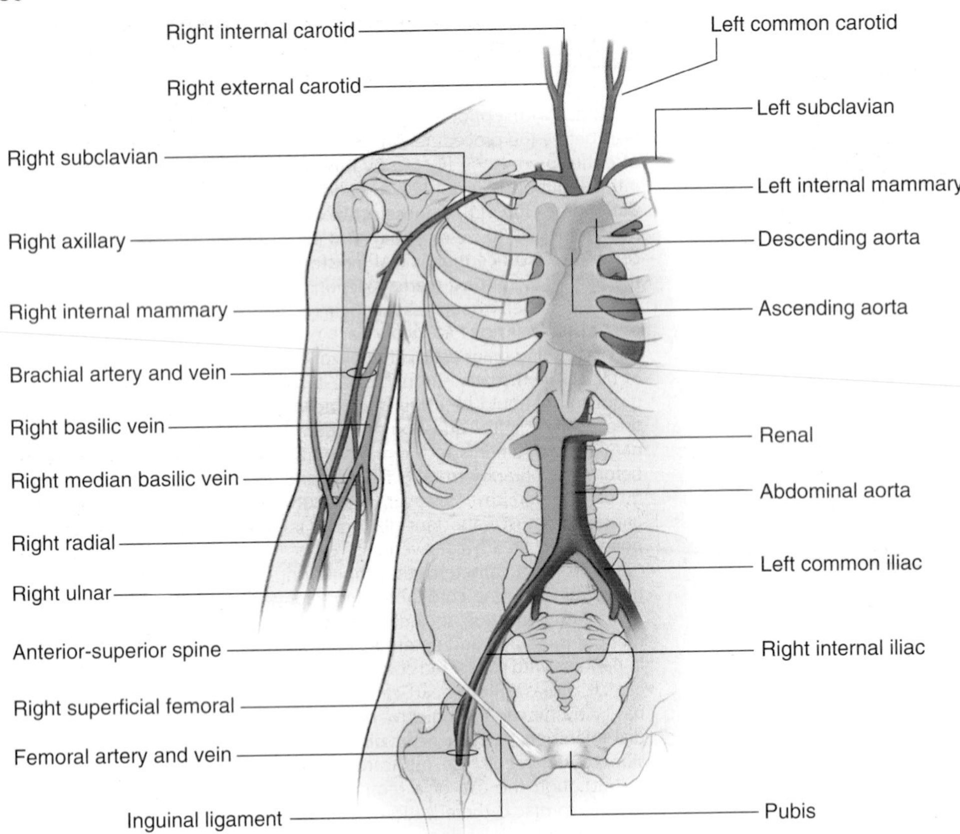

FIGURE 20-2 Principal arteries used for access during cardiac catheterization. Only the superficial veins are shown on the forearm. *(Modified from Thibodeau GA, Patton KT [eds]: Anthony's Textbook of Anatomy and Physiology. 17th ed. St. Louis, CV Mosby, 2002.)*

freely through the inner diameter of the sheath rather than its outer diameter. Therefore, a 7F introducer sheath accepts a 7F catheter (7F = 2.31 mm) but has an outer diameter of more than 2.31 mm.

The choice of the size of the catheters to be used is made by balancing the needs to opacify the coronary arteries and cardiac chambers adequately, to have adequate catheter manipulation, to limit vascular complications, and to permit early ambulation. Although the larger catheters allow greater catheter manipulation and excellent visualization, the most commonly used catheters (4F to 6F) permit earlier ambulation after catheterization and generally provide adequate visualization. Smaller catheters require greater technical skill of manipulation and have lower flow rates. Thus, their use in tortuous anatomy, large body habitus, or high coronary flow states (e.g., aortic regurgitation) may be limited. The relationship between sheath size and vascular complications is not clear. Rather, the arterial puncture technique, anticoagulation status including use of thienopyridines and glycoprotein IIb/IIIa receptor inhibitors, and coagulopathies are more important factors related to vascular complications.[15]

Right-Heart Catheterization

Right-heart catheterization allows measurement and analysis of right atrial, right ventricular (RV), pulmonary artery, and pulmonary capillary wedge pressures; determination of cardiac output; and screening for intracardiac shunts. Screening blood samples for oximetry should be obtained from the superior vena cava (SVC) and pulmonary artery in all patients. Right-heart catheterization is performed antegrade through either the inferior vena cava (IVC) or SVC. Percutaneous entry is achieved through the femoral, internal, jugular, subclavian, or antecubital vein. The anatomy of the major arteries and veins used for cardiac catheterization is shown in **Figure 20-2**.

When left-heart catheterization is performed by the Judkins technique (see later), the femoral vein is used most often for access to the right side of the heart. However, when the right-heart catheter is left indwelling after the procedure, the internal jugular approach is preferable. This approach allows the patient to sit up in bed. The internal jugular approach is preferred to the subclavian to lessen the risk of pneumothorax. The use of a micropuncture kit with a 21-gauge needle and introducer can minimize potential trauma from inadvertent puncture of the carotid artery. When the jugular vein has been entered, the micropuncture assembly can be exchanged for a larger sheath (e.g., 7F) necessary for the right-heart catheterization. Also, the adjunctive use of portable vascular ultrasound probes can help locate and establish the patency of the jugular vein, particularly in patients with short, thick necks or after multiple previous catheterizations.

BALLOON FLOTATION CATHETERS. Balloon flotation catheters are the simplest and most widely used right-heart catheters. If thermodilution cardiac outputs must be determined, catheters that contain thermistors, such as Swan-Ganz catheters, are used (see Fig. 20-1). Intracardiac right-heart pressures and oxygen saturation to evaluate intracardiac shunts can also be obtained. They are both flexible and flow directed, but when the femoral approach is used, fluoroscopic guidance is almost always necessary to cannulate the pulmonary artery and to obtain pulmonary capillary wedge position. Right-heart catheters have either a J-shaped or S-shaped curvature distally to facilitate passage from the SVC to the pulmonary artery or an S-shaped distal end for femoral insertion. Other right-heart balloon flotation end-hole catheters are more rigid and torquable and allow passage of conventional 0.035- or 0.038-inch guidewires. Although these lack the ability to obtain thermodilution cardiac outputs, they yield better pressure fidelity because of less catheter whip artifact and a larger end hole.

There are two methods for advancing a balloon flotation catheter from the femoral vein. Often, the catheter can be advanced directly through the right atrium and across the tricuspid valve. Once it is in the right ventricle, the catheter is clockwise rotated to point superiorly and directly into the RV outflow tract. Once it is in the outflow tract, the balloon tip should allow flotation into the pulmonary artery and wedge positions (**Fig. 20-3**). When necessary, deep inspiration or cough can facilitate this maneuver and assist in crossing of the pulmonic valve. If the catheter continues to point inferiorly toward the RV apex, another technique should be used because further advancement can risk perforation of the RV apex.

Another technique for performing right-heart catheterization with a balloon flotation catheter is shown in Figure 20-3. A loop is formed in the right atrium, with the catheter tip directed laterally. The loop can be created by hooking the catheter tip on the hepatic vein or by advancing the catheter while it is directed laterally in the right atrium. Once the loop is formed, the catheter should be advanced farther, which directs the tip inferiorly and then medially across the tricuspid valve. Antegrade blood flow should then direct the catheter into the pulmonary artery. After the catheter is placed into the wedge position, the redundant loop can be removed with the balloon inflated by slow withdrawal.

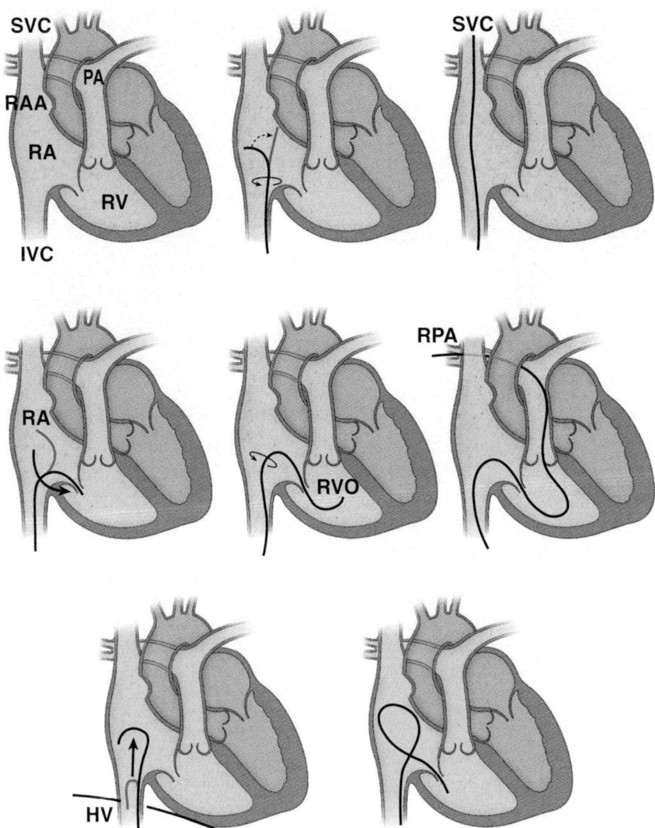

FIGURE 20-3 Right-heart catheterization from the femoral vein, shown in cartoon form. **Top row,** The right-heart catheter is initially placed in the right atrium (RA) aimed at the lateral atrial wall. Counterclockwise rotation aims the catheter posteriorly and allows advancement into the superior vena cava (SVC). Although it is not evident in the figure, clockwise catheter rotation into an anterior orientation would lead to advancement into the right atrial appendage (RAA), precluding SVC catheterization. **Center row,** The catheter is then withdrawn back into the right atrium and aimed laterally. Clockwise rotation causes the catheter tip to sweep anteromedially and to cross the tricuspid valve. With the catheter tip in a horizontal orientation just beyond the spine, it is positioned below the right ventricular outflow (RVO) tract. Additional clockwise rotation causes the catheter to point straight up, allowing advancement into the main pulmonary artery and from there into the right pulmonary artery (RPA). **Bottom row,** Two maneuvers useful in catheterization of a dilated right heart. A larger loop with a downward-directed tip may be required to reach the tricuspid valve and can be formed by catching the catheter tip in the hepatic vein (HV) and advancing the catheter quickly into the right atrium. The reverse loop technique **(bottom right)** gives the catheter tip an upward direction, aimed toward the outflow tract. IVC = inferior vena cava; PA = pulmonary artery; RV = right ventricle. *(From Baim DS, Grossman W: Percutaneous approach, including transseptal and apical puncture.* In *Baim DS, Grossman W [eds]: Cardiac Catheterization, Angiography, and Intervention. 7th ed. Philadelphia, Lea & Febiger, 2006, p 86.)*

NONFLOTATION CATHETERS. When an end-hole catheter (e.g., Cournand or multipurpose) that does not have a balloon tip is used, the technique for cannulation of the pulmonary artery is markedly different. Manipulation and torquing of the nonflotation catheter are necessary to advance it into the pulmonary artery. The catheter should be directed inferiorly across the tricuspid valve and then superiorly into the RV outflow tract. It is generally recommended that one attempt be made to form a loop in the right atrium before advancement into the right ventricle to lessen the risk of perforation.

PATENT FORAMEN OVALE CANNULATION. A probe-patent foramen ovale that allows access to the left atrium is present in 20% to 30% of adult patients. It can be entered by use of a multipurpose catheter with the tip directed medially and slightly posterior. This technique can be used in patients undergoing patent foramen ovale closures. The catheter is withdrawn slowly from the SVC or high right atrium until a slight forward and medial motion is observed. The catheter then prolapses into the left atrium with gentle pressure against the interatrial septum in patients with a probe-patent foramen ovale. Left atrial position can be verified by the pressure waveform, by blood samples demonstrating arterial saturation, or by hand injection of contrast medium. If left atrial access is necessary and cannot be obtained with this technique, a transseptal catheterization should be undertaken (see Transseptal Catheterization).

Left-Heart Catheterization and Coronary Arteriography

THE JUDKINS TECHNIQUE. Because of its relative ease, speed, reliability, and low complication rate,[1,10] the Judkins technique has become the most widely used method of left-heart catheterization and coronary arteriography. After local anesthesia with 1% lidocaine (Xylocaine), percutaneous entry of the femoral artery is achieved by puncturing the vessel 1 to 3 cm (or one to two fingerbreadths) below the inguinal ligament (**Fig. 20-4**). The ligament can be palpated as it courses from the anterior superior iliac spine to the superior pubic ramus. This ligament, not the inguinal crease, should be used as the landmark. The inguinal crease can be misleading, particularly in the obese patient. A hemostatic clamp can be used under fluoroscopy to verify that the nick is made over the inferior edge of the femoral head. A transverse skin incision is made over the femoral artery with a scalpel. With a modified Seldinger technique (**Fig. 20-5**), an 18-gauge thin-walled needle (**Fig. 20-6**) is inserted at a 30- to 45-degree angle into the femoral artery, and a 0.035- or 0.038-inch J-tip polytetrafluoroethylene (Teflon)–coated guidewire is advanced through the needle into the artery. The wire should pass freely up the aorta without tactile resistance and feel like a hot knife passing through butter.

After arterial access is obtained, a sheath at least equal in size to the coronary catheter is usually inserted into the femoral artery. The routine use of heparin for diagnostic cardiac catheterization has not been established. However, in prolonged procedures, such as in patients with bypass grafts or stenotic valve disease, it may be administered at 2000 to 3000 units by intravenous push. The routine administration of protamine after the procedure to reverse heparin is not recommended. Although rare, hypotensive reactions to protamine can be severe and are more common in patients with diabetes. In patients receiving heparin before arrival in the laboratory, an activated clotting time should be obtained after access. Sheath removal is usually not recommended until the activated clotting time is less than 170 seconds unless a vascular closure device is being used.

LV systolic and end-diastolic pressures can be obtained by advancing a pigtail catheter into the left ventricle (**Fig. 20-7**). In assessing valvular aortic stenosis, LV and aortic or femoral artery pressures should be recorded simultaneously with two transducers. The aortic catheter should be placed at least into the abdominal aorta rather than into the femoral artery. The attenuation of pressure can be severe in older adults with peripheral arterial disease, and the estimation of aortic pressure from the femoral artery pressure will be inaccurate for determination of valvular severity. Alternatively, pigtail catheters with both a distal and a proximal lumen can be used. These specially designed catheters measure supravalvular aortic and LV pressure simultaneously when two transducers are used. In suspected mitral stenosis, LV and wedge or left atrial pressures should be obtained simultaneously with two transducers.

Left ventriculography is performed in the 30-degree right anterior oblique and 45- to 50-degree left anterior oblique views. A pigtail catheter is most commonly used for this purpose. Power injection of 30 to 40 mL of contrast medium into the ventricle at 12 to 15 mL/sec is used to assess LV function and the severity of mitral regurgitation. After ventriculography, LV systolic and end-diastolic pressure measurements may be repeated and the systolic pressure recorded as the catheter is withdrawn from the left ventricle into the aorta. If an aortic transvalvular gradient is present, obtaining both of these pressures can detect it. For measurement of suspected intraventricular gradients, a

CH 20

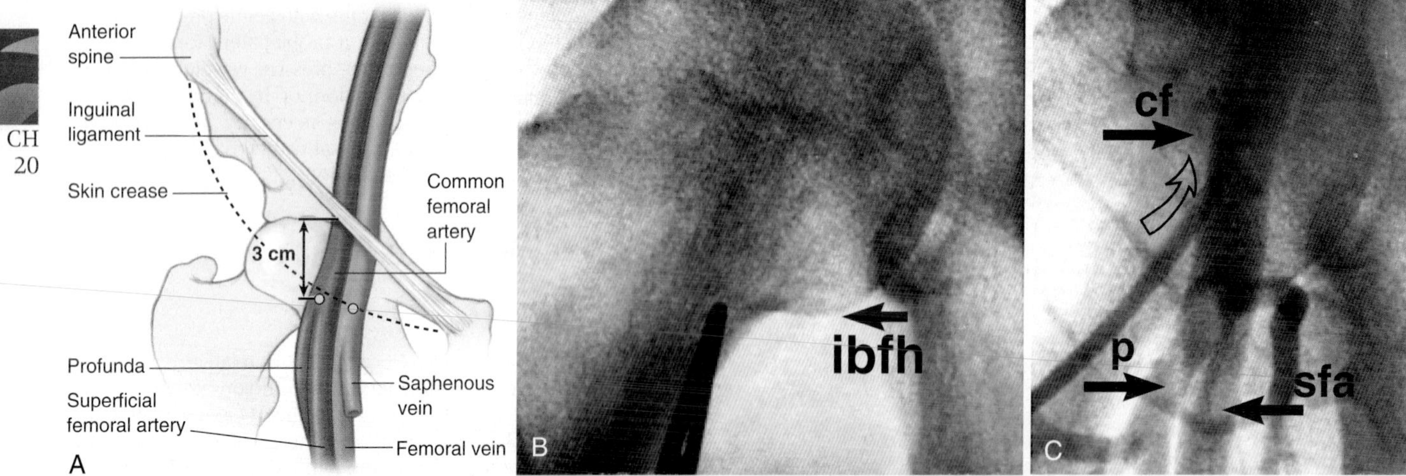

FIGURE 20-4 Regional anatomy relevant to percutaneous femoral arterial and venous catheterization. **A,** Schematic diagram showing the right femoral artery and vein coursing underneath the inguinal ligament, which runs from the anterior superior iliac spine to the pubic tubercle. The arterial skin nick should be placed approximately 3 cm below the ligament and directly over the femoral arterial pulsation; the venous skin nick should be placed at the same level but approximately one fingerbreadth more medial. Although this level corresponds roughly to the skin crease in most patients, anatomic localization relative to the inguinal ligament provides a more constant landmark. **B,** Fluoroscopic localization of skin nick (marked by clamp tip) to the inferior border of the femoral head (ibfh). **C,** Catheter (open arrow) inserted through this skin nick has entered the common femoral artery (cf), above its bifurcation into the superficial femoral artery (sfa) and profunda (p) branches. *(From Baim DS, Grossman W: Percutaneous approach, including transseptal and apical puncture.* In *Baim DS, Grossman W [eds]: Cardiac Catheterization, Angiography, and Intervention. 7th ed. Philadelphia, Lea & Febiger, 2006, p 81.)*

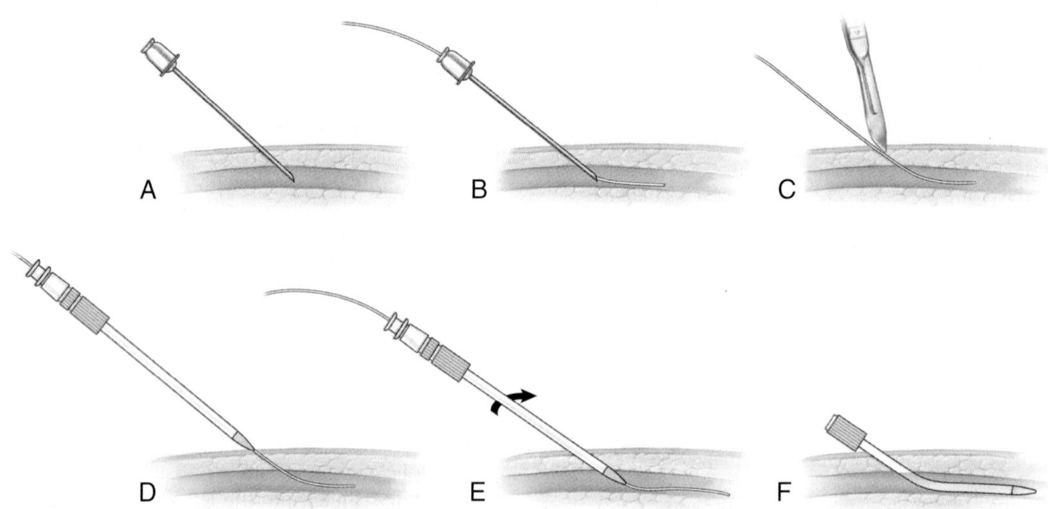

FIGURE 20-5 Modified Seldinger technique for percutaneous catheter sheath introduction. **A,** Vessel punctured by needle. **B,** Flexible guidewire placed into the vessel through the needle. **C,** The needle removed, the guidewire left in place, and the hole in the skin around the wire enlarged with a scalpel. **D,** Sheath and dilator placed over the guidewire. **E,** Sheath and dilator advanced over the guidewire and into the vessel. **F,** Dilator and guidewire removed while the sheath remains in the vessel. *(From Hill JA, Lambert CR, Vlietstra RE, Pepine CJ: Review of general catheterization techniques.* In *Pepine CJ, Hill JA, Lambert CR [eds]: Diagnostic and Therapeutic Cardiac Catheterization. 3rd ed. Baltimore, Williams & Wilkins, 1998, p 107.)*

multipurpose catheter with an end hole is desirable to localize the gradient in the left ventricle. Pigtail catheters contain side holes, which obscure the capacity to define whether the gradient is intraventricular, subvalvular, or transvalvular.

POSTPROCEDURE CARE. After coronary arteriography and left-heart catheterization have been completed, the catheters are removed and firm pressure is applied to the femoral area for 10 minutes by hand. The patient should be instructed to lie in bed for several hours, with the leg remaining straight to prevent hematoma formation. With 4F to 6F catheters, 2 hours of bed rest is usually sufficient, whereas use of catheters larger than 6F usually involves at least 3 to 4 hours.

Alternatively, vascular closure devices may be used. Four types are currently commercially available: collagen plugs, suture closure, metallic clips, and hemostatic patches. Each allows early ambulation of the patients, within 1 to 2 hours after the procedure, and a shorter time to hemostasis than with manual compression.[16,17] They also permit early sheath removal in patients receiving anticoagulation. Although one meta-analysis raised concern about the increased risk of pseudoaneurysm and hematoma with arterial puncture closure devices,[18] another study demonstrated reduced vascular complications compared with manual compression.[19] The ultimate success of any means of achieving hemostasis often relies on a single front-wall puncture of the common femoral artery.

The main advantage of the Judkins technique is speed and ease of selective catheterization. These attributes do not, however, preclude the importance of extensive operator experience to ensure quality studies with acceptable safety. The main disadvantage of this technique

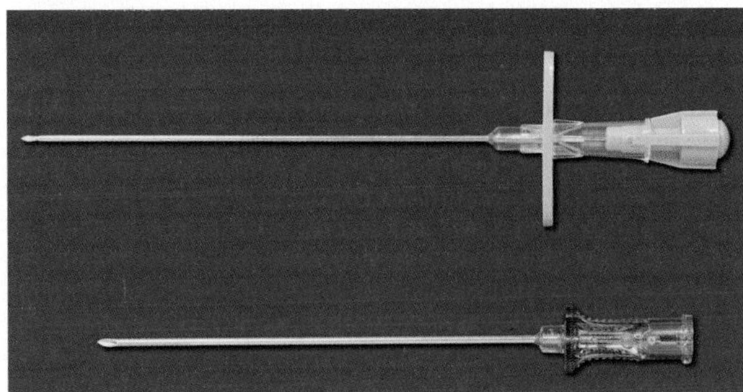

FIGURE 20-6 Two most commonly used needle types for vascular access. **Top,** A two-component, thin-walled Seldinger needle. **Bottom,** A single-piece, thin-walled "front-wall needle."

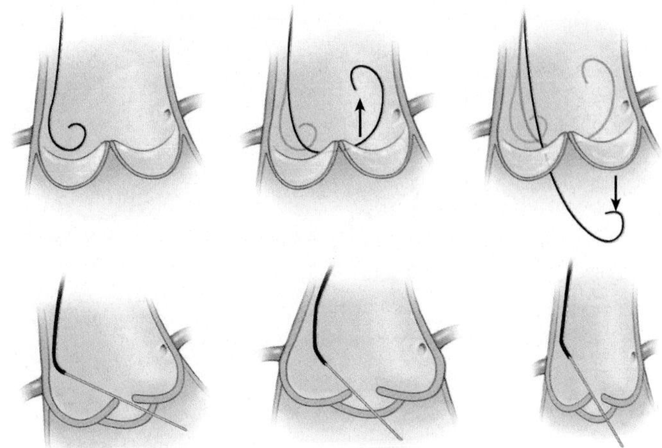

FIGURE 20-7 Technique for retrograde crossing of an aortic valve by a pigtail catheter. The **upper row** shows the technique for crossing of a normal aortic valve. In the **bottom row (left),** the use of a straight guidewire and pigtail catheter in combination is shown. Increasing the length of protruding guidewire straightens the catheter curve and causes the wire to point more toward the right coronary ostium; reducing the length of protruding wire restores the pigtail contour and deflects the guidewire tip toward the left coronary artery. When the correct length of wire and the correct rotational orientation of the catheter have been found, repeated advancement and withdrawal of catheter and guidewire together allow retrograde passage across the valve. In a dilated aortic root **(bottom row, middle),** the angled pigtail catheter is preferable. In a small aortic root **(bottom row, right),** a right coronary Judkins catheter may have advantages. In patients with bicuspid valves, an Amplatz left catheter is often used as it directs the wire more superiorly. *(From Baim DS, Grossman W: Percutaneous approach including transseptal and apical puncture. In Baim DS, Grossman W [eds]: Cardiac Catheterization, Angiography, and Intervention. 6th ed. Philadelphia, Lea & Febiger, 2006, p 93.)*

is its use in patients with severe iliofemoral atherosclerotic disease, in whom retrograde passage of catheters through areas of extreme narrowing or tortuosity may be difficult or impossible. However, with careful technique, fluoroscopic guidance, and torquable floppy-tipped wires (e.g., Wholey wires), passage through synthetic aortofemoral grafts can be achieved with low complication rates.

Brachial Artery Technique–Sones Technique. Sones and colleagues introduced the first technique for coronary artery catheterization by means of a brachial artery cutdown. The technically demanding Sones technique is still used in some centers and is described in Chap. 21.

Percutaneous Brachial Artery Technique. A modification of the Sones technique is the percutaneous brachial artery technique using preformed Judkins catheters. This technique uses the Seldinger method of percutaneous brachial artery entry. A 4F to 6F sheath is placed into the brachial artery, and 3000 to 5000 units of heparin is infused into the side port. A guidewire is then advanced to the ascending aorta under fluoroscopic control. Judkins left, right, and pigtail catheters are passed over the guidewire for routine arteriography and ventriculography. The guidewire may occasionally be necessary to direct the left coronary catheter into the left sinus of Valsalva and the ostium of the left main coronary artery. Alternatively, an Amplatz left or multipurpose catheter is used to intubate the coronary ostium. After removal of the sheath, the arm should be maintained straight with an arm board for 4 to 6 hours with observation of radial and brachial pulses.

The main advantage of the percutaneous brachial technique is that it avoids a brachial artery cutdown and repair. The main disadvantage is that manipulation of catheters can be difficult. Compared with the femoral technique, patients' comfort, hemostasis time, and time to ambulation favor the brachial technique, whereas procedural efficiency, time of radiation exposure, and diagnostic image quality are favorable with the femoral approach. The complication rates appear similar.

Percutaneous Radial Artery Technique. Left-heart catheterization by the radial artery approach was developed as an alternative to the percutaneous transbrachial approach in an attempt to limit vascular complications. The inherent advantages of the transradial approach are that the hand has a dual arterial supply connected through the palmar arches and that there are no nerves or veins at the site of puncture. In addition, bed rest is unnecessary after the procedure, allowing more efficient outpatient angiography.

The procedure requires a normal Allen test result. The Allen test consists of manual compression of both the radial and ulnar arteries during fist clenching until the hand is blanched. Normal color returns to the opened hand within 10 seconds after release of pressure over the ulnar artery, and significant reactive hyperemia is absent on release of pressure over the radial artery.

In the radial technique, the arm is abducted and the wrist hyperextended over a gauze roll. Routine skin anesthesia is used. A micropuncture needle or a 20-gauge Angiocath is introduced at a 30- to 45-degree angle into the radial artery 2 to 3 cm proximal to the flexor crease of the wrist. A 7- to 16-cm-long 4F or 5F sheath is then introduced over a short 0.025-inch wire. Next, about 10 mL of blood is drawn into a syringe containing heparin (3000 to 5000 units IAO) and vasodilators (e.g., 200 μg of nicardipine plus 100 μg of nitroglycerin) to prevent radial artery spasm. The cocktail is mixed with blood to minimize the burning sensation and is then injected into the side arm of the sheath. Coronary catheters are then advanced over a standard 0.035-inch J-tip exchange wire into the ascending aorta. The left and right coronary arteries are intubated in a manner similar to the brachial approach. Hemostasis is obtained at the end of the procedure after sheath removal by use of direct pressure or an inflatable balloon cuff. It is recommended that the arterial puncture site be allowed to bleed for several beats before maintaining direct pressure. The radial pulse should be monitored regularly for several hours after the procedure.

The potential limitations of this procedure include the inability to cannulate the radial artery because of its smaller size and propensity to develop spasm, poor visualization of the coronary arteries resulting from the small-caliber catheters, limited manipulation potential, and risk of radial arterial occlusion caused by dissection or thrombus formation. If intervention is contemplated, device selection may be limited by guide catheter size. Although there is little debate that the femoral approach is the simplest technique for left-heart catheterization, the transradial approach for left-heart catheterization has gained in popularity.[20-22] A recent registry and meta-analysis have demonstrated improvement in bleeding rates compared with the femoral approach.[21-22] However, large-scale randomized trials are lacking.

TRANSSEPTAL CATHETERIZATION. Transseptal left-heart catheterization has increased in popularity as a result of percutaneous balloon mitral commissurotomy as a preferential option to surgical commissurotomy (see Chap. 66), electrophysiologic procedures requiring access to pulmonary veins (see Chap. 40), and use of percutaneous mitral valve repair (see Chap. 59). Transseptal heart catheterization can be performed with a complication rate of less than 1% in experienced centers.[23-25]

An 8F Mullins or transseptal sheath and dilator combination is used. The Brockenbrough needle is 18-gauge that tapers to 21-gauge at the distal tip (**Fig. 20-8**). The needle is placed in the transseptal sheath. One commonly used approach is to place a 0.032-inch guidewire through the femoral vein, through the right atrium, and into the SVC. The Mullins or transseptal sheath and dilator are then advanced over the wire into the SVC. The guidewire is removed and replaced with a Brockenbrough needle. The distal port is connected to a pressure

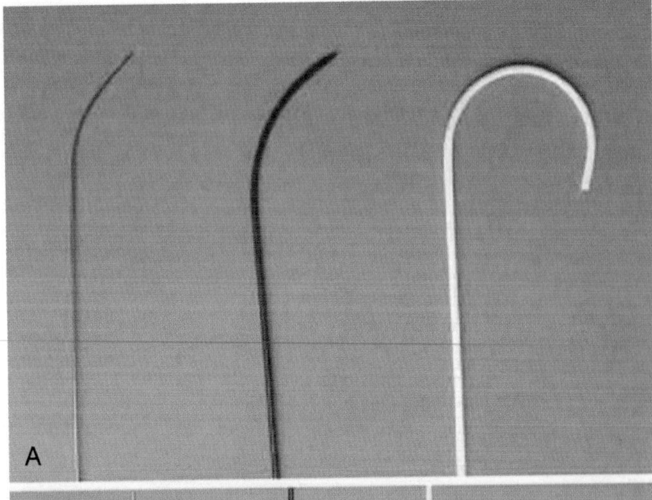

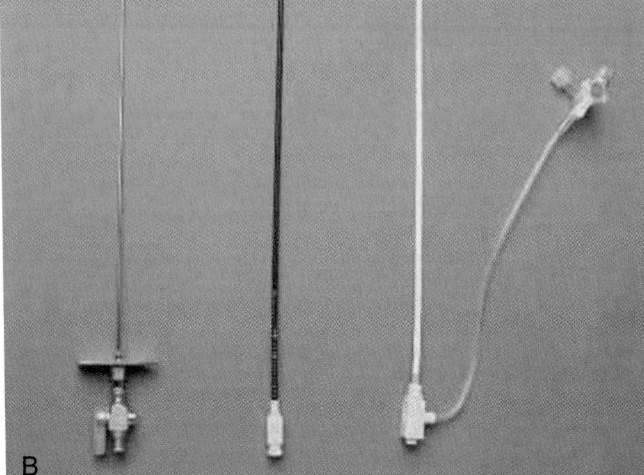

FIGURE 20-8 Transseptal catheters. **A,** Distal catheter. **B,** Proximal catheter. Right, Mullins transseptal sheath. Middle, Introducer (dilator) that is placed inside sheath to add stiffness to the catheter. Left, Brockenbrough transseptal needle that is placed inside the sheath and is used to penetrate the septum.

manifold. With the needle tip just proximal to the Mullins sheath tip, the entire catheter system is withdrawn. The catheter is simultaneously rotated from a 12 o'clock to a 5 o'clock position. The operator observes two abrupt rightward movements. The first occurs as the catheter descends from the SVC to the right atrium. The second occurs as the transseptal dilator tip passes over the limbic edge into the fossa ovalis. The dilator and needle are then advanced gently as a unit. Steady gentle pressure is sometimes adequate to advance the system through the fossa ovalis into the left atrium. If not, the needle should be advanced across the interatrial septum while the sheath is held in place. In cases in which transseptal puncture is technically difficult because of a large right atrium, postsurgical condition, or anatomic variant, intracardiac echocardiography can be useful to localize the fossa ovalis and interatrial septum.[26] (See Intracardiac Echocardiography.)

Left atrial position can be confirmed by the overall increase in pressure with left atrial *a* and *v* waveforms, hand injection of contrast medium, or measurement of arterial oxygen saturation. When the position is confirmed, the catheter should be rotated toward 3 o'clock and the dilator and sheath safely advanced 2 to 3 cm into the left atrium. The sheath is held firmly, and the dilator and needle are removed. Left atrial pressure measurements should then be repeated. If measurement of LV pressure or left ventriculography is necessary, the catheter can usually be advanced easily into the left ventricle after slight counterclockwise rotation. The major risk of transseptal catheterization lies in inadvertent puncture of atrial structures, such as the atrial free wall, left atrial appendage, and coronary sinus, or entry into the aortic root or pulmonary artery.

DIRECT TRANSTHORACIC LEFT VENTRICULAR PUNCTURE. The sole diagnostic indication for direct LV puncture is to measure LV pressure and to perform ventriculography in patients with mechanical prosthetic valves in both the mitral and aortic positions, preventing retrograde arterial and transseptal catheterization. Crossing of tilting disc valves with catheters should be avoided because catheter entrapment, occlusion of the valve, or possible dislodgment of the disc with embolization may result.

The procedure is performed after localization of the LV apex by palpation or, preferably, by echocardiography.[27,28] After local anesthesia is administered, an 18- or 21-gauge 6-inch Teflon catheter system is inserted at the upper rib margin and directed slightly posteriorly and toward the right second intercostal space until the impulse is encountered. The needle and sheath are advanced into the left ventricle The stylet and needle are removed, and the sheath is connected for pressure measurement.

The risks of this procedure include cardiac tamponade, hemothorax, pneumothorax, laceration of the left anterior descending coronary artery, embolism of LV thrombus, vagal reactions, and ventricular arrhythmias. The risk of pericardial tamponade, however, is limited in patients who have undergone prior cardiac surgery because mediastinal fibrosis is present. With current noninvasive imaging techniques including transesophageal echocardiography, this procedure is rarely indicated. Transapical aortic valve implantation uses this technique when femoral access is limited by vessel size (see Chap. 59). Direct visualization of the LV apex is accomplished through intercostal incision followed by apical puncture with the Seldinger technique.

ENDOMYOCARDIAL BIOPSY. Endomyocardial biopsy is performed most commonly with various disposable or, less frequently, reusable bioptomes. The most popular devices used for the internal jugular vein approach include preshaped 50-cm bioptomes. RV biopsy may be performed with use of the internal jugular vein (see Right-Heart Catheterization for internal jugular technique), the subclavian vein, or the femoral vein. LV biopsy is performed with the femoral arterial approach.

When RV biopsy is performed through the right internal jugular vein, a 7F short straight sheath or long curved sheath is introduced by the usual Seldinger technique. If a short sheath is used, a 7F bioptome is advanced under fluoroscopic guidance to the lateral wall of the right atrium. With counterclockwise rotation, the device is advanced across the tricuspid valve and toward the interventricular septum. When a long preshaped sheath is used, it is positioned against the RV septum. RV pressure should be continuously monitored. The bioptome is passed through the sheath, and samples are obtained. Alternatively, two-dimensional echocardiography rather than fluoroscopy has been used to guide the position of the bioptome.

Contact with the myocardium is confirmed by the presence of premature ventricular contractions, resistance to further advancement, and transmission of the ventricular impulse to the operator. The bioptome is then slightly withdrawn from the septum, the forceps jaws are opened, the bioptome is readvanced to make contact with the myocardium, and the forceps is closed. A slight tug is felt on removal of the device. Four to six samples of myocardium are usually required for adequate pathologic analysis. Preprocedure consultation with a pathologist or transplant cardiologist should be obtained to ensure appropriate specimen collection and processing.

RV biopsy from the femoral vein requires insertion of a long 7F sheath directed toward the portion of the ventricle to be sampled. Various configurations of sheaths are used for RV biopsy. The conventional sheath has a 45-degree angle on its distal end to allow access to the right ventricle. However, specifically designed sheaths have dual curves. These catheters possess the usual 180-degree curve and an additional distal perpendicular septal plane curve of 90 degrees, which allows improved manipulation and positioning toward the interventricular septum. This sheath configuration can also be used from the internal jugular approach.

Whatever access is used, the bioptome is advanced through the sheath and should be visualized in both the 30-degree right anterior oblique and 40-degree left anterior oblique views. The right anterior oblique view ensures that the catheter is in the midventricle away from the apex. The left anterior oblique view verifies that the sheath tip is oriented toward the interventricular septum. Contrast medium infusion through the side port of the sheath can be confirmatory. Samples of myocardium are taken in a manner similar to that described earlier.

If LV biopsy is to be performed, the biopsy sheath is generally inserted through the femoral artery and positioned over a multipurpose or pigtail catheter that has been placed in the ventricle. The sheath is advanced below the mitral apparatus and away from the posterobasal wall. The catheter is then withdrawn, and a long LV bioptome is inserted. Care must be taken when LV biopsy is performed to prevent air embolism while the bioptome is introduced into the sheath. A constant infusion of flush solution through the sheath minimizes the risk of air or thrombus embolism.

Complications of endomyocardial biopsy include cardiac perforation with cardiac tamponade, emboli (air, tissue, or thromboembolus), arrhythmias, electrical conduction disturbances, injury to the tricuspid valve, vasovagal reactions, and pneumothorax. The overall complication rate is between 1% and 3%; the risk of cardiac perforation with tamponade is generally reported as less than 0.05%.[29,30] Endomyocardial biopsy is the most common cause of severe tricuspid regurgitation after cardiac transplantation.[31] The use of longer sheaths dramatically decreases the incidence of anatomic disruption of the valve during biopsy.

Systemic embolization and ventricular arrhythmias are more common with LV biopsy. LV biopsy should generally be avoided in patients with right bundle branch block because of the potential for development of complete atrioventricular block as well as in patients with known LV thrombus.

The role of endomyocardial biopsy in the management of cardiovascular disease has been recently defined.[30] There are two Class I indications for endomyocardial biopsy for clinical scenarios (**Table 20-2**). The first is new-onset heart failure of less than 2 weeks' duration associated with either normal or enlarged LV size and hemodynamic compromise. The second is new-onset heart failure of up to 3 months' duration complicated by LV dilation, new ventricular arrhythmias, advanced heart block, or failure to respond to usual care within 2 weeks. The use of biopsy for suspected anthracycline toxicity or restrictive disease is considered a Class IIa indication.[30] Cardiac transplant monitoring for rejection is the most common indication for biopsy (see Chap. 31).

Percutaneous Intra-Aortic Balloon Pump Insertion. Intra-aortic balloon counterpulsation devices are positioned in the descending thoracic aorta. They have a balloon volume of 30 to 50 mL, use helium as the inflation gas, and are timed to inflate during diastole and to deflate during systole. Balloon size is based on the patient's height. The device is inserted through the femoral artery by the standard Seldinger technique so that the tip is 2 to 3 cm below the level of the left subclavian artery. 7F to 8F systems are used. Optimal positioning requires fluoroscopic guidance. Timing of the balloon is adjusted during 1 : 2 (one inflation for each two beats) pumping so that inflation of the balloon occurs at the aortic dicrotic notch and deflation occurs immediately before systole. This timing ensures maximal augmentation of diastolic flow and maximal systolic unloading. **Figure 20-9** displays the optimal timing of an intra-aortic balloon pump (IABP).[32]

Favorable hemodynamic effects include reduction in LV afterload and improvement in myocardial oxygenation.[33] IABP insertion is indicated for patients with angina refractory to medical therapy, cardiogenic shock, or mechanical complications of myocardial infarction (including severe mitral regurgitation and ventricular septal defect) or for those who have severe left main coronary artery stenosis. IABP may also be valuable in patients undergoing high-risk percutaneous coronary intervention or after primary angioplasty in the setting of acute myocardial infarction.[34] IABP insertion is contraindicated in patients with moderate or severe aortic regurgitation, aortic dissection, aortic aneurysm, patent ductus arteriosus, severe peripheral vascular disease, bleeding disorders, or sepsis.

Complications of IABP insertion include limb ischemia requiring early balloon removal or vascular surgery, balloon rupture, balloon entrapment, hematomas, and sepsis.[32,34] The incidence of vascular complications ranges from 12% to greater than 40%. Most patients in whom limb ischemia develops after insertion of a balloon pump device have resolution of the ischemia on balloon removal and do not require surgical

TABLE 20-2 The Role of Endomyocardial Biopsy in 14 Clinical Scenarios

CLINICAL SCENARIO	CLASS OF RECOMMENDATION (I, IIa, IIb, III)	LEVEL OF EVIDENCE (A, B, C)
New-onset heart failure of *<2 weeks'* duration associated with a normal-sized or dilated left ventricle and hemodynamic compromise	I	B
New-onset heart failure of *2 weeks' to 3 months'* duration associated with a dilated left ventricle and new ventricular arrhythmias, second- or third-degree heart block, or failure to respond to usual care within 2 weeks	I	B
Heart failure *>3 months'* duration associated with a dilated left ventricle and new ventricular arrhythmias, second- or third-degree heart block, or failure to respond to usual care within 2 weeks	IIa	C
Heart failure associated with a dilated cardiomyopathy of any duration associated with suspected allergic reaction and/or eosinophilia	IIa	C
Heart failure associated with suspected anthracycline cardiomyopathy	IIa	C
Heart failure associated with unexplained restrictive cardiomyopathy	IIa	C
Suspected cardiac tumors	IIa	C
Unexplained cardiomyopathy in children	IIa	C
New-onset heart failure of *2 weeks' to 3 months'* duration associated with a dilated left ventricle, without new ventricular arrhythmias or second- or third-degree heart block, that responds to usual care within 2 weeks	IIb	B
Heart failure *>3 months'* duration associated with a dilated left ventricle, without new ventricular arrhythmias or second- or third-degree heart block, that responds to usual care within 2 weeks	IIb	C
Heart failure associated with unexplained hypertrophic cardiomyopathy	IIb	C
Suspected arrhythmogenic RV dysplasia	IIb	C
Unexplained ventricular arrhythmias	IIb	C
Unexplained atrial fibrillation	III	C

From Cooper LT, Baughman K, Feldman AM, et al: The role of endomyocardial biopsy in the management of cardiovascular disease. J Am Coll Cardiol 50:1914, 2007.

CH 20

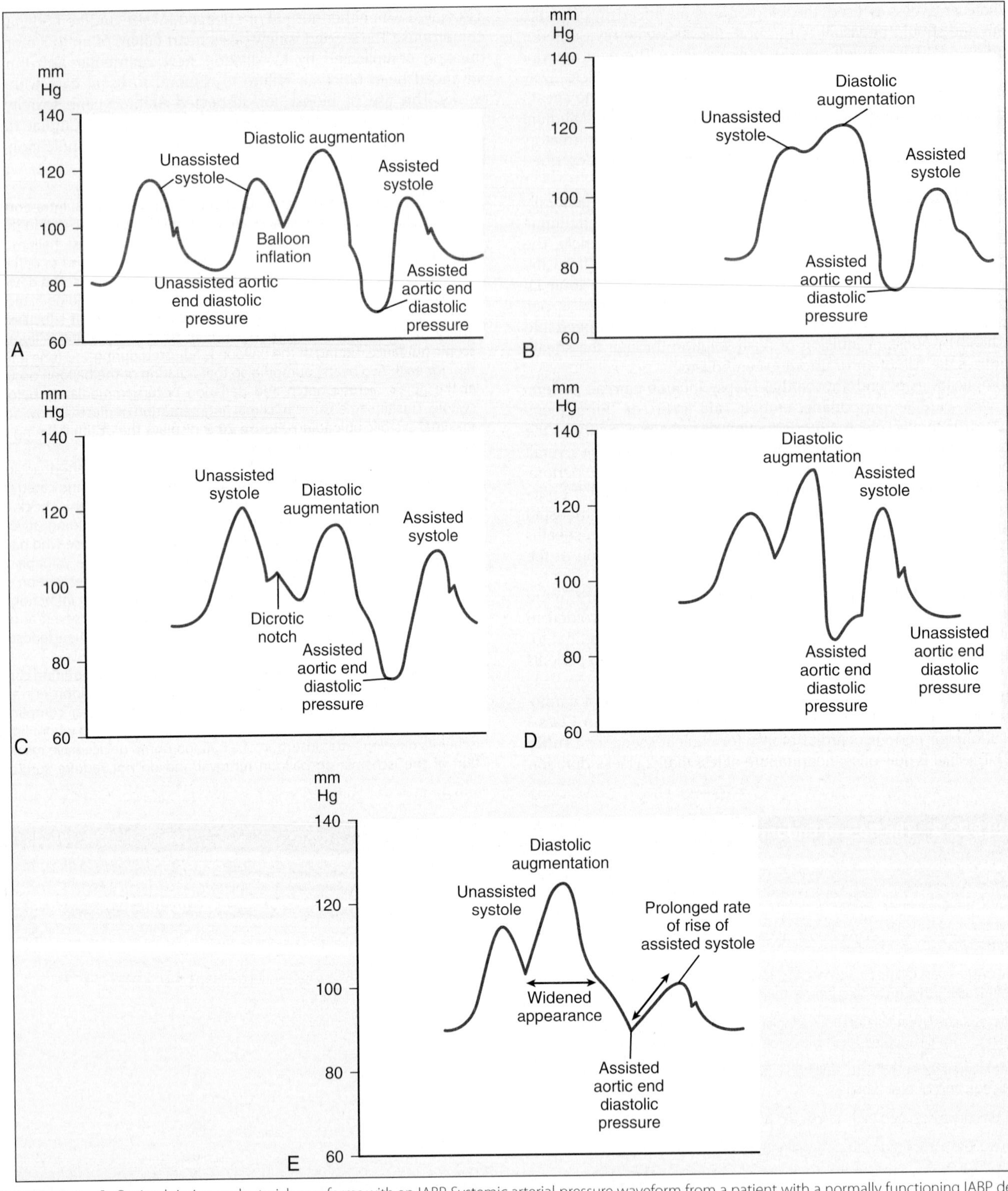

FIGURE 20-9 **A,** Optimal timing and arterial waveforms with an IABP. Systemic arterial pressure waveform from a patient with a normally functioning IABP device in whom the IABP device is programmed to inflate during every other cardiac cycle (commonly referred to as 1:2 inflation). With the first beat, aortic systolic and end-diastolic pressures are shown without IABP support and are therefore unassisted. With the second beat, the balloon inflates with the appearance of the dicrotic notch, and peak-augmented diastolic pressure is inscribed. With balloon deflation, assisted end-diastolic pressure and assisted systolic pressure are observed. To confirm that IABP is producing maximal hemodynamic benefit, the peak diastolic augmentation should be greater than the unassisted systolic pressure, and the two assisted pressures should be less than the unassisted values. **B,** Systemic arterial pressure waveform from a subject in whom balloon inflation occurs too early, before aortic valve closure. Consequently, the left ventricle is forced to empty against an inflated balloon; the corresponding increase in afterload may increase myocardial oxygen demands and worsen systolic function. **C,** Systemic arterial pressure waveform from a patient in whom balloon inflation occurs too late, well after the beginning of diastole, thereby minimizing diastolic pressure augmentation. **D,** Systemic arterial pressure waveform from a patient in whom balloon deflation occurs too early, before the end of diastole. This may shorten the period of diastolic pressure augmentation. A corresponding transient decrease in aortic pressure may promote retrograde arterial flow from the carotid or coronary arteries, possibly inducing cerebral or myocardial ischemia. **E,** Systemic arterial pressure waveform from a subject in whom balloon deflation occurs too late, after the end of diastole, thereby producing the same deleterious consequences as early balloon inflation (increased left ventricular afterload, with a resultant increase in myocardial oxygen demands and a worsening of systolic function). *(From Trost JC, Hillis LD: Intra-aortic balloon counterpulsation. Am J Cardiol 97:1391, 2006.)*

intervention (thrombectomy, vascular repair, fasciotomy, or amputation). The risk of limb ischemia is heightened in patients with diabetes or peripheral arterial disease, in women, and in patients with a postinsertion ankle-brachial index of less than 0.8. However, with the use of smaller catheters (7F), vascular complications are reduced.

Hemodynamic Data

The hemodynamic component of the cardiac catheterization procedure focuses on pressure measurements, the measurement of flow (e.g., cardiac output, shunt flows, flow across a stenotic orifice, regurgitant flows, and coronary blood flow), and the determination of vascular resistances. Simply stated, flow through a blood vessel is determined by the pressure difference within the vessel and the vascular resistance as described by Ohm's law: $Q = \Delta P/R$.

Pressure Measurements

Accurate recording of pressure waveforms and correct interpretation of physiologic data derived from these waveforms are major goals of cardiac catheterization. A pressure wave is the cyclical force generated by cardiac muscle contraction, and its amplitude and duration are influenced by various mechanical and physiologic parameters. The pressure waveform from a particular cardiac chamber is influenced by the force of the contracting chamber and its surrounding structures, including the contiguous chambers of the heart, pericardium, lungs, and vasculature. Physiologic variables of heart rate and the respiratory cycle also influence the pressure waveform. An understanding of the components of the cardiac cycle is essential to the correct interpretation of hemodynamic data obtained in the catheterization laboratory.

PRESSURE MEASUREMENT SYSTEMS

Fluid-Filled Systems

Intravascular pressures are typically measured with use of a fluid-filled catheter that is attached to a pressure transducer. The pressure wave is transmitted from the catheter tip to the transducer by the fluid column within the catheter. The majority of pressure transducers used currently are disposable electrical strain gauges. The pressure wave distorts the diaphragm or wire within the transducer. This energy is then converted to an electrical signal proportional to the pressure being applied using the principle of the Wheatstone bridge. This signal is then amplified and recorded as an analog signal.[35]

There are a number of sources of error when pressures are measured with a fluid-filled catheter-transducer system. Distortion of the output signal occurs as a result of the frequency response characteristics and damping characteristics of the system. The frequency response of the system is the ratio of the output amplitude to input amplitude over a range of frequencies of the input pressure wave. The natural frequency is the frequency at which the system oscillates when it is shock-excited in the absence of friction. Dissipation of the energy of the system, such as by friction, is called damping. To ensure a high-frequency response range, the pressure measurement system should have the highest possible natural frequency and optimal damping. With optimal damping, the energy is dissipated gradually, thus maintaining the frequency response curve as close as possible to an output/input ratio of 1 as it approaches the system's natural frequency. Optimal damping is achieved by use of a short, wide-bore, noncompliant catheter-tubing system that is directly connected to the transducer with use of a low-density liquid from which all air bubbles have been removed.[35]

The pressure transducer must be calibrated against a known pressure, and the establishment of a zero reference must be undertaken at the start of the catheterization procedure. To "zero" the transducer, the transducer is placed at the level of the atria, which is approximately midchest. If the transducer is attached to the manifold and variable positions during the procedure, a second fluid-filled catheter system should be attached to the transducer and positioned at the level of the midchest. All transducers being used during the procedure should be zeroed and calibrated simultaneously. Because of possible variable drift during the procedure, all transducers should be rebalanced immediately before simultaneous recordings for transvalvular gradient or simultaneous pressure determinations are obtained.

Potential sources of error include catheter whip artifact (motion of the tip of the catheter within the measured chamber), end-pressure artifact (an end-hole catheter measures an artificially elevated pressure because of streaming or high velocity of the pressure wave), catheter impact artifact (when the catheter is struck by the walls or valves of the cardiac chambers), and catheter tip obstruction within small vessels or valvular orifices occurring because of the size of the catheter itself. The operator must be aware of the many sources of potential error, and when there is a discrepancy between the observed data and the clinical scenario, all components of the system should be examined for errors or artifacts.

Micromanometer Catheters

The use of these catheters, which have the pressure transducer mounted at the tip, greatly reduces many of the errors inherent to fluid-filled systems. However, their utility is limited by the additional cost and time needed for proper calibration and use of the system. These catheters have higher natural frequencies and more optimal damping characteristics because the interposing fluid column is eliminated. In addition, there is a decrease in catheter whip artifact. The pressure waveform is less distorted and is without the 30- to 40-millisecond delay seen in the fluid-filled catheter-transducer system. Commercially available high-fidelity micromanometer systems have both an end hole and side holes to allow over-the-wire insertion into the circulation while also permitting angiography. Catheters that have two transducers separated by a short distance are useful for accurate measurement of gradients across valvular structures and within ventricular chambers. The micromanometer system has been used for research purposes to assess rate of ventricular pressure rise (dP/dt), wall stress, rate of ventricular pressure decay (−dP/dt), time constant of relaxation (τ), and ventricular pressure-volume relationships (see Chap. 24).

NORMAL PRESSURE WAVEFORMS. An understanding of the normal pressure waveform morphologies is necessary to comprehend the abnormalities that characterize certain pathologic conditions. Normal pressures in the cardiac chambers and great vessels are listed in **Table 20-3**. Simply stated, whenever fluid is added to a chamber or compressed within a chamber, the pressure usually rises; conversely, whenever fluid exits from a chamber or the chamber relaxes, the pressure usually falls. One exception to this rule is the early phase of ventricular diastolic filling, when ventricular volume increases after mitral valve opening but ventricular pressure continues to decrease because of active relaxation. Examples of normal-pressure waveforms are shown in **Figure 20-10**.

Atrial Pressure

The right atrial pressure waveform has three positive deflections, the *a*, *c*, and *v* waves. The *a* wave is due to atrial systole and follows the P wave of the ECG. The height of the *a* wave depends on atrial contractility and the resistance to RV filling. The *x* descent follows the *a* wave and represents relaxation of the atrium and downward pulling of the tricuspid annulus by RV contraction. The *x* descent is interrupted by the *c* wave, which is a small positive deflection caused by protrusion of the closed tricuspid valve into the right atrium. Pressure in the atrium rises after the *x* descent as a result of passive atrial filling. The atrial pressure then peaks as the *v* wave, which represents RV systole. The height of the *v* wave is related to atrial compliance and the amount of blood returning to the atrium from the periphery. The right atrial *v* wave is generally smaller than the *a* wave. The *y* descent occurs after the *v* wave and reflects tricuspid valve opening and right atrial emptying into the right ventricle. During spontaneous respiration, right atrial pressure declines during inhalation as intrathoracic pressure falls. Right atrial pressure rises during exhalation as intrathoracic pressures increase. The opposite effect is seen when patients are mechanically ventilated.

CH 20

The left atrial pressure waveform is similar to that of the right atrium, although normal left atrial pressure is higher, reflecting the high-pressure system of the left side of the heart. In the left atrium, as opposed to the right atrium, the *v* wave is generally higher than the *a* wave. This difference occurs because the left atrium is constrained posteriorly by the pulmonary veins, whereas the right atrium can easily decompress throughout the IVC and SVC. The height of the left atrial *v* wave most accurately reflects left atrial compliance.

Pulmonary Capillary Wedge Pressure

The pulmonary capillary wedge pressure waveform is similar to the left atrial pressure waveform but is slightly damped and delayed as a result of transmission through the lungs. The *a* and *v* waves with both *x* and *y* descents are visible, but *c* waves may not be seen. In the normal state, the pulmonary artery diastolic pressure is similar to the mean pulmonary capillary wedge pressure because the pulmonary circulation has low resistance. In certain disease states that are associated with elevated pulmonary vascular resistance (hypoxemia, pulmonary embolism, and chronic pulmonary hypertension) and occasionally after mitral valve surgery, the pulmonary capillary wedge pressure may overestimate true left atrial pressure. In this circumstance, accurate measurement of the mitral valve gradient may require the direct left atrial pressure to be obtained.[36]

Ventricular Pressure

RV and LV waveforms are similar in morphology. They differ mainly with respect to their magnitudes. The durations of systole and isovolumic contraction and relaxation are longer and the ejection period is shorter in the left than in the right ventricle. There may be a small (5 mm Hg) systolic gradient between the right ventricle and the pulmonary artery. Ventricular diastolic pressure is characterized by an early rapid filling wave, during which most of the ventricle fills; a slow filling phase; and the *a* wave, denoting atrial systolic activity. End-diastolic pressure is generally measured at the C point, which is the rise in ventricular pressure at the onset of isovolumic contraction. When the C point is not well seen, a line is drawn from the R wave on the simultaneous ECG to the ventricular pressure waveform, and this is used as the end-diastolic pressure.

Great Vessel Pressures

The contour of the central aortic pressure and the pulmonary artery pressure tracing consists of a systolic wave, the incisura (indicating closure of the semilunar valves), and a gradual decline in pressure until the following systole. The pulse pressure reflects the stroke volume and compliance of the arterial system. The mean aortic pressure more accurately reflects peripheral resistance. As the systemic pressure wave is transmitted through the length of the aorta, the systolic wave increases in amplitude and becomes more triangular, and the diastolic wave decreases until it reaches the midthoracic aorta and then increases. The mean aortic pressures, however, are usually similar; the mean peripheral arterial pressure is typically ≤5 mm Hg lower than the mean central aortic pressure.

The difference in systolic pressures between the central aorta and the periphery (femoral, brachial, or radial arteries) is greatest in younger patients because of their increased vascular compliance. These potential differences between proximal aorta and peripheral artery must be considered to measure and to interpret the peak systolic pressure gradient between the left ventricle and the systemic arterial system in patients with suspected aortic stenosis. When a transvalvular gradient is present, the most accurate measure of the aortic pressure is obtained at the level of the coronary arteries. This measurement avoids the effect of pressure recovery, which is defined

TABLE 20-3 Normal Pressures and Vascular Resistances

PRESSURES	AVERAGE (mm Hg)	RANGE (mm Hg)
Right atrium		
a wave	6	2-7
v wave	5	2-7
Mean	3	1-5
Right ventricle		
Peak systolic	25	15-30
End-diastolic	4	1-7
Pulmonary artery		
Peak systolic	25	15-30
End-diastolic	9	4-12
Mean	15	9-19
Pulmonary capillary wedge		
Mean	9	4-12
Left atrium		
a wave	10	4-16
v wave	12	6-21
Mean	8	2-12
Left ventricle		
Peak systolic	130	90-140
End-diastolic	8	5-12
Central aorta		
Peak systolic	130	90-140
End-diastolic	70	60-90
Mean	85	70-105
VASCULAR RESISTANCES	**MEAN (DYNE-SEC • CM^{-5})**	**RANGE (DYNE-SEC • CM^{-5})**
Systemic vascular resistance	1100	700-1600
Total pulmonary resistance	200	100-300
Pulmonary vascular resistance	70	20-130

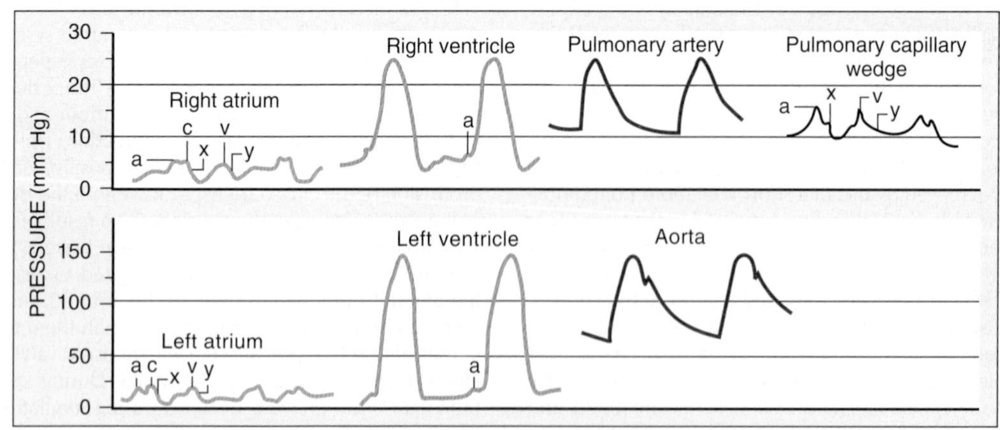

FIGURE 20-10 Normal right- and left-heart pressures recorded from fluid-filled catheter systems in a human. *(From Pepine C, Hill JA, Lambert CR [eds]: Diagnostic and Therapeutic Cardiac Catheterization. 3rd ed. Baltimore, Williams & Wilkins, 1998.)*

as the variable increase in lateral pressure downstream from a stenotic orifice (see Chaps. 15 and 66). This approach can become clinically important in cases of mild to moderate aortic stenosis, particularly when the aorta is small.[37] There will be an underestimation of the transvalve gradient and overestimation of aortic valve area because of higher pressure in the femoral artery in younger patients when supraventricular pressure is not obtained. This can be avoided with a dual-lumen pigtail catheter, which measures pressure in the left ventricle and ascending aorta simultaneously.

ABNORMAL PRESSURE CHARACTERISTICS. Abnormal pressure waveforms may be diagnostic of specific pathologic conditions. **Table 20-4** summarizes the more commonly encountered waveforms.

TABLE 20-4 Pathologic Waveforms

I. Right atrial pressure waveforms
   A. Low mean atrial pressure
      1. Hypovolemia
      2. Improper zeroing of the transducer
   B. Elevated mean atrial pressure
      1. Intravascular volume overload states
      2. Right ventricular failure due to valvular disease (tricuspid or pulmonic stenosis or regurgitation)
      3. Right ventricular failure due to myocardial disease (right ventricular ischemia, cardiomyopathy)
      4. Right ventricular failure due to left-sided heart failure (mitral stenosis or regurgitation, aortic stenosis or regurgitation, cardiomyopathy, ischemia)
      5. Right ventricular failure due to increased pulmonary vascular resistance (pulmonary embolism, chronic obstructive pulmonary disease, primary pulmonary hypertension)
      6. Pericardial effusion with tamponade physiology
      7. Obstructive atrial myxoma
   C. Elevated *a* wave (any increase to ventricular filling)
      1. Tricuspid stenosis
      2. Decreased ventricular compliance due to ventricular failure, pulmonic valve stenosis, or pulmonary hypertension
   D. Cannon *a* wave
      1. Atrial-ventricular asynchrony (atria contract against a closed tricuspid valve, as during complete heart block, following premature ventricular contraction, during ventricular tachycardia, with ventricular pacemaker)
   E. Absent *a* wave
      1. Atrial fibrillation or atrial standstill
      2. Atrial flutter
   F. Elevated *v* wave
      1. Tricuspid regurgitation
      2. Right ventricular heart failure
      3. Reduced atrial compliance (restrictive myopathy)
   G. *a* wave equal to *v* wave
      1. Tamponade
      2. Constrictive pericardial disease
      3. Hypervolemia
   H. Prominent *x* descent
      1. Tamponade
      2. Subacute constriction and possibly chronic constriction
      3. Right ventricular ischemia with preservation of atrial contractility
   I. Prominent *y* descent
      1. Constrictive pericarditis
      2. Restrictive myopathies
      3. Tricuspid regurgitation
   J. Blunted *x* descent
      1. Atrial fibrillation
      2. Right atrial ischemia
   K. Blunted *y* descent
      1. Tamponade
      2. Right ventricular ischemia
      3. Tricuspid stenosis
   L. Miscellaneous abnormalities
      1. Kussmaul sign (inspiratory rise or lack of decline in right atrial pressure): constrictive pericarditis, right ventricular ischemia
      2. Equalization (≤5 mm Hg) of mean right atrial ventricular diastolic, pulmonary artery diastolic, pulmonary capillary wedge, and pericardial pressures in tamponade
      3. M or W patterns: right ventricular ischemia, pericardial constriction, congestive heart failure
      4. Ventricularization of the right atrial pressure: severe tricuspid regurgitation
      5. Sawtooth pattern: atrial flutter
      6. Dissociation between pressure recording and intracardiac electrocardiogram: Ebstein anomaly

II. Left atrial pressure–pulmonary capillary wedge pressure waveforms
   A. Low mean pressure
      1. Hypovolemia
      2. Improper zeroing of the transducer
   B. Elevated mean pressure
      1. Intravascular volume overload states
      2. Left ventricular failure due to valvular disease (mitral or aortic stenosis or regurgitation)
      3. Left ventricular failure due to myocardial disease (ischemia or cardiomyopathy)
      4. Left ventricular failure due to systemic hypertension
      5. Pericardial effusion with tamponade physiology
      6. Obstructive atrial myxoma
   C. Elevated *a* wave (any increased resistance to ventricular filling)
      1. Mitral stenosis
      2. Decreased ventricular compliance due to ventricular failure, aortic valve stenosis, or systemic hypertension
   D. Cannon *a* wave
      1. Atrial-ventricular asynchrony (atria contract against a closed mitral valve, as during complete heart block, following premature ventricular contraction, during ventricular tachycardia, or with ventricular pacemaker)
   E. Absent *a* wave
      1. Atrial fibrillation or atrial standstill
      2. Atrial flutter
   F. Elevated *v* wave
      1. Mitral regurgitation
      2. Left ventricular heart failure
      3. Ventricular septal defect
   G. *a* wave equal to *v* wave
      1. Tamponade
      2. Constrictive pericardial disease
      3. Hypervolemia
   H. Prominent *x* descent
      1. Tamponade
      2. Subacute constriction and possibly chronic constriction
   I. Prominent *y* descent
      1. Constrictive pericarditis
      2. Restrictive myopathies
      3. Mitral regurgitation
   J. Blunted *x* descent
      1. Atrial fibrillation
      2. Atrial ischemia
   K. Blunted *y* descent
      1. Tamponade
      2. Ventricular ischemia
      3. Mitral stenosis
   L. Pulmonary capillary wedge pressure not equal to left ventricular end-diastolic pressure
      1. Mitral stenosis
      2. Left atrial myxoma
      3. Cor triatriatum
      4. Pulmonary venous obstruction
      5. Decreased ventricular compliance
      6. Increased pleural pressure
      7. Placement of catheter in a nondependent zone of the lung

III. Pulmonary artery pressure waveforms
   A. Elevated systolic pressure
      1. Primary pulmonary hypertension
      2. Mitral stenosis or regurgitation
      3. Congestive heart failure
      4. Restrictive myopathies
      5. Significant left-to-right shunt
      6. Pulmonary disease (pulmonary embolism, hypoxemia, chronic obstructive pulmonary disease)

Continued

TABLE 20-4 Pathologic Waveforms—cont'd

B. Reduced systolic pressure
1. Hypovolemia
2. Pulmonary artery stenosis
3. Subvalvular or supravalvular stenosis
4. Ebstein anomaly
5. Tricuspid stenosis
6. Tricuspid atresia

C. Reduced pulse pressure
1. Right-heart ischemia
2. Right ventricular infarction
3. Pulmonary embolism
4. Tamponade

D. Bifid pulmonary artery waveform
1. Large left atrial *v* wave transmitted backward (i.e., mitral regurgitation)

E. Pulmonary artery diastolic pressure higher than pulmonary capillary wedge pressure
1. Pulmonary disease
2. Pulmonary embolus
3. Tachycardia

IV. Ventricular pressure waveforms

A. Systolic pressure elevated
1. Pulmonary or systemic hypertension
2. Pulmonary valve or aortic stenosis
3. Ventricular outflow tract obstruction
4. Supravalvular obstruction
5. Right ventricular pressure elevation with significant
   a. Atrial septal defect
   b. Ventricular septal defect
6. Right ventricular pressure elevation due to factors that increase pulmonary vascular resistance (see factors that increase right atrial pressure)

B. Systolic pressure reduced
1. Hypovolemia
2. Cardiogenic shock
3. Tamponade

C. End-diastolic pressure elevated
1. Hypervolemia
2. Congestive heart failure
3. Diminished compliance
4. Hypertrophy
5. Tamponade
6. Regurgitant valvular disease
7. Pericardial constriction

D. End-diastolic pressure reduced
1. Hypovolemia
2. Tricuspid or mitral stenosis

E. Diminished or absent *a* wave
1. Atrial fibrillation or flutter
2. Tricuspid or mitral stenosis
3. Tricuspid or mitral regurgitation when ventricular compliance is increased

F. Dip and plateau in diastolic pressure wave
1. Constrictive pericarditis
2. Restrictive myopathies
3. Right ventricular ischemia
4. Acute dilation associated with
   a. Tricuspid regurgitation
   b. Mitral regurgitation

G. Left ventricular end-diastolic pressure higher than right ventricular end-diastolic pressure
1. Restrictive myopathies

V. Aortic pressure waveforms

A. Systolic pressure elevated
1. Systemic hypertension
2. Arteriosclerosis
3. Aortic insufficiency

B. Systolic pressure reduced
1. Aortic stenosis
2. Heart failure
3. Hypovolemia

C. Widened pulse pressure
1. Systemic hypertension
2. Aortic insufficiency
3. Significant patent ductus arteriosus
4. Significant ruptures of sinus of Valsalva aneurysm

D. Reduced pulse pressure
1. Tamponade
2. Congestive heart failure
3. Cardiogenic shock
4. Aortic stenosis

E. Pulsus bisferiens
1. Aortic insufficiency
2. Obstructive hypertrophic cardiomyopathy

F. Pulsus paradoxus
1. Tamponade
2. Obstructive airway disease
3. Pulmonary embolism

G. Pulsus alternans
1. Congestive heart failure
2. Cardiomyopathy

H. Pulsus parvus et tardus
1. Aortic stenosis

I. Spike-and-dome configuration
1. Obstructive hypertrophic cardiomyopathy

Cardiac Output Measurements

There is no completely accurate method of measuring cardiac output in all patients, but it can be estimated on the basis of various assumptions. The two most commonly used methods are the Fick method and the thermodilution method. For comparison among patients, cardiac output is often corrected for the patient's size on the basis of the body surface area and expressed as cardiac index.

THERMODILUTION TECHNIQUES. The thermodilution procedure requires injection of a bolus of liquid (usually normal saline) into the proximal port of the catheter. The resultant change in temperature in the liquid is measured by a thermistor mounted in the distal end of the catheter. The change in temperature versus time is graphed. The cardiac output is then calculated by use of an equation that considers the temperature and specific gravity of the injectate and the temperature and specific gravity of the blood along with the injectate volume. A calibration factor is also used. The cardiac output is inversely related to the area under a thermodilution curve, shown as a function of temperature versus time, with a smaller area under the curve indicative of a higher cardiac output (**Fig. 20-11**). Temperature fluctuation in the circuit can affect accuracy,[38] however, and the use of two thermistors can significantly improve the accuracy of this technique.[39]

The thermodilution method has several advantages. It obviates the need for withdrawal of blood from an arterial site and is less affected by recirculation. Perhaps its greatest advantage is the rapid display of results with computerized methods. However, a significant error occurs in patients with severe tricuspid regurgitation. Also, in patients with low outputs (especially <2.5 liter/min), thermodilution tends to overestimate the cardiac output.

FICK METHOD. The Fick principle assumes that the rate at which oxygen is consumed is a function of the rate of blood flow times the rate of oxygen pick-up by the red blood cells. The basic assumption is that the flow of blood in a given period is equal to the amount of substance entering the stream of flow in the same period divided by the difference between the concentrations of the substance in the blood upstream and downstream from its point of entry into the circulation (**Fig. 20-12**). The same number of red blood cells that enter the lung must leave the lung if no intracardiac shunt is present. Thus, if certain parameters are known (the number of oxygen molecules

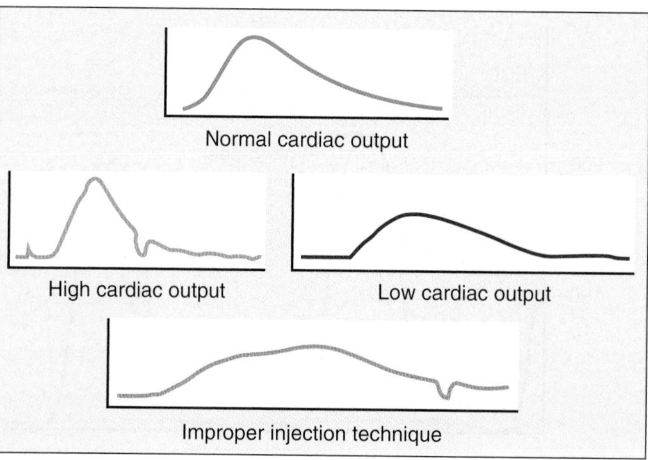

FIGURE 20-11 Thermodilution cardiac output curves. A normal curve has a sharp upstroke after an injection of saline. A smooth curve with a mildly prolonged downslope occurs until it is back to baseline. The area under the curve is inversely related to the cardiac output. At low cardiac output, a prolonged period is required to return to baseline. Therefore, there is a larger area under the curve. In a high cardiac output state, the cooler saline injectate moves faster through the right side of the heart, and temperature returns to baseline more quickly. The area under the curve is smaller and the output is higher.

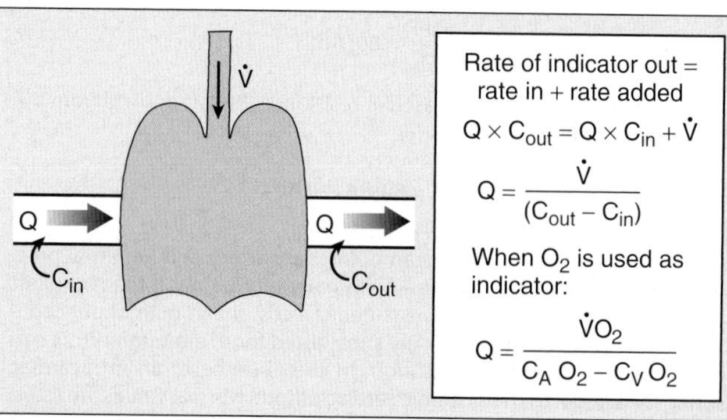

FIGURE 20-12 Schematic illustration of flow measurement by the Fick principle. Fluid containing a known concentration of an indicator (C_{in}) enters a system at flow rate Q. As the fluid passes through the system, indicator is continuously added at rate $\dot{V}$, raising the concentration in the outflow to C_{out}. In a steady state, the rate of indicator leaving the system (QC_{out}) must equal the rate at which it enters (QC_{in}) plus the rate at which it is added ($\dot{V}$). When oxygen is used as the indicator, cardiac output can be determined by measuring oxygen consumption ($\dot{V}O_2$), arterial oxygen content (C_AO_2), and mixed venous oxygen content (C_VO_2). *(From Winniford MD, Kern MJ, Lambert CR: Blood flow measurement.* In *Pepine CJ, Hill JA, Lambert CR [eds]: Diagnostic and Therapeutic Cardiac Catheterization. 3rd ed. Baltimore, Williams & Wilkins, 1998, p 400.)*

that are attached to the red blood cells entering the lung, the number of oxygen molecules that are attached to the red blood cells leaving the lung, and the number of oxygen molecules consumed during travel through the lung), the rate of flow of these red blood cells as they pass through the lung can be determined. This can be expressed in the following terms:

$$\text{Fick cardiac output (liter/min)} = \frac{\text{oxygen consumption (mL/min)}}{\text{A-VO}_2 \times 1.36 \times \text{Hgb} \times 10}$$

where A-VO_2 is the arterial-venous oxygen saturation difference, Hgb is the hemoglobin concentration (mg/dL), and the constant 1.36 is the oxygen-carrying capacity of hemoglobin (expressed in mL O_2/g Hgb).

Measurements must be made in the steady state. Automated methods can accurately determine the oxygen content within the blood samples. Thus, the greatest source of measurement variability is the oxygen consumption. In the original Fick determinations, expiratory gas samples were collected in a large bag during a specified period. By measurement of the expiratory oxygen concentration and knowing the concentration of oxygen in room air, the quantity of oxygen consumed over time could be determined. Currently, measurement of the expired oxygen concentration is quantified by use of a polarograph. This device can be connected to the patient by a plastic hood or by a mouthpiece and tubing.

The advantage of the Fick method is that it is the most accurate method in patients with low cardiac output and thus is preferred to the thermodilution method in these circumstances. It is also independent of the factors that affect curve shape and cause errors in thermodilution cardiac output (e.g., tricuspid regurgitation). The Fick method suffers primarily from the difficulty in obtaining accurate oxygen consumption measurements and the inability to obtain a steady state under certain conditions. Because the method assumes mean flow over time, it is not suitable during rapid changes in flow. Also, the patient cannot be receiving supplemental oxygen during blood sample collection. In patients with significant mitral or aortic regurgitation, the Fick cardiac output should not be used.

Many laboratories use an "assumed" Fick method, in which the oxygen consumption index is assumed on the basis of the patient's age, gender, and body surface area or an estimate is made (125 mL/m^2) on the basis of body surface area. However, when assumed oxygen consumption rather than measured oxygen consumption is used, large errors can occur.[40]

Angiographic Cardiac Output. Angiographic stroke volume can be calculated by tracing the LV end-diastolic and end-systolic images. Stroke volume is the quantity of blood ejected with each beat. End-diastolic volume is the maximum LV volume and occurs immediately before the onset of systole. It occurs immediately after atrial contraction in patients in sinus rhythm. End-systolic volume is the minimum LV volume during the cardiac cycle. Calibration of the images with grids or ventricular phantoms is necessary to obtain accurate ventricular volumes. Angiographic cardiac output and stroke volume are derived from the following equations:

$$\text{Stroke volume} = \text{EDV} - \text{ESV}$$

$$\text{Cardiac output} = (\text{EDV} - \text{ESV}) \times \text{heart rate}$$

where EDV is end-diastolic volume and ESV is end-systolic volume.

The inherent inaccuracies of calibrating angiographic volumes often make this method of measurement unreliable. In cases of valvular regurgitation or atrial fibrillation, angiographic cardiac output does not accurately measure true systemic outputs. However, the angiographic cardiac output is preferred to the Fick or thermodilution output for calculation of stenotic valve areas in patients with significant aortic or mitral regurgitation.

Determination of Vascular Resistance. Vascular resistance calculations are based on hydraulic principles of fluid flow, in which resistance is defined as the ratio of the decrease in pressure between two points in a vascular segment and the blood flow through the segment. Although this straightforward analogy to Ohm's law represents an oversimplification of the complex behavior of pulsatile flow in dynamic and diverse vascular beds, the calculation of vascular resistance based on these principles has proved to be of value in a number of clinical settings.

Determination of the resistance in a vascular bed requires measurement of the mean pressure of the proximal and distal ends of the vascular bed and accurate measurement of cardiac output. Vascular resistance (R) is usually defined in absolute units (dyne-sec • cm^{-5}) and is defined as R = [mean pressure gradient (dyne/cm^2)]/[mean flow (cm^3/sec)]. Hybrid units (Wood units) are less often used.[41]

Systemic vascular resistance (SVR) in absolute units is calculated by the following equation:

$$\frac{\text{SVR}}{Q_s} = 80(\text{Ao}_m - \text{RA}_m)$$

where Ao_m and RA_m are the mean pressures (in mm Hg) in the aorta and right atrium, respectively, and Q_s is the systemic cardiac output (in liters/min). The constant 80 is used to convert units from mm Hg/liter/min (Wood units) to the absolute resistance units dyne-sec • cm^{-5}. If the right atrial pressure is not known, the term RA_m can be dropped, and the resulting value is called the total peripheral resistance (TPR):

$$\frac{TPR}{Q_s} = 80(Ao_m)$$

Similarly, the pulmonary vascular resistance (PVR) is derived from the following equation:

$$\frac{PVR}{Q_p} = 80(PA_m - LA_m)$$

where PA_m and LA_m are the mean pulmonary artery and left atrial pressures, respectively, and Q_p is the pulmonary blood flow. If the mean left atrial pressure has not been measured directly, mean pulmonary capillary wedge pressure is commonly substituted for it, although errors can occur because of this substitution. In the absence of an intracardiac shunt, Q_p is equal to the systemic cardiac output. Normal values are listed in Table 20-3.

Elevated resistances in the systemic and pulmonary circuits may represent reversible abnormalities or may be permanent because of irreversible anatomic changes. In several clinical situations, such as congestive heart failure, valvular heart disease, primary pulmonary hypertension, and congenital heart disease with intracardiac shunting, determination of whether elevated SVR or PVR can be lowered transiently in the catheterization laboratory may provide important insights into potential management strategies. Interventions that may be used in the laboratory for this purpose include administration of vasodilating drugs (e.g., sodium nitroprusside), exercise, and (in patients with pulmonary hypertension) nitric oxide inhalation or intravenous epoprostenol (Flolan), a pulmonary and systemic vasodilator (see Chap. 78).

Vascular impedance measurements account for blood viscosity, pulsatile flow, reflected waves, and arterial compliance. Hence, vascular impedance has the potential to describe the dynamic relation between pressure and flow more comprehensively than is possible with the simpler calculations of vascular resistance. However, because the simultaneous pressure and flow data required for the calculation of impedance are complex and difficult to obtain, the concept of impedance has failed to gain widespread acceptance, and vascular impedance has not been adopted as a routine clinical index.

Evaluation of Valvular Stenosis

Determination of the severity of valvular stenosis on the basis of the pressure gradient and flow across the valve is one of the most important aspects of evaluation of patients with valvular heart disease (see Chap. 66). In many patients, the magnitude of the pressure gradient alone is sufficient to distinguish clinically significant from insignificant valvular stenosis.

DETERMINATION OF PRESSURE GRADIENTS

Aortic Stenosis

In patients with aortic stenosis, the transvalvular pressure gradient is best measured with a catheter in the left ventricle and another in the proximal aorta. Although it is convenient to measure the gradient between the left ventricle and the femoral artery, downstream augmentation of the pressure signal and delay in pressure transmission between the proximal aorta and femoral artery may alter the pressure waveform substantially and introduce errors into the measured gradient.[37]

LV–femoral artery pressure gradients may suffice in many patients as an estimate of the severity of aortic stenosis to confirm the presence of a severely stenotic valve. If the side port of the arterial introducing sheath is used to monitor femoral pressure, the inner diameter of the sheath should be at least 1F size larger than the outer diameter of the LV catheter.

The operator should obtain simultaneous ascending aortic and femoral artery pressures to verify similarity between the two sites. The LV–femoral artery pressure gradient may not always be relied on in the calculation of valve orifice area in patients with moderate valve gradients. A careful single catheter pull-back from left ventricle to aorta is often preferable to simultaneous measurement of LV and femoral artery pressures.

A single catheter with a distal and a proximal lumen or a micromanometer catheter with distal and proximal transducers is preferable for simultaneous measurement of LV pressure and central aortic

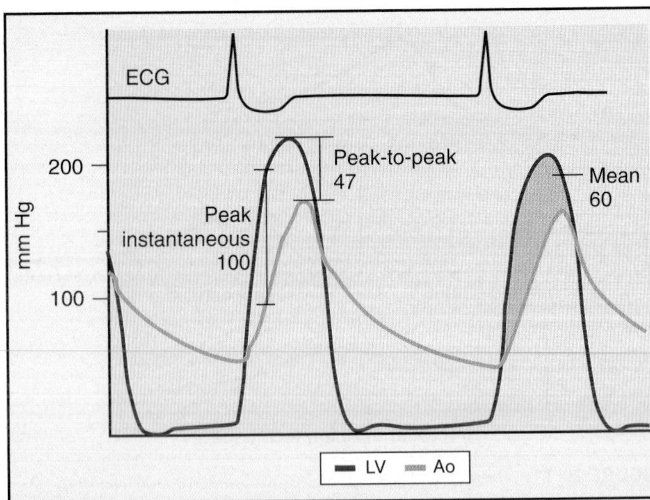

FIGURE 20-13 Various methods of describing an aortic transvalvular gradient. The peak-to-peak gradient (47 mm Hg) is the difference between the maximal pressure in the aorta (Ao) and the maximal left ventricle (LV) pressure. The peak instantaneous gradient (100 mm Hg) is the maximal pressure difference between the Ao and LV when the pressures are measured in the same moment (usually during early systole). The mean gradient (green shaded area) is the integral of the pressure difference between the LV and Ao during systole (60 mm Hg). *(From Bashore TM: Invasive Cardiology: Principles and Techniques. Philadelphia, BC Decker, 1990.)*

pressure. Another method is to use a long arterial catheter in the aorta and the second in the left ventricle.

The mean pressure gradient across the aortic valve is determined by planimetry of the area separating the LV and aortic pressures using multiple beats (**Fig. 20-13**), and it is this gradient that is applied to calculation of the valve orifice area. The peak-to-peak gradient, measured as the difference between peak LV pressure and peak aortic pressure, is commonly used to quantify the valve gradient because this measurement is rapidly obtained and can be estimated visually. However, there is no physiologic basis for the peak-to-peak gradient because the maximum LV and aortic pressures rarely occur simultaneously. The peak-to-peak gradient measured in the catheterization laboratory is generally lower than the peak instantaneous gradient measured in the echocardiography laboratory. This is because the peak instantaneous gradient represents the maximum pressure difference between the left ventricle and aorta when pressures are measured simultaneously. This maximum pressure difference occurs on the upslope of the aortic pressure tracing (see Fig. 20-13). Mean aortic transvalvular gradient and aortic valve area are well correlated with both techniques.[42] In patients with low-gradient low-output aortic stenosis, pharmacologic maneuvers can be helpful (see section on **pharmacologic maneuvers**).

Mitral Stenosis

In patients with mitral stenosis, the most accurate means of determining the mitral valve gradient is measurement of left atrial pressure by the transseptal technique with simultaneous measurement of LV pressure and with planimetry of the area bounded by the LV and left atrial pressures in diastole using several cardiac cycles (**Fig. 20-14**). The pulmonary capillary wedge pressure is usually substituted for the left atrial pressure, as the pulmonary wedge pressure is more readily obtained. The pulmonary wedge pressure tracing must be realigned with the LV tracing for accurate mean gradient determination. Although it has been generally accepted that pulmonary capillary wedge pressure is a satisfactory estimate of left atrial pressure, studies indicate that the pulmonary wedge pressure may systematically overestimate the left atrial pressure by 2 to 3 mm Hg, thereby increasing the measured mitral valve gradient.[36] Improperly wedged catheters, resulting in damped pulmonary artery pressure recordings, further overestimate the severity of mitral stenosis. If there is doubt about accurate positioning of the catheter in the wedge position, the position

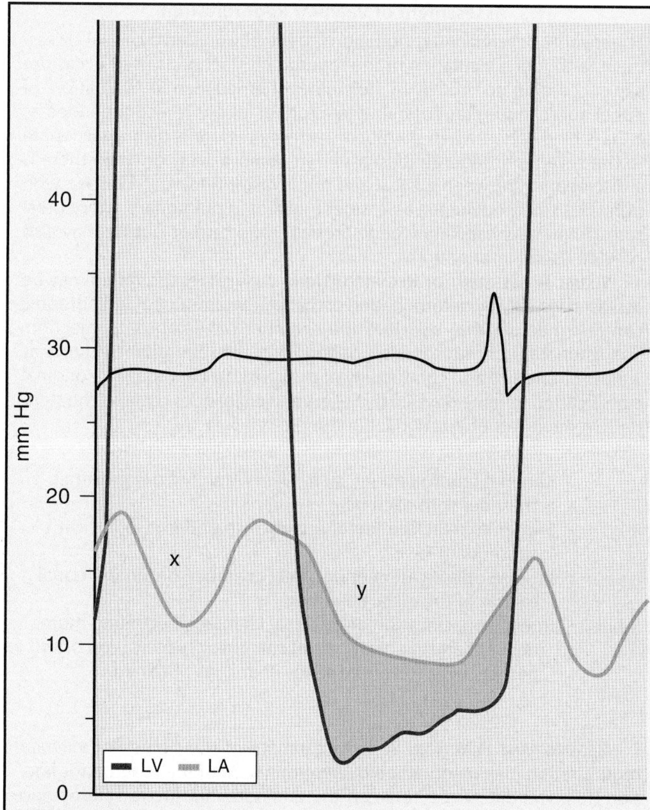

FIGURE 20-14 Pressure gradient in a patient with mitral stenosis. The pressure in the left atrium (LA) exceeds the pressure in the left ventricle (LV) during diastole, producing a diastolic pressure gradient (green shaded area). *(From Bashore TM: Invasive Cardiology: Principles and Techniques. Philadelphia, BC Decker, 1990.)*

can be confirmed by slow withdrawal of blood for oximetric analysis. An oxygen saturation equal to that of the systemic circulation confirms the wedge position.

Right-Sided Valvular Stenosis

In pulmonic stenosis, the valve gradient is obtained by a catheter pullback from the pulmonary artery to the right ventricle or by placement of separate catheters in the right ventricle and pulmonary artery. Multilumen catheters can also be used for simultaneous pressure recordings. Tricuspid valve gradients should be assessed with simultaneous recording of right atrial and RV pressures.

CALCULATION OF STENOTIC VALVE ORIFICE AREAS. The stenotic orifice area is determined from the pressure gradient and cardiac output with the formula developed by Gorlin and Gorlin from the fundamental hydraulic relationships linking the area of an orifice to the flow and pressure drop across the orifice. Flow (F) and orifice area (A) are related by the fundamental formula

$$F = cAV$$

where V is velocity of flow and c is a constant accounting for central streaming of fluid through an orifice, which tends to reduce the effective orifice size. Hence,

$$A = F/cV$$

Velocity is related to the pressure gradient through the relation $V = k(2g\Delta P)^{1/2}$, where k is a constant accounting for frictional energy loss, g is the acceleration due to gravity (980 cm/sec^2), and ΔP is the mean pressure gradient (mm Hg). Substituting for V in the orifice area equation and combining c and k into one constant C,

$$A = \frac{F}{44.3C\sqrt{(\Delta P)}}$$

Gorlin and Gorlin determined the value of the constant C by comparing the calculated valve area with actual valve area measured at autopsy or at surgery in 11 mitral valves. The maximal discrepancy between the actual mitral valve area and calculated values was only 0.2 cm^2 when the constant 0.85 was used. No data were obtained for aortic valves, a limitation noted by the Gorlins, and a constant of 1.0 was assumed.

Because flow across the aortic valve occurs only in systole, the flow value for calculating aortic valve area is the cardiac output in milliliters per minute divided by the systolic ejection period (SEP) in seconds per beat times the heart rate (HR) in beats per minute. The systolic ejection period is defined from aortic valve opening to closure. Hence, the aortic valve area (AVA) is calculated from the Gorlin formula by the following equation:

$$\text{AVA}(\text{cm}^2) = \frac{\text{cardiac output (liters/min)} \times 1000}{(44.3)(\text{HR})(\text{SEP})\sqrt{\text{mean gradient}}}$$

Similarly, as mitral flow occurs only in diastole, the cardiac output is corrected for the diastolic filling period (DFP) in seconds per beat in the equation for mitral valve area (MVA), where the diastolic filling period is defined from mitral valve opening to mitral valve closure:

$$\text{MVA}(\text{cm}^2) = \frac{\text{cardiac output (liters/min)} \times 1000}{(37.7)(\text{HR})(\text{DFP})\sqrt{\text{mean gradient}}}$$

The normal aortic valve area is 2.6 to 3.5 cm^2 in adults. Valve areas of less than 1.0 cm^2 represent severe aortic stenosis (see Chap. 66). The normal mitral valve area is 4 to 6 cm^2, and severe mitral stenosis is present with valve areas of less than 1.0 cm^2.

The calculated valve area is often crucial in management decisions for patients with aortic stenosis or mitral stenosis. Hence, it is essential that accurate and simultaneous pressure gradient and cardiac output determinations be made, especially in patients with borderline or low-pressure gradients.

There are limitations of the Gorlin-derived orifice area. As the square root of the mean gradient is used in the Gorlin formula, the valve area calculation is more strongly influenced by the cardiac output than the pressure gradient. Thus, errors in measuring cardiac output may have profound effects on the calculated valve area, particularly in patients with low cardiac outputs, in whom the calculated valve area is often of greatest importance.

As noted previously, the thermodilution technique may provide inaccurate cardiac output data when cardiac output is reduced or when concomitant aortic, mitral, or tricuspid regurgitation is present. Thus, the Fick method of determining cardiac output is the most accurate for assessing cardiac output, especially in low-output states. In patients with mixed valvular disease (stenosis and regurgitation) of the same valve, the use of forward flow as determined by the Fick method or thermodilution technique overestimates the severity of the valvular stenosis. This overestimation occurs because the Gorlin formula depends on total forward flow across the stenotic valve, not net forward flow. If valvular regurgitation is present, the angiographic cardiac output is the most appropriate measure of flow. If both aortic and mitral regurgitation are present, flow across a single valve cannot be determined, and neither aortic valve area nor mitral valve area can be assessed accurately.

Other potential errors and limitations are inherent in the use of the Gorlin formula, related both to inaccuracies in measurement of valve gradients and to more fundamental issues regarding the validity of the assumptions underlying the formula. In low-output states, the Gorlin formula may systematically predict smaller valve areas than are actually present. Several lines of evidence indicate that the aortic valve area from the Gorlin formula increases with increases in cardiac output. Although this may represent an actual greater opening of stenotic valves by the higher proximal opening pressures that result from increases in transvalvular flow, the flow dependence of the calculated valve area may also reflect inherent errors in the assumptions underlying the Gorlin formula, particularly with respect to the aortic valve.

The increase in Gorlin valve area with increases in transvalvular flow is not associated with alterations in direct planimetry of the aortic valve area by transesophageal echocardiography. This suggests that flow-related variation in the Gorlin aortic valve area is due to disproportional flow dependence of the formula and not a true change in the valve area.[43]

An alternative simplified formula to determine valve areas has been proposed. The effects of the systolic ejection period and the diastolic filling period are relatively constant at normal heart rates, and these terms can be eliminated from the equation. This assumes that (44.3 × HR × SEP) ≈ 1000 in most circumstances. In this modified approach, the aortic valve area can be quickly estimated from the following formula:

$$\text{AVA}\left(\text{cm}^2\right) = \frac{\text{cardiac output (liters/min)}}{\sqrt{\text{peak to peak or mean gradient (mm Hg)}}}$$

Use of either the mean aortic transvalvular gradient or the peak-to-peak gradient produces similar correlation with the Gorlin formula.

Patients with low-output, low-gradient aortic stenosis remain a challenge for accurate determination of valve area by either cardiac catheterization or echocardiography (see Chaps. 15 and 66). Whether afterload mismatch or intrinsic contractility dysfunction is the primary problem in ventricular impairment can be difficult to ascertain. Thus, the use of pharmacologic stress with low-dose dobutamine infusion has been advocated to distinguish moderate from severe aortic stenosis.[44-46] The concept is that patients without true anatomic severe aortic stenosis will have an increase in valve areas with little change in transvalvular gradient.[2] If dobutamine increases the aortic valve area more than 0.2 cm^2 with no change in gradient, it is likely that the baseline evaluation overestimated the severity of aortic stenosis.[2] It has also been shown that patients who increase stroke volume by less than 20% lack contractile reserve and have a poor prognosis with either medical or surgical therapy.[45]

Despite theoretical limitations, the Gorlin formula has proved to be a reliable clinical determination for evaluation of patients with suspected aortic stenosis.

Measurement of Intraventricular Pressure Gradients

The demonstration of an intracavitary pressure gradient is among the most interesting yet challenging aspects of diagnostic catheterization (see Chap. 69). Simultaneous pressure measurements are obtained in either the central aorta or femoral artery and from within the ventricular cavity. Pull-back of a multipurpose end-hole catheter from the ventricular apex to a posterior position just beneath the aortic valve demonstrates an intracavitary gradient. An erroneous intracavitary gradient may be seen if the catheter becomes entrapped by the hypertrophic myocardium.

The intracavitary gradient is distinguished from aortic valvular stenosis by the loss of the aortic–LV gradient when the catheter is still within the left ventricle yet proximal to the myocardial obstruction. In addition, careful analysis of the upstroke of the aortic pressure waveform distinguishes a valvular from a subvalvular stenosis, as the aortic pressure waveform demonstrates a slow upstroke in aortic stenosis. Other methods to localize intracavitary gradients include the use of a dual-lumen catheter, use of a double-sensor micromanometer catheter, or placement of an end-hole catheter in the LV outflow tract while a transseptal catheter is advanced into the left ventricle, with pressure measured simultaneously. An intracavitary gradient may be increased by various provocative maneuvers including the Valsalva maneuver, inhalation of amyl nitrate, introduction of a premature ventricular beat, or isoproterenol infusion (see Physiologic and Pharmacologic Maneuvers).

Assessment of Valvular Regurgitation

The severity of valvular regurgitation is generally graded by visual assessment, although calculation of the regurgitant fraction is used occasionally. According to ACC/AHA guidelines, hemodynamic evaluation of either aortic regurgitant or mitral regurgitant lesions is recommended as a Class I indication when pulmonary artery pressure is disproportionate to the severity of regurgitation assessed noninvasively or when there is a discrepancy between clinical and noninvasive findings.[2] Exercise with right-heart hemodynamic assessment including pulmonary artery pressure, pulmonary capillary wedge pressure, and cardiac output may also provide useful information.

Visual Assessment of Regurgitation. Valvular regurgitation may be assessed visually by determination of the relative amount of radiographic contrast medium that opacifies the chamber proximal to its injection. The estimation of regurgitation depends on the regurgitant volume as well as on the size and contractility of the proximal chamber. The original classification scheme devised by Sellers and colleagues remains the standard in most catheterization laboratories:

+	Minimal regurgitant jet seen. Clears rapidly from proximal chamber with each beat.
++	Moderate opacification of proximal chamber, clearing with subsequent beats.
+++	Intense opacification of proximal chamber, becoming equal to that of the distal chamber.
++++	Intense opacification of proximal chamber, becoming more dense than that of the distal chamber. Opacification often persists over the entire series of images obtained.

Regurgitant Fraction. A gross estimate of the degree of valvular regurgitation may be obtained by determination of the regurgitant fraction (RF). The difference between the angiographic stroke volume and the forward stroke volume can be defined as the regurgitant stroke volume.

$$\text{Regurgitant stroke volume} = \text{angiographic stroke volume} - \text{forward stroke volume}$$

The RF is that portion of the angiographic stroke volume that does not contribute to the net cardiac output. Forward stroke volume is the cardiac output determined by the Fick or thermodilution method divided by the heart rate. Thermodilution cardiac output cannot be used if there is significant concomitant tricuspid regurgitation.

Compared with visual interpretation, 1+ regurgitation is roughly equivalent to an RF of 20% or less, 2+ to an RF of 21% to 40%, 3+ to an RF of 41% to 60%, and 4+ to an RF of more than 60%.

The assumption underlying the determination of RF is that the angiographic and forward cardiac outputs are accurate and comparable, a state requiring similar heart rates, stable hemodynamic states between measurements, and only a single regurgitant valve. Given these conditions, the equation yields only a gross approximation of regurgitant flow.

Shunt Determinations

Normally, pulmonary blood flow and systemic blood flow are equal. With an abnormal communication between intracardiac chambers or great vessels, blood flow is shunted from the systemic circulation to the pulmonary circulation (left-to-right shunt), from the pulmonary circulation to the systemic circulation (right-to-left shunt), or in both directions (bidirectional shunt). The most commonly used method for shunt determination in the cardiac catheterization laboratory is the oximetric method. Although many shunts are suspected before cardiac catheterization, physicians performing the procedure should be vigilant in determining the cause of unexpected findings. For example, an unexplained pulmonary artery oxygen saturation exceeding 80% should raise the operator's suspicion of a left-to-right shunt, whereas unexplained arterial desaturation (<93%) may indicate a right-to-left shunt.[47] Arterial desaturation commonly results from alveolar hypoventilation and associated "physiologic shunting," the causes of which include oversedation from premedication, pulmonary disease, pulmonary venous congestion, pulmonary edema, and cardiogenic shock. If arterial desaturation persists after the patient takes several deep breaths or after administration of 100% oxygen, a right-to-left shunt is likely.

Oximetric Method. The oximetric method is based on blood sampling from various cardiac chambers for the determination of oxygen saturation. A left-to-right shunt is detected when a significant increase in blood oxygen saturation is found between two right-sided vessels or chambers.

A screening oxygen saturation measurement for any left-to-right shunt is often performed with right-heart catheterization by sampling of blood in the SVC and the pulmonary artery. If the difference in oxygen saturation between these samples is 8% or more, a left-to-right shunt may be present, and an oximetry "run" should be performed. This run obtains blood samples from all right-sided locations, including the SVC, IVC, right atrium, right ventricle, and pulmonary artery. In cases of interatrial or interventricular shunts, it is recommended to obtain multiple samples from the high, middle, and low right atrium or the RV inflow tract, apex, and outflow tract to localize the level of the shunt. One may miss a small left-to-right shunt using the right atrium for screening purposes rather than the SVC because of incomplete mixing of blood in the right atrium, which receives blood from the IVC, SVC, and coronary sinus. Oxygen saturation in the IVC is higher than in the SVC because the kidneys use less oxygen relative to their blood flow than do other organs, whereas coronary sinus blood has very low oxygen saturation. Mixed venous saturation is most accurately measured in the pulmonary artery after complete mixing has occurred or can be calculated by IVC + SVC samples (see Shunt Quantification).

A full saturation run obtains samples from the high and low IVC; high and low SVC; high, middle, and low right atrium; RV inflow and outflow tracts and midcavity; main pulmonary artery; left or right pulmonary artery; pulmonary vein and left atrium, if possible; left ventricle; and distal aorta. When a right-to-left shunt must be localized, oxygen saturation samples must be taken from the pulmonary veins, left atrium, left ventricle, and aorta. Although the major weakness of the oxygen step-up method is its lack of sensitivity, clinically significant shunts are generally detected by this technique. Obtaining multiple samples from each chamber can improve sampling error and variability. Another method of oximetric determination of intracardiac shunts uses a balloon-tipped fiberoptic catheter that allows continuous registration of oxygen saturation as it is withdrawn from the pulmonary artery through the right-heart chambers into the SVC and IVC.

SHUNT QUANTIFICATION. The principles used to determine Fick cardiac output are also used to quantify intracardiac shunts. To determine the size of a left-to-right shunt, pulmonary blood flow (PBF) and systemic blood flow (SBF) determinations are required. PBF is simply oxygen consumption divided by the difference in oxygen content across the pulmonary bed, whereas SBF is oxygen consumption divided by the difference in oxygen content across the systemic bed. The effective blood flow (EBF) is the fraction of mixed venous return received by the lungs without contamination by the shunt flow. In the absence of a shunt, PBF, SBF, and EBF all are equal. These equations are as follows:

$$\text{PBF} = \frac{\text{O}_2\ \text{consumption (mL/min)}}{(\text{PVO}_2 - \text{PAO}_2)}$$

$$\text{SBF} = \frac{\text{O}_2\ \text{consumption (mL/min)}}{(\text{SAO}_2 - \text{MVO}_2)}$$

$$\text{EBF} = \frac{\text{O}_2\ \text{consumption (mL/min)}}{(\text{PVO}_2 - \text{MVO}_2)}$$

where PVO_2, PAO_2, SAO_2, and MVO_2 are the oxygen contents (in milliliters of oxygen per liter of blood) of pulmonary venous, pulmonary arterial, systemic arterial, and mixed venous bloods, respectively. The oxygen content is determined as outlined in the section on Fick cardiac output.

If a pulmonary vein is not sampled, systemic arterial oxygen content may be substituted, assuming systemic arterial saturation is 95% or more. As discussed earlier, if systemic arterial saturation is less than 93%, a right-to-left shunt may be present. If arterial desaturation is present but not secondary to a right-to-left shunt, systemic arterial oxygen content is used. If a right-to-left shunt is present, pulmonary venous oxygen content is calculated as 98% of the oxygen capacity.

The mixed venous oxygen content is the average oxygen content of the blood in the chamber proximal to the shunt. When assessing a left-to-right shunt at the level of the right atrium, one must calculate mixed venous oxygen content on the basis of the contributing blood flow from the IVC, SVC, and coronary sinus. The most common method used is the Flamm formula:

$$\text{MVO}_2 = \frac{3(\text{SVC O}_2\ \text{content}) + 1(\text{IVC O}_2\ \text{content})}{4}$$

Assuming conservation of mass, the size of a left-to-right shunt, when there is no associated right-to-left shunt, is simply

$$\text{L} \rightarrow \text{R shunt} = \text{PBF} - \text{SBF}$$

When there is evidence of a right-to-left shunt in addition to a left-to-right shunt, the approximate left-to-right shunt size is

$$\text{L} \rightarrow \text{R shunt} = \text{PBF} - \text{EBF}$$

and the approximate right-to-left shunt size is

$$\text{R} \rightarrow \text{L shunt} = \text{SBF} - \text{EBF}$$

The flow ratio PBF/SBF (or Q_p/Q_s) is used clinically to determine the significance of the shunt. A ratio of less than 1.5 indicates a small left-to-right shunt, and a ratio of 1.5 to 2.0, a moderate-sized shunt. A ratio of 2.0 or more indicates a large left-to-right shunt and generally requires percutaneous or surgical repair to prevent future pulmonary or RV complications. A flow ratio of less than 1.0 indicates a net right-to-left shunt. If oxygen consumption is not measured, the pulmonic-to-systemic blood flow ratio may be calculated as follows:

$$Q_p/Q_s = \text{PBF/SBF} = \frac{(\text{SAO}_2 - \text{MVO}_2)}{(\text{PVO}_2 - \text{PAO}_2)}$$

where SAO_2, MVO_2, PVO_2, and PAO_2 are systemic arterial, mixed venous, pulmonary venous, and pulmonary arterial blood oxygen saturations, respectively.

INDICATOR-DILUTION METHOD. Although the indicator-dilution method is more sensitive than the oximetric method in detection of small shunts, it cannot be used to localize the level of a left-to-right shunt. An indicator such as indocyanine green dye is injected into a proximal chamber while a sample is taken from a distal chamber with a densitometer, and the density of dye is displayed over time. To detect a left-to-right shunt, dye is injected into the pulmonary artery and sampling is performed in a systemic artery. Presence of a shunt is indicated by early recirculation of the dye on the downslope of the curve.

Physiologic and Pharmacologic Maneuvers

Potentially significant cardiac abnormalities may be absent in the resting condition but may be unmasked by stress. Therefore, if the physician performing a cardiac catheterization procedure cannot elucidate the cause of a patient's symptoms at rest, various physiologic and pharmacologic maneuvers can be considered.

Dynamic Exercise

Dynamic exercise in the catheterization laboratory is performed by supine bicycle ergometry, upright bicycle exercise, or straight arm raises. Upright treadmill exercise can be performed outside the catheterization laboratory by use of a balloon flotation catheter inserted through an antecubital or internal jugular vein to measure pulmonary artery and wedge pressures and cardiac output. The associated changes in the heart rate, cardiac output, oxygen consumption, and intracardiac pressures are monitored at rest and during progressive stages of exercise. Normally, the increased oxygen requirements of exercise are met by an increase in cardiac output and an increase in oxygen extraction from arterial blood. Patients with cardiac dysfunction are unable to increase their cardiac output appropriately in response to exercise and must meet the demands of the exercising muscle groups by increasing the extraction of oxygen from arterial blood, thereby increasing the arteriovenous oxygen difference. The relationship between cardiac output and oxygen consumption is linear, and a regression formula can be used to calculate the predicted cardiac index at a given level of oxygen consumption. The actual cardiac index divided by the predicted cardiac index is defined as the exercise index (see Chap. 14). A value of 0.8 or more indicates a normal cardiac output response to exercise. The exercise factor is another method of describing the same relationship between the cardiac output and oxygen consumption. The exercise factor is the increase in cardiac output divided by the increase in oxygen consumption. Normally, for every 100 mL/min increase in oxygen consumption with exercise, the cardiac output should increase by at least 600 mL/min. Therefore, a normal exercise factor should be 6 or more.[48]

Supine exercise normally causes a rise in mean systemic and pulmonary arterial pressures. There is a proportionately greater decrease in SVR compared with PVR and an increase in heart rate. Myocardial contractility increases from both increased sympathetic tone and the increase in heart rate. LV ejection fraction rises. During early levels of exercise, increased venous return augments LV end-diastolic volume, leading to an increase in stroke volume. At progressively higher levels of exercise, both LV end-systolic and end-diastolic volumes decrease so that there is a negligible rise in stroke volume. Thus, the augmentation in cardiac output during peak exercise in the catheterization laboratory is generally caused by an increase in heart rate. For this reason, all agents that may impair the chronotropic response should be discontinued before catheterization if exercise is contemplated during the procedure.

Exercise may provoke symptoms in a patient who had been found to have valvular disease of borderline significance in the resting state (see Chap. 66). Exercise increases transvalvular mitral gradient and pulmonary artery pressures in mitral stenosis.

The hemodynamic response to exercise is also useful in evaluating regurgitant valvular lesions. Clinically important valvular regurgitation exists if an increase occurs in LV end-diastolic pressure, pulmonary capillary wedge pressure, and SVR, in conjunction with a reduced exercise index (<0.8) and abnormal exercise factor (<0.6). Simultaneous echocardiographic evaluation of valvular regurgitation is also useful in equivocal cases. Patients with myocardial disease, ischemic or otherwise, may have pronounced increases in LV end-diastolic pressure with exercise.

Pacing Tachycardia

Rapid atrial or ventricular pacing increases myocardial oxygen consumption and myocardial blood flow. With pacing, in contradistinction to dynamic exercise, LV end-diastolic volume decreases, and there is little change in cardiac output.[49] This method may be used to determine the significance of coronary artery disease or valvular abnormalities. For example, the gradient across the mitral valve increases with rapid atrial pacing because of the increase in heart rate. Pacing has the advantage of allowing greater control and rapid termination of the induced stress.

Physiologic Stress

Various physiologic stresses alter the severity of obstruction in hypertrophic cardiomyopathy (see Chap. 69). The Valsalva maneuver (forcible expiration against a closed glottis) increases the systolic subaortic pressure gradient in the strain phase, during which there is a decrease in venous return and decreased LV volume. This maneuver is also abnormal in patients with congestive heart failure. Another useful maneuver in patients with hypertrophic obstructive cardiomyopathy is the introduction of a premature ventricular beat (Brockenbrough maneuver). Premature ventricular contractions normally increase the pulse pressure of the subsequent ventricular beat. In obstructive hypertrophic cardiomyopathy, the outflow gradient is increased during the post-premature beat with a decrease in the pulse pressure of the aortic contour. A premature ventricular beat may also accentuate the spike-and-dome configuration of the aortic pressure waveform.

Rapid volume loading may reveal occult pericardial constriction (see Chap. 75), when atrial and ventricular filling pressures are relatively normal under baseline conditions as a result of hypovolemia, and can help distinguish pericardial constriction from myocardial restriction. The Kussmaul sign occurs in pericardial constriction. With inspiration, it is demonstrated when mean right atrial pressure fails to decrease or actually increases in relation to impaired RV filling. The ratio of RV to LV systolic pressure–time area during inspiration compared with expiration is called the systolic area index.[50] This is a measure of enhanced ventricular interdependence[51] (**Fig. 20-15**). The index is significantly higher in those with proven constrictive pericarditis compared with restrictive cardiomyopathy (1.4 ± 0.2 versus 0.92 ± 0.019; $P < 0.0001$), with a sensitivity of 97% and predicted accuracy of 100% for identification of constriction.

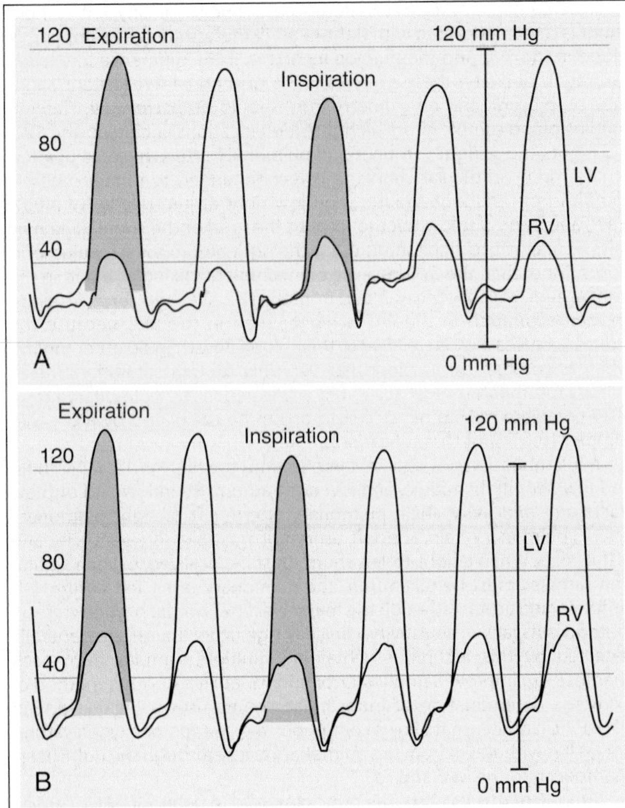

FIGURE 20-15 Left ventricular (LV) and right ventricular (RV) high-fidelity manometer pressure traces from two patients during expiration and inspiration. Both patients have early rapid filling and elevation and end-equalization of the LV and RV pressures at end-expiration. **A,** A patient with surgically documented constrictive pericarditis. During inspiration, there is an increase in the area of the RV pressure curve (yellow shaded area) compared with expiration. The area of the LV pressure curve (green shaded area) decreases during inspiration compared with expiration. **B,** A patient with restrictive myocardial disease documented by endomyocardial biopsy. During inspiration, there is a decrease in the area of the RV pressure curve (yellow shaded area) compared with expiration. The area of the LV pressure curve (green shaded area) is unchanged during inspiration compared with expiration.

Pharmacologic Maneuvers

Dobutamine infusion during cardiac catheterization is indicated in patients with low-flow, low-gradient aortic stenosis (see Chaps. 15 and 66).[2,46] In patients with a mean gradient below 30 mm Hg, low cardiac output, and low ejection fraction (<40%), the Gorlin formula may not reflect the true valve area. Provocation with dobutamine infusion can assist in distinguishing intrinsic contractile dysfunction versus afterload mismatch from valvular stenosis. Up to one third of patients with low-output severe aortic stenosis as calculated by the Gorlin formula may have pseudosevere aortic stenosis.[52]

Resting hemodynamics including transvalvular gradient, cardiac output, and aortic valve area should be determined. Dobutamine is infused at 5 µg/kg/min and increased by 3 to 10 µg/kg/min every 5 minutes with a maximum of 40 µg/kg/min, mean gradient above 40 mm Hg, 50% increase in the cardiac output, or heart rate above 140 beats per minute. Patients with a final aortic valve area smaller than 1.2 cm^2 and mean gradient above 30 mm Hg are considered to have severe aortic stenosis.[44]

Nitric oxide is an endothelium-derived vasodilator with selective pulmonary vasodilator properties that is useful in evaluating patients with pulmonary hypertension (see Chap. 78). Inhaled nitric oxide is rapidly inactivated, in contrast to intravenous vasodilators, which can cause severe systemic hypotension.[53] It has been well established that lowering of pulmonary artery pressure with vasodilators predicts a favorable clinical outcome.

Inhaled nitric oxide can safely and effectively assess the capacity of a patient for pulmonary vasodilator response without causing systemic hypotension. It can accurately predict a response to subsequent medical therapy.[54] Doses of 10, 20, 40, or 80 parts per million can be tested during 5- to 10-minute intervals with serial sampling of mean pulmonary artery pressure and calculation of PVR and cardiac output. The definition of an acute response that may warrant initiation of long-term therapy with oral calcium channel blockers is a decrease in the mean pulmonary artery pressure of at least 10 mm Hg to an absolute mean pulmonary artery pressure of less than 40 mm Hg without a decrease in cardiac output.

Sodium nitroprusside infusion may improve the cardiac output and filling pressures in patients with dilated cardiomyopathies and in patients with mitral regurgitation by lowering SVR and PVR. A favorable response to sodium nitroprusside infusion may predict a good clinical outcome.

Agents that increase SVR, such as phenylephrine, reduce the gradient in obstructive hypertrophic cardiomyopathy. This can be used to improve acute systemic hypertension in patients with hypertrophic cardiomyopathy (see Chap. 69).

Isoproterenol infusion may be used to simulate supine dynamic exercise, although untoward side effects limit its applicability. This drug's positive inotropic and chronotropic effects can increase the gradient in obstructive hypertrophic cardiomyopathy and mitral stenosis. Nitroglycerin and amyl nitrate decrease preload and accentuate the systolic gradient in patients with obstructive hypertrophic cardiomyopathy. Amyl nitrate is generally inhaled, and its onset and offset of action are rapid.

Adjunctive Diagnostic Techniques

Left Ventricular Electromechanical Mapping

Advances in catheter design and navigational technology have resulted in catheter-based three-dimensional mapping systems for evaluation of regional and global LV function. The system provides simultaneous electrical, mechanical, and anatomic information.[55]

Electromechanical LV maps can distinguish viable from nonviable myocardium and ischemic from nonischemic myocardium and correlate with thallium uptake.[56]

The mapping system can predict recovery of function after revascularization, providing on-line assessment of viability.[57] This technique holds promise for guiding local delivery of myocardial regeneration therapies, such as stem cell injection.[58]

Intracardiac Echocardiography

Intracardiac echocardiography (ICE) is used for transvenous imaging within the cardiac chambers. It consists of an 8F or 10F, 90-cm-long catheter that permits two planes of bidirectional steering in the anterior-posterior and left-right direction. The transducer has variable frequencies of 5 to 10 MHz with multiple phased array features, including two-dimensional imaging and color and spectral Doppler analysis.

ICE provides imaging of interatrial or interventricular septum and left-heart structures from either the right atrium or ventricle, with penetration up to 15 cm. Applications include guidance of percutaneous atrial septal defect and patent foramen ovale closures, thus mitigating the need for transesophageal echocardiography and anesthesia (**Fig. 20-16**). In patients requiring transseptal puncture, ICE can facilitate

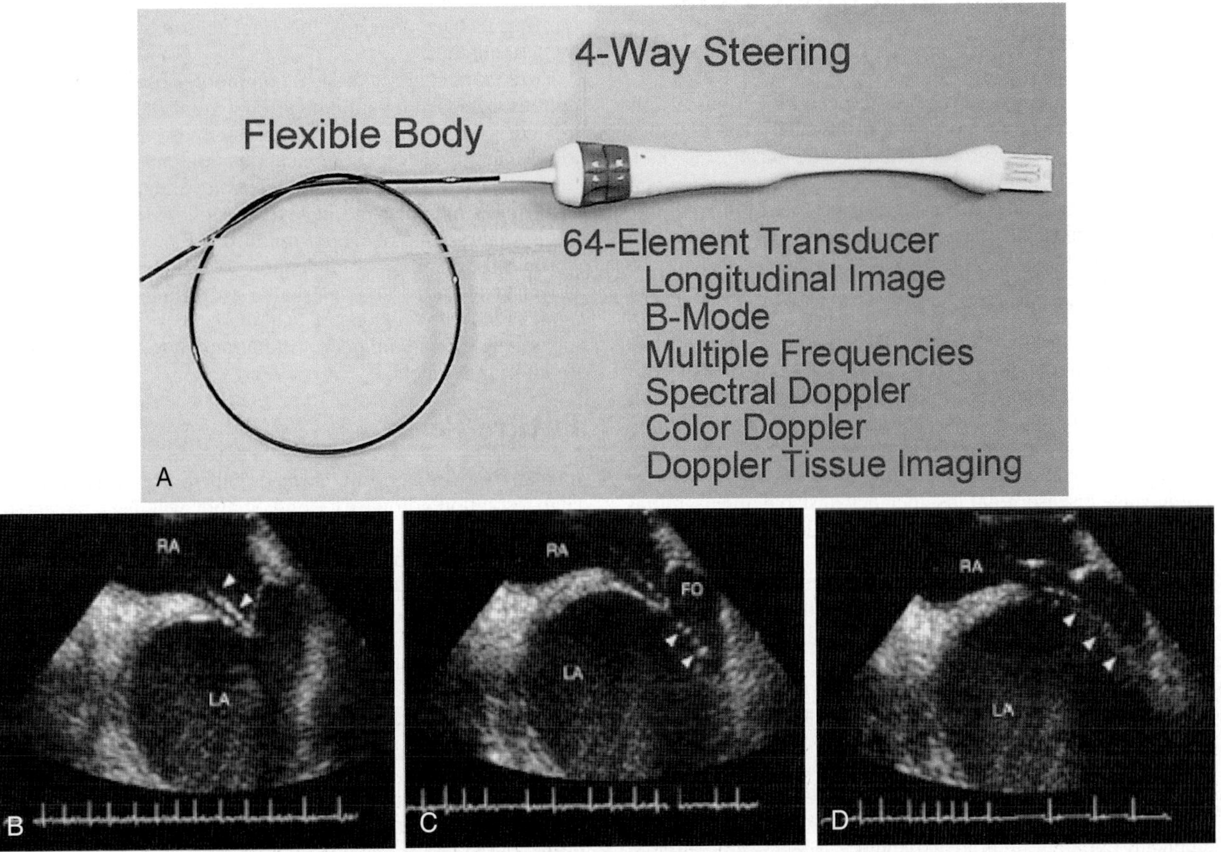

FIGURE 20-16 **A,** Intracardiac echocardiography disposable transducer (Acuson, Inc.), with steering apparatus on proximal end and flexible body with transducer on distal tip of catheter. **B,** Tenting of the membranous fossa by the dilator-needle assembly. The transseptal needle assembly (arrowheads) is advanced to indent the fossa membrane. **C,** Advancement of the transseptal needle across the membranous fossa. Here the needle (arrowheads) is seen near the posterosuperior left atrial wall. The membrane remains tented because the dilator has not yet crossed the septum. **D,** Dilator and sheath passage across the interatrial septum. The dilator and sheath assembly has now advanced into the left atrium, releasing the tenting of the membranous fossa. FO = fossa ovalis; LA = left atrium; RA = right atrium. *(From Johnson SB, Seward JB, Packer DL: Phased-array intracardiac echocardiography for guiding transseptal catheter placement: Utility and learning curve. Pacing Clin Electrophysiol 25:402, 2002.)*

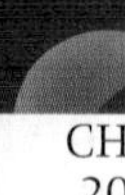

TABLE 20-5 Risk of Cardiac Catheterization and Coronary Angiography

COMPLICATION	RISK (%)*
Mortality	0.11
Myocardial infarction	0.05
Cerebrovascular accident	0.07
Arrhythmia	0.38
Vascular complications	0.43
Contrast reaction	0.37
Hemodynamic complications	0.26
Perforation of heart chamber	0.03
Other complications	0.28
Total of major complications	1.70

*No. of patients = 59,792.

From Scanlon PJ, Faxon DP, Audet AM, et al: ACC/AHA guidelines for coronary angiography: A report of the American College of Cardiology/American Heart Association Task Force on Practice Guidelines (Committee on Coronary Angiography). J Am Coll Cardiol 33:1760, 1999.

localization of the fossa ovalis. ICE is also used to guide electrophysiologic procedures with identification of anatomic structures difficult to view by fluoroscopy (e.g., pulmonary veins or fossa ovalis for transseptal puncture).[26]

Complications Associated with Cardiac Catheterization

Cardiac catheterization is a relatively safe procedure but has a well-defined risk of morbidity and mortality (**Table 20-5**). The potential risk of major complications during cardiac catheterization is often related to comorbid disease. The use of low-osmolar and isosmolar contrast media, lower profile diagnostic catheters, and reduced anticoagulation and extensive operator experience have reduced the incidence of complications. Several large studies provide insight into the incidence of major events and delineate cohorts of patients that are at increased risk.[59,60]

Death related to diagnostic cardiac catheterization occurs in 0.08% to 0.75% of patients, depending on the population studied. Data from the Society for Cardiac Angiography identified subsets of patients with an increased mortality rate.[60] In an analysis of 58,332 patients, multivariate predictors of significant complications were moribund status, advanced New York Heart Association functional class, hypotension, shock, aortic valve disease, renal insufficiency, unstable angina, mitral valve disease, acute myocardial infarction within 24 hours, congestive heart failure, and cardiomyopathy. The risk of any complication during cardiac catheterization is further increased in octogenarians. Although the overall mortality is approximately 0.8% in this cohort, the risk of nonfatal major complications, which are primarily peripheral vascular, is approximately 5%.

The risk of myocardial infarction varies from 0.03% to 0.06%; of significant bradyarrhythmias or tachyarrhythmias, from 0.56% to 1.3%[60]; and of neurologic complications, from 0.03% to 0.2%.[56] One study using serial cranial magnetic resonance imaging demonstrated a 22% incidence of focal acute cerebral embolic events after retrograde crossing of stenotic aortic valves, and 3% of patients demonstrated clinically apparent neurologic deficits.[61] However, this study is in contradistinction to previously published large clinical series and requires additional validation.

Stroke can be periprocedural in the laboratory or occur within a few hours after the procedure. Whether the mechanism is different is unclear. Stroke should be distinguished from other conditions, including seizure, migraine, hypoglycemia, and encephalopathy. The standard stroke management with a multidisciplinary team is important to improve prognosis. Predictors of stroke include diabetes mellitus, hypertension, prior stroke, and renal failure. The procedure length, contrast volume, urgent indications, and use of intra-aortic balloon pumps are known to increase the risk of stroke.[62]

The most common complication is arterial access site bleeding, which is usually manifested by minor oozing or small hematomas. The incidence of major vascular complications in most series has suggested a slightly higher frequency when the Sones brachial approach is used. The incidence of major vascular complications has decreased during the last decade and is currently reported as approximately 0.20%.[60,63] Major vascular complications include occlusion requiring arterial repair or thrombectomy, retroperitoneal bleeding, hematoma formation, pseudoaneurysm, arteriovenous fistula formation, and infection. In a patient with unexplained hypotension or back pain, retroperitoneal hematoma should be suspected. Evaluation should include serial complete blood count determinations, evaluation of anticoagulation status, and either CT or ultrasound evaluation of the groin, pelvis, and abdomen. The risk of requiring surgical repair for vascular injury is related to advanced age, congestive heart failure, and larger body surface area. With ultrasound guidance, many pseudoaneurysms can be successfully treated percutaneously with directed infusion of thrombin, and surgical repair can often be avoided.

The proper management of the arterial sheath is important in avoiding complications. Because dwell times correlate with hematoma formation, all sheaths should be removed as soon as possible with an activated clotting time below 170. Frequent blood pressure and pulse monitoring is essential.

Systemic complications can vary from mild vasovagal responses to severe vagal reactions that lead to prolonged hypotension. Minor complications occur in approximately 4% of patients undergoing routine cardiac catheterization.[63] The most common untoward effects are transient hypotension and brief episodes of angina lasting less than 10 minutes.

Hives can occur but are less commonly observed with low-osmolar contrast agents and with intra-arterial administration. They are readily treated with intravenous corticosteroids and diphenhydramine. Rarely, anaphylactoid complications are observed. These are also treated with intravenous corticosteroid and diphenhydramine. Epinephrine is administered in severe reactions; the dilution of 0.1 mg/mL is administered at 1.4 μg/min during 5 minutes.

The most common complications of right-heart catheterization are nonsustained atrial and ventricular arrhythmias. Major complications associated with right-heart catheterization are infrequent. These include pulmonary infarction, pulmonary artery or right ventricle perforation, and infection.

Future Perspectives

In many ways, diagnostic cardiac catheterization is at a crossroads. High-resolution coronary CT angiography will likely replace the need for cardiac catheterization in low-risk patients in whom coronary artery disease can be excluded with noninvasive testing. On the other hand, the widespread availability of multiple noninvasive screening modalities will provide early detection of cardiovascular disease that will require cardiac catheterization to precisely define the extent and severity of coronary, vascular, and valvular disease. Transcatheter imaging, diagnostic technologies, and provocative testing expand the catheterization laboratory beyond conventional radiographic imaging and hemodynamic assessment.

The expansion of transcatheter repair of coronary, valvular, and structural heart disease will also stimulate the growth of cardiac catheterization in conjunction with the percutaneous therapeutic procedures (see Chaps. 58 and 59). Safety of the technique is well established and continues to improve with experience, standardized quality assurance programs, and advances in imaging technology.

ACKNOWLEDGMENT

The authors would like to thank Robert Fishman, MD, for his contribution to a previous edition of this chapter.

REFERENCES

Indications for Diagnostic Cardiac Catheterization

1. Scanlon PJ, Faxon DP, Audet AM, et al: ACC/AHA guidelines for coronary angiography: A report of the American College of Cardiology/American Heart Association Task Force on Practice Guidelines (Committee on Coronary Angiography). J Am Coll Cardiol 33:1756, 1999.
2. Bonow RO, Carabello BA, Chatterjee K, et al: AHA/ACC 2006 guidelines for the management of patients with valvular heart disease. (http://www.acc.org/clinical/guidelines/valvular/index.pdf).
3. Hunt SA, Abraham WT, Chin MH, et al: ACC/AHA 2005 guidelines update for the diagnosis and management of chronic heart failure in the adult. Circulation 112:e154, 2005.
4. Antman EM, Anbe DT, Armstrong PW, et al: ACC/AHA guidelines for the management of patients with ST-elevation myocardial infarction. Circulation 110:e82, 2004.
5. Smith SC, Hirshfeld JW, Jacobs AK: ACC/AHA/SCAI 2005 guideline update for percutaneous coronary intervention. J Am Cardiol 47:e1, 2006.
6. Eagle KA, Guyton RA, Davidoff R, et al: ACC/AHA 2004 guideline update for coronary artery bypass graft surgery 2004. Available at http://www.americanheart.org/presenter.jhtml?indentifier=9181.
7. Anderson JL, Adams CD, Antman EM, et al: ACC/AHA 2007 guidelines for the management of patients with unstable angina/non–ST-elevation myocardial infarction. J Am Coll Cardiol 50:e1, 2007.
8. Warnes CA, William RG, Bashore TM, et al: ACC/AHA guidelines for management of adults with congenital heart disease. J Am Coll Cardiol 52:e143, 2008.

Technical Aspects

9. Jacobs AK, Faxon DP, Hirshfeld JW, Holmes DR: Task force 3: Training in diagnostic cardiac catheterization and interventional cardiology. Revision of the 1995 COCATS training statement. J Am Coll Cardiol 39:1242, 2002.
10. Bashore TM, Bates ER, Berger PB, et al: ACC/SCAI Clinical expert consensus document on cardiac catheterization laboratory standards. J Am Coll Cardiol 37:2170, 2001.
11. Hirshfeld JW Jr, Balter S, Brinker JA, et al: ACCF/AHA/HRS/SCAI clinical competence statement of physician knowledge to optimize patient safety and image quality in fluoroscopically guided invasive cardiovascular procedures. J Am Coll Cardiol 44:2259, 2004.
12. Heupler FA Jr: Guidelines for performing angiography in patients taking metformin. Members of the Laboratory Performance Standards Committee of the Society for Cardiac Angiography and Interventions. Cathet Cardiovasc Diagn 43:121, 1998.
13. Schweiger MJ, Chambers CE, Davidson CJ, et al: Prevention of contrast induced nephropathy: Recommendations for the high risk patients undergoing cardiovascular procedures. Catheter Cardiovasc Interv 69:135, 2007.
14. Goss JE, Chambers CE, Heupler FA: Systemic anaphylactoid reactions to iodinated contrast media during cardiac catheterization procedures: Guidelines for prevention, diagnosis, and treatment. Laboratory Performance Standards Committee for the Society for Cardiac Angiography and Interventions. Cathet Cardiovasc Diagn 34:99, 1995.
15. Piper WD, Malenka DJ, Ryan TR Jr: Predicting vascular complications in percutaneous coronary interventions. Am Heart J 145:1022, 2003.
16. Kussmaul WG, Buchbinder M, Whitlow P, et al: Rapid arterial hemostasis after cardiac catheterization and percutaneous transluminal angioplasty—results of a randomized trial of a novel hemostatic device. J Am Coll Cardiol 25:1685, 1995.
17. Baim DS, Knopf WDD, Hinohara T, et al: Suture mediated closure of the femoral access site after cardiac catheterization. Am J Cardiol 85:864, 2000.
18. Koreny M, Riedmuller E, Nikfardjam M, et al: Arterial puncture closing devices compared with standard manual compression after cardiac catheterization. JAMA 291:350, 2004.
19. Arora N, Matheny ME, Sepke C, Resnic F: A propensity analysis of the risk of vascular complications after cardiac catheterization procedures with the use of vascular closure devices. Am Heart J 153:606, 2007.
20. Archbold RA, Robinson NM, Schilling RJ: Radial artery access for coronary angiography and percutaneous coronary intervention. BMJ 329:443, 2004.
21. Jolly SS, Amlani S, Hamon N, et al: Radial versus femoral access for coronary angiography or intervention and the impact on major bleeding and ischemic events: A systematic review and meta-analysis of randomized trials. Am Heart J 157:132, 2009.
22. Pristipino C, Trani C, Nazzaro MS, et al: Major improvement of percutaneous cardiovascular procedure outcomes with radial artery catheterization: Results from the PREVAIL study. Heart 95:476, 2009.
23. Baim DS: Percutaneous approach, including transseptal and apical puncture. *In* Baim DS, Grossman W (eds): Cardiac Catheterization, Angiography, and Intervention. 7th ed. Philadelphia, Lippincott Williams & Wilkins, 2006, p 79.
24. DePonti R, Cappato R, Curnis A, et al: Trans-septal catheterization in the electrophysiology laboratory. Data from a multicenter survey spanning 12 years. J Am Coll Cardiol 47:1037, 2006.
25. Liu TJ, Lai HC, Lee WL, et al: Immediate and late outcomes of patients undergoing transseptal left-sided heart catheterization for symptomatic valvular and arrhythmic diseases. Am Heart J 151:235, 2006.
26. Jongbloed MRM, Schalij MJ, Zeppenfeld K, et al: Clinical applications of intracardiac echocardiography in interventional procedures. Heart 91:981, 2005.
27. Zuguchi M, Shindoh C, Chida K, et al: Safety and clinical benefits of transsubxiphoidal left ventricular puncture. Catheter Cardiovasc Interv 55:58, 2001.
28. Walters DL, Sanchez PL, Rodriguez-Alemparte M, et al: Transthoracic left ventricular puncture for the assessment of patients with aortic and mitral valve prosthesis. The Massachusetts General experience 1989-2000. Catheter Cardiovasc Interv 58:539, 2003.
29. Wu LA, Lapeyre AC 3rd, Cooper LT: Current role of endomyocardial biopsy in the management of dilated cardiomyopathy and myocarditis. Mayo Clin Proc 76:1030, 2001.
30. Cooper LT, Baughman K, Feldman AM, et al: The role of endomyocardial biopsy in the management of cardiovascular disease. J Am Cardiol 50:1914, 2007.
31. Wong RC, Abrahams Z, Hanna M, et al: Tricuspid regurgitation after cardiac transplantation: An old problem revisited. J Heart Lung Transplant 27:247, 2008.
32. Trost JC, Hillis LD: Intra-aortic balloon counterpulsation. Am J Cardiol 97:1391, 2006.
33. O'Rourke MF: Augmentation of coronary blood flow with intra-aortic balloon pump counterpulsation. Circulation 103:e129, 2001.
34. Stone GW, Ohman EM, Miller MF: Contemporary utilization and outcomes of intra-aortic balloon counterpulsation in acute myocardial infarction: The Benchmark registry. J Am Coll Cardiol 41:1940, 2003.

Hemodynamic Data

35. Grossman W: Pressure measurement. *In* Grossman W, Baim DS (eds): Cardiac Catheterization, Angiography, and Intervention. 7th ed. Philadelphia, Lea & Febiger, 2006, p 13.
36. Hildick-Smith DJ, Walsh JT, Shapiro LM: Pulmonary capillary wedge pressure in mitral stenosis accurately reflects mean left atrial pressure but overestimates transmitral gradient. Am J Cardiol 85:512, 2000.
37. Schobel WA, Voelker W, Haase KK: Extent, determinants and clinical importance of pressure recovery in patients with aortic valve stenosis. Eur Heart J 20:1355, 1999.
38. Moise SF, Sinclair CJ, Scott DHT: Pulmonary artery blood temperature and the measurement of cardiac output by thermodilution. Anaesthesia 57:562, 2002.
39. Lehmann, KG, Platt MS: Improved accuracy and precision of thermodilution cardiac output measurement using a dual thermistor catheter system. J Am Coll Cardiol 33:883, 1999.
40. Fakler U, Pauli C, Hennig M, et al: Assumed oxygen consumption frequently results in large errors in the determination of cardiac output. J Thorac Cardiovasc Surg 130:272, 2005.
41. Nichols WW, O'Rourke MF (eds): McDonald's Blood Flow in Arteries. 4th ed. New York, Oxford University Press, 1998.
42. Otto CM: Cardiac catheterization and angiography. *In* Otto CM (ed): Valvular Heart Disease. 2nd ed. Philadelphia, WB Saunders, 2004, p 93.
43. Tardif JC, Rodrigues AG, Hardey JF, et al: Simultaneous determination of aortic valve area by the Gorlin formula and by transesophageal echocardiography under different transvalvular flow conditions. J Am Coll Cardiol 29:1296, 1997.
44. Nishimura RA, Grantham JA, Connolly HM, et al: Low-output, low-gradient aortic stenosis in patients with depressed left ventricular systolic function: The clinical utility of the dobutamine challenge in the catheterization laboratory. Circulation 106:809, 2002.
45. Monin JL, Quere JP, Monchi M, et al: Low-gradient aortic stenosis: Operative risk stratification and predictors for long-term outcome: A multicenter study using dobutamine stress hemodynamics. Circulation 108:319, 2003.
46. Burwash IG: Low-flow, low-gradient aortic stenosis: From evaluation to treatment. Curr Opin Cardiol 22:84, 2007.
47. Grossman W: Shunt detection and quantification. *In* Grossman W, Baim DS (eds): Cardiac Catheterization, Angiography, and Intervention. 7th ed. Philadelphia, Lea & Febiger, 2006, p 163.

Physiologic and Pharmacologic Maneuvers

48. Grossman W: Stress testing during cardiac catheterization: Exercise and pacing tachycardia. *In* Grossman W, Baim DS (eds): Cardiac Catheterization, Angiography, and Intervention. 7th ed. Philadelphia, Lea & Febiger, 2006, p 283.
49. Udelson JE, Bacharach SL, Cannon RO, Bonow RO: Minimum left ventricular pressure during beta-adrenergic stimulation in human subjects: Evidence for elastic recoil and diastolic "suction" in the normal heart. Circulation 82:1174, 1990.
50. Higano ST, Azrak E, Tahirkheli NK, Kern MJ: Hemodynamic rounds series II: Hemodynamics of constrictive physiology: Influence of respiratory dynamics on ventricular pressures. Catheter Cardiovasc Interv 46:473, 1999.
51. Talreja DR, Nichimura RA, Oh JK, Homes DR: Constrictive pericarditis in the modern era. J Am Coll Cardiol 51:315, 2008.
52. Blais C, Burwash IG, Mundigler G, et al: Projected valve area at normal flow rate improves the assessment of stenosis severity in patients with low-flow, low-gradient aortic stenosis. The multicenter TOPAS (Truly or Pseudo-Severe Aortic Stenosis) study. Circulation 113:711, 2006.
53. Ichinose F, Roberts JD, Zapol WM: Inhaled nitric oxide: A selective pulmonary vasodilator: Current uses and therapeutic potential. Circulation 109:3106, 2004.
54. Krasuski RA, Warner JJ, Wang A, et al: Inhaled nitric oxide selectively dilates pulmonary vasculature in adult patients with pulmonary hypertension, irrespective of etiology. J Am Coll Cardiol 36:2204, 2000.

Adjunctive Diagnostic Techniques

55. Underwood SR, Bax JJ, Vom Dahl J, et al: Imaging techniques for the assessment of myocardial hibernation. Report of a study group of the European Society of Cardiology. Eur Heart J 25:815, 2004.
56. Gyongyosi M, Sochor H, Khorsand A, et al: Online myocardial viability assessment in the catheterization laboratory via NOGA electroanatomic mapping. Circulation 104:1005, 2001.
57. Koch KC, Wenderdel M, Stellbrink C, et al: Electromechanical assessment of left ventricular function following successful percutaneous coronary revascularization. Catheter Cardiovasc Interv 54:466, 2001.
58. Vale PR, Losordo DW, Milliken CE, et al: Left ventricular electromechanical mapping to assess efficacy of $phVEGF_{165}$ gene transfer for therapeutic angiogenesis in chronic myocardial ischemia. Circulation 102:965, 2000.

Complications Associated with Cardiac Catheterization

59. Davidson CJ, Mark DB, Pieper KS, et al: Thrombotic and cardiovascular complications related to nonionic contrast media during cardiac catheterization. Analysis of 8517 patients. Am J Cardiol 65:1481, 1990.
60. Laskey W, Boyle J, Johnson LW, and the Registry Committee of the Society for Cardiac Angiography and Interventions: Multivariable model for prediction of risk of significant complication during diagnostic cardiac catheterization. Cathet Cardiovasc Diagn 30:185, 1993.
61. Omran H, Schmidt H, Hackenbroch M, et al: Silent and apparent cerebral embolism after retrograde catheterisation of the aortic valve in valvular stenosis: A prospective, randomised study. Lancet 361:1241, 2003.
62. Hamon M, Baron J, Viader F, Hamon M: Periprocedural stroke and cardiac catheterization. Circulation 118:678, 2008.
63. Davidson CJ, Hlatky M, Morris GG, et al: Cardiovascular and renal toxicity of a nonionic radiographic contrast agent after cardiac catheterization. Ann Intern Med 110:119, 1989.

CHAPTER 21 Coronary Arteriography

Jeffrey J. Popma

Coronary arteriography remains the standard for identifying the presence or absence of arterial narrowings related to atherosclerotic coronary artery disease (CAD) and provides the most reliable anatomic information for determining the appropriateness of medical therapy, percutaneous coronary intervention (PCI), or coronary artery bypass graft (CABG) surgery in patients with ischemic CAD. First performed by Sones in 1959, coronary arteriography has subsequently become one of the most widely used invasive procedures in cardiovascular medicine.[1] It is performed by direct injection of radiopaque contrast material into the coronary arteries and recording of digital radiographic images. Approximately 2 million patients will undergo coronary arteriography in the United States this year, and coronary arteriography is now available in 25% of acute care hospitals in this country.

The methods used to perform coronary arteriography have improved substantially since 1959. Smaller (4F to 5F), high-flow injection catheters have replaced larger (8F) thick-walled catheters, and the reduced sheath size has allowed same-day coronary arteriography, ambulation, and discharge. Transradial access has further reduced the vascular complication rates and allowed early ambulation after the procedure. Complication rates associated with coronary arteriography have fallen as a result of a better understanding of the periprocedural management of patients undergoing cardiac catheterization. "Filmless" digital laboratories now permit high-quality image acquisition, electronic storage (rather than the historic 35-mm cinefilm), and rapid image transfer and dissemination.[2]

This chapter reviews the indications for and techniques of coronary arteriography, the normal coronary anatomy and pathologic coronary variants, the qualitative and quantitative angiographic methods to assess severity of stenoses, and the limitations of use of angiography alone to assess the extent of CAD.

Indications for Coronary Arteriography

(see Guidelines for Coronary Arteriography)

Coronary arteriography establishes the presence or absence of coronary stenoses, defines therapeutic options, and determines the prognosis of patients with symptoms or signs of ischemic CAD.[3] Coronary arteriography can also be used as a research tool to evaluate serial changes that occur after PCI or pharmacologic therapy. The American College of Cardiology/American Heart Association (ACC/AHA) Task Force established indications for coronary arteriography in patients with known or suspected CAD (**Table 21-1**).[4] More recently, these indications for cardiac catheterization have supported the appropriateness criteria for coronary revascularization[5] (see Chap. 58).

Patients with suspected CAD who have severe stable angina (Canadian Cardiovascular Society class III or IV) or those who have less severe symptoms or are asymptomatic but demonstrate high-risk criteria for an adverse outcome on noninvasive testing should undergo coronary arteriography. High-risk features include resting or exercise-induced left ventricular dysfunction (left ventricular ejection fraction <35%) or a standard exercise treadmill test demonstrating hypotension or 1 to 2 mm or more of ST-segment depression associated with decreased exercise capacity.[4] Stress imaging that demonstrates a moderate or large perfusion defect (particularly in the anterior wall), multiple defects, a large fixed perfusion defect with left ventricular dilation or increased lung uptake (see Chap. 17), or extensive stress or dobutamine-induced wall motion abnormalities (see Chap. 15) also indicates high risk for an adverse outcome. Patients resuscitated from sudden cardiac death, particularly those with residual ventricular arrhythmias (see Chap. 41), are also candidates for coronary arteriography, given the favorable outcomes associated with revascularization in these patients. In the absence of symptoms and signs of ischemia, the presence of coronary calcification on fluoroscopy and a high calcium score by cardiac computed tomography (see Chap. 19) are not indications for coronary arteriography.

Patients with unstable angina (see Chap. 56) who have recurrent symptoms despite medical therapy or who are at intermediate or high risk for subsequent death or myocardial infarction are also candidates for coronary arteriography.[6] High-risk features include prolonged ongoing (>20 minutes) chest pain, pulmonary edema, worsening mitral regurgitation, dynamic ST-segment depression of 1 mm or more, and hypotension.[4] Intermediate-risk features include angina at rest (>20 minutes) relieved with rest or sublingual nitroglycerin, angina associated with dynamic electrocardiographic changes, recent-onset angina with a high likelihood of CAD, pathologic Q waves or ST-segment depression less than 1 mm in multiple leads, and age older than 65 years.[4,5]

Patients who should undergo coronary arteriography are patients with ST-segment elevation myocardial infarction, non–ST-segment elevation myocardial infarction, or unstable angina who develop spontaneous ischemia; patients with ischemia at a minimal workload; and patients who have myocardial infarction complicated by congestive heart failure, hemodynamic instability, cardiac arrest, mitral regurgitation, or ventricular septal rupture (see Chap. 55). Patients with angina or provocable ischemia after myocardial infarction should also undergo coronary arteriography because revascularization may reduce the high risk of reinfarction in these patients.[7]

Patients who present with chest pain of unclear cause, particularly those who have high-risk criteria on noninvasive testing, may benefit from coronary arteriography for diagnosis or exclusion of significant CAD. Patients who have undergone prior revascularization should undergo coronary arteriography if there is suspicion of abrupt vessel closure or when recurrent angina develops that meets high-risk noninvasive criteria.

Coronary arteriography should be performed in patients scheduled to undergo noncardiac surgery who demonstrate high-risk criteria on noninvasive testing, have angina unresponsive to medical therapy, develop unstable angina, or have equivocal noninvasive test results and are scheduled to undergo high-risk surgery (see Chap. 85 and its Guidelines). Coronary arteriography is also recommended for patients

TABLE 21-1 Indications for Coronary Arteriography

CLASS I	CLASS IIA	CLASS IIB	CLASS III
Asymptomatic or Stable Angina			
CCS class III and IV on medical therapy High-risk criteria on noninvasive testing irrespective of angina Successfully resuscitated from sudden cardiac death with sustained monomorphic VT or nonsustained polymorphic VT	CCS class III or IV that improves to class I or II with medical therapy Worsening abnormalities on noninvasive testing Patients with angina and severe illness that precludes risk stratification CCS class I or II angina with intolerance to medical therapy Individuals whose occupation affects the safety of others	CCS class I or II angina with demonstrable ischemia but no high-risk criteria on noninvasive testing Asymptomatic men or postmenopausal women with ≥2 major clinical risks with low-risk criteria on noninvasive testing and no prior CAD Asymptomatic patients with prior MI, normal LV function, and no high-risk criteria on noninvasive testing	Angina in patients who prefer to avoid revascularization Angina in patients who are not candidates for revascularization or in whom it will not improve QOL As a screening test for CAD After CABG when there is no evidence of ischemia on noninvasive testing Coronary calcification on fluoroscopy or EBCT
Unstable Angina			
High or intermediate risk for adverse outcome in patients refractory to medical therapy High or intermediate risk that stabilizes after initial treatment Initially low short-term risk that is high risk on noninvasive testing Suspected Prinzmetal variant angina	None	Low short-term risk unstable angina without high-risk criteria on noninvasive testing	Recurrent chest discomfort suggestive of unstable angina but without objective signs of ischemia and with a normal coronary angiogram within the past 5 years Unstable angina in patients who are not candidates for revascularization
Postrevascularization Ischemia			
Suspected abrupt closure or subacute stent thrombosis after PCI Recurrent angina and high-risk criteria on noninvasive evaluation within 9 months of PCI	Recurrent symptomatic ischemia within 12 months of CABG Noninvasive evidence of high-risk criteria occurring anytime after CABG Recurrent angina inadequately controlled by medications	Asymptomatic post-PCI patient suspected of having restenosis within the first months after PCI because of an abnormal but not high-risk noninvasive test Recurrent angina without high-risk criteria on noninvasive testing occurring 1 year postoperatively Asymptomatic post-CABG patient in whom a deteriorating noninvasive test is found	Symptoms in a post-CABG patient who is not a candidate for revascularization Routine angiography after PCI or CABG unless part of an approved research protocol
After STEMI or Non-STEMI			
Spontaneous myocardial ischemia or ischemia provoked with minimal exertion Before surgical therapy for acute MR, VSD, true aneurysm or pseudoaneurysm Persistent hemodynamic instability	Suspected MI due to coronary embolism, arteritis, trauma, certain metabolic diseases, or coronary spasm Survivors of acute MI with LVEF <0.40, CHF, prior PCI or CABG, or malignant ventricular arrhythmias	For a suspected persistent occlusion of the IRA to perform delayed PCI Coronary arteriography performed without risk stratification to identify the presence of left main or three-vessel CAD All patients after NQWMI Recurrent ventricular tachycardia despite antiarrhythmic therapy without ongoing ischemia	Patients who are not candidates for or refuse revascularization
Nonspecific Chest Pain			
High-risk features on noninvasive testing	None	Patients with recurrent hospitalizations for chest pain who have abnormal or equivocal findings on noninvasive testing	All other patients with nonspecific chest pain

Class I: conditions for which there is agreement that the procedure is useful and effective. Class IIa: weight of the evidence is in favor of usefulness and efficacy. Class IIb: weight of the evidence is less well established by evidence and opinion. Class III: conditions for which there is general agreement that the procedure is not useful and effective and in some cases may be harmful.
CABG = coronary artery bypass graft surgery; CAD = coronary artery disease; CCS = Canadian Cardiovascular Society; CHF = congestive heart failure; EBCT = electron beam computed tomography; IRA = infarct-related artery; LV = left ventricular; LVEF = left ventricular ejection fraction; MI = myocardial infarction; MR = mitral regurgitation; PCI = percutaneous coronary intervention; QOL = quality of life; STEMI = ST-elevation MI; VSD = ventricular septal defect; VT = ventricular tachycardia.
From Scanlon P, Faxon D, Audet A, et al: ACC/AHA guidelines for coronary angiography. J Am Coll Cardiol 33:1756, 1999.

scheduled to undergo surgery for valvular heart disease or congenital heart disease, particularly those with multiple cardiac risk factors and those with infective endocarditis and evidence of coronary embolization[4] (see Chaps. 65, 66, and 67). One study has suggested that coronary arteriography improves the prognosis of patients undergoing medium- to high-risk peripheral vascular surgery.[8] Coronary arteriography may also improve prognosis in patients hospitalized with acute left ventricular decompensation.[9]

Coronary arteriography should be performed annually in patients after cardiac transplantation in the absence of clinical symptoms because of the characteristically diffuse and often asymptomatic nature of graft atherosclerosis (see Chap. 31). Coronary arteriography is useful in potential donors for cardiac transplantation whose age or cardiac risk profile increases the likelihood of CAD. The arteriogram often provides important diagnostic information about the presence of CAD in patients with intractable arrhythmias before electrophysiologic testing or in patients who present with a dilated cardiomyopathy of unknown cause.

Contraindications. Although there are no absolute contraindications to coronary arteriography, relative contraindications include unexplained fever, untreated infection, severe anemia with hemoglobin concentration less than 8 mg/dL, severe electrolyte imbalance, severe active bleeding, uncontrolled systemic hypertension, digitalis toxicity, previous reaction to contrast material but no pretreatment with corticosteroids, and ongoing stroke.[4] Other disease states that are relative contraindications to coronary arteriography include acute renal failure,

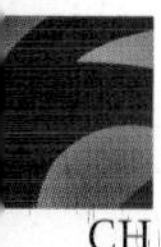

CH 21

TABLE 21-2 Patients at Increased Risk for Complications After Coronary Arteriography

Increased General Medical Risk
Age >70 years
Complex congenital heart disease
Morbid obesity
General debility or cachexia
Uncontrolled glucose intolerance
Arterial oxygen desaturation
Severe chronic obstructive lung disease
Renal insufficiency with creatinine concentration >1.5 mg/dL
Increased Cardiac Risk
Three-vessel coronary artery disease
Left main coronary artery disease
NYHA functional Class IV
Significant mitral or aortic valve disease or mechanical prosthesis
Ejection fraction <35%
High-risk exercise treadmill testing (hypotension or severe ischemia)
Pulmonary hypertension
Pulmonary artery wedge pressure >25 mm Hg
Increased Vascular Risk
Anticoagulation or bleeding diathesis
Uncontrolled systemic hypertension
Severe peripheral vascular disease
Recent stroke
Severe aortic insufficiency

NYHA = New York Heart Association.
Modified from Scanlon P, Faxon D, Audet A, et al: ACC/AHA guidelines for coronary angiography. J Am Coll Cardiol 33:1756, 1999.

TABLE 21-3 Risk of Cardiac Catheterization

COMPLICATION	SCAI REGISTRY (%)
Mortality	0.11
Myocardial infarction	0.05
Cerebrovascular accident	0.07
Arrhythmias	0.38
Vascular complications	0.43
Contrast agent reaction	0.37
Hemodynamic complications	0.26
Perforation of heart chamber	0.03
Other complications	0.28
Total of major complications	1.70

SCAI = Society for Cardiovascular Angiography and Interventions.
Modified from Scanlon P, Faxon D, Audet A, et al: ACC/AHA guidelines for coronary angiography. J Am Coll Cardiol 33:1756, 1999.

decompensated congestive heart failure, severe intrinsic or iatrogenic coagulopathy (international normalized ratio [INR] >2.0), and active endocarditis.[4] Risk factors for significant complications after catheterization include advanced age and several general medical, vascular, and cardiac characteristics (**Table 21-2**).

Given that the majority of these conditions are self-limited, deferral of coronary arteriography until important comorbidities have been stabilized is generally preferred unless there is evidence of ongoing myocardial necrosis. It is recognized that coronary arteriography performed under emergency conditions is associated with a higher risk of procedural complication. The risks and benefits of the procedure and its alternatives should be carefully reviewed with the patient and family in all circumstances before coronary arteriography is undertaken in the presence of relative contraindications.

Complications of Coronary Arteriography

Major complications are uncommon (<2%) after coronary arteriography (**Table 21-3**)[10,11] and include death (0.10% to 0.14%), myocardial infarction (0.06% to 0.07%), contrast agent reactions (0.23%), stroke (0.07% to 0.14%), and local vascular complications (0.24% to 1%).[12] In a retrospective study of more than 6000 patients undergoing diagnostic angiography, the use of vascular closure devices reduced the complication rates from 1.1% to 0.5% ($P = 0.01$)[13] ; their occurrence was also predicted by the presence of chronic renal insufficiency, procedure duration, and female gender.[13] The incidence of death during coronary arteriography is higher in the presence of left main coronary artery (LMCA) disease (0.55%), with left ventricular ejection fraction less than 30% (0.30%), and with New York Heart Association functional Class IV disease (0.29%). Stroke may develop from embolization of atherosclerotic debris into the cerebral circulation or embolization of clot that formed on the injection catheters, particularly in patients with prior CABG who have a diseased ascending aorta. More recently, acute stroke complicating diagnostic catheterization has been amenable to neurovascular intervention.[14] Recent series have shown no increase and, in one study, a decline[11] in the major complication rates associated with coronary arteriography, despite increased morbidity of patients and higher lesion complexity.[11] With the recommendations for universal precautions during cardiac catheterization, including the use of gowns, caps, masks, and protective eyewear, the occurrence of infections after the procedure is low.[15]

Minor complications are also uncommon (<2%) after coronary arteriography. Air embolus is rare (0.1%) during diagnostic coronary arteriography and is generally preventable with meticulous flushing and elimination of air within the manifold.[16] If an air embolus and air lock do occur, 100% oxygen should be administered, which allows resorption of smaller amounts of air within 2 to 4 minutes. Larger air emboli have been treated with direct aspiration of air from the coronary artery.[17,18] Ventricular arrhythmias associated with air embolus can be treated with lidocaine and direct-current cardioversion. Reduced anterograde flow, also called no-reflow, occurs in 0.17% of cases, primarily attributable to air embolism, spasm, or dissection.[19-22] Cholesterol embolization is also uncommon but may occur with catheter manipulation in a diffusely diseased abdominal or thoracic aorta[23,24] (see Chap. 61). Nerve pain after diagnostic catheterization is infrequent and generally resolves spotaneously.[25] Although lactic acidosis may develop after coronary angiography in diabetic patients taking metformin, this complication has been minimized with metformin discontinuation before the administration of contrast material and withholding of metformin after coronary arteriography until renal function has recovered. The presence of chronic kidney disease is also an important predictor of prognosis in patients undergoing coronary angiography[26] (see Chap. 93).

With the expanded use of complex PCI (see Chap. 58), patients may now return for multiple procedures during their lifetime that may subject them to the risk of cumulative radiation injury.[27] An average PCI procedure imparts 150 times the radiation exposure received with a single chest radiograph and 6 times the annual radiation received by background environmental radiation.[27] Radiation dosage may vary by up to 10-fold in patients undergoing coronary arteriography and intervention.[28] Reports of radiodermatitis related to prolonged x-ray exposure have led to the recommendation that patients who receive fluoroscopy for more than 60 minutes be counseled about the delayed effects of radiation injury to the skin, although proportionately more radiation is received with digital cineangiography than with fluoroscopy alone.[29,30] Radiation-induced lesions are generally identified by their location in the region of the x-ray tube and are manifested by an acute erythema, delayed pigmented telangiectasia, and indurated or ulcerated plaques in the upper back or below the axilla.

Technique of Coronary Arteriography

PREPARATION OF THE PATIENT. Elective coronary arteriography should be performed alone or in conjunction with right-heart catheterization or contrast-enhanced left ventriculography (see Chap. 20) when comorbid conditions, such as congestive heart failure, diabetes mellitus, or renal insufficiency, are stable. A baseline electrocardiogram, electrolyte and renal function tests, complete blood cell count, and coagulation panel should be reviewed before coronary arteriography. Patients who may undergo PCI should receive aspirin, 162 to 325 mg, at least 2 hours before the procedure if PCI is planned. Warfarin should be discontinued 2 days before elective coronary arteriography, and the INR should be less than 2.0 before arterial puncture when the femoral artery access is used. Higher INR (up to 2.5) may be acceptable when transradial access is performed.[31,32] Patients at increased risk for systemic thromboembolism on withdrawal of warfarin, such as those with atrial fibrillation, mitral valve disease, or prior history of systemic thromboembolism, may be treated with intravenous unfractionated heparin or subcutaneous low-molecular-weight heparin in the periprocedural period.

VASCULAR ACCESS. A variety of vascular approaches are available for coronary arteriography. The selection of the vascular access depends on operator and patient preferences, anticoagulation status, and presence of peripheral vascular disease.

Femoral Artery Approach

The right and left femoral arteries are the most commonly used access sites for coronary arteriography (see Chap. 20). The common femoral artery courses medially to the femoral head, and the bifurcation of the common femoral artery into its branches is generally distal to the middle third of the femoral head, which can be localized by fluoroscopy before arterial puncture (see also Fig. 20-4). The anterior wall of the common femoral artery should be punctured several centimeters below the inguinal ligament but proximal to the bifurcation of the superficial femoral and profunda arterial branches. If the puncture site is proximal to the inguinal ligament, hemostasis after the procedure may be difficult with manual compression, leading to an increased risk of retroperitoneal hemorrhage. If the puncture site is at or distal to the femoral bifurcation, there is a higher risk of pseudoaneurysm formation after sheath removal. Ipsilateral cannulation of the femoral artery and femoral vein also increases the risk of arteriovenous fistula formation.

Brachial Artery Approach

Although Sones first introduced the cutdown approach to the brachial artery for coronary arteriography, percutaneous access to the brachial and radial arteries is now most often used.[33] These approaches are preferred to the femoral approach in the presence of severe peripheral vascular disease and morbid obesity,[34] and radial artery access is generally preferred to brachial catheterization because of its ease of catheter entry and removal. The brachial artery easily accommodates an 8F (1F = 0.33 mm in diameter) sheath.[33]

Radial Artery Approach

The radial artery is an increasingly used access site, although it is used in less than 3% of diagnostic procedures in the United States (see Chaps. 20 and 58). An Allen test should be carried out to ensure that the ulnar artery is patent in the event of radial artery occlusion.[35] Systemic anticoagulation with intravenous or intra-arterial unfractionated heparin (2000 to 5000 units) or bivalirudin is used for both brachial and radial artery approaches to prevent catheter thrombosis.[36] Use of a hydrophilic sheath and intra-arterial administration of verapamil and nitroglycerin reduce the occurrence of radial artery spasm, although rare episodes of radial artery trauma and avulsion have been reported. The long-term radial artery patency rate may also be improved with the use of a compression device that allows perfusion of the hand during hemostasis.[37] Several anatomic factors relate to transradial success, including a high-bifurcation radial origin (7.0%), full radial loop (2.3%), and extreme radial artery tortuosity (2.5%).[38]

The radial artery approach allows immediate ambulation after coronary arteriography with lower cost (compared with femoral closure devices), improved coronary visualization (compared with smaller 4F-diameter femoral catheters), and reduced bleeding complications (compared with femoral access).[39] Saphenous vein grafts (SVGs) can be engaged with use of either radial artery, but cannulation of the internal mammary artery (IMA) is best performed from the left radial artery. Engagement of the left IMA from the right radial artery is technically challenging but may be performed by use of a "headhunter" or another shaped catheter for selective entry into the left subclavian artery. A 0.035-inch angled hydrophilic guidewire is the most useful support wire for access to the subclavian artery. The radial artery will generally accommodate 4F to 6F catheters.

CATHETERS. Diagnostic catheters developed for coronary arteriography are generally constructed from polyethylene or polyurethane with a fine wire braid within the wall to allow advancement and directional control (torque) and to prevent kinking. The outer diameter size of the catheters ranges from 4F to 8F, but 5F and 6F catheters are used most commonly for diagnostic arteriography.

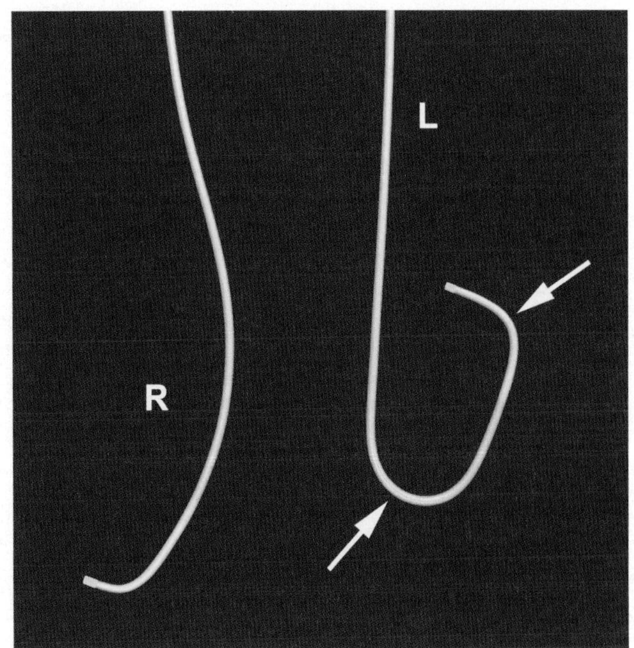

FIGURE 21-1 Right (R) and left (L) Judkins catheters. The primary (upper arrow) and secondary (lower arrow) curves of the Judkins left catheter are shown. *(Courtesy of Charles J. Davidson, Northwestern University.)*

JUDKINS CATHETERS. The Judkins left catheter is preshaped to allow entry into the left coronary ostium from the femoral approach with minimal catheter manipulation (**Figs. 21-1 and 21-2**). A preformed Judkins left catheter can also be used from the left brachial or radial artery, but a catheter with 0.5 cm less curvature than required for the femoral approach is generally better suited for coronary cannulation. The Judkins right catheter is shaped to permit entry into the right coronary artery (RCA) with a small amount of rotational (clockwise) catheter manipulation from any vascular approach.

Selection of Judkins catheter shape is based on the body habitus of the patient and size of the aortic root. The left coronary artery (LCA) is easily engaged with the Judkins left 4.0 catheter from the femoral approach in most patients, whereas patients with a dilated ascending aorta (e.g., in the setting of congenital aortic stenosis and aortic root dilation) may require the use of a Judkins left 5.0 or 6.0 catheter. Patients with large ascending aortic aneurysms may require arteriography with heat-modified catheters to achieve Judkins left 7.0 to 10.0 shapes. Use of a Judkins shape that is too small for the ascending aorta often leads to folding of the catheter within the aortic root. The best technique for removal of a folded Judkins left catheter from the body involves withdrawing the folded catheter into the descending aorta and advancing a guidewire anterograde in the contralateral common iliac artery. On withdrawal of the catheter and guidewire together, the catheter straightens and can be removed safely from the body without disruption of the arterial access site.

AMPLATZ CATHETERS. Amplatz catheters can be used for the femoral or brachial approach to coronary arteriography (**Fig. 21-3**). The Amplatz catheters are an excellent alternative in cases in which the Judkins catheter is not appropriately shaped to enter the coronary arteries. The Amplatz L-1 or L-2 catheter may be used for coronary angiography from the right brachial or radial approach. A modified Amplatz right catheter (AR-1 or AR-2) can be used for engagement of a horizontal or upward takeoff RCA or SVG.

OTHER CATHETERS. Other catheters used for coronary arteriography include the IMA left catheter with an angulated tip that allows engagement of the IMA or an upward takeoff RCA. Catheter shapes that permit engagement of SVGs include the multipurpose catheter (**Fig. 21-4**) and the Judkins right, modified Amplatz right, and hockey stick catheters. Specially designed catheters for engagement of the coronary arteries from the radial artery have also been developed.

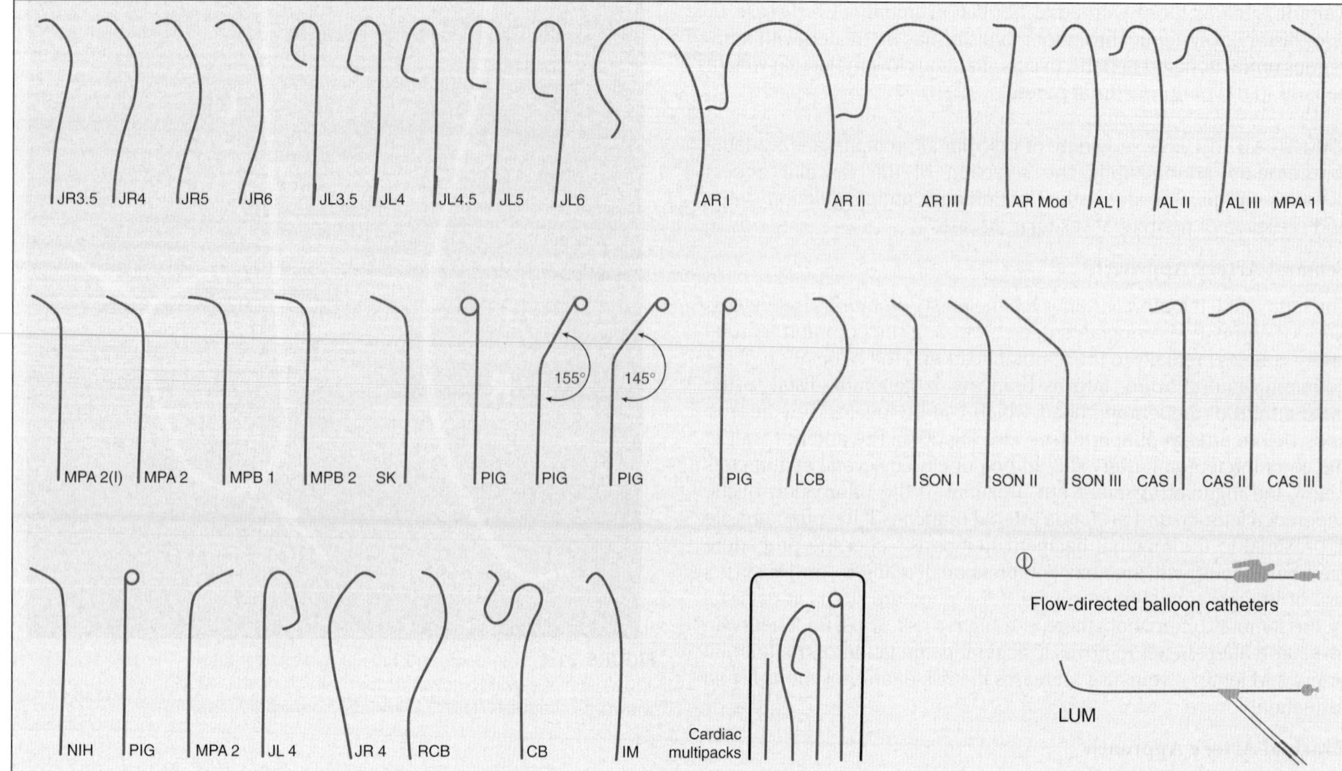

FIGURE 21-2 Tip configurations for several catheters useful in coronary arteriography. AL = Amplatz left; AR = Amplatz right; CAS = Castillo; CB = coronary bypass catheter; IM = internal mammary; JL = Judkins left; JR = Judkins right; LCB = left coronary bypass graft; LUM = lumen; Mod = modified; MP = multipurpose; NIH = National Institutes of Health; PIG = pigtail; RCB = right coronary bypass graft; SON = Sones. *(Courtesy of Cordis Corporation.)*

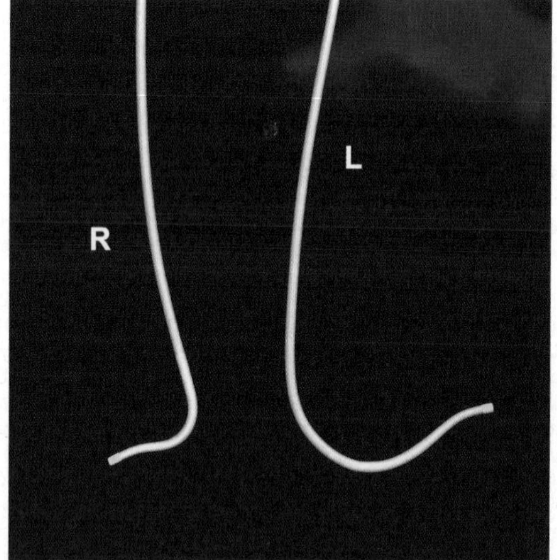

FIGURE 21-3 Amplatz right (R) and left (L) catheters. *(Courtesy of Charles J. Davidson, MD, Northwestern University.)*

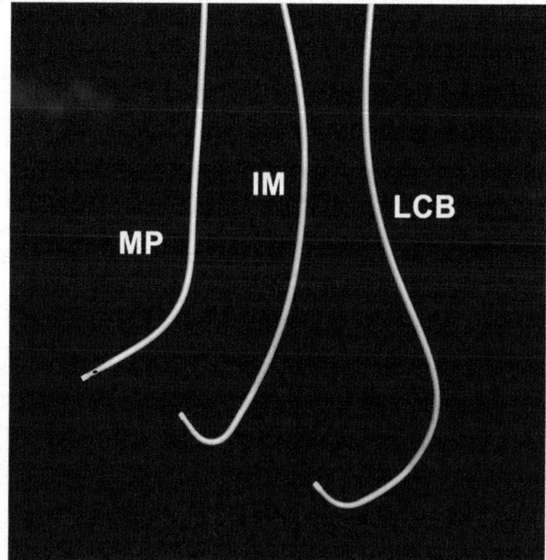

FIGURE 21-4 Multipurpose (MP), internal mammary (IM), and left coronary bypass (LCB) catheters. *(Courtesy of Charles J. Davidson, Northwestern University.)*

Drugs Used During Coronary Arteriography

ANALGESICS. The goal of analgesic use is to achieve a state of conscious sedation, defined by a minimally depressed level of consciousness that allows a patient to respond appropriately to verbal commands and to maintain a patent airway.[40,41] Several different sedation regimens are recommended, but depending on the patient's comorbid conditions, most use diazepam, 2.5 to 10 mg orally, and diphenhydramine, 25 to 50 mg orally, 1 hour before the procedure. Intravenous midazolam, 0.5 to 2 mg, and fentanyl, 25 to 50 μg, are useful agents to provide sedation during the procedure. Patients undergoing conscious sedation should have continuous hemodynamic, electrocardiographic, and oximetry monitoring as well as access to oxygen and suction ports and a resuscitation cart.

ANTICOAGULANTS. Intravenous unfractionated heparin is no longer required during routine coronary arteriography. Patients at increased risk for thromboembolic complications, including those with severe aortic stenosis, critical peripheral arterial disease, or arterial atheroembolic disease, and those undergoing procedures in

TABLE 21-4 Characteristics of Radiocontrast Agents

COMPOUND	BRAND NAME	OSMOLALITY (MOSM/KG H_2O)	VISCOSITY AT 37°C	IODINE (MG/ML)	SODIUM (MEQ/LITER)	ADDITIVES	SIDE EFFECT PROFILE
High-Osmolar Ionic Agents							
Sodium diatrizoate	Hypaque	1690	9.0	37.0	160	Calcium disodium EDTA	Electrophysiologic (++++) Hemodynamic (++++) Anticoagulant (++++) Nephrotoxicity (+++) Allergic (+++)
Sodium meglumine diatrizoate	Renografin	1940	8.4	370	160	Sodium citrate, disodium EDTA	
Nonionic or Low-Osmolar Agents							
Ioxaglate	Hexabrix	600	7.5	320	150	Calcium disodium EDTA	Electrophysiologic (+) Hemodynamic (+) Anticoagulant (+) Nephrotoxicity (+) Allergic (+)
Iohexol	Omnipaque	844	10.4	350	5	Tromethamine calcium disodium EDTA	
Iopamidol	Isovue	790	9.4	370	2	Tromethamine calcium disodium EDTA	
Ioversol	Optiray	702	5.8	320	2	Tromethamine calcium disodium EDTA	
Iodixanol	Visipaque	290	11.8	320	19	Tromethamine calcium disodium EDTA + 0.15 mEq/liter calcium	

++++ = common;+++ = occasional; ++ = infrequent;+ = rare; EDTA=ethylenediaminetetraacetic acid (a divalent cation chelating agent).
Modified from Hill J, Lambert C, Pepine C: Radiographic contrast agents. In Pepine C, Hill J, Lambert C (eds): Diagnostic and Therapeutic Cardiac Catheterization. Baltimore, Williams & Wilkins, 1994, pp 182-194.

which there is a need for prolonged (>1 to 2 minutes) use of guidewires in the central circulation may be given intravenous unfractionated heparin, 2000 to 5000 units. Patients undergoing brachial or radial artery catheterization should also receive systemic anticoagulation with unfractionated heparin or bivalirudin. Frequent flushing of all diagnostic and guiding catheters with heparinized saline prevents the formation of microthrombi within the catheter tip. A continuous flush through the arterial access sheath may also lower the occurrence of distal thromboembolism.

The anticoagulant effect of unfractionated heparin can be reversed with protamine, 1 mg for every 100 units of heparin. Protamine causes anaphylaxis or serious hypotensive episodes in approximately 2% of patients, and protamine should not be administered to patients with prior exposure to NPH insulin, to those with a history of unstable angina or high-risk coronary anatomy, or to patients who have undergone coronary arteriography by means of the brachial or radial artery. Femoral sheaths can be removed after the anticoagulant effect of unfractionated heparin has dissipated, as assessed by an activated clotting time of less than 150 to 180 seconds.

TREATMENT OF PERIPROCEDURAL ISCHEMIA. Patients may develop angina during coronary arteriography because of ischemia induced by tachycardia, hypertension, contrast agents, microembolization, coronary spasm or enhanced vasomotor tone, or dynamic platelet aggregation. Sublingual (0.3 mg), intracoronary (50 to 200 μg), or intravenous (10 to 25 μg/min) nitroglycerin can be given to patients with a systolic blood pressure above 100 mm Hg. Patients without contraindications to beta blockers, such as bradycardia, bronchospasm, or left ventricular dysfunction, can be given intravenous metoprolol, 2.5 to 5.0 mg, or propranolol, 1 to 4 mg. Intra-aortic balloon counterpulsation is also a useful adjunct in patients with coronary ischemia and left main CAD, cardiogenic shock, or refractory pulmonary edema.

CONTRAST AGENTS. All radiographic contrast agents contain iodine, which effectively absorbs x-rays in the energy range of the angiographic imaging system. Radiographic contrast agents currently used for coronary arteriography may also produce a number of adverse hemodynamic, electrophysiologic, and renal effects. The frequency of these side effects varies among the different radiocontrast agents because of differences in their ionic content, osmolality, and viscosity (**Table 21-4**).

IONIC CONTRAST AGENTS. The monomeric ionic contrast agents initially used for coronary arteriography were the high-osmolar meglumine and sodium salts of diatrizoic acid. These substances dissociate into cations and iodine-containing anions that have a higher serum osmolality (>1500 mOsm) than human plasma (300 mOsm). The hypertonicity of these compounds produced sinus bradycardia, heart block, QT interval and QRS prolongation, ST-segment depression, giant T wave inversion, decreased left ventricular contractility, decreased systolic pressure, and increased left ventricular end-diastolic pressure, owing in part to the calcium-chelating properties of these agents. Ventricular tachycardia and fibrillation occurred in 0.5% of cases and developed more often when ionic contrast agents were injected into a damped (ventricularized) coronary catheter, were given too rapidly, or were administered in too great a volume. Because of the availability of other, less toxic contrast agents, ionic contrast agents are now rarely used for coronary arteriography. When ionic agents are selected, additional precautions are needed to avoid complications. Patients should be counseled about coughing, which helps clear contrast material from within the coronary artery, before the first selective coronary arteriogram is performed, and the minimal amount of contrast agent needed to fill the entire coronary artery should be given.

NONIONIC AND LOW-OSMOLAR CONTRAST AGENTS. Nonionic agents do not ionize in solution and provide more iodine-containing particles per milliliter of contrast material than ionic agents. Their osmolality is substantially reduced (<850 mOsm) because these agents exist in solution as single neutral molecules and do not chelate calcium, potentially leading to fewer side effects.

SIDE EFFECTS. Unwanted reactions may also occur after use of nonionic radiocontrast agents, related in part to the hyperosmolality of these agents. These reactions include hot flushing, nausea, vomiting, and arrhythmia. Hypotension after contrast medium administration may be due to an anaphylactoid reaction, a direct toxic effect, or a vasovagal reaction. Ionic radiocontrast agents may inhibit clot formation when they

CH 21

TABLE 21-5 Toxicities Associated with Radiocontrast Agents

Allergic (anaphylactoid) reactions
Grade I: single episode of emesis, nausea, sneezing, or vertigo
Grade II: hives; multiple episodes of emesis, fevers, or chills
Grade III: clinical shock, bronchospasm, laryngospasm or edema, loss of consciousness, hypotension, hypertension, cardiac arrhythmia, angioedema, or pulmonary edema
Cardiovascular toxicity
Electrophysiologic
Bradycardia (asystole, heart block)
Tachycardia (sinus, ventricular)
Ventricular fibrillation
Hemodynamic
Hypotension (cardiac depression, vasodilation)
Heart failure (cardiac depression, increased intravascular volume)
Nephrotoxicity
Discomfort
Nausea, vomiting
Heat and flushing
Hyperthyroidism

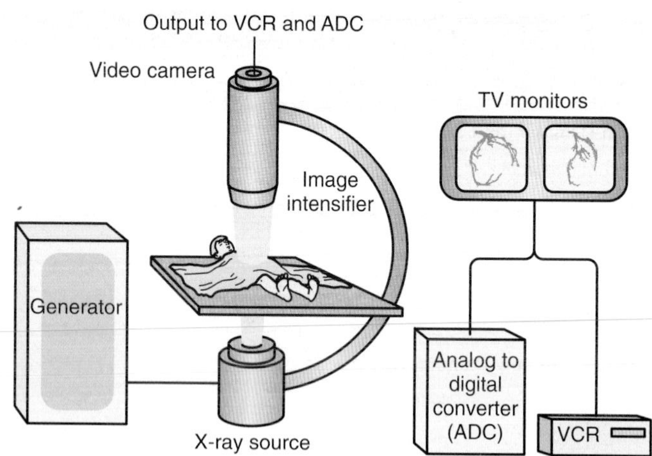

FIGURE 21-5 Cineangiographic equipment. The major components include a generator, x-ray tube, image intensifier attached to a positioner such as a C-arm, optical system, video camera, videocassette recorder (VCR), analog to digital converter (ADC), and television monitors. The x-ray tube is the source of the x-ray beam, which passes superiorly through the patient.

are mixed with blood, and although nonionic agents exhibit less of an anticoagulant effect, the clinical manifestations of clot formation and embolization are uncommon with both classes of contrast agents. The low-osmolality ionic dimer methylglucamine–sodium ioxaglate retains most of the anticoagulant properties of diatrizoate sodium but has complications similar to those of the isosmolar, nonionic dimer contrast agent iodixanol in clinical study.[42] No selective advantage on the prevention of contrast-induced nephropathy has been shown with any of the class of nonionic agents.

CONTRAST-INDUCED NEPHROPATHY. Worsening of renal function may occur after contrast agent administration in 13% to 20% of patients, particularly in those with prior renal insufficiency, diabetes mellitus, dehydration before the procedure, congestive heart failure, larger volumes of contrast material, and recent (<48 hours) exposure to contrast material[43] (see Chap. 93). Fluid administration and limitation of contrast load are useful in preventing contrast nephropathy. Controversy remains whether the use of sodium bicarbonate has benefit over normal saline alone as the agent for volume expansion before administration of contrast material.[44-46] Preprocedural administration of *N*-acetylcysteine may also be useful to prevent this contrast nephropathy after coronary angiography, but large-scale randomized trials are lacking.

CONTRAST REACTION PROPHYLAXIS. Reactions to radiocontrast agents (**Table 21-5**) are classified as mild (grade I: single episode of emesis, nausea, sneezing, or vertigo), moderate (grade II: hives; multiple episodes of emesis, fevers, or chills), or severe (grade III: clinical shock, bronchospasm, laryngospasm or edema, loss of consciousness, hypotension, hypertension, cardiac arrhythmias, angioedema, or pulmonary edema). Although mild or moderate reactions occur in approximately 9.0% of patients, severe reactions are uncommon (0.2% to 1.6%).[47,48] Reactions to contrast agents may be more difficult to manage in patients receiving beta blocker therapy. Recurrence rates may approach 50% on reexposure to contrast agents, and prophylactic use of H1 and H2 histamine-blocking agents and aspirin therapy has been advocated. In a meta-analysis of nine trials addressing the value of premedication in patients with a history of reactions to contrast agents, a 70% reduction in the occurrence of grade III reactions was associated with pretreatment with corticosteroids (from 0.9% to 0.2% in premedicated patients; odds ratio, 0.28; 95% confidence intervals, 0.13 to 0.60). Although these reductions appear clinically relevant, 100 to 150 patients would require pretreatment to prevent a single contrast agent–related event, which has led to the recommendation by one group that premedication is not routinely needed.[47] Nevertheless, patients with a suspected severe prior reaction to a contrast agent should receive two doses of prednisone, 60 mg (or its equivalent), the night before and again at 2 hours before the procedure. Diphenhydramine, 50 mg, and cimetidine, 300 mg, may also be given before the procedure.

Anatomy and Variations of the Coronary Arteries

The basic principle of radiographic coronary imaging is that radiation produced by the x-ray tube is attenuated as it passes through the body and is detected by the image intensifier (**Fig. 21-5**). Iodinated contrast medium injected into the coronary arteries enhances the absorption of x-rays and produces a sharp contrast with the surrounding cardiac tissues. The x-ray shadow is then converted into a visible light image by an image intensifier, displayed on fluoroscopic monitors, and stored on 35-mm cinefilm or a digital storage system. Although 35-mm cinefilm has better image resolution (4 line pairs/mm) than digital imaging (2.5 line pairs/mm) archived in a standard DICOM3 512 × 512 × 8 bit pixel matrix format, digital imaging has largely replaced 35-mm cinefilm for coronary angiography because of its versatility with respect to image transfer, low-cost acquisition and storage, and capability for image enhancement after image acquisition. More recently, direct digital imaging systems, termed flat panel catheterization laboratories, have eliminated the analog to digital converters of the conventional image intensifiers without compromise of the image integrity.[49] This has resulted in reduced radiation exposure and enhanced image quality.[50]

The major epicardial branches and their second- and third-order branches can be visualized by coronary arteriography. The network of smaller intramyocardial branches is generally not seen because of their size, cardiac motion, and limitations in resolution of cineangiographic systems. These fourth-order and higher "resistance" vessels play a major role in autoregulation of coronary blood flow (see Chap. 52), may limit myocardial perfusion during stress, and contribute to ischemia in patients with left ventricular hypertrophy or systemic hypertension. Coronary perfusion in these smaller branch vessels can be quantitatively assessed by use of the myocardial blush score, which has important prognostic significance in patients with ST-segment elevation myocardial infarction and those undergoing PCI.[51]

ARTERIAL NOMENCLATURE AND EXTENT OF DISEASE. The Coronary Artery Surgery Study (CASS) investigators established the nomenclature most commonly used to describe the coronary anatomy, defining 27 segments in three major coronary arteries (**Table 21-6**). The Bypass Angioplasty Revascularization Investigators (BARI) modified these criteria by addition of two segments for the ramus intermedius and the third diagonal branch. In this system, the three major coronary arteries include the left

TABLE 21-6 Classification System for Coronary Segments

NUMBER	MAP LOCATION	NUMBER	MAP LOCATION	NUMBER	MAP LOCATION
Right Coronary Artery (RCA)		**Left Main Coronary Artery**		**Left Circumflex Artery (LCx)**	
1	Proximal RCA	11	Left main coronary artery	18	Proximal LCx
2	Mid RCA	**Left Anterior Descending (LAD)**		19	Distal LCx
3	Distal RCA	12	Proximal LAD	20	First obtuse marginal
4	Right posterior descending branch	13	Mid LAD	21	Second obtuse marginal
5	Right posterior atrioventricular	14	Distal LAD	22	Third obtuse marginal
6	First right posterolateral	15	First diagonal	23	LCx atrioventricular groove
7	Second right posterolateral	16	Second diagonal	24	First left posterolateral
8	Third right posterolateral	17	LAD septal perforators	25	Second left posterolateral
9	Posterior descending septals	29	Third diagonal	26	Third left posterolateral
10	Acute marginal segment	27	Left posterior descending branch		
		28	Ramus intermedius branch		

From CASS Principal Investigators and their Associates: Coronary Artery Surgery Study (CASS): A randomized trial of coronary artery surgery: Survival data. Circulation 68:939, 1983.

anterior descending (LAD) artery, left circumflex (LCx) artery, and RCA with a right-dominant, balanced, or left-dominant circulation (see later). CAD is defined as a more than 50% diameter stenosis in one or more of these vessels, although it is clear that stenoses of less than 50% have major prognostic implications because these lesions most commonly lead to plaque rupture and acute myocardial infarction. Subcritical stenoses of less than 50% are best characterized as nonobstructive CAD; obstructive CAD is classified as one-, two-, or three-vessel disease.

A number of "jeopardy scores" were developed to quantitate plaque burden, to predict patient-based clinical outcomes, and to identify risk factors for the presence of atherosclerosis and its progression.[52] The Califf scoring system divided the coronary circulation into six segments with two points allotted for each coronary stenosis of 75% or more (score range: 0 to 12). The Gensini scoring system used an ordinal ranking based on stenosis severity in 11 coronary segments (score range: 0 to 72). The Candell-Riera scoring system used an ordinal ranking (from 1 to 5) of 13 coronary segments (score range: 0 to 65). Differences between these scoring systems were primarily related to definitions rather than to their ability to provide unique prognostic information; one comparative study found that 80% of the prognostic information in one jeopardy index was obtained with other indices using subtly different methodologies. In CASS, the major determinants of 6-year outcome included the number of diseased vessels, the number of diseased proximal segments, and the global left ventricular function; these three factors accounted for 80% of the prognostic information.

Angiographic Projections. The major coronary arteries traverse the interventricular and atrioventricular grooves, aligned with the long and short axes of the heart, respectively. Because the heart is oriented obliquely in the thoracic cavity, the coronary circulation is generally visualized in the right anterior oblique (RAO) and left anterior oblique (LAO) projections to furnish true posteroanterior and lateral views of the heart, but these views are limited by vessel foreshortening and superimposition of branches. Simultaneous rotation of the x-ray beam in the sagittal plane provides a better view of the major coronary arteries and their branches. A simple nomenclature has evolved for the description of these sagittal views that characterizes the relationship between the image intensifier and the patient. Assuming that the x-ray tube is under the patient's table and the image intensifier is over the patient's table, the projection is referred to as the cranial view if the image intensifier is tilted toward the head of the patient (**Figs. 21-6 and 21-7**). The projection is referred to as the caudal view if the image intensifier is tilted down toward the feet of the patient.

It is difficult to predict which angulated views will be most useful for any particular patient because the "optimal" angiographic projection depends largely on body habitus, variation in the coronary anatomy, and location of the lesion. It is recommended that the coronary arteries be visualized in both the LAO and RAO projections with both cranial and caudal angulation.

LEFT CORONARY ARTERY

Cannulation

The Judkins left 4.0 coronary catheter is used most often to engage the LCA (**Fig. 21-8**). If the Judkins left catheter begins to turn out of profile (so that one or both curves of the catheter are no longer visualized en face), it can be rotated clockwise very slightly and advanced slowly to enter the left sinus of Valsalva, permitting the catheter tip to engage the ostium of the LCA. When the ascending aorta is dilated or the aortic arch is unfolded, advancement of the Judkins left 4.0 coronary catheter may result in the formation of an acute secondary angle of the catheter, pointing the tip of the catheter upward, away from the left coronary ostium. Further advancement of the Judkins left catheter in this position should be avoided because the catheter then prolapses on itself and becomes folded in the ascending aortic arch. In the event this occurs, a guidewire can be temporarily reinserted into the catheter to straighten the secondary bend and to permit the catheter to be advanced to the left sinus of Valsalva. If the ascending aorta is significantly dilated, the Judkins left 4.0 catheter should be exchanged for a larger size (e.g., Judkins left 5.0 or 6.0). If the tip of the Judkins left catheter advances beyond the ostium of the LCA without engagement, the primary bend of the catheter can be reshaped within the patient's body by further careful advancement and prompt withdrawal of the catheter, allowing the tip to "pop into" the ostium of the LCA. This maneuver, along with gentle clockwise or counterclockwise rotation, frequently permits selective engagement of the LCA when the initial attempt has failed. If the catheter tip is located below the origin of the LCA, as in the case of a smaller aortic root, a shorter Judkins left 3.5 catheter can be used to allow coaxial engagement of the LCA.

Use of the Amplatz left catheters to cannulate the LCA requires more catheter manipulation than with the standard Judkins left catheter. In this circumstance, the broad secondary curve of the Amplatz left 1 or 2 catheter is positioned so that it rests on the right aortic cusp with its tip pointing toward the left aortic cusp. Alternating advancement and retraction of the catheter with slight clockwise rotation allows the catheter tip to advance slowly and superiorly along the left sinus of Valsalva to enter the left coronary ostium. When the tip enters the ostium, the position of the catheter can usually be stabilized with slight retraction of the catheter. After the left coronary ostium has been cannulated, the pressure at the tip of the catheter should be checked immediately to ensure that there is no damping or ventricularization of the pressure contour. If a damped or ventricularized pressure tracing is obtained, the catheter should be removed immediately from the LCA, and an attempt at repositioning should be made. If abnormal

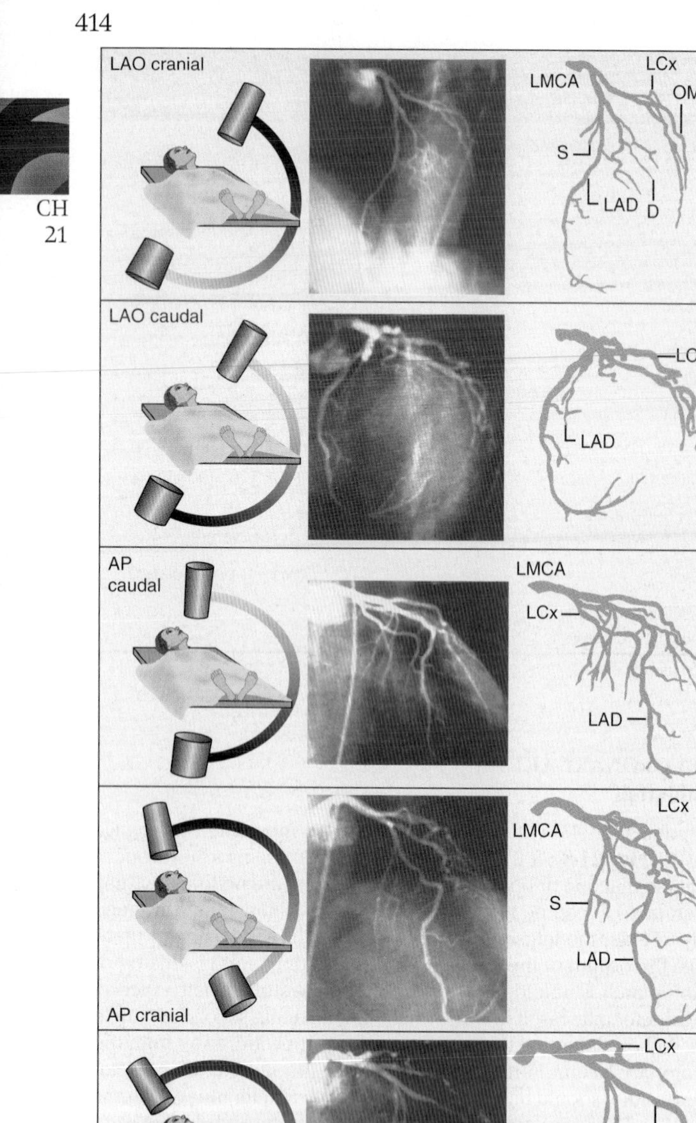

FIGURE 21-6 Angiographic views of the left coronary artery. The approximate positions of the x-ray tube and image intensifier are shown for each of the commonly used angiographic views. The 60-degree left anterior oblique view with 20 degrees of cranial angulation (LAO cranial) shows the ostium and distal portion of the left main coronary artery (LMCA), the middle and distal portions of the left anterior descending (LAD) artery, septal perforators (S), diagonal branches (D), and the proximal left circumflex (LCx) and superior obtuse marginal branch (OMB). The 60-degree left anterior oblique view with 25 degrees of caudal angulation (LAO caudal) shows the proximal LMCA and the proximal segments of the LAD and LCx arteries. The anteroposterior projection with 20 degrees of caudal angulation (AP caudal) shows the distal LMCA and proximal segments of the LAD and LCx arteries. The anteroposterior projection with 20 degrees of cranial angulation (AP cranial) also shows the midportion of the LAD artery and its septal (S) branches. The 30-degree right anterior oblique projection with 20 degrees of cranial angulation (RAO cranial) shows the course of the LAD artery and its septal (S) and diagonal branches. The 30-degree right anterior oblique projection with 25 degrees of caudal angulation (RAO caudal) shows the LCx and obtuse marginal branches (OMB).

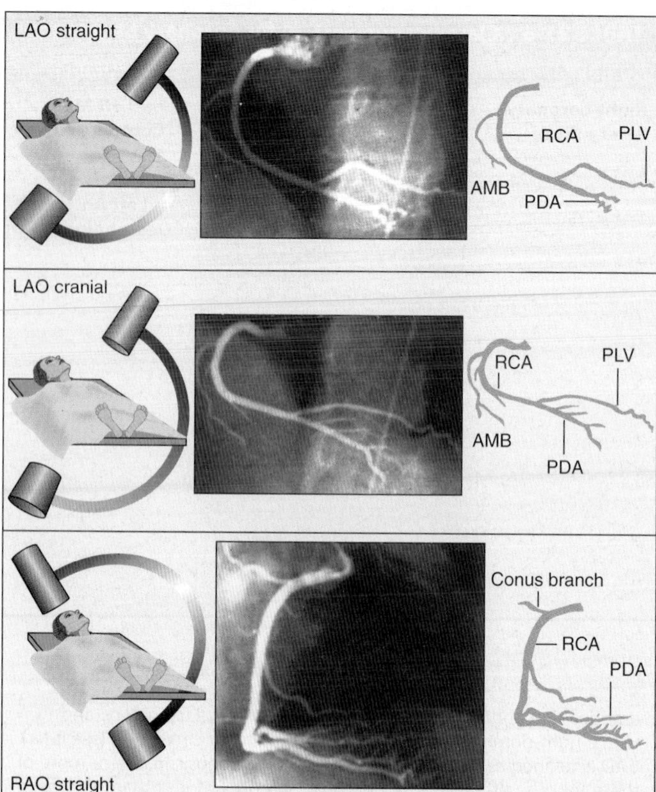

FIGURE 21-7 Angiographic views of the right coronary artery (RCA). The approximate positions of the x-ray tube and image intensifier are shown for each of the commonly used angiographic views. The 60-degree left anterior oblique view (LAO straight) shows the proximal and middle portions of the RCA as well as the acute marginal branches (AMB) and termination of the RCA in the posterior left ventricular branches (PLV). The 60-degree left anterior oblique view with 25 degrees of cranial angulation (LAO cranial) shows the midportion of the RCA and the origin and course of the posterior descending artery (PDA). The 30-degree right anterior oblique view (RAO straight) shows the midportion of the RCA, the conus branch, and the course of the PDA.

pressure recording persists, the catheter should be withdrawn from the coronary artery, and a nonselective injection of contrast medium into the LCA should be performed in the anteroposterior (AP) view to evaluate the LMCA. If the pressure measured at the catheter tip is normal and a test injection of contrast agent suggests the absence of LMCA disease, left coronary arteriography is then performed by standard techniques. To remove the Amplatz left catheter from the coronary artery, the catheter should be advanced forward in the body to disengage the catheter tip superiorly from the coronary ostium. Simply withdrawing the Amplatz left catheter results in deep seating of the catheter tip within the coronary artery, potentially resulting in catheter-induced arterial dissection.

LEFT MAIN CORONARY ARTERY. The LMCA arises from the superior portion of the left aortic sinus, just below the sinotubular ridge of the aorta, which defines the border separating the left sinus of Valsalva from the smooth (tubular) portion of the aorta. The LMCA ranges from 3 to 6 mm in diameter and may be up to 10 to 15 mm in length. The LMCA courses behind the right ventricular outflow tract and usually bifurcates into the LAD artery and LCx branches. Rarely, the LMCA is absent, and there are separate ostia of the LAD and LCx arteries. The LMCA is best visualized in the AP projection with slight (0 to 20 degrees) caudal angulation, but it should be viewed in several projections with the vessel off the spine to exclude LMCA stenosis (**Figs. 21-9 and 21-10**).

LEFT ANTERIOR DESCENDING ARTERY. The LAD courses along the epicardial surface of the anterior interventricular groove toward

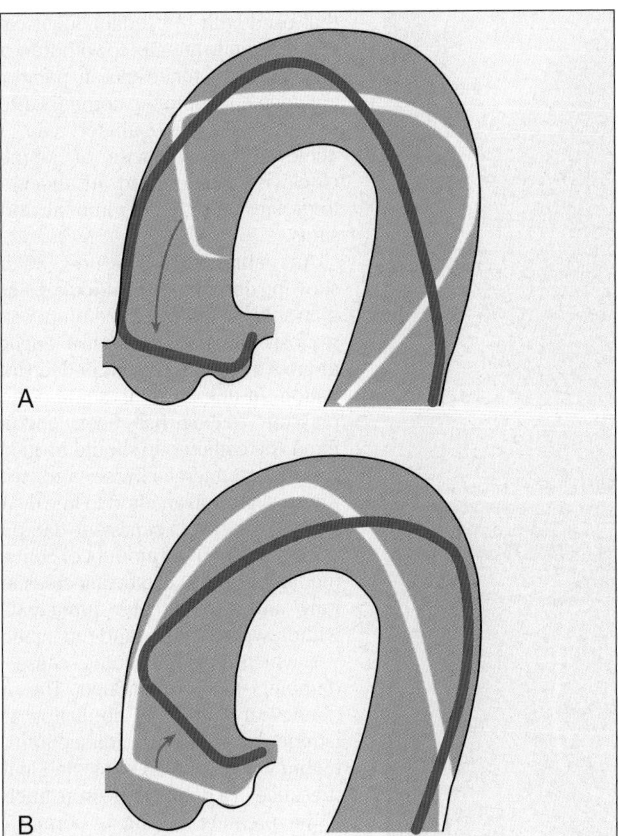

FIGURE 21-8 **A,** Push-pull technique for catheterization of the left coronary artery with the Judkins left catheter. In the left anterior oblique view, the coronary catheter is positioned in the ascending aorta over a guidewire, and the guidewire is removed. The catheter is advanced so that the tip enters the left sinus of Valsalva. **B,** If the catheter does not selectively engage the ostium of the left coronary artery, further slow advancement into the left sinus of Valsalva imparts a temporary acute angle at the catheter. Prompt withdrawal of the catheter allows easy entry into the left coronary artery.

the cardiac apex. In the RAO projection, it extends along the anterior aspect of the heart; in the LAO projection, it passes down the cardiac midline, between the right and left ventricles (see Fig. 21-6).

The major branches of the LAD are the septal and diagonal branches. The septal branches arise from the LAD at approximately 90-degree angles and pass into the interventricular septum, varying in size, number, and distribution. In some cases, there is a large first septal branch that is vertically oriented and divides into a number of secondary "pitchforking" branches that ramify throughout the septum. In other cases, a more horizontally oriented, large first septal branch is present that passes parallel to the LAD itself within the myocardium. In still other cases, a number of septal arteries are roughly comparable in size. These septal branches interconnect with similar septal branches passing upward from the posterior descending branch of the RCA to produce a network of potential collateral channels. The interventricular septum is the most densely vascularized area of the heart.

The diagonal branches of the LAD pass over the anterolateral aspect of the heart. Although virtually all patients have a single LAD in the anterior interventricular groove, there is wide variability in the number and size of diagonal branches. Most patients (90%) have one to three diagonal branches, and acquired atherosclerotic occlusion of the diagonal branches should be suspected if no diagonal branches are seen, particularly if there are unexplained contraction abnormalities of the anterolateral left ventricle. Visualization of the origin of the diagonal branches often requires very steep (50 to 60 degrees) LAO and angulated cranial (20 to 40 degrees) skews.

In some patients, the LMCA trifurcates into the LAD, LCx, and ramus intermedius. When it is present, the ramus intermedius arises between the LAD and LCx arteries. This vessel is analogous to either a diagonal branch or an obtuse marginal branch, depending on its anterior or posterior course along the lateral aspect of the left ventricle. In most patients (80%), the LAD courses around the left ventricular apex and terminates along the diaphragmatic aspect of the left ventricle. In the remaining patients, the LAD fails to reach the diaphragmatic surface, terminating instead either at or before the cardiac apex. In this circumstance, the posterior descending branch (PDA) of the RCA or LCx is larger and longer than usual and supplies the apical portion of the ventricle.

The best angiographic projections for viewing the course of the LAD are the cranially angulated LAO, AP, and RAO views. The LAO cranial view displays the midportion of the LAD and separates the diagonal and septal branches. The RAO cranial view displays the proximal, middle, and distal segment of the LAD and allows separation of the diagonal branches superiorly and the septal branches inferiorly. The AP view requiring cranial (20 to 40 degrees) skew often projects the midportion of the LAD, separating the vessel from its diagonal and septal branches. The LAO caudal view also displays the origin of the LAD in a horizontally oriented heart, and the AP caudal or shallow RAO caudal view visualizes the proximal LAD as it arises from the LMCA. The RAO caudal projection is also useful for visualization of the distal LAD and its apical termination.

In some patients with no LMCA but separate ostia for the LAD and LCx, the LAD generally has a more anterior origin than the LCx. The LAD can be engaged with the Judkins left catheter in this setting with paradoxical counterclockwise rotation, which rotates the secondary bend of the catheter to a posterior position in the aorta and turns the primary bend and tip of the catheter to an anterior position. The opposite maneuver may be used to engage the LCx selectively in the setting of separate LAD and LCx ostia. A Judkins catheter with a larger curve, such as a Judkins left 5.0, selectively engages the downward coursing LCx, and a catheter with a shorter curve, such as a Judkins left 3.5, tends to engage selectively the more anterior and superior LAD.

LEFT CIRCUMFLEX ARTERY. The LCx artery originates from the LMCA and courses within the posterior (left) atrioventricular groove toward the inferior interventricular groove (see Fig. 21-6). The LCx artery is the dominant vessel in 15% of patients, supplying the left PDA from the distal continuation of the LCx. In the remaining patients, the distal LCx varies in size and length, depending on the number of posterolateral branches supplied by the distal RCA. The LCx usually gives off one to three large obtuse marginal branches as it passes down the atrioventricular groove. These are the principal branches of the LCx because they supply the lateral free wall of the left ventricle. Beyond the origins of the obtuse marginal branches, the distal LCx tends to be small. The actual position of the LCx can be determined on the late phase of a left coronary injection when the coronary sinus becomes opacified with diluted contrast material.

The RAO caudal and LAO caudal projections are best for visualization of the proximal and middle LCx and obtuse marginal branches. The AP (or 5- to 15-degree RAO) caudal projections also show the origins of the obtuse marginal branches. More severe rightward angulation often superimposes the origins of the obtuse marginal branches on the LCx. If the LCA is dominant, the optimal projection for the left PDA is the LAO cranial view. The LCx artery also gives rise to one or two left atrial circumflex branches. These branches supply the lateral and posterior aspects of the left atrium.

RIGHT CORONARY ARTERY. Cannulation of the origin of the RCA is also performed in the LAO position but requires maneuvers different from those for cannulation of the LCA. Whereas the Judkins left catheter naturally seeks the ostium of the LCA, the Judkins right or modified Amplatz catheters must be rotated to engage the vessel. This is usually accomplished by first passing the catheter to a point just superior to the aortic valve in the left sinus of Valsalva with the tip of the catheter facing rightward and then rotating the catheter clockwise while the catheter is withdrawn slightly, which forces the tip to move anteriorly from the left sinus of Valsalva to the right sinus of Valsalva along the sinotubular ridge (**Fig. 21-11**). Sudden rightward and downward movement of the catheter tip signifies the entry into the right coronary ostium. If the ostium of the RCA is not easily located, the most common reason is that the ostium has a more superior and anterior origin than anticipated. Repeated attempts to engage the RCA should be made at a level slightly more distal to the aortic valve. Nonselective contrast agent injections in the right sinus of Valsalva may reveal the site of the origin of the RCA. Positioning of an Amplatz left catheter in the ostium of the RCA requires a technique similar to

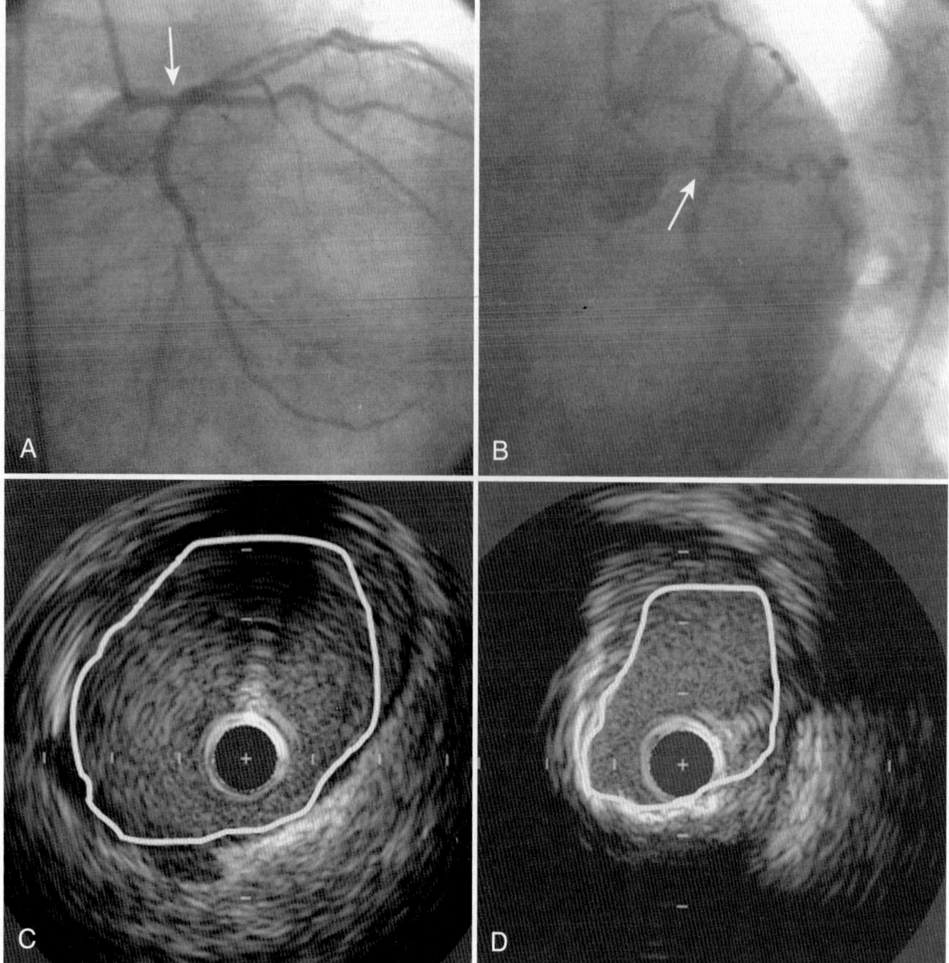

FIGURE 21-9 Intermediate left main coronary artery (LMCA) stenosis evaluated with intravascular ultrasound (IVUS [see Chap. 22]). **A,** Left coronary arteriography in the standard right anterior oblique projection with caudal angulation (arrow indicates distal left main coronary artery). **B,** The left anterior oblique projection with caudal angulation shows a tapered stenosis of the LMCA (arrow). **C,** IVUS of the proximal LMCA shows a minimal cross-sectional area 16 mm^2 (white circle). **D,** IVUS of the distal LMCA shows LMCA stenosis with a luminal cross-sectional area of 6.5 mm^2 (white outline), which is consistent with a hemodynamically significant LMCA stenosis.

that used with the Judkins right catheter. If a gentle attempt to withdraw the Amplatz catheter results in paradoxical deep entry into the coronary artery, removal of the catheter can be achieved by clockwise or counterclockwise rotation and advancement to prolapse the catheter into the aortic sinus.

An abnormal pressure tracing showing damping or ventricularization may suggest the presence of an ostial stenosis or spasm, selective engagement of the conus branch, or deep intubation of the RCA. If an abnormal pressure tracing has been encountered, the catheter tip should be gently rotated counterclockwise and withdrawn slightly in an effort to free the tip of the catheter. If persistent damping occurs, a very small amount of contrast medium (<1 mL) can be injected carefully and the catheter immediately withdrawn in a "shoot-and-run" maneuver, which may allow the cause of damping to be identified. The frequency of ventricular fibrillation and iatrogenic coronary dissection is higher when the RCA is injected in the presence of a damped pressure tracing. If the pressure tracing is normal on entry into the RCA, the vessel should be imaged in at least two projections. The initial injection should be gentle because of the possibility that forceful injection through a catheter whose tip is immediately adjacent to the vessel wall may also lead to dissection. Coronary spasm of the RCA ostium may also occur as a result of catheter intubation. When an ostial stenosis of the RCA is seen, intracoronary nitroglycerin or calcium channel antagonists may be useful in excluding catheter-induced spasm as a cause of the coronary artery narrowing.

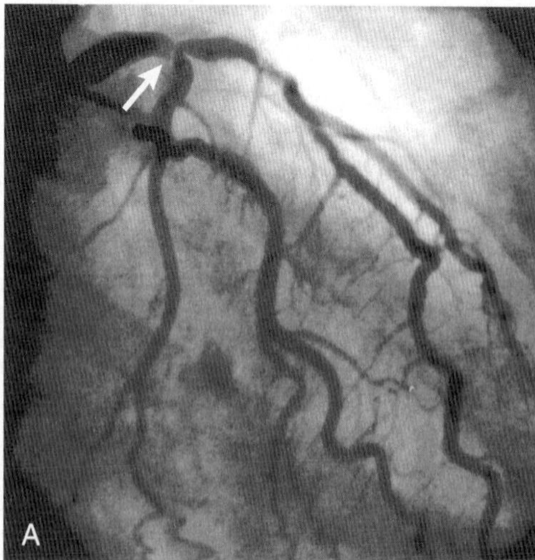

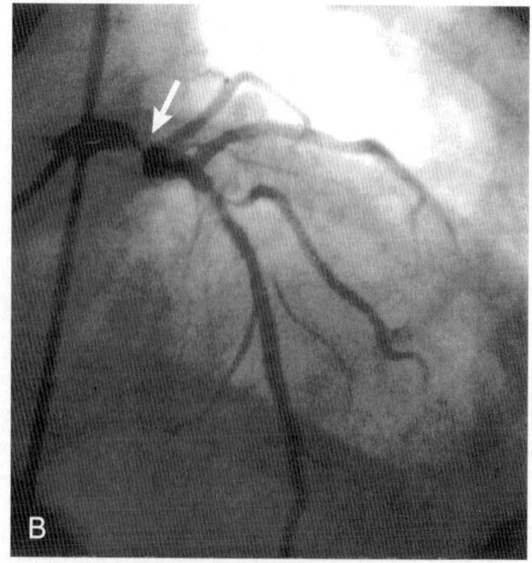

FIGURE 21-10 Severe stenosis of the distal left main coronary artery. **A,** Right anterior oblique projection with caudal angulation demonstrates a severe ulcerated stenosis in the distal portion of the left main coronary artery (arrow). **B,** An anteroposterior view with cranial angulation demonstrates this stenosis in a second view. Limited coronary arteriography should be performed when severe left main coronary artery stenosis (arrow) has been demonstrated.

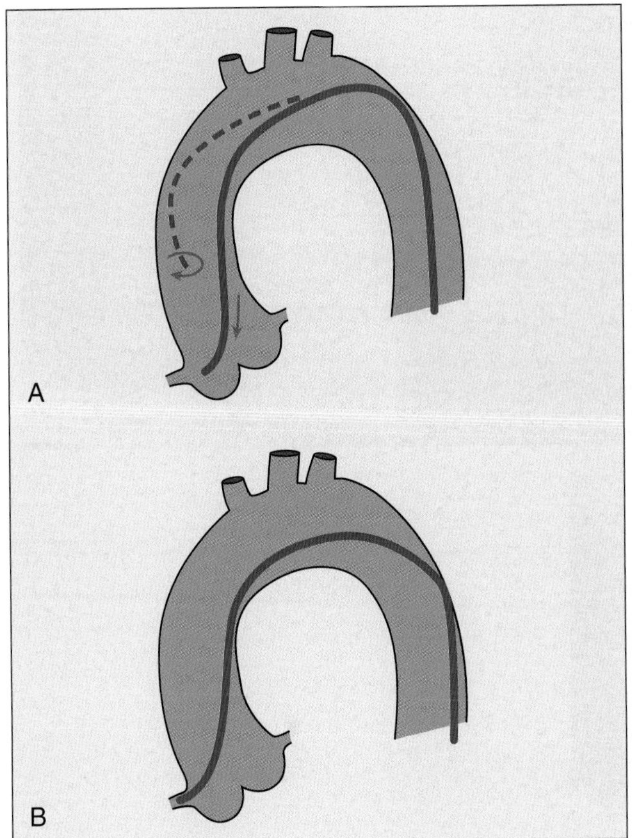

FIGURE 21-11 Cannulation of the right coronary artery with the Judkins right catheter. **A,** The catheter is advanced to a point just superior to the aortic valve in the left sinus of Valsalva with the tip of the catheter facing rightward, and then the catheter is rotated clockwise while the catheter is withdrawn slightly. **B,** Sudden rightward and downward movement of the catheter tip signifies the entry into the right coronary ostium.

The RCA originates from the right anterior aortic sinus somewhat inferior to the origin of the LCA (see Fig. 21-7). It passes along the right atrioventricular groove toward the crux (a point on the diaphragmatic surface of the heart where the anterior atrioventricular groove, the posterior atrioventricular groove, and the inferior interventricular groove coalesce). The first branch of the RCA is generally the conus artery, which arises at the right coronary ostium or within the first few millimeters of the RCA in about 50% of patients. In the remaining patients, the conus artery arises from a separate ostium in the right aortic sinus just above the right coronary ostium. The second branch of the RCA is usually the sinoatrial node artery. It has been found that this vessel arises from the RCA in just under 60% of patients, from the LCx artery in just under 40%, and from both arteries with a dual blood supply in the remaining cases. The midportion of the RCA usually gives rise to one or several medium-sized acute marginal branches. These branches supply the anterior wall of the right ventricle and may provide collateral circulation in patients with LAD occlusion. The RCA terminates in a PDA and one or more right posterolateral branches.

Because the RCA traverses both the atrioventricular and the interventricular grooves, multiple angiographic projections are needed to visualize each segment of the RCA. The ostium of the RCA is best evaluated in the LAO views, with or without cranial or caudal angulation. The left lateral view is also useful for visualization of the ostium of the RCA in difficult cases. The ostium is identified by the reflux of contrast material from the RCA that also delineates the aortic root with swirling of contrast material in the region of the ostium. The proximal RCA is generally evaluated in the LAO cranial or LAO caudal projection but is markedly foreshortened in the RAO projections. The midportion of the RCA is best seen in the LAO cranial, RAO, and left lateral projections. The origin of the PDA and the posterolateral branches are best evaluated in the LAO cranial or AP cranial view, whereas the midportion of the PDA can be shown in the AP cranial or RAO projection.

Right Coronary Artery Dominance (Figs. 21-12 to 21-14). The RCA is dominant in 85% of patients, supplying the PDA and at least one posterolateral branch (right dominant). The PDA courses in the inferior interventricular groove and gives rise to a number of small inferior septal branches, which pass upward to supply the lower portion of the interventricular septum and interdigitate with superior septal branches passing down from the LAD artery. After giving rise to the PDA, the dominant RCA continues beyond the crux cordis (the junction of the atrioventricular and interventricular grooves) as the right posterior atrioventricular branch along the distal portion of the posterior (left) atrioventricular groove, terminating in one or several posterolateral branches that supply the diaphragmatic surface of the left ventricle. The RCA is nondominant in 15% of patients. One half of these patients have a left PDA and left posterolateral branches that are provided by the distal LCx artery (left dominant circulation). In these cases, the RCA is very small, terminates before reaching the crux, and does not supply any blood to the left ventricular myocardium. The remaining patients have an RCA that gives rise to the PDA, with the LCx artery providing all the posterolateral branches (balanced or codominant circulation). In about 25% of patients with RCA dominance, there are significant anatomic variations in the origin of the PDA. These variations include partial supply of the PDA territory by acute marginal branches, double PDA, and early origin of the PDA proximal to the crux. At or near the crux, the dominant artery gives rise to a small atrioventricular node artery, which passes upward to supply the atrioventricular node.

CORONARY BYPASS GRAFTS. Selective cannulation of bypass grafts may be more challenging than cannulation of the native coronary arteries because the locations of graft ostia are more variable, even when surgical clips or ostia markers are used. Knowledge of the number, course, and type of bypass grafts obtained from the operative report is invaluable for the identification of the location of the bypass grafts during arteriography.

SAPHENOUS VEIN GRAFTS. SVGs from the aorta to the distal RCA or PDA originate from the right anterolateral aspect of the aorta approximately 5 cm superior to the sinotubular ridge. SVGs to the LAD artery (or diagonal branches) originate from the anterior portion of the aorta about 7 cm superior to the sinotubular ridge. SVGs to the obtuse marginal branches arise from the left anterolateral aspect of the aorta 9 to 10 cm superior to the sinotubular ridge. In most patients, all SVGs can be engaged with a single catheter, such as a Judkins right 4.0 or a modified Amplatz right 1 or 2. Other catheters useful for engaging SVGs include the right and left bypass graft catheters. Amplatz left 1 and 2 catheters are useful for superiorly oriented SVGs (see Fig. 21-3). A multipurpose catheter may also be useful for the cannulation of the downward takeoff SVG to the RCA or PDA.

Viewed in the LAO projection, the Judkins right 4 or Amplatz right 2 catheter rotates anteriorly from the leftward position as the catheter is rotated in a clockwise direction. The relation between the movement of catheter shaft at the femoral artery and the response of catheter tip on fluoroscopy immediately indicates whether the catheter tip is anteriorly positioned in the aorta and likely to enter an SVG ostium or posteriorly positioned and unlikely to engage an SVG. Steady advancement and withdrawal of the catheter tip proximal and distal in the ascending aorta, 5 to 10 cm above the sinotubular ridge, with varying degrees of rotation, usually result in entry into the SVG. Entry into the SVG is associated with abrupt outward motion of the tip of the catheter. When this occurs, a small test injection of contrast material verifies that the catheter is in the SVG. A well-circumscribed "stump" is almost always present if the SVG is occluded. Each SVG or stump must be viewed in nearly orthogonal views. The relation between the origin of the SVGs and surgical clips confirms whether all targeted SVGs have been visualized. If neither a patent SVG nor a stump can be located, it may be necessary to perform an ascending aortogram (preferably in biplane) in an attempt to visualize all SVGs and their course to the coronary arteries.

The goal of SVG angiography is to assess the ostium of the SVG, its entire course, and the distal insertion ("touchdown") site at the anastomosis between the bypass SVG and the native coronary vessel. The ostium of the SVG must be evaluated by achieving a coaxial engagement of the catheter tip and the origin of the SVG. The midportion (body) of the SVG must be evaluated with complete filling of the SVG by contrast material because inadequate opacification produces an

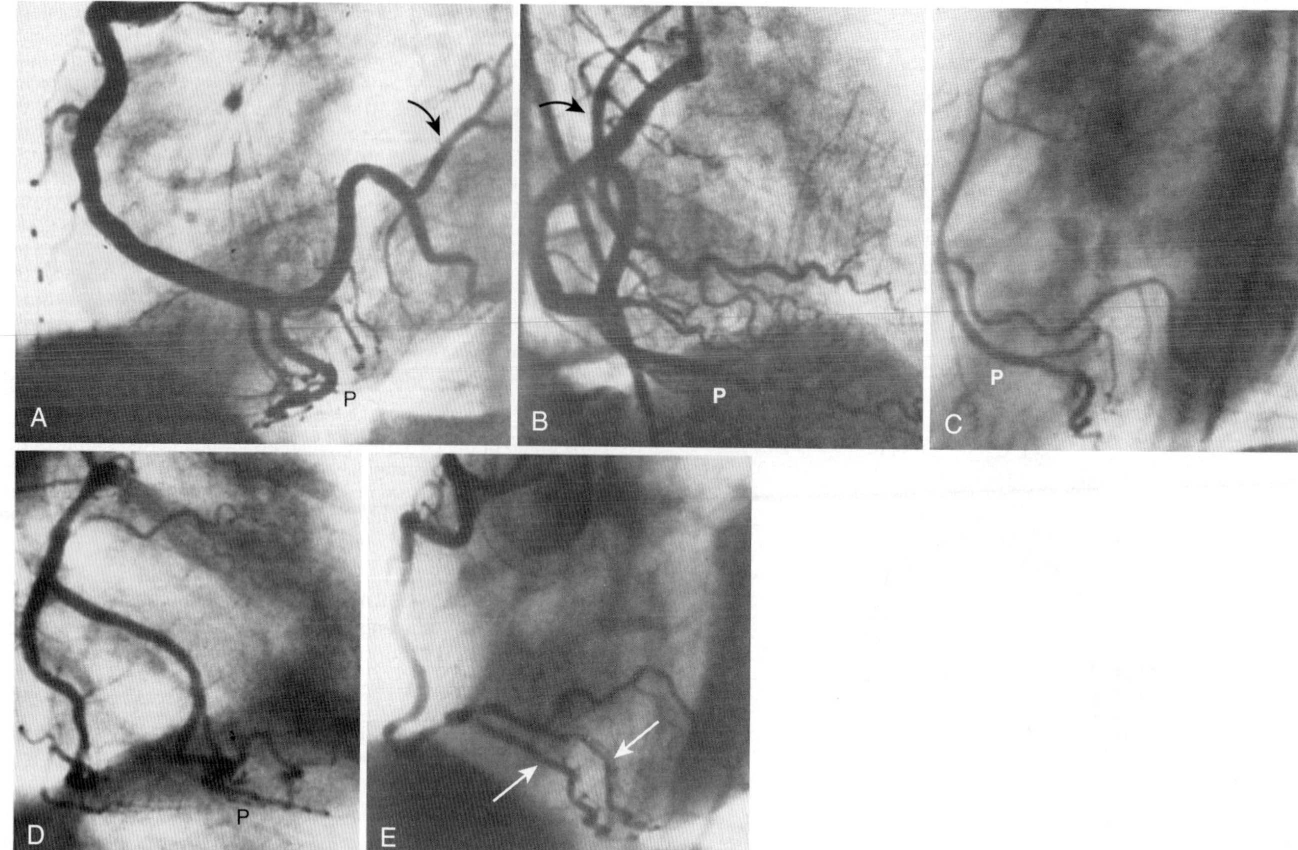

FIGURE 21-12 Strongly dominant right coronary artery (RCA). **A, B,** Left anterior oblique and right anterior oblique views of the RCA show that the distal segment (arrows) extends to the left atrioventricular groove. After giving rise to the posterior descending artery (P), the RCA gives rise to multiple posterior left ventricular branches. **C,** A variation in the origin of the posterior descending artery, which originates early from the RCA, runs parallel to it, and enters the posterior interventricular groove. **D,** Right anterior oblique right coronary arteriogram showing the posterior descending artery arising from a right ventricular branch of the RCA. **E,** Left anterior oblique right coronary arteriogram showing duplicated posterior descending arteries (arrows). *(From Levin DC, Baltaxe HA: Angiographic demonstration of important anatomic variations of the posterior descending artery. AJR Am J Roentgenol 116:41, 1972.)*

angiographic artifact suggestive of friable filling defects. It is critical to assess the SVG insertion or anastomotic site in full profile without any overlap of the distal SVG or the native vessel. Angiographic assessment of the native vessels beyond SVG anastomotic sites requires views that are conventionally used for the native segments themselves. Sequential grafts are those that supply two different epicardial branches in a side-to-side fashion (for the more proximal epicardial artery) and terminate in an end-to-side anastomosis (for the more distal epicardial artery). A Y graft is one in which there is a proximal anastomosis in an end-to-side fashion to another saphenous vein or arterial graft with two distal end-to-side anastomoses to the two epicardial grafts from these two grafts.

INTERNAL MAMMARY ARTERY. The left IMA arises inferiorly from the left subclavian artery approximately 10 cm from its origin. Catheterization of the left IMA is performed with a specially designed J-tip IMA catheter (see Fig. 21-2, bottom row). The catheter is advanced into the aortic arch distal to the origin of the left subclavian artery in the LAO projection and then rotated counterclockwise and is gently withdrawn with the tip pointing in a cranial direction, allowing entry into the left subclavian artery (**Fig. 21-15**). A 0.035 J or angled Terumo guidewire is advanced to the left subclavian artery under fluoroscopy, and the catheter is advanced into the subclavian artery. The RAO or AP projection then can be used to cannulate the IMA selectively by withdrawing and slightly rotating the catheter anteriorly (counterclockwise) with the tip down. The right IMA can also be cannulated with the IMA catheter. The innominate artery is entered in the LAO projection, and the guidewire is advanced cautiously to avoid entry into the right common carotid artery. When the guidewire is positioned in the distal right subclavian artery, the IMA catheter is advanced to a point distal to the expected origin of the right IMA. The catheter is withdrawn in the LAO view and rotated to cannulate the right IMA.

The IMA itself is rarely affected by atherosclerosis. Angiographic studies of the IMAs should assess not only the patency of the graft itself but also the distal anastomosis, where most IMA graft compromise occurs. Although the LAO cranial view may be limited in its ability to demonstrate the anastomosis of the IMA and the LAD because of vessel overlap, the left lateral or AP cranial projection usually provides adequate visualization of the left IMA–LAD anastomotic site. The risk of catheter-induced dissection of the origin of the IMA can be reduced by careful manipulation of the catheter tip and avoidance of forceful advancement without the protection of the guidewire. If the IMA cannot be selectively engaged because of tortuosity of the subclavian artery, nonselective arteriography can be enhanced by placing a blood pressure cuff on the ipsilateral arm and inflating it to a pressure above systolic arterial pressure. Alternatively, the ipsilateral brachial or radial artery may be used to facilitate coaxial IMA engagement. IMA spasm can be treated with 50 to 200 μg of intra-arterial nitroglycerin or 50 to 100 μg of intra-arterial verapamil. The patient may feel chest warmth or discomfort with injection of contrast material because of injection into small IMA branches supplying the chest wall.

GASTROEPIPLOIC ARTERY. The right gastroepiploic artery (GEA) is the largest terminal artery of the gastroduodenal artery and was briefly used as an alternative in situ arterial conduit to the PDA in patients undergoing CABG. The gastroduodenal artery arises from the common hepatic artery in 75% of cases, but it may also arise from the

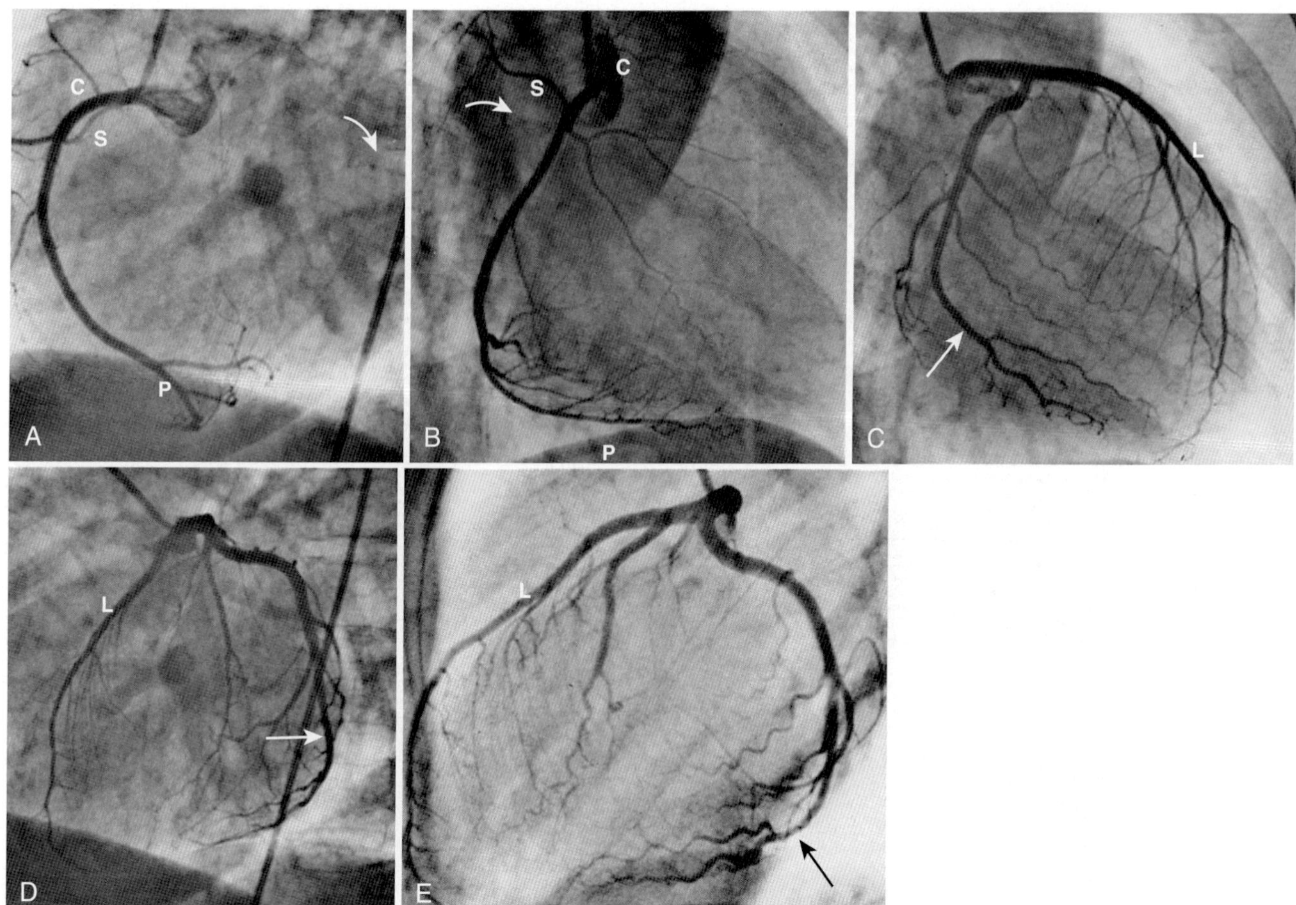

FIGURE 21-13 Weakly dominant right coronary artery (RCA). **A, B,** Left anterior oblique and right anterior oblique views of the RCA. Both the conus and sinoatrial node artery arise from the RCA. The distal portion of the RCA beyond the origin of the posterior descending artery is short and gives rise to a single small posterior left ventricular branch (arrow indicates left atrium). **C-E,** Left coronary artery in the right anterior oblique, left anterior oblique, and left lateral projections. Note that the circumflex artery gives rise to four obtuse marginal branches, the most distal of which (arrow) supplies some of the diaphragmatic surface of the left ventricle. The left anterior descending artery gives rise to two small and one medium-sized diagonal branches. C = conus branch; L = left anterior descending artery; P = posterior descending artery; S = sinoatrial nodal artery.

right or left hepatic artery or the celiac trunk. Catheterization of the right GEA is carried out by first entering the common hepatic artery with a cobra catheter (**Fig. 21-16**). A torquable, hydrophilic-coated guidewire is advanced to the gastroduodenal artery and then to the right GEA. The cobra catheter is then exchanged for a multipurpose or Judkins right coronary catheter, which then permits selective arteriography of the right GEA.

STANDARDIZED PROJECTION ACQUISITION. Although general recommendations can be made for sequences of angiographic image acquisition that are applicable to most patients, tailored views may be needed to accommodate individual variations in anatomy. As a general rule, each coronary artery should be visualized with a number of different projections that minimize vessel foreshortening and overlap (**Fig. 21-17**). An AP view with shallow caudal angulation is often performed first to evaluate the possibility of LMCA disease. Other important views include the LAO cranial view to evaluate the middle and distal LAD, which should have sufficient leftward positioning of the image intensifier to allow separation of the LAD, diagonal, and septal branches; the LAO caudal view to evaluate the LMCA, origin of the LAD, and proximal segment of the LCx; the RAO caudal view to assess the LCx and marginal branches; and a shallow RAO or AP cranial view to evaluate the midportion and distal portion of the LAD. The RCA should be visualized in at least two views, including an LAO cranial view that demonstrates the RCA and origin of the PDA and posterolateral branches and an RAO view that demonstrates the mid-RCA and proximal, middle, and distal termination of the PDA. An AP cranial projection may also be useful for the demonstration of the distal termination of the RCA, and a left lateral view is useful to visualize the ostium of the RCA and midportion of the RCA with separation of the RCA and its right ventricular branches.

Congenital Anomalies of the Coronary Circulation

Coronary anomalies are defined as those angiographic findings in which the number, origin, course, and termination of the arteries are rarely encountered in the general population. Coronary anomalies may occur in 1% to 5% of patients undergoing coronary arteriography, depending on the threshold for defining an anatomic variant (**Table 21-7**).[53-56]

The major reason for appropriate identification and classification of coronary anomalies is to determine their propensity for development of fixed or dynamic myocardial ischemia and sudden cardiac death, particularly in young and otherwise healthy individuals.[57] Documentation of precise ischemia risk for some of these anomalies by conventional exercise stress testing or intravascular Doppler flow studies is poorly predictive and may fail to detect significant anatomic abnormalities.[58] Accordingly, coronary artery anomalies are divided into those that cause and those that do not cause myocardial ischemia (**Table 21-8**).

ANOMALOUS PULMONARY ORIGIN OF THE CORONARY ARTERIES (APOCA). This syndrome is characterized by the origin of the coronary artery arising from the pulmonary artery. The most common variant is an anomalous origin of the LCA from the pulmonary artery (ALCAPA),[59] although single-vessel origins of the RCA, LCx coronary artery, or LAD

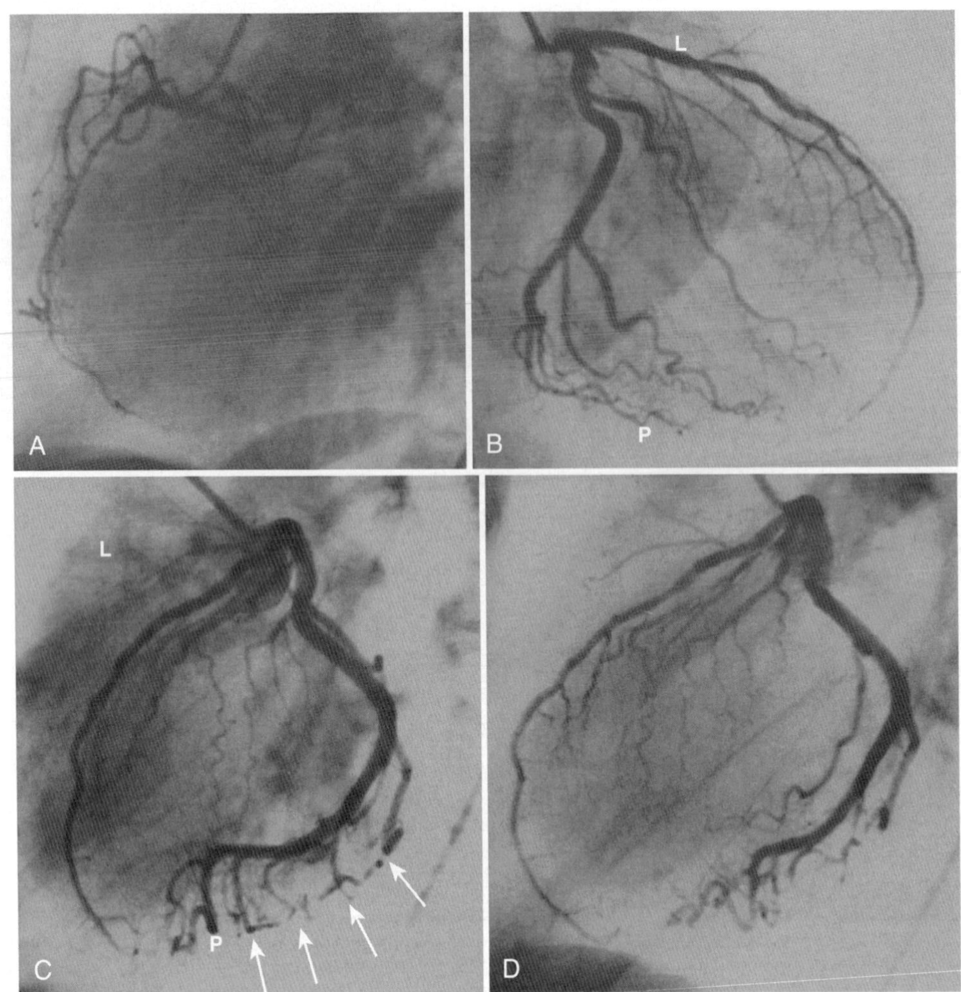

FIGURE 21-14 Dominant left coronary system. **A,** The left anterior oblique projection shows that the right coronary artery is small and terminates before reaching the crux. **B-D,** The right anterior oblique, left anterior oblique, and left lateral projections show that the left circumflex artery is large and gives rise to the posterior descending artery at the crux of the heart and to several posterior descending arteries. Arrows indicate posterolateral branches. L = left anterior descending coronary artery; P = posterior descending artery.

TABLE 21-7 Incidence of Coronary Anomalies Among 1950 Angiograms

VARIABLE	NUMBER	PERCENT
Coronary anomalies	110	5.64
Split RCA	24	1.23
Ectopic RCA (right cusp)	22	1.13
Ectopic RCA (left cusp)	18	0.92
Fistulas	17	0.87
Absent left main coronary artery	13	0.67
LCx arising from right cusp	13	0.67
LCA arising from right cusp	3	0.15
Low origin of RCA	2	0.1
Other anomalies	3	0.15

From Angelini P (ed): Coronary Artery Anomalies: A Comprehensive Approach. Philadelphia, Lippincott Williams & Wilkins, 1999, p 42.

TABLE 21-8 Ischemia Occurring in Coronary Anomalies

TYPE OF ISCHEMIA	CORONARY ANOMALY
Absence of ischemia	Majority of anomalies (split RCA, ectopic RCA from right cusp, ectopic RCA from left cusp)
Episodic ischemia	Anomalous origin of a coronary artery from the opposite sinus (ACAOS); coronary artery fistulas; myocardial bridge
Obligatory ischemia	Anomalous left coronary artery from the pulmonary artery (ALCAPA); coronary ostial atresia or severe stenosis

Modified from Angelini P (ed): Coronary Artery Anomalies: A Comprehensive Approach. Philadelphia, Lippincott Williams & Wilkins, 1999, p 42.

artery from the pulmonary artery have also been reported. Untreated, and in the absence of an adequate collateral network, most (95%) infants with APOCA die within the first year. In the presence of an extensive collateral network, patients may survive into adulthood. Aortography typically shows a large RCA with absence of a left coronary ostium in the left aortic sinus. During the late phase of the aortogram, patulous LAD and LCx branches fill by means of collateral circulation from RCA branches. Still later in the filming sequence, retrograde flow from the LAD and LCx arteries opacifies the LMCA and its origin from the main pulmonary artery (**Fig. 21-18**). Once it is detected, CABG surgery is recommended because of the high incidence of sudden death, cardiomyopathy, and arrhythmias associated with APOCA.

Anomalous Coronary Artery from the Opposite Sinus (ACAOS). Origin of the LCA from the proximal RCA or the right aortic sinus with subsequent passage between the aorta and the right ventricular outflow tract has been associated with sudden death during or shortly after exercise in young persons (**Figs. 21-19 to 21-21**).[60-62] The increased

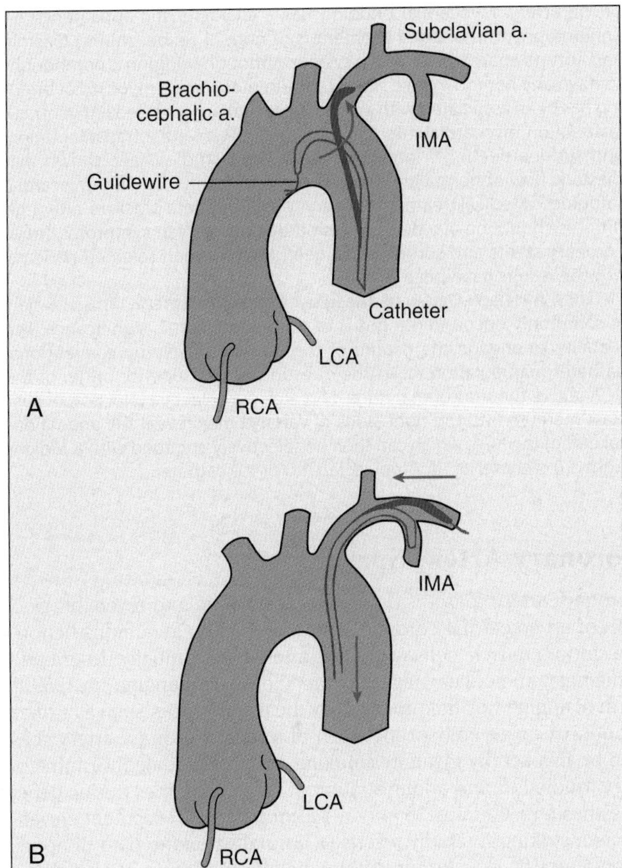

FIGURE 21-15 Catheterization of the left internal mammary artery (IMA). The IMA is positioned in the aortic arch and visualized in the left anterior oblique position. The catheter tip is rotated so that it engages the origin of the left subclavian artery immediately subjacent to the head of the clavicle **(A)**. This is followed by gentle advancement of the guidewire into the left subclavian artery to a point distal to the origin of the left IMA. After the guidewire is removed, the left subclavian artery is visualized in the right anterior oblique projection, the catheter is withdrawn, and the catheter tip engages the ostium of the left IMA selectively **(B)**. LCA = left coronary artery; RCA = right coronary artery. *(From Judkins MW: Coronary arteriography. In Douglas JS Jr, King SB III [eds]: Coronary Arteriography and Intervention. New York, McGraw-Hill, 1985, p 231.)*

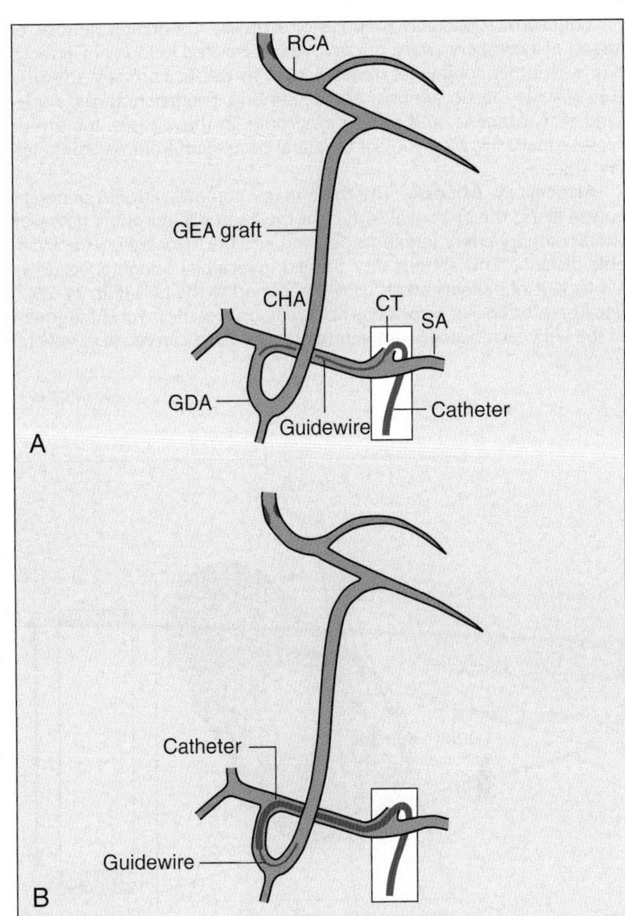

FIGURE 21-16 Catheterization of the right gastroepiploic artery (GEA) graft. The celiac trunk (CT) is selectively engaged with a cobra catheter, and a guidewire is gently advanced to the gastroduodenal artery (GDA) and the GEA. The catheter is advanced over the guidewire for selective arteriography of the GEA graft. CHA = common hepatic artery; RCA = right coronary artery; SA = splenic artery.

risk of sudden death may be due to a slitlike ostium, a bend with acute takeoff angles of the aberrant coronary arteries, or arterial compression between the pulmonary trunk and aorta when there is increased blood flow through these vessels with exercise and stress. Origin of the RCA from the LCA or left aortic sinus with passage between the aorta and the right ventricular outflow tract is also associated with myocardial ischemia and sudden death. In rare cases of anomalous origin of the LCA from the right sinus, myocardial ischemia may occur even if the LCA passes anterior to the right ventricular outflow tract or posterior to the aorta (i.e., not through a tunnel between the two great vessels). Although CABG surgery has been the traditional revascularization approach in patients with ACAOS, coronary stenting has also been reported with acceptable medium-term success.

The course of the anomalous coronary arteries is easily assessed by angiography in the RAO view. The four common courses for the anomalous LCA arising from the right sinus of Valsalva include a septal, anterior, interarterial, and posterior course. The posterior course of the anomalous LCA arising from the right sinus of Valsalva is similar to the course of the anomalous LCx artery arising from the right sinus of Valsalva (see Fig. 21-20), whereas the common interarterial course of the anomalous RCA from the left sinus of Valsalva is similar to the interarterial course of the anomalous LCA arising from the right sinus of Valsalva.

When either the LCA or the LAD arises anomalously from the right sinus, another angiographic method to identify the course of the anomalous vessel is to pass a catheter into the main pulmonary artery and then perform an arteriogram of the aberrant coronary artery in the steep AP caudal projection. This places the aberrant coronary artery, the rightward and anterior pulmonary valve, and the leftward and posterior aortic valve all in one plane. From this "laid-back" aortogram, which can be used even in mapping the course of anomalous coronary arteries in transposition of the great vessels, it is usually possible to confirm whether the course of the aberrant coronary artery is between the great vessels. Although angiography is useful to establish the presence of anomalous coronary arteries, coronary computed tomography angiography may also be an important adjunctive diagnostic tool to establish the course of the vessels (see Chap. 19).[63]

Coronary Artery Fistulas. Coronary artery fistulas are defined as abnormal communications between a coronary artery and a cardiac chamber or major vessel, such as the vena cava, right or left ventricle, pulmonary vein, or pulmonary artery.[64,65] Coronary artery fistulas are rare findings, identified in 10 (0.05%) of 18,272 diagnostic cardiac catheterizations.[66] Fistulas arise from the RCA or its branches in about half of the cases, and drainage generally occurs into the right ventricle, right atrium, and pulmonary arteries; coronary artery fistulas terminating in the left ventricle are uncommon (3%)[64] (**Figs. 21-22 to 21-24**). Coronary arteriography is the best method for demonstration of the origin of these fistulas.

The clinical presentation associated with coronary artery fistulas is dependent on the type of fistula, shunt volume, site of the shunt, and presence of other cardiac conditions, although patients (50%) often remain asymptomatic.[64] Dyspnea on exertion, fatigue, congestive heart failure, pulmonary hypertension, bacterial endocarditis, and arrhythmias are common presentations in symptomatic patients. Myocardial ischemia may also occur, but the mechanism remains speculative.[64] Symptomatic patients or those with severe shunts may be treated with surgical closure, although percutaneous closure with coil embolization may also be tried.

Congenital Coronary Stenosis or Atresia. Congenital stenosis or atresia of a coronary artery can occur as an isolated lesion or in association with other congenital diseases, such as calcific coronary sclerosis, supravalvular aortic stenosis, homocystinuria, Friedreich ataxia, Hurler syndrome, progeria, and rubella syndrome. In these cases, the atretic vessel usually fills by means of collateral circulation from the contralateral side.

Myocardial Bridging. The three major coronary arteries generally course along the epicardial surface of the heart. On occasion, however, short coronary artery segments descend into the myocardium for a variable distance. This abnormality, termed myocardial bridging, occurs in 5% to 12% of patients and is usually confined to the LAD (**Fig. 21-25**).[67] Because a "bridge" of myocardial fibers passes over the involved segment of the LAD, each systolic contraction of these fibers can cause narrowing of the artery. Myocardial bridging has a characteristic appearance on angiography; the bridged segment is of normal caliber during diastole and abruptly narrows with each systole. Although bridging is not thought to have any hemodynamic significance in most cases, myocardial bridging has been associated with angina, arrhythmia, depressed left ventricular function, myocardial stunning, early death after cardiac transplantation, and sudden death.[67,68] Intracoronary Doppler studies have shown that diastolic flow abnormalities may be present in patients with myocardial bridging.[67] Medical treatment generally includes beta blockers, although nitrates should be avoided because they may worsen symptoms. Intracoronary stents and surgery have been attempted in selected patients, but the results have been mixed.[67]

High Anterior Origin of the Right Coronary Artery. This anomaly is commonly encountered but is of no hemodynamic significance. The inability to engage the ostium of the RCA selectively by conventional catheter manipulation raises the question of this superior origin of the RCA above the sinotubular ridge. Forceful, nonselective injection of contrast medium into the right sinus of Valsalva may reveal the anomalous takeoff of the RCA, which can then be selectively engaged with a Judkins right 5.0 catheter or an Amplatz left 1.0 or 2.0 catheter.

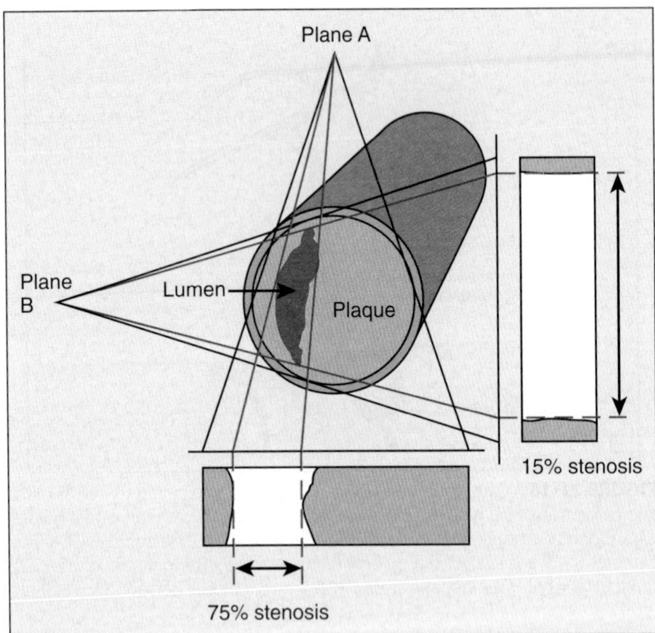

FIGURE 21-17 Importance of orthogonal projections. Each vascular segment of the coronary artery must be recorded in two orthogonal or nearly orthogonal views to avoid missing important diagnostic information about eccentric stenoses. In plane A, the image is associated with 75% stenosis; but in plane B, the image results in 10% stenosis.

Coronary Artery Spasm

Coronary artery spasm is defined as a dynamic and reversible occlusion of an epicardial coronary artery caused by focal constriction of the smooth muscle cells within the arterial wall. Initially described by Prinzmetal and colleagues (Prinzmetal or variant angina) in 1959, this form of angina was not provoked by the usual factors, such as exercise, emotional upset, cold, or ingestion of a meal. Coronary artery spasm can be invoked by cigarette smoking, cocaine use, alcohol, intracoronary irradiation, and administration of catecholamines during general anesthesia (see Chaps. 56 and 57). Although the ST-segment elevation is often striking, it rapidly reverts to normal when the pain disappears spontaneously or is terminated by the administration of nitroglycerin (**Figs. 21-26 and 21-27**; see Fig. 56-20). Coronary artery spasm may be accompanied by atrioventricular block, ventricular ectopic activity, ventricular tachycardia, or ventricular fibrillation. Myocardial infarction and death are rare manifestations of coronary artery spasm. Coronary artery spasm can also be superimposed on the presence of an intramyocardial bridge.[69] On rare occasions, there may be reduced velocity of coronary flow in the absence of a fixed coronary obstruction or coronary vasospasm.[70]

Coronary arteriography is useful in patients with suspected coronary artery spasm to exclude the presence of concomitant CAD and to document an episode of coronary artery spasm by use of provocative intravenous medications. Three provocative tests can be

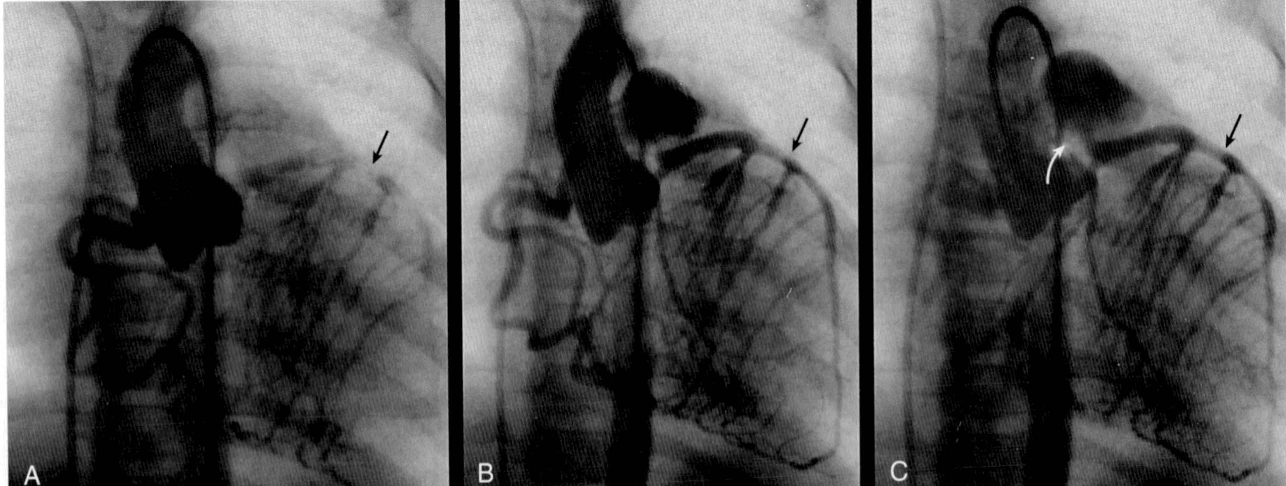

FIGURE 21-18 Anomalous origin of the left coronary artery (LCA) from the pulmonary artery. **A-C,** The thoracic aortogram shows a large right coronary artery (RCA) and no anterograde filling of the LCA. The LCA fills primarily through extensive collaterals from the RCA to the LAD artery (straight arrows). The anomalous origin of the LCA from the pulmonary artery is demonstrated in late phases of the aortogram (**C,** curved arrow).

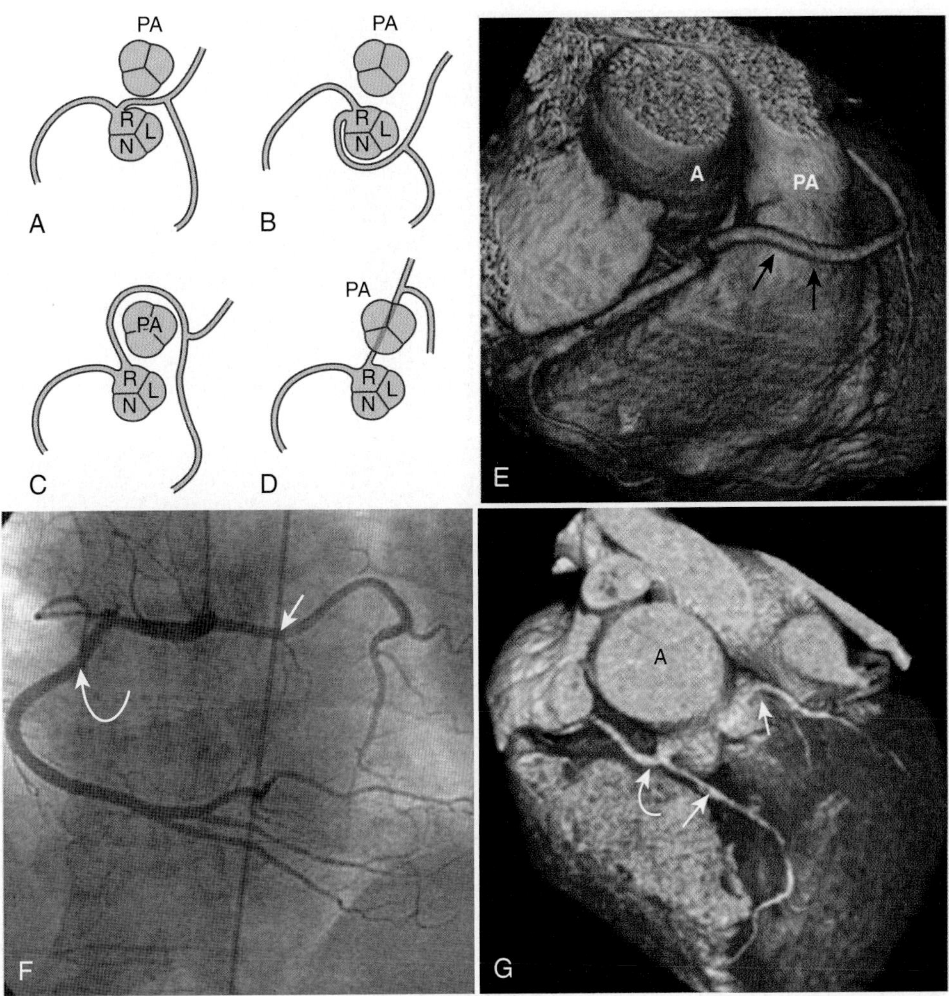

FIGURE 21-19 Four possible pathways of the anomalous left coronary artery arising from the right coronary sinus (R): **A,** interarterial, between the aorta and the pulmonary artery (PA); **B,** retroaortic; **C,** prepulmonic; and **D,** septal, beneath the right ventricular outflow tract. **E,** Computed tomography angiography showing the left coronary artery taking a prepulmonic course (arrows), passing anterior to the pulmonary artery (PA). A = aorta. **F,** The left anterior descending artery arising from the right coronary sinus and taking a septal (subpulmonic) course. The right coronary artery has a normal origin from the right coronary sinus (curved arrow), but the left anterior descending artery arises from the right coronary cusp and courses beneath the pulmonary artery (straight arrow). **G,** Computed tomography angiography showing the left circumflex coronary artery (short straight arrow) arising from its normal location in the left coronary sinus. The curved arrow represents the right coronary artery arising from the right coronary sinus. The aberrant left anterior descending artery arises from the right coronary sinus and takes a subpulmonic course (large straight arrow). A = aorta; L = left coronary sinus; N = noncoronary sinus. *(Reproduced from Kim SY, Seo JB, Do KH, et al: Coronary artery anomalies: Classification and ECG-gated multi-detector row CT findings with angiographic correlation. Radiographics 26:317; discussion 333, 2006.)*

performed to detect the presence of coronary artery spasm. Intravenous ergonovine maleate can elicit two types of responses. A diffuse coronary vasoconstriction that occurs in all the epicardial arteries is a physiologic response to ergonovine not diagnostic of coronary artery spasm. The second response to ergonovine is a focal, occlusive spasm of the epicardial artery that is associated with chest pain and ST-segment elevation. Nitroglycerin should be administered directly into the coronary artery to relieve the coronary spasm. A second provocative test is the use of intravenous acetylcholine. Although it is more sensitive than ergonovine, it may be less specific because of the positive response in patients with atherosclerotic CAD. The final provocative test is hyperventilation during coronary arteriography, which is less sensitive but highly specific for the presence of coronary artery spasm.

In the absence of a positive stimulation test result, the diagnosis of coronary artery spasm must rely instead on clinical features and response to treatment with nitrates and calcium channel blockers. Sole therapy with beta blockers should be avoided because it can worsen the occurrence of coronary artery spasm. Coronary artery spasm that is refractory to conventional therapy with long-acting calcium channel blockers and nitrates can be treated with coronary stenting.

Lesion Complexity

Heterogeneity of the composition, distribution, and location of atherosclerotic plaque within the native coronary artery results in unique patterns of stenosis morphology in patients with CAD. These patterns have been used to identify risk factors for procedural outcome and complications after PCI and to assess the risk for recurrent events in patients who present with an acute coronary syndrome.[71] Criteria established by a joint ACC/AHA Task Force suggested that procedure success and complication rates were related to a number of different lesion characteristics (**Table 21-9**). During the decade after the publication of these criteria, despite substantial improvements in the techniques used for coronary intervention, the most complex lesion morphologies (i.e., type C lesions) remain associated with reduced procedural success in patients with ischemic CAD (**Table 21-10**).

The predictive value of two other risk scores has been compared with the ACC/AHA lesion complexity score.[72,73] The Society for Cardiovascular Angiography and Interventions (SCAI) risk score used an ordinal ranking of two composite criteria (vessel patency and complex morphology) to classify lesions into four groups: non–type C—patent, type C—patent, non–type C—occluded, and type C—occluded.[72] For correct classification of lesions, the ACC/AHA classification had a

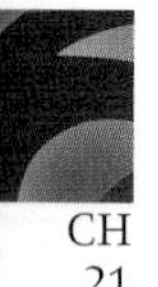

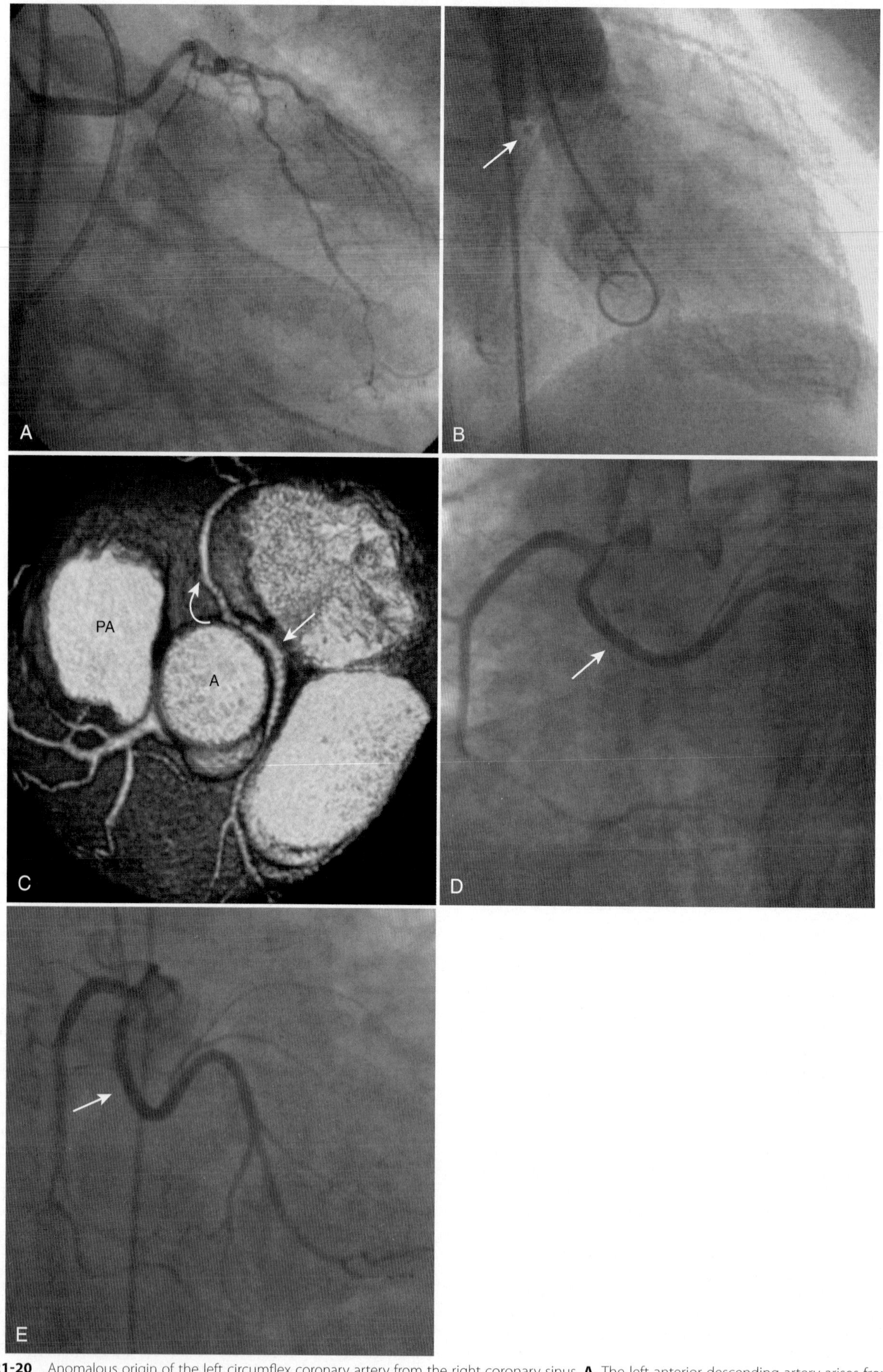

FIGURE 21-20 Anomalous origin of the left circumflex coronary artery from the right coronary sinus. **A,** The left anterior descending artery arises from the left coronary sinus in the usual location, but there is absence of the left circumflex artery. **B,** A left ventriculogram in the right anterior oblique projection shows the "button sign" (arrow) of the anomalous left circumflex artery coursing behind the aorta. **C,** Computed tomography angiography shows the origin of the left circumflex artery from the right coronary sinus and passing behind the aorta (A, arrow). **D, E,** Angiographic demonstration of the anomalous left circumflex artery (arrows) from the right coronary sinus shown in the left anterior oblique projection **(D)** and the right anterior oblique projection **(E)**. PA = pulmonary artery.

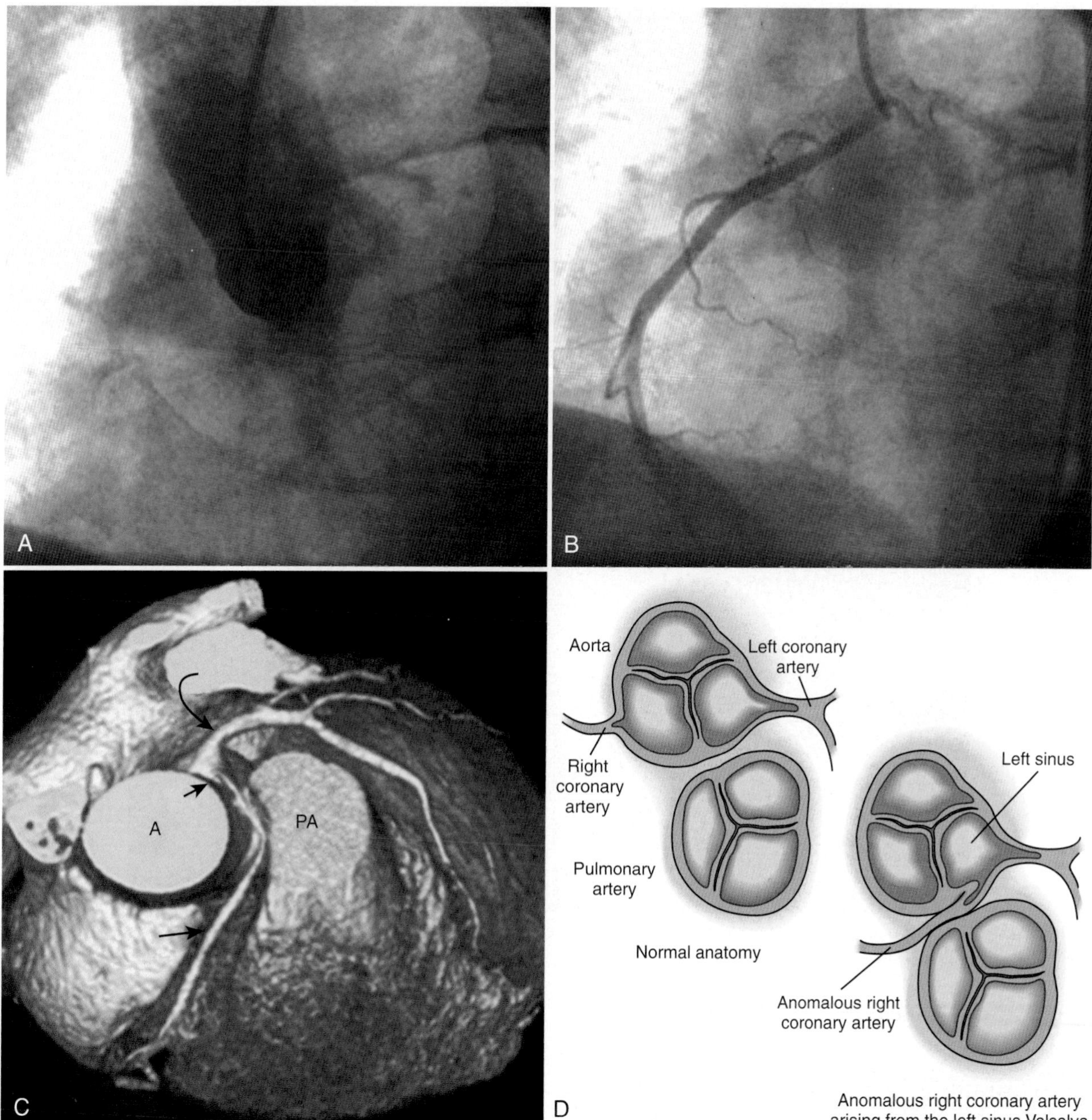

FIGURE 21-21 Anomalous origin of the right coronary artery from the left coronary sinus. **A,** An aortogram in left oblique projection shows the absence of the right coronary artery from the right coronary sinus. **B,** Selective injection of the right coronary artery from the left coronary sinus. **C,** Computed tomography angiography shows the slitlike origin of the right coronary artery (straight arrow) from the left coronary sinus and normal origin of the left coronary artery (curved arrow). The right coronary artery courses between the aorta (A) and pulmonary artery (PA). **D,** The normal anatomy of the right and left coronary arteries is shown in the left plane, and the anomalous origin of the right coronary artery is shown coursing between the aorta and pulmonary artery. *(Reproduced from Kim SY, Seo JB, Do KH, et al: Coronary artery anomalies: Classification and ECG-gated multi-detector row CT findings with angiographic correlation. Radiographics 26:317; discussion 333, 2006; and Qayyum U, Leya F, Steen L, et al: New catheter design for cannulation of the anomalous right coronary artery arising from the left sinus of Valsalva. Catheter Cardiovasc Interv 60:382, 2003.)*

C-statistic of 0.69; the modified ACC/AHA system had a C-statistic of 0.71; and the SCAI classification had a C-statistic of 0.75. The Mayo Clinic Risk Score added the integer scores for the presence of eight morphologic variables and provided a better risk stratification than the ACC/AHA lesion classification for the prediction of cardiovascular complications, whereas the ACC/AHA lesion classification was a better system for identification of angiographic success.[73]

Lesion Length. Lesion length may be measured by a number of methods, including measurement of the "shoulder-to-shoulder" extent of atherosclerosis narrowed by more than 20%, quantification of the lesion length more than 50% narrowed, and estimation of the distance between the proximal and distal angiographically "normal" segment; the last method is used most commonly in clinical practice and provides a longer length than more quantitative methods. Diffuse (>20 mm) lesions are associated with reduced procedural success with drug-eluting stents, primarily related to large degrees of late lumen loss and more extensive underlying atherosclerosis[74] (see Chap. 58).

Ostial Location. Ostial lesions are defined as those arising within 3 mm of origin of the vessel or branch and can be further characterized into aorto-ostial and non–aorto-ostial. Aorto-ostial lesions are often fibrocalcific and rigid, requiring additional ablative devices, such as rotational atherectomy in the presence of extensive calcification, to obtain adequate stent expansion. Positioning of the proximal portion of the stent in the aorto-ostial location so that no more than 1 mm of stent extends into the aorta requires meticulous care. Ostial stenoses that do

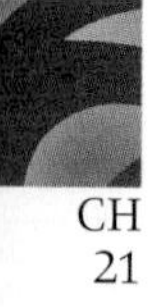

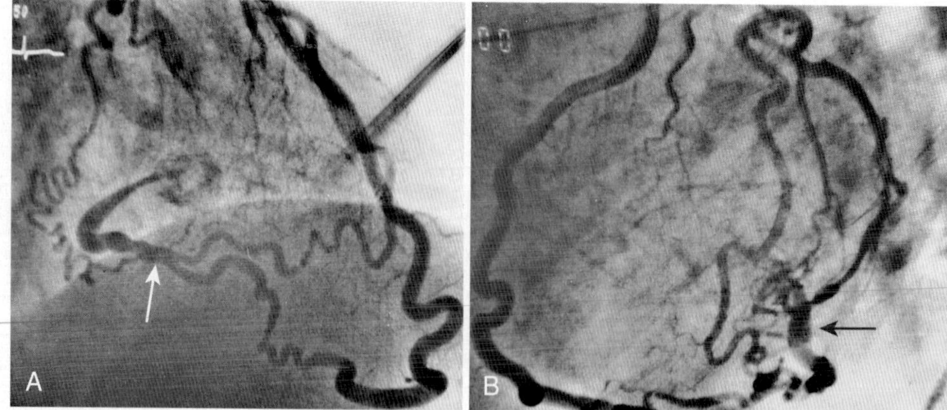

FIGURE 21-22 Congenital fistula to the left ventricle. **A,** Right anterior oblique cranial view of the left coronary arteriogram shows a congenital fistula (arrow) arising from branches of both the left anterior descending and left circumflex arteries and draining into the left ventricle. **B,** Left anterior oblique view of the left coronary arteriogram shows the fistula (arrow).

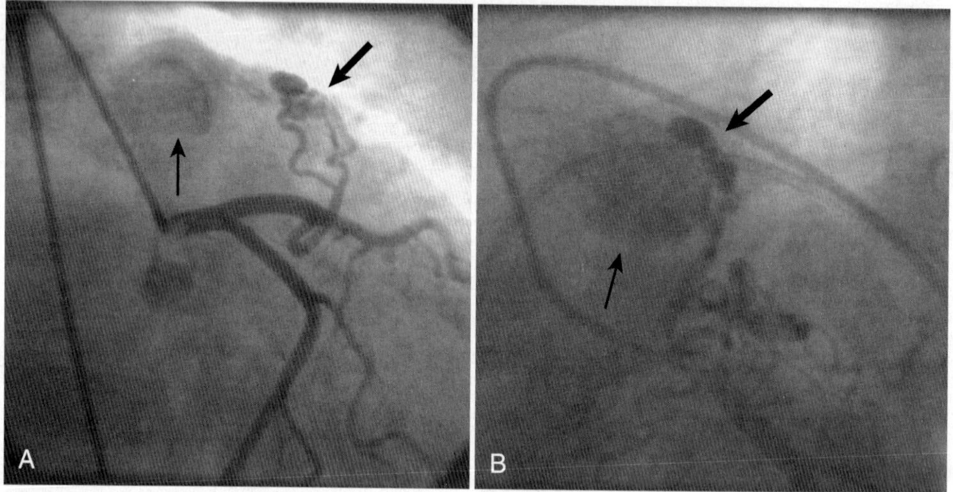

FIGURE 21-23 Congenital fistula to the pulmonary artery. The left coronary arteriogram shows a congenital fistula arising from the left anterior descending (large arrow) and terminating (small arrow) in the pulmonary artery demonstrated in the right anterior oblique **(A)** and left anterior oblique with caudal angulation **(B)**.

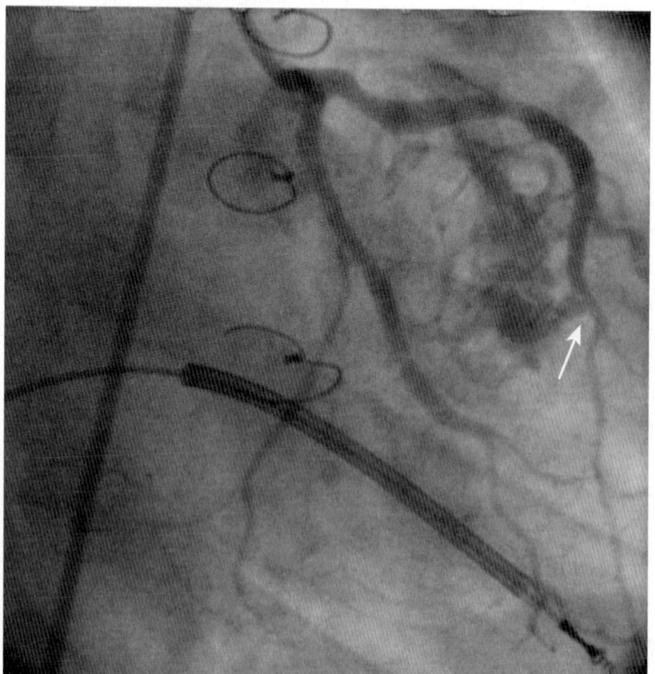

FIGURE 21-24 Iatrogenic fistula of the left anterior descending artery. This patient had undergone prior cardiac transplantation and developed a fistula between the left anterior descending artery and the right ventricle after right ventricular biopsy (arrow).

not involve the aorta may also be more elastic than nonostial lesions and require the same principles for treatment as bifurcation lesions.

Angulated Lesions. Vessel angulation should be measured in the most unforeshortened projection at the site of maximum stenosis using a length of curvature that approximates the balloon length. Balloon angioplasty of angulated lesions increased the risk for dissections, although with the advent of coronary stenting, the inability to deliver the stent and subsequent straightening of the vessel that may predispose to late stent fracture are the largest challenges of highly angulated lesions.

Bifurcation Lesions. The optimal strategic approach for bifurcation lesions remains controversial, and the risk for side branch occlusion during PCI relates to the relative size of the parent and branch vessel, the location of the disease in the parent vessel, and the stenosis severity in the origin of the side branch. In general, placement of one stent is preferable to stent placement in both the parent vessel and side branch (see Chap. 58).

Degenerated Saphenous Vein Grafts. A serial angiographic study in patients undergoing coronary bypass surgery showed that 25% of SVGs occlude within the first year after coronary bypass surgery.[75] Although a drug-eluting stent may reduce the recurrence rate due to restenosis, only embolic protection devices have reduced procedural complications (see Chap. 58).

The extent of graft degeneration and estimated volume of plaque in the target lesion are independent correlates of increased 30-day major adverse cardiac event rates.

Lesion Calcification. Coronary artery calcium is an important marker for coronary atherosclerosis. Conventional angiography is moderately sensitive for the detection of extensive lesion calcification but is less sensitive for detection of milder degrees of lesion calcification. Severely calcified lesions tend to be more rigid and undilatable than

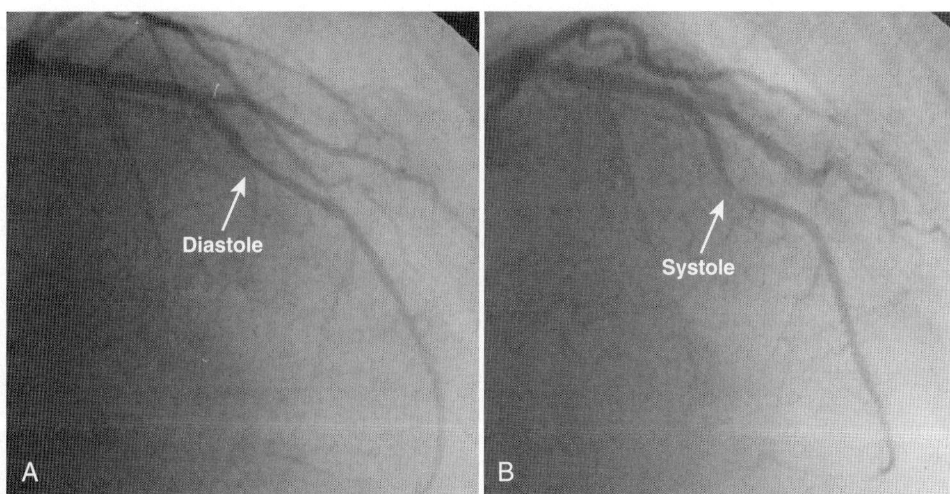

FIGURE 21-25 Intramyocardial bridge. The left anterior descending artery courses into the myocardium shown in diastole **(A)** and systole **(B)**. Note compression of the lumen caliber of the artery during systole.

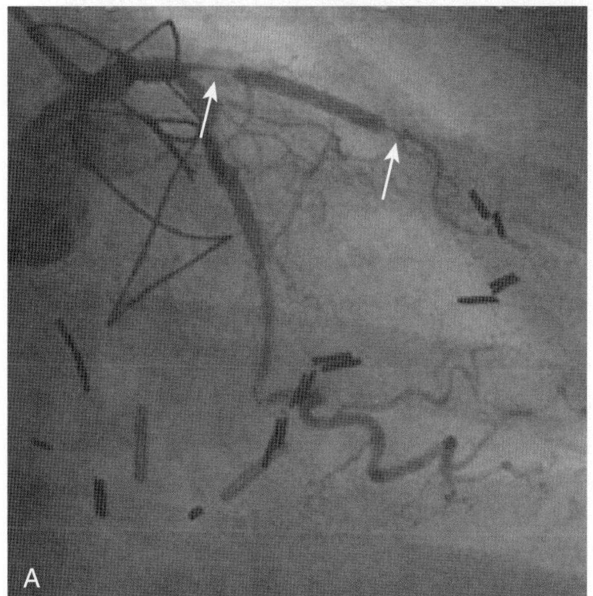

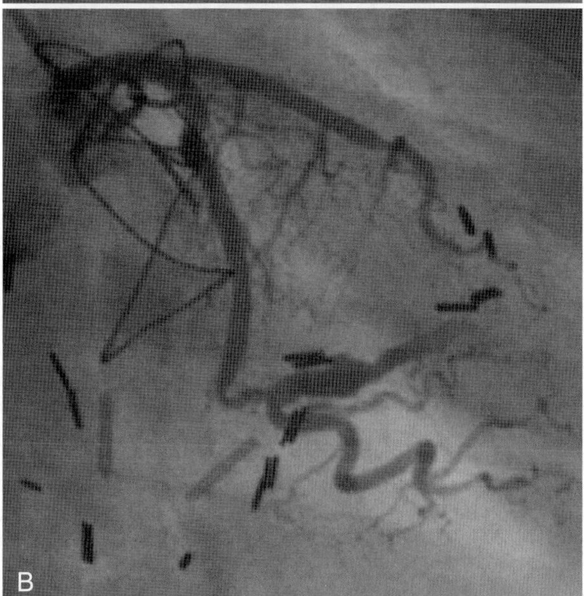

FIGURE 21-26 Coronary artery spasm. Proximal and distal coronary artery spasm was found after stent placement in the left anterior descending coronary artery (**A,** arrows) that was relieved with intracoronary nitroglycerin **(B)**.

TABLE 21-9 Characteristics of Type A, B, and C Coronary Lesions

LESION-SPECIFIC CHARACTERISTICS	
Type A Lesions (high success, >85%; low risk)	
Discrete (<10 mm)	Little or no calcium
Concentric	Less than totally occlusive
Readily accessible	Not ostial in locations
Nonangulated segment, <45 degrees	No major side branch involvement
Smooth contour	Absence of thrombus
Type B Lesions (moderate success, 60%-85%; moderate risk)	
Tubular (10 to 20 mm in length)	Moderate to heavy calcification
Eccentric	Total occlusions <3 months old
Moderate tortuosity of proximal segment	Ostial in location
Moderately angulated segment, ≥45 degrees, <90 degrees	Bifurcation lesion requiring double guidewire
Irregular contour	Some thrombus present
Type C Lesions (low success, <60%; high risk)	
Diffuse (>2 cm in length)	Total occlusion >3 months old
Excessive tortuosity of proximal segment	Inability to protect major side branches
Extremely angulated segments, ≥90 degrees	Degenerated vein grafts with friable lesions

From Ryan TJ, Bauman WB, Kennedy JW, et al: Guidelines for percutaneous coronary angioplasty. A report of the AHA/ACC Task Force on Assessment of Diagnostic and Therapeutic Cardiovascular Procedures (Subcommittee on Percutaneous Transluminal Coronary Angioplasty). Circulation 88:2987, 1993.

noncalcified lesions, and rotational atherectomy may be useful before stenting to ensure stent delivery and complete stent expansion.

Thrombus. Although conventional angiography is a relatively insensitive method for detection of coronary thrombus, its presence is associated with a higher risk of procedural complications, primarily relating to embolization of thrombotic debris into the distal circulation. Large, intracoronary thrombi may be treated with a combination of pharmacologic agents (e.g., glycoprotein IIb/IIIa inhibitors) and mechanical devices (e.g., passive aspiration and rheolytic thrombectomy) (see Chap. 58).

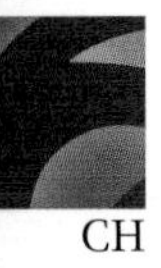

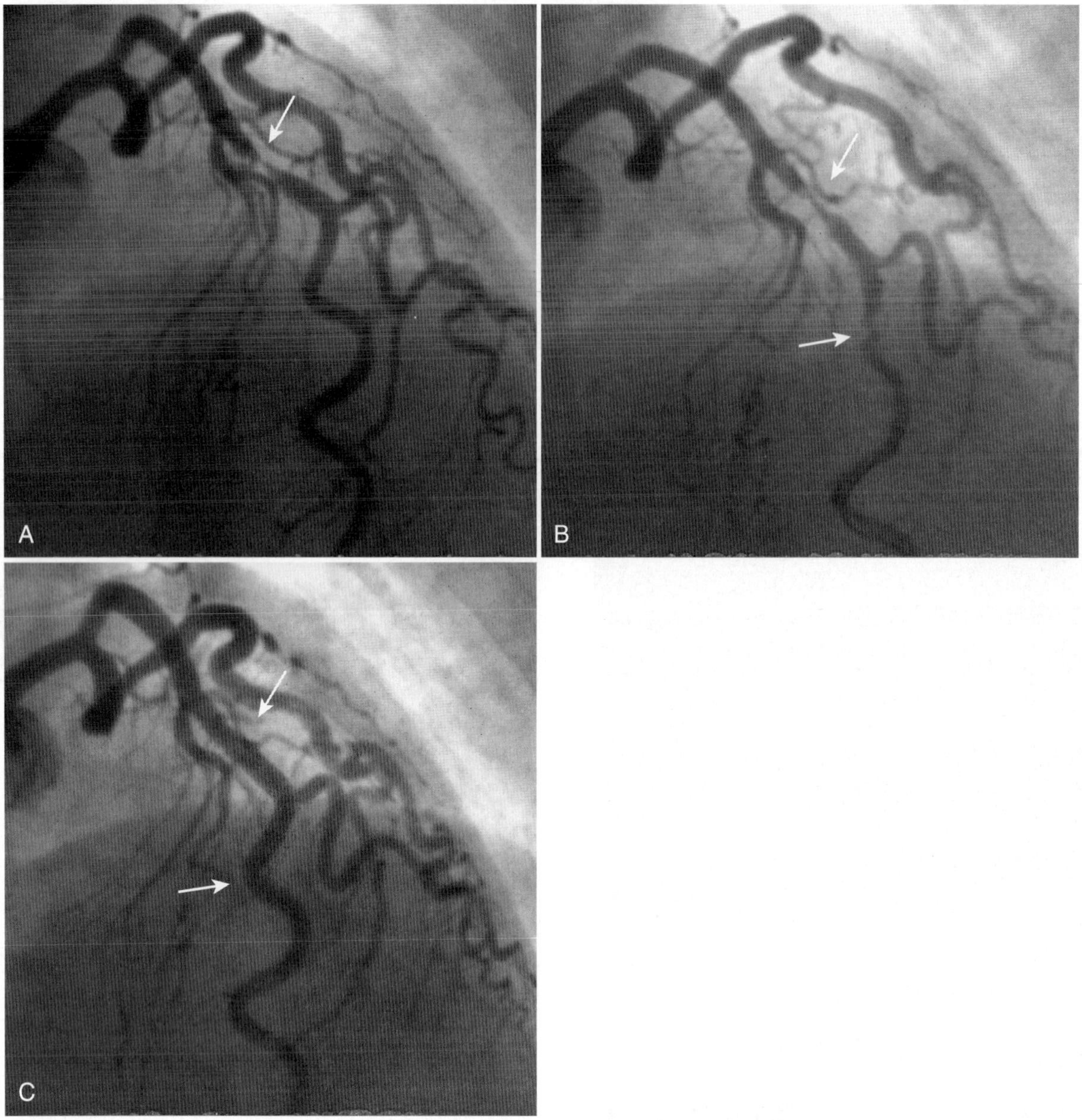

FIGURE 21-27 "Wire pleating." **A,** A focal stenosis (arrow) is shown in the left anterior descending artery. **B,** A 0.014-inch coronary guidewire was advanced across the stenosis but straightened the vessel, resulting in downstream wire pleating, mimicking a coronary stenosis or dissection (bottom arrow). **C,** After a stent was placed in the proximal left anterior descending artery (top arrow), the pseudostenosis was no longer present (bottom arrow).

TOTAL OCCLUSION. Total coronary occlusion is identified as an abrupt termination of the epicardial vessel; anterograde and retrograde collaterals may be present and are helpful in quantifying the length of the totally occluded segment. Success in passage of a coronary guidewire across the occlusion depends on the occlusion duration and on certain lesion morphologic features, such as bridging collaterals, occlusion length of more than 15 mm, and absence of a "nipple" to guide advancement of the guidewire. Newer guidewires and improved operator experience have improved procedural success rates, although the presence of a total occlusion remains one of the major reasons for referral of patients for coronary bypass surgery.

CORONARY PERFUSION. Perfusion distal to a coronary stenosis can occur anterograde by means of the native vessel, retrograde through collaterals, or through a coronary bypass graft. The rate of anterograde coronary flow is influenced by both the severity and complexity of the stenosis and the status of the microvasculature. The Thrombolysis in Myocardial Infarction (TIMI) study group established criteria to assess the degree of anterograde coronary reperfusion in patients with acute myocardial infarction and found that complete restoration of anterograde perfusion by TIMI 3 flow was associated with the lowest mortality rate (**Table 21-11**). TIMI frame count and the TIMI myocardial perfusion grade permit further quantification of anterograde flow and assessment of distal microvascular perfusion.

Coronary Collateral Circulation

Networks of small anastomotic branches interconnect the major coronary arteries and serve as precursors for the collateral circulation that maintains myocardial perfusion despite the development of severe proximal atherosclerotic narrowings. Collateral channels may not be seen in patients with normal or mildly diseased coronary arteries because of their small (<200 μm) caliber, but as CAD progresses and becomes more severe (>90% stenosis), a pressure gradient is generated between the anastomotic channels and the distal vessel that is hypoperfused. The trans-stenosis pressure gradient facilitates blood flow through the anastomotic channels, which progressively dilate and eventually become visible as collateral vessels (**Fig. 21-28**).

TABLE 21-10 Definitions of Preprocedural Lesion Morphology

FEATURE	FREQUENCY (%)	DEFINITION
Eccentricity	48.0	Stenosis that is noted to have one of its luminal edges in the outer quarter of the apparent normal lumen
Irregularity	17.9	Characterized by lesion ulceration, intimal flap, aneurysm, or sawtooth pattern
Ulceration	12.1	Lesions with a small crater consisting of a discrete luminal widening in the area of the stenosis
Intimal flap	3.22	A mobile, radiolucent extension of the vessel wall into the arterial lumen
Aneurysm	5.49	Segment of arterial dilation larger than the dimensions of the normal arterial segment
Sawtooth	0.84	Multiple, sequential stenosis irregularities
Length		Measured "shoulder to shoulder" in an unforeshortened view
Discrete	55.0	Lesion length <10 mm
Tubular	34.8	Lesion length 10-20 mm
Diffuse	10.2	Lesion length >20 mm
Ostial location	10.0	Origin of the lesion within 3 mm of the vessel origin
Angulation		Vessel angle formed by the centerline through the lumen proximal and distal to the stenosis
Moderate	15.3	Lesion angulation ≥45 degrees
Severe	0.93	Lesion angulation ≥90 degrees
Bifurcation stenosis	6.05	Stenosis involving the parent and daughter branch if a medium or large branch (>1.5 mm) originates within the stenosis and if the side branch is completely surrounded by stenotic portions of the lesion to be dilated
Proximal tortuosity		
Moderate	15.3	Lesion is distal to two bends >75 degrees
Severe	NR	Lesion is distal to three bends >75 degrees
Degenerated SVG	7.1	Graft characterized by luminal irregularities or ectasia constituting >50% of the graft length
Calcification	34.3	Readily apparent densities noted within the apparent vascular wall at the site of the stenosis
Total occlusion	6.4	TIMI 0 or 1 flow
Thrombus	3.4	Discrete, intraluminal filling defect is noted with defined borders and is largely separated from the adjacent wall; contrast staining may or may not be present

NR = not reported; SVG = saphenous vein graft; TIMI = Thrombolysis in Myocardial Infarction.
Data obtained from 846 lesions undergoing qualitative angiographic analysis at the Washington Hospital Center Angiographic Core Laboratory.

TABLE 21-11 Thrombolysis in Myocardial Infarction (TIMI) Flow

TIMI FLOW	
Grade 3 (complete reperfusion)	Anterograde flow into the terminal coronary artery segment through a stenosis is as prompt as anterograde flow into a comparable segment proximal to the stenosis. Contrast material clears as rapidly from the distal segment as from an uninvolved, more proximal segment.
Grade 2 (partial reperfusion)	Contrast material flows through the stenosis to opacify the terminal artery segment. However, contrast material enters the terminal segment perceptibly more slowly than more proximal segments. Alternatively, contrast material clears from a segment distal to a stenosis noticeably more slowly than from a comparable segment not preceded by a significant stenosis.
Grade 1 (penetration with minimal artery perfusion)	A small amount of contrast material flows through the stenosis but fails to opacify fully beyond the area of obstruction.
Grade 0 (no perfusion)	No contrast flow through the stenosis

Modified from Sheehan F, Braunwald E, Canner P, et al: The effect of intravenous thrombolytic therapy on left ventricular function: A report on the tissue-type plasminogen activator and streptokinase from the Thrombolysis in Myocardial Infarction (TIMI Phase I) trial. Circulation 75:817, 1987.

The visible collateral channels arise from the contralateral coronary artery, from the ipsilateral coronary artery through intracoronary collateral channels, or through "bridging" channels that have a serpiginous course from the proximal coronary artery to the coronary artery distal to the occlusion. These collaterals may provide up to 50% of anterograde coronary flow in chronic total occlusions and may allow the development of a "protected" region of myocardial perfusion that does not develop ischemia during enhanced myocardial oxygen demands. Recruitment of collateral channels may occur quickly in patients who develop an acute ST-segment elevation myocardial infarction caused by a sudden thrombotic occlusion. Other factors that affect collateral development are patency of the arteries supplying the collateral and the size and vascular resistance of the segment distal to the stenosis. Grading of flow of collaterals can be classified by the Rentrop criteria, including Rentrop grade 0 (no filling), Rentrop grade 1 (small side branches filled), Rentrop grade 2 (partial epicardial filling of the occluded artery), and Rentrop grade 3 (complete epicardial filling of the occluded artery).

Quantitative Angiography

Although visual estimations of coronary stenosis severity are used by virtually all clinicians to guide clinical practice, "eyeball" estimates of percentage diameter stenosis are limited by substantial observer variability and bias. More reliable and objective "on-line" quantitative coronary measurements have had limited clinical use, however, being largely supplanted by more physiologic measures of stenosis severity, such as direct measurements of fractional and coronary flow reserve in regions of intermediate (40% to 70%) stenosis severity. Nevertheless, a number of angiographic measures have been developed to more quantitatively assess early and late procedural outcome after PCI for research protocols and registry reports (**Table 21-12**); these methods have been used to determine the value of new devices and drugs for the treatment of patients with ischemic CAD.

Quantitative coronary angiography was initially performed by Greg Brown and colleagues at the University of Washington nearly 30 years ago. By use of hand-drawn arterial contours that corrected for

CH 21

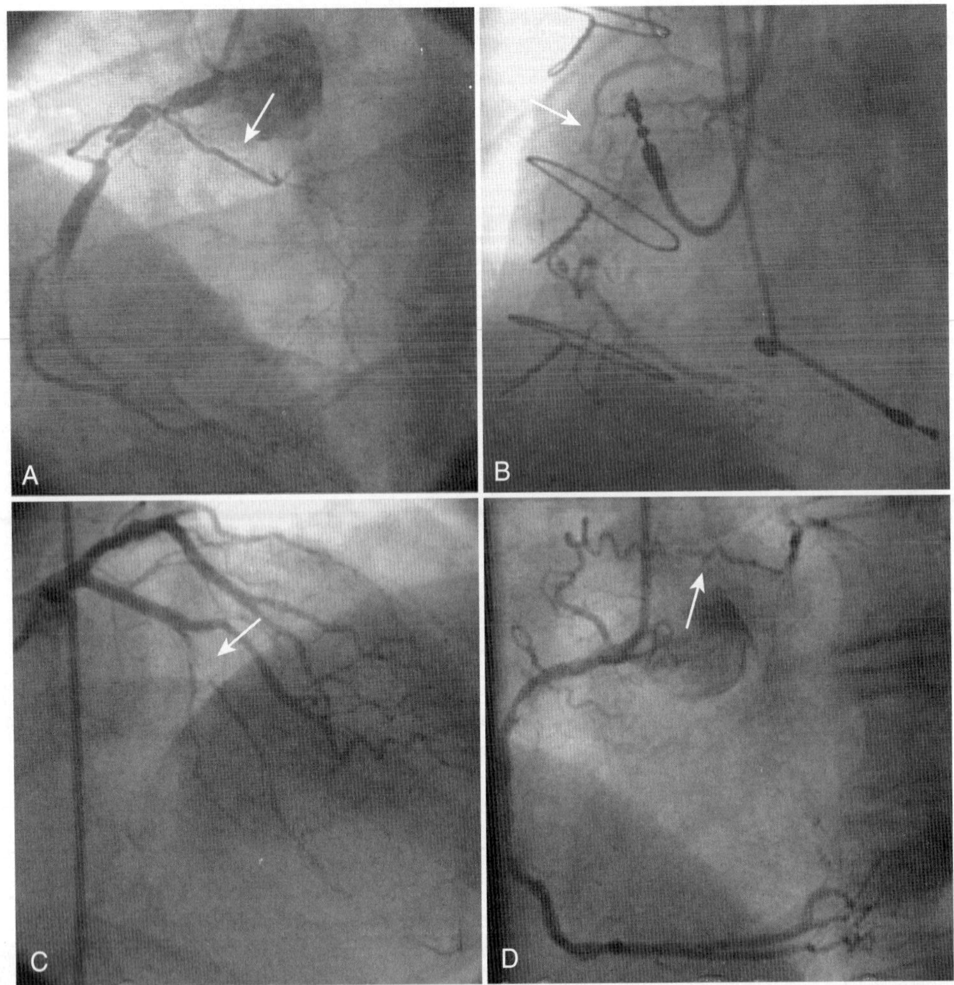

FIGURE 21-28 Coronary collaterals. **A,** A Kugel branch arises from the proximal right coronary artery and extends to the distal posterior descending branch of the right coronary artery (arrow). **B,** Bridging collaterals (arrow) connecting the proximal and distal right coronary artery. **C,** A microchannel in the mid–left anterior descending artery (arrow). **D,** A Vieussens collateral extends from the proximal right coronary artery to the left anterior descending artery (arrow).

TABLE 21-12 Standardized Criteria for Postprocedural Lesion Morphology

FEATURE	DEFINITION
Abrupt closure	Obstruction of contrast flow (TIMI 0 or 1) in a dilated segment with previously documented anterograde flow
Ectasia	A lesion diameter greater than the reference diameter in one or more areas
Luminal irregularities	Arterial contour that has a sawtooth pattern consisting of opacification but not fulfilling the criteria for dissection or intracoronary thrombus
Intimal flap	A discrete filling defect in apparent continuity with the arterial wall
Thrombus dissection*	Discrete, mobile angiographic filling defect with or without contrast staining
A	Small radiolucent area within the lumen of the vessel
B	Linear, nonpersisting extravasation of contrast material
C	Extraluminal, persisting extravasation of contrast material
D	Spiral filling defect
E	Persistent lumen defect with delayed anterograde flow
F	Filling defect accompanied by total coronary occlusion
Dissection, length (mm)	Measure end to end for type B through F dissections
Dissection, staining	Persistence of contrast within the dissection after washout of contrast material from the remaining portion of the vessel
Perforation	
Localized	Extravasation of contrast material confined to the pericardial space immediately surrounding the artery and not associated with clinical tamponade
Nonlocalized	Extravasation of contrast material with a jet not localized to the pericardial space, potentially associated with clinical tamponade
Side branch loss	TIMI 0, 1, or 2 flow in a side branch >1.5 mm in diameter that previously had TIMI 3 flow
Distal embolization	Migration of a filling defect or thrombus to distally occlude the target vessel or one of its branches
Coronary spasm	Transient or permanent narrowing >50% when a <25% stenosis has been previously noted

*National Heart, Lung, and Blood Institute classification system for coronary dissection.

pincushion distortion and reconstructed a three-dimensional representation of the arterial contour, reference vessel and minimal lumen diameters were measured and were used to evaluate the effect of pharmacologic intervention for a number of angiographic plaque regression studies. These initial quantitative angiographic methods were time-consuming and cumbersome and have now been largely replaced with computer-assisted methods for automated arterial contour detection that have used improved microprocessor speed and storage capacity.

Quantitative angiographic analysis is divided into several distinct processes, including film digitization (when needed), image calibration, and arterial contour detection. The contrast-filled diagnostic or guiding catheter can be used as a scaling device for determination of absolute vessel dimensions, yielding a calibration factor in millimeters per pixel. Catheter and arterial contours are obtained by drawing a center line through the segment of interest. Linear density profiles are then constructed perpendicular to the center line, and a weighted average of the first and second derivative function is used to define the catheter or arterial edges. Individual edge points are then connected by an automated algorithm, and outliers are discarded and the edges are smoothed. The automated algorithm is then applied to a selected arterial segment, and absolute coronary dimensions and percentage diameter stenosis are obtained.

The measures obtained by quantitative angiography are used to document angiographic success, defined as <50% residual diameter stenosis after balloon angioplasty or <20% diameter stenosis after coronary stent placement. Long-term results after stent placement and, more recently, drug-eluting stent placement are described using binary angiographic restenosis, defined as 50% or greater follow-up diameter stenosis, and late lumen loss, defined as the loss in lumen diameter during the intermediate (6- to 9-month) period of follow-up. Both the follow-up percentage diameter stenosis and late lumen loss have been correlated with clinical restenosis, manifested by ischemia-driven target lesion revascularization.

Pitfalls of Coronary Arteriography

Errors in image acquisition and interpretation can have a major impact on management strategies in patients with ischemic CAD, particularly when there is disagreement between angiographic, physiologic, and clinical findings. Attention to those factors that affect angiographic image quality at the time of image acquisition will improve the ultimate course selected for patients who undergo arteriography.

INADEQUATE VESSEL OPACIFICATION. Inadequate filling of the coronary artery with contrast medium results in incomplete vessel opacification or "streaming," which may misrepresent the degree of ostial and side branch disease and overestimate the amount of thrombus or the stenosis severity. The causes of contrast streaming include increased native coronary blood flow in the setting of left ventricular hypertrophy, aortic insufficiency, or anemia; competitive filling from collateral branches or bypass graft conduits; diagnostic catheter positioning that is not coaxial (or "in line") with the coronary ostium; and dislodgment of the diagnostic catheter during injection of the contrast agent. Contrast streaming can be overcome by a more forceful injection of the contrast agent as long as catheter tip position and pressure recording confirm the safety of such a maneuver. Switching to an angioplasty-guiding catheter with a soft, short tip and a larger lumen than a diagnostic catheter may allow more complete opacification of the target coronary artery or bypass graft. Superselective injection of contrast medium into the LCx artery (or LAD) through a short LMCA may give the impression of total occlusion of the LAD (or LCx).

ECCENTRIC STENOSES. By its nature, coronary atherosclerosis is a ubiquitous process that leads to asymmetric plaque distribution within the coronary artery. Although most segments of the artery wall are involved in the atherosclerotic process, eccentric or slitlike lesions may be seen by angiography in regions of more focal plaque accumulation. The hemodynamic significance of eccentric lesions is dependent on the percentage area stenosis rather than on the "worst" percentage diameter stenosis. A related problem is that of the hazy bandlike or membranous stenosis, which may be exceedingly difficult to characterize by standard angiographic views. These unique lesions may simply represent atherosclerosis or they may be caused by congenital membranous bands. Because of the difficulty in ascertaining the hemodynamic significance of these eccentric and bandlike lesions, measurement of a fractional flow reserve with a micromanometer-tip guidewire across the region of abnormality during intravenous administration of adenosine may be useful in identifying those patients with hemodynamically significant narrowings (see Chap. 52).

SUPERIMPOSITION OF BRANCHES. Superimposition of major branches of the left and right arteries can result in failure to detect significant stenoses or total occlusions of these branches. Although this problem most commonly affects the LAD artery and parallel diagonal branches, side branch overlap may also occur with the ostium of the obtuse marginal branch lesion of the LCx and the origin of the right ventricular branch of the RCA. Moreover, when the LAD is occluded beyond the origin of the first septal branch, this branch often becomes quite enlarged in an attempt to provide collateral circulation to the vascular bed of the distal LAD. It is important to obtain sufficient angulation for these views to identify the exact anatomy at the origin of the side branch, such as cranial projections for the LAD artery, caudal projections for the LCx, and left lateral projection for the RCA.

MICROCHANNEL RECANALIZATION. It is sometimes difficult to differentiate very severe (>90%) coronary stenoses (with an anterograde lumen) from total occlusions (with no anterograde lumen) that have been recanalized with microchannels and bridging collaterals. Pathologic studies suggest that approximately one third of totally occluded coronary arteries ultimately recanalize, resulting in the development of multiple tortuous channels that are quite small and close to one another and creating the impression on angiography of a single, slightly irregular channel. As angiography lacks sufficient spatial resolution to demonstrate this degree of detail in most patients with recanalized total occlusions, wire crossing may not be possible in some cases unless advanced wire techniques are used.

REFERENCES

1. Bruschke AV, Sheldon WC, Shirey EK, et al: A half century of selective coronary arteriography. J Am Coll Cardiol 54:2139, 2009.
2. Holmes DR, Laskey WK, Wondrow MA, et al: Flat-panel detectors in the cardiac catheterization laboratory: Revolution or evolution—what are the issues? Catheter Cardiovasc Interv 63:324, 2004.
3. Conti R: The continuing value of invasive coronary arteriography. Clin Cardiol 31:345, 2008.

Indications for Coronary Arteriography

4. Scanlon P, Faxon D, Audet A, et al: ACC/AHA Guidelines for coronary angiography. J Am Coll Cardiol 33:1756, 1999.
5. Patel MR, Dehmer GJ, Hirshfeld JW, et al: ACCF/SCAI/STS/AATS/AHA/ASNC 2009 Appropriateness Criteria for Coronary Revascularization. J Am Coll Cardiol 53:530, 2009.
6. Anderson JL, Adams CD, Antman EM, et al: ACC/AHA 2007 guidelines for the management of patients with unstable angina/non ST-elevation myocardial infarction: A report of the ACC/AHA Task Force on Practice Guidelines. J Am Coll Cardiol 50:e1, 2007.
7. Kushner FG, Hand M, Smith SC Jr, et al: 2009 Focused Updates: ACC/AHA Guidelines for the Management of Patients With ST-Elevation Myocardial Infarction and ACC/AHA/SCAI Guidelines on Percutaneous Coronary Intervention. A report of the ACC/AHA Task Force on Practice Guidelines. J Am Coll Cardiol 54:2205, 2009.
8. Monaco M, Stassano P, Di Tommaso L, et al: Systematic strategy of prophylactic coronary angiography improves long-term outcome after major vascular surgery in medium- to high-risk patients: A prospective, randomized study. J Am Coll Cardiol 54:989, 2009.
9. Flaherty JD, Rossi JS, Fonarow GC, et al: Influence of coronary angiography on the utilization of therapies in patients with acute heart failure syndromes: Findings from Organized Program to Initiate Lifesaving Treatment in Hospitalized Patients with Heart Failure (OPTIMIZE-HF). Am Heart J 157:1018, 2009.

Complications of Coronary Arteriography

10. Bulum J, Strozzi M, Smalcelj A: Spontaneous and catheter-induced secondary coronary artery dissection: A single-centre experience. Acta Cardiol 63:203, 2008.
11. West R, Ellis G, Brooks N: Complications of diagnostic cardiac catheterisation: Results from a confidential inquiry into cardiac catheter complications. Heart 92:810, 2006.
12. Samal A, White C: Percutaneous management of access site complications. Catheter Cardiovasc Interv 57:12, 2002.

13. Arora N, Matheny ME, Sepke C, et al: A propensity analysis of the risk of vascular complications after cardiac catheterization procedures with the use of vascular closure devices. Am Heart J 153:606, 2007.
14. Khatri P, Kasner SE: Ischemic strokes after cardiac catheterization: Opportune thrombolysis candidates? Arch Neurol 63:817, 2006.
15. Chambers CE, Eisenhauer MD, McNicol LB, et al: Infection control guidelines for the cardiac catheterization laboratory: Society guidelines revisited. Catheter Cardiovasc Interv 67:78, 2006.
16. Dib J, Boyle AJ, Chan M, et al: Coronary air embolism: A case report and review of the literature. Catheter Cardiovasc Interv 68:897, 2006.
17. Dudar BM, Kim HE: Massive air embolus treated with rheolytic thrombectomy. J Invasive Cardiol 19:E182, 2007.
18. Patterson MS, Kiemeneij F: Coronary air embolism treated with aspiration catheter. Heart 91:e36, 2005.
19. Zavala-Alarcon E, Cecena F, Little R, et al: The no-flow phenomenon during diagnostic coronary angiography. Cardiovasc Revasc Med 6:126, 2005.
20. Sohrabi B, Kazemi B, Aslanabadi N: Percutaneous treatment of catheter-induced dissection of the right coronary artery and adjacent aortic wall. J Invasive Cardiol 19:E199, 2007.
21. Khalid MR, Morris DC, Rab ST: Emergency stenting of the left main coronary artery after diagnostic coronary angiography. J Am Coll Cardiol Intv 2:577, 2009.
22. de Jong J, Piek J, van der Wal A: Multifocal arterial fibromuscular dysplasia causing coronary artery dissection following coronary angiography. EuroIntervention 5:166, 2009.
23. Rana O, McCrea W: Images in clinical medicine. Cholesterol emboli after coronary angioplasty. N Engl J Med 354:1294, 2006.
24. Hussein A, Kasmani R, Irani F, et al: Athero-embolic isolated splenic infarction following left cardiac catheterization. J Cardiovasc Med (Hagerstown) 10:271, 2009.
25. Azuelos A, Coro L, Alexandre A: Femoral nerve entrapment. Acta Neurochir Suppl 92:61, 2005.
26. Na KY, Kim CW, Song YR, et al: The association between kidney function, coronary artery disease, and clinical outcome in patients undergoing coronary angiography. J Korean Med Sci 24(Suppl):S87, 2009.
27. Efstathopoulos EP, Karvouni E, Kottou S, et al: Patient dosimetry during coronary interventions: A comprehensive analysis. Am Heart J 147:468, 2004.
28. Kocinaj D, Cioppa A, Ambrosini G, et al: Radiation dose exposure during cardiac and peripheral arteries catheterisation. Int J Cardiol 113:283, 2006.
29. Hirshfeld JW Jr, Balter S, Brinker JA, et al: ACCF/AHA/HRS/SCAI clinical competence statement on physician knowledge to optimize patient safety and image quality in fluoroscopically guided invasive cardiovascular procedures: A report of the ACC/AHA/ACP Task Force on Clinical Competence and Training. Circulation 111:511, 2005.
30. Klein LW, Miller DL, Balter S, et al: Occupational health hazards in the interventional laboratory: Time for a safer environment. Catheter Cardiovasc Interv 73:432, 2009.

Technique of Coronary Arteriography

31. Helft G, Dambrin G, Zaman A, et al: Percutaneous coronary intervention in anticoagulated patients via radial artery access. Catheter Cardiovasc Interv 73:44, 2009.
32. Lo TS, Buch AN, Hall IR, et al: Percutaneous left and right heart catheterization in fully anticoagulated patients utilizing the radial artery and forearm vein: A two-center experience. J Interv Cardiol 19:258, 2006.
33. Alvarez-Tostado JA, Moise MA, Bena JF, et al: The brachial artery: A critical access for endovascular procedures. J Vasc Surg 49:378, 2009.
34. Cox N, Resnic FS, Popma JJ, et al: Comparison of the risk of vascular complications associated with femoral and radial access coronary catheterization procedures in obese versus nonobese patients. Am J Cardiol 94:1174, 2004.
35. Greenwood MJ, Della-Siega AJ, Fretz EB, et al: Vascular communications of the hand in patients being considered for transradial coronary angiography: Is the Allen's test accurate? J Am Coll Cardiol 46:2013, 2005.
36. Pancholy SB: Comparison of the effect of intra-arterial versus intravenous heparin on radial artery occlusion after transradial catheterization. Am J Cardiol 104:1083, 2009.
37. Pancholy SB: Impact of two different hemostatic devices on radial artery outcomes after transradial catheterization. J Invasive Cardiol 21:101, 2009.
38. Lo TS, Nolan J, Fountzopoulos E, et al: Radial artery anomaly and its influence on transradial coronary procedural outcome. Heart 95:410, 2009.
39. Jolly SS, Amlani S, Hamon M, et al: Radial versus femoral access for coronary angiography or intervention and the impact on major bleeding and ischemic events: A systematic review and meta-analysis of randomized trials. Am Heart J 157:132, 2009.
40. Shook DC, Savage RM: Anesthesia in the cardiac catheterization laboratory and electrophysiology laboratory. Anesthesiol Clin 27:47, 2009.
41. Beddoes L, Botti M, Duke MM: Patients' experiences of cardiology procedures using minimal conscious sedation. Heart Lung 37:196, 2008.
42. Mehran R, Nikolsky E, Kirtane AJ, et al: Ionic low-osmolar versus nonionic iso-osmolar contrast media to obviate worsening nephropathy after angioplasty in chronic renal failure patients: The ICON (Ionic versus non-ionic Contrast to Obviate worsening Nephropathy after angioplasty in chronic renal failure patients) study. J Am Coll Cardiol Intv 2:415, 2009.
43. Caixeta A, Nikolsky E, Mehran R: Prevention and treatment of contrast-associated nephropathy in interventional cardiology. Curr Cardiol Rep 11:377, 2009.
44. Zoungas S, Ninomiya T, Huxley R, et al: Systematic review: Sodium bicarbonate treatment regimens for the prevention of contrast-induced nephropathy. Ann Intern Med 151:631, 2009.
45. Brar SS, Shen AY, Jorgensen MB, et al: Sodium bicarbonate vs sodium chloride for the prevention of contrast medium–induced nephropathy in patients undergoing coronary angiography: A randomized trial. JAMA 300:1038, 2008.
46. Navaneethan S, Singh S, Appasamy S, et al: Sodium bicarbonate therapy for prevention of contrast-induced nephropathy: A systematic review and meta-analysis. Am J Kidney Dis 53:617, 2009.
47. Tramèr MR, von Elm E, Loubeyre P, Hauser C: Pharmacological prevention of serious anaphylactic reactions due to iodinated contrast media: Systematic review. BMJ 333:675, 2006.
48. Thomsen HS, Morcos SK: Management of acute adverse reactions to contrast media. Eur Radiol 14:476, 2004.

Anatomy and Variations of the Coronary Arteries

49. Van Herck PL, Gavit L, Gorissen P, et al: Quantitative coronary arteriography on digital flat-panel system. Catheter Cardiovasc Interv 63:192, 2004.
50. Tsapaki V, Kottou S, Kollaros N, et al: Comparison of a conventional and a flat-panel digital system in interventional cardiology procedures. Br J Radiol 77:562, 2004.
51. Gibson CM, Morrow DA, Murphy SA, et al: A randomized trial to evaluate the relative protection against post-percutaneous coronary intervention microvascular dysfunction, ischemia, and inflammation among antiplatelet and antithrombotic agents: The PROTECT-TIMI-30 trial. J Am Coll Cardiol 47:2364, 2006.
52. Schwartz L, Kip KE, Alderman E, et al: Baseline coronary angiographic findings in the Bypass Angioplasty Revascularization Investigation 2 Diabetes trial (BARI 2D). Am J Cardiol 103:632, 2009.

Congenital Anomalies of the Coronary Circulation

53. Ouali S, Neffeti E, Sendid K, et al: Congenital anomalous aortic origins of the coronary arteries in adults: A Tunisian coronary arteriography study. Arch Cardiovasc Dis 102:201, 2009.
54. Baskurt M, Yyldyz A, Caglar IM, et al: Right coronary artery arising from the pulmonary trunk. Thorac Cardiovasc Surg 57:424, 2009.
55. Angelini P: Coronary artery anomalies—current clinical issues: Definitions, classification, incidence, clinical relevance, and treatment guidelines. Tex Heart Inst J 29:271, 2002.
56. Angelini P, Velasco JA, Flamm S: Coronary anomalies: Incidence, pathophysiology, and clinical relevance. Circulation 105:2449, 2002.
57. Eckart RE, Jones SO, Shry EA, et al: Sudden death associated with anomalous coronary origin and obstructive coronary disease in the young. Cardiol Rev 14:161, 2006.
58. von Kodolitsch Y, Franzen O, Lund GK, et al: Coronary artery anomalies. Part II: Recent insights from clinical investigations. Z Kardiol 94:1, 2005.
59. Hofmeyr L, Moolman J, Brice E, et al: An unusual presentation of an anomalous left coronary artery arising from the pulmonary artery (ALCAPA) in an adult: Anterior papillary muscle rupture causing severe mitral regurgitation. Echocardiography 26:474, 2009.
60. Porto I, MacDonald ST, Selvanayagam JB, et al: Intravascular ultrasound to guide stenting of an anomalous right coronary artery coursing between the aorta and pulmonary artery. J Invasive Cardiol 17:E33, 2005.
61. Gambetta K, Cui W, el-Zein C, et al: Anomalous left coronary artery from the right sinus of Valsalva and noncompaction of the left ventricle. Pediatr Cardiol 29:434, 2008.
62. Park JS, Shin DG, Kim YJ, et al: Left ventricular noncompaction with a single coronary artery of anomalous origin. Int J Cardiol 119:e35, 2007.
63. Kim SY, Seo JB, Do KH, et al: Coronary artery anomalies: Classification and ECG-gated multi-detector row CT findings with angiographic correlation. Radiographics 26:317, 2006.
64. Luo L, Kebede S, Wu S, et al: Coronary artery fistulae. Am J Med Sci 332:79, 2006.
65. Cheng TO: Left coronary artery–to–left ventricular fistula. A follow-up report. Int J Cardiol 118:233, 2007.
66. Cebi N, Schulze-Waltrup N, Fromke J, et al: Congenital coronary artery fistulas in adults: Concomitant pathologies and treatment. Int J Cardiovasc Imaging 24:349, 2008.
67. Alegria JR, Herrmann J, Holmes DR, et al: Myocardial bridging. Eur Heart J 26:1159, 2005.
68. Ishikawa Y, Akasaka Y, Suzuki K, et al: Anatomic properties of myocardial bridge predisposing to myocardial infarction. Circulation 120:376, 2009.
69. Rozenberg V, Nepomnyashchikh L: Pathomorphology of myocardial bridges and their role in the pathogenesis of coronary disease. Bull Exp Biol Med 134:593, 2002.

Lesion Complexity

70. Wozakowska-Kaplon B, Niedziela J, Krzyzak P, et al: Clinical manifestations of slow coronary flow from acute coronary syndrome to serious arrhythmias. Cardiol J 16:462, 2009.
71. Smith S, Feldman T, Hirshfeld J, et al: ACC/AHA/SCAI 2005 Guideline Update for Percutaneous Coronary Intervention. A report of the ACC/AHA. Circulation 113:156, 2006.
72. Krone RJ, Shaw RE, Klein LW, et al: Evaluation of the ACC/AHA/SCAI lesion classification system in the current "stent era" of coronary interventions (from the ACC–National Cardiovascular Data Registry). Am J Cardiol 92:389, 2003.
73. Singh M, Rihal CS, Lennon RJ, et al: Comparison of Mayo Clinic risk score and ACC/AHA lesion classification in the prediction of adverse cardiovascular outcome following percutaneous coronary interventions. J Am Coll Cardiol 44:357, 2004.
74. Popma J, Leon M, Moses J, et al: Quantitative assessment of angiographic restenosis after sirolimus-eluting stent implantation in native coronary arteries. Circulation 110:3773, 2004.
75. Alexander JH, Hafley G, Harrington RA, et al: Efficacy and safety of edifoligide, an E2F transcription factor decoy, for prevention of vein graft failure following coronary artery bypass graft surgery: PREVENT IV: A randomized controlled trial. JAMA 294:2446,2005.

GUIDELINES Jeffrey J. Popma

Coronary Arteriography

The American College of Cardiology (ACC) and the American Heart Association (AHA) first published guidelines for coronary angiography in 1987.[1] These were updated in 1999, in collaboration with the Society for Cardiac Angiography and Interventions.[2] Although these guidelines have not been revised since then, recommendations for the use of coronary angiography are included in several more recent practice guidelines, including those for stable angina,[3] unstable angina and non–ST elevation myocardial infarction,[4] acute ST elevation myocardial infarction,[5] noncardiac surgery,[6,7] heart failure,[8] and valvular disease.[9] The text and tables that follow present an amalgam of recommendations from the 1999 ACC/AHA coronary angiography guidelines and from more recent condition-specific guidelines.

Like other ACC/AHA guidelines, these use the standard ACC/AHA classification system for indications:

Class I: conditions for which there is evidence and/or general agreement that the test is useful and effective

Class II: conditions for which there is conflicting evidence and/or a divergence of opinion about the usefulness or efficacy of performing the test

Class IIa: weight of evidence or opinion is in favor of usefulness or efficacy

Class IIb: usefulness or efficacy is less well established by evidence or opinion

Class III: conditions for which there is evidence and/or general agreement that the test is not useful or effective and in some cases may be harmful

Three levels are used to rate the evidence on which recommendations have been based. Level A recommendations are derived from data from multiple randomized clinical trials; level B recommendations are derived from a single randomized trial or nonrandomized studies; and level C recommendations are based on the consensus opinion of experts.

CORONARY ARTERIOGRAPHY IN ASYMPTOMATIC PATIENTS OR THOSE WITH STABLE ANGINA

The ACC/AHA guidelines recommend that coronary angiography is indicated (Class I) for patients with chest pain who have survived a sudden cardiac arrest, for patients with known chronic coronary disease who have disabling symptoms and high-risk criteria on noninvasive testing, and for those with clinical evidence of heart failure (**Table 21G-1**). The guidelines do not support routine use of coronary angiography as a first-line test for asymptomatic patients with significant comorbidity, in whom the risks outweigh the benefits, and in those patients with minimal symptoms who respond to medical therapy and have no evidence of ischemia on noninvasive testing (see Table 21G-1).

CORONARY ARTERIOGRAPHY IN PATIENTS WITH ST ELEVATION MYOCARDIAL INFARCTION

The ACC/AHA guidelines on coronary angiography[2] and ST-segment elevation myocardial infarction[5] recommend that coronary angiography be performed in candidates for primary or rescue coronary intervention and in patients with cardiogenic shock or other structural cardiac injury (e.g., ventricular septal rupture or severe mitral regurgitation) or other major complications (**Table 21G-2**). Coronary arteriography should not be performed in patients with extensive comorbidities, in whom the risks of revascularization likely outweigh the benefits. After initial reperfusion therapy or in patients who are not treated with primary coronary intervention, coronary arteriography should be performed in patients with spontaneous episodes of myocardial ischemia or ischemia provoked by minimal exertion or those with intermediate or high-risk features on noninvasive testing. Coronary arteriography is also indicated in those patients with mechanical complications of their infarction.

CORONARY ARTERIOGRAPHY IN PATIENTS WITH UNSTABLE ANGINA/NON–ST ELEVATION MYOCARDIAL INFARCTION

Although coronary angiography is not generally recommended as part of the routine evaluation for unstable angina/non–ST elevation myocardial infarction (UA/NSTEMI),[4] the ACC/AHA guidelines recommend a low threshold for angiography as part of an early invasive strategy for patients with high-risk indicators, such as recurrent symptoms of ischemia despite adequate medical therapy, high-risk noninvasive test results, depressed left ventricular systolic function, severe arrhythmia, and prior revascularization (**Table 21G-3**).

CORONARY ARTERIOGRAPHY IN PATIENTS WITH NONSPECIFIC CHEST PAIN

The 1999 ACC/AHA guidelines on coronary angiography[2] as well as the 2007 guidelines update on UA/NSTEMI[4] discourage use of coronary angiography for patients with nonspecific chest pain unless they have high-risk findings on noninvasive testing. The guidelines do support angiography for patients with chest pain after cocaine use if ST segments remain elevated after medical therapy (**Table 21G-4**). Coronary angiography is also endorsed for patients with clinical evidence of coronary spasm.

CORONARY ARTERIOGRAPHY FOR PATIENT FOLLOW-UP

Coronary angiography is supported for patients with marked limitations of functional status despite maximal medical therapy or who have evidence of ongoing ischemia after revascularization procedures, such as those with abrupt closure or restenosis after coronary intervention (**Table 21G-5**). Coronary angiography is not supported as part of routine follow-up of patients who have no change in clinical status (see Table 21G-5).

CORONARY ARTERIOGRAPHY FOR THE EVALUATION AND ASSESSMENT OF HEART FAILURE

The 2009 ACC/AHA guidelines on heart failure[8] recommend that clinicians proceed directly to coronary angiography in patients who have heart failure or impaired left ventricular function and clinical evidence of ischemia, given the benefits of revascularization in this high-risk population (see Table 21G-5). There is weaker support for the use of angiography for patients with heart failure in the absence of clear-cut cardiac chest pain because revascularization has not been shown to improve clinical outcomes in patients without angina.

CORONARY ARTERIOGRAPHY IN PATIENTS WITH VALVULAR DISEASE

Coronary angiography for patients with valvular heart disease is generally used as a prelude to surgery to provide insight into whether the patient has coexisting coronary disease that might warrant concomitant revascularization (**Table 21G-6**). Cardiac catheterization is occasionally needed to obtain hemodynamic data, but advances in noninvasive testing have greatly reduced the role of catheterization for that purpose. The ACC/AHA guidelines on valvular heart disease[9] recommend preoperative coronary angiography in men older than 35 years, premenopausal women older than 35 years with coronary risk factors, and postmenopausal women who have symptoms of coronary artery disease or left ventricular dysfunction. Routine coronary angiography is not indicated in younger patients (younger than 45 years) undergoing surgery for mitral regurgitation caused by mitral valve degeneration in the absence of symptoms and without risk factors.

CORONARY ARTERIOGRAPHY BEFORE AND AFTER NONCARDIAC SURGERY

In general, indications for preoperative coronary angiography are similar to those identified for the nonoperative setting. The ACC/AHA guidelines on perioperative cardiovascular evaluation for noncardiac surgery[6,7] indicate that coronary angiography is an appropriate intervention for patients with high-risk criteria on noninvasive testing as well as for those with angina symptoms that would warrant consideration of revascularization even if they were not candidates for noncardiac surgery (**Table 21G-7**). The ACC/AHA guidelines also recommend coronary arteriography in patients with equivocal noninvasive test results at high clinical risk undergoing high-risk surgery.

CORONARY ARTERIOGRAPHY IN PATIENTS WITH CONGENITAL HEART DISEASE

In patients with congenital heart disease, there are two main indications for coronary angiography: assessment of the hemodynamic impact of

TABLE 21G-1 ACC/AHA Recommendations for Coronary Arteriography in Asymptomatic Patients or Those with Stable Angina

INDICATION	CLASS	RECOMMENDATION	LOE
Establishing a diagnosis in patients with suspected angina or a significant change in anginal symptoms	Class I	Patients with known or possible angina pectoris who have survived sudden cardiac death	B
	Class IIa	Patients with an uncertain diagnosis after noninvasive testing in whom the benefit of a more certain diagnosis outweighs the risk and cost of coronary angiography	C
		Patients who cannot undergo noninvasive testing because of disability, illness, or morbid obesity	C
		Patients with an occupational requirement for a definitive diagnosis	C
		Patients who by virtue of young age at onset of symptoms, noninvasive imaging, or other clinical parameters are suspected of having a nonatherosclerotic cause for myocardial ischemia (e.g., coronary artery anomaly, Kawasaki disease, primary coronary artery dissection, radiation-induced vasculopathy)	C
		Patients in whom coronary artery spasm is suspected and provocative testing may be necessary	C
		Patients with a high pretest probability of left main or three-vessel CAD	C
	Class IIb	Patients with recurrent hospitalization for chest pain in whom a definite diagnosis is judged necessary	C
		Patients with an overriding desire for a definitive diagnosis and a greater than low probability of CAD	C
	Class III	Not recommended in patients with significant comorbidity in whom the risk of coronary arteriography outweighs the benefit of the procedure	C
		Not recommended in patients with an overriding personal desire for a definitive diagnosis and a low probability of CAD	C
Risk stratification in patients with chronic stable angina	Class I	Patients with disabling (CCS classes III and IV) chronic stable angina, despite medical therapy	B
		Patients with high-risk criteria on noninvasive testing regardless of angina severity	B
		Patients with angina who have survived sudden cardiac death or serious ventricular arrhythmia	B
		Patients with angina and symptoms and signs of heart failure	C
		Patients with clinical characteristics that indicate a high likelihood of severe CAD	C
	Class IIa	Patients with significant left ventricular dysfunction (ejection fraction <0.45), CCS class I or II angina, and demonstrable ischemia but less than high-risk criteria on noninvasive testing	C
		Patients with inadequate prognostic information after noninvasive testing	C
	Class IIb	Patients with CCS class I or II angina, preserved left ventricular function (ejection fraction >0.45), and less than high-risk criteria on noninvasive testing	C
		Patients with CCS class III or IV angina, which improves with medical therapy to class I or II	C
		Patients with CCS class I or II angina but intolerance (unacceptable side effects) to adequate medical therapy	C
	Class III	Not recommended in patients with CCS class I or II angina who respond to medical therapy and who have no evidence of ischemia on noninvasive testing	C
		Not recommended in patients who prefer to avoid revascularization	C
Risk stratification in asymptomatic patients	Class IIa	Patients with high-risk criteria suggesting ischemia on noninvasive testing	C
	Class IIb	Patients with inadequate prognostic information after noninvasive testing	C
		Patients with clinical characteristics that indicate a high likelihood of severe CAD	C
	Class III	Not recommended in patients who prefer to avoid revascularization	C
Monitoring of symptoms and antianginal therapy	Class I	Patients with marked limitation of ordinary activity (CCS class III), despite maximal medical therapy	C

CAD = coronary artery disease; CCS = Canadian Cardiovascular Society ; LOE = level of evidence.

From Fraker TD Jr, Fihn SD, Gibbons RJ, et al: ACC/AHA 2007 chronic angina focused update of the ACC/AHA 2002 guidelines for the management of patients with chronic stable angina: A report of the American College of Cardiology/American Heart Association Task Force on Practice Guidelines Writing Group to Develop the Focused Update of the 2002 Guidelines for the Management of Patients With Chronic Stable Angina. J Am Coll Cardiol 50:2264, 2007.

congenital coronary lesions and assessment of the presence of coronary anomalies that potentially could compromise the heart during correction of other congenital heart lesions (**Table 21G-8**). The ACC/AHA guidelines indicate that it is prudent to perform coronary angiography in patients being considered for repair of congenital heart disease if angina, ischemia on noninvasive testing, or multiple coronary risk factors are present. The ACC/AHA guidelines also recommend coronary angiography in young patients with an unexplained cardiac arrest.

OTHER USES OF CORONARY ARTERIOGRAPHY

The ACC/AHA guidelines[2] recommend coronary angiography for patients with aortic aneurysm, hypertrophic cardiomyopathy, and other conditions when knowledge of coronary artery involvement or the presence of coronary artery disease is necessary (**Table 21G-9**).

TABLE 21G-2 ACC/AHA Recommendations for Coronary Arteriography in Patients with ST Elevation Myocardial Infarction

INDICATION	CLASS	RECOMMENDATION	LOE
Diagnosis of STEMI	Class I	Diagnostic coronary angiography should be performed:	
		In candidates for primary or rescue percutaneous coronary intervention	A
		In patients with cardiogenic shock who are candidates for revascularization	A
		In candidates for surgical repair of VSR or severe mitral regurgitation	B
		In patients with persistent hemodynamic and/or electrical instability	C
	Class III	Coronary angiography should not be performed in patients with extensive comorbidities in whom risks of revascularization are likely to outweigh benefits	C
Treatment of STEMI		See Guidelines, Chap. 55	
Hospital management of STEMI	Class I	Patients with spontaneous episodes of myocardial ischemia or episodes of myocardial ischemia provoked by minimal exertion during recovery from STEMI	A
		Patients with intermediate- or high-risk findings on noninvasive testing after STEMI	B
		Patients who are sufficiently stable before definitive therapy for a mechanical complication of STEMI, such as acute mitral regurgitation, VSR, pseudoaneurysm, or LV aneurysm	B
		Patients with persistent hemodynamic instability	B
		Patients who are survivors of STEMI who had clinical heart failure during the acute episode but subsequently demonstrated well-preserved LV function	C
	Class IIa	Patients in whom STEMI is suspected to have occurred by mechanisms other than thrombotic occlusion of an atherosclerotic plaque, including coronary embolism, certain metabolic or hematologic diseases, and coronary artery spasm	C
		Patients with any of the following: diabetes mellitus, LV ejection fraction <0.40, congestive heart failure, prior revascularization, or life-threatening ventricular arrhythmias	C
	Class IIb	May be considered part of strategy of routine coronary arteriography for risk assessment after fibrinolytic therapy	B
	Class III	Should not be performed in survivors of STEMI thought not to be candidates for coronary revascularization	A

LOE = level of evidence; LV = left ventricular; STEMI = ST elevation myocardial infarction; VSR = ventricular septal rupture.

From Fraker TD Jr, Fihn SD, Gibbons RJ, et al: ACC/AHA 2007 chronic angina focused update of the ACC/AHA 2002 guidelines for the management of patients with chronic stable angina: A report of the American College of Cardiology/American Heart Association Task Force on Practice Guidelines Writing Group to Develop the Focused Update of the 2002 Guidelines for the Management of Patients With Chronic Stable Angina. J Am Coll Cardiol 50:2264, 2007.

TABLE 21G-3 ACC/AHA Recommendations for Coronary Arteriography in Patients with Unstable Angina/Non–ST Elevation Myocardial Infarction

INDICATION	CLASS	RECOMMENDATION	LOE
Management of UA/NSTEMI	Class I	An early invasive strategy in patients with UA/NSTEMI and any of the following high-risk indicators:	A
		Recurrent angina or ischemia at rest or with low-level activities despite intensive anti-ischemic therapy	
		Elevated troponin T or troponin I level	
		New or presumably new ST-segment depression	
		Recurrent angina/ischemia with CHF symptoms, an S_3 gallop, pulmonary edema, worsening rales, or new or worsening MR	
		High-risk findings on noninvasive stress testing	
		Depressed LV systolic function (e.g., ejection fraction <0.40 on noninvasive study)	
		Hemodynamic instability	
		Sustained ventricular tachycardia	
		PCI within 6 months	
		Prior CABG	
		In the absence of these findings, either an early conservative or an early invasive strategy in hospitalized patients without contraindications for revascularization	B
	Class IIa	An early invasive strategy in patients with repeated presentations for ACS despite therapy and without evidence for ongoing ischemia or high risk	C
	Class III	Should not be performed in patients with extensive comorbidities (e.g., liver or pulmonary failure, cancer), in whom the risks of revascularization are likely to outweigh the benefits	C
		Should not be performed in patients with acute chest pain and a low likelihood of ACS	C
		Should not be performed in patients who will not consent to revascularization, regardless of the findings	C
Postdischarge follow-up	Class I	Patients managed initially with a conservative strategy who experience recurrent unstable angina or severe (CCS class III) chronic stable angina despite medical management who are suitable for revascularization	B

ACS = acute coronary syndrome; CABG = coronary artery bypass grafting; CAD = coronary artery disease; CCS = Canadian Cardiovascular Society; CHF = congestive heart failure; LOE = level of evidence; LV = left ventricular; MR = mitral regurgitation; NSTEMI = non–ST elevation myocardial infarction; PCI = percutaneous coronary intervention; UA = unstable angina.

From Anderson JL, Adams CD, Antman EM, et al: ACC/AHA 2007 guidelines for the management of patients with unstable angina/non–ST-elevation myocardial infarction. Executive summary: A report of the American College of Cardiology/American Heart Association Task Force on Practice Guidelines (Writing Committee to Revise the 2002 Guidelines for the Management of Patients With Unstable Angina/Non–ST-Elevation Myocardial Infarction). Developed in collaboration with the American College of Emergency Physicians, the Society for Cardiovascular Angiography and Interventions, and the Society of Thoracic Surgeons Endorsed by the American Association of Cardiovascular and Pulmonary Rehabilitation and the Society for Academic Emergency Medicine. J Am Coll Cardiol 50:652, 2007.

CH 21

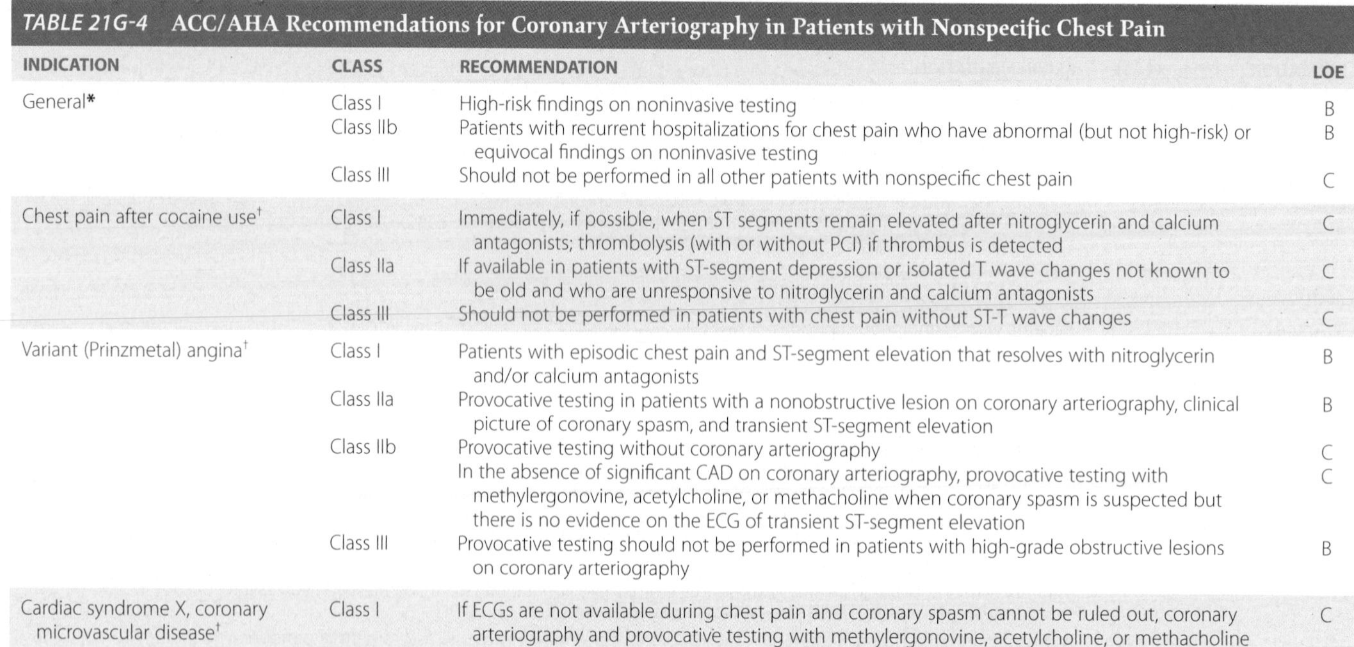

TABLE 21G-4 ACC/AHA Recommendations for Coronary Arteriography in Patients with Nonspecific Chest Pain

INDICATION	CLASS	RECOMMENDATION	LOE
General*	Class I	High-risk findings on noninvasive testing	B
	Class IIb	Patients with recurrent hospitalizations for chest pain who have abnormal (but not high-risk) or equivocal findings on noninvasive testing	B
	Class III	Should not be performed in all other patients with nonspecific chest pain	C
Chest pain after cocaine use†	Class I	Immediately, if possible, when ST segments remain elevated after nitroglycerin and calcium antagonists; thrombolysis (with or without PCI) if thrombus is detected	C
	Class IIa	If available in patients with ST-segment depression or isolated T wave changes not known to be old and who are unresponsive to nitroglycerin and calcium antagonists	C
	Class III	Should not be performed in patients with chest pain without ST-T wave changes	C
Variant (Prinzmetal) angina†	Class I	Patients with episodic chest pain and ST-segment elevation that resolves with nitroglycerin and/or calcium antagonists	B
	Class IIa	Provocative testing in patients with a nonobstructive lesion on coronary arteriography, clinical picture of coronary spasm, and transient ST-segment elevation	B
	Class IIb	Provocative testing without coronary arteriography	C
		In the absence of significant CAD on coronary arteriography, provocative testing with methylergonovine, acetylcholine, or methacholine when coronary spasm is suspected but there is no evidence on the ECG of transient ST-segment elevation	C
	Class III	Provocative testing should not be performed in patients with high-grade obstructive lesions on coronary arteriography	B
Cardiac syndrome X, coronary microvascular disease†	Class I	If ECGs are not available during chest pain and coronary spasm cannot be ruled out, coronary arteriography and provocative testing with methylergonovine, acetylcholine, or methacholine	C

CAD = coronary artery disease; ECG = electrocardiogram; LOE = level of evidence; PCI = percutaneous coronary intervention.

*From Scanlon PJ, Faxon DP, Audet AM, et al: ACC/AHA guidelines for coronary angiography: Executive summary and recommendations. A report of the American College of Cardiology/American Heart Association Task Force on Practice Guidelines (Committee on Coronary Angiography) developed in collaboration with the Society for Cardiac Angiography and Interventions. Circulation 99:2345, 1999.

†From Kushner FG, Hand M, Smith SC Jr, et al: 2009 Focused Updates: ACC/AHA guidelines for the management of patients with ST-elevation myocardial infarction (updating the 2004 guideline and 2007 focused update) and ACC/AHA/SCAI guidelines on percutaneous coronary intervention (updating the 2005 guideline and 2007 focused update): A report of the American College of Cardiology Foundation/American Heart Association Task Force on Practice Guidelines. J Am Coll Cardiol 54:2205, 2004.

TABLE 21G-5 ACC/AHA Recommendations for Coronary Arteriography for Patient Follow-Up

INDICATION	CLASS	RECOMMENDATION	LOE
Monitoring of symptoms and antianginal therapy*	Class I	Patients with marked limitation of ordinary activity (CCS class III) despite maximal medical therapy	C
	Class III	Repeated coronary angiography is not recommended in patients with no change in clinical status, no change on repeated exercise testing or stress imaging, and insignificant CAD on initial evaluation	C
After CABG in patients with UA/NSTEMI†	Class I	Maintain a low threshold for angiography, given the many anatomic possibilities that might be responsible for recurrent ischemia	B
		Patients managed initially with a conservative strategy who experience recurrent unstable angina or severe (CCS class III) chronic stable angina, despite medical management, who are suitable for revascularization should undergo coronary arteriography	B
Postrevascularization ischemia‡	Class I	Suspected abrupt closure or subacute stent thrombosis after percutaneous revascularization	B
		Recurrent angina or high-risk criteria on noninvasive evaluation (see Table 21G-1) within 9 months of PCI	C
	Class IIa	Recurrent symptomatic ischemia within 12 months of CABG	B
		Noninvasive evidence of high-risk criteria at any time post-CABG	B
		Recurrent angina inadequately controlled by medical means after revascularization	C
		For patients undergoing PCI for unprotected left main coronary obstructions, coronary angiography follow-up between 2 and 6 months after PCI is reasonable§	C
	Class IIb	Asymptomatic post-PCI patient suspected of having restenosis within the first months after angioplasty because of an abnormal noninvasive test result but without noninvasive high-risk criteria	B
		Recurrent angina without high-risk criteria on noninvasive testing occurring more than 1 year post-CABG	C
		Asymptomatic post-CABG patient in whom a deterioration in serial noninvasive testing has been documented but who is not at high risk on noninvasive testing	C
	Class III	Not recommended in symptomatic post-CABG patients who are not candidates for repeated revascularization	C
		Routine angiography is not indicated in asymptomatic patients after PCI, CABG, or other surgery, unless as part of an approved research protocol	C
Initial and serial clinical assessment of patients presenting with heart failure**	Class I	Patients presenting with heart failure who have angina or significant ischemia unless the patient is not eligible for revascularization of any kind	B
	Class IIa	Reasonable for patients presenting with heart failure who have chest pain that may or may not be of cardiac origin who have not had evaluation of their coronary anatomy and who have no contraindications to coronary revascularization	C
		Reasonable for patients presenting with heart failure who have known or suspected CAD but who do not have angina unless the patient is not eligible for revascularization of any kind	C

CABG = coronary artery bypass grafting; CAD = coronary artery disease; CCS = Canadian Cardiovascular Society; LOE = level of evidence; NSTEMI = non–ST elevation myocardial infarction; PCI = percutaneous coronary intervention; UA = unstable angina.

*From Fraker TD Jr, Fihn SD, Gibbons RJ, et al: ACC/AHA 2007 chronic angina focused update of the ACC/AHA 2002 guidelines for the management of patients with chronic stable angina: A report of the American College of Cardiology/American Heart Association Task Force on Practice Guidelines Writing Group to Develop the Focused Update of the 2002 Guidelines for the Management of Patients With Chronic Stable Angina. J Am Coll Cardiol 50:2264, 2007.

†From Kushner FG, Hand M, Smith SC Jr, et al: 2009 Focused Updates: ACC/AHA guidelines for the management of patients with ST-elevation myocardial infarction (updating the 2004 guideline and 2007 focused update) and ACC/AHA/SCAI guidelines on percutaneous coronary intervention (updating the 2005 guideline and 2007 focused update): A report of the American College of Cardiology Foundation/American Heart Association Task Force on Practice Guidelines. J Am Coll Cardiol 54:2205, 2004.

‡From Scanlon PJ, Faxon DP, Audet AM, et al: ACC/AHA guidelines for coronary angiography: Executive summary and recommendations. A report of the American College of Cardiology/American Heart Association Task Force on Practice Guidelines (Committee on Coronary Angiography) developed in collaboration with the Society for Cardiac Angiography and Interventions. Circulation 99:2345, 1999.

§From Smith SC Jr, Feldman TE, Hirshfeld JW Jr, et al: ACC/AHA/SCAI 2005 guideline update for percutaneous coronary intervention: A report of the American College of Cardiology/American Heart Association Task Force on Practice Guidelines (ACC/AHA/SCAI Writing Committee to Update the 2001 Guidelines for Percutaneous Coronary Intervention). J Am Coll Cardiol 47:e1, 2006.

** From Hunt SA, Abraham WT, Chin MH, et al: 2009 Focused update incorporated into the ACC/AHA 2005 Guidelines for the Diagnosis and Management of Heart Failure in Adults: A Report of the American College of Cardiology Foundation/American Heart Association Task Force on Practice Guidelines Developed in Collaboration With the International Society for Heart and Lung Transplantation. J Am Coll Cardiol 53:e1, 2009.

TABLE 21G-6 ACC/AHA Recommendations for Coronary Arteriography in Patients with Valvular Disease

INDICATION	CLASS	RECOMMENDATION	LOE
Aortic stenosis	Class I	Before AVR for patients with AS at risk for CAD	B
		Cardiac catheterization for hemodynamic assessment of severity of AS for symptomatic patients when noninvasive tests are inconclusive or when there is discrepancy between noninvasive tests and clinical findings regarding severity of AS	C
		Before AVR for patients with AS for whom a pulmonary autograft (Ross procedure) is contemplated and if origin of coronary arteries was not identified by noninvasive technique	C
	Class III	Cardiac catheterization for hemodynamic measurements not recommended for assessment of severity of AS before AVR when noninvasive tests are adequate and concordant with clinical findings	C
		Cardiac catheterization for hemodynamic measurements not recommended for assessment of LV function and severity of AS in asymptomatic patients	C
Aortic regurgitation	Class I	Before AVR for patients at risk for CAD	C
		Cardiac catheterization with aortic root angiography and measurement of LV pressure indicated for assessment of severity of AR, LV function, or aortic root size when noninvasive tests are inconclusive or discordant with clinical findings	B
	Class III	Cardiac catheterization with aortic root angiography and measurement of LV pressure not indicated for assessment of LV function, aortic root size, or severity of AR before AVR when noninvasive tests are adequate and concordant with clinical findings and coronary angiography is not needed	C
		Cardiac catheterization with aortic root angiography and measurement of LV pressure not indicated for assessment of LV function and severity of regurgitation for asymptomatic patients when noninvasive tests are adequate	C
Mitral regurgitation	Class I	Before mitral valve repair or mitral valve replacement for patients at risk for CAD	C
		Left ventriculography and hemodynamic measurements indicated when noninvasive tests are inconclusive regarding severity of MR, LV function, or need for surgery	C
		Hemodynamic measurements indicated when pulmonary artery pressure is out of proportion to severity of MR as assessed by noninvasive testing	C
		Left ventriculography and hemodynamic measurements indicated when there is a discrepancy between clinical and noninvasive findings regarding severity of MR	C
	Class III	Left ventriculography and hemodynamic measurements not indicated for patients with MR in whom valve surgery is not contemplated	C
Diagnosis of concurrent CAD	Class I	Before valve surgery (including infective endocarditis) or mitral balloon commissurotomy for patients with chest pain, other objective evidence of ischemia, decreased LV systolic function, history of CAD, or coronary risk factors (including age)	C
		Patients undergoing mitral balloon valvotomy need not undergo coronary angiography solely on basis of coronary risk factors	
		Patients with apparently mild to moderate valvular heart disease but with progressive angina (CCS class II or greater), objective evidence of ischemia, decreased LV systolic function, or overt congestive heart failure	C
		Before valve surgery in men 35 years or older, premenopausal women 35 years or older who have coronary risk factors, and postmenopausal women	C
	Class IIa	Surgery without coronary angiography reasonable for patients having emergency valve surgery for acute valve regurgitation, aortic root disease, or infective endocarditis	C
	Class IIb	Coronary angiography may be considered for patients undergoing catheterization to confirm severity of valve lesions before valve surgery without preexisting evidence of CAD, multiple coronary risk factors, or advanced age	C
	Class III	Coronary angiography not indicated for young patients undergoing nonemergency valve surgery when no further hemodynamic assessment by catheterization is deemed necessary and there are no coronary risk factors, no history of CAD, and no evidence of ischemia	C
		Patients should not undergo coronary angiography before valve surgery if severely hemodynamically unstable	C

AR = aortic regurgitation; AS = aortic stenosis; AVR = aortic valve replacement; CAD = coronary artery disease; CCS = Canadian Cardiovascular Society; LOE = level of evidence; LV = left ventricular; MR = mitral regurgitation.

From Bonow RO, Carabello BA, Chatterjee K, et al: 2008 focused update incorporated into the ACC/AHA 2006 guidelines for the management of patients with valvular heart disease: A report of the American College of Cardiology/American Heart Association Task Force on Practice Guidelines (Writing Committee to revise the 1998 guidelines for the management of patients with valvular heart disease). Endorsed by the Society of Cardiovascular Anesthesiologists, Society for Cardiovascular Angiography and Interventions, and Society of Thoracic Surgeons. J Am Coll Cardiol 52:e1, 2008.

TABLE 21G-7 ACC/AHA Recommendations for Coronary Arteriography Before and After Noncardiac Surgery

CLASS	RECOMMENDATION
Class I	Evidence for high risk of adverse outcome based on noninvasive test results Angina unresponsive to adequate medical therapy Unstable angina, particularly when facing intermediate- or high-risk noncardiac surgery Equivocal noninvasive test results in patients at high clinical risk undergoing high-risk surgery
Class IIa	Multiple markers of intermediate clinical risk and planned vascular surgery (noninvasive testing should be considered first) Moderate to large region of ischemia on noninvasive testing but without high-risk features and without lower LV ejection fraction Nondiagnostic, noninvasive test results in patients of intermediate clinical risk undergoing high-risk noncardiac surgery Urgent noncardiac surgery while convalescing from acute myocardial infarction
Class IIb	Medically stabilized class III or IV angina and planned low-risk or minor surgery
Class III	Not recommended for low-risk noncardiac surgery with known CAD and no high-risk results on noninvasive testing Not recommended for asymptomatic patients after CABG or PCI with excellent exercise capacity (≥7 METs) Not recommended for patients with mild stable angina with good LV function and no high-risk noninvasive test results Not recommended for patients who are not candidates for coronary revascularization because of concomitant medical illness, severe LV dysfunction (e.g., LV ejection fraction <0.20), or refusal to consider revascularization Not recommended for patients who are candidates for liver, lung, or renal transplantation older than 40 years, as part of evaluation for transplantation, unless noninvasive testing reveals high risk for adverse outcome

CABG = coronary artery bypass grafting; CAD = coronary artery disease; LV = left ventricular; PCI = percutaneous coronary intervention.
From Eagle KA, Berger PB, Calkins H, et al: ACC/AHA guideline update for perioperative cardiovascular evaluation for noncardiac surgery—executive summary: A report of the American College of Cardiology/American Heart Association Task Force on Practice Guidelines (Committee to Update the 1996 Guidelines on Perioperative Cardiovascular Evaluation for Noncardiac Surgery). J Am Coll Cardiol 39:542, 2002.

TABLE 21G-8 ACC/AHA Recommendations for Coronary Arteriography in Patients with Congenital Heart Disease

CLASS	RECOMMENDATION	LOE
Class I	Before surgical correction of congenital heart disease when chest discomfort or noninvasive evidence suggests associated CAD	C
	Before surgical correction of suspected congenital anomalies such as congenital coronary artery stenosis, coronary arteriovenous fistula, and anomalous origin of left coronary artery	C
	Forms of congenital heart disease frequently associated with coronary artery anomalies that may complicate surgical management	C
	Unexplained cardiac arrest in a young patient	B
Class IIa	Before corrective open heart surgery for congenital heart disease in an adult whose risk profile increases the likelihood of coexisting CAD	C
Class IIb	During left-heart catheterization for hemodynamic assessment of congenital heart disease in an adult in whom the risk of CAD is not high	C
Class III	Not recommended in the routine evaluation of congenital heart disease in asymptomatic patients for whom heart surgery is not planned	C

CAD = coronary artery disease; LOE = level of evidence.
From Scanlon PJ, Faxon DP, Audet AM, et al: ACC/AHA guidelines for coronary angiography: Executive summary and recommendations. A report of the American College of Cardiology/American Heart Association Task Force on Practice Guidelines (Committee on Coronary Angiography) developed in collaboration with the Society for Cardiac Angiography and Interventions. Circulation 99:2345, 1999.

TABLE 21G-9 ACC/AHA Recommendations for Other Uses of Coronary Arteriography

CLASS	RECOMMENDATION	LOE
Class I	Diseases affecting the aorta when knowledge of the presence or extent of coronary artery involvement is necessary for management (e.g., aortic dissection or aneurysm with known CAD)	B
	Hypertrophic cardiomyopathy with angina, despite medical therapy, when knowledge of coronary anatomy might affect therapy	C
	Hypertrophic cardiomyopathy with angina when heart surgery is planned	B
Class IIb	High risk for CAD when other cardiac surgical procedures are planned (e.g., pericardiectomy or removal of chronic pulmonary emboli)	C
	Prospective immediate cardiac transplant donors whose risk profile increases the likelihood of CAD	B
	Asymptomatic patients with Kawasaki disease who have coronary artery aneurysms on echocardiography	B
	Before surgery for aortic aneurysm/dissection in patients without known CAD	C
	Recent blunt chest trauma and suspicion of acute myocardial infarction, without evidence of preexisting CAD	C

CAD = coronary artery disease; LOE = level of evidence.
From Scanlon PJ, Faxon DP, Audet AM, et al: ACC/AHA guidelines for coronary angiography: Executive summary and recommendations. A report of the American College of Cardiology/American Heart Association Task Force on Practice Guidelines (Committee on Coronary Angiography) developed in collaboration with the Society for Cardiac Angiography and Interventions. Circulation 99:2345, 1999.

REFERENCES

1. Guidelines for coronary angiography. A report of the American College of Cardiology/American Heart Association Task Force on Assessment of diagnostic and therapeutic cardiovascular procedures (subcommittee on coronary angiography). J Am Coll Cardiol 10:935, 1987.
2. Scanlon PJ, Faxon DP, Audet AM, et al: ACC/AHA guidelines for coronary angiography: Executive summary and recommendations. A report of the American College of Cardiology/American Heart Association Task Force on Practice Guidelines (Committee on Coronary Angiography) developed in collaboration with the Society for Cardiac Angiography and Interventions. Circulation 99:2345, 1999.
3. Fraker TD Jr, Fihn SD, Gibbons RJ, et al: ACC/AHA 2007 chronic angina focused update of the ACC/AHA 2002 guidelines for the management of patients with chronic stable angina: A report of the American College of Cardiology/American Heart Association Task Force on Practice Guidelines Writing Group to Develop the Focused Update of the 2002 Guidelines for the Management of Patients With Chronic Stable Angina. J Am Coll Cardiol 50:2264, 2007.
4. Anderson JL, Adams CD, Antman EM, et al: ACC/AHA 2007 guidelines for the management of patients with unstable angina/non–ST-elevation myocardial infarction. Executive summary: A report of the American College of Cardiology/American Heart Association Task Force on Practice Guidelines (Writing Committee to Revise the 2002 Guidelines for the Management of Patients With Unstable Angina/Non–ST-Elevation Myocardial Infarction). Developed in collaboration with the American College of Emergency Physicians, the Society for Cardiovascular Angiography and Interventions, and the Society of Thoracic Surgeons Endorsed by the American Association of Cardiovascular and Pulmonary Rehabilitation and the Society for Academic Emergency Medicine. J Am Coll Cardiol 50:652, 2007.
5. Kushner FG, Hand M, Smith SC Jr, et al: 2009 Focused Updates: ACC/AHA guidelines for the management of patients with ST-elevation myocardial infarction (updating the 2004 guideline and 2007 focused update) and ACC/AHA/SCAI guidelines on percutaneous coronary intervention (updating the 2005 guideline and 2007 focused update): A report of the American College of Cardiology Foundation/American Heart Association Task Force on Practice Guidelines. J Am Coll Cardiol 54:2205, 2004.
6. Eagle KA, Berger PB, Calkins H, et al: ACC/AHA guideline update for perioperative cardiovascular evaluation for noncardiac surgery—executive summary: A report of the American College of Cardiology/American Heart Association Task Force on Practice Guidelines (Committee to Update the 1996 Guidelines on Perioperative Cardiovascular Evaluation for Noncardiac Surgery). J Am Coll Cardiol 39:542, 2002.
7. Fleisher LA, Beckman JA, Brown KA, et al: 2009 ACCF/AHA focused update on perioperative beta blockade incorporated into the ACC/AHA 2007 guidelines on perioperative cardiovascular evaluation and care for noncardiac surgery. A report of the American College of Cardiology Foundation, American Heart Association Task Force on Practice Guidelines, American Society of Echocardiography, American Society of Nuclear Cardiology, Heart Rhythm Society, Society of Cardiovascular Anesthesiologists, Society for Cardiovascular Angiography and Interventions, Society for Vascular Medicine, and Society for Vascular Surgery. J Am Coll Cardiol 54:e13, 2009.
8. Hunt SA, Abraham WT, Chin MH, et al: 2009 Focused update incorporated into the ACC/AHA 2005 Guidelines for the Diagnosis and Management of Heart Failure in Adults: A Report of the American College of Cardiology Foundation/American Heart Association Task Force on Practice Guidelines Developed in Collaboration With the International Society for Heart and Lung Transplantation. J Am Coll Cardiol 53:e1, 2009.
9. Bonow RO, Carabello BA, Chatterjee K, et al: 2008 focused update incorporated into the ACC/AHA 2006 guidelines for the management of patients with valvular heart disease: A report of the American College of Cardiology/American Heart Association Task Force on Practice Guidelines (Writing Committee to revise the 1998 guidelines for the management of patients with valvular heart disease). Endorsed by the Society of Cardiovascular Anesthesiologists, Society for Cardiovascular Angiography and Interventions, and Society of Thoracic Surgeons. J Am Coll Cardiol 52:e1, 2008.

CHAPTER 22 Intravascular Ultrasound Imaging

Jean-Claude Tardif and Philippe L. L'Allier

Atherosclerosis is currently the leading cause of death in the world, but the burden of atherosclerotic disease is expected to rise even further in the coming decades (see Chap. 1). Although lifestyle modifications and pharmacologic therapy including cholesterol-lowering medication have been effective, they have failed to keep pace with the expanding population at risk. Atherosclerosis is a chronic inflammatory disease of the arterial wall that secondarily affects the arterial lumen (see Chap. 43). Vascular imaging is an integral part of the diagnostic and therapeutic strategies for patients with suspected or proven clinical manifestations of coronary atherosclerosis.[1] Angiography, the traditional approach used to evaluate coronary artery disease, provides only a planar perspective of the vessel lumen and does not permit direct visualization of the arterial wall. In contrast, intravascular ultrasound (IVUS) provides cross-sectional images of both the arterial lumen and wall, allowing correct assessment of true lumen dimensions and architecture as well as atherosclerotic plaque burden and vessel wall abnormalities.[2] The additional knowledge brought by IVUS imaging has led to its increased use for research applications and clinical indications during the last two decades.

Intravascular Ultrasound Examination

IVUS imaging is conducted by experienced interventional physicians in the cardiac catheterization laboratory (see Chaps. 20 and 21) and requires full anticoagulation. A 0.014-inch guidewire is first advanced to the distal segment of the coronary artery of interest. IVUS imaging is then performed with 2.5F to 3.5F catheters with miniaturized (<1 mm in diameter) ultrasound transducers at their tips. Mechanical catheters, in which a single ultrasound element is in rotation at 1800 rpm within the sheath, are most often used, but a solid-state (multielement) design is also available. Because better spatial resolution is obtained at higher ultrasound frequencies but deeper penetration occurs at lower frequencies, 40 to 45 MHz IVUS catheters are preferable for intracoronary examination. Intracoronary nitroglycerin (150 to 300 μg) should be administered (unless contraindicated) before IVUS examination to minimize dynamic fluctuations in vasomotor tone. The IVUS catheter is advanced distally to a recognizable landmark (arterial branch) that will serve as a distal fiduciary site. The IVUS transducer is then typically withdrawn by automated pull-back at 0.5 mm/sec up to the guiding catheter, but a manual pull-back is also possible when a specific site needs to be examined. The guiding catheter should be disengaged from the coronary ostium when the aorto-ostial junction specifically needs to be evaluated. In this situation, it is important to position the guiding catheter (in the aorta) in the prolongation of the long axis of the proximal segment of the vessel to avoid geometric distortion associated with IVUS probe obliquity. A detailed running audio commentary describing the location of the transducer is useful for off-line analyses. The IVUS procedure typically takes 10 to 15 minutes when it is performed after diagnostic angiography.

Although IVUS is an invasive imaging modality, major clinical complications are rare. When it is performed by experienced operators, most major and acute procedural complications associated with (but not necessarily caused by) IVUS imaging occur during interventional cases.[2] The most frequently encountered complication is coronary spasm, which occurs in approximately 2% of patients and usually responds rapidly to administration of intracoronary nitroglycerin. In one multicenter registry involving more than 2000 patients, there was no occurrence of myocardial infarction associated with IVUS imaging performed for diagnostic indications. The longer term safety of IVUS imaging has been assessed by serial quantitative coronary angiography in patients participating in an IVUS trial conducted for the assessment of a novel pharmacologic agent.[3] There was no significant difference between the imaged and nonimaged vessels in the same patients, in terms of the change in lumen diameter or the incidence of new lesions up to 2 years after the initial IVUS examination. The short-term and long-term safety of IVUS has therefore been adequately demonstrated.

Evaluation of Atheroma Burden and Vascular Remodeling

IVUS provides tomographic, cross-sectional images of both the arterial lumen and wall with excellent axial resolution (≤125 μm at an ultrasound frequency of 40 MHz). Measurements obtained with IVUS imaging have been validated with phantoms and arterial segments, and their reproducibility has been well characterized. Atherosclerotic plaque area at any given cross section is determined by subtracting the lumen area (measured at the blood-intima interface) from the total vessel area (defined by the area circumscribed by the external elastic membrane or the media-adventitia interface) (**Fig. 22-1**).[4]

Whereas most patients with coronary artery disease become symptomatic after 40 years of age, several necropsy studies and more recently IVUS imaging studies have demonstrated that atherosclerosis often begins much earlier.[2] IVUS readily reveals the diffuse nature of atherosclerosis, even if there is no or minimal luminal irregularity on the coronary angiogram (**Fig. 22-2**). This discrepancy can occur because the presence and severity of coronary artery disease are evaluated on angiography by comparing an abnormal site with a reference segment.[1] Because atherosclerosis is a diffuse inflammatory disease, the reference segments are frequently narrowed by atherosclerotic plaque, which causes an underestimation of stenosis severity with angiography. Indeed, relatively uniform disease at a given lesion site and its "reference segment" will not allow detection of a narrowing of the coronary arterial lumen. The absolute change over time in luminal dimension also cannot be perfectly correlated with changes in plaque burden because of vascular remodeling, the process that leads to chronic changes in total vessel dimensions. IVUS imaging takes into account vascular remodeling by allowing direct visualization of the external elastic membrane, which is taken to represent total vessel area.[4]

Positive vascular remodeling was initially described by Glagov and colleagues, when it was observed in a postmortem study that adaptive vessel enlargement allowed the arterial lumen to remain normal until at least 40% of total vessel area was occupied by plaque.[5] IVUS imaging provides confirmation of the ubiquitous nature of this phenomenon in atherosclerosis, either by comparing proximal and distal sites in one examination of the coronary artery or by following a given cross

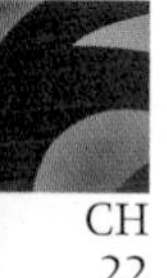

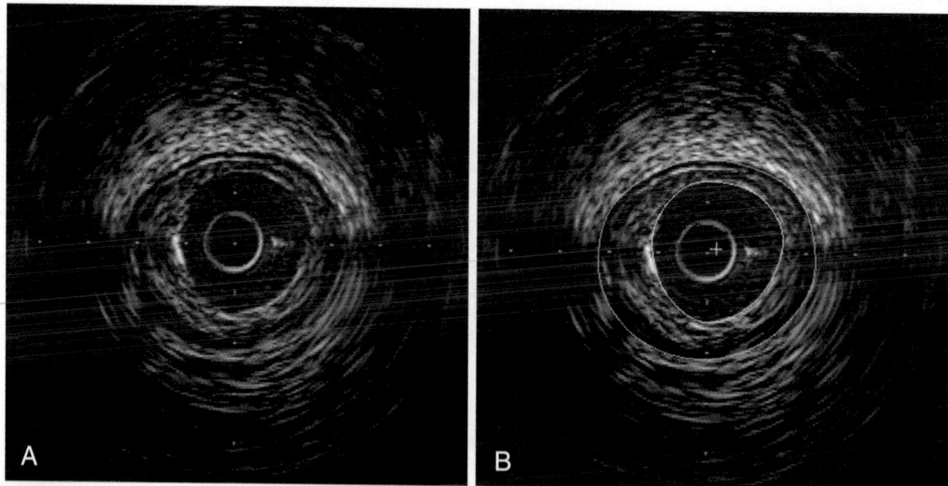

FIGURE 22-1 IVUS image **(A)** and the corresponding measurements **(B)** of lumen area (at the blood-intima interface in yellow) and total vessel area (at the media-adventitia interface, or area circumscribed by the external elastic membrane, in green).

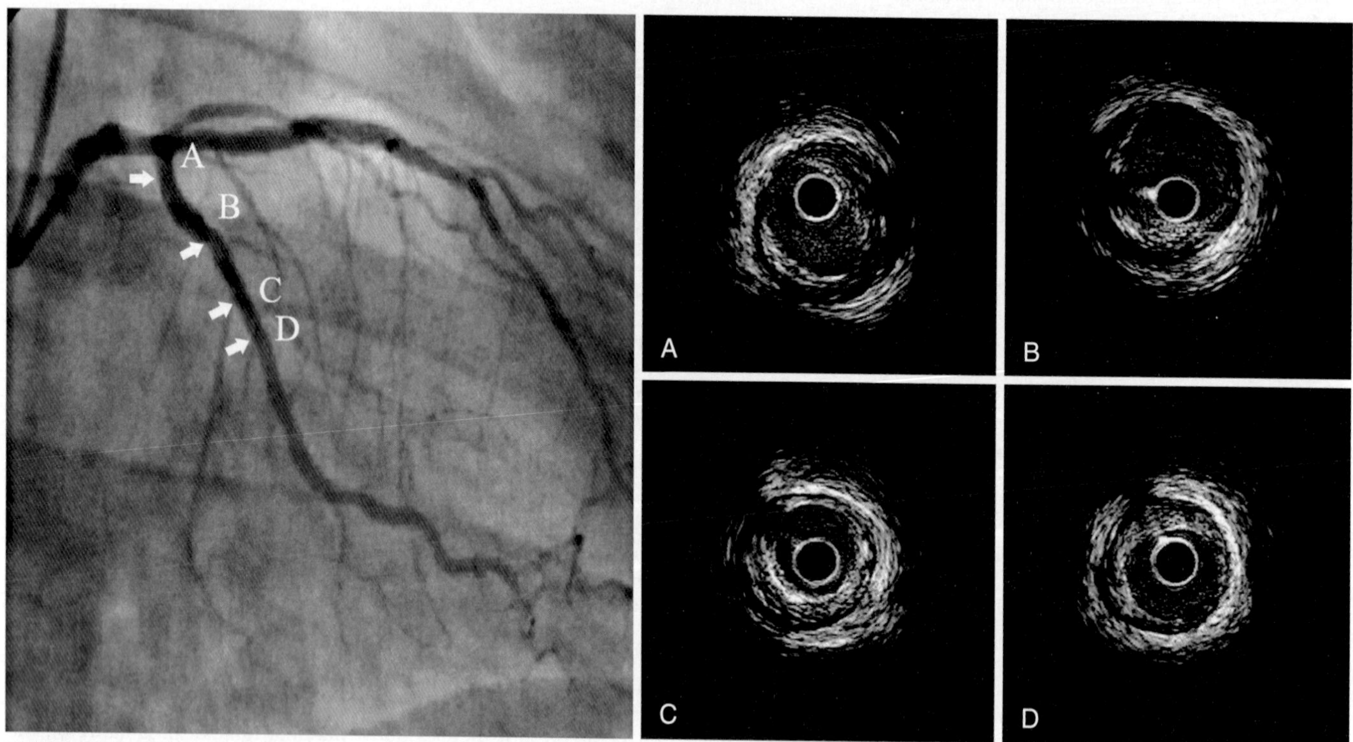

FIGURE 22-2 Multiple IVUS images demonstrating the diffuse nature of coronary atherosclerosis in a coronary artery with minimal lumen narrowing. The coronary angiogram shows the sites of the IVUS cross sections in the left circumflex artery.

section over time in serial examinations (**Fig. 22-3**).[2] Such IVUS studies have demonstrated that negative remodeling or chronic vessel shrinkage can contribute, in addition to increasing plaque burden, to a reduction in luminal dimensions. In addition, IVUS studies have shown that a decrease in atheroma burden can often be accompanied by negative remodeling and therefore relatively unchanged luminal dimensions (**Fig. 22-4**).[6] When regression of atherosclerosis occurs, most often because of intensive multifaceted risk factor treatment, the reduction in atheroma burden correlates much better with the change in vascular remodeling than with that in arterial lumen dimensions.[6]

Clinical Indications for Intravascular Ultrasound Imaging

The cross-sectional images of the vascular lumen and wall provided by IVUS imaging can often be helpful clinically by complementing the information provided by angiography (**Table 22-1**). One extremely important application of IVUS during diagnostic catheterization is the evaluation of left main coronary artery disease when doubt persists about the severity of stenosis on angiography (**Fig. 22-5**).[7] This particularly occurs when a diagnostic catheter repetitively wedges in the left coronary artery, when the left main trunk is diffusely small without any discrete lesion, or when an ostial lesion or a stenosis at the bifurcation is suspected. Although IVUS provides anatomic depiction of narrowings and not a physiologic assessment such as that of fractional flow reserve (see Chap. 52), it nevertheless clarifies the majority of problematic angiographic images of the left main coronary artery.[8] Indeed, IVUS imaging in this context often shows minimal plaque accumulation or severe narrowing. In truly intermediate cases with at least moderate disease, a minimum lumen area of less than 6.0 mm^2 is usually taken to represent significant left main coronary artery stenosis (**Fig. 22-6**).[7]

Other ambiguous lesions on angiography can also be clarified with IVUS. The accuracy of angiography is often limited at coronary artery

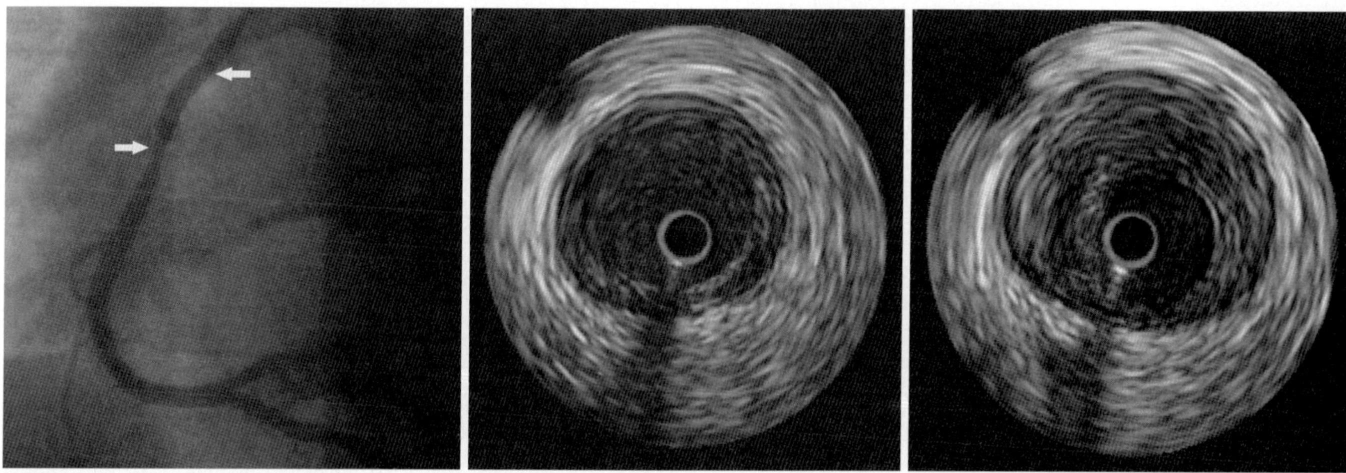

FIGURE 22-3 Angiographic image **(left)** of a stenosis of the right coronary artery and its proximal reference segment (arrows). IVUS imaging reveals mild disease of the reference segment **(center)** and large atheroma with positive vascular remodeling at the site of angiographic stenosis **(right)**. This positive remodeling, or adaptive vascular enlargement, is identified by the larger total vessel dimensions at the site of stenosis than those at the more proximal site of reference.

bifurcations. Unfortunately, atherosclerotic plaques preferentially accumulate at bifurcation points, related to turbulent blood flow. Thus, bifurcation lesions of uncertain severity are another potential diagnostic application of IVUS.[9] IVUS imaging can also provide valuable information for the problematic lesions that are visualized well in only a single angiographic projection or when there is discordance between symptoms or noninvasive test results and the coronary angiogram. A lumen area of less than 4.0 mm^2 on IVUS imaging usually causes a flow-limiting stenosis as determined by nuclear perfusion imaging (see Chap. 17) or flow reserve assessment (see Chap. 52) in coronary vessels other than the left main coronary artery.[2]

IVUS can also help characterize other clinical coronary syndromes, such as syndrome X, myocardial bridging, and coronary artery spasm. The majority of patients with syndrome X (see Chaps. 57 and 81) have abnormal coronary arteries on IVUS imaging manifested by atheroma or marked intimal thickening, despite the absence of angiographic abnormalities. Similarly, a very high incidence of atherosclerotic plaque is detected proximal to bridging segments on IVUS imaging.[10] Furthermore, the "half-moon" sign is characteristically seen on IVUS at the site of a myocardial bridge.[10] Finally, marked atherosclerotic thickening is generally identified by IVUS at the site of focal coronary spasm in the absence of angiographically significant disease.

IVUS imaging can also be helpful in patients undergoing coronary interventions.[11] Confirmation of adequate stent deployment and strut apposition

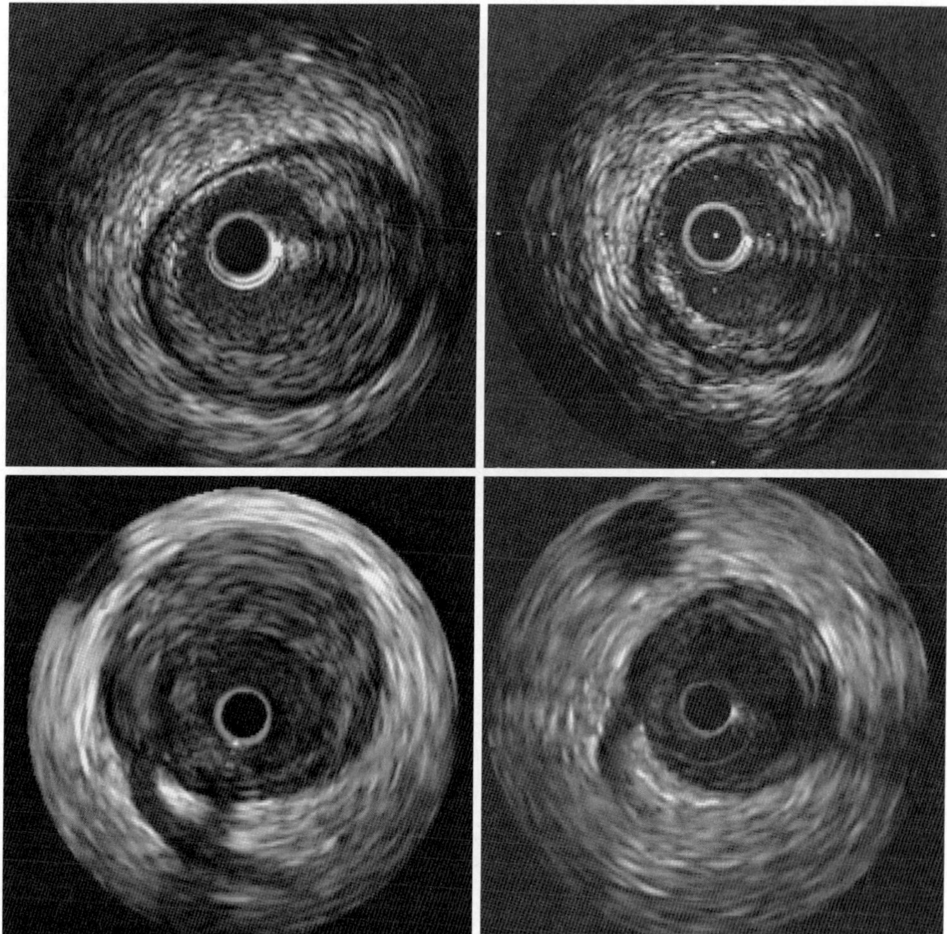

FIGURE 22-4 Serial IVUS images at baseline **(left, upper)** and after 2 years of intensive lipid-lowering therapy and risk factor modification **(right, upper)**, showing regression of coronary atherosclerosis (plaque area was 12.78 mm^2 at baseline and 9.12 mm^2 at follow-up) and accompanying negative vascular remodeling (total vessel area was 18.38 mm^2 at baseline and 15.94 mm^2 at follow-up). The increase in lumen area (from 5.60 mm^2 at baseline to 6.82 mm^2 at 2 years) was smaller than if there had not been a decrease in total vessel dimensions at follow-up. The two lower panels demonstrate major reduction in plaque burden (from 20.34 to 7.59 mm^2) and negative vascular remodeling (from 27.32 to 14.92 mm^2) with minimal change in lumen area (from 6.98 to 7.33 mm^2) from baseline **(left, lower)** to follow-up **(right, lower)**. In these lower panels, a small branch at 7 o'clock and a larger branch at 11 o'clock confirm that the same cross section is assessed at both time points.

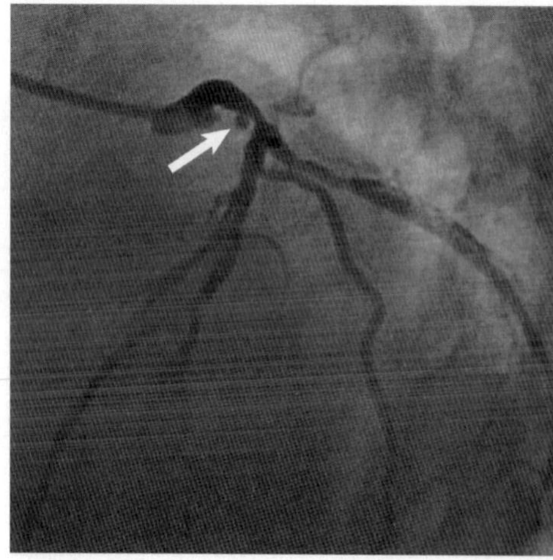

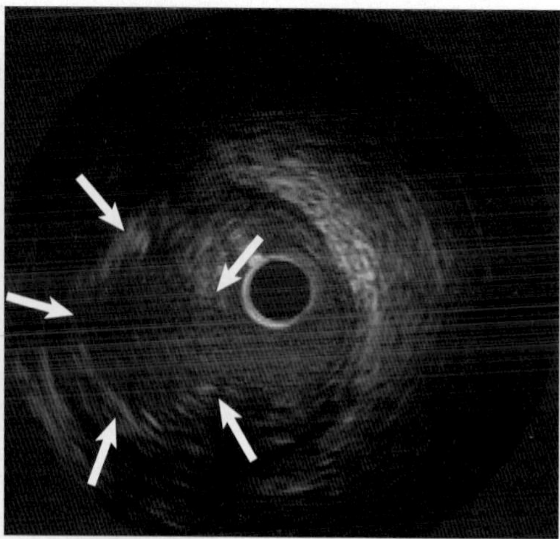

FIGURE 22-5 Coronary angiogram **(left)** of a left main coronary lesion (**left**, arrow). IVUS **(right)** shows evidence of plaque rupture in the left main coronary artery (**right**, arrows).

TABLE 22-1 Clinical Indications for Intravascular Ultrasound

Left main coronary artery disease
Discordance between symptoms or noninvasive test results and coronary angiogram
Ambiguous lesions
Ostial lesion
Bifurcation lesion
Aneurysm
Hazy lesion
Transplant vasculopathy
In-stent restenosis or thrombosis
Stent implantation in medium-sized (2.5-3.25 mm) arteries
Unsatisfactory angiographic or symptomatic results of percutaneous coronary intervention

can readily be obtained with IVUS at the end of the procedure (**Fig. 22-7**).[12] IVUS can be particularly helpful in patients presenting with stent thrombosis or in-stent restenosis to determine if technical issues such as significant stent underexpansion or residual dissection are involved (**Fig. 22-8**).

Coronary artery disease is the leading cause of late mortality after cardiac transplantation (see Chap. 31). A high prevalence of false-negative coronary arteriograms has been documented with the use of IVUS during routine serial catheterization in cardiac transplant recipients.[13] Concentric intimal thickening associated with immunologic transplant arteriopathy is often not detected by angiography because of the diffuse nature of this process. In contrast, IVUS imaging offers early detection and quantification of coronary vasculopathy in patients who have undergone cardiac transplantation. The presence of significant intimal thickening on IVUS has been shown to be predictive of future cardiac events in these patients, even in the absence of angiographically apparent disease.[13] IVUS therefore has the potential to identify cardiac transplant recipients who require more aggressive treatment strategies.[14] IVUS imaging performed within a few weeks of transplantation has also revealed the presence of angiographically silent focal atherosclerotic plaques in 25% to 30% of patients, which most likely result from disease transferred from the donor.

Intravascular Ultrasound Assessment of Novel Antiatherosclerotic Treatments

Most of the large clinical trials that have demonstrated the ability of lipid-modifying agents to decrease cardiovascular morbidity and mortality have involved long-term (3 to 5 years) therapy. Further studies of these agents using atherosclerosis imaging have been able to detect benefit with shorter treatment durations.[1] Several of the newer classes of antiatherosclerotic agents in development do not significantly lower LDL cholesterol and hence do not have a validated surrogate plasma marker. This creates a challenge that is compounded by the fact that these novel agents need to show effectiveness in trials of reasonable sample size on top of modern therapies (including statins) that already provide proven benefit. For that reason, atherosclerosis imaging becomes very helpful to demonstrate the efficacy of such medications.

IVUS imaging has been widely used as the primary efficacy assessment measure of several antiatherosclerotic approaches in randomized clinical trials.[15-18] Volumetric measurements are generally used in this context to integrate changes over an arterial segment. For volume measurements, the lumen and external elastic membrane borders are traced (or determined by an automated edge-detection algorithm) on digitized cross sections at every 1 mm in the segment of interest at baseline and follow-up. Plaque, lumen, and total vessel volumes are computed for the entire length of the analyzed segment by multiplying the corresponding areas of each cross section by the distance between neighboring slices and then adding all the products. The precise assessment of both plaque burden and vascular remodeling with IVUS, as well as its excellent resolution, makes it an ideal imaging modality for clinical trials of atherosclerosis progression and regression.[1]

IVUS has shown that intensive statin therapy can halt progression of coronary atherosclerosis and even induce its regression and also that the effects appear to be more rapid in patients initially naive to such treatment.[19,20] IVUS is also used as a primary efficacy measure to assess novel therapeutic approaches administered to patients already receiving statin therapy. Despite some encouraging preclinical data with acyl-CoA acyltransferase (ACAT) inhibition, IVUS imaging showed in two randomized clinical trials that agents from this class failed to slow atherosclerosis progression and even had deleterious effects on coronary atheroma burden.[15,21] The development of these ACAT inhibitors was abandoned, but the IVUS data generated in one of these trials (A-PLUS) were used to correlate changes over time on IVUS and on quantitative coronary angiography.[22] Patients with angiographic evidence of coronary atherosclerosis progression exhibited on IVUS imaging both larger plaque burden at baseline and greater disease progression at follow-up. The angiographic changes over time in lumen dimensions correlated significantly, albeit modestly, with the change in percent atheroma volume on IVUS.[22] These results are important because disease progression determined by quantitative coronary angiography has been shown to predict long-term cardiovascular outcomes up to 5 years.[1,2] Although robust evidence of the prognostic value of the changes over time detected by coronary IVUS imaging is still lacking, an indirect link can be established between the favorable results obtained on IVUS in stable patients (the REVERSAL study) and cardiovascular outcomes in patients with a recent acute coronary syndrome (the PROVE-IT trial) with more intensive statin therapy (atorvastatin 80 mg) compared with a moderate lipid-lowering approach (pravastatin 40 mg).[19,23]

IVUS has also been used to test the effects of other emerging antiatherosclerotic therapies. IVUS imaging has provided provocative data suggesting that reconstituted HDL particles containing mutant (Milano) or wild-type forms of apoprotein A-I infused on a weekly basis might induce rapid regression of coronary atherosclerosis after less than 6 weeks of therapy.[17,24] The two studies (AIM and ERASE) investigating these two different reconstituted HDL particles both yielded similar results that were highly statistically significant, demonstrating reduction in plaque volume compared with baseline but not compared with placebo given the relatively small sample sizes.[25] These results are exciting because they show the ability of IVUS to demonstrate true atherosclerosis regression and represent a proof of concept for the potential benefits of HDL-based therapies in patients with coronary artery disease. Multicenter IVUS studies evaluating other HDL raising drugs, including peptides and small molecules, are at different stages of preparation.

IVUS imaging was also used to study the cholesteryl ester transfer protein (CETP) inhibitor torcetrapib in the ILLUSTRATE study.[16] Despite large increases (mean, 61%) in HDL cholesterol, torcetrapib failed to improve the primary endpoint of coronary atherosclerosis progression on IVUS. These results are concordant with those of noninvasive carotid imaging (intimal-medial thickness) as well as with worsened clinical outcomes in the large ILLUMINATE trial.[26] Torcetrapib-induced off-target toxicity, manifested by activation of the renin-angiotensin-aldosterone system and an increase in blood pressure, may have been in part responsible for these disappointing clinical results. Because these off-target effects appear to be drug specific and not related to the class itself, atherosclerosis imaging is now in use to assess the effects of dalcetrapib, a CETP inhibitor devoid of such toxicity.

Other lipid-modifying agents, such as a lipoprotein-associated phospholipase A_2 inhibitor, as well as antihypertensive and hypoglycemic agents have also been assessed with IVUS.[27,28]

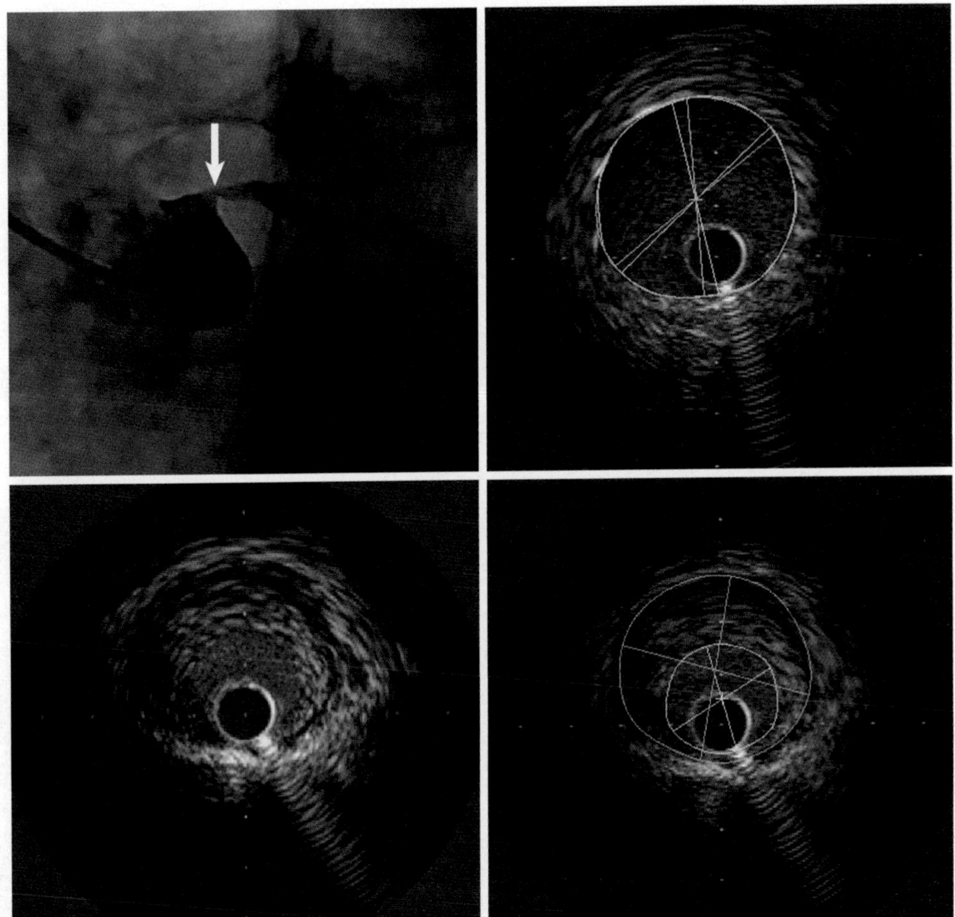

FIGURE 22-6 IVUS imaging performed because of an intermediate lesion of the left main coronary artery on the coronary angiogram (**left upper,** arrow). IVUS shows a severe lesion of the proximal left main coronary artery **(left, lower)** with lumen area equal to 3.68 mm^2, plaque area of 6.91 mm^2, and vessel area of 10.59 mm^2 **(right, lower)**. A normal site in the more distal left main coronary artery is shown for reference **(right, upper)**.

Conclusion

IVUS provides cross-sectional images of both the arterial wall and lumen with excellent resolution, reveals the diffuse nature of atherosclerosis and the involvement of reference segments, and takes into account vessel wall remodeling. Clinical indications of IVUS imaging include the assessment of left main coronary artery disease, ambiguous lesions on angiography, coronary narrowings for which there is discordance between symptoms or noninvasive test results and angiographic findings, and unsatisfactory results of coronary intervention. IVUS is also widely used as the primary efficacy assessment measure of potential antiatherosclerotic approaches in randomized clinical trials.

Future Perspectives

IVUS is an excellent imaging modality for the precise determination of atherosclerotic plaque burden. However, long-term follow-up in large studies linking changes over time in IVUS measurements at 2 years with future clinical vascular outcomes at 5 to 7 years are needed to determine its prognostic value and potential role as a surrogate marker of cardiovascular events. Plaques are typically described on processed IVUS images as being calcified (echobright plaque with distal acoustic shadowing), fibrotic (echobright plaque without shadowing), or lipid laden (echolucent plaque).[29] This classification on IVUS has been shown to correlate well with that on histology but is limited by its nonquantitative nature and the loss of information when data are transformed into two-dimensional images. The value of spectral analysis of IVUS radiofrequency data, an approach also called virtual histology (**Fig. 22-9**), is presently being investigated to identify different plaque types and the size of the lipid core and to determine the significance of changes over time.[30] This line of investigation is important in light of the role of plaque vulnerability and rupture in the

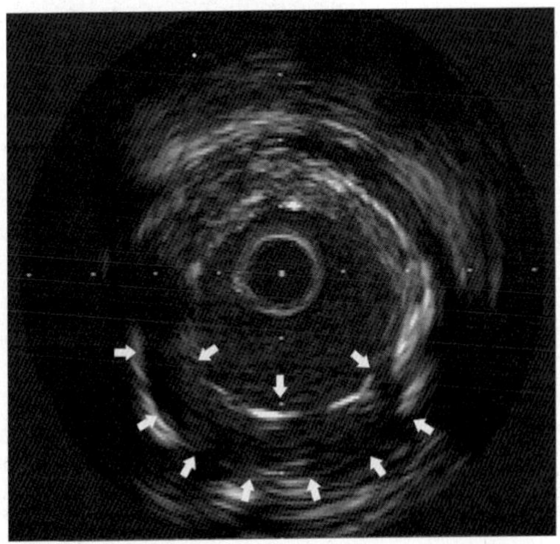

FIGURE 22-7 IVUS image demonstrating malapposition of the stent struts (three arrows pointing downward) to the coronary arterial wall (seven arrows pointing upward) from 5 o'clock to 8 o'clock.

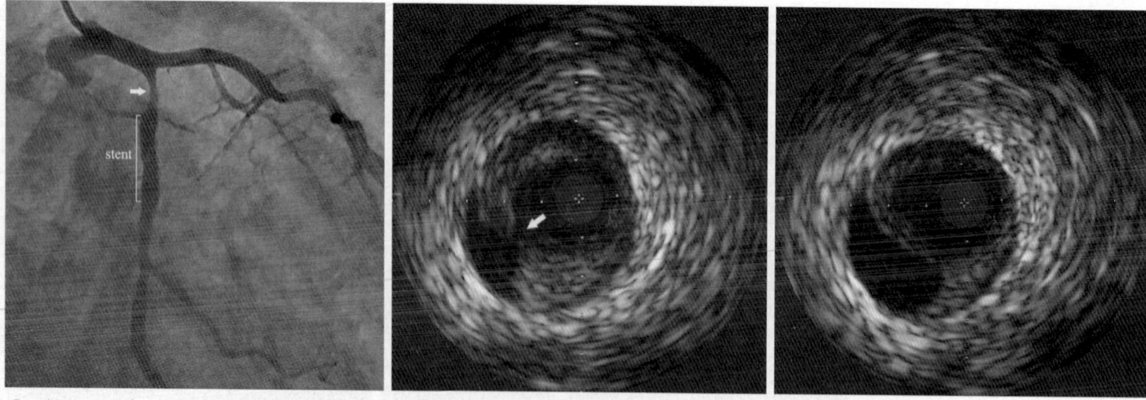

FIGURE 22-8 Angiographic narrowing and haziness (arrow) are observed proximal to the site of stent deployment **(left)**, where IVUS images show a large dissection (**center,** arrow) and intramural hematoma **(right)**.

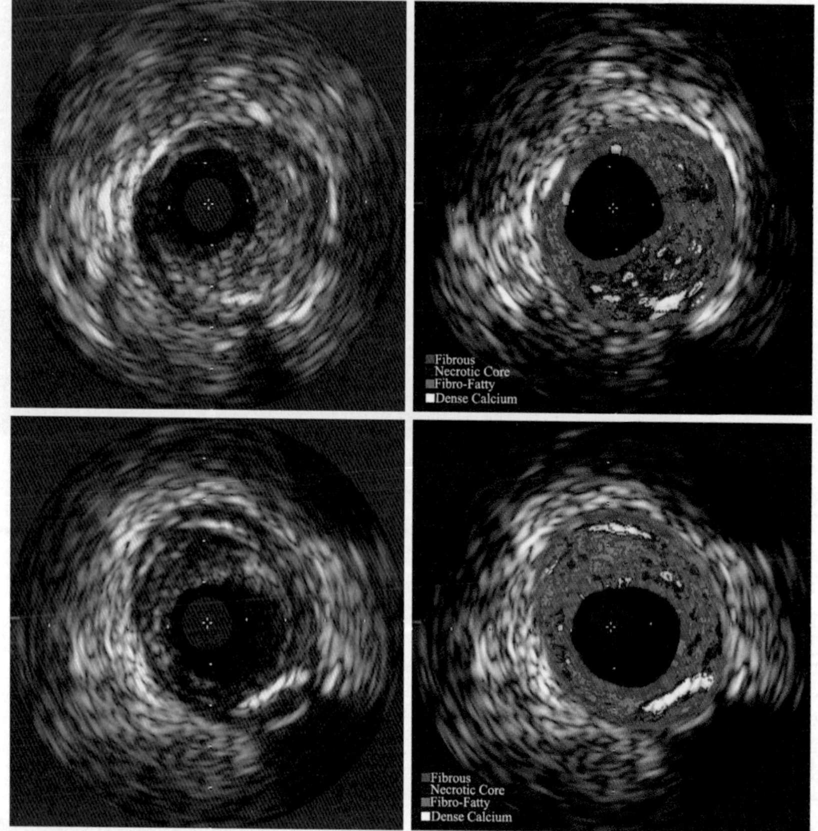

FIGURE 22-9 IVUS two-dimensional image **(left)** with corresponding virtual histology image **(right)** to characterize plaque composition by spectral analysis of radiofrequency data. The color coding for plaque composition is as follows: dark green = fibrous; red = necrotic core; light green = fibrofatty; white = dense calcium.

pathophysiologic process of acute coronary syndromes and death of cardiovascular origin.

REFERENCES

1. Tardif JC, Heinonen T, Orloff D, Libby P: Vascular biomarkers and surrogates in cardiovascular disease. Circulation 113:2936, 2006.
2. Guédès A, Tardif JC: Intravascular ultrasound assessment of atherosclerosis. Curr Atheroscler Rep 6:219, 2004.

Intravascular Ultrasound Examination

3. Guèdès A, Keller PF, L'Allier PL, Tardif JC: Long-term safety of intravascular ultrasound in non-transplant, non-intervened, atherosclerotic coronary arteries. J Am Coll Cardiol 45:559, 2005.
4. Mintz GS, Nissen SE, Anderson WD, et al: American College of Cardiology Clinical Expert Consensus Document on Standards for Acquisition, Measurement and Reporting of Intravascular Ultrasound Studies (IVUS). A report of the American College of Cardiology Task Force on Clinical Expert Consensus Documents. J Am Coll Cardiol 37:1478, 2001.
5. Schoenhagen P, Tuzcu EM, Apperson-Hansen C, et al: Determinants of arterial wall remodeling during lipid-lowering therapy: Serial intravascular ultrasound observations from the Reversal of Atherosclerosis with Aggressive Lipid Lowering Therapy (REVERSAL) trial. Circulation 113:2826, 2006.
6. Tardif JC, Grégoire J, L'Allier PL, et al: Effect of atherosclerotic regression on total luminal size of coronary arteries as determined by intravascular ultrasound. Am J Cardiol 98:23, 2006.

Clinical Indications for Intravascular Ultrasound Imaging

7. Sano K, Mintz GS, Carlier SG, et al: Assessing intermediate left main coronary lesions using intravascular ultrasound. Am Heart J 154:983, 2007.
8. Leesar MA, Mintz GS: Hemodynamic and intravascular ultrasound assessment of an ambiguous left main coronary artery stenosis. Catheter Cardiovasc Interv 70:721, 2007.
9. Van der Waal EC, Mintz GS, Garcia-Garcia HM, et al: Intravascular ultrasound and 3D angle measurements of coronary bifurcations. Catheter Cardiovasc Interv 73:910, 2009.
10. Bourassa MG, Butnaru A, Lespérance J, Tardif JC: Symptomatic myocardial bridges: Overview of ischemic mechanisms and current diagnostic and treatment strategies. J Am Coll Cardiol 41:351, 2003.
11. Roy P, Steinberg DH, Sushinsky SJ, et al: The potential clinical utility of intravascular ultrasound guidance in patients undergoing percutaneous coronary intervention with drug-eluting stents. Eur Heart J 29:1851, 2008.
12. Bertrand OF, De Larochellière R, Joyal M, Tardif JC: Incidence of stent under-deployment as a cause of in-stent restenosis in long stents. Int J Cardiovasc Imaging 20:279, 2004.

13. Tuzcu EM, Kapadia SR, Sachar R, et al: Intravascular ultrasound evidence of angiographically silent progression in coronary atherosclerosis predicts long-term morbidity and mortality after cardiac transplantation. J Am Coll Cardiol 45:1538, 2005.
14. Eisen HJ, Tuzcu EM, Dorent R, et al: Everolimus for the prevention of allograft rejection and vasculopathy in cardiac-transplant recipients. N Engl J Med 349:847, 2003.

Intravascular Ultrasound Assessment of Novel Antiatherosclerotic Treatments

15. Tardif JC, Grégoire J, L'Allier PL, et al: Effects of the acyl coenzyme A:cholesterol acyltransferase inhibitor avasimibe on human atherosclerotic lesions. Circulation 110:3372, 2004.
16. Nissen SE, Tardif JC, Nicholls SJ, et al: Effect of torcetrapib on the progression of coronary atherosclerosis. N Engl J Med 356:1304, 2007.
17. Tardif JC, Grégoire J, L'Allier PL, et al: Effects of reconstituted high-density lipoprotein infusions on coronary atherosclerosis: A randomized controlled trial. JAMA 297:1675, 2007.
18. Nissen SE, Nicholls SJ, Sipahi I, et al: Effect of very high-intensity statin therapy on regression of coronary atherosclerosis. JAMA 295:1556, 2006.
19. Nissen SE, Tuzcu EM, Schoenhagen P, et al: Effect of intensive compared with moderate lipid-lowering therapy on progression of coronary atherosclerosis: A randomized controlled trial. JAMA 291:1071, 2004.
20. Rodes-Cabau J, Tardif JC, Cossette M, et al: Acute effects of statin therapy on coronary atherosclerosis following an acute coronary syndrome. Am J Cardiol 104:750, 2009.
21. Nissen SE, Tuzcu EM, Brewer HB, et al: Effect of ACAT inhibition on the progression of coronary atherosclerosis. N Engl J Med 354:1253, 2006.
22. Berry C, L'Allier PL, Grégoire J, Tardif JC: Comparison of intravascular ultrasound and quantitative coronary angiography for the assessment of coronary artery disease progression. Circulation 115:1851, 2007.
23. Cannon CP, Braunwald E, McCabe CH, et al: Intensive versus moderate lipid lowering with statins after acute coronary syndromes. N Engl J Med 350:1495, 2004.
24. Nissen SE, Tsunoda T, Tuzcu M, et al: Effect of recombinant ApoA-I Milano on coronary atherosclerosis in patients with acute coronary syndromes. JAMA 290:2292, 2003.
25. Tardif JC, Heinonen T, Noble S: High-density lipoprotein/apolipoprotein A-I infusion therapy. Curr Atheroscler Rep 11:58, 2009.
26. Barter P, Caulfield M, Eriksson M, et al: Effects of torcetrapib in patients at high risk for coronary events. N Engl J Med 357:2109, 2007.
27. Serruys PW, Garcia-Garcia HM, Buszman P, et al: Effects of the direct lipoprotein-associated phospholipase A_2 inhibitor darapladib on human coronary atherosclerotic plaque. Circulation 118:1172, 2008.
28. Nissen SE, Nicholls SJ, Wolski K, et al: Comparison of pioglitazone vs glimepiride on progression of coronary atherosclerosis in patients with type 2 diabetes: The PERISCOPE randomized controlled trial. JAMA 299:1561, 2008.

Future Perspectives

29. Heinonen T, Waters DD, Libby P, Tardif JC: A winter's tale: Report from the First Annual Canadian Biomarkers and Surrogate Endpoints Symposium. Can J Cardiol 25:527, 2009.
30. Qian J, Maehara A, Mintz GS, et al: Relation between individual plaque components and overall plaque burden in the prospective, multicenter virtual histology intravascular ultrasound registry. Am J Cardiol 104:501, 2009.

CHAPTER 23 Molecular Imaging in Cardiovascular Disease

Peter Libby, Farouc A. Jaffer, and Ralph Weissleder

Recently, unraveling of the molecular and cellular bases of cardiovascular disease has accelerated. We now possess sufficient knowledge to identify numerous cellular behaviors, as well as molecular signaling and regulatory pathways that participate in the pathogenesis of many cardiovascular diseases. These advances in our understanding of the biology of cardiovascular diseases open a new vista on processes that might serve as targets for imaging. Reaching beyond structural and anatomic information and beyond physiologic variables such as perfusion and flow, the term *molecular imaging* refers to visualization of such cellular and molecular targets in living subjects.

The conjunction of nanotechnology and targeted imaging opens the possibility of "theranostic" approaches to local drug delivery based on biologic attributes. The notion of theranostics embeds the concept of targeted drug delivery confirmed by imaging modalities with parallel evaluation of biologic efficacy using multimodality strategies.

Although cardiovascular molecular imaging as yet has achieved only limited clinical applicability, given its potential and the burgeoning work in this field, this chapter provides a brief introduction to its principles.

Principles of Molecular Imaging

Targeting based on a molecular or cellular interaction constitutes the key concept of molecular imaging. Achievement of this goal requires a targeting moiety that will provide specificity and an imaging moiety that permits visualization (**Fig. 23-1** and **Table 23-1**).

Efficient targeting relies heavily on optimizing pharmacokinetics and binding properties of a given molecular imaging agent (**Fig. 23-2**), the timing of imaging, and adjunct procedures to improve delivery. Pharmacokinetics are important because an agent needs to reach its target before being excreted (or metabolized), and also because any unbound, "nonspecific" agent needs to be cleared to minimize background "noise." Binding, the traditional "lock and key" of biologic recognition, applies to a receptor and its ligand, an enzyme and its substrate, an antibody and its antigen, an extracellular matrix molecule and its interactor, or a transporter and its cargo. A number of strategies can achieve lock and key complementarity. For example, small molecules can interact with binding sites on receptors or enzymes (as do many drugs). Several high-throughput platforms exist for selection of peptides or small molecules complementary to various targets. Antibodies have a high degree of structural selectivity and binding affinity for their cognate antigens. Effective and efficient chemical strategies exist to link these categories of targeting ligands with imaging moieties. Small molecules, peptides, and antibodies each have their strengths and weaknesses (see Table 23-1). In particular, antibodies, with a molecular weight of about 150,000, are large compared with peptides or small molecules, and thus may have less favorable stoichiometry or may present steric constraints when they are used for targeting. Many more targeting peptides than antibodies can reside on a nanoparticle, for example.

Given these challenges of optimizing pharmacokinetics and specific binding, alternative strategies can amplify signals. These strategies include the development of activatable (turn-on) probes and exploiting of biologic properties such as sequestration or cellular trapping.[1-7]

Imaging Strategies

Molecular imaging can harness almost every modality used in cardiovascular diagnosis. Each of these modalities offers advantages and has limitations (**Table 23-2**). For example, radionuclides offer very high sensitivity and the widespread availability of suitable clinical imaging platforms (see Chap. 17). Signals from radionuclides in isolation present a challenge in terms of anatomic colocalization. Hybrid methodologies combining computed tomography (CT) or magnetic resonance imaging (MRI)[8] in coregistration can, however, define the anatomic source of an isotope or fluorescence signal. Other potential limitations of nuclear approaches include the exposure to radiation and the lower spatial resolution than that offered by other approaches.

MRI offers clear-cut definition of anatomy, good spatial resolution, and multicontrast capabilities (see Chap. 18), but it has lower sensitivity than radionuclide or optical approaches. MRI avoids radiation risk but has familiar limitations in individuals with metallic implants. The currently clinically available paramagnetic contrast agents (not molecularly targeted) based on gadolinium have potential toxic effects, particularly in patients with impaired renal function (see Chap. 18).

Contrast-enhanced ultrasound (CEU) uses targeted microbubbles (see Chap. 15).[7,9,10] Advantages of CEU include the widespread availability of suitable imaging platforms (the "installed base"), the familiarity of the technique to clinicians, the lack of ionizing radiation, and the relatively low cost of the imaging infrastructure. Disadvantages of microbubbles include lower inherent sensitivity and limits to tissue penetration.

Optical techniques also have promise for cardiovascular molecular imaging. In particular, near-infrared fluorescence (NIRF) imaging has reasonable signal-to-noise ratio, avoids radiation, has tissue penetration of several centimeters in tomographic mode, and is amenable to adaptation for a variety of targeting strategies, including generation of fluorescence by enzymatic hydrolysis of appropriately designed reporters. Disadvantages of optical techniques include the lack of turnkey clinical imaging platforms and insufficient tissue penetration for noninvasive visualization of very deep or small structures, such as the coronary arteries in humans, although intravascular optical approaches are emerging.[11]

These examples have considered imaging modalities one by one. Multimodality imaging provides a promising approach by combining

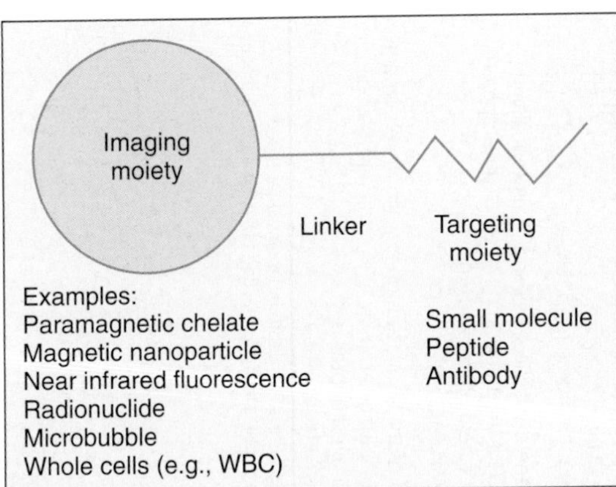

FIGURE 23-1 The design of molecular imaging agents. The fundamental concept of molecular imaging in many cases requires the construction of a bifunctional imaging agent. This diagram schematizes an idealized bifunctional imaging agent. The imaging moiety on the left links chemically to a targeting moiety on the right. The imaging moiety permits visualization by a variety of modalities. The targeting moiety provides the molecular specificity through complementarity or as a substrate for a cellular uptake mechanism, such as phagocytosis or a specific transporter. The imaging moiety might also consist of a nanoparticle that can carry multiple targeting moieties, and/or a therapeutic payload. The latter bifunctional agents open the possibility of theranostics, the ability to combine an imaging agent with targeted delivery of a therapeutic agent.

several modalities in one targeted imaging agent (e.g., magneto-optical probes that yield both fluorescence and magnetic contrast). Trifunctional agents, combining magnetic, optical, and radionuclide imaging functionality, likewise exist.[12-15] Such multimodality agents may prove useful in simultaneously tracking delivery of an imaging probe and the biologic function that it interrogates. For example, a magneto-optical probe could show delivery of the imaging agent to the tissue of interest and report on enzymatic activity using the optical properties of a substrate probe simultaneously.

Biologic Processes Amenable to Molecular Targeting for Imaging

Among the biologic processes potentially amenable to molecular imaging, a number have already undergone exploration. This section considers several categories of potential targets for molecular imaging and illustrates them with examples.[16]

Cell Trafficking: Leukocytes and Stem Cells

Inflammation contributes to a number of acute and chronic cardiovascular diseases. Leukocytes accumulate in the myocardium

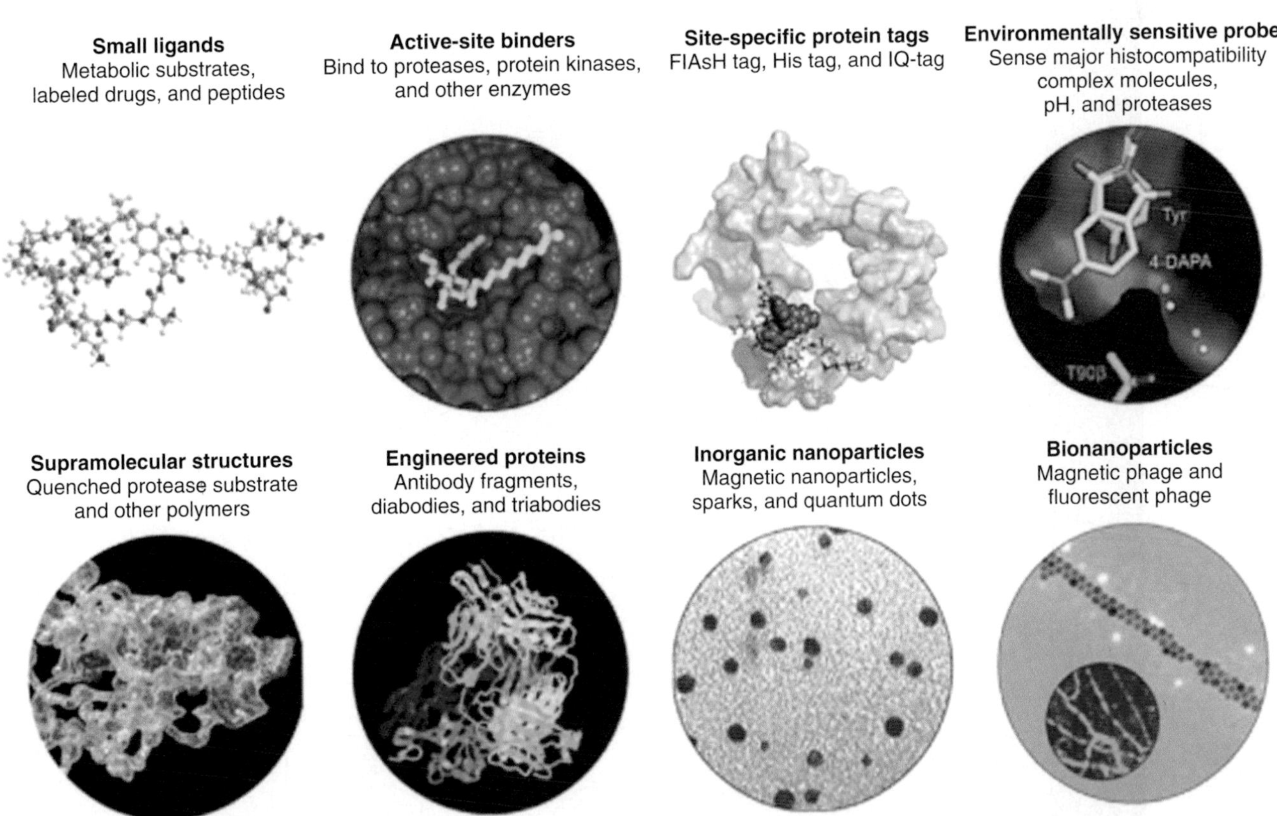

FIGURE 23-2 High-affinity imaging agents with appropriate pharmacokinetics are essential for imaging at the molecular level. Different strategies have been pursued to develop agents for molecular imaging. This figure indicates the various types of available agents and provides examples of each. Small molecules are shown in the top row, and macromolecular agents and nanotechnology-derived agents are shown in the bottom row. Four main types of small molecules are used. Small ligands are imageable small molecules (e.g., ^{18}F-labeled drugs and fluorescent peptides), whereas active-site binders (green) attach to specific protein pockets in enzymes (blue) either covalently or noncovalently. Site-specific protein tags (pink) achieve a similar function, but at sites of interest in engineered proteins (white). Environmentally sensitive probes (e.g., 4-*N,N*-dimethylaminophthalimidoalanine [4-DAPA], yellow) change their physicochemical properties on interaction with the target (in this case, Tyr and T90ß). Two main types of macromolecule are used. Supramolecular structures are synthetic agents that have been useful as enzyme substrates for the imaging of cathepsins and proteases or for delineation of new microvasculature; the figure shows part of a poly-L-lysine backbone (blue) derivatized with protease-cleavable side chains (red) and polyethylene glycol (grey). Engineered proteins (with optimized pharmacokinetics) refer to other macromolecules that have been used for some targets. Finally, a host of nanomaterials that can be used for imaging of phagocytic cells or cell surface targets (green), including inorganic nanoparticles (gray) and bionanoparticles, is emerging. *(Reproduced with permission from Weissleder R, Pittet MJ: Imaging in the era of molecular oncology. Nature 452:580, 2008.)*

TABLE 23-1 Overview of Imaging Systems

TECHNIQUE	RESOLUTION	DEPTH	TIME	QUANTITATION	MULTICHANNEL IMAGING	IMAGING AGENTS	TARGET	COST	PRIMARY SMALL ANIMAL USE	CLINICAL USE
MR imaging	10-100 μm	No limit	Minutes to hours	Absolute	Multiple	Paramagnetic chelates, magnetic particles	A, P, M	$$$	Versatile imaging modality with high soft tissue contrast	Yes
CT imaging	50 μm	No limit	Minutes	Absolute	Multiple	Iodine	A, P, M*	$$	Primarily for vascular, lung, and bone imaging	Yes
Ultrasound imaging	50 μm	Centimeters	Seconds to minutes	Absolute	Multiple	Microbubbles	A, P, M*	$$	Vascular and interventional imaging	Yes
PET imaging	1-2 mm	No limit	Minutes to hours	Absolute	No	^{18}F-, ^{64}Cu-, ^{11}C-, and ^{68}Ga- labeled compounds	P, M	$$$	Versatile imaging modality with many different tracers	Yes
SPECT imaging	1-2 mm	No limit	Minutes to hours	Absolute	Two	^{99m}Tc-, ^{111}In-, ^{131}I-labeled compounds; ^{67}Ga, ^{201}Tl	P, M	$$	Commonly used to image labeled antibodies, peptides, or perfusion	Yes
Fluorescence reflectance imaging	1 mm	<1 cm	Seconds to minutes	Relative	Multiple	Photoproteins, fluorochromes	P, M	$	Rapid screening of molecular events in surface-based disease	Yes
Fluorescence-mediated tomography	1 mm	<10 cm	Minutes	Absolute	Multiple	Near-infrared fluorochromes	P, M	$$	Quantitative imaging of targeted or "smart" fluorochrome reporters	In development
Bioluminescence imaging	Several millimeters-centimeters	Centimeters	Minutes	Relative	Multiple	Luciferins, coelenterazines, luminol	M	$$	Gene expression, cell and bacterial tracking, protein processing, and MPO activity	Potentially in development
Intravital microscopy (e.g., confocal, multiphoton)	1 μm	<400-800 μm	Seconds to hours	Relative	Multiple	Photoproteins, fluorochromes	A, P, M	$$$	All of the above at higher resolutions but at limited depths and coverage	In development (endoscopy, skin)

The Resolution and Cost columns refer to high-resolution, small animal imaging systems and are different for clinical imaging systems. Quantitation: absolute and relative refer to techniques that generate signals that are depth independent and depth dependent, respectively. Relative quantitation techniques typically require extensive controls; however, some of them (e.g., multiphoton microscopy) can be used to derive truly quantitative parameters (e.g., cell velocity, interaction time). Target: area that a given imaging modality interrogates: A = anatomic; P = physiologic; M = molecular. Cost of system: $: <$100,000; $$: $100,000-$300,000; $$$: >$300,000.

CT = computed tomography; MR = magnetic resonance; PET = positron emission tomography; SPECT = single photon emission computed tomography.

*A limited number of molecularly targeted agents have been described.

Modified from Weissleder R, Pittet MJ: Imaging in the era of molecular oncology. Nature 452:580, 2008.

TABLE 23-2 Overview of Agents

CLASS	SUBTYPE	EXAMPLES	SUBSTRATE	PRIMARY USE	EX/EM	TURN-ON/ SHIFT	CLINICAL	MODALITY	LIMITATIONS
Genetic tags	GFP	eGFP	NA	Fusion, reporter	484/507	Yes	No	IVM	Limited to proteins; no human use
	RFP	mCherry	NA	Fusion, reporter	587/610	Yes	No	IVM	Lower QY compared with GFP
		mRaspberry	NA	Fusion, reporter	598/625	Yes	No	IVM, FMT	Lower QY compared with GFP
		IFP	Biliverdin	Fusion, reporter	684/708		No	IVM, FMT	Emerging
	Photoconversion	Dendra	NA	Cytoplasmic	490/507 green		No	IVM	No human use
	Luciferases	Firefly	Luciferin	Reporter	Broad em	Yes	No	BLI	Limited to proteins; no human use
		Renilla	Coelenterazine	Reporter	Broad em	Yes	No	BLI	Limited to proteins; no human use
		Gausia	Coelenterazine	Reporter	Broad em	Yes	No	BLI	Limited to proteins; no human use
Antibodies	Immunoglobulin G	EGFR	NA	Cell surface marker	TD	Possible	Yes	PET, IVM, FMT	Delivery barriers; limited efficacy in vivo
		HER2/neu	NA	Cell surface marker	TD	Possible	Yes	PET, IVM, FMT	Delivery barriers; limited efficacy in vivo
	Fragments	Fab	NA	Cell surface marker	TD	Possible	Yes	PET, IVM, FMT	Delivery barriers; kinetics
		Diabody	NA	Cell surface marker	TD	Possible	Yes	PET, IVM, FMT	Delivery barriers; kinetics
		Minibody	NA	Cell surface marker	TD	Possible	Yes	PET, IVM, FMT	Delivery barriers; kinetics
Small molecules	Metabolites	FDG, FLT, acetate	NA	Metabolism	TD	No	Yes	PET	Limited number of agents
		Steroids	NA	Reporter	TD	No	Yes	PET	Limited number of agents
		Hyperpolarized molecules	NA	Metabolism	—	—	Yes	MRI	Time limitation
	Drugs	Taxol-NBD	NA	Intracellular targets	TD	Possible	No	PET, IVM, FMT	Limited number of high-affinity agents
	Prodrugs	Cathepsins, luminol	NA	Enzymes	TD	Yes	Yes	FMT, BLI	Limited number of high-affinity agents
	Peptides	RGD, collagen	NA	Receptors	TD	No	Yes	PET, IVM, FMT	Limited number of high-affinity agents
	Tags	CFSE, VT680	NA	Cell tags	TD	Yes	No	IVM, FMT	Ex vivo labeling
		Cy dyes	NA	Generic labeling	TD	Yes	Planned	IVM, FMT	
	Environment	pH	NA	Hypoxia, endosomes	TD	Yes	No	IVM, FMT	Limited number of high-affinity agents
Nanotechnology	Q-dot	CdSe	NA	Cell surface marker	TD	Yes	No	IVM, FMT	Possible delivery barriers
	Magnetic	MION	NA	Macrophages	TD	DMR	Yes	MRI	Possible delivery barriers
		CLIO	NA	Cell surface marker	TD	DMR	No	MRI	Experimental use only
		Ferumoxytol	NA	Macrophages	TD	DMR	Yes	MRI	Possible delivery barriers
	Polymers	Prosense	NA	Proteases	TD	Yes	Planned	FMT	Possible delivery barriers
		Angiosense	NA	Vascularity	TD	No	No	FMT	Experimental use only
	Bionano	Phage	NA	Cell surface marker	TD	No	No	FMT, MRI	Experimental use only
Bioorthogonal	Staudinger	Triarylphosphine	Azide	Proteins, carbohydrate	TD	No	No	IVM	Limited in vivo experience
	Click	Alkyne	Azide	Proteins	TD	No	No	FMT, IVM, PET	Limited in vivo experience; reaction slow
	BIND, BOND	Norbornene	Tetrazine	Many targets	TD	No	No	FMT, IVM, PET	Emerging
		TCO	Tetrazine	All targets	TD	Yes	Planned	FMT, IVM, PET	Emerging

BIND = Bioorthogonal in vivo detection; BLI = bioluminescence imaging; BOND = bioorthogonal nanoparticle detection; Click = click chemistry; DMR = diagnostic magnetic resonance; EX/EM = excitation and emission wavelengths; FMT = fluorescence molecular tomography; GFP = green fluorescent protein; IVM = intravital microscopy; MRI = magnetic resonance imaging; PET = positron emission tomography; QY = quantum yield; RFP = red fluorescent protein; TD = depends on attached fluorochrome (VT, Alexa, Cy) or other tracer (^{18}F, ^{11}C).

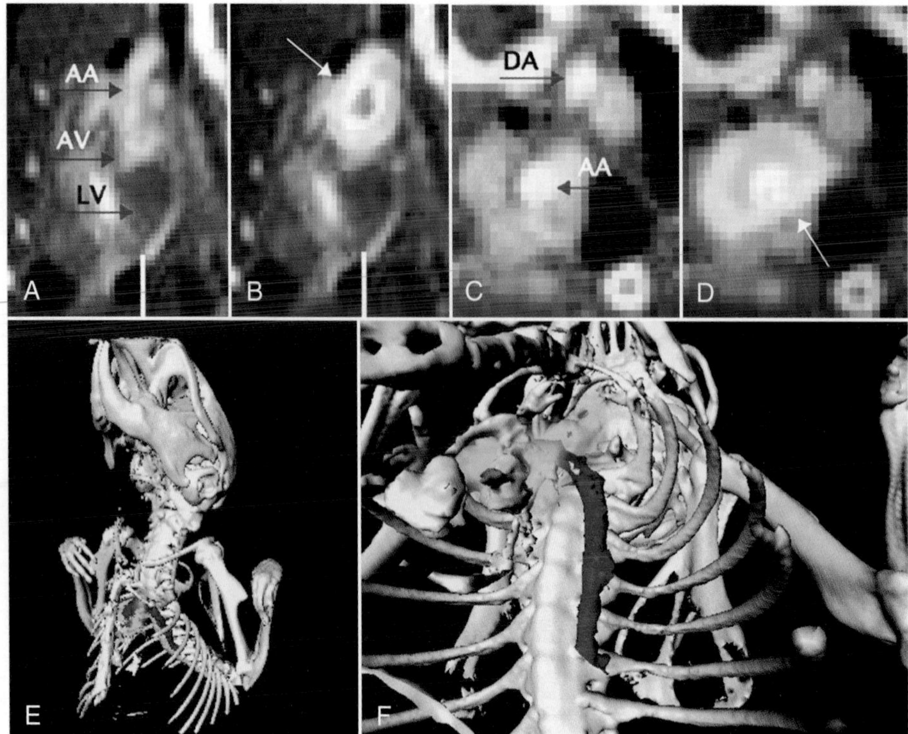

FIGURE 23-3 ^{111}In-labeled monocytes were transferred into apoE$^{-/-}$ mice. **A** and **C** depict CT data only; **B** and **D,** SPECT-CT overlay. **A** and **B** show sagittal views of the heart. AA = ascending aorta; AV = aortic valve region; LV = left ventricle. Note the SPECT signal (white arrow) indicating monocyte recruitment to the ascending aorta in **B**. **C** and **D** depict axial views of ascending (AA) and descending (DA) aorta. Note the SPECT signal in **D** in the ascending aorta, correlating with the location in **B**. **E** and **F,** Three-dimensional rendering; bone structures rendered in white, aorta in red, and monocyte recruitment in blue-green scale. *(From Kircher MF, Grimm J, Swirski FK, et al: Noninvasive in vivo imaging of monocyte trafficking to atherosclerotic lesions. Circulation 117:388, 2008.)*

undergoing infarction, during acute rejection after transplantation, and in various types of myocarditides. Chronic inflammation characterizes active atherosclerotic plaques (see Chap. 43). An early hallmark of the inflammatory response, recruitment of leukocytes of various classes, characterizes the inflammatory response.

Most studies of molecular imaging of leukocytes in the cardiovascular arena have labeled mononuclear phagocytes. Although T lymphocytes may participate more proximally in myocardial immune responses such as parenchymal rejection or viral myocarditis, recruited mononuclear phagocytes soon outnumber the T cells in such lesions and provide a more abundant target for imaging.[17-21] Moreover, their phagocytic properties provide an avenue for labeling them with phagocytosable nanoparticles (see later). Endothelial adhesion molecules capture blood leukocytes and thus participate in their recruitment. The targeting of leukocyte adhesion molecules is considered later.

Ex vivo labeling of leukocytes and their readministration has undergone experimental validation in several contexts. Isolation of monocytes by use of negative selection, which avoids their ex vivo activation, and subsequent labeling with radionuclides such as indium-111 (^{111}In) furnishes one such example.[22] Labeled leukocytes accumulate in areas of atherosclerotic lesions in mice (**Fig. 23-3**).

Transgenic mice expressing green fluorescent protein (GFP) under the direction of cell-selective promoters provide populations of cells traceable by optical imaging. Adoptive transfer of these labeled cells to syngeneic congenic mice with various pathologic conditions furnishes another avenue for the study of leukocyte uptake.[23]

The administration of stem cells derived from bone marrow and other sources has captivated the cardiovascular community (see Chap. 11). The "homing" of stem cells to organs such as the myocardium has become a goal of molecular and cellular imaging in the context of cardiovascular regenerative medicine. Various tagging strategies may permit tracking of stem cells to determine their accumulation within target tissues (see also Fig. 17-45).[24-27]

Phagocytosis

Mononuclear phagocytes that accumulate at a site of injury or inflammation usually mature into tissue macrophages. Macrophages exposed to local inflammatory mediators increase their expression of receptors that mediate endocytosis of various ligands. Activated tissue macrophages also increase bulk pinocytosis and receptor-independent phagocytosis, resulting in intracellular accumulation of cargo and amplification of signal.

Nanometer-sized magnetic particles have proven useful in tracking phagocytosis by MRI. These particles comprise a superparamagnetic core, typically iron oxide coated with a biocompatible layer of dextran. Varying the chain length and the quantity of dextran coating can control the plasma half-life, disposition, and phagocytic potential of such paramagnetic nanoparticles. Such magnetic nanoparticles can monitor phagocytic function in experimental cardiovascular diseases. For example, clinical administration of dextran-coated magnetic nanoparticles leads to suppression of signal in T2-weighted images of human atherosclerotic arteries (**Fig. 23-4A**).[28,29] Histologic studies show colocalization of the iron with mononuclear phagocytes (Fig. 23-4B). Other types of labeling strategies can extend the assessment of phagocytic capacity to nuclear and optical techniques.[15] A therapeutic intervention (e.g., statin treatment) can attenuate this phagocytosis-related signal in experimental atherosclerotic plaques (**Fig. 23-5**).[30] Preliminary clinical data indicate the ability of clinical ultrasmall particulate iron oxide (USPIO) nanoparticles to distinguish high-dose versus low-dose statin anti-inflammatory effects.[31] In addition to imaging atheromas and sites of myocardial infarction, phagocytosable nanoparticles can visualize macrophage accumulation in rejecting myocardium in experimental heart transplantation.[20,21] Iodinated nanoparticles may also permit imaging of phagocytically active macrophages by CT.[32]

Myocardial Injury

Attempts to visualize myosin in damaged myocardial cells provided an early example of molecular imaging in the cardiovascular system. A labeled antibody approach has visualized myosin in injured hearts through nuclear[33] or MRI techniques.[34] In normal cardiocytes, myosin resides intracellularly, inaccessible to tagged antibodies. Under conditions that impair the integrity of the sarcolemma, labeled antibody can gain access to the intracellular compartment and bind to myosin, or to myosin that has leaked into the extracellular space.

Cell Surface Structures: Receptors, Integrins, Adhesion Molecules

The selective expression of cell surface structures such as receptors, integrins, and adhesion molecules furnishes another tempting target category for molecular imaging. In the cardiovascular arena, leukocyte adhesion molecules have undergone fairly extensive experimental exploration. Cell surface–associated integrins can also report on angiogenesis.

Vascular cell adhesion molecule 1 (VCAM-1) represents one well-validated target for atherosclerosis. Normal endothelial cells, as well as most other cell types, do not constitutively express VCAM-1. Stimulation with proinflammatory cytokines in vitro augments the expression of VCAM-1 on endothelial and many other cell types. VCAM-1 recruits just those cell types recruited to the nascent atherosclerotic lesions (see Chap. 43). Moreover, some evidence supports receptor-mediated endocytosis by VCAM-1, yielding intracellular accumulation of ligands. Panning techniques using libraries of peptides generated by bacteriophages have identified VCAM-1 ligands useful for targeting of molecular imaging agents. Optimization of these peptides has yielded several generations of targeting ligands of increasing affinity and efficiency of targeting. The preparation of labeled nanoparticles bearing VCAM ligands has resulted in the ability to image VCAM-1 by several modalities.[35] Magneto-optical VCAM probes can visualize atheromas in mice.[17] A tetrameric peptide that interacts with VCAM-1 can direct radionuclide-targeted VCAM ligand to atheromas, facilitating the clinical translatability of this approach.[36] Statin treatment can decrease VCAM signal in plaque (**Fig. 23-6**).[36]

Scavenger receptors on macrophages also have served as molecular MRI targets in atherosclerosis. Gadolinium-carrying micelles conjugated to a high-affinity macrophage scavenger receptor A antibody have enabled a positive-contrast approach for macrophage imaging.[37]

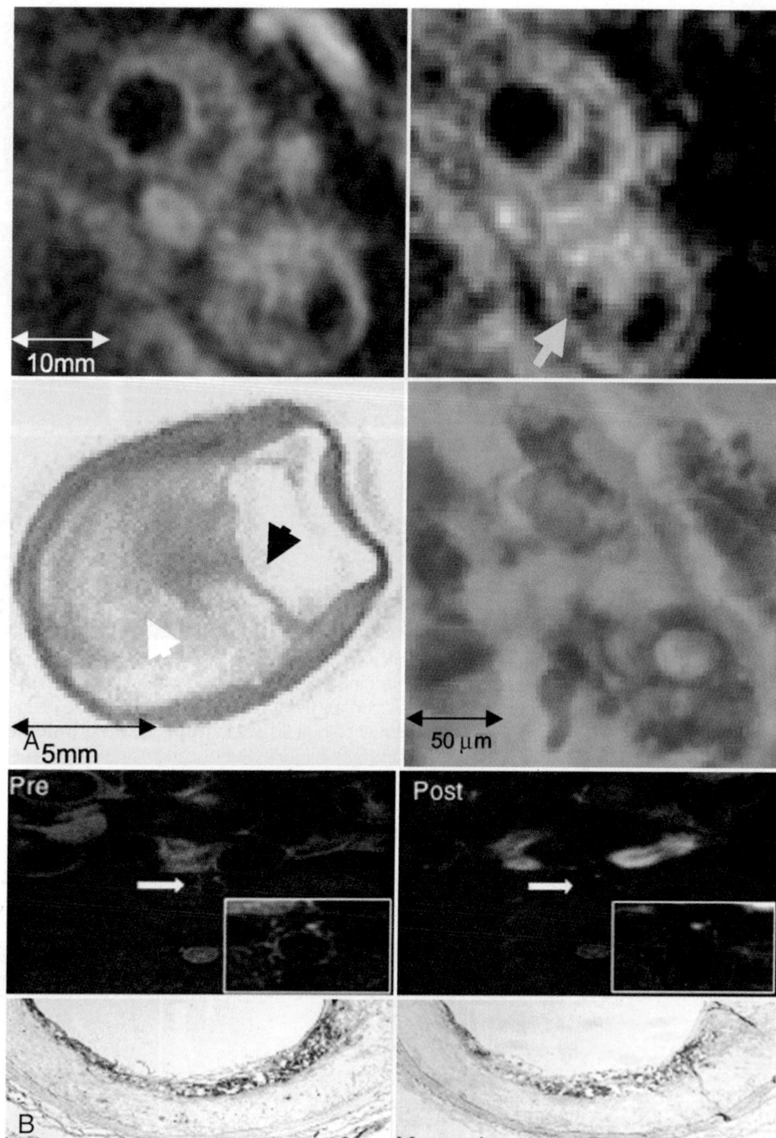

FIGURE 23-4 **A,** Clinical imaging of carotid arterial plaque inflammation with ultrasmall superparamagnetic iron oxide (USPIO) magnetic nanoparticles. Pre-USPIO (top left) and post-USPIO (top right) axial magnetic resonance images, localized 3 mm above the left carotid artery division. USPIO particles induced T2*-mediated signal loss within the plaque (yellow arrow), compared with the baseline (preinjection) image. Bottom left, Plaque histology revealed a thin fibrous cap (black arrowhead) housing a large lipid core (white arrowhead). Bottom right, High-power double Perls/MAC387 stain for USPIO and macrophages demonstrated colocalization of USPIO (blue) with plaque macrophages (brown) near the fibrous cap (magnification ×40). *(From Trivedi RA, U-King-Im JM, Graves MJ, et al: Noninvasive imaging of carotid plaque inflammation. Neurology 63:187, 2004.)* **B,** The reduction of MRI signal intensity in aortic atherosclerosis of hyperlipidemic rabbits in vivo, mediated by venous injection of iron nanoparticles, associates with macrophage accumulation. Top, 3T MRI detected the thickened aortic wall in a hypercholesterolemic rabbit 4 months after mechanical injury and the initiation of high-cholesterol feeding (Pre). Injection of iron nanoparticles as an MRI contrast agent decreased T2-weighted signal intensity in vivo in the aortic wall of hypercholesterolemic rabbits (Post, 72 hours after injection). Bottom, Histologic analyses colocalized iron accumulation (DAB-enhanced Perls Prussian blue, lower left panel) in macrophages (RAM-11, lower right panel) in the luminal surface of atherosclerotic aorta at the level shown in the in vivo magnetic resonance images (top left). Bar = 100 μm. *(From Morishige K, Kacher DF, Libby P, et al: High-resolution MRI enhanced with superparamagnetic nanoparticles measures macrophage burden in atherosclerosis. Circulation 122:1708, 2010.)*

Angiogenesis

Repair of the infarcted myocardium and evolution of the atherosclerotic plaque involve formation of new vessels. In addition, therapeutic angiogenesis has become of interest in cardiovascular therapy (see Chap. 11). Imaging of angiogenesis has garnered considerable attention for these reasons. Newly formed microvessels exhibit heightened expression of the vitronectin receptor, an integrin known as $\alpha_v\beta_3$ on the cell surface. Several groups have targeted $\alpha_v\beta_3$ integrins for molecular imaging by a variety of modalities. Integrins generally bind to the tripeptide sequence arginine-glycine-aspartic acid (RGD) or derived synthetic small molecules. The peptide sequence presented on a peptide can direct magnetically labeled nanoparticles to neovessels forming in the experimental atherosclerotic plaques.[38] Labeled constrained peptides such as knottins can also bind to and visualize α_v integrins.[39] Such strategies have also been used to direct microbubbles visualized by CEU to atherosclerotic plaques[19] and to visualize angiogenesis in experimental hind limb ischemia.[40] CEU targeting the ligand for an adhesion molecule, sialyl

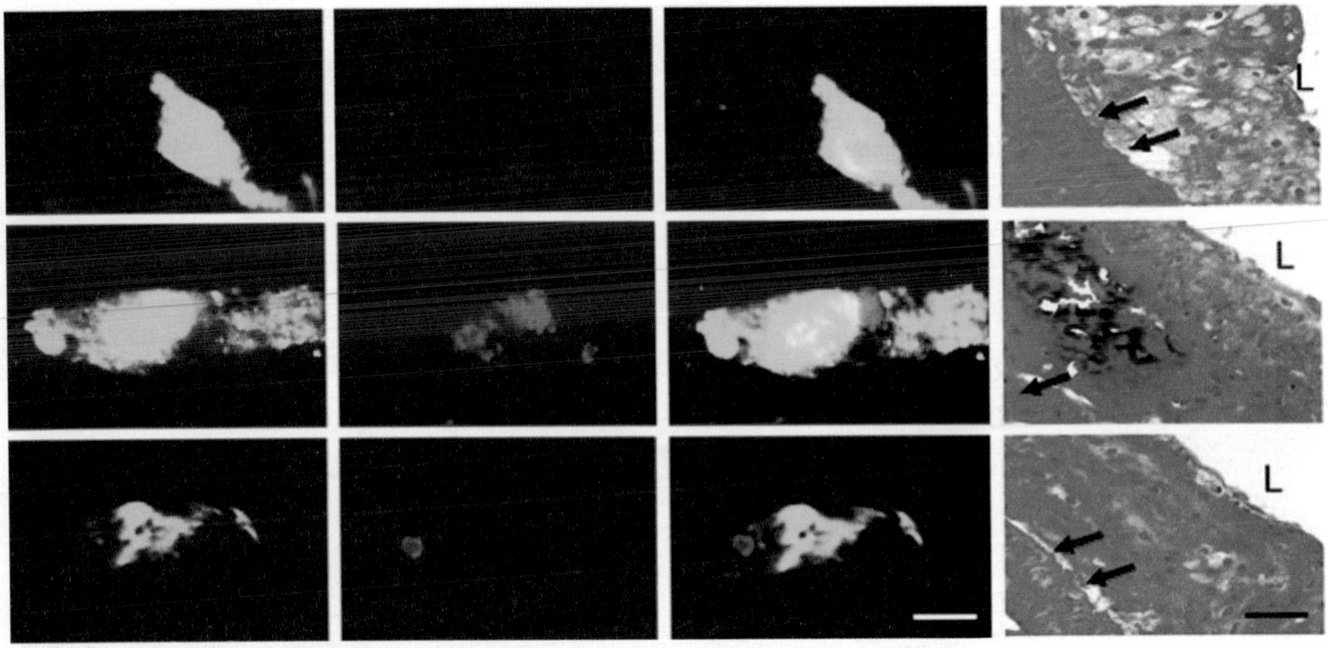

FIGURE 23-5 Sequential intravital fluorescence microscopy was used to monitor concomitant changes in inflammation and osteogenesis in mouse carotid atherosclerotic plaques. At 20 weeks, mice were randomized either to continue with the high-cholesterol diet, or to consume the high-cholesterol diet with or without a statin for 10 more weeks. Intravital microscopy (IVM), fluorescence reflectance imaging, and histopathologic analyses were performed at 20 and 30 weeks in treated and untreated mice. IVM was done sequentially at 20 weeks **(top)**, 30 weeks **(middle)**, and 30 weeks on statin diet **(bottom)**. Image stacks simultaneously visualized two different biologic processes: inflammation (green fluorescence) and osteogenesis (red fluorescence). Bar = 500 μm. Representative hematoxylin and eosin (H&E) images were used to correlate IVM with histopathologic changes **(right panels)**. L = lumen; arrows depict internal elastic lamina. Bar = 50 μm. *(From Aikawa E, Nahrendorf M, Figueiredo JL, et al: Osteogenesis associates with inflammation in early-stage atherosclerosis evaluated by molecular imaging in vivo. Circulation 116:2841, 2007.)*

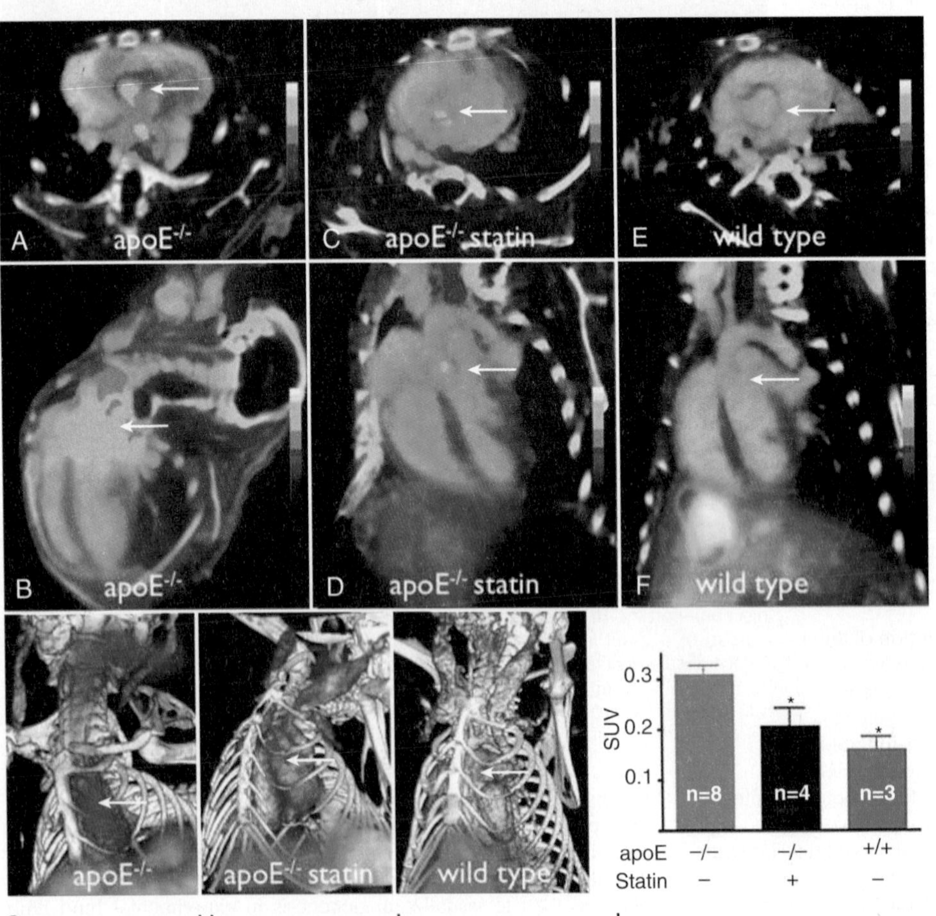

FIGURE 23-6 PET-CT imaging in apoE$^{-/-}$ and statin-treated mice. **A, C, E,** Short-axis PET-CT images of the aortic root (arrows). **B, D, F,** Long-axis views. **G, H, I,** Three-dimensional maximum intensity projection (bone = white, vasculature = blue, ^{18}F-4V = red). **J,** PET signal as standard uptake value (SUV), *$P < 0.05$. *(From Nahrendorf M, Keliher E, Panizzi P, et al: 18F-4V for PET-CT imaging of VCAM-1 expression in inflammatory atherosclerosis. J Am Coll Cardiol Img 2:1213, 2009.)*

Lewis^x, has also been used to monitor ischemic memory experimentally in myocardium (**Fig. 23-7**).[41] VCAM-1 expression can also target vasculogenesis and arteriogenesis.[42]

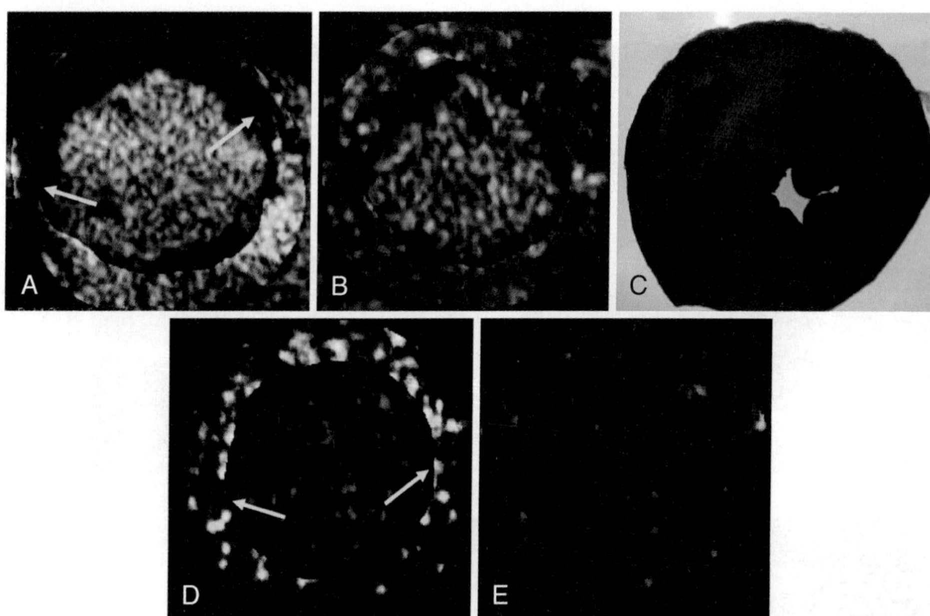

FIGURE 23-7 Ischemic memory imaging at 30 minutes after reflow in one rat undergoing 15 minutes of ischemia but sustaining no infarction **(C).** The myocardial contrast echocardiograms are represented as subtraction images, with values for contrast change color coded for each pixel. The risk area during occlusion (contrast-deficient region between arrows in **A**) resolves after reperfusion **(B).** For the myocardial contrast echocardiography images in **D** and **E,** the image at 4 minutes after injection of contrast material has been subtracted from the 3.5-minute image to yield the signals attributable to adhesion. After injection of sLe^x-conjugated microbubbles, there is persistent contrast enhancement (region between arrows in **D**) within the previously ischemic area **(A),** which is not seen after injection of control microbubbles **(E).** *(Modified from Villanueva FS, Lu E, Bowry S, et al: Myocardial ischemic memory imaging with molecular echocardiography. Circulation 115:345, 2007.)*

Apoptosis

Programmed cell death or apoptosis characterizes the myocardial response to ischemic injury and also occurs in atheromatous plaques, helping to generate the lesion's core. Cells undergoing apoptosis exteriorize phosphatidylcholine on their externally disposed cell membrane. This phospholipid ligand binds a protein known as annexin V. Thus, annexin V may serve as a targeting ligand for visualization of apoptosis. Several groups have used radiolabeled or fluorescent annexin V to visualize apoptosis in vivo in myocardial injury[43,44] and in atherosclerotic plaques.[45,46] Small molecules with specificity for apoptotic cells are also emerging.

Proteolytic Enzymes

Tissue remodeling requires the participation of enzymes capable of degrading the macromolecular constituents of extracellular matrix. Examples include expansion of the infarcted myocardium, outward remodeling of atheromas, and in the extreme, aneurysm formation. Degradation of the collagenous extracellular matrix of the plaque's protective fibrous cap can impair its biomechanical strength. Fracture of the plaque's fibrous cap causes a majority of fatal acute myocardial infarctions by precipitating thrombus formation (see Chap. 54). Thus, proteolytic enzymes specialized in degrading constituents of the extracellular matrix play a pivotal role in important aspects of cardiac and vascular pathophysiology. For such reasons, molecular imaging of matrix-degrading proteinases has generated considerable interest.

Many extracellular matrix–degrading enzymes belong to the family of matrix metalloproteinases (MMPs). Various strategies for molecular imaging of matrix metalloproteinases have undergone exploration. The labeling of selective MMP inhibitors provides one such approach.[47] The use of enzyme-activatable selective fluorescent probes provides another approach that makes use of the catalytic capacity of enzymes.[48] Such quenched fluorescent substrates, when cleaved, can augment their fluorescence by several powers of 10. As one active enzyme molecule can process many substrate molecules, this optical approach to assessment of MMP activity has considerable appeal. The amplification of signal provided by enzymatic catalysis offers a considerable advantage over the 1:1 stoichiometry of a labeled inhibitor.[49,50] Proof-of-concept work has demonstrated the ability to visualize activity of the MMP gelatinases (MMP-2 and MMP-9) in atherosclerotic plaques of mice (**Fig. 23-8**).[51] MMP-9 also possesses elastolytic activity, making it a candidate for extracellular matrix remodeling during aneurysm formation.

The cysteinyl proteinases, some denoted cathepsins, can also exert potent elastolytic activity. NIRF probes that report on members of this class of enzymes have also undergone evaluation in experimental cardiovascular disease. Such sulfhydryl proteinases (e.g., cathepsin B) localize in atherosclerotic plaques and can be imaged experimentally.[11,48,52] As inhibitors of matrix-degrading enzymes are under development, methods to visualize their activity in vivo could help validate targeting in intact subjects and help choose the dose of such an inhibitor for eventual clinical trials in an informed manner.

Oxidative Stress

Regeneration of reactive oxygen species commonly characterizes sites of tissue injury. In particular, the enzyme myeloperoxidase (MPO), which generates the reactive oxygen species hypochlorous acid (HOCl), localizes in atherosclerotic plaques. Circulating levels of this enzyme serve as a biomarker of cardiovascular risk in some studies. Various approaches have successfully visualized HOCl in vivo at sites of inflammation[53] or experimental myocardial infarction.[54] A polymerizable gadolinium-based sensor can enable MPO activity detection by MRI.[55]

Lipoproteins

Receptor-mediated endocytosis of lipoproteins characterizes macrophage foam cells. Efforts to image atherosclerotic lesions with use of labeled lipoproteins date back several decades.[56] Current interest has focused on visualizing accumulation of oxidatively modified lipoproteins by antibody-based targeting strategies for MRI.[57] Experimental data provide intriguing proof-of-principle observations regarding the ability to visualize atherosclerotic plaques by such a strategy. The uptake of radioiodinated or other tagged lipoprotein particles, although explored for many years, has not yielded clinically practical methods thus far.

Glucose Metabolism

Activated phagocytes increase their uptake of glucose. In oncology, heightened glucose transport and use monitored by uptake of fluorodeoxyglucose (FDG) has considerable current clinical utility. Some atherosclerotic plaques show accumulation of FDG as well.[58] Sites of augmented FDG accumulation colocalize with sites of experimental atherosclerotic plaque formation. The FDG signal correlates with the number of macrophages in experimental lesions and also in human atheromas.[59] Statin treatment can lower FDG signals in humans.[60] As myocardial glucose uptake under usual nutritional circumstances in humans can obscure coronary arterial signals, current clinical investigation has evaluated FDG uptake in the carotid arteries and the aorta. A number of alternative explanations beyond mere accumulation of mononuclear phagocytes could underlie enhanced FDG uptake in atheromas. For example, increased microvasculature could enhance the delivery of labeled substrate for glucose uptake locally. As FDG already has widespread clinical use, it has elicited much interest for use as a biomarker in clinical trials. Understanding the precise biologic mechanisms that underlie enhanced glucose

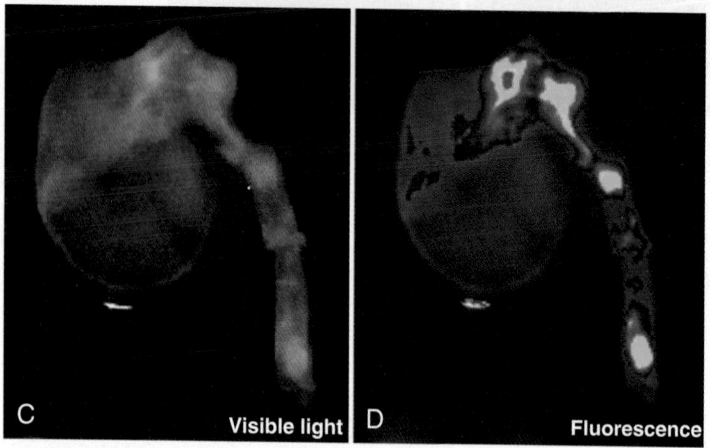

FIGURE 23-8 In vivo fluorescence molecular tomography (FMT) shows MMP activity in mouse atherosclerotic plaques. In vivo FMT after injection of the imaging probe that elaborates near-infrared fluorescence (NIRF) signal on cleavage by gelatinases (MMP-2 and MMP-9) enables the action of these matrix-degrading enzymes to be visualized. An image on an atherosclerosis-prone hypercholesterolemic mouse (apolipoprotein E–deficient or apo$E^{-/-}$ mouse) with no probe injection, superimposed by pseudocolor analysis, detected low NIRF signals **(A),** serving as a control. In vivo FMT on the apo$E^{-/-}$ mouse, 24 hours after the gelatinase probe injection, exhibited substantially more intense NIRF signals **(B)** compared with control. After ex vivo reflectance, imaging with visible light indicated atherosclerotic changes in the excised aorta from the same apo$E^{-/-}$ mouse **(C).** Ex vivo NIRF imaging further showed signals on the aortic root and arch of the same mouse **(D).** *(From Deguchi J, Aikawa M, Tung CH, et al: Inflammation in atherosclerosis: Visualizing matrix metalloproteinase action in vivo. Circulation 114:55, 2006.)*

uptake in atheromatous plaques will require considerable future effort.

Imaging of Transcriptional Activity

Gene transcription represents another biologic process susceptible to visualization by molecular imaging. By introducing into cells plasmids containing promoters that drive genes that encode luciferase, transcriptional activity can yield light output. Bioluminescence imaging can thus track selectively transcriptional activity in vivo. Whereas sensitivity issues may limit this approach, amplification strategies exist to enhance signals.[61] Although translation to humans may prove daunting, imaging of transcriptional activity may provide a useful tool in laboratory investigations.

Neurotransmitter Labeling of Autonomic Activity

An early application of molecular imaging in the cardiovascular system employed radiolabeled analogues of neurotransmitters to track autonomic nerve activity. Given the importance of cardiac autonomic neuropathy in diabetic disease and other circumstances, this approach has considerable investigative interest. Although methods have been available for many years, the use of labeled neurotransmitter analogues to track autonomic nerve function has not yet become routine in clinical practice.[62]

Uses for Molecular Imaging

As molecular imaging methods become clinically applicable, their appropriate use will require rigorous evaluation. Molecular imaging should certainly prove useful for investigative purposes. The ability to probe specific molecular and cellular pathways noninvasively or minimally invasively in intact human subjects will provide an enormous opportunity to translate experimental work into humans. Also, from an investigative standpoint, the ability to distinguish plaques with varying types of biologic activation will no doubt aid understanding of the mechanisms of disease and of clinical complications. The availability of validated molecular imaging strategies should also assist drug development, by helping to choose doses for endpoint trials and to verify delivery of agents to the intended tissue, and by affirming the ability to interfere with the targeted process in some cases. Thus, the use of biomarkers based on molecular imaging could contribute importantly to the development and evaluation of novel therapeutics.

The use of such advanced modalities in routine cardiovascular diagnosis presents several hurdles. First, most of these approaches will require expensive platforms or reagents, rendering them costly for routine screening purposes. Much interest has centered on the identification of so-called vulnerable atherosclerotic plaques. Although this quest has obvious appeal from a research perspective, dealing with the clinical consequences of the ability to identify such lesions remains much more speculative. We already possess much simpler biomarkers of prospective cardiovascular risk (see Chap. 44). Plaques with characteristics of vulnerability appear numerous in a given coronary tree and may coexist with high-risk lesions in other arterial beds, such as the carotid arteries. Systemic therapies rather than local therapies have proven effective in forestalling future cardiovascular events in individuals with established atherosclerosis. Therefore, the use of imaging to define vulnerable plaques to direct local therapies to single or few lesions in a particular arterial bed may prove quixotic. Finally, the design and execution of studies to show the clinical utility and cost-effectiveness of local intervention on atheromatous plaques guided by molecular imaging could prove daunting.

Molecular imaging, like other advanced imaging strategies as they mature into clinical readiness, will likely prove cost-beneficial as part of a tiered strategy for gauging cardiovascular risk or directing therapy. For example, traditional risk algorithms, perhaps modified by the inclusion of emerging less expensive nonimaging biomarkers, will furnish a first approach to risk assessment in screening, particularly in populations of unknown risk (see Chap. 44). Individuals with indications of heightened cardiovascular risk based on an initial level of noninvasive tools may undergo selective imaging to refine prognosis and to direct therapies.

The Future of Molecular Imaging of the Cardiovascular System

This chapter has provided a brief overview on the development of cardiovascular molecular imaging. Many of these modalities—for example, NIRF imaging and the development of sophisticated chemical targeting probes—entail considerable barriers to clinical translation. Imaging platforms suitable for human use will require continued development. Fluorescence molecular tomography, well developed in mice, may require the development of intravascular probes or handheld devices for interrogation of NIRF signals over superficial arteries, such as the carotid or femoral arteries, for initial clinical implementation. High-resolution MRI of carotid arteries now generally requires highly specialized coils not currently widely available for routine clinical application. Each novel imaging agent, even those that use established imaging platforms such as ultrasound, will require regulatory approval both at the level of local institutional review boards for initial development and by federal regulatory authorities. The approval of novel radionuclide-tagged imaging agents requires review with scrutiny that may increase in the future.[16] Overcoming these substantial challenges will require considerable commitment.

The pace of development of other imaging strategies suggests that these barriers will prove superable. MRI and CT imaging have shown remarkable increase in technical sophistication during the last several decades. There is no fundamental reason that molecular imaging could not follow this path, extending cardiovascular imaging beyond the domain of anatomy and physiologic function to interrogate specific molecular targets as described earlier.

REFERENCES

Principles of Molecular Imaging

1. Jaffer FA, Libby P, Weissleder R: Molecular imaging of cardiovascular disease. Circulation 116:1052, 2007.
2. Sanz J, Fayad ZA: Imaging of atherosclerotic cardiovascular disease. Nature 451:953, 2008.
3. McCarthy JR, Weissleder R: Multifunctional magnetic nanoparticles for targeted imaging and therapy. Adv Drug Deliv Rev 60:1241, 2008.
4. Wickline SA, Neubauer AM, Winter P, et al: Applications of nanotechnology to atherosclerosis, thrombosis, and vascular biology. Arterioscler Thromb Vasc Biol 26:435, 2006.
5. Fayad ZA: Cardiovascular molecular imaging. Arterioscler Thromb Vasc Biol 29:981, 2009.
6. Sinusas AJ: Cardiovascular molecular imaging. J Nucl Med 48:26N, 2007.
7. Kaul S: Myocardial contrast echocardiography: A 25-year retrospective. Circulation 118:291, 2008.
8. Judenhofer MS, Wehrl HF, Newport DF, et al: Simultaneous PET-MRI: A new approach for functional and morphological imaging. Nat Med 14:459, 2008.
9. Kaufmann BA, Lindner JR: Molecular imaging with targeted contrast ultrasound. Curr Opin Biotechnol 18:11, 2007.
10. Villanueva FS: Molecular imaging of cardiovascular disease using ultrasound. J Nucl Cardiol 15:576, 2008.
11. Jaffer FA, Vinegoni C, John MC, et al: Real-time catheter molecular sensing of inflammation in proteolytically active atherosclerosis. Circulation 118:1802, 2008.
12. Sinusas AJ, Bengel F, Nahrendorf M, et al: Multimodality cardiovascular molecular imaging, part I. Circ Cardiovasc Imaging 1:244, 2008.
13. Jaffer FA, Libby P, Weissleder R: Optical and multimodality molecular imaging: Insights into atherosclerosis. Arterioscler Thromb Vasc Biol 29:1017, 2009.
14. Silvera SS, Aidi HE, Rudd JH, et al: Multimodality imaging of atherosclerotic plaque activity and composition using FDG-PET/CT and MRI in carotid and femoral arteries. Atherosclerosis 207:139, 2009.
15. Nahrendorf M, Zhang H, Hembrador S, et al: Nanoparticle PET-CT imaging of macrophages in inflammatory atherosclerosis. Circulation 117:379, 2008.

Biologic Processes Amenable to Molecular Targeting for Imaging

16. Libby P, Di Carli MF, Weissleder R: The vascular biology of atherosclerosis and imaging targets. J Nucl Med 51(Suppl):1S, 2010.
17. Nahrendorf M, Jaffer FA, Kelly KA, et al: Noninvasive vascular cell adhesion molecule-1 imaging identifies inflammatory activation of cells in atherosclerosis. Circulation 114:1504, 2006.
18. Sadeghi MM, Schechner JS, Krassilnikova S, et al: Vascular cell adhesion molecule-1–targeted detection of endothelial activation in human microvasculature. Transplant Proc 36:1585, 2004.
19. Kaufmann BA, Sanders JM, Davis C, et al: Molecular imaging of inflammation in atherosclerosis with targeted ultrasound detection of vascular cell adhesion molecule-1. Circulation 116:276, 2007.
20. Christen T, Nahrendorf M, Wildgruber M, et al: Molecular imaging of innate immune cell function in transplant rejection. Circulation 119:1925, 2009.
21. Christen T, Shimizu K, Libby P: Advances in imaging of cardiac allograft rejection. Curr Cardiovasc Imaging Rep 2010; in press.
22. Swirski FK, Pittet MJ, Kircher MF, et al: Monocyte accumulation in mouse atherogenesis is progressive and proportional to extent of disease. Proc Natl Acad Sci U S A 103:10340, 2006.
23. Contag CH: In vivo pathology: Seeing with molecular specificity and cellular resolution in the living body. Annu Rev Pathol 2:277, 2007.
24. Narsinh KH, Cao F, Wu JC: Molecular imaging of human embryonic stem cells. Methods Mol Biol 515:13, 2009.
25. Sun N, Lee A, Wu JC: Long term non-invasive imaging of embryonic stem cells using reporter genes. Nat Protoc 4:1192, 2009.
26. Rodriguez-Porcel M, Brinton TJ, Chen IY, et al: Reporter gene imaging following percutaneous delivery in swine moving toward clinical applications. J Am Coll Cardiol 51:595, 2008.
27. Li Z, Lee A, Huang M, et al: Imaging survival and function of transplanted cardiac resident stem cells. J Am Coll Cardiol 53:1229, 2009.
28. Kooi ME, Cappendijk VC, Cleutjens KB, et al: Accumulation of ultrasmall superparamagnetic particles of iron oxide in human atherosclerotic plaques can be detected by in vivo magnetic resonance imaging. Circulation 107:2453, 2003.
29. Trivedi RA, U-King-Im JM, Graves MJ, et al: In vivo detection of macrophages in human carotid atheroma: Temporal dependence of ultrasmall superparamagnetic particles of iron oxide–enhanced MRI. Stroke 35:1631, 2004.
30. Aikawa E, Nahrendorf M, Figueiredo JL, et al: Osteogenesis associates with inflammation in early-stage atherosclerosis evaluated by molecular imaging in vivo. Circulation 116:2841, 2007.
31. Tang TY, Howarth SP, Miller SR, et al: The ATHEROMA (Atorvastatin Therapy: Effects on Reduction of Macrophage Activity) Study. Evaluation using ultrasmall superparamagnetic iron oxide–enhanced magnetic resonance imaging in carotid disease. J Am Coll Cardiol 53:2039, 2009.
32. Hyafil F, Cornily JC, Feig JE, et al: Noninvasive detection of macrophages using a nanoparticulate contrast agent for computed tomography. Nat Med 13:636, 2007.
33. Khaw BA, Gold HK, Yasuda T, et al: Scintigraphic quantification of myocardial necrosis in patients after intravenous injection of myosin-specific antibody. Circulation 74:501, 1986.
34. Weissleder R, Lee AS, Khaw BA, et al: Antimyosin-labeled monocrystalline iron oxide allows detection of myocardial infarct: MR antibody imaging. Radiology 182:381, 1992.
35. McAteer MA, Sibson NR, von Zur Muhlen C, et al: In vivo magnetic resonance imaging of acute brain inflammation using microparticles of iron oxide. Nat Med 13:1253, 2007.
36. Nahrendorf M, Keliher E, Panizzi P, et al: ^{18}F-4V for PET-CT imaging of VCAM-1 expression in inflammatory atherosclerosis. J Am Coll Cardiol Img 2:1213, 2009.
37. Amirbekian V, Lipinski MJ, Briley-Saebo KC, et al: Detecting and assessing macrophages in vivo to evaluate atherosclerosis noninvasively using molecular MRI. Proc Natl Acad Sci U S A 104:961, 2007.
38. Winter PM, Morawski AM, Caruthers SD, et al: Molecular imaging of angiogenesis in early-stage atherosclerosis with alpha$_v$beta$_3$-integrin–targeted nanoparticles. Circulation 108:2270, 2003.
39. Miao Z, Ren G, Liu H, et al: An engineered knottin peptide labeled with ^{18}F for PET imaging of integrin expression. Bioconjug Chem 20:2342, 2009.
40. Leong-Poi H, Christiansen J, Heppner P, et al: Assessment of endogenous and therapeutic arteriogenesis by contrast ultrasound molecular imaging of integrin expression. Circulation 111:3248, 2005.
41. Villanueva FS, Lu E, Bowry S, et al: Myocardial ischemic memory imaging with molecular echocardiography. Circulation 115:345, 2007.
42. Behm CZ, Kaufmann BA, Carr C, et al: Molecular imaging of endothelial vascular cell adhesion molecule-1 expression and inflammatory cell recruitment during vasculogenesis and ischemia-mediated arteriogenesis. Circulation 117:2902, 2008.
43. Sosnovik DE, Schellenberger EA, Nahrendorf M, et al: Magnetic resonance imaging of cardiomyocyte apoptosis with a novel magneto-optical nanoparticle. Magn Reson Med 54:718, 2005.
44. Sosnovik DE, Garanger E, Aikawa E, et al: Molecular MRI of cardiomyocyte apoptosis with simultaneous delayed-enhancement MRI distinguishes apoptotic and necrotic myocytes in vivo: Potential for midmyocardial salvage in acute ischemia. Circ Cardiovasc Imaging 2:460, 2009.
45. Kietselaer BL, Reutelingsperger CP, Heidendal GA, et al: Noninvasive detection of plaque instability with use of radiolabeled annexin A5 in patients with carotid-artery atherosclerosis. N Engl J Med 350:1472, 2004.
46. Isobe S, Tsimikas S, Zhou J, et al: Noninvasive imaging of atherosclerotic lesions in apolipoprotein E–deficient and low-density-lipoprotein receptor–deficient mice with annexin A5. J Nucl Med 47:1497, 2006.
47. Schafers M, Riemann B, Kopka K, et al: Scintigraphic imaging of matrix metalloproteinase activity in the arterial wall in vivo. Circulation 109:2554, 2004.
48. Chen J, Tung CH, Mahmood U, et al: In vivo imaging of proteolytic activity in atherosclerosis. Circulation 105:2766, 2002.
49. Ohshima S, Petrov A, Fujimoto S, et al: Molecular imaging of matrix metalloproteinase expression in atherosclerotic plaques of mice deficient in apolipoprotein E or low-density-lipoprotein receptor. J Nucl Med 50:612, 2009.
50. Zhang J, Nie L, Razavian M, et al: Molecular imaging of activated matrix metalloproteinases in vascular remodeling. Circulation 118:1953, 2008.
51. Deguchi J, Aikawa M, Tung C-H, et al: Inflammation in atherosclerosis: Visualizing matrix metalloproteinase action in macrophages in vivo. Circulation 114:55, 2006.
52. Jaffer FA, Kim DE, Quinti L, et al: Optical visualization of cathepsin K activity in atherosclerosis with a novel, protease-activatable fluorescence sensor. Circulation 115:2292, 2007.
53. Shepherd J, Hilderbrand SA, Waterman P, et al: A fluorescent probe for the detection of myeloperoxidase activity in atherosclerosis-associated macrophages. Chem Biol 14:1221, 2007.
54. Panizzi P, Nahrendorf M, Wildgruber M, et al: Oxazine conjugated nanoparticle detects in vivo hypochlorous acid and peroxynitrite generation. J Am Chem Soc 131:15739, 2009.
55. Ronald JA, Chen JW, Chen Y, et al: Enzyme-sensitive magnetic resonance imaging targeting myeloperoxidase identifies active inflammation in experimental rabbit atherosclerotic plaques. Circulation 120:592, 2009.
56. Choi SH, Chae A, Chen CH, et al: Emerging approaches for imaging vulnerable plaques in patients. Curr Opin Biotechnol 18:73, 2007.

57. Briley-Saebo KC, Shaw PX, Mulder WJ, et al: Targeted molecular probes for imaging atherosclerotic lesions with magnetic resonance using antibodies that recognize oxidation-specific epitopes. Circulation 117:3206, 2008.
58. Davies JR, Rudd JH, Fryer TD, et al: Identification of culprit lesions after transient ischemic attack by combined ^{18}F fluorodeoxyglucose positron-emission tomography and high-resolution magnetic resonance imaging. Stroke 36:2642, 2005.
59. Tawakol A, Migrino RQ, Bashian GG, et al: In vivo ^{18}F-fluorodeoxyglucose positron emission tomography imaging provides a noninvasive measure of carotid plaque inflammation in patients. J Am Coll Cardiol 48:1818, 2006.
60. Tahara N, Kai H, Ishibashi M, et al: Simvastatin attenuates plaque inflammation: Evaluation by fluorodeoxyglucose positron emission tomography. J Am Coll Cardiol 48:1825, 2006.
61. Chen IY, Gheysens O, Ray S, et al: Indirect imaging of cardiac-specific transgene expression using a bidirectional two-step transcriptional amplification strategy. Gene Ther 17:827, 2010.
62. Koutelou M, Katsikis A, Flevari P, et al: Predictive value of cardiac autonomic indexes and MIBG washout in ICD recipients with mild to moderate heart failure. Ann Nucl Med 23:677, 2009.

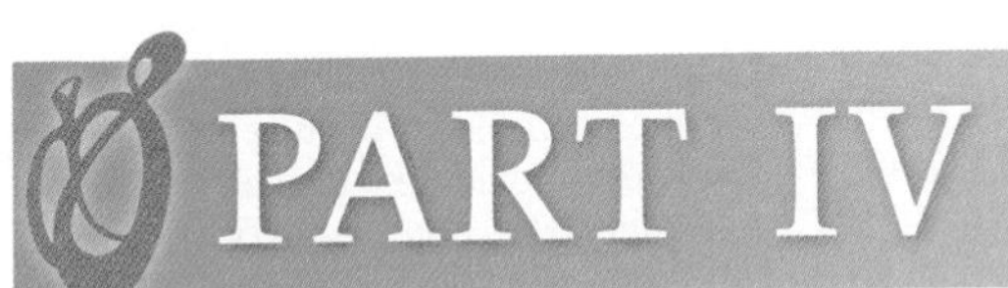

PART IV HEART FAILURE

CHAPTER 24 Mechanisms of Cardiac Contraction and Relaxation

Lionel H. Opie and Gerd Hasenfuss

Microanatomy of Contractile Cells and Proteins

Ultrastructure of Contractile Cells

The major function of myocardial muscle cells (cardiomyocytes or myocytes) is to execute the cardiac contraction-relaxation cycle. The contractile proteins of the heart lie within these myocytes, which constitute about 75% of the total volume of the myocardium although only about one third of all the cells in number. About half of each ventricular cell is occupied by the myofibrils of the myofibers (**Fig. 24-1**) and about one quarter to one third by mitochondria (**Table 24-1**). A myofiber is a group of myocytes (see Fig. 24-1) held together by surrounding collagen connective tissue, the major component of the extracellular matrix. Further strands of collagen connect myofibers to each other. Excess collagen, one cause of left ventricular (LV) diastolic dysfunction, accumulates as part of the growth response to LV pressure overload.

The individual contractile myocytes that account for more than half of the heart's weight are roughly cylindrical (**Fig. 24-2**). Those in the atrium are quite small, being less than 10 μm in diameter and about 20 μm in length. Relative to atrial cells, human ventricular myocytes are large, measuring about 17 to 25 μm in diameter and 60 to 140 μm in length (see Table 24-1).

When they are examined under the light microscope, the atrial and ventricular myocytes have cross striations and are branched. Each myocyte is bounded by a complex cell membrane, the sarcolemma (*sarco,* flesh; *lemma,* thin husk), and is filled with rodlike bundles of myofibrils, the contractile elements (see Fig. 24-1). The sarcolemma of the myocyte invaginates to form an extensive tubular network (the T tubules) that extends the extracellular space into the interior of the cell (see Figs. 24-1 and 24-2). The nucleus, which contains almost all of the cell's genetic information, is often centrally located. Some myocytes have several nuclei. Interspersed between the myofibrils and immediately beneath the sarcolemma are many mitochondria, the main function of which is to generate the energy in the form of adenosine triphosphate (ATP) needed to maintain the heart's contractile function and the associated ion gradients. Of the other organelles, the sarcoplasmic reticulum (SR) is most important (see Fig. 24-1). When the wave of electrical excitation reaches the closely approximated T tubules, the tubular calcium channels open to a relatively small amount of calcium to trigger the release of much more calcium from the calcium release channels of the SR. This is the calcium that initiates myocardial contraction. When the calcium is once again taken up into the SR, relaxation ensues.

The SR is a fine network spreading throughout the myocytes, demarcated by its lipid bilayer, which is similar to that of the sarcolemma. The calcium release channels (also called the ryanodine receptors) are found in the expanded parts of the SR that lie in close apposition to the T tubules. These are called subsarcolemmal cisternae (Latin, boxes or baskets) or the junctional SR. The second part of the SR, the longitudinal or network SR, consists of ramifying tubules (see Fig. 24-1) and is concerned with the uptake of calcium that initiates relaxation. This uptake is achieved by the ATP-requiring calcium pump, also called SERCA (sarcoendoplasmic reticulum Ca^{2+}-ATPase), that increases its activity in response to beta-adrenergic stimulation. Calcium taken up into the SR is then stored at high concentration in

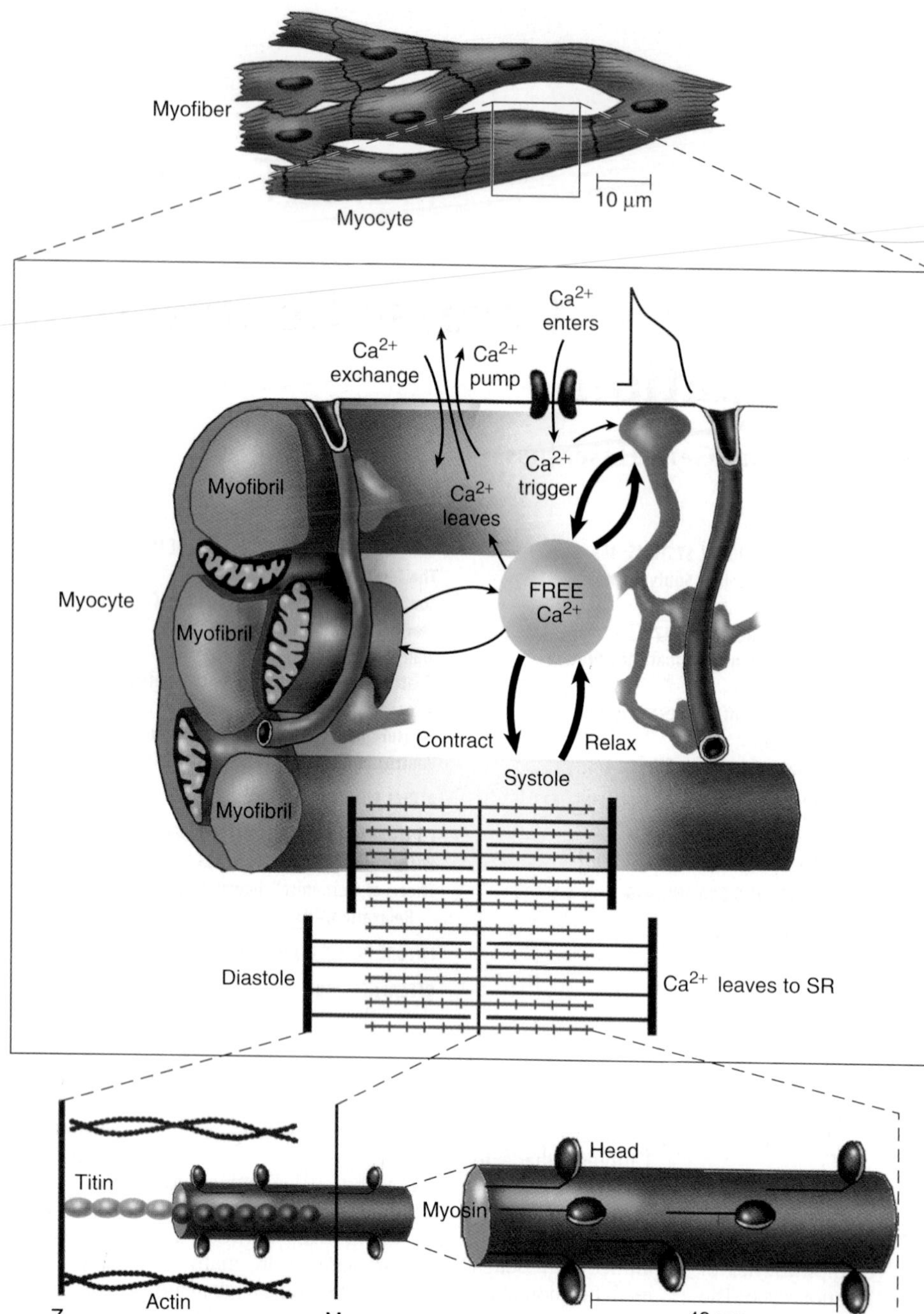

FIGURE 24-1 The crux of the contractile process lies in the changing concentrations of Ca^{2+} ions in the myocardial cytosol. The **upper panel** shows the difference between the myocardial cell or myocyte and the myofiber, composed of many myocytes. In the **middle and lower panels,** Ca^{2+} ions are schematically shown as entering via the calcium channel that opens in response to the wave of depolarization that travels along the sarcolemma. These Ca^{2+} ions "trigger" the release of more calcium from the sarcoplasmic reticulum (SR) and thereby initiate a contraction-relaxation cycle. The small amount of calcium that has entered the cell will eventually leave predominantly by a Na^+/Ca^{2+} exchanger, with a lesser role for the sarcolemmal calcium pump. The varying actin-myosin overlap is shown for systole, when calcium ions arrive, and for diastole, when calcium ions leave. The myosin heads, attached to the thick filaments, interact with the thin actin filaments, as shown in Figure 24-5. For the role of titin, see Figure 24-4. *(Upper panel reproduced from Braunwald E, Ross J Jr, Sonnenblick EH: Mechanisms of Contraction of the Normal and Failing Heart. 2nd ed. Boston, Little Brown, 1976. Middle and lower panels reprinted from Opie LH: Heart Physiology, From Cell to Circulation. Philadelphia Lippincott Williams & Wilkins, 2004. © L. H. Opie, 2004.)*

a number of storage proteins, including calsequestrin, before being released again in response to the next wave of depolarization.

The cytoplasm is the intracellular fluid and the proteins therein contained within the sarcolemma but excluding the contents of organelles, such as mitochondria and the SR. The fluid component of the cytoplasm minus the proteins is called the cytosol. It is in the cytosol that the concentrations of calcium ions rise and fall to cause cardiac contraction and relaxation. The proteins of the sarcoplasm include myriad specialized molecules, the enzymes that accelerate the conversion of one chemical form to another, thereby stimulating crucial metabolic or signaling paths and thereby eventually promoting energy production.

SUBCELLULAR MICROARCHITECTURE. The molecular signal systems that convey messages from surface receptors to intracellular organelles may be directed to specific sites by molecules that "anchor" components of the internal messenger chain to specific organelles, as when the beta-adrenergic chain must link up with the calcium pump of the SR (see later). Scaffolding proteins bring interacting molecules close together, as in the case of the signaling chain, leading to myocyte growth. An example of physiologic subcellular compartmentalization is the local unloading of ATP where it is needed, by the exact location of the enzyme creatine kinase that converts creatine phosphate to ATP.

Contractile Proteins

The major molecules involved in the contraction-relaxation cycle are the two chief contractile proteins, the thin actin filament and the thick myosin filament (see Fig. 24-1). Calcium ions initiate the contraction cycle by interacting with troponin C to relieve the inhibition otherwise exerted by troponin I (**Fig. 24-3**). Titin is a newly discovered large elastic molecule that supports myosin (**Fig. 24-4**). During contraction, the filaments slide over each other without the individual molecules of actin or myosin actually shortening. As they slide, they pull together the two ends of the fundamental contractile unit called the sarcomere. On electron microscopy, the sarcomere is limited on either side by the Z-line (Z, abbreviation for German *Zuckung*, contraction) to which the actin filaments are attached (see Fig. 24-2). Conversely, the myosin filaments extend from the center of the sarcomere in either direction toward but not actually reaching the Z-lines (see Fig. 24-1).

The interaction of the myosin heads with actin filaments when sufficient calcium arrives from the SR (see Fig. 24-1) is called cross-bridge cycling. As the actin filaments move inward toward the center of the sarcomere, they draw the Z-lines closer together, so that the sarcomere shortens. The energy for this shortening is provided by the breakdown of ATP, chiefly made in the mitochondria.

TITIN AND LENGTH SENSING. Titin is a giant molecule, the largest protein yet described. It is an extraordinarily long, flexible, and slender myofibrillar protein (see Fig. 24-4). Titin acts as a third filament to provide elasticity. Being between 0.6 and 1.2 μm in length, the titin molecule extends from the Z-line, stopping just short of the M-line (see Fig. 24-1).

TABLE 24-1 Characteristics of Cardiac Cells, Organelles, and Contractile Proteins

Microanatomy of Heart Cells			
	VENTRICULAR MYOCYTE	**ATRIAL MYOCYTE**	**PURKINJE CELLS**
Shape	Long and narrow	Elliptical	Long and broad
Length, μm	60-140	About 20	150-200
Diameter, μm	About 20	5-6	35-40
Volume, μm^3	15,000-45,000	About 500	135,000-250,000
T tubules	Plentiful	Rare or none	Absent
Intercalated disc	Prominent end-to-end transmission	Side-to-side as well as end-to-end transmission	Very prominent abundant gap junctions; fast; end-to-end transmission
General appearance	Mitochondria and sarcomeres abundant; rectangular branching bundles with little interstitial collagen	Bundles of atrial tissue separated by wide areas of collagen	Fewer sarcomeres, paler

Composition and Function of Ventricular Cells		
ORGANELLE	**% OF CELL VOLUME**	**FUNCTION**
Myofibril	About 50-60	Interaction of thick and thin filaments during contraction cycle
Mitochondria	16 in neonate 33 in adult rat 23 in adult man	Provide ATP chiefly for contraction
T system	About 1	Transmission of electrical signal from sarcolemma to cell interior
Sarcoplasmic reticulum (SR)	33 in neonate 2 in adult	Takes up and releases Ca^{2+} during contraction cycle
Terminal cisternae of SR	0.33 in adult	Site of calcium storage and release
Rest of network of SR	Rest of volume	Site of calcium uptake en route to cisternae
Sarcolemma	Very low	Control of ionic gradients; channels for ions (action potential); maintenance of cell integrity; receptors for drugs and hormones
Nucleus	About 5	Protein synthesis
Lysosomes	Very low	Intracellular digestion and proteolysis
Sarcoplasm (cytoplasm) (plus nuclei and other structures)	About 12 in adult rat 18 in humans	Provides cytosol in which rise and fall of ionized calcium occurs; contains other ions and small molecules

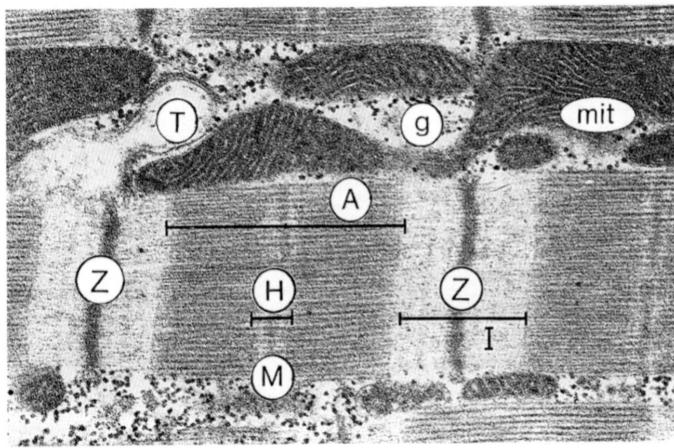

FIGURE 24-2 The sarcomere is the distance between the two Z-lines. Note the presence of numerous mitochondria (mit) sandwiched between the myofibrils and the presence of T tubules (T), which penetrate into the muscle at the level of the Z-lines. This two-dimensional picture should not disguise the fact that the Z-line is really a disc, as is the M-line (M), also shown in Figure 24-1. H = central clear zone containing only myosin filament bodies and the M-line; A = band of actin-myosin overlap; I = band of actin filaments, titin, and Z-line; g = glycogen granules. (×32,000, rat papillary muscle.) *(Courtesy of Dr. J. Moravec, Dijon, France.)*

It has two distinct segments: an inextensible anchoring segment and an extensible elastic segment that stretches as sarcomere length increases. Titin has multiple functions. First, it tethers the myosin molecule to the Z-line, thereby stabilizing the contractile proteins. Second, as it stretches and relaxes, its elasticity explains the stress-strain relation of cardiac and skeletal muscle. At short sarcomere lengths, the elastic domain is folded on itself to generate restoring forces (see Fig. 24-4). These changes in titin help explain the series elastic element, which postulates that there is elasticity in series between the contractile elements and the ends of the muscle. Third, increased diastolic stretch of titin as the sarcomere length of cardiac muscle is increased causes the enfolded part of the titin molecule to straighten. This stretched molecular spring then contracts more vigorously in systole.[1] Such enhanced systolic contraction helps explain the Frank-Starling mechanism (see later). Fourth, titin may transduce mechanical stretch into growth signals. In sustained diastolic stretch as in volume overload, the elastic segment of titin is constantly under strain and transmits this mechanical signal to the muscle LIM protein (MLP) attached to the terminal part of titin that forms part of the Z-disc complex.[2] The MLP protein is proposed as the stretch sensor that transmits the signals resulting in the myocyte growth pattern characteristic of volume overload.[2] This signal system may be defective in a subset of human dilated cardiomyopathy.[2]

Strong and Weak Binding States. Although the events underlying the cross-bridge cycle are exceedingly complex at a molecular level, one simple current hypothesis is that the cross bridges exist in either a strong or a weak binding state (**Fig. 24-5**). The arrival of calcium ions at the contractile proteins is a crucial link in the series of events known as excitation-contraction coupling. The ensuing interaction of calcium with troponin C and the deinhibition of troponin I put the cross bridges in the strong binding state. As long as enough calcium ions are present, the strong binding state potentially dominates (see Fig. 24-5). If, however, the strong binding state were continuously present, the contractile proteins could never relax. Thus, the proposal is that the binding of ATP to the myosin head puts the cross bridges into a weak binding state even when calcium is high. Conversely, when ATP is hydrolyzed to ADP and P_i, the strong binding state again predominates (see Fig. 24-5). Thus, the ATP-induced changes in the molecular configuration of the myosin head result in corresponding variations in the physical properties (a similar concept is common in metabolic regulation). Length activation also promotes the strong binding state (see section on length-dependent activation). Conversely, the weak binding state predominates when cytosolic calcium levels fall at the start of diastole. As the calcium ions leave troponin C, a master switch is turned off, and tropomyosin again assumes the inhibitory configuration.

Actin and Troponin Complex. Although calcium ions provide the essential switch-on signal to the cross-bridge cycle by binding to troponin C, current evidence suggests more than an on-off signaling process. Rather, the arrival of calcium initiates a series of interactions between the troponin components of the thin filament to allow movement of the tropomyosin molecule, which in turn promotes the strong binding state (see Fig. 24-5) so that contraction takes place. To understand the role of calcium first requires a brief description of the molecular structure of actin and the troponin complex. Thin filaments are composed of two actin units, which intertwine in a helical pattern, both being carried on a heavier tropomyosin molecule that functions as a backbone (see Fig. 24-5A). At regular intervals of 38.5 nm along this twisting structure is a closely bound group of three regulatory proteins called the troponin complex. Of these three, it is troponin C that responds to the calcium ions

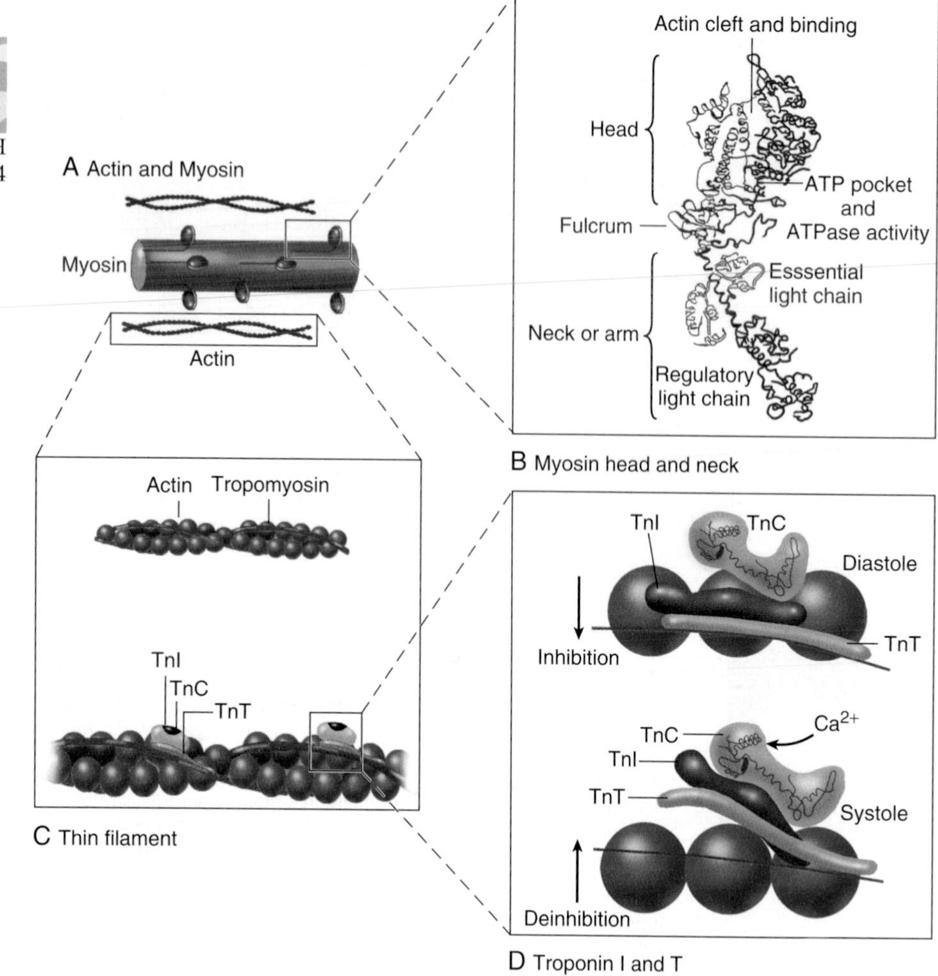

FIGURE 24-3 The major molecules of the contractile system. The thin actin filament **(A)** interacts with the myosin head **(B)** when Ca^{2+} ions arrive at troponin C **(C)**. A complex interaction between TnC and the other troponins moves tropomyosin to "uncover" an actin site to which a myosin head can attach (see Fig. 24-5). The molecular aspects are as follows. **A,** The thin actin filament contains troponin C (TnC) and its Ca^{2+} binding sites. When TnC is not activated by Ca^{2+}, troponin I (TnI) inhibits the actin-myosin interaction. Troponin T (TnT) is an elongated protein that interacts with all the other components of the thin filament,[7] thereby participating in the activation cycle **(D). B,** Myosin head molecular structure (based on Rayment and associates[3]) is composed of heavy and light chains. The heavy head chain in turn has two major domains: one of 70 kDa (i.e., 70,000 molecular weight) that interacts with actin at the actin cleft and has an ATP-binding pocket. The neck domain of 20 kDa, also called the lever, is an elongated alpha helix that extends and bends and has two light chains surrounding it as a collar. The essential light chain is part of the structure. The other regulatory light chain may respond to phosphorylation to influence the extent of the actin-myosin interaction. **C,** Troponin C with sites in the regulatory domain for activation by calcium and for interaction with troponin I. **D,** Calcium binding to TnC induces a conformational change in TnC that elongates (compare systole with diastole). TnI closes up to TnC, and the normal inhibition of TnI on actin-tropomyosin is lessened. There is a strengthening of the interaction between TnC and TnT. These changes allow repositioning of tropomyosin in relation to actin, with lessening of its normal inhibitory effects, as shown in the bottom panel. Now the contractile cycle can start. *(**A-C** modified from Opie LH: Heart Physiology, From Cell to Circulation. Philadelphia, Lippincott Williams & Wilkins, 2004. © L. H. Opie, 2004. **D** modified from Solaro RJ, Van Eyk J: Altered interactions among thin filament proteins modulate cardiac function. J Mol Cell Cardiol 28:217, 1999.)*

that are released in large amounts from the SR to start the cross-bridge cycle.

When the cytosolic calcium level is low, the tropomyosin molecule is twisted in such a way that the myosin heads cannot interact with actin (see Fig. 24-3). Thereby, most cross bridges are in the "blocked position," although some are still in the weakly binding state.[1] As calcium ions increasingly arrive at the start of the contractile cycle and interact with troponin C, the activated troponin C binds tightly to the inhibitory molecule troponin I, which moves to a new position on the thin filament, thereby weakening the interaction between troponin T and tropomyosin (see Fig. 24-3). Ultimately, tropomyosin is repositioned on the thin filament,[1] thereby removing most of the inhibition exerted by tropomyosin on the actin-myosin interaction. Thus, weakly bound or blocked cross bridges enter the strongly bound state, and the cross-bridge cycle is initiated. As the strong cross bridges form, they activate near neighbors and thereby spread the activation process.[1] They also promote further tropomyosin movement to cause more forceful cross-bridge interaction.

MYOSIN AND MOLECULAR BASIS OF MUSCLE CONTRACTION. Each myosin head is the terminal part of a heavy chain. The bodies of two of these chains intertwine and each terminates in a short neck that carries the elongated myosin head (see Fig. 24-3). According to the Rayment model, it is the base of the head, also sometimes called the neck, that changes configuration in the contractile cycle.[3] Together with the bodies of all the other heads, the myosin thick filament is formed. Each lobe of the bilobed head has an ATP-binding pocket (also called nucleotide pocket) and a narrow cleft that extends from the base of this pocket to the actin-binding face.[3] ATP and its breakdown products ADP and P_i bind to the nucleotide pocket close to the myosin ATPase activity that breaks down ATP to its products (see Fig. 24-3). Currently, there is controversy about the role in the contractile cycle of the narrow actin-binding cleft that splits the central 50-kDa segment of the myosin head. According to the revised Rayment model,[1] this cleft responds to the binding of ATP or its breakdown products to the nucleotide pocket in such a way that the conformational changes necessary for movement of the head are produced. According to Dominguez and coworkers,[1] the cleft is closed in the weakly attached states before the power stroke (**Fig. 24-6**) but opens when inorganic phosphate is released through the cleft, whereupon the myosin head attaches strongly to actin to induce the power stroke (see Fig. 24-5D, E).

Starting with the rigor state (see Fig. 24-5A), the binding of ATP to its pocket changes the molecular configuration of the myosin head so that the head detaches from actin to terminate the rigor state (see Fig. 24-5B). Next, the ATPase activity of the myosin head splits ATP into ADP and P_i, and the head flexes (see Fig. 24-5C). As ATP is hydrolyzed, the myosin head binds to an adjacent actin unit. Then P_i is released from the head through the cleft, and there is strong binding of the myosin head to actin (see Fig. 24-5D). Next, the head extends (i.e., straightens). A power stroke takes place, the actin molecule moves by about 10 nm,[1] and the myosin head is now in the rigor state. The pocket then releases ADP, ready for acceptance of ATP and repetition of the cycle. The Rayment model[3] postulates straightening and not flexion of the light chain region of the head (i.e., the neck) that produces the power stroke. The lever arm model[1] is more applicable to many cells and organelles that depend on movement of myosin rather than of actin, for example, for intracellular transport. By contrast, in contracting cardiomyocytes, myosin is fixed and tethered by titin and myosin-binding protein C. The lever arm model proposes that movements of the neck, which is the lever arm, produce large displacements that translate into movement of the whole myosin

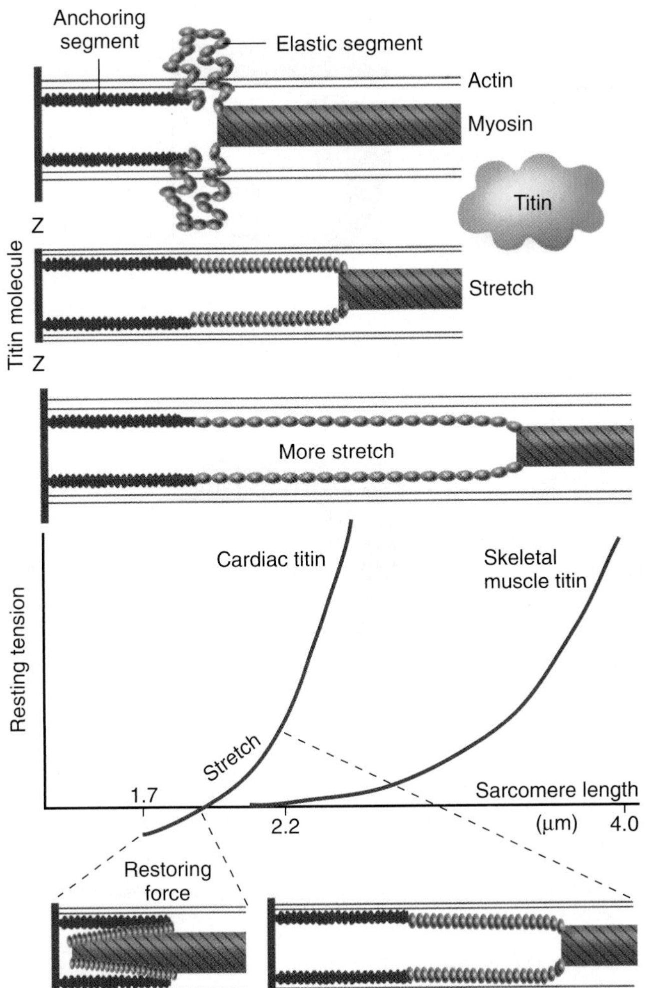

FIGURE 24-4 Titin, a very large elongated protein with elasticity, binds myosin to the Z-line. It may act as a bidirectional spring that develops passive forces in stretched sarcomeres and resting forces in shortened sarcomeres. As the sarcomere is stretched to its maximum physiologic diastolic length of 2.2 μm (see Fig. 24-20), titin first undergoes straightening (up to 2 μm) and then elongation, the latter rapidly increasing the passive forces generated. At low sarcomere lengths, when sarcomeres are slack at about the diastolic limit of 1.85 μm (see Fig. 24-20), the mechanically active elastic domain is folded on top of itself. At even shorter lengths, which may not be physiologic in the intact heart, substantial restoring forces are generated. *(Modified with permission of the American Heart Association from Trombitas K, Jian-Ping J, Granzier H: The mechanically active domain of titin in cardiac muscle. Circ Res 77:856, 1995; and Helmes M, Trombitas K, Granzier H: Titin develops restoring force in rat cardiac myocytes. Circ Res 79:619, 1996.)*

molecule. This model provides evolutionary data that reinforce the crucial nature of movements of the myosin neck (shown as the flexible domain in Fig. 24-5C).

Myosin ATPase activity normally responds to calcium in such a way that increases in calcium concentrations associated with the contraction cycle in the whole heart increase the myosin ATPase activity several-fold in addition to increasing calcium binding to troponin C and force development (see Fig. 24-6).[1]

Myosin heavy chain isoforms help regulate myosin ATPase activity. Each myosin filament consists of two heavy chains (the bodies of which are intertwined, each ending in one head) and four light chains (two in apposition to each head). The heavy chains, containing the myosin ATPase activity on the heads, occur in two isoforms, β and α, of the same molecular weight but with substantially different ATPase activities. The beta–heavy chain (β-MHC) isoform has lower ATPase activity and is the predominant form in the adult human. In small animals, the faster α-MHC form changes to a predominant β-MHC pattern in heart failure.[1]

MYOSIN HEADS: TWO ARE BETTER THAN ONE. The double-headed structure is required to produce the full displacement of actin, about 10 nm, versus only 6 nm with single-headed myosin.[1] The myosin neck is chiefly formed by a long alpha helix (see Fig. 24-3B), surrounded by two light chains (four per bilobed head) that act as a cervical collar. The light chain that is more proximal to the myosin head, the essential light chain (MLC-1), may inhibit the contractile process by interaction with actin. The other regulatory light chain (MLC-2) is a potential site for phosphorylation, for example, in response to beta-adrenergic stimulation. Such phosphorylation (i.e., the gaining of a phosphate grouping) may promote cross-bridge cycling by increasing the affinity of myosin for actin.[1] Mutation of this light chain in one type of human cardiomyopathy impairs the contractile response to tachycardia.[1] In vascular smooth muscle, the phosphorylation that occurs under the influence of the enzyme myosin light chain kinase (MLCK) is an obligatory step in the initiation of the contractile process.

Myosin-binding protein C runs at approximately right angles to the myosin molecules to tether myosin molecules by linking the structures that lie around subfragments of the myosin heads. This binding protein, which stabilizes the myosin head, itself flexes and extends at the level of the light chains. Defects in the binding protein C may be involved in some types of hypertrophic cardiomyopathy.

GRADED EFFECTS OF INCREASED CYTOSOLIC CALCIUM LEVELS ON CROSS-BRIDGE CYCLE. Calcium ions play a crucial role in linking external neurohumoral control of the heart to stimulation of the contractile process by acting at multiple control sites.[1] Calcium interaction with troponin C is essential for cross-bridge cycling. Does calcium act as an on-off switch to regulate the total number of cycling cross bridges? According to this proposal, the enhanced force development in response to a greater calcium ion concentration must be due to recruitment of additional cross bridges. Alternatively, to explain the graded model, there may be (1) a graded response of troponin C to calcium ions, including altered rates of calcium binding and release; (2) a graded response of myosin ATPase to calcium; (3) near-neighbor self-activation, whereby actin-myosin interaction activates additional cross bridges even in the absence of increased binding of calcium to the troponin C of those cross bridges[1]; or (4) alterations in the extent of myosin light chain phosphorylation.[1] Of specific interest is the proposal that tightly bound cross bridges act to spread activation on the thin filament to near-neighbor units to achieve full activation.[1] By such mechanisms, one calcium-troponin complex could turn on as many as 14 actin molecules.

LENGTH-DEPENDENT ACTIVATION. In addition to the cytosolic calcium concentration, the other major factor influencing the strength of contraction is the length of the muscle fiber at the end of diastole, just before the onset of systole. Starling observed that the greater the volume of the heart in diastole, the more forceful the contraction. The increased heart volume translates into an increased muscle length, which acts by a length-sensing mechanism.[1] This relation was previously ascribed to a more optimal overlap between actin and myosin. The current view is that an increased sarcomere length leads to greater sensitivity of the contractile apparatus to the prevailing cytosolic calcium ion concentration.[1] A plausible mechanism for this regulatory change may reside in the decreasing interfilament spacing as the heart muscle is stretched.[1] This satisfactory lattice-dependent explanation for the Frank-Starling relationship has been dealt a setback by the careful x-ray diffraction studies of de Tombe's group.[1] Reducing sarcomere lattice spacing by osmotic compression failed to influence calcium sensitivity. Alternatively, sarcomere stretch increases the passive forces built up by titin,[1] which could in turn hypothetically influence the position of myosin heads. Another proposal, that troponin C is the length sensor, is currently less favored.[1] Probably several mechanisms are at work.

CROSS-BRIDGE CYCLING DIFFERS FROM CARDIAC CONTRACTION-RELAXATION CYCLE. The cardiac cycle of Wiggers (see later) must be distinguished from the cross-bridge cycle.

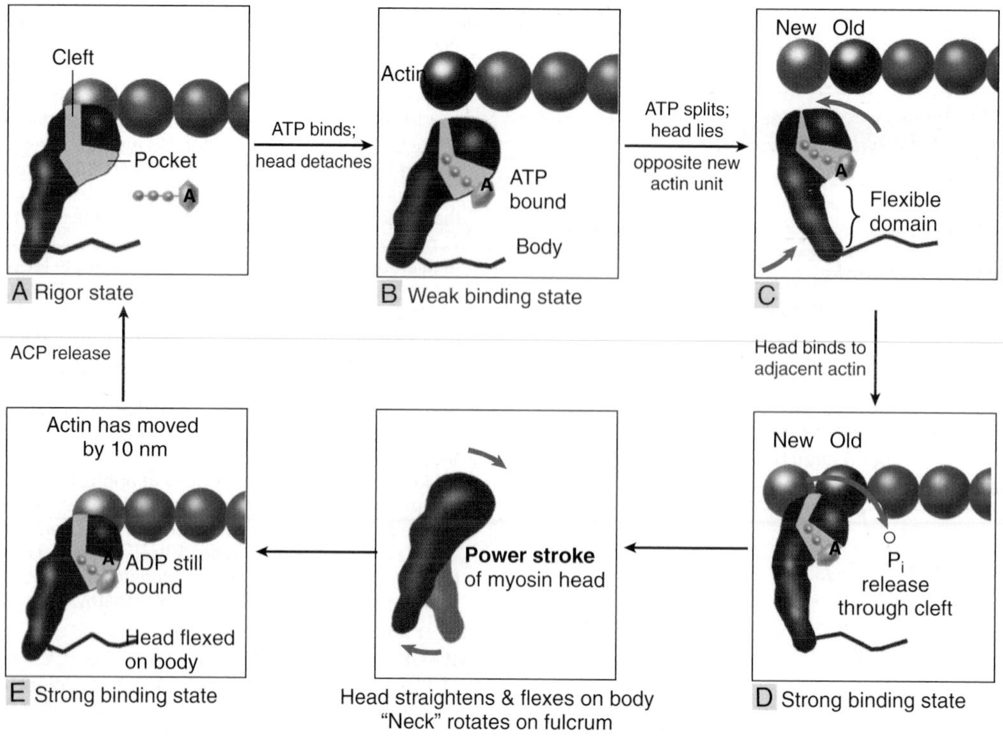

FIGURE 24-5 Cross-bridge cycling molecular model updated from the original Rayment five-step model for interaction between the myosin head and the actin filament,[3] taking into account other models. The cross bridge (only one myosin head depicted) is pear shaped and consists of the catalytic motor domain that interacts with the actin molecule and an extended alpha-helical neck region acting as a lever arm. The nucleotide pocket receiving and binding ATP is a depression near the center of the catalytic domain. The actin-binding cleft bisects the catalytic motor domain. During the cross-bridge cycle, the width of the actin-binding cleft changes in size, although details remain controversial. Starting with the rigor state **(A),** the binding of ATP to the pocket **(B)** is followed by ATP hydrolysis **(C)** that partly closes the actin-binding cleft. The cleft opens when phosphate is released (through the cleft rather than through the pocket), and the myosin head strongly attaches to actin to induce the power stroke **(D, E).** During the power stroke, the myosin head rotates about a fulcrum in the region where the helix terminates within the catalytic motor domain. As the head flexes, the actin filament is displaced by about 10 nm **(E).** In the process, ADP is also released so that the binding pocket becomes vacant. Finally, the rigor state is reached again **(A),** when the myosin head is again ready to receive ATP to reinitiate the cross-bridge cycle. Throughout, the actin monomer with which the myosin head is interacting is speckled with dots. *(Professor J. C. Rüegg of Heidelberg University, Germany, gave valuable advice. For references to Cooke, Holmes, and Dominguez, see Opie.[1])*

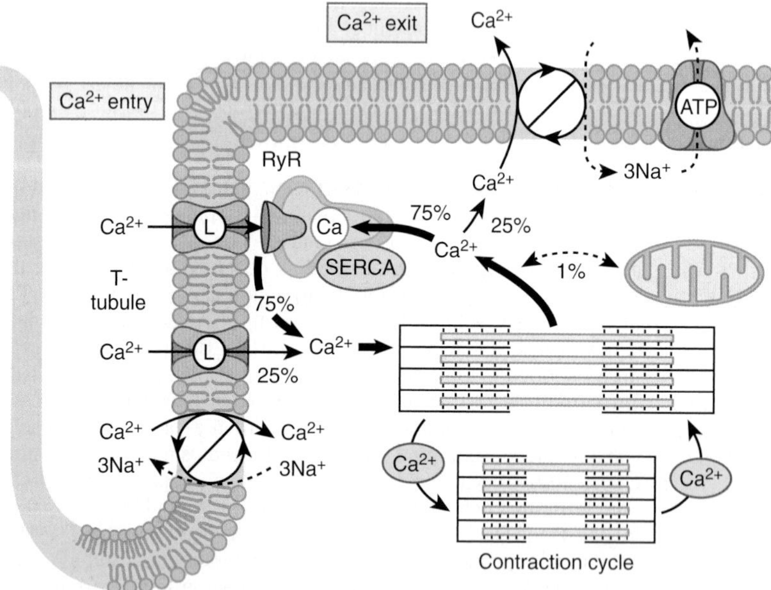

FIGURE 24-6 Calcium fluxes in the myocardium. Crucial features are (1) entry of Ca^{2+} ions via the voltage-sensitive L-type Ca^{2+} channels, acting as a trigger to the release of Ca^{2+} ions from the sarcoplasmic reticulum (SR); (2) the effect of beta-adrenergic stimulation with adenylyl cyclase forming cAMP, the latter helping both to open the Ca^{2+} channel and to increase the rate of uptake of Ca^{2+} into the SR; and (3) exit of Ca^{2+} ions chiefly via the Na^+/Ca^{2+} exchanger, with the sodium pump thereafter extruding the Na^+ ions thus gained. The latter process requires ATP. Note the much higher extracellular (10^{-3} M) than intracellular cytosolic Ca^{2+} values, with much higher calcium values in the SR because of its storage function. Mitochondria can act as a buffer against excessive changes in the free cytosolic calcium concentration. *(From Opie LH: Heart Physiology, From Cell to Circulation. Philadelphia, Lippincott Williams & Wilkins, 2004. © D. M. Bers and L. H. Opie, 2004; also see Bers DM: Cardiac excitation-contraction coupling. Nature 415:198, 2002.)*

The Wiggers cycle reflects the overall pressure changes in the left ventricle, whereas the cross-bridge cycle is the repetitive interaction between myosin heads and actin. According to the Rayment model, the binding of ATP or ADP regulates in part whether the cross bridges would be weak or strong in nature (see Fig. 24-5). So long as enough calcium ions are bound to troponin C, many repetitive cycles of this nature occur. Thus, at any given moment, some myosin heads will be flexing or flexed, some will be extending or extended, some will be attached to actin, and some will be detached from actin. Numerous such cross-bridge cycles, each lasting only a few microseconds, actively move the thin actin filaments toward the central bare area of the thick myosin filaments, thereby shortening the sarcomere. The sum total of all the shortening sarcomeres leads to systole, which is the contraction phase of the cardiac cycle. When calcium ions depart from their binding sites on troponin C, cross-bridge cycling cannot occur, and the diastolic phase of the cardiac cycle sets in.

Myofilament Response to Hemodynamic Demands

Myofilament activity is coupled to the prevailing hemodynamic demands of the circulation. In addition to length-dependent activation, there are two other chief mechanisms. First, there may be variable rates of calcium binding and release from troponin C (as discussed in a previous section). Second, phosphorylation and dephosphorylation of the contractile proteins may help control the extent of activation of the myofilaments. Thus, increased beta-adrenergic–dependent phosphorylation of troponin I reduces the myofilament sensitivity to calcium and thereby leads to an increased rate of relaxation during beta-adrenergic stimulation.[1] Hypothetically, this mechanism enhances the relaxant (lusitropic) effect of increased uptake rates of calcium into the SR. The effects of phosphorylation of other proteins, such as the myosin essential light chains and C protein, still imperfectly understood, may also be important.[1]

FORCE TRANSMISSION. Volume and pressure overload may owe their different effects on myocardial growth to different patterns of force transmission. Whereas increased diastolic forces are transmitted longitudinally via titin to reach the postulated sensor, the MLP protein (see section on titin), increased systolic forces may be transmitted laterally (i.e., at right angles) via the Z-disc and cytoplasmic actin to reach the proteins of the cell-to-matrix junctions, such as the focal adhesion complex. How these mechanical forces become translated into signals that activate the growth pathways, such as those leading to MAP (mitogen-activated protein) kinase, still remains to be discovered.

Current proposals for the onward transmission of mechanical forces from sarcomere show different patterns for systole and diastole, which could explain why greater end-systolic stress leads to thicker myocytes and greater end-diastolic stress to longer myocytes. During systole, the sarcomere shortens as a result of myosin head flexion and movement of actin filaments toward the M-line. Increased horizontal force is exerted on the Z-line, which in turn transmits lateral forces to the sarcolemma by the thin and intermediate filaments, cytoplasmic actin and desmin. Further transmission is to the integrins of the costameres and associated cytoskeletal proteins that connect the stress generated in the Z-lines of the sarcomeres to the extracellular matrix, from where the intracellular hypertrophy program is activated.[4]

During diastole, as the sarcomere stretches, the elastic segment of titin expands and transmits force via MLP, the muscle LIM protein that acts as a mechanical sensor. When long-continued, as in sustained volume overload, MLP-induced stimuli may induce myocyte lengthening as in the dilated failing heart. Further signaling is not clear. Pressure and volume overload may induce distinctly different signal transduction paths; pressure load rapidly activates Akt and the expected downstream kinases, whereas volume loading gives delayed Akt activation not involving the same downstream signals.[5] This clear distinction is consistent with the observation in isolated muscle strip preparations that only afterload (pressure overload) but not preload (volume overload) activates ventricular expression of brain natriuretic peptide (BNP).[6]

CONTRACTILE PROTEINS AND CARDIOMYOPATHY. The concept is that genetic-based hypertrophic and dilated cardiomyopathies produce hearts that not only look and behave differently but have diverse molecular causes. Hypertrophic cardiomyopathy is, in general, linked to mutant genes that cause abnormalities in the force-generating system, such as β-MHC. Less commonly, there may be defects in the genes encoding troponin T, myosin light chain isoforms, troponin I and C isoforms, myosin-binding protein C, and alpha-tropomyosin (see Chaps. 8 and 69). The current hypothesis is that the mutations increase the contractile performance or the energy demand.[7] How such defects translate into hypertrophic cardiomyopathy is still obscure.[7] In contrast, dilated cardiomyopathy can be related to mutations in non–force-generating cytoskeletal proteins, such as dystrophin, nuclear lamin, cytoplasmic actin, and titin, as well as to defects in the enzymes that control the integrity of the matrix (see Chaps. 8 and 25).[8] This distinction between the two types of cardiomyopathy remains useful but is oversimplified, with several examples of overlapping mechanisms.[9]

Calcium Ion Fluxes in Cardiac Contraction-Relaxation Cycle

Calcium Movements and Excitation–Contraction Coupling

Calcium has a crucial role in regulating the contraction and relaxation phases of the cardiac cycle. The details of the associated calcium ion fluxes that link contraction to the wave of excitation (excitation–contraction coupling) are now reasonably well clarified.[1] The generally accepted hypothesis is based on the crucial role of calcium-induced calcium release from the SR. Relatively small amounts of calcium ions, the trigger calcium ions, actually enter and leave the cardiomyocyte during each cardiac cycle, whereas much larger amounts move in and out of the SR (see Fig. 24-6). The basic proposal is that each wave of depolarization traveling down the T tubules opens the L-type calcium channels, which are physically closely approximated to that part of the SR lying close to the T tubule, to activate the calcium release channels, collectively called the ryanodine receptors. Thereby, depolarization releases relatively large amounts of calcium ions into the cytosol in response to the much smaller amounts entering the cardiomyocyte.[1] This process greatly elevates by about 10-fold the concentration of calcium ions in the cytosol. The result is the increasing interaction of calcium ions with troponin C to trigger the contractile process. This theory has received strong support from several sources: (1) the tight proximity of the ryanodine receptors on the SR to the L-type calcium channels of the T tubules, the estimated distance being only 15 nm[10]; (2) the molecular characterization of the calcium-releasing ryanodine receptor on the SR (**Fig. 24-7**); (3) proof of the control of this receptor not only by calcium ions but by beta-adrenergic–mediated phosphorylation and by binding proteins of the FKBP family[11]; and (4) electrophysiologic evidence closely linking the duration of the action potential with the extent of Ca^{2+} release.[1]

Calcium Release and Uptake by the Sarcoplasmic Reticulum

RYANODINE RECEPTORS. Each L-type calcium channel of the sarcolemma controls a cluster of possibly 6 to 20 SR release channels by virtue of anatomic proximity of the calcium channels on the T tubules to the calcium release channels, situated on the SR. The calcium release channel is part of the complex structure known as the ryanodine receptor, so called because it coincidentally binds the potent insecticide ryanodine; it is often abbreviated to RyR2 to indicate the cardiac isoform. Ryanodine receptors have a dual function, both containing the calcium release channels of the SR and acting as scaffolding proteins that localize numerous key regulatory proteins to the junctional complexes.[1] These proteins include the important stabilizing protein (technical term: FKBP-12.6) that responds to phosphorylation to coordinate opening of neighboring ryanodine calcium channels by the process of coupled gating. Phosphatases (see Fig. 24-7) work in the opposite direction. The anatomic basis of the scaffolding function is that part of the ryanodine receptor extends from the membrane of the SR toward the T tubule to constitute the junctional calcium release complex that bridges the gap between the SR and the T tubule. Here the ryanodine receptors are packed in large organized arrays of perhaps 50 to 300 per junction. The ryanodine receptor is very large, and four of these link to form a megacomplex containing one calcium release channel (**Fig. 24-8**). Added to this are all the proteins adhering to the complex via their binding sites, so that the total megacomplex has a molecular weight approximating that of titin. After the wave of depolarization has reached the T tubule and opened the voltage-operated L-type calcium channels, the trigger calcium ions enter the cardiomyocyte to reach the junctional regions

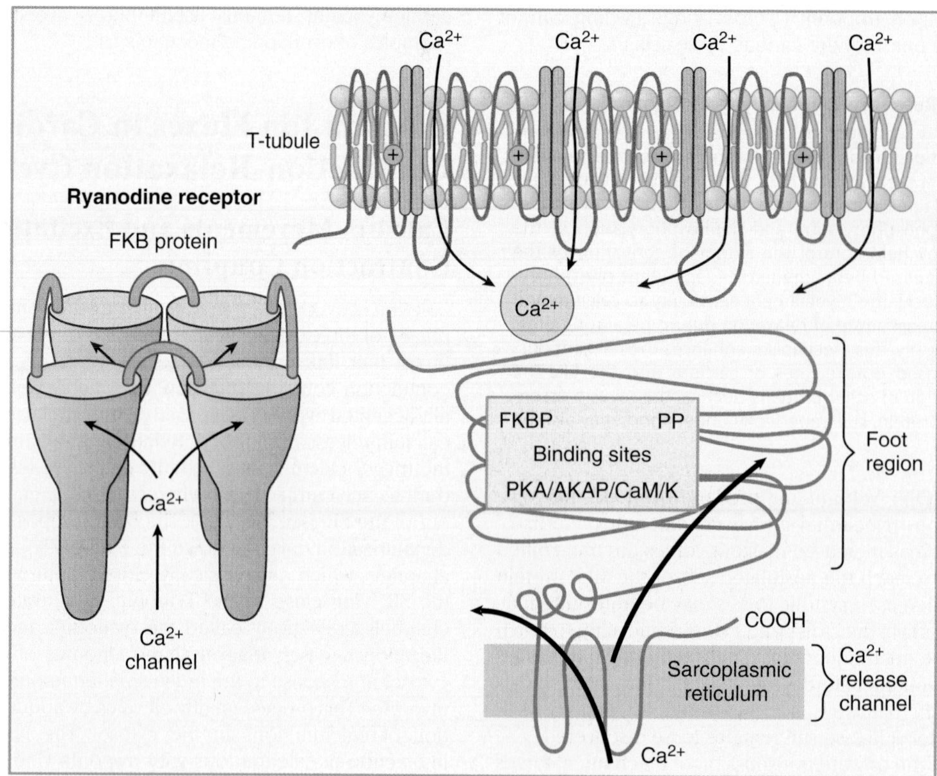

FIGURE 24-7 Role of ryanodine receptor (RyR) in calcium-induced calcium release. The RyR protein forms a link between the T tubule and the SR and is a scaffolding protein (which binds other proteins such as kinases and phosphatases). This makes a macromolecular complex, also called the foot region. One high-affinity RyR is composed of four RyR monomer proteins. The molecular model of one RyR is schematically shown on the right. The four RyR proteins make a single calcium release channel, in a manner similar to the formation of some other ion channels (schematic, left). Depolarization stimulates the L-type calcium channel of the T tubule to allow calcium ion entry. The incoming calcium binds to the RyR to cause molecular conformational changes that result in opening of the calcium release channel and calcium release from the SR. AKAP = anchoring protein for PKA; CaM/K = calmodulin or calmodulin kinase; FKBP = FKBP-12.6 channel stabilizing subunit; PKA = protein kinase A; PP = protein phosphatases. *(From Opie LH: Heart Physiology, From Cell to Circulation. Philadelphia, Lippincott Williams & Wilkins, 2004. © L. H. Opie, 2004.)*

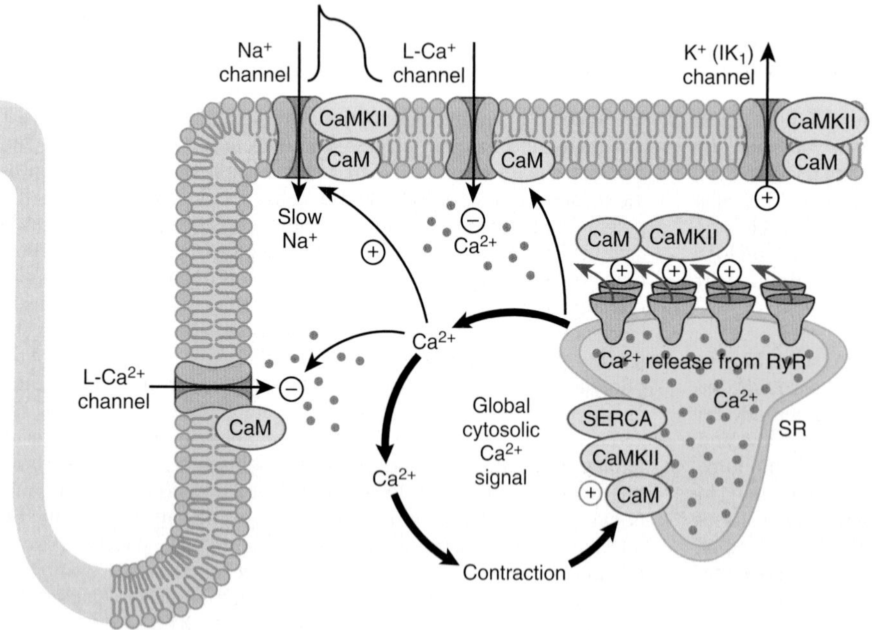

FIGURE 24-8 Role of calmodulin and its kinase in regulating intracellular calcium ion (Ca^{2+}) concentration. The rising cytosolic Ca^{2+} concentration in systole activates the counterbalancing calcium regulator system whereby calcium-calmodulin (CaM) inhibits the inward flow of Ca^{2+} ions through the L-type Ca^{2+} channels and from the ryanodine receptors. This mechanism appears to be a negative feedback system to limit cellular Ca^{2+} gain. The effects of Ca^{2+}/calmodulin-dependent protein kinase II (CaMKII) are less well understood. Some current proposals are that this enzyme helps promote the positive inotropic response during acute beta-adrenergic stimulation when CaMKII (1) limits the extent of Ca^{2+}-dependent inactivation and enhances Ca^{2+} current amplitude and (2) increases the fraction of SR Ca^{2+} released from ryanodine receptors (RyR) in response to the Ca^{2+} current trigger. When CaMKII expression and activity are chronically increased, as may occur during chronic beta-adrenergic stimulation[13] and in heart failure, proposed adverse consequences include proarrhythmic effects.[14] *(Dr. Donald M. Bers is thanked for valuable assistance.)*

of the SR with their ryanodine receptors. The result is a change in the molecular configuration of the ryanodine receptor that opens the calcium release channel of the SR to discharge calcium ions into the subsarcolemmal space between the foot and the T tubule and thence into the cytosol.

PHYSIOLOGIC IMPLICATIONS: FIGHT OR FLIGHT VERSUS HEART RATE–INDUCED CALCIUM RELEASE. An interesting proposal is that there are different sites of phosphorylation for the catecholamine-mediated fight-or-flight reaction versus the heart rate–induced increase in contraction. During fight or flight, protein kinase A (PKA), linked to its anchoring protein, AKAP (see Fig. 24-7), targets the stabilizing protein FKBP-12.6 (that binds FK-506, also called calstabin2) at a specific site, serine 2809. Thus, FKBP-12.6 is detached from the RyR, which is now temporally destabilized to allow a greater calcium efflux from the SR through the RyR channel.[12] A refined study on isolated single L-type calcium channels proves that physiologic beta-adrenergic acceleration of calcium release from the SR can proceed by this PKA-mediated mechanism.[11] An alternative mechanism for calcium leakage from the SR is provided by activation of the calcium-dependent enzyme calmodulin-dependent protein kinase II (CaMKII).[13,14] Yet other data suggest that PKA can activate CaMKII.[13]

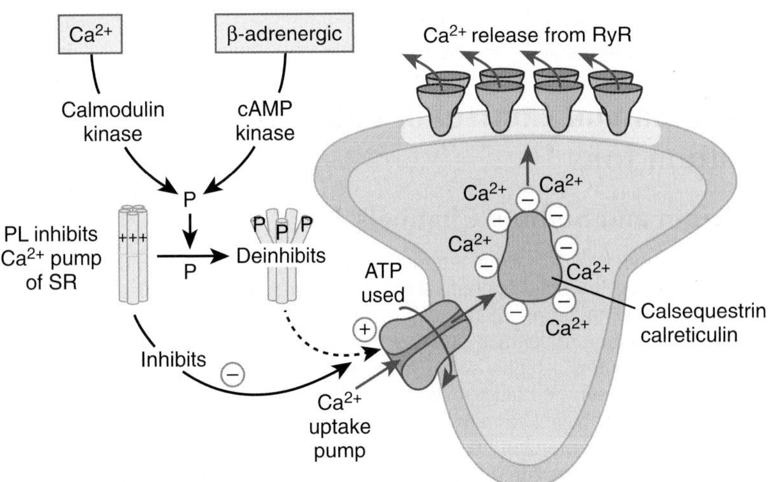

FIGURE 24-9 Mechanism of calcium uptake into the sarcoplasmic reticulum (SR) by the energy-requiring calcium pump SERCA2a. An increased rate of uptake of calcium into the SR enhances the rate of relaxation (lusitropic effect). Phospholamban (PL), when phosphorylated (P), removes the inhibition exerted on the calcium pump by its dephosphorylated form (positively charged hypothetical molecule on the left). Thereby, calcium (Ca^{2+}) uptake is increased either in response to an enhanced cytosolic calcium or in response to beta-adrenergic stimulation. Note the proposal that calmodulin kinase (CaMKII) can be a second messenger of the beta-adrenergic system.[13] Thus, there are two phosphorylations activating phospholamban at two distinct sites, and their effects are additive. cAMP = cyclic adenosine monophosphate; RyR = ryanodine receptor. *(Modified from Opie LH: Heart Physiology, From Cell to Circulation. Philadelphia, Lippincott Williams & Wilkins, 2004. © L. H. Opie, 2004.)*

TURNING OFF CALCIUM RELEASE: ROLE OF CALMODULIN KINASE. The rise of cytosolic calcium that triggers contraction comes to an end as the wave of excitation passes, no more calcium ions enter, and the release of calcium from the SR ceases. This turn-off of release is not as well understood as control of calcium release from the SR, but it is important in avoiding cytosolic calcium overload with potentially serious consequences such as arrhythmias and impaired contraction-relaxation cycles. There are several proposals to explain turn-off, but the best documented implicates the role of the calcium regulator protein calmodulin, which is a small but ubiquitously distributed protein of 16,700 Da that is activated when calcium binds to its high-affinity binding sites to become calcium-calmodulin (CaM) (see Fig. 24-8). The latter in turn also activates the calmodulin kinase II (CaMKII) system. The overall effects are complex and not yet well understood. Activation of CaM closes the previously open L channels to help shut off calcium ion entry into the cell.[10] Because calcium is continuously removed from the cytosol by SERCA and Na^+/Ca^{2+} exchange, the overall effect is that the cytosolic calcium ion concentration starts to fall and diastole is initiated. As the cytosolic calcium decreases, calcium binding to troponin C lessens, tropomyosin again starts to inhibit the interaction between actin and myosin, and relaxation proceeds. On the other hand, the effects of CaMKII are much more complex and appear to play a physiologic role in acute beta-adrenergic stimulation.[13,14] There is a converse pathologic role especially in chronic heart failure,[13,14] when the major effects appear to include (1) increased inflow of the slow sodium current, (2) promotion of calcium leak through the ryanodine receptors to promote release of calcium ions (although this is controversial),[15] and (3) enhancement of calcium entry into the SR by stimulation of the Ca uptake pump, SERCA.[10] The overall effect is calcium dysregulation, especially in chronic beta-adrenergic stimulation.[13] Furthermore, such chronic stimulation can promote several proarrhythmic changes in several of the ion channels.[14]

Calcium Uptake by SERCA into the Sarcoplasmic Reticulum

Calcium ions are taken up into the SR by the activity of the calcium pump called SERCA (sarcoendoplasmic reticulum Ca^{2+}-ATPase) that constitutes nearly 90% of the protein component of the SR. It is about 115 kDa, and it straddles the SR membrane in such a way that part of it actually protrudes into the cytosol. It exists in several isoforms, of which the dominant cardiac form is SERCA2a. For each mole of ATP hydrolyzed by this enzyme, two calcium ions are taken up to accumulate within the SR (**Fig. 24-9**). The source of the energy is at least in part from cytosolic generation of ATP through glycolysis.[16] Important links between SERCA and cardiac contractile activity are found in a variety of animal and human studies. For example, in heart failure, the expression or functional activity of SERCA2a is downregulated (see Chap. 25).

Phospholamban was so named by its discoverers, Tada and Katz, to mean "phosphate receiver."[17] The activity of phospholamban is governed by a state of phosphorylation, a process that alters the molecular configuration of SERCA to promote its activity (see Fig. 24-9). There are two major protein kinases involved: PKA, activated by beta-adrenergic stimulation and cyclic adenosine monophosphate (cAMP); and CaMKII, activated by calcium ions and beta-adrenoceptor stimulation. Phosphorylation of phospholamban enhances the uptake of calcium by SERCA, thus increasing the rate of relaxation. Two major protein kinases involved, the one activated by PKA in response to beta-adrenergic stimulation and cAMP and the other by calcium ions and calcium–calmodulin kinase, act at two different phosphorylation sites.[1] When phospholamban responds to beta-adrenergic stimulation of the cardiomyocyte by enhancing the uptake of calcium by SERCA into the SR, thus increasing the rate of relaxation, the major activation is phosphorylation of the PKA site. The further proposal is that the enhanced store of calcium in the SR correspondingly increases the amount of calcium released by the ryanodine receptor in response to subsequent waves of depolarization to give an increased rate and force of contraction.[1] This sequence is strongly supported by a transgenic mouse model, totally deficient in phospholamban, in which hyperdynamic hearts with maximal rates of contraction and relaxation have attenuated responses to added beta-adrenergic stimulation by isoproterenol. Conversely, in hearts overexpressing phospholamban, cardiac function is depressed.[1]

Calcium, taken up into the SR by the calcium uptake pump, is stored within the SR before further release. The highly charged storage protein calsequestrin is found in that part of the SR that lies near the T tubules. Calcium stored with calsequestrin becomes available for the release process as calsequestrin discharges Ca^{2+} into the inner mouth of the calcium release channel. This process replaces those calcium ions liberated from the outer mouth into the cytosol. Calreticulin is another Ca^{2+}-storing protein, similar in structure to calsequestrin and probably similar in function. Hypothetically, calsequestrin and two other proteins located in the SR membrane (junctin and triadin) may help regulate the properties of the ryanodine receptor.[1]

Sarcolemmal Control of Calcium and Sodium Ions

Calcium and Sodium Channels

All current models of excitation-contraction coupling ascribe a crucial role to the voltage-induced opening of the sarcolemmal L-type calcium channels in the initiation of the contractile process. Channels are pore-forming macromolecular proteins that span the sarcolemmal lipid bilayer to allow a highly selective pathway for ion transfer into the heart cell when the channel changes from a closed to an open state. Ion channels have two major properties, gating and permeation. Guarding each channel are two or more hypothetical gates that control its opening. Ions can permeate through the channel only when both gates are open. In the case of the sodium and calcium channels, which are best understood, the activation gate is shut at the normal resting membrane potential and the inactivation gate is open, so that the channels are voltage gated. Depolarization opens the activation gate.

MOLECULAR STRUCTURE OF L-TYPE CALCIUM CHANNELS. There is a superfamily of voltage-gated ion channels that includes both the sodium and calcium channels and some of the potassium channels. The potassium channels have the simpler structure, from which it is thought that the more complex sodium and calcium channels evolved. Both sodium and calcium channels contain a major alpha subunit with four transmembrane subunits or domains, very similar to each other in structure.[16] In addition, both sodium and calcium channels include in their overall structure a number of other subunits whose function is less well understood, such as the alpha subunit. Each of the four transmembrane domains of the alpha subunit is made up of six helices, folded in on itself, so that the four S5-S6 spans structurally combine to form the single functioning pore of each calcium channel (see Fig. 1-11 of Opie[16]). Activation is now understood in molecular terms as the change in charge on the fourth transmembrane segment, S4, called the voltage sensor, of each of the four subunits of the sodium or calcium channel.[16] Inactivation is the process whereby the current initially elicited by depolarization decreases with time despite continuation of the original stimulus. The alpha subunit acts to enhance the calcium current flow through the beta-subunit pores. Channels are not simply open or closed. Rather, the open state is the last of a sequence of many molecular states, varying from a fully closed to a fully open configuration. Therefore, it is more correct to speak of the probability of channel opening.

CURRENT ACTIVATION AND DEACTIVATION. Having been activated by depolarization, the L-type calcium current is inactivated by (1) the rising voltage during depolarization, at a more positive potential than for activation, and (2) the rising internal calcium ion concentration. Especially the calcium flowing from the ryanodine receptor that pushes up the subsarcolemmal internal calcium ion concentration near the mouth of the L channels of the T tubules terminates current flow.[16]

T- AND L-TYPE CALCIUM CHANNELS. There are two major subpopulations of sarcolemmal calcium channels relevant to the cardiovascular system, namely, the T channels and the L channels. The T (transient) channels open at a more negative voltage, have short bursts of opening, and do not interact with conventional calcium antagonist drugs.[16] The T channels presumably account for the earlier phase of the opening of the calcium channel, which may also give them a special role in the early electrical depolarization of the sinoatrial node and hence in initiation of the heart beat. Although T channels are found in atrial cells, their existence in normal ventricular cells is controversial. T channels are not found in T tubules.[1]

L-CALCIUM CHANNEL REGULATION. The sarcolemmal L (long-lasting) channels, the standard calcium channels found in the myocardium and the T tubules, are involved in calcium-induced calcium release and are inhibited by calcium channel blockers such as verapamil, diltiazem, and the dihydropyridines. During beta-adrenergic stimulation, cAMP increases within the cell, and phosphate groups are transferred from ATP to the alpha$_1$ subunit.[16] Thereby, the electrical charges near the inner mouth of the nearby pores are altered to induce changes in the molecular conformation of the pores, so that there is an increased probability of opening of the L calcium channels. The L channels are also part of the cellular cardiac protective pathway leading from insulin-like growth factor (IGF-1) via phosphatidylinositol 3-kinase and Akt to physiologic hypertrophy and protection from ischemia-reperfusion injury.[18]

SODIUM CHANNELS: ROLE OF CALMODULIN KINASE. Voltage-gated sodium channels are activated on depolarization of the cell membrane, which leads to rapid influx of Na^+, generating the fast upstroke of the action potential. Under normal conditions, Na^+ channels inactivate a few milliseconds after depolarization. However, some Na^+ channels remain open (or reopen), and a small but persistent influx of Na^+ occurs through the plateau of the action potential, generating the late sodium current (I_{Na}). This current is characterized by an ultraslow, voltage-independent inactivation and reactivation.[19,20] Although the amplitude of late I_{Na} is small compared with peak I_{Na}, because of its prolonged duration over hundreds of milliseconds, a substantial sodium influx occurs. CaMKII seems to play a significant role in promoting the late sodium current under conditions of calcium overload, ischemia, heart failure, and excess free radicals (see Fig. 24-8).[19]

Ion Exchangers and Pumps

To balance the small amount of calcium ions entering the heart cell with each depolarization, a similar quantity must leave the cell by one of two processes. First, calcium can be exchanged for sodium ions entering by the Na^+/Ca^{2+} exchanger. Second, an ATP-consuming sarcolemmal calcium pump can transfer calcium into the extracellular space against a concentration gradient.

SODIUM-CALCIUM EXCHANGER. During relaxation, the sarcoplasmic calcium uptake pump and the Na^+/Ca^{2+} exchanger compete for the removal of cytosolic calcium, with the SR pump normally being dominant.[1] Restitution of calcium balance takes place by the activity of a series of transsarcolemmal exchangers, the chief of which is the Na^+/Ca^{2+} exchanger. The direction of ion exchange is responsive to the membrane potential and to the concentrations of sodium and calcium ions on either side of the sarcolemma. Because sodium and calcium ions can exchange either inward or outward in response to the membrane potential, there must be a specific membrane potential, called the reversal or equilibrium potential, at which the ions are so distributed that they can move as easily the one way as the other. The reversal potential may lie about halfway between the resting membrane potential and the potential of the fully depolarized state.

The major factor influencing the activity of the exchanger is the concentration of sodium and calcium ions on either side of the sarcolemma. Thus, of the calcium entering the cardiomyocyte with each depolarization-induced opening of the calcium channel, normally about 25% is extruded by this exchanger. This is basically all the calcium that enters the cell through the L-type calcium channel (see Fig. 24-6). In this situation, the exchanger is operating in the forward mode (Na^+ in, Ca^{2+} out). However, changing the membrane potential from the resting value of, say, −85 mV to +20 mV in the phase of rapid depolarization of the action potential and entry of sodium ions will therefore briefly reverse the direction of Na^+/Ca^{2+} exchange. Thus, the sodium ions that have just entered during the opening of the sodium channel will tend to leave, and calcium ions will tend to enter. This process is called reverse mode exchange. Such transsarcolemmal calcium entry may participate in calcium-induced calcium release.[1] As discussed in Chap. 25, there is evidence that enhanced reversed exchange contributes to the slow decline of the Ca^{2+} transient,[16] which may help explain delayed diastolic relaxation (see section on ventricular relaxation). Prolongation of the action potential duration also provokes reverse mode exchange, with risk of ventricular arrhythmias.[1] Also relevant is the influence of phospholemman, a newly discovered sarcolemmal protein that, when it is phosphorylated by PKA, as during the excess beta-adrenergic stimulation of heart failure, limits the Na^+/Ca^{2+} exchanger.[21] Such inhibition of normal forward exchange could potentially retain calcium within the myocyte and exaggerate diastolic calcium overload of heart failure.

Heart Rate and Na^+/Ca^{2+} Exchanger

This exchanger may participate in the force-frequency relationship (treppe or Bowditch phenomenon). According to the sodium pump lag hypothesis, the rapid accumulation of calcium ions during fast stimulation of the myocardium outstrips the ability of the Na^+/Ca^{2+} exchanger and the sodium pump to achieve return to ionic normality. The result is an accumulation of calcium ions within the SR and an increased force of contraction.

SODIUM PUMP (NA^+,K^+-ATPASE). The sarcolemma becomes highly permeable to Na^+ only during the opening of the Na^+ channel during early depolarization, and Na^+ will also enter during the exit of Ca^{2+} by Na^+/Ca^{2+} exchange. Most of this influx of Na^+ across the sarcolemma must be corrected by the activity of the Na^+/K^+ pump, also called the Na^+,K^+-ATPase or simply the Na^+ pump. The pump is activated by internal Na^+ or external K^+.[1] One ATP molecule is used per transport cycle. The ions are first secluded within the pump protein and then extruded to either side. Although there has been some dispute about the exact ratio of Na^+ to K^+ ions that are pumped, a generally accepted model is that for each three Na^+ exported, two K^+ are imported. During this process, one positive charge must leave the cell. Hence, the pump is electrogenic and is also called the electrogenic Na^+ pump.[1] The current induced by sustained activity of the pump may contribute about −10 mV to the resting membrane potential.[16] Because the pump must extrude Na^+ ions entering either by Na^+/Ca^{2+} exchange or by the Na^+ channel, its sustained activity is essential for the maintenance of normal ion balance.

Beta-Adrenergic Signal Systems

During the sympathetic adrenergic response, norepinephrine is released into the synaptic cleft from small swellings, the terminal varicosities, lying on minute end branches of the neurons of the adrenergic nervous system (**Fig. 24-10**). Norepinephrine is synthesized in the varicosities via two compounds called dopa and dopamine and ultimately from the amino acid tyrosine, which is taken up from the circulation. The norepinephrine thus synthesized is stored within the terminals in storage granules (or vesicles) to be released on stimulation by an adrenergic nervous impulse. Thus, when central stimulation increases during excitement or exercise, an increased number of adrenergic impulses liberate an increased amount of norepinephrine from the terminals into the synaptic cleft. Most of the released norepinephrine is taken up again by the nerve terminal varicosities to reenter the storage vesicles or to be metabolized. The norepinephrine remaining in the synaptic cleft interacts with the postsynaptic beta-adrenergic receptors in the heart and alpha-adrenergic receptors in the arterioles. From these receptors, the messages are passed on by a series of messengers, with two major physiologic end results. Neuromodulation is the process whereby the release of norepinephrine from the terminal neurons is either increased or decreased. Increased beta-adrenergic activity causes the heart to beat faster with stronger contractions, whereas increased alpha-adrenergic activity causes arteriolar constriction to increase the blood pressure (**Table 24-2**). Norepinephrine release is lessened when there is increased vagally mediated cholinergic activity, as at night or in highly trained persons, when the muscarinic presynaptic receptors on the terminal neurons are stimulated (see Fig. 24-10). In these conditions, the heart rate and blood pressure fall. Other negative neuromodulators, decreasing the release of norepinephrine, include the local messengers adenosine and nitric oxide

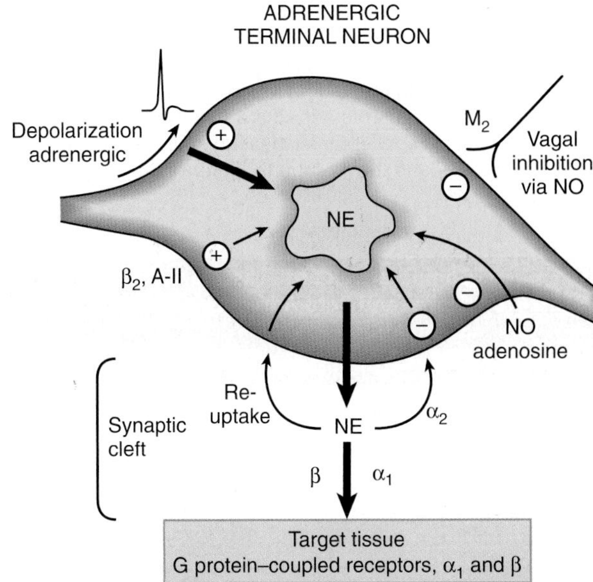

FIGURE 24-10 Control of release of norepinephrine (NE) from terminal neuron. NE is released from the storage granules of the terminal sympathetic neurons into the narrow synaptic cleft that separates the terminals from the G protein–coupled receptors (GPCRs) located in the sarcolemma of the myocytes of the heart or arterial wall. In cardiomyocytes, beta-adrenergic receptors dominate so that their stimulation increases heart rate and contractile force. In arterioles, NE has predominantly vasoconstrictive effects acting via postsynaptic $alpha_1$ receptors (see Fig. 24-17). In addition, NE stimulates presynaptic $alpha_2$ receptors to invoke feedback inhibition of its own release, thereby modulating excess release of NE. Parasympathetic cholinergic stimulation, acting via nitric oxide (NO, see Fig. 24-16), inhibits the release of NE and thereby indirectly reduces the heart rate or causes vasodilation. Circulating epinephrine (E) stimulates vascular vasodilatory $beta_2$ receptors but also presynaptic receptors on the nerve terminal that promote release of NE. Angiotensin II is also powerfully vasoconstrictive, acting by stimulation of NE release (presynaptic receptors, schematically shown to the left of the terminal neuron) and also directly on arteriolar receptors. A-II or angio-II = angiotensin II; M_2 = muscarinic receptor, subtype 2. *(Modified from Opie LH: Heart Physiology, From Cell to Circulation. Philadelphia, Lippincott Williams & Wilkins, 2004. © L. H. Opie, 2004.)*

formed during exercise. Conversely, a powerful positive neuromodulator stimulating the release of norepinephrine and vasoconstriction is angiotensin II.

Beta-Adrenergic Receptor Subtypes

Cardiac beta-adrenergic receptors are chiefly the $beta_1$ subtype, whereas most noncardiac receptors are $beta_2$. There are also $beta_2$ receptors in the human heart, about 20% of the total beta receptor population in the left ventricle and about twice as high a percentage in the atria. Whereas the $beta_1$ receptors are linked to the stimulatory G protein G_s, a component of the G protein–adenylyl cyclase system, $beta_2$ receptors are linked to both G_s and the inhibitory G_i, so that controversially their signaling pathway bifurcates at the very first postreceptor step.[1] Hypothetically, $beta_2$ receptors are normally more strongly coupled to G_s; but in heart failure, this coupling is weakened and that to G_i is strengthened.[1] The beta-adrenergic receptor site is highly stereospecific, the best fit among catecholamines being obtained with the synthetic agent isoproterenol (ISO) rather than with the naturally occurring catecholamines norepinephrine (NE) and epinephrine (E). In the case of $beta_1$ receptors, the order of agonist activity is ISO > E = NE, whereas in the case of $beta_2$ receptors, the order is ISO > E > NE. Human $beta_1$ and $beta_2$ receptors have now both been cloned.[1] The transmembrane domains are held to be the sites of agonist and antagonist binding, whereas the cytoplasmic domains interact with G proteins.

G Proteins

THE STIMULATORY G PROTEIN G_S. G proteins are a superfamily of proteins that bind guanine triphosphate (GTP) and other guanine nucleotides. G proteins are crucial in carrying the signal onward from the first messenger and its receptor to the activity of the membrane-bound enzyme system that produces the second messenger, cAMP (**Figs. 24-11 and 24-12**).[1] The triple combination of the beta receptor, the G protein complex, and adenylyl cyclase is termed the beta-adrenergic system. The G protein itself is a heterotrimer composed of G_α, G_β, and G_γ, which on receptor stimulation splits into the α subunit that is bound to GTP and the $\beta\gamma$ subunit. Either of these subunits may regulate differing effectors, such as adenylyl cyclase, phospholipase C, and ion channels. The activity of adenylyl cyclase is controlled by two different G protein complexes, namely, G_s, which stimulates, and G_i, which inhibits. The α subunit of G_s (α_s) combines with GTP and then separates from the other two subunits to enhance activity of adenylyl cyclase. The β and γ subunits appear to be linked structurally and in function.

TABLE 24-2 Comparative Cardiovascular Effects of Alpha- and Beta-Adrenergic Receptor Stimulation

	ALPHA$_1$ MEDIATED	BETA MEDIATED
Electrophysiologic effects	±	++ Conduction Pacemaker Heart rate
Myocardial mechanics	±	++ Contractility Stroke volume Cardiac output
Myocardial metabolism	± Glycolysis	++ O_2 uptake↑ ATP
Signal systems	GPCR coupled, can activate MAP kinase	GPCR coupled, can activate MAP kinase
Coronary arterioles	++ Constriction	+ Direct dilation +++ Indirect dilation (metabolic)
Peripheral arterioles	+++ Constriction SVR↑ SBP↑	+ Dilation SVR↓ SBP↓

GPCR = G protein–coupled receptor; SBP = systolic blood pressure; SVR = systemic vascular resistance.

Modified from Opie LH: Heart Physiology, From Cell to Circulation. 4th ed. Philadelphia, Lippincott Williams & Wilkins, 2004.

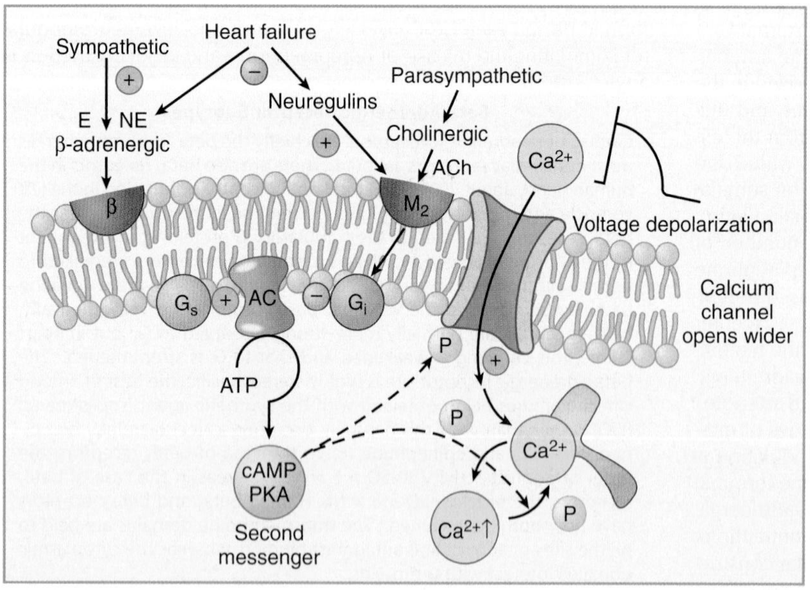

FIGURE 24-11 Interaction between sympathetic and parasympathetic systems could best be explained by countervailing influences on the second messenger, cAMP, mediated respectively by the stimulatory or inhibitory G proteins G_s and G_i. In response to M_2 receptor stimulation, note formation of G_i, with inhibitory effects on the formation of cAMP. AC = adenylyl cyclase; ACh = acetylcholine; E = epinephrine; M_2 = muscarinic receptor, subtype 2; NE = norepinephrine; P = phosphate group; PKA = protein kinase A. *(Modified from Opie LH: Heart Physiology, From Cell to Circulation. Philadelphia, Lippincott Williams & Wilkins, 2004. © L. H. Opie, 2004.)*

THE INHIBITORY G PROTEIN G_i. In contrast, a second trimeric GTP-binding protein, G_i, is responsible for inhibition of adenylyl cyclase.[1] During cholinergic signaling, the muscarinic receptor is stimulated, and GTP binds to the inhibitory α subunit, α_i. The latter then dissociates from the other two components of the G protein complex, which are, as in the case of G_s, the combined $\beta\gamma$ subunits. The $\beta\gamma$ subunits act as follows. By stimulating the enzyme GTPase, they break down the active α_s subunit (α_s-GTP) so that the activation of adenylyl cyclase in response to alpha stimulation becomes less. Furthermore, the $\beta\gamma$ subunit activates the K_{ACh} channel, which in turn can inhibit the sinoatrial node to contribute to the bradycardic effect of cholinergic stimulation. The α_i subunit activates another potassium channel (K_{ATP}), whose physiologic function in the myocardium is still unclear. Preconditioning may link pathophysiologically to this channel (see Chap. 52).

THE THIRD G PROTEIN, G_q. This links a group of heptahelical (*hepta*, seven) myocardial receptors, including the alpha-adrenergic receptor and those for angiotensin II and endothelin, to another membrane-associated enzyme, phospholipase C, and thence to protein kinase C (see later). G_q has at least four isoforms, of which two have been found in the heart. This G protein, unlike G_i, is not susceptible to inhibition by the pertussis toxin. Overexpression of G_q in mice induces a dilated cardiomyopathy,[1] which is of interest because angiotensin II and endothelin, which act through G_q, are overactive in human heart failure. Conversely, when the activity of G_q is genetically inhibited, the hypertrophic response to pressure overload is attenuated, wall stress increases, but cardiac function is relatively well maintained.

Alpha-Adrenergic Receptors

There are two types of alpha-adrenergic receptors. Those situated on the sarcolemma are the postsynaptic or postjunctional vasoconstrictor alpha$_1$ receptors; those situated on the terminal varicosities are called the presynaptic or prejunctional alpha$_2$ receptors (see Fig. 24-10). Norepinephrine can inhibit its own release from the terminal neurons, acting on the presynaptic alpha$_2$-adrenergic receptors, whereas the postsynaptic alpha$_1$-adrenergic receptors act on the arteriolar sarcolemma to regulate arterial tone. An alpha$_1$-adrenergic receptor mediates the response in which the effects resemble those of the pharmacologic agent phenylephrine. Among catecholamines, alpha$_1$-agonist potencies are NE > E > ISO. It is norepinephrine liberated from nerve terminals that is the chief physiologic stimulus to vascular alpha$_1$-adrenergic activity. Both alpha$_1$ and alpha$_2$ receptors are also found in the myocardium, yet despite extensive research, their physiologic function remains much more clearly defined in the peripheral vasculature than in the myocardium.[22] The alpha$_1$ receptor subtype 1A is pathologically involved in cardiac remodeling, partially acting through the sarcolemmal transient receptor potential (Trp) channel family, which promotes calcium ion entry that links to calcineurin and growth pathways.[22]

COUPLING OF ALPHA$_1$ RECEPTOR BY G PROTEINS. This is another example of a G protein–coupled receptor. When an agonist occupies the

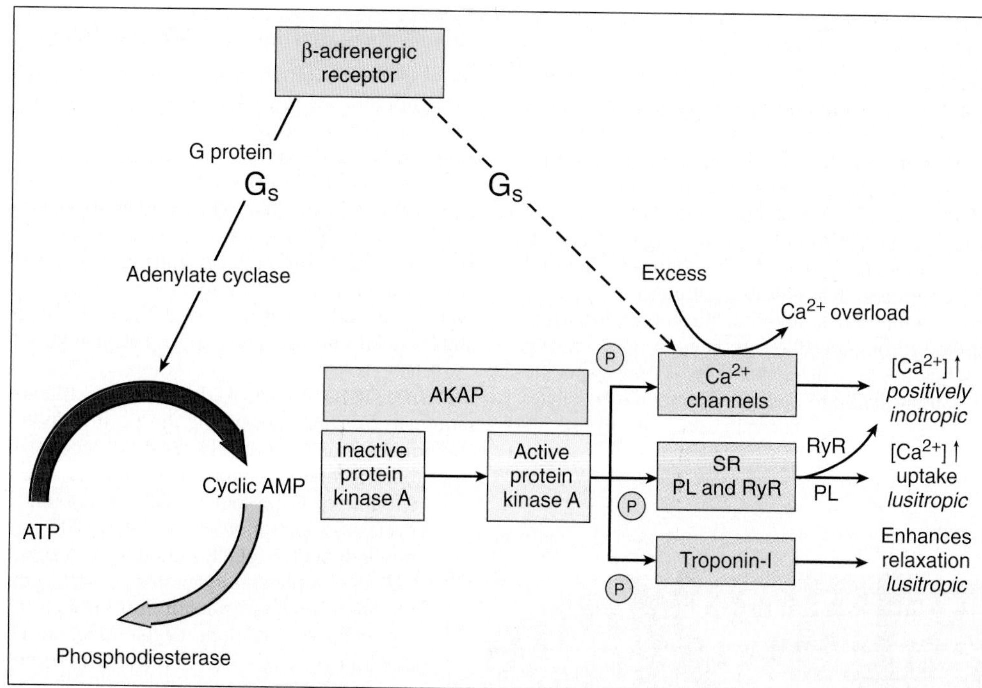

FIGURE 24-12 Key role of protein kinase A in the beta-adrenergic response. The major intracellular effects of beta-agonist catecholamines are by formation of cAMP, which increases the activity of the cAMP-dependent protein kinase A (PKA). PKA achieves its optimal intracellular site by localizing to the scaffolding protein AKAP (A-kinase anchoring protein), whereupon PKA phosphorylates various proteins concerned with contraction and relaxation. SR = sarcoplasmic reticulum; PL = phospholamban; RyR = ryanodine receptor. For inotropic and lusitropic mechanisms, see Figure 21-13. *(From Opie LH: Heart Physiology, From Cell to Circulation. Philadelphia, Lippincott Williams & Wilkins, 2004. © L. H. Opie, 2004.)*

alpha$_1$ receptor, members of the G protein family, such as G_h and G_q, couple the receptor to the activity of the sarcolemmal enzyme system phospholipase C to form phosphatidyl inositol. The latter in turn is split into two components, inositol triphosphate (IP_3) and 1,2-diacylglycerol (DAG), each a second messenger. IP_3 stimulates the release of calcium from the SR, which explains why alpha receptor stimulation can cause vascular smooth muscle to contract without any entry of calcium from the outside. DAG is the messenger that activates protein kinase C and hence eventually the MAP kinase complex, which in turn helps regulate growth (see later, Fig. 24-26).

Positive Inotropic Effect of Alpha$_1$ Stimulation

This effect is not thought to be of major importance in the normal myocardium, when the prime regulation of contraction is through the beta-adrenergic system. Nonetheless, the small positive inotropic effect associated with the formation of IP_3 could come into play in heart failure as a supportive positive inotropic mechanism.

Cyclic Adenosine Monophosphate and Protein Kinase A

ADENYLYL CYCLASE. This is a transmembrane enzyme system, also called adenylate or adenyl cyclase, that responds to input from G proteins. When stimulated by G_s, adenylyl cyclase produces the second messenger cAMP, which then acts through a further series of intracellular signals and specifically the third messenger, protein kinase A (PKA), to increase cytosolic calcium transients. In contrast, cholinergic stimulation exerts inhibitory influences, largely on the heart rate but also on contraction, acting at least in part by decreasing the rate of formation of cAMP.

Adenylyl cyclase is the only enzyme system producing cAMP and specifically requires low concentrations of ATP (and magnesium) as substrate. Surprisingly, the proposed molecular structure resembles certain channel proteins, such as that of the calcium channel. Most of the protein is located on the cytoplasmic side, the presumed site of interaction with the G protein. Another cyclic nucleotide, cyclic guanosine monophosphate (cGMP), acts as a second messenger for some aspects of vagal activity. In vascular smooth muscle, cGMP is the second messenger of the nitric oxide messenger system. These messenger chemicals are present in the heart cell in minute concentrations, that of cAMP being roughly about 10^{-9} M and that of cGMP about 10^{-11} M. cAMP has a rapid turnover as a result of a constant dynamic balance between its formation by adenylyl cyclase and its removal by another enzyme, phosphodiesterase. In general, directional changes in the tissue content of cAMP can be related to directional changes in cardiac contractile activity. For example, beta-adrenergic stimulation increases both, whereas beta blockade inhibits the increases induced by beta-agonists. Forskolin, a direct stimulator of adenylyl cyclase, increases cAMP and contractile activity. Adenosine, acting through A_1 receptors, inhibits adenylyl cyclase, decreases cAMP, and lessens contractile activity. A number of hormones or peptides can couple to myocardial adenylyl cyclase independently of the beta-adrenergic receptor. These are glucagon, thyroid hormone, prostacyclin (PGI_2), and calcitonin gene–related peptide.

Inhibition of Adenylyl Cyclase

The major physiologic stimulus to G_i is thought to be vagal muscarinic receptor stimulation. In addition, adenosine, by interaction with A_1 receptors, couples to G_i to inhibit contraction and heart rate. The adenosine A_2 receptor paradoxically increases cAMP; this effect, of only ancillary significance in the myocardium, is of major importance in vascular smooth muscle, where it induces vasorelaxation. Inhibitory G_i is increased in experimental postinfarction heart failure[1] and in donor hearts before cardiac transplantation.[1]

CYCLIC ADENOSINE MONOPHOSPHATE–DEPENDENT PROTEIN KINASES. It is now clear that most if not all of the effects of cAMP are ultimately mediated by PKA, which phosphorylates various key proteins and enzymes.[1] Phosphorylation is the donation of a phosphate group to the enzyme concerned, acting as a fundamental metabolic switch that can extensively amplify the signal.

Each protein kinase is composed of two subunits, regulatory (R) and catalytic (C). When cAMP interacts with the inactive protein kinase, it binds to the R subunit to liberate the active kinase, which is the C subunit:

$$(R_2 + C_2) + 2cAMP \rightarrow 2RcAMP + 2C$$

At a molecular level, this active kinase catalyzes the transfer of the terminal phosphate of ATP to serine and threonine residues of the protein substrates, leading to phosphorylation and modification of the properties of the proteins concerned, thereby promoting further key reactions. PKA occurs in different cells in two isoforms; PKA II predominates in cardiac cells. The proposed anchorage of this kinase by A-kinase anchoring proteins (AKAPs) to specific organelles, such as the SR, explains the phenomenon of cAMP compartmentalization[1] because anchored PKA requires focal elevation of cAMP even at an unchanged cytosolic concentration. In addition, the G protein system may not be evenly spread throughout the sarcolemma but localized to certain focal areas. Thus, it is very likely that there is only a specific subcompartment of cAMP available to increase contractile activity.

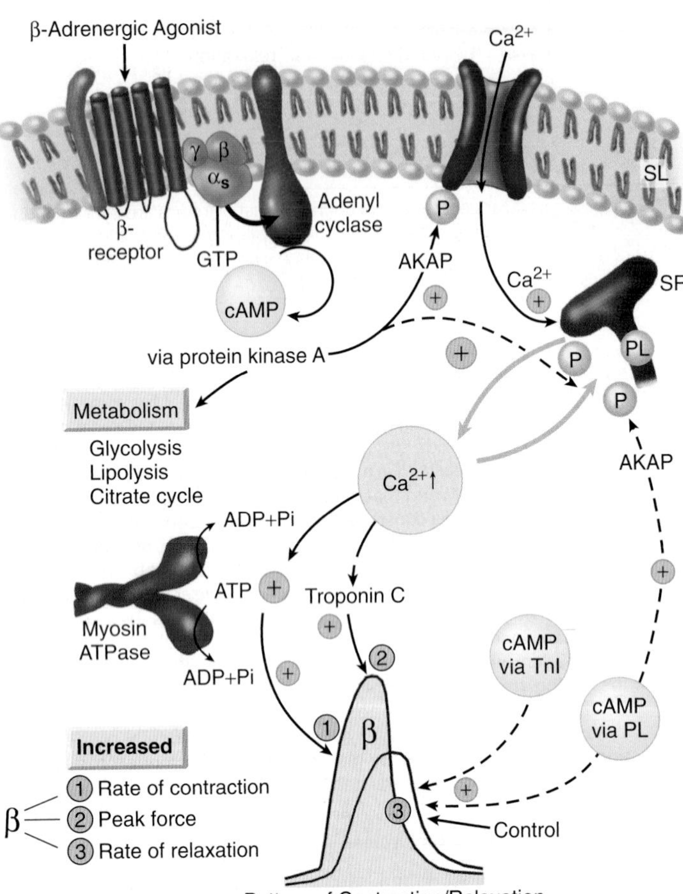

FIGURE 24-13 Signal systems involved in positive inotropic and lusitropic (enhanced relaxation) effects of beta-adrenergic stimulation. When the beta-adrenergic agonist interacts with the beta receptor, a series of G protein–mediated changes (see Fig. 24-12) lead to activation of adenylyl cyclase and formation of cAMP. The cAMP acts via protein kinase A to stimulate metabolism (on the left) and to phosphorylate the calcium channel protein. The result is an enhanced opening probability of the calcium channel, thereby increasing the inward movement of Ca^{2+} ions through the sarcolemma (SL) of the T tubule. These Ca^{2+} ions release more calcium from the sarcoplasmic reticulum (SR) (see Fig. 24-6) to increase cytosolic calcium and to activate troponin C. Calcium ions also increase the rate of breakdown of ATP to ADP and inorganic phosphate (P_i). Enhanced myosin ATPase activity explains the increased rate of contraction with increased activation of troponin C, explaining increased peak force development. An increased rate of relaxation is explained because cAMP also activates the protein phospholamban, situated on the membrane of the SR that controls the rate of uptake of calcium into the SR (see Fig. 24-9). The latter effect explains enhanced relaxation (lusitropic effect). P = phosphorylation; PL = phospholamban; SL = sarcolemma; SR = sarcoplasmic reticulum. AKAP = A-kinase anchoring proteins. *(From Opie LH: Heart Physiology, From Cell to Circulation. Philadelphia, Lippincott Williams & Wilkins, 2004. © L. H. Opie, 2004.)*

Compartmentalization of cAMP and Protein Kinase A

These second and third messengers are not simply evenly distributed throughout the cytosol. Rather, there is increasing evidence for subcellular compartmentalization of cAMP and its further messenger, PKA, in which the scaffolding or anchoring protein AKAP plays an important role (see Fig. 24-12), so that PKA is colocalized with its target.[23] Thus, during beta-adrenergic stimulation, there is subsarcolemmal formation of cAMP with a multimolecular signaling complex involving PKA, PKA anchoring proteins, and the phosphodiesterase 4 (PDE-4) isoform, the last breaking down PKA.[24] Furthermore, this sequence of events is linked to activation of the cardiac L-type calcium channels and thence indirectly also to phosphorylation of the RyR receptor.

PHYSIOLOGIC BETA$_1$-ADRENERGIC EFFECTS. The probable sequence of events describing the positive inotropic effects of catecholamines is as follows (**Fig. 24-13**): catecholamine stimulation → beta receptor → molecular changes → binding of GTP to α_s subunit of G protein → GTP–α_s subunit stimulates adenylyl cyclase → formation of cAMP from ATP → activation of cAMP-dependent PKA, locally bound by an A-kinase anchoring protein (AKAP) → phosphorylation of a sarcolemmal protein p27 → increased entry of calcium ion through increased opening of the voltage-dependent L-type calcium channels → greater calcium-induced calcium release via ryanodine receptor of SR, coupled with phosphorylation of the ryanodine receptor → greater and more rapid rise of intracellular free calcium ion concentration → increased calcium–troponin C interaction with deinhibition of tropomyosin effect on actin-myosin interaction → increased rate and number of cross bridges interacting with increased myosin ATPase activity → increased rate and peak of force development.

The increased lusitropic (relaxant) effect is the consequence of increased PKA-mediated phosphorylation of phospholamban. Also, increased phosphorylation of troponin I may help desensitize the contractile apparatus to calcium ions (see Fig. 24-12).

Physiologic Switch-Off and Beta-Arrestin Signaling

There is a potent and rapid feedback mechanism whereby the degree of postreceptor response to a given degree of beta-adrenergic receptor stimulation can be muted so that an activation of this receptor is not perpetuated (**Fig. 24-14**). This mechanism helps terminate the beta receptor signal by a rapid desensitization of the beta receptor within minutes to seconds. Sustained beta-agonist stimulation rapidly induces the activity of the beta-agonist receptor kinase (βARK1), also called G protein–coupled receptor kinase (GRK2), which is involved in the transfer of the phosphate group to the phosphorylation site on the terminal COOH tail of the receptor, a process that of itself does not markedly affect the signaling properties. Rather, βARK-GRK2 increases the affinity of the beta receptor for another protein family, the arrestins, which cause the dissociation. Beta-arrestin is a scaffolding and signaling protein that links to one of the cytoplasmic loops of the G protein–coupled beta-adrenergic receptor,[1] lessening activation of adenylyl cyclase to inhibit the functioning of this receptor. Furthermore, beta-arrestin switches the agonist coupling from G_s to inhibitory G_i.[25] Resensitization of the receptor occurs if the phosphate group is split off by a phosphatase, and the receptor may then more readily be linked to G_s. Beta-arrestin signaling can also evoke an alternative counterbalancing protective path by activating the epidermal growth factor receptor, which leads to the protective ERK/MAPK path (see Fig. 24-14).[26] Although the GRK2-arrestin effects are best described for the beta$_2$ receptor, they also occur to a lesser extent with the beta$_1$ receptor.[1]

Prolonged beta receptor stimulation as in hyperadrenergic conditions is linked to adverse end results, both impairing contractile function and enhancing adverse signaling. As discussed in Chap. 25, this mechanism also plays a role in long-term desensitization of the beta-adrenergic receptor, as occurs in chronic heart failure.[27] Conversely, transgenic mice with GRK2 overexpression are protected from heart failure.[27] Of note, the desensitization process is reversible, as occurs during experimental cardiac resynchronization therapy, when the specific suppressors of the inhibitor G protein (G_i in Fig. 24-11) are much increased in activity so that beta-adrenergic signaling becomes more normal.[28]

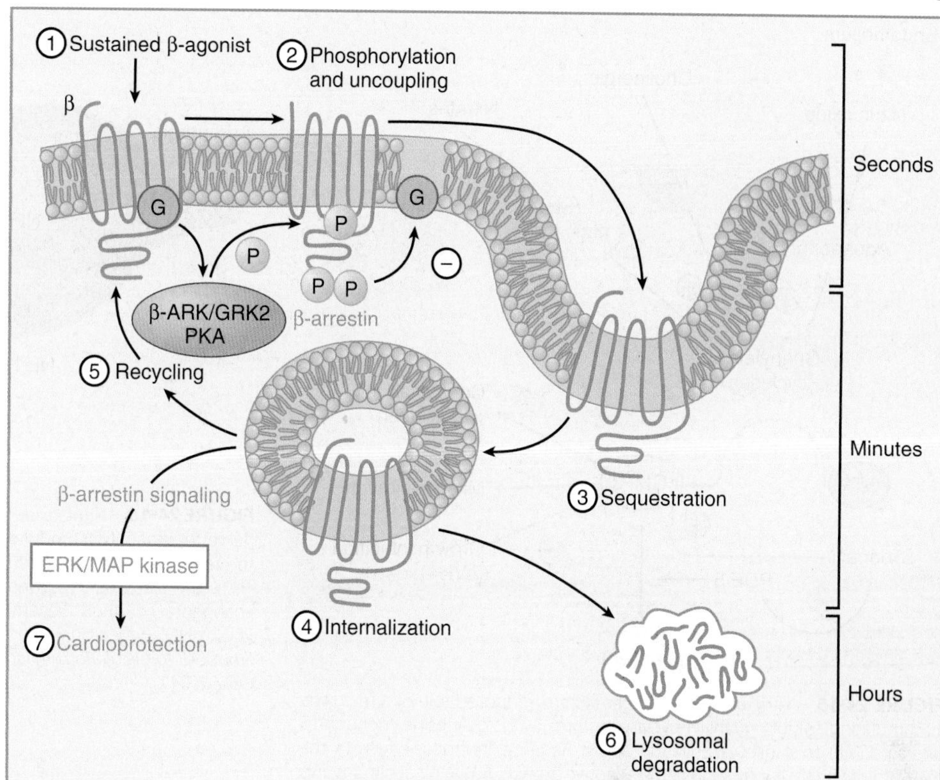

FIGURE 24-14 Mechanisms of beta-adrenergic receptor desensitization and internalization. Note links between the internalized receptor complex with growth stimulation via MAP kinase. βARK = GRK2 = beta-agonist receptor kinase or G protein–coupled receptor kinase 2; ERK = extracellular signal-regulated kinase; MAP = mitogen-activated protein kinase; PKA = protein kinase A. *(Updated from Hein L, Kobilka BK: Adrenergic receptors. From molecular structures to in vivo function. Trends Cardiovasc Med 7:137, 1997.)*

Beta$_2$- and Beta$_3$-Adrenergic Effects

In the normal ventricle, about 20% of the receptors are beta$_2$ in nature; yet in heart failure, this percentage of the whole can double because of beta$_1$ receptor downregulation (see section on heart failure). The beta$_2$ postreceptor signaling involves both the stimulatory and the inhibitory G proteins.[1] In humans, the positive inotropic response to beta$_2$ stimulation by salbutamol occurs, at least in part, through beta$_2$ receptors on the terminal neurons of the cardiac sympathetic nerves, thereby releasing norepinephrine, which in turn exerts dominant beta$_1$ effects.[1] Indirect evidence suggests that the G_i inhibitory path is relatively augmented in heart failure, whereas the strength of the stimulatory G_s path is lessened because of uncoupling of G_s from the beta$_2$ receptor.

Regarding beta$_3$-adrenergic receptors, earlier data proposed a negative inotropic effect through nitric oxide and formation of inhibitory cGMP.[1] By contrast, in recent studies, these receptors are associated with formation of cAMP and with negative modulation by cGMP.[29] Thus, the physiologic role of the beta$_3$ receptors remains in doubt.

Cholinergic and Nitric Oxide Signaling

Cholinergic Signaling

Parasympathetic stimulation reduces heart rate and is negatively inotropic. The key features of its signaling system are similar to the beta$_1$-adrenergic system. There is again an extracellular first messenger (acetylcholine), a receptor system (the cholinergic muscarinic receptor), a sarcolemmal signaling system (the G protein system, specifically the inhibitory G_i), and a second messenger (cGMP). The myocardial muscarinic receptor (M_2) is associated specifically with the activity of the vagal nerve endings. Receptor stimulation produces a negative chronotropic response that is inhibited by atropine. Nitric oxide (NO) facilitates cholinergic signaling at two levels, the nerve terminal and the activity of the enzyme system that produces cGMP. Neuregulins are growth factors that maintain the activity of the muscarinic receptor, thereby indirectly helping to balance the normal parasympathetic modulation of excess beta-adrenergic stimulation.[30]

The mechanisms of vagal heart rate–lowering are multiple. cGMP acts as a second messenger to vagal stimulation just as cAMP does to beta-adrenergic stimulation. Of note, cell-permeable analogues of cGMP have antiadrenergic effects. Cholinergic stimulation of the M_2 receptor activates guanylyl (guanylate, guanyl) cyclase to form cGMP with consequent stimulation of the protein kinase G (PKG), which results in inhibitory cardiac effects such as a decreased heart rate and negative inotropic response.[31] These effects are largely achieved by modulation of calcium ion entry through the L calcium channel and through inhibition of internal calcium cycling.[32] In addition, muscarinic M_2 stimulation acts via G_i to lessen the G_s activation that results from beta receptor occupation. Thus, the vagus has a dual effect on second messengers, inhibiting the formation of cAMP and increasing that of cGMP, thereby providing one of several explanations for sympathetic-parasympathetic interaction. In the sinus node, formation of cGMP may occur not only by guanylyl cyclase (**Fig. 24-15**) but also by a muscarinic-mediated formation of nitric oxide.

COMPARTMENTALIZATION OF cGMP. So far, two compartments of cGMP have been localized, the particulate or subsarcolemmal pool and the soluble or cytosolic pool.[24] Particulate cGMP is activated by the natriuretic peptides such as BNP, whereas the soluble pool is activated by nitric oxide and cholinergic stimulation (see Fig. 24-15). cGMP is broken down by PDE-5, which has achieved prominence as a result of its inhibition by sildenafil and related compounds that enhance penile vasodilation. Emerging data show wider therapeutic potential. Thus, sildenafil, by accumulation of cGMP, combats harmful excessive adrenergic stimulation of contractile function.[33] Furthermore, sildenafil via cGMP can inhibit excess LV growth in response to aortic constriction.[34] The next messenger of cGMP, PKG, like its counterpart PKA, colocalizes with its targets to control substrate phosphorylation.[23] The anchoring protein for PKG may be the same AKAP as for cAMP, allowing tight subcellular colocalization and regulation of the counterpoised activities of cAMP and cGMP and hence of the balance between adrenergic and cholinergic regulation.

Regarding the negative inotropic effect of vagal stimulation (see Fig. 24-11), the mechanisms include (1) heart rate slowing (negative treppe phenomenon), (2) inhibition of the formation of cAMP, and (3) direct negative inotropic effect mediated by cGMP. It has been controversial whether ventricular tissue is as responsive to muscarinic

CH 24

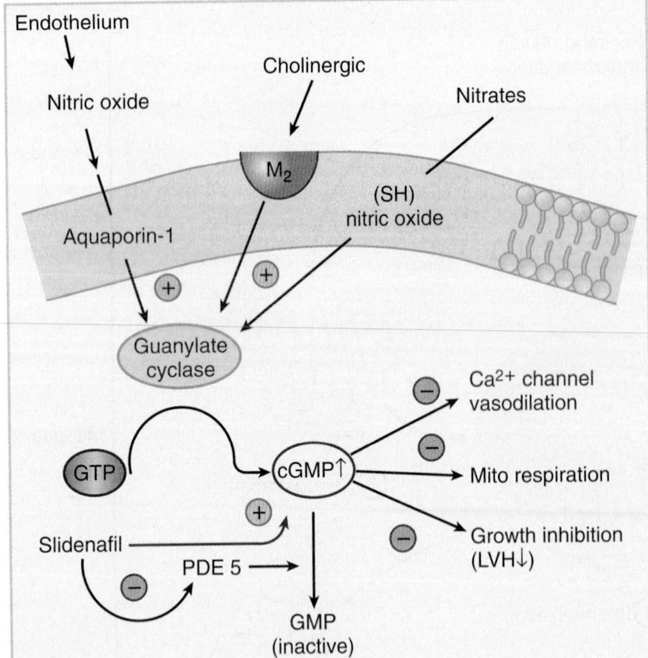

FIGURE 24-15 Nitric oxide messenger system. Proposed role of nitric oxide in stimulating soluble guanylyl cyclase to form cyclic guanosine monophosphate (cGMP) to cause vasodilation and a negative inotropic effect. In the myocardium, there is inhibition of maladaptive growth. Antianginal nitrates also cause coronary vasodilation by this mechanism. Cholinergic stimulation, by acting on the muscarinic receptors (M), also increases vascular and myocardial cGMP. For inhibition by nitric oxide–cGMP of cardiomyocyte hypertrophy via RhoA-ROCK pathway, see Hunter JC et al: Cardiovasc Res 437:810, 2009; LVH = left ventricular hypertrophy; Mito = mitochondrial; PDE = phosphodiesterase. *(Modified from Opie LH: Heart Physiology, From Cell to Circulation. Philadelphia, Lippincott Williams & Wilkins, 2004. © L. H. Opie, 2004.)*

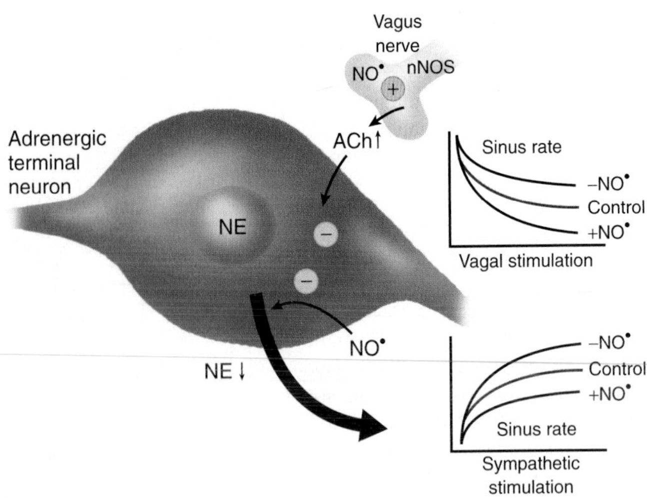

FIGURE 24-16 Nitric oxide (NO) mediates release of acetylcholine from vagal nerve terminals. NO, produced in the terminal vagal nerve endings, increases the release of acetylcholine (ACh) and decreases that of norepinephrine (NE). Thus, the sinus rate response to either vagal or sympathetic stimulation is changed accordingly. Schematics adapted from Paterson D: Exp Physiol 86:1, 2001. nNOS = neuronal nitric oxide synthase. *(From Opie LH: Heart Physiology, From Cell to Circulation. Philadelphia, Lippincott Williams & Wilkins, 2004. © L. H. Opie, 2004.)*

agonists as atrial tissue is, although the receptor populations are similar in density. However, using pressure-volume loops and the slope of the pressure-volume relationship (see later, E_s in Fig. 24-24) as an index of contractile function, vagal stimulation in humans markedly decreases this load-independent measure.[1]

The sympathetic terminal neurons are another site of parasympathetic-sympathetic interaction. There, the presynaptic muscarinic M_2 receptor inhibits the release of norepinephrine. In addition, both adrenergic and cholinergic stimuli exert important and often opposing effects on ion channels and cardiac function (see Fig. 24-11). Such multiple mechanisms for the inhibitory effects of vagal stimulation on the heart rate, the inotropic state, and arrhythmogenicity suggest that "braking" of beta-adrenergic stimulation is desirable (see Fig. 24-14). Otherwise, the risk may be that intense beta-adrenergic stimulation would excessively increase the heart rate or inotropic state or provoke potentially fatal arrhythmias.

Nitric Oxide, the Ubiquitous Messenger

Nitric oxide (NO), the focus of the Nobel Prize for 1998, is a unique messenger in that it is formed in so many tissues, is a gas, and is a physiologic free radical that should more correctly (but infrequently) be written as ·NO (**Fig. 24-16**). Nonetheless, the standard abbreviation is NO. Although it is usually thought to be freely diffusible through cell membranes, a new discovery is that an integral membrane protein, aquaporin 1, facilitates and may regulate diffusion of NO into cells.[35] NO is generated in the heart by one of three isoenzymes.[32] Vasodilatory NO is generated in the vascular endothelium by endothelial nitric oxide synthase (eNOS, also called NOS3), in response to increased blood flow or increased cardiac load or bradykinin (see Chap. 52). Excess NO is generated in cardiomyocytes in diseased states such as cardiogenic or septic shock by the inducible enzyme (iNOS, also called NOS2). Generation of NO by neuronal NOS (nNOS, also called NOS1), the form of the synthase found in vagal nerve terminals, enhances the release of acetylcholine.[36] The enhanced vagal activity of exercise training depends on increased expression of nNOS.[36] Exercise also acts peripherally to enhance the expression of vasodilatory eNOS in humans with coronary disease.[37] Because the activity of guanylyl cyclase, promoted by cholinergic stimulation, is sensitive to and enhanced by NO,[31] previous concepts are revised in that NO is now seen as augmenting parasympathetic simulation both upstream and downstream from acetylcholine. Furthermore, the increase of cGMP induced by eNOS-derived NO potentially adds to that of cholinergic stimulation (see Fig. 24-15). Such increases of cGMP are potentially protective from adverse excess adrenergic stimulation.[33] Whereas physiologic amounts of NO are cardioprotective, as noted in Chap. 25, excessive levels of nitric oxide are harmful.

REACTIVE OXYGEN SPECIES AS SIGNALING MOLECULES. Although excess reactive oxygen species (ROS) production is linked to many cardiovascular diseases, it is often forgotten that ROS probably have important physiologic roles. Pathways for formation are many, as are the endogenous antioxidants and antioxidant enzymes (see Chap. 25).[38] Thus, ROS are part of a protective oxygen-sensing mechanism, allowing cells to adapt to hypoxia.[38] Increased contraction frequency of cardiomyocytes also gives rise to ROS, of unknown physiologic function.[38] As discussed in Chap. 25, excessive ROS production in the heart has numerous consequences (see Fig. 25-5).

OTHER INHIBITORY SIGNAL SYSTEMS. Adenosine, in addition to being a physiologic vasodilator, acts on myocardial A_1 receptors that are coupled to adenylyl cyclase by the inhibitory G protein (α_i subunit). Opioids released in the central nervous system are known to participate in cardiovascular regulation by inhibiting sympathetic and promoting parasympathetic outflow. In the heart, the delta receptors inhibit the adrenergic system by coupling to G_i, thereby inhibiting the activation of adenylyl cyclase by beta-adrenergic stimulation and stimulating the protein kinase C pathway (see later).[39]

Vasoconstrictive Signaling

VASCULAR G PROTEIN–COUPLED RECEPTORS. Agonists with vasoconstriction as their major physiologic role are alpha$_1$-adrenergic catecholamines, angiotensin II, and endothelin (**Fig. 24-17**). By regulation of the degree of vasoconstriction, the peripheral vascular resistance can be tuned to the needs of the circulation with, for example, vasoconstriction occurring in response to alpha$_1$-adrenergic stimulation during the stress of blood loss. Each of these agonists is coupled to its appropriate seven transmembrane–spanning receptor, linked via the G protein G_q to effectors different from those of adrenergic and cholinergic signaling. Specifically, a different calcium release signal system is involved to achieve vasoconstrictive calcium release in vascular tissue. The myocardial ryanodine receptor is replaced by that for IP_3. This IP_3 receptor has a high degree of molecular homology with the ryanodine receptor, although it is only about half its size. This IP_3 messenger system is of fundamental importance in regulating the release of calcium from the SR and thereby regulating arterial tone and hence the afterload against which the heart must work. In cardiac muscle, the role of IP_3 is still sufficiently controversial for its role in the inotropic response to be questioned.

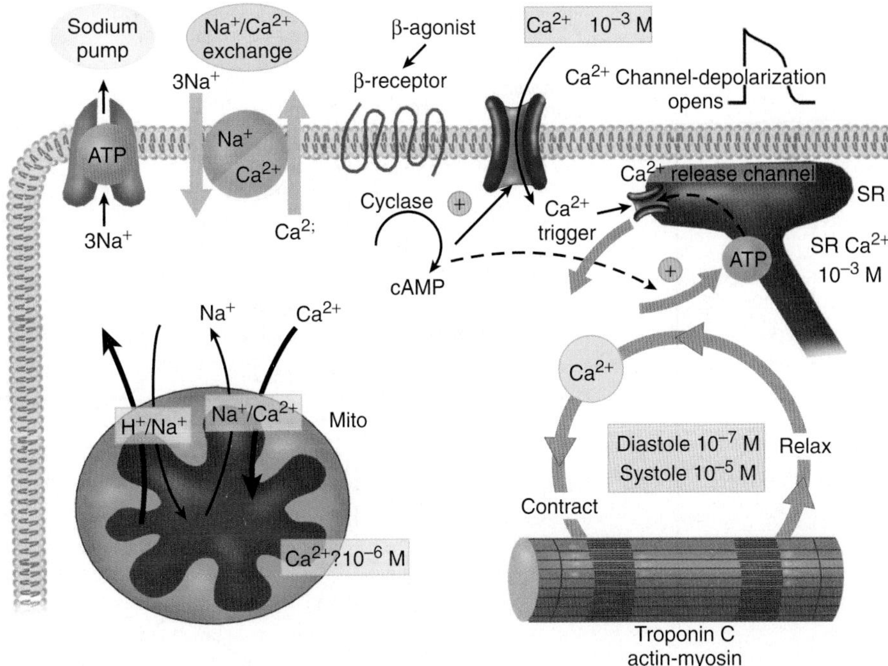

FIGURE 24-17 Patterns of contraction and relaxation in vascular smooth muscle. The angiotensin II (A-II) signaling system is coupled via a G protein to phospholipase C (PLC), which breaks down phosphatidylinositol to 1,2-diacylglycerol (DAG) and IP_3 (inositol triphosphate). DAG translocates protein kinase C (PKC) from cytosol to the sarcolemma, thereby activating PKC. Signals beyond PKC are not clear. It may phosphorylate ion channels to give the sustained vasoconstrictive response. IP_3 releases calcium from the sarcoplasmic reticulum to initiate vascular smooth muscle contraction. Other vasoconstrictors, such as endothelin (ET receptor), act by the same signal system. In response to norepinephrine (NE), an alpha$_1$-agonist, a similar sequence of events occurs to promote contraction. Relaxation is achieved by inhibition of myosin kinase, when either cGMP or cAMP is formed in response, respectively, to nitric oxide (NO) or adenosine (Ado). AC = adenylyl cyclase; GC = guanylyl cyclase. *(From Opie LH: Heart Physiology, From Cell to Circulation. Philadelphia, Lippincott Williams & Wilkins, 2004. © L. H. Opie, 2004.)*

Cytokine Signaling

TUMOR NECROSIS FACTOR-α AND INTERLEUKINS. Tumor necrosis factor (TNF) is one of the family of peptide cytokines that form part of the innate immune system. These cytokines are not normally found in the myocardium but, being stress responsive, are formed during challenge by hypoxia, ischemia-reperfusion, myocardial infarction,[40] or mechanical loading. The cytokine group includes the interleukins IL-1 and IL-6, often formed in concert with TNF. The MAP kinase signaling path is also stress activated (see later, Fig. 24-26) and appears to be required for formation of TNF and IL-6 in cardiomyocytes.[41] Such cytokines mediate local events and are distinct from circulating neurotransmitters or hormones. TNF stimulation has concentration-dependent bifunctional effects; low concentrations mediate protective signals, and high values exert adverse signaling.[1] These paths are neither simple nor completely understood (see section on beneficial survival paths).

CARDIOTROPHIN. This member of the IL-6 family of cytokines is briskly released from the perfused heart in response to ventricular stretch.[42] It interacts with the glycoprotein 130 receptor, which in turn can activate the paths leading to physiologic hypertrophy (see later, Fig. 24-26).

Contractile Performance of the Intact Heart

There are three main determinants of myocardial mechanical performance, namely, the loading conditions (preload and afterload; Frank-Starling mechanism), the contractile state, and the heart rate. This section describes the cardiac cycle and then the determinants of LV function.

TABLE 24-3 The Cardiac Cycle

LV Contraction
Isovolumic contraction (b)
Maximal ejection (c)
LV Relaxation
Start of relaxation and reduced ejection (d)
Isovolumic relaxation (e)
LV Filling
Rapid phase (f)
Slow filling (diastasis) (g)
Atrial systole or booster (a)

The letters a-g refer to the phases of the cardiac cycle shown in Wiggers' diagram (Fig. 24-18). These letters are arbitrarily allocated so that atrial systole (a) coincides with the *a* wave and (c) with the *c* wave of the jugular venous pressure.

The Cardiac Cycle

The cardiac cycle, fully assembled by Lewis[43] but first conceived by Wiggers,[44] yields important information on the temporal sequence of events in the cardiac cycle. The three basic events are LV contraction, LV relaxation, and LV filling (**Table 24-3**). Although similar mechanical events occur on the right side of the heart, it is those on the left side that are focused on.

LEFT VENTRICULAR CONTRACTION. LV pressure starts to build up when the arrival of calcium ions at the contractile proteins starts to trigger actin-myosin interaction. On the electrocardiogram, the

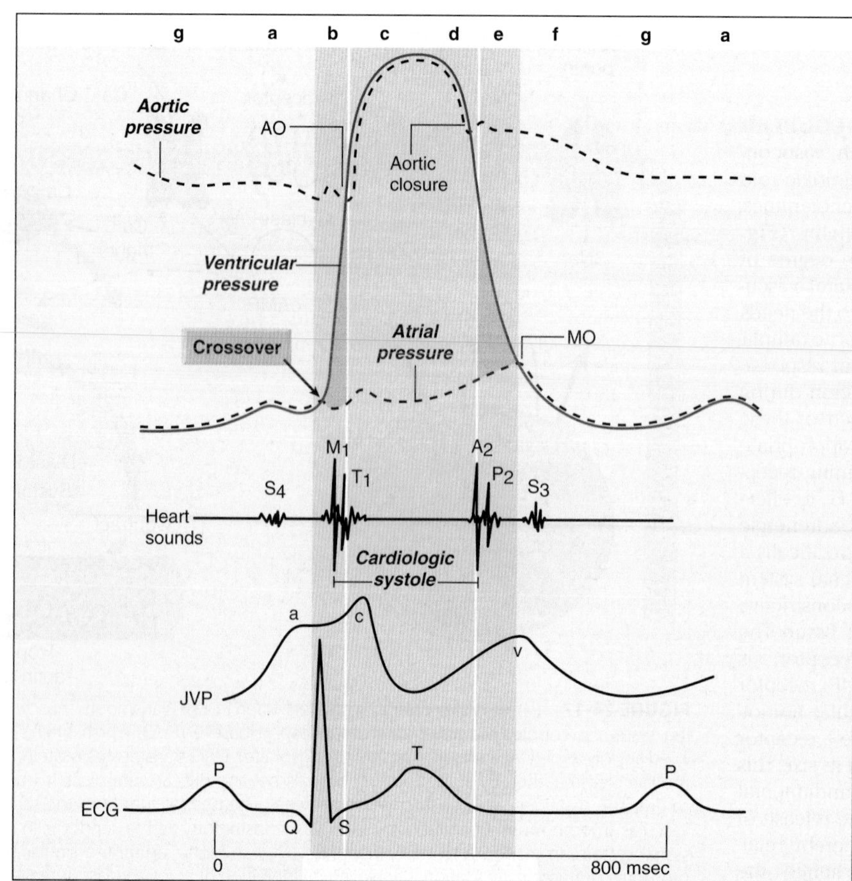

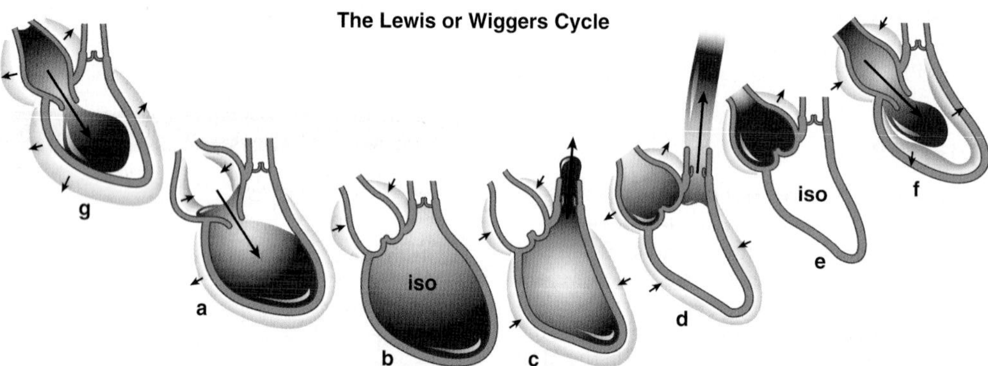

FIGURE 24-18 The mechanical events in the cardiac cycle, first assembled by Lewis[43] in 1920 but first conceived by Wiggers[44] in 1915. Note that mitral valve closure occurs *after* the crossover point of atrial and ventricular pressures at the start of systole. The visual phases of the ventricular cycle on the bottom are modified from Shepherd and Vanhoutte *(Shepherd JT, Vanhoutte PM: The Human Cardiovascular System. New York, Raven Press, 1979, p 68)*. For explanation of phases a to g, see Table 24-3. ECG = electrocardiogram; JVP = jugular venous pressure; M_1 = mitral component of first sound at time of mitral valve closure; T_1 = tricuspid valve closure, second component of first heart sound; AO = aortic valve opening, normally inaudible; A_2 = aortic valve closure, aortic component of second sound; MO = mitral valve opening, may be audible in mitral stenosis as the opening snap; P_2 = pulmonary component of second sound, pulmonary valve closure; S_3 = third heart sound; S_4 = fourth heart sound; a = wave produced by right atrial contraction; c = carotid wave artifact during rapid LV ejection phase; v = venous return wave, which causes pressure to rise while tricuspid valve is closed. Cycle length of 800 milliseconds for 75 beats/min. *(From Opie LH: Heart Physiology, From Cell to Circulation. Philadelphia, Lippincott Williams & Wilkins, 2004. © L. H. Opie, 2004.)*

advance of the wave of depolarization is indicated by the peak of the R wave (**Fig. 24-18**). Soon after, LV pressure in the early contraction phase builds up and exceeds that in the left atrium (normally 10 to 15 mm Hg), followed about 20 milliseconds later by M_1, the mitral component of the first sound, M_1. The exact relation of M_1 to mitral valve closure is open to dispute. Although mitral valve closure is often thought to coincide with the crossover point at which the LV pressure starts to exceed the left atrial pressure,[1] in reality mitral valve closure is delayed because the valve is kept open by the inertia of the blood flow. Shortly thereafter, pressure changes in the right ventricle, similar in pattern to but lesser in magnitude than those in the left ventricle, cause the tricuspid valve to close, thereby creating T_1, which is the second component of the first heart sound. During this phase of contraction between mitral valve closure and aortic valve opening, the LV volume is fixed (isovolumic contraction) because both aortic and mitral valves are shut. As more and more myofibers enter the contracted state, pressure development in the left ventricle proceeds. The interaction of actin and myosin increases, and cross-bridge cycling is augmented. When the pressure in the left ventricle exceeds that in the aorta, the aortic valve opens, usually a clinically silent event. Opening of the aortic valve is followed by the phase of rapid ejection. The rate of ejection is determined not only by the pressure gradient across the aortic valve but also by the elastic properties of the aorta and the arterial tree, which undergoes systolic expansion. LV pressure rises to a peak and then starts to fall.

LEFT VENTRICULAR RELAXATION. As the cytosolic calcium ion concentration starts to decline because of uptake of calcium into the SR under the influence of activated phospholamban, more and more myofibers enter the state of relaxation, and the rate of ejection of blood from the left ventricle into the aorta falls (phase of reduced ejection). During this phase, blood flow from the left ventricle to the aorta rapidly diminishes but is maintained by aortic recoil, the Windkessel effect. The pressure in the aorta exceeds the falling pressure in the left ventricle. The aortic valve closes, creating the first component of the second sound, A_2 (the second component, P_2, results from closure of the pulmonary valve as the pulmonary artery pressure exceeds that in the right ventricle). Thereafter, the ventricle continues to relax. Because the mitral valve is closed during this phase, the LV volume cannot change (isovolumic relaxation). When the LV pressure falls to below that in the left atrium, the mitral valve opens (normally silent), and the filling phase of the cardiac cycle restarts (see Fig. 24-18).

LEFT VENTRICULAR FILLING PHASES. As LV pressure drops below that in the left atrium, just after mitral valve opening, the phase of rapid or early filling occurs to account for most of ventricular filling.[1] Active diastolic relaxation of the ventricle may also contribute to early filling (see section on ventricular suction). Such rapid filling may cause the physiologic third heart sound (S_3), particularly when there is a hyperkinetic circulation.[1] As pressures in the atrium and ventricle equalize, LV filling virtually stops (*diastasis*, separation). Renewed filling requires that the pressure gradient from the atrium to the ventricle increase. This is achieved by atrial systole (or the left atrial booster), which is especially important when a high cardiac output is required, as during exercise, or when the left ventricle fails to relax normally, as in LV hypertrophy.[1]

DEFINITIONS OF SYSTOLE AND DIASTOLE. In Greek, *systole* means contraction and *diastole* means to send apart. The start of systole can be regarded as (1) the beginning of isovolumic contraction when LV pressure exceeds the atrial pressure or (2) mitral valve closure (M_1). These correspond reasonably well because mitral valve closure actually occurs only about 20 milliseconds after the crossover point of the pressures. Thus, in practice, the term *isovolumic contraction* often also includes this brief period of early systolic contraction even before the mitral valve shuts, when the heart volume does not change substantially. Physiologic systole lasts from the start of isovolumic contraction (where LV pressure crosses over atrial pressure, Fig. 24-18) to the peak of the ejection phase, so that physiologic diastole commences as the LV pressure starts to fall (**Table 24-4**). This concept fits well with the standard pressure-volume curve. Physiologic diastole commences as calcium ions are taken up into the SR, so that myocyte relaxation dominates over contraction, and the LV pressure starts to fall as shown on the pressure-volume curve. In contrast, cardiologic systole is demarcated by the interval between the first and second heart sounds, lasting from the first heart sound (M_1) to the closure of the aortic valve (A_2). The remainder of the cardiac cycle automatically becomes cardiologic diastole. Thus, cardiologic systole, demarcated by heart sounds rather than by physiologic events, starts fractionally later than physiologic systole and ends significantly later. For the cardiologist, protodiastole is the early phase of rapid filling, the time when the third heart sound (S_3) can be heard. This sound probably reflects ventricular wall vibrations during rapid filling and becomes audible with an increase in LV diastolic pressure, wall stiffness, or rate of filling.

TABLE 24-4 Physiologic Versus Cardiologic Systole and Diastole

PHYSIOLOGIC SYSTOLE	CARDIOLOGIC SYSTOLE
Isovolumic contraction Maximal ejection	From M_1 to A_2, including: Major part of isovolumic contraction* Maximal ejection Reduced ejection
PHYSIOLOGIC DIASTOLE	**CARDIOLOGIC DIASTOLE**
Reduced ejection Isovolumic relaxation Filling phases	A_2-M_1 interval (filling phases included)

*Note that M_1 occurs with a definite albeit short delay after the start of LV contraction.

Contractile Function Versus Loading Conditions

CONTRACTILE FUNCTION. Contractile function is the inherent capacity of the myocardium to contract independently of changes in the preload or afterload. It is a key word in our cardiologic language. At a molecular level, an increased inotropic state can be explained by enhanced interaction between calcium ions and the contractile proteins. Increased contractile function means a greater rate of contraction, to reach a greater peak force. An increased contractile function is often associated with enhanced rates of relaxation, called the lusitropic effect. Alternative names for contractile function are the inotropic state (*ino*, fiber; *tropos*, to move) and the contractile state. Contractile function is an important regulator of the myocardial oxygen uptake. Factors that increase contractile function include exercise, adrenergic stimulation, digitalis, and other inotropic agents.

PRELOAD AND AFTERLOAD. Any change in the contractile state should be independent of the loading conditions. The preload is the load present before contraction has started, at the end of diastole (the afterload is discussed later). The preload reflects the venous filling pressure that fills the left atrium, which in turn fills the left ventricle during diastole. When the preload increases, the left ventricle distends during diastole, and the stroke volume rises according to Starling's law (next section). The heart rate also increases by stimulation of the atrial mechanoreceptors that enhance the rate of discharge of the sinoatrial node. Thus, the cardiac output (stroke volume × heart rate) rises.

Starling's Law of the Heart

VENOUS FILLING PRESSURE AND HEART VOLUME. Starling, in 1918, related the venous pressure in the right atrium to the heart volume in the dog heart-lung preparation (see Fig. 12-3 in Opie[16]). He proposed that within physiologic limits, the larger the volume of the heart, the greater the energy of its contraction and the amount of chemical change at each contraction. Starling did not, however, measure sarcomere length. He could relate only LV volume to cardiac output. This holds in normal, compliant hearts. One modern version of Starling's law is that stroke volume is related to the end-diastolic volume. The LV volume can now be directly measured with two-dimensional echocardiography; yet the value found depends on a number of simplifying assumptions, such as a spherical LV shape, and neglects the confounding influence of the complex anatomy of the left ventricle. From the investigational point of view, real-time three-dimensional echocardiographic records can now yield both global LV volume and endocardial function.[45] In practice, the LV volume is not often measured; rather, a variety of surrogate measures, such as LV end-diastolic pressure and the pulmonary capillary wedge pressure, are used. The relation between LV end-diastolic volume and LV end-diastolic pressure is curvilinear, depending on the LV compliance.

The LV diastolic filling pressure (the difference between the left atrial pressure and the LV diastolic pressure) is easier to measure and in diseased, noncompliant hearts may be taken as a surrogate for heart volume. The venous filling pressure can be measured in humans albeit indirectly by the technique of Swan-Ganz catheterization, as can the stroke volume. The LV pressure and volume are, however, not linearly related because of variations in the compliance of the myocardium. Therefore, a jump from pressure to volume is required to apply the Starling concept to the hemodynamic management of those critically ill and receiving a Swan-Ganz catheter.

FRANK AND ISOVOLUMIC CONTRACTION. If a larger heart volume increases the initial length of the muscle fiber to increase the stroke volume and hence the cardiac output, diastolic stretch of the left ventricle actually increases contractile function. Frank, in 1895, had already reported that the greater the initial LV volume, the more rapid the rate of rise, the greater the peak pressure reached, and the faster the rate of relaxation (see Fig. 24-6 in Opie[16]). He described both a positive inotropic effect and an increased lusitropic effect. These complementary findings of Frank and Starling are often combined into the Frank-Starling law, which can account for two of the mechanisms underlying the increased stroke volume of exercise, namely, the increased diastolic filling (Starling's law) and the increased inotropic state (Frank's findings).

AFTERLOAD. This is the systolic load on the left ventricle after it has started to contract. In the nonfailing heart, the left ventricle can overcome any physiologic acute increase in load. Chronically, however, the left ventricle must hypertrophy to overcome sustained arterial hypertension or significant aortic stenosis. In clinical practice, the arterial blood pressure is often taken to be synonymous with the afterload while ignoring the aortic compliance, the extent to which the aorta can "yield" during systole. A stiff aorta, as in isolated systolic hypertension of the elderly, increases the afterload.

PRELOAD AND AFTERLOAD ARE INTERLINKED. The distinctions between preload and afterload do not allow for those situations when the two change concurrently. By the Frank-Starling law, an increased LV volume leads to increased contractile function, which in turn will increase the systolic blood pressure and hence the afterload. Nonetheless, in general, the preload is related to the degree to which the myocardial fibers are stretched at the end of diastole, and the afterload is related to the wall stress generated by those fibers during systole.

FORCE-LENGTH RELATIONSHIPS AND CALCIUM TRANSIENTS. Proof that there is no increase in the calcium transient as the sarcomere length increases is provided by direct measurements (**Fig. 24-19**). The favored explanation for the steep length-tension relation of cardiac muscles is length-dependent activation, whereby an increase in calcium sensitivity is the major factor explaining the steep increase of force development as the initial sarcomere length increases. This change may be explained by stretch of the titin molecule (see Fig. 24-4). Is the degree of overlap of actin and myosin also involved? Whereas the overlap theory explains the force-length relationship in skeletal muscle, the situation is different in cardiac muscle. In cardiac muscle, even at 80% of the maximal length, only 10% or less of the maximal force is developed. Thus, it can be predicted that cardiac sarcomeres must function near the upper limit of their maximal length (L_{max}). Rodriguez and colleagues[46] have tested this prediction by relating sarcomere length changes to volume changes of the intact heart. By implantation of small radiopaque beads in only about 1 cm^3 of the LV free wall and with biplane cineradiography, the motion of the markers could be tracked through various cardiac cycles, with allowances made for local myocardial deformation. Thus, the change in sarcomere length from approximately 85% of L_{max} to L_{max} itself is able to effect physiologic LV volume changes (**Fig. 24-20**). This estimate is remarkably close to the normal fiber shortening of 15% in the human heart in situ.[1]

PRELOAD AND SERCA2a. When LV muscle is stretched acutely (such as in LV overload), expression of SERCA is increased.[47] This may be a protective system to increase contractile performance in situations of increased load (see Fig. 24-19).

ANREP EFFECT: ABRUPT INCREASE IN AFTERLOAD. When the aortic pressure is elevated abruptly, a positive inotropic effect rapidly follows. This used to be called homeometric autoregulation (*homeo*, the same; *metric*, length) because it was apparently independent of muscle length and by definition a true inotropic effect. A reasonable speculation would be that increased LV wall tension could increase cytosolic sodium and then, by Na^+/Ca^{2+} exchange, the cytosolic calcium. Thus, this effect would be different from that of an increase in preload (which acts by length activation).

Wall Stress

A more exact definition of the afterload is the wall stress during LV ejection. Technically, wall stress develops when tension is applied to

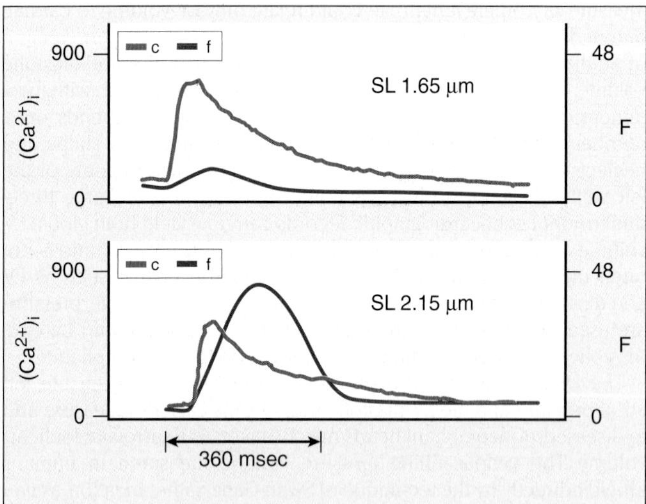

FIGURE 24-19 Length sensitization of the sarcomere. **Top,** The sarcomere length (SL) is 1.65 μm, which gives very little force (f) development (see Fig. 24-20). **Bottom,** At a nearly maximum sarcomere length (see Fig. 24-20), the same Ca^{2+} transient (c) with the same peak value and overall pattern causes a much greater force development. Therefore, there has been length-induced calcium sensitization. *(Modified from Backx PH, ter Keurs HE: Fluorescent properties of rat cardiac trabeculae microinjected with fura-2 salt. Am J Physio. 264:H1098, 1993.)*

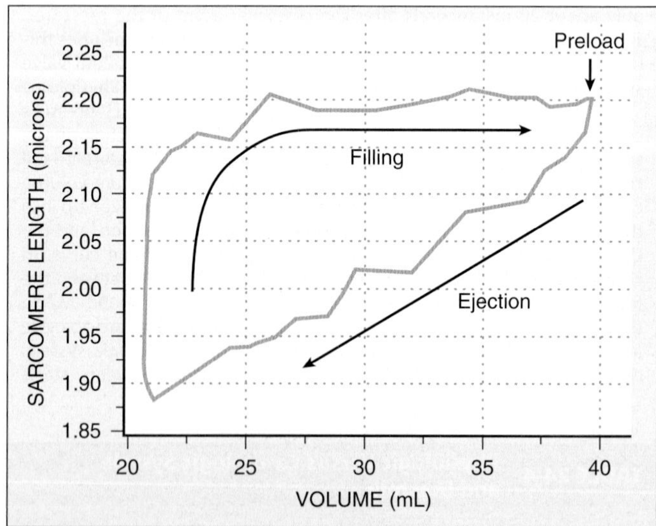

FIGURE 24-20 Changes in sarcomere length during a typical cardiac contraction-relaxation cycle. During diastole, the sarcomere length is 2.2 μm, reducing to 1.90 μm during systole in the intact dog heart. Starting at the top right, the preload is the maximum sarcomere length just before the onset of contraction. As ejection decreases the LV volume, by somewhat more than half, sarcomere length falls from 2.20 to 1.90 μm. Then, during the rapid phase of filling (see Fig. 24-18), the sarcomere length increases from 1.90 to 2.15 μm to be followed by the phase of constant sarcomere length (diastasis). *(Modified from Rodriguez EK, Hunter WC, Royce MJ, et al: A method to reconstruct sarcomere lengths and orientations to transmural sites in beating canine hearts. Am J Physiol 263:H293, 1992, with permission of the American Physiological Society.)*

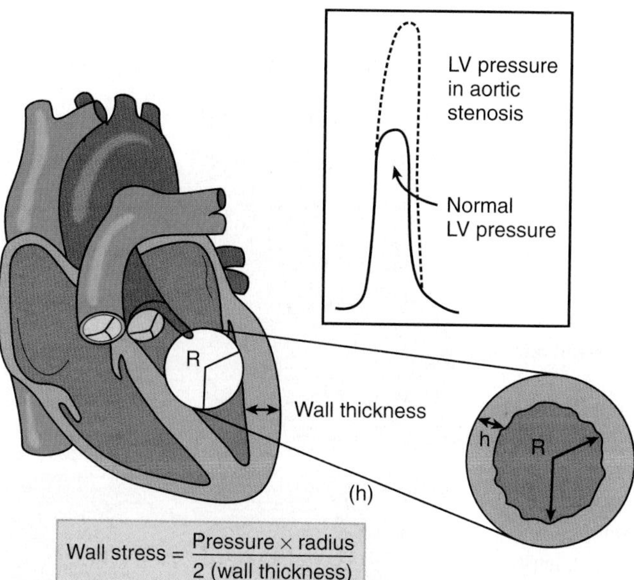

FIGURE 24-21 Wall stress increases as the afterload increases. The formula shown is derived from the Laplace law. The increased LV pressure in aortic stenosis is compensated for by LV wall hypertrophy, which decreases the denominator on the right side of the equation. R = radius. *(From Opie LH: Heart Physiology, From Cell to Circulation. Philadelphia, Lippincott Williams & Wilkins, 2004. © L. H. Opie, 2004.)*

a cross-sectional area, and the units are force per unit area. According to the Laplace law (**Fig. 24-21**):

$$\text{Wall stress} = \frac{\text{pressure}}{2} \times \frac{\text{radius}}{\text{wall thickness}}$$

This equation, although it is an oversimplification, emphasizes two points. First, the bigger the left ventricle and the greater its radius, the more is the wall stress. Second, at any given radius (LV size), the greater the pressure developed by the left ventricle, the greater the wall stress. An increase in wall stress achieved by either of these mechanisms (LV size or intraventricular pressure) will increase myocardial oxygen uptake. This is because a greater rate of ATP use is required, as the myofibrils develop greater tension.

In cardiac hypertrophy, Laplace's law explains the effects of changes in wall thickness on wall stress (see Fig. 24-21). The increased wall thickness caused by hypertrophy balances the increased pressure, and the wall stress remains unchanged during the phase of compensatory hypertrophy. This change was previously regarded as compensatory and beneficial, but this view has been seriously challenged by a mouse model in which the process of hypertrophy was genetically inhibited so that wall stress increased in response to a pressure load, yet these mice had better cardiac mechanical function than did the wild type that developed compensatory hypertrophy.[1] Despite this "mighty mouse" challenge, it is difficult to see how a patient with significant aortic stenosis could develop the required intraventricular pressure to eject blood through the stenosed valve without the development of LV hypertrophy. Another clinically useful concept is that in congestive heart failure, the heart dilates so that the increased radius elevates wall stress. Furthermore, because ejection of blood is inadequate, the radius stays too large throughout the contractile cycle, and both end-diastolic and end-systolic tensions are higher. Compensation for the LV enlargement may be that myocytes need to contract less to maintain stroke volume. Overall reduction of heart size decreases wall stress and improves LV function.

WALL STRESS, PRELOAD, AND AFTERLOAD. This definition brings in both the volume and the fiber length that define the radius. Preload can now be defined more exactly as the wall stress at the end of diastole and therefore at the maximal resting length of the sarcomere (see Fig. 24-20). Measurement of wall stress in vivo is difficult because the radius of the left ventricle (see preceding sections) neglects the confounding influence of the complex anatomy of the left ventricle. Surrogate measurements of the indices of preload include LV end-diastolic pressure and dimensions (the latter being the major and minor axes of the heart in a two-dimensional echocardiographic view). The afterload, being the load on the contracting myocardium, is also the wall stress during LV ejection. Increased afterload means that an increased intraventricular pressure has to be generated first to open the aortic valve and then during the ejection phase. These increases will be translated into an increased myocardial wall stress, which can be measured as an average value or at end-systole. Peak systolic wall stress reflects the three major components of the afterload, namely, the peripheral resistance, the arterial compliance, and the peak intraventricular pressure. Decreased arterial compliance and increased afterload can be anticipated when there is aortic dilation, as in severe systemic hypertension or in the elderly. In general, in clinical practice, it is a sufficient approximation to take the systolic blood pressure as an indirect measure of the afterload (reflecting both peripheral resistance and peak intraventricular pressure), provided there is neither significant aortic stenosis nor change in arterial compliance.

Aortic impedance (arterial input impedance) gives another accurate measure of the afterload. The aortic impedance is the aortic pressure divided by the aortic flow at that instance, so that this index of the afterload varies at each stage of the contraction cycle. Factors reducing aortic flow, such as high arterial blood pressure, aortic stenosis, and loss of aortic compliance, will increase impedance and hence the afterload. During systole, when the aortic valve is open, an increased afterload will be communicated to the ventricles by increasing wall stress. In LV failure, aortic impedance is augmented not only by peripheral vasoconstriction but by decreases in aortic compliance. The problem with the clinical measurement of aortic impedance is that invasive instrumentation is required. An approximation can be found by using transesophageal echocardiography to determine aortic blood flow at, for example, the time of maximal increase of aortic flow just after aortic valve opening.

Heart Rate and Force-Frequency Relation

TREPPE OR BOWDITCH EFFECT. An increased heart rate progressively enhances the force of ventricular contraction, even in an isolated papillary muscle preparation (Bowditch staircase phenomenon). Alternative names are the treppe (German, steps) phenomenon, positive inotropic effect of activation, and force-frequency relationship (**Fig. 24-22**). Conversely, a decreased heart rate has a negative staircase effect. When stimulation becomes too rapid, force decreases. The proposal is that during rapid stimulation, more sodium and calcium ions enter the myocardial cell than can be handled by the sodium pump and the mechanisms for calcium exit. Opposing the force-frequency effect is the negative contractile influence of the decreased duration of ventricular filling at high heart rates. The longer the filling interval, the better the ventricular filling and the stronger the subsequent contraction. This phenomenon can be shown in patients with atrial fibrillation with a variable filling interval. In heart failure, the phenomenon is muted or lost.

Post-extrasystolic potentiation and the inotropic effect of paired pacing can be explained by the same model, again assuming an enhanced contractile state after the prolonged interval between beats. Nonetheless, the exact cellular mechanism remains to be clarified.

FORCE-FREQUENCY RELATIONSHIP AND OPTIMAL HEART RATE. Normally, peak contractile force at a fixed muscle length (isometric contraction) increases and a peak is reached at about 150 to 180 stimuli per minute.[1] This is the human counterpart of the treppe phenomenon. In situ, the optimal heart rate is the rate that would give maximal mechanical performance of an isolated muscle strip and is also determined by the need for adequate time for diastolic filling. In normal humans, it is not possible to attach exact values to the heart rate required to decrease rather than to increase cardiac output or to keep it steady. Pacing rates of up to 150 beats/min can be tolerated, whereas higher rates cannot because of the development of AV block.

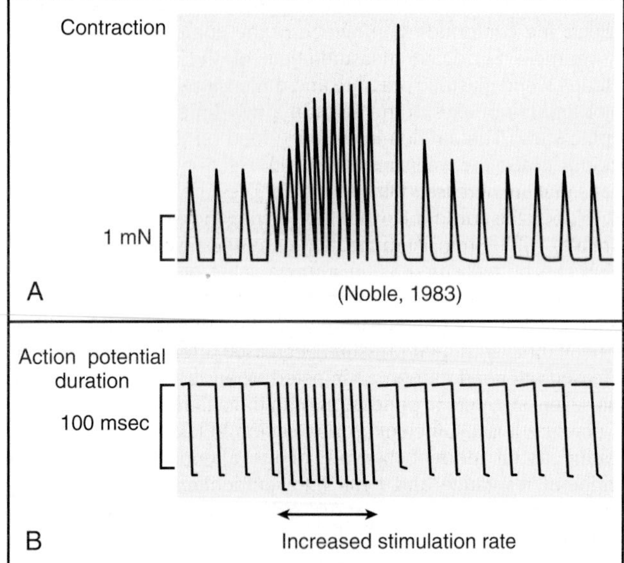

FIGURE 24-22 Bowditch or treppe phenomenon. A faster stimulation rate **(B)** increases the force of contraction **(A).** The stimulus rate is shown as the action potential duration (milliseconds) on an analog analyzer. The tension developed by papillary muscle contraction is shown in millinewtons (mN) in **A.** On cessation of rapid stimulation, the contraction force gradually declines. Hypothetically, the explanation for the increased contraction during the increased stimulation is repetitive Ca^{2+} entry with each depolarization and, hence, an accumulation of cytosolic calcium. *(From Noble MIM: Excitation-contraction coupling.* In *Drake-Holland AJ, Noble MIM [eds]: Cardiac Metabolism. Chichester, UK, John Wiley, 1983, pp 49-71.)*

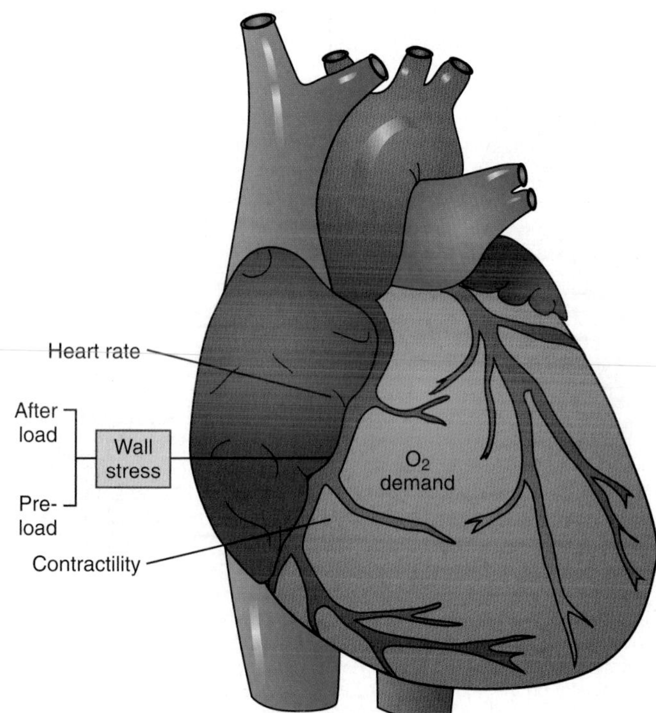

FIGURE 24-23 Major determinants of the oxygen (O_2) demand of the normal heart. These are heart rate, wall stress, and contractile function. For use of pressure-volume area as index of oxygen uptake, see Figure 24-24. *(Modified from Opie LH: The Heart: Physiology, From Cell to Circulation. Philadelphia, Lippincott Raven, 1998. © L. H. Opie, 2000.)*

In contrast, during exercise, indices of LV function still increase up to a maximum heart rate of about 170 beats/min, presumably because of enhanced contractile function and peripheral vasodilation.[1] In patients with severe LV hypertrophy, the critical heart rate is between 100 and 130 beats/min, with a fall off in LV function at higher rates (see Fig. 15-3 in Opie[16]).

Myocardial Oxygen Uptake

The myocardial oxygen demand can be increased by heart rate, preload, or afterload (**Fig. 24-23**), factors that can precipitate myocardial ischemia in those with coronary artery disease. The oxygen uptake can also be augmented by increased contractile function as during beta-adrenergic stimulation. Because myocardial oxygen uptake ultimately reflects the rate of mitochondrial metabolism and of ATP production, any increase of ATP requirement will be reflected in an increased oxygen uptake. In general, factors increasing wall stress will increase the oxygen uptake. An increased afterload causes an increased systolic wall stress, which needs a greater oxygen uptake. An increased diastolic wall stress, resulting from an increased preload, will also require more oxygen because the greater stroke volume must be ejected against the afterload. In states of enhanced contractile function, the rate of change of wall stress is increased. Thus, thinking in terms of wall stress provides a comprehensive approach to the problem of myocardial oxygen uptake. Because the systolic blood pressure is an important determinant of the afterload, a practical index of the oxygen uptake is systolic blood pressure × heart rate, the double-product. In addition, the metabolic component to the oxygen uptake is usually small but may be prominent in certain special conditions, such as the "oxygen wastage" found during abnormally high circulating free fatty acid values in hyperadrenergic conditions such as severe heart failure.[48] The concept of wall stress in relation to oxygen uptake also explains why heart size is such an important determinant of the myocardial oxygen uptake (because the larger radius increases wall stress).

WORK OF THE HEART. External work is done when, for example, a mass is lifted a certain distance. In terms of the heart, the cardiac output is the mass moved, and the resistance against which it is moved is the blood pressure. Because volume work needs less oxygen than pressure work does, it might be supposed that external work is not an important determinant of the myocardial oxygen uptake. However, three determinants of the myocardial oxygen uptake are involved: preload (because this helps determine the stroke volume), afterload (in part determined by the blood pressure), and heart rate, as can be seen from the following formula:

$$\text{Minute work} = \text{SBP} \times \text{SV} \times \text{heart rate}$$

where SBP is systolic blood pressure and SV is stroke volume. Thus, it is not surprising that heart work is related to oxygen uptake. The pressure-work index takes into account both the double-product (SBP × heart rate) and the heart rate × SV (i.e., cardiac output). The pressure-volume area, another index of myocardial oxygen uptake, requires invasive monitoring for accurate measurements. External cardiac work can account for up to 40% of the total myocardial oxygen uptake.

INTERNAL WORK (POTENTIAL ENERGY). The total oxygen consumption is related to the total work of the heart (area abcd in **Fig. 24-24**), meaning both the external work (the area abce) and the volume-pressure triangle joining the end-systolic volume-pressure point to the origin (the area cde; marked PE).[49] Although this area has been called internal work, more strictly it should be called potential energy that is generated within each contraction cycle but not converted to external work. Such potential energy at the end of systole (point c) may be likened to the potential energy of a compressed spring.

KINETIC WORK. In strict terms, the work performed (power production) needs to take into account not only pressure but kinetic components. It is the pressure work that has been discussed (product of cardiac output and peak systolic pressure). The kinetic work is the component required to move the blood against the afterload. Normally, kinetic work is less than 1% of the total. In aortic stenosis, kinetic work increases sharply as the cross-sectional area of the aortic valve narrows, whereas

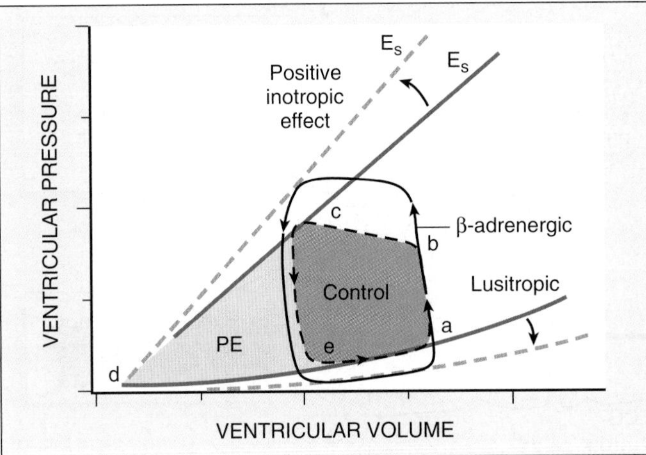

FIGURE 24-24 Pressure-volume loop of left ventricle. Note the effects of beta-adrenergic catecholamines with both positive inotropic (increased slope of line E_s) and increased lusitropic (relaxant) effects. E_s is the slope of the pressure-volume relationship. The total pressure-volume area (for control area, see abcd) is closely related to the myocardial oxygen uptake. The area cde is that component of work spent in generating potential energy (PE). *(Modified from Opie LH: Heart Physiology, From Cell to Circulation. Philadelphia, Lippincott Williams & Wilkins, 2004. © L. H. Opie, 2004.)*

pressure work increases as the gradient across the aortic valve rises. Noninvasive measures of peak power production are being assessed as indices of cardiac contractile function.

Efficiency of work is the relation between the work performed and the myocardial oxygen uptake. Exercise increases the efficiency of external work, an improvement that offsets any metabolic cost of the increased contractile function.[1] Efficiency is metabolically increased by promotion of glucose rather than of fatty acids as major myocardial fuel.[1] Conversely, heart failure decreases the efficiency of work, possibly by beta-adrenergic–promoted fatty acid metabolism.[1] The subcellular basis for changes in efficiency of work is not fully understood. Because as little as 12% to 14% of the oxygen uptake may be converted to external work,[1] it is probably the internal work that becomes less demanding. Internal ion fluxes ($Na^+/K^+/Ca^{2+}$) account for about 20% to 30% of the ATP requirement of the heart, so that most ATP is spent on actin-myosin interaction, and much of that on generation of heat rather than on external work. An increased initial muscle length sensitizes the contractile apparatus to calcium (see Fig. 24-19), thereby theoretically increasing the efficiency of contraction by diminishing the amount of calcium flux required.

Measurements of Contractile Function

FORCE-VELOCITY RELATIONSHIP AND MAXIMUM CONTRACTILE FUNCTION IN MUSCLE MODELS. If the concept of contractile function is truly independent of the load and the heart rate, unloaded heart muscle stimulated at a fixed rate should have a maximum value of contractile function for any given magnitude of the cytosolic calcium transient. This value, the V_{max} of muscle contraction, is defined as the maximal velocity of contraction when there is no load on the isolated muscle or no afterload to prevent maximal rates of cardiac ejection. Beta-adrenergic stimulation increases V_{max}, and converse changes are found in the failing myocardium. V_{max} is also termed V_0 (the maximum velocity at zero load). The problem with this relatively simple concept is that V_{max} cannot be measured directly but is extrapolated from the peak rates of shortening in unloaded muscle obtained from the intercept on the velocity axis. In another extreme condition, there is no muscle shortening at all (zero shortening), and all the energy goes into development of pressure (P_0) or force (F_0). This situation is an example of isometric shortening (*iso,* the same; *metric,* length). Because the peak velocity is obtained at zero load when there is no external force development, the relationship is usually termed the force-velocity relationship.

The concept of V_{max} has been subject to much debate over many years chiefly because of the technical difficulties in obtaining truly unloaded conditions. Braunwald and colleagues[50] used cat papillary muscle to define a hyperbolic force-velocity curve, with V_{max} relatively independent of the initial muscle length but increased by the addition of norepinephrine. The force-velocity relation is hyperbolic, suggesting the existence of intracellular passive elastic elements such as those generated by titin (see Fig. 24-4) that contribute to the load on the isolated myocyte.

ISOMETRIC VERSUS ISOTONIC CONTRACTION. Data for P_0 are obtained under isometric conditions (length unchanged). When muscle is allowed to shorten against a steady load, the conditions are isotonic (*iso,* same; *tonic,* contractile force). Thus, the force-velocity curve may be a combination of initial isometric conditions followed by isotonic contraction, then the abrupt and total unloading to measure V_{max}. Although isometric conditions can be found in the whole heart as an approximation during isovolumic contraction, isotonic conditions cannot prevail because the load is constantly changing during the ejection period, and complete unloading is impossible. Therefore, the application of force-velocity relations to the heart in vivo is limited.

PRESSURE-VOLUME LOOPS. Accordingly, measurements of pressure-volume loops are among the best of the current approaches to the assessment of the contractile behavior of the intact heart (see Fig. 24-24). A crucial measurement is E_s, the pressure-volume relationship. When the loading conditions are changed, changes in the slope of this line joining the different E_s points (the ESPV or end-systolic pressure-volume relationship) are generally a good load-independent index of the contractile performance of the heart. In clinical practice, the need to change the loading conditions and the invasive monitoring required for the full pressure-volume loop lessen the usefulness of this index. To measure LV volume adequately and continuously throughout the cardiac cycle is not easy. During a positive inotropic intervention, the pressure-volume loop reflects a smaller end-systolic volume and a higher end-systolic pressure, so that the slope of the pressure-volume relationship (E_s) has moved upward and to the left (see Fig. 24-24). When the positive inotropic intervention is by beta-adrenergic stimulation, enhanced relaxation (lusitropic effect) results in a lower pressure-volume curve during ventricular filling than in controls.

POWER PRODUCTION AND CONTRACTILE FUNCTION. Power production is the basis of another approach to contractile function. Power is defined as work per unit time, where F equals force:

$$\text{Power} = \text{work/time} = (\text{F} \times \text{cm})/\text{time} = \text{pressure}(\text{F/cm}^2) \times \text{CO}(\text{cm}^3/\text{time})$$

Power is composed of kinetic and pressure components.[16] The peak power index is the maximal power divided by the end-diastolic volume, which is proposed as a load-independent index of contractile function.[33] Maximum power in turn is approximated by peak aortic flow and systolic pressure, which in practice can be measured invasively as the maximal instantaneous product of pressure and flow.[33]

DEFECTS IN THE CONTRACTILE FUNCTION CONCEPT. Despite all these procedures that can be adopted to attempt to measure true contractile function, the concept has at least two serious defects: (1) the absence of any potential index that can be measured in situ and is free of significant criticism and, in particular, the absence of any acceptable noninvasive index; and (2) the impossibility of separating the cellular mechanisms of contractile function changes from those of load or heart rate. Thus, an increased heart rate through the sodium pump lag mechanism gives rise to an increased cytosolic calcium, which is thought to explain the treppe phenomenon. An increased preload involves increased fiber stretch, which in turn causes length activation, explicable by sensitization of the contractile proteins to the prevailing cytosolic calcium concentration. An increased afterload may increase cytosolic calcium through stretch-sensitive channels. Thus, there is a clear overlap between contractile function, which should be independent of load or heart rate, and the effects of load and heart rate on the cellular mechanisms. Hence, the traditional separation of inotropic state from load and heart rate effects as two independent regulators of cardiac muscle performance is no longer simple now that the underlying cellular mechanisms have been uncovered. An example of this dilemma is in humans with atrial fibrillation and a constantly varying force-frequency relationship. Contractile function as measured in situ by pressure-volume loops constantly changes from beat to beat, and the explanation could be either a true change in contractile function or the operation of the Frank-Starling mechanism because of varying diastolic filling times.[1]

Left Ventricular Twist Motion and Noninvasive Measurement of Contractility

Whatever the defects of the concept and the problems of measuring it, contractile function remains an essential cardiac concept to separate the effects of a primary change in loading conditions or heart rate from an intrinsic change in the force of contraction. A standard index of contractility is the maximal positive dP/dt (dP/dt_{max}), an index measured during the isovolumic phase of contraction that is relatively load independent. This index, however, requires invasive and highly accurate LV pressure measurements. Optimal measurement of LV function should assess LV twist motion, which results from apical counterclockwise and basal clockwise rotation of the left ventricle, both essential for generation of LV pumping power.[51] The extent of the twist can now be measured noninvasively by speckle tracking echocardiography, which closely correlates with dP/dt_{max} in a variety of experimental conditions and is superior to the global ejection fraction.[51]

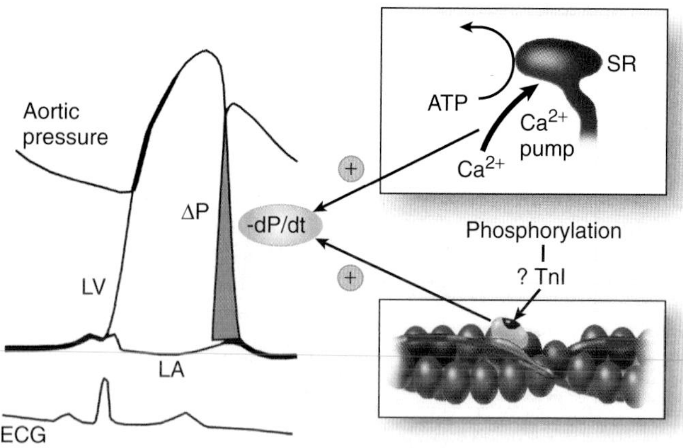

FIGURE 24-25 Factors governing the isovolumic relaxation phase of the cardiac cycle. This period of the cycle extends from the aortic second sound (A_2) to the crossover point between the left ventricular and left atrial pressures (see Fig 24-18). The maximum negative rate of pressure development ($-dP/dt_{max}$), which gives the isovolumic relaxation rate, is measured either invasively or by a continuous-wave Doppler velocity spectrum in aortic regurgitation. Isovolumic relaxation is increased (plus sign) when the rate of calcium uptake into the sarcoplasmic reticulum (SR) is enhanced, for example, during beta-adrenergic stimulation (see Fig. 24-11). Isovolumic relaxation may also be enhanced when phosphorylation of troponin I (TnI), as in response to beta-adrenergic stimulation, may decrease the affinity of the contractile system for calcium (see Fig. 24-3). *(From Opie LH: Heart Physiology, From Cell to Circulation. Philadelphia, Lippincott Williams & Wilkins, 2004. © L. H. Opie, 2004.)*

Ventricular Relaxation and Diastolic Dysfunction

That diastolic dysfunction and diastolic heart failure can occur in the presence of normal or relatively normal systolic function (now often referred to as a preserved ejection fraction) is now widely accepted (see Chap. 30). Indeed, approximately 40% to 50% of patients with heart failure will have a preserved ejection fraction. Among the many complex physiologic and pathologic factors influencing relaxation, four are of chief interest. First, the cytosolic calcium level must fall to cause the relaxation phase, a process requiring ATP and phosphorylation of phospholamban for uptake of calcium into the SR. Second, the inherent viscoelastic properties of the myocardium are of importance. In the hypertrophied heart with increased fibrosis, relaxation occurs more slowly. Particularly in the early stages of the hypertrophied heart of hypertension and aortic stenosis, a situation arises in which systolic function is relatively well preserved but diastolic relaxation is impaired. The probable explanation is that hypertrophy is accompanied by increasing fibrosis.[52] Third, increased phosphorylation of troponin I enhances the rate of relaxation.[1] Fourth, relaxation is influenced by the systolic load.[1] Thus, the history of contraction affects cross-bridge relaxation. Within limits, the greater the systolic load, the faster the rate of relaxation. This complex relationship has been explored in detail by Brutsaert's group[53] but could perhaps be simplified as follows. When the workload is high, peak cytosolic calcium is also high. Thus, the rate of fall of calcium is also greater, provided the diastolic uptake mechanisms function effectively. In this way, a systolic pressure load and the rate of diastolic relaxation can be related. Furthermore, a greater muscle length (when the workload is high) at the end of systole should produce a more rapid rate of relaxation by the opposite of length-dependent sensitization. When the afterload exceeds a certain limit, the rate of relaxation is delayed,[16] with diastolic dysfunction. Thus, in congestive heart failure caused by an excess systolic load, relaxation becomes increasingly afterload dependent, so that therapeutic reduction of the systolic load should improve LV relaxation.

IMPAIRED RELAXATION AND CYTOSOLIC CALCIUM (see Chap. 30). For these purposes, this chapter uses the clinical definition of diastole, according to which diastole extends from aortic valve closure to the start of the first heart sound. The first phase of diastole is the isovolumic phase, which, by definition, does not contribute to ventricular filling. The second phase of rapid filling provides most of ventricular filling. The third phase of slow filling or diastasis accounts for only 5% of the total filling. The final atrial booster phase accounts for the remaining 15%.

Isovolumic relaxation is energy dependent, requiring ATP for the uptake of calcium ions by the SR (**Fig. 24-25**), which is an active, not a passive, process. Impaired relaxation is an early event in angina pectoris. A proposed metabolic explanation is that there is impaired generation of energy, which diminishes the supply of ATP required for the early diastolic uptake of calcium by the SR. The result is that the cytosolic calcium level, at a peak in systole, delays its return to normal in the early diastolic period. In other conditions, too, there is a relationship between the rate of diastolic decay of the calcium transient and diastolic relaxation, with a relation to impaired function of the SR.[16] Also, regional nonuniformity of contraction may impair isovolumic relaxation. When the rate of relaxation is prolonged by hypothyroidism, the rate of return of the systolic calcium elevation is likewise delayed, whereas opposite changes occur in hyperthyroidism. In congestive heart failure, diastolic relaxation also is delayed and irregular, as is the rate of decay of the cytosolic calcium elevation. Most patients with coronary artery disease have a variety of abnormalities of diastolic filling, probably related to those also found in angina pectoris. Theoretically, such abnormalities of relaxation are potentially reversible because they depend on changes in patterns of calcium ion movement.

MEASUREMENT OF ISOVOLUMIC RELAXATION. The rate of isovolumic relaxation is best measured by negative dP/dt_{max} at invasive catheterization. Tau, the time constant of relaxation, describes the rate of fall of LV pressure during isovolumic relaxation and also requires invasive techniques for precise determination. Tau is increased as the systolic LV pressure rises. Other indices of isovolumic relaxation can be obtained echocardiographically or from tissue Doppler measurements to monitor the peak rate of wall thinning.

VENTRICULAR SUCTION DURING EARLY DIASTOLE. The idea that the LV suction by active relaxation could increase the pressure gradient from left atrium to left ventricle during the early filling phase is now well supported by data.[54] The suction effect can be found by carefully comparing LV and left atrial pressures, and it occurs especially in the early diastolic phase of rapid filling as a result of the LV elastic recoil. During catecholamine stimulation, the rate of relaxation increases to enhance the sucking effect and to prolong the period of filling. In mitral stenosis, the mitral valve does not respond as it otherwise should in response to diastolic suction, hence impairing diastolic filling. In dilated cardiomyopathy, there is a double defect. The impaired elastic recoil of the left ventricle lessens the diastolic suction, while the pattern of blood flow from the mitral valve to the apex is abnormal, deviating from the longitudinal axis of the ventricle with formation of vortices.[54]

The proposed molecular mechanism of sucking is as follows. In early diastole, myosin is pulled into the space between the two anchoring segments of titin to lower the intraventricular pressure to below that in the atrium.[1] Ventricular suction, by propagating a dominant backward pressure wave, is also responsible for diastolic coronary filling and attenuated in LV hypertrophy.[55]

Atrial Function

The left atrium has five main functions.[1,56] The best known function is that of a blood-receiving reservoir chamber. Second, it also is a contractile chamber that, by presystolic contraction and its atrial booster function, helps complete LV filling. Third, it functions as a conduit that empties its contents into the left ventricle down a pressure gradient after the mitral valve opens. Fourth, it is the volume sensor of the heart, releasing atrial natriuretic peptide (ANP) in response to intermittent stretch, so that an ANP-induced diuresis can help restore blood volume to normal. Fifth and finally, the atrium contains receptors for the afferent arms of various reflexes including mechanoreceptors that increase sinus discharge rate, thereby contributing to the tachycardia of exercise as the venous return increases (Bainbridge reflex).

The atrial pressure-volume loop is very different in shape from that of the ventricles, resembling a figure-of-8. During atrial pacing, the preload is increased and the atria are distended, so that the volume part of the loop is small and the pressure part of the loop is much enlarged.[57] The atria have a number of differences in structure and function from the ventricles, including smaller myocytes, a shorter action potential duration, and a more fetal type of myosin (both in heavy and light chains). The more rapid atrial repolarization is thought to be due to increased outward potassium currents, such as I_{to} and $I_{K.ACh}$. In general, these histologic and physiologic changes can be related to the decreased need for the atria to generate high intrachamber pressures, rather being sensitive to volume changes while retaining enough contractile action to help with LV filling and to respond to inotropic stimuli. Atrial remodeling refers to a variety of ionic, structural, contractile, and metabolic changes that are induced by insults such as chronic atrial tachyarrhythmias, including atrial fibrillation,[57] or by left atrial stretch and enlargement. The cellular mechanisms include decreased L-type calcium channel activity,[57] increased abnormal collagen,[58] and probably adverse stretch-induced signaling. The results include poor contractile performance and an increased initiation and perpetuation of atrial fibrillation.

Contractile Patterns in Physiologic and Pathologic Hypertrophy

Effects of Mechanical Load on Contraction and Relaxation

WALL STRESS AND COMPENSATED LEFT VENTRICULAR HYPERTROPHY. Meerson, in 1962, studied the cardiac hypertrophic response to experimental constriction of the aorta (for concept, see Fig. 21-6, Braunwald, 7th edition).[59] He described the prolonged protective state of "compensatory hyperfunction" of the heart. Thereafter, if the pressure load were continued, the left ventricle developed fibrosis with a transition to the "decompensated" state with failure and dilation. To explain the mechanism of the LV hypertrophy, Grossman, in 1975, proposed that the hypertrophic response was evoked by increased wall stretch, the result of an increased intraventricular LV pressure (**Fig. 24-26**). According to his systolic stress correction hypothesis, pressure overload caused myocytes to grow in width and to thicken (see Fig. 24-26). Then, according to the Laplace law, the

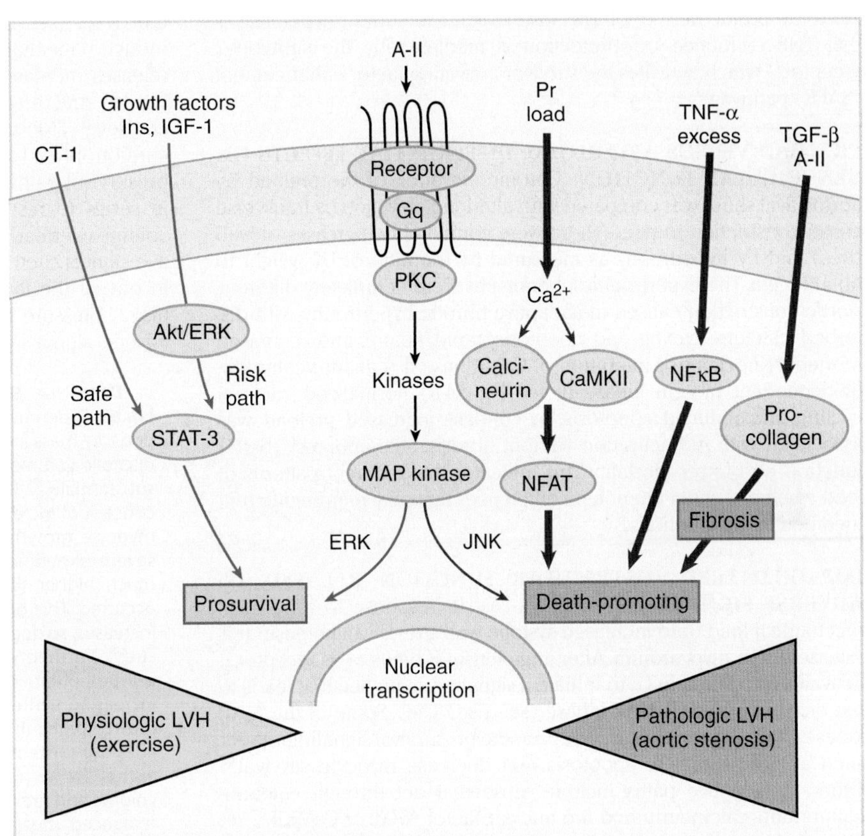

FIGURE 24-26 Consequences of physiologic versus pathologic signaling for mechanical function. Pathways on the left side of figure lead predominantly to myocyte survival and adaptive hypertrophy with enhanced contraction-relaxation function, whereas those on the right lead to death-promoting fibrosis and apoptosis. Angiotensin II (A-II) released from myocardial cells by biomechanical stress, such as prolonged stretch or pressure, leads to both prosurvival (on the left) and death-promoting pathways (on the right), the former via ERK (extracellular signal-regulated kinase) and the later via JNK (Jun N-terminal kinase). Tumor necrosis factor-α (TNF-α) acting physiologically, as on the left, is prosurvival; but in excess, it probably acts adversely via NF-κB (nuclear factor κ-B), which is also where prolonged pressure (Pr) loading acts. Calmodulin kinase II (CaMKII) is a newly recognized step on the pathologic pressure-overload path.[69] Transforming growth factor-β (TGF-β) promotes the conversion of procollagen to fibrosis. Thus, depending on the nature of the biomechanical stress, the myocardium can adapt in such a way that mechanical function is either enhanced (left side of figure) or depressed (right side of figure). Akt = protein kinase B/Akt; CT-1 = cardiotrophin-1; IGF-1 = insulin-like growth factor; Ins = insulin; MAP = mitogen-activated protein; NFAT= nuclear factor of activated T cells; PKC = protein kinase C; SAFE = survivor activating factor enhancement; RISK = reperfusion injury survival kinases; STAT = signal transducer and activator of transcription. *(Updated from Opie LH: Heart Physiology, From Cell to Circulation. Philadelphia, Lippincott Williams & Wilkins, 2004. © L. H. Opie, 2004.)*

increased wall thickness would decrease and even normalize the increased wall stress (for review, see Opie[59]). This hypothesis is currently under challenge from studies on transgenic mice, yet the compensated hypertrophic state remains an oft-cited clinical entity.[52] An examination of the signaling paths involved in LV hypertrophy can explain such apparent contradictions.

LEFT VENTRICULAR RESPONSE TO MECHANICAL STRESS. There are two basic patterns of response to a sustained LV pressure load hypothetically associated with adaptive and maladaptive signals (see Fig. 24-26). According to the signaling stimulus invoked by the load, the myocyte can either survive, leading to "beneficial hypertrophy," or undergo adverse patterns of signaling that lead to hypertrophy-associated apoptosis (programmed cell death) and related degenerative patterns. Thus, in adverse signaling, LV hypertrophy is associated with varying degrees of LV failure and dilation.[59]

The "beneficial" survival paths include the prosurvival extracellular signal–regulated kinase (ERK), which, when genetically activated,[59] yields an adaptive hypertrophy with normalized wall stress and fully compensated for an increased load (see Fig. 24-26). Likewise, exercise-induced heart hypertrophy (see later) involves the closely related enzyme Akt, also known as protein kinase B (see Fig. 24-26).[60] The Akt path can also be activated by IGF-1. Two groups have recently emphasized the protective role of low-dose TNF-α. The current hypothesis is that TNF-α–induced cytoprotection is mediated by the subtype 2 receptor,[61] which activates the survivor activating factor enhancement (SAFE) pathway.[62]

PRELOAD VERSUS AFTERLOAD: DIFFERENTIAL EFFECTS ON VENTRICULAR FUNCTION. Chronic elevation of the preload by aorto-caval shunt was compared with afterload elevation by transverse aortic constriction in mice. There were comparable increases of wall stress and LV hypertrophy, as measured by the ratio of LV weight to tibial length. The hypertrophic phenotypes were completely different. Aortic constriction caused maladaptive fibrotic hypertrophy with disturbed calcium cycling and apoptosis, rapid failure, and increased mortality. Knockout or inhibition of CaMKinase II (calcium/calmodulin-dependent protein kinase II; see Fig. 24-8) normalized calcium cycling and reduced apoptosis. In contrast, increased preload was associated with Akt activation without fibrosis, little apoptosis, better function, and lower mortality. This indicates that different patterns of load result in distinct phenotype differences that may require different therapeutic interventions.[62a]

IMPAIRED LEFT VENTRICULAR FUNCTION RELATED TO ADVERSE SIGNALING (see Chap. 25). In response to an abrupt mechanical load or to increased systolic wall stress,[59] angiotensin II is released from myocardium. After angiotensin II binds to its receptor, it activates the G protein G_q to initiate a signaling sequence that leads to the enzyme complex MAP kinase (see Fig. 24-26). Some of the MAP kinase components, such as ERK, promote prosurvival signaling; others, such as JNK, stimulate apoptosis and decrease myocyte survival.[59] Other maladaptive paths include those that act through calcium-calmodulin, calcineurin and the nuclear factor NFAT, or CaMKII.[63] Yet others promote fibrosis in response to angiotensin II, aldosterone, and transforming growth factor-β.

If pressure-induced angiotensin II stimulation leads to more maladaptive than adaptive growth and more apoptosis, genetic interruption of the angiotensin II path would lessen hypertrophy yet protect the myocardium. In a mouse model in which part of the angiotensin II receptor–related signaling system was transgenically inactivated by elimination of the G protein G_q, pressure loading gave less than predicted hypertrophy with decreased correction of wall stress,[64] yet contractile function was better than in the wild type that had more LV hypertrophy. This finding shows that the wall stress model is not infallible, rather depending on which is the signaling path that promotes the hypertrophy.

LEFT VENTRICULAR HYPERTROPHY AND DIASTOLIC DYSFUNCTION (see Chap. 30). In hearts with concentric hypertrophy, as in chronic hypertension or severe aortic stenosis, abnormalities of diastole are common and may precede systolic failure. Regarding the signaling paths involved in aortic stenosis with LV hypertrophy, there is strong evidence for growth signals such as angiotensin II and transforming growth factor-β being associated not only with myocyte growth but also with maladaptive fibrosis, myocyte degeneration, and eventual myocyte loss.[52] Overall, taking both experimental and limited patient data into account, a sustained pressure load, as in aortic stenosis, is a mixed stimulus that produces both beneficial adaptive and adverse maladaptive remodeling. The latter could explain why the wall stress correction hypothesis does not always apply and why, in patients with aortic stenosis, increased LV mass predicts systolic dysfunction and heart failure.[65]

LEFT VENTRICULAR DYSFUNCTION IN INSULIN RESISTANCE. In conditions such as diabetes type 2, an accumulation of myocardial triglyceride (cardiac steatosis) is related to diastolic dysfunction rather than to systolic failure. The proposed mechanism is related to excess circulating free fatty acids and impaired glucose tolerance associated with insulin resistance.[66]

LEFT VENTRICULAR VOLUME LOADING AND THE SIGNALS INVOLVED. Volume differs from pressure loading in several important ways (see Fig. 25-9). From the signaling point of view, volume-induced mechanical stress with progressively greater LV volumes releases increasing amounts of TNF from the normal myocardium. Passive stretch of ventricular muscle promotes TNF mRNA synthesis. Low-level TNF stimulation interlinks with other cytokines, such as cardiotrophin 1 acting on the glycoprotein 130 receptor, to promote prosurvival pathways (see Fig. 24-26) so that the sarcomere units form in series to result in eccentric hypertrophy.[59] Remodeling in early volume overload may be related to stretch-induced signaling via adaptive signals such as cardiotrophin 1, low-level TNF-α, cGMP, and IGF-1. In one of the few direct comparisons with pressure-loading mechanisms, pressure but not volume overload increased the potentially adverse signal JNK,[67] compatible with the scheme in Figure 24-26.

DOES THE STRESS CORRECTION HYPOTHESIS HOLD FOR A VOLUME LOAD? Experimentally, after 3 months of severe mitral regurgitation in dogs, LV mass increased with cardiomyocyte lengthening, whereas end-diastolic volume and wall stress (both diastolic and systolic) increased substantially.[68] Overall, the data are compatible with the Grossman concept of increased diastolic wall stress as the initiator of longitudinal myocyte growth in response to a chronic volume load.[59] However, in severe experimental mitral regurgitation, end-diastolic wall stress is much higher (by about fourfold) so that stress correction has not occurred. This problem could be predicted because as myocyte length increases, so does the radius, thus increasing rather than decreasing wall stress. Furthermore, volume-induced ventricular enlargement may be self-perpetuating by promotion of increasing mitral regurgitation and increasing ventricular sphericity.[59] At this late stage, it is likely that the growth paths that are stimulated would be chiefly those with the maladaptive patterns (right side of Fig. 24-26), for example, in response to excess TNF-α. Conversely, athletic training may induce pathways of volume and pressure loading in a manner that produces an enlarged but "balanced" heart (**Table 24-5**; see Chap. 24 Online Supplement for further details about physiologic hypertrophy of the athlete's heart).

Future Perspectives

There will be an increasing focus on the multiple abnormalities of contraction and relaxation and the regulation of calcium cycles, especially in relation to ventricular dysfunction. On the basis of the increasing trend to deeper understanding and better treatment of the sub-subcellular aspects of human disease, calcium ion movements will be more specifically manipulated at new controlling microdomain sites. The key intracellular regulators will be found to be snuggling up to their molecular partners in a very localized way. Similar arguments hold for subcellular affinity domains for cGMP, which is coming to the fore as the major counterregulator of pathologic increased adrenergic activity. Likewise, further therapeutic targets might be the protein kinases and their scaffolding proteins and the relevant paths for their

TABLE 24-5 Contractile Patterns in Physiologic Versus Pathologic Hypertrophy

	PHYSIOLOGIC	PATHOLOGIC
Example	Athletic training	Aortic stenosis, severe
Signaling pattern	Prosurvival	Proapoptotic Profibrotic
Key signals	IGF-1; PI3K-Akt (also inhibits pathologic growth) STAT-3	P38 MAP kinase JNK TGF-β Angio-II
Fetal gene program	No	Yes
Interstitial fibrosis	No	Yes
Myocyte apoptosis	No	Yes
Systolic contraction	Normal or increased	Decreased
Diastolic relaxation	Normal or increased	Decreased
Doppler LV filling	Normal	Impaired

For sources, see references 59, 60, 70.
IGF = insulin-like growth factor; PI3K-Akt = phosphatidylinositol-3-phosphate kinase–Akt, where Akt is another term for protein kinase B; STAT-3 = signal transducer and activator of transcription; MAP kinase = mitogen-activated protein kinase; JNK = Jun N-terminal kinase; TGF-β = transforming growth factor-β; angio-II = angiotensin II.

synthesis and degradation. In the therapy for heart failure, two of the most successful current therapies relate to the beta receptor, namely, the therapeutic efficacy of beta-adrenergic blockers and the benefit of an exercise training program that increases vagal tone, hence being antiadrenergic. Two of the major basic science issues will be how to overcome beta receptor downregulation and how to stabilize the ryanodine receptor despite a beta-adrenergic assault. New drugs will sooner or later make feasible this jump from bench to bedside.

ACKNOWLEDGMENT

With regrets, many earlier references found in the previous edition (reference 1) had to be omitted.

REFERENCES

Cellular and Molecular Mechanisms

1. Opie LH: Mechanisms of cardiac contraction and relaxation. *In* Libby P, Bonow RO, Mann DL, Zipes DP (eds): Heart Disease: A Textbook of Cardiovascular Medicine. 8th ed. Philadelphia, Elsevier Saunders, 2008, pp 509-539.
2. Knoll R, Hoshijima M, Hoffman HM, et al: The cardiac mechanical stretch sensor machinery involves a Z disc complex that is defective in a subset of human dilated cardiomyopathy. Cell 111:943, 2002.
3. Rayment I, Holden HM, Whittaker M: Structure of the actin-myosin complex and its implications for muscle contraction. Science 261:58, 1993.
4. Brancaccio M, Hirsch E, Notte A, et al: Integrin signalling: The tug-of-war in heart hypertrophy. Cardiovasc Res 70:422, 2006.
5. Miyamoto T, Takeishi Y, Takahashi H, et al: Activation of distinct signal transduction pathways in hypertrophied hearts by pressure and volume overload. Basic Res Cardiol 99:328, 2004.
6. Toischer K, Kögler H, Tenderich G, et al: Elevated afterload, neuroendocrine stimulation, and human heart failure increase BNP levels and inhibit preload-dependent SERCA upregulation. Circ Heart Fail 1:265, 2008.
7. Ertz-Berger BR, He H, Dowell C, et al: Changes in the chemical and dynamic properties of cardiac troponin T cause discrete cardiomyopathies in transgenic mice. Proc Natl Acad Sci U S A 102:18219, 2005.
8. Fedak PW, Smookler DS, Kassiri Z, et al: TIMP-3 deficiency leads to dilated cardiomyopathy. Circulation 110:2401, 2004.
9. Chien KR: Genotype, phenotype: Upstairs, downstairs in the family of cardiomyopathies [commentary]. J Clin Invest 111:175, 2003.
10. Anderson ME, Mohler PJ: Rescuing a failing heart: Think globally, treat locally. Nat Med 15:25, 2009.
11. Zhou P, Zhao YT, Guo YB, et al: Beta-adrenergic signaling accelerates and synchronizes cardiac ryanodine receptor response to a single L-type Ca^{2+} channel. Proc Natl Acad Sci U S A 106:18028, 2009.
12. Wehrens XH, Lehnart SE, Reiken SR, Marks AR: Ca^{2+}/calmodulin-dependent protein kinase II phosphorylation regulates the cardiac ryanodine receptor. Circ Res 94:e61, 2004.
13. Grimm M, Brown J: Beta-adrenergic receptor signaling in the heart: Role of CaMKII. J Mol Cell Cardiol 48:322, 2010.
14. Bers DM, Grandi E: Calcium/calmodulin-dependent kinase II regulation of cardiac ion channels. J Cardiovasc Pharmacol 54:180, 2009.
15. Yang D, Zhu WZ, Xiao B, et al: Ca^{2+}/calmodulin kinase II–dependent phosphorylation of ryanodine receptors suppresses Ca^{2+} sparks and Ca^{2+} waves in cardiac myocytes. Circ Res 100:399, 2007.
16. Opie LH: Heart Physiology, From Cell to Circulation. 4th ed. Philadelphia, Lippincott Williams & Wilkins, 2004.
17. Tada M, Katz AM: Phosphorylation of the sarcoplasmic reticulum and sarcolemma. Annu Rev Physiol 44:401, 1982.
18. Kamp TJ, Chiamvimonvat N: Mission impossible: IGF-1 and PTEN specifically "Akt"ing on cardiac L-type Ca^{2+} channels. Circ Res 98:1349, 2006.
19. Aiba T, Hesketh GG, Liu T, et al: Na^+ channel regulation by Ca^{2+}/calmodulin and Ca^{2+}/calmodulin-dependent protein kinase II in guinea-pig ventricular myocytes. Cardiovasc Res 85:454, 2010.
20. Maltsev VA, Reznikov V, Undrovinas NA, et al: Modulation of late sodium current by Ca^{2+}, calmodulin, and CaMKII in normal and failing dog cardiomyocytes: Similarities and differences. Am J Physiol Heart Circ Physiol 294:H1597, 2008.
21. Zhang XQ, Ahlers BA, Tucker AL, et al: Phospholemman inhibition of the cardiac Na^+/Ca^{2+} exchanger. Role of phosphorylation. J Biol Chem 281:7784, 2006.

Cell Signaling

22. Woodcock EA, Du XJ, Reichelt ME, Graham RM: Cardiac $alpha_1$-adrenergic drive in pathological remodelling. Cardiovasc Res 77:452, 2008.
23. Dodge-Kafka KL, Langeberg L, Scott JD: Compartmentation of cyclic nucleotide signaling in the heart: The role of A-kinase anchoring proteins. Circ Res 98:993, 2006.
24. Castro LR, Verde I, Cooper DM, Fischmeister R: Cyclic guanosine monophosphate compartmentation in rat cardiac myocytes. Circulation 113:2221, 2006.
25. Baillie GS, Sood A, McPhee I, et al: Beta-arrestin–mediated PDE4 cAMP phosphodiesterase recruitment regulates beta-adrenoceptor switching from G_s to G_i. Proc Natl Acad Sci U S A 100:940, 2003.
26. Engelhardt S: Alternative signaling: Cardiomyocyte $beta_1$-adrenergic receptors signal through EGFRs. J Clin Invest 117:2396, 2007.
27. Penela P, Murga C, Ribas C, et al: Mechanisms of regulation of G protein–coupled receptor kinases (GRKs) and cardiovascular disease. Cardiovasc Res 69:46, 2006.
28. Chakir K, Daya SK, Aiba T, et al: Mechanisms of enhanced beta-adrenergic reserve from cardiac resynchronization therapy. Circulation 119:1231, 2009.
29. Sterin-Borda L, Bernabeo G, Ganzinelli S, et al: Role of nitric oxide/cyclic GMP and cyclic AMP in $beta_3$ adrenoceptor–chronotropic response. J Mol Cell Cardiol 40:580, 2006.
30. Okoshi K, Nakayama M, Yan X, et al: Neuregulins regulate cardiac parasympathetic activity: Muscarinic modulation of beta-adrenergic activity in myocytes from mice with neuregulin-1 gene deletion. Circulation 110:713, 2004.
31. Friebe A, Koesling D: Regulation of nitric oxide–sensitive guanylyl cyclase. Circ Res 93:96, 2003.
32. Ziolo MT, Bers DM: The real estate of NOS signaling. Location, location, location. Circ Res 92:1279, 2003.
33. Borlaug BA, Melenovsky V, Marhin T, et al: Sildenafil inhibits beta-adrenergic–stimulated cardiac contractility in humans. Circulation 112:2642, 2005.
34. Takimoto E, Champion HC, Li M, et al: Chronic inhibition of cyclic GMP phosphodiesterase 5A prevents and reverses cardiac hypertrophy. Nat Med 11:214, 2005.
35. Kone BC: NO break-ins at water gate. Hypertension 48:29, 2006.
36. Danson EJ, Paterson DJ: Enhanced neuronal nitric oxide synthase expression is central to cardiac vagal phenotype in exercise-trained mice. J Physiol 546:225, 2003.
37. Hambrecht R, Adams V, Erbs S, et al: Regular physical activity improves endothelial function in patients with coronary artery disease by increasing phosphorylation of endothelial nitric oxide synthase. Circulation 107:3152, 2003.
38. Shah AM, Sauer H: Transmitting biological information using oxygen: Reactive oxygen species as signalling molecules in cardiovascular pathophysiology. Cardiovasc Res 71:191, 2006.
39. Gross GJ: Role of opioids in acute and delayed preconditioning. J Mol Cell Cardiol 35:709, 2003.
40. Valgimigli M, Ceconi C, Malagutti P, et al: Tumor necrosis factor-alpha receptor 1 is a major predictor of mortality and new-onset heart failure in patients with acute myocardial infarction: The Cytokine-Activation and Long-Term Prognosis in Myocardial Infarction (C-ALPHA) study. Circulation 111:863, 2005.
41. Li M, Georgakopoulos D, Lu G, et al: p38 MAP kinase mediates inflammatory cytokine induction in cardiomyocytes and extracellular matrix remodeling in heart. Circulation 111:2494, 2005.
42. Pemberton CJ, Raudsepp SD, Yandle TG, et al: Plasma cardiotrophin-1 is elevated in human hypertension and stimulated by ventricular stretch. Cardiovasc Res 68:109, 2005.

Contractile Performance of the Heart

43. Lewis T: The Mechanism and Graphic Registration of the Heart Beat. London, Shaw and Sons, 1920.
44. Wiggers CJ: Modern Aspects of Circulation in Health and Disease. Philadelphia, Lea & Febiger, 1915.
45. Corsi C, Lang RM, Veronesi F, et al: Volumetric quantification of global and regional left ventricular function from real-time three-dimensional echocardiographic images. Circulation 112:1161, 2005.
46. Rodriguez EK, Hunter WC, Royce MJ: A method to reconstruct myocardial sarcomere lengths and orientations at transmural sites in beating canine hearts. Am J Physiol 263:H293, 1992.
47. Kogler H, Schott P, Toischer K, et al: Relevance of brain natriuretic peptide in preload-dependent regulation of cardiac sarcoplasmic reticulum Ca^{2+} ATPase expression. Circulation 113:2724, 2006.
48. Opie LH, Knuuti J: The adrenergic-fatty acid load in heart failure. J Am Coll Cardiol 54:1637, 2009.
49. Suga H, Hisano R, Hirata S, et al: Mechanism of higher oxygen consumption rate: Pressure-loaded vs volume-loaded heart. Am J Physiol 242:H942, 1982.
50. Braunwald E, Sonnenblick EH, Ross J: Normal and abnormal circulatory function. *In* Braunwald E (ed): Heart Disease: A Textbook of Cardiovascular Medicine. 4th ed. Philadelphia, WB Saunders, 1992.
51. Kim WJ, Lee BH, Kim YJ, et al: Apical rotation assessed by speckle-tracking echocardiography as an index of global left ventricular contractility. Circ Cardiovasc Imaging 2:123, 2009.
52. Hein S, Amon E, Kostin S, et al: Progression from compensated hypertrophy to failure in the pressure-overloaded human heart. Structural deterioration and compensatory mechanisms. Circulation 107:984, 2003.
53. Zile MR, Brutsaert DL: New concepts in diastolic dysfunction and diastolic heart failure: Part 1. Circulation 105:1387, 2002.

54. Little WC: Diastolic dysfunction beyond distensibility: Adverse effects of ventricular dilatation. Circulation 112:2888, 2005.
55. Davies JE, Whinnett ZI, Francis DP, et al: Evidence of a dominant backward-propagating "suction" wave responsible for diastolic coronary filling in humans, attenuated in left ventricular hypertrophy. Circulation 113:1768, 2006.
56. Pagel PS, Kehl F, Gare M, et al: Mechanical function of the left atrium: New insights based on analysis of pressure-volume relations and Doppler echocardiography. Anesthesiology 98:975, 2003.
57. Schotten U, Duytschaever M, Ausma J, et al: Electrical and contractile remodeling during the first days of atrial fibrillation go hand in hand. Circulation 107:1433, 2003.
58. Xu J, Cui G, Esmailian F, et al: Atrial extracellular matrix remodeling and the maintenance of atrial fibrillation. Circulation 109:363, 2004.
59. Opie LH, Commerford PJ, Gersh BJ, Pfeffer MA: Controversies in ventricular remodelling. Lancet 367:356, 2006.
60. Walsh K: Akt signaling and growth of the heart. Circulation 113:2032, 2006.
61. Burchfield JS, Dong JW, Sakata Y, et al: The cytoprotective effects of tumor necrosis factor are conveyed through tumor necrosis factor receptor–associated factor 2 in the heart. Circ Heart Fail 3:157, 2010.
62. Lacerda L, Somers S, Opie LH, Lecour S: Ischaemic postconditioning protects against reperfusion injury via the SAFE pathway. Cardiovasc Res 84:201, 2009.
62a. Toischer K, Rokita AG, Unsöld B, et al: Differential cardiac remodeling in preload versus afterload. Circulation 122:993, 2010.
63. Dorn GW 2nd, Force T: Protein kinase cascades in the regulation of cardiac hypertrophy. J Clin Invest 115:527, 2005.
64. Esposito G, Rapacciuolo A, Prasad SVN, et al: Genetic alterations that inhibit in vivo pressure-overload hypertrophy prevent cardiac dysfunction despite increased wall stress. Circulation 105:85, 2002.
65. Kupari M, Turto H, Lommi J: Left ventricular hypertrophy in aortic valve stenosis: Preventive or promotive of systolic dysfunction and heart failure? Eur Heart J 26:1790, 2005.
66. McGavock JM, Lingvay I, Zib I, et al: Cardiac steatosis in diabetes mellitus: A ^{1}H-magnetic resonance spectroscopy study. Circulation 116:1170, 2007.
67. Sopontammarak S, Aliharoob A, Ocampo C, et al: Mitogen-activated protein kinases (p38 and c-Jun NH_2-terminal kinase) are differentially regulated during cardiac volume and pressure overload hypertrophy. Cell Biochem Biophys 43:61, 2005.
68. Perry GJ, Wei CC, Hankes GH, et al: Angiotensin II receptor blockade does not improve left ventricular function and remodeling in subacute mitral regurgitation in the dog. J Am Coll Cardiol 39:1374, 2002.
69. Derumeaux G, Mulder P, Richard V, et al: Tissue Doppler imaging differentiates physiological from pathological pressure-overload left ventricular hypertrophy in rats. Circulation 105:1602, 2002.
70. Backs J, Backs T, Neef S, et al: The delta isoform of CaM kinase II is required for pathological cardiac hypertrophy and remodeling after pressure overload. Proc Natl Acad Sci U S A 106:2342, 2009.

CHAPTER 25 Pathophysiology of Heart Failure

Douglas L. Mann

Overview

Despite repeated attempts to delineate the quintessential mechanism(s) that explains the clinical syndrome of heart failure (HF), no single conceptual paradigm has withstood the test of time. Whereas clinicians initially viewed HF as a problem of excessive salt and water retention caused by abnormalities of renal blood flow (the cardiorenal model) or abnormal pumping capacity of the heart (cardiocirculatory or hemodynamic model),[1] these models do not adequately explain the relentless "disease progression" that occurs in this syndrome. Accordingly, in this chapter, the focus is on the molecular and cellular changes that underlie HF with depressed systolic function, with an emphasis on the role of neurohormonal activation and left ventricular (LV) remodeling as the primary determinants of disease progression in HF. The hemodynamic, contractile, and wall motion disorders in systolic HF are discussed in the chapters on echocardiography (see Chap. 15), cardiac catheterization (see Chap. 20), radionuclide imaging (see Chap. 17), and the clinical assessment of the patient with HF (see Chap. 26). The pathogenesis of HF with a normal ejection fraction is discussed elsewhere (see Chap. 30).

Pathogenesis

As shown in **Figure 25-1A**, HF may be viewed as a progressive disorder that is initiated after an index event either damages the heart muscle, with a resultant loss of functioning cardiac myocytes, or disrupts the ability of the myocardium to generate force, thereby preventing the heart from contracting normally. This index event may have an abrupt onset, as in the case of a myocardial infarction; it may have a gradual or insidious onset, as in the case of hemodynamic pressure or volume overloading; or it may be hereditary, as in the case of many of the genetic cardiomyopathies. Regardless of the nature of the inciting event, the feature that is common to each of these index events is that they all, in some manner, produce a decline in pumping capacity of the heart. In most instances, patients will remain asymptomatic or minimally symptomatic after the initial decline in pumping capacity of the heart or will develop symptoms only after the dysfunction has been present for some time. Although the precise reason that patients with LV dysfunction remain asymptomatic is not certain, one potential explanation is that a number of compensatory mechanisms become activated in the setting of cardiac injury or depressed cardiac output; these appear to modulate LV function within a physiologic-homeostatic range, such that the functional capacity of the patient is preserved or is depressed only minimally. However, as patients transition to symptomatic HF, the sustained activation of neurohormonal and cytokine systems leads to a series of end-organ changes within the myocardium referred to collectively as LV remodeling. As will be discussed later, LV remodeling is sufficient to lead to disease progression in HF independent of the neurohormonal status of the patient.

Heart Failure as a Progressive Model

Neurohormonal Mechanisms

A growing body of experimental and clinical evidence suggests that HF progresses as a result of the overexpression of biologically active molecules that are capable of exerting deleterious effects on the heart and circulation (Fig. 25-1B).[1] The portfolio of compensatory mechanisms that have been described thus far includes activation of the adrenergic nervous system and renin-angiotensin system (RAS), which are responsible for maintaining cardiac output through increased retention of salt and water, peripheral arterial vasoconstriction, and increased contractility, and activation of inflammatory mediators, which are responsible for cardiac repair and remodeling. The term *neurohormone* is largely a historical term, reflecting the original observation that many of the molecules elaborated in HF are produced by the neuroendocrine system and thus act on the heart in an endocrine manner. However, it has since become apparent that a great many of the so-called classical neurohormones, such as norepinephrine (NE) and angiotensin II, are synthesized directly within the myocardium and thus act in an autocrine and paracrine manner. Nonetheless, the important unifying concept that arises from the neurohormonal model is that the overexpression of portfolios of biologically active molecules contributes to disease progression by virtue of the deleterious effects these molecules exert on the heart and circulation.

ACTIVATION OF THE SYMPATHETIC NERVOUS SYSTEM. The decrease in cardiac output in HF activates a series of compensatory adaptations that are intended to maintain cardiovascular homeostasis. One of the most important adaptations is activation of the sympathetic (adrenergic) nervous system, which occurs early in the course of HF. Activation of the sympathetic nervous system in HF is accompanied by a concomitant withdrawal of parasympathetic tone (see Fig. 25-e1 on website). Although these disturbances in autonomic control were initially attributed to loss of the inhibitory input from arterial or cardiopulmonary baroreceptor reflexes, there is increasing evidence that excitatory reflexes may also participate in the autonomic imbalance that occurs in HF.[2] Under normal conditions, inhibitory inputs from the high-pressure carotid sinus and aortic arch baroreceptors and the low-pressure cardiopulmonary mechanoreceptors are the principal inhibitors of sympathetic outflow, whereas discharge from the nonbaroreflex peripheral chemoreceptors and muscle metaboreceptors are the major excitatory inputs to sympathetic outflow. The vagal limb of the baroreceptor heart rate reflex is also responsive to arterial baroreceptor afferent inhibitory input. Healthy individuals display low sympathetic discharge at rest and have a high heart rate variability. However, in HF patients, inhibitory input from baroreceptors and mechanoreceptors decreases and excitatory input increases, with the net result that there is a generalized increase in sympathetic nerve traffic and blunted parasympathetic nerve traffic, with a resultant loss of heart rate variability and increased peripheral vascular resistance.[2]

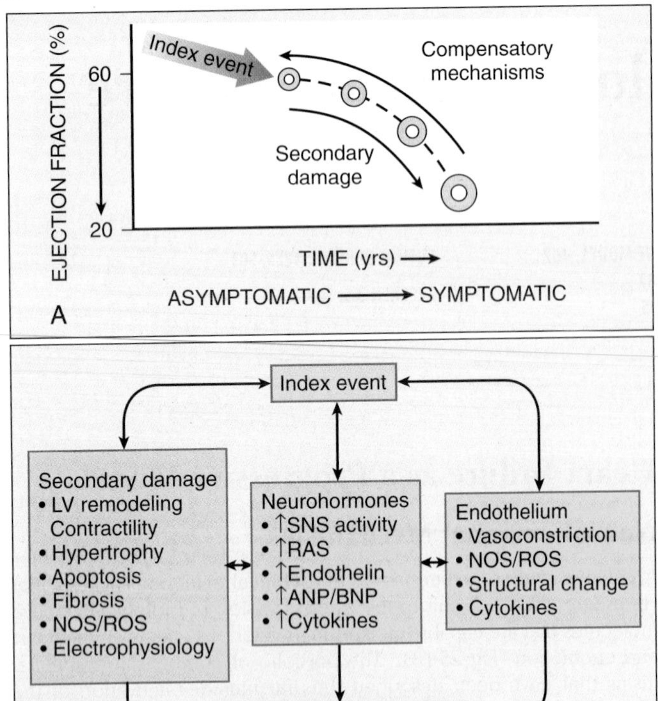

FIGURE 25-1 Pathogenesis of HF. **A,** HF begins after an index event produces an initial decline in pumping capacity of the heart. **B,** Following this initial decline in pumping capacity of the heart, a variety of compensatory mechanisms are activated, including the adrenergic nervous system, the renin-angiotensin system, and the cytokine systems. In the short term, these systems are able to restore cardiovascular function to a normal homeostatic range with the result that the patient remains asymptomatic. However, with time, the sustained activation of these systems can lead to secondary end-organ damage within the ventricle, with worsening LV remodeling and subsequent cardiac decompensation. As a result of worsening LV remodeling and cardiac decompensation, patients undergo the transition from asymptomatic to symptomatic HF. *(From Mann DL: Mechanisms and models in HF: A combinatorial approach. Circulation 100:99, 1999; and Kaye DM, Krum H: Drug discovery for heart failure: A new era or the end of the pipeline? Nat Rev Drug Discov 6:127, 2007.)*

As a result of the increase in sympathetic tone, there is an increase in circulating levels of NE, a potent adrenergic neurotransmitter. The elevated levels of circulating NE result from a combination of increased release of NE from adrenergic nerve endings, and its consequent "spillover" into the plasma, with reduced uptake of NE by adrenergic nerve endings. In patients with advanced HF, the circulating levels of NE in resting patients are two to three times those found in normal subjects. Indeed, plasma levels of NE predict mortality in patients with HF. Whereas the normal heart usually extracts NE from the arterial blood, in patients with moderate HF, the coronary sinus NE concentration exceeds the arterial concentration, indicating increased adrenergic stimulation of the heart. However, as HF progresses, there is a significant decrease in the myocardial concentration of NE. The mechanism responsible for cardiac NE depletion in severe HF is not clear and may relate to an "exhaustion" phenomenon resulting from the prolonged adrenergic activation of the cardiac adrenergic nerves in HF. In addition, there is decreased activity of myocardial tyrosine hydroxylase, which is the rate-limiting enzyme in the synthesis of NE. In patients with cardiomyopathy, iodine-131–labeled metaiodobenzylguanidine (MIBG), a radiopharmaceutical that is taken up by adrenergic nerve endings, is not taken up normally, suggesting that NE reuptake is also impaired in HF.

The ADMIRE-HF study (Prognostic Significance of ^{123}I-MIBG Myocardial Scintigraphy in Heart Failure) examined the prognostic usefulness of the assessment of myocardial sympathetic innervation, as determined by the heart to mediastinum (H/M) ratio on planar ^{123}I-MIBG imaging as either normal (>1.6) or abnormal (<1.6), for identifying NYHA class II/III HF patients with an EF < 35% who were at increased risk of experiencing an adverse cardiac event. Results showed that the composite endpoint, the first occurrence of NYHA heart-failure class progression, potentially life-threatening arrhythmic event, or cardiac death, occurred significantly ($P < 0.0001$) more frequently in patients who had low uptake of the tracer, suggesting that molecular imaging might be one day be used to guide defibrillator therapy in the future.[2a]

Increased sympathetic activation of the beta$_1$-adrenergic receptor results in increased heart rate and force of myocardial contraction, with a resultant increase in cardiac output (see Chap. 24). In addition, the heightened activity of the adrenergic nervous system leads to stimulation of myocardial alpha$_1$-adrenergic receptors, which elicits a modest positive inotropic effect, as well as peripheral arterial vasoconstriction (**Fig. 25-2**). Although NE enhances both contraction and relaxation and maintains blood pressure, myocardial energy requirements are augmented, which can intensify ischemia when myocardial oxygen delivery is restricted. The augmented adrenergic outflow from

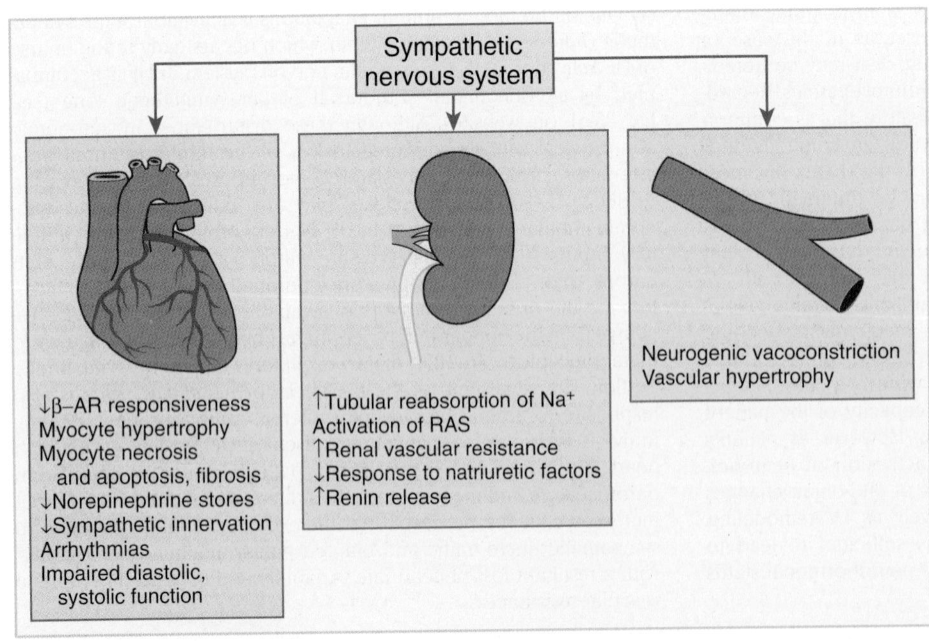

FIGURE 25-2 Activation of the sympathetic nervous system. Increased sympathetic nervous system activity may contribute to the pathophysiologic process of congestive heart failure by multiple mechanisms involving cardiac, renal, and vascular function. In the heart, increased sympathetic nervous system outflow may lead to desensitization of β-adrenergic receptors (β-AR), myocyte hypertrophy, necrosis, apoptosis, and fibrosis. In the kidneys, increased sympathetic activation induces arterial and venous vasoconstriction, activation of the renin-angiotensin system, increase in salt and water retention, and attenuated response to natriuretic factors. In the peripheral vessels, neurogenic vasoconstriction and vascular hypertrophy are induced by increased sympathetic nervous activity. *(From Nohria A, Cusco JA, Creager MA: Neurohormonal, renal and vascular adjustments in heart failure. In Colucci WS [ed]: Atlas of Heart Failure. 4th ed. Philadelphia, Current Medicine, 2005, p 106.)*

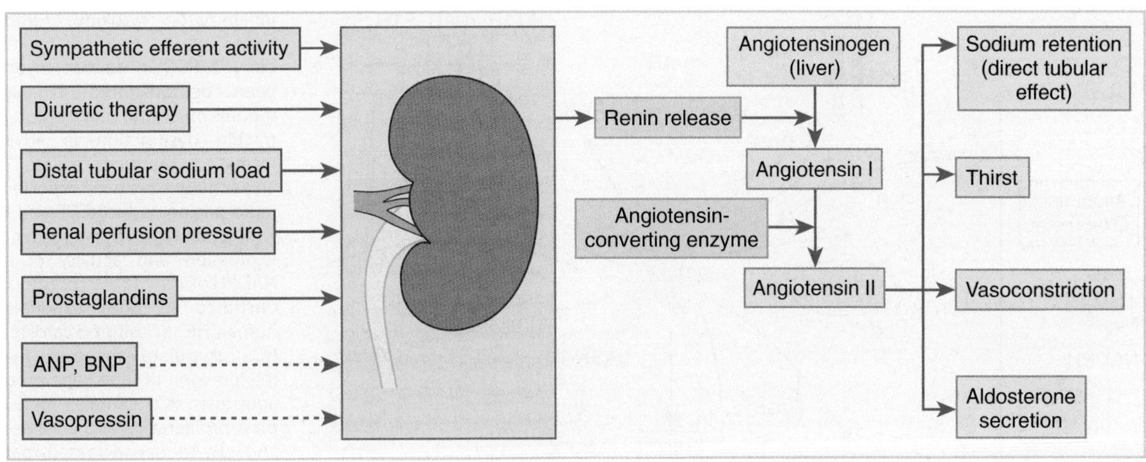

FIGURE 25-3 Activation of the renin-angiotensin system. The renin-angiotensin system is activated in patients with heart failure. The major site of release of circulating renin is the juxtaglomerular apparatus of the kidney, where multiple stimuli may contribute to renal release of renin into the systemic circulation, including renal sympathetic efferent activity, decreased distal sodium delivery, reduced renal perfusion pressure, and diuretic therapy. Natriuretic peptides (ANP, BNP) and vasopressin (dashed arrows) may inhibit the release of renin. Renin enzymatically cleaves angiotensinogen to form angiotensin II from angiotensin I. Angiotensin II is a potent vasoconstrictor and promotes sodium resorption by increasing aldosterone secretion and by a direct effect on the tubules. Angiotensin II also stimulates water intake by directly acting on the thirst center. *(From Nohria A, Cusco JA, Creager MA: Neurohormonal, renal and vascular adjustments in heart failure.* In *Colucci WS [ed]: Atlas of Heart Failure. 4th ed. Philadelphia, Current Medicine, 2005, p 107.)*

the central nervous system may also trigger ventricular tachycardia or even sudden cardiac death, particularly in the presence of myocardial ischemia. Thus, activation of the sympathetic nervous system provides short-term support that has the potential to become maladaptive in the long term (see Fig. 25-2).

ACTIVATION OF THE RENIN-ANGIOTENSIN SYSTEM. In contrast to the sympathetic nervous system, the components of the RAS are activated comparatively later in HF. The presumptive mechanisms for RAS activation in HF include renal hypoperfusion; decreased filtered sodium reaching the macula densa in the distal tubule; and increased sympathetic stimulation of the kidney, leading to increased renin release from the juxtaglomerular apparatus (**Fig. 25-3**). As shown in **Figure 25-4**, renin cleaves four amino acids from circulating angiotensinogen, which is synthesized in the liver, to form the biologically inactive decapeptide angiotensin I. Angiotensin-converting enzyme (ACE) cleaves two amino acids from angiotensin I to form the biologically active octapeptide (1-8) angiotensin II. The majority (~90%) of ACE activity in the body is found in tissues; the remaining 10% of ACE activity is found in a soluble (non–membrane bound) form in the interstitium of the heart and vessel wall. The importance of tissue ACE activity in HF is suggested by the observation that ACE mRNA, ACE binding sites, and ACE activity are increased in explanted human hearts.[3] Angiotensin II can also be synthesized through renin-independent pathways, through the enzymatic conversion of angiotensinogen to angiotensin I by kallikrein and cathepsin G (see Fig. 25-4). The tissue production of angiotensin II may also occur through ACE-independent pathways, through the activation of chymase; this pathway may be of major importance in the myocardium, particularly when the levels of renin and angiotensin I are increased by the use of ACE inhibitors. Angiotensin II itself can undergo further proteolysis to generate three biologically active fragments, angiotensin III (2-8) and angiotensin IV (3-8), which promote vasconstriction,[4] and angiotensin (1-7), which may act to counteract the deleterious effects of angiotensin II on endothelial function.

Angiotensin II exerts its effects by binding to two G protein–coupled receptors termed the angiotensin type 1 (AT_1) and angiotensin type 2 (AT_2) receptors. The predominant angiotensin receptor in the vasculature is the AT_1 receptor. Although both the AT_1 and AT_2 receptor subtypes are present in human myocardium, the AT_2 receptor predominates in a 2:1 molar ratio. Cellular localization of the AT_1 receptor in the heart is most abundant in nerves distributed in the myocardium; the AT_2 receptor is localized more highly in fibroblasts and the interstitium. Activation of the AT_1 receptor leads to vasoconstriction, cell growth, aldosterone secretion, and catecholamine release; activation of the AT_2 receptor leads to vasodilation, inhibition of cell growth, natriuresis, and bradykinin release. Studies have shown that the AT_1 receptor and mRNA levels are downregulated in failing human hearts, whereas AT_2 receptor density is increased or unchanged, with the result that the ratio of AT_1 to AT_2 receptors decreases.[3]

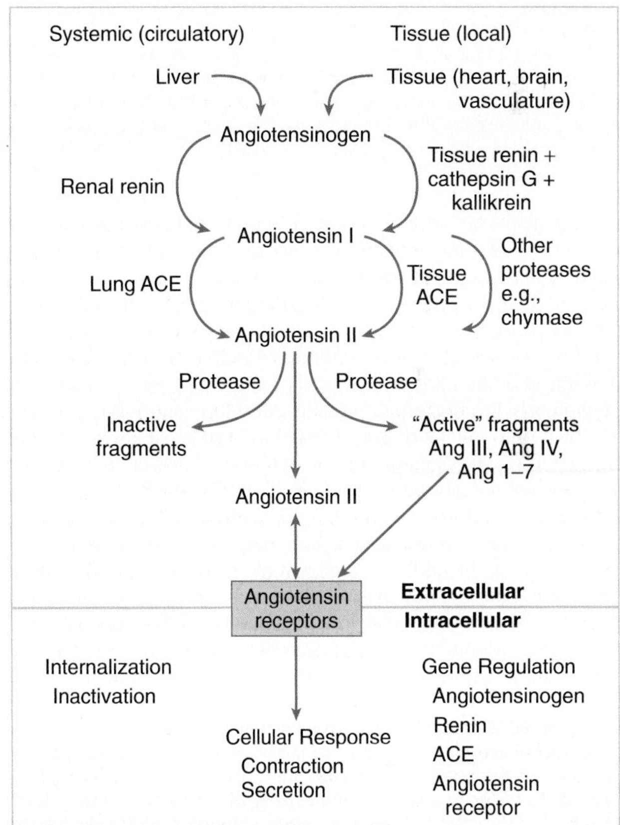

FIGURE 25-4 The systemic and tissue components of the renin-angiotensin system. Several tissues, including myocardium, vasculature, kidney, and brain, have the capacity to generate angiotensin II independent of the circulating renin-angiotensin system. Angiotensin II produced at the tissue level may play an important role in the pathophysiology of HF. ACE = angiotensin-converting enzyme. *(Modified from Timmermans PB, Wong PC, Chiu AT, et al: Angiotensin II receptors and angiotensin II receptor antagonists. Pharmacol Rev 45:205, 1993.)*

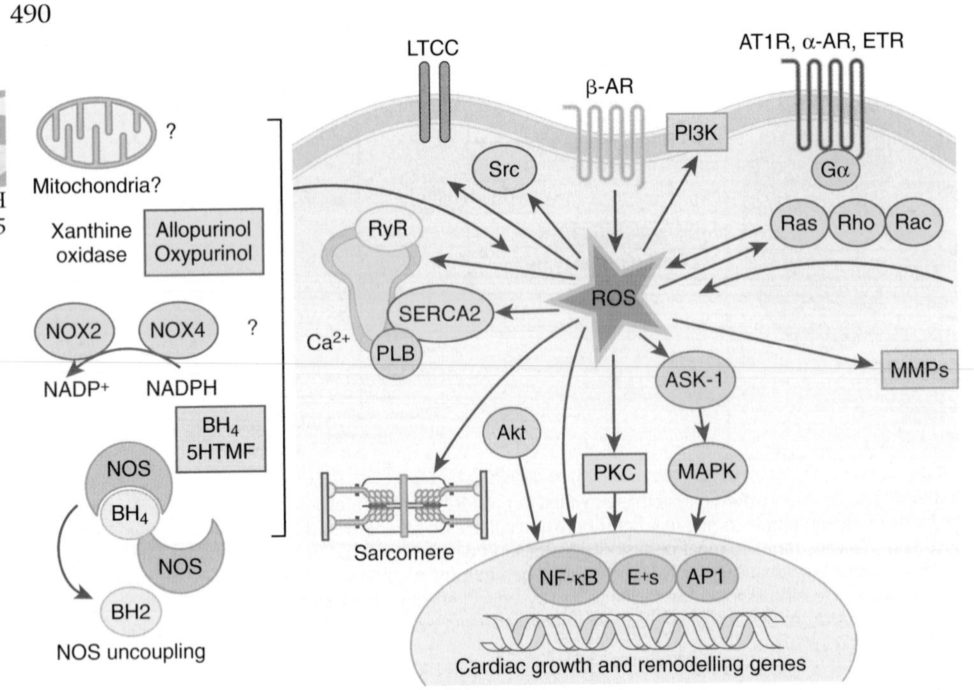

FIGURE 25-5 Cellular sources of ROS and ROS signaling in cardiac hypertrophy. ROS-generating systems are shown on the left and include xanthine oxidase, NADPH oxidases (NOX2, NOX4), nitric oxide synthase (NOS), and mitochondrial complexes. ROS activation has protean effects on calcium handling, myofilament function, matrix activation, kinase and phosphatase stimulation, and transcriptional regulation. NF-κB = nuclear factor-κB; PKC = protein kinase C; PI3K = phosphatidylinositol 3-kinase; PLB = phospholamban; RyR = ryanodine receptor; SERCA2 = sarcoplasmic reticular ATPase 2. *(Modified from McKinsey TA, Kass DA: Small-molecule therapies for cardiac hypertrophy: Moving beneath the cell surface. Nat Rev Drug Discov 6:617, 2007.)*

Angiotensin II has several important actions that are critical to maintenance of short-term circulatory homeostasis (see later). However, the sustained expression of angiotensin II is maladaptive and leads to fibrosis of the heart, kidneys, and other organs. Angiotensin II can also lead to worsening neurohormonal activation by enhancing the release of NE from sympathetic nerve endings as well as stimulating the zona glomerulosa of the adrenal cortex to produce aldosterone. Analogous to angiotensin II, aldosterone provides short-term support to the circulation by promoting the reabsorption of sodium in exchange for potassium in the distal segments of the nephron. However, the sustained expression of aldosterone may exert harmful effects by provoking hypertrophy and fibrosis within the vasculature and the myocardium, thus contributing to reduced vascular compliance and increased ventricular stiffness. In addition, aldosterone provokes endothelial cell dysfunction, baroreceptor dysfunction, and inhibition of NE uptake, any or all of which may lead to worsening of HF. The mechanism of action of aldosterone in the cardiovascular system appears to involve oxidative stress with resultant inflammation in target tissues.

Oxidative Stress. Reactive oxygen species (ROS) are a normal byproduct of aerobic metabolism. In the heart, the potential sources for ROS include the mitochondria, xanthine oxidase, and NADPH oxidase (**Fig. 25-5**). ROS can modulate the activity of a variety of intracellular proteins and signaling pathways, including essential proteins involved in myocardial excitation-contraction coupling, such as ion channels, sarcoplasmic reticulum calcium release channels, and myofilament proteins, as well as signaling pathways that are coupled to myocyte growth.[5] Oxidative stress occurs when the production of ROS exceeds the buffering capacity of antioxidant defense systems, leading to an excess of ROS within the cell. In the heart, the important antioxidants are manganese superoxide dismutase (MnSOD), which converts O_2^- to H_2O_2; catalase and glutathione peroxidase, which convert reduced glutathione (GSH) and H_2O_2 to H_2O and oxidized glutathione (GSSG); and glutathione reductase (GR), which reduces GSSG back to GSH. There is substantial evidence that the level of oxidative stress is increased both systemically and in the myocardium of HF patients. Oxidative stress in the heart may be due to reduced antioxidant capacity or the increased production of ROS, which may arise secondary to mechanical strain of the myocardium, neurohormonal stimulation (angiotensin II, alpha-adrenergic agonists, ET-1), or inflammatory cytokines (tumor necrosis factor, IL-1). Excessive mitochondria-derived ROS in cardiac myocytes have been demonstrated in experimental models of HF and may contribute to contractile dysfunction in advanced HF. Increased xanthine oxidase expression and activity have been reported in canine rapid pacing–induced HF and in patients with end-stage HF. Moreover, increased expression and activity of myocardial NADPH oxidases have recently been demonstrated in both experimental and human HF.[5] In cultured cardiac myocytes, ROS stimulate myocyte hypertrophy, reexpression of fetal gene programs, and apoptosis. ROS can also modulate fibroblast proliferation and collagen synthesis and can trigger increased matrix metalloproteinase abundance and activation. ROS can also affect the peripheral vasculature in HF by decreasing the bioavailability of nitric oxide (NO). These and other observations have led to the suggestion that strategies to reduce ROS may be of therapeutic value in HF. The OPT-CHF (Oxypurinol Therapy in Congestive Heart Failure) study with oxypurinol (a xanthine oxidase inhibitor) failed to alter the primary composite endpoint of hospitalization or cardiovascular death, although there was a trend toward improvement for the subgroup of patients with the highest levels of uric acid (a biomarker for oxidative stress), suggesting that this therapy may benefit the patients with the highest degree of oxidative stress.[6]

The importance of aldosterone, independent of angiotensin II, has been demonstrated by clinical trials (see Chap. 28) showing that low-dose spironolactone increased the survival of patients with systolic HF as well as improved survival after myocardial infarction, independent of changes in volume or electrolyte status.[7]

NEUROHORMONAL ALTERATIONS OF RENAL FUNCTION. One of the signatures of advancing HF is increased salt and water retention by the kidneys. Traditional theories have ascribed this increase to either "forward" failure, which attributes sodium retention to inadequate renal perfusion as a consequence of impaired cardiac output, or "backward" failure, which emphasizes the importance of increased venous pressure in favoring transudation of salt and water from the intravascular to the extracellular compartment. These mechanisms have largely been supplanted by the concept of decreased effective arterial blood volume, which postulates that despite blood volume expansion in HF, inadequate cardiac output sensed by baroreceptors in the vascular tree leads to a series of compensatory neurohormonal adaptations that resemble the homeostatic response to acute blood loss.[8] As illustrated in **Figure 25-6**, a falling cardiac output or redistribution of the circulating blood volume is sensed by baroreceptors in the LV, the aortic arch, the carotid sinus, and the renal afferent arterioles. The loss of inhibitory input from arterial or cardiopulmonary baroreceptor reflexes leads to sustained activation of the sympathetic nervous system and the RAS.

There is little evidence to suggest that a primary renal abnormality is responsible for excessive sodium retention in HF. Rather, volume overload in HF is likley to be secondary to a functional derangement of renal physiology in response to several factors that have the potential to cause increased sodium reabsorption, including activation of the sympathetic nervous system, activation of the RAS, reduced renal perfusion pressures, and blunting of renal responsiveness to natriuretic peptides. Increased renal sympathetic nerve–mediated vasconstriction leads to decreased renal blood flow as well as increased renal tubular sodium and water reabsorption throughout the nephron. Renal sympathathetic stimulation can also lead to the nonosmotic release of arginine vasopressin (AVP) from the posterior pituitary, which reduces the excretion of free water and contributes to worsening peripheral vasoconstriction as well as increased endothelin production.[8]

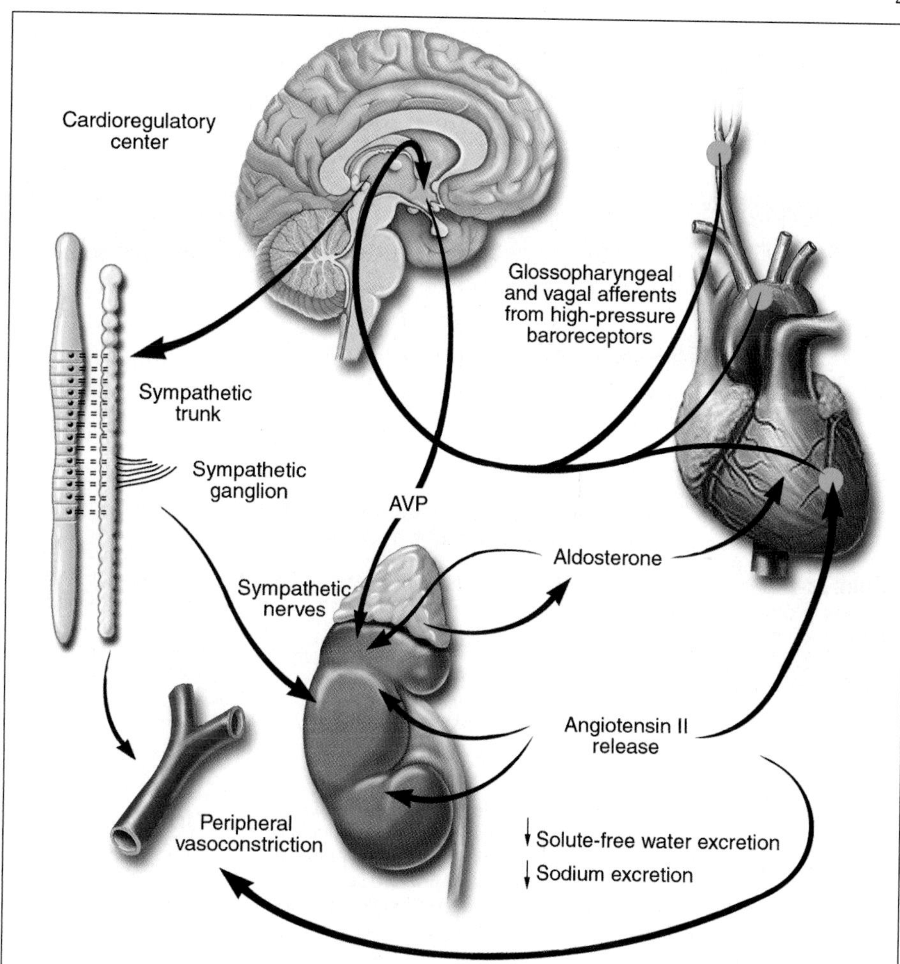

FIGURE 25-6 Unloading of high-pressure baroreceptors (circles) in the left ventricle, carotid sinus, and aortic arch generates afferent signals that stimulate cardioregulatory centers in the brain, resulting in the activation of efferent pathways in the sympathetic nervous system. The sympathetic nervous system appears to be the primary integrator of the neurohumoral vasoconstrictor response to arterial underfilling. Activation of renal sympathetic nerves stimulates the release of arginine vasopressin (AVP). Sympathetic activation also causes peripheral and renal vasoconstriction, as does angiotensin II. Angiotensin II constricts blood vessels and stimulates the release of aldosterone from the adrenal gland, and it also increases tubular sodium reabsorption and causes remodeling of cardiac myocytes. Aldosterone may also have direct cardiac effects, in addition to increasing the reabsorption of sodium and the secretion of potassium and hydrogen ions in the collecting duct. The lines designate circulating hormones. *(Modified from Schrier RW, Abraham WT: Hormones and hemodynamics in heart failure. N Engl J Med 341:577, 1999.)*

ARGININE VASOPRESSIN. AVP is a pituitary hormone that plays a central role in the regulation of free water clearance and plasma osmolality (see Fig. 25-6). Under normal circumstances, AVP is released in response to an increase in plasma osmolality, leading to increased retention of water from the proximal duct. Of note, circulating AVP is elevated in many patients with HF, even after correction for plasma osmolality (i.e., nonosmotic release),[9] and may contribute to the hyponatremia that occurs in HF. The cellular effects of AVP are mediated mainly by interactions with three types of receptors, termed V_{1a}, V_{1b}, and V_2. The V_{1a} receptor is the most widespread subtype and is found primarily in vascular smooth muscle cells. The V_{1b} receptor has a more limited distribution and is located mainly in the central nervous system. The V_2 receptors are found primarily in the epithelial cells in the renal collecting duct and the thick ascending limb. AVP receptors are members of the G protein–coupled receptors. The V_{1a} receptor mediates vasoconstriction, platelet aggregation, and stimulation of myocardial growth factors; the V_{1b} receptor modulates adrenocorticotropic hormone secretion from the anterior pituitary; and the V_2 receptor mediates antidiuretic effects by stimulating adenylyl cyclase to increase the rate of insertion of vesicles containing water channels into the apical membrane. Because the water channels contain preformed functional water channels, termed aquaporins, their localization in the apical membranes in response to V_2 stimulation increases the water permeability of the apical membrane, leading to water retention. In dogs with pacing-induced HF, the selective inhibition of V_1 receptors increased cardiac output without affecting electrolytes or hormone levels. In contrast, inhibition of V_2 receptors increased serum sodium concentration, plasma renin activity, and plasma AVP levels but did not affect hemodynamics. When the two inhibitors were combined, the hemodynamic effects were potentiated.[10] The vaptans, vasopressin receptor antagonists with V_{1a} (relcovaptan) or V_2 (tolvaptan, lixivaptan) selectivity or nonselective V_{1a}/V_2 activity (conivaptan), have been shown to reduce body weight and to reduce hyponatremia in clinical trials (see Chaps. 27 and 28).

Increased renal sympathetic activity leads to increased renin production by the kidneys, with a resultant sustained activation of the RAS, despite an expanded extracellular volume (see Fig. 25-3). Angiotensin II facilitates retention of sodium and water by multiple renal mechanisms, including a direct proximal tubular effect, as well as through activation of aldosterone, which leads to increased sodium resorption in the distal tubule. Angiotensin II also stimulates the thirst center of the brain and provokes the release of AVP and aldosterone, which can both lead to further dysregulation of salt and water homeostasis.

A number of counterregulatory neurohormonal systems become activated in HF to offset the deleterious effects of the vasoconstricting neurohormones (see Table 25-e1 on website). Metabolites of vasodilatory prostaglandins, including prostaglandin E_2 (PGE_2) and prostacyclin (PGI_2), are elevated in patients with HF. In addition to being a vasodilator, PGE_2 enhances renal sodium excretion and modulates the antidiuretic action of AVP. The natriuretic peptides, including atrial natriuretic peptide (ANP) and brain-type natriuretic peptide (BNP), are one of the most important counterregulatory neurohormonal systems that become activated in HF. Under physiologic conditions, ANP and BNP function as natriuretic hormones that are released in response to increases in atrial or myocardial stretch, often secondary to excessive sodium intake. Once released, these cardiac peptides act on the kidney and peripheral circulation to unload the heart, through increased excretion of sodium and water, while inhibiting the release of renin and aldosterone. In the setting of RAS activation, the release of ANP and BNP may serve as an important counterregulatory mechanism that maintains sodium and water homeostasis. However, for reasons that are not entirely clear, the renal effects of the natriuretic peptides appear to become blunted with advancing HF, leaving the effects of RAS unopposed.[11] Potential reasons for this blunting include low renal perfusion pressure, relative deficiency or altered molecular forms of the natriuretic peptides, and decreased levels of natriuretic peptide receptors.

NATRIURETIC PEPTIDES. The natriuretic peptide system consists of five structurally similar peptides, termed ANP, urodilantin (an isoform of ANP), BNP, C-type natriuretic peptide (CNP), and dendroaspis natriuretic

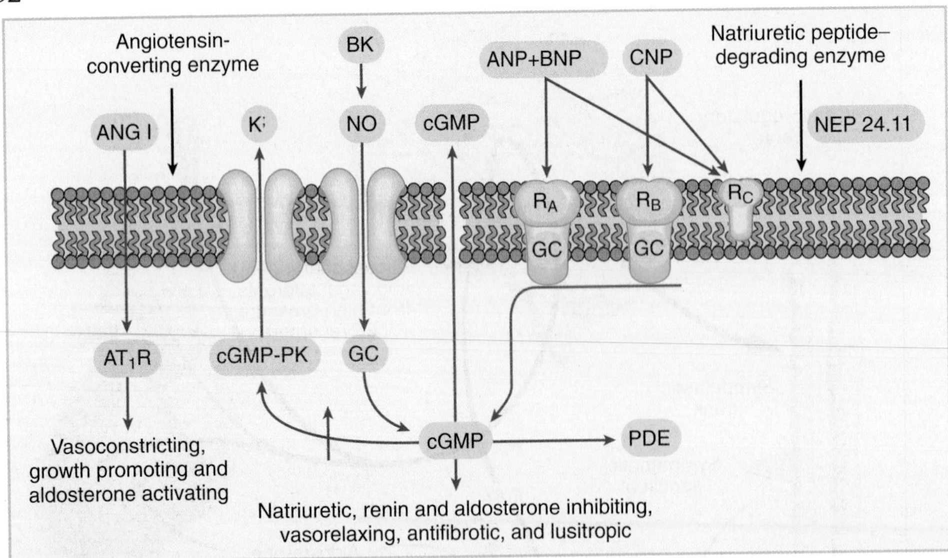

FIGURE 25-7 Cellular actions in signaling of the natriuretic peptide system. Ang I = angiotensin I; ANP = atrial natriuretic peptide; AT_1R = angiotensin type 1 receptor; BK = bradykinin; BNP = brain natriuretic peptide; cGMP = cyclic guanosine monophosphate; CNP = C-type natriuretic peptide; GC = guanylate cyclase; NEP = neutral endopeptidase; PDE = phosphodiesterase; PK = phosphokinase; R_A = particulate guanylate cyclase A receptor; R_B = particulate guanylate cyclase B receptor; R_C = particulate guanylate cyclase C receptor. *(From Burnett JC, Costello-Boerrigter L, Boerrigter G: Alterations in the kidney in heart failure: The cardiorenal axis in the regulation of sodium homeostasis.* In *Mann DL [ed]: Heart Failure: A Companion to Braunwald's Heart Disease. Philadelphia, Elsevier, 2004, pp 279-289.)*

peptide (DNP).[12] ANP, a 28–amino acid peptide hormone, is produced principally in the cardiac atria; BNP, a 32–amino acid peptide originally isolated from porcine brain, was later identified as a hormone primarily produced in the cardiac ventricles.[13] Both ANP and BNP are secreted in response to increasing cardiac wall tension; however, other factors, such as neurohormones (e.g., angiotensin II, ET-1) and physiologic factors (e.g., age, gender, renal function), may also play a role in their regulation. The biosynthesis, secretion, and clearance of BNP differ from those of ANP, suggesting that these two natriuretic peptides have discrete physiologic and pathophysiologic roles. Whereas ANP is secreted in short bursts in response to acute changes in atrial pressure, the activation of BNP is regulated transcriptionally in response to chronic increases in atrial or ventricular pressure. ANP and BNP are initially synthesized as prohormones that are subsequently proteolytically cleaved, respectively, by corin and furin to yield large biologically inactive N-terminal fragments (NT-ANP or NT-BNP) and smaller biologically active peptides (ANP or BNP). ANP has a relatively short half-life of approximately 3 minutes, whereas BNP has a plasma half-life of approximately 20 minutes. CNP, which is located primarily in the vasculature, is also released as a prohormone that is cleaved into a biologically inactive form (NT-CNP) and a 22–amino acid biologically active form (CNP).

Figure 25-7 illustrates the signaling pathway of the natriuretic peptide system. The natriuretic peptides stimulate the production of the intracellular second messenger cyclic guanosine monophosphate (cGMP), via binding to the natriuretic peptide A receptor (NPR-A), which preferentially binds ANP and BNP, and the natriuretic peptide B receptor (NPR-B), which preferentially binds CNP. Both NPR-A and NPR-B receptors are coupled to particulate guanylate cyclase. Activation of NPR-A and NPR-B results in natriuresis, vasorelaxation, inhibition of renin and aldosterone, inhibition of fibrosis, and increased lusitropy. The natriuretic peptide C receptor (NPR-C) is not linked to cGMP and serves as a clearance receptor for the natriuretic peptides. Natriuretic peptides are degraded by neutral endopeptidase 24.11 (NEP), which is widely expressed in multiple tissues, where it is often colocalized with ACE. Inhibition of NEP may further potentiate the renal actions of ANP and BNP. The infusion of the endopeptidase inhibitor candoxatrilat into patients with HF resulted in a reduction of left- and right-sided filling pressures that was associated with suppression of plasma NE levels and a transient reduction in plasma vasopressin.[14] Vasopeptidase inhibitors, such as omapatrilat, that inhibit both neutral endopeptidase and ACE were developed with the intent of inhibiting the RAS while concurrently elevating natriuretic peptide levels. Although some early trials suggested that neutral endopeptidase inhibition would have a greater benefit than ACE inhibition, more recent trials have found the two classes of drug to exert similar effects on survival.[15]

The biologic importance of the natriuretic peptides in renal sodium handling has been demonstrated in multiple studies employing natriuretic peptide receptor antagonists as well as overexpression of ANP or BNP.[11] In experimental HF models, either acute blockade of the natriuretic A and B receptors or chronic genetic disruption of the natriuretic peptide A receptor blunts the renal natriuretic response to acute volume expansion, demonstrating the renal protective action of natriuretic peptide activation.[16] The infusion of a recombinant human BNP (rhBNP) exerts beneficial hemodynamic effects that are characterized by decreases in arterial and venous pressures, increase in cardiac output, and suppression of neurohormonal activation. Indeed, the unique properties of the natriuretic peptides have resulted in their clinical development as therapeutic agents for human HF. rhBNP has been approved by the Food and Drug Administration for use in acute decompensated HF (see Chap. 27). In addition to their important biologic role, the natriuretic peptides have provided important diagnostic and prognostic information in HF (see Chap. 26).

NEUROHORMONAL ALTERATIONS IN THE PERIPHERAL VASCULATURE. In patients with HF, the complex interactions between the autonomic nervous system and local autoregulatory mechanisms tend to preserve circulation to the brain and heart while decreasing blood flow to the skin, skeletal muscles, splanchnic organs, and kidneys. This intense visceral vasoconstriction during exercise helps divert the limited cardiac output to exercising muscle but contributes to hypoperfusion of the gut and kidneys. The most powerful stimulus for peripheral vasoconstriction is sympathetic activation, which releases the potent vasoconstrictor NE. Other vasoconstrictors that contribute to maintenance of circulatory homeostasis include angiotensin II, endothelin, neuropeptide Y, urotensin II, thromboxane A_2, and AVP (see Table 25-e1 on website). The increased sympathetic adrenergic stimulation of the peripheral arteries and the increased concentrations of circulating vasoconstrictors contribute to the arteriolar vasoconstriction and to the maintenance of arterial pressure; the sympathetic stimulation of the veins contributes to an increase in venous tone, which helps to maintain venous return and ventricular filling and to support cardiac performance by Starling's law of the heart (see Chap. 24).

ENDOTHELIN. There are three endothelin peptides (ET-1, ET-2, and ET-3), all of which are potent vasoconstrictors (see Chap. 52). Although it is primarily released by endothelial cells, endothelin can also be synthesized and released by a variety of other cell types, such as cardiac myocytes. ET-1 is the predominant isoform of the endothelin peptide family and is ubiquitously expressed. ET-1 is synthesized as a protein precursor, termed preproET-1. PreproET-1 is processed by multiple proteases in a process that involves the proteolytic release of proET-1 (big endothelin), followed by C-terminal trimming by a carboxypeptidase and further processing by endothelin-converting enzyme (ECE) to generate the biologically active 21–amino acid ET-1 peptide. However, studies in ECE knockout mice show that significant levels of mature ET-1 exist, suggesting that there may be alternative ECE-independent (e.g., chymase, non-ECE metalloproteinases) pathways for generation of ET-1. At least two subtypes of endothelin receptors (A and B) have been identified in human myocardium. Endothelin ET_A receptors mediate vasoconstriction, cell proliferation, pathologic hypertrophy, fibrosis, and increased contractility; ET_B receptors are involved in the clearance of ET-1 and the release of NO and prostacyclin. The release of endothelin from endothelial cells in vitro can be enhanced by several vasoactive agents (e.g., NE, angiotensin II, thrombin) and cytokines (e.g., transforming growth factor-β, tumor necrosis factor, and IL-1). Several reports have documented an increase in circulating levels of ET-1 in patients with HF and have shown that endothelin levels correlate with patient outcomes. Further, plasma endothelin concentrations correlate directly with pulmonary artery pressure and pulmonary vascular resistance. On the basis of the biologic properties of endothelin, endothelin receptor antagonists were developed for the treatment of patients with HF. Although early experimental studies showed that ET_A receptor antagonists inhibited myocardial hypertrophy in rats with pressure overload–induced hypertrophy caused by aortic banding and prevented cardiac remodeling in rats with myocardial infarction,[17] and although early clinical studies confirmed the ability of these new agents to improve hemodynamics, the effect of chronic endothelin receptor antagonism has not been beneficial in clinical HF trials and has led to worsening outcomes in some settings.[18] This statement notwithstanding, endothelin receptor antagonists have been shown to be beneficial in the setting of pulmonary hypertension and are currently approved by the Food and Drug Administration for the treatment of pulmonary artery hypertension in patients with moderate disability (functional Class III).

NEUROPEPTIDE Y. Neuropeptide Y (NPY) is a vasoconstricting peptide that is released together with NE from sympathetic nerve endings. NPY is abundant in cerebral cortex, hippocampus, thalamus, hypothalamus, and brainstem. Of note, the inhibitory effects of NPY on NE release in the paraventricular nucleus are blunted in animals with HF after an acute infarction, leading to an increase in sympathetic nerve activity and peripheral NE levels. NPY elicits peripheral vasoconstriction by interacting with Y_1 receptors, which are located postjunctionally at the sympathetic neuroeffector junction in blood vessels. In addition, NPY potentiates the vasoconstrictor effects of other extracellular messengers, including alpha-adrenergic agonists and angiotensin II, and inhibits acetylcholine release from parasympathetic nerve endings in the heart. Although the role of NPY in HF is not known, circulating concentrations of NPY-like immunoreactivity are significantly increased in moderate to severe forms of HF and correlated with circulating levels of NE.[19]

UROTENSIN II. Mammalian urotensin II is the most potent endogenous cardiostimulatory peptide identified thus far, with an 8- to 110-fold greater potency than ET-1. The effects of urotensin II are mediated by binding to the urotensin receptor. Urotensin II mediates vascular tone and increased contractile force in human atrium and ventricle. Analogous to ET-1, urotensin II provokes trophic and mitogenic actions in vascular smooth muscle cells, cardiac myocytes, and cardiac fibroblasts. However, unlike ET-1, which uniformly constricts most blood vessels, the vasoactive effects of urotensin II are both species and vascular bed dependent. Urotensin receptor expression is increased in cardiac myocytes, endothelial cells, and fibroblasts in the rat heart after coronary artery ligation. Urotensin II treatment increased collagen mRNA and protein levels in cardiac fibroblasts and cardiac hypertrophy in cultured neonatal cardiomyocytes after transfection with recombinant urotensin II receptor.[20] Plasma levels of urotensin II have been found to be elevated in some but not all studies in HF patients. Interestingly, iontophoresis of urotensin II into the skin showed that urotensin II mediated a dose-dependent vasodilator response in normal subjects, whereas urotensin II mediated a dose-dependent vasoconstrictor response in patients with HF, suggesting that urotensin II may contribute to the increased peripheral vascular tone that occurs in HF.[21]

As noted before, the vasoconstricting neurohormones activate counterregulatory vasodilator responses, including release of natriuretic peptides, NO, bradykinin, adrenomedullin, apelin, and vasodilating prostaglandins PGI_2 and PGE_2 (see Table 25-e1 on website). Under normal circumstances, the continuous release of NO from the endothelium counteracts the vasoconstricting factors and allows appropriate vasodilatory responses during exercise. However, as HF advances, there is loss of the endothelium-mediated vasodilatory responsiveness, which contributes to the excessive peripheral arterial vasoconstriction that is emblematic of advanced HF. Of interest, the vasodilator response can be restored by the administration of L-arginine, a precursor of endothelium-derived NO.[22]

NITRIC OXIDE. The free radical gas NO is produced by three isoforms of NO synthase (NOS). All three isoforms are present in the heart, including NOS1 (nNOS, neuronal NOS), NOS2 (iNOS, inducible NOS), and NOS3 (eNOS, endothelial-constitutive NOS). NOS1 has been detected in cardiac conduction tissue, intracardiac neurons, and the sarcoplasmic reticulum of cardiac myocytes; NOS2 is an inducible isoform that is not normally expressed in the myocardium but is synthesized de novo in virtually all cells in the heart in response to inflammatory cytokines; NOS3 is expressed in coronary endothelium, endocardium, and the sarcolemma and T-tubule membranes of cardiac myocytes. NOS1 and NOS3 can be activated by calcium or calmodulin, whereas the induction of NOS2 is calcium independent. NO activates soluble guanylate cyclase (see Fig. 25-7). This activation leads to the production of cGMP, which in turn activates protein kinase G and cascade of different signaling events. In normal subjects, NO released by endothelial cells mediates vasodilation in the peripheral vasculature through cGMP-mediated relaxation of vascular smooth muscle. In patients with HF, endothelium-dependent NO-mediated dilation of the peripheral vasculature is blunted, which has been attributed to decreased NOS3 expression and activity. The actions of NO on the myocardium are complex and include both short-term alterations in function and energetics and longer term effects on structure. NO modulates the activity of several key calcium channels involved in excitation-contraction coupling as well as mitochondrial respiratory complexes. This type of regulation is accomplished by spatial localization of different NOS isoforms in distinct cellular microdomains involved in excitation-contraction coupling. Specifically, NOS1 localizes to the sarcoplasmic reticulum in proximity to the ryanodine receptor and the sarcoplasmic reticulum Ca^{2+}-ATPase (SERCA2a), and NOS3 is found in sarcolemmal caveolae compartmentalized with cell surface receptors and the L-type Ca^{2+} channel. There is evidence that the subcellular location of NO becomes disrupted in HF (see Fig. 25-e2 on website).[23] NO also participates in mitochondrial respiration, the process that fuels excitation-contraction coupling. The different NOS isoforms may also participate in the process of cardiac remodeling. LV remodeling was ameliorated and survival improved after myocardial infarction in transgenic mice deficient in NOS2.[24] In contrast, overexpression of NOS3 resulted in improved remodeling after myocardial infarction. These contrasting effects of NOS2 and NOS3 may reflect the differences in amount of NO produced, which is much higher with NOS2.

Emerging evidence suggests that there is an imbalance between free radical production and NO generation in HF (nitroso-redox imbalance) (**Fig. 25-8**).[25] Within the heart, xanthine oxidase activity stimulates cardiac myocyte hypertrophy and apoptosis and impairs matrix structure. The underpinnings of these derangements can be linked not solely to oxidative stress but also to reduced NO generation. In this regard, xanthine oxidase interacts with NO signaling at numerous levels, including a direct protein-protein interaction with neuronal NO synthase (NOS1) in the sarcoplasmic reticulum. Deficiency or translocation of NOS1 away from this microdomain leads to increased activity of xanthine oxidoreductase, which in turn impairs excitation-contraction coupling and myofilament calcium sensitivity (see Fig 25-8).[25] Studies have also suggested that NOS uncoupling secondary to a deficiency of tetrahydrobiopterin may also play a role in hypertrophy and HF (see Fig. 25-7).[26]

BRADYKININ. Kinins are vasodilators released from inactive protein precursors (kininogens) through the action of proteolytic enzymes termed kallikreins. The biologic actions of the kinins are mediated by binding to B_1 and B_2 receptors. Most cardiovascular actions are initiated by the B_2 receptor, which is distributed widely in tissues, where it binds bradykinin and kallidin. The B_1 receptor binds the metabolites of bradykinin and kallidin. Stimulation of the B_2 receptor leads to vasodilation, which is mediated by the activation of NOS3, phospholipase A_2, and adenylyl cyclase. Studies suggest that bradykinin plays an important role in the regulation of vascular tone in HF.[27] The breakdown of bradykinin is catalyzed by ACE, so that this enzyme not only leads to the formation of a potent vasoconstrictor (angiotensin II) but also mediates the breakdown of a vasodilator (bradykinin). The augmentation of bradykinin levels probably contributes to the beneficial actions of ACE inhibitors (see Chap. 28).

ADRENOMEDULLIN. Adrenomedullin is a 52–amino acid vasodilatory peptide that was originally discovered in human pheochromocytoma tissue. Subsequently, high levels of adrenomedullin immunoreactivity were detected in cardiac atrium and adrenal and pituitary glands, with lower levels detected in the ventricle, kidney, and vasculature.[28] Adrenomedullin binds to a number of G protein–coupled receptors, including the calcitonin receptor–like receptor and one specific for the adrenomedullin peptide. Adrenomedullin receptors are present in multiple

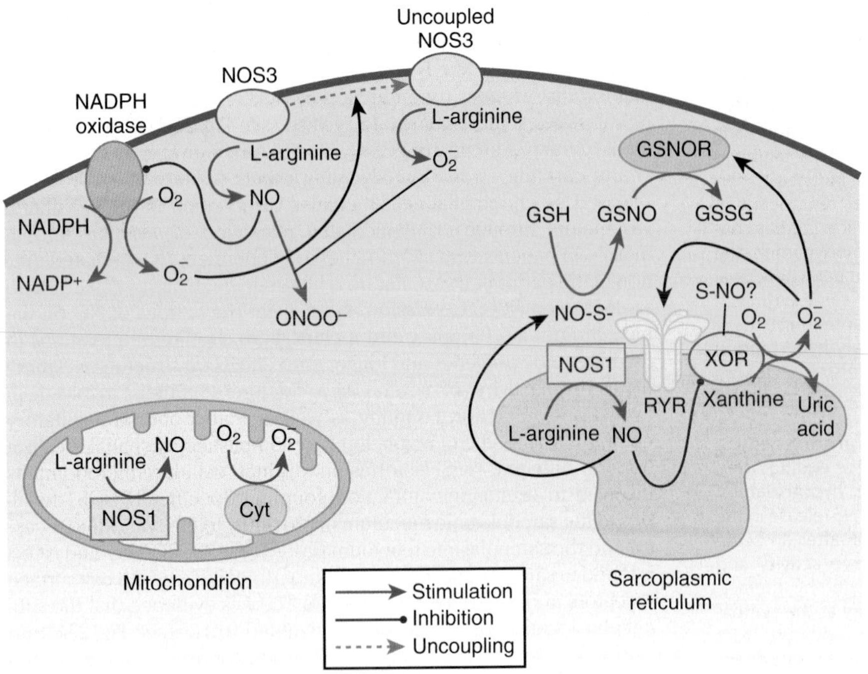

FIGURE 25-8 Interaction of oxidative and nitrosative pathways in heart failure. The principal sources of reactive oxygen species in the cardiomyocyte are xanthine oxidoreductase (XOR), nicotinamide adenine dinucleotide phosphate oxidase (NADPH), and the mitochondria. Nitric oxide (NO) is produced by neuronal nitric oxide synthase (NOS1), situated in the sarcoplasmic reticulum (SR) and in the mitochondria, and endothelial nitric oxide synthase (eNOS), situated in the caveolae in the cell membrane. XOR and NOS1 colocalize in the SR, and this allows the inhibition of XOR by NOS1, possibly through *S*-nitrosylation. In turn, XOR reduces *S*-nitrosoglutathione (GSNO), leading to the regeneration of glutathione (GSH), the enzyme that reduces SNO moieties in proteins and preserves the *S*-nitrosylation equilibrium. In SR, NOS1 regulates the activity of the ryanodine receptor (RyR) through *S*-nitrosylation; in contrast, XOR-generated superoxide (O_2^-) irreversibly activates RyR, precluding this regulatory action of NO. In the cell membrane, NOS3 suppresses NADPH activity, whereas NADPH-produced O_2^- can induce NOS3 uncoupling, resulting in O_2^- production and reduced NO synthesis. O_2^- interacts with NO and generates peroxynitrite ($ONOO^-$). GSSG = oxidized GSH; GSNOR = GSNO reductase; Cyt = cytochrome. *(From Tziomalos K, Hare JM: Role of xanthine oxidoreductase in cardiac nitroso-redox imbalance. Front Biosci 14:237, 2009.)*

TABLE 25-1 Effects of Inflammatory Mediators on Left Ventricular Remodeling

Alterations in the Biology of the Myocyte
Myocyte hypertrophy
Fetal gene expression
Negative inotropic effects
Increased oxidative stress
Alterations in the Biology of the Nonmyocytes
Conversion of fibroblasts to myofibroblasts
Upregulation of AT_1 receptors on fibroblasts
Increased MMP secretion by fibroblasts
Alterations in the Extracellular Matrix
Degradation of the matrix
Myocardial fibrosis
Progressive Myocyte Loss
Necrosis
Apoptosis

tissue beds as well as in endothelial and vascular smooth muscle cells. Circulating concentrations of adrenomedullin are elevated in cardiovascular disease and HF in proportion to the severity of cardiac and hemodynamic impairment. There is increasing evidence that adrenomedullin may play a compensatory role in HF by offsetting the deleterious effects of excessive peripheral vasoconstriction. Administration of adrenomedullin in experimental and human HF leads to a decrease in blood pressure and cardiac filling pressures, improves cardiac output, and leads to improved renal function and suppression of plasma aldosterone.[28]

APELIN. Apelin is a recently discovered (1993) vasoactive peptide that is an endogenous ligand for the G protein–coupled receptor APJ. In the cardiovascular system, apelin elicits endothelium-dependent, NO-mediated vasorelaxation and reduces arterial blood pressure. In addition, apelin demonstrates potent and inotropic activity without stimulating concomitant cardiac myocyte hypertrophy. Apelin also produces diuresis by inhibition of AVP activity. In experimental animals, apelin concentrations are significantly lower in failing hearts and are increased after treatment with an angiotensin receptor blocker. Further, apelin levels are significantly reduced in HF patients compared with controls and are significantly increased after cardiac resynchronization.

ADIPOKINES. Although adipose tissue was once considered a simple storage for fat, adipose tissue is now known to produce and to secrete an ever-increasing range of factors, collectively referred to as adipokines (see Fig. 25-e3 on website). Adipokines include adiponectin, tumor necrosis factor, plasminogen activator inhibitor type 1, transforming growth factor-β, and resistin. Leptin is the product of the obese (*ob*) gene, which is predominantly synthesized and secreted by adipocytes, although the heart is also a site of leptin synthesis. The initial role of leptin was thought to be as a signal of adiposity to decrease food intake via hypothalamic stimulation. However, elevated circulating levels of leptin, which acts via a family of receptor (ob.R) isoforms, appear to play an important role in hypertension, hypertrophy, and HF.[29] Leptin may have an impact on myocardial function via direct peripheral effects or via secondary central nervous system–mediated responses. Lack of leptin or leptin resistance may lead to an accumulation of lipids in nonadipose peripheral tissues and a variety of lipotoxic effects, including cardiac myocyte apoptosis. Several studies suggest that leptin directly induces hypertrophy in both human and rodent cardiac myocytes.[29] Adiponectin was also initially thought to be exclusively produced by adipose tissue. However, studies have demonstrated adiponectin expression in the heart. Studies in adiponectin-deficient mice showed that there was progressive cardiac remodeling after a superimposed pressure overload. Moreover, administration of adiponectin diminished the infarct size, apoptosis, and tumor necrosis factor production induced by ischemia-reperfusion in both wild-type and adiponectin-deficient mice. Of interest, many studies have correlated decreased adiponectin levels with the development of obesity-linked HF. Thus, adiponectin has been proposed as a potential biomarker of HF as well as a potential therapeutic target in the treatment of HF.[29]

INFLAMMATORY MEDIATORS. One of the recent conceptual advances with respect to our understanding of the pathogenesis of HF has been the insight that proinflammatory cytokines, such as tumor necrosis factor and IL-1, may contribute to the progressive cardiac remodeling that occurs in HF. Whereas proinflammatory cytokines have traditionally been thought to be produced by the immune system, it is now recognized that these molecules are produced locally within the myocardium by cells that reside within the myocardium, including cardiac myocytes, in direct response to one or more different forms of cardiac injury. Although the primary role for these molecules is to initiate repair of the injured myocardium, when they are expressed for protracted periods or at high levels, these molecules are sufficient to recapitulate virtually all aspects of the HF phenotype by provoking deleterious changes in cardiac myocytes and nonmyocytes as well as changes in the myocardial extracellular matrix (**Table 25-1**).[30] Moreover, in experimental models, there is substantial crosstalk between proinflammatory cytokines and the RAS, such that angiotensin II upregulates the expression of tumor necrosis factor through an NF-κB–dependent pathway, and the expression of inflammatory mediators leads to upregulation of the RAS through increased activation of myocardial ACE and chymase. Circulating levels of proinflammatory cytokines including tumor necrosis factor and IL-6 are increased in patients with HF and correlate with adverse patient outcomes.[31] Conversely, the plasma concentrations of anti-inflammatory cytokines such as IL-10 are reduced in patients with HF and are decreased more in direct relation to the degree of

TABLE 25-2 Overview of Left Ventricular Remodeling

Alterations in Myocyte Biology
Excitation-contraction coupling
Myosin heavy chain (fetal) gene expression
Beta-adrenergic desensitization
Hypertrophy
Myocytolysis
Cytoskeletal proteins
Myocardial Changes
Myocyte loss
Necrosis
Apoptosis
Autophagy
Alterations in extracellular matrix
Matrix degradation
Myocardial fibrosis
Alterations in Left Ventricular Chamber Geometry
LV dilation
Increased LV sphericity
LV wall thinning
Mitral valve incompetence

severity of HF, suggesting that the imbalance between proinflammatory and anti-inflammatory cytokine expression may contribute to progressive HF.

Left Ventricular Remodeling

Although the neurohormonal model explains many aspects of disease progression in the failing heart, there is increasing clinical evidence to suggest that our current neurohormonal models fail to completely explain disease progression in HF. That is, whereas neurohormonal antagonists stabilize HF and in some cases reverse certain aspects of the disease process, HF will progress in the overwhelming majority of patients, albeit at a slower rate. It has recently been suggested that the process of LV remodeling is directly related to future deterioration in LV performance and a less favorable clinical course in patients with HF (reviewed in reference 32). Whereas the complex changes that occur in the heart during LV remodeling have traditionally been described in anatomic terms, the process of LV remodeling also importantly affects the biology of the cardiac myocyte, the volume of myocyte and nonmyocyte components of the myocardium, and the geometry and architecture of the LV chamber (**Table 25-2**).

ALTERATIONS IN THE BIOLOGY OF THE CARDIAC MYOCYTE. Numerous studies have suggested that failing human cardiac myocytes undergo a number of important changes that might be expected to lead to a progressive loss of contractile function, including decreased α-MHC gene expression with a concomitant increase in β-MHC expression, progressive loss of myofilaments in cardiac myocytes, alterations in cytoskeletal proteins, alterations in excitation-contraction coupling, and desensitization of beta-adrenergic signaling (see Table 25-2).

Cardiac Myocyte Hypertrophy

Two basic patterns of cardiac hypertrophy occur in response to hemodynamic overload (**Fig. 25-9**). In pressure overload hypertrophy (e.g., with aortic stenosis or hypertension), the increase in systolic wall stress leads to the addition of sarcomeres in parallel, an increase in myocyte cross-sectional area (Fig. 25-9A), and an increase in LV wall thickening. This pattern of remodeling has been referred to as concentric hypertrophy (Fig. 25-9A). In contrast, in volume overload hypertrophy (e.g., with aortic and mitral regurgitation), increased diastolic wall stress leads to an increase in myocyte length with the addition of sarcomeres in series (Fig. 25-9A), thereby engendering increased LV ventricular dilation (Fig. 25-9A). This pattern of remodeling has been referred to

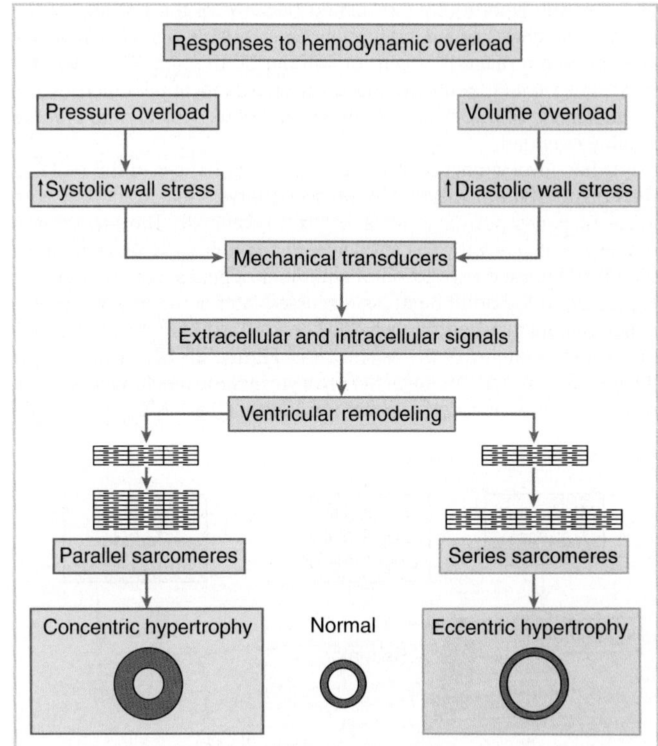

FIGURE 25-9 The pattern of cardiac and cellular remodeling that occurs in response to hemodynamic overloading depends on the nature of the inciting stimulus. **A,** When the overload is predominantly caused by an increase in pressure (e.g., with systemic hypertension or aortic stenosis), the increase in systolic wall stress leads to the parallel addition of sarcomeres and widening of the cardiac myocytes, resulting in concentric cardiac hypertrophy. When the overload is predominantly caused by an increase in ventricular volume, the increase in diastolic wall stress leads to the series addition of sarcomeres, lengthening of cardiac myocytes, and LV dilation, which is referred to as eccentric chamber hypertrophy. *(From Colucci WS [ed]: Heart Failure: Cardiac Function and Dysfunction. 2nd ed. Philadelphia, Current Medicine, 1999, p 42)* **B,** Phenotypically distinct changes occur in the morphology of the myocyte in response to the type of hemodynamic overload that is superimposed. When the overload is predominantly caused by an increase in pressure, the increase in systolic wall stress leads to the parallel addition of sarcomeres and widening of the cardiac myocytes. When the overload is predominantly caused by an increase in ventricular volume, the increase in diastolic wall stress leads to the series addition of sarcomeres and thus lengthening of cardiac myocytes. The expression of maladaptive embryonic genes (see Table 25-2) is increased in both eccentric and concentric hypertrophy but not in physiologic myocyte hypertrophy that occurs with exercise. *(Modified from Hunter JJ, Chien KR: Signaling pathways for cardiac hypertrophy and failure. N Engl J Med 341:1276, 1999.)*

as eccentric hypertrophy (so named because of the position of the heart in the chest) or a dilated phenotype. Patients with HF classically present with a dilated LV with or without LV thinning. The myocytes from these failing ventricles have an elongated appearance that is characteristic of myocytes obtained from hearts subjected to chronic volume overload.

Cardiac myocyte hypertrophy also leads to changes in the biologic phenotype of the myocyte that are secondary to reactivation of portfolios of genes normally not expressed postnatally. The reactivation of these fetal genes, the so-called fetal gene program, is also accompanied by decreased expression of a number of genes that are normally expressed in the adult heart. As discussed later, activation of the fetal gene program may contribute to the contractile dysfunction that develops in the failing myocyte. As shown in **Figure 25-10**, the stimuli for the genetic reprogramming of the myocyte include mechanical stretch-strain of the myocyte, neurohormones (e.g., NE, angiotensin II), inflammatory cytokines (e.g., tumor necrosis factor, IL-6), other peptides and growth factors (e.g., endothelin), and ROS (e.g., superoxide, NO). These stimuli occur locally within the myocardium, where they exert autocrine or paracrine effects, as well as systemically, where they exert endocrine effects.

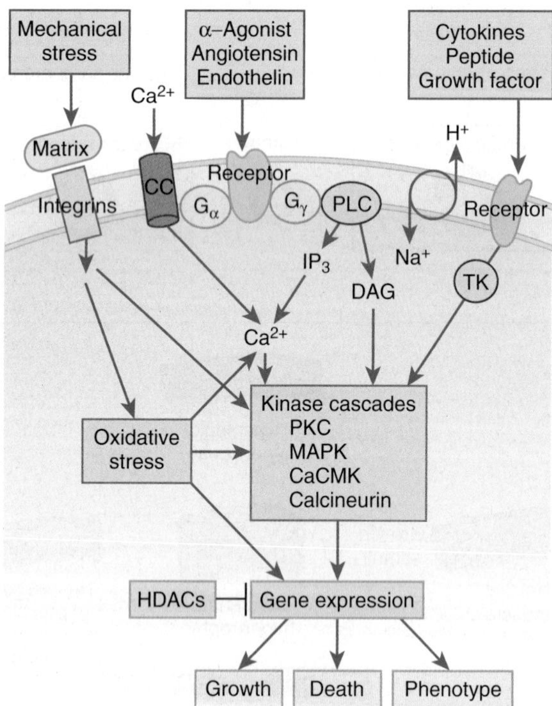

FIGURE 25-10 Cellular signaling pathways in cardiac hypertrophy and failure. Many signaling pathways have the potential to regulate the growth of cardiac cells acting through an increasingly complex network of intracellular signaling cascades. Agonists for α-adrenergic, angiotensin, and endothelin receptors couple to phospholipase C (PLC) and calcium influx channels (CC) by way of G proteins (G_x and G_y). Activation of PLC results in the generation of two second messengers, inositol triphosphate (IP_3) and diacylglycerol (DAG). IP_3 causes the release of calcium from intracellular stores, and DAG activates protein kinase C (PKC). Changes in intracellular calcium stores can activate calcium/calmodulin-dependent kinases (CaCMK) as well as calcineurin, which can affect gene expression in multiple ways. PKC can affect gene expression directly or indirectly by its effects on Na^+/H^+ exchange (to regulate cellular pH) or by activating mitogen-activated protein kinase (MAPK) cascades. Histone deacetylase complexes (HDACs) are emerging as important negative regulators of genes involved in cardiac hypertrophy. Cytokines and peptide growth factors can be elaborated by various cells within the heart and may act in an autocrine or paracrine manner. These growth factors activate cellular receptors that usually possess tyrosine kinase (TK) activity and are coupled to a cascade of protein kinases (ras, Raf, MAPKK, MAPK). Mechanical deformation of cardiac myocytes through matrix-integrin interactions can lead to activation or modulation of several signaling pathways, at least in part through autocrine action of released agonists such as angiotensin. Both nitric oxide and oxidative stress may be induced after stimulation of signaling pathways and modulate the activity of kinase cascades and transcription factors, leading to alterations in contractile phenotype, growth, and death of myocytes. *(From Sawyer DB, Colucci WS: Molecular and cellular events in myocardial hypertrophy and failure.* In Colucci WS [ed]: *Atlas of Heart Failure. 4th ed. Philadelphia, Current Medicine, 2005, p 62.)*

The early stage of cardiac myocyte hypertrophy is characterized morphologically by increases in the number of myofibrils and mitochondria as well as by enlargement of mitochondria and nuclei (see Fig. 25-e4 on website). At this stage, the cardiac myocytes are larger than normal and have preserved cellular organization. As hypertrophy continues, there is an increase in the number of mitochondria as well as the addition of new contractile elements in localized areas of the cell. Cells subjected to longstanding hypertrophy show more obvious disruptions in cellular organization, such as markedly enlarged nuclei with highly lobulated membranes, accompanied by the displacement of adjacent myofibrils with loss of the normal registration of the Z-bands. The late stage of hypertrophy is characterized by loss of contractile elements (myocytolysis) with marked disruption of Z-bands and severe disruption of the normal parallel arrangement of the sarcomeres, accompanied by dilation and increased tortuosity of T tubules (see Fig. 25-e4 on website).

Alterations in Excitation-Contraction Coupling

As discussed in Chap. 24, excitation-contraction coupling refers to the cascade of biologic events that begins with the cardiac action potential and ends with myocyte contraction and relaxation (see Fig. 24-6). Classic studies from explanted failing hearts have shown that patients with end-stage HF exhibit abnormal prolongation of the action potential as well as depressed developed force and impaired relaxation.[33] The intracellular Ca^{2+} transient, as assessed by the fluorescent indicator fura-2, demonstrates a blunted rise after depolarization, reflecting slower delivery of Ca^{2+} to the contractile apparatus (causing slower activation), followed by a slowed rate of fall during repolarization (causing slowed relaxation). Changes in the abundance or phosphorylation state of critical Ca^{2+} regulatory proteins are likely to play an important role in the contractile dysfunction of failing cardiac myocytes.

SARCOPLASMIC RETICULUM IN THE FAILING HEART. The normal function of the sarcoplasmic reticulum (SR) is described in detail in Chap. 24. As shown in **Table 25-3**, there are a number of alterations in SR proteins and function in the failing heart. Given the central role for SERCA2a (sarcoendoplasmic reticulum Ca^{2+}) in excitation-contraction coupling, it has been suggested that the reduced activity of SERCA2 may play an important role in the pathogenesis of HF. Indeed, several (but not all) studies have reported that the levels of SERCA2 mRNA and protein are reduced in animal models of HF as well as in myocardium samples obtained from patients with end-stage HF. The downregulation in SERCA2 expression was associated with a corresponding reduction in SR Ca^{2+} reuptake in some (but not all) myocardial samples obtained from patients with severe failure. This reduction in the abundance or functional activity of SERCA2a could explain the slow decay of the Ca^{2+} transient and the reduced SR Ca^{2+} storage and release that have been observed in failing myocytes.[33] Importantly, overexpression of SERCA2a improves myocardial performance in the senescent heart, prevents the development of HF after aortic banding, and improves the contractile performance of human cardiac myocytes taken from the explanted hearts of HF patients. However, SERCA2a abundance (or Ca^{2+} uptake rate) has also been reported to be normal in some failing hearts with depressed contractility, suggesting that there may also be functional abnormalities in other molecules that regulate SR function. For example, decreases in phospholamban phosphorylation or activity in the failing human heart could disrupt normal SR function or alternatively could exacerbate the effect of decreased SERCA abundance. As a case in point, transgenic mice with a defect in muscle LIM protein ($MLP^{-/-}$), a structural protein involved in muscle development, develop a dilated cardiomyopathy that can be completely repaired by knocking out phospholamban.[34] Another mechanism that has been proposed relates to the leakage of the ryanodine receptor, which is closed during diastole and thus allows Ca^{2+} that is transported into the SR to accumulate until activation by the L-type Ca^{2+} leads to SR Ca^{2+} release. Studies in experimental models of HF and failing human myocardium suggest that the ryanodine receptor is hyperphosphorylated on serine residue

TABLE 25-3 Changes in the Biology of the Failing Myocyte

PROTEIN	CHANGE IN HUMAN HEART FAILURE
Plasma Membrane	
L-type calcium channels	Decreased*,†
Sodium/calcium exchanger	Increased*,†
Sodium pump	Reexpression of fetal isoforms
Beta$_1$-adrenergic receptor	Decreased*,†
Beta$_2$-adrenergic receptor	Increased*
Alpha$_1$-adrenergic receptor	Increased*
Contractile Proteins	
Myosin heavy chain	Reversion to fetal isoform
Myosin light chain	Reversion to fetal isoform
Actin	Normal*
Troponin I	Normal*
Troponin T	Reversion to isoform
Troponin C	Normal*
Tropomyosin	Normal*
Sarcoplasmic Reticulum	
SERCA2a	Normal or decreased*,†
Phospholamban	Decreased*,†
Ryanodine receptor	Hyperphosphorylated†
Calsequestrin	Normal*
Calreticulin	Normal*

*Refers to protein level.
†Refers to functional activity.
Modified from Katz AM: Physiology of the Heart. Philadelphia, Lippincott Williams & Wilkins, 2001.

2809 and that this hyperphosphorylation leads to loss of calstabin2 (FKBP-12.6) from the ryanodine receptor complex and increases the open probability of the receptor, causing a persistent leak of Ca^{2+} from the SR.[35]

L-Type Calcium Channel. The L-type calcium channel opens when the membrane depolarizes during the upstroke of the cardiac action potential. The subsequent Ca^{2+} influx helps produce the plateau phase of the action potential and elevates $[Ca^{2+}]$ in the cytosol. Studies have shown that there is a reduction in the mRNA and protein levels and an increased level of phosphorylation of the L-type Ca^{2+} channels in HF.[33] Both of these abnormalities would reduce both the magnitude and the homogeneity of the inward Ca^{2+} current and thus adversely affect SR Ca^{2+}release.

Na^+/Ca^{2+} Exchanger. Under normal conditions, Ca^{2+} enters myocytes from the extracellular space down a large electrochemical gradient. At a normal resting potential of −80 mV and with normal intracellular Na^+ levels, energy in the Na^+ electrochemical gradient is sufficient to remove approximately 20% of the Ca^{2+} from the cytoplasm via the Na^+/Ca^{2+} exchanger (forward mode conductance; see Chap. 24). In HF mRNA, protein levels and activity levels of the Na^+/Ca^{2+} exchanger have been reported to be increased.[36] It has been suggested that the increased expression of the Na^+/Ca^{2+} exchanger compensates for decreased Ca^{2+} uptake because of the reduction in SERCA2a activity in HF. However, this seems unlikely to be the case in human HF, insofar as SERCA2a Ca^{2+} uptake occurs when forward mode conductance is minimal. It has recently been suggested that Ca^{2+} entry via reverse mode Na^+/Ca^{2+} exchanger activity contributes to abnormal Ca^{2+} handling in HF.[36]

Abnormalities in Contractile and Regulatory Proteins (see Table 25-3)

Early studies showed that the activity of myofibrillar ATPase was reduced in the hearts of patients who died of HF. Furthermore, reductions in the activities of myofibrillar ATPase, actomyosin ATPase, or myosin ATPase have been demonstrated in several animal models of HF. Subsequent studies showed that these abnormalities in ATPase activity could be explained by a shift to the fetal isoform of myosin heavy chain (MHC) in cardiac hypertrophy and failure. In rodents, the predominant MHC is the "fast" V1 isoform (α-MHC), which has high ATPase activity. With pressure-induced hypertrophy or after myocardial infarction in rodents, there is reexpression of the "slow" V3 fetal isoform of MHC that has low ATPase activity (β-MHC) and decreased expression of the V1 isoform. Although translating this information to human HF proved to be more challenging, insofar as the predominant MHC isoform in humans is the slower V3 isoform (β-MHC), it has been possible with the development of the polymerase chain reaction to demonstrate that the α-MHC accounts for approximately 33% of MHC mRNA in normal human myocardium, whereas α-MHC mRNA abundance decreases to about 2% in failing heart. Further, in human studies in which myocardial biopsy specimens were obtained in patients who were taking beta blockers, there were reciprocal changes in the levels of α-MHC (increase) and β-MHC (decrease) mRNA and an increase in the ratio of α/β-MHC in the patients who had an improvement in LV function; these changes in myosin isoform shifts did not occur in HF patients in whom there was no improvement in LV function with beta blockers.[37] Thus, the decreased expression of α-MHC may play a significant role in the pathophysiologic process of dilated cardiomyopathy. Another important modification of contractile proteins that contributes to contractile dysfunction is proteolysis of the myofilaments themselves (myocytolysis). Myocardial biopsy samples from patients with advanced LV dysfunction show a significant reduction in the volume of myofibrils per cell, which may contribute to the development of cardiac decompensation.

Alteration in the expression or activity of myofilament regulatory proteins has also been proposed as a potential mechanism for the decrease in cardiac contractile function in HF (see Table 25-3), including the myosin light chains and the troponin-tropomyosin complex in HF. Changes in myosin light chain isoforms have been observed in the atria and ventricles of patients whose hearts have been subjected to mechanical overload. Although changes in the abundance or isoforms of troponin I and troponin C (see Chap. 24) have not been reported in HF, isoform shifts have been reported in troponin T. In normal adult myocardium, troponin T is expressed as a single isoform (cTnT3). However, in myocardium samples from patients with end-stage HF, both the fetal cTnT1 and the cTnT4 isoforms are expressed at increased levels, which might be expected to lead to a decrease in maximal active tension.[38]

Abnormalities in Cytoskeletal Proteins

The cytoskeleton of cardiac myocytes consists of actin, the intermediate filament desmin, the sarcomeric protein titin (see Chap. 24), and alpha- and beta-tubulin that form the microtubules by polymerization. Vinculin, talin, dystrophin, and spectrin represent a separate group of membrane-associated proteins. In numerous experimental studies, the role of cytoskeletal or membrane-associated proteins has been implicated in the pathogenesis of HF. In patients with dilated cardiomyopathy, titin is downregulated; the cytoskeletal protein desmin and membrane-associated proteins such as vinculin and dystrophin are upregulated. Proteolytic digestion of the dystrophin molecule was recently identified as a possible reversible cause of HF.[39] Loss of integrity of the cytoskeleton and its linkage of the sarcomere to the sarcolemma and extracellular matrix would be expected to lead to contractile dysfunction at the myocyte level as well as at the myocardial level.

Beta-Adrenergic Desensitization

Ventricles obtained from HF patients demonstrate a marked reduction in beta-adrenergic receptor density, isoproterenol-mediated adenylyl cyclase stimulation, and contractile response to beta-adrenergic agonists (see Fig. 25-e5 on website).[40] The downregulation of beta-adrenergic receptors is likely to be mediated by increased levels of NE in the vicinity of the receptor. In patients with dilated cardiomyopathy, this reduction in receptor density involves primarily the beta$_1$ receptor protein and mRNA and is proportional to the severity of HF. In contrast, the level of beta$_2$-adrenergic receptor protein and mRNA is unchanged. In addition, there are increases in the expression of beta-adrenergic receptor kinase 1 (βARK1, also called G protein–coupled receptor kinase 2), a member of the family of G protein–coupled receptor kinases, in failing human hearts. As noted in Chap. 24, βARK phosphorylates the cytoplasmic loops of both beta$_1$- and beta$_2$-adrenergic receptors and increases the affinity of these receptors for a scaffolding protein termed beta-arrestin (see Fig. 24-14). The binding of beta-arrestins to the cytoplasmic tail of the beta receptor not only uncouples the receptor from heterotrimeric G proteins but also targets the receptor for internalization in clathrin-coated vesicles. Although this internalization fosters receptor dephosphorylation and serves as a prelude to recycling of the beta receptor to the surface for reactivation, at some point receptor entry via endocytosis is not followed by recycling but rather leads to receptor trafficking to lysosomes and receptor degradation. Increased βARK (also known as GRK2) activity may therefore contribute to the desensitization of both $beta_1$- and $beta_2$-adrenergic receptors in patients with HF. Desensitization of the beta receptors can be both beneficial and deleterious in HF. By reducing LV contractility, desensitization may be deleterious; however, by reducing energy expenditure of the energy-starved myocardium and protecting the myocyte from the deleterious effects of sustained adrenergic stimulation, this adaptive response is beneficial. Of interest, transgenic mice that overexpress βARK are protected from development of HF.[41]

ALTERATIONS IN THE MYOCARDIUM IN HEART FAILURE. The alterations that occur in failing myocardium may be categorized broadly into those that occur in the volume of cardiac myocytes and changes that occur in the volume and composition of the extracellular matrix. With respect to the changes that occur in the cardiac myocyte component of the myocardium, there is increasing evidence to suggest that progressive myocyte loss, through necrotic, apoptotic, or autophagic cell death pathways, may contribute to progressive cardiac dysfunction and LV remodeling.

NECROSIS. Necrosis is an "accidental" form of cell death that follows extreme myocyte injury. The hallmark of necrosis is cell rupture, which is generally preceded by distention of various cellular organelles, clumping and random degradation of nuclear DNA, and cell swelling, culminating in disruption of the plasma membrane barrier. In the heart, increased plasma membrane permeability allows calcium to leak into the cell, exposing the contractile proteins to very high concentrations of this activator, which in turn initiates extreme interactions between the myofilaments (contraction bands), which further contributes to disruption of the cellular membrane. Necrotic myocyte death occurs in ischemic heart disease, myocardial injury, toxin exposure (e.g., daunorubicin [see Chap. 90]), infection, and inflammation. Neurohormonal activation can also lead to necrotic cell death. For example, concentrations of NE that are available within myocardial tissue as well as circulating levels in patients with advanced HF are sufficient to provoke myocyte necrosis in experimental model systems. Moreover, excessive stimulation with either angiotensin II or endothelin has been shown to provoke myocyte necrosis in experimental models. Myocyte necrosis was sevenfold greater than apoptosis in explanted hearts from male and female HF patients. Interestingly, necrotic cell death was twofold higher in men than in women.[42] Additional evidence for the existence of ongoing myonecrosis in patients with HF is suggested by studies showing that levels of circulating troponin I and troponin T are increased significantly in patients with advanced HF. In contrast to apoptosis (see next), the rupture of cell membranes with cell necrosis releases intracellular contents that evoke an intense inflammatory reaction, leading to the influx of granulocytes, macrophages, and collagen-secreting fibroblasts into the area of injury. The final result is a fibrotic scar, which may alter the structural and functional properties of the myocardium (see later).

APOPTOSIS. Apoptosis, or programmed cell death, is an evolutionarily conserved process that allows multicellular organisms to selectively remove cells through a highly orchestrated program of cell suicide. The ensemble of proteins that are responsible for activating apoptosis is preprogrammed into the genetic code of the cells that are destined to die. However, under pathologic circumstances, such as acute ischemia and dilated cardiomyopathy, the apoptotic program can be triggered inappropriately, resulting in inadvertent cell death. Apoptosis requires energy and activation of specific biochemical steps that are involved in triggering and execution of cell death through activation of intrinsic (mitochondrial) and extrinsic (death receptor mediated) pathways that lead to the activation of executioner caspases (**Fig. 25-11**). In contrast to the cell swelling that characterizes necrosis, the cell shrinks during apoptosis and eventually breaks up into small, membrane-surrounded fragments. These often contain bits of condensed chromatin, referred to as apoptotic bodies. Maintenance of plasma membrane integrity until late in the apoptotic process allows the dying cell to be engulfed by macrophages, which prevents the release of the reactive intracellular contents, thereby preventing an inflammatory reaction. An important distinction between necrosis and apoptosis is the manner in which DNA is degraded. In necrosis, DNA is broken down into randomly sized fragments, whereas the endonuclease-mediated breakdown of DNA in apoptosis leads to the generation of multiples of 180– to 200–base pair fragments that resemble a ladder (DNA laddering) when they are run out on electrophoretic gels. Another characteristic feature of apoptosis is that the type of DNA cleavage has a characteristic single 3′ overhang that can be readily detected by a number of molecular probes (see later).

The gold standard for identification of apoptotic cells is ultrastructural evidence of chromatin condensation, the earliest characteristic morphologic feature. However, although ultrastructural evidence of chromatin condensation is highly reliable, the routine use of electron microscopy to detect chromatin condensation is impractical because it is labor-intensive and costly. The terminal deoxynucleotidyl transferase (TUNEL) method is the most widely used technique because the microscopic evaluation of myocardial samples is relatively easy and inexpensive (see Fig. 25-e6 on website). The TUNEL method uses a molecular probe that anneals to DNA with double-stranded breaks characteristic of apoptosis (i.e., with 3′ overhangs). The *Taq* polymerase method follows a similar principle.[43] However, the TUNEL technique not only labels apoptotic nuclei but can also label necrotic and oncotic nuclei as well as nuclei undergoing DNA repair. Similar limitations apply to the *Taq* polymerase method, albeit to a lesser extent.

Cardiac myocyte apoptosis has been shown to occur in failing human hearts.[44] Indeed, many of the factors that have been implicated in the pathogenesis of HF, including catecholamines acting through $beta_1$-adrenergic receptor, angiotensin II, ROS, NO, inflammatory cytokines, and mechanical strain, have been shown to trigger apoptosis in vitro. Moreover, activation of either the extrinsic or intrinsic cell death pathways provokes progressive LV dilation and decompensation in transgenic mice.[45] Nonetheless, the exact physiologic significance and consequences of apoptosis in human HF have been difficult to determine because of the tremendous uncertainty with respect to the actual rate of cardiac myocyte apoptosis in the failing human heart (reviewed in reference 1). This statement notwithstanding, the aggregate clinical and experimental data suggest that apoptosis is likely to play an important role in HF.

AUTOPHAGY. Autophagy refers to the homeostatic cellular process of sequestering organelles and long-lived proteins in a double-membrane vesicle inside the cell (autophagosome), where the contents are subsequently delivered to the lysosome for degradation. When autophagy involves the total destruction of the cell, it is referred to as autophagic cell death. Studies have demonstrated the existence of autophagic cell death in hypertrophied, failing, and hibernating myocardium.[46] Approximately 0.3% of the cardiac myocytes in explanted hearts from patients with HF exhibited autophagic cell death,[47] whereas the predominant form of cell death in pressure-overloaded human hearts was mainly by autophagy and oncosis.[48]

The distinction between necrosis and apoptosis is obvious in certain circumstances, but the dividing line between these two conditions is often less clear in the failing heart. Indeed, similar mechanisms can operate in both types of cell death. For example, cell death that begins as apoptosis can also lead to necrosis if the decline in adenosine triphosphate (ATP) content results in cell rupture (secondary necrosis) before the cell can be engulfed by macrophages. Moreover, cardiac myocytes can undergo either necrotic or apoptotic cell death in response to different stimuli (e.g., NE). Ultimately, what determines cell fate in the failing heart is the intensity or rapidity of the injury, the expression levels of the downstream proapoptotic and antiapoptotic proteins, and the extent of the calcium overload and the intracellular ATP levels. Thus, instead of the existence of distinct types of cell death in HF, there is likely to be a continuum of cell death responses that contribute to progressive myocyte loss and disease progression.

Changes within the extracellular matrix constitute the second important myocardial adaptation that occurs during cardiac remodeling. The myocardial extracellular matrix consists of a basement membrane, a fibrillar collagen network that surrounds the myocytes, proteoglycans and glycosaminoglycans, and biologically active signaling molecules. The major fibrillar collagens in the heart are type I and type III, with a ratio of type I to type III of approximately 1.3 to 1.9:1. The organization of myocardial fibrillar type I and type III collagen ensures the structural integrity of adjoining myocytes and

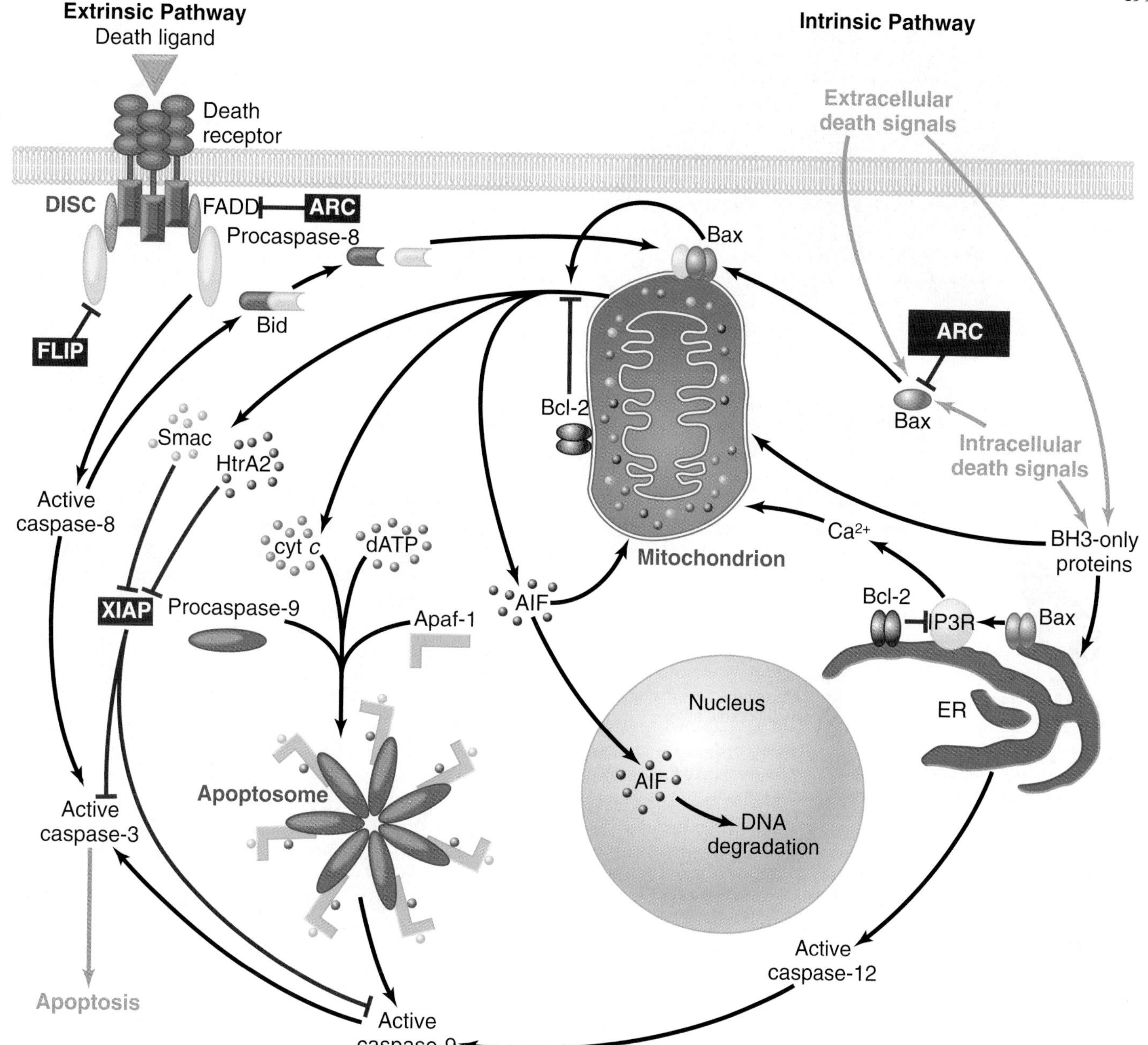

FIGURE 25-11 Intrinsic and extrinsic cell death pathways in cardiac myocytes. In the extrinsic pathway, ligand binding induces death receptors to recruit FADD, which recruits procaspase-8. Within this complex (DISC), procaspase-8 dimerizes and activates. Caspase-8 proteolytically activates procaspase-3, which cleaves cellular proteins, causing cell death. In the intrinsic pathway, extracellular and intracellular stimuli signal to the mitochondria through a variety of BH3-only proteins (e.g., Bid) and through Bax, which translocates to and inserts into the outer mitochondrial membrane. Bax and Bak (not shown) stimulate the release of cytochrome *c* (cyt *c*) and other apoptogens. Once released, cytochrome *c* binds Apaf-1 along with dATP. This triggers oligomerization of Apaf-1 and recruitment of procaspase-9. Within this complex (apoptosome), procaspase-9 dimerizes and activates. Caspase-9 proteolytically activates procaspase-3. Caspase-8 also cleaves Bid, and its C-terminal fragment translocates to the mitochondria, where it activates Bax and Bak, stimulating apoptogen release. Activation of the extrinsic pathway is prevented by the antiapoptotic proteins c-FLIP and ARC, whereas activation of the intrinsic pathway is prevented by the antiapoptotic proteins ARC, Bcl-2, or Bcl-X_L (not shown). The X-linked inhibitor of apoptosis (XIAP) blocks the activation of caspase-3. AIF translocates to the nucleus and, in conjunction with a presumed endonuclease, mediates large-scale DNA fragmentation in a caspase-independent manner. *(Modified from Foo RS, Mani K, Kitsis RN: Death begets failure in the heart. J Clin Invest 115:565, 2005.)*

is essential for maintaining alignment of myofibrils within the myocyte through the interaction of collagen and integrins with the cytoskeletal proteins (**Fig. 25-12**). During cardiac remodeling, there are important changes in the extracellular matrix, including changes in fibrillar collagen synthesis and degradation (**Fig. 25-13**), changes in the degree of collagen cross-linking, and loss of collagen struts that connect the individual cardiac myocytes.[49] Markers of collagen turnover have been shown to be increased in patients with dilated cardiomyopathy compared with age-matched control subjects.[49] In patients with idiopathic or ischemic dilated cardiomyopathy, serum N-terminal type III collagen peptide (PIIINP) levels have been shown to be independent predictors of mortality.[50] In the RALES trial (see Chap. 28), serum PIP and PIIINP were assessed at baseline and at 6 months. At 6 months, both PIIINP and PINP were decreased in the spironolactone-treated patients, whereas they were increased or remained unchanged in the placebo group, suggesting that aldosterone may play an important role in extracellular matrix synthesis.

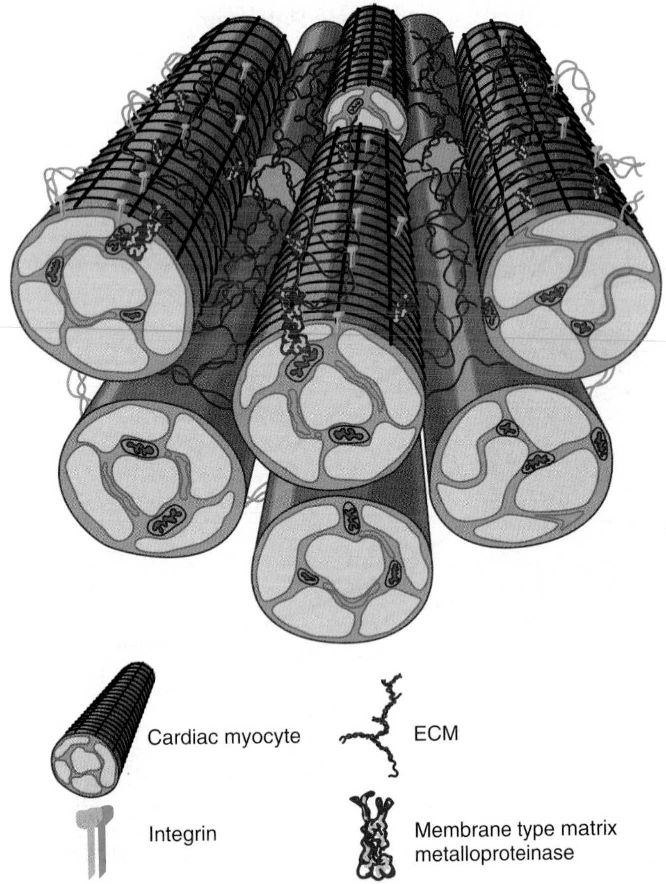

FIGURE 25-12 Relationship between the fibrillar collagen extracellular matrix (ECM) and cardiac myocytes. The myocytes are interconnected by a complex of fibrillar collagen weave and extracellular matrix proteins, such as fibronectin. As shown, the myocyte adheres to the extracellular matrix through a family of transmembrane proteins referred to as integrins. Integrins are composed of alpha and beta subunits that each contain a single transmembrane domain. The engagement of the integrins allows the transduction of sarcomere shortening into myocyte shortening, which in turn facilitates muscle fiber shortening. In addition, the integrins form an important intracellular signaling role by activation of intracellular signaling pathways. The membrane-type matrix metalloproteinase (MT-MMP) is an important proteolytic enzyme that is responsible for extracellular matrix degradation and remodeling. As shown, MT-MMPs may colocalize with the integrins. The activation of the MT-MMPs may cause local extracellular matrix degradation and in turn alter the degree of integrin engagement and ultimately intracellular signaling pathways. *(Modified from Deschamps AM, Spinale FG: Extracellular matrix. In Walsh RA [ed]: Molecular mechanisms of cardiac hypertrophy and failure. Boca Raton, Fla, Taylor and Francis, 2005, pp 101-116.)*

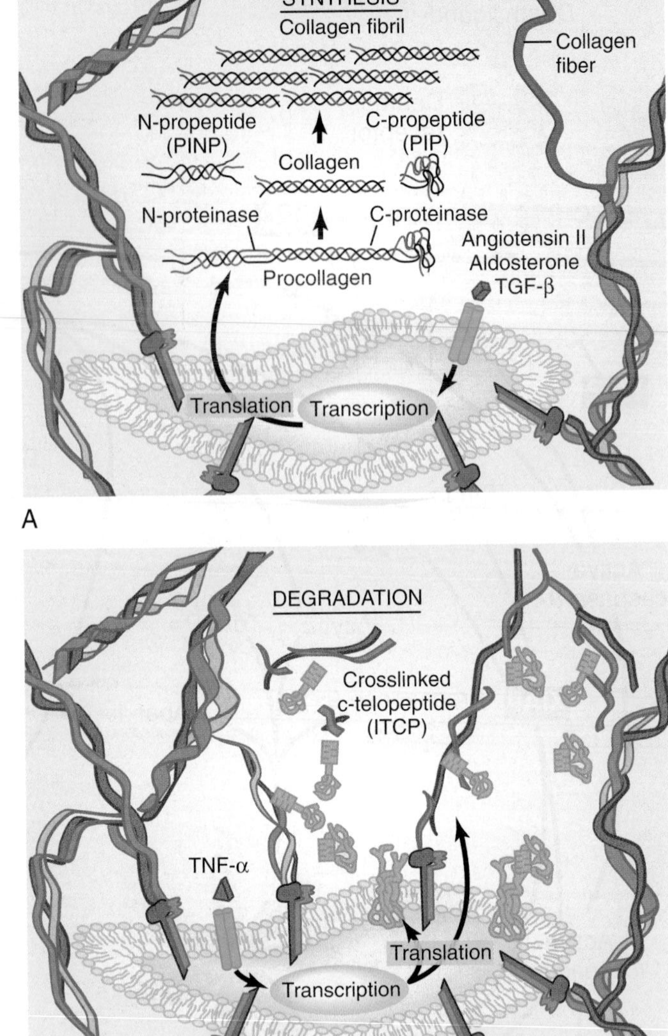

FIGURE 25-13 Collagen synthesis and degradation. **A,** Intracellular signals generated by neurohormonal or mechanical stimulation of cardiac fibroblasts result in transcription and translation of nascent collagen proteins containing amino-terminal (N-terminal) and carboxyl-terminal (C-terminal) propeptides that prevent collagen from assembling into mature fibrils. Once secreted into the interstitium, these propeptides are cleaved by N- and C-proteinases, yielding two procollagen fragments and a mature triple-stranded collagen molecule. In the case of collagen type I, these propeptides are referred to as N-terminal peptide collagen type I propeptide (PINP) and C-terminal peptide type I collagen propeptide (PIP). Removal of the propeptide sequences allows the secreted collagen molecule to integrate into growing collagen fibrils, which can then further assemble into collagen fibers. After the collagen fibrils form in the extracellular space, their tensile strength is greatly strengthened by the formation of covalent cross-links between the lysine residues on the collagen molecules. **B,** The degradation of the collagen matrix within the myocardium involves a number of biochemical events in a number of protease systems. Degradation of collagen fibrils occurs through catalytic cleavage of the three collagen alpha chains at a single locus by interstitial collagenase, yielding 36-kDa and 12-kDa collagen telopeptides that maintain their helical structure and hence are resistant to further proteolytic degradation. The big 36-kDa telopeptide spontaneously denatures into nonhelical gelatin derivatives, which in turn are completely degraded by interstitial gelatinases. The small 12-kDa pyridinoline cross-linked C-terminal telopeptide resulting from the cleavage of collagen type I (ICTP) is found intact in blood, where it appears to be derived from tissues with a stoichiometric ratio of 1:1 between the number of collagen type I molecules degraded and ITCP released. *(From Deschamps AM, Spinale FG: Extracellular matrix. In Walsh RA [ed]: Molecular Mechanisms of Cardiac Hypertrophy and Failure. Boca Raton, Fla, Taylor and Francis, 2005, pp 101-116.)*

Cardiac Fibroblasts and Mast Cells

The cardiac fibroblast, which represents most (>90%) of the nonmyocyte cells in the heart, is the primary cell type responsible for the secretion of the majority of extracellular matrix components in the heart, such as collagens I, III, and IV and laminin and fibronectin. In response to mechanical stress or neurohormonal activation, a subset of fibroblasts undergo phenotypic conversion to myofibroblasts that are characterized by increased expression of alpha-smooth muscle actin and enhanced secretory activity. Myofibroblasts migrate into the area surrounding tissue injury, where they are responsible for the collagen secretion and contraction-realignment of the nascent collagen fibers and thus play an important role in the final scar formation at the site of injury. There is increasing evidence that mast cells, which are bone marrow–derived cells that "home" to and reside in the myocardium, also play an important role in remodeling of the extracellular matrix. Myocardial mast cells are located mainly around blood vessels and between myocytes, where they are capable of releasing profibrotic cytokines and growth factors that influence extracellular matrix remodeling. Experimental studies have shown that mast cell proliferation and degranulation contribute to the remodeling process.[51]

As noted before, one of the histologic signatures of advancing HF is the progressive increase in collagen content of the heart (myocardial fibrosis). Studies in failing human myocardium have shown that there is a quantitative increase in collagens I, III, VI, and IV and in fibronectin, laminin, and vimentin and that the ratio of type I collagen to type III collagen is decreased in patients with ischemic cardiomyopathy. Moreover, clinical studies suggest that there is a progressive loss of cross-linking of collagen in the failing heart as well as loss of connectivity of the collagen network with individual myocytes, which would be expected to result in profound alterations in LV structure and function. Further, loss of cross-linking of the fibrillar collagen has been associated with progressive LV dilation after myocardial injury. The accumulation of collagen can occur on a "reactive" basis around intramural coronary arteries and arterioles (perivascular fibrosis) or in the interstitial space (interstitial fibrosis) and does not require myocyte cell death (see Fig. 25-e7 on website). Alternatively, collagen accumulation can be a result of microscopic scarring (replacement fibrosis) that develops in response to cardiac myocyte cell necrosis. This scarring or "replacement fibrosis" is an adaptation to the loss of parenchyma and is therefore critical to preserve the structural integrity of the heart. The increased fibrous tissue would be expected to lead to increased myocardial stiffness, which would presumably result in decreased myocardial shortening for a given degree of afterload. In addition, myocardial fibrosis may provide the structural substrate for atrial and ventricular arrhythmias, thus potentially contributing to sudden death (see Chap. 41). Although the full complement of molecules that are responsible for fibroblast activation is not known, many of the classical neurohormones (e.g., angiotensin II, aldosterone) and cytokines (endothelin, transforming growth factor-β, cardiotrophin 1) that are expressed in HF are sufficient to provoke fibroblast activation. Indeed, the use of ACE inhibitors, beta blockers, and aldosterone receptor antagonists has been associated with a decrease in myocardial fibrosis in experimental HF models.[1]

Although the fibrillar collagen matrix was initially considered to form a relatively static complex, it is now recognized that these structural proteins can undergo rapid turnover. One of the more exciting developments with respect to understanding of the pathogenesis of cardiac remodeling has been the discovery that a family of collagenolytic enzymes, collectively referred to as matrix metalloproteinases (MMPs), are activated within the failing myocardium. Conceptually, disruption of the extracellular matrix would be expected to lead to LV dilation and wall thinning as a result of mural realignment (slippage) of myocyte bundles or individual myocytes within the LV wall (see Fig. 25-e8 on website) as well as to LV dysfunction as a result of dyssynchronous contraction of the LV. Whereas the precise biochemical triggers responsible for activation of MMPs are not known, tumor necrosis factor and other cytokines and peptide growth factors that are expressed within the failing myocardium are capable of activating MMPs. However, the biology of matrix remodeling in HF is likely to be much more complex than the simple presence or absence of MMP activation, insofar as degradation of the matrix is also controlled by glycoproteins, termed tissue inhibitors of matrix metalloproteinases (TIMPs), that are capable of regulating the activation of MMPs by binding to and preventing these enzymes from degrading the collagen matrix of the heart. The TIMP family presently consists of four distinct members known as TIMP-1, TIMP-2, TIMP-3, and TIMP-4, each of which is constitutively expressed in the heart by fibroblasts as well as by myocytes. TIMP-1, TIMP-2, TIMP-3, and TIMP-4 are secreted proteins that act as the natural inhibitors of active forms of all MMPs, although the efficiency of MMP inhibition varies among the different members. The extant literature suggests that MMP activation can lead to progressive LV dilation, whereas TIMP expression favors progressive myocardial fibrosis.

Matrix Metalloproteinases. The MMPs represent a family of zinc-dependent proteases that play an important role in normal tissue remodeling as well as in pathologic processes such as inflammation, tumor invasion, and metastasis. The MMPs are secreted as inactive zymogens that must be activated by cleavage of the N-terminal sequence of the propeptide domain, which allows the Zn^{2+} binding site of the catalytic domain to become exposed. The exception is membrane-type 1 MMP (MT-MMP1), which is cell surface bound and is processed before cell surface localization by a furin-dependent mechanism. The MMPs can be classified into subgroups on the basis of substrate specificity or structure (**Table 25-4**). This classification includes the collagenases (e.g., MMP-1 and MMP-13), the stromelysins (e.g., MMP-3), the gelatinases (e.g., MMP-9 and MMP-2), and the membrane-type MMPs. Once activated, the MMPs are capable of degrading all of the extracellular matrix components.[52] Myocardial MMP abundance and activation have been assessed in end-stage human HF (see Table 25-4).[52] Although the majority of MMP species are increased in HF (see Table 25-4), the abundance of MMP-1 is significantly reduced in HF patients.[52] Furthermore, different levels of MMP-2 abundance and activity have been observed in congestive HF myocardium of ischemic or nonischemic origin. Loss of TIMP-mediated inhibitory control has been suggested as a reason for enhanced MMP activity in patients with dilated cardiomyopathy, in whom a reduction in relative myocardial levels of TIMP-1 and TIMP-3 or alterations in MMP-TIMP binding have been reported. This disparity between MMP and TIMP levels favors a persistent MMP activation, enhanced extracellular matrix proteolysis, and progressive LV dilation.[52] The role of MMP inhibition in the postinfarction setting was examined in humans in the PREMIER (Prevention of Myocardial Infarction Early Remodeling) trial, in which 253 patients with ST-segment elevation myocardial infarction and an ejection fraction between 15% and 40% were randomized in a 1:1 ratio to placebo or an MMP inhibitor (PG-116800) with high affinity for MMPs 1, 3, 8, 9, 13, and 14. In this small study, MMP inhibition failed to reduce LV remodeling or to improve clinical outcomes after myocardial infarction. The failure to show a benefit may have been related to inadequate dosing of the MMP inhibitor.[53]

TABLE 25-4 Classes of Matrix Metalloproteinases That Have Been Identified in Human Myocardium

NAME	NUMBER	SUBSTRATE/ FUNCTION	ABUNDANCE/ ACTIVITY IN HEART FAILURE
Collagenase			
Interstitial collagenases	MMP-1	Collagens I, II, III, VII; basement membrane components	Decreased
Collagenase 3	MMP-13	Collagens I, II, III	Increased
Neutrophil collagenase	MMP-8	Collagens I, II, III; basement membrane components	
Gelatinase			
Gelatinase A	MMP-2	Gelatins; collagens I, IV, V, VII; basement membrane components	Increased or unchanged
Gelatinase B	MMP-9	Gelatins; collagens IV, V, XIV; basement membrane components	Increased
Stromelysin			
Stromelysin 1	MMP-3	Fibronectin; laminin; collagens III, IV, IX; MMP activation	Increased
Membrane-type MMP			
MT1-MMP	MMP-14	Collagens I, II, III; fibronectin; laminin-1; activates pro-MMP-2 and pro-MMP-13	Increased

Modified from Deschamps AM, Spinale FG: Extracellular matrix. *In* Walsh RA (ed): Molecular Mechanisms of Cardiac Hypertrophy and Failure. Boca Raton, Fla, Taylor and Francis, 2005, pp 101-116.

CH 25

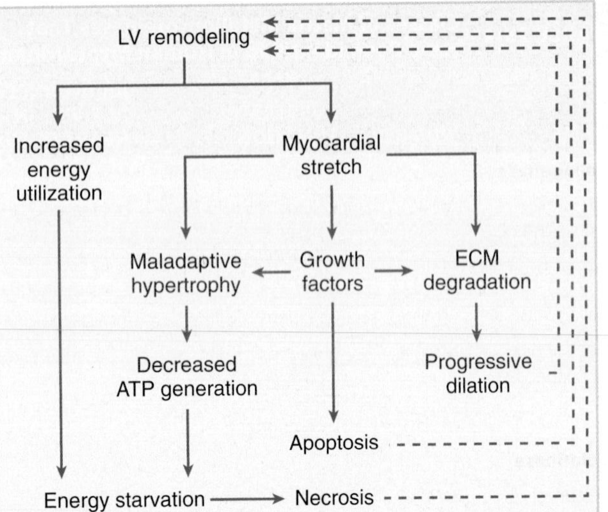

FIGURE 25-14 Self-amplifying nature of LV remodeling. LV remodeling results in increased afterload on the heart, which increases energy use and further stimulates cardiac growth through stretch-mediated activation of growth factors. The former contributes directly to a state of energy starvation, whereas the latter contributes to further cardiac remodeling including increased myocyte hypertrophy and further matrix remodeling. The sustained activation of growth stimuli also promotes apoptosis and myocardial fibrosis, which contribute to LV dysfunction and LV remodeling. ECM = extracellular matrix. *(Modified from Katz AM: Heart Failure. Philadelphia, Lippincott Williams & Wilkins, 2000.)*

ALTERATIONS IN THE LEFT VENTRICULAR STRUCTURE IN HEART FAILURE. The aforementioned changes in the biology of the failing myocyte as well as of the failing myocardium are largely responsible for the progressive LV dilation and LV dysfunction that occur during cardiac remodeling. As discussed later, many of the structural changes of LV remodeling may contribute to worsening HF (see Table 25-e2 on website). Indeed, one of the first observations with respect to the abnormal geometry of remodeled ventricle was the consistent finding that the remodeled heart is not only larger but also more spherical.[32] A change in LV shape from a prolate ellipse to a more spherical shape results in an increase in meridional wall stress of the LV, thereby creating a de novo energetic burden for the failing heart (see Fig. 25-e9 on website). Inasmuch as the load on the ventricle at end-diastole contributes importantly to the afterload that the ventricle faces at the onset of systole, it follows that LV dilation itself will increase mechanical energy expenditure of the ventricle, which exacerbates the underlying problems with energy use in the failing ventricle (**Fig. 25-14**). See Chap. 25 Online Supplement for further details about cardiac energetics.

In addition to the increase in LV end-diastolic volume, LV wall thinning also occurs as the ventricle begins to remodel. The increase in wall thinning along with the increase in afterload created by LV dilation leads to a functional "afterload mismatch" that may further contribute to a decrease in forward cardiac output. Increased LV wall stress can also lead to sustained expression of stretch-activated genes (angiotensin II, endothelin, and tumor necrosis factor) or stretch activation of hypertrophic signaling pathways. Moreover, the high end-diastolic wall stress might be expected to lead to episodic hypoperfusion of the subendocardium, with resultant worsening of LV function, as well as increased oxidative stress, with the resultant activation of families of genes that are sensitive to free radical generation (e.g., tumor necrosis factor and IL-1β). Another important mechanical problem that results from progressive LV dilation is that the papillary muscles are pulled apart, resulting in incompetence of the mitral valve and the development of functional mitral regurgitation (see Fig. 15-53). In addition to the loss of forward blood flow, mitral regurgitation results in further hemodynamic volume overloading of the ventricle. Taken together, the mechanical burdens engendered by LV remodeling might be expected to lead to increased LV

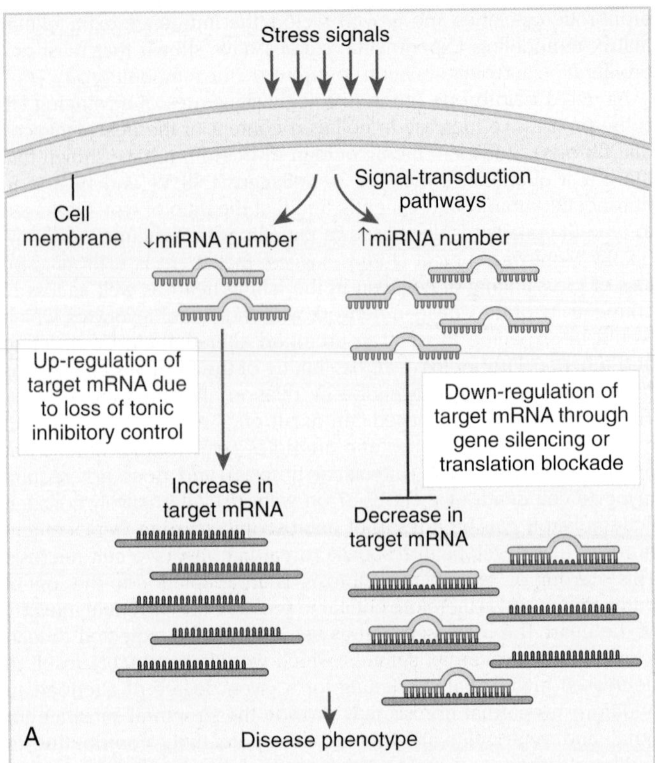

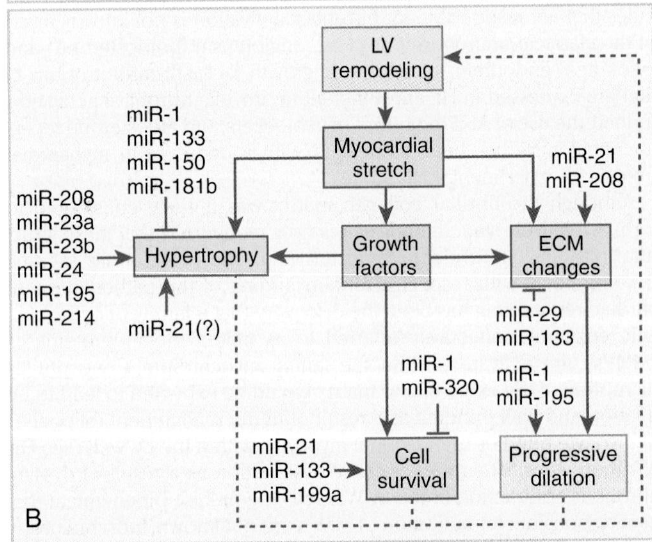

FIGURE 25-15 Role of microRNAs in cardiac remodeling. **A,** Mechanism for miRNA regulation of target mRNA levels. Stress signals (such as hemodynamic overload) activate signal transduction pathways that lead to either the upregulation or downregulation of specific microRNAs (miRNAs). Stress signals that increase the expression levels of miRNAs can result in the downregulation of several target mRNAs through gene silencing or, more commonly, translational blockade of the target mRNA. Alternatively, a stress-induced decrease in the expression levels of inhibitory miRNAs can lead to upregulation of previously suppressed target genes. Ultimately, it is the miRNA-induced pattern of change in gene expression that contributes to the resultant disease phenotype. **B,** Role of miRNAs in LV remodeling. Candidate miRNAs that have been reported or suggested to have roles in cardiac remodeling are depicted in relation to the components of the remodeling process that they affect. Postulated mechanisms with limited evidence are represented by question marks. *(Reproduced from Mann DL: MicroRNAs and the failing heart. N Engl J Med 356:2644, 2007; and Divakaran V, Mann DL: The emerging role of microRNAs in cardiac remodeling and heart failure. Circ Res 103:1072, 2008.)*

dilation, decreased forward cardiac output, and increased hemodynamic overloading (see Fig. 25-14), any or all of which are sufficient to contribute to worsening LV function independently of the neurohormonal status of the patient.

MicroRNAs. Experimental studies from several laboratories have recently shown that microRNAs (miRNAs or miRs) have a profound effect on cardiac remodeling. miRNAs are noncoding RNAs that pair with specific "target" mRNAs and negatively regulate their expression through translational repression or mRNA degradation (gene silencing). The binding specificity of miRNAs depends on complementary base pairing of a region of about six nucleotides at the 5′ end of the microRNA with the 3′ untranslated region of the corresponding mRNA target. As shown in **Figure 25-15**A, binding of miRNAs to their cognate target mRNAs commonly leads to decreased expression of target genes. Studies have suggested that miRNAs contribute to adverse or pathologic remodeling in experimental HF models.[54] As shown in Figure 25-15B, miRNAs regulate key components of the remodeling process, including cardiac myocyte biology, cell fate, extracellular matrix remodeling, and neurohormonal activation. Given that miRNAs are coordinately upregulated in response to stress signals, and given that miRNAs regulate the expression levels of gene networks that determine the so-called HF phenotype, it is tempting to speculate that miRNAs, acting singly or in combination, may be responsible for modulating the transition from adaptive to pathologic cardiac remodeling. Moreover, it is possible that certain miRNAs may themselves become therapeutic targets by use of chemically modified oligonucleotides to target specific miRNAs or to disrupt the binding between a specific miRNA and a specific mRNA target.

REVERSIBILITY OF LEFT VENTRICULAR REMODELING (MYOCARDIAL RECOVERY). Currently available medical and device therapies for HF have consistently demonstrated the reversibility of the abnormal biology of the failing cardiac myocyte, the unfavorable changes in the composition of the extracellular matrix, and the adverse geometry of the failing heart, indicating that the HF phenotype exhibits remarkable plasticity. For want of a better term, this process of myocardial recovery, which encompasses myriad changes at the molecular, cellular, tissue, and organ levels, has been referred to as reverse remodeling. Although the precise cellular and molecular mechanisms responsible for the remarkable return toward normal LV size and shape are not fully known, there is a fairly consistent theme with respect to the parameters that return toward baseline after pharmacologic or device therapy (see Table 25-e3 on website). For example, studies in patients who have been treated with beta blockers showed that patients who had an improvement in ejection fraction also had an increase in SERC2a mRNA and α-MHC mRNA and a decrease in β-MHC mRNA, thus demonstrating that the functional improvement in ventricular function after treatment with beta blockers is associated with favorable changes in myocardial gene expression.[37] Similar findings have been obtained when myocardial recovery is examined after pharmacologic support with ACE inhibitors, LV assist devices, or cardiac support devices, suggesting that there may be specific gene programs that accompany myocardial recovery (see Table 25-e3 on website). However, although many of the individual elements of recovery have been identified, it is still not clear how the decrease in LV chamber mass and LV chamber dilation are coordinated during the process of myocardial recovery. Moreover, it is unclear which of the changes in the biology of the myocyte is essential for the return of function in isolated failing cardiac myocytes and which of the changes are unrelated to recovery. The impetus for addressing these important questions extends well beyond simple intellectual curiosity about the biology of HF. Indeed, the answers to these questions may allow the development of therapies that directly target myocardial recovery rather than continuing to target signaling pathways that attenuate remodeling.

Future Perspectives

In this chapter, the clinical syndrome of HF is described in terms of several different clinical model systems, including a cardiorenal model, a hemodynamic model, and a neurohormonal model. As noted, each of the models has strengths and weaknesses in terms of understanding the mechanisms responsible for HF as well as developing effective new therapies for HF. Nonetheless, as noted, our current models for understanding the mechanisms for HF are inadequate and do not adequately describe disease progression in HF. Moreover, they do not provide an adequate scaffold for understanding newer device therapies that appear to work through neurohormonal independent mechanisms. For this reason, the importance of cardiac remodeling has been emphasized as a neurohormonal independent mechanism that fosters worsening LV function and disease progression in HF. Together, these observations suggest that HF can be viewed as a biomechanical model, in which HF develops and progresses as a result of the deleterious changes in cardiac function and cardiac remodeling that occur from sustained neurohormonal activation.[1] Whereas this point of view does not obviate the importance of neurohormonal activation in the setting of HF, it suggests that future therapies will likely be focused on reversal or stabilization of the downstream biologic consequences of neurohormonal activation (e.g., antagonizing upregulation of miRs) rather than on neurohormonal activation per se.

REFERENCES

Neurohormonal Mechanisms

1. Mann DL, Bristow MR: Mechanisms and models in heart failure: The biomechanical model and beyond. Circulation 111:2837, 2005.
2. Floras JS: Sympathetic activation in human heart failure: Diverse mechanisms, therapeutic opportunities. Acta Physiol Scand 177:391, 2003.

2a. Jacobson A.F, Senior R, Cerqueira MD, et al: Myocardial iodine-123 meta-iodobenzylguanidine imaging and cardiac events in heart failure. Results of the prospective ADMIRE-HF (AdreView Myocardial Imaging for Risk Evaluation in Heart Failure) study. J Am Coll Cardiol 55:2212, 2010.

3. Dell'Italia L, Sabri A: Activation of the renin-angiotensin system in hypertrophy and heart failure. *In* Mann DL (ed): Heart Failure: A Companion to Braunwald's Heart Disease. Philadelphia, Saunders, 2004, pp 129-143.
4. Haulica I, Petrescu G, Slatineanu SM, et al: New bioactive angiotensins formation pathways and functional involvements. Rom J Intern Med 42:27, 2004.
5. Grieve DJ, Shah AM: Oxidative stress in heart failure. More than just damage. Eur Heart J 24:2161, 2003.
6. Hare JM, Mangal B, Brown J, et al: Impact of oxypurinol in patients with symptomatic heart failure. Results of the OPT-CHF study. J Am Coll Cardiol 51:2301, 2008.
7. Pitt B, Remme W, Zannad F: Eplerenone, a selective aldosterone blocker, in patients with left ventricular dysfunction after myocardial infarction. N Engl J Med 348:1309, 2003.
8. Schrier RW, Abraham WT: Hormones and hemodynamics in heart failure. N Engl J Med 341:577, 1999.
9. Tang WH, Bhavnani S, Francis GS: Vasopressin receptor antagonists in the management of acute heart failure. Expert Opin Investig Drugs 14:593, 2005.
10. Naitoh M, Suzuki H, Murakami M, et al: Effects of oral AVP receptor antagonists OPC-21268 and OPC-31260 on congestive heart failure in conscious dogs. Am J Physiol 267:H2245, 1994.
11. Burnett JC Jr, Costello-Boerrigter L, Boerriger G: Alterations in the kidney in heart failure: The cardiorenal axis in the regulation of sodium homeostasis. *In* Mann DL (ed): Heart Failure: A Companion to Braunwald's Heart Disease. Philadelphia, Saunders, 2004, pp 279-289.
12. Cea LB: Natriuretic peptide family: New aspects. Curr Med Chem Cardiovasc Hematol Agents 3:87, 2005.
13. Rademaker MT, Richards AM: Cardiac natriuretic peptides for cardiac health. Clin Sci (Lond) 108:23, 2005.
14. Munzel T, Kurz S, Holtz J, et al: Neurohormonal inhibition and hemodynamic unloading during prolonged inhibition of ANF degradation in patients with severe chronic heart failure. Circulation 86:1089, 1992.
15. Packer M, Califf RM, Konstam MA, et al: Comparison of omapatrilat and enalapril in patients with chronic heart failure: The Omapatrilat Versus Enalapril Randomized Trial of Utility in Reducing Events (OVERTURE). Circulation 106:920, 2002.
16. Cataliotti A, Burnett JC Jr: Natriuretic peptides: Novel therapeutic targets in heart failure. J Investig Med 53:378, 2005.
17. Podesser BK, Siwik DA, Eberli FR, et al: ET_A-receptor blockade prevents matrix metalloproteinase activation late postmyocardial infarction in the rat. Am J Physiol Heart Circ Physiol 280:H984, 2001.
18. Teerlink JR: Recent heart failure trials of neurohormonal modulation (OVERTURE and ENABLE): Approaching the asymptote of efficacy? J Card Fail 8:124, 2002.
19. Feng QP, Hedner T, Andersson B, et al: Cardiac neuropeptide Y and noradrenaline balance in patients with congestive heart failure. Br Heart J 71:261, 1994.
20. Onan D, Pipolo L, Yang E, et al: Urotensin II promotes hypertrophy of cardiac myocytes via mitogen-activated protein kinases. Mol Endocrinol 18:2344, 2004.
21. Lim M, Honisett S, Sparkes CD, et al: Differential effect of urotensin II on vascular tone in normal subjects and patients with chronic heart failure. Circulation 109:1212, 2004.
22. Scherrer-Crosbie M, Ullrich R, Bloch KD, et al: Endothelial nitric oxide synthase limits left ventricular remodeling after myocardial infarction in mice. Circulation 104:1286, 2001.
23. Damy T, Ratajczak P, Shah AM, et al: Increased neuronal nitric oxide synthase–derived NO production in the failing human heart. Lancet 363:1365, 2004.
24. Sam F, Sawyer DB, Xie Z, et al: Mice lacking inducible nitric oxide synthase have improved left ventricular contractile function and reduced apoptotic cell death late after myocardial infarction. Circ Res 89:351, 2001.
25. Tziomalos K, Hare JM: Role of xanthine oxidoreductase in cardiac nitroso-redox imbalance. Front Biosci 14:237, 2009.

26. Moens AL, Takimoto E, Tocchetti CG, et al: Reversal of cardiac hypertrophy and fibrosis from pressure overload by tetrahydrobiopterin: Efficacy of recoupling nitric oxide synthase as a therapeutic strategy. Circulation 117:2626, 2008.
27. Sharma JN, Sharma J: Cardiovascular properties of the kallikrein-kinin system. Curr Med Res Opin 18:10, 2002.
28. Rademaker MT, Cameron VA, Charles CJ, et al: Adrenomedullin and heart failure. Regul Pept 112:51, 2003.
29. Abel ED, Litwin SE, Sweeney G: Cardiac remodeling in obesity. Physiol Rev 88:389, 2008.
30. Mann DL: Inflammatory mediators and the failing heart: Past, present, and the foreseeable future. Circ Res 91:988, 2002.
31. Deswal A, Petersen NJ, Feldman AM, et al: Cytokines and cytokine receptors in advanced heart failure: An analysis of the cytokine database from the Vesnarinone trial (VEST). Circulation 103:2055, 2001.

Left Ventricular Remodeling

32. Mann DL: Left ventricular size and shape: Determinants of mechanical signal transduction pathways. Heart Fail Rev 10:95, 2005.
33. Houser SR, Margulies KB: Is depressed myocyte contractility centrally involved in heart failure? Circ Res 92:350, 2003.
34. Minamisawa S, Hoshijima M, Chu G, et al: Chronic phospholamban–sarcoplasmic reticulum calcium ATPase interaction is the critical calcium cycling defect in dilated cardiomyopathy. Cell 99:313, 1999.
35. Zalk R, Lehnart SE, Marks AR: Modulation of the ryanodine receptor and intracellular calcium. Annu Rev Biochem 76:367, 2007.
36. Margulies K, House SR: Myocyte abnormalities. *In* Mann DL (ed): Heart Failure: A Companion to Braunwald's Heart Disease. Philadelphia, Saunders, 2004, pp 41-56.
37. Lowes BD, Gilbert EM, Abraham WT, et al: Myocardial gene expression in dilated cardiomyopathy treated with beta-blocking agents. N Engl J Med 346:1357, 2002.
38. Nassar R, Malouf NN, Mao L, et al: cTnT1, a cardiac troponin T isoform, decreases myofilament tension and affects the left ventricular pressure waveform. Am J Physiol Heart Circ Physiol 288:H1147, 2005.
39. Vatta M, Stetson SJ, Perez-Verdia A, et al: Molecular remodelling of dystrophin in patients with end-stage cardiomyopathies and reversal in patients on assistance-device therapy. Lancet 359:936, 2002.
40. Bristow MR: Beta-adrenergic receptor blockade in chronic heart failure. Circulation 101:558, 2000.
41. Penela P, Murga C, Ribas C, et al: Mechanisms of regulation of G protein–coupled receptor kinases (GRKs) and cardiovascular disease. Cardiovasc Res 69:46, 2006.
42. Guerra S, Leri A, Wang X, et al: Myocyte death in the failing human heart is gender dependent. Circ Res 85:856, 1999.
43. Rodriguez M, Schaper J: Apoptosis: Measurement and technical issues. J Mol Cell Cardiol 38:15, 2005.
44. Garg S, Narula J, Chandrashekhar Y: Apoptosis and heart failure: Clinical relevance and therapeutic target. J Mol Cell Cardiol 38:73, 2005.
45. Haudek SB, Taffet GE, Schneider MD, et al: TNF provokes cardiomyocyte apoptosis and cardiac remodeling through activation of multiple cell death pathways. J Clin Invest 117:2692, 2007.
46. Kostin S, Pool L, Elsasser A, et al: Myocytes die by multiple mechanisms in failing human hearts. Circ Res 92:7154, 2003.
47. Knaapen MW, Davies MJ, De Bie M, et al: Apoptotic versus autophagic cell death in heart failure. Cardiovasc Res 51:304, 2001.
48. Hein S, Arnon E, Kostin S, et al: Progression from compensated hypertrophy to failure in the pressure-overloaded human heart: Structural deterioration and compensatory mechanisms. Circulation 107:984, 2003.
49. Deschamps AM, Spinale FG: Matrix modulation and heart failure: New concepts question old beliefs. Curr Opin Cardiol 20:211, 2005.
50. Zannad F, Dousset B, Alla F: Treatment of congestive heart failure: Interfering the aldosterone-cardiac extracellular matrix relationship. Hypertension 38:1227, 2001.
51. Shiota N, Rysa J, Kovanen PT, et al: A role for cardiac mast cells in the pathogenesis of hypertensive heart disease. J Hypertens 21:1935, 2003.
52. Spinale FG: Matrix metalloproteinases: Regulation and dysregulation in the failing heart. Circ Res 90:520, 2002.
53. Hudson MP, Armstrong PW, Ruzyllo W, et al: Effects of selective matrix metalloproteinase inhibitor (PG-116800) to prevent ventricular remodeling after myocardial infarction: Results of the PREMIER (Prevention of Myocardial Infarction Early Remodeling) trial. J Am Coll Cardiol 48:15, 2006.
54. van Rooij E, Olson EN: MicroRNAs: Powerful new regulators of heart disease and provocative therapeutic targets. J Clin Invest 117:2369, 2007.

CHAPTER 26 Clinical Assessment of Heart Failure

Barry Greenberg and Andrew M. Kahn

Heart failure prevalence is rising throughout the world.[1] The reasons for this pandemic include the aging populations of both industrialized and developing nations; a growing incidence of obesity, diabetes, and hypertension (related to changes in traditional patterns of exercise and diet) in many countries; improved survival after myocardial infarction; and success in preventing sudden cardiac death (see Chap. 28). Fortunately, therapies that have emerged during the past few decades can greatly improve outcomes in heart failure patients. The most effective use of these therapies, however, requires a thorough clinical assessment.

In assessing patients with heart failure, it is important to recognize that they have a complex clinical syndrome in which damage to the heart or increased myocardial stress activates a systemic response that provides short-term support of the cardiovascular system but that adversely affects cardiac structure and function over time (see Chap. 25). The clinical phenotype that evolves in an individual heart failure patient is determined by the interplay between the underlying cause, compensatory changes that develop in response to altered cardiac function, genetic and environmental factors, and comorbid diseases. The goals of the clinical assessment are to determine whether heart failure is present, to define the underlying cause, to assess severity of the disease and the patient's prognosis, and to identify comorbidities that can influence the clinical course and response to treatment.

Whereas the diagnosis of heart failure can be straightforward when the patient presents with a constellation of the classic signs and symptoms (**Tables 26-1 and 26-2**) in the appropriate clinical setting, attribution of causality to an atypical or inconsistent clinical pattern can be challenging. The reason for this is that none of these signs or symptoms can, by themselves, define the presence or severity of heart failure. Moreover, recitation of symptoms by the patient (or the patient's family) is a subjective process that is open to interpretation by all involved, and the detection of physical findings is an imprecise science. Thus, as depicted in **Figure 26-1**, the clinical assessment of heart failure most often depends on information that is gleaned from a variety of sources, including the history (both past and present), physical examination, laboratory tests, cardiac imaging, and functional studies.

Medical History and Physical Examination

A complete medical history and carefully focused physical examination serve as the core of the diagnostic process (see Chap. 12). The information obtained guides the further direction of the patient's evaluation and enables the clinician to make the most judicious use of additional tests. It helps determine the value of incongruent and conflicting results that can emerge during the diagnostic process, and it can obviate the need for tests that are costly or expose the patient to discomfort or risk. The deep understanding of the patient that can be obtained only through the immediacy of the history and physical examination also plays a pivotal role in treatment decisions that must be addressed at various points throughout the patient's lifetime.

Heart Failure Symptoms

Patients with heart failure may complain of a vast array of symptoms, the most common of which are listed in Table 26-1. Although none of these is specific, some are more reliable than others for defining the presence and severity of heart failure. Dyspnea (the subjective complaint of discomfort while breathing), shortness of breath, and fatigue are common complaints of heart failure patients. Patients with worsening heart failure frequently experience exertional dyspnea, and this symptom often triggers a visit to the clinic or emergency department. The absence of significant dyspnea that limits exercise, however, does not necessarily exclude the diagnosis of heart failure because patients may accommodate symptoms by substantially modifying their lifestyle. Probing more deeply into the current level of activity by asking patients to compare themselves with age-matched peers or with their own level of activity 3 or 6 months ago may uncover a decline in exercise capacity that is not immediately apparent. Dyspnea at rest is often mentioned by elderly patients hospitalized with heart failure, and it has a high diagnostic sensitivity in this population. However, it is also cited by patients with many other medical conditions so that the specificity and positive predictive value of this symptom alone are low.[2] Patients may sleep with their heads elevated to relieve symptoms of pulmonary congestion, but they may also sleep upright because of an enlarged abdominal pannus, esophageal reflux, or orthopedic problems. A history of weight gain, increasing abdominal girth, and the onset of edema in dependent organs (extremities or scrotum) is helpful when it is present but also is nonspecific. Gastrointestinal tract symptoms such as loss of appetite, early satiety, and right upper quadrant pain are common in heart failure patients and are often attributed to other conditions. Cachexia (seen with advanced heart failure) may lead to an extensive workup for malignant disease. In contrast to many of the nonspecific symptoms listed in Table 26-1, the authors have found the complaint of paroxysmal nocturnal dyspnea to be a highly reliable indicator of the presence of heart failure. Classically, the patient experiences nocturnal awakenings usually occurring at a fixed time after retiring (often in the range of 1 to 2 hours) precipitated by

TABLE 26-1 Use of the Medical History to Assess the Heart Failure Patient

Symptoms Associated With Heart Failure
Fatigue
Shortness of breath at rest or during exercise
Dyspnea
Tachypnea
Cough
Diminished exercise capacity
Orthopnea
Paroxysmal nocturnal dyspnea
Nocturia
Weight gain or weight loss
Edema (of the extremities, scrotum, or elsewhere)
Increasing abdominal girth or bloating
Abdominal pain (particularly confined to the right upper quadrant)
Loss of appetite or early satiety
History of Cheyne-Stokes respirations during sleep (often reported by the family rather than by the patient)
Somnolence or diminished mental acuity
Historical Information That Is Helpful in Determining if Symptoms Are Due to Heart Failure
A past history of heart failure
Cardiac disease (e.g., coronary artery, valvular, or congenital disease; previous myocardial infarction)
Risk factors for heart failure (e.g., diabetes, hypertension, obesity)
Systemic illnesses that can involve the heart (e.g., amyloidosis, sarcoidosis, inherited neuromuscular diseases)
Recent viral illness or history of human immunodeficiency virus infection or Chagas disease
Family history of heart failure or sudden cardiac death
Environmental or medical exposure to cardiotoxic substances
Substance abuse
Noncardiac illnesses that could affect the heart indirectly (including high-output states such as anemia, hyperthyroidism, arteriovenous fistulas)

TABLE 26-2 Physical Findings of Heart Failure

Physical Findings
Tachycardia
Extra beats or irregular rhythm
Narrow pulse pressure or thready pulse*
Pulsus alternans*
Tachypnea
Cool or mottled extremities*
Elevated jugular venous pressure
Dullness and diminished breath sounds at one or both lung bases
Rales, rhonchi, or wheezes
Apical impulse displaced leftward or inferiorly
Sustained apical impulse
Parasternal lift
S_3 or S_4 (either palpable or audible)
Tricuspid or mitral regurgitant murmur
Hepatomegaly (often accompanied by right upper quadrant discomfort)
Ascites
Presacral edema
Anasarca*
Pedal edema
Chronic venous stasis changes

*Indicative of more severe disease.

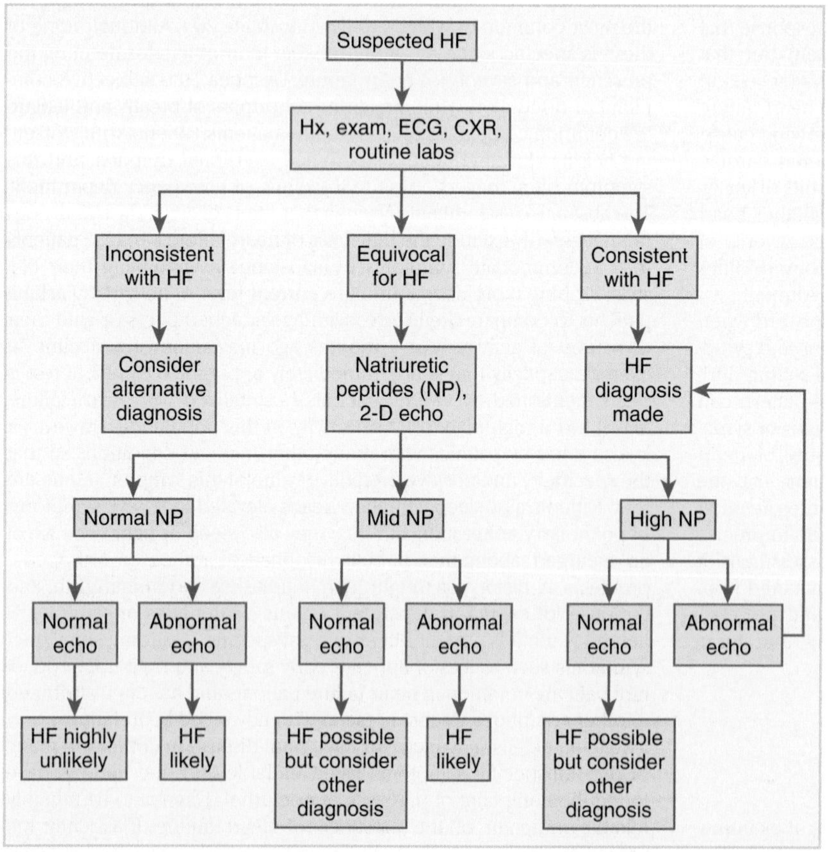

the subjective feeling of air hunger, smothering, or drowning that causes the patient to sit upright (sometimes seeking fresh air from an open window) for a period of 15 to 30 minutes before resolution. This must be differentiated from nocturnal awakenings due to myriad other conditions, most prominently anxiety and insomnia, musculoskeletal complaints, and the need to void (particularly in patients receiving diuretics).

Quantification of heart failure symptoms is useful for assessing the adequacy of therapy and determining prognosis. The New York Heart Association (NYHA) functional classification (summarized in **Table 26-3**) is most often used for this purpose. It provides a shorthand means of detecting changes in the patient's symptomatic status that occur over time or in response to treatment, and it facilitates communication between various providers about the patient's clinical status. Evaluation of the NYHA functional class also provides important prognostic information as there is a stepwise increase in morbidity and mortality risk with increasing functional class. Whereas some objective measures of symptomatic limitation (e.g., cardiopulmonary exercise testing) can more accurately determine whether subjective complaints are due to heart failure and can provide a more precise indication of the patient's limitation, the ease and economy of determining NYHA functional class have made it a standard means of assessing and communicating symptomatic status.

FIGURE 26-1 Flow chart for the evaluation of patients with heart failure. CXR = chest radiography; ECG = electrocardiography; echo = echocardiography; HF = heart failure; Hx = history; NP = natriuretic peptides.

Other Historical Information

Information about a patient's past and current medical problems and the patient's family and social history provides the background on which symptoms are interpreted and a management plan is designed. The likelihood of a given constellation of symptoms being due to heart failure will increase when there is a history of heart failure or risk factors known to be associated with cardiac disease. The presence of hypertension, coronary artery disease, or diabetes is particularly helpful because these conditions account for approximately 90% of the population's attributable risk for heart failure in the United States.[3] The medical history should also focus on whether there have been environmental or toxic exposures, alcohol or drug abuse, or a

TABLE 26-3 New York Heart Association Functional Classification of Heart Failure

CLASS	SYMPTOMS
Class I (mild)	No limitation of physical activity Ordinary physical activity does not cause undue fatigue, palpitation, or dyspnea (shortness of breath)
Class II (mild)	Slight limitation of physical activity Comfortable at rest, but ordinary physical activity results in fatigue, palpitation, or dyspnea
Class III (moderate)	Marked limitation of physical activity Comfortable at rest, but less than ordinary activity causes fatigue, palpitation, or dyspnea
Class IV (severe)	Unable to carry out any physical activity without discomfort Symptoms of cardiac insufficiency at rest If any physical activity is undertaken, discomfort is increased

family history of heart failure (or sudden cardiac death). Information about the presence of comorbidities (as described later) is essential in devising management plans. Whereas most causes of heart failure are cardiac, some systemic illnesses (e.g., anemia, hyperthyroidism) can cause this syndrome without direct cardiac involvement.

Physical Examination

The physical findings listed in Table 26-2 complement information from the medical history in defining the presence and severity of heart failure (see Chap. 12). The typical (and atypical) signs of heart failure have been extensively described.[4,5] An evaluation for the presence and severity of heart failure should include consideration of the patient's general appearance, measurement of vital signs, examination of the heart and pulses, and assessment of other organs for evidence of congestion, hypoperfusion, or indications of comorbid conditions.

The patient's general appearance conveys vital information that may greatly influence the direction of the evaluation. The examiner should assess the patient's body habitus (noting the presence of obesity or muscle wasting), level of hygiene, state of alertness, and appropriateness of emotions as well as whether the patient is comfortable, short of breath (either while talking or moving about in the examining room), coughing, or in pain.

By observing or palpating the apical impulse and percussing the left cardiac border, the examiner can determine heart size before results of chest radiography or echocardiography are available. Palpable filling waves in the apical impulse occurring early or late in diastole correlate with a third or fourth heart sound, respectively. Palpable pulmonary artery pulsations, pulmonic valve closure, or a parasternal lift (particularly if it is accompanied by pulsations in the subxiphoid region) suggests pulmonary hypertension. Precordial thrills are generated by turbulent flow due to valvular lesions or intracardiac shunts.

A characteristic holosystolic murmur of mitral insufficiency is heard in many heart failure patients. Tricuspid insufficiency, which is also common, can be differentiated from mitral insufficiency by the location of the murmur at the left sternal border, an increased intensity of the murmur during inspiration, and the presence of prominent *v* waves in the jugular venous pulse (JVP). Both mitral and tricuspid insufficiency murmurs may become softer as volume overload is treated and a reduction in ventricular size improves valve competency. Aortic stenosis is an important cause of heart failure, particularly because its presence greatly alters management. The presentation can be subtle, however, because the intensity of the murmur depends on blood flow across the valve, and this may be reduced as heart failure develops. The delay in time until the murmur peaks is a much better indicator of the severity of aortic stenosis than is the intensity of the murmur. In elderly patients who have aortic stenosis due to "senile calcification" of a tricuspid aortic valve, the murmur may have a high-pitched "sawing" sound that is best heard at the cardiac apex, and it may be mistaken for mitral regurgitation. Recognition of this pattern and detection of a low-volume, slow-rising carotid pulse will help make the diagnosis at the bedside. The presence of a third heart sound suggests increased ventricular filling volume or diminished relaxation; a fourth heart sound usually indicates ventricular stiffening. An increase in the intensity of either gallop sound during inspiration indicates that it originated in the right ventricle.

A key objective of the examination is to detect and to quantify pulmonary or systemic congestion. As with symptoms, evidence of congestion does not always indicate with certainty that heart failure is present. Pedal edema, a common finding in volume-overloaded heart failure patients, may be the result of venous insufficiency (particularly after saphenous veins have been harvested for coronary artery bypass grafts), a side effect of medications (e.g., calcium channel blockers, thiazolidinediones), or a consequence of portal hypertension in a cirrhotic patient. A more definitive test for assessment of a patient's volume status is by the measurement of JVP. Not only does an elevated JVP detect systemic congestion, but there is good sensitivity (70%) and specificity (79%) between high JVP and elevated left-sided filling pressure.[6] Moreover, changes in JVP with therapy usually parallel changes in left-sided filling pressure. Significant interobserver variability regarding the extent of JVP elevation, however, has been noted.[7] An acute increase in left ventricular filling pressures as occurs in the setting of myocardial ischemia or myocardial infarction may not result in increased JVP unless pulmonary artery pressure is increased to the extent that right ventricular failure or tricuspid insufficiency occurs. Conversely, right atrial pressures can be elevated without an increase in left ventricular filling pressures in patients with pulmonary arterial hypertension on the basis of abnormalities in the lung or pulmonary vasculature itself or when injury (such as an infarct) to the right ventricle occurs.

Measurement of JVP is best performed with the patient comfortably seated on an examining table in a warm, well-lighted room with the neck fully exposed from the clavicle to the ear. Assessment of JVP is usually initiated with the patient's upper torso elevated at a 30- to 45-degree angle, but it can be performed at virtually any angle so long as the true height of the meniscus of the venous pulse can be identified. The vertical distance of the venous pulse above the angle of Louis at the second intercostal space of the sternum is then determined, and 5 cm (to account for the vertical distance to the midportion of the right atrium) is added to determine right atrial pressure. Arterial pulsations in the neck can be differentiated from venous pulsations on the basis of contour; an arterial pulse has its predominant (more rapid) motion directed outward, whereas a venous pulse tends to collapse inward. Both sensitivity and specificity of the JVP in detecting congestion can be improved by exerting pressure on the right upper quadrant of the abdomen while assessing venous pulsations in the neck (i.e., hepatojugular or abdominojugular reflux).[8]

Pulmonary congestion is detected on physical examination from signs indicating the presence of fluid in the pleural space or lung parenchyma. Dullness to percussion and diminished breath sounds at one or both lung bases suggest the presence of a pleural effusion. Bilateral pleural effusions are most common, but when an effusion is present unilaterally, it is usually right sided; only ~10% occur exclusively on the left side. The presence of a pleural effusion is usually indicative of increased filling pressures on both the right and left sides of the heart. Leakage of fluid from pulmonary capillaries into the lung parenchyma can be manifested as rales, rhonchi, or wheezes. Pulmonary rales due to heart failure are usually fine in nature and extend from the base upward; those due to other causes (e.g., atelectasis, bronchiectasis) tend to be coarser or may exclude the basilar portion of the lungs (e.g., pneumonia). Rales may be absent, however, when left ventricular filling pressure is markedly elevated in patients with chronic elevations of left-sided filling pressure who, over time, develop compensatory changes in lymphatic drainage and perivascular tissue that prevent excess fluid from accumulating in the lung. In some patients, wheezing and diminished airflow may be the predominant pulmonary findings. The occurrence of so-called cardiac asthma is

TABLE 26-4 Physical Findings Consistent with Reduced Cardiac Output

Fatigue
Somnolence or loss of mental acuity
Low body temperature
Tachycardia
Low systolic blood pressure with narrow pulse pressure
Diminished volume or low-amplitude central arterial (i.e., femoral or carotid) pulses
Cool, mottled extremities

due to the physical presence of fluid in the bronchial wall as well as secondary bronchospasm.

Detection of reduced cardiac output (CO) and systemic hypoperfusion is a key component of the examination. Whereas patients with poor systemic perfusion due to low CO usually have low systolic and narrow pulse pressures, this relationship is not exact. Many patients with systolic blood pressure in the range of 80 mm Hg (or even lower) may have adequate perfusion; others with reduced CO maintain blood pressure in the normal range at the expense of tissue perfusion by greatly increasing systemic vascular resistance. **Table 26-4** lists findings that help determine whether tissue hypoperfusion is present.

Routine Tests

An algorithm for the diagnosis of heart failure or left ventricular dysfunction is presented in Figure 26-1. The diagnosis of heart failure alone is not sufficient; it is important to establish the cause of heart failure, insofar as some forms of heart failure may be correctable or may require special treatment that goes beyond the conventional treatment strategies discussed in Chaps. 28 and 30. The laboratory testing and imaging modalities described here provide important information for the diagnosis and management of patients with heart failure.

Chest Radiography (see Chap. 16)

Despite dependence on echocardiography to determine cardiac chamber size and function and on biomarkers to distinguish heart failure from other causes of dyspnea, chest radiography remains a useful component of the assessment, particularly when the clinical presentation is ambiguous. A "butterfly" pattern of alveolar opacities that fan out bilaterally from engorged hilar pulmonary arteries to the periphery of the lungs is the classic pattern of congestion seen in decompensated heart failure (see Fig. 16-16). Many patients, however, present with a more subtle picture in which increased interstitial markings including Kerley B lines (thin horizontal linear opacities extending to the pleural surface caused by accumulation of fluid in the interstitial space), peribronchial cuffing, and evidence of prominent upper lobe vasculature (indicating pulmonary venous hypertension) are the most prominent chest radiographic findings. Pleural effusions or fluid in the right minor fissure may also be seen. Cardiomegaly is usually determined from the posteroanterior projection with the beam source at a standard distance of 6 feet from the patient's back. Radiographs obtained in the anteroposterior projection or with the beam source closer to the patient than usual (both of which are common with portable chest radiography) will magnify the cardiac silhouette, making determination of cardiac size problematic. A lateral film helps detect ventricular enlargement and differentiate between anterior right ventricular and posterior left ventricular enlargement. The chest radiograph can provide clues about the cause of heart failure. For instance, the absence of cardiomegaly suggests that ejection fraction is preserved or that the onset of systolic dysfunction has been recent. Disproportionate enlargement of the left atrium raises the possibility of mitral valve disease or (when there is biatrial enlargement) an infiltrative process. Prominence of the right ventricle without enlargement of other chambers should raise the suspicion of pulmonary hypertension as a cause of right-sided heart failure. The chest radiograph may also provide an indication that heart failure is due to coronary, valvular, or pericardial disease when calcification is noted in the appropriate position.

Electrocardiography (see Chap. 13)

The electrocardiogram (ECG) is a standard part of the initial evaluation of a patient with suspected heart failure and also when previously diagnosed patients experience an episode of decompensation. Sinus tachycardia due to sympathetic nervous system activation is seen with advanced heart failure or during episodes of decompensation. Treatment with beta blockers, however, may blunt this response. The presence of atrial arrhythmias on the ECG may explain why heart failure has worsened as well as provide a target for therapeutic interventions. A QRS complex exceeding 120 milliseconds in a patient with systolic dysfunction is a useful indicator of ventricular dyssynchrony and is the major electrocardiographic criterion for deciding if cardiac resynchronization therapy is indicated. A biphasic P wave in lead V_1 is a sensitive indicator of left atrial enlargement; increased P wave duration in lead II is specific for left atrial enlargement. Increased P wave amplitude in lead II suggests right atrial enlargement. The presence of left ventricular hypertrophy can provide clues about the cause (e.g., hypertension or valvular disease). If right ventricular hypertrophy is present, conditions that cause primary or secondary pulmonary hypertension should be considered. The presence of Q waves suggests that heart failure may have been caused by a myocardial infarction; new or reversible repolarization changes raise concerns that clinical deterioration may be due to worsening myocardial ischemia even when chest pain is absent. Low QRS voltage suggests the presence of an infiltrative disease or pericardial effusion.

Measurement of Blood Chemistry and Hematologic Variables

Blood chemistries and hematologic variables are routinely measured as part of the initial heart failure evaluation. The results provide information that is essential in considering management strategies as well as for the detection of comorbidities that could complicate evaluation and treatment. Repeated determination of electrolyte values, renal function, and other variables is also required as the clinical course develops over time. Electrolyte levels in blood are determined intermittently, with the frequency dictated by the clinical situation. Hyponatremia is common in heart failure patients, particularly during periods of decompensation. Registry data suggest that ~20% have values below 135 mmol/liter.[9] Although hyponatremia is associated with significantly higher in-hospital and follow-up mortality and longer hospital stays,[9] strategies to correct serum sodium levels have not been shown to improve the clinical course.[10] Hyponatremia, however, has been associated with impaired cognitive and neuromuscular function, an issue that is of particular importance in elderly heart failure patients.[11] Hypokalemia occurs commonly in heart failure patients who are treated with diuretics. Besides increasing the risk of cardiac arrhythmias, it can cause further muscle weakness. An elevated bicarbonate level should alert the clinician to the possibility of carbon dioxide retention or a contraction alkalosis due to excessive diuresis; low levels may indicate a metabolic acidosis. Additional electrolyte abnormalities include hypomagnesemia and hypophosphatemia.

Renal function should be measured as part of the initial evaluation and periodically during follow-up as abnormalities commonly result from the hemodynamic perturbations seen in heart failure or as a consequence of comorbid conditions such as atherosclerosis, hypertension, and diabetes. In addition, heart failure therapies, including most notably diuretics and angiotensin-converting enzyme inhibitors or angiotensin receptor blockers, can increase blood urea nitrogen and creatinine levels. Dronedarone, an agent used to treat intermittent or recurrent atrial fibrillation, can also increase creatinine levels.[12] In patients hospitalized with decompensated heart failure, registry data suggest that 60% to 70% have a reduced estimated glomerular filtration rate,[13] and 20% to 30% increase serum creatinine concentration by

>0.3 mg/dL during hospitalization.[14] Impaired renal function at baseline and worsening during hospitalization are both potent predictors of poor outcome.

Diabetes is common in heart failure patients. High plasma glucose levels indicate the presence of this disease as well as the failure of glycemic control. Because diuretics can cause gout, measurement of uric acid levels can help in management of the patient. Abnormalities in aspartate aminotransferase and alanine aminotransferase may occur in heart failure patients as a consequence of either hemodynamic derangements or medications, and it is important to follow levels periodically. An unexpected increase in prothrombin time in patients receiving warfarin therapy may be an early harbinger of decompensation as it may reflect impaired synthetic capacity of a congested liver. Albumin levels are an indication of the patient's nutritional status, and they may be depressed because of poor appetite or impaired absorption across an engorged bowel wall. Elevations in bilirubin are most often seen during episodes of severe decompensation.

A recent meta-analysis reported that 37.2% of heart failure patients were anemic.[15] Low hemoglobin levels have been associated with more severe symptoms, reduced exercise capacity and quality of life, and increased mortality.[15,16] Although anemia may be a consequence of chronic disease in heart failure patients, a low hemoglobin level should trigger an evaluation to detect treatable causes. The white blood cell count and differential are helpful in detecting the presence of infection that is responsible for destabilizing a previously well-compensated patient and could provide a clue that heart failure is due to an uncommon cause, such as eosinophilic infiltration of the myocardium.

Biomarkers

Measurement of biomarkers has emerged during the past decade as an important means of distinguishing heart failure from other conditions, particularly when there is ambiguity in the clinical presentation. Biomarkers also provide useful prognostic information in heart failure patients, and there is considerable interest in determining their ability to guide therapy in both the acute and chronic settings. An array of enzymes, hormones, and markers of myocardial stress, structural changes in the heart, and myocardial malfunction and injury are currently being used for these purposes. As shown in **Table 26-5**, Braunwald has proposed that heart failure biomarkers be divided into six distinct categories, with an additional one reserved for biomarkers that have not yet been classified.[17] As noted by Morrow and de Lemos,[18] clinically useful biomarkers should (1) be accurate, affordable, and have a short turn-around period; (2) provide information that is not available from clinical assessment; and (3) aid in making medical decisions. The extent to which an individual biomarker (or panel of biomarkers) meets these criteria ultimately determines its usefulness in the assessment of heart failure patients.

The natriuretic peptides, mainly brain natriuretic peptide (BNP) and N-terminal pro-BNP (NT-proBNP), approach the criteria of Morrow and de Lemos and have been the subject of excellent reviews.[17,19,20] Release of these peptides is enhanced by increased hemodynamic stress due to either ventricular hypertrophy or dilation or by increased wall stress. Natriuretic peptide levels increase progressively with worsening NYHA functional class. Whereas BNP and NT-proBNP are elevated in patients with dyspnea due to decompensated heart failure, the levels tend to be greater in patients with systolic dysfunction than in patients with heart failure and preserved ejection fraction. Although natriuretic peptide levels increase with age and worsening renal function, there is uncertainty about whether this is due to increased myocardial wall stress or other factors, such as diminished renal clearance. This is particularly true of NT-proBNP, which is more dependent than BNP on renal clearance. Women also tend to have higher levels than their age-matched male counterparts do. Natriuretic peptide levels have an inverse relationship with body mass index, a finding that may be related to an increase in clearance receptors in adipocytes. An elevated natriuretic peptide level does not necessarily indicate that decompensation is present or even imminent because high levels are often seen in clinically stable heart failure patients. Levels can also be elevated in patients with acute coronary syndromes and various hyperdynamic states, including sepsis, hyperthyroidism, and cirrhosis. Patients who have right ventricular dysfunction as a result of pulmonary embolus, pulmonary hypertension, or severe lung disease may have elevated natriuretic peptides levels, although they tend to be lower than with conditions affecting the left ventricle. Conversely, patients with flash pulmonary edema may not have elevated levels because they are often evaluated before natriuretic peptides are released from the left ventricle. Patients with pericardial restriction do not have increased natriuretic peptides as left ventricular wall stress is only minimally elevated.

Knowledge of natriuretic peptide levels has proven to be of greatest value in the emergency department, particularly when there is uncertainty about the cause of dyspnea in a patient (see Fig. 26-1). In the Breathing Not Properly Study, which evaluated more than 1500 patients presenting to the emergency department complaining of shortness of breath, BNP was more accurate than the emergency department physician in diagnosing the presence of heart failure.[21]

TABLE 26-5 Biomarkers Used in Assessment of Patients with Heart Failure

Inflammation*†‡
C-reactive protein
Tumor necrosis factor
Fas (APO-1)
Interleukins 1, 6, and 18
Oxidative Stress*†§
Oxidized low-density lipoproteins
Myeloperoxidase
Urinary biopyrrins
Urinary and plasma isoprostanes
Plasma malondialdehyde
Extracellular Matrix Remodeling*§
Matrix metalloproteinases
Tissue inhibitors of metalloproteinases
Collagen propeptides
Propeptide procollagen type I
Plasma procollagen type III
Neurohormones*†§
Norepinephrine
Renin
Angiotensin II
Aldosterone
Arginine vasopressin
Endothelin
Myocyte Injury*†§
Cardiac-specific troponins I and T
Myosin light chain kinase I
Heart-type fatty acid protein
Creatine kinase MB fraction
Myocyte Stress†‡§¶
Brain natriuretic peptide
N-terminal pro-BNP
Midregional fragment of proadrenomedullin
ST2
New Biomarkers†
Chromogranin
Galectin 3
Osteoprotegerin
Adiponectin
Growth differentiation factor 15

*Biomarkers in this category aid in elucidating the pathogenesis of heart failure.
†Biomarkers in this category provide prognostic information and enhance risk stratification.
‡Biomarkers in this category can be used to identify subjects at risk for heart failure.
§Biomarkers in this category are potential targets of therapy.
¶Biomarkers in this category are useful in the diagnosis of heart failure and in monitoring therapy.
From Braunwald E: Biomarkers in heart failure. N Engl J Med 358:2148, 2008.

The area under the receiver operating characteristic curve (AUC) was 0.91, and a BNP cut point of 100 pg/mL was 90% sensitive and 76% specific for diagnosis of heart failure as the cause of dyspnea. A BNP level above 400 pg/mL in this setting made the diagnosis of heart failure likely. Similar results were found in the PRIDE (ProBNP Investigation of Dyspnea in the Emergency Department) study,[22] in which patients with acute heart failure were found to have a median NT-proBNP above 4000 pg/mL compared with 130 pg/mL in those without heart failure. A level of NT-proBNP of 300 pg/mL has been proposed to exclude a diagnosis of heart failure, and age-dependent cut points have been suggested to "rule in" the diagnosis. Knowledge of natriuretic peptide levels in the emergency department has also been associated with more rapid diagnosis, lower admission rate, shorter length of hospital stay, and reduced cost.[23,24] For patients with less acute presentations of dyspnea in settings other than the emergency department, the value of the natriuretic peptide levels is not well established because there is limited information in the medical literature describing their discriminatory power in nonacute settings.

Natriuretic peptide levels also provide useful prognostic information in heart failure patients. Measurements obtained at the time of hospital admission for decompensated heart failure predict the likelihood of in-hospital mortality, and those obtained in the outpatient setting have been shown to predict morbidity and mortality risk.[25,26] Although use of natriuretic peptide levels to guide heart failure therapy has been advocated, clinical trial results, thus far, have been conflicting; some but not all show improved outcomes when they are used to guide management.[27,28]

Other promising biomarkers for detection of heart failure and assessment of risk have been identified. These include the midregional fragment of proadrenomedullin and ST2, a member of the interleukin receptor family.[17] Both are increased by stretch on the myocardium, and each is increased in the setting of decompensation.[29] Galectin 3, produced by activated macrophages and believed to play an important role in promoting cardiac fibrosis, also appears to be able to predict adverse outcomes in heart failure patients.[30] The myofibrillar proteins troponin T and troponin I are indicators of cardiomyocyte injury and may be elevated in heart failure patients in the absence of an acute coronary syndrome or even significant coronary artery disease. Troponin release into the circulation is likely to indicate myocardial injury on the basis of ischemia related to an imbalance between myocardial oxygen supply and demand. Elevated troponin levels in patients with either acutely decompensated heart failure or compensated heart failure in the outpatient setting are associated with increased mortality risk.[31,32] High-sensitivity assays indicate that a substantial portion of heart failure patients have detectable troponin T levels and that the prognostic information obtained from this assay is additive to that of the natriuretic peptides.[33] In fact, several of the biomarkers listed in Table 26-5 have been shown to yield prognostic information that is supplementary to that obtained from measurement of the natriuretic peptides. It seems likely that a combination or panel of biomarkers will prove to be the most useful way of assessing prognosis in heart failure.

Right-Heart Catheterization

Measurement of intracardiac pressures and CO by right-heart catheterization is less commonly performed now than in the past either as part of the diagnostic workup or for guiding therapy because biomarkers and noninvasive imaging techniques provide much of the information that was previously available only by heart catheterization. When there is uncertainty about the cause of a patient's symptoms and in situations in which precise measurements are required to guide therapy or decision making (e.g., selection of patients for heart transplantation), right-heart catheterization is still of considerable value. Whereas determination of hemodynamic variables at rest suffices in most patients, there are cases in which exercise helps reveal the presence or magnitude of abnormal intracardiac pressures and flow. Mitral regurgitation, for example, can be highly dynamic, and exercise measurements may be needed to fully define the severity of this lesion. Similarly, the magnitude of pulmonary hypertension may not be apparent unless the patient is exercised. Unfortunately, many laboratories lack either the equipment or the experience needed to obtain reliable measurements during exercise.

When right-heart catheterization is performed, pressure (both mean and phasic) and flow measurements are obtained. The waveforms in the pressure tracing can provide useful information. Large A waves in the right atrial or pulmonary artery wedge pressure tracing may indicate a constrictive or restrictive process in either of the ventricles; a large V wave is most often caused by tricuspid or mitral regurgitation. Increased flow due to high CO or intracardiac shunts, however, can also increase V wave amplitude. The response of mitral regurgitation to vasodilator therapy can be assessed by changes in V wave amplitude and level of pulmonary artery wedge pressure. Similarly, when pulmonary artery pressures are elevated, the response to pulmonary arterial vasodilating agents can be determined. Demonstration that high pulmonary artery pressures and resistance can be reduced to an acceptable range is essential information in determining whether a patient with pulmonary hypertension will be acceptable for cardiac transplantation. Although CO is usually determined by thermodilution, it is also helpful to measure mixed venous oxygen ($M\text{v}O_2$) saturation in pulmonary artery blood. This measurement alone is a good indicator of the adequacy of CO for ambient tissue oxygen requirements, and it can be used to determine or to estimate CO. Patients with heart failure often have reduced $M\text{v}O_2$ saturation levels. A profound reduction into the 40% to 50% range may help explain symptoms of fatigue and limited exercise capacity. Furthermore, thermodilution measurement of CO, which relies on changes in the temperature of blood in the pulmonary artery produced by delivery of a bolus of injectate of known temperature into the right atrium, loses accuracy when there is recycling of the injectate due to tricuspid insufficiency or when CO is very low and the tracer is warmed by surrounding tissue.

Use of hemodynamic monitoring to guide therapy was evaluated in patients with advanced heart failure in the Evaluation Study of Congestive Heart Failure and Pulmonary Artery Catheterization Effectiveness (ESCAPE) trial.[34] The results did not show any clear-cut benefit on morbidity and mortality of this approach compared with careful clinical assessment. Pulmonary artery catheterization was, however, associated with an increased incidence of anticipated adverse effects. The failure to affect postdischarge outcomes appears to be related to the fact that the hemodynamic improvements that were affected during hospitalization reverted back toward baseline within a relatively short time.[35] Consequently, "tailored therapy" of heart failure is used less commonly now than in the past.

Endomyocardial Biopsy

The role of endomyocardial biopsy in evaluating patients with heart failure is discussed in Chap. 70. In general, it is performed if a disorder with a unique prognosis or one that would benefit from a specific treatment regimen is suspected and the diagnosis cannot be made by conventional methods. The incremental diagnostic, therapeutic, and prognostic benefit offered by the information obtained from a biopsy must be weighed against the risks of the procedure.

Detection of Comorbidities

The incidence of heart failure rises sharply from the sixth decade onward, which is coincident with the time when other chronic diseases begin to be manifested. In addition, many of the conditions leading to the development of heart failure (e.g., diabetes, hypertension, atherosclerosis) affect organs other than the heart. Thus, comorbidities are common in heart failure patients. Insight into the prevalence and range of comorbidities comes from registry data for patients hospitalized with decompensated heart failure outlined in **Table 26-6**. Recognition of these comorbidities and understanding of their impact on heart failure presentation, response to treatment, and prognosis are critical components of the assessment process. The importance of comorbid illness in determining the course of patients can be gleaned from a recent survey of the Olmsted County, Minnesota, population.[36] Whereas hospital admissions were common in heart failure patients in this population, the causes were non–heart

TABLE 26-6 Comorbidities in Patients Hospitalized with Heart Failure (N = 48,612)

COMORBIDITY	NO. (%)
Insulin-treated diabetes mellitus	8089 (16.6)
Non–insulin-treated diabetes mellitus	12,104 (24.9)
Hypertension	34,479 (70.9)
Atrial arrhythmia	14,970 (30.8)
Ventricular arrhythmia	2681 (5.5)
Previous cerebrovascular accident or transient ischemic attack	7558 (15.5)
Hyperlipidemia	15,621 (32.1)
Liver disease	791 (1.6)
Chronic renal insufficiency	9515 (19.6)
Chronic obstructive pulmonary disease	13,395 (27.6)
Peripheral vascular disease	6648 (13.6)
Anemia	8552 (17.6)

From Fonarow GC, Abraham WT, Albert NM, et al: Factors identified as precipitating hospital admissions for heart failure and clinical outcomes: Findings from OPTIMIZE-HF. Arch Intern Med 168:847, 2008.

failure related in most cases and were not precipitated by a cardiac condition in more than half of them.

Information about the most common of these comorbidities can be obtained from the history (supplemented by available hospital notes and tests), physical examination, and routine laboratory tests that are performed when the patient is initially evaluated. Additional testing is dictated by the presence or suspicion of a specific comorbidity. Sleep apnea is frequently overlooked during the clinical assessment but has been reported in more than 50% of heart failure patients.[37] Recognition of the obstructive form of sleep apnea is of great importance because appropriate therapy can have a significant effect on the patient's symptomatic status and also improve ejection fraction in patients with systolic dysfunction.[38] Clues to the presence of sleep apnea come from the patient's body habitus (e.g., obesity or a thick neck) and a history of snoring or daytime somnolence. The spouse or significant other often provides the description of these symptoms and the presence of apneic periods and Cheyne-Stokes respirations that occur while the patient sleeps.

Assessment of Exercise Capacity

Although heart failure patients often complain of reduced exercise capacity, both the significance and cause of this symptom may be difficult to interpret and to quantify. Many heart failure patients have comorbidities that influence their ability to exercise. Patients may also overestimate or underestimate their exercise capacity for a variety of reasons. Thus, having an objective measure of exercise capacity can help determine the cause and extent of impairment. The six-minute walk test is a valuable tool in this regard. It is simple to perform, safe to administer, and quantifies the patient's subjective complaints. The results have also been shown to predict outcomes.[39] It does not, however, discriminate between the causes (e.g., cardiac, pulmonary, orthopedic) of impaired exercise capacity, determine if low levels of exercise are influenced by motivational issues, or account for the effects of conditioning or age. Nonetheless, given the simplicity of administration, the six-minute walk test is an excellent tool for assessing heart failure patients. When more precise information is needed, cardiopulmonary exercise testing is often used because it provides better quantification of exercise capacity and can determine whether the cause of exercise limitation is cardiac.[40] The results of cardiopulmonary exercise testing are good prognostic indicators, and they are used routinely to determine whether patients will derive benefit from advanced therapies such as cardiac transplantation.

TABLE 26-7 Potential Imaging Targets in Heart Failure Patients

Structural
Chamber sizes
Left ventricular mass
Congenital or acquired morphologic abnormalities
Pericardial disease
Valvular disease
Myocardial tissue characterization

Functional
Ventricular systolic and diastolic function
Ventricular dyssynchrony
Cardiac output

Hemodynamic
Intracardiac pressures
Valvular gradients
Valvular regurgitation

Myocardial Blood Supply
Epicardial coronary arteries
Perfusion
Ischemia
Viability

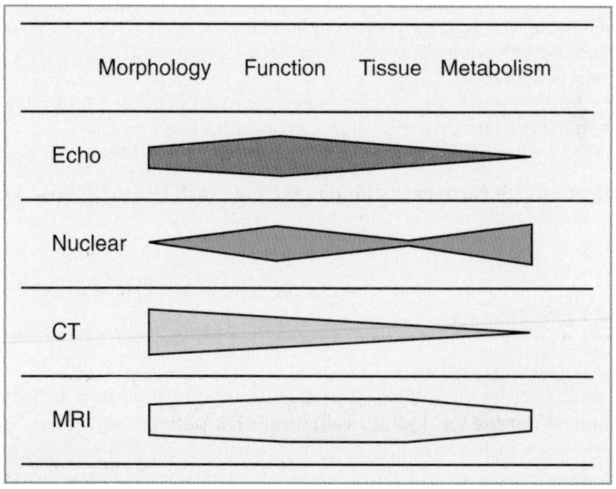

FIGURE 26-2 Relative strengths of noninvasive cardiac imaging modalities. *(Modified from Friedrich MG: Tissue characterization of acute myocardial infarction and myocarditis by cardiac magnetic resonance. J Am Cardiol Img 1:652, 2008.)*

Use of Imaging Modalities in the Diagnosis and Management of Patients with Heart Failure (see Chaps. 15, 17-19)

Noninvasive cardiac imaging serves a vital role in the assessment of patients with heart failure. As part of the initial evaluation, it is used to help confirm the diagnosis of heart failure by assessing the presence and severity of structural and functional changes in the heart, to determine (or provide clues about) the cause of cardiac dysfunction (i.e., congenital heart disease, valvular abnormalities, pericardial disease, coronary artery disease), to risk stratify patients, and to guide treatment strategies. Imaging modalities can also be used to help assess the efficacy of therapeutic interventions, to provide ongoing prognostic information, and to further guide treatment. **Table 26-7** summarizes potential targets of noninvasive imaging in patients with heart failure. The primary noninvasive cardiac imaging modalities used to evaluate heart failure patients are echocardiography, magnetic resonance imaging (MRI), computed tomography (CT), and nuclear imaging. Attributes of these modalities are summarized in Table 26-e1 on the website, and their relative strengths are summarized in **Figure 26-2**.[41] These modalities often provide complementary data,

CH 26

TABLE 26-8 Indications for MRI, CT, and Nuclear Imaging in Heart Failure Patients

Indications for Cardiac MRI in Patients with Heart Failure
Differentiate ischemic from nonischemic cause
Evaluate for ischemia
Evaluate for potentially viable segments of myocardium
Determine left ventricular systolic function in patients with poor-quality echocardiograms
Evaluate presence and pattern of wall thickness and assess for fibrosis in patients with suspected hypertrophic cardiomyopathy
Detect the presence of pericardial or acquired structural disease
Determine the presence and nature of congenital heart disease
Evaluate for myocarditis
Evaluate for the presence of an intracardiac mass or thrombus
Characterize myocardium in patients with suspected cardiomyopathies, including
Amyloidosis
Sarcoidosis
Noncompaction
Iron deposition
Arrhythmogenic right ventricular dysplasia
Chagas disease
Anderson-Fabry disease
Hypereosinophilic syndrome
Stress-induced cardiomyopathy
Indications for Cardiac CT in Patients with Heart Failure
Differentiate ischemic from nonischemic cause
Determine left ventricular systolic function in patients with poor-quality echocardiograms
Detect the presence of suspected pericardial or acquired structural disease
Determine the presence and nature of congenital heart disease
Evaluate for the presence of an intracardiac mass or thrombus
Indications for Nuclear Imaging in Patients with Heart Failure
Differentiate ischemic from nonischemic cause
Evaluate for ischemia
Evaluate for viability
Determine left ventricular systolic function in patients with poor-quality echocardiograms

and each has the capacity to provide unique information in individual patients. Whereas the initial evaluation of a patient with newly diagnosed heart failure should include transthoracic echocardiography, further imaging with MRI, CT, or nuclear techniques may be considered, depending on the need to further address questions about cardiac structure and function, etiology, and issues such as the potential for reversibility of systolic dysfunction with revascularization. The specific indications for each of these imaging modalities are summarized in **Table 26-8**.

Echocardiography (see Chap. 15)

Transthoracic echocardiography can be performed without risk to the patient, does not involve radiation exposure, and can be performed at the bedside if necessary. It is particularly well suited for evaluating the structure and function of both the myocardium and heart valves and providing information about intracardiac pressures and flows. Echocardiography may be limited in some patients because available imaging planes and image quality depend on acoustic windows, which may be suboptimal as a result of obesity, emphysema, or other causes.

For heart failure patients with a depressed ejection fraction, left ventricular volumes and systolic function can be assessed semiquantitatively or quantified by the biplane method and the modified Simpson rule.[42] Information about the morphology and relative sizes of the cardiac chambers may suggest specific diagnoses. For example, concentric left ventricular hypertrophy with severe biatrial enlargement raises the possibility that heart failure is due to an infiltrative process such as amyloidosis (as shown in **Fig. 26-3**; see Figs. 15-68 to 15-78). Diastolic function is easily assessed by echocardiography with Doppler measurements (see Figs. 15-26 to 15-28): analyses of the mitral valve inflow pattern, including measurement of early (E) and atrial (A) waveforms; tissue velocities at the mitral valve annulus; pulmonary vein flows; and left atrial volume indexed to body surface area (see Chap. 30). Diastolic dysfunction can be further classified as grade I to grade III on the basis of these measurements (see Fig. 30-7).[43] Pulmonary hypertension in patients without significant systolic dysfunction or pulmonary disease suggests that diastolic dysfunction may be present.[44] Left ventricular filling pressures are estimated primarily on the basis of the ratio of the peak mitral inflow E wave velocity (Fig. 26-3B) to that of the tissue Doppler e′ wave velocity (Fig. 26-3D).[45] This index, however, may be less reliable in the setting of acute decompensated heart failure with left ventricular systolic dysfunction.[46]

Echocardiographic measurements are also used to estimate right-sided heart pressures noninvasively, which may be useful in assessing and managing heart failure patients. For example, right atrial pressures are estimated by the inferior vena cava (IVC) diameter and the relative change in diameter on inspiration. Normal IVC diameter and inspiratory collapse of at least 50% are associated with normal right atrial pressures; increased IVC diameter and smaller inspiratory changes indicate elevated right atrial pressure. Right ventricular and pulmonary arterial systolic pressures can usually be estimated from the estimated right atrial pressure and peak tricuspid valve regurgitant velocity. The right atrial pressure can be important in the determination of pulmonary hypertension as it may be elevated to as much as 25 mm Hg or more in heart failure patients. Similarly, pulmonary artery end-diastolic pressures can be assessed by use of the right atrial pressure and the end-diastolic regurgitant jet velocity through the pulmonic valve.

Magnetic Resonance Imaging (see Chap. 18)

MRI involves no radiation, and diagnostic images can be obtained in nearly all patients, provided they can be accommodated in the scanner and are not claustrophobic. Unlike with echocardiography, images can be obtained in arbitrary tomographic planes. MRI is excellent for evaluation of cardiac morphology, chamber sizes, and cardiac function. Using different pulse sequences with and without gadolinium contrast, MRI can characterize myocardial tissue, assess myocardial viability, and help diagnose specific cardiomyopathies (e.g., left ventricular noncompaction; **Fig. 26-4** (see Fig. 18-16)). Cine MRI imaging without contrast enhancement provides highly accurate and reproducible assessment of myocardial mass, chamber volumes, and left ventricular and right ventricular systolic function[44] without the need for geometric assumptions. MRI is particularly useful for evaluation of left ventricular function in patients with limited acoustic windows and poor-quality echocardiograms. MRI is also useful in evaluating and quantifying right ventricular systolic function, and this measurement can provide important prognostic information in heart failure patients.[45] A major limitation is that the current implanted pacemakers or defibrillators are not compatible with MRI, although this limitation may be obviated by the development of newer devices that are MRI compatible. Also, the risk of nephrogenic sclerosing fibrosis must be considered in deciding whether to administer gadolinium-based contrast agents to patients with renal dysfunction.

Cardiac Computed Tomography (see Chap. 19)

Cardiac CT provides isotropic volumetric data with excellent spatial resolution. Currently, its primary role in heart failure is to help determine whether obstructive coronary artery disease is present. This is done by CT angiography, which does expose the patient to ionizing radiation, an issue that has generated a good deal of concern in the medical and lay press. Exposure, however, may be reduced significantly by use of prospective gating to image only during diastole. Cardiac CT angiography generally also involves administration of iodinated contrast material, which is of concern in patients who are at risk for development of nephrotoxicity.

Nuclear Imaging (see Chap. 17)

A wide array of nuclear imaging techniques have been developed with use of different radionuclide tracers and protocols. In particular, single-photon emission computed tomography (SPECT) and positron emission tomography (PET) technologies are well suited for assessment of myocardial ischemia and viability and for evaluation of myocardial function. Nuclear imaging also involves radiation but does not require the administration of iodinated or other contrast agents, and diagnostic images can be obtained in virtually all patients. The use of nuclear imaging to determine myocardial viability is discussed in Chap. 17.

Cardiac Imaging to Differentiate Between Ischemic and Nonischemic Causes of Heart Failure

In patients with heart failure and depressed left ventricular systolic function, differentiation of ischemic from nonischemic causes has important therapeutic and prognostic implications. Cardiac catheterization with coronary angiography is the "gold standard" for determining the presence and severity of coronary artery disease (see Chap. 20). It is often used to evaluate patients with left ventricular systolic dysfunction, especially when there is a high degree of suspicion from the clinical presentation that there is an ischemic cause. Noninvasive imaging is particularly valuable in patients with lower pretest probability of coronary disease because the invasive procedure can be avoided in many of these cases. The decision to proceed to heart catheterization or to study the patient noninvasively depends on a variety of factors, including historical information and symptoms, clinical presentation, the patient's age and comorbidities, presence and severity of risk factors for coronary artery disease, and electrocardiographic findings. Patients with ischemic cardiomyopathy often have regional myocardial thinning and contractile dysfunction on the resting echocardiogram; hypokinesis tends to be more global with nonischemic cardiomyopathies. This differentiation is not precise, however, and patients with ischemic causes may have diffuse hypokinesis, whereas others with nonischemic cardiomyopathies may have regional wall motion abnormalities.

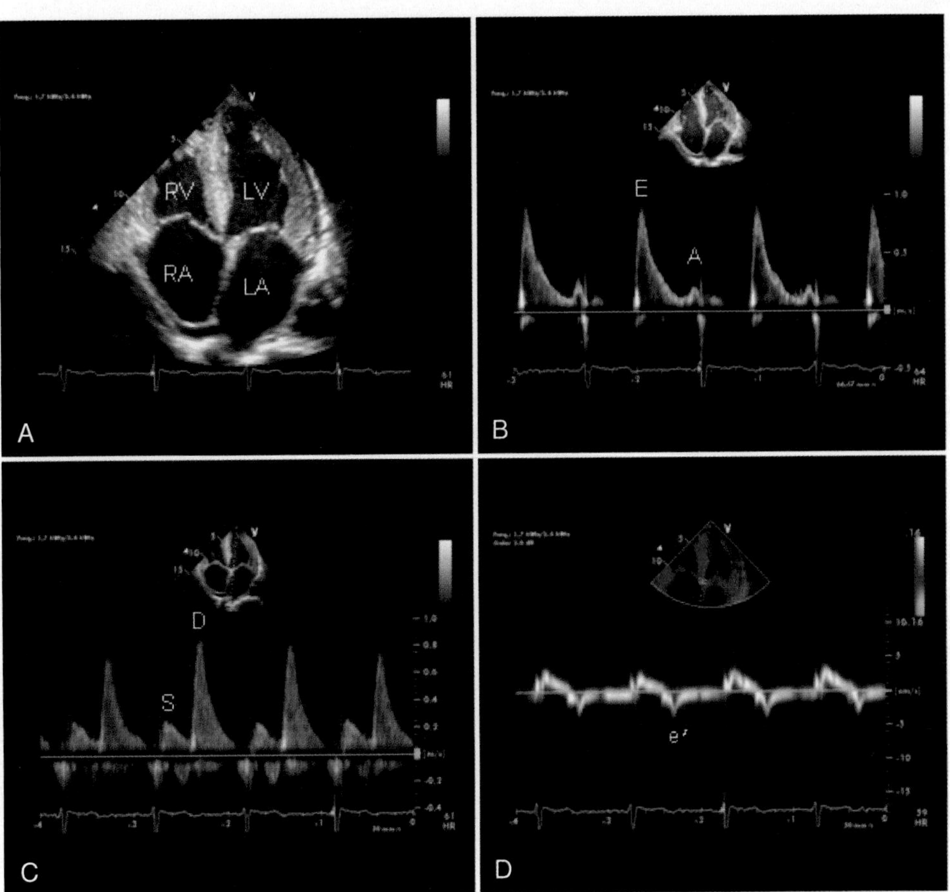

FIGURE 26-3 Echocardiographic images from a patient with cardiac amyloidosis and severe diastolic dysfunction. **A,** Apical four-chamber view showing biventricular hypertrophy, biatrial enlargement, and a small pericardial effusion. **B,** Mitral valve inflow pattern showing large E wave, rapid deceleration, and small A wave. **C,** Pulmonary venous inflow pattern showing large D wave. **D,** Tissue Doppler recording from the mitral annulus showing small E′ wave. Note that the E/e′ ratio equals approximately 25, consistent with elevated filling pressures.

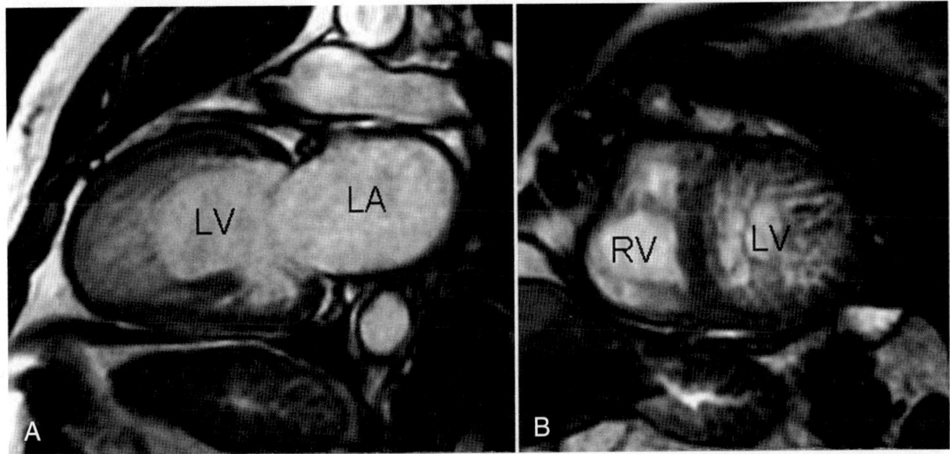

FIGURE 26-4 Cardiac MRI steady-state free precession long-axis **(A)** and short-axis **(B)** views showing an abnormal degree of trabeculation consistent with noncompaction cardiomyopathy in a patient with heart failure and severe left ventricular systolic dysfunction. LA = left atrium; LV = left ventricle; RA = right atrium; RV = right ventricle.

As summarized in Table 26-e2 on the website, the four major cardiac imaging modalities have different diagnostic sensitivity and specificity with regard to differentiating between ischemic and nonischemic causes of heart failure. Stress echocardiography can be used to assess for inducible regional ischemia and associated wall motion abnormalities.[47] CT angiography has a high negative predictive value and is highly sensitive in identifying obstructive coronary artery disease. A single-center study that used CT angiography with retrospective gating to evaluate patients with cardiomyopathies of unknown origin found that this test had a sensitivity of 98.1% and a specificity of 99.9% to detect stenoses of 50% or greater.[48] Alternatively, cardiac MRI can distinguish ischemic from nonischemic cardiomyopathies on the basis of the pattern of delayed enhancement from T1-weighted images taken minutes after the intravenous administration of gadolinium-based contrast material (see Chap. 18). Ischemic cardiomyopathies usually show characteristic subendocardial enhancement at the sites of prior infarctions; nonischemic dilated cardiomyopathies most commonly have no enhancement, midwall enhancement, or other patterns, depending on the cause, as exemplified in **Figure 26-5**. Therefore, delayed enhancement in a subendocardial distribution that matches coronary artery territories is a relatively sensitive method of noninvasively identifying patients with ischemic cardiomyopathies.[49] Nuclear stress testing using rest and stress perfusion and wall motion has been shown to be sensitive but less specific (see Chap. 17).[50] Of the noninvasive techniques, direct visualization of the coronary arteries by CT has excellent negative predictive value and is an attractive means of excluding coronary disease. MRI has the benefit of not involving radiation and the potential to obtain additional diagnostic data about viability and

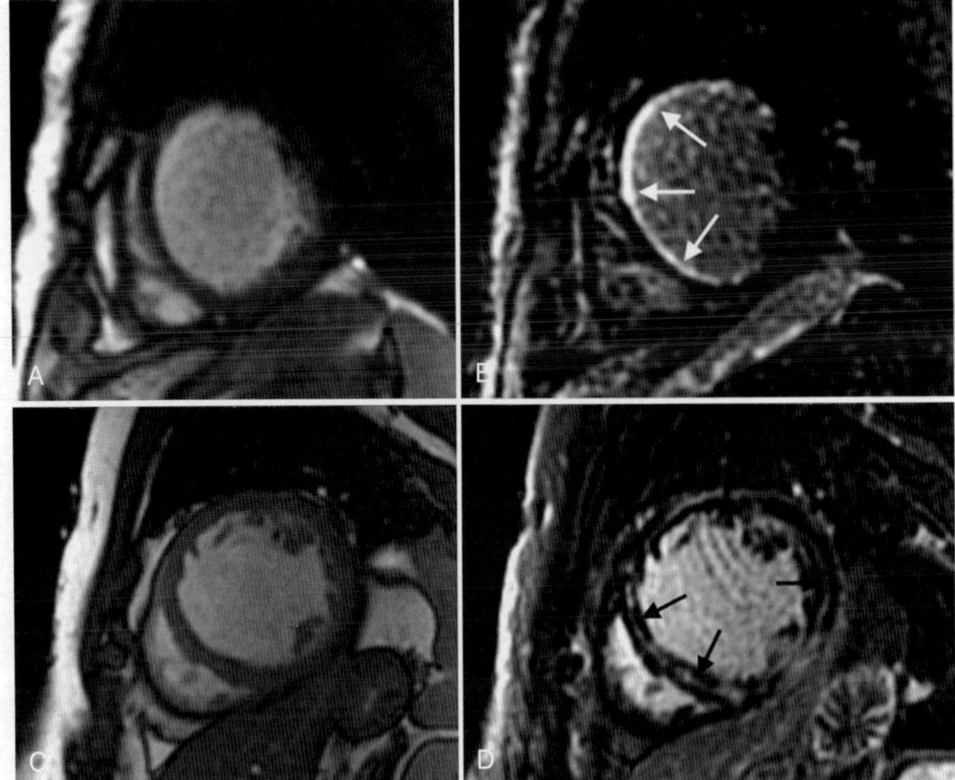

FIGURE 26-5 Cardiac MRI of two patients with heart failure and severe left ventricular dysfunction, one with an ischemic cardiomyopathy (**A** and **B**) and one with a nonischemic cardiomyopathy (**C** and **D**). Steady-state free precession images in the short-axis plane are shown in **A** and **C**. Delayed gadolinium enhancement in the short-axis plane shows evidence of extensive subendocardial delayed enhancement (**B**, arrows) consistent with scar from myocardial infarction and midwall delayed enhancement (**D**, arrows) consistent with nonischemic cardiomyopathy.

nonischemic causes during the same study. The choice of modality is often appropriately influenced by the degree of local experience and expertise with these imaging techniques. Patients identified by noninvasive testing as having evidence of obstructive coronary artery disease can then be referred for invasive coronary angiography. The presence of obstructive coronary artery disease, however, does not necessarily imply that ischemia or previous infarction is the cause of left ventricular dysfunction. The clinician must determine if the anatomic distribution and burden of coronary artery disease is consistent with the degree of systolic dysfunction, as patients may have nonischemic cardiomyopathies with coexisting coronary artery disease or cardiomyopathies with both ischemic and nonischemic contributions.

In patients with nonischemic cardiomyopathy, imaging techniques can further characterize myocardial tissue and provide additional diagnostic information that may be useful in determining the cause of nonischemic cardiomyopathies. By use of selected MRI sequences and parameters, the relative image intensities with different magnetic relaxation time (T1 and T2) weightings and the relative early and late enhancement after contrast administration can be assessed.[51] By combining these data with the data from cine imaging, specific pathologic processes can be detected and characterized. In addition to detection of ischemic cardiomyopathy, the pattern of delayed enhancement may differ for different causes of nonischemic cardiomyopathy (**Fig. 26-6**). For example, when delayed enhancement images are obtained in patients with cardiac amyloidosis, the myocardium may be difficult to null, the difference between myocardial and blood pool signals may be less pronounced than usual, and there can be relatively diffuse subendocardial and midwall delayed enhancement (see Fig. 18-14). Furthermore, patterns of late enhancement seen with MRI can provide additional prognostic data. In patients with dilated nonischemic cardiomyopathies, midwall enhancement, as shown in Figure 26-5, is associated with increased cardiac morbidity.[52]

Cardiac Imaging to Assess Myocardial Viability

(see Chaps. 17, 18, 31 and 52)

As noted in Chap. 31, myocardial revascularization is associated with improved survival in patients with viable myocardium but offers no mortality benefit beyond medical treatment in patients who do not have evidence of viable myocardium.[53] Insofar as the risk of percutaneous and surgical revascularization is increased in patients with heart failure, it is important to determine the likelihood of benefit from these approaches. As noted in Chaps. 31 and 52, patients with ischemic cardiomyopathy have several possible mechanisms for reversible myocardial dysfunction, including myocardial stunning and hibernation. Imaging can help identify viable segments of myocardium that have greater likelihood of improving functionally when adequate blood supply is restored. See Chap. 26 Online Supplement for further details on myocardial viability.

Summary and Future Perspectives

As treatment options (and the health care system itself) continue to evolve, there will be increased emphasis on more rapid, accurate, and cost-effective assessment of patients, with the goal being to provide unambiguous information about the presence, severity, and cause of heart failure. New insights into the biology of cardiac dysfunction are likely to lead to the development of therapeutic approaches that are specific to the underlying cause. Advances in the use of biomarkers and imaging techniques to diagnose, stage, and determine cause of heart failure will be needed to meet these future demands. Even as these diagnostic modalities increase in their precision and accuracy, the information obtained through the history and physical examination will remain at the core of our ability to understand how to employ these tests most judiciously and to treat patients most effectively.

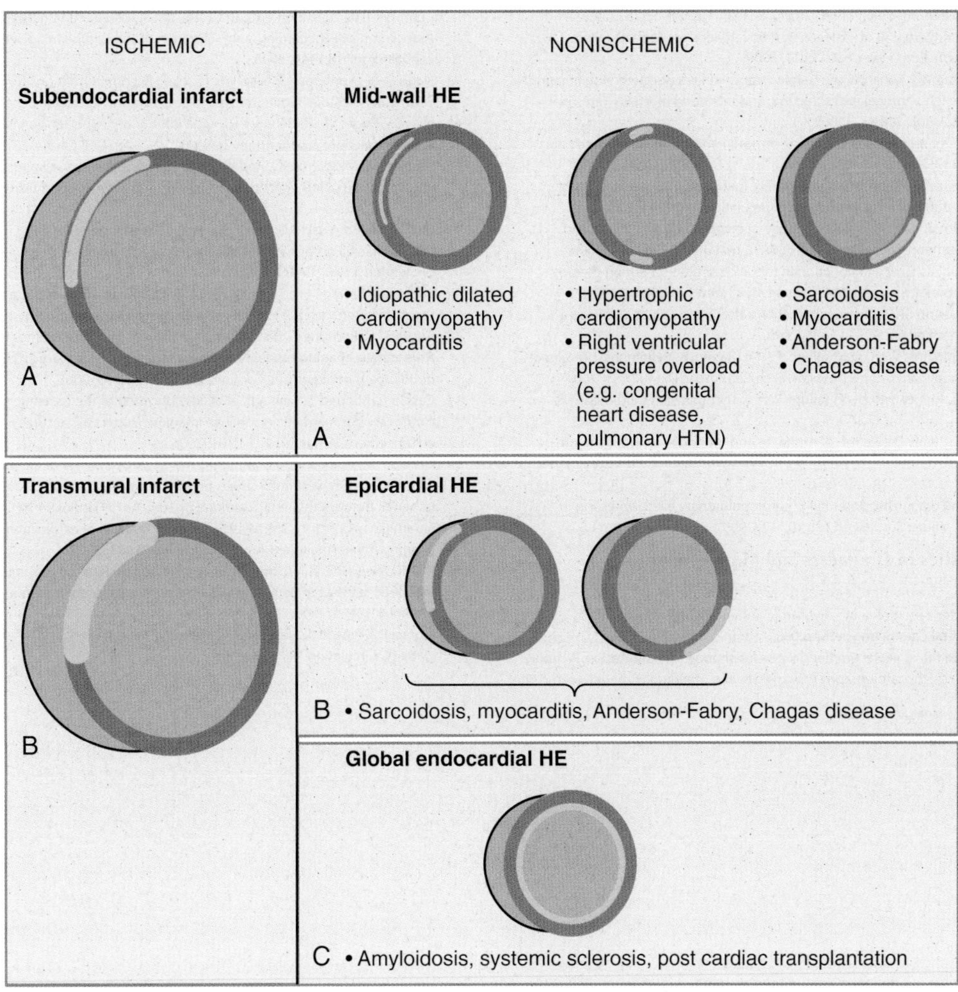

FIGURE 26-6 Patterns of hyperenhancement (HE) with MRI in different myocardial diseases. HTN = hypertension. *(Modified from Mahrholdt H, Wagner A, Judd RM, et al: Delayed enhancement cardiovascular magnetic resonance assessment of non-ischaemic cardiomyopathies. Eur Heart J 26:1461, 2005.)*

REFERENCES

Medical History and Physical Examination

1. Schocken DD, Benjamin EJ, Fonarow GC, et al: Prevention of heart failure: A scientific statement from the American Heart Association Councils on Epidemiology and Prevention, Clinical Cardiology, Cardiovascular Nursing, and High Blood Pressure Research; Quality of Care and Outcomes Research Interdisciplinary Working Group; and Functional Genomics and Translational Biology Interdisciplinary Working Group. Circulation 117:2544, 2008.
2. Ahmed A, Allman RM, Aronow WS, DeLong JF: Diagnosis of heart failure in older adults: Predictive value of dyspnea at rest. Arch Gerontol Geriatr 38:297, 2004.
3. Levy D, Larson MG, Vasan RS, et al: The progression from hypertension to congestive heart failure. JAMA 275:1557, 1996.
4. Leier CV, Chatterjee K: The physical examination in heart failure—Part I. Congest Heart Fail 13:41, 2007.
5. Leier CV, Chatterjee K. The physical examination in heart failure—Part II. Congest Heart Fail 13:99, 2007.
6. Chakko S, Woska D, Martinez H, et al: Clinical, radiographic, and hemodynamic correlations in chronic congestive heart failure: Conflicting results may lead to inappropriate care. Am J Med 90:353, 1991.
7. McGee SR: Physical examination of venous pressure: A critical review. Am Heart J 136:10, 1998.
8. Butman SM, Ewy GA, Standen JR, et al: Bedside cardiovascular examination in patients with severe chronic heart failure: Importance of rest or inducible jugular venous distension. J Am Coll Cardiol 22:968, 1993.

Laboratory Testing, Right-Heart Catheterization, Endomyocardial Biopsy, and Exercise Testing

9. Gheorghiade M, Abraham WT, Albert NM, et al: Relationship between admission serum sodium concentration and clinical outcomes in patients hospitalized for heart failure: An analysis from the OPTIMIZE-HF registry. Eur Heart J 28:980, 2007.
10. Konstam MA, Gheorghiade M, Burnett JC Jr, et al: Effects of oral tolvaptan in patients hospitalized for worsening heart failure: The EVEREST Outcome Trial. JAMA 297:1319, 2007.
11. Pereira AF, Simões do Couto F, de Mendonça A: The use of laboratory tests in patients with mild cognitive impairment. J Alzheimers Dis 10:53, 2006.
12. Tschuppert Y, Buclin T, Rothuizen LE, et al: Effect of dronedarone on renal function in healthy subjects. Br J Clin Pharmacol 64:785, 2007.
13. Heywood JT, Fonarow GC, Costanzo MR, et al: High prevalence of renal dysfunction and its impact on outcome in 118,465 patients hospitalized with acute decompensated heart failure: A report from the ADHERE database. J Card Fail 13:422, 2007.
14. Damman K, Navis G, Voors AA, et al: Worsening renal function and prognosis in heart failure: Systematic review and meta-analysis. J Card Fail 13:599, 2007.
15. Groenveld HF, Januzzi JL, Damman K, et al: Anemia and mortality in heart failure patients a systematic review and meta-analysis. J Am Coll Cardiol 52:818, 2008.
16. Adams KF Jr, Piña IL, Ghali JK, et al: Prospective evaluation of the association between hemoglobin concentration and quality of life in patients with heart failure. Am Heart J 158:965, 2009.
17. Braunwald E: Biomarkers in heart failure. N Engl J Med 358:2148, 2008.
18. Morrow DA, de Lemos JA: Benchmarks for the assessment of novel cardiovascular biomarkers. Circulation 115:949, 2007.
19. Daniels LB, Maisel AS: Natriuretic peptides. J Am Coll Cardiol 50:2357, 2007.
20. Maisel A, Mueller C, Adams K Jr, et al: State of the art: Using natriuretic peptide levels in clinical practice. Eur J Heart Fail 10:824, 2008.
21. Maisel AS, Krishnaswamy P, Nowak RM, et al: Rapid measurement of B-type natriuretic peptide in the emergency diagnosis of heart failure N Engl J Med 347:161, 2002.
22. Januzzi JL Jr, Camargo CA, Anwaruddin S, et al: The N-terminal pro-BNP investigation of dyspnea in the emergency department (PRIDE) study. Am J Cardiol 95:948, 2005.
23. Mueller C, Scholer A, Laule-Kilian K, et al: Use of B-type natriuretic peptide in the evaluation and management of acute dyspnea. N Engl J Med 350:647, 2004.
24. Moe GW, Howlett J, Januzzi JL, Zowall H: N-terminal pro-B-type natriuretic peptide testing improves the management of patients with suspected acute heart failure: Primary results of the Canadian prospective randomized multicenter IMPROVE-CHF study. Circulation 115:3103, 2007.
25. Fonarow GC, Peacock WF, Phillips CO, et al: Admission B-type natriuretic peptide levels and in-hospital mortality in acute decompensated heart failure. J Am Coll Cardiol 49:1943, 2007.
26. Sugiura T, Takase H, Toriyama T, et al: Circulating levels of myocardial proteins predict future deterioration of congestive heart failure. J Card Fail 11:504, 2005.
27. Jourdain P, Jondeau G, Funck F, et al: Plasma brain natriuretic peptide–guided therapy to improve outcome in heart failure: The STARS-BNP Multicenter Study. J Am Coll Cardiol 49:1733, 2007.
28. Pfisterer M, Buser P, Rickli H, et al: BNP-guided vs symptom-guided heart failure therapy: The Trial of Intensified vs Standard Medical Therapy in Elderly Patients With Congestive Heart Failure (TIME-CHF) randomized trial. JAMA 301:383, 2009.

29. Kakkar R, Lee RT: ST2 and adrenomedullin in heart failure. Heart Fail Clin 5:515, 2009.
30. de Boer RA, Voors AA, Muntendam P, et al: Galectin-3: A novel mediator of heart failure development and progression. Eur J Heart Fail 11:811, 2009.
31. Horwich TB, Patel J, MacLellan WR, Fonarow GC: Cardiac troponin I is associated with impaired hemodynamics, progressive left ventricular dysfunction, and increased mortality rates in advanced heart failure. Circulation 108:833, 2003.
32. Peacock WF IV, De Marco T, Fonarow GC, et al: Cardiac troponin and outcome in acute heart failure. N Engl J Med 358:2117, 2008.
33. Latini R, Masson S, Anand IS, et al: Prognostic value of very low plasma concentrations of troponin T in patients with stable chronic heart failure. Circulation 116:1242, 2007.
34. Binanay C, Califf RM, Hasselblad V, et al: Evaluation study of congestive heart failure and pulmonary artery catheterization effectiveness: The ESCAPE trial. JAMA 294:1625, 2005.
35. Palardy M, Stevenson LW, Tasissa G, et al: Reduction in mitral regurgitation during therapy guided by measured filling pressures in the ESCAPE trial. Circ Heart Fail 2:181, 2009.
36. Dunlay SM, Redfield MM, Weston SA, et al: Hospitalizations after heart failure diagnosis a community perspective. J Am Coll Cardiol 54:1695, 2009.
37. Bordier P: Sleep apnoea in patients with heart failure. Part I: Diagnosis, definitions, prevalence, pathophysiology and haemodynamic consequences. Arch Cardiovasc Dis 102:651, 2009.
38. Bordier P: Sleep apnoea in patients with heart failure. Part II: Therapy. Arch Cardiovasc Dis 102:711, 2009.
39. Bittner V, Weiner DH, Yusuf S, et al: Prediction of mortality and morbidity with a 6-minute walk test in patients with left ventricular dysfunction. SOLVD Investigators. JAMA 270:1702, 1993.
40. Ingle L: Prognostic value and diagnostic potential of cardiopulmonary exercise testing in patients with chronic heart failure. Eur J Heart Fail 10:112, 2008.

Use of Imaging Modalities in Diagnosis and Management of Heart Failure

41. Friedrich MG: Tissue characterization of acute myocardial infarction and myocarditis by cardiac magnetic resonance. J Am Coll Cardiol Img 1:652, 2008.
42. Lang RM, Bierig M, Devereux RB, et al: Recommendations for chamber quantification: A report from the American Society of Echocardiography's Guidelines and Standards Committee and the Chamber Quantification Writing Group, developed in conjunction with the European Association of Echocardiography, a branch of the European Society of Cardiology. J Am Soc Echocardiogr 18:1440, 2005.
43. Nagueh SF, Appleton CP, Gillebert TC, et al: Recommendations for the evaluation of left ventricular diastolic function by echocardiography. J Am Soc Echocardiogr 22:107, 2009.
44. Lam CS, Roger VL, Rodeheffer RJ, et al: Pulmonary hypertension in heart failure with preserved ejection fraction: A community-based study. J Am Coll Cardiol 53:1119, 2009.
45. Nagueh SF, Middleton KJ, Kopelen HA, et al: Doppler tissue imaging: A noninvasive technique for evaluation of left ventricular relaxation and estimation of filling pressures. J Am Coll Cardiol 30:1527, 1997.
46. Mullens W, Borowski AG, Curtin RJ, et al: Tissue Doppler imaging in the estimation of intracardiac filling pressure in decompensated patients with advanced systolic heart failure. Circulation 119:62, 2009.
47. Sharp SM, Sawada SG, Segar DS, et al: Dobutamine stress echocardiography: Detection of coronary artery disease in patients with dilated cardiomyopathy. J Am Coll Cardiol 24:934, 1994.
48. Andreini D, Pontone G, Bartorelli AL, et al: Sixty-four-slice multidetector computed tomography: An accurate imaging modality for the evaluation of coronary arteries in dilated cardiomyopathy of unknown etiology. Circ Cardiovasc Imaging 2:199, 2009.
49. Casolo G, Minneci S, Manta R, et al: Identification of the ischemic etiology of heart failure by cardiovascular magnetic resonance imaging: Diagnostic accuracy of late gadolinium enhancement. Am Heart J 151:101, 2006.
50. Danias PG, Papaioannou GI, Ahlberg AW, et al: Usefulness of electrocardiographic-gated stress technetium-99m sestamibi single-photon emission computed tomography to differentiate ischemic from nonischemic cardiomyopathy. Am J Cardiol 94:14, 2004.
51. Karamitsos TD, Francis JM, Myerson S, et al: The role of cardiovascular magnetic resonance imaging in heart failure. J Am Coll Cardiol 54:1407, 2009.
52. Wu KC, Weiss RG, Thiemann DR, et al: Late gadolinium enhancement by cardiovascular magnetic resonance heralds an adverse prognosis in nonischemic cardiomyopathy. J Am Coll Cardiol 51:2414, 2008.
53. Camici PG, Prasad SK, Rimoldi OE: Stunning, hibernation, and assessment of myocardial viability. Circulation 117:103, 2008.

CHAPTER 27 Diagnosis and Management of Acute Heart Failure Syndromes

Mihai Gheorghiade, Gerasimos S. Filippatos, and G. Michael Felker

Acute heart failure syndromes (AHFS) are among the most common causes for hospitalization in patients older than 65 years. In the United States alone, approximately 3 million patients are admitted each year with a primary or secondary diagnosis of heart failure (HF).[1,2] The direct and indirect costs associated with HF are estimated at more than $37 billion in 2009 in the United States and are mainly related to hospitalizations. The number of admissions for HF has tripled during the last three decades and will continue to grow because of a convergence of several epidemiologic trends: the aging of the population, because the incidence of HF is age related; the greatly improved survival after myocardial infarction, resulting in more patients living with chronic left ventricular (LV) dysfunction; and the availability of effective therapy for prevention of sudden death. Previously considered part of the clinical history of chronic HF, AHFS have been increasingly recognized during the last decade as a group of distinct disorders with unique epidemiology, pathophysiology, need for specific treatments, and outcomes.

Nomenclature and Definition

As is evident from the plural terminology *acute heart failure syndromes*, acute HF (AHF) is not a single disease but rather a family of related disorders. A variety of other overlapping terms have been used in the literature, including AHF, acute decompensated HF (ADHF), and acute decompensation of chronic HF (ADCHF). We prefer the broader term AHFS, insofar as it encompasses the heterogeneity of these disorders. In general, AHFS can be defined as the new onset or recurrence of gradually or rapidly developing symptoms and signs of HF requiring urgent or emergent therapy and resulting in hospitalization.

Epidemiology

AHFS represent a major burden in the developed world. In the United States, HF is the primary diagnosis for more than 1 million hospitalized patients annually, which represents an expenditure of $39 billion per year. Similar numbers of hospitalizations are reported in Europe, with geographical variations in the length of stay, rehospitalization rate, and mortality. In the last decade, large AHFS registries from both the United States (Acute Decompensated Heart Failure National Registry Database [ADHERE][3] and Organized Program to Initiate Lifesaving Treatment in Hospitalized Patients with Heart Failure [OPTIMIZE-HF][4]) and Europe (EuroHeart Failure Survey I and II[5]) have provided a detailed characterization of this population of patients. AHFS disproportionally affect elderly people, with a mean age of 75 years in large registries. AHFS affect men and women almost equally, but women tend to be older and are more likely to have a history of hypertension and preserved systolic function (**Table 27-1**). With regard to race and ethnicity, in OPTIMIZE-HF, approximately 17% of patients were African American.[6] They tended to be substantially younger (64 versus 75 years) and to have a higher proportion of hypertension and a lower incidence of ischemic heart disease than white patients. Both cardiovascular and noncardiovascular comorbid conditions are extremely common in AHFS. About 60% to 70% of patients have a history of coronary artery disease (CAD); 70% have a history of hypertension; 40% have diabetes; 30% to 40% have atrial fibrillation; and 20% to 30% have significant renal dysfunction.[4] On the basis of the registry data, 40% to 50% of patients hospitalized with AHFS have normal or nearly normal systolic function; this condition is commonly referred to as HF with preserved ejection fraction (HFpEF; see Chap. 30). Compared with patients with HF and low ejection fraction, those with HFpEF are more likely to be older, to be female, and to have a history of hypertension while being less likely to have CAD (**Table 27-2**). The in-hospital mortality of patients with HFpEF appears to be lower compared with that of patients with depressed LV ejection fraction (2.8% versus 3.9%). However, the duration of intensive care unit stay and total hospital length of stay appear similar. Although postdischarge rehospitalization and mortality rates are high and similar for both groups, the mode of death and reason for rehospitalization may be very different.

Classification

The heterogeneity of AHFS makes the development of a comprehensive classification scheme difficult. Although no single classification system has garnered universal acceptance, many of the classifications reviewed here have substantial similarities and provide tools for understanding the overall epidemiology of AHFS. One useful method of classification is based on the presence or absence of a prior history of HF.[7] The 2008 European Society of Cardiology (ESC) guidelines have embraced this approach and emphasize the importance of history and time course of presentation.[8] Accordingly, we categorize patients with AHFS by the following:

CH 27

TABLE 27-1 Demographics and Comorbidities of Patients Hospitalized with Acute Heart Failure from Various Registries

	ADHERE N = 105,388	OPTIMIZE-HF N = 48,612	EHFS II N = 3580	ARGENTINA N = 2974	JAPAN
Mean age, years	72	73	70	68	73
Women, %	52	52	39	41	41
Prior HF, %	76	88	63	50	—
Preserved EF, %	40	49	52	26	43
Medical history, %					
CAD	57	50	54	—	—
Hypertension	73	71	62	66	71
Myocardial infarction	31	—	—	22	—
Atrial fibrillation	31	31	39	27	40
Diabetes	44	42	33	23	34
Renal insufficiency	30	20	17	10	—
COPD/asthma	31	34	19	15	9

CAD = coronary artery disease; COPD = chronic obstructive pulmonary disease; EF = ejection fraction; HF = heart failure.

Data compiled from Yancy CW, Lopatin M, Stevenson LW, et al: Clinical presentation, management, and in-hospital outcomes of patients admitted with acute decompensated heart failure with preserved systolic function: A report from the Acute Decompensated Heart Failure National Registry (ADHERE) Database. J Am Coll Cardiol 47:76, 2006; Gheorghiade M, Abraham WT, Albert NM, et al: Systolic blood pressure at admission, clinical characteristics, and outcomes in patients hospitalized with acute heart failure. JAMA 296:2217, 2006; Nieminen MS, Brutsaert D, Dickstein K, et al: EuroHeart Failure Survey II (EHFS II): A survey on hospitalized acute heart failure patients: Description of population. Eur Heart J 27:2725, 2006; Perna ER, Barbagelata A, Grinfeld L, et al: Overview of decompensated heart failure in Argentina: Lessons learned from five registries during the last decade. Am Heart J 151:84, 2006; Sato N, Kajimoto K, Asai K, et al: Acute decompensated heart failure sydromes (ATTEND) registry. A prospective observational multicenter cohort study: Rationale, design, and preliminary data. Am Heart J 159:949, 2010.

TABLE 27-2 Characteristics of Patients Admitted with Preserved Ejection Fraction Versus Reduced Ejection Fraction in the OPTIMIZE Registry

CHARACTERISTICS AT ADMISSION	PATIENTS WITH LVSD (N = 20,118)	PATIENTS WITH HFPEF (N = 21,149)
Demographics		
Mean age (yr)	70.4 ± 14.3	75.1 ± 13.1
Male	62%	38%
White	71%	77%
African American	21%	15%
Medical history		
Diabetes, insulin treated	15%	17%
Diabetes, non–insulin treated	24%	26%
Hypertension	66%	76%
Hyperlipidemia	34%	32%
Atrial arrhythmia	28%	33%
Vital signs on admission		
Median body weight (kg [25th, 75th percentile])	78.5 [65.8, 94.0]	78.9 [64.0, 97.5]
Mean heart rate (beats/min)	89 ± 22	85 ± 21
Mean SBP (mm Hg)	135 ± 31	149 ± 33
Mean DBP (mm Hg)	77 ± 19	76 ± 19
Etiology		
Ischemic	54%	38%
Hypertensive	17%	28%
Idiopathic	18%	21%
Findings on admission		
Acute pulmonary edema	3%	2%
Chest pain	23%	24%
Uncontrolled hypertension	9%	12%
Dyspnea at rest	44%	44%
Dyspnea on exertion	63%	62%
Rales	63%	65%
Lower extremity edema	62%	68%
Jugular venous pulsation	33%	26%
Left ventricular EF (mean)	24.3% ± 7.7%	54.7% ± 10.2%
Laboratory values		
Mean serum sodium (mEq/liter)	137.7 ± 4.6	137.9 ± 4.8
Median serum creatinine (mg/dL [25th, 75th percentile])	1.4 [1.1, 1.9]	1.3 [1.0, 1.8]
Mean serum hemoglobin (g/dL)	12.5 ± 2.0	11.9 ± 2.0
Median BNP (pg/mL [25th, 75th percentile])	1170.0 [603.0, 2280.0]	601.5 [320.0, 1190.0]
Median troponin I (ng/mL [25th, 75th percentile])	0.1 [0.1, 0.3]	0.1 [0.0, 0.3]

BNP = B-type natriuretic peptide; DBP = diastolic blood pressure; EF = ejection fraction; HFpEF = heart failure with preserved ejection fraction; LVSD = left ventricular systolic dysfunction; SBP = systolic blood pressure.

Modified from Fonarow GC, Stough WG, Abraham WT, et al: Characteristics, treatments, and outcomes of patients with preserved systolic function hospitalized for heart failure: A report from the OPTIMIZE-HF Registry. J Am Coll Cardiol 50:768, 2007.

1. New-onset or de novo HF (approximately 20% of all AHFS admissions). Patients in this group present for the first time with symptoms of HF. They may have no prior history of cardiovascular disease or risk factors (e.g., acute myocarditis); but more commonly, they have a background of risk factors for HF (HF stage A according to the ACC/AHA guidelines) or pre-existing structural heart disease (HF stage B according to the ACC/AHA guidelines). A substantial portion of these patients develop AHFS in the setting of acute coronary syndromes (ACS).
2. Worsening chronic HF. These patients have a history of chronic HF (HF stage C according to the ACC/AHA guidelines) and present with an episode of decompensation. This group accounts for the majority (approximately 80%) of patients hospitalized with AHFS. Such patients may have easily identifiable precipitants (see later) or no clear explanation for decompensation. A subgroup of these patients (10% to 15%) has advanced or end-stage HF defined as refractoriness to available therapies (ACC/AHA stage D). In these advanced HF patients, hospitalization may be triggered by severe chronic symptoms rather than by an abrupt change in clinical condition.

Several additional clinical profiles or scenarios that are based on clinical presentation and that may have implications for therapy have also been proposed recently. The schema of clinical profiles or scenarios[7] that have been adopted by the ESC 2008 guidelines subdivides AHFS into different clinical scenarios (**Table 27-3**),[8] including elevated blood pressure (>160 mm Hg), normal or moderately elevated blood pressure, low blood pressure (<90 mm Hg), flash pulmonary edema, cardiogenic shock, ACS, and isolated right-sided HF. Some of these clinical profiles or scenarios, such as pulmonary edema, hypertensive HF, and ACS, may overlap.

The EuroHeart Failure Survey II (EHFS II) quantified the proportion of patients hospitalized with HF who fit into different clinical scenarios[5]:

1. Worsening or decompensated chronic HF. This group is composed of patients with worsening signs and symptoms of congestion before hospitalization. They can have either preserved or reduced ejection fraction. In EHFS II, 65% of AHFS patients were included in this category.
2. Clinical pulmonary edema. Patients present with severe respiratory distress, hypoxemia, and radiographic congestion on chest radiography. In EHFS II, 16% of AHFS fit this profile. Much lower numbers were reported in the United States.
3. Hypertensive HF. In this group, hypertension can be triggered by a high sympathetic tone (reactive hypertension) due to worsening HF or hypertension may be the cause of HF. Patients in whom hypertension is the cause of HF are more likely to have a preserved systolic function and are less likely to have signs of congestion. They

TABLE 27-3 Clinical Scenarios at the Time of Presentation with Acute Heart Failure Syndromes

CLINICAL PRESENTATION	INCIDENCE	CHARACTERISTICS	TARGETS AND THERAPIES
Elevated blood pressure (>160 mm Hg)	~25%	Predominantly pulmonary (radiographic or clinical) with or without systemic congestion Many patients have preserved ejection fraction	Target: blood pressure and volume management Therapy: vasodilators (e.g., nitrates, nesiritide, nitroprusside) and loop diuretics
Normal or moderately elevated blood pressure	~50%	Develop gradually (days or weeks) and are associated with systemic congestion Radiographic pulmonary congestion may be minimal in patients with advanced HF	Target: volume management Therapy: loop diuretics ± vasodilators
Low blood pressure (<90 mm Hg)	<8%	Mostly related to low cardiac output and associated with decreased renal function	Target: cardiac performance Therapy: inotropes with vasodilatory properties (e.g., milrinone, dobutamine, levosimendan) Consider digoxin (IV or PO) ± vasopressor medications ± mechanical assist devices
Flash pulmonary edema	3%*	Abrupt onset Precipitated by severe systemic hypertension; uncorrected, respiratory failure and death ensue Patients are easily treated with vasodilators and diuretics After blood pressure normalization and reinstitution of routine medications, patients can be discharged within 24 hr	Target: blood pressure, volume management Therapy: vasodilators, diuretics, invasive or noninvasive ventilation, morphine
Cardiogenic shock	1%	Rapid onset Primarily complicating acute MI, fulminating myocarditis, acute valvular disease	Target: improve cardiac pump function Therapy: inotropes ± vasoactive medications ± mechanical assist devices (e.g., IABP), corrective surgery
ACS and AHFS	Approximately 25% of ACS have HF signs or symptoms	Rapid or gradual onset Many such patients may have signs and symptoms of HF that resolve after initial therapy or resolution of ischemia	Target: coronary thrombosis, plaque stabilization, correction of ischemia Therapy: reperfusion (e.g., PCI, lytics, nitrates, antiplatelet agents)
Isolated right-sided HF from pulmonary HTN or intrinsic RV failure (e.g., infarction)	?	Rapid or gradual onset due to primary or secondary pulmonary arterial hypertension or RV disease (e.g., RV infarction) Not well characterized; there are no epidemiologic data	Target: pulmonary artery pressure Therapy: epoprostenol, phosphodiesterase inhibitors, endothelin blocking agents

*The percentage in Europe is reported to be higher.
ACS = acute coronary syndromes; AHFS = acute heart failure syndromes; HF = heart failure; HTN = hypertension; IABP = intra-aortic balloon pump; MI = myocardial infarction; PCI = percutaneous coronary intervention; RV = right ventricular.
Modified from Gheorghiade M, Zannad F, Sopko G, et al: Acute heart failure syndromes: Current state and framework for future research. Circulation 112:3958, 2005.

respond rapidly to therapy and have low in-hospital mortality. In EHFS II, 11% of patients fit this profile.
4. Cardiogenic shock. This group presents with low blood pressure and signs of organ hypoperfusion in spite of adequate LV diastolic pressure. This presentation is uncommon (4% of AHFS presentations in EHFS II).
5. Isolated right-sided HF is characterized by systemic congestion, defined as jugular venous distention and edema and the absence of pulmonary radiographic or clinical congestion. Like cardiogenic shock, this is a relatively rare presentation of AHFS (3% of patients in EHFS II).
6. ACS and HF. The majority of patients present with chest discomfort, electrocardiographic changes suggestive of ischemia, and often a troponin level elevation. Among patients with ACS, approximately 10% to 20% have signs and symptoms of HF.

A similar classification with fewer categories has been proposed in the 2009 American College of Cardiology/American Heart Association (ACC/AHA) guidelines,[9] in which three clinical profiles describe the patient hospitalized with HF. These categories do not directly map to the categories proposed by the ESC guidelines, although similar general concepts are applicable in both sets of guidelines:

1. The patient with volume overload, manifested by pulmonary or systemic congestion, frequently precipitated by an acute increase in chronic hypertension.
2. The patient with profound depression of cardiac output, manifested by hypotension, renal insufficiency, or a shock syndrome.
3. The patient with signs and symptoms of both fluid overload and systemic hypoperfusion.

The Heart Failure Society of America guidelines do not provide a definition or classification of AHFS patients, given the ongoing changes in our understanding of the pathophysiology of these syndromes.[9b]

Finally, after the initial management and stabilization, it may be useful to classify patients on the basis of disease severity and the potential reversibility of cardiac abnormalities. One practical advantage of such a framework is that it has obvious and direct implications for therapy. This divides patients into those with (1) a correctable or partially correctable problem that had led to the development of AHFS (e.g., myocardial ischemia, primary valvular abnormalities, arrhythmias, dyssynchrony), (2) underlying chronic HF in which the trigger of the AHFS can be identified and treated, and (3) advanced or refractory HF. None of these classification schemes encompasses all potential causes of AHFS. Because HF is a "final common pathway" of many cardiovascular disorders, a variety of specific disorders (tachyarrhythmias or bradyarrhythmias, tamponade, ventricular septal defect) may lead to the development of AHF (**Table 27-4**). In each of these cases, the therapy is directed primarily at the underlying cause rather than at HF per se.

TABLE 27-4 Causes and Precipitating Factors of Acute Heart Failure Syndromes

Ischemic Heart Disease
Acute coronary syndromes
Mechanical complications of acute myocardial infarction
Right ventricular infarction
Valvular
Valve stenosis
Valvular regurgitation
Endocarditis
Aortic dissection
Myopathies
Postpartum cardiomyopathy
Acute myocarditis
Hypertension, Arrhythmia
Hypertension
Acute arrhythmia
Circulatory Failure
Septicemia
Thyrotoxicosis
Anemia
Shunts
Tamponade
Pulmonary embolism
Decompensation of Pre-existing Chronic HF
Lack of adherence
Volume overload
Pulmonary emboli
Infections, especially pneumonia
Cerebrovascular insult
Surgery
Renal dysfunction
Asthmas, chronic obstructive pulmonary disease
Drug abuse
Alcohol abuse

From Dickstein K, Cohen-Solal A, Filippatos G, et al: ESC Guidelines for the diagnosis and treatment of acute and chronic heart failure 2008. Eur Heart J 29:2388, 2008.

Pathophysiology

AHFS are not a single disease but a family of related disorders. The pathophysiology of AHFS is notably heterogeneous, with many overlapping pathogenetic mechanisms that may be operative in any given patient to a greater or lesser degree. This fundamental heterogeneity complicates the attempt to create a simple and unified conceptual model. Rather, the pathophysiology of AHF can be best understood as a variety of potential mechanisms that may contribute to varying degrees in an individual patient, resulting in a common set of clinical signs and symptoms (primarily related to congestion due to a very high LV filling pressure) that define the AHF. A potentially useful framework for understanding of the pathophysiology of AHF is to consider it as the result of the interaction of underlying substrate, initiating mechanisms, and amplifying mechanisms.

In this context, substrate refers to cardiac structure and function. The underlying substrate may be one of normal ventricular function, for example, patients without a prior history of HF who develop AHF because of sudden changes in ventricular function from an acute insult such as myocardial infarction or acute myocarditis. Alternatively, some patients may have no prior history of HF but abnormal substrate (e.g., stage B patients with asymptomatic LV dysfunction) with a first presentation of HF (de novo HF). Finally, most patients with AHF have a substrate of chronic compensated HF and then develop decompensation. Understanding of the underlying substrate is key to defining targets for therapy. Patients can be divided into those in whom causes of AHF are totally reversible, partially reversible, or mostly irreversible. It is reasonable to postulate that the majority of patients have at least some correctable cardiac problems when they are properly assessed with both noninvasive and invasive methods, such as echocardiography and cardiac catheterization.

Initiating mechanisms vary according to and interact with the underlying substrate and may be cardiac or extracardiac. For patients with normal substrate (normal myocardium), a substantial insult to cardiac performance (e.g., acute myocarditis) is required to lead to HF. For patients with abnormal substrate at baseline (asymptomatic LV dysfunction), smaller perturbations (e.g., poorly controlled hypertension, atrial fibrillation, or ischemia) may precipitate an AHF episode. For patients with a substrate of compensated or stable chronic HF, medical or dietary noncompliance, drugs such as nonsteroidal anti-inflammatory agents, and infectious processes are common triggers for decompensation.

Regardless of the substrate or initiating factors, a variety of "amplifying mechanisms," such as the neurohormonal activation, inflammatory mediators, ongoing myocardial injury, and worsening renal function, may contribute to the propagation and worsening of the AHF episode (**Fig. 27-1**).

Congestion in Acute Heart Failure Syndromes

Systemic or pulmonary congestion most often due to a high LV diastolic pressure is the hallmark of the clinical presentation of most patients hospitalized for AHF.[10] In this sense, congestion can be seen as a final common pathway by which mechanisms described in this section produce clinical symptoms leading to hospitalization. A simplified view of AHF pathophysiology is that gradual increases in intravascular volume lead to symptoms of congestion and clinical presentation, and normalization of volume status with diuretic therapy results in restoration of homeostasis. Whereas this mechanism may be operative in some patients (particularly those with frank noncompliance with sodium restriction or diuretic therapy), this model is a vast oversimplification. Congestion often occurs even in the absence of such nonadherence, and the same degree of nonadherence may not lead to decompensation in a given patient. Although some data suggest that increases in body weight often precede decompensation and hospitalization for HF,[11] careful studies using implantable hemodynamic monitors suggest that increases in invasively measured LV filling pressures could occur without substantial changes in body weight.[12] Although patients present with systemic or pulmonary "clinical congestion," defined as rales, elevated jugular venous pressure, and edema, this state is often preceded or followed after initial therapy by "hemodynamic congestion," defined as high LV diastolic pressures without overt clinical signs. Of note, in chronic HF, there is a poor correlation between hemodynamic and clinical congestion. In fact, the majority of patients with a high LV diastolic pressure do not have radiographic or clinical congestion. It has been postulated that hemodynamic congestion may contribute to the progression of HF because it may result in wall stress as well as in renin-angiotensin-aldosterone system (RAAS) activation. This may trigger a variety of molecular responses in the myocardium, including myocyte loss and increased fibrosis of the extracellular matrix. In addition, elevated diastolic filling pressures may decrease coronary perfusion pressure, resulting in subendocardial ischemia that may further exacerbate cardiac dysfunction.[10,13] This may be particularly deleterious in patients with arterial hypotension and epicardial obstructive CAD. Increased LV filling pressures can also lead to acute changes in ventricular architecture (more spherical shape), contributing to worsening mitral regurgitation. These mechanisms also play an important role in pathologic remodeling of the ventricle, a chronic process that may be accelerated by each episode of decompensation. Consistent with this paradigm is the well-established clinical observation that each hospitalization for AHF heralds a substantial worsening of the long-term prognosis,[14] an effect that appears additive with recurrent hospitalizations (**Fig. 27-2**).[15]

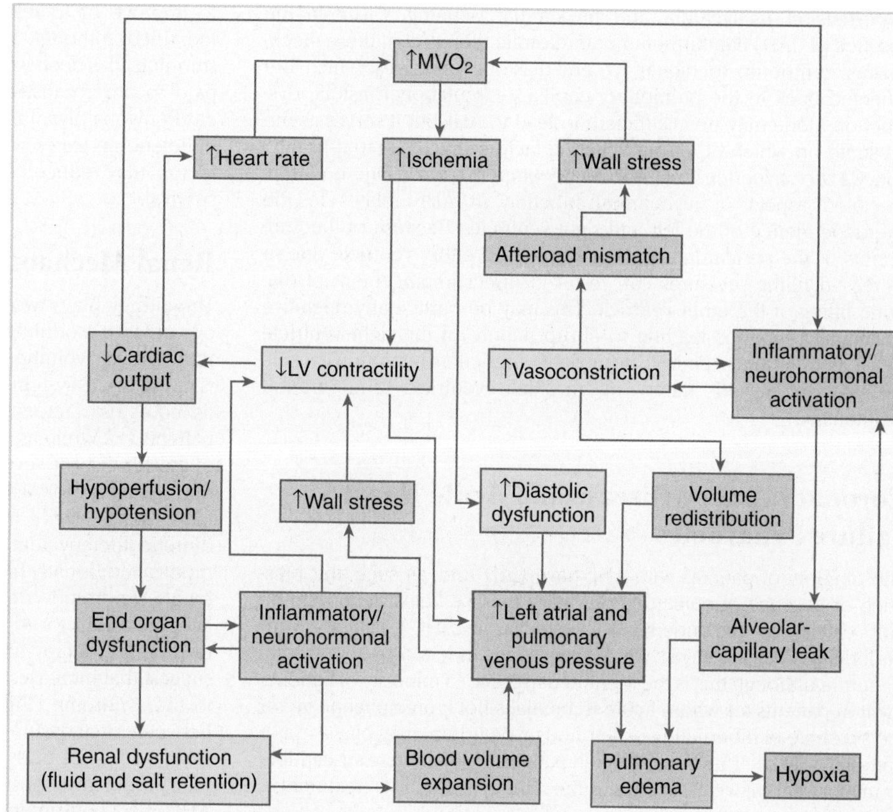

FIGURE 27-1 A schematic representation of the pathophysiology of acute heart failure. Cardiac (decreased contractility or increased diastolic dysfunction), vascular, or renal abnormalities are central to the pathophysiologic process, and each can independently cause acute heart failure. MVO_2 = myocardial oxygen consumption. *(From Teerlink J: Diagnosis and management of heart failure. In Libby P, Bonow RO, Mann DL, Zipes DP [eds]: Braunwald's Heart Disease. 8th ed. Philadelphia, Elsevier, 2008, pp 583-607.)*

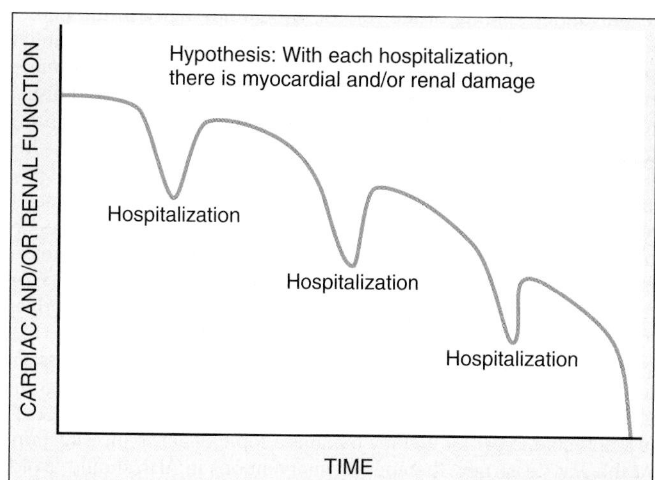

FIGURE 27-2 Acute heart failure syndromes and progression of heart failure. *(From Gheorghiade M, De Luca L, Fonarow GC, et al: Pathophysiologic targets in the early phase of acute heart failure syndromes. Am J Cardiol 96[Suppl]:11G, 2005.)*

Myocardial Function in Acute Heart Failure Syndromes (see Chaps. 24, 26, 28, and 30)

Although a variety of extracardiac factors play important roles in AHF, impairments of cardiac function (systolic, diastolic, or both) remain central to our understanding of this disorder. Changes in systolic function can initiate a cascade of deleterious effects including activation of the sympathetic nervous system and RAAS axis. This results in vasoconstriction, total body volume increase and redistribution from the periphery, increases in diastolic filling pressures, and clinical symptoms. Excessive and continuous neurohormonal activation contributes to ventricular remodeling and disease progression due to loss of myocytes (see Chap. 25). In patients with underlying ischemic heart disease, initial defects in systolic function may initiate a vicious circle of decreasing coronary perfusion and progressively worsening cardiac performance. If changes in myocardial systolic function are sudden or severe or if baseline systolic function is already severely impaired, patients may present with hypotension and end-organ hypoperfusion.

Although decreases in systolic function clearly play a role in the development of AHF in some cases, observational data show that approximately half of patients with AHF present with relatively preserved systolic function.[4,16] Abnormalities in diastolic function are present in patients with both preserved and impaired ejection fraction. The impairment of the diastolic phase may be related to passive stiffness, abnormal active relaxation of the left ventricle, or both.

Hypertension, tachycardia, and myocardial ischemia (even in the absence of CAD) can further impair diastolic filling. All of these mechanisms contribute to higher LV end-diastolic pressures, which are reflected back to the pulmonary capillary circulation. Diastolic dysfunction alone may be insufficient to lead to AHF, but it serves as the substrate on which other precipitating factors (such as atrial fibrillation, CAD, or hypertension) lead to decompensation.[17] One underappreciated aspect of myocardial function in AHF relates to the interdependence of the left and right ventricles. Because of the constraints of the pericardial space, distention of either ventricle due to increased filling pressures can result in direct impingement of diastolic filling of the other ventricle. This may be particularly operative in clinical scenarios leading to abrupt failure of the right ventricle (such as pulmonary embolism or right ventricular infarction), resulting in diminished filling of the left ventricle and arterial hypotension.

Coronary Artery Disease and Acute Heart Failure Syndromes (see Chaps. 52, 54, 56, and 57)

The majority of patients with AHF have CAD and, as such, the presence or absence of epicardial coronary disease helps define important categories of underlying substrates in AHF.[13] Patients with underlying CAD are at risk for AHF episodes induced by myocardial ischemia, although this is the identified trigger in a minority of patients. Even in patients for whom acute ischemia is not a precipitating factor, the substrate of hibernating or stunned myocardium may play a major pathophysiologic role because such patients may be more susceptible to myocardial injury as a result of the AHF episode or its treatment.

Myocardial Injury and Acute Heart Failure Syndromes

The availability of sensitive assays for circulating contractile proteins (such as troponin T and troponin I) has led to substantial evolution of our understanding of the role of myocardial injury in the pathophysiology of HF. Circulating troponins are elevated in a substantial proportion of patients with acute and chronic HF, even in the absence of clinically overt myocardial ischemia.[18-21] The precise mechanisms mediating myocardial injury in AHF are poorly defined, but increased myocardial wall stress, decreased coronary perfusion pressure, increased myocardial oxygen demand, endothelial dysfunction, activation of the neurohormonal and inflammatory axes, and platelet activation may all contribute to myocyte injury even in the absence of epicardial CAD. Specific therapeutic interventions that may increase myocardial oxygen demand (such as positive inotropic agents)[22] or decrease coronary artery perfusion pressure (such as some vasodilators)[23] may exacerbate myocardial injury and further contribute to the cycle of decompensation. The development of more sensitive assays for circulating troponin[18] will provide new insights into the significance of troponin elevation in HF. Whether myocardial injury in AHF is a potential target for therapy remains a topic of active investigation. At the very least, new therapeutic interventions in AHF should avoid exacerbating myocardial injury and contributing to the cycle of cardiac decompensation. The maintenance of adequate coronary perfusion is of paramount importance if injury is to be prevented.[24]

Viable but Dysfunctional Myocardium (see Chap. 52)

Patients with chronic HF and reduced ejection fraction are known to have variable degrees of viable but dysfunctional myocardium (VDM). Myocytes in VDM are potentially salvageable because they have not lost integrity of the cell membrane and mitochondria, and they exhibit preserved glucose metabolism and contractile reserve. Thus, partial or complete return of function can occur with appropriate therapy. For example, beta blockers and revascularization have been shown to improve or to restore contractility in patients in whom VDM is identified. Although VDM due to chronic ischemia (hibernation or stunning) has been well studied (see Chap. 52), less attention has been paid to other causes of VDM, particularly in patients with primary cardiomyopathies. In these conditions, it is possible that metabolic deficiencies, excessive sympathetic stimulation, and hemodynamic factors may reduce contractility without affecting short-term myocyte survival.

Renal Mechanisms in Acute Heart Failure

The kidney plays two fundamental roles relative to the pathophysiology of HF: it modulates loading conditions of the heart by controlling intravascular volume and is responsible for neurohormonal outputs (i.e., the RAAS system). Abnormalities of renal function are well established as risk factors for the progression and decompensation of HF patients.[25,26] Whereas impaired renal function may serve as a marker of greater disease severity, it is apparent that changes in renal function during therapy for AHF (cardiorenal syndrome) may also play a pathophysiologic role.[27] Impaired cardiac output and excessive loop diuretic therapy that may result in further activation of neurohormones traditionally have been considered major causes of the cardiorenal syndrome, defined as worsening renal function during hospitalization for AHF in spite of clinical improvement in response to diuretic therapy and adequate intravascular volume. Recent data suggest that increases in central venous pressures may also contribute to the syndrome (**Fig. 27-3**).[28,29] It may be important to distinguish between renal dysfunction (a potentially transient phenomenon often related to local or systemic hemodynamic factors) and frank renal injury. Both myocardial and renal injury during hospitalizations for AHFS may contribute to the progression of HF (see Fig. 27-1).

Vascular Mechanisms in Acute Heart Failure

Clinically, it is now well recognized that most patients with AHFS present with hypertension rather than with low blood pressure (see Table 27-3). In many, the increase in blood pressure is most likely driven by an increased LV filling pressure and further activation of the sympathetic nervous system and RAAS. In fact, there is a relatively rapid normalization and improvement of blood pressure in response to diuretic therapy. This type of hypertension, which has been called reactive hypertension, is an indirect measure of cardiac reserve and is associated with better prognosis. In contrast, in other patients, severe hypertension may be the cause rather than the result of AHF and may precipitate pulmonary edema. This "acute hypertensive emergency" occurs most frequently in patients with susceptible underlying substrate (e.g., diastolic dysfunction due to LV hypertrophy). In a given patient, the extent to which elevation of systemic vascular resistance is the cause or the effect of AHFS remains uncertain.[30]

Emerging Mechanisms in the Pathophysiology of Acute Heart Failure Syndromes

Inflammation. Like the neurohormonal pathways, inflammatory activation also appears to play a pathogenic role in the progression of HF, although this has not yet led to new therapies.[31] In animal models, changes in the balance of circulating proinflammatory and anti-inflammatory mediators can lead to increased diastolic stiffness and pulmonary capillary leakage, recapitulating many of the aspects of AHF.[32,33] In addition, inflammatory activation can lead to increases in vascular stiffness,[34] a known precipitant of AHF as described before. Clinical observations suggest that inflammatory markers are increased in AHF and can persist beyond apparent clinical stabilization.[35] Infections (in particular pulmonary infections) are a well-described clinical precipitant of HF hospitalizations.[36]

Abnormalities of the Natriuretic Peptide System. The natriuretic peptides (NP) type A (ANP) and B (BNP) play an important counterregulatory role in the pathogenesis of HF, with actions on the kidney, heart, and vasculature. Measurements of NP levels now play a pivotal role in the diagnosis and prognosis of patients with AHF.[37,38] Recent observations have shown that abnormal high-molecular-weight forms of NP with reduced biologic activity are identifiable in the circulation and may be the predominant circulating form in some patients with HF.[39-41] These findings suggest the hypothesis (not yet confirmed experimentally) that transition from a compensated to a decompensated state could be triggered by alterations of the NP system with progression of HF.

Platelet Activation. Platelet activation is central to the current understanding of the pathogenesis of the ACS. Platelet activation in HF may be due to a combination of factors, including enhanced sympathetic nervous system activity, RAAS activation, and inflammation. Pilot studies have suggested that various markers of platelet activation are increased in HF regardless of etiology, including increases in platelet aggregation and circulating levels of beta-thromboglobulin and P-selectin.[42,43] In addition to platelet activation, the known hypercoagulable state noted in patients with HF may contribute to the pathophysiology of AHFS by causing not only systemic embolic events, known to be rare, but also pulmonary emboli and coronary events that often are undetected clinically in this population of patients. This is the subject of ongoing investigations with newer and possibly safer antithrombotic agents.

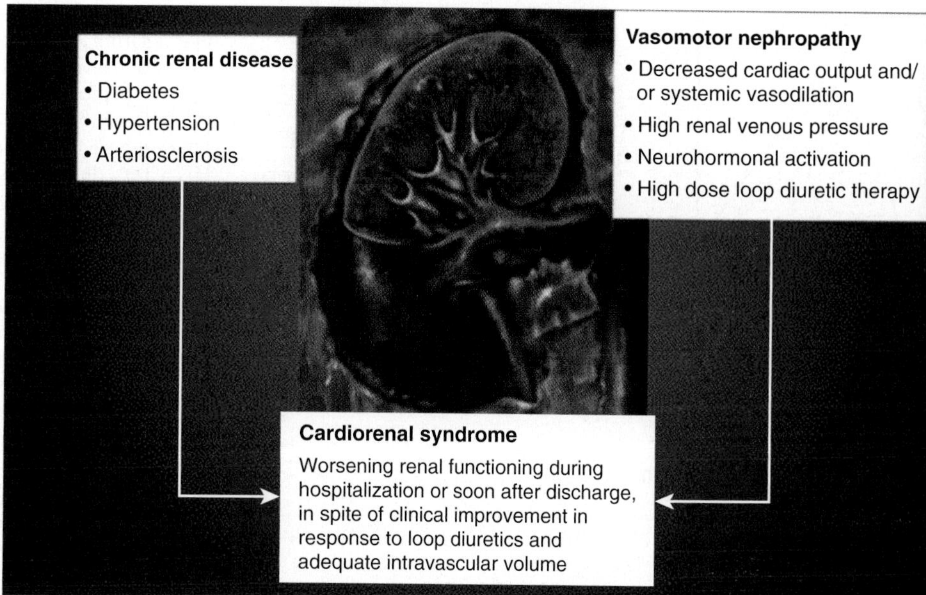

FIGURE 27-3 Cardiorenal syndrome in acute heart failure syndromes. *(From Gheorghiade M, Pang PS: Acute heart failure syndromes. J Am Coll Cardiol 53:557, 2009.)*

Clinical Triggers of Acute Heart Failure Syndromes

Whereas the preceding section focused on intrinsic mechanisms involved in the pathophysiology of AHF, a variety of specific identifiable clinical triggers may be identified as well (see Table 27-4). Although some of these triggers have long been recognized, only the recent advent of large observational registries has provided more definitive data on their relative contribution in the broader HF population. In the OPTIMIZE-HF registry comprising 48,612 patients, approximately 60% had an identifiable clinical precipitant, with pulmonary processes (15%), myocardial ischemia (15%), and arrhythmias (14%) being the most common.[36] Similar observational data from Europe show an even higher incidence of ischemia as a trigger, especially in patients presenting with low-output states and cardiogenic shock.[44]

Clinical Outcomes in Acute Heart Failure Syndromes

Hospital Course

Most available data suggest that inpatient mortality in AHFS ranges between 3% and 7%. One notable exception is in patients who present with cardiogenic shock, who have an extremely high in-hospital mortality rate (40% in EHFS II). There appear to be substantial geographic differences in level of care and hospital course between the United States and European countries.[45,46] Median length of stay in the United States is approximately 4 days, whereas lengths of stay in Europe are generally markedly longer (median of 9 days in EHFS II). In the U.S. ADHERE registry comprising 105,388, patients, 23% of patients were admitted to an intensive care unit setting, whereas a substantially higher proportion (51%) had an intensive care unit stay in EHFS II. Although systemic and pulmonary congestion is the main reason for hospitalization in most patients, many do not have a decrease in body weight during their hospital stay and are discharged with signs and symptoms of HF.[47] Often, a comprehensive assessment is not performed (e.g., cardiac catheterization), which may result in underuse of evidence-based therapies.[48] In patients admitted with worsening HF, introduction of new evidence-based therapies (e.g., angiotensin-converting enzyme [ACE] inhibitors) is less than 10%.[45]

Postdischarge Course

Mortality and rehospitalization rates postdischarge in patients admitted with HF may be as high as 15% and 30% within 60 to 90 days, respectively. Recent claims data using the U.S. Medicare sample suggest an even more striking rate of rehospitalization in elderly patients, with a 30-day rehospitalization rate of 27%.[49] Approximately 30% of patients hospitalized with HF and reduced ejection fraction die suddenly within several months after discharge, and 40% die of progressive HF in spite of receiving evidence-based therapy (**Fig. 27-4**).[50] Of note, approximately half of the rehospitalizations are not HF related.[50] Rates of early postdischarge events in patients with HFpEF appear to be similar to those in patients with reduced ejection fraction. However, the modes of death and reasons for rehospitalization have not been studied in the former group. It is possible that a significant number of morbid events in the HFpEF population are related to coexisting cardiac or noncardiac comorbidities, such as CAD, hypertension, atrial fibrillation, renal insufficiency, or stroke.[17]

Prognostic Models in Acute Heart Failure Syndromes

Given that rehospitalization drives much of the cost associated with AHFS, there has been increased interest in predicting risk of rehospitalization among payers and policy makers as a means to control health care costs. These risk stratification models can serve as important clinical tools by helping to identify those patients at both ends of the spectrum of risk; patients who are at very high risk may be observed more closely or treated more intensively, whereas patients at low risk may need less rigorous follow-up and monitoring.[51-51b] In addition to being clinical tools, these risk stratification models can serve to identify pathophysiologic targets for therapy. Important caveats in comparing risk models are that differences in populations, follow-up, and granularity of baseline data (e.g., claims data versus registries versus clinical trials) can all have substantial effects on the results obtained.

Predictive Models of In-Hospital Mortality

Data from the ADHERE registry have been used to develop a classification and regression tree (CART) analysis to identify the best predictors of in-hospital mortality and to develop a risk stratification model. Of

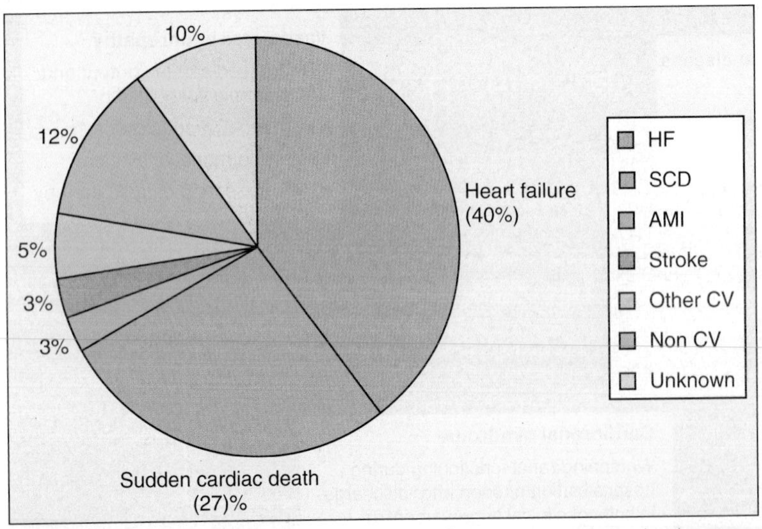

FIGURE 27-4 Postrandomization causes of death of 4,133 patients admitted with worsening HF and reduced ejection fraction in the EVEREST trial. The overall mortality at 9.9 months was 26%. *(From O'Connor CM, Miller AB, Blair JE, et al: Causes of death and rehospitalization in patients hospitalized with worsening heart failure and reduced left ventricular ejection fraction: Results from Efficacy of Vasopressin Antagonism in Heart Failure Outcome Study with Tolvaptan [EVEREST] program. Am Heart J 159:841, 2010.)*

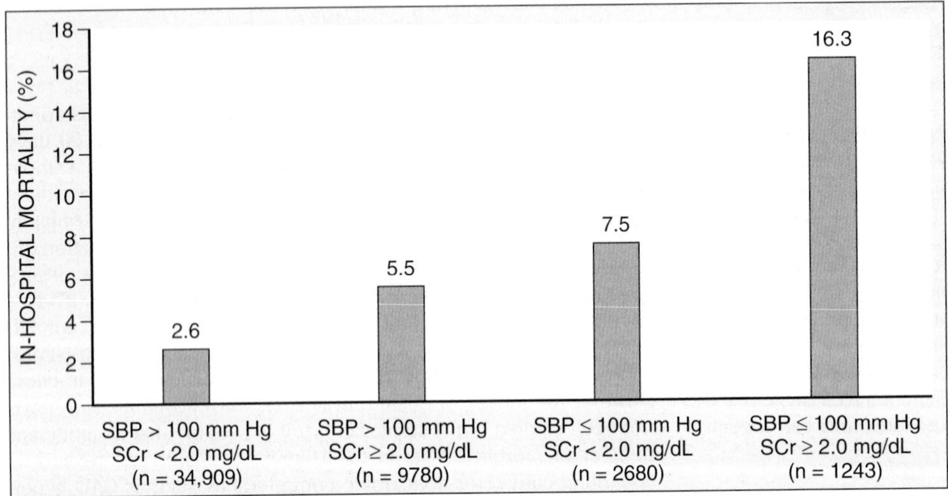

FIGURE 27-5 In-hospital mortality by serum creatinine (SCr) concentration and systolic blood pressure (SBP) in the ADHERE registry. *(From Abraham WT, Fonarow GC, Albert NM, et al: Predictors of in-hospital mortality in patients hospitalized for heart failure: Insights from the Organized Program to Initiate Lifesaving Treatment in Hospitalized Patients With Heart Failure [OPTIMIZE-HF]. J Am Coll Cardiol 52:347, 2008.)*

the 39 variables evaluated, the CART method identified elevated blood urea nitrogen (BUN), lower systolic blood pressure (SBP), and higher serum creatinine at the time of admission to be the best discriminators between hospital survivors and nonsurvivors. A similar model from the OPTIMIZE registry identified serum creatinine, SBP, age, heart rate, and serum sodium as the most powerful predictors of in-hospital mortality in AHFS.[52] A combination of two variables (creatinine concentration and SBP) that were powerful predictors in both ADHERE and OPTIMIZE-HF was able to risk stratify patients into risk groups (**Fig. 27-5**).

Predictive Models of Postdischarge Events

As noted before, there is a substantial risk of mortality or rehospitalization in the first 60 to 90 days after discharge in AHF patients. Some variables may predict mortality but not rehospitalization, and vice versa. In the cohort from the OPTIMIZE-HF study with 60- to 90-day follow-up data, the most important predictors for the combined endpoint of death or rehospitalization were admission serum creatinine concentration, SBP, admission hemoglobin level, discharge use of ACE inhibitor or angiotensin receptor blocker (ARB), and pulmonary disease.[53] In the EVEREST trial, composed of patients admitted with worsening HF and reduced ejection fraction, independent predictors during hospitalization of readmission and mortality included low admission Kansas City Cardiomyopathy Questionnaire (KCCQ) score, high BNP, hyponatremia, tachycardia, hypotension, absence of beta blocker therapy, and history of diabetes and arrhythmias.[54] When patients were examined at 1 week after discharge, patients not receiving a beta-blocker, or those with rales, pedal edema, hyponatremia, lower creatinine clearance, higher brain natriuretic peptide, and worse health status were at significant risk for rehospitalization and death.[51]

Specific Prognostic Indicators

Blood Pressure. In a detailed analysis of SBP in patients from the OPTIMIZE-HF study, there was a relatively monotonic relationship between blood pressure and mortality across the spectrum of blood pressure (**Table 27-5**), with no evidence of increased risk even at very high levels of blood pressure (>180 mm Hg).[30] One notable feature of this analysis is that even SBP in the "normal range" (120 to 139 mm Hg) was associated with increased risk compared with patients with higher blood pressure, with a combined in-hospital and postdischarge mortality of 12%. However, the readmission rate was approximately 30% and was independent of admission pressure.

Renal Function. Renal function (estimated by BUN, creatinine, and glomerular filtration rate) is an important predictor of prognosis in patients with AHFS. There appears to be a substantial increase in risk of both mortality and rehospitalization in patients who develop worsening of renal function during hospitalization. Worsening renal function soon after discharge, which occurs in about 15% to 20% of patients, also is an important predictor of early readmission and mortality.[55]

Natriuretic Peptides and Troponins. BNP and N-terminal pro-BNP (NT-proBNP) have been demonstrated to be powerful predictors of risk in HF. In the setting of AHFS, NP levels at initial presentation are important predictors of both short-term and long-term outcomes. In the PRIDE study of patients presenting to the emergency department with unexplained dyspnea, a single NT-proBNP value at initial presentation was an independent predictor of mortality out to 1 year.[56] In the ADHERE registry, admission BNP level was a significant predictor of in-hospital mortality in patients with reduced or preserved ejection fraction.[57]

Cardiac troponins also provide prognostic information in patients with AHFS. The ADHERE registry demonstrated a marked increase in in-hospital mortality (8.0% versus 2.7%) in patients with an elevated troponin level by any clinical assay at the time of hospitalization.[58] Similarly, You and colleagues[59] reported data from the EFFECT study showing that elevated troponin (troponin I > 0.5 ng/mL) is associated with increased mortality even after multivariate adjustment and demonstrated a dose-response relationship between the magnitude of circulating troponin and outcomes. The combination of elevation in NP levels and troponin elevation appears to portend a particularly poor prognosis.[60] To date, attempts to improve outcomes by targeting HF prognostic markers, such as BNP, with therapies not known to affect outcomes have not proved effective.[61]

Hyponatremia. Approximately 25% of patients admitted with HF have mild, usually dilutional or hypervolemic hyponatremia, defined as a serum sodium concentration <135 mmol/liter, independent of their ejection fraction.[62] Hyponatremia is not usually corrected during hospitalization. In spite of a similar clinical response during hospitalization,

TABLE 27-5 Outcomes in Patients Admitted with Acute Heart Failure Syndromes by Systolic Blood Pressure

	Admission Systolic Blood Pressure			
	<120 mm Hg (N = 10,525)	120-139 mm Hg (N = 10,276)	140-161 mm Hg (N = 10,263)	>161 mm Hg (N = 10,161)
In-Hospital Mortality (%)				
LVSD	6.6	3.1	2.5	1.6
No LVSD	6.2	3.2	2.0	1.4
Mean/Median Length of Stay (days)				
LVSD	6.8/5.0	5.8/4.0	5.6/4.0	5.1/4.0
No LVSD	6.5/5.0	5.9/5.0	5.6/4.0	5.3/4.0
	(N = 1336)*	(N = 1259)*	(N = 1397)*	(N = 1113)*
Postdischarge Mortality (%)				
LVSD	13.0	6.8	6.3	4.1
No LVSD	14.9	10.0	4.7	4.7
60- to 90-Day Rehospitalization (%)				
LVSD	31.5	28.6	32.4	25.5
No LVSD	29	31.6	28.4	28.2

LVSD = left ventricular systolic dysfunction.
Modified from Gheorghiade M, Abraham WT, Albert NM, et al: Systolic blood pressure at admission, clinical characteristics, and outcomes in patients hospitalized with acute heart failure. JAMA 296:2217, 2006.
*Only a subset of patients (12%) were followed after hospital discharge.

patients discharged with hyponatremia have a significantly high risk for mortality and rehospitalization after discharge.[63]

BODY WEIGHT. Increased body weight is an important contributor to hospitalization in ambulatory patients with HF. Although the majority of patients, once admitted with AHF, have a significant decrease in body weight during hospitalization, many increase their body weight soon after discharge. It appears that an increase in body weight early or late after the discharge period is an independent major predictor for rehospitalization but not for mortality.[64] Improved outcomes as a result of body weight reduction will likely depend on the mechanisms used to remove the fluid and will need to balance potential adverse effects of the therapeutic intervention.

QRS DURATION. Between 30% and 40% of patients admitted with AHFS and a reduced ejection fraction have a prolonged QRS, defined as a duration ≥120 milliseconds. Prolonged QRS is a marker of LV dyssynchrony and is an independent predictor of increased postdischarge morbidity and mortality in spite of optimal medical therapy including ACE inhibitors or ARBs.[65]

CORONARY ARTERY DISEASE (see Chaps. 28 and 57)**.** Patients with CAD have a worse prognosis compared with non-CAD patients. It appears that revascularization and therapies for CAD may cancel those differences during the postdischarge period. Knowledge of the extent and severity of CAD and the presence of ischemic, stunned, or hibernating myocardium may influence the initial and in-hospital management of the patient.[48,66]

ARRHYTHMIAS. The incidence of new ventricular or supraventricular arrhythmias during hospitalizations of HF patients has not been well characterized. Of the 949 patients in the OPTIME-HF study, approximately 6% developed new, sustained arrhythmias; of these, 50% were atrial fibrillation or flutter and the remaining sustained ventricular arrhythmias. The mortality during index hospitalization was 26% in the arrhythmias group and 1.8% in the group with no new arrhythmias. Similarly, death or rehospitalization at 60 days was 35% in the new arrhythmias group compared with 8.2% in the remaining patients.[67]

UNTOWARD EFFECTS OF PHARMACOLOGIC TREATMENT OF AHFS. Data from registries and clinical trials have shown that the use of high-dose diuretics and of inodilators such as milrinone, levosimendan, and dobutamine, even for short periods, may be associated with an increased postdischarge mortality.[1] This occurred particularly in patients with CAD, in whom these agents caused a significant reduction of blood pressure.

Assessment of Acute Heart Failure Syndromes

A thorough assessment including physical examination, laboratory data, and the performance of ancillary tests is critical to optimize the management of AHFS (see Chap. 26). As discussed later, AHFS encompass multiple conditions and require in-depth diagnostic workup for successful treatment to be achieved.

Initial Presentation

SYMPTOMS. The most common symptoms in patients presenting with AHFS relate to systemic and pulmonary congestion, and dyspnea is usually the main reason to seek medical attention. In the ADHERE registry, dyspnea was the presenting symptom in 89% of the patients, whereas fatigue was the cause of hospitalization in only 31% of patients. The URGENT registry has shown that dyspnea improves relatively rapidly but not completely with the initial management. However, many patients continue to have orthopnea or dyspnea with minimal exertion during the first days of hospitalization, which can be missed if not provoked.[68]

BLOOD PRESSURE. Measurement of blood pressure is one of the most important steps in the initial assessment of AHFS patients. Blood pressure defines the clinical profiles that guide management strategies (see Chap. 27 Online Supplement). Systolic and diastolic blood pressure, pulse pressure, and orthostatic changes are relevant in the evaluation of patients and may provide valuable insights into the pathophysiology of AHFS. SBP is usually normal or high (≥140 mm Hg); approximately 10% of patients have values of SBP ≥180 mm Hg. Only a minority of patients have systolic hypotension, defined as <90 mm Hg. In patients presenting with high SBP, the pressure increase may be related to an enhanced sympathetic tone triggered by elevated LV filling pressure (reactive hypertension). In fact, these patients are relatively normotensive soon after the initial therapy. In contrast, a minority of patients will be resistant to initial therapy and require arterial vasodilators. Elevated diastolic blood pressure (DBP) suggests the presence of enhanced sympathetic tone. In contrast, low DBP is usually an index of peripheral vasodilation, suggesting the presence of high-output HF caused by conditions such as hyperthyroidism and arteriovenous fistula. Pulse pressure is usually elevated in patients with aortic insufficiency, anemia, and other high-output states. When it is decreased, it reflects a low cardiac output associated with systemic vasoconstriction and predicts a 2.5-fold increase in risk of death in patients with AHFS.[69]

BLOOD PRESSURE IN RESPONSE TO PROVOCATIVE TESTING. In patients with severely reduced ejection fraction and elevated LV filling pressure, there may be no decrease or even an increase in blood pressure when they assume an upright position. This may be explained by an improvement in LV performance, probably as a result of improved subendocardial perfusion or reduced mitral regurgitation due to a decreased LV diastolic pressure. Orthostatic hypotension (defined by a fall >20 mm Hg in SBP or >10 mm Hg in DBP in response to moving from a supine to a standing position within 3 minutes) is suggestive of volume depletion. This may be a useful tool to monitor diuretic therapy and to prevent excessive diuresis. The specificity of this sign is reduced in patients with autonomic neuropathy. Blood pressure measurements during a Valsalva maneuver may suggest the presence of elevated LV filling pressure.[70]

EXAMINATION (see Chap. 26). The general examination and vital signs will give important clues about the presence of respiratory distress, oxygenation, volume status, nutritional status, or stigmata from an underlying disorder. An altered mental status may be a marker of brain hypoperfusion. The patient is usually tachypneic, looks pale and diaphoretic, and is unable to lie flat.

Examination of the neck should focus on jugular pulse, which allows the estimation of venous pressure. Jugular venous pressure (JVP) is a direct measure of right atrial pressure and is expressed in centimeters of water. The majority of patients admitted with AHFS have elevated JVP, which usually reflects elevated LV filling pressure. However, the JVP is not an indicator of increased LV diastolic pressure in patients with isolated right-sided HF. Visual inspection of the anterior chest may reveal a dyskinetic area over the precordium, which may suggest the presence of an LV aneurysm. On palpation, the point of maximal impulse may be displaced, reflecting an enlarged heart. A late diastolic sound (S_4) can often be heard in patients with HF and preserved systolic function, when in sinus rhythm. In contrast, an early diastolic sound (S_3) is highly specific for a reduced ejection fraction. A systolic murmur is often present in patients with dilated left ventricle and low ejection fraction and is usually related to secondary mitral insufficiency. However, the severity of mitral regurgitation, particularly in the acute setting, may not correlate with the intensity of the murmur. Lung examination may reveal important clues about the patient's volume status and the presence of pulmonary congestion. Percussion of the posterior chest may elicit dullness at one or both lung bases, although more often on the right than on the left, indicating pleural effusion secondary to HF rather than to other causes. Inspiratory crackles are heard in a majority of patients with AHFS, which suggests elevated LV filling pressure and alveolar transudation.[47] Crackles or rales may be absent in patients admitted with longstanding and severe HF in spite of a high LV diastolic pressure.

Examination of the abdomen may also yield important findings in support of a diagnosis of volume overload. Inspection may reveal the presence of ascites, usually associated with severe right-sided HF. At palpation, hepatomegaly may be present and is usually secondary to liver congestion due to an increase in central venous pressure. At presentation, the majority of patients with AHFS are found to have peripheral edema. The edema should be considered a sign of HF only when it is associated with an elevated JVP. During hospitalization, lower extremity edema often may appear to improve or to disappear even though the body weight does not substantially decrease. This may be due to fluid redistribution to other dependent areas of the body, such as the sacrum, secondary to prolonged bed rest. In this setting, lower extremity edema may not necessarily correlate with the intravascular volume.

A grading tool has recently been introduced to help in the initial evaluation and in the follow-up of congestion in patients with AHF (**Table 27-6**).

Diagnostic Aids in the Evaluation of Patients with Suspected Acute Heart Failure Syndromes

Given the complexity of the pathophysiology of AHFS, the frequent occurrence of comorbidities, and the need for an accurate differential diagnosis, a number of laboratory and diagnostic tests are often employed in the initial evaluation and management of patients presenting with AHFS, as suggested by the existing guidelines.[8]

COMMON LABORATORY TESTS

Serum Electrolytes

Mild abnormalities in serum electrolytes are a frequent occurrence in patients with AHFS and can be related to neurohormonal imbalance or side effects from medications. Hyponatremia is commonly encountered, and about 25% of patients are found to have a serum sodium concentration <135 mEq/liter. More marked decreases in sodium levels are less prevalent, and only about 5% of patients present with sodium levels <130 mEq/liter. Despite the widespread use of diuretics, potassium levels are found to be <3.6 mEq/liter in only approximately 3% of presenting patients. A slightly higher proportion of patients (approximately 8%) have hyperkalemia, defined as serum potassium concentration >5.5 mEq/liter.[71] Diabetes, chronic kidney disease, ACE inhibitors, ARBs, and aldosterone blocking agents may all increase the risk for hyperkalemia.

Renal Function Tests

Renal function tests are among the most important laboratory evaluations in the assessment of patients with AHFS. A disproportionate increase in BUN levels compared with serum creatinine concentration is often a sign of renal hypoperfusion due to a low cardiac output in

TABLE 27-6 Grading of Congestion

	Score				
VARIABLE	−1	0	1	2	3
Bedside Assessment					
Orthopnea*		None	Mild	Moderate	Severe or worst
JVP (cm)	<8 and no hepatojugular reflux		8-10 or hepatojugular reflux	11-15	>16
Hepatomegaly	Absent in the setting of normal JVP	Absent	Liver edge	Moderate pulsatile enlargement	Massive tender enlargement extending to midline
Edema		None	1+	2+	3+/4+
Laboratory					
Natriuretic peptides (one)					
BNP		<100	100-299	300-500	>500
NT-proBNP		<400	400-1500	1500- 3000	>3000
Dynamic Maneuvers					
Orthostatic testing	Significant decrease in SBP or increase in heart rate	No change in SBP or heart rate			
6-minute walk test		No difficulty	Mild	Moderate	Severe or worst
6-minute walk test	>400 m	300-400 m	200-300 m	100-200 m	<100 m
Valsalva maneuver	Normal response		Absent overshoot pattern	Square wave pattern	

Congestion grade: <1, none; 1-7, mild; 8-14, moderate; 15-20, severe. Edema: in the absence of other cause of edema.

*Orthopnea: 0, absent; 1, mild (use of one pillow); 2, moderate (use of more than one pillow); 3, severe: sleeps in an armchair on in a sitting position.

Modified from Gheorghiade M, Follath F, Ponikowski P, et al: Assessing and grading congestion in acute heart failure. A Scientific Statement from the Acute Heart Failure Committee of the Heart Failure Association of the European Society of Cardiology and endorsed by the European Society of Intensive Care Medicine. Eur J Heart Fail 12:423, 2010.

the setting of a high LV filling pressure. This ratio may also be a sign of decreased intravascular volume in response to large doses of diuretics. Renal hypoperfusion may be the result of marked neurohormonal activation leading to increases in proximal sodium reabsorption and a parallel rise in urea reabsorption. Because creatinine handling is not affected, the BUN/creatinine ratio is increased. Plasma creatinine levels will increase only if the degree of hypovolemia is severe enough to lower the glomerular filtration rate. Abnormal renal function may develop as a result of therapies with ACE inhibitors or ARBs and in patients receiving nonsteroidal anti-inflammatory agents.

Liver Function Tests

Approximately 30% of patients admitted with HF have abnormal liver function test results. These abnormalities appear not to change or to improve slightly during hospitalization, in spite of improvement in congestion as reflected by significant decreases in body weight and edema.[72,73] The presence of liver dysfunction may have a significant impact on AHFS because it can be associated with reduced metabolism of aldosterone.

Hematologic Parameters

In the OPTIMIZE registry, low hemoglobin (<12.1 g/dL) was present in about 50% of patients.[74] Approximately half of them had hemoglobin levels between 5 and 10.7 g/dL. Patients in this group were older, were more often women, and had preserved systolic function and elevated creatinine. Hemodilution may also contribute to low hemoglobin concentration.

Natriuretic Peptides and Other Neurohormones (see Chap. 26)

The NPs are a family of important counterregulatory hormones in HF with vasodilatory, lusitropic, antifibrotic, and natriuretic effects.[75,76] These actions antagonize the vasoconstrictive and profibrotic effects of other neurohormones. The prohormone pro-BNP is secreted from myocytes in response to stretch and then cleaved in the plasma into active peptide (BNP) and a biologically inert N-terminal fragment (NT-proBNP). Circulating levels of NPs generally mirror elevation of ventricular filling pressures in HF patients. Data from national registries show that levels of BNP and NT-proBNP are markedly elevated at the time of admission.[3] Both markers may aid in the differential diagnosis of patients presenting in the emergency department with dyspnea. Data regarding use of NT-proBNP as a diagnostic tool in patients with dyspnea mirror those for BNP. NT-proBNP levels of <300 pg/mL have a 98% negative predictive value for a diagnosis of HF. Reductions in BNP >30% during hospitalization have been associated with an improvement in postdischarge outcomes.[77] NP levels may be low in obesity, very early presentation with AHFS, and acute mitral regurgitation. Bearing these potential pitfalls in mind, BNP testing should not be approached as a stand-alone marker but should be interpreted within a comprehensive clinical evaluation. Besides the NPs, the circulating levels of a number of other hormones, such as aldosterone and copeptin, have been found to be elevated in patients presenting with AHFS.[78] The clinical value of measuring hormones other than NPs has yet to be determined.

COMMON DIAGNOSTIC TESTS

Chest Radiography (see Chap. 16)

Chest radiography is a standard test in the emergency department evaluation of patients with dyspnea or other respiratory symptoms. Radiographic pulmonary congestion is present in approximately 80% of patients presenting with AHFS.[79] However, the absence of radiographic pulmonary congestion does not exclude the presence of a high pulmonary capillary wedge pressure (PCWP).

Electrocardiography (see Chap. 13)

The electrocardiogram is abnormal in most AHF patients, with sinus tachycardia being the most common finding. Approximately 20% to 30% of patients present with atrial fibrillation. A significant proportion of electrocardiograms show conduction abnormalities with wide QRS complex, mostly due to left bundle branch block.[65]

Echocardiography (see Chaps. 15 and 26)

Echocardiography with Doppler study is one of the most important noninvasive tests in the in-hospital evaluation of AHF patients. It allows the accurate assessment of chamber size, left and right ventricular systolic function, LV diastolic function, wall motion abnormalities, valvular structure and function, pericardial effusion, and hemodynamics. In combination with exercise or pharmacologic stress testing, it can evaluate functional capacity and the presence of ischemia, and it can assess contractile reserve in patients with depressed ejection fraction. An important aspect of contractile reserve is its ability to predict the potential for improvement in LV function in response to different treatments.[80] In patients with obstructive CAD, it allows identification of hibernating or stunned myocardium due to chronic ischemia, directing clinicians toward the use of invasive strategies when feasible.

Cardiac Magnetic Resonance Imaging (see Chaps. 18 and 26)

Cardiac magnetic resonance imaging (MRI) has become a valuable complement to echocardiography in the evaluation of cardiac anatomy and function. Because of its ability to detect myocardial scarring and infiltration, MRI has become the imaging modality of choice for the differential diagnosis of cardiomyopathies. In addition, when the intravenous administration of gadolinium is not contraindicated by renal impairment, areas of infarction can be detected with high resolution, and the extent of residual myocardial viability can be determined. A major current limitation of MRI is that this method cannot be used in patients who have implanted electrical devices, such as implantable cardiac defibrillators (ICDs) or pacemakers.[81]

Nuclear Studies (see Chaps. 17 and 26)

Nuclear studies may have a role in the evaluation of AHFS patients in whom an ischemic etiology is suspected. In addition, rest-redistribution studies may identify areas of VDM. Exercise or pharmacologic stress nuclear SPECT imaging with thallium Tl 201 or technetium Tc 99 may detect ischemia or previous myocardial infarction and also assess LV function.

Pulmonary Artery Catheter

Despite the advances of noninvasive modalities to assess hemodynamic parameters, the use of a pulmonary artery catheter (PAC) may be necessary in selected patients to obtain a more accurate and comprehensive hemodynamic profile during hospitalization. The PAC allows direct measurement of right atrial and ventricular pressures, pulmonary artery pressure, and PCWP and calculation of cardiac output and systemic vascular resistance. The Evaluation Study of Congestive Heart Failure and Pulmonary Artery Catheterization Effectiveness (ESCAPE) evaluated the role of a PAC in patients hospitalized with AHFS.[82] Patients who were deemed by the investigator to require a PAC were not entered in this study. Although the use of a PAC was not associated with major complications, this intervention did not contribute to a decrease in length of hospital stay, postdischarge readmission rate, or mortality. The results of this trial have sparked a considerable debate and have led to a significant decline in PAC use. Nevertheless, invasive hemodynamic monitoring with a PAC still represents a valuable tool and should be considered in the setting of a myocardial infarction complicated by HF, hypotension (particularly in the presence of renal hypoperfusion), and patients refractory to therapy. It should be considered in patients receiving intravenous vasodilators such as sodium nitroprusside or intravenous inotropes other than digoxin.

Management of Acute Heart Failure Syndromes

A patient's hospital stay provides an opportunity to identify and to treat correctable causes of HF and to alter its downhill course. A summary of the concepts that should guide the management of AHF patients is depicted in **Table 27-7**. As described in detail in previous sections, the hemodynamic abnormalities characteristic of AHFS are

CH 27

TABLE 27-7 Concepts in the Management of Acute Heart Failure Syndromes

1. The severity of clinical presentation of AHFS does not always correlate with long-term outcomes.
   Patients with preserved ejection fraction presenting with severe symptoms, such as pulmonary edema, once treated may have an excellent prognosis; in contrast, other patients presenting with minimal symptoms but severely compromised left ventricular ejection fraction may have very poor overall prognosis.
2. LV dysfunction and its progression are the main cause of the high rehospitalization rates and of the mortality observed in HF.
   Accordingly, the main goal of management is to improve or to restore LV function or at least to prevent further worsening.
3. Hemodynamic improvement should result from amelioration of myocardial dysfunction rather than from myocardial stimulation that may result in myocardial injury.
   Inotropic therapies should therefore be used only when absolutely necessary.
4. Viable but dysfunctional myocardium, which may potentially be salvageable, is presumably present in a number of patients with AHFS and may represent an important target for therapy.
5. Myocardial or kidney injury may occur during an episode of AHF and may contribute to the progression of HF.
   Accordingly, in addition to achieving clinical and hemodynamic improvement, AHFS management should also prevent or limit cardiac or renal injury.
6. Hospitalization for AHFS often represents a turning point in the clinical course of HF patients and portends high risk of readmission and poor prognosis.
   This may be due in part to persistence of hemodynamic and neurohormonal abnormalities after treatment, in spite of significant clinical improvement.
7. Limitations of current management include the following:
   Therapies aiming to improve signs, symptoms, and hemodynamics, such as diuretics, vasodilators, and inotropes, may theoretically precipitate or aggravate myocardial and kidney injury.
   Proven therapies for chronic HF, such as beta blockers, ACE inhibitors, and ARBs, may worsen hemodynamics and kidney function.
8. The implementation of current performance measures does not always appear to improve postdischarge outcomes.

the result of complex cardiac and noncardiac abnormalities. Accordingly, the in-hospital management of AHFS not only should improve hemodynamics but also should identify and treat the reversible causes of myocardial dysfunction and prevent further myocyte damage, diagnose and treat the initiating mechanisms (e.g., atrial fibrillation, myocardial ischemia), and identify amplifying mechanisms (e.g., inflammation) and implement strategies to limit their negative effects.

Phases of Management

There are three phases of AHFS management. Phase I deals primarily with urgent treatment and stabilization, most often occurring in the emergency department. Phase II consists of the continued in-hospital management. Phase III, often referred to as the vulnerable phase, focuses on close monitoring during the early postdischarge period, the importance of which is becoming increasingly recognized.[51a] The overall goals of AHFS management are a prompt diagnostic workup and safe and effective treatment with rapid resolution of symptoms and signs (phase I), followed by identification and treatment of correctable causes of HF and implementation of evidence-based treatments known to improve outcomes (phases II and III; see also Guidelines: Management of Heart Failure). To achieve these goals, a seamless integration of the various phases of management with a high level of coordination between the in-hospital and postdischarge caregivers is necessary.

Phase I: Management in the Emergency Department

The main therapeutic goals of the initial phase of management are to promptly recognize and treat life-threatening conditions, to identify and correctly diagnose the initiating mechanisms and provide specific treatment, and to provide symptom relief rapidly and safely (**Fig. 27-6**). For most patients, this phase occurs in the emergency department.[83] Early management should take into consideration whether a given patient presents with worsening chronic HF or with the first episode of HF. In the latter case, a patient is more likely to have a specific cause of HF, such as an acute myocardial infarction. Given that measurement of blood pressure is readily available at the time of initial evaluation and is important for both management and prognostication, patients may be divided into three groups: hypertensive, defined as SBP >160 mm Hg; normotensive; and hypotensive, defined as SBP <90 mm Hg. Within each group, on the basis of blood pressure at presentation, patients may present with different clinical scenarios, such as pulmonary edema, ACS, or isolated right-sided failure. For each scenario, specific therapies may be required (**Fig. 27-7**; see Chap. 27 Online Supplement). Insofar as dyspnea is the most common complaint in AHFS patients, the initial management of uncomplicated AHFS usually starts with treatment of these respiratory issues.

OXYGEN AND INTRAVENOUS MORPHINE. These therapies can be effective in relieving dyspnea, particularly when pulmonary edema and hypertension are present. Oxygen should be administered as early as possible by a nasal cannula or facemask. In patients with obstructive pulmonary disease, high concentrations of oxygen should not be used to avoid the risk of respiratory depression and worsening hypercapnia. For more severe forms of hypoxia (Sa_{O_2} <90%) and in the presence of acute cardiogenic pulmonary edema, noninvasive ventilation with positive end-expiratory pressure (PEEP) should be started as early as possible. Morphine may be particularly useful in the early stage of the treatment of severe AHF, especially if the patients are anxious or have chest discomfort.[84] However, morphine use has been associated with increased likelihood of mechanical ventilation, intensive care unit admission, and prolonged hospital stay in some retrospective analyses. The ESC guidelines recommend the administration of an intravenous bolus of 2.5 to 5 mg as soon as an intravenous line is inserted; the same doses can be repeated as required. Morphine should be used cautiously or avoided in the presence of hypotension, bradycardia, advanced atrioventricular block, or carbon dioxide retention.[8]

NONINVASIVE VENTILATION. Noninvasive ventilation has been shown to reduce respiratory distress and to improve LV function by reducing afterload. Either continuous positive airway pressure (CPAP) or noninvasive intermittent positive-pressure ventilation (NIPPV) can be used. Initial clinical studies and a meta-analyses suggest that in patients with cardiogenic pulmonary edema, treatment with CPAP or NIPPV improves symptoms and physiologic variables and markedly reduces need for invasive ventilation and mortality.[85] The Three Interventions in Cardiogenic Pulmonary Oedema (3CPO) trial enrolled patients with pulmonary edema who were randomized to standard oxygen therapy, CPAP, or NIPPV (**Table 27-8**).[86] At 7 days, noninvasive ventilation with CPAP or NIPPV was not associated with a mortality benefit or a decreased need for intubation compared with standard oxygen therapy. However, noninvasive ventilation was associated with greater improvement in patient-reported dyspnea, heart rate, acidosis, and hypercapnia. The ESC guidelines recommend the use of CPAP with an initial PEEP of 5 to 7.5 cm H_2O with uptitration to 10 cm H_2O if needed; the Fi_{O_2} should be ≥0.40 for cardiogenic pulmonary edema. This therapy may be repeated until the improvement in the patient's dyspnea and oxygen saturation remains stable off treatment.[8] Contraindications to the use of noninvasive ventilation include immediate need for endotracheal intubation (inability to protect the airways, life-threatening hypoxia) and lack of cooperation by the patient (altered sensorium, unconsciousness, anxiety, inability to tolerate mask). Caution should be used in patients with cardiogenic shock, right ventricular failure, and severe obstructive airways disease. Potential side effects and complications include anxiety, claustrophobia, dry mucous membranes, worsening right ventricular failure, hypercapnia, pneumothorax, and aspiration.

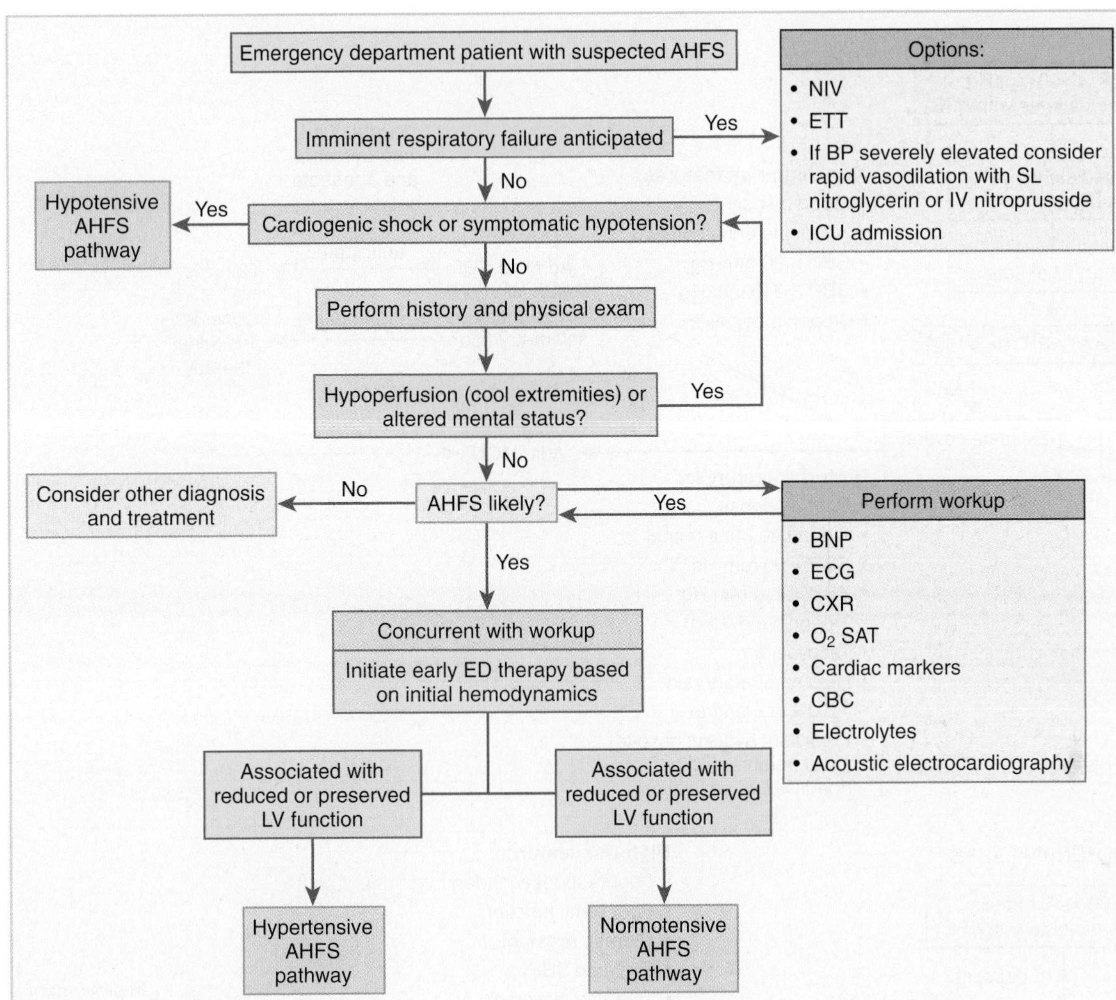

FIGURE 27-6 Initial management of patients presenting with AHFS. Suggested initial triage in patients with suspected acute heart failure syndromes. AHFS = acute heart failure syndromes; BNP = b-type natriuretic peptide; BP = blood pressure; CXR = chest x-ray; ETT = endotracheal intubation; LV = left ventricular; NIV = non-invasive ventilation; O_2sat = oxygen saturation; SL = sublingual. *(From Collins S, Storrow AB, Kirk JD, et al: Beyond pulmonary edema: Diagnostic, risk stratification, and treatment challenges of acute heart failure management in the emergency department. Ann Emerg Med 51:45, 2008.)*

DIURETICS (Table 27-9; see Table 28-7**).** Diuretics are among the most important drugs in the treatment of patients with AHFS and volume overload and are discussed in detail in Chap. 28. Large initial diuresis induced by a high dose of a potent diuretic may cause hypotension and worsening renal function. Loop diuretics (furosemide, torsemide, bumetanide, and ethacrynic acid; see Table 28-7) are the single most effective diuretics and can lead to excretion of up to 25% of the filtered sodium. They are routinely used as initial therapy for patients with AHFS, and they may rapidly improve symptoms. Even if they are frequently administered as intravenous boluses in the acute setting, small studies have suggested that intravenous infusion may be more effective and safer.[87] Thiazide-type diuretics (thiazides, chlorthalidone, metolazone) have a less marked natriuretic effect and are not considered first-line agents in patients with AHFS. As noted in Chap. 28, thiazide diuretics can have synergistic effects with loop diuretics and can significantly increase sodium excretion and urine output in patients who have reduced response to loop agents alone. Potassium-sparing diuretics (triamterene, amiloride, spironolactone, and eplerenone) have relatively weak natriuretic effects and are mainly used in patients with hypokalemia or with refractory edema.

The use of diuretics, particularly at the high doses given in the setting of AHFS management, is often associated with hemodynamic, renal, or electrolyte abnormalities. The rapid reduction in effective circulating volume may result in hypotension and a decrease in renal perfusion. This is often manifested by a disproportionate increase of BUN over creatinine. Although these abnormalities are reversible, repeated episodes may potentially lead to kidney injury.[88] Electrolyte abnormalities, including hypokalemia, hypomagnesemia, and hyponatremia, frequently occur. Therefore, frequent monitoring (at least daily) with aggressive repletion should be instituted. Observational data have suggested that the use of high-dose diuretics may be associated with worsening renal function and higher mortality.[88] These data are supported by the evidence that furosemide accelerates LV systolic dysfunction, elevates serum aldosterone levels, and alters calcium handling in an animal model of HF.[89] According to ESC guidelines,[8] on admission, furosemide should be initially given in an intravenous bolus dose of 20 to 40 mg; alternatively, 0.5 to 1 mg of bumetanide or 10 to 20 mg of torsemide can be administered. The patient's urine output should be closely followed. In patients with evidence of volume overload, the dose of loop diuretic may be titrated according to renal function, and continuous infusion may also be considered after the initial dose. The total furosemide dose should not exceed 100 mg in the first 6 hours and 240 mg during the first 24 hours. Combination with thiazides or aldosterone antagonists (spironolactone or eplerenone, 25 to 50 mg orally) may be useful in patients with diuretic resistance (see Table 27-9). The optimal dose and means of administration of loop diuretics have recently been evaluated in the Diuretic Optimal Strategy Evaluation in Acute Heart Failure (DOSE) trial (ClinicalTrials.gov Identifier: NCT00577135), sponsored by the National Heart, Lung and Blood Institute.[90] Initial results from the DOSE study have demonstrated that bolus dosing every 12 hours and continuous infusion appear to be equivalent in terms of symptom relief, changes in renal function, and measures of congestion. Although high-dose therapy (2.5× the oral dose given intravenously) was not superior to

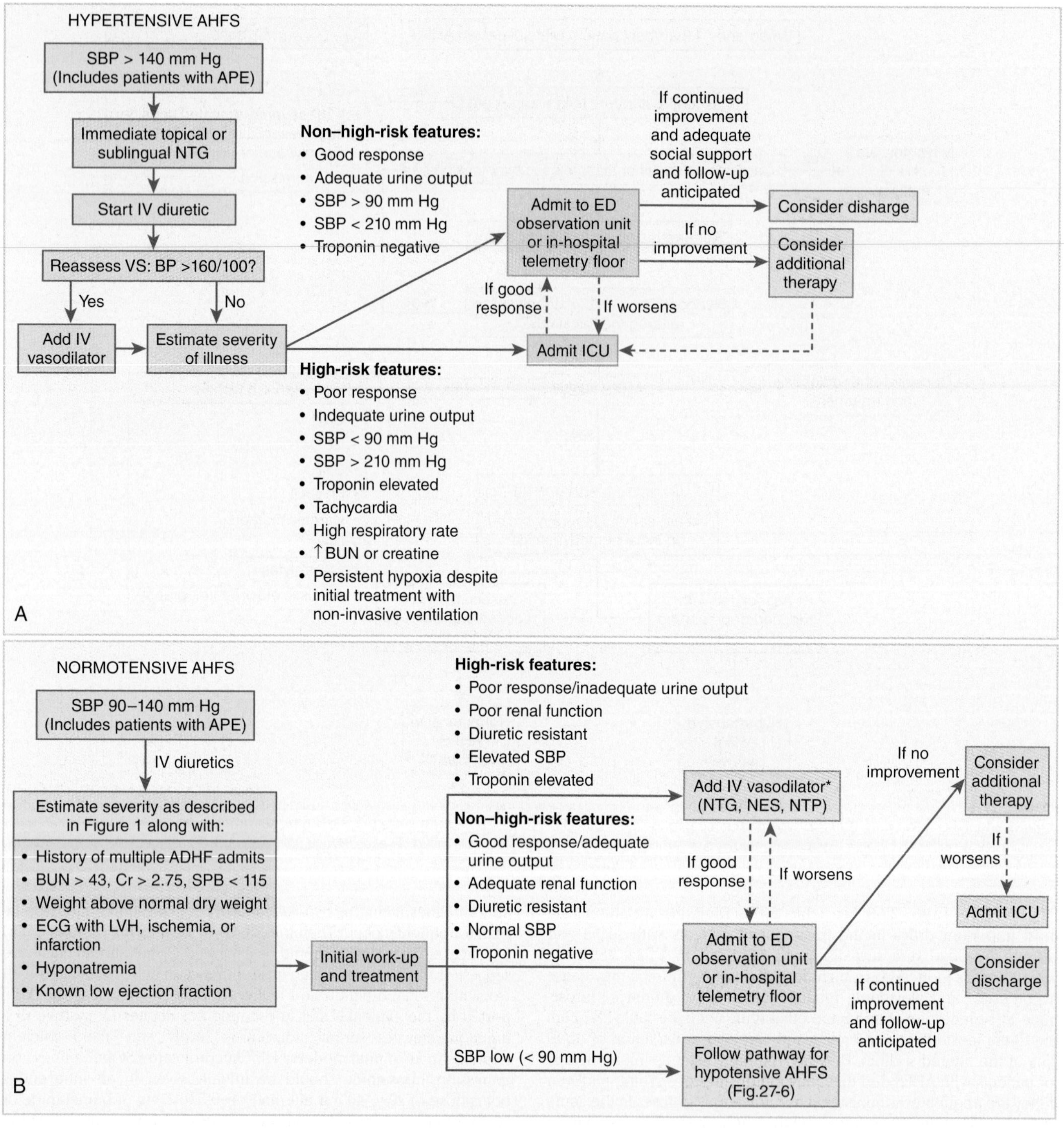

FIGURE 27-7 Management of patients with AHFS based on systolic blood pressure at presentation. **A,** Algorithm for treatment of AHFS patients presenting with hypertension. **B,** Algorithm for treatment of AHFS patients presenting with normal blood pressure.

low dose (1× the oral dose given intravenously) on the basis of the primary efficacy endpoint of global symptom relief during 72 hours, high dose was associated with improvements in dyspnea, resolution of signs and symptoms of congestion, net fluid loss, and greater decrease in NT-proBNP. These potentially beneficial findings were balanced against a modest worsening of renal function in the high-dose arm, although these differences in renal function were transient and did not persist until discharge or day 60.[90]

VASODILATORS (see Table 27-9). Vasodilators can be used in combination with diuretics in the management of AHFS patients. They can be classified as predominantly venous dilators, with consequent reduction in preload; arterial dilators, leading to a decrease in afterload; and balanced vasodilators, with combined action on both the venous and the arterial system. Currently available vasodilators include the organic nitrates (nitroglycerin and isosorbide dinitrate), sodium nitroprusside, and nesiritide. All of these drugs act by activating soluble guanylate cyclase in the smooth muscle cells, leading to higher intracellular concentrations of cyclic guanosine monophosphate (cGMP) and consequent vessel relaxation. They should be used with caution in patients with HFpEF and in patients with CAD because they may cause severe hypotension. According to Heart Failure Society of

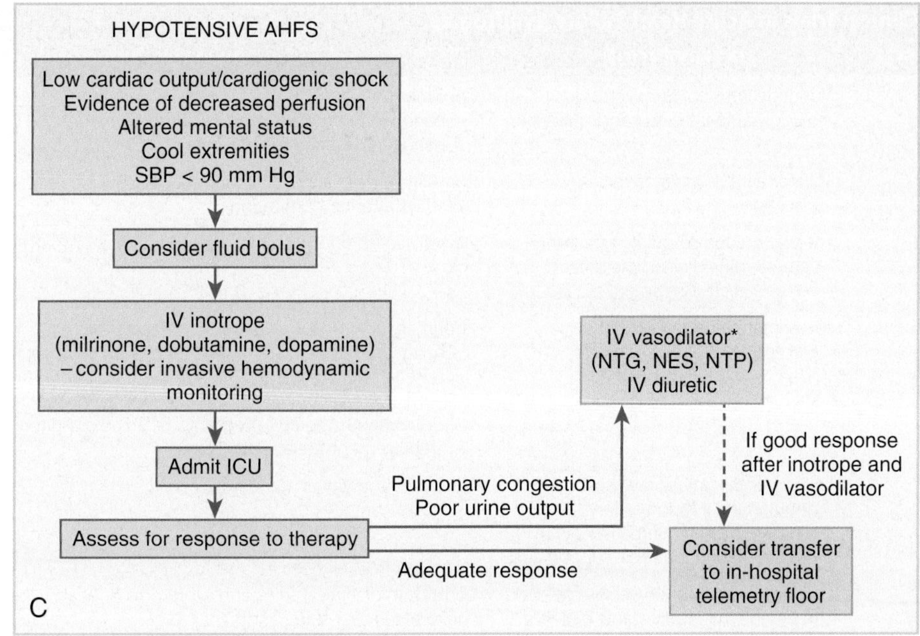

FIGURE 27-7, cont'd C, Algorithm for treatment of AHFS patients presenting with hypotension. APE = acute pulmonary edema; NES = nesiritide; NTG = nitroglycerin; NTP = sodium nitroprusside. *(From Collins S, Storrow AB, Kirk JD, et al: Beyond pulmonary edema: Diagnostic, risk stratification, and treatment challenges of acute heart failure management in the emergency department. Ann Emerg Med 51:45, 2008.)*

America guidelines,[91] intravenous nitroglycerin, sodium nitroprusside, or nesiritide may be added to diuretic treatment in the absence of hypotension to improve congestive symptoms. Blood pressure should be monitored frequently and the drug discontinued if symptomatic hypotension develops.

Nitrates

Nitroglycerin can be given sublingually, transdermally, or intravenously. When given at the lower doses, nitrates have a prevalent venodilatory effect resulting in rapid decline of pulmonary venous and LV filling pressure, with improvement in pulmonary congestion, reduction of dyspnea, and decrease in myocardial oxygen consumption. With the higher doses, they also exhibit arterial vasodilation in the systemic and coronary circulation. In the coronary circulation, the vasodilatory effects of nitroglycerin are exerted particularly on the epicardial vessels, which may lead to increased blood flow. Except for the Vasodilatation in the Management of Acute Congestive Heart Failure (VMAC) study,[92] no large studies have investigated the clinical effects of nitroglycerin in treatment of AHFS. Serious side effects of nitrates are uncommon. However, hypotension can develop in patients whose cardiac output is preload dependent, such as in the case of right ventricular infarction and severe aortic stenosis. Given the risk of severe hypotension with potentially catastrophic consequences, the recent use of phosphodiesterase 5 inhibitors (sildenafil, tadalafil, and vardenafil) should be ruled out before administration of nitrates. A limitation of these drugs is tolerance, which can develop within 24 hours. Approximately 20% of patients do not have significant hemodynamic response. The ESC guidelines recommend the early use of nitrates in AHFS patients (see Table 27-9).[8] To reduce the risk of significant hypotension, nitrates should be titrated slowly and blood pressure monitored closely.

Sodium Nitroprusside

Sodium nitroprusside is a potent balanced vasodilator, acting through its active metabolite nitric oxide. It has a short half-life that allows fine titration and extremely rapid onset and offset of action. It is useful in the treatment of conditions that require rapid reduction of preload or afterload, such as hypertensive crises and acute mitral regurgitation. Sodium nitroprusside rapidly reduces LV filling pressures, but it may cause severe hypotension and may require blood pressure monitoring with an arterial line. Its arterial vasodilatory actions are mainly at the level of resistance vessels, which may lead to coronary steal syndrome in patients with CAD. In patients with chronic obstructive pulmonary disease, sodium nitroprusside may cause hypoxemia due to ventilation-perfusion mismatch. Cyanide toxicity may occur, particularly in patients with impaired renal function. Given the potential for these significant side effects, sodium nitroprusside is not commonly used in patients admitted with AHFS (<1% in both the United States and Europe). The Veterans Administration Cooperative Study examined the effect of short-term sodium nitroprusside infusion on mortality in patients with acute myocardial infarction complicated by LV failure.[23] In retrospect, the early use (within 9 hours of onset of symptoms) of sodium nitroprusside was associated with a significant increase in mortality within the first 3 months after myocardial infarction. This may have been the result of the acute decrease in coronary perfusion and further myocardial injury, a hypothesis that remains to be tested. According to the ESC, intravenous sodium nitroprusside should be used with caution and with invasive blood pressure monitoring. It should not be used in patients with SBP <100 mm Hg[8] (see Table 27-9).

Nesiritide

Nesiritide is a recombinant form of human BNP available as an intravenous agent and is currently approved in the United States but not in the majority of European countries for the treatment of AHFS. Its main effects include balanced vasodilation, with an increase in cardiac output independent of changes in cardiac contractility and heart rate and less consistently natriuresis and diuresis. The VMAC trial was conducted to compare the hemodynamic and clinical effects and safety of intravenous nesiritide versus intravenous nitroglycerin versus placebo when added to standard care in patients hospitalized with AHFS.[92] This study included patients with both preserved and depressed systolic function, with or without ischemia. Nesiritide improved dyspnea at 3 hours compared with placebo but not compared with nitroglycerin. After 24 hours, the mean reduction in PCWP was significantly greater in the nesiritide group than in the nitroglycerin group, but there was no significant difference in dyspnea between the two groups. Subsequent retrospective analyses suggest that nesiritide may increase mortality and worsen renal function.[93,93a] The effects of nesiritide on mortality in AHFS are being prospectively investigated in the ASCEND-HF (Acute Study of Clinical Effectiveness of Nesiritide in Decompensated Heart Failure) trial (see Table 27-8; ClinicalTrials.gov Identifier: NCT00475852), in which patients with ADHF will be randomly assigned to receive either intravenous nesiritide or matching

TABLE 27-8 Large Clinical Trials in Acute Heart Failure Syndromes

ACRONYM	SAMPLE SIZE	INTERVENTION	PRIMARY ENDPOINTS
VMAC	489	Nesiritide infusion 48 hr versus nitroglycerin infusion versus placebo	Coprimary: Change in pulmonary capillary wedge pressure at 3 hr Change in dyspnea (Likert) at 3 hr
OPTIME	951	Milrinone infusion 48 hr versus placebo	Cumulative days of hospitalization for cardiovascular cause or days dead within 60 days after randomization
ESCAPE	433	Therapy guided by pulmonary artery catheter plus clinical assessment versus clinical assessment alone	Days alive and out of hospital during the first 6 months
VERITAS	1435	Tezosentan infusion 24-72 hr versus placebo	Coprimary: Change in dyspnea (at 3, 6, and 24 hr with visual analog scale 0-100) for 24 hr (area under the curve) Death or worsening heart failure (pulmonary edema, shock, new or ↑ intravenous therapy, mechanical cardiac or pulmonary support, renal replacement therapy) at 7 days
SURVIVE	1327	Levosimendan infusion versus dobutamine infusion as long as clinically indicated in patients with AHFS requiring inotropic support	All-cause mortality at 180 days
REVIVE II	600	Levosimendan infusion versus placebo in hemodynamically stable patients with AHFS	Composite of clinical signs and symptoms of heart failure during 5 days expressed as 3-stage endpoint: Better (moderately or markedly improved global assessment at 6 hr, 24 hr, and 5 days with no worsening) Same Worse (death from any cause; persistent or worsening HF requiring intravenous diuretics, vasodilators, or inotropes at any time; or moderately or markedly worse patient global assessment at 6 hr, 24 hr, or 5 days)
3CPO	1069	Standard oxygen therapy versus noninvasive intermittent positive-pressure ventilation (NIPPV) versus continuous positive airway pressure (CPAP) ventilation in acute pulmonary edema	Death within 7 days (oxygen therapy versus NIPPV) or death or intubation within 7 days (NIPPV versus CPAP)
EVEREST	4133	Tolvaptan versus placebo up to 112 wk	Short-term composite: changes in global clinical status (by visual analog scale) and body weight at day 7 or discharge Long-term dual endpoints: All-cause mortality (superiority and noninferiority) Cardiovascular death or HF hospitalization (superiority only)
ASCEND-HF	7000	Nesiritide infusion versus placebo	Coprimary: Composite of all-cause mortality and heart failure rehospitalization through 30 days Dyspnea at 6 and 24 hr
PROTECT I and II	2033	Rolofylline infusion versus placebo	Composite of clinical signs and symptoms of heart failure during 7 days expressed as 3-stage endpoint: Better (moderately or markedly improved global assessment at 24 and 48 hr with no worsening) Same Worse (death from any cause, persistent or worsening heart failure through day 7, or creatinine increase ≥0.3 mg/dL at 7 and 14 days)

From Felker GM , Pang PS, Adams KF, et al: Clinical trials of pharmacological therapies in acute heart failure syndromes: Lessons learned and directions forward. Circ Heart Fail 3:314, 2010.

placebo for 24 hours to 7 days. The two coprimary endpoints were (1) assessment of acute dyspnea at 6 or 24 hours and (2) death or rehospitalization for HF within 30 days (**Fig. 27-8**). Nesiritide did not reduce the rate of recurrent HF hospitalization or death. Although nesiritide reduced dyspnea to a modest degree, it did not meet the pre-specified protocol endpoint. However, the trial proved conclusively that nesiritide does not increase mortality or worsen renal function, as suggested by prior meta-analysis. Nesiritide has a longer effective half-life than nitroglycerin or sodium nitroprusside, and its negative effects on blood pressure may persist longer. As a general rule, the risk of hypotension may be reduced by avoiding bolus administration and strictly following the recommended doses (see Table 27-9).

INOTROPES WITH VASODILATORY PROPERTIES (Table 27-10). These drugs are known to significantly decrease PCWP and to increase cardiac output. However, retrospective data from both registries and trials of AHF patients suggest that even the short-term use (hours to a few days) of intravenous inotropes (except for digoxin) is associated with significant side effects, such as hypotension and atrial or ventricular arrhythmias, and possibly an increase in long-term mortality. In particular, patients with CAD are at high risk for development of adverse events because a decrease in blood pressure may reduce coronary perfusion, with possible myocardial ischemia and injury; this may be further compounded by the increased myocardial oxygen requirements triggered by the enhanced contractile state and increased heart rate. This may be particularly deleterious in patients with hibernating or ischemic myocardium because they are known experimentally to cause myocardial necrosis in this setting.[94] Despite these considerations, several intravenous inotropes are available, including dobutamine, dopamine, milrinone, enoximone, and levosimendan, and

TABLE 27-9 Pharmacologic Agents Used in Acute Heart Failure Syndromes

INDICATION	DIURETIC	DOSING*	COMMENTS
Moderate volume overload	Furosemide *or*	20-40 mg	Oral or IV according to clinical symptoms
	Bumetanide *or*	0.5-1 mg	Titrate dose according to clinical response
	Torsemide	10-20 mg	Monitor potassium, sodium, and creatinine concentrations and blood pressure
Severe volume overload	Furosemide	40-100 mg	IV; increase dose
	Furosemide infusion	(5-40 mg/hr)	
	Bumetanide	1-4 mg	Oral or IV
	Torsemide	20-100 mg	Oral
Refractory to diuretics	*Add* Hydrochlorothiazide *or*	50-100 mg	Combination better than very high dose of loop diuretics
	Metolazone *or*	2.5-10 mg	More potent if creatinine clearance <30 mL/min
	Spironolactone	25-50 mg	Spironolactone best choice if no renal failure and normal or low potassium concentration
With alkalosis	Acetazolamide	0.5 mg	IV
Refractory to loop diuretics and thiazides	Add dopamine (renal vasodilation) or dobutamine		Consider ultrafiltration or hemodialysis if coexisting renal failure
INDICATION	**VASODILATOR**	**DOSING**	**COMMENTS**
Pulmonary congestion or edema BP >90 mm Hg	Nitroglycerin	Start 10-20 μg/min, increase up to 200 μg/min	Hypotension, headache Tolerance on continuous use
	Isosorbide dinitrate	Start with 1 mg/hr, increase up to 10 mg/hr	Hypotension, headache Tolerance on continuous use
	Nitroprusside (hypertensive HF)	Start with 0.3 μg/kg/min and increase up to 5 μg/kg/min	Hypotension, isocyanate toxicity Light sensitive
	Nesiritide	Bolus 2 μg/kg + infusion 0.015-0.03 μg/kg/min	Hypotension

*Patients on chronic diuretic therapy or who have kidney disease may need higher doses.
Modified from Dickstein K, Cohen-Solal A, Filippatos G, et al: ESC Guidelines for the diagnosis and treatment of acute and chronic heart failure 2008. Eur Heart J 29:2388, 2008.

TABLE 27-10 Inotropic Agents Used in Acute Heart Failure Syndromes

INOTROPIC AGENT	BOLUS	INFUSION RATE
Dobutamine	No	2-20 μg/kg/min (β+)
Dopamine	No	<3 μg/kg/min: renal effect (δ+) 3-5 μg/kg/min: inotropic (β+) >5 μg/kg/min: (β+), vasopressor (α+)
Milrinone	25-75 μg/kg during 10-20 min (optional)	0.375-0.75 μg/kg/min
Enoximone	0.25-0.75 mg/kg	1.25-7.5 μg/kg/min
Levosimendan	12 μg/kg during 10 min (optional)	0.1 μg/kg/min, which can be decreased to 0.05 or increased to 0.2 μg/kg/min
Norepinephrine	No	0.2-1.0 μg/kg/min
Epinephrine	Bolus: 1 mg can be given IV during resuscitation, repeated every 3-5 min	0.05-0.5 μg/kg/min

α+ = alpha-adrenergic agonist; β+ = beta-adrenergic agonist, δ+ = dopaminergic agonist.
Modified from Dickstein K, Cohen-Solal A, Filippatos G, et al: ESC Guidelines for the diagnosis and treatment of acute and chronic heart failure 2008. Eur Heart J 29:2388, 2008.

are still frequently used. In North American (ADHERE and OPTIMIZE-HF) and European registries, approximately 15% and 25% of patients were treated with inotropes.[3,30] For these reasons, a number of recommendations have been issued regarding the indications for inotropes in treatment of AHFS.[8,91] The use of these drugs should be limited to patients with dilated ventricles and reduced ejection fraction, who present with low SBP (<90 mm Hg) or low measured cardiac output in the presence of signs of congestion and organ hypoperfusion such as decreased mentation and reduced urine output. Inotropic agents should be started as early as possible with close hemodynamic and telemetry monitoring and should be stopped as soon as adequate organ perfusion is restored or congestion reduced. All these agents may increase conduction through the atrioventricular node, and this is particularly deleterious in patients presenting with atrial fibrillation and uncontrolled ventricular response. In addition, intravenous inotropes may be employed in cardiogenic shock as a temporary therapy to prevent hemodynamic collapse or as a life-sustaining bridge to more definitive therapy for those patients awaiting mechanical circulatory support, ventricular assist devices, or cardiac transplantation.

Dobutamine

Dobutamine, a nonselective $beta_1$- and $beta_2$-adrenergic receptor agonist with variable activity on the $alpha_1$ receptor, is the most commonly used inotropic agent in the United States and Europe.[5,95] Its

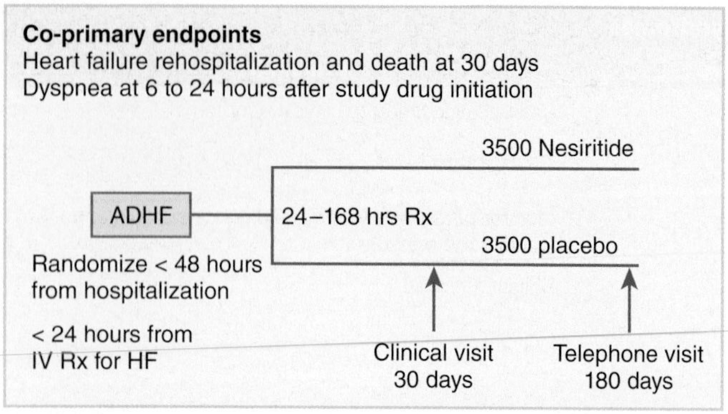

Co-primary endpoints
Heart failure rehospitalization and death at 30 days
Dyspnea at 6 to 24 hours after study drug initiation

3500 Nesiritide
ADHF
24–168 hrs Rx
3500 placebo
Randomize < 48 hours from hospitalization
< 24 hours from IV Rx for HF
Clinical visit 30 days
Telephone visit 180 days

FIGURE 27-8 Clinical trial design for the ASCEND-HF trial. Patients with acute decompensated heart failure (ADHF) will be randomly assigned to receive either intravenous nesiritide or matching placebo for 24 hours to 7 days. The two coprimary endpoints are (1) assessment of acute dyspnea at 6 or 24 hours and (2) death or rehospitalization for heart failure within 30 days. A total of 7000 patients will be enrolled worldwide. *(Modified from Hernandez AF, O'Connor CM, Starling RC: Rationale and design of the Acute Study of Clinical Effectiveness of Nesiritide in Decompensated Heart Failure Trial [ASCEND-HF]. Am Heart J 157:271, 2009.)*

actions depend on the net effect of the dose-dependent activation of the various adrenoceptor subtypes.[96] At low doses, there is prevalent $beta_1$ and $beta_2$ stimulation, with positive inotropic and chronotropic responses as well as vasorelaxation. These effects result in a reduced afterload, with increase in stroke volume, heart rate, and cardiac output. At higher doses, $alpha_1$ activation becomes more evident and leads to venous and arterial constriction. The ESC guidelines recommend starting dobutamine at an infusion rate of 2 to 3 μg/kg/min without a loading dose (see Table 27-10). The infusion rate may then be adjusted on the basis of the clinical status symptoms, response to diuretics, and symptoms, and it should not normally exceed 15 μg/kg/min. However, if a patient has received beta blockers, the rate of infusion may have to be increased to as high as 20 μg/kg/min to restore its inotropic effect. Dobutamine should not be discontinued abruptly, and the dose should be tapered by steps of 2 μg/kg/min.

Dopamine

The cardiovascular actions of dopamine represent the sum effects of dose-dependent activation of types of receptors in a dose-dependent manner.[97] At low doses (≤2 μg/kg/min), dopamine primarily binds to vascular D_1 receptors in the coronary, renal, and mesenteric beds, with vasodilation and natriuresis. At intermediate doses (2 to 5 μg/kg/min), dopamine activates myocardial $beta_1$ receptors, with positive inotropic effects. Dopamine usually increases SBP and heart rate, with no or minor changes in diastolic pressure and peripheral vascular resistance. At high doses (5 to 15 μg/kg/min), dopamine also binds to $alpha_1$ receptors and triggers vasoconstriction. Dopamine and dobutamine should not be used in patients with atrial fibrillation and a rapid ventricular response because it may result in a decrease in cardiac output that may be rate related. Low-dose dopamine (1 to 2 μg/kg/min) has been used together with dobutamine because dobutamine may decrease renal perfusion.

Milrinone

Milrinone is a phosphodiesterase 3 inhibitor approved for short-term circulatory support in patients with advanced HF.[96,97] In the Outcomes of a Prospective Trial of Intravenous Milrinone for Exacerbations of Chronic Heart Failure (OPTIME-HF; see Table 27-8),[98] the addition of milrinone without a bolus in those patients admitted with HF and a reduced ejection fraction who did not require an inotrope did not improve hospital mortality rate, 60-day mortality rate, or the composite incidence of death or readmission. However, more patients in the milrinone group developed severe hypotension as well as atrial and ventricular arrhythmias. In retrospect,[22] it appeared that patients with CAD had an increase in postdischarge mortality (42% versus 36%) compared with placebo in spite of its short-term use of milrinone. Accordingly, milrinone should be used with extreme caution in patients with CAD and should be used only in patients with a low cardiac output state not responding to other noninotropic therapy. Because of its hypotensive effects, a loading dose should not be used.

Levosimendan

Levosimendan is a calcium sensitizer and ATP-dependent potassium channel opener that has positive inotropic and vasodilatory effect.[99] Levosimendan has been extensively studied in patients with AHFS. In the Randomized, Multicenter Evaluation of Intravenous Levosimendan Efficacy Versus Placebo in the Short-term Treatment of Decompensated Chronic HF trial, the REVIVE II study (see Table 27-8), an improvement in patient self-assessment, a decrease in levels of BNP, and a shorter hospital stay were noted in response to levosimendan when it was added to standard therapy in patients admitted with HF and reduced ejection fraction.[100] However, compared with placebo, levosimendan use was associated with more hypotension (50% versus 34%), ventricular tachycardia (25% versus 17%), and atrial fibrillation (9% versus 2%). A trend toward increase in early mortality was also observed in the levosimendan-treated patients. The SURVIVE study was a randomized, double-blind trial comparing short-term use of intravenous levosimendan with dobutamine in 1327 patients hospitalized with AHFS requiring inotropic support (see Table 27-8).[101] At 6 months of follow-up, mortality was 26% in the levosimendan group and 28% in the dobutamine group. In addition, there were no differences between treatment groups in all-cause mortality at 31 days, number of days alive and out of the hospital, patient global assessment, or patient assessment of dyspnea at 24 hours. However, levosimendan use was associated with more atrial fibrillation and hypokalemia and fewer episodes of HF compared with dobutamine. Levosimendan is approved in several European countries but not in the United States. According to the ESC guidelines, levosimendan should be considered for patients with low cardiac output states despite the use of other therapies. Levosimendan should be started with a bolus dose (3 to 12 mg/kg) during 10 minutes, unless SBP <100 mm Hg, followed by a continuous infusion (0.05 to 0.2 mg/kg/min for 24 hours; see Table 27-10).[8] In spite of the ESC recommendation, the loading dose is avoided by many clinicians to minimize the potential development of hypotension that has been reported with this drug.

VASOPRESSOR AGENTS

Phenylephrine

Phenylephrine is a selective $alpha_1$ receptor agonist with direct arterial vasoconstrictor effects. This agent may be used in case of severe hypotension to preserve coronary perfusion. It may be useful when the hypotension is related to systemic vasodilation rather than to a decrease in cardiac output.

Norepinephrine

Norepinephrine is a catecholamine with high affinity for alpha receptors and is generally used to increase systemic vascular resistance. Norepinephrine may improve coronary perfusion in the presence of severe hypotension and can and should be used as a rescue agent in those patients to maintain blood pressure until other therapies to improve cardiac function can be instituted. Norepinephrine also may be particularly useful in patients with low blood pressure and "inappropriate" vasodilation (low blood pressure in the presence of normal or high cardiac output). It should be administered only through a central venous line because extravasation may cause tissue necrosis.

Digoxin

Digoxin was approved by the Food and Drug Administration in 1997 for the treatment of atrial fibrillation and chronic HF. However, its use in North America and Europe has been on the decline in the last decade.[102] Although digoxin displays many of the properties of an ideal drug for the treatment of AHFS in patients with reduced ejection fraction with or without atrial fibrillation, no trials have investigated its role in this setting.[102] Digoxin rapidly improves hemodynamics without increasing heart rate or decreasing blood pressure[103] and should be considered in patients with a low blood pressure due to a low cardiac output. Although digoxin may be used intravenously, the oral route is preferable. When used intravenously, it should be given slowly because rapid administration may cause vasoconstriction. The average loading dose is 0.75 mg. This should be given slowly because a rapid administration may cause systemic vasoconstriction. The initial bolus should be followed by an oral or intravenous dose of 0.25 mg at least 12 hours after the initial dose. The dose should be adjusted according to renal function and should result in a trough serum concentration of < 1 ng/mL. In patients with reduced ejection fraction who continue to have signs and symptoms of HF, digoxin therapy should be continued in addition to other therapies during hospitalization and after discharge. Ischemia, hypokalemia, and hypomagnesemia may increase the likelihood for development of digitalis intoxication, even at the therapeutic doses. Digoxin should not be used in patients with moderate to severe renal impairment, ongoing ischemia, or advanced atrioventricular block.

Arginine Vasopressin Antagonists (see Chaps. 25 and 28)

As discussed in Chap. 25, arginine vasopressin, also known as antidiuretic hormone, is the main regulator of plasma osmolality. Arginine vasopressin exerts its physiologic actions by binding to three types of receptors, V_{1a}, V_{1b}, and V_2. The V_{1a} receptor is the most widespread subtype and is found in vascular smooth muscle, where it mediates vasoconstriction; V_2 receptors are located predominantly in the renal collecting duct system and are the main mediators of antidiuretic hormone effects of water reabsorption (see Fig. 28-12); and V_{1b} receptors are mainly found in the anterior pituitary and the brain, where they regulate neural pathways.[104] Vasopressin levels are inappropriately high in both acute and chronic HF and are thought to have a major role in the pathophysiology of HF. In particular, vasopressin appears to be the major contributor to the development of the hyponatremia observed in patients with HF. Currently available vasopressin antagonists are tolvaptan (an oral, selective V_2 receptor antagonist) and conivaptan (a V_{1a} and V_2 receptor antagonist for intravenous use). Tolvaptan improves PCWP but not cardiac output.[105] In patients with hyponatremia related to chronic HF, cirrhosis, or the syndrome of inappropriate antidiuretic hormone secretion and not fluid-restricted, tolvaptan rapidly improved or normalized serum sodium concentration.[106] The Efficacy of Vasopressin Antagonism in Heart Failure Outcome Study with Tolvaptan (EVEREST) was an international trial that evaluated 4,133 patients admitted with AHF and reduced ejection fraction. EVEREST was composed of 2 short-term A and B studies embedded in a large outcome postdischarge study. In the outcome study, the coprimary endpoints for the trial were all-cause mortality (superiority and noninferiority) and cardiovascular death or hospitalization for HF (superiority only). In the short-term A and B study, secondary endpoints included changes in dyspnea, body weight, and edema. During a median follow-up of 9.9 months, death occurred in 25.9% in the tolvaptan group and 26.3% in the placebo group (hazard ratio [HR], 0.98; 95% confidence interval [CI], 0.87-1.11; $P = 0.68$). The upper confidence limit for the mortality difference was within the prespecified noninferiority margin of 1.25 ($P < 0.001$; **Fig. 27-9A**). The composite of cardiovascular death or hospitalization for HF was not significantly different in the placebo- and the tolvaptan-treated patients (HR, 1.04; 95% CI, 0.95-1.14; $P = 0.55$). Tolvaptan, however, in the short-term studies, when added to standard therapy modestly improved signs and symptoms during hospitalization and reduced body weight without affecting heart rate, or blood pressure (Fig. 27-9B).[72,73] It is important to note postdischarge survival and readmission rates were not affected by chronic postdischarge therapy with tolvaptan in spite of the fact that this therapy resulted in a sustained decrease in body weight and an improvement or normalization in serum sodium concentration in the patients with hyponatremia and in the absence of significant side effects.[72] In patients with AHF, the addition of conivaptan to standard therapy increased urine output without a significant improvement in signs or symptoms or decrease in body weight.[107] Although tolvaptan and conivaptan have been approved for the treatment of clinically significant hypervolemic and euvolemic hyponatremia, their value in the management of AHFS, with or without hyponatremia, remains to be determined.

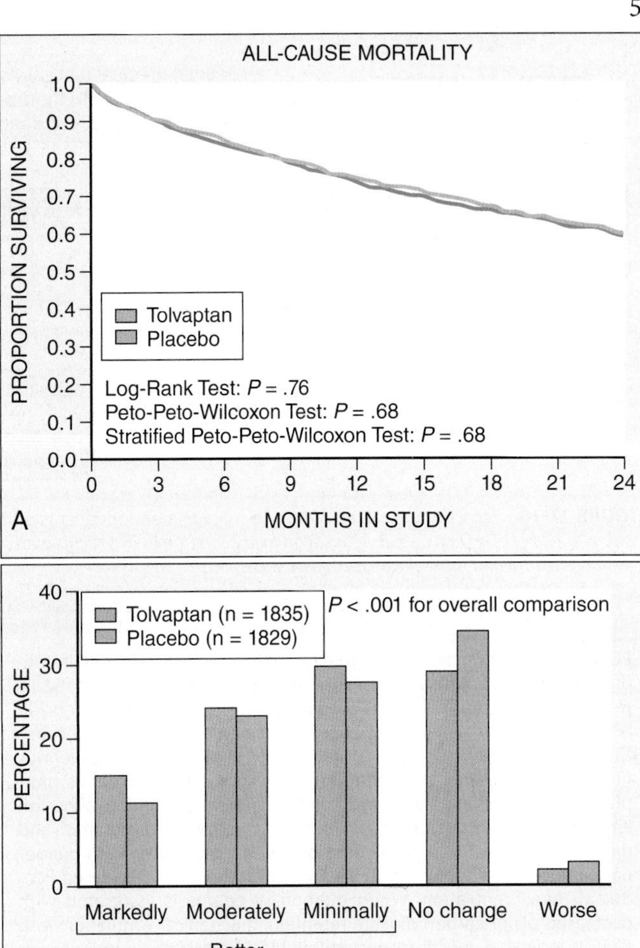

FIGURE 27-9 Clinical outcomes in the EVEREST trial. **A,** Kaplan-Meier analyses of all-cause mortality (coprimary endpoint). **B,** Change in patient-assessed dyspnea at day 1 for patients manifesting dyspnea at baseline (secondary endpoint). *(From Konstam MA, Gheorghiade M, Burnett JC Jr, et al: Effects of oral tolvaptan in patients hospitalized for worsening heart failure: The EVEREST Outcome Trial. JAMA 297:1319, 2007.)*

Intravenous Beta Blockers

As a general rule, de novo therapy with beta blockers should not be started during the initial phase of AHFS because beta blockers acutely decrease cardiac contractility. However, a short-acting intravenous beta blocker such as esmolol may be considered when AHF is precipitated by atrial fibrillation or flutter with a rapid ventricular response. These agents should be continued during hospitalization in patients already receiving chronic beta blocker therapy unless shock, severe hypotension, or bradycardia is present.

Other Intravenous Agents

Calcium channel blockers such as nicardipine,[108] ACE inhibitors, such as enalapril, and hydralazine can be given intravenously, have relatively rapid effects, and result in improved hemodynamics; however, they have not been studied and are rarely used in the early management phase of AHFS. Nevertheless, these agents may be potentially useful in patients presenting with severe hypertension refractory to other therapies.

Specific Clinical Scenarios

In the early stages of phase I clinical management, there are a series of specific clinical presentations that require special attention. These include cardiogenic pulmonary edema, predominantly right-sided HF, ACS, CAD without ACS, and cardiogenic shock.

CARDIOGENIC PULMONARY EDEMA. Cardiogenic pulmonary edema is the result of interstitial and alveolar transudation secondary to elevated

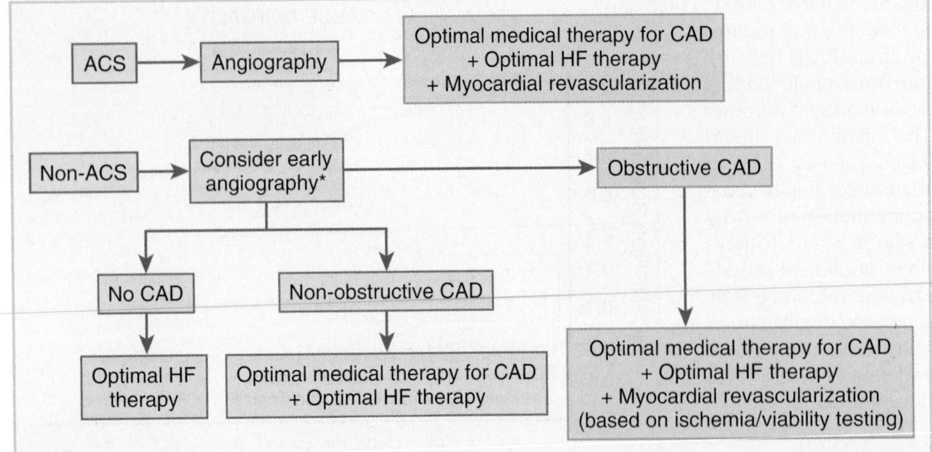

FIGURE 27-10 Algorithm for assessment and management of patients admitted with AHFS and CAD. *(From Flaherty JD, Bax JJ, De Luca L, et al: Acute heart failure syndromes in patients with coronary artery disease early assessment and treatment. J Am Coll Cardiol 53:254, 2009.)*

PCWP and is accompanied by severe respiratory distress requiring immediate intervention. When untreated, it may result in death. These patients may present with any level of blood pressure, although hypertension predominates. The patient should be placed in a seated position because this decreases venous return. In addition to sublingual or intravenous nitrates and diuretics, administration of oxygen and intravenous morphine may also relieve the symptoms. Noninvasive ventilation, although it may not improve outcomes, is beneficial for restoring oxygenation and decreasing symptoms. The majority of patients presenting with pulmonary edema have hypoxia with a slightly raised pH and decreased P_{CO_2} due to hyperventilation. When pulmonary edema is associated with decreased pH or carbon dioxide retention, mechanical ventilation with PEEP is indicated. In the setting of low blood pressure, an intravenous inodilator such as dobutamine should be considered. It is important also to treat precipitating factors such as atrial fibrillation with a rapid ventricular response or ischemia.

Right-Sided Heart Failure. The most common cause of right-sided HF in AHFS is related to left-sided failure. Isolated right-sided HF (which is relatively rare) may be caused by an acute right ventricular infarction. Pulmonary arterial hypertension, defined as a high pulmonary artery pressure without an elevation in the PCWP (usually <15 mm Hg), may also be a cause and may be primary or secondary. The secondary form may be related to chronic obstructive pulmonary disease, chronic or acute pulmonary embolism, pulmonary fibrosis, or connective tissue disorders such as scleroderma. For acute right ventricular infarction resulting in right-sided HF, early reperfusion is the mainstay of treatment. For primary pulmonary hypertension, selective pulmonary arterial vasodilators such as sildenafil, epoprostenol, and bosentan may be used; however, they are contraindicated when left-sided failure is the cause. The agents have not been studied in the area of AHFS. For secondary pulmonary arterial hypertension, the treatment should be directed toward the cause.

Acute Coronary Syndromes. ACS may be the underlying trigger in patients presenting with AHFS (see Table 27-3). In these situations, patients commonly present with chest discomfort, electrocardiographic changes consistent with ischemia, and often serum troponin elevation. The therapy for these patients, particularly those presenting with ST-segment elevation, is antiplatelet therapy with immediate coronary reperfusion with percutaneous coronary intervention (**Fig. 27-10**). Maintenance of a mean blood pressure >70 mm Hg is essential. Patients with ACS and AHFS may also benefit from intravenous nitrates and a short-acting beta blocker such as esmolol, particularly when HF is exacerbated by elevated blood pressure or heart rate. Intravenous inodilators should be avoided because experimental data have shown that they can cause necrosis of ischemic or hibernating myocardium.[94] Urgent surgery is indicated in patients with mechanical complications after ACS, such as ventricular septal defect or severe mitral regurgitation due to ruptured papillary muscle.

Coronary Artery Disease Without Acute Coronary Syndromes. The majority of patients admitted with AHFS have CAD, although for many, its extent and severity have not been previously established.[13] Even when ACS is not suspected, CAD patients commonly have an elevation of serum troponins.[21] Therapies with antiplatelet agents, and intravenous nitroglycerin should be considered, and maintenance of an adequate perfusion pressure (mean blood pressure >70 mm Hg) may be particularly important in this group of patients. Intravenous inodilators should be avoided if possible[24] (see Fig. 27-10).

Cardiogenic Shock. Cardiogenic shock is characterized by marked hypotension (SBP <80 mm Hg) lasting more than 30 minutes, associated with severe reduction of cardiac index (usually <1.8 liter/min/m^2) in spite of elevated LV filling pressure (PCWP >18 mm Hg), resulting in organ hypoperfusion. Despite the improvement in critical care management in the last 30 years, mortality can be as high as 50% to 60% in patients with large acute myocardial infarctions,[109] usually with a loss of ≥40% of LV mass, which accounts for the majority of patients presenting in cardiogenic shock. However, mechanical complications of acute myocardial infarction, such as mitral insufficiency, cardiac rupture with ventricular septal defect or tamponade, and isolated right ventricular infarction, may also be causes in this setting. The exact mechanism for cardiogenic shock is important for optimization of therapies. In addition to vasopressor agents that may be used to bridge the patients to more definitive therapy, pulmonary artery catheter insertion, echocardiographic evaluation with Doppler study, intra-aortic balloon counterpulsation, and urgent cardiac catheterization are indicated. Intra-aortic balloon counterpulsation has become a standard component of initial treatment in patients with cardiogenic shock who do not respond rapidly to vasodilation and inotropic support or have acute severe mitral regurgitation, rupture of the interventricular septum, or ongoing myocardial ischemia and need stabilization for diagnostic studies and further therapies. For suitable patients, coronary angiography and revascularization should be performed as soon as possible. Temporary mechanical circulatory assistance may be indicated in patients with AHFS who are not responding to conventional therapy as a bridge to heart transplantation or other mechanical intervention.[110]

Phase II: Management in the Hospital

After initial management in the emergency department (phase I), patients are usually transferred to an inpatient unit for continuation of treatment, for completion of the diagnostic workup, and for postdischarge management planning (phases II and III). Registry data show that in the United States, 65% of patients are admitted to a telemetry unit, 13% to an intensive care unit, 9% to a step-down unit, and 11% to a regular ward in phase II.[3] Whereas the initial treatment usually achieves symptomatic relief of dyspnea at rest, at the time of transition into phase II, the majority of patients continue to have symptoms during exertion as well as signs of volume overload (e.g., jugular venous distention, pulmonary rales, peripheral edema), very abnormal hemodynamics (high PCWP or low cardiac output), and significant neurohormonal abnormalities (e.g., high BNP). In fact, a significant number do not decrease their body weight during hospitalization and are being discharged with persisting symptoms and signs.[47]

During the in-hospital phase, the goals are to continue treatment to improve signs and symptoms of congestion and to achieve euvolemia without worsening renal function; to perform a thorough assessment of myocardial structure and function to stratify and treat patients according to whether recovery of myocardial function is possible; and to implement evidence-based interventions that are known to improve outcomes in patients with HF (see Guidelines: Management of Heart Failure).

TREATMENT OF CLINICAL AND HEMODYNAMIC CONGESTION. In the beginning of phase II, an accurate reassessment of the patient's status should be performed while the initial therapies addressing congestion and respiratory and hemodynamic status are continued. To maximize the efficacy of management and to reduce the risk of deleterious effects, close monitoring of the patient should be continued, including vital signs at baseline and during provocative tests (e.g., orthostatic blood pressure), physical examination to assess systemic perfusion and to detect signs of congestion, daily fluid balance (with temporary use of urinary catheter if needed), and body weight (using the same accurate scale at the same time each day). Daily laboratory tests should include serum electrolyte (K^+, Mg^+, Na^+), BUN, and creatinine determinations as well as additional analyses if clinically appropriate (e.g., troponin in patients with ACS, arterial blood gas analysis in patients with hypoxia). In patients with congestion, diuretics are usually continued during this phase and often switched from an intravenous to an oral form. In this setting, oral diuretics (usually loop diuretics) should be given at least twice a day, and therapies should be maximized to achieve euvolemia without worsening renal function. In patients not responding to loop diuretics, thiazide-like drugs such as metolazone should be considered. Also, potassium-sparing agents such as spironolactone and eplerenone may be added in patients with hypokalemia. Useful clinical endpoints for titration of diuretic therapy include the persistence or resolution of signs and symptoms of congestion, the onset of orthostatic changes that usually reflect intravascular depletion, and the trend of renal function.

PERIPHERAL ULTRAFILTRATION (see Chap. 28). Peripheral ultrafiltration is an available modality to remove sodium and water in hospitalized HF patients who are refractory to pharmacologic therapy. The Ultrafiltration Versus Intravenous Diuretics for Patients Hospitalized for Acute Decompensated Heart Failure (UNLOAD) trial enrolled 200 patients with AHFS and reduced or preserved ejection fraction. The patients randomized to the venovenous ultrafiltration arm showed a greater reduction in their body weight at 48 hours compared with standard diuretic therapy. However, dyspnea and renal function were not improved. There was a decreased need for vasoactive drug use and reduced rate of hospital readmission at 90 days.[111] Given the relatively small number of patients studied and the fact that this was not a blinded trial, the clinical value of this approach in improving outcomes for patients with fluid overload remains to be determined. This intervention, however, should be considered in patients who continue to have severe congestion and are refractory to pharmacologic therapy.

IMPLEMENTATION OF EVIDENCE-BASED INTERVENTIONS KNOWN TO IMPROVE OUTCOMES IN HEART FAILURE. As discussed in detail in Chap. 28, several therapies (ACE inhibitors or ARBs, beta blockers, aldosterone blocking agents, and the combination hydralazine-isosorbide) have been shown to decrease mortality and hospitalizations in ambulatory HF patients with reduced ejection fraction. Although these therapies have not been studied in the setting of hospitalizations for HF, they are frequently continued in patients who are receiving the therapy before admission or are implemented for the first time during hospitalization or soon after discharge.

Both the ACC/AHA[9] and ESC[8] guidelines support continuation of ACE inhibitors or ARBs, beta blockers, and aldosterone antagonists during hospitalization for AHFS unless hemodynamic instability or other contraindications are present. For those AHFS patients with low ejection fraction who are not on a chronic evidence-based regimen, therapy with ACE inhibitors or ARBs and beta blocker should be started in stable patients before discharge. Before initiation of a beta blocker, the patient should be hemodynamically stable and volume status should be optimized. In addition, patients should no longer be dependent on intravenous inotropic agents or vasodilators. The initial dose should be low, and particular caution should be exerted in patients who have required inotropic therapy during admission.[112] Patients should be closely monitored for supine and orthostatic hypotension, recurrence of HF symptoms, and worsening renal function and electrolyte abnormalities. The majority of patients admitted with AHFS, particularly in the United States, are not receiving aldosterone antagoniststs.[113] Given the high postdischarge event rate in this population, it may be appropriate to consider the addition of an aldosterone blocking agent before discharge. However, caution should be exercised in patients with diabetes and renal insufficiency and in those receiving ACE inhibitors or ARBs as the addition of this treatment may result in hyperkalemia. Aldosterone blocking agents are contraindicated for patients with a potassium concentration >5 mEq/liter or creatinine >2.2 mg/dL.

The DIG trial showed that the addition of digoxin to ACE inhibitors and diuretics reduces rehospitalizations and, in retrospect, mortality in patients with serum concentration of the drug <1 ng/mL.[114] In addition, studies showing clinical benefits with ACE inhibitors, beta blockers, or aldosterone blocking agents were conducted in patients often receiving digoxin.[115] These benefits were observed particularly in patients with a very low ejection fraction, increased cardiothoracic ratio, or severe signs and symptoms.[103] On the basis of this evidence, it is reasonable to add low-dose digoxin to standard therapy, particularly in patients who continue to have signs and symptoms of HF in spite of taking ACE inhibitors or ARBs, beta blockers, or aldosterone blocking agents. In addition, digoxin may be particularly useful in controlling ventricular response in patients with atrial fibrillation. Digoxin can be started with a maintenance dose and adjusted in order to not exceed a trough serum concentration of > 1.0 ng/mL; however, it should not be used in patients with severe renal failure or atrioventricular blocks. Retrospective data from the DIG trial suggest that women are more likely to have an adverse event. Accordingly, digoxin doses for women should be lower than those for men and not exceed the level of 1 ng/mL.[103]

The combination of hydralazine and nitrates has been shown to be beneficial when it is added to standard therapy in African Americans with a depressed ejection fraction. This therapy should be considered before or soon after discharge, particularly if there are any residual signs and symptoms of HF. The use of this combination appears to be less effective in other ethnic groups.[116]

The efficacy of an ICD device that is placed at the time of admission has not been evaluated in patients with AHFS. Moreover, patients may not be candidates for ICD implantation after 3 to 6 months of evidence-based medical therapies for HF. Retrospective data suggest that the ICD status does not decrease event rate after discharge.[117] Similarly, because approximately 40% of AHFS patients with reduced ejection fraction have a wide QRS complex, cardiac resynchronization therapy should be considered after discharge if the patient remains symptomatic after an appropriate trial of evidence-based therapies for HF.[118]

REVASCULARIZATION (see Chaps. 31, 52, and 57). Patients with obstructive CAD may benefit from revascularization procedures, particularly when there is ischemia or hibernating myocardium.[119] The role of coronary artery bypass grafting in patients with chronic HF and CAD is being investigated in the multicenter, international, randomized Surgical Treatment for Ischemic Heart Failure (STICH; ClinicalTrials.gov Identifier: NCT00023595; see Chaps. 31 and 57).[119]

RECOMMENDATIONS PRIOR TO DISCHARGE. Before discharge, all the potential therapies for the patient's HF should be addressed, implemented, or planned. Clear communication with the patient, family, and outpatient providers is critical to ensure a smooth transition from hospital to home. Exercise capacity with simple maneuvers such as climbing one flight of stairs or walking down the corridor may be a simple and valuable tool to use before discharge. Education of the patient and family should be started during hospitalization and should continue during outpatient follow-up. Lifestyle modification should be reviewed with the patient, and achievable goals should be set and reviewed during scheduled follow-up. The potential need for micronutrients and macronutrients during the follow-up period should also be addressed.[120,121]

Phase III: Management After Discharge and During the Vulnerable Phase

Early recurrence of signs and symptoms of HF suggestive of worsening volume overload or neurohormonal activation is likely to contribute to the high rates of readmission that are observed in AHFS. Prompt interventions may therefore correct the causes of the hemodynamic abnormalities and prevent the progression of volume overload and new admissions. A follow-up appointment is typically scheduled within approximately 1 month after discharge. However, closer follow-up (in a week or less) should be considered for patients with one or more of the predictors of rehospitalization or death (see earlier). These patients have a high risk of worsening of their clinical and hemodynamic status as well as of their renal function and neurohormonal profile early after discharge. This critical period is known as the vulnerable phase and may represent a critical window of time for intervention to prevent rehospitalization and death. Accordingly, every effort should be made to identify those patients before discharge; to ensure early follow-up with monitoring of blood pressure, body weight, renal function, and possibly BNP; and finally to modify postdischarge therapy if needed.[51a]

Potential New Therapies

All large clinical trials conducted to date that use intravenous agents in patients admitted with AHFS have been negative in terms of efficacy and/or safety (see Table 27-8), possibly owing to lack of drug efficacy, patient selection, or wrong clinical endpoints, and/or study execution.[7,46,121a] Nonetheless, given the diverse pathophysiology of AHFS, it is unrealistic to expect that a single drug would exert beneficial effects in all or even a majority of patients with AHFS.[7,46] A number of promising compounds are undergoing development or clinical evaluation.

SOLUBLE GUANYLATE CYCLASE ACTIVATORS. Cinaciguat (BAY 58-2667) is a soluble guanylate cyclase (sGC) activator that is being developed as a first-in-class treatment for AHFS. In contrast to organic nitrates Cinaciguat acts independently of the sGC ligand nitric oxide and activates the soluble form of guanylate cyclase in smooth muscle cells, thus leading to the synthesis of cGMP and subsequent vasodilation.[122] During periods of increased oxidative stress, such as AHFS, a significant proportion of heme-bound iron may become oxidized, potentially blunting the effects of nitric oxide donors.[123] In contrast, cinaciguat appears to be a heme-independent soluble guanylate cyclase activator, with more predictable vasodilator response in conditions of elevated oxidative stress. In accord with pharmacologic data, cinaciguat has been shown to improve hemodynamics in patients with AHFS[122-122b]; however, at high doses, it has been associated with significant hypotension. The hypotension was not associated with other major adverse events, nor did it affect mortality at 30-days postdischarge. The effects of cinaciguat on hemodynamics and dyspnea are now being investigated in the COMPOSE program that includes three phase II trials in patients admitted with AHFS (ClinicalTrials.gov Identifier NCT01064037).

CHIMERIC NATRIURETIC PEPTIDES. These compounds have been molecularly engineered to optimize the beneficial aspects of different natriuretic peptides into a single molecule while attempting to minimize any potential negative side effects. Chimeric Natriuretic Peptide (CD-NP) combines the beneficial aspects of C-type natriuretic peptide (CNP) with dendroaspis NP (DNP).[124] CNP lacks the natriuretic effects of ANP or BNP but has the benefit of less hypotension because it is a primary venodilator, as opposed to BNP, which dilates both arteries and veins. DNP has significant natriuretic effects but also causes hypotension. CD-NP ideally combines the lack of unwanted arterial vasodilation of CNP with the positive natriuretic effects of DNP.[125] Preliminary studies in AHFS are ongoing (ClinicalTrials.gov Identifier NCT00839007).

DIRECT RENIN INHIBITORS (see Chap. 28). The mechanism of action of this class of drugs consists of the inhibition of the first enzymatic step in the RAAS cascade, leading to a profound suppression of this neurohormonal system.[126] Given the role of RAAS in the pathogenesis of HF and its complications as well as the improved survival associated with its inhibition, further blockade of this system may confer additional survival benefits. Aliskiren, the first oral direct renin inhibitor on the market and currently approved for the treatment of hypertension, is undergoing a phase III trial (ASTRONAUT) to test whether the addition of a direct renin inhibitor to standard therapy delays time to events, including cardiovascular death or HF rehospitalization within 6 months in patients hospitalized for AHFS and ejection fraction <40%.[127] (ClinicalTrials.gov Identifier NCT00894387).

ADENOSINE ANTAGONISTS. The glomerular filtration rate of the kidney is adapted to changes in the sodium concentration in the early distal tubule through the mechanism termed tubuloglomerular feedback. Tubuloglomerular feedback refers to a series of events whereby changes in the Na^+, Cl^-, and K^+ concentrations in the tubular fluid are sensed by the macula densa through the Na^+-K^+-$2Cl^-$ cotransporter. An increase or decrease in Na^+, Cl^-, and K^+ uptake elicits inverse changes in glomerular filtration rate by altering the vascular tone, predominantly of the afferent arteriole. Studies indicate that adenosine (through activation of the adenosine A_1 receptor) and possibly ATP mediate this mechanism, which is increased in HF. Given that adenosine levels are increased in HF patients and may contribute to the progression of renal dysfunction, adenosine A_1 receptor antagonists have been developed to increase renal blood flow and to enhance diuresis without activating the tubuloglomerular feedback. Rolofylline is a highly selective adenosine A_1 receptor antagonist that has been studied in patients with HF. Despite the positive trends seen in the PROTECT pilot study,[128] the phase III PROTECT II trial showed only a mild benefit on symptoms, but no effects on renal protection and other prespecified outcomes, and was associated with more central nervous system events compared with placebo (ClinicalTrials.gov Identifier: NCT00354458).[129] Given these results, it is doubtful that these agents will undergo further evaluation in AHFS.

ULARITIDE. Ularitide is a synthetic analogue of urodilatin, a natriuretic and diuretic hormone of the family of A-type natriuretic peptides produced by tubular renal cells.[130] Besides the effects on sodium and water handling, ularitide induces peripheral arterial vasodilation by activating the cGMP pathway. The effects of a short-term infusion of ularitide in patients with ADHF have been investigated in the SIRIUS (Safety and Efficacy of an Intravenous Placebo-Controlled Randomized Infusion of Ularitide in a Prospective Double-Blind Study in Patients with Symptomatic Decompensated Chronic Heart Failure) trials I and II. Compared with placebo, ularitide improved clinical status, hemodynamics, and neurohormonal profile; however, it was associated with significant hypotension.[131]

ENDOTHELIN ANTAGONISTS. Endothelin 1 is the most powerful endogenous vasoconstrictor and is produced by the vascular endothelial cells. It exerts its effects by binding to two receptors, ET_A and ET_B, located on the vascular smooth muscle cells, resulting in significant systemic arterial vasoconstriction. Tezosentan, a nonselective ET_{A-B} antagonist, has been shown to improve hemodynamics in patients with AHFS. The Value of Endothelin Receptor Inhibition with Tezosentan in Acute Heart Failure Study (VERITAS) studied more than 1400 patients admitted with AHF in an international trial (see Table 27-8). The addition of intravenous tezosentan to standard therapy did not improve symptoms or decrease mortality at 7 days after randomization.[132]

CARDIAC MYOSIN ACTIVATORS. Cardiac myosin activators (CMA) increase, specifically, cardiac myosin ATPase, enhancing the release of inorganic phosphate, which strengthens binding between myosin and actin, the fundamental power-stroke leading to shortening of the cardiac sarcomere. CMAs increase the efficiency with which ATP is utilized without increasing ATP consumption by increasing the number and duration of actin-myosin crossbridges for each ATP molecule consumed. This prolongs systole but not the rate at which force is developed. This is unlike conventional inotropic agents that generally increase ATP consumption, increase the velocity of contraction, and rate of force generation, but may shorten the duration of systole. Importantly, CMAs do not possess phosphodiesterase activity, do not increase diastolic calcium concentrations and can increase cardiac performance in patients receiving beta-blockers.[133,133a] Preliminary data from studies of the CMA, omecamtiv mecarbil (CK-1827452), given intravenously either to healthy volunteers or to patients with stable, mild-to-moderate HF show marked dose-dependent increases in systolic ejection time, with a reflex decline in heart rate at higher concentrations. Concentration-dependent increases were also observed in Doppler-derived stroke volume, fractional shortening, and ejection fraction. OM was well tolerated with no serious adverse events at intended doses in this group of HF patients.[133a] OM is well absorbed from the gut and an oral formulation is being developed (Clinical Trials.gov Identifier NCT01077167).

ISTAROXIME. Istaroxime, the prototype of a new class of drugs, has dual action on the myocyte: by inhibition of the membrane-bound Na^+,K^+-ATPase and by enhancing the activity of the sarcoendoplasmic reticulum Ca^{2+}-ATPase type 2a (SERCA-2a). These distinct mechanisms respectively result in increased cytosolic calcium accumulation during systole, with positive inotropic effects, and rapid sequestration of cytosolic calcium into the sarcoplasmic reticulum during diastole, leading to an enhanced lusitropic effect.[134] Experimentally, istaroxime appears to improve both systolic and diastolic function, to reduce LV dimension in diastole, and to increase SBP. These beneficial effects were not associated with an increase in myocardial oxygen consumption.[135] The HORIZON-HF (A Phase II Trial to Assess Hemodynamic Effects of Istaroxime in Patients with Worsening HF and Reduced LV Systolic Function) studied 120 patients admitted with AHF and decreased ejection fraction (ClinicalTrial.gov identifier NCT00616161). The addition of istaroxime to standard therapy lowered PCWP and heart rate and increased SBP. The higher infusion dose (1.5 μg/k/min) increased cardiac index and reduced LV end-diastolic volume. There were no changes in neurohormones, renal function, or troponin I levels during the short 6-hour infusion.[136,137] This agent is being developed for patients presenting with AHFS and low cardiac output because the majority of inotropes that are often required for these patients tend to decrease blood pressure and have significant side effects.

STRESSCOPIN. The peptide human urocortin 2 (h-UCN2) is a member of the urocortin family, a recently discovered group of peptide hormones of the corticotropin-releasing factor family. They bind with a strong affinity to the corticotropin-releasing hormone receptor 2, which is highly expressed in the myocardium and in the vascular endothelium. Urocortins exhibit potent inotropic and lusitropic effects on rat and sheep heart and activate a group of myocyte protective pathways collectively known as reperfusion injury salvage kinase (RISK).[138] Studies in healthy volunteers and HF patients showed that brief intravenous infusions of urocortin 2 induced pronounced dose-related increases in cardiac output, heart rate, and LV ejection fraction while decreasing systemic vascular resistance.[139,139a] The hemodynamic effects of stresscopin in patients admitted with AHFS is being studied now in a Phase IIa trial.

Human stresscopin (h-SCP), another member of the urocortin family, is a 40-amino-acid peptide, is related to h-UCN2 and both are members of the corticotrophin releasing hormone (CRH) peptide family. The biological actions of the CRH peptide family are elicited by two 7 transmembrane G-protein coupled receptors—CRH receptor type 1 (CRHR1) and CRH receptor type 2 (CRHR2). This molecule is presently being studied for its hemodynamic effects in patients admitted with AHFS (ClihicalTrials.gov NCT01120210).

RELAXIN. Relaxin was first identified as a major hormone of pregnancy with powerful systemic and renal vascular effects.[140] The recent dose-finding phase IIb study Pre-RELAX-AHF assessed the dose-response effects of 48-hour infusion of relaxin versus placebo on symptom relief, other clinical outcomes, and safety in patients with AHF and normal to increased blood pressure. Relaxin therapy was associated with improvement in dyspnea and other clinical outcomes, with an acceptable safety profile.[141] Relaxin is currently being evaluated in the RELAX-AHF (Efficacy and Safety of Relaxin for the Treatment of Acute Heart Failure) phase II/III clinical trial (ClinicalTrials.gov Identifier: NCT00520806).

Future Perspectives

Hospitalizations for AHFS are associated with unacceptably high post-discharge mortality and rehospitalization rates. Although this may be related to severe progressive and irreversible HF in a proportion of these patients, it is possible that many have potential targets for therapies that have not been identified and addressed. A thorough understanding of the specific pathophysiology associated with the diverse syndromes of AHF resulting in appropriate therapies is necessary to achieve improved outcomes. At present, this understanding is lacking, and our management consists of treating the manifestations rather than the pathophysiologic processes. For example, the success achieved in the treatment of ACS has stemmed from the discovery of the specific mechanism of arterial thrombosis secondary to plaque rupture.

It appears that myocardial dysfunction is the major contributor to the progression of HF and that a significant number of patients with AHFS have viable but dysfunctional myocardium that is potentially salvageable. Currently, the extent of "viability" is not being systematically assessed in patients with those syndromes. Although some causes for dysfunctional myocardium, such as chronic ischemia and excessive sympathetic stimulation, are known, there may be many others that have not been identified. For example, failing hearts have abnormal energy use probably due to metabolic abnormalities. Thus, a better understanding of cardiac metabolism of the dysfunctional but viable myocardium will allow development of specific therapies. Because we are dealing with a heterogeneous population of patients, it is unlikely that a "one therapy fits all" approach will lead to an improvement in outcomes. In fact, the trials conducted in AHFS have been to a large extent unsuccessful when this approach was used. Patient characterization and classification based on a pathophysiologic approach will be key for a successful therapy. The importance of this approach has been confirmed in the management of patients presenting with an acute myocardial infarction, when the same therapy may result in different outcomes based on the presence of ST-segment elevation or depression on the electrocardiogram.

REFERENCES

Nomenclature, Definition, Epidemiology, and Classification

1. Gheorghiade M, Pang PS: Acute heart failure syndromes. J Am Coll Cardiol 53:557, 2009.
2. Pang PS, Komajda M, Gheorghiade M: The current and future management of acute heart failure syndromes. Eur Heart J 31:784, 2010.
3. Adams KF Jr, Fonarow GC, Emerman CL, et al: Characteristics and outcomes of patients hospitalized for heart failure in the United States: rationale, design, and preliminary observations from the first 100,000 cases in the Acute Decompensated Heart Failure National Registry (ADHERE). Am Heart J 149:209, 2005.
4. Fonarow GC, Stough WG, Abraham WT, et al: Characteristics, treatments, and outcomes of patients with preserved systolic function hospitalized for heart failure: A report from the OPTIMIZE-HF Registry. J Am Coll Cardiol 50:768, 2007.
5. Cleland JG, Swedberg K, Cohen-Solal A, et al: The Euro Heart Failure Survey of the EUROHEART survey programme. A survey on the quality of care among patients with heart failure in Europe. The Study Group on Diagnosis of the Working Group on Heart Failure of the European Society of Cardiology. The Medicines Evaluation Group Centre for Health Economics University of York. Eur J Heart Fail 2:123, 2000.
6. Albert NM, Fonarow GC, Abraham WT, et al: Predictors of delivery of hospital-based heart failure patient education: A report from OPTIMIZE-HF. J Card Fail 13:189, 2007.
7. Gheorghiade M, Zannad F, Sopko G, et al: Acute heart failure syndromes: Current state and framework for future research. Circulation 112:3958, 2005.
8. Dickstein K, Cohen-Solal A, Filippatos G, et al: ESC guidelines for the diagnosis and treatment of acute and chronic heart failure 2008: The Task Force for the diagnosis and treatment of acute and chronic heart failure 2008 of the European Society of Cardiology. Developed in collaboration with the Heart Failure Association of the ESC (HFA) and endorsed by the European Society of Intensive Care Medicine (ESICM). Eur J Heart Fail 10:933, 2008.
9. Hunt SA, Abraham WT, Chin MH, et al: 2009 Focused update incorporated into the ACC/AHA 2005 Guidelines for the Diagnosis and Management of Heart Failure in Adults A Report of the American College of Cardiology Foundation/American Heart Association Task Force on Practice Guidelines Developed in Collaboration With the International Society for Heart and Lung Transplantation. J Am Coll Cardiol 53:e1, 2009.

9a. Lindenfeld J, Albert NM, Boehmer JP, et al: Executive Summary: Heart Failure Society of America 2010 Comprehensive Heart Failure Practice Guideline. J Card Fail 16:475, 2010.

Pathophysiology

10. Gheorghiade M, Filippatos G, De Luca L, Burnett J: Congestion in acute heart failure syndromes: An essential target of evaluation and treatment. Am J Med 119:S3, 2006.
11. Chaudhry SI, Wang Y, Concato J, et al: Patterns of weight change preceding hospitalization for heart failure. Circulation 116:1549, 2007.

12. Zile MR, Bennett TD, St. John Sutton M, et al: Transition from chronic compensated to acute decompensated heart failure: Pathophysiological insights obtained from continuous monitoring of intracardiac pressures. Circulation 118:1433, 2008.
13. Flaherty JD, Bax JJ, De Luca L, et al: Acute heart failure syndromes in patients with coronary artery disease early assessment and treatment. J Am Coll Cardiol 53:254, 2009.
14. Solomon SD, Wang D, Finn P, et al: Effect of candesartan on cause-specific mortality in heart failure patients: The Candesartan in Heart failure Assessment of Reduction in Mortality and morbidity (CHARM) program. Circulation 110:2180, 2004.
15. Lee DS, Austin PC, Stukel TA, et al: "Dose-dependent" impact of recurrent cardiac events on mortality in patients with heart failure. Am J Med 122:162, 2009.
16. Yancy CW, Lopatin M, Stevenson LW, et al: Clinical presentation, management, and in-hospital outcomes of patients admitted with acute decompensated heart failure with preserved systolic function: A report from the Acute Decompensated Heart Failure National Registry (ADHERE) Database. J Am Coll Cardiol 47:76, 2006.
17. Shah SJ, Gheorghiade M: Heart failure with preserved ejection fraction: Treat now by treating comorbidities. JAMA 300:431, 2008.
18. Latini R, Masson S, Anand IS, et al: Prognostic value of very low plasma concentrations of troponin T in patients with stable chronic heart failure. Circulation 116:1242, 2007.
19. Metra M, Nodari S, Parrinello G, et al: The role of plasma biomarkers in acute heart failure. Serial changes and independent prognostic value of NT-proBNP and cardiac troponin-T. Eur J Heart Fail 9:776, 2007.
20. Peacock WF, De Marco T, Fonarow GC, et al: Cardiac troponin and outcome in acute heart failure. N Engl J Med 358:2117, 2008.
21. Gheorghiade M, Gattis Stough W, et al: The Pilot Randomized Study of Nesiritide Versus Dobutamine in Heart Failure (PRESERVD-HF). Am J Cardiol 96:18G, 2005.
22. Felker GM, Benza RL, Chandler AB, et al: Heart failure etiology and response to milrinone in decompensated heart failure: Results from the OPTIME-CHF study. J Am Coll Cardiol 41:997, 2003.
23. Cohn JN, Franciosa JA, Francis GS, et al: Effect of short-term infusion of sodium nitroprusside on mortality rate in acute myocardial infarction complicated by left ventricular failure: Results of a Veterans Administration cooperative study. N Engl J Med 306:1129, 1982.
24. Beohar N, Erdogan AK, Lee DC, et al: Acute heart failure syndromes and coronary perfusion. J Am Coll Cardiol 52:13, 2008.
25. Damman K, Navis G, Voors AA, et al: Worsening renal function and prognosis in heart failure: Systematic review and meta-analysis. J Card Fail 13:599, 2007.
26. Hillege HL, Nitsch D, Pfeffer MA, et al: Renal function as a predictor of outcome in a broad spectrum of patients with heart failure. Circulation 113:671, 2006.
27. Forman DE, Butler J, Wang Y, et al: Incidence, predictors at admission, and impact of worsening renal function among patients hospitalized with heart failure. J Am Coll Cardiol 43:61, 2004.
28. Mullens W, Abrahams Z, Francis GS, et al: Importance of venous congestion for worsening of renal function in advanced decompensated heart failure. J Am Coll Cardiol 53:589, 2009.
29. Damman K, van Deursen VM, Navis G, et al: Increased central venous pressure is associated with impaired renal function and mortality in a broad spectrum of patients with cardiovascular disease. J Am Coll Cardiol 53:582, 2009.
30. Gheorghiade M, Abraham WT, Albert NM, et al: Systolic blood pressure at admission, clinical characteristics, and outcomes in patients hospitalized with acute heart failure. JAMA 296:2217, 2006.
31. Bozkurt B, Mann DL, Deswal A: Biomarkers of inflammation in heart failure. Heart Fail Rev 15:331, 2010.
32. Janssen SPM, Gayan-Ramirez G, Van Den Bergh A, et al: Interleukin-6 causes myocardial failure and skeletal muscle atrophy in rats. Circulation 111:996, 2005.
33. Pagani FD, Baker LS, Hsi C, et al: Left ventricular systolic and diastolic dysfunction after infusion of tumor necrosis factor-alpha in conscious dogs. J Clin Invest 90:389, 1992.
34. Vlachopoulos C, Dima I, Aznaouridis K, et al: Acute systemic inflammation increases arterial stiffness and decreases wave reflections in healthy individuals. Circulation 112:2193, 2005.
35. Milo O, Cotter G, Kaluski E, et al: Comparison of inflammatory and neurohormonal activation in cardiogenic pulmonary edema secondary to ischemic versus nonischemic causes. Am J Cardiol 92:222, 2003.
36. Fonarow GC, Abraham WT, Albert NM, et al: Factors identified as precipitating hospital admissions for heart failure and clinical outcomes: Findings from OPTIMIZE-HF. Arch Intern Med 168:847, 2008.
37. Maisel AS, Krishnaswamy P, Nowak RM, et al: Rapid measurement of B-type natriuretic peptide in the emergency diagnosis of heart failure. N Engl J Med 347:161, 2002.
38. Anand IS, Fisher LD, Chiang YT, et al: Changes in brain natriuretic peptide and norepinephrine over time and mortality and morbidity in the Valsartan Heart Failure Trial (Val-HeFT). Circulation 107:1278, 2003.
39. Heublein DM, Huntley BK, Boerrigter G, et al: Immunoreactivity and guanosine 3′,5′-cyclic monophosphate activating actions of various molecular forms of human B-type natriuretic peptide. Hypertension 49:1114, 2007.
40. Waldo SW, Beede J, Isakson S, et al: Pro-B-type natriuretic peptide levels in acute decompensated heart failure. J Am Coll Cardiol 51:1874, 2008.
41. Lam CS, Burnett JC Jr, Costello-Boerrigter L, et al: Alternate circulating pro-B-type natriuretic peptide and B-type natriuretic peptide forms in the general population. J Am Coll Cardiol 49:1193, 2007.
42. Gurbel PA, Gattis WA, Fuzaylov SF, et al: Evaluation of platelets in heart failure: Is platelet activity related to etiology, functional class, or clinical outcomes? Am Heart J 143:1068, 2002.
43. O'Connor CM, Gurbel PA, Serebruany VL: Usefulness of soluble and surface-bound P-selectin in detecting heightened platelet activity in patients with congestive heart failure. Am J Cardiol 83:1345, 1999.
44. Nieminen MS, Brutsaert D, Dickstein K, et al: EuroHeart Failure Survey II (EHFS II): A survey on hospitalized acute heart failure patients: Description of population. Eur Heart J 27:2725, 2006.

Outcomes in Acute Heart Failure Syndromes

45. Blair JE, Zannad F, Konstam MA, et al: Continental differences in clinical characteristics, management, and outcomes in patients hospitalized with worsening heart failure results from the EVEREST (Efficacy of Vasopressin Antagonism in Heart Failure: Outcome Study with Tolvaptan) program. J Am Coll Cardiol 52:1640, 2008.
46. Gheorghiade M, Adams KF, Cleland JG, et al: Phase III clinical trial end points in acute heart failure syndromes: A virtual roundtable with the Acute Heart Failure Syndromes International Working Group. Am Heart J 157:957, 2009.
47. Fonarow G, Albert N, Curtis A, et al: Improving evidence-based care for heart failure in outpatient cardiology practices. Primary results of the Registry to Improve the Use of Evidence-Based Heart Failure Therapies in the Outpatient Setting (IMPROVE HF). Circulation 2010 Jul 26. [Epub ahead of print]
48. Flaherty JD, Rossi JS, Fonarow GC, et al: Influence of coronary angiography on the utilization of therapies in patients with acute heart failure syndromes: Findings from Organized Program to Initiate Lifesaving Treatment in Hospitalized Patients with Heart Failure (OPTIMIZE-HF). Am Heart J 157:1018, 2009.
49. Jencks SF, Williams MV, Coleman EA: Rehospitalizations among patients in the Medicare fee-for-service program. N Engl J Med 360:1418, 2009.
50. O'Connor CM, Miller AB, Blair JE, et al: Mode of death and re-hospitalization in patients hospitalized with worsening heart failure and reduced left ventricular ejection fraction: Results from Efficacy of Vasopressin Antagonism in Heart Failure Outcome Study with Tolvaptan (EVEREST) program. Am Heart J 159:841, 2010.
51. Dunlay S, Gheorghiade M, Reid K, et al: Critical elements of clinical follow-up after hospital discharge for heart failure: Insights from the EVEREST trial. Eur J Heart Fail 12:367, 2010.
51a. Gheorghiade M, Bonow RO: Heart failure: early follow-up after hospitalization for heart failure. Nat Rev Cardiol 7:422, 2010.
51b. Hernandez AF, Greiner MA, Fonarow GC, et al: Relationship between early physician follow-up and 30-day readmission among Medicare beneficiaries hospitalized for heart failure. JAMA 303:1716, 2010.
52. Abraham WT, Fonarow GC, Albert NM, et al: Predictors of in-hospital mortality in patients hospitalized for heart failure: Insights from the Organized Program to Initiate Lifesaving Treatment in Hospitalized Patients With Heart Failure (OPTIMIZE-HF). J Am Coll Cardiol 52:347, 2008.
53. O'Connor CM, Abraham WT, Albert NM, et al: Predictors of mortality after discharge in patients hospitalized with heart failure: An analysis from the Organized Program to Initiate Lifesaving Treatment in Hospitalized Patients with Heart Failure (OPTIMIZE-HF). Am Heart J 156:662, 2008.
54. Allen LA, Reid KJ, Dunlay SM, et al: Predictors of persistently low health status following hospitalization for heart failure. Abstract presentation. AHA Quality of Care and Outcome Conference. 2009 April 23; Washington, D.C.
55. Blair JE, Burnett JC, Konstam MA, et al: Prognostic value and changes in renal function in patients admitted with acute heart failure—results from the EVEREST program. Eur Heart J 29(Abstract Suppl):270, 2008.
56. Januzzi JL Jr, Sakhuja R, O'Donoghue M, et al: Utility of amino-terminal pro-brain natriuretic peptide testing for prediction of 1-year mortality in patients with dyspnea treated in the emergency department. Arch Intern Med 166:315, 2006.
57. Fonarow GC, Peacock WF, Phillips CO, et al: Admission B-type natriuretic peptide levels and in-hospital mortality in acute decompensated heart failure. J Am Coll Cardiol 49:1943, 2007.
58. Peacock WF, De Marco T, Fonarow GC, et al: Cardiac troponin and outcome in acute heart failure. N Engl J Med 358:2117, 2008.
59. You JJ, Austin PC, Alter DA, et al: Relation between cardiac troponin I and mortality in acute decompensated heart failure. Am Heart J 153:462, 2007.
60. Fonarow GC, Peacock WF, Horwich TB, et al: Usefulness of B-type natriuretic peptide and cardiac troponin levels to predict in-hospital mortality from ADHERE. Am J Cardiol 101:231, 2008.
61. Gheorghiade M, Pang PS: Are BNP changes during hospitalization for heart failure a reliable surrogate for predicting the effects of therapies on post-discharge mortality? J Am Coll Cardiol 53:2349, 2009.
62. Gheorghiade M, Abraham WT, Albert NM, et al: Relationship between admission serum sodium concentration and clinical outcomes in patients hospitalized for heart failure: An analysis from the OPTIMIZE-HF registry. Eur Heart J 28:980, 2007.
63. Gheorghiade M, Rossi JS, Cotts W, et al: Characterization and prognostic value of persistent hyponatremia in patients with severe heart failure in the ESCAPE Trial. Arch Intern Med 167:1998, 2007.
64. Blair JE, Khan S, Konstam MA, et al: Weight changes after hospitalization for worsening heart failure and subsequent re-hospitalization and mortality in the EVEREST trial. Eur Heart J 30:1666, 2009.
65. Wang NC, Maggioni AP, Konstam MA, et al: Clinical implications of QRS duration in patients hospitalized with worsening heart failure and reduced left ventricular ejection fraction. JAMA 299:2656, 2008.
66. Rossi JS, Flaherty JD, Fonarow GC, et al: Influence of coronary artery disease and coronary revascularization status on outcomes in patients with acute heart failure syndromes: A report from OPTIMIZE-HF (Organized Program to Initiate Lifesaving Treatment in Hospitalized Patients with Heart Failure). Eur J Heart Fail 10:1215, 2008.
67. Benza RL, Tallaj JA, Felker GM, et al: The impact of arrhythmias in acute heart failure. J Card Fail 10:279, 2004.

Assessment of Acute Heart Failure Syndromes

68. Mebazaa A, Pang PS, Tavares M, et al: The impact of early standard therapy on dyspnoea in patients with acute heart failure: The URGENT-dyspnoea study. Eur Heart J 31:832, 2010.
69. Aronson D, Burger AJ: Relation between pulse pressure and survival in patients with decompensated heart failure. Am J Cardiol 93:785, 2004.
70. Felker GM, Cuculich PS, Gheorghiade M: The Valsalva maneuver: A bedside "biomarker" for heart failure. Am J Med 119:117, 2006.
71. Tavazzi L, Maggioni AP, Lucci D, et al: Nationwide survey on acute heart failure in cardiology ward services in Italy. Eur Heart J 27:1207, 2006.
72. Konstam MA, Gheorghiade M, Burnett JC Jr, et al: Effects of oral tolvaptan in patients hospitalized for worsening heart failure: The EVEREST Outcome Trial. JAMA 297:1319, 2007.
73. Gheorghiade M, Konstam MA, Burnett JC Jr, et al: Short-term clinical effects of tolvaptan, an oral vasopressin antagonist, in patients hospitalized for heart failure: The EVEREST Clinical Status Trials. JAMA 297:1332, 2007.
74. Young JB, Abraham WT, Albert NM, et al: Relation of low hemoglobin and anemia to morbidity and mortality in patients hospitalized with heart failure (insight from the OPTIMIZE-HF registry). Am J Cardiol 101:223, 2008.

75. Hobbs RE, Mills RM: Endogenous B-type natriuretic peptide: A limb of the regulatory response to acutely decompensated heart failure. Clin Cardiol 31:407, 2008.
76. Maisel A, Mueller C, Adams K Jr, et al: State of the art: using natriuretic peptide levels in clinical practice. Eur J Heart Fail 10:824, 2008.
77. Cohen-Solal A, Logeart D, Huang B, et al: Lowered B-type natriuretic peptide in response to levosimendan or dobutamine treatment is associated with improved survival in patients with severe acutely decompensated heart failure. J Am Coll Cardiol 53:2343, 2009.
78. Maisel A, Mueller C, Nowak R, et al: Mid-region pro-hormone markers for diagnosis and prognosis in acute dyspnea: results from the BACH (Biomarkers in Acute Heart Failure) trial. J Am Coll Cardiol 55:2062, 2010.
79. Collins SP, Lindsell CJ, Storrow AB, Abraham WT: Prevalence of negative chest radiography results in the emergency department patient with decompensated heart failure. Ann Emerg Med 47:13, 2006.
80. Seghatol FF, Shah DJ, Diluzio S, et al: Relation between contractile reserve and improvement in left ventricular function with beta-blocker therapy in patients with heart failure secondary to ischemic or idiopathic dilated cardiomyopathy. Am J Cardiol 93:854, 2004.
81. Shors SM, Cotts WG, Pavlovic-Surjancev B, et al: Non-invasive cardiac evaluation in heart failure patients using magnetic resonance imaging: A feasibility study. Heart Fail Rev 10:265, 2005.
82. ESCAPE Investigators and ESCAPE Study Coordinators: Evaluation study of congestive heart failure and pulmonary artery catheterization effectiveness: The ESCAPE trial. JAMA 294:1625, 2005.

Management of Acute Heart Failure Syndromes

83. Fonarow GC, Heywood JT, Heidenreich PA, et al: Temporal trends in clinical characteristics, treatments, and outcomes for heart failure hospitalizations, 2002 to 2004: Findings from Acute Decompensated Heart Failure National Registry (ADHERE). Am Heart J 153:1021, 2007.
84. Peacock WF, Hollander JE, Diercks DB, et al: Morphine and outcomes in acute decompensated heart failure: An ADHERE analysis. Emerg Med J 25:205, 2008.
85. Masip J, Roque M, Sanchez B, et al: Noninvasive ventilation in acute cardiogenic pulmonary edema: Systematic review and meta-analysis. JAMA 294:3124, 2005.
86. Masip J, Mebazaa A, Filippatos GS: Noninvasive ventilation in acute cardiogenic pulmonary edema. N Engl J Med 359:2068, 2008.
87. Salvador DR, Rey NR, Ramos GC, Punzalan FE: Continuous infusion versus bolus injection of loop diuretics in congestive heart failure. Cochrane Database Syst Rev (3):CD003178, 2005.
88. Felker GM, O'Connor CM, Braunwald E: Loop diuretics in acute decompensated heart failure: Necessary? Evil? A necessary evil? Circ Heart Fail 2:56, 2009.
89. McCurley JM, Hanlon SU, Wei SK, et al: Furosemide and the progression of left ventricular dysfunction in experimental heart failure. J Am Coll Cardiol 44:1301, 2004.
90. Stiles S: How to diurese in acute HF: Dosing strategies get an evidence base. Available at: http://www.theheart.org/article/1058939.do. Accessed March 23, 2010.
91. Lindenfeld J, Albert NM, Boehmer JP, et al: HFSA 2010 comprehensive heart failure practice guideline. J Card Fail 16:e1, 2010.
92. Intravenous nesiritide vs nitroglycerin for treatment of decompensated congestive heart failure: A randomized controlled trial. JAMA 287:1531, 2002.
93. Sackner-Bernstein JD, Kowalski M, Fox M, Aaronson K: Short-term risk of death after treatment with nesiritide for decompensated heart failure: A pooled analysis of randomized controlled trials. JAMA 293:1900, 2005.
93a. Sackner-Bernstein JD, Skopicki HA, Aaronson KD: Risk of worsening renal function with nesiritide in patients with acutely decompensated heart failure. Circulation 111:1487, 2005.
94. Schulz R, Rose J, Martin C, et al: Development of short-term myocardial hibernation. Its limitation by the severity of ischemia and inotropic stimulation. Circulation 88:684, 1993.
95. Abraham WT, Adams KF, Fonarow GC, et al: In-hospital mortality in patients with acute decompensated heart failure requiring intravenous vasoactive medications: An analysis from the Acute Decompensated Heart Failure National Registry (ADHERE). J Am Coll Cardiol 46:57, 2005.
96. Shin DD, Brandimarte F, De Luca L, et al: Review of current and investigational pharmacologic agents for acute heart failure syndromes. Am J Cardiol 99:4A, 2007.
97. Bayram M, De Luca L, Massie MB, Gheorghiade M: Reassessment of dobutamine, dopamine, and milrinone in the management of acute heart failure syndromes. Am J Cardiol 96:47G, 2005.
98. Gheorghiade M, Gattis WA, Klein L: OPTIME in CHF trial: Rethinking the use of inotropes in the management of worsening chronic heart failure resulting in hospitalization. Eur J Heart Fail 5:9, 2003.
99. De Luca L, Colucci WS, Nieminen MS, et al: Evidence-based use of levosimendan in different clinical settings. Eur Heart J 27:1908, 2006.
100. Packer M: REVIVE II: Multicenter placebo-controlled trial of levosimendan on clinical status in acutely decompensated heart failure. American Heart Association Scientific Sessions 2005 Late Breaking Clinical Trials II; November 13-16, 2005; Dallas, Texas.
101. Mebazaa A, Nieminen MS, Packer M, et al: Levosimendan vs dobutamine for patients with acute decompensated heart failure: The SURVIVE Randomized Trial. JAMA 297:1883, 2007.
102. Gheorghiade M, Braunwald E: Reconsidering the role for digoxin in the management of acute heart failure syndromes. JAMA 302:2146, 2009.
103. Gheorghiade M, van Veldhuisen DJ, Colucci WS: Contemporary use of digoxin in the management of cardiovascular disorders. Circulation 113:2556, 2006.
104. Goldsmith SR, Gheorghiade M: Vasopressin antagonism in heart failure. J Am Coll Cardiol 46:1785, 2005.
105. Udelson JE, Orlandi C, Ouyang J, et al: Acute hemodynamic effects of tolvaptan, a vasopressin V_2 receptor blocker, in patients with symptomatic heart failure and systolic dysfunction: An international, multicenter, randomized, placebo-controlled trial. J Am Coll Cardiol 52:1540, 2008.
106. Schrier RW, Gross P, Gheorghiade M, et al: Tolvaptan, a selective oral vasopressin V_2-receptor antagonist, for hyponatremia. N Engl J Med 355:2099, 2006.
107. Goldsmith SR, Elkayam U, Haught WH, et al: Efficacy and safety of the vasopressin V_{1A}/V_2-receptor antagonist conivaptan in acute decompensated heart failure: A dose-ranging pilot study. J Card Fail 14:641, 2008.
108. Burlew BS, Gheorghiade M, Jafri SM, et al: Acute and chronic hemodynamic effects of nicardipine hydrochloride in patients with heart failure. Am Heart J 114:793, 1987.
109. Reynolds HR, Hochman JS: Cardiogenic shock: Current concepts and improving outcomes. Circulation 117:686, 2008.
110. O'Connell JB, McCarthy PM, Sopko G, et al: Mechanical circulatory support devices for acute heart failure syndromes: Considerations for clinical trial design. Heart Fail Rev 14:101, 2009.
111. Costanzo MR, Guglin ME, Saltzberg MT, et al: Ultrafiltration versus intravenous diuretics for patients hospitalized for acute decompensated heart failure. J Am Coll Cardiol 49:675, 2007.
112. Gattis WA, O'Connor CM, Gallup DS, et al: Predischarge initiation of carvedilol in patients hospitalized for decompensated heart failure: Results of the Initiation Management Predischarge: Process for Assessment of Carvedilol Therapy in Heart Failure (IMPACT-HF) trial. J Am Coll Cardiol 43:1534, 2004.
113. Albert NM, Yancy CW, Liang L, et al: Use of aldosterone antagonists in heart failure. JAMA 302:1658, 2009.
114. Ahmed A, Rich MW, Love TE, et al: Digoxin and reduction in mortality and hospitalization in heart failure: A comprehensive post hoc analysis of the DIG trial. Eur Heart J 27:178, 2006.
115. McMurray JJ: Clinical practice. Systolic heart failure. N Engl J Med 362:228, 2010.
116. Taylor AL, Ziesche S, Yancy C, et al: Combination of isosorbide dinitrate and hydralazine in blacks with heart failure. N Engl J Med 351:2049, 2004.
117. Wang NC, Piccini JP, Konstam MA, et al: Post-discharge outcomes based on implantable cardioverter-defibrillator status in patients hospitalized for heart failure with chronically reduced left ventricular ejection fraction. Am J Ther 17:e78, 2010.
118. Cleland JG, Freemantle N, Coletta AP, Clark AL: Clinical trials update from the American Heart Association: REPAIR-AMI, ASTAMI, JELIS, MEGA, REVIVE-II, SURVIVE, and PROACTIVE. Eur J Heart Fail 8:105, 2006.
119. Gheorghiade M, Sopko G, De Luca L, et al: Navigating the crossroads of coronary artery disease and heart failure. Circulation 114:1202, 2006.
120. Soukoulis V, Dihu JB, Sole M, et al: Micronutrient deficiencies an unmet need in heart failure. J Am Coll Cardiol 54:1660, 2009.
121. Tavazzi L, Maggioni AP, Marchioli R, et al: Effect of n-3 polyunsaturated fatty acids in patients with chronic heart failure (the GISSI-HF trial): A randomised, double-blind, placebo-controlled trial. Lancet 372:1223, 2008.
121a. Felker GM, Pang PS, Adams KF, et al: Clinical trials of pharmacological therapies in acute heart failure syndromes: Lessons learned and directions forward. Circ Heart Fail 3:314, 2010. PubMed PMID: 20233993.

Potential New Therapies and Future Perspectives

122. Lapp H, Mitrovic V, Franz N, et al: Cinaciguat (BAY 58-2667) improves cardiopulmonary hemodynamics in patients with acute decompensated heart failure. Circulation 119:2781, 2009.
122a. Erdmann E, Semigran MJ, Nieminen MS, et al: Cinaciguat, a soluble guanylate cyclase activator, unloads the heart in acute decompensated heart failure. JACC 55; A16. E147(10)60148, 2010.
122b. Mitrovic V, Hernandez AF, Meyer M, Gheorghiade M: Role of guanylate cyclase modulators in decompensated heart failure. Heart Fail Rev 14:309, 2009. Review.
123. Evgenov OV, Pacher P, Schmidt PM, et al: NO-independent stimulators and activators of soluble guanylate cyclase: Discovery and therapeutic potential. Nat Rev Drug Discov 5:755, 2006.
124. Lisy O, Huntley BK, McCormick DJ, et al: Design, synthesis, and actions of a novel chimeric natriuretic peptide: CD-NP. J Am Coll Cardiol 52:60, 2008.
125. Lee CY, Chen HH, Lisy O, et al: Pharmacodynamics of a novel designer natriuretic peptide, CD-NP, in a first-in-human clinical trial in healthy subjects. J Clin Pharmacol 49:668, 2009.
126. Andersen K, Weinberger MH, Egan B, et al: Comparative efficacy and safety of aliskiren, an oral direct renin inhibitor, and ramipril in hypertension: A 6-month, randomized, double-blind trial. J Hypertens 26:589, 2008.
127. Gheorghiade M, Albaghdadi M, Zannad F, et al: Rationale and Design of the Multicenter, Randomized, Double-Blind, Placebo-Controlled Aliskiren Trial on Acute Heart Failure Outcomes (ASTRONAUT). European Journal of HF. In press.
128. Cotter G, Dittrich HC, Weatherley BD, et al: The PROTECT pilot study: A randomized, placebo-controlled, dose-finding study of the adenosine A_1 receptor antagonist rolofylline in patients with acute heart failure and renal impairment. J Card Fail 14:631, 2008.
129. Massie BM, O'Connor CM, Marco M, et al: Rolofylline, an adenosine a_1–receptor antagonist, in acute heart failure. N Engl J Med 363:1419, 2010.
130. De Luca L, Mebazaa A, Filippatos G, et al: Overview of emerging pharmacologic agents for acute heart failure syndromes. Eur J Heart Fail 10:201, 2008.
131. Mitrovic V, Seferovic PM, Simeunovic D, et al: Haemodynamic and clinical effects of ularitide in decompensated heart failure. Eur Heart J 27:2823, 2006.
132. McMurray JJ, Teerlink JR, Cotter G, et al: Effects of tezosentan on symptoms and clinical outcomes in patients with acute heart failure: The VERITAS randomized controlled trials. JAMA 298:2009, 2007.
133. Teerlink JR: A novel approach to improve cardiac performance: Cardiac myosin activators. Heart Fail Rev 14:289, 2009.
134. Khan H, Metra M, Blair JE, et al: Istaroxime, a first in class new chemical entity exhibiting SERCA-2 activation and Na-K-ATPase inhibition: A new promising treatment for acute heart failure syndromes? Heart Fail Rev 14:277, 2009.
135. Sabbah HN, Imai M, Cowart D, et al: Hemodynamic properties of a new-generation positive luso-inotropic agent for the acute treatment of advanced heart failure. Am J Cardiol 99:41A, 2007.
136. Shah SJ, Blair JE, Filippatos GS, et al: Effects of istaroxime on diastolic stiffness in acute heart failure syndromes: Results from the Hemodynamic, Echocardiographic, and Neurohormonal Effects of Istaroxime, a Novel Intravenous Inotropic and Lusitropic Agent: A Randomized Controlled Trial in Patients Hospitalized with Heart Failure (HORIZON-HF) trial. Am Heart J 157:1035, 2009.
137. Gheorghiade M, Blair JE, Filippatos GS, et al: Hemodynamic, echocardiographic, and neurohormonal effects of istaroxime, a novel intravenous inotropic and lusitropic agent: A randomized controlled trial in patients hospitalized with heart failure. J Am Coll Cardiol 51:2276, 2008.

138. Rademaker MT, Cameron VA, Charles CJ, Richards AM: Integrated hemodynamic, hormonal, and renal actions of urocortin 2 in normal and paced sheep: Beneficial effects in heart failure. Circulation 112:3624, 2005.
139. Davis ME, Pemberton CJ, Yandle TG, et al: Urocortin 2 infusion in healthy humans: Hemodynamic, neurohormonal, and renal responses. J Am Coll Cardiol 49:461, 2007.
139a. Davis ME, Pemberton CJ, Yandle TG, et al: Urocortin 2 infusion in human heart failure. Eur Heart J 28:2589. Epub 2007 Aug 25. PubMed PMID: 17720993.
140. Du XJ, Bathgate RA, Samuel CS, et al: Cardiovascular effects of relaxin: From basic science to clinical therapy. Nat Rev Cardiol 7:48, 2010.
141. Teerlink JR, Metra M, Felker GM, et al: Relaxin for the treatment of patients with acute heart failure (Pre-RELAX-AHF): A multicentre, randomised, placebo-controlled, parallel-group, dose-finding phase IIb study. Lancet 373:1429, 2009.

CHAPTER 28 Management of Heart Failure Patients with Reduced Ejection Fraction

Douglas L. Mann

Epidemiology

The worldwide prevalence and incidence rates of heart failure (HF) are approaching epidemic proportions, as evidenced by the relentless increase in the number of HF hospitalizations, the growing number of HF-attributable deaths, and the spiraling costs associated with the care of HF patients. Worldwide, HF affects almost 23 million people. In the United States, HF affects approximately 4.7 million persons (1.5% to 2% of the total population), with approximately 550,000 incident cases of HF diagnosed annually. Estimates of the prevalence of symptomatic HF in the general European population is similar to that in the United States, and ranges from 0.4% to 2%.[1] The prevalence of HF follows an exponential pattern, rising with age, and affects 6% to 10% of people older than 65 years (**Fig. 28-1**). Data from the Framingham Heart Study suggest that the overall incidence of HF has declined among women but not among men.[2] However, although the relative incidence of HF is lower in women than in men, women constitute at least 50% of cases of HF because of their longer life expectancy. In North America and Europe, the lifetime risk of developing HF is approximately one in five for a 40-year-old. The overall prevalence of HF is thought to be increasing, in part because our current therapies of cardiac disorders, such as myocardial infarction, valvular heart disease, and arrhythmias, are allowing patients to survive longer. Very little is known with respect to the prevalence or risk of developing HF in emerging nations because of the lack of population-based studies in these countries.[3] Although HF was once thought to arise primarily in the setting of a depressed left ventricular ejection fraction (LVEF), epidemiologic studies have shown that approximately 50% of patients who develop HF have a normal or preserved EF (EF > 40% to 50%). Accordingly, HF patients are now broadly categorized into one of two groups: (1) HF with a reduced (depressed) EF, commonly referred to as systolic failure; or (2) HF with a preserved EF, commonly referred to as diastolic failure. The epidemiology of HF with a normal EF is discussed in Chap. 30.

Based on population-attributable risks, hypertension has the greatest impact on the development of HF, accounting for 39% of HF events in men and 59% in women. Despite its much lower prevalence in the population (3% to 10%), myocardial infarction also has a high attributable risk in men (34%) and women (13%). Valvular heart disease only accounted for 7% to 8% of HF (**Table 28-1**). Dyslipidemia characterized by a high total high-density lipoprotein (HDL) cholesterol ratio, but not the total cholesterol alone, was also a risk factor for the development of HF.

Studies from the Framingham Study have suggested that obesity is a potential risk factor for the development of HF in men and women (**Fig. 28-2**).[4] However, although obesity is a risk factor for the development of HF, obese patients with HF seem to have a more favorable clinical prognosis. The association between obesity, a traditional cardiovascular risk factor, and improved clinical outcomes in HF patients (i.e., reverse epidemiology) has been termed the *obesity paradox*.

Causative Factors

As shown in **Table 28-2**, any condition that leads to an alteration in LV structure or function can predispose a patient to developing HF. Although the cause of HF in patients with a preserved EF differs from that of patient with depressed EF (see Chap. 30), there is considerable overlap between the causes of these two conditions. In industrialized countries, coronary artery disease (CAD) has become the predominant cause in men and women, and is responsible for 60% to 75% of cases of HF. Hypertension contributes to the development of HF in 75% of patients, including most patients with CAD. Both CAD and hypertension interact to augment the risk of HF. Rheumatic heart disease remains a major cause of HF in Africa and Asia, especially in the young. Hypertension is an important cause of HF in the African and African American population. Chagas disease is still a major cause of HF in South America.[3] Not surprisingly, anemia is a frequent concomitant factor in HF in many developing nations. As developing nations undergo socioeconomic development, the epidemiology of HF is becoming similar to that of Western Europe and North America, with CAD emerging as the single most common cause of HF. Although the contribution of diabetes mellitus to HF is not well understood, diabetes accelerates atherosclerosis and is often associated with hypertension.

In 20% to 30% of the cases of HF with a depressed EF, the exact causative basis is not known. These patients are referred to as having nonischemic, dilated, or idiopathic cardiomyopathy if the cause is unknown (see Chap. 68). Prior viral infection (see Chap. 70) or toxin exposure (e.g., alcohol [see Chap. 73] or use of chemotherapeutic agents [see Chap. 90]) may also lead to a dilated cardiomyopathy. Although excessive alcohol consumption can promote cardiomyopathy, alcohol consumption per se is not associated with increased risk for HF, and may protect against the development of HF when consumed in moderation.[5] It is also becoming increasingly clear that a large number of the cases of dilated cardiomyopathy are secondary to specific genetic defects, most notably those in the

CH 28

TABLE 28-1 Risk Factors for Cardiac Failure: Framingham Offspring and Cohort Study*

	Age- and Risk Factor–Adjusted Hazard Ratio		*Prevalence (%)*		*Population-Attributable Risk (%)*	
PARAMETER	MEN	WOMEN	MEN	WOMEN	MEN	WOMEN
High blood pressure (≥140/90 mm Hg)	2.1	3.4	60	62	39	59
Myocardial infarction	6.3	6.0	10	3	34	13
Angina	1.4	1.7	11	9	5	5
Diabetes	1.8	3.7	8	5	6	12
Left ventricular hypertrophy	2.2	2.9	4	3	4	5
Valvular heart disease	2.5	2.1	5	8	7	8

*Subjects aged 40-89; 18-year follow-up.

From Levy D, Larson MG, Vasan RS, et al: The progression from hypertension to congestive heart failure. JAMA 275:1557, 1996.

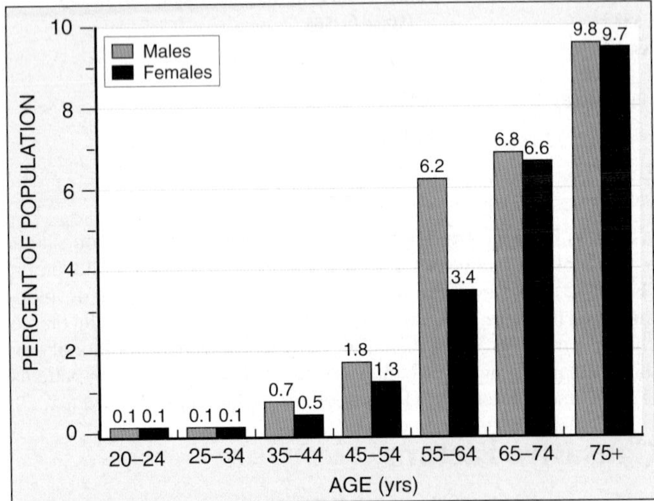

FIGURE 28-1 Prevalence rates of heart failure by gender and age in the United States, 1988-1994—the Third National Health and Nutrition Examination Survey (NHANES III). In men (blue), the prevalence increased from 18 cases/1000 in those aged 45 to 54 years to 98 cases/1000 in those aged 75 years and older. In women (purple), the prevalence increased from 13 cases/1000 in those aged 45 to 54 years to 97 cases/1000 in those aged 75 years and older. *(Data from American Heart Association: Heart Disease and Stroke Statistics—2003 Update. Dallas, American Heart Association, 2002.)*

TABLE 28-2 Causes of Chronic Heart Failure

- Myocardial disease
- Coronary artery disease
  - Myocardial infarction*
  - Myocardial ischemia*
- Chronic pressure overload
  - Hypertension*
  - Obstructive valvular disease*
- Chronic volume overload
  - Regurgitant valvular disease
  - Intracardiac (left-to-right) shunting
  - Extracardiac shunting
- Nonischemic dilated cardiomyopathy
  - Familial or genetic disorders
  - Infiltrative disorders*
  - Toxic or drug-induced damage
  - Metabolic disorder*
  - Viral or other infectious agents
- Disorders of rate and rhythm
  - Chronic bradyarrhythmias
  - Chronic tachyarrhythmias
- Pulmonary heart disease
  - Cor pulmonale
  - Pulmonary vascular disorders
- High-output states
- Metabolic disorders
  - Thyrotoxicosis
  - Nutritional disorders (beriberi)
- Excessive blood flow requirements
  - Systemic arteriovenous shunting
  - Chronic anemia

*Indicates conditions that can also lead to HF with a preserved EF.

cytoskeleton (see Chaps. 8 and 68). Most forms of familial dilated cardiomyopathy are inherited in an autosomal dominant fashion. Mutations of genes encoding cytoskeletal proteins (desmin, cardiac myosin, vinculin) and nuclear membrane proteins (lamin) have been identified thus far. Dilated cardiomyopathy is also associated with Duchenne, Becker, and limb girdle muscular dystrophies. Conditions that lead to a high cardiac output (e.g., arteriovenous fistula, anemia) are seldom responsible for the development of HF in a normal heart. However, in the presence of underlying structural heart disease, these conditions often lead to overt congestive failure.

Prognosis

Although several reports have suggested that the mortality for HF patients is improving, the overall mortality rate remains higher than for many cancers, including those involving the bladder, breast, uterus, and prostate. In the Framingham Study, the median survival was 1.7 years for men and 3.2 years for women, with only 25% of men and 38% of women surviving 5 years. European studies have confirmed a similarly poor long-term prognosis (**Fig. 28-3**).[1] More recent data from the Framingham Study have examined long-term trends in the survival of patients with HF and shown improved survival in men and women, with an overall decline in mortality of approximately 12%/decade from 1950 to 1999.[2] Moreover, reports from Scotland, Sweden, and the United Kingdom have also suggested that survival rates may be improving following hospital discharge.[1,6] Of note, the mortality of HF in epidemiologic studies is substantially higher than that reported in clinical HF trials involving drug and/or device therapies, in which the mortality figures are often deceptively low because the patients enrolled in these trials are younger and more stable and tend to be followed more closely clinically.

The role of gender and HF prognosis remains a controversial issue with respect to HF outcomes. Nonetheless, the aggregate data suggest that women with HF have a better overall prognosis than men.[2] However, women appear to have a greater degree of functional incapacity for the same degree of LV dysfunction and also have a higher prevalence of HF with a normal EF (see Chap. 30). Controversy has also arisen regarding the impact of race on outcome, with higher mortality rates being reported in blacks in some but not all studies. In the United States, HF affects approximately 3% of blacks, whereas in the general population the prevalence is about 2%.[7] Blacks with HF present at an earlier age and have more advanced LV dysfunction and

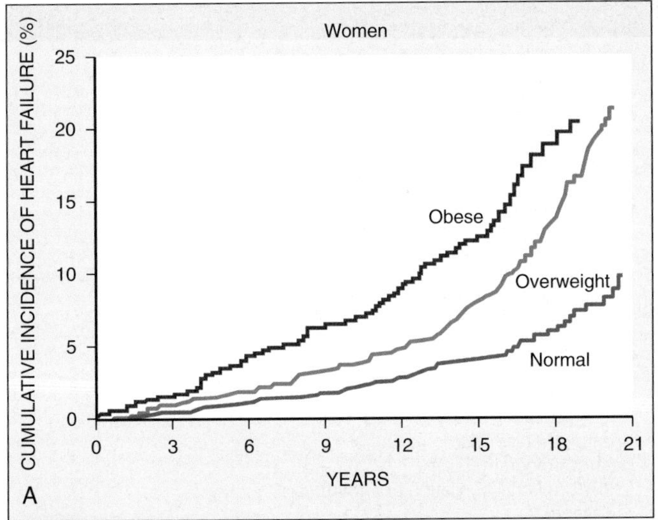

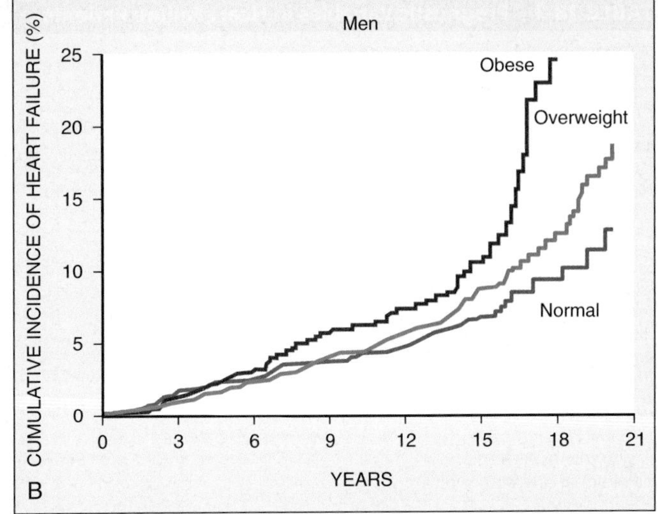

FIGURE 28-2 Cumulative incidence of heart failure in women **(A)** and men **(B)** according to body mass index (BMI) at the baseline examination. The BMI was 18.5 to 24.9 in normal subjects, 25.0 to 29.9 in overweight subjects, and 30.0 or more in obese subjects. *(Modified from Kenchaiah S, Evans JC, Levy D, et al: Obesity and the risk of heart failure. N Engl J Med 347:305, 2002.)*

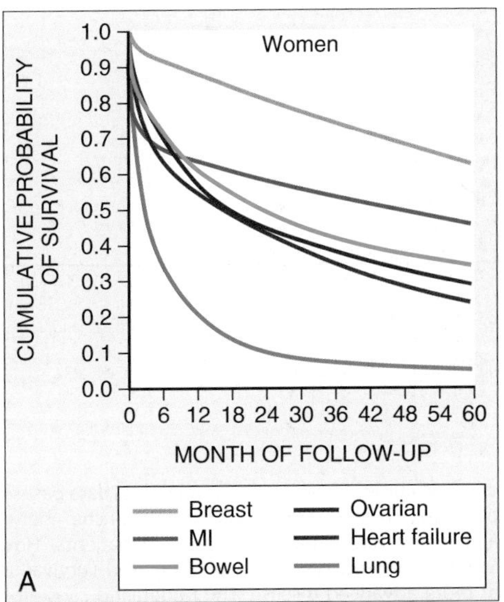

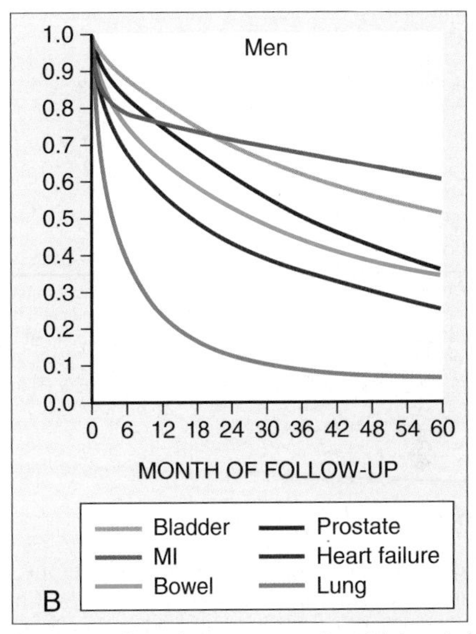

FIGURE 28-3 Survival in HF patients compared with cancer patients. Shown is 5-year survival following a first admission to any Scottish hospital in 1991 for HF, MI, and the four most common sites of cancer specific to women **(A)** and men **(B)**. *(Modified from Stewart S, MacIntyre K, Hole DJ, et al: More 'malignant' than cancer? Five-year survival following a first admission for heart failure. Eur J Heart Fail 3:315, 2001.)*

a worse New York Heart Association (NYHA) class at the time of diagnosis. Although the reasons for these differences are not known, differences in HF etiology might explain some of these observations. In the registry for the Studies on Left Ventricular Dysfunction (SOLVD), 73% of whites had coronary heart disease as a cause for their HF compared to only 36% of black participants. On the other hand, 32% of blacks in the SOLVD registry had HF that was attributed to hypertension, with only 4% of whites having hypertension as a primary cause. When compared in the SOLVD registry, cardiovascular and total mortality were no different in the black and white cohorts, although the black cohort was younger and had a higher proportion of females than the white group.[8] There may also be additional socioeconomic factors that may influence outcomes in black patients, such as geographic location and access to health care. Age is one of the stronger and most consistent predictors of adverse outcome in HF (see later, "Special Populations").[2]

Many other factors have been associated with increased mortality in HF patients (**Table 28-3**). Most factors listed as outcome predictors have survived at least univariate analysis, with many standing out independently when multifactorial analysis techniques were used. Nonetheless, it is extraordinarily difficult to determine which prognostic variable is most important to predict individual patient outcome in either clinical trials or, more importantly, during the daily management of an individual patient. To this end, a multivariate model for predicting the HF prognosis has been developed and validated. The Seattle Heart Failure Model was derived by retrospectively investigating predictors of survival among HF patients in clinical trials.[9] The Seattle Heart Failure Model provides an accurate estimate of 1-, 2-, and 3-year survival with the use of easily obtained clinical, pharmacologic, device, and laboratory characteristics, and is accessible free of charge to all health care providers as an interactive Internet-based program (http://depts.washington.edu/shfm).

TABLE 28-3 Prognostic Variables in Heart Failure Patients

Demographics	Exercise testing
Gender	Metabolic assessment
Race	BP response
Age	Heart rate response
Heart failure cause	6-min walk
CAD	Peak Vo_2
IDCM	Anaerobic threshold
Valvular heart disease	VE/Vco_2
Myocarditis	Oxygen uptake slope
Hypertrophy	Metabolic factors
Alcohol	Serum sodium level
Anthracyclines	Thyroid dysfunction
Amyloidosis	Anemia
Hemachromatosis	Acidosis, alkalosis
Genetic factors	Chest x-ray
Comorbidities	Congestion
Diabetes	Cardiothoracic ratio
Systemic hypertension	Electrocardiogram (ECG)
Pulmonary hypertension	Rhythm (atrial fibrillation or arrhythmias)
Sleep apnea	Voltage
Obesity, cachexia (body mass)	QRS width
Renal insufficiency	QT interval
Hepatic abnormalities	Signal-averaged ECG (T wave alternans)
COPD	HR variability
Clinical assessment	Biomarkers
NYHA class (symptoms)	NE, PRA, AVP, aldosterone
Syncope	ANP, BNP, endothelin-1
Angina pectoris	TNF, IL-1, IL-6, IL-10, CRP, ESR
Systolic versus diastolic dysfunction	Cardiac troponins, hematocrit
Hemodynamics	Endomyocardial biopsy
LVEF	Inflammatory states
RVEF	Degree of fibrosis
PAP	Degree of cellular disarray
PCWP	Infiltrative processes
CI	
PAP-PCWP	
Exercise hemodynamics	

ANP = atrial natriuretic peptide; AVP = arginine vasopressin; BNP = brain natriuretic peptide; BP = blood pressure; CAD = coronary artery disease; CI = cardiac index; COPD = chronic obstructive pulmonary disease; CRP = C-reactive protein; ESR = erythrocyte sedimentation rate; IDCM = idiopathic dilated cardiomyopathy; LVEF = left ventricular ejection fraction; NE = norepinephrine; NYHA = New York Heart Association; PAP = pulmonary artery pressure; PAP-PCWP = gradient across lung; PCWP = pulmonary capillary wedge pressure; PRA = plasma renin activity; RVEF = right ventricular ejection fraction; TNF = tumor necrosis factor, IL = interleukin.

Modified from Young JB: The prognosis of heart failure. *In* Mann DL (ed): Heart Failure: A Companion to Braunwald's Heart Disease. Philadelphia, Elsevier, 2004, pp 489-506.

Biomarkers and Prognosis

The observation that the renin angiotensin-aldosterone, adrenergic, and inflammatory systems are activated in HF (see Chap. 25) has prompted the examination of the relationships between a variety of biochemical measurements and clinical outcomes (see Table 28-3 and Chap. 26). Strong inverse correlations have been reported between survival and plasma levels of norepinephrine, renin, arginine vasopressin, aldosterone, atrial and brain natriuretic peptides (BNPs), and endothelin-1, and inflammatory markers such as tumor necrosis factor (TNF) and TNF receptors, C-reactive protein, and erythrocyte sedimentation rate. Markers of oxidative stress, such as oxidized low-density lipoprotein and serum uric acid, have also been associated with worsening clinical status and impaired survival in patients with chronic HF. Cardiac troponin T and I levels, sensitive markers of myocyte damage, may be elevated in patients with nonischemic and predict adverse cardiac outcomes. The association between low hemoglobin and hematocrit values and adverse HF outcomes has also long been recognized, but has garnered considerable attention after studies illustrated the independent prognostic value of anemia in patients with HF with reduced or normal EF.[10]

Published estimates of the prevalence of anemia in HF patients vary widely, ranging from 4% to 50% depending on the population studied and definition of anemia that is used.[10] In general, the prevalence of anemia is significantly greater in patients with more advanced disease. Furthermore, the severity of anemia may contribute to the increasing severity of HF. Multiple reports from observational data bases and clinical trial populations have demonstrated a relationship between lower hemoglobin levels and impaired survival in patients. However, it is unclear whether anemia is a cause of decreased survival, or simply a marker of more advanced disease. The underlying cause for anemia is likely multifactorial, including reduced sensitivity to erythropoietin receptors, the presence of a hematopoiesis inhibitor, and/or a defective iron supply for erythropoiesis given as possible explanations. Potential treatments for anemia include the use of red blood cell transfusions and treatment with erythropoietin analogues to increase red blood cell production, and intravenous iron.

At present, the role for blood transfusions in patients with cardiovascular disease is controversial. Although a transfusion threshold for maintaining the hematocrit higher than 30% in patients with cardiovascular disease has generally been accepted, this clinical practice has been based more on expert opinion rather than on direct evidence that documents the efficacy for this form of therapy. Given the risks and costs of red blood cell transfusion, the evanescent benefits of blood transfusions in patients with a chronic anemia, and the unclear benefit in HF patients, the routine use of blood transfusion cannot be recommended for treating the anemia that occurs in stable HF patients. In a randomized double-blind study,[11] intravenous iron (ferric carboxymaltose) improved patient symptoms (odds ratio for improvement, 2.51; 95% confidence interval [CI], 1.75 to 3.61), NYHA functional class (primary endpoints), and quality of life (secondary endpoint) when compared with placebo in patients with NYHA functional Class II (LVEF < 40%) or III (LVEF < 45%) HF iron deficiency (**Fig. 28-4**). The total iron dose for repletion was calculated at baseline; patients were administered intravenous ferric carboxymaltose until iron repletion was achieved, and then every 4 weeks during the maintenance phase of the study (total of 24 weeks of therapy). Of note,

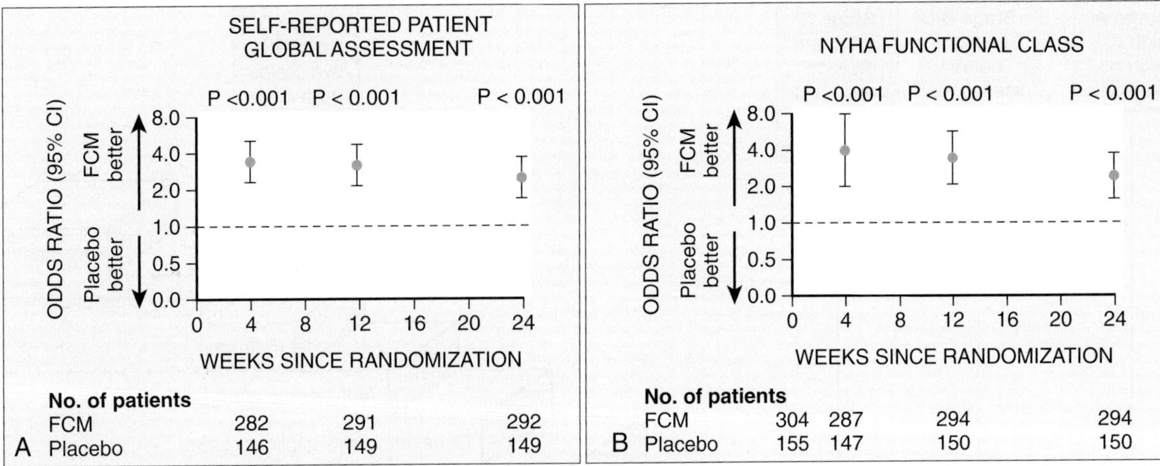

FIGURE 28-4 Effect of treatment with intravenous iron (ferric carboxymaltose) on patient symptoms and functional status. **A,** Effect of ferric carboxymaltose (FCM) on the self-reported Patient Global Assessment and NYHA functional status **(B)**. The data in **A** and **B** are presented as odds ratios for the FCM group compared with the placebo group, and being in an improved or worsened self-assessment category or improved or worsened NYHA functional class. Patients who were hospitalized at each time point were given an assessment of much worse, or NYHA Class IV. Patients who died before week 24 were categorized as dead (in **B**, corresponding to NYHA Class V). *(Modified from Anker SD, Comin CJ, Filippatos G, et al: Ferric carboxymaltose in patients with heart failure and iron deficiency. N Engl J Med 361:2436, 2009.)*

several small studies have suggested benefit from the use of erythropoietin analogues for the treatment of mild anemia in HF.[10] However, there is concern that thromboembolic events may be increased with this strategy. Treatment of anemic HF patients with the erythropoietin analogue darbepoetin alpha is undergoing further investigation in a large international study, Reduction of Events with Darbepoetin in Heart Failure (RED-HF; ClinicalTrials.gov identifier, NCT00358215).

Renal Insufficiency

Renal insufficiency is associated with poorer outcomes in patients with HF; however, it is uncertain whether renal impairment is a simply a marker for worsening HF or whether renal impairment might be causally linked to worsening HF. Although more common in patients hospitalized for HF, at least some degree of renal impairment is still present in about 50% of stable HF outpatients. Patients with renal hypoperfusion or intrinsic renal disease show an impaired response to diuretics and angiotensin-converting enzyme inhibitors (ACEIs) and are at increased risk of adverse effects during treatment with digitalis. In a recent meta-analysis, most HF patients had some degree of renal impairment. These patients represented a high-risk group with an approximately 50% increased relative mortality risk when compared with patients who had normal renal function.[12] Similar findings were observed in the Second Prospective Randomized Study of Ibopamine on Mortality and Efficacy, in which impaired renal function was a stronger predictor of mortality than impaired LV function and NYHA class in patients with advanced HF (**Fig. 28-5**).[13] Thus, renal insufficiency is emerging as a strong independent predictor of adverse outcomes in HF patients.

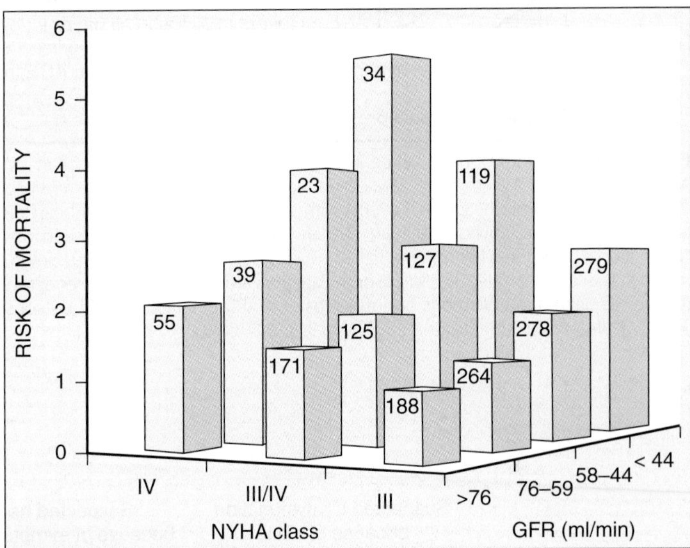

FIGURE 28-5 Effect of renal function on outcomes in HF patients. This three-dimensional bar graph shows the risk of mortality (vertical axis) in relation to decreasing NYHA class (horizontal axis) and decreasing quartiles of glomerular filtration rate (GFR; diagonal axis). *(From Hillege HL, Girbes AR, de Kam PJ, et al: Renal function, neurohormonal activation, and survival in patients with chronic heart failure. Circulation 102:203, 2000.)*

Approach to the Patient

Stages of Heart Failure

HF should be viewed as a continuum that comprises four interrelated stages (**Fig. 28-6**).[14] Stage A includes patients who are at high risk for developing HF, but without structural heart disease or symptoms of HF (e.g., patients with diabetes or hypertension). Stage B includes patients who have structural heart disease but without symptoms of HF (e.g., patients with a previous myocardial infarction [MI] and asymptomatic LV dysfunction). Stage C includes patients who have structural heart disease who have developed symptoms of HF (e.g., patients with a previous MI with shortness of breath and fatigue). Stage D includes patients with refractory HF requiring special interventions (e.g., patients with refractory HF who are awaiting cardiac transplantation). A simplified algorithm for approaching patients with HF is illustrated in **Figure 28-7**. The diagnosis and clinical assessment of patients with HF with a reduced EF is discussed in detail in Chap. 26, and the diagnosis and management of patients with HF with a normal or preserved EF is discussed in detail in Chap. 30.

PATIENTS AT HIGH RISK FOR DEVELOPING HEART FAILURE (STAGE A). For patients at high risk of developing HF, every effort should be made to prevent HF using standard practice guidelines to treat preventable conditions that are known to lead to HF, including hypertension (see Chap. 45), hyperlipidemia (see Chap. 49) and diabetes (see Chap. 64). In this regard, ACEIs are particularly useful for preventing HF in patients who have a history of atherosclerotic vascular disease, diabetes mellitus, or hypertension with associated cardiovascular risk factors.

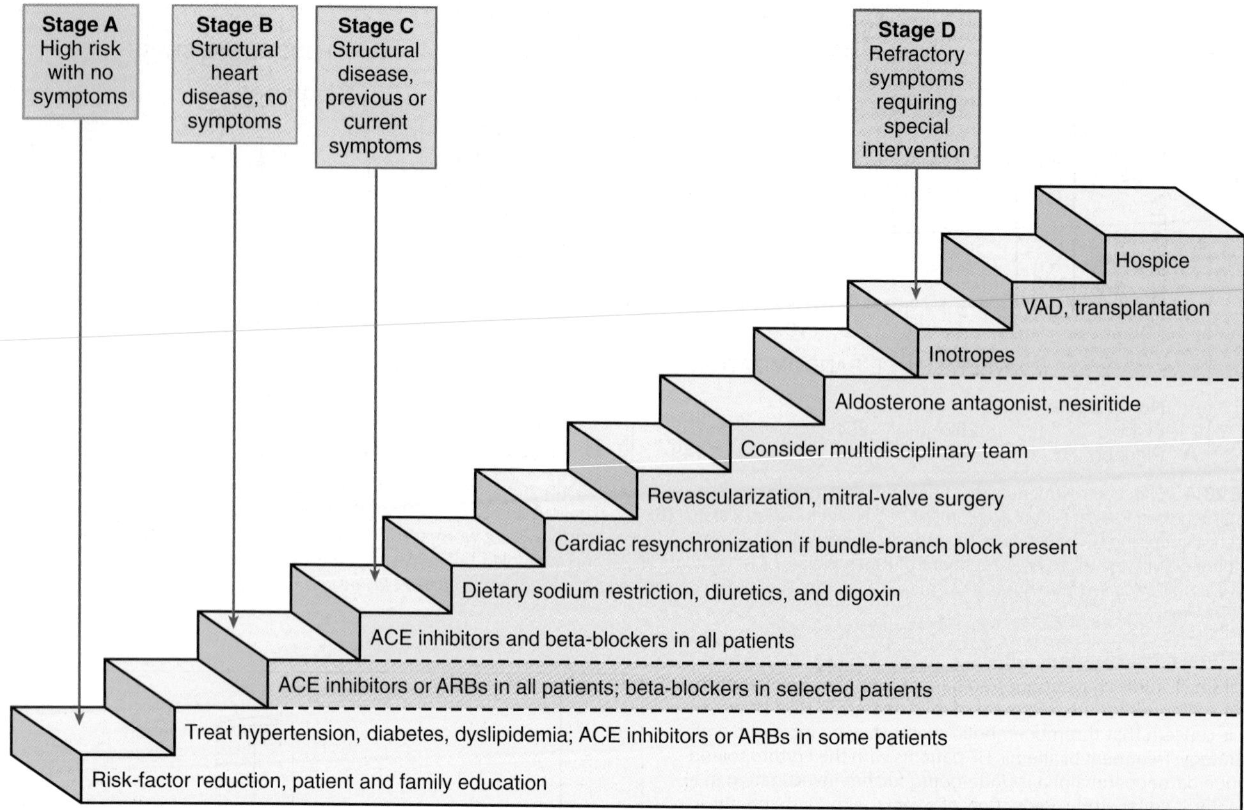

FIGURE 28-6 Stages of heart failure and treatment options for systolic heart failure. Patients with stage A HF are at high risk for HF but do not have structural heart disease or symptoms of HF. This group includes patients with hypertension, diabetes, coronary artery disease, previous exposure to cardiotoxic drugs, or a family history of cardiomyopathy. Patients with stage B HF have structural heart disease but no symptoms of HF. This group includes patients with left ventricular hypertrophy, previous myocardial infarction, left ventricular systolic dysfunction, or valvular heart disease, all of whom would be considered to have New York Heart Association (NYHA) Class I symptoms. Patients with stage C heart failure have known structural heart disease and current or previous symptoms of HF. Their symptoms may be classified as NYHA Class I, II, III, or IV. Patients with stage D HF have refractory symptoms of HF at rest despite maximal medical therapy, are hospitalized, and require specialized interventions or hospice care. All these patients would be considered to have NYHA Class IV symptoms. VAD = ventricular assist device. *(From Jessup M, Brozena S: Heart failure. N Engl J Med 348:2007, 2003.)*

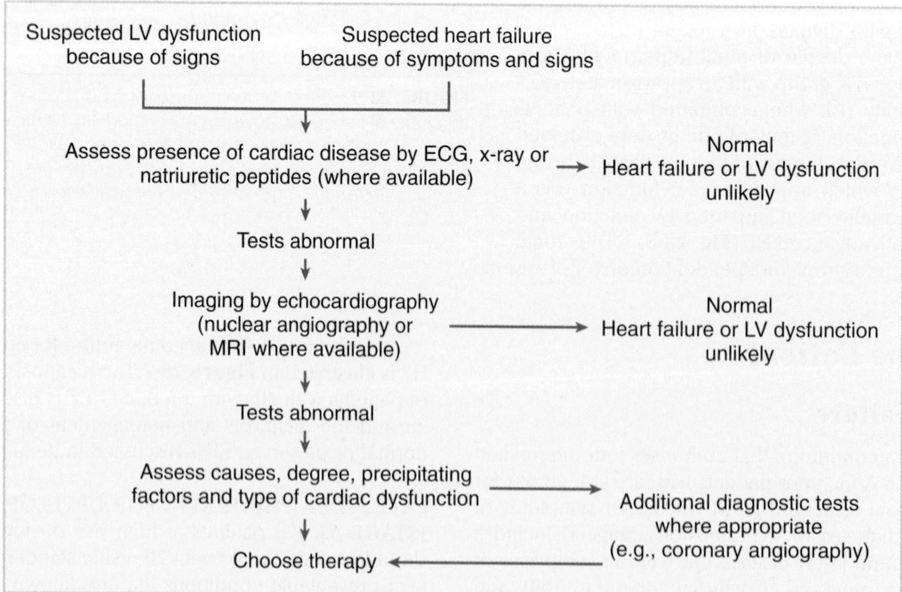

FIGURE 28-7 Relationships among cardiac dysfunction, symptomatic HF, and asymptomatic HF following appropriate treatment. *(From Swedberg K, Cleland J, Dargie H, et al: Guidelines for the diagnosis and treatment of chronic heart failure: Executive summary (update 2005): The Task Force for the Diagnosis and Treatment of Chronic Heart Failure of the European Society of Cardiology. Eur Heart J 26:1115, 2005.)*

TABLE 28-4 Diagnostic Criteria for Heart Failure in Population-Based Studies

Framingham Criteria		
MAJOR CRITERIA	**MINOR CRITERIA**	**MAJOR OR MINOR CRITERIA**
Paroxysmal nocturnal dyspnea or orthopnea Neck-vein distention Rales Cardiomegaly Acute pulmonary edema S_3 gallop Increased venous pressure, >16 cm H_2O Hepatojugular reflux	Ankle edema Night cough Dyspnea on exertion Hepatomegaly Pleural effusion Vital capacity decreased by one third from maximal capacity Tachycardia (rate > 120 beats /min)	Weight loss > 4.5 kg in 5 days in response to treatment

NHANES Criteria		
CATEGORY	**CRITERIA**	**POINTS**
History	Dyspnea	
	• Does patient have shortness of breath when hurrying on flat ground or a slight elevation?	1
	• Does patient have shortness of breath when walking on flat ground?	1
	• Does patient stop for breath when walking at an ordinary pace?	2
	• Does patient stop for breath after 100 yards when on flat ground?	2
Physical examination	Heart rate	
	• 91-110 beats/min	1
	• >110 beats/min	2
	Jugular venous pressure > 6 cm H_2O alone	1
	Plus hepatomegaly or edema	2
	Rales—basilar crackles	1
	Crackles—more than basilar crackles	2
Chest radiography	Upper zone flow redistribution	1
	Interstitial pulmonary edema	2
	Interstitial edema plus pleural fluid	3
	Alveolar fluid plus pleural fluid	3

The diagnosis of HF using the Framingham criteria requires the simultaneous presence of at least two major criteria or one major criterion in conjunction with two minor criteria. Minor criteria are acceptable only if they cannot be attributed to another medical condition (e.g. pulmonary hypertension, chronic lung disease, cirrhosis, ascites, nephrotic syndrome).

NHANES criteria—diagnosis of HF if score ≥ 3 points.

Modified from Ho KK, Pinsky JL, Kannel WB et al: The epidemiology of heart failure: The Framingham Study. J Am Coll Cardiol 22:6A, 1993; and Schocken DD, Arrieta MI, Leaverton PE, et al: Prevalence and mortality rate of congestive heart failure in the United States. J Am Coll Cardiol 20:301, 1992.

POPULATION SCREENING. At present, there is limited information available to support the screening of broad populations to detect undiagnosed HF and/or asymptomatic LV dysfunction. A study has suggested that elevated levels of BNP (see Chap. 26) can be used as a cost-effective strategy for screening asymptomatic people older than 60 years with an EF lower than 40%.[15] However, screening general populations with BNP is not recommended at this time. Patients who are at very high risk of a developing cardiomyopathy (e.g., those with a strong family history of cardiomyopathy or those receiving cardiotoxic interventions; see Chap. 90) are appropriate targets for more aggressive screening, such as two-dimensional echocardiography, to assess LV function. However, the routine periodic assessment of LV function in other patients is not currently recommended. Several sophisticated clinical scoring systems have been developed to screen for HF in population based studies, including the Framingham Criteria, which screens for HF on the basis of clinical criteria, and the National Health and Nutrition Survey (NHANES), which uses self-reporting of symptoms to identify HF patients (**Table 28-4**). As discussed in Chap. 26, additional laboratory testing is usually necessary to make the diagnosis of HF definitively when these methodologies are used.

Management of Patients with Symptomatic and Asymptomatic Heart Failure

Transient Left Ventricular Dysfunction

As noted in Chap. 25, the clinical syndrome of HF with reduced EF begins after an initial index event produces a decline in ejection performance of the heart. However, it is important to recognize that LV dysfunction may develop transiently in various different clinical settings, which may not lead invariably to the development of the clinical syndrome of HF. **Figure 28-8** illustrates the important relationship between LV dysfunction (transient and sustained) and the clinical syndrome of HF (asymptomatic and symptomatic). LV dysfunction with pulmonary edema may develop acutely in patients with previously normal LV structure and function. This occurs most commonly postoperatively following cardiac surgery, in the setting of severe brain injury, or after a systemic infection. The general pathophysiologic mechanism involved is some form of "stunning" of functional myocardium (see Chap. 52) or activation of proinflammatory cytokines that are capable of suppressing LV function (see Chap. 25). Emotional stress can also precipitate severe reversible LV dysfunction that is accompanied by chest pain, pulmonary edema, and cardiogenic shock in patients without coronary disease (takotsubo syndrome). In this setting, LV dysfunction is thought to occur secondary to the deleterious effects of catecholamines following heightened sympathetic stimulation.[16] It is also important to note that exercise-induced LV dysfunction, usually caused by myocardial ischemia, may lead to symptoms by causing a rise in LV filling pressure and a fall in cardiac output in the absence of discernable LV dysfunction at rest. If LV dysfunction persists following the initial cardiac injury, patients may remain asymptomatic for a period of months to years; however, the weight of epidemiologic and clinical evidence suggests that at some point these patients will undergo the transition to overt symptomatic HF.

Defining the Appropriate Strategy

The main goals of treatment are to reduce symptoms, prolong survival, improve the quality of life, and prevent disease progression.

CH 28

TABLE 28-5 Pharmacologic and Device Therapy in Patients with Chronic Heart Failure

INDICATION	ACEI	ARB	DIURETIC	BETA BLOCKER	ALDOSTERONE ANTAGONISTS	CARDIAC GLYCOSIDES	CRT	ICD
Asymptomatic LV dysfunction (NYHA I)	Indicated	If ACEI-intolerant	Not indicated	Post-MI indicated*	Recent MI	With atrial fibrillation	Not indicated	Not indicated
Symptomatic HF (NYHA II)	Indicated	Indicated with or without ACEI	Indicated with fluid retention	Indicated	Recent MI	1. With atrial fibrillation 2. When improved from more severe HF in sinus rhythm	Not indicated	Indicated
Worsening HF (NYHA III, IV)	Indicated	Indicated with or without ACEI	Indicated, combination of diuretics	Indicated (under specialist's care)	Indicated	Indicated	Indicated if QRS > 0.12 msec†	Indicated
End-stage HF (NYHA IV)	Indicated	Indicated with or without ACEI	Indicated, combination of diuretics	Indicated (under specialist's care)	Indicated	Indicated	Indicated if QRS > 0.12 msec†	Not indicated

*Represents expert opinion.
†Patients must be in sinus rhythm.
Modified from Swedberg K, Cleland J, Dargie H, et al: Guidelines for the diagnosis and treatment of chronic heart failure: Executive summary (update 2005): The Task Force for the Diagnosis and Treatment of Chronic Heart Failure of the European Society of Cardiology. Eur Heart J 26:1115, 2005.

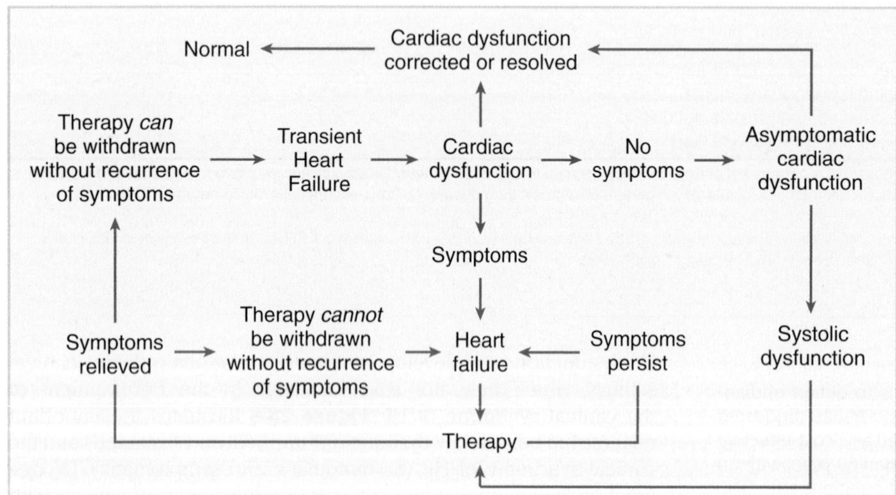

FIGURE 28-8 Algorithm for the diagnosis of heart failure or LV dysfunction. *(From Swedberg K, Cleland J, Dargie H, et al: Guidelines for the diagnosis and treatment of chronic heart failure: Executive summary (update 2005): The Task Force for the Diagnosis and Treatment of Chronic Heart Failure of the European Society of Cardiology. Eur Heart J 26:1115, 2005.)*

As discussed later, the current pharmacologic, device, and surgical therapeutic armamentarium for the management of patients with a reduced EF permits health care providers to achieve each of these goals in the great majority of patients. As shown in **Table 28-5**, once patients have developed structural heart disease (stages B to D), the choice of therapy for patients with HF with a reduced EF depends on their NYHA functional classification (see Chap. 26 and Table 26-3). Although this classification system is notoriously subjective, and has large interobserver variability, it has withstood the test of time and continues to be widely applied to patients with HF. For patients who have developed LV systolic dysfunction, but who remain asymptomatic (Class I), the goal should be to slow disease progression by blocking neurohormonal systems that lead to cardiac remodeling (see Chap. 25). For patients who have developed symptoms (Classes II to IV), the primary goal should be to alleviate fluid retention, lessen disability, and reduce the risk of further disease progression and death. As will be discussed subsequently, these goals generally require a strategy that combines diuretics (to control salt and water retention) with neurohormonal interventions (to minimize cardiac remodeling).

General Measures

Identification and correction of the condition(s) responsible for the cardiac structural and/or functional abnormalities are critical (see Table 28-2), insofar as some conditions that provoke LV structural and functional abnormalities are potentially treatable and/or reversible. Furthermore, clinicians should aim to screen for and treat aggressively comorbidities such as hypertension and diabetes, which are thought to underlie the structural heart disease. In addition to searching for reversible causes and comorbidities that contribute to the development of HF, it is equally important to identify factors that provoke worsening HF in stable patients (**Table 28-6**). Among the most common causes of acute decompensation in a previously stable patient are dietary indiscretion and inappropriate reduction of HF therapy, either from patient self-discontinuation of medication or from physician withdrawal of effective pharmacotherapy (e.g., because of concern over azotemia). HF patients should be advised to stop smoking and to limit daily alcohol consumption to two standard drinks in men or one standard drink in women. Patients suspected of having an alcohol-induced cardiomyopathy should be advised to abstain from alcohol consumption indefinitely. Excessive temperature extremes and heavy physical exertion should be avoided. Certain drugs are known to make HF worse and should also be avoided. For example, nonsteroidal anti-inflammatory drugs (NSAIDs), including cyclooxygenase 2 (COX-2) inhibitors, are not recommended in patients with chronic HF because the risk of renal failure and fluid retention is markedly increased in the setting of reduced renal function and/or ACEI use. Patients should be advised to weigh themselves on a regular basis to monitor weight gain and alert a health care provider or adjust their diuretic dose in the case of a sudden unexpected weight gain of more than 3 to 4 pounds over a 3-day period. Although there is no documented evidence of the effects of immunization in HF patients, they are at high risk of developing pneumococcal pneumonia and influenza. Accordingly, clinicians should consider recommending influenza and pneumococcal vaccines to their HF patient to prevent respiratory infections.

It is equally important to educate the patient and family about HF, the importance of proper diet, and the importance of compliance with the medical regimen. Supervision of outpatient care by a specially trained nurse or physician assistant and/or specialized HF clinics have all been found to be helpful, particularly in patients with advanced disease (see later, "Disease Management").

ACTIVITY. Although heavy physical labor is not recommended in HF, routine modest exercise has been shown to be beneficial in select patients with NYHA Classes I to III HF. The HF-ACTION trial[17] a controlled trial investigating outcomes of exercise training) was a large, multicenter, randomized controlled study whose primary endpoint was a composite of all-cause mortality and all-cause hospitalization. Secondary end points included all-cause mortality, all-cause hospitalization, and the composite of cardiovascular mortality or cardiovascular hospitalization. HF-ACTION failed to show a significant improvement in all-cause mortality or all-cause hospitalization (hazard ratio [HR], 0.93; 95% CI, 0.84 to 1.02; $P = 0.13$) in patients who received a 12-week (three times/week) exercise training program followed by a 25- to 30-minute, home-based, self-monitored exercise workout on a treadmill or stationary bicycle 5 days/week (**Fig. 28-9A**). Moreover, there was no difference in all-cause mortality (HR, 0.96; 95% CI, 0.79 to 1.17; $P = 0.70$; see Fig. 28-9B). However, there was a trend toward decreased cardiovascular mortality or HF hospitalizations (HR, 0.87; 95% CI, 0.74 to 0.99; $P = 0.06$) and quality of life was significantly improved in the exercise group. For euvolemic patients, regular isotonic exercise such as walking or riding a stationary bicycle with an ergometer may be useful as an adjunctive therapy to improve clinical status after patients have undergone exercise testing to determine suitability for exercise training (i.e., patient does not develop significant ischemia or arrhythmias). Exercise training is not recommended, however, for HF patients with a reduced EF who have had a major cardiovascular event or procedure within the last 6 weeks, patients with cardiac devices that limit the ability to achieve target heart rates, and patients with significant arrhythmia or ischemia during baseline cardiopulmonary exercise testing.

TABLE 28-6 Potential Precipitating Factors of Acute Decompensation in Patients with Chronic Heart Failure

Dietary indiscretion
Inappropriate reduction in HF medications
Myocardial ischemia, infarction
Arrhythmias (tachycardia, bradycardia)
Infection
Anemia
Initiation of medications that worsen the symptoms of HF
- Calcium antagonists (verapamil, diltiazem)
- Beta blockers
- Nonsteroidal anti-inflammatory drugs
- Thiazolidinediones
- Antiarrhythmic agents (all Class I agents, sotalol [Class III])
- Anti-TNF antibodies

Alcohol consumption
Pregnancy
Worsening hypertension
Acute valvular insufficiency

From Mann DL: Heart failure and cor pulmonale. *In* Kasper DL, Braunwald E, Fauci AS, Hauser SL, et al (eds): Harrison's Principles of Internal Medicine. 17th ed. New York, McGraw-Hill, 2007, p 1448.

DIET. Dietary restriction of sodium (2 to 3 g daily) is recommended for all patients with the clinical syndrome of HF and preserved or depressed EF. Further restriction (<2 g daily) may be considered in moderate to severe HF. Fluid restriction is generally unnecessary unless the patient is hyponatremic (<130 mEq/liter), which may develop because of activation of the renin angiotensin system, excessive secretion of arginine vasopressin (AVP), or loss of salt in excess of water from prior diuretic use. Fluid restriction (<2 liters/day) should be considered in hyponatremic patients (<130 mEq/liter) or for those patients whose fluid retention is difficult to control despite high doses of diuretics and sodium restriction. Caloric supplementation is recommended for patients with advanced HF and unintentional weight loss or muscle wasting (cardiac cachexia); however, anabolic steroids are not recommended for these patients because of potential problems with volume retention. The measurement of nitrogen balance, caloric intake, and prealbumin level may be useful in determining appropriate nutritional supplementation. The use of dietary supplements (nutraceuticals) should be avoided in the management of symptomatic HF because of the lack of proven benefit and the potential for significant interactions with effective HF therapeutics (see Chap. 33).

Management of Fluid Status

Many clinical manifestations result from excessive salt and water retention that leads to an inappropriate volume expansion of the

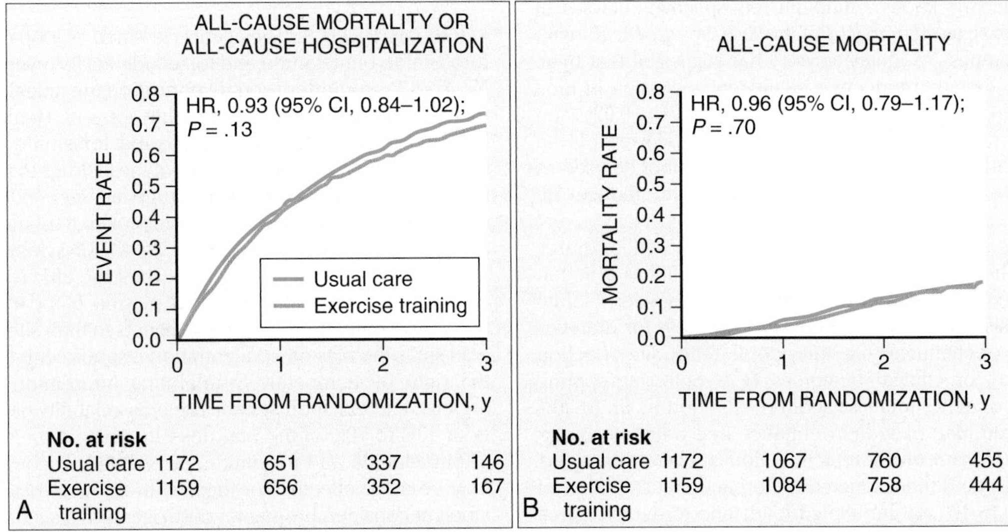

FIGURE 28-9 Kaplan-Meier analysis of the effect of exercise versus usual care on HF morbidity and mortality. **A,** Time to all-cause hospitalization and all-cause mortality and time to all-cause mortality **(B)** in the HF-ACTION trial. *(From O'Connor CM, Whellan DJ, Lee KL, et al: Efficacy and safety of exercise training in patients with chronic heart failure: HF-ACTION randomized controlled trial. JAMA 301:1439, 2009.)*

CH 28

TABLE 28-7 Diuretics for Treating Fluid Retention in Chronic Heart Failure

DRUG	INITIAL DAILY DOSAGE	MAXIMUM TOTAL DAILY DOSAGE	DURATION OF ACTION (HR)
Loop diuretics*			
Bumetanide	0.5-1.0 mg qd or bid	10 mg	4-6
Furosemide	20-40 mg qd or bid	600 mg	6-8
Torsemide	10-20 mg qd	200 mg	12-16
Ethacrynic acid	25-50 mg qd or bid	200 mg	6
Thiazide diuretics†			
Chlorothiazide	250-500 mg qd or bid	1000 mg	6-12
Chlorthalidone	12.5-25 mg qd	100 mg	24-72
Hydrochlorothiazide	25 mg qd or bid	200 mg	6-12
Indapamide	2.5 mg qd	5 mg	36
Metolazone	2.5-5 mg qd	20 mg	12-24
Potassium-sparing diuretics			
Amiloride	12.5-25 mg qd	20 mg	24
Triamterene	50-75 mg bid	200 mg	7-9
AVP antagonists			
Satavaptan	25 mg qd	50 mg qd	NS
Tolvaptan	15 mg qd	60 mg qd	NS
Lixivaptan	125 mg qd	250 mg bid	NS
Conivaptan (IV)	20-mg IV loading dose, followed by 20-mg continuous IV infusion/day	40-mg IV infusion/day	7-9
Sequential nephron blockade			
Metolazone	2.5 to 10 mg qd plus loop diuretic		
Hydrochlorothiazide	25 to 100 mg qd or bid plus loop diuretic		
Chlorothiazide (IV)	500 to 1000 mg qd plus loop diuretic		

NOTE: Unless indicated, all doses are for oral diuretics.
*Equivalent doses: 40 mg furosemide = 1 mg bumetanide = 20 mg torsemide = 50 mg of ethacrynic acid.
†Do not use if estimated glomerular filtration is <30 mL/min or with cytochrome 3A4 inhibitors.
NS = not specified.
Modified from Hunt SA, Abraham WT, Chin MH, et al: ACC/AHA 2005 Guideline Update for the Diagnosis and Management of Chronic Heart Failure in the Adult: a report of the American College of Cardiology/American Heart Association Task Force on Practice Guidelines. Circulation 112:e154, 2005.

vascular and extravascular space. Although both digitalis and low doses of ACEIs enhance urinary sodium excretion, few volume-overloaded HF patients can maintain proper sodium balance without the use of diuretic drugs. Attempts to substitute ACEIs for diuretics have been shown to lead to pulmonary edema and peripheral congestion. In short-term clinical trials, diuretic therapy has led to a reduction in jugular venous pressure, pulmonary congestion, peripheral edema, and body weight, all of which were observed within days of initiation of therapy. In intermediate-term studies, diuretics have been shown to improve cardiac function, symptoms, and exercise tolerance in HF patients.[18] To date, there have been no long-term studies of diuretic therapy in HF; thus, their effects on morbidity and mortality are not clearly known. Although retrospective analyses of clinical trials have suggested that diuretic use is associated with worse clinical outcomes,[19] a meta-analysis[18] has suggested that treatment with diuretic therapy produces a significant reduction in mortality (odds ratio [OR], 0.24; 95% CI, 0.07 to 0.83; $P = 0.02$) and worsening HF (OR, 0.07; 95% CI, 0.01 to 0.52; $P = 0.01$). However, given the retrospective nature of this review, this analysis cannot be used as formal evidence to recommend the use diuretics to reduce HF mortality.

A number of classification schemes have been proposed for diuretics on the basis of their mechanism of action, anatomic locus of action within the nephron, and the form of diuresis that they elicit (solute versus water diuresis). The most common classification for diuretics uses an admixture of chemical (e.g., thiazide diuretic), site of action (e.g., loop diuretic), or clinical outcomes (e.g., potassium-sparing diuretic). The loop diuretics increase sodium excretion by up to 20% to 25% of the filtered load of sodium, enhance free water clearance, and maintain their efficacy unless renal function is severely impaired. In contrast, the thiazide diuretics increase the fractional excretion of sodium to only 5% to 10% of the filtered load, tend to decrease free water clearance, and lose their effectiveness in patients with impaired renal function (creatinine clearance less than 40 mL/min). Consequently, the loop diuretics have emerged as the preferred diuretic agents for use in most patients with HF. Diuretics that induce a water diuresis (aquaretics) include demeclocycline, lithium, and vasopressin V_2 receptor antagonists, each of which inhibits the action of AVP on the collecting duct through different mechanisms, thereby increasing free water clearance. Drugs that cause solute diuresis are subdivided into two types—osmotic diuretics, which are nonresorbable solutes that osmotically retain water and other solutes in the tubular lumen, and drugs that selectively inhibit ion transport pathways across tubular epithelia, which constitute the majority of potent, clinically useful diuretics. The classes of diuretics and individual class members are listed in **Table 28-7** and their renal sites of action are depicted in **Figure 28-10**.

LOOP DIURETICS. The agents classified as loop diuretics, including furosemide, bumetanide, and torsemide, act by reversibly inhibiting the Na^+-K^+-$2Cl^-$ symporter (cotransporter) on the apical membrane of epithelial cells in the thick ascending loop of Henle (see Fig. 28-10). Because furosemide, bumetanide, and torsemide are bound extensively to plasma proteins, delivery of these drugs to the tubule by filtration is limited. However, these drugs are secreted efficiently by the organic acid transport system in the proximal tubule and thereby gain access to their binding sites on the Na^+-K^+-$2Cl^-$ symporter in the luminal membrane of the ascending limb. Thus, the efficacy of loop diuretics is dependent on sufficient renal plasma blood flow and proximal tubular secretion to deliver these agents to their site of action. Probenecid shifts the plasma concentration-response curve for furosemide to the right by competitively inhibiting furosemide excretion by the organic acid transport system. The bioavailability of furosemide ranges from 40% to 70% of the oral dose. In contrast, the oral bioavailability of bumetanide and torsemide exceed 80%. Accordingly, these agents may be more effective for those with advanced HF or right-sided HF, albeit at considerably greater cost. Agents in a second functional class of loop diuretics (e.g., ethacrynic acid) exhibit a slower onset of action and have delayed and only partial reversibility. Ethacrynic acid may be safely used in sulfa-allergic HF patients.

Mechanisms of Action. Loop diuretics are believed to improve symptoms of congestion by several mechanisms. First, loop diuretics reversibly bind to and reversibly inhibit the action of the Na^+,K^+-$2Cl^-$ cotransporter, thereby preventing salt transport in the thick ascending loop of Henle. Inhibition of this symporter also inhibits Ca^{2+} and Mg^{2+} resorption by abolishing the transepithelial potential difference that is the driving force for absorption of these cations. By inhibiting the concentration of solute within the medullary interstitium, these drugs also reduce the driving force for water resorption in the collecting duct, even in the presence of AVP (see Chaps. 25 and 27). The decreased resorption of water by the collecting duct results in the production of urine that is almost isotonic with plasma. The increase in delivery of Na^+ and water to the distal nephron segments also markedly enhances K^+ excretion, particularly in the presence of elevated aldosterone levels.

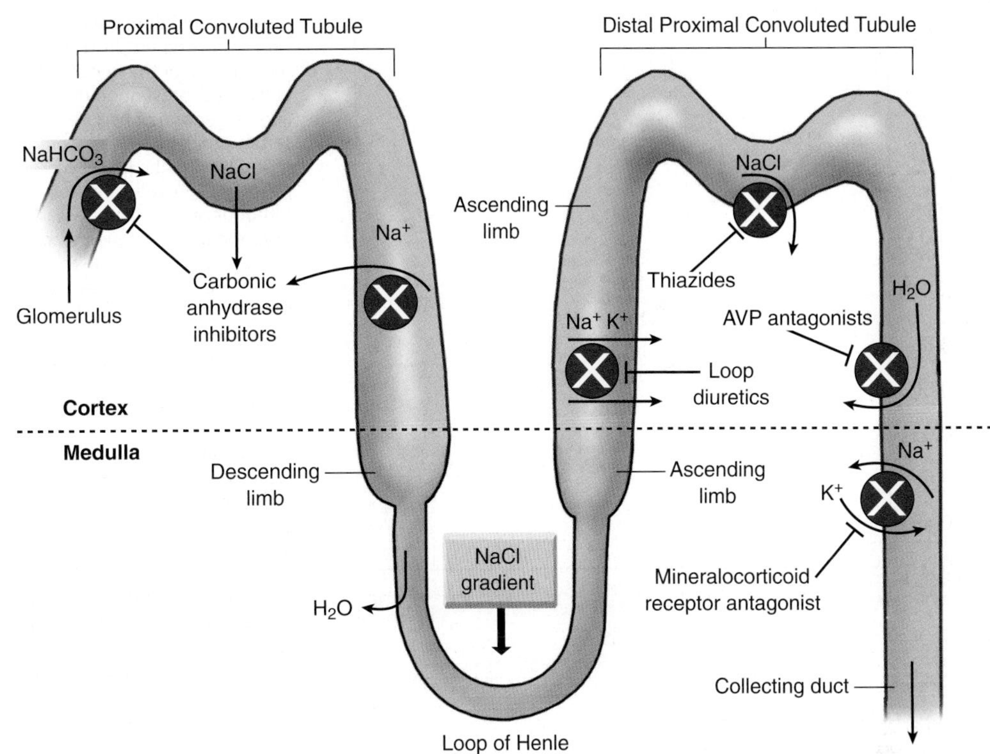

FIGURE 28-10 Sites of action of diuretics in the kidney. AVP = arginine vasopressin. *(From Bristow MR, Linas S, Port DJ: Drugs in the treatment of heart failure. In Zipes DP, Libby P, Bonow RO, Braunwald E [eds]: Braunwald's Heart Disease. 7th ed. Philadelphia, Elsevier, 2004, p 573.)*

Loop diuretics also exhibit several characteristic effects on intracardiac pressure and systemic hemodynamics. Furosemide acts as a venodilator and reduces right atrial and pulmonary capillary wedge pressure within minutes when given intravenously (0.5 to 1.0 mg/kg). Similar data, although not as extensive, have accumulated for bumetanide and torsemide. This initial improvement in hemodynamics may be secondary to the release of vasodilatory prostaglandins, insofar as studies in animals and humans have demonstrated that the venodilatory actions of furosemide are inhibited by indomethacin. There have also been reports of an acute rise in systemic vascular resistance in response to loop diuretics, which has been attributed to the transient activation of the systemic or intravascular renin-angiotensin system (RAS). The potentially deleterious rise in LV afterload reinforces the importance of initiating vasodilator therapy with diuretics in patients with acute pulmonary edema and adequate blood pressure (see Chap. 27).

THIAZIDE AND THIAZIDE-LIKE DIURETICS. The benzothiadiazides, also known as thiazide diuretics, were the initial class of drugs synthesized to block the Na^+-Cl^- transporter in the distal nephron. Subsequently, drugs that share similar pharmacologic properties became known as thiazide-like diuretics, even though they were technically not benzothiadiazine derivatives. Because thiazide and thiazide-like diuretics prevent maximal dilution of urine, they decrease the kidney's ability to increase free water clearance, and may therefore contribute to the development of hyponatremia. Thiazides increase Ca^{2+} resorption in the distal nephron (see Fig. 28-10) by several mechanisms, occasionally resulting in a small increase in serum Ca^{2+} levels. In contrast, Mg^{2+} resorption is diminished and hypomagnesemia may occur with prolonged use. Increased delivery of NaCl and fluid into the collecting duct directly enhances K^+ and H^+ secretion by this segment of the nephron, which may lead to clinically important hypokalemia.

Mechanisms of Action. The site of action of these drugs within the distal convoluted tubule has been identified as the Na^+-Cl^- symporter of the distal convoluted tubule. Although this cotransporter shares approximately 50% amino acid homology with the Na^+-K^+-$2Cl^-$ symporter of the ascending limb of the loop of Henle, it is insensitive to the effects of furosemide. This cotransporter (or related isoforms) is also present on cells within the vasculature and many cell types in other organs and tissues, and may contribute to some of the other actions of these agents, such as their usefulness as antihypertensive agents. Similar to the loop diuretics, the efficacy of thiazide diuretics is dependent, at least in part, on proximal tubular secretion to deliver these agents to their site of action. However, unlike the loop diuretics, the plasma protein binding varies considerably among the thiazide diuretics; accordingly, this parameter will determine the contribution that glomerular filtration makes to tubular delivery of a specific diuretic.

MINERALOCORTICOID RECEPTOR ANTAGONISTS. Mineralocorticoids such as aldosterone cause retention of salt and water and increase the excretion of K^+ and H^+ by binding to specific mineralocorticoid receptors. Early studies indicated that spirolactones block the effects of mineralocorticoids, which subsequently led to the development of specific antagonists for the mineralocorticoid receptor. Spironolactone and eplerenone are synthetic mineralocorticoid receptor antagonists that act on the distal nephron to inhibit Na^+-K^+ excretion at the site of aldosterone action (see Fig. 28-10). Spironolactone has antiandrogenic and progesterone-like effects, which may cause gynecomastia or impotence in men and menstrual irregularities in women. To overcome these side effects, eplerenone was developed by replacing the 17-alpha thioacetyl group of spironolactone with a carbomethoxy group. As a result of this modification, eplerenone has greater selectivity for the mineralocorticoid receptor than for steroid receptors, and has less sex hormone side effects than spironolactone. Eplerenone is further distinguished from spironolactone by its shorter half-life and the fact that it does not have any active metabolites. Although spironolactone and eplerenone are both weak diuretics, clinical trials have shown that both of these agents have profound effects on cardiovascular morbidity and mortality (**Fig. 28-11**) by virtue of their ability to antagonize the deleterious effects of aldosterone in the cardiovascular system (see Chap. 25). Hence, these agents are used in patients more for their ability to antagonize the renin angiotensin aldosterone system (see later) than for their diuretic properties.

Mechanisms of Action. Spironolactone (see Table 28-7) and its active metabolite, canrenone, competitively inhibit the binding of aldosterone to mineralocorticoid or type I receptors in many tissues, including

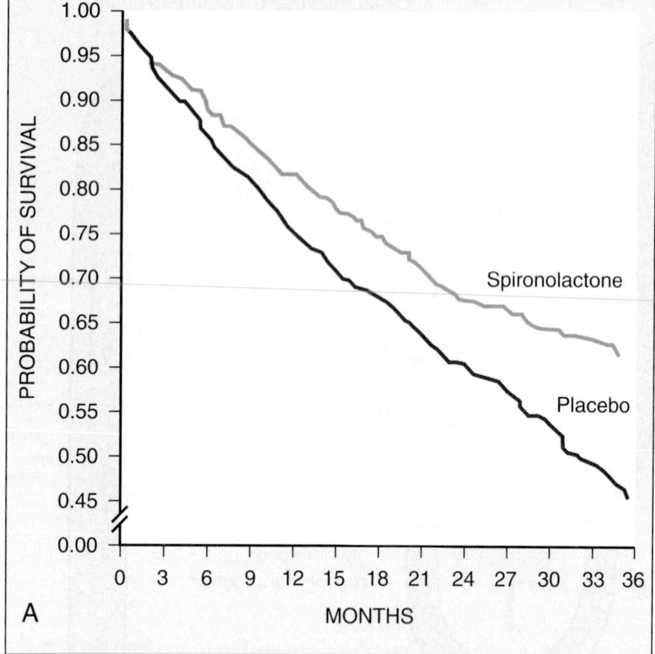

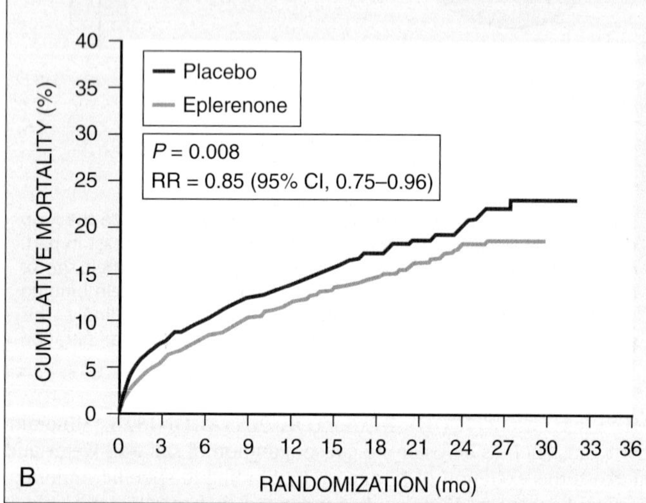

FIGURE 28-11 Kaplan-Meier analysis of the probability of survival in patients in the placebo and treatment groups in the RALES trial **(A)** with spironolactone, and probability of mortality in patients in the placebo and treatment groups in the EPHESUS **(B)** trial using eplerenone. *(Modified from Pitt B, Zannad F, Remme WJ, et al: The effect of spironolactone on morbidity and mortality in patients with severe heart failure. N Engl J Med 341:709, 1999; and Pitt B, Remme W, Zannad F, et al: Eplerenone, a selective aldosterone blocker, in patients with left ventricular dysfunction after myocardial infarction. N Engl J Med 348:1309, 2003.)*

epithelial cells of the distal convoluted tubule and collecting duct. These cytosolic receptors are ligand-dependent transcription factors, which, on binding of the ligand (e.g., aldosterone), translocate to the nucleus, where they bind to hormone response elements present in the promoter of some genes, including several involved in vascular and myocardial fibrosis, inflammation, and calcification. The first evidence that aldosterone antagonists could produce a major clinical benefit was shown by the Randomized Aldactone Evaluation Study (RALES) trial,[20] which evaluated spironolactone (25 mg/day initially, titrated to 50 mg/day for signs of worsening HF) versus placebo in NYHA Class III or IV HF patients with a LVEF lower than 35%, who were being treated with an ACEI, loop diuretic and, in most cases, digoxin. The primary endpoint was death from all causes. As shown in Figure 28-11A, spironolactone led to a 30% reduction in total mortality when compared with placebo ($P = 0.001$), which was attributed to a lower risk of death from progressive pump failure and sudden death. The frequency of hospitalization for worsening was also 35% lower in the spironolactone group than in the placebo group. In addition, patients who received spironolactone had a significant improvement in NYHA functional class ($P < 0.001$). Although the mechanism for the beneficial effect of spironolactone has not been fully elucidated, prevention of extracellular matrix remodeling (see Chap. 25) and prevention of hypokalemia are plausible mechanisms. In RALES, the serum potassium levels were 0.3 mEq/liter higher in the spironolactone group than in the placebo group ($P = 0.001$), which could have played a major role in reducing sudden or even pump failure-related deaths. Although spironolactone was well tolerated in RALES, gynecomastia was reported in 10% of men who were treated with spironolactone, as compared with 1% of men in the placebo group ($P < 0.001$). In the RALES trial, the incidence of serious hyperkalemia was minimal in both groups of patients; however, there have been several subsequent reports of severe hyperkalemia. In addition to the RALES trial, which was confined to patients with NYHA Classes III and IV HF, a retrospective analysis of a cohort of patients with mild to moderate HF suggested a favorable trend toward improved mortality when spironolactone was added to the HF regimen.

The second line of evidence that aldosterone antagonists could produce a major clinical benefit independent of the their diuretic effects came from the Eplerenone Post-Acute Myocardial Infarction Heart Failure Efficacy and Survival Study (EPHESUS; see Fig. 28-11B), a double-blind, placebo-controlled study that evaluated the effect of eplerenone on morbidity and mortality in patients with acute MI (AMI) complicated by LV dysfunction and HF. Patients were randomly assigned to eplerenone (25 mg/day initially, titrated to a maximum of 50 mg/day) or placebo in addition to optimal medical therapy. The primary end points were death from any cause and death from cardiovascular causes or hospitalization for HF, AMI, stroke, or ventricular arrhythmia. As shown in Figure 28-11B, there was a significant decrease in all-cause death in the patients randomized to receive eplerenone (relative risk [RR], 0.83; 95% CI, 0.72 to 0.94; $P = 0.005$). The rate of the other primary endpoint, death from cardiovascular causes or hospitalization for cardiovascular events, was reduced by eplerenone (RR, 0.85; 95% CI, 0.75 to 0.96; $P = 0.006$), as was the secondary endpoint of death from any cause or any hospitalization. There was also a reduction in the rate of sudden death from cardiac causes.[21] The role of eplerenone in mild HF (NYHA Class II) is being examined prospectively in the Eplerenone in Mild Patients Hospitalization and Survival Study in Heart Failure (EMPHASIS-HF) trial (ClinicalTrials.gov identifier, NCT00232180). This trial was halted prematurely on May 27, 2010, because the trial had met its primary endpoints, which was cardiovascular death or HF hospitalization.

POTASSIUM-SPARING DIURETICS. Triamterene and amiloride are referred to as potassium-sparing diuretics. These agents share the common property of causing a mild increase in NaCl excretion, as well as having antikaluretic properties. Triamterene is a pyrazinoylguanidine derivative, whereas amiloride is a pteridine. Both drugs are organic bases that are transported into the proximal tubule, where they block Na^+ reabsorption in the late distal tubule and collecting duct. However, because Na^+ retention occurs in more proximal nephron sites in HF, neither amiloride nor triamterene is effective in achieving a net negative Na^+ balance when given alone in HF patients. Both amiloride and triamterene appear to share a similar mechanism of action. Considerable evidence suggests that amiloride blocks Na^+ channels in the luminal membrane of the principal cells in the late distal tubule and collecting duct, perhaps by competing with Na^+ for negatively charged areas within the pore of the Na^+ channel. Blockade of Na^+ channels leads to hyperpolarization of the luminal membrane of the tubule, which reduces the electrochemical gradient that provides the driving force for K^+ secretion into the lumen. Amiloride and its congeners also inhibit Na^+-H^+ antiporters in renal epithelial cells and in many other cell types, but only at concentrations higher than those used clinically.

CARBONIC ANHYDRASE INHIBITORS. The zinc metalloenzyme carbonic anhydrase plays an essential role in the $NaHCO_3$ resorption and acid secretion in the proximal tubule. Although weak diuretics, carbonic anhydrase inhibitors (see Table 28-7) such as acetazolamide potently inhibit carbonic anhydrase, resulting in almost complete loss of $NaHCO_3$ resorption in the proximal tubule. The use of these agents in patients with HF is confined to temporary administration to correct the metabolic alkalosis that occurs as a contraction phenomenon in response to the administration of other diuretics. When used

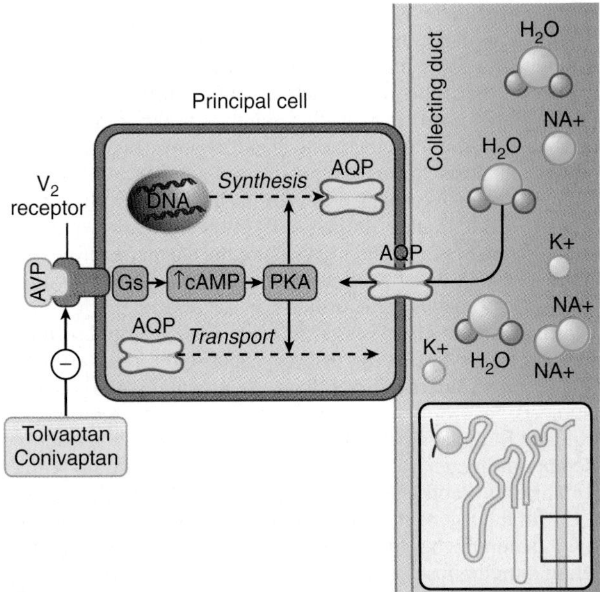

FIGURE 28-12 Mechanism of action of vasopressin antagonists. The binding of AVP to V_2 receptors stimulates the synthesis of aquaporin-2 (AQP) water channel proteins and promotes their transport to the apical surface. At the cell membrane, aquaporin-2 permits selective free water reabsorption down the medullary osmotic gradient, ultimately decreasing serum osmolarity and increasing fluid balance. V_2 antagonists work by preventing AVP from binding to its cognate receptor. *(Modified from deGoma EM, Vagelos RH, Fowler MB, Ashley EA: Emerging therapies for the management of decompensated heart failure: From bench to bedside. J Am Coll Cardiol 48:2397, 2006.)*

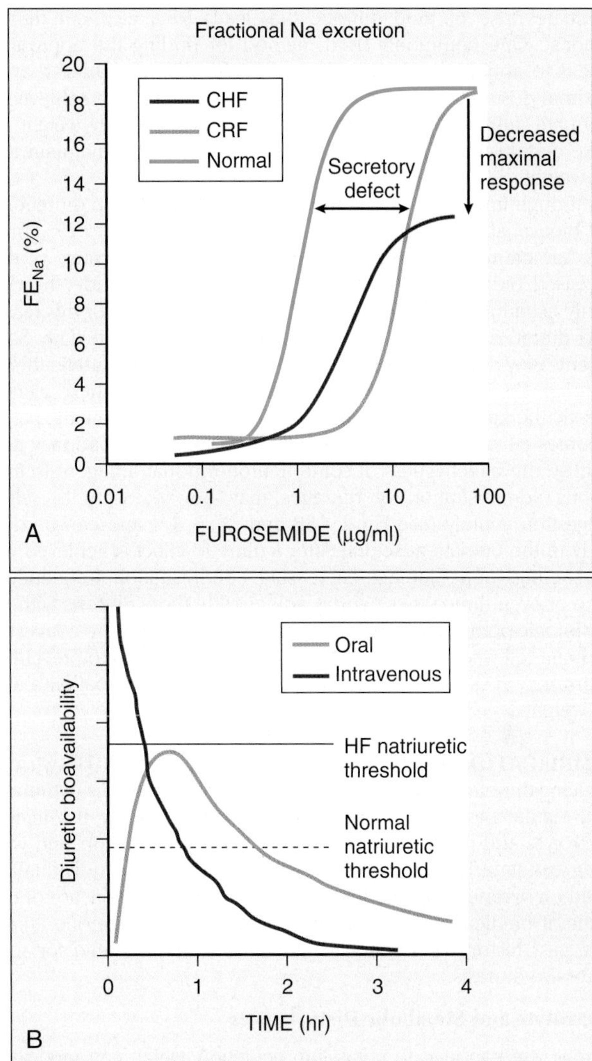

FIGURE 28-13 Dose-response curves for loop diuretics. **A,** Fractional Na excretion (FE_{Na}) as a function of loop diuretic concentration. Compared with normal patients, patients with chronic renal failure (CRF) show a rightward shift in the curve because of impaired diuretic secretion. The maximal response is preserved when expressed as FE_{Na}, but not when expressed as absolute Na excretion. Patients with HF demonstrate a rightward and downward shift, even when the response is expressed as FE_{Na}, and thus are relatively diuretic-resistant. **B,** Comparison of the response to intravenous and oral doses of loop diuretics in normal subjects and HF patients. Diuretic bioavailability is shown for normal and HF patients. The natriuretic threshold necessary to produce a diuresis is shown for normal subjects (dotted line) and for HF patients (solid line). In a normal individual, an oral dose may be as effective as an intravenous dose because the diuretic bioavailability (area under the curve) above the natriuretic threshold for intravenous and oral diuretics is approximately equal. However, if the natriuretic threshold increases in a patient with HF, the oral dose may not provide a high enough serum level to elicit a significant natriuresis. *(Modified from Ellison DH: Diuretic therapy and resistance in congestive heart failure. Cardiology 96:132, 2001.)*

repeatedly, these agents can lead to metabolic acidosis and severe hypokalemia.

VASOPRESSIN ANTAGONISTS. As discussed in Chap. 25, increased circulating levels of the pituitary hormone AVP contribute to the increased systemic vascular resistance and positive water balance in HF patients. The cellular effects of AVP are mediated by interactions with three types of receptors, V_{1a}, V_{2a}, and V_2. Selective V_{1a} antagonists block the vasoconstricting effects of AVP in peripheral vascular smooth muscle cells, whereas V_2 selective receptor antagonists inhibit recruitment of aquaporin water channels into the apical membranes of collecting duct epithelial cells, thereby reducing the ability of the collecting duct to resorb water (**Fig. 28-12**). Combined V_{1a}/V_2 antagonists lead to a decrease in systemic vascular resistance and prevent the dilutional hyponatremia that occurs in HF patients.[22]

The AVP antagonists, or vaptans, (see Table 28-7) were developed to block the V_2 receptors (e.g., tolvaptan, lixivaptan, satavaptan) selectively or nonselectively block both the V_{1a} and V_2 receptors (e.g., conivaptan). All four AVP antagonists increase urine volume, decrease urine osmolarity, and have no effect on 24-hour sodium excretion (see Chap. 27).[22] Long-term therapy with the V_2 selective vasopressin antagonist tolvaptan did not improve mortality but appeared to be safe in patients with advanced HF (see Chap. 27).[23] Currently, two vasopressin antagonists are U.S. Food and Drug Administration (FDA)–approved (conivaptan and tolvaptan) for the treatment of clinically significant hypervolemic and euvolemic hyponatremia (serum $Na^+ \leq 125$ mEq/liter) that is symptomatic and resisted correction with fluid restriction. However, neither of these agents is currently approved for the treatment of HF. Use of these agents is appropriate after traditional measures to treat hyponatremia have been tried, including water restriction and maximization of medical therapies such as ACEIs or angiotensin receptor blockers (ARBs), which block or decrease angiotensin II. Lixivaptan is currently being evaluated in a phase II study in hypervolemic HF patients (ClinicalTrials.gov identifier, NCT01055912).

DIURETIC TREATMENT OF HEART FAILURE. Patients with evidence of volume overload or a history of fluid retention should be treated with a diuretic to relieve their symptoms. In symptomatic patients, diuretics should always be used in combination with neurohormonal antagonists known to prevent disease progression (see later, Table 28-9). When patients have moderate to severe symptoms or renal insufficiency, a loop diuretic is generally required. Diuretics should be initiated in low doses (see Table 28-7) and then titrated upward to relieve signs and symptoms of fluid overload. A typical starting dose of furosemide for patients with systolic HF and normal renal function is 40 mg, although doses of 80 to 160 mg are often necessary to achieve adequate diuresis. Because of the steep dose-response curve and effective threshold for loop diuretics (**Fig. 28-13**), it is critical to find an adequate dose of loop diuretic that leads to a clear-cut diuretic response. One commonly used method for finding the appropriate dose is to double the dose until the desired effect is achieved or the maximal dose of diuretic is reached. Once patients have achieved an adequate diuresis, it is important to document their dry weight and make certain that patients weigh themselves daily to maintain their dry weight.

Although furosemide is the most commonly used loop diuretic, the oral bioavailability of furosemide is approximately 40% to 79%. Therefore, bumetanide or torsemide may be preferable because of their increased bioavailability. With the exception of torsemide, the commonly used loop diuretics are short acting (<3 hours). For this reason, loop diuretics usually need to be given at least twice daily. Some patients may develop hypotension or azotemia during diuretic therapy. Although the rapidity of diuresis should be slowed in these patients, diuretic therapy should be maintained at a lower level until the patient becomes euvolemic, insofar as persistent volume overload may compromise the effectiveness of some neurohormonal antagonists. Intravenous administration of diuretics may be necessary to relieve congestion acutely (see Fig. 25-13B and Chap. 27), and can be done safely in the outpatient setting. After a diuretic effect is achieved with short-acting loop diuretics, increasing administration frequency to twice or even three times per day will provide more diuresis with less physiologic perturbation than larger single doses. Once the congestion has been relieved, treatment with diuretics is continued to prevent the recurrence of salt and water retention to maintain the patient's ideal dry weight.

COMPLICATIONS OF DIURETIC USE. Patients with HF who are receiving diuretics should be monitored for complications of diuretics on a regular basis. The major complications of diuretic use include electrolyte and metabolic disturbances, volume depletion, and worsening azotemia. The interval for reassessment should be individualized based on severity of illness and underlying renal function, use of concomitant medications such as ACEIs, ARBs, and aldosterone antagonists, past history of electrolyte imbalances, and/or need for more aggressive diuresis.

Electrolyte and Metabolic Disturbances

Diuretic use can lead to potassium depletion, which can predispose the patient to significant cardiac arrhythmia. Renal potassium losses from diuretic use can also be exacerbated by the increase in circulating levels of aldosterone observed in patients with advanced HF, as well by the marked increases in distal nephron Na^+ delivery that follows the use of loop or distal nephron diuretics. The level of dietary salt intake may also contribute to the extent of renal K^+ wasting with diuretics.

In the absence of formal guidelines with respect to the level of maintenance of serum K^+ levels in HF patients, many experienced HF clinicians have advocated that the serum K^+ level be maintained between 4.0 and 5.0 mEq/liter because HF patients are often treated with pharmacologic agents likely to provoke proarrhythmic effects in the presence of hypokalemia (e.g., digoxin, type III antiarrhythmics, beta agonists, phosphodiesterase inhibitors). Hypokalemia can be prevented by increasing the oral intake of KCl. The normal daily dietary K^+ intake is approximately 40 to 80 mEq. Therefore, to increase this by 50% requires 20 to 40 mEq K^+ daily. However, in the presence of alkalosis, hyperaldosteronism, or Mg^{2+} depletion, hypokalemia is unresponsive to increased dietary intake of KCl, and more aggressive replacement is necessary. If supplementation is necessary, oral potassium supplements in the form of KCl extended-release tablets or liquid concentrate should be used whenever possible. Intravenous potassium is potentially hazardous and should be avoided except in emergencies. Where appropriate, the use of an aldosterone receptor antagonist may also prevent the development of hypokalemia.

The use of aldosterone receptor antagonists is often associated with the development of life-threatening hyperkalemia, particularly when they are combined with ACEIs and/or ARBs.[24] Potassium supplementation is generally stopped after the initiation of aldosterone antagonists, and patients should be counseled to avoid high potassium-containing foods. However, patients who have required large amounts of potassium supplementation may need to continue receiving supplementation, albeit at a lower dose, particularly when previous episodes of hypokalemia have been associated with ventricular arrhythmias. Diuretics may be associated with a number of other metabolic and electrolyte disturbances, including hyponatremia, hypomagnesemia, metabolic alkalosis, hyperglycemia, hyperlipidemia, and hyperuricemia. Hyponatremia is usually observed in HF patients with a very high degree of RAS activation and/or AVP levels. Aggressive diuretic use can also lead to hyponatremia. Hyponatremia can generally be treated by more stringent water restriction. Both loop and thiazide diuretics can cause hypomagnesemia, which can aggravate muscle weakness and cardiac arrhythmias. Magnesium replacement should be administered for signs or symptoms of hypomagnesemia (e.g., arrhythmias, muscle cramps), and can be routinely given, with uncertain benefit, to all subjects receiving large doses of diuretics or requiring large amounts of K^+ replacement. The modest hyperglycemia and/or hyperlipidemia produced by thiazide diuretics is not usually clinically important, and blood glucose and lipid levels are usually easily controlled with the use of standard practice guidelines. Metabolic alkalosis can generally be treated by increasing KCl supplementation, lowering diuretic doses, or transiently using acetazolamide.

Hypotension and Azotemia

The excessive use of diuretics can lead to decreased blood pressure, decreased exercise tolerance, and increased fatigue, as well as impaired renal function. Hypotensive symptoms usually resolve after a decrease in the dose or frequency of diuretics in patients who are volume-depleted. However, in most cases, the use of diuretics is associated with the decrease in blood pressure and/or mild azotemia that do not lead to patient symptoms. In this case, reductions in the diuretic dose are not necessary, particularly if the patient remains edematous. In some patients with advanced chronic HF, elevated blood urea nitrogen (BUN) and creatinine concentrations may be necessary to maintain control of congestive symptoms.

Neurohormonal Activation

Diuretics may increase the activation of endogenous neurohormonal systems in HF patients, which can lead to disease progression unless patients are receiving treatment with a concomitant neurohormonal antagonist (e.g., ACEI or beta blocker).

Ototoxicity

Ototoxicity, which is more frequent with ethacrynic acid than the other loop diuretics, can manifest as tinnitus, hearing impairment, and deafness. Hearing impairment and deafness are usually, but not invariably, reversible. Ototoxicity occurs most frequently with rapid intravenous injections, and least frequently with oral administration.

DIURETIC RESISTANCE AND MANAGEMENT. One of the inherent limitations of diuretics is that they achieve water loss via excretion of solute at the expense of glomerular filtration, which in turn activates a set of homeostatic mechanisms that ultimately limit their effectiveness. In normal subjects, the magnitude of natriuresis following a given dose of diuretic declines over time as a result of the so-called braking phenomenon (**Fig. 28-14**). Studies have shown that the time-dependent decline in natriuresis for a given diuretic dose is critically dependent on reduction of the extracellular fluid volume, which leads to an increase in solute and fluid reabsorption in the proximal tubule. In addition, contraction of the extracellular volume can lead to stimulation of efferent sympathetic nerves, which reduces urinary Na^+ excretion by reducing renal blood flow, stimulating renin (and ultimately aldosterone) release, which in turn stimulates Na^+ reabsorption along the nephron (see Chap. 25). The magnitude of the natriuretic effect of potent loop diuretics may also decline in HF patients, particularly as HF progresses. Although the bioavailability of these diuretics is generally not decreased in HF, the potential delay in their rate of absorption may result in peak drug levels in the tubular lumen in the ascending loop of Henle that are insufficient to induce maximal natriuresis (see Fig. 28-13). The use of intravenous formulations may obviate this

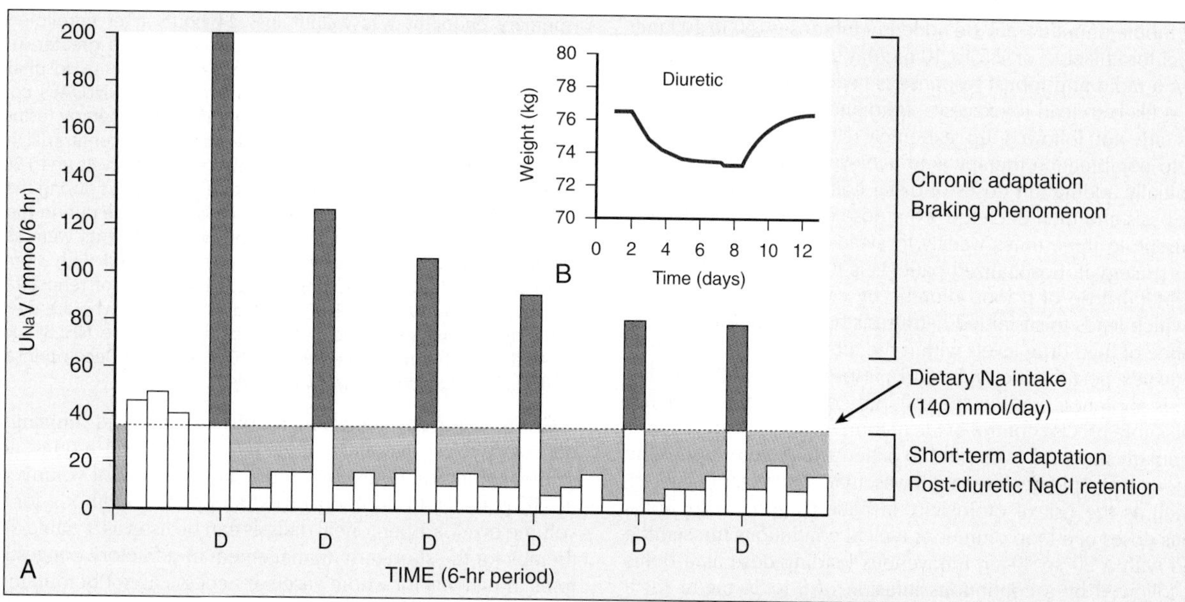

FIGURE 28-14 Effects of diuretics on urinary Na excretion and extracellular fluid (ECF) volume. **A,** Effects of a loop diuretic on urinary Na excretion ($U_{Na}V$). Bars represent 6-hour periods of Na balance before and after doses of loop diuretic (D). The dashed line indicates dietary Na intake. The shaded portion of the bars indicates the amount whereby Na excretion exceeds intake during natriuresis. The solid shaded area beneath the dashed line indicates the amount of positive Na balance after the diuretic effect has worn off. Net Na balance during 24 hours is the difference between the shaded area beneath the dashed line (postdiuretic NaCl retention) and the shaded portion within the bars. (diuretic-induced natriuresis). Chronic adaptation is indicated by progressively smaller peak natriuretic effects (the braking phenomenon) and is mirrored by a return to neutral balance. **Inset (B),** Effect of a diuretic on body weight, taken as an index of ECF volume. Note that a steady state is reached within 6-8 days despite continued diuretic administration. *(Modified from Ellison DH: Diuretic therapy and resistance in congestive heart failure. Cardiology 96:132, 2001.)*

problem (see Chap. 27). However, even with intravenous dosing, a rightward shift of the dose-response curve is observed between the diuretic concentration in the tubular lumen and its natriuretic effect in HF (see Fig. 28-13A). Moreover, the maximal effect (ceiling) is lower in HF. This rightward shift has been referred to as diuretic resistance and is likely caused by several factors in addition to the braking phenomenon described. First, most loop diuretics, with the exception of torsemide, are short-acting drugs. Accordingly, after a period of natriuresis, the diuretic concentration in plasma and tubular fluid declines below the diuretic threshold. In this situation, renal Na^+ reabsorption is no longer inhibited and a period of antinatriuresis or postdiuretic NaCl retention ensues. If dietary NaCl intake is moderate to excessive, postdiuretic NaCl retention may overcome the initial natriuresis in patients, with excessive activation of the adrenergic nervous system and RAS. This observation forms the rationale for administering short-acting diuretics several times daily to obtain consistent daily salt and water loss. Second, there is a loss of renal responsiveness to endogenous natriuretic peptides as HF advances (see Chap. 25). Third, diuretics increase solute delivery to distal segments of the nephron, causing epithelial cells to undergo hypertrophy and hyperplasia. Although the diuretic-induced signals that initiate changes in distal nephron structure and function are not well understood, chronic loop diuretic administration increases the Na^+,K^+-ATPase activity in the distal collecting duct and cortical collecting tubule, and increases the number of thiazide-sensitive NaCl cotransporters in the distal nephron, which increases the solute resorptive capacity of the kidney as much as threefold.

In patients with HF, an abrupt decline in cardiac and/or renal function or patient noncompliance with the diuretic regimen or diet may lead to diuretic resistance. Apart from these more obvious causes, it is important to query the patient about the use of concurrent use of drugs that adversely affect renal function (e.g., NSAIDs and COX inhibitors; see Table 28-6). The insulin-sensitizing thiazolidinediones (TZDs) have also been linked to increased fluid retention in patients with HF, although the clinical significance of this finding is unknown. It has been suggested that thiazolidinediones activate proliferator-activated receptor gamma expression in the renal collecting duct, which enhances the expression of cell surface epithelial Na^+ channels. Moreover, studies in healthy men have shown that pioglitazone stimulates plasma renin activity that may contribute to increased Na^+ retention. Rarely, drugs such as probenecid or high plasma concentrations of some antibiotics may compete with the organic ion transporters in the proximal tubule responsible for the transfer of most diuretics from the recirculation into the tubular lumen. The use of increasing doses of vasodilators, with or without a marked decline in intravascular volume as a result of concomitant diuretic therapy, may lower renal perfusion pressure below that necessary to maintain normal autoregulation and glomerular filtration in patients with renal artery stenosis from atherosclerotic disease. Accordingly, a reduction in renal blood flow may occur, despite an increase in cardiac output, thereby leading to a decrease in diuretic effectiveness.

A patient with HF may be considered to be resistant to diuretic drugs when moderate doses of a loop diuretic do not achieve the desired reduction of the extracellular fluid volume. In outpatients, a common and useful method for treating the diuretic-resistant patient is to administer two classes of diuretic concurrently. Adding a proximal tubule diuretic or a distal collecting tubule diuretic to a regimen of loop diuretics is often dramatically effective. As a general rule, when adding a second class of diuretic, the dose of loop diuretic should not be altered because the shape of the dose-response curve for loop diuretics is not affected by the addition of other diuretics, and the loop diuretic must be given at an effective dose for it to be effective. The combination of loop and distal collecting tubule diuretics has been shown to be effective through several mechanisms.[25] One is that distal collecting tubule diuretics have longer half-lives than loop diuretics and may thus prevent or attenuate postdiuretic NaCl retention. A second mechanism whereby distal collecting tubule diuretics potentiate the effects of loop diuretics is by inhibiting Na^+ transport along the proximal tubule, insofar as most thiazide diuretics also inhibit carbonic anhydrase, and by inhibiting NaCl transport along the distal renal tubule, which may counteract the increased solute resorptive effects of the hypertrophied and hyperplastic distal epithelial cells.

The selection of which distal collecting tubule diuretic to use as a second diuretic is a matter of choice. Many clinicians choose metolazone because its half-life is longer than that of some other distal collecting tubule diuretics, and because it has been reported to remain effective even when the glomerular filtration rate is low. However, direct comparisons between metolazone and several traditional thiazides have shown little difference in natriuretic potency when they are included in a regimen with loop diuretics in HF patients.[25] Distal collecting tubule diuretics may be added in full doses (50 to 100 mg/day hydrochlorothiazide or 2.5 to 10 mg/day metolazone; see Table 28-7) when a rapid and robust response is needed. However, such an approach is likely to lead to excessive fluid and electrolyte depletion if patients are not followed up extremely closely. One reasonable approach to combination therapy is to achieve control of fluid overload by initially adding full doses of distal collecting tubule diuretic on a daily basis and then decreasing the dose of the distal collecting tubule diuretic to three times weekly to avoid excessive diuresis. An alternative strategy in hospitalized patients is to administer the same daily parenteral dose of a loop diuretic by continuous intravenous infusion, which leads to sustained natriuresis because of the continuous presence of high drug levels within the tubular lumen (see Chap. 27), and avoids postdiuretic (rebound) resorption of Na^+ (see Fig. 28-14B). This approach requires the use of a constant infusion pump but permits more precise control of the natriuretic effect achieved over time, particularly in carefully monitored patients. It also diminishes the potential for a too rapid decline in intravascular volume and hypotension, as well as the risk of ototoxicity in patients given large bolus intravenous doses of a loop diuretic. A typical continuous furosemide is initiated with a 20- to 40-mg intravenous loading dose as a bolus injection, followed by a continuous infusion of 5 to 10 mg/hr for a patient who had been receiving 200 mg of oral furosemide/day in divided doses. The usefulness of continuous versus bolus IV furosemide was evaluated in the National Heart, Lung and Blood Institute (NHLBI)–sponsored phase IV DOSE (Diuretic Optimal Strategy Evaluation in Acute Heart Failure) study (ClinicalTrials.gov identifier, NCT00577135). The provisional results of this study suggest that high-dose IV q12hr dosing and continuous IV dosing appear to be equivalent (see Chap. 27).

Another common reason for diuretic resistance in advanced HF is the development of the cardiorenal syndrome, which is recognized clinically as worsening renal function that limits diuresis in patients with obvious clinical volume overload.[26] In patients with advanced HF, the cardiorenal syndrome is frequently present in patients who have repeated HF hospitalizations, and in whom adequate diuresis is difficult to obtain because of worsening indices of renal function. This impairment in renal function often is dismissed as prerenal; however, when measured carefully, neither cardiac output nor renal perfusion pressure have been shown to be reduced in diuretic-treated patients who develop the cardiorenal syndrome. Importantly, worsening indices of renal function contribute to longer hospital stays, and predict higher rates of early rehospitalization and death (see Fig. 28-5). The mechanisms for and treatment of the cardiorenal syndrome remain poorly understood.

DEVICE-BASED THERAPIES FOR MANAGEMENT OF FLUID STATUS. The use of mechanical methods of fluid removal, such as extracorporeal ultrafiltration, may be needed to achieve adequate control of fluid retention, particularly in patients who become resistant and/or refractory to diuretic therapy (see Chap. 27). Extracorporeal ultrafiltration (UF) removes salt and water isotonically by driving the patient's blood through a highly permeable filter via an extracorporeal circuit in an arteriovenous or venovenous mode. Alternative extracorporeal methods include continuous hemofiltration, continuous hemodialysis, and continuous hemodiafiltration. With slow continuous UF, the patient's intravascular fluid volume remains stable as fluid shifts from the extravascular space into the intravascular space, so there is no deleterious activation of neurohormonal systems. UF has been shown to reduce right atrial and pulmonary artery wedge pressures and increase cardiac output, diuresis, and natriuresis without changes in heart rate, systolic blood pressure, renal function, electrolytes, or intravascular volume.[27]

The Relief for Acutely Fluid-Overloaded Patients with Decompensated Congestive Heart Failure (RAPID-CHF) trial, which was the first randomized controlled trial of UF for acute decompensated HF, enrolled 40 patients who were randomized to receive usual care (diuretic) or a single 8-hour UF (using a proprietary device) in addition to usual care.[27] The primary endpoint was weight loss 24 hours after enrollment. Fluid removal after 24 hours was approximately twofold greater in the UF group. The Ultrafiltration versus IV Diuretics for Patients Hospitalized for Acute Decompensated Congestive Heart Failure (UNLOAD) compared the long-term safety and efficacy of ultrafiltration therapy (using a proprietary device) with intravenous diuretics in a multicenter trial involving 200 patients, who were assessed at entry and at intervals up to 90 days.[28] The primary endpoint of the trial was total weight loss during the first 48 hours of randomization and change in dyspnea score during the first 48 hours of randomization. Although the two treatments were similar in their ability to relieve dyspnea, UF was associated with significantly greater fluid loss over 48 hours and a lower rate of rehospitalization during the next 90 days. The use of UF in patients who are developing the cardiorenal syndrome is being explored in the NHLBI-sponsored CARRESS trial (Cardiorenal Rescue Study in Acute Decompensated HF; ClinicalTrials.gov identifier, NCT00608491).

Given the cost, need for venous access, and nursing support necessary to implement UF, this intervention will require additional studies to determine its role in the management of volume overload in HF patients. In addition to extracorporeal methods for relieving volume overload, peritoneal dialysis can be used as a viable alternative therapy for the short-term management of refractory congestive symptoms in patients for whom vascular access cannot be obtained, or for whom appropriate extracorporeal therapies are not available.

Preventing Disease Progression

Drugs that interfere with the excessive activation of renin angiotensin-aldosterone system and the adrenergic nervous system can relieve the symptoms of HF with a depressed EF by stabilizing and/or reversing cardiac remodeling (see Chap. 25; **Table 28-8**). In this regard ACEIs, ARBs, and beta blockers have emerged as cornerstones of modern HF therapy for patients with a depressed EF.

ANGIOTENSIN-CONVERTING ENZYME INHIBITORS. There is overwhelming evidence that ACEIs should be used in symptomatic and asymptomatic patients with a reduced EF (<40%). ACEIs interfere with the RAS by inhibiting the enzyme that is responsible for the conversion of angiotensin I to angiotensin II (see Chap. 25). However, because ACEIs also inhibit kininase II, they may lead to the upregulation of bradykinin, which may further enhance the effects of angiotensin suppression. ACEIs stabilize LV remodeling, improve patient symptoms, prevent hospitalization, and prolong life. Because fluid retention can attenuate the effects of ACEIs, it is preferable to optimize the dose of diuretic first, before starting the ACEI. However, it may be necessary to reduce the dose of diuretic during the initiation of an ACEI to prevent symptomatic hypotension. ACEIs should be initiated in low doses, followed by increments in dose if lower doses have been well tolerated. Titration is generally achieved by doubling the dosage every 3 to 5 days. The dose of ACE inhibitor should be increased until the doses used are similar to those that have been shown to be effective in clinical trials (see Table 28-8). Higher doses are more effective than lower doses in preventing hospitalization. For stable patients, it is acceptable to add therapy with beta-blocking agents before full target doses of ACEIs are reached. Blood pressure (including postural changes), renal function, and potassium level should be evaluated within 1 to 2 weeks after initiation of ACEIs, especially in patients with preexisting azotemia, hypotension, hyponatremia, or diabetes mellitus, or in those taking potassium supplements. Abrupt withdrawal of treatment with an ACEI may lead to clinical deterioration and should therefore be avoided in the absence of life-threatening complications (e.g., angioedema, hyperkalemia).

The efficacy of ACEIs has been consistently demonstrated in clinical trials with patients with asymptomatic and symptomatic LV dysfunction (**Fig. 28-15**).[29,30] These trials recruited a broad variety of patients, including women and older patients, as well as patients with a wide range of causes and severity of LV dysfunction. The consistency of data from the SOLVD Prevention Trial, Survival and Ventricular Enlargement (SAVE), and Trandolapril Cardiac Evaluation (TRACE) has shown that asymptomatic patients with LV dysfunction will have less development of symptomatic

TABLE 28-8 Drugs for the Prevention and Treatment of Chronic Heart Failure

AGENTS	INITIATING DOSAGE	MAXIMAL DOSAGE
Angiotensin-Converting Enzyme Inhibitors		
Captopril	6.25 mg tid	50 mg tid
Enalapril	2.5 mg bid	10 mg bid
Lisinopril	2.5-5.0 mg qd	20 mg qd
Ramipril	1.25-2.5 mg qd	10 mg qd
Fosinopril	5-10 mg qd	40 mg qd
Quinapril	5 bid	40 mg bid
Trandolapril	0.5 mg qd	4 mg qd
Angiotensin Receptor Blockers		
Valsartan	40 mg bid	160 mg bid
Candesartan	4-8 mg qd	32 mg qd
Losartan	12.5-25 mg qd	50 mg qd
Beta Receptor Blockers		
Carvedilol	3.125 mg bid	25 mg bid (50 mg bid if body weight > 85 kg)
Carvedilol-CR	10 mg qd	80 mg qd
Bisoprolol	1.25 mg bid	10 mg qd
Metoprolol succinate CR	12.5-25 mg qd	200 mg qd
Aldosterone Antagonists		
Spironolactone	12.5-25 mg qd	25-50 mg qd
Eplerenone	25 mg qd	50 mg qd
Other Agents		
Combination of hydralazine/ isosorbide dinitrate	10-25 mg/10 mg tid	75 mg/40 mg tid
Fixed dose of hydralazine/ isosorbide dinitrate	37.5 mg/20 mg (one tablet) tid	75 mg/40 mg (two tablets) tid
Digoxin*	0.125 mg qd	≤0.375 mg/day[†]

*Dosing should be based on ideal body weight, age and renal function

[†]Trough level should be 0.5-1 ng/mL, although absolute levels have not been established.

Modified from Mann DL: Heart failure and cor pulmonale. *In* Kasper DL, Braunwald E, Fauci AS, Hauser SL, et al (eds): Harrison's Principles of Internal Medicine. 17th ed. New York, McGraw-Hill, 2007, p 1449.

HF and fewer hospitalizations when treated with an ACEI. ACEIs have also consistently shown benefit for patients with symptomatic LV dysfunction. As shown in **Table 28-9**, all placebo-controlled chronic HF trials have demonstrated a reduction in mortality. Furthermore, the absolute benefit is greatest in patients with the most severe HF. The patients with NYHA Class IV HF in the Cooperative North Scandinavian Enalapril Survival Study (CONSENSUS I) had a much larger effect size than the SOLVD Treatment Trial, which in turn had a larger effect size than the SOLVD Prevention Trial. Although only three placebo-controlled mortality trials have been conducted in patients with chronic HF, the aggregate data suggest that ACEIs reduce mortality in direct relation to the degree of severity of chronic HF. The Vasodilator in Heart Failure II (V-HeFT-II) trial provided evidence that ACEIs improve the natural history of HF through mechanisms other than vasodilation, inasmuch as subjects treated with enalapril had significantly lower mortality than subjects treated with the vasodilatory combination of hydralazine plus isosorbide dinitrate, which does not directly inhibit neurohormonal systems. Although enalapril is the only ACEI that has been used in placebo-controlled mortality trials in chronic HF, as shown in Table 28-9, a number of ACEIs have proven to be more or less equally effective when administered orally within the first week of the ischemic event in MI trials. ACEIs markedly enhance survival in patients with signs or symptoms of HF after MI. In addition to these effects on mortality, ACEIs improve the functional status of patients with HF. In contrast, ACEIs only produce small benefits in exercise capacity. Taken together, these observations support the conclusion that the effects of ACEIs on the natural history of chronic HF, post-MI LV dysfunction, or patients at high risk of developing HF represent a class effect of these agents. Nonetheless, it should be emphasized that patients with low blood pressure (<90 mm Hg systolic) or impaired renal function (serum creatinine level > 2.5 mg/mL) were not recruited and/or represent a small proportion of patients who participated in these trials. Thus, the efficacy of these agents for this latter patient population is less well established.

Complications of Angiotensin-Converting Enzyme Inhibitor Use

Most adverse effects of ACEIs are related to suppression of the RAS. The decreases in blood pressure and mild azotemia often seen during the initiation of therapy are, in general, well tolerated and do not require a decrease in the dose of the ACEI. However, if hypotension is accompanied by dizziness or if the renal dysfunction becomes severe, it may be necessary to decrease the dose of the diuretic if significant fluid retention is not present or, alternatively, decrease the dose of the ACEI if significant fluid retention is present. Potassium retention may also become problematic if the patient is receiving potassium supplements or a potassium-sparing diuretic. Potassium retention that is not responsive to these measures may require a reduction in the dose of ACEI. The side effects of ACEIs that are related to kinin potentiation include a nonproductive cough (10% to 15% of patients) and angioedema (1% of patients). In patients who cannot tolerate ACEIs because of cough or angioedema, ARBs are the next recommended line of therapy. Patients intolerant to ACEIs because of hyperkalemia or renal insufficiency are likely to experience the same side effects with ARBs. The combination of hydralazine and an oral nitrate should be considered for these latter patients (see Table 28-8).

ANGIOTENSIN RECEPTOR BLOCKERS. ARBs are well tolerated in patients who are intolerant of ACEIs because of the development of cough, skin rash, and angioedema and should therefore be used in symptomatic and asymptomatic patients with an EF less than 40% who are ACE-intolerant for reasons other than hyperkalemia or renal insufficiency (see Table 28-9). Although ACEIs and ARBs inhibit RAS, they do so by a different mechanism. Whereas ACEIs block the enzyme responsible for converting angiotensin I to angiotensin II, ARBs block the effects of angiotensin II on the angiotensin type 1 receptor, the receptor subtype responsible for almost all the adverse biologic effects relevant to angiotensin II on cardiac remodeling (see Chap. 25). ARBs approved for the treatment of hypertension are now available to clinicians. Three of these, losartan, valsartan and candesartan, have been extensively evaluated in the setting of HF (see Table 28-8). Some clinical trials have demonstrated that ARBs are as effective as ACEIs in reversing the process of LV remodeling, improving patient symptoms, preventing hospitalization, and prolonging life. Moreover, several studies have shown that there is added therapeutic benefit for the addition of ARB to an ACEI in patients with chronic HF. ARBs should be initiated with the starting doses shown in Table 28-8, which can be uptitrated every 3 to 5 days by doubling the dose of ARB. As with ACEIs, blood pressure, renal function, and potassium level should be reassessed within 1 to 2 weeks after initiation and followed closely after changes in dosage.

In studies of symptomatic HF patients who were intolerant to ACEIs, the aggregate clinical data suggest that ARBs are as effective as ACEIs in reducing HF morbidity and mortality.[30] Candesartan significantly reduced all-cause mortality, cardiovascular death, and/or hospital admission in the Candesartan Heart Failure: Assessment of Reduction in Mortality and Morbidity trial (CHARM-Alternative Trial; **Fig. 28-16A**).[31] Importantly, candesartan reduced all-cause mortality, irrespective of background ACEI or beta blocker therapy. Similar findings were shown with valsartan in the small subgroup of patients not receiving an ACEI in the Valsartan Heart Failure Trial (Val-HeFT).[32] A direct comparison of ACEIs and ARBs was assessed in the Losartan Heart Failure Survival Study (ELITE-II), which showed that losartan was not associated with improved survival in older HF patients when compared with captopril, but was significantly better tolerated. Two trials have compared ARBs with ACEIs in post-MI patients

CH 28

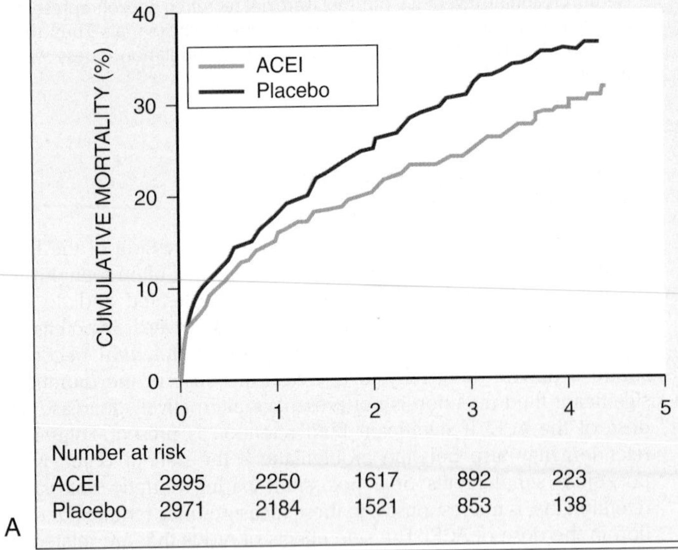

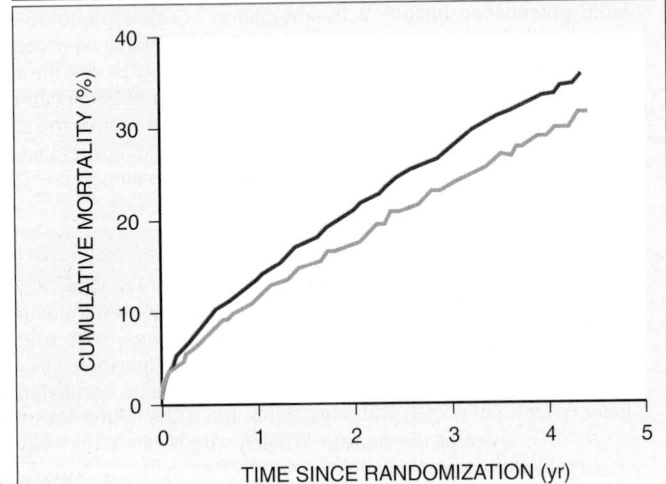

FIGURE 28-15 Meta-analysis of ACE inhibitors in HF patients with a depressed EF. **A,** Kaplan-Meier curves for mortality for HF patients with a depressed EF treated with an ACEI following an acute AMI (three trials). **B,** Kaplan-Meier curves for mortality for HF patients with a depressed EF treated with an ACEI in five clinical trials, including postinfarction trials. The benefits of ACEIs were observed early and persisted long term. *(Modified from Flather MD, Yusuf S, Kober L, et al: Long-term ACE-inhibitor therapy in patients with heart failure or left ventricular dysfunction: A systematic overview of data from individual patients. Lancet 355:1575, 2000.)*

who developed LV dysfunction or signs of HF. The direct comparison of losartan with captopril indicated that losartan is not as effective as captopril on all-cause mortality, whereas valsartan was shown to be noninferior to captopril on all-cause mortality in the Valsartan in Acute Myocardial Infarction Trial (VALIANT).[33] The combination of captopril and valsartan produced no further reduction in mortality in VALIANT, although the number of adverse events increased. When given in addition to ACEIs in general cohorts of patients with symptomatic HF, the ARBs were shown to have a modest beneficial effect in the CHARM-Added trial (see Fig. 28-16B).[34] However, the addition of valsartan to ACEIs had no beneficial effect on mortality in Val-HeFT, although the combined endpoint of mortality and morbidity was significantly lower (13.2%) with valsartan than with placebo because of a reduction in the number of patients hospitalized for HF.[32] The question of high-dose versus low-dose angiotensin receptor antagonism on clinical outcomes was evaluated in the Heart Failure Endpoint Evaluation of Angiotensin II Antagonist Losartan (HEAAL) trial.[35] This study showed that the use of high-dose losartan was not associated with a significant reduction in the primary endpoint of all-cause death or admission for heart failure (HR, 0.94; 95% CI, 0.84 to 1.04; $P = 0.24$) when compared to low-dose losartan, but was associated with a significant reduction in HF admissions (HR, 0.94; 95% CI, 0.84 to 1.04; $P = 0.24$), suggesting that uptitration of ARBs may confer clinical benefit.

Although one meta-analysis has suggested that ARBs and ACEIs have similar effects on all-cause mortality and heart failure hospitalizations,[36] and although ARBs may be considered as initial therapy rather than ACEIs following MI, the general consensus is that ACEIs remain first-line therapy for the treatment of HF, whereas ARBs are recommended for ACE-intolerant patients (see Chap. 30, Guidelines).

Complications of Angiotensin Receptor Blocker Use

Both ACEIs and ARBs have similar effects on blood pressure, renal function, and potassium levels. Therefore, the problems of symptomatic hypotension, azotemia, and hyperkalemia will be similar for both these agents. Although angioedema is less frequent than with ACEIs, it has also been reported in some patients who receive ARBs. In patients who are intolerant to ACEIs and ARBs, the combined use of hydralazine and isosorbide dinitrate may be considered as a therapeutic option (see Table 28-8). However, compliance with this combination has generally been poor because of the large number of tablets required and the high incidence of adverse reactions.

RENIN INHIBITORS. Aliskiren is an orally active renin inhibitor that appears to suppress RAS to a similar degree as ACE-inhibitors. Aliskiren is a nonpeptide inhibitor that binds to the active site (S1/S3 hydrophobic binding pocket) of renin, preventing the conversion of angiotensinogen to angiotensin I (see Fig. 25-4). The Aliskiren Observation of Heart Failure Treatment (ALOFT) study evaluated aliskiren in addition to an ACEI in patients with NYHA Classes II to IV heart failure. The primary endpoint was the change from baseline to 3 months in N-terminal pro BNP (NT-proBNP). In this study, NT-proBNP was significantly ($P < 0.01$) lower in patients who were randomized to aliskiren when compared with placebo.[37] Aliskiren is currently being evaluated in a phase III study that will evaluate the efficacy and safety of both aliskiren monotherapy and aliskiren-enalapril combination therapy as compared with enalapril monotherapy in regard to cardiovascular death and heart failure hospitalizations in NYHA Classes II to IV HF patients in the ATMOSPHERE (Efficacy and Safety of Aliskiren and Aliskiren/Enalapril Combination on Morbi-mortality in Patients With Chronic Heart Failure) study (ClinicalTrials.gov identifier, NCT00853658).

BETA-ADRENERGIC RECEPTOR BLOCKERS. Beta blocker therapy represents a major advance in the treatment of HF patients with a depressed EF. Beta blockers interfere with the harmful effects of sustained activation of the nervous system by competitively antagonizing one or more adrenergic receptors ($alpha_1$, $beta_1$, and $beta_2$). Although there are a number of potential benefits to blocking all three receptors, most of the deleterious effects of sympathetic activation are mediated by the $beta_1$-adrenergic receptor.[38] When given in concert with ACEIs, beta blockers reverse the process of LV remodeling, improve patient symptoms, prevent hospitalization, and prolong life. Therefore, beta blockers are indicated for patients with symptomatic or asymptomatic HF and a depressed EF (<40%). Three beta blockers have been shown to be effective in reducing the risk of death in patients with chronic HF; bisoprolol and sustained-release metoprolol succinate both competitively block the $beta_1$-adrenergic receptor, and carvedilol competitively blocks the $alpha_1$-, $beta_1$-, and $beta_2$-adrenergic receptors. Analogous to the use of ACEIs, beta blockers should be initiated in low doses (see Table 28-8), followed by gradual increments if lower doses have been well tolerated. The dose of beta blocker should be increased until the doses used are similar to those that have been reported to be effective in clinical trials. However, unlike ACEIs, which may be uptitrated relatively rapidly, the dose titration of beta blockers should proceed no sooner than at 2-week intervals, because the initiation and/or increased dosing of these agents may lead to worsening fluid retention because of the abrupt withdrawal of adrenergic support to the heart and the circulation. Therefore, it is important to optimize the dose of diuretic before starting therapy with beta blockers. If worsening fluid retention

TABLE 28-9 Mortality Rates in Placebo-Controlled Trials*

TRIAL NAME	AGENT	NYHA CLASS	NO. OF PATIENTS IN STUDY	12-MO PLACEBO MORTALITY (%)	12-MO EFFECT SIZE (%)	*P* VALUE AT 12 MO (FULL FOLLOW-UP)
ACEIs						
HF						
CONSENSUS-1	Enalapril	IV	253	52	↓31	0.01(0.0003)
SOLVD-Rx	Enalapril	I-III	2569	15	↓21	0.02 (0.004)
SOLVD-Asx	Enalapril	I, II	4228	5	0	0.82 (0.30)
Post-MI						
SAVE	Captopril	—	2231	12	↓18	0.11 (0.02)
AIRE	Ramipril	—	1986	20	↓22	0.01 (0.002)
TRACE	Trandolapril	—	1749	26	↓16	0.046 (0.001)
ARBs						
HF						
VAL-HeFT	Valsartan	II-IV	5010	9	0	NS (0.80)
CHARM-Alternative	Candesartan	II-IV	2028	8	↓14	NS
CHARM-Added	Candesartan	II-IV	2548	8	↓12	NS
Aldosterone Antagonists						
HF						
RALES	Spironolactone	III, IV	1663	24	↓25	NS (<0.001)
Post-MI						
EPHESUS	Eplerenone	I	6632	12	↓15	NS (0.005)
Beta Blockers						
HF						
CIBIS-I	Bisoprolol	III, IV	641	21	↓20†	NS (0.22)
U.S. Carvedilol	Carvedilol	II, III	1094	8	↓66†	NS (< 0.001)
ANZ-Carvedilol	Carvedilol	I-III	415	NS	NS	NS (>0.1)
CIBIS-II	Bisoprolol	III, IV	2647	12	↓34†	NS (0.001)
MERIT-HF	Metoprolol CR	II-IV	3991	10	↓35†	NS (0.006)
BEST	Bucindolol	III, IV	2708	23	↓10†	NS (0.16)
COPERNICUS	Carvedilol	Severe	2289	28	↓38†	NS (0.0001)
Post-MI						
CAPRICORN	Carvedilol	I	1959		↓23†	NS (0.03)
BEAT	Bucindolol	I	343	NS	↓12†	NS (0.06)

NOTE: Twelve-month mortality rates were taken from the survival curves when data were not directly available in published material.

*Conducted in patients with chronic HF (EF < 40%) or patients with AMI or at risk for HF.

†Effect size at the conclusion of the trial.

AIRE = Acute Infarction Ramipril Efficacy; BEAT = Bucindolol Evaluation in Acute Myocardial Infarction Trial; BEST = Beta Blocker Evaluation of Survival Trial; CAPRICORN = Carvedilol Post-Infarct Survival Control in Left Ventricular Dysfunction; CHARM = Candesartan in Heart Failure—Assessment of Reduction in Mortality and Morbidity; CIBIS = Cardiac Insufficiency Bisoprolol Study; CONSENSUS = Cooperative North Scandinavian Enalapril Survival Study; COPERNICUS = Carvedilol Prospective Randomized Cumulative Survival; EPHESUS = Eplerenone Post-Acute Myocardial Infarction Heart Failure Efficacy and Survival Study; MERIT-HF = Metoprolol CR/XL Randomized Interventional Trial in Congestive Heart Failure; NS = not specified; RALES = Randomized Aldactone Evaluation Study; SAVE = Survival and Ventricular Enlargement; SOLVD = Studies of Left Ventricular Dysfunction; TRACE = Trandolapril Cardiac Evaluation; Val-HeFT = Valsartan Heart Failure Trail.

Modified from Bristow MR, Linas S, Port DJ: Drugs in the treatment of heart failure. *In* Zipes DP, Libby P, Bonow RO, Braunwald E (eds): Braunwald's Heart Disease. 7th ed. Philadelphia, Elsevier, 2004, p 573.

does occurs, it is likely to occur within 3 to 5 days of initiating therapy, and will be manifested as an increase in body weight and/or symptoms of worsening HF. The increased fluid retention can usually be managed by increasing the dose of diuretics. Patients need not be taking high doses of ACEIs before being considered for treatment with a beta blocker, because most patients enrolled in the beta blocker trials were not taking high doses of ACEIs. Furthermore, in patients taking a low dose of an ACEI, the addition of a beta blocker produces a greater improvement in symptoms and reduction in the risk of death than an increase in the dose of the ACEI. It has been shown that beta blockers can be safely started before discharge, even in patients hospitalized for HF, provided that the patient is stable and does not require intravenous HF therapy. Contrary to early reports, the aggregate results of clinical trials suggest that beta blocker therapy is well tolerated by the great majority of HF patients (>85%), including patients with comorbid conditions such as diabetes mellitus, chronic obstructive lung disease, and peripheral vascular disease. Nonetheless, there is a subset of patients (10% to 15%) who remain intolerant to beta blockers because of worsening fluid retention or symptomatic hypotension.

The first placebo-controlled multicenter trial with a beta-blocking agent was the Metoprolol in Dilated Cardiomyopathy (MDC) trial, which used the shorter-acting tartrate preparation at a target dose of 50 mg three times daily in symptomatic HF patients with idiopathic dilated cardiomyopathy. Metoprolol tartrate at an average dose of 108 mg/day reduced the prevalence of the primary endpoint of death or need for cardiac transplantation by 34%, which did not quite reach statistical significance ($P = 0.058$). The benefit was entirely the result of a reduction in the morbidity component of the primary endpoint by metoprolol, with no favorable trends in the mortality component of the primary endpoint. A more efficacious formulation of metoprolol was subsequently developed, metoprolol succinate CR/XL, which has a better pharmacologic profile than metoprolol tartrate because of its controlled-release profile and longer half-life. In the Metoprolol CR/XL Randomized Intervention Trial in Congestive Heart Failure (MERIT-HF), metoprolol CR/XL provided a significant relative risk reduction of 34% reduction in mortality in subjects with mild to moderate HF and moderate to severe systolic dysfunction when compared with the placebo group (**Fig. 28-17**).[30] Importantly, metoprolol CR/X reduced mortality from both sudden death and progressive pump failure. Furthermore, mortality was reduced across most demographic groups, including older versus younger subjects, nonischemic versus ischemic cause, and lower versus higher ejection fractions.

Bisoprolol is a second-generation $beta_1$ receptor–selective blocking agent, with approximately 120-fold higher affinity for human $beta_1$ versus $beta_2$ receptors. The first trial performed with bisoprolol was the Cardiac Insufficiency Bisoprolol Study I (CIBIS-I) trial, which examined the

CH 28

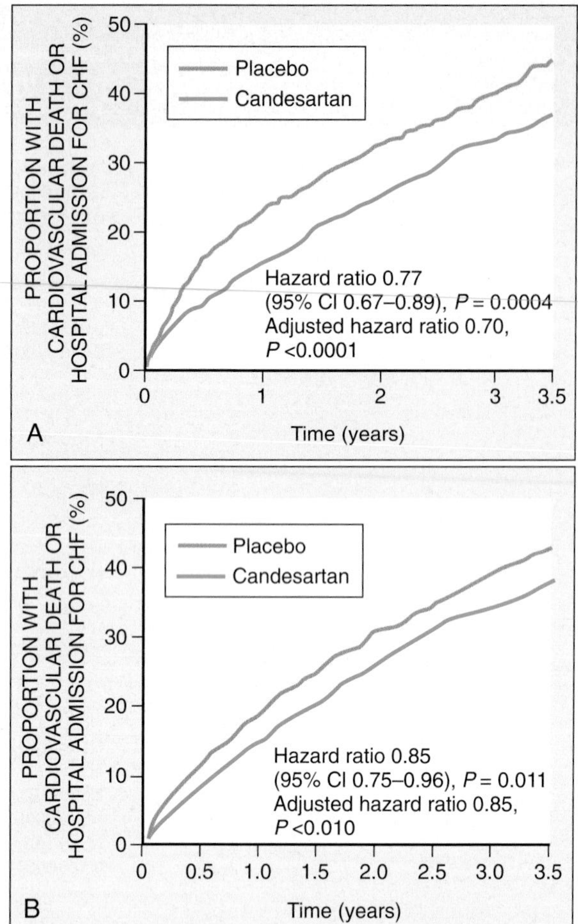

FIGURE 28-16 Effect of candesartan on cardiovascular mortality or hospital admission for heart failure in the CHARM-Alternative trial **(A)** and the CHARM-Added trial **(B)**. Two groups of patients who were randomized to candesartan or placebo are depicted—patients who were not receiving an ACEI **(A)** and patients who were receiving an ACEI **(B)**. The effect size of candesartan was reduced in the group of patients who were receiving an ACEI. *(Modified from Granger CB, McMurray JJ, Yusuf S, et al: Effects of candesartan in patients with chronic heart failure and reduced left-ventricular systolic function intolerant to angiotensin-converting-enzyme inhibitors: The CHARM-Alternative trial. Lancet 362:772, 2003; and McMurray JJ, Ostergren J, Swedberg K, et al: Effects of candesartan in patients with chronic heart failure and reduced left-ventricular systolic function taking angiotensin-converting-enzyme inhibitors: The CHARM-Added trial. Lancet 362:767, 2003.)*

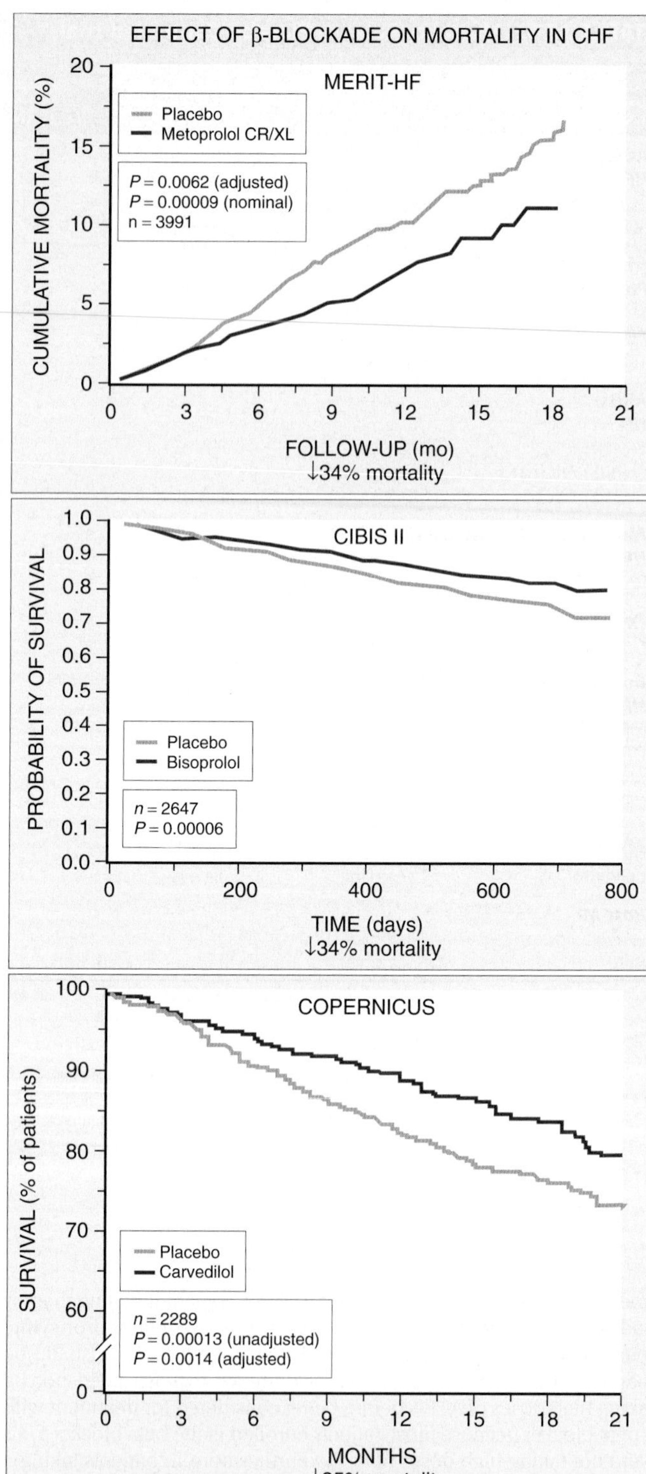

FIGURE 28-17 Kaplan-Meier analysis of the probability of survival in patients in the placebo and beta blocker groups in the MERIT-HF (top), CIBIS II (middle), and COPERNICUS (bottom) trials. CHF = chronic heart failure. *(Data from The Cardiac Insufficiency Bisoprolol Study II [CIBIS-II]: A randomised trial. Lancet 353:9, 1999; Effect of metoprolol CR/XL in chronic heart failure: Metoprolol CR/XL Randomised Intervention Trial in Congestive Heart Failure [MERIT-HF]. Lancet 353:2001, 1999; and Packer M, Coats AJ, Fowler MB, et al: Effect of carvedilol on survival in severe chronic heart failure. N Engl J Med 344:1651, 2001.)*

effects of bisoprolol on mortality in subjects with symptomatic ischemic or nonischemic cardiomyopathy. CIBIS-I showed a nonsignificant (P = 0.22) 20% risk reduction for mortality at 2-year follow-up. Because the sample size for CIBIS-I was based on an unrealistically high expected event rate in the control group, a follow-up trial with more conservative effect size estimates and sample size calculations was conducted. In CIBIS-II, bisoprolol reduced all-cause mortality by 32% (11.8% versus 17.3%; $P = 0.002$), sudden cardiac death by 45% (3.6% versus 6.4%; $P = 0.001$), HF hospitalizations by 30% (11.9% bisoprolol versus 17.6% placebo; $P < 0.001$), and all-cause hospitalizations by 15% (33.6% versus 39.6%; $P = 0.002$; see Fig. 28-17). The CIBIS-III trial addressed the important question of whether an initial treatment strategy using the beta blocker bisoprolol was noninferior to a treatment strategy of using an ACEI (enalapril) first in patients with newly diagnosed mild to moderate HF. The two strategies were compared in a blinded manner with regard to the combined primary endpoint of all-cause mortality or hospitalization, and with regard to each of the components of the primary endpoint individually. In the per-protocol primary endpoint analysis (the most conservative approach with regard to noninferiority), death or rehospitalization occurred in 32.4% of the bisoprolol-first strategy and 33.1% of the enalapril-first strategy (HR, 0.97; 95% CI, 0.78 to 1.21; $P = 0.046$ for noninferiority), which missed the prespecified criteria for noninferiority of an

HR 1.17. However, when the data were analyzed using an intent to treat analysis, bisoprolol was shown to be noninferior to enalapril (HR, 0.94; 95% CI, 0.77 to 1.16; $P = 0.019$ for noninferiority). Although CIBIS-III did not provide clear-cut evidence to justify starting with a beta blocker first, the overall safety profile of the two strategies was similar. Current guidelines continue to recommend starting with an ACEI first, followed by the subsequent addition of a beta blocker.

Of the three beta blockers that are approved for the treatment of HF, carvedilol has been studied most extensively (see Table 28-9). The phase III U.S. Trials Program, composed of four individual trials managed by a single Steering and Data and Safety Monitoring Committee, was stopped prematurely because of a highly significant ($P < 0.0001$) 65% reduction in mortality by carvedilol observed across all four trials. This was followed by a second study, the Australia-New Zealand Heart Failure Research Collaborative Group Carvedilol Trial (ANZ-Carvedilol), which showed that there was a significant improvement in LVEF ($P < 0.0001$) and a significant reduction ($P = 0.0015$) in LV end-diastolic volume index in the carvedilol-treated group at 12 months, as well as a significant relative risk reduction of 26% in the clinical composite of death or hospitalization for the carvedilol group at 19 months. Rates of hospitalization were also significantly lower for patients treated with carvedilol (48%) compared with placebo (58%). The Carvedilol Prospective Randomized Cumulative Survival (COPERNICUS) study extended these benefits to patients with more advanced HF. In COPERNICUS patients with advanced HF, symptoms had to be clinically euvolemic and the LVEF less than 25%. When compared with placebo, carvedilol reduced the mortality risk at 12 months by 38% (see Table 28-9) and the relative risk of death or HF hospitalization by 31% (see Fig. 28-17). Carvedilol has also been evaluated in a post-MI trial in which patients had to exhibit LV dysfunction. The Carvedilol Post-Infarct Survival Controlled Evaluation (CAPRICORN) trial was a randomized, placebo-controlled trial designed to test the long-term efficacy of carvedilol on morbidity and mortality in patients with post-MI LV dysfunction already treated with ACEIs.[39] Although carvedilol did not reduce the prespecified primary end point of mortality plus cardiovascular hospitalization, it did significantly reduce total mortality by 23% ($P = 0.03$), cardiovascular mortality by 25% ($P < 0.05$), and nonfatal MI by 41% ($P = 0.014$). Finally, in the Carvedilol or Metoprolol European Trial (COMET), carvedilol (target dose, 25 mg twice daily) was compared with immediate-release metoprolol tartrate (target dose, 50 mg twice daily) with respect to the primary endpoint of all-cause mortality. In COMET, carvedilol was associated with a significant 33% reduction in all-cause mortality when compared with metoprolol tartrate (33.9% versus 39.5%; HR, 0.83; 95% CI, 0.74 to 0.93; $P = 0.0017$).[40] Based on the results of the COMET trial, short-acting metoprolol tartrate is not recommended for use in the treatment of HF. The results of the COMET trial emphasize the importance of using doses and formulations of beta blockers that have been shown to be effective in clinical trials. There have been no trials to ascertain whether the survival benefits of carvedilol are greater than those of metoprolol succinate CR/XL when both drugs are used at the appropriate target doses.

Not all studies with beta blockers have been universally successful, suggesting that the effects of beta blockers should not necessarily be viewed broadly as a class effect. Early studies with the first generation of non-specific $beta_1$ and $beta_2$ receptors without ancillary vasodilating properties (e.g., propranolol) resulted in significant worsening of HF and death. The Beta blocker Evaluation of Survival Trial (BEST) evaluated the third-generation beta-blocking agent bucindolol, which is a completely nonselective $beta_1$ and $beta_2$ blocker with some $alpha_1$ receptor blockade. In the BEST trial, bucindolol produced a statistically nonsignificant ($P = 0.10$) 10% reduction in total mortality that was heterogeneous with respect to race. That is, the 76% of subjects in BEST who were not black had a statistically significant ($P = 0.01$), 19% reduction in mortality, whereas the 24% who were black had a nonsignificant trend for an increase (by 17%) in mortality (interaction P value < 0.05). The differential response of bucindilol in white patients has been suggested to be secondary to a polymorphism (arginine 389) in the $beta_1$-adrenergic receptor (see Chap. 33).[41] Bucindolol is not currently approved for clinical use at this time.

Furthermore, not all antiadrenergic strategies are beneficial in HF patients. For example, moxonidine is a centrally acting imidazoline receptor antagonist that powerfully lowers adrenergic activity. In the Moxonidine in Heart Failure (MOXCON) trial, moxonidine SR or matching placebo was titrated to a target dose of 1.5 mg twice daily.[42] This trial was stopped prematurely because of early increase in death rate (~50% increase) and adverse events in the moxonidine SR group when compared with placebo. Analysis of norepinephrine (NE) levels showed that NE levels were significantly less in the moxonidine treatment arm, suggesting that generalized sympathetic inhibition (withdrawal) may be deleterious in patients with HF. Nebivolol is a selective $beta_1$ receptor antagonist, not yet approved for the treatment of HF, with ancillary vasodilatory properties that are mediated, at least in part, by nitric oxide. In the Study of Effects of Nebivolol Intervention on Outcomes and Rehospitalization in Seniors with Heart Failure (SENIORS), nebivolol significantly (HR, 0.86; 95% CI, 0.74 to 0.99; $P < 0.04$) reduced the composite outcome of death or cardiovascular hospitalizations in older patients comparing nebivolol with placebo ($P < 0.04$) with a known EF $\leq$ 35% or a previous hospitalization for HF within 1 year (35% had an EF > 35%).[43] In a prespecified subgroup analysis, the effects of nebivolol versus placebo on death or cardiovascular hospitalizations were found to be of similar magnitude in HF patients with depressed and preserved EF.

Side Effects of Beta Blockers

The adverse affects of beta blockers are generally related to the predictable complications that arise from interfering with the adrenergic nervous system. These reactions generally occur within several days of initiating therapy and are generally responsive to adjusting concomitant medications (see earlier). The problem of fluid retention has been discussed. Treatment with a beta blocker can be accompanied by feelings of general fatigue or weakness. In most cases, the increased fatigue spontaneously resolves within several weeks or months; however, in some patients, it may be severe enough to limit the dose of beta blocker or require the withdrawal or reduction of treatment. Therapy with beta blockers can lead to bradycardia and/or exacerbate heart block. Moreover, beta blockers (particularly those that block the $alpha_1$ receptor) can lead to vasodilatory side effects. Accordingly, the dose of beta blockers should be decreased if the heart rate decreases to less than 50 beats/min and/or second- or third-degree heart block or symptomatic hypotension develops. Beta blockers are not recommended for patients with asthma with active bronchospasm

ALDOSTERONE ANTAGONISTS. Although classified as potassium-sparing diuretics, drugs that block the effects of aldosterone (e.g., spironolactone) have beneficial effects that are independent of the effects of these agents on sodium balance (see Fig. 28-11). Although ACEIs may transiently decrease aldosterone secretion, with chronic therapy there is a rapid return of aldosterone to levels similar to those before ACEIs. The administration of an aldosterone antagonist is recommended for patients with NHA Class III (previously Class IV) or IV HF who have a depressed EF (<35%), and are receiving standard therapy, including diuretics, ACEIs, and beta blockers.[30] It is possible that the indications for the use of aldosterone antagonists will be expanded when the results of the EMPHASIS-HF trial are published. The dose of aldosterone antagonist should be increased until the doses used are similar to those that have been shown to be effective in clinical trials (see Table 28-8). Spironolactone should be initiated at a dose of 12.5 to 25 mg daily or, occasionally, on alternate days. Eplerenone was used after MI in one study at doses of 25 mg/day, increasing to 50 mg daily (see Table 28-9). As noted, potassium supplementation is generally stopped after the initiation of aldosterone antagonists, and patients should be counseled to avoid high potassium-containing foods. Potassium levels and renal function should be rechecked within 3 days and again at 1 week after initiation of an aldosterone antagonist. Subsequent monitoring should be dictated by the general clinical stability of renal function and fluid status but should be done at least monthly for the first 6 months.

Side Effects of Aldosterone Antagonists

The major problem with the use of aldosterone antagonists is the development of life-threatening hyperkalemia, which is more prone to occur in patients who are receiving potassium supplements or who have underlying renal insufficiency. Aldosterone antagonists are not recommended when the serum creatinine level is higher than 2.5 mg/dL (or creatinine clearance < 30 mL/min) or the serum potassium level is higher than 5.5 mmol/liter. The development of worsening renal function should lead to consideration of stopping aldosterone antagonists because of the potential risk of hyperkalemia. Painful gynecomastia may develop in 10% to 15% of patients who use spironolactone, in which case eplerenone may be substituted.

CH 28

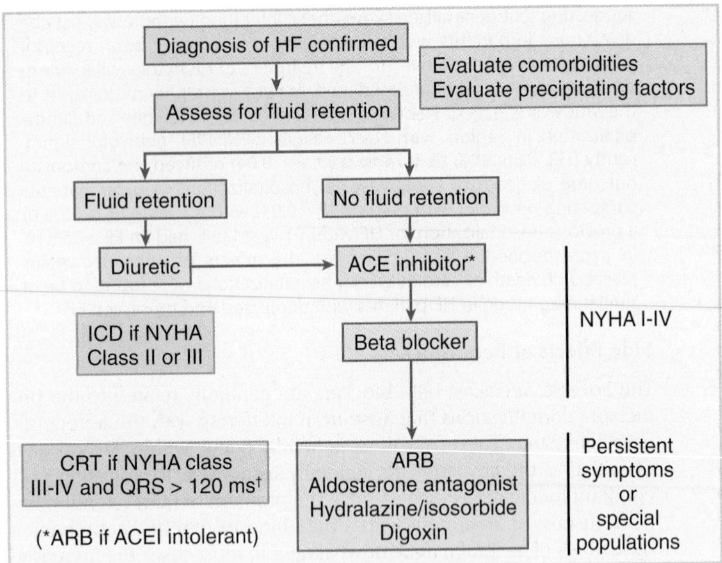

FIGURE 28-18 Treatment algorithm for patients with chronic heart failure with a reduced EF. After the clinical diagnosis of HF is made, it is important to treat the fluid retention that the patient experienced before starting an ACEI (or an ARB if the patient is ACEI-intolerant). Beta blockers should be started after the fluid retention has been treated and/or the ACEI has been uptitrated. If the patient remains symptomatic, an ARB or aldosterone antagonist or digoxin can be added as triple therapy. The fixed-dose combination of hydralazine and isosorbide dinitrate should be added to an ACEI and beta blocker in African American patients with NYHA Classes II-IV HF. Device therapy should be considered in addition to pharmacologic therapy in appropriate patients. †The Centers for Medicare & Medicaid Services (CMS) has expanded the coverage for CRT-defibrillators (CRT-D) to include patients with left bundle branch block with a QRS ≥130 ms, an EF ≤30% and mild (NYHA Class II) ischemic or nonischemic heart failure or asymptomatic (NYHA Class I) ischemic heart failure. Updated practice guidelines will likely reflect the expanded CMS indications for use of CRT-D. *(Modified from Mann DL: Heart failure and cor pulmonale.* In *Kasper DL, Braunwald E, Fauci AS, et al: Harrison's Principles of Internal Medicine. 17th ed. New York, McGraw-Hill, 2007, p 1450.)*

Management of Patients Who Remain Symptomatic

As noted, an ACEI (or an ARB) plus a beta blocker should be standard background therapy for HF patients with a depressed LVEF. Additional pharmacologic therapy (polypharmacy) or device therapy (see later) should be considered in patients who have persistent symptoms or progressive worsening despite optimized therapy with an ACEI and beta blocker (**Fig. 28-18**; see Table 28-9). Agents that may be considered as part of additional therapy include an ARB (NYHA Classes II to IV), spironolactone (NYHA Classes III to IV), the combination of hydralazine and isosorbide dinitrate (NYHA Classes III to IV), or digitalis.[30] The optimal choice of additional drug therapy to improve outcome further in patients has not been firmly established. Thus, the choice of specific agent will be influenced by clinical considerations, including renal function, serum potassium concentration, blood pressure, and race (see later). The triple combination of an ACE inhibitor, ARB, and aldosterone antagonist is not recommended because of the risk of hyperkalemia. Digoxin is recommended for patients with symptomatic LV systolic dysfunction who have concomitant atrial fibrillation, and should be considered for patients who have signs or symptoms of HF while receiving standard therapy, including ACEIs and beta blockers.

CARDIAC GLYCOSIDES. Digoxin and digitoxin are the most frequently used cardiac glycosides. Given that digoxin is most commonly used, and is the only glycoside that has been evaluated in placebo-controlled trials, there is little reason to prescribe other cardiac glycosides for the management of patients with chronic HF. Digoxin exerts its effects by inhibiting the Na^+,K^+-ATPase pump in cell membranes, including the sarcolemmal Na^+, K^+-ATPase pump of cardiac myocytes (see Chap. 25). Inhibition of the Na^+,K^+-ATPase pump leads to an increase in intracellular calcium and hence increased cardiac contractility, which has led to the suggestion that beneficial effects of digoxin are secondary to its inotropic properties. However, the more likely mechanism of digoxin in HF patients is to sensitize Na^+,K^+-ATPase activity in vagal afferent nerves, leading to an increase in vagal tone that counterbalances the increased activation of the adrenergic system in advanced HF. Digoxin also inhibits Na^+,K^+-ATPase activity in the kidney and may therefore blunt renal tubular resorption of sodium. Therapy with digoxin is commonly initiated and maintained at a dose of 0.125 to 0.25 mg daily. For most patients, the dose should be 0.125 mg daily and the serum digoxin level should be less than 1.0 ng/mL, especially in older patients, patients with impaired renal function, and patients with a low lean body mass. Higher doses (e.g., digoxin > 0.25 mg daily) are rarely used and/or not recommended for the management of HF patients in sinus rhythm or those who have atrial fibrillation. Further details about digitalis, including details about mechanism of action, pharmacokinetics, and interaction with other commonly used drugs can be found in the online supplement (see digitalis supplement on the website).

Although clinicians have used cardiac glycosides to treat patients with chronic HF for more than 200 years, there is still considerable debate regarding the effectiveness of the cardiac glycosides for HF patients. Whereas small and medium-sized trials conducted in the 1970s and 1980s yielded equivocal results, two relatively large digoxin withdrawal studies in the early 1990s, the Randomized Assessment of Digoxin and Inhibitors of Angiotensin-Converting Enzyme (RADIANCE) and the Prospective Randomized Study of Ventricular Function and Efficacy of Digoxin (PROVED), provided strong support for clinical benefit from digoxin.[44] In these studies, worsening HF and HF hospitalizations developed in more patients who were withdrawn from digoxin than in patients who were maintained on digoxin.

Insofar as withdrawal studies are difficult to interpret with respect to the efficacy of a given therapeutic agent, the Digoxin Investigator Group (DIG) trial was conducted to address the role of digitalis in chronic HF prospectively. Although the DIG trial showed that digoxin had a neutral effect on the primary endpoint of mortality, digoxin reduced hospitalizations and favorably affected the combined endpoints of death or hospitalization caused by worsening HF. Data from the DIG trial have indicated a strong trend ($P = 0.06$) toward a decrease in deaths secondary to progressive pump failure, which was offset by an increase in sudden and other non–pump failure cardiac deaths ($P = 0.04$). One of the most important findings to emerge from the DIG trial was that mortality is directly related to the digoxin serum level.[44] In men enrolled in the DIG trial, trough levels between 0.6 and 0.8 ng/mL were associated with decreased mortality, suggesting that trough levels of digitalis should be maintained between 0.5 and 1.0 ng/mL. There is also evidence that digoxin may be potentially harmful in women. In a post hoc multivariable analysis of the DIG trial, digoxin was associated with a significantly higher risk (23%) of death from any cause among women, but not men, possibly because of the relatively lower body weights in women, who were prescribed doses of digoxin on the basis of a nomogram rather than on trough levels.[45] The DIG trial was conducted prior to the widespread use of beta blockers, and no large trial of digoxin in addition to therapy with both ACEIs and beta blockers is available.

Complications of Digoxin Use

The principal adverse effects of digoxin are as follows: (1) cardiac arrhythmias, including heart block (especially in older patients) and ectopic and reentrant cardiac rhythms; (2) neurologic complaints such as visual disturbances, disorientation, and confusion; and (3) gastrointestinal symptoms such as anorexia, nausea, and vomiting. As noted, these side effects can generally be minimized by maintaining trough levels of 0.5 to 1.0 ng/mL. In patients with HF, overt digitalis toxicity tends to emerge at serum concentrations greater than 2.0 ng/mL; however, digitalis toxicity may occur with lower digoxin levels, particularly if hypokalemia or hypomagnesemia coexist. Oral potassium administration is often useful for atrial, AV junctional, or ventricular ectopic rhythms, even when the serum potassium level is in the normal range, unless high-grade AV block is also present. However, serum K^+ levels must be monitored carefully to avoid hyperkalemia, especially in patients with renal failure or those taking aldosterone receptor antagonists. Potentially life-threatening digoxin toxicity can be reversed by antidigoxin immunotherapy using purified Fab fragments (see website for details). The concomitant use of quinidine, verapamil, spironolactone, flecainide, propafenone, and/or amiodarone can increase serum digoxin levels and may increase the risk of adverse reactions (see website). Patients with advanced heart block should not be given digitalis unless a pacemaker is in place.

N-3 POLYUNSATURATED (OMEGA-3) FATTY ACIDS. There is a large body of experimental evidence suggesting that n-3 polyunsaturated fatty acids (n-3 PUFAs; omega-3 fatty acids) have favorable effects on inflammation, including a reduction of endothelial activation and production of inflammatory cytokines, platelet aggregation, autonomic tone, blood pressure, heart rate, and LV function. The GISSI-HF (Gruppo Italiano per lo Studio della Sopravvivenza nell'Insufficienza Cardiaca-Heart Failure) study has shown that long-term administration of 1 g/day of omega-3 fatty acids results in a significant reduction in both all-cause mortality (adjusted HR, 0.91; 95.5% CI, 0.83 to 0.99; $P = 0.041$) and all-cause mortality and cardiovascular admissions (adjusted HR, 0.92; 99% CI, 0.85 to 0.99; $P = 0.009$) in all the predefined subgroups, including HF patients with nonischemic cardiomyopathy.[46] Although omega-3 fatty acids are not endorsed by current practice guidelines, their use may be considered for patients who remain symptomatic despite optimal medical therapy.

Management of Atherosclerotic Disease

The clinical evaluation of atherosclerotic cardiovascular heart disease in HF patients is discussed in Chap. 26. In patients with a prior MI and HF without angina, the use of ACEIs and beta blockers has been shown to decrease the risk of reinfarction and death. Although aspirin has been shown to reduce the risk of major ischemic events in patients without HF, the role of aspirin in patients with HF has not been clearly established.[30] Prior studies have suggested that the use of aspirin may attenuate the beneficial effects of ACEIs in HF patients. For these reasons, the role of aspirin in preventing ischemic events in patients with chronic HF remains controversial. Alternative antiplatelet agents (e.g., clopidogrel) may not interact adversely with ACEIs and may have superior effects in preventing clinical events; however, their ability to affect outcomes favorably in HF has not been demonstrated. Although some clinicians recommend the use of coronary revascularization in patients with HF and CAD who do not have symptoms of angina, coronary revascularization has not been shown to improve cardiac function or symptoms or prevent reinfarction or death in HF patients without angina. In contrast, coronary artery bypass grafting has been shown to improve symptoms and survival in patients with modestly reduced EF and angina, although patients with clinical HF or markedly depressed ventricular function have generally been excluded from these studies. To this end, an ongoing National Institutes of Health–funded trial is evaluating the usefulness of surgical revascularization in such patients (see Chap. 31). Until the results of randomized clinical trials are forthcoming, it is reasonable to consider coronary artery revascularization with coronary artery bypass surgery or percutaneous coronary intervention for HF patients who have suitable coronary anatomy and angina or for patients who have demonstrable evidence of myocardial viability in areas of significant obstructive coronary disease and/or the presence of inducible ischemia.[30] The surgical management of patients with CAD disease and HF is discussed in Chap. 31.

Special Populations

WOMEN. Although women account for a significant proportion of those affected by the growing heart failure epidemic, they have been poorly represented in clinical trials (see Chap. 81). Women with heart failure are more likely to be older (see Fig. 28-1) and to have a preserved HF (see Chap. 30) and nonischemic cause for their HF. Although clinical trials have demonstrated improved outcomes among HF patients with a depressed EF, they have mainly included men and have been often been powered inadequately to detect a benefit in women. Nonetheless, pooled analyses of several large-scale prospective clinical trials with beta blockers and ACEIs have suggested that these agents provide similar survival benefits in women with systolic dysfunction, as in men.[47] In addition, some studies have suggested that ARBs may result in improved survival in women when compared with ACEIs.

RACE. Epidemiologic (see earlier) and clinical trial data have raised awareness of potential areas of concern regarding the evaluation and treatment of HF in blacks (see Chap. 2). A retrospective analysis, the Vasodilator in Heart Failure Trial I (V-HeFT I) has suggested that overall mortality and HF hospitalization are significantly reduced in black patients who receive combination therapy with hydralazine and isosorbide, whereas white patients show no treatment effect when compared with placebo. In contrast, in V-HeFT II, only white patients showed a significant mortality reduction from ACEI therapy (enalapril) when compared with treatment with hydralazine and isosorbide, whereas black patients had no apparent treatment benefit from ACEIs.[7] To address the role of hydralazine plus isosorbide treatment in blacks, the African-American Heart Failure Trial (A-HeFT) compared the adjunctive use of a proprietary formulation of isosorbide dinitrate and hydralazine to a standard HF regimen of ACEIs, beta blockers, and diuretics in blacks with NYHA Class III or IV HF.[48] The primary endpoint was a composite score made up of weighted values for death from any cause, a first hospitalization for HF, and change in the quality of life. The study was terminated early because there was a significant 43% reduction in the rate of death from any cause (see Fig. 2-6). and a significant 33% relative reduction in the rate of first hospitalization for HF. The mechanism for the beneficial effect of the hydralazine and isosorbide regimen may be related to improved nitric oxide bioavailability; however, the combination therapy group also had a small (but significant) effect of blood pressure lowering. The effect of this combination of isosorbide dinitrate and hydralazine in other HF patients who are being treated with standard therapy is not known because the population studied in A-HeFT was limited to blacks. However, there is no reason to believe that this benefit is limited to blacks. The results of the A-HeFT trial have suggested that the addition of isosorbide dinitrate and hydralazine to a standard medical regimen for HF, including ACEIs and beta blockers, is reasonable and can be effective in blacks with NYHA functional Class III or IV HF (see Fig. 28-18). The emerging field of genomic medicine has begun to suggest that important variances in the expression of certain high-risk, single-nucleotide polymorphisms may be evident along racial lines and may provide a physiologic basis for differences in the natural history of HF and in drug responsiveness (see Chaps. 10 and 33).

OLDER PATIENTS. As noted, the prevalence of HF increases with age (see Fig. 28-1) and is the most common reason for hospitalization in older patients (see Chap. 80). Of note, the presentation of HF may differ in older patients. Although they commonly present with the classic symptoms of dyspnea and fatigue, they are more likely than younger patients to present with atypical symptoms such as altered mental status, depression, or poor executive functioning.[49] The therapeutic approach to HF with a reduced EF in older patients should be, in principal, identical to that in younger patients with respect to the choice of pharmacologic therapy. However, altered pharmacokinetic and pharmacodynamic properties of cardiovascular drugs in older patients may require that these therapies be applied more cautiously, with reductions in drug dosages when appropriate. Other complicating factors may include blunting of baroreceptor function and orthostatic dysregulation of blood pressure, which may make it difficult to use target doses of some neurohormonal antagonists. Multidisciplinary HF programs have been successful in decreasing the rate of readmission and associated morbidity in older patients (see later).

CANCER PATIENTS. Patients with cancer are particularly predisposed to the development of HF as a result of the cardiotoxic effects of many cancer chemotherapeutic agents. The management of these patients is discussed in Chap. 90.

Anticoagulation and Antiplatelet Therapy

Patients with HF have an increased risk for arterial or venous thromboembolic events. In clinical HF trials, the rate of stroke ranges from 1.3% to 2.4%/year. Depressed LV function is believed to promote relative stasis of blood in dilated cardiac chambers with increased risk of thrombus formation. Treatment with warfarin (goal international normalized ratio [INR] = 2.0 to 3.0) is recommended for all patients with HF and chronic or paroxysmal atrial fibrillation and a history of systemic or pulmonary emboli, including stroke or transient ischemic attack. Patients with symptomatic or asymptomatic ischemic cardiomyopathy and a documented, recent, large anterior MI or recent MI with documented LV thrombus should be treated with warfarin (goal INR, 2.0 to 3.0) for the initial 3 months after MI unless there are contraindications. In the absence of these indications, the optimal strategy to prevent stroke in individuals with HF is less certain.

Although warfarin was associated with a reduction in cardiovascular events and death in a retrospective analysis of the SOLVD studies, no difference in antiplatelet or anticoagulant therapy has been observed in other retrospective analyses. To date, two prospective randomized trials of anticoagulation in HF have been published; however, both of these trials were underpowered to show a difference in clinical outcomes. The Warfarin/Aspirin Study in Heart Failure (WASH) showed no differences in the combined primary outcomes of death, MI, or stroke for HF patients who were randomized to receive warfarin (INR target, 2.5), 300 mg aspirin, or no treatment.[50] In the Warfarin and Antiplatelet Therapy in Chronic Heart Failure (WATCH) trial, patients with symptomatic heart failure and reduced EF were randomized to aspirin, 162 mg/day, clopidogrel, 75 mg/day, or open-label warfarin to achieve an INR of 2.5 to 3.[50] There was no difference in the primary outcome measure of death, nonfatal MI, or nonfatal stroke, although warfarin was associated with fewer nonfatal strokes compared with aspirin or clopidogrel. To address this important question more effectively, the National Institutes of Neurological Disorders and Stroke (NINDS) is conducting the WARCEF (Warfarin Versus Aspirin in Reduced Cardiac Ejection Fraction) trial (ClinicalTrials.gov identifier, NCT00041938), to determine whether there are differences between warfarin (INR = 2.5 to 3) and aspirin (325 mg) with respect to event-free survival for the composite endpoint of all-cause mortality and stroke or stroke (ischemic or hemorrhagic). At present, in the absence of strong data, the decision to anticoagulate must be an individual one in patients with dilated cardiomyopathy and EF ≤35%. Currently, aspirin is recommended in HF patients with ischemic heart disease for the prevention of MI and death. However, lower doses of aspirin (75 or 81 mg) may be preferable because of the concern of worsening of HF at higher doses, as noted above.

Management of Cardiac Arrhythmias

The management of atrial arrhythmias is discussed in detail in Chaps. 39 and 40. Briefly, atrial fibrillation occurs in 15% to 30% of patients with HF, and is a frequent cause of cardiac decompensation (see Table 28-6). Most antiarrhythmic agents, with the exception of amiodarone and dofetilide, have negative inotropic effects and are proarrhythmic. Amiodarone is a Class III antiarrhythmic that has little or no negative inotropic and/or proarrhythmic effects, and is effective against most supraventricular arrhythmias. Amiodarone is the preferred drug for restoring and maintaining sinus rhythm, and may improve the success of electrical cardioversion in patients with HF. Amiodarone increases the level of phenytoin and digoxin and will prolong the INR in patients taking warfarin. Therefore, it is often necessary to reduce the dose of these drugs by as much as 50% when initiating therapy with amiodarone. The risk of adverse events such as hyperthyroidism, hypothyroidism, pulmonary fibrosis, and hepatitis is relatively low, particularly when lower doses of amiodarone are used (100 to 200 mg/day). Dronedarone is a novel antiarrhythmic drug that reduces the incidence of atrial fibrillation and atrial flutter and has electrophysiologic effects similar to those of amiodarone but does not contain iodine, and thus does not cause iodine-related adverse reactions. Although dronedarone was significantly more effective than placebo in maintaining sinus rhythm in several studies, the ANDROMEDA trial (European Trial of Dronedarone in Moderate to Severe Congestive Heart Failure) had to be terminated prematurely because of a twofold increase in mortality (HR, 2.13; 95% CI, 1.07 to 4.25; $P = 0.167$) in the dronedarone-treated HF patients.[51] The excess mortality was predominantly related to worsening of heart failure. As a result of this study, dronedarone is contraindicated in patients with Class IV heart failure or those with Class II or III heart failure who have had a recent heart failure decompensation. Because of the risk of proarrhythmic effects of antiarrhythmic agents in patients with LV dysfunction, it is preferable to treat ventricular arrhythmias with implantable cardiac defibrillators (ICDs), either alone or in combination with amiodarone (see Chap. 29).

Device Therapy

CARDIAC RESYNCHRONIZATION. Cardiac resynchronization therapy (CRT) is discussed in detail in Chaps. 29 and 38. When CRT is added to optimal medical therapy in patients in sinus rhythm, there is a significant decrease in patient mortality and hospitalization, a reversal of LV remodeling, and improved quality of life and exercise capacity.[52] Implantation of a biventricular pacing device should be considered for patients with NYHA Class III or IV HF with a depressed EF (<30% to 35%) who are already on optimal background therapy, including an ACEI, ARB, beta blocker, or aldosterone antagonist for several months (see Fig. 28-18).

IMPLANTABLE CARDIOVERTER DEFIBRILLATORS. ICDs are discussed in detail in Chaps. 29, 38, and 41. Briefly, the prophylactic implantation of ICDs in patients with mild to moderate HF (NYHA Class II or III) has been shown to reduce the incidence of sudden cardiac death in patients with ischemic or nonischemic cardiomyopathy. Accordingly, implantation of an ICD should be considered for patients with NYHA Class II or III HF with a depressed EF (<30% to 35%) who are already on optimal background therapy including an ACEI, ARB, beta blocker, or aldosterone antagonist for several months, and who have a reasonable expectation of survival with good functional status for longer than 1 year (see Fig. 28-18).

Sleep-Disordered Breathing

The general topic of sleep disorders in cardiovascular disease is discussed in detail in Chap. 79. HF patients with a reduced EF (<40%) commonly exhibit sleep-disordered breathing; approximately 40% of patients exhibit central sleep apnea (CSA), commonly referred to as Cheyne-Stokes breathing (see Chap. 26), whereas another 10% exhibit obstructive sleep apnea (OSA). CSA associated with Cheyne-Stokes respiration is a form of periodic breathing in which central apnea and hypopnea alternate with periods of hyperventilation that have a waxing-waning pattern of tidal volume. Risk factors for the development of CSA in HF patients include male gender, age older than 60 years, presence of atrial fibrillation, and hypocapnia.[53] **Figure 28-19** illustrates the proposed mechanisms that underlie periodic oscillations in ventilation in HF. The main clinical significance of CSA in HF is its association with increased mortality. Whether this is because Cheyne-Stokes respiration with CSA is a reflection of advanced disease with poor LV function or whether its presence constitutes a separate additional adverse influence on outcomes is not clear. Nevertheless, multivariate analyses have suggested that CSA remains an independent risk factor for death or cardiac transplantation, even after controlling for potentially confounding risk factors. The potential mechanism(s) for adverse outcomes in HF patients with CSA may be attributed to marked neurohumoral activation, especially norepinephrine. Studies have suggested that Cheyne-Stokes respirations can resolve with proper treatment of HF. However, if the patient continues to have symptoms related to sleep-disordered breathing (sleep onset or sleep maintenance insomnia), despite optimization of HF therapies (see Fig. 28-19), the patient should undergo a comprehensive overnight sleep study (polysomnography).

At present, there is no consensus as to how CSA should be treated, or whether CSA should be treated at all. Insofar as CSA is to some extent a manifestation of advanced HF, the first consideration is to optimize drug therapy, including aggressive diuresis to lower cardiac filling

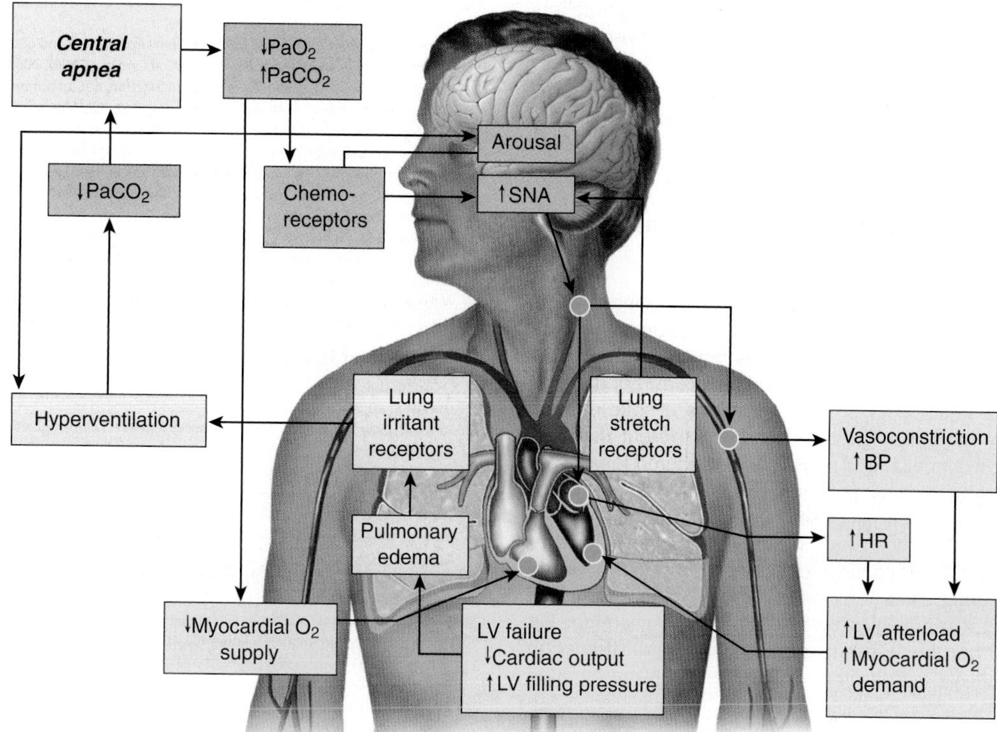

FIGURE 28-19 Pathophysiology of CSA and Cheyne-Stokes respiration in HF. HF leads to increased LV filling pressure. The resulting pulmonary congestion activates lung vagal irritant receptors, which stimulate hyperventilation and hypocapnia. Superimposed arousals cause further abrupt increases in ventilation and drive the partial pressure of carbon dioxide in arterial blood ($Paco_2$) below the threshold for ventilation, triggering a central apnea. CSAs are sustained by recurrent arousal resulting from apnea-induced hypoxia and the increased effort to breathe during the ventilatory phase because of pulmonary congestion and reduced lung compliance. Increased sympathetic activity causes increases in blood pressure (BP) and heart rate (HR) and increases myocardial oxygen (O_2) demand in the presence of reduced supply. Pao_2 = partial pressure of oxygen in arterial blood; SNA = sympathetic nervous system activity. *(Modified from Bradley TD, Floras JS: Sleep apnea and heart failure. Part II: Central sleep apnea. Circulation 107:1822, 2003.)*

pressure, along with the use of ACEIs, ARBs, and beta blockers, which may lessen the severity of CSA. In some cases, however, metabolic alkalosis arising from diuretic use may predispose to CSA by narrowing the difference between the circulating $Paco_2$ level and the $Paco_2$ threshold necessary for apnea to develop.[53] The use of nocturnal oxygen and devices that provide continuous positive airway pressure has been reported to alleviate CSA, abolish apnea-related hypoxia, decrease nocturnal norepinephrine levels, and produce symptomatic and functional improvement in HF patients when used in the short term (up to 1 month). However, the effects of supplemental oxygen on cardiovascular endpoints over more prolonged periods have not been assessed. Although there is no direct evidence that treatment of sleep-disturbed breathing prevents the development of HF, treatment of established LV dysfunction with continuous positive airway pressure (CPAP) breathing has been shown to improve LV structure and function in patients with OSA or CSA disturbed breathing syndrome. Despite these objective measurements of improvement with CPAP, this treatment modality did not lead to a prolongation of life in the Canadian Continuous Positive Airway Pressure for Patients with Central Sleep Apnea and Heart Failure (CANPAP) trial.[54] In CANPAP, patients with HF and central sleep apnea were randomly assigned to receive CPAP or no CPAP for a mean duration of 2 years. The trial was discontinued early after the event rate for death or transplantation observed in the trial was too low to detect a difference based on the expected event rate used to determine the sample size for the trial. There was no difference in the primary endpoint of death or transplantation ($P = 0.54$), nor was there a significant difference in the frequency of hospitalization between groups (0.56 versus 0.61 hospitalizations/patient year; $P = 0.45$). Additional studies will be needed to evaluate the efficacy of these types of interventions in HF patients.

Disease Management

Despite the compelling scientific evidence that ACEIs, ARBs, beta blockers, and aldosterone antagonists reduce hospitalizations and mortality in patients with HF, these life-prolonging therapies continue to be underused outside the highly artificial environment of clinical trials. Numerous studies in a variety of different clinical settings have documented that a significant proportion of patients with HF are not receiving treatment with guideline-recommended, evidence-based therapies.[55] The failure to deliver optimal medical care to HF patients is almost certainly multifactorial, as for other complex chronic conditions that have substantial morbidity and mortality. Furthermore, because many HF patients are older and often have a myriad of comorbidities, health care providers face a special challenge. Optimal HF care includes the following: (1) a trained network of providers for the delivery of HF management and interventions, including nurses, case managers, physicians, pharmacists, case workers, dietitians, physical therapists, psychologists, and information systems specialists; (2) a method for communicating this knowledge to the patient, including patient education, education of caregivers and family members, medication management, peer support, or some form of postacute care; (3) a method of ensuring that the patient has received and understood the knowledge; and (4) a system for encouraging adherence to the recommended regimen and patient compliance. Studies have shown that many of the challenges to delivering optimal care to HF patients can be met through an integrated, specialized HF clinical approach that uses nurse and physician extenders to deliver and ensure the implementation of care.[56] Technology-driven strategies that use low-cost telemonitoring also appear promising in terms of improving HF management and outcomes (see Chap. 29),[57] emphasizing the importance of team management in the care of these complex patients. A disease management approach to HF has been shown to reduce hospitalizations and increase the percentage of patients who receive ideal guideline-recommended therapy.[58] Recent studies have demonstrated that disease management programs need not be confined to the outpatient setting; hospital-based disease management systems can also improve medical care and education of hospitalized

HF patients and accelerate the use of evidence-based guideline-recommended therapies by administering them before hospital discharge.[30] Although disease management strategies can lead to improved survival, it is not clear that these strategies are necessarily more cost-effective. Accordingly, the biggest challenge to disease management programs will be to determine how to support the additional personnel required to implement this model of care.

Patients with Refractory End-Stage Heart Failure (Stage D)

Most patients with HF caused by reduced LVEF respond well to evidence-based pharmacologic and nonpharmacologic treatments, and enjoy a good quality of life with a meaningful prolongation. However, for reasons that are not clear, some patients do not improve or will experience a rapid recurrence of symptoms, despite optimal medical and device therapies. These individuals represent the most advanced stage of HF (stage D) and should be considered for specialized treatment strategies, such as mechanical circulatory support (see Chap. 32), continuous intravenous positive inotropic therapy, referral for cardiac transplantation (see Chap. 31), or hospice care. However, before a patient is considered to have refractory HF, physicians should identify any contributing conditions (see Table 28-6) and ensure that all conventional medical strategies have been optimally used (see Fig. 28-18). When no further therapies are appropriate, careful discussion of the prognosis and options for end-of-life care should be initiated (see Chap. 34).

Future Perspectives

As noted, ACEIs, ARBs, aldosterone antagonists, beta blocker therapy, and cardiac devices have substantially improved quality and quantity of life for patients with HF with a reduced EF. Unfortunately, we appear to be limited with regard to further antagonism of neurohormonal-cytokine systems inasmuch as most trials attempting to add additional neurohormonal-cytokine inhibition to the background therapy of ACE inhibition and beta blockade have been unsuccessful. These failures include certain endothelin antagonists, tumor necrosis factor antagonists, and neutral endopeptidase inhibitors, which indicates the potential limits of neurohormonal inhibitory strategies and strongly signals that different drug development approaches are needed. Currently, these approaches are underway, with newer small molecules, cell replacement therapy (see Chap. 11), and gene therapy (see Chap. 33), accompanied by growing appreciation of the role of pharmacogenetics (see Chaps. 10 and 33). Further refinement of device technology and appropriate patient selection may allow device therapies, especially CRT, to be extended to more eligible patients. It is likely that one or more of these therapies that target maladaptive mechanisms and/or cardiac remodeling will soon be successful.

REFERENCES

Epidemiology and Prognosis

1. Swedberg K, Cleland J, Dargie H, et al: Guidelines for the diagnosis and treatment of chronic heart failure: Executive summary (update 2005): The Task Force for the Diagnosis and Treatment of Chronic Heart Failure of the European Society of Cardiology. Eur Heart J 26:1115, 2005.
2. Levy D, Kenchaiah S, Larson MG, et al: Long-term trends in the incidence of and survival with heart failure. Eur Heart J 347:1397, 2002.
3. Mendez GF, Cowie MR: The epidemiological features of heart failure in developing countries: A review of the literature. Int J Cardiol 80:213, 2001.
4. Kenchaiah S, Evans JC, Levy D, et al: Obesity and the risk of heart failure. N Engl J Med 347:305, 2002.
5. Walsh CR, Larson MG, Evans JC, et al: Alcohol consumption and risk for congestive heart failure in the Framingham Heart Study. Ann Intern Med 136:181, 2002.
6. Murray-Thomas T, Cowie MR: Epidemiology and clinical aspects of congestive heart failure. J Renin Angiotensin Aldosterone Syst 4:131, 2003.
7. Yancy CW: Heart failure in African Americans. Am J Cardiol 96:3i, 2005.
8. Young JB: The prognosis of heart failure. *In* Mann DL (ed): Heart Failure: A Companion to Braunwald's Heart Disease. Philadelphia, WB Saunders, 2003, pp 489-506.
9. Levy WC, Mozaffarian,D, Linker DT, et al: The Seattle Heart Failure Model: Prediction of survival in heart failure. Circulation 113:1424, 2006.
10. Tang YD, Katz SD: Anemia in chronic heart failure: Prevalence, cause, clinical correlates, and treatment options. Circulation 113:2454, 2006.
11. Anker SD, Comin CJ, Filippatos G, et al: Ferric carboxymaltose in patients with heart failure and iron deficiency. N Engl J Med 361:2436, 2009.
12. Smith GL, Lichtman JH, Bracken MB, et al: Renal impairment and outcomes in heart failure: Systematic review and meta-analysis. J Am Coll Cardiol 47:1987, 2006.
13. Hillege HL, Girbes AR, de Kam PJ, et al: Renal function, neurohormonal activation, and survival in patients with chronic heart failure. Circulation 102:203, 2000.
14. Hunt SA, Abraham WT, Chin MH, et al: 2009 focused update incorporated into the ACC/AHA 2005 Guidelines for the Diagnosis and Management of Heart Failure in Adults: A report of the American College of Cardiology Foundation/American Heart Association Task Force on Practice Guidelines: Developed in collaboration with the International Society for Heart and Lung Transplantation. Circulation 119:e391, 2009.
15. Heidenreich PA, Gubens MA, Fonarow GC, et al: Cost-effectiveness of screening with B-type natriuretic peptide to identify patients with reduced left ventricular ejection fraction. J Am Coll Cardiol 43:1019, 2004.
16. Wittstein IS, Thiemann DR, Lima JA, et al: Neurohumoral features of myocardial stunning due to sudden emotional stress. N Engl J Med 352:539, 2005.

Management of Heart Failure

17. O'Connor CM, Whellan DJ, Lee KL, et al: Efficacy and safety of exercise training in patients with chronic heart failure: HF-ACTION randomized controlled trial. JAMA 301:1439, 2009.
18. Faris R, Flather MD, Purcell H, et al: Diuretics for heart failure. Cochrane Database Syst Rev (1):CD003838, 2006.
19. Domanski M, Tian X, Haigney M, et al: Diuretic use, progressive heart failure, and death in patients in the DIG study. J Card Fail 12:327, 2006.
20. Pitt B, Zannad F, Remme WJ, et al: The effect of spironolactone on morbidity and mortality in patients with severe heart failure. Randomized Aldactone Evaluation Study Investigators. N Engl J Med 341:709, 1999.
21. Pitt B, Remme W, Zannad F: Eplerenone, a selective aldosterone blocker, in patients with left ventricular dysfunction after myocardial infarction. N Engl J Med 348:1309, 2003.
22. Finley JJ, Konstam MA, Udelson, JE: Arginine vasopressin antagonists for the treatment of heart failure and hyponatremia. Circulation 118:410, 2008.
23. Konstam MA, Gheorghiade M, Burnett JC Jr, et al: Effects of oral tolvaptan in patients hospitalized for worsening heart failure: The EVEREST Outcome Trial. JAMA 297:1319, 2007.
24. Juurlink DN, Mamdani MM, Lee DS, et al: Rates of hyperkalemia after publication of the Randomized Aldactone Evaluation Study. N Engl J Med 351:543, 2004.
25. Ellison DH: Diuretic therapy and resistance in congestive heart failure. Cardiology 96:132, 2001.
26. Stevenson LW, Nohria A, Mielniczuk L: Torrent or torment from the tubules? Challenge of the cardiorenal connections. J Am Coll Cardiol 45:2004, 2005.
27. Costanzo MR: Ultrafiltration in the management of heart failure. Curr Opin Crit Care 14:524, 2008.
28. Costanzo MR, Guglin ME, Saltzberg MT, et al: Ultrafiltration versus intravenous diuretics for patients hospitalized for acute decompensated heart failure. J Am Coll Cardiol 49:675, 2007.
29. Flather MD, Yusuf S, Kober L, et al: Long-term ACE-inhibitor therapy in patients with heart failure or left ventricular dysfunction: A systematic overview of data from individual patients. ACE-Inhibitor Myocardial Infarction Collaborative Group. Lancet 355:1575, 2000.
30. Jessup ML, Abraham WT, Casey DE, et al: 2009 focused update: ACCF/AHA Guidelines for the Diagnosis and Management of Heart Failure in Adults: A report of the American College of Cardiology Foundation/American Heart Association Task Force on Practice Guidelines: Developed in collaboration with the International Society for Heart and Lung Transplantation. Circulation 119:1977, 2009.
31. Granger CB, McMurray JJ, Yusuf S, et al: Effects of candesartan in patients with chronic heart failure and reduced left ventricular systolic function intolerant to angiotensin-converting-enzyme inhibitors: The CHARM-Alternative trial. Lancet 362:772, 2003.
32. Cohn JN, Tognoni G: A randomized trial of the angiotensin-receptor blocker valsartan in chronic heart failure. N Engl J Med 345:1667, 2001.
33. Pfeffer MA, McMurray JJ, Velazquez EJ, et al: Valsartan, captopril, or both in myocardial infarction complicated by heart failure, left ventricular dysfunction, or both. N Engl J Med 349:1893, 2003.
34. McMurray JJ, Ostergren J, Swedberg K, et al: Effects of candesartan in patients with chronic heart failure and reduced left-ventricular systolic function taking angiotensin-converting-enzyme inhibitors: The CHARM-Added trial. Lancet 362:767, 2003.
35. Konstam MA, Neaton JD, Dickstein K, et al: Effects of high-dose versus low-dose losartan on clinical outcomes in patients with heart failure (HEAAL study): A randomised, double-blind trial. Lancet 374:1840, 2009.
36. Lee VC, Rhew DC, Dylan M, et al: Meta-analysis: Angiotensin-receptor blockers in chronic heart failure and high-risk acute myocardial infarction. Ann Intern Med 141:693, 2004.
37. Cleland JG, Abdellah AT, Khaleva O, et al: Clinical trials update from the European Society of Cardiology Congress 2007: 3CPO, ALOFT, PROSPECT and statins for heart failure. Eur J Heart Fail 9:1070, 2007.
38. Mann DL, Bristow MR: Mechanisms and models in heart failure: The biomechanical model and beyond. Circulation 111:2837, 2005.
39. Dargie HJ: Effect of carvedilol on outcome after myocardial infarction in patients with left-ventricular dysfunction: The CAPRICORN randomised trial. Lancet 357:1385, 2001.
40. Poole-Wilson PA, Swedberg K, Cleland JG, et al: Comparison of carvedilol and metoprolol on clinical outcomes in patients with chronic heart failure in the Carvedilol Or Metoprolol European Trial (COMET): Randomised controlled trial. Lancet 362:7, 2003.
41. Liggett SB, Mialet-Perez J, Thaneemit-Chen S, et al: A polymorphism within a conserved β_1-adrenergic receptor motif alters cardiac function and beta blocker response in human heart failure. Proc Natl Acad Sci U S A 103:11288, 2006.
42. Cohn JN, Pfeffer MA, Rouleau J, et al: Adverse mortality effect of central sympathetic inhibition with sustained-release moxonidine in patients with heart failure (MOXCON). Eur J Heart Fail 5:659, 2003.
43. Flather MD, Shibata MC, Coats AJ, et al: Randomized trial to determine the effect of nebivolol on mortality and cardiovascular hospital admission in elderly patients with heart failure (SENIORS). Eur Heart J 26:215, 2005.
44. Gheorghiade M, Adams KF Jr, Colucci WS: Digoxin in the management of cardiovascular disorders. Circulation 109:2959, 2004.
45. Rathore SS, Wang Y, Krumholz HM: Sex-based differences in the effect of digoxin for the treatment of heart failure. N Engl J Med 347:1403, 2002.

46. Gissi-HF Investigators; Tavazzi L, Maggioni AP, Marchioli R, et al: Effect of n-3 polyunsaturated fatty acids in patients with chronic heart failure (the GISSI-HF trial): A randomised, double-blind, placebo-controlled trial. Lancet 372:1223, 2008.
47. Hsich EM, Pina IL: Heart failure in women: A need for prospective data. J Am Coll Cardiol 54:491, 2009.
48. Taylor AL, Ziesche S, Yancy C, et al: Combination of isosorbide dinitrate and hydralazine in blacks with heart failure. N Engl J Med 351:2049, 2004.
49. Rich MW: Epidemiology, clinical features, and prognosis of acute myocardial infarction in the elderly. Am J Geriatr Cardiol 15:7, 2006.
50. Kohsaka S, Homma S: Anticoagulation for heart failure: Selecting the best therapy. Expert Rev Cardiovasc Ther 7:1209, 2009.
51. Kober L, Torp-Pedersen C, McMurray JJ, et al: Increased mortality after dronedarone therapy for severe heart failure. N Engl J Med 358:2678, 2008.
52. Cleland JG, Daubert JC, Erdmann E, et al: The effect of cardiac resynchronization on morbidity and mortality in heart failure. N Engl J Med 352:1539, 2005.
53. Wolk R, Gami AS, Garcia-Touchard A, et al: Sleep and cardiovascular disease. Curr Probl Cardiol 30:625, 2005.
54. Bradley TD, Logan AG, Kimoff RJ, et al: Continuous positive airway pressure for central sleep apnea and heart failure. N Engl J Med 353:2025, 2005.
55. Fonarow GC, Yancy CW, Albert NM, et al: Improving the use of evidence-based heart failure therapies in the outpatient setting: The IMPROVE HF performance improvement registry. Am Heart J 154:12, 2007.
56. Granger BB, Swedberg K, Ekman I, et al: Adherence to candesartan and placebo and outcomes in chronic heart failure in the CHARM programme: Double-blind, randomised, controlled clinical trial. Lancet 366:2005, 2005.
57. Maric B, Kaan A, Ignaszewski A, et al: A systematic review of telemonitoring technologies in heart failure. Eur J Heart Fail 11:506, 2009.
58. Fonarow GC: How well are chronic heart failure patients being managed? Rev Cardiovasc Med 7(Suppl 1):S3, 2006.

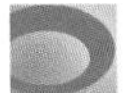

GUIDELINES DOUGLAS L. MANN

Management of Heart Failure

A joint task force of the American College of Cardiology and the American Heart Association (ACC/AHA) published guidelines for the evaluation and management of heart failure in 2005[1] and subsequently updated them in 2009.[2] These guidelines superseded previous sets of recommendations issued by the ACC/AHA in 2001[3] and 1995[4] as well as guidelines from the Agency for Health Care Policy and Research in 1994[5] and the Heart Failure Society of America in 1999.[6] New guidelines from the Heart Failure Society were published in 2006,[7] and a complete revision of the Heart Failure Society guidelines will be published in 2010. The most recent European Society of Cardiology (ESC) guidelines for the diagnosis and treatment of chronic heart failure were published in 2008.[8] The current ACC/AHA guidelines classify patients according to four stages, which reflects the growing appreciation for the importance of the prevention of heart failure:

Stage A: patients at high risk for developing heart failure but without structural disorders of the heart

Stage B: patients with a structural disorder of the heart but no symptoms of heart failure

Stage C: patients with past or current symptoms of heart failure associated with underlying structural heart disease

Stage D: patients with end-stage disease who require specialized treatment strategies such as mechanical circulatory support, continuous inotropic infusions, cardiac transplantation, or hospice care

The advantage of the four-stage system is that it recommends interventions for asymptomatic patients with the goal of preventing signs or symptoms of heart failure. In contrast, the traditional New York Heart Association (NYHA) functional classification system primarily gauges the severity of symptoms in patients who are in stage C or stage D. **Figure 28G-1** summarizes the guideline recommendations for therapy by stage.

Like other ACC/AHA guidelines, these recommendations classify interventions into one of three classes as follows, including two levels of the intermediate group:

Class I: conditions for which there is evidence and/or general agreement that a given procedure/therapy is useful and effective

Class II: conditions for which there is conflicting evidence and/or a divergence of opinion about the usefulness/efficacy of performing the procedure/therapy

Class IIa: weight of evidence and opinion in favor of usefulness/efficacy

Class IIb: usefulness/efficacy is less well established by evidence and opinion

Class III: conditions for which there is evidence and/or general agreement that a procedure or therapy is not useful or effective and in some cases may be harmful

The ACC/AHA guidelines also adopt a convention for rating levels of evidence on which recommendations have been based. Level A recommendations are derived from data from multiple randomized clinical trials; level B recommendations are derived from a single randomized trial or nonrandomized studies; and level C recommendations are based on the consensus opinion of experts. The guidelines emphasize that the strength of evidence does not necessarily reflect the strength of a recommendation. A treatment may be controversial despite having been evaluated in controlled clinical trials; conversely, a strong recommendation may be supported only by historical data or by no data at all.

INITIAL PATIENT EVALUATION

The ACC/AHA guidelines state that a complete history and physical examination should be the first step in the evaluation of patients with heart failure (**Table 28G-1**). This evaluation may provide insight into the cause of the patient's heart failure and the presence or absence of structural cardiovascular abnormalities. Other issues to be addressed include the presence or absence of history of diabetes, rheumatic fever, chest irradiation, or exposure to cardiotoxic drugs and the use or abuse of alcohol, illicit drugs, or alternative therapies. The patient's functional and hemodynamic status should also be evaluated to assess prognosis and to guide management.

The guidelines recommend that the initial evaluation include a complete blood count; urinalysis; serum electrolyte determinations, plus calcium and magnesium concentrations; renal and hepatic function tests; fasting blood glucose concentration and HbA1c level; lipid profile; thyroid function tests; chest radiography; 12-lead electrocardiography; two-dimensional echocardiography with Doppler study; and coronary arteriography in patients with angina or significant ischemia (unless the patient is ineligible for revascularization).

Measurements of serum ferritin level and transferrin saturation are considered potentially useful for the detection of hemochromatosis because this condition is a treatable cause of heart failure. Screening for the human immunodeficiency virus, sleep-disturbed breathing, connective tissue diseases, amyloidosis, or pheochromocytoma is also reasonable in selected patients.

The updated guidelines reflect recent research on B-type natriuretic peptide (BNP). In the 2009 guidelines, the ACC/AHA supports its use in the urgent care setting when the diagnosis of heart failure is uncertain as well as for risk stratification but does not recommend that BNP be used to guide therapy.

Echocardiography to assess left ventricular function and to detect underlying myocardial, valvular, or pericardial disease is considered a more valuable initial test than radionuclide ventriculography or magnetic resonance imaging.

Screening for and assessment of coronary artery disease in patients with heart failure are given considerable attention in these guidelines, reflecting the frequent coexistence of these conditions and the survival benefit of revascularization of patients with severe coronary disease and left ventricular dysfunction. Coronary arteriography is recommended (Class I indication) for patients with angina or significant ischemia and heart failure unless they are not eligible for revascularization. For patients who have chest pain and heart failure, the guidelines provide support for bypassing the step of noninvasive testing and proceeding directly to coronary angiography (Class IIa indication). For patients without chest pain, the guidelines consider coronary angiography "reasonable" for excluding the diagnosis of coronary disease. Maximal exercise testing is

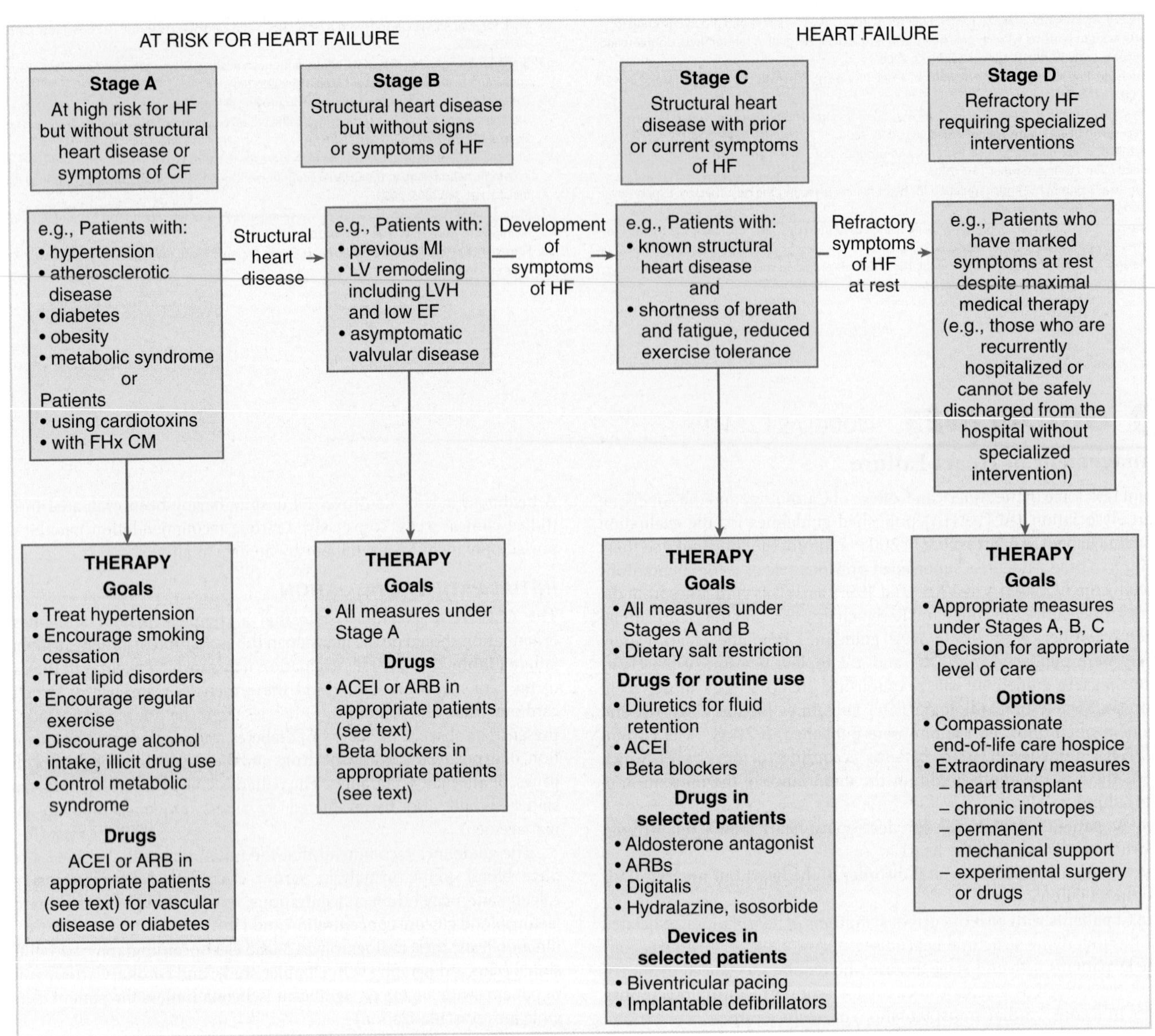

FIGURE 28G-1 Stages in the evolution of heart failure (HF) and recommended therapy by stage. ACEI = angiotensin-converting enzyme inhibitor; ARB = angiotensin receptor blocker; EF = ejection fraction; FHx CM = family history of cardiomyopathy; IV = intravenous; LV = left ventricular; LVH = left ventricular hypertrophy; MI = myocardial infarction. *(From Hunt SA, Baker DW, Chin MH, et al: ACC/AHA guidelines for the evaluation and management of chronic heart failure in the adult: Executive summary. A report of the American College of Cardiology/American Heart Association Task Force on Practice Guidelines [Committee to Revise the 1995 Guidelines for the Evaluation and Management of Heart Failure]. J Am Coll Cardiol 104:2996, 2001.)*

recommended to help determine if heart failure is the cause of exercise limitation or to identify high-risk patients with heart failure who may be candidates for cardiac transplantation or other advanced therapy.

The guidelines offered only weak support for noninvasive testing to define the likelihood of coronary artery disease in patients with heart failure and left ventricular dysfunction and for Holter monitoring in patients with a history of myocardial infarction who might be susceptible to ventricular tachycardia.

Routine use of endomyocardial biopsy or signal-averaged electrocardiography and routine measurement of circulating levels of neurohormones such as norepinephrine and endothelin are not recommended.

ONGOING ASSESSMENT OF PATIENTS WITH HEART FAILURE

The guidelines support routine assessment of functional and volume status in patients with heart failure along with assessment of potentially harmful behaviors or habits (see Table 28G-1). They discourage routine serial measurement of ejection fraction at regular intervals and instead recommend that ejection fraction be reassessed if patients have had a change in clinical status, recovered from a significant clinical event, or received treatment that might affect left ventricular function. The value of serial measurements of BNP remains uncertain.

TREATMENT OF PATIENTS AT HIGH RISK OF DEVELOPING HEART FAILURE (STAGE A)

The ACC/AHA guidelines provide strong recommendations (Class I) for control of risk factors for coronary disease and other causes of cardiomyopathy, including hypertension, hyperlipidemia, diabetes, alcohol abuse, cigarette smoking, supraventricular tachycardia, and thyroid disorders (**Table 28G-2**). Patients at risk for heart failure should also be assessed frequently for evidence that this condition is developing, particularly those with a strong family history of cardiomyopathy and those receiving cardiotoxic interventions. Attention should be paid to secondary prevention efforts in patients with atherosclerotic vascular disease.

The guidelines suggest a low threshold for use of angiotensin-converting enzyme (ACE) inhibitors or angiotensin II receptor blockers (Class IIa). The ACC/AHA Task Force recommends advising patients not to use nutritional supplements solely to prevent the development of heart failure.

TABLE 28G-1 ACC/AHA Guidelines for Initial and Serial Evaluation of Heart Failure

CLASS	INDICATION	LEVEL OF EVIDENCE*
	ACC/AHA Guidelines for initial Evaluation of Patients with Heart Failure	
I (indicated)	1. Thorough history and physical examination to identify cardiac and noncardiac disorders or behaviors that might cause heart failure or accelerate its development or progression	C
	2. Obtain a careful history of current and past use of alcohol, illicit drugs, current or past standard or "alternative therapies," and chemotherapy drugs	C
	3. Initial assessment of the patient's ability to perform routine and desired activities of daily living	C
	4. Initial examination should include assessment of volume status, orthostatic blood pressure changes, measurement of weight and height, and calculation of body mass index	C
	5. Initial laboratory evaluation should include complete blood count, urinalysis, serum electrolytes (including calcium and magnesium), blood urea nitrogen, serum creatinine, fasting blood glucose (glycohemoglobin), lipid profile, liver function tests, and thyroid-stimulating hormone	C
	6. Initial 12-lead electrocardiogram and chest radiograph (posteroanterior and lateral)	C
	7. Initial two-dimensional echocardiography with Doppler to assess left ventricular size and ejection fraction, wall thickness, and valve function; radionuclide ventriculography can be performed to assess left ventricular ejection fraction and volumes	C
	8. Coronary arteriography in patients with angina or significant ischemia except those who are not eligible for revascularization	B
IIa (good supportive evidence)	1. Coronary arteriography in patients with chest pain whose coronary anatomy has not been evaluated and who do not have contraindications to coronary revascularization	C
	2. Coronary arteriography in patients with known or suspected coronary artery disease but without angina except those who are not eligible for revascularization	C
	3. Noninvasive imaging to detect myocardial ischemia and viability in patients with known coronary artery disease and without angina except those who are not eligible for revascularization	B
	4. Maximal exercise testing with or without measurement of respiratory gas exchange and/or blood oxygen saturation to help determine whether heart failure is the cause of exercise limitation when the contribution of heart failure is uncertain	C
	5. Maximal exercise testing with measurement of respiratory gas exchange to identify high-risk patients who are candidates for cardiac transplantation or other advanced treatments	B
	6. Screening for hemochromatosis, sleep-disturbed breathing, or human immunodeficiency virus in selected patients	C
	7. Tests for rheumatologic diseases, amyloidosis, or pheochromocytoma in patients in whom there is a clinical suspicion of these diseases	C
	8. Endomyocardial biopsy in patients when a specific diagnosis is suspected that would influence therapy	C
	9. Measurement of B-type natriuretic peptide in the urgent care setting when the clinical diagnosis of heart failure is uncertain, as well as in prognostication	A
IIb (weak supportive evidence)	1. Noninvasive imaging to define the likelihood of coronary artery disease in patients with left ventricular dysfunction	C
	2. Holter monitoring in patients with a history of myocardial infarction who are being considered for electrophysiologic study to document inducibility of ventricular tachycardia	C
III (not indicated)	1. Routine evaluation with endomyocardial biopsy	C
	2. Routine use of signal-averaged electrocardiography	C
	3. Routine measurement of circulating levels of neurohormones (e.g., norepinephrine or endothelin)	C
	ACC/AHA Guidelines for Serial Clinical Assessment of Patients with Heart Failure	
I (indicated)	1. Assess at each visit the patient's ability to perform routine and desired activities of daily living	C
	2. Assess at each visit the patient's volume status and weight	C
	3. Ask at each visit about the patient's current use of alcohol, tobacco, illicit drugs, "alternative therapies," and chemotherapy drugs as well as about diet and sodium intake	C
IIa (good supportive evidence)	1. Repeat measurements of ejection fraction and structural remodeling in patients who have had a change in clinical status, who have experienced or recovered from a clinical event, or who have received treatment that might have had a significant effect on cardiac function	C
IIb (weak supportive evidence)	1. Serial measurement of B-type natriuretic peptide to guide therapy is not well established	C

*See guidelines text for definition of level of evidence categories.

TREATMENT OF PATIENTS WITH LEFT VENTRICULAR DYSFUNCTION WHO HAVE NOT DEVELOPED SYMPTOMS (STAGE B)

In this population, the goal of therapy is to reduce the risk of further damage to the left ventricle and to minimize the rate of progression of left ventricular dysfunction. The same risk factor modifications supported for stage A patients are also recommended for stage B patients (**Table 28G-3**). As is true for virtually all patients with heart failure, no evidence was found to support the use of nutritional supplements.

In the absence of contraindications, beta blockers and ACE inhibitors (or angiotensin receptor blockers [ARBs] in those intolerant of ACE inhibitors) are recommended for all patients with histories of myocardial infarction, regardless of ejection fraction, and for all patients with diminished ejection fraction, regardless of history of myocardial infarction. In contrast, the guidelines discourage use of digoxin and calcium channel blockers with negative inotropic action in this population.

The guidelines support the use of coronary revascularization in appropriate patients as well as surgery to correct valvular disease in patients with hemodynamically significant valvular stenosis or regurgitation that causes heart failure.

The guidelines indicate that placement of an implantable cardioverter-defibrillator (ICD) is reasonable in patients with ischemic cardiomyopathy who have had a recent (>40 days) myocardial infarction, have compromised left ventricular ejection fraction, and have reasonable expectation of

TABLE 28G-2 ACC/AHA Guidelines for Treating Patients at High Risk of Developing Heart Failure (Stage A)

CLASS	INDICATION	LEVEL OF EVIDENCE*
I (indicated)	1. Control of systolic and diastolic hypertension in accordance with contemporary guidelines	A
	2. Treatment of lipid disorders in accordance with contemporary guidelines	A
	3. Control of blood glucose in patients with diabetes mellitus in accordance with contemporary guidelines	C
	4. Avoidance of behaviors that may increase the risk of heart failure, such as smoking, excessive alcohol consumption, and illicit drug use	C
	5. Control of ventricular rate or restoration of sinus rhythm in patients with supraventricular tachyarrhythmias	B
	6. Treatment of thyroid disorders in accordance with contemporary guidelines	C
	7. Perform periodic evaluation for signs and symptoms of heart failure in high-risk patients	C
	8. Follow current guidelines for secondary prevention for patients with known atherosclerotic vascular disease	C
	9. Noninvasive evaluation of left ventricular function in patients with a strong family history of cardiomyopathy or in those receiving cardiotoxic interventions	C
IIa (good supportive evidence)	1. ACE inhibition in patients with a history of atherosclerotic vascular disease, diabetes mellitus, or hypertension with associated cardiovascular risk factors	A
	2. Angiotensin II receptor blockers in patients with a history of atherosclerotic vascular disease, diabetes mellitus, or hypertension with associated cardiovascular risk factors	C
III (not indicated)	1. Use of nutritional supplements to prevent the development of structural heart disease	C

*See guidelines text for definition of level of evidence categories.

TABLE 28G-3 ACC/AHA Guidelines for Treatment of Asymptomatic Left Ventricular Systolic Dysfunction (Stage B)

CLASS	INDICATION	LEVEL OF EVIDENCE*
I (indicated)	1. Apply all Class I recommendations for stage A	A, B, C
	2. Beta blockade and ACE inhibition in all patients with a recent or remote history of myocardial infarction regardless of ejection fraction or presence of heart failure	A
	3. Beta blockade in all patients without a history of myocardial infarction who have a reduced left ventricular ejection fraction but no heart failure symptoms	C
	4. ACE inhibition in patients with a reduced ejection fraction whether or not they have experienced a myocardial infarction	A
	5. Angiotensin II receptor blockers (ARBs) for post–myocardial infarction patients without heart failure but with a low left ventricular ejection fraction who are intolerant of ACE inhibitors	B
	6. Treat post–myocardial infarction patients according to contemporary guidelines	C
	7. Recommend coronary revascularization in accordance with contemporary guidelines	A
	8. Valve replacement or repair for patients with hemodynamically significant valvular stenosis or regurgitation	B
IIa (good supportive evidence)	1. ACE inhibition or ARBs for patients with hypertension and left ventricular hypertrophy	B
	2. ARBs for patients with low ejection fraction who are intolerant of ACE inhibitors	C
	3. Placement of an ICD in patients with ischemic cardiomyopathy who are at least 40 days post–myocardial infarction, have a left ventricular ejection fraction ≤30%, are NYHA functional Class I on chronic optimal medical therapy, and have reasonable expectation of survival with a good functional status for more than 1 year	A
III (not indicated)	1. Use of digoxin in patients with low ejection fraction, sinus rhythm, and no history of heart failure symptoms (risk of harm not balanced by known benefit)	C
	2. Use of nutritional supplements to treat structural heart disease or to prevent the development of symptoms of heart failure	C
	3. Calcium channel blockers with negative inotropic effects may be harmful in asymptomatic patients with low left ventricular ejection fraction after myocardial infarction	C

*See guidelines text for definition of level of evidence categories.

survival with good functional status for more than 1 year. There was less support for ICD placement in similar patients with nonischemic cardiomyopathy, although the recently completed MADIT-CRT trial (Multicenter Automatic Defibrillator Implantation Trial with Cardiac Resynchronization Therapy), which demonstrated beneficial outcomes in patients with NYHA Class I heart failure (ejection fraction <30%) and prolonged QRS duration (>130 milliseconds) who received an ICD with cardiac resynchronization therapy (CRT), may lead to stronger recommendation in subsequent guidelines to implant ICD/CRT in patients with less symptomatic heart failure.[9]

TREATMENT OF PATIENTS WITH LEFT VENTRICULAR DYSFUNCTION AND CURRENT OR PRIOR SYMPTOMS (STAGE C)

Application of the same measures recommended for preventing or minimizing progression of left ventricular dysfunction for stage A and stage B patients is supported for stage C patients who have current or prior symptoms attributable to left ventricular dysfunction (**Table 28G-4**). However, in contrast to the recommendations for stage B patients, the guidelines support use of moderate sodium restriction as well as daily measurement of weight.

Physical activity is recommended for stage C patients. More detailed recommendations are provided in an AHA Scientific Statement on Exercise and Heart Failure, published in 2003.[10] The updated guidelines also reflect the results of the recent HF-ACTION trial, in which exercise training did not have a favorable impact on all-cause mortality or heart failure hospitalization (see Fig. 28-9). Maximal exercise testing with or without measurement of respiratory gas exchange to facilitate an appropriate exercise program has been changed from a Class I recommendation to a Class IIa indication.

The 2009 ACC/AHA updated guidelines support the use of beta blockers (bisoprolol, carvedilol, and sustained-release metoprolol succinate) and ACE inhibitors (ARBs for patients who cannot tolerate ACE inhibitors) for all stage C patients, in the absence of contraindications, and the use of diuretics for patients with fluid overload. Addition of an aldosterone antagonist is recommended in selected patients who can be carefully monitored for preserved renal function and normal potassium concentration. The use of hydralazine was recommended in patients who

TABLE 28G-4 ACC/AHA Guidelines for Treatment of Symptomatic Left Ventricular Systolic Dysfunction (Stage C)

CLASS	INDICATION	LEVEL OF EVIDENCE*
I (indicated)	1. Apply all Class I recommendations for Stage A	A, B, C
	2. Diuretics and salt restriction in patients with evidence of fluid retention	C
	3. ACE inhibition in all patients unless contraindicated	A
	4. Beta blockade with one of the three proven to reduce mortality (bisoprolol, carvedilol, or sustained-release metoprolol succinate) in all patients unless contraindicated	A
	5. Angiotensin II receptor blockers approved for the treatment of heart failure (candesartan or valsartan) in patients who cannot tolerate ACE inhibitors	A
	6. Avoid or withdraw drugs known to adversely affect heart failure whenever possible, such as nonsteroidal anti-inflammatory drugs, most antiarrhythmic drugs, and most calcium channel blocking drugs	B
	7. Exercise training as an adjunctive approach to improve clinical status in ambulatory patients	B
	8. Placement of an implantable cardioverter-defibrillator (ICD) for secondary prevention to prolong survival in patients with a history of cardiac arrest, ventricular fibrillation, or hemodynamically destabilizing ventricular tachycardia	A
	9. ICD therapy to prevent sudden cardiac death in patients with ischemic heart disease who are at least 40 days post–myocardial infarction, have a left ventricular ejection fraction ≤35%, with NYHA functional Class II or III symptoms while undergoing chronic optimal medical therapy, and have reasonable expectation of survival for more than 1 year with good functional status	A
	10. ICD therapy to prevent sudden cardiac death in patients with nonischemic cardiomyopathy who are at least 40 days post–myocardial infarction, have a left ventricular ejection fraction ≤35%, with NYHA functional Class II or III symptoms while undergoing chronic optimal medical therapy, and have reasonable expectation of survival for more than 1 year with good functional status	B
	11. Cardiac resynchronization therapy in patients with cardiac dyssynchrony (a QRS duration > 0.12 msec), a left ventricular ejection fraction ≤35% who are in sinus rhythm and are in NYHA functional Class III or ambulatory Class IV in spite of optimal medical therapy, unless contraindicated	A
	12. Addition of an aldosterone antagonist in selected patients who can be carefully monitored for preserved renal function and normal potassium concentration; creatinine should be ≤2.5 mg/dL in men or ≤2.0 mg/dL in women and potassium should be ≤5.0 mEq/L.	B
IIa (good supportive evidence)	1. ARBs are a reasonable alternative to ACE inhibitors as first-line therapy, especially for patients already taking ARBs for other indications	A
	2. Digitalis to decrease hospitalizations for heart failure	B
	3. The addition of a combination of hydralazine and a nitrate for patients who have persistent symptoms in spite of already taking an ACE inhibitor and beta blocker	A
	4. In patients with cardiac dyssynchrony (a QRS duration > 0.12 msec), a left ventricular ejection fraction ≤35%, and atrial fibrillation, cardiac resynchronization therapy with or without an ICD is reasonable for the treatment of NYHA functional Class III or ambulatory Class IV patients on optimal medical therapy	B
IIb (weak supportive evidence)	1. A combination of hydralazine and a nitrate in patients who cannot tolerate an ACE inhibitor or ARB because of drug intolerance, hypotension, or renal insufficiency	C
	2. Adding an ARB in persistently symptomatic patients who are already being treated with conventional therapy	B
III (not indicated)	1. Routinely combining an ACE inhibitor, an ARB, and an aldosterone antagonist	C
	2. Routine use of calcium channel blocking drugs	A
	3. Long-term use of an infusion of a positive inotropic drug may be harmful and is not recommended except as palliation for patients with end-stage disease who cannot be stabilized with standard medical treatment	C
	4. Use of nutritional supplements as treatment for heart failure	C
	5. Hormonal therapies other than to replete deficiencies may be harmful	C

*See guidelines text for definition of level of evidence categories.

are intolerant of an ACE inhibitor or an ARB. A new Class I recommendation in the updated guidelines is the use of hydralazine isosorbide in self-identified African Americans who remain symptomatic despite optimal therapy.

The recommendations regarding the use of ICDs were simplified in the 2009 ACC/AHA updated guidelines and were harmonized with the 2008 ACC/AHA/Heart Rhythm Society Device-Based Therapy guidelines.[11,12] Class I recommendations support the use of ICDs in nonischemic dilated cardiomyopathy, ischemic cardiomyopathy at least 40 days after myocardial infarction, left ventricular ejection fraction <35% (previously 30%), and NYHA Class II-III symptoms despite optimal medical therapy. As in the 2005 ACC/AHA guidelines, Class I recommendations support the use of ICDs in stage C patients with a history of cardiac arrest, ventricular fibrillation, or hemodynamically destabilizing ventricular tachycardia. Guidelines covering patient selection for CRT were published in 2005.[13] CRT is a Class I indication in patients with a left ventricular ejection fraction <35% who are in sinus rhythm and NYHA functional Class III or ambulatory Class IV despite optimal medical therapy. The 2009 updated ACC/AHA also consider CRT reasonable (Class IIa) in NYHA Class III-IV heart failure patients with an ejection fraction <35% who are in atrial fibrillation or who have a frequent dependence on ventricular pacing. As discussed in Chap. 29, the Centers for Medicare & Medicaid Services (CMS) has expanded the coverage for CRT-defibrillators (CRT-D) to include patients with left bundle branch block with a QRS ≥130 ms, an EF ≤30% and mild (NYHA Class II) ischemic or nonischemic heart failure or asymptomatic (NYHA Class I) ischemic heart failure. It is anticipated that updated practice guidelines will reflect the expanded CMS indications for use of CRT-D in subsequent updates.

The guidelines offer qualified support (Class IIa) for the use of ARBs in place of ACE inhibitors as first-line therapy, especially in patients already taking an ARB for another indication. Digitalis is a reasonable approach to decrease hospitalizations in symptomatic patients.

The guidelines explicitly discourage the routine use of a combination of an ACE inhibitor, ARB, and aldosterone antagonist; calcium channel blockers; long-term infusion of positive inotropic drugs (except as palliation in patients with end-stage disease; see Table 28G-10); nutritional supplements as treatment; and hormonal therapies other than those needed to replete deficiencies.

TREATMENT OF PATIENTS WITH REFRACTORY END-STAGE HEART FAILURE (STAGE D)

The ACC/AHA guidelines emphasize the importance of meticulous application of the measures listed as Class I recommendations for patients in stages A, B, and C (see Tables 28G-2 to 28G-4) and consider these patients

CH 28

TABLE 28G-5 ACC/AHA Guidelines for Treatment of Patients with End-Stage Heart Failure (Stage D)

CLASS	INDICATION	LEVEL OF EVIDENCE*
I (indicated)	1. Meticulous identification and control of fluid retention	B
	2. Refer potentially eligible patient for cardiac transplantation	B
	3. Refer patients to a heart failure program with expertise in the management of refractory heart failure	A
	4. Discuss options for end-of-life care with the patient and family when severe symptoms persist despite application of all recommended therapies	C
	5. Offer patients with implantable defibrillators and end-stage disease the option to inactivate defibrillation	C
IIa (good supportive evidence)	1. Consider a left ventricular assist device as permanent or "destination" therapy in highly selected patients with refractory end-stage heart failure and an estimated 1-year mortality >50% with medical therapy	B
IIb (weak supportive evidence)	1. Pulmonary artery catheter placement to guide therapy in patients with persistently severe symptoms	C
	2. Mitral valve repair or replacement is not established for severe secondary mitral regurgitation	C
	3. Continuous intravenous infusion of a positive inotropic agent may be considered for palliation	C
III (not indicated)	1. Partial left ventriculectomy is not recommended in patients with nonischemic cardiomyopathy	C
	2. Routine intermittent infusions of positive inotropic agents are not recommended	A

*See guidelines text for definition of level of evidence categories.

TABLE 28G-6 ACC/AHA Guidelines: Indications for Cardiac Transplantation

Absolute Indications
For hemodynamic compromise due to heart failure
Refractory cardiogenic shock
Documented dependence on intravenous inotropic support to maintain adequate organ perfusion
Peak $\dot{V}O_2$ <10 mL/kg/min with achievement of anaerobic metabolism
Severe symptoms of ischemia that consistently limit routine activity and are not amenable to coronary artery bypass surgery or percutaneous coronary intervention
Recurrent symptomatic ventricular arrhythmias refractory to all therapeutic modalities
Relative Indications
Peak $\dot{V}O_2$ 11 to 14 mL/kg/min (or 55% of predicted) and major limitation of the patient's daily activities
Recurrent unstable ischemia not amenable to other intervention
Recurrent instability of fluid balance/renal function not due to patient noncompliance with medical regimen
Insufficient Indications
Low left ventricular ejection fraction
History of functional Class III or IV symptoms of heart failure
Peak $\dot{V}O_2$ >15 mL/kg/min (and >55% of predicted) without other indications

$\dot{V}O_2$ = oxygen consumption per unit time.

candidates for specialized treatment strategies, such as referral for cardiac transplantation, mechanical circulatory support, continuous intravenous positive inotropic therapy, or hospice care (**Table 28G-5**). The guidelines also endorse the use of team management approaches, such as heart failure programs. Detailed specifications of the components of such heart failure programs are provided in an AHA Scientific Statement published in 2000.[14]

The guidelines include explicit cautionary notes about the use of ACE inhibitors and beta blockers in this population. Although consideration of these agents is supported, the guidelines state, "Treatment with either type of drug should not be initiated in patients who have systolic blood pressures less than 80 mm Hg or who have signs of peripheral hypoperfusion. In addition, patients should not be started on a beta blocker if they have significant fluid retention or if they recently required treatment with an intravenous positive inotropic agent." When these medications are used, very low doses should be prescribed at initiation, and patients should be monitored closely for evidence of intolerance. The guidelines note that spironolactone has been shown to be beneficial in patients with advanced heart failure, but they emphasize that these data are derived from patients with preserved renal function and that spironolactone may induce hyperkalemia in patients with impaired renal function.

According to the updated 2009 guidelines, there is limited evidence to support the placement of a pulmonary artery catheter to guide therapy or mitral valve repair or replacement for severe mitral regurgitation.

The ACC/AHA guidelines recognize the value of continuous intravenous inotropic support for some patients who require a "bridge" strategy while awaiting cardiac transplantation or who cannot otherwise be discharged from the hospital. However, the guidelines directly discourage routine intermittent intravenous infusion of inotropic agents. Similarly, the guidelines did not encourage use of partial left ventriculectomy.

The guidelines also include a summary of indications for cardiac transplantation (**Table 28G-6**). These indications make explicit that low left ventricular ejection fraction and poor functional status are insufficient indications in the absence of demonstrated peak oxygen consumption less than 15 mL/kg/min.

THE HOSPITALIZED PATIENT

The most significant addition to the 2009 ACC/AHA updated guidelines is inclusion of specific new recommendations regarding the hospitalized patient (**Table 28G-7**). Although a number of new Class I indications involve the diagnosis of heart failure, use of BNP and N-terminal pro-BNP (NT-proBNP), recognition of acute coronary syndromes, recognition of potential precipitating factors, use of supplemental oxygen, use of intravenous inotropic or pressure agents in patients with clinical evidence of hypotension with hypoperfusion, use of pulmonary artery catheters, and transition from intravenous to oral diuretics, the level of evidence supporting each of these recommendations is based on consensus opinion or standard use of care (i.e., level C). Stronger Class I recommendations (level of evidence B) are provided for the use of intravenous diuretics to decongest patients, initiation of ACE inhibitors/ARBs and beta blockers before hospital discharge, and postdischarge systems of care.

TABLE 28G-7 ACC/AHA Recommendations for the Hospitalized Patient

CLASS	INDICATION	LEVEL OF EVIDENCE*
I (indicated)	1. Evaluate for adequacy of systemic perfusion, volume status, the contribution of precipitating factors and/or comorbidities, and whether heart failure is associated with preserved ejection fraction	C
	2. B-type natriuretic peptide (BNP) or N-terminal pro-BNP (NT-proBNP) should be measured to evaluate dyspnea if the contribution of heart failure is not known	A
	3. Acute coronary syndromes precipitating hospitalization for heart failure should be promptly evaluated and treated	C
	4. Identify potential precipitating factors for acute heart failure	C
	5. Oxygen therapy should be administered to relieve symptoms related to hypoxemia	C
	6. Rapidly improve systemic perfusion in patients who present with rapid decompensation and hypoperfusion associated with decreasing urine output and other manifestations of shock	C
	7. Treatment of significant fluid overload with intravenous loop diuretics; the diuretic dose should be titrated to relieve symptoms and to reduce extracellular fluid volume excess	B, C
	8. Monitor the effects of therapy with careful measurement of fluid intake and output, vital signs, body weight, and symptoms of systemic perfusion and congestion	C
	9. Intensify the diuretic regimen (higher dose, add second diuretic, continuous infusion) when the diuresis is inadequate to relieve congestion	C
	10. Intravenous inotropic or vasopressor drugs should be administered to maintain systemic perfusion and preserve end-organ performance in patients with clinical evidence of hypotension associated with hypoperfusion and elevated cardiac filling pressures	C
	11. Invasive hemodynamic monitoring to guide therapy in patients who are in respiratory distress or with clinical evidence of impaired perfusion if filling pressures cannot be determined from clinical assessment	C
	12. Medications should be reconciled and adjusted as appropriate on admission to and discharge from the hospital	C
	13. Maintenance treatment with oral therapies known to improve outcomes (ACE inhibitors or ARBs and beta blocker therapy) in the absence of hemodynamic instability or contraindications	C
	14. Initiation of treatment with oral therapies known to improve outcomes (ACE inhibitors or ARBs and beta blocker therapy) in stable patients prior to hospital discharge	B
	15. During the transition from intravenous to oral diuretic therapy, the patient should be monitored carefully for supine and upright hypotension, worsening renal function, and heart failure signs or symptoms	C
	16. Comprehensive written discharge instructions for patients and their caregivers are strongly recommended	C
	17. Postdischarge systems of care, if available, should be used to facilitate the transition to effective outpatient care	B
IIa (good supportive evidence)	1. Urgent cardiac catheterization and revascularization in patients with acute heart failure with known or suspected acute myocardial ischemia due to occlusive coronary disease when there are signs and symptoms of inadequate systemic perfusion and revascularization is likely to prolong meaningful survival	C
	2. Intravenous nitroglycerin, nitroprusside, or nesiritide for patients with evidence of severely symptomatic fluid overload in the absence of systemic hypotension	C
	3. Ultrafiltration for patients with refractory congestion not responding to medical therapy	B
IIb (weak supportive evidence)	1. Intravenous inotropic drugs (dopamine, dobutamine, or milrinone) for patients presenting with documented severe systolic dysfunction, low blood pressure, and evidence of low cardiac output, with or without congestion, to maintain systemic perfusion and preserve end-organ performance	C
III (not indicated)	1. Use of parenteral inotropes in normotensive patients with acute decompensated heart failure without evidence of decreased organ perfusion	B
	2. Routine use of invasive hemodynamic monitoring in normotensive patients with acute decompensated heart failure and congestion with symptomatic response to diuretics and vasodilators	B

*See guidelines text for definition of level of evidence categories.

The updated guidelines offer qualified support (Class IIa) for the use of urgent catheterization and revascularization, the use of vasodilators (intravenous nitroglycerin, nitroprusside, nesiritide), invasive hemodynamic monitoring, and ultrafiltration. More muted support (Class IIb) is given to the use of inotropic agents (dopamine, dobutamine, or milrinone) in patients with severe left ventricular dysfunction, low blood pressure, and evidence of low cardiac output. In contrast, the use of inotropic agents in patients without evidence of decreased organ perfusion as well as the routine use of invasive hemodynamic monitoring is not recommended (Class III indication).

SPECIAL POPULATIONS AND CONCOMITANT DISORDERS

The ACC/AHA guidelines support consideration of patient-specific needs and coexisting medical conditions. Clinicians are reminded that even though heart failure has traditionally been considered to be a disease of men, women—particularly elderly women—make up the majority of the general population with heart failure. Yet women have not been included in sufficient numbers in most large trials to allow conclusions about the efficacy of the treatments under study. In addition, women, minorities, and the elderly are less likely to receive interventions supported by clinical trials, and differences in the natural history of heart failure and response to treatment exist among various patient subsets.

Patients from high-risk ethnic minority groups, such as blacks, as well as from groups underrepresented in clinical trials and those believed to be underserved should receive the same clinical screening and therapy as received by the broader population, in the absence of specific evidence to the contrary. As noted before, the 2009 update of the guidelines recommends the addition of a fixed dose of isosorbide dinitrate and hydralazine to a standard medical regimen for heart failure that includes ACE inhibition and beta blockade to improve outcomes for self-described African American patients who have NYHA functional Class III or IV heart failure (changed from a Class IIa to Class I indication). The guidelines acknowledge that other groups of patients may also benefit, but this has not been tested.

Specific clinical recommendations for the management of patients with concomitant disorders (**Table 28G-8**) emphasize the importance of meticulous management of hypertension, ischemic heart disease, anticoagulation, and supraventricular and ventricular arrhythmias. The use of digitalis, particularly in combination with a beta blocker, to control the ventricular response rate in patients with atrial fibrillation and of amiodarone to decrease the recurrence of atrial arrhythmias and the likelihood of an ICD discharge is considered reasonable. The updated 2009 guidelines suggest that although verapamil and diltiazem can effectively suppress the ventricular response during exercise, they should be avoided because of

TABLE 28G-8 ACC/AHA Guidelines for Management of Concomitant Diseases in Patients with Heart Failure

CLASS	INDICATION	LEVEL OF EVIDENCE*
I (indicated)	1. Apply all other recommendations in the absence of specific exceptions	C
	2. Control systolic and diastolic hypertension and diabetes mellitus in accordance with recommended guidelines	C
	3. Nitrates and beta blockers for the treatment of angina	B
	4. Coronary revascularization according to recommended guidelines in patients with both angina and heart failure	A
	5. Anticoagulants in patients with heart failure who have paroxysmal or persistent atrial fibrillation or a previous thromboembolic event	A
	6. Beta blockade (or amiodarone, if beta blockers are contraindicated or not tolerated) to control the ventricular response rate in patients with atrial fibrillation	A
	7. Treat patients with coronary artery disease and heart failure in accordance with recommended guidelines for chronic stable angina	C
	8. Antiplatelet agents for prevention of myocardial infarction and death in patients with heart failure and underlying coronary artery disease	B
IIa (good supportive evidence)	1. Digitalis to control the ventricular response rate in patients with heart failure and atrial fibrillation	A
	2. Amiodarone to decrease recurrence of atrial arrhythmias and recurrence of ICD discharge for ventricular arrhythmias	C
IIb (weak supportive evidence)	1. Current strategies to restore and to maintain sinus rhythm in patients with heart failure and atrial fibrillation are not well established	C
	2. Anticoagulation in patients with heart failure who do not have atrial fibrillation or a previous thromboembolic event is not well established	B
	3. Enhancing erythropoiesis in patients with heart failure and anemia is not established	C
III (not indicated)	1. Class I or III antiarrhythmic drugs are not recommended for the prevention of ventricular arrhythmias	A
	2. Antiarrhythmic medication is not indicated for primary treatment of asymptomatic ventricular arrhythmias or to improve survival	A

*See guidelines text for definition of level of evidence categories.

TABLE 28G-9 ACC/AHA Guidelines for Treatment of Patients with Heart Failure and Normal Left Ventricular Ejection Fraction

CLASS	INDICATION	LEVEL OF EVIDENCE*
I (indicated)	1. Control systolic and diastolic hypertension in accordance with published guidelines	A
	2. Control ventricular rate in patients with atrial fibrillation	C
	3. Diuretics to control pulmonary congestion and peripheral edema	C
IIa (good supportive evidence)	1. Coronary revascularization in patients with coronary artery disease in whom symptomatic or demonstrable myocardial ischemia is judged to be having an adverse effect on cardiac function	C
IIb (weak supportive evidence)	1. Restoration and maintenance of sinus rhythm in patients with atrial fibrillation	C
	2. Use of beta blockade, ACE inhibitors, ARBs, or calcium antagonists may minimize heart failure symptoms	C
	3. Use of digitalis to minimize symptoms is not well established	C

*See guidelines text for definition of level of evidence categories.

their propensity to depress left ventricular function and to worsen heart failure.

There is insufficient evidence to recommend for or against the use of current strategies to restore and to maintain sinus rhythm in patients with atrial fibrillation, the usefulness of anticoagulation in patients without atrial fibrillation or a prior myocardial infarction, or the improvement of erythropoiesis in anemia patients.

The guidelines do not support routine use of Class I or III antiarrhythmic drugs, except amiodarone, or the use of antiarrhythmic drugs for primary treatment of asymptomatic ventricular arrhythmias.

DIASTOLIC DYSFUNCTION

Recommendations for management of patients with heart failure in the absence of left ventricular systolic dysfunction reflect the lack of conclusive data on effective therapies and are unchanged in the 2009 ACC/AHA update of the heart failure guidelines. The major strategies are control of hypertension, control of ventricular rate in patients with atrial fibrillation, and use of diuretics to control pulmonary congestion and peripheral edema (**Table 28G-9**). Because myocardial ischemia can cause diastolic dysfunction, the guidelines offer support for consideration of use of coronary revascularization in patients with coronary disease (Class IIa indication). Possibly useful therapies include restoration and maintenance of sinus rhythm in patients with atrial fibrillation and the use of beta blockers, ACE inhibitors, ARBs, or calcium channel blockers to minimize symptoms in patients with controlled hypertension.

END-OF-LIFE CARE

Despite significant advances in the diagnosis and management of heart failure, approximately half of individuals die within 5 years of its diagnosis. For many patients, there is an abrupt transition from the period of aggressive intervention to one of palliation and comfort. Addressing end-of-life issues relatively early in the course of heart failure, before the patient becomes unable to participate in decision making, is important for all involved (**Table 28G-10**). The guidelines recommend discussing treatment preferences, living wills, and advance directives, the formulation of which can be more difficult than for patients with cancer or other conditions. Heart failure can be characterized by periods of good quality of life even after hospitalization for intensive care or the approach of death. In addition to resuscitation, discussions should cover the possible deactivation of an ICD.

Hospice services, once available primarily for cancer patients, are being extended to those dying of heart failure. In such patients, compassionate care may include the use of intravenous diuretics and positive inotropic agents as well as pain medications.

TABLE 28G-10 ACC/AHA Guidelines on End-of-Life Care for Patients with Heart Failure

CLASS	INDICATION	LEVEL OF EVIDENCE*
I (indicated)	1. Ongoing education of the patient and family regarding prognosis for functional capacity and survival	C
	2. Patient and family education about options for formulating and implementing advance directives and the role of palliative and hospice care services with reevaluation for changing clinical status	C
	3. Discussion regarding the option of inactivating implantable cardioverter-defibrillators	C
	4. Ensure continuity of medical care between inpatient and outpatient settings	C
	5. Palliation at the end of life should include standard components of hospice care, such as opiates for pain control, and should not preclude the use of inotropes and intravenous diuretics	C
	6. Examine current end-of-life processes and work toward improvement in approaches to palliation and end-of-life care	C
III (not indicated)	1. Aggressive procedures performed within the final days of life (including intubation and implantation of a cardioverter-defibrillator in patients with NYHA functional Class IV symptoms who are not anticipated to experience clinical improvement from available treatments)	C

*See guidelines text for definition of level of evidence categories.

The guidelines explicitly discourage the performance of aggressive procedures, such as intubation and ICD implantation, within the final days of life in patients with severe end-stage symptoms who are not expected to experience clinical improvements.

REFERENCES

1. Hunt SA, Abraham WT, Chin MH, et al: ACC/AHA 2005 Guideline Update for the Diagnosis and Management of Chronic Heart Failure in the Adult: A report of the American College of Cardiology/American Heart Association Task Force on Practice Guidelines (Writing Committee to Update the 2001 Guidelines for the Evaluation and Management of Heart Failure): Developed in collaboration with the American College of Chest Physicians and the International Society for Heart and Lung Transplantation: Endorsed by the Heart Rhythm Society. Circulation 112:e154, 2005.
2. Jessup M, Abraham WT, Casey DE, et al: 2009 Focused update: ACCF/AHA Guidelines for the Diagnosis and Management of Heart Failure in Adults: A report of the American College of Cardiology Foundation/American Heart Association Task Force on Practice Guidelines: Developed in collaboration with the International Society for Heart and Lung Transplantation. Circulation 119:1977, 2009.
3. Hunt SA, Baker DW, Chin MH, et al: ACC/AHA guidelines for the evaluation and management of chronic heart failure in the adult: Executive summary. A report of the American College of Cardiology/American Heart Association Task Force on Practice Guidelines (Committee to revise the 1995 Guidelines for the Evaluation and Management of Heart Failure). J Am Coll Cardiol 38:2101, 2001.
4. Guidelines for the evaluation and management of heart failure. Report of the American College of Cardiology/American Heart Association Task Force on Practice Guidelines (Committee on Evaluation and Management of Heart Failure). J Am Coll Cardiol 26:1376, 1995.
5. Konstam M, Dracup K, Baker D, et al: Heart Failure: Management of Patients with Left-Ventricular Systolic Dysfunction. Quick Reference Guide for Clinicians No. 11. AHCPR Publication No. 94-0613. Rockville, Md, Agency for Health Care Policy and Research, Public Health Service, U.S. Department of Health and Human Services, June 1994.
6. Roberts JM, D'Urso G: An origin unwinding activity regulates initiation of DNA replication during mammalian cell cycle. Science 241:1486, 1988.
7. Heart Failure Society of America: HFSA 2006 Comprehensive Heart Failure Practice Guideline. J Card Fail 12:e1, 2006.
8. Dickstein K, Cohen-Solal A, Filippatos G, McMurray JJ, et al: ESC guidelines for the diagnosis and treatment of acute and chronic heart failure 2008: the Task Force for the diagnosis and treatment of acute and chronic heart failure 2008 of the European Society of Cardiology. Developed in collaboration with the Heart Failure Association of the ESC (HFA) and endorsed by the European Society of Intensive Care Medicine (ESICM). Eur J Heart Fail 10:933, 2008.
9. Moss AJ, Hall WJ, Cannom DS, et al: Cardiac-resynchronization therapy for the prevention of heart-failure events. N Engl J Med 361:1329, 2009.
10. Pina IL, Apstein CS, Balady GJ, et al: Exercise and heart failure: A statement from the American Heart Association Committee on exercise, rehabilitation, and prevention. Circulation 107:1210, 2003.
11. Zipes DP, Camm AJ, Borggrefe M, et al: ACC/AHA/ESC 2006 Guidelines for Management of Patients With Ventricular Arrhythmias and the Prevention of Sudden Cardiac Death: A report of the American College of Cardiology/American Heart Association Task Force and the European Society of Cardiology Committee for Practice Guidelines (writing committee to develop Guidelines for Management of Patients With Ventricular Arrhythmias and the Prevention of Sudden Cardiac Death): Developed in collaboration with the European Heart Rhythm Association and the Heart Rhythm Society. Circulation 114:e385, 2006.
12. Epstein AE, DiMarco JP, Ellenbogen KA, et al: ACC/AHA/HRS 2008 Guidelines for Device-Based Therapy of Cardiac Rhythm Abnormalities: Executive summary. Heart Rhythm 5:934, 2008.
13. Strickberger SA, Conti J, Daoud EG, et al: Patient selection for cardiac resynchronization therapy: From the Council on Clinical Cardiology Subcommittee on Electrocardiography and Arrhythmias and the Quality of Care and Outcomes Research Interdisciplinary Working Group, in collaboration with the Heart Rhythm Society. Circulation 111:2146, 2005.
14. Grady KL, Dracup K, Kennedy G, et al: Team management of patients with heart failure: A statement for healthcare professionals from The Cardiovascular Nursing Council of the American Heart Association. Circulation 102:2443, 2000.

CHAPTER 29 Devices for Monitoring and Managing Heart Failure

William T. Abraham

In 2001, a new era of implantable device therapies for the management of heart failure was initiated with the U.S. Food and Drug Administration (FDA) approval of the first cardiac resynchronization therapy (CRT) device. Over the subsequent few years, implantable cardioverter-defibrillators (ICDs) and combined CRT-ICD devices were also FDA-approved for the management of heart failure (see Chaps. 28 and 38). ICDs became indicated for the primary prevention of all-cause mortality through a reduction in the incidence of sudden cardiac death in patients with heart failure and reduced ejection fractions. Combined CRT-ICD devices were shown to reduce morbidity and mortality in heart failure patients with ventricular dysynchrony, with a suggestion of additive benefit compared with a CRT device alone. In acknowledgment of the evidence-based benefits of these devices, the 2005 update to the American College of Cardiology/American Heart Association (ACC/AHA) heart failure guideline strongly supported, with Class I indications, the use of ICD and/or CRT devices for the management of eligible heart failure patients[1]; these indications were updated in 2009 (see Chap. 28 Guidelines).[2]

In addition to these therapeutic devices, implantable devices that monitor physiologic parameters, such as patient activity level, heart rate variability, intrathoracic impedance, and/or hemodynamics, have been developed. In some cases, these data are already available in currently implantable CRT and ICD devices. The usefulness of such device-based diagnostic or monitoring information is unknown and currently under investigation. This chapter reviews the use of CRT and ICDs for the management of heart failure and discusses the potential use of implantable heart failure monitoring devices. The medical management of patients with heart failure is discussed in Chaps. 28 and 30.

Ventricular Dysynchrony: The Target of Cardiac Resynchronization Therapy

Several conduction abnormalities are commonly seen in association with chronic heart failure. Among these are abnormalities of ventricular conduction, such as bundle branch blocks, that alter the timing and pattern of ventricular contraction so as to place the already failing heart at a further mechanical disadvantage. These ventricular conduction delays produce suboptimal ventricular filling, a reduction in left ventricular contractility, prolonged duration of mitral regurgitation, and paradoxical septal wall motion.[3-6] Taken together, these mechanical manifestations of altered ventricular conduction have been termed *ventricular dysynchrony*. Ventricular dysynchrony has been defined by a prolonged QRS duration, generally longer than 120 milliseconds, on the surface electrocardiogram (ECG). By this definition, about one third of patients with systolic heart failure have ventricular dysynchrony.[7,8] In addition to reducing the ability of the failing heart to eject blood, ventricular dysynchrony has also been associated with increased mortality in heart failure patients.[9-12]

Ventricular dysynchrony may now be addressed with pacing therapy through the implantation of pacing leads to both the right and left ventricles. This form of pacing therapy has come to be known as CRT. Favorable single-case experiences with CRT in the mid-1990s led to small observational studies evaluating the acute effects of CRT on hemodynamics and other measures of cardiac performance.[5,13] These studies provided additional proof of concept supporting the use of CRT. Several uncontrolled or unblinded studies soon followed to evaluate the acute and longer term effects of CRT on clinical status in heart failure patients further.[14-22] The results of these trials were equally encouraging, with patients demonstrating consistent, sustained improvement in exercise tolerance, quality of life, and New York Heart Association (NYHA) functional Class. Finally, large-scale randomized controlled trials have confirmed the beneficial effects of CRT on functional status and outcomes, leading to the initial indications for this therapy. More recent and ongoing trials promise to expand current indications for CRT.

Randomized Controlled Trials of Cardiac Resynchronization Therapy

More than 4000 patients have been evaluated in randomized controlled trials of CRT in NYHA functional Class III and IV heart failure. The following randomized controlled trials are considered among the landmark studies of CRT in this patient population: Multisite Stimulation in Cardiomyopathy (MUSTIC) studies[23,24]; Multicenter InSync Randomized Clinical Evaluation (MIRACLE) trial[25,26]; MIRACLE ICD trial[27]; CONTAK CD trial[28]; Cardiac Resynchronization in Heart Failure (CARE HF) trial[29,30]; and Comparison of Medical Therapy, Pacing and Defibrillation in Heart Failure (COMPANION) trial.[31,32] To understand the clinical benefits, risks, and limitations of CRT with or without an ICD, these studies will be reviewed.

MULTISITE STIMULATION IN CARDIOMYOPATHY TRIALS. The MUSTIC trials were designed to evaluate the safety and efficacy of CRT in patients with advanced heart failure, ventricular dysynchrony, and either normal sinus rhythm[23] or atrial fibrillation.[24] They represent the first randomized single-blinded trials of CRT for heart failure. The first study involved 58 randomized patients with NYHA Class III heart failure, normal sinus rhythm, and a QRS duration of at least 150 milliseconds. All patients were implanted with a CRT device and, after a run-in period, patients were randomized to active pacing or to no pacing. After 12 weeks, patients were crossed over and remained in the alternate study assignment for 12 weeks. The second MUSTIC study involved fewer patients (only 37 completers) with atrial fibrillation and a slow ventricular rate (either spontaneously or from radiofrequency ablation). A VVIR biventricular pacemaker and leads for each ventricle were implanted and the same randomization procedure described earlier was applied. However, biventricular VVIR pacing versus single-site right ventricular VVIR pacing (rather than no pacing) were compared in this group of patients with atrial fibrillation.

The primary endpoints for MUSTIC were exercise tolerance assessed by measurement of peak $\dot{V}O_2$ or the 6-minute hall walk test and quality of life determined using the Minnesota Living with Heart Failure (MLWHF) questionnaire. Secondary endpoints included rehospitalizations and/or drug therapy modifications for worsening heart failure. Results from the normal sinus rhythm arm of MUSTIC provided strong evidence of benefit. The mean distance walked in 6 minutes was 23% greater with CRT than without CRT ($P < 0.001$). Significant improvement was also seen in quality of life and NYHA functional Class ranking. There were fewer hospitalizations during active resynchronization therapy. The atrial fibrillation cohort evaluated in MUSTIC demonstrated similar improvements, although the magnitude of benefit was slightly less.

MULTICENTER INSYNC RANDOMIZED CLINICAL EVALUATION. MIRACLE was the first prospective, randomized, double-blind, parallel-controlled clinical trial designed to evaluate the benefits of CRT.[25,26] Primary endpoints were NYHA Class, quality of life score (using the MLWHF questionnaire), and 6-minute hall walk distance. Secondary endpoints included assessments of a composite clinical response, cardiopulmonary exercise performance, cardiac structure and function, a variety of measures of worsening heart failure, and combined morbidity and mortality.

The MIRACLE trial was conducted between 1998 and 2000. It included 453 patients with moderate to severe symptoms of heart failure associated with a left ventricular ejection fraction less than or equal to 35% and a QRS duration of at least 130 milliseconds. They were randomized (double-blind) to CRT ($n = 228$) or to a control group ($n = 225$) for 6 months while conventional therapy for heart failure was maintained.[36] Compared with the control group, patients randomized to CRT demonstrated a significant improvement in quality of life score (−8.0 versus −9.0 points, p = 0.001), 6-minute walk distance (+39 versus +10 m; $P = 0.005$), NYHA functional Class ranking (−1.0 versus 0.0 Class; $P < 0.001$), treadmill exercise time (+81 versus +19 seconds; $P = 0.001$), peak $\dot{V}O_2$ (+1.1 versus 0.1 mL/kg/min; $P < 0.01$), and left ventricular ejection fraction (+4.6% versus −0.2%; $P < 0.001$). Patients randomized to CRT demonstrated a highly significant improvement in a composite clinical heart failure response endpoint compared with control subjects, suggesting an overall improvement in heart failure clinical status (**Fig. 29-1**). In addition, when compared with the control group, fewer patients in the CRT group required hospitalization (8% versus 15%) or intravenous medications (7% and 15%) for the treatment of worsening heart failure (both, $P < 0.05$). In the resynchronization group, the 50% reduction in hospitalization was accompanied by a significant reduction in length of stay, resulting in a 77% decrease in total days hospitalized over 6 months compared with the control group. The major limitation of the therapy was caused by the unsuccessful implantation of the device in 8% of patients. The results of this trial led to FDA approval of the InSync system in August 2001, the first approved CRT system in the United States, allowing the introduction of CRT into clinical practice.

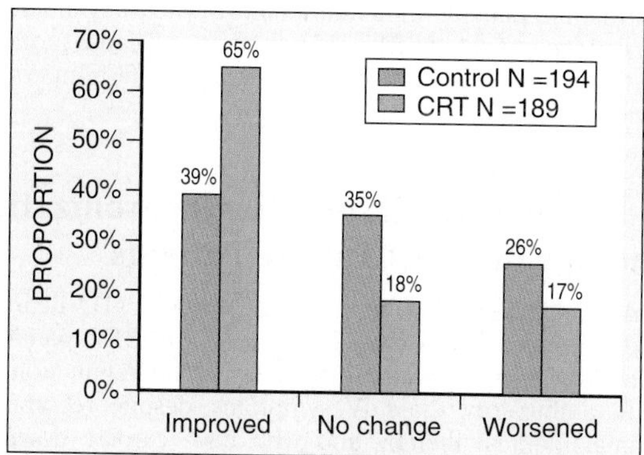

FIGURE 29-1 Effect of cardiac resynchronization therapy on a composite clinical response endpoint in the MIRACLE trial. Worsened: Patient dies or is hospitalized because of or associated with worsening heart failure, or demonstrates worsening in NYHA class at last observation carried forward (LOCF) or moderate-marked worsening of patient global assessment score at LOCF. Improved: Patient has not worsened (as defined above) and demonstrates improvement in NYHA class at LOCF and/or moderate-marked improvement in patient global assessment score at LOCF. Unchanged: Patient is neither improved nor worsened; $P < 0.001$ for chi square analysis. *(Modified from Abraham WT, Fisher WG, Smith AL, et al: Multicenter InSync Randomized Clinical Evaluation: Double-blind, randomized controlled trial of cardiac resynchronization in chronic heart failure. N Engl J Med 346:1845, 2002.)*

The MIRACLE trial also provided persuasive evidence supporting the occurrence of reverse left ventricular remodeling (see Chap. 25) with chronic CRT. In the MIRACLE trial, serial Doppler echocardiograms were obtained at baseline, 3, and 6 months in a subset of 323 patients.[33] CRT for 6 months was associated with reduced end-diastolic and end-systolic volumes (both, $P < 0.001$), reduced left ventricular mass ($P < 0.01$), increased ejection fraction ($P < 0.001$), reduced mitral regurgitant blood flow ($P < 0.001$), and improved myocardial performance index ($P < 0.001$) as compared with controls. These effects are similar to those seen with beta blockade in heart failure but were seen in MIRACLE in patients already receiving beta blocker therapy.

MULTICENTER INSYNC–IMPLANTABLE CARDIOVERTER-DEFIBRILLATOR RANDOMIZED CLINICAL EVALUATION. The MIRACLE ICD study was designed to be almost identical to the MIRACLE trial. MIRACLE ICD was a prospective, multicenter, randomized, double-blind, parallel-controlled clinical trial intended to assess the safety and efficacy of a combined CRT-ICD system in patients with dilated cardiomyopathy (left ventricular ejection fraction [LVEF] ≤ 35%; left ventricular end-diastolic diameter [LVEDD] ≥ 55 mm), NYHA Class III or IV heart failure, ventricular dysynchrony (QRS ≥ 130 milliseconds), and an indication for an ICD. Primary and secondary efficacy measures were essentially the same as those evaluated in the MIRACLE trial, but also included measures of ICD function.

Of 369 patients receiving devices and randomized, 182 were controls (ICD activated, CRT inactive) and 187 were in the resynchronization group (ICD activated, CRT active). At 6 months, patients assigned to active CRT had a greater improvement in median quality of life score (−17.5 versus −11.0; $P = 0.02$) and functional Class (−1 versus 0; $P = 0.007$) than controls, but were no different than controls in the change in distance walked in 6 minutes (55 versus 53 m; $P = 0.36$).[27] Peak oxygen consumption increased by 1.1 mL/kg/min in the resynchronization group, versus 0.1 mL/kg/min in controls ($P = 0.04$); treadmill exercise duration increased by 56 seconds in the CRT group and decreased by 11 seconds in controls ($P = 0.0006$). The magnitude of improvement was comparable to that seen in the MIRACLE trial, suggesting that heart failure patients with an ICD indication benefit as much from cardiac resynchronization therapy as those patients without an indication for an ICD. The combined CRT-ICD device used in this study was approved by the FDA in June 2002for use in NYHA Class III or IV systolic heart failure patients with ventricular dysynchrony and an ICD indication.

CONTAK CD. The CONTAK CD trial enrolled 581 symptomatic heart failure patients with ventricular dysynchrony and malignant ventricular tachyarrhythmias who were all candidates for an ICD.[28] Following unsuccessful implant attempts and withdrawals, 490 patients were available for analysis. The study did not meet its primary endpoint of a reduction in disease progression, defined by a composite endpoint of heart failure hospitalization, all-cause mortality, and ventricular arrhythmia requiring defibrillator therapies, although the trends were in a direction favoring improved outcomes with CRT. However, the CONTAK CD trial did demonstrate statistically significant improvements in peak oxygen uptake and quality of life in the resynchronization group compared with control subjects, although quality of life was improved only in NYHA Class III and IV patients without right bundle branch block. Left ventricular dimensions were also reduced, and LVEFs increased, as seen in other trials of CRT. Importantly, the improvement seen in peak $\dot{V}O2$ WITH cardiac resynchronization was again comparable to that observed in the MIRACLE trial. Improvements in NYHA functional Class were not observed in this study. The CONTAK CD device was approved by the FDA in May 2002 for use in NYHA Class III and IV systolic heart failure patients with ventricular dysynchrony and an ICD indication.

CARDIAC RESYNCHRONIZATION IN HEART FAILURE TRIAL. The CARE-HF trial was designed to evaluate the effects of resynchronization therapy without an ICD on morbidity and mortality in patients with NYHA Class III or IV heart failure and ventricular dysynchrony.[29,30] In this trial, 819 patients with an LVEF of 35% or less and ventricular dysynchrony, defined as a QRS duration of 150 milliseconds or longer or a QRS duration between 120 and 150 milliseconds, with echocardiographic evidence of dysynchrony, were enrolled in this randomized, unblinded, controlled trial and followed for an average of 29.4 months.[30] Of these, 404 patients were assigned to receive optimal medical therapy alone and 409 patients were randomized to optimal medical therapy plus resynchronization therapy alone. The risk of death from any cause or unplanned hospitalization for a major cardiac event, the primary endpoint analyzed as time to first event, was significantly reduced by 37% in the treatment group compared with control subjects (hazard ratio [HR], 0.63; 95% confidence interval [CI], 0.51 to 0.77; P < 0.001). In the CRT group, 82 patients (20%) died during follow-up compared with120 patients (30%) in the medical group, yielding a significant 36% reduction in all-cause mortality with resynchronization therapy (HR, 0.64; 95% CI, 0.48 to 0.85; P < 0.002; **Fig. 29-2**). Resynchronization therapy also significantly reduced the risk of unplanned hospitalization for a major cardiac event by 39%, all-cause mortality plus heart failure hospitalization by 46%, and heart failure hospitalization by 52%.

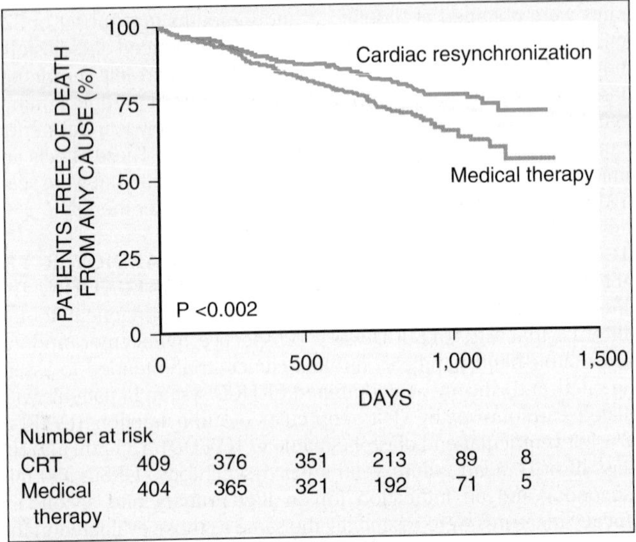

FIGURE 29-2 Kaplan-Meier estimates of all cause survival in patients randomized to CRT compared with conventional medical therapy in the CARE-HF trial *(Modified from Cleland JGF, Daubert J-C, Erdmann E, et al; Cardiac Resynchronization–Heart Failure (CARE-HF) Study Investigators: The effect of cardiac resynchronization on morbidity and mortality in heart failure. N Engl J Med 352:1539, 2005.)*

COMPARISON OF MEDICAL THERAPY, PACING, AND DEFIBRILLATION IN HEART FAILURE. Begun in early 2000, the COMPANION trial was a multicenter, prospective, randomized, controlled clinical trial designed to compare drug therapy alone with drug therapy in combination with cardiac resynchronization in patients with dilated cardiomyopathy, a wide QRS (≥ 120 msec), NYHA Class III or IV heart failure, and no indication for a device.[31,32] The COMPANION trial randomized 1520 patients into one of three treatment groups in a 1:2:2 allocation—group I (308 patients) received optimal medical care only, group II (617 patients) received optimal medical care and the Guidant CONTAK TR (biventricular pulse generator), and group III (595 patients) received optimal medical care and the CONTAK CD (combined heart failure–bradycardia–tachycardia device). The primary endpoint of the COMPANION trial was a composite of all-cause mortality and all-cause hospitalization, measured as time to first event beginning from time of randomization. Secondary endpoints included all-cause mortality and a variety of measures of cardiovascular morbidity. When compared with optimal medical therapy alone, the combined endpoint of mortality or heart failure hospitalization was reduced by 35% for patients receiving CRT and 40% for patients receiving CRT-ICD (both, $P < 0.001$). For the mortality endpoint alone, CRT patients had a 24% risk reduction ($P = 0.060$) and CRT-ICD patients experienced a risk reduction of 36% ($P < 0.003$) when compared with optimal medical therapy (**Fig. 29-3**). The COMPANION trial confirmed the results of earlier resynchronization therapy trials in improving symptoms, exercise tolerance, and quality of life for heart failure patients with ventricular dysynchrony. In addition, it showed the impact of CRT-ICD on reducing all-cause mortality for the first time and suggested incremental benefit from combined device therapies.

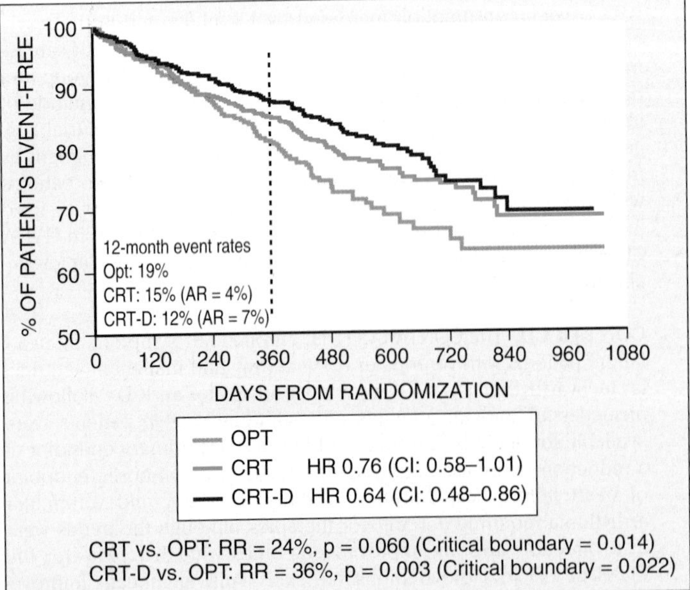

FIGURE 29-3 Kaplan–Meier estimates of the time to death from any cause in patients randomized to optimal medical therapy (OPT) alone versus OPT with CRT alone versus OPT with a combined CRT-ICD device (CRT-D) in the COMPANION trial. *(Modified from Bristow MR, Saxon LA, Boehmer J, et al: Cardiac-resynchronization therapy with or without an implantable defibrillator in advanced chronic heart failure. N Engl J Med 350:2140, 2004.)*

Indications for Cardiac Resynchronization Therapy in Heart Failure Patients

As noted in Chap. 28 Guidelines, the 2009 ACC/AHA heart failure guidelines proposed a Class I indication for CRT in patients with an LVEF of 35% or less, sinus rhythm, and NYHA Functional Class III or ambulatory Class IV symptoms, despite recommended optimal medical therapy and who have cardiac dysynchrony, which is currently defined as a QRS interval of 0.120 second or longer (level of evidence: A). The guidelines also now recommend CRT for similar patients with atrial fibrillation, although the strength of that recommendation is weaker (Class IIa), and states that for patients who have an LVEF of 35% or less, a QRS duration of 0.12 second or longer, and atrial fibrillation, CRT with or without an ICD is reasonable for the treatment of NYHA functional Class III ambulatory or Class IV heart failure symptoms on optimal recommended medical therapy. Importantly, the updated guidelines finally recommend CRT as "reasonable" for pacemaker-dependent patients for patients with an LVEF of 35% or less with

NYHA functional Class III or ambulatory Class IV symptoms who are receiving optimal recommended medical therapy and who have frequent dependence on ventricular pacing (level of evidence: C).

Currently, the guideline defines ventricular dysynchrony as a QRS duration of at least 0.120 second (120 milliseconds). Although echocardiography appears to be a promising way to define ventricular dysynchrony in the future (see Fig. 15-64), the Predictors of Response to Cardiac Resynchronization Therapy (PROSPECT) trial did not support the use of echocardiographic measures of dysynchrony as selection criteria for CRT in patients with a QRS duration of 120 milliseconds or longer.[34,35] Other ongoing trials of CRT are evaluating the usefulness of this therapy in NYHA Class I and II patients and in patients with narrow QRS durations but with echocardiographic evidence of ventricular dysynchrony.

Limitations of Cardiac Resynchronization Therapy

The success rate for placement of a transvenous cardiac resynchronization system has ranged from about 88% to 92% in clinical trials, although in contemporary clinical experience it is as high as 97% to 98% in some centers (e.g., Ohio State University). Thus, some patients undergoing an implant procedure will not receive a functioning system using this approach. Implant-related complications are similar to those seen with standard pacemakers and defibrillators, with the additional risk of dissection or perforation of the coronary sinus. This is a rare event but may lead to substantial morbidity and even mortality in heart failure patients.

Despite the results of randomized controlled CRT trials, some patients do not respond to this therapy. The nonresponder rate for cardiac resynchronization therapy appears to be about 25%, a rate similar to the nonresponder rate for heart failure drug therapies. A variety of factors have been proposed as contributing to the nonresponder rate associated with CRT, including suboptimal left ventricular lead placement, suboptimal atrioventricular (AV) and ventricle-to-ventricle (V-V) timing, ventricular scar, and heart failure disease progression.

Future Directions in Cardiac Resynchronization Therapy

The most recent clinical trials in CRT have focused on delaying progression of heart failure in asymptomatic or less symptomatic patients. The MIRACLE-ICD II trial suggested such a benefit in a small cohort of NYHA Class II subjects.[36] The impact of CRT on NYHA Class I and II heart failure has now been addressed in two larger clinical trials, the Resynchronization Reverses Remodeling in Systolic Left Ventricular Dysfunction Trial (REVERSE) and Multicenter Automatic Defibrillator Implantation Trial with Cardiac Resynchronization Therapy (MADIT-CRT).

RESYNCHRONIZATION REVERSES REMODELING IN SYSTOLIC LEFT VENTRICULAR DYSFUNCTION TRIAL. The REVERSE trial was a randomized, double-blinded, controlled trial designed to address the benefit of CRT on heart failure morbidity in mild heart failure patients when compared with optimal medical therapy alone.[37,38] In this trial, 610 with NYHA Class I or II heart failure, QRS of 120 milliseconds or longer, an LVEF of 40% or less, and an LVEDD of 55 mm or more were randomized. All patients received a CRT device with or without an ICD, and 191 were assigned to the control of optimal medical therapy alone (CRT off) and 419 to the CRT group combined with optimal medical therapy. The primary endpoint was a clinical composite heart failure score. Because the goal of the study was to determine the effect on preventing disease progression, a "worsened" status was considered a negative outcome.

Although the percentage worsened in the clinical composite response endpoint was not significantly reduced in the CRT group compared with control subjects (16% versus 21%; $P = 0.10$), a significant benefit of CRT was seen in improvement in ventricular structure and function and in heart failure morbidity, which was also significantly improved, with a 53% relative risk reduction in the time to first heart failure hospitalization (HR, 0.47; $P = 0.03$). Thus, REVERSE was the first large, randomized, multicenter trial to demonstrate the potential for CRT to slow progression of disease through reverse remodeling in NYHA Class I and II heart failure patients with ventricular dysynchrony.

MULTICENTER AUTOMATIC DEFIBRILLATOR IMPLANTATION TRIAL WITH CARDIAC RESYNCHRONIZATION THERAPY. The MADIT-CRT trial was a multicenter, randomized clinical trial designed to address the potential survival and morbidity benefit of CRT in NYHA Class I and II heart failure patients by assessing the reduction in the risk of death and nonfatal heart failure events in this population.[39,40] Prophylactic CRT combined with an ICD was compared with ICD only in 1820 patients with an LVEF of 30% or less, QRS of 130 milliseconds, and either an ischemic (Class I patients) or any (Class II patients) cause. The study was not blinded because the treating physicians were aware of the study group assignments.

During the average follow-up of 2.4 years, the primary endpoint of death from any cause or nonfatal heart failure event occurred in 17.2% of the CRT-ICD group versus 25.2% of the ICD-only group, with a relative risk reduction of 34% (HR, 0.66: 95% CI, 0.52 to 0.84; $P = 0.001$; **Fig. 29-4**). This significant benefit was driven by a 41% reduction in heart failure events (13.9% versus 22.8%; HR, 0.59; 95% CI, 0.47 to 0.74; $P < 0.001$). In terms of prespecified subgroups, both ischemic and nonischemic groups showed benefit with CRT; however, a greater benefit was noted for women versus men and in patients with a QRS interval of 150 milliseconds or longer. Another factor predicting CRT responsiveness in this trial was QRS morphology; patients benefiting the most had left bundle branch block (LBBB).[41] Based on an analysis of the MADIT-CRT patients with LBBB, the Centers for Medicare & Medicaid Services (CMS) has altered labeling for certain CRT-defibrillator (CRT-D) devices. Under the most recent labeling, CRT-D is now indicated for patients with LBBB with QRS ≥130 ms, EF ≤30% and mild (NYHA Class II) ischemic or nonischemic heart failure or asymptomatic (NYHA Class I) ischemic heart failure. It is anticipated that updated practice guidelines will reflect the expanded CMS indications for use of CRT-D in subsequent updates.

Finally, the Echocardiographic-guided CRT (EchoCRT) trial is evaluating whether CRT will improve all-cause mortality or first hospitalization for worsening heart failure in narrow QRS patients (<130 milliseconds) with NYHA Class III and IV symptoms who meet predefined echocardiographic criteria for ventricular dyssynchrony (ClinicalTrials.gov identifier: NCT00683696). Ventricular dyssynchrony will be defined by one of the two following criteria: (1) intra–left

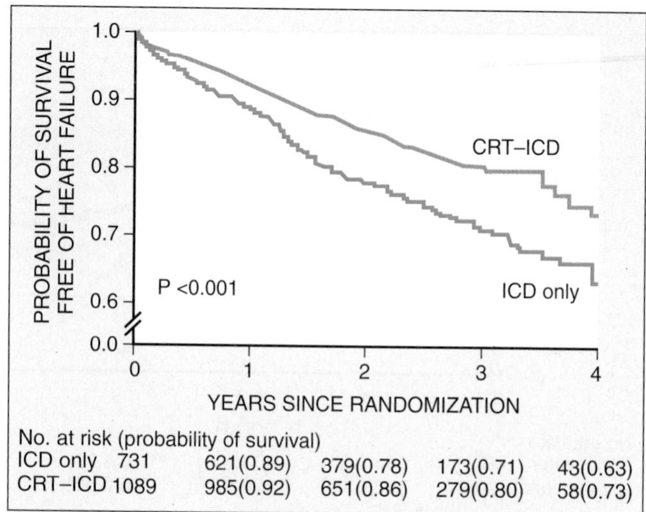

FIGURE 29-4 Kaplan-Meier estimates of the probability of survival free of heart failure in MADIT-CRT. There was a significant difference in the estimate of survival free of heart failure between the group that received CRT-ICD and the group that received an ICD only (unadjusted $P < 0.001$ by the log-rank test). *(Modified from Moss AJ, Hall WJ, Cannom DS, et al: Cardiac resynchronization therapy for the prevention of heart failure events. N Engl J Med 361:1329, 2009.)*

ventricular dyssynchrony measured by color tissue Doppler imaging (TDI) with an opposing wall delay of 80 milliseconds or longer in the four-chamber or apical long-axis view; or (2) speckle-tracking radial strain septal-posterior wall delay of 130 milliseconds or longer (see Chap. 15).

Sudden Cardiac Death in Heart Failure

Patients with heart failure and left ventricular systolic dysfunction are at increased risk for sudden cardiac death (SCD; see Chap. 41).[42,43] Sudden cardiac death is the leading cause of mortality in patients with heart failure and occurs at a rate six to nine times that seen in the general population. A randomized controlled trial of beta blockade in heart failure demonstrated that patients with NYHA)Class II or III symptoms die most frequently as a result of SCD.[44] This study estimated the proportion of total mortality attributable to SCD at 64% and 59% for NYHA Class II and III patients, respectively. In contrast, the major cause of death in Class IV patients was worsening heart failure. Given this high incidence of SCD in heart failure, it was easy to hypothesize that an ICD used as prophylactic therapy would reduce total mortality by reducing the incidence of SCD. A series of studies have considered this hypothesis.[45-50]

Randomized Controlled Trials of Implantable Cardioverter Defibrillators in Heart Failure

Several early studies, including the Multicenter Automatic Defibrillator Implantation Trial (MADIT), CABG-Patch trial, and the Multicenter Unsustained Tachycardia Trial (MUSTT)[45-47] have supported the benefit of prophylactic ICD implantation for the prevention of sudden cardiac trials; however, none of these trials were conclusive with respect to the benefit of prophylactic ICD implantation on sudden cardiac death. The landmark trials establishing a role for ICDs as primary prevention of mortality in heart failure patients are the Multicenter Automatic Defibrillator Implantation II Trial (MADIT II), Prophylactic Defibrillator Implantation in Patients with Nonischemic Dilated Cardiomyopathy (DEFINITE) trial, and National Institutes of Health–sponsored Sudden Cardiac Death-Heart Failure Trial (SCD-HeFT).[48-50]

MULTICENTER AUTOMATIC DEFIBRILLATOR IMPLANTATION II TRIAL. MADIT II, a randomized controlled trial, was prospectively designed and powered to assess the survival benefit of ICDs in a population of post-MI patients with reduced ejection fractions (<30%). Importantly, this trial included no arrhythmic markers such as nonsustained or inducible ventricular tachycardia for inclusion. A total of 1232 patients were randomly assigned in a 3:2 ratio to receive an ICD (742 patients) or conventional medical therapy (490 patients).[48] During an average follow-up of 20 months, the all-cause mortality rates were 19.8% in the conventional therapy arm and 14.2% in the ICD group (31% relative risk reduction; $P = 0.016$; **Fig. 29-5**). The effect of ICD therapy on survival was similar in subgroup analyses stratified according to age, gender, ejection fraction, NYHA class, and QRS interval. Moreover, beta blocker use was 72% in these patients and was well balanced between the ICD and conventional therapy groups.

Of note, most patients enrolled into MADIT II were classified in NYHA Class II or III. Class IV patients were excluded and the Class I cohort was relatively small. The average LVEF was 23%. These findings suggest that heart failure patients with mild to moderate symptoms and moderate to severe reductions in LVEF may benefit the most from a prophylactic ICD. Moreover, the survival benefit observed in MADIT II began approximately 9 months after the device was implanted. This observation may be important when considering the timing of device placement in eligible patients.

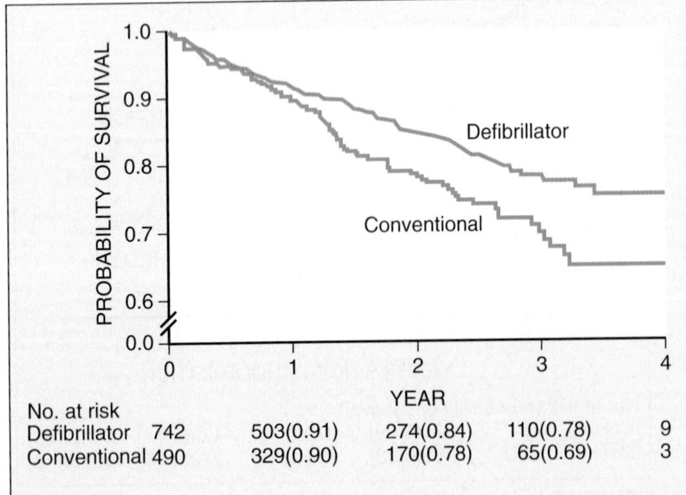

FIGURE 29-5 Kaplan-Meier estimates of all-cause survival in patients randomized to an ICD compared with conventional medical therapy in the MADIT II trial. There was a relative risk reduction of 31% with the ICD; $P = 0.007$ by the log-rank test. *(Modified from Moss AJ, Hall WJ, Cannom DS, et al: Cardiac resynchronization therapy for the prevention of heart failure events. N Engl J Med 361:1329, 2009.)*

PROPHYLACTIC DEFIBRILLATOR IMPLANTATION IN PATIENTS WITH NONISCHEMIC DILATED CARDIOMYOPATHY TRIAL. Whereas MADIT II enrolled exclusively post-MI patients with an ischemic cause of left ventricular systolic dysfunction and heart failure, the DEFINITE trial was the first randomized trial of primary prevention therapy with an ICD in nonischemic cardiomyopathy patients.[49] Such patients also exhibit high rates of SCD; however, until recently, there has been little consensus regarding the management of SCD risk in such patients. This may be the result, in part, of limitations in objective risk assessment, in that no invasive or noninvasive testing procedure has been shown to determine accurately which nonischemic heart failure patient is likely to die suddenly. Also clouding the picture were older observations suggesting that the prophylactic administration of an antiarrhythmic agent, amiodarone, might prolong survival in nonischemic cardiomyopathy patients.[51]

The DEFINITE trial was a prospective evaluation of 458 patients with nonischemic dilated cardiomyopathy. Entry criteria included an ejection fraction of 35% or less, a history of symptomatic heart failure, and the presence of ambient arrhythmias defined as an episode of nonsustained ventricular tachycardia or at least ten premature ventricular contractions per 24-hour period on continuous ambulatory electrocardiographic monitoring. In this trial, 229 patients were randomized to each arm of the study to receive either an ICD and standard medical therapy or standard medical therapy alone. Compliance with medical therapy was excellent and included an angiotensin-converting enzyme inhibitor (ACEI) in 86% of the cohort and a beta blocker in 85%. The patients were followed for a mean of 29.0 ± 14.4 months, with a primary endpoint of all-cause mortality.

There were 68 deaths reported in DEFINITE, 28 in the ICD group and 40 in the standard therapy group. The implantation of an ICD yielded a nonsignificant 35% reduction in death from any cause (HR, 0.65; 95% CI, 0.40 to 1.06; $P = 0.08$) and significantly reduced the risk of sudden death by a remarkable 80% (HR, 0.20; 95% CI, 0.06 to 0.71; $P = 0.006$). In the subgroup of NYHA Class III patients, all-cause mortality was significantly decreased in the ICD arm (HR, 0.37, 95% CI 0.15 to 0.90; $P = 0.02$). Although this study was underpowered and did not reach statistical significance with respect to the primary endpoint of all-cause mortality for the entire randomized cohort, the results demonstrated a strong trend toward a survival advantage for patients receiving an ICD.

SUDDEN CARDIAC DEATH–HEART FAILURE TRIAL. The results of the SCD-HeFT trial were published in 2005 and have had a substantial impact on current practice guidelines for ICDs.[50] This landmark randomized controlled trial enrolled 2521 patients between 1997 and 2001. Patients with NYHA Class II (70%) or III (30%) heart failure and reduced LVEF (≤35%; mean, ≈25%) of ischemic or nonischemic cause were eligible for the study. SCD-HeFT was a three-arm trial, comparing treatment with an ICD to amiodarone and placebo. Thus, SCD-HeFT addressed at least two important issues in heart failure management: (1) whether empirical amiodarone therapy saved lives in well-treated NYHA Class II and III heart failure patients with no arrhythmic indication for the drug; and (2) whether a prophylactic ICD saved lives in these patients with heart failure from an ischemic or nonischemic cause.

In SCD-HeFT, patients received standard heart failure therapy, if tolerated, which included an ACEI or angiotensin receptor blocker in 85%, beta blocker in 69%, and aldosterone antagonists in 19%, compatible with guideline recommendations at the time the study was conducted. The median follow-up was 45.5 months. Importantly, the cohort was equally divided between ischemic and nonischemic causes of heart failure, allowing an important subgroup analysis of these cohorts to be carried out.

Mortality rates in the ICD, amiodarone, and placebo groups were 17.1%, 24%, and 22.3% at 3 years and 28.9%, 34.1%, and 35.9%, respectively, at 5 years (**Fig. 29-6**). The ICD was associated with a statistically significant 23% reduction in all-cause mortality compared with placebo (HR, 0.77; 97.5% CI, 0.62 to 0.96; $P = 0.007$). Mortality in the amiodarone arm was not significantly different from placebo across all subgroups (HR, 1.06; 97.5% CI, 0.86 to 1.30). Similar degrees of benefit with the ICD were noted in patients with ischemic (21% mortality reduction) and nonischemic (27% mortality reduction) heart failure, thus confirming the findings of MADIT II and DEFINITE, respectively. The SCD-HeFT trial provides the most robust evidence to date supporting the prophylactic use of an ICD in patients with NYHA Class II or III systolic heart failure.

Indications for Prophylactic Cardioverter-Defibrillator Implantation in Heart Failure Patients

As noted in Chap. 28 Guidelines, the 2009 ACC/AHA heart failure guidelines simplified prior recommendations by combining three separate recommendations for prophylactic ICDs in heart failure into one.[2] The most recent version of the guidelines suggest that ICD therapy is recommended for primary prevention of sudden cardiac death to reduce total mortality in patients with nonischemic dilated cardiomyopathy or ischemic heart disease at least 40 days post-MI, an LVEF of 35% or less, NYHA functional Class II or III symptoms while receiving chronic optimal medical therapy, and who have reasonable expectation of survival, with a good functional status for longer than 1 year (level of evidence: A).

Implantable Devices to Monitor Heart Failure

Implantable devices can provide substantial physiologic information about heart failure patients. Such information may be useful for evaluating heart failure clinical status and/or in predicting episodes of heart failure decompensation. If these devices are reliable in the latter sense, the use of this information may improve heart failure outcomes by reducing the risk of worsening heart failure. For example, many implantable CRT and ICD devices can provide information on atrial heart rate and rhythm, ventricular heart rate and rhythm, patient activity level, heart rate variability (HRV) and, in some cases, intrathoracic impedance, which has been proposed as a measure of lung "wetness."

Many implantable devices record an activity trend, providing an objective record of the number of hours that patients are physically active each day. The activity level may serve as a useful teaching and reinforcement tool to the patient and family about the importance and level of activity. Because exercise intolerance is a manifestation of worsening heart failure, a decrease in patient activity level may provide one objective clue to disease progression or decompensation.

HRV reflects the balance between sympathetic and parasympathetic nervous system activity in the heart; a decrease in HRV is as a marker of increased sympathetic and decreased parasympathetic tone. A study by Adamson and colleagues[52] has shown that HRV decreases in the days to -weeks leading up to a hospitalization for worsening heart failure, suggesting that decreases in HRV may predict episodes of worsening heart failure. Given our understanding of the changes in the neurohormonal milieu that occur as heart failure worsens, this approach to heart failure monitoring may ultimately prove useful.

Because most patients with decompensation exhibit pulmonary congestion caused by an elevated left ventricular filling pressure, indirect measurement of lung water or direct measurement of left ventricular filling pressure or its surrogate may be useful for managing heart failure patients on an outpatient basis. Implantable devices can monitor fluid status by assessing changes in intrathoracic impedance. In a small study of 33 patients, intrathoracic impedance changes demonstrated the ability to predict hospitalizations for decompensated heart failure 10 to 14 days in advance of the event.[53] A more recent and larger study, the Fluid Accumulation Status Trial (FAST), confirmed this observation and demonstrated the superiority of intrathoracic impedance versus daily weight monitoring in predicting worsening heart failure events (ClinicalTrials.gov Identifier: NCT00289276).[54] Finally, a new generation of even more sophisticated implantable monitoring devices is under investigation. These devices allow continuous or intermittent assessment of hemodynamics, generally focused on the estimation or direct measurement of left atrial pressure (LAP). Preliminary observations have supported the usefulness of these devices,[55-58] but definitive data from adequately powered prospective randomized controlled trials is pending. The COMPASS-HF (Chronicle Offers Management to Patients with Advanced Signs and Symptoms of Heart Failure) trial was a randomized controlled study of an implantable continuous hemodynamic monitor that was placed in the right ventricular outflow tract (the Chronicle) in patients with advanced heart failure. The primary efficacy end point of COMPASS-HF, which was a reduction in the rate of HF-related events (hospitalizations and emergency or urgent care visits requiring intravenous therapy), was not met insofar as the group with the implantable hemodynamic device had a nonsignificant ($P = 0.33$) 21% lower rate of all HF-related

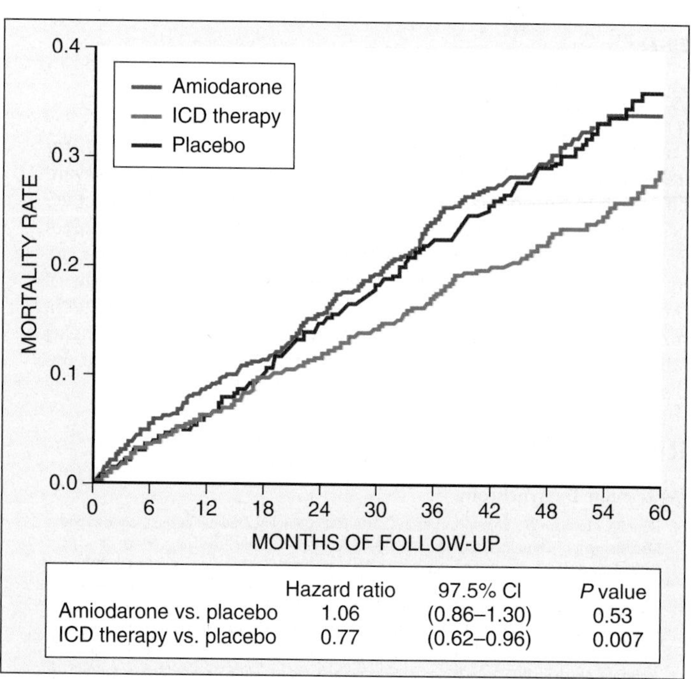

	Hazard ratio	97.5% CI	*P* value
Amiodarone vs. placebo	1.06	(0.86–1.30)	0.53
ICD therapy vs. placebo	0.77	(0.62–0.96)	0.007

FIGURE 29-6 Kaplan-Meier estimates of survival in patients randomized to an ICD compared with conventional medical therapy or conventional medical therapy plus amiodarone in the SCD-HeFT trial. *(Modified from Bardy GH, Lee KL, Mark DB, et al: Amiodarone or an implantable cardioverter-defibrillator for congestive heart failure. N Engl J Med 352:225, 2005.)*

CH 29

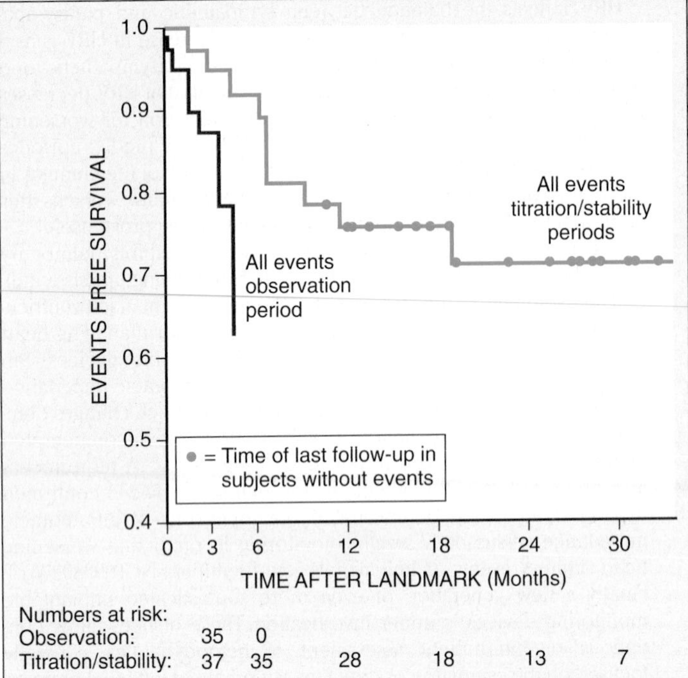

FIGURE 29-7 Modified landmark analysis showing time to first event during the initial observation period. Management was by standard heart failure therapy in comparison to the titration and stability periods, when LAP-guided therapy was implemented. *(Modified from Ritzema J, Troughton R, Melton I, et al: Physician-directed patient self-management of left atrial pressure in advanced chronic heart failure. Circulation 121:106, 2010.)*

events compared with the control group.[57] Another of these systems, an implantable LAP monitoring system, may radically change the way heart failure patients are chronically managed by promoting a physician-directed, patient self-management paradigm for use. The use of this system is similar to how diabetics self-titrate insulin with the aid of a glucometer. Preliminary data have demonstrated the feasibility and potential usefulness of this approach in heart failure patients (**Fig. 29-7**).[58]

Summary and Future Directions

Cardiac resynchronization therapy offers a therapeutic approach for treating patients with ventricular dysynchrony and moderate to severe heart failure. Substantial experience suggests that it is safe and effective, with patients demonstrating significant improvement in clinical symptoms and multiple measures of functional status, exercise capacity, and outcomes. Prophylactic implantation of an ICD is also now of proven benefit in heart failure patients. Implantable monitoring technologies promise to improve our ability to avoid episodes of heart failure decompensation and may improve the natural history of the disease.

REFERENCES

Ventricular Dyssynchrony

1. Hunt SA, Abraham WT, Chin MH, et al: ACC/AHA 2005 Guideline Update for the Diagnosis and Management of Chronic Heart Failure in the Adult: A report of the American College of Cardiology/American Heart Association Task Force on Practice Guidelines (Writing Committee to Update the 2001 Guidelines for the Evaluation and Management of Heart Failure): Developed in collaboration with the American College of Chest Physicians and the International Society for Heart and Lung Transplantation: Endorsed by the Heart Rhythm Society. Circulation 112:e154, 2005.
2. Jessup M, Abraham WT, Casey DE, et al: 2009 focused update: ACCF/AHA Guidelines for the Diagnosis and Management of Heart Failure in Adults: A report of the American College of Cardiology Foundation/American Heart Association Task Force on Practice Guidelines developed in collaboration with the International Society for Heart and Lung Transplantation. Circulation 119:1977, 2009.
3. Xiao HB, Brecker SJ, Gibson DG: Effects of abnormal activation on the time course of the left ventricular pressure pulse in dilated cardiomyopathy. Br Heart J 68:403, 1992.
4. Littmann L, Symanski JD: Hemodynamic implications of left bundle branch block. J Electrocardiol 33(Suppl):115, 2000.
5. Saxon LA, Kerwin WF, Cahalan MK, et al: Acute effects of intraoperative multisite ventricular pacing on left ventricular function and activation/contraction sequence in patients with depressed ventricular function. J Cardiovasc Electrophysiol 9:13, 1998.
6. Kerwin WF, Botvinick EH, O'Connell JW, et al: Ventricular contraction abnormalities in dilated cardiomyopathy: Effect of biventricular pacing to correct interventricular dyssynchrony. J Am Coll Cardiol 35:1221, 2000.
7. Farwell D, Patel NR, Hall A, et al: How many people with heart failure are appropriate for biventricular resynchronization? Eur Heart J 21:1246, 2000.
8. Aaronson KD, Schwartz JS, Chen TM, et al: Development and prospective validation of a clinical index to predict survival in ambulatory patients referred for cardiac transplant evaluation. Circulation 95:2660, 1997.
9. Xiao HB, Roy C, Fujimoto S, et al: Natural history of abnormal conduction and its relation to prognosis in patients with dilated cardiomyopathy. Int J Cardiol 53:163, 1996.
10. Unverferth DV, Magorien RD, Moeschberger ML, et al: Factors influencing the one-year mortality of dilated cardiomyopathy. Am J Cardiol 54:147, 1984.
11. Shamim W, Francis DP, Yousufuddin M, et al: Intraventricular conduction delay: A prognostic marker in chronic heart failure. Int J Cardiol 70:171, 1999.
12. Brophy JM, Deslauriers G, Rouleau JL: Long-term prognosis of patients presenting to the emergency room with decompensated congestive heart failure. Can J Cardiol 10:543, 1994.
13. Foster AH, Gold MR, McLaughlin JS: Acute hemodynamic effects of atrio-biventricular pacing in humans. Ann Thorac Surg 59:294, 1995.
14. Cazeau S, Ritter P, Lazarus A, et al: Multisite pacing for end-stage heart failure: Early experience. Pacing Clin Electrophysiol 19:1748, 1996.
15. Blanc JJ, Etienne Y, Gilard M, et al: Evaluation of different ventricular pacing sites in patients with severe heart failure: Results of an acute hemodynamic study. Circulation 96:3273, 1997.
16. Leclercq C, Cazeau S, Le Breton H, et al: Acute hemodynamic effects of biventricular DDD pacing in patients with end-stage heart failure. J Am Coll Cardiol 32:1825, 1998.
17. Kass DA, Chen CH, Curry C, et al: Improved left ventricular mechanics from acute VDD pacing in patients with dilated cardiomyopathy and ventricular conduction delay. Circulation 99:1567, 1999.
18. Gras D, Mabo P, Tang T, et al: Multisite pacing as a supplemental treatment of congestive heart failure: Preliminary results of the Medtronic Inc. InSync Study. Pacing Clin Electrophysiol 21:2249, 1998.
19. Auricchio A, Stellbrink C, Sack S, et al: The Pacing Therapies for Congestive Heart Failure (PATH-CHF) Study: Rationale, design, and endpoints of a prospective randomized multicenter study. Am J Cardiol 1999; 83:130D, 1999.
20. Auricchio A, Stellbrink C, Block M, et al: Effect of pacing chamber and atrioventricular delay on acute systolic function of paced patients with congestive heart failure. Circulation 99:2993, 1999.
21. Auricchio A, Klein H, Spinelli J: Pacing for heart failure: Selection of patients, techniques, and benefits. Eu J Heart Fail 1:275, 1999.
22. Gras D, Leclercq C, Tang A, et al: Cardiac resynchronization therapy in advanced heart failure: The multicenter InSync clinical study. Eur J Heart Fail 4:311, 2002.
23. Cazeau S, Leclercq C, Lavergne T, et al: Effects of multisite biventricular pacing in patients with heart failure and intraventricular conduction delay. N Engl J Med 344:873, 2001.
24. Leclercq C, Walker S, Linde C, et al: Comparative effects of permanent biventricular and right-univentricular pacing in heart failure patients with chronic atrial fibrillation. Eur Heart J 23:1780, 2002.
25. Abraham WT: Rationale and design of a randomized clinical trial to assess the safety and efficacy of cardiac resynchronization therapy in patients with advanced heart failure: The Multicenter InSync Randomized Clinical Evaluation (MIRACLE). J Card Fail 6:369, 2000.
26. Abraham WT, Fisher WG, Smith AL, et al: Double-blind, randomized controlled trial of cardiac resynchronization in chronic heart failure. N Engl J Med 346:1845, 2002.
27. Young JB, Abraham WT, Smith AL, et al: Safety and efficacy of combined cardiac resynchronization therapy and implantable cardioversion defibrillation in patients with advanced chronic heart failure. The Miracle ICD trial. JAMA 289:2685, 2003.
28. Higgins SL, Hummel JD, Niazi IK, et al: Cardiac resynchronization therapy for the treatment of heart failure in patients with intraventricular conduction delay and malignant ventricular tachyarrhythmias. J Am Coll Cardiol 42:1454, 2003.
29. Cleland JGF, Daubert JC, Erdmann E, et al: The CARE-HF study (CArdiac REsynchronisation in Heart Failure study): Rationale, design and end-points. Eur J Heart Fail 3:481, 2001.
30. Cleland JGF, Daubert J-C, Erdmann E, et al: The effect of cardiac resynchronization on morbidity and mortality in heart failure. N Engl J Med 352:1539, 2005.
31. Bristow MR, Feldman AM, Saxon LA: Heart failure management using implantable devices for ventricular resynchronization: Comparison of Medical Therapy, Pacing, and Defibrillation in Chronic Heart Failure (COMPANION) trial. J Card Fail 6:276, 2000.
32. Bristow MR, Saxon LA, Boehmer J, et al: Cardiac-resynchronization therapy with or without an implantable defibrillator in advanced chronic heart failure. N Engl J Med 350:2140, 2004.
33. St. John-Sutton MG, Plappert T, Abraham WT, et al: Effect of cardiac resynchronization therapy on left ventricular size and function in chronic heart failure. Circulation 107:1985, 2003.
34. Yu CM, Abraham WT, Bax JJ, et al: Predictor of response to cardiac resynchronization therapy (PROSPECT)—study design. Am Heart J 149:600, 2005.
35. Chung ES, Leon AR, Tavazzi A, et al: Results of the predictors of response to CRT (PROSPECT) trial. Circulation 117:2608, 2008.
36. Abraham WT, Young JB, Leon AR, et al: Effects of cardiac resynchronization on disease progression in patients with left ventricular systolic dysfunction, an indication for an implantable cardioverter defibrillator, and mildly symptomatic chronic heart failure. Circulation 110:2864, 2004.
37. Linde C, Gold M, Abraham WT, Daubert JC: Rationale and design of a randomized controlled trial to assess the safety and efficacy of cardiac resynchronization therapy in patients with asymptomatic left ventricular dysfunction with previous symptoms or mild heart failure—the REsynchronization reVErses Remodeling in Systolic left vEntricular dysfunction (REVERSE) study. Am Heart J 151:288, 2006.

38. Linde C, Abraham WT, Gold MR, et al: Randomized trial of cardiac resynchronization in mildly symptomatic heart failure patients and in asymptomatic patients with left ventricular dysfunction and previous heart failure symptoms. J Am Coll Cardiol 52:1834, 2008.
39. Moss AJ, Brown MW, Cannom DS, et al: Multicenter automatic defibrillator implantation trial—cardiac resynchronization therapy (MADIT-CRT): Design and clinical protocol. Ann Noninvasive Electrocardiol 10:34, 2005.
40. Moss AJ, Hall WJ, Cannom DS, et al: Cardiac resynchronization therapy for the prevention of heart failure events. N Engl J Med 361:1329, 2009.

Sudden Cardiac Death

41. Sponsor's Executive Summary: Multicenter Automatic Defibrillator Implantation Trial with Cardiac Resynchronization Therapy (MADIT-CRT), February 15, 2010. (http://www.fda.gov/downloads/AdvisoryCommittees/CommitteesMeetingMaterials/MedicalDevices/MedicalDevicesAdvisoryCommittee/CirculatorySystemDevicesPanel/UCM204607.pdf).
42. Uretsky B, Sheahan R: Primary prevention of sudden cardiac death in heart failure: will the solution be shocking? J Am Coll Cardiol 30:1589, 1997.
43. Stevenson WG, Stevenson LW, Middlekauff HR, Saxon LA: Sudden death prevention in patients with advanced ventricular dysfunction. Circulation 88:2953, 1993.
44. Effects of metoprolol CR/XL in chronic heart failure: Metoprolol CR/XL Randomised Intervention Trial in Congestive Heart Failure (MERIT-HF). Lancet 353:2001, 1999.
45. Moss AJ, Hall WJ, Cannom DS, et al: Improved survival with an implanted defibrillator in patients with coronary disease at high risk for ventricular arrhythmia. N Engl J Med 335:1933, 1996.
46. Bigger JT: Prophylactic use of implanted cardiac defibrillators in patients at high risk for ventricular arrhythmia after coronary artery bypass graft surgery. N Engl J Med 337:1569, 1997.
47. Buxton AE, Lee KL, Fisher JD, et al: A randomized study of the prevention of sudden death in patients with coronary artery disease. N Engl J Med 341:1882, 1999.
48. Moss AJ, Zareba W, Hall J, et al: Prophylactic implantation of a defibrillator in patients with myocardial infarction and reduced ejection fraction. N Engl J Med 346:877, 2002.
49. Kadish A, Dyer A, Daubert JP, et al: Prophylactic defibrillator implantation in patients with nonischemic dilated cardiomyopathy. N Engl J Med 350:2151, 2004.
50. Bardy GH, Lee KL, Mark DB, et al: Amiodarone or an implantable cardioverter-defibrillator for congestive heart failure. N Engl J Med 352:225, 2005.
51. Doval HC, Nul DR, Grancelli HO, et al: Randomized trial of low-dose amiodarone in severe congestive heart failure. Lancet 344:493, 1994.

Implantable Devices to Monitor Heart Failure

52. Adamson P, Smith A, Abraham W, et al: Continuous autonomic assessment in patient with symptomatic heart failure: Prognostic value of heart rate variability measured by an implanted cardiac resynchronization device. Circulation 110:2389, 2004.
53. Yu CM, Wang L, Chau E, et al: Intrathoracic impedance monitoring in patients with heart failure. Correlation with fluid status and feasibility of early warning preceding hospitalization. Circulation 112:841, 2005.
54. Stiles S: FAST Enough? Intrathoracic monitor bests weight gain in predicting worsening heart failure (http://www.theheart.org/article/1003313.do).
55. Magalski A, Adamson P, Gadler F, et al: Continuous ambulatory right heart pressure measurements with an implantable hemodynamic monitor: A multicenter 12-month follow-up study of patients with chronic heart failure. J Card Fail 8:63, 2002.
56. Adamson PB, Magalski A, Braunschweig F, et al: Ongoing right ventricular hemodynamics in heart failure: Clinical value of measurements derived from an implantable monitoring system. J Am Coll Cardiol 41:565, 2003.
57. Bourge RC, Abraham WT, Adamson PB, et al: Randomized controlled trial of an implantable continuous hemodynamic monitor in patients with advanced heart failure: The COMPASS-HF study. J Am Coll Cardiol 51:1073, 2008.
58. Ritzema J, Troughton R, Melton I, et al: Physician-directed patient self-management of left atrial pressure in advanced chronic heart failure. Circulation 121:1086, 2010.

CHAPTER 30 Heart Failure with Normal Ejection Fraction

Margaret M. Redfield

Historical Perspective

Until the last two decades, the possibility that large numbers of patients with heart failure (HF) might have a normal ejection fraction (EF) was not considered. As numerous studies have now demonstrated, heart failure with a normal ejection fraction (HFnlEF) is common; why it was not previously recognized is unclear. It may be that HFnlEF was always common but that the cardiology community failed to recognize it. It is also possible that the prevalence of HFnlEF has increased over time, leading to more widespread recognition. Support for this concept comes from a study showing that the prevalence of HFnlEF among patients admitted for HF at a single large institution had increased dramatically during a 15-year period from 1987 to 2001 (**Fig. 30-1**).[1] The emergence of this "new" form of HF engendered considerable early skepticism, despite growing epidemiologic evidence of its importance. Controversy about the significance of HFnlEF has largely but not completely abated. This chapter summarizes much of what is currently known about HFnlEF; our understanding of this syndrome is incomplete and will continue to evolve as the field advances.

Nomenclature and Classification

As recognition of the importance of HFnlEF as a public health problem increased, controversy arose over the proper term to use for HFnlEF. Most early studies referred to HFnlEF as diastolic HF, a term implying that diastolic dysfunction is the key pathophysiologic mechanism responsible for hemodynamic perturbations and symptoms in these patients. Similarly, systolic HF was commonly used to refer to patients with HF with reduced or depressed EF. Because of the paucity of studies measuring diastolic function in patients with HFnlEF, some have argued that HF with preserved (HFpEF) or normal (HFnlEF) EF be used. The term HFnlEF has been used in current HF management guidelines[2,3] and thus is used in this chapter. **Figure 30-2** serves to define the population of patients that is the focus of this chapter and emphasizes consideration of an appropriate differential diagnosis for patients with clinical evidence of HF and normal EF. EF is a continuous variable with a fairly normal distribution within the population,[4] and the threshold value to define normal versus reduced EF is arbitrary. Although consensus seems to be building toward use of an EF higher than 50% to designate HFnlEF, the approach to patients with borderline reduction in EF (EF of 40% to 50%) adds to the complexity of the classification.

Epidemiology

Numerous epidemiologic studies and national HF registries have defined the prevalence of HFnlEF in various HF populations and have documented a prevalence of 50% to 55%.[1,5-8] The prevalence of HF increases with age (**Fig. 30-3A**) and is similar in men and women (Fig. 30-3B). The prevalence of HF with a depressed EF increases with age but is more common in men than in women at any age (Fig. 30-3D), whereas the prevalence of HFnlEF increases even more dramatically with age (more than HF with a reduced EF) and is much more common in women than in men at any age (Fig. 30-3C).[9]

Natural History

Mortality

Most large contemporary studies have now suggested that all-cause mortality for HFnlEF is similar to that of HF with a reduced EF (see Chap. 28).[1,5-7] Survival curves from two large studies comparing survival in HF patients with preserved or reduced EF are shown in **Figure 30-4**.[1,7] Differences in survival between the two forms of HF are variably reported but generally minimal. Although survival has improved over time for patients with HF with a reduced EF, it has not changed for patients with HFnlEF (**Fig. 30-5**).[1] In the Digitalis Investigation Group (DIG) study, which included HF patients with normal and reduced EF[10] (**Fig. 30-6A**), and in a community-based HF surveillance study[11] (Fig. 30-6B), compared with patients with reduced EF, HF patients with normal EF more often died of noncardiovascular causes, whereas deaths due to coronary disease were less frequent.

Morbidity

Patients with HFnlEF have morbidity comparable to that of patients with HF with a reduced EF, with minimal differences in HF readmission rates.[6,7] A community-based HF surveillance study reported the lifetime burden of hospitalization after a diagnosis of HF. Whereas the lifetime burden of all-cause hospitalization is high and nearly equivalent among patients with preserved or reduced EF, in either form of HF, a minority (16.5%) of hospitalizations are due to HF. These data underscore the fact that HF is a disease of the elderly, in whom comorbidities influence morbidity and mortality.[12] Rates of progressive functional decline after an admission for HF are also similar in patients with preserved or reduced EF.[13]

Clinical Features

Patients with HFnlEF were shown to have pathophysiologic characteristics similar to those of HF patients with a reduced EF, including severely reduced exercise capacity, neuroendocrine activation, and impaired quality of life (see also Chap. 28).[14] Pertinent clinical features in HFnlEF are reviewed in **Table 30-1**, with particular emphasis on

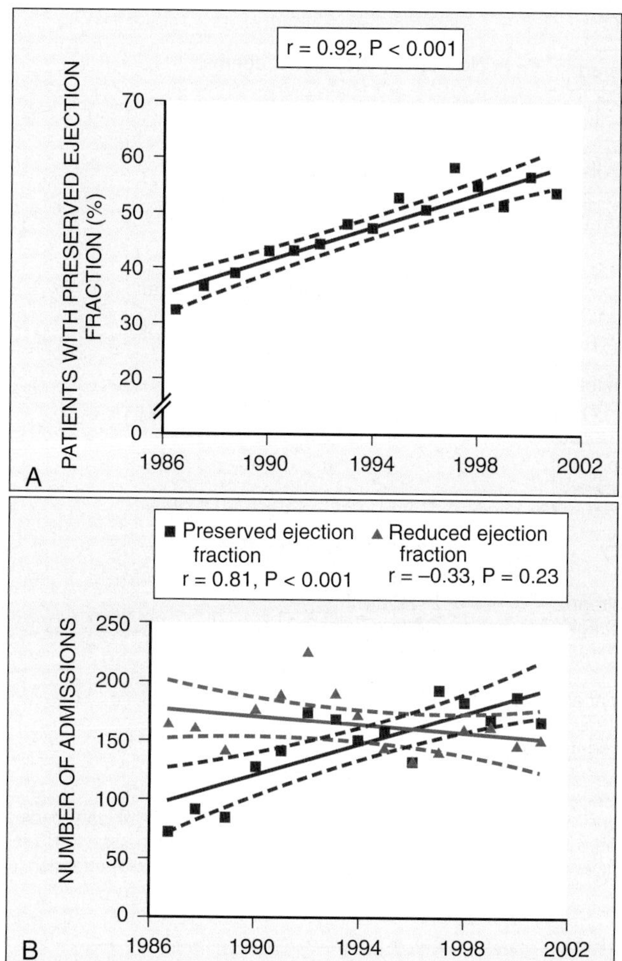

FIGURE 30-1 Increased prevalence of HFnlEF. **A,** A large study of patients hospitalized with HF at a single institution during a 15-year period from 1987 to 2001 demonstrated that the percentage of HF patients who have normal EF has increased over time. **B,** This was the result of an increased number of admissions for HFnlEF; the number of admissions for HF with reduced EF remained stable. *(From Owan T, Hodge D, Herges D, et al: Heart failure with preserved ejection fraction: Trends in prevalence and outcomes. N Engl J Med 355:308, 2006.)*

establishing the diagnosis of HF. There are minimal differences between clinical symptoms, signs, or radiographic findings in HF patients with normal or reduced EF, and no clinical features (symptoms, signs, or chest radiography) can be used to reliably distinguish between the two. Thus, assessment of EF with cardiac imaging is required in all patients with new-onset HF.

Demographic Features and Comorbid Conditions

Patients with HFnlEF are generally older than 65 years, with many older than 80 years, and they are prominently although not predominantly women (50% to 70%). A history of hypertension is present in most patients and may have developed only later in life. Obesity is seen in 30% to 50% of patients, diabetes in 30% to 50%, and atrial fibrillation in up to 20% to 40%. The prevalence of renal disease is high and similar to that noted in patients with HF and a reduced EF. The reported medications at diagnosis in patients with HFnlEF have included diuretics, digoxin, angiotensin-converting enzyme (ACE) inhibitors, beta blockers, calcium channel blockers and various other vasodilators, and antihypertensive and antiarrhythmic drugs. The reported prevalence of coronary artery disease varies widely but is lower in HFnlEF than in HF with reduced EF.[15] The demographic features and comorbid conditions that are highly prevalent in HFnlEF are discussed in more detail.

Aging. Although cardiovascular disease may contribute to diastolic dysfunction in older people, studies have also suggested that diastolic function deteriorates with normal aging (see Chap. 80).[16] The speed of left ventricular (LV) relaxation declines with age in men and women, even in the absence of cardiovascular disease. Vascular, LV systolic, and LV diastolic stiffness increase with aging.[16,17] Increases in vascular stiffness have been shown to be related to effort intolerance in patients with HFnlEF. Structural cardiac changes with aging (e.g., increased cardiomyocyte size, increased apoptosis with decreased myocyte number, altered growth factor regulation, focal collagen deposition) and functional changes at the cellular level involving blunted beta-adrenergic responsiveness, excitation-contraction coupling, and altered calcium-handling proteins may contribute to diastolic dysfunction with normal aging. Some studies have suggested that prolonged, sustained endurance training may preserve LV compliance with aging and help prevent HF in the elderly.[18]

Gender. Along with age, female gender is a potent risk factor for HFnlEF (see Chap. 81). Indeed, there appear to be important age-gender interactions, such that the prevalence of HFnlEF increases more sharply with age in women than the prevalence of HF with a reduced EF (see Fig. 30-4).[9] The reasons for the female prominence in HFnlEF are not entirely clear, but women have higher vascular and LV systolic and diastolic stiffness than men do, and vascular and ventricular stiffness increases more dramatically with age in women.[16] Unique coronary vascular functional changes in women may also play a role in the pathophysiologic process of HFnlEF.

Hypertension (see Chaps. 45 and 46)**.** Hypertension is the most commonly associated cardiac condition in patients with HFnlEF. Chronically increased blood pressure is an important stimulus for cardiac structural remodeling and functional changes. The resultant hypertensive heart disease is characterized by LV hypertrophy (LVH), increasing vascular and ventricular systolic stiffness, impaired relaxation, and increased diastolic stiffness, all factors linked to the pathogenesis of HFnlEF.[19] In the presence of hypertensive heart disease, ischemia produces exaggerated increases in filling pressures, and hypertensive heart disease and ischemic heart disease are often present in combination in patients with HFnlEF. Elucidating which factors mediate transition to HFnlEF in persons with hypertensive heart disease is an area of active investigation.

Coronary Artery Disease (see Chap. 57)**.** The reported prevalence of coronary artery disease or myocardial ischemia in patients with HFnlEF varies widely.[15] Although acute ischemia is known to cause diastolic dysfunction (see later), the role of coronary artery disease and ischemia in contributing to chronic diastolic dysfunction and symptoms in patients with HFnlEF remains speculative. Despite uncertainty about the role of ischemia in the pathophysiologic process of HFnlEF and a lack of data documenting that revascularization improves outcomes in patients with HFnlEF, HF management guidelines recommend revascularization in those HFnlEF patients in whom "ischemia is felt to contribute to diastolic dysfunction."[2,3] Whether unique features (e.g., diffuse disease, more endothelial dysfunction) play a role in the pathophysiologic process of HFnlEF in women remains to be determined. Even in the absence of epicardial coronary disease, aging, hypertension, and diabetes are associated with vascular rarefaction and reduced coronary microvascular density, which can lead to impaired coronary flow reserve and diastolic dysfunction during stress.[20]

Atrial Fibrillation and Other Rhythm Disturbances (see Chap. 40)**.** Atrial fibrillation is recognized as a frequent precipitant of acute decompensation in patients with HFnlEF. Potential mechanisms responsible for this frequent presentation are discussed more fully later. Whereas atrial fibrillation may cause decompensated HF in patients with diastolic dysfunction, diastolic dysfunction (in the absence of HF) is also a risk factor for atrial fibrillation.[21] Thus, diastolic dysfunction, atrial fibrillation, and HFnlEF are common and related conditions that probably share common pathogenic mechanisms in the elderly. The prevalence of ventricular arrhythmias in HFnlEF is poorly defined. Although tachycardia caused by atrial arrhythmias is a recognized precipitant of acute decompensation in HFnlEF, bradycardia and adverse atrioventricular timing caused by first-degree heart block may also adversely affect LV filling in some patients.

Obesity. Obesity is associated with an increased risk for HF. In general, patients with HFnlEF are more often obese than are patients with HF with a reduced EF, and the prevalence of diastolic dysfunction is increased in obese persons. Increased adiposity not only imposes an adverse hemodynamic load on the heart but also is a source of a large number of biologically active peptide and nonpeptide mediators, many

CH 30

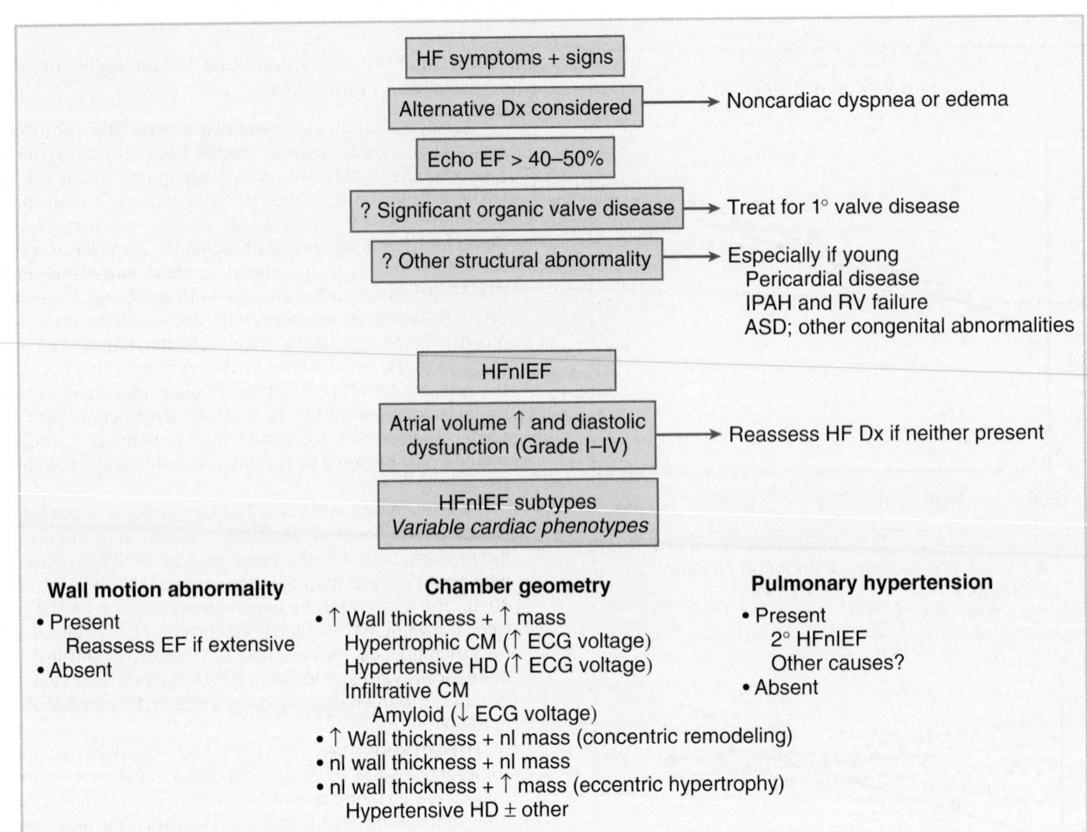

FIGURE 30-2 HFnlEF classification, differential diagnosis, and variable cardiac phenotype. When the term HFnlEF is used, care must be taken to exclude conditions attributable to noncardiac processes or to other recognized specific cardiac abnormalities for which effective therapy exists. The cardiac phenotype in HFnlEF is variable. ASD = atrial septal defect; CM = cardiomyopathy; ECG = electrocardiogram; HD = heart disease; IPAH = idiopathic pulmonary arterial hypertension; nl = normal; RV = right ventricular.

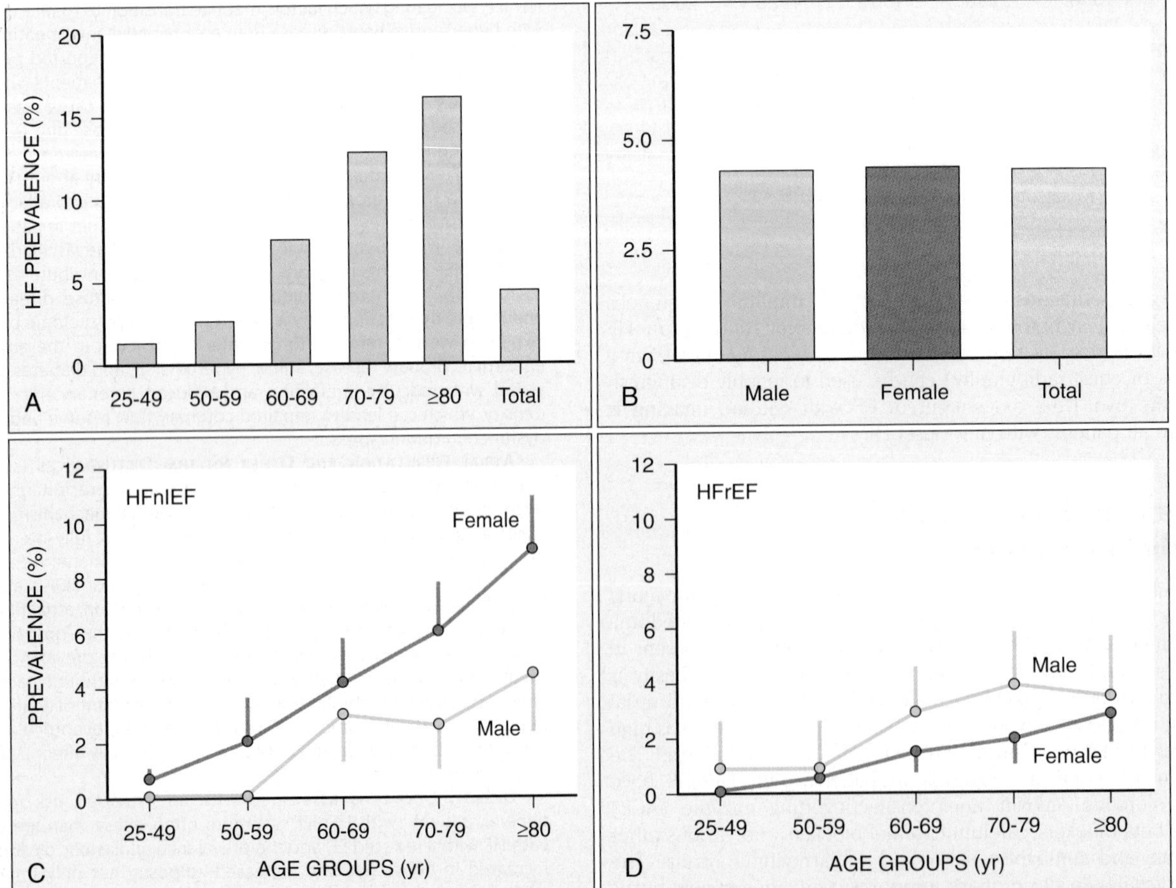

FIGURE 30-3 The age- and gender-specific prevalence of HFnlEF and HF with reduced EF. **A,** HF prevalence by age. **B,** HF prevalence by gender. **C,** HFnlEF prevalence by age. **D,** HF with reduced EF (HFrEF) prevalence by gender. As demonstrated in this study and others,[1,5-7] although the prevalence of both forms of HF increases dramatically with age, the prevalence of HFnlEF increases more steeply with age and, in contrast to HF with reduced EF, is more common in women at any age. *(Modified from Ceia F, Fonseca C, Mota T, et al: Prevalence of chronic heart failure in Southwestern Europe: The EPICA study. Eur J Heart Fail 4:531, 2002.)*

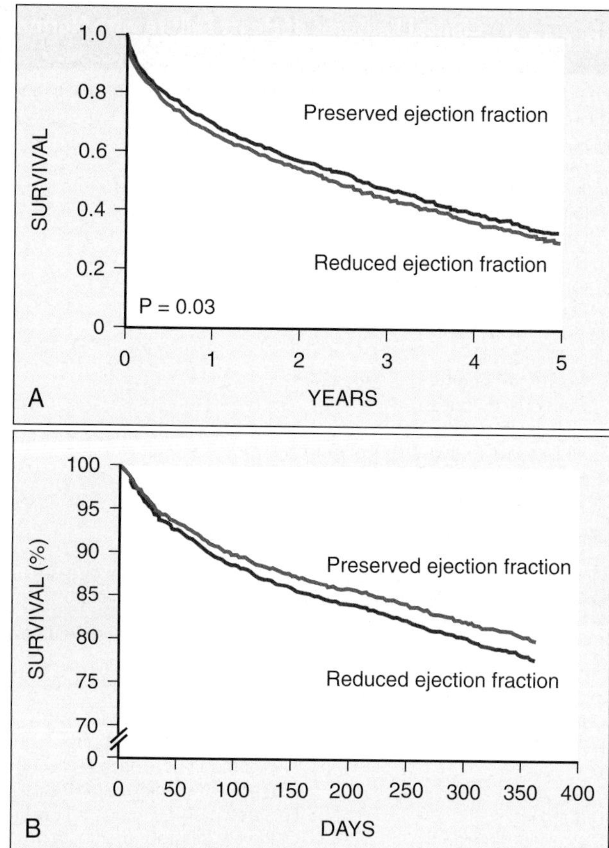

FIGURE 30-4 A, B, Kaplan-Meier survival curves comparing survival in patients with HFnlEF to that of patients with HF with reduced EF. As in most previous studies,[5,6] both studies showed only small differences in survival between the two types of HF. Note that the study in **B** compared survival in those patients with an EF of less than 40% to those with an EF of higher than 50%, whereas the study in **A** compared survival between those with an EF of less than 50% and those with an EF of higher than 50%. *(**A** from Owan T, Hodge D, Herges D, et al: Heart failure with preserved ejection fraction: Trends in prevalence and outcomes. N Engl J Med 355:308, 2006. **B** from Bhatia RS, Tu JV, Lee DS, et al: Outcome of heart failure with preserved ejection fraction in a population-based study. N Engl J Med 355:260, 2006.)*

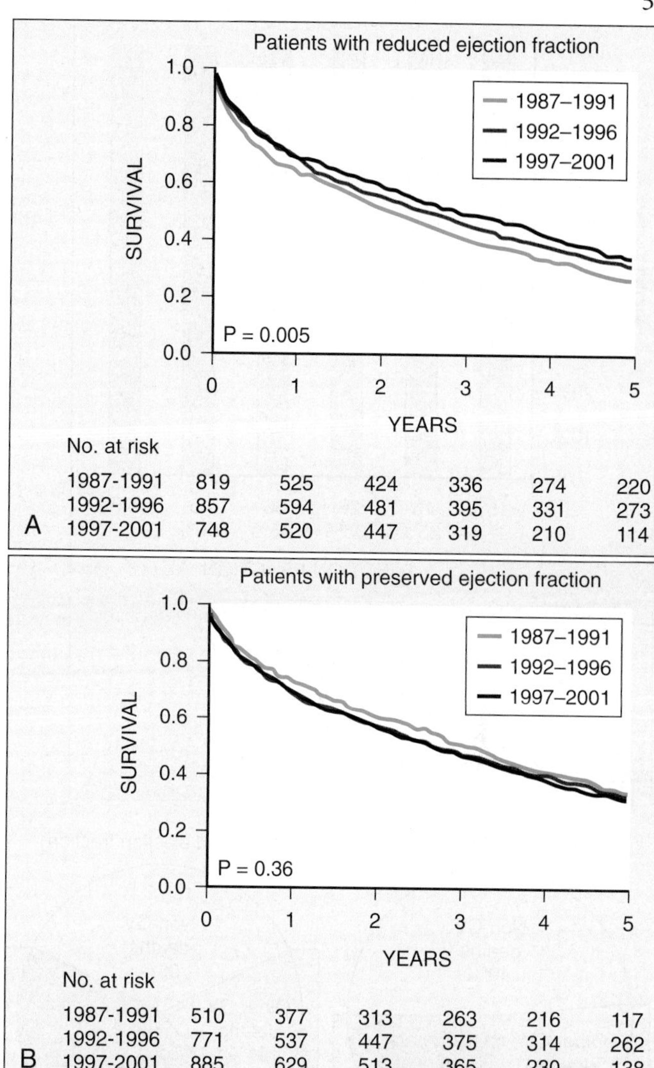

FIGURE 30-5 Survival curves for patients with HFnlEF have not improved. Whereas survival for patients with HF with reduced EF was shown to be improving over time in this study from Olmsted County, Minnesota **(A)**, no such improvement was observed for patients with HFnlEF **(B)**. *(From Owan T, Hodge D, Herges D, et al: Heart failure with preserved ejection fraction: Trends in prevalence and outcomes. N Engl J Med 355:308, 2006.)*

linked to chronic inflammation. Increased body mass index is a risk factor for hypertension, diabetes mellitus, coronary artery disease, and atrial fibrillation, all of which are associated with HFnlEF. Studies using tissue Doppler imaging or invasive LV pressure measurement have reported an association between diastolic dysfunction, elevated filling pressures, and obesity, even in the absence of a diagnosis of HF.[22]

Diabetes Mellitus (see Chap. 64)**.** Diabetes is a potent risk factor for HF, and the prevalence of diabetes is similar in patients with HF and reduced or preserved EF, suggesting that diabetes contributes to the pathophysiologic process of both forms of HF. Although diabetes predisposes to coronary artery disease, renal dysfunction, and hypertension, numerous direct effects of diabetes and hyperglycemia on myocardial structure and function have been described. The morphologic changes in the diabetic heart include myocyte hypertrophy, increased extracellular matrix (fibrosis), and intramyocardial microangiopathy. Functional changes, which may represent a continuum, include impaired endothelium-dependent and endothelium-independent vasodilation, impaired LV relaxation, increased passive diastolic stiffness, and contractile dysfunction. Mechanisms contributing to structural and functional coronary vascular and myocardial changes are diverse and include metabolic disturbances, activation of proinflammatory and profibrotic mediators, cardiac autonomic neuropathy, and increases in advanced glycation end products, which promote increased collagen accumulation and increased collagen stiffness. Accumulation of advanced glycation end products may play a role in age-related cardiac and vascular stiffening.

Renal Dysfunction (see Chap. 93)**.** The critical impact of renal function on morbidity and mortality in HF is well established.[23] Studies have shown no difference in the severity of renal dysfunction in patients with reduced or preserved EF.[1,6,7] Furthermore, the incidence of worsening renal function during HF therapy is similar in patients with preserved or reduced EF.[24] Although the prevalence of renal vascular disease in HF has been poorly delineated, it is probably high, and bilateral renal artery stenosis with rapid-onset pulmonary edema is a well-recognized cause of HFnlEF. Evaluation of the renal arteries should be considered in patients presenting with the triad of hypertension, renal dysfunction, and HFnlEF.

Sleep Apnea (see Chap. 79)**.** Obstructive sleep apnea is common in patients with HFnlEF risk factors (obesity, atrial fibrillation, hypertension) and in HFnlEF and can contribute to symptom severity and probably promote progression of HF. Central sleep apnea can occur in association with severe HFnlEF.

Rarer Causes of Heart Failure with a Normal Ejection Fraction. Hypertrophic cardiomyopathy, infiltrative cardiomyopathies such as amyloidosis, valvular disease, and constrictive pericarditis should always be considered in young patients with HFnlEF or patients with other suggestive features (see Fig. 30-2; see Chaps. 68, 69, and 71). However, these diseases account for a minority of patients with HFnlEF. Idiopathic restrictive cardiomyopathy in young persons without the factors discussed earlier may represent a distinct group, particularly if a family history is present. However, the clinical presentation and echocardiographic appearance in older persons with HFnlEF may be identical to those of patients previously described as having restrictive cardiomyopathy. An important consideration in patients with previous malignant disease treated with mediastinal irradiation is radiation heart disease (see Chap. 90). Radiation can cause pericardial and concomitant myocardial

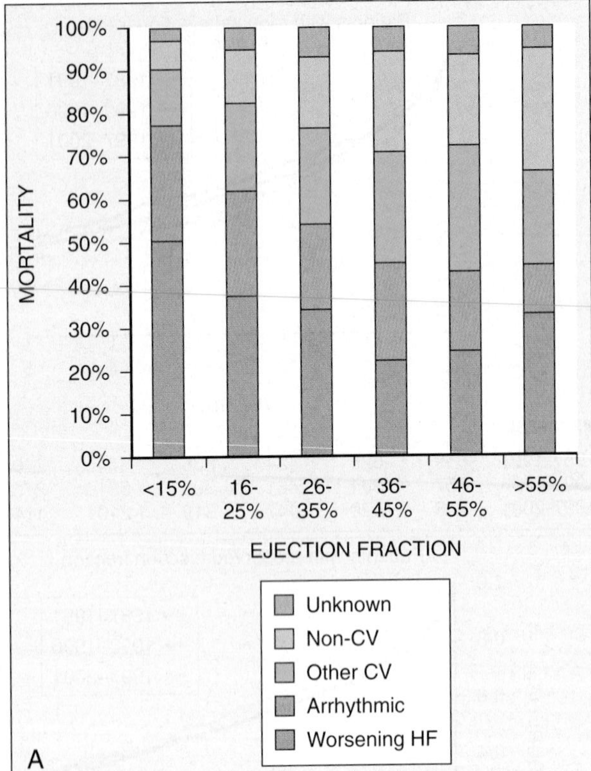

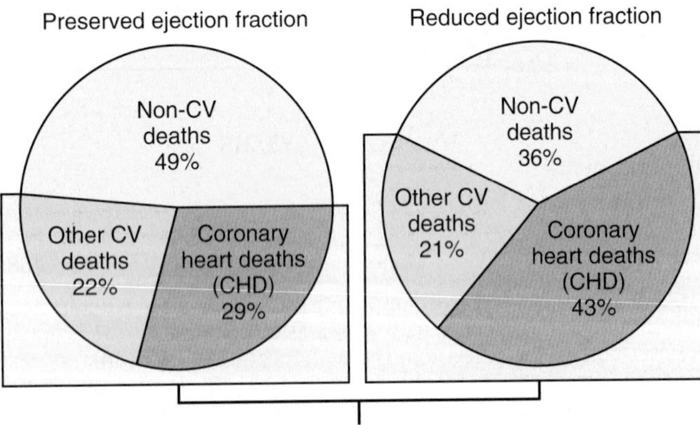

FIGURE 30-6 Cause of death in patients with HFnlEF. In a post hoc analysis from the Digitalis Investigation Group (DIG) trial **(A)**, which included a subgroup of patients with HFnlEF, the cause of death in different EF groups was assessed. Patients with normal EF had more deaths from noncardiovascular causes and more deaths from cardiovascular (CV) causes other than arrhythmia or HF. *(From Curtis JP, Sokol SI, Wang Y, et al: The association of left ventricular ejection fraction, mortality, and cause of death in stable outpatients with heart failure. J Am Coll Cardiol 42:736, 2003.)* In a community-based study **(B)**, the cause of death in HF patients with normal or reduced EF was assessed. HFnlEF patients were more likely to die of noncardiovascular causes and less likely to die of coronary disease than were patients with HF and reduced EF. *(From Henkel DM, Redfield MM, Weston SA, et al: Death in heart failure: A community perspective. Circ Heart Fail 1:91, 2008.)*

TABLE 30-1 Clinical Features of Heart Failure with Normal Ejection Fraction

Framingham criteria for diagnosis of heart failure (two major or one major and two minor criteria)	
Major	
Paroxysmal nocturnal dyspnea or orthopnea	
Jugular venous distention (or central venous pressure > 16 mm Hg)	
Rales or acute pulmonary edema	
Cardiomegaly	
Hepatojugular reflex	
Circulation time > 25 seconds	
Response to diuretic (weight loss > 4.5 kg in 5 days)	
Minor	
Ankle edema	
Nocturnal cough	
Exertional dyspnea	
Pleural effusion	
Vital capacity < two thirds of normal	
Hepatomegaly	
Tachycardia (>120 beats/min)	
Demographic features	Elderly; female > male
Underlying cardiovascular disease	Hypertension, coronary disease, diabetes, atrial fibrillation
Comorbidities	Obesity, renal dysfunction, multiple other
Doppler echocardiography	
Left ventricle size	Normal to ↓ (small subset with ↑)
Left ventricle mass	Left ventricular hypertrophy common but *frequently* absent; ↑ relative wall thickness (>0.45)
Left atrium	Enlarged
Diastolic dysfunction	Grade I-IV (diastolic dysfunction severity, blood pressure, volume status)
Other features	Pulmonary hypertension, wall motion abnormality, right ventricle enlargement
Pertinent negatives	Rule out valve disease, pericardial disease, atrial septal defect
BNP or NT-proBNP	Normal to ↑, but HFnlEF < HF with reduced EF
Exercise testing	↓ Vo_2max Exaggerated hypertensive response in many Chronotropic incompetence in subset
Chest radiography	Similar to HF with reduced EF, cardiomegaly, pulmonary venous hypertension, edema, pleural effusion
Electrocardiography	Variable

damage, and persistent HF after pericardiectomy is frequent because of concomitant myocardial disease. Concomitant valvular disease and premature coronary artery disease are also common in patients with previous mediastinal irradiation and may contribute to the pathophysiologic changes of HFnlEF in patients with radiation heart disease.

The Elderly Patient with Exertional Dyspnea, Normal Ejection Fraction, and Pulmonary Hypertension. An increasingly common clinical scenario relates to elderly patients with dyspnea who are referred to echocardiography, when a normal EF and significant pulmonary hypertension are found. These patients are often referred to pulmonary hypertension clinics for consideration of pulmonary arterial vasodilator therapy. Guidelines mandate that the severity and cause of pulmonary hypertension be defined by right-heart catheterization,[25] and many of these elderly patients have pulmonary hypertension due to resting or exertional pulmonary venous hypertension with normal or only mildly elevated pulmonary vascular resistance.[26,27] Chronic pulmonary venous hypertension in HF has a direct hemodynamic effect on pulmonary pressure and causes reactive pulmonary arterial vasoconstriction, which can be slow to resolve after HF treatment and reduction of LV filling pressures. With time, chronic pulmonary venous hypertension causes pulmonary vascular remodeling (congestive pulmonary vasculopathy) and irreversible pulmonary hypertension. These changes are well described in HF with a reduced EF and mitral valvular disease but commonly occur in HFnlEF as well. The prevalence of significant pulmonary hypertension in HFnlEF is as high as 86% and is associated with poorer survival.[28,29] An approach to the evaluation of such patients has recently been published,[25] and empiric pulmonary arterial vasodilator therapy based on echocardiography-derived evidence of pulmonary hypertension should be avoided.

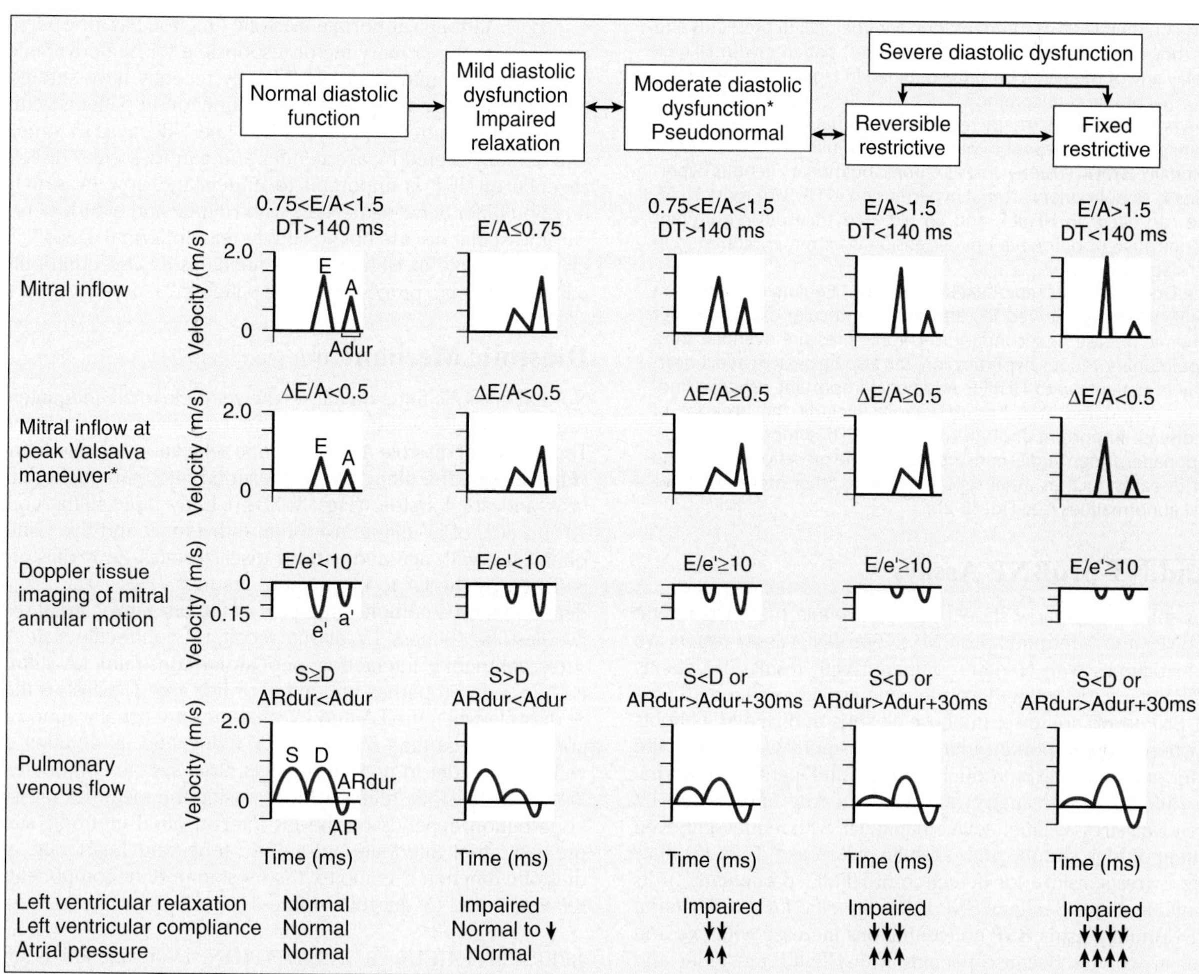

FIGURE 30-7 Proposed progression of diastolic function abnormalities as assessed with comprehensive Doppler echocardiography, with correlation of invasively measured diastolic properties (see text at bottom). A comprehensive Doppler assessment as outlined here can yield useful information about relaxation, filling pressures, and (indirectly) diastolic stiffness in most patients but requires careful data acquisition and informed interpretation. A = transmitral flow velocity with atrial contraction; a′ = velocity of mitral annulus motion with atrial systole; Adur = duration of A; AR = flow from left atrium to pulmonary veins during atrial contraction; ARdur = duration of AR; D = diastolic; DT = deceleration time; E = early diastolic transmitral flow velocity; e′ = velocity of early diastolic mitral annular motion; S = systolic. *Corrected for E/A fusion. *(From Redfield MM, Jacobsen SJ, Burnett JC Jr, et al: Burden of systolic and diastolic ventricular dysfunction in the community: Appreciating the scope of the heart failure epidemic. JAMA 289:194, 2003.)*

Clinical Features Associated with Acute Decompensation

Uncontrolled hypertension, dietary or medication noncompliance, atrial arrhythmias, ischemia, and concomitant processes such as infection, anemia, or other medical illness are common in patients presenting with acutely decompensated HFnlEF. It is likely that in many older sedentary patients with multiple comorbidities, the stress imposed by a comorbidity may trigger the acute HF episode. After volume status is restored, the inciting comorbid condition remains and influences the subsequent clinical course. This may contribute to the high rate of non-HF rehospitalization observed after an episode of HF.[12,30] In contrast, patients with chronic, stable HF are likely to have fewer reversible features.

Findings on Doppler Echocardiography

Comprehensive Doppler echocardiography is invaluable in the evaluation of HF patients (see Chap. 15). Beyond the presence of a normal EF, expected or possible findings in patients with HFnlEF are outlined here and in Table 30-1.

Left Ventricular Size. Most patients with HFnlEF have normal chamber dimensions, although a small subset may have variable degrees of LV enlargement.

Left Ventricular Hypertrophy. Although HFnlEF has been thought to occur primarily in patients with LVH, studies that have carefully quantified LV mass report that echocardiographic criteria for LVH are met in less than 50% of patients.[14,31-33] Patients with HFnlEF have, on average, increased relative wall thickness and an increased mass-to-volume ratio,[14] but these findings often occur in the setting of normal LV mass. Thus, despite traditional teaching, severe LVH is not invariably present in HFnlEF, in which the cardiac phenotype is variable (see Fig. 30-2). There is some evidence that the prevalence of LVH may be higher in African American HFnlEF patients.[34,35]

Doppler Echocardiographic Assessment of Diastolic Function and Filling Pressures. The Doppler assessment of diastolic function and filling pressures requires careful acquisition of data and informed interpretation. Assessment of diastolic function begins with the transmitral flow velocity profile. Decreases in the ratio of early to late diastolic filling (E/A), increases in the deceleration time, or increases in the isovolumic relaxation time indicate impaired relaxation. However, in the presence of impaired relaxation, increases in filling pressure progressively modify the transmitral gradient and mitral inflow pattern (**Fig. 30-7**; see Figs. 15-26 and 15-29). A comprehensive Doppler assessment must be used to determine diastolic function and filling pressures.[4] Patients studied at various times during their presentation (e.g., acutely decompensated, after initial treatment of an acute decompensation episode, or as stable outpatients) will display a spectrum of filling patterns, including abnormal relaxation and pseudonormal or restrictive patterns. Such a spectrum has also been reported in patients with HF with a depressed EF and reflects the potent effect of filling pressures and blood pressure and their interaction with underlying diastolic dysfunction on the Doppler patterns. Thus, depending on their level of compensation and their filling pressures and whether they have exertional or rest symptoms, patients with HFnlEF may display any of the filling patterns outlined in Figure 30-7, although a truly normal profile is uncommon.[36]

LEFT ATRIAL ENLARGEMENT. Increases in left atrial (LA) dimension or volume are commonly present in patients with HFnlEF.[28,35,37]

PULMONARY HYPERTENSION. Just as chronic pulmonary venous hypertension leads to pulmonary arterial hypertension in HF with reduced EF, the same can occur in HFnlEF, and an elevated tricuspid regurgitant velocity indicative of pulmonary hypertension is extremely common in HFnlEF[28,29] (see earlier).

OTHER DOPPLER ECHOCARDIOGRAPHIC FINDINGS. Regional wall motion abnormalities (with preserved EF) and right ventricular dilation, either from ischemic disease or secondary to chronic pressure overload from chronic pulmonary venous hypertension, can also be present at echocardiography in patients with HFnlEF. Additional important *negative* findings to be considered at echocardiography include the absence of valvular disease important enough to cause the HF symptoms, pericardial tamponade, or pericardial constriction and the presence of congenital heart diseases such as atrial septal defect or other more extensive structural abnormalities (see Fig. 30-2).

BNP and NT-proBNP Assays

Numerous studies have now shown that on average, brain natriuretic peptide (BNP) and N-terminal pro-BNP (NT-proBNP) assay results are elevated in patients with HFnlEF compared with results in persons without HF but are lower than levels in patients with reduced EF (see Chap. 26). BNP levels are lower in obese persons, and HFnlEF patients are often obese. More important, increased transmural wall stress is the stimulus for enhanced BNP production. As HFnlEF patients have dramatically different LV geometry (smaller LV cavity and thicker LV walls), their wall stress is much lower than in HF with reduced EF, even in the setting of high systolic and diastolic pressures.[38] Thus, for diagnosis, BNP is less sensitive for detection of HFnlEF, particularly in its early or milder stages. Similarly, BNP is less specific for the detection of HFnlEF. Normal plasma BNP concentrations increase with age and are higher in women. Because patients with HFnlEF are older and more often female than are patients with HF and a reduced EF, the standard partition value of 100 pg/mL suggested for the diagnosis of HF may not be appropriate in HFnlEF. However, the *prognostic* value of NT-proBNP was shown to be robust in a large clinical trial of HFnlEF patients.

Exercise Testing (see Chap. 14)

Cardiopulmonary exercise testing (CPET) is useful in the diagnostic evaluation of exercise intolerance of unclear cause, and thus in select patients with suspected HFnlEF, CPET may play a role in the diagnostic evaluation. Objective measures of exercise tolerance are similarly impaired in HF (of similar clinical severity) with reduced and preserved EF. Exaggerated exertional hypertension can cause load-dependent diastolic dysfunction and recognition, and treatment of exercise-induced hypertension is important in the treatment of HFnlEF. Importantly, stress testing also allows assessment of the heart rate response to exercise. Whereas past recommendations have focused on the potential use of negative chronotropic agents to allow a longer diastolic filling period in patients with impaired relaxation, recent studies have suggested that chronotropic incompetence is also relatively common (higher than 20%) in patients with HFnlEF (although not more common than in HF with a reduced EF), even in the absence of beta blocker therapy. CPET can also reveal poor motivation and pulmonary limitation as alternative explanations for dyspnea in patients with HF symptoms and normal EF.

Pathophysiology

Understanding of the pathophysiologic mechanisms in HFnlEF mandates a clear understanding of LV diastolic and systolic function and the manner in which LV function is influenced by volume status, which together with LV geometry determines preload, and of the arterial system, which together with LV geometry affects afterload (see Chap. 24). Although abnormal diastolic function has long been hypothesized to be the primary factor responsible for hemodynamic perturbations and symptoms in HFnlEF, only recently have studies proved this hypothesis by studying diastolic function in patients with HFnlEF and relevant control populations (see later). Because LV structure and function are altered by age, gender, and cardiovascular disease in the absence of HF, it is important to understand how LV structure and function differ between persons with HFnlEF and elderly persons with cardiovascular disease but no HF. Whereas abnormal diastolic function plays a key role in HFnlEF, other mechanisms also contribute to the pathophysiologic process in many patients.

Diastolic Mechanisms (see Chap. 24)

Normal diastolic function allows the ventricle to fill adequately during rest and exercise, without an abnormal increase in diastolic pressures. The phases of diastole are isovolumic relaxation and the filling phase (**Fig. 30-8A**). The filling phase is divided into early rapid filling, diastasis, and atrial systole (Figs. 30-8B-D). Early rapid filling contributes 70% to 80% of LV filling in normal individuals, and this contribution diminishes with age and various disease states. Early diastolic filling is driven by the LA to LV pressure gradient (Figs. 30-8C, D), which is dependent on a complex interplay of factors—myocardial relaxation, LV diastolic stiffness, LV elastic recoil, LV contractile state, LA pressures, ventricular interaction, pericardial constraint, LA stiffness, pulmonary vein properties, and mitral orifice area. Diastasis is the period of diastole when the LA and LV pressures are usually almost equal. It contributes less than 5% of the LV filling, and its duration shortens with tachycardia. In normal subjects, atrial systole contributes 15% to 25% of LV diastolic filling without raising the mean LA pressure. This contribution depends on the PR interval, atrial inotropic state, atrial preload, atrial afterload, autonomic tone, and heart rate. Although diastolic function is complex, the most important components are LV relaxation and LV diastolic stiffness.

LEFT VENTRICULAR RELAXATION. LV relaxation is an active, energy-dependent process that begins during the ejection phase of systole and continues through isovolumic relaxation and the rapid filling phase. In normal hearts, catecholamine-induced enhancement of relaxation during exercise lowers LV pressures in early diastole; thus, enhanced relaxation increases the LA-LV pressure gradient without increasing LA pressures and enhances filling during exercise without the need for elevated LA pressures.

Invasive and Noninvasive Assessment of Left Ventricular Relaxation

The time constant of relaxation (tau, τ) describes the rate of LV pressure decay during isovolumic relaxation. Measurement of tau requires high-fidelity manometer-tipped LV catheters for precise determination. The pressure (P) and time (t) data during the period from end-systole (peak + dP/dt) to the onset of LV filling (determined from LA to LV crossover pressure, or estimated as 5 mm Hg above the end-diastolic pressure) are used to calculate tau (**Fig. 30-9**). The pressure-time data during isovolumic relaxation are fitted to various equations to derive the value of tau. The equations used make different assumptions about the LV minimum pressure obtained. The Weiss equation

$$\text{LV P} = P_0 e^{-t/t}$$

where P_0 is LV P at end ejection, assumes a zero asymptote (or that the LV minimum pressure must be positive) and thus derives tau as the negative inverse of the slope of the relationship between the natural log (ln) of LV pressure and time during isovolumic relaxation (see Fig. 30-9). Use of a non-zero asymptote or fitting the data to a logistic equation may provide a better assessment of lusitropy. With all methods, the larger the value of tau, the longer it takes for the LV to relax and the more impaired is relaxation. A normal value for tau is less than 40 milliseconds in most age groups, and relaxation is complete by 3.5 × tau (less than 140 milliseconds).

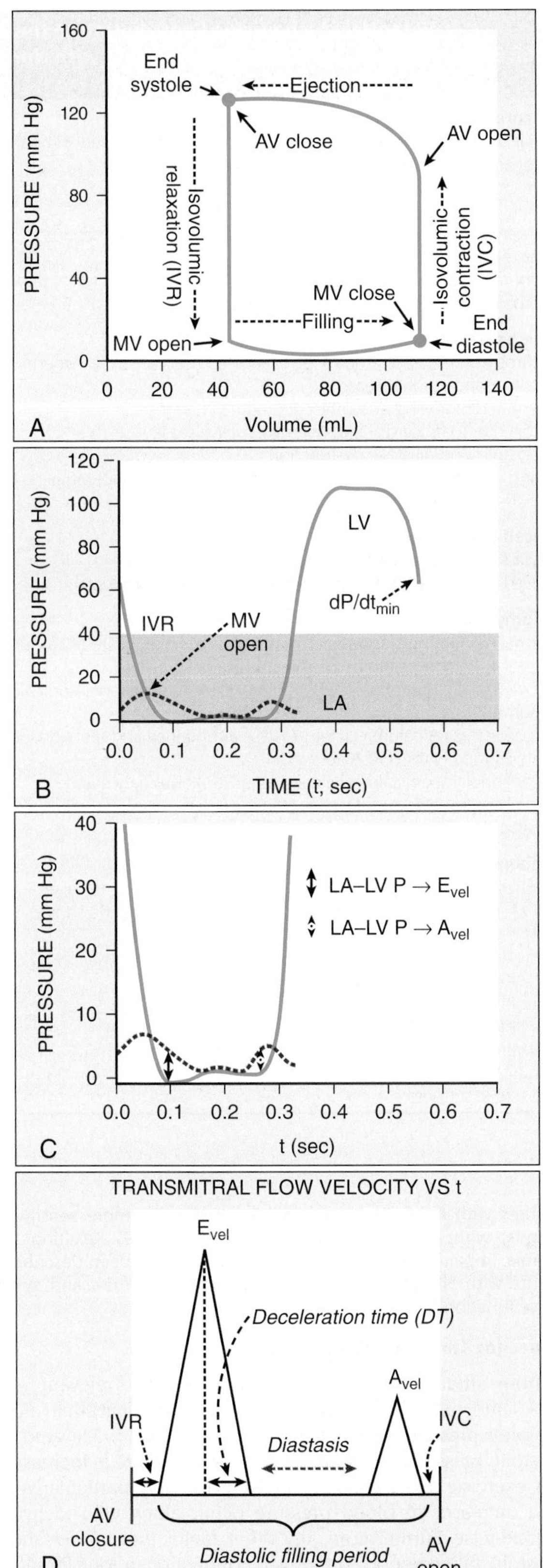

FIGURE 30-8 Assessment of ventricular diastolic function and filling in the pressure (P)–volume, pressure-time, and flow velocity–time domains. **A,** Cardiac cycle in the pressure-volume domain. Diastole includes isovolumic relaxation and the filling phase. **B,** Left ventricular (LV) and left atrial (LA) pressures during diastole, expanded to emphasize diastole **(C)**. **D,** LA to LV pressure gradient determines the velocity of LV filling during early rapid filling, diastasis, and atrial systole. See text for details. A_{vel} = transmitral flow velocity with atrial contraction; AV = aortic valve; E_{vel} = early diastolic transmitral flow velocity; IVC = isovolumic contraction; IVR = isovolumic relaxation; MV = mitral valve; t = time.

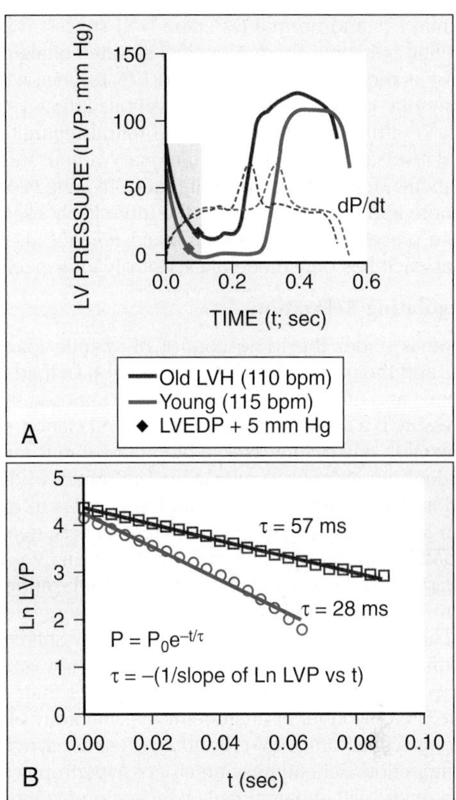

FIGURE 30-9 Invasive assessment of ventricular relaxation time constant of isovolumic relaxation (tau, τ). **A,** Pressure (P)–time (t) curves starting at the peak negative dP/dt (dotted lines) obtained with a high-fidelity manometer-tipped catheter in a young normal canine (blue) and an elderly canine (red) with chronic hypertension and left ventricular hypertrophy (LVH). Despite similar heart rates and peak positive dP/dt, contraction duration is increased in the elderly dog and filling pressures are increased. **B,** The highlighted area is expanded, and data are graphed as the natural log (ln) of LV pressure versus time during the period from the peak negative dP/dt to 5 mm Hg above the LV end-diastolic pressure (LVEDP). The negative inverse of the slope of this relationship is the time constant of isovolumic relaxation, tau (τ), expressed in milliseconds (ms). Relaxation is impaired (slowed) in the elderly canine. P_0 = LV P at end ejection.

Doppler echocardiography may also be used to assess relaxation. The transmitral flow velocity versus time profile is affected by impaired relaxation in a variable manner. If relaxation is impaired but LA pressures are not elevated, the slower LV pressure decay and the higher LV minimum pressure associated with impaired relaxation will decrease the early diastolic LA to LV pressure gradient, decrease the velocity of early diastolic filling (E_{vel}), and prolong the duration of early diastolic filling (deceleration time; see Figs. 30-7 and 30-8). Reduced LA emptying during early diastole increases atrial preload, and the velocity of filling with atrial contraction (A_{vel}) increases while the E/A ratio decreases. This produces an "impaired relaxation" pattern. However, if LA pressures are elevated, the LA to LV pressure gradient is restored, and the filling velocity profile will resume a normal configuration (pseudonormalization) with a normal E_{vel}, deceleration time, and E/A ratio despite the presence of impaired relaxation. With marked increases in passive LV diastolic stiffness and further elevation of LA pressures, E_{vel} increases further. In this setting, atrial afterload increases (because of the noncompliant LV), A_{vel} decreases, and deceleration time decreases (reflecting rapid equalization of LV diastolic pressures during early diastolic filling), yielding a "restrictive" pattern (see Fig. 30-7). Thus, the transmitral flow pattern alone cannot be used to assess relaxation in patients with HF. Measurement of the velocity of mitral annular ascent during early diastole (e'_{vel}) with tissue Doppler imaging provides a relatively preload-independent measure of LV relaxation that correlates inversely with tau.

Thus, a normal e'_{vel} and normal E/e′ ratio (<8) suggest normal relaxation and filling pressures. The presence of elevated filling pressures is supported by a very high (>15) E/e′ ratio, E/A reversal with Valsalva maneuver, systolic < diastolic pulmonary venous inflow velocities (in the absence of atrial fibrillation or severe mitral regurgitation), prolonged atrial reversal duration in the pulmonary venous inflow profile, LA enlargement, and presence of pulmonary hypertension (see Fig. 30-7). The more abnormalities present, the more likely elevated filling pressures are present, and one should avoid reliance on any single parameter as each has only moderate sensitivity and specificity.

Factors Regulating Relaxation

LV relaxation is under the triple control of systolic load, myofiber inactivation, and the uniformity of the distribution of load and inactivation in space and time. Thus, the systolic load imposed by increases in blood pressure is a critical factor influencing relaxation, and impairment of relaxation due to increases in blood pressure is referred to as load-dependent impairment in relaxation. Uniformity of the distribution of load and inactivation in space and time refers to the fact that increases in systolic load may have different effects, depending on when the load is imposed during systole. Increases in LV pressure late in systole hasten the onset of LV relaxation, but relaxation occurs at a slower rate (increased tau). Increases in LV pressure late in systole occur with aging because of age-related vascular stiffening, which alters the timing of the reflected pressure wave in the vascular tree so that the reflected wave arrives in late systole rather than in diastole. Furthermore, on a myofiber or chamber level, synchrony of relaxation in all segments will enhance LV relaxation, whereas asynchrony (e.g., caused by infarction, ischemia, asymmetry of hypertrophy, or conduction abnormalities) will impair global LV relaxation. Myofiber inactivation refers to the many cellular processes (see Chap. 24) that ultimately influence the rate and extent of detachment of actin-myosin cross bridges, allowing myofiber lengthening during diastole. Mechanisms of particular current or emerging clinical interest in HFnlEF are briefly summarized (**Table 30-2**).

Actin-myosin cross-bridge detachment requires prompt decreases in cytosolic calcium concentrations during diastole. Prolongation of the calcium transient may be caused by several mechanisms (see Chap. 24) but particularly by reduced reuptake of calcium into the sarcoplasmic reticulum as a result of decreases in the amount or activity of the sarcoplasmic reticulum calcium ATPase (SERCA). Beta-adrenergic stimulation activates protein kinase A (PKA), which phosphorylates phospholamban and removes its tonic inhibition of SERCA activity, hastening calcium reuptake and LV relaxation. Beta-adrenergic/PKA-mediated phosphorylation of troponin I also hastens relaxation by decreasing calcium sensitivity, and reduced troponin I phosphorylation may accentuate afterload-induced changes in relaxation.[39] Impaired beta-adrenergic signaling is well established in HF with reduced EF (see Chap. 25) and in animal models of pressure overload with relevance to HFnlEF.[40] Chronic catecholamine activation contributes to beta-adrenergic receptor downregulation and desensitization, and catecholamine levels are elevated in HFnlEF,[14] suggesting that impaired beta-adrenergic signaling may contribute to relaxation impairment in HFnlEF. More recently, chronotropic incompetence and impaired systolic and lusitropic reserve function have been reported in HFnlEF, findings that further support a role for impaired beta-adrenergic signaling in HFnlEF.[34,41-45] Phospholamban phosphorylation may also be reduced by increases in protein kinase C (PKC) via effects on protein phosphatases.[46] PKC activity is increased in HF with reduced EF and in animal models of pressure overload with relevance to HFnlEF. Impaired beta-adrenergic/PKA signaling, reduced SERCA amount and activity, and increased PKC activity all may provide potential therapeutic targets for novel HFnlEF therapies.

Energy (ATP) supply influences relaxation by regulating calcium reuptake via SERCA and by influencing cross-bridge detachment at the myosin heads, where the phosphocreatine shuttle mechanism ensures delivery of ATP from the mitochondria and removal of ADP and inorganic phosphate (P_i) from the site of cross-bridge formation (see Chap. 24). Inadequate ATP and increased levels of ADP at the cross-bridge sites impair cross-bridge detachment and slow relaxation. Impaired relaxation is the first functional abnormality to occur during acute ischemia and with persistent ischemia is accompanied by parallel upward shifts of the diastolic pressure-volume relationship (decreased distensibility) due to rigor bonds. Both features may contribute to the elevated filling pressures with ischemia. Hypertrophied hearts are more sensitive to ischemia, with greater increases in filling pressures resulting from ischemia. Impaired creatine kinase ATP kinetics have been described in patients with HFnlEF and linked to impaired relaxation and systolic reserve function.[43]

TABLE 30-2 Potential Mechanisms Contributing to the Pathophysiology of Heart Failure with Normal Ejection Fraction

Extracardiac
- Vascular dysfunction (arterial stiffening; endothelial dysfunction; impaired coronary, pulmonary, and peripheral flow reserve)
- Extrinsic forces (RV-LV interaction and pericardial constraint)
- Peripheral muscle and ergoreflex dysfunction
- Pulmonary hypertension (secondary to chronic pulmonary venous hypertension)
- Neurohumoral activation
- Comorbidities (renal dysfunction, anemia)

Whole heart
- Asynchrony of relaxation due to regional infarction, ischemia, hypertrophy, fibrosis, conduction disease
- Concentric remodeling and other geometric changes
- Ischemia due to epicardial and microvascular disease
- Atrial systolic and diastolic dysfunction
- Rate and rhythm abnormalities (chronotropic incompetence, atrial fibrillation, supraventricular tachycardia)

Extracellular matrix
- Increased extracellular matrix (collagen)
- Increased collagen stiffness (advanced glycation end products)

Cardiomyocyte
- Abnormal calcium homeostasis (↑ diastolic calcium or ↓ rate of calcium reuptake → incomplete or impaired relaxation)
  - Sarcolemmal calcium channels (sodium/calcium exchanger and calcium pump)
  - Sarcoplasmic reticulum calcium ATPase abundance and function (SERCA)
  - Proteins modifying SERCA activity
    - Phospholamban, calmodulin, calsequestrin abundance and phosphorylation state
    - Sarcoplasmic reticulum calcium release channels

Myofilaments
- Energetics (↓ATP or ↑ADP slows actin-myosin cross-bridge release)
  - ADP/ATP ratio, ADP and P_i concentration, phosphocreatine shuttle function
- Proteins regulating cross-bridge formation and calcium sensitivity
  - Troponin C calcium binding
  - Troponin I phosphorylation state
- Cytoskeletal proteins
  - Microtubules (increased density) → ↑ diastolic stiffness
  - Titin isoforms (↑ noncompliant isoform and phosphorylation state) → ↑ diastolic stiffness

Evidence for Impaired Relaxation

Data from studies of humans with HFnlEF,[32,33,37] relevant animal models,[47] and mathematical modeling systems[48] indicate that impaired relaxation is present in HFnlEF and may contribute to elevated mean LV diastolic pressures in HFnlEF when the heart rate is increased (as during exercise; see Fig. 30-e1 on website) and particularly when marked increases in blood pressure occur along with tachycardia during exercise. Furthermore, any other factor that further shortens the diastolic filling period (prolonged contraction or long PR interval) will enhance the effect of impaired relaxation on LV diastolic pressures during filling and thus affect the mean LA pressure needed to fill the LV. Studies in patients with HFnlEF have reported average resting values of tau of approximately 60 milliseconds (heart rate, approximately 70 beats/min), with values increasing to approximately 86 milliseconds during exercise.[32,33] Whether therapies to enhance relaxation directly and specifically can be developed, and whether such therapies will relieve symptoms, remains an area of active investigation.

Patients with HFnlEF and impaired relaxation display increased dependence on atrial contraction for filling[49] and thus are at risk for development of HF with the onset of atrial fibrillation. The acute reduction in filling associated with loss of atrial systolic activity, coupled with the increased heart rate, mandates acute elevation of LA pressures to maintain filling. In contrast, in normal individuals with normal relaxation and brisk early diastolic filling, dependence on diastasis flow and atrial filling is minimal, and rapid atrial fibrillation is much less likely to induce acute pulmonary edema.

LEFT VENTRICULAR DIASTOLIC STIFFNESS. Stiffness or elastance is defined as the relationship between the change in stress and the resulting strain. On the chamber level, the elastance of the LV varies over the cardiac cycle (time-varying elastance), and end-systolic and end-diastolic elastance are defined by the changes in systolic or diastolic pressure associated with a change in end-systolic or end-diastolic volume (**Fig. 30-10**). Increases in LV diastolic stiffness will mandate higher LA pressures to maintain filling and thus promote elevated pulmonary venous pressures and pulmonary congestion when LA pressures are elevated or reduced cardiac output when LA pressures are not elevated.

Invasive and Noninvasive Assessment of Left Ventricular Diastolic Stiffness. Measurement of LV diastolic stiffness requires the simultaneous assessment of pressure and volume during acute alteration in preload to define the end-diastolic pressure-volume relationship (EDPVR) over a range of preloads, the multiple-beat method (see Fig. 30-10). Alternatively, pressure and volume can be assessed over a single-beat, steady-state measurement, and the diastolic portion of the pressure-volume curve can be used to estimate stiffness. This single-beat method is subject to three important limitations. First, the EDPVR is curvilinear, and the stiffness measured at a higher operating volume (operant stiffness) will be higher than that obtained when the single beat is taken at a lower operating volume (Fig. 30-10B). Second, impaired relaxation may also influence the pressure during mid-diastole (Fig. 30-10C). In the normal ventricle, relaxation is brisk and the LV minimum pressure occurs early in diastole, yielding an exponential contour to the mid to late diastolic pressure-volume relationship. Here, only the passive stiffness of the ventricle influences the pressure-volume relationship in mid to late diastole, and the pressure and volume data measured over a single cardiac cycle will fit an exponential relationship that allows calculation of a stiffness constant:

$$P = \alpha \times e^{\beta V}$$

where β is the stiffness constant and α is a curve-fitting constant. However, when relaxation is markedly impaired (Fig. 30-10B), relaxation may continue into mid-diastole to an extent determined by the degree of relaxation impairment (tau), heart rate, and duration of contraction (see earlier). Thus, the LV minimum pressure occurs later in diastole, and the diastolic pressure-volume relationship over the single beat is influenced by relaxation and passive stiffness. This limitation is best addressed by use of preload reduction to define the EDPVR, avoiding measurements in other portions of diastole that may be influenced by relaxation (Fig. 30-10C). Alternatively, mathematical methods to correct for the effect of relaxation on diastolic pressures in the single-beat method have been used.[32,50] Finally, the single-beat method cannot separate the effect

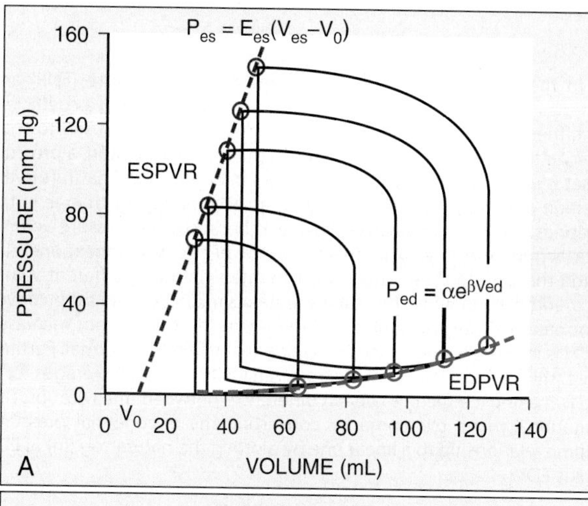

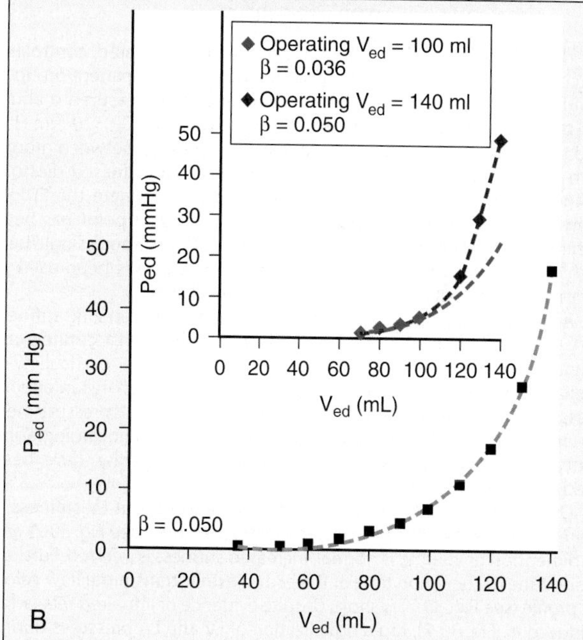

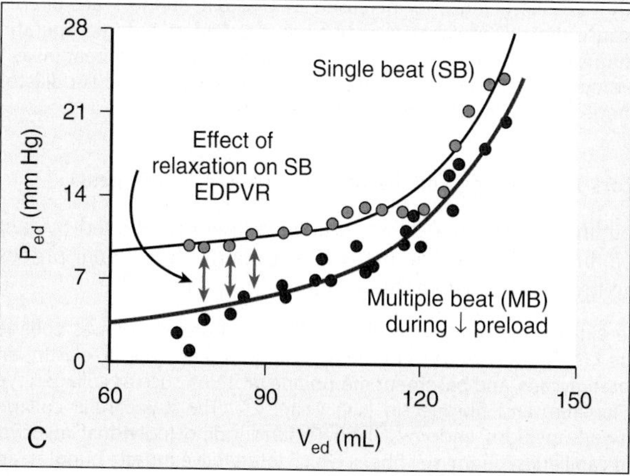

FIGURE 30-10 Invasive assessment of LV diastolic stiffness. **A,** LV pressure-volume loops during acute reduction in preload produced by sudden transient inferior vena cava occlusion. The relationship between pressure and volume at end-systole (ESPVR, red) and end-diastole (EDPVR, blue) defines end-systolic (E_{es}) and end-diastolic stiffness. **B,** Curvilinear EDPVR. Thus, at lower operating volumes (inset, blue), diastolic stiffness as reflected by the diastolic stiffness constant (β) will be lower than when stiffness is assessed at higher operating volumes (inset, red). This is true whether stiffness is assessed by a single-beat or multiple-beat method (see text). **C,** Limitations of using the single-beat method of assessing diastolic stiffness. When diastolic pressure and volume data are collected over a single beat (black) and used to calculate stiffness, the pressure data can be affected by relaxation as well as by the passive properties of the ventricle (see text). The diastolic pressure-volume curves shown here were collected with the single-beat (gray) and multiple-beat (red) methods. This effect is most dramatic in the presence of markedly impaired relaxation, as is present in HFnlEF patients. Thus, accurate assessment of diastolic stiffness using a single steady-state beat without preload reduction requires use of methods to correct for the effect of impaired relaxation on the diastolic pressure-volume relationship (see text). P_{ed} = end-diastolic pressure; P_{es} = end-systolic pressure; V_0 = *x* intercept of the ESPVR; V_{ed} = end-diastolic volume; V_{es} = end-systolic volume. *(**C** modified from Kawaguchi M, Hay I, Fetics B, et al: Combined ventricular systolic and arterial stiffening in patients with heart failure and preserved ejection fraction: Implications for systolic and diastolic reserve limitations. Circulation 107:714, 2003.)*

of external forces (pericardial constraint and ventricular interdependence) on LV diastolic pressures.

Another important limitation to both the single- and multiple-beat methods for assessment of diastolic stiffness involves the desire to express the position and contour of the exponential EDPVR as a single number and to compare that parameter between groups (i.e., HFnlEF and control populations). In the multiple-beat method, the end-diastolic pressure-volume data points during preload reduction are fitted to one of two frequently used exponential equations:

$$EDP = \alpha \times e^{\beta \times EDV}$$

or

$$EDP = P_0 + \alpha \times (e^{\beta \times EDV} - 1)$$

In these equations, which relate end-diastolic pressure (EDP) and end-diastolic volume (EDV), a curve-fitting constant (α) and a coefficient of stiffness (β) are calculated, and the stiffness constant is used to characterize the stiffness of the ventricle. In the second equation, a pressure offset is also calculated (P_0), which allows quantification of a shift in the position of the EDPVR with or without an accompanying change in the steepness of the relationship. However, because the pressure-volume data acquired in any experiment are not perfectly monoexponential, fitting the data to these equations can often yield very different values for α and β, even when the curves appear similar. Both α and β convey information about the stiffness of the ventricle, so if β is not increased but α is increased, one cannot conclude that stiffness is normal. Furthermore, this can result in considerable variability in group averages for α and β, making it difficult to detect differences between small groups. This limitation can be overcome by converting the exponential pressure-volume relationship to a linear one by plotting the natural log (ln) of EDP versus EDV:

$$\ln EDP = \ln \alpha + \beta (EDV)$$

The slope of this relationship (β) can then be compared, controlling for concomitant changes in the offset (ln α) and for the patient group in multiple linear regression analysis. Alternatively, the measured α and β can be used to calculate the volume at a given EDP (e.g., EDP = 20 mm Hg), and that volume (EDV at 20 mm Hg) can be compared between groups with smaller volumes at a common EDP, reflecting increased diastolic stiffness.[51] More recently, a theoretical method to estimate the EDPVR from a single end-diastolic pressure and volume data point has been described, which allows estimates of diastolic stiffness from a single beat with use of invasive or noninvasive data,[52] and this has been used to estimate LV diastolic stiffness in large patient cohorts.[37]

A final limitation to either invasive method of characterizing stiffness with pressure-volume data is the considerable difficulty in accurately and instantaneously measuring volume along with pressure, particularly in clinical studies. Use of a conductance catheter allows such instantaneous pressure-volume measurements. Alternatively, invasive LV pressure measurements, coupled with simultaneously acquired echocardiography, contrast ventriculography, and radionuclide angiography, have been used in clinical studies.

Doppler data can provide indirect information about LV stiffness. If there is Doppler evidence of elevated filling pressures (see Fig. 30-7) and LV dimension or volume is normal, increased stiffness is inferred. Furthermore, if the deceleration time of the early diastolic transmitral flow velocity profile (see Fig. 30-7) is short, despite evidence of impaired relaxation (reduced e′, Fig. 30-7), rapid equalization of LV and LA pressures during early diastolic filling and increased LV diastolic stiffness are inferred. Because these Doppler parameters are acquired at a single operating volume, they are subject to the same limitations as single-beat invasive methods; that is, they reflect operating stiffness at a particular diastolic volume and are influenced by external forces.

Factors Influencing Left Ventricular Diastolic Stiffness

As outlined in Table 30-2, LV diastolic stiffness is affected by factors that influence the cardiac extracellular matrix, the cellular processes at the myocyte level, and the myofibers themselves.[53-56]

The extracellular matrix consists of fibrillar proteins, such as collagen type I (predominant form in the myocardium) and type III, elastin, and proteoglycans, and basement membrane proteins, such as collagen type IV, laminin, and fibronectin (see Chap. 25). The myocardial collagen network includes endomysial fibers surrounding individual myocytes and capillaries; perimysial fibers, which interweave muscle bundles; and epimysium fibers, which form a matrix adjacent to the epicardial and endocardial surfaces. The extracellular matrix is dynamic, with its abundance regulated by many physical, humoral, and inflammatory mediators that modulate collagen production and breakdown (see Chap. 25). The extracellular matrix is increased in conditions associated with HFnlEF, such as hypertensive heart disease and coronary artery disease. Experimental studies have shown that destruction of perimysial fibers by collagenase perfusion results in decreased LV stiffness. Animal models have demonstrated that interventions associated with increases or decreases in myocardial fibrosis are associated with increased or decreased LV diastolic stiffness. Thus, evidence that the extracellular matrix contributes to diastolic dysfunction by increasing diastolic stiffness or contributes to impairment in relaxation by altering regional loading or uniformity is strong and supports the potential therapeutic efficacy of preventing or reducing fibrosis in therapy for HFnlEF. Also, as mentioned earlier, post-translational modification of collagen fibers through formation of nonenzymatic collagen cross-linking (advanced glycation end products) has been shown to increase diastolic stiffness.

As discussed in Chap. 24, the giant molecular spring titin also contributes to myocardial diastolic tension. A number of factors, including titin isoform switches (to a less compliant N2B isoform) and titin phosphorylation state, can affect passive myofiber stiffness, and perturbations in both have been described in HFnlEF.[57-59] Interaction of titin with other signaling molecules and with ion channels may also contribute to the effect of titin on diastolic stiffness. It is believed that alterations in titin may occur in concert with changes in the extracellular matrix, but this interaction is not well defined. Unfortunately, our understanding of the role of alteration in titin and titin interactions in patients with HFnlEF is extremely limited, and much remains to be clarified.

Relaxation is clearly recognized to be sensitive to alterations in energetics and is thus characterized as active, whereas diastolic stiffness is characterized as passive. This distinction is probably inaccurate because reduction in energy supply (as in ischemia) can result in decreased diastolic distensibility, phosphorylation of titin and other myofilament proteins can be acutely regulated, and other factors leading to persistent cross-bridge formation during diastole can occur acutely.

Other structural changes in the myocyte, such as T-tubule density, may also occur in disease states associated with hypertrophy and alter diastolic stiffness.

Evidence for Increased Left Ventricular Diastolic Stiffness

The difficulties inherent in characterizing LV diastolic stiffness in patients have limited studies characterizing ventricular diastolic stiffness in patients with HFnlEF. However, several studies using both invasive and noninvasive estimates of LV stiffness have shown increased LV stiffness in HFnlEF[32,37,58,60-62] compared with age-matched (but not always disease-matched) control cohorts without HF.

Other Contributing Factors

Whereas impaired relaxation and increased diastolic stiffness are now well proven to be present in patients with HFnlEF, other important perturbations in cardiovascular function accompany these impairments in diastolic function and contribute to the HFnlEF phenotype.

Left Ventricular Systolic Dysfunction. Whereas LV *chamber* systolic function (EF and end-systolic elastance) is normal in patients with HFnlEF, numerous studies have shown that at rest, *myocardial* systolic function is impaired in many if not most patients with HFnlEF. Some of these studies have used load-dependent measures, such as Doppler-derived systolic strain[63,64]; others have used load-independent measures of contractility, such as preload recruitable stroke work or stress-corrected midwall fiber shortening[34,65,66] or measures of LV torsion or "twist."[41] Myocardial systolic dysfunction can occur in the setting of a normal EF because concentric remodeling and cross-fiber shortening preserve the extent of endocardial motion relative to the diastolic cavity despite myofiber shortening.[67,68] Although subtle at rest, these abnormalities are associated with impaired prognosis.[65] Perhaps more important, the ability to enhance systolic function with exercise is dramatically impaired,[41,43,44] contributing to impaired reserve function (see later) in HFnlEF.

Vascular Dysfunction. Vascular stiffness increases with age, diabetes, and hypertension and is higher in women, all risk factors for HFnlEF.[16,17] Impaired endothelial function is common in hypertension, diabetes, and atherosclerosis (all common in HFnlEF) and may contribute to impaired ability to dilate systemic, pulmonary, and coronary vasculature during exercise. As mentioned earlier, vascular rarefaction results in decreased microvascular density with aging, hypertension, and diabetes and may further impair flow reserve in the heart and periphery. Thus, vascular dysfunction predisposes to impaired diastolic and systolic dysfunction in HFnlEF. As discussed before, pulmonary vascular function is abnormal in HFnlEF because of chronic pulmonary venous hypertension and age-related changes.[26,28,69]

VENTRICULAR-VASCULAR COUPLING. Chronic changes in vascular stiffness are met by increases in LV systolic stiffness to maintain optimal ventricular-vascular matching (EF) and thus optimal cardiac performance. Vascular stiffening and LV systolic stiffening (end-systolic elastance, E_{es}) are increased in HFnlEF compared with normal disease-free subjects but are similar in HFnlEF and patients with hypertension but no HF.[34,37] The mechanisms whereby LV systolic stiffness increases to maintain EF in HFnlEF are not fully understood. A study showed that LV systolic stiffening is driven by increases in myocardial contractility in patients with hypertension but by increases in passive stiffening in HFnlEF.[65] Whereas ventricular-vascular coupling helps maintain stroke volume and mechanical efficiency, increases in E_{es} may have adverse effects. Increases in E_{es} indicate increased sensitivity of systolic pressure to changes in volume (as demonstrated by the steeper slope of the end-systolic pressure-volume relationship). Thus, volume overload in such individuals could be associated with greater increases in systolic blood pressure. Together, increases in arterial and systolic stiffness promote load-induced impairment in LV relaxation.[33] Whereas coupling of vascular and ventricular systolic stiffness is preserved at rest in HFnlEF, such coupling may not be preserved during exercise.

IMPAIRED RESERVE FUNCTION. In its advanced stages or in the setting of marked volume overload, HFnlEF patients may have resting symptoms. However, many patients have only exertional symptoms, and HF is, fundamentally, a condition characterized by exercise intolerance. Impaired vascular reserve (ability to vasodilate during exercise), ventricular systolic reserve, ventricular diastolic reserve, and ventricular-vascular coupling reserve have now been established in HFnlEF and contribute to exertional intolerance.[41,43,44]

ATRIAL DYSFUNCTION. Although most discussion has centered on ventricular function in HFnlEF, atrial function may also play an important role in the pathophysiologic process of HFnlEF. Early- and mid-diastolic LV (and thus LA) pressures as well as systolic atrial pressures (atrial V wave) are important contributors to mean LA pressure, which is therefore the resistance to filling that the pulmonary venous system faces. Whereas LA systolic function compensates for reduced early filling in the earlier stages of HFnlEF,[49] atrial failure eventually occurs. Indeed, an often forgotten hemodynamic hallmark of restrictive cardiomyopathy is the presence of large V waves in the LA pressure waveform in the absence of mitral regurgitation, reflecting reduced LA compliance. Reduced LA compliance has been shown to potently influence the development of pulmonary arterial hypertension in mitral valve disease and may play a similar role in HFnlEF. Reduced LA systolic function limits LV filling in the setting of impaired relaxation and necessitates higher mean LA pressures to augment early diastolic filling. Thus, enlarged and dysfunctional atria may contribute to the pathophysiologic process of HFnlEF.

NEUROHUMORAL ACTIVATION. Neurohumoral activation plays a fundamental role in the progression of HF with reduced EF. Activation of the sympathetic nervous system, aldosterone, and the natriuretic peptide system occurs in HF regardless of EF,[14,70] and although natriuretic peptide levels are lower in HFnlEF, levels of catecholamines and aldosterone are similar in the limited study to date. Whether other counterregulatory hormones such as renin, angiotensin II, and endothelin are activated in HFnlEF remains to be determined.

PERIPHERAL FACTORS AND ERGOREFLEX CONTROL. Ventilatory drive and vascular tone are affected by alterations in mechanical and metabolic sensor stimulation in peripheral muscle during exercise, and perturbations in reflex control during exercise (ergoreflex) have been well described in HF with reduced EF, in which the magnitude of the disruption is greater in subjects with reduced muscle mass.[71] Although impaired ergoreflex control has not yet been studied in HFnlEF, such factors may well contribute to effort intolerance in the elderly HFnlEF population.

VOLUME OVERLOAD WITHOUT DIASTOLIC DYSFUNCTION. On average, LV cavity dimensions or volumes are normal in patients with HFnlEF. However, the potential for a subgroup of HFnlEF patients to have LV dilation has been previously reported.[31,72] In persons with LV dilation and normal EF, cardiac output is increased, and there may be a "high-output" subset of patients with HFnlEF with increased LV diastolic pressures due to volume overload without underlying diastolic dysfunction. Whereas the potential for increased volumes in a subset of patients and the importance of volume overload should be acknowledged, most studies indicate that this is a small subset of the HFnlEF population.

Therapy

In general, the management of HFnlEF has two objectives. The first is to treat the presenting syndrome of HF—relieve resting or exercise-associated venous congestion and eliminate precipitating factors. The second is to reverse the factors responsible for diastolic dysfunction or other perturbations that lead to HFnlEF. Both nonpharmacologic and pharmacologic strategies may be used to achieve these objectives. Present treatment strategies for HFnlEF are largely based on assumptions of its pathophysiologic mechanisms and on extrapolations from proven strategies used in HF with a reduced EF.

Nonpharmacologic Therapy

General measures that may be used in the management of patients with chronic HFnlEF are not different from those pursued in patients with HF with a reduced EF. They include daily monitoring of weight, attention to diet and lifestyle, patient education, and close medical follow-up. In patients with HFnlEF, aggressive control of hypertension, tachycardia, and other potential precipitants of HF decompensation should be emphasized. The role of exercise training in patients with HFnlEF has also been explored.[73] Although there are no adequate clinical trials with appropriate outcome endpoints, such as increased longevity, decreased symptoms, or improved quality of life, to prove the benefits of exercise training in patients with HFnlEF definitively, several clinical and experimental studies have suggested that exercise training would be beneficial for such patients.[2,3,18]

Medical and Surgical Therapy

In contrast to the treatment of HF with reduced EF (see Chap. 28), information to guide the pharmacologic therapy for patients with HFnlEF is lacking. Limited available data from clinical studies and randomized controlled clinical trials are reviewed here, followed by largely empiric recommendations for therapy.

CLINICAL STUDIES. Small controlled studies have been performed with various standard HF drugs in patients with HFnlEF. The drugs used have included ACE inhibitors, angiotensin receptor antagonists, beta blockers, and calcium channel blockers. These trials have, however, been small or have produced inconclusive results.[74]

Randomized Controlled Clinical Trials

The Digitalis Investigation Group (DIG) trial included a small subgroup of patients with HFnlEF. In the HFnlEF group, digoxin did not alter the primary endpoint of HF hospitalization or cardiovascular mortality (**Fig. 30-11A**) but did reduce HF hospitalizations.[75] Unfortunately, total cardiovascular hospitalizations were not reduced because of an increased rate of admissions for unstable angina, which completely negated the beneficial effect of reduced HF hospitalizations.

In the CHARM-Preserved Trial,[76] HF patients with an EF higher than 40% were randomized to candesartan (an angiotensin receptor antagonist) or placebo in addition to standard therapy. Fewer patients in the candesartan group than in the placebo group reached the primary endpoint of cardiovascular death or HF hospitalization, a finding that reached statistical significance only after adjustment for nonsignificant differences in baseline characteristics (Fig. 30-11B).

The I-PRESERVE trial tested the angiotensin receptor blocker irbesartan in 4128 patients who were at least 60 years of age and had New York Heart Association Class II, III, or IV HF and an EF of at least 45%.[77] The primary composite outcome was death from any cause or hospitalization for a cardiovascular cause (HF, myocardial infarction, unstable angina, arrhythmia, or stroke). Secondary outcomes included death from HF or hospitalization for HF, death from any cause and from cardiovascular causes, and quality of life. Irbesartan had no effect on any of the prespecified outcome measures (Fig. 30-11C).

In the PEP-CHF trial, patients older than 70 years with chronic HF and normal or near-normal EF were randomized to perindopril (an

CH 30

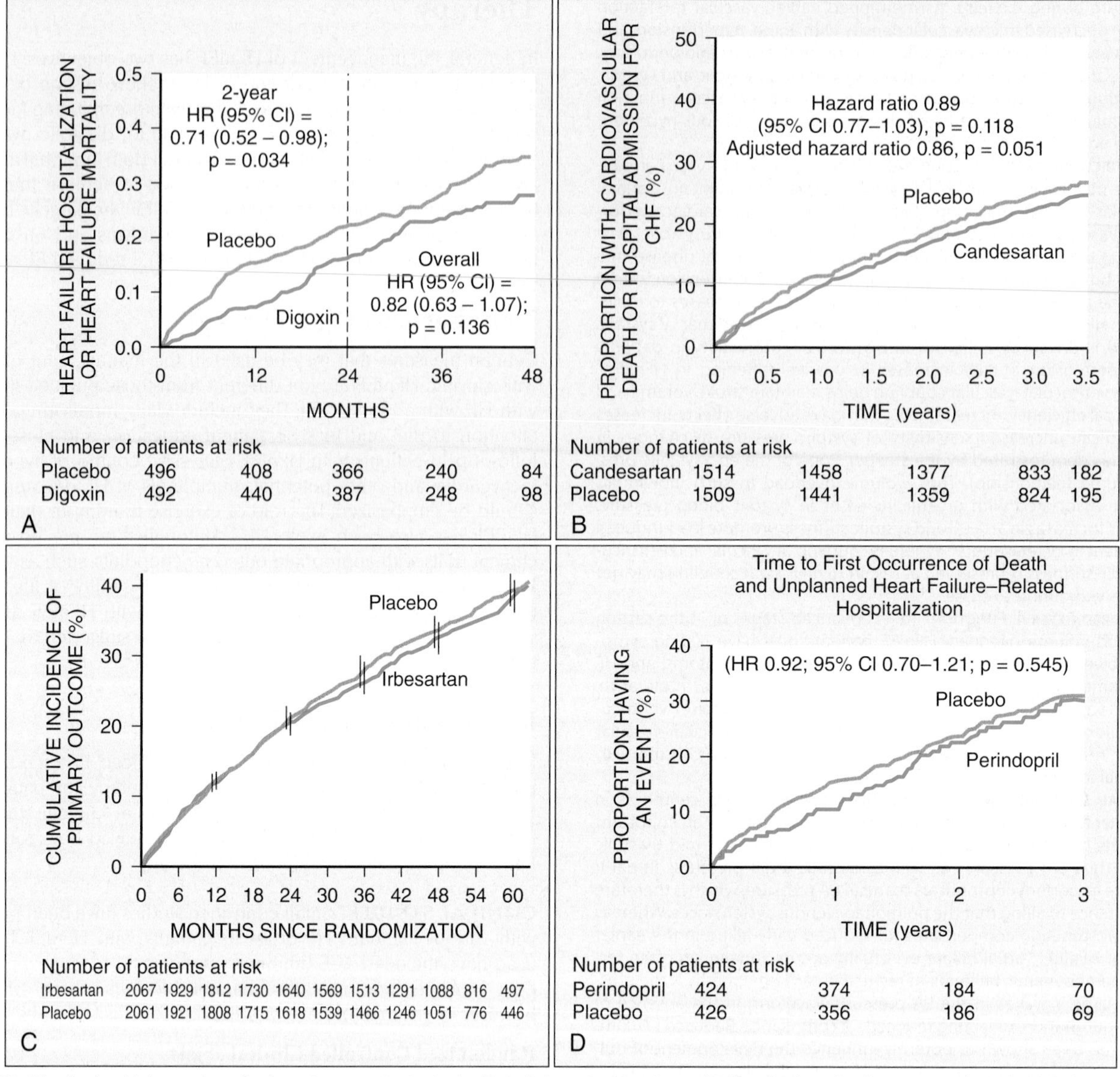

FIGURE 30-11 Kaplan-Meier analyses for the primary endpoint in the Digitalis Investigation Group (DIG) trial substudy of patients with HFnlEF **(A)**, the Candesartan in Heart Failure: Assessment of Reduction in Morbidity and Mortality (CHARM)–Preserved trial **(B)**, the Irbesartan in patients with heart failure and preserved ejection fraction (I-PRESERVE) trial **(C)**, and the perindopril in elderly people with chronic heart failure (PEP-CHF) trial **(D)**. See text for discussion. CI = confidence interval; HR = hazard ratio. *(**A** from Ahmed A, Rich MW, Fleg JL, et al: Effects of digoxin on morbidity and mortality in diastolic heart failure: The ancillary digitalis investigation group trial. Circulation 114:397, 2006. **B** from Yusuf S, Pfeffer MA, Swedberg K, et al: Effects of candesartan in patients with chronic heart failure and preserved left-ventricular ejection fraction: The CHARM-Preserved Trial. Lancet 362:777, 2003. **C** from Massie BM, Carson PE, McMurray JJ, et al: Irbesartan in patients with heart failure and preserved ejection fraction. N Engl J Med. 359:2456, 2008. **D** from Cleland JG, Tendera M, Adamus J, et al: The perindopril in elderly people with chronic heart failure [PEP-CHF] study. Eur Heart J 27:2338, 2006.)*

ACE inhibitor) or placebo.[78] The primary endpoint was a composite of all-cause mortality or unplanned HF-related hospitalization. Both enrollment and event rates were lower than anticipated, and there was a high rate of cessation of blinded therapy, with crossover to open-label ACE inhibitor use in both groups. These factors limited the strength of the study, which did not show significant reduction in the primary endpoint (Fig. 30-11D). Some trends toward benefit, primarily driven by reduction in HF-related hospitalizations, were observed at 1 year, when crossover therapy rates were lower.

The SENIORS trial tested the effect of the beta$_1$-selective blocker nebivolol in patients with HF.[79] Nebivolol also has vasodilator properties thought to be related to its effects on nitric oxide release. This trial was not restricted to those with normal EF. There was a modest but significant reduction in the primary endpoint of all-cause mortality or cardiovascular hospitalizations, which was driven primarily by the effect on hospitalizations. Prespecified subgroup analysis in patients with EF less than versus more than 35% did not detect any trends toward reduced benefit in those with higher EF. Unfortunately, there were very few patients with EF higher than 50% in the trial.

The Hong Kong diastolic heart failure study[80] randomized 150 patients with HFnlEF (EF > 45%) to diuretics alone, diuretics plus irbesartan, or diuretics plus ramipril. Quality of life assessment, 6-minute walk test, and Doppler echocardiography were performed at baseline and at 12, 24, and 52 weeks. The quality of life score and 6-minute walk test increased similarly, and hospitalizations were similar in all three groups. Modest improvements in Doppler systolic and diastolic indices and NT-proBNP levels were seen only in the irbesartan and ramipril groups.

A number of ongoing clinical trials in HFnlEF are testing novel treatment strategies, including (but not limited to) endothelin antagonists, aldosterone antagonists (TOPCAT trial), sildenafil (RELAX trial), atrial pacing (RESET trial), and baroreflex control devices (Rheos diastolic heart failure trial). (See www.clinicaltrials.gov.)

Current Therapeutic Recommendations

Current recommendations for treatment of patients with HFnlEF are outlined in Table 28G-9 in the Heart Failure Guidelines).[2,3] In addition, it is important to treat other contributing comorbidities and risk factors aggressively, such as diabetes, hyperlipidemia, renal dysfunction, and renal vascular disease. One retrospective study has shown that statin use, but not the use of beta blockers, ACE inhibitors, or calcium channel blockers, is associated with improved survival in patients with HFnlEF.[81] Until more clinical trials are performed in patients with HFnlEF, the empiric nature of therapeutic recommendations and their uncertain benefit must be recognized.

Future Perspectives

Better information on regional and ethnic variation in the characteristics and outcomes of patients with HFnlEF is needed. A better understanding of the earlier phases of the syndrome (when therapy might be more effective) is needed. A better understanding of how diastolic dysfunction and other contributors interact to result in the syndrome of HFnlEF is needed as it may be possible that only pluripotent therapies will have beneficial effects. Careful consideration needs to be given to treatment goals and clinical trial outcomes. Mortality endpoints may be less relevant in the elderly patients, in whom mortality may be driven by comorbidities, and endpoints such as improved reserve function, exercise capacity, quality of life, and reduced lifetime medical resource use may be more meaningful endpoints in some populations of patients. The potential therapeutic effect of beta blockers remains uncertain despite the SENIORS trial, and there should be equipoise for a randomized clinical trial. Concerns remain about overdiagnosis and underdiagnosis of HFnlEF, and better diagnostic tools, particularly surrogates for rest and exercise hemodynamics, are needed because available biomarkers are of limited value as outlined before. More work in humans and relevant animal models is needed to better define the basic mechanisms influencing cardiac remodeling and diastolic function in the elderly. Most basic studies are done in young rodents, and these observations may or may not be relevant to this syndrome, in which the interaction between age and cardiovascular disease plays such an obvious role.

REFERENCES

Historical Perspective, Nomenclature and Classification

1. Owan T, Hodge D, Herges D, et al: Heart failure with preserved ejection fraction: Trends in prevalence and outcomes. N Engl J Med 355:308, 2006.
2. Heart Failure Society of America: Executive summary: HFSA 2006 Comprehensive Heart Failure Practice Guideline. J Card Fail 12:10, 2006.
3. Hunt SA, Abraham WT, Chin MH, et al: ACC/AHA 2005 Guideline Update for the Diagnosis and Management of Chronic Heart Failure in the Adult—Summary Article: A Report of the American College of Cardiology/American Heart Association Task Force on Practice Guidelines (Writing Committee to Update the 2001 Guidelines for the Evaluation and Management of Heart Failure): Developed in Collaboration With the American College of Chest Physicians and the International Society for Heart and Lung Transplantation: Endorsed by the Heart Rhythm Society. Circ Heart Fail 112:1825, 2005.

Epidemiology and Natural History

4. Redfield MM, Jacobsen SJ, Burnett JC Jr, et al: Burden of systolic and diastolic ventricular dysfunction in the community: Appreciating the scope of the heart failure epidemic. JAMA 289:194, 2003.
5. Owan TE, Redfield MM: Epidemiology of diastolic heart failure. Prog Cardiovasc Dis 47:320, 2005.
6. Hogg K, Swedberg K, McMurray J: Heart failure with preserved left ventricular systolic function; epidemiology, clinical characteristics, and prognosis. J Am Coll Cardiol 43:317, 2004.
7. Bhatia RS, Tu JV, Lee DS, et al: Outcome of heart failure with preserved ejection fraction in a population-based study. N Engl J Med 355:260, 2006.
8. Yancy CW, Lopatin M, Stevenson LW, et al: Clinical presentation, management, and in-hospital outcomes of patients admitted with acute decompensated heart failure with preserved systolic function: A report from the Acute Decompensated Heart Failure National Registry (ADHERE) Database. J Am Coll Cardiol 47:76, 2006.
9. Ceia F, Fonseca C, Mota T, et al: Prevalence of chronic heart failure in Southwestern Europe: The EPICA study. Eur J Heart Fail 4:531, 2002.
10. Curtis JP, Sokol SI, Wang Y, et al: The association of left ventricular ejection fraction, mortality, and cause of death in stable outpatients with heart failure. J Am Coll Cardiol 42:736, 2003.
11. Henkel DM, Redfield MM, Weston SA, et al: Death in heart failure: A community perspective. Circ Heart Fail 1:91, 2008.
12. Dunlay SM, Redfield MM, Weston SA, et al: Hospitalizations after heart failure diagnosis a community perspective. J Am Coll Cardiol 54:1695, 2009.
13. Smith GL, Masoudi FA, Vaccarino V, et al: Outcomes in heart failure patients with preserved ejection fraction: Mortality, readmission, and functional decline. J Am Coll Cardiol 41:1510, 2003.

Clinical Features

14. Kitzman DW, Little WC, Brubaker PH, et al: Pathophysiological characterization of isolated diastolic heart failure in comparison to systolic heart failure. JAMA 288:2144, 2002.
15. Choudhury L, Gheorghiade M, Bonow RO: Coronary artery disease in patients with heart failure and preserved systolic function. Am J Cardiol 89:719, 2002.
16. Redfield MM, Jacobsen SJ, Borlaug BA, et al: Age- and gender-related ventricular-vascular stiffening: A community-based study. Circ Heart Fail 112:2254, 2005.
17. Chen CH, Nakayama M, Nevo E, et al: Coupled systolic-ventricular and vascular stiffening with age: Implications for pressure regulation and cardiac reserve in the elderly. J Am Coll Cardiol 32:1221, 1998.
18. Arbab-Zadeh A, Dijk E, Prasad A, et al: Effect of aging and physical activity on left ventricular compliance. Circ Heart Fail 110:1799, 2004.
19. Diamond JA, Phillips RA: Hypertensive heart disease. Hypertens Res 28:191, 2005.
20. Hoenig MR, Bianchi C, Rosenzweig A, et al: The cardiac microvasculature in hypertension, cardiac hypertrophy and diastolic heart failure. Curr Vasc Pharmacol 6:292, 2008.
21. Tsang TS, Gersh BJ, Appleton CP, et al: Left ventricular diastolic dysfunction as a predictor of the first diagnosed nonvalvular atrial fibrillation in 840 elderly men and women. J Am Coll Cardiol 40:1636, 2002.
22. Powell BD, Redfield MM, Bybee KA, et al: Association of obesity with left ventricular remodeling and diastolic dysfunction in patients without coronary artery disease. Am J Cardiol 98:116, 2006.
23. Smith GL, Lichtman JH, Bracken MB, et al: Renal impairment and outcomes in heart failure: Systematic review and meta-analysis. J Am Coll Cardiol 47:1987, 2006.
24. Forman DE, Butler J, Wang Y, et al: Incidence, predictors at admission, and impact of worsening renal function among patients hospitalized with heart failure. J Am Coll Cardiol 43:61, 2004.
25. Hoeper MM, Barbera JA, Channick RN, et al: Diagnosis, assessment, and treatment of non-pulmonary arterial hypertension pulmonary hypertension. J Am Coll Cardiol 54:S85, 2009.
26. Tolle JJ, Waxman AB, Van Horn TL, et al: Exercise-induced pulmonary arterial hypertension. Circ Heart Fail 118:2183, 2008.
27. Shapiro BP, McGoon MD, Redfield MM: Unexplained pulmonary hypertension in elderly patients. Chest 131:94, 2007.
28. Lam CS, Roger VL, Rodeheffer RJ, et al: Pulmonary hypertension in heart failure with preserved ejection fraction: A community-based study. J Am Coll Cardiol 53:1119, 2009.
29. Kjaergaard J, Akkan D, Iversen KK, et al: Prognostic importance of pulmonary hypertension in patients with heart failure. Am J Cardiol 99:1146, 2007.
30. Jencks SF, Williams MV, Coleman EA: Rehospitalizations among patients in the Medicare fee-for-service program. N Engl J Med 360:1418, 2009.
31. Chen HH, Lainchbury JG, Senni M, et al: Diastolic heart failure in the community: Clinical profile, natural history, therapy, and impact of proposed diagnostic criteria. J Card Fail 8:279, 2002.
32. Zile MR, Baicu CF, Gaasch WH: Diastolic heart failure—abnormalities in active relaxation and passive stiffness of the left ventricle. N Engl J Med 350:1953, 2004.
33. Kawaguchi M, Hay I, Fetics B, et al: Combined ventricular systolic and arterial stiffening in patients with heart failure and preserved ejection fraction: Implications for systolic and diastolic reserve limitations. Circ Heart Fail 107:714, 2003.
34. Borlaug BA, Melenovsky V, Russell SD, et al: Impaired chronotropic and vasodilator reserves limit exercise capacity in patients with heart failure and a preserved ejection fraction. Circ Heart Fail 114:2138, 2006.
35. Melenovsky V, Borlaug BA, Rosen B, et al: Cardiovascular features of heart failure with preserved ejection fraction versus nonfailing hypertensive left ventricular hypertrophy in the urban Baltimore community: The role of atrial remodeling/dysfunction. J Am Coll Cardiol 49:198, 2007.
36. Bursi F, Weston SA, Redfield MM, et al: Systolic and diastolic heart failure in the community. JAMA 296: 2209, 2006.
37. Lam CS, Roger VL, Rodeheffer RJ, et al: Cardiac structure and ventricular-vascular function in persons with heart failure and preserved ejection fraction from Olmsted County, Minnesota. Circ Heart Fail 115:1982, 2007.
38. Iwanaga Y, Nishi I, Furuichi S, et al: B-type natriuretic peptide strongly reflects diastolic wall stress in patients with chronic heart failure: Comparison between systolic and diastolic heart failure. J Am Coll Cardiol 47:742, 2006.

Pathophysiology

39. Bilchick KC, Duncan JG, Ravi R, et al: Heart failure–associated alterations in troponin I phosphorylation impair ventricular relaxation-afterload and force-frequency responses and systolic function. Am J Physiol Heart Circ Physiol 292:H318, 2007.
40. Perrino C, Naga Prasad SV, Mao L, et al: Intermittent pressure overload triggers hypertrophy-independent cardiac dysfunction and vascular rarefaction. J Clin Invest 116:1547, 2006.
41. Tan YT, Wenzelburger F, Lee E, et al: The pathophysiology of heart failure with normal ejection fraction: Exercise echocardiography reveals complex abnormalities of both systolic and diastolic ventricular function involving torsion, untwist, and longitudinal motion. J Am Coll Cardiol 54:36-46, 2009.
42. Phan TT, Nallur Shivu G, Abozguia K, et al: Impaired heart rate recovery and chronotropic incompetence in patients with heart failure with preserved ejection fraction. Circ Heart Fail 3:29, 2010.
43. Phan TT, Abozguia K, Nallur Shivu G, et al: Heart failure with preserved ejection fraction is characterized by dynamic impairment of active relaxation and contraction of the left ventricle on exercise and associated with myocardial energy deficiency. J Am Coll Cardiol 54:402, 2009.
44. Ennezat PV, Lefetz Y, Marechaux S, et al: Left ventricular abnormal response during dynamic exercise in patients with heart failure and preserved left ventricular ejection fraction at rest. J Card Fail 14:475, 2008.
45. Chattopadhyay S, Alamgir MF, Nikitin NP, et al: Lack of diastolic reserve in patients with heart failure and normal ejection fraction. Circ Heart Fail 3:35, 2010.
46. Braz JC, Gregory K, Pathak A, et al: PKC-alpha regulates cardiac contractility and propensity toward heart failure. Nat Med 10:248, 2004.
47. Munagala VK, Hart CY, Burnett JC Jr, et al: Ventricular structure and function in aged dogs with renal hypertension: A model of experimental diastolic heart failure. Circ Heart Fail 111:1128, 2005.

48. Hay I, Rich J, Ferber P, et al: Role of impaired myocardial relaxation in the production of elevated left ventricular filling pressure. Am J Physiol Heart Circ Physiol 288:H1203, 2005.
49. Phan TT, Abozguia K, Shivu GN, et al: Increased atrial contribution to left ventricular filling compensates for impaired early filling during exercise in heart failure with preserved ejection fraction. J Card Fail 15:890, 2009.
50. Jaber WA, Lam CS, Meyer DM, et al: Revisiting methods for assessing and comparing left ventricular diastolic stiffness: Impact of relaxation, external forces, hypertrophy, and comparators. Am J Physiol Heart Circ Physiol 293:H2738, 2007.
51. Burkhoff D, Mirsky I, Suga H: Assessment of systolic and diastolic ventricular properties via pressure-volume analysis: A guide for clinical, translational, and basic researchers. Am J Physiol Heart Circ Physiol 289:H501, 2005.
52. Klotz S, Hay I, Dickstein ML, et al: Single-beat estimation of end-diastolic pressure-volume relationship: A novel method with potential for noninvasive application. Am J Physiol Heart Circ Physiol 291:H403, 2006.
53. Zile MR, Brutsaert DL: New concepts in diastolic dysfunction and diastolic heart failure: Part I: Diagnosis, prognosis, and measurements of diastolic function. Circ Heart Fail 105:1387, 2002.
54. Zile MR, Brutsaert DL: New concepts in diastolic dysfunction and diastolic heart failure: Part II: Causal mechanisms and treatment. Circulation 105:1503, 2002.
55. Katz AM, Zile MR: New molecular mechanism in diastolic heart failure. Circ Heart Fail 113:1922, 2006.
56. Kass DA, Bronzwaer JG, Paulus WJ: What mechanisms underlie diastolic dysfunction in heart failure? Circ Res 94:1533, 2004.
57. Borbely A, Falcao-Pires I, van Heerebeek L, et al: Hypophosphorylation of the Stiff N2B titin isoform raises cardiomyocyte resting tension in failing human myocardium. Circ Res 104:780, 2009.
58. Borbely A, van der Velden J, Papp Z, et al: Cardiomyocyte stiffness in diastolic heart failure. Circ Heart Fail 111:774, 2005.
59. Borbely A, van Heerebeek L, Paulus WJ: Transcriptional and posttranslational modifications of titin: Implications for diastole. Circ Res 104:12, 2009.
60. Liu C-P, Ting C-T, Lawrence W, et al: Arrhythmias/drugs: Diminished contractile response to increased heart rate in intact human left ventricular hypertrophy: Systolic versus diastolic determinants. Circ Heart Fail 88:1893, 1993.
61. van Heerebeek L, Hamdani N, Handoko ML, et al: Diastolic stiffness of the failing diabetic heart: Importance of fibrosis, advanced glycation end products, and myocyte resting tension. Circ Heart Fail 117:43, 2008.
62. Westermann D, Kasner M, Steendijk P, et al: Role of left ventricular stiffness in heart failure with normal ejection fraction. Circ Heart Fail 117:2051, 2008.
63. Yip G, Wang M, Zhang Y, et al: Left ventricular long axis function in diastolic heart failure is reduced in both diastole and systole: Time for a redefinition? Heart 87:121, 2002.
64. Yu CM, Lin H, Yang H, et al: Progression of systolic abnormalities in patients with "isolated" diastolic heart failure and diastolic dysfunction. Circ Heart Fail 105:1195, 2002.
65. Borlaug BA, Lam CS, Roger VL, et al: Contractility and ventricular systolic stiffening in hypertensive heart disease insights into the pathogenesis of heart failure with preserved ejection fraction. J Am Coll Cardiol 54:410, 2009.
66. Vinch CS, Aurigemma GP, Simon HU, et al: Analysis of left ventricular systolic function using midwall mechanics in patients >60 years of age with hypertensive heart disease and heart failure. Am J Cardiol 96:1299, 2005.
67. Shimizu G, Hirota Y, Kita Y, et al: Left ventricular midwall mechanics in systemic arterial hypertension. Circ Heart Fail 83:1676, 1991.
68. de Simone G, Devereux RB: Rationale of echocardiographic assessment of left ventricular wall stress and midwall mechanics in hypertensive heart disease. Eur J Echocardiogr 3:192, 2002.
69. Lam CS, Borlaug BA, Kane GC, et al: Age-associated increases in pulmonary artery systolic pressure in the general population. Circ Heart Fail 119:2663, 2009.
70. Guder G, Bauersachs J, Frantz S, et al: Complementary and incremental mortality risk prediction by cortisol and aldosterone in chronic heart failure. Circ Heart Fail 115:1754, 2007.
71. Piepoli MF, Kaczmarek A, Francis DP, et al: Reduced peripheral skeletal muscle mass and abnormal reflex physiology in chronic heart failure. Circ Heart Fail 114:126, 2006.
72. Maurer MS, King DL, El-Khoury Rumbarger L, et al: Left heart failure with a normal ejection fraction: Identification of different pathophysiologic mechanisms. J Card Fail 11:177, 2005.

Therapy

73. Pina IL, Apstein CS, Balady GJ, et al: Exercise and heart failure: A statement from the American Heart Association Committee on exercise, rehabilitation, and prevention. Circ Heart Fail 107:1210, 2003.
74. Little WC, Brucks S: Therapy for diastolic heart failure. Prog Cardiovasc Dis 47:380, 2005.
75. Ahmed A, Rich MW, Fleg JL, et al: Effects of digoxin on morbidity and mortality in diastolic heart failure: The ancillary digitalis investigation group trial. Circ Heart Fail 114:397, 2006.
76. Yusuf S, Pfeffer MA, Swedberg K, et al: Effects of candesartan in patients with chronic heart failure and preserved left-ventricular ejection fraction: The CHARM-Preserved Trial. Lancet 362:777, 2003.
77. Massie BM, Carson PE, McMurray JJ, et al: Irbesartan in patients with heart failure and preserved ejection fraction. N Engl J Med 359:2456, 2008.
78. Cleland JG, Tendera M, Adamus J, et al: The perindopril in elderly people with chronic heart failure (PEP-CHF) study. Eur Heart J 27:2338, 2006.
79. Flather MD, Shibata MC, Coats AJ, et al: Randomized trial to determine the effect of nebivolol on mortality and cardiovascular hospital admission in elderly patients with heart failure (SENIORS). Eur Heart J 26:215, 2005.
80. Yip GW, Wang M, Wang T, et al: The Hong Kong diastolic heart failure study: A randomised controlled trial of diuretics, irbesartan and ramipril on quality of life, exercise capacity, left ventricular global and regional function in heart failure with a normal ejection fraction. Heart 94:573, 2008.
81. Fukuta H, Sane DC, Brucks S, et al: Statin therapy may be associated with lower mortality in patients with diastolic heart failure: A preliminary report. Circ Heart Fail 112:357, 2005.

CHAPTER 31 Surgical Management of Heart Failure

Michael A. Acker and Mariell Jessup

In the current era of managing patients with heart failure with a depressed ejection fraction, clinicians frequently encounter optimally treated patients who remain symptomatic. Indeed, despite the variety of available medical therapies and electrophysiologic interventions, such as biventricular pacemakers and implantable cardiac defibrillators (see Chap. 29), many heart failure patients are still left with a reduced quality of life and a poor prognosis. In a subpopulation of these patients, surgical intervention may be appropriate to alleviate ischemia, to attenuate valvular dysfunction, to reverse or to reduce mechanical disadvantages caused by ventricular remodeling, and finally to perform cardiac transplantation when all other treatment options have failed. In this chapter, we discuss the surgical management of patients with heart failure secondary to a low ejection fraction. The medical management of patients with a reduced ejection fraction is discussed in Chap. 28, and the role of circulatory assist devices is discussed in Chap. 32.

Coronary Artery Revascularization

Ischemic Cardiomyopathy

The term *ischemic cardiomyopathy* is used to describe the myocardial dysfunction that arises secondary to occlusive or obstructive coronary artery disease (see Chap. 57). Although ischemic cardiomyopathy was considered the second most common cause of heart failure (after hypertension) in the Framingham Study (see Chap. 28), ischemic cardiomyopathy is now recognized as the most common cause of heart failure in clinical trials. This section focuses on the impact and outcome of surgical coronary artery revascularization in patients with ischemic cardiomyopathy.

Ischemic cardiomyopathy can be envisioned as three interrelated pathophysiologic processes: *myocardial hibernation,* defined as persistent contractile dysfunction at rest, caused by reduced coronary blood flow that can be partially or completely restored to normal by myocardial revascularization; *myocardial stunning,* wherein the viable myocardium may demonstrate prolonged but reversible postischemic contractile dysfunction caused by the generation of oxygen-derived free radicals on reperfusion and by a loss of sensitivity of contractile filaments to calcium; and irreversible *myocyte cell death,* leading to ventricular remodeling and contractile dysfunction.

Selection of Patients for Coronary Artery Revascularization

No randomized clinical trials have evaluated the outcomes of revascularization in patients with advanced ischemic cardiomyopathy. As discussed in Chap. 57, the three major randomized clinical trials that have compared coronary artery bypass grafting (CABG) with medical management (the Veterans Administration Cooperative Study, the European Coronary Surgery Study, and the Coronary Artery Surgery Study) have all excluded patients with heart failure or severe left ventricular (LV) dysfunction.[1] Several clinical factors play a major role in the decision-making process with respect to selection of suitable heart failure patients to undergo coronary artery revascularization, including the presence of angina, severity of heart failure symptoms, LV dimensions, degree of hemodynamic compromise, and comorbidities. Other major technical issues to be considered are the adequacy of target vessels for revascularization and an adequate conduit strategy. The most important determinant, however, is the extent of jeopardized but still viable myocardium (see Chap. 57). Current studies have suggested that for a significant improvement in heart failure symptoms and LV function as well as for improvement in survival to occur after coronary revascularization, at least 25% of the myocardium should be viable.[2]

Risks of Coronary Artery Bypass Grafting

The perioperative risks in patients with severe LV dysfunction range from 2% to nearly 10%, depending on the availability of targets and their viability, right ventricular dysfunction, advanced heart failure symptoms (New York Heart Association [NYHA] Class IV), increased LV end-diastolic pressure, comorbidities of advanced age, peripheral vascular disease, and chronic obstructive pulmonary disease.[3,4] The Society of Thoracic Surgeons (STS)–predicted mortality for a 70-year-old patient with no comorbidities but with a 20% LV ejection fraction (LVEF) in 2006 was 1.6%. This is compared with a 0.9% risk for a same-aged man with a normal ejection fraction. Compared with patients with an LVEF of 40% or higher, patients with LVEFs between 20% and 39% or below 20% had 1.5- and 3.4-fold increases in perioperative mortality, respectively.[1] Furthermore, mortality rates increase substantially when the LVEF is below 20% or when the heart failure is severe (NYHA Class IV).

Studies have indicated that for patients with clinical heart failure, perioperative mortality rates will range from approximately 2.6% to 8.7%, depending on age and presence of one or more comorbid conditions.[1] Pocar and associates[3] found a 30-day mortality of 4.4% in 45 consecutive angina-free patients with NYHA Class III-IV, LVEF below 35%, and significant viability by positron emission tomography (PET). Predictors of death included LV end-diastolic pressure above 25 mm Hg, age older than 70 years, and significant peripheral vascular disease. In the CABG Patch trial, patients without angina or heart failure had a perioperative mortality of 1.3%. The mortality increased to 4.8% for patients with no angina and mild heart failure, NYHA Class I or II, and 7.4% with no angina and NYHA Class III or IV heart failure.[5] Importantly, viability imaging was not used to stratify these outcomes. For cardiogenic shock after myocardial infarction, the results of emergent CABG are poor but still better than medical therapy. The SHOCK Trial (Should We Emergently Revascularize Occluded Coronaries for Cardiogenic Shock?) gave 1-year mortality after CABG of 42% and 56% for patients in cardiogenic shock. This is compared with 56% and 75% with medical therapy alone.[6] Stabilization of the patients with the use of an intra-aortic balloon pump decreased in-hospital mortality but had no effect on 1-year survival. More recently, smaller experiences with percutaneous partial pumps, such as the Impella and TandemHeart devices, suggest that perioperative mortality can be improved after revascularization, but these results have not yet been confirmed with a larger experience.

Benefits of Coronary Artery Bypass Grafting

The beneficial effect of revascularization should, theoretically, result from improved blood flow to hypoperfused but viable myocardium, with a subsequent improvement in LV function and clinical outcomes. Alleviation of ischemia may also lessen the tendency toward proarrhythmias, thereby reducing the incidence of sudden cardiac death. Accordingly, coronary artery revascularization has the potential to improve symptoms of heart failure, LV function, and survival.

IMPROVEMENT IN LEFT VENTRICULAR FUNCTION. A review of pooled viability data demonstrated that significant viability (25% to 30%) predicted an improvement in LVEF. Nuclear studies, PET, and dobutamine echocardiography predict improvement of LV function of approximately 8% to 10% when viability of the myocardium is present. Similarly, PET, nuclear studies, or dobutamine echocardiography images that demonstrate the absence of viability are likewise useful to predict the absence of improvement in LVEF (**Fig. 31-1**). The presence of hibernating or viable myocardium is essential for improvement in LVEF after surgical revascularization.[2] Similarly, the likelihood of future adverse LV remodeling decreases as the number of viable segments, demonstrated by dobutamine echocardiography, increases. Reverse remodeling occurred in patients with viable myocardium. In contrast, LV volumes significantly increased after surgical revascularization in patients without significant viability.[7] Thus, recovery of LV function after revascularization is related to the degree of reversible myocardial ischemia, severity of the LV dysfunction, LV chamber dimensions, and LV geometry. There may be continuing improvements in LVEF as late as 6 to 12 months after surgery.[1]

SYMPTOMATIC IMPROVEMENT. Several studies have reported marked improvement in heart failure symptoms after revascularization. In a study from Verona, 167 patients with an average LVEF of 28%, with angina and heart failure symptoms, demonstrated significant freedom from angina after surgery, 98% and 81% at 1 and 5 years. Freedom from heart failure was 78% and 47% at 1 and 5 years. Only 54% of patients were symptom free of both angina and heart failure at follow-up.[8] Di Carli and colleagues have studied 36 patients with LVEF of 28% by PET imaging.[9] They found a significant correlation between the total extent of a PET mismatch and percentage improvement in functional class after CABG. A blood flow–metabolism mismatch of more than 18% was associated with a sensitivity of 76% and a specificity of 78% for predicting a change in functional status after revascularization. A substantial objective improvement in physical activity was noted in patients with presurgical mismatches that occupied at least 20% of the ventricular myocardium. Thus, patients with large perfusion-metabolism mismatch exhibited the greatest clinical benefit after revascularization. Another study has shown a similar significant improvement in functional capacity after revascularization, as reflected by a 34% increase in exercise capacity from 5.6 to 7.5 METs (metabolic equivalents) in the group of patients with revascularization PET mismatch.[1]

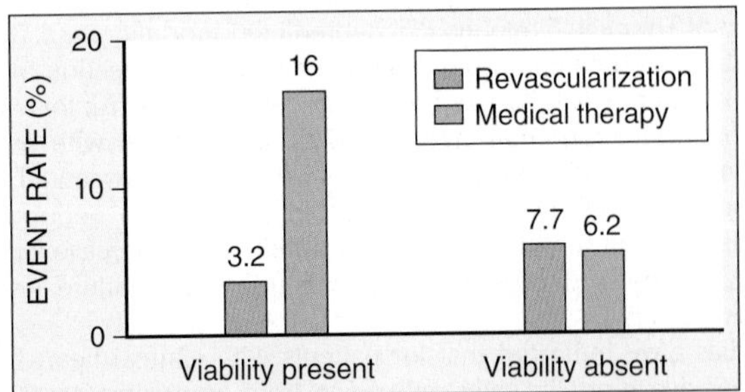

FIGURE 31-1 Analysis of pooled data from 24 prognostic studies that used different viability techniques and that showed 3.2% annual death rate in patients who had viable myocardium and who were undergoing revascularization compared with 16% annual death rate in patients who had viable myocardium and who were treated medically. Intermediate event rates (7.7% and 6.2%) were observed in patients with nonviable myocardium. *(From Allman KC, Shaw LJ, Hachamovitch R, Udelson JE: Myocardial viability testing and impact of revascularization on prognosis in patients with coronary artery disease and left ventricular dysfunction: A meta-analysis. J Am Coll Cardiol 39:1151, 2002.)*

SURVIVAL BENEFIT. In the absence of large, randomized, prospective clinical trials, registry and data bases have been used to guide decision making in patients with ischemic cardiomyopathy. The Duke database compared CABG with medical therapy during a 25-year period. Medical therapy was used in 1052 patients and CABG in 339 patients.[10] Unadjusted and adjusted survival (Cox proportional hazards model) strongly favored CABG after 30 days and at 10 years with one-, two-, or three-vessel disease (**Fig. 31-2**). CABG was better than medical therapy in patients with heart failure regardless of age, LVEF, NYHA class, or presence of angina (**Fig. 31-3**). Adjusted overall survival at 1, 5, and 10 years was 83% versus 74%, 61% versus 37%, and 42% versus 13% for CABG versus medical therapy, respectively ($P < 0.0001$).[10] Several studies have shown that overall survival and cardiac events (including cardiac death, infarction, and hospitalization for heart failure) are directly related to the presence of myocardial viability in heart failure patients. In a meta-analysis of 24 studies involving a total of 3088 patients with ischemic cardiomyopathy, revascularization decreased the risk of death by 79.6% in patients with evidence of viable myocardial tissue, yielding an annual mortality of 3.2% compared with 16.0% for patients who did not undergo revascularization.[11] This analysis showed that the type of viability study (thallium perfusion imaging, PET, or dobutamine echocardiography) did not affect the clinical outcomes. Furthermore, the results were proportionately better the worse the ventricular function. In contrast, patients without viability showed no survival benefit with revascularization.[11] A study of 908 CABG patients with ischemic cardiomyopathy looking at mid- and long-term results after surgical revascularization for ischemic cardiomyopathy showed that independent risk factors for short- and long-term event-free survival are quality of coronary arteries, degree of myocardial viability, completeness of revascularization, number of grafts, and elective operation.[12] Elefteriades and Edwards[13] reported the short- and long-term results of 188 consecutive patients, with an ejection fraction of 30% or less, undergoing CABG by a single surgeon at their institution. They demonstrated an overall mortality of 5.3% (2.8% in elective patients); improvement in ejection fraction from 23.3% to 33.2%; improvement in NYHA functional class from 3.1 to 1.4; and survival at 1, 3, and 5 years of 88%, 77%, and 60%, respectively.

A reasonable management strategy for patients who present with heart failure secondary to coronary artery disease (i.e., ischemic cardiomyopathy) includes coronary angiography (see Chaps. 21 and 28). Viability studies are appropriate for those patients with severe disease and adequate surgical targets. If significant viability is present (≥25%), the weight of currently available clinical evidence suggests that CABG may improve survival and quality of life over medical therapy alone.[14] Current American College of Cardiology/American Heart Association (ACC/AHA) guidelines for CABG in patients with poor LV function recommend surgery as a Class I indication for those patients with left main or equivalent disease, Class IIa for patients with viable noncontracting muscle, and Class III for those without evidence of ischemia or viability.[15,16]

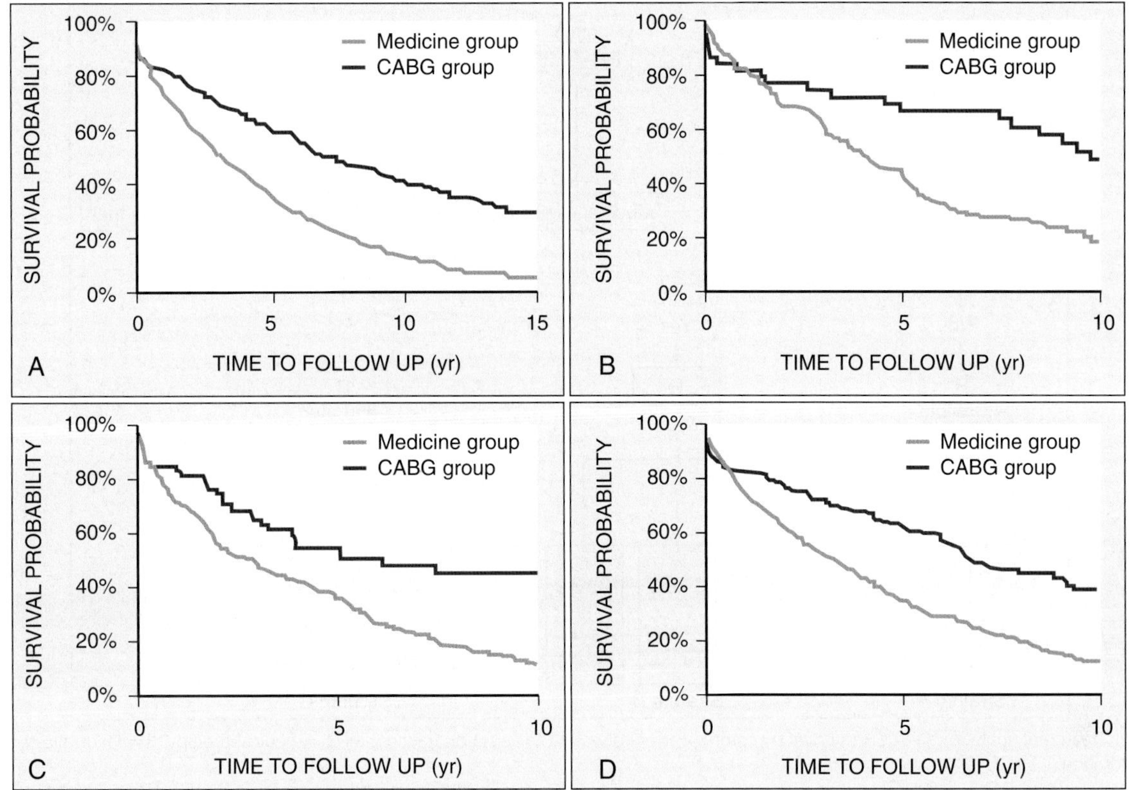

FIGURE 31-2 Coronary artery revascularization versus medical therapy in patients with heart failure. **A,** Overall cohort. **B,** One-vessel disease. **C,** Two-vessel disease. **D,** Three-vessel disease. *(Modified from O'Connor CM, Velazquez EJ, Gardner LH, et al: Comparison of coronary artery bypass grafting versus medical therapy on long-term outcome in patients with ischemic cardiomyopathy: A 25-year experience from the Duke Cardiovascular Disease Databank. Am J Cardiol 90:101, 2002.)*

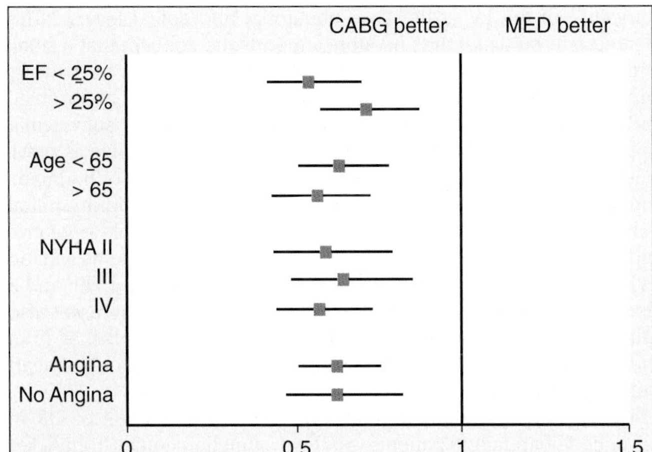

FIGURE 31-3 Subgroup analysis of coronary artery revascularization versus medical therapy (MED) in patients with heart failure. Hazard ratios (95% confidence interval) for mortality for a number of baseline characteristics all favored CABG. *(Modified from O'Connor CM, Velazquez EJ, Gardner LH, et al: Comparison of coronary artery bypass grafting versus medical therapy on long-term outcome in patients with ischemic cardiomyopathy: A 25-year experience from the Duke Cardiovascular Disease Databank. Am J Cardiol 90:101, 2002.)*

Because of the importance of the question of coronary artery revascularization in heart failure patients, the National Institutes of Health funded the STICH (Surgical Treatment of Ischemic Heart Failure) trial in 2002. STICH, a prospective, randomized study, included 2800 patients randomized from 100 centers. Patients with LV dysfunction and coronary artery disease amenable to CABG were randomized to a combination of three different treatment strategies: CABG, CABG plus surgical ventricular reconstruction (SVR), or intense medical therapy. This trial was powered to address two primary hypotheses: (1) CABG combined with medical therapy improves long-term survival compared with medical therapy alone; and (2) SVR provides additional long-term survival benefit when it is combined with CABG and medical therapy (**Fig. 31-4**). Secondary endpoints of the trial include cardiac morbidity and mortality, economic impact of various treatments, quality of life of the patient, and usefulness of biochemical imaging modalities for predicting optimal treatment strategies. Patients were included in the trial on the basis of an ejection fraction below 35% and coronary anatomy that was suitable for revascularization. The results of Stratum C of the STICH trial have been reported[17] and are discussed later (see Left Ventricular Reconstruction).

Valve Surgery in Patients with Left Ventricular Dysfunction

As discussed in Chap. 66, the surgical treatment of valvular heart disease that leads to LV dysfunction or heart failure is now widely accepted. However, patients who have valvular dysfunction *secondary* to a primary cardiomyopathy pose a much more difficult management problem. The following section focuses on the impact and outcome of valve repair or replacement for patients with a dilated cardiomyopathy and secondary mitral regurgitation. The indications for valve replacement in ischemic mitral regurgitation are discussed in Chap. 66.

Mitral Valve

Mitral regurgitation (MR) is commonly observed in patients with heart failure and associated with a poor prognosis.[18] Progressive LV remodeling characterized by progressive LV dilation and a change to a more spherical shape can result in functional MR as a result of annular dilation, papillary muscle displacement, and chordal tethering (see Chap. 66). The functional MR leads to an increased preload, increased wall

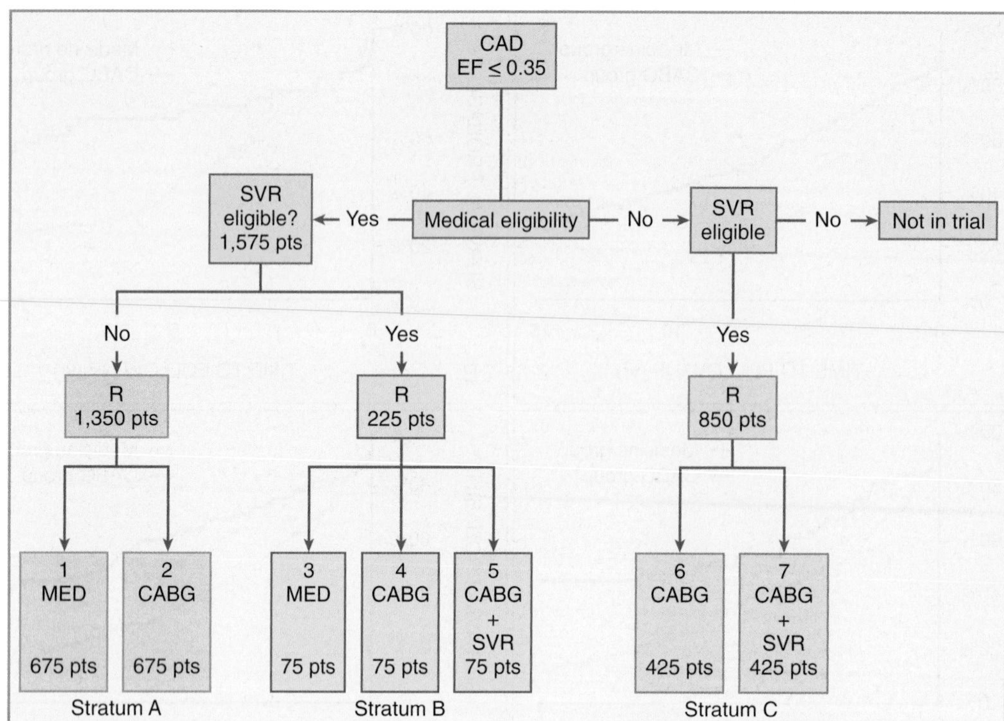

FIGURE 31-4 Treatment strata in the STICH trial. CAD = coronary artery disease; EF = ejection fraction; MED = medical therapy; R = randomized; SVR = surgical ventricular restoration.

tension, and increased LV workload, all of which contribute in a positive feedback loop to progressive heart failure. The presence of MR itself is the independent risk factor of poor outcome, in both nonischemic and ischemic causes.[18] Even uncorrected mild MR, as well as moderate to severe MR associated with ischemic cardiomyopathy, is associated with reduced long-term survival. In addition, it is a progressive disorder in which MR related to LV volume overload promotes further LV remodeling, leading to worsening MR.

Mitral valve repair or replacement to restore valve competency is a well-established procedure when there are symptoms of heart failure and the primary disease is of the valve leaflets (see Chap. 66). However, recent interest has focused on functional or secondary mitral insufficiency, in which the valve leaflets are anatomically normal but do not fully coapt because of annular dilation and restricted leaflet motion secondary to increased ventricular size and sphericity. Such a remodeled ventricle is often associated with an LVEF of 40% or less and heart failure symptoms of NYHA Class III or Class IV. Surgery in this situation is controversial as the MR is the consequence and not the cause of LV dysfunction, and the prognosis, therefore, is more related to the underlying cardiomyopathic process.

Although it is clear that the advent of secondary mitral insufficiency is associated with a worse prognosis, it is unclear whether the worse outcomes stem from the MR itself or whether MR is simply a marker for worsening heart failure and the correction of MR will improve symptoms or survival. Specifically, can surgery be done in patients with advanced heart failure and LV dysfunction with an acceptable operative mortality? Is there evidence that the elimination of MR results in LV reverse remodeling or improved survival?

Conventional teaching has been that surgical correction of MR in advanced heart failure patients with poor LV function is associated with prohibitive operative mortality. This view was challenged by Bolling and others more than 10 years ago.[19] The traditional hypothesis held that the mitral valve functions as a "pop-off valve" for the failing ventricle and surgical correction results in prohibitive mortality. The Bolling hypothesis is that there is an "annular solution for a ventricular problem . . . such that reconstruction of the mitral valve annulus' geometric abnormality by an undersized ring restores valvular competency, alleviates excessive ventricular workload, improves ventricular geometry and improves ventricular function." Miller and his Stanford colleagues have reported, in an ischemic sheep model of MR, that the reduction of the annulus by a small ring reduces a radius of curvature of the LV at the base equatorial and apical levels.[20] This decrease in radius of the curvature supports the concept that a small ring can restore a more elliptical ventricular shape. It is now recognized that the surgical mortality of mitral valve replacement observed in the past was most likely the result of the loss of the subvalvular apparatus and not secondary to the loss of the pop-off valve as previously thought, underscoring the paramount importance of maintaining the integrity of annular and subvalvular continuity during mitral valve surgery. Bolling was the first to show an acceptable operative mortality (5%) in a series of 140 Class III and Class IV patients with an LVEF of less than 25%. He demonstrated improvement in LVEF and a decrease in end-diastolic volumes during 3 to 5 years.[19] There was also improvement in functional class in his series of patients. Bishay from the Cleveland Clinic had comparable results in a similar group of heart failure patients.[21]

The most comprehensive analysis to date of correction of MR in advanced heart failure patients with LV dysfunction comes from Acker and colleagues in the Acorn trial.[22] This trial evaluated the safety and efficacy of mitral valve surgery with and without the CorCap cardiac support device. The Acorn clinical trial, although not randomized to study the efficacy of mitral valve repair, did prospectively assess the safety and efficacy of mitral valve surgery in advanced heart failure patients performed in multiple trial centers. Of 193 entered, 73% were in Class III. Most of the patients were idiopathic or valvular patients; only 6% had ischemic cardiomyopathy. The duration of heart failure was nearly 5 years; 97% of patients were taking angiotensin-converting enzyme inhibitors, and 80% were taking beta blockers. The mean LVEF was 23.9%, peak $\dot{V}O_2$ was 14 mL/kg/min, and LV end-diastolic dimension was nearly 70 mm. Remarkably, the operative mortality rate was only 1.6%, one of the lowest mortality rates of any series[19,21] and especially noteworthy because it represents the outcome of nearly 30 different centers. Twelve-month cumulative survival was 86.5%; at 2 years, the cumulative survival was 85.2%. The majority of patients received a complete, small annuloplasty repair. Mitral valve insufficiency was reduced from 2.7 at baseline to 0.6 at 18 months and was

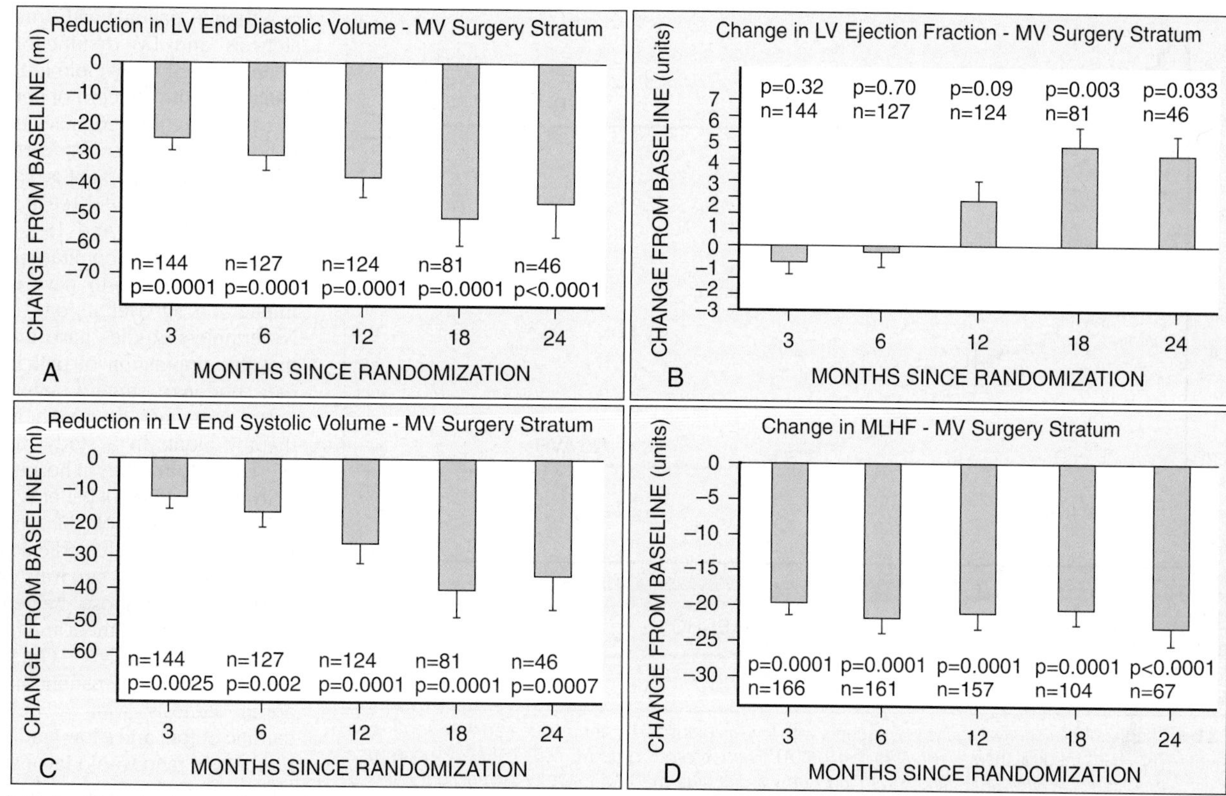

FIGURE 31-5 Clinical outcomes in mitral surgery treatment arm in the Acorn trial. **A,** Change in LV end-diastolic volume. **B,** Change in LVEF. **C,** Change in LV end-systolic volume. **D,** Change in Minnesota Living with Heart Failure (MLHF) score. *(From Acker MA, Bolling S, Shemin R, et al: Mitral valve surgery in heart failure: Insights from the Acorn Clinical Trial. J Thorac Cardiovasc Surg 132:568, 2006.)*

accompanied by evidence of reverse remodeling. A significant decrease in LV end-diastolic volume, LV end-systolic volume, and LV mass was observed at 2 years (**Fig. 31-5**). Moreover, the sphericity index increased and remained significant at 2 years, consistent with a more ellipsoid shape of the left ventricle. Finally, the baseline NYHA class of 2.8 was reduced significantly to 2.2 at 2 years. In summary, for the patients with primarily nonischemic advanced heart failure and severe LV dysfunction, mitral valve surgery was shown to be safe, with a low operative mortality rate and associated with significant reversal of LV remodeling compared with baseline as well as improvement in NYHA functional class.[22]

LV reverse remodeling has also been demonstrated in several studies as a result of mitral valve repair either alone or in combination with coronary artery revascularization for patients with ischemic disease. Acker and colleagues[23] demonstrated, in patients with primarily nonischemic cardiomyopathies, a significant decrease in LV end-diastolic volume as a result of mitral repair, and this reversal has remained significant up to 5 years. In ischemic cardiomyopathy patients, Bax and Braun have shown that the combination of mitral valve repair and coronary artery bypass resulted in a significant decrease in LV end-diastolic volume up to 4 years after surgery.[24,25] In addition, Fattouch has recently demonstrated, in a randomized study of coronary artery bypass versus coronary artery bypass and mitral valve repair, that the addition of mitral valve repair improves postoperative NYHA functional class and ventricular remodeling, decreases pulmonary arterial pressure, and leads to a decrease in hospitalization for heart failure.[25] In addition, these same studies also showed low operative mortality rates for combined mitral valve surgery and coronary artery bypass procedures in patients with significant LV dysfunction and advanced heart failure symptoms. There is also accumulating evidence in patients with ischemic mitral insufficiency that the combination of surgical revascularization and mitral valve repair will improve quality of life significantly.[24-26] In multiple retrospective series, NYHA class improved from greater than NYHA Class III to less than Class II with up to 4 years of follow-up.[24,25]

Review of the literature shows that ischemic patients can also undergo mitral valve surgery with mortality rates of less than 5%, and many series suggest operative mortality of less than 2%. Clearly, the old theory that the mitral valve in heart failure patients functions as a pop-off valve has been disproven.[24-26] As Miller from Stanford states, "We now recognize that ignoring an important degree of ischemic MR at the time of coronary artery bypass surgery is not prudent because it will only limit the potential functional benefits to be obtained from the operation and compound the patient's poor life expectancy."[27]

Multiple studies suggest that the recurrent rates of MR after repair are approximately 30% to 40%. These studies generally fail to address ring selection and amount of downsizing as an important consideration for durable results in the ischemic MR population. Early failure with recurrent MR, reported by McGee[28] and Mihaljevic[29] in ischemic heart failure patients after coronary artery bypass surgery and annuloplasty ring, was likely due to the use of a flexible band or ring. These results stand in sharp contrast to little recurrent MR seen up to 4 years when a rigid ring has been downsized by two to four sizes.[24] Spoor and colleagues[30] found that the MR recurrence rate was 9.5% with a flexible ring versus 2.5% with a nonflexible ring in patients with a preoperative LVEF of less than 30% and no primary mitral disease. The failure of a flexible band in ischemic MR can be explained by the fact that the intratrigonal distance is subject to dilation for which a band does not provide protection. In addition, fixation of the septal lateral dimension is most important in preventing return of MR, and an undersized rigid ring will address that.[27] The ACC/AHA Guidelines 2006 as well as the European Society of Cardiology Guidelines 2007 suggest that "mitral annuloplasty alone with a downsized annuloplasty ring is often effective in relieving ischemic MR," and the European Society of Cardiology Guidelines 2007 state that most patients with ischemic MR seem to benefit from valve repair with use of an undersized rigid ring annuloplasty.

Currently, there are no randomized studies comparing mitral valve repair with medical management in patients with advanced heart failure and LV dysfunction. Wu and coworkers,[31] between

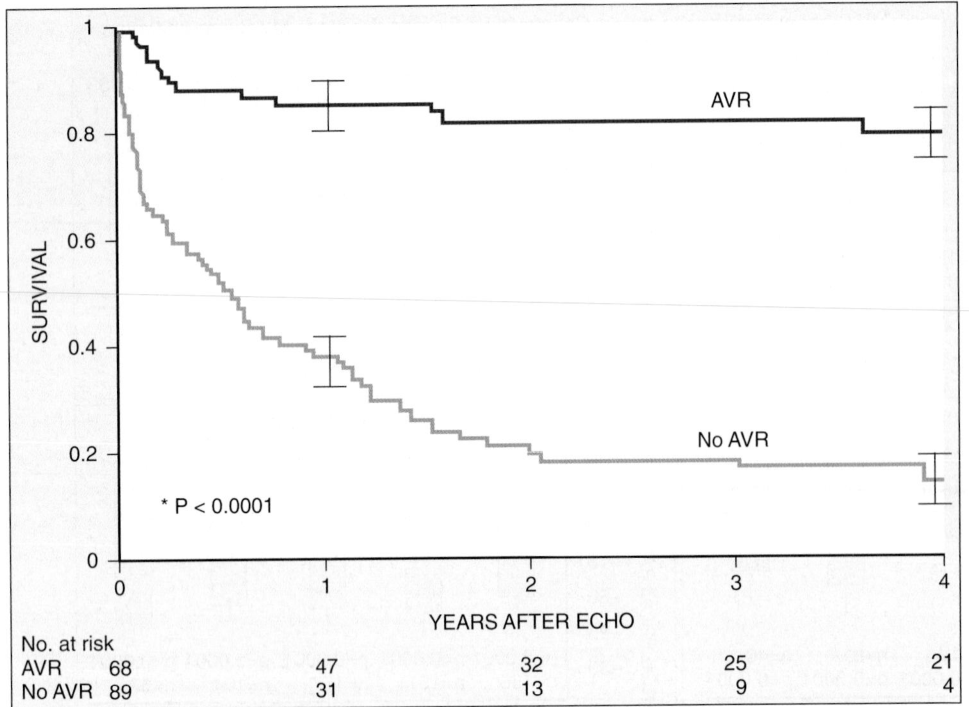

FIGURE 31-6 Kaplan-Meier survival analysis of patients with low-gradient aortic stenosis treated with aortic valve replacement (AVR) versus medical therapy (No AVR) ($P < 0.0001$). *(From Pereira JJ, Lauer MS, Bashir M, et al: Survival after aortic valve replacement for severe aortic stenosis with low transvalvular gradients and severe LV dysfunction. J Am Coll Cardiol 39:1356, 2002.)*

1995 and 2002, published a retrospective propensity-matched analysis of consecutive patients with significant MR and LV dysfunction. They compared the 126 patients who underwent mitral valve annuloplasty with the medical patients who did not undergo surgery. Valve repair did not predict the clinical outcome (survival, transplant, or ventricular assist device). However, this study was limited in that it did not report changes in LV size or function or quality of life improvement. In addition, there were no data on the presence of recurrent MR at the follow-up, nor was the type of annuloplasty ring noted.

In summary, the current literature suggests that functional mitral insufficiency in patients with advanced heart failure and LV dysfunction can be corrected with a low operative mortality in either ischemic or nonischemic cardiomyopathies. There are multiple prospective but nonrandomized series that suggest a symptomatic benefit as well as a remodeling benefit in patients who undergo mitral valve repair in idiopathic dilated cardiomyopathies and coronary revascularization with mitral valve repair in ischemic cardiomyopathies. There is currently no evidence that elimination of mitral insufficiency in heart failure patients conveys a survival benefit.

Aortic Valve

The indications for valve replacement in aortic stenosis and regurgitation are discussed in Chap. 66. This section focuses on aortic valve replacement for patients with aortic valve disease and ventricular dysfunction or heart failure. Patients with aortic stenosis may develop ventricular dysfunction with a low gradient across the aortic valve[32] (see Chap. 66). Aortic valve replacement is warranted in these patients if the LV dysfunction is secondary to the aortic stenosis. Accordingly, it is important to differentiate between pseudo-obstruction, with poor ventricular function leading to reduced opening of the aortic valve, and true aortic stenosis. In the latter case, there is a primary valve obstruction that leads to LV dysfunction in patients with aortic stenosis and a low cardiac output. Dobutamine echocardiography is useful to make this determination (see Chaps. 15 and 66).

Although patients with true aortic stenosis and LV dysfunction have been deemed inoperable in the past because of the concern of perioperative mortality, the prognosis of these patients, if they do not receive an aortic valve replacement, is extremely poor, with 1-, 5-, and 10-year survival rates of 62%, 32%, and 18%, respectively. Moreover, concomitant pharmacotherapy appears to have had no impact on survival in one series.[33] Nevertheless, studies have indicated that this population of patients also can undergo surgery safely, with better outcomes than with medical therapy alone. In a study from the Cleveland Clinic, the in-hospital mortality for this group of patients was 8%, with 1-year survival of 82% versus 41% for those treated with medical therapy alone and 4-year survival of 78% versus 15% for those treated with aortic valve replacement and medical therapy, respectively[32] (**Fig. 31-6**). Assuming that the patient has true aortic stenosis with a depressed cardiac output and a low gradient, the risk-benefit ratio would favor surgical interventions in those patients who are otherwise healthy enough to undergo surgery.[32-34]

Patients with severe aortic regurgitation and LV dysfunction pose a different problem. Some patients develop advanced heart failure and have been considered for cardiac transplantation because the LV dysfunction was considered to be irreversible. Although the operative mortality in this group has been high historically, a study from the Cleveland Clinic has indicated that for patients with pure aortic regurgitation, the operative mortality has been negligible since 1985.[35] In this series, there was a regression in LV mass and improvement in LV volumes in most patients after aortic valve replacement surgery.[36] Although late survival may not be as good for patients with normal preoperative LV function with severe aortic insufficiency, the outcomes are better than the option of cardiac transplantation or continued medical therapy. The ACC/AHA guidelines now endorse surgery in this group of patients (Class I recommendation).[37]

In summary, in experienced centers, mitral valve repair for patients with LV dysfunction and MR may be appropriate for those undergoing CABG as well as for selected patients with idiopathic dilated cardiomyopathy who remain symptomatic despite optimal medical therapy. Aortic valve surgery can be performed safely, albeit at higher operative risk, in patients with severe LV dysfunction and heart failure, and it appears to have a better clinical outcome than current medical therapy in observational studies.

Left Ventricular Reconstruction

Revascularization and valve operations improve many patients, but in others, ventricular dilation and dysfunction are so severe that direct ventricular surgery is needed to optimize cardiac function. Patients who have a transmural myocardial infarction may develop ventricular dilation and remodeling that lead to changes in increased LV wall stress and LV dysfunction (see Table 25-2).[38] A host of adverse events are initiated, including increased myocardial oxygen consumption secondary to increased wall stress, increased neurohormone and cytokine levels, afterload mismatch, and subendocardial hypoperfusion. The goals of ventricular reconstruction are to remove or to exclude the infarcted segment to restore an elliptical ventricular chamber, to diminish remote wall stress, to promote helical fiber

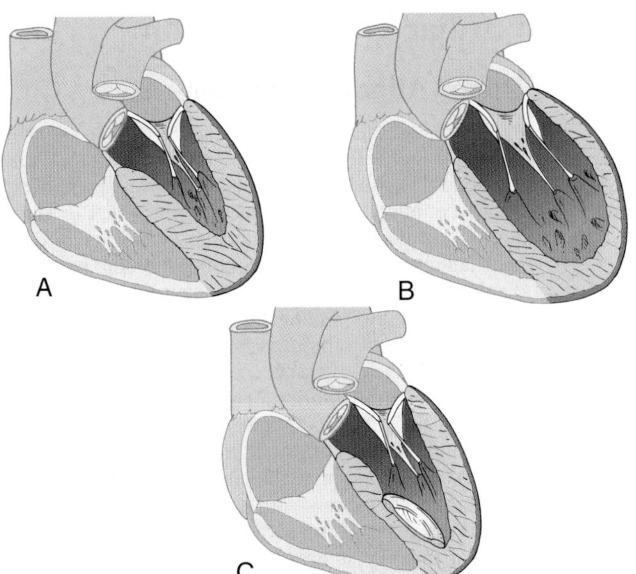

FIGURE 31-7 **A,** Normal left ventricle. **B,** Remodeled left ventricle after anteroseptal myocardial infarction. **C,** SVR (Dor) procedure: Dacron patch exclusion of infarcted anteroseptum restoring normal shape and size.

orientation and to increase thickening of the akinetic or dyskinetic portion of the chamber, to reduce end-systolic volume, to diminish mitral insufficiency, and to eliminate residual ischemia.[39] Concomitant CABG is often necessary, and if more than moderate MR is present, this should be corrected separately. This type of operation is variously named surgical ventricular reconstruction (SVR) or the Dor procedure (after Vincent Dor), in which the aneurysm or akinetic segment is reconstructed, typically with a patch (endoventricular patch plasty) (**Fig. 31-7**).

The operation is performed through the area of scar. A purse-string suture is placed between the infarcted and normal myocardium. An endoventricular Dacron patch is usually used to exclude the infarcted segment, with closure of the aneurysm sac over the patch. A mandrel is often used to ensure that adequate ventricular volume is maintained. This operation is typically reserved for patients who have had a large anterior-apical infarct that involves the apex, anterior wall, and septum with resulting LV remodeling. The goal of the operation is to reduce end-systolic volumes by at least 30% while ensuring that the ventricle is not too small.

The RESTORE (Reconstructive Endoventricular Surgery returning Torsion Original Radius Elliptical shape to the left ventricle) multicenter study investigated various techniques for LV reconstruction in a registry of 1198 post–anterior infarction heart failure patients operated on between 1998 and 2003. Concomitant procedures included CABG in 95% and mitral valve repair in 22%. The operative mortality in patients who underwent LV reconstruction was 5.3%. At 5 years, the overall survival was 68% ± 2.8%, and freedom from hospital readmission for heart failure was 78%. Logistic regression analysis identified LVEF less than 30%, LV end-systolic volume index 80 mL/m^2 or higher, advanced NYHA functional class, and age older than 75 years as risk factors for death. LV reconstruction resulted in a significant decrease in LV end-systolic volume index (from 80.0 ± 5.1 to 56.0 ± 34.3 mL/m^2) and a significant increase in LVEF (from 29% ± 11.0% to 39% ± 12.3%). Preoperatively, 67% of patients were in NYHA Class III or IV, whereas postoperatively, 85% were in NYHA Class I or II. The study has reported a 30-day mortality of 1% and 1-, 3-, and 5-year survival of 92%, 90%, and 80%, respectively.[40]

Mathematical modeling has indicated that the effect of volume reduction surgery on overall ventricular pumping characteristics is determined by the differential effects on end-systolic and end-diastolic properties, which in turn are determined by the material properties of the region being removed or excluded surgically. In this analysis, there was a beneficial effect on this relationship by resection of dyskinetic tissue, an equivocal effect of akinetic scar resection (typically, at surgery, these have the appearance of marbled muscle and scar that are mixed together), and a negative effect of removal of contracting myocardium.[41] Preoperative and postoperative pressure-volume loop analysis demonstrated a significant reduction in end-diastolic and end-systolic volume and unchanged stroke volume, indicating improved LVEF. The end-systolic pressure-volume relationship showed a leftward shift of the increased slope, indicating improved systolic function. The end-diastolic pressure-volume relationship, however, showed a leftward shift, also indicating increased diastolic stiffness after surgery. Heterogeneity in operative mortality in late outcomes observed in clinical experience to date may relate the balance of these two factors.[42]

The SVR portion of the STICH trial results were recently published.[17] The study tested the hypothesis that adding SVR to CABG in ischemic heart failure patients would decrease death or cardiac rehospitalization compared with CABG alone. One thousand heart failure patients (operated on between 2002 and 2006) with coronary artery disease, ejection fraction of less than 35%, and anterior LV wall scar amenable to SVR were randomized. Bypass surgery alone was done in 499 patients, and CABG plus SVR was performed in 501 patients. They were studied for a median follow-up of 48 months. There were no differences in deaths from any cause or hospitalization for cardiac causes during the 5 years of the study[17] (**Fig. 31-8**). The results of the study have been criticized because the average percentage reduction in end-systolic volume after CABG plus SVR was only 19%. This is below the accepted criterion for successful LV reconstruction of a minimum of 30% reduction in end-systolic volume.[43,44] In addition, the absolute end-systolic volume index (mL/m^2) in the STICH patients undergoing CABG plus SVR was 67. The results of Menicanti demonstrated that patients who were left with a residual end-systolic volume index of >60 had a worse survival compared with a more optimal end-systolic volume index of <30 (**Fig. 31-9**). An additional limitation of the STICH trial is that 13% of patients did not have an infarct before development of LV dysfunction. Another criticism is that there was an ongoing selection bias so that the study did not include patients thought to clearly benefit from SVR. Important subgroup analyses of preoperative viability and baseline volume and regional LV function characteristics are pending. There are significant concerns that because of many limitations, STICH did not prove or disprove the original hypothesis.[43]

Passive Cardiac Support Devices

The preceding sections have outlined direct surgical reconstruction of coronary arteries, valves, or the left ventricle. This section describes novel surgical approaches to inhibit or to reverse LV remodeling. The current generation of passive cardiac support devices was developed out of original observations with dynamic cardiomyoplasty, which was initially intended to act as an auxiliary pump for the failing heart.[1] Subsequent hemodynamic assessments in animals and humans have suggested that much of the observed benefit of dynamic cardiomyoplasty appeared to be derived from the passive girdling effect of the muscle wrap, which limits ventricular dilation, reduces LV wall stress, and prevents LV remodeling.[1] These early experiences with dynamic cardiomyoplasty and the insights into its biologic effects have led to the ongoing development of surgical therapies specifically aimed at inhibiting LV remodeling.

The CorCap cardiac support device (CSD; Acorn Cardiovascular, St. Paul, Minn) is a fabric mesh sock that is surgically implanted around the heart. The CSD is designed to provide circumferential diastolic support and to reduce LV wall stress, thereby leading to reverse cardiac remodeling. The original device was planted via a sternotomy, but a second-generation device is placed through a minimally invasive left thoracotomy on a beating heart without cardiopulmonary bypass. The Acorn trial was a randomized, prospective, multicenter clinical trial involving 300 patients. In this trial, CSD-treated patients had significantly fewer cardiac procedures indicative of worsening

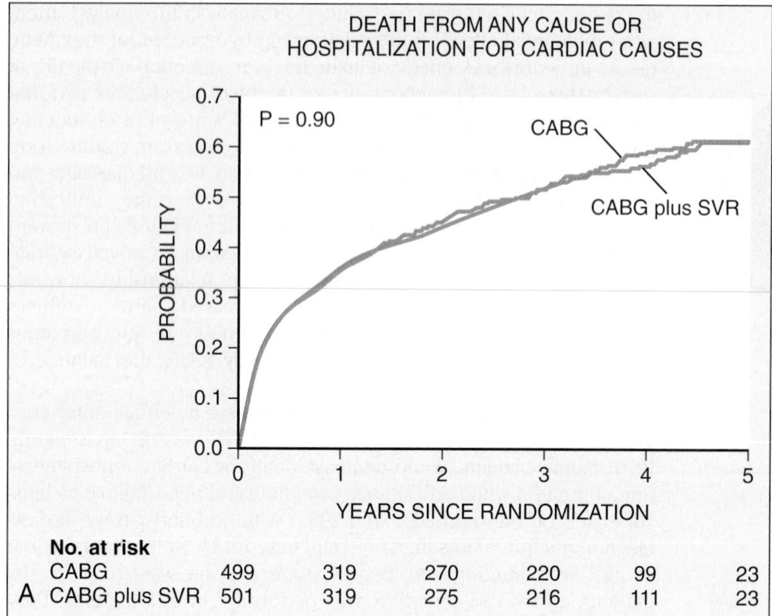

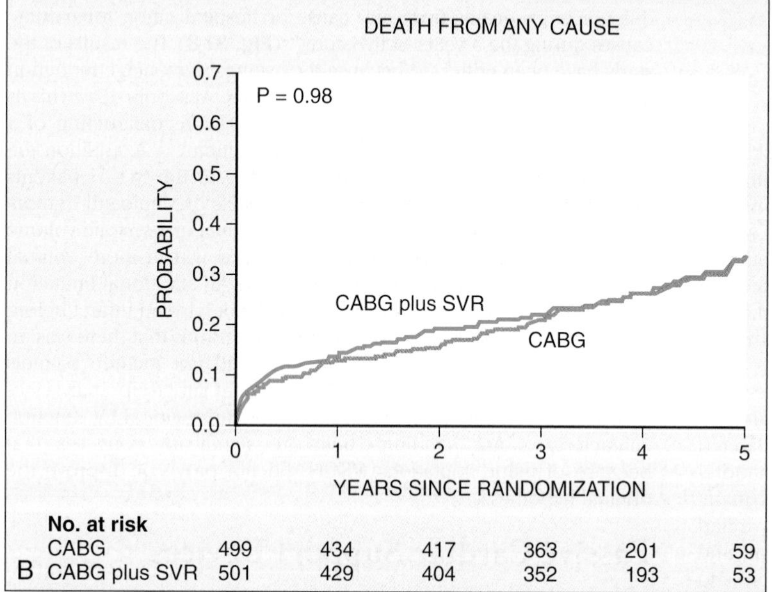

FIGURE 31-8 Results of STICH trial showing no benefit for SVR and CABG over CABG alone. *(From Jones RH, Velazquez EF, Michler RE, et al: Coronary bypass surgery with or without surgical ventricular reconstruction. N Engl J Med 360:1705, 2009.)*

heart failure (cardiac transplantation and LV assist device) and experienced an improvement in NYHA class. Treatment with the CSD also led to a decrease in LV end-diastolic and end-systolic volumes, indicative of reverse cardiac remodeling, and an increase in the LV sphericity index, indicative of a more elliptically shaped ventricle (**Fig. 31-10**). CSD-treated patients also had a significant improvement in quality of life scores.[45,46] The addition of the CSD device to standard mitral repair or replacement has provided significant additive benefits compared with mitral valve surgery alone and resulted in greater reductions in LV volume and a notable improvement in sphericity index.[22,23] The benefits of reducing LV remodeling have continued up to 5 years, with a significant added benefit both in patients who had CorCap and mitral valve repair versus mitral valve repair alone and in patients who had CorCap alone versus medical therapy. Importantly, there has been no evidence of constrictive physiology now up to 5 years.[23] This device is not currently approved by the Food and Drug Administration.

Cardiac Transplantation

Donor Allocation System

In the United States, the allocation of donor organs is accomplished under the supervision of the United Network of Organ Sharing (UNOS), a private organization under contract to the federal government. The United States is divided geographically into 11 regions for donor heart allocation. Under UNOS policy, thoracic organs are distributed on the basis of blood type, medical urgency, and time on the waiting list. The physiologic limit of approximately 4 hours of ischemic out-of-body time for hearts precludes a national sharing of donor hearts. Currently, the highest priority for patients to receive donor organs is assigned according to the severity of illness. Each candidate awaiting heart transplantation is assigned a status corresponding to the medical urgency of the candidate who is to receive a heart transplant. For a candidate who is 18 years of age or older at the time of listing, medical urgency is assigned as follows (UNOS policy 3.73). Status 1A refers to patients who are hospitalized and have a left or right ventricular assist device, a total artificial heart, extracorporeal membrane oxygenation, or a balloon pump; this is valid for 30 days unless relisted. Patients have only a one-time window of 30 days after receiving an implantable ventricular assist device unless they develop device-related infection or device failure; a patient with invasive hemodynamic monitoring and two or more inotropic drugs also meets requirement for status 1A. Status 1B refers to hospitalized patients who are being treated with a right or left ventricular circulatory assist device after their initial 30-day window as status 1A or a continuous intravenous infusion of inotropes. A candidate who does not meet the criteria for status 1A or 1B is listed as status 2; status 2 patients are often those outpatients who are stable on a medical regimen. A candidate who is listed as status 7 is considered temporarily unsuitable to receive a thoracic organ transplant (see also policies of the Organ Procurement and Transplantation Network, http://www.optn.org).

Evaluation of the Potential Recipient

Figure 31-11 outlines the questions that must be answered to evaluate a potential patient for cardiac transplantation. Patients estimated to have less than a 1-year life expectancy are the usual candidates. Typically, patients for consideration have (1) cardiogenic shock requiring mechanical support or high-dose inotropic or vasopressor drugs (in which case the irreversibility of their course is usually clear); (2) chronic progressive, refractory, or stage D heart failure symptoms despite optimal therapy[47]; (3) recurrent life-threatening arrhythmias despite maximal interventions, including implanted defibrillators; or, rarely, (4) refractory angina without potential for revascularization.[48] More recently, adult patients with repaired congenital heart disease are developing progressive heart failure and are being increasingly considered for heart transplantation.[49] Several models have been proposed to assist in the risk stratification of patients with heart failure by use of both invasive and noninvasive methods.[50,51] The most potent predictor of outcome in ambulatory patients with heart failure is a symptom-limited metabolic stress test to calculate peak oxygen consumption, or peak $\dot{V}O_2$. A peak $\dot{V}O_2$ of less than 12 mL/kg/min indicates a poor prognosis, with a survival that is less than that of a transplant.[52] Nonambulatory patients requiring continuous intravenous inotropic support who cannot be weaned or requiring mechanical support to maintain adequate cardiac index are more obviously at risk for a poor outcome without transplantation, but signs and symptoms of end-organ failure of the pulmonary, hepatic, and renal systems that may signal an ominous prognosis even with a transplant procedure are often manifested.

Each patient must then undergo an extensive medical and psychosocial evaluation by the transplant team to exclude contraindications to transplantation, to further efforts at prognosis, to determine the urgency of transplantation, and to determine immunologic status. There are a number of relative contraindications to heart transplantation; one of the most debated and variable among centers is the upper age limit for consideration. In general, patients older than 70 years are ineligible and are more often assigned to high-risk reparative surgery, permanent cardiac assist devices, or investigational therapies, such as cell transplantation, or to receive hearts from an alternate list of less than optimal donors. An active or recent malignant neoplasm and diabetes with severe end-organ damage limit life expectancy after transplantation and are common reasons to exclude potential recipients. Significant lung disease complicates postoperative management and precludes the possibility of normal physical functioning; extremes of weight, as measured by body mass index (BMI), have also been shown to worsen posttransplantation prognosis.[48] Advanced heart failure patients with renal dysfunction are generally excluded from heart transplantation because abnormal renal function increases morbidity after transplantation. Thus, it is important to clearly distinguish patients with potentially reversible renal failure from those patients in whom renal dysfunction is associated with advanced, irreversible end-stage renal disease.

Pulmonary arterial hypertension, with a pulmonary vascular resistance of more than 6 Wood units that cannot be reduced by medical therapy or after the placement of a ventricular assist device, is considered an absolute contraindication to cardiac transplantation. In the setting of fixed pulmonary hypertension, the donor right ventricle will often fail, leading to a high rate of early postoperative mortality.[53] In patients with irreversible pulmonary pressures, some centers may consider individual patients for a combined heart-lung transplant procedure. There are other comorbidities that may have a negative impact on a transplant team's decision to further consider a potential recipient, including hepatitis C or cirrhosis, peripheral or cerebral vascular disease, advanced neuropathy, human immunodeficiency virus (HIV) status, addictions to alcohol or illicit drugs, and social or psychiatric disorders.

An increasingly sophisticated immunologic evaluation of each patient is done for ABO blood typing and antibody screening, panel reactive antibody (PRA) level determination, and human leukocyte antigen (HLA) typing. The PRA test can identify the presence of circulating anti-HLA antibody but not the specificity or strength of antibody. Enzyme-linked immunoassay and flow cytometry can also determine PRA level and are more sensitive than the cytotoxic test.[54] Virtual crossmatch methods, in which flow cytometry–based single-antigen bead assays allow the clear identification of antibody specificities, are now being used with some success. Prospective donors with these antigens can be avoided and a compatible donor can be selected without the need for a prospective crossmatch. This allows an increased donor match outside the geographic area of the local organ procurement organization.

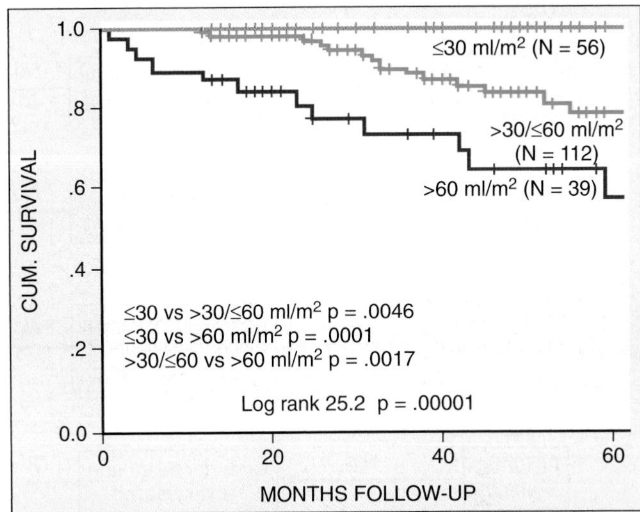

FIGURE 31-9 Cumulative survival after SVR and CABG depends on end-systolic volume index after the procedure. *(From DiDonato M, Toso A, Maioli M, et al: Intermediate survival and predictors of death after surgical ventricular restoration. Semin Thorac Cardiovasc Surg 13:468, 2001.)*

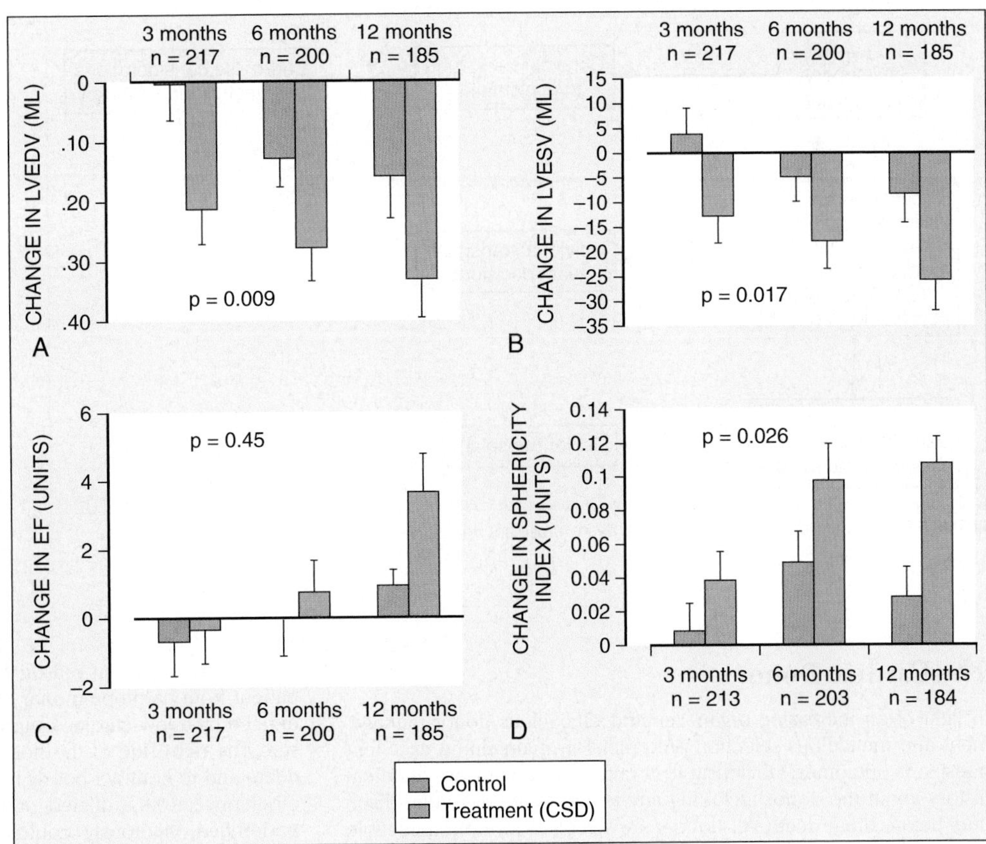

FIGURE 31-10 Change in LV structure in cardiac support device (CSD) treatment and control groups in the Acorn trial. **A,** Change in LV end-diastolic volume (LVEDV) from baseline. **B,** Change in LV end-systolic volume (LVESV) from baseline. **C,** Change in LV ejection fraction (EF) from baseline. **D,** Change in LV sphericity index (ratio of LV long axis to LV short axis) at 3, 6, and 12 months.

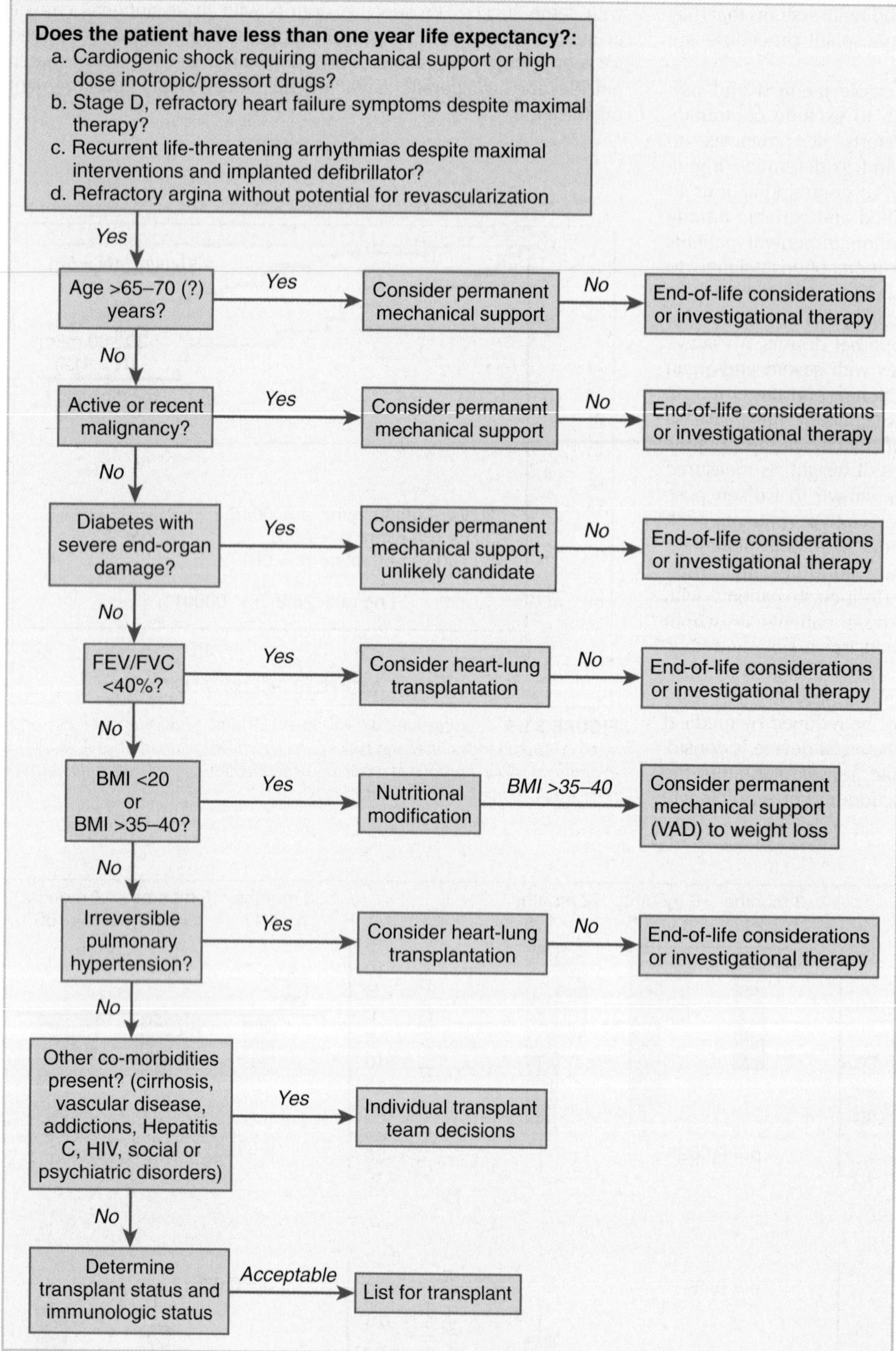

FIGURE 31-11 Evaluation of the potential heart transplant recipient.

The Cardiac Donor

In light of an increasing organ demand, efficacious donor management and meticulous selection are crucial in maintaining excellent transplant outcomes. Obviously, it is critical to obtain any medical history about the donor, including any relevant cardiovascular disorders before brain death. All donors are screened for communicable diseases, including viral disorders such as hepatitis and HIV infection. Specific information that is relevant for the assessment of cardiac donor suitability also includes the presence or absence of thoracic trauma, donor hemodynamic stability, pressor and inotropic requirements, duration of cardiac arrest, and need for cardiopulmonary resuscitation. Some cardiac donors undergo hemodynamic deterioration caused by brain death. Cardiac echocardiography is required on all donors, and coronary arteriography is required to evaluate the presence of coronary artery disease in donors older than 45 to 50 years, depending on other risk factors.

The acceptable cold ischemia time for cardiac transplantation is approximately 4 hours. Prolonged ischemic time has been shown to be a significant risk factor for mortality after cardiac transplantation, especially when it is coupled with other risk factors, such as older donor age. Donors up to the age of 60 to 65 years are currently considered, depending on distance and other donor risk factors. The final decision to accept a heart for transplantation is made at the time of harvesting after direct examination of the heart for coronary calcification, as well as LV hypertrophy or dilation.

Surgical Considerations

The two most common surgical approaches for the implantation of the donor heart are the biatrial and the bicaval anastomoses. The bicaval anastomosis technique was introduced in the early 1990s with the intention to reduce right atrial size, to minimize distortion of the recipient heart, to preserve atrial conduction pathways, and to decrease tricuspid regurgitation. In this alternative procedure, there are five anastomoses: left atrium, pulmonary artery, aorta, inferior vena cava, and superior vena cava. Although there has been no prospective trial to establish the superiority of either technique, the bicaval technique is now being done most often in the United States, primarily because it appears to decrease the need for permanent pacemakers in transplanted recipients.[55] Most important, the number of patients coming to transplantation with ventricular assist devices in place has steadily increased, so that transplant procedures are riskier and result in more bleeding.

The most common reason for failure to wean a heart transplant patient from cardiopulmonary bypass is right-sided heart failure, evidenced by a low cardiac output despite a rising central venous pressure. The right side of the heart can be seen in the surgical field to dilate and to contract poorly. Intraoperative transesophageal echocardiography shows a dilated, poorly contracting right ventricle and an underfilled, vigorously contracting left ventricle. Right ventricular function may be enhanced with inotropes and pulmonary vasodilators, but the prognostic importance of preoperative pulmonary vascular resistance becomes obvious in these first few hours after surgery.[56]

Immunosuppression

Immunosuppressive regimens begin with the simultaneous use of three classes of drugs: glucocorticoids, calcineurin inhibitors, and antiproliferative agents. In a subset of patients, transplant teams use a variety of drugs for induction therapy to rapidly enhance immune tolerance. In the immediate postoperative period, immunosuppressive agents are given parenterally with a quick transition to oral formulations. Corticosteroids are nonspecific anti-inflammatory agents that work primarily by lymphocyte depletion. Patients initially receive high doses of intravenous, then oral corticosteroids that are gradually tapered during the next 6 months; the goal is often to withdraw corticosteroid therapy completely. At many centers, corticosteroids are given several hours before the transplant surgery. Side effects include cushingoid appearance, hypertension, dyslipidemia, weight gain with central obesity, peptic ulcer formation and gastrointestinal bleeding, pancreatitis, personality changes, cataract formation, hyperglycemia progressing to corticosteroid diabetes, and osteoporosis with avascular necrosis of bone. The well-appreciated adverse profile of the corticosteroids has led to a number of innovative strategies to eliminate them as early as possible after the transplant surgery. Corticosteroids are usually the drug of first choice to treat acute rejection as well.[57]

There are two calcineurin inhibitors, cyclosporine and tacrolimus. Their main mechanism of action involves binding to specific proteins to form complexes that block the action of calcineurin, a key participant in T-cell activation. The calcineurin inhibitors serve to block the signal transduction pathways responsible for T-cell and B-cell activation and therefore act specifically on the immune system and do not affect other rapidly proliferating cells. Critical and often limiting adverse effects include nephrotoxicity in as many as 40% to 70% of patients and hypertension with the development of LV hypertrophy; both drugs cause a roughly equivalent incidence of these untoward events.[58] Hirsutism, gingival hyperplasia, and hyperlipidemia are more frequent with cyclosporine, and diabetes and neuropathy are more frequent with tacrolimus. There is also an increased incidence of deep venous thrombosis, tremor, headache, convulsions, and paresthesias of the limbs with both drugs.[57]

Antiproliferative agents work to either directly or indirectly inhibit the expansion of alloactivated T-cell and B-cell clones. Azathioprine was the earlier agent used in this class and served as the mainstay of immunosuppression even before the routine use of cyclosporine. In the past decade, mycophenolate mofetil (MMF) has replaced azathioprine as the first-line antiproliferative drug, with several randomized trials demonstrating superiority compared with azathioprine.[59] MMF is hydrolyzed to mycophenolic acid, which inhibits de novo purine synthesis. Both azathioprine and MMF cause leukopenia as their major adverse effect; the use of MMF can be limited by debilitating diarrhea or nausea. It is likely that the combination of MMF and tacrolimus potentiates their individual adverse effects.

Sirolimus (often called rapamycin) and everolimus are two newer agents that block activation of T cells after autocrine stimulation by interleukin-2. They also are known to inhibit proliferation of endothelial cells and fibroblasts. Their action is complementary to calcineurin inhibitors, and both sirolimus and everolimus have been used as maintenance immunosuppression, as alternatives to standard immunosuppression, and as rescue drugs for rejection. Sirolimus, an m-TOR inhibitor, has been shown to slow progression of cardiac allograft vasculopathy with established disease,[60] and everolimus has been demonstrated to reduce both acute rejection and cardiac allograft vasculopathy.[61] In one randomized trial, sirolimus, compared to azathioprine, with cyclosporine and corticosteroids, decreased by half the number of patients with acute rejection, which resulted in less subsequent development of cardiac allograft vasculopathy.[62] Because the drugs inhibit the proliferation of fibroblasts, they may cause significant difficulties with wound healing, and most centers do not use them as initial therapy immediately after the transplant surgery. The drugs have also been associated with the development of significant pericardial effusions. Sirolimus has been increasingly used to replace the calcineurin inhibitors as a strategy to improve renal dysfunction or to reverse LV hypertrophy.[58,62]

The longstanding use of the maintenance combination of cyclosporine, azathioprine, and corticosteroids has been challenged in a number of trials. Tacrolimus plus MMF, or tacrolimus plus sirolimus, was evaluated against cyclosporine plus MMF in a multicenter trial.[59] Overall 1-year survival did not differ between the three regimens, but there was statistically less significant rejection with or without hemodynamic compromise in the tacrolimus plus MMF arm compared with the cyclosporine plus MMF arm. Overall, the tacrolimus plus MMF group had better renal function and triglyceride levels at 1 year. This trial has been pivotal in moving tacrolimus as the primary calcineurin inhibitor used worldwide. Later studies have explored the use of converting a calcineurin inhibitor to sirolimus or everolimus for a renal-sparing effect.[63]

Rejection

Rejection involves cell- or antibody-mediated cardiac injury resulting from recognition of the cardiac allograft as non-self. By histologic and immunologic criteria, this process is categorized into three major types of rejection: hyperacute, acute, and chronic.[64] Hyperacute rejection results when an abrupt loss of allograft function occurs within minutes to hours after circulation is reestablished in the donor heart and is rare in modern-day transplantation. The phenomenon is mediated by preexisting antibodies to allogeneic antigens on the vascular endothelial cells of the donor organ, which is now avoided with current HLA typing techniques. These antibodies fix complement that promotes intravascular thrombosis. Subsequently, there is rapid occlusion of graft vasculature and swift and overwhelming failure of the cardiac graft.

Acute cellular rejection or cell-mediated rejection is a mononuclear inflammatory response, predominantly lymphocytic, directed against the donor heart; it is most common from the first week to several years after transplantation, and it occurs in up to 40% of patients during the first year after surgery. The key event in both the initiation and the coordination of the rejection response is T-cell activation, moderated by interleukin-2, a cytokine. Interleukin-2 is produced by CD4 cells and to a lesser extent by CD8 cells and exerts both an autocrine and a paracrine response. Unlike in renal and liver transplants, there are no reliable serologic markers for rejection in the cardiac transplant. Therefore, the endomyocardial biopsy remains the gold standard for the diagnosis of acute rejection. Biopsies are performed via a transjugular approach weekly, then every other week for several months; monthly biopsies continue for 6 to 12 months in many programs and for years thereafter in some. Cell-mediated rejection is graded according to a universally agreed on system that is periodically reviewed, as shown in **Table 31-1**.[65]

Risk factors for early rejection include younger recipient age, female gender, female donor, positive cytomegalovirus (CMV) serology, prior infections, black recipient race, and number of HLA mismatches.[66] Most important, patients who fail to take or to tolerate their immunosuppressant drugs, especially early in the postoperative course, are at very high risk for severe or recurrent cellular rejection. The occurrence of one or more episodes of treated rejections during the first year is a risk factor for both 5-year survival and development of transplant coronary disease.[67] Likewise, treatment of acute rejection in the first 6 months after transplantation contributes to a slower overall rehabilitation of the patient.

The aggressiveness of treatment for cell-mediated rejection depends on the biopsy grade, clinical correlation, patient risk factors, rejection history, length of time after transplantation, and whether or not target levels of the immunosuppressant drugs are achieved. For example, an asymptomatic, early moderate rejection soon after transplantation in a patient who is at or above target levels of immunosuppressants, or who has one or more risk factors for early rejection, would be treated more aggressively than in a low-risk patient with no prior history of cell-mediated rejection.

Another form of acute rejection is acute humoral rejection, or antibody-mediated rejection, which occurs days to weeks after transplantation and is initiated by antibodies rather than by T cells. The alloantibodies are directed against donor HLA or endothelial cell

CH 31

TABLE 31-1 Current Grading System for Cell-Mediated Rejection in Heart Transplantation Compared with an Earlier System

2004		1990	
Grade 0 R	No rejection	Grade 0	No rejection
Grade 1 R, mild	Interstitial and/or perivascular infiltrate with up to one focus of myocyte damage	Grade 1, mild	
		A—focal	Focal perivascular and/or interstitial infiltrate without myocyte damage
		B—diffuse	Diffuse infiltrate without myocyte damage
Grade 2 R, moderate	Two or more foci of infiltrate with associated myocyte damage	Grade 2, moderate (focal)	One focus of infiltrate with associated myocyte damage
Grade 3 R, severe	Diffuse infiltrate with multifocal myocyte damage ± edema, ± hemorrhage, ± vasculitis	Grade 3, moderate	
		A—focal	Multifocal infiltrate with myocyte damage
		B—diffuse	Diffuse infiltrate with myocyte damage
		Grade 4, severe	Diffuse, polymorphous infiltrate with extensive myocyte damage ± hemorrhage ± vasculitis

From Stewart S, Winters GL, Fishbein MC, et al: Revision of the 1990 working formulation for the standardization of nomenclature in the diagnosis of heart rejection. J Heart Lung Transplant 24:1710, 2005.

TABLE 31-2 Diagnostic Criteria for Antibody-Mediated Rejection

CRITERIA	FINDING	COMMENT
Clinical	Graft dysfunction	
Histologic	Capillary endothelial changes: swelling, denudation, congestion	Required
	Macrophages in capillaries	Required
	Neutrophils in capillaries	More severe cases
	Interstitial changes: edema and/or hemorrhage	More severe cases
Immunopathologic	Immunoglobulin (G, M, and/or A) plus C3d and/or C4d or C1q staining (2–2+) in capillaries by immunofluorescence	One immunopathologic criterion is required
	CD68 positivity for macrophages in capillaries and/or C4D staining of capillaries with 2–3+ intensity by paraffin immunohistochemistry	
	Fibrin in vessels	More severe cases
Serologic	Evidence of anti-HLA class I and/or class II antibodies or other antidonor antibody at time of biopsy	Supports other findings

antigens. Antibody-mediated rejection is a serious complication after heart transplantation and is manifested as "graft dysfunction" or hemodynamic abnormalities in the absence of cellular rejection on biopsy. Antibody-mediated rejection is now recognized as a distinct clinical entity, and strict histopathologic and immunologic criteria for its diagnosis have been established, as shown in **Table 31-2**.[65] Patients at greatest risk for antibody-mediated rejection are women and patients with a high PRA level or a positive crossmatch. It is estimated that significant antibody-mediated rejection occurs in about 7% of patients, but it may be as high as 20%. As antibody assays are becoming more precise, it is probable that more antibody-mediated rejection will be recognized, with a correlating need for newer treatment algorithms.[64]

Chronic rejection, or late graft failure, is an irreversible gradual deterioration of graft function that occurs in many allografts months to years after transplantation. Current concepts suggest that donor heart dysfunction in the chronic stages of maintenance immunosuppression is either related to chronic rejection, mediated by antibodies, or a result of progressive graft loss from ischemia. The latter process is characterized by intimal thickening and fibrosis, leading to luminal occlusion of the graft vasculature, and is often referred to as cardiac allograft vasculopathy or transplant coronary artery disease. An approach to the patient with nonspecific graft dysfunction is outlined in **Figure 31-12** and is primarily focused on the diagnosis of antibody-mediated rejection versus the presence of cardiac allograft vasculopathy.[68]

Infection

Despite the advances in immunosuppressive management, a major untoward consequence remains the occurrence of life-threatening

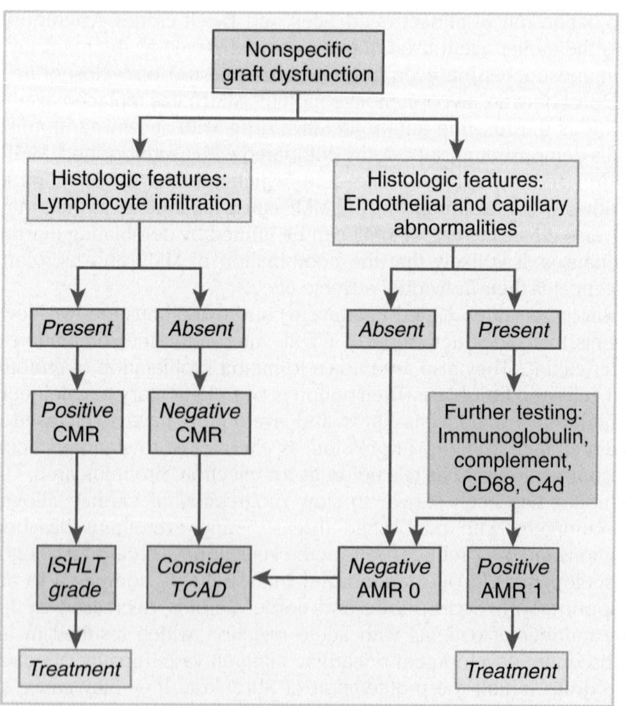

FIGURE 31-12 Diagnostic algorithm for the heart transplant patient with nonspecific graft dysfunction. AMR = antibody-mediated rejection; CMR = cell-mediated rejection; ISHLT = International Society of Heart and Lung Transplantation; TCAD = transplant coronary artery disease. *(From Jessup M, Brozena S: State-of-the-art strategies for immunosuppression. Curr Opin Organ Transplant 12:536, 2007.)*

TABLE 31-3 Post–Heart Transplantation Morbidity for Adults*

OUTCOME	WITHIN 5 YEARS	TOTAL N WITH KNOWN RESPONSE	WITHIN 10 YEARS	TOTAL N WITH KNOWN RESPONSE
Hypertension	93.8%	N = 8266	98.5%	N = 1586
Renal dysfunction	32.6%	N = 8859	38.7%	N = 1829
Abnormal creatinine <2.5 mg/dL	21.2%		24.4%	
Creatinine >2.5 mg/dL	8.4%		8.2%	
Chronic dialysis	2.5%		4.9%	
Renal transplant	0.5%		1.2%	
Hyperlipidemia	87.1%	N = 9237	93.3%	N = 1890
Diabetes	34.8%	N = 8219	36.7%	N = 1601
Cardiac allograft vasculopathy	31.5%	N = 5944	52.7%	N = 896

*Cumulative prevalence in survivors at 5 and 10 years after transplantation (follow-ups: April 1994-June 2005).
From Hertz MI, Aurora P, Christie JD, et al: Registry of the International Society for Heart and Lung Transplantation: A quarter century of thoracic transplantation. J Heart Lung Transplant 27:937, 2008.

infections. Infections cause approximately 20% of deaths within the first year after transplantation and continue to be a common cause of morbidity and mortality throughout the recipient's life. The most common infections in the first month after surgery are nosocomial, bacterial, and fungal infections related to mechanical ventilation, catheters, and the surgical site. Mortality is highest for fungal infections, followed by protozoal, bacterial, and viral infections. Aspergillosis and candidiasis are the most common fungal infections after heart transplantation. Viral infections, especially CMV, can enhance immunosuppression, resulting in additional opportunistic infections. Accordingly, patients are typically given a prophylactic regimen against CMV, *Pneumocystis carinii*, herpes simplex virus, and oral candidiasis to be used during the first 6 to 12 months after transplantation. Prophylactic intravenous ganciclovir or oral valganciclovir is generally given for variable amounts of time in the CMV-seronegative recipient of a CMV-positive donor.

TABLE 31-4 Type and Cumulative Prevalence of Malignant Neoplasia After Heart Transplantation*

MALIGNANCY/ TYPE	1-YEAR SURVIVORS	5-YEAR SURVIVORS	10-YEAR SURVIVORS
No malignancy	20,441 (97.1%)	7780 (84.9%)	1264 (68.1%)
Malignancy (all types combined	612 (2.9%)	1389 (15.1%)	592 (31.9%)
Malignancy type			
Skin	282	937	360
Lymph	142	127	38
Other	132	359	108
Type not reported	56	39	126

*Cumulative prevalence in survivors (follow-ups: April 1994-June 2006).
From Hertz MI, Aurora P, Christie JD, et al: Registry of the International Society for Heart and Lung Transplantation: A quarter century of thoracic transplantation. J Heart Lung Transplant 27:937, 2008.

Medical Complications and Comorbidities

The complications that follow heart transplantation reflect, in part, the premorbid status of the majority of transplant recipients who have vascular disease and other significant medical conditions. After 5 years, more than 90% of recipients have hypertension, at least 80% have hyperlipidemia, and more than 30% have diabetes, as shown in **Table 31-3**.[69] Each year after transplantation, a larger number of patients will develop clinically significant cardiac allograft vasculopathy, which is the major limitation to long life after transplantation. By 5 years, almost 30% of recipients will have cardiac allograft vasculopathy, and at least half will be so afflicted at 10 years. Likewise, progressive renal insufficiency is an insidious problem that is only recently being addressed by substitution protocols to limit the administration of calcineurin inhibitors.[62]

MALIGNANT NEOPLASIA. The magnitude of over-immunosuppression in many transplant recipients is illustrated by the prediction of a 30% to 40% incidence of neoplasia in transplant patients during the past 30 years. The risk of fatal malignant disease progressively increases in the years after transplantation, and there is a substantially higher risk in immunosuppressed patients compared with the normal population. Post-transplantation lymphoproliferative disease and lung cancer are the most common fatal malignant neoplasms, as shown in **Table 31-4**.[69]

DIABETES. Patients who develop new-onset diabetes mellitus after transplantation are at increased risk for morbidity and mortality. Accumulating evidence suggests that their long-term outcomes, including patient survival and graft survival, may be adversely affected. Much of the diabetes that occurs is attributed to the high-dose corticosteroids used early after transplant surgery, but it is now appreciated that the calcineurin inhibitors play an important role as well. Impaired B-cell function appears to be the primary mechanism of calcineurin inhibitor–induced new-onset diabetes.[70]

The risk factors for the development of diabetes after transplantation include obesity, increased age, family history of diabetes, abnormal glucose tolerance, and African American or Hispanic descent. Changing trends in the demographics of transplant patients, such as increased age and increased BMI, suggest that these patients may now be at a greater risk for new-onset diabetes than in the past. Increased BMI increases risk of insulin resistance, and corticosteroids can cause glucose intolerance, insulin resistance, and frank hyperglycemia. African Americans are more likely to develop new-onset diabetes mellitus regardless of the immunosuppression used but are particularly susceptible after treatment with tacrolimus.

HYPERTENSION. The excess risk of hypertension is primarily related to the use of calcineurin inhibitors because of both direct effects of the drugs on the kidney and the associated renal insufficiency that is also highly prevalent. The incidence of hypertension may be lower with tacrolimus compared with cyclosporine.[71] Post-transplantation hypertension is difficult to control and often requires a combination of several antihypertensive agents.

RENAL INSUFFICIENCY. In a large registry of almost 70,000 nonrenal solid organ transplant recipients, the risk for development of chronic renal failure was 16% at 10 years.[72] There are a variety of postulated causes of calcineurin inhibitor–associated early renal insufficiency, including direct calcineurin inhibitor–mediated renal arteriolar vasoconstriction, increased levels of endothelin 1 (a potent vasoconstrictor), decreased nitric oxide production, and alterations in the kidney's ability to adjust to changes in serum tonicity. Once early renal insufficiency occurs, progressive renal failure has appeared to be inexorable, until recently. A number of new trials are in progress to evaluate the effects on renal function as well as rejection episodes of substituting an m-TOR inhibitor, sirolimus or everolimus, for a calcineurin inhibitor.[73]

HYPERLIPIDEMIA. Hyperlipidemia is common after transplantation, as it is in the general population. The concern has been that many studies have associated hyperlipidemia with the development of cardiac allograft vasculopathy and cerebrovascular and peripheral vascular disease, with the attendant morbidity and mortality of these vascular disorders. Typically, total cholesterol, LDL-cholesterol, and triglycerides increase by 3 months after transplantation and then generally fall somewhat after the first year. A number of drugs commonly used after transplantation contribute to the hyperlipidemia observed. Corticosteroids may lead to insulin resistance, increased free fatty acid synthesis, and increased very low-density lipoprotein production. Cyclosporine increases serum LDL-cholesterol and binds to the LDL receptor, decreasing its availability to absorb cholesterol from the bloodstream; tacrolimus probably causes less hyperlipidemia. Sirolimus and MMF also have unfavorable effects on lipids. Sirolimus in escalating doses has been shown to result in prominent elevation of triglyceride levels.[57]

Lipid-lowering therapy with any statin, or HMG-CoA reductase inhibitor, was strongly associated with a marked improvement in 1-year survival in the Heart Transplant Lipid registry.[74] In heart transplant recipients, pravastatin and simvastatin have been associated with outcome benefits in survival, severity of rejection, and cardiac allograft vasculopathy.[66]

CARDIAC ALLOGRAFT VASCULOPATHY. The development of transplant vasculopathy remains the most disheartening long-term complication of heart transplantation, with an annual incidence rate of 5% to 10%. The prognosis of heart transplant recipients is largely determined by the occurrence of cardiac allograft vasculopathy (CAV); after the first postoperative year, CAV becomes increasingly important as a cause of death. CAV can develop as early as 3 months after transplantation and is detected angiographically in 20% of grafts at 1 year and in 40% to 50% at 5 years.[70,75] In contrast to eccentric lesions seen in atheromatous disease, CAV results from neointimal proliferation of vascular smooth muscle cells, so that it is a generalized process. Typically, the condition is characterized by concentric narrowing that affects the entire length of the coronary tree, from the epicardial to intramyocardial segments, leading to rapid tapering, pruning, and obliteration of third-order branch vessels. The majority of patients will not experience anginal symptoms because of denervation of coronary arteries. The first clinical manifestation of CAV may include myocardial ischemia and infarction, heart failure, ventricular arrhythmia, or sudden death.

The causes of transplant vasculopathy are multifactorial. The risk for CAV increases as the number of HLA mismatches and the number and duration of rejection episodes increase. Various nonimmunologic factors, including CMV infection of the recipient, donor or recipient factors (e.g., age, gender, pretransplantation diagnosis), and factors related to surgery (ischemia-reperfusion injury), have been associated with development of CAV and increase the risk for CAV. Classic risk factors for vascular disease, such as smoking, obesity, diabetes, dyslipidemia, and hypertension, increase CAV as well.

In an effort to detect the development of CAV, transplant teams must devise an approach to screen for the disease and, when it is found, to control its progression. Coronary angiography is limited by the fact that CAV produces concentric lesions that affect the distal and small vessels, often before it becomes apparent in the main epicardial vessels. Intravascular ultrasound (IVUS) is currently the most sensitive imaging technique to study early transplant vasculopathy. IVUS provides quantitative information on vessel wall morphology and lumen dimensions. An increase in intimal thickness of at least 0.5 mm in the first year after transplantation is a reliable indicator of both CAV development and 5-year mortality.[76] However, increased invasiveness and cost of IVUS preclude its widespread application. Dobutamine stress echocardiography has a high sensitivity (83% to 95%) and specificity (between 53% and 91%) compared with angiographic evaluation of CAV and even greater specificity compared with IVUS-detected disease.[76,77] Most transplant centers do one of these screening tests on an annual basis to assess the risk of new CAV.

Recently, there have been an increased number of trials examining the efficacy of sirolimus or everolimus to prevent the development or progression of CAV in heart transplant recipients. The precise role of the two drugs in maintenance immunosuppression has not yet been determined, but they are frequently used and are promising in their reduction of coronary intimal thickening once CAV has been detected.[70]

Outcomes After Heart Transplantation

SURVIVAL. **Figure 31-13** depicts the latest data from the International Society for Heart and Lung Transplantation on overall transplant survival.[78] During the first year after transplantation, early causes of death are graft failure, infection, and rejection, with an overall survival at 1 year of 87%. Interestingly, although worldwide approaches to the management of the cardiac transplant recipient are substantially different from center to center, the outcomes are surprisingly similar. For example, the 5-, 10-, and 15-year survival rates after heart transplantation were comparable in two centers, one from Nantes, France,[79] and one from Utrecht, the Netherlands.[80] Indeed, this phenomenon of similar outcomes despite marked differences in programmatic management may be regarded as a testament to the overall antirejection strategy. Nonspecific graft failure accounted for 41% of deaths during the first 30 days after transplantation, whereas non-CMV infection was the primary cause of death during the first year. After 5 years, CAV and late graft failure (31% together), malignant neoplasia (24%), and non-CMV infection (10%) are the most prominent causes of death.[66,81]

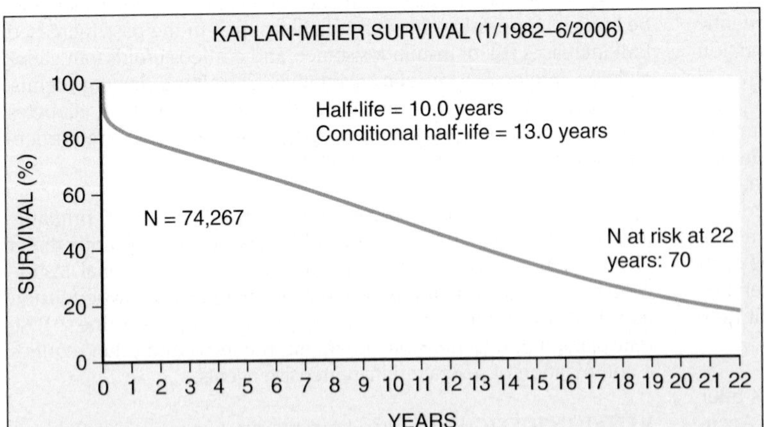

FIGURE 31-13 Overall heart transplant survival in 74,267 first-time recipients, showing a 10-year survival of at least 50%. *(From Hertz MI, Aurora P, Christie JD, et al: Registry of the International Society for Heart and Lung Transplantation: A quarter century of thoracic transplantation. J Heart Lung Transplant 27:937, 2008.)*

FUNCTIONAL OUTCOMES. By the first year after transplantation surgery, 90% of surviving patients report no functional limitations and approximately 35% return to work.[82] These figures may change as the demographics of cardiac transplant recipients evolve. There are numerous challenges to ensure optimal functional outcomes, not the least of which is non-reimbursement for cardiac rehabilitation programs by many third-party payers in the United States and reluctance of employers in the United States to hire the transplant survivor.

The heart transplant procedure markedly reduces cardiac filling pressures observed in the recipient before transplantation and augments cardiac output. There may be an abnormal maximal cardiac output during exercise secondary to denervation, limited atrial function, decreased myocardial compliance from rejection or ischemic injury, and donor-recipient size mismatch. Much of this hemodynamic abnormality may be normalized with regular exercise.[83] Immediately after surgery, a restrictive hemodynamic pattern is frequently observed that gradually improves during a few days to weeks. Some 10% to 15% of recipients develop a chronic restrictive-type response during exercise that may produce fatigue and breathlessness. In the absence of parasympathetic innervation that normally lowers the heart rate, the resting heart rate of a recipient is typically 90 to 115 beats/min. Likewise, beta blockers may further impair exercise response in the transplant patient and should not be first-line therapy for hypertension in this group.

Future Perspectives

There are many potential surgical "targets" in heart failure patients, especially for patients with ischemic cardiomyopathy. The most widely used surgery for heart failure is coronary artery bypass, and with the aid of viability studies, this appears to be effective therapy to reduce the risk of death versus medical therapy. Overall, heart surgery is not as dangerous as it used to be in this population of patients. Furthermore, recent randomized trials in mitral valve surgery and patients with low LVEF indicate that this is more widely applicable than at just a handful of specialized centers. Despite the discouraging results of the STICH trial, there may be a discrete population of patients with localized LV infarction and dilation that may benefit from LV reconstruction. As surgical and anesthesia management of heart failure continues to improve, maximizing the surgical options for patients referred for heart transplantation may help diminish the wait times for cardiac transplant candidates who truly have no other surgical or medical options left.

REFERENCES

Coronary Artery Revascularization

1. Starling RC, McCarthy PM, Yamini MH: Surgical treatment of chronic congestive heart failure. *In* Mann D (ed): Heart Failure: A Companion to Braunwald's Heart Disease. Philadelphia, WB Saunders, 2003, pp 717-736.
2. Shinkle AFL, Poldermans D, Elhendy A, Bax JJ: Assessment of myocardial viability in patients with heart failure. J Nucl Med 48:1135, 2007.
3. Pocar M, Moneta A, Grossi A, Donatelli F: Coronary artery bypass for heart failure in ischemic cardiomyopathy: 17-year follow-up. Ann Thorac Surg 83:468, 2007.
4. Hillis GS, Zehr KJ, Williams AW, et al: Outcome of patients with low ejection fraction undergoing coronary artery bypass grafting: Renal function and mortality after 3.8 years. Circulation 114:I414, 2006.
5. Argenziano M, Spotnitz HM, Whang W, et al: Risk stratification for coronary artery bypass surgery in patients with left ventricular dysfunction: Analysis of the coronary artery bypass grafting patch trial database. Circulation 100(Suppl II):II119, 1999.
6. Hochman JS, Sleeper LA, Webb JG, et al: Early revascularization in acute myocardial infarction complicated by cardiogenic shock. N Engl J Med 341:625, 1999.
7. Rizzello, V, Poldermans D, Boersma E, et al: Opposite patterns of left ventricular remodeling after coronary artery revascularization in patients with ischemic cardiomyopathy. Circulation 110:2383, 2004.
8. Pagano D, Bonser RS, Camici PG: Myocardial revascularization for the treatment of post-ischemic heart failure. Curr Opin Cardiol 14:506, 1999.
9. Di Carli MF, Asgarzadie F, Schelbert HR, et al: Quantitative relation between myocardial viability and improvement in heart failure symptoms after revascularization in patients with ischemic cardiomyopathy. Circulation 92:3436, 1995.
10. O'Connor CM, Velazquez EJ, Gardner LH, et al: Comparison of coronary artery bypass grafting versus medical therapy on long-term outcome in patients with ischemic cardiomyopathy: A 25-year experience from the Duke Cardiovascular Disease Databank. Am J Cardiol 90:101, 2002.
11. Allman KC, Shaw LJ, Hachamovitch R, et al: Myocardial viability testing and impact of revascularization on prognosis in patients with coronary artery disease and left ventricular dysfunction: A meta-analysis. J Am Coll Cardiol 39:1151, 2002.
12. Kleikamp G. Maleszka A, Reiss N, et al: Determinants of mid and long-term results in patients after surgical revascularization for ischemic cardiomyopathy. Ann Thorac Surg 75:1406, 2003.
13. Elefteriades J, Edwards R: Coronary bypass in left heart failure. Semin Thorac Cardiovasc Surg 14:125, 2002.
14. Carnici PG, Prasad SK, Rinoldi OE: Stunning, hibernation, and assessment of myocardial viability. Circulation 117:103, 2008.
15. Hunt SA, Abraham WT, Chin MH, et al: ACC/AHA 2005 Guideline Update for the Diagnosis and Management of Chronic Heart Failure in the Adult: A report of the American College of Cardiology/American Heart Association Task Force on Practice Guidelines (Writing Committee to Update the 2001 Guidelines for the Evaluation and Management of Heart Failure): Developed in collaboration with the American College of Chest Physicians and the International Society for Heart and Lung Transplantation: Endorsed by the Heart Rhythm Society. Circulation 112:e154, 2005.
16. Eagle KA, Guyton RA, Davidoff R, et al: ACC/AHA guidelines for coronary artery bypass graft surgery: Executive summary and recommendations: A report of the American College of Cardiology/American Heart Association Task Force on Practice Guidelines (Committee to revise the 1991 guidelines for coronary artery bypass graft surgery). Circulation 100:1464, 1999.
17. Jones RH, Velazquez EJ, Michler RE, et al: STICH Hypothesis 2 Investigators: Coronary bypass surgery with or without surgical ventricular reconstruction. N Engl J Med 360:1705, 2009.

Valve Surgery in Patients with Left Ventricular Dysfunction

18. Trichon BH, Felker GM, Shaw LK, et al: Relation of frequency and severity of mitral regurgitation to survival among patients with left ventricular systolic dysfunction and heart failure. Am J Cardiol 91:538, 2003.
19. Bach DS, Bolling SF: Improvement following correction of secondary mitral regurgitation in end-stage cardiomyopathy with mitral annuloplasty. Am J Cardiol 78:966, 1996.
20. Tibayan FA, Rodriguez F, Langer F, et al: Undersized mitral annuloplasty alters left ventricular shape during acute ischemic mitral regurgitation. Circulation 110:II98, 2004.
21. Bishay ES, McCarthy PM, Cosgrove DM, et al: Mitral valve surgery in patients with severe left ventricular dysfunction. Eur J Cardiothorac Surg 17:213, 2000.
22. Acker MA, Bolling S, Shemin R, et al: Mitral valve surgery in heart failure: Insights from the Acorn clinical trial. J Thorac Cardiovasc Surg 132:568, 2006.
23. Acker MA, Jessup M, Bolling SF, et al: Mitral valve repair in heart failure: 5-year follow-up from the MVR Stratum of the Acorn Randomized Trial. J Thorac Cardiovasc Surg (In press).
24. Braun J, van de Veire NR, Klautz RJM, et al: Restrictive mitral annuloplasty cures ischemic mitral regurgitation and heart failure. Ann Thorac Surg 85:430, 2008.
25. Fattouch K, Guccione F, Sampognaro R, et al: Efficacy of adding mitral valve restrictive annuloplasty to coronary artery bypass grafting in patients with moderate ischemic mitral valve regurgitation: A randomized trial. J Thorac Cardiovasc Surg 138:278, 2009.
26. Westenberg JJ, van der Geest RJ, Lamb HL, et al: MRI to evaluate left atrial and ventricular reverse remodeling after restrictive mitral annuloplasty in dilated cardiomyopathy. Circulation 112(Suppl):I437, 2005.
27. Miller DC: Ischemic mitral regurgitation redux—to repair or to replace? J Thorac Cardiovasc Surg 122:1059, 2001.
28. McGee EC, Gillinov AM, Blackstone EH, et al: Recurrent mitral regurgitation after annuloplasty for functional ischemic MR. J Thorac Cardiovasc Surg 128:916, 2004.
29. Mihaljevic T, Lam BK, Rajeswaran J, et al: Impact of mitral valve annuloplasty combined with revascularization in patients with functional ischemic MR. J Am Coll Cardiol 49:2191, 2007.
30. Spoor MT, Geltz A, Bolling SF: Flexible versus nonflexible mitral valve rings for congestive heart failure: Differential durability of repair. Circlation 114(Suppl 1):I67, 2006.
31. Wu AH, Aaronson KD, Bolling SF, et al: Impact of mitral valve annuloplasty on mortality risk in patients with mitral regurgitation and left ventricular systolic dysfunction. J Am Coll Cardiol 45:381, 2005.
32. Pereira JJ, Lauer MS, Bashir M, et al: Survival after aortic valve replacement for severe aortic stenosis with low transvalvular gradients and severe left ventricular dysfunction. J Am Coll Cardiol 39:1356, 2002.
33. Varadarajan P, Kapoor N, Bansal RC, et al: Clinical profile and natural history of 453 nonsurgically managed patients with severe aortic stenosis. Ann Thorac Surg 82:2111, 2006.
34. Quere JP, Monin JL, Levy F, et al: Influence of preoperative left ventricular contractile reserve on postoperative ejection fraction in low-gradient aortic stenosis. Circulation 113:1738, 2006.
35. Bhudia SK, McCarthy PM, Kumpati GS, et al: Improved outcomes after aortic valve surgery for chronic aortic regurgitation with severe left ventricular dysfunction. J Am Coll Cardiol 49:1465, 2007.
36. McCarthy PM: Valve surgery for patients with left ventricular dysfunction. *In* Young J, McCarthy PM (eds): Heart Failure: A Combined Medical and Surgical Approach. Malden, Mass, Blackwell Futura, 2006, pp 153-173.
37. Bonow RO, Carabello BA, Chatterjee K, et al: ACC/AHA 2006 guidelines for the management of patients with valvular heart disease: A report of the American College of Cardiology/American Heart Association Task Force on Practice Guidelines (writing Committee to Revise the 1998 guidelines for the management of patients with valvular heart disease) developed in collaboration with the Society of Cardiovascular Anesthesiologists; endorsed by the Society for Cardiovascular Angiography and Interventions and the Society of Thoracic Surgeons. J Am Coll Cardiol 48:e1, 2006.

Left Ventricular Reconstruction

38. Mann DL: Mechanisms and models in heart failure: A combinatorial approach. Circulation 100:999, 1999.
39. McCarthy PM, McGee EC: Ventricular reconstruction and device therapies for cardiomyopathy patients. *In* Young J, McCarthy PM (eds): Heart Failure: A Combined Medical and Surgical Approach. Malden, Mass, Blackwell Futura, 2006, pp 174-191.
40. Athanasuleas CL, Buckberg GD, Stanley AW, et al: Surgical ventricular restoration in the treatment of congestive heart failure caused by post-infarction ventricular dilation. J Am Coll Cardiol 44:1439, 2004.
41. Artrip JH, Oz MC, Burkhoff D: Left ventricular volume reduction surgery for heart failure: A physiologic perspective. J Thorac Cardiovasc Surg 122:775, 2001.
42. Tulner SA, Steendijk P, Klautz RJ, et al: Surgical ventricular restoration in patients with ischemic dilated cardiomyopathy: Evaluation of systolic and diastolic ventricular function, wall stress, dyssynchrony and mechanical efficiency by pressure-volume loop. J Thorac Cardiovasc Surg 132:610, 2006.
43. Athanasuleas CL, Buckberg GD, Conte JV, et al: Surgical ventricular reconstruction. N Engl J Med 361:529, 2009; author reply 531-532.
44. Athanasuleas CL, Buckberg GD, Menicanti L, Ghasib M; the RESTORE Group: Optimizing ventricular shape in anterior restoration. Semin Thorac Cardiovasc Surgery 13:459, 2001.

Passive Cardiac Support Devices

45. Starling RC, Jessup M, Oh JK, et al: Sustained benefits of the CorCap Cardiac Support Device on left ventricular remodeling: Three year follow-up results from the Acorn clinical trial. Ann Thorac Surg 84:1236, 2007.
46. Mann DL, Acker MA, Jessup M, et al: Clinical evaluation of the CorCap Cardiac Support Device in patients with dilated cardiomyopathy. Ann Thorac Surg 84:1226, 2007.

Cardiac Transplantation

47. Stevenson LW, Pagani FD, Young JB, et al: INTERMACS profiles of advanced heart failure: The current picture. J Heart Lung Transplant 28:535, 2009.
48. Mehra MR, Kobashigawa J, Starling R, et al: Listing criteria for heart transplantation: International Society for Heart and Lung Transplantation guidelines for the care of cardiac transplant candidates—2006. J Heart Lung Transplant 25:1024, 2006.
49. Simmonds J, Burch M, Dawkins H, et al: Heart transplantation after congenital heart surgery: Improving results and future goals. Eur J Cardiothorac Surg 34:313, 2008.
50. Goldberg LR, Jessup M: A time to be born and a time to die. Circulation 116:360, 2007.
51. Levy WC, Mozaffarian D, Linker DT, et al: Can the Seattle heart failure model be used to risk-stratify heart failure patients for potential left ventricular assist device therapy? J Heart Lung Transplant 28:231, 2009.
52. Lund LH, Aaronson KD, Mancini DM, et al: Validation of peak exercise oxygen consumption and the Heart Failure Survival Score for serial risk stratification in advanced heart failure. Am J Cardiol 2005:734, 95.
53. Klotz S, Wenzelburger F, Stypmann J, et al: Reversible pulmonary hypertension in heart transplant candidates: To transplant or not to transplant. Ann Thorac Surg 82:1770, 2006.
54. Kobashigawa J, Mehra M, West L, et al: Report from a consensus conference on the sensitized patient awaiting heart transplantation. J Heart Lung Transplant 28:213, 2009.
55. Grande AM, Gaeta R, Campana C, et al: Comparison of standard and bicaval approach in orthotopic heart transplantation: 10-year follow-up. J Cardiovasc Med 9:493, 2008.
56. Ramakrishna H, Jaroszewski DE, Arabia FA: Adult cardiac transplantation: A review of perioperative management Part-I. Ann Card Anaesth 12:71, 2009.
57. Lindenfeld J, Miller GG, Shakar SF, et al: Drug therapy in the heart transplant recipient: Part I: Cardiac rejection and immunosuppressive drugs. Circulation 110:3734, 2004.
58. Flechner SM, Kobashigawa J, Klintmalm G: Calcineurin inhibitor–sparing regimens in solid organ transplantation: Focus on improving renal function and nephrotoxicity. Clin Transplant 22:1, 2008.
59. Kobashigawa JA, Miller LW, Russell SD, et al: Tacrolimus with mycophenolate mofetil (MMF) or sirolimus vs. cyclosporine with MMF in cardiac transplant patients: 1-year report. Am J Transplant 6:1377, 2006.
60. Raichlin E, Bae JH, Khalpey Z, et al: Conversion to sirolimus as primary immunosuppression attenuates the progression of allograft vasculopathy after cardiac transplantation. Circulation 116:2726, 2007.
61. Sanchez-Fructuoso AI: Everolimus: An update on the mechanism of action, pharmacokinetics and recent clinical trials. Expert Opin Drug Metab Toxicol 4:807, 2008.
62. Groetzner J, Kaczmarek I, Schulz U, et al: Mycophenolate and sirolimus as calcineurin inhibitor–free immunosuppression improves renal function better than calcineurin inhibitor–reduction in late cardiac transplant recipients with chronic renal failure. Transplantation 87:726, 2009.
63. Rothenburger M, Zuckermann A, Bara C, et al: Recommendations for the use of everolimus (Certican) in heart transplantation: Results from the second German-Austrian Certican Consensus Conference. J Heart Lung Transplant 26:305, 2007.
64. Singh N, Pirsch J, Samaniego M: Antibody-mediated rejection: Treatment alternatives and outcomes. Transplant Rev 23:34, 2009.
65. Stewart S, Winters GL, Fishbein MC, et al: Revision of the 1990 working formulation for the standardization of nomenclature in the diagnosis of heart rejection. J Heart Lung Transplant 24:1710, 2005.
66. Kobashigawa JA, Starling RC, Mehra MR, et al: Multicenter retrospective analysis of cardiovascular risk factors affecting long-term outcome of de novo cardiac transplant recipients. J Heart Lung Transplant 25:1063, 2006.
67. Taylor DO, Edwards LB, Boucek MM, et al: Registry of the International Society for Heart and Lung Transplantation: Twenty-second official adult heart transplant report—2005. J Heart Lung Transplant 24:945, 2005.
68. Jessup M, Brozena S: State-of-the-art strategies for immunosuppression. Curr Opin Organ Transplant 12:536, 2007.
69. Hertz MI, Aurora P, Christie JD, et al: Registry of the International Society for Heart and Lung Transplantation: A quarter century of thoracic transplantation. J Heart Lung Transplant 27:937, 2008.
70. Russo MJ, Chen JM, Hong KN, et al: Survival after heart transplantation is not diminished among recipients with uncomplicated diabetes mellitus: An analysis of the United Network of Organ Sharing database. Circulation 114:2280, 2006.
71. Ye F, Ying-Bin X, Yu-Guo W, et al: Tacrolimus versus cyclosporine microemulsion for heart transplant recipients: A meta-analysis. J Heart Lung Transplant 28:58, 2009.
72. Lonze BE, Warren DS, Stewart ZA, et al: Kidney transplantation in previous heart or lung recipients. Am J Transplant 9:578, 2009.
73. Gonzalez-Vilchez F, de Prada JA, Exposito V, et al: Avoidance of calcineurin inhibitors with use of proliferation signal inhibitors in de novo heart transplantation with renal failure. J Heart Lung Transplant 27:1135, 2008.
74. Wu AH, Ballantyne CM, Short BC, et al: Statin use and risks of death or fatal rejection in the Heart Transplant Lipid Registry. Am J Cardiol 95:367, 2005.
75. Schmauss D, Weis M, Schmauss D, Weis M: Cardiac allograft vasculopathy: Recent developments. Circulation 117:2131, 2008.
76. Kobashigawa JA, Tobis JM, Starling RC, et al: Multicenter intravascular ultrasound validation study among heart transplant recipients: Outcomes after five years. J Am Coll Cardiol 45:1532, 2005.
77. Bacal F, Moreira L, Souza G, et al: Dobutamine stress echocardiography predicts cardiac events or death in asymptomatic patients long-term after heart transplantation: 4-year prospective evaluation. J Heart Lung Transplant 23:1238, 2004.
78. Delgado JF, Manito N, Segovia J, et al: The use of proliferation signal inhibitors in the prevention and treatment of allograft vasculopathy in heart transplantation. Transplant Rev 23:69, 2009.
79. Roussel JC, Baron O, Perigaud C, et al: Outcome of heart transplants 15 to 20 years ago: Graft survival, post-transplant morbidity, and risk factors for mortality. J Heart Lung Transplant 27:486, 2008.
80. Tjang YS, van der Heijden GJ, Tenderich G, et al: Survival analysis in heart transplantation: Results from an analysis of 1290 cases in a single center. Eur J Cardiothorac Surg 33:856, 2008.
81. Weiss ES, Nwakanma LU, Patel ND, et al: Outcomes in patients older than 60 years of age undergoing orthotopic heart transplantation: An analysis of the UNOS database. J Heart Lung Transplant 27:184, 2008.
82. Grady KL, Naftel DC, Young JB, et al: Patterns and predictors of physical functional disability at 5 to 10 years after heart transplantation. J Heart Lung Transplant 26:1182, 2007.
83. Haykowsky M, Taylor D, Kim D, et al: Exercise training improves aerobic capacity and skeletal muscle function in heart transplant recipients. Am J Transplant 9:734, 2009.

CHAPTER 32 Assisted Circulation in the Treatment of Heart Failure

Mandeep R. Mehra and Bartley P. Griffith

The remarkable success of pharmacologic management (see Chap. 28) and percutaneous long-term implantable devices (cardiac resynchronization therapy and implantable cardioverter-defibrillators; see Chap. 29) has yielded a population of advanced heart failure patients who transition to a stage manifested by a poor quality of life, frequent rehospitalization, and eventual hemodynamic collapse. Cardiac transplantation (see Chap. 31) cannot be applied to most such individuals, largely because of donor organ scarcity and the requirement of noncardiac organ physiologic stability. Furthermore, as time to acquisition of a suitable organ donor is prolonged, these patients may need temporary hemodynamic support to facilitate the process of transplantation. It is in this context and to address the overt treatment gap that the concept of mechanical assistance of the failing circulation has emerged.

History of Permanent Mechanical Circulatory Support

The National Heart, Lung and Blood Institute (NHLBI) initiated a total artificial heart program in 1964. Although a practical total artificial heart that can pump 100,000 times daily for a lifetime remains elusive, the follow-on NHLBI left ventricular assist device program begun in 1972 spawned clinical success and commercially viable devices that continue to evolve. First-generation left ventricular assist devices were possible because of advances in tested artificial valves and durable membranes in the total artificial heart program. Engineers designed bladder-type ventricles from biocompatible elastic polymers. These blood pumps attempted to duplicate a functional ventricle that would fully eject in systole and fill completely in diastole. Variations combined an inlet "mitral" type valve, a compliant flexing blood sac "ventricle," and an outlet valve. In 1974, a prototype nuclear total artificial heart with plutonium-238 and a 10-year life cycle was developed, but regulatory hurdles led to pneumatic and battery-driven electrical systems and percutaneous drivelines. The patients adapted well to the left ventricular assist devices and, as early as 1988, were discharged from hospitals to wait for a donor heart. Considerable progress has ensued in miniaturizing the early drive consoles, and shoulder-holstered battery plus drive systems are now the norm.

Theory and Definitions of Mechanical Circulatory Support

Early on, mechanical circulatory support in chronic heart failure evolved as a means of supporting patients awaiting transplantation, and this indication provided successful transition to heart transplantation and enhanced post-transplantation outcomes. Although it was initially proposed as a means to "bridge" patients to heart transplantation, it became recognized that this therapy could be considered for treatment of those patients ineligible for transplantation, which led to the notion of "destination therapy" to provide palliative support for patients with severe irreversible refractory heart failure. As experience developed, it became clear that many patients initially ineligible for transplantation could be transformed into eventual transplant candidates by virtue of chronic hemodynamic support, which resulted in improvement in end-organ hypoperfusion and recovery of heart failure–initiated comorbidity. Traditionally, advanced renal dysfunction and pharmacologically irreversible pulmonary hypertension render patients ineligible for transplantation because of the well-defined observation of increased post-transplantation morbidity and mortality. However, the application of chronic mechanical circulatory support improves pulmonary and renal hemodynamics, allowing eligibility for transplantation. Thus, the notion of a "bridge to candidacy" surfaced. In contemporary thinking, the dichotomous decision of either a bridge to transplantation or destination therapy is no longer tenable, and one could consider mechanical circulatory support in the context of a "bridge to decision."[1] It has recently been recognized that a small subset of patients may have sufficient cardiac structural and functional improvement to allow removal of implanted mechanical support devices, a notion now referred to as "bridge to recovery" (**Table 32-1**).

Classification and Description of Devices

A mechanical circulatory support pump may be positioned extracorporeally (outside the body) or intracorporeally (contained within the body) as a biventricular assist device (BiVAD), a right ventricular assist device (RVAD), or more commonly a left ventricular assist device (LVAD). In addition, the pump characteristic further substratifies it into a pulsatile or nonpulsatile device. The first-generation mechanical circulatory devices used volume displacement to invoke pulsatility (HeartMate XVE and Novacor; **Fig. 32-1**). The newer second-generation devices are continuous-flow axial pumps (HeartMate II, **Fig. 32-2**; Jarvik 2000, **Fig. 32-3**). Pulsatile volume displacement pumps are large in profile, preload dependent, and associated with decreased durability. The continuous-flow pumps are smaller, capable of similar degrees of pumping support (10 liters/min), more durable, and functionally dependent on both preload and afterload.[2]

Third-generation mechanical circulatory support devices represent the emerging future of this technology. These devices are uniformly continuous-flow devices but may be axial or centrifugal. In addition, these devices use an impeller pump that is either magnetically or hydrodynamically levitated. The net result is a smaller profile, lower weight, and potential for greater durability, and early evidence suggests improvements in right ventricular failure and infection rates.[2]

HeartWare HVAD. This small, centrifugal, rotary pump has a non–contact-bearing design and is placed completely within the pericardial cavity at the apex of the left ventricle. The impeller has no bearings, which obviated the need for abdominal surgery. The device is commercially available in Europe, and clinical trials for a bridge to transplantation indication are ongoing in the United States.

VentrAssist Device. This centrifugal pump used a magnetically levitated internal impeller, and despite initial favorable data, the device development was discontinued because of lack of financial viability of the company. Furthermore, although the device engineering was laudable, surgeons raised concerns with the intracardiac cannula and its angulation that caused mechanical problems.

DuraHeart Device. This continuous-flow, centrifugal rotary pump is designed with active magnetic levitation of the impeller along with hydrodynamic bearings to support impeller levitation in case of failure of the magnetic levitation system. Rather than fixed-speed devices, this pump can achieve a flow rate of 2 to 8 liters/min, and the flow rate can vary with physiologic changes. In the European experience of 68 patients eligible for transplantation, 6-month survival was 81% and 12-month survival 77%. However, device-related infections were seen in 61%; stroke, bleeding, and right-sided heart failure occurred in a fourth of patients. Device failures were not noted, pointing to the durability of these devices.

Levacor Device. This small, bearingless, centrifugal pump has a magnetically levitated impeller. The pump is implanted in a left subcostal, preperitoneal space, with a titanium inflow cannula and a woven polyester outflow graft anastomosed to the ascending aorta. Clinical trials are under way.

INCOR Device. This axial continuous-flow pump uses a free-floating impeller that is magnetically levitated. This pump is bearingless and has no mechanical wear. This pump is associated with a low infection rate but exhibits a high thromboembolic event incidence.

Synergy Micro-Pump. This pump has the smallest profile of any device and weighs a mere 25 g. By a right-sided mini-thoracotomy, this device is inserted into a pacemaker-like pocket. Uniquely, the inflow cannula is attached to the left atrium and the outflow cannula to the right subclavian artery. The device provides only partial flow (up to 3 liters/min). This device is anticipated to provide support to those with milder stages of heart failure, in whom partial support will be all that is required (**Fig. 32-4**).

TABLE 32-1 Mechanical Circulatory Support

INDICATION NOMENCLATURE	DEFINITION
Bridge to transplantation	Patient is listed for heart transplantation
Bridge to candidacy	Patient initially deemed ineligible for heart transplantation because of comorbidity (cardiorenal syndrome or pulmonary hypertension), which improves during mechanical support
Bridge to recovery	Patient with a potentially reversible cause of cardiac decompensation (acute myocarditis, postcardiotomy syndrome, peripartum cardiomyopathy)
Bridge to decision	Patient in whom the potential for transplantation or recovery is yet unclear
Destination therapy	Patient in whom recovery or transplantation is not feasible

Hemodynamic Unloading and Cardiac Structural Recovery

The weight of evidence with mechanical unloading by use of assist devices suggests that hemodynamic restoration is accompanied by regression of cellular hypertrophy, normalization of the neuroendocrine axis, improved expression of contractile proteins, enhanced cellular respiratory control, and decreases in markers of apoptosis and cellular stress (**Table 32-2**; see Chap. 25).[3]

Clinical Cardiac Recovery

In aggregate, structural recovery from hemodynamic unloading leads to functional recovery (see Chap. 25); however, translation of this recovery to sustainable function permitting device removal remains uncertain. Early investigations suggested that structural myocardial improvements that allowed exercise despite reduced device support were insufficient to result in meaningful functional recovery. Others have demonstrated more success by evaluating not only structural improvements in the ventricle but also regression of circulating autoantibodies to the beta$_1$-adrenergic receptor. In the series by Dandel and coworkers, 32 nonischemic patients who were weaned demonstrated a survival rate of 78% at 5 years after device explantation. Clinical heart failure recurred during the first 3 years after weaning in 31.3%, and two died of heart failure. More recently, the same group has updated their experience and defined characteristics associated with successful long-term survival after explantation. They suggested that left ventricular ejection fraction >45% at an end-diastolic diameter of <55 mm carries a predictive value for 5-year cardiac stability of 87.5%. In predominantly reversible causes of severe heart failure, such as myocarditis,

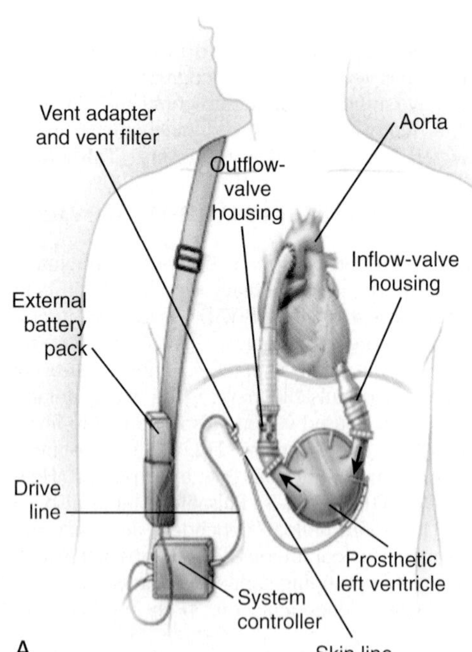

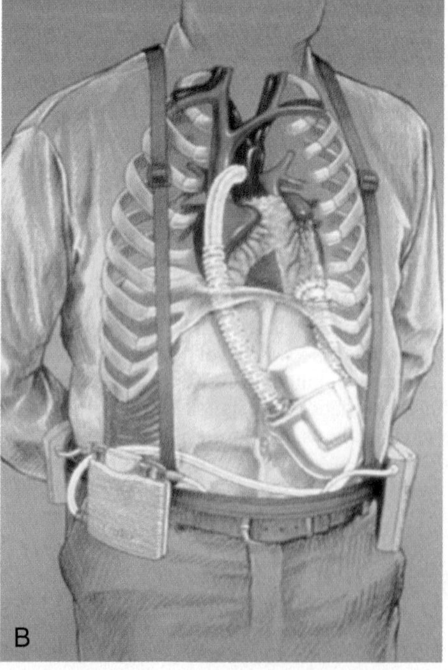

FIGURE 32-1 First-generation pulsatile devices. The HeartMate VE/XVE **(A)** shown here as the electric version and the Novacor LVAS **(B)** emerged as the most successful implanted LVADs in the late 1980s and 1990s.

peripartum cardiomyopathy, and post–cardiac surgery, the success of recovery after device explantation is more meaningfully demonstrated.[4]

Birks and colleagues[5] implanted LVADs in 15 patients with severe heart failure due to nonischemic cardiomyopathy and no histologic evidence of active myocarditis. The patients were treated with lisinopril, carvedilol, spironolactone, and losartan to enhance reverse remodeling. Once regression of left ventricular enlargement had been achieved, the $beta_2$-adrenergic receptor agonist clenbuterol was administered to prevent myocardial atrophy. Of the 15 patients, 11 had sufficient myocardial recovery to undergo explantation of the LVAD at 10 months after implantation of the device. One patient died of intractable arrhythmias 24 hours after explantation; another died of carcinoma of the lung 27 months after explantation. The cumulative rate of freedom from recurrent heart failure among the surviving patients was 100% and 88.9% at 1 year and 4 years, respectively. This investigation suggests long-term recovery with pharmacologic support; however, the absence of a control group precludes conclusive statements about the precise role of quadruple therapy and in particular raises doubts about the true impact of the agent clenbuterol. These data require confirmation in randomized controlled trials.

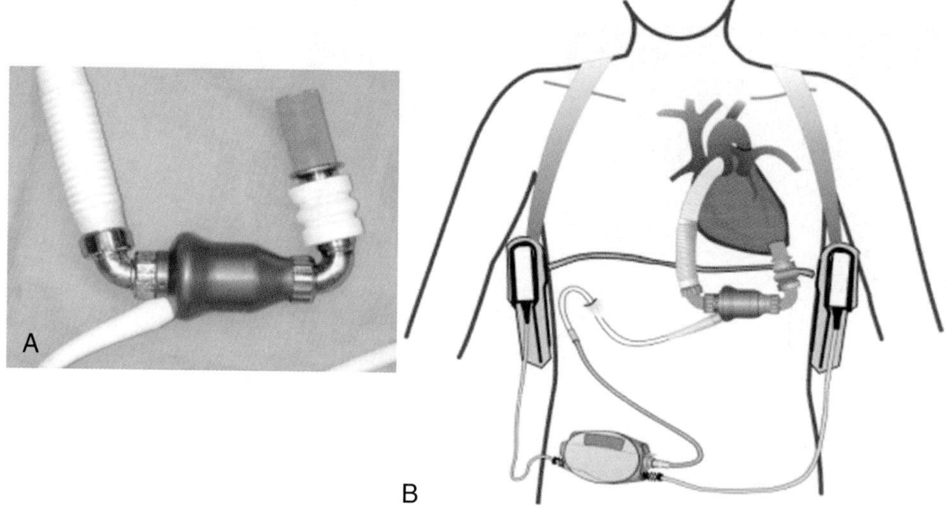

FIGURE 32-2 The second-generation HeartMate II device has an inlet cannula of sintered titanium and a Dacron outflow cannula shown here with bend relief to reduce kinking and injury at resternotomy **(A)**. The system provides mobility for the patient **(B)**.

Clinical Outcomes with Chronic Mechanical Assistance

Even in otherwise initially moribund patients awaiting transplantation or those who are ineligible, the portable battery-powered ventricular assist devices stabilize clinical parameters and allow patients to be discharged from the hospital after they are rehabilitated, typically while waiting for heart transplantation. In patients who are deemed permanently or currently ineligible for transplantation, the use of such devices has achieved a level of evidence that supports increased survival. The Randomized Evaluation of Mechanical Assistance for the Treatment of Congestive Heart Failure (REMATCH) trial, a multicenter study supported by the NHLBI to compare long-term implantation of LVADs with optimal medical management for patients with refractory heart failure, was conducted to test the hypothesis of destination therapy for patients ineligible for transplantation.[6] Briefly, 129 patients with severe heart failure (New York Heart Association Class IV, left ventricular ejection fraction ≤25%) were randomized to a control group or implantation of an LVAD, in addition to optimal medical therapy, between 1998 and 2001. Baseline medical therapy included digoxin, loop diuretics, spironolactone, angiotensin-converting enzyme inhibitors, angiotensin II antagonists, amiodarone, beta blockers, and intravenous inotropic agents (>70% of patients). This trial demonstrated that compared with best medical therapy (continuous inotropic support and oral pharmacologic measures), device-implanted patients had an average extension of life of 8 months, of which 3 months were spent in the hospital (see Fig. 32e-1 on website). This particular trial demonstrated that when they are appropriately selected, patients with a futile outlook can achieve clinically meaningful benefits. However, patients with devices were more than twice as likely to develop an adverse event and had a higher median number of days spent in and out of the hospital. Thus, at 2 years, only 23% in the ventricular assist device group were alive (compared with 8% in the medical group). The probability of infection with the device was 28%; bleeding, 42%; and device failure, 35%, requiring device replacement. This early proof-of-concept trial did not result in an aggressive widespread translation into community application because of concerns of cost, lack of device durability, and complications related to infection and thromboembolism.

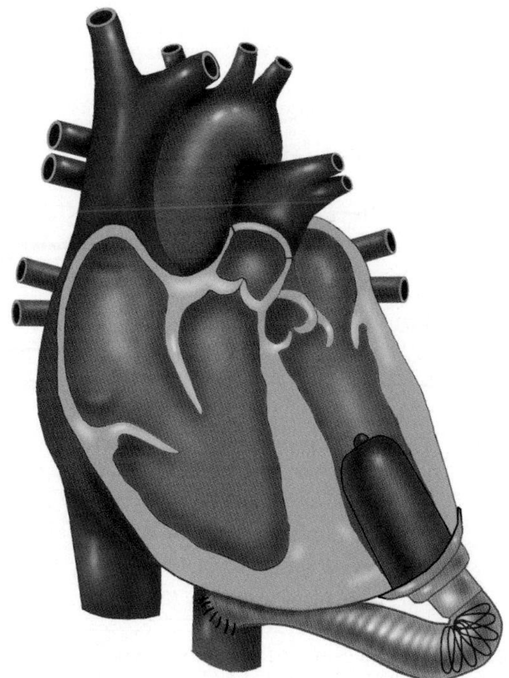

FIGURE 32-3 The Jarvik 2000 LVAD with unique intraventricular position, which avoids an inlet cannula. Outflow attachment is to either ascending or descending aorta (as shown). *(Courtesy of Texas Heart Institute, Houston, Texas.)*

The first continuous-flow device to complete clinical trials for bridge to transplantation and for destination therapy is the HeartMate II LVAD. The bridge to transplantation clinical trial for this device resulted in market approval by the Food and Drug Administration (FDA) in April 2008.[7] The pivotal destination therapy trial with the HeartMate II, completed as a randomized comparison between the HeartMate II and the HeartMate XVE (first-generation pulsatile device), demonstrated that the HeartMate II had a significantly greater percentage of patients who reached the primary endpoint of survival at 2 years, free of disabling stroke and reoperation for pump replacement, compared with the XVE.[8] The actuarial survival was 68% and 58% at

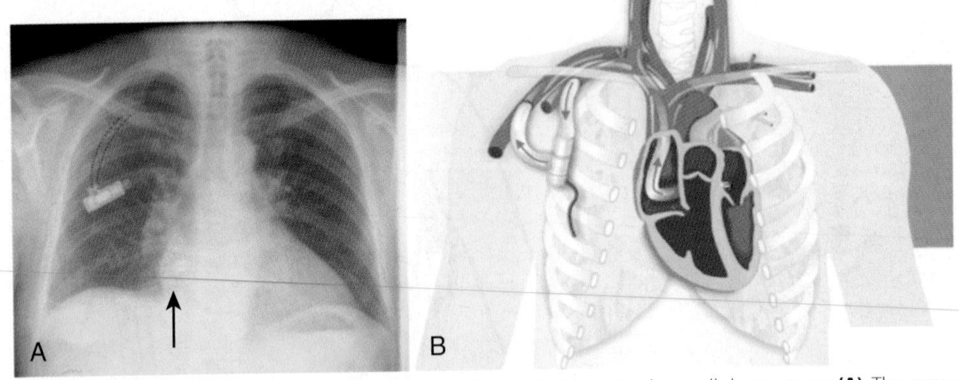

FIGURE 32-4 The CircuLite Synergy system shown after surgical insertion by small thoracotomy **(A)**. The arrow marks the tip of the inlet cannula in the left atrium, and dotted lines follow the outflow cannula fixed onto the side of the axillary artery. The pump rests subcuticularly in a pacemaker-type subclavicular pocket. An interventionally applied system **(B)** is undergoing large animal testing.

TABLE 32-2 Effects of Chronic Hemodynamic Unloading with Ventricular Assist Devices

Structural
Regression of myocyte hypertrophy
Reduction in neurohormonal activation
Normalization in expression of contractile proteins (SERCA-2a)
Enhanced electron transport chain respiratory function
Decreased apoptosis and cellular stress markers
Functional
Improvement in left ventricular ejection fraction and diastolic and systolic dimension
Recovery from spherical to more elliptical left ventricular shape
Improvement in heart failure–specific indices of quality of life
Improvement in peak aerobic capacity

1 year and 2 years, significantly improved over the 55% and 24% for the HeartMate XVE (**Fig. 32-5**). The evidence accrued from this investigation led to the FDA approval of this device for destination therapy in January 2010. However, the rates of disabling strokes were similar between these two devices and point to further work that is needed to improve on this critical adverse effect.

Selection of Patients and Prediction of Heart Failure Survival

Critical factors in achieving optimal outcomes after implantation of a newer generation ventricular assist device include severity of the patient's illness, underlying comorbidity, and timing of device implantation. It is imperative that surgery be undertaken at a time in the stage of the patient's illness that is neither too early nor too late. The INTERMACS registry,[9] which follows all long-term ventricular assist device implantations performed in the United States, has defined patient profiles purported to distinguish various categories of risk among the subset of advanced heart failure patients (**Table 32-3**).

The INTERMACS profiles are used to classify disease severity, and most patients receiving implantable ventricular assist devices were initially in profiles 1 and 2 with high perioperative mortality. As experience has accrued and with the recognition of the importance of the patient's illness that can result in futility, a gradual shift to less sick profiles is being noted. The most recent INTERMACS report analyzed 1092 primary LVAD implants, which included 48% pulsatile-flow and 52% continuous-flow pumps.[10] At the time of implantation, 85% of patients were in INTERMACS level 1 or 2 or 3, and less than 5% were higher than level 4. The spectrum of INTERMACS levels changed during the course of the study; the proportion of profile 1 decreased from 38% during the first half of the study to 27% during the second half.

The Heart Failure Survival Score and the Seattle Heart Failure Model can be used to estimate a heart failure patient's expected survival during the next 1 to 2 years with medical management and to identify patients at high risk of death who might benefit from LVAD support. In a recent study, the Seattle Heart Failure Model was used to analyze patients in the REMATCH trial, which concluded that patients could be stratified into high, medium, and low risk for LVAD support.[11] The Toronto model, which includes comorbidities like cerebrovascular disease, lung disease, dementia, cancer, and cirrhosis, is online at *www.ccort.ca/CHFriskmodel.asp*; the Seattle Heart Failure Model is online at *SeattleHeartFailureModel.org*. A clinical algorithm that takes into account clinical features of an evolving nature that can be used to initiate consideration for implantable devices is depicted in **Figure 32-6**.

Patient Factors Influencing Outcome

A risk factor analysis of data from the HeartMate XVE destination therapy registry was conducted by Lietz and associates.[12] This risk variable investigation demonstrated that perioperative death in those receiving a destination therapy implant was influenced by a confluence of deficiencies in nutritional status, hematologic abnormalities, end-organ and right-sided heart dysfunction, and lack of inotropic use. Lietz and associates' multivariate analysis produced nine risk factors for 90-day mortality, which were assigned a weighted score (**Table 32-4**). The cumulative scores for each patient were used to assign a risk category: 0 to 8, low risk; 9 to 16, medium risk; 17 to 19, high risk.

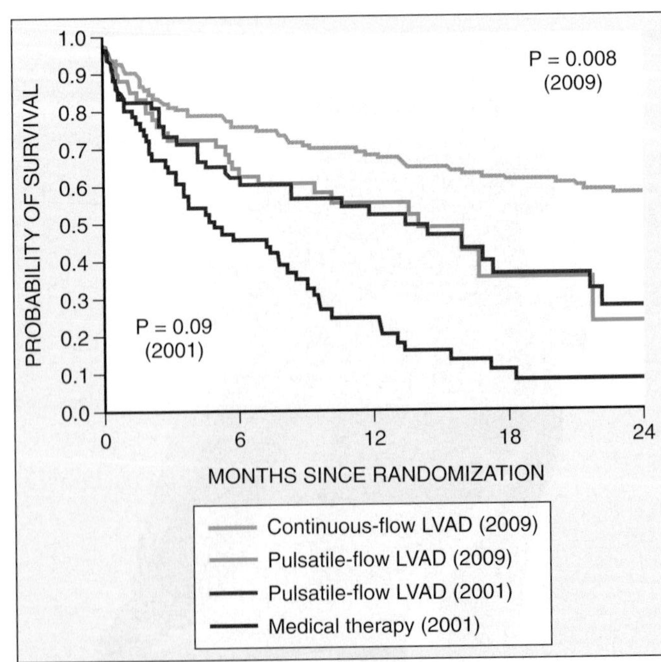

FIGURE 32-5 Survival rates in two trials of LVADs as destination therapy. The curves labeled 2009 are those reported by Slaughter and colleagues[8]; those labeled 2001 were reported for the REMATCH trial.[6] *(From Fang J: Rise of the machines—left ventricular assist devices as permanent therapy for advanced heart failure. N Engl J Med 361:2282, 2009.)*

TABLE 32-3 INTERMACS Patient Profile Descriptions

Profile 1: Critical cardiogenic shock *"Crash and burn"*
Patients with life-threatening hypotension despite rapidly escalating inotropic support, critical organ hypoperfusion. Definitive intervention needed within hours.

Profile 2: Progressive decline *"Sliding on inotropes"*
Patient with declining function despite intravenous inotropic support; may be manifested by worsening renal function, nutritional depletion, inability to restore volume balance. Also describes declining status in patients unable to tolerate inotropic therapy. Definitive intervention needed within few days.

Profile 3: Stable but inotrope dependent *"Dependent stability"*
Patient with stable blood pressure, organ function, nutrition, and symptoms on continuous intravenous inotropic support (or a temporary circulatory support device or both) but demonstrating repeated failure to be weaned from support due to recurrent symptomatic hypotension or renal dysfunction. Definitive intervention elective during a period of weeks to few months.

Profile 4: Resting symptoms *"Persistent advanced symptoms"*
Patient can be stabilized close to normal volume status but experiences daily symptoms of congestion at rest or during daily activities. Doses of diuretics generally fluctuate at very high levels. Some patients may shuttle between 4 and 5. Definitive intervention elective during a period of weeks to few months.

Profile 5: Exertion intolerant *"Minimal activity intolerant"*
Comfortable at rest but unable to engage in any other activity, housebound. Patients are comfortable at rest without congestive symptoms but may have underlying refractory elevated volume status, often with renal dysfunction. If underlying nutritional status and organ function are marginal, patient may be more at risk than INTERMACS 4 and require definitive intervention. Variable urgency, depends on maintenance of nutrition, organ function, and activity level.

Profile 6: Exertion limited *"Walking wounded"*
Patient without evidence of fluid overload is comfortable at rest and with activities of daily living and minor activities outside the home but fatigues after the first few minutes of any meaningful activity. Attribution to cardiac limitation requires careful measurement of peak oxygen consumption, in some cases with hemodynamic monitoring to confirm severity of cardiac impairment. Variable urgency, depends on maintenance of nutrition, organ function, and activity level.

Profile 7: Advanced NYHA III
A placeholder for more precise specification in future, this level includes patients who are without current or recent episodes of unstable fluid balance, living comfortably with meaningful activity limited to mild physical exertion. Transplantation or circulatory support may not currently be indicated.

MODIFIERS FOR PROFILES	POSSIBLE PROFILES TO MODIFY
TCS: temporary circulatory support—can modify only patients in the hospital (other devices would be INTERMACS devices); includes IABP, ECMO, TandemHeart, Levitronix, BVS 5000 or AB5000, Impella	1, 2, 3 in hospital
A: arrhythmia—can modify any profile; recurrent ventricular tachyarrhythmias that have recently contributed substantially to clinical compromise; this includes frequent ICD shock or requirement for external defibrillator, usually more than twice weekly	Any profile
FF: frequent flyer—can modify only outpatients, designating a patient requiring frequent emergency visits or hospitalizations for diuretics, ultrafiltration, or temporary intravenous vasoactive therapy	3 if at home; 4, 5, 6. A frequent flyer would rarely be profile 7.

Modified from Stevenson LW, Pagani FD, Young JB, et al: INTERMACS profiles of advanced heart failure: The current picture. J Heart Lung Transplant 28:535, 2009.

More than 19 was very high risk. The survival to hospital discharge in the four groups was 87.5%, 70.5%, 26%, and 13.7% for low, medium, high, and very high risk, respectively. Although not proven, patients with initial high or very high risk scores could benefit from a period of optimization therapy to attempt to lower their risk score (e.g., coagulation, nutrition, renal function, hemodynamics). Similarly, those with a low risk should be considered for prompt elective device implantation before their condition worsens. This risk model has not yet been validated with continuous-flow devices implanted for destination therapy. Several important comorbidities and hemodynamic factors may influence outcomes with LVAD support, including nutrition, hemodynamics, renal function, hepatic function, hematologic parameters, pulmonary function, and neuropsychiatric and psychological considerations.[13]

Nutrition. Malnutrition is often overlooked and remains a potentially modifiable risk factor for outcomes in mechanical support candidates. The presence of nutritional abnormalities increases the risk of infection, delays wound healing, and is generally associated with poor outcomes. Stable patients with cachexia and without worsening organ function should undergo nutrition optimization before implantation if possible, generally with enteral feeding. **Table 32-5** lists markers of significant malnutrition. Prealbumin is a risk marker for death during the postoperative phase of mechanical circulatory support device implantation and should be checked twice weekly. It should ideally be >15 mg/dL before implantation.

Hemodynamics. A major hemodynamic objective is to reduce the right atrial pressure to 15 mm Hg or less. This goal is suggested to decrease hepatic congestion and, it is hoped, to defray the need for right ventricular device support. A low pulmonary arterial pressure (mean <25 mm Hg) often reflects significant right ventricular failure and a low right ventricular stroke work index and is associated with increased mortality. Those patients presenting in cardiogenic shock may require optimization with temporary support by a short-term device as a bridge to decision. Recent reports suggest that the planned use of biventricular support, with either a left-sided implantable device and temporary right ventricular support or bilateral paracorporeal devices versus delayed right-sided support after LVAD implantation, improves outcomes in selected patients with right-sided heart failure or pulmonary hypertension.

Renal Function. In general, a urine output as low as 20 to 30 mL/hr for 6 to 8 hours, baseline creatinine concentration >2.5 mg/dL, and blood urea nitrogen concentration >40 mg/dL or chronic dialysis are associated with poor outcomes. Renal dysfunction generally improves after hemodynamic support if decreased glomerular flow rate is due to preoperative low cardiac output. However, renal function may not improve in patients who have sustained acute or chronic renal injury from poor perfusion or, more commonly, in patients with underlying renal disease such as diabetes or chronic hypertension.

Hepatic Function. The presence of cirrhosis is predictive of poor outcome. Liver dysfunction is associated with greater need for intraoperative and perioperative blood transfusion, which can result in worsened right-sided heart function. If cirrhosis has been excluded, hepatic function improves after implantation of a continuous-flow LVAD, typically normalizing by 6 months. Hepatic decongestion, by addressing right-sided heart function before device implantation, is important. Administration of vitamin K to normalize coagulation and stopping of all anticoagulant and antiplatelet agents well in advance of surgery are critical to minimization of perioperative bleeding.

Hematologic Parameters. Thrombocytopenia and a low hematocrit are associated with poor outcomes. Preoperative abnormal coagulation is common in heart failure patients because of hepatic dysfunction and the use of anticoagulant or antiplatelet medications. When possible, these medications should be stopped before implantation. Vitamin K may be given to reverse the effects of warfarin. For patients who are at high risk of preoperative thrombosis, a continuous infusion of heparin should be given as the effects of warfarin are reversed. Infusion of fresh frozen plasma may also be used to improve coagulation defects. Heparin-induced thrombocytopenia (HIT) is a clotting abnormality that warrants consideration for patients undergoing mechanical circulatory support. Although it is not measured routinely in all patients, it should be assessed preoperatively in those with platelet counts <150,000 or in those who had a recent drop of platelets by >20%. Clinical manifestations of HIT include any thrombotic event while heparin is being taken. The serotonin release assay is the most reliable test to establish the diagnosis of HIT.

Pulmonary Function. Patients with severe obstructive or restrictive pulmonary disease are not eligible for LVAD therapy. When pulmonary

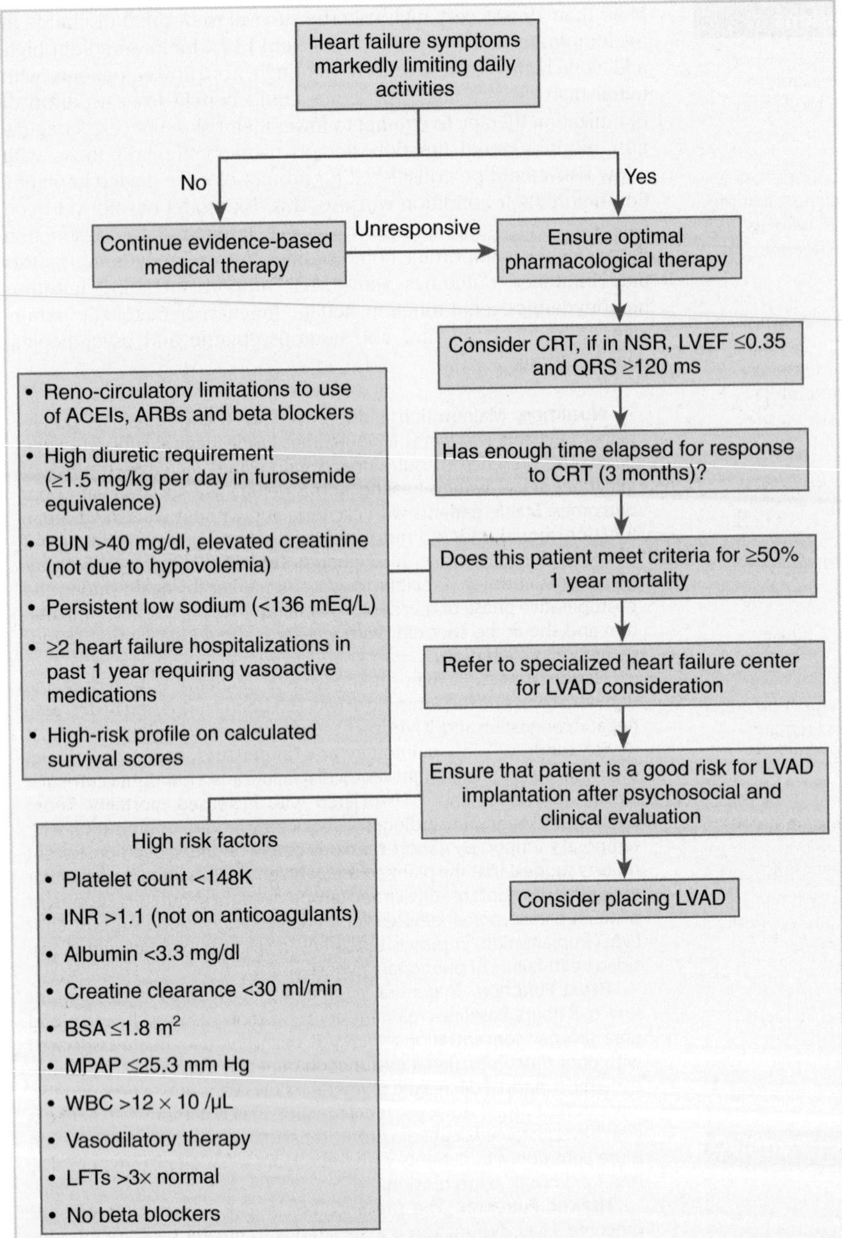

FIGURE 32-6 A proposed clinical algorithm to initiate mechanical circulatory support consideration. (This algorithm has not been validated in trials.) ACEI = angiotensin-converting enzyme inhibitor; ARB = angiotensin II receptor blocker; BSA = body surface area; BUN = blood urea nitrogen; CRT = cardiac resynchronization therapy; INR = international normalized ratio; LFT = liver function test; LVAD = left ventricular assist device; LVEF = left ventricular ejection fraction; MPAP = mean pulmonary artery pressure; NSR = normal sinus rhythm; WBC = white blood cell count.

TABLE 32-4 Risk Factors for Mortality (90-Day) After Ventricular Assist Device Implantation

RISK FACTORS	WEIGHTED SCORES
Platelet count <148 ×10³/μL	7
Serum albumin <3.3 g/dL	5
International normalized ratio >1.1	4
Vasodilator therapy	4
Mean pulmonary artery pressures <25 mm Hg	3
Aspartate aminotransferase >45 units/mL	2
Hematocrit <34%	2
Blood urea nitrogen >51 units/dL	2
No intravenous inotropes	2

function testing can be performed reliably and the forced vital capacity, forced expiratory volume at 1 second, and carbon monoxide diffusing capacity are all less than 50% predicted, exclusion from surgical implantation should be considered. There are no definitive cut points to guide mandated prohibition from device use.

Neuropsychiatric and Psychosocial Considerations. Patients with neurologic or psychiatric disease that compromises their ability to use and to care for external system components or to ambulate and exercise are poor candidates for mechanical support. Patients with known recent drug abuse or a history of noncompliance may not be suitable. Adequate family and caregiver support, housing, and community infrastructure are additional determining factors for potential candidates.

Surgical Considerations

The continuous-flow pumps are smaller than the preceding generations of pulsatile devices. Whereas cardiopulmonary bypass (CPB) is still recommended, the corresponding invasiveness of the surgical implantation has been reduced because the pump pocket is small and the outlet graft is reduced in diameter. The inlet connection to the left ventricular apex is unchanged and requires a cup or sewing ring to be attached by interrupted, nearly full left ventricle thickness sutures. In general, a circular coring tool is used to remove the apical muscle within the sutured fixation ring. These plugs have provided fresh myocardium for a variety of analyses useful in study of end-stage myopathy. With the left ventricle decompressed and empty on CPB, the chambers may be examined for thrombus or trabeculae that might interfere with the inflow to the pump. The inflow cannula with its usually metal tip is secured 3 to 5 cm in the left ventricle and aligned parallel to the septum. The proper alignment reduces the likelihood of obstruction by the septum or free wall. The pump is connected between the inflow cannula and one previously sutured to the right lateral side of the ascending aorta. The Jarvik 2000 is the only pump that is sutured within the left ventricular chamber, thereby eliminating an inflow cannula per se. This pump also is designed to be positioned into the descending or ascending aorta. For the former, a left thoracotomy is used and sternotomy avoided. This is particularly useful when the patient has had previous sternotomy. The downside of the descending aortic outflow is that the proximal aortic sinus does not wash well if the aortic valve remains closed because of poor left ventricular function. The supravalvular aortic sinus becomes a cul-de-sac, and there are reports of spontaneous thrombus in this area of the aortic valve and coronary arteries. Special concerns occur for thrombosis of saphenous vein grafts, if attached nearby. The Jarvik 2000 speed algorithm now includes a speed reduction for 8 of every 60 seconds to encourage the left ventricle to eject through the aortic valve. The HeartWare pump is positioned intrapericardially, like the

TABLE 32-5 Markers of Severe Malnutrition

Body mass index <20 kg/m²
Albumin <3.2 g/dL
Prealbumin <15 mg/dL
Total cholesterol <130 mg/dL
Lymphocyte count <100 ×10/μL
Tuberculin skin test anergy

Jarvik, avoiding an abdominal wall pocket altogether. It is small, and its inflow is short to permit the pump to be positioned on the apical fixation ring. Each of the current devices has small drivelines that are tunneled from the mediastinum, or left subcostal pump pocket in the case of HeartMate II, across the subcutaneous layer to exit the skin above the waist on the left lateral subcostal area.

It is important to eliminate air from the left ventricle, the pump, and the outflow graft before permitting the pump to flow freely. Air embolism can cause neurologic injury, and even a small amount caught in the anterior right coronary artery will predispose to right ventricular failure. In weaning from CPB, the surgeon will observe the function of the right ventricle directly and by transesophageal echocardiography. The pulmonary artery pressure is observed, and a temporary flowmeter is applied to the outflow graft. The echocardiogram also provides essential information about the degree of left ventricular filling. As the CPB is reduced, the pump speed is slowly increased to ensure that the left ventricle is moderately decompressed. The speed cannot exceed the ability of the right ventricle to deliver preload across the lungs. The inflow cannula is observed for its proper alignment. Malalignment is suspected if pump flows are low and the left ventricle is distended. Usually, if mitral valve regurgitation has been present preoperatively, it is significantly reduced after activation of the LVAD. In general, patients are begun on a modest dose of inotrope to assist the weaning process, and this is continued for a number of days postoperatively. When the patient has a high pulmonary vascular resistance, a pulmonary vasodilator-like inhaled nitric oxide or prostaglandin E is useful to help unload the right ventricle. A long period is spent in the operating room before wound closure in an attempt to gain complete hemostasis. In the situation in which pre-existing liver congestion causes a postsurgical coagulopathy, the wound can be packed and covered with a sterile dressing for closure 24 to 48 hours later when hemostasis is improved. Few problems arise from the delayed closure option, whereas many patients aggressively closed without dry drainage tubes require urgent reopening of the sternum or resuscitation from tamponade.

Principles of Perioperative and Postoperative Care

Important principles of preimplantation echocardiography to be kept in mind by the cardiologist are the delineation of interatrial communications and the detection of left ventricular and left atrial appendage thrombi.[13] The surgeon needs guidance on closure of a patent foramen ovale and removal of left-sided thrombi to prevent postoperative strokes. During positioning of the mechanical circulatory support device, the surgeon must be careful to direct the inflow cannula away from the septum and toward the posterior aspect of the mitral valve. This is important to prevent extreme septal shifts that obstruct inflow into the device. Knowledge of valvular disease in the aortic and mitral valves is essential for optimal surgical technique. As an example, aortic regurgitation and mitral stenosis require correction before completion of a successful device implantation. The use of echocardiography after implantation is critical to evaluate for septal suction events, opening of the aortic valve, and left ventricular chamber dimension. Evaluation of optimal left ventricular device function can be ascertained by use of a 3-point approach that includes (1) assessment of right ventricular function, (2) left ventricular imaging (to assess ventricular chamber size, opening of the aortic valve, septal function), and (3) functioning characteristics of the pump.

Early in the course of a left ventricular device implantation, attention must be focused on prevention of worsening right ventricular failure. Clinically mild right ventricular failure preoperatively can be worsened immediately postoperatively. The underlying reason for this is the need by the dysfunctional right ventricle to adjust to a higher cardiac output after LVAD implantation, resulting in increased right-sided flow. Furthermore, decompression of the left ventricle by the assist device results in a decrease in the septal contribution to ventricular interdependence. Right ventricular dysfunction is typically treated by adjunctive inotropic support and a decrease in the pumping power of the LVAD to prevent excessive suction pressure on the interventricular septum. When these measures are insufficient, reoperation for temporary or permanent RVAD support may be required. In rare situations, the inflow cannula of the left ventricular device may need to be redirected away from the septum and repositioned to prevent inflow obstruction. The vacuum effect on the septum is more common with continuous-flow devices, which tend to operate at speeds that are not necessarily sensitive to preload. A decreased preload, a small left ventricular cavity size, and excessive power and speed of the device provide a perfect constellation of factors that provoke a septal "suck down" effect. Imaging of the left ventricle will typically reveal a decompressed left ventricle, little or no evidence of aortic valve opening, and a septum that is close to the inflow cannula. Although a decrease in the mechanical device power and speed should be entertained, one must remain vigilant for causes of a low preload, including pericardial tamponade, hypovolemia, and severe right ventricular failure. Special issues of concern in the perioperative period include HIT, anticoagulation, right ventricular function, and infection.

Heparin-Induced Thrombocytopenia and Optimal Anticoagulation

HIT is a clinical and laboratory syndrome of thromboembolism, reduced platelet numbers, and antiplatelet factor 4 (PF4) antibodies (see Chap. 87). Patients undergoing mechanical circulatory support commonly are exposed to prolonged anticoagulation with heparin preoperatively and postoperatively. A multimolecular complex of the CXC cytokine subfamily binds to polyanionic domains on heparin. Immunoglobulin G antibodies can form that are directed against the PF4-heparin complexes, which induce activation of platelets. Arterial and venous thromboses can occur, and with consumption, platelet counts fall to at least 50% of baseline. In general, a combination of a 5- to 10-day immunization period before platelet counts fall and the development of pathogenic heparin-dependent platelet-activating antibodies can be used to distinguish HIT from thrombocytopenia observed in critically ill patients. Whereas HIT occurs in less than 3% of patients after coronary artery bypass, anti-PF4 antibodies can be detected in more than 50%. Most of the antiplatelet antibodies selected by enzyme immunoassay do not activate platelets. Even in the presence of specific serologic evidence, HIT may not occur, probably because platelets are partially responsive to the antibodies due to low density of Fc receptors or low expression of PF4. The type of thromboembolism observed in LVAD patients with HIT stresses transient and permanent ischemic cerebral insults. In LVAD patients, the risk of heparin-induced immunization is likely to approach 65% and clinical thrombosis 10%. However, the ventricular assist device population has confounding heart failure and shock, and the true incidence may not in fact be as high as claimed. The diagnosis is complex in ventricular assist device patients who demonstrate a high incidence of thrombocytopenia and clinically irrelevant anti-PF4 antibodies.[14]

The anticoagulation management of the ventricular assist device patient in whom HIT is highly suspected or proven is a challenge because postoperative surgical bleeding complications are high and the risk of thromboembolism is significant. Direct and indirect thrombin inhibitors are available, and most centers employ the hirudin analogue bivalirudin because it has a 30-minute half-life and its elimination is enzymatic by thrombin, thus not dependent on renal (hirudin) or liver (argatroban) excretion. LVAD patients frequently have liver and renal dysfunction, and bivalirudin is begun at 0.25 mg/kg per hour and titrated to activated partial thromboplastin time target values. Some have advocated for elimination of heparin postoperatively in all ventricular assist device patients and implementation of a direct thrombin inhibitor.[14]

Optimal anticoagulation after left ventricular device implantation is a critical management facet. First, antiplatelets and anticoagulants must be started only after meticulous control of postoperative bleeding has ensued. Second, use of intravenous heparin is often not required to bridge these patients to oral anticoagulation and may increase the risk of postoperative bleeding. Third, the optimal international normalized ratio with the newer continuous-flow devices (HeartMate II) is in the range of 1.5 to 2.5, beyond which the risk of thrombosis and bleeding escalates.[13] Lower anticoagulation may not always be appropriate; in situations of atrial fibrillation, prior thromboembolic events, or known left atrial or ventricular thrombi, and if low assist device flow rates (<3 liter/min) are anticipated, higher degrees of anticoagulation must be targeted.

Right Ventricular Failure

Attempts to identify patients with biventricular failure, who are at significant risk of persisting right ventricular failure after insertion of an LVAD, have generally cobbled together preoperative clinical and hemodynamic variables. With an LVAD, the right ventricle receives more venous return and, assuming a prompt drop in left atrial pressure, works against a reduced afterload. A clarifying analysis of this problem for a continuous-flow pump was recently made in 484 patients who enrolled in the Heart-Mate II pivotal bridge to transplantation trial.[15] Of these patients, 6% required an immediate RVAD, another 7% needed early inotropic support that persisted beyond 14 days, and 7% more developed the need for inotropes after 14 days. Multivariate analysis determined that central venous pressure/pulmonary capillary pressure ratio >0.63, blood urea nitrogen concentration >39 mg/dL, and preoperative mechanical ventilator support were univariate predictors of right ventricular failure at odds ratio of 2.1, 2.3, and 5.5, respectively. Insertion of an RVAD for right ventricular failure after insertion of an LVAD not only prolongs hospitalization but reduces survival to transplantation. To close this survival gap, an argument can be made for more elective placement of an RVAD when the prospects for development of multiorgan failure are high and mechanical ventilation is nearly ensured. This may be particularly advantageous if a donor organ is not likely to be available soon on the basis of blood type O, HLA sensitization, the patient's size, or local competition for organs.

The pneumatic Thoratec provides excellent long-term right ventricular support, but because most right ventricular failure is reversible or ultimately responds to inotropes or phosphodiesterase inhibition, there has been a trend to adopt short-term centrifugal pumps like the CentriMag. This pump is less expensive and easier to implant and can be explanted in 2 or 3 weeks. The presence of a long-term LVAD system and a short-term RVAD requires technical expertise at the bedside and an understanding that even a short episode of LVAD failure (for reasons including electromechanical failure, malpositioning of the left ventricular inlet cannula, or obstructing thrombus) without reducing the RVAD flow will result in sudden and overwhelming pulmonary edema and suffocating bronchorrhea. As patients may develop renal failure preoperatively or postoperatively and have tissue edema, management of BiVAD speeds and flows can be difficult. It is particularly important as pulmonary artery catheters are removed that the physician team have a good feel for the patient's intravascular volume, echocardiography-based degree of left ventricular decompression versus LVAD pump speed, and relative left versus right atrial pressures as indicated by atrial septal shift. In general, in time, patients settle into a mated pattern with their BiVADS, management becomes routine, and the right ventricle improves.[13]

Infection

A recent review of 593 patients entered into the INTERMACS data base has summarized the problem, and the findings suggest where improvements may be made.[16] Bacterial pathogens dominate fungal organisms at a ratio of nearly 9:1. Infection presents most commonly in the blood (32%) or driveline (21%). There were nearly 2.5 cumulative infections per patient at 18 months, but most occurred within the 3-month perioperative period ($P < .0001$). INTERMACS level 1, age older than 60 years, high blood urea nitrogen concentration, and need for biventricular support were predictors of infection. Specialists have described the problem of recurrent blood infections as "VADitis" and stress the life-long need for antibiotics. Clearly, small flexible drivelines that gain greater likelihood of fixation to the skin and near elimination of pump pockets within the abdominal wall will have a positive impact on the incidence of infection. Advanced transcutaneous energy transfer systems will ultimately be employed for the patient's convenience and reduced risk of infection.

Special Issues in Long-term Management

Gastrointestinal bleeding is more commonly encountered with the newer continuous-flow pumps.[17] Although the exact reason for this occurrence is uncertain, one hypothesis implicates the development of acquired von Willebrand disease caused by increased shear stress and reduced pulsatility of these devices with an increased prevalence of arteriovenous malformations. The risk/benefit of reducing or discontinuing anticoagulation should be thoroughly assessed and discussed with the patient. Lowering of the device power and speed to decrease shear stress is advocated to decrease such bleeding episodes but remains to be proven as a viable treatment option.

Infection remains a serious complication after device implantation and affects success of bridging to transplantation and overall survival. Commonly, device infection occurs within the driveline, in the device pocket site, or in the interior of the device itself. Bloodstream infections in these patients may emerge from within the device or can be the result of a non–device-related source, such as a urinary tract infection, pneumonia, or indwelling line–related infection. Device endocarditis can be treated with systemic antibiotics as well as with emergent heart transplantation, device explantation, or device replacement. Infection follows cardiac failure as the second leading cause of death in mechanical circulatory support irrespective of device intent, whether it is a bridge to transplantation, bridge to decision, or destination therapy.[13]

Immune interactions and allosensitization are two unique complications of permanently implantable mechanical support devices.[18] The pulsatile devices are associated with significant T-cell activation on the device surface and in the circulation but demonstrate defective responses to proliferative stimulation. Circulating T cells also develop a heightened activation-induced cell death. In contrast to T-cell responses, B-cell hyperreactivity is also noted. The net result of these two defects is an increased proclivity for infection due to the T-cell abnormality and increased allosensitization due to the B-cell activation profile. Indeed, circulating anti-HLA class I and II antibodies (sensitization) occur commonly in these patients before transplantation, and this phenomenon is associated with a significant risk for early graft failure and poor patient survival. Allosensitization also is due to the number of necessary blood product transfusions (especially platelet), and this must be minimized. Strategies to desensitize patients are advocated, but the best approach remains uncertain. Prospective crossmatching of donor and recipient blood is required, and in those unable to match blood physically, virtual crossmatching is advocated.

Blood pressure management is of particular importance for the newer generation continuous-flow devices. Even with the first-generation devices, hypertension and consequent increased afterload were associated with device cannula bioprosthetic valve destruction. In the continuous-flow devices, hypertension decreases device function because the difference in the left ventricular cavity to aortic pressure is a primary determinant of device flow. Thus, every effort is made to keep aortic pressure low because suboptimal device flow can result in thromboembolic events. If beta blockers are used, particular attention to the right ventricular function must be maintained. Because pulsatility is low, a Doppler-derived blood pressure is most reliable, and one should not necessarily focus on a systolic or diastolic pressure component.[13]

Hemolysis may potentially occur, especially with the continuous-flow devices using an impeller pump design, and therefore the lactate dehydrogenase and plasma free hemoglobin values should be determined if anemia or hemoglobinuria ensues. The development of hemolysis may indicate a thrombus within the continuous-flow device. In such cases, the device indicates a gradual increase in power, a reduction in the pulsatility index, and lack of decompression of the left ventricle.[13]

Total Artificial Heart

This complete cardiac replacement system is designed to provide biventricular support. In this context, the CardioWest SynCardia is the only total artificial heart approved by the U.S. FDA as a bridge to transplantation.[19] The CardioWest total artificial heart consists of two pneumatically driven pumps with tilting disc valves and short outflow grafts that replace both native ventricles, the proximal segment of the aorta and pulmonary artery, and all four of the associated valves. Thus, this device can be used in situations of profound right ventricular failure, severe bivalvular disease, myocardial rupture, or severe arrhythmias that would render a univentricular device nonfunctional. However, the size requirements are precise, and insertion of this device requires a large body surface area (>1.7 m^2) and a chest anteroposterior diameter of at least 10 cm as assessed by computed tomography scan. The current device does not allow discharge to the ambulatory setting (**Fig. 32-7**).

Percutaneous Mechanical Support

The ability to deploy rapid and bedside support is often needed in the context of expected recovery (myocardial stunning) or as a bridge to

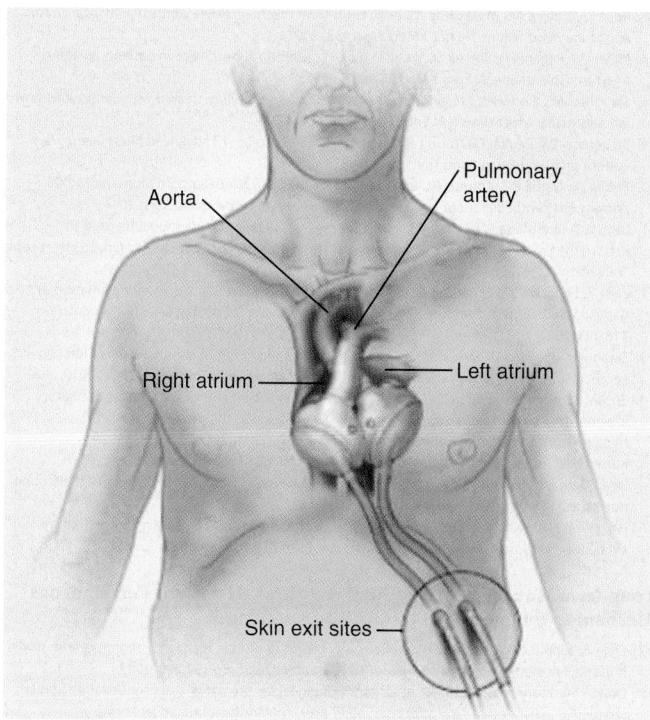

FIGURE 32-7 The CardioWest total artificial heart.

permanent support. Intra-aortic balloon counterpulsation uses the concept of systolic unloading and diastolic augmentation and is commonly used in cardiogenic shock due to myocardial infarction as an initial mechanical support. Further use in those with ongoing ischemia, unstable angina, deteriorating hemodynamics, or ischemic arrhythmias is generally advocated but has been recently challenged.[20] However, care must be taken to avoid insertion of an intra-aortic balloon pump in the setting of aortic insufficiency and aortic dissection. Similarly, care must be taken to avoid local vascular complications from cannulation. More recently, two percutaneous LVADs have been clinically introduced: the TandemHeart and the Impella Recover LP system.[21] Compared with the intra-aortic balloon pump, the TandemHeart has been shown to significantly reduce preload and to augment cardiac output. In two randomized comparisons between the TandemHeart and intra-aortic balloon pump support in patients with cardiogenic shock and in one such study with the Impella pump, the LVAD improved cardiac index and pulmonary hemodynamics; however, no significant differences with respect to 30-day mortality were noted, and complications including limb ischemia and severe bleeding were more frequent with LVADs than with intra-aortic balloon pump support (**Fig. 32-8**).

The Emerging Future of Mechanical Circulatory Support

LVADs have improved because of more than 35 years of clinical experience and a steady development of technology. This has prompted a consideration of LVADs to an earlier stage of heart failure

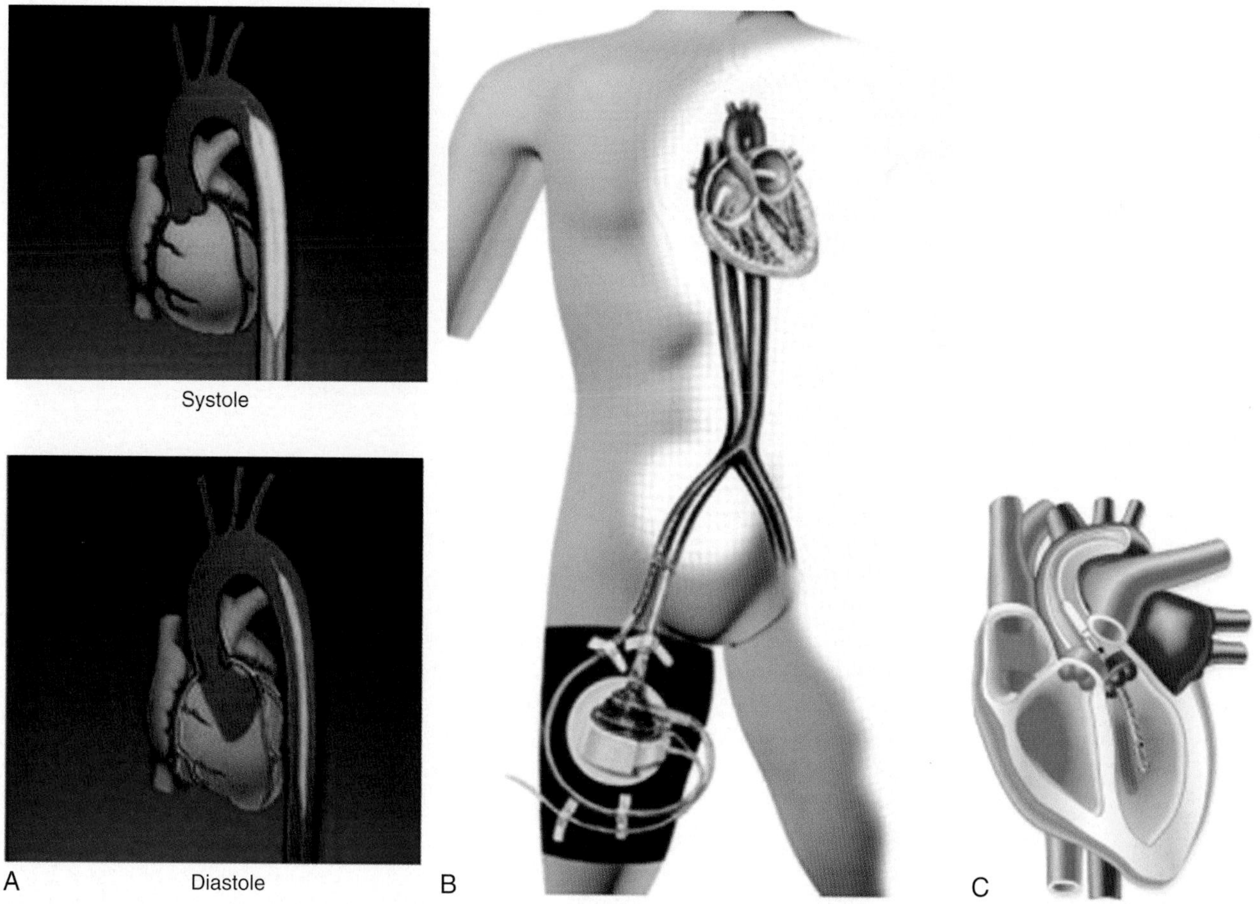

FIGURE 32-8 Percutaneous left ventricular support devices. **A,** Intra-aortic balloon counterpulsation device inflating in systole and deflating during diastole. **B,** The TandemHeart inflow cannula enters the left atrium transseptally; its outflow cannula is inserted into the arterial circulation. **C,** The Impella 2.5 liter/min device enters the ventricle in a retroaortic manner.

when candidates with the highest risk can be avoided. By ratcheting back on the severity of illness, it is believed that perioperative mortality and complications will be reduced to a minimum, and the treatment will be a test of the pump's reliability and biocompatibility versus the best available medical therapy. A number of micropumps are under development to target less ill patients. They are designed for implantation either by a minimally invasive surgical procedure or, remarkably, by interventional catheter-based techniques. Their small size places the optimal rates of flow in the range of 2 to 3 liters/min. These devices, unlike larger pumps that replace left ventricular function, are designed to assist and more correctly are defined as ventricular assist devices. One can only conjecture as to whether these types of devices will reduce progression of heart failure or even reverse remodel early-stage disease. Futurists believe the micropumps that can be implanted without mortality and with acceptable biocompatibility and that can function with an adverse event profile similar to that of a prosthetic valve will change the paradigms for accepted treatment of advanced heart failure.

REFERENCES

History, Definitions, Classification, and Recovery

1. Felker GM, Rogers JG: Same bridge, new destinations: Rethinking paradigms for mechanical cardiac support in heart failure. J Am Coll Cardiol 47:930, 2006.
2. Krishnamani R, DeNofrio D, Konstam MA: Emerging ventricular assist devices for long-term cardiac support. Nat Rev Cardiol 7:71, 2010.
3. Drakos SG, Terrovitis JV, Anastasiou-Nana MI, Nanas JN: Reverse remodeling during long-term mechanical unloading of the left ventricle. J Mol Cell Cardiol 43:231, 2007.
4. Dandel M, Weng Y, Siniawski H, et al: Prediction of cardiac stability after weaning from left ventricular assist devices in patients with idiopathic dilated cardiomyopathy. Circulation 118(Suppl):S94, 2008.

Clinical Outcomes, Selection of Patients and Prediction, Outcomes, and Surgical Considerations

5. Birks EJ, Tansley PD, Hardy J, et al: Left ventricular assist device and drug therapy for the reversal of heart failure. N Engl J Med 355:1873, 2006.
6. Rose EA, Gelijns AC, Moskowitz AJ, et al: Long-term mechanical left ventricular assistance for end-stage heart failure. N Engl J Med 345:1435, 2001.
7. Miller LW, Pagani FD, Russell SD, et al: Use of a continuous-flow device in patients awaiting heart transplantation. N Engl J Med 357:885, 2007.
8. Slaughter MS, Rogers JG, Milano CA, et al: Advanced heart failure treated with continuous-flow left ventricular assist device. N Engl J Med 361:2241, 2009.
9. Stevenson LW, Pagani FD, Young JB, et al: INTERMACS profiles of advanced heart failure: The current picture. J Heart Lung Transplant 28:535, 2009.
10. Kirklin JK, Naftel DC, Kormos RL, et al: Second INTERMACS annual report: More than 1,000 primary left ventricular assist device implants. J Heart Lung Transplant 29:1, 2010.
11. Levy WC, Mozaffarian D, Linker DT, et al: Can the Seattle heart failure model be used to risk-stratify heart failure patients for potential left ventricular assist device therapy? J Heart Lung Transplant 28:231, 2009.
12. Lietz K, Long JW, Kfoury AG, et al: Outcomes of left ventricular assist device implantation as destination therapy in the post-REMATCH era: Implications for patient selection. Circulation 116:497, 2007.
13. Slaughter MS, Pagani FD, Rogers JG, et al: Clinical management of continuous-flow left ventricular assist devices in advanced heart failure. J Heart Lung Transplant 29:S1, 2010.
14. Zucker MJ, Sabnani I, Baran DA, et al: Cardiac transplantation and/or mechanical circulatory support device placement using heparin anti-coagulation in the presence of acute heparin-induced thrombocytopenia. J Heart Lung Transplant 29:53, 2010.
15. Kormos RL, Teuteberg JJ, Pagani FD, et al: Right ventricular failure in patients with the HeartMate II continuous-flow left ventricular assist device: Incidence, risk factors, and effect on outcomes. J Thorac Cardiovasc Surg 139:1316, 2010.
16. Holman WL, Kirklin JK, Naftel DC, et al: Infection after implantation of pulsatile mechanical circulatory support devices. J Thorac Cardiovasc Surg 139:1632, 2010.

Long-term Management, the Total Artificial Heart, and Percutaneous Mechanical Support

17. Crow S, John R, Boyle A, et al: Gastrointestinal bleeding rates in recipients of nonpulsatile and pulsatile left ventricular assist devices. J Thorac Cardiovasc Surg 137:208, 2009.
18. Drakos SG, Kfoury AG, Kotter JR, et al: Prior human leukocyte antigen-allosensitization and left ventricular assist device type affect degree of post-implantation human leukocyte antigen-allosensitization. J Heart Lung Transplant 28:838, 2009.
19. Copeland JG, Smith RG, Arabia FA, et al: Cardiac replacement with a total artificial heart as a bridge to transplantation. N Engl J Med 351:859, 2004.
20. Sjauw KD, Engström AE, Vis MM, et al: A systematic review and meta-analysis of intra-aortic balloon pump therapy in ST-elevation myocardial infarction: Should we change the guidelines? Eur Heart J 30:459, 2009.
21. Sarkar K, Kini AS: Percutaneous left ventricular support devices. Cardiol Clin 28:169, 2010.

CHAPTER 33 Emerging Therapies and Strategies in the Treatment of Heart Failure

Stefanie Dimmeler, Douglas L. Mann, and Andreas M. Zeiher

Our current therapeutic approach to heart failure (HF) relies on treatment of the patient's symptoms with digitalis and diuretics and the use of neurohormonal antagonists such as angiotensin-converting enzyme (ACE) inhibitors, angiotensin receptor blockers, beta blockers, and aldosterone antagonists to prevent disease (see Chap. 28) as well as biventricular pacemakers and defibrillators in appropriate populations of patients (see Chaps. 29 and 38). Nonetheless, despite these pharmacologic and device interventions, HF remains a progressive disease with an unacceptably high mortality and morbidity. Thus, there is an ongoing need for new and improved therapeutic approaches to HF. In this chapter, we review some of the new therapeutic approaches that are being evaluated in patients with HF. The organization of this chapter focuses first on new nonpharmacologic strategies in HF, including the exciting concept of myocardial repair and regeneration, followed by a review of emerging pharmacologic strategies, such as pharmacogenomics, and a discussion of novel targets in HF. New and emerging surgical approaches to HF are reviewed in Chap. 31.

Nonpharmacologic Strategies

Myocardial Repair and Regeneration

As noted in Chap. 25, HF may develop as a consequence of myocyte loss or dysfunction, eventually leading to left ventricular (LV) remodeling and cardiac decompensation. Replacement of dead or dysfunctional cardiac myocytes through cell-based therapies represents a logical and novel option for the treatment of HF. As will be discussed later, cell-based therapies may achieve true cardiac regeneration by renewing the pool of functionally active cardiac myocytes or may lead to cardiac repair by supporting neovascularization, supplementing or augmenting the cytoprotective mechanisms that occur naturally, or by favorably influencing the remodeling processes. The promise of cellular cardiomyogenesis, neovascularization, and additional cell-mediated beneficial effects, individually or in combination, offers altogether novel opportunities for tailored treatment of the underlying pathobiologic process.

STEM AND PROGENITOR CELLS (see Chap. 11). Three types of stem cells should be discussed separately: embryonic stem (ES) cells, inducible pluripotent stem cells, and adult stem cells (**Fig. 33-1**). Whereas ES cells clearly have the capacity to give rise to all cell types of the body and are capable of forming tissues and organs, most adult stem cells are more specified (more lineage committed); hence, the use of adult stem cells for organogenesis has not been explored so far. ES cells are derived from the inner cell layer of the early embryonic trophoblast and can be propagated in cell culture in an undifferentiated state infinitely. By changing the cultivation conditions (the so-called hanging drop technique), ES cells aggregate and form embryoid bodies, an early embryonic tissue consisting of all three germ layers. Within an embryoid body, approximately 5% to 10% of ES cells spontaneously differentiate into cardiomyocytes. Functionally active cardiomyocytes (ESC-CM) have been generated from mouse as well as from human ES cells (hESC-CM), although the excitation-contraction coupling properties of hESC-CM differ from the adult myocardium.[1] ES cell–derived cardiomyocytes show macromolecular sarcomeric organization, calcium sparks, ionic currents, functional and anatomic integration with surrounding cardiomyocytes, and propagation of electrical activity as well as pacemaker activity.[1] Collectively, these data demonstrate that ES cells spontaneously differentiate into fully functionally active, fetal-like cardiomyocytes in vitro. Although these in vitro data would suggest that ES cells are ideal candidates for in vivo cardiac repair, animal studies have shown a dose-dependent incidence of tumor formation, in particular teratocarcinoma formation, after transplantation of ES cells into mice. Several strategies aiming to specifically select differentiated cardiomyocytes to exclude highly proliferating ES cells with a tumor-forming capacity are currently being tested. An additional question relates to the immunogenic activity of ES cells in an allogeneic setting. It is unclear whether the low immune privilege proposed by experimental studies is maintained when the ES cells are differentiated and functionally integrated into the human heart for a long time. Therefore, the safety of ES cell transplantation remains an unsolved question.[2]

The seminal observation by Yamanaka and coworkers that differentiated adult cells can be reprogrammed to become pluripotent stem cells by replenishment with pluripotency genes or their gene product in mice and humans has sparked great interest in the use of these so-called induced pluripotent stem cells (iPS) for true cardiac regeneration (see Chap. 11).[3] iPS cells were shown to differentiate into all cardiovascular lineages, and transplantation of iPS cells improved heart function in experimental models.[4] Whereas the use of patient-specific iPS cells for cardiac regeneration would clearly circumvent both the problems of immunogenicity and ethical concerns regarding ES cells, the safety of iPS cells with respect to tumor formation and potential genetic instability remains an unsolved problem. Moreover, because iPS cells have to be cultivated and propagated for weeks, their use in acute situations (e.g., acute myocardial infarction) is limited.

Adult stem cells comprise at least three different groups: the bone marrow–derived stem cells, the circulating pool of stem or progenitor cells (which at least in part is derived from the bone marrow), and the tissue-resident stem cells (see Fig. 33-1). Bone marrow–derived stem cells are the best studied and were used in most of the clinical trials performed thus far. Bone marrow contains a complex assortment of progenitor cells, including hematopoietic stem cells, the so-called side population cells (SP cells, defined by the expression of the Abcg2 transporter allowing export of Hoechst dye), mesenchymal stem cells or stromal cells as well as subsets thereof, and very small embryonic-like stem cells.

Circulating blood-derived progenitor cells were initially discovered in searching for proangiogenic cells for therapeutic vasculogenesis. Asahara and Isner isolated endothelial progenitor cells, which were defined by their ability to form new blood vessels and to enhance neovascularization after ischemia (for review, see references 5 and 6). On the basis of the assumption that these cells may represent adult hemangioblasts, these cells were characterized by the expression of

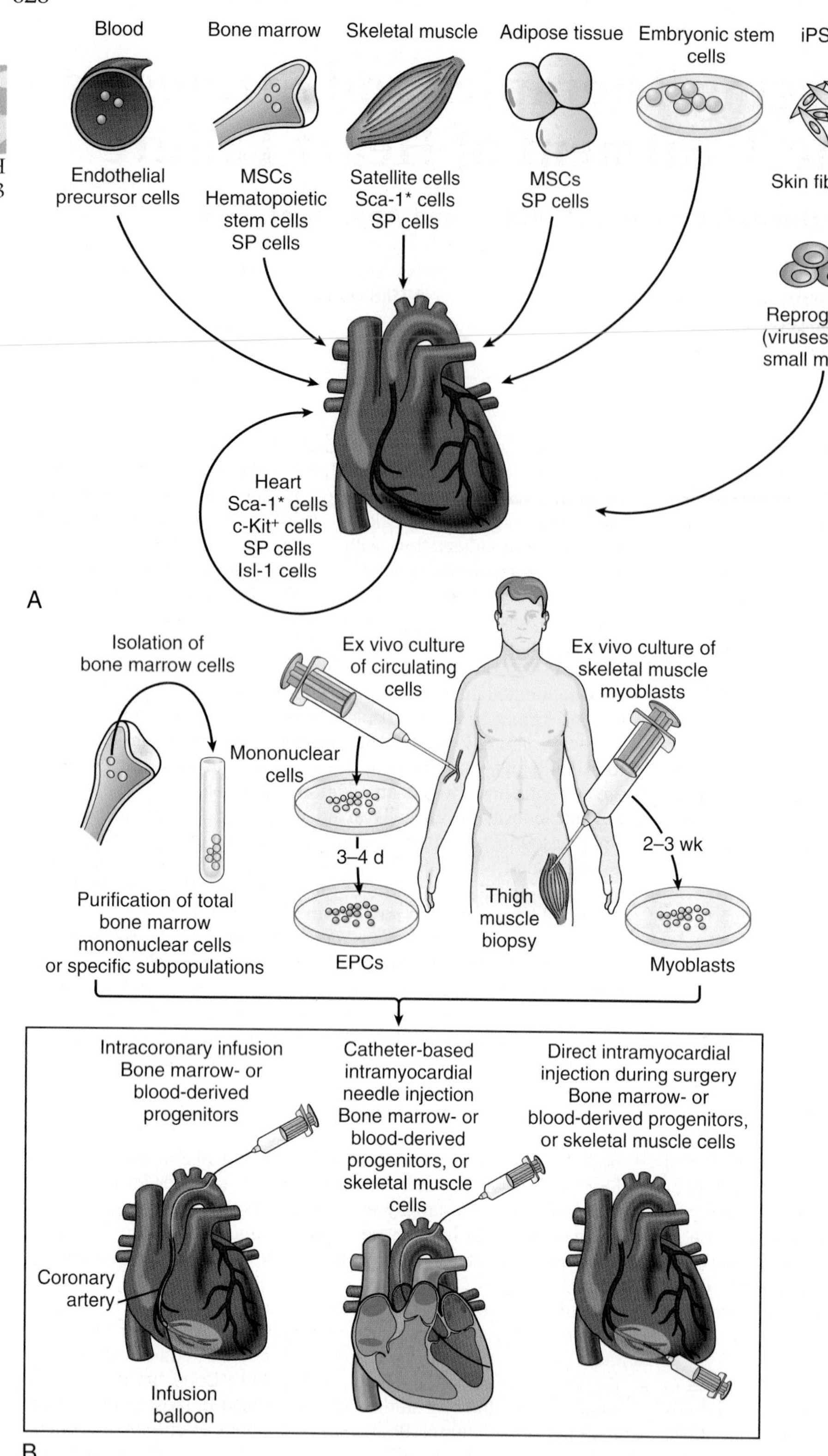

FIGURE 33-1 Cell types and mode of delivery of cells for cardiac repair. **A,** Cell types used for cardiovascular repair. **B,** Delivery strategies used in the clinical setting for cell therapy. EPCs = endothelial progenitor cells; iPS cells = induced pluripotent stem cells; MSCs = mesenchymal stem cells; SP cells = side population cells. *(From Dimmeler S, Zeiher AM, Schneider MD: Unchain my heart: The scientific foundations of cardiac repair. J Clin Invest 115:572, 2005.)*

hematopoietic markers, such as CD133+ and CD34+, and endothelial markers for vascular endothelial growth factor (VEGF) receptor 2 (KDR or Flk-1). However, it is evident that these circulating progenitor cells (particularly when they are cultured in vitro) comprise several different entities.[5] Individual cells may indeed have clonal potential and stem cell characteristics. Others, including distinct myeloid subpopulations, may preferentially act as proangiogenic cells[7] in addition to their capacity to differentiate to endothelial cells. Myeloid cells also have been shown to contribute to muscle regeneration by fusion, indicating that myeloid subpopulations may act diversely. An interesting source of endothelial progenitor cells is placental cord blood, which is enriched in clonally expandable endothelial progenitor cells.

Mesoangioblasts are vessel-associated multipotent progenitors that express the key marker of angiopoietic progenitors, VEGF receptor 2, but are distinct from hematopoietic endothelial progenitor cells. In vitro, mesoangioblasts differentiate into many mesoderm cell types, such as smooth, cardiac, and striated muscle and bone and endothelium, and improve skeletal muscle dystrophy and heart function.[8,9] Importantly, studies have revealed that mesoangioblast-like cells are mobilized into the blood in cardiovascular stress situations and might thereby be harvested for therapeutic purposes.[10]

The discovery of tissue-resident stem cells in the heart, the cardiac stem cell, offers the potential to harvest cells that are primed to acquire a cardiac phenotype and therefore might be optimally suited for cardiac repair. Several different populations have been identified and characterized: c-Kit+ cells,[11] Sca-1+ cells,[12] SP cells, and cells expressing the protein Islet-1.[13] Whereas c-Kit+ cells, Sca-1+ cells, and cardiac SP cells are isolated from adult hearts, cells expressing Islet-1 so far have been detected only in the postnatal stage. Whether c-Kit+, Sca-1+, and cardiac SP cells represent three different cell populations is not entirely resolved. At least Sca-1+ cells contain a fraction of SP cells, and among cardiac SP cells, the greatest potential for cardiomyogenic differentiation is restricted to cells positive for Sca-1 expression (but negative for CD31),[14] indicating that the two cell populations may share some common features. Cardiac stem cells also were obtained by growing of self-adherent clusters (termed cardiospheres) from subcultures of murine or human biopsy specimens. Others have generated cardiac SP cell–derived cardiospheres by adaptation of a method used to create a neurosphere and claimed that cardiac neural crest cells contribute to cardiac SP cells.[15] Cardiosphere-derived cardiac stem cells as well as c-Kit+ cardiac stem cells are capable of long-term self-renewal and can differentiate into the major specialized cell types of the heart, myocytes and vascular cells (i.e., cells with endothelial or smooth muscle markers). So far, the origin of and the mechanisms maintaining the cardiac stem cell pool are unclear. Whereas two studies suggested that c-Kit+ and cardiac SP cells may derive from the bone marrow,[16,17] these studies cannot entirely exclude that specific subpopulations of cardiac stem cells originate from distinct sources and may represent remnants from embryonic development in selected niches within the heart.

Adipose tissue is another rich source of distinct subsets of stem and progenitor cells that are potentially useful for cardiac repair and neovascularization improvement (see later).[18] Both mesenchymal stem cells and endothelial progenitor cells have been isolated after enzymatic digestion of adipose tissue and showed beneficial effects in experimental studies. Very recently, pluripotent spermatogonial stem cells from adult mouse testis that possess the capacity to differentiate to fully active cardiac myocytes in vitro have been identified.[19]

In summary, the identification and characterization of stem and progenitor cell populations with potential therapeutic properties for the treatment of heart disease is an emerging field. Because direct side-by-side comparisons are missing, it is impossible to estimate what might be the best cells for cardiac repair. Clearly, a ranking not only will be based on the assessment of the functional capacities of the cells to differentiate into cardiac myocytes but also will include other aspects of progenitor cell functions. Particularly for the clinical application, the safety of the treatment and the feasibility will be of major importance.

MECHANISMS OF ACTION OF STEM CELLS. In contrast to ES cells, most adult stem or progenitor cells do not spontaneously differentiate into cardiomyocytes but rather require an adequate stimulus to do so. The local microenvironment plays an important role in inducing cell fate changes by physical cell-to-cell interaction or by providing paracrine factors (see Fig. 33-e1 on website). On the basis of this concept, a co-culture technique was developed whereby stem or progenitor cells are cultured together with rat neonatal ventricular cardiomyocytes to simulate a cardiac-like surrounding in vitro.[20] Use of such a co-culture system to induce differentiation of adult stem or progenitor cells from various species and organs demonstrated that the physical contact with beating neighboring cardiomyocytes is indeed required for the differentiation process to occur. Alternatively, the nonspecific transcriptional activators neurohormones or cytokines of the Wnt or platelet-derived growth factor family have been employed to induce or to enhance differentiation of adult stem cells (for review, see reference 21). However, experimental studies addressing the capacity of bone marrow–derived stem cells to differentiate into the cardiomyogenic lineage yielded conflicting results, and the extent to which differentiation into cardiac myocytes occurs in vivo varies dramatically between the different experimental studies. The identification of subsets of adult stem cells with a higher capacity to differentiate into cardiac myocytes and the enhancement of cardiac differentiation by interaction with the pathways controlling differentiation are currently under investigation. Interestingly, functional improvement of the heart was even seen in experimental studies in which no formation of new cardiomyocytes was detected. Therefore, additional mechanisms initiated by cell therapy most likely contribute to functional cardiac repair (**Fig. 33-2**).

In addition to transdifferentiation of stem cells, several other mechanisms should be considered, including enhanced neovascularization, alterations in scar formation, and cytoprotection (see Fig. 33-2). Of these, most obviously, progenitor cells may improve neovascularization and thereby augment nutrients and oxygen supply. This mode of action is expected to contribute to cardiac regeneration particularly in situations in which blood supply is limited (e.g., as in chronic ischemic HF with angina pectoris) or alternatively in the presence of hibernating myocardium. Neovascularization can be mediated by the physical incorporation of progenitor cells into new capillaries[22] or by perivascular accumulation of cells. Incorporated progenitor cells of most if not all types may release growth factors that promote angiogenesis by acting on mature endothelial cells.[23] Paracrine factors may also beneficially influence cardiac repair by protecting cardiac myocytes from apoptotic stimuli or activate cardiac-resident stem cells to enhance the endogenous repair capacity.[23,24] Finally, the release of various cytokines will affect cardiac remodeling processes by altering the development of fibrosis during scar formation or by modulating inflammatory processes. The extent to which progenitor cells contribute to vasculogenesis by becoming physical elements of newly formed vessels versus acting through secreted factors may depend on the environment to which the cell is exposed. Importantly, recent studies using human bone marrow–derived mononuclear cells engineered with a suicide vector to specifically kill administered cells within weeks after therapeutic application in an animal model of acute myocardial infarction demonstrated that persistence of the administered cells for at least 3 weeks contributes to the beneficial effects on recovery of cardiac function. Moreover, lineage commitment to the endothelial cell phenotype, as evidenced by activation of the endothelial nitric oxide synthase promoter, mediated the recovery of cardiac function, whereas lineage commitment to vascular smooth muscle cells or cardiomyocytes plays only a minor role.[25] Thus, it is currently assumed that the beneficial effects of bone marrow–derived mononuclear cells administered in acute myocardial infarction mainly comprise improved neovascularization, recovery of microvascular function, and increased blood supply to ischemic areas, either directly or indirectly.

CLINICAL APPLICATION OF PROGENITOR CELLS

Clinically Used Cell Types

A variety of autologous adult progenitor cells are currently undergoing clinical evaluation (**Fig. 33-3** and **Table 33-1**). The first clinically relevant cells proposed for cardiac myocytes were skeletal muscle myoblasts, undifferentiated proliferation-competent cells that serve as

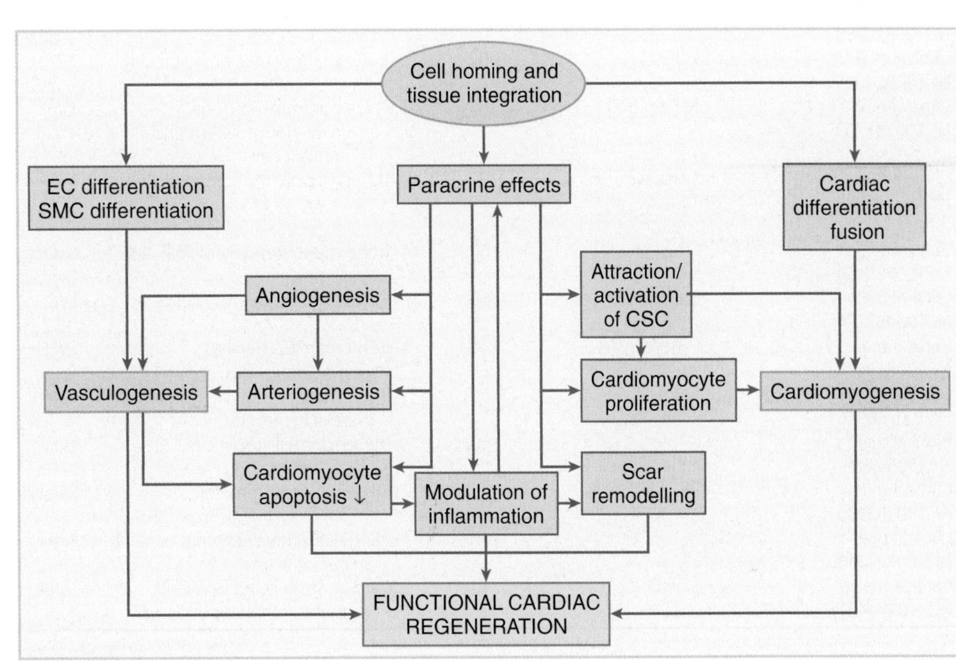

FIGURE 33-2 Proposed mechanisms of action of stem and progenitor cells in cardiovascular repair. CSC = cardiac stem cell; EC = endothelial cell; SMC = smooth muscle cell.

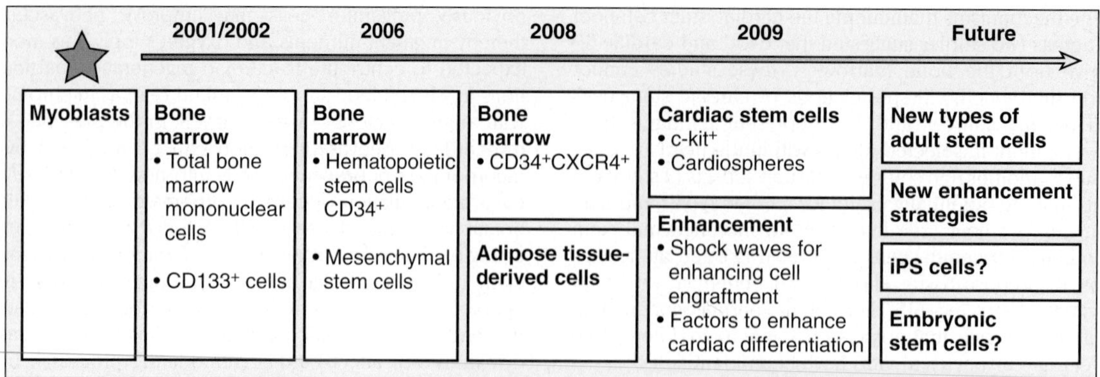

FIGURE 33-3 Cells used for cell therapy of heart disease and future perspective. *(Modified from Chavakis E, Koyanagi M, Dimmeler S: Enhancing the outcome of cell therapy for cardiac repair: Progress from bench to bedside and back. Circulation 121:325, 2010.)*

TABLE 33-1 Ongoing Cell Therapy Trials in Patients with Coronary Heart Disease

STUDY IDENTIFIER	TRIAL NAME	NUMBER OF PATIENTS	CELLS	PRIMARY ENDPOINT	ROUTE OF CELL DELIVERY
Non–ST Elevation Acute Coronary Syndrome					
Clinical trial NCT00711542	REPAIR-ACS	100	Bone marrow–derived progenitor cells	Coronary flow reserve	Intracoronary
Acute Myocardial Infarction					
Controlled trial ISRCTN17457407	BOOST-2	200	Bone marrow cells Low versus high cell number Nonirradiated versus irradiated cells	LVEF	Intracoronary
Clinical trial NCT00355186	SWISS-AMI	150	Bone marrow–derived stem cells	LVEF	Intracoronary Day 5-7 versus day 21-28
Clinical trial NCT00684021	TIME	120	Bone marrow mononuclear cells	LVEF	Intracoronary Day 3 versus day 7 post AMI
Clinical trial NCT00684060	Late TIME	87	Bone marrow mononuclear cells	LVEF	Intracoronary 2-3 weeks post AMI
Clinical trial NCT00501917	MAGIC Cell-5	116	Peripheral blood stem cells mobilized with G-CSF versus G-CSF with darbepoetin	LVEF	Intracoronary
Clinical trial NCT00877903	—	220	Allogeneic mesenchymal stem cells	LVESV	Intravenous
Clinical trial NCT00677222	—	28	Allogeneic mesenchymal stem cells	Safety	Perivascular
Ischemic Heart Failure					
Clinical trial NCT00526253	MARVEL	390	Skeletal myoblasts	6-minute walk test, quality of life, LVEF	Transendocardial
Clinical trial NCT00824005	FOCUS	87	Bone marrow mononuclear cells	$M\dot{V}O_2$, LVESV, ischemic area	Transendocardial
Clinical trial NCT00747708	REGEN-IHD	165	G-CSF–stimulated bone marrow–derived stem and progenitor cells	LVEF	Transendocardial versus intracoronary
Clinical trial NCT00326989	Cellwave	100	Bone marrow mononuclear cells	LVEF	Extracorporeal shock wave, then intracoronary cell therapy
Clinical trial NCT00285454	—	60	Bone marrow mononuclear cells	Safety, perfusion Systolic function	Retrograde coronary venous delivery
Clinical trial NCT00462774	Cardio133	60	CD1331 bone marrow cells	LVEF	Transepicardial during CABG
Clinical trial NCT00810238	C-Cure	240	Bone marrow–derived cardiopoietic cells	LVEF	Transendocardial
Clinical trial NCT00768066	TAC-HFT	60	Bone marrow cells versus mesenchymal stem cells	Safety	Transendocardial
Clinical trial NCT00644410	—	60	Mesenchymal stem cells	LVEF	Transendocardial
Clinical trial NCT00587990	PROMETHEUS	45	Mesenchymal stem cells	Safety	Transepicardial during CABG
Clinical trial NCT00721045	—	60	Allogeneic mesenchymal precursor cells	Safety	Transendocardial
Clinical trial NCT00474461	SCIPIO	40	Cardiac stem cells harvested from right atrial appendage	Safety	Intracoronary

Unless otherwise stated, autologous cell sources are used. AMI = acute myocardial infarction; CABG = coronary artery bypass grafting; G-CSF = granulocyte colony-stimulating factor; LVEF = left ventricular ejection fraction; LVESV = left ventricular end-systolic volume; $M\dot{V}O_2$ = maximal oxygen consumption.

Modified from Wollert KC, Drexler HC: Cell therapy for the treatment of coronary heart disease: A critical appraisal. Nat Rev Cardiol 7:204, 2010. See *www.clinicaltrials.gov* for additional description of the clinical trials by NCT registry number.

precursors to skeletal muscle (for review, see reference 26). For clinical use, autologous human myoblasts are isolated from skeletal muscle biopsy specimens, propagated and expanded ex vivo for a few days or weeks, and then injected directly into the ventricular wall. Bone marrow is, at present, the most frequent source of stem cells used clinically for cardiac repair. The rapid transition from the bench to the clinic was facilitated by the more than 30 years of clinical experience and the excellent safety profile of infused bone marrow–derived mononuclear cells for bone marrow transplantation. Bone marrow is aspirated under local anesthesia in most of the studies; the entire mononuclear cell fraction is obtained (a heterogeneous mixture of cells with varying percentage of hematopoietic stem cells, endothelial progenitor cells, mesenchymal stem cells, and SP cells). So far, isolated bone marrow–derived cells have been injected into the heart without further ex vivo expansion. In a few studies, specific subpopulations, such as a fraction of hematopoietic and endothelial progenitor cells expressing the marker protein CD133 or CD34 as well as cells coexpressing CD34 and the homing receptor CXCR4, were purified and used.[27] Last, peripheral blood-derived ex vivo–cultured proangiogenic cells (early endothelial progenitor cells) are used for both clinical cardiac repair and peripheral ischemia.[28,29] Alternatively, a specific subfraction, the hematopoietic CD34^{+} progenitor cell, is enriched from whole blood after G-CSF–mediated mobilization from the bone marrow into the blood.[30]

Routes of Application

Progenitor cells for cardiac repair can be delivered in different ways (see Fig. 33-1). Intracoronary infusion by standard balloon catheters has been used in all clinical trials treating patients with acute myocardial infarction. This technique offers the advantage that cells can travel directly only into myocardial regions in which nutrient blood flow and oxygen supply are preserved, thereby ensuring a favorable environment for survival of the cells, a prerequisite for stable engraftment. Conversely, homing of intra-arterially applied progenitor cells requires migration out of the vasculature into the surrounding tissue, which may mean that unperfused regions of myocardium will be targeted far less efficiently if at all. Moreover, whereas bone marrow–derived and blood-derived progenitor cells are known to extravasate and to migrate to ischemic areas, other cell types may not and may even obstruct the microcirculation after intra-arterial administration, leading to embolic myocardial damage, thus limiting the use of intracoronary delivery.

Injection of cells into the ventricular wall by a percutaneous endocardial or surgical epicardial approach is an alternative delivery strategy circumventing some of these limitations. Direct delivery of progenitor cells into scar tissue or areas of hibernating myocardium by catheter-based needle injection, direct injection during open heart surgery, and minimally invasive thoracoscopic procedures are not limited by cell uptake from the circulation or by embolic risk. An offsetting consideration is the risk for ventricular perforation, which may limit direct needle injection into freshly infarcted hearts. In addition, it is difficult to envisage that progenitor cells injected into uniformly necrotic tissue—lacking the syncytium of live muscle cells that may furnish instructive signals and lacking blood flow for the delivery of oxygen and nutrients—would receive the necessary cues and environment to engraft and to differentiate. Most cells, if injected directly, simply die. For this reason, electromechanical mapping of viable but hibernating myocardium may be useful to pinpoint the preferred regions for injection. Finally, in diffuse disease like dilated nonischemic cardiomyopathy, focal deposits of directly injected cells might be poorly matched to the underlying anatomy and physiology. Thus, it is likely that the nature of the patient's cardiomyopathy will ultimately influence if not dictate the source and route chosen among potential progenitor cell therapies. Additional strategies to augment cell homing and to promote homogeneous integration of cells may be required, particularly in patients with chronic healed infarcts or diffuse nonischemic cardiomyopathy lacking active recruitment signals.

Intravenous administration of cells may be hampered by trapping of the cells in the pulmonary circulation. Indeed, in clinical trials with labeled bone marrow–derived cells, no homing to the heart in acute myocardial infarction was observed after intravenous cell administration.[31] However, intravenous application of allogeneic mesenchymal stem cells was used safely[32] and is currently being tested in a clinical phase II study.

Results of Clinical Trials

The results of clinical trials published to date, aimed at progenitor cell–based myocardial repair, are summarized in two recent meta-analyses,[33,34] which suggest that intracoronary cell therapy after percutaneous coronary intervention for acute myocardial infarction appears to provide statistically significant and clinically relevant benefits with respect to LV function and LV remodeling. It is essential to distinguish between studies performed in patients with acute myocardial infarction and those performed in patients with chronic HF because fundamentally different pathophysiologic processes are targeted with each clinical scenario. In patients with acute myocardial infarction, progenitor cell transplantation aims to prevent or to ameliorate postinfarction LV remodeling, thereby reducing postinfarction HF. Such an effect might even be achieved by enhanced neovascularization and reduced cardiomyocyte apoptosis, irrespective of long-term engraftment and transdifferentiation. Conversely, the first two mechanisms acting alone may have limited benefit in patients with long-established scars, absent hibernating myocytes and end-stage HF, when cardiomyogenesis in its pure sense would be desirable.

CELL THERAPY IN ACUTE MYOCARDIAL INFARCTION. On the basis of meta-analyses summarizing the results of the initial studies, the infusion of autologous bone marrow–derived cells (BMCs) is safe and feasible in patients with acute myocardial infarction.[33,34] These analyses suggest that there is an overall improvement (absolute) in global LV ejection fraction (LVEF) by 3% to 4%, a reduction in LV end-systolic volume by 5 mL, and improved perfusion in the infarcted area 4 to 6 months after cell transplantation.

Currently, there are six published randomized controlled trials assessing the effects of intracoronary administration of BMCs in patients with acute myocardial infarction: BOOST (intracoronary autologous bone-marrow cell transfer after myocardial infarction)[35]; REPAIR-AMI (Reinfusion of Enriched Progenitor Cells and Infarct Remodeling in Acute Myocardial Infarction)[36]; Leuven-AMI (autologous bone marrow–derived stem cell transfer in patients with ST-segment elevation myocardial infarction)[37]; REGENT (Myocardial Regeneration by Intracoronary Infusion of Selected Population of Stem Cells in Acute Myocardial Infarction)[27]; FINCELL (effects of intracoronary injection of mononuclear bone marrow cells on LV function, arrhythmia risk profile, and restenosis after thrombolytic therapy of acute myocardial infarction)[38]; and ASTAMI (Autologous Stem Cell Transplantation in Acute Myocardial Infarction).[39] Three of the trials were placebo controlled. The primary endpoint common to all these trials was change in LVEF at 4 to 6 months. In four of the trials, recovery of global LVEF was significantly greater in the BMC-treated patient group compared with the placebo or control group; one trial demonstrated only regional contractile improvement in the infarcted segments, and one trial did not show any differences between the treatment and the control groups. The Leuvin-AMI, which showed only regional contractile improvement in the infarcted segment, differed importantly from the other trials with respect to the timing of BMC administration, which was performed within 24 hours after reperfusion therapy for acute myocardial infarction. Although not yet published in manuscript form, the results of the HEBE trial (bone marrow cell therapy after acute myocardial infarction) have been presented recently in abstract form.[40] In this study, 200 patients with acute myocardial infarction were randomly assigned either to receive an infusion of mononucleated BMCs or mononucleated cells isolated from peripheral blood (PBMCs) or to primary percutaneous angioplasty alone (1:1:1 ratio). Despite promising results in the pilot trial, intracoronary infusion of mononucleated BMCs or PBMCs did not improve regional LV systolic function (primary endpoint) or global LV function and LV remodeling (secondary endpoints) at 4 months, assessed by magnetic resonance imaging. The reasons that the ASTAMI and HEBE trials failed to show a benefit of cell therapy are unclear. However, preclinical work suggested that the processing techniques used to isolate the cells may have affected outcome of the ASTAMI trial.[41] The reasons for these negative findings of the HEBE trial are unclear and will remain speculative until publication of the full trial.

Overall, absolute recovery of global LVEF in these trials was improved by 2.5% to 6% in the BMC group compared with the placebo (or control) group at 4 to 6 months. The enhanced recovery of LV function was accompanied by less of an increase in end-systolic volume, suggesting that there was less adverse LV remodeling after stem cell therapy. In addition, analysis of regional LV function revealed the most prominent differences between BMC administration and placebo (control) to occur in the infarct and infarct border zone. Remarkably, the studies consistently demonstrated that those patients with a lower LVEF at inclusion showed the greatest benefit with respect to the recovery of LVEF by the administration of BMCs compared with placebo administration or the control group. Indeed, as illustrated in **Figure 33-4**, the entire effect of improved contractile recovery by BMC administration was confined to the patients with an LVEF below the median at the time of inclusion into the study.

Studies using serial cardiac magnetic resonance imaging revealed some mechanistic insights into why intracoronary BMC administration appears to be specifically effective in the patients with the most severely depressed LV function at inclusion into the studies. Adverse LV remodeling as measured by assessment of increases in end-systolic LV volumes at 1 year was essentially confined to patients with the most severely depressed LV function 3 to 8 days after reperfusion therapy for acute myocardial infarction, at which time BMCs were administered. In these patients, BMC administration abrogated LV end-systolic volume expansion, thereby contributing to improved global contractile recovery compared with the placebo (control) group. In contrast, when LVEF recovered close to normal values within 3 to 8 days after reperfusion therapy for acute myocardial infarction, no adverse remodeling was observed at 1 year of follow-up, and no effect of BMC administration could be detected. Thus, it appears that the beneficial effects of BMC administration in patients with acute myocardial infarction are most pronounced in those patients at risk for adverse LV remodeling.

Importantly, because patients who are at risk for adverse LV remodeling after acute myocardial infarction are also at a profoundly increased risk to suffer from major adverse clinical events over time, it is reassuring to see that the incidence of the cumulative clinical endpoints death, myocardial reinfarction, and rehospitalization for HF was significantly lower in the BMC-treated patients compared with placebo after 2 years of follow-up in REPAIR-AMI (see Fig. 33-e2 on website).[42] However, none of the studies performed so far was powered to detect a potential clinical benefit in terms of reducing adverse events. Therefore, large-scale clinical trials are still mandatory to document a clinical benefit of intracoronary BMC administration in patients with acute myocardial infarction. However, the phase II trials provided extremely valuable information to identify the patient cohort at risk that would derive the most clinical profit from BMC administration after an acute myocardial infarction.

What additional variables might influence outcome? The large number of patients enrolled in the phase II trials allowed the evaluation of several predefined secondary endpoints to generate hypotheses for the next-generation trials. Besides the significant interaction between the baseline ejection fraction and the improvement seen after BMC therapy, the timing of BMC delivery appears to affect outcome. Surprisingly, patients who had been treated up to 4 days after the myocardial infarction showed no benefit, whereas later treatment (days 4 to 8) provided an enhanced improvement of ejection fraction during follow-up. Given that several experimental studies demonstrated that the cells provide a cytoprotective activity coinciding with a reduction of cardiomyocyte apoptosis, one would have expected early timing of cell infusion to have been the most efficient. On the basis of the data of the REPAIR-AMI trial, one may speculate that the microenvironment after acute myocardial infarction changes during the first week after reperfusion, thereby modulating the homing or the subsequent functional activity of the infused cells.[36] It is well known that ischemia-reperfusion induces a transient change in the expression of chemoattractant factors such as VEGF and SDF-1, which are known to be essential for stimulating the recruitment and retention of cells in the tissue. Moreover, the initial edema formation is followed by a transient invasion of different "waves" of cells. Therefore, it is conceivable that cell homing might be best a few days after reperfusion rather than immediately. Further studies are currently under way to prospectively address this

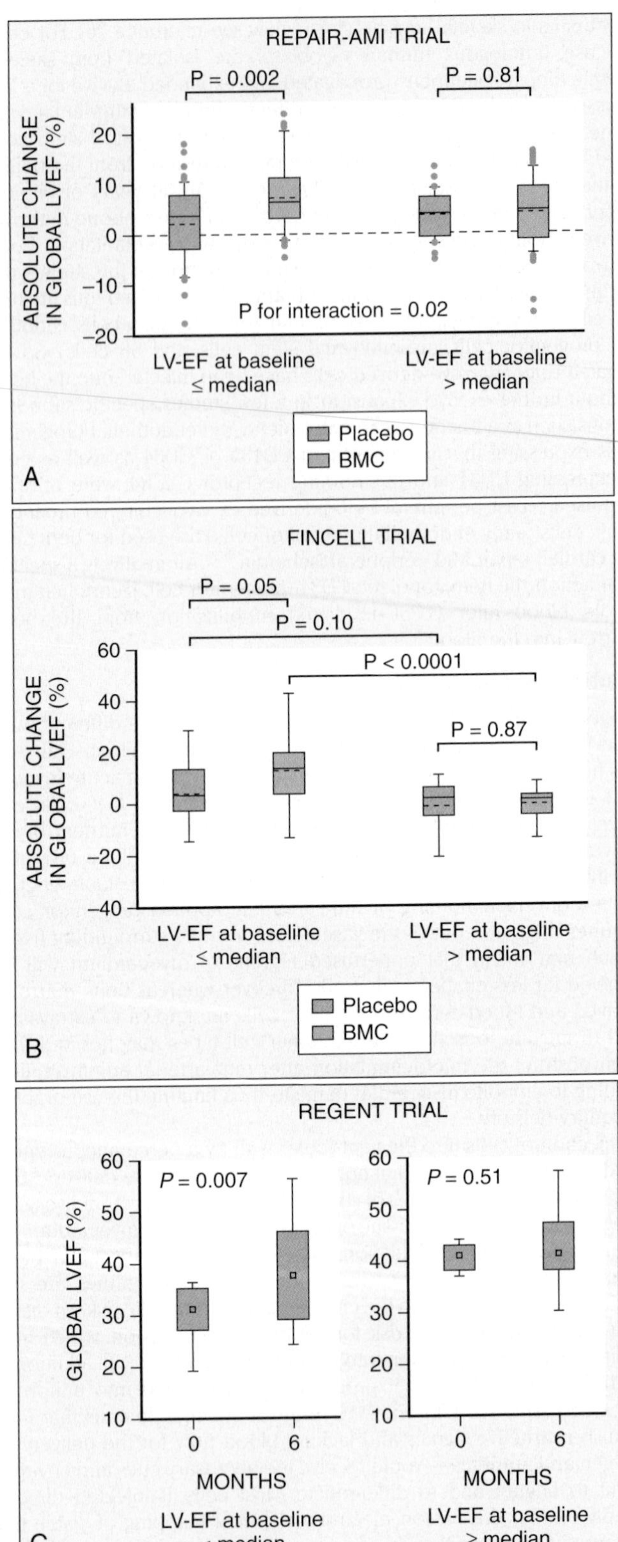

FIGURE 33-4 Interaction between baseline left ventricular ejection fraction (LV-EF) and the absolute change in left ventricular ejection fraction after administration of bone marrow–derived progenitor cells. **A,** Results of the REPAIR-AMI trial. *(From Schachinger V, Erbs S, Elsasser A, et al: Intracoronary bone marrow–derived progenitor cells in acute myocardial infarction. N Engl J Med 355:1210, 2006.)* **B,** Results of the FINCELL trial. *(Modified from Miettinen JA, Ylitalo K, Hedberg P, et al: Determinants of functional recovery after myocardial infarction of patients treated with bone marrow–derived stem cells after thrombolytic therapy. Heart 96:362, 2010.)* **C,** Results of the REGENT trial. *(Modified from Tendera M, Wojakowski W, Ruzyllo W, et al: Intracoronary infusion of bone marrow–derived selected $CD34^+CXCR4^+$ cells and non-selected mononuclear cells in patients with acute STEMI and reduced left ventricular ejection fraction: Results of randomized, multicentre Myocardial Regeneration by Intracoronary Infusion of Selected Population of Stem Cells in Acute Myocardial Infarction [REGENT] Trial. Eur Heart J 30:1313, 2009.)*

question (SWISS-AMI trial [SWiss Multicenter Intracoronary Stem Cells Study in Acute Myocardial Infarction; ClinicalTrials.gov Identifier: NCT00355186]; TIME Study [Use of Adult Autologous Stem Cells in Treating People Who Have Had a Heart Attack; ClinicalTrials.gov Identifier: NCT00684021]). Finally, recent data from REPAIR-AMI documented that the quality of cell processing and specifically the contamination of the final cell product with red blood cells are major determinants of a beneficial effect on contractile recovery.[41,42] These data also provide clinical evidence for a bioactivity-response relationship of BMC therapy much like a dose-response relationship in drug trials.

Overall, the clinical data available at present indicate that cell therapy with BMCs is feasible and safe at least for the follow-up available (up to 5 years in the pioneering studies). None of the studies so far reported an increased incidence of arrhythmias (as has been seen in some of the myoblast trials). Moreover, restenosis, which was considered a potential side effect by progenitor cell–mediated plaque angiogenesis or plaque inflammation, was increased in only one study using $CD133^+$ cells.[43] Because $CD133^+$ cells were isolated by use of a mouse antibody, one may speculate that the remaining antibody might have elicited a local proinflammatory reaction despite the failure to detect systemic anti-mouse antibodies in the patients. All other studies did not observe an augmented risk for restenosis, if anything; there was a significantly decreased necessity for revascularization procedures in the REPAIR-AMI trial.

Mobilization Strategies in Acute Myocardial Infarction. Progenitor cell mobilization from the bone marrow is controlled by various cytokines including colony-stimulating factors and various angiogenic cytokines (for review, see reference 44). Colony-stimulating factors such as granulocyte colony-stimulating factor (G-CSF) and granulocyte-monocyte colony-stimulating factor (GM-CSF) are established mobilizers of hematopoietic progenitor cells and are clinically used for reconstitution of hematopoiesis. G-CSF and GM-CSF additionally mobilize $CD34^+CD133^+$ cells and cultured proangiogenic cells[45] and improve the recovery after myocardial ischemia.[46,47] On the basis of these experimental findings, clinical trials addressed whether G-CSF improves LVEF in patients with acute myocardial ischemia. The results of these clinical trials have been variable and overall showed that G-CSF therapy appears safe but did not lead to a significant improvement of cardiac function (for review, see reference 48). The reason for the lack of clinical benefit may be that the design of the clinical trials might have been suboptimal because subanalysis indicated that very early treatment of patients with lower ejection fraction provides some benefit.[48] In addition, G-CSF was shown to reduce the activity of the homing receptor CXCR4, thereby potentially impairing the migration and retention of the mobilized progenitor cells and proangiogenic cells to the infarcted tissue.[49,50] Despite the disappointing clinical results with G-CSF therapy, G-CSF was successfully used to mobilize $CD34^+$ cells for cell therapy of patients with refractory angina,[30] and the injection of G-CSF–mobilized cells induced a better improvement of cardiac function in patients with acute myocardial infarction compared with therapy with G-CSF alone.[51] These trials indicate that G-CSF might be useful to augment the number of circulating progenitor cells for intravascular or intramyocardial injection. The REGEN-HD trial (Bone Marrow Derived Adult Stem Cells for Chronic Heart Failure; ClinicalTrials.gov Identifier: NCT00747708) is being conducted to determine whether direct intracoronary administration of G-CSF–mobilized autologous bone marrow–derived stems cells will confer an additional improvement in cardiac function above that derived from G-CSF infusion alone. Furthermore, an experimental study showed that G-CSF effectively improved the recovery of cardiac function after myocardial infarction if coadministrated with a CD26/dipeptidyl peptidase 4 inhibitor that reduces the cleavage of SDF-1 in the heart and thereby augments recruitment of progenitor cells.[52] This approach is currently being tested in the SITAGRAMI trial (Sitagliptin Plus Granulocyte-colony Stimulating Factor in Acute Myocardial Infarction; ClinicalTrials.gov Identifier: NCT00650143).[53]

An alternative cytokine that might be useful for progenitor cell mobilization is erythropoietin (Epo). Epo significantly increased mobilization of hematopoietic and proangiogenic cells.[54] In addition, Epo is also protective for cardiac myocytes after ischemia-reperfusion in patients with HF because it decreases the number of apoptotic myocytes, thereby limiting infarct expansion and attenuating the deterioration of hemodynamic function after acute myocardial infarction.[55] These beneficial effects of Epo, which may override potential Epo-related side effects such as elevated blood pressure and the incidence of thrombosis, led to the initiation of clinical trials using recombinant Epo for the treatment of patients with large infarcts or cardiac ischemia.

CELL THERAPY AND CELL MOBILIZATION STRATEGIES IN PATIENTS WITH CHRONIC HEART FAILURE. In patients with chronic ischemic heart disease and a prior myocardial infarction, the results of the initial attempts at cell-based myocardial repair have been more heterogeneous, and the number of patients that have been treated has been less compared with acute myocardial infarction trials. The first cell-based therapy trial used skeletal muscle–derived progenitor cells, which were directly injected into the scarred region of the left ventricle during open heart surgery for coronary artery bypass grafting. Global and regional LV function was significantly and persistently improved. However, the concomitant coronary artery revascularization confounded the assessment of true benefit in these studies. A recent randomized, placebo-controlled trial using myoblast injections combined with coronary bypass surgery did not demonstrate a significant improvement in heart function, although high-dose injections of myoblasts appeared to revert end-diastolic LV volume increases.[56] In patients not undergoing simultaneous revascularization, the transcatheter injection of myoblasts into the preexisting (5- to 6-year-old) postinfarction scar tissue led to a reduction in the symptoms of HF without any objective evidence of an improvement in global LV function. Unfortunately, even though extensive previous animal experiments provided no hint of increased arrhythmias, the enthusiasm for injection of myoblasts into scar tissue for cardiac repair was dampened by development of life-threatening arrhythmias in the patients who were treated.[57] Mechanistically, these arrhythmias may be related to the lack of electrical coupling of skeletal muscle to neighboring cardiac myocytes, or alternatively, it may be contingent on coupling by the few hybrid cells formed by fusion with adjacent cardiac myocytes, which generate spatially heterogeneous calcium transients. Therefore, currently, the implantation of skeletal myoblasts requires the implantation of an implantable cardioverter-defibrillator as a mandatory adjunct to therapy.

Bone marrow–derived progenitor cells have been employed in several smaller, nonrandomized trials for chronic ischemic HF with use of different strategies for cell delivery. Three studies have used electromechanical mapping of the LV endocardial surface to identify sites for injection of cells into areas of myocardial hibernation.[58,59] Each of these studies has shown a significant increase in global LVEF associated with decreased end-systolic volumes as well as an improvement in exercise capacity. Whereas this functional improvement might be secondary to an improved blood supply to hibernating cardiomyocytes, it is also conceivable that hibernating myocardium may provide a more favorable microenvironment for the survival or engraftment of the injected cells compared with an injection in scar tissue. Others have used a surgical approach to inject BMCs during coronary artery bypass graft surgery (CABG). Again, an increase in ejection fraction was documented. Whereas the effects of CABG and BMCs cannot be dissociated in these pilot trials, a study showed a more profound effect in patients being treated with CABG and cells in comparison to CABG or cells alone.[60]

Three published studies addressed the possibility of intracoronary delivery of BMCs by a balloon catheter. The IACT (Regeneration of Human Infarcted Heart Muscle by Intracoronary Autologous Bone Marrow Cell Transplantation in Chronic Coronary Artery Disease) study tested the feasibility of BMC infusion in patients with chronic HF and demonstrated a substantial increase in ejection fraction (+15%) in patients with healed (>3 months old) myocardial infarction.[61] Smaller but significant improvements were also seen in the randomized controlled trials by Erbs and coworkers and the TOPCARE-CHF study. Erbs and coworkers infused G-CSF–mobilized, ex vivo–cultivated endothelial progenitor cells in a recanalized coronary artery.[29] Coronary flow reserve in response to adenosine and global ejection fraction were improved in the cell-treated patients compared with recanalization without cell therapy. A smaller but significant improvement was also observed in the TOPCARE-CHF study.[62] Interestingly, this study was the first to examine a direct side-by-side comparison of two different cell types in patients with old myocardial infarctions. In this patient cohort, BMCs were shown to be significantly better compared with circulating progenitor cells. This is in contrast to the TOPCARE-AMI trial, in which BMCs and endothelial progenitor cells showed a similar effectiveness in acute myocardial infarction patients.[28] The reason for this discrepancy is unclear. One may speculate that the number and function of circulating cells are further impaired in HF patients and that an additional mobilization step is required to yield a sufficiently high number of functionally active cells (as done by Erbs and colleagues[29]). Another potential explanation may relate to the combination of a lower number of endothelial progenitor cells applied (22×10^6 compared with 205×10^6 BMCs) or a reduced homing capacity in the chronic setting, which might limit the efficiency of endothelial progenitor cells.

Finally, as discussed extensively before, different cell types may activate different mechanisms that may be more or less beneficial in acute versus chronic ischemic HF. Mobilization of progenitor cells with G-CSF without intracoronary reinfusion did not result in any measurable benefit on LV function but was associated with adverse coronary events in two studies.[63,64]

CELL THERAPY FOR REFRACTORY ANGINA. So-called no-option patients with refractory angina, in whom revascularization procedures have been fully exploited, represent an attractive target for cell therapy. Three placebo-controlled small trials have addressed a potential effect of catheter-based intramyocardial injections of either G-CSF–mobilized $CD34^+$ cells obtained from the blood by leukopheresis[30] or BMCs harvested from bone marrow aspirates in patients with preserved LV function but refractory angina. All three trials used electromagnetic mapping to identify underperfused areas of the left ventricle for direct cell injections. All three trials demonstrated a significant reduction in ischemic symptoms as well as in the extent of stress-induced ischemia quantified by SPECT imaging. These data further support a beneficial effect of cell therapy on coronary microcirculatory function, as has also been directly shown by intracoronary flow measurements using Doppler wires in patients with acute myocardial infarction and in patients after reopening of a chronic total coronary occlusion.[29,65] Taken together, these observations corroborate the hypothesis that a major effect of cell therapy in the clinical setting is related to improved coronary vascular function, by either direct or indirect mechanisms.

DEFINING THE BEST CELL TYPE FOR CARDIAC REPAIR. Direct side-by-side clinical effectiveness trials comparing different cell types have been limited, as noted before. The ongoing TAC-HFT trial (Transendocardial Autologous Cells in Ischemic Heart Failure Trial; ClinicalTrials.gov Identifier: NCT00768066) will compare the clinical effectiveness of mesenchymal stem cells versus bone marrow–derived stem cells in patients with chronic ischemic LV dysfunction and HF secondary to myocardial infarction. As noted before, although BMCs have provided beneficial effects in various studies, the effects on LV function are relatively modest. This has set the stage for broader clinical testing with a variety of different autologous cell types. A rapid and relatively simple purification procedure has been developed to isolate a mixed mononuclear progenitor cell population from adipose tissue, which had a promising profile in preclinical testing.[66] Despite early enthusiasm for adipose tissue–derived stems cells, enrollment in early-phase clinical protocols has been halted in the APOLLO trial (Randomized Clinical Trial of Adipose-Derived Stem Cells in the Treatment of Patients With ST-Elevation Myocardial Infarction; ClinicalTrials.gov Identifier: NCT00442806) in patients with acute myocardial infarction and in the PRECISE trial (A Randomized Clinical Trial of Adipose-Derived Stem Cells in Treatment of Non Revascularizable Ischemic Myocardium; ClinicalTrials.gov Identifier: NCT00426868) in patients with chronic ischemic cardiomyopathy.[66] On the basis of preclinical research suggesting that aldehyde dehydrogenase–bright stem cells might stimulate the growth of new vessels, selected aldehyde dehydrogenase–expressing cells are being isolated from the bone marrow and then injected back into the heart in patients with ischemic cardiomyopathy (FOCUS [Intramyocardial Injection of Autologous Aldehyde Dehydrogenase–Bright Stem Cells for Therapeutic Angiogenesis]; ClinicalTrials.gov Identifier: NCT00314366).

Cardiosphere-derived stem cells and cardiac-resident progenitor cells, which presumably have a heightened predisposition to adopt the cardiac muscle fate, are currently undergoing clinical evaluation in pilot trials. The CADUCEUS trial (Cardiosphere-Derived Autologous Stem Cells to Reverse Ventricular Dysfunction; ClinicalTrials.gov Identifier: NCT00893360) is examining the effects of cardiospheres derived from myocardial biopsy samples in patients with ischemic LV dysfunction, whereas the SCIPIO trial (Cardiac Stem Cell Infusion in Patients With Ischemic Cardiomyopathy; ClinicalTrials.gov Identifier: NCT00474461) is examining the effects of cardiac progenitor cells harvested from the right atrial appendage in patients with ischemic cardiomyopathy. Moreover, there is also an ongoing phase II multicenter trial to examine the safety and feasibility of transendocardial delivery of three different doses of allogeneic mesenchymal stem cells in patients with acute myocardial infarction (ClinicalTrials.gov Identifier: NCT00721045; see Table 33-1), based on the encouraging results of a small pilot trial that demonstrated safety after intravenous injection.[32] Whether the promise of augmented cardiac myogenesis suggested by experimental studies will translate into enhanced contractile function in HF is unknown.

Another challenging area of stem cell biology relates to the potential inability of autologous stem cells to migrate and to survive within an ischemic milieu in their naive and unmanipulated state. Cell enhancement strategies to improve patient-derived cells by pretreatment with small molecules or genetic modification may contribute to an augmented recruitment as well as enhance differentiation or other beneficial functions of stem cells. Thus far, several potential primary strategies have been used, including PPAR-γ modulators, endothelial nitric oxide synthase enhancers, integrin activators, and statins, to improve homing, engraftment, and other stem cell functions.[66] The ENACT-AMI trial (Enhanced Angiogenic Cell Therapy–Acute Myocardial Infarction; ClinicalTrials.gov Identifier: NCT00936819) is examining the effects of endothelial progenitor cells in patients with large myocardial infarctions. Circulating mononuclear cells are obtained by apheresis and subjected to differential culture for 3 days to select a population of highly regenerative, endothelial-like, culture-modified mononuclear cells (referred to as early progenitor cells), including one group of culture-modified mononuclear cells that have been transfected with human endothelial nitric oxide synthase.

FUTURE PERSPECTIVES IN MYOCARDIAL REPAIR AND REGENERATION. Thus far, cell transplantation has been performed days, months, or years after myocardial infarction. In acute myocardial infarction, the established safety and proof-of-concept studies provide a cogent rationale for larger, randomized trials addressing the question of whether cellular therapy aimed at cardiac repair not only improves pump function but also reduces mortality and morbidity. Moreover, several open questions are likely to be answered in the future: What is the optimal time of delivery after acute myocardial infarction? Is there a dose-response relationship? How do different cell types compare? One of the most urgent questions in basic science, to elucidate the mechanism by which stem and progenitor cells achieve a functional improvement, is difficult to test in the clinical scenario. Although clinicians can measure flow reserve and heart function, the underlying detailed mechanism cannot be determined with an ethically applicable technology in the near future. In chronic ischemic HF, a superimposed question is whether identification of hibernating myocardium to direct cell therapy is essential to an effective outcome. For established scar tissue late in the disease, specific strategies might be needed. The treatment of nonischemic heart disease is not yet addressed in controlled trials, but initial pilot studies have been performed with moderate effects on improved contractile function. An overview of currently ongoing clinical trials of progenitor cell application for cardiac regeneration is depicted in Table 33-1.

Clearly, the use of stem and progenitor cells for cardiac repair is currently not at a stage for routine clinical practice. Despite a wealth of experimental and clinical data suggesting feasibility, safety, and even early clinical efficacy in patients with acute myocardial infarction, progression to widespread clinical application of progenitor cell administration to promote functional cardiac regeneration must be balanced against the inherent risk of testing a novel therapy. As such, attempts of regenerative therapeutic interventions in patients with significant cardiac dysfunction should proceed in controlled trials with the utmost rigorous scientific and ethical standards, paralleled by further extensive in vitro and animal studies. Such a strategy not only will maximize patient safety, which is of paramount interest, but also will generate reciprocal insights into mechanisms and potential shortcomings of cell-based therapies aimed at functional cardiac regeneration. Specific attention should be given to the processing of the cells and to ascertainment of their functionality for regenerative purposes before initiation of their clinical application. The promise of functional cardiac regeneration by cell-based therapies offers novel opportunities to address the large, unmet clinical need of treating patients with severe cardiac dysfunction.

Gene Therapy

Gene therapy represents another emerging approach to the treatment of HF. Improvements in gene transfer vectors and gene transfer methodology have enabled recombinant genes to be expressed at robust levels in cardiac myocytes.[67] Furthermore, recent advances in the field of RNA interference (RNAi) suggest that it may also be possible to use gene therapy to "silence" key pathogenetic genes or pathways that are activated in the failing heart.[68,69]

Three elements are necessary for the successful clinical application of any gene therapeutic approach.[70] First, a vector or packaging system is necessary to deliver the genetic material. Although naked DNA can be taken up into muscle cells, this method is not very efficient. Coupling of the naked DNA to various compounds, such as liposomes, poloaxime nanospheres, gelatin, or cholesterol lipopolymers, has improved transfection efficiency but has not resulted in sufficiently high levels of expression for clinical use. Viruses are designed to circumvent many of the problems that contribute to the low efficiency of plasmid DNA expression (**Fig. 33-5A, B**). Only a few of the currently available viral vectors are able to achieve efficient, high-level transgene expression in postmitotic cells such as cardiac myocytes (Fig. 33-5C). These include recombinant adenoviruses, adeno-associated viruses, and possibly retroviruses and lentiviruses. Recombinant adenoviruses have been used most commonly because of their ability to "package" large DNA constructs as well as their ability to transduce nonreplicating cells. However, the robust immune response that these vectors evoke suggests that clinical applications will likely require other vectors or further refined adenoviral systems. Newer generations of adenoviral vectors that are devoid of more of the immunogenic vital epitopes (so-called gutted adenoviral vectors) may obviate this problem. Second, the vector needs to be adequately delivered to the affected tissues. The ideal model of gene delivery would be a vector that could be administered intravenously and that would be taken up efficiently in the heart. Although several of the adeno-associated viruses have tropism for cardiac muscle, this goal may not be achievable because of the large blood volume in humans. The feasibility of in vivo cardiac gene transfer by viral vectors has been consistently demonstrated in experimental studies. As illustrated in **Figure 33-6**, a number of mechanical approaches have been used to achieve cardiac gene transfer. Intracoronary catheter delivery of an adenovirus encoding the reporter gene beta-galactosidase achieved transduction of approximately 30% of the cardiac myocytes in the distribution of the injected coronary artery. Direct injection of adenovirus into the ventricular wall by an epicardial approach has also been shown to induce significant expression of reporter constructs; however, the expression was focal, and the needle injections within the heart resulted in myocardial damage. Intramyocardial delivery of adenovirus by an intraventricular approach with retroinfusion of coronary veins has also been used in larger animals, yielding regional areas of transduction. Injection of an adenovirus carrying beta-galactosidase into the pericardial sac transduced only the pericardial cell layers.[70] The third element that is necessary for a successful gene therapeutic approach is to identify the appropriate gene targets to be modulated. **Table 33-2** summarizes potential targets for gene therapy in HF based on experimental studies. The major promising targets for gene transfer have been those genes that regulate the beta-adrenergic receptor signaling pathway and genes that regulate calcium handling in the heart.[69]

As noted in Chap. 24, the beta-adrenergic receptor signaling pathway is critical for modulation of myocardial contractility. Studies have shown that alterations in the myocardial beta-adrenergic receptor both precede and accompany the development of HF in humans, including downregulation of the beta-adrenergic receptor, functional uncoupling of beta-adrenergic receptors from second-messenger systems, and increased levels of inhibitory G proteins that blunt beta-adrenergic receptor signaling (see Chap. 25).[71] Indeed, transgenic mice with cardiac-restricted overexpression of the beta$_2$-adrenergic receptor have enhanced myocardial contractility.[72] However, as noted in Chap. 25, excessive or sustained stimulation of the beta-adrenergic receptor signaling can also lead to activation of maladaptive signaling pathways in the heart (e.g., activation of the fetal gene program) as well as myocyte death through both necrosis and apoptosis. For example, transgenic mice that overexpress the beta$_1$-adrenergic receptor develop a dilated cardiomyopathy.[73] Viewed together, these types of experimental studies have generated considerable interest in use of selective genetic approaches to modulate beta-adrenergic receptor signaling pathways in HF models. Thus far, adenovirus-mediated gene transfer of the human beta$_2$-adrenergic receptor resulted in an improvement in contractility in myocytes isolated from a rabbit model of HF[70] and in myocytes from failing hearts.[69] Similarly, adenovirus-mediated gene transfer of a peptide inhibitor of beta-adrenergic receptor kinase (see Chaps. 24 and 25) resulted in restoration of beta-adrenergic receptor signaling, increased cAMP, and reversal of ventricular dysfunction in rabbit HF models.[70]

Enhancement of myocardial contractility through manipulation of intracellular calcium signaling has garnered considerable enthusiasm as a potential target for gene therapy in HF. Several studies suggest that functional suppression of sarcoplasmic reticulum Ca^{2+}-ATPase (SERCA2a) activity, or an absolute reduction in the amount of SERCA2a protein, may contribute significantly to the abnormalities in Ca^{2+} handling and myocardial contraction observed in failing hearts (see Chap. 25). In an animal model of pressure-overload hypertrophy that transitions to failure, overexpression of SERCA2a by gene transfer in vivo restored both systolic and diastolic function to normal levels.[74] Similarly, overexpression of SERCA2a through gene targeting resulted in normalization of LV volumes, improved energetics, and prolonged survival in an experimental model of pressure-overload hypertrophy.[75] Overexpression of an antisense phospholamban construct or a dominant-negative mutant of phospholamban (see Chap. 24) has recently been shown to enhance SERCA2a activity, consistent with the prior observation that genetic ablation of phospholamban prevents the functional abnormalities otherwise seen in a mouse model of dilated cardiomyopathy.[70] Similar beneficial effects on cardiac contractility, including normalized calcium handling and enhanced SERCA2a activity, have been observed in experimental and human HF models after gene transfer of S100A1 (a calcium-binding protein).[76] A clinical gene therapy trial using adeno-associated virus–mediated gene transfer of SERCA2a (AAV1/SERCA2a), the CUPID trial (Efficacy and Safety Study of Genetically Targeted Enzyme Replacement Therapy for Advanced Heart Failure), has been initiated in patients with ischemic or nonischemic New York Heart Association (NYHA) Class II-IV HF (ClinicalTrials.gov Identifier: NCT00454818). The primary outcome variable was patient safety as measured by the incidence and severity of adverse events, all-cause mortality, progression of HF leading to hospitalization, and intravenous inotrope, vasodilator, or diuretic administration; the secondary outcome variables are changes from baseline to 3, 6, 9, and 12 months in $\dot{V}O_2$ max, 6-minute walk test, echocardiographic assessments, NT-proBNP level, NYHA classification, and quality of life assessed by Minnesota Living with Heart Failure questionnaire. The results of the CUPID trial have been presented in preliminary form, and suggest that gene therapy appeared to improve symptoms, functional status, and ventricular volumes in patients with severe systolic heart failure, supporting the rationale for larger clinical trials.

In addition to modulating myocardial contractility, gene therapeutic approaches may also be used to target myocyte viability or pluripotential stem cells within the myocardium (see Chap. 11). Morphologic and biologic markers of programmed cell death or apoptosis have been identified in human HF, suggesting that these pathways may contribute to cardiomyocyte loss and cardiac dysfunction in HF (see Chap. 25). The potential to block cardiomyocyte apoptosis through somatic gene transfer is therefore another area of ongoing investigation.[77] Also, the ability to use gene therapeutic approaches to reprogram fibroblasts into pluripotential stem cells that have a potential to differentiate into cardiac myocytes is being explored.[78]

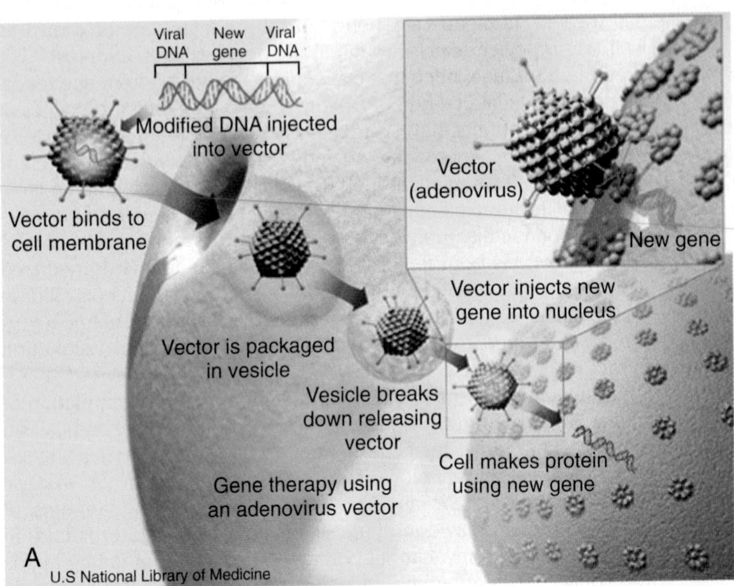

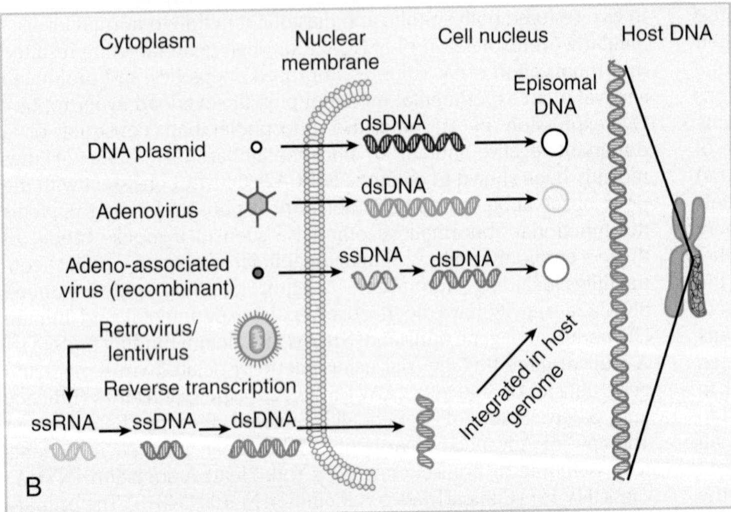

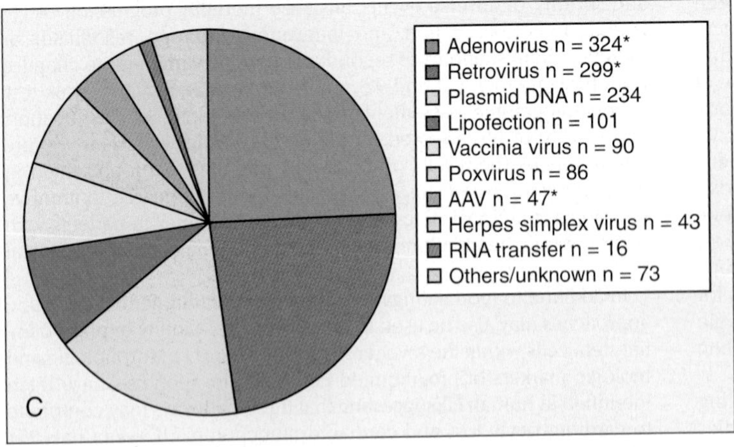

FIGURE 33-5 Viral gene therapy. **A,** Viral gene therapy vector entry into the mammalian cell. Viral vectors bind to cell surface receptors, initiating endocytosis by the clathrin-dependent process. Once they are internalized, the viral particles avoid degradation through the lysosomal pathway and direct endosome trafficking to the cell nucleus. Adenoviruses and adeno-associated viruses are released from the endosome in the perinuclear region, and the viral particles "dock" on the nuclear envelope membrane pores. The viral particle capsid coat dissociates, and the genome is delivered into the cell nucleus. Retroviral and lentiviral vectors require further processing in the cytoplasm, including reverse transcription, before arrival in the nucleus. *(Created by the U.S. National Library of Medicine.)* **B,** A comparison of the nucleic acid processing steps required by gene therapy vectors for successful expression of their therapeutic gene. Plasmid DNA (black) is delivered as double-stranded DNA. The delivery of the naked DNA macromolecule to the nuclear envelope and import into the nucleus are extremely inefficient. Adenoviral vectors deliver to the nucleus double-stranded DNA (light blue), which remains separate from the host genome as an episomal ring of DNA. Gene expression can commence rapidly. Recombinant adeno-associated viral vectors (rAAV) deliver single-stranded DNA (red), which must be converted to double-stranded DNA (pink) before gene expression can commence. The rAAV genome also remains episomal. Retroviral and lentiviral vectors contain single-stranded RNA (yellow). This must be converted to single-stranded DNA (red) by reverse transcription in the cell cytoplasm. The single-stranded DNA is then converted to double-stranded DNA (green) before import into the cell nucleus. For gene expression to occur, the retroviral and lentiviral dsDNA must integrate into the host genome (dark blue), creating the possibility of insertional mutagenesis. dsDNA = double-stranded deoxyribonucleic acid; ssDNA = single-stranded deoxyribonucleic acid; ssRNA = single-stranded ribonucleic acid. **C,** Vectors used in clinical gene therapy trials registered with the international gene therapy clinical trial registry up to January 2007. *Candidate vectors for myocardial gene therapy.

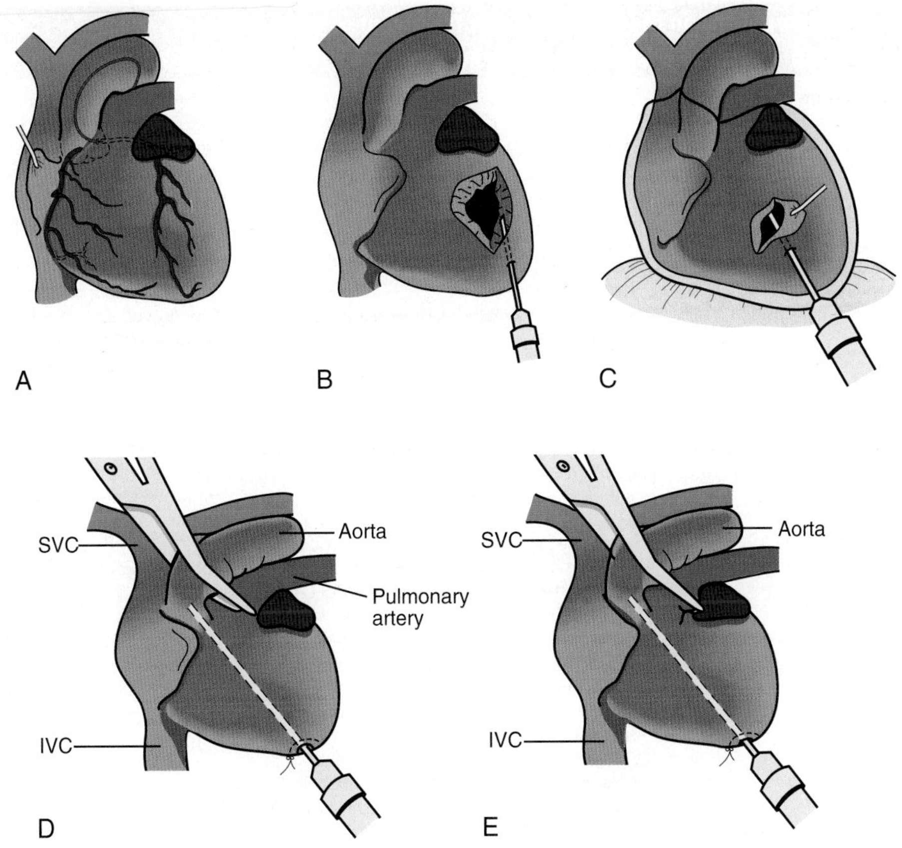

FIGURE 33-6 Different techniques for in vivo cardiac gene transfer. **A,** Coronary perfusion. **B,** Intramyocardial injection. **C,** Pericardial injection. **D,** Aortic clamping. **E,** Cross-clamping of the aorta and pulmonary artery. IVC = inferior vena cava; SVC = superior vena cava. *(Modified from Hajjar RJ, del Monte F, Matsui T, Rosenzweig A: Prospects for gene therapy for heart failure. Circ Res 86:616, 2000.)*

TABLE 33-2 Potential Therapeutic Targets for Gene Therapy in Heart Failure

TARGET	FUNCTION
Beta-adrenergic receptor kinase inhibitor (βARKct)	Inhibits phosphorylation of β-adrenergic receptor, thus preventing its desensitization
Adenylyl cyclase	Synthesizes cAMP to activate PKA, which then phosphorylates substrates to regulate calcium handling
Sarcoplasmic reticulum Ca^{2+}-ATPase (SERCA2)	Responsible for the reuptake of calcium from cytoplasm into the SR lumen Critical determinant of both relaxation and contractility through calcium sequestration into SR and by control of SR calcium loading, respectively
Phospholamban	Inhibits SERCA2, inactivated by phosphorylation by PKA and CaMKII
Parvalbumin	Rapidly removes calcium in myofilaments, naturally abundant in skeletal muscle (not cardiac), results in enhanced relaxation
S100 protein	A calcium-binding protein, a positive inotropic regulator of cardiac function that enhances calcium cycling and cardiac contractile performance in vitro and in vivo

SR = sarcoplasmic reticulum; PKA = protein kinase A; CaMKII = Ca^{2+}/calmodulin-dependent protein kinase.
Modified from Nayak L, Rosengart TK: Gene therapy for heart failure. Semin Thorac Cardiovasc Surg 17:343, 2005.

FUTURE PERSPECTIVES IN GENE THERAPY. In summary, gene transfer strategies that result in improvements in myocardial contractility or cardiac remodeling appear promising in experimental models of HF. However, considerable work remains to be done with respect to improvements in vector technology, methods for cardiac gene delivery, and perhaps most important, understanding what gene targets are safe to target in clinical trials in HF patients.

Pharmacologic Strategies

Pharmacogenetics

As discussed in Chap. 10, the field of pharmacogenetics attempts to define common gene polymorphisms, or sets of polymorphisms, that underlie variability in drug action. Given the tremendous heterogeneity that exists in HF patients, it is likely that genetic variations play a significant role in determining drug metabolism, disposition, and functional activity in HF patients. As noted, current HF practice guidelines (see Chap. 28 Guidelines) recommend titration of ACE inhibitors, angiotensin receptor blockers, aldosterone antagonists, and beta blockers to doses that have been shown to be beneficial in clinical trials (**Table 33-3**). Although this approach tends to work well for most patients, it has two major shortcomings. The most obvious is that basing of drug dosing on the doses selected in clinical trials does not allow dose optimization in patients in whom the drug may be metabolized or distributed differently. The second problem is that clinical trials are generally designed to yield "binary" results. That is, a drug under investigation is either deemed beneficial or not beneficial because the patients in the treatment arm have or have not reached a prespecified endpoint (e.g., death or hospitalization). A beneficial effect in a positive clinical trial implies that all patients will receive the same degree of benefit from the drug that is given. However, a more likely outcome is that a given therapy will have a markedly

CH 33

TABLE 33-3 Effect of Gene Polymorphisms on the Pharmacologic Treatment of Heart Failure

PATHWAY/GENE	POLYMORPHISM	FUNCTIONAL IMPACT	IMPACT ON PHARMACOLOGIC THERAPY
Renin-Angiotensin-Aldosterone System			
ACE	287-bp insertion (I) or deletion (D) in intron 16	DD genotype has increased ACE activity and worse clinical outcomes in some but not all studies	Use of beta-blockers and ACE inhibitors attenuates adverse outcomes of DD genotype but has no effect on II and ID genotypes; II or ID genotype predicts reverse LV remodeling in response to spironolactone
Angiotensinogen	Methionine (Met) to threonine (Thr) switch at amino acid 235	Increased angiotensinogen levels with hypertension	Modest risk of hypertension in whites; effect on drug responsiveness in HF not known
Aldosterone synthase	C to T transition at position −344 (T/C)	−344C allele associated with higher aldosterone levels	TT genotype associated with greater impact of fixed combination of isosorbide dinitrate and hydralazine on the event-free survival in A-HeFT
Adrenergic Nervous System			
beta$_1$-AR	Arginine (Arg) to glycine (Gly) switch at amino acid 389	Arg389 polymorphism has increased 3× greater adenylyl cyclase activity in response to agonist than Gly389 variant	Arg389Arg genotype greatest improvement in ejection fraction with beta blockers and improved mortality with bucindolol treatment in BEST
beta$_1$-AR	Serine (Ser) to glycine (Gly) switch at amino acid 49	In vitro, the Gly49 variant shows decreased receptor expression compared with Ser49 variant after exposure to isoproterenol (24 hours)	Ser49Ser genotype requires higher doses of beta blocker to achieve a mortality benefit
beta$_2$-AR	Threonine (Thr) to isoleucine (Ile) switch at amino acid 164	Ile164 beta$_2$-AR has decreased affinity for catecholamine binding, decreased basal and epinephrine-stimulated adenylyl cyclase activity, and impaired agonist-promoted sequestration Ile164 transgenic mice display depressed resting and agonist-stimulated contractile function in vivo compared with Thr164 mice	Associated with decreased $\dot{V}O_2$max and worse HF outcomes Effect on drug responsiveness in HF not known
GRK5	Glutamine (Gln) to leucine (Leu) switch at amino acid 41	GRK5-Leu41 uncouples isoproterenol-stimulated responses >GRK5-Gln41 in transfected cells and transgenic mice and protects against experimental catecholamine-induced cardiomyopathy	GRK5-Leu41 is associated with decreased mortality in African Americans with heart failure or cardiac ischemia
alpha$_{2C}$-AR	alpha$_{2C}$Del322-325	Decreased NE uptake	Increased likelihood for development of HF in patients with the beta$_1$-AR Arg389 polymorphism Effect on drug responsiveness in HF not known

ACE = angiotensin converting enzyme; AR = adrenergic receptor; GRK = G-coupled receptor kinase; HF = heart failure; NE = norepinephrine.

positive impact for some patients, may have a more modest effect in others, and may be completely ineffective or perhaps even harmful in a smaller group of treated patients. Thus, even though a drug is deemed beneficial in a clinical trial, there is no guarantee that an individual patient will benefit from the treatment. For example, beta blockers have been shown consistently to reduce the risk of death in HF patients by approximately 35% (see Fig. 28-17); however, clinical trials have also shown that beta blockers will need to be discontinued in 8% to 25% of HF patients because of significant adverse effects, including worsening HF.[79] Recent advances in the field of pharmacogenetics suggest that a careful analysis of underlying gene polymorphisms within a given patient may enable clinicians to develop personalized therapeutic regimens for HF patients. Given the central role of the renin-angiotensin-aldosterone (RAS) and adrenergic systems in the pathophysiology (see Chap. 25) and treatment of HF (see Chap. 28), it is perhaps not surprising that polymorphisms in the genes that regulate these pathways appear to influence the therapeutic efficacy of ACE inhibitors and beta blockers. Table 33-3 provides an overview of the major genetic variations in these pathways, the proposed functional impact of these polymorphisms, and how these genetic polymorphisms influence traditional pharmacotherapeutic approaches in HF.

One of the most widely studied genetic variants is the ACE insertion/deletion polymorphism (I/D) that involves a 287–base pair insertion or deletion within intron 16 of the ACE gene. Although the clinical significance of this polymorphism remains controversial, the physiologic association with ACE enzymatic activity has consistently been demonstrated. Studies have shown that individuals with the DD genotype have the highest ACE activity and angiotensin II levels, heterozygotes (ID) have intermediate levels, and individuals who are homozygous for the I allele (II) have the lowest levels of ACE activity. The relationship of ACE I/D has been explored with respect to numerous conditions including atherosclerosis, myocardial infarction, LV hypertrophy, hypertrophic cardiomyopathy, and HF. Although, the current weight of evidence does not allow definitive conclusions to be made with respect to the overall contribution of the ACE I/D polymorphism to the clinical outcome in these conditions, there is growing evidence that the ACE I/D polymorphism may predict drug responsiveness to both beta blockers and ACE inhibitors in HF patients. In one study of patients with chronic HF, the ACE DD polymorphism was significantly associated with death or the need for transplantation compared with patients with II or ID genotypes. Within the ACE DD group, patients treated with beta blockers had significantly improved transplant-free survival compared with patients not receiving beta blocker therapy, whereas beta blocker treatment had no effect on clinical outcomes in the II or ID groups.[80] In a similar study, patients with the DD genotype had better clinical outcomes when receiving high-dose ACE inhibitor therapy compared with low-dose ACE inhibitor therapy, whereas the ACE dose had no effect on clinical outcomes in patients with either the II or ID genotype. In this study, the regimen of high-dose ACE inhibitors and beta blockers had the greatest impact on transplant-free survival in patients with the DD variant.[80] Taken together, these studies suggest a differential clinical response to standard HF therapy based on the ACE I/D polymorphism.

Whereas the impact of genetic heterogeneity on HF outcomes has been extensively studied in predominantly white cohorts, few studies have investigated the impact of genomic variation in blacks. In a genetic substudy of the African-American Heart Failure Trial (A-HeFT; see Chap. 28), a single nucleotide polymorphism within the promoter region of the aldosterone synthase gene (C to T transition at position −344) was shown to predict responsiveness to the fixed combination of hydralazine isosorbide dinitrate.[81] In A-HeFT, treatment with the fixed combination of hydralazine isosorbide dinitrate was associated with a markedly improved clinical outcome (mortality, HF hospitalization, and change in quality of life at 6 months) in the TT homozygotes but had no significant impact among subjects with the −344C allele, suggesting that genetic variations in aldosterone production may play an important role in disease progression in blacks with HF.

Polymorphisms that affect the function of beta- or alpha-adrenergic receptors may also influence the pharmacologic response in HF patients (see Table 33-3). Patients with a common polymorphism of the $beta_1$-adrenergic receptor that results in either an arginine (Arg) or glycine (Gly) substitution at amino acid position 389 have different clinical responses to beta blockers. In the Bucindolol Evaluation of Survival Trial (BEST), bucindolol-treated patients who were homozygous for the Arg389 polymorphism (Arg389Arg) had improved clinical outcomes compared with "glycine carriers" (Arg389Gly and Gly389Gly) who were treated with bucindolol (**Fig. 33-7**), suggesting that the therapeutic response to beta blockers differs by genotype.[82] The Arg389Arg genotype was also associated with significantly greater reductions in LV end-diastolic and end-systolic diameters after treatment with beta blockers compared with identically treated Gly389 carriers.[83] The $alpha_{2C}$-adrenergic receptor inhibits norepinephrine release at cardiac presynaptic nerve endings through a negative feedback mechanism. The deletion of four consecutive amino acids (322 to 325) in the $alpha_{2C}$-adrenergic receptor results in loss of the normal synaptic autoinhibitory feedback mechanism and hence enhanced presynaptic release of norepinephrine. There appears to be an increased risk for development of HF (see Fig. 33-e3 on website) when the $alpha_{2C}$Del322-325 and the Arg389 $beta_1$-adrenergic receptor polymorphisms are both present (i.e., a diplotype).[84] Although the impact of the $alpha_{2C}$Del322-325 and Arg389 $beta_1$-adrenergic receptor synergism on beta blocker responsiveness is not known, it is likely that patients with this diplotype may have increased responsiveness to beta blockers, based on what has been reported thus far for the Arg389 polymorphism. A nonsynonymous polymorphism in which leucine (Leu) is substituted for glutamine (Gln) at amino acid position 41 of G protein receptor kinase 5 (GRK5-Leu41), which desensitizes beta-adrenergic receptor signaling, was recently shown to uncouple beta-adrenergic receptor signaling more effectively than did the GRK5 polymorphism. Human association studies showed a pharmacogenomic interaction between GRK5-Leu41 and beta blocker treatment, in which the presence of the GRK5-Leu41 polymorphism was associated with decreased mortality in African Americans (in whom this polymorphism is more prevalent) with HF or cardiac ischemia. Subsequent studies showed that among patients not taking beta blockers, GRK5-Leu41 was associated with improved survival in African Americans, suggesting that GRK5-Leu41 provides a "genetic beta blockade" that improves survival in African Americans with HF.[85] In addition to contributing to the functional response to beta blockers, genetic polymorphisms that affect drug metabolism may also influence the therapeutic response to beta blockers. For example, genetic variants in the cytochrome P-450 (CYP) 2D6 gene have a marked effect on plasma concentrations of metoprolol and carvedilol. In subjects with a nonfunctional CYP2D6 enzyme (poor metabolizers), the peak plasma concentration of metoprolol is sixfold higher than in subjects with a normally functioning enzyme.[79]

FUTURE PERSPECTIVES IN PHARMACOGENETICS. Although previous studies have explored the role of single-gene polymorphisms with the renin-angiotensin-aldosterone and adrenergic systems in HF patients, it is likely that future investigations will explore the functional role of multiple genetic variations within a given pathway (i.e., polygenic phenotypes). Given the wealth of data emerging from the Human Genome Project and Human Haplotype Mapping Program (HapMap), it will soon be possible to analyze complex phenotypes in relation to drug responsiveness in individual HF patients to better predict outcomes. This statement notwithstanding, the concept of personalizing therapeutic approaches in HF based on genetic background is far from fully developed and will need to be carefully evaluated prospectively in suitable populations of patients before this type of information can be used to guide clinical practice.

Metabolic Modulation

Optimization of myocardial energy use represents another unique approach for the treatment of HF. As will be discussed, there are a

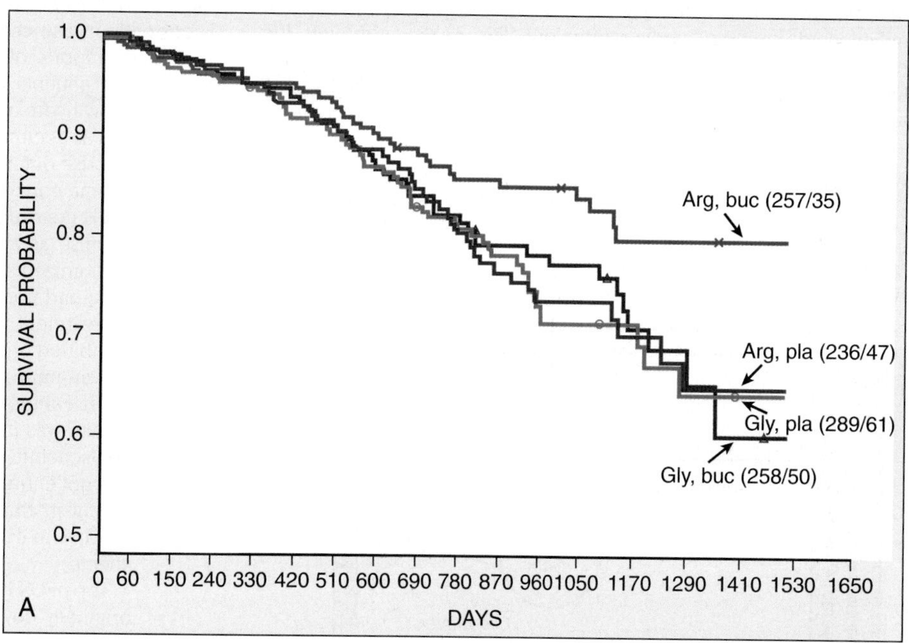

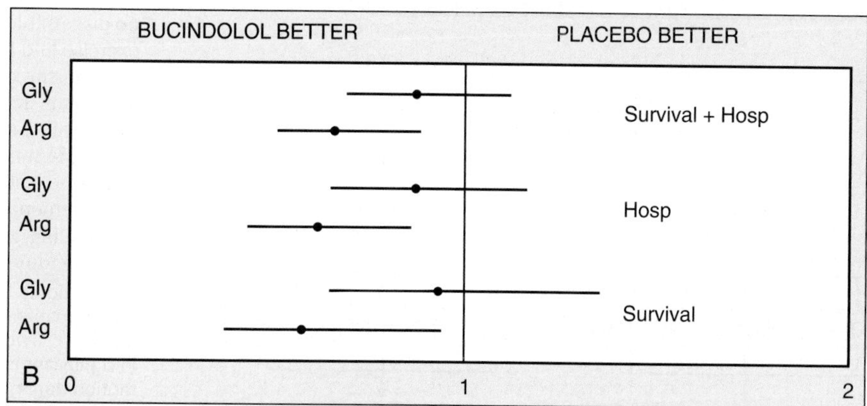

FIGURE 33-7 Kaplan-Meier analysis of endpoints in the Bucindolol Evaluation of Survival Trial (BEST) stratified by treatment (placebo or bucindolol) and $beta_1$-adrenergic receptor genotype. **A,** For survival, Arg homozygotes had an HR = 0.62, 95% CI = 0.40-0.96, $P = 0.03$. In contrast, for $beta_1$-Gly-389 carriers, the HR = 0.90, 95% CI = 0.62-1.30, $P = 0.57$. **B,** Graphic representation of hazard ratios and confidence intervals by bucindolol and placebo. Hosp = hospitalization. *(From Liggett SB, Mialet-Perez J, Thaneemit-Chen S, et al: A polymorphism within a conserved $beta_1$-adrenergic receptor motif alters cardiac function and beta-blocker response in human heart failure. Proc Natl Acad Sci U S A 103:11288, 2006.)*

number of derangements in myocardial metabolism that may explain partially the decrease in high-energy phosphates and phosphocreatine that have been reported in the failing heart (see Chap. 25). In the normal heart, free fatty acids are the preferred fuel, producing roughly four times the ATP per mole of substrate used compared with glucose. However, fatty acid oxidation is less efficient than glucose oxidation, requiring 10% to 12% more oxygen consumption to produce equivalent amounts of ATP. Under conditions wherein oxygen is the limiting substrate, such as occurs in the failing heart (see Chap. 25), glycolysis becomes the more efficient pathway, requiring less oxygen compared with oxidation of free fatty acids. Fatty acid oxidation is physiologically regulated at several levels, including the concentration of circulating free fatty acid substrate, at the level of entry into the mitochondrion, and by the activity of several of the mitochondrial matrix enzymes that compose the beta-oxidation pathway.[86] On the other hand, the rate of glucose oxidation is regulated primarily, although not exclusively, by the rate of fatty acid oxidation, which inhibits the pyruvate dehydrogenase complex, the activity of which is rate limiting for glucose oxidation (**Fig. 33-8A**). Inhibition of pyruvate dehydrogenase can lead to increased glucose use through conversion of pyruvate to lactate, resulting in progressive tissue acidosis and impaired myocyte contractility (Fig. 33-8A). From a theoretical perspective, shifting of energy use from free fatty acids to glucose would optimize metabolic efficiency, reverse abnormalities in the cellular milieu, and improve cardiac function (Fig. 33-8B). Although the results of the studies on substrate use in HF have often yielded conflicting results, the aggregate data support the concept that rates of fatty acid oxidation are normal or slightly increased in pathologic hypertrophy early in HF, whereas fatty acid oxidation is decreased during the latter stages of HF, accompanied by an absolute or relative increase in glucose use during late stages of HF.[87]

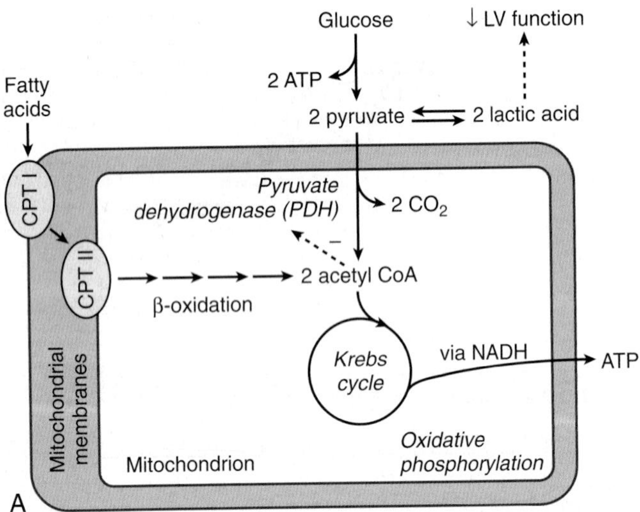

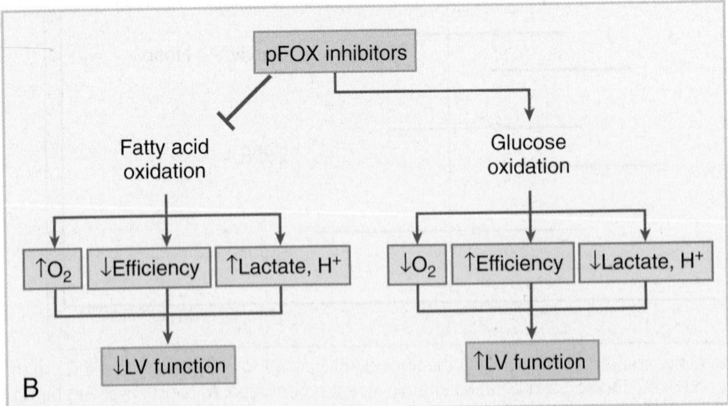

FIGURE 33-8 Metabolism of free fatty acids and glucose. **A,** Metabolic pathway for glucose metabolism and fatty acid oxidation. **B,** Effects of switching metabolism from fatty acid beta-oxidation to glucose oxidation (under conditions wherein oxygen supply is rate limiting) using partial inhibitors of fatty acid oxidation (pFOX).

The prototype partial inhibitors of fatty acid oxidation (pFOX), etomoxir, oxfenicine, and perhexiline, act by inhibiting carnitine palmitoyltransferase I (CPT I), the gatekeeper of fatty acid entry to the mitochondrion (Fig. 33-8A). These agents shift energy use from free fatty acids to glucose by decreasing oxidation of free fatty acids. However, because there is no apparent feedback from CPT I activity to sarcolemmal fatty acid import, CPT I inhibitors can lead to accumulation of unmetabolized lipids in cardiac myocytes, which may lead to lipotoxicity-induced cardiac myocyte cell death. Etomoxir is an oxirane carboxylic acid derivative that indirectly promotes increased glucose oxidation through inhibition of CPT I. In an open-label, uncontrolled trial conducted in 10 patients with NYHA Class II-III HF, treatment with etomoxir for 3 months was associated with a significant improvement in LVEF, cardiac output at peak exercise, and clinical status.[88] Subsequent phase II studies with etomoxir were halted because the compound did have the expected efficacy in the treatment of HF (data obtained from MediGene 2002 Annual Report [March 26, 2003]). Although oxfenicine was shown to be beneficial in the canine rapid pacing model of HF, treatment with oxfenicine in other animal models resulted in a dose-related increase in cardiac mass as well as an increase in liver and kidney weights. Perhexiline is currently in use clinically as an antianginal agent. Although there were early reports of hepatotoxicity with this agent, hepatotoxicity occurred in patients with a genetic variant of a cytochrome P-450 enzyme (slow hydroxylation), which resulted in drug accumulation as well as accumulation of phospholipids in the liver and nerves. The risk of toxic effects is virtually eliminated by maintaining plasma concentrations between 150 and 600 ng/mL, at which levels the drug still remains effective.[88] Perhexiline has shown promise as adjunctive therapy for HF in a small short-term randomized double-blind clinical trial in patients with ischemic and nonischemic cardiomyopathy. In this study, 8 weeks of treatment with perhexiline resulted in an increase in the combined primary endpoint of peak oxygen uptake and LVEF and an improvement in quality of life (Minnesota Living with Heart Failure questionnaire). Importantly, maximum oxygen uptake was increased significantly in both the ischemic and nonischemic groups, suggesting that the benefit of perhexiline was not entirely anti-ischemic.[89] Although there remains some optimism that CPT I inhibitors can be used as adjunctive therapy in HF, other pFOX inhibitors may have fewer side effects.

The pFOX inhibitors trimetazidine and ranolazine were also originally developed as antianginal agents. Trimetazidine is a piperazine compound that has been widely used outside of the United States as an antianginal agent. Trimetazidine has no discernible vasodilator properties at rest or during dynamic exercise and has a very favorable side effect profile. The exact mechanism of action of trimetazidine is not known, but it appears to work, at least in part, through inhibition of long-chain 3-ketoacyl coenzyme A thiolase, a crucial enzyme in the terminal steps of mitochondrial beta-oxidation. As discussed later, several small clinical trials have shown improvements in ejection performance, reverse cardiac remodeling, and improvement in NYHA functional class with trimetazadine.[88]

Trimetazidine has been evaluated in a number of small clinical trials in patients with both ischemic and nonischemic cardiomyopathy.[86,88] Two months of treatment with trimetazidine resulted in significant improvement in LVEF at rest and enhanced LV wall motion during a dobutamine stress test compared with placebo in NYHA Class II and III HF patients.[86] In two small clinical studies, trimetazidine was shown to improve systolic LV function in patients with diabetes and ischemic cardiomyopathy compared with placebo.[86,90] In contrast, another study that assessed the effects of trimetazidine in patients with HF who were diabetic demonstrated no significant effect on exercise capacity and only minor effects on LV systolic function.[88] In a study that specifically enrolled elderly patients with coronary artery disease and LVEF <50%, the group that received 6 months of trimetazidine on top of standard therapy showed a significantly greater improvement in LVEF (~7%) as well as smaller LV end-diastolic and systolic dimensions. In addition, the trimetazidine group had improved NYHA functional class and quality of life scores (Minnesota Living with Heart Failure questionnaire). These findings have been confirmed in recent larger trials with longer follow-up (18 to 24 months), which have also shown improvements in LVEF, reduction in LV volumes, and improvement in NYHA functional class in patients with ischemic cardiomyopathy (LVEF <50%).[88] Given the antianginal effects of trimetazidine, it is perhaps not surprising that this agent led to improvements in LV function and NYHA functional class in patients with ischemic cardiomyopathy. However, a study with trimetazidine also included patients with nonischemic cardiomyopathy and showed similar increases in LVEF, reductions in LV end-systolic volume, and similar trends for improved quality of life and exercise capacity in both the ischemic and nonischemic groups.[91] Thus, it appears that trimetazidine has both functional and physiologic benefits regardless of the HF etiology.

Ranolazine (Ranexa) is a novel anti-ischemic drug that prolongs the QT interval and is the first pFOX inhibitor approved by the Food and Drug Administration for the treatment of angina. The principal mechanism of action for this drug as an antianginal remains controversial, although studies suggest that the antianginal effects of ranolazine may be related to decreased sodium entry into cells by inhibition of the rapid component of the delayed rectifier K^+ current, I_{Kr} (see Chap. 35). Ranolazine also increases the activity of pyruvate decarboxylase, a key regulator of glucose metabolism, most likely because of loss of inhibition of the end products of the beta-oxidation (NADH, acetyl-CoA). Although no clinical trials have yet been reported with use of ranolazine in patients with dilated cardiomyopathy, there is an ongoing study with ranolazine that is examining the effects of this agent on diastolic filling in NYHA Class I-II patients with moderate to severe diastolic dysfunction (ClinicalTrials.gov Identifier: NCT00574756).

GLUCAGON-LIKE PEPTIDE 1. Sustained activation of the sympathetic nervous system (see Chap. 25) in HF leads to increased lipolysis, with a subsequent rise in levels of circulating fatty acids and a resultant insulin resistance. Although the exact role of insulin resistance in HF is not known, studies with the incretin hormone glucagon-like peptide 1 (GLP-1), which increases postprandial insulin secretion and improves insulin sensitivity, have demonstrated improvements in contractility in both experimental and human HF. In a study of 12 patients with NYHA functional Class III-IV HF, a continuous infusion of GLP-1 for 12 weeks improved LVEF (21% to 27%) and functional capacity, even in nondiabetic patients.[92] Similarly, in a study of 10 patients with acute myocardial infarction and LV systolic dysfunction (LVEF <40%), a 72-hour continuous infusion of GLP-1 was associated with a significant improvement in LVEF as well as global and regional wall motion.[93] In contrast to these early encouraging findings, there was no improvement in cardiac index, LVEF, or brain natriuretic peptide levels in a small study of 20 nondiabetic patients with NYHA Class II-III HF after a 48-hour infusion of GLP-1. Moreover, there was a small but potentially concerning rise in heart rate and diastolic blood pressure in this study.[94] At present, GLP-1 has to be given as an infusion and has a very short half-life, which may limit its clinical applicability. Alternative GLP-1 agonists with longer half-lives or agents that inhibit the catabolism of GLP-1 by dipeptidyl peptidase 4 may need to be developed for this approach to be useful clinically in HF patients.

MICRONUTRIENT SUPPLEMENTATION. The heart requires a continuous supply of energy-providing substrates and amino acids to maintain normal structure and function. In HF, alterations in substrate metabolism, the tricarboxylic acid cycle, or oxidative phosphorylation may contribute to contractile dysfunction (**Fig. 33-9**). For example, deficiencies in coenzyme Q10, L-carnitine, amino acids, thiamine, and other B vitamins have been documented in the failing heart,[95] raising the interesting possibility that micronutrient supplementation might improve the abnormal energetic milieu of the failing heart. Although a number of supplementation trials of key micronutrients involved in cardiac metabolism, such as coenzyme Q10, L-carnitine,

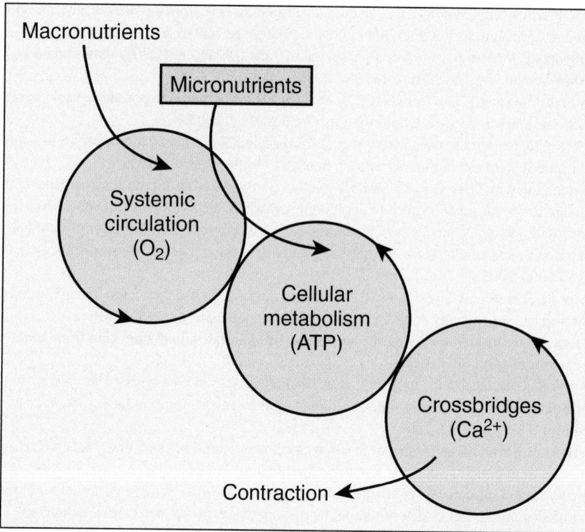

FIGURE 33-9 Cycles of energy transfer and the place of micronutrients. Energy transfer in the heart as a system of interconnected cycles. Micronutrients are essential components of moiety-conserved cycles in the cell. *(Modified from Soukoulis V, Dihu JB, Sole M, et al: Micronutrient deficiencies an unmet need in heart failure. J Am Coll Cardiol 54:1660, 2009.)*

thiamine, and taurine, have yielded promising results in patients with HF, none of these clinical trials has yielded conclusive results (reviewed in reference 95). Because of the absence of definitive clinical trial data in this area, the updated American College of Cardiology/American Heart Association practice guidelines (see Chap. 28 Guidelines) do not recommend the use of nutritional supplements for treatment of HF in patients with current or prior HF symptoms.

FUTURE PERSPECTIVES IN METABOLIC MODULATION. In summary, modulation of substrate metabolism using pFOX inhibitors represents an attractive therapeutic target in patients with HF. Conceptually, another means to impair substrate metabolism would be to directly stimulate glucose uptake or pyruvate oxidation; however, pharmacologic agents are not available to accomplish this. Although the use of pFOX inhibitors and micronutrients appears promising, all of the clinical studies to date are small and have design flaws that are inherent to early-phase clinical trials, not the least of which is a lack of long-term outcomes data. Accordingly, additional studies will be required before this therapy can be used in HF patients.

REFERENCES

Myocardial Regeneration

1. Kehat I, Kenyagin-Karsenti D, Snir M, et al: Human embryonic stem cells can differentiate into myocytes with structural and functional properties of cardiomyocytes. J Clin Invest 108:407, 2001.
2. Dai W, Kloner RA: Myocardial regeneration by embryonic stem cell transplantation: Present and future trends. Expert Rev Cardiovasc Ther 4:375, 2006.
3. Takahashi K, Tanabe K, Ohnuki M, et al: Induction of pluripotent stem cells from adult human fibroblasts by defined factors. Cell 131:861, 2007.
4. Nelson TJ, Martinez-Fernandez A, Yamada S, et al: Repair of acute myocardial infarction by human stemness factors induced pluripotent stem cells. Circulation 120:408, 2009.
5. Urbich C, Dimmeler S: Endothelial progenitor cells: Characterization and role in vascular biology. Circ Res 95:343, 2004.
6. Rafii S, Lyden D: Therapeutic stem and progenitor cell transplantation for organ vascularization and regeneration. Nat Med 9:702, 2003.
7. Grunewald M, Avraham I, Dor Y, et al: VEGF-induced adult neovascularization: Recruitment, retention, and role of accessory cells. Cell 124:175, 2006.
8. Galvez BG, Sampaolesi M, Brunelli S, et al: Complete repair of dystrophic skeletal muscle by mesoangioblasts with enhanced migration ability. J Cell Biol 174:231, 2006.
9. Galli D, Innocenzi A, Staszewsky L, et al: Mesoangioblasts, vessel-associated multipotent stem cells, repair the infarcted heart by multiple cellular mechanisms: A comparison with bone marrow progenitors, fibroblasts, and endothelial cells. Arterioscler Thromb Vasc Biol 25:692, 2005.
10. Koyanagi M, Iwasaki M, Rupp S, et al: Sox2 transduction enhances cardiovascular repair capacity of blood-derived mesoangioblasts. Circ Res 106:1290, 2010.
11. Beltrami AP, Barlucchi L, Torella D, et al: Adult cardiac stem cells are multipotent and support myocardial regeneration. Cell 114:763, 2003.

12. Oh H, Bradfute SB, Gallardo TD, et al: Cardiac progenitor cells from adult myocardium: Homing, differentiation, and fusion after infarction. Proc Natl Acad Sci U S A 100:12313, 2003.
13. Laugwitz KL, Moretti A, Lam J, et al: Postnatal isl1+ cardioblasts enter fully differentiated cardiomyocyte lineages. Nature 433:647, 2005.
14. Pfister O, Mouquet F, Jain M, et al: CD31− but not CD31+ cardiac side population cells exhibit functional cardiomyogenic differentiation. Circ Res 97:52, 2005.
15. Tomita Y, Matsumura K, Wakamatsu Y, et al: Cardiac neural crest cells contribute to the dormant multipotent stem cell in the mammalian heart. J Cell Biol 170:1135, 2005.
16. Fazel S, Cimini M, Chen L, et al: Cardioprotective c-kit+ cells are from the bone marrow and regulate the myocardial balance of angiogenic cytokines. J Clin Invest 116:1865, 2006.
17. Mouquet F, Pfister O, Jain M, et al: Restoration of cardiac progenitor cells after myocardial infarction by self-proliferation and selective homing of bone marrow–derived stem cells. Circ Res 97:1090, 2005.
18. Fraser JK, Schreiber R, Strem B, et al: Plasticity of human adipose stem cells toward endothelial cells and cardiomyocytes. Nat Clin Pract Cardiovasc Med 3(Suppl 1):S33, 2006.
19. Guan K, Nayernia K, Maier LS, et al: Pluripotency of spermatogonial stem cells from adult mouse testis. Nature 440:11993, 2006.
20. Condorelli G, Borello U, De Angelis L, et al: Cardiomyocytes induce endothelial cells to trans-differentiate into cardiac muscle: Implications for myocardium regeneration. Proc Natl Acad Sci U S A 98:10733, 2001.
21. Chavakis E, Koyanagi M, Dimmeler S: Enhancing the outcome of cell therapy for cardiac repair: Progress from bench to bedside and back. Circulation 121:325, 2010.
22. Kawamoto A, Tkebuchava T, Yamaguchi J, et al: Intramyocardial transplantation of autologous endothelial progenitor cells for therapeutic neovascularization of myocardial ischemia. Circulation 107:461, 2003.
23. Urbich C, Aicher A, Heeschen C, et al: Soluble factors released by endothelial progenitor cells promote migration of endothelial cells and cardiac resident progenitor cells. J Mol Cell Cardiol 39:733, 2005.
24. Gnecchi M, He H, Liang OD, et al: Paracrine action accounts for marked protection of ischemic heart by Akt-modified mesenchymal stem cells. Nat Med 11:367, 2005.
25. Yoon CH, Koyanagi M, Iekushi K, et al: Mechanism of improved cardiac function after bone marrow mononuclear cell therapy: Role of cardiovascular lineage commitment. Circulation 121:2001, 2010.
26. Menasche P: Skeletal myoblast for cell therapy. Coron Artery Dis 16:105, 2005.
27. Tendera M, Wojakowski W, Ruzyllo W, et al: Intracoronary infusion of bone marrow–derived selected CD34+CXCR4+ cells and non-selected mononuclear cells in patients with acute STEMI and reduced left ventricular ejection fraction: Results of randomized, multicentre Myocardial Regeneration by Intracoronary Infusion of Selected Population of Stem Cells in Acute Myocardial Infarction (REGENT) Trial. Eur Heart J 30:1313, 2009.
28. Assmus B, Schachinger V, Teupe C, et al: Transplantation of Progenitor Cells and Regeneration Enhancement in Acute Myocardial Infarction (TOPCARE-AMI). Circulation 106:3009, 2002.
29. Erbs S, Linke A, Schuler G, et al: Intracoronary administration of circulating blood-derived progenitor cells after recanalization of chronic coronary artery occlusion improves endothelial function. Circ Res 98:e48, 2006.
30. Losordo DW, Schatz RA, White CJ, et al: Intramyocardial transplantation of autologous CD34+ stem cells for intractable angina: A phase I/IIa double-blind, randomized controlled trial. Circulation 115:3165, 2007.
31. Hofmann M, Wollert KC, Meyer GP, et al: Monitoring of bone marrow cell homing into the infarcted human myocardium. Circulation 111:2198, 2005.
32. Hare JM, Traverse JH, Henry TD, et al: A randomized, double-blind, placebo-controlled, dose-escalation study of intravenous adult human mesenchymal stem cells (prochymal) after acute myocardial infarction. J Am Coll Cardiol 54:2277, 2009.
33. Abdel-Latif A, Bolli R, Tleyjeh IM, et al: Adult bone marrow–derived cells for cardiac repair: A systematic review and meta-analysis. Arch Intern Med 167:989, 2007.
34. Lipinski MJ, Biondi-Zoccai GG, Abbate A, et al: Impact of intracoronary cell therapy on left ventricular function in the setting of acute myocardial infarction: A collaborative systematic review and meta-analysis of controlled clinical trials. J Am Coll Cardiol 50:1761, 2007.
35. Wollert KC, Meyer GP, Lotz J, et al: Intracoronary autologous bone-marrow cell transfer after myocardial infarction: The BOOST randomised controlled clinical trial. Lancet 364:141, 2004.
36. Schachinger V, Erbs S, Elsasser A, et al: Intracoronary bone marrow–derived progenitor cells in acute myocardial infarction. N Engl J Med 355:1210, 2006.
37. Janssens S, Dubois C, Bogaert J, et al: Autologous bone marrow–derived stem-cell transfer in patients with ST-segment elevation myocardial infarction: Double-blind, randomised controlled trial. Lancet 367:113, 2006.
38. Huikuri HV, Kervinen K, Niemela M, et al: Effects of intracoronary injection of mononuclear bone marrow cells on left ventricular function, arrhythmia risk profile, and restenosis after thrombolytic therapy of acute myocardial infarction. Eur Heart J 29:2723, 2008.
39. Lunde K, Solheim S, Aakhus S, et al: Intracoronary injection of mononuclear bone marrow cells in acute myocardial infarction. N Engl J Med 355:11999, 2006.
40. Wollert KC, Drexler HC: Cell therapy for the treatment of coronary heart disease: A critical appraisal. Nat Rev Cardiol 7:204, 2010.
41. Seeger FH, Tonn T, Krzossok N, et al: Cell isolation procedures matter: A comparison of different isolation protocols of bone marrow mononuclear cells used for cell therapy in patients with acute myocardial infarction. Eur Heart J 28:766, 2007.
42. Assmus B, Rolf A, Erbs S, et al: Clinical outcome 2 years after intracoronary administration of bone marrow–derived progenitor cells in acute myocardial infarction. Circ Heart Fail 3:89, 2010.
43. Mansour S, Vanderheyden M, De Bruyne B, et al: Intracoronary delivery of hematopoietic bone marrow stem cells and luminal loss of the infarct-related artery in patients with recent myocardial infarction. J Am Coll Cardiol 47:1727, 2006.
44. Dimmeler S: Regulation of bone marrow–derived vascular progenitor cell mobilization and maintenance. Arterioscler Thromb Vasc Biol 30:1088, 2010.
45. Takahashi T, Kalka C, Masuda H, et al: Ischemia- and cytokine-induced mobilization of bone marrow–derived endothelial progenitor cells for neovascularization. Nat Med 5:434, 1999.
46. Harada M, Qin Y, Takano H, et al: G-CSF prevents cardiac remodeling after myocardial infarction by activating the Jak-Stat pathway in cardiomyocytes. Nat Med 11:305, 2005.
47. Orlic D, Kajstura J, Chimenti S, et al: Mobilized bone marrow cells repair the infarcted heart, improving function and survival. Proc Natl Acad Sci U S A 98:10344, 2001.
48. Abdel-Latif A, Bolli R, Zuba-Surma EK, et al: Granulocyte colony-stimulating factor therapy for cardiac repair after acute myocardial infarction: A systematic review and meta-analysis of randomized controlled trials. Am Heart J 156:216, 2008.
49. Honold J, Lehmann R, Heeschen C, et al: Effects of granulocyte colony simulating factor on functional activities of endothelial progenitor cells in patients with chronic ischemic heart disease. Arterioscler Thromb Vasc Biol 26:2238, 2006.
50. Petit I, Szyper-Kravitz M, Nagler A, et al: G-CSF induces stem cell mobilization by decreasing bone marrow SDF-1 and up-regulating CXCR4. Nat Immunol 3:687, 2002.
51. Kang HJ, Kim HS, Koo BK, et al: Intracoronary infusion of the mobilized peripheral blood stem cell by G-CSF is better than mobilization alone by G-CSF for improvement of cardiac function and remodeling: 2-year follow-up results of the Myocardial Regeneration and Angiogenesis in Myocardial Infarction with G-CSF and Intra-Coronary Stem Cell Infusion (MAGIC Cell) 1 trial. Am Heart J 153:237, 2007.
52. Zaruba MM, Theiss HD, Vallaster M, et al: Synergy between CD26/DPP-IV inhibition and G-CSF improves cardiac function after acute myocardial infarction. Cell Stem Cell 4:313, 2009.
53. Theiss HD, Brenner C, Engelmann MG, et al: Safety and efficacy of SITAgliptin plus GRanulocyte-colony-stimulating factor in patients suffering from Acute Myocardial Infarction (SITAGRAMI-Trial)—rationale, design and first interim analysis. Int J Cardiol 2010 Jan 3. [Epub ahead of print.]
54. Bahlmann FH, De Groot K, Spandau JM, et al: Erythropoietin regulates endothelial progenitor cells. Blood 103:921, 2004.
55. Calvillo L, Latini R, Kajstura J, et al: Recombinant human erythropoietin protects the myocardium from ischemia-reperfusion injury and promotes beneficial remodeling. Proc Natl Acad Sci U S A 100:4802, 2003.
56. Menasche P, Alfieri O, Janssens S, et al: The Myoblast Autologous Grafting in Ischemic Cardiomyopathy (MAGIC) trial: First randomized placebo-controlled study of myoblast transplantation. Circulation 117:1189, 2008.
57. Smits PC: Myocardial repair with autologous skeletal myoblasts: A review of the clinical studies and problems. Minerva Cardioangiol 52:525, 2004.
58. Perin EC, Dohmann HF, Borojevic R, et al: Transendocardial, autologous bone marrow cell transplantation for severe, chronic ischemic heart failure. Circulation 107:2294, 2003.
59. Fuchs S, Satler LF, Kornowski R, et al: Catheter-based autologous bone marrow myocardial injection in no-option patients with advanced coronary artery disease: A feasibility study. J Am Coll Cardiol 41:1721, 2003.
60. Galinanes M, Loubani M, Davies J, et al: Autotransplantation of unmanipulated bone marrow into scarred myocardium is safe and enhances cardiac function in humans. Cell Transplant 13:7, 2004.
61. Strauer BE, Brehm M, Zeus T, et al: Regeneration of human infarcted heart muscle by intracoronary autologous bone marrow cell transplantation in chronic coronary artery disease: The IACT Study. J Am Coll Cardiol 46:1651, 2005.
62. Assmus B, Honold J, Schachinger V, et al: Transcoronary transplantation of progenitor cells after myocardial infarction. N Engl J Med 355:1222, 2006.
63. Hill JM, Syed MA, Arai AE, et al: Outcomes and risks of granulocyte colony-stimulating factor in patients with coronary artery disease. J Am Coll Cardiol 46:1643, 2005.
64. Huttmann A, Duhrsen U, Stypmann J, et al: Granulocyte colony-stimulating factor–induced blood stem cell mobilisation in patients with chronic heart failure—feasibility, safety and effects on exercise tolerance and cardiac function. Basic Res Cardiol 101:78, 2006.
65. Erbs S, Linke A, Schachinger V, et al: Restoration of microvascular function in the infarct-related artery by intracoronary transplantation of bone marrow progenitor cells in patients with acute myocardial infarction: The Doppler Substudy of the Reinfusion of Enriched Progenitor Cells and Infarct Remodeling in Acute Myocardial Infarction (REPAIR-AMI) trial. Circulation 116:366, 2007.
66. Janssens S: Stem cells in the treatment of heart disease. Annu Rev Med 61:287, 2010.

Gene Therapy

67. Nayak L, Rosengart TK: Gene therapy for heart failure. Semin Thorac Cardiovasc Surg 17:343, 2005.
68. Li CX, Parker A, Menocal E, et al: Delivery of RNA interference. Cell Cycle 5:2103, 2006.
69. Nordlie MA, Wold LE, Simkhovich BZ, et al: Molecular aspects of ischemic heart disease: Ischemia/reperfusion-induced genetic changes and potential applications of gene and RNA interference therapy. J Cardiovasc Pharmacol Ther 11:17, 2006.
70. Hajjar RJ, del Monte F, Matsui T, et al: Prospects for gene therapy for heart failure. Circ Res 86:616, 2000.
71. Hata JA, Williams ML, Koch WJ: Genetic manipulation of myocardial beta-adrenergic receptor activation and desensitization. J Mol Cell Cardiol 37:11, 2004.
72. Milano CA, Allen LF, Rockman HA, et al: Enhanced myocardial function in transgenic mice overexpressing the $beta_2$-adrenergic receptor. Science 264:582, 1994.
73. Engelhardt S, Hein L, Wiesmann F, et al: Progressive hypertrophy and heart failure in $beta_1$-adrenergic receptor transgenic mice. Proc Natl Acad Sci U S A 96:7059, 1999.
74. Miyamoto MI, del Monte F, Schmidt U, et al: Adenoviral gene transfer of SERCA2a improves left-ventricular function in aortic-banded rats in transition to heart failure. Proc Natl Acad Sci U S A 97:793, 2000.
75. del Monte F, Harding SE, Dec GW, et al: Targeting phospholamban by gene transfer in human heart failure. Circulation 105:904, 2002.
76. Vinge LE, Raake PW, Koch WJ: Gene therapy in heart failure. Circ Res 102:1458, 2008.
77. Haunstetter A, Izumo S: Toward antiapoptosis as a new treatment modality. Circ Res 86:371, 2000.
78. Freund C, Mummery CL: Prospects for pluripotent stem cell–derived cardiomyocytes in cardiac cell therapy and as disease models. J Cell Biochem 107:592, 2009.

Pharmacogenetics

79. Muszkat M, Stein CM: Pharmacogenetics and response to beta-adrenergic receptor antagonists in heart failure. Clin Pharmacol Ther 77:123, 2005.
80. McNamara DM, Holubkov R, Janosko K, et al: Pharmacogenetic interactions between beta-blocker therapy and the angiotensin-converting enzyme deletion polymorphism in patients with congestive heart failure. Circulation 103:1644, 2001.
81. McNamara DM, Tam SW, Sabolinski ML, et al: Aldosterone synthase promoter polymorphism predicts outcome in African Americans with heart failure: Results from the A-HeFT Trial. J Am Coll Cardiol 48:1277, 2006.

82. Liggett SB, Mialet-Perez J, Thaneemit-Chen S, et al: A polymorphism within a conserved $beta_1$-adrenergic receptor motif alters cardiac function and beta-blocker response in human heart failure. Proc Natl Acad Sci U S A 103:11288, 2006.
83. Terra SG, Hamilton KK, Pauly DF, et al: $Beta_1$-adrenergic receptor polymorphisms and left ventricular remodeling changes in response to beta-blocker therapy. Pharmacogenet Genomics 15:227, 2005.
84. Small KM, Wagoner LE, Levin AM, et al: Synergistic polymorphisms of $beta_1$- and $alpha_{2C}$-adrenergic receptors and the risk of congestive heart failure. N Engl J Med 347:1135, 2002.
85. Cresci S, Kelly RJ, Cappola TP, et al: Clinical and genetic modifiers of long-term survival in heart failure. J Am Coll Cardiol 54:432, 2009.

Metabolic Modulation

86. Stanley WC, Recchia FA, Lopaschuk GD: Myocardial substrate metabolism in the normal and failing heart. Physiol Rev 85:1093, 2005.
87. Revenco D, Morgan JP: Metabolic modulation and cellular therapy of cardiac dysfunction and failure. J Cell Mol Med 13:811, 2009.
88. Abozguia K, Clarke K, Lee L, et al: Modification of myocardial substrate use as a therapy for heart failure. Nat Clin Pract Cardiovasc Med 3:490, 2006.
89. Lee L, Campbell R, Scheuermann-Freestone M, et al: Metabolic modulation with perhexiline in chronic heart failure: A randomized, controlled trial of short-term use of a novel treatment. Circulation 112:3280, 2005.
90. Fragasso G, Piatti Md PM, Monti L, et al: Short- and long-term beneficial effects of trimetazidine in patients with diabetes and ischemic cardiomyopathy. Am Heart J 146:E18, 2003.
91. Fragasso G, Palloshi A, Puccetti P, et al: A randomized clinical trial of trimetazidine, a partial free fatty acid oxidation inhibitor, in patients with heart failure. J Am Coll Cardiol 48:992, 2006.
92. Sokos GG, Nikolaidis LA, Mankad S, et al: Glucagon-like peptide-1 infusion improves left ventricular ejection fraction and functional status in patients with chronic heart failure. J Card Fail 12:694, 2006.
93. Nikolaidis LA, Mankad S, Sokos GG, et al: Effects of glucagon-like peptide-1 in patients with acute myocardial infarction and left ventricular dysfunction after successful reperfusion. Circulation 109:962, 2004.
94. Halbirk M, Norrelund H, Moller N, et al: Cardiovascular and metabolic effects of 48-h glucagon-like peptide-1 infusion in compensated chronic patients with heart failure. Am J Physiol Heart Circ Physiol 298:H1096, 2010.
95. Soukoulis V, Dihu JB, Sole M, et al: Micronutrient deficiencies an unmet need in heart failure. J Am Coll Cardiol 54:1660, 2009.

CHAPTER 34 Care of Patients with End-Stage Heart Disease

Linda L. Emanuel and Robert O. Bonow

Care for the incurable has been a defining part of medicine from its earliest origins, as reflected in the emphasis on comfort in the writings of the Greek physician Hippocrates (fifth century BC).[1] In recent history, the fields of palliative care and cardiology have developed in parallel and tacit partnership. When English physician William Harvey first described circulation in *Exercitatio anatomica de motu cordis et sanguinis in animalibus* in 1628, hospice meant an alms house for the poor. However, at the time French physician René Laennec developed the stethoscope in the early 1800s, two prominent Massachusetts General Hospital physicians were writing on end-of-life care. Jacob Bigelow urged withholding of bloodletting from those for whom it would merely "embitter the approach of death when it is inevitable," and John Warren wrote in *Etherization; with Surgical Remarks* (1848) that ether should be used to relieve the suffering of "mortification." In recent decades, advances in cardiopulmonary resuscitation, cardiovascular surgery, and implantable devices have stimulated medical ethics discussions of who should receive resuscitation, who should undergo life-prolonging procedures, and when life really ends. End-of-life care and palliative care more generally remain a defining part of the practice of cardiology. For instance, a primary indication for coronary artery bypass, stents, and other procedures is symptom control and quality of life; in this sense, a significant amount of care provided by cardiologists is quality palliative care.

With the advent of palliative care as a subspecialty, this focus has been able to develop further.[2-4] The 2005 American College of Cardiology/American Heart Association (ACC/AHA) guidelines on chronic heart failure[5] included a Class I recommendation for educating patients and their families about the role of palliative and hospice care services. This is also emphasized in the 2009 ACC/AHA guideline update.[6] Recent consensus statements made similar recommendations,[7,8] and leading opinions note that the nature of cardiac disease makes it particularly important for cardiologists to integrate palliative care into cardiac care services so that it can be tailored to the unpredictable illness course that characterizes advanced heart disease and to the needs of the individual patient.[9] By explicitly integrating palliative care considerations into all patient assessment, treatment decision making, continuity of care planning, and systems of care delivery, cardiovascular medicine can further advance the quality of care it provides.[10]

Epidemiology

Of the approximate 2,426,264 deaths in the United States in 2006, 1,347,000 or 56% were primarily or secondarily caused by cardiovascular disease.[11] Cardiovascular disease was the primary cause of death in every year of the 20th century except 1918. Whereas cardiovascular disease, and particularly heart failure, is more common with advancing age, it is not restricted to the elderly; more than 151,000 Americans younger than 65 years die of cardiovascular disease each year.[11] The characteristic cardiovascular decompensation and the characteristic death are sudden. Both are predictable during months to years but not in a more precise time frame. However, cardiovascular conditions are also chronic and may afflict children and young adults as well as the elderly. Roughly 81.1 million Americans are living with one or more chronic forms of cardiovascular disease; hypertension afflicts roughly 74.5 million Americans, coronary heart disease 17.6 million, and congestive heart failure 5.8 million. Some 6.4 million are living with the aftermath of a stroke.

The site of death has also evolved in an important way. Nearly 60% of Americans died as inpatients in hospitals in 1980; by 2005, about 37% died in hospitals as inpatients.[12] Although this trend corresponds with patient and family preferences, patients with cardiovascular disease are least represented among those receiving home care and hospice care. Referrals for hospice care for heart failure are infrequent.[13,14] In 2008, approximately 39% of all decedents received hospice care, with cancer patients constituting 38% of hospice users.[15] Among nine cancer diagnoses, 15% to 34% of decedents used hospice; among myocardial infarction and congestive heart failure diagnoses, 7% and 8%, respectively, of decedents used hospice.[16] In one estimate, only 4% of heart failure patients receive palliative care. Patients in need of palliative care may be ambulatory, in long-term care, on the hospital ward, or in an intensive care unit. Consequently, palliative care is needed in a full range of settings.

Palliative Care

Because terminally ill patients have a wide variety of advanced diseases, often with multiple symptoms demanding relief, and require a noninvasive therapeutic regimen to be delivered in a commodious care setting, their care requires some of the most complex and demanding cognitive skills for assessments and interventions. Fundamental to ensuring quality palliative end-of-life care is a focus on four broad domains of the illness experience: (1) physical symptoms; (2) mental or psychological symptoms; (3) social needs—relationships, practical issues, and economic; and (4) existential or spiritual needs. Palliative care also includes support for the family, including for their bereavement. Studies have confirmed that these domains coincide with the experiences and preferences for care of patients with advanced illness, including heart disease,[17] and their families. A whole-person assessment screens for and evaluates needs in each of these four domains. Goals for care are discerned and decided on in discussion with the patient and family on the basis of the assessment in each of these domains. Although physicians are responsible for certain (especially technical) interventions and for coordinating the interventions, they depend on an interdisciplinary team and the family to provide all of them. Importantly, failure to address any one of the domains is likely to preclude a good death, and hence a well-coordinated, effectively communicating interdisciplinary team takes on special importance in end-of-life care.

Assessment, Goals, and Care Planning

Whole-Person Assessment

The assessment of physical and mental symptoms should follow a modified version of the traditional history and physical examination that emphasizes symptoms. Questions should be included that discern sources of suffering and how much these symptoms interfere with the patient's life. Standardized assessment questions are available from clinically relevant scales, such as the Memorial Symptom Assessment Scale; these have the advantage of ensuring that the assessment is comprehensive. For a patient with late end-stage disease for whom the care goal is quality of being, aspects of the physical examination that are uncomfortable and tests should be evaluated for their benefit-to-burden ratio for the patient. Because a focused physical examination may be all that is reasonable, these skills need to be well developed.

In the area of social needs, health care providers should screen for financial needs, the status of important relationships, caregiving needs, and access to medical care. Relevant questions may include these: *How often is there someone to feel close to? How much help do you need with things like getting meals or getting around? How much trouble do you have getting the medical care you need?* In the area of existential needs, providers should assess distress and the patient's sense of being emotionally and existentially settled and of finding purpose or meaning.[18] A helpful assessment question is, *How much are you able to find meaning since your illness began?* It is helpful to ask about the patient's perception of his or her care: *How much do you feel your doctors and nurses respect you? How clear is the information from us about what to expect regarding your illness? How much do you feel that the medical care you are getting fits with your goals?* If concern is detected in any areas, deeper evaluation questions are warranted.[19]

Communication

Communication is arguably as powerful an intervention in medicine as any invasive procedure. Several studies involving patients with advanced heart failure indicate that communication with patients and their families is not always optimal.[20-22] Compared with patients with cancer, patients with heart failure have less information about their condition, and they are also less involved in decision making.[22] Continued focus on correcting hemodynamic abnormalities or improving symptoms often takes precedence over communication about prognosis and options for care. This focus may be only partly physician led; contributing factors from patients who may have less inclination to think of or to talk of dying, compared with cancer patients, for instance, also exist.[23] Nonetheless, poor communication has significant adverse consequences, and quality communication allows navigating of difficult situations in the best available fashion. Because communication requires both effective "signal output" and effective reception, the clinician must assist the patient and family with their ability to receive difficult information as well as offer ways to think about the options they have.

A seven-step guide for communicating important information has been developed by Buckman[24]: (1) Prepare, mentally and physically, by (2) setting up a quiet environment with room for face-to-face discussion and accommodating items, such as a chair, a box of tissues, a pen and paper to write down information, and perhaps a beverage. (3) Begin by asking what the patient and family know or understand and then (4) ask how they prefer to receive new information and how much they want to know. (5) Give the new information according to their preferences. (6) Allow emotional responses and (7) plan for the next steps in care, including by identifying the next concrete steps. See **Table 34-1** for suggested wording and the rationale behind each step.

Prognosis

Among patients with an equally poor prognosis, 75% of cancer patients reported that they knew they would likely die, whereas only 54% of noncancer patients, many of whom had cardiac diagnoses, reported the same.[25] The established gap between prognosis in late-stage cardiovascular conditions and the patient's expectation of death, the continuous stream of life-prolonging cardiovascular therapies and devices, the difficulty in establishing accurate prognoses in individual cases,[26] and the need to sustain hope may be only four of multiple factors that conspire to keep poor prognosis from triggering appropriate forms of palliative care.

Clinicians should provide population-based statistics about prognosis to patients and families and allow these statistics rather than individual predictions to trigger the kinds of whole-patient assessments and continuous goal assessment conversations that follow palliative care guidelines. This in turn will allow patients and families not only to follow plans for care that are appropriate but also to achieve the kinds of psychological, social, and existential engagements that people tend to seek when going through the last stages of life.[27-30] In general, clinicians should share population-based prognosis at the time of diagnosis and then introduce a palliative care framework of whole-patient assessment and continuous goal adjustment from the time when clinical indicators suggest a prognosis of 6 months or less. When sharing prognostic information, use language such as this, for example: *Of all the people with your condition in America, about half will go on to live for more than 3 years and about half will die within 3 years.* Go on to say something like this: *We will hope for the best but also plan for the worst so that we are not caught unprepared and you can live your life with a positive attitude.* And further: *Many people have special things they want to accomplish in this phase of their life—such as a project, a trip, or coming to terms in a personal relationship. I encourage you to think about what that might be for you so that I can do my best to tailor our medical care to your goals.* For patients with cardiovascular illnesses, it is often helpful to point out: *The good news is that we can expect you to feel well and to function pretty normally. Often people with cardiac disease avoid the long phases of disability and suffering that other illnesses can cause. The counterpart is that people sometimes do not engage in the growth that often comes near the end of life or they become overly fearful of dying suddenly. Preparation of the kind we just mentioned can bring the best of both worlds. So let's keep an open discussion about your goals for care.*

Continuous Goal Assessment

Goals for care are numerous. They range from cure of a specific condition to delaying the course of an incurable disease, adapting to progressive disability without disrupting the family, finding peace of mind or personal meaning, and dying in a manner that leaves loved ones with a positive "departure memory." Discernment of goals for care can be approached through a seven-step protocol:

1. Ensure that information is as complete as reasonably possible and understood by all relevant parties (see sections on Whole-Patient Assessment and on Communication).
2. Explore what the patient and family are hoping for.
3. Share all the options with the patient and family. Delineate some relevant goals that are also realistic.
4. Respond empathically to the patient and family as they adjust to declining realistic expectations.
5. Make a plan, emphasizing what can be done toward the realistic goals.
6. Follow through with the plan.
7. Review and revise this plan periodically, considering at every encounter whether the goals of care should be reviewed with the patient and family.

If a patient or family member has difficulty letting go of an unrealistic goal, suggest that while hoping for the best, it is still prudent to have a plan for other outcomes as well.

TABLE 34-1 Elements of Communicating Bad News—The P-SPIKES Approach

ACRONYM	STEPS	AIM OF THE INTERACTION	PREPARATIONS, QUESTIONS, OR PHRASES
P	Preparation	• Mentally prepare for the interaction with the patient and/or family.	• Review what information needs to be communicated. • Plan how you will provide emotional support. • Rehearse key steps and phrases in the interaction.
S	Setting of the interaction	• Ensure the appropriate setting of a serious and emotionally charged discussion.	• Ensure that patient, family, and appropriate social supports are present. • Devote sufficient time—do not squeeze in a discussion. • Ensure privacy and prevent interruptions by people or beeper. • Bring a box of tissues.
P	Patient's perception and preparation	• Begin the discussion by establishing the baseline and whether the patient and family can grasp the information. • Ease tension by having the patient and family contribute.	• Start with open-ended questions to encourage participation. • Possible phrases to use: *What do you understand about your illness?* *When you first had symptom X, what did you think it might be?* *What did Dr. X tell you when he sent you here?* *What do you think is going to happen?*
I	Invitation and information needs	• Discover what information needs the patient and/or family have and what limits they want regarding the bad information.	• Possible phrases to use: *If this condition turns out to be something serious, do you want to know?* *Would you like me to tell you the full details of your condition? If not, then to whom would you like me to talk?*
K	Knowledge of the condition	• Provide the bad news or other information to the patient and/or family sensitively.	• Do not just dump the information on the patient and family. • Interrupt and check that the patient and family understand. • Possible phrases to use: *I feel bad to have to tell you this, but … Unfortunately, the tests showed …* *I'm afraid the news is not good …*
E	Empathy and exploration	• Identify the cause of the emotions, e.g., poor prognosis. • Empathize with the patient and/or family's feeling. • Explore by asking open-ended questions.	• Strong feelings in reaction to bad news are normal. • Acknowledge what the patient and family are feeling. • Remind them that such feelings are normal even if frightening. • Give them time to respond. • Remind the patient and family that you will not abandon them. • Possible phrases to use: *I imagine this is very hard for you.* *You must be upset. Tell me how you are feeling.* *I wish the news were different.* *I'll do whatever I can to help you.*
S	Summarize and plan a strategy	• Delineate for the patient and the family the next steps, including additional tests or interventions.	• It is the unknown and uncertain that increase anxiety. • Recommend a schedule with goals and landmarks. Provide your rationale for the patient and/or family to accept (or to reject). • If the patient and/or family are not ready to discuss the next steps, schedule a follow-up visit.

Modified from Buckman R: How to Break Bad News: A Guide for Health Care Professionals. Baltimore, Md, Johns Hopkins University Press, 1992.

Advance Care Planning

Advance care planning is a process of planning for future medical care in the case that the patient becomes incapable of making medical decisions (see Chap. 3). Ideally, it starts before a health care crisis or the terminal phase of an illness. However, although 80% of Americans endorse advance care planning, only 20% have actually done so. A similarly small proportion of health care providers have completed their advance care planning. A good first step is for health care providers to start with themselves. Personal planning makes the providers aware of the critical and charged choices in the process and allows them to truthfully tell their patients that they have done this themselves. With experience, advance care planning discussions need not take long.

Steps in effective advance care planning involve (1) introducing the topic, (2) structuring a discussion, (3) reviewing plans that have been discussed by the patient and family, (4) documenting the plans, (5) updating them periodically, and (6) implementing the advance care directive (**Table 34-2**). Raising the topic can be done efficiently as a routine matter, analogous to insurance or estate planning, that is recommended for all patients. Structuring a focused discussion (step 2) is the central skill. Identify the health care proxy and recommend his or her involvement in the discussion. Select a worksheet, preferably one that has been evaluated and demonstrated to produce reliable and valid expressions of patient preferences, and orient the patient and proxy to it. Discuss with the patient and proxy one scenario as an example to demonstrate how to think about the issues. It is often helpful to begin with a scenario in which the patient is likely to have settled preferences, such as being in a persistent vegetative state. Ask the patient and proxy to discuss and to complete the worksheet for the other scenarios. If appropriate, suggest that they involve family members in the discussion. On a return visit, go over the patient's preferences, checking and resolving any medical or logical inconsistencies. After having the patient and proxy sign the document, place it in the medical chart and be sure that copies are provided to relevant family members and care sites. Because patients' preferences can change, review these documents periodically or after an illness episode or personal experience.

A most useful thing to discern in advance care planning is the patient's individual threshold for making quality of life a priority over longevity. Most patients have a discernible threshold that becomes evident during review of illness scenarios. Try to identify and to feed that back to the patient and family for verification and include that in the record. Patients, health proxies, and clinicians can all be considerably aided by knowledge of that single feature about a patient.

Types of Documents. Two broad types of advance care planning documents exist. The first includes living wills and instructional directives; these advisory documents describe the types of decisions that should direct care. Some are specific, delineating scenarios and interventions. Among these, some are for general use and others are for a specific type of disease, such as cancer or human immunodeficiency virus (HIV) infection; some are available in multiple languages.[31] Less specific directives can be general statements or may describe the values that should guide decisions. Health care proxy forms appoint an individual to make decisions. A combined directive that both directs care and designates a proxy is generally recommended, and the directive should clearly indicate whether the patient's preferences or the proxy's choice should take precedence if they conflict.

The U.S. Supreme Court has established that patients have a constitutional right to refuse or to terminate life-sustaining interventions and that mentally incompetent patients may do so by having previously

TABLE 34-2 Steps in Advance Care Planning

STEP	GOALS TO BE ACHIEVED AND MEASURES TO COVER	USEFUL PHRASES OR POINTS TO MAKE
Introducing advance care planning	• Ask the patient what he or she knows about advance care planning and if he or she has already completed an advance care directive. • Indicate that you as a physician have completed advance care planning. • Indicate that you try to perform advance care planning with all patients regardless of prognosis. • Explain the goals of the process as empowering the patient and ensuring that you and the proxy understand the patient's preferences. • Provide the patient relevant literature, including the advance care directive that you prefer to use. • Recommend that the patient identify a proxy decision-maker who should attend the next meeting.	• *I'd like to talk with you about something I try to discuss with all my patients. It's called advance care planning. In fact, I feel that this is such an important topic that I have done this myself. Are you familiar with advance care planning or living wills?* • *Have you thought about the type of care you would want if you ever became too sick to speak for yourself? That is the purpose of advance care planning.* • *There is no change in health that we have not discussed. I am bringing this up now because it is sensible for everyone, no matter how well or ill, old or young.* • Have many copies of advance care directives available, including in the waiting room, for patients and families.
Structured discussion of scenarios and patient preferences	• Affirm that the goal of the process is to follow the patient's wishes if the patient loses decision-making capacity. • Elicit the patient's overall goals related to health care. • Elicit the patient's preferences for specific interventions in a few salient and common scenarios. • Help the patient define the threshold for withdrawing and withholding interventions. • Define the patient's preference for the role of the proxy.	• Use a structured worksheet with typical scenarios. • Begin the discussion with persistent vegetative state and consider other scenarios, such as recovery from an acute event with serious disability, asking the patient about his or her preferences regarding specific interventions, such as ventilators, nasogastric feedings, and CPR, and then proceeding to less invasive interventions, such as blood transfusions and antibiotics.
Review the patient's preferences	• After the patient has made choices of interventions, review them to ensure that they are consistent and medically sensible and that the proxy is aware of them.	
Document the patient's preferences	• Formally complete the advance care directive and have a witness sign it. • Provide a copy for the patient and the proxy. • Insert a copy into the patient's medical record.	
Update the directive	• Periodically, and with major changes in health status, review with the patient the existing choice made and make any modifications.	
Apply the directive	• The directive goes into effect only when the patient becomes unable to make medical decisions for himself or herself. • Re-read the directive to be sure about its content. • Discuss your proposed actions on the basis of the directive with the proxy.	

provided "clear and convincing evidence" of their advance preferences.[32] As of 2003, all states and the District of Columbia also have living will or health care proxy legislation. State variations exist but are less important than they could be because the Constitution has been interpreted to require states to honor any clear advance care directive. A potentially misleading distinction relates to statutory as opposed to advisory documents. Statutory documents are drafted to fit relevant state statutes. They tend to be written with the goal of protecting clinicians from legal action if they follow the patient's stated wishes. Advisory documents are drafted to reflect the patient's wishes. Both are legal, the first under state and the second under common or constitutional law. However, it is simpler to honor a statement that complies with all laws, so if a patient is not using a statutory form, it is appropriate to attach a statutory form to the advance care directive being used.

Interventions

Physical and Psychological Symptoms and Their Management

Advanced heart disease is widely associated with fatigue and breathlessness; many patients also experience pain, nausea, sleep disturbances, palpitations, anorexia, dry mouth, cough, and limb swelling, to name just the more common ones.[33,34] Psychological symptoms, which patients find at least as distressing and as compromising of quality of life as physical symptoms, are also common, including depression, anxiety, and irritability.[35,36]

Symptom management skills have been mostly developed for cancer and other illnesses in palliative care, but some are well developed in cardiovascular disease, and both are well described elsewhere,[37] including, for the latter, in this textbook (see Chap. 28). A rational approach to symptom management is being developed for advanced heart failure; cardiologists and palliative care clinicians should expect advances in symptom management in the coming years.[38]

These approaches include the following. Angiotensin-converting enzyme inhibitors improve symptoms. Beta blockers also do but affect quality of life more. Spironolactone provides more variable improvement. Loop diuretics are particularly useful during acute exacerbations. Dietary control of fluid and sodium intake reduces fatigue and edema. Exercise improves dyspnea, strength, and breathing and reduces limb swelling.

Continuous positive airway pressure applied through a mask improves some sleep disordered breathing, including sleep apnea and Cheyne-Stokes breathing, as does oxygen supplementation in some patients. Oral nitrates may relieve dyspnea as well as angina. Opioids improve dyspnea.

Pain is a problem for about half of patients with advanced cardiac disease, including chest pain, osteoarthritis and musculoskeletal pain, and pain from edema. Nonsteroidal anti-inflammatory drugs are detrimental to renal function and sodium retention, but other medications, including opioids, can be used.

For patients with depression and renal impairment, serotonin reuptake inhibitors may be the antidepressant of choice, although tricyclic antidepressants are appropriate for some. Methylphenidate has a more rapid effect and may be the optimal choice for faster relief. Benzodiazepines are useful for anxiety, as are support groups and other psychosocial interventions.

Social Needs and Their Management

FINANCIAL BURDENS. Dying can impose substantial economic strains on patients and families. In the United States, about 20% of terminally ill patients and their families have to spend more than 10% of family income on health care costs over and above health insurance premiums. Between 10% and 30% of families have sold assets, used savings, or taken out a mortgage to pay for the patient's health care costs. Nearly 40% of terminally ill patients report that the cost of their illness was a moderate or great economic hardship for their family.

One source of economic burden is related to medical costs; medical costs correlate with personal bankruptcy even among the medically insured. The second, more universal source of economic burden is a decline in the patient's income. In 20% of cases, a family member stopped working to provide care. Economic burden is associated with poor physical functioning and needs for housekeeping, nursing, and personal care. That is, more debilitated and less well-off patients experience greater economic burdens. Economic burdens tend to increase the psychological distress of families and patients. Assistance from a social worker, early on if possible, to ensure access to available benefits may be helpful. Many people are unaware of options including insurance benefits, the Family Medical Leave Act, and other sources of assistance.

Importantly, palliative care, by reducing symptom burden and supporting the family, may well reduce the financial blow to households of serious and terminal illness. Because illness and poverty correlate, clinicians should consider serious financial burden an adverse event associated with medical interventions and seek the approaches of early and coordinated palliative care to mitigate and preempt the impact as much as possible.[39]

RELATIONSHIPS. Closing the narrative of lived relationships is a nearly universal need. When asked if sudden death or death after an illness is preferable, respondents often initially select the former but soon change to the latter as they reflect on the importance of saying goodbye. Bereaved family members who have not had the chance to say goodbye often have a difficult grief process. Because many of the deaths in cardiology are sudden, this is of particular importance. Patients and their families should be encouraged to settle what they would like to, even though it is more difficult to anticipate the time of death. Family and close friends may need to be accommodated with unrestricted visiting hours for inpatients, including, in some cases, sleeping near the patient even in institutional settings. Assistance for patients and family members who are unsure about how to create or help preserve memories can be deeply appreciated, such as by providing raw materials like a scrapbook, a memory box, or a guide to creating an ethical will or by offering suggestions and informational resources. Taking photographs and creating videos or audiotapes can be especially helpful to patients with life-shortening illness who have younger children. Dignity Therapy is an effective several-day psychotherapeutic intervention for patients near death; although it is primarily an intervention for patients, it is also helpful for families.[40]

FAMILY CAREGIVERS. Caring for seriously ill patients places a heavy burden on families.[29] Families are required to provide transportation, homemaking, and other services. Typically, paid professionals, such as home health nurses and hospice, supplement family caregiving; only about a quarter of all caregiving is provided exclusively by paid professional assistance. The trend toward more out-of-hospital deaths will increase reliance on families for end-of-life care. About three quarters of the caregivers of terminally ill patients are female—wives, daughters, and even sisters. Consequently, female patients tend to be able to rely less on family for caregiving assistance and may need more paid assistance. About 20% of terminally ill patients report substantial unmet needs for nursing and personal care. Caregiving is particularly difficult for heart disease, as patients often do not accept the seriousness of the illness at early stages, and they have unpredictable needs and high medical noncompliance.[41] Spousal caregivers report marital distress more; financial burdens are particularly high; and caregivers of transplant patients report major depression, adjustment disorders, and even post-traumatic stress disorders.[42]

All this makes it imperative to inquire about unmet needs and to facilitate family or paid professional services. Assistance from religious or community groups can often be mobilized by one or two phone calls from the medical team to someone the patient or family identifies.

Existential Needs and Their Management

Dying is one of the ultimate existential challenges. Religion and spirituality are important to dying patients, including cardiac patients.[43,44] Approximately 70% of patients report becoming more religious or spiritual when they became terminally ill, and many find comfort in practices such as prayer. Some studies suggest that women and older patients are more likely to experience greater interest in religion and spirituality. On the other hand, about 20% of terminally ill patients become less religious, frequently feeling alienated by becoming terminally ill. For other patients, the need is for existential meaning and purpose that is distinct from spirituality and may even be an antireligious form of spirituality. Among patients with cardiovascular conditions, clinical experience suggests that fear of sudden death is common. Furthermore, the well-recognized accomplishment of personal growth and relationship resolution characteristic among patients who foresee death in the near future is less apparent among patients with cardiovascular illnesses.[45] However, patients with end-stage heart failure do engage in life cycle–appropriate roles, including "biographical work" and "arrangement work," and creating a legacy document may be of significant help in the spiritual domain.[40,46]

Health care providers are often hesitant about involving themselves in the religious, spiritual, and existential experiences of their patients because it may seem private, related to alternative lifestyles, or "soft." However, physicians and other members of the interdisciplinary team should be able at least to detect spiritual need. Screening questions have been developed for a physician's spiritual history taking. Spiritual distress can amplify other types of suffering and even masquerade as, for instance, intractable physical pain or anxiety. The screening questions in the whole-person assessment are usually sufficient. Deeper evaluation and intervention are rarely appropriate for the physician unless no other member of the team is available or suitable. Pastors, whether from the medical institution or the patient's community, may be helpful.

Precisely how religious practices, spirituality, and existential explorations can be facilitated and improve end-of-life care is not well established. In one study, only 36% of respondents indicated that a clergy member would be comforting. Dignity Therapy is a nondenominational intervention that invites the patient to make a legacy document for his or her loved ones; provided by a trained therapist, this intervention meets with strong personal satisfaction scores.[40]

Managing the Last Stages

Withdrawing and Withholding Life-Sustaining Treatment

For centuries, it has been deemed ethical to withhold or to withdraw life-sustaining interventions. For patients who are incompetent and terminally ill but have not completed an advance care directive, next of kin can exercise this right, although this may be restricted in some states, depending on how clear and convincing the evidence is of the patient's preferences. In theory, a patient's right to refuse medical therapy can be limited by four countervailing interests: (1) preservation of life; (2) prevention of suicide; (3) protection of third parties, such as children; and (4) preservation of the integrity of the medical profession. In practice, these interests almost never override the right of competent patients or incompetent patients who have left explicit advance care directives. Regarding incompetent patients whose wishes are not clear, two criteria can help guide decisions. First, many courts have advocated use of the substituted-judgment criterion, which holds that the proxy decision-makers should try to imagine what the incompetent patient would do if he or she were competent. However, most proxies, even close family members, cannot accurately predict what the patient would have wanted. The second criterion is that of best interests and holds that proxies should decide on the basis of the likely best outcome for the patient. Yet, as many family conflicts reveal, different people can have very different views of what is in the patient's best interests. As a matter of practice, physicians rely on family members to make decisions that they think are best and object only if these decisions seem to demand treatments that the physicians consider nonbeneficial.

PHYSICIANS' ORDERS REGARDING CARDIOPULMONARY RESUSCITATION AND OTHER LIFE-SUSTAINING TREATMENTS. In the SUPPORT Project, only 25% of patients hospitalized with heart failure recalled having discussions with their physicians about resuscitation preferences.[21] Whenever a patient is a suitable candidate for a do not resuscitate (DNR) order, he or she deserves to have had a comprehensive discussion about the goals of care, the plan of care, and possibly also the advance care planning. Use of predesigned forms, such as the Physician Orders for Life-Sustaining Treatments (POLST), in place of limited DNR forms can encourage these more comprehensive and coherent approaches to creating plans of care. In general, an isolated DNR order with no reference to other life-sustaining treatment preferences can be considered a red flag that should prompt a physician to include or to return to a whole-patient assessment and a comprehensive plan for care with goal-tailored treatment choices.

IMPLANTABLE CARDIOVERTER-DEFIBRILLATORS. With increasing indications for implantable cardioverter-defibrillators (ICDs) in patients with left ventricular dysfunction (see Chaps. 29 and 38), the number of patients receiving these devices will undoubtedly continue to increase.[47] The difficult ethical dilemmas include not only the indications for implanting ICDs and the impact on health care finances but also the issues regarding when these devices should be deactivated.[48] These issues also include the need to discuss these decisions with patients and their families.[5] These discussions should be an essential component of overall advance care planning.

The thorny issues of ICD management are highlighted by a study of family members' views of ICDs in end-of-life care.[49] Among 100 family members of patients who died with ICDs in place, only 27 family members reported discussions of possible deactivation and often only in the last few days of life.

MECHANICAL VENTILATION. Perhaps the most challenging intervention to withdraw is mechanical ventilation. There are two approaches: terminal extubation, which is the removal of the endotracheal tube; and terminal wean, which is the gradual reduction of the FIO_2 or ventilator rate. Some physicians recommend the terminal wean because patients do not develop upper airway obstruction and the distress caused by secretions or stridor, but it is reported that terminal weaning can prolong the dying process. To ensure comfort for conscious or semiconscious patients, a common practice is to inject a bolus of lorazepam (1 to 2 mg) before withdrawal followed by 5 to 10 mg of morphine and continuous infusion of morphine (50% of the bolus dose per hour). (Higher doses will be needed for patients already receiving anxiolytics and opioids.) Remove any neuromuscular blocking agents so that patients can show any discomfort, which can in turn allow medication titration or additional boluses of morphine or midazolam. Families need to be warned that up to 10% of patients unexpectedly survive for 1 day or more after mechanical ventilation is stopped.

FUTILE CARE. Beginning in the late 1980s, some commentators argued that physicians could terminate futile treatments demanded by families of terminally ill patients. There is no objective definition or standard of futility. The term conceals subjective value judgments about when a treatment is not beneficial. A more practical approach acknowledges that many cases in which futility concerns are raised overlie communication gaps or unresolved personal issues that are best dealt with in team or family meetings. On occasion, true value differences exist; these may be best handled with assistance from an ethics committee.

Euthanasia and Physician-Assisted Suicide

Terminating life-sustaining intervention and providing opioids to manage symptoms are not to be confused with euthanasia or physician-assisted suicide. Both the first two, unlike the last, have long been considered ethical by the medical profession and legal by courts.

A growing body of data indicates that depression, hopelessness, and worries about loss of dignity or autonomy are the primary factors motivating a desire for euthanasia or physician-assisted suicide. Whereas any of these can occur in patients with cardiovascular conditions, there appear to be fewer requests in this population than in cancer and AIDS patients. Perhaps the characteristic sudden death among cardiac patients helps avoid some of the fears of indignity and dependence associated with a slow, highly symptomatic decline. Nonetheless, multiple symptoms and chronic disability do occur in patients with end-stage heart disease, and requests for physician-assisted suicide or euthanasia also occur. Cardiologists should know how to respond to such requests.

After receiving a request for euthanasia or physician-assisted suicide, probe with empathic, open-ended questions to help elucidate the underlying cause for the request, such as, "What makes you want to consider this option?" Endorsing either moral opposition or moral support for the act tends to be counterproductive, lending an impression of being judgmental or of endorsing the worthlessness of the patient's life. Health care providers must reassure the patient of continued care and commitment. Simultaneously, the patient should be educated about (1) the alternative, less controversial options, such as symptom management and withdrawal of any unwanted treatments; (2) the reality of euthanasia and physician-assisted suicide because the patient is likely to have misconceptions about its effectiveness; and (3) the legal implications of the choice. As indicated, depression, hopelessness, and other symptoms of psychological distress as well as physical suffering and economic burdens are likely factors motivating the request. Health care providers should identify the factors motivating the request and aggressively treat those factors. Most patients, after these interventions and clarification of options, proceed with a less controversial approach of declining life-sustaining interventions, possibly including refusal of nutrition and hydration.

Care During the Last Hours

Most lay people have limited experiences with the actual dying process and death. They frequently do not know what to expect of the final hours and afterward. There is no rehearsal and no second chance. Therefore, the family and other caregivers must be prepared, especially if the plan is for the patient to die at home.

For patients with heart failure, there may be several last days of life with characteristic pathophysiologic changes, such as increased orthopnea and nocturnal dyspnea. Patients experience extreme weakness and fatigue and become bed bound. This can lead to bedsores. If the end is near and the sores are causing less distress than dressing changes and frequent turning, it is reasonable to drop these usual types of care. Dry mucosal membranes should be cared for with frequent oral swabbing, lip lubricants, and artificial tears. These activities can provide the family with a form of care to substitute for those that no longer help, such as feeding. With loss of the gag reflex and dysphagia, patients may also accumulate airway and pharyngeal secretions, producing noises during respiration sometimes called the death rattle. Scopolamine can reduce this. They also have changes in respiration with periods of apnea or Cheyne-Stokes breathing. Decreased intravascular volume and cardiac output causes tachycardia, hypotension, peripheral coolness, and livedo reticularis (skin mottling). Patients can also have urinary and fecal incontinence at death as the sphincters lose their tone. Most important, changes occur in

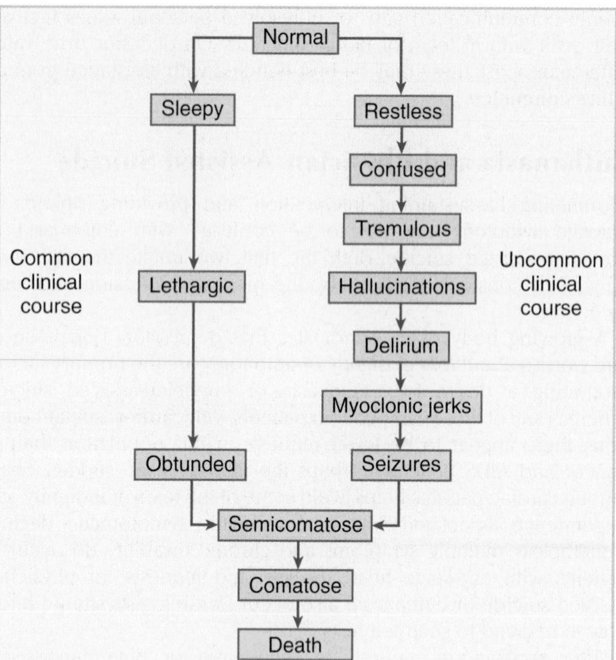

FIGURE 34-1 Common and uncommon clinical courses of the last days of terminally ill patients. *(Modified from Mount Sinai Hospital and Casey House Hospice: Advance planning.* In *Ferris FD, Flannery JS, McNeal HB, et al [eds]: A Comprehensive Guide for the Care of Persons with HIV Disease. Module 4: Palliative Care. Toronto, Mount Sinai Hospital and Casey House Hospice, 1995 [http://www.cpsonline.info/content/resources/hivmodule4.html.])*

consciousness and neurologic function, leading to two very different paths to death (**Fig. 34-1**).

Each of these terminal changes can cause patients and families distress. Most lay people have limited experiences with the dying process and do not know what to expect. Informing families, even by providing an information sheet, can help. For instance, it can be calming to know that patients stop eating because they are dying, not dying because they have stopped eating, or that the death rattle is not a sign of suffocation, or that mottling tends to mean that death is near.

It is claimed that hearing and touch are the last senses to stop functioning. Families should be encouraged to communicate with and touch the patient, even if he or she is unconscious.

When the plan is for the patient to die at home, the family needs to know how to determine when death has occurred, including the cardinal signs of cessation of cardiac function and respiration, fixed pupils, coolness, changes in skin color and texture, and incontinence. Remind the family that the eyes may remain open. It helps to have a plan of who the family and caregivers will contact when the patient is dying or has died. Without a plan, they may panic and call 911, unleashing a cascade of unwanted events from arrival of emergency personnel and resuscitation to hospital admission. Family and caregivers should be instructed to contact hospice, the covering physician, or the on-call member of the palliative care team. There is no reason to contact the coroner, unless the state requires it for all deaths. Similarly, unless foul play is suspected, the health care team need not contact the coroner either.

Just after the patient dies, even the best prepared family may experience shock and bereavement and be distraught. They need time to assimilate the event and be comforted. Health care providers should write a bereavement card or letter to the family. It can be appropriate, although it is not obligatory, to attend the funerals of patients to lend support to the grieving family and to find an opportunity for closure for the physician.

Death is a strong predictor of poor health, and even mortality, for the surviving spouse. It may be important to alert the spouse's physician about the death to be aware of symptoms that might require professional attention.

Sudden Death

Sudden death may "shortchange" patients from the growth that often happens in the last phase of life and that may make it easier for bereaved family members to go on. Children of patients who have died suddenly may be excessively influenced by the sudden disappearance of their parent, without a chance to say goodbye, and by the fear of suffering the same fate. Preparedness through discussion, planning, and engaging the benefits of the consciously trodden last paths in life can help, as can extended bereavement counseling. The services of a social worker or other professional with expertise in the area should almost always be considered.

PALLIATIVE CARE SERVICES

How and Where. For nearly two decades, hospice has been a leading model of palliative care services. Patients who use hospice tend to appreciate the care, and their families tend to do better than others in similar situations.[50] In 1983, Medicare began paying for hospice services under Part A, the hospital insurance part of reimbursement. To be eligible, a patient must be certified by two physicians as having a prognosis of 6 months or less if the disease runs its usual course. Prognoses are probabilistic by their nature; patients are not required to die within 6 months but rather to have a condition from which half the people with it would be deceased within 6 months. Patients sign a hospice enrollment form that states their intent to forgo curative services related to their terminal illness but can still receive medical services for other comorbid conditions. Patients can also dis-enroll and re-enroll later; that is, the hospice Medicare benefit can be reinvoked later to secure traditional Medicare benefits. Payments to hospice are per diem rather than fee-for-service and are intended to cover comprehensive care, including physician services for the medical direction of the interdisciplinary team, regular home care visits by registered nurses and licensed practical nurses, home health aide and homemaker services, dietary counseling, chaplain services, social work services, and bereavement counseling as well as medical equipment, supplies, and medications. Additional clinical care, including that by the primary physician, is covered by Medicare Part B even while the hospice Medicare benefit is in place.

Physicians should initiate earlier referrals to hospice to allow more time for patients to receive palliative care. By 1996, the mean length of enrollment in hospice was 65 days, with the median being less than 24 days. Since then, the length of enrollment has declined. The hospice length of stay tends to be longer for heart failure patients than for other patients.[51] In two surveys, the mean length of stay of patients with heart failure was 43.5 and 60 days.[51,52]

Until relatively recently, hospice had been the main way of securing palliative services for terminally ill patients. Efforts are now directed at ensuring continuity of palliative care across settings and through time, and this is particularly important for heart patients, who often have multiple comorbid conditions and transition across many care settings. Increasingly, these same types of palliative care services are available as consultative services in hospitals, in day care and other outpatient settings, and in nursing homes. For instance, in the United States, although most hospice care is provided in residential homes, just more than 10% now occurs in nursing homes. In addition, palliative care consultations for non-hospice patients can be billed as for other consultations under Medicare Part B, the physician reimbursement part. Many believe that palliative care should be offered to patients regardless of their prognosis. A patient and his or her family should not have to make an "either curative care or palliative care" choice, in large part because it can be psychologically stressful to embrace mortality. Provision of palliative care as needed from the onset of illness onward is ideal,[53] but discontinuities in care can make this challenging. Documentation of goals, orders for life-sustaining treatment that are comprehensive and standardized,[54] and advance care planning and the date of the most recent update can help coordinate care across care sites, among members of the care team, and along the illness trajectory of changing goals for care.

Outcome Measures

Care near the end of life cannot be measured by most of the available validated outcome measures because palliative care does not consider death a bad outcome. Similarly, the family and patients receiving end-of-life care may not seek or appreciate the elements of quality of life measurements and may seek different elements of quality that are not included in standard measures when their active engagement is with dying well. Symptom control, enhanced family relationships, and quality of bereavement are difficult to measure and are rarely the primary focus of carefully developed or widely used outcome measures. Nevertheless, outcomes are as important in end-of-life care as in any other field of medical care. Specific end-of-life care instruments are being developed both for assessment, such as the Brief Hospice Inventory and Needs and the End-of-life Screening Tool (NEST), and for outcome measures, such as the Palliative Care Outcome Scale and the QUAL-E.[55] The field of end-of-life care is ready to enter an era of evidence-based practice and continuous improvement within established institutions.

RESOURCES

Education in Palliative and End-of-Life Care (EPEC) Project, Northwestern University's Feinberg School of Medicine (www.epec.net).

End of Life/Palliative Education Resource Center, Medical College of Wisconsin (www.eperc.mcw.edu).

National Comprehensive Cancer Network (NCCN): Palliative Care Guidelines, 2002 (www.nccn.org).

REFERENCES

1. Asimov I: Asimov's Biographical Encyclopedia of Science and Technology. 2nd revised ed. Garden City, NY, Doubleday, 1982.
2. Hanratty B, Hibbert D, Mair F, et al: Doctor's perceptions of palliative care for heart failure: Focus group study. BMJ 325:581, 2002.
3. Easson AM, Crosby JA, Librach SL: Discussion of death and dying in surgical textbooks. Am J Surg 182:34, 2001.
4. Rabow MW, McPhee SJ: Deficiencies in end-of-life care content in medical textbooks. J Am Geriatr Soc 50:397, 2002.
5. Hunt SA, Abraham WT, Chin MH, et al: ACC/AHA 2005 guideline update for the management of chronic heart failure in the adult: A report of the American College of Cardiology/American Heart Association Task Force on Practice Guidelines (Writing Committee to Update the 2001 Guidelines for the Evaluation and Management of Heart Failure). Available at: http://www.acc.org/clinical/guidelines/failure/index.pdf.
6. Jessup M, Abraham WT, Casey DE, et al: 2009 Focused Update: ACCF/AHA Guidelines for the Diagnosis and Management of Heart Failure in Adults: A Report of the American College of Cardiology Foundation/American Heart Association Task Force on Practice Guidelines. Developed in Collaboration With the International Society for Heart and Lung Transplantation. Circulation 119:1977, 2009.
7. Goodlin SJ, Hauptman PJ, Arnold R, et al: Consensus statement: Palliative and supportive care in advanced heart failure. J Card Fail 10:200, 2004.
8. Jaarsma T, Beattie JM, Ryder M, et al: Palliative care in heart failure: A position statement from the palliative care workshop of the Heart Failure Association of the European Society of Cardiology. Eur J Heart Fail 11:433, 2009.
9. Selman LE, Beattie JM, Murtagh FE, Higginson IJ: Palliative care: Based on neither diagnosis nor prognosis, but patient and family need. Soc Sci Med 69:154, 2009.
10. Emanuel L, Alexander C, Arnold R, et al: Integrating palliative care into disease management guidelines. J Palliat Med 7:774, 2004.
11. Lloyd-Jones D, Adams RJ, Brown TM, et al: Heart disease and stroke statistics—2010 update. A report from the American Heart Association. Circulation 121:948, 2010.
12. Worktable 309: Deaths by place of death, age, race, and sex: United States, 2005. Centers for Disease Control. Available at: http://www.cdc.gov/nchs/data/dvs/Mortfinal2005_worktable_309.pdf. Accessed February 9, 2010.

Palliative Care

13. Gibbs JSR, McCoy ASM, Gibbs LME, et al: Living with and dying from heart failure: The role of palliative care. Heart 88(Suppl II):ii36, 2002.
14. Davis MP, Albert NM, Young JB: Palliation of heart failure. Am J Hosp Palliat Care 22:211, 2005.
15. NHPCO Facts and Figures: Hospice Care in America. 2009 ed. National Hospice and Palliative Care Organization. Available at: http://www.nhpco.org/files/public/Statistics_Research/NHPCO_facts_and_figures.pdf. Accessed February 9, 2010.
16. Iwashyna T, Zhang JX, Christakis NA: Disease-specific patterns of hospice and related healthcare use in an incidence cohort of seriously ill elderly patients. J Palliat Med 5:531, 2002.
17. Selman L, Beynon T, Higginson IJ, Harding R: Psychological, social and spiritual distress at the end of life in heart failure patients. Curr Opin Support Palliat Care 1:260, 2007.
18. Lo B, Ruston D, Kates LW, et al: Discussing religious and spiritual issues at the end of life: A practical guide for physicians. JAMA 287:749, 2002.

Assessment, Goals, and Care Planning

19. Emanuel LL, Alpert H, Emanuel EJ: Concise screening questions for clinical assessments of terminal care: The needs near the end of life care screening tool (NEST). J Palliat Med 4:465, 2001.
20. Rogers AE, Addington-Hall JM, Abery AJ, et al: Knowledge and communication difficulties for patients with chronic heart failure: Qualitative study. BMJ 321:605, 2000
21. Krumholtz HM, Phillips RS, Hamel MB, et al: Resuscitation preferences among patients with severe congestive heart failure: Results from the SUPPORT Project. Circulation 98:648, 1998.
22. Murray SA, Boyd K, Kendall M, et al: Dying of lung cancer or cardiac failure: Prospective qualitative interview study of patients and their carers in the community. BMJ 325:929, 2002.
23. Gott M, Small N, Barnes S, et al: Older people's views of a good death in heart failure: Implications for palliative care provision. Soc Sci Med 67:1113, 2008.
24. Buckman R: How to Break Bad News: A Guide for Health Care Professionals. Baltimore, Md, The Johns Hopkins University Press, 1992, pp 65-97.
25. Lamont EB, Christakis NA: Complexities in prognostication in advanced cancer: "To help them live their lives the way they want to." JAMA 290:98, 2003.
26. Gott M, Barnes S, Parker C, et al: Dying trajectories in heart failure. Palliat Med 21:95, 2007.
27. Emanuel EJ, Emanuel LL: The promise of a good death. Lancet 351(Suppl II):SII21, 1998.
28. Singer PA, Martin DK, Kelner M: Quality end-of-life care: Patients' perspectives. JAMA 281:163, 1999.
29. Thorns AR, Gibbs LME, Gibbs JSR: Management of severe heart failure by specialist palliative care. Heart 85:93, 2001.
30. Krumholtz HM, Phillips RS, Hamel MB, et al: Resuscitation preferences among patients with severe congestive heart failure: Results from the SUPPORT Project. Circulation 98:648, 1998.
31. Emanuel LL: The Health Care Directive: Learning how to draft advance care documents. J Am Geriatr Soc 39:1221, 1991 (www.medicaldirective.org).
32. President's Commission for the Study of Ethical Issues in Medicine and Biomedical and Behavioral Research: Deciding to Forego Life-Sustaining Treatment. Washington, DC, U.S. Government Printing Office, 1983.
33. O'Leary N: The comparative palliative care needs of those with heart failure and cancer patients. Curr Opin Support Palliat Care 3:241, 2009.
34. Opasich C, Gualco A: The complex symptom burden of the aged heart failure population. Curr Opin Support Palliat Care 1:255, 2007.
35. Janssen DJ, Spruit MA, Woulters EF, Schols JM: Daily symptom burden in end-stage chronic organ failure: A systematic review. Palliat Med 22:938, 2008.
36. Blinderman CD, Homel P, Billings JA, et al: Symptom distress and quality of life in patients with advanced congestive heart failure. J Pain Symptom Manage 35:594, 2008.
37. An ASCO Curriculum: Optimizing Cancer Care—The Importance of Symptom Management, vols I and II. Dubuque, Iowa, Kendall/Hunt Publishing Company, 2001.
38. Goodlin SJ: Palliative care in congestive heart failure. J Am Coll Cardiol 54:386, 2009.
39. Cross ER, Emanuel L: Providing inbuilt economic resilience options: An obligation of comprehensive cancer care. Cancer 113(Suppl):3548, 2008.
40. Chochinov HM: Dignity and the essence of medicine: The A, B, C, and D of dignity conserving care. BMJ 335:184, 2007.
41. Hooley PJ, Butler G, Howlett GJ: The relationship of quality of life, depression, and caregiver burden in outpatients with congestive heart failure. Congest Heart Fail 11:303, 2005.
42. Usher BM, Cammarata K: Heart failure and family caregiver burden: An update. Prog Cardiovasc Nurs 24:113, 2009.
43. Bekelman DB: Symptom burden, depression, and spiritual well-being: A comparison of heart failure and advanced cancer patients. J Gen Intern Med 5:592, 2009.
44. Murray SA: Patterns of social, psychological, and spiritual decline. J Pain Symptom Manage 34:393, 2007.
45. Byock I: Dying Well: The Prospect for Growth at the End of Life. New York, Putnam/Riverhead, 1998.
46. Willems DL, Hak A, Visser FC, et al: Patient work in end-stage heart failure: A prospective longitudinal multiple case study. Palliat Med 20:25, 2006.
47. McClellan MB, Tunis SR: Medicare coverage of ICDs. N Engl J Med 352:222, 2005.
48. Berger JT: The ethics of deactivating implanted cardioverter defibrillators. Ann Intern Med 142:631, 2005.
49. Goldstein NE, Lampert R, Bradley E, et al: Management of implantable cardioverter defibrillators in end-of-life care. Ann Intern Med 141:835, 2004.
50. Christakis NA, Iwashyna TJ: The health impact of health care on families: A matched cohort study of hospice use by decedents and mortality outcomes in surviving, widowed spouses. Soc Sci Med 57:465, 2003.
51. Christakis N, Escarce J: Survival of Medicare patients after enrollment in hospice programs. N Engl J Med 335:172, 1996.
52. Goodlin SJ, Kutner JS, O'Conner SR, et al: Hospice care for patients with heart failure. J Pain Symptom Manage 29:525, 2005.
53. Goodlin SJ: Palliative care for end-stage heart failure. Curr Heart Fail Rep 2:1550, 2005.
54. Physician Orders for Life-Sustaining Treatment (POLST) forms. Center for Ethics in Health Care, Oregon Health Sciences University, 3181 SW Sam Jackson Park Road, L101, Portland OR 97201-3098, 1997.
55. Steinhauser KE, Clipp EC, Bosworth HB, et al: Measuring quality of life at the end of life: Validation of the QUAL-E. Palliat Support Care 2:3, 2004.

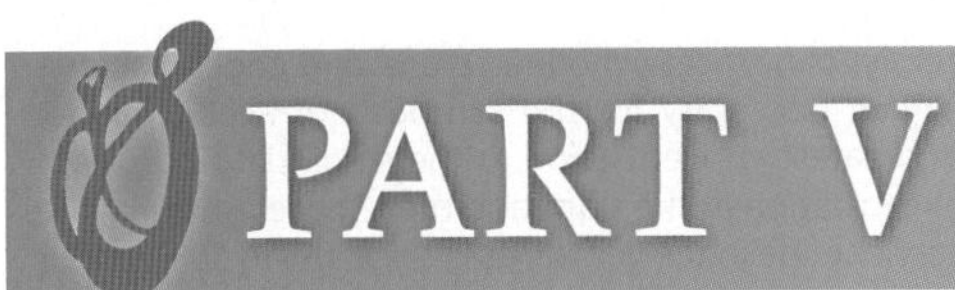

ARRHYTHMIAS, SUDDEN DEATH, AND SYNCOPE

CHAPTER 35 Genesis of Cardiac Arrhythmias: Electrophysiologic Considerations

Michael Rubart and Douglas P. Zipes

Anatomy of the Cardiac Conduction System

Sinoatrial Node

In humans, the sinoatrial node is a spindle-shaped structure composed of a fibrous tissue matrix with closely packed cells. It is 10 to 20 mm long, 2 to 3 mm wide, and thick, tending to narrow caudally toward the inferior vena cava. It lies less than 1 mm from the epicardial surface, laterally in the right atrial sulcus terminalis at the junction of the superior vena cava and right atrium (**Figs. 35-1** and **35-2**). The artery supplying the sinoatrial node branches from the right (55% to 60% of the time) or the left (40% to 45%) circumflex coronary artery and approaches the node from a clockwise or counterclockwise direction around the superior vena cava–right atrium junction.

Cellular Structure. Cells from the sinoatrial node region exhibit a wide variety of morphologic features, including spindle- and spider-shaped cells, rod-shaped atrial cells with clear striations, and small round cells corresponding to endothelial cells.[1] Only the spindle- and spider-shaped cells exhibit the typical electrophysiologic characteristics of pacemaker cells, including hyperpolarization-activated current, I_f,[1] and spontaneous beating under physiologic conditions.[2]

Function. The ionic mechanism underlying sinoatrial node cell automaticity has been controversial, but a large body of experimental evidence supports the notion that it involves rhythmic oscillations of intracellular free calcium levels, which then, via modulation of calcium-sensitive ion channels and transporters in the outer membrane, give rise to diastolic depolarizations, culminating in triggering of a propagating sinoatrial node cell action potential (see later). Similarly, the mechanism of entrainment that enables synchronization of the electrical activity of multiple individual sinoatrial node cells to give rise to a sinoatrial node discharge has been uncertain. Very probably, no single cell in the sinoatrial node serves as *the* pacemaker. Rather, sinoatrial nodal cells function as electrically coupled oscillators that discharge synchronously. The interaction depends on the degree of coupling and the electrophysiologic characteristics of the individual sinoatrial node cell. The resulting rate is not just a simple average of each of the cells. With an individual pacemaker cell coupled to an average of five other cells, each with potentially different electrophysiologic properties, the resulting discharge rate is not obvious. The function of the sinoatrial node as pacemaker requires a delicate balance of intercellular electrical coupling. Excess electrical coupling depresses sinoatrial node automaticity because the sinoatrial node membrane potential is damped by the surrounding atrial myocardium to a more negative potential than the normal maximal diastolic potential, thereby inhibiting spontaneous diastolic depolarization (see Fig. 35-6). Too little coupling can prevent impulse transmission to the adjacent atrial muscle. Restriction of the hyperpolarizing influence of the atrial muscle on the sinoatrial node while maintaining impulse exit into the adjacent atrial myocardium is achieved by the composition and spatial organization of connexins, proteins that form gap junction channels responsible for intercellular ion fluxes (see later, Intercalated Discs). Connexin40 and connexin45, but not connexin43, are expressed in the central sinoatrial node (**Fig. 35-3**). The major part of the crista terminalis–sinoatrial node border exhibits a sharp demarcation boundary of connexin43-expressing atrial myocytes and connexin40/connexin45-expressing myocytes. On the endocardial side, a transitional zone (paranodal area; see Fig. 35-2) exists between the crista terminalis and the peripheral node, in which connexin45 and connexin43 are colocalized. This colocalization of different connexin isoforms raises the possibility that individual gap junctional channels in the transitional zone are formed by more than one connexin isoform.[2]

These disparate connexin phenotypes may create specific types of hybrid channels with rectifying electrical properties that ensure the maintenance of sinoatrial node pacemaker activity but diminish electrotonic interference from the atrial muscle.[3] At the level of the intact sinoatrial node in situ, more recent studies combining immunohistochemistry and high-resolution optical mapping of action potentials have provided structural and functional evidence for the existence of discrete exit pathways that electrically connect the sinoatrial node and atria in canines, whose three-dimensional sinoatrial node structure closely resembles that of humans. In this model (**Fig. 35-4**), electrical excitation during sinoatrial rhythm originates in the central portion of the sinoatrial node and spreads bidirectionally at low speed (1 to 14 cm/sec) within the sinoatrial node, failing to conduct laterally to the crista terminalis and interatrial septum (see Fig. 35-4). After a conduction delay of ~50 milliseconds within the sinoatrial node, the impulse reaches the atrial myocardium via two main superior or inferior exit pathways located a few millimeters from the leading pacemaker site. The ellipsoidal sinoatrial node is thus functionally insulated from the adjacent working myocardium. This insulation coincides with the lack of connexin43 expression and the presence of connective tissue and coronary arteries at the sinoatrial border (see Fig. 35-4, C-F).[4] The intranodal location of the primary pacemaking site is not fixed but rather appears to shift under varying conditions (e.g., sympathetic stimulation; see later in this chapter).

Innervation. The sinoatrial node is densely innervated, with postganglionic adrenergic and cholinergic nerve terminals.[5] Discrete vagal efferent pathways innervate both the sinoatrial and atrioventricular (AV) regions of the dog and nonhuman primate. Most efferent vagal fibers to the atria appear to converge first at a single fat pad between the medial portion of the superior vena cava and the aortic root, superior to the right pulmonary artery; the fibers then project onto two other fat pads found at the inferior vena cava–left atrium junction and the right pulmonary vein–atrium junction and subsequently project to both atria. Vagal fibers to the sinoatrial and AV nodes also converge at the superior vena cava–aortic root fat pad before projection to the right pulmonary vein and inferior vena cava fat pads.[5] Although the sinoatrial nodal region contains amounts of norepinephrine equivalent to those in other parts of the right atrium, acetylcholine, acetylcholinesterase, and choline acetyltransferase (the enzyme necessary for the synthesis of acetylcholine) have been found in greatest concentration in the sinoatrial node, with the next highest concentration in the right and then the left atrium. The concentration of acetylcholine in the ventricles is only 20% to 50% of that in the atria.

Neurotransmitters modulate the sinoatrial node discharge rate by stimulation of beta-adrenergic and muscarinic receptors. Both beta$_1$- and beta$_2$-adrenoceptor subtypes are present in the sinoatrial node. Human sinoatrial nodes contain a more than threefold greater density of beta-adrenergic and muscarinic cholinergic receptors than adjacent atrial tissue. The functional significance of beta-adrenoceptor subtype diversity in the sinoatrial node is unclear. Binding of receptor agonists released from sympathetic nerve terminals causes a positive chronotropic response through a beta$_1$ receptor–activated pathway involving the stimulatory guanosine triphosphate (GTP) regulatory protein (G_s), activation of adenylyl cyclase, intracellular accumulation of cyclic adenosine monophosphate (cAMP), stimulation of cAMP-dependent protein kinase A, and phosphorylation of target proteins (including the L-type Ca^{2+} channel, the channels underlying I_f, and the ryanodine-sensitive Ca^{2+} release channel [ryanodine receptor] in the sarcoplasmic reticulum [SR] membrane). Heart rate increases after beta$_2$-receptor stimulation involve a positive shift of the I_f activation curve, possibly resulting from increases

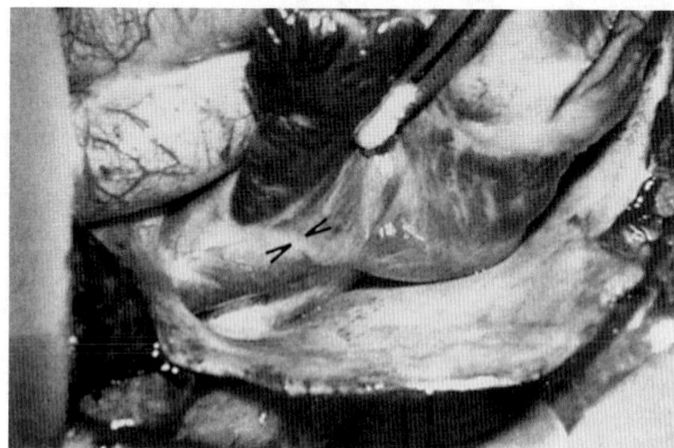

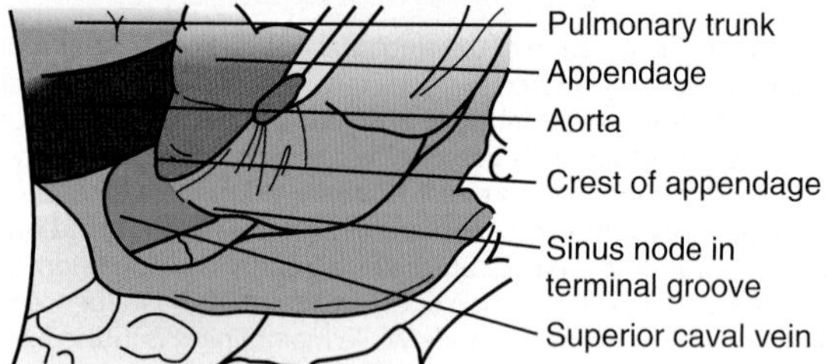

FIGURE 35-1 The human sinus node. This photograph, taken in the operating room, shows the location of the normal cigar-shaped sinus node along the lateral border of the terminal groove at the superior vena cava–atrium junction (arrowheads). *(From Anderson RH, Wilcox BR, Becker AE: Anatomy of the normal heart.* In *Hurst JW, Anderson RH, Becker AE, Wilcox BR [eds]: Atlas of the Heart. New York, Gower, 1988, p 1.2.)*

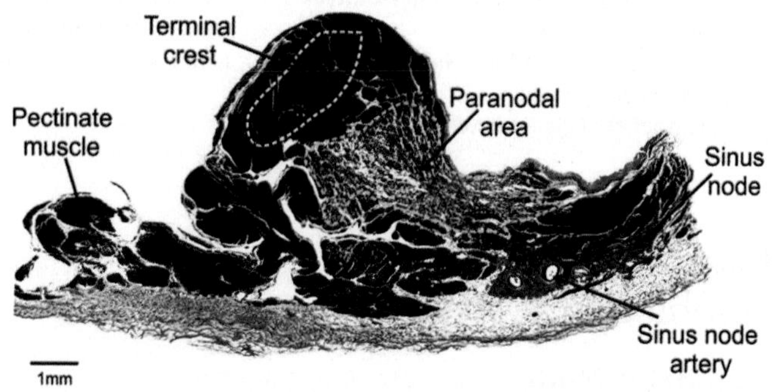

FIGURE 35-2 Masson trichrome–stained section through the human sinus node region. The node (red dashed line) is identified on the basis of the presence of the sinus node artery and the large amount of connective tissue (stained blue; myocytes stained purple-pink). The section also reveals the presence of a paranodal area (green dashed line), which is composed of loosely packed myocytes and sandwiched between the crista terminalis (yellow dashed line) and the sinus node. *(From Chandler NJ, Greener ID, Tellez JO, et al: Molecular architecture of the human sinus node. Circulation 119:1562, 2009. By permission of the American Heart Association.)*

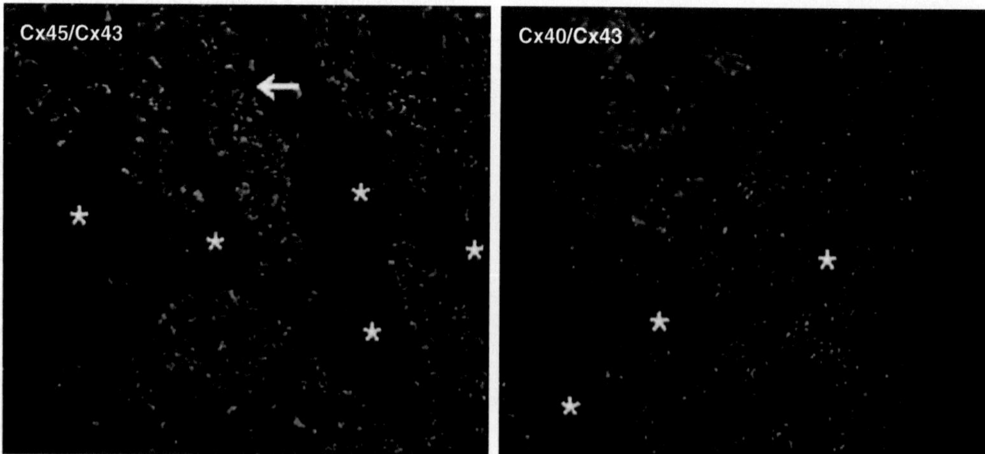

FIGURE 35-3 Sections through the sinoatrial node double-labeled with connexin45/connexin43 **(left)** and connexin40/connexin43 **(right)**. Regions positive for connexin40/connexin45 (small punctate green signals) showing no detectable connexin43 signal (red) are sharply demarcated from adjacent connexin43-expressing regions of the crista terminalis. A zone of connective tissue (asterisks) contributes to separation between the zones, although elsewhere (arrow) the zones seem to be more closely approximated. *(From Coppen SR, Kodama I, Boyett MR, et al: Connexin45, a major connexin of the rabbit sino-atrial node, is co-expressed with connexin43 in a restricted zone at the nodal–crista terminalis border. J Histochem Cytochem 47:907, 1999.)*

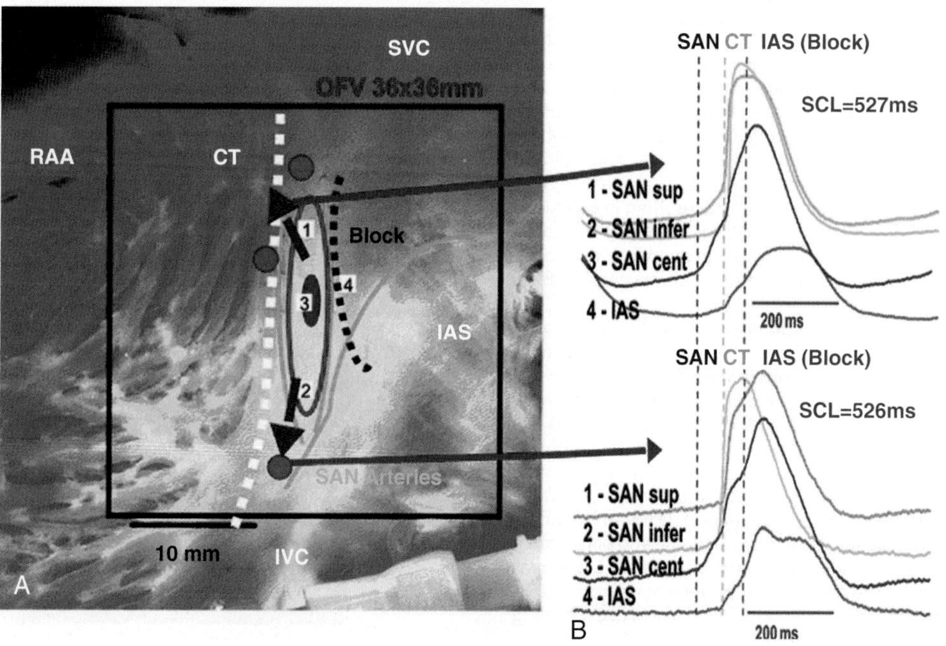

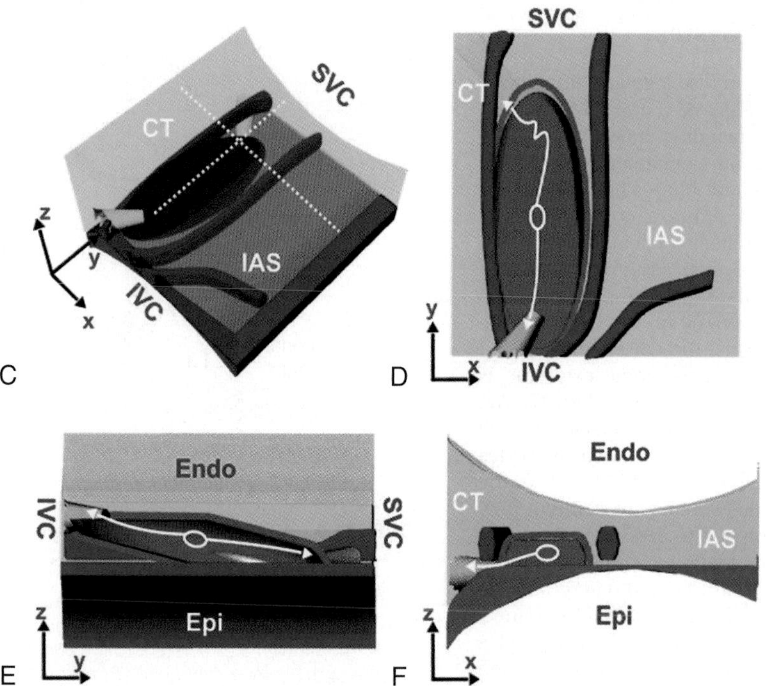

FIGURE 35-4 Endocardial optical voltage mapping in a canine right atrial preparation. **A,** Photograph of the endocardial aspect of the preparation. CT = crista terminalis; IAS = interatrial septum. OFV = optical field of view from which the optical recordings were taken; RAA = right atrial appendage; SVC and IVC = superior and inferior vena cava, respectively. The sinoatrial node (SAN; red oval) is flanked by branches of the SAN artery (drawn schematically in light blue). **B,** Optical action potentials recorded during sinus rhythm from sites 1 through 4 depicted in the photograph in **A**. Sites 1 and 2 are from the superior (SAN sup) and inferior (SAN infer) part of the SAN, near the SAN exit pathways. Site 3 is from the leading pacemaker site (SAN cent), and site 4 is from the IAS block zone. Electrical excitation originates in the central portion of the SAN (dark blue oval in **A**) and spreads bidirectionally within the SAN, failing to conduct in a perpendicular direction into the IAS and CT. After a conduction delay of ~50 milliseconds within the SAN, excitation reaches the atrial myocardium via superior (upper tracings in panel **B**) or inferior (lower tracings in panel **B**) sinoatrial exit pathways ~9 mm from the leading pacemaker site. The ellipsoidal SAN structure (red line in **A**) is functionally insulated from the atrial myocardium, as indicated by the dashed white and black lines in **A**, respectively, except for two (inferior and superior) exit pathways. Vertical dashed lines indicate the beginning of the SAN, CT, and IAS activation. SCL denotes sinus cycle length. Numbers to the left of the optical action potential tracings correspond to the respective recording sites in the photograph in **A**. **C-F,** Three-dimensional model of the SAN. The green area represents the myocardium. The fibrotic tissue (purple) and coronary arteries (blue) enclose the SAN (red). The initial excitation during sinus rhythm is shown by a white oval. The white arrows denote the two main directions of the impulse propagation within the SAN. The yellow bundles show the sinus node exit pathways. **C** and **D** show side and top projections, respectively. **E** and **F** show cross sections in the *z-y* and *z-x* plane, respectively. *(From Fedorov VV, Schuessler RB, Hemhill M, et al: Structural and functional evidence for discrete exit pathways that connect the canine sinoatrial node and atria. Circ Res 104:915-923, 2009. By permission of the American Heart Association.)*

in cytosolic cAMP levels.[6] The negative chronotropic response of vagal stimulation is mediated by acetylcholine binding to and ensuing activation of M_2 muscarinic receptors. Membrane currents regulated by muscarinic receptor activation include the acetylcholine- and adenosine-sensitive K^+ current ($I_{K(Ach,Ade)}$; see Table 35-3), $I_{Ca.L}$, and I_f. The effect of muscarinic receptor agonist in activating $I_{K(Ach,Ade)}$ is mediated by direct interaction of a G protein subunit with the $K_{(Ach,Ade)}$ channel and does not require second messengers. Activation of $I_{K(Ach,Ade)}$ causes hyperpolarization of the sinoatrial node cell membrane, resulting in a reduced rate of diastolic depolarization. Muscarinic receptor activation–mediated effects on $I_{Ca.L}$ and I_f are primarily caused by a reduction in the intracellular cAMP level, thereby antagonizing the positive chronotropic effects of beta-adrenoceptor stimulation.

In addition to its negative chronotropic effect, acetylcholine also prolongs intranodal conduction time, at times to the point of sinoatrial nodal exit block. Acetylcholine increases whereas norepinephrine decreases refractoriness in the center of the sinoatrial node. The phase (timing) in the cardiac cycle at which vagal discharge occurs and the background sympathetic tone importantly influence vagal effects on the sinus rate and conduction (see later). After cessation of vagal stimulation, sinoatrial nodal automaticity may accelerate transiently (postvagal tachycardia). The neurotransmitters neuropeptide Y (NPY) and vasoactive intestinal peptide (VIP) are localized in sympathetic and parasympathetic nerve terminals, respectively. VIP reversibly increases I_f, whereas NPY reversibly decreases I_f.[6] The role of other peripheral neurotransmitters (such as calcitonin gene–related peptide, substance P) in controlling sinoatrial node electrophysiology is unclear.

Atrioventricular Junctional Area and Intraventricular Conduction System

ATRIOVENTRICULAR NODE. Based on histology and immunolabeling, the normal AV junctional area (**Figs. 35-5** and **35-6**) is composed of multiple distinct structures, including transitional tissue, inferior nodal extension, compact portion, penetrating bundle, His bundle, atrial and ventricular muscle, central fibrous body, tendon of Todaro, and valves.[7,8] **Figure 35-7A, B** shows a computer three-dimensional reconstruction of the AV junctional area in a rabbit heart. At the level of the AV junction, the tract of nodal tissue is divided into two major components, the inferior nodal extension and the penetrating bundle (red and purple areas, respectively, in Fig. 35-7A, B). The inferior nodal extension is located between the coronary sinus and the tricuspid valve, and the end of the inferior nodal extension is covered by transitional tissue (light green area in Fig. 35-7A, B). The small myocytes in the inferior nodal extension are dispersed among connective tissue and do not express connexin43, whereas myocytes in the transitional zone do express connexin43; but unlike the connexin43-positive atrial myocytes in the working myocardium, they are loosely packed between collagen septa. The inferior nodal extension is continuous with the penetrating bundle, which penetrates the fibrous tissue separating the atria and ventricles, and emerges in the ventricles as the bundle of His. Both structures are covered by connective tissue (sheaths in Fig. 35-7A) and are therefore enclosed. Myocytes in the penetrating bundle express connexin43 and are dispersed among connective tissue. A tract of connexin43-positive nodal tissue projects into the connexin43-negative inferior nodal extension.

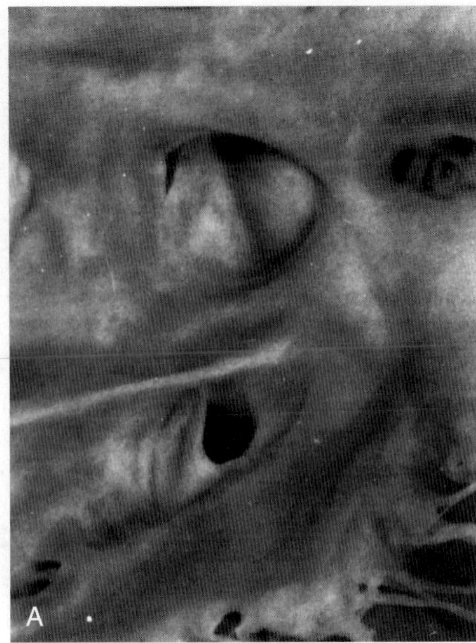

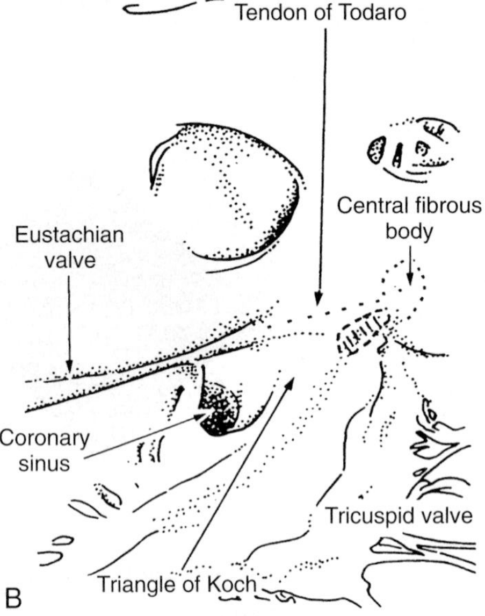

FIGURE 35-5 **A,** Photograph of a normal human heart showing the anatomic landmarks of the triangle of Koch. This triangle is delimited by the tendon of Todaro superiorly, the fibrous commissure of the flap guarding the openings of the inferior vena cava and coronary sinus, by the attachment of the septal leaflet of the tricuspid valve inferiorly, and by the mouth of the coronary sinus at the base. **B,** The stippled area adjacent to the central fibrous body is the approximate site of the compact AV node. *(From Janse MJ, Anderson RH, McGuire MA, et al: "AV nodal" reentry: I. "AV nodal" reentry revisited. J Cardiovasc Electrophysiol 4:561, 1993.)*

The compact portion of the AV node (yellow area in Fig. 35-7A, B) is a superficial structure lying just beneath the right atrial endocardium, anterior to the ostium of the coronary sinus, and directly above the insertion of the septal leaflet of the tricuspid valve. It is at the apex of a triangle formed by the tricuspid annulus and the tendon of Todaro (blue area in Fig. 35-7A, B), which originates in the central fibrous body and passes posteriorly through the atrial septum to continue with the eustachian valve (see Figs. 35-5 and 35-6A). The term *triangle of Koch,* however, has to be used with caution because histologic studies of anatomically normal adult hearts have demonstrated that the tendon of Todaro, which forms one side of the triangle of Koch, is absent in about two thirds of hearts. The compact node is located at the junction where the connexin43-negative nodal tissue (red area in Fig. 35-7A, B) meets the connexin43-positive nodal tissue (purple area in Fig. 35-7A, B). Myocytes in the nodal portion are small and weakly positive for connexin43. In 85% to 90% of human hearts, the arterial supply to the AV node is a branch from the right coronary artery that originates at the posterior intersection of the AV and interventricular grooves (crux). A branch of the circumflex coronary artery provides the AV nodal artery in the remaining hearts. Fibers in the lower part of the AV node may exhibit automatic impulse formation.[8] The main function of the AV node is delaying atrial impulse transmission to the ventricles, thereby coordinating atrial and ventricular contractions (Fig. 35-7C, D).

During normal anterograde AV conduction, the action potential propagates from the sinoatrial node through atrial working myocardium (the existence of specialized internodal conduction pathways has been controversial) and enters the tract of nodal tissue at two points (see Fig. 35-7C; see also Video 35-1 on website). The first point is at the end of the inferior nodal extension (next to the penetrating bundle) via the transitional tissue. This conduction pathway most likely corresponds to the fast pathway route previously observed in electrical mapping experiments.[8]

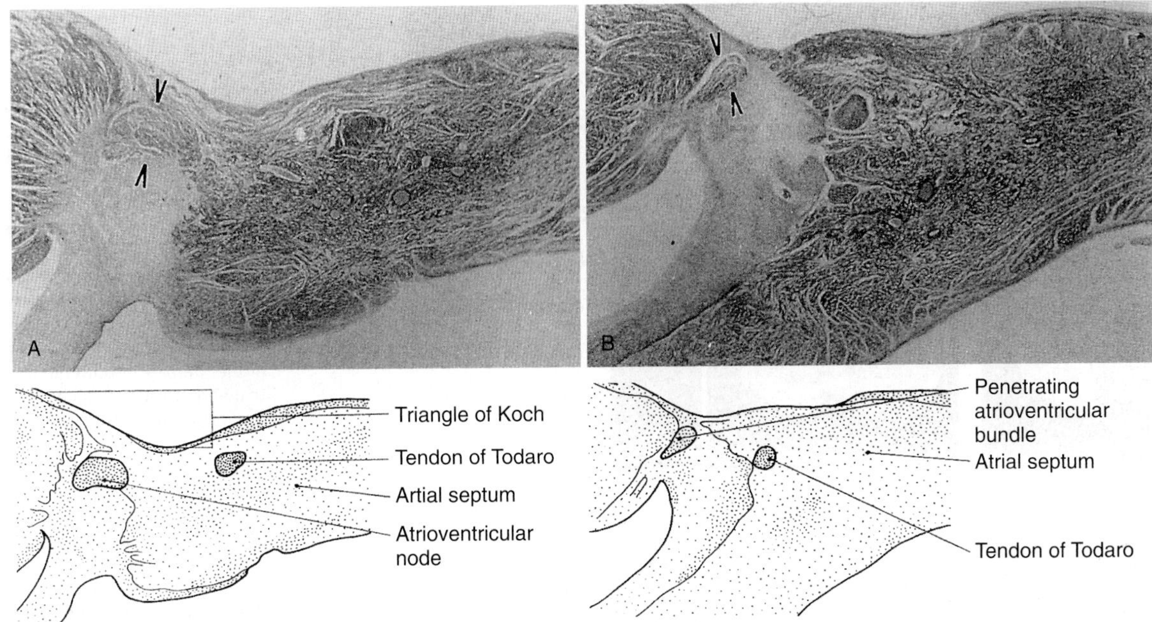

FIGURE 35-6 Sections through the AV junction show the position of the AV node (arrowheads) within the triangle of Koch **(A)** and the penetrating AV bundle of His (arrowheads) within the central fibrous body **(B)**.

Second, the action potential enters toward the beginning of the inferior nodal extension. This conduction pathway likely constitutes the slow pathway route. The action potential cannot enter the nodal tissue at other tissue points because nodal and atrial tissues are isolated from each other by a vein along this length of tissue (dark green area in Fig. 35-7B, C). From the two entry points, the action potentials propagate both anterogradely and retrogradely along the inferior nodal extension and eventually annihilate each other. The action potential entering the nodal tract via the transitional zone also propagates into the compact node and then reaches the His bundle and propagates down the left and right bundle branches. Transmembrane action potentials recorded from in situ cardiomyocytes at various locations within the nodal tract exhibit distinct shapes and time courses (Fig. 35-7D). Action potentials from extranodal atrial tissue and His bundle (locations 1 and 5, respectively, in Fig. 35-7C) have more hyperpolarized diastolic potentials and faster upstrokes than myocytes in the transitional zone (location 3) and penetrating bundle (location 4). This smaller rate of depolarization results in conduction slowing across the compact portion and penetrating bundle (conduction velocity, <10 cm/sec versus 35 cm/sec in atrial working myocardium), giving rise to AV conduction delay.

BUNDLE OF HIS (PENETRATING PORTION OF THE ATRIOVENTRICULAR BUNDLE). This structure is the continuation of the penetrating bundle on the ventricular side of the AV junction before it divides to form the left and right bundle (see Fig. 35-6A). Myocytes in the His bundle are small and connexin43 positive (see Fig. 35-7C). However, large, well-formed fasciculoventricular connections between the penetrating portion of the AV bundle and the ventricular septal crest are rarely found in adult hearts (see Chap. 39). Branches from the anterior and posterior descending coronary arteries supply the upper muscular interventricular septum with blood, which makes the conduction system at this site more impervious to ischemic damage unless the ischemia is extensive.

BUNDLE BRANCHES (BRANCHING PORTION OF THE ATRIOVENTRICULAR BUNDLE). These structures begin at the superior margin of the muscular interventricular septum, immediately beneath the membranous septum, with the cells of the left bundle branch cascading downward as a continuous sheet onto the septum beneath the noncoronary aortic cusp (**Fig. 35-8A**). The AV bundle may then give off other left bundle branches, sometimes constituting a true bifascicular system with an anterosuperior branch, in other hearts giving rise to a group of central fibers, and in still others appearing more as a network without a clear division into a fascicular system (Fig. 35-8B). The right bundle branch continues intramyocardially as an unbranched extension of the AV bundle down the right side of the interventricular septum to the apex of the right ventricle and base of the anterior papillary muscle. In some human hearts, the His bundle traverses the right interventricular crest and gives rise to a right-sided narrow stem origin of the left bundle branch. The anatomy of the left bundle branch system can be variable and not conform to a constant bifascicular division. However, the concept of a trifascicular system remains useful to both the electrocardiographer and the clinician (see Chap. 13).

TERMINAL PURKINJE FIBERS. These fibers connect with the ends of the bundle branches to form interweaving networks on the endocardial surface of both ventricles, which transmit the cardiac impulse almost simultaneously to the entire right and left ventricular endocardium. Purkinje fibers tend to be less concentrated at the base of the ventricle and at the papillary muscle tips. They penetrate the myocardium for varying distances, depending on the animal species. In humans, they apparently penetrate only the inner third of the endocardium, whereas in the pig, they almost reach the epicardium. Such variations could influence changes produced by myocardial ischemia, for example, because Purkinje fibers appear to be more resistant to ischemia than ordinary myocardial fibers are. Purkinje myocytes are found in the His bundle and bundle branches, cover much of the endocardium of both ventricles (Fig. 35-8B), and align to form multicellular bundles in longitudinal strands separated by collagen. Although conduction of the cardiac impulse appears to be their major function, free-running Purkinje fibers, sometimes called false tendons, which are composed of many Purkinje cells in a series, are capable of contraction. Action potentials propagate within thin Purkinje fiber bundles from base to apex before activation of the surrounding myocytes occurs. Purkinje myocytes largely lack transverse tubules (see Fig. 35-e1 on website), reducing membrane capacitance and thus accelerating action potential propagation.[9] Action potential propagation within the His-Purkinje system and the working myocardium is mediated by connexins. Ventricular myocytes express mainly connexin43, and Purkinje fibers express connexin40 and connexin45. The molecular identity of the connexin type that enables impulse transmission at the Purkinje fiber–myocyte junction (PMJ) is unclear. It is also still not clear how the small amount of depolarizing current provided

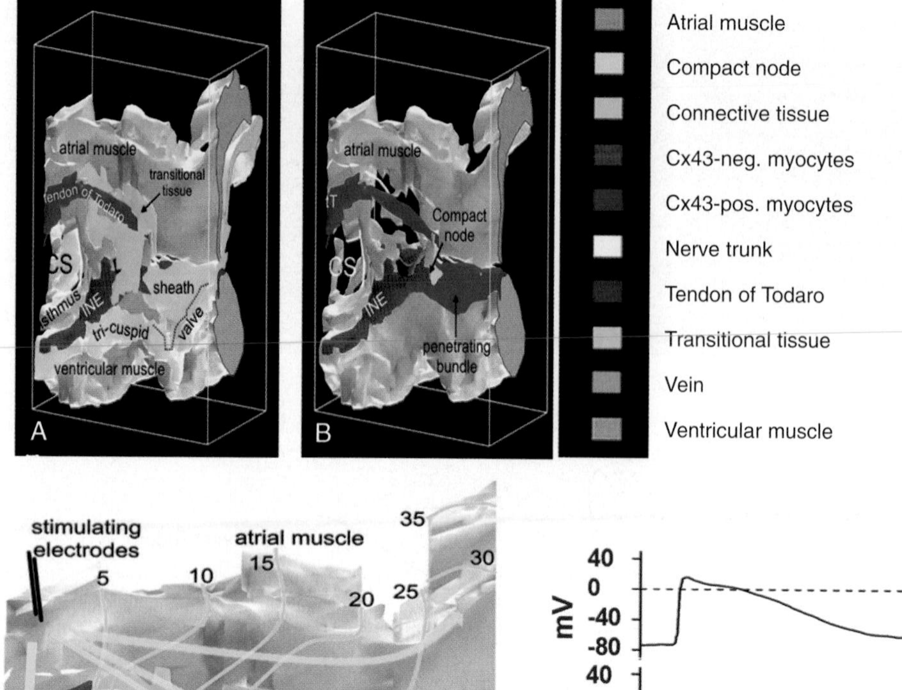

FIGURE 35-7 **A, B,** Computer three-dimensional anatomic model of the AV node as viewed from the right atrium–ventricle. **A** shows all cell types. **B** shows the model after removal of transitional and connective tissues. The inferior nodal extension (INE) is located between the coronary sinus (CS) and the tricuspid valve, the end of the INE is covered by transitional tissue, the penetrating bundle begins at the apex of the triangle of Koch (formed by the CS, tendon of Todaro [tT], and tricuspid valve), and the penetrating bundle and His bundle are covered by connective tissue ("sheath"). After removal of the transitional and connective tissues, one sees the protraction of a connexin(Cx)43-positive portion of nodal tissue into the Cx43-negative INE. The compact node is located at the junction of Cx43-negative and Cx43-positive nodal tissue. **C, D,** Structure-function relationships of the AV node. **C,** Schematic representation of the sequence of anterograde AV conduction, using a combination of mathematical modeling and experimental mapping of action potential propagation. The preparation is electrically stimulated at the crista terminalis. The activation sequence is shown as isochrones at 5-millisecond intervals. Yellow arrows delineate the conduction pathways. (See also Video 35-1 on website.) **D,** Transmembrane action potentials recorded at locations demarked by black dots in **A** (numbered 1 through 5). *(Modified from Li J, Greener ID, Inada S, et al: Computer three dimensional reconstruction of the atrioventricular node. Circ Res 102:975, 2008. By permission of the American Heart Association.)*

by the thin bundle of Purkinje fibers can activate a much larger mass of ventricular muscle (current to load mismatch).[10] It is possible that individual gap junctional channels at the PMJ are formed by more than one connexin isoform. These disparate connexin phenotypes may create specific types of hybrid channels with unique properties that ensure safe conduction at the PMJ. Because Purkinje cells have markedly longer repolarization times than surrounding myocytes (see Fig. 35-17E), these connexin hybrids could also decrease entrainment of repolarization at the PMJ and thereby increase repolarization gradients.

Innervation of the Atrioventricular Node, His Bundle, and Ventricular Myocardium

Pathways of Innervation. The AV node and His bundle region are innervated by a rich supply of cholinergic and adrenergic fibers with densities exceeding those found in the ventricular myocardium.[11] Immunolabeling with markers for sympathetic and parasympathetic nerves revealed nonuniform innervation density in the AV junctional area. For example, the inferior nodal extension has been shown to exhibit a higher density of both nerve types than the working atrial myocardium, whereas the opposite is true for the compact node.[12] Ganglia, nerve fibers, and nerve nets lie close to the AV node. Parasympathetic nerves to the AV node region enter the canine heart at the junction of the inferior vena cava and the inferior aspect of the left atrium, adjacent to the coronary sinus entrance. Nerves in direct contact with AV nodal fibers have been noted, along with agranular and granular vesicular processes, presumably representing cholinergic and adrenergic processes.

In general, autonomic neural input to the heart exhibits some degree of "sidedness," with the right sympathetic and vagal nerves affecting the sinoatrial node more than the AV node, and the left sympathetic and vagal nerves affecting the AV node more than the sinoatrial node. The distribution of the neural input to the sinoatrial and AV nodes is complex because of substantial overlapping innervation. Despite the overlap, specific branches of the vagal and sympathetic nerves can be shown to innervate certain regions preferentially. Supersensitivity to acetylcholine follows vagal denervation. Stimulation of the right stellate ganglion produces sinus tachycardia with less effect on AV nodal conduction, whereas stimulation of the left stellate ganglion generally produces a shift in the sinus pacemaker to an ectopic site and consistently shortens AV nodal conduction time and refractoriness but inconsistently speeds the sinoatrial nodal discharge rate. Stimulation of the right cervical vagus nerve primarily slows the sinoatrial nodal discharge rate, and stimulation of the left vagus primarily prolongs AV nodal conduction time and refractoriness when sidedness is present. Neither sympathetic nor vagal stimulation affects normal conduction in the His bundle. The negative dromotropic response of the heart to vagal stimulation is mediated by the activation of $I_{K(Ach,Ade)}$, which results in hyperpolarization of the AV nodal cells, thereby influencing the conductive properties of the node. The positive dromotropic effect of sympathetic stimulation arises as a consequence of increase in cytosolic cAMP levels and ensuing activation of the L-type Ca^{2+} current, $I_{Ca.L}$ (see Table 35-3).

Most efferent sympathetic impulses reach the canine ventricles over the ansae subclaviae, branches from the stellate ganglia. Sympathetic nerves then synapse primarily in the caudal cervical ganglia and form individual cardiac nerves that innervate relatively localized parts of the ventricles. The major route to the heart is the recurrent cardiac nerve on the right side and the ventrolateral cardiac nerve on the left. In general,

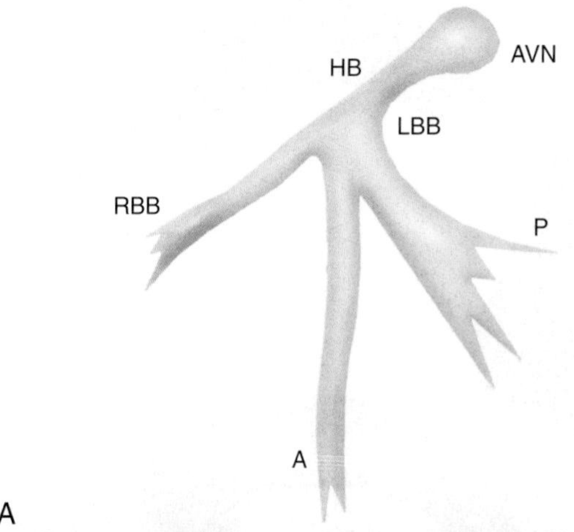

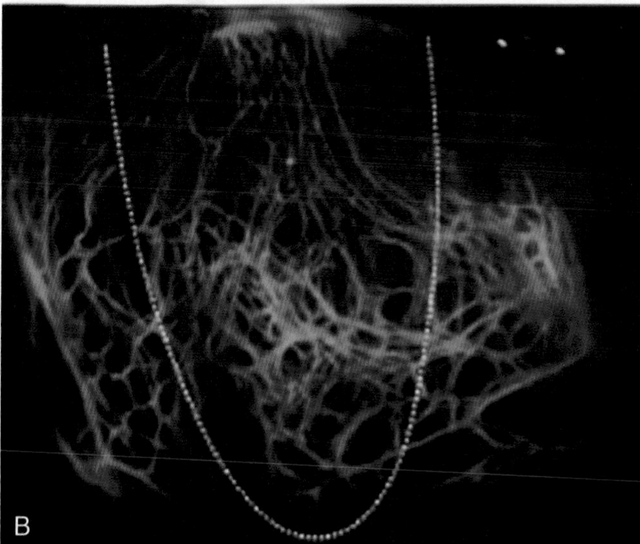

FIGURE 35-8 **A,** Schematic representation of the trifascicular bundle branch system. **B,** Structural organization of the His-Purkinje system in mouse heart. Expression of a green fluorescent protein was specifically targeted to cells of the His-Purkinje system in mice. Green fluorescent cell networks in the left ventricular chamber are shown. The left ventricular free wall (LVW) was incised from base to apex, and then the two parts of the LVW were pulled back to expose the left flank of the interventricular septum (LF). The dotted line demarcates the border between the LF and the LVW. A = anterosuperior fascicle of the left bundle branch; AVN = atrioventricular node; HB = His bundle; LBB = left bundle branch; P = posteroinferior fascicle of the left bundle branch; PF = Purkinje fiber; RBB = right bundle branch. *(**A** modified from Rosenbaum MB, Elizari MV, Lazzari JO: The Hemiblocks. Oldsmar, Fla, Tampa Tracings, 1970, cover illustration. **B** from Micquerol L, Meysen S, Mangoni M, et al: Architectural and functional asymmetry of the His-Purkinje system of the murine heart. Cardiovasc Res 63:77, 2004.)*

the right sympathetic chain shortens refractoriness primarily of the anterior portion of the ventricles, and the left affects primarily the posterior surface of the ventricles, although overlapping areas of distribution occur.

The intraventricular route of sympathetic nerves generally follows coronary arteries. Functional data have suggested that afferent and efferent sympathetic nerves travel in the superficial layers of the epicardium and dive to innervate the endocardium, and anatomic observations have supported this conclusion. Vagal fibers travel intramurally or subendocardially and rise to the epicardium at the AV groove (**Fig. 35-9**). Sympathetic nerve density in the left ventricle appears to be higher in the epicardial than in the endocardial portion of the left ventricle, which at least in part results from differential expression of cytokines during cardiac development that attract and repel, respectively, sympathetic nerve growth.[11]

Effects of Vagal Stimulation. The vagus modulates cardiac sympathetic activity at prejunctional and postjunctional sites by regulating the amount of norepinephrine released and by inhibiting cAMP-induced phosphorylation of cardiac proteins, including ion channels and calcium pumps. The latter inhibition occurs at more than one level in the series of reactions constituting the adenylate cyclase–, cAMP-dependent protein kinase system. Neuropeptides released from nerve fibers of both autonomic limbs also modulate autonomic responses. For example, NPY released from sympathetic nerve terminals inhibits cardiac vagal effects.

Tonic vagal stimulation produces a greater absolute reduction in sinoatrial rate in the presence of tonic background sympathetic stimulation, a sympathetic-parasympathetic interaction termed *accentuated antagonism*. In contrast, changes in AV conduction during concomitant sympathetic and vagal stimulation are essentially the algebraic sum of the individual AV conduction responses to tonic vagal and sympathetic stimulation alone. Cardiac responses to brief vagal bursts begin after a short latency and dissipate quickly; in contrast, cardiac responses to sympathetic stimulation commence and dissipate slowly. The rapid onset and offset of responses to vagal stimulation allow dynamic beat-to-beat vagal modulation of heart rate and AV conduction, whereas the slow temporal response to sympathetic stimulation precludes any beat-to-beat regulation by sympathetic activity. Periodic vagal bursting, as may occur each time a systolic pressure wave arrives at the baroreceptor regions in the aortic and carotid sinuses, induces phasic changes in sinus cycle length and can entrain the sinus node to discharge faster or slower at periods identical to those of the vagal burst. In a similar phasic manner, vagal bursts prolong AV nodal conduction time and are influenced by background levels of sympathetic tone. Because the peak vagal effects on sinus rate and AV nodal conduction occur at different times in the cardiac cycle, a brief vagal burst can slow the sinus rate without affecting AV nodal conduction or can prolong AV nodal conduction time and not slow the sinus rate. Bilateral but not unilateral vagal nerve stimulation increases and reverses spatial dispersion of ventricular repolarization as the direction of repolarization from apex → base in sinus rhythm shifts to base → apex. This effect is attributable to a more pronounced action potential prolongation at the apex compared with the base of the heart (see Fig. 35-e2 on website).[13]

Effects of Sympathetic Stimulation. Similar to bilateral vagal nerve stimulation, sympathetic nerve stimulation also increases and reverses spatial gradients of ventricular repolarization from apex → base in sinus rhythm to base → apex. The reversal results from a marked shortening of action potential duration at the base, with no or very little effect on the repolarization time course at the apex of the heart (see Fig. 35-e2 on website).[13] Nonuniform distribution of sympathetic nerves, and thus norepinephrine levels, may in part contribute to some of the nonuniform electrophysiologic effects because the ventricular content of norepinephrine is greater at the base than at the apex of the heart.[11] Afferent vagal activity appears to be higher in the posterior ventricular myocardium, which may account for the vagomimetic effects of inferior myocardial infarction.

The vagi exert minimal but measurable effects on ventricular tissue, decreasing the strength of myocardial contraction and prolonging refractoriness. Under some circumstances, acetylcholine can cause a positive inotropic effect. It is now clear that the vagus (acetylcholine) can exert direct effects on some types of ventricular fibers as well as indirect effects by modulating sympathetic influences.

Beyond the beat-to-beat regulation of rate and contractile force, sympathetic input to the heart, through both translational and post-translational modifications, also exerts long-term regulation of adrenergic receptor sensitivity and ionic channels. These long-term changes in autonomic responsiveness and cardiac electrical properties appear to be mediated, at least in part, by highly localized signaling cascades involving neurally released molecules, such as NPY.[14]

Arrhythmias and the Autonomic Nervous System

Alterations in vagal and sympathetic innervation (autonomic remodeling) can influence the development of arrhythmias and sudden cardiac death from ventricular tachyarrhythmias.[15] Damage to nerves extrinsic to the heart, such as the stellate ganglia, as well as to intrinsic cardiac nerves from diseases that may affect primarily nerves, such as viral infections, or from diseases that secondarily cause cardiac damage may produce cardioneuropathy. Although the mechanisms by which altered sympathetic innervation modulates cardiac electrical properties are largely unknown, spatially heterogeneous sympathetic hyperinnervation could result in enhanced dispersion of

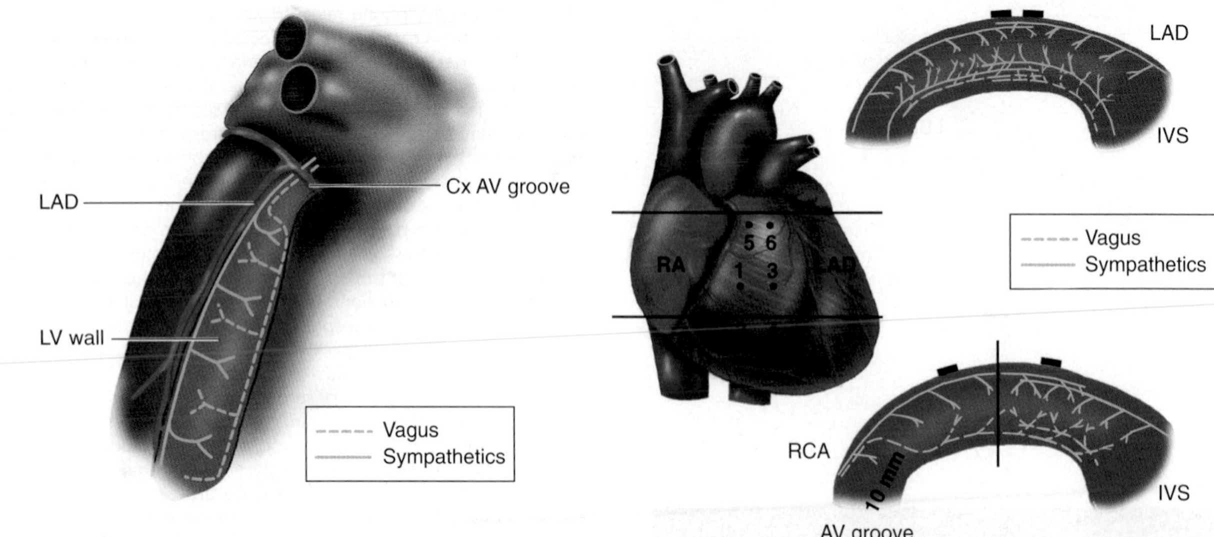

FIGURE 35-9 **Left,** Intraventricular route of sympathetic and vagal nerves to the left ventricle (LV). **Right,** Schematic of the transverse views of the right ventricular (RV) wall showing functional pathways of the efferent sympathetic and vagal nerves. **Top right,** Transverse view of the RV outflow tract at the upper horizontal line on the left. **Bottom right,** Transverse view of the anterolateral wall at the lower horizontal line on the left. The vertical solid line indicates the center of the RV anterolateral wall. Closed circles indicate positions of plunge electrodes (labeled 1 to 6). AV = atrioventricular; Cx = circumflex; IVS = interventricular septum; LAD = left anterior descending coronary artery; RA = right atrium; RCA = right coronary artery. *(From Ito M, Zipes DP: Efferent sympathetic and vagal innervation of the canine right ventricle. Circulation 90:1459, 1994. By permission of the American Heart Association.)*

myocardial excitability and refractoriness via patchy adrenergic stimulation of ionic currents, including $I_{Ca.L}$, I_{Ks}, and I_{Cl} (see Table 35-3). Sympathetic hypoinnervation has been shown to increase the sensitivity of adrenergic receptors to activation by circulating catecholamines (denervation supersensitivity).[11]

Numerous studies have suggested a primary role of altered cardiac sympathetic innervation in arrhythmogenesis. Chronic infusion of nerve growth factor (NGF) to the left stellate ganglion in dogs with chronic myocardial infarction and complete AV block caused spatially heterogeneous sympathetic cardiac hyperinnervation (nerve sprouting) and dramatically increased the incidence of sudden death from ventricular tachyarrhythmias.[15] Ambulatory long-term recordings of left stellate ganglion nerve activity in these dogs revealed that the majority of malignant ventricular arrhythmias were preceded by increased neuronal discharge, suggesting a causal role of sympathetic input in triggering arrhythmogenic sudden cardiac death.[16] A high-cholesterol diet was reported to result in cardiac sympathetic hyperinnervation in rabbits and a marked increase in the incidence of ventricular fibrillation (**Fig. 35-10A**).[17] Explanted human hearts from transplant recipients with a history of arrhythmias exhibited a significantly higher and also more heterogeneous density of sympathetic nerve fibers than those from patients without arrhythmias (Fig. 35-10B). Whether neural remodeling also involved parasympathetic nerve fibers in the heart was not examined in these studies. The junctions between pulmonary veins and left atrium are highly innervated structures. Both sympathetic and parasympathetic nerves are colocated and concentrated in "ganglionated plexi" around the pulmonary veins.[18] Selective ablation of ganglionated plexi as well as extensive regional ablation targeting anatomic areas containing ganglionated plexi has been shown to reduce the incidence of paroxysmal atrial fibrillation in both clinical and experimental studies, further supporting a causal involvement of autonomic nerve activity in atrial arrhythmogenesis.[19,20] On the other hand, spatially heterogeneous sympathetic denervation was similarly associated with an increased risk of atrial and ventricular arrhythmias. Mutations in genes encoding cardiac ion channel subunits also affect channel function in the central and peripheral autonomic nervous system, resulting in abnormal firing properties of affected neurons.[21,22] This observation may partially explain the clinical finding that sudden cardiac death in some variants of the long-QT syndrome (see Chaps. 9, 36, and 39) is typically preceded by a sympathetic arousal.

BASIC ELECTROPHYSIOLOGIC PRINCIPLES

Physiology of Ion Channels

Electrical signaling in the heart involves the passage of ions through ionic channels. The Na^+, K^+, Ca^{2+}, and Cl^- ions are the major charge carriers, and their movement across the cell membrane creates a flow of current that generates excitation and signals in cardiac myocytes. Ion channels are macromolecular pores that span the lipid bilayer of the cell membrane (**Fig. 35-11**). Conformational transitions change (gate) a single ion channel from closed to open, which allows selected ions to flow passively down the electrochemical activity gradient at a very high rate (>10^6 ions per second). The high transfer rates and restriction to "downhill" fluxes not stoichiometrically coupled to the hydrolysis of energy-rich phosphates distinguish ionic channel mechanisms from those of other ion-transporting structures, such as the sarcolemmal Na^+,K^+-adenosine triphosphatase (ATPase) or the sarcoplasmic reticular Mg^{2+},Ca^{2+}-ATPase (SERCA). Ion channels may be gated by extracellular and intracellular ligands, changes in transmembrane voltage, or mechanical stress (see Table 35-3). Gating of single ion channels can best be studied by means of the patch-clamp technique.

Ion channels are usually named after the strongest permeant ion—Na^+, K^+, Ca^{2+}, and Cl^-—but some channels are less selective or are not selective, as in gap junctional channels. Channels have also been named after neurotransmitters, as in acetylcholine-sensitive K^+ channels, $I_{K.Ach}$.

The ionic permeability ratio is a commonly used quantitative index of a channel's selectivity. It is defined as the ratio of the permeability of one ion type to that of the main permeant ion type. Permeability ratios of voltage-gated K^+ and Na^+ channels for monovalent and divalent (e.g., Ca^{2+}) cations are usually less than 1:10. Voltage-gated Ca^{2+} channels exhibit a more than 1000-fold discrimination against Na^+ and K^+ ions (e.g., P_K/P_{Ca} = 1/3000) and are impermeable to anions.

Because ions are charged, net ionic flux through an open channel is determined by both the concentration and electrical gradient across the membrane (electrodiffusion). The potential at which the passive flux of ions along the chemical driving force is exactly balanced by the electrical driving force is called the reversal or Nernst potential of the channel. In the case of a channel that is perfectly selective for one ion species, the reversal potential equals the thermodynamic equilibrium potential of that ion, E_S, which is given by the Nernst equation in the form

$$E_S = (RT/zF)\ln([S_o]/[S_i])$$

where $[S_i]$ and $[S_o]$ are the intracellular and extracellular concentrations of the permeant ion, respectively, z is the valence of the ion, R is the gas constant, F is the Faraday constant, T is the temperature (kelvin), and ln is the logarithm to the base e. At membrane voltages more positive to the reversal potential of the channel, passive ion movement is outward, whereas it is inward at membrane potentials more negative to the Nernst potential of that channel. If the current through an open channel is carried by more than one permeant ion, the reversal potential becomes a weighted mean of all Nernst potentials.

Membrane voltages during a cardiac action potential are in the range of −94 to +30 mV (see **Table 35-1**). With physiologic external K^+ (4 mM), E_K is approximately −91 mV, and passive K^+ movement during an action potential is out of the cell. On the other hand, because the calculated reversal potential of a cardiac Ca^{2+} channel is +64 mV (assuming P_K/P_{Ca} = 1/3000, K_i = 150 mM, K_o = 4 mM, Ca_i = 100 nM, Ca_o = 2 mM), passive Ca^{2+} flux is into the cell. With physiologic internal and external chloride concentrations, E_{Cl} is −83 to −36 mV, and passive movement of Cl^- ions through open chloride channels can be both inward and outward at membrane potentials typically occurring during a cardiac action potential. In more general terms, the direction and magnitude of passive ion flux through a single open channel at any given transmembrane voltage are governed by the reversal potential of that ion and its concentration on the two sides of the membrane, with the net flux being larger when ions move from the more concentrated side.

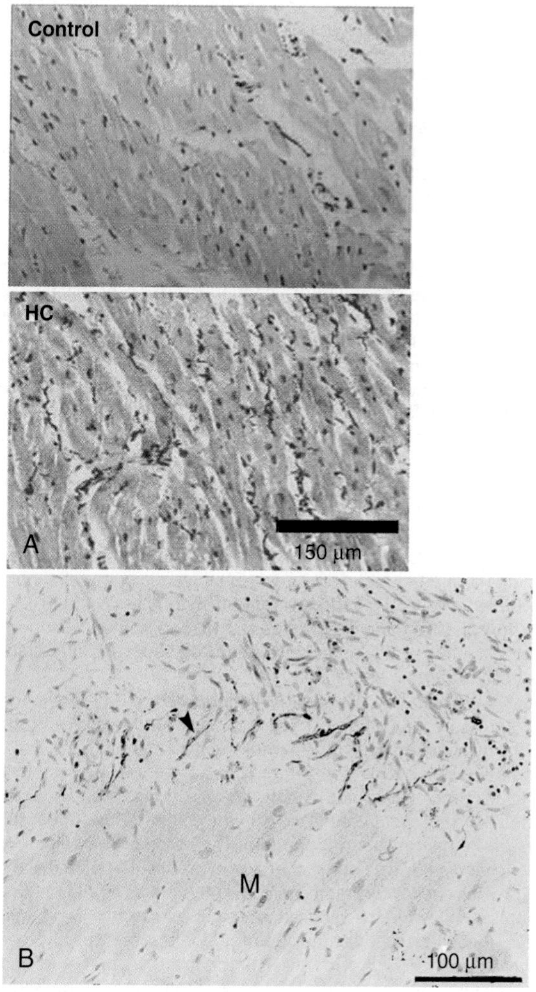

Ion Flux Through Voltage-Gated Channels. Changes in transmembrane potential determine ion flux through voltage-gated channels, not only through the voltage dependence of the electrochemical driving force on the permeant ion but also through the voltage dependence of channel activation, that is, the fraction of time that a channel permits ions to permeate is determined by the membrane voltage. If the probability of a channel's being activated (i.e., the open-state probability of that channel) exhibits voltage dependence, as is the case with the fast Na^+ channel or voltage-dependent K^+ channels in cardiac myocytes, activation increases with membrane depolarization. Note that channels do not have a sharp voltage threshold for opening. The dependence of channel activation on membrane potential is rather a continuous function of voltage and follows a sigmoidal curve (**Fig. 35-12**, green curve). The potential at which activation is half-maximal and the steepness of

FIGURE 35-10 Sympathetic neural remodeling in diseased heart. **A,** Left ventricular myocardium exhibiting normal **(upper panel)** and increased sympathetic nerve density (red). Sections were obtained from a control rabbit (Control) and a rabbit with experimentally induced hypercholesterolemia (HC). *(From Liu Y, Lee Y, Pak H, et al: Effects of simvastatin on cardiac neural and electrophysiologic remodeling in rabbits with hypercholesterolemia. Heart Rhythm 6:69, 2009.)* **B,** Regional hyperinnervation (arrowhead) at the junction between necrotic and normal, surviving myocardium (M) in a patient with cardiomyopathy and ventricular tachyarrhythmias. *(From Cao J, Fishbein MC, Han JB, et al: Relationship between regional cardiac hyperinnervation and ventricular arrhythmia. Circulation 101:1960, 2000. By permission of the American Heart Association.)*

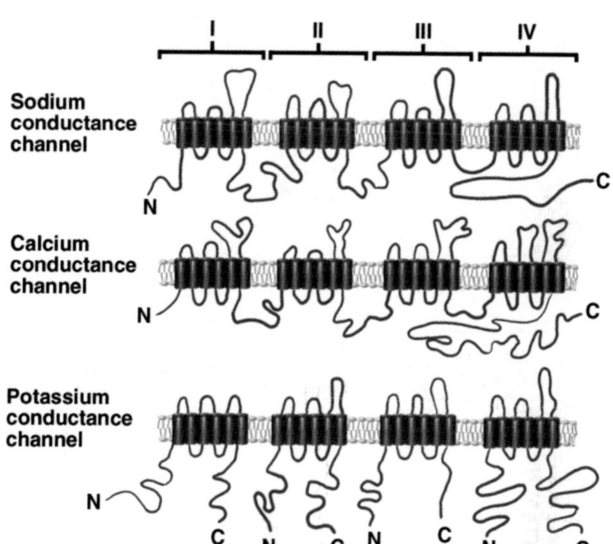

FIGURE 35-11 Structure of ion channels. Voltage-gated Na^+ and Ca^{2+} channels are composed of a single tetramer consisting of four covalently linked repeats of the six transmembrane-spanning motifs, whereas voltage-gated K^+ channels are composed of four separate subunits, each containing a single six transmembrane-spanning motif. Inwardly rectifying K^+ channels are formed by inward rectifier K^+ channel pore-forming (alpha) subunits. In contrast to voltage-gated K^+ channel alpha subunits, the Kir alpha subunits have only two (not six) transmembrane domains. *(Modified from Katz AM: Molecular biology in cardiology, a paradigmatic shift. J Mol Cell Cardiol 20:355, 1988; and from Shivkumar K, Weiss JN: Adenosine triphosphate–sensitive potassium channels.* In *Zipes DP, Jalife J [eds]: Cardiac Electrophysiology: From Cell to Bedside. Philadelphia, WB Saunders, 1999, pp 86-93.)*

TABLE 35-1 Intracellular and Extracellular Ion Concentrations in Cardiac Muscle

ION	EXTRACELLULAR CONCENTRATION	INTRACELLULAR CONCENTRATION	RATIO OF EXTRACELLULAR TO INTRACELLULAR CONCENTRATION	E_I (MV)
Na^+	145 mM	15 mM	9.7	+60
K^+	4 mM	150 mM	0.027	−94
Cl^-	120 mM	5-30 mM	4-24	−83 to −36
Ca^{2+}	2 mM	10^{-7} M	2×10^4	+129

Although intracellular Ca^{2+} content is about 2 mM, most of this Ca^{2+} is bound or sequestered in intracellular organelles (mitochondria and sarcoplasmic reticulum).

E_I = equilibrium potential for a particular ion at 37°C.

Modified from Sperelakis N: Origin of the cardiac resting potential. *In* Berne RM, Sperelakis N, Geiger SR (eds): Handbook of Physiology: The Cardiovascular System. Bethesda, Md, American Physiological Society, 1979, p 193.

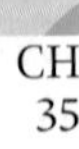

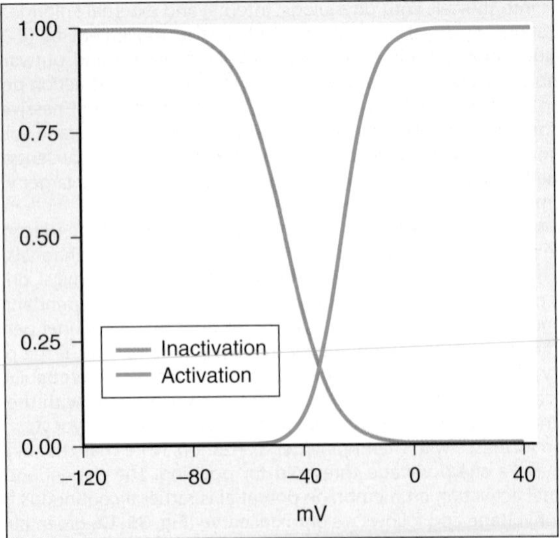

FIGURE 35-12 Voltage dependence of fast Na^+ current steady-state activation (blue) and steady-state inactivation (gold). Fractional activation and inactivation (*y* axis) are plotted as a function of membrane potential. The inactivation and activation curves overlap within a voltage range from ~−60 to ~0 mV, demarcating the voltage range of the noninactivating Na^+ window current.

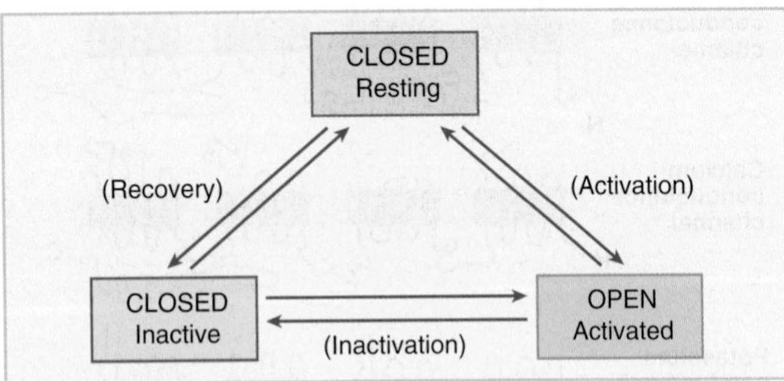

FIGURE 35-13 Simplest scheme for gating of voltage-gated ion channels.

the activation curve determine the channel's activity during changes in membrane potential. Shifting the activation curve to potentials positive to the midpoint of activation and reducing the steepness of the channel's activation curve are two possible mechanisms by which ion channel blockers can inhibit ion channel activity.

As indicated in **Figure 35-13**, open channels enter a nonconducting conformation after a depolarizing change in membrane potential, a process termed *inactivation.* If membrane depolarization persists, the channel remains inactivated and cannot reopen. This steady-state inactivation increases with membrane depolarization in a sigmoidal fashion (Fig. 35-12, red curve). Inactivation curves of the various voltage-gated ion channel types in the heart differ in their slopes and midpoints of inactivation. For example, sustained cardiomyocyte membrane depolarization to −50 mV (as may occur in acutely ischemic myocardium) causes almost complete inactivation of the fast, voltage-gated Na^+ channel (Fig. 35-12, red curve), whereas the L-type Ca^{2+} channel exhibits only little inactivation at this membrane potential. Activation and inactivation curves can overlap, in which case a steady-state or noninactivating current flows. The existence of such a "window" current has been verified for both the voltage-gated Na^+ current[23] and the L-type Ca^{2+} current. The L-type Ca^{2+} current and the fast Na^+ window current have been implicated in the genesis of triggered activity arising from early and delayed afterdepolarizations.[24]

Channels recover from inactivation and then enter the closed state, from which they can be reactivated (see Fig. 35-13). Rates of recovery from inactivation vary among the different types of voltage-dependent channels and usually follow monoexponential or multiexponential time courses, with the longest time constants ranging from a few milliseconds, for example, as for the fast sodium channel, to several seconds, as for some subtypes of K^+ channels (see Table 35-3). Together, the activity of voltage-dependent ion channels in cardiomyocytes over the course of an action potential is tightly regulated by the orchestrated interplay of a number of time- and voltage-dependent gating mechanisms, including activation, inactivation, and recovery from inactivation. All these mechanisms represent potential targets for pharmacologic interventions.

PRINCIPLES OF IONIC CURRENT MODULATION. The whole-cell current amplitude, I, is the product of the number of functional channels in the membrane available for opening (N), the probability that a channel will open (P_o), and the single-channel current amplitude (i), or $I = N \cdot P_o \cdot i$. Modulation of current amplitudes in single cardiomyocytes therefore results from alterations in N, P_o, i, or any combination of these. Changes in the number of available channels in the cell membrane may result from changes in the expression of ion channel–encoding genes. The magnitude of the single-channel current amplitude is dependent, among other factors, on the ionic concentration gradient across the membrane. For example, an increase in the extracellular Ca^{2+} concentration increases current through a single Ca^{2+} channel. Changes in channel activation can result from phosphorylation or dephosphorylation of the channel protein by second messenger–mediated activation of protein kinases and protein phosphatases, respectively. Channel phosphorylation or dephosphorylation causes a shift in the membrane potential dependence of a channel's activation or availability curve, or both, or modification of the sensitivity of channel activation or inactivation to changes in membrane potential. For example, Ca^{2+}/calmodulin kinase II–mediated phosphorylation shifts the activation curve of the cardiac sodium current to more negative potentials.[25]

MOLECULAR STRUCTURE OF ION CHANNELS. Electrophysiologic studies have detailed the functional properties of Na^+, Ca^{2+}, and K^+ currents in cardiomyocytes, and molecular cloning has revealed a large number of pore-forming (alpha) and auxiliary (beta, delta, and gamma) subunits thought to contribute to the formation of the cell surface ion channels. These studies have demonstrated that distinct molecular entities give rise to the various cardiac ion channels and shape the myocardial action potential. It has also been demonstrated that mutations in the genes encoding subunits underlying functional cardiac ion channels are responsible for several inherited cardiac arrhythmias (see Chap. 9).[26] The expression and functional properties of myocardial ion channels also change in a number of acquired disease states, and these alterations can predispose to cardiac arrhythmias.[27,28]

VOLTAGE-GATED NA^+ CHANNELS. Voltage-gated Na^+ (Nav) channel pore-forming (alpha) subunits have four homologous domains (I to IV), each of which contains six transmembrane–spanning regions, and these four domains come together to form the Na^+ permeable pore (see Fig. 35-11).[29] Among the multiple Nav alpha subunits, Nav1.5 (which is encoded by the *SCN5A* gene) is the prominent Nav alpha subunit expressed in mammalian myocardium. The name of the voltage-gated sodium channel consists of the chemical symbol of the principal permeating ion (Na), and v indicates its principal physiologic regulator (voltage). The number following the v indicates the gene subfamily (Nav1), and the number following the decimal point identifies the specific channel isoform (e.g., Nav1.1). An identical nomenclature applies to voltage-gated calcium and potassium channels. Mutations in the sequence linking domains III and IV in *SCN5A,* associated with the LQT3 syndrome (see Chap. 9), disrupt Nav channel inactivation, which gives rise to a sustained inward Na^+ current during the plateau phase of the action potential and to action potential prolongation. Cases of sudden infant death syndrome (SIDS) in African Americans have been linked to a polymorphism in the *SCN5A* gene, encoding a variant cardiac sodium channel with diminished channel inactivation in the presence of lowered intracellular pH.[30] Mutations in *SCN5A* are also linked to Brugada syndrome. Brugada syndrome mutations result in reduced Nav current amplitude, which leads to slowing of phase 0 action potential upstroke, reduced action potential amplitude, and altered phase 1 repolarization (see Chap. 9).

Nav1.5 pore-forming alpha subunits coassemble with one to two auxiliary Nav beta subunits to form functional cell surface Nav channels in cardiomyocytes. Nav beta subunits appear to play an important role in anchoring ion channel proteins to the outer cell membrane.

VOLTAGE-GATED CA^{2+} CHANNELS. Like Nav channels, cardiac voltage-gated Ca^{2+} (Cav) channels are assemblies of a pore-forming alpha subunit and auxiliary Cav beta or Cav $alpha_2$-delta subunits (see Fig. 35-11).[28] Among the various alpha subunits, Cav1.2 encoded by the *CACNA1C* gene is the prominent Cav alpha subunit expressed in mammalian myocardium. Cav1.2 channels exhibit many of the time- and voltage-dependent properties and pharmacologic sensitivities of cardiac L-type Ca^{2+} currents (see Table 35-3). Accessory subunits modulate the functional properties of Cav channels.

Cav3.1/$alpha_{1G}$ alpha subunits form a Ca^{2+}-selective channel with time- and voltage-dependent characteristics and pharmacologic sensitivities that resemble those of the low-voltage activated T-type Ca^{2+}

channel. Disruption of the gene encoding Cav3.1/alpha$_{1G}$ alpha subunits (*CACNA1G*) in mice has been demonstrated to slow sinus node rate and AV conduction consistent with its role in sinoatrial and AV node function.[31]

Voltage-Gated K$^+$ Channels. Voltage-gated K$^+$ channels (Kv) are composed of four *separate* pore-forming (alpha) subunits, each containing six regions (S1 through S6) of hydrophobic amino acids that are thought to form membrane-spanning domains (see Fig. 35-11).[29] Kv alpha subunits expressed in the human heart include members of the Kv1, Kv4, hERG, and KvLQT subfamilies. In addition, Kv channel alpha subunit proteins interact with Kv channel accessory subunits, including minK, KiChIP2, and MiRP1 (see Table 35-3), to form functional cell surface channels with distinct time- and voltage-dependent properties. Coassembly of the Kv4.3 alpha subunits and the accessory subunit KChIP2 gives rise to the cardiac transient outward Kv channel, I_{to}. ERG1 alpha subunits, together with MiRP1 accessory subunits, contribute to the generation of functional cardiac I_{Kr} channels. Mutations in the gene encoding ERG1 (*KCNH2*) have been shown to underlie the congenital LQT2 syndrome. These LQT2 syndrome mutations are loss of function mutations and lead to reduced functional I_{Kr} channel expression or to alterations in channel processing or trafficking.[32]

KvLQT1 alpha subunits associate with minK accessory subunits to form functional channels that resemble slowly activating, noninactivating K$^+$ currents, referred to as I_{Ks}, in human myocardium. Mutations in the minK-encoding gene, *KCNE1,* are associated with the LQT5 syndrome. Mutations in the gene encoding KvLQT1 alpha subunits, *KCNQ1,* have been linked to the LQT1 syndrome. These mutations are all loss-of-function mutations, resulting in reduced expression of functional I_{Ks} channels in the outer membrane.

Kv1.5 alpha subunits contribute to K$^+$-selective channels with time- and voltage-dependent characteristics that resemble the rapidly activating and slowly inactivating I_{Kur} in human atrial myocytes. I_{Kur} densities are markedly downregulated in atria of patients with chronic atrial fibrillation.

Small-conductance, Ca^{2+}-sensitive K$^+$ channels are tetrameric assemblies of SK alpha subunits and underlie a Ca^{2+}-activated K$^+$ current, $I_{K.Ca}$, in human cardiomyocytes.[33]

Inwardly Rectifying Cardiac K$^+$ (Kir) Channels. Kir channels in cardiac myocytes, as in other cells, conduct inward current at membrane potentials negative to E_K and smaller outward currents at membrane potentials positive to E_K. The activity of Kir channels is a function of both the membrane potential and the extracellular K$^+$ concentration ($[K^+]_o$). As $[K^+]_o$ changes, the channel conducts inward current at potentials negative to the new E_K while a small outward current within a certain potential range positive to the new E_K remains. Inwardly rectifying K$^+$ channels are formed by inward rectifier K$^+$ channel pore-forming alpha subunits (see Fig. 35-11). In contrast to Kv alpha subunits, Kir alpha subunits have only two (not six) transmembrane domains (see Fig. 35-11). Molecular studies have provided direct evidence that alpha subunits of the Kir2 subfamily (Kir2.1 and Kir2.2) encode the strongly inwardly rectifying Kir channel I_{K1} in cardiomyocytes.

In cardiomyocytes, Kir6.2 alpha subunits assemble with sulfonylurea receptor proteins to form K$^+$-selective sarcolemmal $I_{K.ATP}$ channels. $I_{K.ATP}$ channels are thought to play a pivotal role in myocardial ischemia and preconditioning. For example, opening of cardiac sarcolemmal $I_{K.ATP}$ channels underlies electrocardiographic ST-segment elevation during acute myocardial ischemia. Drugs such as nicorandil and diazoxide open ATP-sensitive K$^+$ channels, whereas sulfonylurea compounds (such as glibenclamide) inhibit the activity of $I_{K.ATP}$.

The molecular basis of the acetylcholine-activated K$^+$ channel, $I_{K.Ach}$, is a heteromultimer of two inwardly rectifying potassium channel subunits, Kir3.1 and Kir3.4. Stimulation of $I_{K.Ach}$ by vagally secreted acetylcholine decreases spontaneous depolarization in the sinoatrial node and slows the velocity of conduction in the AV node. Adenosine, through type 1 purinergic receptor–mediated G protein activation, also increases $I_{K.Ach}$ activity in atrial, sinoatrial node, and AV node cells, thus making this compound a treatment of choice for AV reentry tachycardia.

Cardiac Pacemaker Channel. The channels underlying the pacemaker ("funny") current, I_f, of sinoatrial myocytes are encoded by the hyperpolarization-activated, cyclic nucleotide–gated (HCN) channel gene family. Of the four known HCN pore-forming alpha subunits, HCN4 is the most highly expressed in the mammalian myocardium.[34] A mutation in the human *HCN4* gene has been linked to familial sinus bradycardia.[35]

Intercalated Discs

Another family of ion channel proteins is that containing the gap junctional channels. These dodecameric channels are found in the intercalated discs between adjacent cells. Three types of specialized junctions make up each intercalated disc. The macula adherens or desmosome and fascia adherens form areas of strong adhesion between cells and may provide a linkage for the transfer of mechanical energy from one cell to the next. The nexus, also called the tight or gap junction, is a region in the intercalated disc where cells are in functional contact with each other. Membranes at these junctions are separated by only about 10 to 20 Å and are connected by a series of hexagonally packed subunit bridges. Gap junctions provide biochemical and low-resistance electrical coupling between adjacent cells by establishing aqueous pores that directly link the cytoplasm of these adjacent cells. Gap junctions allow movement of ions (e.g., Na$^+$, Cl$^-$, K$^+$, Ca^{2+}) and small molecules (e.g., cAMP, cGMP, IP_3) between cells, thereby linking the interiors of adjacent cells.

Gap junctions permit a multicellular structure such as the heart to function electrically like an orderly, synchronized, interconnected unit and are probably responsible in part for the fact that conduction in the myocardium is anisotropic; that is, its anatomic and biophysical properties vary according to the direction in which they are measured. Usually, conduction velocity is two to three times faster longitudinally, in the direction of the long axis of the fiber, than it is transversely, in the direction perpendicular to this long axis.[36] Resistivity is lower longitudinally than transversely. Interestingly, the safety factor for propagation is greater transversely than horizontally. The safety factor for conduction determines the success of action potential propagation and has been defined as the ratio of electrical charge that is generated to charge that is consumed during the excitation cycle of a single myocyte in tissue.[36] Conduction delay or block occurs more commonly in the longitudinal direction than it does transversely. Cardiac conduction is discontinuous because of resistive discontinuities created by the gap junctions, which have an anisotropic distribution on the cell surface.[36] Because of anisotropy, propagation is discontinuous and can be a cause of reentry.

Gap junctions also provide "biochemical coupling," which permits cell-to-cell movement of ATP (or other high-energy phosphates), cyclic nucleotides, and inositol triphosphate (IP_3, the activator of the IP_3-sensitive SR Ca^{2+} release channel),[37] demonstrating that diffusion of second-messenger substances through gap junctional channels constitutes a mechanism enabling coordinated responses of the myocardial syncytium to physiologic stimuli.

Gap junctions can also change their electrical resistance. When the intracellular calcium level rises, as in myocardial infarction, the gap junction may close to help seal off the effects of injured from noninjured cells. Acidosis increases and alkalosis decreases gap junctional resistance. Increased gap junctional resistance tends to slow the rate of action potential propagation, a condition that could lead to conduction delay or block. Cardiac-restricted inactivation of gap junctions decreases transverse conduction velocity to a greater degree than longitudinal conduction, resulting in an increased anisotropic ratio that may play a role in premature sudden death from ventricular arrhythmias.[38]

Connexins are the proteins that form the intercellular channels of gap junctions. An individual channel is created by two hemichannels (connexons), each located in the plasma membrane of adjacent cells and composed of six integral membrane protein subunits (connexins). The hemichannels surround an aqueous pore and thereby create a transmembrane channel (**Fig. 35-14**). Connexin43, a 43-kDa polypeptide, is the most abundant cardiac connexin, with connexin40 and connexin45 found in smaller amounts. Ventricular muscle expresses connexin43 and connexin45, whereas atrial muscle and components of the specialized conduction system express connexin43, connexin45, and connexin40. Expression of connexin30.2 appears to be confined to the cardiac conduction system.[39] Individual cardiac connexins form gap junctional channels with characteristic unitary conductances, voltage sensitivities, and permeabilities. Tissue-specific connexin expression and spatial distribution of gap junctions determine the disparate conduction properties of cardiac tissue (see Fig. 35-7). The functional diversity of cardiac gap junctions is further enhanced by the ability of different connexin isoforms to form hybrid gap junctional channels with unique electrophysiologic properties. These channel chimeras appear to have a major function in controlling impulse transmission at the sinoatrial node–atrium border, the atrium–AV node transitional zone, and the Purkinje-myocyte border.[3]

Alterations in distribution and function of cardiac gap junctions are associated with increased susceptibility to arrhythmias. Conduction slowing and arrhythmogenesis have been associated with redistribution of connexin43 gap junctions from the end of the cardiomyocytes to the lateral borders and with decreased phosphorylation of connexin43 in a dog model of nonischemic dilated cardiomyopathy.[40,41] Adult mice genetically engineered to express progressively decreasing levels of cardiac connexin43 exhibited increased susceptibility to the induction of

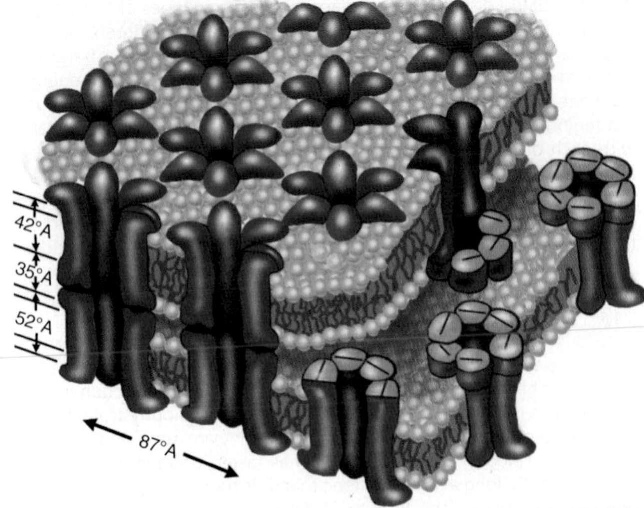

FIGURE 35-14 Model of the structure of a gap junction based on results of x-ray diffraction studies. Individual channels are composed of paired hexamers that travel in the membranes of adjacent cells and adjoin in the extracellular gap to form an aqueous pore that provides continuity of the cytoplasm of the two cells. *(From Saffitz JE: Cell-to-cell communication in the heart. Cardiol Rev 3:86, 1995.)*

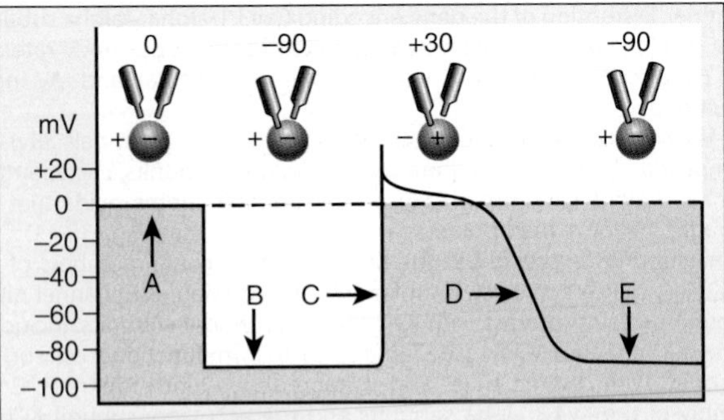

FIGURE 35-15 Demonstration of action potentials recorded during impalement of a cardiac cell. **Upper row,** Shown are a cell (circle), two microelectrodes, and stages during impalement of the cell and its activation and recovery. Both microelectrodes are extracellular (A), and no difference in potential exists between them (0 potential). The environment inside the cell is negative and the outside is positive because the cell is polarized. One microelectrode has pierced the cell membrane (B) to record the intracellular resting membrane potential, which is −90 mV with respect to the outside of the cell. The cell has depolarized (C), and the upstroke of the action potential is recorded. At its peak voltage, the inside of the cell is about +30 mV with respect to the outside of the cell. The repolarization phase (D) is shown, with the membrane returning to its former resting potential (E). *(From Cranefield PF: The Conduction of the Cardiac Impulse. Mount Kisco, NY, Futura, 1975.)*

fatal tachyarrhythmias.[42,43] Side-to-side electrical coupling between cardiomyocytes from the epicardial border zone of healing infarcts has been shown to be reduced, exaggerating anisotropy and facilitating reentrant activity.[44] Finally, a rare single nucleotide polymorphism in the atrial-specific connexin40 gene has been found to increase the risk of idiopathic atrial fibrillation.[45] Studies have suggested that normal electrical coupling of cardiomyocytes via gap junctions depends on normal mechanical coupling via cell-cell adhesion junctions.[46] A defect in cell-cell adhesion or a discontinuity in the linkage between intercellular junctions and the cytoskeleton prevents normal localization of connexins in gap junctions, which in turn could contribute to sudden death from tachyarrhythmias. For example, Carvajal syndrome is caused by recessive mutation in desmoplakin, a protein that links desmosomal adhesion molecules to desmin, a filament protein of the cardiomyocyte cytoskeleton.[47] Naxos disease is caused by a recessive mutation in plakoglobin, a protein that connects N-cadherins to actin and desmosomal cadherins to desmin.[48] Approximately 70% of the mutations linked to familial arrhythmogenic right ventricular cardiomyopathy are in the gene encoding the desmosomal protein plakophilin2. Recent experiments have demonstrated that loss of plakophilin2 expression leads to redistribution of connexin43 to the intracellular space of cardiomyocytes, loss of gap junction plaques, and reduced functional coupling between cells.[49] Further demonstration of the important role of other adhesion proteins in stabilizing gap junctions comes from a study wherein conditional loss of N-cadherin expression in mouse hearts resulted in a decrease in connexin43 gap junctions and changes in conduction velocity with concomitant increase in arrhythmogenicity (see Fig. 35-e3 on website).[50]

Phases of the Cardiac Action Potential

The cardiac transmembrane action potential consists of five phases: phase 0, upstroke or rapid depolarization; phase 1, early rapid repolarization; phase 2, plateau; phase 3, final rapid repolarization; and phase 4, resting membrane potential and diastolic depolarization (**Figs. 35-15 and 35-16**). These phases are the result of passive ion fluxes moving down electrochemical gradients established by active ion pumps and exchange mechanisms. Each ion moves primarily through its own ion-specific channel. The following discussion explains the electrogenesis of each of these phases.

General Considerations

Ionic fluxes regulate membrane potential in cardiac myocytes in the following fashion. When only one type of ion channel opens, assuming that this channel is perfectly selective for that ion, the membrane potential of the entire cell would equal the Nernst potential of that ion. Solving the Nernst equation for the four major ions across the plasma membrane,

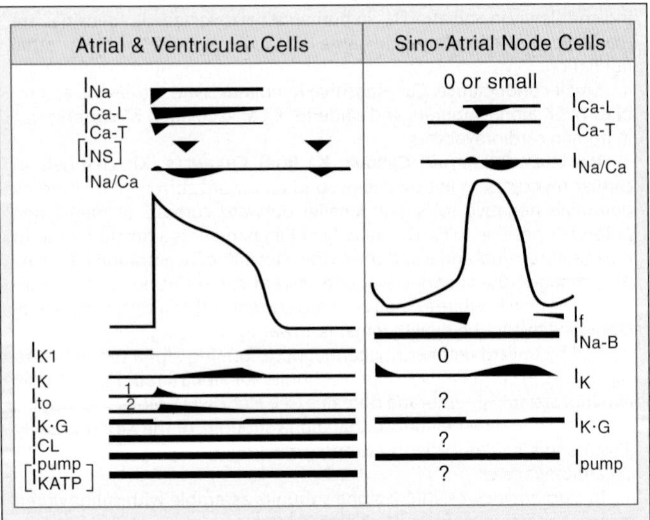

FIGURE 35-16 Currents and channels involved in generating resting and action potentials. The time course of a stylized action potential of atrial and ventricular cells is shown on the left, and that of sinoatrial node cells is on the right. Above and below are the various channels and pumps that contribute the currents underlying the electrical events. See Table 35-3 for identification of the symbols and description of the channels or currents. Where possible, the approximate time courses of the currents associated with the channels or pumps are shown symbolically, without trying to represent their magnitudes relative to each other. I_K incorporates at least two currents, I_{Kr} and I_{Ks}. There appears to be an ultrarapid component as well, designated I_{Kur}. The heavy bars for I_{CL}, I_{pump}, and I_{KATP} indicate only the presence of these channels or pump without implying magnitude of currents because that would vary with physiologic and pathophysiologic conditions. The channels identified by brackets (I_{NS} and I_{KATP}) are active only under pathologic conditions. I_{NS} may represent a swelling-activated cation current. For the sinoatrial node cells, I_{NS} and I_{K1} are small or absent. Question marks indicate that experimental evidence is not yet available to determine the presence of these channels in sinoatrial cell membranes. Although it is likely that other ionic current mechanisms exist, they are not shown here because their roles in electrogenesis are not sufficiently well defined. *(From Members of the Sicilian Gambit: Antiarrhythmic Therapy: A Pathophysiologic Approach. Mount Kisco, NY, Futura, 1994, p 13.)*

TABLE 35-2 Properties of Transmembrane Potentials in Mammalian Hearts

PROPERTY	SINUS NODAL CELL	ATRIAL MUSCLE CELL	AV NODAL CELL	PURKINJE FIBER	VENTRICULAR MUSCLE CELL
Resting potential (mV)	−50 to −60	−80 to −90	−60 to −70	−90 to −95	−80 to −90
Action potential					
Amplitude (mV)	60-70	110-120	70-80	120	110-120
Overshoot (mV)	0-10	30	5-15	30	30
Duration (msec)	100-300	100-300	100-300	300-500	200-300
$\dot{V}max$ (V/sec)	1-10	100-200	5-15	500-700	100-200
Propagation velocity (m/sec)	<0.05	0.3-0.4	0.1	2-3	0.3-0.4
Fiber diameter (μm)	5-10	10-15	1-10	100	10-16

$\dot{V}max$ = maximal rise of membrane potential.

Modified from Sperelakis N: Origin of the cardiac resting potential. *In* Berne RM, Sperelakis N, Geiger SR (eds): Handbook of Physiology: The Cardiovascular System. Bethesda, Md, American Physiological Society, 1979, p 190.

the following equilibrium potentials are obtained: sodium, +60 mV; potassium, −94 mV; calcium, +129 mV; and chloride, −83 to −36 mV (Table 35-1). Therefore, if a single K^+-selective channel opens, such as the inwardly rectifying K^+ channel, the membrane potential approaches E_K (−94 mV). If a single Na^+-selective channel opens, the transmembrane potential becomes E_{Na} (+60 mV). A quiescent cardiac myocyte (phase 4) has many more open potassium than sodium channels, and the cell's transmembrane potential is close to E_K (**Table 35-2**). When two or more types of ion channel open simultaneously, each type tries to make the membrane potential go to the equilibrium potential of that channel. The contribution of each ion type to the overall membrane potential at any given moment is determined by the instantaneous permeability of the plasma membrane to that ion. For example, deviation of the measured resting membrane potential from E_K (see Table 35-1) would predict that other ion types with equilibrium potentials positive to E_K contribute to the resting membrane potential in cardiac myocytes. If it is assumed that Na^+, K^+, and Cl^- are the permeant ions at resting potential, their individual contributions to the resting membrane potential V can be quantified by the GHK *voltage* equation of the form

$$V=(RT/F)\ln[(P_K[K]_o+P_{Na}[Na]_o+P_{Cl}[Cl]_i)/(P_K[K]_i+P_{Na}[Na]P_{Cl}[Cl]_o)]$$

where the symbols have the meanings outlined previously. With only one permeant ion, V becomes the Nernst potential for that ion. With several permeant ion types, V is a weighted mean of all the Nernst potentials.

Intracellular electrical activity can be recorded by inserting a glass microelectrode filled with an electrolyte solution and with a tip diameter smaller than 0.5 μm into a single cell. The electrode produces minimal damage, its entry point apparently being sealed by the cell. The transmembrane potential is recorded by using this electrode in reference to an extracellular ground electrode placed in the tissue bath near the cell membrane and represents the potential difference between intracellular and extracellular voltage (see Fig. 35-15). Alternatively, the patch-clamp technique in current clamp mode can be used to measure transmembrane potentials.

Phase 4: The Resting Membrane Potential

The intracellular potential during electrical quiescence in diastole is −50 to −95 mV, depending on the cell type (see Table 35-2). Therefore, the inside of the cell is 50 to 95 mV negative relative to the outside of the cell because of the distribution of ions such as K^+, Na^+, and Cl^-.

Because cardiac myocytes have an abundance of open K^+ channels at rest, the cardiac transmembrane potential (in phase 4) is close to E_K. Potassium outward current through open, inwardly rectifying K^+ channels, I_{K1}, mainly contributes to the resting membrane potential in atrial and ventricular myocytes, as well as in Purkinje cells, under normal conditions. Deviation of the resting membrane potential from E_K is the result of movement of monovalent ions with an equilibrium potential greater than the E_K, for example, Cl^- efflux through activated chloride channels, such as $I_{Cl.cAMP}$, $I_{Cl.Ca}$, and $I_{Cl.swell}$. Calcium does not contribute directly to the resting membrane potential, but changes in intracellular free calcium concentration can affect other membrane conductance values. For example, an increase in SR Ca^{2+} load can cause spontaneous intracellular Ca^{2+} waves, which in turn activate the Ca^{2+}-dependent chloride conductance $I_{Cl.Ca}$ and thereby lead to spontaneous transient inward currents and concomitant membrane depolarization.[51] Increases in $[Ca^{2+}]_i$ can also stimulate the Na^+/Ca^{2+} exchanger $I_{Na/Ca}$. This protein exchanges three Na^+ ions for one Ca^{2+} ion; the direction is dependent on the sodium and calcium concentrations on the two sides of the membrane and the transmembrane potential difference. At resting membrane potential and during a spontaneous SR Ca^{2+} release event, this exchanger would generate a net Na^+ influx, possibly causing transient membrane depolarizations (see Fig. 35-22).[50] $[Ca^{2+}]_i$ has also been shown to activate I_{K1} in cardiac myocytes, thereby indirectly contributing to cardiac resting membrane potential.[50] Because of the Na-K pump, which pumps Na^+ out of the cell against its electrochemical gradient and simultaneously pumps K^+ into the cell against its chemical gradient, the intracellular K^+ concentration remains high and the intracellular Na^+ concentration remains low. This pump, fueled by an Na^+,K^+-ATPase enzyme that hydrolyzes ATP for energy, is bound to the membrane. It requires both Na^+ and K^+ to function and can transport three Na^+ ions outward for two K^+ ions inward. Therefore, the pump can be electrogenic and generate a net outward movement of positive charges. The rate of Na^+-K^+ pumping to maintain the same ionic gradients must increase as the heart rate increases because the cell gains a slight amount of Na^+ and loses a slight amount of K^+ with each depolarization. Cardiac glycoside–induced block of the Na^+,K^+-ATPase increases contractility through an increase in intracellular Na^+ concentration, which in turn reduces Ca^{2+} extrusion through the Na^+/Ca^{2+} exchanger (see later), ultimately increasing myocyte contractility.[52]

Phase 0: Upstroke or Rapid Depolarization

A stimulus delivered to excitable tissue evokes an action potential characterized by a sudden voltage change caused by transient depolarization followed by repolarization. The action potential is conducted throughout the heart and is responsible for initiating each heartbeat. Electrical changes in action potential follow a relatively fixed time and voltage relationship that differs according to specific cell types (**Fig. 35-17**). In nerve, the entire process takes several milliseconds, whereas action potentials in human cardiac fibers last several hundred milliseconds. Normally, the action potential is independent of the size of the depolarizing stimulus if the latter exceeds a certain threshold potential. Small subthreshold depolarizing stimuli depolarize the membrane in proportion to the strength of the stimulus. However, when the stimulus is sufficiently intense to reduce membrane potential to a threshold value in the range of −70 to −65 mV for normal Purkinje fibers, more intense stimuli do not produce larger action potential responses, and an "all-or-none" response results. In contrast, hyperpolarizing pulses, stimuli that render the membrane potential more negative, elicit a response proportional to the strength of the stimulus.

MECHANISM OF PHASE 0. The upstroke of the cardiac action potential in atrial and ventricular muscle and His-Purkinje fibers is the result of a sudden increase in membrane conductance to Na^+. An externally applied stimulus or a spontaneously generated local membrane circuit current in advance of a propagating action potential depolarizes a sufficiently large area of membrane at a sufficiently rapid rate to open the Na^+ channels and depolarize the membrane further. When the stimulus activates enough Na^+ channels, Na^+ ions enter the cell, down their electrochemical gradient. The excited membrane no longer behaves like a K^+ electrode, that is, exclusively permeable to K^+, but more closely approximates a Na^+ electrode, and the membrane moves toward the Na^+ equilibrium potential.

The rate at which depolarization occurs during phase 0, that is, the maximum rate of change of voltage over time, is indicated by the expression dV/dt_{max} or $\dot{V}max$ (see Table 35-2), which is a reasonable approximation of the rate and magnitude of Na^+ entry into the cell and a determinant of conduction velocity for the propagated action potential. The transient increase in sodium conductance lasts 1 to 2 milliseconds. The action

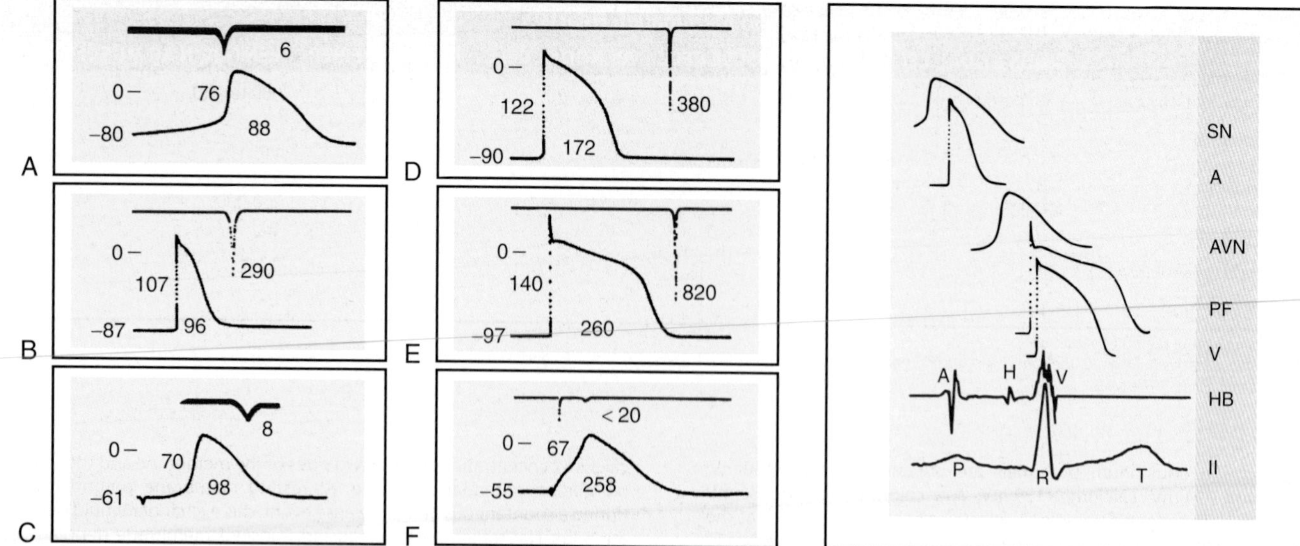

FIGURE 35-17 Action potentials recorded from different tissues in the heart **(left)** remounted along with a His bundle recording and scalar electrocardiogram from a patient **(right)** to illustrate the timing during a single cardiac cycle. In panels **A** to **F,** the top tracing is dV/dt of phase 0 and the second tracing is the action potential. For each panel, the numbers (from left to right) indicate maximum diastolic potential (mV), action potential amplitude (mV), action potential duration at 90% of repolarization (milliseconds), and V̇max of phase 0 (V/sec). Zero potential is indicated by the short horizontal line next to the zero on the upper left of each action potential. **A,** Rabbit sinoatrial node. **B,** Canine atrial muscle. **C,** Rabbit AV node. **D,** Canine ventricular muscle. **E,** Canine Purkinje fiber. **F,** Diseased human ventricle. Note that the action potentials recorded in **A, C,** and **F** have reduced resting membrane potentials, amplitudes, and V̇max compared with the other action potentials. A = atrial muscle potential; AVN = atrioventricular nodal potential; HB = His bundle recording; II = lead II; PF = Purkinje fiber potential; SN = sinus nodal potential; V = ventricular muscle potential. Horizontal calibration on the left: 50 milliseconds for **A** and **C,** 100 milliseconds for **B, D, E,** and **F;** 200 milliseconds on the right. Vertical calibration on the left, 50 mV. Horizontal calibration on the right, 200 milliseconds. *(Modified from Gilmour RF Jr, Zipes DP: Basic electrophysiology of the slow inward current.* In *Antman E, Stone PH [eds]: Calcium Blocking Agents in the Treatment of Cardiovascular Disorders. Mount Kisco, NY, Futura, 1983, pp 1-37.)*

potential, or more properly the Na^+ current (I_{Na}), is said to be regenerative; that is, intracellular movement of a little Na^+ depolarizes the membrane more, which increases conductance to Na^+ more, which allows more Na^+ to enter, and so on. As this process is occurring, however, $[Na^+]_i$ and positive intracellular charges increase and reduce the driving force for Na^+. When the equilibrium potential for Na^+ (E_{Na}) is reached, Na^+ no longer enters the cell; that is, when the driving force acting on the ion to enter the cell balances the driving force acting on the ion to exit the cell, no current flows. In addition, Na^+ conductance is time dependent, so that when the membrane spends some time at voltages less negative than the resting potential, Na^+ conductance decreases (inactivation; see earlier). Therefore, an intervention that reduces membrane potential for a time (acute myocardial ischemia), but not to threshold, partially inactivates Na^+ channels, and if threshold is now achieved, the magnitude and rate of Na^+ influx are reduced, causing the conduction velocity to slow.

In cardiac Purkinje fibers, sinoatrial cells, and, to a lesser extent, ventricular muscle, two different populations of Na^+ channels exist: the TTX-sensitive, neuronal Na^+ channel isoform (Nav1.1) and the TTX-resistant Nav1.5 isoform, the latter being the predominant isoform in cardiac muscle. Whereas the precise role of Nav1.1 channels in ventricular or atrial cardiomyocytes has not been defined, this channel is an important modulator of sinoatrial node pacemaking[53] and in determining Purkinje myocyte action potential duration.

Upstroke of the Action Potential. In normal atrial and ventricular muscle and in fibers in the His-Purkinje system, action potentials have very rapid upstrokes, with a large V̇max, and are called fast responses. Action potentials in the normal sinoatrial and AV nodes and many types of diseased tissue have very slow upstrokes with a reduced V̇max and are called slow responses (**Table 35-3**; see Figs. 35-4, 35-7, and 35-17). Upstrokes of slow responses are mediated by a slow inward, predominantly L-type voltage-gated (Cav) Ca^{2+} current ($I_{Ca.L}$) rather than by the fast inward I_{Na}. These potentials have been termed *slow response* potentials because the time required for activation and inactivation of the slow inward current ($I_{Ca.L}$) is approximately an order of magnitude slower than that for the fast inward Na^+ current (I_{Na}). Recovery from inactivation also takes longer. Calcium entry and $[Ca^{2+}]_i$ help promote inactivation. The slow channel requires more time after a stimulus to be reactivated. In fact, recovery of excitability outlasts full restoration of maximum diastolic potential, which means that even though the membrane potential has returned to normal, the cell has not recovered excitability completely because the latter depends on the elapse of a certain amount of time (i.e., is time dependent) and not just on recovery of a particular membrane potential (i.e., voltage dependent), a phenomenon termed *postrepolarization refractoriness.*

The threshold for activation of $I_{Ca.L}$, that is, the voltage that the cell must reach to "turn on" the slow inward current, is about −30 to −40 mV. In fibers of the fast response type, $I_{Ca.L}$ is normally activated during phase 0 by the regenerative depolarization caused by the fast sodium current. Current flows through both fast and slow channels during the latter part of the action potential upstroke. However, $I_{Ca.L}$ is much smaller than the peak Na^+ current and therefore contributes little to the action potential until the fast Na^+ current is inactivated, after completion of phase 0. Thus, $I_{Ca.L}$ affects mainly the plateau of action potentials recorded in atrial and ventricular muscle and His-Purkinje fibers. In addition, $I_{Ca.L}$ may play a prominent role in partially depolarized cells in which the fast Na^+ channels have been inactivated if conditions are appropriate for slow channel activation.

Ca^{2+} entry through activated L-type Cav channels triggers Ca^{2+} release from the SR stores and is an essential component of cardiac excitation-contraction coupling in atrial and ventricular myocardium (see Chap. 24). L-type Cav channels are also expressed in sinoatrial and AV nodal cells, where they play a role in controlling automaticity and action potential propagation, respectively. Cardiac L-type Cav channels undergo rapid voltage- and Ca^{2+}-dependent inactivation, the time course of which importantly affects the action potential waveform and time course of repolarization. Although T-type Cav channels have not been detected in human myocardium, experimental evidence in animals has suggested that these channels play an important role in determining sinoatrial node automaticity and AV nodal conduction.[30] Whether Ca^{2+} influx through open T-type channels provides a sufficient trigger for Ca^{2+} release from the SR is controversial. The density of T-type Ca^{2+} channels has been found to be increased in myocytes from hearts with experimentally induced hypertrophy, but the role of enhanced T-type channel density under these conditions remains to be determined.

Other significant differences exist between the fast and slow channels. Drugs that elevate cAMP levels, such as beta-adrenoceptor agonists, phosphodiesterase inhibitors such as theophylline, and the lipid-soluble derivative of cAMP, dibutyryl cAMP, increase $I_{Ca.L}$. Binding of the beta-adrenoceptor agonist to specific sarcolemmal receptors facilitates the dissociation of two subunits of a regulatory protein (G protein; see Chap. 24), one of which (G_s) activates adenylate cyclase and thus increases intracellular levels of cAMP. The latter binds to a regulatory subunit of a cAMP-dependent protein kinase that promotes phosphorylation of specific phosphorylation sites on the channel protein, ultimately resulting in

TABLE 35-3 Synopsis of Transsarcolemmal Ionic Currents in Mammalian Cardiac Myocytes

CURRENT	SUBUNIT	FUNCTIONAL PROPERTIES
I_{Na}	Nav1.5, Nav1.1, Nav1.3, Nav1.6 (alpha subunits)	Tetrodotoxin-resistant (Nav1.5) and tetrodotoxin-sensitive (Nav1.1, Nav1.3, Nav1.6) voltage-gated currents; Nav1.5 is the major cardiac isoform; neuronal Na^+ channel isoforms contribute to sinoatrial node pacemaking
$I_{Ca.L}$	Cav1.2 (alpha subunit)	L-type (*l*ong lasting, *l*arge conductance) Ca^{2+} currents through voltage-gated Ca^{2+} (Cav) channels blocked by dihydropyridine-type antagonists (e.g., nifedipine), phenylalkylamines (e.g., verapamil), benzothiazepines (e.g., diltiazem), and various divalent ions (e.g., Cd^{2+}); activated by dihydropyridine-type agonists (e.g., Bay K 8644); responsible for phase 0 depolarization and propagation in sinoatrial and AV nodal tissue and contributing to plateau of atrial, His-Purkinje, and ventricular cells; main trigger of Ca^{2+} release from the sarcoplasmic reticulum (Ca^{2+}-induced Ca^{2+} release); noninactivating or "window" component may underlie early afterdepolarizations
$I_{Ca.T}$	Cav3.1/alpha$_{1G}$ (alpha subunit)	T-type (*t*ransient current, *t*iny conductance) Ca^{2+} currents through Cav channels blocked by mibefradil but insensitive to dihydropyridines; may contribute inward current to later phase of phase 4 depolarization in pacemaker cells and action potential propagation in AV nodal cells; role in triggering Ca^{2+}-induced Ca^{2+} release uncertain
I_f	HCN4 (alpha subunit)	Hyperpolarization-activated current carried by Na^+ and K^+ in sinoatrial and AV nodal cells and His-Purkinje cells; involved in generating phase 4 depolarization; increases rate of impulse initiation in pacemaker cells
I_{K1}	Kir2.1 (alpha subunit)	K^+ current through inwardly rectifying K^+ (Kir) channels, voltage-dependent block by Ba^{2+} at micromolar concentrations; responsible for maintaining resting membrane potential in atrial, His-Purkinje, and ventricular cells; channel activity is function of both membrane potential and $[K^+]_o$; inward rectification appears to result from depolarization-induced internal block by Mg^{2+} and neutral or positively charged amino acid residues in the cytoplasmic channel pore
$I_{K.G}$ ($I_{K.Ach}$, $I_{K.Ade}$)	Kir3.1/Kir3.4 (alpha subunit)	Inwardly rectifying K^+ current activated by muscarinic (M_2) and purinergic (type 1) receptor stimulation via GTP regulatory (G) protein signal transduction; expressed in sinoatrial and AV nodal cells and atrial cells, where it causes hyperpolarization and action potential shortening; activation causes negative chronotropic and dromotropic effects
I_{Ks}	KvLQT1 (alpha subunit)/minK (beta subunit)	K^+ current carried by a voltage-gated K^+ (Kv) channel (delayed rectifier K^+ channel); plays a major role in determining phase 3 of the action potential
I_{Kr}	hERG (alpha subunit)/MiRP1 (beta subunit)	Rapidly activating component of delayed rectifier K^+ current; I_{Kr} specifically blocked by dofetilide and sotalol in a reverse use–dependent manner; inward rectification of I_{Kr} results from depolarization-induced fast inactivation; plays a major role in determining action potential duration
I_{Kur}	Kv1.5 (alpha subunit)	K^+ current through a Kv channel with ultrarapid activation but ultraslow inactivation kinetics; expressed in atrial myocytes; determines action potential duration
$I_{K.Ca}$	SK2 (alpha subunit)	K^+ current through small-conductance Ca^{2+}-activated channels; blocked by apamine and dequalinium chloride; expressed in human atrial myocytes; determines action potential duration
I_{to} (I_{to1}, I_A)	Kv4.3 (alpha subunit)/KChIP2 (beta subunit)	Transient outward K^+ current through voltage-gated (Kv) channels; exhibits fast activation and inactivation and recovery kinetics; blocked by 4-aminopyridine in a reverse use–dependent manner; contributes to time course of phase 1 repolarization; transmural differences in I_{to} properties contribute to regional differences in early repolarization
$I_{Cl.Ca}$ (I_{to2})	?	4-Aminopyridine–resistant transient outward current carried by Cl^- ions; activated by increase in intracellular calcium level; blocked by stilbene derivatives (SITS, DIDS); contributes to time course of phase 1 repolarization; may underlie spontaneous transient inward currents under conditions of Ca^{2+} overload; molecular correlate uncertain
$I_{Cl.cAMP}$	?	Time-independent chloride current regulated by cAMP/adenylate cyclase pathway; slightly depolarizes resting membrane potential and significantly shortens action potential duration; antagonizes action potential prolongation associated with beta-adrenergic stimulation of $I_{Ca.L}$
$I_{Cl.swell}$ or $I_{Cl.vol}$	?	Outwardly rectifying, swelling-activated Cl^- current; inhibited by 9-anthracene carboxylic acid; activation causes resting membrane depolarization and action potential shortening
$I_{K.ATP}$	Kir6.2 (alpha subunit)/SUR	Time-independent K^+ current through Kir channels activated by a fall in intracellular ATP concentration; inhibited by sulfonylurea drugs, such as glibenclamide; activated by pinacidil, nicorandil, cromakalim; causes shortening of action potential duration during myocardial ischemia or hypoxia
$I_{Cir.swell}$	?	Inwardly rectifying, swelling-activated cation current; permeable to Na^+ and K^+ ($P_{Na}/P_K = 8$); inhibited by Gd^{3+}; depolarizes resting membrane potential and prolongs terminal (phase 3) repolarization
$I_{Na/Ca}$	NCX1.1	Current carried by Na^+/Ca^{2+} exchanger; causes net Na^+ outward current and Ca^{2+} inward current (reverse mode) or net Na^+ inward and Ca^{2+} outward current (3 Na^+ for 1 Ca^{2+}); direction of Na^+ flux depends on membrane potential and intracellular and extracellular concentrations of Na^+ and Ca^{2+}; Ca^{2+} influx mediated by $I_{Na/Ca}$ can trigger sarcoplasmic reticulum Ca^{2+} release; underlies I_{ti} (transient inward current) under conditions of intracellular Ca^{2+} overload
$I_{Na/K}$	Alpha subunit/beta subunit	Na^+ outward current generated by Na^+,K^+-ATPase (stoichiometry: 3 Na^+ leave and 2 K^+ enter); inhibited by digitalis
I_{ti}	?	Transient inward current activated by Ca^{2+} waves; I_{ti} possibly reflects 3 Ca^{2+}-dependent components: I_{NCX}, $I_{Cl.Ca}$, and a TRPM4 (transient receptor potential cation channel, member 4 gene)–mediated current

Continued

TABLE 35-3 Synopsis of Transsarcolemmal Ionic Currents in Mammalian Cardiac Myocytes—cont'd

CURRENT	SUBUNIT	FUNCTIONAL PROPERTIES
Electroneutral Ion-Exchanging Proteins		
Ca^{2+}-ATPase		Extrudes cytosolic calcium
Na/H	Cardiac myocytes express isoform NHE1	Exchanges intracellular H^+ for extracellular Na^+; Specifically inhibited by benzoylguanidine derivatives HOE 694 and HOE 642; inhibition causes intracellular acidification
Cl^--HCO_3^-		Exchanges intracellular HCO_3^- for external Cl^-; inhibited by SITS
Na^+-K^+-$2Cl^-$		Cotransporter blocked by amiloride

DIDS = 4,4′-diisothiocyanatostilbene-2,2′-disulfonic acid; SITS = 4-acetamido-4′-isothiocyanatostilbene-2,2′-disulfonic acid.

enhanced open-state probability of the channel. Although Nav channels are sensitive to increases in cAMP, the net effect (decrease versus increase) appears to be species dependent.

Acetylcholine reduces $I_{Ca.L}$ by decreasing adenylate cyclase activity. However, acetylcholine stimulates cyclic guanosine monophosphate (cGMP) accumulation. cGMP has negligible effects on basal $I_{Ca.L}$ but decreases $I_{Ca.L}$ levels that have been elevated by beta-adrenoceptor agonists. This effect is mediated by cAMP hydrolysis through a cGMP-stimulated cyclic nucleotide phosphodiesterase.

Differences Between Channels. Fast and slow channels can be differentiated on the basis of their pharmacologic sensitivity. Drugs that block the slow channel with a *fair* degree of specificity include verapamil, nifedipine, diltiazem, and D-600 (a methoxy derivative of verapamil). Antiarrhythmic agents such as lidocaine, quinidine, procainamide, and disopyramide (see Chap. 37) affect the fast channel and not the slow channel.

Normal action potentials recorded from the sinus node and the compact node of the AV junction have a reduced resting membrane potential, action potential amplitude, overshoot, upstroke, and conduction velocity compared with action potentials in muscle or Purkinje fibers (see Figs. 35-7 and 35-17).

Slow channel blockers suppress sinus and AV nodal action potentials. The prolonged time for reactivation of $I_{Ca.L}$ probably accounts for the fact that sinoatrial and AV nodal cells remain refractory longer than the time that it takes for full voltage repolarization to occur. Thus, premature stimulation immediately after the membrane potential reaches full repolarization leads to action potentials with reduced amplitudes and upstroke velocities. Therefore, slow conduction and prolonged refractoriness are characteristic features of nodal cells. These cells also have a reduced "safety factor for conduction" (see earlier), which means that the stimulating efficacy of the propagating impulse is low and conduction block occurs easily.

Inward Currents. Thus, I_{Na} and $I_{Ca.L}$ represent two important inward currents. Another important inward current is I_f, also called the pacemaker or "funny" current.[54] This current is activated by hyperpolarization and is carried by Na^+ and K^+. It generates phase 4 diastolic depolarization in the sinoatrial node. I_f modulation is one major mechanism whereby beta-adrenergic and cholinergic neurotransmitters regulate cardiac rhythm under physiologic conditions. Catecholamines increase the probability of channel opening by shifting the channel's activation curve to more positive potentials, which leads to increased current availability for the generation of diastolic depolarization, hence steepening its rate. Cholinergic action, in general, exerts the opposite effect.[54] Fish oil depresses I_f.[55] The electrophysiologic changes accompanying *acute* myocardial ischemia may represent a depressed form of a fast response in the center of the ischemic zone and a slow response in the border area. Probable slow-response activity has been shown in myocardium resected from patients undergoing surgery for recurrent ventricular tachyarrhythmias (see Fig. 35-17F). Whether and how slow responses play a role in the genesis of ventricular arrhythmias in these patients have not been established.

Phase 1: Early Rapid Repolarization

Following phase 0, the membrane repolarizes rapidly and transiently to almost 0 mV (early notch), partly because of the inactivation of I_{Na} and concomitant activation of several outward currents.

I_{to}. The 4-aminopyridine–sensitive transient outward K^+ current, commonly termed I_{to} (or I_{to1}), is turned on rapidly by depolarization and then rapidly inactivates. Both the density and recovery of I_{to} from inactivation exhibit transmural gradients in the left ventricular free wall, with the density decreasing and reactivation becoming progressively prolonged from epicardium to endocardium.[29] Transmural differences in expression of KChIP2, the auxiliary subunit to Kv4.3 pore-forming alpha subunits, appears to be the primary determinant of the transmural gradient in I_{to} properties and densities in the human heart.[56] This gradient gives rise to regional differences in action potential shape, with increasingly slower phase 1 restitution kinetics and diminution of the notch along the transmural axis (**Fig. 35-18**). These regional differences might create transmural voltage gradients, specifically at higher rates, thereby increasing dispersion of repolarization, a putative arrhythmogenic factor (Brugada syndrome; see Chap. 39). However, elimination of the physiologic repolarization gradient appears to be similarly arrhythmogenic.[56] Downregulation of I_{to} is at least partially responsible for slowing of phase 1 repolarization in failing human myocytes. Studies have demonstrated that these changes in the phase 1 notch of the cardiac action potential cause a reduction in the kinetics and peak amplitude of the action potential–evoked intracellular Ca^{2+} transient because of failed recruitment and synchronization of the SR Ca^{2+} release through $I_{Ca.L}$ (**Fig. 35-19**; see Fig. 35-18C). Thus, modulation of I_{to} appears to play a significant physiologic role in controlling cardiac excitation-contraction coupling,[57] and it remains to be determined whether transmural differences in phase 1 repolarization translate into similar differences in regional contractility.

$I_{Cl.Ca}$. The 4-aminopyridine–resistant, Ca^{2+}-activated chloride current $I_{Cl.Ca}$ (or I_{to2}) also contributes a significant outward current during phase 1 repolarization.[58] This current is activated by the action potential–evoked intracellular Ca^{2+} transient. Therefore, interventions that augment the amplitude of the Ca^{2+} transient associated with the twitch (such as beta-adrenergic receptor stimulation) also enhance outward $I_{Cl.Ca}$. It is not currently known whether human cardiac myocytes express Ca^{2+}-activated chloride channels. Other, time-*independent* chloride currents may also play a role in determining the time course of early repolarization, such as the cAMP- or swelling-activated chloride conductances $I_{Cl.cAMP}$ and $I_{Cl.swell}$.

Na/Ca Exchanger. A third current contributing to early repolarization is Na^+ outward movement through the Na^+/Ca^{2+} exchanger operating in reverse mode (see Fig. 35-16).[59] Overexpression of the exchanger in transgenic mice caused accentuation of the early notch in left ventricular myocytes.

Sometimes, a transient depolarization follows phase 1 repolarization. This notch is well defined and separated from phase 2 in Purkinje fibers and left ventricular epicardial and midmyocardial myocytes (see Fig. 35-18).

Phase 2: Plateau

During the plateau phase, which may last several hundred milliseconds, membrane conductance to all ions falls to rather low values. Thus, less change in current is required near plateau levels than near resting potential levels to produce the same changes in transmembrane potential. The plateau is maintained by the competition between outward current carried by K^+ and Cl^- ions and inward current carried by Ca^{2+} moving through open L-type Ca^{2+} channels and Na^+ being exchanged for internal

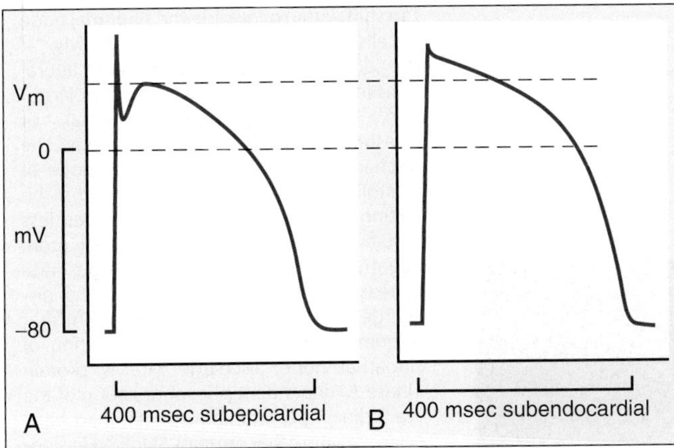

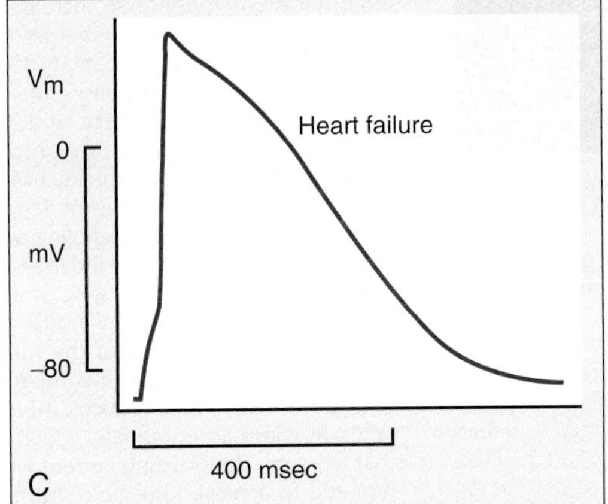

FIGURE 35-18 Action potential plots demonstrating differences in the action potential shape of human ventricular myocytes of subepicardial **(A)** and subendocardial **(B)** origin. Subepicardial myocytes present a prominent notch during phase 1 repolarization of the action potential, most likely caused by a larger I_{to} in these cells. The notch is absent in subendocardial cells. The peak plateau potential is higher in subendocardial than in subepicardial myocytes, and the action potential duration tends to be shorter in subepicardial cells. **C,** Transmembrane action potential in a human ventricular cardiomyocyte of a failing heart. Note loss of the prominent phase 1 notch and delayed repolarization. Recording temperature = 35°C; V_m = membrane potential. *(**A** and **B** from Näbauer M, Beuckelmann DJ, Uberfuhr P, Steinbeck G: Regional differences in current density and rate-dependent properties of the transient outward current in subepicardial and subendocardial myocytes of human left ventricle. Circulation 93:168, 1996. By permission of the American Heart Association. **C** from Priebe L, Beuckelmann DJ: Simulation studies of cellular electrical properties in heart failure. Circ Res 82:1206-1223, 1998.)*

Ca^{2+} by the Na^+/Ca^{2+} exchanger operating in forward mode. After depolarization, potassium conductance falls to plateau levels as a result of inward rectification in spite of the large electrochemical driving force on K^+ ions.

Rectification simply means that membrane conductance changes with voltage. Specifically, inward rectification means that K^+ channels are open at negative potentials but closed at less negative or positive voltages. Membrane depolarization-induced internal block by intracellular ionized magnesium is thought to underlie inward rectification of cardiac I_{KI} channels. Inward rectification can also be induced by neutral and positively charged amino acid residues in the cytoplasmic channel pore that is formed by four Kir2.1 subunits.[60] The mechanism underlying rectification of the rapid component of the delayed rectifier K^+ current (I_{Kr}) in cardiac cells is the inactivation that channels rapidly undergo during depolarizing pulses. More I_{Kr} channels enter the inactivated state with stronger depolarizations, thereby causing inward rectification. This fast inactivation mechanism is sensitive to changes in extracellular K^+ in the physiologic range, with inactivation more accentuated at low extracellular K^+ concentrations. Thus, hypokalemia would decrease outward I_{Kr}, thereby prolonging action potential duration.

Outward K^+ movement carried by the slow component of the delayed rectifier K^+ current (I_{Ks}) also contributes to plateau duration: (1) I_{Ks} density has been shown to be correlated with action potential duration; and (2) isolated defects in the KvLQT1 subunit, which in combination with the IsK subunit (minK) reconstitutes the cardiac I_{Ks} current, are associated with abnormally prolonged ventricular repolarization (long-QT syndrome, type 1; see Chaps. 9 and 39). Although I_{Ks} activates slowly compared with action potential duration, it is only slowly inactivated. Therefore, increases in heart rate can cause this activation to accumulate during successive depolarizations, and cumulative activation can determine the contribution to repolarization of K^+ currents that are active during the plateau of the action potential. In conditions of reduced intracellular ATP concentration (e.g., hypoxia, ischemia), K^+ efflux through activated K_{ATP} channels is enhanced, thereby shortening the plateau phase of the action potential. Other ionic mechanisms that control plateau potential and duration include the kinetics of inactivation of the L-type Ca^{2+} current. Reduced efficiency of intracellular free Ca^{2+} to induce Ca^{2+}-dependent inactivation, such as in myocytes from hypertrophic hearts, can result in delayed repolarization. Steady-state components of both I_{Na} and $I_{Ca.L}$ (window currents) also shape the plateau phase.[24] Na^+,K^+-ATPase generates a net outward current by pumping out three Na^+ ions in exchange for two K^+ ions. Noninactivating chloride currents, such as $I_{Cl.swell}$ and $I_{Cl.cAMP}$, may produce significant outward currents during the plateau phase under certain conditions, thereby significantly shortening action potential duration. A nonselective, swelling-induced cation current has been shown to cause action potential prolongation in myocytes from failing ventricles.

Phase 3: Final Rapid Repolarization

In this portion of the action potential, repolarization proceeds rapidly at least in part because of two currents: time-dependent inactivation of $I_{Ca.L}$, with a decrease in the intracellular movement of positive charges, and activation of repolarizing K^+ currents, including the slow and rapid components of the delayed rectifier K^+ current I_{Ks} and I_{Kr} and the inwardly rectifying K^+ currents I_{KI} and $I_{K.Ach}$, which all cause an increase in the movement of positive charges out of the cell. The net membrane current becomes more outward, and the membrane potential shifts to the resting potential. A small-conductance Ca^{2+}-activated K^+ current, $I_{K.Ca}$, is expressed in human atrial myocytes, where it controls the time course of phase 3 repolarization.[61] Loss-of-function mutations in the human ether-a-go-go–related gene (*HERG*), which is responsible for I_{Kr}, prolong phase 3 repolarization, thereby predisposing to the development of torsades de pointes. Macrolide antibiotics such as erythromycin, antihistamines such as terfenadine, and antifungal drugs such as ketoconazole inhibit I_{Kr} and have been implicated in the acquired form of long-QT syndrome (see Chaps. 9 and 39). A decrease in I_{KI} activity, as is the case in left ventricular myocytes from failing hearts, causes action potential prolongation by slowing of phase 3 repolarization and resting membrane depolarization. Reduction in the outward potassium current through open inward rectifier K^+ channels renders the failing cardiomyocyte more susceptible to the induction of delayed afterdepolarizations triggered by spontaneous intracellular Ca^{2+} release events and therefore plays a major role in arrhythmogenesis in the failing heart (see Fig. 35-21).

Phase 4: Diastolic Depolarization

Under normal conditions, the membrane potential of atrial and ventricular muscle cells remains steady throughout diastole. I_{KI} is the current responsible for maintaining the resting potential near the K^+ equilibrium potential in atrial, His-Purkinje, and ventricular cells. I_{KI} is the inward rectifier and shuts off during depolarization. In other fibers found in certain parts of the atria, in the muscle of the mitral and tricuspid valves, in His-Purkinje fibers, and in the sinoatrial node and portions of the AV nodal tract, the resting membrane potential does not remain constant in diastole but gradually depolarizes (see Figs. 35-4, 35-7, and 35-17A). The property possessed by spontaneously discharging cells is called phase 4 diastolic depolarization; when it leads to initiation of action potentials, automaticity results. The discharge rate of the sinoatrial node normally exceeds the discharge rate of other potentially automatic pacemaker sites and thus maintains dominance of the cardiac rhythm. The discharge rate of the sinoatrial node is normally more sensitive than the discharge rate of ventricular muscle cells to the effects of norepinephrine and acetylcholine. Normal or abnormal automaticity at other sites can cause discharge at rates faster than the sinoatrial nodal discharge rate and can usurp control of the cardiac rhythm for one cycle or many (see Chap. 36).

Normal Automaticity

Robust experimental evidence supports the notion that rhythmic oscillations in the level of intracellular free calcium ($[Ca^{2+}]_i$) constitute an essential component of the pacemaking mechanism not only in sinoatrial nodal cells[1] but also in Purkinje cells,[62] AV nodal cells, and embryonic cells.[63] In fact, rhythmic $[Ca^{2+}]_i$ elevations are the formal cause for spontaneous action potentials and normal automaticity in these cell

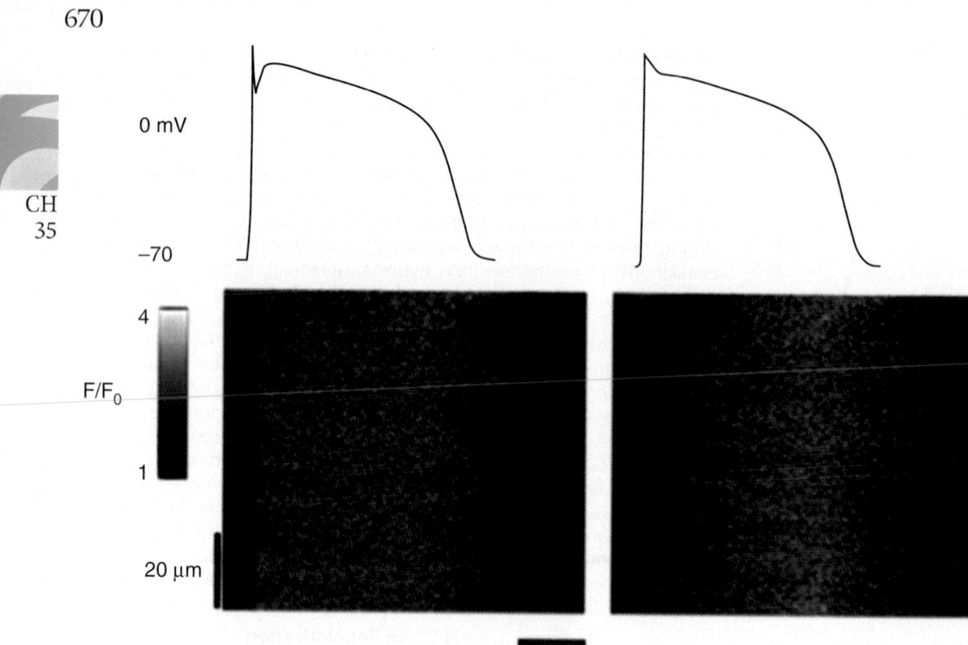

FIGURE 35-19 Diminution of phase 1 amplitude ("notch") causes asynchronous sarcoplasmic reticulum Ca^{2+} release. Normal cardiomyocytes were voltage clamped with action potential profiles with a normal or congestive heart failure wave shape, and local changes in intracellular calcium were recorded simultaneously. When the myocyte was clamped with a normal action potential profile having the early phase 1 repolarization notch **(left),** there was uniform Ca^{2+} release. However, when a congestive heart failure action potential profile without early rapid phase 1 repolarization was used, Ca^{2+} release was dyssynchronous. This dyssynchrony causes a slowing in the rate of rise of the Ca^{2+} transient and a loss of spatial and temporal release uniformity. F/F_0 = fluorescence of Ca^{2+} indicator normalized to its baseline fluorescence. *(From Harris DM, Mills GD, Chen X, et al: Alterations in early action potential repolarization causes localized failure of sarcoplasmic reticulum Ca^{2+} release. Circ Res 96:543, 2005. By permission of the American Heart Association.)*

types, that is, periodic increases in $[Ca^{2+}]_i$ serve as an internal generator ("calcium clock") of rhythmic signals that are transformed into changes in membrane voltage via modulation of calcium-sensitive ion channels and transporters in the outer membrane ("membrane clock"). This novel concept is illustrated in **Figure 35-20**, using simultaneous $[Ca^{2+}]_i$ and action potential measurements in isolated sinoatrial myocytes as an example. Local submembrane increases in $[Ca^{2+}]_i$ (denoted by the white arrows in Fig. 35-20A, B) occurring during the later part of the spontaneous diastolic depolarization (transmembrane action potentials are shown in blue) precede the rapid upstroke of the action potential. These local submembrane increases in $[Ca^{2+}]_i$ are abolished by the specific blocker of the SR Ca^{2+} release channel, ryanodine (ryan), concurrent with a slowing of the beating frequency by this drug. The periodic SR Ca^{2+} release events rhythmically activate the Na^+/Ca^{2+} exchange inward (i.e., depolarizing) current (I_{NCX}; Fig. 35-20C), which then results in an exponential increase in membrane potential, prompting activation of surface membrane L-type Ca^{2+} channels to initiate an action potential (Fig. 35-20C). Thus, the Na^+/Ca^{2+} exchanger operating in forward mode plays an essential role in converting the primary intracellular Ca^{2+} signals into membrane (i.e., voltage) signals. In this novel model of sinoatrial node pacemaking, spontaneous SR Ca^{2+} release–induced membrane excitation initiates the sinoatrial node cell duty cycle, as schematically illustrated in Figure 35-20C. Once an action potential has been initiated, two highly interacting, concurrent series of events proceed during a normal sinoatrial node cell cycle (Fig. 35-20C). In one event series (delimited to the outer membrane), depolarization-induced activation of the delayed rectifier K^+ current, I_K (see Table 35-3), leads to membrane hyperpolarization, which is followed by slow diastolic depolarization via activation of a number of inward currents, including I_f and $I_{Ca,T}$ (see Table 35-3). In a second, parallel cycle of events, action potential–induced SR Ca^{2+} release is followed by Ca^{2+} reuptake into the SR, which subsequently gives rise to multifocal, synchronized spontaneous Ca^{2+} release events culminating in an increase in inward I_{NCX}. The role of late diastolic spontaneous SR Ca^{2+} release events in triggering the sinoatrial node action potential has recently been confirmed in canine hearts in situ (see Fig. 35-e4 on website).[64]

The rate of sinoatrial nodal discharge can be varied by several mechanisms in response to autonomic or other influences. The pacemaker locus can shift within or outside the sinoatrial node to cells discharging faster or more slowly.[64] If the pacemaker site remains the same, alterations in the slope of the diastolic depolarization, maximum diastolic potential, or threshold potential can speed or slow the discharge rate. For example, if the slope of diastolic depolarization steepens and if the resting membrane potential becomes less negative or the threshold potential more negative (within limits), discharge rate increases. Opposite changes slow the discharge rate. The molecular mechanism that is primarily responsible for acceleration of sinoatrial node discharge rate is protein kinase A–dependent phosphorylation of the ryanodine receptor phospholamban (see Chap. 24) and other proteins involved in sinoatrial node Ca^{2+} cycling: an increase in the level of cAMP (after beta-adrenergic receptor stimulation) augments the activity of protein kinase A, which then increases the rate of spontaneous SR Ca^{2+} release and SR Ca^{2+} reuptake via synergistic activation of these proteins, whereas a reduction in cAMP levels (after muscarinic receptor stimulation) has the opposite effect.[1] Acetylcholine activates K^+ efflux through acetylcholine-sensitive inward rectifier K^+ channels, which are expressed in both sinoatrial nodal and AV nodal cells, thereby shifting the maximum diastolic potential to more negative values. The same mechanism reduces input resistance at diastolic potentials, which means that a greater depolarizing current would be required to achieve "threshold" for firing an action potential.

PASSIVE MEMBRANE ELECTRICAL PROPERTIES. Passive membrane properties, including membrane resistance, capacitance, and cable properties, play an important role in cardiac electrophysiology. Although the cardiac cell membrane is resistant to current flow, it also has capacitative properties, which means that it behaves like a battery and can store charges of opposite signs on its two sides—an excess of negative charges inside the membrane balanced by equivalent positive charges outside the membrane. These resistive and capacitative properties cause the membrane to take a certain amount of time to respond to an applied stimulus, rather than responding instantly, because the charges across the capacitative membrane must be altered first. A subthreshold rectangular current pulse applied to the membrane produces a slowly rising and decaying membrane voltage change rather than a rectangular voltage change. A value called the time constant of the membrane reflects this property. The time constant, tau, is equal to the product of membrane resistance R_m and cell capacitance C_m:

$$tau = R_m \cdot C_m$$

This is the time taken by the membrane voltage to reach 63% of its final value after application of a steady current. The time course of changes in membrane potential after application of a hyperpolarizing or depolarizing subthreshold current step is typically monoexponential in all myocyte types, indicating that the entire sarcolemma (including the T-tubular membrane; see Fig. 35-e1 on website) is charging uniformly.

When aligned end to end, cardiac cells, particularly the His-Purkinje system, behave like a long cable in which current flows more easily inside the cell and to the adjacent cell across the gap junction than it does across the cell membrane to the outside. When current is injected at a point, most of it flows along inside the cell, but some leaks out. Because of this loss of current, the voltage change of a cell at a site distant from the point of applied current is less than the change in membrane voltage where the stimulus was given. A measure of this property of a cable is called the space or length constant lambda (λ), which is the distance along the cable from the point of stimulation at which the voltage at steady state is 1/e (37%) of its value at the point of introduction.

Restated, λ describes how far current flows before leaking passively across the surface membrane to a value about one third of its initial value. This distance is normally about 2 mm for Purkinje fibers, 0.5 mm

Abnormal Automaticity. Mechanisms responsible for normal automaticity were described earlier. Abnormal automaticity can arise from cells that have reduced maximum diastolic potentials, often at membrane potentials positive to −50 mV, when I_K and $I_{Ca.L}$ may be operative.

Automaticity at membrane potentials more negative than −70 mV may be caused by I_f. When the membrane potential is between −50 and −70 mV, the cell may be quiescent. Electrotonic effects from surrounding normally polarized or more depolarized myocardium influence the development of automaticity.[65] Abnormal automaticity has been found in Purkinje fibers removed from dogs subjected to myocardial infarction, in rat myocardium damaged by epinephrine, in human atrial samples, and in ventricular myocardial specimens from patients undergoing aneurysmectomy and endocardial resection for recurrent ventricular tachyarrhythmias.

Abnormal automaticity can be produced in normal muscle or Purkinje fibers by appropriate interventions, such as current passage that reduces diastolic potential. An automatic discharge rate speeds up with progressive depolarization, and hyperpolarizing pulses slow the spontaneous firing. It is possible that partial depolarization and failure to reach normal maximal diastolic potential can induce automatic discharge in most if not all cardiac fibers. Although this type of spontaneous automatic activity has been found in human atrial and ventricular fibers, its relationship to the genesis of clinical arrhythmias has not been established. Abnormal automaticity in Purkinje cells can also originate secondary to spontaneous, submembrane Ca^{2+} elevations via activation of calcium-sensitive membrane conductances, a process identical to that previously identified in sinoatrial nodal myocytes. The occurrence of such spontaneous localized $[Ca^{2+}]_i$ transients has recently been confirmed in canine Purkinje cells (see Video 35-2 on website).[62]

Rhythms resulting from automaticity may be slow atrial, junctional, and ventricular escape rhythms; certain types of atrial tachycardias (e.g., those produced by digitalis or perhaps those coming from the pulmonary veins); accelerated junctional (nonparoxysmal junctional tachycardia) and idioventricular rhythms; and parasystole (see Chap. 39).

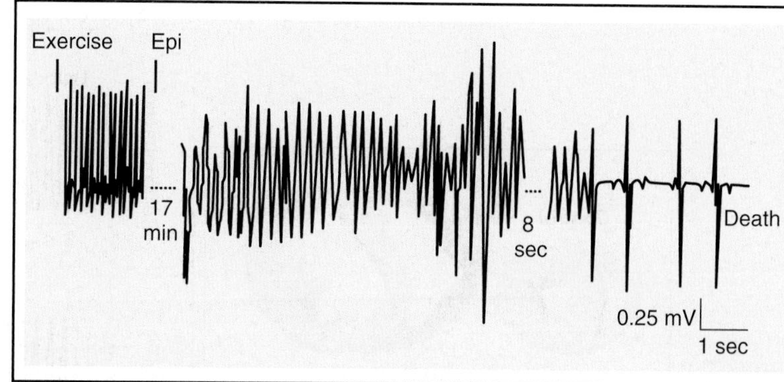

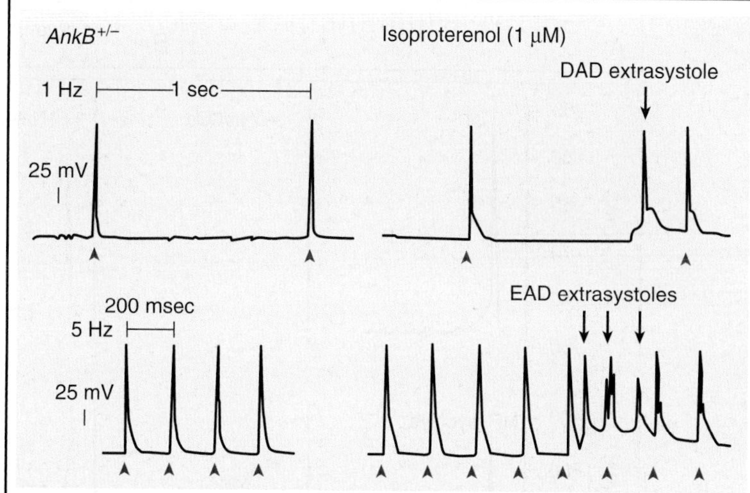

FIGURE 35-21 Polymorphic ventricular tachycardia and sudden death in an animal model of type 4 long-QT syndrome. **A,** Electrocardiogram after exercise and administration of epinephrine in a mouse heterozygous for a loss-of-function mutation in the gene encoding ankyrin-B ($AnkB^-$). Polymorphic ventricular tachycardia (torsades de pointes) occurred within about 17 minutes of epinephrine administration, followed by marked bradycardia and death 2 minutes after the arrhythmia. **B,** Transmembrane action potentials in single cardiomyocytes from $AnkB^{+/-}$ mice at the frequencies indicated. Acute exposure to isoproterenol induced both delayed and early afterdepolarizations that led to extra beats. *(From Mohler PJ, Schott J, Gramolini AO, et al: Ankyrin-B mutation causes type 4 long-QT cardiac arrhythmia and sudden cardiac death. Nature 421:634, 2003.)*

TRIGGERED ACTIVITY. Automaticity is the property of a fiber to initiate an impulse spontaneously, without need for prior stimulation, so that electrical quiescence does not occur. Triggered activity is initiated by afterdepolarizations, which are depolarizing oscillations in membrane voltage induced by one or more preceding action potentials. Thus, triggered activity is pacemaker activity that results consequent to a preceding impulse or series of impulses, without which electrical quiescence occurs (**Fig. 35-21**). This triggering activity is not caused by an automatic self-generating mechanism, and the term *triggered automaticity* is therefore contradictory. These depolarizations can occur before or after full repolarization of the fiber and are best termed *early afterdepolarizations* (EADs), when they arise from a reduced level of membrane potential during phases 2 (type 1) and 3 (type 2) of the cardiac action potential, or *late* or *delayed afterdepolarizations* (DADs), when they occur after completion of repolarization (phase 4), generally at a more negative membrane potential than that from which EADs arise. Not all afterdepolarizations may reach threshold potential, but if they do, they can trigger another afterdepolarization and thus self-perpetuate.

Delayed Afterdepolarizations. DADs and triggered activity have been demonstrated in Purkinje fibers, specialized atrial fibers and ventricular muscle fibers exposed to digitalis preparations, pulmonary veins, normal Purkinje fibers exposed to Na-free superfusates from the endocardium of the intact heart, ventricular myocardial cells from failing hearts (**Fig. 35-22**) and from mouse hearts with ankyrin-B mutations (see Fig. 35-21) during beta-adrenergic stimulation, and endocardial preparations 1 day after a myocardial infarction.[66,67] When fibers in the rabbit, canine, simian, and human mitral valves and in the canine tricuspid valve and coronary sinus are superfused with norepinephrine, they exhibit the capability for sustained triggered rhythmic activity.

Triggered activity caused by DADs has also been noted in diseased human atrial and ventricular fibers studied in vitro. Left stellate ganglion stimulation can elicit DADs in canine ventricles. In vivo, atrial and ventricular arrhythmias apparently caused by triggered activity have been reported in the dog and possibly in humans. It is tempting to ascribe certain clinical arrhythmias to DADs, such as some arrhythmias precipitated by digitalis or some atrial fibrillations arising from DADs in pulmonary veins. The accelerated idioventricular rhythm 1 day after experimental canine myocardial infarction may be caused by DADs, and some evidence has suggested that certain ventricular tachycardias, such as those arising in the right ventricular outflow tract, may be caused by DADs, whereas other data suggest that EADs are responsible.[68]

Major Role of Intracellular Ca^{2+} Handling Abnormalities in DAD Generation. It is well recognized that DADs result from activation of a calcium-sensitive inward current elicited by spontaneous increases in intracellular free calcium concentration. Acquired or inherited abnormalities in the properties of the SR calcium release channels or SR calcium-binding proteins underlie these spontaneous calcium release events.

Rapid mobilization of Ca^{2+} from the SR into the cytosol is mediated by the synchronous opening of ryanodine-sensitive Ca^{2+} release channels (ryanodine receptors, RyRs). The cardiac RyR is composed of four equivalent subunits (homotetramer), each encoded by the *RYR2* gene. During cardiac systole, the small influx of calcium ions through L-type Cav channels triggers a massive release of Ca^{2+} from the SR via synchronous opening of RyR2 channels, a process called Ca^{2+}-induced Ca^{2+} release (see Chap. 24). During diastole, RyR2 channels close and Ca^{2+} is

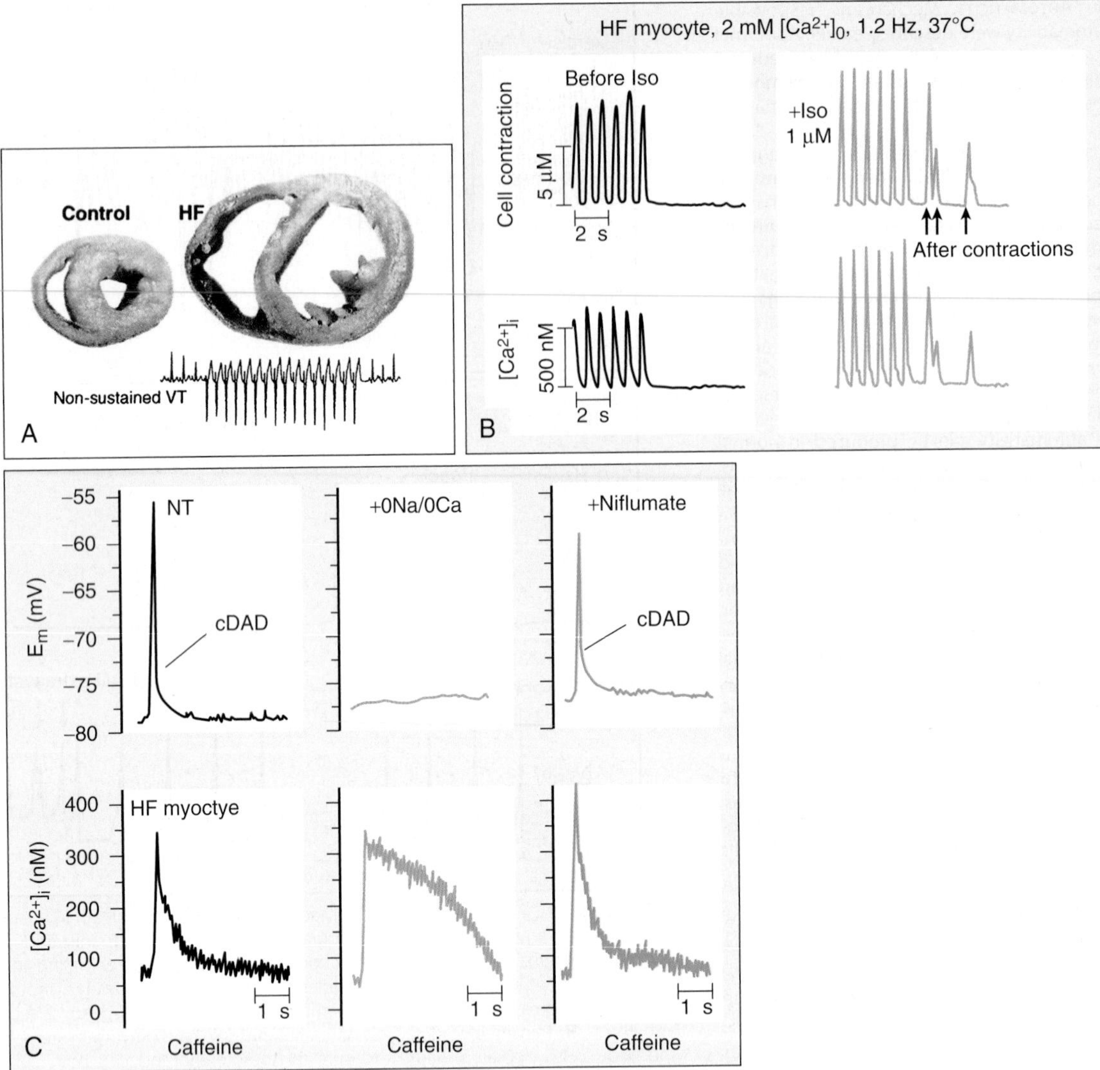

FIGURE 35-22 Ventricular arrhythmia in an animal model of heart failure (aortic constriction-insufficiency in rabbit). **A,** Cross sections of a control and failing heart (HF) and Holter recording of nonsustained ventricular tachycardia (VT) seen in a failing heart. **B,** Spontaneous aftercontractions and increases in $[Ca^{2+}]_i$ in a failing cardiomyocyte after exposure to isoproterenol. **C,** Induction of a DAD by application of caffeine (cDAD) in a cardiomyocyte isolated from a failing rabbit heart. In normal Tyrode (NT) solution, caffeine causes rapid release of Ca^{2+} from the sarcoplasmic reticulum that leads to increases in intracellular free calcium concentration **(bottom tracing),** which in turn causes membrane depolarization. Blocking of the Na^+/Ca^{2+} exchange current in Na^+-free and Ca^{2+}-free solution (0Na/0Ca) abolished DADs despite a similar increase in $[Ca^{2+}]_i$, whereas blocking of the Ca^{2+}-activated Cl^- current with niflumate did not prevent DADs. E_m = membrane voltage. *(From Pogwizd SM, Schlotthauer K, Li L, et al: Arrhythmogenesis and contractile dysfunction in heart failure. Circ Res 88:1159, 2001. By permission of the American Heart Association.)*

recycled into the SR via calcium pumps, thereby refilling SR Ca^{2+} stores for the next release cycle. The duration and amplitude of Ca^{2+} efflux from the SR are therefore tightly controlled by the gating of RyR2 channels. RyR2 interacts with a number of accessory proteins to form a macromolecular Ca^{2+} release complex (see Fig. 35-e5 on website). Proteins interact with the RyR2 at multiple sites within the cytosolic domains of RyR2 (e.g., protein phosphatases) or at the SR level (e.g., calsequestrin, the major calcium-binding protein in the SR lumen). Among the cytosolic ligands, FKBP-12.6 (calstabin2) has been implicated in stabilizing the closed state of the RyR2 channel, preventing diastolic Ca^{2+} leakage.[69]

Mutations in the human *RYR2* gene and in the gene *CASQ2* that encodes calsequestrin (see Fig. 35-e5 on website) have been linked to catecholaminergic polymorphic ventricular tachycardia (CPVT). Experimental studies have revealed that *RYR2* and *CASQ2* mutations that underlie CPVT cause an increase in the sensitivity of the RyR2 channel to luminal Ca^{2+} activation on adrenergic stimulation (e.g., from emotional or physical stress) and enhance the propensity for spontaneous, diastolic Ca^{2+} release from the SR, resulting in DAD-triggered arrhythmias (see later).[20,70-72] It is also possible that CPVT mutants exhibit reduced affinity for the binding of the regulatory protein FKBP-12.6, resulting in diastolic Ca^{2+} leakage from the SR.[73] Reduced FKBP-12.6 binding caused by protein kinase A–mediated hyperphosphorylation has been implicated in cardiac arrhythmogenesis associated with heart failure.[74] FKBP-12.6–deficient mice develop polymorphic ventricular tachycardia on adrenergic stimulation.[75] Treatment with the 1,4-benzothiazepine derivatives JTV519 and S107, which restore FKBP-12.6 affinity for RyR2, has been shown to suppress catecholamine-induced polymorphic ventricular tachycardia in FKBP-12.6–deficient mice.[20,76]

The inositol 1,4,5-trisphosphate (IP_3) receptor (IP_3R) is another Ca^{2+} release channel in cardiomyocytes that is activated by binding of the second messenger IP_3. The type 2 IP_3 receptor (IP_3R2) is the predominant subtype in atrial myocytes, where they are located near RyR2 channels at the SR Ca^{2+} release sites and contribute to altered excitation-contraction coupling and arrhythmogenesis in atria.[77] In Purkinje myocytes, type 1 IP_3 receptors colocalize with type 3 RyR in the subsarcolemmal space to form a functional dyad that critically determines electrical excitability.[62,78] IP_3-dependent Ca^{2+} signaling has been implicated in cardiac arrhythmias attributable to ischemia and reperfusion injury, inflammatory processes, and developing cardiac failure.[79] IP_3 receptors are upregulated in heart failure and atrial fibrillation.[80] In atrial and Purkinje myocytes, IP_3 causes spontaneous $[Ca^{2+}]_i$ transients, Ca^{2+} waves, and Ca^{2+} alternans and facilitates the generation of afterdepolarizations.[79]

The cascade of events linking cellular Ca^{2+} handling abnormalities to cardiac arrhythmias is illustrated in **Figure 35-23**. Ca^{2+} leaking through SR Ca^{2+} release channels during diastole gives rise to localized increases in the cytosolic calcium level in a single cardiomyocyte. The focally elevated Ca^{2+} then causes a propagating Ca^{2+} wave, which depolarizes the cardiomyocyte membrane, triggering a DAD via transient activation of the inward Na^+/Ca^{2+} exchange current ($I_{Na/Ca}$).[21] Inhibition of calmodulin kinase eliminates transient inward $I_{Na/Ca}$ in isolated rabbit ventricular myocytes, indicating that activation of this enzyme plays an important role in cardiac arrhythmogenesis. In addition, drugs that reduce I_{Na} also reduce the transient inward current, relieve Ca^{2+} overload, and can abolish DADs. DADs most likely play a causative role in arrhythmogenesis in the failing heart, where upregulation of $I_{Na/Ca}$, in combination with downregulation of the inward rectifier K^+ current, I_{K1}, facilitates DAD generation (see Fig. 35-22).[51]

Although the causal role of spontaneous SR Ca^{2+} release events in triggering DADs in isolated cardiomyocytes is generally accepted, little is known about whether or how calcium waves within the heart actually produce arrhythmogenic membrane depolarizations. A study using simultaneous optical mapping of changes in $[Ca^{2+}]_i$ and membrane potential with cellular resolution in intact, isolated perfused rat heart demonstrated that the occurrence of triggered activity required the synchronous appearance of Ca^{2+} waves in multiple, adjacent cardiomyocytes. In contrast, sporadic Ca^{2+} waves in individual cardiomyocytes never gave rise to triggered activity (see Fig. 35-e6 on website).[81]

Short coupling intervals and pacing at rates more rapid than the triggered activity rate (overdrive pacing) increase the amplitude and shorten the cycle length of the DAD after cessation of pacing (overdrive acceleration), rather than suppressing and delaying the escape rate of the afterdepolarization, as in normal automatic mechanisms. Premature stimulation exerts a similar effect; the shorter the premature interval, the larger the amplitude and the shorter the escape interval of the triggered event.

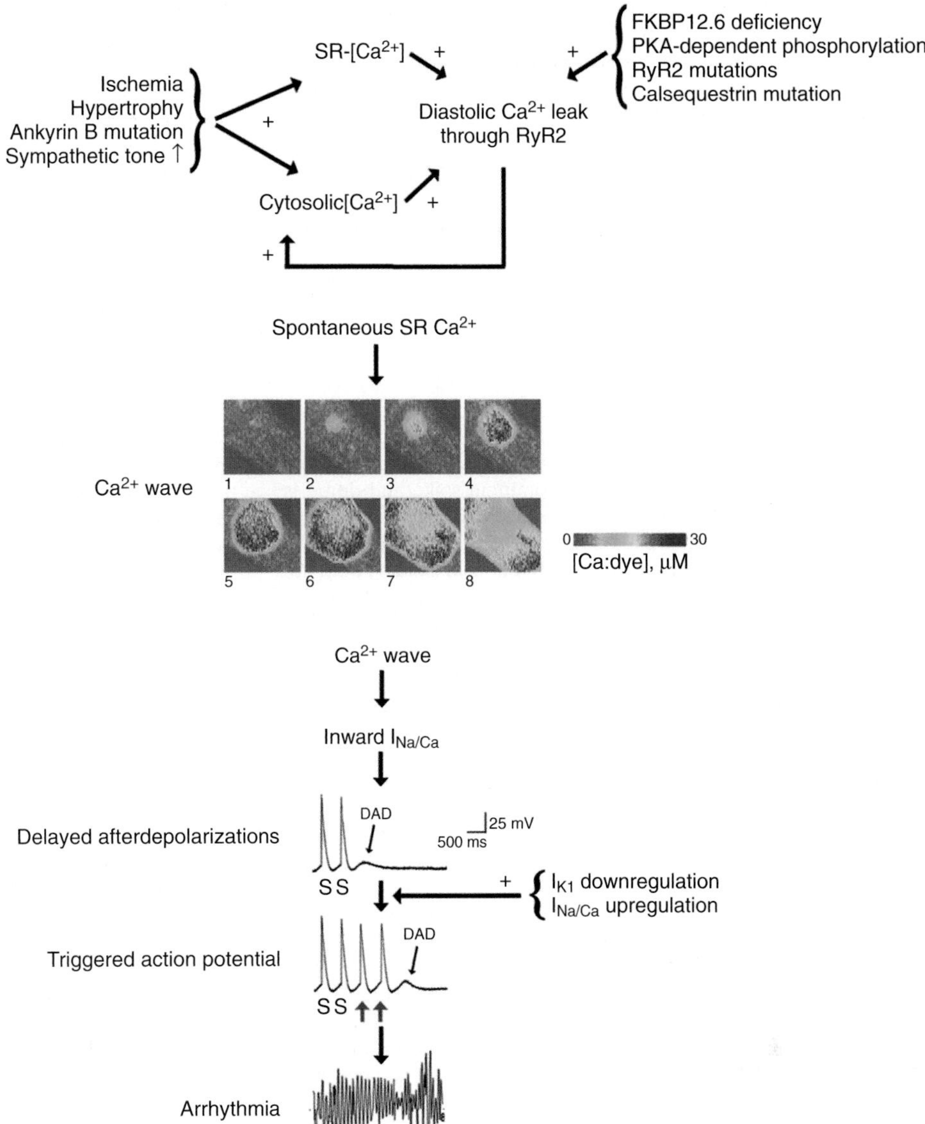

FIGURE 35-23 Proposed scheme of events leading to delayed afterdepolarizations and triggered tachyarrhythmia. **Top panel,** Congenital (e.g., gain-of-function mutations in the *RyR2* or *CASQ2* genes) or acquired factors (e.g., ischemia, hypertrophy, increased sympathetic tone, heart failure) will cause a diastolic Ca^{2+} leak through RyR2, resulting in localized and transient increases in $[Ca^{2+}]_i$ in cardiomyocytes. **Middle panel,** Representative series of images showing changes in $[Ca^{2+}]_i$ during a Ca^{2+} wave in a single cardiomyocyte loaded with a Ca^{2+}-sensitive fluorescent dye. Images were obtained at 117-millisecond intervals. Focally elevated Ca^{2+} (2) diffuses to adjacent junctional sarcoplasmic reticulum (SR), where it initiates more Ca^{2+} release events, resulting in a propagating Ca^{2+} wave (3-8). **Bottom panel,** The Ca^{2+} wave, through activation of inward $I_{Na/Ca}$, will depolarize the cardiomyocyte (DAD). If of sufficient magnitude, the DAD will depolarize the cardiomyocyte above threshold, resulting in a single or repetitive premature heartbeat (red arrows), which can trigger an arrhythmia. Downregulation of the inward rectifier potassium current (I_{K1}) or upregulation of $I_{Na/Ca}$ can promote the generation of DAD-triggered action potentials. S = stimulus. *(Modified from Rubart M, Zipes DP: Mechanisms of sudden cardiac death. J Clin Invest 115:2305, 2005. With permission from Journal of Clinical Investigation.)*

The clinical implication might be that tachyarrhythmias caused by DAD-triggered activity may not be suppressed easily or indeed may be precipitated by rapid rates, either spontaneously (such as a sinus tachycardia) or induced by pacing. Finally, because a single premature stimulus can both initiate and terminate triggered activity, differentiation from reentry (see later) becomes difficult. The response to overdrive pacing may help separate triggered arrhythmias from reentrant arrhythmias.

EARLY AFTERDEPOLARIZATIONS. Various interventions, each of which results in an increase in intracellular positivity, can cause EADs. EADs may be responsible for the lengthened repolarization time and ventricular tachyarrhythmias seen in several clinical situations, such as the acquired and congenital forms of the long-QT syndrome (see Fig. 35-21; see Chap. 39).[82] Left ansa subclavian stimulation increases the amplitude of cesium-induced EADs in dogs and the prevalence of ventricular tachyarrhythmias more than right ansa subclavian stimulation does, possibly because of a greater quantitative effect of the left than of the right stellate ganglion on the left ventricle.

LONG-QT SYNDROME. Patients with the heritable long-QT syndrome have abnormally prolonged cardiac action potential duration and are at increased risk for sudden cardiac death from ventricular tachyarrhythmias (see Chaps. 9 and 39). The genesis of long-QT syndrome–associated ventricular tachycardia or fibrillation is uncertain. There is mounting evidence that increased intracellular Ca^{2+}

concentration related to spontaneous Ca^{2+} release from the SR in cardiomyocytes, coupled with dispersion of repolarization, plays a causative role in long-QT syndrome–associated cardiac arrhythmia and sudden cardiac death. Action potential prolongation may increase Ca^{2+} influx through L-type Ca^{2+} channels during a cardiac cycle, causing excessive Ca^{2+} accumulation in the SR and spontaneous sarcoplasmic reticular Ca^{2+} release. The ensuing elevation of intracellular free calcium can depolarize cardiomyocyte membrane potential by activation of Ca^{2+}-dependent chloride currents, the electrogenic Na^+/Ca^{2+} exchange current, or both, thereby evoking EADs. EADs can trigger a propagated response and thereby elicit an extra beat, potentially launching a tachycardia.

Experimental observations have also suggested an important role of transmural or longitudinal heterogeneity of repolarization. Marked transmural dispersion of repolarization can create a vulnerable window for the development of reentry. A number of studies of isolated ventricular myocytes or tissue preparations have demonstrated spatial dispersion of repolarization along the transmural axes of the left and right ventricular free walls. A prominent spike and dome is apparent in myocytes from epicardium and the M region but not in myocytes from endocardium.[83] Action potential duration–rate relationships are considerably more pronounced in cells isolated from the M region in some studies. The ionic basis for electrophysiologic distinctions between epicardial, midmyocardial, and endocardial myocytes is a large gradient in both the density- and rate-dependent properties of the transient outward K^+ current and a smaller density of the slow component of the delayed rectifier K^+ current I_{Ks} as well as larger late Na^+ currents and inward $I_{Na/Ca}$ in midmyocardial cells than in endocardial and epicardial myocytes.

Sympathetic stimulation, primarily left, can increase the EAD amplitude to provoke ventricular tachyarrhythmias. Alpha-adrenoceptor stimulation also increases the amplitude of cesium-induced EADs and the prevalence of ventricular tachyarrhythmias, both of which are suppressed by magnesium.

In patients with the acquired long-QT syndrome and torsades de pointes from drugs such as quinidine, *N*-acetylprocainamide, cisapride, erythromycin, and some class III antiarrhythmic agents, EADs can also be responsible (see Chaps. 10 and 37). Such drugs easily elicit EADs experimentally and clinically, whereas magnesium suppresses them. It is possible that multiple drugs can cause summation effects to provoke EADs and torsades de pointes in patients. Activators of ATP-dependent potassium channels, such as pinacidil and nicorandil, can eliminate EADs.

PARASYSTOLE. Classically, parasystole has been likened to the function of a fixed-rate asynchronously discharging pacemaker—its timing is not altered by the dominant rhythm, it produces depolarization when the myocardium is excitable, and the intervals between discharges are multiples of a basic interval (see Chaps. 38 and 39). Complete entrance block, constant or intermittent, insulates and protects the parasystolic focus from surrounding electrical events and accounts for such behavior. On occasion, the focus can exhibit exit block, during which it may fail to depolarize excitable myocardium. In fact, the dominant cardiac rhythm may modulate parasystolic discharge to speed up or to slow down its rate. Brief subthreshold depolarizations induced during the first half of the cardiac cycle of a spontaneously discharging pacemaker delay the subsequent discharge, whereas similar depolarizations induced in the second half of the cardiac cycle accelerate it (see Fig. 35-e7 on website).

Disorders of Impulse Conduction

Conduction delay and block can result in bradyarrhythmias or tachyarrhythmias. Bradyarrhythmias occur when the propagating impulse is blocked and is followed by asystole or a slow escape rhythm; tachyarrhythmias occur when the delay and block produce reentrant excitation (see later). Various factors involving both active and passive membrane properties determine the conduction velocity of an impulse and whether conduction is successful. Among these factors are the stimulating efficacy of the propagating impulse, related to the amplitude and rate of rise of phase 0; the excitability of the tissue into which the impulse is conducted; and the geometry of the tissue.

DECELERATION-DEPENDENT BLOCK. Diastolic depolarization has been suggested as a cause of conduction block at slow rates, so-called bradycardia- or deceleration-dependent block (see Chap. 39). However, excitability and speed of impulse propagation *increase* as the membrane depolarizes until about −70 mV, despite a reduction in action potential amplitude and $\dot{V}max$. Experiments in Purkinje fiber bundles have demonstrated that diastolic (phase 4) depolarization is not a necessary condition for the occurrence of deceleration-dependent block.[84] Evidently, depolarization-induced inactivation of fast Na^+ channels is offset by other factors, such as reduction in the difference between membrane potential and threshold potential and increase in membrane excitability.

TACHYCARDIA-DEPENDENT BLOCK. More commonly, impulses are blocked at rapid rates or short cycle lengths as a result of incomplete recovery of refractoriness (postrepolarization refractoriness) caused by incomplete time- or voltage-dependent recovery of excitability (see Chap. 36).[84] For example, such incomplete recovery is the usual mechanism responsible for a nonconducted premature P wave or one that conducts with a functional bundle branch block.

DECREMENTAL CONDUCTION. Decremental conduction is a term used commonly in the clinical literature but is often misapplied to describe any Wenckebach-like conduction block, that is, responses similar to block in the AV node during which progressive conduction delay precedes the nonconducted impulse. Correctly used, decremental conduction refers to a situation in which the properties of the fiber change along its length so that the action potential loses its efficacy as a stimulus to excite the fiber ahead of it. Thus, the stimulating efficacy of the propagating action potential diminishes progressively, possibly as a result of its decreasing amplitude and decreasing $\dot{V}max$.

REENTRY. Electrical activity during each normal cardiac cycle begins in the sinoatrial node and continues until the entire heart has been activated. Each cell becomes activated in turn, and the cardiac impulse dies out when all fibers have been discharged and are completely refractory. During this absolute refractory period, the cardiac impulse has "no place to go." It must be extinguished and restarted by the next sinus impulse. If, however, a group of fibers not activated during the initial wave of depolarization recovers excitability in time to be discharged before the impulse dies out, the fibers may serve as a link to reexcite areas that were just discharged and have now recovered from the initial depolarization. Such a process has been given various names, all meaning approximately the same thing—reentry, reentrant excitation, circus movement, reciprocal or echo beat, or reciprocating tachycardia.

ENTRAINMENT. Entraining the tachycardia (i.e., increasing the rate of the tachycardia by pacing), with resumption of the intrinsic rate of the tachycardia when pacing is stopped, establishes the presence of reentry (**Fig. 35-24A**). Entrainment represents capture or continuous resetting of the reentrant circuit of the tachycardia by the pacing-induced activation. Each pacing stimulus creates a wave front that travels in an anterograde direction (orthodromic) and resets the tachycardia to the pacing rate. A wave front propagating retrogradely in the opposite direction (antidromic) collides with the orthodromic wave front of the previous beat (Fig. 35-24B). These wave front interactions create electrocardiographic and electrophysiologic features that can be explained only by reentry. Therefore, the criteria of entrainment can be used to prove the reentrant mechanism of a clinical tachycardia and form the basis for localizing the pathway traveled by the tachycardia wave front. Such localization is essential for ablation therapy.

ANATOMIC REENTRY. Studies on reentry have used models that had anatomically defined separate pathways in which it could be shown that they had an area of unidirectional block and recirculation of the impulse to its point of origin. An example is illustrated in **Figure 35-25** using AV nodal reentry. Because the two pathways have different electrophysiologic properties (e.g., shorter refractory period and slower conduction in one pathway versus longer refractory period and faster conduction of the other), the impulse is first blocked in one pathway with longer refractory period (green area in Fig. 35-25) and then propagates slowly in the adjacent pathway whose refractory period is shorter (red area in Fig. 35-25A, right panel). If conduction in this alternative route is sufficiently depressed, the slowly propagating impulse excites tissue beyond the blocked pathway (see Fig. 35-25A right panel, dashed yellow arrow) and returns in a reversed direction along the pathway initially blocked to reexcite tissue proximal to the site of block. A clinical arrhythmia caused by anatomic reentry is most likely to have a monomorphic contour (see Video 35-3 on website).[8]

For reentry of this type to occur, the time for conduction within the depressed but unblocked area and for excitation of the distal segments must exceed the refractory period of the initially blocked pathway (see Fig. 35-25) and the tissue proximal to the site of block. Stated another way, continuous reentry requires the anatomic length of the circuit traveled to equal or to exceed the reentrant wavelength. The latter is equal to the mean conduction velocity of the impulse multiplied by the longest refractory period of the elements in the circuit. Both values can be different at different points along the reentry pathway, and thus the wavelength value is somewhat contrived.

Conditions for Reentry

The length of the pathway is fixed and determined by the anatomy. Conditions that depress conduction velocity or abbreviate the refractory period promote the development of reentry in this model, whereas prolonging refractoriness and speeding conduction velocity can hinder it. For example, if conduction velocity (0.30 m/sec) and refractoriness (350 milliseconds) for ventricular muscle were normal, a pathway of 105 mm (0.30 m/sec × 0.35 sec) would be necessary for reentry to occur. However, under certain conditions, conduction velocity in ventricular muscle and Purkinje fibers can be very slow (0.03 m/sec), and if refractoriness is not greatly prolonged (600

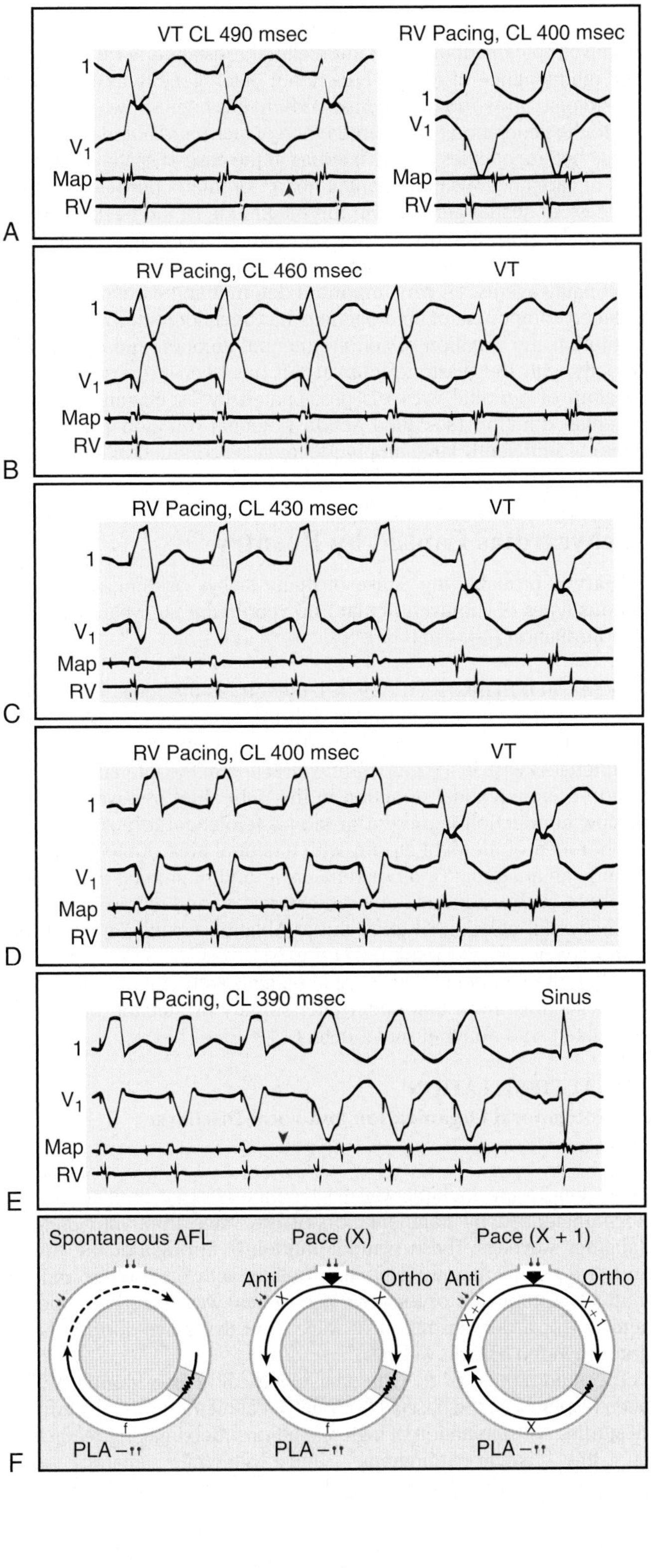

FIGURE 35-24 **A-E,** Criteria for entrainment exemplified in a case of postinfarction ventricular tachycardia (VT). **A, left,** Two leads of the electrocardiogram of a VT and intracardiac recordings from a mapping catheter (Map) at a left ventricular site critical for VT continuation as well as from the right ventricular apex (RV). Note the diastolic potential (red arrowhead) during VT. Recordings are similarly arranged in all subsequent panels. **A, right,** RV pacing in the setting of sinus rhythm. **B,** RV pacing at a cycle length (CL) slightly shorter than VT produces a QRS complex that is a blend between fully VT and fully paced ("fusion") complexes. All recordings are accelerated to the paced CL, and after pacing ceases, the same VT resumes. Each fused QRS complex is identical and the last beat is entrained, but surface fusion is absent. **C, D,** The same phenomena, but at shorter paced CLs. Note that the fused QRS complex appears more similar to pacing than it does to VT as the pacing CL shortens. **B-D,** Progressive degrees of fusion in the electrocardiogram. The Map recording of **B** through **D** also shows a progression of fusion, with both the morphology and timing of a portion of the electrogram changing with faster pacing. **E,** Finally, a still shorter paced CL results in a sudden change in both the Map electrogram (block in the small diastolic potential, red arrowhead) and the surface electrocardiogram, which is now fully paced. When pacing ceases, VT has been interrupted. **F,** Diagrammatic representation of the reentrant circuit during spontaneous atrial flutter (AFL) and transient entrainment of the AFL. **Left,** The reentrant circuit during spontaneous type I AFL. f = circulating wave front of the AFL. **Center,** Introduction of the first pacing impulse (X) during rapid pacing from a high atrial site during AFL. The large arrow indicates entry of the pacing impulse into the reentrant circuit, whereupon it is conducted orthodromically (Ortho) and antidromically (Anti). The antidromic wave front of the pacing impulse (X) collides with the previous beat, in this case the circulating wave front of the spontaneous AFL (f), which results in an atrial fusion beat and, in effect, terminates the AFL. However, the orthodromic wave front from the pacing impulse (X) continues the tachycardia and resets it to the pacing rate. **Right,** Introduction of the next pacing impulse (X + 1) during rapid pacing from the same high atrial site. The large arrow again indicates the entry of the pacing impulse into the reentrant circuit, whereupon it is conducted orthodromically and antidromically. Once again, the antidromic wave front from the pacing impulse (X + 1) collides with the orthodromic wave front of the previous beat. In this case, it is the orthodromic wave front of the previous paced beat (X), and an atrial fusion beat results. The orthodromic wave front from the pacing impulse (X + 1) continues the tachycardia and resets it to the pacing rate. In all three parts, arrows indicate the direction of spread of the impulses; the serpentine line indicates slow conduction through a presumed area of slow conduction (stippled region) in the reentrant circuit, and the red dots with tails indicate bipolar electrodes at the high atrial pacing site, the posteroinferior portion of the left atrium (PLA), and another atrial site. *(**A-E** from Zipes DP: A century of cardiac arrhythmia: In search of Jason's golden fleece. J Am Coll Cardiol 34:959, 1999. **F** from Waldo AL: Atrial flutter. Entrainment characteristics. J Cardiovasc Electrophysiol 8:337, 1997.)*

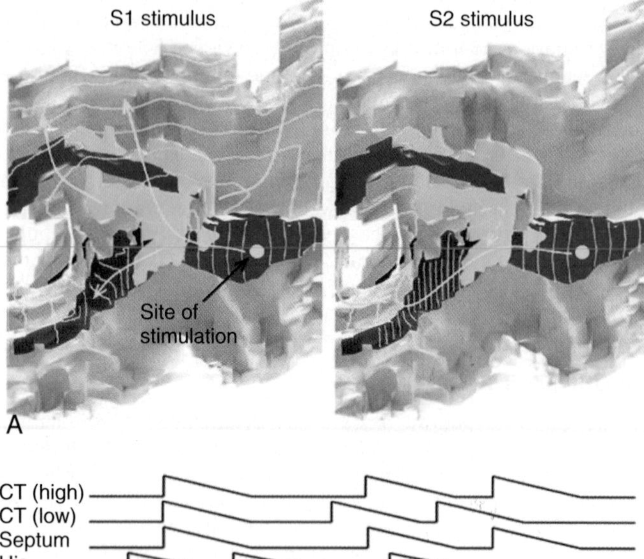

FIGURE 35-25 Simulation of reentry in a model of the AV node. **A**, Electrical stimuli are applied to the His bundle (yellow point), using an S1-S2 protocol (S1-S2 interval, 96 milliseconds). The activation sequences (shown as isochrones at 5-millisecond intervals) in response to S1 and S2 stimuli are shown. Arrows highlight the conduction pathways. Two stimuli are delivered. The S1 action potential exits into the atrial muscle via the transitional tissue (green area), the putative fast pathway. The premature S2 action potential fails to exit via the transitional tissue because the S1-S2 interval is shorter than the refractory period of the transitional tissue. Instead, the S2 action potential exits into the atrial muscle via the inferior nodal extension (INE, the putative slow pathway; red area) because the refractory period of the INE is shorter. The conduction velocity within the INE is low, as indicated by the isochrone crowding within the red area. The action potential then propagates anterogradely along the fast pathway (transitional tissue is no longer refractory) back into the His bundle. **B**, Simulated action potentials (at high and low crista terminalis, interatrial septum, and His bundle) at different time points on the reentry circuit during S1-S2 stimulation. The S2 action potential retrogradely excites atrial tissue (the action potential at the low crista terminalis appears first) and then anterogradely the His bundle, completing one reentry cycle. The reentry beat propagates along the INE and out into the atrial muscle once more but then fails to reexcite anterogradely the His bundle. Color coding of the various tissue types is the same as in Figure 35-7. *(From Li J, Greener ID, Inada S, et al: Computer three-dimensional reconstruction of the atrioventricular node. Circ Res 102:975, 2008. By permission of the American Heart Association.)*

milliseconds), a pathway of only 18 mm (0.03 m/sec × 0.60 sec) may be necessary. Such reentry frequently exhibits an excitable gap, that is, a time interval between the end of refractoriness from one cycle and the beginning of depolarization in the next, when tissue in the circuit is excitable. This condition results because the wavelength of the reentrant circuit is less than the pathway length. Electrical stimulation during this time period can invade the reentrant circuit and reset its timing or terminate the tachycardia. Although "microanatomic" reentry (confinement of the reentrant circuit to a few adjacent myocytes) has been postulated to occur in fibrotic myocardium,[85] its occurrence in intact heart muscle has not been demonstrated directly. This difficulty results from the inability to unambiguously distinguish microreentry from triggered activity with currently available techniques.

Rapid pacing can entrain the tachycardia, that is, continuously reset it by entering the circuit and propagating around it in the same way as the reentrant impulse, which increases the tachycardia rate to the pacing rate without terminating the tachycardia (see Fig. 35-24). In reentrant circuits with an excitable gap, conduction velocity determines the revolution time of the impulse around the circuit and therefore the rate of the tachycardia. Prolongation of refractoriness, unless it is long enough to eliminate the excitable gap and make the impulse propagate in relatively refractory tissue, does not influence the revolution time around the circuit or the rate of the tachycardia. Anatomic reentry occurs in patients with the Wolff-Parkinson-White syndrome, in AV nodal reentry, in some atrial flutters, in some ventricular tachycardias, and in ventricular fibrillation. For example, mapping studies in isolated ovine atria have demonstrated key roles of anatomic structures (e.g., fibrotic patches) in the maintenance of reentry during fibrillation.[86]

FUNCTIONAL REENTRY. Functional reentry lacks confining anatomic boundaries and can occur in contiguous fibers that exhibit functionally different electrophysiologic properties caused by local differences in transmembrane action potential (e.g., Purkinje-myocyte transition). Dispersion of excitability, refractoriness, or both, as well as anisotropic distributions of intercellular resistance, permit initiation and maintenance of reentry. Functional heterogeneity in the electrophysiologic properties of the myocardium has been shown to contribute to the generation and maintenance of tachycardia and fibrillation. These heterogeneities can be fixed, as in the case of spatial redistribution of gap junctions in the failing heart[39] or infarct border zone or in the case of spatial gradients in the magnitude of the background K^+ current, I_{K1} (**Fig. 35-26B**).[87] They can also change dynamically, as in the acutely ischemic myocardium[88] or in the presence of repolarization-prolonging agents.[89] A very important determinant of the dynamically induced component of heterogeneity has been identified as electrical restitution, the variation of action potential duration and conduction velocity with the diastolic interval.[90] It has been proposed that the breakup of periodic waves is precipitated by oscillations of action potential duration (so-called action potential duration [APD] alternans) of sufficiently large amplitude to cause conduction block along a spiral wave front (see Fig. 35-29).

Tachycardias Caused by Reentry

Reentry is probably the cause of many tachyarrhythmias, including various types of supraventricular and ventricular tachycardias, flutter, and fibrillation (see Chap. 39).

ATRIAL FLUTTER (see Chap. 39). Reentry is the most likely cause of the usual form of atrial flutter, with the reentrant circuit confined to the right atrium in typical atrial flutter, where it usually travels counterclockwise in a caudocranial direction in the interatrial septum and in a craniocaudal direction in the right atrial free wall. An area of slow conduction is present in the posterolateral to posteromedial inferior area of the right atrium, with a central area of block that can include an anatomic (inferior vena cava) and functional component. This area of slow conduction is rather constant and represents the site of successful ablation of atrial flutter. Ablation results are consistent with a macroreentry circuit (see Chap. 37).

Different reentrant circuits exist in patients with other types of atrial flutter, such as those that occur after surgery or ablation or that are associated with an atrial septal defect (see Chap. 65).

ATRIAL FIBRILLATION

Spatiotemporal Organization and Focal Discharge
(see Chap. 40)

According to the multiple-wavelet hypothesis, atrial fibrillation (AF) is characterized by fragmentation of the wave front into multiple daughter wavelets. These wander randomly throughout the atrium and give rise to new wavelets that collide with each other and are mutually annihilated or that give rise to new wavelets in a perpetual activity (for a demonstration of wave front dynamics during fibrillation, see Video 35-4 on website).

The randomness of the irregular electrical activity during AF has been disputed on the basis of both statistical methods and experimental studies. A combination of high-resolution video imaging, recordings of the electrocardiogram, and spectral analysis was used to demonstrate that reentry in anatomically or functionally determined circuits forms the basis of spatiotemporal periodicity during acute AF. The cycle length of the source in the left atrium determines the dominant peak in the frequency spectra. The underlying periodicity may stem from a repetitive focal source of activity propagated from an individual pulmonary vein or left atrial site to the remainder of the atrium as fibrillating waves. If a single repetitive focal source of activity that undergoes fractionation underlies the maintenance of AF, ablation of this focal source should interrupt AF. Indeed, delivery of radiofrequency energy to discrete sites in the distal pulmonary veins in humans has been shown to eliminate or to reduce recurrence of AF. In a large animal model of inducible AF associated with heart failure, it was recently demonstrated that AF dynamics was characterized by rapid repetitive activation (resulting from either microanatomic reentry or triggered activity) revolving around fibrotic obstacles in the posterior left atrium or pulmonary vein ostia. Furthermore, fibrillatory activity was maintained by intramural reentry centered on fibrotic patches and appeared as endocardial breakthroughs at the posterior left atrium (endocardial breakthroughs are considered sudden and unexpected appearances of localized electrical activity not related to activation or slow conduction in the surrounding regions.). In heart failure atria, AF waves changed origin and direction of propagation on a beat-to-beat basis; whereas in normal left atria, the breakthrough sites and direction of activation of AF wave fronts were highly recurrent from one AF wave to the next (see Fig. 35-e8 and Video 35-5 on website). Interestingly, numerical simulations of AF dynamics best recapitulated the experimental observations in this study when cardiomyocytes were assumed to be electrotonically coupled to myofibroblasts, supporting a role of heterocellular electrical coupling in atrial arrhythmogenesis.[86]

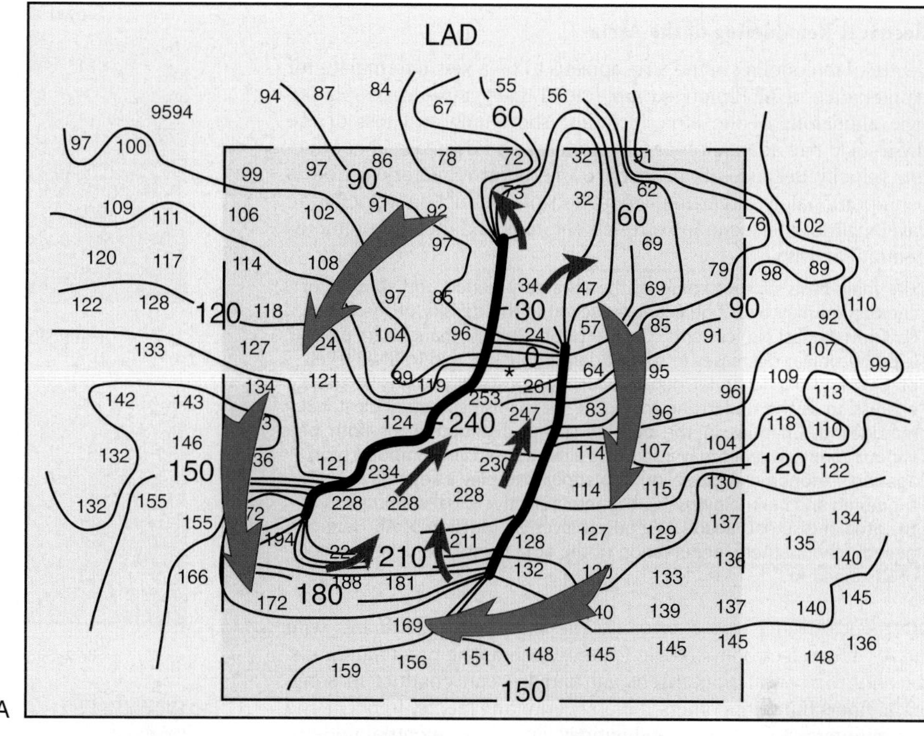

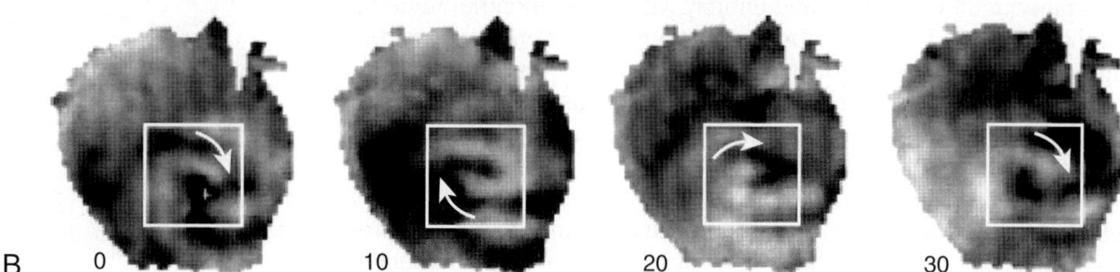

FIGURE 35-26 Functional models of reentry. **A,** Figure-of-8 reentry in anisotropic myocardium. Maps of activation times of a stable reentrant circuit during ventricular tachycardia in the epicardial border zone of a 4-day-old anterior infarct in a dog. The activation times (in milliseconds, small numbers) are shown, as are lines of isochronal activation, at 10-millisecond intervals (larger numbers). The lines of functional block are shown in bold. The circuit consists of clockwise and counterclockwise wave fronts around two functional arcs of block that merge into a central common pathway that usually represents the slow zone of the reentrant circuit. The localization of the functional arcs of block coincides with the spatial disarray of connexin43 gap junctions. **B,** Spiral wave model. Recording of spiral wave reentry during ventricular fibrillation in a Langendorff-perfused guinea pig heart using a potentiometric fluorophore. Shown are the distributions of membrane potentials at four different times during one rotation on the left ventricular epicardial surface, with white and black being the most positive and most negative membrane potentials, respectively. Numbers are time in milliseconds. Arrows denote direction of wave front propagation. *(**A** from Peters NS, Coromilas J, Severs NJ, et al: Disturbed connexin43 gap junction distribution correlates with the location of reentrant circuits in the epicardial border zone of healing canine infarcts that cause ventricular tachycardia. Circulation 95:988, 1997. By permission of the American Heart Association. **B** from Samie FH, Berenfeld O, Anumonwo J, et al: Background potassium current. A determinant of rotor dynamics in ventricular fibrillation. Circ Res 89:1216, 2001. By permission of the American Heart Association.)*

Several experimental models have been used to study the structural and basic electrophysiologic properties of pulmonary veins that are thought to play a role in initiation and maintenance of AF. Morphologic studies have demonstrated the presence of complex anatomic structures and phenotypically different cardiomyocytes in pulmonary veins.[91,92] Electrophysiologic studies have shown that the combination of reentrant and nonreentrant mechanisms (automaticity and triggered activity) is the underlying arrhythmogenic mechanism for AF initiation from the pulmonary veins.[92,93] Abnormal intracellular calcium handling probably plays a pivotal role in the pulmonary vein electrical activity. Dual mapping of cardiomyocyte membrane potential and intracellular free calcium has demonstrated the appearance of spontaneous calcium release events, resulting in focal discharge.[93] The role of dysfunctions of calcium-handling proteins (e.g., Na^+/Ca^{2+} exchanger, ryanodine receptor calcium release channels) in AF awaits further investigation.

Primary Ion Channel Abnormalities in Atrial Fibrillation. A number of studies have revealed a primary role of abnormalities in ion channel expression or properties in causing AF. Rapid pacing–induced AF in dogs causes a decrease in FKBP-12.6 binding to the ryanodine receptor Ca^{2+} release channel (see Fig. 35-e5 on website), resulting in diastolic SR Ca^{2+} leakage, which in turn, through activation of Ca^{2+}-sensitive currents, can initiate electrical instability and contribute to fibrillation.[94] Mice with a genetic gain-of-function defect in the gene encoding the type 2 ryanodine receptor exhibit increased susceptibility to inducible AF. AF induction in this animal model may involve triggered activity arising from EADs, whereas maintenance of AF requires reentrant activity.[72] Cav1.3 Ca^{2+} channel–deficient mice exhibit increased susceptibility to inducible atrial flutter and fibrillation.[95] Mice in which the gene encoding KCNE1, an auxiliary subunit of the pore-forming K^+ channel alpha subunit KCNQ1, has been knocked out display frequent spontaneous episodes of AF.[96] Finally, a human connexin40 gene polymorphism is associated with increased vulnerability to AF induction.[97]

Electrical Remodeling of the Atria

Electrical remodeling of the atria appears to be a key determinant for maintenance of AF. Prolonged rapid atrial rates cause electrophysiologic alterations of the atria, including shortening and loss of the physiologic rate adaptation of refractoriness and decrease in conduction velocity. Because abbreviation of the atrial refractory period is disproportionately larger than reduction of conduction velocity, the wavelength of the reentrant wavelets shortens and thereby promotes reentrant activity.

The ionic basis of shortening of the refractory period and slowing of conduction may be a significant reduction in the density of the L-type Ca^{2+} and the fast Na^{+} currents. The electrophysiologic changes are paralleled by similar decreases in messenger ribonucleic acid (mRNA) levels of Ca^{2+} and Na^{+} channel genes, which suggests alterations in gene expression as the underlying molecular mechanisms of atrial electrical remodeling. Changes in the density, spatial distribution, or both of various connexin types may also cause alterations in atrial impulse propagation. Autonomic remodeling also appears to play a key role in both triggering and maintaining AF. Long-term selective vagal denervation of the atria and sinoatrial and AV nodes prevents induction of AF. Heterogeneous sympathetic denervation of the atria favors the development of sustained AF.

SINUS REENTRY (see Chap. 39). The sinoatrial node shares with the AV node electrophysiologic features such as the potential for dissociation of conduction, that is, an impulse can conduct in some nodal fibers but not in others, thereby permitting reentry to occur. The reentrant circuit can be located entirely within the sinoatrial node or involve both the sinoatrial node and atrium. Supraventricular tachycardias caused by sinus node reentry are generally less symptomatic than other supraventricular tachycardias because of slower rates. Ablation of the sinoatrial node may be necessary in an occasional refractory tachycardia.

ATRIAL REENTRY (see Chap. 39). Reentry within the atrium, unrelated to the sinoatrial node, can be a cause of supraventricular tachycardia in humans. Distinguishing atrial tachycardia caused by automaticity or afterdepolarizations from atrial tachycardia sustained by reentry over small areas (i.e., microanatomic reentry) is difficult.

ATRIOVENTRICULAR NODAL REENTRY (see Chap. 39). Differences in the electrical properties of the various tissue types that contribute to the AV node are responsible for AV nodal reentrant tachycardia (AVNRT; see Figs. 35-7 and 35-25). Optical mapping of AV nodal transmembrane action potentials during echo beats reveals the reentrant pathways underlying various types of AVNRT (**Fig. 35-27**; see also Fig. 35-7 for nomenclature of AV nodal regions). The reentrant pathway of the slow-fast type starts counterclockwise with block in the fast pathway (the transitional zone; see light green area in Fig. 35-7), delay in conduction across the slow pathway (the inferior nodal extension; see red area in Fig. 35-7) to the compact AV node (see yellow area in Fig. 35-7), exit from the AV node to the fast pathway, and rapid return to the slow pathway through atrial tissue located at the base of the triangle of Koch. The reentrant circuit of the fast-slow type is clockwise. In the slow-slow type, anterograde conduction is over the intermediate pathway and retrograde conduction is over the slow pathway. Because slow pathway conduction is involved in each type of AVNRT, ablation of the slow pathway is effective in all types of AVNRT. These results also demonstrate that atrial tissue surrounding the triangle of Koch is clearly involved in all three types of AV nodal reentry in these examples.

PREEXCITATION SYNDROME (see Chap. 39). In most patients who have reciprocating tachycardias associated with Wolff-Parkinson-White syndrome, the accessory pathway conducts more rapidly than the normal AV node but takes a longer time to recover excitability; that is, the anterograde refractory period of the accessory pathway exceeds that of the AV node at long cycles. Consequently, a premature atrial complex that occurs sufficiently early is blocked anterogradely in the accessory pathway and continues to the ventricle over the normal AV node and His bundle. After the ventricles have been excited, the impulse is able to enter the accessory pathway retrogradely and return to the atrium. A continuous conduction loop of this type establishes the circuit for the tachycardia. The usual (orthodromic) activation wave during such a reciprocating tachycardia in a patient with an accessory pathway occurs anterogradely over the normal AV node–His-Purkinje system and retrogradely over the accessory pathway, which results in a normal QRS complex (**Fig. 35-28**).

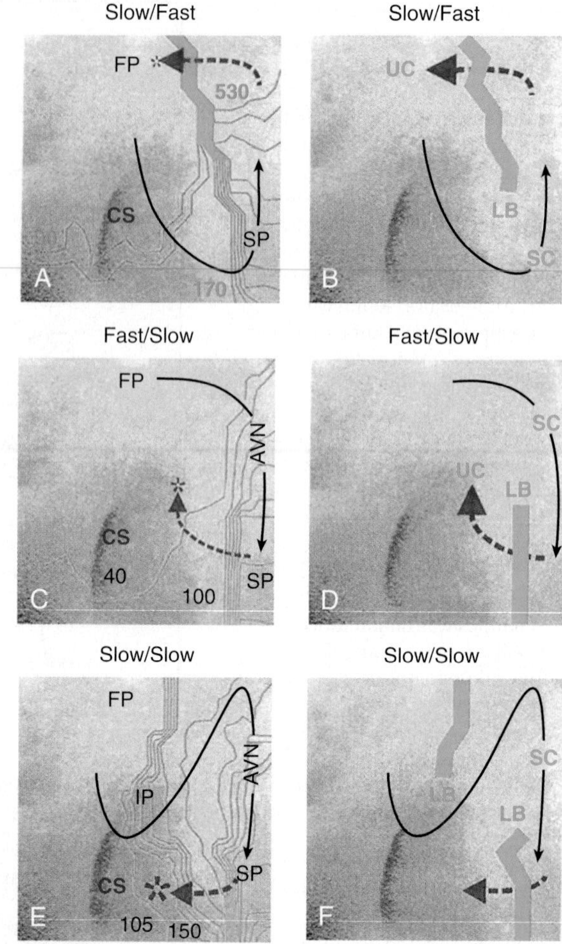

FIGURE 35-27 Reentrant circuits of different types of AV nodal reentrant tachycardia. Pictures of the optical activation maps of A_2 obtained from three different experiments at A_2 coupling intervals of 190, 220, and 190 milliseconds, respectively, were merged with the pictures of the mapping area to show the initiation of echo beats in **A** (Slow/Fast), **C** (Fast/Slow), and **E** (Slow/Slow). The numbers in the maps indicate the activation times in reference to the A_2 stimulus. The black arrow indicates anterograde conduction, and the asterisk and the dashed red arrow represent the site of earliest retrograde atrial activation. The corresponding locations of the lines of block (LB, green), slow anterograde conduction (SC, black arrow), and unidirectional conduction (UC, red) are shown in **B, D,** and **F,** respectively. CS, coronary sinus; FP, fast pathway; IP, intermediate pathway; SP =slow pathway. *(From Wu J, Zipes DP: Mechanisms underlying atrioventricular nodal conduction and the reentrant circuit of atrioventricular nodal reentrant tachycardia using optical mapping. J Cardiovasc Electrophysiol 13:831, 2002.)*

Because the circuit requires both atria and ventricles, the term *supraventricular tachycardia* is not precisely correct, and the tachycardia is more accurately termed *atrioventricular reciprocating tachycardia* (AVRT). The reentrant loop can be interrupted by ablation of the normal AV node–His bundle pathway *or* the accessory pathway. On occasion, the activation wave travels in a reverse (antidromic) direction to the ventricles over the accessory pathway and to the atria retrogradely up the AV node. Two accessory pathways can form the circuit in some patients with antidromic AVRT. In some patients, the accessory pathway may be capable of only retrograde conduction ("concealed"), but the circuit and mechanism of AVRT remain the same. Less

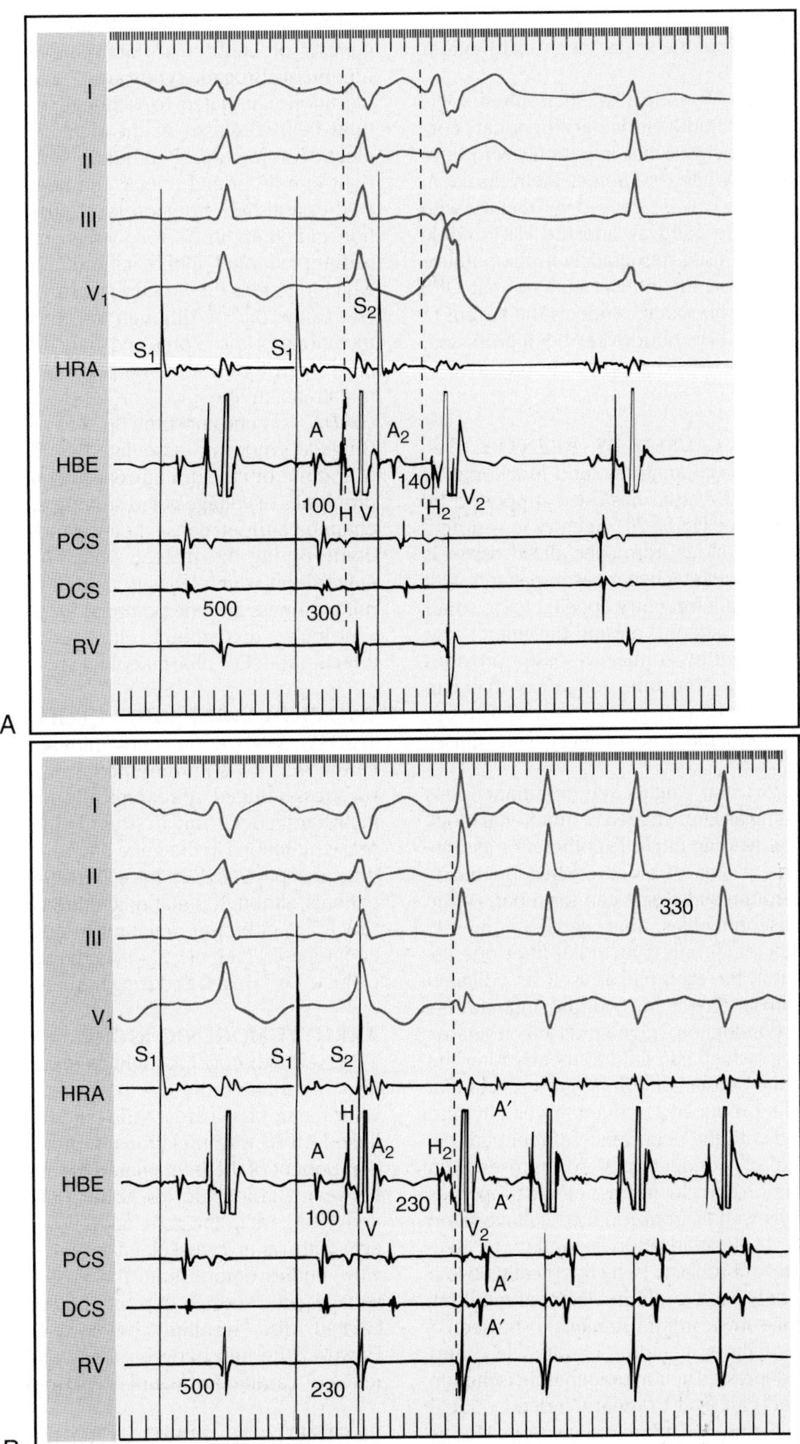

FIGURE 35-28 **A,** Wolff-Parkinson-White syndrome. Following high right atrial pacing at a cycle length of 500 milliseconds (S_1-S_1), premature stimulation at a coupling interval of 300 milliseconds (S_1-S_2) produces physiologic delay in AV nodal conduction, resulting in an increase in the A-H interval from 100 to 140 milliseconds but no delay in the AV interval. Consequently, activation of the His bundle follows activation of the QRS complex (second interrupted line), and the QRS complex becomes more anomalous in appearance because of increased ventricular activation over the accessory pathway. **B,** Induction of reciprocating AV tachycardia. Premature stimulation at a coupling interval of 230 milliseconds prolongs the A-H interval to 230 milliseconds and results in anterograde block in the accessory pathway and normalization of the QRS complex (a slight functional aberrancy in the nature of incomplete right bundle branch block occurs). Note that H_2 precedes onset of the QRS complex (interrupted line). Following V_2, the atria are excited retrogradely (A′) beginning in the distal coronary sinus, followed by atrial activation in leads recording from the proximal coronary sinus, His bundle, and high right atrium. A supraventricular tachycardia is initiated at a cycle length of 330 milliseconds. I, II, III, and V_1 indicate scalar electrocardiographic leads. DCS = distal coronary sinus electrogram; HBE = His bundle electrogram; HRA = high right atrium; PCS = proximal coronary sinus electrogram; RV = right ventricular electrogram. Time lines are in 50- and 10-millisecond intervals. S_1, stimulus of the drive train; S_2, premature stimulus. A, H-V, atrial, His bundle, and ventricular activation during the drive train; A_2, H_2, V_2, atrial, His bundle, and ventricular activation during the premature stimulus. *(From Zipes DP, Mahomed Y, King RD, et al: Wolff-Parkinson-White syndrome: Cryosurgical treatment. Indiana Med 89:432, 1986.)*

commonly, the accessory pathway can conduct only anterogradely. The pathway can be localized by analysis of the scalar electrocardiogram. Patients can have AF as well as AVRT.

Unusual accessory pathways with AV node–like electrophysiologic properties, that is, nodofascicular or nodoventricular fibers, can constitute the circuit for reciprocating tachycardias in patients who have some form of the Wolff-Parkinson-White syndrome. Tachycardia in patients with nodoventricular fibers can be caused by reentry, with these fibers used as the anterograde pathway and the His-Purkinje fibers and a portion of the AV node used retrogradely. In the putative Lown-Ganong-Levine syndrome (short PR interval and normal QRS complex), conduction over a James fiber that connects the atrium to the distal portion of the AV node and His bundle has been proposed, although little functional evidence exists to support the presence of this entity.

VENTRICULAR TACHYCARDIA CAUSED BY REENTRY (see Chap. 39). Reentry in the ventricle, both anatomic and functional, as a cause of sustained ventricular tachycardia has been supported by many animal and clinical studies (see Fig. 35-26). Reentry in ventricular muscle, with or without contributions from specialized tissue, is responsible for many or most ventricular tachycardias in patients with ischemic heart disease. The area of microreentry appears to be small, and less commonly, a macroreentry is found around the infarct scar. Surviving myocardial tissue separated by connective tissue provides serpentine routes of activation traversing infarcted areas that can establish reentry pathways. Bundle branch reentry can cause sustained ventricular tachycardia, particularly in patients with dilated cardiomyopathy.

Both figure-of-8 (see Fig. 35-26) and single-circle reentrant loops have been described as circulating around an area of functional block in a manner consistent with the leading circle hypothesis or as conducting slowly across an apparent area of block created by anisotropy.[98] When intramural myocardium survives, it can form part of the reentrant loop. Structural discontinuities that separate muscle bundles—as a result of naturally occurring myocardial fiber orientation and anisotropic conduction, for example, as well as collagen matrices formed from the fibrosis after a myocardial infarction—establish the basis for slowed conduction, fragmented electrograms, and continuous electrical activity, which can lead to reentry. After the infarction, the surviving epicardial border zone undergoes substantial electrical remodeling,[99] including reduced conduction velocity and increased anisotropy associated with the occurrence of reentrant circuits and ventricular tachycardia.[41] Conduction slowing arises from alterations in the spatial distribution and electrophysiologic properties of connexin43 gap junctions[41] as well as from reduced voltage-gated sodium current. Whether myocyte depolarization secondary to electrotonic coupling to adjacent myofibroblasts (which typically have a much more depolarized potential) plays a role in electrical remodeling in postinfarction border zone myocardium remains to be seen.[65] During acute ischemia, various factors, including elevated $[K]_o$ and reduced pH, combine to create depressed action potentials in ischemic cells that retard conduction and can lead to reentry. Indeed, optical mapping studies in arterially perfused canine wedge preparations during global no-flow ischemia have demonstrated reentry initiation during initial ischemia and subsequent reperfusion caused by the unidirectional block of conduction resulting from the spatiotemporal dispersion in tissue responses to stimulation.[88] The rapidly changing combination of the transmural dispersion in response to endocardial pacing stimuli and velocity of conduction creates a dynamic substrate in which reentry can be initiated and sustained. The results of this study are compatible with previous observations that fibrillation during reperfusion can be caused by intramural reentry. Interestingly, transmural reentry under these experimental conditions could be triggered by epicardial, but not endocardial, stimulation, at a time when there was epicardial conduction delay or block with preserved endocardial conduction due to the increased susceptibility of the epicardium to the effects of ischemia. Clinically, this might facilitate tachycardia induction by a premature ventricular complex arising in the epicardium but not in the endocardium.

BRUGADA SYNDROME. Phase 2 reentry has been implicated in the genesis of ventricular tachycardia-fibrillation associated with the inheritable Brugada syndrome,[100] which is characterized by ST-segment elevation (unrelated to ischemia, electrolyte abnormalities, or structural heart disease) in the right precordial (V_1 to V_3) leads of the electrocardiogram, often but not always accompanied by an apparent right bundle branch block. The hereditary nature of the syndrome is well established. Brugada syndrome has been linked to loss-of-function mutations in *SCN5A*, which encodes the pore-forming cardiac sodium channel alpha subunit Nav1.5, and mutations in *SCN1B*, which encodes the function-modifying sodium channel $beta_1$ subunit (see Chap. 9).[101,102] Although Na^+ channel mutations are most common, mutations in the alpha and beta subunits of the Ca^{2+} channel gene have been found in some patients with Brugada syndrome, as have mutations in the glycerol-3-phosphate dehydrogenase 1–like gene (*GPD1L*) on chromosome 3p22-25 (BS2), reducing the Na^+ current, I_{Na}. Brugada syndrome–associated gene defects cause reduction or loss of sodium or calcium current in combination with altered functional properties of voltage-gated sodium channels. Alterations in the sodium channel current cause heterogeneous loss of the action potential dome during the plateau phase (phase 2) in the right ventricular epicardium, which leads to a marked dispersion of repolarization and refractoriness and the potential for phase 2 reentry.[103] Ablation of right ventricular epicardium eliminates ventricular arrhythmias in an animal model of pharmacologically induced Brugada syndrome.[100]

CATECHOLAMINERGIC POLYMORPHIC VENTRICULAR TACHYCARDIA. Catecholaminergic polymorphic ventricular tachycardia (CPVT) is an inherited arrhythmogenic disease characterized by stress-induced, adrenergically mediated polymorphic ventricular tachycardia occurring in structurally normal hearts. Heterozygous missense mutations in the gene encoding the Ca^{2+} release channel ryanodine receptor (RyR2) have been reported in the majority of CPVT patients, although mutations in the calsequestrin gene can also cause CPVT.[104] A common mechanism underlying RyR2-associated CPVT is an increased leak of Ca^{2+} from the SR during diastole, leading to intracellular Ca^{2+} waves and triggered activity.[105,106]

ARRHYTHMOGENIC RIGHT VENTRICULAR CARDIOMYOPATHY. Arrhythmogenic right ventricular cardiomyopathy (ARVC) is also an inherited disease that presents with sustained monomorphic ventricular tachycardia and sudden death. Previous studies have linked ARVC with mutations in proteins of the cardiac desmosome, a component of the intercalated disc essential for mechanical coupling between cardiomyocytes. About 70% of the mutations linked to inherited ARVC are in the gene encoding plakophilin2 (*PKP2*), which interacts with other cytoskeletal proteins to stabilize the desmosome. In vitro studies demonstrate that loss of *PKP2* expression reduces the voltage-gated sodium current and connexin43 expression at the intercalated disc, resulting in slowed action potential propagation. However, the link between these molecular changes and the occurrence of cardiac arrhythmias will have to be defined.[107,108]

VENTRICULAR FIBRILLATION: INITIATION AND MAINTENANCE (see Chap. 39). Previous experimental and simulation investigations have suggested that ventricular fibrillation (VF) is maintained solely by reentry. This reentry was thought to be unstable, maintained by wandering wavelets of activation following constantly changing paths of activation and exhibiting frequent conduction block caused by nonuniform dispersion of refractoriness. More recent investigations have suggested other mechanisms of fibrillation maintenance and have introduced the concepts of restitution kinetics, wave front, wave break, focal discharge, and rotor as replacement for the classic reentry theory.[109]

The hallmark of cardiac fibrillation is ongoing wave break (or wave splitting).[110] Wave break is caused by conduction block occurring at a specific site along the wave front while the remaining portions of the front continue to propagate. This localized block, wave break, causes splitting of the mother wave front into two daughter wavelets. Two hypotheses exist in regard to the genesis of wave breaks during fibrillation. The mother

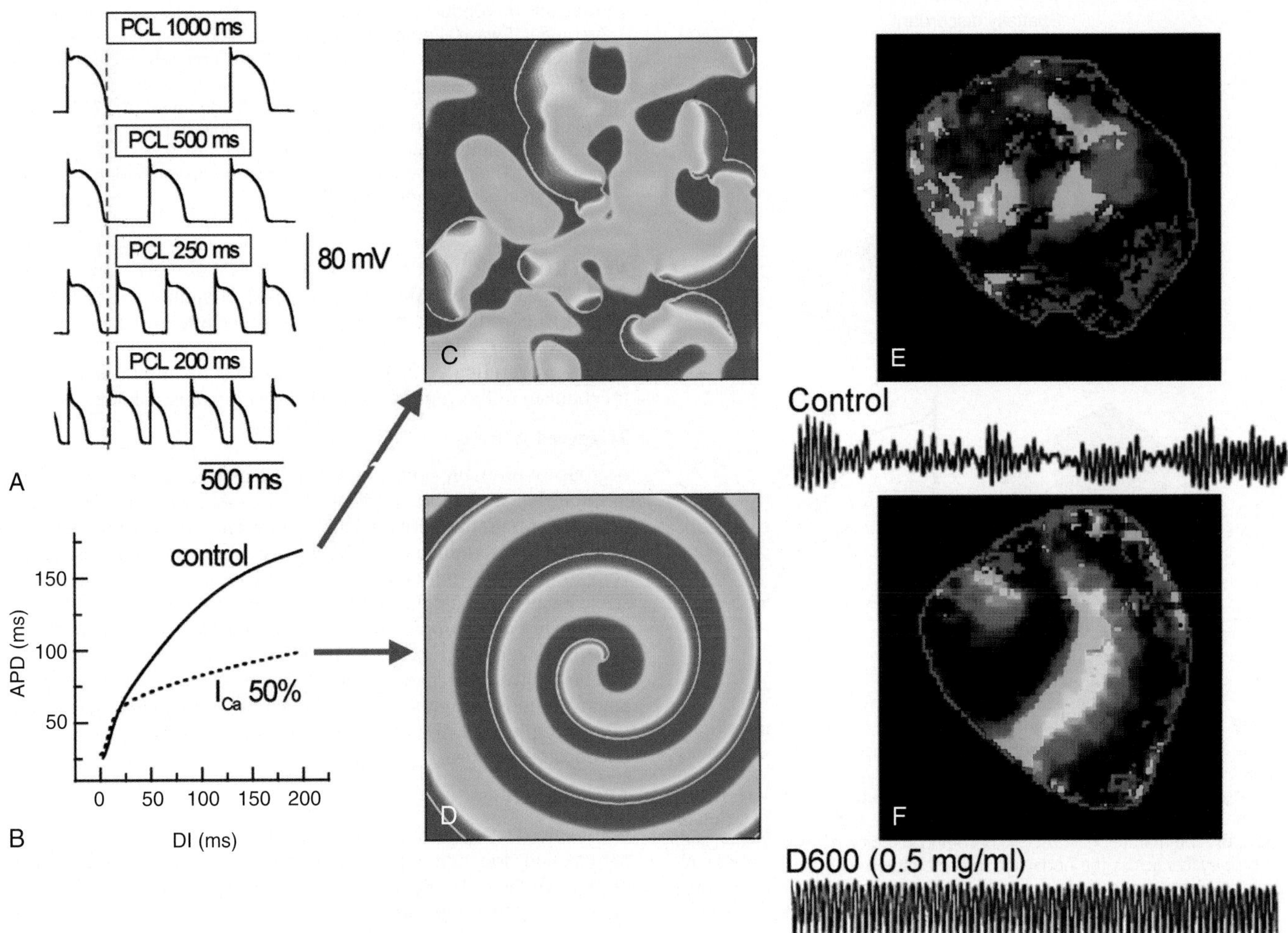

FIGURE 35-29 Action potential duration restitution slope and rotor stability. **A**, Action potential duration (APD) shortening and APD alternans as pacing cycle length (PCL) decreases (computer simulations). **B**, APD restitution curves, with slope >1 (solid line) or <1 (dashed line, obtained with 50% block of the calcium current). **C, D**, Spiral wave behavior several seconds after initiating a rotor in homogeneous two-dimensional tissue. All myocytes are assumed identical, with either a steep **(C)** or shallow **(D)** APD restitution slope. **E, F**, Conversion of multiple-wavelet VF to mother rotor VF. Optically measured surface voltage maps obtained from an intact Langendorff-perfused rabbit heart before **(E)** and after **(F)** partially blocking the L-type calcium current to flatten the APD restitution slope to <1. In **E,** multiple wavefronts move in a complex VF pattern. In **F,** VF has converted to ventricular tachycardia, manifested as a stable rotor. Black tracings below color panels in **E** and **F** are corresponding electrograms. *(From Weiss JN, Qu Z, Chen PS, et al: The dynamics of cardiac fibrillation. Circulation 112:1232, 2005. By permission of the American Heart Association.)*

rotor hypothesis states that VF is maintained by a single, stationary, intramural stable reentrant circuit (i.e., the mother rotor) in a dominant domain, which has the shortest refractory period from which activations propagate into the more slowly activating domains with longer refractory periods. Wave breaks result from Wenckebach-like conduction as high-frequency impulses emanating from the dominant domain are unable to sustain 1:1 conduction through heterogeneous tissue. In this case, the fastest activating (i.e., dominating) rotor, rather than ongoing wave break, is the engine driving cardiac fibrillation, and wave break occurs only secondarily.[109,111] Evidence supporting this concept is that frequency analyses have shown (1) single, stable (both in space and time), dominant frequencies in the power spectra of membrane voltage signals obtained from various regions of the heart; (2) correlation of dominant frequencies and the frequency of reentry; (3) relative infrequency of reentry on the surface of the heart during fibrillation, favoring an intramural location of the mother rotor, such as the Purkinje network; and (4) Wenckebach-like conduction at the borders between different dominant frequency domains. These borders can result from preexisting structural or functional heterogeneities. For example, high-resolution electrical mapping has suggested that fast activation during VF is driven by Purkinje fibers. Spatial heterogeneity in the magnitude of ionic currents has been implicated in the generation of spatial gradients in activation rates and in maintaining rotor stability in the fastest activating regions. For example, the magnitude of the inward rectifying K^+ current, I_{K1} (see Table 35-3), was larger in the rapidly activating left ventricular myocytes than in the slower activating right ventricular myocytes.[87] Furthermore, regions with larger I_{K1} had faster activation rates and more stable rotors than did regions with smaller I_{K1}.[87]

In contrast to the stable mother rotor theory, other experimental evidence has supported the idea that dynamic wave break plays a fundamental role in the initiation and maintenance of short-duration VF (wandering wavelet hypothesis).[109,110,112,113] According to this hypothesis, VF is maintained by wandering wavelets with constantly changing, evanescent, reentrant circuits. The experimental evidence favoring the multiple wavelet hypothesis includes (1) inability to detect a single dominant frequency in power spectra of mapping data from fibrillating hearts; (2) spatiotemporal instability of frequency domain distributions during VF, with the exception of anatomic borders, such as Purkinje-myocyte transition; (3) failure to demonstrate stable intramural reentry at higher frequencies than at the surface; and (4) boundaries dynamically generated by wavelet behavior rather than by anatomic conduction block. To reproduce the dynamic spatiotemporal instability of dominant frequency domains, a combination of dynamically changing and fixed tissue heterogeneity is required.[109] The most important determinant of the dynamically induced component of heterogeneity has been identified as electrical restitution, the variation of action potential duration and conduction velocity with the diastolic interval. For example, it has been proposed that the breakup of periodic waves is precipitated by oscillations of action potential duration (so-called APD alternans) that are sufficiently large enough to cause conduction block along the spiral wave front. Simulations (**Fig. 35-29**) have shown that a reentrant rotor becomes unstable and breaks down into multiple rotors when the slope of the

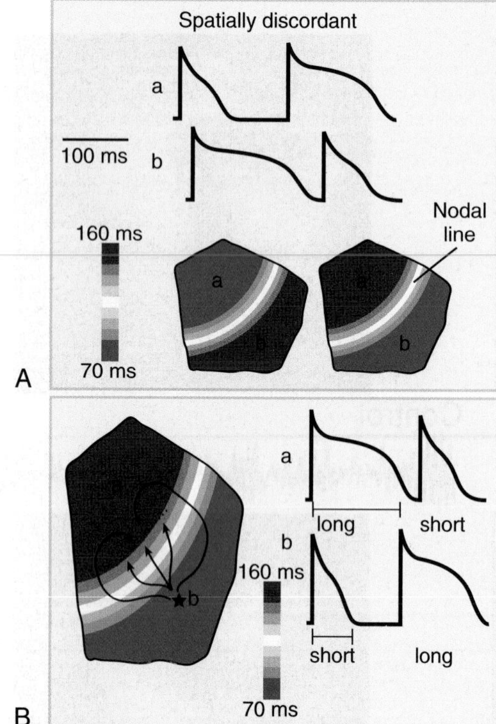

FIGURE 35-30 Initiation of reentry by a premature beat during spatially discordant alternans. **A, upper panel,** At rapid rates, action potentials at site *a* alternate short-long, whereas at the same time, action potentials at site *b* alternate long-short, creating a steep gradient of APD distribution, with a nodal line with no APD alternation separating the out-of-phase regions *a* and *b* **(lower panel). B,** A premature beat (asterisk) occurring in region *b* blocks (dotted line) as it propagates across the nodal line into the region with long APD (*a*). The premature beat propagates laterally along the nodal line, waiting for the long APD region to repolarize, and then reenters the blocked region to initiate figure-of-8 reentry. *(From Weiss JN, Karma A, Shiferaw Y, et al: From pulsus to pulseless: The saga of cardiac alternans. Circ Res 98:1244, 2006. By permission of the American Heart Association.)*

restitution curve for action potential duration versus the diastolic interval is >1. Pharmacologic blockade of the L-type calcium current can terminate VF via reducing the action potential duration restitution slope (see Fig. 35-29).[114] If it is occurring in a spatially discordant pattern, alternans is considered a key arrhythmogenic factor predisposing the heart to reentry and fibrillation.[115] At the cellular level, the origin of APD alternans appears to be primarily determined by alternations in cardiomyocyte calcium transient amplitude or duration (calcium alternans).

During spatially discordant alternans, the action potential duration alternates out of phase in different regions of the heart, thereby increasing dispersion of refractoriness so that ectopic beats have a high probability of inducing reentry. This mechanism is illustrated in **Figure 35-30**; some regions of the heart alternate in a long-short-long pattern, whereas other regions at the same time alternate in a short-long-short pattern. These out-of-phase regions are separated by a nodal line, in which no alternans is present, but spatial gradients in action potential duration are steepest along this line. Thus, spatially discordant alternans creates gradients in tissue refractoriness, which in turn favor the development of reentry by a premature beat (Fig. 35-30B). At the cellular level, the steepness of the action potential duration restitution curve and intracellular calcium level ($[Ca^{2+}]_i$) dynamics cause action potential duration and the $[Ca^{2+}]_i$ transient to alternate. Given the bidirectional coupling between changes in $[Ca^{2+}]_i$ and membrane potential—for example, membrane potential determines the activity of L-type Cav channels, and conversely, the $[Ca^{2+}]_i$ transient amplitude strongly modulates action potential duration through its effects on Ca^{2+}-sensitive currents (e.g., $I_{Na/Ca}$) during the action potential plateau—alternation in $[Ca^{2+}]_i$ transient amplitude can cause secondary alternation in action potential duration. Indeed, experimental evidence has strongly suggested that the onset of APD alternans is primarily attributable to instabilities of $[Ca^{2+}]_i$ cycling dynamics, thus defining a causal role of intracellular Ca^{2+} handling abnormalities in initiating electrical instability. At the tissue level, alternans combines with instabilities in conduction velocity to cause alternans to become spatially discordant. T wave alternans is the electrocardiographic manifestation of APD/$[Ca^{2+}]_i$ alternans and thus is a clinical predictor of future arrhythmic events.

In addition to a role of Purkinje fibers in the initiation of VF, other studies have suggested involvement of Purkinje fibers in the maintenance of VF, either as part of a reentrant circuit or as a source of focal activations. Their role appears to be more important during later (>1 minute) than earlier stages of VF.[109]

VENTRICULAR TACHYCARDIAS CAUSED BY NONREENTRANT MECHANISMS. In some cases of ventricular tachycardia related to coronary artery disease, but especially in patients without coronary artery disease, nonreentrant mechanisms are important causes of ventricular tachycardias. However, in many patients, the mechanism of the ventricular tachycardia remains unknown.

Triggered Activity

A group of probably nonreentrant ventricular tachycardias occurring in the absence of structural heart disease can be initiated and terminated by programmed stimulation. They are catecholamine dependent and are terminated by the Valsalva maneuver, adenosine, and verapamil. These ventricular tachycardias are generally but not exclusively located in the right ventricular outflow tract and may be caused by triggered activity, possibly DADs that are cAMP dependent.[68] EADs have been recorded in this tachycardia as well. Left ventricular fascicular tachycardias can be suppressed by verapamil but not generally by adenosine, and some may be caused by triggered activity and others by reentry. EADs and triggered activity may be responsible for torsades de pointes.

Automaticity

Automatic discharge can be responsible for some ventricular tachycardias and does not appear to be suppressed by adenosine. Unless invasive studies are undertaken, mechanisms of ventricular tachycardia can only be conjectured.

REFERENCES

Anatomy of the Cardiac Conduction System

1. Maltsev VA, Vinogradova TM, Lakatta EG: The emergence of a general theory of the initiation and strength of the heartbeat. J Pharmacol Sci 100:338, 2006.
2. Chandler NJ, Greener ID, Tellez JO, et al: Molecular architecture of the human sinus node. Circulation 119:1562, 2009.
3. Boyett MR, Inada S, Yoo S, et al: Connexins in the sinoatrial and atrioventricular nodes. Adv Cardiol 42:175, 2006.
4. Fedorov VV, Schuessler RB, Hemhill M, et al: Structural and functional evidence for discrete exit pathways that connect the canine sinoatrial node and atria. Circ Res 104:915, 2009.
5. Schwartz PJ, Zipes DP: Autonomic modulation of cardiac arrhythmias. *In* Zipes DP, Jalife J (eds): Cardiac Electrophysiology: From Cell to Bedside. 3rd ed. Philadelphia, WB Saunders, 1999, pp 300-314.
6. Barbuti A, Terragni B, Brioschi C, et al: Localization of f-channels to caveolae mediates specific β_2-adrenergic receptor modulation of rate in sinoatrial myocytes. J Mol Cell Cardiol 42:71, 2007.
7. Ko Y, Yeh H, Ko Y, et al: Three-dimensional reconstruction of the rabbit atrioventricular conduction axis by combining histological, desmin, and connexin mapping data. Circulation 109:1172, 2004.
8. Li J, Greener ID, Inada S, et al: Computer three dimensional reconstruction of the atrioventricular node. Circ Res 102:975, 2008.
9. Di Maio, Ter Keurs HE, Franzini-Armstrong C: T-tubule profiles in Purkinje fibres of mammalian myocardium. J Muscle Res Cell Motil 28:115, 2007.
10. Rohr S, Kucera JP, Fast VG, et al: Paradoxical improvement of impulse conduction in cardiac tissue by partial uncoupling. Science 275:841, 1997.
11. Ieda M, Kanazawa H, Kimura K, et al: Sema3a maintains normal heart rhythm through sympathetic innervation patterning. Nat Med 13:604, 2007.
12. Hucker WJ, Nikolski VP, Efimov IR: Autonomic control and innervation of the atrioventricular junctional pacemaker. Heart Rhythm 4:1326, 2007.
13. Mantravadi R, Gabris B, Liu T, et al: Autonomic nerve stimulation reverses ventricular repolarization sequence in rabbit hearts. Circ Res 100:e72, 2007.
14. Jacques D, Abdel-Samad D: Neuropeptide Y (NPY) and NPY receptors in the cardiovascular system: Implication in the regulation of intracellular calcium. Can J Physiol Pharmacol 85:43, 2007.
15. Oh YS, Jong AY, Kim DT, et al: Spatial distribution of nerve sprouting after myocardial infarction in mice. Heart Rhythm 3:728, 2006.
16. Zhou S, Jung BC, Tan AY, et al: Spontaneous stellate ganglion nerve activity and ventricular arrythmias in a canine model of sudden death. Heart Rhythm 5:131, 2008.
17. Liu Y, Lee Y, Pak H, et al: Effects of simvastatin on cardiac neural and electrophysiologic remodeling in rabbits with hypercholesterolemia. Heart Rhythm 6:69, 2009.

18. Tan AY, Chen PS: Autonomic nerves in pulmonary veins. Heart Rhythm 4:S57, 2007.
19. Pokushalov E, Romanov A, Shugayev P, et al: Selective ganglionated plexi ablation for paroxysmal atrial fibrillation. Heart Rhythm 6:1257, 2009.
20. Scanavacca M, Pisani C, Hachul D, et al: Selective atrial vagal denervation guided by evoked vagal reflex to treat patients with paroxysmal atrial fibrillation. Circulation 114:876, 2006.
21. Lehnart SE, Mongillo M, Belinger A, et al: Leaky Ca^{2+} release channel/ryanodine receptor 2 causes seizures and sudden cardiac death in mice. J Clin Invest 118:2230, 2008.
22. Scornik FS, Desai M, Brugada R, et al: Functional expression of "cardiac-type" Nav1.5 sodium channel in canine intracardiac ganglia. Heart Rhythm 3:842, 2006.

Basic Electrophysiologic Principles

23. Song Y, Shryock JC, Belardinelli L, et al: A slowly-inactivating sodium current contributes to spontaneous diastolic depolarization of atrial myocytes. Am J Physiol Heart Circ Physiol 297:H1254, 2009.
24. Song Y, Shryock JC, Belardinelli L: An increase of late sodium current induces delayed afterdepolarizations and sustained triggered activity in atrial myocytes. Am J Physiol Heart Circ Physiol 294:H2031, 2008.
25. Wagner S, Dybkova N, Rasenack ENL, et al: Ca^{2+}/calmodulin-dependent protein kinase II regulates cardiac sodium channels. J Clin Invest 116:3127, 2006.
26. Kass RS, Moss AJ: Long QT syndrome: Novel insights into the mechanisms of cardiac arrhythmias. J Clin Invest 112:810, 2003.
27. Shah M, Akar FG, Tomaselli GF: Molecular basis of arrhythmias. Circulation 112:2517, 2005.
28. Zipes DP, Tomaselli GF: What causes sudden death in heart failure? Circ Res 95:754, 2004.
29. Nerbonne JM, Kass RS: Molecular physiology of cardiac repolarization. Physiol Rev 85:1205, 2005.
30. Plant LD, Bowers PN, Liu Q, et al: A common cardiac sodium channel variant associated with sudden infant death in African Americans, SCN5A S1103Y. J Clin Invest 116:430, 2006.
31. Mangoni ME, Traboulsie A, Leoni AL, et al: Bradycardia and slowing of the atrioventricular conduction in mice lacking CaV3.1/alpha1G T-type calcium channels. Circ Res 98:1422, 2006.
32. Anderson CL, Delisle BP, Anson BD, et al: Most LQT2 mutations reduce Kv11.1 (hERG) current by a class 2 (trafficking-deficient) mechanism. Circulation 113:365, 2006.
33. Li N, Timofeyev V, Tuteja D, et al: Ablation of a Ca^{2+}-activated K^+ channel (SK2 channel) results in action potential prolongation in atrial myocytes and atrial fibrillation. J Physiol 587:1087, 2009.
34. Baruscotti M, Bucchi A, DiFrancesco D: Physiology and pharmacology of the cardiac pacemaker ("funny") current. Pharmacol Ther 107:59, 2005.
35. Milanesi R, Baruscotti M, Gnecchi-Ruscone T, et al: Familial sinus bradycardia associated with a mutation in the cardiac pacemaker channel. N Engl J Med 354:151, 2006.
36. Kleber A, Rudy Y: Basic mechanisms of cardiac impulse propagation and associated arrhythmias. Physiol Rev 84:431, 2004.
37. Kanaporis G, Mese G, Valiuniene L, et al: Gap junction channels exhibit connexin-specific permeability to cyclic nucleotides. J Gen Physiol 131:293, 2008.
38. Li J, Patel VV, Kostetskii I, et al: Cardiac-specific loss of N-cadherin leads to alteration in connexins with conduction slowing and arrhythmogenesis. Circ Res 97:474, 2005.
39. Kreuzberg MM, Söhl G, Kim J: Functional properties of mouse connexin30.2 expressed in the conduction system of the heart. Circ Res 96:1169, 2005.
40. Akar FG, Spragg DD, Tunin RS, et al: Mechanisms underlying conduction slowing and arrhythmogenesis in nonischemic dilated cardiomyopathy. Circ Res 95:717, 2004.
41. Kieken F, Mutsaers N, Dolmatova E, et al: Structural and molecular mechanisms of gap junction remodeling in epicardial border zone myocytes following myocardial infarction. Circ Res 104:1103, 2009.
42. Danik SB, Liu F, Zhang F, et al: Modulation of cardiac gap junction expression and arrhythmic susceptibility. Circ Res 95:1035, 2004.
43. Morley GE, Danik SB, Bernstein S, et al: Reduced intercellular coupling leads to paradoxical propagation across the Purkinje-ventricular junction and aberrant myocardial activation. Proc Natl Acad Sci U S A 102:4126, 2005.
44. Yao JA, Gutstein DE, Liu F, et al: Cell coupling between ventricular myocyte pairs from connexin43-deficient murine hearts. Circ Res 93:736, 2003.
45. Firouzi M, Ramanna H, Kok B, et al: Association of human connexin40 gene polymorphisms with atrial vulnerability as a risk factor for idiopathic atrial fibrillation. Circ Res 95:e29, 2004.
46. Gard JJ, Yamada K, Green KG, et al: Remodeling of gap junctions and slow conduction in a mouse model of desmin-related cardiomyopathy. Cardiovasc Res 67:539, 2005.
47. Kaplan SR, Gard JJ, Carvajal-Huerta L, et al: Structural and molecular pathology of the heart in Carvajal syndrome. Cardiovasc Pathol 13:26, 2004.
48. Kaplan SR, Gard JJ, Protonotarios N, et al: Remodeling of gap junctions in arrhythmogenic right ventricular cardiomyopathy due to a deletion in plakoglobin (Naxos disease). Heart Rhythm 1:3, 2004.
49. Oxford EM, Musa H, Maass K, et al: Connexin43 remodeling caused by inhibition of plakophilin-2 expression in cardiac cells. Circ Res 101:703, 2007.
50. Li J, Patel VV, Kostetskii I, et al: Cardiac-specific loss of N-cadherin leads to alteration in connexins with conduction slowing and arrhythmogenesis. Circ Res 97:474, 2005.
51. Rubart M, Zipes DP: Mechanisms of sudden cardiac death. J Clin Invest 115:2305, 2005.
52. Reuter H, Henderson SA, Han T, et al: The Na^+-Ca^{2+} exchanger is essential for the action of cardiac glycosides. Circ Res 90:305, 2002.
53. Lei M, Jones SA, Liu J, et al: Requirement of neuronal- and cardiac-type sodium channels for murine sinoatrial node pacemaking. J Physiol 559(pt 3):835, 2004.
54. Baruscotti M, Bucchi A, DiFrancesco D: Physiology and pharmacology of the cardiac pacemaker ("funny") current. Pharmacol Ther 107:59, 2005.
55. Verkerk AO, den Ruijter HM, Bourier J, et al: Dietary fish oil reduces pacemaker current and heart rate in rabbit. Heart Rhythm 6:1485, 2009.
56. Costantini DL, Arruda EP, Agarwal P, et al: The homeodomain transcription factor Irx5 establishes the mouse cardiac ventricular repolarization gradient. Cell 123:347, 2005.
57. Harris DM, Mills GD, Chen X, et al: Alterations in early action potential repolarization causes localized failure of sarcoplasmic reticulum Ca^{2+} release. Circ Res 96:543, 2005.
58. Zygmunt AC, Goodrow RJ, Weigel CM: I_{NaCa} and $I_{Cl(Ca)}$ contribute to isoproterenol-induced delayed afterdepolarizations in midmyocardial cells. Am J Physiol 275:H1979, 1998.
59. Bers DM, Ginsburg KS: Na:Ca stoichiometry and cytosolic Ca-dependent activation of NCX in intact cardiomyocytes. Ann N Y Acad Sci 1099:326, 2007.
60. Yeh S, Chang H, Shieh R: Electrostatics in the cytoplasmic pore produce intrinsic inward rectification in the Kir2.1 channels. J Gen Physiol 126:551, 2005.
61. Li N, Timofeyev V, Tuteja D, et al: Ablation of a Ca^{2+}-activated K^+ channel (SK2 channel) results in action potential prolongation in atrial myocytes and atrial fibrillation. J Physiol 587:1087, 2009.
62. Stuyvers BD, Dun W, Matkovich S, et al: Ca^{2+} sparks and waves in canine Purkinje cells: A triple layered system of Ca^{2+} activation. Circ Res 97:35, 2005.
63. Sasse P, Zhang J, Cleemann L, et al: Intracellular Ca^{2+} oscillations, a potential pacemaking mechanism in early embryonic heart cells. J Gen Physiol 130:133, 2007.
64. Joung B, Tang L, Maruyama M, et al: Intracellular calcium dynamics and acceleration of sinus rhythm by β-adrenergic stimulation. Circulation 119:788, 2009.
65. Miragoli M, Salvarami N, Rohr S: Myofibroblasts induce ectopic activity in cardiac tissue. Circ Res DOI:10.1161/CIRCRESAHA.107.160549, 2007.

Mechanisms of Arrhythmogenesis

66. Patterson E, Po SS, Scherlag BJ, et al: Triggered firing in pulmonary veins initiated by in vitro autonomic nerve stimulation. Heart Rhythm 2:624, 2005.
67. Mohler PJ, Schott J, Gramolini AO, et al: Ankyrin-B mutation causes type 4 long-QT cardiac arrhythmia and sudden cardiac death. Nature 421:634, 2003.
68. Lerman BB, Stein KM, Markowitz SM, et al: Ventricular tachycardia in patients with structurally normal hearts. *In* Zipes DP, Jalife J (eds): Cardiac Electrophysiology: From Cell to Bedside. 3rd ed. Philadelphia, WB Saunders, 1999, pp 640-656.
69. Lehnart SE, Wehrens XH, Marks AR: Calstabin deficiency, ryanodine receptors, and sudden cardiac death. Biochem Biophys Res Commun 322:1267, 2004.
70. Cerrone MM, Colombi B, Santoro M, et al: Bidirectional ventricular tachycardia and fibrillation elicited in a knock-in mouse model carrier of a mutation in the cardiac ryanodine receptor. Circ Res 96:77, 2005.
71. Terentyev D, Nori A, Santoro M, et al: Abnormal interactions of calsequestrin with the ryanodine receptor calcium release channel complex linked to exercise-induced sudden cardiac death. Circ Res 98:1151, 2006.
72. Chelu MG, Sarma S, Sood S, et al: Calmodulin kinase II–mediated sarcoplasmic reticulum Ca^{2+} leak promotes atrial fibrillation in mice. J Clin Invest 119:1940, 2009.
73. Lehnart SE, Mongillo M, Belinger A, et al: Leaky Ca^{2+} release channel/ryanodine receptor 2 causes seizures and sudden cardiac death in mice. J Clin Invest 118:2230, 2008.
74. Yano M, Ikeda Y, Matsuzaki M: Altered intracellular Ca^{2+} handling in heart failure. J Clin Invest 115:556, 2005.
75. Wehrens XH, Lehnart SE, Reiken SR, et al: Protection from cardiac arrhythmia through ryanodine receptor–stabilizing protein calstabin2. Science 304:292, 2004.
76. Lehnart SE, Terrenoire C, Reiken S, et al: Stabilization of cardiac ryanodine receptor prevents intracellular calcium leak and arrhythmias. Proc Natl Acad Sci USA 103:7906, 2006.
77. Li X, Zima AV, Sheikh F, et al: Endothelin-1–induced arrhythmogenic Ca^{2+} signaling is abolished in atrial myocytes of inositol-1,4,5-trisphosphate(IP3)-receptor type 2–deficient mice. Circ Res 96:1274, 2005.
78. Hirose M, Stuyvers BD, Dun W, et al: Wide long lasting perinuclear calcium release events generated by an interaction between ryanodine and IP3 receptors in canine Purkinje cell. J Mol Cell Cardiol 45:176, 2008.
79. Zima AV, Blatter LA: Inositol-1,4,5-trisphosphate–dependent Ca^{2+} signalling in cat atrial excitation-contraction coupling and arrhythmias. J Physiol 555:607, 2004.
80. Zhao ZH, Zhang HC, Xu Y: Inositol-1,4,5-trisphosphate and ryanodine-dependent Ca^{2+} signaling in a chronic dog model of atrial fibrillation. Cardiology 107:269, 2007.
81. Fujiwara K, Tanaka H, Mani H, et al: Burst emergence of intracellular Ca^{2+} waves evokes arrhythmogenic oscillatory depolarization via the Na^+-Ca^{2+} exchanger. Circ Res 103:509, 2008.
82. Kass RS, Moss AJ: Long QT syndrome: Novel insights into the mechanisms of cardiac arrhythmias. J Clin Invest 112:810, 2003.
83. Antzelevitch C, Shimizu W, Yan G, et al: The M cell: Its contribution to the ECG and to normal and abnormal electrical function of the heart. J Cardiovasc Electrophysiol 10:1124, 1999.
84. El-Sherif N, Jalife J: Paroxysmal atrioventricular block: Are phase 3 and phase 4 block mechanisms or misnomers? Heart Rhythm 6:1514, 2009.
85. Spach M: Mounting evidence that fibrosis generates a major mechanism for atrial fibrillation. Circ Res 101:743, 2007.
86. Tanaka K, Zlochiver S, Vikstrom KL, et al: Spatial distribution of fibrosis governs fibrillation wave dynamics in the posterior left atrium during heart failure. Circ Res 101:839, 2007.
87. Muñoz V, Grzeda KR, Desplantez T, et al: Adenoviral expression of IKs contributes to wavebreak and fibrillatory conduction in neonatal rat ventricular cardiomyocyte monolayers. Circ Res 101:475, 2007.
88. Wu J, Zipes DP: Transmural reentry triggered by epicardial stimulation during acute ischemia in canine ventricular muscle. Am J Physiol Heart Circ Physiol 283:H2004, 2002.
89. Ueda N, Zipes DP, Wu J: Functional and transmural modulation of M cell behavior in canine ventricular wall. Am J Physiol Heart Circ Physiol 287:H2569, 2004.
90. Weiss JN, Qu Z, Chen PS, et al: The dynamics of cardiac fibrillation. Circulation 112:1232, 2005.
91. Chen Y, Chen S: Electrophysiology of pulmonary veins. J Cardiovasc Electrophysiol 17:220, 2006.
92. Chou CC, Nihei M, Zhou S, et al: Intracellular calcium dynamics and anisotropic reentry in isolated canine pulmonary veins and left atrium. Circulation 111:2889, 2005.
93. Chou CC, Zhou S, Tan AY, et al: High-density mapping of pulmonary veins and left atrium during ibutilide administration in a canine model of sustained atrial fibrillation. Am J Physiol Heart Circ Physiol 289:H2704, 2005.
94. Vest JA, Wehrens XH, Reiken SR, et al: Defective cardiac ryanodine receptor regulation during atrial fibrillation. Circulation 111:2025, 2005.
95. Zhang Z, He Y, Tuteja D, et al: Functional roles of Cav1.3(α_{1D}) calcium channels in atria: Insights gained from gene-targeted null mutant mice. Circulation 112:1936, 2005.
96. Temple J, Frias P, Rottman J, et al: Atrial fibrillation in KCNE1-null mice. Circ Res 97:62, 2005.
97. Firouzi M, Ramanna H, Kok B, et al: Association of human connexin40 gene polymorphisms with atrial vulnerability as a risk factor for idiopathic atrial fibrillation. Circ Res 95:e29, 2004.

98. Ciaccio EJ, Ashikaga H, Kaba RA, et al: Model of reentrant ventricular tachycardia based upon infarct border zone geometry predicts reentrant circuit features as determined by activation mapping. Heart Rhythm 4:1034, 2007.
99. Cabo C, Boyden PA: Heterogeneous gap junction remodeling stabilizes reentrant circuits in the epicardial border zone of the healing canine infarct: A computational study. Am J Physiol Heart Circ Physiol 291:H2606, 2006.
100. Morita H, Zipes DP, Morita ST, et al: Epicardial ablation eliminates ventricular arrhythmias in an experimental model of Brugada syndrome. Heart Rhythm 6:665, 2009.
101. Watanabe H, Koopmann TT, Scouarnec SL, et al: Sodium channel β1 subunit mutations associated with Brugada syndrome and cardiac conduction disease in humans. J Clin Invest 118:2260, 2008.
102. Chen Q, Glenn E, Zhang D, et al: Genetic basis and molecular mechanism for idiopathic ventricular fibrillation. Nature 392:293, 1998.
103. Morita H, Zipes DP, Wu J: Brugada syndrome: Insights of ST elevation, arrhythmogenicity, and risk stratification from experimental observations. Heart Rhythm DOI: 10.1016/j.hrthm.2009.07.018.
104. ter Keurs HEDJ, Boyden PA: Calcium and arrhythmogenesis. Physiol Rev 87:457, 2007.
105. Fernandez-Velasco M, Rueda A, Rizzi N, et al: Increased Ca^{2+} sensitivity of the ryanodine receptor mutant $RyR2^{R4496C}$ underlies catecholaminergic polymorphic ventricular tachycardia. Circ Res 104:201, 2009.
106. Lehnart SE, Mongillo M, Belinger A, et al: Leaky Ca^{2+} release channel/ryanodine receptor 2 causes seizures and sudden cardiac death in mice. J Clin Invest 118:2230, 2008.
107. Sato PY, Musa H, Coombs W, et al: Loss of plakophilin-2 expression leads to decreased sodium current and slower conduction velocity in cultured cardiac myocytes. Circ Res 105:523, 2009.
108. Oxford EM, Musa H, Maass K, et al: Connexin43 remodeling caused by inhibition of plakophilin-2 expression in cardiac cells. Circ Res 101:703, 2007.
109. Tabereaux PB, Dosdall DJ, Ideker RE, et al: Mechanisms of VF maintenance: Wandering wavelets, mother rotors, or foci. Heart Rhythm 6:405, 2009.
110. Ten Tusscher KH, Hren R, Panfilov AV: Organization of ventricular fibrillation in the human heart. Circ Res 100:e87, 2007.
111. Newton JC, Smith WM, Ideker RE: Estimated global transmural distribution of activation rate and conduction block during porcine and canine ventricular fibrillation. Circ Res 94:836, 2004.
112. Choi B, Nho W, Liu T, et al: Life span of ventricular fibrillation frequencies. Circ Res 91:339, 2002.
113. Roger JM, Huang J, Melnick SB, et al: Sustained reentry in the left ventricle of fibrillating pig hearts. Circ Res 92:539, 2003.
114. Weiss JN, Qu Z, Chen PS, et al: The dynamics of cardiac fibrillation. Circulation 112:1232, 2005.
115. Weiss JN, Karma A, Shiferaw Y, et al: From pulsus to pulseless: The saga of cardiac alternans. Circ Res 98:1244, 2006.

CHAPTER 36 Diagnosis of Cardiac Arrhythmias

John M. Miller and Douglas P. Zipes

In the management of clinical arrhythmias, the physician must evaluate and treat the whole patient, not just the rhythm disturbance.[1] Some arrhythmias are hazardous to the patient, regardless of the clinical setting (e.g., ventricular fibrillation, VF), whereas others are hazardous because of the clinical setting (e.g., rapidly conducted atrial fibrillation in a patient with severe coronary artery stenoses). Some arrhythmias, such as premature ventricular complexes (PVCs), may be highly symptomatic and may not be associated with any adverse outcome, whereas some patients with atrial fibrillation have no symptoms at all but may still be at significant risk of stroke. Evaluation of the patient begins with a careful history and physical examination and should usually progress from the simplest to the most complex test, from the least invasive and safest to the most invasive and risky, and from the least expensive out-of-hospital evaluations to those that require hospitalization and sophisticated, costly procedures. On occasion, depending on the clinical circumstances, the physician may wish to proceed directly to a high-risk, expensive procedure, such as an electrophysiologic study (EPS), before obtaining a 24-hour electrocardiographic recording.

History

Patients with cardiac rhythm disturbances can present with various complaints, but symptoms such as palpitations, syncope, presyncope, or congestive heart failure commonly cause them to seek a physician's help. Their awareness of palpitations and of a regular or irregular cardiac rhythm varies greatly.[2] Some patients perceive slight variations in their heart rhythm with uncommon accuracy, whereas others are oblivious even to sustained episodes of ventricular tachycardia (VT); still others complain of palpitations when they actually have regular sinus rhythm.

In assessing a patient with known or suspected arrhythmia, several key pieces of information should be obtained that can help determine a diagnosis or guide further diagnostic testing. The *mode of onset* of an episode may provide clues about the type of arrhythmia or preferred treatment option. For example, palpitations that occur in the setting of exercise, fright, or anger are often caused by catecholamine-sensitive automatic or triggered tachycardias that may respond to adrenergic blocking agents (see Chap. 37); palpitations that occur at rest or that awaken the patient may be caused by vagal initiation, such as atrial fibrillation. Lightheadedness or syncope occurring in the setting of a tightly fitting collar, shaving the neck, or turning the head suggests carotid sinus hypersensitivity. The triggering event may help establish the presence of an inherited ion channel abnormality (see Chap. 9). The *mode of termination* of episodes can also be helpful: if palpitations can be reliably terminated by breath-holding, Valsalva, or other vagal maneuvers, it is likely that the atrioventricular (AV) node is an integral part of a tachycardia circuit; on occasion, focal atrial tachycardias or VTs terminate with vagal maneuvers. Patients should be asked how frequently episodes occur, how long they last, and how severe the symptoms are. These features can help guide how aggressively and quickly the physician needs to pursue a diagnostic or therapeutic plan (a patient with daily episodes associated with near-syncope or severe dyspnea warrants a more expeditious evaluation than one with infrequent episodes of mild palpitations and no other symptoms). Patients can sometimes report the heart rate during an episode (either rapid or slow, regular or irregular) by counting the pulse directly or using an automatic blood pressure or heart rate monitor. Characteristics of mode of onset and frequency of episodes can guide the choice of diagnostic tests (see later).

A careful drug and dietary history should also be sought; some nasal decongestants can provoke tachycardia episodes, whereas beta-adrenergic blocking eye drops for treatment of glaucoma can drain into tear ducts, be absorbed systemically, and precipitate syncope caused by bradycardia. Dietary supplements, particularly those containing ephedrine-like compounds, can cause arrhythmias. A growing list of drugs can directly or indirectly affect ventricular repolarization and produce long-QT interval–related tachyarrhythmias (see Chap. 10). The patient should be questioned about the presence of systemic illnesses that may be associated with arrhythmias, such as chronic obstructive pulmonary disease, thyrotoxicosis (see Chap. 86), pericarditis (see Chap. 26), or congestive heart failure (see Chaps. 27 and 28). A family history of rhythm disturbances is often present in long-QT syndrome or other inherited arrhythmia syndromes (see Chap. 9), hypertrophic cardiomyopathy (see Chap. 69), and muscular or myotonic dystrophies (see Chap. 92).

Physical Examination

Examination of the patient during a symptomatic episode can be revealing. Clearly, heart rate and blood pressure are key measurements to make. Assessment of the jugular venous pressure and waveform can disclose the rapid oscillations of atrial flutter or "cannon" A waves indicative of contraction of the right atrium against a closed tricuspid valve in patients with AV dissociation in disorders such as complete heart block or VT. Variations in the intensity of the first heart sound and systolic blood pressure have the same implications.

Physical maneuvers during a tachycardia can have diagnostic and therapeutic value. The Valsalva maneuver or carotid sinus massage causes a transient increase in vagal tone; tachyarrhythmias that depend on the AV node for continuation can terminate or slow with these maneuvers but may also show no change. Focal atrial tachycardias occasionally terminate in response to vagal stimulation, as do rare VTs. Sinus tachycardia slows slightly after vagal stimulation, returning to its original rate soon thereafter; the ventricular response during atrial flutter and fibrillation and other atrial tachycardias can decrease briefly. During wide QRS tachycardias with a 1:1 relationship between P waves and QRS complexes, vagal influence can terminate or slow a supraventricular tachycardia (SVT) that depends on the AV node for perpetuation; on the other hand, vagal effects on the AV node

CH
36

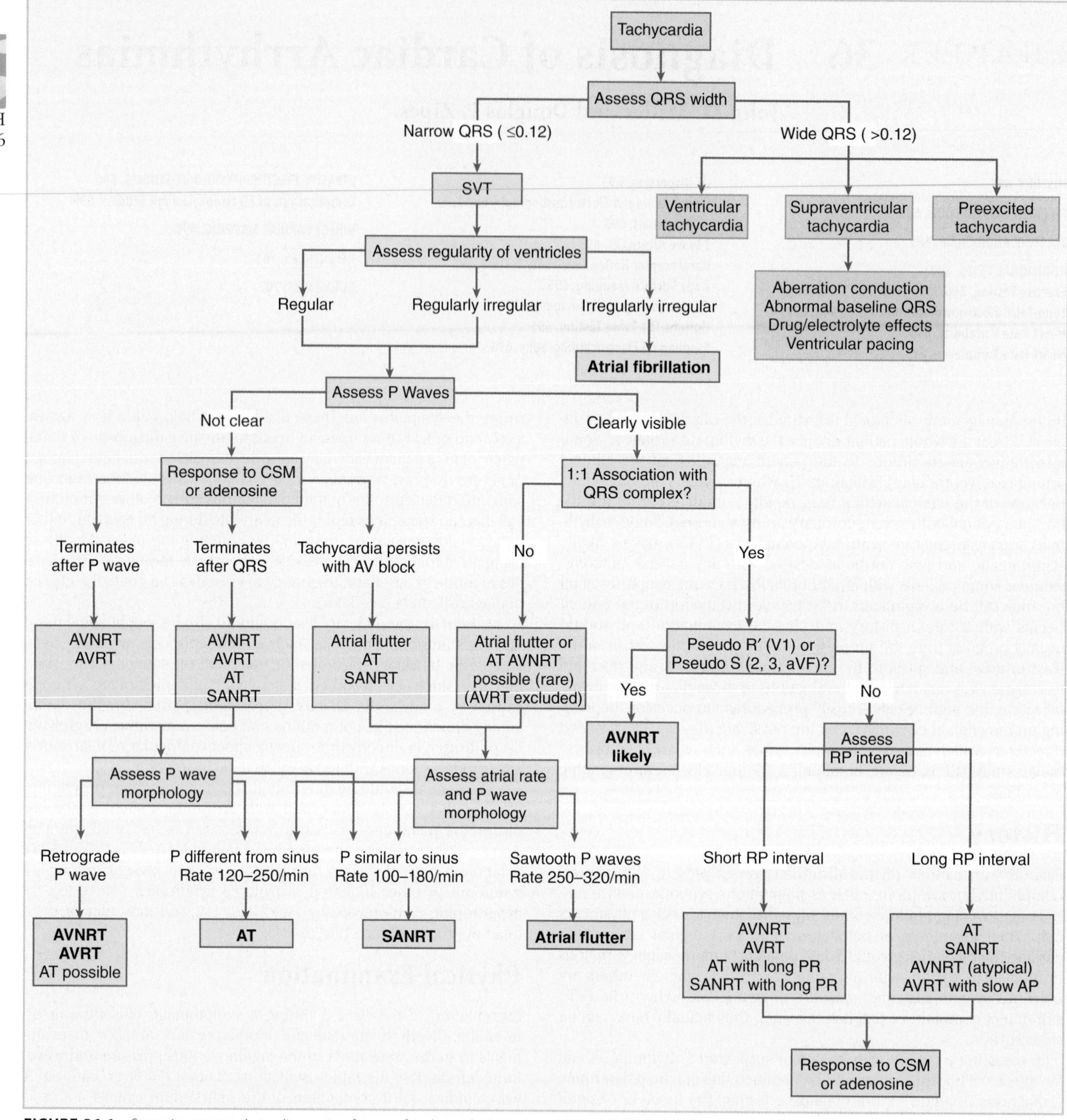

FIGURE 36-1 Stepwise approach to diagnosis of type of tachycardia based on 12-lead ECG during the episode. The initial step is to determine whether the tachycardia has a wide or narrow QRS complex. For wide-complex tachycardia, see Table 36-1; the remainder of the algorithm is helpful in diagnosis of the type of narrow-complex tachycardia. AP = accessory pathway; AT = atrial tachycardia; AVNRT = AV nodal reentrant tachycardia; AVRT = AV reciprocating tachycardia; CSM = carotid sinus massage; SANRT = sinoatrial nodal reentry tachycardia; SVT = supraventricular tachycardia.

can transiently block retrograde conduction and thus establish the diagnosis of VT by demonstrating AV dissociation. The effect of either of these physical maneuvers typically lasts only seconds; the physician must be ready to observe or record any changes in rhythm on an electrocardiogram (ECG) when the maneuver is performed or the response may not be appreciated.

Carotid massage is performed with the patient supine and comfortable, with the head tipped away from the side being stimulated. Careful auscultation for carotid bruits must always precede any attempt at carotid massage because there have been reports of embolic events associated with massage. The area of the carotid sinus, at the artery's bifurcation, is palpated with two fingers at the angle of the jaw until a good pulse is felt. Even this minimal amount of pressure can induce a hypersensitive response in affected individuals. If there is no initial effect, a side-to-side or rotating motion of the fingers over the site is performed for up to 5 seconds. A negative response is lack of effect on the ECG after 5 seconds of pressure adequate to cause mild discomfort. Because responses to carotid massage may differ on the two sides, the maneuver can be repeated on the opposite side; however, both sides should never be stimulated simultaneously.

Physical findings can suggest the presence of structural heart disease (and thus generally a clinically more serious situation with a worse overall prognosis), even in the absence of an arrhythmia episode. For example, a laterally displaced or dyskinetic apical impulse, a regurgitant or stenotic murmur, or a third heart sound in an older adult can denote significant myocardial or valvular dysfunction or damage.

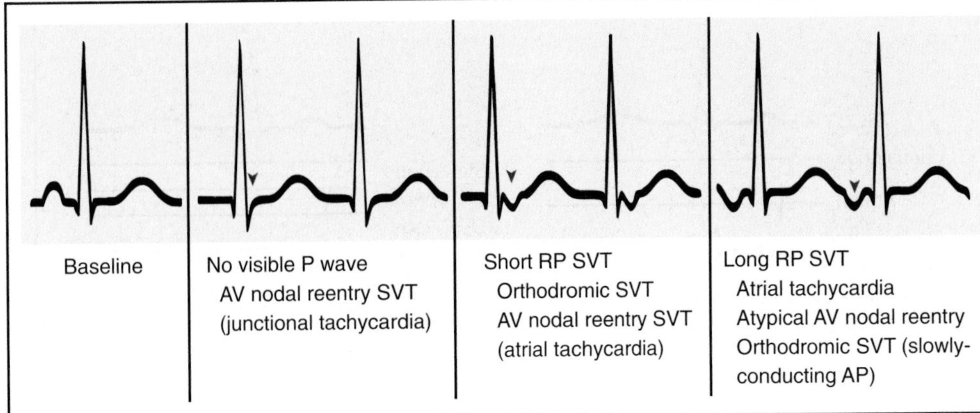

FIGURE 36-2 Differential diagnosis of different types of supraventricular tachycardia (SVT) based on timing of atrial activity (RP and PR intervals). Left, Normal beat. Different types of tachycardia are listed below the representative electrocardiographic patterns that they can produce, categorized by P wave position relative to the QRS complex. Red arrowhead shows the location of the P wave in each example. AV = atrioventricular; AP = accessory pathway.

Electrocardiogram

The ECG is the primary tool in arrhythmia analysis (see Chap. 13); an EPS, in which intracardiac catheters are used to record activity from several regions of the heart at one time, is more definitive. Initially, a 12-lead ECG is recorded. In addition, a long continuous recording with use of the lead that shows distinct P waves is often helpful for closer analysis; most commonly, this is one of the inferior leads (2, 3, aVF), V_1, or aVR. The ECG obtained during an episode of arrhythmia may be diagnostic by itself, obviating the need for further diagnostic testing. **Figure 36-1** depicts an algorithm for diagnosis of specific tachyarrhythmias from the 12-lead ECG (see Chap. 39). A major branch point in the differential diagnosis concerns the QRS duration: wide QRS (more than 0.12 second) tachycardias are often VTs, and narrow QRS (0.12 second or less) tachycardias are almost always SVTs, but there is some overlap (**Table 36-1**).[3] The next most important questions to answer, regardless of QRS width, concern characteristics of P waves. If P waves are not clearly visible, atrial activity can sometimes be recorded by placing the right and left arm leads in various anterior chest positions to discern P waves (so-called Lewis leads) or by applying esophageal electrodes or obtaining intracavitary right atrial recordings; the last methods are not readily available in most clinical situations. An echocardiogram showing atrial contraction can be helpful. The long rhythm strip may yield important clues by revealing P waves if perturbations occur during the arrhythmia (e.g., changes in rate, premature complexes, sudden termination, and effect of physical maneuvers, as noted earlier).

Each arrhythmia should be approached in a systematic manner to answer several key questions; as suggested earlier, many of these relate to P wave characteristics and underscore the importance of assessing the ECG carefully for these. If P waves are visible, are the atrial and ventricular rates identical? Are the P-P and R-R intervals regular or irregular? If irregular, is it a consistent, repeating irregularity? Is there a P wave related to each QRS complex? Does the P wave seem to precede (long RP interval) or follow (short RP interval) the QRS complex (**Fig. 36-2**)? Are the resultant RP and PR intervals constant? Are all P waves and QRS complexes identical? Is the P wave vector normal or abnormal? Are P, PR, QRS, and QT durations normal? Once these questions have been addressed, one needs to assess the significance of the arrhythmia in view of the clinical setting. Should it be treated, and if so, how? For SVTs with a normal QRS complex, a branching decision tree such as that shown in Figure 36-1 may be useful.

TABLE 36-1 Electrocardiographic Distinctions for Diagnosis of Wide QRS Complex Tachycardia

FAVOR SUPRAVENTRICULAR TACHYCARDIA	FAVOR VENTRICULAR TACHYCARDIA
Initiation with premature P wave	Initiation with premature QRS complex
QRS complexes identical to those in resting rhythm	Tachycardia beats identical to PVCs during sinus rhythm
Changes in P-P interval precede changes in R-R interval	Changes in R-R interval precede changes in P-P interval
Long-short sequence preceding initiation	Short-long sequence preceding initiation
QRS contours consistent with aberrant conduction (V_1, V_6)	QRS contours inconsistent with aberrant conduction (V_1, V_6)
QRS duration <0.14 sec	QRS duration >0.14 sec
Slowing or termination with vagal maneuvers	AV dissociation or other non-1:1 AV relationship
	Fusion beats, capture beats
	Left axis deviation (esp. −90 to 180 degrees)
	Concordant R wave progression pattern
	Contralateral bundle branch block pattern from resting rhythm
	Absence of rS complex in any precordial lead
	Poor AV conduction baseline

THE LADDER DIAGRAM

The ladder diagram, derived from the ECG, is used to depict depolarization and conduction schematically to aid understanding of the rhythm. Straight or slightly slanting lines drawn on a tiered framework beneath an ECG represent electrical events occurring in the various cardiac structures (**Fig. 36-3**). Because the ECG and therefore the ladder diagram represent electrical activity against a time base, conduction is indicated by the lines of the ladder diagram sloping in a left-to-right direction. A steep line represents rapid conduction, and more slanting lines depict slower conduction. A short bar drawn perpendicularly to a sloping line represents blocked conduction. Activity originating in an ectopic site such as the ventricle is indicated by lines emanating from that tier. Sinus nodal discharge and conduction and, under certain circumstances, AV junctional discharge and conduction can only be inferred; their activity is not directly recorded on a scalar ECG.

Most patients have only occasional episodes of arrhythmia and spend most of the time in their baseline rhythm (e.g., sinus, atrial fibrillation). The ECG during the patient's resting rhythm can provide clues about the presence of a substrate for arrhythmia (i.e., structural or physiologic abnormalities from which arrhythmias can arise).

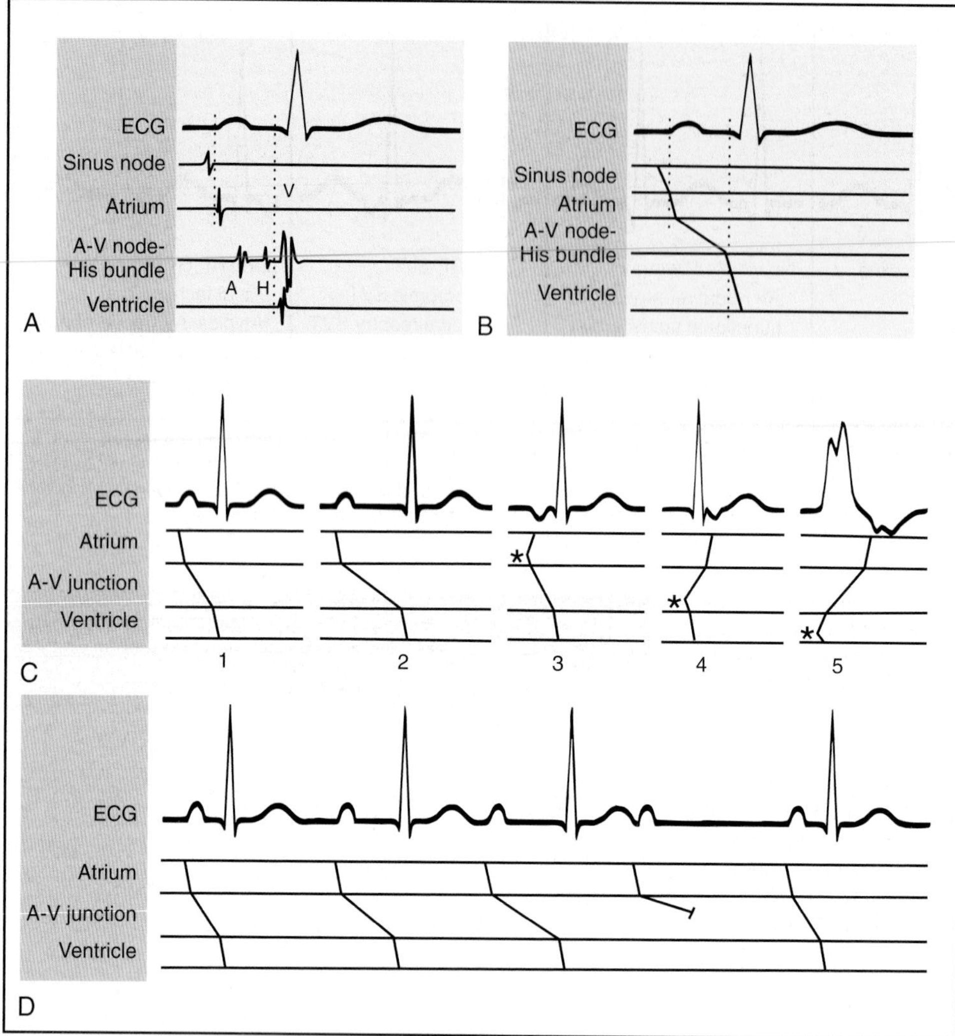

FIGURE 36-3 Intracardiac signals and ladder diagrams. **A,** A single beat is shown with accompanying intracardiac signals from the sinus node, right atrium, AV nodal and His bundle regions, and right ventricle. **B,** The same beat is shown with accompanying ladder diagram below. Cardiac regions have been divided into tiers separated by horizontal lines. Vertical dotted lines denote onset of P wave and QRS complexes. Note the relatively steep lines (rapid conduction through atrium, His bundle, and ventricular muscle) and more gently sloping lines as the impulse traverses the sinus and AV nodes (signifying slow conduction). **C,** Several different situations are depicted with accompanying explanatory ladder diagrams. Beat 1 is normal, as in **B**; beat 2 shows first-degree AV delay, with a more gradual slope than normal in the AV nodal tier, signifying very slow conduction in this region. In beat 3, an atrial premature complex is shown (starting in atrial tier as asterisk) producing an inverted P wave on the ECG. In beat 4, an ectopic impulse arises in the His bundle (asterisk) and propagates to the ventricle as well as retrogradely through the AV node to the atrium. In beat 5, a ventricular ectopic complex (asterisk) conducts retrogradely through the His bundle and AV node and eventually to the atrium. **D,** A Wenckebach AV cycle (type I second-degree block) is shown. As the PR interval progressively increases from left to right in the figure, the slope of the line in the AV nodal region is progressively less steep until it fails to propagate at all after the fourth P wave (small line perpendicular to sloping AV nodal conduction line), after which the cycle repeats. A = atrial recording; H = His recording; V = ventricular recording.

Several of these are shown in **Figure 36-4**. In most patients with SVT (aside from those with Wolff-Parkinson-White syndrome), the resting ECG is normal. This is also true for many patients with ventricular tachyarrhythmias. Thus, although it is capable of showing an abnormality with possible arrhythmic implications, the resting ECG is not a very sensitive tool.

Additional Tests

The following additional tests can be used to evaluate patients who have cardiac arrhythmias. The physician's choice of which test to use depends on the clinical circumstances. For example, a patient with multiple daily episodes of presyncope is likely to have an event recorded on a 24-hour ambulatory electrocardiographic (Holter) monitor, whereas in a patient who complains of infrequent anxiety- or exercise-induced palpitations, exercise stress testing may be more likely to provide a diagnosis.

Exercise Testing (see Chap. 14)

Exercise can induce various types of supraventricular and ventricular tachyarrhythmias and, uncommonly, bradyarrhythmias.[4] About one third of normal subjects develop ventricular ectopy in response to exercise testing. Ectopy is more likely to occur at faster heart rates, usually in the form of occasional PVCs of constant morphology or even pairs of PVCs, and is often not reproducible from one stress test to the next. Three to six beats of nonsustained VT can occur in normal patients, especially the elderly, and its occurrence does not establish the existence of ischemic or other forms of heart disease or predict increased cardiovascular morbidity or mortality. Premature supraventricular complexes are often more common during exercise than at rest and increase in frequency with age; their occurrence does not imply the presence of structural heart disease. A persistent elevation of heart rate after the end of exercise (delay in return to baseline) is associated with a worse cardiovascular prognosis.[5]

Approximately 50% of patients who have coronary artery disease develop PVCs in response to exercise testing. Ventricular ectopy appears in these patients at lower heart rates (less than 130 beats/min) than in the normal population and often occurs in the early recovery period as well. Frequent (more than 7 PVCs/min) or complex ectopy is associated with a worse prognosis.[6] Exercise reproduced sustained VT or VF in only about 10% of patients with spontaneous VT or VF late after myocardial infarction, but those who had it experienced a worse outcome. The relation of exercise to ventricular arrhythmia in patients with structurally normal hearts has no prognostic implications. Stress testing and Holter recording have been used to assess antiarrhythmic drug efficacy.

Patients who have symptoms consistent with an arrhythmia induced by exercise (e.g., syncope, sustained palpitations) should be considered for stress testing. Stress testing may be indicated to uncover more complex grades of ventricular arrhythmia, to provoke supraventricular arrhythmias, to determine the relationship of the arrhythmia to activity, to aid in choosing antiarrhythmic therapy and uncovering proarrhythmic responses, and possibly to provide some insight into the mechanism of the tachycardia. The test can be performed safely and appears more sensitive than a standard 12-lead resting ECG for detection of ventricular ectopy. However, prolonged ambulatory recording is more sensitive than exercise testing in detecting ventricular ectopy. Because either technique can uncover serious arrhythmias that the

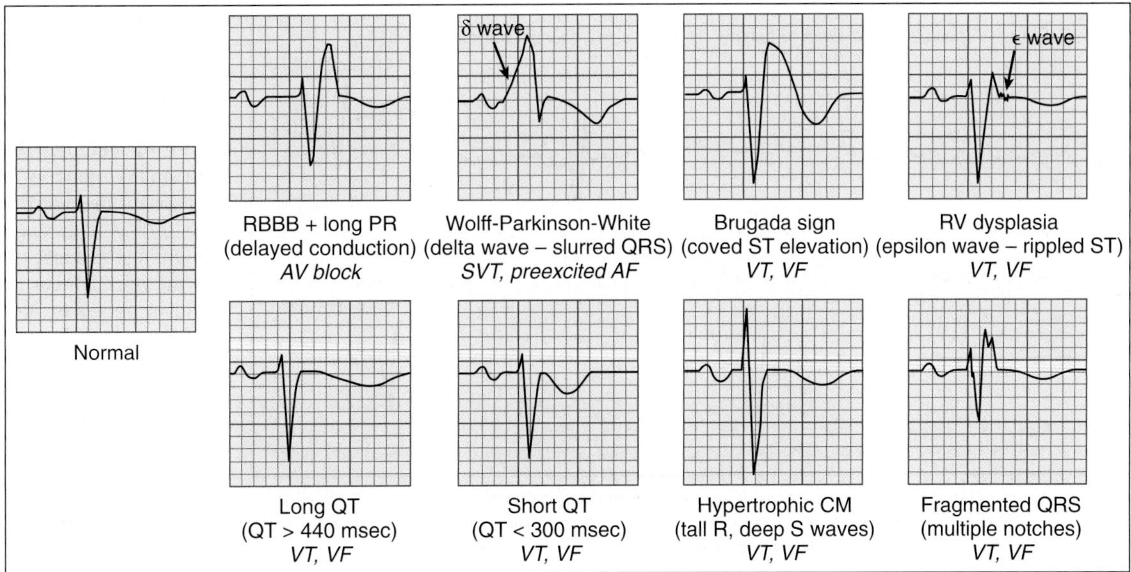

FIGURE 36-4 Electrocardiographic abnormalities in resting rhythm that suggest arrhythmia potential. Lead V_1 is shown in each example; a normal complex is shown at left for reference. AF = atrial fibrillation; AV = atrioventricular; CM = cardiomyopathy; RBBB = right bundle branch block; SVT = supraventricular tachycardia; VF = ventricular fibrillation; VT = ventricular tachycardia.

other technique misses, both examinations may be indicated for selected patients. Stress testing is often useful in long-QT syndrome and catecholaminergic VT (see Chap. 14).

Long-Term Electrocardiographic Recording

Prolonged electrocardiographic recording in patients engaged in normal daily activities is the most useful noninvasive method to document and to quantitate the frequency and complexity of an arrhythmia, to correlate the arrhythmia with the patient's symptoms, and to evaluate the effect of antiarrhythmic therapy on spontaneous arrhythmia. For example, recording normal sinus rhythm during the patient's typical symptomatic episode effectively excludes cardiac arrhythmia as a cause. In addition, some recorders can document alterations in QRS, ST, and T contours (**Fig. 36-5**).

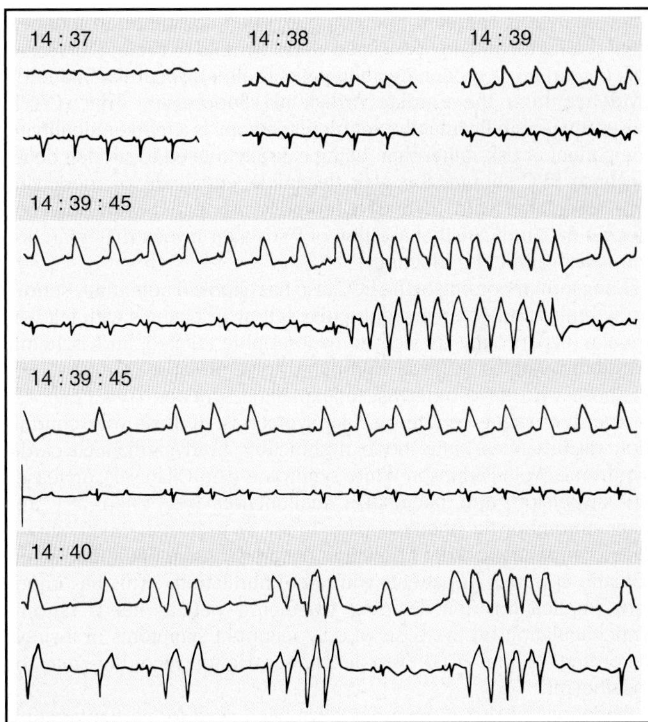

FIGURE 36-5 Long-term electrocardiographic recording in a patient with atypical angina. Top channel, inferior lead. Bottom channel, anterior lead. Note progressive ST-segment elevation in the inferior lead, eventually resembling a monophasic action potential. Bursts of nonsustained ventricular tachycardia result. Sinus slowing and Wenckebach AV block then occur from a vasodepressor reflex response elicited by ischemia of the inferior myocardial wall or possibly caused by ischemia of the sinus and AV nodes. Bottom tracing, both AV block and ventricular arrhythmias are apparent. Numbers indicate time (e.g., 14:37 = 2:37 PM). *(Courtesy of D. A. Chilson, MD.)*

AMBULATORY ELECTROCARDIOGRAPHIC (HOLTER) RECORDING

Continuous electrocardiographic tape recorders represent the traditional Holter monitor and typically record (on analog tape or digital cards) two or three electrocardiographic channels for 24 hours.[7] Interpretative accuracy of long-term recordings varies with the system used, but most computers that scan the recording media are sufficiently accurate to meet clinical needs. All systems can potentially record more information than the physician needs or can assimilate. As long as the system detects important episodes of ectopic activity, VT, or asystolic intervals and semiquantitates these abnormalities, the physician probably receives all the clinical information that is needed. Twenty-five percent to 50% of patients experience a complaint during a 24-hour recording, caused by an arrhythmia in 2% to 15% (**Fig. 36-6**). The ability to correlate symptoms temporally with abnormalities in the ECG is one of the strengths of this technique.

Significant rhythm disturbances are uncommon in healthy young persons. Sinus bradycardia with heart rates of 35 to 40 beats/min, sinus arrhythmia with pauses exceeding 3 seconds, sinoatrial exit block, type I (Wenckebach) second-degree AV block (often during sleep), wandering atrial pacemaker, junctional escape complexes, and premature atrial complexes (PACs) and PVCs can be observed and are not necessarily abnormal. Frequent and complex atrial and ventricular rhythm disturbances are less commonly observed, however, and type II second-degree AV conduction disturbances (see Chap. 39) are not recorded in normal patients. Elderly patients (see Chap. 80) may have a higher prevalence of arrhythmias, some of which may be responsible for neurologic symptoms (see Fig. 36-6; see Chap. 92). The long-term prognosis in asymptomatic healthy subjects with frequent and complex PVCs usually resembles that of the healthy U.S. population, without an increased risk of death. However, frequent PVCs have recently been shown to produce heart failure in some people.[8]

CH 36

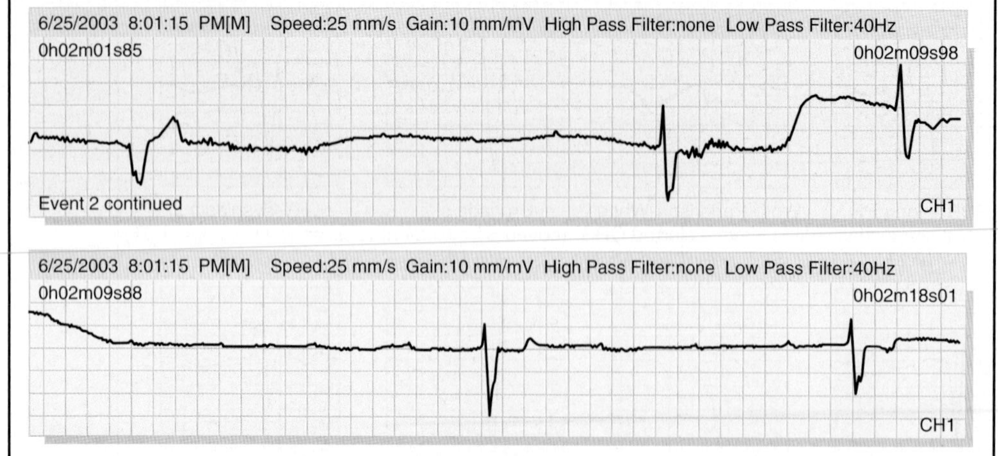

FIGURE 36-6 Continuous electrocardiographic recording from a patient-activated event monitor during an episode of lightheadedness. Sinus rhythm at 75 beats/min with sudden AV block is present with pauses of longer than 4 seconds, and in the bottom strip, there is an effective heart rate of about 8 beats/min.

Most patients who have ischemic heart disease, particularly after myocardial infarction (see Chaps. 54 and 55), exhibit PVCs when they are monitored for 6 to 24 hours. The frequency of PVCs progressively increases during the first several weeks, decreasing at about 6 months after infarction. Frequent and complex PVCs constitute an independent risk factor and are associated with a twofold to fivefold increased risk of cardiac or sudden death in patients after myocardial infarction. Evidence from the Cardiac Arrhythmia Suppression Trial (CAST) raises the possibility that the ventricular ectopy is a marker identifying the patient at risk, rather than being causally related to sudden death, because PVC suppression with flecainide, encainide, or moricizine was associated with increased mortality compared with placebo.[9] Recent data indicate that ablation of PVCs after myocardial infarction improves ventricular function.[10]

Long-term recording of the ECG also has exposed potentially serious arrhythmias and complex ventricular ectopy in patients with left ventricular hypertrophy as well as hypertrophic, dilated, and ischemic cardiomyopathies; in those with mitral valve prolapse (see Chap. 66); in those who have otherwise unexplained syncope (see Chap. 42) or transient vague cerebrovascular symptoms; in those with conduction disturbances, sinus node dysfunction, bradycardia-tachycardia syndrome, Wolff-Parkinson-White syndrome (see Chap. 39), increased QT dispersion, and pacemaker malfunction (see Chap. 38); and after thrombolytic therapy (see Chap. 87). It has been shown that asymptomatic atrial fibrillation occurs far more often than symptomatic episodes in patients with atrial fibrillation.[11] This has important implications for deciding whether a patient needs chronic anticoagulation on the basis of only recurrent symptoms or a single recording of the ECG. Even a 24-hour Holter recording may be insufficient.[12]

Variations of Holter recording have been used for particular applications. Repeated 24-hour recording periods may be needed to obtain enough episodes of PAC triggering atrial fibrillation to warrant proceeding to an EPS and catheter ablation. Some monitoring systems are able to reconstruct a full 12-lead ECG from a 7-electrode recording system. This is especially useful in trying to document the electrocardiographic morphology of VT before an ablation procedure or a consistent morphology of PACs that may arise from an ablatable focus of atrial tachycardia or fibrillation. Most Holter recording and analysis systems can place a clearly recognizable deflection on the recording when a pacemaker stimulus is detected. This greatly facilitates diagnosis of potential pacemaker malfunction. On occasion, artifacts in the ECG caused by alterations in tape recording or playback speed can mimic bradycardias or tachycardias and lead to erroneous therapy. Newer digital Holter systems are less subject to this phenomenon. Finally, most systems can also provide heart rate variability and QT data (see later). Use of these systems for detection of myocardial ischemia (ST-segment analysis) has yielded mixed results (high specificity but poor sensitivity).

EVENT RECORDING

In many patients, the 24-hour snapshot provided by the Holter recording is incapable of documenting the cause of the patient's symptoms. Longer term monitoring is necessary in these cases, which occur frequently, such as with an event recorder. These devices are about the size of a pager and are kept by the patient for 30 days. During that time, digital recordings can be made during symptomatic episodes and transmitted to a receiving station over standard telephone lines at the patient's convenience (see Fig. 36-6). Some of these recorders store more than 30 seconds of the ECG before the patient activates the recording. These loop recorders record continuously, but only a small window of time is present in memory at any moment; when the event button is pressed by the patient, the current window is frozen while the device continues recording for another 30 to 60 seconds, depending on how it is configured. Event recorders are highly effective in documenting infrequent events, but the quality of the recordings is more variable than with Holter recorders, and usually only one channel can be recorded. With some systems, the patient must be able to press the event button to begin recording; if syncope occurs without warning and the patient is not able to actuate the device, it cannot provide diagnostic information. With other systems, the device automatically begins recording the rhythm when the heart rate falls outside predetermined parameters. One system incorporates cell phone technology that automatically notifies a central monitoring facility when certain conditions are met (e.g., extreme bradycardia or tachycardia). In this way, the time between occurrence and effective treatment of serious arrhythmias can be significantly shortened.

Most currently available pacemakers and implantable defibrillators are capable of providing Holter-like data when premature beats or tachycardia episodes occur and can even store electrograms of these events from the implanted leads. The device can then be interrogated later and the electrograms printed for analysis. Increasingly, implanted device systems incorporate remote monitoring so that if patients develop symptoms, they can perform a limited device interrogation at home; the information is then transmitted via the Internet to the physician's office for more prompt diagnosis and treatment.

IMPLANTABLE LOOP RECORDER

For patients with infrequent and transient symptoms, neither Holter recorders nor 30-day event recorders may yield diagnostic information. In such patients, implantable loop recorders may be used.[13] This device (about the size of a pack of chewing gum) is inserted under the skin at about the second rib on the left front of the chest and is activated by passing a special magnet over the device. It is capable of recording up to 42 minutes of a single channel of the ECG that can be partitioned for one to seven episodes, with up to 20 minutes of the preactivation ECG saved for subsequent downloading to a programming unit for analysis. Both P waves and QRS complexes can usually be identified. The device can be configured to store patient-activated episodes, automatically activated recordings (heart rate outside preset parameters), or a combination of these (**Fig. 36-7**). In one report, this device was implanted in 24 patients with recurrent syncope who had undergone extensive evaluation without determination of a cause of syncope. During a mean 5-month period after implantation, 21 patients had recurrent syncope; the device was instrumental in establishing the diagnosis in 18 patients.[14]

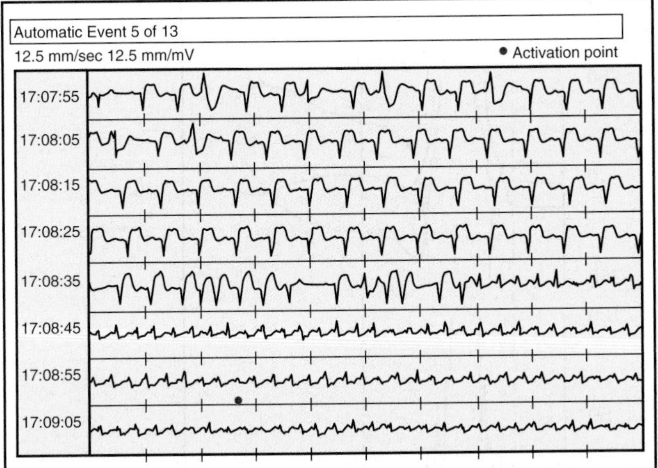

FIGURE 36-7 Recordings from an implantable loop recorder. Each line contains 10 seconds of continuous ECG from the implanted device. The first four lines show sinus rhythm with premature ventricular complexes; during the fifth line, short runs of atrial tachycardia precede an episode of a faster tachycardia with a different complex (ventricular tachycardia). This episode triggered an automatic activation (red circle) of the device recording (no symptoms associated with the episode).

Heart Rate Variability

Heart rate variability is used to evaluate vagal and sympathetic influences on the sinus node (inferring that the same activity is occurring in the ventricles also) and to identify patients at risk for a cardiovascular event or death.[15,16] Frequency domain analysis resolves parasympathetic and sympathetic influences better than time domain analysis, but both types of analysis are useful. R-R variability predicts all-cause mortality as well as left ventricular ejection fraction or nonsustained VT in patients after myocardial infarction and can be added to other measures of risk to enhance predictive accuracy. Similar results have been obtained in patients with dilated cardiomyopathy (see Chap. 68). High-frequency components of R-R interval variability reflect tonic vagal activity. Reduced R-R interval variability, the marker of increased risk, indicates loss or reduction of the physiologic periodic sinus node fluctuations, which can be caused by many different influences and may not necessarily represent a significant shift in autonomic modulation. New indices of heart rate variability are continually being evaluated.[17] Even the simple measure of resting heart rate has been shown to be an independent cardiovascular risk factor, although a target "safe" heart rate has not been established, as has heart rate obtained during and after exercise.

Heart Rate Turbulence

Heart rate turbulence is an index of changes in sinus discharge rate after a PVC that is followed by a compensatory pause.[18] In normal individuals, the sinus rate initially accelerates and then slows; this phenomenon is blunted or absent in patients with various heart diseases. Heart rate turbulence is a measure of reflex vagal control of the heart, whereas heart rate variability is more indicative of overall vagal tone. Abnormal heart rate turbulence is a powerful independent predictor of mortality in patients with coronary artery disease and dilated cardiomyopathy; abnormal indices in some patients can be improved or normalized after treatment with beta blockers and statin drugs.

QT Dispersion

Heterogeneity in refractoriness and conduction velocity is a hallmark of reentrant arrhythmias. One index of heterogeneity of ventricular refractoriness can be found in differences in length of the QT interval in surface leads of the ECG. The most commonly used index to calculate this QT dispersion has been the difference between the longest and shortest QT intervals on the 12-lead ECG, which is often adjusted for heart rate as well as number of leads sampled (when the T wave is flat in some). Other indices have been developed. Abnormally high QT dispersion has been correlated with risk of arrhythmic death in various disorders, although results are not consistent. Its mechanism has been characterized in several disease states.[19] QT dispersion has been correlated with both efficacy and proarrhythmic potential of drug therapy. Different techniques exist for determining dispersion (including automated algorithms), and the results of one study are often difficult to compare with those of another; in addition, the test is sensitive to age, time of day, season of the year, and even body position.[20] Overall, assessment of QT dispersion (from a standard 12-lead ECG) has not gained popularity as a useful clinical tool.

Signal-Averaged Electrocardiography and Late Potentials

Signal averaging is a method that improves signal-to-noise ratio when signals are recurrent and the noise is random.[21] In conjunction with appropriate filtering and other methods of noise reduction, signal averaging can detect cardiac signals of a few microvolts in amplitude, reducing noise amplitude, such as muscle potentials that are typically 5 to 25 mV, to less than 1 mV. With this method, very low amplitude electrical potentials generated by the sinus and AV nodes, His bundle, and bundle branches are detectable at the body surface.

One constituent of reentrant ventricular arrhythmias in patients with prior myocardial damage is slow conduction. Direct cardiac mapping techniques can record myocardial activation from damaged areas that occurs after the end of the surface electrocardiographic QRS complex during sinus rhythm. These delayed signals have a very low amplitude that cannot be discerned by routine electrocardiography and correspond to the delayed and fragmented conduction in the ventricles recorded with direct mapping techniques (**Fig. 36-8**). Signal averaging has been applied clinically most often to detect such late ventricular potentials of 1 to 25 mV. Criteria for late potentials are the following: (1) filtered QRS complex duration longer than 114 to 120 milliseconds; (2) less than 20 mV of root mean square signal amplitude in the last 40 milliseconds of the filtered QRS complex; and (3) terminal filtered QRS complex remains below 40 mV for longer than 39 milliseconds. These late potentials have been recorded in 70% to 90% of patients with spontaneous sustained and inducible VT after myocardial infarction, in only 0% to 6% of normal volunteers, and in 7% to 15% of patients after myocardial infarction who do not have VT. Late potentials can be detected as early as 3 hours after the onset of chest pain, increase in prevalence in the first week after myocardial infarction, and disappear in some patients after 1 year. If they are not present initially, late potentials usually do not appear later. Early use of thrombolytic agents may reduce the prevalence of late potentials after coronary occlusion. Patients with bundle branch block or paced ventricular rhythms already have wide QRS complexes, rendering the technique less useful in these cases.

Late potentials also have been recorded in patients with VT not related to ischemia, such as in dilated cardiomyopathies. Successful surgical resection of the VT can eliminate late potentials but is not necessary to cause tachycardia suppression. The presence of a late potential is a sensitive but not specific marker of arrhythmic risk, and thus its prognostic use is limited.[22] In specific situations, it can be helpful; for example, a patient with a prior inferior wall myocardial infarction (normally the last portion of the heart to be activated) who has no late potential has a very low likelihood of having VT episodes.

The high-pass filtering used to record late potentials meeting the criteria just noted is called *time domain analysis* because the filter output corresponds in time to the input signal. Because late potentials are high-frequency signals, Fourier transform can be applied to extract high-frequency content from the signal-averaged ECG, called *frequency domain analysis*. Some data suggest that frequency domain analysis provides useful information not available in the time domain analysis.

Signal averaging has been applied to the P wave to determine the risk for development of atrial fibrillation (especially after cardiac surgery) as well as maintenance of sinus rhythm after cardioversion.[23,24] The overall use of the technique remains limited at present.

T Wave Alternans

Beat-to-beat alternation in the amplitude or morphology of the electrocardiographic recording of ventricular repolarization, the ST segment and T wave, has been found in conditions favoring the development of ventricular tachyarrhythmias, such as ischemia and long-QT syndrome, and in patients with ventricular arrhythmias. The electrophysiologic basis appears to be the alternation of repolarization of ventricular myocytes. In the presence of a long QT interval, the cellular basis of alternation may be beat-to-beat repolarization changes in midmyocardial cells (so-called M cells). Whether this mechanism applies to different disease states is not known.[25] T wave alternans testing requires exercise or atrial pacing to achieve a heart rate of 100 to 120 beats/min with relatively little atrial or ventricular ectopic activity. The test is less useful in patients with a wide QRS complex (longer than 120 milliseconds). A positive T wave alternans test result (**Fig. 36-9**) is associated with a worse arrhythmic prognosis in various

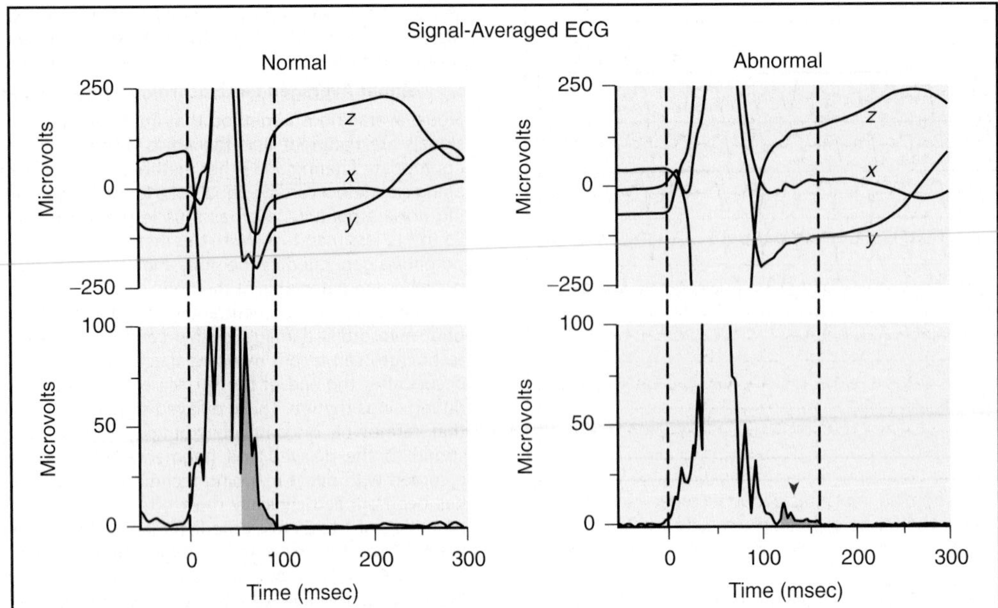

FIGURE 36-8 Signal-averaged ECG. Normal **(left)** and abnormal **(right)** results are shown from a patient with prior myocardial infarction and ventricular tachycardia. **Bottom panels,** Shaded blue areas at the end of each tracing represent voltage content of last 40 milliseconds of the filtered QRS integral. The small shaded area in the abnormal study denotes prolonged, slow conduction and suggests the potential for reentrant ventricular arrhythmias.

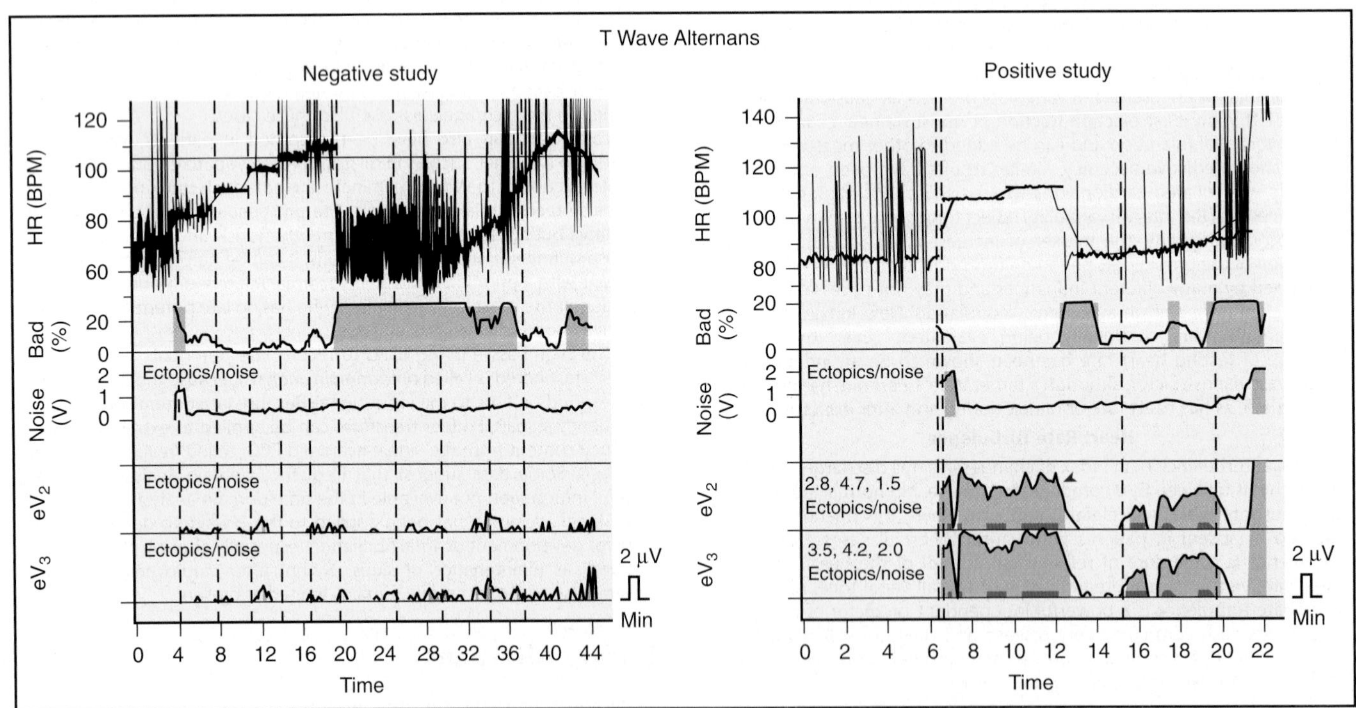

FIGURE 36-9 T wave alternans. Reports of T wave alternans analysis from two patients are shown, displaying heart rate in beats per minute (HR BPM), proportion of beats rejected from analysis (% Bad), ECG noise level (in microvolts), and selected precordial leads (V_2 and V_3) as a function of time. **Left panel,** Records from a patient with no structural heart disease; the amplitude of T wave alternans was minimal. **Right panel,** Records from a patient hospitalized for sustained ventricular tachycardia after myocardial infarction shows T wave alternans (blue shaded area, arrowhead).

disorders, including ischemic heart disease and nonischemic cardiomyopathy.[26,27] The test's greatest usefulness appears to be in the detection of a group of patients with low risk for development of malignant ventricular arrhythmias (negative T wave alternans test result). Although the predictive value of a positive test result varies greatly, depending on the population studied, a negative test result strongly predicts freedom from VT and VF in all group studies thus far, at least during a short follow-up period. This has important implications for implantable cardioverter-defibrillator (ICD) use in high-risk patients who have not yet manifested dangerous arrhythmias (primary prevention or prophylactic devices).[28] A significant proportion of these patients will never benefit from these devices (lack of spontaneous VT or VF), and some investigators have suggested that T wave alternans testing may segregate those who are more likely to benefit from ICD use (positive test result) from those who are not (negative test result) and who should therefore not undergo ICD implantation.[29]

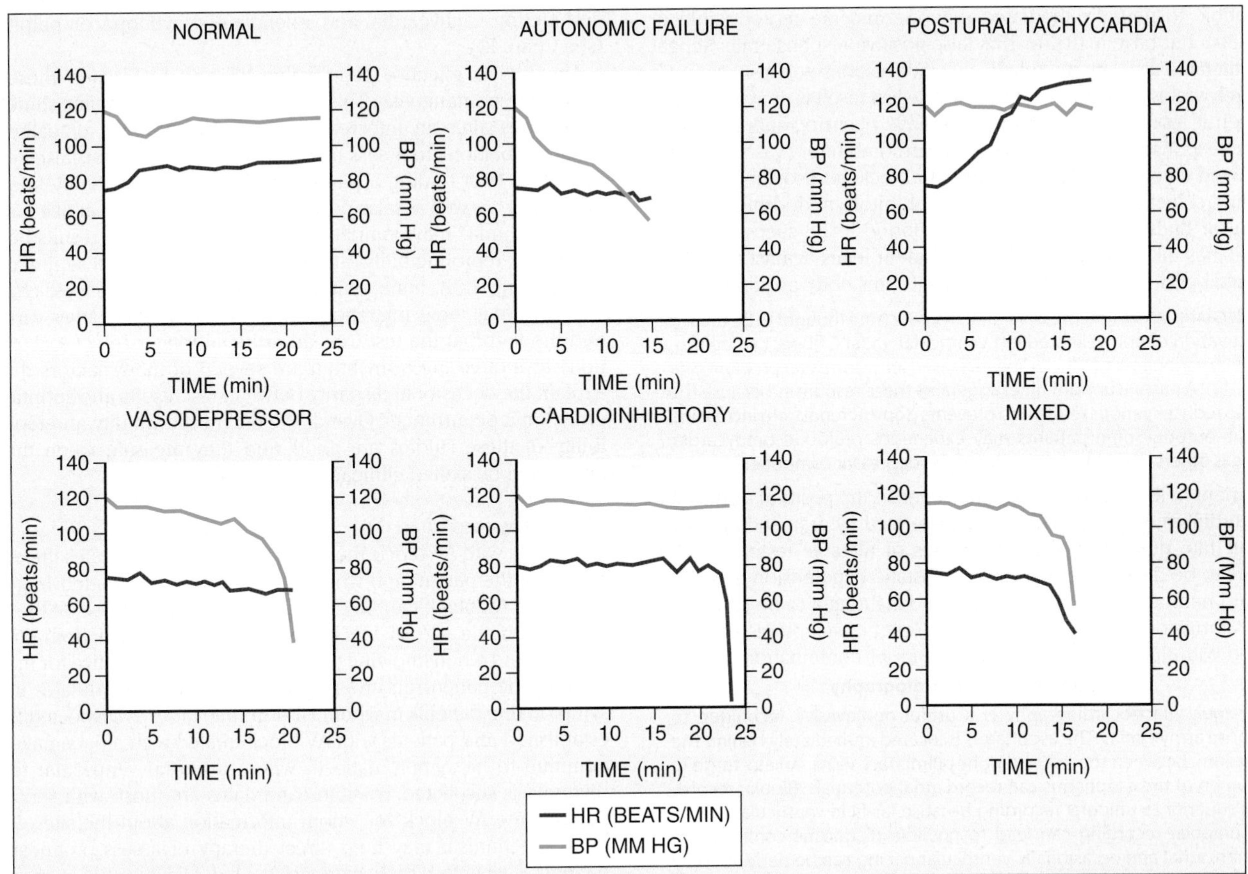

FIGURE 36-10 Head-up tilt-table testing. Several responses to tilt-table testing are shown; heart rate (HR) and systolic blood pressure (BP) are plotted as time functions. A normal response is an early, slight drop in BP with compensatory increase in HR mediated by the autonomic nervous system. With autonomic dysfunction, a progressive fall in BP is not counteracted by HR increase. In the postural tachycardia syndrome, an exaggerated increase in HR is seen. The **bottom panel** depicts findings with neurocardiogenic syncope: a pure vasodepressor response is a relatively sudden drop in BP without marked change in HR, whereas the pure cardioinhibitory response shows a sudden decrease in HR without change in BP. A mixed response shows decreases in both HR and BP.

Further studies are necessary in this area.[30] T wave alternans may represent a fundamental marker of an electrically unstable myocardium prone to development of VT or VF, and as such, ST-T wave analysis for alternans may be increasingly useful in the future as a method to risk-stratify patients. Other methods of analyzing T wave alternans, including time domain and T wave variability, are undergoing study.

Baroreceptor Reflex Sensitivity Testing

Acute blood pressure elevation triggers a baroreceptor reflex that augments vagal tone to the heart and slows the sinus rate. The increase in sinus cycle length per millimeter of mercury systolic blood pressure increase is a measure of the sensitivity of the baroreceptor reflex and, when reduced, identifies patients susceptible to development of VT and VF.[15] The mechanism of the reduction in baroreceptor reflex sensitivity is not certain. However, this test may be useful to identify patients at risk for development of a serious ventricular arrhythmia after myocardial infarction.

Body Surface Mapping

Isopotential body surface maps are used to provide a complete picture of the effects of the currents from the heart on the body surface. The potential distributions are represented by contour lines of equal potential, and each distribution is displayed instant by instant throughout activation, recovery, or both.

Body surface maps have been used clinically to localize and to size areas of myocardial ischemia, to localize ectopic foci or accessory pathways, to differentiate aberrant supraventricular conduction from ventricular origin, to recognize the patient prone to development of arrhythmias, and possibly to understand the mechanisms involved. Although these procedures are of interest, their clinical usefulness has not yet been established. In addition, the technique is cumbersome and the analysis is complex.

Electrocardiographic Imaging

Another promising technology is electrocardiographic imaging, in which cardiac electrical activity recorded at the skin surface is spatially integrated with imaging data (currently, cardiac computed tomography scanning).[31] Using complex mathematical processing of electrical data collected from 224 electrodes on the skin surface, this technique can plot atrial and ventricular electrical activity on an epicardial "shell" of the patient's own heart and thereby follow the course of activation during sinus rhythm or an arrhythmia. Clinical experience is limited thus far but encouraging.[32]

Upright Tilt-Table Testing

The tilt-table test is used to identify patients who have a vasodepressor or cardioinhibitory response as a cause of syncope (see Chap. 42).[33] Patients are positioned on a tilt table in the supine position and are tilted upright to a maximum of 60 to 80 degrees for 20 to 45 minutes or longer if necessary (**Fig. 36-10**). Isoproterenol, as a bolus or infusion, may provoke syncope in patients whose initial upright tilt-table test result shows no abnormalities or after just several minutes of tilt to shorten the time of the test necessary to produce a positive response. An initial intravenous isoproterenol dose of 1 mcg/min can be increased in 0.5-mcg/min steps until symptoms occur or a maximum of 4 mcg/min is given. Isoproterenol induces a vasodepressor response in upright susceptible patients, generally consisting of a decrease in heart rate and blood pressure along with near-syncope or syncope. Intravenous edrophonium chloride, nitroglycerin, and esmolol withdrawal has also been used. Atropine can block the early bradycardia but not the hypotension; beta blockers can inhibit the latter. Tilt-table test results are positive in two thirds to three fourths of patients susceptible to neurally mediated syncope and are reproducible in about 80% but have a 10% to 15% false-positive response rate. Repeat of the tilt-table test with an initially negative response on a subsequent day rarely yields a positive result. A positive test result is more meaningful when it reproduces symptoms that have occurred spontaneously. Positive responses can be divided into cardioinhibitory, vasodepressor, and mixed categories. Therapy with beta blockers, disopyramide, theophylline, selective serotonin reuptake inhibitors, midodrine, and salt loading or fludrocortisone has been reported to be successful with each, as has tilt training, in which the patient leans against a wall for prolonged periods to increase tolerance to this body position.

Mechanism. Vasodepressor reactions, which are thought to be caused by activation of unmyelinated left ventricular vagal C fibers, can be triggered by various events, including increased left ventricular pressure (see Chap. 42). A passive upright tilt exaggerates these responses because the tilt also reduces venous return and prevents isoproterenol from increasing cardiac output. Some patients may experience profound bradycardia, whereas others may have a prominent vasodepressor component.

A variant of the neurocardiogenic response, the postural orthostatic tachycardia syndrome (POTS), is characterized by dramatic increases in heart rate during the first 10 minutes of tilt-table testing.[34] POTS appears to be distinct from simple orthostatic hypotension as well as standard neurocardiogenic responses and is thought to be caused by various forms of autonomic imbalance. Relief of symptoms has been effected with fludrocortisone, beta blockers, or combinations.

Esophageal Electrocardiography

Esophageal electrocardiography is a useful noninvasive technique to diagnose arrhythmias. The esophagus is located immediately behind the left atrium, between the left and right pulmonary veins. An electrode in the lumen of the esophagus can record atrial potentials. Bipolar recording is superior to unipolar recording because far-field ventricular events with unipolar recording can lead to possible diagnostic confusion. In addition, atrial and occasionally ventricular pacing can be performed by means of a catheter electrode inserted into the esophagus, and tachycardias can be initiated and terminated. Optimal electrode position for atrial pacing correlates with the patient's height and is within about 1 cm of the site at which the maximum amplitude of the atrial electrogram is recorded. When it is recorded simultaneously with the surface ECG, the esophageal atrial electrogram can be used to differentiate SVT with aberrancy from VT and to define the mechanism of SVTs. For example, if atrial and ventricular depolarizations occur simultaneously during a narrow QRS tachycardia, reentry using an accessory AV pathway (Wolff-Parkinson-White syndrome) can be excluded, and AV nodal reentry is the most likely mechanism for the tachycardia. Complications of transesophageal recording and pacing are uncommon, but the technique is not comfortable for most patients, and it is therefore not commonly used.

Invasive Electrophysiologic Studies

An invasive EPS involves introducing multipolar catheter electrodes into the venous or arterial system, positioning the electrodes at various intracardiac sites to record or to stimulate cardiac electrical activity. Assessment of AV conduction at rest is made by positioning the catheter along the septal leaflet of the tricuspid valve and measuring the atrial-His interval (an estimate of AV nodal conduction time; normally, 60 to 125 milliseconds) and the His-ventricular (H-V) interval (a measure of infranodal conduction; normally, 35 to 55 milliseconds). The heart is stimulated from portions of the atria or ventricles and from the region of the His bundle, bundle branches, accessory pathways, and other structures. Such studies are performed diagnostically to provide information about the type of clinical rhythm disturbance and insight into its electrophysiologic mechanism. An EPS is used therapeutically to terminate a tachycardia by electrical stimulation or electroshock, to evaluate the effects of therapy by determining whether a particular intervention modifies or prevents electrical induction of a tachycardia or whether an electrical device properly senses and terminates an induced tachyarrhythmia, and to ablate myocardium involved in the tachycardia to prevent further episodes. Finally, these tests have been used prognostically to identify patients at risk for sudden cardiac death. The study may be helpful in patients who have AV block, intraventricular conduction disturbance, sinus node dysfunction, tachycardia, and unexplained syncope or palpitations (see Chap. 42).

The EPS is effective at initiating VT and SVT when these have occurred spontaneously. This enables the use of similar stimulation techniques after an intervention (e.g., drug therapy or catheter or surgical ablation) to assess treatment efficacy. However, false-negative responses (not finding a particular electrical abnormality known to be present) as well as false-positive responses (induction of a nonclinical arrhythmia) may complicate interpretation of the results because many lack reproducibility. Altered autonomic tone in a supine patient undergoing study, hemodynamic or ischemic influences, changing anatomy (e.g., new infarction) after the study, day-to-day variability, and the fact that the test uses an artificial trigger (electrical stimulation) to induce the arrhythmia are several of many factors that can explain the occasional disparity between test results and spontaneous arrhythmia occurrences. Overall, the diagnostic validity and reproducibility of these studies are good, and they are safe when they are performed by skilled clinical electrophysiologists.

AV BLOCK (see Chap. 39)

In patients with AV block, the site of block usually dictates the clinical course of the patient and whether a pacemaker is needed. In general, the site of AV block can be determined from an analysis of the scalar ECG. When the site of block cannot be determined from such an analysis, and when knowing the site of block is imperative for management of the patient, an invasive EPS is indicated. Candidates include symptomatic patients in whom His-Purkinje block is suspected but not established and patients with AV block treated with a pacemaker who continue to be symptomatic, in whom a causal ventricular tachyarrhythmia is suspected. Possible candidates are those with second- or third-degree AV block, for whom information about the site of block or its mechanism may help direct therapy or assess prognosis, and patients suspected of having concealed His bundle extrasystoles. Patients with block in the His-Purkinje system become symptomatic because of periods of bradycardia or asystole and require pacemaker implantation more often than do patients who have AV nodal block. Type I (Wenckebach) AV block in older patients may have clinical implications similar to those for type II AV block. The results of EPS for evaluating the conduction system must be interpreted with caution, however. In rare cases, the process of recording conduction intervals alters their values. For example, catheter pressure on the AV node or His bundle can cause a prolongation of the atrial-His or H-V interval and lead to erroneous diagnosis and therapy.

INTRAVENTRICULAR CONDUCTION DISTURBANCE

For patients with an intraventricular conduction disturbance, an EPS provides information about the duration of the H-V interval, which can be prolonged with a normal PR interval or normal with a prolonged PR interval. A prolonged H-V interval (longer than 55 milliseconds) is associated with a greater likelihood for development of trifascicular block (but the rate of progression is slow, 2% to 3% annually), having structural disease, and higher mortality. The finding of very long H-V intervals (longer than 80 to 90 milliseconds) identifies patients at increased risk for development of AV block. The H-V interval has a high specificity (approximately 80%) but low sensitivity (approximately 66%) for predicting the development of complete AV block. During the study, atrial pacing is used to uncover abnormal His-Purkinje conduction. A positive response is provocation of distal His block during 1:1 AV nodal conduction at rates of 135 beats/min or less. Again, sensitivity is low but specificity is high. Functional His-Purkinje block caused by normal His-Purkinje refractoriness is not a positive response. Drug infusion, such as with procainamide or ajmaline, sometimes exposes abnormal His-Purkinje conduction (**Fig. 36-11**). Ajmaline (not available in the United States) can cause arrhythmias and should be used cautiously.

An EPS is indicated in the patient with symptoms (syncope or presyncope) that appear to be related to a bradyarrhythmia or tachyarrhythmia when no other cause of symptoms is found. For many of these patients, ventricular tachyarrhythmias rather than AV block can be the cause of their symptoms.

SINUS NODE DYSFUNCTION

(see Chap. 39)

The demonstration of slow sinus rates, sinus exit block, or sinus pauses temporally related to symptoms suggests a causal relationship and usually obviates further diagnostic studies. Carotid sinus pressure that results in several seconds of complete cardiac asystole or AV block and reproduces the patient's usual symptoms exposes the presence of a hypersensitive carotid sinus reflex. Carotid sinus massage must be done cautiously. Rarely, carotid sinus massage can precipitate a stroke. Neurohumoral agents, adenosine, or stress testing can be used to evaluate the effects of autonomic tone on sinus node automaticity and sinoatrial conduction time. An EPS should be considered in patients who have symptoms attributable to bradycardia or asystole, such as presyncope or syncope, and for whom noninvasive approaches have provided no explanation for the symptoms.

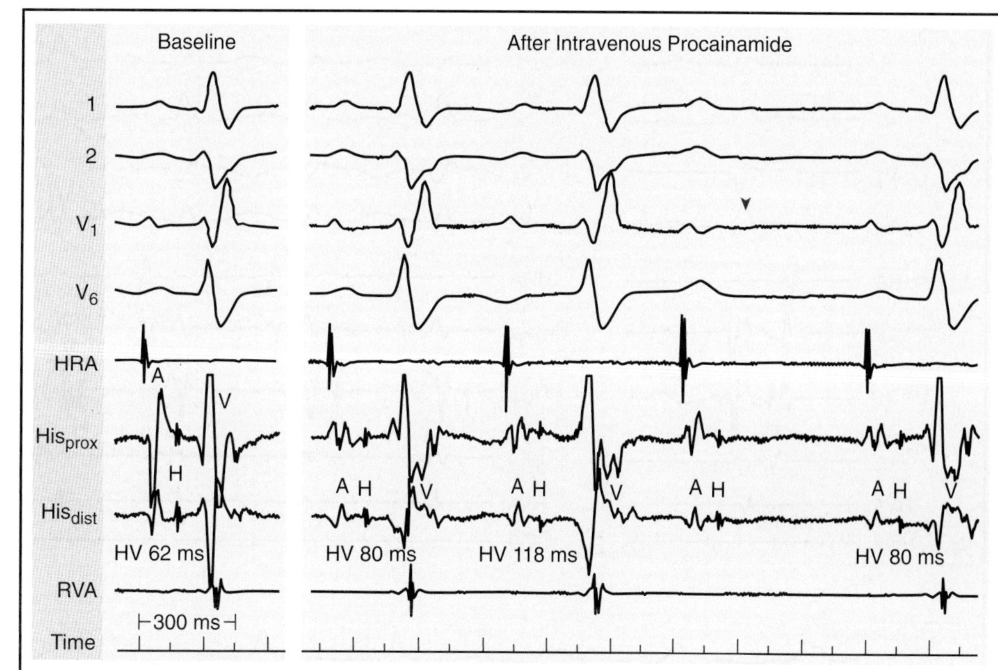

FIGURE 36-11 Testing the His-Purkinje system. A 43-year-old woman with sarcoid underwent EPS after a syncopal episode. Surface leads 1, 2, V_1, and V_6 are shown, with intracardiac recordings from catheters in the high right atrium (HRA), proximal (His_{prox}) and distal (His_{dis}) electrode pairs of a catheter at the AV junction to record the His potential, and right ventricular apex (RVA). During baseline recording, the H-V interval is only slightly prolonged (62 milliseconds). After infusion of intravenous procainamide, the H-V interval is longer and infra-His Wenckebach block is present. The arrowhead denotes the missing QRS complex caused by infra-His block. A = atrial electrogram; H = His potential; V = ventricular electrogram.

Sinus Node Recovery Time. Sinus node recovery time (SNRT) is a technique that can be useful to evaluate sinus node function. The interval between the last paced high right atrial response and first spontaneous (sinus) high right atrial response after termination of pacing is measured to determine the SNRT. Because the spontaneous sinus rate influences the SNRT, the value is corrected by subtracting the spontaneous sinus node cycle length (before pacing) from the SNRT (**Fig. 36-12**). This value, the corrected SNRT (CSNRT), is generally shorter than 525 milliseconds. Prolonged CSNRT has been found in patients suspected of having sinus node dysfunction. Direct recordings of the sinus node electrogram have documented that SNRT is influenced by the prolongation of sinoatrial conduction time (the time from the onset of the sinus impulse to the onset of activation of surrounding atrial myocardium) as well as by changes in sinus node automaticity, especially in the first beat after cessation of pacing. After cessation of pacing, the first return sinus cycle can be normal and can be followed by secondary pauses. Secondary pauses appear to be more common in patients whose sinus node dysfunction is caused by sinoatrial exit block (a potential cause of electrocardiographic sinus pauses). Finally, it is important to evaluate AV node and His-Purkinje function in patients with sinus node dysfunction because many also exhibit impaired AV conduction.

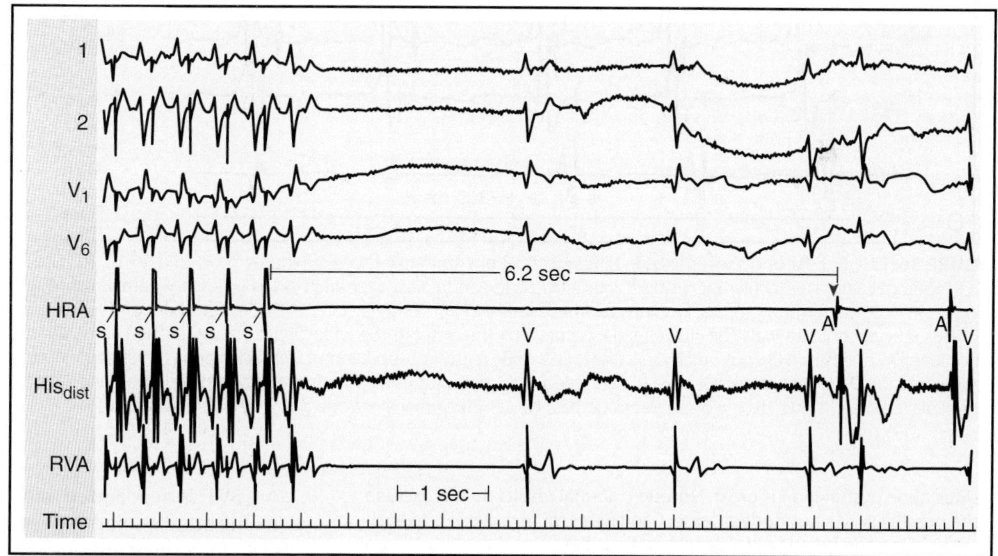

FIGURE 36-12 Abnormal sinus node function. Recordings are similar to those in Figure 36-11. The last five complexes of a 1-minute burst of atrial pacing (S) at a cycle length of 400 milliseconds are shown, after which pacing is stopped. The sinus node does not spontaneously discharge (sinus node recovery time) until 6.2 seconds later (arrowhead). Three junctional escape beats occurred before this time. His_{dis} = distal electrode pair; HRA = high right atrium; RVA = right ventricular apex.

Sinoatrial Conduction Time. The sinoatrial conduction time (SACT) can be estimated by simple pacing techniques based on the assumptions that (1) conduction times into and out of the sinus node are equal, (2) no depression of sinus node automaticity occurs, and (3) the pacemaker site does not shift after premature stimulation (see Chap. 36). These assumptions can be erroneous, particularly in patients with sinus node dysfunction. SACT can also be measured directly with extracellular electrodes placed in the region of the sinus node. This direct measurement correlates well with the SACT measured indirectly in patients with normal sinus node function. The sensitivity of the SACT and SNRT tests is only about 50% for each test alone and about 65% when they are combined. The specificity, combined, is about 88%, with a low predictive value. Thus, if these test results are abnormal, the likelihood of the patient's having

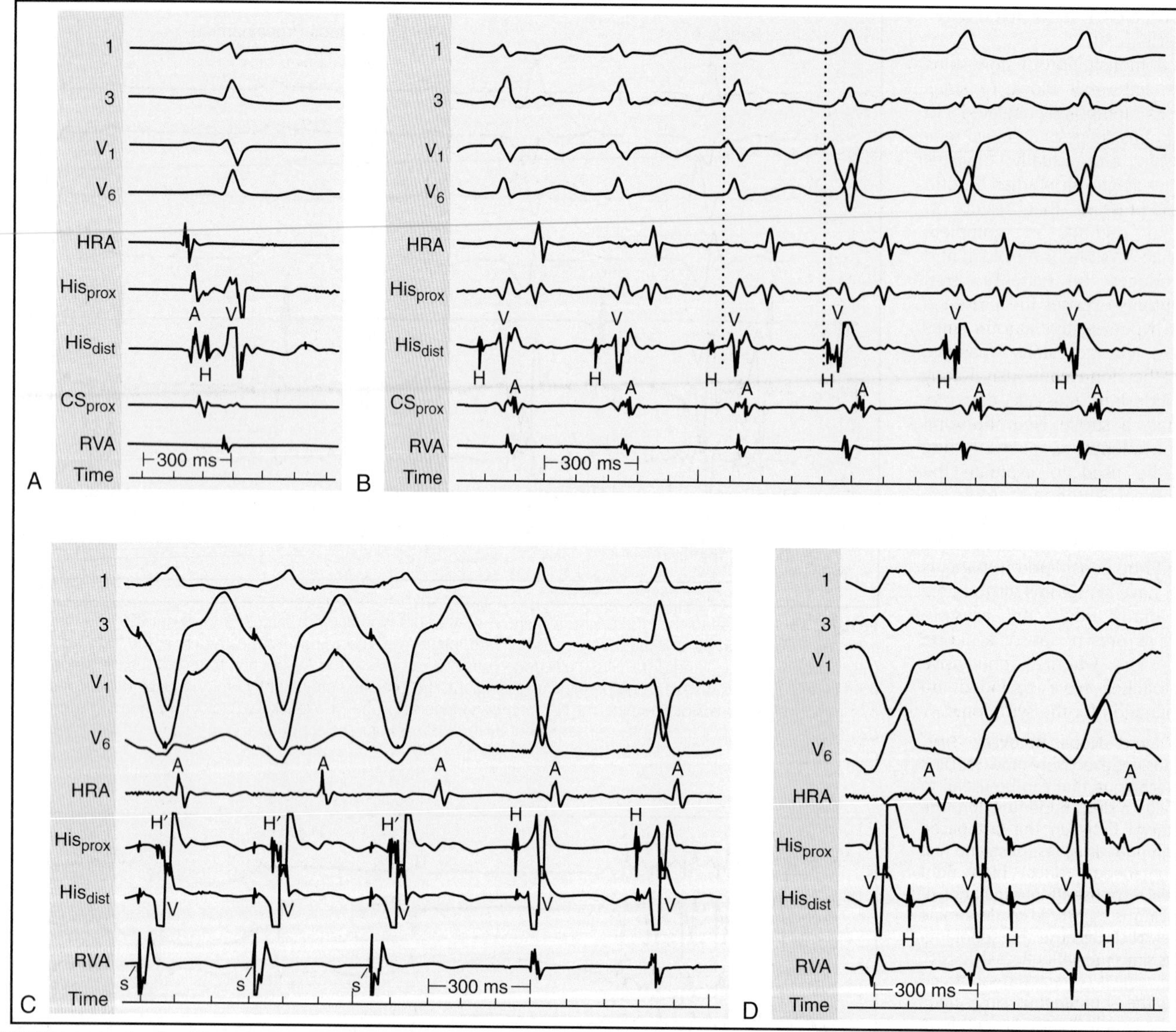

FIGURE 36-13 Bundle of His recordings in different situations similar to those in Figures 36-11 and 36-12. **A,** Baseline sinus rhythm with normal AV conduction. **B,** Orthodromic supraventricular tachycardia with retrograde conduction over a left-sided accessory pathway throughout the tracing. The first three beats have a narrow QRS complex with a normal H-V interval; the last three QRS complexes represent a fusion of conduction over the AV node–His and a slowly conducting right-sided accessory pathway. The His potential occurs after the onset of the wide QRS complex (dashed lines). **C,** Three paced ventricular beats are shown with a retrograde His potential (H′), followed by initiation of AV node reentrant supraventricular tachycardia (atrial depolarization near the end of the QRS complex, as seen in HRA tracing). **D,** Ventricular tachycardia with delayed activation of the His potential and complete retrograde AV node block (dissociated atrial complexes). CS_{prox} = proximal coronary sinus; His_{dis} = distal electrode pair; His_{prox} = proximal electrode pair; HRA = high right atrium; RVA = right ventricular apex.

sinus node dysfunction is great. However, normal results do not exclude the possibility of sinus node disease. Candidates for invasive EPS to evaluate sinus node function are symptomatic patients in whom sinus node dysfunction has not been established as a cause of the symptoms. Potential candidates are those requiring pacemakers to determine the pacing modality, patients with sinus node dysfunction to determine the mechanism and response to therapy, and patients in whom other causes of symptoms (e.g., tachyarrhythmias) are to be excluded.

TACHYCARDIA (see Chap. 39)

In patients with tachycardias, an EPS can be used to diagnose the arrhythmia, to determine and to deliver therapy, to determine the anatomic sites involved in the tachycardia, to identify patients at high risk for development of serious arrhythmias, and to gain insights into mechanisms responsible for the arrhythmia. The study can differentiate aberrant supraventricular conduction from ventricular tachyarrhythmias when standard electrocardiographic criteria are equivocal.

An SVT is recognized electrophysiologically by an H-V interval equaling or exceeding that recorded during normal sinus rhythm (**Fig. 36-13**). In contrast, during VT, the H-V interval is shorter than normal or the His deflection cannot be recorded clearly because of superimposition of the larger ventricular electrogram.[35] Only two situations exist in which a consistently short H-V interval occurs, during retrograde activation of the His bundle from activation originating in the ventricle (i.e., PVC or VT) and during conduction over an accessory pathway (preexcitation syndrome). Atrial pacing at rates exceeding the tachycardia rate can demonstrate the ventricular origin of the wide QRS tachycardia by producing fusion and capture beats and normalization of the H-V interval. The only VT that exhibits an H-V interval equal to or slightly exceeding the normal sinus H-V interval is bundle branch reentry, but His activation will be in the retrograde direction.

An EPS should be considered for the following: (1) in patients who have symptomatic, recurrent, or drug-resistant supraventricular or ventricular tachyarrhythmias to help select optimal therapy; (2) in patients with tachyarrhythmias occurring too infrequently to permit adequate diagnostic or therapeutic assessment; (3) in differentiation of SVT and aberrant conduction from VT; (4) whenever nonpharmacologic therapy, such as the use of electrical devices, catheter ablation, or surgery, is contemplated; (5) in patients surviving an episode of cardiac arrest, occurring more than 48 hours after an acute myocardial infarction or without evidence of an acute Q wave myocardial infarction; and (6) in assessment of the risk of sustained VT in patients with a prior myocardial infarction, ejection fraction of 0.3 to 0.4, and nonsustained VT on an ECG. In general, EPS is not indicated in patients with long-QT syndrome and torsades de pointes.

The process of initiation and termination of SVT or VT with programmed electrical stimulation to test the potential efficacy of pharmacologic, electrical, or surgical therapy represents an important application of EPS in patients with tachycardia. The role of drug therapy in clinically significant arrhythmias continues to diminish; although EPS was once widely used to predict the efficacy of drug therapy in suppressing spontaneous tachycardia recurrences, the technique is now rarely used for this purpose. Noninvasive stimulation from an implanted pacemaker or defibrillator can be used to test the effects of drug therapy given to try to decrease arrhythmia frequency.[36]

UNEXPLAINED SYNCOPE (see Chap. 42)

The three common arrhythmic causes of syncope are sinus node dysfunction, AV block, and tachyarrhythmias. Of the three, tachyarrhythmias are most reliably initiated in the electrophysiology laboratory, followed by sinus node abnormalities and His-Purkinje block.[37]

The cause of syncope remains uncertain in up to 50% of patients, depending in part on the extent of the evaluation. A careful, accurately performed history and physical examination begin the evaluation,[1] followed by noninvasive tests, including a 12-lead ECG, and can lead to a diagnosis in 50% or more of patients. A small percentage (less than 5%) of patients develop an arrhythmia coincident with syncope or presyncope during a 24-hour recording of the ECG, whereas a larger percentage (15%) have symptoms without an arrhythmia, excluding an arrhythmic cause. Prolonged electrocardiographic monitoring with patient-activated transtelephonic event recorders that have memory loops may increase the yield. Tilt-table and stress testing can be useful for selected patients, as can long-term electrocardiographic recordings.

The EPS helps explain the cause of syncope or palpitations when it induces an arrhythmia that replicates the patient's symptoms. Syncopal patients with a nondiagnostic EPS have a low incidence of sudden death and an 80% remission rate. In those with recurrent syncope, the test is falsely negative in 20% because of failure to find AV block or sinus node dysfunction. On the other hand, in many patients with structural heart disease, several abnormalities that could account for syncope can be diagnosed at EPS. Deciding which among these abnormalities is responsible for syncope and therefore requires therapy can be difficult. Mortality and incidence of sudden cardiac death are mainly determined by the presence of underlying heart disease.

Syncopal patients considered for an EPS are those whose spells remain undiagnosed despite general, neurologic, and noninvasive cardiac evaluation, particularly if the patient has structural heart disease. The diagnostic yield is about 70% in that group but only about 12% in patients without structural heart disease.[38] Therapy for a putative cause found during an EPS prevents recurrence of syncope in about 80% of patients. Among arrhythmic causes of syncope, intermittent conduction disturbances are the most difficult to diagnose. EPS is poor at establishing this diagnosis, despite an array of provocative tests that can be used. When tachyarrhythmias have been thoroughly sought and excluded and the clinical suspicion of intermittent heart block is high (e.g., bundle branch block or long H-V interval), empiric permanent pacing may be justified.

PALPITATIONS

An EPS is indicated in patients with palpitations who have had a pulse documented by medical personnel to be inappropriately rapid or slow without electrocardiographic recording and in those suspected of having clinically significant palpitations without electrocardiographic documentation.

In patients with syncope or palpitations, the sensitivity of the EPS may be low but may be increased at the expense of specificity. For example, more aggressive pacing techniques (e.g., use of three or four premature stimuli), administration of drugs (e.g., isoproterenol), or left ventricular pacing can increase the success rate of ventricular arrhythmia induction by precipitating nonclinical ventricular tachyarrhythmias, such as nonsustained polymorphic or monomorphic VT or VF. Similarly, aggressive techniques during atrial pacing can induce nonspecific episodes of atrial flutter or atrial fibrillation. A diagnostic dilemma arises when the patient's clinical, symptom-producing arrhythmia is one of these nonspecific arrhythmias that can be produced in the normal patient who has no arrhythmia. In most patients, these arrhythmias are regarded as nonclinical (i.e., nonspecific responses to intense stimulation). In other patients, such as those with hypertrophic or dilated nonischemic cardiomyopathy, these may be clinically relevant arrhythmias. However, induction of a sustained SVT (e.g., AV nodal reentry, AV reciprocating tachycardia) or monomorphic VT is almost never an artifact of intense stimulation. Initiation of these arrhythmias in patients who have not had known spontaneous episodes of these tachycardias is uncommon and provides important information; for example, the induced tachyarrhythmia may be clinically significant and responsible for the patient's symptoms. In general, other abnormalities, such as prolonged sinus pauses after overdrive atrial pacing or His-Purkinje AV block, are not induced in patients who do not or may not experience these abnormalities spontaneously. Induction of these arrhythmias has a high degree of specificity.

Complications of Electrophysiologic Studies

The risks of undergoing only an EPS are small. Because most procedures do not involve left-sided heart access, risk of stroke, systemic embolism, or myocardial infarction is less than that of coronary arteriography. Myocardial perforation with cardiac tamponade, pseudoaneurysms at arterial access sites, and provocation of nonclinical arrhythmias can occur, each with less than 1 in 500 incidence. The addition of therapeutic maneuvers (e.g., ablation) to the procedure increases the incidence of complications. In a European survey of 4398 patients reported from 68 institutions, ablation procedure–related complications ranged from 3.2% to 8%. Five deaths occurred within the perioperative period of the ablation. In a Heart Rhythm Society (formerly North American Society of Pacing and Electrophysiology) survey,[39] of 164 hospitals reporting in 1998 on more than 3300 patients who had received radiofrequency ablation, complications occurred in 1% to 3%, with procedure-related deaths in about 0.2%. In a study of 1050 patients undergoing temperature-controlled ablation for supraventricular arrhythmias, 32 (3%) had a major complication. Predictors of major complications were ejection fraction less than 0.35 and multiple ablation targets. The improvement in the complication rate probably reflects the learning curve for radiofrequency ablation. In many centers, a diagnostic EPS and even ablation procedures are performed on an outpatient basis. With the increasing use of extensive ablation in the left atrium to treat atrial fibrillation, an increase in systemic thromboembolic complications has been observed, as have pericardial effusion and tamponade, valve damage, and phrenic nerve injury (see Chap. 39).

DIRECT CARDIAC MAPPING: RECORDING POTENTIALS DIRECTLY FROM THE HEART

Cardiac mapping is a method whereby potentials recorded directly from the heart are spatially depicted as a function of time in an integrated manner (**Fig. 36-14**). The location of recording electrodes (e.g., epicardial, intramural, or endocardial) and the recording mode used (unipolar versus bipolar) as well as the method of display (isopotential versus isochronous maps) depend on the problem under consideration. Special electrodes can record monophasic action potentials.

Direct cardiac mapping by catheter electrodes, or less commonly at the time of cardiac surgery, can be used to identify and to localize the areas responsible for rhythm disturbances in patients

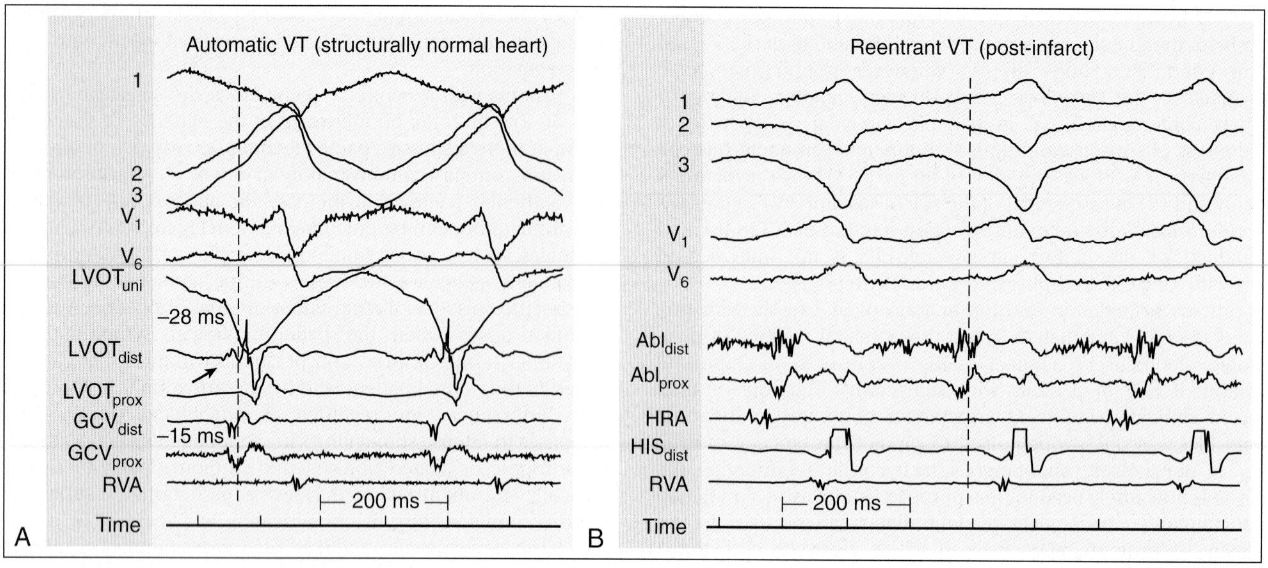

FIGURE 36-14 Endocardial catheter recordings during ventricular tachycardia (VT) in two patients. Dashed lines denote onset of QRS complexes. **A,** A woman without structural heart disease had a sustained VT arising from the left ventricular outflow tract (LVOT). Note unipolar (uni) electrogram with a sharp "QS" complex and the onset (arrow) of the distal bipolar recording ($LVOT_{dist}$) preceding the right ventricular recording. It also precedes recordings from a multielectrode catheter advanced along the coronary sinus and down the great cardiac vein (GCV_{dist} and GCV_{prox}) on the epicardial surface opposite the endocardial recording. Retrograde 1:1 conduction is present. Ablation at this site (LVOT) terminated the VT. **B,** A patient with reentrant VT caused by a prior inferior wall infarction underwent mapping. The ablation catheter (Abl_{dist}) on the inferomedial wall shows a very prolonged, fragmented electrogram indicative of slow conduction. The electrogram spans the entire diastolic interval between QRS complexes. Ablation at this site eliminated the VT. Abl_{prox} = proximal ablation catheter electrodes.

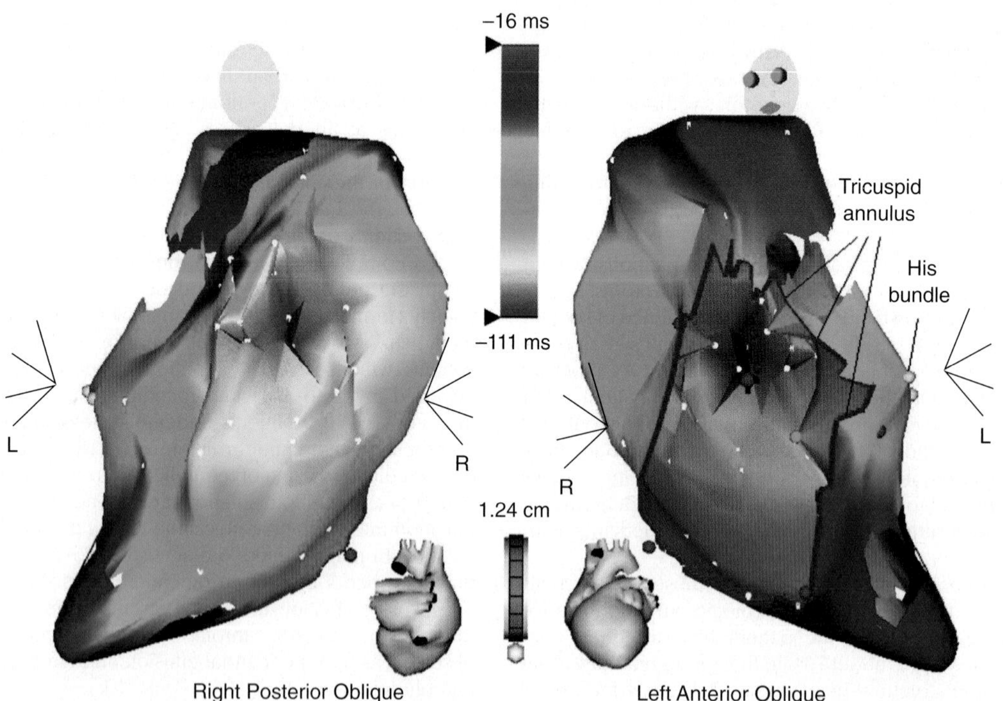

FIGURE 36-15 Electroanatomic map of focal atrial tachycardia. The right atrium is shown in two views (small gray icons at bottom center help with orientation). A color-coded time scale of activation is shown at top center; red indicates earliest activation, purple latest. A distance scale is shown below. This atrial tachycardia arose in the posterolateral right atrium (red spot), with all other areas activated centrifugally. Ablation at this site eliminated the tachycardia.

with supraventricular and ventricular tachyarrhythmias for catheter or surgical ablation, isolation, or resection. Disorders amenable to this approach include accessory pathways associated with Wolff-Parkinson-White syndrome, the pathways in AV node reentry, AV node–His bundle ablation, sites of origin of atrial tachycardia and VTs, isolated pathways essential for the maintenance of reentrant atrial tachycardia or VTs, and various substrates responsible for episodes of atrial fibrillation (see Chap. 40). Mapping can also be used to delineate the anatomic course of the His bundle to avoid injury during catheter ablation or open heart surgery for repair of congenital heart disease.

Early efforts at mapping involved moving an electrode from location to location, acquiring data from a single point at a time, and comparing the timing of local activation with some reference recording as well as other mapped sites. Obtaining enough data points to determine where ablation should be performed relied heavily on the memory of the operator. Specialized mapping systems have now been developed that use computers to log not only the activation times at various points in the heart but the physical locations from which these were obtained. The mapping information acquired in this way can be displayed on a screen, showing relative activation times in a color-coded sequence. By use of such systems, dozens or even hundreds of sites can be sampled relatively quickly, leading to a clear picture of cardiac activation and potential target sites for ablation (**Figs. 36-15** and **36-16**). These systems can also record signal amplitude at each site sampled, allowing differentiation of normal versus scarred myocardium that can help in planning ablation strategies (**Fig. 36-17**). Other mapping systems can acquire data from several thousand points simultaneously, using a multipolar electrode array. This is particularly useful for hemodynamically unstable tachycardias or those that terminate spontaneously within seconds, precluding detailed point-to-point mapping.

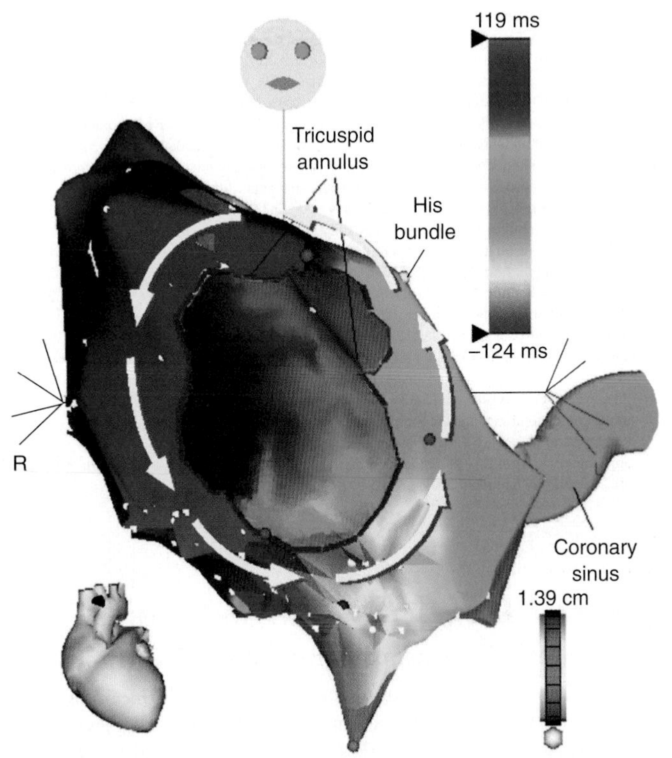

FIGURE 36-16 Electroanatomic map of reentrant atrial flutter. A left anterior oblique view of the right atrium is shown, along with a depiction of the coronary sinus. See Figure 36-15 for other details. The electrical wave front propagates around the tricuspid annulus in a counterclockwise direction; in this complete circuit, early activation (in red) abuts late activation (purple) near the bottom of the tricuspid annulus. The cycle length of the tachycardia was 250 milliseconds, almost completely described by the points shown in the figure (from −124 to +119 milliseconds, a total of 243 milliseconds). A distance scale is shown below.

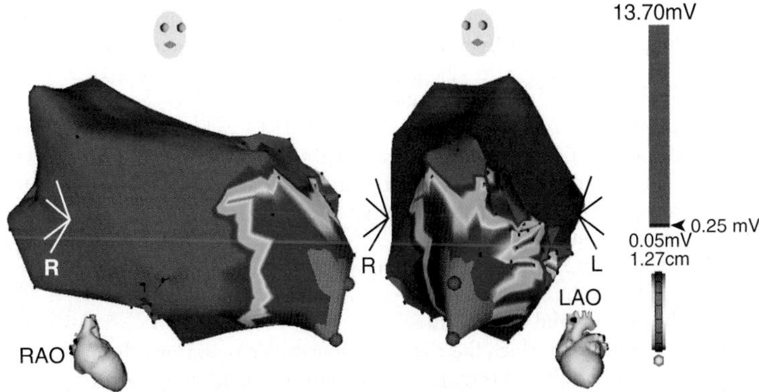

FIGURE 36-17 Electroanatomic left ventricular voltage maps during sinus rhythm. Right and left anterior oblique views are shown; the voltage scale at right indicates normal areas (purple) versus scarred (gray) or very low voltage (red, with gradation to higher voltages through green and blue) areas. The patient had an old anteroapical myocardial infarction leading to reentrant ventricular tachycardia that originated in the border between scar and more normal myocardium, LAO = left anterior oblique; RAO = right anterior oblique.

REFERENCES

1. Das M, Zipes DP: Assessment of the patient with a cardiac arrhythmia. *In* Zipes DP, Jalife J (eds): Cardiac Electrophysiology: From Cell to Bedside. 5th ed. Philadelphia, WB Saunders, 2009, pp 831-836.
2. Barsky AJ: Palpitations, arrhythmias, and awareness of cardiac activity. Ann Intern Med 134:832, 2001.
3. Miller JM, Das M: Differential diagnosis for wide QRS complex tachycardia. *In* Zipes DP, Jalife J (eds): Cardiac Electrophysiology: From Cell to Bedside. 5th ed. Philadelphia, WB Saunders, 2009, pp 823-830.
4. Valderrábano M: Exercise-induced arrhythmias. *In* Zipes DP, Jalife J (eds): Cardiac Electrophysiology: From Cell to Bedside. 5th ed. Philadelphia, WB Saunders, 2009, pp 837-844.
5. Cole CR, Blackstone EH, Pashkow FJ, et al: Heart-rate recovery immediately after exercise as a predictor of mortality. N Engl J Med 341:1351, 1999.
6. Frolkis JP, Pothier CE, Blackstone EH, et al: Frequent ventricular ectopy after exercise as a predictor of death. N Engl J Med 348:781, 2003.
7. Kennedy HL: Use of long-term (Holter) electrocardiographic recordings. *In* Zipes DP, Jalife J (eds): Cardiac Electrophysiology: From Cell to Bedside. 4th ed. Philadelphia, WB Saunders, 2004, pp 772-792.
8. Bogun F, Crawford T, Reich S, et al: Radiofrequency ablation of frequent, idiopathic premature ventricular complexes: Comparison with a control group without intervention. Heart Rhythm 4:863, 2007.
9. The CAST Investigators: Preliminary report: Effect of encainide and flecainide on mortality in a randomized trial of arrhythmia suppression after myocardial infarction. N Engl J Med 321:406, 1989.
10. Sarrazin JF, Labounty T, Kuhne M, et al: Impact of radiofrequency ablation of frequent post-infarction premature ventricular complexes on left ventricular ejection fraction. Heart Rhythm 6:1543, 2009.
11. Page RL, Tilsch TW, Connolly SJ, et al: Asymptomatic or "silent" atrial fibrillation: Frequency in untreated patients and patients receiving azimilide. Circulation 107:1141, 2003.
12. Giada F, Gulizia M, Francese M, et al: Recurrent unexplained palpitations (RUP) study comparison of implantable loop recorder versus conventional diagnostic strategy. J Am Coll Cardiol 49:1951, 2007.
13. Ho RT, Wicks T, Wyeth D, et al: Generalized tonic-clonic seizures detected by implantable loop recorder devices: Diagnosing more than cardiac arrhythmias. Heart Rhythm 3:857, 2006.
14. Brignole M, Sutton R, Menozzi C, et al: Early application of an implantable loop recorder allows effective specific therapy in patients with recurrent suspected neurally mediated syncope. Eur Heart J 27:1085, 2006.
15. Malik M: Electrocardiographic and autonomic testing of cardiac risk. *In* Zipes DP, Jalife J (eds): Cardiac Electrophysiology: From Cell to Bedside. 5th ed. Philadelphia, WB Saunders, 2009, pp 871-880.
16. Tulppo M, Huikuri HV: Origin and significance of heart rate variability. J Am Coll Cardiol 43:2278, 2004.
17. Stein PK, Barzilay JI, Chaves PH, et al: Novel measures of heart rate variability predict cardiovascular mortality in older adults independent of traditional cardiovascular risk factors: The Cardiovascular Health Study (CHS). J Cardiovasc Electrophysiol 19:1169, 2008.
18. Bauer A, Malik M, Schmidt G, et al: Heart rate turbulence: Standards of measurement, physiological interpretation, and clinical use: International Society for Holter and Noninvasive Electrophysiology Consensus. J Am Coll Cardiol 52:1353, 2008.
19. Antzelevitch C, Oliva A: Amplification of spatial dispersion of repolarization underlies sudden cardiac death associated with catecholaminergic polymorphic VT, long QT, short QT and Brugada syndromes. J Intern Med 259:48, 2006.
20. Kinoshita O, Wakamatsu M, Tomita T, et al: Diurnal variation in QT dispersion in patients with chronic heart failure. Congest Heart Fail 11:262, 2005.
21. Berbari E: High-resolution electrocardiography. *In* Zipes DP, Jalife J (eds): Cardiac Electrophysiology: From Cell to Bedside. 5th ed. Philadelphia, WB Saunders, 2009, pp 851-858.
22. Kudaiberdieva G, Gorenek B, Goktekin O, et al: Combination of QT variability and signal-averaged electrocardiography in association with ventricular tachycardia in postinfarction patients. J Electrocardiol 36:17, 2003.
23. Budeus M, Hennersdorf M, Perings C, et al: Prediction of the recurrence of atrial fibrillation after successful cardioversion with P wave signal-averaged ECG. Ann Noninvasive Electrocardiol 10:414, 2005.

24. Budeus M, Hennersdorf M, Rohlen S, et al: Prediction of atrial fibrillation after coronary artery bypass grafting: The role of chemoreflex-sensitivity and P wave signal averaged ECG. Int J Cardiol 106:67, 2006.
25. Pruvot EJ, Katra RP, Rosenbaum DS, et al: Role of calcium cycling versus restitution in the mechanism of repolarization alternans. Circ Res 94:1083, 2004.
26. Chow T, Kereiakes DJ, Bartone C, et al: Prognostic utility of microvolt T-wave alternans in risk stratification of patients with ischemic cardiomyopathy. J Am Coll Cardiol 47:1820, 2006.
27. Hohnloser SH, Klingenheben T, Bloomfield D, et al: Usefulness of microvolt T-wave alternans for prediction of ventricular tachyarrhythmic events in patients with dilated cardiomyopathy: Results from a prospective observational study. J Am Coll Cardiol 41:2220, 2003.
28. Costantini O, Hohnloser SH, Kirk MM, et al: The ABCD (Alternans Before Cardioverter Defibrillator) Trial: Strategies using T-wave alternans to improve efficiency of sudden cardiac death prevention. J Am Coll Cardiol 53:471, 2009.
29. Chan PS, Stein K, Chow T, et al: Cost-effectiveness of a microvolt T-wave alternans screening strategy for implantable cardioverter-defibrillator placement in the MADIT-II–eligible population. J Am Coll Cardiol 48:112, 2006.
30. Verrier RL, Kumar K, Nearing BD: Basis for sudden cardiac death prediction by T-wave alternans from an integrative physiology perspective. Heart Rhythm 6:416, 2009.
31. Ramanathan C, Jia P, Ghanem R, et al: Activation and repolarization of the normal human heart under complete physiological conditions. Proc Natl Acad Sci U S A 103:6309, 2006.
32. Rudy Y, Wang Y, Cuculich P: Noninvasive electrocardiographic imaging (ECGI): Clinical applications. *In* Zipes DP, Jalife J (eds): Cardiac Electrophysiology: From Cell to Bedside. 4th ed. Philadelphia, WB Saunders, 2009, pp 905-912.
33. Benditt DG, Sakaguchi S, Lü F, et al: Head-up tilt table testing. *In* Zipes DP, Jalife J (eds): Cardiac Electrophysiology: From Cell to Bedside. 5th ed. Philadelphia, WB Saunders, 2009, pp 859-870.
34. Low PA, Sandroni P, Joyner M, et al: Postural tachycardia syndrome (POTS). J Cardiovasc Electrophysiol 20:352, 2009.
35. Scheinman MM: Role of the His-Purkinje system in the genesis of cardiac arrhythmia. Heart Rhythm 6:1050, 2009.
36. Zipes DP, Camm AJ, Borggrefe M, et al: ACC/AHA/ESC 2006 Guidelines for the Management of Patients with Sudden Cardiac Arrest and Ventricular Arrhythmia: A report of the American College of Cardiology/American Heart Association Task Force on Practice Guidelines and the European Society of Cardiology Committee for Practice Guidelines (Writing Committee to Revise the 2001 Guidelines for the Management of Patients With Atrial Fibrillation): Developed in collaboration with the European Heart Rhythm Association and the Heart Rhythm Society. Circulation 114:e385, 2006.
37. Calkins H: Syncope. *In* Zipes DP, Jalife J (eds): Cardiac Electrophysiology: From Cell to Bedside. 5th ed. Philadelphia, WB Saunders, 2009, pp 913-922.
38. Goldschlager N, Epstein AE, Grubb BP, et al: Etiologic considerations in the patient with syncope and an apparently normal heart. Arch Intern Med 163:151, 2003.
39. Scheinman MM, Huang S: The 1998 NASPE prospective catheter ablation registry. Pacing Clin Electrophysiol 23:1020, 2000.

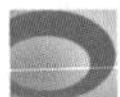

GUIDELINES

John M. Miller and Douglas P. Zipes

Ambulatory Electrocardiographic and Electrophysiologic Testing

Guidelines for the appropriate use of ambulatory electrocardiography (ECG) were first published by the American College of Cardiology/American Heart Association (ACC/AHA) in 1989[1] and updated in 1999.[2] In conjunction with other professional societies, the ACC/AHA issued a statement of requirements for clinical competence in ambulatory ECG in 2001.[3] Guidelines for performance of electrophysiology testing were first published in 1985[4] and updated in 1989 and 1995.[5] A clinical competence statement was issued by the ACC/AHA for electrophysiology studies and catheter ablation in 2000[6]; this was updated by a statement on training in electrophysiology, cardiac pacing, and arrhythmia management in 2006[7] and again in 2008.[8] The AHA and the North American Society of Pacing and Electrophysiology (NASPE, now the Heart Rhythm Society) made recommendations on safety-related topics, such as restrictions on driving, for patients with arrhythmia in 1996[9] and updated them in 2007[10] (covered in the Guidelines to Chap. 38). Since then, efforts to update guidelines have focused on appropriate indications for use of pacemakers and implantable cardioverter-defibrillators (ICDs), reflecting rapid advances in knowledge about the ability of ICDs to improve survival for patients with arrhythmia with or without electrophysiologic testing. These were issued in 2002[11] and updated in 2008.[12] Guidelines on ICD use are further addressed in Chap. 38.

The standard ACC/AHA classification system is used for indications:

Class I: conditions for which there is evidence and/or general agreement that the test is useful and effective

Class II: conditions for which there is conflicting evidence and/or a divergence of opinion about the usefulness or efficacy of performing the test

Class IIa: weight of evidence or opinion is in favor of usefulness or efficacy

Class IIb: usefulness or efficacy is less well established by evidence or opinion

Class III: conditions for which there is evidence and/or general agreement that the test is not useful or effective and in some cases may be harmful

Three levels are used to rate the evidence on which recommendations have been based. Level A recommendations are derived from data from multiple randomized clinical trials; level B recommendations are derived from a single randomized trial or nonrandomized studies; and level C recommendations are based on the consensus opinion of experts.

AMBULATORY ELECTROCARDIOGRAPHY

The evolution of guidelines for use of ambulatory ECG from 1989 to 1999 reflected important progress in several areas, including the following:

Understanding of the limited usefulness of suppression of ventricular ectopy with drug therapy

Solid-state digital technology that facilitates transtelephonic transmission of electrocardiographic data

Technical advances in long-term event recorders

Improved signal quality and interpretation

Improved computer arrhythmia interpretation

Increasingly sophisticated monitoring capacity of pacemakers and ICDs

As a result of progress in these areas, with increased knowledge about arrhythmias, ambulatory ECG is now considered to be of uncertain appropriateness for many indications for which it was once an accepted strategy.

Diagnosis

In the assessment of symptoms that may be caused by arrhythmias, ambulatory ECG (Holter) monitoring is clearly established for the evaluation of syncope (**Table 36G-1**; see Chap. 42). A 2006 American Heart Association/American College of Cardiology Foundation scientific statement on the evaluation of syncope stipulates that the type and duration of ambulatory ECG monitoring are dictated by the frequency of symptoms.[13] Holter monitors (24 to 48 hours) are appropriate for episodes that occur at least daily and event recorders (30 to 60 days) for episodes that occur at least monthly. Implantable loop recorders inserted subcutaneously can record bipolar ECG signals for up to 14 months. In patients with unexplained syncope, use of an implantable loop recorder for 1 year is more likely to identify the mechanism of syncope than is a conventional approach that uses Holter or event monitors and electrophysiologic testing and is cost-effective.

Ambulatory ECG is also supported for the evaluation of recurrent palpitations, particularly if the frequency of these symptoms makes it reasonably likely that they can be correlated with the tracings obtained during a 24-hour monitoring period. The guidelines note that data on the use of ambulatory ECG for near-syncope or dizziness are insufficient to describe the diagnostic performance of this technology for patients with such symptoms.

The ACC/AHA guidelines explicitly discourage ambulatory ECG for patients with syncope or palpitations if other causes have been identified during the clinical evaluation and for patients with cerebrovascular accidents and no other evidence of arrhythmia. The guidelines seek to reduce performance of ambulatory ECG "for completeness" in such cases. Little support is provided for use of ambulatory ECG in cases in which the cause of the patient's symptoms is unclear but in which the likelihood of detecting an unsuspected arrhythmia is low (Class IIb indications).

Assessment of Risk

The ACC/AHA guidelines discouraged the use of ambulatory ECG for either arrhythmia detection or analysis of heart rhythm variability for the purpose of risk assessment in patients without symptoms of arrhythmia,

TABLE 36G-1 ACC/AHA Guidelines for Ambulatory Electrocardiography for Assessment of Symptoms and Arrhythmias

INDICATION	CLASS I (INDICATED)	CLASS IIa (GOOD SUPPORTIVE EVIDENCE)	CLASS IIb (WEAK SUPPORTIVE EVIDENCE)	CLASS III (NOT INDICATED)
Assessment of symptoms possibly related to rhythm disturbances	Patients with unexplained syncope, near-syncope, or episodic dizziness in whom the cause is not obvious Patients with unexplained recurrent palpitation		Patients with episodic shortness of breath, chest pain, or fatigue that is not otherwise explained Patients with neurologic events when transient atrial fibrillation or flutter is suspected Patients with symptoms such as syncope, near-syncope, episodic dizziness, or palpitation in whom a probable cause other than an arrhythmia has been identified but in whom symptoms persist despite treatment of this other cause	Patients with symptoms such as syncope, near-syncope, episodic dizziness, or palpitation in whom other causes have been identified by history, physical examination, or laboratory tests Patients with cerebrovascular accidents, without other evidence of arrhythmia
Arrhythmia detection to assess risk for future cardiac events in patients without symptoms from arrhythmia			Post-MI patients with LV dysfunction (ejection fraction <40%) Patients with CHF Patients with idiopathic hypertrophic cardiomyopathy	Patients who have sustained myocardial contusion Systemic hypertensive patients with LV hypertrophy Post-MI patients with normal LV function Preoperative arrhythmia evaluation of patients for noncardiac surgery Patients with sleep apnea Patients with valvular heart disease
Measurement of heart rate variability to assess risk for future cardiac events in patients without symptoms from arrhythmia			Post-MI patients with LV dysfunction Patients with CHF Patients with idiopathic hypertrophic cardiomyopathy	Post-MI patients with normal LV function Diabetic subjects to evaluate for diabetic neuropathy Patients with rhythm disturbances that preclude HRV analysis (e.g., atrial fibrillation)
Assessment of antiarrhythmic therapy	To assess antiarrhythmic drug response in individuals in whom baseline frequency of arrhythmia has been characterized as reproducible and of sufficient frequency to permit analysis	To detect proarrhythmic responses to antiarrhythmic therapy in patients at high risk	To assess rate control during atrial fibrillation To document recurrent or asymptomatic nonsustained arrhythmias during therapy in the outpatient setting	

CHF = congestive heart failure; HRV = heart rhythm variability; LV = left ventricular; MI = myocardial infarction.

even if they had cardiovascular conditions such as myocardial contusions, left ventricular hypertrophy, or valvular heart disease (see Table 36G-1). Routine use for patients in whom arrhythmia is a common cause of death (left ventricular dysfunction, hypertrophic cardiomyopathy) was considered a Class IIb indication. These recommendations preceded data demonstrating the beneficial impact of ICDs for patients with left ventricular dysfunction after acute myocardial infarction even without symptoms of arrhythmia. These more recent findings are leading to an expanded role for ambulatory ECG in determining which asymptomatic patients most need these expensive devices.

Efficacy of Antiarrhythmic Therapy

In the absence of data demonstrating that oral antiarrhythmic therapy can improve survival through control of ventricular arrhythmias, ambulatory ECG has a diminished role as a test for evaluation of the efficacy of treatment (see Table 36G-1). Oral antiarrhythmic agents are important for control of supraventricular arrhythmias, but most patients with such arrhythmias do not have episodes every day. Event recorders can be useful for documenting the relationship between symptoms and recurrent arrhythmia and the interval between episodes, which can help guide therapy.

The guidelines provide some support for the use of ambulatory ECG for detection of proarrhythmia during initiation of drug therapy, but patients at high risk for such complications tend to have initiation of these medications as inpatients.

Assessment of Pacemaker and Implantable Cardioverter-Defibrillator Function

Ambulatory ECG was considered to be appropriate for evaluation of function of pacemakers and ICDs (see Chap. 38), but the role of ambulatory ECG is being reduced by increasing diagnostic and monitoring functions being built into these devices, especially with the use of remote monitoring. Ambulatory ECG can provide useful information by correlating symptoms with device activity and by detecting abnormalities in sensing and capture during chronic follow-up (**Table 36G-2**). However, the ACC/AHA guidelines emphasize that ambulatory ECG should not be used when data available from device interrogation are sufficient to guide clinical management.

Monitoring for Myocardial Ischemia

The 1999 ACC/AHA guidelines do not provide strong support for any indications for routine clinical use of ambulatory ECG monitoring for myocardial ischemia (**Table 36G-3**). The only indication for which the task force thought there was good supportive evidence was for patients with suspected variant angina. This technology was not considered a first-choice alternative to exercise testing for patients who are unable to exercise.

Clinical Competence

The ACC/AHA statement on clinical competence recommended that trainees interpret at least 150 ambulatory electrocardiograms under

TABLE 36G-2 ACC/AHA Guidelines for Ambulatory Electrocardiography for Assessment of Pacemaker and Implantable Cardioverter-Defibrillator Function

CLASS	INDICATION
Class I (indicated)	Evaluation of frequent symptoms of palpitations, syncope, or near-syncope to assess device function to exclude myopotential inhibition and pacemaker-mediated tachycardia and to assist in the programming of enhanced features, such as rate responsivity and automatic mode switching Evaluation of suspected component failure or malfunction when device interrogation is not definitive in establishing a diagnosis To assess the response to adjunctive pharmacologic therapy in patients receiving frequent ICD therapy
Class IIa (good supportive evidence)	
Class IIb (weak supportive evidence)	Evaluation of immediate postoperative pacemaker function after pacemaker or ICD implantation as an alternative or adjunct to continuous telemetric monitoring Evaluation of the rate of supraventricular arrhythmias in patients with implanted defibrillators
Class III (not indicated)	Assessment of ICD or pacemaker malfunction when device interrogation, electrocardiogram, or other available data (e.g., chest radiograph) are sufficient to establish an underlying cause or diagnosis Routine follow-up in asymptomatic patients

TABLE 36G-3 ACC/AHA Guidelines for Ischemia Monitoring

CLASS	INDICATION
Class I (indicated)	
Class IIa (good supportive evidence)	Patients with suspected variant angina
Class IIb (weak supportive evidence)	Evaluation of patients with chest pain who cannot exercise Preoperative evaluation for vascular surgery of patients who cannot exercise Patients with known coronary artery disease and atypical chest pain syndrome
Class III (not indicated)	Initial evaluation of patients with chest pain who are able to exercise Routine screening of asymptomatic subjects

supervision to acquire minimal competence with this technology.[3] A minimum of 25 test interpretations per year was recommended to maintain competence.

ELECTROPHYSIOLOGIC PROCEDURES FOR DIAGNOSIS

The ACC/AHA guidelines for use of intracardiac electrophysiologic procedures from 1989[4] and 1995[5] reflect the emerging role of catheter ablation as a therapeutic strategy but do not fully reflect the reduced importance of antiarrhythmic medications and the growing role of ICDs that have occurred. Nevertheless, most of the basic themes of these guidelines remain valid. An updated clinical competence statement for performing these procedures was issued in 2006.[14]

Evaluation of Sinus Node Function

Clinical evaluation of sinus node dysfunction is often difficult because of the episodic nature of symptomatic abnormalities and the wide variability in sinus node function in asymptomatic individuals. Invasive tests of sinus function can test the ability of the sinus node to recover from overdrive suppression and assess sinoatrial conduction by introducing atrial extrastimuli or by atrial pacing.

The ACC/AHA guidelines consider electrophysiologic studies of sinus node function most appropriate for patients in whom dysfunction is suspected but not proved after a noninvasive evaluation (**Table 36G-4**). In contrast, the guidelines consider such studies inappropriate when a documented bradyarrhythmia has been found to be correlated with the patient's symptoms and management is unlikely to be influenced by an electrophysiologic study. Studies are also considered inappropriate in asymptomatic patients and those who have sinus pauses only during sleep. When bradyarrhythmias were recognized as the cause of the patient's symptoms, electrophysiologic studies were considered to have possible but uncertain appropriateness (Class II) if such data might refine treatment choices.

Acquired Atrioventricular Block

The ACC/AHA guidelines emphasize that electrophysiologic studies are inappropriate (Class III) when ECG findings correlate with symptoms and the findings from electrophysiologic studies are unlikely to alter management (e.g., documentation of His bundle conduction rarely improves management for a patient whose other clinical data indicate that placement of a permanent pacemaker is warranted because of symptomatic advanced atrioventricular [AV] block). Similarly, electrophysiologic studies are not appropriate for asymptomatic patients with mild degrees of AV block who are not likely to warrant pacemaker implantation. According to these guidelines, electrophysiologic studies of AV conduction should be performed when a relationship between symptoms and AV block is a reasonable possibility but has not been proved.

Chronic Intraventricular Delay

According to ACC/AHA guidelines, the main role of electrophysiologic testing in patients with prolonged H-V intervals is not to predict future complications but to determine whether the symptoms of arrhythmia are caused by conduction delay or block versus some other arrhythmia. The only Class I (clearly appropriate) indication for electrophysiologic testing is in symptomatic patients for whom the cause of symptoms is not known. The guidelines specifically discourage such testing of asymptomatic patients and provide only equivocal support for asymptomatic patients with bundle branch block in whom treatment with drugs that might increase conduction delay is being considered.

Narrow- and Wide-Complex QRS Tachycardia The ACC/AHA guidelines define different roles for electrophysiologic testing in patients with narrow- and wide-complex tachycardias. In narrow QRS tachycardia, the site of abnormal impulse formation or the reentry circuit can often be determined from information from the 12-lead electrocardiogram. Thus, electrophysiologic testing was considered more appropriate as a guide to therapy in this setting than as a tool for diagnosis. Class I indications for electrophysiologic testing include patients with recurrent tachycardia for whom data from testing may help clinicians choose among drug therapy, catheter ablation, pacing, and surgery. However, testing is not considered useful for patients whose tachycardias are controlled by vagal maneuvers or medications and who are not candidates for nonpharmacologic therapy.

TABLE 36G-4 ACC/AHA Guidelines for Clinical Intracardiac Electrophysiologic Studies for Evaluation of Specific Electrocardiographic Abnormalities

INDICATION	CLASS I (APPROPRIATE)	CLASS II (EQUIVOCAL)	CLASS III (INAPPROPRIATE)
Evaluation of sinus node function	Symptomatic patients in whom sinus node dysfunction is suspected as the cause of symptoms but a causal relation between an arrhythmia and the symptoms has not been established after appropriate evaluation	Patients with documented sinus node dysfunction in whom evaluation of atrioventricular (AV) or ventriculoatrial (VA) conduction or susceptibility to arrhythmias may aid in selection of the most appropriate pacing modality Patients with electrocardiographically documented sinus bradyarrhythmias to determine whether abnormalities are caused by intrinsic disease, autonomic nervous system dysfunction, or effects of drugs to help select therapeutic options Symptomatic patients with known sinus bradyarrhythmias to evaluate potential for other arrhythmias as the cause of symptoms	Symptomatic patients in whom an association between symptoms and a documented bradyarrhythmia has been established and choice of therapy would not be affected by results of an electrophysiologic study Asymptomatic patients with sinus bradyarrhythmias or sinus pauses observed only during sleep, including sleep apnea
Acquired AV block	Symptomatic patients in whom His-Purkinje block, suspected as a cause of symptoms, has not been established Patients with second- or third-degree AV block treated with a pacemaker who remain symptomatic and in whom another arrhythmia is suspected as a cause of symptoms	Patients with second- or third-degree AV block in whom knowledge of the site of block or its mechanism or response to pharmacologic or other temporary intervention may help direct therapy or assess prognosis Patients with premature, concealed junctional depolarizations suspected as a cause of second- or third-degree AV block pattern (e.g., pseudo-AV block)	Symptomatic patients in whom the symptoms and presence of AV block are correlated by ECG findings Asymptomatic patients with transient AV block associated with sinus slowing (e.g., nocturnal type I second-degree AV block)
Chronic intraventricular conduction delay	Symptomatic patients in whom the cause of symptoms is not known	Asymptomatic patients with bundle branch block in whom pharmacologic therapy that could increase conduction delay or produce heart block is contemplated	Asymptomatic patients with intraventricular conduction delay Symptomatic patients whose symptoms can be correlated with or excluded by ECG events
Narrow QRS tachycardia (QRS complex < 0.12 sec)	Patients with frequent or poorly tolerated episodes of tachycardia who do not adequately respond to drug therapy and for whom information about site of origin, mechanism, and electrophysiologic properties of pathways of the tachycardia is essential for choosing appropriate therapy (e.g., drugs, catheter ablation, pacing, or surgery) Patients who prefer ablative therapy to pharmacologic treatment	Patients with frequent episodes of tachycardia requiring drug treatment for whom there is concern about proarrhythmia or effects of the antiarrhythmic drug on the sinus node or AV conduction	Patients with tachycardias easily controlled by vagal maneuvers and/or well-tolerated drug therapy who are not candidates for nonpharmacologic therapy
Wide-complex tachycardias	Patients with wide QRS complex tachycardia in whom correct diagnosis is unclear after analysis of available ECG tracings and for whom knowledge of the correct diagnosis is necessary for care	None	Patients with ventricular tachycardia or supraventricular tachycardia with aberrant conduction or preexcitation syndromes diagnosed with certainty by ECG criteria and for whom invasive electrophysiologic data would not influence therapy; however, data obtained at baseline electrophysiologic study in these patients might be appropriate as guide for subsequent therapy
Prolonged QT interval syndrome	None	Identification of proarrhythmic effect of a drug in patients experiencing sustained ventricular tachycardia or cardiac arrest while receiving the drug Patients who have equivocal abnormalities of QT interval duration or TU wave configuration, with syncope or symptomatic arrhythmias, in whom catecholamine effects may unmask a distinct QT abnormality	Patients with clinically manifest congenital QT prolongation, with or without symptomatic arrhythmias Patients with acquired prolonged QT syndrome with symptoms closely related to an identifiable cause or mechanism

Continued

TABLE 36G-4 ACC/AHA Guidelines for Clinical Intracardiac Electrophysiologic Studies for Evaluation of Specific Electrocardiographic Abnormalities—cont'd

INDICATION	CLASS I (APPROPRIATE)	CLASS II (EQUIVOCAL)	CLASS III (INAPPROPRIATE)
Wolff-Parkinson-White syndrome	Patients being evaluated for catheter ablation or surgical ablation of an accessory pathway Patients with ventricular preexcitation who have survived cardiac arrest or who have unexplained syncope Symptomatic patients in whom determination of the mechanism of arrhythmia or knowledge of the electrophysiologic properties of the accessory pathway and normal conduction system would help in determining appropriate therapy	Asymptomatic patients with a family history of sudden cardiac death or with ventricular preexcitation but no spontaneous arrhythmia who engage in high-risk occupations or activities and in whom knowledge of the electrophysiologic properties of the accessory pathway or inducible tachycardia may help determine recommendations for further activities or therapy Patients with ventricular preexcitation who are undergoing cardiac surgery for other reasons	Asymptomatic patients with ventricular preexcitation, except those in Class II
Ventricular premature complexes, couplets, and nonsustained ventricular tachycardia (VT)	None	Patients with other risk factors for future arrhythmic events, such as a low ejection fraction, positive signal-averaged electrocardiogram, and nonsustained VT on ambulatory ECG recordings in whom electrophysiologic studies will be used for further risk assessment and for guiding therapy in patients with inducible VT Patients with highly symptomatic, uniform morphology premature ventricular complexes, couplets, and nonsustained VT who are considered potential candidates for catheter ablation	Asymptomatic or mildly symptomatic patients with premature ventricular complexes, couplets, and nonsustained VT without other risk factors for sustained arrhythmias

In wide-complex tachycardias, correct diagnosis is occasionally not possible from ECG tracings alone. However, electrophysiologic testing permits accurate diagnosis in virtually all patients. Because knowledge of the mechanism of the arrhythmia is essential for selection of optimal therapy, electrophysiologic testing was considered appropriate (Class I) for the diagnosis of wide-complex tachycardias in these guidelines. However, when the diagnosis is clear from other data and electrophysiologic testing is not likely to influence therapy, the guidelines consider it inappropriate.

Prolonged QT Intervals The ACC/AHA guidelines do not consider electrophysiologic testing for any indications for routine use in patients with prolonged QT intervals. Whether catecholamine infusion during testing is useful for revealing patients who are at high risk for complications or whether electrophysiologic testing can be used to evaluate proarrhythmic effects in this population is considered uncertain.

Wolff-Parkinson-White Syndrome Electrophysiologic testing is useful for patients with this syndrome for both diagnosis and planning of therapy. The ACC/AHA guidelines consider electrophysiologic testing appropriate for patients who are candidates for catheter or surgical ablation, for those who have had cardiac arrests or unexplained syncope, or for patients whose management might be altered by knowledge of the electrophysiologic properties of the accessory pathway and normal conduction system. For asymptomatic patients, however, electrophysiologic studies are deemed inappropriate except in special situations, such as patients with high-risk occupations or those with a family history of sudden cardiac death. More recently recognized entities, such as Brugada syndrome, catecholaminergic tachycardia, and right ventricular cardiomyopathy, were not considered.

Nonsustained Ventricular Tachycardia For patients with ventricular premature complexes, couplets, and nonsustained ventricular tachycardia, the usefulness of electrophysiologic testing is compromised by the lack of therapeutic strategies that have been shown to improve outcomes. There are no clearly appropriate indications for electrophysiologic studies in these patients, and the guidelines discourage testing in patients without other risk factors for sustained arrhythmias. Research published since these guidelines suggests that exceptions would include patients who fit the Multicenter Automatic Defibrillator Implantation Trial (MADIT) or Multicenter Unsustained Tachycardia Trial (MUSTT) criteria. For certain patients with other data suggesting an adverse prognosis, electrophysiologic testing is believed to have possible but unproven appropriateness (Class II).

Unexplained Syncope

In patients with unexplained syncope and structural heart disease (see Chap. 42), recent ACC/AHA guidelines on the evaluation of syncope[10] recommend a low threshold for the use of electrophysiologic testing (**Table 36G-5**). In patients without structural heart disease, the yield of electrophysiologic testing is low. Thus, the guidelines recommend a higher threshold for use of electrophysiologic studies in such patients and suggest that head-up tilt testing may be a more useful test. However, given the low risk of electrophysiologic testing and the high risk of potentially harmful recurrent syncope, electrophysiologic testing may be beneficial for patients with a malignant episode of syncope.[13]

Survivors of Cardiac Arrest

The ACC/AHA guidelines consider electrophysiologic testing appropriate for patients who are survivors of cardiac arrest (see Chap. 41) other than in the earliest phase of acute myocardial infarction (see Table 36G-5). Since publication of these guidelines, acceptance of the usefulness of ICDs has become more widespread, and many of these patients receive such a device without electrophysiologic testing or receive limited electrophysiologic testing at device implantation. The guidelines consider electrophysiologic studies inappropriate when cardiac arrest has occurred within the first 48 hours of myocardial infarction or when the cardiac arrest results from clearly definable specific causes.

Unexplained Palpitations

The procedure of choice to determine the cause of palpitations is ambulatory ECG, according to the ACC/AHA guidelines. The guidelines suggest that electrophysiologic testing should be reserved for patients with palpitations that are associated with syncope or for those in whom electrocardiograms have failed to capture a cause of the palpitations but who have been

TABLE 36G-5 ACC/AHA Guidelines for Clinical Intracardiac Electrophysiologic Studies for Evaluation of Clinical Syndromes

INDICATION	CLASS I (APPROPRIATE)	CLASS II (EQUIVOCAL)	CLASS III (INAPPROPRIATE)
Unexplained syncope	Patients with suspected structural heart disease and syncope that remain unexplained after appropriate evaluation	Patients with recurrent unexplained syncope without structural heart disease and a negative head-up tilt test result	Patients with known cause of syncope for whom treatment will not be guided by electrophysiologic testing
Survivors of cardiac arrest	Patients surviving cardiac arrest without evidence of an acute Q wave myocardial infarction (MI) Patients surviving cardiac arrest occurring more than 48 hours after acute phase of MI in absence of recurrent ischemic event	Patients surviving cardiac arrest caused by bradyarrhythmia Patients surviving cardiac arrest thought to be associated with a congenital repolarization abnormality (long-QT syndrome) in whom results of noninvasive diagnostic testing are equivocal	Patients surviving a cardiac arrest that occurred during the acute phase (<48 hours) of MI Patients with cardiac arrest resulting from clearly definable specific causes, such as reversible ischemia, severe valvular aortic stenosis, or noninvasively defined congenital or acquired long-QT syndrome
Unexplained palpitations	Patients with palpitations who have pulse rate documented by medical personnel as inappropriately rapid and in whom ECG recordings fail to document cause of the palpitations Patients with palpitations preceding a syncopal episode	Patients with clinically significant palpitations, suspected to be of cardiac origin, in whom symptoms are sporadic and cannot be documented; studies performed to determine mechanisms of arrhythmias, direct or provide therapy, or assess prognosis	Patients with palpitations documented to be due to extracardiac causes (e.g., hyperthyroidism)

noted to have a rapid pulse rate by medical personnel (see Table 36G-5). Electrophysiologic testing is considered of equivocal value in patients with symptoms so sporadic that they cannot be documented while ambulatory ECG is performed.

ELECTROPHYSIOLOGIC STUDIES FOR THERAPEUTIC INTERVENTION

The 1995 ACC/AHA guidelines for appropriateness of electrophysiologic studies for guidance of drug therapy and implantable electrical devices do not reflect the decline in the role of oral antiarrhythmic therapy and the rise in the use of ICDs for treatment of patients who have had cardiac arrests (**Table 36G-6**). However, the guideline recommendations for the role of catheter ablation remain valid. The characteristics that are common among appropriate indications include supraventricular arrhythmias that are symptomatic; that cannot be controlled with medications because of limited effectiveness, side effects, or inconvenience; or that have caused sudden cardiac death. Catheter ablation is also useful for the same reasons in some patients with ventricular tachycardia when it occurs in the absence of structural heart disease, and ablation is often useful as an adjunct to ICD implantation to limit the episodes of ventricular tachycardia requiring ICD treatment. Left ventricular dysfunction develops in some patients from frequent premature ventricular complexes, with reversal after ablation of the premature ventricular complex.

Clinical Competence

The ACC/AHA statement on clinical competence[8] describes three levels of training: level 1 for every cardiology trainee, level 2 for those wishing to acquire advanced training in arrhythmia management, and level 3 for those intending to specialize in invasive diagnostic and therapeutic cardiac electrophysiology. The level 3 guidelines recommend a minimum of 1 year of specialized training in electrophysiologic studies, during which the physician should be the primary operator and analyze 100 to 150 initial diagnostic studies, at least 50 of which should involve patients with supraventricular arrhythmias. Because antiarrhythmic devices constitute a major part of current electrophysiology practice, the guidelines suggest that a trainee should be the primary operator during at least 25 electrophysiologic evaluations of implantable antiarrhythmic devices. For maintenance of competence, a minimum of 100 diagnostic electrophysiologic studies per year is recommended. The statement also recommends that specialists in electrophysiology attend at least 30 hours of formal continuing medical education every 2 years to remain abreast of changes in knowledge and technology.

For physicians who perform catheter ablation, the NASPE Ad Hoc Committee on Catheter Ablation (now the Heart Rhythm Society) has recommended that training should include at least 75 catheter ablations, of which at least 10 are accessory pathway ablations and 30 to 50 are mentored ablations.[8] The ACC/AHA statement recommends that physicians who perform ablations carry out at least 20 to 50 ablations per year.

Individuals receiving training in pacemaker implantation must participate as the primary operator (under direct supervision) in at least 50 primary implantations of transvenous pacemakers and 20 pacemaker system revisions or replacements. At least half of the implantations should involve dual-chamber pacemakers. The trainee must also participate in the follow-up of at least 100 pacemaker patient visits and acquire proficiency in advanced pacemaker electrocardiography, interrogation, and programming of complex pacemakers.[8]

TABLE 36G-6 ACC/AHA Guidelines for Clinical Intracardiac Electrophysiologic Studies for Therapeutic Intervention

INDICATION	CLASS I (APPROPRIATE)	CLASS II (EQUIVOCAL)	CLASS III (INAPPROPRIATE)
Guidance of drug therapy	Patients with sustained VT or cardiac arrest, especially those with prior MI Patients with AVNRT, AV reentrant tachycardia using an accessory pathway, or atrial fibrillation associated with an accessory pathway, for whom chronic drug therapy is planned	Patients with sinus node reentrant tachycardia, atrial tachycardia, atrial fibrillation, or atrial flutter without ventricular preexcitation syndrome, for whom chronic drug therapy is planned Patients with arrhythmias not inducible during controlled electrophysiologic study for whom drug therapy is planned	Patients with isolated atrial or ventricular premature complexes Patients with ventricular fibrillation with a clearly identified reversible cause
Patients who are candidates for or who have implantable electrical devices	Patients with tachyarrhythmias, before and during implantation, and final (predischarge) programming of an electrical device to confirm its ability to perform as anticipated Patients with an implanted electrical antitachyarrhythmia device in whom changes in status or therapy may have influenced the continued safety and efficacy of the device Patients who have a pacemaker to treat a bradyarrhythmia and receive a cardioverter-defibrillator to test for device interactions	Patients with previously documented indications for pacemaker implantation to test for most appropriate long-term pacing mode and sites to optimize symptomatic improvement and hemodynamics	Patients who are not candidates for device therapy
Indications for catheter ablation procedures	Patients with symptomatic atrial tachyarrhythmias who have inadequately controlled ventricular rates unless primary ablation of the atrial tachyarrhythmia is possible Patients with symptomatic atrial tachyarrhythmias such as those above but in whom drugs are not tolerated or the patient does not wish to take them, even though the ventricular rate can be controlled Patients with symptomatic nonparoxysmal junctional tachycardia that is drug resistant or the patient is drug intolerant or does not wish to take it Patients resuscitated from sudden cardiac death caused by atrial flutter or atrial fibrillation with a rapid ventricular response in the absence of an accessory pathway	Patients with a dual-chamber pacemaker and pacemaker-mediated tachycardia that cannot be treated effectively by drugs or by reprogramming the pacemaker	Patients with atrial tachyarrhythmias responsive to drug therapy acceptable to the patient
Radiofrequency catheter ablation for AVNRT	Patients with symptomatic sustained AVNRT that is drug resistant or the patient is drug intolerant or does not desire long-term drug therapy	Patients with sustained AVNRT identified during electrophysiologic study or catheter ablation of another arrhythmia Finding of dual AV nodal pathway physiology and atrial echoes but without AVNRT during electrophysiologic study in patients suspected of having AVNRT clinically	Patients with AVNRT responsive to drug therapy that is well tolerated and preferred by the patient to ablation Finding of dual AV nodal pathway physiology (with or without echo complexes) during electrophysiologic study in patients in whom AVNRT is not suspected clinically
Ablation of atrial tachycardia, flutter, and fibrillation: atrium/atrial sites	Patients with atrial tachycardia that is drug resistant or the patient is drug intolerant or does not desire long-term drug therapy Patients with atrial flutter that is drug resistant or the patient is drug intolerant or does not desire long-term drug therapy	Atrial flutter or atrial tachycardia associated with paroxysmal atrial fibrillation when the tachycardia is drug resistant or the patient is drug intolerant or does not desire long-term drug therapy Patients with atrial fibrillation and evidence of a localized site of origin when the tachycardia is drug resistant or the patient is drug intolerant or does not desire long-term drug therapy	Patients with atrial arrhythmia responsive to drug therapy, well tolerated, and preferred by the patient to ablation Patients with multiform atrial tachycardia

TABLE 36G-6 ACC/AHA Guidelines for Clinical Intracardiac Electrophysiologic Studies for Therapeutic Intervention—cont'd

INDICATION	CLASS I (APPROPRIATE)	CLASS II (EQUIVOCAL)	CLASS III (INAPPROPRIATE)
Ablation of atrial tachycardia, flutter, and fibrillation: accessory pathways	Patients with symptomatic AV reentrant tachycardia that is drug resistant or the patient is drug intolerant or does not desire long-term drug therapy Patients with atrial fibrillation (or other atria tachyarrhythmia) and a rapid ventricular response through the accessory pathway when the tachycardia is drug resistant or the patient is drug intolerant or does not desire long-term drug therapy	Patients with AV reentrant tachycardia or atrial fibrillation with rapid ventricular rates identified during electrophysiologic study of another arrhythmia Asymptomatic patients with ventricular preexcitation whose livelihood or profession, important activities, insurability, or mental well-being or the public safety would be affected by spontaneous tachyarrhythmias or the presence of the ECG abnormality Patients with atrial fibrillation and a controlled ventricular response through the accessory pathway Patients with a family history of sudden cardiac death	Patients who have accessory pathway–related arrhythmias responsive to drug therapy, well tolerated, and preferred by the patient to ablation
Ablation of VT	Patients with symptomatic sustained monomorphic VT when the tachycardia is drug resistant or the patient is drug intolerant or does not desire long-term drug therapy Patients with bundle branch reentrant VT Patients with sustained monomorphic VT and an ICD who are receiving multiple shocks not manageable by reprogramming or concomitant drug therapy	Nonsustained VT that is symptomatic when the tachycardia is drug resistant or the patient is drug intolerant or does not desire long-term drug therapy	Patients with VT responsive to drug, ICD, or surgical therapy that is well tolerated and preferred by the patient to ablation Asymptomatic and clinically benign nonsustained VT

AVNRT = AV nodal reentrant tachycardia; ICD = implantable cardioverter-defibrillator; MI = myocardial infarction; VT = ventricular tachycardia.

REFERENCES

1. Knoebel SB, Crawford MH, Dunn MI, et al: Guidelines for ambulatory electrocardiography. A report of the American College of Cardiology/American Heart Association Task Force on Assessment of Diagnostic and Therapeutic Cardiovascular Procedures (Subcommittee on Ambulatory Electrocardiography). Circulation 79:206, 1989.
2. Crawford MH, Bernstein SJ, Deedwania PC, et al: ACC/AHA Guidelines for Ambulatory Electrocardiography. A report of the American College of Cardiology/American Heart Association Task Force on Practice Guidelines (Committee to Revise the Guidelines for Ambulatory Electrocardiography). Developed in collaboration with the North American Society for Pacing and Electrophysiology. J Am Coll Cardiol 34:912, 1999.
3. Kadish AH, Buxton AE, Kennedy HL, et al: ACC/AHA clinical competence statement on electrocardiography and ambulatory electrocardiography: A report of the ACC/AHA/ACP-ASIM task force on clinical competence (ACC/AHA Committee to develop a clinical competence statement on electrocardiography and ambulatory electrocardiography) endorsed by the International Society for Holter and noninvasive electrocardiology. Circulation 104:3169, 2001.
4. Akhtar M, Fisher JD, Gillette PC, et al: NASPE Ad Hoc Committee on Guidelines for Cardiac Electrophysiological Studies. Pacing Clin Electrophysiol 8:611, 1985.
5. Zipes DP, DiMarco JP, Gillette PC, et al: Guidelines for clinical intracardiac electrophysiological and catheter ablation procedures. A report of the American College of Cardiology/American Heart Association Task Force on Practice Guidelines (Committee on Clinical Intracardiac Electrophysiologic and Catheter Ablation Procedures), developed in collaboration with the North American Society of Pacing and Electrophysiology. J Am Coll Cardiol 26:555, 1995.
6. Tracy CM, Akhtar M, DiMarco JP, et al: American College of Cardiology/American Heart Association 2006 update of the clinical competence statement on invasive electrophysiology studies, catheter ablation, and cardioversion: A report of the American College of Cardiology/American Heart Association/American College of Physicians Task Force on Clinical Competence and Training developed in collaboration with the Heart Rhythm Society. J Am Coll Cardiol 48:1503, 2006.
7. Naccarelli GV, Conti JB, DiMarco JP, et al: Task Force 6: Training in specialized electrophysiology, cardiac pacing, and arrhythmia management: Endorsed by the Heart Rhythm Society. J Am Coll Cardiol 47:904, 2006.
8. Naccarelli GV, Conti JB, DiMarco JP, et al: Task force 6: Training in specialized electrophysiology, cardiac pacing, and arrhythmia management endorsed by the Heart Rhythm Society. J Am Coll Cardiol 51:374, 2008.
9. Epstein AE, Miles WM, Benditt DG, et al: Personal and public safety issues related to arrhythmias that may affect consciousness: Implications for regulation and physician recommendations. A medical/scientific statement from the American Heart Association and the North American Society of Pacing and Electrophysiology. Circulation 94:1147, 1996.
10. Epstein AE, Baessler CA, Curtis AB, et al: Addendum to "Personal and Public Safety Issues Related to Arrhythmias That May Affect Consciousness: Implications for Regulation and Physician Recommendations. A medical/scientific statement from the American Heart Association and the North American Society of Pacing and Electrophysiology." Public safety issues in patients with implantable defibrillators. A Scientific statement from the American Heart Association and the Heart Rhythm Society. Heart Rhythm 4:386, 2007.
11. Gregoratos G, Abrams J, Epstein AE, et al: ACC/AHA/NASPE 2002 Guideline Update for Implantation of Cardiac Pacemakers and Antiarrhythmia Devices—summary article: A report of the American College of Cardiology/American Heart Association Task Force on Practice Guidelines (ACC/AHA/NASPE Committee to Update the 1998 Pacemaker Guidelines). J Am Coll Cardiol 40:1703, 2002.
12. Epstein AE, DiMarco JP, Ellenbogen KA, et al: ACC/AHA/HRS 2008 Guidelines for Device-Based Therapy of Cardiac Rhythm Abnormalities: A report of the American College of Cardiology/American Heart Association Task Force on Practice Guidelines (Writing Committee to Revise the ACC/AHA/NASPE 2002 Guideline Update for Implantation of Cardiac Pacemakers and Antiarrhythmia Devices): Developed in collaboration with the American Association for Thoracic Surgery and Society of Thoracic Surgeons. Circulation 117:e350, 2008.
13. Strickberger SA, Benson DW, Biaggioni I, et al: AHA/ACCF Scientific Statement on the evaluation of syncope: From the American Heart Association Councils on Clinical Cardiology, Cardiovascular Nursing, Cardiovascular Disease in the Young, and Stroke, and the Quality of Care and Outcomes Research Interdisciplinary Working Group; and the American College of Cardiology Foundation: In collaboration with the Heart Rhythm Society: Endorsed by the American Autonomic Society. Circulation 113:316, 2006.
14. Tracy CM, Akhtar M, DiMarco JP, et al: American College of Cardiology/American Heart Association 2006 update of the clinical competence statement on invasive electrophysiology studies, catheter ablation, and cardioversion: A report of the American College of Cardiology/American Heart Association/American College of Physicians Task Force on Clinical Competence and Training: Developed in collaboration with the Heart Rhythm Society. Circulation 114:1654, 2006.

CHAPTER 37 Therapy for Cardiac Arrhythmias

John M. Miller and Douglas P. Zipes

The treatment of patients with tachyarrhythmias has evolved dramatically in the last 40 years. Antiarrhythmic drugs were the mainstay of therapy until the late 1960s, when surgical therapy to cure, not just suppress, tachyarrhythmias was developed. This mode was replaced by catheter ablation (at first with direct current, then with radiofrequency current) for cure of tachyarrhythmias in the 1980s. This form of therapy has largely replaced surgical and drug therapy for patients who need treatment for supraventricular tachycardia (SVT) and ventricular tachycardia (VT) in the absence of structural heart disease. Other forms of energy have also been developed for ablation of cardiac tissue. The implantable cardioverter-defibrillator (ICD) was introduced in the early 1980s and has become standard therapy for patients with serious ventricular arrhythmias in the presence of structural heart disease. Some patients require a combination of these forms of treatment (hybrid therapy, such as an ICD and antiarrhythmic drugs, or surgery and an ICD); drug therapy can also affect ICD function, either positively or negatively.[1] Drug therapy of arrhythmias, at one time the only option, now plays a supporting role in many cases.

Pharmacologic Therapy

Principles of clinical pharmacokinetics and pharmacodynamics are discussed in Chap. 10.

General Considerations Regarding Antiarrhythmic Drugs

Most of the available antiarrhythmic drugs (**Table 37-1**) can be classified according to whether they exert blocking actions predominantly on sodium, potassium, or calcium channels and whether they block receptors. The commonly used Vaughan Williams classification is limited because it is based on the electrophysiologic effects exerted by an arbitrary concentration of the drug, generally on normal cardiac tissue. In reality, the actions of these drugs are complex and depend on tissue type, degree of acute or chronic damage, heart rate, membrane potential, ionic composition of the extracellular milieu, genetics (see Chap. 9),[2] age (see Chap. 80), and other factors (see Table 37-1). Many drugs exert more than one type of electrophysiologic effect or operate indirectly, such as by altering hemodynamics, myocardial metabolism, or autonomic neural transmission. Some drugs have active metabolites that exert effects different from those of the parent compound. Not all drugs in the same class have identical effects (e.g., amiodarone, sotalol, and ibutilide). Whereas all class III agents are dramatically different, some drugs in different classes have overlapping actions (e.g., class IA and class IC drugs). In vitro studies on healthy myocardium usually establish the properties of antiarrhythmic agents rather than their actual antiarrhythmic properties in vivo.

Despite these limitations, the Vaughan Williams classification is widely known and provides a useful communication shorthand, but the reader is cautioned that drug actions are more complex than those depicted by the classification. A more realistic view of antiarrhythmic agents is provided by the Sicilian Gambit. This approach to drug classification is an attempt to identify the mechanisms of a particular arrhythmia, to determine the vulnerable parameter of the arrhythmia most susceptible to modification, to define the target most likely to affect the vulnerable parameter, and then to select a drug that will modify the target. This concept provides a framework in which to consider antiarrhythmic drugs (**Table 37-2**; see Table 37-1).

DRUG CLASSIFICATION (Table 37-3). According to the Vaughan Williams classification, class I drugs predominantly block the fast sodium channel; they can also block potassium channels. They, in turn, are divided into three subgroups, classes IA, IB, and IC.

Class IA

This class includes drugs that reduce $\dot{V}max$ (rate of rise of action potential upstroke [phase 0]) and prolong action potential duration (see Chap. 35)—quinidine, procainamide, and disopyramide. Their kinetics of onset and offset in blocking the Na^+ channel are of intermediate rapidity (less than 5 seconds) compared with class IB and class IC agents.

Class IB

This class of drugs does not reduce $\dot{V}max$ and shortens action potential duration—mexiletine, phenytoin, and lidocaine. Their kinetics of onset and offset in blocking the sodium channel are rapid (less than 500 milliseconds).

Class IC

This class of drugs can reduce $\dot{V}max$, primarily slow conduction velocity, and prolong refractoriness minimally—flecainide and propafenone. These drugs have slow onset and offset kinetics (10 to 20 seconds).

Class II

These drugs block beta-adrenergic receptors and include propranolol, timolol, and metoprolol.

Class III

This class of drugs predominantly blocks potassium channels (such as I_{Kr}) and prolongs repolarization. Included are sotalol, amiodarone, and bretylium.

Class IV

This class of drugs predominantly blocks the slow calcium channel ($I_{Ca.L}$)—verapamil, diltiazem, nifedipine, and others (felodipine blocks $I_{Ca.T}$).

Antiarrhythmic drugs appear to cross the cell membrane and interact with receptors in the membrane channels when the channels are in the rested, activated, or inactivated state (see Table 37-1; see Chap. 35), and each of these interactions is characterized by different association and dissociation rate constants. Such interactions are voltage and time dependent. Transitions among rested, activated, and inactivated states are governed by standard Hodgkin-Huxley–type equations. When the drug is bound (associated) to a receptor site at or very

TABLE 37-1 Actions of Drugs Used in Treatment of Arrhythmias

	CHANNELS						RECEPTORS				PUMPS	CLINICAL EFFECTS		
	NA*													
DRUG	FAST	MED	SLOW	CA	K_r	K_s	ALPHA	BETA	M_2	P	NA,K-ATPASE	LV FUNCTION	SINUS RATE	EXTRACARDIAC
Quinidine		●A			⊙		○		○			—	↑	⊙
Procainamide		●A			⊙							↓	—	⊙
Disopyramide		●A			⊙				○			↓	—	●
Ajmaline		●A										—	—↓	○
Lidocaine	○											—	—↓	○
Mexiletine	○											—	—	○
Phenytoin	○											—	—	⊙
Flecainide			●A		○							↓	—	○
Propafenone		●A			○			⊙				↓	↓	○
Propranolol	○							●				↓	↓	○
Nadolol								●				↓	↓	○
Amiodarone	○			⊙	●	⊙	⊙	⊙				—	↓	●
Dronedarone	○			⊙	●	⊙	⊙	⊙				—	↓	○
Sotalol					●			●				↓	↓	○
Ibutilide					○							—	↓	○
Dofetilide					●							—	—	○
Verapamil	○			●			⊙					↓	↓	○
Diltiazem				⊙								↓	↓	○
Adenosine										□		—	↓	⊙
Digoxin									○		●	↑	↓	⊙
Atropine									●			—	↑	⊙

*Fast, med (medium), and slow refer to kinetics of recovery from sodium channel blockade.
Relative potency of blockade or extracardiac side effect: ○ = low; ⊙ = moderate; ● = high.
□ = agonist; A = activated state blocker; — = minimal effect; ↑ = increase; ↓ = decrease; K_r = rapid component of delayed rectifier K^+ current; K_s = slow component of delayed rectifier K^+ current; M_2 = muscarinic receptor subtype 2; P = A_1 purinergic receptor.
Modified from Schwartz PJ, Zaza A: Haemodynamic effects of a new multifactoral antihypertensive drug. Eur Heart J 13:26, 1992.

close to the ionic channel (the drug probably does not actually plug the channel), the channel cannot conduct, even in the activated state.

USE DEPENDENCE. Some drugs exert greater inhibitory effects on the upstroke of the action potential at more rapid rates of stimulation and after longer periods of stimulation, a characteristic called use dependence. Use dependence means that depression of $\dot{V}max$ is greater after the channel has been "used" (i.e., after action potential depolarization rather than after a rest period). It is possible that this use dependence results from preferential interaction of the antiarrhythmic drug with the open or the inactive channel, and there is little interaction with the resting channels of the unstimulated cell. Agents in class IB exhibit fast kinetics of onset and offset or use-dependent block of the fast channel; that is, they bind and dissociate quickly from the receptors. Class IC drugs have slow kinetics, and class IA drugs are intermediate. With increased time spent in diastole (slower rate), a greater proportion of receptors become drug free, and the drug exerts less effect. Cells with reduced membrane potentials recover more slowly from drug actions than do cells with more negative membrane potentials.

REVERSE USE DEPENDENCE. Some drugs exert greater effects at slow rates than at fast rates, a property known as reverse use dependence. This is particularly true for drugs that lengthen repolarization. The QT interval becomes more prolonged at slow rather than fast rates. This effect is opposite to what the ideal antiarrhythmic agent would do because prolongation of refractoriness should be increased at fast rates to interrupt or to prevent a tachycardia and should be minimal at slow rates to avoid precipitation of torsades de pointes.

MECHANISMS OF ARRHYTHMIA SUPPRESSION (see Table 37-2). Given the fact that enhanced automaticity, triggered activity, or reentry can cause cardiac arrhythmias (see Chap. 35), mechanisms by which antiarrhythmic agents suppress arrhythmias can be postulated. Antiarrhythmic agents can slow the spontaneous discharge frequency of an automatic pacemaker by depressing the slope of diastolic depolarization, shifting the threshold voltage toward zero, or hyperpolarizing the resting membrane potential. Mechanisms whereby different drugs suppress normal or abnormal automaticity may not be the same. In general, however, most antiarrhythmic agents in therapeutic doses depress the automatic firing rate of spontaneously discharging ectopic sites while minimally affecting the discharge rate of the normal sinus node. Slow channel blockers such as verapamil, beta blockers such as propranolol, and some antiarrhythmic agents such as amiodarone also depress spontaneous discharge of the sinus node, whereas drugs that exert vagolytic effects, such as disopyramide and quinidine, can increase the sinus discharge rate. Drugs can also suppress early or delayed afterdepolarizations and eliminate triggered arrhythmias related to these mechanisms.

Reentry depends critically on the interrelationships between refractoriness and conduction velocity, the presence of unidirectional block in one of the pathways, and other factors that influence refractoriness and conduction, such as excitability (see Chap. 35). An antiarrhythmic agent can stop ongoing reentry that is already present or prevent it from starting if the drug improves or depresses conduction. For example, improving conduction can (1) eliminate the unidirectional block so that reentry cannot begin or (2) facilitate conduction in the reentrant loop so that the returning wave front reenters too quickly, encounters cells that are still refractory, and is extinguished. A drug that depresses conduction can transform the unidirectional block to bidirectional block and thus terminate reentry or prevent it from starting by creating an area of complete block in the reentrant pathway. Conversely, a drug that slows conduction without producing block or lengthening refractoriness significantly can promote reentry. Finally, most antiarrhythmic agents share the ability to

TABLE 37-2 Classification of Drug Actions on Arrhythmias Based on Modification of Vulnerable Parameter

MECHANISM	ARRHYTHMIA	VULNERABLE PARAMETER (EFFECT)	DRUGS (EFFECT)
Automaticity			
Enhanced normal	Inappropriate sinus tachycardia	Phase 4 depolarization (decrease)	Beta-adrenergic blocking agents
	Some idiopathic ventricular tachycardias		Na^+ channel blocking agents
Abnormal	Atrial tachycardia	Maximum diastolic potential (hyperpolarization)	Muscarinic receptor subtype 2 (M_2) agonists
		Phase 4 depolarization (decrease)	Ca^{2+} or Na^+ channel blocking agents; M_2 agonists
	Accelerated idioventricular rhythms	Phase 4 depolarization (decrease)	Ca^{2+} or Na^+ channel blocking agents
Triggered Activity			
Early afterdepolarization (EAD)	Torsades de pointes	Action potential duration (shorten)	Beta-adrenergic agonists; vagolytic agents (increase rate)
		EAD (suppress)	Ca^{2+} channel blocking agents; Mg^{2+}; beta-adrenergic blocking agents
Delayed afterdepolarization (DAD)	Digitalis-induced arrhythmias	Calcium overload (unload)	Ca^{2+} channel blocking agents
		DAD (suppress)	Na^+ channel blocking agents
	Right ventricular outflow tract ventricular tachycardia	Calcium overload (unload)	Beta-adrenergic blocking agents
		DAD (suppress)	Ca^{2+} channel blocking agents; adenosine
Na^+ Channel–Dependent Reentry			
Long excitable gap	Typical atrial flutter	Conduction and excitability (depress)	Types IA, IC Na^+ channel blocking agents
	Circus movement tachycardia in Wolff-Parkinson-White syndrome (WPW)	Conduction and excitability (depress)	Types IA, IC Na^+ channel blocking agents
	Sustained uniform ventricular tachycardia	Conduction and excitability (depress)	Na^+ channel blocking agents
Short excitable gap	Atypical atrial flutter	Refractory period (prolong)	K^+ channel blocking agents
	Atrial fibrillation	Refractory period (prolong)	K^+ channel blocking agents
	Circus movement tachycardia in WPW	Refractory period (prolong)	Amiodarone, sotalol
	Polymorphic and uniform ventricular tachycardia	Refractory period (prolong)	Type IA Na^+ channel blocking agents
	Bundle branch reentry	Refractory period (prolong)	Type IA Na^+ channel blocking agents; amiodarone
	Ventricular fibrillation	Refractory period (prolong)	
Ca^{2+} Channel–Dependent Reentry			
	Atrioventricular nodal reentrant tachycardia	Conduction and excitability (depress)	Ca^{2+} channel blocking agents
	Circus movement tachycardia in WPW	Conduction and excitability (depress)	Ca^{2+} channel blocking agents
	Verapamil-sensitive ventricular tachycardia	Conduction and excitability (depress)	Ca^{2+} channel blocking agents

From the Task Force of the Working Group on Arrhythmias of the European Society of Cardiology: The Sicilian gambit: A new approach to the classification of antiarrhythmic drugs based on their actions on arrhythmogenic mechanisms. Circulation 84:1831, 1991. Copyright 1991, American Heart Association.

prolong refractoriness relative to their effects on action potential duration (APD); that is, the ratio of effective refractory period (ERP) to APD exceeds 1.0. If a drug prolongs refractoriness of fibers in the reentrant pathway, the pathway may not recover excitability in time to be depolarized by the reentering impulse, and reentrant propagation ceases. The different types of reentry (see Chap. 35) influence the effects and effectiveness of a drug.

In considering the properties of a drug, it is important that the situation or model from which conclusions are drawn be defined with care. Electrophysiologic, hemodynamic, autonomic, pharmacokinetic, and adverse effects may all differ in normal subjects compared with patients, in normal tissue compared with abnormal tissue, in cardiac muscle compared with specialized conduction fibers, and in atrium as opposed to ventricular muscle (**Table 37-4**).

Drug Metabolites. Drug metabolites can add to or alter the effects of the parent compound by exerting similar actions, competing with the parent compound, or mediating drug toxicity. Quinidine has at least four active metabolites but none with a potency exceeding that of the parent drug and none implicated in causing torsades de pointes. About 50% of procainamide is metabolized to *N*-acetylprocainamide (NAPA), which prolongs repolarization and is a less effective antiarrhythmic drug but competes with procainamide for renotubular secretory sites and can increase the parent drug's elimination half-life. Lidocaine's metabolite can compete with lidocaine for sodium channels and partially reverse block produced by lidocaine.

Pharmacogenetics (see Chap. 10)**.** Genetically determined metabolic pathways account for many of the differences in patients' responses to some drugs.[3] The genetically determined activity of hepatic *N*-acetyltransferase regulates the development of antinuclear antibodies and development of the lupus syndrome in response to procainamide. Slow acetylator phenotypes appear more prone than rapid acetylators to the development of lupus. About 7% of subjects lack debrisoquin 4-hydroxylase. The enzyme cytochrome P-450 (CYP450) is needed to metabolize debrisoquin (an antihypertensive drug) and propafenone, to hydroxylate several beta blockers, and to biotransform flecainide. Lack of this enzyme reduces metabolism of the parent compound, leading to increased plasma concentrations of the parent drug and reduced concentrations of metabolites. Propafenone is metabolized by CYP450 to a compound with slightly less antiarrhythmic and beta-adrenergic blocking effects as well as fewer central nervous system side effects. Thus, poor metabolizers

TABLE 37-3 In Vitro Electrophysiologic Characteristics of Antiarrhythmic Drugs

DRUG	APD	DV/DT	MDP	ERP	CV	PF PHASE 4	SN AUTO	CONTR	SI CURR	AUTONOMIC NERVOUS SYSTEM
Quinidine	↑	↓	0	↑	↓	↓	0	0	0	Antivagal; alpha blocker
Procainamide	↑	↓	0	↑	↓	↓	0	0	0	Slight antivagal
Disopyramide	↑	↓	0	↑	↓	↓	↓0↑	↓	0	Central: antivagal, antisympathetic
Ajmaline	↑	↓	0	↑	↓	↓	↓0	↓	0	Antivagal
Lidocaine	↓	0↓	0	↓	0↓	↓	0	0	0	0
Mexiletine	↓	0↓	0	↓	↓	↓	0	↓	0	0
Phenytoin	↓	↓0↑	0	↓	0	↓	0		0	0
Flecainide	0↑	↓	0	↑	↓↓	↓	0	↓	0	0
Propafenone	0↑	↓	0	↑	↓↓	↓	0	↓	0↓	Antisympathetic
Propranolol	0↓	0↓	0	↓	0	↓*	↓	↓	0↓	Antisympathetic
Amiodarone	↑	0↓	0	↑	↓	↓	↓	0↑	0	Antisympathetic
Dronedarone	↑	0↓	0	↑	↓	↓	↓	0↓	0	Antisympathetic
Sotalol	↑	0↓	0	↑	0	0↓	↓	↓	0↓	Antisympathetic
Ibutilide	↑	0	0	↑	0	0	↓	0	0	0
Dofetilide	↑	0	0	↑	0	0	0	0	0	0
Verapamil	↓	0	0	0	0	↓*	↓	↓	↓↓	? Block alpha receptors; enhance vagal
Adenosine	↑	0↓	0	↑	0	0↓	↓	0	↓	Vagomimetic

*With a background of sympathetic activity.

APD = action potential duration; dV/dt = rate of rise of action potential; MDP = maximum diastolic potential; ERP = effective refractory period (longest S_1-S_2 interval at which S_2 fails to produce a response); CV = conduction velocity; PF = Purkinje fiber; SN Auto = sinus nodal automaticity; Contr = contractility; SI Curr = slow inward current.

may experience more heart rate slowing and neurotoxicity than extensive metabolizers do.

Understanding of stereoselectivity (whereby two compounds with identical atomic composition but different spatial arrangement can display different pharmacologic effects) and pharmacogenetics can provide major clues to understanding of differences in drug efficacy and toxicity from one patient to the next. Drugs such as rifampin, phenobarbital, and phenytoin induce the synthesis of larger amounts of CYP450, leading to lower concentrations of parent drugs that are extensively metabolized, whereas erythromycin, clarithromycin, fluoxetine, and grapefruit juice inhibit enzyme activity, leading to accumulation of the parent compound. This effect is thought to explain why cisapride, an agent that had been used to increase gastric motility, could cause QT interval prolongation and torsades de pointes in isolated cases. Cisapride blocked the delayed rectifier current I_{Kr} but did not prolong the QT interval significantly in most patients, presumably because of extensive metabolism. In patients who take an inhibitor of CYP450 (such as erythromycin) along with cisapride, the latter drug can accumulate, leading to QT prolongation and torsades de pointes.

CLINICAL USE. In treatment of cardiac rhythm disorders, most drugs are given on a daily basis (in one to three doses) to prevent episodes from occurring or, in the case of atrial fibrillation, to control the ventricular rate. Efficacy can be judged in various ways, depending on the clinical circumstances. Symptom reduction (in the case of benign arrhythmias, such as most premature ventricular complexes [PVCs]) and electrocardiographic monitoring (long term or event; see Chap. 36) are useful; electrophysiologic studies have been used in the past, with suppression of electrical arrhythmia induction as the goal. However, this is rarely used currently. Interrogation of implanted device memory can also provide an indicator of success of drug therapy.

In some patients, tachycardia episodes are infrequent enough (months between occurrences) and symptoms mild enough that reactive drug administration is more reasonable than chronic daily dosing. In this setting, a patient takes a medication only after an episode has started, with the hope that the tachycardia will terminate in response to the drug and a physician's office or emergency department visit can be avoided thereby. This "pill in the pocket" strategy has worked well in some patients with atrial fibrillation who have been given one of various medications orally in a monitored setting to ensure safety as well as efficacy before allowing self-medication at home or elsewhere.

SIDE EFFECTS. Antiarrhythmic drugs produce one group of side effects related to excessive dosage and plasma concentrations, resulting in both noncardiac (e.g., neurologic defects) and cardiac (e.g., heart failure, some arrhythmias) toxicity, and another group of side effects unrelated to plasma concentrations, which is termed *idiosyncratic*. Examples of the latter include procainamide-induced lupus syndrome and some arrhythmias, such as quinidine-induced torsades de pointes, which can occur in individuals with a forme fruste of the long QT syndrome (i.e., normal QT interval at rest but markedly prolonged interval in the presence of certain medications). In the future, it is likely that genetic differences will explain many idiosyncratic reactions.

Proarrhythmia

Drug-induced or drug-exacerbated cardiac arrhythmias (proarrhythmia) constitute a major clinical problem.[4,5] Proarrhythmia can be manifested as an increase in frequency of a preexisting arrhythmia, sustaining of a previously nonsustained arrhythmia (even making it incessant), or development of arrhythmias that the patient has not previously experienced. Electrophysiologic mechanisms are probably related to prolongation of repolarization or increase of its transmural dispersion, development of early afterdepolarizations to cause torsades de pointes, and alterations in reentry pathways to initiate or to sustain tachyarrhythmias (see Chap. 35). Proarrhythmic events can occur in as many as 5% to 10% of patients receiving antiarrhythmic agents. Heart failure increases this risk. Patients with atrial fibrillation treated with antiarrhythmic agents had a 4.7-fold increased risk of cardiac death if they had a history of heart failure compared with patients not so treated, who had a relative risk of arrhythmic death of 3.7. Patients without a history of congestive heart failure had no increased risk of cardiac mortality during antiarrhythmic drug

TABLE 37-4 Clinical Usage Information for Antiarrhythmic Agents

	USUAL DOSAGE RANGES									
	INTRAVENOUS (mg)		ORAL (mg)							
DRUG	LOADING	MAINTENANCE	LOADING	MAINTENANCE	TIME TO PEAK PLASMA CONCENTRATION (ORAL) (hr)	EFFECTIVE SERUM OR PLASMA CONCENTRATION (μg/ml)	HALF-LIFE (hr)	BIOAVAILABILITY (%)	MAJOR ROUTE OF ELIMINATION	PREGNANCY CLASS
Quinidine	6 to 10 mg/kg at 0.3 to 0.5 mg/kg/min	—	800 to 1000	300 to 600 q 6 hr	1.5 to 3.0	3 to 6	5 to 9	60 to 80	Liver	C
Procainamide	6 to 13 mg/kg at 0.2 to 0.5 mg/kg/min	2 to 6 mg/min	500 to 1000	250 to 1000 q 4-6 hr	1	4 to 10	3 to 5	70 to 85	Kidneys	C
Disopyramide	1 to 2 mg/kg over 15 to 45 min*	1 mg/kg/hr		100 to 300 q 6-8 hr	1 to 2	2 to 5	8 to 9	80 to 90	Kidneys	C
Lidocaine	1 to 3 mg/kg at 20 to 50 mg/min	1 to 4 mg/min	N/A	N/A	N/A	1 to 5	1 to 2	N/A	Liver	B
Mexiletine	500 mg*	0.5 to 1.0 g/24 hr	400 to 600	150 to 300 q 8-12 hr	2 to 4	0.75 to 2	10 to 17	90	Liver	C
Phenytoin	100 mg q 5 min for ≤1000 mg		1000	100 to 400 q12-24 hr	8 to 12	10 to 20	18 to 36	50 to 70	Liver	D
Flecainide	2 mg/kg*	100 to 200 q 12 hr		50 to 200 q 12 hr	3 to 4	0.2 to 1.0	20	95	Kidneys	C
Propafenone	1 to 2 mg/kg		600 to 900	150 to 300 q 8-12 hr	1 to 3	0.2 to 3.0	5 to 8	25 to 75	Liver	C
Propranolol	0.25 to 0.5 mg q 5 min to ≤0.20 mg/kg			10 to 200 q 6-8 hr	4	1 to 2.5	3 to 6	35 to 65	Liver	C
Amiodarone	15 mg/min for 10 min 1 mg/min for 3 hr 0.5 mg/min thereafter	1 mg/min	800 to 1600 qd for 7-14 days	200 to 600 qd		0.5 to 1.5	56 days	25	Kidneys	D
Dronedarone	N/A	N/A	N/A	400 mg q 12hr	3 to 4	0.3 to 0.6	13 to 19	70 to 90	Liver	X
Sotalol	10 mg over 1 to 2 min*			80 to 320 q 12 hr	2.5 to 4	2.5	12	90 to 100	Kidneys	B
Ibutilide	1 mg over 10 min	N/A	N/A	N/A	N/A	N/A	6		Kidneys	C
Dofetilide	2 to 5 μg/kg infusion*	N/A	N/A	0.125 to 0.5 q 12 hr			7 to 13	90	Kidneys	C
Verapamil	5 to 10 mg over 1 to 2 min	0.005 mg/kg/min		80 to 120 q 6-8 hr	1 to 2	0.10 to 0.15	3 to 8	10 to 35	Liver	C
Adenosine	6 to 18 mg (rapidly)	N/A	N/A	N/A	N/A					C
Digoxin	0.5 to 1.0 mg	0.125 to 0.25 qd	0.5 to 1.0	0.125 to 0.25 qd	2 to 6	0.0008 to 0.002	36 to 48	60 to 80	Kidneys	C

*Intravenous use investigational.
N/A: not applicable.
Results presented may vary according to doses, disease state, and intravenous or oral administration.
Pregnancy class: A—controlled studies show no fetal risk; B—no controlled studies, but no evidence of fetal risk; fetal harm unlikely; C—fetal risk cannot be excluded; drug should be used only if potential benefits outweigh potential risk; D—definite fetal risk; drug should be avoided unless in a life-threatening situation or safer alternatives do not exist ; X—contraindicated in pregnancy.

TABLE 37-5 In Vivo Electrophysiologic Characteristics of Antiarrhythmic Drugs

	ELECTROCARDIOGRAPHIC MEASUREMENTS					*ELECTROPHYSIOLOGIC INTERVALS*					
DRUG	**SINUS RATE**	**PR**	**QRS**	**QT**	**JT**	**ERP-AVN**	**ERP-HPS**	**ERP-A**	**ERP-V**	**A-H**	**H-V**
Quinidine	0 ↑	↓ 0 ↑	↑	↑	↑	0 ↑	↑	↑	↑	0 ↓	↑
Procainamide	0	0 ↑	↑	↑	↑	0 ↑	↑	↑	↑	0 ↑	↑
Disopyramide	0 ↑	↓ 0 ↑	↑	↑	↑	↑ 0	↑	↑	↑	↓ 0 ↑	↑
Ajmaline	0	0 ↑	↑	↑	↑	0	↑	↑	↑	↓ 0 ↑	↑
Lidocaine	0	0	0	0 ↓	↓	0 ↓	0 ↑	0	0	0 ↓	0 ↑
Mexiletine	0	0	0	0 ↓	↓	0 ↑	0 ↑	0	0	0 ↑	0 ↑
Phenytoin	0	0	0	0	0	0 ↓	↓	0	0	0 ↑	0
Flecainide	0 ↓	↑	↑	0 ↑	0	↑	↑	↑	↑	↑	↑
Propafenone	0 ↓	↑	↑	0 ↑	0	0 ↑	0 ↑	0 ↑	↑	↑	↑
Propranolol	↓	0 ↑	0	0 ↓	0	↑	0	0	0	0	0
Amiodarone	↓	0 ↑	↑	↑	↑	↑	↑	↑	↑	↑	↑
Dronedarone	↓	0 ↑	↑	↑	↑	↑	↑	↑	↑	↑	0
Sotalol	↓	0 ↑	0	↑	↑	↑	↑	↑	↑	↑	0
Ibutilide	↓	0 ↓	0	↑	↑	0	0	↑	↑	0	0
Dofetilide	0	0	0	↑	↑	0	0	↑	↑	0	0
Verapamil	0 ↓	↑	0	0	0	↑	0	0	0	↑	0
Adenosine	↓ then ↑	↑	0	0	0	↑	0	↓	0	↑	0
Digoxin	↓	↑	0	0	↓	↑	0	↓	0	↑	0

Results presented may vary according to tissue type, drug concentration. and autonomic tone. ↑ = increase; ↓ = decrease; 0 = no change; 0 ↑ or 0 ↓ = slight or inconsistent increase or decrease; A = atrium; AVN = AV node; HPS = His-Purkinje system; V = ventricle; A-H = atrio-His interval (an index of AV nodal conduction); H-V = His-ventricular interval (an index of His-Purkinje conduction); ERP = effective refractory period (longest S_1-S_2 interval at which S_2 fails to produce a response).

treatment. Reduced left ventricular function, treatment with digitalis and diuretics, and longer pretreatment QT interval characterize patients who experience drug-induced ventricular fibrillation (VF). The more commonly known proarrhythmic events occur within several days of beginning drug therapy or changing dosage and are represented by such developments as incessant VT, long QT syndrome, and torsades de pointes. However, in the Cardiac Arrhythmia Suppression Trial (CAST), researchers found that encainide and flecainide reduced spontaneous ventricular arrhythmias but were associated with a total mortality of 7.7%, in comparison with 3.0% in the group receiving placebo. Deaths were equally distributed throughout the treatment period, raising the important consideration that another type of proarrhythmic response can occur some time after the beginning of drug therapy. Such late proarrhythmic effects may be related to drug-induced exacerbation of regional myocardial conduction delay caused by ischemia and heterogeneous drug concentrations that can promote reentry.

The availability of catheter ablation (see later) and implantable devices (pacemakers and ICDs; see Chap. 38) to treat a wide variety of arrhythmias has largely relegated drug therapy to a secondary role. Drugs are still useful to prevent or to decrease frequency of recurrences in patients who have relatively infrequent episodes of benign tachycardias, those who have had incomplete success with catheter ablation procedures, and patients with an ICD to decrease frequency of shocks due to ventricular arrhythmia.

Antiarrhythmic Agents

CLASS IA AGENTS

Quinidine

Quinidine and quinine are isomeric alkaloids isolated from cinchona bark. Although quinidine shares the antimalarial, antipyretic, and vagolytic actions of quinine, only quinidine has electrophysiologic effects.[6]

ELECTROPHYSIOLOGIC ACTIONS (Table 37-5; see Tables 37-1, 37-2, and 37-3**).** Quinidine exerts little effect on automaticity of the normal sinus node but suppresses automaticity in normal Purkinje fibers. In patients with the sick sinus syndrome, quinidine can depress sinus node automaticity. Quinidine produces early afterdepolarizations in experimental preparations and in humans, which may be responsible for torsades de pointes. Because of its significant anticholinergic effect and reflex sympathetic stimulation resulting from alpha-adrenergic blockade, which causes peripheral vasodilation, quinidine can increase sinus node discharge rate and can improve atrioventricular (AV) nodal conduction. Quinidine prolongs repolarization, an effect that is more prominent at slow heart rates (reverse use dependence) because of block of I_{Kr} (as well as enhancing late Na current). Faster rates result in more block of sodium channels and less unblocking because of a smaller percentage of time spent in a polarized state (use dependence). Isoproterenol can modulate the effects of quinidine on reentrant circuits in humans. Quinidine at higher doses inhibits the late Na current.

HEMODYNAMIC EFFECTS. Quinidine decreases peripheral vascular resistance and can cause significant hypotension because of its alpha-adrenergic receptor blocking effects. Concomitant administration of vasodilators can exaggerate the potential for hypotension. It does not cause significant direct myocardial depression.

PHARMACOKINETICS (see Table 37-4**).** Although orally administered quinidine sulfate and quinidine gluconate exhibit similar systemic availability, plasma quinidine concentrations peak at about 90 minutes after a dose of the sulfate but at 3 to 4 hours after a dose of the gluconate preparation. Quinidine can be given intravenously if it is infused slowly, but intramuscular dosing should be avoided. Approximately 80% of plasma quinidine is protein bound, especially to alpha$_1$-acid glycoprotein, which increases in heart failure. Both the liver and the kidneys remove quinidine; dose adjustments may be made according to the creatinine clearance. Metabolism is by means of the CYP450 system. Approximately 20% is excreted unchanged in the urine. Because congestive heart failure, hepatic disease, or poor renal function can reduce quinidine elimination and increase plasma concentration, the dosage should be reduced and the drug given cautiously to patients with these disorders while serum quinidine concentration is monitored. Elimination half-life is 5 to 8 hours after oral administration. Quinidine's effect on repolarization and overall efficacy vary directly with left ventricular function; for the same serum concentration, the QT interval is longer in women than in men.

DOSAGE AND ADMINISTRATION (see Table 37-4). The usual oral dose of quinidine sulfate for an adult is 300 to 600 mg four times daily, which results in a steady-state level within about 24 hours. A loading dose of 600 to 1000 mg produces an earlier effective concentration. Oral doses of the gluconate are about 30% higher than those of the sulfate. Important interactions with other drugs occur.

INDICATIONS. Quinidine is a versatile antiarrhythmic agent, with efficacy in treating premature supraventricular and ventricular complexes and sustained tachyarrhythmias. Its benefits are tempered by adverse effects (see later). It may prevent spontaneous recurrences of AV nodal reentrant tachycardia (AVNRT) and other forms of SVT by prolonging atrial and ventricular refractoriness and depressing conduction in the essential portions of reentrant circuits. Quinidine and other antiarrhythmic agents can also prevent recurrences of tachycardia by suppressing the "trigger" (i.e., PVC or premature atrial complex [PAC]) that initiates a sustained tachycardia (see Chap. 39).

Quinidine successfully terminates atrial flutter or atrial fibrillation in 20% to 60% of patients, with higher success rates if the arrhythmia is of more recent onset and if the atria are not enlarged.[7] Before quinidine is administered to these patients, the ventricular response should be slowed sufficiently with a beta or calcium channel blocker because quinidine-induced slowing of the atrial flutter rate (e.g., from 300 to 230 beats/min) and its vagolytic effect on AV nodal conduction can convert a 2:1 AV response (ventricular rate, 150 beats/min) to a 1:1 AV response, with an increase in the ventricular rate (to 230 beats/min). If quinidine is going to be used to try to maintain sinus rhythm after elective cardioversion of patients with atrial fibrillation, it probably should be given for 1 to 2 days before planned cardioversion because this regimen restores sinus rhythm in some patients, thus obviating the need for direct-current cardioversion, and helps maintain sinus rhythm once it has been achieved. In addition, early toxicity or the patient's intolerance of the drug may be observed and changes made in drug therapy before cardioversion is attempted. However, a meta-analysis of six studies testing the effects of quinidine versus control in maintaining sinus rhythm in patients with atrial fibrillation showed that quinidine-treated patients remain in sinus rhythm longer than the control group but have an increased total mortality during the same period.

Quinidine has limited usefulness in the prevention of VT and VF; however, patients with primary VF as well as those with Brugada syndrome (see Chap. 9) and the short-QT syndrome have been treated successfully with this agent.[8] Because it crosses the placenta, quinidine can be used to treat arrhythmias in the fetus.

ADVERSE EFFECTS. The most common adverse effects of chronic oral quinidine therapy are gastrointestinal and include nausea, vomiting, diarrhea, abdominal pain, and anorexia (milder with the gluconate form). Central nervous system toxicity includes tinnitus, hearing loss, visual disturbances, confusion, delirium, and psychosis (cinchonism). Allergic reactions may be manifested as rash, fever, immune-mediated thrombocytopenia, hemolytic anemia, and, rarely, anaphylaxis. Side effects may preclude long-term administration of quinidine in 30% to 40% of patients.

Quinidine can slow cardiac conduction, sometimes to the point of block, manifested as prolongation of the QRS duration or sinoatrial or AV nodal conduction disturbances. Quinidine can produce syncope in 0.5% to 2.0% of patients, most often the result of a self-terminating episode of torsades de pointes. Quinidine prolongs the QT interval in most patients, whether or not ventricular arrhythmias occur, but significant QT prolongation (QT interval of 500 to 600 milliseconds) is often a characteristic of patients with quinidine syncope. Many of these patients are also receiving digitalis or diuretics or have hypokalemia; women are more susceptible than men. Syncope is unrelated to plasma concentrations of quinidine or duration of therapy, although most episodes occur within the first 2 to 4 days of therapy, often after conversion of atrial fibrillation to sinus rhythm. Therapy requires immediate discontinuation of the drug and avoidance of other drugs that have similar pharmacologic effects because cross-sensitivity exists in some patients. Magnesium given intravenously (2 g during 1 to 2 minutes, followed by an infusion of 3 to 20 mg/min) is the initial drug treatment of choice. Atrial or ventricular pacing can be used to suppress the ventricular tachyarrhythmia, perhaps acting by suppressing early afterdepolarizations. When pacing is not available, isoproterenol can be given with caution. The arrhythmia gradually dissipates as quinidine is cleared and the QT interval returns to baseline.

Drugs that induce hepatic enzyme production, such as phenobarbital and phenytoin, can shorten the duration of quinidine's action by increasing its rate of elimination. Quinidine can increase plasma concentrations of flecainide by inhibiting the CYP450 enzyme system. Quinidine may elevate serum digoxin concentrations by decreasing its clearance, volume of distribution, and affinity of tissue receptors.

Procainamide

ELECTROPHYSIOLOGIC ACTIONS (see Tables 37-1, 37-2, 37-3, and 37-5). The cardiac actions of procainamide on automaticity, conduction, excitability, and membrane responsiveness resemble those of quinidine.[6] Procainamide predominantly blocks the inactivated state of I_{Na}. It also blocks I_{Kr} and $I_{K.ATP}$. Like quinidine, procainamide usually prolongs the ERP more than it prolongs the APD and thus may prevent reentry. Procainamide exerts the least anticholinergic effects among type IA drugs. It does not affect normal sinus node automaticity. In vitro, procainamide decreases abnormal automaticity, with less effect on triggered activity or catecholamine-enhanced normal automaticity. The electrophysiologic effects of NAPA, procainamide's major metabolite, differ from those of the parent compound. NAPA, a K^+ channel blocker (I_{Kr}), exerts a class III action and prolongs the APD of ventricular muscle and Purkinje fibers in a dose-dependent manner. High levels can produce early afterdepolarizations, triggered activity, and torsades de pointes.

HEMODYNAMIC EFFECTS. Procainamide can depress myocardial contractility in high doses. It does not produce alpha blockade but can result in peripheral vasodilation, possibly through antisympathetic effects on brain or spinal cord that can impair cardiovascular reflexes.

PHARMACOKINETICS (see Table 37-4). Oral administration produces a peak plasma concentration in about 1 hour. Approximately 80% of oral procainamide is bioavailable; the overall elimination half-life for procainamide is 3 to 5 hours, with 50% to 60% of the drug eliminated by the kidney and 10% to 30% eliminated by hepatic metabolism. The drug is acetylated to NAPA, which is excreted almost exclusively by the kidneys. As renal function decreases and in patients with heart failure, NAPA levels increase and, because of the risk of serious cardiotoxicity, need to be carefully monitored in these situations. NAPA has an elimination half-life of 7 to 8 hours, but the half-life exceeds 10 hours if high doses of procainamide are used. Increased age, congestive heart failure, and reduced creatinine clearance lower the procainamide clearance and necessitate a reduced dosage.

DOSAGE AND ADMINISTRATION (see Table 37-4). Procainamide can be given by the oral, intravenous, or intramuscular route to achieve plasma concentrations in the range of 4 to 10 mg/mL that produce an antiarrhythmic effect. Several intravenous regimens have been used to administer procainamide; 25 to 50 mg can be given during a 1-minute period and then repeated every 5 minutes until the arrhythmia has been controlled, hypotension results, or the QRS complex is prolonged more than 50%. Doses of 10 to 15 mg/kg at 50 mg/min can also be used. With this method, the plasma concentration falls rapidly during the first 15 minutes after the loading dose, with parallel effects on refractoriness and conduction. A constant rate intravenous infusion of procainamide can be given at a dose of 2 to 6 mg/min, depending on the patient's response.

Oral administration of procainamide requires a 3- to 4-hour dosing interval at a total daily dose of 2 to 6 g, with a steady state reached within 1 day. When a loading dose is used, it should be twice the maintenance dose. Frequent dosing is required because of the short elimination half-life in normal subjects. For the extended-release forms of procainamide, dosing is at 6- to 12-hour intervals. Procainamide is well absorbed after intramuscular injection, with almost 100% of the dose bioavailable.

INDICATIONS. Procainamide is used to treat both supraventricular and ventricular arrhythmias in a manner comparable to that of quinidine. Although both drugs have similar electrophysiologic actions, either drug can effectively suppress a supraventricular or ventricular arrhythmia that is resistant to the other drug. Procainamide can be used to convert recent-onset atrial fibrillation to sinus rhythm. As with quinidine, prior treatment with beta or calcium channel blockers is recommended to prevent acceleration of the ventricular response during atrial flutter or fibrillation after procainamide therapy. Procainamide can block conduction in the accessory pathway of patients with the Wolff-Parkinson-White syndrome and may be used in patients with atrial fibrillation and a rapid ventricular response related to conduction over the accessory pathway. It can produce His-Purkinje block (see Fig. 36-11) and is sometimes administered during an electrophysiologic study (EPS) to stress the His-Purkinje system in evaluating the need for a pacemaker. However, it should be used with caution in patients with evidence of His-Purkinje disease (bundle branch block) in whom a ventricular pacemaker is not readily available. Procainamide is more effective than lidocaine in acutely terminating sustained VT. Most consistently, procainamide slows the VT rate, a change correlated with the increase in QRS duration. The electrophysiologic response to procainamide given intravenously appears to predict the response to the drug given orally. It has been used to facilitate VT induction at EPS when the arrhythmia could not be initiated in the baseline state.

ADVERSE EFFECTS. Noncardiac adverse effects from procainamide administration include rashes, myalgias, digital vasculitis, and Raynaud phenomenon. Fever and agranulocytosis may be the result of hypersensitivity reactions, and white blood cell and differential counts should be assessed at regular intervals. Gastrointestinal side effects are less frequent than with quinidine, and adverse central nervous system side effects are less frequent than with lidocaine. Toxic concentrations of procainamide can diminish myocardial performance and promote hypotension. Various conduction disturbances or ventricular tachyarrhythmias can occur that are similar to those produced by quinidine, including prolonged QT syndrome and polymorphic VT. NAPA can also cause QT prolongation and torsades de pointes. In the absence of sinus node disease, procainamide does not adversely affect sinus node function. In patients with sinus node dysfunction, procainamide can prolong sinus node recovery time and worsen symptoms in some patients who have the bradycardia-tachycardia syndrome.

Arthralgia, fever, pleuropericarditis, hepatomegaly, and hemorrhagic pericardial effusion with tamponade have been described in a systemic lupus erythematosus (SLE)–like syndrome related to procainamide administration. The syndrome occurs more frequently and earlier in patients who are slow acetylators of procainamide and is genetically influenced (see Chap. 10). Acetylation of an aromatic amino group on procainamide to form NAPA appears to block the SLE-inducing effect. Sixty percent to 70% of patients who receive procainamide on a chronic basis develop antinuclear antibodies, with clinical symptoms in 20% to 30%, but this is reversible when procainamide is stopped. Positive serologic test results are not necessarily a reason to discontinue drug therapy; however, the development of symptoms or a positive anti-DNA antibody indicates that drug therapy should be discontinued. Corticosteroid administration in these patients may eliminate the symptoms. In this syndrome, in contrast to naturally occurring SLE, the brain and kidney are spared, and there is no predilection for women.

Disopyramide

Disopyramide has been approved in the United States for oral administration to treat patients with ventricular and supraventricular arrhythmias.

ELECTROPHYSIOLOGIC ACTIONS (see Tables 37-1, 37-2, 37-3, and 37-5). Although it is structurally different from quinidine and procainamide, disopyramide produces similar electrophysiologic effects, causing use-dependent block of I_{Na} and non–use-dependent block of I_{Kr}. Disopyramide also inhibits $I_{K,ATP}$; it does not affect calcium-dependent action potentials, except possibly at very high concentrations.

Disopyramide is a muscarinic blocker and can increase the sinus node discharge rate and shorten AV nodal conduction time and refractoriness when the nodes are under cholinergic (vagal) influences. Disopyramide can also slow the sinus node discharge rate by a direct action when it is given in a high concentration and can significantly depress sinus node activity in patients with sinus node dysfunction. It exerts greater anticholinergic effects than quinidine and does not appear to affect alpha or beta adrenoceptors. The drug prolongs atrial and ventricular refractory periods, but its effect on AV nodal conduction and refractoriness is not consistent. Disopyramide prolongs His-Purkinje conduction time, but infra-His block rarely occurs. It can be administered safely to patients who have first-degree AV delay and narrow QRS complexes.

HEMODYNAMIC EFFECTS. Disopyramide suppresses ventricular systolic performance and is a mild arterial vasodilator. The drug should generally be avoided in patients who have reduced left ventricular systolic function because they tolerate disopyramide's negative inotropic effects poorly.

PHARMACOKINETICS (see Table 37-4). Disopyramide is 80% to 90% absorbed, with a mean elimination half-life of 8 to 9 hours in healthy volunteers but almost 10 hours in patients with heart failure. Renal insufficiency prolongs the elimination time. Thus, in patients who have renal, hepatic, or cardiac insufficiency, loading and maintenance doses need to be reduced. Peak blood levels after oral administration are seen in 1 to 2 hours. It is bound to alpha$_1$-acid glycoprotein and passes through the placenta. About 50% of an oral dose is recovered unchanged in the urine, with about 30% as the mono-*N*-dealkylated metabolite. The metabolites appear to exert less effect than the parent compound. Erythromycin inhibits its metabolism.

DOSAGE AND ADMINISTRATION (see Table 37-4). Doses are generally 100 to 200 mg orally every 6 hours, with a range of 400 to 1200 mg/day. A controlled-release preparation can be given as 200 to 300 mg every 12 hours.

INDICATIONS. Disopyramide appears comparable to quinidine and procainamide in reducing the frequency of PVCs and effectively preventing recurrence of VT in selected patients. Disopyramide has been combined with other drugs, such as mexiletine, to treat patients who do not respond or respond only partially to one drug.

Disopyramide helps prevent recurrence of atrial fibrillation after successful cardioversion as effectively as quinidine and may terminate atrial flutter. In treating patients with atrial fibrillation, particularly atrial flutter, the ventricular rate must be controlled before disopyramide is administered, or the combination of a decrease in atrial rate with vagolytic effects on the AV node can result in 1:1 AV conduction during atrial flutter. Disopyramide may be useful in preventing episodes of neurally mediated syncope. It has been used in patients with hypertrophic cardiomyopathy.

ADVERSE EFFECTS. Three types of adverse effects follow disopyramide administration. The most common effects are related to the drug's potent parasympatholytic properties and include urinary hesitancy or retention, constipation, blurred vision, closed-angle glaucoma, and dry mouth. Symptoms are less with the sustained-release form. Second, disopyramide can produce ventricular tachyarrhythmias that are commonly associated with QT prolongation and torsades de pointes. Some patients can have cross-sensitization to both quinidine and disopyramide and develop torsades de pointes while receiving either drug. When drug-induced torsades de pointes occurs, agents that prolong the QT interval should be used cautiously or not at all. Finally, disopyramide can reduce contractility of the normal ventricle, but the depression of ventricular function is much more pronounced in patients with preexisting ventricular failure. Rarely, cardiovascular collapse can result.

Ajmaline

Ajmaline, a rauwolfia derivative, has been used extensively to treat patients with ventricular and supraventricular arrhythmias in Europe and Asia but is not available in the United States.

ELECTROPHYSIOLOGIC ACTIONS (see Tables 37-1, 37-2, 37-3, and 37-5). Like other type IA drugs, ajmaline produces use-dependent block of I_{Na}; it also weakly blocks I_{Kr}. The drug has mild anticholinergic activity.

HEMODYNAMIC EFFECTS. Ajmaline mildly suppresses ventricular systolic performance but does not affect peripheral resistance. It also inhibits platelet activity more potently than aspirin does.

PHARMACOKINETICS, DOSAGE, AND ADMINISTRATION (see Table 37-4). Ajmaline is well absorbed, with a mean elimination half-life of 13 minutes in most patients, making it poorly suited to long-term oral use. The dose for acute arrhythmia termination is generally 50 mg intravenously during 1 to 2 minutes.

INDICATIONS. Although it is useful for terminating SVTs by intravenous infusion, other medications have largely supplanted ajmaline for this purpose. The drug's use has evolved to that of a diagnostic tool.

When it is administered intravenously at doses of 50 mg during 3 minutes, or 10 mg/min, to a total dose of 1 mg/kg, ajmaline can have the following effects: (1) delta wave disappearance in patients with Wolff-Parkinson-White syndrome (indicating an accessory pathway anterograde ERP more than 250 milliseconds); (2) ST-T abnormalities and interventricular conduction blocks in patients with occult chagasic cardiomyopathy; (3) heart block in patients with bundle branch block and syncope, but in whom no rhythm disturbance had been discovered; and (4) right precordial ST elevation in patients with suspected Brugada syndrome in whom the resting electrocardiogram (ECG) is normal. It is in this last setting that ajmaline is used most frequently.

Adverse Effects. Ajmaline can produce mild anticholinergic side effects as well as mild depression in left ventricular systolic function and can worsen AV conduction in patients with His-Purkinje disease. Rare occurrences of torsades de pointes have been reported. Ajmaline can cause an increase in the defibrillation threshold.

CLASS IB AGENTS

Lidocaine

Electrophysiologic Actions (see Tables 37-1, 37-2, 37-3, and 37-5). Lidocaine blocks I_{Na}, predominantly in the open or possibly inactivated state. It has rapid onset and offset kinetics and does not affect normal sinus node automaticity in usual doses but does depress other normal and abnormal forms of automaticity as well as early and late afterdepolarizations in Purkinje fibers in vitro. Lidocaine has only a modest depressant effect on $\dot{V}max$; however, faster rates of stimulation, reduced pH, increased extracellular K^+ concentration, and reduced membrane potential, all changes that can result from ischemia, increase the ability of lidocaine to block I_{Na}. Lidocaine can convert areas of unidirectional block into bidirectional block during ischemia and prevent development of VF by preventing fragmentation of organized large wave fronts into heterogeneous wavelets.

Except in very high concentrations, lidocaine does not affect slow channel–dependent action potentials, despite its moderate suppression of the slow inward current. Lidocaine has little effect on atrial fibers and does not affect conduction in accessory pathways. Patients with preexisting sinus node dysfunction, abnormal His-Purkinje conduction, or junctional or ventricular escape rhythms can develop depressed automaticity or conduction. Part of its effects may involve inhibition of cardiac sympathetic nerve activity.

Hemodynamic Effects. Clinically significant adverse hemodynamic effects are rarely noted at usual drug concentrations unless left ventricular function is severely impaired.

Pharmacokinetics (see Table 37-4). Lidocaine is used only parenterally because oral administration results in extensive first-pass hepatic metabolism and unpredictable low plasma levels, with excessive metabolites that can produce toxicity. Hepatic metabolism of lidocaine depends on hepatic blood flow; severe hepatic disease or reduced hepatic blood flow, as in heart failure or shock, can markedly decrease the rate of lidocaine metabolism. Beta adrenoceptor blockers can decrease hepatic blood flow and increase lidocaine serum concentration. Prolonged infusion can reduce lidocaine clearance. Its elimination half-life averages 1 to 2 hours in normal subjects, longer than 4 hours in patients after uncomplicated myocardial infarction, longer than 10 hours in patients after myocardial infarction complicated by cardiac failure, and even longer in the presence of cardiogenic shock. Maintenance doses should be reduced by one third to one half for patients with low cardiac output. Lidocaine is 50% to 80% protein bound and binds to $alpha_1$-acid glycoprotein.

DOSAGE AND ADMINISTRATION (see Table 37-4). Although lidocaine can be given intramuscularly, the intravenous route is most commonly used. Intramuscular lidocaine is given in doses of 4 to 5 mg/kg (250 to 350 mg), resulting in effective serum levels at about 15 minutes and lasting for about 90 minutes. Intravenously, lidocaine is given as an initial bolus of 1 to 2 mg/kg body weight at a rate of 20 to 50 mg/min, with a second injection of half the initial dose 20 to 40 minutes later. Patients treated with an initial bolus followed by a maintenance infusion may experience transient subtherapeutic plasma concentrations 30 to 120 minutes after initiation of therapy. A second bolus of about 0.5 mg/kg without increase of the maintenance infusion rate reestablishes therapeutic serum concentrations.

If recurrence of arrhythmia appears after a steady state has been achieved (e.g., 6 to 10 hours after therapy is started), a similar bolus should be given and the maintenance infusion rate increased. Increase of the maintenance infusion rate alone without an additional bolus results in a very slow increase in plasma lidocaine concentrations and is therefore not recommended. Another recommended intravenous dosing regimen is 1.5 mg/kg initially and 0.8 mg/kg at 8-minute intervals for three doses. Doses are reduced by about 50% for patients with heart failure.

If the initial bolus of lidocaine is ineffective, up to two more boluses of 1 mg/kg may be administered at 5-minute intervals. Patients who require more than one bolus to achieve a therapeutic effect have arrhythmias that respond only to higher lidocaine plasma concentrations, and a higher maintenance dose may be necessary to sustain these higher concentrations. Maintenance infusion rates in the range of 1 to 4 mg/min produce steady-state plasma levels of 1 to 5 mg/mL in patients with uncomplicated myocardial infarction, but these rates must be reduced during heart failure or shock because of concomitant reduced hepatic blood flow. Higher doses are unlikely to provide additional benefit but increase the risk of toxicity.

INDICATIONS. Lidocaine has moderate efficacy against ventricular arrhythmias of diverse causes; it is generally ineffective against supraventricular arrhythmias. It rarely terminates monomorphic VT. Although once commonly used to try to prevent VF in the first 2 days after acute myocardial infarction, its efficacy was not great, and because it can produce side effects and a possible increase in the risk for development of asystole, this use is not recommended. Lidocaine has been effective in patients after coronary revascularization and in patients resuscitated from out-of-hospital VF, although amiodarone has been shown to yield higher rates of survival, at least to hospital admission.

ADVERSE EFFECTS. The most commonly reported adverse effects of lidocaine are dose-related manifestations of central nervous system toxicity: dizziness, paresthesias, confusion, delirium, stupor, coma, and seizures. Occasional sinus node depression and His-Purkinje block have been reported. Rarely, lidocaine can cause malignant hyperthermia. Both lidocaine and procainamide can elevate defibrillation thresholds.

Mexiletine

Mexiletine, a local anesthetic congener of lidocaine with anticonvulsant properties, is used for the oral treatment of patients with symptomatic ventricular arrhythmias.

Electrophysiologic Actions (see Tables 37-1, 37-2, 37-3, and 37-5). Mexiletine is similar to lidocaine in many of its electrophysiologic actions. In vitro, mexiletine shortens the APD and ERP of Purkinje fibers and, to a lesser extent, of ventricular muscle. It depresses $\dot{V}max$ of phase 0 by blocking I_{Na}, especially at faster rates, and depresses automaticity of Purkinje fibers but not of the normal sinus node. Its onset and offset kinetics are rapid. Hypoxia or ischemia can increase its effects.

Mexiletine can result in severe bradycardia and abnormal sinus node recovery time in patients with sinus node disease, but not in patients with a normal sinus node. It does not affect AV nodal conduction and can depress His-Purkinje conduction, but not greatly, unless conduction was abnormal initially. Mexiletine does not appear to affect human atrial muscle. It does not affect the QT interval.

Hemodynamic Effects. Mexiletine exerts no major hemodynamic effects on ventricular contractile performance or peripheral resistance.

Pharmacokinetics (see Table 37-4). Mexiletine is rapidly and almost completely absorbed after oral ingestion by volunteers, with peak plasma concentrations attained in 2 to 4 hours. Elimination half-life is approximately 10 hours in healthy subjects but 17 hours in patients after myocardial infarction. Therapeutic plasma levels of 0.5 to 2 mg/mL are maintained by oral doses of 200 to 300 mg every 6 to 8 hours. Absorption with less than a 10% first-pass hepatic effect occurs in the upper small intestine and is delayed and incomplete in patients who have myocardial infarction and in patients receiving narcotics, antacids, or atropine-like drugs that retard gastric emptying. About 70% of the drug is protein bound. The apparent volume of distribution is large, reflecting extensive tissue uptake. Normally, mexiletine is eliminated metabolically by the liver, with less than 10% excreted unchanged in the urine. Doses should be reduced in patients with cirrhosis or left ventricular failure. Renal clearance of mexiletine decreases as the urinary pH increases. Known metabolites exert no electrophysiologic effects. Metabolism can be increased by phenytoin, phenobarbital, and rifampin and reduced by cimetidine.

DOSAGE AND ADMINISTRATION (see Table 37-4). The recommended starting dose is 200 mg orally every 8 hours when rapid arrhythmia control is not essential. Doses may be increased or decreased by 50 to 100 mg every 2 to 3 days and are better tolerated when given with food. Total daily dose should not exceed 1200 mg. In some patients, administration every 12 hours can be effective.

INDICATIONS. Mexiletine is a moderately effective antiarrhythmic agent for treatment of patients with acute and chronic ventricular tachyarrhythmias but not SVTs. Success rates vary from 6% to 60% and can be increased in some patients if mexiletine is combined with other drugs such as procainamide, beta blockers, quinidine, disopyramide, propafenone, or amiodarone. Most studies show no clear superiority of mexiletine over other class I agents. Mexiletine may be very useful in children with congenital heart disease and serious ventricular arrhythmias. In treating patients with a long QT interval, mexiletine may be safer than drugs such as quinidine that increase the QT interval further. Limited experience in treating subsets of patients with long-QT syndrome (LQT3, which is related to the *SCN5A* gene for the cardiac sodium channel) suggests a beneficial role (see Chap. 9).

ADVERSE EFFECTS. Up to 40% of patients may require a change in dose or discontinuation of mexiletine therapy as a result of adverse effects, including tremor, dysarthria, dizziness, paresthesia, diplopia, nystagmus, mental confusion, anxiety, nausea, vomiting, and dyspepsia. Cardiovascular side effects are rare but include hypotension, bradycardia, and exacerbation of arrhythmia. Adverse effects of mexiletine appear to be dose related, and toxic effects occur at plasma concentrations only slightly higher than therapeutic levels. Therefore, effective use of this antiarrhythmic drug requires careful titration of dose and monitoring of plasma concentration. Lidocaine should be avoided, or the dose reduced, in patients receiving mexiletine.

Phenytoin

Phenytoin was used originally to treat seizure disorders. Its value as an antiarrhythmic agent remains limited.

Electrophysiologic Actions (see Tables 37-1, 37-2, 37-3, and 37-5). Phenytoin effectively abolishes abnormal automaticity caused by digitalis-induced delayed afterdepolarizations in cardiac Purkinje fibers and suppresses certain digitalis-induced arrhythmias in humans. The rate of rise of action potentials initiated early in the relative refractory period is increased, as is membrane responsiveness, possibly reducing the chance for impaired conduction and block. Phenytoin minimally affects sinus discharge rate and AV conduction in humans. Some of phenytoin's antiarrhythmic effects may be neurally mediated because it can modulate both sympathetic and vagal efferent activity. It has no peripheral cholinergic or beta-adrenergic blocking actions and minimal hemodynamic effect.

Pharmacokinetics (see Table 37-4). The pharmacokinetics of phenytoin are less than ideal. Absorption after oral administration is incomplete and varies with the brand of drug. Plasma concentrations peak 8 to 12 hours after an oral dose; 90% of the drug is protein bound. Phenytoin has limited solubility at physiologic pH, and intramuscular administration is associated with pain, muscle necrosis, sterile abscesses, and variable absorption. Therapeutic serum concentrations of phenytoin (10 to 20 mg/mL) are similar for treatment of cardiac arrhythmias and epilepsy. Lower concentrations can suppress certain digitalis-induced arrhythmias.

Metabolism. More than 90% of a dose is hydroxylated in the liver to presumably inactive compounds; significant genetically determined variation can occur. Elimination half-time is about 24 hours and can be slowed in the presence of liver disease or when phenytoin is administered concomitantly with drugs such as warfarin, isoniazid, and phenothiazines, which compete with phenytoin for hepatic enzymes. Because of the large number of medications that can increase or decrease phenytoin levels during chronic therapy, phenytoin plasma concentration should be determined frequently when changes are made in other medications. Phenytoin has concentration-dependent kinetics for elimination that can cause unexpected toxicity because disproportionately large changes in plasma concentration can follow dose increases.

Dosage and Administration (see Table 37-4). To achieve a therapeutic plasma concentration rapidly, 100 mg of phenytoin should be administered intravenously every 5 minutes until the arrhythmia is controlled, 1 g has been given, or adverse side effects result. In general, if phenytoin is going to control the arrhythmia, 700 to 1000 mg suffices. A large central vein should be used to avoid pain and development of phlebitis produced by the drug's alkalotic vehicle. Orally, phenytoin is given as a loading dose of 1000 mg the first day, 500 mg on the second and third days, and 300 to 400 mg daily thereafter. Maintenance doses can generally be given once daily because of the long half-life of elimination.

Indications. Phenytoin has been used successfully to treat atrial and ventricular arrhythmias caused by digitalis toxicity but is much less effective in treating ventricular arrhythmias in patients with ischemic heart disease or with atrial arrhythmias not caused by digitalis toxicity. It may be useful in some patients with the long-QT syndrome.

Adverse Effects. The most common manifestations of phenytoin toxicity are central nervous system effects of nystagmus, ataxia, drowsiness, stupor, and coma and correlate with increases in plasma drug concentration. Nausea, epigastric pain, and anorexia are also relatively common effects of phenytoin. Long-term administration can result in hyperglycemia, hypocalcemia, rashes, megaloblastic anemia, gingival hypertrophy, lymph node hyperplasia (a syndrome resembling malignant lymphoma), peripheral neuropathy, pneumonitis, and drug-induced SLE. Birth defects can also result.

CLASS IC AGENTS.

Flecainide

Flecainide is approved by the U.S. Food and Drug Administration (FDA) to treat patients with life-threatening ventricular arrhythmias as well as various supraventricular arrhythmias.[6]

Electrophysiologic Actions (see Tables 37-1, 37-2, 37-3, and 37-5). Flecainide exhibits marked use-dependent depressant effects on the rapid sodium channel, decreasing $\dot{V}max$, with slow onset and offset kinetics. Drug dissociation from the sodium channel is slow, with time constants of 10 to 30 seconds (compared with 4 to 8 seconds for quinidine and less than 1 second for lidocaine). Thus, marked drug effects can occur at physiologic heart rates. Flecainide shortens the duration of the Purkinje fiber action potential but prolongs it in ventricular muscle, actions that, depending on the circumstances, could enhance or reduce electrical heterogeneity and create or suppress arrhythmias. Flecainide profoundly slows conduction in all cardiac fibers and, in high concentrations, inhibits the slow Ca^{2+} channel (see Chap. 35). Conduction time in the atria, ventricles, AV node, and His-Purkinje system is prolonged. Minimal increases in atrial or ventricular refractoriness or in the QT interval result. Anterograde and retrograde refractoriness in accessory pathways can increase significantly in a use-dependent fashion. Sinus node function remains unchanged in normal subjects but may be depressed in patients with sinus node dysfunction. Flecainide can facilitate or inhibit reentry and may transform atrial fibrillation to flutter. Pacing and defibrillation thresholds are characteristically slightly increased.

Hemodynamic Effects. Flecainide depresses cardiac performance, particularly in patients with compromised ventricular systolic function, and should be used cautiously or not at all in patients with moderate or severe ventricular systolic dysfunction.

Pharmacokinetics (see Table 37-4). Flecainide is at least 90% absorbed, with peak plasma concentrations in 3 to 4 hours. Elimination half-life in patients with ventricular arrhythmias is 20 hours, with 85% of the drug being excreted unchanged or as an inactive metabolite in urine. Two major metabolites exert fewer effects than the parent drug. Elimination is slower in patients with renal disease and heart failure, and doses should be reduced in these situations. Men may have a more rapid rate of elimination, lower drug concentrations, and less efficacy than women do.[9] Therapeutic plasma concentrations range from 0.2 to 1.0 mg/mL. About 40% of the drug is protein bound. Increases in serum concentrations of digoxin (15% to 25%) and propranolol (30%) result during coadministration with flecainide. Propranolol, quinidine, and amiodarone may increase flecainide serum concentrations. Five to 7 days of dosing may be required to reach a steady state in some patients.

DOSAGE AND ADMINISTRATION (see Table 37-4). The starting dose is 100 mg every 12 hours, increased in increments of 50 mg twice daily, no sooner than every 3 to 4 days, until efficacy is achieved or an adverse effect is noted or to a maximum of 400 mg/day. Cardiac rhythm and QRS duration should be monitored after dose changes.

INDICATIONS. Flecainide is indicated for the treatment of life-threatening ventricular tachyarrhythmias, SVTs, and paroxysmal atrial fibrillation. Preliminary data suggest that it might be useful in catecholaminergic polymorphic VT (see Chap. 9). Some experts have suggested that therapy should begin in the hospital while the ECG is being monitored because of the possibility of proarrhythmic events (see later). Serum concentration should not exceed 1.0 mg/mL. Flecainide is particularly effective in almost totally suppressing PVCs and short runs of nonsustained VT. As with other class I antiarrhythmic drugs, there are no data from controlled studies to indicate that the drug favorably affects survival or sudden cardiac death, and data from the CAST study have indicated increased mortality in patients with coronary artery disease. Flecainide produces a use-dependent prolongation of VT cycle length that can improve hemodynamic tolerance. Flecainide is also useful in various SVTs, such as atrial tachycardia (AT), flutter, and atrial fibrillation (including oral loading to terminate episodes acutely). When it is administered chronically, isoproterenol can reverse some of these effects. It is important to slow the ventricular rate before treatment of atrial fibrillation with flecainide to avoid 1:1 AV conduction. Flecainide has been used to treat fetal arrhythmias and arrhythmias in children. Flecainide administration may produce ST elevation in lead V_1 characteristic of Brugada syndrome (see Chap. 9) and has been used as a diagnostic tool in patients suspected of having this disorder.[10]

ADVERSE EFFECTS. Proarrhythmic effects are some of the most important adverse effects of flecainide. Its marked slowing of conduction precludes its use in patients with second-degree AV block without a pacemaker and warrants cautious administration in patients with intraventricular conduction disorders. Worsening of existing ventricular arrhythmias or onset of new ventricular arrhythmias can occur in 5% to 30% of patients, especially in patients with preexisting sustained VT, cardiac decompensation, and higher doses of the drug. Failure of the flecainide-related arrhythmia to respond to therapy, including electrical cardioversion-defibrillation, may result in mortality as high as 10% in patients who develop proarrhythmic events. Negative inotropic effects can cause or worsen heart failure. Patients with sinus node dysfunction may experience sinus arrest, and those with pacemakers may develop an increase in pacing threshold. In the CAST study, patients treated with flecainide had 5.1% mortality or nonfatal cardiac arrest compared with 2.3% in the placebo group during 10 months. Mortality was highest in those with non–Q-wave infarction, frequent PVCs, and faster heart rates, raising the possibility of drug interaction with ischemia and electrical instability. Exercise can amplify the conduction slowing in the ventricle produced by flecainide and in some cases can precipitate a proarrhythmic response. Therefore, exercise testing has been recommended to screen for proarrhythmia. Central nervous system complaints, including confusion and irritability, represent the most frequent noncardiac adverse effects. The safety of flecainide during pregnancy has not been determined, although, as noted previously, it is occasionally used to treat fetal arrhythmias. It is concentrated in breast milk to a level 2.5- to 4-fold higher than in plasma.

Propafenone

Propafenone has been approved by the FDA for treatment of patients with life-threatening ventricular tachyarrhythmias as well as atrial fibrillation.[6]

Electrophysiologic Actions (see Tables 37-1, 37-2, 37-3, and 37-5). Propafenone blocks the fast sodium current in a use-dependent manner in Purkinje fibers and to a lesser degree in ventricular muscle. Use-dependent effects contribute to its ability to terminate atrial fibrillation. The dissociation constant from the receptor is slow, similar to that of flecainide. Effects are greater in ischemic than in normal tissue and at reduced membrane potentials. Propafenone decreases excitability and suppresses spontaneous automaticity and triggered activity. The drug is a weak blocker of I_{Kr} and beta-adrenergic receptors. Although ventricular refractoriness increases, conduction slowing is the major effect. Propafenone has several active metabolites that exert electrophysiologic effects. It depresses sinus node automaticity, and A-H, H-V, PR, and QRS intervals increase, as do refractory periods of the atria, ventricles, AV node, and accessory pathways. The QT interval increases only as a function of increased QRS duration.

Hemodynamic Effects. Propafenone and 5-hydroxypropafenone exhibit negative inotropic properties at high concentrations. In patients with left ventricular ejection fractions exceeding 40%, the negative inotropic effects are well tolerated, but patients with preexisting left ventricular dysfunction and congestive heart failure may have symptomatic worsening of their hemodynamic status.

Pharmacokinetics (see Table 37-4). With more than 95% of the drug absorbed, propafenone's maximum plasma concentration occurs in 2 to 3 hours. Systemic bioavailability is dose dependent and ranges from 3% to 40% because of variable presystemic clearance. Bioavailability increases as the dose increases, and plasma concentration is therefore nonlinear. A 3-fold increase in dosage (300 to 900 mg/day) results in a 10-fold increase in plasma concentration, presumably because of saturation of hepatic metabolic mechanisms. Propafenone is 97% bound to alpha$_1$-acid glycoprotein, with an elimination half-life of 5 to 8 hours. Maximum therapeutic effects occur at serum concentrations of 0.2 to 1.5 mg/mL. Marked interpatient variability of pharmacokinetics and pharmacodynamics may be the result of genetically determined differences in metabolism (see Chap. 10). About 7% of the population are poor metabolizers, who have an elimination half-life of 15 to 20 hours for the parent compound and almost no 5-hydroxypropafenone. The (+)-enantiomer provides nonspecific beta-adrenergic receptor blockade with 2.5% to 5% of the potency of propranolol, but because plasma propafenone concentrations may be 50 times or more higher than propranolol levels, these beta-blocking properties may be relevant. Poor metabolizers have a greater beta-adrenergic receptor blocking effect than extensive metabolizers do.

DOSAGE AND ADMINISTRATION (see Table 37-4). Most patients respond to oral doses of 150 to 300 mg every 8 hours, not exceeding 1200 mg/day. Doses are similar for patients of both metabolizing phenotypes. A sustained-release form is available for treatment of atrial fibrillation; dosing is 225 to 425 mg twice daily. Concomitant food administration increases bioavailability, as does hepatic dysfunction. No good correlation between plasma propafenone concentration and arrhythmia suppression has been shown. Doses should not be increased more often than every 3 to 4 days. Propafenone increases plasma concentrations of warfarin, digoxin, and metoprolol.

INDICATIONS. Propafenone is indicated for the treatment of paroxysmal SVT, atrial fibrillation, and life-threatening ventricular tachyarrhythmias and effectively suppresses spontaneous PVCs and nonsustained and sustained VT. Acute termination of atrial fibrillation episodes occurred with a single 600-mg oral dose of propafenone in 76% of patients given the drug (twice the rate of those given placebo). It has been used effectively in the pediatric age group. Propafenone increases the pacing threshold but minimally affects the defibrillation threshold. Sinus rate during exercise is reduced. Propafenone use is associated with higher mortality in cardiac arrest survivors than with use of an implantable defibrillator.

ADVERSE EFFECTS. Minor noncardiac effects occur in about 15% of patients, with dizziness, disturbances in taste, and blurred vision the most common and gastrointestinal side effects next. Exacerbation of bronchospastic lung disease can occur because of mild beta-blocking effects. Cardiovascular side effects occur in 10% to 15% of patients, including AV block, sinus node depression, and worsening of heart failure. Proarrhythmic responses, which occur more often in patients with a history of sustained VT and decreased ejection fractions, appear less commonly than with flecainide (approximately 5%). The applicability of data from the CAST study about flecainide to propafenone is not clear, but limiting propafenone's application in a manner similar to that of other class IC drugs seems prudent. Its beta-blocking actions may make it different, however. The safety of propafenone administration during pregnancy has not been established (class C).

Moricizine

As of December 31, 2007, moricizine (Ethmozine)[11] is no longer available in the United States.

CLASS II AGENTS

Beta Adrenoceptor Blocking Agents

Although many beta adrenoceptor blocking drugs have been approved for use in the United States, metoprolol, carvedilol, atenolol, propranolol, and esmolol have been most widely used to treat supraventricular and ventricular arrhythmias. Acebutolol, nadolol, timolol, betaxolol, pindolol, and bisoprolol have been less extensively used for treatment of arrhythmias. Metoprolol, atenolol, carvedilol, atenolol, timolol, and propranolol decrease overall mortality and sudden death after myocardial infarction (see Chap. 41). It is generally considered that beta blockers possess class effects and that, titrated to the proper dose, all can be used effectively to treat cardiac arrhythmias, hypertension, or other disorders. However, differences in pharmacokinetic or pharmacodynamic properties that confer safety, reduce adverse effects, or affect dosing intervals or drug interactions influence the choice of agent. Also, some beta blockers, such as sotalol, pindolol, and carvedilol, exert unique actions.[12]

Beta receptors can be separated into those that affect predominantly the heart ($beta_1$) and those that affect predominantly blood vessels and the bronchi ($beta_2$). In low doses, selective beta blockers can block $beta_1$ receptors more than they block $beta_2$ receptors and might be preferable for treatment of patients with pulmonary or peripheral vascular diseases. In high doses, the "selective" $beta_1$ blockers also block $beta_2$ receptors. Carvedilol also exerts alpha-blocking effects and is used primarily in patients with heart failure (see Chaps. 26 to 28).

Some beta blockers exert intrinsic sympathomimetic activity; that is, they slightly activate the beta receptor. These drugs appear to be as efficacious as beta blockers without intrinsic sympathomimetic actions and may cause less slowing of heart rate at rest and less prolongation of AV nodal conduction time. They have been shown to induce less depression of left ventricular function than beta blockers without intrinsic sympathomimetic activity. Beta blockers without intrinsic sympathomimetic activity have been shown to reduce mortality in patients after myocardial infarction, with nonselective agents possibly conferring slightly greater benefit (**Fig. 37-1**; see Chaps. 54 and 55).

The following discussion focuses on the use of propranolol as a prototypical antiarrhythmic agent but is generally applicable to other beta blockers.

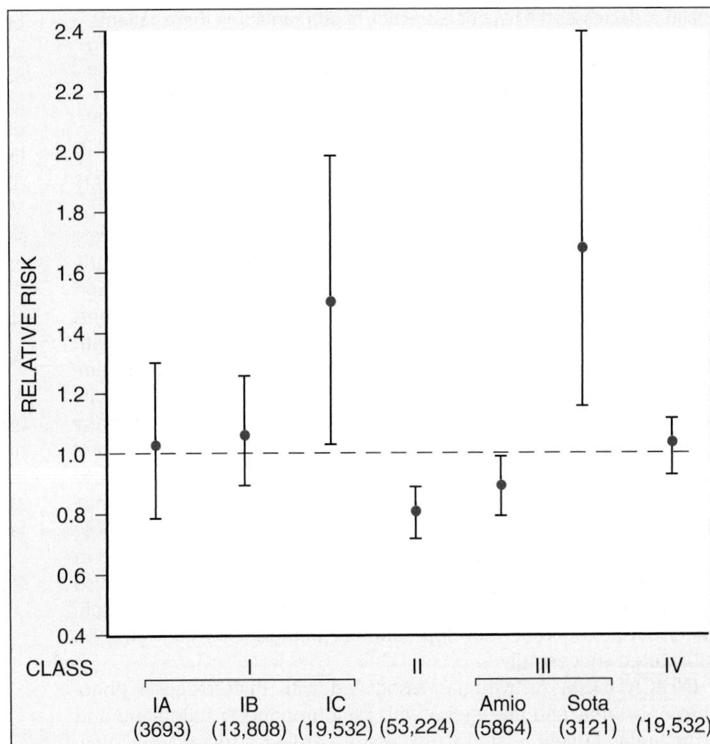

FIGURE 37-1 Meta-analytical data from randomized clinical trials of antiarrhythmic drugs in survivors of acute myocardial infarction. The relative risk is compared with placebo therapy (mean and 95% confidence interval) for death during therapy with various electrophysiologic classes of compounds. Class I agents, particularly IC, and sotalol increase mortality, whereas beta blockers and amiodarone decrease mortality. Numbers under each drug class refer to number of patients involved in the trials. Amio = amiodarone; Sota = sotalol. *(Modified from Teo KK, Yusuf S: In Singh BN, Dzau VJ, Vanhoutte PM, Woosley RL [eds]: Cardiovascular Pharmacology and Therapeutics. New York, Churchill Livingstone, 1994, pp 631-643; and Waldo AL, Camm AJ, deRuyter H, et al: Effect of d-sotalol on mortality in patients with left ventricular dysfunction after recent and remote myocardial infarction: Lancet 348:7, 1996.)*

Electrophysiologic Actions (see Tables 37-1, 37-2, 37-3, and 37-5)**.** Beta blockers exert an electrophysiologic action by competitively inhibiting catecholamine binding at beta adrenoceptor sites, an effect almost entirely the result of the (–)-levorotatory stereoisomer, or by their quinidine-like or direct membrane-stabilizing action. The latter is a local anesthetic effect that depresses I_{Na} and membrane responsiveness in cardiac Purkinje fibers, occurs at concentrations generally 10 times that necessary to produce beta blockade, and most likely plays an insignificant antiarrhythmic role. Thus, beta blockers exert their major effects in cells most actively stimulated by adrenergic actions. At a beta-blocking concentration, propranolol slows spontaneous automaticity in the sinus node or in Purkinje fibers that are being stimulated by adrenergic tone, producing I_f block (see Chap. 35). Beta blockers also block $I_{Ca.L}$ stimulated by beta agonists. In the absence of adrenergic stimulation, only high concentrations of propranolol slow normal automaticity in Purkinje fibers, probably by a direct membrane action.

Concentrations that cause beta receptor blockade but no local anesthetic effects do not alter the normal resting membrane potential, maximum diastolic potential amplitude, $\dot{V}max$, repolarization, or refractoriness of atrial, Purkinje, or ventricular muscle cells in the absence of catecholamine stimulation. However, in the presence of isoproterenol, a relatively pure beta receptor stimulator, beta blockers reverse isoproterenol's accelerating effects on repolarization. Propranolol reduces the amplitude of digitalis-induced delayed afterdepolarizations and suppresses triggered activity in Purkinje fibers.

Concentrations exceeding 3 mg/mL are required to depress $\dot{V}max$ action potential amplitude, membrane responsiveness, and conduction in normal atrial, ventricular, and Purkinje fibers without altering resting membrane potential. These effects probably result from depression of I_{Na}. Long-term administration of propranolol may lengthen APD. Like the effects of lidocaine, acceleration of repolarization of Purkinje fibers is most marked in areas of the ventricular conduction system in which the APD is greatest. At least one beta blocker, sotalol, markedly increases the time course of repolarization in Purkinje fibers and ventricular muscle.

Propranolol slows the sinus discharge rate in humans by 10% to 20%, although severe bradycardia occasionally results if the heart is particularly dependent on sympathetic tone or if sinus node dysfunction is present. The PR interval lengthens, as do AV nodal conduction time and AV nodal effective and functional refractory periods (at a constant heart rate), but refractoriness and conduction in the normal His-Purkinje system remain unchanged, even after high doses of propranolol. Therefore, therapeutic doses of propranolol in humans do not exert a direct depressant or "quinidine-like" action but influence cardiac electrophysiology through a beta-blocking action. Beta blockers do not affect conduction or repolarization in normal ventricular muscle, as evidenced by their lack of effect on the QRS complex and QT interval, respectively.

Because administration of beta blockers that do not have direct membrane action prevents many arrhythmias resulting from activation of the autonomic nervous system, it is thought that the beta-blocking action is responsible for their antiarrhythmic effects. Nevertheless, the possible importance of the direct membrane effect of some of these drugs cannot be discounted totally because beta blockers with direct membrane actions can affect transmembrane potentials of diseased cardiac fibers at much lower concentrations than are needed to affect normal fibers directly. However, indirect actions on arrhythmogenic effects of ischemia are probably most important. Beta blockers reduce myocardial injury during experimental cardiopulmonary resuscitation.

Hemodynamic Effects. Beta blockers exert negative inotropic effects and can precipitate or worsen heart failure. However, beta blockers clearly improve survival in patients with heart failure (see Chap. 33). By blocking beta receptors, these drugs may allow unopposed alpha-adrenergic effects to produce peripheral vasoconstriction and exacerbate coronary artery spasm or pain from peripheral vascular disease in some patients.

Pharmacokinetics (see Table 37-4)**.** Although various types of beta blockers exert similar pharmacologic effects, their pharmacokinetics differ substantially. Propranolol is almost 100% absorbed, but the effects of first-pass hepatic metabolism reduce bioavailability to about 30% and produce significant interpatient variability of plasma concentration for a given dose. Reduction in hepatic blood flow, as in patients with heart failure, decreases the hepatic extraction of propranolol; in these patients, propranolol may further decrease its own elimination rate by reducing cardiac output and hepatic blood flow. Beta blockers eliminated by the kidney tend to have longer half-lives and exhibit less interpatient variability of drug concentration than do beta blockers metabolized by the liver.

DOSAGE AND ADMINISTRATION (see Table 37-4). The appropriate dose of propranolol is best determined by a measure of the patient's physiologic response, such as changes in resting heart rate or prevention of exercise-induced tachycardia, because wide individual differences exist between the observed physiologic effect and plasma concentration. For example, intravenous dosing is best achieved by titration of the dose to a clinical effect, beginning with doses of 0.25 to 0.50 mg, increasing to 1.0 mg if necessary, and administering doses every 5 minutes until either a desired effect or toxicity is produced or a total of 0.15 to 0.20 mg/kg has been given. In many cases, the short-acting effects of esmolol are preferred. Orally, propranolol is given in four divided doses, usually ranging from 40 to 160 mg/day to more than 1 g/day. Some beta blockers, such as carvedilol and pindolol, need to be given twice daily; many are available as once-daily long-acting preparations. In general, if one agent in adequate doses proves to be ineffective, other beta blockers are also ineffective. Conversely, if one agent produces the desired physiologic effect but a side effect develops, another beta blocker can often be substituted successfully.

INDICATIONS. Arrhythmias associated with thyrotoxicosis, pheochromocytoma, and anesthesia with cyclopropane or halothane and arrhythmias largely related to excessive cardiac adrenergic stimulation, such as those initiated by exercise, emotion, or cocaine, often respond to beta blocker therapy. Beta-blocking drugs usually do not convert chronic atrial flutter or atrial fibrillation to normal sinus rhythm but may do so if the arrhythmia is of recent onset and in patients who have recently undergone cardiac surgery. The atrial rate during atrial flutter or fibrillation is not changed, but the ventricular response decreases because beta blockade prolongs AV nodal conduction time and refractoriness. Esmolol can be used intravenously for rapid control of heart rate. For reentrant SVTs using the AV node as one of the reentrant pathways, such as AVNRT and orthodromic reciprocating tachycardias in the Wolff-Parkinson-White syndrome or inappropriate sinus tachycardia, or for ATs, beta blockers can slow or terminate the tachycardia and can be used prophylactically to prevent a recurrence. Combining beta blockers with digitalis, quinidine, or various other agents may be effective when the beta blocker as a single agent fails. Metoprolol and esmolol may be useful in patients with multifocal AT. These agents must be used with caution in this arrhythmia, however, because a common setting for it is advanced lung disease, often with a bronchospastic component.

Beta blockers can be effective for digitalis-induced arrhythmias such as AT, nonparoxysmal AV junctional tachycardia, PVCs, or VT. If a significant degree of AV block is present during a digitalis-induced arrhythmia, lidocaine or phenytoin may be preferable to propranolol. Beta blockers can also be useful to treat ventricular arrhythmias associated with the prolonged QT interval syndrome (see Chap. 9) and with mitral valve prolapse (see Chap. 66). For patients with ischemic heart disease, beta blockers generally do not prevent episodes of recurrent monomorphic VT that occur in the absence of acute ischemia. It is well accepted that several beta blockers reduce the incidence of overall death and sudden cardiac death after myocardial infarction (see Chaps. 54 and 55). The mechanism of this reduction in mortality is not entirely clear and may be related to reduction of the extent of ischemic damage, autonomic effects, a direct antiarrhythmic effect, or combinations of these factors. Beta blockers may have been protective against proarrhythmic responses in CAST.

ADVERSE EFFECTS. Adverse cardiovascular effects from beta blockers include unacceptable hypotension, bradycardia, and congestive heart failure. The bradycardia may be caused by sinus slowing or AV block. Sudden withdrawal of propranolol in patients with angina pectoris can precipitate or worsen angina and cardiac arrhythmias and cause an acute myocardial infarction, possibly because of heightened sensitivity to beta agonists caused by previous beta blockade (receptor upregulation). Heightened sensitivity may begin several days after cessation of beta blocker therapy and can last 5 or 6 days. Other adverse effects of beta blockers include worsening of asthma or chronic obstructive pulmonary disease, intermittent claudication, Raynaud phenomenon, mental depression, increased risk of hypoglycemia in insulin-dependent diabetic patients, easy fatigability, disturbingly vivid dreams or insomnia, and impaired sexual function. Many of these side effects were noted less frequently with use of $beta_1$-selective agents, but even so-called cardioselective beta blockers can exacerbate asthma or diabetic control in individual patients.

CLASS III AGENTS.

Amiodarone

Amiodarone is a benzofuran derivative approved by the FDA for the treatment of patients with life-threatening ventricular tachyarrhythmias when other drugs are ineffective or are not tolerated. Dronedarone, a noniodinated derivative of amiodarone, has recently been approved for use in the United States to treat patients with atrial fibrillation (see later).[13]

Electrophysiologic Actions (see Tables 37-1, 37-2, 37-3, and 37-5). When it is chronically given orally, amiodarone prolongs APD and refractoriness of all cardiac fibers without affecting resting membrane potential (see Chap. 35). When acute effects are evaluated, amiodarone and its metabolite, desethylamiodarone, prolong the APD of ventricular muscle but shorten the APD of Purkinje fibers. Injected into the sinus and AV node arteries, amiodarone reduces sinus and junctional discharge rates and prolongs AV nodal conduction time. It depresses $\dot{V}max$ in ventricular muscle in a rate- or use-dependent manner by blocking of inactivated sodium channels, an effect that is accentuated by depolarized and reduced by hyperpolarized membrane potentials. Amiodarone depresses conduction at fast rates more than at slow rates (use dependence), not only by depressing $\dot{V}max$ but also by increasing resistance to passive current flow. It does not prolong repolarization more at slow than at fast rates (i.e., does not demonstrate reverse use dependence) but does exert time-dependent effects on refractoriness, which may in part explain the high antiarrhythmic efficacy and low incidence of torsades de pointes.

Desethylamiodarone has relatively greater effects on fast channel tissue and probably contributes notably to antiarrhythmic efficacy. The delay in building up adequate concentrations of this metabolite may in part explain the delay in amiodarone's antiarrhythmic action.

Amiodarone noncompetitively antagonizes alpha and beta receptors and blocks conversion of thyroxine (T_4) to triiodothyronine (T_3), which may account for some of its electrophysiologic effects. Amiodarone exhibits slow channel–blocking effects, and chronic oral therapy has been found to slow the spontaneous sinus node discharge rate in anesthetized dogs even after pretreatment with propranolol and atropine. With oral administration, it slows the sinus rate by 20% to 30% and prolongs the QT interval, at times changing the contour of the T wave and producing U waves.

ERPs of all cardiac tissues are prolonged. His-Purkinje conduction time increases and QRS duration lengthens, especially at fast rates. Amiodarone given intravenously modestly prolongs the refractory period of atrial and ventricular muscle. The PR interval and AV nodal conduction time lengthen. The duration of the QRS complex lengthens at increased rates but less than after oral amiodarone. Thus, far less increase in prolongation of conduction time (except for the AV node), duration of repolarization, and refractoriness occurs after intravenous administration compared with the oral route. Considering these actions, it is clear that amiodarone has class I (blocks I_{Na}), class II (antiadrenergic), and class IV (blocks $I_{Ca.L}$) actions in addition to its class III effects (blocks I_K). Amiodarone's actions approximate those of a theoretically ideal drug that exhibits use-dependent Na^+ channel blockade with fast diastolic recovery from block and use-dependent prolongation of APD. It does not increase and may decrease QT dispersion. Catecholamines can partially reverse some of the effects of amiodarone.

Hemodynamic Effects. Amiodarone is a peripheral and coronary vasodilator. When it is administered intravenously (150 mg during 10 minutes, then 1-mg/min infusion), amiodarone decreases heart rate, systemic vascular resistance, left ventricular contractile force, and left ventricular dP/dt. Oral doses of amiodarone sufficient to control cardiac arrhythmias do not depress the left ventricular ejection fraction, even in patients with reduced ejection fractions, and ejection fraction and cardiac output may increase slightly. However, because of antiadrenergic actions of amiodarone and because it does exert some negative inotropic action, it should be given cautiously, particularly intravenously, to patients with marginal cardiac compensation.

PHARMACOKINETICS (see Table 37-4). Amiodarone is slowly, variably, and incompletely absorbed, with a systemic bioavailability of 35% to 65%. Plasma concentrations peak 3 to 7 hours after a single oral dose. There is a minimal first-pass effect, indicating little hepatic extraction. Elimination is by hepatic excretion into bile with some enterohepatic recirculation. Extensive hepatic metabolism occurs with desethylamiodarone as a major metabolite. Both accumulate extensively in the liver, lung, fat, "blue" skin, and other tissues. Myocardium develops a concentration 10 to 50 times that found in the plasma. Plasma clearance of amiodarone is low, and renal excretion is negligible. Doses need not be reduced in patients with renal disease. Amiodarone and desethylamiodarone are not dialyzable. The volume of distribution is large but variable, averaging 60 liter/kg. Amiodarone is highly protein bound (96%), crosses the placenta (10% to 50%), and is found in breast milk.

The onset of action after intravenous administration is generally within 1 to 2 hours. After oral administration, the onset of action may require 2 to 3 days, often 1 to 3 weeks, and, on occasion, even longer. Loading doses reduce this time interval. Plasma concentrations relate well to oral doses during chronic treatment, averaging about 0.5 mg/mL for each 100 mg/day at doses between 100 and 600 mg/day. Elimination half-life is multiphasic, with an initial 50% reduction in plasma concentration 3 to 10 days after cessation of drug ingestion (probably representing elimination from well-perfused tissues), followed by a terminal half-life of 26 to 107 days (mean, 53 days), with most patients in the 40- to 55-day range. To achieve steady state without a loading dose takes about 265 days. Interpatient variability of these pharmacokinetic parameters mandates close monitoring of the patient. Therapeutic serum concentrations range from 1 to 2.5 mg/mL. Greater suppression of arrhythmias may occur up to 3.5 mg/mL, but the risk of side effects increases.

DOSAGE AND ADMINISTRATION (see Table 37-4). An optimal dosing schedule for all patients has not been achieved. One recommended approach is to treat with 800 to 1200 mg/day for 1 to 3 weeks, reduced to 400 mg/day for the next several weeks and finally, after 2 to 3 months of treatment, a maintenance dose of 300 mg or less per day. Maintenance drug can be given once or twice daily and should be titrated to the lowest effective dose to minimize the occurrence of side effects. Doses as low as 100 mg/day can be effective in some patients. Regimens must be individualized for a given patient and clinical situation. Amiodarone can be administered intravenously to achieve more rapid loading and effect in emergencies, at initial doses of 15 mg/min for 10 minutes, followed by 1 mg/min for 6 hours, and then 0.5 mg/min for the remaining 18 hours and for the next several days, as necessary. Supplemental infusions of 150 mg during 10 minutes can be used for breakthrough VT or VF. Intravenous infusions can be continued safely for 2 to 3 weeks. Intravenous amiodarone is generally well tolerated, even in patients with left ventricular dysfunction. Patients with depressed ejection fractions should receive intravenous amiodarone with great caution because of hypotension. High-dose oral loading (800 to 2000 mg/day to maintain trough serum concentrations of 2 to 3 mg/mL) may suppress ventricular arrhythmias in 1 to 2 days.

INDICATIONS. Amiodarone has been used to suppress a wide spectrum of supraventricular and ventricular tachyarrhythmias in utero, in adults, and in children, including AV node and AV entry, junctional tachycardia, atrial flutter and fibrillation, VT and VF associated with coronary artery disease, and hypertrophic cardiomyopathy. Success rates vary widely, depending on the population of patients, arrhythmia, underlying heart disease, length of follow-up, definition and determination of success, and other factors. In general, however, amiodarone's efficacy equals or exceeds that of all other antiarrhythmic agents and may be in the range of 60% to 80% for most supraventricular tachyarrhythmias and 40% to 60% for ventricular tachyarrhythmias. Amiodarone may be useful in improving survival in patients with hypertrophic cardiomyopathy, nonischemic dilated cardiomyopathy, asymptomatic ventricular arrhythmias after myocardial infarction, and ventricular tachyarrhythmia during and after resuscitation from cardiac arrest. Amiodarone given before open heart surgery as well as postoperatively has been shown to decrease the incidence of postoperative atrial fibrillation. Amiodarone is superior to class I antiarrhythmic agents and sotalol in maintaining sinus rhythm in patients with recurrent atrial fibrillation.

Patients who have an ICD receive fewer shocks if they are treated with amiodarone compared with conventional drugs.[14] Amiodarone has little effect on pacing threshold but typically increases the electrical defibrillation threshold slightly.

Several prospective, randomized, controlled trials and a meta-analysis have demonstrated improved survival with amiodarone therapy compared with placebo; however, amiodarone has been proved to result in inferior survival compared with ICD therapy, and in the SCD-HeFT population (class II or III heart failure; ejection fraction, 35%), survival of amiodarone-treated patients was no different from that of those treated with placebo.[15] The drug may still be used adjunctively in ICD-treated patients to decrease the frequency of shocks from VT and VF episodes or to control supraventricular tachyarrhythmias that elicit device therapy (see Chap. 39). The drug can slow the rate of spontaneous VT episodes beneath the detection rate of the device; careful patient assessment and, occasionally, device reprogramming and testing are necessary.

Because of the serious nature of the arrhythmias being treated, the unusual pharmacokinetics of the drug, and its adverse effects, amiodarone therapy should generally be started with the patient hospitalized and monitored for at least several days. Combining other antiarrhythmic agents with amiodarone may improve efficacy in some patients.

ADVERSE EFFECTS. Adverse effects are reported by about 75% of patients treated with amiodarone for 5 years, but these compel stopping of the drug in 18% to 37%.[16] The most frequent side effects requiring drug discontinuation involve pulmonary and gastrointestinal complaints. Most adverse effects are reversible with dose reduction or cessation of treatment. Adverse effects are more common when therapy is continued in the long term and at higher doses. Of the noncardiac adverse reactions, pulmonary toxicity is the most serious; in one study, it occurred in 33 of 573 patients between 6 days and 60 months of treatment, with three deaths. The mechanism is unclear but may involve a hypersensitivity reaction, widespread phospholipidosis, or both. Dyspnea, nonproductive cough, and fever are common symptoms, with crackles on examination, hypoxia, abnormal gallium scan, reduced diffusion capacity, and radiographic evidence of pulmonary infiltrates. Amiodarone must be discontinued if such pulmonary inflammatory changes occur. Corticosteroids can be tried, but no controlled studies have been done to support their use. A 10% mortality results in patients with pulmonary inflammatory changes, often in patients with unrecognized pulmonary involvement that is allowed to progress. Chest radiography and pulmonary function testing, including carbon monoxide diffusion capacity (DLCO), at 3-month intervals for the first year and then twice a year for several years has been recommended. At maintenance doses less than 300 mg/day, pulmonary toxicity is uncommon but can occur. Advanced age, high drug maintenance dose, and reduced predrug diffusion capacity are risk factors for development of pulmonary toxicity. An unchanged DLCO on therapy may be a negative predictor of pulmonary toxicity.

Although asymptomatic elevations of liver enzyme levels are found in most patients, the drug is not stopped unless values exceed two or three times normal in a patient with initially normal values. Cirrhosis occurs uncommonly but may be fatal. Neurologic dysfunction, photosensitivity (perhaps minimized by sunscreens), bluish skin discoloration, gastroenterologic disturbances, and hyperthyroidism (1% to 2%) or hypothyroidism (2% to 4%) can occur. Amiodarone appears to inhibit the peripheral conversion of T_4 to T_3 so that chemical changes result; these are characterized by a slight increase in T_4, reverse T_3, and thyroid-stimulating hormone (TSH) and a slight decrease in T_3 levels. Reverse T_3 concentration has been used as an index of drug efficacy. During hypothyroidism, the TSH level increases greatly, whereas the level of T_3 increases in hyperthyroidism. Thyroid function tests should be performed approximately every 3 months for the first year while amiodarone is taken and once or twice yearly thereafter, sooner if symptoms develop that are consistent with thyroid dysfunction. Corneal microdeposits occur in almost 100% of adults receiving the drug longer than 6 months. More serious ocular reactions, including optic neuritis and atrophy with visual loss, have been reported but are rare, and causation by amiodarone has not been established.

Cardiac side effects include symptomatic bradycardias in about 2% of patients; worsening of ventricular tachyarrhythmias, with occasional development of torsades de pointes in 1% to 2%, possibly higher in women; and worsening of congestive heart failure in 2%. Possibly because of interactions with anesthetics, complications after open heart surgery, including pulmonary dysfunction, hypotension, severe bradycardia, hepatic dysfunction, and low cardiac output, have been noted by some investigators.

In general, the lowest possible maintenance dose of amiodarone that is still effective should be used to avoid significant adverse effects. Many supraventricular arrhythmias can be successfully managed with daily dosages of 200 mg or less, whereas ventricular arrhythmias generally require higher doses. Adverse effects are uncommon at dosages of 200 mg/day or less but still occur. Because of potential toxicity in various organ systems, special multidisciplinary amiodarone clinics have been used by some to attempt to prevent adverse outcomes when the drug is used.

Important interactions with other drugs occur, and when given concomitantly with amiodarone, the doses of warfarin, digoxin, and other antiarrhythmic drugs should be reduced by one third to one half and the patient observed closely. Drugs with synergistic actions, such as beta blockers or calcium channel blockers, must be given cautiously. Amiodarone's safety during pregnancy has not been established, and it should be used in the pregnant patient only if no alternatives exist.

Dronedarone

Dronedarone has recently been approved by the FDA to facilitate maintenance of sinus rhythm in patients with atrial flutter and fibrillation.[17]

Electrophysiologic Actions (see Tables 37-1, 37-2, 37-3, and 37-5). Like amiodarone, dronedarone alters activity of multiple cardiac ion channels. It is a more potent blocker of the rapid sodium current than amiodarone and exhibits similar effects on L-type calcium current. Dronedarone's blockade of both rapid and slow components of the delayed rectifier potassium current is likewise similar to that of amiodarone, whereas its effect on the atrial acetylcholine-activated potassium current and antiadrenergic effects (via noncompetitive binding) are significantly more potent than amiodarone's. Sinus node function is depressed to a minor degree. Pacing and defibrillation thresholds are slightly increased.

Hemodynamic Effects. Dronedarone has little effect on cardiac performance except in patients with compromised ventricular systolic function and should not be used in patients with clinical signs of heart failure.

Pharmacokinetics (see Table 37-4). Dronedarone is 70% to 90% absorbed after oral administration, with peak plasma concentrations in 3 to 4 hours; absorption is enhanced by food. Unlike amiodarone's very long half-life, dronedarone's elimination half-life is 13 to 19 hours, with 85% of the drug being excreted unchanged in feces and the remainder in urine. Dronedarone is metabolized by and slightly inhibits the activity of CYP3A4 (as well as CYP2D6) and should not be used in conjunction with other agents that strongly inhibit these enzyme systems.

DOSAGE AND ADMINISTRATION (see Table 37-4). The standard recommended dose is 400 mg every 12 hours with food. There is currently no parenteral form.

INDICATIONS. Dronedarone is indicated to facilitate cardioversion of atrial flutter or fibrillation or to maintain sinus rhythm after restoration of sinus rhythm. It is slightly less effective than amiodarone in these regards. In the Antiarrhythmic Trial with Dronedarone in Moderate-to-Severe Congestive Heart Failure Evaluating Morbidity Decrease (ANDROMEDA) study, dronedarone-treated patients had a mortality rate more than twice that of placebo (8.1% versus 3.8%).[18] Thus, the medication should not be used in patients with current or recent episodes of clinical heart failure.

ADVERSE EFFECTS. A transient, predictable increase in serum creatinine, without adversely affecting actual glomerular filtration or other measures of renal function, occurs with standard dosing and is not a reason to alter dose or to discontinue the drug. Patients with New York Heart Association Class III or IV heart failure should not be given the drug because these patients had a higher mortality when taking dronedarone in one study. Patients with severe liver dysfunction should not receive the drug. The QT interval predictably is prolonged, but proarrhythmic effects from this or other mechanisms are rare (although sinus bradycardia is sometimes seen). Rash, photosensitivity, nausea, diarrhea, and asthenia have occurred among treated patients in higher frequency than in controls. The absence of the iodine molecule appears to account for the low prevalence of lung and thyroid toxicity among dronedarone-treated patients compared with those taking amiodarone. Dronedarone should not be used during pregnancy (category X, evidence or risk of fetal harm) and is possibly unsafe for breast feeding.

Bretylium Tosylate

Bretylium is a quaternary ammonium compound that had been used parenterally in patients with life-threatening ventricular tachyarrhythmias[11] (see Chap. 41). It is no longer manufactured or available in the United States.

Sotalol

Sotalol is a nonspecific beta adrenoceptor blocker without intrinsic sympathomimetic activity that prolongs repolarization. It is approved by the FDA to treat patients with life-threatening ventricular tachyarrhythmias and those with atrial fibrillation.[13]

Electrophysiologic Actions (see Tables 37-1, 37-2, 37-3, and 37-5). Both *d* and *l* isomers have similar effects on prolonging repolarization, whereas the *l* isomer is responsible for almost all the beta-blocking activity. Sotalol does not block alpha adrenoceptors and does not block the sodium channel (no membrane-stabilizing effects) but does prolong atrial and ventricular repolarization times by reducing I_{Kr}, thus prolonging the plateau of the action potential. Action potential prolongation is greater at slower rates (reverse use dependence). Resting membrane potential, action potential amplitude, and $\dot{V}max$ are not significantly altered. Sotalol prolongs atrial and ventricular refractoriness, A-H and QT intervals, and sinus cycle length (see Chap. 39).

Hemodynamics. Sotalol exerts a negative inotropic effect only through its beta-blocking action. It can increase the strength of contraction by prolonging repolarization, which occurs maximally at slow heart rates. In patients with reduced cardiac function, sotalol can decrease cardiac index, increase filling pressure, and precipitate overt heart failure. Therefore, it must be used cautiously in patients with marginal cardiac compensation but is well tolerated in patients with normal cardiac function.

Pharmacokinetics (see Table 37-4). Sotalol is completely absorbed and not metabolized, making it 90% to 100% bioavailable. It is not bound to plasma proteins, is excreted unchanged primarily by the kidneys, and has an elimination half-life of 10 to 15 hours. Peak plasma concentrations occur 2.5 to 4 hours after oral ingestion, with a steady state attained after five or six doses. Over the dose range of 160 to 640 mg, sotalol displays dose proportionality with plasma concentration (usually in the range of 2.5 μg/mL). The dose must be reduced in patients with renal disease. The beta-blocking effect is half-maximal at 80 mg/day and maximal at 320 mg/day. Significant beta-blocking action occurs at 160 mg/day.

DOSAGE (see Table 37-4). The typical oral dose is 80 to 160 mg every 12 hours, allowing 2 to 3 days between dose adjustments to attain a steady state and to monitor the ECG for arrhythmias and QT prolongation. Doses exceeding 320 mg/day can be used in patients when the potential benefits outweigh the risk of proarrhythmia.

INDICATIONS. Approved by the FDA to treat patients with ventricular tachyarrhythmias and atrial fibrillation, sotalol is also useful to prevent recurrence of a wide variety of SVTs, including atrial flutter, AT, AV node reentry, and AV reentry (see Chap. 39). It also slows the ventricular response to atrial tachyarrhythmias. It appears to be more effective than conventional antiarrhythmic drugs and may be comparable to amiodarone in treatment of patients with ventricular tachyarrhythmias as well as in prevention of atrial fibrillation recurrences after cardioversion.[19] It has been used successfully to decrease the incidence of atrial fibrillation after cardiac surgery. Sotalol may be effective in fetal and pediatric patients. Unlike most other antiarrhythmic drugs, it may decrease the frequency of ICD discharges and reduce the defibrillation threshold.

ADVERSE EFFECTS. Proarrhythmia is the most serious adverse effect. Overall, new or worsened ventricular tachyarrhythmias occur in about 4% of patients; this response is the result of torsades de pointes in about 2.5%. The incidence of torsades de pointes increases to 4% in patients with a history of sustained VT and is dose related, only 1.6% at 320 mg/day but 4.4% at 480 mg/day. This proarrhythmic effect was probably the cause of excess mortality in patients given *d*-sotalol (the enantiomer lacking a beta-blocking effect) after an acute myocardial infarction in the Survival With Oral *d*-Sotalol (SWORD) trial. Other adverse effects commonly seen with other beta blockers also apply to sotalol. Sotalol should be used with caution or not at all in combination with other drugs that prolong the QT interval. However, such combinations have been used successfully.

Ibutilide

Ibutilide is an agent released for use in acute termination of episodes of atrial flutter and fibrillation (see Chap. 39).[13]

Electrophysiologic Actions (see Tables 37-1, 37-2, 37-3, and 37-5). Like other class III agents, ibutilide prolongs repolarization. Although it is similar to other class III agents that block outward potassium currents, such as I_{Kr}, ibutilide is unique in that it also activates a slow inward sodium current. Administered intravenously, ibutilide causes mild slowing of the sinus rate and has minimal effects on AV conduction or QRS duration, but the QT interval is characteristically prolonged. Ibutilide has no significant effect on hemodynamics.

Pharmacokinetics (see Table 37-4). Ibutilide is administered intravenously and has a large volume of distribution. Clearance is predominantly renal, with a drug half-life averaging 6 hours, but with considerable interpatient variability. Protein binding is approximately 40%. One of the drug's metabolites has weak class III effects.

DOSAGE AND ADMINISTRATION (see Table 37-4). Ibutilide is given as an intravenous infusion of 1 mg during 10 minutes. It should not be given in the presence of a QTc interval longer than 440 milliseconds or other drugs that prolong the QT interval or when uncorrected hypokalemia or bradycardia exists. A second 1-mg dose may be given after the first dose is finished if the arrhythmia persists. Patients must have continuous electrocardiographic monitoring throughout the dosing period and for 6 to 8 hours thereafter because of the risk of ventricular arrhythmias. Pretreatment with intravenous magnesium may decrease ventricular arrhythmia risk. Up to 60% of patients with atrial fibrillation and 70% of those with atrial flutter convert to sinus rhythm after 2 mg of ibutilide has been administered.

INDICATIONS. Ibutilide is indicated for termination of an established episode of atrial flutter or fibrillation. It should not be used in patients with frequent short paroxysms of atrial fibrillation because it merely terminates episodes and is not useful for prevention. Patients whose condition is hemodynamically unstable should proceed to direct-current cardioversion. Ibutilide has been used safely and effectively in patients who were already taking amiodarone or propafenone.[20] Ibutilide has been administered at the time of transthoracic electrical cardioversion to increase the likelihood of termination of atrial fibrillation. In one study, all 50 patients given ibutilide before attempted electrical cardioversion achieved sinus rhythm, whereas only 34 of 50 who did not receive the drug converted to sinus rhythm. Of note, all 16 patients who did not respond to electrical cardioversion without ibutilide were successfully electrically cardioverted to sinus rhythm when a second attempt was made after ibutilide pretreatment.

Ibutilide prolongs accessory pathway refractoriness and can temporarily slow the ventricular rate during preexcited atrial fibrillation. The drug can also terminate episodes of organized AT as well as sustained uniform morphology VT.

ADVERSE EFFECTS. The most significant adverse effects of ibutilide are QT prolongation and torsades de pointes, which occur in approximately 2% of patients given the drug (twice as often in women as in men). This effect occurs within the first 4 to 6 hours of dosing, after which the risk is negligible. Thus, patients in whom the drug is used must undergo electrocardiographic monitoring for up to 8 hours after dosing. This requirement can make ibutilide's use in emergency departments or private offices problematic. Ibutilide's safety during pregnancy has not been well studied, and its use in this setting should be restricted to patients in whom no safer alternative exists.

Dofetilide

Dofetilide is approved for acute conversion of atrial fibrillation to sinus rhythm as well as for chronic suppression of recurrent atrial fibrillation.

Electrophysiologic Actions (see Tables 37-1, 37-2, 37-3, and 37-5). The sole electrophysiologic effect of dofetilide is block of the rapid component of the delayed rectifier potassium current (I_{Kr}), important in repolarization. This effect is more prominent in the atria than in the ventricles—30% increase in atrial refractory period versus 20% in the ventricle. Dofetilide's effect on I_{Kr} prolongs refractoriness without slowing conduction, which is believed to be largely responsible for its antiarrhythmic effect. It is also responsible for the prolongation of the QT interval on the ECG, which averages 11% but can be much greater. This effect on the QT interval is dose dependent and linear. No other important electrocardiographic changes are observed with the drug. It has no significant hemodynamic effects. Dofetilide is more effective than quinidine at converting atrial fibrillation to sinus rhythm. Long-term efficacy is similar to that of other agents.[21]

Pharmacokinetics (see Table 37-4). Orally administered dofetilide is absorbed well, with more than 90% bioavailability. Fifty percent to 60% of the drug is excreted unchanged in urine, with a mean elimination half-life of 7 to 13 hours. The remainder of the drug undergoes hepatic metabolism to inert compounds. Significant drug-drug interactions have been reported in patients using dofetilide; cimetidine, verapamil, ketoconazole, and trimethoprim, alone or in combination with sulfamethoxazole, cause a significant elevation in the dofetilide serum concentration and should not be used with this drug.

DOSAGE AND ADMINISTRATION (see Table 37-4). Dofetilide is available only as an oral preparation. Dosing is from 0.125 to 0.5 mg twice daily and must be initiated in a hospital setting with continuous electrocardiographic monitoring to ensure that inordinate QT prolongation and torsades de pointes do not develop. Physicians must be specially certified to prescribe the drug. Dosage must be decreased in the presence of impaired renal function or an increase in the QT interval of more than 15%, or 500 milliseconds. The drug should not be given to patients with a creatinine clearance of less than 20 mL/min or a baseline corrected QT interval longer than 440 milliseconds.

INDICATIONS. Oral dofetilide is indicated for prevention of episodes of supraventricular tachyarrhythmias, particularly atrial flutter and fibrillation. Dofetilide's role in therapy for ventricular arrhythmias is less clear. Dofetilide has been shown to have a neutral effect on mortality when it is given to patients after myocardial infarction.

ADVERSE EFFECTS. The most significant adverse effect of dofetilide is QT interval prolongation with torsades de pointes, occurring in 2% to 4% of patients given the drug. Risk is highest in patients with a baseline prolonged QT interval, in those who are hypokalemic, in those taking some other agent that prolongs repolarization, and after conversion from atrial fibrillation to sinus rhythm. The drug is otherwise well tolerated, with few side effects. Its use in pregnancy has not been studied extensively, and it should probably be avoided in this setting if possible.

CLASS IV AGENTS

Calcium Channel Antagonists: Verapamil and Diltiazem

Verapamil, a synthetic papaverine derivative, is the prototype of a class of drugs that block the slow calcium channel and reduce $I_{Ca.L}$ in cardiac muscle (see Chap. 35). Diltiazem has electrophysiologic actions similar to those of verapamil.[12] Nifedipine and other dihydropyridine agents exhibit minimal electrophysiologic effects at clinically used doses; these drugs are not discussed here.

Electrophysiologic Actions (see Tables 37-1, 37-2, 37-3, and 37-5). By blocking $I_{Ca.L}$ in all cardiac fibers, verapamil reduces the plateau height of the action potential, slightly shortens muscle action potential, and slightly prolongs total Purkinje fiber action potential. It does not appreciably affect the action potential amplitude, $\dot{V}max$ of phase 0, or resting membrane voltage in cells that have fast-response characteristics related to I_{Na} (e.g., atrial and ventricular muscle, the His-Purkinje system). Verapamil suppresses slow responses elicited by various experimental methods as well as sustained triggered activity and early and late afterdepolarizations. Verapamil and diltiazem suppress electrical activity in the normal sinus and AV nodes. Verapamil depresses the slope of diastolic depolarization in sinus node cells, $\dot{V}max$ of phase 0, and maximum diastolic potential and prolongs conduction time and refractory periods of the AV node. The AV node blocking effects of verapamil and diltiazem are more apparent at faster rates of stimulation (use dependence) and in depolarized fibers (voltage-dependence). Verapamil slows the activation and delays recovery from inactivation of the slow channel.

Verapamil does exert some local anesthetic activity because the dextrorotatory stereoisomer of the clinically used racemic mixture exerts slight blocking effects on I_{Na}. The levorotatory stereoisomer blocks the slow inward current carried by calcium, as well as other ions, traveling through the slow channel. Verapamil does not affect calcium-activated adenosine triphosphatase, nor does it block beta receptors, but it may block alpha receptors and potentiate vagal effects on the AV node. Verapamil may also cause other effects that indirectly alter cardiac electrophysiology, such as decreasing platelet adhesiveness or reducing the extent of myocardial ischemia.

In humans, verapamil prolongs conduction time through the AV node (the A-H interval) without affecting the P wave or QRS duration or H-V interval and lengthens AV nodal anterograde and retrograde refractory periods. The spontaneous sinus rate may decrease slightly, an effect only partially reversed by atropine. More commonly, the sinus rate does not change significantly because verapamil causes peripheral vasodilation, transient hypotension, and reflex sympathetic stimulation that mitigates any direct slowing effect that verapamil exerts on the sinus node. If verapamil is given to a patient who is also receiving a beta blocker, the sinus node discharge rate may slow because reflex sympathetic stimulation is blocked. Verapamil does not exert a significant direct effect on atrial or ventricular refractoriness or on anterograde or retrograde properties of accessory pathways. However, reflex sympathetic stimulation after intravenous verapamil administration may increase the ventricular response over the accessory pathway during atrial fibrillation in patients with the Wolff-Parkinson-White syndrome.

Hemodynamic Effects. Because verapamil interferes with excitation-contraction coupling, it inhibits vascular smooth muscle contraction and causes marked vasodilation in coronary and other peripheral vascular beds. Propranolol does not block the vasodilation produced by verapamil. Reflex sympathetic effects may reduce the marked negative inotropic action of verapamil on isolated cardiac muscle, but the direct myocardial depressant effects of verapamil may predominate when the drug is given in high doses. In patients with well-preserved left ventricular function, combined therapy with propranolol and verapamil appears to be well tolerated, but beta blockade can accentuate the hemodynamic depressant effects produced by oral verapamil. Patients who have reduced left ventricular function may not tolerate the combined blockade of beta receptors and slow channels; thus, in these patients, verapamil and propranolol should be used in combination either cautiously or not at all. Verapamil decreases myocardial oxygen demand while decreasing coronary vascular resistance. Such changes may be indirectly antiarrhythmic.

Peak alterations in hemodynamic variables occur 3 to 5 minutes after completion of a verapamil injection, with the major effects dissipating within 10 minutes. Systemic resistance and mean arterial pressure decrease, as does left ventricular dP/dt_{max}, and left ventricular end-diastolic pressure increases. Heart rate, cardiac index, left ventricular minute work, and mean pulmonary artery pressure do not change significantly. Thus, afterload reduction produced by verapamil significantly counterbalances its negative inotropic action, so that the cardiac index may not be reduced. In addition, when verapamil slows the ventricular rate in a patient with a tachycardia, hemodynamics may also improve. Nevertheless, caution should be exercised in giving verapamil to patients with severe myocardial depression or those receiving beta blockers or disopyramide because hemodynamic deterioration may progress in some patients.

Pharmacokinetics (see Table 37-4). After single oral doses of verapamil, measurable prolongation of AV nodal conduction time occurs in 30 minutes and lasts 4 to 6 hours. After intravenous administration, AV nodal conduction delay occurs within 1 to 2 minutes and A-H interval prolongation is still detectable after 6 hours. After oral administration, absorption is almost complete, but an overall bioavailability of 20% to 35% suggests substantial first-pass metabolism in the liver, particularly of the *l* isomer. The elimination half-life of verapamil is 3 to 7 hours, with up to 70% of the drug excreted by the kidneys. Norverapamil is a major metabolite that may contribute to verapamil's electrophysiologic actions. Serum protein binding is approximately 90%. With diltiazem, the percentage of heart rate reduction in atrial fibrillation is related to plasma concentration.

DOSAGE AND ADMINISTRATION (see Table 37-4). For acute termination of SVT or rapid achievement of ventricular rate control during atrial fibrillation, the most commonly used intravenous dose of verapamil is 10 mg infused during 1 to 2 minutes while cardiac rhythm and blood pressure are monitored. A second injection of an equal dose may be given 30 minutes later. The initial effect achieved with the first bolus injection, such as slowing of the ventricular response during atrial fibrillation, can be maintained by a continuous infusion of the drug at a rate of 0.005 mg/kg/min. The oral dose is 240 to 480 mg/day in divided doses. Diltiazem is given intravenously at a dose of 0.25 mg/kg as a bolus during 2 minutes, with a second dose in 15 minutes if necessary; because it is generally better tolerated (less hypotension) for long-term administration, such as for control of ventricular rate during atrial fibrillation, diltiazem is preferred to verapamil in this setting. Orally, doses must be adjusted to the patient's needs, with a 120- to 360-mg range. Various long-acting preparations (once daily) are available for verapamil and diltiazem.

INDICATIONS. After simple vagal maneuvers have been tried and adenosine has been given, intravenous verapamil or diltiazem is the next treatment of choice for termination of sustained AV node reentry or orthodromic AV reciprocating tachycardia associated with an accessory pathway (see Chap. 39). Verapamil is as effective as adenosine for termination of these arrhythmias. Assuming the patient is stable, verapamil should definitely be tried before termination is attempted by digitalis administration, pacing, electrical direct-current cardioversion, or acute blood pressure elevation with vasopressors. Verapamil and diltiazem terminate 60% to 90% or more episodes of paroxysmal SVTs within several minutes. Verapamil may also be of use in some fetal SVTs. Although intravenous verapamil has been given along with intravenous propranolol, this combination should be used only with great caution.

Verapamil and diltiazem decrease the ventricular response over the AV node during atrial fibrillation or atrial flutter, possibly converting a small number of episodes to sinus rhythm, particularly if the atrial flutter or fibrillation is of recent onset. In addition, verapamil may prevent early recurrence of atrial fibrillation after cardioversion. Some patients with atrial flutter may develop atrial fibrillation after verapamil administration. As noted earlier, in patients with preexcited ventricular complexes during atrial fibrillation associated with the Wolff-Parkinson-White syndrome, intravenous verapamil may accelerate the ventricular response; therefore, the intravenous route is contraindicated in this situation. Verapamil can terminate some ATs. Even though verapamil can often terminate an idiopathic left septal VT, hemodynamic collapse can occur if intravenous verapamil is given to patients with the more common forms of VT because they generally occur in the setting of decreased left ventricular systolic function. A general rule for avoiding complications, however, is not to administer verapamil intravenously to any patient with wide QRS tachycardia unless one is absolutely certain of the nature of the tachycardia and its likely response to verapamil.

Orally, verapamil or diltiazem can prevent the recurrence of AV node reentrant and orthodromic AV reciprocating tachycardias associated with an accessory pathway as well as help maintain a decreased ventricular response during atrial flutter or atrial fibrillation in patients without an accessory pathway. Verapamil generally has not been effective in treating patients who have recurrent ventricular tachyarrhythmias, although it may suppress some forms of VT, such as a left septal VT (noted earlier). It may also be useful in about two thirds of patients with idiopathic VT that has a left bundle branch block morphology (right ventricular outflow tract origin), patients with hypertrophic cardiomyopathy who have experienced cardiac arrest, patients with a short-coupled variant of polymorphic VT, and patients with ventricular arrhythmias related to coronary artery spasm. Calcium channel blockers have not been shown to reduce mortality or to prevent sudden cardiac death in patients after acute myocardial infarction, except for diltiazem in patients with non–Q-wave infarctions.

ADVERSE EFFECTS. Verapamil must be used cautiously in patients with significant hemodynamic impairment or in those receiving beta blockers, as noted earlier. Hypotension, bradycardia, AV block, and asystole are more likely to occur when the drug is given to patients who are already receiving beta-blocking agents. Hemodynamic collapse has been noted in infants, and verapamil should be used cautiously in patients younger than 1 year. Verapamil should also be used with caution in patients with sinus node abnormalities because marked depression of sinus node function or asystole can result in some of these patients. Intravenous isoproterenol, calcium, glucagon, dopamine, or atropine, which may be only partially effective, or temporary pacing may be necessary to counteract some of the adverse effects of verapamil. Isoproterenol may be more effective for treatment of bradyarrhythmias, and calcium may be used for treatment of hemodynamic dysfunction secondary to verapamil. AV node depression is common in overdoses. Contraindications to the use of verapamil and diltiazem include the presence of advanced heart failure, second- or third-degree AV block without a pacemaker in place, atrial fibrillation and anterograde conduction over an accessory pathway, significant sinus node dysfunction, most VTs, cardiogenic shock, and other hypotensive states. Although these drugs probably should not be used in patients with overt heart failure, if it is caused by one of the supraventricular tachyarrhythmias noted earlier, verapamil or diltiazem may restore sinus rhythm or significantly decrease the ventricular rate, leading to hemodynamic improvement. Finally, verapamil can decrease the excretion of digoxin by about 30%. Hepatotoxicity may occur on occasion. Verapamil crosses the placental barrier; its use in pregnancy has been associated with impaired uterine contraction, fetal bradycardia, and possibly fetal digital defects. It should therefore be used only if no effective alternatives exist.

OTHER ANTIARRHYTHMIC AGENTS

Adenosine

Adenosine is an endogenous nucleoside present throughout the body and has been approved by the FDA to treat patients with SVTs.[22]

Electrophysiologic Actions (see Tables 37-1, 37-2, 37-3, and 37-5). Adenosine interacts with A_1 receptors present on the extracellular surface of cardiac cells, activating K^+ channels ($I_{K.Ach}$, $I_{K.Ade}$) in a fashion similar to that produced by acetylcholine. The increase in K^+ conductance shortens atrial APD, hyperpolarizes the membrane potential, and decreases atrial contractility. Similar changes occur in the sinus and AV nodes. In contrast to these direct effects mediated through the guanine nucleotide regulatory proteins G_i and G_o, adenosine antagonizes catecholamine-stimulated adenylate cyclase to decrease cyclic adenosine monophosphate accumulation and to decrease $I_{Ca.L}$ and the pacemaker current I_f in sinus node cells along with a decrease in $\dot{V}max$. Shifts in pacemaker site within the sinus node and sinus exit block may occur. Adenosine slows the sinus rate in humans, which is followed by a reflex increase in sinus rate. In the N region of the AV node, conduction is depressed, along with decreases in action potential amplitude, duration, and $\dot{V}max$. Transient prolongation of the A-H interval results, often with transient first-, second-, or third-degree AV node block. Delay in AV nodal conduction is rate dependent. His-Purkinje conduction is generally not directly affected. Adenosine does not affect conduction in normal accessory pathways. Conduction may be blocked in accessory pathways that have long conduction times or decremental conduction properties. Patients with heart transplants exhibit a supersensitive response to adenosine. Adenosine may mediate the phenomenon of ischemic preconditioning.

Pharmacokinetics (see Table 37-4). Adenosine is removed from the extracellular space by washout, enzymatically by degradation to inosine, by phosphorylation to adenosine monophosphate, or by reuptake into cells through a nucleoside transport system. The vascular endothelium and the formed blood elements contain these elimination systems, which result in very rapid clearance of adenosine from the circulation. Elimination half-life is 1 to 6 seconds. Most of adenosine's effects are produced during its first passage through the circulation. Important drug interactions occur; methylxanthines are competitive antagonists, and therapeutic concentrations of theophylline totally block the exogenous adenosine effect. Dipyridamole is a nucleoside transport blocker that blocks reuptake of adenosine, delaying its clearance from the circulation or interstitial space and potentiating its effect. Smaller adenosine doses should be used in patients receiving dipyridamole.

DOSAGE AND ADMINISTRATION (see Table 37-4). To terminate tachycardia, a bolus of adenosine is rapidly injected intravenously at doses of 6 to 12 mg, followed by a flush. Pediatric dosing should be 0.1 to 0.3 mg/kg. When it is given into a central vein and in patients after heart transplantation or those receiving dipyridamole, the initial dose should be reduced to 3 mg. Transient sinus slowing or AV node block results, lasting less than 5 seconds. Doses of more than 18 mg are unlikely to revert a tachycardia and should not be used.

INDICATIONS. Adenosine has become the drug of first choice to terminate an SVT acutely, such as AV node or AV reentry (see Chap. 39). It is useful in pediatric patients and to judge the effectiveness of ablation of accessory pathways. Adenosine can produce AV block or terminate ATs and sinus node reentry. It results in only transient AV block during atrial flutter or fibrillation and is thus useful only for diagnosis, not therapy. Adenosine terminates a group of VTs whose maintenance depends on adrenergic drive, which is most often located in the right ventricular outflow tract but found at other sites as well; idiopathic left septal VT rarely responds, however. Adenosine has less potential than verapamil for lowering the blood pressure should tachycardia persist after injection.

Doses as low as 2.5 mg terminate some tachycardias; doses of 12 mg or less terminate 92% of SVTs, usually within 30 seconds. Successful termination rates with adenosine are comparable to those achieved with verapamil. Because of its effectiveness and extremely short duration of action, adenosine is preferable to verapamil in most cases, particularly in patients who have previously received intravenous beta adrenoceptor blockers, in those having poorly compensated heart failure or severe hypotension, and in neonates. Verapamil might be chosen first in patients receiving drugs such as theophylline (which is known to interfere with adenosine's actions or metabolism), in patients with active bronchoconstriction, and in those with inadequate venous access.

Adenosine may be useful to help differentiate among causes of wide QRS tachycardias because it terminates many SVTs with aberrancy or reveals the underlying atrial mechanism, and it does not block conduction over an accessory pathway or terminate most VTs. Adenosine in rare cases terminates some VTs, characteristically those of right ventricular outflow tract origin, and therefore tachycardia termination is not completely diagnostic for an SVT. This agent may predispose to the development of atrial fibrillation and might increase the ventricular response in patients with atrial fibrillation conducting over an accessory pathway. Adenosine may also be useful in differentiating conduction over the AV node from that over an accessory pathway during ablative procedures designed to interrupt the accessory pathway. However, this distinction is not absolute because adenosine can block conduction in slowly conducting accessory pathways and does not always produce block in the AV node. Endogenously released adenosine may be important in ischemia and hypoxia-induced AV node block and in postdefibrillation bradyarrhythmias.

ADVERSE EFFECTS. Transient side effects occur in almost 40% of patients with SVT given adenosine and are most commonly flushing, dyspnea, and chest pressure. These symptoms are fleeting, lasting less than 1 minute, and are well tolerated. PVCs, transient sinus bradycardia, sinus arrest, and AV block are common when an SVT is abruptly terminated. Atrial fibrillation is occasionally observed (12% in one study) with adenosine administration, perhaps because of the drug's effect in shortening atrial refractoriness. Induction of atrial fibrillation can be problematic in patients with the Wolff-Parkinson-White syndrome and rapid AV conduction over the accessory pathway.

Digoxin

Cardiac actions of digitalis glycosides have been recognized for centuries. Digoxin is used for control of supraventricular arrhythmias, mainly control of ventricular rate during atrial fibrillation. The use of digoxin has decreased because of the availability of agents with greater potency and a wider therapeutic to toxic drug concentration range.[22]

Electrophysiologic Actions (see Tables 37-1, 37-2, 37-3, and 37-5). Digoxin acts mainly through the autonomic nervous system, in particular by enhancing both central and peripheral vagal tone. These actions are largely confined to slowing of the sinus node discharge rate, shortening of atrial refractoriness, and prolongation of AV nodal refractoriness. Electrophysiologic effects on the His-Purkinje system and ventricular muscle are minimal, except in toxic concentrations. In studies of denervated hearts, digoxin has relatively little effect on the AV node and causes a mild increase in atrial refractoriness.

The sinus rate and P wave duration are minimally changed in most patients taking digoxin. The sinus rate may decrease in patients with heart failure whose left ventricular performance is improved by the drug; individuals with significant underlying sinus node disease also have slower sinus rates or even sinus arrest. Similarly, the PR interval is generally unchanged, except in patients with underlying AV node disease. QRS and QT intervals are unaffected. The characteristic ST and T wave abnormalities seen with digoxin use do not represent toxicity.

Pharmacokinetics (see Table 37-4). Intravenously administered digoxin yields some electrophysiologic effect within minutes, with a peak effect occurring after 1.5 to 3 hours. After oral dosing, the peak effect occurs in 4 to 6 hours. The extent of digoxin absorption after oral administration varies according to the preparation; tablet forms are 60% to 75% absorbed, whereas encapsulated gel forms are almost completely absorbed. Ingestion of cholestyramine or an antacid preparation at the same time as digoxin ingestion decreases its absorption. The serum half-life of digoxin is 36 to 48 hours, and the drug is excreted unchanged by the kidneys.

DOSAGE AND ADMINISTRATION (see Table 37-4). In acute loading doses of 0.5 to 1.0 mg, digoxin may be given intravenously or by mouth. Chronic daily oral dosing should be adjusted on the basis of clinical indications and the extent of renal dysfunction. Most patients require 0.125 to 0.25 mg/day as a single dose. However, as little as 0.125 mg every other day is needed in some patients receiving renal dialysis, whereas young patients may require as much as 0.5 mg/day. Serum digoxin levels may be used to monitor compliance with therapy as well as to determine whether digitalis toxicity is the cause of new symptoms compatible with the diagnosis. However, routine monitoring of digoxin levels is not warranted in patients whose ventricular rate is controlled during atrial fibrillation and who have no symptoms of toxicity.

INDICATIONS. Digoxin can be used intravenously to slow the ventricular rate during atrial fibrillation and flutter; it was formerly used to attempt to convert SVTs to sinus rhythm, but its onset of action is much slower and its success rate less than that of adenosine, verapamil, or beta blockers. Thus, it is now rarely used in this way. Digoxin is more commonly used orally to control the ventricular rate in chronic atrial fibrillation. When the patient with atrial fibrillation is at rest and vagal tone predominates, the ventricular rate can be maintained between 60 and 100 beats/min in 40% to 60% of cases. However, when the patient begins to exercise, the decrease in vagal tone and increase in adrenergic tone combine to diminish digoxin's beneficial effects on AV nodal conduction. Patients may experience a marked increase in ventricular rate with even mild exertion. Digoxin is therefore rarely used as a single agent to control the ventricular rate in chronic atrial fibrillation. The drug has little ability to prevent episodes of paroxysmal atrial fibrillation or to control ventricular rate during the episodes. Finally, digoxin is no more effective than placebo at terminating episodes of acute- or recent-onset atrial fibrillation.

ADVERSE EFFECTS. One major reason that digoxin use has decreased is its potential for serious adverse effects and the narrow window between therapeutic and toxic concentrations. Digitalis toxicity produces various symptoms and signs, including headache, nausea and vomiting, altered color perception, halo vision, and generalized malaise. More serious than these are digitalis-related arrhythmias, which include bradycardias related to a markedly enhanced vagal effect (e.g., sinus bradycardia or arrest, AV node block) and tachyarrhythmias that may be caused by delayed afterdepolarization-mediated triggered activity (e.g., atrial, junctional, and fascicular or ventricular tachycardia). Worsening renal function, advanced age, hypokalemia, chronic lung disease, hypothyroidism, and amyloidosis increase a patient's sensitivity to digitalis-related arrhythmias. The diagnosis can be confirmed by determination of the serum digoxin level. Therapy for most bradycardias consists of withdrawal of digoxin; atropine or temporary pacing may be needed in symptomatic patients. Phenytoin can be used for control of atrial tachyarrhythmias, whereas lidocaine has been successful in treating infranodal tachycardias. Life-threatening arrhythmias can be treated with digoxin-specific antibody fragments. Electrical direct-current cardioversion should be performed only when absolutely necessary in the digitalis-toxic patient because life-threatening VT or VF can result, which can be very difficult to control.

ANTIARRHYTHMIC EFFECTS OF NON-ANTIARRHYTHMIC DRUGS. Several medications commonly used for other indications also have some degree of antiarrhythmic effect. In some cases, physicians can use these drugs for their standard indications and achieve additional, although often small, amounts of benefit in treating the patient's rhythm disturbance. Among these drugs are angiotensin-converting enzyme inhibitors and angiotensin receptor blocking agents, aldosterone antagonists, statins and omega-3 fatty acids (prevention of sudden death),[23,24] and these same classes of drugs with the addition of nondihydropyridine calcium channel blockers and ranolazine (less atrial fibrillation).[25] The mechanisms whereby these drugs exert their attenuating effect on arrhythmias is not clear in most cases, and they should not be relied on as the sole form of antiarrhythmic therapy. Ranolazine appears to block a late sodium current, which may account for its antiarrhythmic effects. In patients who have arrhythmias as well as another disorder that requires drug therapy (hypertension, heart failure), one of these medications may be preferable to agents that treat the primary disorder but do not possess antiarrhythmic effects.

Electrotherapy of Cardiac Arrhythmias

Direct-Current Electrical Cardioversion

Electrical cardioversion offers obvious advantages over drug therapy in terminating tachycardia. Under conditions optimal for close supervision and monitoring, a precisely regulated "dose" of electricity can restore sinus rhythm immediately and safely. The distinction between supraventricular and ventricular tachyarrhythmias, crucial to the proper medical management of arrhythmias, becomes less significant, and the time-consuming titration of drugs with potential side effects is obviated.

Mechanisms. Electrical cardioversion appears most effective in terminating tachycardias related to reentry, such as atrial flutter and many cases of atrial fibrillation, AV node reentry, reciprocating tachycardias associated with the Wolff-Parkinson-White syndrome, most forms of VT, ventricular flutter, and VF. The electrical shock, by depolarizing all excitable myocardium and possibly by prolonging refractoriness, interrupts reentrant circuits and establishes electrical homogeneity, which terminates reentry. The mechanism by which a shock successfully terminates VF has not been completely explained. If the precipitating factors are no longer present, interruption of the tachyarrhythmia for only the brief time produced by the shock may prevent its return for long periods, even though the anatomic and electrophysiologic substrates required for the tachycardia are still present.

Tachycardias thought to be caused by disorders of impulse formation (automaticity) include parasystole, some forms of AT, ectopic junctional tachycardia (with or without digitalis toxicity), accelerated idioventricular rhythm, and rare forms of VT (see Chaps. 35 and 39). An attempt to cardiovert these tachycardias electrically is not indicated in most cases because they typically recur within seconds after the shock; release of endogenous catecholamines consequent to the shock may further exacerbate the arrhythmia. It has not been established whether cardioversion can terminate tachycardias caused by enhanced automaticity or triggered activity.

Technique. Before *elective* cardioversion, a careful physical examination, including palpation of limb pulses, should be performed. A 12-lead ECG is obtained before and after cardioversion, as well as a rhythm strip during the electroshock. The patient, who should be informed completely about what to expect, is in a fasting state and metabolically balanced; that is, blood gas, pH, and electrolyte values should be normal, with no evidence of drug toxicity. Withholding of digitalis for several days

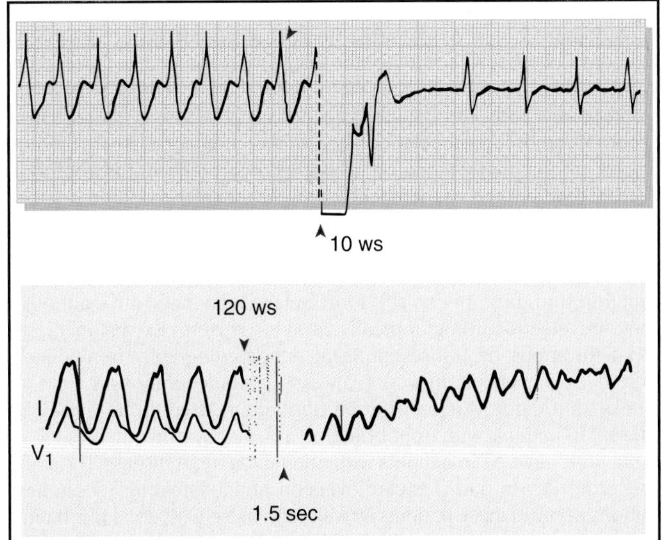

FIGURE 37-2 **Top,** A synchronized shock (note synchronization mark in the apex of the QRS complex [arrowhead]) during ventricular tachycardia is followed by a single repetitive ventricular response and then normal sinus rhythm. **Bottom,** A shock synchronized to the terminal portion of the QRS complex (arrowhead) in a patient with atrial fibrillation and conduction to the ventricle over an accessory pathway (Wolff-Parkinson-White syndrome) resulted in ventricular fibrillation that was promptly terminated by a 400-J shock. Recording was lost for 1.5 seconds (arrowhead) because of baseline drift after the shock. ws = watt seconds.

before elective cardioversion in patients without clinical evidence of digitalis toxicity is not necessary, although patients in whom digitalis toxicity is suspected should not be electrically cardioverted until this situation has been corrected. Maintenance antiarrhythmic drug administration 1 to 2 days before electrical cardioversion of patients with atrial fibrillation can revert some patients to sinus rhythm, help prevent recurrence of atrial fibrillation once sinus rhythm is restored, and help determine the patient's tolerance for the drug. There is also evidence that angiotensin-converting enzyme inhibitor and receptor blockers may prevent recurrence of fibrillation, especially in patients with ventricular dysfunction.[26]

Self-adhesive pads applied in the standard apicoanterior or apicoposterior paddle positions have transthoracic impedances similar to those of paddles and are useful in elective cardioversions or other situations in which there is time for their application. Paddles 12 to 13 cm in diameter can be used to deliver maximum current to the heart, but the benefits of these paddles compared with those of paddles 8 to 9 cm in diameter have not been clearly established. Larger paddles may distribute the intracardiac current over a wider area and may reduce shock-induced myocardial injury.

A synchronized shock (i.e., one delivered during the QRS complex) is used for all cardioversions except for very rapid ventricular tachyarrhythmias, such as ventricular flutter or VF (**Fig. 37-2**). Although generally minimal, shock-related myocardial damage increases directly with increases in applied energy, and so the minimum effective shock should be used. Therefore, shocks are "titrated" when the clinical situation permits. Except for atrial fibrillation, shocks in the range of 25 to 50 J successfully terminate most SVTs and should be tried initially. If the shock is unsuccessful, a second shock of higher energy can be delivered. The starting level to terminate atrial fibrillation with older monophasic machines should be no less than 100 J, but with newer biphasic systems, a shock as low as 25 J may succeed. Delivered energy can be increased in a stepwise fashion; up to 360 J can be used safely. It is critical to remember to resynchronize the defibrillator to the QRS complex after an unsuccessful shock before delivery of another shock to avoid initiation of VF (machines typically revert to asynchronous mode after each shock). Anteroposterior pads may have a higher efficacy rate by placing more of the atrial mass in the shock vector than is the case for apicoanterior pads. If a shock of 360 J fails to convert the rhythm, repeated shocks at the same energy may succeed by decreasing chest wall impedance; reversing pad polarity can occasionally help as well. Administration of ibutilide has been shown to facilitate electrical cardioversion of atrial fibrillation to sinus rhythm.[20] Intracardiac defibrillation can be tried if all attempts at external cardioversion fail. For patients with stable VT, starting levels in the range of 25 to 50 J can be used. If there is some urgency to terminate the tachyarrhythmia, one can begin with higher energies. To terminate VF, 100 to 200 J (biphasic; 200 to 360 J with monophasic machines) is generally used, although much lower energies (less than 50 J) terminate VF when the shock is delivered soon after the onset of the arrhythmia, for example, using adhesive pads in the electrophysiology laboratory.

During elective cardioversion, a short-acting barbiturate such as methohexital, a sedative such as propofol, or an amnesic such as diazepam or midazolam can be used. A physician skilled in airway management should be in attendance; an intravenous route should be established; and pulse oximetry, the ECG, and blood pressure should be monitored. All equipment necessary for emergency resuscitation should be immediately accessible. Before cardioversion, 100% oxygen may be administered for 5 to 15 minutes by nasal cannula or face mask and is continued throughout the procedure. Manual ventilation of the patient may be necessary to avoid hypoxia during periods of deepest sedation. Adequate sedation of the patient undergoing even urgent cardioversion is essential; some patients who have needlessly been shocked while awake, perhaps because of uneasiness of the physician with the arrhythmia, have declined further medical care for their arrhythmias because of concern that they would again undergo cardioversion without proper sedation.

In up to 5% of patients with atrial fibrillation, sinus rhythm cannot be restored by external countershock despite all the preceding measures, including ibutilide pretreatment and biphasic shocks. It is important to distinguish between inability to attain sinus rhythm, indicating inadequate energy delivery to the atria, and inability to maintain sinus rhythm after transient termination of fibrillation; the latter condition (early reinitiation of atrial fibrillation) does not respond to higher energy shocks because fibrillation has already been terminated but quickly recurs. Pretreatment with an antiarrhythmic drug may help maintain sinus rhythm after subsequent shocks. Patients in whom atrial fibrillation simply cannot be terminated with external shock tend to be very obese or have severe obstructive lung disease. In such cases, internal cardioversion can be performed by use of specially configured catheters, with multiple large electrodes covering several centimeters of the distal portion of the catheter for distributing shock energy. By standard percutaneous access, these catheters can be situated in the lateral right atrium and coronary sinus to achieve a shock vector across most of the atrial mass. With such configurations, internal shocks of 2 to 15 J can terminate atrial fibrillation in more than 90% of patients whose arrhythmia is refractory to transthoracic shock. Esophageal cardioversion has also been reported.

INDICATIONS. As a rule, any tachycardia that produces hypotension, congestive heart failure, mental status changes, or angina and does not respond promptly to medical management should be terminated electrically. Very rapid ventricular rates in patients with atrial fibrillation and Wolff-Parkinson-White syndrome are often best treated by electrical cardioversion. In almost all cases, the patient's hemodynamic status improves after cardioversion. Rarely, a patient may experience hypotension, reduced cardiac output, or congestive heart failure after the shock. This problem may be related to complications of the cardioversion, such as embolic events, myocardial depression resulting from the anesthetic agent or the shock itself, hypoxia, lack of restoration of left atrial contraction despite return of electrical atrial systole, or postshock arrhythmias. Direct-current countershock of digitalis-induced tachyarrhythmias is contraindicated.

Favorable candidates for electrical cardioversion of atrial fibrillation include patients who (1) have symptomatic atrial fibrillation of less than 12 months' duration, (2) continue to have atrial fibrillation after the precipitating cause has been removed (e.g., after treatment of thyrotoxicosis), (3) have a rapid ventricular rate that is difficult to slow, or (4) have symptoms of decreased cardiac output (e.g., fatigue, lightheadedness, dyspnea) attributable to lack of atrial contraction's contribution to ventricular filling. In patients who have indications for chronic warfarin therapy to prevent stroke, the hope of avoiding anticoagulation by restoring sinus rhythm is not a reason to attempt cardioversion because these patients are still at increased risk for thromboembolic events. Several large trials have shown that maintenance of sinus rhythm confers no survival advantage over rate control and anticoagulation; thus, not all patients with newly discovered atrial fibrillation warrant an attempt at restoration of sinus rhythm. Treatment must be determined individually.

Unfavorable candidates include patients with (1) digitalis toxicity; (2) no symptoms and a well-controlled ventricular rate without therapy; (3) sinus node dysfunction and various unstable supraventricular tachyarrhythmias or bradyarrhythmias—often the bradycardia-tachycardia syndrome—who finally develop and maintain atrial fibrillation, which in essence represents a cure for the sick sinus syndrome; (4) little or no symptomatic improvement with normal sinus rhythm who promptly revert to atrial fibrillation after cardioversion despite drug therapy; (5) a large left atrium and longstanding atrial fibrillation; (6) episodes of atrial fibrillation that revert spontaneously to sinus rhythm; (7) no mechanical atrial systole after the return of electrical atrial systole; (8) atrial fibrillation and advanced heart block; (9) cardiac surgery planned in the near future; and (10) antiarrhythmic drug intolerance. Atrial fibrillation is more likely to recur after cardioversion in patients who have significant chronic obstructive lung disease, congestive heart failure, mitral valve disease (particularly mitral regurgitation), atrial fibrillation present longer than 1 year, and enlarged left atrium (echocardiographic diameter more than 4.5 cm).

In patients with atrial flutter, slowing the ventricular rate by administration of beta or calcium channel blockers or terminating the flutter with an antiarrhythmic agent may be difficult, and electrical cardioversion is often the initial treatment of choice. For the patient with other types of SVT, electrical cardioversion may be used when (1) vagal maneuvers or simple medical management (e.g., intravenous adenosine and verapamil) has failed to terminate the tachycardia and (2) the clinical setting indicates that fairly prompt restoration of sinus rhythm is desirable because of hemodynamic decompensation or electrophysiologic consequences of the tachycardia. Similarly, in patients with VT, the hemodynamic and electrophysiologic consequences of the arrhythmias determine the need for and urgency of direct-current cardioversion. Electrical countershock is the initial treatment of choice for ventricular flutter or VF. Speed is essential (see Chap. 41).

If, after the first shock, reversion of the arrhythmia to sinus rhythm does not occur, a higher energy level should be tried. When transient ventricular arrhythmias result after an unsuccessful shock, a bolus of lidocaine can be given before delivery of a shock at the next energy level. If sinus rhythm returns only transiently and is promptly supplanted by the tachycardia, a repeated shock can be tried, depending on the tachyarrhythmia being treated and its consequences. Administration of an antiarrhythmic agent intravenously may be useful before delivery of the next cardioversion shock (such as ibutilide in resistant atrial fibrillation). After cardioversion, the patient should be monitored, at least until full consciousness has been restored and preferably for several hours thereafter, depending on the duration of recovery from the particular form of sedation or anesthesia used. If ibutilide has been given, the ECG should be monitored for up to 8 hours because torsades de pointes can develop in the first few hours after administration.

RESULTS. Cardioversion restores sinus rhythm in 70% to 95% of patients, depending on the type of tachyarrhythmia. However, sinus rhythm remains after 12 months in less than one third to one half of patients with chronic atrial fibrillation. Thus, maintenance of sinus rhythm, once established, is the difficult problem, not the immediate termination of the tachycardia. The likelihood of maintaining sinus rhythm depends on the particular arrhythmia, the presence of underlying heart disease, and the response to antiarrhythmic drug therapy. Atrial size often decreases after termination of atrial fibrillation and restoration of sinus rhythm, and functional capacity improves.

COMPLICATIONS. Arrhythmias induced by electrical cardioversion are generally caused by inadequate synchronization, with the shock occurring during the ST segment or T wave. On occasion, a properly synchronized shock can produce VF (see Fig. 37-2). Postshock arrhythmias are usually transient and do not require therapy. Embolic episodes are reported to occur in 1% to 3% of patients converted from atrial fibrillation to sinus rhythm. Prior therapeutic anticoagulation (international normalized ratio, 2.0 to 3.0) consistently for at least 3 weeks should be used for patients who have no contraindication to such therapy and have had atrial fibrillation present for longer than 2 to 3 days or of indeterminate duration. This approach is particularly valid for those who are at high risk for emboli, such as those with mitral stenosis and atrial fibrillation of recent onset, a history of recent or recurrent emboli, a prosthetic mitral valve, an enlarged heart (including left atrial enlargement), or congestive heart failure. It is important to note that 3 weeks of therapeutic anticoagulation is not the same as simply administering warfarin for 3 weeks. Anticoagulation with warfarin for at least 4 weeks afterward is recommended because restoration of atrial mechanical function lags behind that of electrical systolic function, and thrombi can still form in largely akinetic atria, although they are electrocardiographically in sinus rhythm. Exclusion of left atrial thrombus by transesophageal echocardiography immediately before cardioversion may not always preclude embolism days or weeks after cardioversion of atrial fibrillation. Atrial thrombi may be present in patients with nonfibrillation atrial tachyarrhythmias, such as atrial flutter and AT in patients with congenital heart disease. The same precardioversion and postcardioversion anticoagulation recommendations apply to these patients as well as to those with atrial fibrillation. Although direct-current shock has been demonstrated in animals to cause myocardial injury, studies in humans have indicated that elevations of myocardial enzymes after cardioversion are not common. ST-segment elevation, sometimes dramatic, can occur immediately after elective direct-current cardioversion and last for 1 to 2 minutes, although cardiac enzymes and myocardial scintigraphy may be unremarkable. ST elevation lasting longer than 2 minutes usually indicates myocardial injury unrelated to the shock. A decrease in serum K^+ and Mg^{2+} levels can occur after cardioversion of VT.

Cardioversion of VT can also be achieved by a chest thump. Its mechanism of termination is probably related to a mechanically induced PVC that interrupts a tachycardia and may be related to commotio cordis (see Chap. 83). The thump cannot be timed very well and is probably effective only when it is delivered during a nonrefractory part of the cardiac cycle. The thump can alter a VT and possibly induce ventricular flutter or VF if it occurs during the vulnerable period of the T wave. Because there may be a slightly greater likelihood of converting a stable VT to VF than of terminating VT to sinus rhythm, chest thump cardioversion should not be attempted unless a defibrillator is simply unavailable.

Implantable Electrical Devices for Treatment of Cardiac Arrhythmias

Implantable devices that monitor the cardiac rhythm and can deliver competing pacing stimuli and low- and high-energy shocks have been used effectively in selected patients (see Chap. 38).

Ablation Therapy for Cardiac Arrhythmias

The purpose of catheter ablation is to destroy myocardial tissue by delivery of electrical energy through electrodes on a catheter placed next to an area of the myocardium integrally related to the onset or maintenance of the arrhythmia. For tachycardias with an apparent focal origin (e.g., automatic, triggered activity, microreentry), the focus itself is targeted. In macroreentrant atrial and ventricular tachycardias, inexcitable scar tissue typically separates strands of remaining myocardium, and wave fronts propagate around these scars. The target for ablation is a narrow portion of myocardium between inexcitable areas (e.g., scar, valve annulus; **Fig. 37-3**). The first catheter ablation procedures were performed with direct-current shocks, but this energy source has been supplanted by radiofrequency (RF) energy, which is delivered from an external generator and destroys tissue by controlled heat production.[27] Lasers and microwave energy sources have been used, but not commonly; cryothermal catheter ablation has been approved for use in humans. When a target tissue has been identified by an EPS, the tip of the ablation catheter is maneuvered into apposition with this tissue. After stable catheter position and recordings have been ensured, RF energy is delivered between the catheter tip and an indifferent electrode, usually an electrocautery-type grounding pad on the skin of the patient's thigh. Because energies in the RF portion of the electromagnetic spectrum are poorly conducted by cardiac tissue, RF energy instead causes resistive heating in the cells close to the catheter tip (i.e., these cells transduce the electrical energy into thermal energy). When the tissue temperature exceeds 50°C, irreversible cellular damage and tissue death occur. An expanding front of conducted heat emanates from the region of resistive heating while RF delivery continues, resulting in production of a homogeneous, roughly hemispheric lesion of coagulative necrosis 3 to 5 mm in diameter (**Fig. 37-4**). RF-induced heating of tissue that has inherent automaticity (e.g., His bundle, foci of automatic tachycardias) results in initial acceleration of a rhythm, whereas RF delivery during a reentrant arrhythmia typically causes slowing and termination of the arrhythmia. In most cases, RF delivery is painless, although ablation of atrial or RV tissue can be uncomfortable for some patients.

Cooled-Tip Radiofrequency Ablation. There are situations in which the catheter can be delivered to the correct location but conventional RF energy delivery cannot eliminate the tachycardia. In some of these cases, the amount of damage—depth or breadth—caused by standard RF energy is inadequate. With use of standard RF energy, power delivery is usually regulated to maintain a preset catheter tip temperature (typically, 55°C to 70°C). Tip temperatures higher than 90°C are associated with coagulation of blood elements on the electrode that preclude further energy delivery and that could also become detached and embolize. Cooling of the catheter tip by internal circulation of liquid or continuous fluid infusion through small holes in the tip electrode can prevent excessive heating of the tip and allow greater power delivery, thus producing a larger lesion and potentially enhancing efficacy. Cooled-tip ablation has been used to good advantage in cases in which standard (4-mm tip) catheter ablation has failed as well as for primary therapy in atrial flutter and VT associated with structural heart disease, in which additional damage to already diseased areas is not harmful and may be required to achieve the desired result.[28]

Catheter-delivered cryoablation causes tissue damage by freezing cellular structures. Nitrous oxide is delivered to the catheter tip, where it is allowed to boil, cooling the tip electrode, after which the gas is circulated back to the delivery console. The catheter tip temperature can be regulated, cooling to as low as −80°C. Cooling to 0°C causes reversible loss of function and can be used as a diagnostic test (i.e., termination of a tachycardia when the catheter is in contact with a group of cells critical to its perpetuation). The catheter tip can then be cooled more deeply to produce permanent damage and thus cure of the arrhythmia. Cryoablation appears to cause less endocardial damage than RF and may thus engender less risk of thromboemboli after ablation as well as less chance of esophageal injury with ablation of atrial fibrillation.[29]

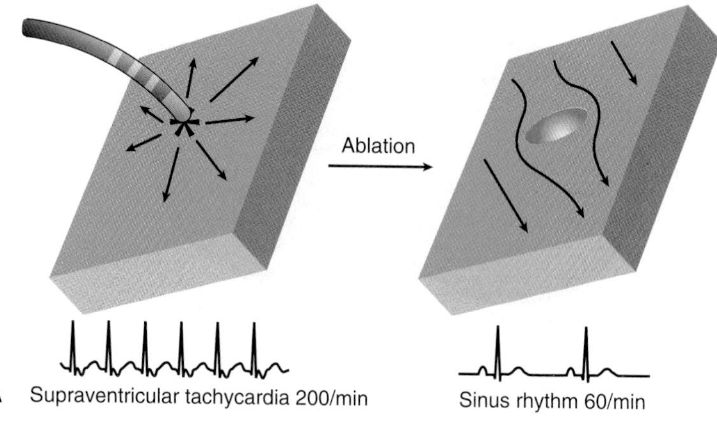

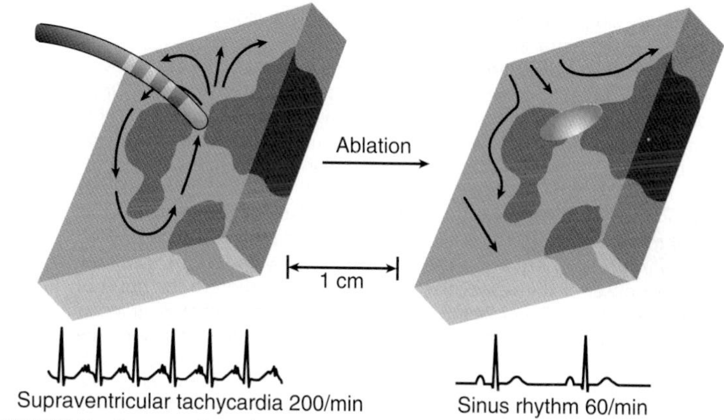

FIGURE 37-3 Strategies for catheter ablation. **A,** Focal tachycardia. At left, SVT is caused by an atrial focus, with activation emanating in all directions. Ablation of the focus (right) eliminates the arrhythmia with minimal disruption of normal activation. **B,** Macroreentrant SVT in setting of prior atrial damage, resulting in scar formation. During SVT (left), a wave front circulates around a scarred area and through a narrow isthmus between this and another area of scar. Ablation at this critical site (right) prevents further reentry.

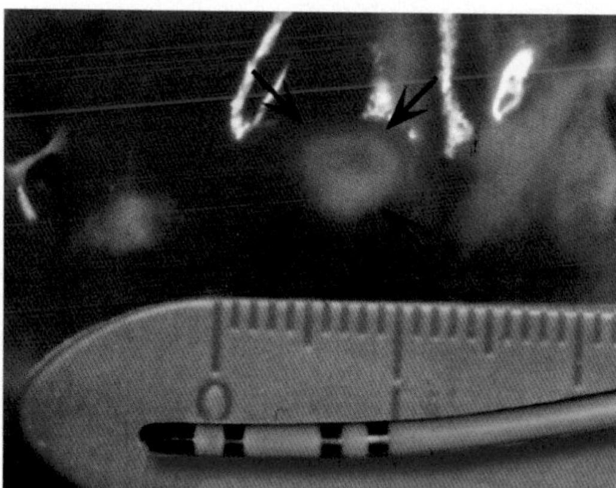

FIGURE 37-4 Radiofrequency lesion in human ventricular myocardium (explanted heart at the time of transplantation). A 30-second application of energy was made at the location denoted by arrows with the tip of the catheter shown. The lesion is 5 mm in diameter and has a well-demarcated border. A central depression in the lesion results from partial desiccation of tissue.

Radiofrequency Catheter Ablation of Accessory Pathways

Location of Pathways. The safety, efficacy, and cost-effectiveness of RF catheter ablation of an accessory AV pathway have made ablation the treatment of choice in most adult and many pediatric patients who have AV reentrant tachycardia (AVRT) or atrial flutter or fibrillation associated with a rapid ventricular response over the accessory pathway (see Chap. 39). When RF energy is delivered to an immature heart, the lesion size can increase as the heart grows; however, this has not been shown to cause problems later in life.

An EPS is performed initially to determine that the accessory pathway is part of the tachycardia circuit or capable of rapid AV conduction during atrial fibrillation and to localize the accessory pathway, the optimal site for ablation. Pathways can exist in the right or left free wall or septum of the heart (**Fig. 37-5**). Septal accessory pathways are further classified as superoparaseptal, midseptal, and posteroseptal. Pathways classified as posteroseptal are posterior to the central fibrous body within the so-called pyramidal space, which is bounded by the posterior superior process of the left ventricle and inferomedial aspects of both atria. Superoparaseptal pathways are found near the His bundle, and accessory pathway activation potential as well as His bundle potential can be recorded simultaneously from a catheter placed at the His bundle region. Midseptal pathways are close to the AV node and can usually be ablated from a right-sided approach; rarely, a left atrial approach is needed. Right posteroseptal pathways insert along the tricuspid ring in the vicinity of the coronary sinus ostium, whereas left posteroseptal pathways are further into the coronary sinus and may be located at a subepicardial site around the proximal coronary sinus, within a middle cardiac vein or

Anterior
Anterolateral
Anteroseptal
His
Anterior
Anterolateral
AV node
Mitral Orifice
Lateral
Lateral
Tricuspid Orifice
Midseptal
Coronary sinus
Posterolateral
Posterolateral
Posteroseptal
Posterior
Posterior

FIGURE 37-5 Locations of accessory pathways by anatomic region. Tricuspid and mitral valve annuli are depicted in a left anterior oblique view. Locations of coronary sinus, AV node, and bundle of His are shown. Accessory pathways may connect atrial to ventricular myocardium in any of the regions shown.

coronary sinus diverticulum, or subendocardially along the ventricular aspect of the mitral annulus.

Pathways at all locations and in all age groups can be ablated successfully. Multiple pathways are present in about 5% of patients. Occasional epicardial locations may be more easily approached from within the coronary sinus. Rarely, pathways may connect an atrial appendage with adjacent ventricular epicardium, 2 cm or more from the AV groove.

Ablation Site. The optimal ablation site can be found by direct recordings of the accessory pathway (**Fig. 37-6**), although deflections that mimic accessory pathway potentials can be recorded at other sites. The ventricular insertion site can be determined by finding the site of the earliest onset of the ventricular electrogram in relation to the onset of the delta wave. Other helpful guidelines include unfiltered unipolar recordings that register a QS wave and the shortest AV conduction time during maximal preexcitation. A major ventricular potential synchronous with the onset of the delta wave can be a target site in left-sided preexcitation, whereas earlier ventricular excitation in relation to the delta wave can be found for right-sided preexcitation. The atrial insertion site of manifest or concealed pathways (i.e., delta wave present or absent, respectively) can be found by locating the site showing the earliest atrial activation during retrograde conduction over the pathway. Reproducible mechanical inhibition of accessory pathway conduction during catheter manipulation and subthreshold stimulation has also been used to determine the optimal site. Accidental catheter trauma should be avoided, however, because it can hide the target for prolonged periods. Right free wall and superoparaseptal pathways are particularly susceptible to catheter trauma.

Left-sided accessory pathways often cross the mitral annulus obliquely. Consequently, the earliest site of retrograde atrial activation and the earliest site of anterograde ventricular activation are not directly across the AV groove from each other. Identification of the earliest site of atrial activation is usually performed during orthodromic AVRT or relatively rapid ventricular pacing, so that retrograde conduction using the AV node does not confuse assessment of the location of the earliest atrial activation.

Successful ablation sites should exhibit stable fluoroscopic and electrical characteristics. During sinus rhythm, the local ventricular activation at the successful ablation site precedes the onset of the delta wave on the ECG by 10 to 35 milliseconds; during orthodromic AVRT, the interval between the onset of ventricular activation in any lead and local atrial activation is usually 70 to 90 milliseconds (see Fig. 37-5). When temperature-measuring ablation catheters are used, a stable rise in catheter tip temperature is a helpful indicator of catheter stability and adequate contact between the electrode and tissue. In such a case, the tip temperature generally exceeds 50°C. The retrograde transaortic and transseptal approaches have been used with equal success to ablate accessory pathways located along the mitral annulus. A routine EPS performed weeks after the ablation procedure is generally not indicated but may be considered in patients who have recurrent delta wave or symptoms of tachycardia. Catheter-delivered cryoablation can be useful in patients with septal accessory pathways (located near AV node or His bundle). With use of this system, the catheter tip and adjacent tissue can be reversibly cooled to test a potential site. If accessory pathway conduction fails while normal AV conduction is preserved, deeper cooling can be performed at the site to complete the ablation. If, however, normal AV conduction is worsened, permanent damage is almost always averted by quickly allowing the catheter to rewarm.

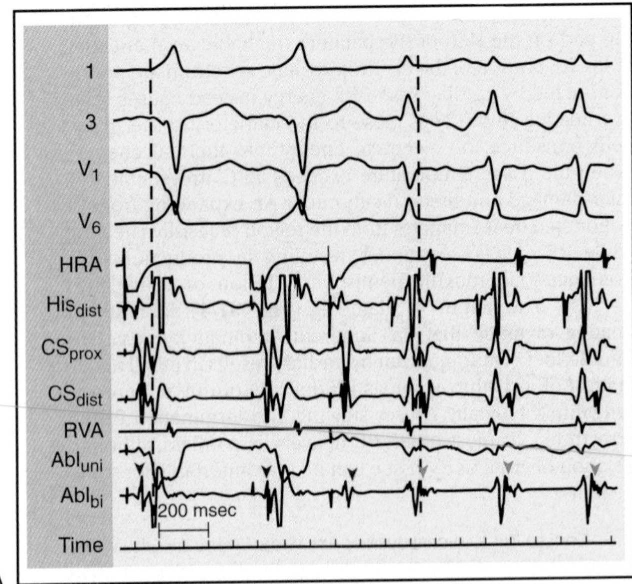

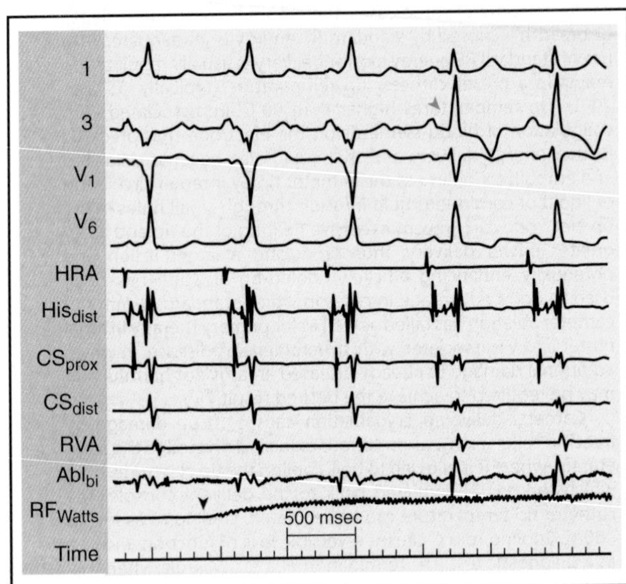

FIGURE 37-6 Wolff-Parkinson-White syndrome. Surface ECG leads 1, 3, V_1, and V_6 are shown, with intracardiac recordings from high right atrium (HRA), distal His (His_{dist}) bundle region, proximal (CS_{prox}) and distal (CS_{dist}) coronary sinus, right ventricular apex (RVA), and unipolar (Abl_{uni}) and bipolar (Abl_{bi}) tip electrodes of ablation catheter. Radiofrequency power in watts (RF_{Watts}) is also shown. **A,** Two beats of atrial pacing are conducted over the accessory pathway (blue arrowheads in Abl_{bi} recording, from the site of the accessory pathway), resulting in a delta wave on the ECG; a premature atrial stimulus (center) encounters accessory pathway refractoriness (red arrowhead), instead conducting over the AV node and bundle of His, resulting in a narrow QRS complex and starting an episode of AV reentrant tachycardia. After each narrow QRS complex is an atrial deflection, the earliest portion of which is recorded at the ablation site (green arrowheads). **B,** Ablation of this pathway is accomplished by delivery of RF energy from the ablation catheter tip. The blue arrowhead denotes onset of RF energy delivery; two QRS complexes later, the delta wave is abruptly lost (green arrowhead in lead 3) because of elimination of conduction over the accessory pathway.

Atriofascicular accessory pathways have connections consisting of a proximal portion, responsible for conduction delay and decremental conduction properties, and a long distal segment located along the endocardial surface of the right ventricular free wall that has electrophysiologic properties similar to those of the right bundle branch. The distal end of the right atriofascicular accessory pathway can insert into the apical region of the right ventricular free wall, close to the distal right bundle branch, or can actually fuse with the latter. Right atriofascicular accessory pathways might represent a duplication of the AV conduction system and can be localized for ablation by recording potentials from the rapidly conducting distal component, which crosses the tricuspid annulus (analogous to the His bundle) and extends to the apical region of the right ventricular free wall. Ablation at such a site on the annulus is usually successful; these pathways are very sensitive to catheter trauma, and the operator must use great care to avoid this.

Indications

Ablation of accessory pathways is indicated in patients with symptomatic AVRT that is drug resistant or who are drug intolerant or do not desire long-term drug therapy. It is also indicated in patients with atrial fibrillation, or other atrial tachyarrhythmias, and a rapid ventricular response by means of an accessory pathway when the tachycardia is drug resistant or who are drug intolerant or do not desire long-term drug therapy. Other potential candidates include the following: (1) patients with AVRT or atrial fibrillation with rapid ventricular rates identified during an EPS for another arrhythmia; (2) asymptomatic patients with ventricular preexcitation whose livelihood, profession, important activities, insurability, or mental well-being and the public's safety would be affected by spontaneous tachyarrhythmias or by the presence of the electrocardiographic abnormality; (3) patients with atrial fibrillation and a controlled ventricular response by means of the accessory pathway; and (4) patients with a family history of sudden cardiac death. Controversy remains as to whether all patients with accessory pathways need treatment; however, ablation has such a high success rate and low complication rate that in most centers, patients who need any form of therapy are referred for catheter ablation.

Results

Currently, in the hands of an experienced operator, the success rate for accessory pathway ablation is more than 95% (slightly less for right free wall pathways, in which stable catheter-tissue contact is more problematic), with a 2% recurrence rate after an apparently successful procedure. There is a 1% to 2% complication rate, including bleeding, vascular damage, myocardial perforation with cardiac tamponade, valve damage, stroke, and myocardial infarction. Heart block occurs in less than 3% of septal pathways. Procedure-related death is very rare.

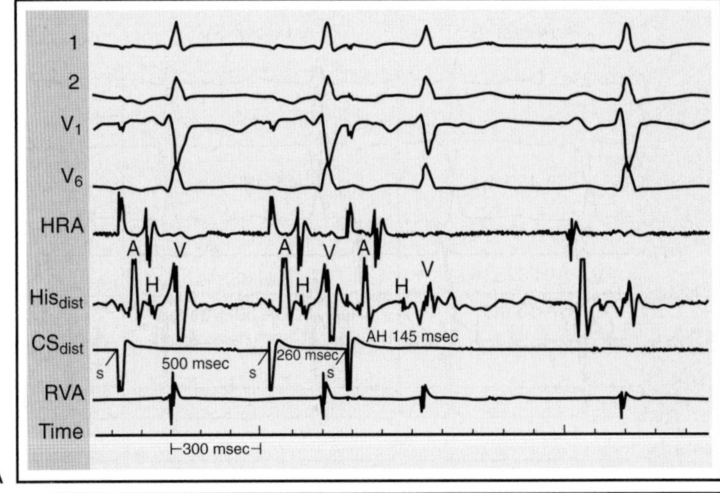

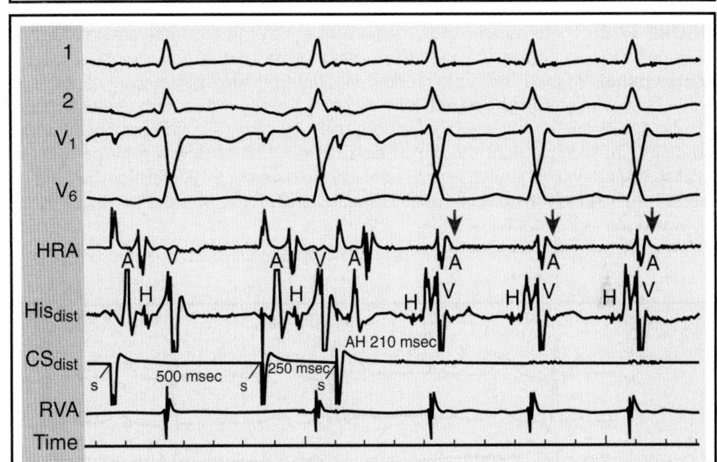

FIGURE 37-7 AV node reentry. **A,** Two atrial paced complexes from the coronary sinus (CS) are followed by an atrial premature stimulus at a coupling interval of 260 milliseconds, resulting in an A-H interval of 145 milliseconds. **B,** The same atrial drive train is followed by an atrial extrastimulus 10 milliseconds earlier than before (250 milliseconds). This results in a marked increase in the A-H interval to 210 milliseconds, after which AV nodal reentrant tachycardia ensues because the extrastimulus encounters block in a "fast" AV node pathway, conducts down a "slow" pathway, and then conducts back up the fast pathway in a repeating fashion. Red arrowheads denote atrial electrograms coincident with QRS complexes, characteristic of the most common type of AV node reentry. Recording was done as in prior figures.

RADIOFREQUENCY CATHETER MODIFICATION OF THE AV NODE FOR AV NODAL REENTRANT TACHYCARDIAS. AV node reentry is a common cause of SVT episodes (see Chaps. 35 and 39). Although controversy still exists about the exact nature of the tachycardia circuit, abundant evidence has indicated that two pathways in the region of the AV node participate, one with relatively fast conduction but long refractoriness, and the other with shorter refractoriness but slower conduction. PACs can encounter refractoriness in the fast pathway, conduct down the slow pathway, and reenter the fast pathway retrogradely, initiating AV nodal reentrant SVT (**Fig. 37-7**). Although this is the most common presentation of AV node reentry, some patients have what appears to be propagation in the opposite direction in this circuit (anterograde fast, retrograde slow) as well as a "slow-slow" variant. Other, far less common types have been described. Two or more of these variants can exist in the same patient (**Fig. 37-8**).

FAST PATHWAY ABLATION. Ablation can be performed to eliminate conduction in the fast pathway or the slow pathway. Currently, fast pathway ablation is rarely performed because it is associated with a prolonged PR interval, a higher recurrence rate (10% to 15%), and a slightly higher risk of complete AV block (2% to 5%) compared with slow pathway ablation. One uncommon situation in which fast pathway ablation may be preferred is for patients who have a markedly prolonged PR interval at rest and no evidence of anterograde fast pathway conduction. In such cases, ablation of the anterograde slow pathway may produce complete AV block, whereas retrograde fast pathway ablation can eliminate SVT without altering AV conduction.

SLOW PATHWAY ABLATION. The slow pathway can be located by mapping along the posteromedial tricuspid annulus close to the coronary sinus os. Electrographic recordings are obtained with an atrial-to-ventricular electrogram ratio less than 0.5 and either a multicomponent atrial electrogram or a recording of possible slow pathway potential. In the anatomic approach, target sites are selected fluoroscopically. A single RF application suffices in many cases; but in others, serial RF lesions may be needed, starting at the most posterior site (near the coronary sinus os) and progressing to the more anterior locus (closer to the His bundle recording site). An accelerated junctional rhythm (**Fig. 37-9**) usually occurs when RF energy is applied at a site that will result in successful elimination of SVT. The success rate is equivalent with the anatomic or electrographic mapping approach, and most often, combinations of both are used, yielding success rates approaching 100%, with less than a 1% chance of complete heart block. Catheter-delivered cryoablation has been used for treatment of AVNRT with excellent results.

Slow pathway ablation results in an increase in the anterograde AV block cycle length and AV node ERP without a change in the A-H interval or retrograde conduction properties of the AV node. Patients in whom slow pathway conduction is completely eliminated almost never have

CH 37

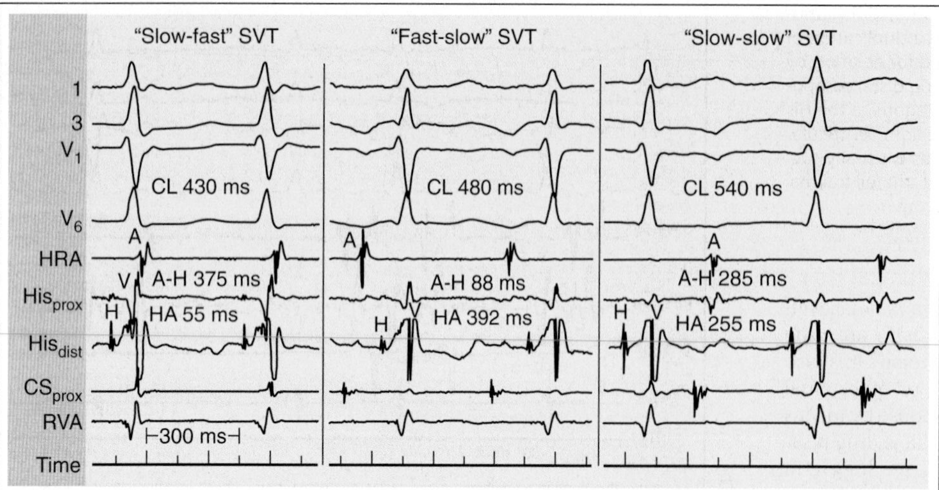

FIGURE 37-8 Three variants of AV node reentrant SVT in the same patient. **Left panel,** Most common type of AV node SVT (anterograde slow pathway, retrograde fast); atrial activation is coincident with ventricular activation. **Center panel,** "Atypical" AV node reentry, with anterograde fast pathway conduction and retrograde conduction over a slow pathway. **Right panel,** Rare variety is shown, with anterograde conduction over a slow pathway and retrograde conduction over a second slow pathway. Note the similar atrial activation sequences in the last two (coronary sinus before right atrium), as distinct from that of slow-fast AV node reentry (coronary sinus and right atrial activation nearly simultaneous). Note also the different P-QRS relationships, from simultaneous activation (left, short RP interval) to P in front of the QRS (middle, long RP interval) and P midway in the cardiac cycle (right). Recording was done as in prior figures. CL = cycle length.

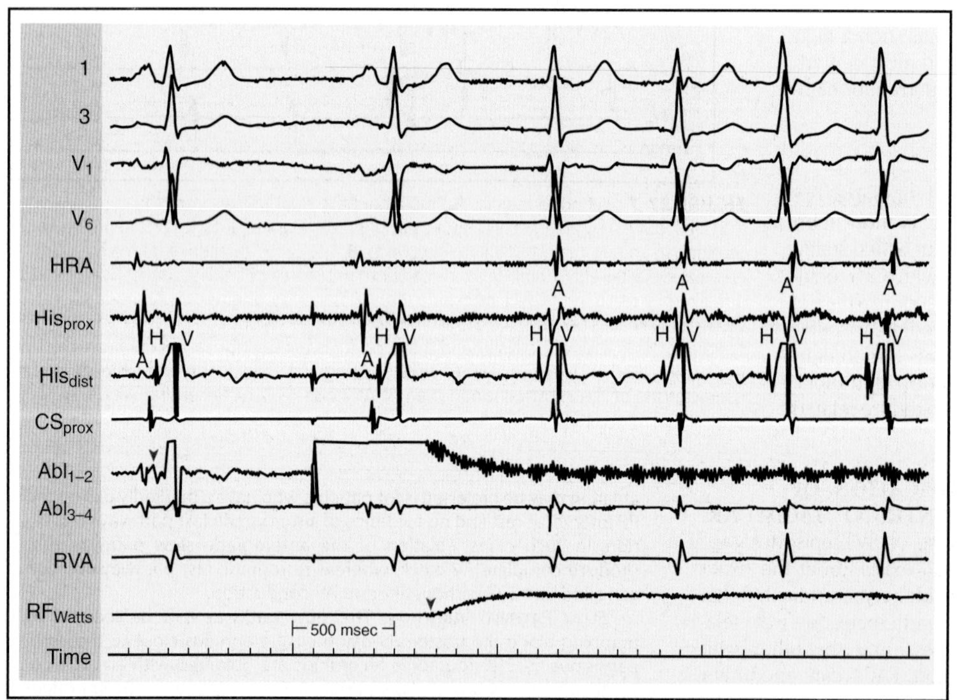

FIGURE 37-9 AV node slow pathway modification for cure of AV node reentrant SVT. The ablation recording (arrowhead in $Abl_{1\text{-}2}$) shows a slurred deflection between atrial and ventricular electrogram components; this may represent the AV node slow pathway deflection (but it is not the bundle of His deflection, which is instead recorded from a separate catheter 15 mm away). Shortly after the onset of radiofrequency delivery (arrowhead in RF_{Watts}), an accelerated junctional rhythm begins and gradually speeds up further. Retrograde conduction is present during the junctional rhythm. $Abl_{3\text{-}4}$ = proximal electrode recording from ablation catheter. Recording was done as in prior figures.

recurrent SVT episodes; approximately 40% percent of patients can have evidence of residual slow pathway function after successful elimination of sustained AVNRT, usually manifested as persistent dual AV node physiology and single AV node echoes during atrial extrastimulation. The surest endpoint for slow pathway ablation is the elimination of sustained AVNRT, with and without an infusion of isoproterenol.

AVNRT recurs in about 5% of patients after slow pathway ablation. In some patients, the ERP of the fast pathway decreases after slow pathway ablation, possibly because of electrotonic interaction between the two pathways. Atypical forms of reentry can result after ablation, as can apparent parasympathetic denervation, resulting in inappropriate sinus tachycardia.

At present, the slow pathway approach is the preferred method for ablation of typical AVNRT. Ablation of the slow pathway is also a safe and effective means for treatment of atypical forms of AVNRT. In patients with AVNRT undergoing slow pathway ablation, junctional ectopy during application of RF energy is a sensitive but nonspecific marker of successful ablation, occurring in longer bursts at effective target sites than at ineffective sites. Ventriculoatrial conduction should be expected during the junctional ectopy, and poor ventriculoatrial conduction or actual block may herald subsequent *anterograde* AV block. Junctional ectopic rhythm is caused by heating of the AV node and does not occur with cryoablation.

Indications

RF catheter ablation for AVNRT can be considered for patients with recurrent, symptomatic, sustained AVNRT that is drug resistant or who are drug intolerant or do not desire long-term drug treatment. The procedure can also be considered for a patient with sustained AVNRT identified during EPS or catheter ablation of another arrhythmia or when there is a finding of dual AV node pathway physiology and atrial echoes but without AVNRT during EPS in a patient suspected of having AVNRT clinically.

Results

Most centers currently use slow pathway ablation, resulting in a procedural success rate of 98%, recurrence rate of less than 2%, and incidence of heart block requiring permanent pacing of less than 1%.

ECTOPIC JUNCTIONAL TACHYCARDIA. Ectopic junctional tachycardia is a rare form of SVT in which the ECG resembles that in AVNRT but is distinct in that (1) the mechanism is automatic, not reentrant, and (2) the atrium is clearly not involved in the tachycardia. This disorder is most commonly observed in young healthy individuals, in women more often than in men, and is usually catecholamine dependent. Ablation must be carried out close to the His bundle, and the risk of heart block requiring pacemaker insertion exceeds 5%.

RADIOFREQUENCY CATHETER ABLATION OF ARRHYTHMIAS RELATED TO THE SINUS NODE. Reentry in or around the sinus node is an uncommon arrhythmia, characterized by episodes of

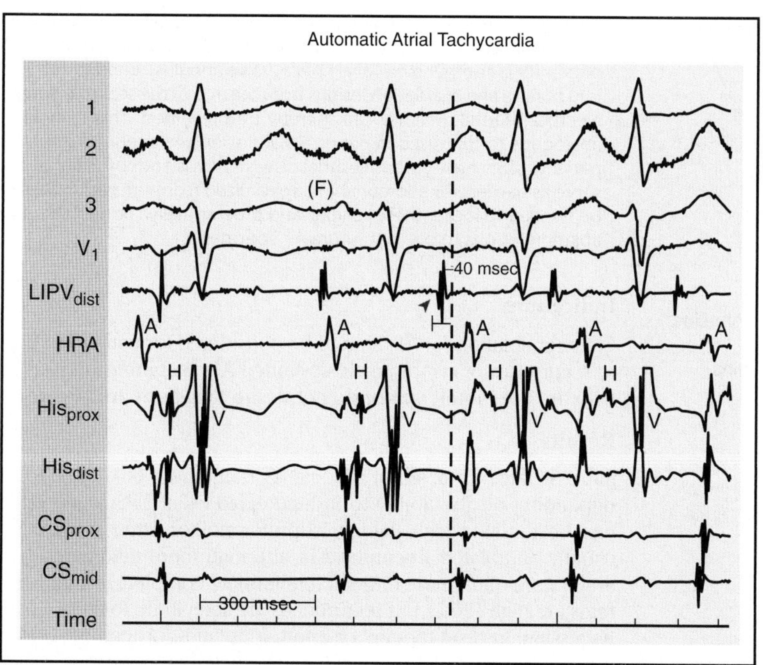

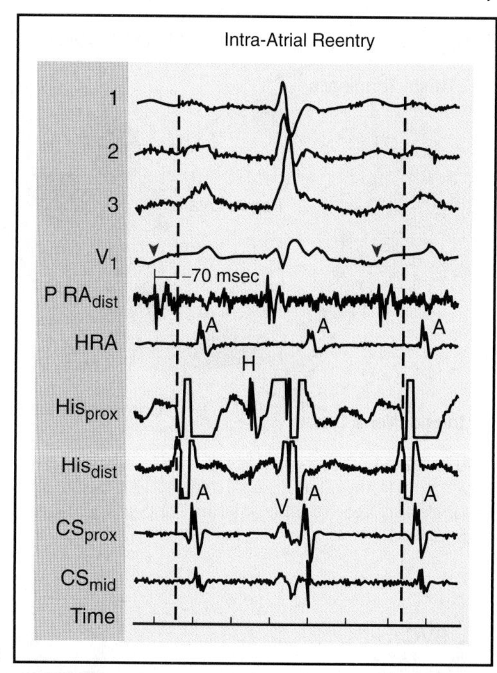

FIGURE 37-10 Atrial tachycardias. **A,** Automatic atrial tachycardia arising in the left inferior pulmonary vein (LIPV). A sinus beat is shown at left, followed by a fusion beat (F) of sinus and tachycardia activation. The last three beats in the panel are atrial tachycardia. The ablation catheter was within the LIPV and recorded a sharp potential (arrowhead) 40 milliseconds before the P wave onset (dashed line). Ablation at this site terminated the tachycardia. **B,** Intra-atrial reentrant tachycardia in a patient who had undergone atrial septal defect repair years earlier. The ablation catheter is in the posterior right atrium (P RA), where a fragmented signal is recorded. A portion of this electrogram (arrowheads) precedes the P wave onset during tachycardia (dashed line) by 70 milliseconds. Ablation at this site terminated the tachycardia. Recording was done as in prior figures.

tachycardia with a P wave identical to the sinus P wave, usually with a PR interval longer than in sinus; in physiologic sinus tachycardia, the PR interval remains normal or shortens because of catecholamine effects on the AV node as well as on the sinus node. RF applications are placed around the region of the sinus node at sites of early activation, before P wave onset, until tachycardia terminates.

Inappropriate sinus tachycardia is a syndrome characterized by high sinus rates with exercise and at rest. Patients complain of palpitations at all times of day that correlate with inappropriately high sinus rates. They may not respond well to beta blocker therapy because of lack of desired effect or occurrence of side effects. When the sinus node area is to be ablated, it can be identified anatomically and electrophysiologically, and ablation lesions are usually placed between the superior vena cava and crista terminalis at sites of early atrial activation. Intracardiac echocardiography can help in defining anatomy and positioning the ablation catheter. Isoproterenol may be helpful in "forcing" the site of impulse formation to cells with the most rapid discharge rate. Care must be taken to apply RF energy at the most cephalad sites first; initial ablation performed farther down the crista terminalis does not alter the atrial rate at the time but can damage subsidiary pacemaker regions that may be needed after the sinus node has eventually been ablated.

Indications

Catheter ablation for sinus node reentrant tachycardia can be performed in patients with recurrent symptomatic episodes of sustained SVT that is drug resistant or who are drug intolerant or do not desire long-term drug treatment. Patients with inappropriate sinus tachycardia should be considered for ablation only after clear failure of medical therapy because ablation results are often less than completely satisfactory. Whenever ablation is performed in the region of the sinus node, the patient should be apprised of the risk of needing a pacemaker after the procedure. Phrenic nerve damage is also a possibility.

Results

Sinus node reentrant tachycardia can be successfully ablated in more than 90% of candidates. Results are not as good for inappropriate sinus tachycardia; although a good technical result may be obtained at the time of the procedure, symptoms often persist because of recurrence of rapid sinus rates (at or near preablation rates) or for nonarrhythmic reasons. Multiple ablation sessions are needed in some patients, and about 20% eventually undergo pacemaker implantation; however, not all these patients have relief of palpitations, despite a normal heart rate.

RADIOFREQUENCY CATHETER ABLATION OF ATRIAL TACHYCARDIA (See Chap. 39). ATs are a heterogeneous group of disorders; causative factors include rapid discharge of a focus (focal tachycardia) and reentry. The former can occur in anyone, irrespective of the presence of structural abnormalities of the atria, whereas reentrant ATs almost always occur in the setting of structurally damaged atria. Symptoms vary from none, in relatively infrequent or slow ATs in patients without heart disease, to syncope (rapid AT with compromised cardiac function) or heart failure (incessant AT during a period of weeks or months). All forms of AT are amenable to catheter ablation.

FOCAL ATRIAL TACHYCARDIA. In focal ATs (automatic or triggered foci or microreentry), activation mapping is used to determine the site of the AT by recording the earliest onset of local activation. These tachycardias can behave capriciously and be practically noninducible in an EPS, despite the patient's complaining of multiple daily episodes before EPS. Ten percent to 15% of patients can have multiple atrial foci. Sites tend to cluster near the pulmonary veins in the left atrium and the mouths of the atrial appendages and along the crista terminalis on the right (**Figs. 37-10A and 37-11**; see Fig. 36-15).[30] Activation times of these sites typically occur only 15 to 40 milliseconds before the onset of the P wave on the ECG. Care must be taken to avoid inadvertent damage to the phrenic nerve; its location can be determined by pacing at high current at a potential site of ablation, observing for diaphragmatic contraction. Ablation should not be performed at a site at which this is seen, if at all possible.

REENTRANT ATRIAL TACHYCARDIA. As noted, these ATs occur more commonly in the setting of structural heart disease, especially after prior surgery involving an atrial incision (repair of congenital heart disease such as atrial septal defect, Mustard or Senning repair of transposed great vessels, or one of a variety of Fontan repairs for tricuspid atresia

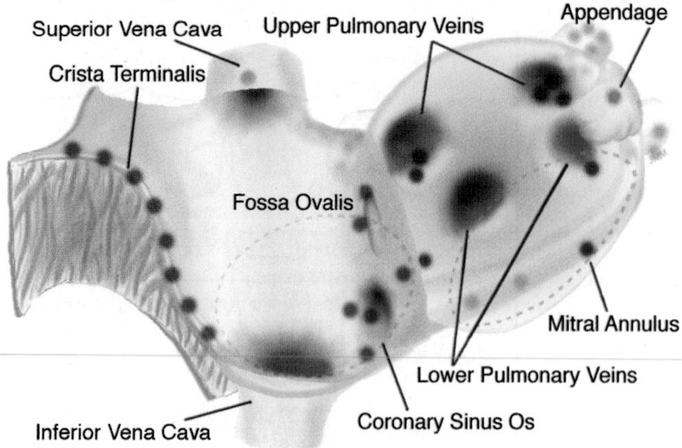

FIGURE 37-11 Locations of origins of focal atrial tachycardias. The atria are viewed from front with right atrial free wall retracted to show interior. Structures are labeled as shown; right atrial foci appear in shades of blue, left atrial in shades of red.

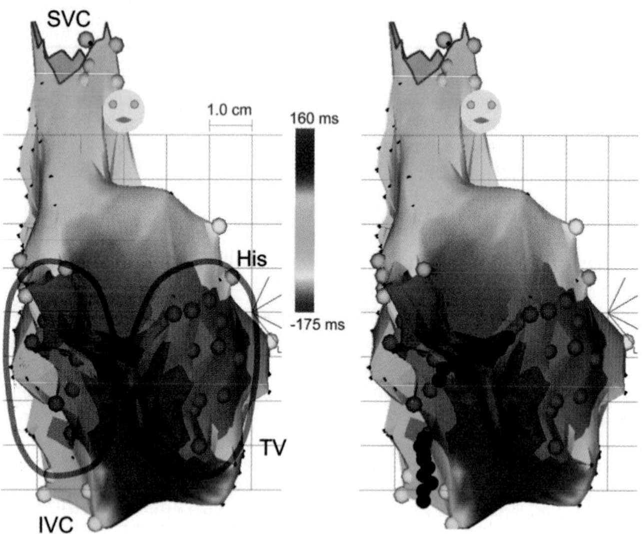

FIGURE 37-12 Reentrant atrial tachycardia. At left, an electroanatomic activation map of the right atrium is shown in a patient with a prior right atrial incision for atrial septal defect closure. Scar is shown as gray areas; arrows depict a double loop of reentry around scars with a common diastolic pathway between scars. Color bar at center shows progression of activation times during atrial tachycardia (from red through green, blue, and purple). The tachycardia cycle length (350 milliseconds) is almost entirely represented in the range of colors. At right, red dots are ablation sites connecting scars (transecting diastolic pathway) and connecting one scar to the inferior vena cava (IVC) to preclude reentry around all barriers. His = His bundle; SVC = superior vena cava; TV = tricuspid valve.

and other disorders) or prior atrial ablation (e.g., for atrial fibrillation).[31] The region of slow conduction is typically related to an end of an atriotomy or prior ablation scar; this is, however, not in a constant anatomic location but varies from patient to patient. Therefore, preprocedural review of operative and ablation procedure reports and careful electrophysiologic mapping are essential. Because reentry within a complete circuit is occurring, activation can be recorded throughout the entire cardiac cycle. The ablation strategy is to identify regions with mid-diastolic atrial activation during tachycardia that can be proved by pacing techniques to be integral to the tachycardia (Fig. 37-10B and **Fig. 37-12**).[32] Such sites are attractive ablation targets because they are composed of relatively few cells—hence, electrical silence on the surface ECG in diastole—and are thus more easily ablated by a typical application of RF energy than other areas might be. Focal ablation of these sites can then be performed, but often tachycardia can still be initiated (usually at a slower rate) or recurs after the procedure. Because these sites are typically located at a relatively narrow zone between the ends of prior scars or surgical incisions or ablation lines and another nonconducting barrier (e.g., another scar, caval orifice, valve annulus), another technique is to make a line of ablation lesions from the end of the scar to the nearest electrical barrier. Reentry can thereby be prevented. This technique is analogous to that used in curing atrial flutter (see later). Because these patients often have extensive atrial disease with islands of scar that could serve as barriers for additional ATs, specialized mapping techniques may be needed to locate these regions and preemptively connect them with ablation lesions to prevent future AT episodes.

Indications

Catheter ablation for ATs should be considered for patients with recurrent episodes of symptomatic sustained ATs that are drug resistant or who are drug intolerant or do not desire long-term drug treatment.

Results

Success rates for ablation of focal AT range from 80% to 95%, largely depending on the ability to induce episodes at EPS; when episodes can be initiated with pacing, isoproterenol, or other means, AT can usually be ablated. Reentrant ATs, although more readily induced by an EPS, are often more difficult to eliminate completely; initial success rates are high (90%), but recurrences are seen in up to 20% of patients, necessitating drug therapy or another ablation procedure. Complications, occurring in 1% to 2% of patients, include phrenic nerve damage, cardiac tamponade, and heart block (with rare perinodal ATs).

Radiofrequency Catheter Ablation of Atrial Flutter (see Chap. 39). Atrial flutter may be defined electrocardiographically (most typically, negative sawtooth waves in leads II, III, and aVF, at a rate of about 300 beats/min) or electrophysiologically (a rapid, organized macroreentrant AT, the circuit for which is anatomically determined). Understanding of the reentrant pathway for all forms of atrial flutter is essential for development of an ablation approach. Reentry in the right atrium, with the left atrium passively activated, constitutes the mechanism of the typical electrocardiographic variety of atrial flutter, with caudocranial activation along the right atrial septum and craniocaudal activation of the right atrial free wall (**Fig. 37-13A**). In some cases, a zone of slow conduction exists in the low right atrium, which is typically bounded by the tricuspid annulus, inferior vena cava, and coronary sinus. In other cases, conduction velocity is more uniform throughout the large circuit. Placement of an ablative lesion between any two anatomic barriers that transects a portion of the circuit necessary for perpetuation of reentry can be curative. Typically, this is across the isthmus of atrial tissue between the inferior vena caval orifice and tricuspid annulus (the cavotricuspid isthmus), a relatively narrow point in the circuit. Successful ablation can be accomplished where the advancing flutter wave front enters this zone in the low inferolateral right atrium, near the exit of this zone at the inferomedial right atrium, or in between these sites. Locations for RF delivery can be guided anatomically or electrophysiologically. Less commonly, the direction of wave front propagation in this large right atrial circuit is reversed ("clockwise" flutter proceeding cephalad up the right atrial free wall and caudad down the septum, with upright flutter waves in the inferior leads; Fig. 37-13A). This arrhythmia, which has been called *atypical atrial flutter,* may also be ablated by the same techniques as with more typical atrial flutter. These two arrhythmias constitute cavotricuspid isthmus–dependent flutter and are distinct from other rapid atrial arrhythmias that may have a similar appearance on the ECG but use different (and often multiple) circuits in other parts of the right or left atrium. Ablation can be more difficult in these cases, which often occur in the setting of advanced lung disease or prior cardiac surgery or ablation. A common theme in these complex reentrant arrhythmias is the presence of an anatomically determined zone of inexcitability, around which an electrical wave front can circulate. Specialized mapping tools and skills are necessary to produce successful ablation in these cases.

In patients with atrial fibrillation, an antiarrhythmic drug can slow intra-atrial conduction to such an extent that atrial flutter results and fibrillation is no longer observed. In some of these patients, ablation of atrial flutter and having them continue to take the antiarrhythmic drug can prevent recurrences of these atrial arrhythmias.

The endpoint of atrial flutter ablation procedures was initially termination of atrial flutter, with RF application accompanied by noninducibility of the arrhythmia. However, by use of these criteria, up to 30% of patients had recurrent flutter because of lack of complete and permanent conduction block in the cavotricuspid isthmus. In the last several

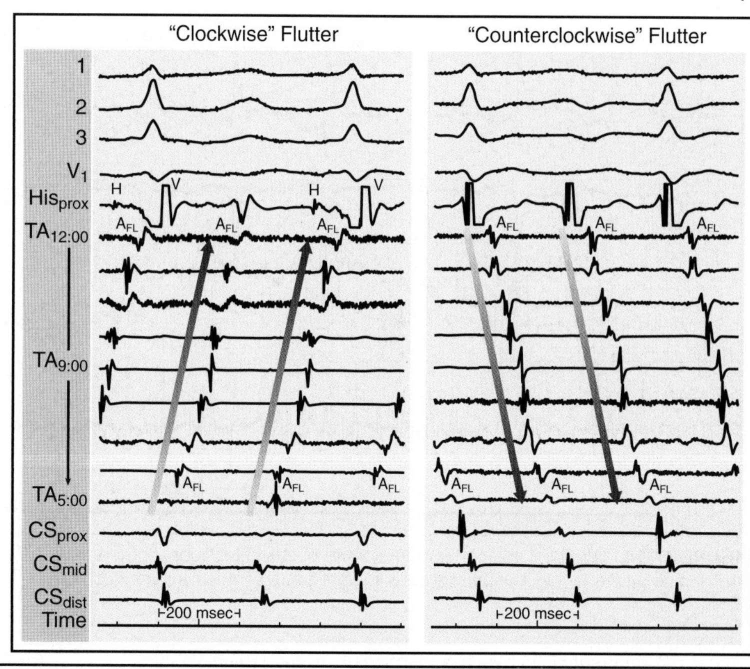

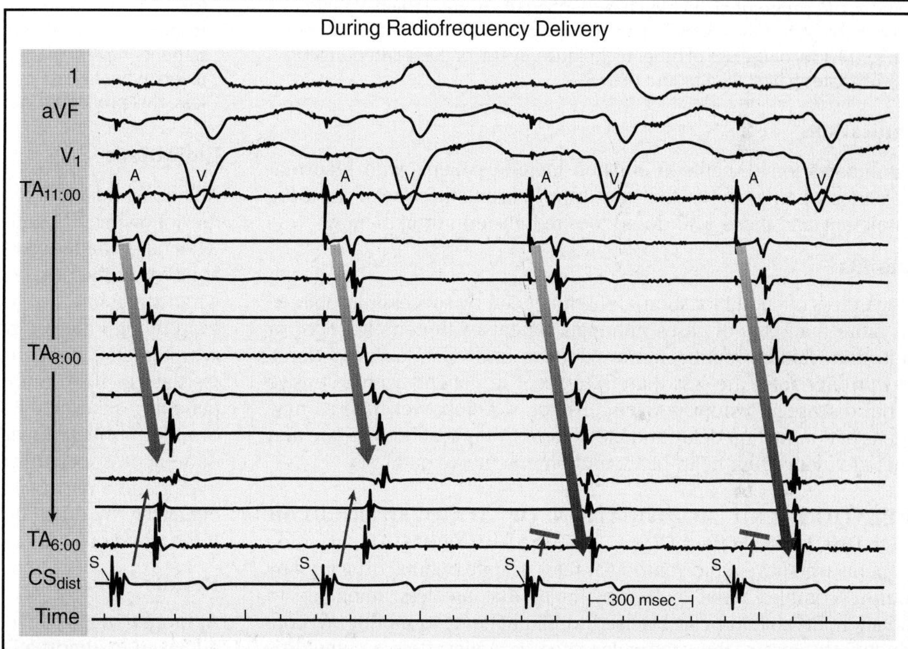

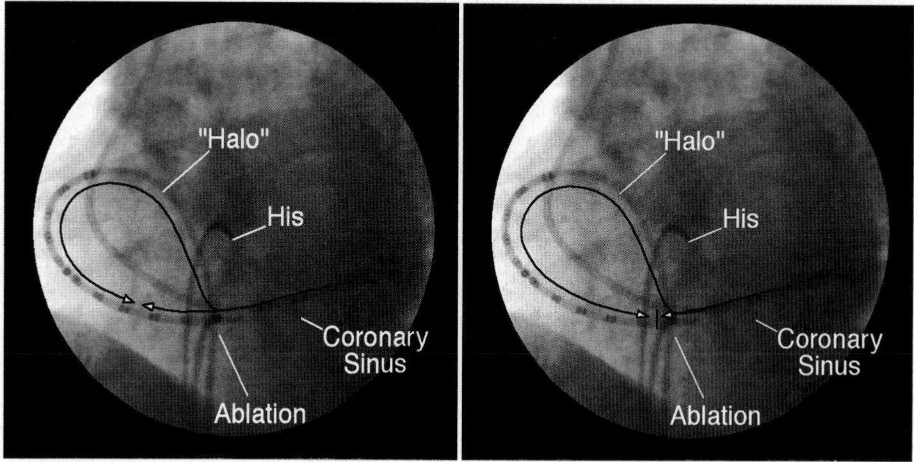

FIGURE 37-13 **A,** Two forms of atrial flutter in the same patient are shown. A halo catheter with 10 electrode pairs is situated on the atrial side of the tricuspid annulus (TA), with recording sites displayed from the top of the annulus (12:00) to the inferomedial aspect (5:00), as shown in fluoroscopic views in **B**. On the left, the wave front of atrial activation proceeds in a clockwise fashion (arrows) along the annulus, whereas on the right, the direction of propagation is the reverse. **B,** Ablation of the isthmus of atrial tissue between the tricuspid annulus and inferior vena caval orifice for cure of atrial flutter. Recordings are displayed from the multipolar catheter around much of the circumference of the tricuspid annulus (see left anterior oblique fluoroscopy images). Ablation of this isthmus is performed during coronary sinus pacing. In the two beats on the left, atrial conduction proceeds in two directions around the tricuspid annulus, as indicated by arrows and recorded along the halo catheter. In the two beats on the right, ablation has interrupted conduction in the floor of the right atrium, eliminating one path for transmission along the tricuspid annulus. The halo catheter now records conduction, proceeding all the way around the annulus. This finding demonstrates unidirectional block in the isthmus; block in the other direction may be demonstrated by pacing from one of the halo electrodes and observing a similar lack of isthmus conduction. (The bundle of His recording in the right panel is lost because of catheter movement.)

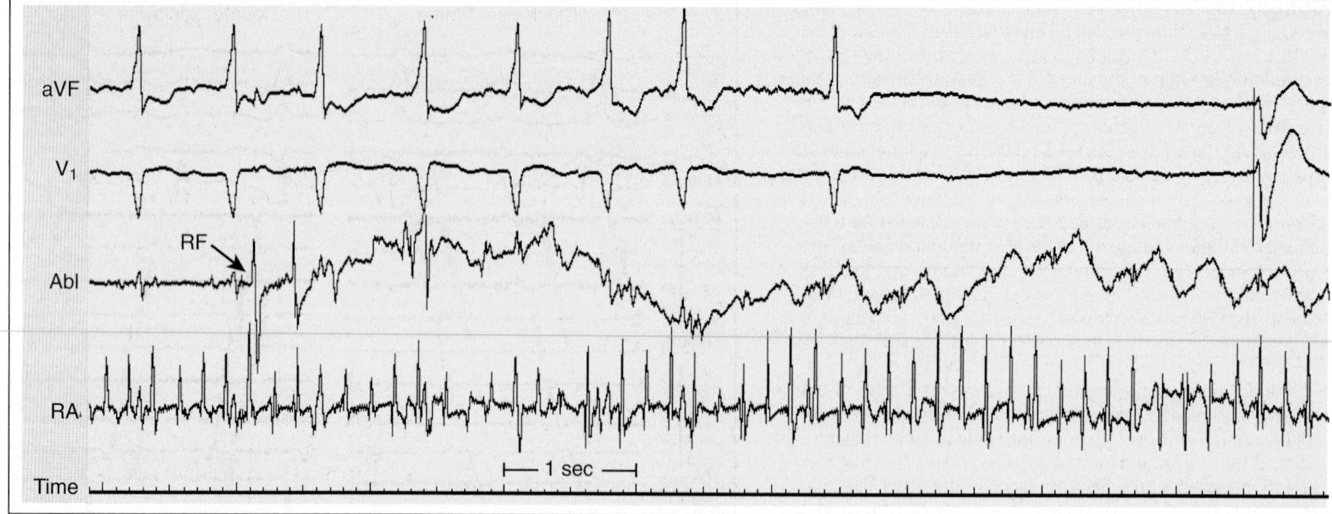

FIGURE 37-14 AV nodal ablation for rate control of atrial fibrillation. ECG shows rapidly conducted atrial fibrillation; radiofrequency energy application (arrow) results in complete AV block within seconds, followed by a ventricular paced complex.

years, the endpoint of ablation has changed to ensuring a line of bidirectional block in this region by pacing from opposite sides of the isthmus (Fig. 37-13B) or the use of other techniques. By use of these criteria, recurrence rates have fallen to less than 5%.

Indications

Candidates for RF catheter ablation include patients with recurrent episodes of atrial flutter that are drug resistant, those who are drug intolerant, and those who do not desire long-term drug therapy.

Results

Regardless of circuit location, atrial flutter can be successfully ablated in more than 90% of cases, although patients with complex right or left atrial flutters require more extensive and complex procedures. Recurrence rates are less than 5%, except in patients with extensive atrial disease, in whom new circuits can develop over time as new areas of conduction delay and block form. Complications are rare and include inadvertent heart block and phrenic nerve paralysis.

ABLATION AND MODIFICATION OF ATRIOVENTRICULAR CONDUCTION FOR ATRIAL TACHYARRHYTHMIAS. In some patients who have rapid ventricular rates despite optimal drug therapy during complex atrial tachyarrhythmias that are less amenable to ablation, RF ablation can be used to eliminate or to modify AV conduction to control the ventricular rates. To achieve this, a catheter is placed across the tricuspid valve and positioned to record a small His bundle electrogram associated with a large atrial electrogram. RF energy is applied until complete AV block has been achieved and is continued for an additional 30 to 60 seconds (**Fig. 37-14**). If no change in AV conduction is observed after 15 seconds of RF ablation despite good contact, the catheter is repositioned and the attempt repeated. In occasional patients, attempts at RF ablation by this right-sided heart approach fail to achieve heart block. These patients can undergo an attempt from the left ventricle with a catheter positioned along the posterior interventricular septum, just beneath the aortic valve, to record a large His bundle electrogram. Energy is applied between the catheter electrode and skin patch or between catheters in the left and right ventricles. Success rates currently approach 100%, with recurrence of AV conduction in less than 5% of cases. Improved left ventricular function can result from control of ventricular rate during atrial fibrillation and withdrawal of rate-controlling medications with negative inotropic action. Permanent ventricular or AV pacing is required after ablation.

In some cases, the AV junction can be modified to slow the ventricular rate without producing complete AV block by ablation in the region of the slow pathway, as described in connection with AV node modification for AV node reentry. Initial success rates for slowing of the ventricular response are good; however, long-term results are less consistent. Some patients have a gradual increase in ventricular rate to near-preablation levels, whereas late complete heart block may occur in others. Nonetheless, this procedure can be tried before producing complete AV block.

Indications

Ablation and modification of AV conduction can be considered in the following: (1) patients with symptomatic atrial tachyarrhythmias who have inadequately controlled ventricular rates unless primary ablation of the atrial tachyarrhythmia is possible; (2) similar patients when drugs are not tolerated or patients do not wish to take them, even though the ventricular rate can be controlled; (3) patients with symptomatic, nonparoxysmal, junctional tachycardia that is drug resistant or in whom drugs are not tolerated or are not desired; (4) patients resuscitated from sudden cardiac death related to atrial flutter or atrial fibrillation with a rapid ventricular response in the absence of an accessory pathway; and (5) patients with a dual-chamber pacemaker and a pacemaker-mediated tachycardia that cannot be treated effectively by drugs or by reprogramming of the pacemaker. The last three situations are rarely encountered.

Results

As noted before, successful interruption of AV conduction can be achieved in almost all cases; recurrent conduction is observed in less than 5%. Significant complications occur in 1% to 2%. In early studies, up to 4% of patients had an episode of sudden death after AV junction ablation despite adequate pacemaker function, presumably because of relative bradycardia after long periods of rapid ventricular rates serving as the setting for repolarization-related ventricular arrhythmias. In one study, 6 of 100 patients died suddenly when the initial pacing rate was set to 60 beats/min, but none of 135 died suddenly when the rate was set to 90 beats/min for 1 to 3 months after ablation. Improvements in quality of life indices as well as cost-effectiveness have been demonstrated for this procedure.

Radiofrequency Catheter Ablation of Atrial Fibrillation. See Chaps. 39 and 40.

RADIOFREQUENCY CATHETER ABLATION OF VENTRICULAR TACHYCARDIA. In general, the success rate for ablation of VTs is lower than that for AV node reentry or AV reentry. This lower success rate may be related to the fact that this procedure is often a last resort in patients with drug-resistant VTs who have extensive structural heart disease, but it is also related to more difficult mapping in the ventricles. Furthermore, in the ideal case, the VT induction must be reproducible, with uniform QRS morphology from beat to beat, and VT

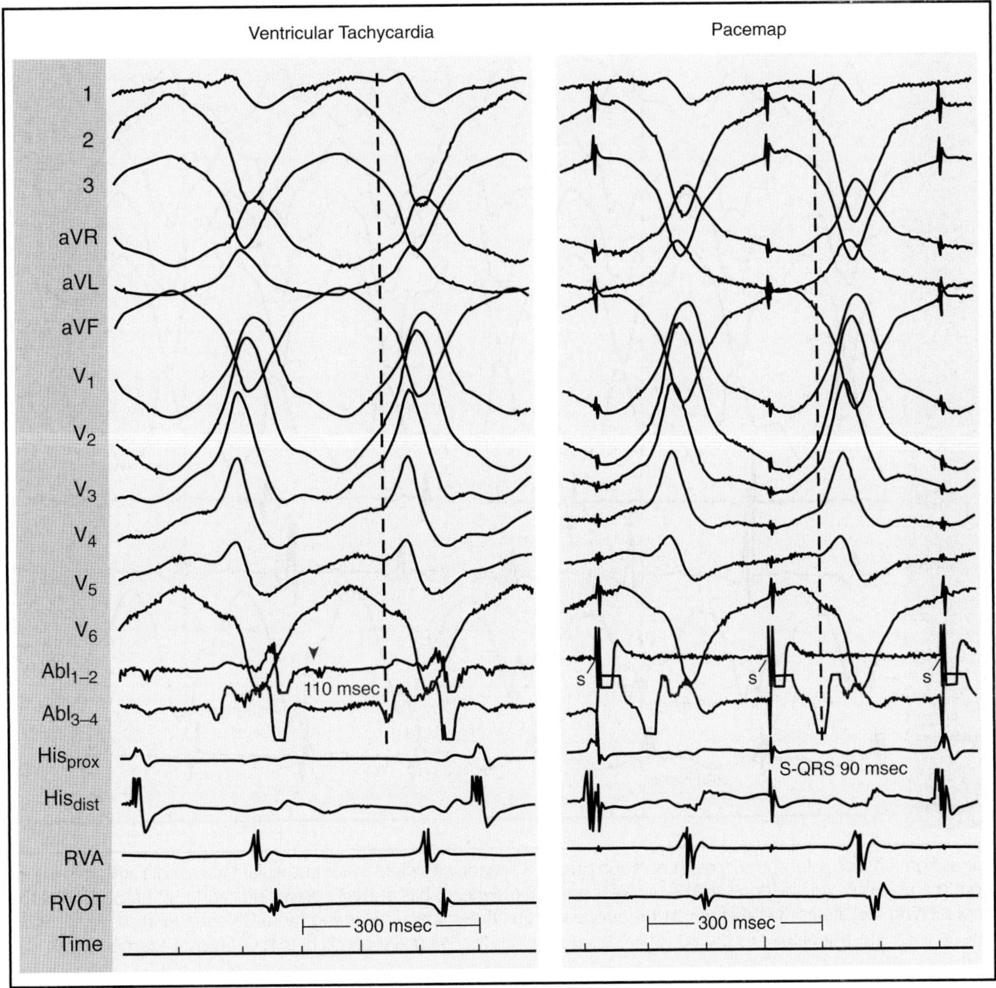

FIGURE 37-15 Ventricular tachycardia and pace mapping. All 12 surface ECG leads are shown, along with intracardiac recordings during VT. The Abl_{1-2} recording shows a small deflection occurring early in electrical diastole (arrowhead) 110 milliseconds before the onset of the QRS (dashed line). In the right panel, pacing is performed from this site. This produces an identical QRS complex in each lead, with a stimulus-QRS onset interval similar to the electrogram-QRS onset interval during VT. Ablation at this site eliminated VT in 2 seconds. RVOT = right ventricular outflow tract.

must be sustained and hemodynamically stable so that the patient can tolerate the VT long enough during the procedure to undergo the extensive mapping necessary to localize optimal ablation target sites. Patients with several electrocardiographically distinct, uniform morphologies of VT can still be candidates for ablation because, in many cases, a common reentrant pathway is shared by two or more VT morphologies. Also, the target for ablation must be fairly circumscribed and endocardially situated, although cases of successful ablation only from the epicardial aspect have become more common.[33] Very rapid VT, polymorphic VT, and infrequent, nonsustained episodes are less well suited to this form of therapy at this time (see later).

Location and Ablation. RF catheter ablation of VT can be divided into idiopathic VT, which occurs in patients with essentially structurally normal hearts; VT that occurs in various disease settings but without coronary artery disease; and VT in patients with coronary artery disease and usually prior myocardial infarction. In the first group, VTs can arise in either ventricle. Right ventricular tachycardias most commonly originate in the outflow tract and have a characteristic left bundle branch block–like, inferior axis morphology (see Chap. 39); less often, VTs arise in the inflow tract or free wall. Initiation of tachycardia can often be facilitated by catecholamines. Most left ventricular tachycardias are septal in origin and have a characteristic QRS configuration (i.e., right bundle branch block, superior axis); other VTs occur less commonly and arise from different areas of the left ventricle, including the left ventricular outflow tract and aortic sinuses of Valsalva, and are similar in electrocardiographic appearance and clinical behavior to those arising in the right ventricular outflow tract.[34] Abnormal patterns of sympathetic innervation may be present in some. VTs in abnormal hearts without coronary artery disease can be the result of bundle branch reentry (see Chap. 39), most typically observed in patients with dilated cardiomyopathies. In these patients, ablation of the right bundle branch eliminates the tachycardia. VT can occur in right ventricular dysplasia (see Chap. 9), sarcoidosis, Chagas disease, hypertrophic cardiomyopathy (see Chap. 69), and a host of other noncoronary disease states.

Activation mapping and pace mapping are effective in patients with idiopathic VTs to locate the site of origin of the VT. In activation mapping, the timing of endocardial electrograms sampled by the mapping catheter is compared with the onset of the surface QRS complex. Sites that are activated before the surface QRS onset are near the origin of the VT (**Fig. 37-15**; see Fig. 36-14). In idiopathic VT, ablation at a site at which the unipolar electrogram shows a QS complex may yield greater success than if an rS potential is observed (**Fig. 37-16**). Pace mapping involves stimulation of various ventricular sites to produce a QRS contour that duplicates the QRS contour of the spontaneous VT, thus establishing the apparent site of origin of the arrhythmia (see Fig. 37-15). This technique is limited by several methodologic problems but may be useful when the tachycardia cannot be initiated and when a 12-lead ECG has been obtained during the spontaneous VT. Presystolic Purkinje potentials as well as very low amplitude mid-diastolic signals can be recorded during VT from sites at which ablation cures VT in most patients with left ventricular VTs that have a right bundle branch block superior axis. Localization of optimal ablation sites for VT in patients with coronary artery disease and prior infarction can be more challenging than in patients with structurally normal hearts because of the altered anatomy and electrophysiology. Pace mapping has lower sensitivity and specificity than for idiopathic VT. Furthermore, reentry circuits can sometimes be large and resistant to the relatively small lesions produced by RF catheter ablation in scarred endocardium.

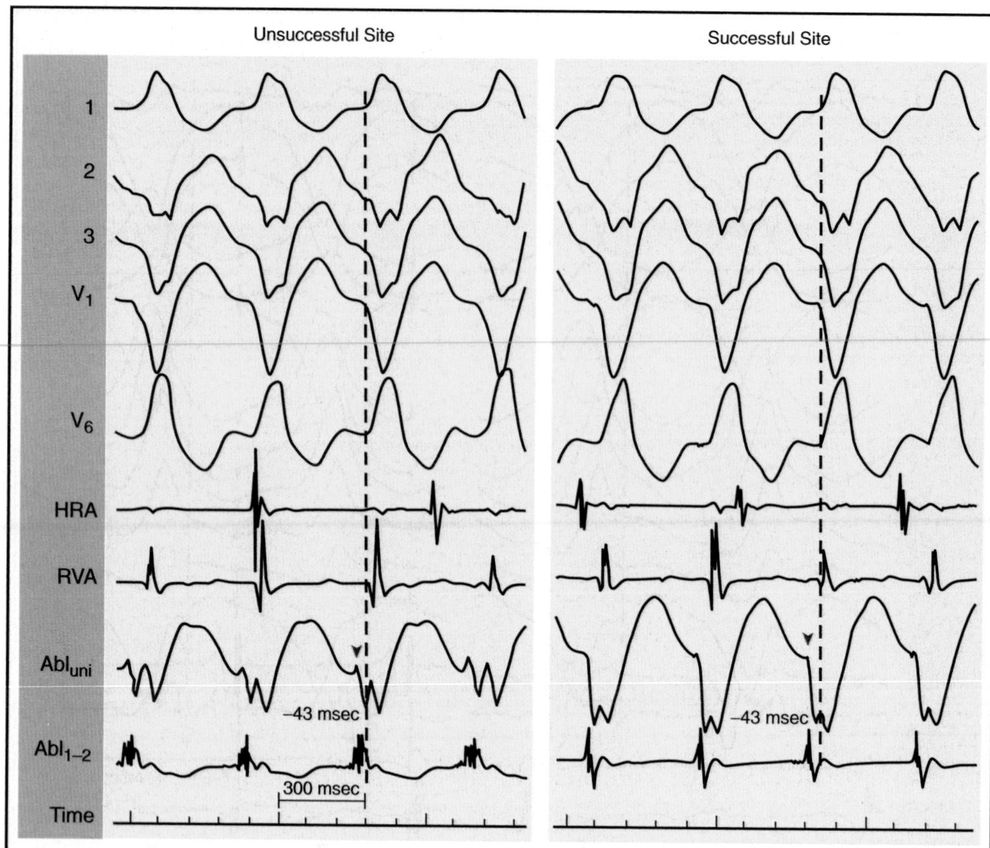

FIGURE 37-16 Recordings from unsuccessful and successful ablation sites in a patient with idiopathic ventricular tachycardia arising in the inferior right ventricular wall. In the recordings from the unsuccessful ablation site, the unipolar signal (arrowhead) has a small r wave, indicating that a portion of the wave front from the focus of tachycardia is approaching the site from elsewhere. At the successful site, the unipolar recording has a QS configuration, indicating that all depolarization is emanating from this site. In each site, the bipolar recording (Abl_{1-2}) occurs an identical 43 milliseconds before QRS onset (dashed lines).

In scar-based VT (e.g., postinfarction, cardiomyopathies), finding of a protected region of diastolic activation used as a critical part of the reentrant circuit is desirable because ablation at this site has a good chance of eliminating the tachycardia (**Fig. 37-17**). Because of the extensive derangement in electrophysiology caused by the previous damage (e.g., infarct, myopathy), many areas of the ventricle may have diastolic activation but may not be relevant to the perpetuation of the VT. These "bystander sites" make activation mapping more difficult. Pacing techniques such as entrainment can be used to test whether a site is actually part of a circuit or a bystander. Entrainment involves pacing for several seconds during a tachycardia at a rate slightly faster than the VT rate; after pacing is stopped and the same tachycardia resumes, the timing of the first complex relative to the last paced beat is an indicator of how close the pacing site is to a part of the VT circuit. During entrainment, part of the ventricle is activated by the paced wave front and part by the VT wave front being forced to exit earlier than it ordinarily would, resulting in a fusion complex on the ECG. Pacing from within a critical portion of the circuit itself produces an exact QRS match with the VT; fusion occurs only within the circuit and is "concealed" on the surface ECG. Sites with a low-amplitude, isolated, mid-diastolic potential that cannot be dissociated from the tachycardia by pacing perturbations, at which entrainment with concealed fusion can be demonstrated, are highly likely to be successful ablation sites.[35]

In a significant proportion of patients with VT in the presence of structural heart disease, activation mapping and entrainment cannot be performed because of poor hemodynamic tolerance of the arrhythmia or inability to initiate sustained tachycardia during an EPS. In these situations, additional methods can be used that are categorized as *substrate mapping,* in which areas of low electrical voltage or from which very delayed potentials are recorded during sinus rhythm, or at which pacing closely replicates a known VT 12-lead ECG morphology (pace mapping), are targeted for ablation without performance of any mapping during VT. These methods have yielded very good results in many cases.

In patients without structural heart disease, only a single VT is usually present, and catheter ablation of that VT is most often curative. In patients with extensive structural heart disease, especially those with prior myocardial infarction, multiple VTs are usually present. Catheter ablation of a single VT in such patients may be only palliative and may not eliminate the need for further antiarrhythmic therapy. The genesis of multiple tachycardia morphologies is not clear, although in some cases they are merely different manifestations of one circuit (e.g., different directions of wave front propagation or exit to the ventricle as a whole), and ablation of one may prevent recurrence of others. The presence of multiple VT morphologies contributes to the difficulties in mapping and ablation of VT in these patients because pacing techniques used to validate recordings at potential sites of ablation may result in a change in morphology to another VT that does not arise in the same region.

After ablation of VT, ventricular stimulation is repeated to assess efficacy. In some cases, rapid polymorphic VT or fibrillation is initiated. The clinical significance of these arrhythmias is unclear, but some evidence has suggested that they have a low likelihood of spontaneous occurrence during follow-up.

As noted earlier, most cases of polymorphic VT and VF are not currently amenable to ablation because of hemodynamic instability and beat-to-beat changes in activation sequence. However, some cases appear to have a focal source (similar to focal sources of atrial fibrillation), and if the focus can be identified and ablated, further arrhythmia episodes can be prevented. In such cases, repeated episodes of arrhythmia have constant electrocardiographic features of the initiating beat or beats, suggesting a consistent source, which may be in either ventricle.[36] The electrogram at sites of successful ablation often has very sharp presystolic potentials reminiscent of Purkinje potentials, with a 50- to 100-millisecond delay to the QRS onset.

Indications

Patients considered for RF catheter ablation of VT in the absence of structural heart disease are those with symptomatic, sustained, monomorphic VT when the tachycardia is drug resistant, when the patient is drug intolerant, or when the patient does not desire long-term drug

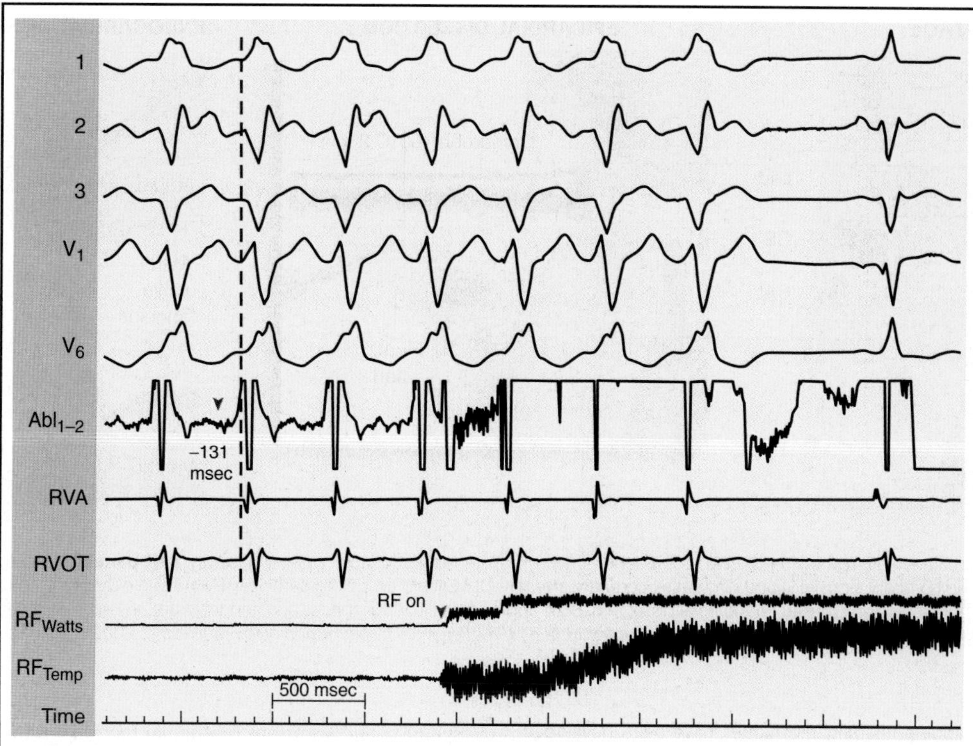

FIGURE 37-17 RF ablation of postinfarction VT. The electrogram in the ablation recording (Abl_{1-2}, arrowhead) precedes the QRS onset (dashed line) by 131 milliseconds. Ablation here (RF on) results in slight deceleration of VT before termination in 1.3 seconds. Temperature monitored from the catheter tip had just peaked (approximately 70°C) at the time VT terminated. Recording was done as in prior figures.

therapy. Patients with structural heart disease who are candidates for ablation include those with bundle branch reentrant VT and those with sustained monomorphic VT and an ICD who are receiving multiple shocks not manageable by reprogramming or concomitant drug therapy. On occasion, nonsustained VT or even severely symptomatic PVCs require RF catheter ablation. In some of these cases, in which the ventricular ectopy occurs frequently, significant left ventricular systolic dysfunction has occurred (presumably a form of tachycardia-related cardiomyopathy). After successful ablation, ventricular function may significantly improve or even normalize.[37,38]

Results

In patients with structurally normal hearts, the success rate of VT ablation is about 85%. In patients with postinfarction VT, more than 70% no longer have recurrences of VT after the ablation procedure, despite inducibility of rapid VT or VF (only about 30% of patients will have no inducible ventricular arrhythmia of any type and no spontaneous recurrences). Almost all these patients have an ICD, regardless of outcome. Significant complications occur in up to 3%, including vascular damage, heart block, worsening of heart failure, cardiac tamponade, stroke, and valve damage; death is rare but can occur in patients with severe coronary artery disease and systolic dysfunction.

New Mapping and Ablation Technologies

Multielectrode Mapping Systems. As noted earlier, many limitations of ablation are related to inadequate mapping. These problems include only isolated premature complexes during the EPS as opposed to sustained tachycardias (in idiopathic atrial and ventricular tachycardias), nonsustained episodes of VT, poor hemodynamic tolerance of VT, and multiple VT morphologies. Standard mapping techniques sample single sites sequentially and are poorly suited to these situations. New mapping systems are available that enable sampling of many sites simultaneously and incorporate sophisticated computer algorithms for analysis and display of global maps. These mapping systems use various technologies, ranging from multiple electrodes situated on each of several splines of a basket catheter, to the use of low-intensity electrical or magnetic fields to localize the catheter tip in the heart and record and plot activation times on a contour map of the chamber, to the use of complex mathematics to compute "virtual" electrograms recorded from a mesh electrode situated in the middle of a chamber cavity. Some of these systems are capable of generating activation maps of an entire chamber using only one cardiac complex, an obvious advantage in patients with only rare premature complexes, nonsustained arrhythmias, or poor hemodynamic tolerance of sustained arrhythmias.

Epicardial Catheter Mapping. Although most VTs can be ablated from the endocardium, occasional cases are resistant to this therapy. In some of these, epicardial ablation may be successful. Much of the work in this area has been performed in patients with VT related to Chagas disease, most of whom appear to require epicardial mapping and ablation; it is often needed in VT due to cardiomyopathy but less frequently in postinfarction patients and those without structural heart disease.

The technique for gaining access to the epicardium differs slightly from that for pericardiocentesis. A long spinal anesthesia needle is introduced from a subxiphoid approach under fluoroscopic guidance. As the pericardial surface is approached, a small amount of a radiocontrast agent is injected. If the needle tip is still outside the pericardium, the dye stays where it is injected; when the pericardial space has been entered, the dye disperses, outlining the heart. A guidewire is introduced through the needle and a standard vascular introducer sheath exchanged over the wire. The pericardial space is accessible for a mapping/ablation catheter. Usual mapping techniques can then be applied. When a site is selected for possible ablation, coronary arteriography may be warranted to avoid delivery of RF energy near a coronary artery. This is less important in cases of postinfarction VT because the VT substrate is typically in a region of prior transmural infarction. The technique can be used for patients who have had prior cardiac surgery, although adhesions may obliterate portions of the pericardial space; on occasion, a small incision in the subxiphoid region is needed for better access and visualization of the space. The most frequent complication of epicardial mapping is pericarditis related to the ablation; cardiac tamponade is rare.

Chemical Ablation. Chemical ablation with alcohol or phenol of an area of myocardium involved in a tachycardia has been used to create AV block in patients not responding to catheter ablation and to eliminate atrial and ventricular tachycardias. Recurrences of tachycardia several days after apparently successful ablation are common. Excessive myocardial necrosis is the major complication, and alcohol ablation should be considered only when other ablative approaches fail or cannot be done.

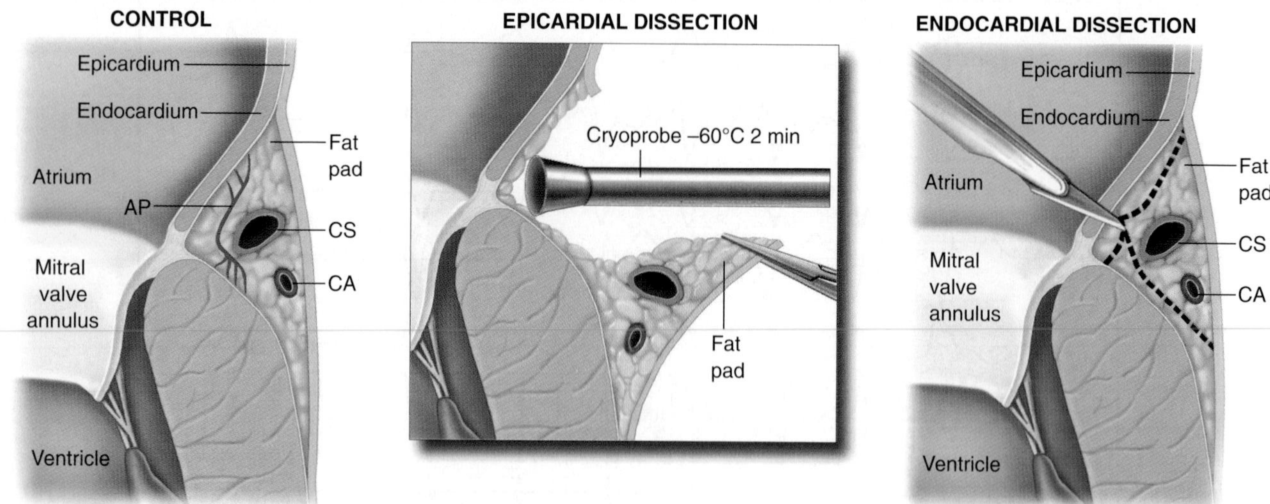

FIGURE 37-18 Schematic diagram showing the two approaches for surgical interruption of an accessory pathway. **Left panel,** Left atrioventricular groove and its vascular contents, the coronary sinus (CS) and circumflex coronary artery (CA). Multiple accessory pathways (APs) course through the fat pad. **Middle panel,** Epicardial dissection approach. **Right panel,** Endocardial dissection. Both approaches clear out the fat pad and interrupt any accessory pathways. *(From Zipes DP: Cardiac electrophysiology: Promises and contributions. J Am Coll Cardiol 13:1329, 1989. Reprinted by permission of the American College of Cardiology.)*

Several other mapping/imaging techniques have been developed recently, including integration of a previously obtained computed tomography or magnetic resonance imaging study into computerized mapping systems and use of intracardiac ultrasound to construct a facsimile of intracardiac anatomy in any chamber during ablation procedures to guide placement of anatomic ablation and reduce fluoroscopic exposure; use of algorithms to select complex fractionated atrial electrograms for ablation in patients with atrial fibrillation; and impedance mapping to avoid unnecessary ablation in pulmonary veins or areas of dense scar. Aside from the image integration techniques, these have not yet gained widespread application.

Surgical Therapy for Tachyarrhythmias

The objectives of a surgical approach to treatment of a tachycardia are to excise, isolate, or interrupt tissue in the heart critical for the initiation, maintenance, or propagation of the tachycardia while preserving or even improving myocardial function. In addition to a direct surgical approach to the arrhythmia, indirect approaches such as aneurysmectomy, coronary artery bypass grafting, and relief of valvular regurgitation or stenosis can be useful for selected patients by improving cardiac hemodynamics and myocardial blood supply. Cardiac sympathectomy alters adrenergic influences on the heart and has been effective in some patients, particularly those who have recurrent VT with the long-QT syndrome despite beta blockade.

Supraventricular Tachycardias

Surgical procedures exist for patients (adults and children) with ATs, atrial flutter and fibrillation (see Chap. 40), AV node reentry, and AV reentry (**Fig. 37-18**). RF catheter ablation adequately treats most of these patients and has thus replaced direct surgical intervention, except for the occasional patient in whom RF catheter ablation fails or who is having concomitant cardiovascular surgery. In some cases, a prior attempt at RF catheter ablation complicates surgery by obliterating the normal tissue planes that exist in the AV groove of the heart or by rendering tissues friable. On occasion, patients with ATs have multiple foci that require surgical intervention. Several surgical procedures have been developed to treat atrial fibrillation; these are reviewed in Chap. 40.

Ventricular Tachycardia

In contrast to patients with supraventricular arrhythmias, candidates for surgical therapy for ventricular arrhythmias often have severe left ventricular dysfunction, generally the result of coronary artery disease. The cause of the underlying heart disease influences the type of surgery performed. Candidates are patients with drug-resistant, symptomatic, recurrent ventricular tachyarrhythmias who ideally have a segmental wall motion abnormality (scar or aneurysm) with preserved residual left ventricular function, have not benefited from prior attempts at catheter ablation, or are not candidates for catheter ablation because of hemodynamic instability during VT or the presence of left ventricular thrombus. Poorer surgical results are obtained in patients with nonischemic cardiomyopathy.

ISCHEMIC HEART DISEASE. In almost all patients who have VT associated with ischemic heart disease, the arrhythmia, regardless of its configuration on the surface ECG, arises in the left ventricle or on the left ventricular side of the interventricular septum. The electrocardiographic contour of the VT can change from a right bundle branch block to a left bundle branch block pattern without a change in the site of earliest diastolic activation, suggesting that the site of the circuit within the left ventricle remains the same, often near the septum, but its exit pathway is altered.

Indirect surgical approaches, including cardiothoracic sympathectomy, coronary artery revascularization, and ventricular aneurysm or infarct resection with or without coronary artery bypass grafting, have been successful in no more than 20% to 30% of reported cases. Coronary artery bypass grafting as a primary therapeutic approach has generally been successful only in patients who experience rapid VT during ischemia as well as in patients with ischemia-related VF, but it can sometimes be useful in patients with coronary disease resuscitated from sudden death who have no inducible arrhythmias at EPS. These patients generally have a clear relationship between episodes of ventricular arrhythmia and immediately antecedent severe ischemia and have no evidence of infarction or minimal wall motion abnormalities, with preserved overall left ventricular function. Patients with sustained monomorphic VT or only polymorphic VT rarely have their arrhythmias affected by coronary bypass surgery, although it can reduce the frequency of the arrhythmic episodes in some patients and prevent new ischemic events. An ICD may not be required after the surgical procedure.

SURGICAL TECHNIQUES. In general, two types of direct surgical procedures are used, resection and ablation (**Fig. 37-19**).[39] The first direct surgical approach to VT was encircling endocardial ventriculotomy, using a transmural ventriculotomy to isolate areas of endocardial fibrosis that were recognized visually; this procedure is rarely used now. Another procedure, subendocardial resection, is based on animal and clinical data indicating that arrhythmias after myocardial infarction arise mostly at the subendocardial borders between normal and infarcted tissues.

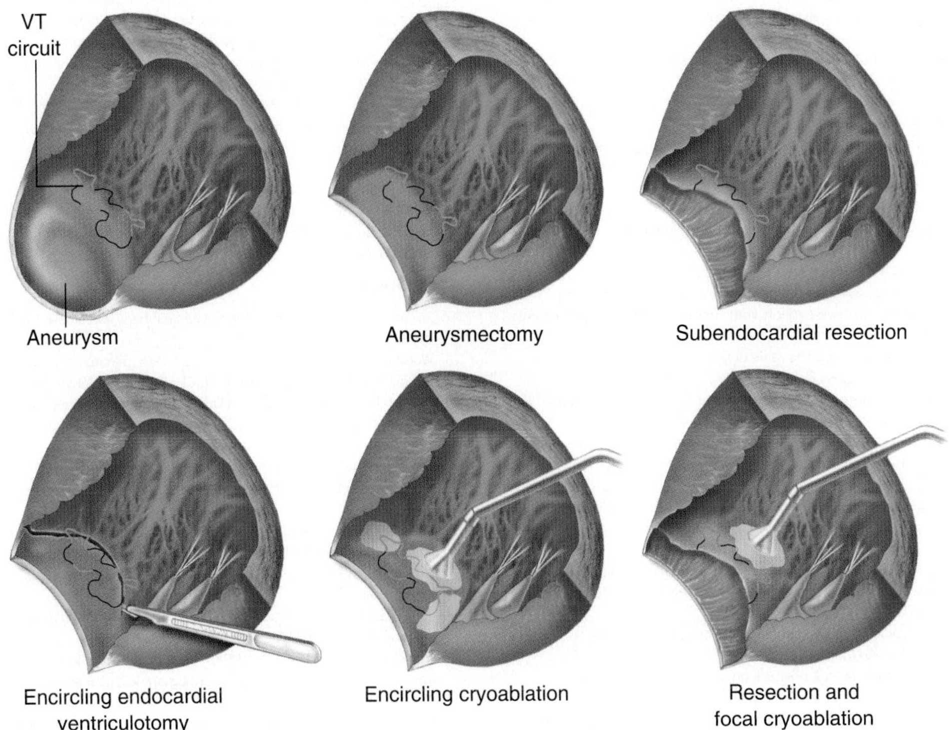

FIGURE 37-19 Schematic diagram showing surgical procedures for treatment of postinfarction VT with left ventricular aneurysm. A damaged left ventricle is depicted as opened along the lateral wall and viewing the septum and papillary muscles. The tachycardia circuit (upper left) takes a meandering course near where the aneurysm meets normal myocardium and at times is superficial and at other times coursing deeper (green lines). Simple aneurysmectomy that leaves a portion of the aneurysm for suturing often misses the circuit and thus does not cure the arrhythmia. By subendocardial resection, a layer of endocardium and subjacent tissue is removed, including at least some of the tachycardia circuit. This resection results in elimination of tachycardia. Encircling endocardial ventriculotomy attempts to isolate the circuit electrically without removal of tissue, but it probably actually works by incising portions of the circuit. Cryoablation can be used to encircle the infarct zone or in combination with resection to damaged tissue too deep in the wall to be resected safely.

Subendocardial resection entails peeling off a 1- to 3-mm-thick layer of endocardium, often near the rim of an aneurysm, that has been demonstrated by mapping procedures to contain sites of mid-diastolic activation recorded during VT. Some VTs can arise from the epicardium. Tachycardias arising from near the base of the papillary muscles are treated with a cryoprobe cooled to −70°C. Cryoablation can also be used to isolate areas of the ventricle that cannot be resected and is often combined with resection. The neodymium: yttrium-aluminum-garnet laser has also been used with good success, but the equipment is expensive and difficult to work with.

Results. For ventricular tachyarrhythmias, operative mortality ranges from 5% to 10%; success rates, defined as absence of recurrence of spontaneous ventricular arrhythmias, range from 59% to 98%. In experienced centers, operative mortality can be as low as 5% in stable patients undergoing elective procedures, with 85% to 95% of survivors free of inducible or spontaneous ventricular tachyarrhythmias. Long-term recurrence rates range from 2% to 15% and correlate with results of the patient's postoperative electrophysiologic stimulation study. Operative survival is strongly influenced by the degree of left ventricular dysfunction.

Operative mortality for nonthoracotomy ICD implantation is far less than 1%, with an annual sudden cardiac death mortality rate less than 2%. Because of the difference in operative survival and shorter hospital stay with ICD insertion compared with direct surgery for VT and the success rates for catheter ablation in patients who have an ICD but experience frequent episodes of VT, few curative surgical procedures are now performed.

Electrophysiologic Studies

Preoperative Electrophysiologic Study. In patients for whom direct surgical therapy for VT is planned, a preoperative EPS is usually warranted. This study involves initiation of the VT and electrophysiologic mapping to localize the area to be resected, as is done with catheter ablation. A resolution of 4 to 8 cm^2 of ventricular endocardium is thereby achieved, although more accurate anatomic localization of the mapping electrode tip in the ventricle may be possible. Tachycardias that are too rapid, short in duration, or polymorphic cannot be mapped accurately unless multiple catheters or a multielectrode array is used. Administration of a drug such as procainamide may slow the VT and transform a nonsustained polymorphic VT into a sustained VT of uniform contour that can be mapped. Preoperative catheter mapping is contraindicated in patients who have known left ventricular thrombus that might be dislodged by the mapping catheter.

Intraoperative Ventricular Mapping. Electrophysiologic mapping is also performed at the time of surgery, with the surgeon using a handheld probe or an electrode array coupled with computer techniques that instantaneously provide an overall activation map, cycle by cycle. The sequence of activation during VT can be plotted and the area of earliest activation determined. Resection or cryoablation of tissue from which these recordings are made usually cures the VT, indicating that they represent a critical portion of the reentrant circuit. However, it is clear that such electrical activity can be late following the preceding cycle or early in advance of the next cycle. When the earliest recordable endocardial electrical activity occurs less than 30 milliseconds before the onset of the QRS complex, the critical portions of the circuit may be in the interventricular septum or near the epicardium of the free wall. In some patients, intramural mapping using a plunge needle electrode can be useful. Most centers have used a strategy of "sequential" subendocardial resection, in which VT is initiated, mapped, and ablated (resected or cryoablated) while the heart is warm and beating and stimulation is immediately repeated. If VT can still be initiated, mapping and resection are also repeated until VT can no longer be initiated. Reentry around an inferior scar, with a critical diastolic pathway confined to an isthmus of ventricular muscle between the scar and mitral valve annulus, can be cured by cryoablation of this isthmus. Cure rates in this situation exceed 93%.

REFERENCES

Pharmacologic Therapy

1. Dopp AL, Miller JM, Tisdale JE: Effect of drugs on defibrillation capacity. Drugs 68:607, 2008.
2. Darbar D, Roden DM: Pharmacogenetics of antiarrhythmic therapy. Expert Opin Pharmacother 7:1583, 2006.

3. Roden DM: Pharmacogenetics of cardiac arrhythmias and impact on drug therapy. *In* Zipes DP, Jalife J (eds): Cardiac Electrophysiology: From Cell to Bedside. 5th ed. Philadelphia, WB Saunders, 2009, pp 471-478.
4. Hondeghem LM: Relative contributions of TRIaD and QT to proarrhythmia. J Cardiovasc Electrophysiol 18:655, 2007.
5. Heist EK, Ruskin JN: Drug-induced proarrhythmia and use of QTc-prolonging agents: Clues for clinicians. Heart Rhythm 2:S1, 2005.
6. Gillis AM: Class I antiarrhythmic drugs: Quinidine, procainamide, disopyramide, flecainide and propafenone. *In* Zipes DP, Jalife J (eds): Cardiac Electrophysiology: From Cell to Bedside. 5th ed. Philadelphia, WB Saunders, 2009, pp 911-917.
7. Schwaab B, Katalinic A, Boge UM, et al: Quinidine for pharmacological cardioversion of atrial fibrillation: A retrospective analysis in 501 consecutive patients. Ann Noninvasive Electrocardiol 14:128, 2009.
8. Yang F, Hanon S, Lam P, et al: Quinidine revisited. Am J Med 122:317, 2009.
9. Doki K, Homma M, Kuga K, et al: Gender-associated differences in pharmacokinetics and anti-arrhythmic effects of flecainide in Japanese patients with supraventricular tachyarrhythmia. Eur J Clin Pharmacol 63:951, 2007.
10. Meregalli PG, Ruijter JM, Hofman N, et al: Diagnostic value of flecainide testing in unmasking SCN5A-related Brugada syndrome. J Cardiovasc Electrophysiol 17:857, 2006.
11. Miller JM, Zipes DP: Therapy for cardiac arrhythmias. *In* Zipes DP, Libby P, Bonow RO, Braunwald E (eds): Braunwald's Heart Disease. 8th ed. Philadelphia, Elsevier, 2008, pp 779-859.
12. Singh BN: Beta blockers and calcium channel blockers as antiarrhythmic drugs. *In* Zipes DP, Jalife J (eds): Cardiac Electrophysiology: From Cell to Bedside. 5th ed. Philadelphia, WB Saunders, 2009, pp 918-931.
13. Smith TW, Cain ME: Class III antiarrhythmic drugs: Amiodarone, ibutilide and sotalol. *In* Zipes DP, Jalife J (eds): Cardiac Electrophysiology: From Cell to Bedside. 5th ed. Philadelphia, WB Saunders, 2009, pp 932-941.
14. Connolly SJ, Dorian P, Roberts RS, et al: Comparison of beta-blockers, amiodarone plus beta-blockers, or sotalol for prevention of shocks from implantable cardioverter defibrillators: The OPTIC Study: A randomized trial. JAMA 295:165, 2006.
15. Bardy GH, Lee KL, Mark DB, et al: Amiodarone or an implantable cardioverter-defibrillator for congestive heart failure. N Engl J Med 352:225, 2005.
16. Goldschlager N, Epstein AE, Naccarelli GV, et al: A practical guide for clinicians who treat patients with amiodarone: 2007. Heart Rhythm 4:1250, 2007.
17. Hohnloser SH, Crijns HJ, van Eickels M, et al: Effect of dronedarone on cardiovascular events in atrial fibrillation. N Engl J Med 360:668, 2009.
18. Kober L, Torp-Pedersen C, McMurray JJ, et al: Increased mortality after dronedarone therapy for severe heart failure. N Engl J Med 358:2678, 2008.
19. Singh BN, Singh SN, Reda DJ, et al: Amiodarone versus sotalol for atrial fibrillation. N Engl J Med 352:1861, 2005.
20. Fragakis N, Papadopoulos N, Papanastasiou S, et al: Efficacy and safety of ibutilide for cardioversion of atrial flutter and fibrillation in patients receiving amiodarone or propafenone. Pacing Clin Electrophysiol 28:954, 2005.
21. Mykytsey A, Bauman JL, Razminia M, et al: Observations on the safety and effectiveness of dofetilide in patients with paroxysmal atrial fibrillation and normal left ventricular function. J Cardiovasc Pharmacol Ther 12:36, 2007.
22. DiMarco JP: Adenosine and digoxin. *In* Zipes DP, Jalife J (eds): Cardiac Electrophysiology: From Cell to Bedside. 5th ed. Philadelphia, WB Saunders, 2009, pp 942-949.
23. Boriani G, Valzania C, Diemberger I, et al: Potential of non-antiarrhythmic drugs to provide an innovative upstream approach to the pharmacological prevention of sudden cardiac death. Expert Opin Investig Drugs 16:605, 2007.
24. Goldberger J, Weinberg KM, Kadish AH: Impact of nontraditional antiarrhythmic drugs on sudden cardiac death. *In* Zipes DP, Jalife J (eds): Cardiac Electrophysiology: From Cell to Bedside. 5th ed. Philadelphia, WB Saunders, 2009, pp 950-958.
25. Lozano HF, Conde CA, Florin T, et al: Treatment and prevention of atrial fibrillation with non-antiarrhythmic pharmacologic therapy. Heart Rhythm 2:1000, 2005.
26. Belluzzi F, Sernesi L, Preti P, et al: Prevention of recurrent lone atrial fibrillation by the angiotensin-II converting enzyme inhibitor ramipril in normotensive patients. J Am Coll Cardiol 53:24, 2009.

Electrotherapy

27. Morady F: Radio-frequency ablation as treatment for cardiac arrhythmias. N Engl J Med 340:534, 1999.
28. Wood MA, Parvez B, Ellenbogen AL, et al: Determinants of lesion sizes and tissue temperatures during catheter cryoablation. Pacing Clin Electrophysiol 30:644, 2007.
29. Evonich RF 3rd, Nori DM, Haines DE: A randomized trial comparing effects of radiofrequency and cryoablation on the structural integrity of esophageal tissue. J Interv Card Electrophysiol 19:77, 2007.
30. Teh AW, Kistler PM, Kalman JM: Using the 12-lead ECG to localize the origin of ventricular and atrial tachycardias: Part 1. Focal atrial tachycardia. J Cardiovasc Electrophysiol 20:706; quiz 705, 2009.
31. Morady F, Oral H, Chugh A: Diagnosis and ablation of atypical atrial tachycardia and flutter complicating atrial fibrillation ablation. Heart Rhythm 6:S29, 2009.
32. Anselme F: Macroreentrant atrial tachycardia: Pathophysiological concepts. Heart Rhythm 5:S18, 2008.
33. Sosa E, Scanavacca M: Epicardial mapping and ablation techniques to control ventricular tachycardia. J Cardiovasc Electrophysiol 16:449, 2005.
34. Ouyang F, Fotuhi P, Ho SY, et al: Repetitive monomorphic ventricular tachycardia originating from the aortic sinus cusp: Electrocardiographic characterization for guiding catheter ablation. J Am Coll Cardiol 39:500, 2002.
35. Bogun F, Kim HM, Han J, et al: Comparison of mapping criteria for hemodynamically tolerated, postinfarction ventricular tachycardia. Heart Rhythm 3:20, 2006.
36. Haïssaguerre M, Shoda M, Jaïs P, et al: Mapping and ablation of idiopathic ventricular fibrillation. Circulation 106:962, 2002.
37. Yarlagadda RK, Iwai S, Stein KM, et al: Reversal of cardiomyopathy in patients with repetitive monomorphic ventricular ectopy originating from the right ventricular outflow tract. Circulation 112:1092, 2005.
38. Bogun F, Crawford T, Reich S, et al: Radiofrequency ablation of frequent, idiopathic premature ventricular complexes: Comparison with a control group without intervention. Heart Rhythm 4:863, 2007.
39. Miller JM, Mahomed Y: Antiarrhythmic surgery. *In* Camm AJ, Saksena S (eds): Electrophysiological Disorders of the Heart. Philadelphia, Elsevier, 2005, pp 981-991.

CHAPTER 38 Pacemakers and Implantable Cardioverter-Defibrillators

Charles D. Swerdlow, David L. Hayes, and Douglas P. Zipes

Background: Cardiac Electrical Stimulation

Electrical therapy for cardiac arrhythmias includes low-voltage pulses, which are used to treat bradycardia or to provide antitachycardia pacing to terminate reentrant tachycardias, and high-voltage shocks, which are used to defibrillate atrial fibrillation (AF) or ventricular fibrillation (VF) or to cardiovert ventricular tachycardia (VT).

An applied electrical stimulus interacts with cardiac electrical activity via its resultant electrical field, which is proportional to the local rate of change of the applied voltage with respect to distance (spatial derivative). The response of the heart is mediated by the passive and active (ion channel) properties of cell membranes, by the properties of electrical connections between cardiac cells, and possibly by direct intracellular electrical effects.

Local and Global Effects of Cardiac Electrical Stimulation

Local. Cardiac pacing requires a local stimulus sufficient to depolarize (reduce the membrane potential of) local myocardium during diastole to initiate a self-propagating wave front of depolarization. To achieve this local effect, pacing pulses are delivered from electrodes with small surface area (1 to 6 mm^2). The required local field strength is about 1 V/cm. A stimulus that successfully stimulates local myocardium is said to capture it.

Bradycardia pacing requires propagation of the stimulated wave front to most or all of the myocardium, resulting in mechanical contraction. In contrast, antitachycardia pacing requires capture of the specific reentrant circuit driving the tachycardia. This circuit may be small or large, but it is usually remote from the site of pacing. Thus, successful antitachycardia pacing requires that the stimulus capture local myocardium during the relative refractory period, propagate to the reentry circuit, enter the circuit during an excitable gap in refractoriness, and terminate the tachycardia by causing bidirectional block (see Chap. 35). The stimulus strength for local capture by antitachycardia pacing is higher than that for bradycardia pacing because antitachycardia pacing pulses are delivered during the relative refractory period rather than during diastole.

Global. In contrast to pacing, initiation and termination of AF or VF by shocks require global field effects. Defibrillation shocks are delivered from electrodes with large surface areas (400 to 800 mm^2 for transvenous electrodes, 35 to 70 cm^2 for subcutaneous or epicardial electrodes) separated by 10 to 40 cm. The minimum global field strength required for ventricular defibrillation is 3 to 4 V/cm using biphasic shocks and 5 to 6 V/cm using monophasic shocks. Although the field strength required for defibrillation is only a few multiples of that required for pacing, defibrillation requires achievement of these field strengths throughout both ventricles, whereas pacing requires achievement of them only locally, within a few millimeters of the tip electrode.

Principles of Bioelectrical Stimulation

Thresholds for Pacing and Defibrillation. A threshold stimulus is the minimum stimulus required to evoke a response. Stimuli weaker than the threshold never evoke a response, and stimuli stronger than the threshold always evoke a response. Thus, the threshold for pacing is the minimum stimulus strength required to depolarize local myocardium and to initiate a propagated response. Defibrillation is best described by a probability of success curve (**Fig. 38-1**) rather than by a threshold.[1] Shock strength is plotted on the abscissa and probability of successful defibrillation on the ordinate. The probabilistic nature of defibrillation ensures that over the clinically relevant range of shock strengths, the same shock strength may either succeed or fail on successive attempts. Nevertheless, the term *defibrillation threshold* (DFT) is used as the minimum shock strength that defibrillates during a sequence of fibrillation episodes in which defibrillation test shocks of different strengths are delivered.

Waveforms. The waveform of an electrical pulse is the temporal pattern of its amplitude, measured by voltage (or current). Voltage is a critical parameter for pacing or defibrillation because it determines the electrical field that interacts with the heart. In general, current is linearly related to voltage by Ohm's law (E = IR, where E is voltage, I is current, and R is resistance). Waveform duration is critical because the shock interacts with the heart for the duration of the waveform. Furthermore, the heart's response to a pacing or defibrillation pulse occurs during a period that depends on time-dependent passive and active ion channel processes, collectively referred to as the time constant of cardiac tissue (see Chap. 35). Both pacing and defibrillation waveforms are most efficient when their durations are close to cardiac time constants (see Strength-Duration Relationship). Thus, the most easily measured electrical parameter relevant to pacing or defibrillation is voltage (or current) as a function of time.[2] Although implantable cardioverter-defibrillator (ICD) shocks are often specified in terms of energy (joules), energy is not a direct determinant of defibrillation.[3]

Pacing waveforms approximate constant voltage pulses with lower amplitude, longer duration afterpotentials of opposite polarity (**Fig. 38-2A**). Defibrillation pulses are capacitive-discharge, truncated exponential waveforms as described in Figure 38-2B. Biphasic waveforms defibrillate more efficiently (lower voltage) than monophasic waveforms (Fig. 38-2C).

Strength-Duration Relationship. The plot of stimulus or shock strength as a function of pulse duration is known as a strength-duration curve (**Fig. 38-3**), in which the effect on threshold of equivalent change in duration is much greater at short durations than at long durations. The long-duration asymptote (essentially the lowest value) is referred to as

CH 38

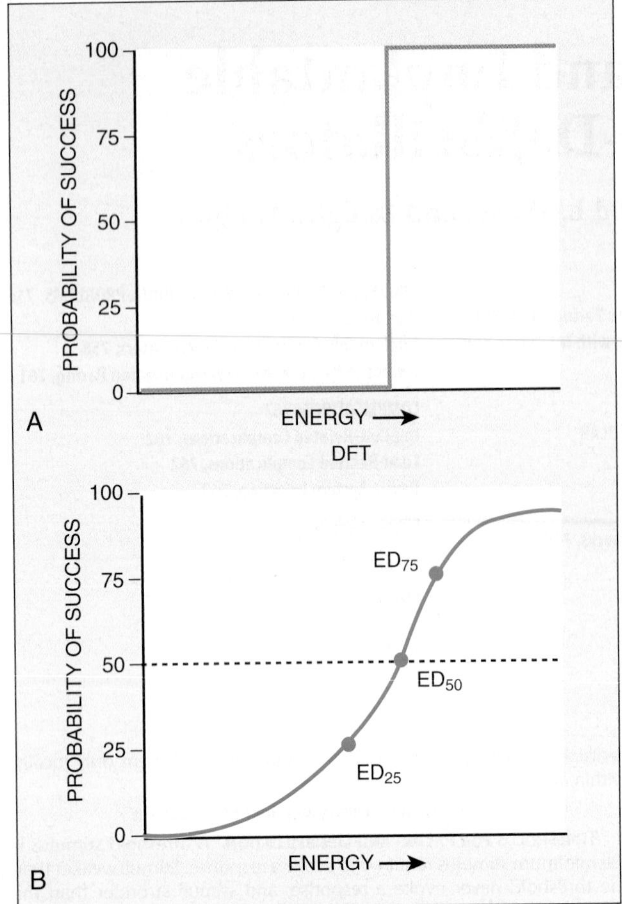

FIGURE 38-1 Defibrillation "threshold." **A,** The expected response to a shock if a true threshold value existed. In reality, the likelihood of success is a sigmoidal dose-response curve, as shown in **B.** ED_{25}, ED_{50}, and ED_{75} indicate the energy dose with 25%, 50%, and 75% probability of success, respectively.

the rheobase. The chronaxie is defined as the threshold duration at twice the rheobase amplitude. For pacing pulses that approximate square waves, the optimal duration that minimizes energy occurs at a pulse duration equal to the chronaxie, which is close to the cell membrane's time constant. For capacitive-discharge defibrillation pulses, the pulse duration for minimum energy is a "compromise" between the optimal duration for response of the cell membrane (chronaxie) and the optimal duration for the capacitor to deliver its charge.[2] Minimizing energy is an important consideration for longevity and size of ICD and pacemaker generators.

Programming Strength and Duration of Pacing and Defibrillation Pulses. The durations of pacing and defibrillation pulses are optimized to achieve the desired physiologic result with the minimum energy consumption from the device's battery. Typically, the voltage output for pacing is set to 1.5 to 2 times the threshold at pulse durations of 0.4 to 0.5 millisecond, 1.5 to 2 times the pacing chronaxie of 0.2 to 0.3 millisecond. Lower safety margins may be programmed for pacemakers that assess automatically. The shock strength for defibrillation typically is programmed near the ICD's maximum output of 700 to 800 V or 30 to 40 J with pulse durations of 3.5 to 6 milliseconds for the first phase of biphasic waveforms, longer than the defibrillation chronaxie of about 3 milliseconds but toward the short end of the range of shock-waveform time constants of 4 to 8 milliseconds.

Various drugs and metabolic effects can alter pacing and defibrillation thresholds. The most clinically important metabolic abnormalities include any marked acidosis or alkalosis and marked electrolyte abnormalities, especially hyperkalemia. The most clinically important drug effects are the alterations in pacing and sensing thresholds that can be seen with class IC drugs (e.g., flecainide) and the effect of amiodarone on defibrillation thresholds.

Polarity. At long coupling intervals used in bradycardia pacing, the pacing threshold is lower if the negative electrode (cathode) is used for stimulation; but at short coupling intervals that may initiate tachyarrhythmias, the stimulation threshold is lower for the positive electrode (anode). Thus, cathodal pacing is preferred for bradycardia pacing to enhance device longevity and to minimize proarrhythmia.

For clinically used biphasic defibrillation waveforms, polarity has little or no effect on defibrillation efficacy.

Hemodynamics

Restoration of rate responsiveness and restoration of atrioventricular (AV) synchrony should be the complementary goals of physiologic pacing.

CHRONOTROPIC RESPONSE. Appropriate heart rate response during exercise (i.e., chronotropic competence) is the most important contributor to cardiac output, especially at moderate or extreme degrees of exercise (**Fig. 38-4**).

ATRIOVENTRICULAR SYNCHRONY. At rest and at lower levels of activity, AV synchrony also contributes significantly. It is estimated to increase stroke volume by as much as 50% and in normal hearts may decrease left atrial pressure and increase cardiac index by as much as 25% to 30%. Because many paced patients may depend on adequate preload owing to decreased ventricular compliance, AV synchrony is probably as important as rate responsiveness for achieving optimal cardiovascular hemodynamics in the typical patient. Mitral valve closure and diastolic filling are influenced by the timing of atrial and ventricular contraction. If the AV interval is too long, ventricular contraction does not immediately follow atrial emptying. If it is too short, ventricular contraction and closure of the AV valves occur before completion of atrial emptying. In patients with cardiomyopathy and heart failure, the timing of right ventricular (RV) and left ventricular (LV) contraction and relaxation may differ sufficiently that optimal AV timing for one may not be ideal for the other. Patients with severe diastolic dysfunction may benefit most from AV synchrony because they depend on optimal preload.

Lack of AV synchrony as a result of exclusive ventricular pacing can result in hemodynamic impairment caused by ventriculoatrial conduction and atrial contraction against a closed AV valve. The constellation of physical signs and symptoms that can result from this abnormal physiologic state is known as pacemaker syndrome, causing malaise, lightheadedness, and atypical chest discomfort. Pacemaker syndrome was initially identified as a complication of VVI pacing; however, it can occur with any pacing mode when there is effective AV dissociation, such as a sufficiently prolonged AV delay in dual-chamber pacing causing atrial systole to time with or after ventricular systole.

The Mode Selection Trial (MOST), which compared DDD with VVI pacing in sinus node disease, demonstrated a lower incidence of AF and heart failure with DDD pacing.[4] Unnecessary RV pacing is associated with an increased incidence of heart failure in patients with LV dysfunction[5] and AF,[6] even if AV synchrony is preserved. These studies led to the use of pacing algorithms that avoid unnecessary RV pacing in patients with normal intraventricular conduction, such as prolongation of the AV interval to allow intrinsic ventricular depolarization.

RATIONALE FOR CARDIAC RESYNCHRONIZATION THERAPY. In patients with abnormal intraventricular conduction, dyssynchronous diastolic filling and systolic contraction patterns may cause or exacerbate ventricular dysfunction, especially in patients with left bundle branch block or those who depend on RV pacing (see Chap. 13). In such patients, biventricular or LV pacing may normalize the ventricular activation sequence, thereby improving cardiac efficiency[7] (see Chap. 33).

Dyssynchronous LV activation in the cardiomyopathic patient increases isovolumic contraction and relaxation times, thereby increasing the duration of mitral regurgitation and shortening LV filling time, with the net effect of decreasing preload. Regionally diminished myocardial function or disturbed temporal sequence of

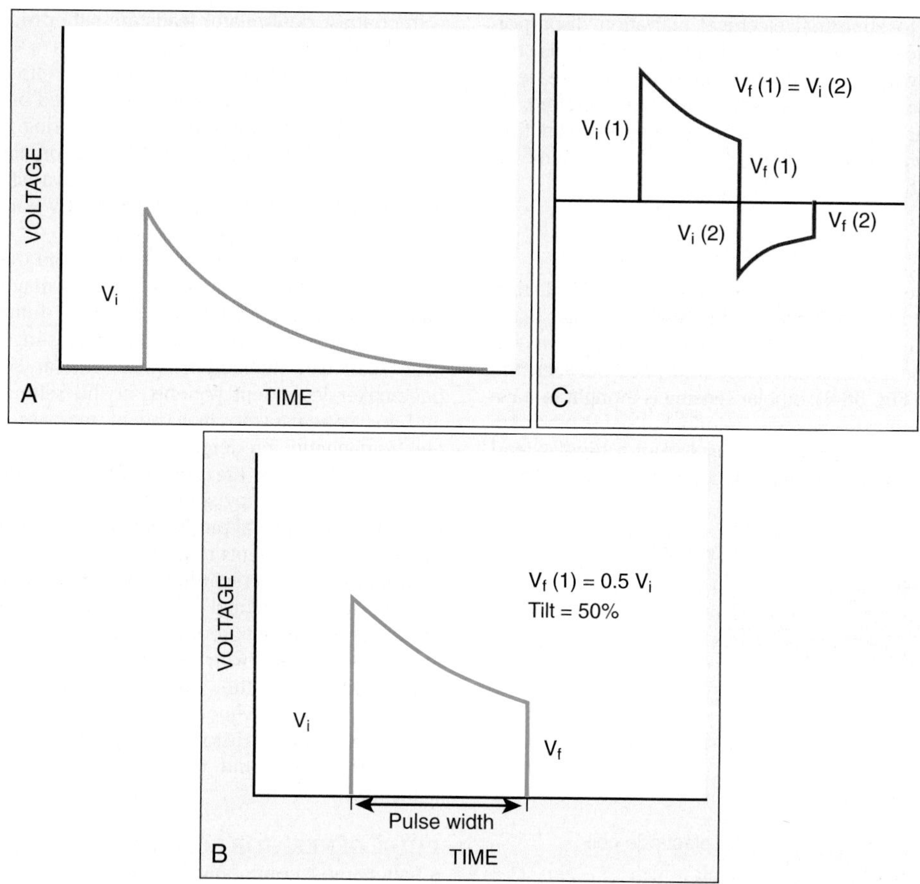

FIGURE 38-2 Defibrillation waveforms. **A,** Exponential capacitor discharge with initial voltage V_i and final voltage zero. **B,** Monophasic truncated exponential waveform with initial voltage V_i and final voltage V_f. The pulse width is the time from the onset of the discharge to truncation. In this case $V_f = 0.5\ V_i$ so that tilt ($V_i - V_f/VF$) equals 50%. The duration of the waveform may be specified directly by duration (pulse width) or tilt. **C,** Biphasic truncated exponential waveform with initial voltage of the second phase (V_i (2)) equal to the final voltage of the first phase (V_f (1)). Biphasic waveforms in which the initial voltage of the second phase equals the final voltage of the first phase are referred to as single-capacitor biphasic waveforms because they can be generated by reversing the polarity of a single capacitor after the first phase is truncated and then continuing the discharge.

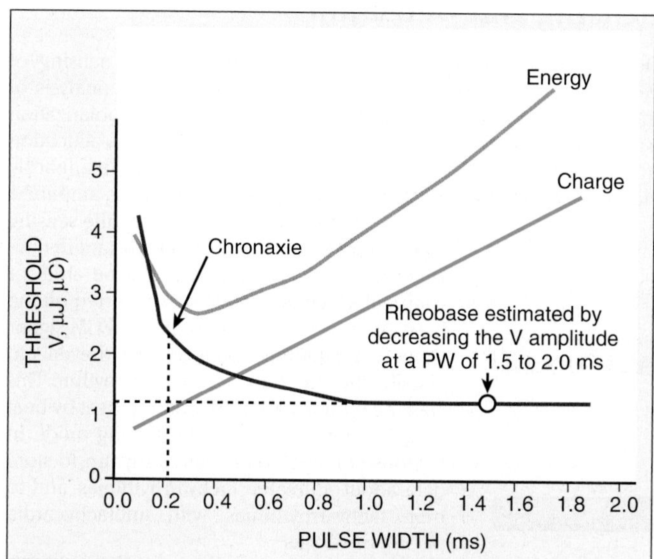

FIGURE 38-3 Relationships among chronic ventricular strength-duration curves from a canine, expressed as potential (V), charge (µC), and energy (µJ). Rheobase is the threshold at infinitely long pulse duration. Chronaxie is the pulse duration at twice rheobase. *(From Stokes K, Bornzin G: The electrode-biointerface stimulation. In Barold SS [ed]: Modern Cardiac Pacing. Mount Kisco, NY, Futura Publishing Company, 1985, pp 33-77. By permission of the publisher.)*

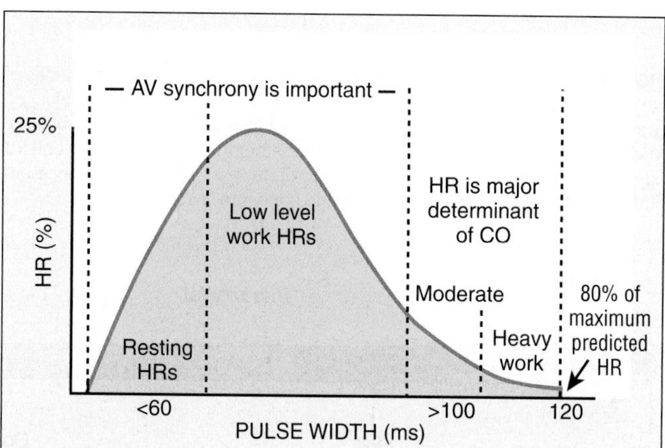

FIGURE 38-4 Schematic representation of the AV interval response when both differential AV interval and rate-adaptive AV interval are activated. The solid lines represent paced atrial events and the dashed lines sensed atrial events. CO, cardiac output; HR, heart rate.

contraction secondary to abnormal electrical activation disproportionately worsens systolic dysfunction in cardiomyopathy because the remaining myocardium cannot provide the compensatory increase in fiber shortening necessary to maintain stroke volume. Therefore, LV pacing and biventricular (RV and LV) pacing are used to resynchronize ventricular electrical and mechanical activation sequence in patients with symptomatic LV dysfunction.

Hardware

LEADS. The choice of leads for transvenous pacing and defibrillation depends on the patient and application (**Fig. 38-5**). Unipolar leads sense and pace between a tip electrode and the housing ("can") of the pulse generator. Bipolar leads can sense and pace between the tip and ring electrodes (**Fig. 38-6**). Bipolar sensing is thought to have a lower susceptibility to electromagnetic interference and other far-field signals compared with unipolar sensing. Use of a bipolar lead permits programming of either bipolar or unipolar pacing and sensing.

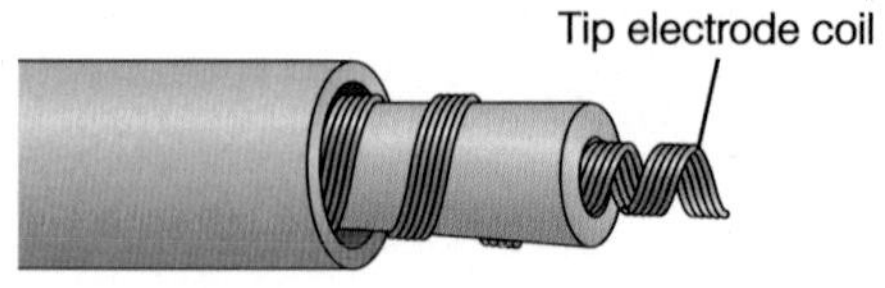

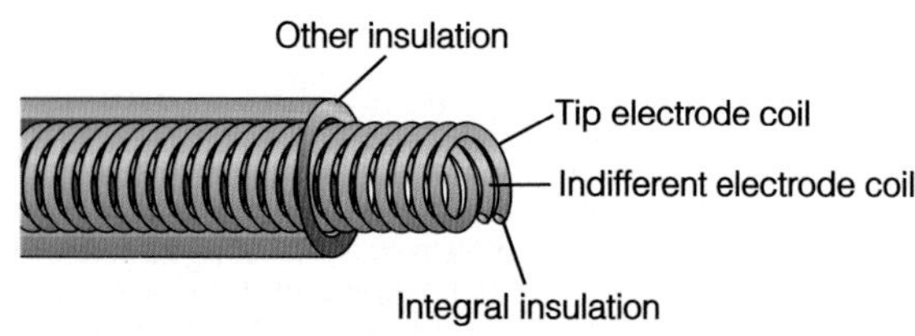

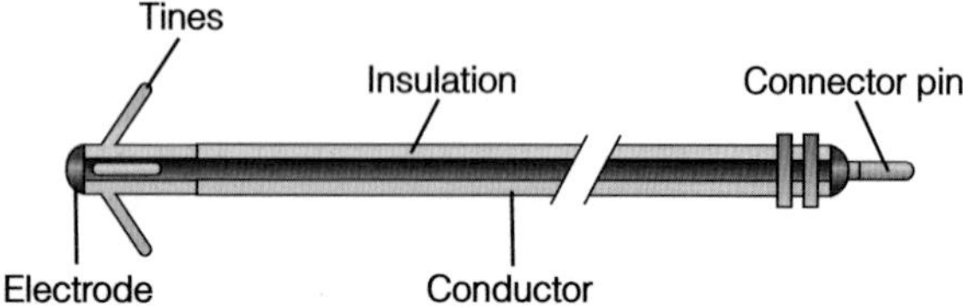

FIGURE 38-5 Basic components of a passive fixation pacing lead. Varieties of conductor construction. ***Top,*** Bipolar coaxial design with an inner multifilar coil surrounded by insulation (inner), an outer multifilar coil, and outer insulation. **Middle,** Individually coated wires wound together in a single multifilar coil for bipolar pacing. **Bottom,** Schematic of passive fixation lead with identification of the electrode, insulation, conductor and connector pin.

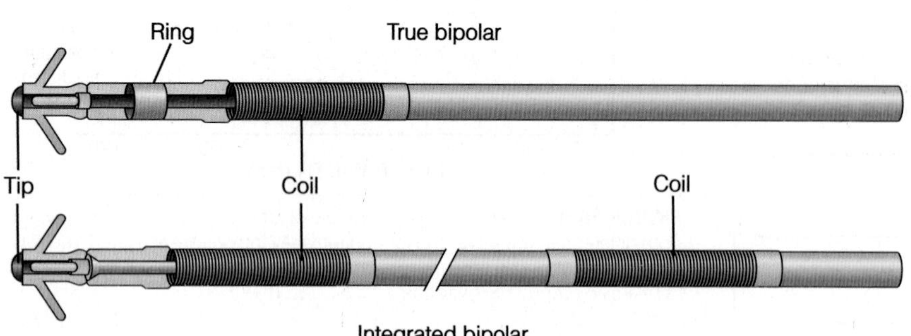

FIGURE 38-6 True bipolar **(top)** and integrated bipolar **(bottom)** leads. The true bipolar lead senses between the distal tip and the proximal ring, which are dedicated for pacing and sensing. True bipolar leads have a single coil. In contrast, integrated bipolar leads pace and sense between the tip and the distal coil. The distal coil is used for sensing, pacing, and defibrillation. Integrated bipolar leads also contain a second, proximal coil, increasing the lead surface area for defibrillation.

In contrast, defibrillator leads are either tripolar or quadripolar. All include a pace/sense tip electrode and a RV coil electrode. True bipolar leads sense and pace between the tip electrode and a closely spaced dedicated ring electrode. Integrated bipolar sensing leads use the RV defibrillation coil as the anodal ring for sensing and pacing. Dual-coil defibrillation leads have a proximal defibrillation coil intended to rest in the superior vena cava when the tip is in the RV apex. Most ICD systems shock from the RV coil to the pulse generator can and the superior vena cava coil.

For most patients, dual- or single-coil and true or integrated bipolar systems are effective. Single-coil systems may be favored in younger patients who have a potential need for future extraction or as an additional lead in patients with a preexisting dual-coil lead to minimize lead-lead interactions. True bipolar sensing is preferred in pacemaker-dependent patients, in the setting of abandoned leads, and for patients who may be at increased risk for exposure to electromagnetic interference. Dual-coil systems may be preferable when higher DFTs are anticipated (hypertrophic cardiomyopathy, antiarrhythmic therapy, some inherited sodium channel abnormalities), although clinical predictors of high DFTs have been limited, and less than 5% of patients require system revision.[1]

Nontransvenous, epicardial (myocardial) leads can be necessary in patients with congenital cardiac anomalies associated with univentricular hearts or that prevent the access needed for transvenous leads as well as in patients with tricuspid valve conditions that preclude lead placement across the valve (e.g., mechanical prosthetic valve). However, coronary venous pacing can obviate the need for some epicardial pacing. Historically, epicardial leads have had higher pacing thresholds and more conductor failures than transvenous leads have.

PULSE GENERATOR COMPONENTS. All pulse generators include a battery, most commonly lithium-iodine in pacemakers and lithium–silver vanadium oxide in ICDs. Located adjacent to the battery is the "hybrid" or circuit board, which is the mini-computer that processes bidirectional information between incoming signals from the heart and the programmer and responds to cardiac signals as programmed. The hybrid also stores information that can be retrieved via the programmer. An ICD also includes a high-voltage transformer and a bulky system of high-voltage capacitors that allow the device to develop and to store the charge adequate for defibrillation.

Sensing and Detection

Delivery of appropriate electrical therapy depends on sensing of cardiac depolarizations and detection of arrhythmias by analysis of the timing and morphology of sensed events. When a depolarization wave front passes the tip electrode of an intracardiac lead, a deflection in the continuous electrogram (EGM) signal travels instantaneously via the electrode to the pulse generator. There, the signal is amplified, filtered, digitized, and processed by the sensing electronics. A sensed event is an instant in time when the device determines that an atrial or ventricular depolarization has occurred on the basis of processing the continuous EGM signal. Detection algorithms process sensed events to classify the atrial or ventricular rhythm. This classification is used to control beat-by-beat paced events, to change the pacing mode in response to a pathologic atrial rhythm, to store data about untreated tachyarrhythmias, and to treat tachyarrhythmias with antitachycardia pacing or shocks.

Intracardiac Electrogram

An EGM displays the electrical potential difference between two points in space over time. The electrocardiogram (ECG), recorded from two electrodes on the body's surface, records electrical activity from the entire heart. In contrast, EGMs recorded from endocardial or epicardial pacing electrodes record only local activity.

Unipolar EGMs are recorded between a small tip electrode in the heart and a large remote (indifferent) electrode, typically the pulse generator metal device housing or can. The location of the remote electrode has little effect on the cardiac EGM, but it may record noncardiac potentials, such as pectoral myopotentials. True bipolar EGMs are recorded between the tip and ring electrodes on a lead. Integrated bipolar EGMs are recorded between the tip of a RV defibrillation lead and the large RV coil. Compared with true bipolar electrodes (tip to ring), integrated bipolar EGMs have a wider field of view and are thus more likely to oversense nonphysiologic signals or physiologic signals that do not reflect local myocardial depolarization (see Fig. 38-6). Signals that do not originate in the local myocardium are called far-field signals. They include signals originating in a different cardiac chamber.

The typical amplitude of transvenous atrial and ventricular EGMs is in the range of 1.0 to 5 mV and 5 to 20 mV, respectively. The frequency content of ventricular and atrial EGMs is similar (5 to 50 Hz). T waves have lower frequency content (1 to 10 Hz), whereas most noncardiac myopotentials and electromagnetic interference have higher frequencies. This permits use of electronic band pass filters to reduce oversensing (**Fig. 38-7**). Low-amplitude local EGMs can result in failure to sense (undersensing).

Sensing

Sensing and detection in ICDs and pacemakers share many features. One major difference is that ICDs need reliable sensing and detection during VF, whereas pacemakers do not. A second is that pacemakers can use unipolar or bipolar sensing, whereas ICDs always use bipolar sensing.

BLANKING AND REFRACTORY PERIODS. The primary functional operations within the sensing system of a pacemaker or ICD are shown in **Figure 38-8**. A sensed event occurs when the processed signal exceeds the sensing threshold voltage. The sense amplifier is turned off for a short blanking period (20 to 250 milliseconds) after each sensed event to prevent multiple sensed events during a single depolarization. During the refractory period that follows the blanking period, events may be sensed for tachyarrhythmia detection algorithms but do not alter pacemaker timing cycles (**Fig. 38-9**). Same-chamber blanking and refractory periods after sensed events reduce double counting of intrinsic cardiac depolarizations. The blanking and refractory periods in the ventricle after atrial sensed or paced events and in the atrium after ventricular sensed or paced events are called cross-chamber blanking and refractory periods. Cross-chamber blanking periods reduce oversensing of the pacing artifact after a paced event in the opposite chamber. The atrial blanking period after ventricular events (postventricular atrial blanking) is designed to avoid oversensing of ventricular pacing stimuli and far-field R waves.

Devices that incorporate tachyarrhythmia detection such as ICDs and atrial therapy devices typically have shorter blanking and refractory periods than standard pacemakers do so that short cardiac cycles can be sensed reliably. The duration of the total atrial refractory period

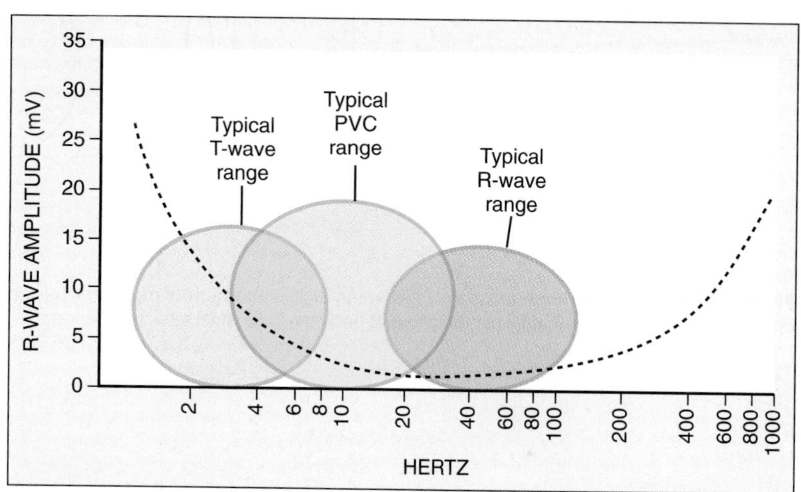

FIGURE 38-7 Electromagnetic frequency spectrum of intracardiac events. PVC, premature ventricular contraction.

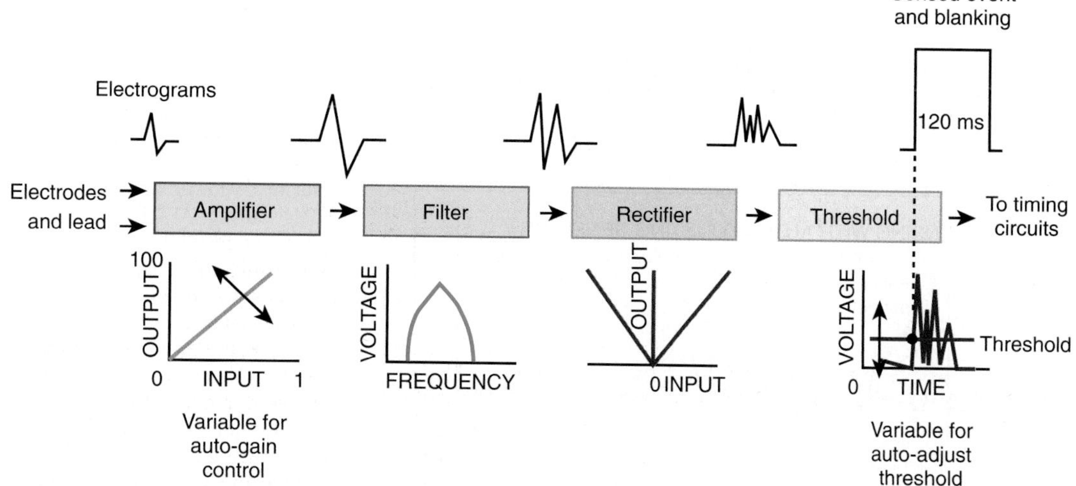

FIGURE 38-8 A functional block diagram for a pacemaker or ICD sense amplifier. The EGM signal from the two implanted electrodes is first amplified for subsequent processing. Band pass filtering reduces the amplitude of lower frequency signals, such as T waves and far-field R waves, and higher frequency signals, such as myopotentials and electromagnetic interference. After band pass filtering, the signal is rectified to make polarity unimportant. The thresholding operation compares the amplified, filtered, or rectified signal with the sensing threshold voltage. At the instant the processed signal exceeds the sensing threshold voltage, the sense amplifier is blanked (turned off) for a short time (about 20 to 120 milliseconds, depending on the ICD model) so that each depolarization is sensed only once, and a sensed event is declared to pacemaker or ICD timing circuits. For pacemakers, the programmed sensitivity controls the constant sensing threshold voltage. For ICDs, the amplifier gain may be controlled by the input EGM amplitude. The programmable sensing threshold for ICDs controls the high and low limits on the sensing threshold that automatically adjusts on a beat-by-beat basis. In actual circuits, some functions, such as amplification and filtering, may be integrated.

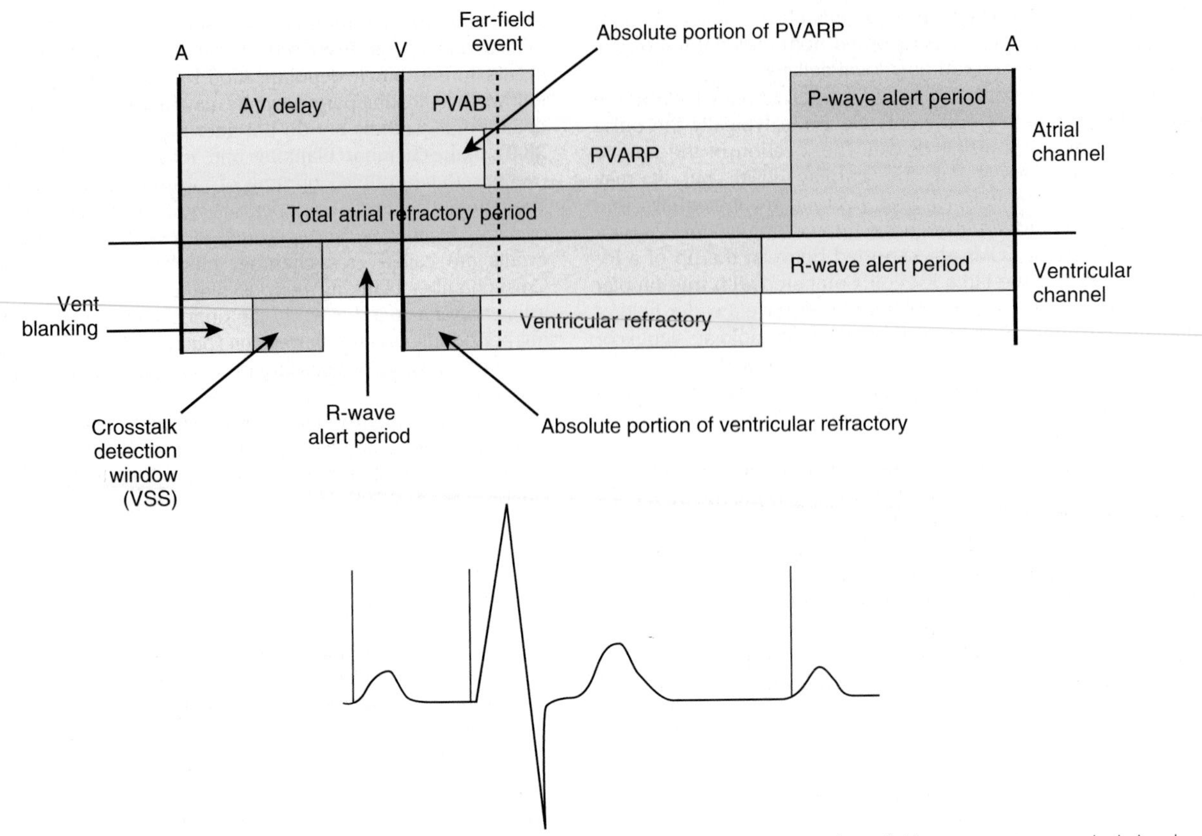

FIGURE 38-9 Schematic representation of the timing cycle interactions of most refractory and blanking periods available on contemporary dual-chamber pacemakers. PVAB, postventricular atrial blanking; PVARP, postventricular atrial refractory period.

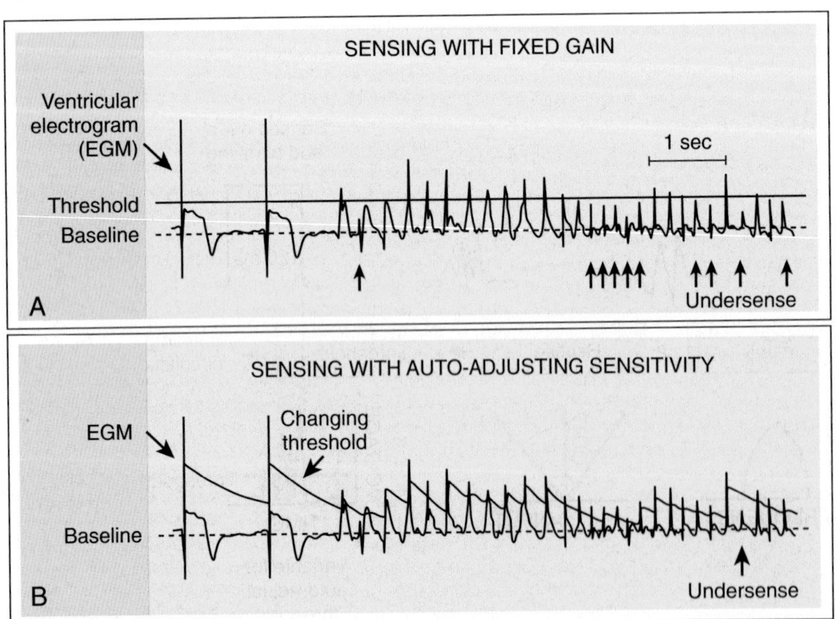

FIGURE 38-10 ICD sensing systems. **A,** Fixed gain (and sensitivity) requires that the sensed potential exceed a fixed threshold. Because of the highly variable amplitude during VF, undersensing occurs (arrows). If the threshold is lowered, T wave oversensing may occur (note that the threshold is just above the T wave amplitude during sinus rhythm, first two complexes). **B,** Autoadjusting sensitivity. The gain is fixed, but the threshold for sensing changes throughout the cardiac cycle. Undersensing is diminished. *(Modified from Olson WH: Tachyarrhythmia sensing and detection. In Singer I [ed]: Implantable Cardioverter-Defibrillator. Armonk, NY, Futura Publishing Company, 1994, pp 71-107. By permission of the publisher.)*

(TARP) is defined as the AV delay plus the postventricular atrial refractory period (PVARP). In dual-chamber pacing modes with atrial sensing, the TARP limits atrial tracking of the atrium at high sinus rates without affecting atrial sensing.

SENSING THRESHOLDS. Sensing thresholds in most pacemakers usually are programmable to fixed values. Ventricular channels in pacemakers typically operate at thresholds of 2.0 to 3.5 mV, about 10 times less sensitive than those in ICDs. Thus, pacemakers can undersense VF. Atrial sensing thresholds typically are 0.3 to 0.6 mV to allow sensing of lower amplitude P waves and atrial EGMs during AF. Highly sensitive programmed values can result in oversensing of far-field cardiac and extracardiac signals, causing inappropriate pacemaker inhibition or tracking, especially with unipolar sensing.

In ICDs, the principal guiding design of sensing circuits is that sensing of VF should be sufficiently reliable that clinically significant delays in detection do not occur. Although high sensitivity is required to ensure reliable sensing in VF despite variable and low-amplitude EGMs, continuous high sensitivity can result in oversensing of cardiac or extracardiac signals during regular rhythm. To minimize both undersensing during VF and oversensing during regular rhythms, ICDs use feedback mechanisms based on R wave amplitude to adjust the sensing threshold dynamically (automatic adjustment of sensitivity; **Fig. 38-10**).

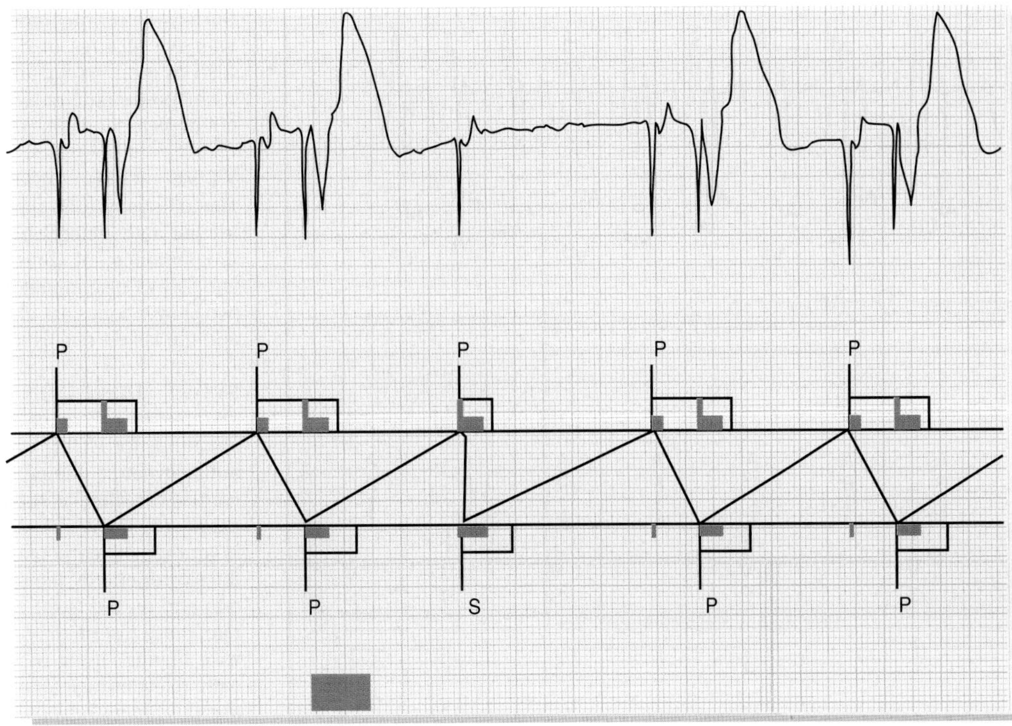

FIGURE 38-11 Electrocardiographic example of crosstalk. Although crosstalk appears to be the most likely cause of ventricular failure to output when the surface ECG is assessed, it is confirmed by the telemetered ladder diagram. The ladder diagram, a type of diagnostic channel that is not commonly seen with contemporary devices, confirms that the atrial output was detected almost simultaneously on the ventricular sensing channel and that ventricular output was inhibited. P, paced; S, sensed.

AUTOMATIC OPTIMIZATION OF PACEMAKER FUNCTION BASED ON SENSING. Pacemakers and ICDs incorporate algorithms to prevent inhibition during oversensing, inappropriately high pacing rates due to tracking of atrial tachyarrhythmias, unnecessary ventricular pacing in patients with intact AV conduction, and loss of pacemaker capture. Ventricular safety pacing prevents inappropriate pacemaker inhibition caused by ventricular oversensing of atrial pacing stimuli or crosstalk (**Fig. 38-11**). Noise reversion to fixed-rate asynchronous pacing prevents pacemaker inhibition during continuous ventricular oversensing. Automatic mode switching in dual-chamber pacing systems initiates a temporary mode change to a nontracking pacing mode during paroxysmal atrial tachyarrhythmias to prevent rapid ventricular pacing while tracking high atrial rates. When the atrial rhythm again meets the defined criteria for a physiologic rhythm, the mode switches back to an atrial tracking mode (**Fig. 38-12**).

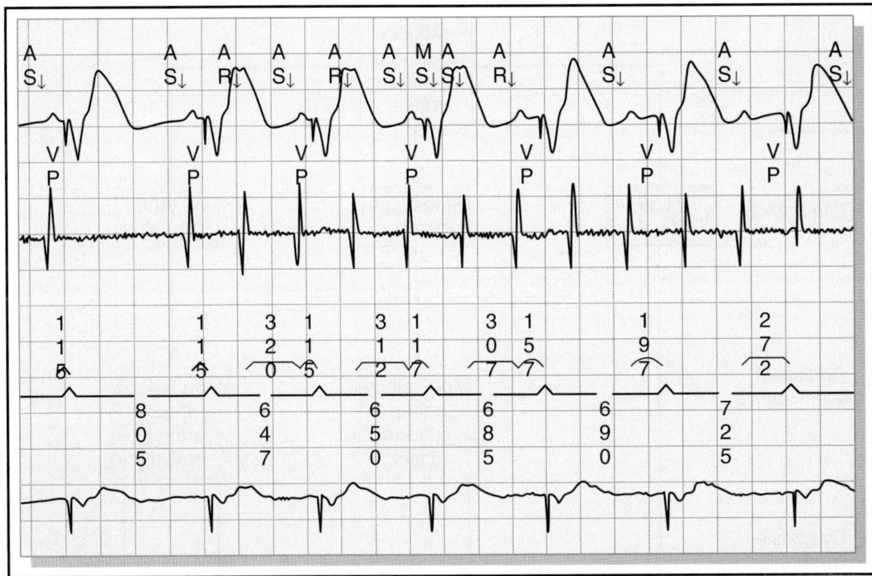

FIGURE 38-12 Mode switch from DDDR to DDIR mode. MS = mode switch.

Conventional DDD pacing can result in an unnecessarily high percentage of ventricular pacing, which may contribute to adverse clinical outcomes, such as heart failure hospitalizations and increased risk of AF.[4,5] To reduce unnecessary ventricular pacing, pacemaker algorithms adaptively lengthen AV intervals to promote intrinsic conduction (**Fig. 38-13A**). Alternatively, the pacemaker may effectively operate in AAI mode during normal operation with mode switching to DDD if AV block occurs or the AR or PR interval is prolonged beyond a specified duration (AAIR ⇔ DDDR mode; Fig. 38-13B).

VT/VF Detection

Figure 38-14 shows an overview of the structure of VT/VF detection algorithms. Initial detection of tachycardia is based on rate and duration. The minimum duration required for detection is programmable, either directly (in seconds) or indirectly by setting the number of ventricular intervals required for detection. A tachycardia episode begins when the minimum rate and duration criteria are satisfied.

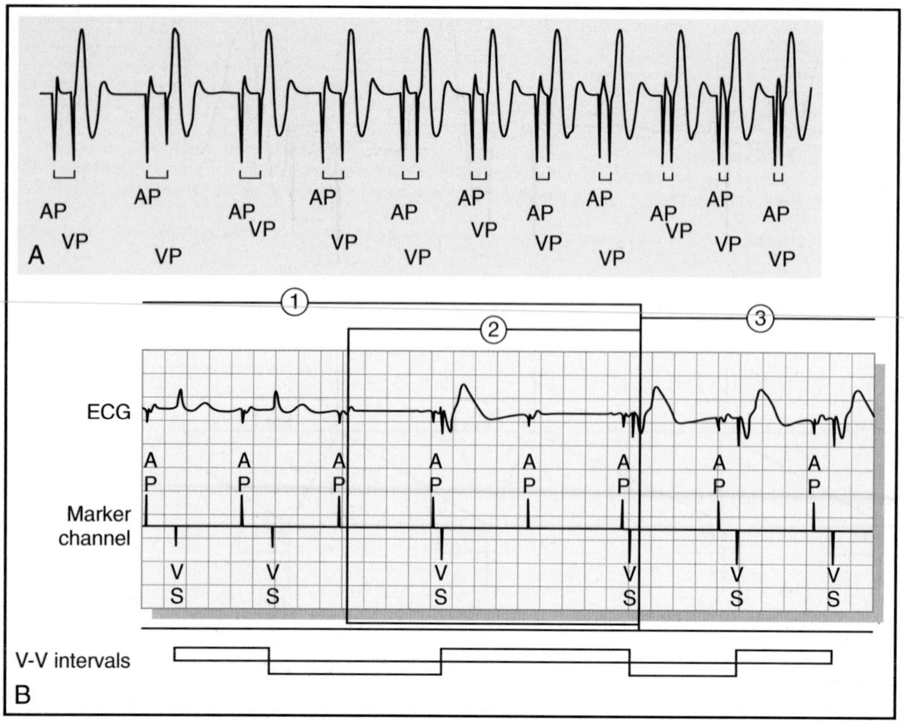

FIGURE 38-13 **A,** Schematic example of AV search hysteresis, which successfully demonstrates intrinsic AV conduction. **B,** Example of managed ventricular pacing. Initially, AAIR pacing is seen; if an atrial pace event occurs without a ventricular sensed event, a ventricular backup output occurs and the pacemaker then switches to DDDR mode.

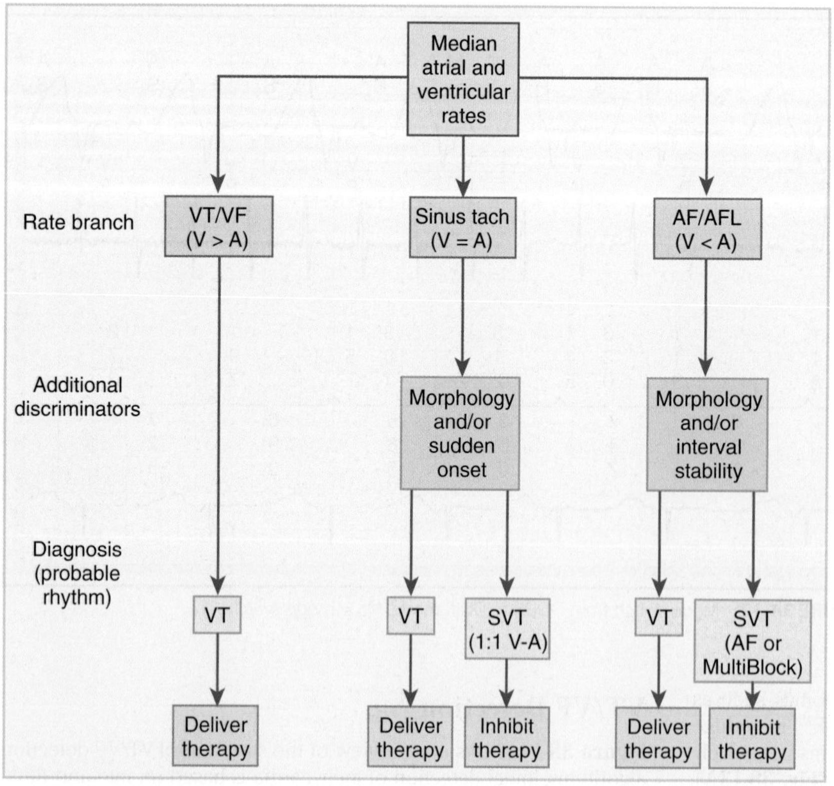

FIGURE 38-14 Rate Branch logic used in St. Jude Medical dual-chamber ICDs.

During detection, more computationally intensive features of detection algorithms, such as morphology analysis, are activated so the power required to operate them does not deplete the ICD's battery.

VT/VF RATE DETECTION ZONES. Tiered-therapy ICDs have up to three ventricular rate detection zones that permit programming of zone-specific therapies and SVT-VT discriminators (**Fig. 38-15**). The two slower zones are classified as VT zones and the fastest one as a VF zone.

SVT-VT DISCRIMINATORS. This programmable subset of an ICD's detection algorithm for VT/VF withholds ventricular antitachycardia pacing or shocks for tachycardias classified as supraventricular tachycardia (SVT). SVT-VT discriminators apply in a range of ventricular rates bounded on the slower end by the slowest VT detection rate and on the faster end by an SVT limit rate. These discriminators operate in a stepwise manner using a series of physiologically relevant logical "building blocks" that use the timing relationships and morphology of sensed EGMs. Single-chamber ventricular building blocks include regularity of rate, abruptness of tachycardia onset, and similarity of the EGM to a template EGM stored in baseline rhythm. Dual-chamber building blocks include comparison of atrial and ventricular rates, patterns of AV relationships (indicating anterograde conduction, retrograde conduction, or AV dissociation), and chamber in which the tachycardia originates.

CONFIRMATION, REDETECTION, AND EPISODE TERMINATION. Once a tachycardia has been classified as VT or VF, therapy that is appropriate for the detection zone (**Fig. 38-16**) is delivered. Antitachycardia pacing is delivered immediately, but shocks require capacitor charging, which takes 6 to 15 seconds for maximum energy shocks. The first shock in a shock sequence is synchronized to the ventricular sensing EGM whether it is delivered for device-detected VT or VF. It is "noncommitted," meaning that it may be aborted if the detection algorithm identifies termination of the arrhythmia during or immediately after charging of the high-energy capacitors (see Fig. 38-16). Confirmation or reconfirmation is the brief process that occurs after charging by which ICDs determine whether to deliver or to abort the first shock in a sequence. Subsequent shocks are synchronized if possible but may be delivered asynchronously because undersensing of VF may occur after shocks (committed shocks).

Redetection is the process by which ICDs determine whether VT or VF detection criteria remain satisfied after therapy is delivered. Episodes continue after each tiered therapy until either a tachyarrhythmia is redetected to initiate the next therapy or the rhythm is classified as normal (sinus), resulting in episode termination. Episode termination is based on slow rate for sufficient duration.

Pacemaker Modes and Timing Cycles

Table 38-1 describes the accepted nomenclature for pacing modes. In general, the DDD(R) or AAI(R) ⇔ DDD(R) mode is appropriate for dual-chamber pacemakers with adequate atrial sensing. DDI(R) mode can be used for patients with sinus bradycardia if atrial undersensing prevents appropriate mode switching during AF. Rate-responsive pacing is indicated in patients with chronotropic incompetence, but it is unnecessary in patients with AV block and a normally functioning sinus node.

Magnet application results in an asynchronous mode of operation for pacemakers (DOO, AOO, or VOO). For ICDs, magnets inhibit ICD detection of VT/VF but do not alter programmed pacing functions.

The timing cycle of each pacing mode determines its advantages and disadvantages and the characteristics of the resultant paced ECG.

Ventricular Inhibited Pacing (VVI)

VVI is a pacing mode that incorporates sensing on the ventricular channel, enabling a sensed ventricular event to inhibit pacemaker output (**Fig. 38-17**). VVI pacemakers are refractory for an interval after a paced or sensed ventricular event, the ventricular refractory period. Any ventricular event occurring within the ventricular refractory period is not sensed and does not reset timing. VVI pacing protects the patient from lethal bradycardias, but it does not restore or maintain AV synchrony.

Atrial Inhibited Pacing (AAI)

AAI pacing mode incorporates the same timing cycles, with the obvious difference that pacing and sensing occur from the atrium and pacemaker output is inhibited by a sensed atrial event (**Fig. 38-18**). An atrial paced or sensed event initiates a refractory period during which no spontaneous event alters delivery of the next pacing stimulus. When the atrial timing cycle ends, the atrial pacing stimulus is delivered regardless of ventricular events because an AAI pacemaker should not sense ventricular events. The single exception to this rule is far-field sensing; that is, the ventricular signal is large enough to be inappropriately sensed by the atrial lead. In this situation, the atrial timing cycle is reset by events sensed in the ventricle. This abnormality can sometimes be corrected by making the atrial channel less sensitive or by lengthening the atrial refractory period.

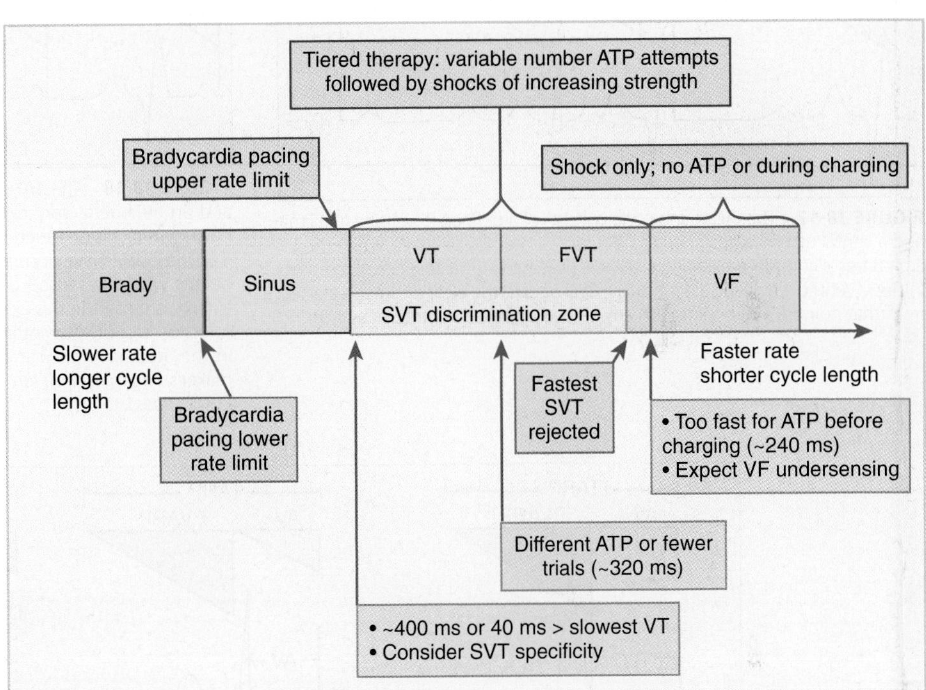

FIGURE 38-15 ICD rate zones. See text for details. ATP = antitachycardia pacing; FVT = fast VT; SVT = supraventricular tachycardia. Some ICDs permit programming of an additional monitor-only zone.

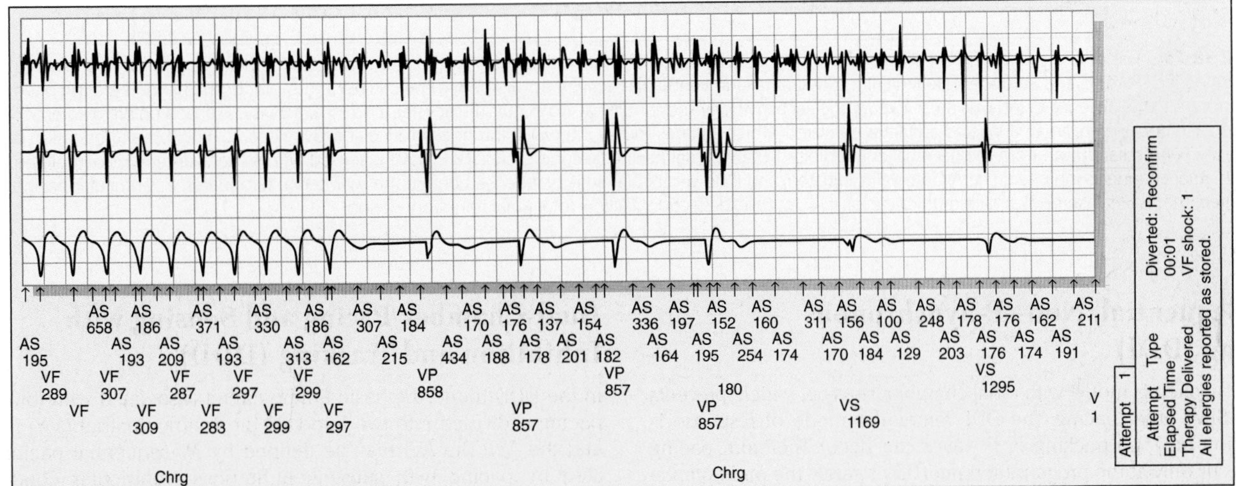

FIGURE 38-16 Noncommitted shocks. Stored episode on a nonsustained VT in a noncommitted device. From top to bottom are atrial EGM, near-field ventricular EGM, and far-field ventricular EGM. Continuing atrial fibrillation is present. During capacitor charge, the VT terminates. Slow sensed events (VS) after charge completion (at the second Chrg marker) indicate arrhythmia termination, so that the shock is withheld (Diverted-Reconfirm in the box at far right). Note that during the charge, pacing support (VP) is provided.

TABLE 38-1 NASPE/BPEG Generic Code for Antibradycardia Pacing

POSITION	I	II	III	IV	V
Category	Chamber(s) paced O = None A = Atrium V = Ventricle D = Dual (A + V)	Chamber(s) sensed O = None A = Atrium V = Ventricle D = Dual (A + V)	Response to sensing O = None T = Triggered I = Inhibited D = Dual (T + I)	Rate modulation O = None R = Rate modulation	Multisite pacing O = None A = Atrium V = Ventricle D = Dual (A + V)
Manufacturers' designation only	S = Single (A or V)	S = Single (A or V)			

See text for explanation of use of the code.
BPEG = British Pacing and Electrophysiology Group; NASPE = North American Society of Pacing and Electrophysiology.
From Bernstein AD, Daubert JC, Fletcher RD, et al: The revised NASPE/BPEG generic code for antibradycardia, adaptive-rate, and multisite pacing. Pacing Clin Electrophysiol 25:260, 2002.

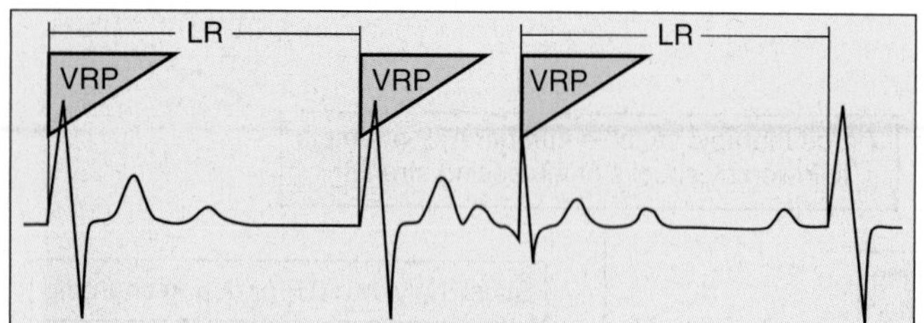

FIGURE 38-17 The VVI timing cycle consists of a defined lower rate (LR) limit and a ventricular refractory period (VRP, represented by triangle). When the LR limit timer is complete, a pacing artifact is delivered in the absence of a sensed intrinsic ventricular event. If an intrinsic QRS occurs, the LR limit timer is started from that point. A VRP begins with any sensed or paced ventricular activity.

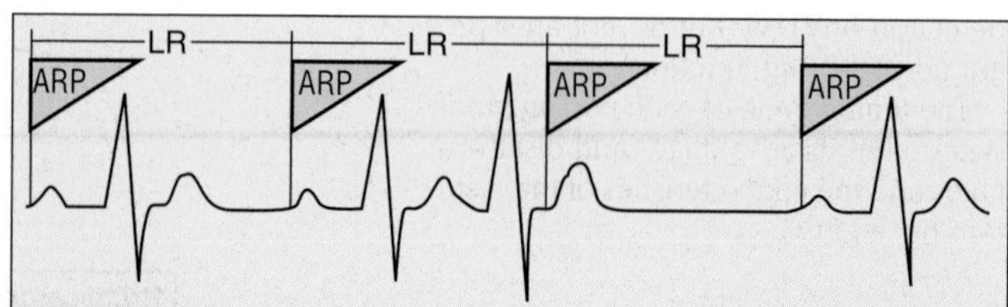

FIGURE 38-18 The AAI timing cycle consists of a defined lower rate (LR) limit and an atrial refractory period (ARP). When the LR limit timer is complete, a pacing artifact is delivered in the atrium in the absence of a sensed atrial event. If an intrinsic P wave occurs, the LR limit timer is started from that point. An ARP begins with any sensed or paced atrial activity. In the AAI mode, only atrial activity is sensed. In this example, it may appear unusual for paced atrial activity to occur so soon after intrinsic ventricular activity. Because sensing occurs only in the atrium, ventricular activity would not be expected to reset the pacemaker's timing cycle. *(From Hayes and Levine. By permission of Blackwell Scientific Publications.)*

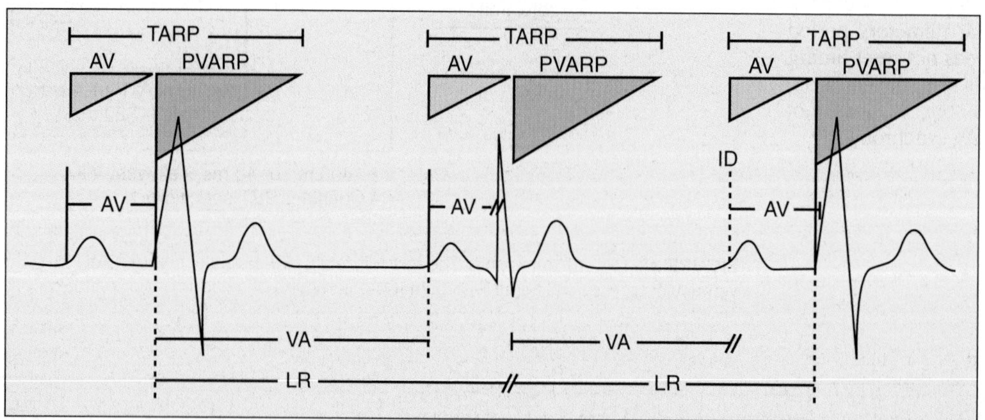

FIGURE 38-19 The timing cycle in DDD consists of a lower rate (LR) limit, an atrioventricular (AV) interval, a ventricular refractory period, a postventricular atrial refractory period (PVARP), and an upper rate limit. If intrinsic atrial and ventricular activity occurs before the LR limit times out, both channels are inhibited and no pacing occurs. In the absence of intrinsic atrial and ventricular activity, AV sequential pacing occurs (first cycle). If no atrial activity is sensed before the ventriculoatrial (VA) interval is completed, an atrial pacing artifact is delivered, which initiates the AV interval. If intrinsic ventricular activity occurs before the termination of the AV interval, the ventricular output from the pacemaker is inhibited, that is, atrial pacing (second cycle). If a P wave is sensed before the VA interval is completed, output from the atrial channel is inhibited. The AV interval is initiated, and if no ventricular activity is sensed before the AV interval terminates, a ventricular pacing artifact is delivered, that is, P-synchronous pacing (third cycle). ID = intrinsic deflection; TARP = total atrial refractory period.

AV Sequential, Non–P-Synchronous Pacing (DDI)

DDI is a pacing mode with dual-chamber sensing, which prevents competitive atrial pacing. The DDI ventricular mode of response is inhibition only; no tracking of P waves can occur. Therefore, pacing can occur only at the programmed rate. DDI is rarely the preimplantation mode of choice but remains a programmable option in most dual-chamber pacemakers. The DDI pacing mode could be considered atrial undersensing during intermittent atrial tachyarrhythmias and prevents mode switching.

Dual-Chamber Pacing and Sensing with Inhibition and Tracking (DDD)

In the DDD mode, the basic timing circuit associated with lower rate pacing is divided into two intervals: the ventriculoatrial (VA) interval and the AVI. The AVI may be defined by AV sequential pacing initiated by pacing with subsequent intrinsic ventricular conduction or initiated by a native P wave with subsequent ventricular pacing (**Fig. 38-19**).

As discussed, the sum of the PVARP and the AV interval defines the total atrial refractory period (TARP). In DDD pacing, if the intrinsic atrial rate exceeds the programmed upper rate limit, the pacemaker will not allow the upper rate limit to be violated; the electrocardiographic appearance depends on the intrinsic atrial rate. Wenckebach-like behavior can occur as spontaneous P waves intermittently timed in the PVARP and are thus not tracked. This can be followed by 2:1 pacing, that is, every other P wave falls in the PVARP (**Fig. 38-20**). The PVARP is especially important for the prevention of endless loop, or pacemaker-mediated, tachycardia (**Fig. 38-21**).

Rate-Adaptive Sensors

If a rate-adaptive sensor is incorporated in the pacemaker, the device will provide rate responsiveness when the sensor is on. Any pacing mode is designated rate adaptive by the addition of an R in the fourth position of the code (e.g., VVIR, AAIR, DDIR, and DDDR). The most common sensors used are the accelerometer, based on activity, and minute ventilation, which is based on transthoracic impedance measurements. Many other sensors have been used.[8]

Electrical Therapy for Ventricular Tachyarrhythmias

Tiered Therapy

Once VT or VF is detected, the ICD delivers a progression of up to six therapies, consisting of trains of antitachycardia pacing or individual high-voltage shock therapies. After each delivered therapy, the ICD's redetection algorithm monitors the rhythm for termination of VT/VF and resumption of sinus rhythm, persistence of the same VT/VF, or change in VT/VF. In the tiered therapy strategy, therapies escalate from low-power antitachycardia pacing to high-power shocks as the sequence progresses. Therapy sequences are programmable independently for up to three detection zones based on ventricular rate: slow VT, fast VT, and VF.

Antitachycardia Pacing

To be successful, at least one antitachycardia pacing pulse must enter the reentry circuit, terminate the VT, and not reinitiate VT (see Chap. 35). Approximately 80% to 90% of slower monomorphic VTs (cycle length >320 milliseconds) and 60% to 70% of faster VTs can be terminated by antitachycardia pacing. Antitachycardia pacing consists of short (3- to 10-beat) trains of pulses at a cycle length shorter than the VT cycle length. Monomorphic VT accounts for approximately 90% of all VT/VF treated by ICDs. Antitachycardia pacing is rarely effective for polymorphic VT or VF.

In contrast to bradycardia pacing, antitachycardia pacing is applied in an adaptive mode with the first pulse set to a percentage of VT cycle length, typically 85% to 90% for faster VTs and 75% to 85% for slower VTs. In burst mode, pulses within a train have a fixed cycle length, which may be decremented by 10 to 30 milliseconds between successive trains if the first train does not terminate VT. In ramp mode, sequential pulses within each train are delivered at progressively shorter cycle lengths until a minimum value is reached. Whereas comparison of the effectiveness of burst and ramp modes is difficult, burst mode typically is at least as effective as ramp mode and has a lower risk of accelerating VT to VF.

Painless termination of VT improves the quality of life in ICD patients

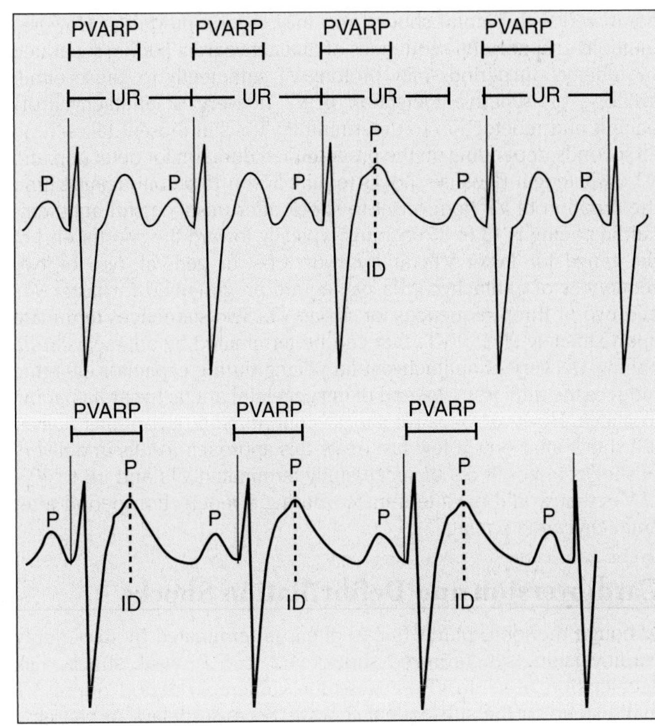

FIGURE 38-20 When the sinus rate exceeds the programmed maximum tracking rate, several upper rate (UR) behaviors can occur. In the top panel, pseudo-Wenckebach behavior is seen. If a P wave occurs outside the postventricular atrial refractory period (PVARP) and is sensed, the atrioventricular interval (AVI) is initiated. However, a ventricular pacing artifact cannot be delivered at the end of the programmed AVI if this would violate the programmed maximum tracking rate. Instead, the AVI would be lengthened and the ventricular pacing artifact would occur when the maximum tracking rate had "timed out." For example, if the maximum tracking rate is 120 beats/min or an interval of 500 milliseconds, the AVI is 150 milliseconds, the PVARP is 250 milliseconds, and the P wave is sensed 10 milliseconds after completion of the PVARP, or 260 milliseconds after the preceding ventricular event, the next ventricular pacing artifact could not be delivered for 240 milliseconds (500 − 260). In the bottom panel, 2:1 UR behavior occurs when every other sinus beat falls in the PVARP. ID = intrinsic deflection. *(From Hayes DL: DDDR timing cycles: Upper rate behavior. In Barold SS, Mugica J [eds]: New Perspectives in Cardiac Pacing, 3. Mount Kisco, NY, Futura Publishing Company, 1993, pp 233-257. By permission of the publisher.)*

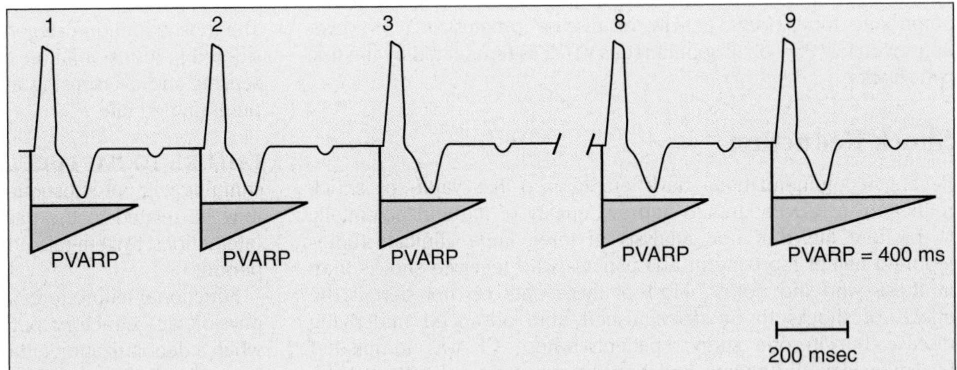

FIGURE 38-21 Schematic representation of pacemaker-mediated tachycardia. The intrinsic conduction system acts as the retrograde pathway and the pacemaker as the anterograde pathway. In this schematic, assumed to be from a patient at rest with a maximum tracking rate of 120 ppm (500 milliseconds), with beats 1 through 8, the retrograde P wave occurs outside the PVARP or imitates the AV interval. On beat 9, an algorithm to limit endless loop tachycardia extends the PVARP to 400 milliseconds. The retrograde P wave after beat 9 occurs within the PVARP and will terminate the endless loop tachycardia.

compared with painful shocks and may reduce mortality.[9] However, multiple unsuccessful sequences of antitachycardia pacing separated by redetection periods may prolong VT sufficiently to cause either syncope or ischemia. Detection of VT, delivery of antitachycardia pacing, and redetection to determine if VT is still present takes 10 to 20 seconds, depending on the programmed duration for detection and VT cycle length. Because shocks require a 5- to 15-second charge time, the duration of VT from onset to shock after unsuccessful antitachycardia pacing is 15 to 35 seconds, typically toward the shorter end of the range for faster VTs and newer ICDs. In general, one or two sequences of antitachycardia pacing are programmed for faster VTs and two or three sequences for slower VTs. Two sequences terminate approximately 90% of VTs that can be terminated by antitachycardia pacing. Delivery of antitachycardia pacing during capacitor charging reduces the time from the end of unsuccessful antitachycardia pacing to shock. However, because shock "confirmation" algorithms deliver the shock after only a few fast beats, this approach results in delivery of shocks to about 5% of successfully terminated VTs and up to 30% of VTs that would have terminated during a redetection period after antitachycardia pacing.[10]

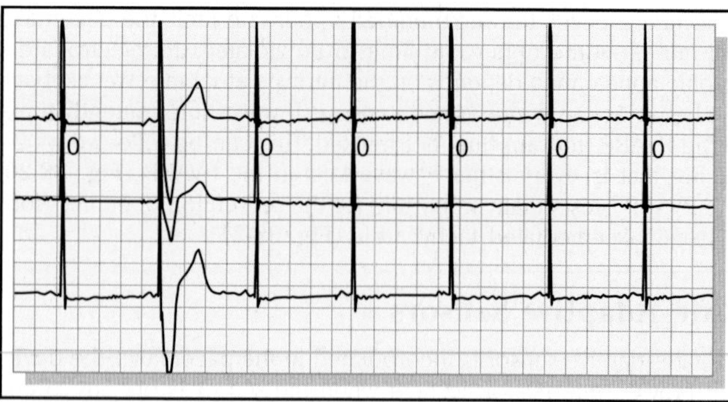

FIGURE 38-22 Three-channel tracing from an ambulatory monitor that was obtained because the patient had recurrent symptoms after pacemaker implantation. The tracing demonstrates intermittent failure to capture, and the pacemaker malfunction correlated with symptoms. The patient was found to have developed excessively high pacing thresholds on epicardial pacing leads.

Cardioversion and Defibrillation Shocks

Although monomorphic VTs can often be terminated by low-energy cardioversion (synchronized shocks = 2 to 5 J), weak shocks risk acceleration of VT to VF because the vulnerable period during VT may extend to the subsequent R wave. Because delays in charging the capacitor are not less significant clinically during VT than during VF and shock pain is not dependent on shock strength, we generally recommend programming high-energy (20 J) shocks for all VTs.

The first defibrillation shock is programmed either to a patient-specific value determined in relation to the weakest shock strength judged to be effective on the basis of implant testing or to maximum output. In adults, subsequent shocks usually are programmed to maximum output of 30 to 40 J. A patient-specific strategy reduces charge times and minimizes long-term adverse effects of excessive programmed shock strength, such as myocardial depression. However, modern ICDs charge sufficiently rapidly (at least near the beginning of service) that charge times are rarely an issue, and clinical benefit of lower shock strengths has not been established.

Maximum output shocks terminate induced VF in more than 95% of patients with modern ICD systems, including intraoperative system revisions if necessary; but first ICD shocks at the same shock strengths terminate only 80% to 90% of rhythms detected as VF during clinical follow-up, despite the fact that most of these rhythms are VT.[1] Thus, the success of shocks for clinical VT/VF may depend on factors that are not evaluated at implantation (e.g., ischemia, autonomic tone, drugs, activity, or disease progression). However, approximately 98% of all spontaneous VT/VF is terminated by the first two shocks.

Shock Reduction

Recent recommendations have emphasized the value of shock reduction in ICD patients to improve quality of life and potentially to prolong life. Post hoc analysis of three large clinical studies reported higher mortality in ICD patients who received shocks than in those who did not.[11-13] Most of these data do not permit the effects of shocks to be distinguished from advanced underlying disease, but in one study,[13] patients whose VT was terminated by antitachycardia pacing had better survival than did those who had shocks for VT. Present approaches to minimization of shocks include (1) program a sufficient duration for detection of VT to minimize delivery of shocks for VT that would stop spontaneously; (2) program antitachycardia pacing for all VTs, unless specifically contraindicated; (3) program SVT-VT discriminators to minimize inappropriate therapy of SVT; and (4) confirm reliable sensing to minimize inappropriate detection of VT/VF caused by oversensing.

Indications

Guidelines for pacemakers, ICDs, and cardiac resynchronization therapy were most recently updated in 2008.[14] Guidelines for management of patients with ventricular arrhythmias and the prevention of sudden cardiac death were presented in 2006.[15] Similar guidelines for cardiac pacing and cardiac resynchronization therapy were published in 2007.[16] See Guidelines: Cardiac Pacemakers and Cardioverter-Defibrillators.

Troubleshooting Common Clinical Problems

Noninvasive troubleshooting tools include history, chest radiography, surface electrocardiography, stored device data (programming, lead impedance values and trends, stored EGMs, and marker channels), and real-time device data (pacing and sensing thresholds, real-time EGMs during pocket manipulation or arm motion). For ICDs, they include induction of VF to sense testing and defibrillation and induction of VT to test antitachycardia pacing. For resynchronization pacing, they also include measures of heart failure and LV function (including the echocardiogram).

Pacemakers

The most common categories of pacemaker malfunction can be considered in terms of failure to capture, failure to pace or output, undersensing and oversensing, and pacing at a rate not consistent with the programmed rate.

FAILURE TO CAPTURE. Failure to capture is defined as a pacing stimulus without subsequent cardiac depolarization (**Fig. 38-22**). It may be related to the pacing system, the patient, or patient-system interactions. System-related causes are common in the perioperative period.

Functional failure to capture results when a stimulus occurs in the physiologic refractory period of a depolarization. This may occur when a depolarization either is not sensed because it times in a blanking period or is not used to adjust pacemaker timing (e.g., an asynchronous pacing mode).

FAILURE TO PACE. Failure to output an appropriate pacing stimulus is most commonly due to oversensing of physiologic (**Fig. 38-23**) or nonphysiologic signals, resulting in inhibition of the pacing output. (See also later discussion of oversensing in ICDs.) Rarely, it may be caused by failure of the pulse generator or an open circuit (e.g., a lead fracture or a loose set screw).

Crosstalk is a specific form of oversensing in which the atrial pacing stimulus is sensed on the ventricular channel, resulting in inhibition of ventricular output (see Fig. 38-11). Settings that promote crosstalk include high atrial output, ventricular sensing parameter programmed to a very sensitive value, and short duration of ventricular blanking after atrial pacing. Pacemakers have features to prevent crosstalk, including ventricular blanking after atrial pacing and triggered ventricular pacing in response to a sensed event in the AV interval.

Lead or header-connector problems can cause oversensing of noncardiac signals or open circuits. Lead insulation failures are manifested with low pacing impedance. Lead fractures can present with high pacing impedance or oversensing with a normal impedance. The most common header-connector problems are failure to insert the lead fully into the connector block and failure to tighten the set screw. The combination of failure to capture and failure to pace usually indicates a problem with the pacing system as opposed to a physiologic problem.

PACING AT A RATE NOT CONSISTENT WITH THE PROGRAMMED RATE. Pacing with a shorter than expected escape interval indicates undersensing of myocardial depolarizations (**Fig. 38-24**). Like failure to capture, undersensing can be related to the pacing system, the patient, or patient-system interactions. Premature atrial and ventricular complexes can have different local EGMs than normal beats. A pacing system that undersenses only during premature beats rarely requires revision.

Pacing consistently at a rate slower than the programmed lower rate limit usually indicates either oversensing of a constant signal during each cardiac cycle (most commonly T wave oversensing; **Fig. 38-25**) or battery depletion. Rarely, it can be caused by electronic component failure.

Nonphysiologic rapid pacing (i.e., not a result of tracking an intrinsic atrial rhythm or appropriate sensor activation with exertion) can have several causes. Rapid pacing, usually at or near the upper rate limit, can represent pacemaker-mediated tachycardia. Sometimes, this term is restricted to endless loop tachycardia, in which the pacemaker functions as the anterograde limb of AV reentrant tachycardia and the normal conduction system functions as the retrograde limb (see Fig. 38-21). Unexpected pacing at or near the upper rate limit can also be caused by inappropriate sensor-driven pacing in single- or dual-chamber pacemakers or by ventricular tracking of pathologic atrial tachyarrhythmias. High sensed atrial rates can be caused by

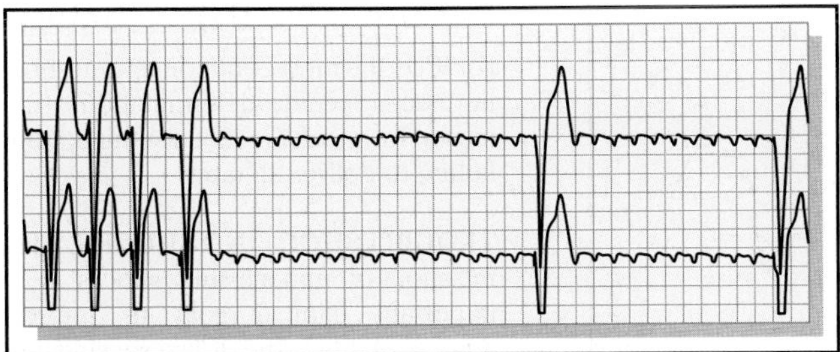

FIGURE 38-23 Electrocardiographic tracing from a patient with a single-chamber pacemaker. The tracing was obtained when the patient was exposed to an external source of electromagnetic interference, which profoundly inhibited ventricular output, that is, ventricular oversensing.

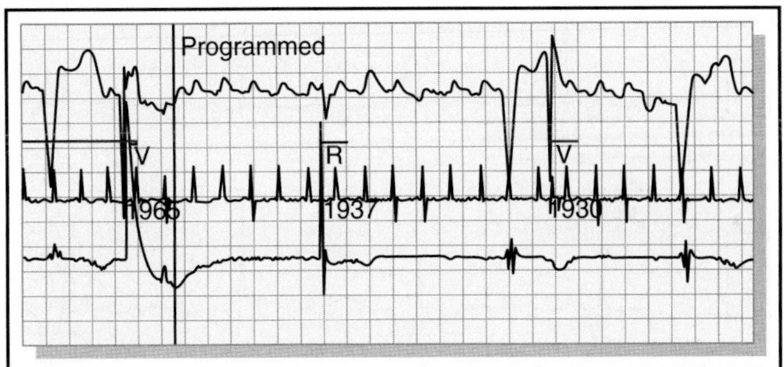

FIGURE 38-24 Telemetry with surface ECG (top), atrial EGM (middle), and ventricular EGM (bottom). Markers are present on the ventricular channel. There are six ventricular events but only three with marker annotation. The first ventricular event is not sensed and not annotated. The second ventricular event is labeled as a paced ventricular (V) event; the third is an intrinsic ventricular event (R); the fourth is not sensed and is followed approximately 360 milliseconds later by a paced ventricular event (V); and the final event is not sensed.

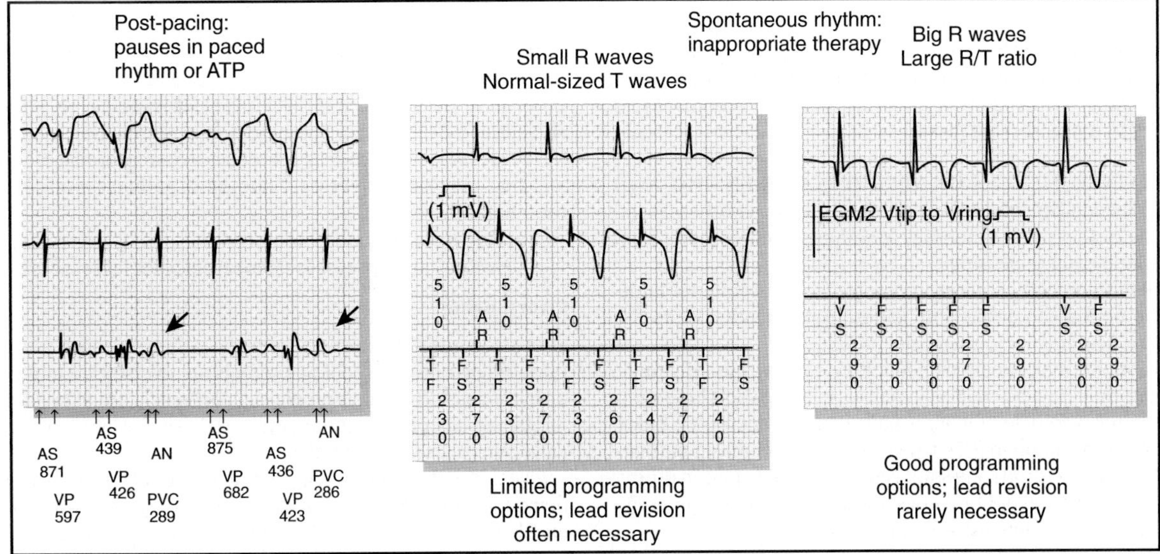

FIGURE 38-25 Classification of T wave oversensing. During pacing (left panel), T wave oversensing may cause a pause. From top to bottom in the left panel are shown the surface ECG, atrial EGM, ventricular EGM, and marker annotations. The oversensed T wave is indicated with an arrow on the ventricular EGM. The middle panel shows T wave oversensing with a very small R wave–to–T wave ratio, in this case due to small R waves and normal-sized T waves. From top to bottom are atrial EGM, near-field ventricular EGM, and markers. Reprogramming options are limited in this situation, and lead revision is often necessary. It is important that the near-field ventricular EGM be reviewed (as opposed to far-field) as this represents the signal the ICD uses for rate detection. The right panel shows T wave oversensing in the setting of a large R/T ratio; this is typically corrected with device reprogramming. From top to bottom are the ventricular near-field EGM and markers. ATP = antitachycardia pacing. *(From Swerdlow CD, Friedman PA: Advanced ICD troubleshooting: Part I. Pacing Clin Electrophysiol 28:1322, 2005.)*

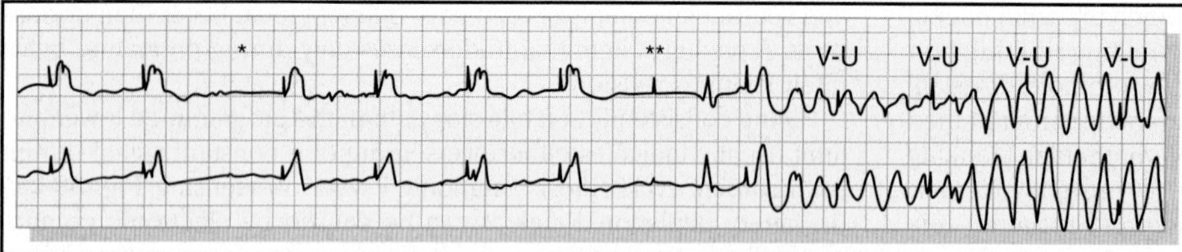

FIGURE 38-26 Electrocardiographic tracing from a patient with a pacemaker programmed to VVI at approximately 70 ppm. There is a longer V-V interval representing oversensing (*); there is a subsequent pacing spike with failure to capture (**); and in the terminal portion of the tracing, the patient develops VT and the pacemaker does not sense the tachyarrhythmia. Pacing artifacts can be seen to march through the tachyarrhythmia, labeled V-U (ventricular undersensing).

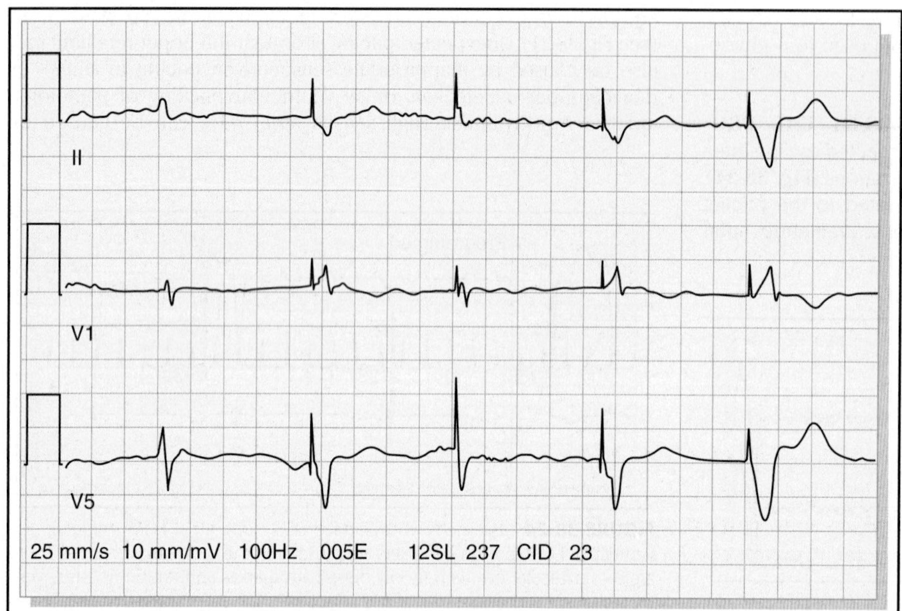

FIGURE 38-27 Three-channel tracing from an ambulatory monitor. The first QRS is intrinsic. The second and fourth beats represent fusion; the third beat is pseudofusion, that is, the underlying morphology is nearly identical to the intrinsic QRS; and the final QRS represents paced depolarization.

atrial tachyarrhythmias or atrial oversensing of pectoral myopotentials or by electromagnetic interference. Sensor-driven, pacemaker-mediated tachycardia can be terminated by altering the rate-response parameters or programming to rate-response off. Endless loop tachycardia or tracking of high sensed atrial rates can be terminated by programming to a nontracking mode.

ADVERSE CONSEQUENCES OF APPROPRIATE SENSING AND CAPTURE. Pacemaker syndrome, described before, can be caused by VVI pacing or loss of AV synchrony in a dual-chamber mode from failure of atrial pacing or sensing.

Extracardiac stimulation can occur as a result of unwanted stimulation from the pocket or cardiac stimulation from a lead close to the phrenic nerve, diaphragm, or intercostal muscle.

On occasion, normal pacemaker function can be proarrhythmic, especially if normal function results in pauses causing short-long-short sequences in the ventricle, initiating pause-dependent VT/VF. Proarrhythmia is more common in ICD patients than in pacemaker patients (**Fig. 38-26**).[6] Because short-long-short sequences are common during programming, an external defibrillator should be available in programming of pacemaker patients whose underlying rhythm is slow.

MISINTERPRETATION OF NORMAL PACEMAKER FUNCTION. Historically, fusion and pseudofusion beats on the ECG have been a source of confusion. Fusion indicates that depolarization occurs partially as a result of intrinsic activation and partially as a result of capture from the pacemaker stimulus (**Fig. 38-27**). Pseudofusion indicates that the pacemaker stimulus does not alter intrinsic QRS morphology on the surface ECG. This occurs when local activation around the sensing electrode is delayed relative to the surface ECG. The pacing pulse is thus delivered at the appropriate escape interval into the absolute refractory period of almost the entire paced chamber, except for a small region around the electrode. At times, the surface ECG may not permit determination of the chamber paced. For example, atrial undersensing during AF can result in functional failure of atrial capture but can be misinterpreted as failure of ventricular capture.

Contemporary pacemakers have features that may not be inferred from basic timing cycles without detailed knowledge of specific programming. Algorithms that promote intrinsic AV conduction to reduce unnecessary ventricular pacing can be especially confusing (see Fig. 38-14).

Implantable Cardioverter-Defibrillators

For ICDs, the most common troubleshooting issues include determination of the reason for shocks, ineffective therapy, and failure to deliver therapy.

TROUBLESHOOTING SHOCKS. Minimization of unnecessary shocks is an important clinical goal to improve quality of life.[9] The ICD's sensing and detection is imperfect. ICDs can detect VT/VF if either a true tachycardia (SVT or VT) occurs or nonarrhythmic electrical signals are oversensed. ICDs also discriminate tachycardias imperfectly; true SVT episodes may be classified as VT or VF, and true VT may be classified as SVT. An ICD may correctly classify VT but not detect that VT has terminated during capacitor charging, thus delivering a shock for self-terminating nonsustained VT. Inappropriate shocks usually are defined as shocks delivered for rhythms other than VT/VF and can be a result of oversensing, incorrect classification of SVT or AF, or failure to detect termination of nonsustained VT. However, even if shocks are delivered "appropriately" for ongoing VT, they may be unnecessary shocks if antitachycardia pacing can terminate VT.

The first step in troubleshooting shocks is to determine if therapy was delivered in response to oversensing or a tachycardia.

Oversensing

Shocks occur in the absence of tachycardias because nonarrhythmic physiologic or nonphysiologic signals are oversensed and detected as arrhythmias.[3,17] Nonphysiologic signals usually are extracardiac. Physiologic signals can be intracardiac (P, R, or T waves) or extracardiac (myopotentials) (**Fig. 38-28**).

Oversensing of physiologic intracardiac signals can result in two device-detected R waves for each cardiac cycle. P wave oversensing and R wave double counting present as alternating cycle lengths of sensed R-R intervals. T wave oversensing presents as alternating morphologies.[18] P wave oversensing can occur if the distal coil of an integrated bipolar lead is too close to the tricuspid valve. R wave double counting occurs if the duration of the sensing EGM exceeds the ventricular blanking period of 120 to 140 milliseconds. T wave oversensing often occurs in the setting of low-amplitude R waves. Whereas oversensing of native T waves causes inappropriate therapy,

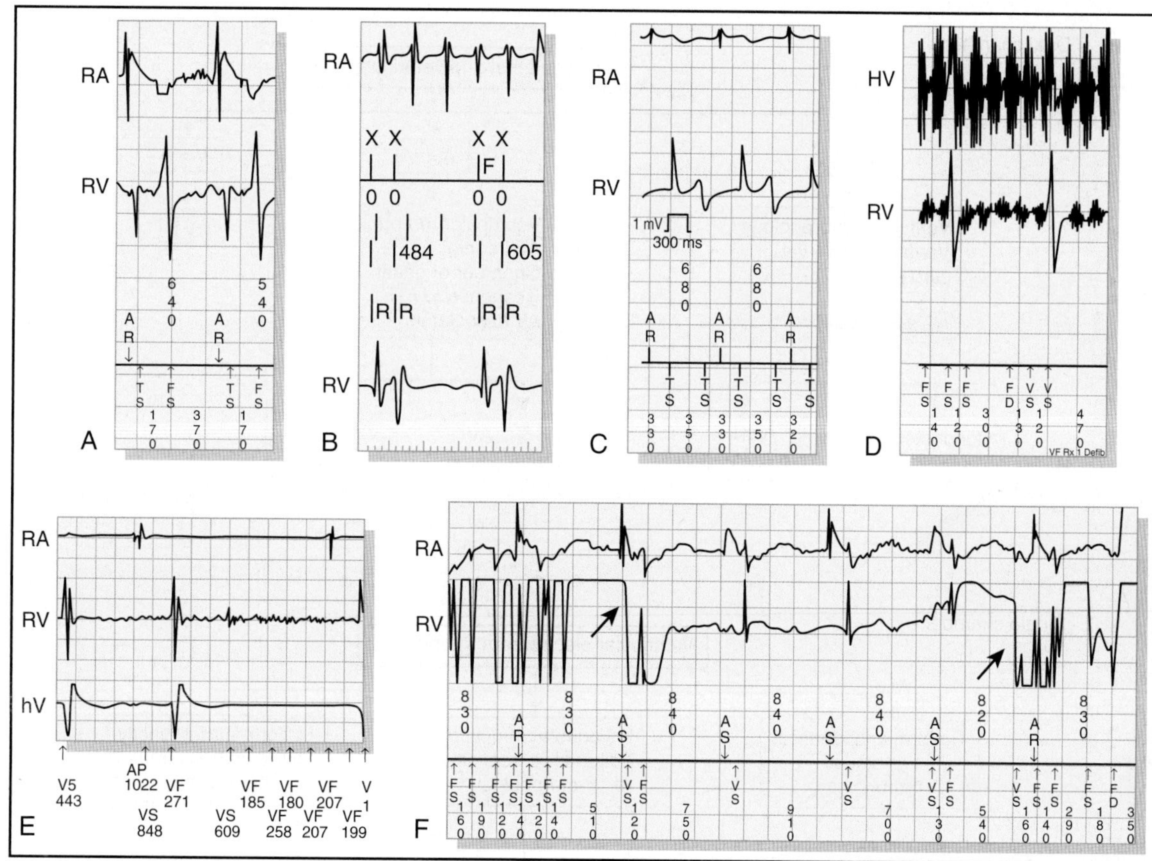

FIGURE 38-28 Types of oversensing resulting in inappropriate detection of VT or VF. **A-C,** Oversensing of physiologic, intracardiac signals. **D-F,** Oversensing of extracardiac signals. **A,** P wave oversensing in sinus rhythm from integrated bipolar lead with distal coil near the tricuspid valve. **B,** R wave double counting during conducted AF in a biventricular sensing ICD. **C,** T wave oversensing in patient with low-amplitude R wave (note mV calibration marker). **D,** Electromagnetic interference from a power drill has higher amplitude on widely spaced high-voltage EGM than on closely spaced true bipolar sensing EGM. **E,** Diaphragmatic myopotential oversensing in a patent with an integrated bipolar lead at the RV apex. Note that noise level is constant, but oversensing does not occur until automatic gain control increases the gain sufficiently, about 600 milliseconds after the sensed R waves. **F,** Lead fracture noise results in intermittent saturation of amplifier range denoted by arrow. RA = right atrium; RV = right ventricular sensing electrogram; HV = high-voltage electrogram. *(Reprinted with permission from Swerdlow C, Shivkumar K: Implantable cardioverter defibrillators: Clinical aspects. In Zipes DP, Jalife J [eds]: Cardiac Electrophysiology: From Cell to Bedside. 4th ed. Philadelphia, WB Saunders, 2004, pp 980-993.)*

oversensing of paced T waves causes bradycardia or antitachycardia pacing at the wrong rate.

When extracardiac signals are oversensed, the isoelectric baseline is replaced by high-frequency noise that has no fixed relationship to the cardiac cycle (see Fig. 38-28). External electromagnetic interference usually is continuous. Signal amplitude is greater on the high-voltage EGM recorded from widely spaced electrodes than on the sensing EGM recorded from closely spaced electrodes. Oversensing due to lead or connector (header, adapter, or set screw) problems is intermittent, occurring only during a small fraction of the cardiac cycle, and is often associated with abnormal pacing-lead impedance. It can be limited to the sensing EGM and can saturate the amplifier range. This type of oversensing is the most important, both because the ICD system may not deliver pacing and shocks and because an inappropriate shock into a faulty lead can be sufficiently strong to induce VF (if it is applied in the vulnerable period) but insufficient to defibrillate. Myopotential oversensing has variable duration. Pectoral myopotentials are more prominent on the high-voltage EGM, whereas diaphragmatic myopotentials are more prominent on the sensing EGM.

VT Versus SVT

If stored EGMs indicate that a shock was delivered in response to a true tachycardia, the second step in diagnosis is to determine if the rhythm is VT or SVT. Established principles of ECG and EGM analysis usually lead to the correct diagnosis (**Fig. 38-29**)[3,17] (see Chap. 36). For single-chamber ICDs, diagnosis is based on analysis of the tachycardia onset and the morphology and regularity of the ventricular EGM. A real-time, reference sinus EGM should be recorded with the patient in the same posture in which the episode occurred to facilitate analysis of EGM morphology. For dual-chamber ICDs, analyses of the chamber of onset, atrial and ventricular rates, and AV relationships improve diagnostic accuracy. Inappropriate therapy due to SVT can be reduced by optimal programming of VT and VF detection rates, optimal programming of SVT-VT discriminators, appropriate use of beta blockers and antiarrhythmic drugs for SVT, and catheter ablation of SVT.

Nonsustained VT

Shocks delivered in response to self-terminating VT can be prevented by increasing the duration for detection (**Fig. 38-30**) or altering specific programming relating to shock confirmation or episode termination.[19]

Unnecessary Shocks for Sustained VT

Approximately 80% to 90% of monomorphic VTs slower than 190/min and 60% to 70% of faster monomorphic VTs can be terminated by painless antitachycardia pacing (**Fig. 38-31**). The frequency of shocks for VT can be reduced by programming antitachycardia pacing for monomorphic VT slowed by antiarrhythmic drugs.[9,20]

Approach to the Patient Experiencing an ICD Shock

If a patient experiences single or infrequent shocks, the ICD should be interrogated within 24 to 48 hours unless the necessary

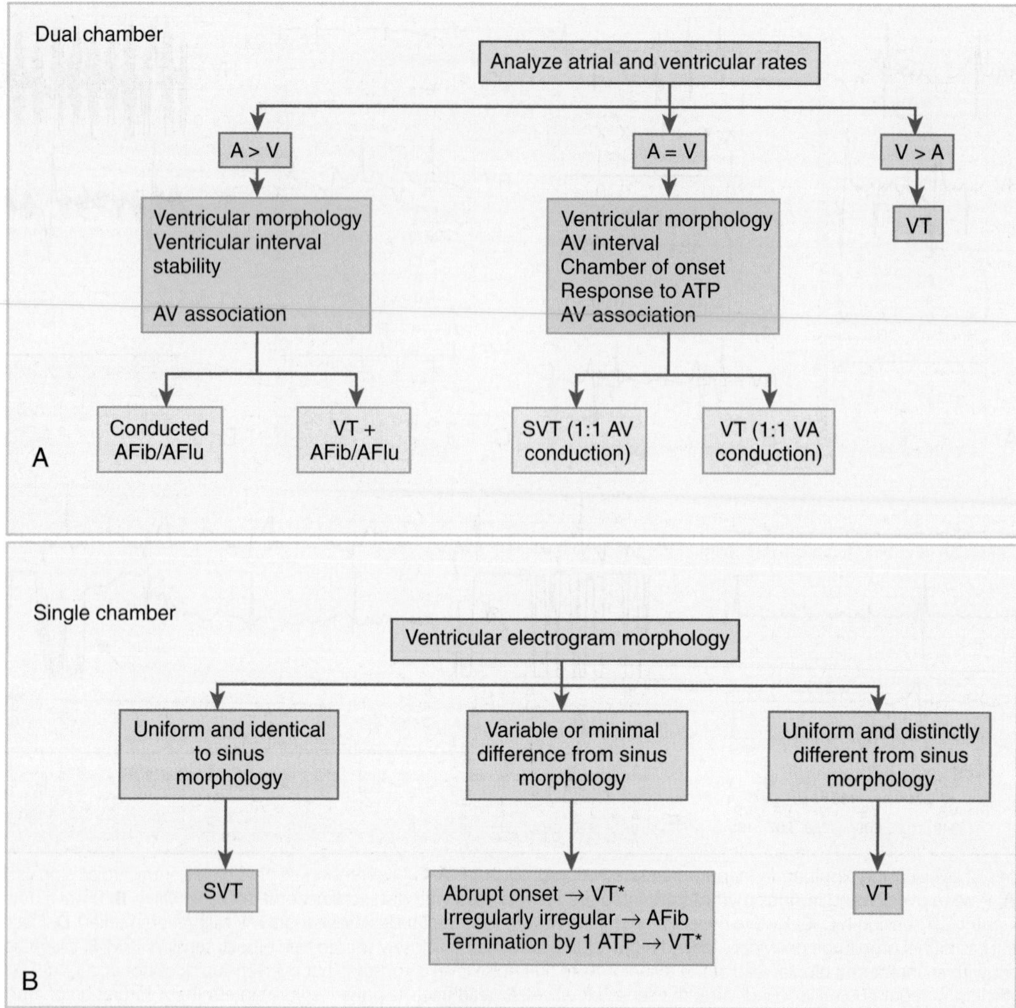

FIGURE 38-29 Method for analysis of stored EGMs in dual-chamber ICDs **(A)** and single-chamber ICDs **(B)**. Asterisks denote weaker criteria. ATP = antitachycardia pacing; AFib = atrial fibrillation, AFlu = atrial flutter. See text for details. *(Reproduced with permission from Swerdlow C, Friedman P: Advanced ICD troubleshooting: Part I. Pacing Clin Electrophysiol 28:1322, 2005, Blackwell Publishing.)*

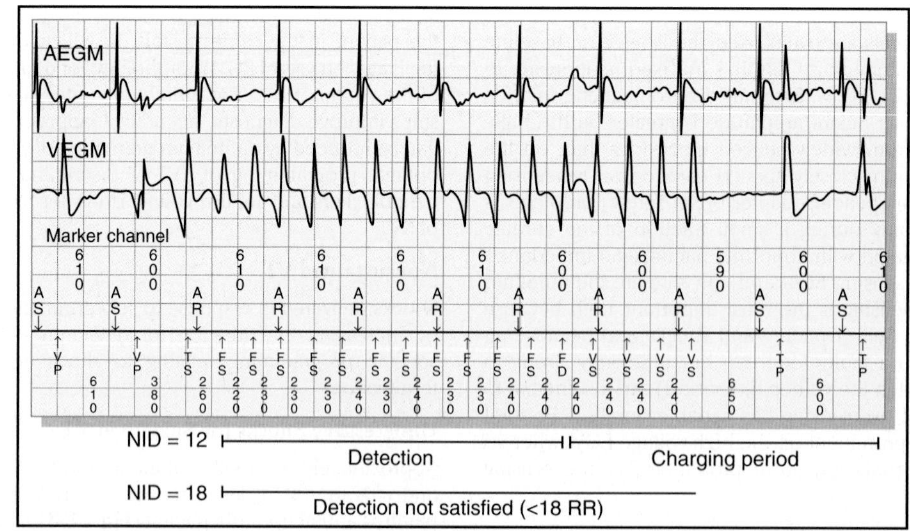

FIGURE 38-30 Nonsustained VT. Rapid VT detected in the VF detection zone with 12 intervals but terminated spontaneously during the ICD charging period. AEGM = atrial electrogram; VEGM = far-field ventricular electrogram; FS = fibrillation sense; FD = fibrillation detected; TS = tachycardia sense; AR = atrial refractory sense; VP = ventricular pace; TP = ventricular pace during charging; VS = ventricular sense. *(From Gunderson BD, Abeyratne AI, Olson WH, Swerdlow CD: Effect of programmed number of intervals to detect ventricular fibrillation on implantable cardioverter-defibrillator aborted and unnecessary shocks. Pacing Clin Electrophysiol 30:157, 2007.)*

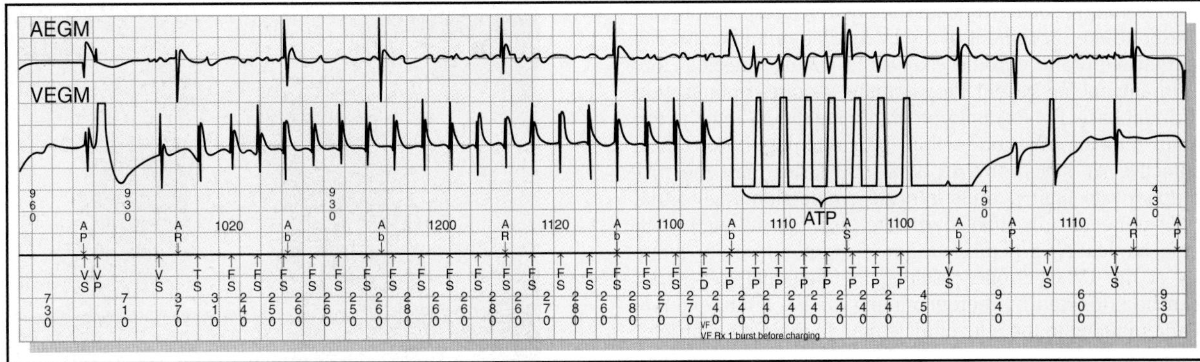

FIGURE 38-31 Antitachycardia pacing (ATP) for monomorphic VT. Stored atrial (AEGM) and ventricular (VEGM) electrograms and atrial and ventricular marker channels from an episode of rapid monomorphic VT (cycle length, 240 to 270 milliseconds; rate, 220 to 250 beats/min). VT with AV dissociation begins with the second ventricular electrogram. After 18 intervals shorter than the programmed VF detection interval of 320 milliseconds, adaptive ATP is delivered at cycle length 240 milliseconds, 88% of the VT cycle length, terminating the VT. On the marker channel, VS, TS, and FS indicate intervals classified in the sinus, VT, and VF rate zones, respectively. TP = ATP. FD = detection of VF. Note that a burst of ATP is delivered even though the intervals are in the VF zone. AP = atrial paced events. Ab and AR indicate atrial intervals in the postventricular atrial blanking and refractory periods, respectively.

clinical information is available from a remote monitoring system.

Frequent or repetitive shocks constitute an emergency. If a patient receives repetitive inappropriate shocks caused by SVT or oversensing during sinus rhythm, VT/VF detection can be disabled by a programmer or magnet. Repetitive shocks for VT can be caused by recurring episodes of VT after successful shock termination of VT (VT storm, cluster shocks) or by multiple unsuccessful shocks for a single episode. Therapeutic approaches differ. VT storm can be caused by acute ischemia, exacerbation of heart failure, metabolic abnormalities (e.g., hypokalemia, amiodarone-induced hyperthyroidism), and drug effects (e.g., proarrhythmia, change in prescribed drugs, or noncompliance). Diagnosis of acute coronary syndromes during VT storm is difficult because multiple shocks can cause changes in repolarization and elevations of troponin I. Therapy may include reversal of the precipitating cause, beta blockers, antiarrhythmic drugs (e.g., sotalol, amiodarone), and catheter ablation. Rarely, ICDs deliver unnecessary repetitive shocks for recurring self-terminating episodes of VT. Increasing the duration required for detection and redetection of VT or VF may prevent these shocks.

TABLE 38-2 Causes of Unsuccessful ICD Shocks

Misclassified Therapy
VT/VF recurs before the ICD determines the VT/VF episode has terminated
Failure to terminate SVT (e.g., sinus tachycardia)
Post-shock rhythm is SVT in the VT rate zone
Patient-Related Factors
Metabolic (hyperkalemia)
Ischemia
Progression of heart failure
Some antiarrhythmic drugs (e.g., amiodarone, type IC)
Pleural or pericardial effusions
ICD System–Related Reasons
Insufficient programmed shock strength
Battery depletion
Failure of generator component or lead
Incorrect device-lead connection
Lead dislodgment
Delayed detection resulting in a prolonged episode that increases required shock strength

UNSUCCESSFUL SHOCKS. Because defibrillation success is probabilistic, occasional shocks fail; but failure of two maximum-output shocks is rare if the safety margin is adequate.[1,21] If an ICD classifies a shock as unsuccessful, stored EGMs should be reviewed to determine if the shock was delivered during true VT/VF and if the shock failed to terminate VT/VF.

ICDs misclassify effective therapy as ineffective if VT/VF recurs before the ICD determines that the VT/VF episode has terminated or if the post-shock rhythm is SVT in the VT rate zone (e.g., catecholamine-induced sinus tachycardia or shock-induced AF).

Shocks from chronic ICD systems that defibrillated reliably at implantation may fail to terminate true VT or VF because of patient-related or ICD system–related reasons. In chronically implanted systems, most patient-related causes of unsuccessful shocks can be reversed, but most system-related causes require operative intervention (**Table 38-2**). Failure of multiple high-output shocks to terminate a regular tachycardia suggests sinus tachycardia because monomorphic VT and non-sinus SVT usually are terminated by one or two shocks.

FAILURE TO DELIVER THERAPY OR DELAYED THERAPY. These can be caused by problems with either ICD programming (including human error) or the ICD system. VT or VF will not be detected if the ICD is inactivated, VT is slower than the programmed detection interval, SVT-VT discriminators diagnose SVT, or sensing is impaired by device-device or intradevice interactions. VF may be undersensed because of combinations of programming (sensitivity, rate, or duration), low-amplitude EGMs, rapidly varying EGM amplitude, drug effects, or post-shock tissue changes.[3] Lead, connector, or generator malfunction may also prevent therapy from being delivered.

Failure to Respond to Resynchronization Pacing

This can be caused by patient-related factors, system-related factors, or an interaction between the patient and the system. In the context of this chapter, failure to respond refers to objective measures of LV performance because failure of clinical response alone can be due to noncardiac factors such as depression.

Response to resynchronization pacing requires effective resynchronization of at least 90% of R-R intervals,[22] and the clinical goal should be biventricular pacing at or near 100%. For properly selected patients (see Chap. 33), the most common patient-related cause of nonresponse is resynchronization of less than 90% of R-R intervals caused by conducted AF or frequent premature ventricular complexes.

The most common system-related cause is loss of LV capture due to lead dislodgment, which can be identified by the surface ECG and confirmed by lead threshold testing. If the LV lead captures, sensing errors can prevent delivery of effective resynchronization. For example, atrial undersensing permits intrinsic conduction, and atrial oversensing can result in reversion to a nontracking mode.

The most common patient-system interactions responsible for failure to respond are placement of the LV lead at an ineffective site for resynchronization and chronic changes in pacing threshold that can occur in any pacing system. Programming requires optimization on an individual basis. For example, programming the AV interval too long permits intrinsic AV conduction; programming it too short reduces effective AV synchrony. An atrial rate faster than the programmed upper rate limit permits intrinsic conduction. Right atrial pacing at an unnecessarily high lower rate limit can interfere with left-sided mechanical AV synchrony. Failure to respond due to stimulus latency at the LV electrode, resulting in functional loss of LV capture, can be corrected by reprogramming the V-V timing interval to allow earlier pacing in the left ventricle than in the right ventricle.

Complications

Complications can be divided into early complications of a component of the implanted system and late complications related to the patient or system.

Implant-Related Complications

Most patients have some discomfort at the site of the incision, and many will have mild ecchymoses. Hematomas occur most commonly when the patient is taking clopidogrel or when heparin or heparin equivalents are used in the early postimplantation period. Anticoagulation with warfarin is usually less of a problem, and many implanters perform device implantation on the warfarin-anticoagulated patient with an international normalized ratio below about 2.5.[23] Most hematomas resolve without evacuation, but evacuation can be required to relieve severe pain, to maintain integrity of the suture line, or to permit reinitiation of anticoagulation.

Complications of subclavian puncture include traumatic pneumothorax and hemopneumothorax, inadvertent arterial puncture, air embolism, arteriovenous fistula, thoracic duct injury, subcutaneous emphysema, and brachial plexus injury. These complications are minimized with an extrathoracic puncture technique or with direct cephalic access.

Introduction of the lead or leads into the subclavian artery, the aorta, and the left ventricle usually is readily recognized because of the pulsatile flow of saturated blood. A pacing lead can also be placed in the left ventricle by passing it across an unsuspected atrial or ventricular septal defect or patent foramen ovale. LV lead placement should be recognized by a posteriorly positioned lead on lateral fluoroscopy. A right bundle branch block pattern during ventricular pacing should raise suspicion of LV pacing.

Patients should be made aware of the potential for lead perforation. Although cardiac tamponade is the most dramatic outcome from perforation, asymptomatic ventricular perforation can occur. Signs can include elevation of pacing or sensing thresholds, right bundle branch block pattern from a lead placed in the right ventricle, intercostal muscle or diaphragmatic contraction, friction rub, pericarditis, or pericardial effusion.

Partial or silent venous thrombosis of the subclavian vein is not uncommon after transvenous lead placement and is usually clinically insignificant. Symptomatic thrombosis of the subclavian vein, with an edematous, painful upper extremity, is uncommon. Management includes elevation and anticoagulation for most patients.

Lead-Related Complications

Lead-related complications include dislodgment, header-connector pin problems, conductor/cable (lead) fracture, and insulation break.

Acceptable dislodgment rates should be less than 1% for ventricular leads and 2% to 3% for atrial leads. On radiographic examination, dislodgment may be evident (macrodislodgment; **Fig. 38-32**) or not detectable (microdislodgment).

Intermittent or complete failure of output can occur because of a loose or inadequate connection between the lead and connector block, usually because the lead was incorrectly connected to the header at the time of implantation (**Fig. 38-33**). When a connection is loose, manipulation of the pulse generator or pocket may reproduce the problem. The poor connection may be evident radiographically.

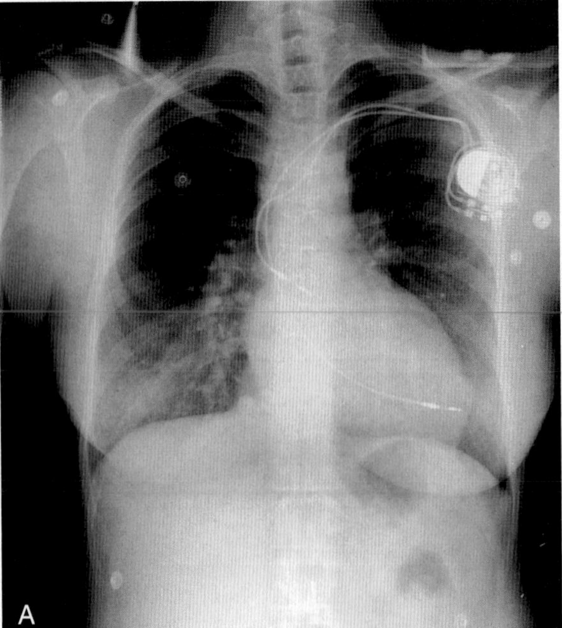

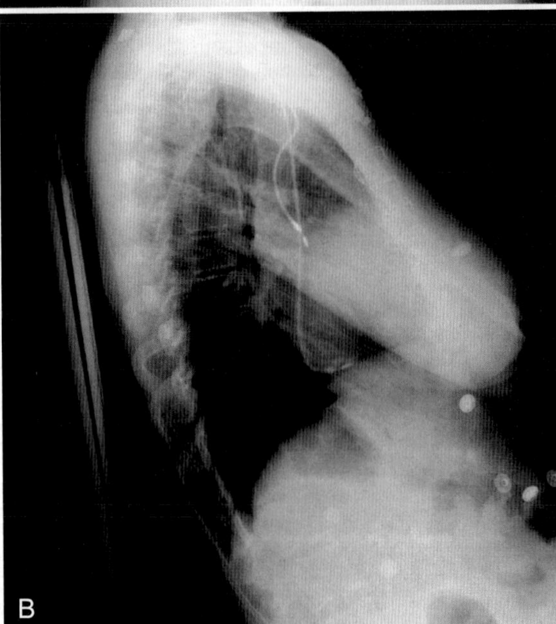

FIGURE 38-32 Posteroanterior **(A)** and lateral **(B)** chest radiograph demonstrating a grossly dislodged (macrodislodgment) atrial lead.

Lead or connector problems present as oversensing "noise" or impedance abnormalities. In pacemaker-dependent patients, oversensing presents as inhibition of pacing. In ICD patients, they may present as inappropriate shocks. Failures involving the defibrillation coils may present as ineffective defibrillation.

Acute device proarrhythmia presents most commonly as ventricular extrasystoles morphologically similar to the paced beats because they originate at the same site as the paced beats. They usually resolve spontaneously and almost never require pharmacologic suppression.

Extracardiac stimulation usually involves the diaphragm or the pectoral or intercostal muscles. Diaphragmatic contractions can be caused by direct stimulation of the diaphragm (usually stimulation of the left hemidiaphragm by the RV lead) or stimulation of the phrenic nerve (on the right by the atrial lead and on the left by the LV lead).

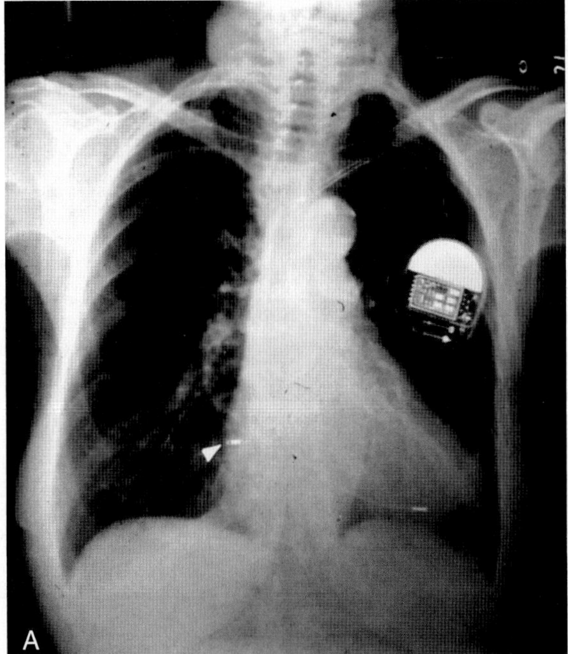

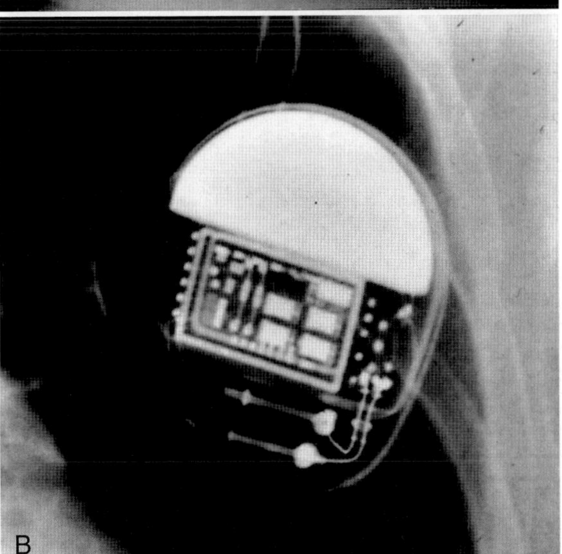

FIGURE 38-33 Posteroanterior **(A)** and close-up **(B)** views from a patient with intermittent failure to pace. Comparison of the upper and lower pins reveals that the lower of the two unipolar leads is not completely advanced. This difference is more evident on the close-up view. By convention, the lower of the two leads in the connector block is the ventricular lead, so that this patient must have had intermittent or permanent ventricular failure to output. An unrelated observation, noted by the arrowhead, is shallow positioning of the atrial lead, that is, the J is much wider than 90 degrees. *(From Hayes DL: Pacemaker radiography.* In *Furman S, Hayes DL, Holmes DR Jr [eds]: A Practice of Cardiac Pacing. 3rd ed. Mount Kisco, NY, Futura Publishing, 1993, pp 361-400. Used with permission of Mayo Foundation for Medical Education and Research.)*

Diaphragmatic stimulation occurring during the early postimplantation period can be due to either microdislodgment or macrodislodgment. Stimulation can be minimized or alleviated by decreasing the voltage, but an adequate pacing margin of safety must be maintained after the output parameters are decreased. If the problem cannot be resolved by reprogramming, lead repositioning will be required.

Device System Infection

Erosion is an uncommon complication that usually occurs because of an indolent infection, although it may also be the result of a device pocket that is too small for the pulse generator, particularly in a thin patient. If the pulse generator is too superficial or if the patient has minimal subcutaneous tissue and the overlying skin is stretched very tight, to the point that skin integrity is compromised, the pulse generator can erode or extrude through the skin. If there is impending erosion in an uninfected pocket, it may be possible to revise the pocket and reimplant the device. Impending erosion should be dealt with as an emergency because once any portion of the device has eroded through the skin, removal of the device system and placement of a new system in another site are usually required.

The incidence of infection after initial device implantation should be less than 1%. Preoperative antibiotics reduce the incidence of infection.[24] Careful attention to surgical details and sterile procedures is critical. Device infection can present as local inflammation or abscess formation in the pocket, erosion of part of the pacing system with secondary infection, or sepsis with or without a focus of infection elsewhere.

The most common clinical presentation is localized pocket infection; sepsis is uncommon. Many infectious agents can be responsible, but early infections are most commonly caused by *Staphylococcus aureus,* are aggressive, and are often associated with fever and systemic symptoms. Late infections commonly caused by *Staphylococcus epidermidis* are more indolent, usually without fever or systemic manifestation. Treatment of device-related septicemia requires removal of the entire infected pacing system, device, and leads. A consensus statement on transvenous lead extraction has recently been developed.[25]

Follow-up

Patients with an implantable cardiac device must be observed on a regular schedule, including office visits with or without remote monitoring of device function by transtelephonic or Internet-based systems. Follow-up of the patient with an ICD is increasingly done by Internet-based remote monitoring with less frequent in-office visits than previously required (**Fig. 38-34**). Patients may require interim assessment if there are concerns about the appropriateness of delivered therapy or other changes in the patient's medical status or drug regimen that could affect ICD therapy and require device reprogramming.

Aspects of ICD follow-up include history suggesting delivered therapy or tachyarrhythmic events; inspection of the pocket; device interrogation; assessment of battery status and charge time; retrieval and assessment of stored diagnostic data; radiographic assessment, when indicated, for troubleshooting; and DFT assessment when it is deemed necessary because of a change in medications or system revision.[26]

Internet-based remote monitoring is gaining widespread acceptance, resulting in revolutionary change in the follow-up of all implantable devices. Presently, remote monitoring permits essentially complete device interrogation but not reprogramming. Potential benefits include reduction of paperwork, direct communication with the electronic medical record, potential for daily or real-time monitoring of patients, and prevention of some trips to the emergency department or office. Diagnostic information in cardiac resynchronization therapy devices may allow early detection of and intervention for decompensation of heart failure, reducing hospitalizations.

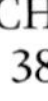

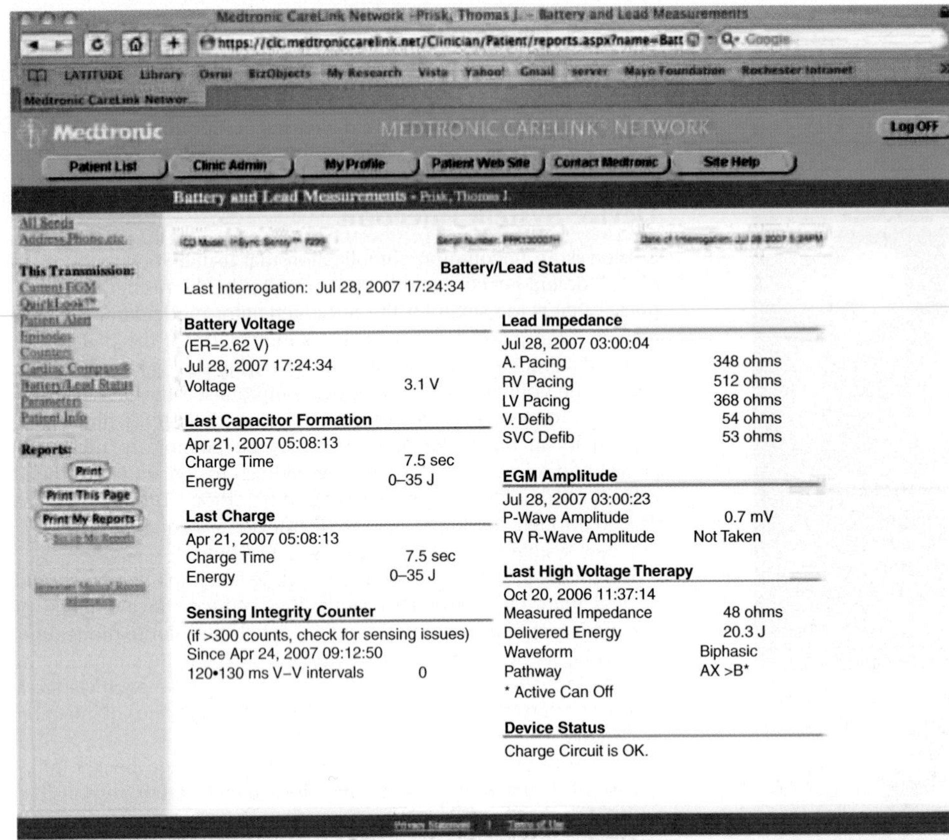

FIGURE 38-34 Remote access ICD report using the Medtronic CareLink Network showing battery voltage, capacitor information, and lead status (impedance and EGM information). The sensing integrity counter records V-V intervals that are too short to be physiologic, indicating electrical noise such as that due to lead fracture or loose set screw. In this patient, there is no lead fracture, and the counter reports zero short V-V intervals.

REFERENCES

Principles of Bioelectrical Stimulation

1. Swerdlow C, Russo A, Degroot P: The dilemma of ICD implant testing. Pacing Clin Electrophysiol 30:675, 2007.
2. Kroll M, Swerdlow C: Optimizing defibrillation waveforms for ICDs. J Interv Card Electrophysiol 18:247, 2007.
3. Swerdlow CD, Friedman PA: Advanced ICD troubleshooting: Part II. Pacing Clin Electrophysiol 29:70, 2006.

Hemodynamics

4. Sweeney MO, Hellkamp AS, Ellenbogen KA, et al: Adverse effect of ventricular pacing on heart failure and atrial fibrillation among patients with normal baseline QRS duration in a clinical trial of pacemaker therapy for sinus node dysfunction. Circulation 107:2932, 2003.
5. Wilkoff BL, Cook JR, Epstein AE, et al: Dual-chamber pacing or ventricular backup pacing in patients with an implantable defibrillator: The Dual Chamber and VVI Implantable Defibrillator (DAVID) Trial. JAMA 288:3115, 2002.
6. Sweeney MO, Ruetz LL, Belk P, et al: Bradycardia pacing-induced short-long-short sequences at the onset of ventricular tachyarrhythmias: A possible mechanism of proarrhythmia? J Am Coll Cardiol 50:614, 2007.
7. Kass DA, Chen CH, Curry C, et al: Improved left ventricular mechanics from acute VDD pacing in patients with dilated cardiomyopathy and ventricular conduction delay. Circulation 99:1567, 1999.

Pacemaker Modes and Timing Cycles

8. Leung SK, Lau CP: Developments in sensor-driven pacing. Cardiol Clin 18:113, 2000.

Electrical Therapy for Ventricular Tachyarrhythmias

9. Wathen MS, DeGroot PJ, Sweeney MO, et al: Prospective randomized multicenter trial of empirical antitachycardia pacing versus shocks for spontaneous rapid ventricular tachycardia in patients with implantable cardioverter-defibrillators: Pacing Fast Ventricular Tachycardia Reduces Shock Therapies (PainFREE Rx II) trial results. Circulation 110:2591, 2004.
10. Wathen MS, Sweeney MO, DeGroot PJ, et al: Shock reduction using antitachycardia pacing for spontaneous rapid ventricular tachycardia in patients with coronary artery disease. Circulation 104:796, 2001.
11. Daubert JP, Zareba W, Cannom DS, et al: Inappropriate implantable cardioverter-defibrillator shocks in MADIT II: Frequency, mechanisms, predictors, and survival impact. J Am Coll Cardiol 51:1357, 2008.
12. Poole JE, Johnson GW, Hellkamp AS, et al: Prognostic importance of defibrillator shocks in patients with heart failure. N Engl J Med 359:1009, 2008.
13. Sweeney MO, Sherfesee L, DeGroot PJ, et al: Differences in effects of electrical therapy for ventricular arrhythmias on mortality in implantable cardioverter-defibrillator patients. Heart Rhythm 7:353, 2010.

Indications

14. Epstein AE, DiMarco JP, Ellenbogen KA, et al: ACC/AHA/HRS 2008 guidelines for device-based therapy of cardiac rhythm abnormalities: A report of the ACC/AHA Task Force on Practice Guidelines. J Am Coll Cardiol 51:e1, 2008.
15. Zipes DP, Camm AJ, Borggrefe M, et al: ACC/AHA/ESC 2006 guidelines for management of patients with ventricular arrhythmias and the prevention of sudden cardiac death: A report of the ACC/AHA Task Force and the ESC Committee for Practice Guidelines. Circulation 114:e385, 2006.
16. Vardas PE, Auricchio A, Blanc JJ, et al: Guidelines for cardiac pacing and cardiac resynchronization therapy: The Task Force for Cardiac Pacing and Cardiac Resynchronization Therapy of the European Society of Cardiology. Eur Heart J 28:2256, 2007.

ICDs

17. Swerdlow CD, Friedman PA: Advanced ICD troubleshooting: Part I. Pacing Clin Electrophysiol 28:1322, 2005.
18. Gunderson B, Patel A, Bounds C: Automatic identification of implantable cardioverter-defibrillator lead problems using intracardiac electrograms. Comput Cardiol 29:121, 2002.
19. Glikson M, Swerdlow CD, Gurevitz OT, et al: Optimal combination of discriminators for differentiating ventricular from supraventricular tachycardia by dual-chamber defibrillators. J Cardiovasc Electrophysiol 16:732, 2005.
20. Sweeney M: Antitachycardia pacing for ventricular tachycardia using implantable cardioverter defibrillators. Pacing Clin Electrophysiol 27:1292, 2004.
21. Swerdlow CD, Shehata M, Chen PS: Using the upper limit of vulnerability to assess defibrillation efficacy at implantation of ICDs. Pacing Clin Electrophysiol 30:258, 2007.

Failure to Respond to Resynchronization Pacing

22. Koplan BA, Kaplan AJ, Weiner S, et al: Heart failure decompensation and all-cause mortality in relation to percent biventricular pacing in patients with heart failure: Is a goal of 100% biventricular pacing necessary? J Am Coll Cardiol 53:355, 2009.

Complications

23. Giudici MC, Paul DL, Bontu P, Barold SS: Pacemaker and implantable cardioverter defibrillator implantation without reversal of warfarin therapy. Pacing Clin Electrophysiol 27:358, 2004.
24. de Oliveira JC, Martinelli M, Nishioka SA, et al: Efficacy of antibiotic prophylaxis before the implantation of pacemakers and cardioverter-defibrillators: Results of a large, prospective, randomized, double-blinded, placebo-controlled trial. Circ Arrhythm Electrophysiol 2:29, 2009.
25. Wilkoff BL, Love CJ, Byrd CL, et al: Transvenous lead extraction: Heart Rhythm Society Expert Consensus on Facilities, Training, Indications, and Patient Management. Heart Rhythm 6:1085, 2009.
26. Heidbuchel H, Lioen P, Foulon S, et al: Potential role of remote monitoring for scheduled and unscheduled evaluations of patients with an implantable defibrillator. Europace 10:351, 2008.

GUIDELINES Charles D. Swerdlow, David L. Hayes, and Douglas P. Zipes

Cardiac Pacemakers and Cardioverter-Defibrillators

The American College of Cardiology/American Heart Association/Heart Rhythm Society (ACC/AHA/HRS) guidelines for the use of cardiac pacemakers, implantable cardioverter-defibrillators (ICDs), and cardiac resynchronization therapy (CRT) were most recently updated in 2008.[1] The ACC, AHA, and ESC, along with the HRS collaborated on guidelines for management of patients with ventricular arrhythmias and the prevention of sudden cardiac death in 2006.[2] Similar guidelines for cardiac pacing and CRT were published by the ESC in 2007.[3]

Like other ACC/AHA guidelines, these use the standard ACC/AHA classification system for indications:

Class I: conditions for which there is evidence and/or general agreement that the test is useful and effective

Class II: conditions for which there is conflicting evidence and/or a divergence of opinion about the usefulness or efficacy of performing the test

Class IIa: weight of evidence/opinion is in favor of usefulness or efficacy

Class IIb: usefulness or efficacy is less well established by evidence/opinion

Class III: conditions for which there is evidence and/or general agreement that the test is not useful or effective and in some cases may be harmful

Three levels are used to rate the evidence on which recommendations have been based. Level A recommendations are derived from data from multiple randomized clinical trials; level B recommendations are derived from a single randomized trial or nonrandomized studies; and level C recommendations are based on the consensus opinion of experts.

INDICATIONS FOR PERMANENT PACING (Tables 38G-1 to 38G-10)

Acquired AV Block For patients with complete or second-degree atrioventricular (AV) block, the ACC/AHA guidelines consider permanent pacing to be appropriate when the abnormality causes symptoms and is not precipitated by a drug that can be discontinued (**Table 38G-1**) or a condition that is likely to be reversible, such as acute inferior myocardial infarction with a narrow QRS. Examples of symptoms include fatigue, syncope or presyncope, seizures, congestive heart failure, and confusional states. For asymptomatic patients, pacing is indicated for patients at high risk for development of complications, such as those with periods of asystole of 3 seconds or longer or an escape rate less than 40 beats/min, or patients who have specific high-risk conditions.

The guidelines do not support pacing for patients with asymptomatic first-degree or type I second-degree AV block, and they do not support the use of pacing for patients with hypoxia and sleep apnea syndrome in the absence of symptoms.

Chronic Bifascicular and Trifascicular Block Syncope is common in these patients, but the risk of sudden death or progression to complete heart block varies in patient subsets. The guidelines for pacing in these settings (**Table 38G-2**) include alternating bundle branch block as a Class I indication because it indicates abnormal and unstable conduction in all three fascicles. The guidelines also support pacing in patients with markedly abnormal conduction infranodal at electrophysiologic studies, even if patients are asymptomatic (Class IIa). Pacing is not supported for patients without symptoms even if first-degree AV block is also present.

Acute Myocardial Infarction Symptoms do not play a role in appropriateness for pacing in patients with acute myocardial infarction because of the high risk for sudden death in some postinfarction patients with conduction system disturbances (**Table 38G-3**). The guidelines emphasize that the requirement for temporary pacing after acute myocardial

TABLE 38G-1 Indications for Pacing in AV Block

Class I

1. Third-degree or advanced second-degree AV block at any anatomic level associated with any one of the following conditions:
   a. Symptoms (including heart failure) attributable to AV block *(Level of Evidence: C)*
   b. Arrhythmias and other medical conditions that require drugs that result in symptomatic bradycardia *(Level of Evidence: C)*
   c. Documented periods of asystole >3.0 seconds, any escape rate <40 beats/min, or any escape rhythm below the AV junction (e.g., a wide QRS morphology) in awake, asymptomatic patients in sinus rhythm) *(Level of Evidence: C)*
   d. A documented period of asystole >5 seconds in awake, asymptomatic patients in atrial fibrillation *(Level of Evidence: C)*
   e. After catheter ablation of the AV junction *(Level of Evidence: C)*
   f. Postoperative AV block that is not expected to resolve after cardiac surgery *(Level of Evidence: C)*
   g. Neuromuscular diseases, such as myotonic muscular dystrophy, Kearns–Sayre syndrome, Erb (limb-girdle) dystrophy, and peroneal muscular atrophy, with or without symptoms of bradycardia *(Level of Evidence: B)*
2. Asymptomatic third-degree AV block at any anatomic site with an average awake ventricular rate >40 beats/min in patients with cardiomegaly or left ventricular dysfunction
3. Second-degree or third-degree AV block during exercise in the absence of myocardial ischemia *(Level of Evidence: C)*
4. Symptomatic second-degree AV block regardless of type or site of block *(Level of Evidence: B)*

Class IIa

1. Advanced second-degree or third-degree AV block at any anatomic site with an average ventricular rate >40 beats/min in the absence of cardiomegaly *(Level of Evidence: C)*
2. Asymptomatic second-degree AV block at intra- or infra-His levels found at electrophysiologic study *(Level of Evidence: B)*
3. First-degree or second-degree AV block with symptoms similar to those of pacemaker syndrome *(Level of Evidence: B)*
4. Asymptomatic type II second-degree AV block with a narrow QRS. When type II second-degree AV block occurs with a wide QRS, including isolated right bundle branch block, pacing becomes a Class I recommendation. *(Level of Evidence: B)*

Class IIb

1. AV block due to drug use or toxicity when the block is expected to recur even after withdrawal of the drug *(Level of Evidence: B)*
2. Neuromuscular diseases, such as myotonic muscular dystrophy, Kearns–Sayre syndrome, Erb (limb-girdle) dystrophy, and peroneal muscular atrophy with any degree of AV block (including first-degree AV block), with or without symptoms of bradycardia *(Level of Evidence: B)*

Class III

1. Asymptomatic first-degree AV block *(Level of Evidence B)*
2. Asymptomatic type I second-degree AV block at a site above the His (i.e., the AV node) level or not known to be intra- or infra-Hisian by electrophysiologic study *(Level of Evidence: B)*
3. AV block expected to resolve and unlikely to recur (e.g., drug toxicity, Lyme disease, nocturnally in sleep apnea, early postoperative status, transient increases in vagal tone) *(Level of Evidence: B)*

TABLE 38G-2 Indications for Pacing in Chronic Bifascicular and Trifascicular Block

Class I

1. Intermittent third-degree or advanced second-degree AV block *(Level of Evidence: B)*
2. Type II second-degree AV block *(Level of Evidence: B)*
3. Alternating bundle branch block *(Level of Evidence: C)*

Class IIa

1. Syncope not demonstrated to be due to AV block when other likely causes, specifically ventricular tachycardia, have been excluded *(Level of Evidence: B)*
2. Incidental finding at electrophysiologic study of markedly prolonged HV interval (≥100 msec) in asymptomatic patients *(Level of Evidence: B)*
3. Incidental finding at electrophysiologic study of pacing-induced infra-His block that is not physiologic *(Level of Evidence: B)*

Class IIb

1. Neuromuscular diseases, such as myotonic muscular dystrophy, Kearns–Sayre syndrome, Erb (limb-girdle) dystrophy, and peroneal muscular atrophy with any degree of fascicular block, with or without symptoms of bradycardia *(Level of Evidence: C)*

Class III

1. Fascicular block without AV block or symptoms *(Level of Evidence: B)*
2. Fascicular block with first-degree AV block without symptoms *(Level of Evidence: B)*

TABLE 38G-3 Indications for Permanent Pacing After Acute Myocardial Infarction

Class I

1. Third-degree AV block within or below the His-Purkinje system after ST-segment elevation myocardial infarction or persistent second-degree AV block in the His-Purkinje system with alternating bundle branch block *(Level of Evidence: B)*
2. Transient second- or third-degree infranodal AV block and associated bundle branch block. If the site of block is uncertain, an electrophysiologic study may be necessary. *(Level of Evidence: B)*
3. Persistent and symptomatic second- or third-degree AV block *(Level of Evidence: C)*

Class IIb

1. Persistent second- or third-degree transient AV block at the AV node level, with or without symptoms *(Level of Evidence: B)*

Class III

1. Transient AV block without intraventricular conduction defects *(Level of Evidence: B)*
2. Transient AV block with isolated left anterior fascicular block *(Level of Evidence: B)*
3. Acquired left anterior fascicular block without AV block *(Level of Evidence: B)*
4. Asymptomatic first-degree AV block with bundle branch or fascicular block *(Level of Evidence: B)*

TABLE 38G-4 Indications for Pacing in Sinus Node Dysfunction

Class I

1. Symptomatic bradycardia or frequent symptomatic sinus pauses *(Level of Evidence: C)*
2. Symptomatic chronotropic incompetence (Level of Evidence: C)
3. Symptomatic bradycardia that results from required drug therapy (Level of Evidence: C)

Class IIa

1. Sinus node dysfunction occurring spontaneously or as a result of necessary drug therapy, with heart rate <40 beats/min, when a clear association between significant symptoms consistent with bradycardia and the actual presence of bradycardia has not been documented *(Level of Evidence: C)*
2. Syncope of unknown etiology when sinus node dysfunction is provoked or discovered during electrophysiologic testing that is thought to be clinically significant *(Level of Evidence: C)*

Class IIb

1. In minimally symptomatic patients, chronic heart rate <40 beats/min while awake *(Level of Evidence: C)*

Class III

1. Sinus node dysfunction in asymptomatic patients *(Level of Evidence: C)*
2. Sinus node dysfunction in patients with symptoms that are clearly documented in the absence of bradycardia *(Level of Evidence: C)*
3. Sinus node dysfunction with symptomatic bradycardia due to nonessential drug therapy *(Level of Evidence: C)*

TABLE 38G-5 Indications for Pacemakers to Terminate Tachycardia

Class IIa

1. Symptomatic recurrent supraventricular tachycardia that is reproducibly terminated by pacing in the unlikely event that catheter ablation and/or drugs fail to control the arrhythmia or produce intolerable side effects *(Level of Evidence: C)*

Class III

1. The presence of accessory pathways with the capacity for rapid anterograde conduction *(Level of Evidence: C)*

infarction does not automatically indicate a need for permanent pacing. However, permanent pacemakers are supported in patients with transient (presumed) infranodal AV block and associated bundle branch block, one of the rare times that transient AV block is judged an indication for permanent pacing. The usefulness of permanent pacemakers for patients with advanced AV block at the AV node level is less clear (Class IIb).

Sinus Node Dysfunction As for patients with acquired AV block, pacing is indicated for patients with symptoms caused by bradycardia that is not the result of a drug that can be discontinued (**Table 38G-4**). Pacing is discouraged in asymptomatic patients, even when resting heart rates are lower than 40 beats/min, and in symptomatic patients when symptoms cannot be proved to be caused by bradycardia. A Class IIa recommendation supports pacing in patients with syncope of unexplained origin when major abnormalities of sinus node function are demonstrated at electrophysiologic testing.

Prevention and Termination of Tachyarrhythmias In some patients with long-QT syndrome, continuous pacing can prevent recurrent tachyarrhythmias. In addition, paroxysmal reentrant tachyarrhythmias can be terminated in some patients through programmed stimulation and short bursts of rapid pacing. However, the guidelines do not provide support for the routine use of antitachycardia pacemakers without extensive testing before implantation (**Table 38G-5**), but they continue to consider bradycardia pacing appropriate (Class I indication) for patients with sustained pause-dependent ventricular tachycardia (unrelated to a drug that can be discontinued), with or without prolonged QT, if the efficacy of temporary pacing has been demonstrated (**Table 38G-6**). However, some patients have or are at risk for other types of ventricular tachycardia. In these patients, an ICD may be more appropriate.

Carotid Sinus Syndrome and Neurocardiogenic Syncope The only Class I indication for permanent pacing is recurrent syncope caused by

TABLE 38G-6 Indications for Pacemakers to Prevent Tachycardia

Class I

1. Pause-dependent sustained ventricular tachycardia with or without prolonged QT *(Level of Evidence: C)*

Class IIa

1. Pacing is reasonable for patients with congenital long-QT syndrome considered to be high risk *(Level of Evidence: C)*

Class IIb

1. Prevention of symptomatic, drug-refractory recurrent atrial fibrillation in patients with coexisting sinus node dysfunction *(Level of Evidence: B)*

Class III

1. Frequent or complex ventricular ectopic activity without sustained ventricular tachycardia in patients without long-QT syndrome *(Level of Evidence: C)*
2. Torsades de pointes ventricular tachycardia due to reversible causes *(Level of Evidence: A)*

TABLE 38G-7 Indications for Pacing in Neurally Mediated Reflex Syncope

Class I

1. Recurrent syncope caused by carotid sinus hypersensitivity, defined as minimal carotid sinus pressure inducing ventricular asystole of >3 seconds in patients not receiving medications that depress the sinus node or AV conduction *(Level of Evidence: C)*

Class IIa

1. Syncope in the absence of definite provocative event with a pause of ≥3 seconds with carotid massage *(Level of Evidence: C)*

Class IIb

1. Recurrent symptomatic neurocardiogenic syncope with a cardioinhibitory response during tilt-table testing *(Level of Evidence: B)*

Class III

1. A cardioinhibitory response during carotid sinus stimulation without symptoms or with vague symptoms *(Level of Evidence: C)*
2. Situational vasovagal syncope in which avoidance behavior is effective *(Level of Evidence: C)*

carotid sinus stimulation in the absence of any drug that depresses the sinus node or AV conduction (**Table 38G-7**). Pacing is discouraged in patients without symptoms or who have syncope without bradycardia.

Hypertrophic Cardiomyopathy The guidelines minimize indications for pacing in patients with hypertrophic cardiomyopathy unless they have associated sinus node dysfunction or AV block that would fulfill related indications for pacing (**Table 38G-8**). A Class IIb indication permits pacing in medically refractory symptomatic patients with hypertrophic cardiomyopathy and significant resting or provoked left ventricular (LV) outflow tract gradient. Pacing should really only be considered if the patient is truly refractory to pharmacologic therapy.

Cardiac Transplantation **Table 38G-9** details these indications.

Cardiac Resynchronization Therapy The evidence base for CRT has expanded substantially and is reflected in significant changes in the 2008 guidelines (**Table 38G-10**). Based on an analysis of the MADIT-CRT patients with LBBB, CMS has altered labeling for certain CRT-D devices. Under the recent labeling, CRT-D would be indicated for patients with LBBB with QRS ≥ 130 ms, EF ≤ 30%, and mild (NYHA Class II) ischemic or nonischemic heart failure or asymptomatic (NYHA Class I) ischemic heart failure (see Chap. 33).

Selection of Pacemakers

The guidelines provide recommendations (**Table 38G-11**) and decision trees to help physicians match patients' needs to the technology implanted

TABLE 38G-8 Pacing in Hypertrophic Cardiomyopathy

Class I

1. Indicated in the presence of sinus node dysfunction or AV block as previously described *(Level of Evidence: C)*

Class IIb

1. Medically refractory symptomatic patients and significant LV outflow tract obstruction at rest or provocable *(Level of Evidence: A)*

Class III

1. Asymptomatic patients or those whose symptoms are medically controlled *(Level of Evidence: C)*
2. Symptomatic patients in the absence of LV outflow tract obstruction *(Level of Evidence: C)*

TABLE 38G-9 Indications for Pacing After Cardiac Transplantation

Class I

1. Persistent symptomatic or inappropriate bradycardia that is not expected to resolve *(Level of Evidence: C)*

Class IIb

1. Relative bradycardia is recurrent or prolonged, limiting rehabilitation or hospital discharge *(Level of Evidence: C)*
2. Syncope after transplantation even in the absence of a documented bradyarrhythmia *(Level of Evidence: C)*

TABLE 38G-10 Indications for Cardiac Resynchronization Therapy

Class I

1. For patients with LVEF ≤35%, a QRS duration ≥0.12 second, and sinus rhythm, CRT with or without an ICD is indicated for the treatment of NYHA functional Class III or ambulatory Class IV heart failure symptoms with optimal recommended medical therapy. *(Level of Evidence: A)*

Class IIa

1. For patients with LVEF ≤35%, a QRS duration ≥0.12 second, and atrial fibrillation, CRT with or without an ICD is reasonable for the treatment of NYHA functional Class III or ambulatory Class IV heart failure symptoms on optimal recommended medical therapy. *(Level of Evidence: B)*
2. For patients with LVEF ≤35% with NYHA functional Class III or ambulatory Class IV symptoms who are receiving optimal recommended medical therapy and who have frequent dependence on ventricular pacing, CRT is reasonable. *(Level of Evidence: C)*

Class IIb

1. For patients with LVEF ≤35% with NYHA functional Class I or II symptoms who are receiving optimal recommended medical therapy and who are undergoing implantation of a permanent pacemaker and/or ICD with anticipated frequent ventricular pacing, CRT may be considered. *(Level of Evidence: C)*

Class III

1. CRT is not indicated for asymptomatic patients with reduced LVEF in the absence of other indications for pacing. *(Level of Evidence: B)*
2. CRT is not indicated for patients whose functional status and life expectancy are limited predominantly by chronic noncardiac conditions. *(Level of Evidence: C)*

TABLE 38G-11 ACC/AHA Guidelines for Choice of Pacemaker

TYPE OF PACEMAKER	SINUS NODE DYSFUNCTION	AV BLOCK	NEURALLY MEDIATED SYNCOPE OR CAROTID SINUS HYPERSENSITIVITY
Single-chamber atrial	No suspected abnormality of AV conduction and not at increased risk for future AV block Maintenance of AV synchrony during pacing desired Rate response available if desired	Not appropriate	Not appropriate
Single-chamber ventricular	Maintenance of AV synchrony during pacing not necessary Rate response available if desired	Chronic atrial fibrillation or other atrial tachyarrhythmia or maintenance of AV synchrony during pacing not necessary Rate response available if desired	Chronic atrial fibrillation or other atrial tachyarrhythmia Rate response available if desired
Dual-chamber	AV synchrony during pacing desired Suspected abnormality of AV conduction or increased risk for future AV block Rate response available if desired	Rate response available if desired AV synchrony during pacing desired Atrial pacing desired	Sinus mechanism present Rate response available if desired
Single-lead, atrial-sensing ventricular	Not appropriate	Normal sinus node function and no need for atrial pacing Desire to limit number of pacemaker leads	Not appropriate

TABLE 38G-12 Indications for Permanent Pacemaker in Children, Adolescents, and Patients with Congenital Heart Disease

Class I

1. Advanced second- or third-degree AV block associated with symptomatic bradycardia, ventricular dysfunction, or low cardiac output *(Level of Evidence: C)*
2. Sinus node dysfunction with correlation of symptoms during age-inappropriate bradycardia. The definition of bradycardia varies with the patient's age and expected heart rate. *(Level of Evidence: B)*
3. Postoperative advanced second- or third-degree AV block that is not expected to resolve or that persists at least 7 days after cardiac surgery *(Level of Evidence: B)*
4. Congenital third-degree AV block with a wide QRS escape rhythm, complex ventricular ectopy, or ventricular dysfunction *(Level of Evidence: B)*
5. Congenital third-degree AV block in the infant with a ventricular rate <55 beats/min or with congenital heart disease and a ventricular rate <70 beats/min *(Level of Evidence: C)*

Class IIa

1. Congenital heart disease and sinus bradycardia for the prevention of recurrent episodes of intra-atrial reentrant tachycardia; sinus node dysfunction may be intrinsic or secondary to antiarrhythmic treatment *(Level of Evidence: C)*
2. Congenital third-degree AV block beyond the first year of life with an average heart rate <50 beats/min and abrupt pauses in ventricular rate that are 2 or 3 times the basic cycle length or associated with symptoms due to chronotropic incompetence *(Level of Evidence: B)*
3. Sinus bradycardia with complex congenital heart disease with a resting heart rate <40 beats/min or pauses in ventricular rate >3 seconds *(Level of Evidence: C)*
4. Congenital heart disease and impaired hemodynamics due to sinus bradycardia or loss of AV synchrony *(Level of Evidence: C)*
5. Unexplained syncope in the patient with prior congenital heart surgery complicated by transient complete heart block with residual fascicular block after a careful evaluation to exclude other causes of syncope *(Level of Evidence: B)*

Class IIb

1. Transient postoperative third-degree AV block that reverts to sinus rhythm with residual bifascicular block *(Level of Evidence: C)*
2. Congenital third-degree AV block in asymptomatic children or adolescents with an acceptable rate, a narrow QRS complex, and normal ventricular function *(Level of Evidence: B)*
3. Asymptomatic sinus bradycardia after biventricular repair of congenital heart disease with a resting heart rate <40 beats/min or pauses in ventricular rate >3 seconds *(Level of Evidence: C)*

Class III

1. Transient postoperative AV block with return of normal AV conduction in the otherwise asymptomatic patient *(Level of Evidence: B)*
2. Asymptomatic bifascicular block with or without first-degree AV block after surgery for congenital heart disease in the absence of prior transient complete AV block *(Level of Evidence: C)*
3. Asymptomatic type I second-degree AV block *(Level of Evidence: C)*
4. Asymptomatic sinus bradycardia with the longest relative risk interval <3 seconds and a minimum heart rate >40 beats/min *(Level of Evidence: C)*

and to anticipate future needs of the patient. Elderly patients should receive devices according to the same indications as for younger patients, according to the guidelines (**Table 38G-12**).

IMPLANTABLE CARDIOVERTER-DEFIBRILLATOR THERAPY

The 2008 guidelines group all indications together, that is, they no longer separate primary and secondary indications (**Table 38G-13**). The strongest evidence for "secondary prevention" use of ICDs exists among patients with LV dysfunction who have been resuscitated from ventricular fibrillation or hemodynamically unstable ventricular tachycardia or ventricular tachycardia with syncope and who remain at risk for future cardiac arrests. There is also strong evidence supporting "primary prevention" use of ICDs for patients who are at least 40 days post–myocardial infarction and have depressed LV function with ejection fractions less than 30% to 40% and patients with nonischemic dilated cardiomyopathy who have an ejection fraction less than 30% to 35%.

TABLE 38G-13 Indications for ICD Therapy

Class I

1. Survivors of cardiac arrest due to ventricular fibrillation (VF) or hemodynamically unstable sustained ventricular tachycardia (VT) after evaluation to define the cause of the event and to exclude any completely reversible causes *(Level of Evidence: A)*
2. Structural heart disease and spontaneous sustained VT, whether hemodynamically stable or unstable *(Level of Evidence: B)*
3. Syncope of undetermined origin with clinically relevant, hemodynamically significant sustained VT or VF induced at electrophysiologic study *(Level of Evidence: B)*
4. LVEF <35% due to prior myocardial infarction in patients who are at least 40 days post–myocardial infarction and are in NYHA functional Class II or III *(Level of Evidence: A)*
5. Nonischemic dilated cardiomyopathy in patients who have an LVEF ≤35% and who are in NYHA functional Class II or III *(Level of Evidence: B)*
6. LV dysfunction due to prior myocardial infarction in patients who are at least 40 days post–myocardial infarction, have an LVEF <30%, and are in NYHA functional Class I *(Level of Evidence: A)*
7. Nonsustained VT due to prior myocardial infarction, LVEF <40%, and inducible VF or sustained VT at electrophysiologic study *(Level of Evidence: B)*

Class IIa

1. Unexplained syncope, significant LV dysfunction, and nonischemic dilated cardiomyopathy *(Level of Evidence: C)*
2. Sustained VT and normal or near-normal ventricular function *(Level of Evidence: C)*
3. Hypertrophic cardiomyopathy in patients who have 1 or more major risk factors for sudden cardiac death *(Level of Evidence: C)*
4. Arrhythmogenic right ventricular dysplasia/cardiomyopathy in patients who have 1 or more risk factors for sudden cardiac death *(Level of Evidence: C)*
5. Long-QT syndrome in patients who are experiencing syncope and/or VT while receiving beta blockers *(Level of Evidence: B)*
6. Nonhospitalized patients awaiting transplantation *(Level of Evidence: C)*
7. Brugada syndrome in patients who have had syncope *(Level of Evidence: C)*
8. Brugada syndrome in patients who have documented VT that has not resulted in cardiac arrest *(Level of Evidence: C)*
9. Catecholaminergic polymorphic VT in patients who have syncope and/or documented sustained VT while receiving beta blockers *(Level of Evidence: C)*
10. Cardiac sarcoidosis, giant cell myocarditis, or Chagas disease *(Level of Evidence: C)*

Class IIb

1. Nonischemic heart disease in patients who have an LVEF of ≤35% and who are in NYHA functional Class I *(Level of Evidence: C)*
2. Long-QT syndrome and risk factors for sudden cardiac death *(Level of Evidence: B)*
3. Syncope and advanced structural heart disease in patients in whom thorough invasive and noninvasive investigations have failed to define a cause *(Level of Evidence: C)*
4. Familial cardiomyopathy associated with sudden death *(Level of Evidence: C)*
5. LV noncompaction *(Level of Evidence: C)*

Class III

1. Patients who do not have a reasonable expectation of survival with an acceptable functional status for at least 1 year, even if they meet ICD implantation criteria specified in the Class I, IIa, and IIb recommendations *(Level of Evidence: C)*
2. Incessant VT or VF *(Level of Evidence: C)*
3. Significant psychiatric illnesses that may be aggravated by device implantation or that may preclude systematic follow-up *(Level of Evidence: C)*
4. Drug-refractory congestive heart failure in patients who are not candidates for cardiac transplantation or CRT-D *(Level of Evidence: C)*
5. Syncope of undetermined cause in a patient without inducible ventricular tachyarrhythmias and without structural heart disease *(Level of Evidence: C)*
6. When VF or VT is amenable to surgical or catheter ablation (e.g., atrial arrhythmias associated with the Wolff-Parkinson-White syndrome, right or left ventricular outflow tract VT, idiopathic VT, or fascicular VT in the absence of structural heart disease) *(Level of Evidence: C)*
7. Ventricular tachyarrhythmias due to a completely reversible disorder in the absence of structural heart disease (e.g., electrolyte imbalance, drugs, or trauma) *(Level of Evidence: B)*

However, it is important to recognize the conceptual difference between Class I indications for pacing ICDs and those for primary prevention ICDs. Many Class I indications for pacing relieve serious symptoms that occur frequently in day-to-day life. In contrast, Class I indications for primary prevention ICDs address the risk of infrequent but catastrophic events, and the decision to implant an ICD should include consideration of the presence of severe comorbidities, which could limit benefit from the ICD. In contrast, pacing is almost never withheld from patients with persistent symptomatic bradycardia because of comorbidities.

PERSONAL AND PUBLIC SAFETY ISSUES

The AHA and the North American Society of Pacing and Electrophysiology (NASPE) published a medical-scientific statement in 1996 regarding personal and public safety issues that arise in the care of patients with arrhythmias.[4] This publication summarized guidelines from other organizations, such as the U.S. Federal Aviation Administration, and the limited data available to estimate the risk of injury to the patient and others related to arrhythmias; it provided recommendations about acceptable activities for patients with arrhythmias that may impair consciousness.

These guidelines divide patients into three classes (**Table 38G-14**):

Class A patients should have no restrictions.

Class B patients are restricted for a defined time if arrhythmia does not recur, usually after a therapeutic intervention. This time period is usually expressed as a subscript indicating the number of months of restriction (e.g., B_3).

Class C patients should have permanent restriction of potentially hazardous activities.

Restrictions were divided into two categories—personal or noncommercial driving and commercial driving or flying, which were generally the same. Recommended restriction for commercial drivers may also be relevant to people in other potentially hazardous occupations, such as operators of heavy equipment.

The restrictions imposed by the guidelines vary according to the severity of the arrhythmia and accompanying symptoms (see Table 38G-14). The duration of the restriction depends on the severity of symptoms and the expected likelihood that treatment will prevent arrhythmia recurrence or symptoms.

It should be noted that these guidelines were published in 1996, before established guidelines for primary prevention.

CH 38

TABLE 38G-14 AHA/NASPE Guidelines for Safe Resumption of Activities (Classes of Restriction)

ARRHYTHMIA	PRIVATE	COMMERCIAL
Nonsustained ventricular tachycardia	B_3 if symptoms of impaired consciousness with arrhythmia before treatment A if no impairment of consciousness with arrhythmia	B_6 if symptoms of impaired consciousness with arrhythmia before treatment A if no impairment of consciousness with arrhythmia
Sustained ventricular tachycardia	B_6 B_3 if idiopathic ventricular tachycardia (normal coronary arteries, normal ventricular function) and no impairment of consciousness	C B_6 if idiopathic ventricular tachycardia (normal coronary arteries, normal ventricular function) and no impairment of consciousness
Ventricular fibrillation	B_6	C
Asymptomatic or minimally symptomatic SVT (including WPW syndrome)	A	A
Symptomatic (evidence of hemodynamic compromise) SVT	B until after initiation of therapy that eliminates symptoms	B until after initiation of therapy that eliminates symptoms
Atrial fibrillation treated by catheter ablation of AV node	B	B
SVT with uncontrolled symptoms	C	C
Bradycardia without a pacemaker—no symptoms	A	A
Bradycardia without a pacemaker—syncope or near-syncope	C	C
Bradycardia with a pacemaker—not pacemaker dependent*	A	A
Bradycardia with a pacemaker—pacemaker dependent*	B—1 wk	B—4 wk
Vasovagal syncope, mild	A	B_1
Vasovagal syncope, severe		
Treated vasovagal syncope	B_3	B_6
Untreated vasovagal syncope	C	C
Carotid sinus syncope, mild	A	A
Carotid sinus syncope, severe, treated with control	B_1	B_1
Carotid sinus syncope, severe, treated with uncertain control	B_3	B_6
Untreated	C	C

*Patients who are pacemaker dependent are defined as those who have lost consciousness in the past because of bradyarrhythmias. This group may also include patients immediately after atrioventricular junction ablation or any other patient in whom sudden pacemaker failure would be likely to result in alteration of consciousness.
Class A = no restriction. Class B = restricted for months (in subscript). Class C = total restriction. SVT = supraventricular tachycardia; WPW = Wolff-Parkinson-White.
From Epstein AE, Miles WM, Benditt DG, et al: Personal and public safety issues related to arrhythmias that may affect consciousness: Implications for regulation and physician recommendations. Circulation 94:1147, 1996.

REFERENCES

1. Epstein AE, DiMarco JP, Ellenbogen KA, et al: ACC/AHA/HRS 2008 guidelines for device-based therapy of cardiac rhythm abnormalities: A report of the ACC/AHA Task Force on Practice Guidelines. Circulation 117:e350, 2008.
2. Zipes DP, Camm AJ, Borggrefe M, et al: ACC/AHA/ESC 2006 guidelines for management of patients with ventricular arrhythmias and the prevention of sudden cardiac death: A report of the ACC/AHA Task Force and the ESC Committee for Practice Guidelines. Circulation 114:e385, 2006.
3. Vardas PE, Auricchio A, Blanc JJ, et al: Guidelines for cardiac pacing and cardiac resynchronization therapy: The task force for cardiac pacing and cardiac resynchronization therapy of the european society of cardiology. Eur Heart J 28:2256, 2007.
4. Epstein AE, Miles WM, Benditt DG, et al: Personal and public safety issues related to arrhythmias that may affect consciousness: Implications for regulation and physician recommendations. Circulation 94:1147, 1996.

CHAPTER 39 Specific Arrhythmias: Diagnosis and Treatment

Jeffrey Olgin and Douglas P. Zipes

Normal Sinus Rhythm

Normal sinus rhythm is arbitrarily limited to impulse formation beginning in the sinus node at rates between 60 and 100 beats/min. Infants and children generally have faster heart rates than adults do, both at rest and during exercise. The P wave is upright in electrocardiographic leads I, II, and aVF and negativf9005e in lead aVR, with a vector in the frontal plane between 0 and +90 degrees. In the horizontal plane, the P vector is directed anteriorly and slightly leftward and can therefore be negative in leads V_1 and V_2 but positive in V_3 to V_6. The PR interval exceeds 120 milliseconds and can vary slightly with the rate. If the pacemaker site (site of impulse origin) shifts, a change in morphology of the P wave can occur. The rate of sinus rhythm varies significantly and depends on many factors, including age, gender, and physical activity.

The sinus nodal discharge rate responds readily to autonomic stimuli and depends on the effect of the two opposing autonomic influences—sympathetics and parasympathetics. Steady vagal (parasympathetic) stimulation decreases the spontaneous sinus nodal discharge rate and predominates over steady sympathetic stimulation, which increases the spontaneous sinus nodal discharge rate. A given vagal stimulus produces a greater absolute reduction in heart rate when the basal heart rate has been increased by sympathetic stimulation, a phenomenon known as accentuated antagonism.

Rates below 50 beats/min are considered to be bradycardia, and rates above 100 beats/min are considered to be tachycardia. As described in Chap. 35, the normal sequence of electrical activation of the heart is from the sinus node through the atria to the atrioventricular (AV) node and His-Purkinje system and to the ventricular myocardium. Arrhythmias resulting in bradycardia or tachycardia can be thought of as specific disorders of each of these components. Specific tachyarrhythmias and bradyarrhythmias presented as disorders of this electrophysiologic hierarchy and their characteristics are summarized in **Table 39-1**.

Tachyarrhythmias

Tachyarrhythmias are broadly characterized as supraventricular tachycardia (SVT), defined as a tachycardia in which the driving circuit or focus originates, at least in part, in tissue above the level of the ventricle (i.e., sinus node, atria, AV node, or His bundle), and ventricular tachycardia (VT), defined as a tachycardia in which the driving circuit or focus solely originates in ventricular tissue or Purkinje fibers. Because of differences in prognosis and management, the distinction between SVT and VT is critical early in the acute management of a tachyarrhythmia.[1] In general (with the exception of idiopathic VT, described later), VT often carries a much graver prognosis, usually implies the presence of significant heart disease, results in more profound hemodynamic compromise, and therefore requires immediate attention and measures to revert to sinus rhythm. On the other hand, SVT is usually not lethal and often does not result in hemodynamic collapse; therefore, more conservative measures can be applied initially to convert to sinus rhythm.[2-4]

The distinction between SVT and VT can usually be made on the basis of the electrocardiogram (ECG) obtained during tachycardia (see Chap. 36). It is important to obtain a 12-lead ECG during tachycardia if possible and to obtain 12-lead (or at least multilead) rhythm strips during any intervention aimed at termination of the tachycardia because this information is the best way to identify the specific arrhythmia (discussed later) at the bedside. In general, if the QRS is narrow (duration less than 120 milliseconds, often referred to as narrow-complex tachycardias) during the tachycardia, the ventricle is being activated via the normal His-Purkinje system, and thus the origin of the tachycardia is supraventricular (**Fig. 39-1**). In contrast, a wide QRS (duration exceeding 120 milliseconds) during tachycardia suggests VT; however, there are common scenarios in which SVT can produce a wide QRS complex. Therefore, a more descriptive term, *wide-complex tachycardia,* is often used when the precise arrhythmia mechanism cannot be determined. For example, SVT with a concurrent bundle branch block or intraventricular conduction defect can produce wide-complex tachycardias despite a supraventricular origin. In addition, preexcited tachycardias (tachycardias in which the ventricle is activated in whole or in part over an accessory pathway) produce wide QRS complexes, despite their being supraventricular in origin. Therefore, although a narrow-complex tachycardia almost always makes the diagnosis of SVT, a wide-complex tachycardia can be supraventricular or ventricular. Fusion or capture beats and AV dissociation are diagnostic of VT (discussed later, Ventricular Tachycardia, Electrocardiographic Recognition) but are often not present or are difficult to detect. Criteria have been developed on the basis of the 12-lead ECG (**Table 39-2**) that can be helpful in determining whether a wide-complex tachycardia is more likely to be SVT or VT.[5]

Sinus Tachycardia

ELECTROCARDIOGRAPHIC RECOGNITION. Tachycardia (**Fig. 39-2**) in an adult is defined as a rate of 100 beats/min. During sinus tachycardia, the sinus node exhibits a discharge frequency between 100 and 180 beats/min, but it can be higher with extreme exertion and in young individuals. The maximum heart rate achieved during strenuous physical activity decreases with age from about 200 beats/min at 20 years to less than 140 beats/min at 80 years. Sinus tachycardia generally has a gradual onset and termination. The P-P interval can vary slightly from cycle to cycle, especially at slower rates. P waves

TABLE 39-1 Arrhythmia Characteristics*

	P WAVES			QRS COMPLEXES				PHYSICAL EXAMINATION			
TYPE OF ARRHYTHMIA	RATE (BEATS/MIN)	RHYTHM	CONTOUR	RATE (BEATS/MIN)	RHYTHM	CONTOUR	VENTRICULAR RESPONSE TO CAROTID SINUS MASSAGE	INTENSITY OF S_1	SPLITTING OF S_2	A WAVES	TREATMENT
Sinus rhythm	60-100	Regular[†]	Normal	60-100	Regular	Normal	Gradual slowing and return to former rate	Constant	Normal	Normal	None
Sinus bradycardia	<60	Regular	Normal	<60	Regular	Normal	Gradual slowing and return to former rate	Constant	Normal	Normal	None, unless symptomatic; atropine
Sinus tachycardia	100-180	Regular	May be peaked	100-180	Regular	Normal	Gradual slowing[‡] and return to former rate	Constant	Normal	Normal	None, unless symptomatic; treat underlying disease
AV nodal reentry	150-250	Very regular except at onset and termination	Retrograde; difficult to see; lost in QRS complex	150-250	Very regular except at onset and termination	Normal	Abrupt slowing caused by termination of tachycardia, or no effect	Constant	Normal	Constant cannon *a* waves	Vagal stimulation, adenosine, verapamil, digitalis, propranolol, DC shock, pacing
Atrial flutter	250-350	Regular	Sawtooth	75-175	Generally regular in absence of drugs or disease	Normal	Abrupt slowing and return to former rate; flutter remains	Constant; variable if AV block changing	Normal	Flutter waves	DC shock, digitalis, quinidine, propranolol, verapamil, adenosine
Atrial fibrillation	400-600	Grossly irregular	Baseline undulation, no P waves	100-160	Grossly irregular	Normal	Slowing; gross irregularity remains	Variable	Normal	No *a* waves	Digitalis, quinidine, DC shock, verapamil, adenosine
Atrial tachycardia with block	150-250	Regular; may be irregular	Abnormal	75-200	Generally regular in absence of drugs or disease	Normal	Abrupt slowing and return to normal rate; tachycardia remains	Constant; variable if AV block changing	Normal	More *a* waves than *c-v* waves	Stop digitalis if toxic; digitalis if not toxic; possibly verapamil
AV junctional rhythm	40-100[§]	Regular	Normal	40-60	Fairly regular	Normal	None; may be slight slowing	Variable[¶]	Normal	Intermittent cannon waves	None, unless symptomatic; atropine
Reciprocating tachycardias using an accessory (WPW) pathway	150-250	Very regular except at onset and termination	Retrograde; difficult to see; monitor the QRS complex	150-250	Very regular except at onset and termination	Normal	Abrupt slowing caused by termination of tachycardia, or no effect	Constant but decreased	Normal	Constant cannon waves	See AV nodal reentry earlier
Nonparoxysmal AV junctional tachycardia	60-100[¶]	Regular	Normal	70-130	Fairly regular	Normal	None; may be slight slowing	Variable[¶]	Normal	Intermittent cannon waves[¶]	None, unless symptomatic; stop digitalis if toxic

Ventricular tachycardia	60-100¶	Regular	Normal	110-250	Fairly regular; may be irregular	Abnormal, >0.12 sec	None	Variable¶	Abnormal	Intermittent cannon waves¶	Lidocaine, procainamide, DC shock, quinidine, amiodarone
Accelerated idioventricular rhythm	60-100¶	Regular	Normal	50-110	Fairly regular; may be irregular	Abnormal, >0.12 sec	None	Variable¶	Abnormal	Intermittent cannon waves¶	None, unless symptomatic; lidocaine, atropine
Ventricular flutter	60-100¶	Regular	Normal; difficult to see	150-300	Regular	Sine wave	None	Soft or absent	Soft or absent	Cannon waves	DC shock
Ventricular fibrillation	60-100¶	Regular	Normal; difficult to see	400-600	Grossly irregular	Baseline undulations; no QRS	None	None	None	Cannon waves	DC shock
First-degree AV block	60-100**	Regular	Normal	60-100	Regular	Normal	Gradual slowing caused by sinus	Constant, diminished	Normal	Normal	None
Type I second-degree AV block	60-100**	Regular	Normal	30-100	Irregular††	Normal	Slowing caused by sinus slowing and an increase in AV block	Cyclic decrease, then increase after pause	Normal	Normal; increasing *a-c* interval; *a* waves without *c* waves	None, unless symptomatic; atropine
Type II second-degree AV block	60-100**	Regular	Normal	30-100	Irregular††	Abnormal, >0.12 sec	Gradual slowing caused by sinus slowing	Constant	Abnormal	Normal; constant *a-c* interval; *a* waves	Pacemaker
Complete AV block	60-100¶	Regular	Normal	<40	Fairly regular	Abnormal, 0.12 sec	None	Variable**	Abnormal	Intermittent cannon waves**	Pacemaker
Right bundle branch block	60-100	Regular	Normal	60-100	Regular	Abnormal, 0.12 sec	Gradual slowing and return to former rate	Constant	Wide	Normal	None
Left bundle branch block	60-100	Regular	Normal	60-100	Regular	Abnormal, >0.12 sec	Gradual slowing and return to former rate	Constant	Paradoxical	Normal	None

*In an effort to summarize these arrhythmias in tabular form, generalizations have to be made. For example, the response to carotid sinus massage may be slightly different from what is listed. Acute therapy to terminate a tachycardia may be different from chronic therapy to prevent recurrence. Some of the exceptions are indicated in the footnotes; the reader is referred to the text for a complete discussion.

†P waves initiated by sinus node discharge may not be precisely regular because of sinus arrhythmia.

‡Often, carotid sinus massage fails to slow a sinus tachycardia.

§Any independent atrial arrhythmia may exit or the atria may be captured retrogradely.

¶Constant if the atria are captured retrogradely.

** Atrial rhythm and rate may vary, depending on whether sinus bradycardia, sinus tachycardia, or another abnormality is the atrial mechanism.

††Regular or constant if block is unchanging.

DC = direct current; WPW = Wolff-Parkinson-White.

Modified from Zipes DP: Arrhythmias. *In* Andreoli K, Zipes DP, Wallace AG, et al (eds): Comprehensive Cardiac Care. 6th ed. St. Louis, CV Mosby, 1987.

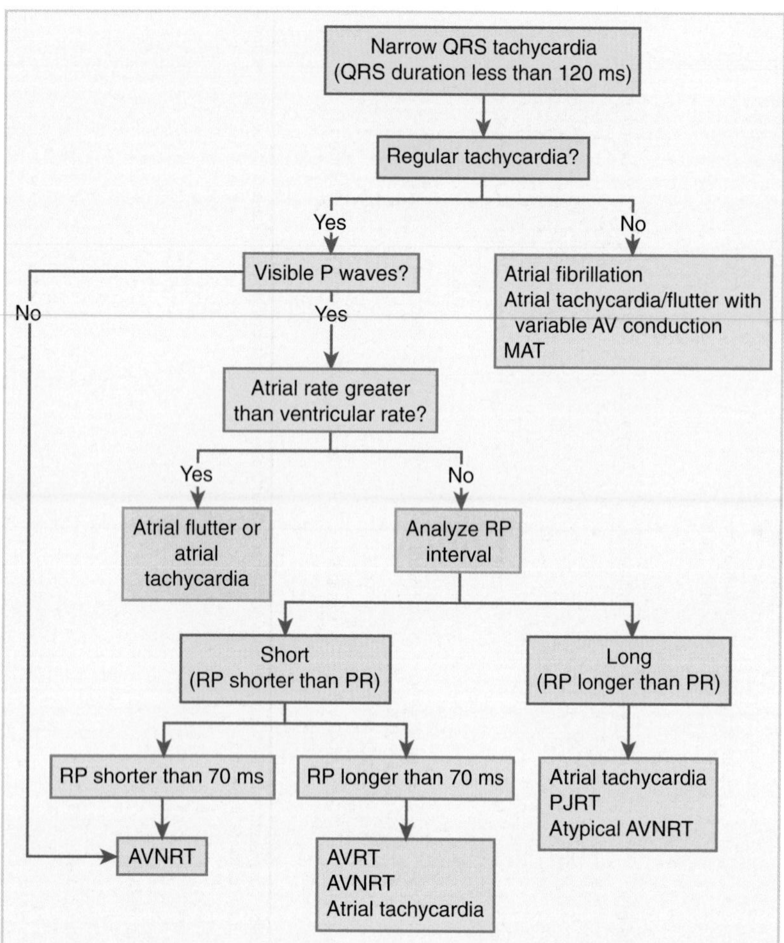

FIGURE 39-1 Algorithm for diagnosis of a narrow QRS tachycardia. AVRT = AV reentrant tachycardia; AVNRT = AV nodal reentrant tachycardia; MAT = multifocal atrial tachycardia; PJRT = permanent form of AV junctional reciprocating tachycardia. *(From Blomstrom-Lundqvist C, Scheinman MM, Aliot EM, et al: ACC/AHA/ESC guidelines for the management of patients with supraventricular arrhythmias—executive summary: A report of the American College of Cardiology/American Heart Association Task Force on Practice Guidelines and the European Society of Cardiology Committee for Practice Guidelines [Writing Committee to Develop Guidelines for the Management of Patients With Supraventricular Arrhythmias]. Circulation 108:1871, 2003.)*

TABLE 39-2 Major Features in the Differential Diagnosis of Wide QRS Beats Versus Tachycardia

SUPPORTS SVT	SUPPORTS VT
Slowing or termination by vagal tone	Fusion beats
Onset with premature P wave	Capture beats
RP interval ≤100 msec	AV dissociation
P and QRS rate and rhythm linked to suggest that ventricular activation depends on atrial discharge, e.g., 2:1 AV block rSR′ V_1	P and QRS rate and rhythm linked to suggest that atrial activation depends on ventricular discharge, e.g., 2:1 VA block
Long-short cycle sequence	"Compensatory" pause Left-axis deviation; QRS duration >140 msec Specific QRS contours (see text)

have a normal contour, a larger amplitude can develop, and the wave can become peaked. They appear before each QRS complex with a stable PR interval unless concomitant AV block ensues.

Accelerated phase 4 diastolic depolarization of sinus nodal cells (see Chap. 35) is generally responsible for sinus tachycardia and is usually caused by elevated adrenergic tone or withdrawal of parasympathetic tone. Carotid sinus massage and Valsalva or other vagal maneuvers gradually slow sinus tachycardia, which then accelerates to its previous rate on cessation of enhanced vagal tone. More rapid sinus rates can fail to slow in response to a vagal maneuver, particularly those driven by high adrenergic tone.

CLINICAL FEATURES. Sinus tachycardia is common in infancy and early childhood and is the normal reaction to various physiologic or pathophysiologic stresses, such as fever, hypotension, thyrotoxicosis, anemia, anxiety, exertion, hypovolemia, pulmonary emboli, myocardial ischemia, congestive heart failure, and shock. Drugs such as atropine, catecholamines, and thyroid medications as well as alcohol, nicotine, caffeine, and amphetamines or other stimulants can produce sinus tachycardia. Persistent sinus tachycardia can be a manifestation of heart failure.

In patients with structural heart disease, sinus tachycardia can result in reduced cardiac output or angina or can precipitate another arrhythmia, in part related to the abbreviated ventricular filling time and compromised coronary blood flow. Sinus tachycardia can be a cause of inappropriate defibrillator discharge in patients with an implantable cardioverter-defibrillator (ICD; see Chap. 38). Chronic inappropriate sinus tachycardia (also known as the syndrome of inappropriate sinus tachycardia) has been described in otherwise healthy persons, possibly secondary to increased automaticity of the sinus node or an automatic atrial focus near the sinus node.[6,7] The abnormality can result from a defect in either sympathetic or vagal nerve control of sinoatrial (SA) automaticity or from an abnormality of the intrinsic heart rate. In postural orthostatic tachycardia syndrome, a related syndrome with orthostatic hypotension and sinus tachycardia, the cause of the orthostatic decrease in blood pressure is not hypovolemia or drugs. Both syndromes can result from autonomic neuropathy (either peripheral, as in diabetic patients, or central, from spinal cord injury).[6,7] Sinus node reentry (see Fig. 39-e1 on website) is an atrial tachycardia originating from tissue near the sinus node and thus has a P wave morphology similar to sinus rhythm. The mechanism and management of this tachycardia are discussed later in more detail in the section on focal atrial tachycardias.

MANAGEMENT. Management should focus on the cause of the sinus tachycardia. In the hospital inpatient setting, this is usually obvious (e.g., hemorrhage, sepsis, agitation). In the outpatient setting, the cause may be more elusive. The most common reversible causes include hyperthyroidism, anemia, infection or inflammation, and hypovolemia. Diabetic neuropathy is also common but not reversible. Elimination of tobacco, alcohol, coffee, tea, or other stimulants, such as the sympathomimetic agents in nose drops and cold medications, may be helpful. Drugs such as propranolol and verapamil, fluid replacement in a hypovolemic patient, or fever reduction in a febrile patient can help slow the sinus nodal discharge rate. Treatment of inappropriate sinus tachycardia requires beta blockers or calcium channel blockers, alone or in combination. In severe cases, sinus node radiofrequency (RF) or surgical ablation may be indicated; however, these approaches are usually only temporarily palliative (see Chap. 37). A specific blocker of the pacemaker current (I_f), ivabradine, has been developed (currently available in some European countries and Australia) and may be useful treatment in some patients with inappropriate or refractory sinus tachycardia.

Premature Atrial Complexes

Premature complexes are among the most common causes of an irregular pulse. They can originate from any area in the heart—most frequently from the ventricles, less often from the atria and the AV junctional area, and rarely from the sinus node. Although premature complexes arise commonly in normal hearts, they are more often associated with structural heart disease and increase in frequency with age.

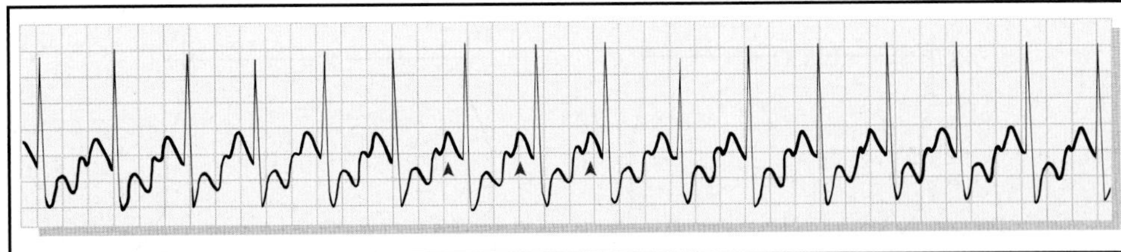

FIGURE 39-2 Sinus tachycardia (150 beats/min) in a patient during acute myocardial ischemia; note the ST-segment depression. P waves are indicated by arrowheads.

ELECTROCARDIOGRAPHIC RECOGNITION. The diagnosis of premature atrial complexes (PACs) is made on the ECG (**Fig. 39-3**) by the presence of a premature P wave with a PR interval of 120 milliseconds (except in Wolff-Parkinson-White syndrome, in which case the PR interval is usually shorter than 120 milliseconds). Although the contour of a premature P wave can resemble that of a normal sinus P wave, it generally differs. Whereas variations in the basic sinus rate can at times make the diagnosis of prematurity difficult, differences in the contour of the P waves are usually apparent and indicate a different focus of origin. When a PAC occurs early in diastole, conduction may not be completely normal. The AV junction may still be refractory from the preceding beat and prevent propagation of the impulse (blocked or nonconducted PAC; Fig. 39-3A) or cause conduction to be slowed (PAC with a prolonged PR interval). As a general rule, the RP interval is inversely related to the PR interval; thus, a short RP interval produced by an early PAC occurring close to the preceding QRS complex is followed by a long PR interval. When PACs occur early in the cardiac cycle, the premature P waves can be difficult to discern because they are superimposed on T waves. Careful examination of tracings from several leads may be necessary before the PAC is recognized as a slight deformity of the T wave. Often, such PACs are blocked before reaching the ventricle and can be misinterpreted as a sinus pause or sinus exit block (Fig. 39-3A).

The length of the pause that follows any premature complex or series of premature complexes is determined by the interaction of several factors. If the PAC occurs when the sinus node and perinodal tissue are not refractory, the impulse can be conducted into the sinus node, discharge it prematurely, and cause the next sinus cycle to begin from that time. The interval between the two normal P waves flanking a PAC that has reset the timing of the basic sinus rhythm is less than twice the normal P-P interval, and the pause

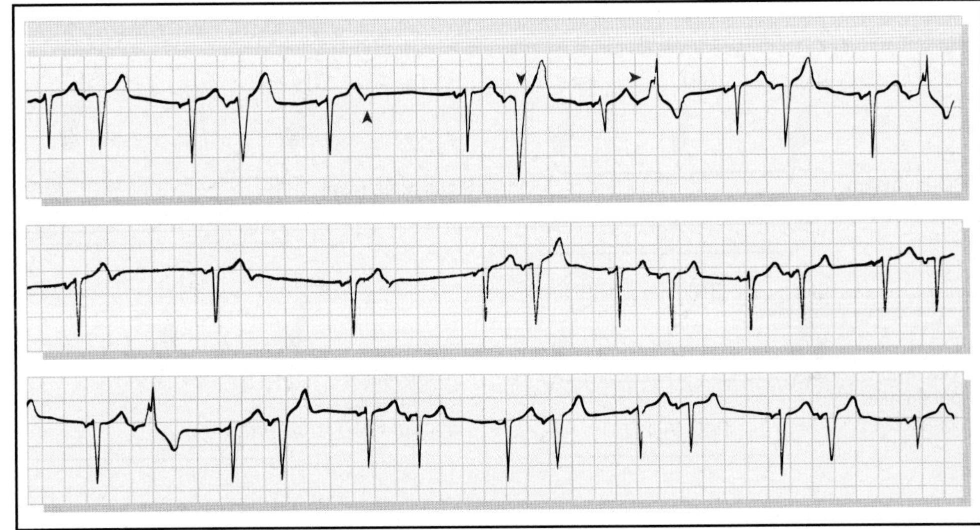

A

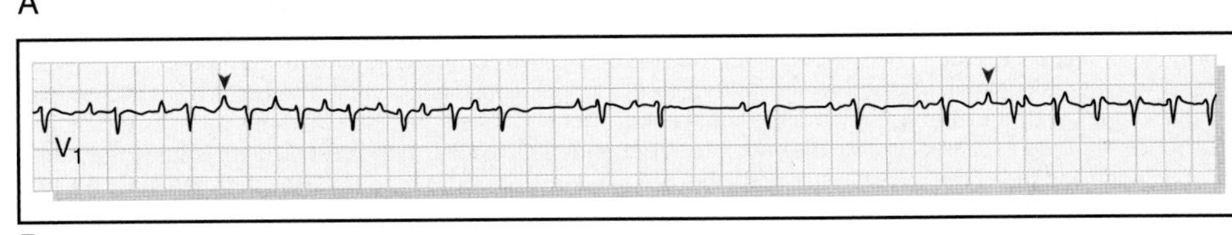

B

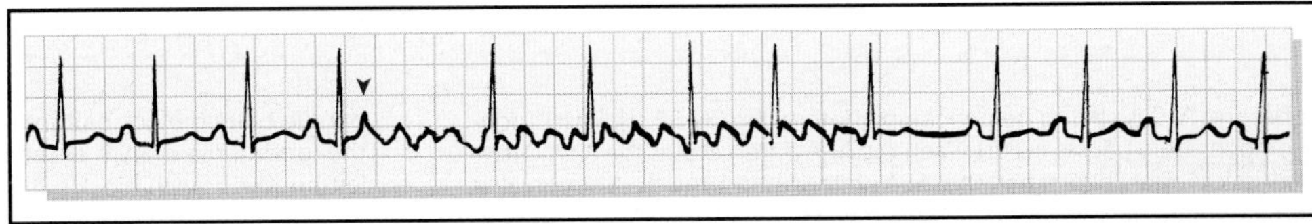

C

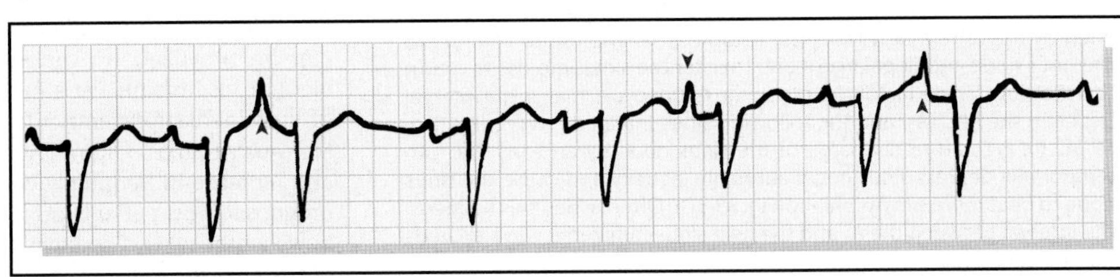

D

FIGURE 39-3 **A,** PACs that block conduction entirely or conduct with a functional right or functional left bundle branch block. Depending on the preceding cycle length and coupling interval of the PAC, the PAC blocks conduction entirely in the AV node (arrowhead ↑) or conducts with a functional left bundle branch block (arrowhead ↓) or functional right bundle branch block (arrowhead →). **B,** A PAC on the left (arrowhead) initiates AV nodal reentry that is caused by reentry anterogradely and retrogradely over two slow AV nodal pathways, with a retrograde P wave produced midway in the cardiac cycle. On the right, a PAC (arrowhead) initiates AV nodal reentry as a result of anterograde conduction over the slow pathway and retrograde conduction over the fast pathway (see Fig. 39-8A), which produces a retrograde P wave in the terminal portion of the QRS complex that simulates an r′ wave. **C, D,** A PAC (arrowhead ↓) initiating a short run of atrial flutter **(C)** and a PAC (arrowhead ↑) depressing return of the next sinus nodal discharge **(D)**. A slightly later PAC (arrowhead ↓) in **D** does not depress sinus nodal automaticity. **B-D,** Monitor leads.

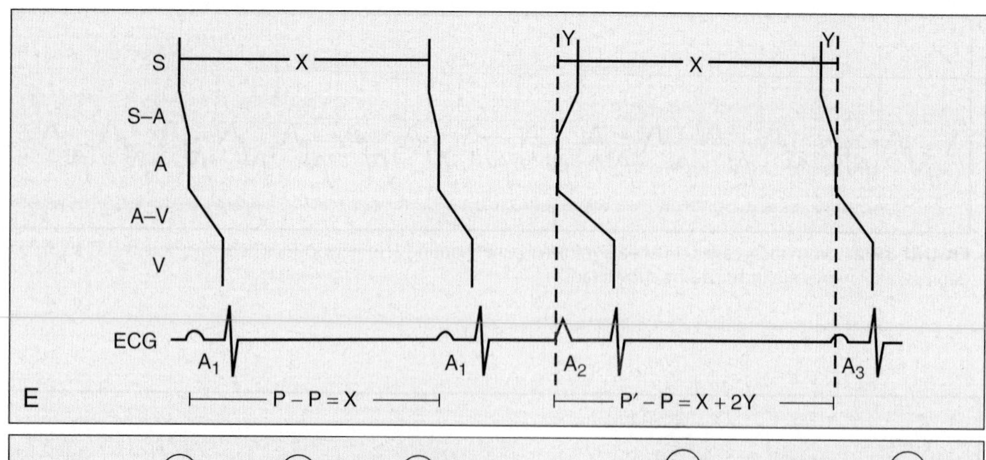

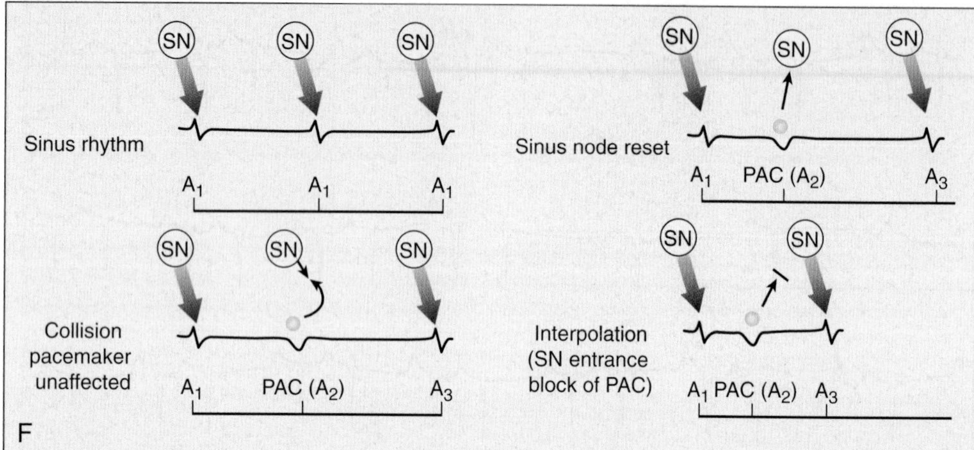

FIGURE 39-3, cont'd E, Diagrammatic example of the effects of a PAC. The sinus interval (A_1-A_1) equals X. The third P wave represents a PAC (A_2) that reaches and discharges the SA node, which causes the next sinus cycle to begin at that time. Therefore, the P-P (A_2-A_3) interval equals X + 2Y milliseconds, assuming no depression of SA nodal automaticity. **F,** Diagram of interactions of a PAC (yellow circles indicate origin; QRS complexes omitted) with the sinus node (SN) depending on the degree of prematurity. The top represents spontaneous sinus rhythm. The bottom is a late coupled PAC that collides with the exiting sinus impulse and therefore does not affect (or reset) the sinus pacemaker. The next sinus impulse (S_3) occurs at exactly twice the sinus interval. An early coupled PAC in the next diagram is able to penetrate the sinus node and resets the pacemaker, thereby resulting in resetting of the sinus node (as depicted in **E**). An even earlier coupled PAC in the lower figure reaches refractory tissue around the sinus node and is thus unable to penetrate the sinus node (SN entrance block); therefore, it does not affect sinus node discharge. The next spontaneous sinus beat (S_3) arrives exactly at the sinus interval. ***(E** modified from Zipes DP, Fisch C: Premature atrial contraction. Arch Intern Med 128:453, 1971.)*

after the PAC is said to be noncompensatory (Fig. 39-3E, F). Reset (noncompensatory pause) occurs when the A_1-A_2 interval plus the A_2-A_3 interval is less than two times the A_1-A_1 interval and the A_2-A_3 interval is greater than the A_1-A_1 interval. The interval between the PAC (A_2) and the following sinus-initiated P wave (A_3) exceeds one sinus cycle but is less than fully compensatory (see later) because the A_2-A_3 interval is lengthened by the time that it takes the ectopic atrial impulse to conduct to the sinus node and depolarize it and then for the sinus impulse to return to the atrium. These factors lengthen the return cycle, that is, the interval between the PAC (A_2) and the following sinus-initiated P wave (A_3) (Fig. 39-3E, F). Premature discharge of the sinus node by an early PAC can temporarily depress sinus nodal automatic activity and cause the sinus node to beat more slowly initially (Fig. 39-3D). Often, when this happens, the interval between the A_3 and the next sinus-initiated P wave exceeds the A_1-A_1 interval.

Less commonly, the PAC encounters a refractory sinus node or perinodal tissue (Fig. 39-3F), in which case the timing of the basic sinus rhythm is not altered because the sinus node is not reset by the PAC and the interval between the two normal sinus-initiated P waves flanking the PAC is twice the normal P-P interval. The interval that follows this premature atrial discharge is said to be a full compensatory pause, that is, of sufficient duration so that the P-P interval bounding the PAC is twice the normal P-P interval. However, sinus arrhythmia can lengthen or shorten this pause. Rarely, an interpolated PAC may occur. In this case, the pause after the PAC is very short, and the interval bounded by the normal sinus-initiated P waves on each side of the PAC is only slightly longer than or is equal to one normal P-P cycle length. The interpolated PAC fails to affect the sinus nodal pacemaker, and the sinus impulse that follows the PAC is conducted to the ventricles, often with a slightly lengthened PR interval. An interpolated atrial or ventricular premature complex of any type represents the only type of premature systole that does not actually replace the normally conducted beat. PACs can originate in the sinus node and are identified by premature P waves that have a contour identical to that of the normal sinus P wave.

On occasion, when the AV node has had sufficient time to repolarize and conduct without delay, the supraventricular QRS complex initiated by the PAC can be aberrant in configuration because the His-Purkinje system or ventricular muscle has not completely repolarized and conducts with a functional delay or block (Fig. 39-3A). The refractory period of cardiac fibers is directly related to cycle length. (In an adult, the AV nodal effective refractory period is prolonged at shorter cycle lengths.) A slow heart rate (long cycle length) produces a longer His-Purkinje refractory period than a faster heart rate. As a consequence, a PAC that follows a long R-R interval (long refractory period) can result in a functional bundle branch block (aberrant ventricular conduction). Because the right bundle branch at long cycles has a longer refractory period than the left bundle branch, aberration with a right bundle branch block pattern at slow rates occurs more commonly than aberration with a left bundle branch block pattern. At shorter cycles, the refractory period of the left bundle branch exceeds that of the right bundle branch, and a left bundle branch block pattern may be more likely to occur.

CLINICAL FEATURES. PACs can occur in various situations, such as during infection, inflammation, or myocardial ischemia, or they can be provoked by various medications, tension states, tobacco, alcohol, or caffeine. PACs can precipitate or presage the occurrence of sustained supraventricular (Fig. 39-3B, C) and, rarely, ventricular tachyarrhythmias. Often, PACs occur without any reversible causes and increase in frequency with aging. In general, PACs have a benign prognosis. Most patients do not have significant symptoms with PACs; however, those who do have symptoms most often feel the pauses that occur after the PAC.

MANAGEMENT. PACs generally do not require therapy. In symptomatic patients or when the PACs precipitate tachycardias, treatment with a beta blocker or a calcium antagonist can be tried. In drug-refractory, highly symptomatic cases, ablation of the PAC focus can be effective when a single focus can be identified.

Atrial Fibrillation

See Chap. 40.

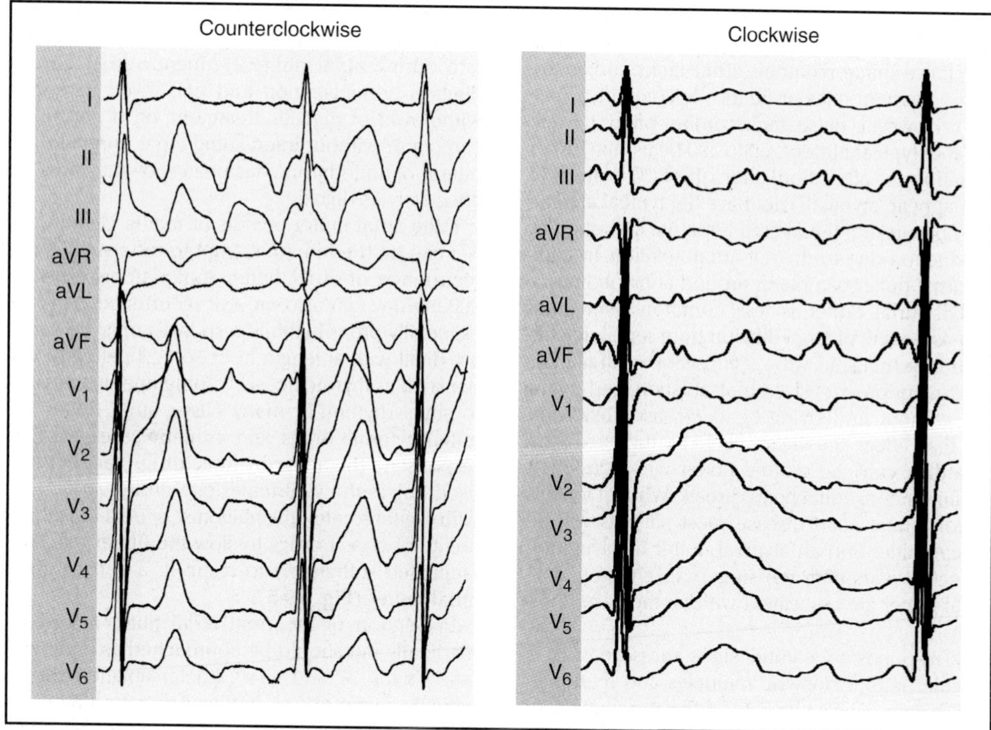

FIGURE 39-4 Twelve-lead ECG of counterclockwise and clockwise atrial flutter. In counterclockwise atrial flutter, the flutter waves are negative in leads II, III, aVF, and V_6 and upright in V_1. In clockwise atrial flutter, the flutter waves are upright in leads II, III, and aVF and often notched.

Atrial Tachycardias

Three types of atrial tachycardia have been distinguished experimentally—automatic, triggered, and reentrant. Entrainment, resetting of curve patterns in response to overdrive pacing, the patient's response to adenosine, and recording of monophasic action potentials and mode of initiation may suggest the presence of one of these mechanisms. However, in most cases, no clear identification of the mechanism can be made clinically because the clinical presentations and electrophysiologic features can overlap, especially when the reentrant circuit is small (i.e., microreentry). For example, adrenergic stimulation can initiate automatic and triggered atrial tachycardias, and burst pacing may initiate triggered and microreentrant atrial tachycardias. Therefore, because it determines the approach to mapping and ablation as well as to management, atrial tachycardias are more broadly characterized as being focal (originating from a small area of the atrium with atrial excitation emanating from this focus) or macroreentrant (a relatively large reentrant circuit using conduction barriers to create the circuit). Atrial flutter is the most common type of macroreentrant atrial tachycardia.

Atrial Flutter and Other Macroreentrant Atrial Tachycardias

Atrial flutter is the prototypic macroreentrant atrial rhythm. Typical atrial flutter (historically called type I by electrocardiographers) is a reentrant rhythm in the right atrium constrained anteriorly by the tricuspid annulus and posteriorly by the crista terminalis and eustachian ridge. The flutter can circulate in a counterclockwise direction around the tricuspid annulus in the frontal plane (typical flutter, counterclockwise flutter) or in a clockwise direction (atypical, clockwise, or reverse flutter). Because both these forms of atrial flutter use the same circuit and are constrained by the same anatomic structures, their rates and flutter wave morphology on the surface ECG are consistent and predictable (see later). Other forms of atrial flutter are now recognized as distinct types and include atrial macroreentry caused by incisional scars from prior atrial surgery, prior atrial ablation, idiopathic fibrosis in areas of the atrium, or other anatomic or functional conduction barriers in the atria. Atrial flutters originating in the left atrium (e.g., circulating around the mitral annulus, involving prior ablation lesions from atrial fibrillation ablations or surgical scars from maze procedures) have also been described.[8,9] Because the barriers that constrain these atrial flutters are variable, the electrocardiographic pattern of these so-called atypical atrial flutters can be varied. Often, flutter wave morphology changes during the same episode of flutter, which indicates multiple circuits or nonfixed conduction barriers.

ELECTROCARDIOGRAPHIC RECOGNITION. The atrial rate during typical atrial flutter is usually 250 to 350 beats/min, although it is occasionally slower, particularly when the patient is treated with antiarrhythmic drugs, which can reduce the rate to about 200 beats/min. If such slowing occurs, the ventricles can respond in a 1:1 fashion to the slower atrial rate. Ordinarily, the atrial rate is about 300 beats/min, and in untreated patients, the ventricular rate is half the atrial rate, that is, 150 beats/min. A significantly slower ventricular rate (in the absence of drugs) suggests abnormal AV conduction. In children, in patients with the preexcitation syndrome, occasionally in patients with hyperthyroidism, and in those whose AV nodes conduct rapidly, atrial flutter can conduct to the ventricle in a 1:1 fashion and produce a ventricular rate of 300 beats/min.

In typical atrial flutter, the ECG reveals identically recurring, regular, sawtooth flutter waves (Fig. 39-3C) and evidence of continual electrical activity (lack of an isoelectric interval between flutter waves), often best visualized in leads II, III, aVF, or V_1 (**Fig. 39-4**). In some cases, transient slowing of the ventricular response, with either carotid sinus massage or adenosine, is necessary to visualize the flutter waves. The flutter waves for type I typical atrial flutter are inverted (negative) in these leads because of a counterclockwise reentrant pathway, and sometimes they are upright (positive) when the reentrant loop is clockwise (see Fig. 39-4). When the flutter waves are upright from clockwise rotation, they are often notched. If the AV conduction ratio remains constant, the ventricular rhythm will be regular; if the ratio of conducted beats varies (usually the result of a Wenckebach AV block), the ventricular rhythm will be irregular. Recurrent alternation of short and long ventricular intervals can be the result of concealed conduction. Various degrees of penetration into the AV junction by flutter impulses can also influence AV conduction. The ratio of flutter waves to conducted ventricular complexes is most often an even number (e.g., 2:1, 4:1).

As mentioned earlier, because the circuits for atypical flutters (not involving the cavotricuspid isthmus) can be variable, the electrocardiographic features of these macroreentrant atrial tachycardias are highly variable, without consistent rates or flutter wave contours (see Fig. 39-e2 on website). However, these tachycardias often have a flutter rate similar to that of typical flutter (250 to 390 beats/min). After extensive left atrial ablation for atrial fibrillation, the ECG pattern of even typical flutter can appear "atypical" (not have the typical appearance described before) because of the altered left atrial activation as a result of altered conduction due to the left atrial ablation. In addition, unusual forms of atrial flutter can occur around ablation lines.

CLINICAL FEATURES. Atrial flutter is less common than atrial fibrillation. It can occur as a result of atrial dilation from septal defects, pulmonary emboli, mitral or tricuspid valve stenosis or regurgitation, chronic ventricular failure, prior extensive atrial ablation, and aging, but it can also occur without underlying heart disease. Toxic and metabolic conditions that affect the heart, such as thyrotoxicosis, alcoholism, and pericarditis, can cause atrial flutter. On occasion, it can follow surgical repair for congenital heart disease. When it follows reparative surgery of congenital heart disease, most patients will be able to have both typical flutter and an atypical flutter involving the atriotomy that often occurs years after the surgery. In children, continued episodes of atrial flutter are associated with an increased possibility of sudden death.

Atrial flutter usually responds to carotid sinus massage with a decrease in the ventricular rate in stepwise multiples and returns in reverse manner to the former ventricular rate at the termination of carotid massage. Physical examination may reveal rapid flutter waves in the jugular venous pulse. If the relationship of flutter waves to conducted QRS complexes remains constant, the first heart sound will have a constant intensity. Sounds caused by atrial contraction can occasionally be auscultated.

MANAGEMENT. Cardioversion (see Chap. 37) is commonly the initial treatment of choice for atrial flutter because it promptly and effectively restores sinus rhythm. Cardioversion can be accomplished with synchronous direct current (DC), which often requires relatively low energies (approximately 50 J). If the electrical shock results in atrial fibrillation, a second shock at a higher energy level is used to restore sinus rhythm; or, depending on clinical circumstances, the atrial fibrillation can be left untreated and can revert to atrial flutter or sinus rhythm. The short-acting antiarrhythmic medication ibutilide can also be given intravenously to convert atrial flutter. Ibutilide appears to successfully cardiovert about 60% to 90% of episodes of atrial flutter. However, because this medication prolongs the QT interval, torsades de pointes is a potential complication during and shortly after the infusion. Other medications, such as procainamide, can be given to convert atrial flutter chemically. Rapid atrial pacing with a catheter in the esophagus or the right atrium can effectively terminate typical and some forms of atypical atrial flutter in most patients and produce sinus rhythm or atrial fibrillation, with a slowing of the ventricular rate and concomitant clinical improvement. Because ablation is highly effective for typical flutter and because of the high relapse rate after cardioversion, ablation is also a reasonable approach for stable patients who do not require immediate cardioversion. Although the risk of thromboembolism is lower than that for atrial fibrillation, patients with atrial flutter do appear to have a risk of thromboembolism immediately after conversion to sinus rhythm.[10] In general, indications for anticoagulation in patients with atrial flutter are similar to those with atrial fibrillation.

As a general rule, atrial flutter is much more difficult to rate-control than atrial fibrillation. Verapamil (see Chap. 37) given as an initial bolus of 2.5 to 10 mg intravenously (may repeat 5-10 mg after 15-30 minutes), or diltiazem 0.25 mg/kg to slow the ventricular response can be tried. Adenosine produces a transient AV block and can be used to reveal flutter waves if diagnosis of the arrhythmias is in doubt. It will not generally terminate the atrial flutter and can provoke atrial fibrillation. Esmolol, a beta-adrenergic blocker with a 9-minute elimination half-life, or other intravenous beta blockers can be used to slow the ventricular rate. If the use of calcium channel blockers and beta blockers in combination is insufficient, digoxin can be added. The dose of digitalis necessary to slow the ventricular response varies and at times can result in toxic levels because it is often difficult to slow the ventricular rate during atrial flutter. Frequently, atrial fibrillation develops after digitalis administration and can revert to normal sinus rhythm on withdrawal of digitalis treatment; on occasion, normal sinus rhythm can occur without intervening atrial fibrillation. Intravenous administration of amiodarone has been shown to slow the ventricular rate as effectively as digoxin.

If the atrial flutter persists or recurs, class IA or IC drugs (see Chap. 37) can be tried in an attempt to restore sinus rhythm and to prevent recurrence of atrial flutter. Amiodarone, especially in low doses of 200 mg/day, can also prevent recurrences. Side effects of these drugs, especially proarrhythmic responses, must be carefully considered and are dealt with at length in Chap. 37. Treatment of the underlying disorder, such as thyrotoxicosis, is sometimes necessary to effect conversion to sinus rhythm. In many cases, atrial flutter can continue despite antiarrhythmic drugs, and in many cases, the flutter rate will slow in response to the antiarrhythmic drug. Class I or III drugs should not be used unless the ventricular rate during atrial flutter has been slowed with digitalis, calcium antagonist, or beta-blocking drug. Because of the ability of class I drugs to slow the flutter rate, AV conduction can be facilitated sufficiently to result in a 1:1 ventricular response to the atrial flutter (**Fig. 39-5**).

Prevention of recurrent atrial flutter is often difficult to achieve medically but should be approached as outlined for atrial fibrillation (see Chaps. 37 and 40). Catheter ablation should be considered in patients refractory to medical therapy. Catheter ablation of typical flutter (counterclockwise and clockwise) is a highly effective cure and has a long-term success rate of 90% to 100%. Because ablation of atrial flutter is so effective, with little risk, it can be offered as an alternative to drug therapy. Ablation of other forms of macroreentrant atrial tachycardia is also effective, although success rates are somewhat lower and more variable. Increasing evidence has indicated that the risk of emboli in atrial flutter may be more significant than once thought.[10] Because of this, and because many patients with atrial flutter also have atrial fibrillation, anticoagulation is usually warranted. However, carefully controlled studies to determine the degree of embolic risk in patients with only atrial flutter are lacking. Long-term anticoagulation, as in atrial fibrillation, should probably be considered until more definitive data are available.

Focal Atrial Tachycardias

ELECTROCARDIOGRAPHIC RECOGNITION. Focal atrial tachycardias (**Fig. 39-6**) generally have atrial rates of 150 to 200 beats/min, with a P wave contour different from that of the sinus P wave. However, atrial tachycardias, with foci near the sinus node, can have P wave contours very similar to those in sinus rhythm. At onset, there may be some warming up of the rate, resulting in a slight increase in heart rate over the initial several complexes. Frequently, atrial tachycardias occur in short, recurrent bursts with spontaneous terminations. However, more incessant forms of atrial tachycardias do occur. P waves are usually found in the second half of the tachycardia cycle (long RP–short PR tachycardia). If the atrial rate is not excessive and AV conduction is not depressed, each P wave can conduct to the ventricles. If the atrial rate increases and AV conduction becomes impaired, a Wenckebach (Mobitz type I) second-degree AV block can ensue. This aberration is sometimes called atrial tachycardia with block. When it is caused by digitalis, other manifestations of digitalis excess are present, such as premature ventricular complexes (PVCs). In nearly half the cases of atrial tachycardia with block, the atrial rate is irregular. Characteristic isoelectric intervals between P waves, in contrast to atrial flutter, are usually present in all leads. However, at rapid atrial rates, the distinction between atrial tachycardia with block and atrial flutter can be difficult. Analysis of P wave configuration during tachycardia indicates that a positive or biphasic P wave in V_1 predicts a right atrial focus, whereas a negative P wave in V_1 predicts a left atrial focus.

CLINICAL FEATURES. Although atrial tachycardia occurs commonly in patients with significant structural heart disease such as coronary artery disease, with or without myocardial infarction, cor

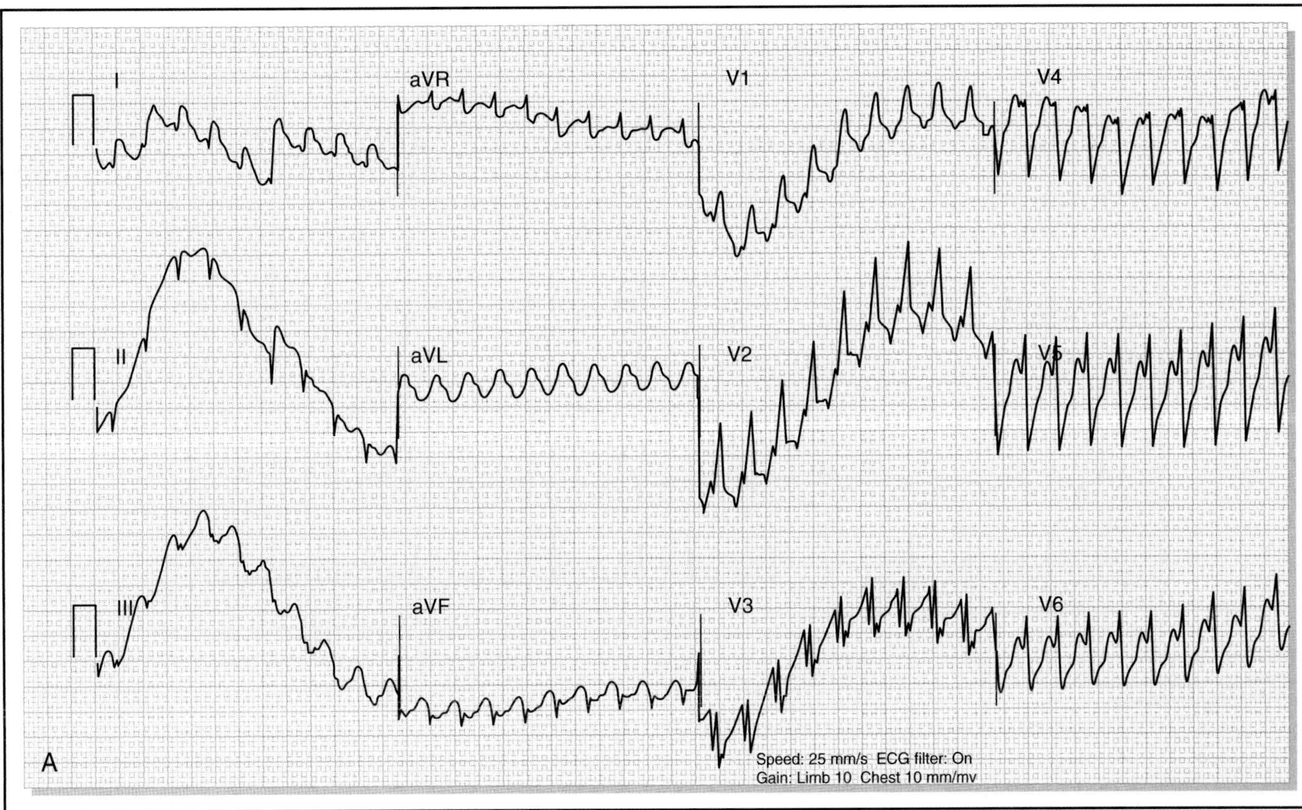

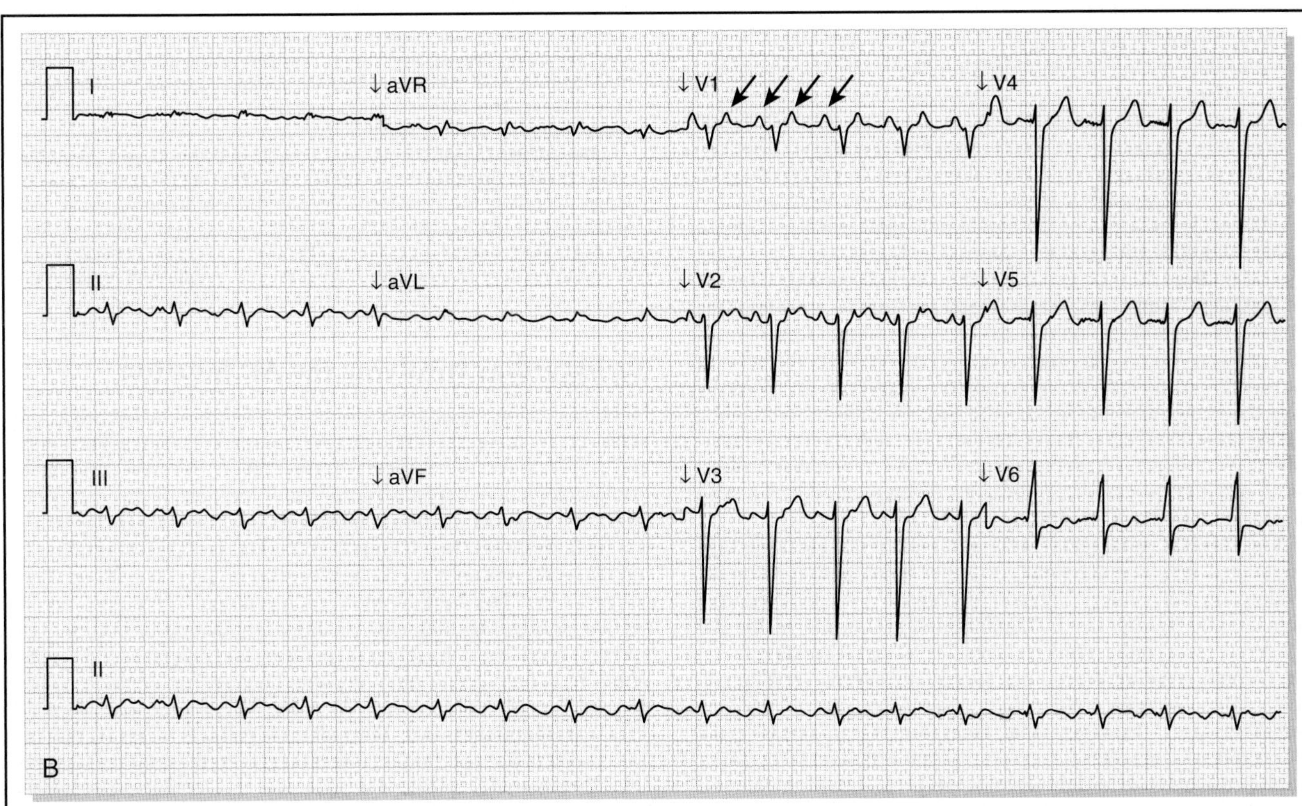

FIGURE 39-5 Atrial flutter with 1:1 conduction and QRS widening caused by flecainide. **A,** Atrial flutter occurs with 1:1 conduction and a widened QRS because of slowing of the atrial flutter rate from the flecainide and acceleration of conduction through the AV node, resulting in a rapid ventricular response. This rapid ventricular response results in a widened QRS complex because of the use dependence of flecainide's sodium channel blocking. **B,** After administration of AV nodal blocking agents (in this case, metoprolol), 2:1 conduction occurs, the ventricular rate is slowed, and the QRS duration shortens. In addition, the flutter waves are now apparent on the ECG (arrows).

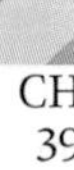

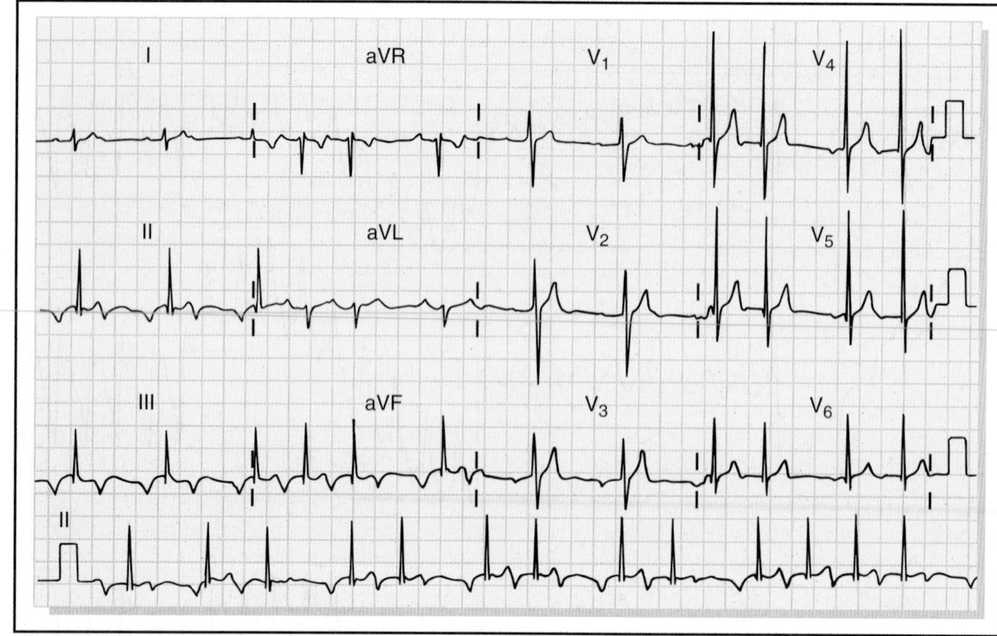

FIGURE 39-6 Atrial tachycardia. This 12-lead ECG and rhythm strip (bottom) demonstrate an atrial tachycardia at a cycle length of approximately 520 milliseconds. Conduction varies between 3:2 and 2:1. Note the negative P waves in leads II, III, and aVF and, when consecutive P waves are conducted, that the RP interval exceeds the PR interval. Note also that the tachycardia persists despite the development of AV block, an important finding that excludes the participation of an AV accessory pathway and sharply differentiates this tachycardia from the one shown in Figure 39-21.

pulmonale, or digitalis intoxication, it is also seen in patients without structural heart disease. Potassium depletion can precipitate the arrhythmia in patients taking digitalis. The signs, symptoms, and prognosis are usually related to the underlying cardiovascular status and the rate of the tachycardia. Atrial tachycardias often occur in short recurrent bursts but on occasion can be incessant. When they are incessant, tachycardia-induced cardiomyopathy can result. This can be partially or totally reversible with elimination of the tachycardia. In some patients, exercise or stress can provoke the tachycardia; in others, the tachycardia can be positional. Stimulants such as caffeine, chocolate, and ephedrine can also provoke episodes.

Physical findings during a variable rhythm include variable intensity of the first heart sound and systolic blood pressure as a result of the varying AV block and PR interval. An excessive number of *a* waves can be seen in the jugular venous pulse. Carotid sinus massage or administration of adenosine increases the degree of AV block by slowing the ventricular rate in stepwise fashion without terminating the tachycardia, as in atrial flutter. It should be performed cautiously in patients with digitalis toxicity because serious ventricular arrhythmias can result. On occasion, carotid sinus massage or adenosine can terminate some forms of atrial tachycardia.

MANAGEMENT. Atrial tachycardia in a patient not receiving digitalis is treated in a manner similar to other atrial tachyarrhythmias. Depending on the clinical situation, digitalis, a beta blocker, or a calcium channel blocker can be administered to slow the ventricular rate; if atrial tachycardia remains, class IA, IC, or III drugs can be added. Catheter ablation procedures are usually effective at eliminating the atrial tachycardia, depending on the mechanism and underlying heart disease.[11] However, atrial tachycardias can occasionally recur at a different site after a successful ablation. If atrial tachycardia appears in a patient receiving digitalis, the drug should initially be assumed to be responsible for the arrhythmia. Therapy includes cessation of digitalis and administration of digitalis antibodies or potassium, if the level is low. Often, the ventricular response is not excessively fast, and simply withholding digitalis is all that is necessary.

Chaotic Atrial Tachycardia

Chaotic (sometimes called multifocal) atrial tachycardia is characterized by atrial rates between 100 and 130 beats/min, with marked variation in P wave morphology and totally irregular P-P intervals (**Fig. 39-7**). In general, at least three P wave contours are noted, with most P waves conducted to the ventricles, although often with variable PR intervals. This tachycardia occurs commonly in older patients with chronic obstructive pulmonary disease and congestive heart failure and may eventually develop into atrial fibrillation. Digitalis appears to be an unusual cause, and theophylline administration has been implicated. Chaotic atrial tachycardia can occur in childhood.

MANAGEMENT. Management is primarily directed toward the underlying disease. Antiarrhythmic agents are often ineffective in slowing either the rate of the atrial tachycardia or the ventricular response. Beta adrenoceptor blockers should be avoided in patients with bronchospastic pulmonary disease but can be effective if tolerated. Verapamil and amiodarone have been useful. Potassium and magnesium replacement may suppress the tachycardia. Ablation may be effective in some cases.[12]

Tachycardias Involving the AV Junction

Much confusion exists about the nomenclature of tachycardias characterized by a supraventricular QRS complex, a regular R-R interval, and no evidence of ventricular preexcitation. Because various electrophysiologic mechanisms can account for these tachycardias (**Fig. 39-8**), the nonspecific term *paroxysmal supraventricular tachycardia* has been proposed to encompass the entire group. This term may be inappropriate because some tachycardias in patients with accessory pathways (see later) are no more supraventricular than they are ventricular in origin as they may require participation of both the atria and the ventricles in the reentrant pathway and exhibit a QRS complex of normal contour and duration, only because anterograde conduction occurs over the normal AV node–His bundle pathways (Fig. 39-8C). If conduction over the reentrant pathway reverses direction and travels in an "antidromic" direction (i.e., to the ventricles over the accessory pathway and to the atria over the AV node–His bundle), the QRS complex exhibits a prolonged duration, although the tachycardia is basically the same. The term *reciprocating tachycardia* has been offered as a substitute for paroxysmal SVT, but use of such a term presumes the mechanism of the tachycardia to be reentrant, which is probably the case for many SVTs. Reciprocating tachycardia is probably the mechanism of many VTs as well. Thus, no universally acceptable nomenclature exists for these tachycardias, but rather descriptive labels for specific arrhythmias, as used throughout this chapter.

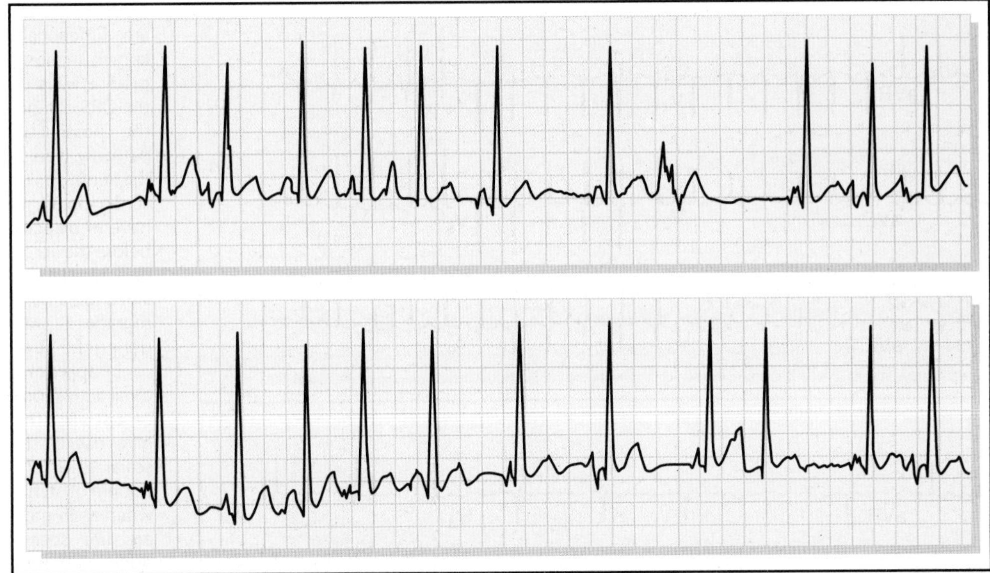

FIGURE 39-7 Chaotic (multifocal) atrial tachycardia. PACs occur at varying cycle lengths and with differing contours.

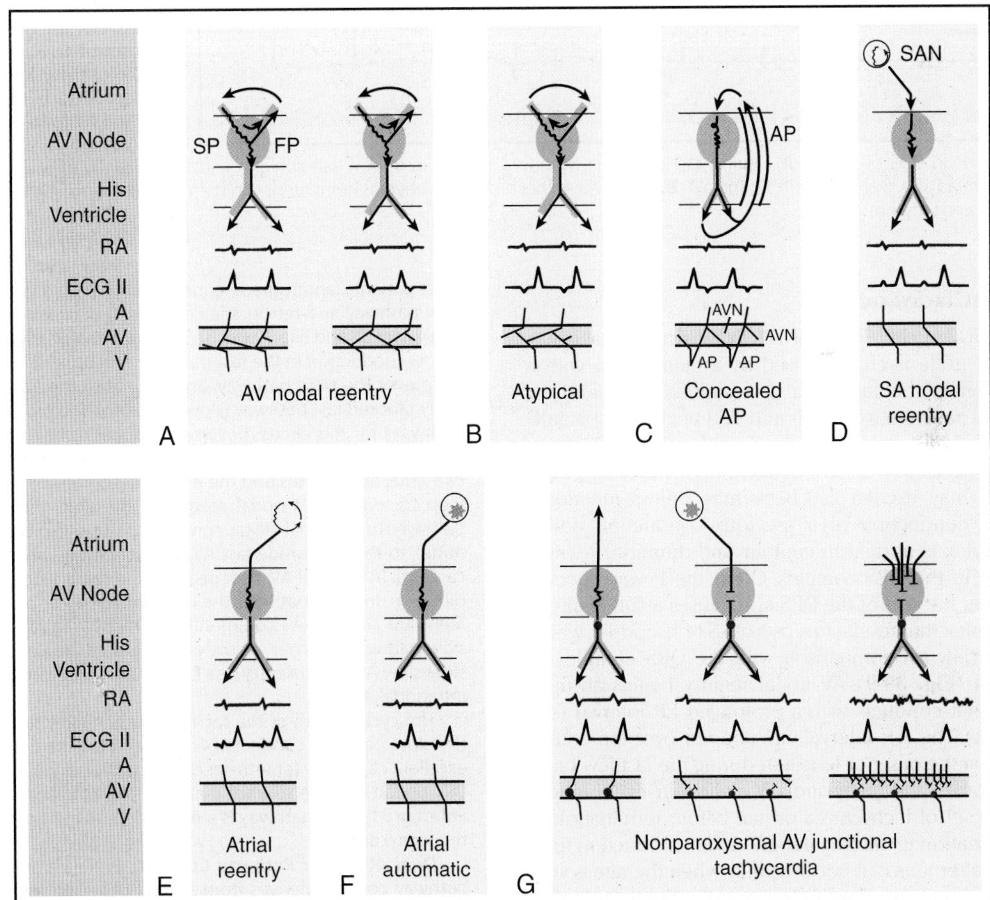

FIGURE 39-8 Diagrammatic representation of various tachycardias. In the upper portion of each example, a schematic of the presumed anatomic pathways is shown; in the lower half, the ECG and explanatory ladder diagram are depicted. **A,** AV nodal reentry. In the left example, reentrant excitation is drawn with retrograde atrial activity occurring simultaneously with ventricular activity as a result of anterograde conduction over the slow AV nodal pathway (SP) and retrograde conduction over the fast AV nodal pathway (FP). In the right example, atrial activity occurs slightly later than ventricular activity because of retrograde conduction delay. **B,** Atypical AV nodal reentry caused by anterograde conduction over a fast AV nodal pathway and retrograde conduction over a slow AV nodal pathway. **C,** Concealed accessory pathway (AP). Reciprocating tachycardia is caused by anterograde conduction over the AV node (AVN) and retrograde conduction over the accessory pathway. Retrograde P waves occur after the QRS complex. **D,** Sinus nodal reentry. The tachycardia is caused by reentry within the sinus node, which then conducts the impulse to the rest of the heart. **E,** Atrial reentry. Tachycardia is caused by reentry within the atrium, which then conducts the impulse to the rest of the heart. **F,** Automatic atrial tachycardia (star indicates origin). Tachycardia is caused by automatic discharge in the atrium, which then conducts the impulse to the rest of the heart; it is difficult to distinguish from atrial reentry. **G,** Nonparoxysmal AV junctional tachycardia. Various manifestations of this tachycardia are depicted with retrograde atrial capture, AV dissociation with the sinus node in control of the atria, and AV dissociation with atrial fibrillation. Star indicates sinus node discharge. Red circles indicate site of junctional discharge. SAN = sinoatrial node.

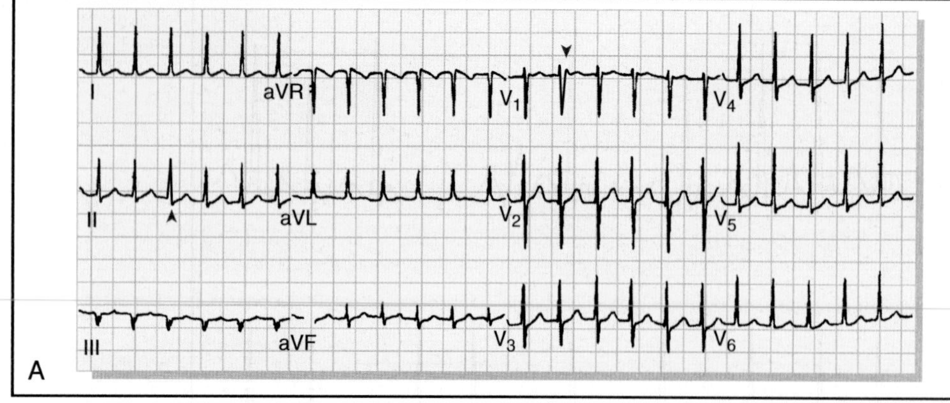

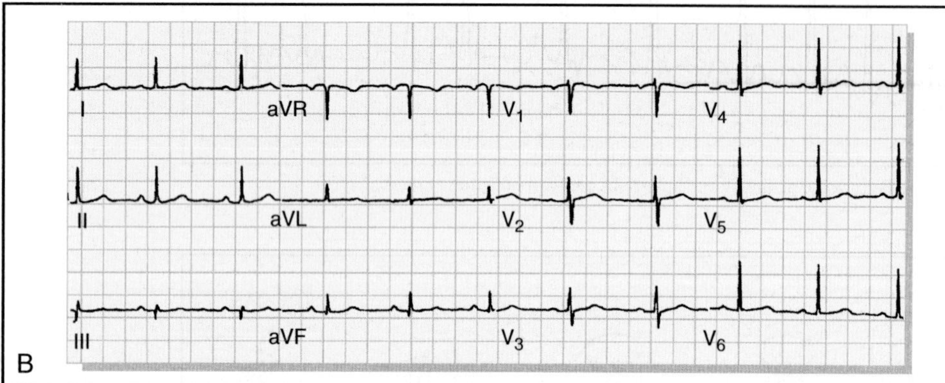

FIGURE 39-9 Twelve-lead ECG of AVNRT. **A,** During tachycardia, a pseudo-r′ is seen in lead V_1 (arrowhead) and pseudo-S waves (arrowhead) are seen in leads II, III, and aVF. **B,** These waves become more obvious compared with the QRS complexes during sinus rhythm.

AV Nodal Reentrant Tachycardia

ELECTROCARDIOGRAPHIC RECOGNITION. Reentrant tachycardia involving the AV node is characterized by a tachycardia with a QRS complex of supraventricular origin, with sudden onset and termination generally at rates between 150 and 250 beats/min (usually 180 to 200 beats/min in adults) and with a regular rhythm. Uncommonly, the rate may be as low as 110 beats/min; occasionally, especially in children, it may exceed 250 beats/min. Unless functional aberrant ventricular conduction or a previous conduction defect exists, the QRS complex is normal in contour and duration. P waves are generally buried in the QRS complex. Often, the P wave occurs just before or just after the end of the QRS and causes a subtle alteration in the QRS complex that results in a pseudo-S or pseudo-r′, which may be recognized only on comparison with the QRS complex in normal sinus rhythm (**Fig. 39-9**). AV nodal reentry begins abruptly, usually after a PAC that conducts with a prolonged PR interval (see Figs. 39-3B and 39-8A). The R-R interval can shorten over the course of the first few beats at the onset or lengthen during the last few beats preceding termination of the tachycardia. Variation in cycle length, particularly at the onset of tachycardia or just before termination, is usually caused by variation in anterograde AV nodal conduction time. Cycle length or QRS alternans can occur, usually when the rate is very fast. Carotid sinus massage can slow the tachycardia slightly before its termination or, if termination does not occur, can produce only slight slowing of the tachycardia.

ELECTROPHYSIOLOGIC FEATURES. An atrial complex that conducts with a critical prolongation of AV nodal conduction time generally precipitates AV nodal reentry (**Figs. 39-10 and 39-11**). Premature ventricular stimulation can also induce AV nodal reentry in about one third of patients. Data from RF catheter ablation results and mapping support the presence of differential atrial inputs into the AV node, the fast and slow pathways, to explain this tachycardia (see Chaps. 35 and 37). In Figure 39-8A and B, the atria are shown as a necessary link between the fast and slow pathways. Whether these pathways are discrete pathways (perhaps caused by anisotropy) or are functional in nature is not known. In most examples, the retrograde P wave occurs at the onset of the QRS complex, clearly excluding the possibility of an accessory pathway. If an accessory pathway in the ventricle were part of the tachycardia circuit, the ventricles would have to be activated anterogradely before the accessory pathway could be activated retrogradely and depolarize the atria, thus placing the retrograde P wave no earlier than during the ST segment.

In approximately 30% of cases, atrial activation begins at the end of or just after the QRS complex and gives rise to a discrete P wave on the scalar ECG (often appearing as a nubbin of an R in V_1; see Fig. 39-8A), whereas in most patients, P waves are not seen because they are buried within the inscription of the QRS complex. In the most common variety of AV nodal reentrant tachycardia (AVNRT), the ventriculoatrial (VA) interval (i.e., the interval between the onset of QRS and the onset of atrial activity) is less than 50% of the R-R interval (a so-called short RP tachycardia), and the ratio of the AV to the VA interval exceeds 1.0. These VA intervals are longer in patients with tachycardia related to accessory pathways as well as in atypical forms of AV nodal reentry (see Fig. 39-8B).

Slow and Fast Pathways. In most patients, anterograde conduction to the ventricle occurs over the slow pathway and retrograde conduction occurs over the fast pathway (see Chap. 35 and Fig. 39-8A, B). To initiate tachycardia, an atrial complex blocks conduction in the fast pathway anterogradely, travels to the ventricle over the slow pathway, and returns to the atrium over the previously blocked fast pathway (slow-fast form). The proximal and distal final pathways for this circus movement appear to be located within the AV node, so as currently conceived, the circus movement occurs over the two atrial approaches and the AV node (see Fig. 39-8A, B). The reentrant loop for typical AV nodal reentry is the anterograde slow AV nodal pathway to the final distal common pathway (probably the distal AV node), to the retrograde fast AV nodal pathway, and then to atrial myocardium. In atypical AV node reentry, the reentry occurs in the opposite direction. In some patients, the His bundle may be incorporated into the reentrant circuit. Less commonly, the reentry pathway can be over two slow pathways or over a slow and intermediate pathway, the so-called slow-slow AV node reentry (see Fig. 39-3B). Some data are consistent with intranodal activity.

The cycle length of the tachycardia generally depends on how well the slow pathway conducts because the fast pathway usually exhibits excellent capability for retrograde conduction and has the shorter refractory period in the retrograde direction. Therefore, conduction time in the anterograde slow pathway is a major determinant of the cycle length of the tachycardia.

Dual AV Nodal Pathway Concept. Evidence supporting the dual-pathway concept derives from several observations, the most compelling of which is that RF catheter ablation of either the slow pathway or the fast pathway eliminates AV nodal reentry without eliminating AV nodal conduction. Other observations provide supporting proof. For example, in these patients, a plot of the A_1-A_2 versus the A_2-H_2 or the A_1-A_2 versus the H_1-H_2 interval shows a discontinuous curve (see Fig. 39-11). The explanation is that at a crucial A_1-A_2 interval, the impulse is suddenly blocked in the fast pathway and is conducted with delay over the slow pathway, with sudden prolongation of the A_2-H_2 (or H_1-H_2) interval. In general, the A-H interval increases at least 50 milliseconds, with only a 10-millisecond decrease in the coupling interval of the PAC. Less commonly, dual pathways may be manifested by different PR or A-H intervals during sinus rhythm or at identical paced rates or by a sudden jump in the A-H interval during atrial pacing at a constant cycle length. Two QRS

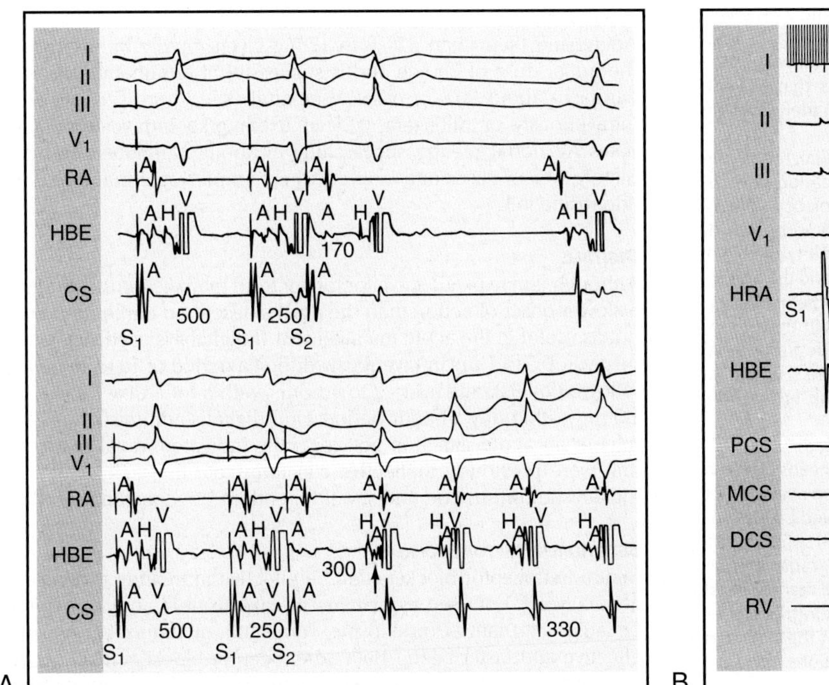

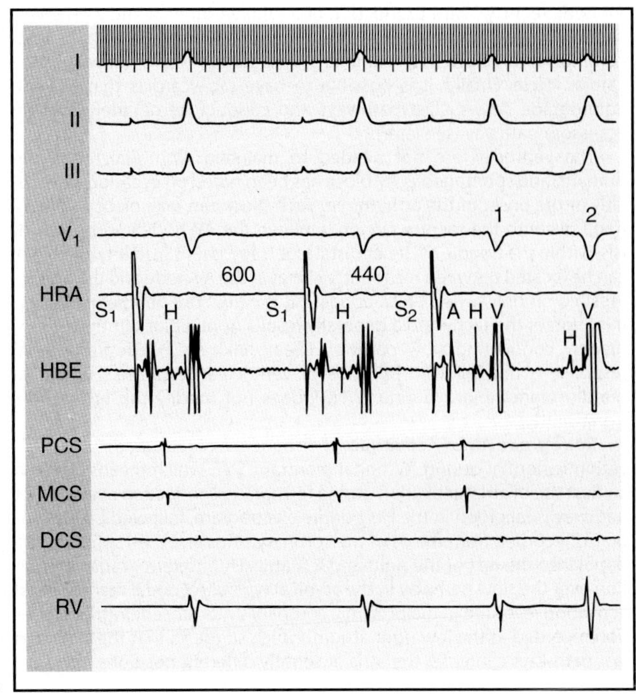

FIGURE 39-10 **A,** Initiation of AVNRT in a patient with dual AV nodal pathways. Upper and lower panels show the last two paced beats of a train of stimuli delivered to the coronary sinus at a pacing cycle length of 500 milliseconds. The results of premature atrial stimulation at an S_1-S_2 interval of 250 milliseconds on two occasions are shown. **Upper panel,** S_2 was conducted to the ventricle with an A-H interval of 170 milliseconds and was then followed by a sinus beat. **Lower panel,** S_2 was conducted with an A-H interval of 300 milliseconds and initiated AV nodal reentry. Note that the retrograde atrial activity occurs (arrow) before the onset of ventricular septal depolarization and is superimposed on the QRS complex. Retrograde atrial activity begins first in the low right atrium (HBE lead) and then progresses to the high right atrium (RA) and coronary sinus (CS) recordings. **B,** Two QRS complexes in response to a single atrial premature complex. After a basic train of S_1 stimuli at 600 milliseconds, an S_2 at 440 milliseconds is introduced. The first QRS complex in response to S_2 occurs after a short A-H interval (95 milliseconds) caused by anterograde conduction over the fast AV nodal pathway. The first QRS complex is labeled 1 (in lead V_1). The second QRS complex in response to the S_2 stimulus (labeled 2) follows a long A-H interval (430 milliseconds) caused by anterograde conduction over the slow AV nodal pathway.

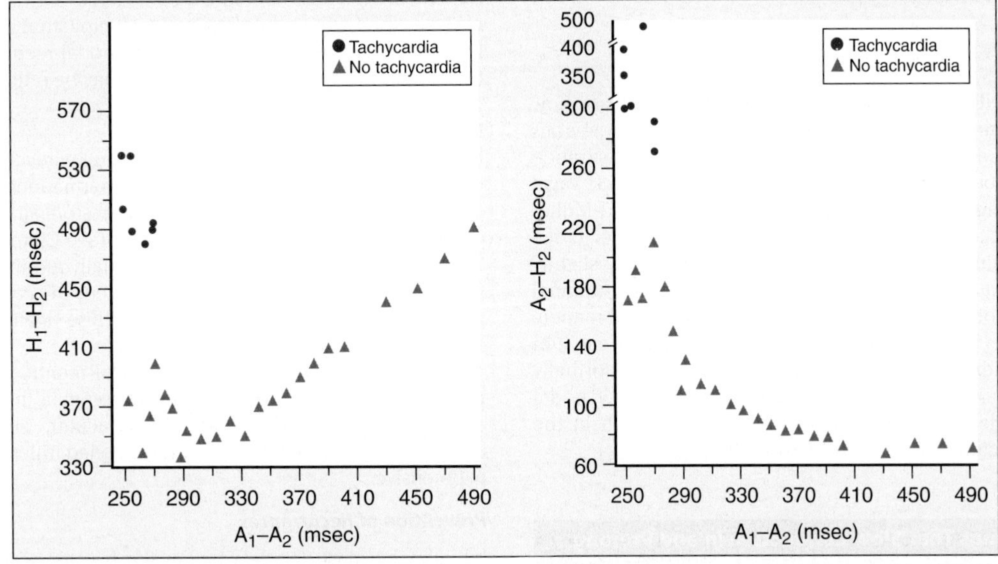

FIGURE 39-11 H_1-H_2 intervals **(left)** and A_2-H_2 intervals **(right)** at various A_1-A_2 intervals with a discontinuous AV nodal curve. At a critical A_1-A_2 interval, the H_1-H_2 and the A_2-H_2 intervals increase markedly. At the break in the curves, AVNRT is initiated.

complexes in response to one P wave provide additional evidence (see Fig. 39-10B).

Some patients with AV nodal reentry may not have discontinuous refractory period curves, and some patients who do not have AV nodal reentry can exhibit discontinuous refractory curves. In the latter patients, dual AV nodal pathways can be a benign finding. Many of these patients also exhibit discontinuous curves retrogradely. Similar mechanisms of tachycardia can occur in children. Triple AV nodal pathways can be demonstrated in occasional patients. Virtually irrefutable proof of dual AV nodal pathways is the simultaneous propagation in opposite directions of two AV nodal wave fronts without collision (see Chap. 35) or the production of two QRS complexes from one P wave (see Fig. 39-10B) or two P waves from one QRS complex.

In less than 5% to 10% of patients with AV nodal reentry, anterograde conduction proceeds over the fast pathway and retrograde conduction over the slow pathway (termed the unusual or atypical form of fast-slow

AV node reentry), with production of a long VA interval and a relatively short AV interval (generally AV/VA less than 0.75; see Fig. 39-8B). The least common form (slow-slow) exhibits a retrograde P wave midway in the cardiac cycle. Finally, it is possible to have tachycardias that use the anterograde slow or fast pathways and conduct retrogradely over an accessory pathway (see later).

The ventricles are not needed to maintain AV nodal reentry in humans, and spontaneous AV block has been noted on occasion, particularly at the onset of the arrhythmia. Such block can take place in the AV node distal to the reentry circuit, between the AV node and bundle of His, within the bundle of His, or distal to it (see Chap. 35). Rarely, the block can be located between the reentry circuit in the AV node and the atrium. Most commonly, when block appears, it is below the bundle of His. Termination of the tachycardia generally results from a block in the anterogradely conducting slow pathway (weak link), so a retrograde atrial response is not followed by a His or ventricular response. Functional bundle branch block during AVNRT does not modify the tachycardia significantly.

Retrograde Atrial Activation. The sequence of retrograde atrial activation is normal during AV nodal reentrant SVT, which means that the earliest site of atrial activation during retrograde conduction over the fast pathway is recorded in the His bundle electrogram, followed by electrograms recorded from the os of the coronary sinus and then spreading to depolarize the rest of the right and left atria. During retrograde conduction over the slow pathway in the atypical type of AV nodal reentry, atrial activation recorded in the proximal coronary sinus precedes atrial activation recorded in the low right atrium, which suggests that the slow and fast pathways can enter the atria at slightly different positions.

CLINICAL FEATURES. AV nodal reentry commonly occurs in patients who have no structural heart disease and, in the adult population, frequently presents in the third or fourth decade of life. Symptoms frequently accompany the tachycardia and range from feelings of palpitations, nervousness, and anxiety to angina, heart failure, syncope, or shock, depending on the duration and rate of the tachycardia and the presence of structural heart disease. Tachycardia can cause syncope because of the rapid ventricular rate, reduced cardiac output, and cerebral circulation or because of asystole when the tachycardia terminates as a result of tachycardia-induced depression of sinus node automaticity. The prognosis for patients without heart disease is usually good.

MANAGEMENT

Acute Attack

Management of AVNRT depends on the underlying heart disease, how well the tachycardia is tolerated, and the natural history of previous attacks in the individual patient. For some patients, rest, reassurance, and sedation may be all that are required to abort an attack. Vagal maneuvers, including carotid sinus massage, the Valsalva and Müller maneuvers, gagging, and occasionally exposure of the face to ice water, serve as the first line of therapy. These maneuvers may slightly slow the tachycardia rate, which then can speed up to the original rate after cessation of the attempt, or can terminate it. If vagal maneuvers fail, adenosine is the initial drug of choice. Digitalis, calcium antagonists, beta adrenoceptor blockers, and adenosine normally depress conduction in the anterogradely conducting slow AV nodal pathway, whereas class IA and IC drugs depress conduction in the retrogradely conducting fast pathway (**Table 39-3**).

TABLE 39-3 Drugs That Slow Conduction in and Prolong Refractoriness of Accessory Pathway and AV Node

AFFECTED TISSUE	DRUGS
Accessory pathway	Class IA
AV node	Class II Class IV Adenosine Digitalis
Both	Class IC Class III (amiodarone)

Adenosine

Adenosine (see Chap. 37), 6 to 12 mg given rapidly intravenously, is the initial drug of choice and is successful at terminating the tachycardia in about 90% of cases. Verapamil (see Chap. 37), 5 to 10 mg intravenously, or diltiazem, 0.25 to 0.39 mg/kg intravenously, terminates AV nodal reentry successfully in about 2 minutes in approximately 90% of cases and is given when simple vagal maneuvers and adenosine fail.

Digitalis

Although it may be effective for longer term management, digitalis has a slower onset of action than the agents described earlier and thus is not as useful in the acute management. If digitalis is used, digoxin can be given, 0.5 to 1 mg intravenously during a period of 10 to 15 minutes, followed by 0.25 mg every 2 to 4 hours, with a total dose of less than 1.5 mg within any 24-hour period. Oral digitalis administration to terminate an acute attack is not generally indicated. Vagal maneuvers that were previously ineffective can terminate the tachycardia after digitalis administration and should therefore be repeated.

Beta Adrenoceptor Blockers

Beta adrenoceptor blockers can be effective in treating episodes but generally are not used as first-line therapy to treat an acute episode because alternatives (adenosine, verapamil, or diltiazem) are more effective and faster acting. Beta adrenoceptor blockers must be used cautiously, if at all, in patients with heart failure, chronic lung disease, or a history of asthma because their beta adrenoceptor blocking action depresses myocardial contractility and can produce bronchospasm.

DC Cardioversion

Rarely, AVNRT results in hemodynamic compromise and is refractory to adenosine. In such cases of hemodynamic compromise, DC cardioversion may be indicated. DC shock administered to patients who have received excessive amounts of digitalis can be dangerous and result in serious postshock ventricular arrhythmias (see Chap. 37). Particularly if signs or symptoms of cardiac decompensation occur, DC electrical shock should be considered early. DC shock, synchronized to the QRS complex to avoid precipitation of ventricular fibrillation (VF), successfully terminates AV nodal reentry, with energies in the range of 10 to 50 J; higher energies may be required in some cases.

Pacing

If DC shock is contraindicated or if pacing wires are already in place (postoperatively, or if the patient has a permanent pacemaker), competitive atrial or ventricular pacing can restore sinus rhythm. In some cases, esophageal pacing can be useful (see Chap. 38).

Classes IA, IC, and III drugs are not usually required to terminate AV nodal reentry. Unless it is contraindicated, DC cardioversion should generally be attempted before use of these agents, which are more often administered to prevent recurrence.

Pressor drugs can terminate AV nodal reentry by inducing reflex vagal stimulation mediated by baroreceptors in the carotid sinus and aorta when systolic blood pressure is acutely elevated to levels of about 180 mm Hg, but they are rarely needed unless the patient is also hypotensive.

Prevention of Recurrences

Initially, one must decide whether the frequency and severity of the attacks warrant long-term therapy. If the attacks of paroxysmal tachycardia are infrequent, well tolerated, and short and either terminate spontaneously or are easily terminated by the patient, no prophylactic therapy may be necessary. If the attacks are sufficiently frequent or long to necessitate therapy, the patient can be treated with drugs empirically. If empiric testing is desirable, a long-acting calcium antagonist, a long-acting beta adrenoceptor blocker, and digitalis are reasonable initial choices. The clinical situation and potential contraindications, such as beta blockers in an asthmatic patient, usually dictate the selection. If digitalis is used, rapid oral digitalization can be accomplished in 24 to 36 hours with digoxin at an initial dose of 1 to 1.5 mg, followed by 0.25 to 0.5 mg every 6 hours, for a total dose of 2 to 3 mg. A less rapid oral regimen induces digitalization in 2 to 3 days with an initial dose of 0.75 to 1 mg, followed by 0.25 to 0.5 mg every 12 hours, for a total dose of 2 to 3 mg. Alternatively, digoxin administered as a maintenance dose of 0.125 to 0.5 mg achieves digitalization in about 1 week. If any of these drugs is ineffective when it is taken singly, combinations can be attempted.

RADIOFREQUENCY ABLATION. RF ablation is more than 95% effective at curing patients long term, with a low incidence of complications. Because it is preferable to cure the patient of the tachycardia rather than to use potentially toxic drugs to suppress it or to implant an antitachycardia device that terminates the tachycardia only after its onset (see Chap. 37), RF catheter ablation should be considered early in the management of patients with symptomatic recurrent episodes of AV node reentry. The procedure can be offered as an alternative to drug therapy in patients with frequent symptomatic episodes. For patients who do not wish to take drugs, patients who are drug intolerant, or those in whom drugs are ineffective, RF catheter ablation is the treatment of choice. It should be considered before long-term therapy with class IA, IC, or III antiarrhythmic drugs. Ablation has replaced surgery in virtually all cases and may be considered the initial treatment of choice in many symptomatic patients.

Accessory AV Pathways

Accessory pathways are fibers that connect the atrium or AV node to the ventricle outside the normal AV nodal–His-Purkinje conduction system. These pathways can conduct impulses in the forward (anterograde from atrium to ventricle) or reverse (retrograde from ventricle to atrium) direction and are potential substrates for reentrant tachycardias (AV reciprocating tachycardia). When the pathway is capable of anterograde conduction, the ventricle can be depolarized in part by the accessory pathway (outside of the normal His-Purkinje system) and produces a QRS complex that is preexcited (i.e., with a delta wave; see later). When a ventricular preexcitation is present and symptoms are compatible with tachycardia, the patient is said to have the Wolff-Parkinson-White (WPW) syndrome. In some cases, the pathways are able to conduct only in the retrograde direction; thus, they do not produce any ventricular preexcitation and are said to be concealed.

Reentry over a Concealed (Retrograde-only) Accessory Pathway

ELECTROCARDIOGRAPHIC RECOGNITION. The presence of an accessory pathway that conducts unidirectionally from the ventricle to the atrium but not in the reverse direction is not apparent by analysis of the scalar ECG during sinus rhythm because the ventricle is not preexcited (**Fig. 39-12**). Therefore, electrocardiographic manifestations of WPW syndrome are absent, and the accessory pathway is said to be concealed. Because the mechanism responsible for most tachycardias in patients who have WPW syndrome is macroreentry caused by anterograde conduction over the AV node–His bundle pathway and retrograde conduction over an accessory pathway, the accessory pathway, even if it conducts only retrogradely, can still participate in the reentrant circuit to cause an AV reciprocating tachycardia. On electrocardiographic examination, a tachycardia resulting from this mechanism can be suspected when the QRS complex is normal and the retrograde P wave occurs after completion of the QRS complex, in the ST segment, or early in the T wave (see Fig. 39-8C). Sometimes the P wave is not clearly visible and can result in depression of the ST segment; when this is seen during tachycardia, the mechanism of the arrhythmia is most often reentry involving an accessory pathway (AV reentrant tachycardia). In addition, in this setting, the ST depression that occurs only during the tachycardia (resolves with tachycardia termination) does not indicate ischemia in the absence of other evidence for ischemia (chest pain, enzyme elevation, known coronary disease).

The P wave follows the QRS complex during tachycardia because the ventricle must be activated before the propagating impulse can enter the accessory pathway and excite the atria retrogradely. Therefore, the retrograde P wave must occur after ventricular excitation, in contrast to AV nodal reentry, in which the atria are usually excited during ventricular

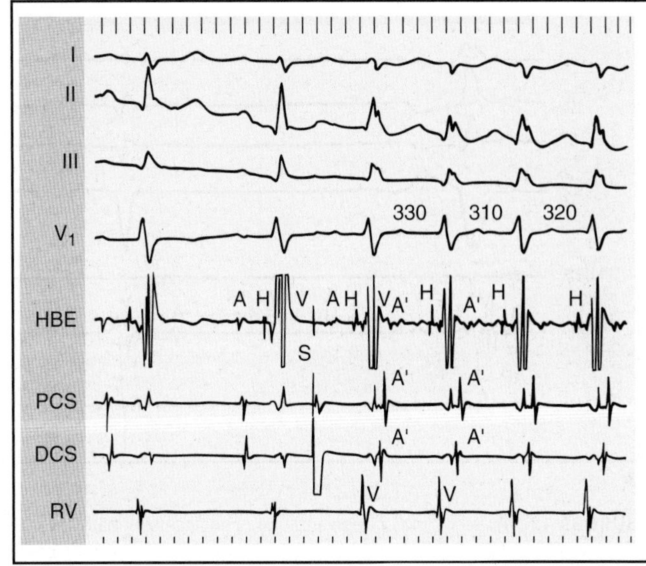

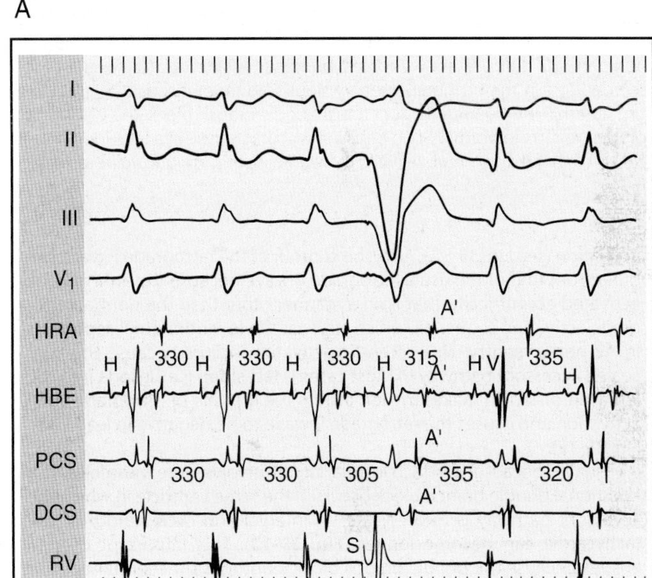

FIGURE 39-12 Atrial preexcitation during AV reciprocating tachycardia in a patient with a concealed accessory pathway. No evidence of accessory pathway conduction is present in the two sinus-initiated beats shown in **A**. A premature stimulus in the coronary sinus (S) precipitates SVT at a cycle length of approximately 330 milliseconds. The retrograde atrial activation sequence begins first in the distal coronary sinus (A′, DCS), followed by activation recorded in the proximal coronary sinus (PCS), low right atrium (HBE), and then high right atrium (not shown). The QRS complex is normal and identical to the sinus-initiated QRS complex. (The terminal portion is slightly deformed by superimposition of the retrograde atrial recording.) Note that the RP interval is short and the PR interval is long. The shortest VA interval exceeds 65 milliseconds, consistent with conduction over a retrogradely conducting AV pathway. **B,** Premature ventricular stimulation at a time when the His bundle is still refractory from anterograde activation during tachycardia shortens the A-A interval from 330 to 305 milliseconds without a change in the retrograde atrial activation sequence. (Note that no change occurs in the H-H interval when the right ventricular stimulus, S, is delivered. H-H intervals are in milliseconds in the HBE lead.) Thus, the ventricular stimulus, despite His bundle refractoriness, still reaches the atrium and produces an identical retrograde atrial activation sequence. The only way that this finding can be explained is by conduction over a retrogradely conducting accessory pathway. Therefore, the patient has a concealed accessory pathway with the WPW syndrome. HRA = high right atrium; RV = right ventricle.

CH 39

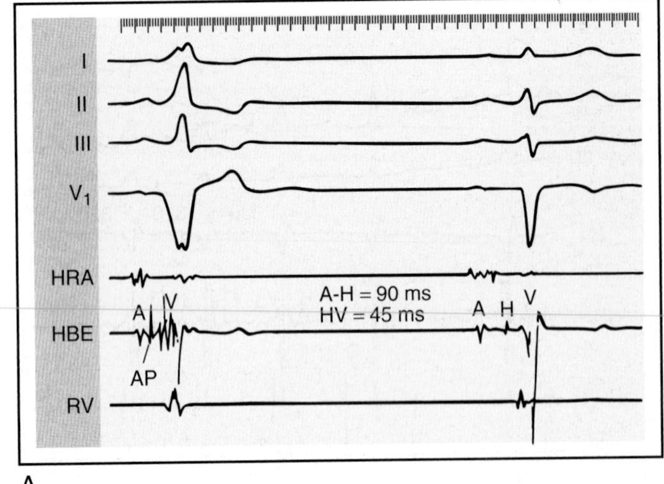

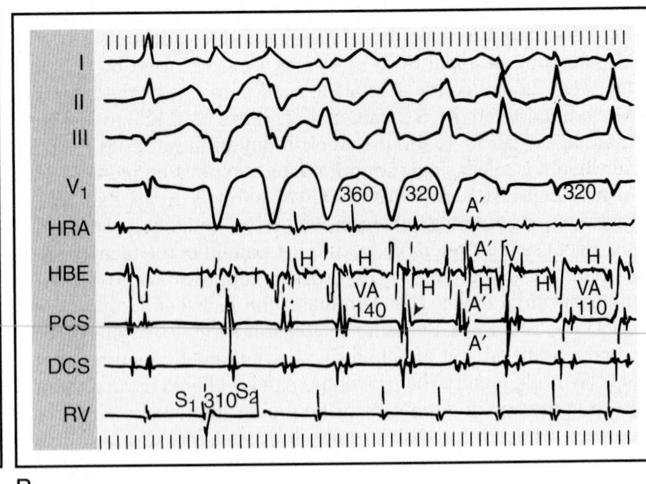

FIGURE 39-13 A, Recording of depolarization of an accessory pathway (AP) with a catheter electrode. The first QRS complex illustrates conduction over the AP. In the scalar ECG, a short PR interval and delta wave (best seen in leads I and V_1) are apparent. His bundle activation is buried within the ventricular complex. In the following complex, conduction has blocked over the AP, and a normal QRS complex results. His bundle activation clearly precedes the onset of ventricular depolarization by 45 milliseconds. The A-H interval for this complex is 90 milliseconds. **B,** Influence of functional ipsilateral bundle branch block on the VA interval during an AV reciprocating tachycardia. Partial preexcitation can be noted in the sinus-initiated complex (first complex). Two premature ventricular stimuli (S_1, S_2) initiate a sustained SVT that persists with a left bundle branch block for several complexes before finally reverting to normal. The retrograde atrial activation sequence is recorded first in the proximal coronary sinus lead (arrowhead, PCS), then in the distal coronary sinus lead (DCS) and low right atrium (HBE), and then high in the right atrium (HRA). During the functional bundle branch block, the VA interval in the PCS lead is 140 milliseconds, which shortens to 110 milliseconds when the QRS complex reverts to normal. Such behavior is characteristic of a left-sided accessory pathway with prolongation of the reentrant pathway by the functional left bundle branch block. (***A** from Prystowsky EN, Browne KF, Zipes DP: Intracardiac recording by catheter electrode of accessory pathway depolarization. J Am Coll Cardiol 1:468, 1983.*)

activation (see Fig. 39-8A). Also, the contour of the retrograde P wave can differ from that of the usual retrograde P wave because the atria may be activated eccentrically, that is, in a manner other than the normal retrograde activation sequence, which starts at the low right atrial septum as in AV nodal reentry. This eccentric activation occurs because the concealed accessory pathway in most cases is left-sided (i.e., inserts into the left atrium), which makes the left atrium the first site of retrograde atrial activation and causes the retrograde P wave to be negative in lead I (see Fig. 39-12).

Finally, because the tachycardia circuit involves the ventricles, if a functional bundle branch block occurs in the same ventricle in which the accessory pathway is located, the VA interval and cycle length of the tachycardia can become longer (**Fig. 39-13**). This important change ensues because the bundle branch block lengthens the reentrant circuit (see Preexcitation Syndrome). For example, the normal activation sequence for a reciprocating tachycardia circuit with a left-sided accessory pathway but without a functional bundle branch block progresses from the atrium to the AV node–His bundle, to the right and left ventricles, to the accessory pathway, and then to the atrium. However, during a functional left bundle branch block, for example, the tachycardia circuit travels from the atrium to the AV node–His bundle, to the right ventricle, to the septum, to the left ventricle, to the accessory pathway, and then back to the atrium. This increase in the VA interval provides definitive proof that the ventricle and accessory pathway are part of the reentry circuit. The additional time required for the impulse to travel across the septum from the right to the left ventricle before reaching the accessory pathway and atrium lengthens the VA interval, which lengthens the cycle length of the tachycardia by an equal amount, assuming that no other changes in conduction times occur within the circuit. Thus, lengthening of the tachycardia cycle length by more than 39 milliseconds during an ipsilateral functional bundle branch block is diagnostic of a free wall accessory pathway if the lengthening can be shown to be caused by VA prolongation only and not by prolongation of the H-V interval (which can develop with the appearance of a bundle branch block). In an occasional patient, the increase in cycle length because of prolongation of VA conduction can be nullified by a simultaneous decrease in the PR (A-H) interval.

The presence of an ipsilateral bundle branch block can facilitate reentry and cause an incessant AV reentrant tachycardia. A functional bundle branch block in the ventricle contralateral to the accessory pathway does not lengthen the tachycardia cycle if the H-V interval does not lengthen.

Septal Accessory Pathway

An exception to these observations occurs in a patient with a concealed septal accessory pathway. First, retrograde atrial activation is normal because it occurs retrogradely up the septum. Second, the VA interval and cycle length of the tachycardia increase 25 milliseconds or less with the development of an ipsilateral functional bundle branch block.

Vagal maneuvers, by acting predominantly on the AV node, produce a response on AV reentry similar to AV nodal reentry, and the tachycardia can transiently slow and sometimes terminate. In general, termination occurs in the anterograde direction, so the last retrograde P wave fails to conduct to the ventricle.

Electrophysiologic Features. Electrophysiologic criteria supporting the diagnosis of tachycardia involving reentry over a concealed accessory pathway include the fact that initiation of tachycardia depends on a critical degree of AV delay (necessary to allow time for the accessory pathway to recover excitability so that it can conduct retrogradely), but the delay can be in the AV node or His-Purkinje system; that is, a critical degree of A-H delay is not necessary (as it is in AV nodal reentry). On occasion, a tachycardia can start with little or no measurable lengthening of AV nodal or His-Purkinje conduction time. The AV nodal refractory period curve is smooth, in contrast to the discontinuous curve found in many patients with AV nodal reentry. Dual AV nodal pathways can occasionally be noted as a concomitant but unrelated finding.

DIAGNOSIS OF ACCESSORY PATHWAYS. Diagnosis can be made by demonstrating that during ventricular pacing, premature ventricular stimulation activates the atria before retrograde depolarization of the His bundle, thus indicating that the impulse reached the atria before it depolarized the His bundle and therefore must have traveled a different pathway. Also, if the ventricles can be stimulated prematurely during tachycardia at a time when the His bundle is refractory and the impulse still conducts to the atrium, retrograde propagation traveled to the atrium over a pathway other than the bundle of His (see Fig. 39-12B). If the PVC depolarizes the atria without lengthening the VA interval and with the same retrograde atrial activation sequence, one assumes that the stimulation site (i.e., ventricle) is within the reentrant circuit without intervening His-Purkinje or AV nodal tissue that might increase the VA interval and therefore the A-A interval. In addition, if a PVC delivered at a time when the His bundle is refractory terminates the tachycardia without activating the atria retrogradely, it most likely invaded and blocked conduction in an accessory pathway.

The VA interval (a measurement of conduction over the accessory pathway) is generally constant over a wide range of ventricular paced rates and coupling intervals of PVCs as well as during the tachycardia in the absence of aberration. Similar short VA intervals can be observed in some patients during AV nodal reentry, but if the VA conduction time or RP interval is the same during tachycardia and ventricular pacing at comparable rates, an accessory pathway is almost certainly present. The VA interval is usually less than 50% of the R-R interval. The tachycardia can be easily initiated after premature ventricular stimulation that conducts retrogradely in the accessory pathway but blocks conduction in the AV node or His bundle. Atria and ventricles are required components of the macroreentrant circuit; therefore, continuation of the tachycardia in the presence of AV or VA block excludes an accessory AV pathway as part of the reentrant circuit.

CLINICAL FEATURES. The presence of concealed accessory pathways is estimated to account for about 30% of patients with apparent SVT referred for electrophysiologic evaluation. Most of these accessory pathways are located between the left ventricle and left atrium or in the posteroseptal area, less commonly between the right ventricle and right atrium. It is important to be aware of a concealed accessory pathway as a possible cause of apparently routine SVT because the therapeutic response may at times not follow the usual guidelines. Tachycardia rates tend to be somewhat faster than those occurring in AV nodal reentry (200 beats/min), but a great deal of overlap exists between the two groups.

Syncope can occur because the rapid ventricular rate fails to provide adequate cerebral circulation or because the tachyarrhythmia depresses the sinus pacemaker and causes a period of asystole when the tachyarrhythmia terminates. Physical examination reveals an unvarying, regular ventricular rhythm, with constant intensity of the first heart sound. Jugular venous pressure can be elevated (large A wave), but the waveform generally remains constant.

MANAGEMENT. The therapeutic approach to terminate this form of tachycardia acutely is as outlined for AV nodal reentry because the AV node is a critical part of the circuit here as well. It is necessary to achieve block of a single impulse from atrium to ventricle or ventricle to atrium. In general, the most successful method is to produce a transient AV nodal block; therefore, vagal maneuvers and intravenous administration of adenosine, verapamil or diltiazem, digitalis, and beta blockers are acceptable choices. RF catheter ablation and conventional antiarrhythmic agents that prolong the activation time or refractory period in the accessory pathway need to be considered for chronic prophylactic therapy, similar to that discussed for reciprocating tachycardias associated with the preexcitation syndrome. RF catheter ablation is curative, has low risk, and should be considered early for symptomatic patients (see Chap. 37). The presence of atrial fibrillation in patients with a concealed accessory pathway should not be a greater therapeutic challenge than in patients who do not have such a pathway because anterograde AV conduction occurs only over the AV node and not over an accessory pathway. Intravenous administration of verapamil and digitalis is not contraindicated. However, under some circumstances, such as catecholamine stimulation, anterograde conduction can occur in the apparently concealed accessory pathway.

Preexcitation Syndrome

ELECTROCARDIOGRAPHIC RECOGNITION. Preexcitation, or the WPW abnormality on the ECG, occurs when the atrial impulse activates the entire ventricle or some part of it or the ventricular impulse activates the entire atrium or some part of it earlier than would be expected if the impulse traveled by way of the normal specialized conduction system only (**Fig. 39-14**). This premature activation is caused by muscle connections composed of working myocardial fibers that exist outside the specialized conducting tissue and connect the atrium and ventricle while bypassing AV nodal conduction delay. They are referred to as accessory AV pathways or connections and are responsible for the most common variety of preexcitation (incidentally noted in other species such as monkeys, dogs, and cats). The term *syndrome* is attached to this disorder when tachyarrhythmias occur as a result of the accessory pathway. Three basic features typify the electrocardiographic abnormalities of patients with the usual form of WPW conduction caused by an AV connection: (1) PR interval less than 120 milliseconds during sinus rhythm; (2) QRS complex duration exceeding 120 milliseconds with a slurred, slowly rising onset of the QRS in some leads (delta wave) and usually a normal terminal QRS portion; and (3) secondary ST-T wave changes that are generally directed in an opposite direction to the major delta and QRS vectors. Analysis of the scalar ECG can be used to localize the accessory pathway (Fig. 39-14D).[13]

In the WPW syndrome, the most common tachycardia is characterized by a normal QRS, a regular rhythm, ventricular rates of 150 to 250 beats/min (generally faster than AV nodal reentry), and sudden onset and termination, in most respects behaving like the tachycardia described for conduction over a concealed pathway (see earlier). The major difference between the two is the capacity for anterograde conduction over the accessory pathway during atrial flutter or atrial fibrillation (see later).

Variants

Various other anatomic substrates exist and provide the basis for different electrocardiographic manifestations of several variations of the preexcitation syndrome, as summarized in **Table 39-4** (**Fig. 39-15**). Fibers from the atrium to the His bundle bypassing the physiologic delay of the AV node are called atriohisian tracts (Fig. 39-15B) and are associated with a short PR interval and a normal QRS complex. Although demonstrated anatomically (see later), the electrophysiologic significance of these tracts in the genesis of tachycardias with a short PR interval and a normal QRS complex (so-called Lown-Ganong-Levine [LGL] syndrome) remains to be established. Indeed, evidence does not support the presence of a specific LGL syndrome consisting of a short PR interval, normal QRS complex, and tachycardias related to an atriohisian bypass tract.

Another variant of accessory pathway conduction is that caused by atriofascicular or nodofascicular accessory pathways. These fibers result in a unique AV conduction pattern, sometimes referred to as Mahaim conduction, characterized by the development of ventricular preexcitation (widened QRS and short H-V interval) with a progressive increase in the AV interval in response to atrial overdrive pacing, as opposed to the behavior of the usual accessory pathway, in which preexcitation occurs with short AV intervals (**Fig. 39-16**). Because the accessory pathways responsible for this conduction pattern usually insert into the right bundle branch, preexcitation generally results in a left bundle branch block pattern. This phenomenon can be caused by fibers passing from the AV node to the ventricle, called nodoventricular fibers (or nodofascicular if the insertion is into the right bundle branch rather than into ventricular muscle; see Fig. 39-15C). For nodoventricular connections, the PR interval may be normal or short, and the QRS complex is a fusion beat. This pattern of preexcitation can also result from atriofascicular accessory pathways. These fibers almost always represent a duplication of the AV node and the distal conducting system and are located in the right ventricular free wall. The apical end lies close to the lateral tricuspid annulus and conducts slowly, with AV node–like properties. After a long course, the distal portion of these fibers, which conducts rapidly, inserts into the distal right bundle branch or the apical region of the right ventricle. No preexcitation is generally apparent during sinus rhythm, but it can be exposed by premature right atrial stimulation. The usual absence of retrograde conduction in these pathways produces only an antidromic AV reentry tachycardia ("preexcited" tachycardia), characterized by anterograde conduction over the accessory pathway and retrograde conduction over the right bundle branch–His bundle–AV node, thus making the atrium a necessary part of the circuit. The preexcited tachycardia has a left bundle branch block pattern, long AV interval (because of the long conduction time over the accessory pathway), and short VA interval. A right bundle branch block can be proarrhythmic by increasing the length of the tachycardia circuit (the VA interval is prolonged because of a delay in retrograde activation of the His bundle), and the tachycardia can become incessant.

In patients who have an atriohisian tract, theoretically, the QRS complex would remain normal and the short A-H interval fixed or show very little increase during atrial pacing at more rapid rates. This response is uncommon. Rapid atrial pacing in patients who have nodoventricular or nodofascicular connections shortens the H-V interval and widens the QRS complex, with production of a left bundle branch block contour, but in contrast to the situation in patients who have an AV connection (**Fig. 39-17**), the AV interval also lengthens. In patients who have

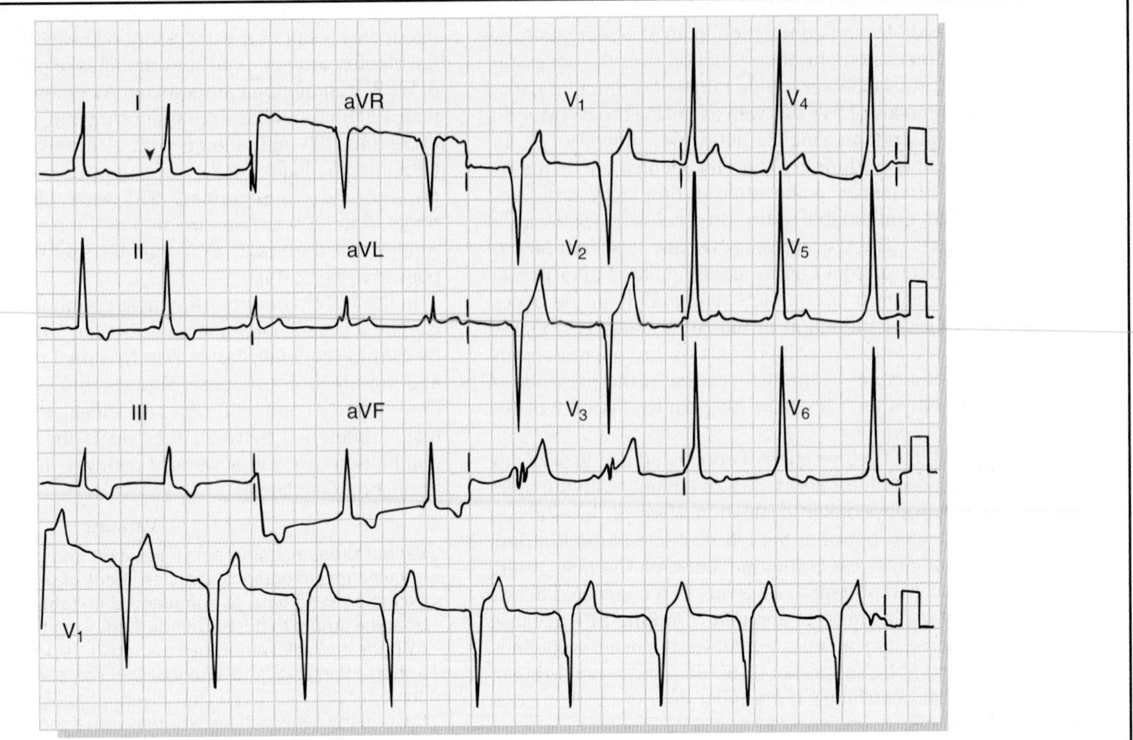

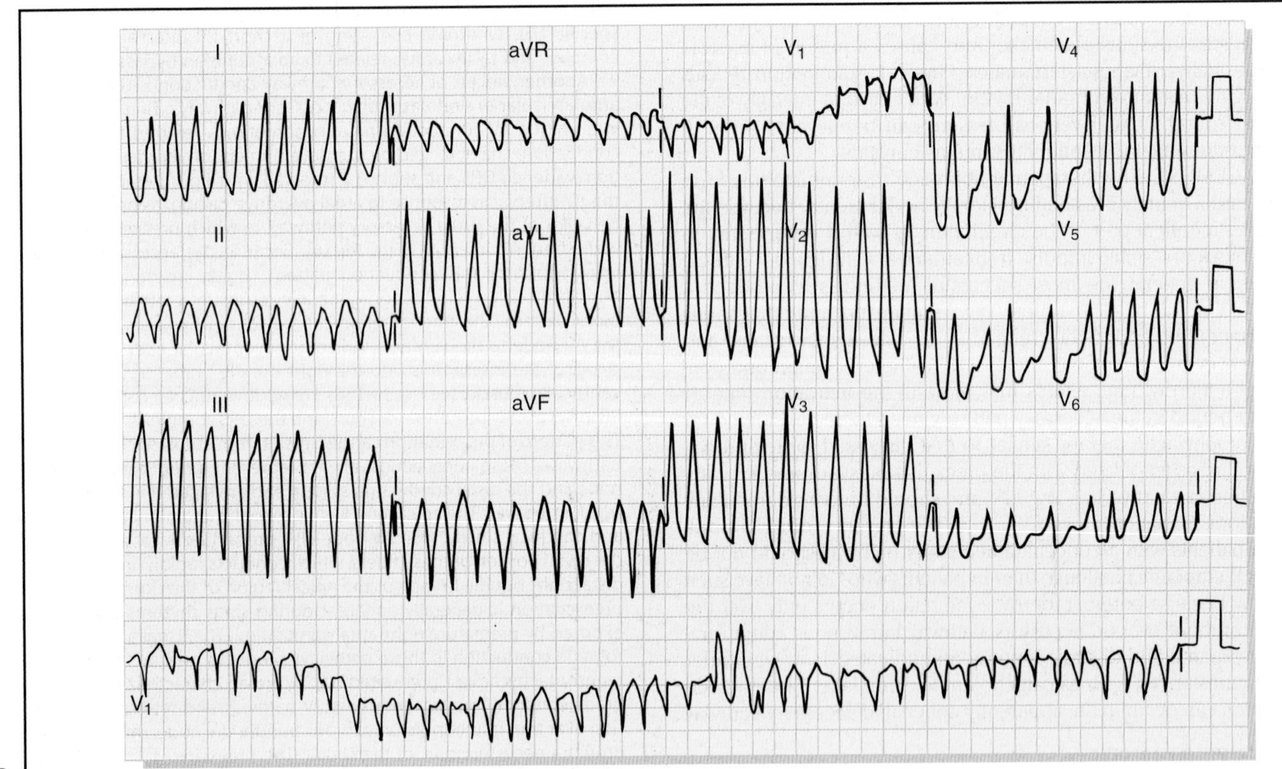

FIGURE 39-14 **A,** Right anteroseptal accessory pathway. The 12-lead ECG characteristically exhibits a normal to inferior axis. The delta wave is negative in V_1 and V_2; upright in leads I, II, aVL, and aVF; isoelectric in lead III; and negative in aVR. Location was verified at surgery. The arrowhead indicates a delta wave (lead I). **B,** Right posteroseptal accessory pathway. Negative delta waves in leads II, III, and aVF, upright in I and aVL, localize this pathway to the posteroseptal region. The negative delta wave in V_1 with sharp transition to an upright delta wave in V_2 pinpoints it to the right posteroseptal area. Atrial fibrillation is present. The location was verified at surgery.

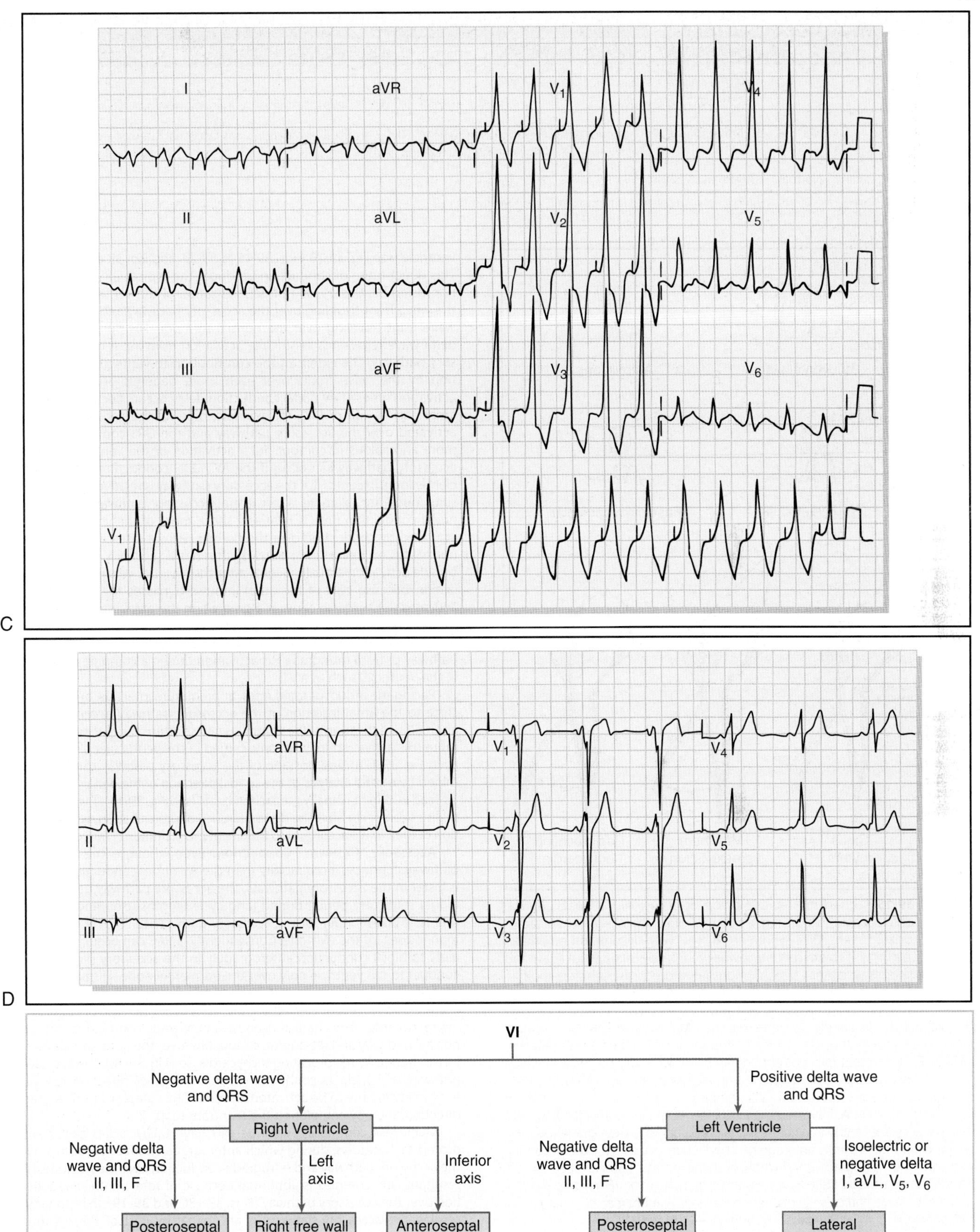

FIGURE 39-14, cont'd **C,** Left lateral accessory pathway. A positive delta wave in the anterior precordial leads and in leads II, III, and aVF, positive or isoelectric in leads I and aVL and isoelectric or negative in leads V_5 and V_6, are typical of a left lateral accessory pathway. Rapid coronary sinus pacing (450-millisecond cycle length) was used to enhance preexcitation (negative P wave in leads I, II, III, aVF, and V_3 through V_6). The location was verified at surgery. **D,** Right free wall accessory pathway. The predominantly negative delta wave in V_1 and the axis more leftward than in **A** indicate the presence of a right free wall accessory pathway. **E,** Logic diagram to determine the location of accessory pathways. Begin with analysis of V_1 to determine whether the delta wave and the QRS complex are negative or positive. That establishes the ventricle in which the accessory pathway is located. Next, determine whether the delta wave and QRS complex are negative in leads II, III, and aVF. If so, the accessory pathway is located in a posteroseptal position. If the accessory pathway is located in the right ventricle, an inferior axis indicates an anteroseptal location, whereas a left axis indicates a right free wall location. If the accessory pathway is located in the left ventricle, an isoelectric or negative delta wave and QRS complex in leads I, aVL, V_5, and V_6 indicate a left lateral (free wall) location.

CH 39

TABLE 39-4 Accessory Pathway Variants

PATHWAY TYPE	PR	QRS	TACHYCARDIA	COMMENTS
Atriohisian	Short	Normal	Unlikely	
Atriofascicular	Normal	Preexcitation (LBBB, superior axis)	Antidromic AVRT	Preexcitation with fast atrial rates or atrial extrastimuli
Nodofascicular	Normal	Preexcitation (LBBB, superior axis)	Antidromic AVRT; AVNRT with bystander activation of AP	Preexcitation with fast atrial rates or atrial extrastimuli
Fasciculoventricular	Normal	Anomalous (short H-V)	?	

AP = accessory pathway; AVNRT = atrioventricular nodal reentrant tachycardia; AVRT = atrioventricular reentrant (reciprocating) tachycardia; LBBB = left bundle branch block.

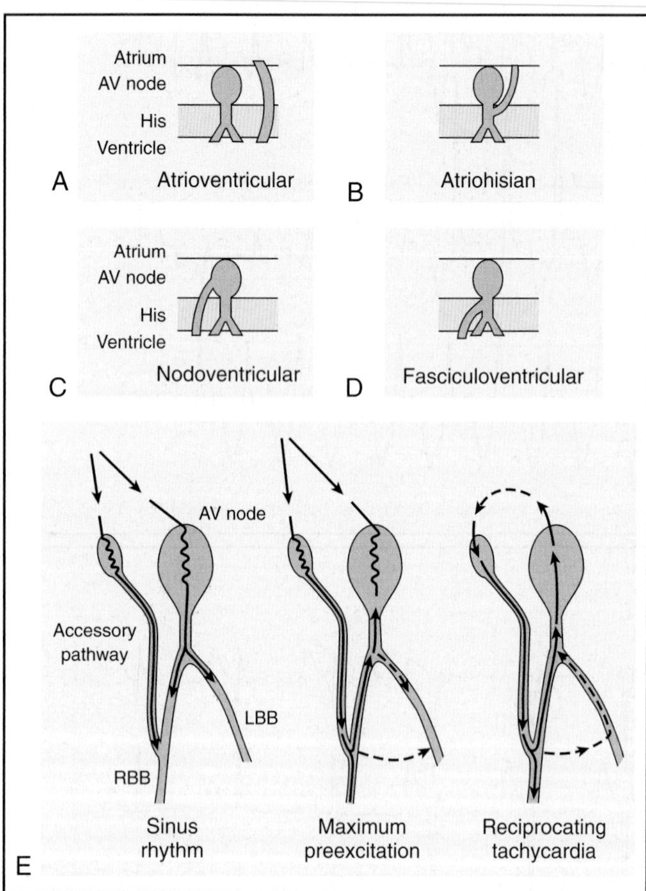

FIGURE 39-15 Schematic representation of accessory pathways. **A,** The "usual" AV accessory pathway giving rise to most clinical manifestations of tachycardia associated with WPW syndrome. **B,** The very uncommon atriohisian accessory pathway. If Lown-Ganong-Levine syndrome exists, it would have this type of anatomy, which has been demonstrated on occasion histopathologically. **C,** Nodoventricular pathways, original concept, in which anterograde conduction travels down the accessory pathway with retrograde conduction in the bundle branch–His bundle–AV node (see later). **D,** Fasciculoventricular connections, which are not thought to play an important role in the genesis of tachycardias. **E,** The current concept of nodofascicular accessory pathway, in which the accessory pathway is an AV communication with AV node–like properties. Sinus rhythm results in a fusion QRS complex, as in the usual form of WPW syndrome shown in **A**. Maximum preexcitation results in ventricular activation over the accessory pathway, and the His bundle is activated retrogradely. During reciprocating tachycardia, anterograde conduction occurs over the accessory pathway, with retrograde conduction over the normal pathway. LBBB = left bundle branch block; RBBB = right bundle branch block. *(**E** from Benditt DG, Milstein S: Nodoventricular accessory connection: A misnomer or a structural/functional spectrum? J Cardiovasc Electrophysiol 1:231, 1990.)*

fasciculoventricular connections, the H-V interval remains short and the QRS complex unchanged and anomalous during rapid atrial pacing.

Electrophysiologic Features of Preexcitation. If the accessory pathway is capable of anterograde conduction, two parallel routes of AV conduction are possible, one subject to physiologic delay over the AV node and the other passing directly without delay from the atrium to the ventricle (see Fig. 39-13, Figs. 39-15 to 39-22, and Fig. 39-e3 on website). This direct route of conduction produces the typical QRS complex that is a fusion beat as a result of depolarization of the ventricle, in part by the wave front traveling over the accessory pathway and in part by the wave front traveling over the normal AV node–His bundle route. The delta wave represents ventricular activation from input over the accessory pathway. The extent of the contribution to ventricular depolarization by the wave fronts over each route depends on their relative activation times. If AV nodal conduction delay occurs because of a rapid atrial pacing rate or PAC, for example, more of the ventricle becomes activated over the accessory pathway and the QRS complex becomes more anomalous in contour. Total activation of the ventricle over the accessory pathway can occur if the AV nodal conduction delay is sufficiently long. In contrast, if the accessory pathway is relatively far from the sinus node, for example, a left lateral accessory pathway, or if the AV nodal conduction time is relatively short, more of the ventricle can be activated by conduction over the normal pathway (see Fig. 39-17). The normal fusion beat during sinus rhythm has a short H-V interval or His bundle activation actually begins after the onset of ventricular depolarization because part of the atrial impulse bypasses the AV node and activates the ventricle early, at a time when the atrial impulse traveling the normal route just reaches the His bundle. This finding of a short or negative H-V interval occurs only during conduction over an accessory pathway or from retrograde His activation during a complex originating in the ventricle, such as a VT.

Pacing the atrium at rapid rates, at premature intervals, or from a site close to the atrial insertion of the accessory pathway accentuates the anomalous activation of the ventricles and shortens the H-V interval even more (His activation may become buried in the ventricular electrogram, as in Fig. 39-17B). The position of the accessory pathway can be determined by careful analysis of the spatial direction of the delta wave in the 12-lead ECG in maximally preexcited beats (see Fig. 39-14). T wave abnormalities can occur after the disappearance of preexcitation, with orientation of the T wave according to the site of preexcitation (T wave memory).

Accessory Pathway Conduction. Even though the accessory pathway conducts more rapidly than the AV node (conduction velocity is faster in the accessory pathway), the accessory pathway usually has a longer refractory period during long cycle lengths (e.g., sinus rhythm); that is, it takes longer for the accessory pathway to recover excitability than it does for the AV node. Consequently, a PAC can occur sufficiently early to block conduction anterogradely in the accessory pathway and conduct to the ventricle only over the normal AV node–His bundle (**Fig. 39-18A, B**). The resultant H-V interval and the QRS complex become normal. Such an event can initiate the most common type of reciprocating tachycardia, one characterized by anterograde conduction over the normal pathway and retrograde conduction over the accessory pathway (orthodromic AV reciprocating tachycardia; see Fig. 39-18). The accessory pathway, which blocks conduction in an anterograde direction, recovers excitability in time to be activated after the QRS complex in a retrograde direction, thereby completing the reentrant loop.

Much less commonly, patients can have tachycardias called antidromic tachycardias, during which anterograde conduction occurs over the accessory pathway and retrograde conduction over the AV node. The resultant QRS complex is abnormal because of total ventricular activation over the accessory pathway (Figs. 39-18C and **39-19**). In both tachycardias, the accessory pathway is an obligatory part of the reentrant circuit. In patients with bidirectional conduction over the accessory pathway, different fibers can be used anterogradely and retrogradely.

A small percentage of patients have multiple accessory pathways, often suggested by various clues on the ECG, and on occasion, tachycardia can be caused by a reentrant loop conducting anterogradely over one accessory pathway and retrogradely over the other. Fifteen percent to 20% of patients may exhibit AV nodal echoes or AV nodal reentry after interruption of the accessory pathway.

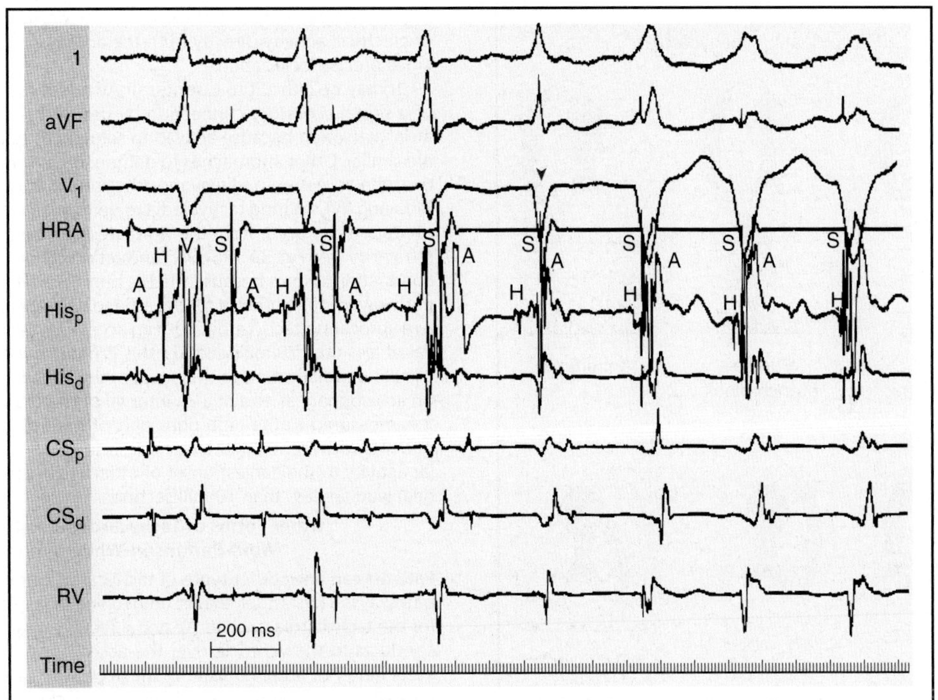

FIGURE 39-16 Development of preexcitation over an atriofascicular accessory pathway. During atrial pacing (S) on the left side of the figure, conduction occurs down the AV node as evidenced by a normal-appearing QRS complex and a normal H-V interval. The stimulus marked by the arrowhead conducts the impulse down an atriofascicular fiber, which results in a preexcited QRS, as evidenced by a widened QRS and short H-V interval.

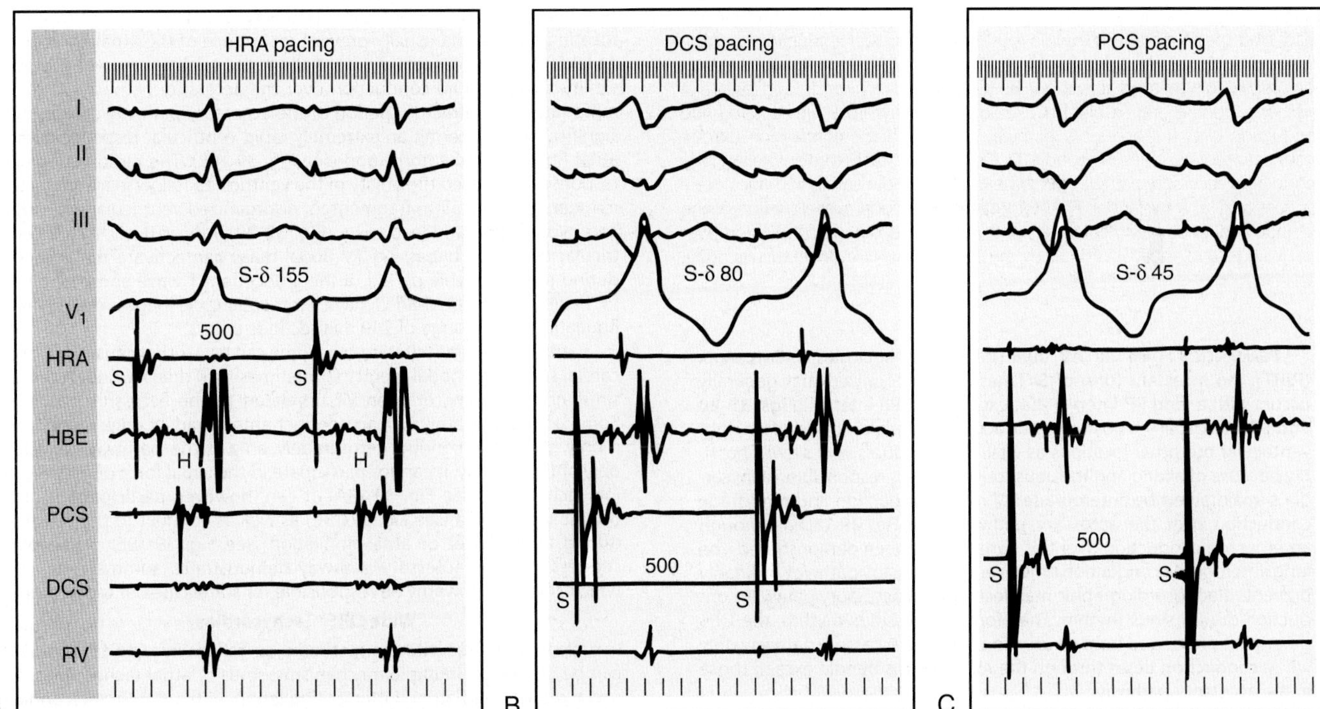

FIGURE 39-17 Atrial pacing at different atrial sites illustrating different conduction over the accessory pathway. **A,** High right atrial (HRA) pacing at a cycle length of 500 milliseconds produces anomalous activation of the ventricle (note the upright QRS complex in V_1) and a stimulus-delta interval of 155 milliseconds (S-δ 155). This interval indicates that the time from the onset of the stimulus to the beginning of the QRS complex is relatively long because the stimulus is delivered at a fairly large distance from the accessory pathway. Note that His bundle activation (H) occurs at about the onset of the QRS complex. **B,** Atrial pacing occurs through the distal coronary sinus electrode (DCS). At the same pacing cycle length, DCS pacing results in more anomalous ventricular activation and a shorter stimulus-delta interval (80 milliseconds). His bundle activation is now buried within the inscription of the ventricular electrogram in the HBE lead. **C,** Pacing from the proximal coronary sinus electrode (PCS) results in the shortest stimulus-delta interval (45 milliseconds); such an interval indicates that the pacing stimulus is being delivered very close to the atrial insertion of the accessory pathway, which is located in the left posteroseptal region of the AV groove.

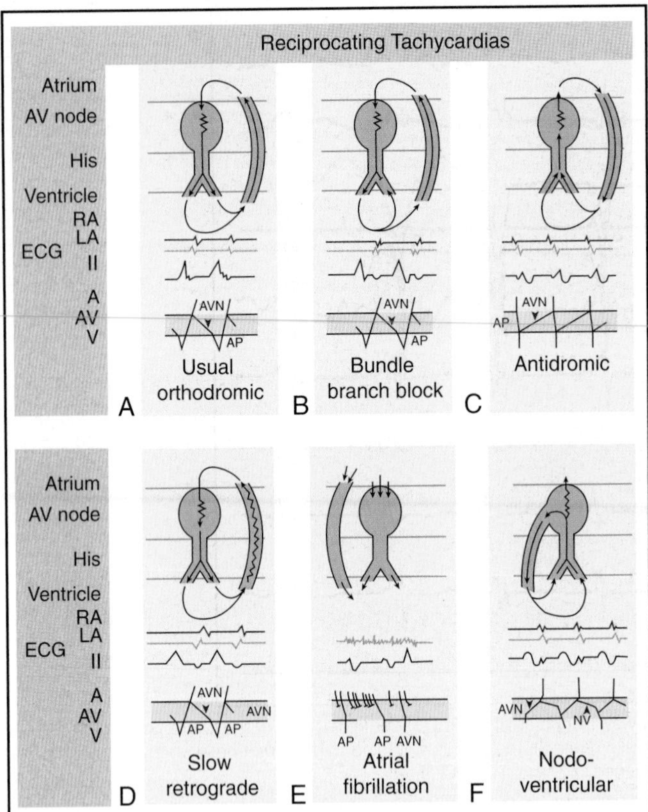

FIGURE 39-18 Schematic diagram of tachycardias associated with accessory pathways. **A,** Orthodromic tachycardia with anterograde conduction (arrowhead) over the AV node–His bundle route and retrograde conduction over the accessory pathway (left-sided for this example, as depicted by left atrial activation preceding right atrial activation). **B,** Orthodromic tachycardia and ipsilateral functional bundle branch block. **C,** Antidromic tachycardia with anterograde conduction over the accessory pathway and retrograde conduction (arrowhead) over the AV node–His bundle. **D,** Orthodromic tachycardia with a slowly conducting accessory pathway (arrowhead). **E,** Atrial fibrillation with the accessory pathway as a bystander. **F,** Anterograde conduction over a portion of the AV node and a nodoventricular (NV) pathway and retrograde conduction over the AV node (arrowheads). AP = accessory pathway; AVN = atrioventricular node.

PERMANENT FORM OF AV JUNCTIONAL RECIPROCATING TACHYCARDIA (PJRT). An incessant form of SVT has been recognized that generally occurs with a long RP interval that exceeds the PR interval (**Figs. 39-20 and 39-21**). Usually, a posteroseptal accessory pathway (most often right ventricular but other locations as well) that conducts very slowly, possibly because of a long and tortuous route, appears responsible. Tachycardia is maintained by anterograde AV nodal conduction and retrograde conduction over the accessory pathway (see Fig. 39-18D). Although anterograde conduction over this pathway has been demonstrated, the long anterograde conduction time over the accessory pathway ordinarily prevents electrocardiographic manifestations of accessory pathway conduction during sinus rhythm. Therefore, during sinus rhythm, the QRS duration is prolonged from conduction over this accessory pathway only when conduction times through the AV node–His bundle exceed those in the accessory pathway.

RECOGNITION OF ACCESSORY PATHWAYS. When retrograde atrial activation during tachycardia occurs over an accessory pathway that connects the left atrium to the left ventricle, the earliest retrograde activity is recorded from a left atrial electrode usually positioned in the coronary sinus (see Fig. 39-12). When retrograde atrial activation during tachycardia occurs over an accessory pathway that connects the right ventricle to the right atrium, the earliest retrograde atrial activity is generally recorded from a lateral right atrial electrode. Participation of a septal accessory pathway creates the earliest retrograde atrial activation in the low right portion of the atrium situated near the septum, anterior or posterior, depending on the insertion site. These mapping techniques provide an accurate assessment of the position of the accessory pathway, which can be anywhere in the AV groove except in the intervalvular trigone between the mitral valve and the aortic valve annuli. Recording of electrical activity directly from the accessory pathway obviously provides precise localization.

It may be difficult to distinguish AV nodal reentry from participation of a septal accessory connection by use of the retrograde sequence of atrial activation because activation sequences during both tachycardias are similar. Other approaches to demonstrate retrograde atrial activation over the accessory pathway must be tried and can be accomplished by inducing PVCs during tachycardia to determine whether retrograde atrial excitation can occur from the ventricle at a time when the His bundle is refractory (see Fig. 39-17B). VA conduction cannot occur over the normal conduction system because the His bundle is refractory, so an accessory pathway must be present for the atria to become excited. No patient with a reciprocating tachycardia from an accessory AV pathway has a VA interval of less than 70 milliseconds; this is measured from the onset of ventricular depolarization to the onset of the earliest atrial activity recorded on an esophageal lead or a VA interval of less than 95 milliseconds when it is measured to the high right part of the atrium. In contrast, in most patients with reentry in the AV node, intervals from the onset of ventricular activity to the earliest onset of atrial activity recorded in the esophageal lead are less than 70 milliseconds.

Other Forms of Tachycardia in Patients with Wolff-Parkinson-White Syndrome

Patients can have other types of tachycardia during which the accessory pathway is a bystander, that is, uninvolved in the mechanism responsible for the tachycardia, such as AV nodal reentry or an atrial tachycardia that conducts to the ventricle over the accessory pathway. In patients with atrial flutter or atrial fibrillation, the accessory pathway is not a requisite part of the mechanism responsible for tachycardia, and the flutter or fibrillation occurs in the atrium unrelated to the accessory pathway (see Fig. 39-18E). Propagation to the ventricle during atrial flutter or atrial fibrillation can therefore occur over the normal AV node–His bundle or accessory pathway. Patients with WPW syndrome who have atrial fibrillation almost always have inducible reciprocating tachycardias as well, which can develop into atrial fibrillation (see Fig. 39-e3 on website). In fact, interruption of the accessory pathway and elimination of AV reciprocating tachycardia usually prevent recurrence of the atrial fibrillation. Atrial fibrillation presents a potentially serious risk because of the possibility for very rapid conduction over the accessory pathway. At more rapid rates, the refractory period of the accessory pathway can shorten significantly and permit an extremely rapid ventricular response during atrial flutter or atrial fibrillation (see Fig. 39-14B). The rapid ventricular response can exceed the ability of the ventricle to follow in an organized manner; it can result in fragmented, disorganized ventricular activation and hypotension and lead to VF (**Fig. 39-22**). Alternatively, a supraventricular discharge bypassing AV nodal delay can activate the ventricle during the vulnerable period of the antecedent T wave and precipitate VF. Patients who have had VF have ventricular cycle lengths during atrial fibrillation in the range of 240 milliseconds or less.

Patients with preexcitation syndrome can have other causes of tachycardia, such as AV nodal reentry (sometimes with dual AV nodal curves), sinus nodal reentry, or even VT unrelated to the accessory pathway. Some accessory pathways can conduct anterogradely only; more commonly, pathways conduct retrogradely only. If the pathway conducts only anterogradely, it cannot participate in the usual form of reciprocating tachycardia (see Fig. 39-18A). It can, however, participate in antidromic tachycardia (see Fig. 39-18C) as well as conduct to the ventricle during atrial flutter or atrial fibrillation (see Fig. 39-18E). Some data suggest that the accessory pathway demonstrates automatic activity, which could conceivably be responsible for some cases of tachycardia.

"Wide QRS" Tachycardias

In patients with preexcitation syndrome, so-called wide QRS tachycardias can be caused by multiple mechanisms: sinus or atrial tachycardias, AV nodal reentry, and atrial flutter or fibrillation with anterograde conduction over the accessory pathway; orthodromic reciprocating tachycardia with functional or preexisting bundle branch block; antidromic reciprocating tachycardia; reciprocating tachycardia with anterograde conduction over one accessory pathway and retrograde conduction over a second one; tachycardias using nodofascicular or atriofascicular fibers; and VT.

CLINICAL FEATURES. The reported incidence of preexcitation syndrome depends in large measure on the population studied and varies from 0.1 to 3/1000 in apparently healthy subjects, with an average of about 1.5/1000. The incidence of the electrocardiographic pattern of WPW conduction in 22,500 healthy aviation personnel was 0.25%, with a prevalence of documented tachyarrhythmias of 1.8%.

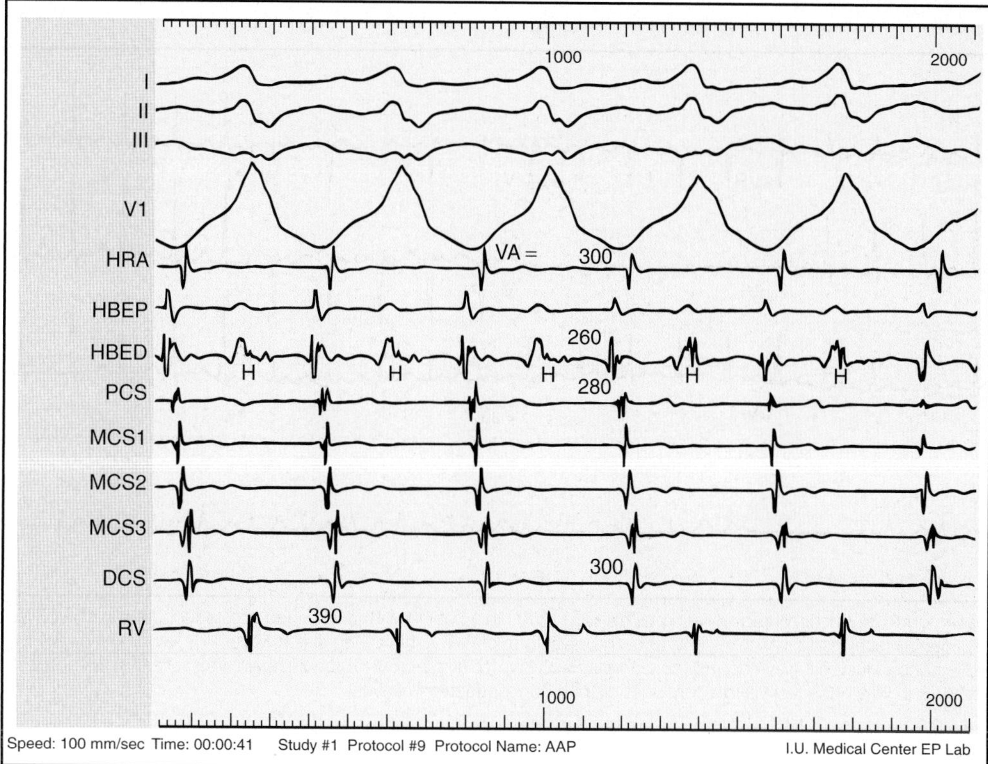

FIGURE 39-19 Antidromic AV reciprocating tachycardia. Tachycardia in this example is caused by anterograde conduction over the accessory pathway (note the abnormal QRS complex of a left posterior accessory pathway) and a normal retrograde atrial activation sequence (beginning first in the HBED lead), which is caused by retrograde conduction over the AV node. Tachycardia cycle length is 390 milliseconds, with a VA interval of 300 milliseconds measured in the high right atrial lead, 260 milliseconds in the distal His lead, and 280 milliseconds in the proximal coronary sinus lead. I, II, III, and V_1 are scalar leads. DCS = distal coronary sinus lead; HBEP and HBED leads = His bundle electrogram, proximal and distal; HRA = high right atrial electrogram; MCS1-3 = midcoronary sinus leads; PCS = proximal coronary sinus; RV = right ventricular electrogram.

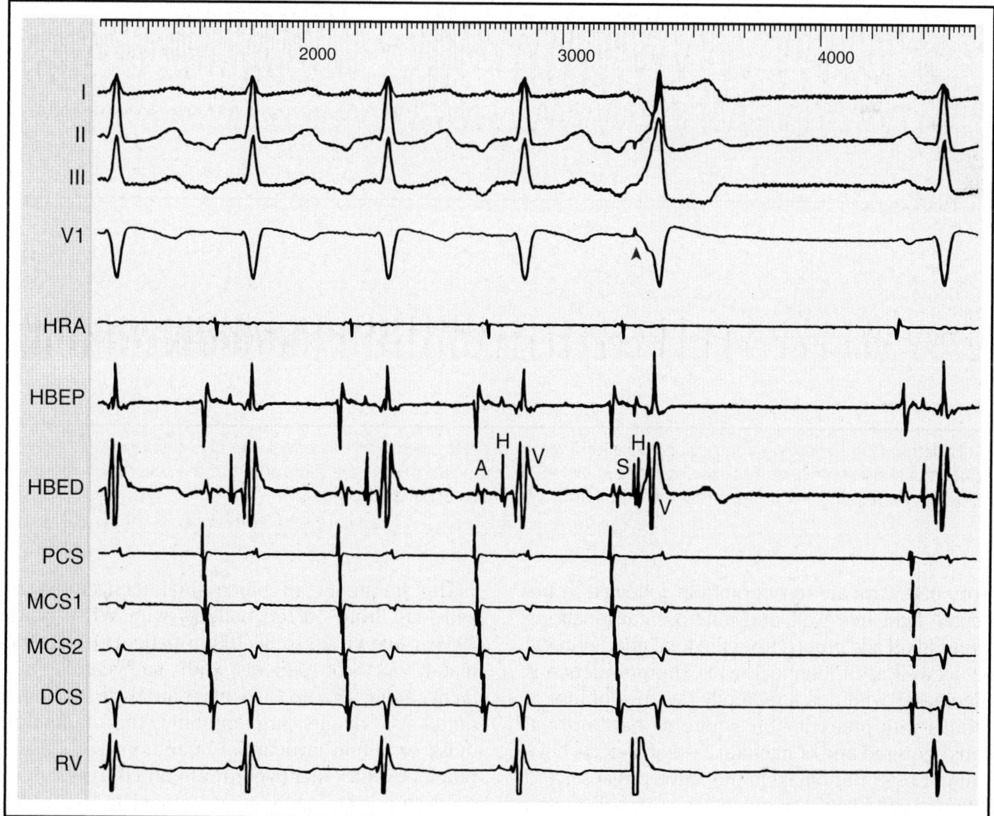

FIGURE 39-20 Termination of the permanent form of AV junctional reciprocating tachycardia (PJRT). In the left portion of this example, PJRT is present. The atrial activation sequence is indistinguishable from atypical AV nodal reentry and atrial tachycardia originating in the low right atrium. The response to premature stimulation identifies the tachycardia as PJRT. Premature ventricular stimulation (arrowhead) occurs at a time when the His bundle is refractory from depolarization during the tachycardia (second labeled H). Therefore, premature ventricular stimulation cannot enter the AV node. Furthermore, premature ventricular stimulation does not reach the atrium. Premature ventricular stimulation, however, terminates the tachycardia. This detail can be explained only by the PVC invading and blocking in a retrogradely conducting accessory pathway. I, II, III, and V_1 are scalar electrocardiographic leads. DCS = distal coronary sinus electrogram; HBEP, HBED = His bundle electrogram, proximal and distal; HRA = high right atrial electrogram; MCS1, MCS2 = midcoronary sinus electrograms; PCS = proximal coronary sinus electrogram; RV = right ventricular electrogram.

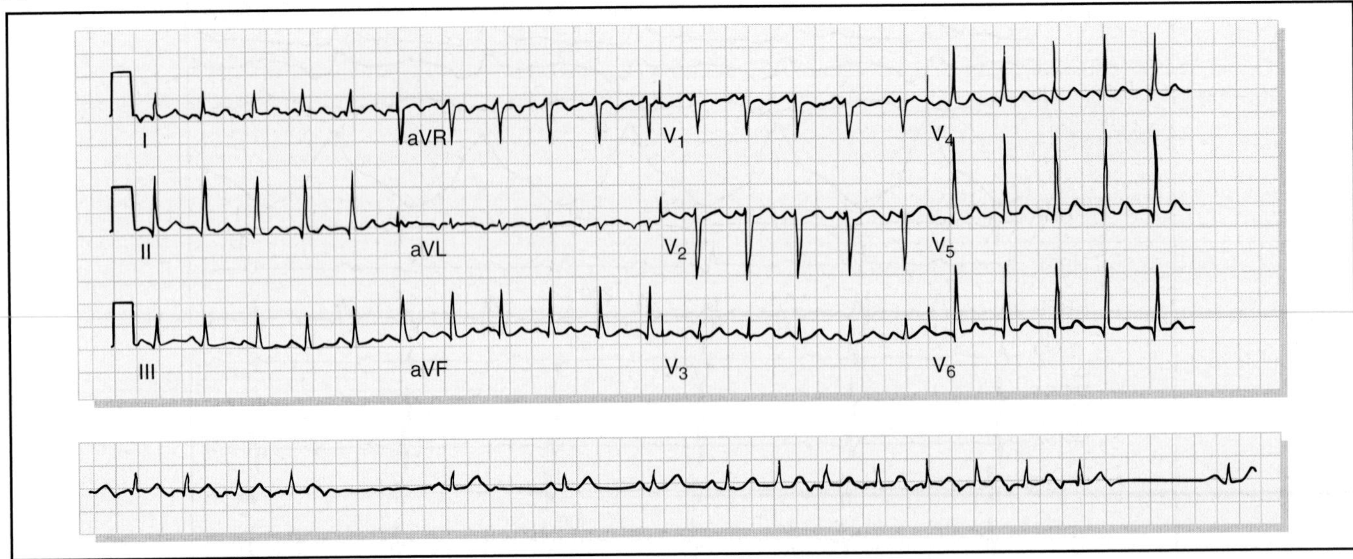

FIGURE 39-21 Permanent form of junctional reciprocating tachycardia (PJRT) in a patient with a left-sided accessory pathway. The 12-lead ECG demonstrates a long RP interval–short PR interval tachycardia, which in contrast to the usual form of PJRT exhibits negative P waves in leads I and aVL. The rhythm strips below (lead I) indicate that whenever a nonconducted P wave occurs, the tachycardia always terminates, only to begin again after several sinus beats. This pattern is in marked contrast to that in Figure 39-6, in which the tachycardia continues despite nonconducted P waves.

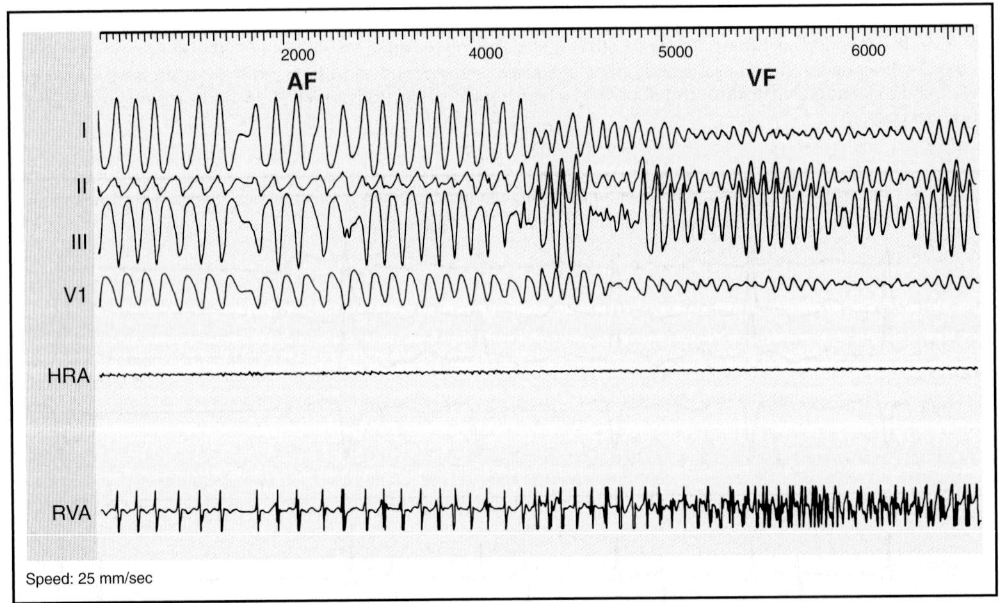

FIGURE 39-22 Atrial fibrillation (AF) becoming ventricular fibrillation (VF). In the left portion of this panel, the ECG demonstrates AF with conduction over an accessory pathway producing a rapid ventricular response, at times in excess of 390 beats/min. In the midportion of the tracing, VF can be seen to develop. I, II, III, and V_1 are scalar ECG leads. HRA = high right atrial electrogram; RVA = right ventricular apex electrogram.

Left free wall accessory pathways are most common, followed in frequency by posteroseptal, right free wall, and anteroseptal locations. WPW syndrome is found in all age groups from the fetal and neonatal periods to the elderly as well as in identical twins. The prevalence is higher in men and decreases with age, apparently because of loss of preexcitation. Most adults with preexcitation syndrome have normal hearts, although various acquired and congenital cardiac defects have been reported, including Ebstein anomaly, mitral valve prolapse, and cardiomyopathies. Patients with Ebstein anomaly (see Chap. 65) often have multiple right-sided accessory pathways, either in the posterior septum or in the posterolateral wall, with preexcitation localized to the atrialized ventricle. They often have reciprocating tachycardia, with a long VA interval and a right bundle branch block morphology.

The frequency of paroxysmal tachycardia apparently increases with age, from 10/100 patients with WPW syndrome in the 20- to 39-year age group to 36/100 in patients older than 60 years. Approximately 80% of patients with tachycardia have a reciprocating tachycardia, 15% to 30% have atrial fibrillation, and 5% have atrial flutter. VT occurs uncommonly. The anomalous complexes can mask or mimic myocardial infarction (see Chap. 54), bundle branch block, or ventricular hypertrophy, and the presence of the preexcitation syndrome can suggest an associated cardiac defect. Although the prognosis was once thought to be excellent in patients without tachycardia or an associated cardiac anomaly, data from Italy suggest that there exists some risk, albeit rare, of VF in asymptomatic children and adults with electrocardiographic evidence of preexcitation.[14] For most patients with recurrent tachycardia, the prognosis is good but sudden death occurs rarely, with an estimated frequency of 0.1%.

It is highly likely that an accessory pathway is congenital, although its manifestations can be detected in later years and appear to be acquired. Relatives of patients with preexcitation, particularly those with multiple pathways, have an increased prevalence of preexcitation, thus suggesting a hereditary mode of acquisition. Some children and adults can lose their tendency for the development of tachyarrhythmias as they grow older, possibly as a result of fibrotic or other changes at the site of the accessory pathway insertion. Pathways can lose their ability to conduct anterogradely. Tachycardia beginning in infancy can disappear but frequently recurs. Tachycardia still present after 5 years of age persists in 75% of patients, regardless of accessory pathway location. Intermittent preexcitation during sinus rhythm and abrupt loss of conduction over the accessory pathway after intravenous administration of procainamide and with exercise suggest that the refractory period of the accessory pathway is long and that the patient is not at risk for a rapid ventricular rate should atrial flutter or fibrillation develop. These approaches are relatively specific but not very sensitive, with a low positive predictive accuracy. Exceptions to these safeguards can occur; the only way to be certain of the accessory pathway's properties and propensity for rapid conduction is by an electrophysiologic study.

TREATMENT. Patients with ventricular preexcitation who have only the electrocardiographic abnormality, without tachyarrhythmias or history of palpitations, do not generally require electrophysiologic evaluation or therapy. Data from randomized trials have, however, questioned this paradigm.[14] However, for patients with frequent episodes of symptomatic tachyarrhythmia, therapy should be initiated.

Two therapeutic options exist, catheter ablation and pharmacologic therapy. Drugs are chosen to prolong conduction time or refractoriness in the AV node, the accessory pathway, or both to prevent rapid rates from occurring. If it is successful, this therapy prevents maintenance of an AV reciprocating tachycardia or a rapid ventricular response to atrial flutter or atrial fibrillation. Some drugs can suppress premature complexes that precipitate the arrhythmias.

Adenosine, verapamil, propranolol, and digitalis prolong conduction time and refractoriness in the AV node. Verapamil and propranolol do not directly affect conduction in the accessory pathway, and digitalis has had variable effects. Because digitalis has been reported to shorten refractoriness in the accessory pathway and to speed the ventricular response in some patients with atrial fibrillation, it is advisable to not use digitalis as a single drug in patients with WPW syndrome who have or may have atrial flutter or atrial fibrillation. Because atrial fibrillation can develop during the reciprocating tachycardia in many patients (see Fig. 39-e3 on website), this caveat probably applies to all patients who have tachycardia and WPW syndrome. Rather, drugs that prolong the refractory period in the accessory pathway should be used, such as classes IA and IC drugs (see Chap. 37).

Class IC drugs, amiodarone, and sotalol can affect both the AV node and the accessory pathway. Lidocaine does not generally prolong refractoriness of the accessory pathway. Verapamil and intravenous lidocaine can increase the ventricular rate during atrial fibrillation in patients with WPW syndrome. Intravenous verapamil can precipitate VF when it is given to a patient with WPW syndrome who has a rapid ventricular rate during atrial fibrillation. This effect does not seem to occur with oral verapamil. Catecholamines can expose WPW syndromes, shorten the refractory period of the accessory pathway, and reverse the effects of some antiarrhythmic drugs.

Termination of an Acute Episode

Termination of an acute episode of reciprocating tachycardia, suspected electrocardiographically from a normal QRS complex, regular R-R intervals, a rate of about 200 beats/min, and a retrograde P wave in the ST segment, should be approached similarly to AV nodal reentry. After vagal maneuvers, adenosine followed by intravenous verapamil or diltiazem is the initial treatment of choice. Atrial fibrillation can occur after drug administration, particularly adenosine, with a rapid ventricular response. An external cardioverter-defibrillator should be immediately available if necessary. For atrial flutter or fibrillation (with atrial fibrillation suspected from an anomalous QRS complex and grossly irregular R-R intervals; see Fig. 39-14B and Fig. 39-e3 on website), drugs must be used that prolong refractoriness in the accessory pathway, often coupled with drugs that prolong AV nodal refractoriness (e.g., procainamide, propranolol). In many patients, particularly those with a very rapid ventricular response and any signs of hemodynamic impairment, electrical cardioversion is the initial treatment of choice.

Prevention

For long-term therapy to prevent recurrence, RF catheter ablation of the accessory pathway has become the first-line therapy for most patients. For those patients with frequent symptomatic arrhythmias that are not fully controlled by drugs or who are drug intolerant, or for those who do not wish to take drugs, ablation is advisable. This option should be considered early in the course of treatment of a symptomatic patient because of its high success rate, low frequency of complications, and potential cost-effectiveness. Ablation is the treatment of choice in those patients with atrial fibrillation and rapid conduction over an accessory pathway. Whereas transvenous catheter ablation is generally very effective, epicardial ablations through a pericardial approach or surgical interruption of the accessory pathway can be necessary in rare cases.

Drug therapy is an alternative to ablation, but it is not always possible to predict which drugs may be most effective for an individual patient. Some drugs can actually increase the frequency of episodes of reciprocating tachycardia by prolonging the duration of anterograde and not retrograde refractory periods of the accessory pathway, thereby making it easier for a PAC to block conduction anterogradely in the accessory pathway and to initiate tachycardia. Oral administration of two drugs, such as flecainide and propranolol, to decrease conduction capability in both limbs of the reentrant circuit can be beneficial. Class IC drugs, amiodarone, and sotalol, which prolong refractoriness in both the accessory pathway and the AV node, can be effective. Depending on the clinical situation, empiric drug trials or serial electrophysiologic drug testing can be used to determine optimal drug therapy for patients with reciprocating tachycardia. For patients who have atrial fibrillation with a rapid ventricular response, induction of atrial fibrillation while the patient is receiving therapy is essential to be certain that the ventricular rate is controlled. Exercise or isoproterenol can be superimposed to be certain that the rate is controlled. Patients who have accessory pathways with very short refractory periods may be poor candidates for drug therapy because the refractory periods may be insignificantly prolonged in response to the standard agents.

Summary of Electrocardiographic Diagnosis of Supraventricular Tachycardias

Electrocardiographic clues that permit differentiation among the various SVTs are often present. P waves during tachycardia that are identical to sinus P waves and occur with a long RP interval and a short PR interval are most likely caused by sinus nodal reentry, sinus tachycardia, or an atrial tachycardia arising from the right atrium near the sinus node. Retrograde (inverted in leads II, III, and aVF) P waves generally represent reentry involving the AV junction, either AV nodal reentry or reciprocating tachycardia using a paraseptal accessory pathway. Depression of the ST segment during a narrow-complex tachycardia usually signifies AV reentrant tachycardia using an accessory pathway. Tachycardia without manifest P waves is probably caused by AV nodal reentry (retrograde P waves buried in QRS), whereas a tachycardia with an RP interval exceeding 90 milliseconds may be caused by an accessory pathway. AV dissociation or AV block during tachycardia excludes the participation of an AV accessory pathway and makes AV nodal reentry less likely. Multiple tachycardias can occur at different times in the same patient. QRS alternans, thought to be a feature of AV reciprocating tachycardia, is more likely a rapid rate–related phenomenon independent of the tachycardia mechanism. RP-PR relationships (**Table 39-5**) help differentiate SVTs. QRS voltage can increase during SVT.

TABLE 39-5 Supraventricular Tachycardias

SHORT RP–LONG PR INTERVAL	LONG RP–SHORT PR INTERVAL
AV node reentry	Atrial tachycardia
AV reentry	Sinus node reentry Atypical AV node reentry AVRT with a slowly conducting accessory pathway (e.g., PJRT)

AVRT = AV reciprocating tachycardia; PJRT = paroxysmal junctional reciprocating tachycardia.

because it is not known whether multiple foci are discharging or whether conduction of the impulse originating from one site is merely changing.

PVCs can exhibit fixed or variable coupling; that is, the interval between the normal QRS complex and the PVC can be relatively stable or variable. Fixed coupling can be caused by reentry, triggered activity (see Chap. 35), or other mechanisms. Variable coupling can be caused by parasystole, changing conduction in a reentrant circuit, or changing discharge rates of triggered activity. Usually, it is difficult to determine the precise mechanism responsible for the PVC on the basis of constant or variable coupling intervals.

Ventricular Rhythm Disturbances

Premature Ventricular Complexes

ELECTROCARDIOGRAPHIC RECOGNITION. A PVC is characterized by the premature occurrence of a QRS complex that is abnormal in shape and has a duration usually exceeding the dominant QRS complex, generally longer than 120 milliseconds. The T wave is usually large and opposite in direction to the major deflection of the QRS. The QRS complex is not preceded by a premature P wave but can be preceded by a nonconducted sinus P wave occurring at its expected time. The diagnosis of a PVC can never be made with unequivocal certainty from the scalar ECG because a supraventricular beat or rhythm can mimic the manifestations of ventricular arrhythmia (**Fig. 39-23**). Retrograde transmission to the atria from the PVC occurs fairly frequently but is often obscured by the distorted QRS complex and T wave. If the retrograde impulse discharges and resets the sinus node prematurely, it produces a pause that is not fully compensatory. More commonly, the sinus node and atria are not discharged prematurely by the retrograde impulse because interference of impulses frequently occurs at the AV junction in the form of a collision between the anterograde impulse conducted from the sinus node and the retrograde impulse conducted from the PVC. Therefore, a fully compensatory pause usually follows a PVC—the R-R interval produced by the two sinus-initiated QRS complexes on either side of the PVC equals twice the normally conducted R-R interval. The PVC may not produce any pause and may therefore be interpolated (Fig. 39-23E). Conversely, it may produce a postponed compensatory pause when an interpolated premature complex causes PR prolongation of the first postextrasystolic beat to such a degree that the P wave of the second postextrasystolic beat occurs at a very short RP interval and is therefore blocked.

Interference within the ventricle can result in ventricular fusion beats caused by simultaneous activation of the ventricle by two foci, one from the supraventricular impulse and the other from the PVC. On occasion, a fusion beat can be narrower than the dominant sinus beat, as when a right bundle branch block pattern of a PVC arising in the left ventricle fuses with the sinus-initiated left bundle branch block complex conducting through the AV junction (see Fig. 39-18) or when a sinus beat with a right bundle branch block pattern fuses with a right ventricular paced beat with a left bundle branch block pattern. Narrow PVCs have also been explained as originating at a point equidistant from each ventricle in the ventricular septum and by arising high in the fascicular system. Whether a compensatory or noncompensatory pause, retrograde atrial excitation, interpolated complex, fusion complex, or echo beat occurs (see Fig. 39-23D) is merely a function of how the AV junction conducts and the timing of the events taking place.

The term *bigeminy* refers to pairs of complexes and indicates a normal and premature complex; *trigeminy* indicates a premature complex that follows two normal beats; a premature complex that follows three normal beats is called *quadrigeminy,* and so on. Two successive PVCs are known as a pair or a couplet, whereas three successive PVCs are called a triplet. Arbitrarily, three or more successive PVCs are termed *ventricular tachycardia.* PVCs can have different contours and are often called multifocal (**Fig. 39-24**). More properly, they should be called multiform, polymorphic, or pleomorphic

CLINICAL FEATURES. The prevalence of premature complexes increases with age; they are associated with male gender and a reduced serum potassium concentration. PVCs are more frequent in the morning in patients after myocardial infarction, but this circadian variation is absent in patients with severe left ventricular (LV) dysfunction. Symptoms of palpitations or discomfort in the neck or chest can result because of the greater than normal contractile force of the postextrasystolic beat or the feeling that the heart has stopped during the long pause after the premature complex. Long runs of frequent PVCs in patients with heart disease can produce angina, hypotension, or heart failure. Frequent interpolated PVCs actually represent a doubling of the heart rate and can compromise the patient's hemodynamic status. In some patients, frequent PVCs alone can cause heart failure that is reversed when the PVC site is ablated. Activity that increases the heart rate can decrease the patient's awareness of the premature systoles or reduce their number. Exercise can increase the number of premature complexes in some patients. Premature systoles can be uncomfortable in patients who have aortic regurgitation because of the large stroke volume. Sleep is usually associated with a decrease in the frequency of ventricular arrhythmias, but some patients can experience an increase.

PVCs occur in association with various stimuli and can be produced by direct mechanical, electrical, and chemical stimulation of the myocardium. Often, they are noted in patients with LV false tendons, during infection, in ischemic or inflamed myocardium, and during hypoxia, anesthesia, or surgery. They can be provoked by various medications, electrolyte imbalance, tension states, myocardial stretch, and excessive use of tobacco, caffeine, or alcohol. Both central and peripheral autonomic stimulation have profound effects on the heart rate and can produce or suppress premature complexes.

Physical examination reveals a premature beat followed by a long pause. A fully compensatory pause can be distinguished from one that is not fully compensatory in that the former does not change the timing of the basic rhythm. The premature beat is often accompanied by a decrease in intensity of the heart sounds, often with auscultation of just the first heart sound, which can be sharp and snapping, and a decreased or absent peripheral (e.g., radial) pulse. The relationship of atrial to ventricular systole determines the presence of normal *a* waves or giant *a* waves in the jugular venous pulse, and the length of the PR interval determines the intensity of the first heart sound. The second heart sound can be abnormally split, depending on the origin of the ventricular complex.

The importance of PVCs depends on the clinical setting. In the absence of underlying heart disease, the presence of PVCs usually has no impact on longevity or limitation of activity; antiarrhythmic drugs are not indicated. Patients should be reassured if they are symptomatic (see Chap. 37).

In patients suffering from acute myocardial infarction, PVCs once considered to presage the onset of VF, such as those occurring close to the preceding T wave, more than five or six per minute, bigeminal or multiform complexes, or those occurring in salvoes of two or three or more, do not occur in about 50% of patients in whom VF develops, and VF does not develop in about 50% of patients who have these PVCs. Thus, these PVCs are not particularly helpful prognostically. The presence of 1 to 10 or more ventricular extrasystoles per hour can identify patients at increased risk for VT or sudden cardiac death after myocardial infarction but is similarly nonspecific.

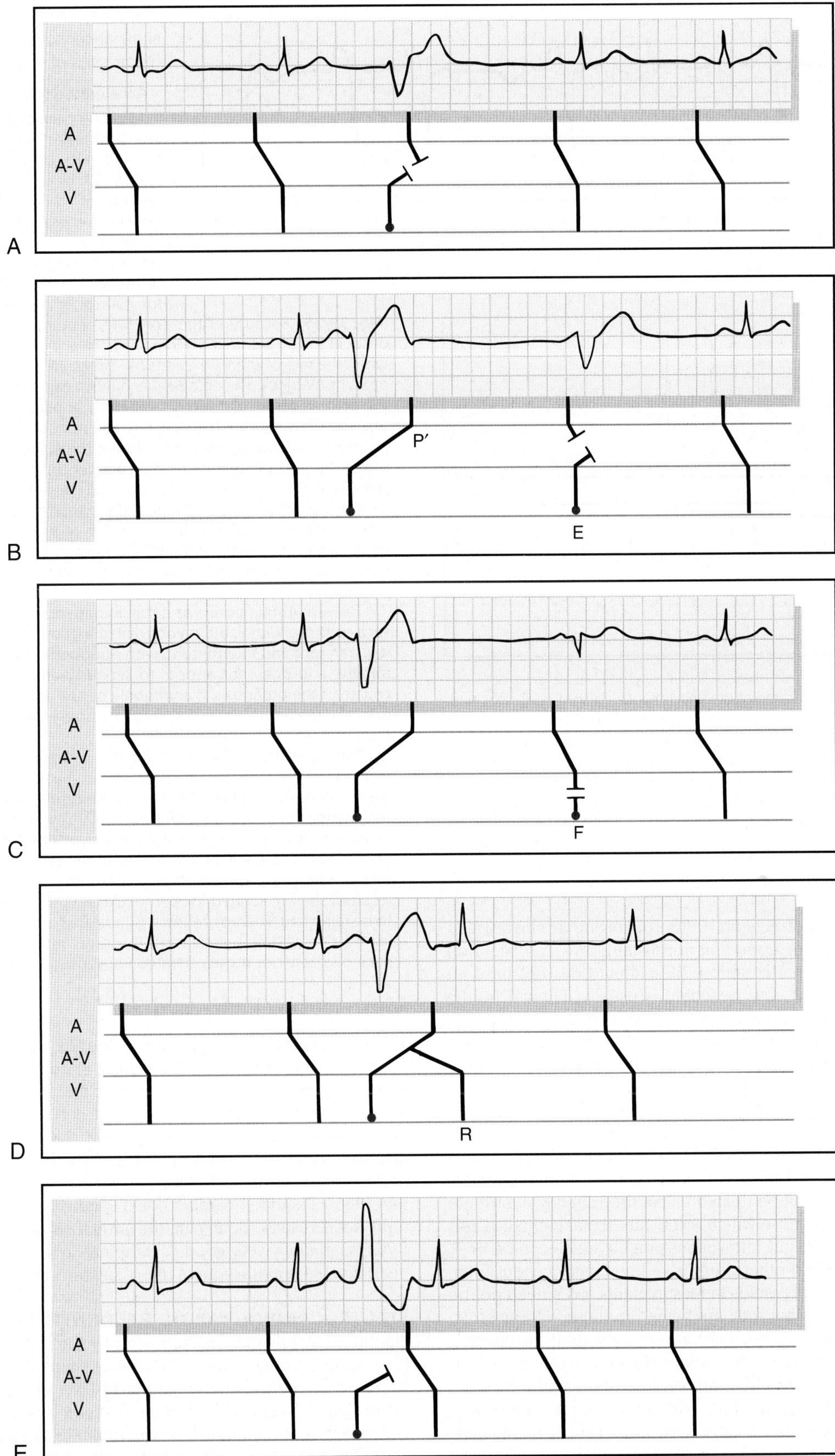

FIGURE 39-23 PVCs. **A** to **D** were recorded in the same patient. **A,** A late PVC results in a compensatory pause. **B,** A slower sinus rate and a slightly earlier PVC result in retrograde atrial excitation (P′). The sinus node is reset, followed by a noncompensatory pause. Before the sinus-initiated P wave that follows the retrograde P wave can conduct the impulse to the ventricle, ventricular escape (E) occurs. **C,** Events are similar to those in **B** except that a ventricular fusion beat (F) results after the PVC because of a slightly faster sinus rate. **D,** The impulse propagating retrogradely to the atrium reverses its direction after a delay and returns to reexcite the ventricles (R) to produce a ventricular echo. **E,** An interpolated PVC is followed by a slightly prolonged PR interval of the sinus-initiated beat. Lead II. ECG is shown. Red circles indicate origin of PVCs.

CH 39

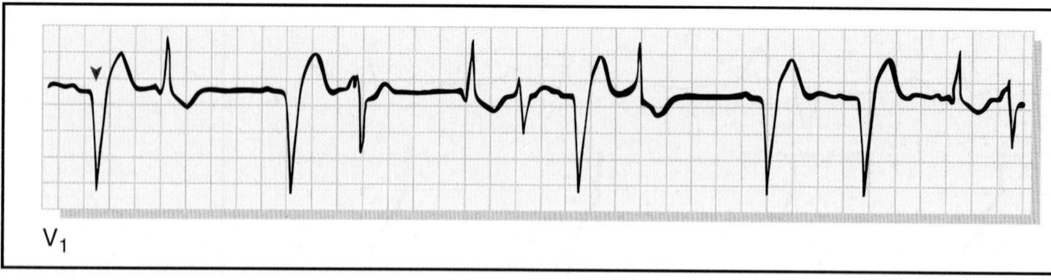

FIGURE 39-24 Multiform PVCs. The normally conducted QRS complexes exhibit a left bundle branch block contour (arrowhead) and are followed by PVCs with three different morphologies.

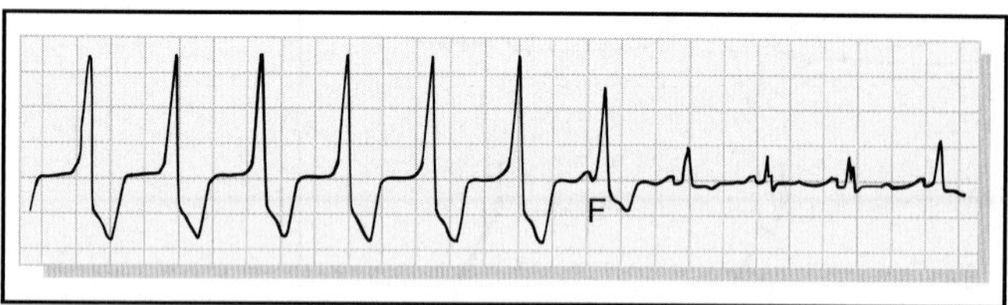

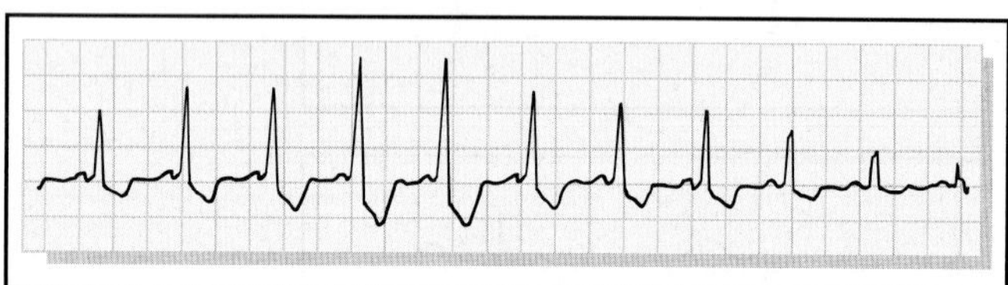

FIGURE 39-25 Accelerated idioventricular rhythm. In this continuous monitor lead recording, an accelerated idioventricular rhythm competes with the sinus rhythm. Wide QRS complexes at a rate of 90 beats/min fuse (F) with the sinus rhythm, which takes control briefly, generates the narrow QRS complexes, and then yields once again to the accelerated idioventricular rhythm as the P waves move "in and out" of the QRS complex. This example of isorhythmic AV dissociation may be caused by hemodynamic modulation of the sinus rate via the autonomic nervous system.

MANAGEMENT. In most patients, PVCs (occurring as single PVCs, bigeminy, or trigeminy but excluding nonsustained VT; see later) do not need to be treated, particularly if the patient does not have an acute coronary syndrome, and treatment is usually dictated by the presence of symptoms attributable to the PVCs. Both fast and slow heart rates can provoke the development of PVCs. PVCs accompanying slow ventricular rates can be abolished by increasing the basic rate with atropine or isoproterenol or by pacing, whereas slowing of the heart rate in some patients with sinus tachycardia can eradicate PVCs. In hospitalized patients, intravenous lidocaine (see Chap. 37) is generally the initial treatment of choice to suppress PVCs but is rarely indicated. Frequent PVCs, even in the setting of an acute myocardial infarction, need not be treated unless they directly contribute to hemodynamic compromise, which is very rare. If maximum dosages of lidocaine are unsuccessful, intravenous procainamide can be tried. Propranolol is suggested if other drugs have been unsuccessful. Intravenous magnesium can be useful. In most patients, PVCs need not be treated, and reassurance that they are benign in those without structural heart disease often is sufficient for most patients. If treatment is warranted (dictated by symptoms), various class I, II, and III drugs can be useful. Beta blockers are often the first line of therapy. If they are ineffective, class IC drugs seem particularly successful in suppressing PVCs, but flecainide and moricizine have been shown to increase mortality in patients treated after myocardial infarction and thus should be reserved for patients without coronary artery disease or LV dysfunction. Amiodarone can be effective, but because of its side effects, it should be reserved for highly symptomatic patients and those with structural heart disease. For patients with significant symptoms, particularly those with reduced cardiac function, RF ablation of the PVC focus can be effective and improve cardiac performance. Low levels of serum potassium and magnesium are associated with higher prevalence rates of ventricular arrhythmias.

Accelerated Idioventricular Rhythm

ELECTROCARDIOGRAPHIC RECOGNITION. The ventricular rate, commonly between 60 and 110 beats/min, usually hovers within 10 beats of the sinus rate, so control of the cardiac rhythm shifts between these two competing pacemaker sites. Consequently, fusion beats often occur at the onset and termination of the arrhythmia as the pacemakers vie for control of ventricular depolarization (**Fig. 39-25**). Because of the slow rate, capture beats are common. The onset of this arrhythmia is generally gradual (nonparoxysmal) and occurs when the rate of the VT exceeds the sinus rate because of sinus slowing or SA or AV block. The ectopic mechanism can also begin after a PVC, or the ectopic ventricular focus can simply accelerate sufficiently to overtake the sinus rhythm. The slow rate and nonparoxysmal onset avoid the problems initiated by excitation during the vulnerable period, and consequently precipitation of more rapid ventricular arrhythmias is rarely seen. Termination of the rhythm generally occurs gradually as the dominant sinus rhythm accelerates or as the ectopic ventricular rhythm decelerates. The ventricular rhythm can be regular or irregular and can occasionally show sudden doubling, which suggests the presence of exit block. Many characteristics incriminate enhanced automaticity as the responsible mechanism.

The arrhythmia occurs as a rule in patients who have heart disease, such as those with acute myocardial infarction or with digitalis toxicity. It is transient and intermittent, with episodes lasting a few seconds to a minute, and does not appear to seriously affect the patient's clinical course or the prognosis. It commonly occurs at the moment of reperfusion of a previously occluded coronary artery and can be found during resuscitation.

MANAGEMENT. Suppressive therapy is rarely necessary because the ventricular rate is generally less than 100 beats/min, but such therapy may be considered when AV dissociation results in loss of sequential AV contraction, an accelerated idioventricular rhythm occurs together with a more rapid VT, an accelerated idioventricular rhythm begins with a PVC discharging in the vulnerable period of the preceding T wave, the ventricular rate is too rapid and produces symptoms, or VF develops as a result of the accelerated idioventricular rhythm. This last event appears to be fairly rare. Therapy, when it is indicated, should be as noted earlier for VT. Often, simply increasing the sinus rate with atropine or atrial pacing suppresses the accelerated idioventricular rhythm.

Ventricular Tachycardia

VT arises distal to the bifurcation of the His bundle in the specialized conduction system, ventricular muscle, or combinations of both tissue types. Mechanisms include disorders of impulse formation (enhanced automaticity or triggered activity) and conduction (reentry) considered earlier (see Chap. 35). In general, the specific type, prognosis, and management of VT depend on whether underlying structural heart disease is present. With the exception of those patients with inherited VT–sudden cardiac death syndromes (see Chap. 9), if structural heart disease is absent, the prognosis in patients with VT and PVCs is generally very good,[15-18] whereas in the presence of structural heart disease, the subsequent risk of sudden cardiac death is increased.

ELECTROCARDIOGRAPHIC RECOGNITION. The electrocardiographic diagnosis of VT is suggested by the occurrence of a series of three or more consecutive, abnormally shaped PVCs whose duration exceeds 120 milliseconds, with the ST-T vector pointing opposite the major QRS deflection. The R-R interval can be exceedingly regular or can vary. Patients can have VTs with multiple morphologies originating at the same or closely adjacent sites, probably with different exit paths. Others have multiple sites of origin. Atrial activity can be independent of ventricular activity, or the atria can be depolarized by the ventricles retrogradely (VA association). Depending on the particular type of VT, rates range from 70 to 250 beats/min, and the onset can be paroxysmal (sudden) or nonparoxysmal. QRS contours during the VT can be unchanging (uniform, monomorphic) and can vary randomly

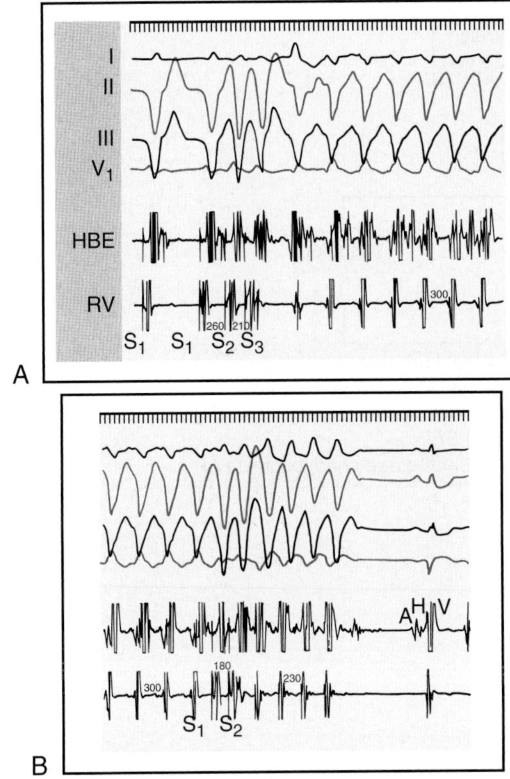

FIGURE 39-26 Initiation and termination of VT by means of programmed ventricular stimulation. The last two ventricular paced beats at a cycle length of 600 milliseconds are shown in **A**. A premature stimulus (S_2) at an S_1-S_2 interval of 260 milliseconds and another premature stimulus (S_3) at a cycle length of 210 milliseconds initiate a sustained monomorphic VT at a cycle length of 300 milliseconds. **B,** Two premature ventricular stimuli (S_1-S_2) create an unstable VT that persists for several beats at a shorter cycle length (230 milliseconds) and then terminates, followed by sinus rhythm. HBE = His bundle electrogram; RV = right ventricle.

(multiform, polymorphic, or pleomorphic) in a more or less repetitive manner (torsades de pointes), in alternate complexes (bidirectional VT), or in a stable but changing contour (i.e., right bundle branch contour changing to a left bundle branch contour). VT can be sustained, defined arbitrarily as lasting longer than 30 seconds or requiring termination because of hemodynamic collapse, or nonsustained, when it stops spontaneously in less than 30 seconds. Most commonly, very premature stimulation is required to initiate VT electrically, whereas late coupled ventricular complexes usually initiate its spontaneous onset (**Fig. 39-26**).

The electrocardiographic distinction between SVT with aberration and VT can be difficult at times because features of both arrhythmias overlap, and under certain circumstances, SVT can mimic the criteria established for VT.[5] Ventricular complexes with an abnormal and prolonged configuration indicate only that conduction through the ventricle is abnormal, and such complexes can occur in supraventricular rhythms as a result of preexisting bundle branch block, aberrant conduction during incomplete recovery of repolarization, conduction over accessory pathways, and several other conditions. These complexes do not necessarily indicate the origin of impulse formation or the reason for the abnormal conduction. Conversely, ectopic beats originating in the ventricle can uncommonly have a fairly normal duration and shape. However, VT is the most common cause of tachycardia with a wide QRS complex. A past history of myocardial infarction makes the diagnosis even more likely.

During the course of a tachycardia characterized by wide, abnormal QRS complexes, the presence of fusion beats and capture beats provides maximum support for the diagnosis of VT but occurs relatively infrequently (**Fig. 39-27**; see Table 39-2). Fusion beats indicate activation of the ventricle from two different foci, with the implication that one of the foci had a ventricular origin. Capture of the ventricle by the supraventricular rhythm with a normal configuration of the captured QRS complex at an interval shorter than the tachycardia in question indicates that the impulse has a supraventricular origin and thus excludes a supraventricular origin of the tachycardia. AV dissociation has long been considered a hallmark of VT. However, retrograde VA conduction to the atria from ventricular beats occurs in at least 25% of patients, and therefore VT may not exhibit AV dissociation. AV dissociation can occur uncommonly during SVTs. Even if a P wave appears to be related to each QRS complex, it is at times difficult to determine whether the P wave is conducted anterogradely to the next QRS complex (i.e., SVT with aberrancy and a long PR interval) or retrogradely from the preceding QRS complex (i.e., a VT). As a general rule, however, AV dissociation during tachycardia with a wide QRS is strong presumptive evidence that the tachycardia is of ventricular origin.

Differentiation Between Ventricular and Supraventricular Tachycardia

Although fusion and capture beats and AV dissociation provide the strongest electrocardiographic evidence for differentiation of VT from SVT with aberrant conduction, these features are not always present. Therefore, other clues from the ECG may be required to help with this differentiation. Features characterizing supraventricular arrhythmia with aberrancy include the following: (1) consistent onset of the tachycardia with a premature P wave; (2) very short RP interval (0.1 second), often requiring an esophageal recording to visualize the P waves; (3) QRS configuration the same as that occurring from known supraventricular conduction at similar rates; (4) P wave and QRS rate and rhythm linked to suggest that ventricular activation depends on atrial discharge (e.g., an AV Wenckebach block); and (5) slowing or termination of the tachycardia by vagal maneuvers.[19]

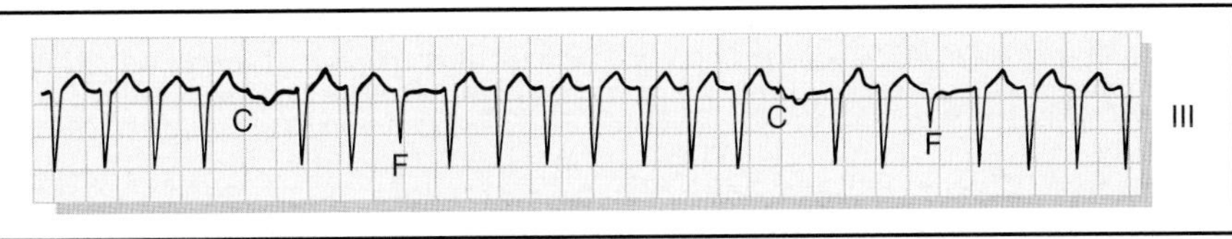

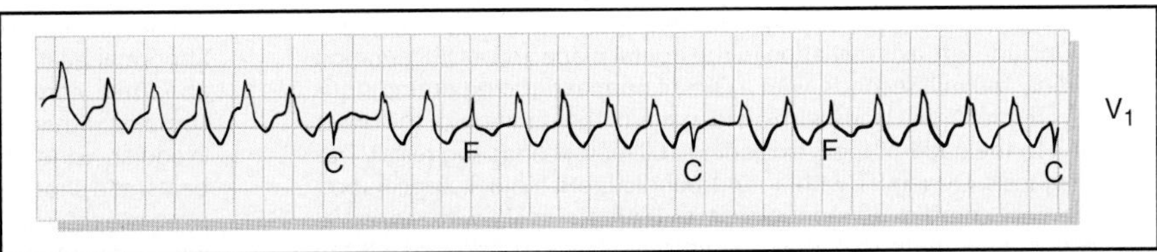

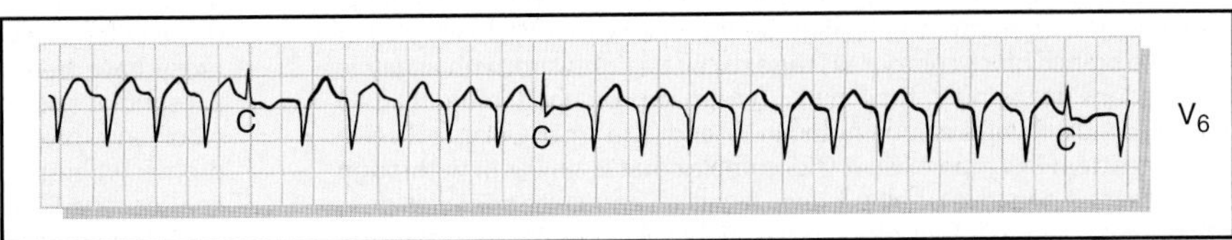

FIGURE 39-27 Fusion and capture beats during VT. The QRS complex is prolonged, and the R-R interval is regular except for occasional capture beats (C) that have a normal contour and are slightly premature. Complexes intermediate in contour represent fusion beats (F). Thus, even though atrial activity is not clearly apparent, AV dissociation is present during VT and produces intermittent capture and fusion beats.

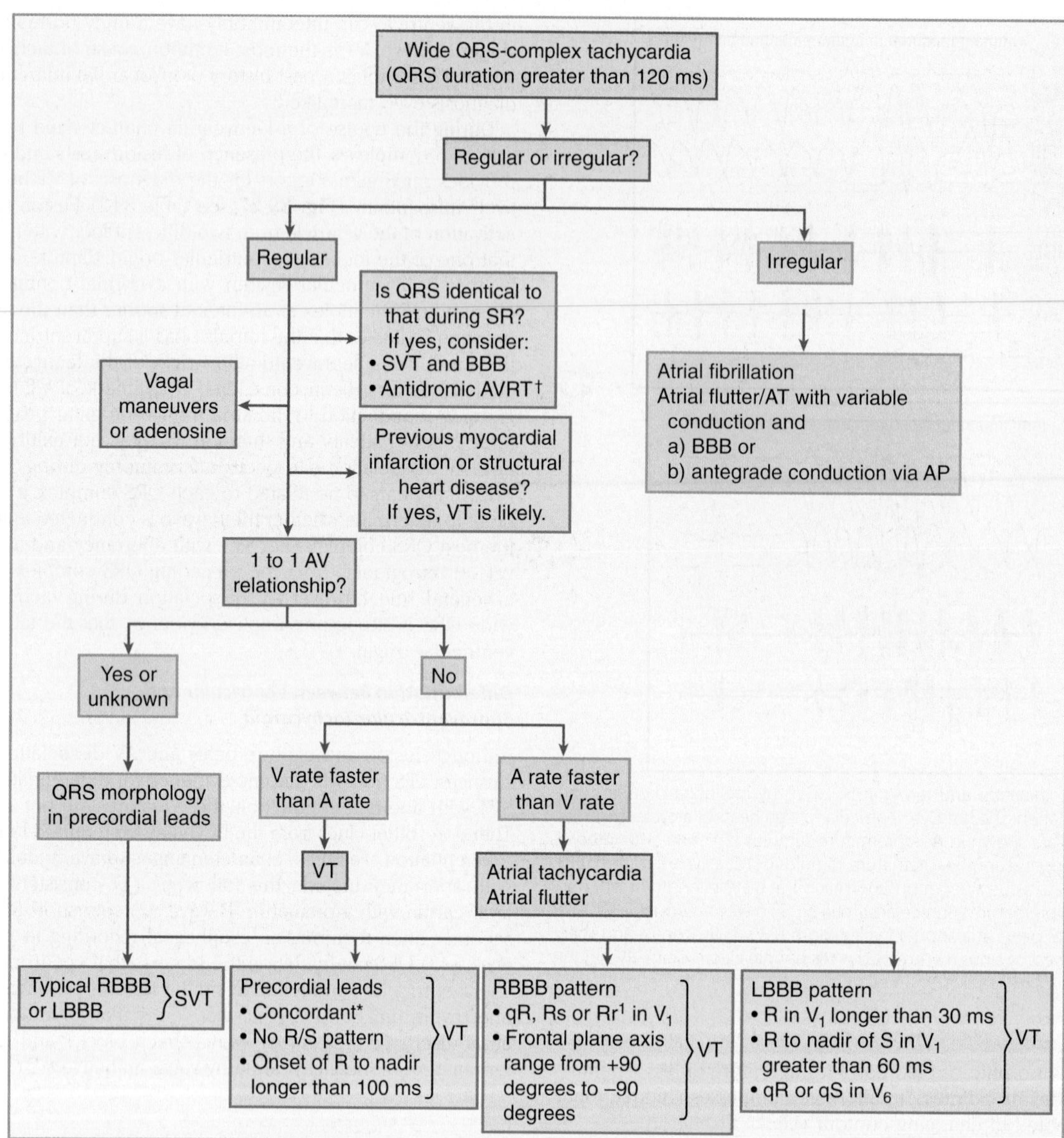

FIGURE 39-28 Algorithm for diagnosis of a wide QRS tachycardia. AP = accessory pathway; AT = atrial tachycardia; AVRT = AV reentrant tachycardia; LBBB = left bundle branch block; RBBB = right bundle branch block; SVT = supraventricular tachycardia; VT = ventricular tachycardia. *(From Blomstrom-Lundqvist C, Scheinman MM, Aliot EM, et al: ACC/AHA/ESC guidelines for the management of patients with supraventricular arrhythmias—executive summary: A report of the American College of Cardiology/American Heart Association Task Force on Practice Guidelines and the European Society of Cardiology Committee for Practice Guidelines [Writing Committee to Develop Guidelines for the Management of Patients With Supraventricular Arrhythmias]. Circulation 108:1871, 2003.)*

Analysis of specific QRS contours can also be helpful in diagnosis of VT and localization of its site of origin. For example, QRS contours suggesting VT include left-axis deviation in the frontal plane and a QRS duration exceeding 140 milliseconds, with a QRS of normal duration during sinus rhythm. In precordial leads with an RS pattern, the duration of the onset of the R to the nadir of the S exceeding 100 milliseconds suggests VT as the diagnosis. During VT with a right bundle branch block appearance, (1) the QRS complex is monophasic or biphasic in V_1, with an initial deflection different from that of the sinus-initiated QRS complex, (2) the amplitude of the R wave in V_1 exceeds the R′, and (3) a small R and large S wave or a QS pattern in V_6 may be present. With a VT having a left bundle branch block contour, (1) the axis can be rightward, with negative deflections deeper in V_1 than in V_6, (2) a broad prolonged (more than 40 milliseconds) R wave can be noted in V_1, and (3) a small Q–large R wave or QS pattern in V_6 can exist. A QRS complex that is similar in V_1 through V_6, either all negative or all positive, favors a ventricular origin, as does the presence of a 2:1 VA block. (An upright QRS complex in V_1 through V_6 can also occur from conduction over a left-sided accessory pathway.) Supraventricular beats with aberration often have a triphasic pattern in V_1, an initial vector of the abnormal complex similar to that of the normally conducted beats, and a wide QRS complex that terminates a short cycle length after a long cycle (long-short cycle sequence). During atrial fibrillation, fixed coupling, short coupling intervals, a long pause after the abnormal beat, and runs of bigeminy rather than a consecutive series of abnormal complexes all favor a ventricular origin of the premature complex rather than a supraventricular origin with aberration. A grossly irregular, wide QRS tachycardia with ventricular rates exceeding 200 beats/min should raise the question of atrial fibrillation with conduction over an accessory pathway (see Fig. 39-22). In the presence of a preexisting bundle branch block, a wide QRS tachycardia with a contour different from the contour during sinus rhythm is most likely a VT. On the basis of these criteria, several algorithms to distinguish VT from SVT with aberrancy have been suggested, one of which is shown in **Figure 39-28**. Exceptions exist to all the aforementioned criteria, especially in patients who have preexisting conduction disturbances or preexcitation syndrome; when in doubt, one must rely on sound clinical judgment and consider the ECG only as one of several helpful ancillary tests.

Termination of a tachycardia by triggering of vagal reflexes is considered diagnostic of SVTs. However, VT, especially if it is originating in the right ventricular outflow tract, can be stopped in a similar manner.

ELECTROPHYSIOLOGIC FEATURES. VT can be distinguished electrophysiologically by a short or negative H-V interval (i.e., H begins after the onset of ventricular depolarization) because of retrograde activation from the ventricles (see Chaps. 35 and 36). His bundle deflections are not usually apparent during VT because they are obscured by simultaneous ventricular septal depolarization or inadequate catheter position. The latter must be determined during supraventricular rhythm before the onset or after the termination of VT (see Fig. 39-26). His bundle deflections dissociated from ventricular activation are diagnostic, with rare exceptions. VT can produce QRS complexes of narrow duration and short H-V interval, most likely when the site of origin is close to the His bundle in the fascicles.

Successful electrical induction of VT by premature ventricular stimulation (see Fig. 39-26) depends on the characteristics of the VT and the anatomic substrate. Patients with sustained, hemodynamically stable VT and VT secondary to chronic coronary artery disease have monomorphic VT induced more frequently (90%) than do patients with nonsustained VT, VT from non–coronary-related causes or acute ischemia, and cardiac arrest (40% to 75%). In general, it is more difficult to induce VT with late premature ventricular stimuli than with early premature stimuli, during sinus rhythm than during ventricular pacing, and with one premature stimulus than with two or three stimuli. The specificity of VT induction using more than two premature ventricular stimuli begins to decrease, whereas the sensitivity increases, and nonsustained polymorphic VT or VF can be induced in patients who have no history of VT. Of patients with stable VT who have inducible sustained monomorphic VT, the latter is induced in about 25% with a single extra stimulus, in 50% with double extra stimuli, and in 25% with triple extra stimuli. On occasion, VT can be initiated only from the left ventricle or from specific sites in the right ventricle. Multiple premature stimuli reduce the need for LV stimulation. Drugs such as isoproterenol can facilitate the induction of VT. Coughing during VT that causes hypotension can help maintain blood pressure.

Termination by pacing depends significantly on the rate of the VT and the site of pacing. Slower VTs are terminated more easily and with fewer stimuli than are more rapid ones. An increasing number of stimuli are required to terminate more rapid VTs, which increases the risks of pacing-induced acceleration of the VT. Subthreshold stimulation and transthoracic stimulation can terminate VT. Atrial pacing, at times, can also induce and terminate VT (see Chap. 35).

CLINICAL FEATURES. Symptoms occurring during VT depend on the ventricular rate, duration of tachycardia, and presence and extent of the underlying heart disease and peripheral vascular disease. VT can occur in several forms: short, asymptomatic, nonsustained episodes; sustained, hemodynamically stable events, generally occurring at slower rates or in otherwise normal hearts; or unstable runs, often degenerating into VF. In some patients who have nonsustained VTs initially, sustained episodes or VF later develops. The location of impulse formation and therefore the way in which the depolarization wave spreads across the myocardium can also be important. Physical findings depend in part on the P-to-QRS relationship. If atrial activity is dissociated from the ventricular contractions, the findings of AV dissociation are present. If the atria are captured retrogradely, regularly occurring cannon *a* waves appear when atrial and ventricular contractions occur simultaneously and signs of AV dissociation are absent.

More than 50% of patients treated for symptomatic recurrent VT have ischemic heart disease. The next largest group has cardiomyopathy (both congestive and hypertrophic; see Chaps. 68 and 69), with lesser percentages divided among those with primary electrical disease such as inherited ion channel abnormalities (see Chap. 9), mitral valve prolapse, valvular heart disease (see Chap. 66), congenital heart disease (see Chap. 65), and miscellaneous causes. LV hypertrophy can lead to ventricular arrhythmias. Coronary artery spasm can cause transient myocardial ischemia with severe ventricular arrhythmias in some patients, during ischemia as well as during the apparent reperfusion period (see Chap. 54). Complex ventricular arrhythmias can occur after coronary artery bypass grafting. In patients resuscitated from sudden cardiac death (see Chap. 41), most (75%) have severe coronary artery disease, and ventricular tachyarrhythmias can be induced by premature ventricular stimulation in approximately 75%. When VT occurs in an ambulatory patient, it is uncommonly induced by R-on-T PVCs. Patients who have sustained VT are more likely to have a reduced ejection fraction, slowed intraventricular conduction and electrographic abnormalities, LV aneurysm, and previous myocardial infarction than are patients who have VF, thus indicating different electrophysiologic and anatomic substrates. Young patients can also suffer cardiac arrest from VT or VF, and persistent electrical inducibility of arrhythmias in these patients connotes a poor prognosis. In patients with coronary artery disease, sustained VT displays a circadian variation, with peak frequency in the morning.

Many approaches have been used to assess prognosis in patients with ventricular arrhythmias. Reduced baroreceptor sensitivity and heart rate variability apparently caused by reduced vagal activity may indicate an increased risk of VT or sudden cardiac death. The presence of nonsustained VT after myocardial infarction often presages sudden cardiac death. Electrophysiologic study findings of reduced LV function, spontaneous ventricular arrhythmias, late potentials on signal-averaged ECG, QT interval dispersion, T wave alternans,[20,21] prolonged QRS duration, heart rate turbulence, and inducible sustained VTs all carry increased risk. Currently, however, no noninvasive technique reliably predicts outcome better than assessment of LV function. LV function and inducibility of VT during electrophysiologic study are the two strongest predictors of poor outcome. Some early studies have suggested that T wave alternans may be a good risk-stratifying modality, but randomized trials are pending.[20-22] New risk factors, such as elevated C-reactive protein level, various cytokines, and genotypes, may provide useful information in the future. In general, the prognosis for patients with idiopathic VT (see later), in the absence of structural heart disease or a prolonged QT interval, is good, and less aggressive treatment is warranted than for patients with structural heart disease. Patients with inherited ion channel abnormalities are an exception to that statement (see Chap. 9).

MANAGEMENT. The dramatic changes in the management of VT and aborted sudden death during the past decade have been fueled by several large clinical trials (**Table 39-6**) and development of the ICD. Management decisions can be stratified into those involved in acute management (or termination) and those involved in long-term therapy (or prevention of recurrence or sudden death; see Chap. 41).

Acute Management of Sustained Ventricular Tachycardia

VT that does not cause hemodynamic decompensation can be treated medically to achieve acute termination by the intravenous administration of amiodarone, lidocaine, or procainamide, followed by an infusion of the successful drug.[19] Lidocaine is often ineffective; amiodarone, sotalol, and procainamide appear to be superior. In patients in whom procainamide is ineffective or in whom procainamide may be problematic (severe heart failure, renal failure), intravenous amiodarone is often effective. In general, an initial amiodarone loading dose of 15 mg/min is given during a 10-minute period. This dose is followed by an infusion of 1 mg/min for 6 hours and then a maintenance dose of 0.5 mg/min for the remaining 18 hours and for the next several days, as necessary. If VT does not terminate, or if it recurs, a repeated loading dose can be given. Rarely, sinus bradycardia or AV block can be seen with intravenous amiodarone. The hypotension associated with intravenous amiodarone, caused largely by the diluent used in earlier formulations, does not seem to be as frequent a problem and is usually related to the rate of infusion.

If the arrhythmia does not respond to medical therapy, electrical DC cardioversion can be used. VT that precipitates hypotension, shock, angina, congestive heart failure, or symptoms of cerebral hypoperfusion should be treated promptly with DC cardioversion (see Chaps. 37 and 41). Very low energies can terminate VT, beginning with a synchronized shock of 10 to 50 J. Digitalis-induced VT is best treated pharmacologically. After conversion of the arrhythmia to a normal rhythm, it is essential to institute measures to prevent recurrence.

Striking the patient's chest, sometimes called thumpversion, can terminate VT by mechanically inducing a PVC that presumably interrupts the reentrant pathway necessary to support it. Chest stimulation at the time of the vulnerable period during the arrhythmia can accelerate the VT or possibly provoke VF.

In some cases, such as VT associated with a remote myocardial infarction (which is caused by reentry), ventricular pacing via a

TABLE 39-6 Clinical Trials in the Treatment of Ventricular Tachycardia and Prevention of Cardiac Arrest

STUDY	PATIENT INCLUSION	ENDPOINTS	TREATMENT ARMS	KEY RESULTS
Primary Prevention Studies				
BHAT[1]	Post MI	Total mortality Sudden cardiac death	Propranolol Placebo	Total mortality, sudden cardiac death reduced in treatment arm
CAST[2,3]	Post MI ≥6 PVCs/hr LVEF ≤40%	Arrhythmic death	Flecainide Encainide Moricizine Placebo	Arrhythmic death increased with all treatment arms
SWORD[4]	Post MI LVEF <40% *or* Remote MI NYHA Class II-III	Total mortality	*d*-Sotalol Placebo	Increased mortality in treatment arm
EMIAT[5]	Post MI LVEF <40%	Total mortality Arrhythmic death	Amiodarone Placebo	Amiodarone reduced arrhythmic death but not total mortality
CAMIAT[6]	Post MI ≥10 PVCs/hr or NSVT	Arrhythmic death Total mortality	Amiodarone Placebo	Amiodarone reduced arrhythmic death but not total mortality
GESICA[7]	CHF LVEF ≤35%	Total mortality	Amiodarone Best therapy	Amiodarone reduced mortality; patients with NSVT had higher mortality
CHF-STAT[8]	CHF LVEF ≤40% ≥10 PVCs/hr (asymptomatic)	Total mortality	Amiodarone Placebo	No effect in ischemic cardiomyopathy but trend toward reduced mortality in nonischemic cardiomyopathy
CABG-PATCH[9]	CAD undergoing CABG LVEF <36% Positive SAECG	Total mortality	CABG CABG + ICD	No difference in total mortality
MADIT[10]	Post MI NSVT LVEF ≤35% NYHA Class I-III Inducible VT not suppressed by procainamide	Total mortality	ICD Antiarrhythmic drug (80% amiodarone)	ICD reduced mortality
MUSTT[11]	Post MI LVEF <40% NSVT	Arrhythmic death or cardiac arrest	ICD in nonsuppressible group Antiarrhythmic drug in suppressible group No therapy	Improved survival in ICD group; no difference between no therapy and antiarrhythmic group
MADIT II[12]	Post MI EF ≤30% >10 PVCs/hr or couplets	Total mortality	ICD No ICD	Improved survival in ICD arm
DINAMIT[13]	Immediate post MI EF ≤35%	Total mortality Arrhythmic mortality	ICD No ICD	No improvement in survival with ICD
COMPANION[14]	Ischemic or nonischemic CM NYHA Class III-IV QRS ≥120 msec	Total mortality	Medical therapy PM-CRT ICD-CRT	Improved survival in ICD-CRT group > PM-CRT > medical therapy
DEFINITE[15]	Nonischemic CM EF ≤36% PVCs or NSVT	Total mortality Arrhythmic mortality	ICD No ICD	Improved survival in the ICD arm
SCD-HeFT[16]	CHF LVEF ≤35% NYHA Class II-III	Total mortality Arrhythmic mortality Cost Quality of life	ICD Amiodarone Placebo	Improved survival with ICD; no effect of amiodarone on survival
Secondary Prevention Studies				
ESVEM[17,18]	Cardiac arrest, sustained VT, or syncope ≥10 PVCs/hr Inducible VT	Recurrence of arrhythmia	EP-guided antiarrhythmics (imipramine, mexiletine, procainamide, quinidine, sotalol, pirmenol, propafenone) Holter-guided antiarrhythmics	No difference between Holter- and EP-guided groups; sotalol group had lowest recurrence rate of VT, arrhythmic death, total death
CASCADE[19]	Cardiac arrest Not associated with acute MI	Cardiac mortality Aborted cardiac arrest	EP- or Holter-guided conventional drug therapy Empiric amiodarone	Amiodarone survival better than conventional guided drug therapy
CASH[20]	Cardiac arrest Not associated with acute MI	Total mortality	Empiric amiodarone Metoprolol Propafenone ICD	Sudden cardiac death mortality lowest in ICD arm; increased mortality in propafenone arm

TABLE 39-6 Clinical Trials in the Treatment of Ventricular Tachycardia and Prevention of Cardiac Arrest—cont'd

STUDY	PATIENT INCLUSION	ENDPOINTS	TREATMENT ARMS	KEY RESULTS
AVID[21]	Cardiac arrest or sustained VT	Total mortality Cost Quality of life	ICD Drug therapy (empiric amiodarone, or EP- or Holter-guided sotalol)	Survival better in ICD group, with most benefit occurring in first 9 months; benefit most pronounced in patients with EF <35%
CIDS[22,23]	Cardiac arrest or sustained VT	Total mortality	ICD Amiodarone	Survival trended better in ICD group

CABG = coronary artery bypass graft; CAD = coronary artery disease; CHF = congestive heart failure; CM = cardiomyopathy; CRT = cardiac resynchronization therapy; EF = ejection fraction; EP = electrophysiologic study; ICD = implantable cardioverter-defibrillator; LVEF = left ventricular ejection fraction; MI = myocardial infarction; NSVT = nonsustained ventricular tachycardia; NYHA = New York Heart Association; PM = pacemaker; PVCs = premature ventricular complexes; SAECG = signal-averaged electrocardiogram; VT = ventricular tachycardia.

1. β-Blocker Heart Attack Trial Research Group: A randomized trial of propranolol in patients with acute myocardial infarction. I. Mortality results. JAMA 247:1707, 1982.
2. Echt DS, Liebson PR, Mitchell LB, et al: Mortality and morbidity in patients receiving encainide, flecainide, or placebo. The Cardiac Arrhythmia Suppression Trial. N Engl J Med 324:781, 1991.
3. The Cardiac Arrhythmia Suppression Trial II Investigators: Effect of the antiarrhythmic agent moricizine on survival after myocardial infarction. N Engl J Med 327:227, 1992.
4. Waldo AL, Camm AJ, deRuyter H, et al: Effect of d-sotalol on mortality in patients with left ventricular dysfunction after recent and remote myocardial infarction. Lancet 348:7, 1996.
5. Julian DG, Camm AJ, Frangin G, et al: Randomised trial of effect of amiodarone on mortality in patients with left-ventricular dysfunction after recent myocardial infarction: EMIAT. Lancet 349:667, 1997.
6. Cairns JA, Connolly SJ, Roberts R, Gent M: Randomised trial of outcome after myocardial infarction in patients with frequent or repetitive ventricular premature depolarisations: CAMIAT. Lancet 349:675, 1997.
7. Doval HC, Nul DR, Grancelli HO, et al: Nonsustained ventricular tachycardia in severe heart failure. Independent marker of increased mortality due to sudden death. Circulation 94:3198, 1996.
8. Singh SN, Fletcher RD, Fisher SG, et al: Amiodarone in patients with congestive heart failure and asymptomatic ventricular arrhythmia. N Engl J Med 333:77, 1995.
9. Bigger JT Jr, Whang W, Rottman JN, et al: Mechanisms of death in the CABG Patch trial: A randomized trial of implantable cardiac defibrillator prophylaxis in patients at high risk of death after coronary artery bypass graft surgery. Circulation 99:1416, 1999.
10. Moss AJ, Hall WJ, Cannom DS, et al: Improved survival with an implanted defibrillator in patients with coronary disease at high risk for ventricular arrhythmia. N Engl J Med 335:1933, 1996.
11. Buxton AE, Lee KL, Fisher JD, et al: A randomized study of the prevention of sudden death in patients with coronary artery disease. N Engl J Med 341:1882, 1999.
12. Moss AJ, Zareba W, Hall WJ, et al: Prophylactic implantation of a defibrillator in patients with myocardial infarction and reduced ejection fraction. N Engl J Med 346:877, 2002.
13. Hohnloser SH, Kuck KH, Dorian P, et al: Prophylactic use of an implantable cardioverter-defibrillator after acute myocardial infarction. N Engl J Med 351:2481, 2004.
14. Bristow MR, Saxon LA, Boehmer J, et al: Cardiac-resynchronization therapy with or without an implantable defibrillator in advanced chronic heart failure. N Engl J Med 350:2140, 2004.
15. Kadish A, Dyer A, Daubert JP, et al: Prophylactic defibrillator implantation in patients with nonischemic dilated cardiomyopathy. N Engl J Med 350:2151, 2004.
16. Bardy GH, Lee KL, Mark DB, et al: Amiodarone or an implantable cardioverter-defibrillator for congestive heart failure. N Engl J Med 352:225, 2005.
17. Mason JW: A comparison of electrophysiologic testing with Holter monitoring to predict antiarrhythmic-drug efficacy for ventricular tachyarrhythmias. N Engl J Med 329:445, 1993.
18. Mason JW: A comparison of seven antiarrhythmic drugs in patients with ventricular tachyarrhythmias. N Engl J Med 329:452, 1993.
19. Greene HL: The CASCADE Study: Randomized antiarrhythmic drug therapy in survivors of cardiac arrest in Seattle. Am J Cardiol 72:70F, 1993.
20. Siebels J, Cappato R, Ruppel R, et al: Preliminary results of the Cardiac Arrest Study Hamburg (CASH). Am J Cardiol 72:109F, 1993.
21. The Antiarrhythmics Versus Implantable Defibrillators (AVID) Investigators: A comparison of antiarrhythmic-drug therapy with implantable defibrillators in patients resuscitated from near-fatal ventricular arrhythmias [see comments]. N Engl J Med 337:1576, 1997.
22. Connolly SJ, Gent M, Roberts RS, et al: Canadian Implantable Defibrillator Study (CIDS): Study design and organization. Am J Cardiol 72:103F, 1993.
23. Cappato R: Secondary prevention of sudden death: The Dutch Study, the Antiarrhythmics Versus Implantable Defibrillator Trial, the Cardiac Arrest Study Hamburg, and the Canadian Implantable Defibrillator Study. Am J Cardiol 83:68D, 1999.

pacing catheter inserted into the right ventricle or transcutaneously at rates faster than the tachycardia can terminate the tachycardia. This procedure incurs the risk of accelerating the VT to ventricular flutter or VF. In patients with recurrent VT, competitive ventricular pacing can be used to prevent recurrence. Intermittent VT, interrupted by several supraventricular beats, is generally best treated pharmacologically.

A search for reversible conditions contributing to the initiation and maintenance of VT should be made and the conditions corrected, if possible. For example, VT related to ischemia, hypotension, or hypokalemia can at times be terminated by antianginal treatment, vasopressors, or potassium, respectively. Correction of heart failure can reduce the frequency of ventricular arrhythmias. Slow ventricular rates caused by sinus bradycardia or AV block can permit the occurrence of PVCs and ventricular tachyarrhythmias, which can be corrected by administration of atropine, temporary isoproterenol administration, or transvenous pacing. SVT can initiate ventricular tachyarrhythmias and should be prevented, if possible.

Long-Term Therapy for Prevention of Recurrences

The goal of long-term therapy is to prevent sudden cardiac death and recurrence of symptomatic VT. Asymptomatic nonsustained ventricular arrhythmias in low-risk populations (i.e., preserved LV function) often need not be treated. In patients with symptomatic nonsustained tachycardia, beta blockers are frequently effective in preventing recurrences. In patients refractory to beta blockers, class IC agents, sotalol, or amiodarone can be effective. However, class IC agents should be avoided in patients with structural heart disease, especially those with coronary artery disease because of the increased mortality associated with these drugs caused by proarrhythmia. Sotalol should be used cautiously because of its potential for prolonging the QT interval and producing torsades de pointes. Patients with nonsustained VT after myocardial infarction and poor LV function are at significant risk for sudden death. The Multicenter Automatic Defibrillator Implantation Trial (MADIT) found that patients with prior myocardial infarction and an ejection fraction of 0.35 or less who had inducible VT that was not suppressed with drugs had better survival with treatment with an ICD, with a hazard ratio of 0.46. In the Multicenter Unsustained Tachycardia Trial (MUSTT), patients with an ejection fraction of 0.40 or less with coronary disease and asymptomatic nonsustained VT who had inducible sustained VT at electrophysiologic study had a 65% relative (31% absolute) reduction in mortality with treatment with an ICD. These studies have suggested that patients with nonsustained VT and an ejection fraction of 0.35 to 0.40 or less should undergo electrophysiologic study and, if they have inducible VT (i.e., not suppressed with procainamide), should have an ICD. The MADIT-II study found that patients with ischemic cardiomyopathy (prior myocardial infarction) with an ejection fraction of 0.30 or less and no requirement for ventricular arrhythmia had improved survival with treatment with an ICD (hazard ratio, 0.69). The Sudden Cardiac Death in Heart Failure Trial (SCD-HeFT) found that patients with nonischemic and ischemic cardiomyopathy, NYHA Class II or III heart failure, and an ejection fraction of 35% had no mortality benefit from amiodarone compared with placebo, but those randomized to receive an ICD had a 24% relative (6.8% absolute) reduction in mortality.[23] Multiple ICD trials have demonstrated the superiority of the ICD over drugs for primary prevention of sudden cardiac death in patients at risk for a life-threatening ventricular arrhythmia (see Chaps. 38 and 41).[24] Additional risk stratifiers (such as T wave alternans) may be beneficial.[25]

For secondary prevention of sustained VT or cardiac arrest (see Table 39-6 and Chaps. 37 and 41) in patients with structural heart disease, it is now clear from several clinical trials that (1) class I antiarrhythmic drugs produce a worse outcome than class III antiarrhythmic drugs, (2) empiric amiodarone results in better survival than electrophysiology-guided antiarrhythmic drugs, and (3) ICDs provide better survival than amiodarone, particularly in patients with a left ventricular ejection fraction less than 0.35. Therefore, in patients who have survived a cardiac arrest or who have sustained VT resulting in hemodynamic compromise and poor LV function, an ICD is the treatment of choice. In patients who refuse an ICD, empiric amiodarone may be the next best therapy, although there was no mortality reduction in SCD-HeFT. The optimal therapy for patients with coronary disease who have preserved LV function with sustained VT is not currently known. Empiric amiodarone appears to be the safest therapy, although Holter-guided sotalol has been advocated. Some patients who receive ICDs have frequent shocks because of recurrent VT. In these patients, concomitant therapy with amiodarone can be required to reduce the frequency of VT or to slow the rate of the VT to allow it to be pace terminated. Other drugs, such as sotalol, procainamide, mexiletine, and flecainide, may be required if amiodarone is not effective. On occasion, a combination of drugs can be effective when a single drug is not. Ablation can also be considered in this situation. Although RF ablation (see Chap. 37) of certain types of idiopathic VT (see later) is very effective, ablation for postinfarction VT or that associated with dilated cardiomyopathy is somewhat less effective. In addition, because of the significant mortality associated with these arrhythmias in patients with structural heart disease and depressed LV function, ablation is generally used as an adjunct to ICD placement to reduce the frequency of VT and ICD shocks. However, in patients with well-tolerated postinfarction VT and well-preserved LV function or in patients refractory to drugs, it can be used as first-line therapy.

Specific Types of Ventricular Tachycardia

A number of fairly specific types of VT have been identified, and distinction is based on a constellation of distinctive electrocardiographic and electrophysiologic features, a specific set of clinical events, and, in some instances, genetics (see Chap. 9). Although our understanding of the electrophysiologic mechanisms responsible for clinically occurring VTs is still developing (see Chap. 35), being able to identify different types of VTs is the first step toward understanding their mechanisms. These different types of VT often carry different prognoses and responses to different therapy. They are distinct from VTs associated with remote myocardial infarction or dilated cardiomyopathies.

Ventricular Arrhythmias in Patients with Cardiomyopathies

(see Chaps. 68 and 69)

ISCHEMIC CARDIOMYOPATHY. Patients with previous myocardial infarction are at risk for development of VT. In the setting of a remote myocardial infarction, the mechanism of VT is reentry, involving the infarct scar and in particular the border zone or other areas of the scar with deranged conduction. As a result, the VT in this setting is typically monomorphic. In some cases, more than one morphology can be seen because of different exit sites from the same circuit resulting in different activation patterns of the rest of the ventricle or reversal of the direction of reentry using the same circuit (and resulting in a different activation of the rest of the ventricle) or other circuits existing in the infarct scar. Polymorphic VT or VF in the setting of ischemic heart disease usually occurs during active ischemia or infarction. Treatment of VT in the setting of ischemic heart disease follows the recommendations described earlier. In general, ICDs are indicated to prevent sudden cardiac death from VT in this group of patients, especially in those with depressed LV function. Monomorphic VT in this setting is often amenable to pace termination. In patients with preserved LV function and no hemodynamic compromise, optimal long-term treatment is still controversial. Primary suppression with antiarrhythmic drugs (e.g., amiodarone), implantation with an ICD, antitachycardia pacing, and ablation are options. Newer approaches to ablation of VT caused by a prior infarct scar have increased the efficacy, but there is a high recurrence rate because of multiple circuits, and it is in general reserved for refractory VT or very well tolerated VT (see Chap. 37). Surgical endocardial resection of the scarred area is also an effective treatment of refractory VT caused by prior infarction.

DILATED CARDIOMYOPATHY. Both dilated and hypertrophic cardiomyopathies can be associated with VTs and an increased risk of sudden cardiac death. Induction of VT by programmed stimulation does not reliably identify high-risk patients. Because it is difficult to predict patients at risk for sudden death or those who might respond favorably to an antiarrhythmic drug, ICDs have been advocated for patients with life-threatening ventricular arrhythmias and dilated cardiomyopathy. This recommendation has been supported by a large multicenter randomized trial (see Table 39-6) comparing amiodarone with ICDs in patients with poor ventricular function and symptomatic sustained VT; the study found improved survival in patients who received a defibrillator. Bundle branch reentry may be the basis of some VTs in this population and can be treated by ablation of the right bundle branch. Asymptomatic ventricular arrhythmias are common. The role of antiarrhythmic drugs and ICDs in the primary prevention of sudden cardiac death in patients with dilated cardiomyopathy may be warranted in certain high-risk patients, as discussed earlier.

HYPERTROPHIC CARDIOMYOPATHY. The risk of sudden death in patients with hypertrophic cardiomyopathy (see Chap. 69) is increased by the presence of syncope, a family history of sudden death in first-degree relatives, a septal thickness of more than 3 cm, or the presence of nonsustained VT on 24-hour electrocardiographic recordings. Asymptomatic or mildly symptomatic patients with brief and infrequent episodes of nonsustained VT have a low mortality. The use of electrophysiologic testing to identify patients at increased risk of ventricular arrhythmias and sudden death is controversial. Amiodarone has been useful in some patients with mildly symptomatic, nonsustained VT but not in improving survival. QT dispersion is increased in those with ventricular arrhythmias and sudden death, as is T wave alternans. Dual-chamber pacing has been useful in reducing the outflow gradient in some studies, but its role in affecting ventricular arrhythmia has not been established. Currently, no totally acceptable way to risk-stratify patients with hypertrophic cardiomyopathy in terms of VT has been identified. In patients believed to be at high risk for sudden death or those with sustained VT or frequent nonsustained VT, an ICD may be indicated.[26] Alcohol ablation of the septum by direct injection into the septal branches of the coronary circulation has been used to improve outflow gradients, but its potential effect on ventricular arrhythmias and sudden cardiac death is of concern.

ARRHYTHMOGENIC RIGHT VENTRICULAR CARDIOMYOPATHY. Patients with arrhythmogenic right ventricular cardiomyopathy have VT that generally has a left bundle branch block contour (because the tachycardia arises in the right ventricle), often with right-axis deviation and T waves inverted over the right precordial leads (**Fig. 39-29A**). The VT may be caused by reentry. Supraventricular arrhythmias can also occur, and exercise can induce the VT in some patients.

Arrhythmogenic right ventricular cardiomyopathy is caused by a type of cardiomyopathy, familial in some patients, with hypokinetic areas involving the wall of the right ventricle. Genetic abnormalities in desmosomal proteins (plakoglobin, desmoplakin, and plakophilin), the ryanodine receptor, and transforming growth factor β3 have been identified in many families; however, the precise pathway and pathogenesis remain unknown in many patients (see Chaps. 9 and 35).[27-30]

Arrhythmogenic right ventricular cardiomyopathy can be an important cause of ventricular arrhythmia in children and young adults with apparently normal hearts as well as in older patients.[30] Initial findings can be subtle and often mimic those of outflow tract VT (see later), that is, manifested only by tachycardia and no symptoms of right-sided heart failure. Right-sided heart failure or asymptomatic right ventricular enlargement can be present with normal pulmonary vasculature. Male patients predominate, and most patients usually show an abnormal right ventricle by echocardiography, computed tomography, right ventricular angiography, or magnetic resonance imaging, although this abnormality may not be apparent on initial evaluation.

Two pathologic patterns have been identified, fatty and fibrofatty infiltration. In the fibrofatty infiltration, myocardial atrophy appears to result from injury and myocyte death (perhaps from apoptosis) and culminates in fibrofatty replacement mediated by patchy myocarditis. The fatty degeneration preferentially occurs in the right ventricular inflow and outflow tracts and the apex. The left ventricle can be involved in advanced forms of the disease in up to 60% of patients. The ECG during sinus rhythm can exhibit complete or incomplete right bundle branch block and T wave inversions in V_1 to V_3. A terminal notch in the QRS, called an epsilon wave, can be present as a result of slowed intraventricular conduction. The signal-averaged ECG can be abnormal because of delayed conduction in the right ventricle. More recently, a measure of ventricular conduction, QRS fragmentation, has also been reported to be present in many of these patients.[31] Although there have been no clinical trials to date, ICDs are generally preferable to pharmacologic approaches because of the progressive nature of the disease and poor prognosis, particularly if the patients have poorly tolerated VT, resulting in syncope or sudden cardiac death. RF catheter ablation can be tried but is often not successful because of the multiple morphologies of VT and the progressive nature of the disease.

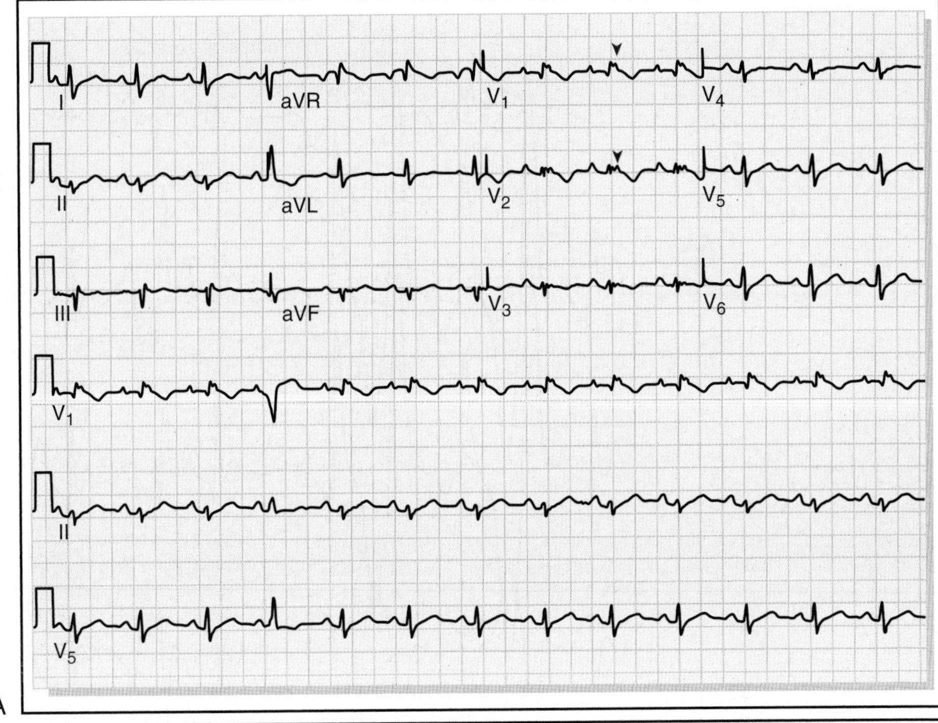

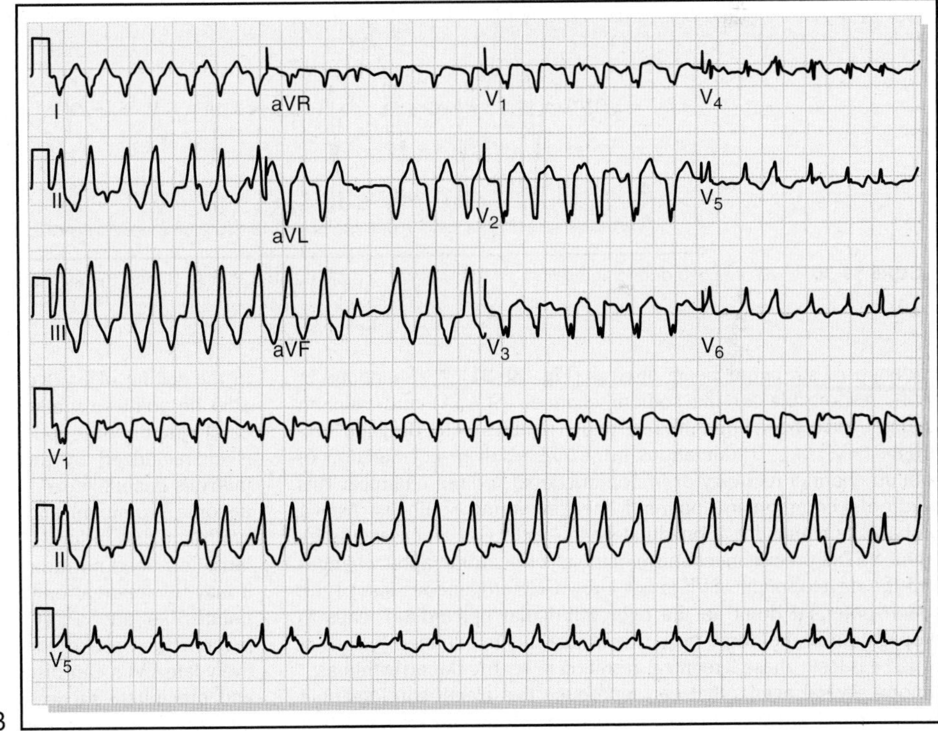

FIGURE 39-29 **A,** Normal sinus rhythm in a patient with arrhythmogenic right ventricular dysplasia. The arrowheads in V_1 and V_2 point to late right ventricular activation called an epsilon wave. **B,** VT in the same patient with right ventricular dysplasia.

Tetralogy of Fallot

Chronic serious ventricular arrhythmias can occur in patients some years after repair of the tetralogy of Fallot (see Chap. 65). Sustained VT after repair can be caused by reentry at the site of previous surgery in the right ventricular outflow tract and can be cured by resection or catheter ablation of this area. The signal-averaged ECG can be abnormal. Decreased cardiac output can occur during VT and residual right ventricular outflow obstruction and lead to VF.

Inherited Arrhythmia Syndromes (see Chap. 9)

CATECHOLAMINERGIC POLYMORPHIC VENTRICULAR TACHYCARDIA. Catecholaminergic polymorphic VT (CPVT) is an uncommon form of inherited VT that occurs in children and adolescents without any overt structural heart disease.[32-34] Patients typically present with syncope or aborted sudden death with highly reproducible, stress-induced VT that is often bidirectional. These patients have no structural heart disease and normal QT intervals. A family history of sudden death or stress-induced syncope is present in about 30% of cases. During exercise, typical responses include initial sinus tachycardia and ventricular extrasystoles followed by salvoes of monomorphic or bidirectional VT, which eventually lead to polymorphic VT as exercise continues (**Fig. 39-30**). Mutations of the ryanodine receptor gene result in an autosomal dominant form of CPVT and account for about 50% of cases; mutations in the calsequestrin gene result in an autosomal recessive form of CPVT and account for about 2% of the cases. The genetic abnormalities, if they exist, in the remainder of the cases are not currently known. The treatment of choice is beta blockers and an ICD, although breakthrough can occur on beta blockade. Sympathectomy has been reported to be effective in a few cases.[35,36] In addition, one study has reported that flecainide inhibited ryanodine receptor–mediated calcium release in mice and prevented CPVT in two patients.[37] Patients with CPVT should be instructed to avoid vigorous exercise.

BRUGADA SYNDROME. Brugada syndrome is a distinct form of idiopathic VF in which patients have right bundle branch block and ST-segment elevation in the anterior precordial leads, without

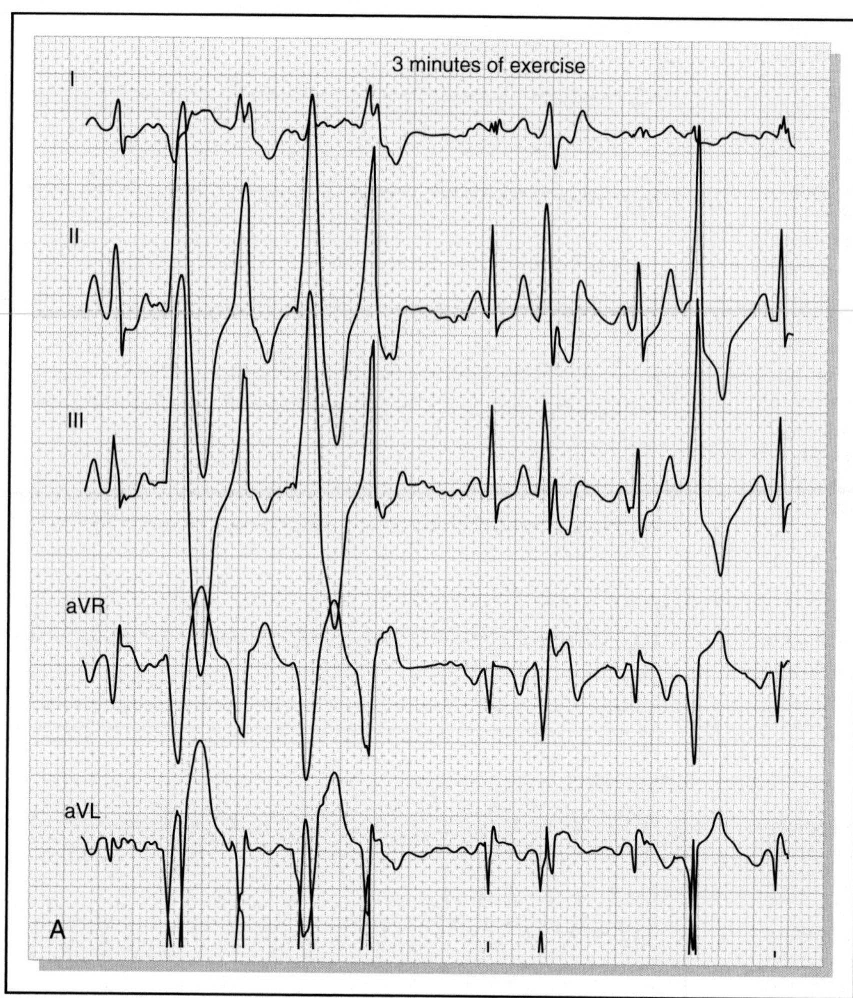

FIGURE 39-30 ECG obtained during an exercise treadmill test in a patient with CPVT. **A,** During the early phase of exercise, short runs of polymorphic VT and PVCs occur.

evidence of structural heart disease (**Fig. 39-31**).[38-40] Mutations in genes responsible for the sodium channel (*SCN5A*) and calcium channel have been identified in many families with Brugada syndrome (see Chap. 9). Mutations in *SCN5A* result in acceleration of sodium channel recovery or in nonfunctional sodium channels. This syndrome, common in apparently healthy young Southeast Asians, probably accounts for approximately 40% to 60% of all cases of idiopathic VF. The precise mechanism of the electrocardiographic changes and the development of VF is not known. Heterogeneous loss of the action potential dome in the right ventricular epicardium leads to propagation of the dome from sites where it is maintained to sites at which it is lost (phase 2 reentry), resulting in ventricular arrhythmias.[41] Among several agents that can reproduce this electrocardiographic phenomenon are sodium channel blockers. They can expose latent electrocardiographic forms of the syndrome and have been proposed as a provocative test. Currently, no pharmacologic treatment reliably prevents VF in these patients. ICDs are the only effective treatment to prevent sudden death. Electrophysiologic studies to determine inducibility of ventricular arrhythmias have been advocated by some as a means to risk stratify; however, this approach remains controversial. Recently, notches in the QRS have identified at-risk individuals.[42] A website (*www.brugadadrugs.org*) has been established to identify drugs causing or interacting with Brugada syndrome.[43]

Torsades de Pointes

ELECTROCARDIOGRAPHIC RECOGNITION. The term *torsades de pointes* refers to a VT characterized by QRS complexes of changing amplitude that appear to twist around the isoelectric line and occur at rates of 200 to 250/min (**Fig. 39-32A**). Originally described in the setting of bradycardia caused by complete heart block, torsades de pointes usually connotes a syndrome, not simply an electrocardiographic description of the QRS complex of the tachycardia. It is characterized by prolonged ventricular repolarization, with QT intervals generally exceeding 500 milliseconds. The U wave can also become prominent and merge with the T wave, but its role in this syndrome and in long-QT syndrome is not clear. The abnormal repolarization need not be present or at least prominent in all beats, but it may be apparent only on the beat before the onset of torsades de pointes (i.e., after a PVC). Long-short R-R cycle sequences commonly precede the onset of torsades de pointes from acquired causes. Relatively late PVCs can discharge during termination of the long T wave and precipitate successive bursts of VT, during which the peaks of the QRS complexes appear successively on one side and then on the other side of the isoelectric baseline; these give the typical twisting appearance, with continuous and progressive changes in QRS contour and amplitude. Torsades de pointes can terminate with progressive prolongation in cycle length and larger and more distinctly formed QRS complexes and culminate in a return to the basal rhythm, a period of ventricular standstill, and a new attack of torsades de pointes or VF.

A less common form, the short-coupled variant of torsades de pointes, is a malignant disease with a high mortality rate and shares several characteristics with idiopathic VF. The ventricular arrhythmia in this setting is initiated with a close-coupled PVC and usually does not involve preceding pauses or bradycardia.

VT that is similar morphologically to torsades de pointes and occurs in patients without QT prolongation, whether spontaneous or electrically induced, should generally be classified as polymorphic VT, not as

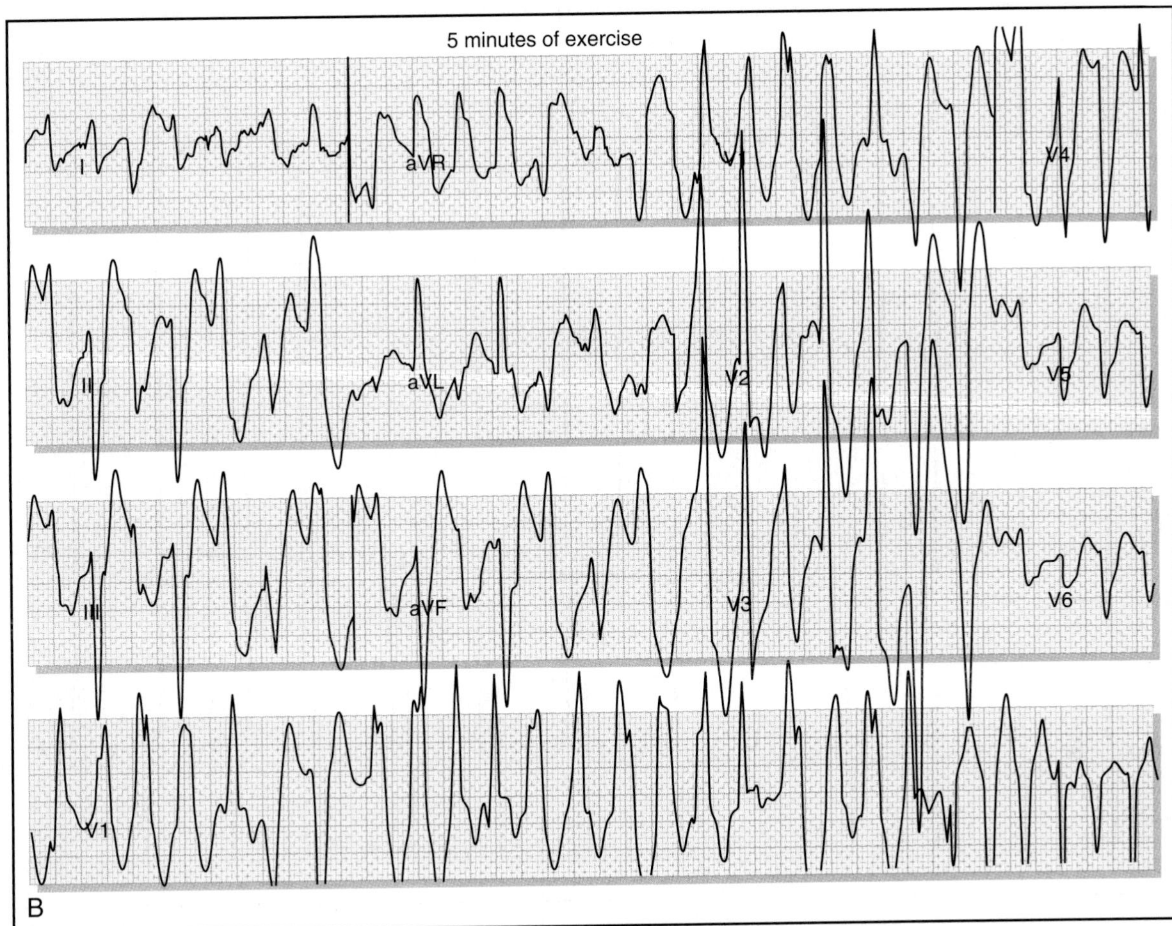

FIGURE 39-30, cont'd **B,** With further exercise, bidirectional VT ensues.

torsades de pointes. The distinction has important therapeutic implications (see later).

ELECTROPHYSIOLOGIC FEATURES. The electrophysiologic mechanisms responsible for torsades de pointes are not completely understood. Most data suggest that early afterdepolarizations (see Chap. 35) are responsible for both long-QT syndrome and the torsades de pointes, or at least its initiation. Perpetuation can be caused by triggered activity, reentry resulting from dispersion of repolarization produced by the early afterdepolarizations, or abnormal automaticity. However, most data currently point to transmural reentry as the most likely mechanism of perpetuation. Putative M cells, located in the midmyocardium, have prolonged repolarization and may play a role in the genesis of torsades de pointes. Their presence is not universally accepted.[44]

CLINICAL FEATURES. Although many predisposing factors have been cited, the most common causes are congenital, severe bradycardia, potassium depletion, and use of antiarrhythmic medications (such as class IA or III antiarrhythmic drugs). More than 50 drugs have been noted to prolong the QT interval (see later, Long-QT Syndrome). Clinical features depend on whether the torsades de pointes is caused by the acquired or congenital (idiopathic) long-QT syndrome (see later). Symptoms from the tachycardia depend on its rate and duration, as with other VTs, and range from palpitations to syncope and death. Women, perhaps because of a longer QT interval, are at greater risk for torsades de pointes than men are.

MANAGEMENT. The approach to management of VT with a polymorphic pattern depends on whether it occurs in the setting of a prolonged QT interval. For this practical reason, and because the mechanism of the tachycardia can differ according to whether a long-QT interval is present, it is important to restrict the definition of torsades de pointes to the typical polymorphic VT in the setting of a long-QT or U wave in the basal complexes. In all patients with torsades de pointes, administration of class IA, possibly some class IC, and class III antiarrhythmic agents (e.g., amiodarone, dofetilide, sotalol) can increase the abnormal QT interval and worsen the arrhythmia. Intravenous magnesium is the initial treatment of choice for torsades de pointes from an acquired cause, followed by temporary ventricular or atrial pacing. Isoproterenol, given cautiously because it can exacerbate the arrhythmia, can be used to increase the rate until pacing is instituted. Lidocaine, mexiletine, or phenytoin can be tried. The cause of the long QT should be determined and corrected, if possible. When the QT interval is normal, polymorphic VT resembling torsades de pointes is diagnosed, and standard antiarrhythmic drugs can be given. In borderline cases, the clinical context may help determine whether treatment should be initiated with antiarrhythmic drugs. Torsades de pointes resulting from congenital long-QT syndrome is treated with beta blockade, surgical sympathetic interruption, pacing, and ICDs (see later). ECGs obtained from close relatives can help secure the diagnosis of long-QT syndrome in borderline cases.

Long-QT Syndrome

ELECTROCARDIOGRAPHIC RECOGNITION. The upper limit for duration of the normal QT interval corrected for heart rate (QTc) is often given as 0.44 second (Fig. 39-32B). However, the normal corrected QT interval may actually be longer (0.46 second for men and 0.47 second for women), with a normal range of ±15% of the mean value. The nature of the U wave abnormality and its relationship to long-QT syndrome is not clear. The probable risk for development of life-threatening ventricular arrhythmias in patients with idiopathic long-QT syndrome is related to the length of the QTc interval. T wave "humps" in the ECG can suggest the presence of long-QT syndrome and can be caused by early afterdepolarizations. Unique T wave contours have been ascribed to specific genotypes causing long-QT syndrome.

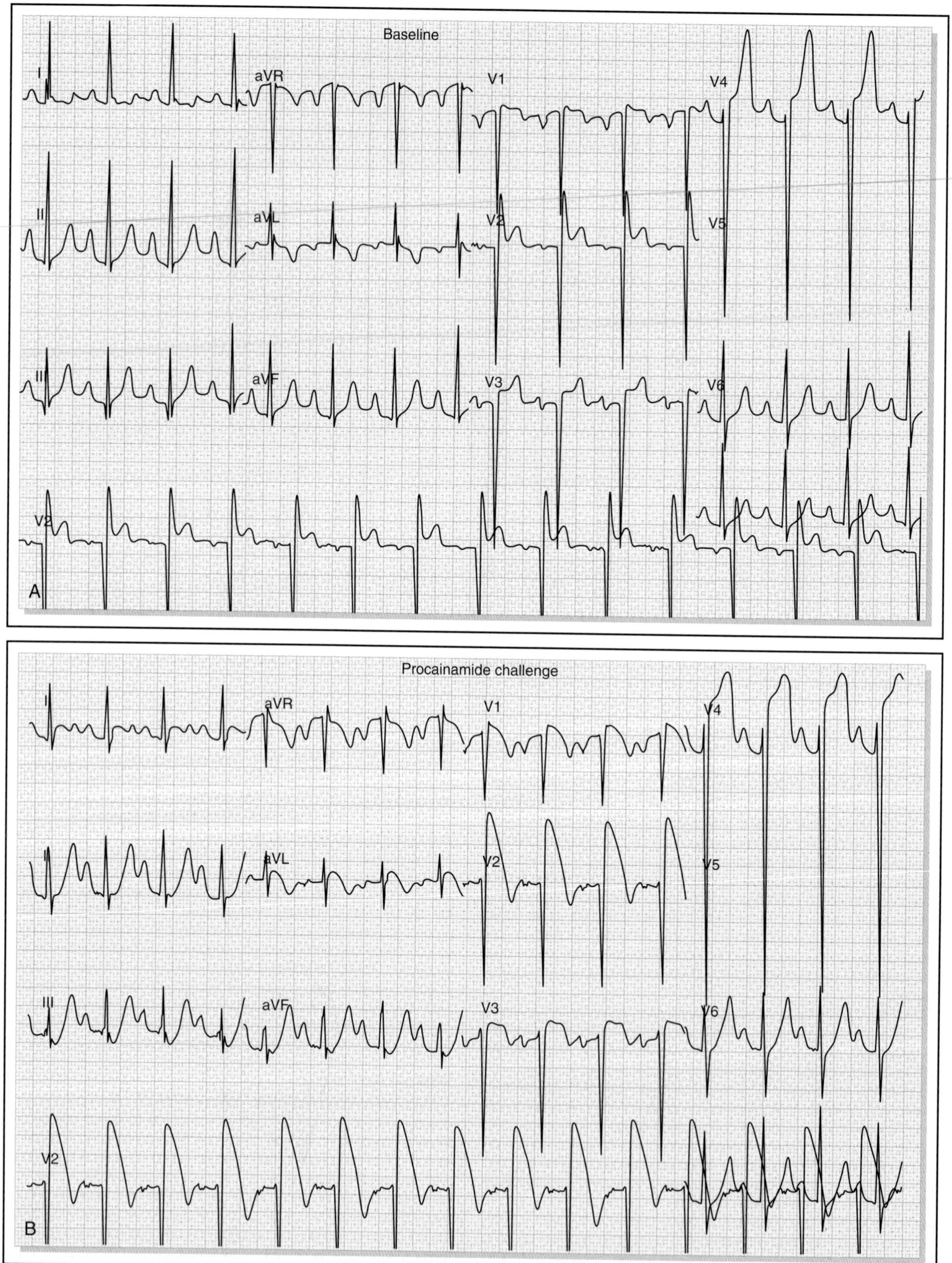

FIGURE 39-31 **A,** Twelve-lead ECG of a patient with Brugada syndrome. The ECG is characterized by a right bundle branch block pattern and persistent ST elevation in leads V_1 through V_3. This ECG shows a type 2 Brugada pattern, with a "saddleback" ST-segment elevation greater than 1 mm and a biphasic T wave in V_1 (positive in V_2-V_3). **B,** After a procainamide challenge, the prototypic ECG changes are exaggerated, with an increase in the ST elevation, and the ECG shows a type 1 pattern, with a downward-sloping coved ST elevation and negative T waves in V_1-V_3.

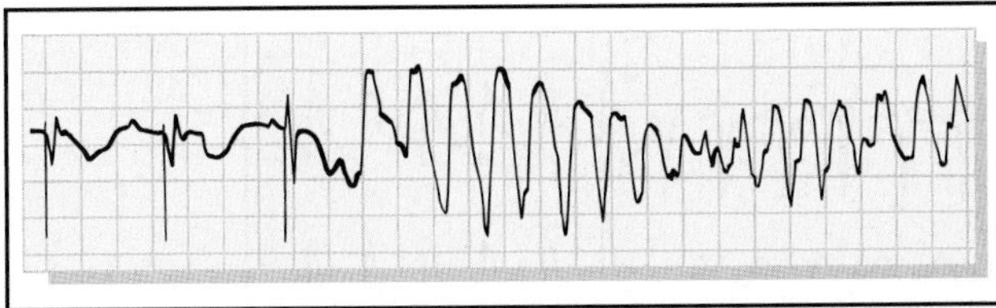

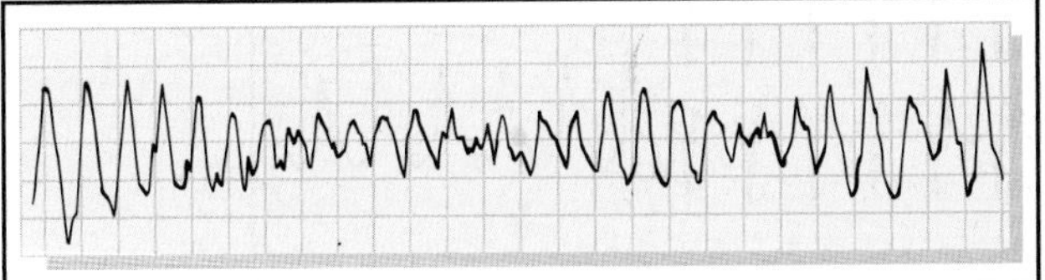

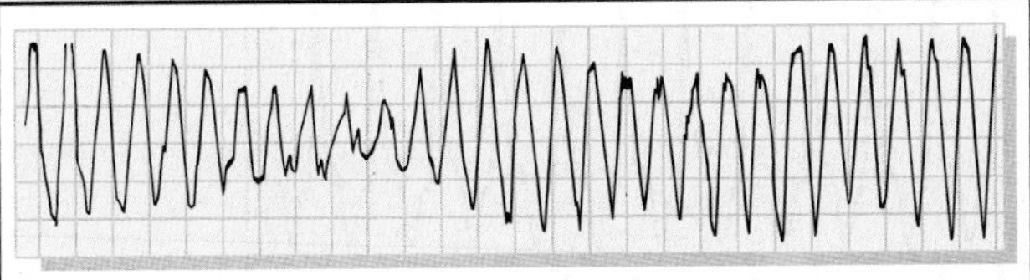

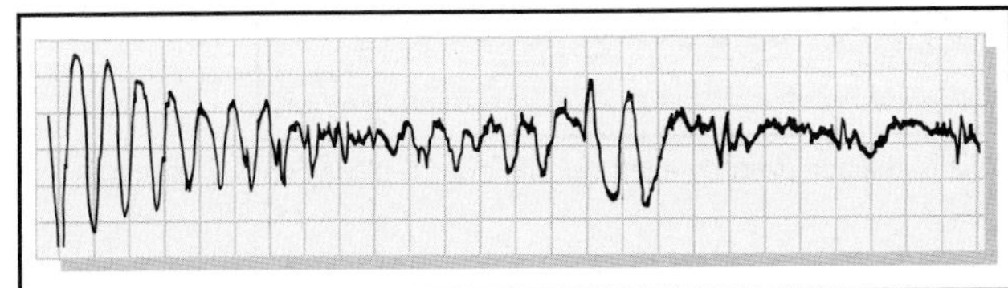

A

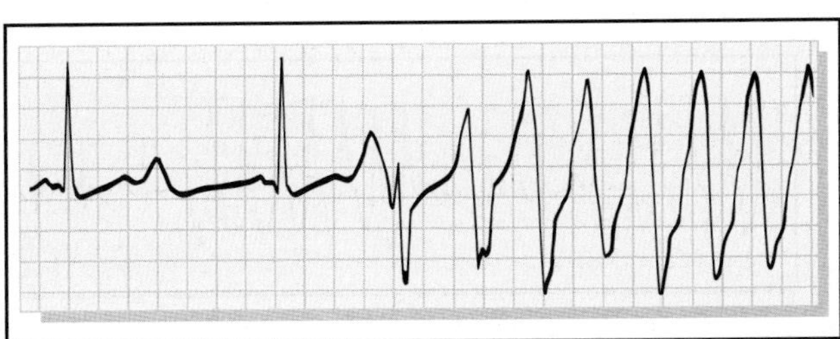

B

FIGURE 39-32 Torsades de pointes. **A,** Continuous monitor lead recording. A demand ventricular pacemaker (VVI) had been implanted because of type II second-degree AV block. After treatment with amiodarone for recurrent VT, the QT interval became prolonged (about 640 milliseconds during paced beats), and episodes of torsades de pointes developed. In this recording, the tachycardia spontaneously terminates and a paced ventricular rhythm is restored. Motion artifact is noted at the end of the recording as the patient lost consciousness. **B,** Tracing from a young boy with congenital long-QT syndrome. The QTU interval in the sinus beats is at least 600 milliseconds. Note TU wave alternans in the first and second complexes. A late premature complex occurring in the downslope of the TU wave initiates an episode of VT.

CLINICAL FEATURES. Long-QT syndrome can be divided into congenital and acquired forms. The congenital form is a familial disorder that can be associated with sensorineural deafness (Jervell and Lange-Nielsen syndrome, autosomal recessive) or normal hearing (Romano-Ward syndrome, autosomal dominant). Most forms of congenital long-QT syndrome are caused by inherited channelopathies created by mutations in one or more genes (see Chap. 9).[45]

The acquired form has a long-QT interval caused by various drugs, such as quinidine, procainamide, *N*-acetylprocainamide, sotalol, amiodarone, disopyramide, phenothiazines, tricyclic antidepressants, erythromycin, pentamidine, some antimalarials, cisapride, and probucol; electrolyte abnormalities, such as hypokalemia and hypomagnesemia; the effects of a liquid protein diet and starvation; central nervous system lesions; significant bradyarrhythmias; cardiac ganglionitis; and mitral valve prolapse. A more comprehensive list that is regularly updated can be found on the Internet *(http://www.azcert.org/medical-pros/drug-lists/drug-lists.cfm)*.

Patients with congenital long-QT syndrome can initially have syncope, at times misdiagnosed as epilepsy, from torsades de pointes. Sudden death can occur in this group of patients; it occurs in about 10% of pediatric patients without preceding symptoms. It is obvious that in some patients, the ventricular arrhythmia becomes sustained and probably results in VF. Patients with idiopathic long-QT syndrome who are at increased risk for sudden death include those with family members who died suddenly at an early age and those who have experienced syncope. Exercise, particularly swimming, and emotional stress appear to be triggers in LQT1, with lethal cardiac events more frequently at rest or during sleep in LQT3. LQT2 has many events occurring with emotional stress or by a sudden loud noise (e.g., telephone or alarm clock) (see Chap. 9).

Stress testing can prolong the QT interval and produce T wave alternans, the latter indicative of electrical instability. ECGs should be obtained for all family members when the proband has symptoms. Patients should undergo prolonged electrocardiographic recording with various stresses designed to evoke ventricular arrhythmias, such as auditory stimuli, psychological stress, cold pressor stimulation, and exercise. The Valsalva maneuver can lengthen the QT interval and cause T wave alternans and VT in patients who have prolonged QT syndromes. Catecholamines can be infused in some patients, but this challenge must be performed cautiously, with resuscitative equipment along with alpha and beta antagonists readily available. Premature ventricular stimulation electrically does not generally induce arrhythmias in this syndrome, and electrophysiologic studies are usually not helpful in the diagnosis. Torsades de pointes commonly develops in patients with the acquired form during periods of bradycardia or after a long pause in the R-R interval, whereas those with the idiopathic form can have a sinus tachycardia preceding the ventricular arrhythmia.

MANAGEMENT. For patients who have idiopathic long-QT syndrome but not syncope, complex ventricular arrhythmias, a family history of sudden cardiac death, or a QTc longer than 500 milliseconds, no therapy or treatment with a beta blocker is generally recommended. In asymptomatic patients with complex ventricular arrhythmias, a family history of early sudden cardiac death, or a QTc longer than 500 milliseconds, beta adrenoceptor blockers at maximally tolerated doses are recommended. Implantation of a permanent pacemaker to prevent the bradycardia or pauses that may predispose to the development of torsades de pointes may be indicated. In patients with syncope caused by ventricular arrhythmias or aborted sudden death, an ICD is warranted. These patients should also be treated with concomitant beta blockers and perhaps overdrive atrial pacing (via the ICD) to minimize the frequency of ICD discharges. The ICD is beneficial in these patients, not simply because of the shocking capabilities but because of the ability to pace continually to prevent bradycardia-induced torsades and algorithms to prevent post-PVC pauses. The use of an ICD in patients without syncope but with a long-QT interval and a strong family history of sudden death is still controversial but may be warranted in these high-risk patients. For patients who continue to have syncope despite maximum drug therapy, left-sided cervicothoracic sympathetic ganglionectomy that interrupts the stellate ganglion and the first three or four thoracic ganglia may be helpful.[36] Most competitive sports are contraindicated for patients with the congenital long-QT syndrome.[46] For patients with the acquired form and torsades de pointes, intravenous magnesium and atrial or ventricular pacing are initial choices. Class IB antiarrhythmic drugs or isoproterenol (cautiously) to increase the heart rate can be tried. Avoidance of precipitating drugs is mandatory.

Short-QT Syndrome

A new inherited syndrome resulting in a short-QT interval has recently been identified to carry an increased risk of sudden death due to VF and likely is one of the syndromes responsible for "idiopathic VF."[47] Patients with the short-QT syndrome are also prone to development of atrial fibrillation. Several genetic abnormalities have been identified, many of which are gain-of-function mutations in the same genes that cause the long-QT syndrome. Although no clear definition of what represents a pathologically short QT as related to outcomes of sudden

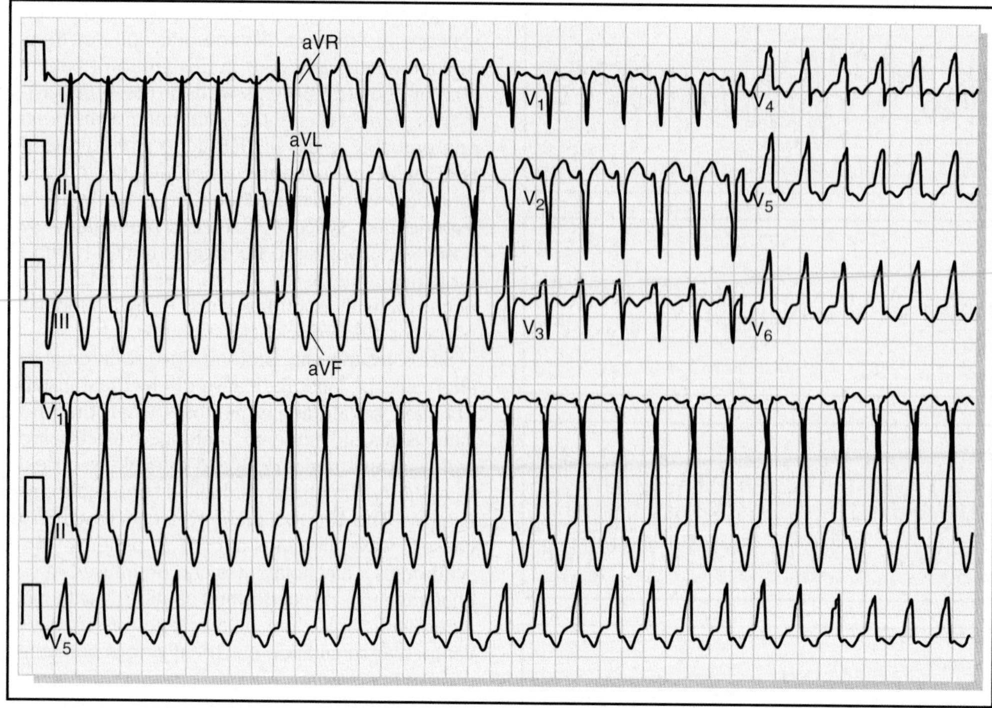

FIGURE 39-33 VT originating from the right ventricular outflow tract. This tachycardia is characterized by a left bundle branch block contour in lead V_1 and an inferior axis.

death exists, a QT of less than 350 milliseconds at rates of less than 100 beats/min (which is more than 2 SD from the mean in a large healthy population) is generally accepted as abnormally short. A short-QT interval on an ECG without a family history of sudden death or history of syncope, palpitations, or atrial fibrillation may not necessarily indicate an increased risk of sudden death. Patients with short-QT syndrome often have persistently short-QT intervals, short or absent ST segments, and tall and narrow T waves in the precordial leads. Other causes of short QT, such as hyperkalemia, hypercalcemia, hyperthermia, acidosis, and digitalis, should be excluded. ICDs are considered the treatment of choice in symptomatic patients to prevent sudden cardiac death. Antiarrhythmic drugs that prolong refractoriness have been reported to be effective in some patients. In particular, quinidine has been shown to be effective in patients with a gain-of-function mutation in the *HERG* (*KCNH2*) gene.[48]

Idiopathic Ventricular Tachycardias

Idiopathic VT is defined as monomorphic VT in patients without any structural heart disease or coronary disease. When more than one morphology of VT is present, one should suspect other disease entities, such as arrhythmogenic right ventricular dysplasia. Idiopathic VTs have any one of several characteristic ECG morphologies representing three distinct entities, based on the location of the VT—outflow tract tachycardias, annular tachycardias, and fascicular tachycardias—each described in the following. Prognosis for all forms of idiopathic monomorphic VT is good. They are amenable to ablation and often respond well to drug therapy.

OUTFLOW TRACT TACHYCARDIAS. Idiopathic VTs with monomorphic contours can be divided into at least three types. Two types, paroxysmal VT and repetitive monomorphic VT, appear to originate from the region of the right ventricular outflow tract (**Figs. 39-33** and **39-34**) or the left ventricular outflow tract. Rarely, the VT can originate from the proximal pulmonary artery (just beyond the pulmonic valve or from the cusps of the aortic valve).[49] Right ventricular outflow tract VTs have a characteristic electrocardiographic appearance of a left bundle branch block contour in V_1 and an inferior axis in the frontal plane. Vagal maneuvers, including adenosine, can terminate the VT, whereas exercise, stress, isoproterenol infusion, and rapid or premature stimulation often initiate or perpetuate the tachycardia. Beta blockers and verapamil can suppress this tachycardia as well. The mechanism responsible may be cyclic adenosine monophosphate–triggered activity resulting from early or delayed afterdepolarizations. The paroxysmal form is exercise or stress induced, whereas the repetitive monomorphic type occurs at rest with sinus beats interposed between runs of

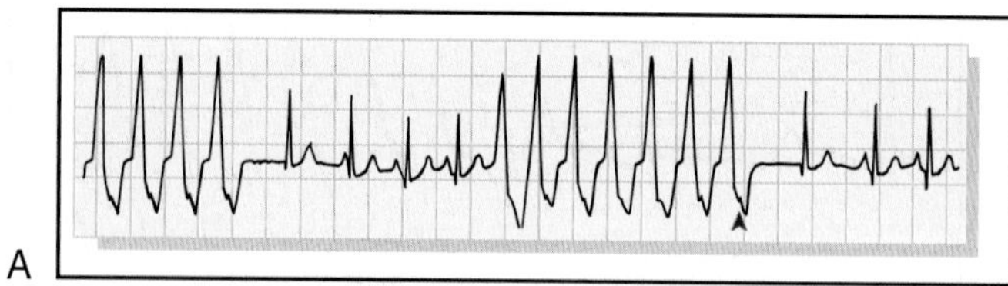

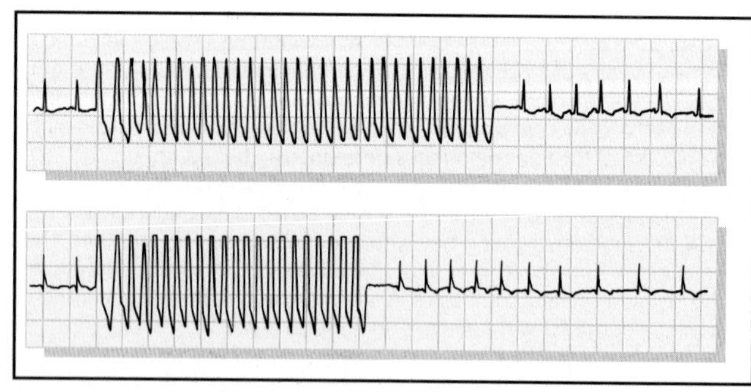

FIGURE 39-34 **A,** Repetitive monomorphic VT. Short episodes of a monomorphic VT at a rate of 160 beats/min repeatedly interrupt the normal sinus rhythm. Retrograde atrial capture probably occurs (the arrowhead points to the deflection in the ST segment), and the retrograde P wave of the last complex of the repetitive monomorphic VT conducts over the normal pathway to produce a QRS complex with a normal contour. **B,** Short runs of a very rapid (260 beats/min) VT of uniform contour. They probably provoke a compensatory sympathetic response because each is followed by a brief period of sinus tachycardia. The sinus pacemaker appears unstable because changes in P wave morphology result.

nonsustained VT that may be precipitated by transient increases in sympathetic activity unrelated to exertion. In a small number of patients, the tachycardia seems to arise in the inflow tract or apex of the right ventricle. A similar tachycardia has been identified in the left ventricular outflow tract and may mimic that of right ventricular outflow tract tachycardia. A distinguishing feature on the ECG is the presence of an S wave in lead I and an early precordial R wave transition (V_1-V_2) during left ventricular outflow tract VT.[50] The prognosis for most patients with outflow tract (right ventricular or left ventricular outflow tract) VT is good. RF catheter ablation effectively eliminates this focal tachycardia in symptomatic patients. In others, antiarrhythmic drugs can be effective.

ANNULAR VENTRICULAR TACHYCARDIAS. VTs arising from the mitral or tricuspid annulus account for between 4% and 7% of idiopathic VTs.[51] Most often, they are of the repetitive monomorphic type. For mitral annular VT, the ECG pattern is typically right bundle branch block pattern (transition in V_1 or V_2), S wave in V_6, and monophasic R or Rs in leads V_2 through V_6. For tricuspid annular VT, the foci generally originate in the septal region, and thus the typical ECG pattern is a left bundle branch block pattern (Qs in lead V_1), an early transition in precordial leads (V_3), and narrower QRS complexes.[52] These VTs behave similarly to outflow tract VT, both in prognosis and in drug response.[53] Annular VTs are amenable to ablation.

FASCICULAR VENTRICULAR TACHYCARDIA (LEFT SEPTAL VENTRICULAR TACHYCARDIA). A left septal VT has been described as arising in the left posterior septum, often preceded by a fascicular potential, and is sometimes called a fascicular tachycardia (**Fig. 39-35**). Entrainment has been demonstrated, which suggests reentry as a cause of some of the tachycardias. Verapamil or diltiazem often suppresses this tachycardia, whereas adenosine does so only rarely. The response to verapamil suggests that the slow inward current may be important, possibly in a reentrant circuit or via delayed afterdepolarizations. Several mechanisms may be operative, and the group may not be homogeneous. Oral verapamil is not as effective as intravenous verapamil. Once it is initiated, the tachycardia is paroxysmal and sustained. It can be started by rapid atrial or ventricular pacing and sometimes by exercise or isoproterenol. The prognosis is generally good. RF catheter ablation is effective in symptomatic patients.

Idiopathic Ventricular Fibrillation

Idiopathic VF can occur in about 1% to 8% of cases of out-of-hospital VF. There is overlap with the short-QT syndrome. Cardiovascular evaluation is normal, except for the arrhythmia. Monomorphic VT is rarely induced at electrophysiologic study. The natural history is incompletely known, but recurrences are not uncommon. It is important in this entity, as well as in patients with idiopathic VTs, to remember that the arrhythmia may at times be an early manifestation of a developing cardiomyopathy, at least in some patients. Idiopathic VF has been associated with early repolarization in one case-control study.[54] However, it is unclear whether early repolarization in the general population carries any additional risk for VF. There is some thought that the early repolarization syndrome is part of the spectrum of disease of channelopathies affecting the J wave portion of the ECG, so-called J wave syndromes, which include the Brugada syndrome.[55] In some instances, short-coupled PVCs can trigger VF (**Fig. 39-36**).[56] In patients with idiopathic VF, ICDs are a useful therapeutic choice. Ablation of short-coupled PVCs that trigger VF, often from Purkinje fibers, has also been shown to be effective at reducing recurrence.[56]

Bidirectional Ventricular Tachycardia

Bidirectional VT is an uncommon type of VT characterized by QRS complexes with a right bundle branch block pattern, an alternating polarity in the frontal plane from −60 to −90 degrees to +120 to +130 degrees, and a regular rhythm. The ventricular rate is between 140 and 200 beats/min. Although the mechanism and site of origin of this tachycardia have remained somewhat controversial, most evidence supports a ventricular origin.

Bidirectional VT can be a manifestation of digitalis excess, typically in older patients and in those with severe myocardial disease. When the tachycardia is caused by digitalis, the extent of toxicity is often advanced, with a poor prognosis. CPVT can present as bidirectional VT.

In addition to digoxin-binding antibodies (digoxin immune Fab, Digibind), drugs useful to treat digitalis toxicity, such as lidocaine, potassium,

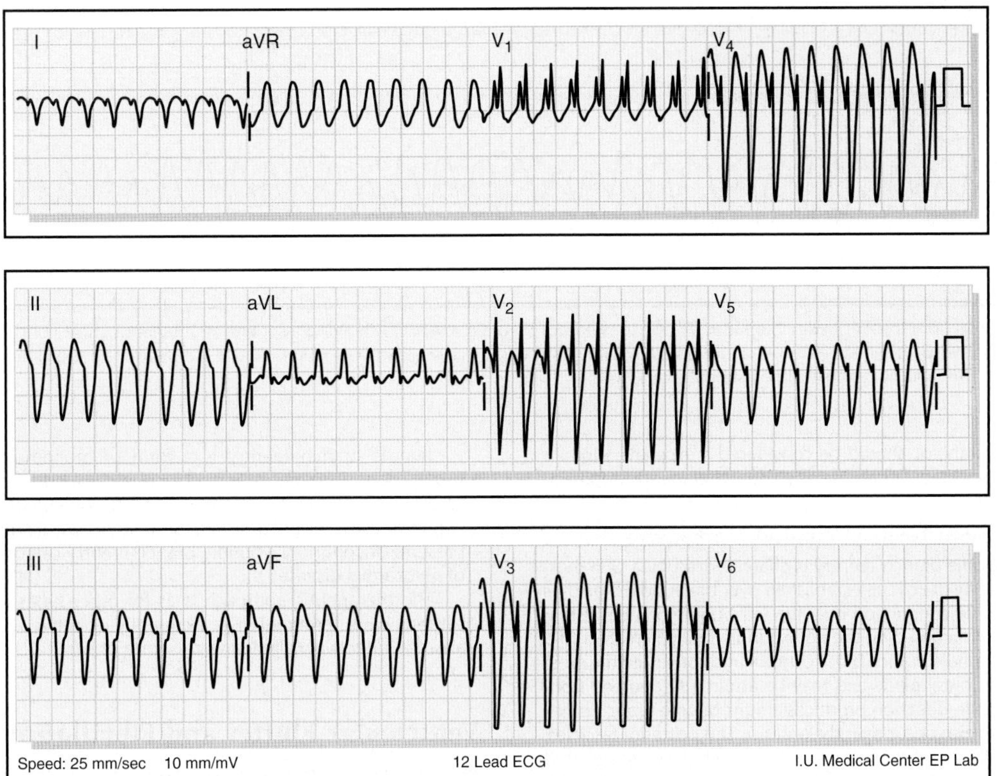

FIGURE 39-35 Left septal VT. This tachycardia is characterized by a right bundle branch block contour. In this instance, the axis was rightward. The site of the VT was established to be in the left posterior septum by electrophysiologic mapping and ablation.

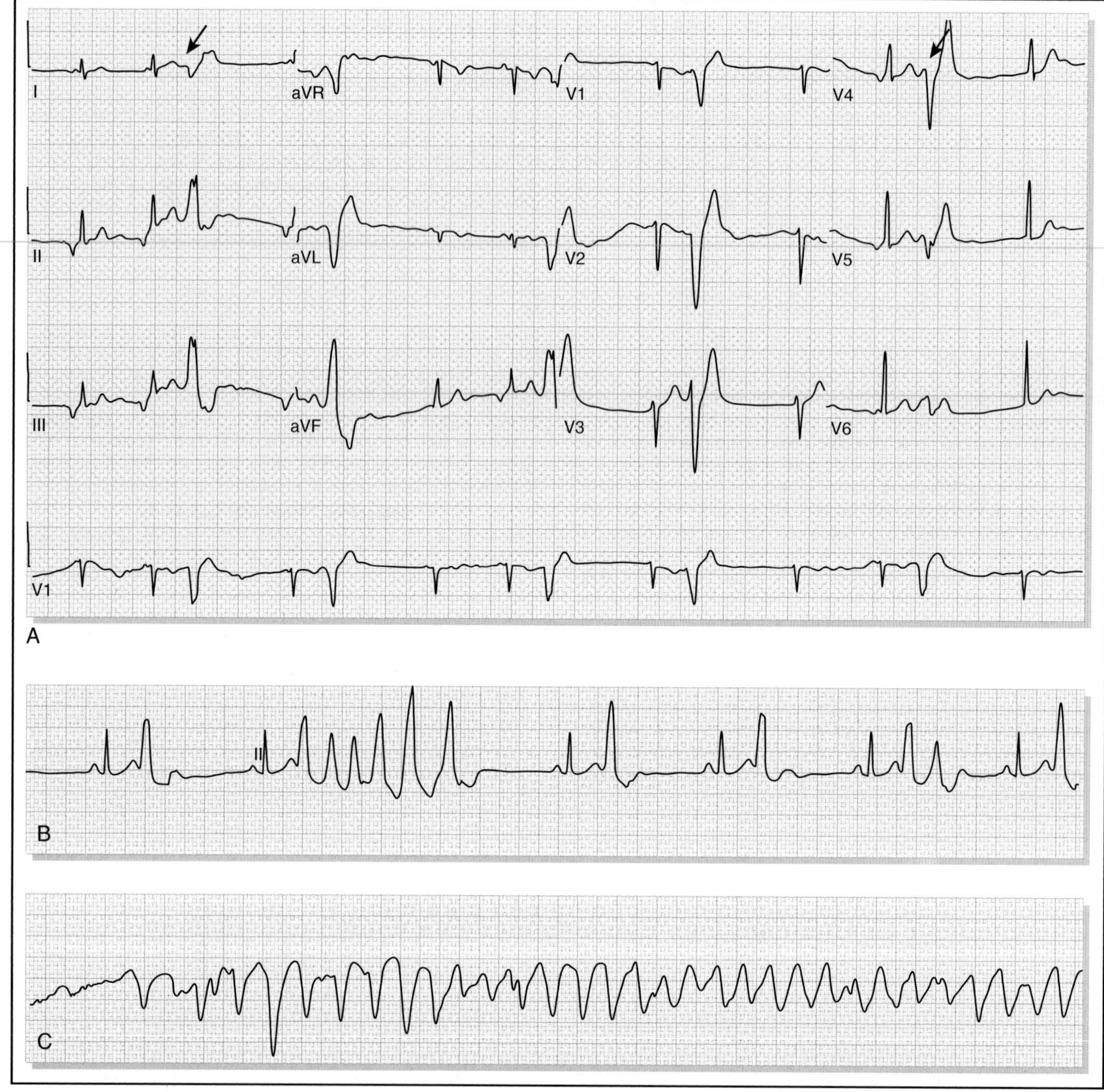

FIGURE 39-36 Tracings from a patient with idiopathic VF due to short-coupled PVCs. **A,** ECG showing frequent, spontaneous short-coupled PVCs, occurring on the late phase of the T wave. **B,** When the PVCs occur during bradycardia, they occur in the early phase of the T wave and produce a short run of VF. **C,** Spontaneous VF in the same patient after another short-coupled spontaneous PVC.

phenytoin, and propranolol, should be considered if excessive digitalis administration is suspected. Otherwise, the usual therapeutic approach to VT is recommended.

Bundle Branch Reentrant Ventricular Tachycardia

VT secondary to bundle branch reentry is characterized by a QRS morphology determined by the circuit established over the bundle branches or fascicles. Retrograde conduction over the left bundle branch system and anterograde conduction over the right bundle branch create a QRS complex with a left bundle branch block contour and constitute the most common form. The frontal plane axis may be about +30 degrees. Conduction in the opposite direction produces a right bundle branch block contour. Reentry can also occur over the anterior and posterior fascicles. Electrophysiologically, bundle branch reentrant complexes are started after a critical S_2-H_2 or S_3-H_3 delay. The H-V interval of the bundle branch reentrant complex equals or exceeds the H-V interval of the spontaneous normally conducted QRS complex.

Bundle branch reentry is a form of monomorphic sustained VT usually seen in patients with structural heart disease, such as dilated cardiomyopathy. During follow-up, congestive heart failure is the most common cause of death in this population. Myocardial VTs can also be present. Uncommonly, bundle branch reentry can occur in the absence of myocardial disease.

The therapeutic approach is as for other types of VT. In the acute setting, pace termination is frequently effective. Long-term catheter ablation effectively eliminates this form of VT.

Ventricular Flutter and Fibrillation (see Chap. 41)

ELECTROCARDIOGRAPHIC RECOGNITION. These arrhythmias represent severe derangements of the heartbeat that usually terminate fatally within 3 to 5 minutes unless corrective measures are

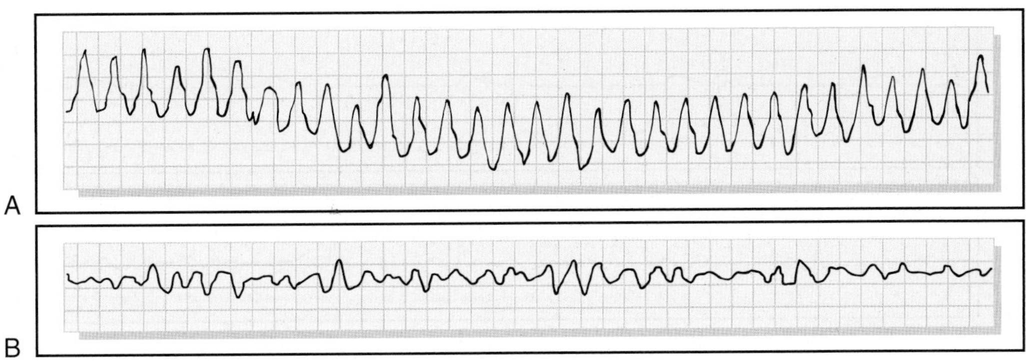

FIGURE 39-37 Ventricular flutter and ventricular fibrillation. **A,** The sine wave appearance of the complexes occurring at a rate of 300 beats/min is characteristic of ventricular flutter. **B,** The irregular undulating baseline typifies ventricular fibrillation.

undertaken promptly. Ventricular flutter is manifested as a sine wave in appearance—regular large oscillations occurring at a rate of 150 to 300 beats/min (usually about 200) (**Fig. 39-37A**). The distinction between rapid VT and ventricular flutter can be difficult and is usually of academic interest only. Hemodynamic collapse is present with both. VF is recognized by the presence of irregular undulations of varying contour and amplitude (Fig. 39-37B). Distinct QRS complexes, ST segments, and T waves are absent. Fine-amplitude fibrillatory waves (0.2 mV) are present with prolonged VF. These fine waves identify patients with worse survival rates and are sometimes confused with asystole.

MECHANISMS. VF occurs in various clinical situations but most commonly in association with coronary artery disease and as a terminal event (see Chap. 35). Thrombolytic agents reduce the incidence of ventricular arrhythmias and inducible VT after myocardial infarction. Cardiovascular events, including sudden cardiac death from VF, but not asystole, occur most frequently in the morning. VF can occur during antiarrhythmic drug administration, hypoxia, ischemia, or atrial fibrillation that results in very rapid ventricular rates in patients with the preexcitation syndrome; after electrical shock administered during cardioversion (see Chaps. 37 and 38) or accidentally by improperly grounded equipment; and during competitive ventricular pacing to terminate VT.

CLINICAL FEATURES. Ventricular flutter or VF results in faintness, followed by loss of consciousness, seizures, apnea, and eventually, if the rhythm continues untreated, death. The blood pressure is unobtainable, and heart sounds are usually absent. The atria can continue to beat at an independent rhythm for a time or in response to impulses from the fibrillating ventricles. Eventually, electrical activity of the heart ceases.

In patients resuscitated from out-of-hospital cardiac arrest, 75% have VF. Bradycardia or asystole, which can occur in 15% to 25% of these patients, is associated with a worse prognosis than VF and is usually associated with more advanced LV dysfunction. VT commonly precedes the onset of VF, although frequently no consistent premonitory patterns emerge.

Although 75% of resuscitated patients exhibit significant coronary artery disease, acute transmural myocardial infarction develops in only 20% to 30%. Those in whom myocardial infarction does not develop have an increased recurrence rate for sudden cardiac death or VF. Predictors of death for resuscitated patients include a reduced ejection fraction, abnormal wall motion, history of congestive heart failure, history of myocardial infarction but no acute event, and presence of ventricular arrhythmias. Patients discharged after an anterior myocardial infarction complicated by VF appear to represent a subgroup at high risk of sudden death. VF can occur in infants, young people, athletes, and persons without known structural heart disease.

MANAGEMENT. Management should follow basic life support and advanced cardiac life support guidelines (see Chap. 41). Immediate nonsynchronized DC electrical shock using 200 to 400 J is mandatory therapy for VF and for ventricular flutter that has caused loss of consciousness. Automatic external defibrillators have facilitated the ability to defibrillate early. Cardiopulmonary resuscitation is used only until the defibrillation equipment is readied. Time should not be wasted with cardiopulmonary resuscitation maneuvers if electrical defibrillation can be done promptly. Defibrillation requires fewer joules if it is done early. If the circulation is markedly inadequate despite return to sinus rhythm, closed-chest massage and artificial ventilation as needed should be instituted. The use of anesthesia during electrical shock is obviously dictated by the patient's condition and is generally not required. After conversion of the arrhythmia to a normal rhythm, it is essential to monitor the rhythm continuously and to institute measures to prevent recurrence. Metabolic acidosis quickly follows cardiovascular collapse. If the arrhythmia is terminated within 30 to 60 seconds, significant acidosis does not occur. Judicious use of sodium bicarbonate to reverse the acidosis may be necessary, but its use should not delay administration of defibrillation shocks (see Chap. 41).

If the resuscitation time is short, artificial ventilation by means of a tightly fitting rubber face mask and an Ambu bag is satisfactory and eliminates the delay attending intubation by inexperienced personnel. If such a mask and bag are not available, mouth-to-mouth or mouth-to-nose resuscitation is indicated. There should be no delay in institution of electrical shock. A search for conditions contributing to the initiation of ventricular flutter or fibrillation should be made and the conditions corrected, if possible. Initial medical approaches to prevent recurrence of VF include intravenous administration of amiodarone, lidocaine, or procainamide. Amiodarone tends to be the most effective and does not produce the ventricular dysfunction and hypotension often seen with procainamide. VF rarely terminates spontaneously, and death results unless countermeasures are instituted immediately. Subsequent therapy is necessary to prevent recurrence. ICDs have become the mainstay of chronic therapy in patients at continued risk for VF or VT from nonreversible causes (see Chaps. 37 and 41).

Bradyarrhythmias

Bradyarrhythmias are arbitrarily defined as a heart rate below 60 beats/min. In some cases, bradyarrhythmias are physiologic, as in well-conditioned athletes with low resting heart rates or type I AV block during sleep, and in other cases are pathologic. Like tachyarrhythmias, bradyarrhythmias can be categorized on the basis of the level of disturbance in the hierarchy of the normal impulse generation and conduction system (from sinus node to AV node to His-Purkinje system).

Sinus Bradycardia

ELECTROCARDIOGRAPHIC RECOGNITION. Sinus bradycardia (**Fig. 39-38A**) exists in an adult when the sinus node discharges at a rate slower than 60 beats/min. P waves have a normal contour and

CH 39

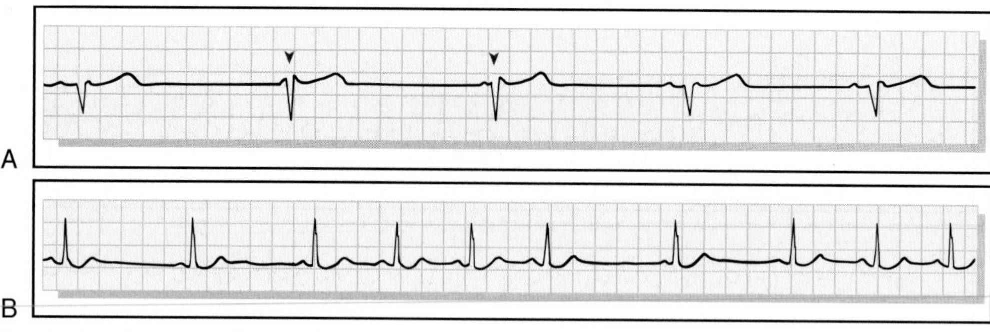

FIGURE 39-38 **A,** Sinus bradycardia at a rate of 40 to 48 beats/min. The second and third QRS complexes (arrowheads) represent junctional escape beats. Note the P waves at the onset of the QRS complex. **B,** Nonrespiratory sinus arrhythmia occurring as a consequence of digitalis toxicity. Monitor leads.

occur before each QRS complex, usually with a constant PR interval longer than 120 milliseconds. Sinus arrhythmia often coexists.

CLINICAL FEATURES. Sinus bradycardia can result from excessive vagal or decreased sympathetic tone, as an effect of medications, or from anatomic changes in the sinus node. In most cases, symptomatic sinus bradycardia is caused by the effects of medication. Asymptomatic sinus bradycardia frequently occurs in healthy young adults, particularly well-trained athletes, and decreases in prevalence with advancing age. During sleep, the normal heart rate can fall to 39 to 40 beats/min, especially in adolescents and young adults, with marked sinus arrhythmia sometimes producing pauses of 2 seconds or longer. Eye surgery, coronary arteriography, meningitis, intracranial tumors, increased intracranial pressure, cervical and mediastinal tumors, and certain disease states (such as severe hypoxia, myxedema, hypothermia, fibrodegenerative changes, convalescence from some infections, gram-negative sepsis, and mental depression) can produce sinus bradycardia. Sinus bradycardia also occurs during vomiting or vasovagal syncope (see Chap. 42) and can be produced by carotid sinus stimulation or by the administration of parasympathomimetic drugs, lithium, amiodarone, beta adrenoceptor blocking drugs, clonidine, propafenone, ivabradine (a specific I_f pacemaker current blocker; see Chap. 35), or calcium antagonists. Conjunctival instillation of beta blockers for glaucoma can produce sinus or AV nodal abnormalities, especially in the elderly.

In most cases, sinus bradycardia is a benign arrhythmia and can actually be beneficial by producing a longer period of diastole and increasing the ventricular filling time. It can be associated with syncope caused by an abnormal autonomic reflex (cardioinhibitory; see Chap. 42). Sinus bradycardia occurs in 10% to 15% of patients with acute myocardial infarction and may be even more prevalent when patients are seen in the early hours of infarction. Unless it is accompanied by hemodynamic decompensation or arrhythmias, sinus bradycardia is generally associated with a more favorable outcome after myocardial infarction than is sinus tachycardia. It is usually transient and occurs more commonly during inferior than anterior myocardial infarction; it has also been noted during reperfusion with thrombolytic agents (see Chap. 55). Bradycardia that follows resuscitation from cardiac arrest is associated with a poor prognosis.

MANAGEMENT. Treatment of sinus bradycardia per se is not usually necessary. For example, if a patient with acute myocardial infarction is asymptomatic, it is probably best to not speed up the sinus rate. If cardiac output is inadequate or if arrhythmias are associated with the slow rate, atropine (0.5 mg intravenously as an initial dose, repeated if necessary) is usually effective. Lower doses of atropine, particularly when it is given subcutaneously or intramuscularly, can exert an initial parasympathomimetic effect, possibly via a central action. For symptomatic episodes of sinus bradycardia that are more than momentary or are recurrent (e.g., as during a myocardial infarction), temporary pacing via a transvenous electrode is usually preferable to repeated or prolonged drug therapy. In some patients who experience congestive heart failure or symptoms of low cardiac output as a result of chronic sinus bradycardia, permanent pacing may be needed (see Chap. 38). Atrial pacing is usually preferable to ventricular pacing to preserve sequential AV contraction and is preferable to drug therapy for long-term management of sinus bradycardia. As a general rule, no available drugs increase the heart rate reliably and safely during long periods without important side effects.

Sinus Arrhythmia

Sinus arrhythmia (Fig. 39-38B) is characterized by a phasic variation in sinus cycle length during which the maximum sinus cycle length minus the minimum sinus cycle length exceeds 120 milliseconds, or the maximum sinus cycle length minus the minimum sinus cycle length divided by the minimum sinus cycle length exceeds 10%. It is the most frequent form of arrhythmia and is considered to be a normal event. P wave morphology does not usually vary, and the PR interval exceeds 120 milliseconds and remains unchanged because the focus of discharge remains relatively fixed within the sinus node. On occasion, the pacemaker focus can wander within the sinus node, or its exit to the atrium may change and produce P waves of a slightly different contour (but not retrograde) and a slightly changing PR interval that exceeds 120 milliseconds.

Sinus arrhythmia commonly occurs in the young, especially those with slower heart rates or after enhanced vagal tone, such as after the administration of digitalis or morphine, and decreases with age or with autonomic dysfunction, such as in diabetic neuropathy. Sinus arrhythmia appears in two basic forms. In the respiratory form, the P-P interval cyclically shortens during inspiration, primarily as a result of reflex inhibition of vagal tone, and slows during expiration; breath-holding eliminates the cycle length variation (see Heart Rate Variability, Chap. 36). Efferent vagal effects alone have been suggested as being responsible for respiratory sinus arrhythmias. Nonrespiratory sinus arrhythmia is characterized by a phasic variation in the P-P interval unrelated to the respiratory cycle and may be the result of digitalis intoxication. Loss of sinus rhythm variability is a risk factor for sudden cardiac death (see Chap. 41).

Symptoms produced by sinus arrhythmia are uncommon, but on occasion, if the pauses between beats are excessively long, palpitations or dizziness may result. Marked sinus arrhythmia can produce a sinus pause sufficiently long to cause syncope if it is not accompanied by an escape rhythm.

Treatment is usually unnecessary. Increasing the heart rate by exercise or drugs generally abolishes sinus arrhythmia. Symptomatic individuals may experience relief from palpitations with sedatives, tranquilizers, atropine, ephedrine, or isoproterenol administration, as for the treatment of sinus bradycardia.

VENTRICULOPHASIC SINUS ARRHYTHMIA. The most common example occurs during complete AV block and a slow ventricular rate, when P-P cycles that contain a QRS complex are shorter than P-P cycles without a QRS complex. Similar lengthening can be present in the P-P cycle that follows a PVC with a compensatory pause. Alterations in the P-P interval are probably caused by the influence of the autonomic nervous system responding to changes in ventricular stroke volume.

SINUS PAUSE OR SINUS ARREST. Sinus pause or sinus arrest (**Fig. 39-39**) is recognized by a pause in the sinus rhythm. The P-P interval delimiting the pause does not equal a multiple of the basic P-P interval. Differentiation of sinus arrest, which is thought to be caused by slowing or cessation of spontaneous sinus nodal automaticity and therefore a disorder of impulse formation, from SA exit block (see later) in patients with sinus arrhythmia can be difficult without direct recordings of sinus node discharge.

Failure of sinus nodal discharge results in the absence of atrial depolarization and in periods of ventricular asystole if escape beats initiated by latent pacemakers do not occur (see Fig. 39-39). Involvement of the sinus node by acute myocardial infarction, degenerative fibrotic changes, effects of digitalis toxicity, stroke, or excessive vagal tone can produce sinus arrest. Transient sinus arrest may have no clinical significance by itself if latent pacemakers promptly escape to prevent ventricular asystole or the genesis of other arrhythmias precipitated by the slow rates. Sinus arrest and AV block have been demonstrated in as many as 30% of patients with sleep apnea (see Chap. 79).

Treatment is as outlined earlier for sinus bradycardia. In patients who have a chronic form of sinus node disease characterized by marked sinus bradycardia or sinus arrest, permanent pacing is often necessary. However, as a general rule, chronic pacing for sinus bradycardia is indicated only in symptomatic patients or those with a sinus pause exceeding 3 seconds.

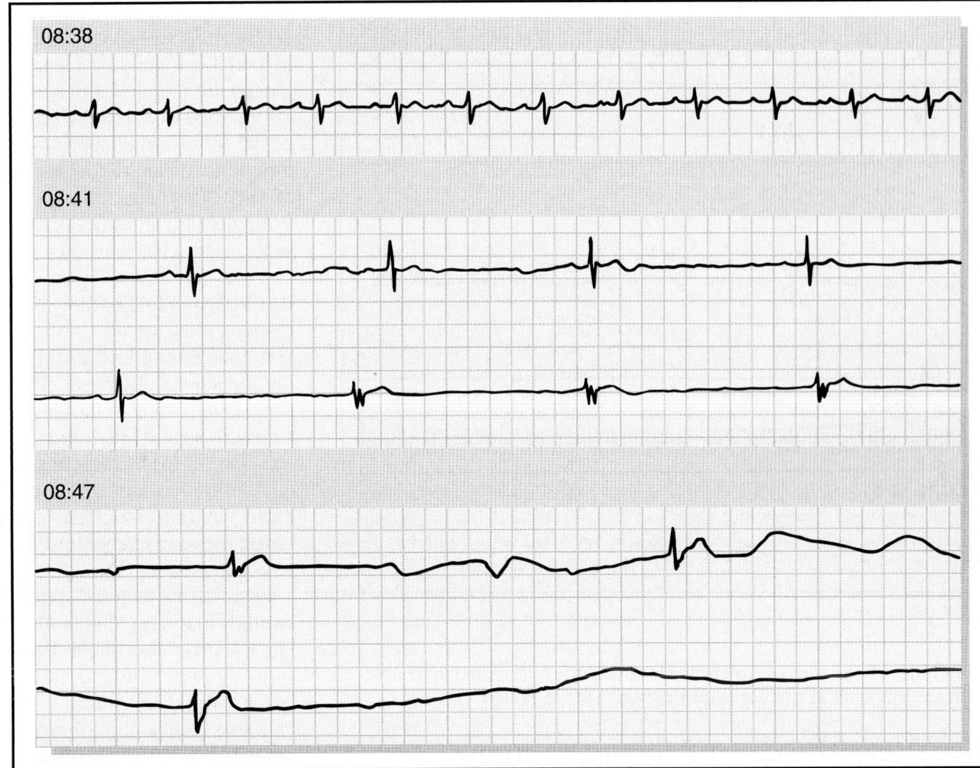

FIGURE 39-39 Sinus arrest. The patient had a long-term electrocardiographic recorder connected when he died suddenly of cardiac standstill. The rhythms demonstrate progressive sinus bradycardia and sinus arrest at 8:41 AM. The rhythm then becomes a ventricular escape rhythm, which progressively slows and finally ceases at 8:47 AM. Monitor lead. The double electrocardiographic strips are continuous recordings.

Sinoatrial Exit Block. This arrhythmia is recognized electrocardiographically by a pause resulting from absence of the normally expected P wave (**Fig. 39-40**). The duration of the pause is a multiple of the basic P-P interval. SA exit block is caused by a conduction disturbance during which an impulse formed within the sinus node fails to depolarize the atria or does so with delay (**Fig. 39-41**). An interval without P waves that equals approximately two, three, or four times the normal P-P cycle characterizes type II second-degree SA exit block. During type I (Wenckebach) second-degree SA exit block, the P-P interval progressively shortens before the pause, and the duration of the pause is less than two P-P cycles. (See Chap. 36 for further discussion of Wenckebach intervals.) First-degree SA exit block cannot be recognized on the ECG because SA nodal discharge is not recorded. Third-degree SA exit block can be manifested as a complete absence of P waves and is difficult to diagnose with certainty without sinus node electrograms.

Excessive vagal stimulation, acute myocarditis, infarction, or fibrosis involving the atrium as well as drugs such as quinidine, procainamide, and digitalis can produce SA exit block. SA exit block is usually transient. It may be of no clinical importance except to prompt a search for the underlying cause. On occasion, syncope can result if the SA block is prolonged and unaccompanied by an escape rhythm. SA exit block can occur in well-trained athletes.

Therapy for patients who have symptomatic SA exit block is as outlined earlier for sinus bradycardia.

Wandering Pacemaker. This variant of sinus arrhythmia involves passive transfer of the dominant pacemaker focus from the sinus node to latent pacemakers that have the next highest degree of automaticity located in other atrial sites (usually lower in the crista terminalis) or in AV junctional tissue. The change occurs in a gradual fashion over the duration of several beats; thus, only one pacemaker at a time controls the rhythm, in sharp contrast with AV dissociation. The ECG (**Fig. 39-42**) displays a cyclical increase in the R-R interval—a PR interval that gradually shortens and can become less than 120 milliseconds and a change in the P wave contour, which becomes negative in lead I or II (depending on the site of discharge) or is lost within the QRS complex. In general, these changes occur in reverse as the pacemaker shifts back to the sinus node. Wandering pacemaker is a normal phenomenon that often occurs in the very young and particularly in athletes, presumably because of augmented vagal tone. Persistence of an AV junctional rhythm (**Fig. 39-43**; see Fig 39-e4 on website) for long periods, however, may indicate

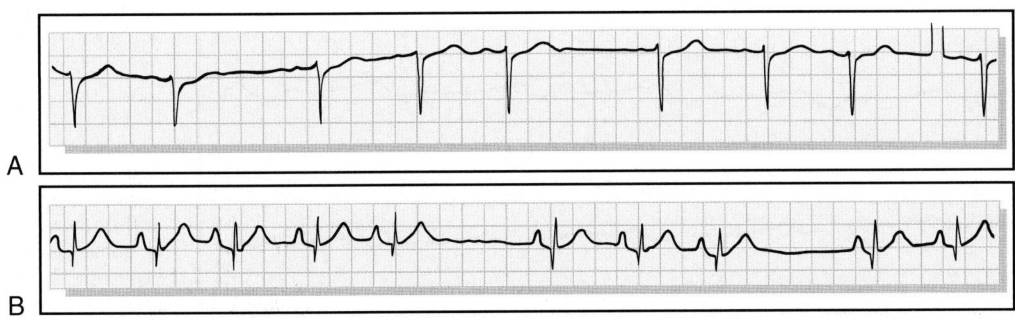

FIGURE 39-40 Sinus nodal exit block. **A,** A type I SA nodal exit block has the following features. The P-P interval shortens from the first to the second cycle in each grouping, followed by a pause. The duration of the pause is less than twice the shortest cycle length, and the cycle after the pause exceeds the cycle before the pause. The PR interval is normal and constant. Lead V_1. **B,** The P-P interval varies slightly because of sinus arrhythmia. The two pauses in sinus nodal activity equal twice the basic P-P interval and are consistent with a type II 2 : 1 SA nodal exit block. The PR interval is normal and constant. Lead III.

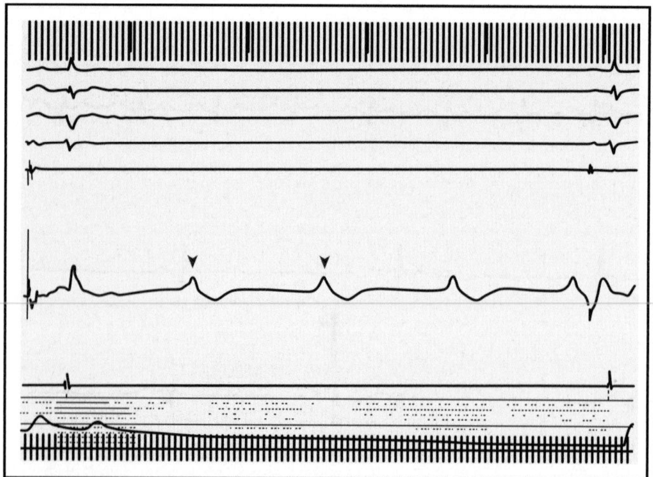

FIGURE 39-41 Sinus node exit block. After a period of atrial pacing (only the last paced cycle is shown), sinus node exit block developed. The tracing demonstrates sinus node potentials (arrowheads), recorded with a catheter electrode, not conducting to the atrium until the last complex. Recordings are leads I, II, III, and V_1, right atrial recording, sinus node recording, and right ventricular apical recording. The bottom tracing is femoral artery blood pressure.

underlying heart disease. Treatment is not usually indicated but, if necessary, is the same as that for sinus bradycardia (see earlier).

Hypersensitive Carotid Sinus Syndrome (see Chap. 42)

ELECTROCARDIOGRAPHIC RECOGNITION. Hypersensitive carotid sinus syndrome (**Fig. 39-44**) is characterized most frequently by ventricular asystole caused by cessation of atrial activity from sinus arrest or SA exit block. AV block is observed less frequently, probably in part because the absence of atrial activity from sinus arrest precludes the manifestations of AV block. However, if an atrial pacemaker maintained an atrial rhythm during the episodes, a higher prevalence of AV block would probably be noted. In symptomatic patients, AV junctional or ventricular escapes generally do not occur or are present at very slow rates, thus suggesting that heightened vagal tone and sympathetic withdrawal can suppress subsidiary pacemakers located in the ventricles as well as in supraventricular structures.

CLINICAL FEATURES. Two types of hypersensitive carotid sinus responses are noted. Cardioinhibitory carotid sinus hypersensitivity is generally defined as ventricular asystole exceeding 3 seconds during carotid sinus stimulation, although normal limits have not been definitively established. In fact, asystole exceeding 3 seconds during carotid sinus massage is not common but can occur in asymptomatic subjects (see Fig. 39-44). Vasodepressor carotid sinus hypersensitivity is generally defined as a decrease in systolic blood pressure of 50 mm Hg or more without associated cardiac slowing or a decrease in systolic blood pressure exceeding 30 mm Hg when the patient's symptoms are reproduced.

Even if a hyperactive carotid sinus reflex is elicited in patients, particularly in older patients who complain of syncope or presyncope, the hyperactive reflex elicited with carotid sinus massage may not necessarily be responsible for these symptoms. Direct pressure or extension of the carotid sinus from head turning, neck tension, and tight collars can also be a source of syncope by reducing blood flow through the cerebral arteries. Hypersensitive carotid sinus reflex is most commonly associated with coronary artery disease. The mechanism responsible for hypersensitive carotid sinus reflex is not known.

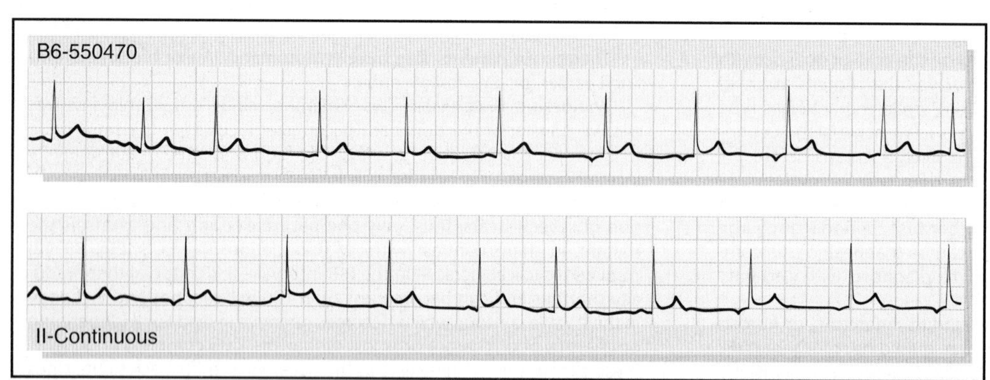

FIGURE 39-42 Wandering atrial pacemaker. As the heart rate slows, the P waves become inverted and then gradually revert toward normal when the heart rate speeds up again. The PR interval shortens to 0.14 second with the inverted P wave and is 0.16 second with the upright P wave. This phasic variation in cycle length with varying P wave contour suggests a shift in pacemaker site and is characteristic of wandering atrial pacemaker.

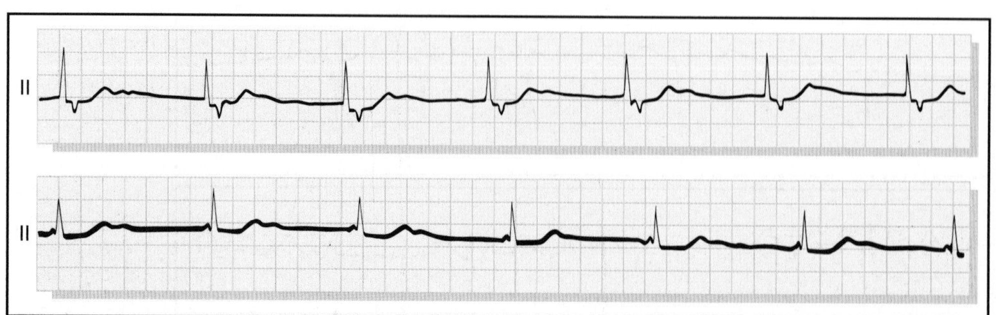

FIGURE 39-43 AV junctional rhythm. **Top,** AV junctional discharge occurs fairly regularly at a rate of approximately 50 beats/min. Retrograde atrial activity follows each junctional discharge. **Bottom,** Recording made on a different day in the same patient. The AV junctional rate is slightly more variable, and retrograde P waves precede onset of the QRS complex. The positive terminal portion of the P wave gives the appearance of AV dissociation, which was not present.

MANAGEMENT. Atropine abolishes cardioinhibitory carotid sinus hypersensitivity. However, most symptomatic patients require pacemaker implantation. Because AV block can occur during periods of hypersensitive carotid reflex, some form of ventricular pacing, with or without atrial pacing, is generally required. Atropine and pacing do not prevent the decrease in systemic blood pressure in the vasodepressor form of carotid sinus hypersensitivity, which may result from inhibition of sympathetic vasoconstrictor nerves and possibly from activation of cholinergic sympathetic vasodilator fibers. Combinations of vasodepressor and cardioinhibitory types can occur, and vasodepression can account for continued syncope after pacemaker implantation in some patients. Patients who have a hyperactive carotid sinus reflex that does not cause symptoms require no treatment. Drugs such as digitalis, methyldopa, clonidine, and propranolol can enhance the response to carotid sinus massage and be responsible for symptoms in some patients. Elastic support hose and sodium-retaining drugs may be helpful in patients with vasodepressor responses.

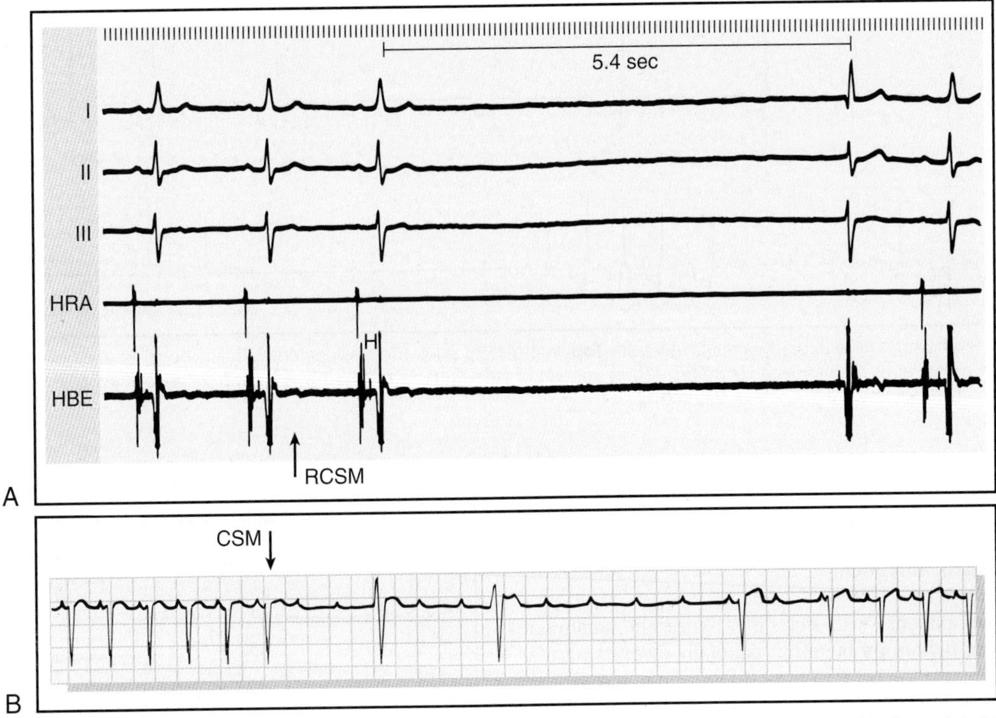

FIGURE 39-44 **A,** Right carotid sinus massage (RCSM, arrow) results in sinus arrest and a ventricular escape beat (probably fascicular) 5.4 seconds later. Sinus discharge then resumes. **B,** Carotid sinus massage (CSM, arrow; monitor lead) results in slight sinus slowing but, more important, advanced AV block. Obviously, an atrial pacemaker without ventricular pacing would be inappropriate for this patient.

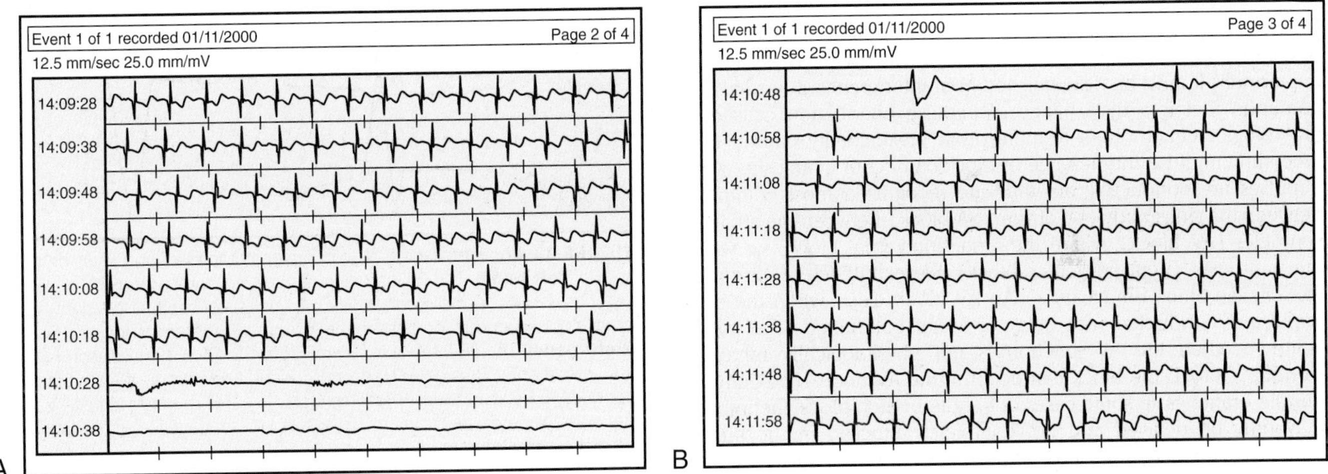

FIGURE 39-45 Continuous recording from an implanted loop recorder in a patient with syncope. The tracing shows paroxysmal sinus node arrest and a sinus pause of nearly 30 seconds. The preceding sinus cycle length appears to lengthen just before the pause, suggesting an autonomic component to the pause. There is also a single ventricular escape complex at 14:10:48.

Sick Sinus Syndrome

ELECTROCARDIOGRAPHIC RECOGNITION. *Sick sinus syndrome* is a term applied to a syndrome encompassing a number of sinus nodal abnormalities, including the following: (1) persistent spontaneous sinus bradycardia not caused by drugs and inappropriate for the physiologic circumstance; (2) sinus arrest or exit block (**Fig. 39-45**); (3) combinations of SA and AV conduction disturbances; and (4) alternation of paroxysms of rapid regular or irregular atrial tachyarrhythmias and periods of slow atrial and ventricular rates (bradycardia-tachycardia syndrome; **Fig. 39-46**). More than one of these conditions can be recorded in the same patient on different occasions, and their mechanisms often can be shown to be causally interrelated and combined with an abnormal state of AV conduction or automaticity.

Patients who have sinus node disease can be categorized as having intrinsic sinus node disease unrelated to autonomic abnormalities or combinations of intrinsic and autonomic abnormalities. Symptomatic patients with sinus pauses or SA exit block frequently show abnormal responses on electrophysiologic testing and can have a relatively high incidence of atrial fibrillation. In children, sinus node dysfunction most commonly occurs in those with congenital or acquired heart disease, particularly after corrective cardiac surgery. Sick sinus syndrome can occur in the absence of other cardiac abnormalities. The course of the disease is frequently intermittent and unpredictable because it is influenced by the severity of the underlying heart disease. Excessive physical training can heighten vagal tone and produce syncope related to sinus bradycardia or AV conduction abnormalities in otherwise normal individuals.

The anatomic basis of sick sinus syndrome can involve total or subtotal destruction of the sinus node, areas of nodal-atrial discontinuity, inflammatory or degenerative changes in the nerves and ganglia surrounding the node, and pathologic changes in the atrial

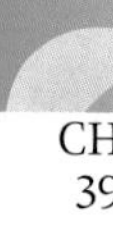

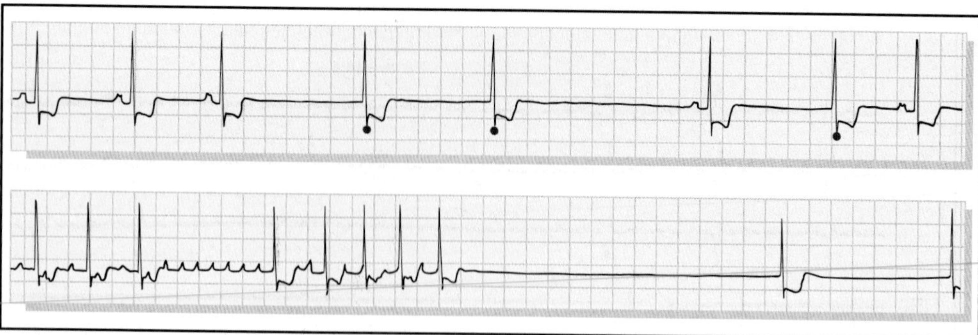

FIGURE 39-46 Sick sinus syndrome with bradycardia-tachycardia. **Top,** Intermittent sinus arrest is apparent with junctional escape beats at irregular intervals (red circles). **Bottom,** In this continuous monitor lead recording, a short episode of atrial flutter is followed by almost 5 seconds of asystole before a junctional escape rhythm resumes. The patient became presyncopal at this point.

wall. Fibrosis and fatty infiltration occur, and the sclerodegenerative processes generally involve the sinus node and the AV node or the bundle of His and its branches or distal subdivisions. Occlusion of the sinus node artery may be important.

MANAGEMENT. For patients with sick sinus syndrome, treatment depends on the basic rhythm problem but generally involves permanent pacemaker implantation when symptoms are manifested (see Chap. 38). Pacing for the bradycardia, combined with drug therapy to treat the tachycardia, is required in those with bradycardia-tachycardia syndrome.

Atrioventricular Block (Heart Block)

Heart block is a disturbance of impulse conduction that can be permanent or transient, depending on the anatomic or functional impairment. It must be distinguished from interference, a normal phenomenon that is a disturbance of impulse conduction caused by physiologic refractoriness resulting from inexcitability caused by a preceding impulse. Interference or block can occur at any site where impulses are conducted, but they are recognized most commonly between the sinus node and atrium (SA block), between the atria and ventricles (AV block), within the atria (intra-atrial block), or within the ventricles (intraventricular block). SA exit block is discussed earlier (see Sinus Bradycardia). An AV block exists when the atrial impulse is conducted with delay or is not conducted at all to the ventricle when the AV junction is not physiologically refractory. During AV block, the block can occur in the AV node, His bundle, or bundle branches. In some cases of bundle branch block, the impulse may only be delayed and not completely blocked in the bundle branch, yet the resulting QRS complex may be indistinguishable from a QRS complex generated by a complete bundle branch block.

The conduction disturbance is classified by severity into three categories. During first-degree heart block, conduction time is prolonged but all impulses are conducted. Second-degree heart block occurs in two forms, Mobitz type I (Wenckebach) and type II. Type I heart block is characterized by a progressive lengthening of the conduction time until an impulse is not conducted. Type II heart block denotes occasional or repetitive sudden block of conduction of an impulse, without prior measurable lengthening of conduction time. When no impulses are conducted, complete or third-degree block is present. The degree of block may depend in part on the direction of impulse propagation. For unknown reasons, normal retrograde conduction can occur in the presence of advanced anterograde AV block. The reverse can also occur. Some electrocardiographers use the term *advanced heart block* to indicate blockage of two or more consecutive impulses.

First-Degree AV Block

During first-degree AV block, every atrial impulse conducts to the ventricles and a regular ventricular rate is produced, but the PR interval exceeds 0.20 second in adults. PR intervals as long as 1.0 second have been noted and can at times exceed the P-P interval, a phenomenon known as skipped P waves. Clinically important PR interval prolongation can result from a conduction delay in the AV node (A-H interval), in the His-Purkinje system (H-V interval), or at both sites. Equally delayed conduction over both bundle branches can uncommonly produce PR prolongation without significant QRS complex aberration. On occasion, an intra-atrial conduction delay can result in PR prolongation. If the QRS complex in the scalar ECG is normal in contour and duration, the AV delay almost always resides in the AV node and rarely within the His bundle itself. If the QRS complex shows a bundle branch block pattern, the conduction delay may be within the AV node or His-Purkinje system (**Fig. 39-47**). In this latter case, a His bundle ECG is necessary to localize the site of conduction delay. Acceleration of the atrial rate or enhancement of vagal tone by carotid massage can cause first-degree AV nodal block to progress to type I second-degree AV block. Conversely, type I second-degree AV nodal block can revert to first-degree block with deceleration of the sinus rate.

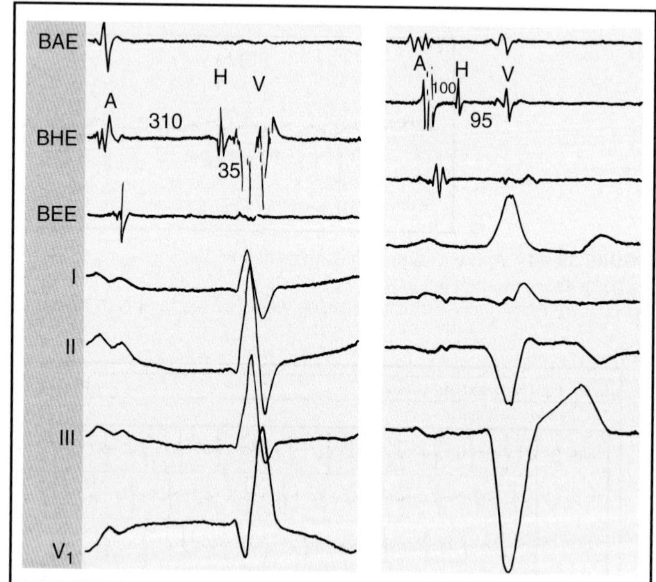

FIGURE 39-47 First-degree AV block. One complex during sinus rhythm is shown. **Left panel,** The PR interval measured 370 milliseconds (PA = 25 milliseconds; A-H = 310 milliseconds; H-V = 39 milliseconds) during a right bundle branch block. Conduction delay in the AV node causes the first-degree AV block. **Right panel,** The PR interval is 230 milliseconds (PA = 39 milliseconds; A-H = 100 milliseconds; H-V = 95 milliseconds) during a left bundle branch block. The conduction delay in the His-Purkinje system causes the first-degree AV block. BAE = bipolar atrial electrogram; BEE = bipolar esophageal electrogram; BHE = bipolar His electrogram.

Second-Degree AV Block

Blocking of some atrial impulses conducted to the ventricle at a time when physiologic interference is not involved constitutes second-degree AV block (**Figs. 39-48** and **39-49**; see 39-e5 on website). The nonconducted P wave can be intermittent or frequent, at regular or irregular intervals, and can be preceded by fixed or lengthening PR intervals. A distinguishing feature is that conducted P waves relate to the QRS complex with recurring PR intervals; that is, the association of P with QRS is not random. Electrocardiographically, typical type I second-degree AV block is characterized by progressive PR prolongation culminating in a nonconducted P wave (see Fig. 39-e5 on website), whereas in type II second-degree AV block, the PR interval remains constant before the blocked P wave (**Fig. 39-50A**). In both cases, the AV block is intermittent and generally repetitive and can block several P waves in a row. Often, the eponyms Mobitz type I and Mobitz type II are applied to the two types of block, whereas Wenckebach block refers to type I block only. A Wenckebach block in the His-Purkinje system in a patient with a bundle branch block can resemble an AV nodal Wenckebach block very closely (Fig. 39-50B).

Certain features of type I second-degree block deserve special emphasis because when actual conduction times are not apparent on the ECG—for example, during SA, junctional, or ventricular exit block (see Fig. 39-48)—a type I conduction disturbance can be difficult to recognize. During a typical type I block, the increment in conduction time is greatest in the second beat of the Wenckebach group, and the absolute increase in conduction time decreases progressively over subsequent beats. These two features serve to establish the characteristics of classic Wenckebach group beating: (1) the interval between successive beats progressively decreases, although the conduction time increases (but by a decreasing function); (2) the duration of the pause produced by the nonconducted impulse is less than twice the interval preceding the blocked impulse (which is usually the shortest interval); and (3) the cycle that follows the nonconducted beat (beginning the Wenckebach group) is longer than the cycle preceding the blocked impulse. Although much emphasis has been placed on this characteristic grouping of cycles, primarily to be able to diagnose a Wenckebach exit block, this typical grouping occurs in less than 50% of patients who have a type I Wenckebach AV nodal block.

Differences in these cycle length patterns can result from changes in pacemaker rate (e.g., sinus arrhythmia), in neurogenic control of conduction, and in the increment of conduction delay. For example, if the PR increment in the last cycle increases, the R-R cycle of the last conducted beat can lengthen rather than shorten. In addition, because the last conducted beat is often at a critical state of conduction, it can become blocked and produce a 5:3 or 3:1 conduction ratio instead of a 5:4 or 3:2 ratio. During a 3:2 Wenckebach structure, the duration

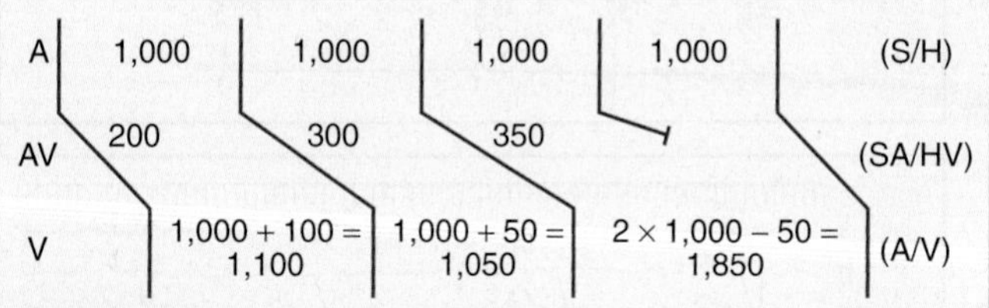

FIGURE 39-48 Typical 4:3 Wenckebach cycle. P waves (A tier) occur at a cycle length of 1000 milliseconds. The PR interval (AV tier) is 200 milliseconds for the first beat and generates a ventricular response (V tier). The PR interval increases by 100 milliseconds in the next complex, which results in an R-R interval of 1100 milliseconds (1000 + 100). The increment in the PR interval is only 50 milliseconds for the third cycle, and the PR interval becomes 350 milliseconds. The R-R interval shortens to 1050 milliseconds (1000 + 50). The next P wave is blocked, and an R-R interval is created that is less than twice the P-P interval by an amount equal to the increments in the PR interval. Thus, the Wenckebach features explained in the text can be found in this diagram. If the increment in the PR interval of the last conducted complex increased rather than decreased (e.g., 150 milliseconds rather than 50 milliseconds), the last R-R interval before the block would increase (1150 milliseconds) rather than decrease and thus become an example of an atypical Wenckebach cycle (see Fig. 39-38). If this were a Wenckebach exit block from the sinus node to the atrium, the sinus node cycle length (S) would be 1000 milliseconds, and the SA interval would increase from 200 to 300 to 350 milliseconds and culminate in a block. These events would be inapparent in the scalar ECG. However, the P-P interval in the ECG would shorten from 1100 to 1050 milliseconds, and, finally, there would be a pause of 1850 milliseconds (A). If this rhythm were a junctional rhythm arising from the His bundle and conducting to the ventricle, the junctional rhythm cycle length would be 1000 milliseconds (H) and the H-V interval would progressively lengthen from 200 to 300 to 350 milliseconds, whereas the R-R interval would decrease from 1100 to 1050 milliseconds and then increase to 1850 milliseconds (V). The only clue to the Wenckebach exit block would be the cycle length changes in the ventricular rhythm.

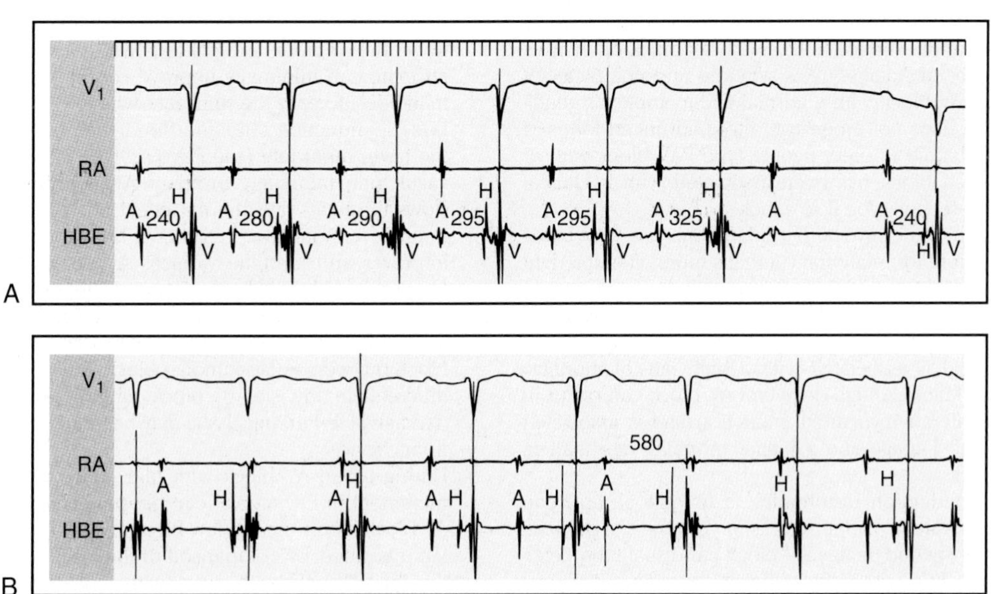

FIGURE 39-49 **A,** Type I (Wenckebach) AV nodal block. During spontaneous sinus rhythm, progressive PR prolongation occurs and culminates in a nonconducted P wave. From the His bundle recording (HBE), it is apparent that the conduction delay and subsequent block occur within the AV node. Because the increment in conduction delay does not consistently decrease, the R-R intervals do not reflect the classic Wenckebach structure. **B,** Recorded 5 minutes after the intravenous administration of atropine 0.6 mg. Atropine has had its predominant effect on sinus and junctional automaticity by this time, with little improvement in AV conduction. Consequently, more P waves are blocked, and AV dissociation, caused by a combination of AV block and an enhanced junctional discharge rate, is present. At 8 minutes (not shown), when atropine finally improved AV conduction, 1:1 AV conduction occurred. RA = right atrium.

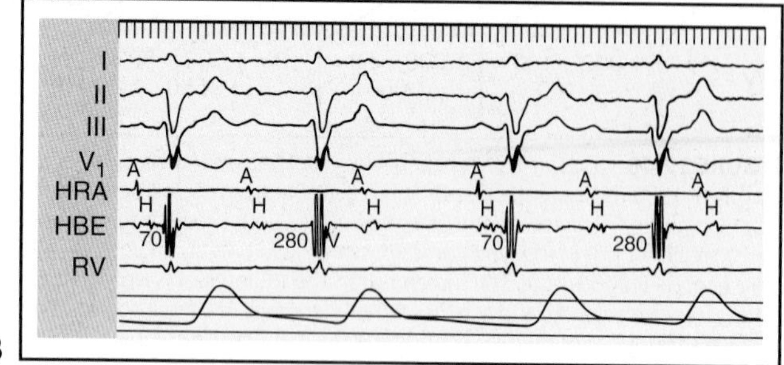

FIGURE 39-50 Type II AV block. **A,** The sudden development of a His-Purkinje block is apparent. The A-H and H-V intervals remain constant, as does the PR interval. Left bundle branch block is present. **B,** Wenckebach AV block in the His-Purkinje system. The QRS complex exhibits a right bundle branch block morphology. However, note that the second QRS complex in the 3:2 conduction exhibits a slightly different contour from the first QRS complex, particularly in V_1. This finding is the clue that the Wenckebach AV block might be in the His-Purkinje system. The H-V interval increases from 70 to 280 milliseconds, and then block distal to the His bundle results. HBE = His bundle electrogram; HRA = high right atrium; RV = right ventricle.

of the cycle that follows the nonconducted beat will be the same as the duration of the cycle that precedes the nonconducted beat.

Although it has been suggested that type I and type II AV block are different manifestations of the same electrophysiologic mechanism that differ only quantitatively in the size of the increments, clinical separation of second-degree AV block into types I and II serves a useful function, and in most cases, the differentiation can be made easily and reliably from the surface ECG. Type II AV block often antedates the development of Adams-Stokes syncope and complete AV block, whereas type I AV block with a normal QRS complex is generally more benign and does not progress to more advanced forms of AV conduction disturbance. In older people, type I AV block with or without bundle branch block has been associated with a clinical picture similar to that seen in type II AV block.

In a patient with an acute myocardial infarction, type I AV block usually accompanies inferior infarction (perhaps more often if a right ventricular infarction also occurs), is transient, and does not require temporary pacing; whereas type II AV block occurs in the setting of an acute anterior myocardial infarction, can require temporary or permanent pacing, and is associated with a high rate of mortality, generally from pump failure. A high degree of AV block can occur in patients with acute inferior myocardial infarction and is associated with more myocardial damage and a higher mortality rate than in those without AV block.

Although type I conduction disturbance is ubiquitous and can occur in any cardiac tissue in vivo as well as in vitro, the site of block for the usual forms of second-degree AV block can usually be determined from the surface ECG with sufficient reliability to permit clinical decisions without requiring invasive electrophysiologic studies. Type I AV block with a normal QRS complex almost always takes place at the level of the AV node, proximal to the His bundle. An exception is the uncommon patient with type I intrahisian block. Type II AV block, particularly in association with a bundle branch block, is localized to the His-Purkinje system. Type I AV block in a patient with a bundle branch block can be caused by a block in the AV node or in the His-Purkinje system. Type II AV block in a patient with a normal QRS complex can be caused by an intrahisian AV block, but the block is likely to be a type I AV nodal block, which exhibits small increments in AV conduction time.

Differentiation of Type I from Type II AV Block

The preceding generalizations encompass most patients with second-degree AV block. However, certain caveats must be heeded to avoid misdiagnosis because of subtle electrocardiographic changes or exceptions.

1. The 2:1 AV block can be a form of type I or type II AV block (**Fig. 39-51**). If the QRS complex is normal, the block is more likely to be type I and located in the AV node, and one should search for transition of the 2:1 block to a 3:2 block, during which the PR interval lengthens in the second cardiac cycle. If a bundle branch block is present, the block can be located in the AV node or His-Purkinje system.
2. AV block can occur simultaneously at two or more levels and cause difficulty in distinguishing between types I and II.
3. If the atrial rate varies, it can alter conduction times and cause a type I AV block to stimulate a type II block or change a type II AV block into type I. For example, if the shortest atrial cycle length that has just achieved 1:1 AV nodal conduction at a constant PR interval is decreased by as little as 10 or 20 milliseconds, the P wave of the shortened cycle can block conduction at the level of the AV node without an apparent increase in the antecedent PR interval. An apparent type II AV block in the His-Purkinje system can be converted to type I in the His-Purkinje system in some patients by increasing the atrial rate.
4. Concealed premature His depolarizations can create electrocardiographic patterns that simulate those of type I or II AV block.
5. Abrupt transient alterations in autonomic tone can cause sudden block of one or more P waves without altering the PR interval of the conducted P wave before or after the block. Thus, an apparent type II AV block would be produced at the AV node. Clinically, a burst of vagal tone usually lengthens the P-P interval as well as producing an AV block.
6. The response of the AV block to autonomic changes, either spontaneous or induced, to distinguish type I from type II AV block can be misleading. Although vagal stimulation generally increases and vagolytic agents decrease the extent of type I AV block, such conclusions are based on the assumption that the intervention acts primarily on the AV node and fail to consider rate changes. For example, atropine can minimally improve conduction in the AV node and markedly increase the sinus rate, which results in an increase in AV nodal conduction time and the degree of AV block as a result of the faster atrial rate (see Fig. 39-49B). Conversely, if an increase in vagal tone minimally prolongs AV conduction time but greatly slows the heart rate, the net effect on type I AV block may be to improve conduction. In general, however, carotid sinus massage improves and atropine worsens AV conduction in patients with His-Purkinje block, whereas the opposite results are to be expected in patients who have AV nodal block. Similarly, exercise or isoproterenol is likely to increase the sinus rate and improve AV nodal block but worsen His-Purkinje block. These interventions can help differentiate the site of block without invasive study, although damaged His-Purkinje tissue may be influenced by changes in autonomic tone.
7. During type I AV block with high ratios of conducted beats, the increment in PR interval can be quite small and suggest a type II AV block if only the last few PR intervals before the blocked P wave are measured. By comparison of the PR interval of the first beat in the long Wenckebach cycle with that of the beats immediately preceding the blocked P wave, the increment in AV conduction becomes readily apparent.
8. The classic AV Wenckebach structure depends on a stable atrial rate and a maximal increment in AV conduction time for the second PR interval of the Wenckebach cycle, with a progressive decrease in subsequent beats. Unstable or unusual alterations in the

increment of AV conduction time or in the atrial rate, often seen with long Wenckebach cycles, result in atypical forms of type I AV block in which the last R-R interval can lengthen because the PR increment increases; these alterations are common.

9. Finally, the PR interval in the scalar ECG is made up of conduction through the atrium, AV node, and His-Purkinje system. An increment in H-V conduction, for example, can be masked in the scalar ECG by a reduction in the A-H interval, and the resulting PR interval will not reflect the entire increment in His-Purkinje conduction time. Very long PR intervals (200 milliseconds) are more likely to result from AV nodal conduction delay (and block), with or without concomitant His-Purkinje conduction delay, although an H-V interval of 390 milliseconds is possible.

First-degree and type I second-degree AV block can occur in normal healthy children, and a Wenckebach AV block can be a normal phenomenon in well-trained athletes, as noted earlier, probably related to an increase in resting vagal tone. On occasion, progressive worsening of the Wenckebach AV conduction disorder can result and the athlete becomes symptomatic and has to decondition. In patients who have chronic second-degree AV nodal block (proximal to the His bundle) without structural heart disease, the course is relatively benign (except in older age groups), whereas in those who have structural heart disease, the prognosis is poor and related to the underlying heart disease.

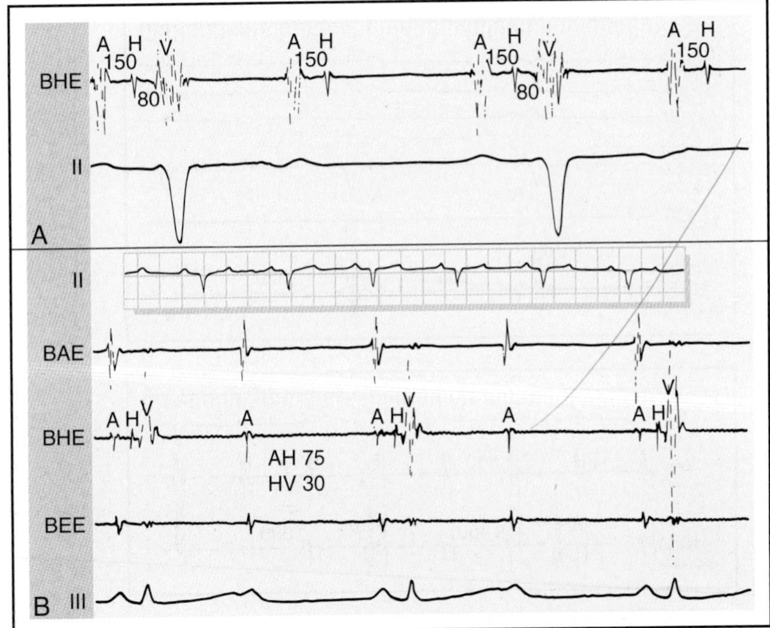

FIGURE 39-51 A 2:1 AV block proximal and distal to the His bundle deflection in two different patients. **A,** A 2:1 AV block seen in the scalar ECG occurs distal to the His bundle recording site in a patient with right bundle branch block and anterior hemiblock. The A-H interval (150 milliseconds) and H-V interval (80 milliseconds) are both prolonged. **B,** A 2:1 AV block proximal to the bundle of His in a patient with a normal QRS complex. The A-H interval (75 milliseconds) and the H-V interval (30 milliseconds) remain constant and normal. BAE = bipolar atrial electrogram; BEE = bipolar esophageal electrogram; BHE = bipolar His electrogram.

Third-Degree (Complete) AV Block

Third-degree or complete AV block occurs when no atrial activity is conducted to the ventricles and therefore the atria and ventricles are controlled by independent pacemakers. Thus, complete AV block is one type of complete AV dissociation. The atrial pacemaker can be sinus or ectopic (tachycardia, flutter, or fibrillation) or can result from an AV junctional focus occurring above the block with retrograde atrial conduction. The ventricular focus is usually located just below the region of the block, which can be above or below the His bundle bifurcation. Sites of ventricular pacemaker activity that are in or closer to the His bundle appear to be more stable and can produce a faster escape rate than can those located more distally in the ventricular conduction system. The ventricular rate in acquired complete heart block is less than 40 beats/min but can be faster in congenital complete AV block. The ventricular rhythm, usually regular, can vary in response to PVCs, a shift in the pacemaker site, an irregularly discharging pacemaker focus, or autonomic influences.

Complete AV block can result from block at the level of the AV node (usually congenital; **Fig. 39-52**), within the bundle of His, or distal to it in the Purkinje system (usually acquired; **Fig. 39-53**). Block proximal to the His bundle generally exhibits normal QRS complexes and rates of 40 to 60 beats/min because the escape focus that controls the ventricle arises in or near the His bundle. In complete AV nodal block, the P wave is not followed by a His deflection, but each ventricular complex is preceded by a His deflection (see Fig. 39-52). His bundle recording can be useful to differentiate AV nodal from intrahisian block because the latter may carry a more serious prognosis than the former. Intrahisian block is recognized infrequently without invasive studies. In patients with AV nodal block, atropine usually speeds both the atrial and ventricular rates. Exercise can reduce the extent of AV nodal block. Acquired complete AV block occurs most commonly distal to the bundle of His because of trifascicular conduction disturbance. Each P wave is followed by a His deflection, and the ventricular escape complexes are not preceded by a His deflection (see Fig. 39-53). The QRS complex is abnormal, and the ventricular rate is usually less than 40 beats/min. A hereditary form caused by degeneration of the His bundle and bundle branches has been linked to the *SCN5A* gene that is also responsible for LQT3 (see Chap. 9).

Paroxysmal AV block[57] in some cases can be caused by hyperresponsiveness of the AV node to vagotonic reflexes. Surgery, electrolyte disturbances, myoendocarditis, tumors, Chagas disease, rheumatoid nodules, calcific aortic stenosis, myxedema, polymyositis, infiltrative processes (e.g., amyloidosis, sarcoidosis, scleroderma), and an almost endless assortment of common and unusual conditions can produce AV block. In adults, rapid rates can sometimes be followed by block (called tachycardia-dependent AV block), which is thought to be due to phase 3 block (block due to incomplete action potential recovery), postrepolarization refractoriness, and concealed conduction in the AV node.[58] Less common than tachycardia-dependent AV block, pause-dependent paroxysmal AV block can also occur, which results in AV block after a pause or during relative bradycardia and thus can be difficult to distinguish from vagal AV block. This form of AV block is often referred to as phase 4 block, as it is thought that spontaneous depolarizations during the resting phase of the action potential result in an inability to depolarize, although other mechanisms may also play a role.[57,58]

In children, the most common cause of AV block is congenital (see Chap. 65). Under such circumstances, the AV block can be an isolated finding or associated with other lesions. Connective tissue disease and the presence of anti-Rh_0 antibodies in the maternal sera of patients with congenital complete AV block raise the possibility that placentally transmitted antibodies play a role in some cases. Anatomic disruption between the atrial musculature and peripheral parts of the conduction system and nodoventricular discontinuity are two common histologic findings. Children are most often asymptomatic; however, in some children, symptoms develop that require pacemaker implantation. Mortality from congenital AV block is highest in the neonatal period, is much lower during childhood and adolescence, and increases slowly later in life. Adams-Stokes attacks can occur in patients with congenital heart block at any age. It is difficult to predict the prognosis in an individual patient. A persistent heart rate at rest of 50 beats/min or less correlates with the incidence of syncope, and extreme bradycardia can contribute to the frequency of Adams-Stokes attacks in children with congenital complete AV block. The site of block may not distinguish symptomatic children who have congenital or surgically induced complete heart block from those without

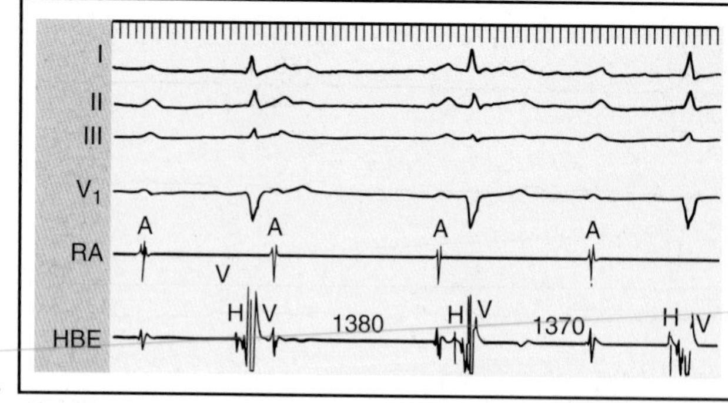

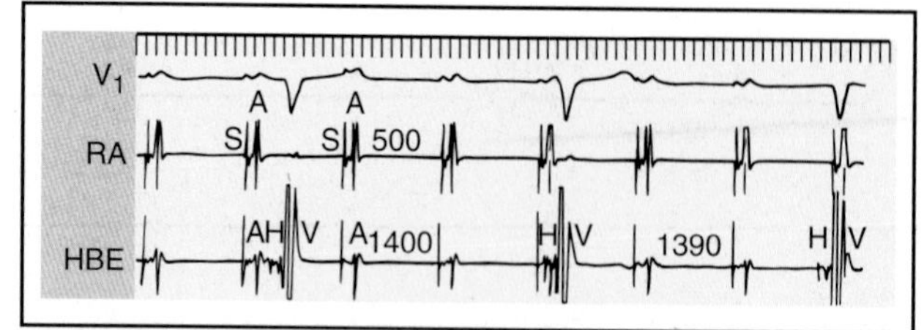

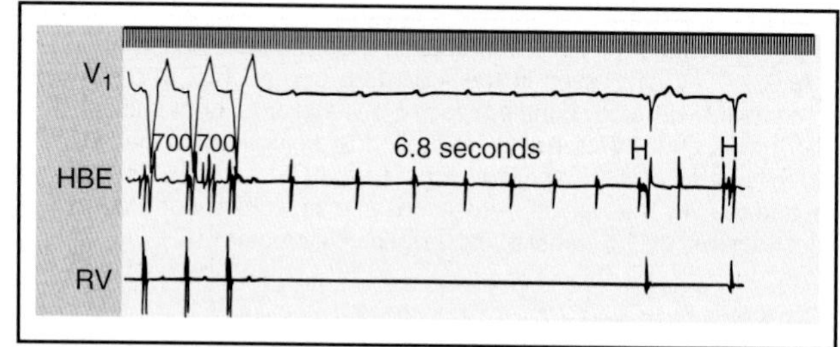

FIGURE 39-52 Congenital third-degree AV block. **A,** Complete AV nodal block is apparent. No P wave is followed by a His bundle potential, whereas each ventricular depolarization is preceded by a His bundle potential. **B,** Atrial pacing (cycle length of 500 milliseconds) fails to alter the cycle length of the functional rhythm. Still, no P wave is followed by a His bundle potential. **C,** After 30 seconds of ventricular pacing (cycle length of 700 milliseconds), suppression of the junctional focus results for almost 7 seconds (overdrive suppression of automaticity). HBE = His bundle electrogram; RA = right atrium; RV = right ventricle.

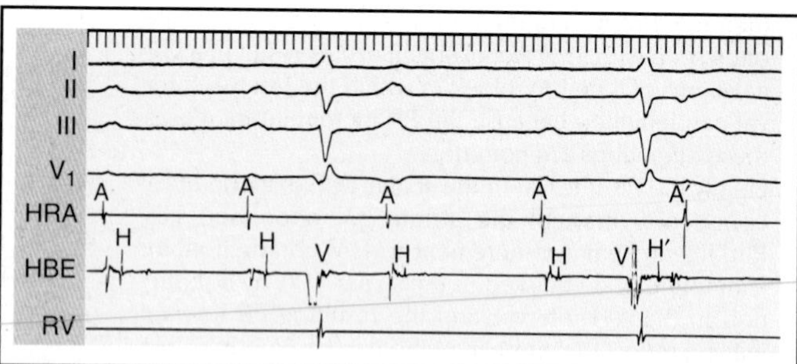

FIGURE 39-53 Complete anterograde AV block with retrograde VA conduction. All the sinus P waves are blocked distal to the His bundle, consistent with acquired complete AV block. The ventricles escape at a cycle length of approximately 1800 milliseconds (33 beats/min) and are not preceded by His bundle activation. The ventricular escape rhythm produces a QRS contour with left-axis deviation and right bundle branch block, possibly caused by impulse origin in the posterior fascicle of the left bundle branch. Of interest is the fact that the second ventricular escape beat conducts retrogradely through His (H) and to the atrium (note the low-high atrial activation sequence and the negative P wave in leads II and III). The first ventricular complex does not conduct retrogradely, probably because the His bundle is still refractory from the immediately preceding atrial impulse. HBE = His bundle electrogram; HRA = high right atrium; RV = right ventricle.

symptoms. Prolonged recovery times of escape foci after rapid pacing (see Fig. 39-52C), slow heart rates on 24-hour ECG recordings, and the occurrence of paroxysmal tachycardias may be predisposing factors to the development of symptoms.

CLINICAL FEATURES. Many of the signs of AV block are evidenced at the bedside. First-degree AV block can be recognized by a long *a-c* wave interval in the jugular venous pulse and by diminished intensity of the first heart sound as the PR interval lengthens. In type I second-degree AV block, the heart rate may increase imperceptibly with gradually diminishing intensity of the first heart sound, widening of the *a-c* interval, terminated by a pause, and an *a* wave not followed by a *v* wave. Intermittent ventricular pauses and *a* waves in the neck not followed by *v* waves characterize type II AV block. The first heart sound maintains a constant intensity. In complete AV block, the findings are the same as those in AV dissociation (see later).

Significant clinical manifestations of first- and second-degree AV block usually consist of palpitations or subjective feelings of the heart's "missing a beat." Persistent 2:1 AV block can produce symptoms of chronic bradycardia. Complete AV block can be accompanied by signs and symptoms of reduced cardiac output, syncope or presyncope, angina, or palpitations from ventricular tachyarrhythmias. It can occur in twins.

MANAGEMENT. For patients with transient or paroxysmal AV block who present with presyncope or syncope, the diagnosis can be elusive. Ambulatory monitoring (Holter or external loop recorders) can be useful, but monitoring for longer periods may be necessary on occasion, and thus an implantable loop recorder may be needed to establish the diagnosis. Drugs cannot be relied on to increase the heart rate for more than several hours to several days in patients with symptomatic heart block without producing significant side effects. Therefore, temporary or permanent pacemaker insertion is indicated for patients with symptomatic bradyarrhythmias. For short-term therapy, when the block is likely to be evanescent but still requires treatment or until adequate pacing therapy can be established, vagolytic agents such as atropine are useful for patients who have AV nodal disturbances, whereas catecholamines such as isoproterenol can be used transiently to treat patients who have heart block at any site (see Sinus Bradycardia). Isoproterenol should be used with extreme caution or not at all in patients who have acute myocardial infarction. The use of transcutaneous or temporary transvenous pacing is preferable. For symptomatic AV block or high-grade AV block (e.g., infrahisian, type II AV block, third-degree heart block not caused by congenital AV block), permanent pacemaker placement is the treatment of choice.

Atrioventricular Dissociation

CLASSIFICATION. As the term indicates, dissociated or independent beating of the atria and ventricles defines AV dissociation. AV dissociation is never a primary disturbance of rhythm but is a "symptom" of an underlying rhythm disturbance produced by one of three causes or a combination of causes (**Fig. 39-54**) that prevent the normal transmission of impulses from atrium to ventricle:

1. Slowing of the dominant pacemaker of the heart (usually the sinus node), which allows escape of a subsidiary or latent pacemaker. AV dissociation by default of the primary pacemaker to a subsidiary one in this manner is often a normal phenomenon. It may occur during sinus arrhythmia or sinus bradycardia and permit an independent AV junction rhythm to arise (see Fig. 39-38A).
2. Acceleration of a latent pacemaker, which usurps control of the ventricles. An abnormally enhanced discharge rate of a usually slower subsidiary pacemaker is pathologic and commonly occurs during nonparoxysmal AV junctional tachycardia or VT without retrograde atrial capture (see Fig. 39-27; also see Fig. 39-e6 on website).
3. Block, generally at the AV junction, that prevents impulses formed at a normal rate in a dominant pacemaker from reaching the

ventricles and allows the ventricles to beat under the control of a subsidiary pacemaker. Junctional or ventricular escape rhythm during AV block, without retrograde atrial capture, is a common example in which block gives rise to AV dissociation. Complete AV block is not synonymous with complete AV dissociation. Patients who have complete AV block have complete AV dissociation, but patients who have complete AV dissociation may or may not have complete AV block (see Figs. 39-52 and 39-53).

4. A combination of causes, for example, when digitalis excess results in the production of nonparoxysmal AV junctional tachycardia associated with SA or AV block.

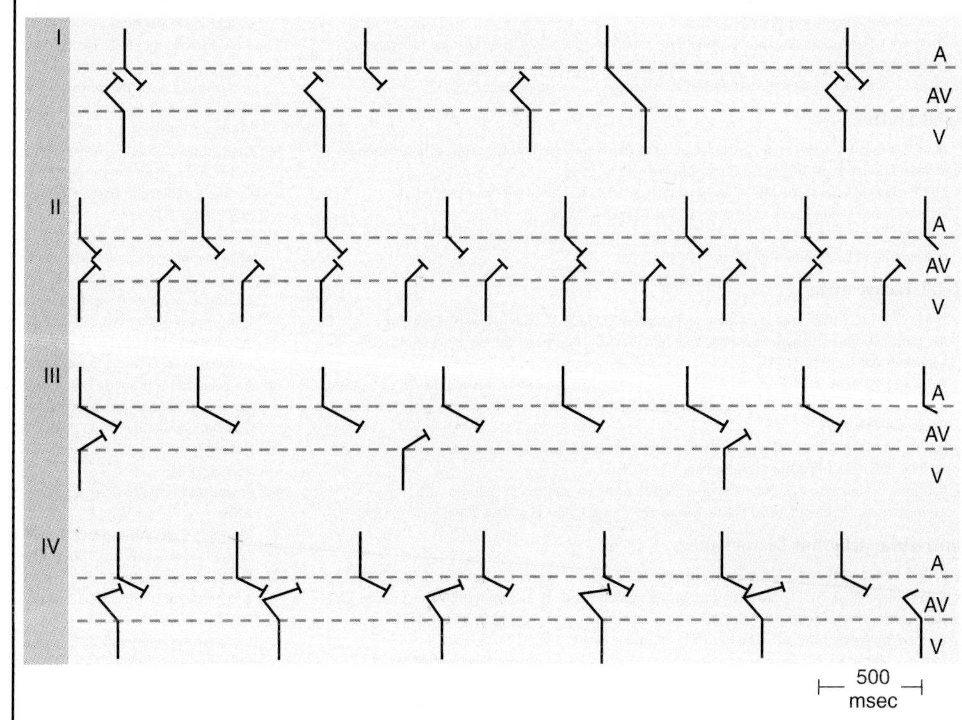

FIGURE 39-54 Diagrammatic illustration of the four causes of AV dissociation. A sinus bradycardia allowing escape of an AV junctional rhythm that does not capture the atria retrogradely illustrates cause I; intermittent sinus captures occur (third P wave) and produce incomplete AV dissociation. For cause II, VT without retrograde atrial capture produces complete AV dissociation (see Fig. 39-27 and Fig 39-e6 on website). As the third cause, complete AV block with a ventricular escape rhythm is diagrammed (see Figs. 39-52 and 39-53). In the bottom panel, the combination of causes II and III is shown, which represents a nonparoxysmal AV junctional tachycardia and some degree of AV block.

MECHANISMS. With this classification in mind, it is important to emphasize that AV dissociation is not a diagnosis and is used in a manner similar to jaundice or fever. One must state that "AV dissociation is present and is caused by . . ." and then give the cause. An accelerated rate of a slower, normally subsidiary pacemaker or a slower rate of a faster, normally dominant pacemaker that prevents conduction because of physiologic collision and mutual extinction of opposing wave fronts (interference) or the manifestations of AV block are the basic disturbances producing AV dissociation. The atria in all these cases beat independently from the ventricles, under control of the sinus node or ectopic atrial or AV junctional pacemakers, and can exhibit any type of supraventricular rhythm. If a single pacemaker establishes control of both atria and ventricles for one beat (capture) or a series of beats (e.g., sinus rhythm, AV junctional rhythm with retrograde atrial capture [see Figs. 39-43 and Fig 39-e4 on website], VT with retrograde atrial capture), AV dissociation is abolished for that period. Conversely, as stated earlier, whenever the atria and ventricles fail to respond to a single impulse for one beat (PVC without retrograde capture of the atrium) or a series of beats (VT without retrograde atrial capture), AV dissociation exists for that period. The interruption of AV dissociation by one or a series of beats under the control of one pacemaker, anterogradely or retrogradely, indicates that the AV dissociation is incomplete. Complete or incomplete dissociation can also occur in association with all forms of AV block. Commonly, when AV dissociation occurs as a result of AV block, the atrial rate exceeds the ventricular rate. For example, a subsidiary pacemaker with a rate of 40 beats/min can escape in the presence of a 2:1 AV block when the atrial rate is 78 beats/min. If the AV block is bidirectional, AV dissociation results.

ELECTROCARDIOGRAPHIC AND CLINICAL FEATURES. The ECG demonstrates the independence of P waves and QRS complexes. The P wave morphology depends on the rhythm controlling the atria—sinus, atrial tachycardia, junctional, flutter, or fibrillation. During complete AV dissociation, both the QRS complex and the P waves appear regularly spaced without a fixed temporal relationship to each other. When the dissociation is incomplete, a QRS complex of supraventricular contour occurs early and is preceded by a P wave at a PR interval exceeding 0.12 second and within a conductible range. This combination indicates ventricular capture by the supraventricular focus. Similarly, a premature P wave with retrograde morphology and a conductible RP interval may indicate retrograde atrial capture by the subsidiary focus.

Physical findings include a variable intensity of the first heart sound as the PR interval changes, atrial sounds, and *a* waves in the jugular venous pulse lacking a consistent relationship to ventricular contraction. Intermittent large (cannon) *a* waves may be seen in the jugular venous pulse when atrial and ventricular contractions occur simultaneously. The second heart sound can split normally or paradoxically, depending on the manner of ventricular activation. A premature beat representing ventricular capture can interrupt a regular heart rhythm. When the ventricular rate exceeds the atrial rate, a cyclical increase in intensity of the first heart sound is produced as the PR interval shortens, climaxed by a very loud sound (bruit de canon). This intense sound is followed by a sudden reduction in intensity of the first heart sound and the appearance of giant *a* waves as the PR interval shortens and P waves "march through" the cardiac cycle.

MANAGEMENT. Management is directed toward the underlying heart disease and precipitating cause. The individual components producing the AV dissociation, not the AV dissociation per se, determine the specific type of antiarrhythmic approach.

REFERENCES

Supraventricular Arrhythmias

1. Goldberger ZD, Rho RW, Page RL: Approach to the diagnosis and initial management of the stable adult patient with a wide complex tachycardia. Am J Cardiol 101:1456, 2008.
2. Lee KW, Badhwar N, Scheinman MM: Supraventricular tachycardia—part I. Curr Probl Cardiol 33:467, 2008.
3. Lee KW, Badhwar N, Scheinman MM: Supraventricular tachycardia—part II: History, presentation, mechanism, and treatment. Curr Probl Cardiol 33:557, 2008.
4. Delacrétaz E: Clinical practice. Supraventricular tachycardia. N Engl J Med 354:1039, 2006.
5. Blomstrom-Lundqvist C, Scheinman MM, Aliot EM, et al: ACC/AHA/ESC guidelines for the management of patients with supraventricular arrhythmias—executive summary: A report of the American College of Cardiology/American Heart Association Task Force on Practice Guidelines and the European Society of Cardiology Committee for Practice Guidelines (Writing

Committee to Develop Guidelines for the Management of Patients With Supraventricular Arrhythmias). Circulation 108:1871, 2003.
6. Brady PA, Low PA, Shen WK: Inappropriate sinus tachycardia, postural orthostatic tachycardia syndrome, and overlapping syndromes. Pacing Clin Electrophysiol 28:1112, 2005.
7. Yusuf S, Camm AJ: Deciphering the sinus tachycardias. Clin Cardiol 28:267, 2005.

Atrial Flutter

8. Jais P, Sanders P, Hsu LF, et al: Flutter localized to the anterior left atrium after catheter ablation of atrial fibrillation. J Cardiovasc Electrophysiol 17:279, 2006.
9. Ishii Y, Gleva MJ, Gamache MC, et al: Atrial tachyarrhythmias after the maze procedure: Incidence and prognosis. Circulation 110(Suppl 1):II164, 2004.
10. Ghali WA, Wasil BI, Brant R, et al: Atrial flutter and the risk of thromboembolism: A systematic review and meta-analysis. Am J Med 118:101, 2005.

Atrial Tachycardia

11. Lee B, Olgin JE: Ablation of focal atrial tachycardias. *In* Wood M, Huang S (eds): Catheter Ablation of Cardiac Arrhythmias: Principles and Practical Approach. 8th ed. Philadelphia, WB Saunders, 2005, pp 181-194.
12. Hillock RJ, Kalman JM, Roberts-Thomson KC, et al: Multiple focal atrial tachycardias in a healthy adult population: Characterization and description of successful radiofrequency ablation. Heart Rhythm 4:435, 2007.
13. Fox DJ, Klein GJ, Skanes AC, et al. How to identify the location of an accessory pathway by the 12-lead ECG. Heart Rhythm 5:1763, 2008.
14. Pappone C, Manguso F, Santinelli R, et al: Radiofrequency ablation in children with asymptomatic Wolff-Parkinson-White syndrome. N Engl J Med 351:1197, 2004.

Ventricular Rhythm Disturbances

15. Latif S, Dixit S, Callans DJ: Ventricular arrhythmias in normal hearts. Cardiol Clin 26:367, 2008.
16. Bala R, Marchlinski FE: Electrocardiographic recognition and ablation of outflow tract ventricular tachycardia. Heart Rhythm 4:366, 2007.
17. Lerman BB: Mechanism of outflow tract tachycardia. Heart Rhythm 4:973, 2007.
18. Mittal S: "Focal" ventricular tachycardia: Insights from catheter ablation. Heart Rhythm 5(Suppl):S64, 2008.
19. Goldberger ZD, Rho RW, Page RL: Approach to the diagnosis and initial management of the stable adult patient with a wide complex tachycardia. Am J Cardiol 101:1456, 2008.
20. Bloomfield DM, Steinman RC, Namerow PB, et al: Microvolt T-wave alternans distinguishes between patients likely and patients not likely to benefit from implanted cardiac defibrillator therapy: A solution to the Multicenter Automatic Defibrillator Implantation Trial (MADIT) II conundrum. Circulation 110:1885, 2004.
21. Chow T, Kereiakes DJ, Bartone C, et al: Prognostic utility of microvolt T-wave alternans in risk stratification of patients with ischemic cardiomyopathy. J Am Coll Cardiol 47:1820, 2006.
22. Tanno K, Ryu S, Watanabe N, et al: Microvolt T-wave alternans as a predictor of ventricular tachyarrhythmias: A prospective study using atrial pacing. Circulation 109:1854, 2004.
23. Bardy GH, Lee KL, Mark DB, et al; Sudden Cardiac Death in Heart Failure Trial (SCD-HeFT) Investigators: Amiodarone or an implantable cardioverter-defibrillator for congestive heart failure. N Engl J Med 352:225, 2005.
24. Zipes DP, Camm AJ, Borggrefe M, et al: ACC/AHA/ESC 2006 guidelines for management of patients with ventricular arrhythmias and the prevention of sudden cardiac death: A report of the American College of Cardiology/American Heart Association Task Force and the European Society of Cardiology Committee for Practice Guidelines (Writing Committee to Develop Guidelines for Management of Patients With Ventricular Arrhythmias and the Prevention of Sudden Cardiac Death). J Am Coll Cardiol 48:e247, 2006.
25. Das MK, Zipes DP: Fragmented QRS: A predictor of mortality and sudden cardiac death. Heart Rhythm 6(3 Suppl):S8-14, 2009. Epub Oct 17, 2008.
26. Almquist AK, Montgomery JV, Haas TS, Maron BJ: Cardioverter-defibrillator implantation in high-risk patients with hypertrophic cardiomyopathy. Heart Rhythm 2:814, 2005.
27. Dokuparti MV, Pamuru PR, Thakkar B, et al: Etiopathogenesis of arrhythmogenic right ventricular cardiomyopathy. J Hum Genet 50:375, 2005.
28. Awad MM, Calkins H, Judge DP; Medscape: Mechanisms of disease: Molecular genetics of arrhythmogenic right ventricular dysplasia/cardiomyopathy. Nat Clin Pract Cardiovasc Med 5:258, 2008.
29. Basso C, Corrado D, Marcus FI, et al: Arrhythmogenic right ventricular cardiomyopathy. Lancet 373:1289, 2009.
30. Marcus FI, Zareba W, Calkins H, et al: Arrhythmogenic right ventricular cardiomyopathy/dysplasia clinical presentation and diagnostic evaluation: Results from the North American Multidisciplinary Study. Heart Rhythm 6:984, 2009.
31. Peters S, Trümmel M, Koehler B: QRS fragmentation in standard ECG as a diagnostic marker of arrhythmogenic right ventricular dysplasia–cardiomyopathy. Heart Rhythm 5:1417, 2008.
32. Liu N, Ruan Y, Priori SG: Catecholaminergic polymorphic ventricular tachycardia. Prog Cardiovasc Dis 51:23, 2008.
33. Napolitano C, Priori SG: Diagnosis and treatment of catecholaminergic polymorphic ventricular tachycardia. Heart Rhythm 4:675, 2007.
34. Györke S: Molecular basis of catecholaminergic polymorphic ventricular tachycardia. Heart Rhythm 6:123, 2009.
35. Wilde AA, Bhuiyan ZA, Crotti L, et al: Left cardiac sympathetic denervation for catecholaminergic polymorphic ventricular tachycardia. N Engl J Med 358:2024, 2008.
36. Collura CA, Johnson JN, Moir C, Ackerman MJ: Left cardiac sympathetic denervation for the treatment of long QT syndrome and catecholaminergic polymorphic ventricular tachycardia using video-assisted thoracic surgery. Heart Rhythm 6:752, 2009.
37. Watanabe H, Chopra N, Laver D, et al: Flecainide prevents catecholaminergic polymorphic ventricular tachycardia in mice and humans. Nat Med 15:380, 2009.
38. Antzelevitch C, Brugada P, Borggrefe M, et al: Brugada syndrome: Report of the second consensus conference: endorsed by the Heart Rhythm Society and the European Heart Rhythm Association. Circulation 111:659, 2005.
39. Boussy T, Paparella G, de Asmundis C, et al: Genetic basis of ventricular arrhythmias. Cardiol Clin 26:335, 2008.
40. Fowler SJ, Priori SG: Clinical spectrum of patients with a Brugada ECG. Curr Opin Cardiol 24:74, 2009.
41. Morita H, Zipes DP, Lopshire J, et al: T wave alternans in an in vitro canine tissue model of Brugada syndrome. Am J Physiol Heart Circ Physiol 291:H421, 2006.
42. Morita H, Kusano KF, Miura D, et al: Fragmented QRS as a marker of conduction abnormality and predictor of prognosis of Brugada syndrome. Circulation 118:1697, 2008.
43. Postema PG, Wolpert C, Amin AS, et al: Drugs and Brugada syndrome patients: Review of the literature, recommendations, and an up-to-date website (www.brugadadrugs.org). Heart Rhythm 6:1335, 2009.
44. Voss F, Opthof T, Marker J, et al: There is no transmural heterogeneity in an index of action potential duration in the canine left ventricle. Heart Rhythm 6:1028, 2009.
45. Goldenberg I, Moss AJ: Long QT syndrome. J Am Coll Cardiol 51:2291, 2008.
46. Maron BJ, Zipes DP: Introduction: Eligibility recommendations for competitive athletes with cardiovascular abnormalities—general considerations. J Am Coll Cardiol 45:1318, 2005.
47. Morita H, Wu J, Zipes DP: The QT syndromes: Long and short. Lancet 372:750, 2008.
48. Gaita F, Giustetto C, Bianchi F, et al: Short QT syndrome: Pharmacological treatment. J Am Coll Cardiol 43:1494, 2004.
49. Yamada T, Yoshida N, Murakami Y, et al: Electrocardiographic characteristics of ventricular arrhythmias originating from the junction of the left and right coronary sinuses of Valsalva in the aorta: The activation pattern as a rationale for the electrocardiographic characteristics. Heart Rhythm 5:184, 2008.
50. Bala R, Marchlinski FE: Electrocardiographic recognition and ablation of outflow tract ventricular tachycardia. Heart Rhythm 4:366, 2007.
51. Tada H, Tadokoro K, Ito S, et al: Idiopathic ventricular arrhythmias originating from the tricuspid annulus: Prevalence, electrocardiographic characteristics, and results of radiofrequency catheter ablation. Heart Rhythm 4:7, 2007.
52. Kumagai K, Yamauchi Y, Takahashi A, et al: Idiopathic left ventricular tachycardia originating from the mitral annulus. J Cardiovasc Electrophysiol 16:1029, 2005.
53. Stevenson WG, Soejima K: Catheter ablation for ventricular tachycardia. Circulation 115:2750, 2007.
54. Haïssaguerre M, Derval N, Sacher F, et al: Sudden cardiac arrest associated with early repolarization. N Engl J Med 358:2016, 2008.
55. Antzelevitch C, Yan GX: J wave syndromes. Heart Rhythm 7:549, 2010 .
56. Knecht S, Sacher F, Wright M, et al: Long-term follow-up of idiopathic ventricular fibrillation ablation: A multicenter study. J Am Coll Cardiol 54:522, 2009.

Atrioventricular Block (Heart Block)

57. Lee S, Wellens HJ, Josephson ME: Paroxysmal atrioventricular block. Heart Rhythm 6:1229, 2009.
58. El-Sherif N, Jalife J: Paroxysmal atrioventricular block: Are phase 3 and phase 4 block mechanisms or misnomers? Heart Rhythm 6:1514, 2009.

CHAPTER 40 Atrial Fibrillation: Clinical Features, Mechanisms, and Management

Fred Morady and Douglas P. Zipes

Electrocardiographic Features

Atrial fibrillation (AF) is a supraventricular arrhythmia characterized electrocardiographically by low-amplitude baseline oscillations (fibrillatory or f waves) and an irregularly irregular ventricular rhythm. The f waves have a rate of 300 to 600 beats/min and are variable in amplitude, shape, and timing. In contrast, flutter waves have a rate of 250 to 350 beats/min and are constant in timing and morphology (**Fig. 40-1**). In lead V_1, f waves sometimes appear uniform and can mimic flutter waves (**Fig. 40-2**). The distinguishing feature from atrial flutter is the absence of uniform and regular atrial activity in the other leads of the electrocardiogram. In some patients, f waves are very small and not perceptible on the electrocardiogram. In such patients, the diagnosis of AF is based on the irregularly irregular ventricular rhythm (**Fig. 40-3**).

The ventricular rate during AF in the absence of negative dromotropic agents typically is 100 to 160 beats/min. In patients with the Wolff-Parkinson-White syndrome, the ventricular rate during AF can exceed 250 beats/min because of conduction over the accessory pathway (see Chap. 39). When the ventricular rate during AF is very rapid (>170 beats/min), the degree of irregularity is attenuated and the rhythm can seem regular (**Fig. 40-4**).

The ventricular rhythm can be regular during AF in patients with a ventricular pacemaker who are fully paced and when there is third-degree atrioventricular (AV) block with a regular escape rhythm. In these cases, the diagnosis of AF is based on the presence of f waves. When there is third-degree AV block with a junctional escape, Wenckebach exit block in the AV junction (as can occur during digitalis toxicity) results in a regularly irregular ventricular rate (see Chaps. 36 and 39).

Classification of Atrial Fibrillation

AF that terminates spontaneously within 7 days is termed paroxysmal, and AF present continuously for more than 7 days is called persistent. AF persistent for more than 1 year is termed longstanding, whereas longstanding AF refractory to cardioversion is termed permanent. However, "permanent AF" is not necessarily permanent in the literal sense because it may be successfully eliminated by surgical or catheter ablation.

Some patients with paroxysmal AF occasionally can have episodes that are persistent, and vice versa. The predominant form of AF determines how it should be categorized.

A confounding factor in the classification of AF is cardioversion and antiarrhythmic drug therapy. For example, if a patient undergoes transthoracic cardioversion 24 hours after the onset of AF, it is unknown whether the AF would have persisted for more than 7 days. Furthermore, antiarrhythmic drug therapy may change persistent AF into paroxysmal AF. It is generally thought that the classification of AF should not be altered on the basis of the effects of electrical cardioversion or antiarrhythmic drug therapy.

Lone AF refers to AF that occurs in patients younger than 60 years who do not have hypertension or any evidence of structural heart disease. This designation is clinically relevant because patients with lone AF are at lower risk of thromboembolic complications, eliminating the necessity for anticoagulation with warfarin. In addition, the absence of structural heart disease allows the safe use of rhythm-control drugs such as flecainide in patients with lone AF.

Paroxysmal AF also can be classified clinically on the basis of the autonomic setting in which it most often occurs. Approximately 25% of patients with paroxysmal AF have "vagotonic AF," in which AF is initiated in the setting of high vagal tone, typically in the evening when the patient is relaxing or during sleep. At least in theory, drugs that have a vagotonic effect (such as digitalis) may aggravate vagotonic AF, and drugs that have a vagolytic effect (such as disopyramide) may be particularly appropriate for prophylactic therapy. "Adrenergic AF" occurs in approximately 10% to 15% of patients with paroxysmal AF in the setting of high sympathetic tone, for example, during strenuous exertion. In patients with adrenergic AF, beta blockers not only may provide rate control but may prevent the onset of AF. Most patients have a mixed or random form of paroxysmal AF, with no consistent pattern of onset.

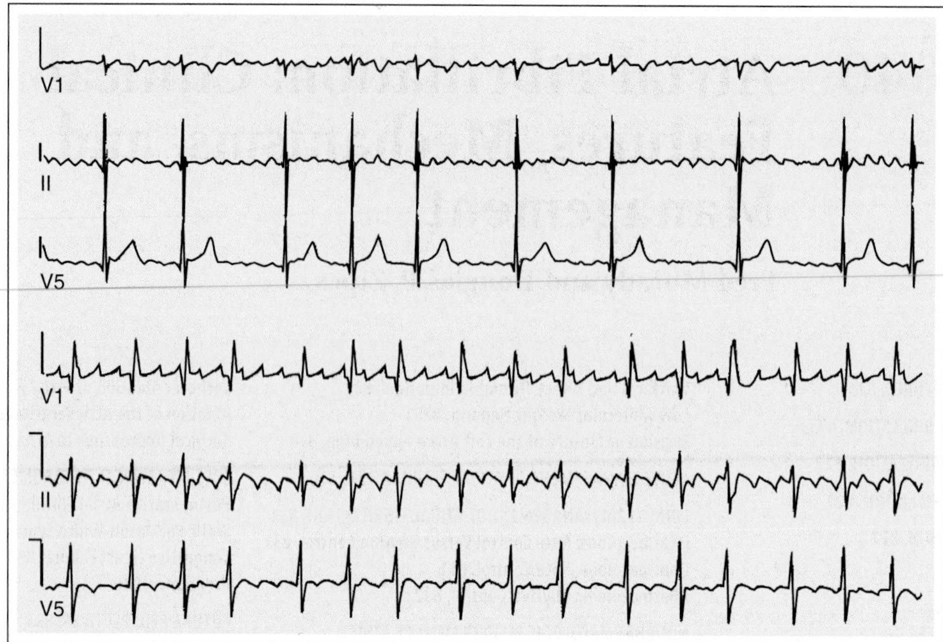

FIGURE 40-1 Comparison between the f waves of AF **(top panel)** and the flutter waves of atrial flutter (**bottom panel)**. Note that f waves are variable in rate, shape, and amplitude, whereas flutter waves are constant in rate and all aspects of morphology. Shown are leads V_1, II, and V_5.

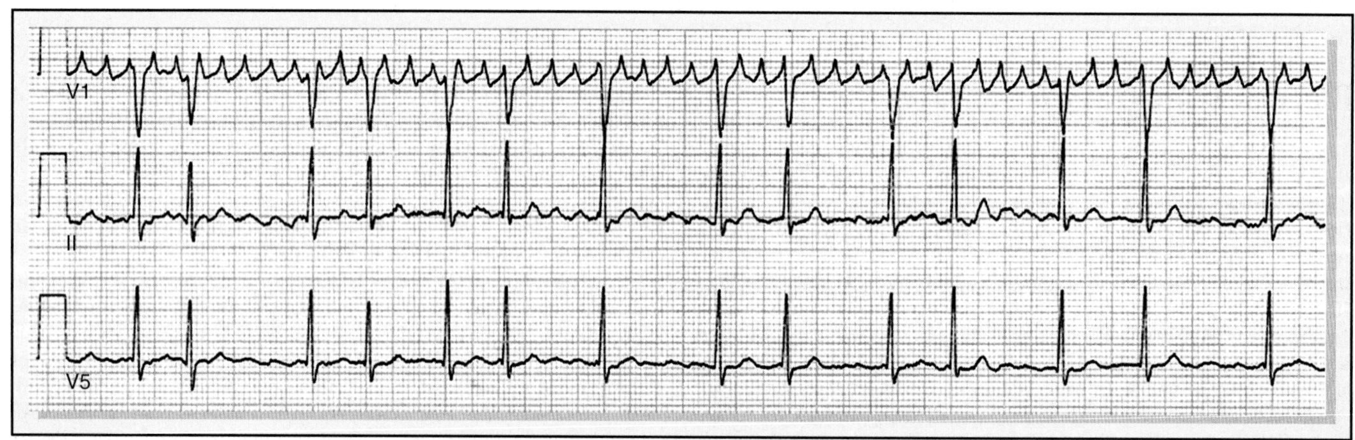

FIGURE 40-2 An example of AF with prominent f waves in V_1 that mimic atrial flutter waves. Note that typical f waves are present in leads II and V_5, establishing the diagnosis of AF.

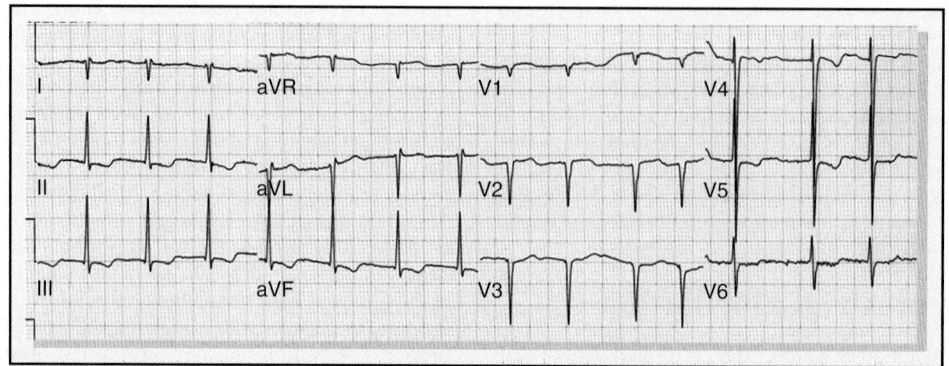

FIGURE 40-3 A 12-lead electrocardiogram of AF in which f waves are not discernible. The irregularly irregular ventricular rate indicates that this is AF and not a junctional rhythm.

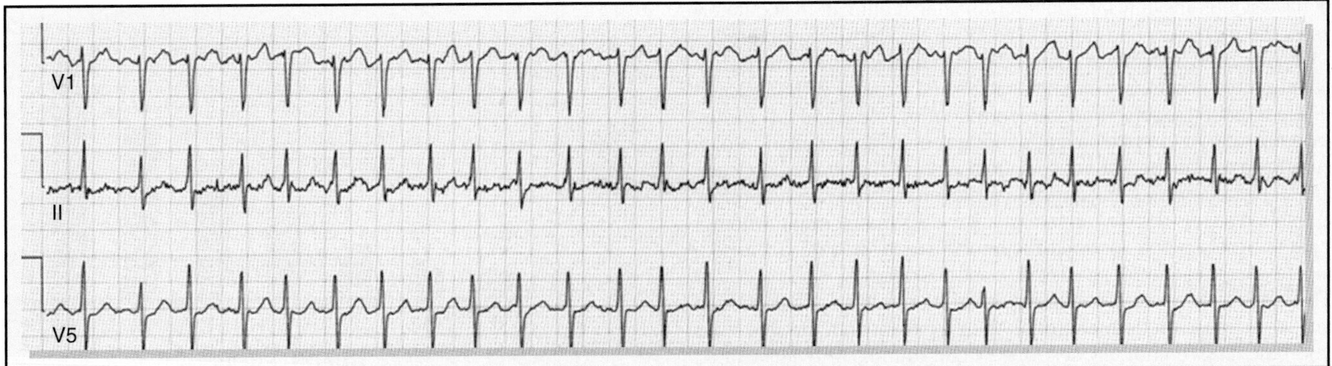

FIGURE 40-4 A recording of AF with a rapid ventricular rate of 160 beats/min. Shown are leads V_1, II, and V_5. On quick review, there may appear to be a regular rate consistent with paroxysmal supraventricular tachycardia. On closer inspection, it is clear that the rate is irregularly irregular.

Epidemiology of Atrial Fibrillation

AF is the most common arrhythmia treated in clinical practice and the most common arrhythmia for which patients are hospitalized; approximately 33% of arrhythmia-related hospitalizations are for AF. AF is associated with approximately a fivefold increase in the risk of stroke and a twofold increase in the risk of all-cause mortality.[1] AF also is associated with the development of heart failure.

It is estimated that at least 1% of the population in the United States has AF. Estimates of the actual number of individuals with AF in the United States range between 2.3 and 5 million in most studies. The incidence of AF is age and gender related, ranging from 0.1%/year before the age of 40 years to more than 1.5%/year in women and more than 2%/year in men older than 80 years. The Framingham Study[2] estimated the lifetime risk for development of AF after the age of 40 years to be 26% for men and 23% for women. Congestive heart failure, aortic and mitral valve disease, left atrial enlargement, hypertension, and advanced age are independent risk factors for the development of AF. Obesity and obstructive sleep apnea (see Chap. 79) also are risk factors for AF.[3,4]

A community-based cohort study in Olmstead County, Minnesota, reported that the age-adjusted incidence of AF per 1000 person-years increased significantly between 1980 and 2000 from 4.4 to 5.4 in men and from 2.4 to 2.8 in women.[5] There was a relative increase of 0.6%/year in the age-adjusted AF incidence. This increase was not accounted for by increased use of electrocardiography. An increase in obesity accounted for 60% of the age-adjusted increase in AF incidence. The number of patients with AF in the United States was estimated to be 3.2 million in 1980 and 5.1 million in 2000 and was projected to be 12.1 to 15.9 million in 2050, all of which are higher than previous estimates.

Mechanisms of Atrial Fibrillation

The mechanisms responsible for AF are complex. Triggering events may differ from maintenance mechanisms. In addition, the clinical phenotypes of paroxysmal, persistent, and longstanding persistent have different electrophysiologic characteristics because of remodeling and different clinical modulators that affect the substrate, such as heart failure, atrial stretch and ischemia, sympathovagal influences, inflammation, and fibrosis.

There probably are two electrophysiologic mechanisms of AF: one or more automatic, triggered, or microreentrant foci, so-called drivers, which fire at rapid rates and cause fibrillation-like activity; and multiple reentrant circuits meandering throughout the atria, annihilating and reforming wavelets that perpetuate the fibrillation. In many studies, the left atrium contains the site of dominant frequency discharge, with a left-to-right gradient. Both mechanisms may be present simultaneously. Rapid discharges from the pulmonary veins are the most common triggers of AF and also may play a perpetuating role, more so in paroxysmal AF than in persistent AF. This is why pulmonary vein isolation is particularly effective for elimination of paroxysmal AF. In persistent AF, changes in the atrial substrate, including interstitial fibrosis that contributes to slow, discontinuous, and anisotropic conduction, may give rise to complex fractionated atrial electrograms (CFAEs) and reentry. Therefore, pulmonary vein isolation is rarely sufficient to eliminate persistent AF, and additional ablation of the atrial substrate usually is necessary (see Chap. 39).

Causes of Atrial Fibrillation

The majority of patients with AF have hypertension (usually with left ventricular hypertrophy; see Chaps. 45 and 46) or some other form of structural heart disease. In addition to hypertensive heart disease, the most common cardiac abnormalities associated with AF are ischemic heart disease (see Chap. 57), mitral valve disease (see Chap. 66), hypertrophic cardiomyopathy (see Chap. 69), and dilated cardiomyopathy (see Chap. 68). Less common causes of AF are restrictive cardiomyopathies such as amyloidosis (see Chap. 68), constrictive pericarditis (see Chap. 75), and cardiac tumors (see Chap. 74). Severe pulmonary hypertension often is associated with AF (see Chap. 78).

Obesity and obstructive sleep apnea (see Chap. 79) are associated with each other, and both have been found to independently increase the risk of AF.[3] Available data suggest that atrial dilation and an increase in systemic inflammatory factors are responsible for the relationship between obesity and AF. The possible mechanisms of AF in patients with sleep apnea include hypoxia, surges in autonomic tone, and hypertension.

AF can be due to causes that are temporary or reversible. The most common temporary causes are excessive alcohol intake (holiday heart), open heart or thoracic surgery, myocardial infarction (see Chap. 55), pericarditis (see Chap. 75), myocarditis (see Chap. 70), and pulmonary embolism (see Chap. 77). The most common correctable cause is hyperthyroidism (see Chap. 86).

AF is sometimes tachycardia induced. Patients with tachycardia-induced AF most often have AV nodal reentrant tachycardia or a tachycardia related to the Wolff-Parkinson-White syndrome that degenerates into AF. If a patient presenting with AF has a history of rapid and regular palpitations before the onset of irregular palpitations or has a Wolff-Parkinson-White electrocardiographic pattern, this should raise the suspicion of tachycardia-induced AF. Treatment of the tachycardia that triggers the AF often but not always prevents recurrences of AF.

Clinical Features

The symptoms of AF vary widely between patients, ranging from none to severe and functionally disabling symptoms. The most common symptoms of AF are palpitations, fatigue, dyspnea, effort intolerance, and lightheadedness. Polyuria can occur because of release of atrial natriuretic hormone. Many patients with symptomatic paroxysmal AF also have asymptomatic episodes, and some patients with persistent

AF have symptoms only intermittently, making it difficult to accurately assess the frequency and duration of AF on the basis of symptoms.

It is estimated that approximately 25% of patients with AF are asymptomatic, more commonly elderly patients and patients with persistent AF. Such patients sometimes are erroneously classified as having asymptomatic AF despite having symptoms of fatigue or effort intolerance. Because fatigue is a nonspecific symptom, it may not be clearly due to persistent AF. A "diagnostic cardioversion" may be helpful by maintaining sinus rhythm for at least a few days to determine whether a patient feels better in sinus rhythm. This can provide a basis to pursue a rhythm-control versus rate-control strategy.

Syncope is an uncommon symptom of AF, most often caused by a long sinus pause on termination of AF in a patient with the sick sinus syndrome. Less commonly, syncope occurs during AF with a rapid ventricular rate either because of neurocardiogenic (vasodepressor) syncope that is triggered by the tachycardia or because of a severe drop in blood pressure due to a sudden reduction in cardiac output. The latter is most likely to occur in patients with structural heart diseases such as hypertrophic cardiomyopathy and aortic stenosis.

Asymptomatic or minimally symptomatic AF patients are not prompted to seek medical care and can present with a thromboembolic complication such as stroke or the insidious onset of heart failure symptoms, eventually presenting in florid congestive heart failure.

The hallmark of AF on physical examination is an irregularly irregular pulse. Short R-R intervals during AF do not allow adequate time for left ventricular diastolic filling, resulting in a low stroke volume and the absence of palpable peripheral pulse. This results in a "pulse deficit," during which the peripheral pulse is not as rapid as the apical rate. Other manifestations of AF on the physical examination are irregular jugular venous pulsations and variable intensity of the first heart sound.

Diagnostic Evaluation

In a patient who describes irregular or rapid palpitations suggestive of paroxysmal AF, ambulatory monitoring is useful to document whether AF is responsible for the symptoms. If the symptoms occur on a daily basis, a 24-hour Holter recording is appropriate. However, extended monitoring for 2 to 4 weeks with an event monitor or by mobile cardiac outpatient telemetry is appropriate for patients whose symptoms are sporadic (see Chap. 36).

The history should be directed at determination of the type and severity of symptoms, the first onset of AF, whether the AF is paroxysmal or persistent, the triggers of AF, whether the episodes are random or occur at particular times (such as during sleep), and the frequency and duration of episodes. When it is unclear from the history, 3 to 4 weeks of ambulatory monitoring with an autotrigger event monitor or by mobile cardiac outpatient telemetry is useful to determine whether AF is paroxysmal or persistent and to quantitate the AF burden in patients with paroxysmal AF. The history also should be directed at identification of potentially correctible causes (e.g., hyperthyroidism, excessive alcohol intake), structural heart disease, and comorbidities.

Laboratory testing should include thyroid function tests, liver function tests, and renal function tests. Echocardiography always is appropriate to evaluate atrial size and left ventricular function and to look for left ventricular hypertrophy, congenital heart disease (see Chap. 65), and valvular heart disease. Chest radiography is appropriate if the history or physical examination is suggestive of pulmonary disease (see Chap. 16). A stress test is appropriate for evaluation of ischemic heart disease in at-risk patients (see Chap. 14).

Prevention of Thromboembolic Complications

Risk Stratification

A major goal of therapy in patients with AF is to prevent thromboembolic complications such as stroke. It is well established that warfarin

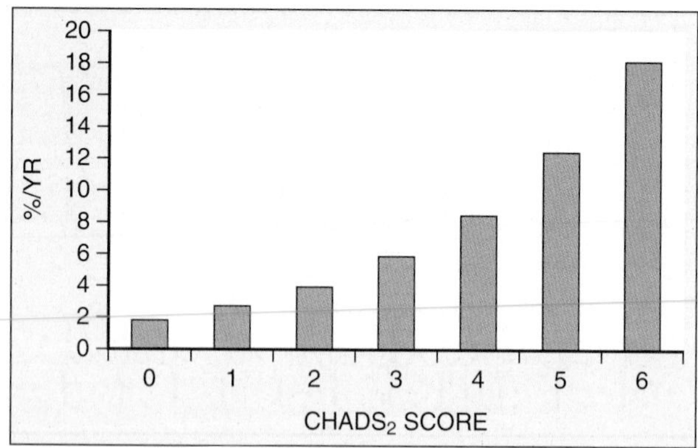

FIGURE 40-5 The annual risk of stroke based on the $CHADS_2$ score. *(Based on data in Table 9 of reference 7.)*

is more effective than aspirin for prevention of thromboembolic complications.[6] However, because of the risk of hemorrhage during warfarin therapy, its use should be limited to patients whose risk of thromboembolic complications is greater than the risk of hemorrhage. Therefore, it is useful to risk stratify patients with AF to identify appropriate candidates for warfarin therapy.

The strongest predictors of ischemic stroke and systemic thromboembolism are a history of stroke or transient ischemic episode and mitral stenosis. When patients with AF and a prior ischemic stroke are treated with aspirin, the risk of another stroke is very high, in the range of 10% to 12%/year. At the other end of the risk spectrum are patients with lone AF, whose cumulative 15-year risk of stroke was reported to be only 1.3%. Aside from prior stroke, the risk factors best established for stroke in patients with nonvalvular AF are diabetes (relative risk, 1.7), hypertension (relative risk, 1.6), heart failure (relative risk, 1.4), and age ≥70 years (relative risk, 1.4 per decade).[7]

A simple clinical scheme to risk stratify patients on the basis of the major risk factors is the $CHADS_2$ (cardiac failure, hypertension, age, diabetes, stroke) score.[8] Each of the first four risk factors is worth 1 point, and a prior stroke or transient ischemic event is worth 2 points. The clinical value of the $CHADS_2$ score lies in its simplicity and predictive value. The score can be calculated on the basis of the initial clinical evaluation of the patient and will range from 0 to 6, depending on the number of risk factors present. There is a direct relationship between the $CHADS_2$ score and the annual risk of stroke in the absence of aspirin or warfarin therapy (**Fig. 40-5**).

A large-scale study demonstrated that renal failure also is an independent risk factor for stroke in patients with AF.[9] The relative risk of a thromboembolic event in the absence of anticoagulation was 1.4 in patients with an estimated glomerular filtration rate <45 mL/min/1.73 m^2. The predictive strength of this degree of renal failure for a thromboembolic event appears to be equivalent to that of heart failure and advanced age. Therefore, it may be appropriate to take renal failure into account in evaluating the risk profile of a patient with AF.

By definition, the burden of AF is greater in patients with persistent AF than in patients with paroxysmal AF. It may seem reasonable to assume that the risk of stroke is lower in patients with occasional episodes of self-limited AF than in patients with AF continuously. However, the available data in fact indicate that the risk of thromboembolic complications is the same in patients with paroxysmal and persistent AF.[10] Even 15 minutes of AF may be long enough to result in local cardiac platelet activation and endothelial dysfunction that predispose to thrombus formation during an acute episode of AF.[11] Therefore, the type of AF should not be taken into account in risk stratifying AF patients for thromboembolic risk.

Modern-day dual-chamber pacemakers and implantable cardioverter-defibrillators (ICDs) are capable of detecting short episodes of asymptomatic AF that otherwise would not have been detected clinically. These episodes can be as short as 30 to 60 seconds.

Retrospective studies have suggested that asymptomatic atrial high-rate events lasting more than 5 minutes a day may double the risk of stroke and death.[12] However, the prognostic significance of short episodes of AF detectable only by an implanted device remains unclear and currently is under investigation in prospective studies.[13]

Aspirin and Other Antithrombotic Agents

Aspirin does not prevent thromboembolic complications as effectively as warfarin in patients with AF. In a meta-analysis of five randomized clinical trials, aspirin reduced the risk of stroke by only 18%.[6] Therefore, aspirin is adequate prophylactic therapy only in patients at lowest risk of thromboembolic complications ($CHADS_2$ score of 0), in whom the risk of stroke (1% to 2%/year) is in the same range as the risk of hemorrhagic complications of warfarin.[14] In patients who have a $CHADS_2$ score >1 and an annual stroke risk of ≥4%, aspirin is inadequate.

In patients with a $CHADS_2$ score of 1, who have an annual stroke risk of approximately 2.8%, the decision to use aspirin or warfarin should be individualized. For example, in patients who have risk factors for hemorrhagic complications or who are averse to long-term warfarin therapy, aspirin would be the appropriate choice for stroke prevention therapy. On the other hand, warfarin may be appropriate for patients with a $CHADS_2$ score of 1 who desire maximum protection from stroke. However, a cohort study of more than 13,000 patients with nonvalvular AF reported that when the annual risk of intracranial hemorrhage attributable to warfarin was taken into account, there was no net clinical benefit from warfarin in patients with a $CHADS_2$ score <2.[15] These data may favor the use of aspirin in patients with a $CHADS_2$ score of 1.

When aspirin is used for stroke prevention in patients with AF, the appropriate daily dose is 81 to 325 mg/day. There are no data that indicate superiority of a particular dose for prevention of thromboembolism.

In patients with a $CHADS_2$ score >1 who are not able to tolerate anticoagulation with warfarin, combination therapy with aspirin and the platelet inhibitor clopidogrel is more efficacious than aspirin alone for prevention of thromboembolic complications. In a recent randomized, double-blind clinical trial (ACTIVE-A), all patients with AF and one or more risk factors for stroke who were not suitable candidates for anticoagulation with warfarin were treated with 75 to 100 mg/day of aspirin.[16] The patients were randomly assigned to also receive either 75 mg/day of clopidogrel or a matching placebo. The primary outcome was a composite of stroke, myocardial infarction, systemic embolism, and vascular death. Compared with placebo, clopidogrel reduced the risk of stroke by 28% and the risk of the primary outcome by 11% but increased the risk of major hemorrhage. The study demonstrated that for every 1000 patients treated with the combination of aspirin plus clopidogrel instead of aspirin alone, 28 strokes (17 fatal or disabling) and 6 myocardial infarctions would be prevented, at a cost of 20 major bleeds (3 fatal). Therefore, in high-risk patients who are not suitable candidates for warfarin, the benefits of combination therapy with aspirin plus clopidogrel outweigh the risk.

Warfarin and Direct Thrombin Inhibitors

A meta-analysis of the major randomized clinical trials that compared warfarin with placebo for prevention of thromboembolism in patients with AF demonstrated that warfarin reduced the risk of all strokes (ischemic and hemorrhagic) by 61%.[6] The target international normalized ratio (INR) should be 2.0 to 3.0. This range of INRs provides the best balance between stroke prevention and hemorrhagic complications.[17] In clinical practice, maintenance of the INR in therapeutic range has been challenging, and a large proportion of patients often have an INR <2.0. A large prospective study of community-based practices demonstrated that the mean time in therapeutic range in patients treated with warfarin was only 66% and that the time in therapeutic range was <60% in 34% of patients.[18] Maintaining the INR at a level of ≥2.0 is important because even a relatively small decrease in INR from 2.0 to 1.7 more than doubles the risk of stroke. Furthermore, available data indicate that the combination of aspirin and low-intensity anticoagulation with warfarin is inferior to warfarin in the standard therapeutic range for stroke prevention.

The annual risk of a major hemorrhagic complication during anticoagulation with warfarin is in the range of 1% to 2%, and a strong predictor of major bleeding events is an INR >3.0. For example, the risk of intracranial bleeding is approximately twice as high at an INR of 4.0 than 3.0.[17] This emphasizes the importance of maintaining the INR in the range of 2.0 to 3.0. Maintaining a diet steady in vitamin K intake, from leafy vegetables, for example, can be helpful.

Some studies have indicated that advanced age can be a risk factor for intracranial hemorrhage in patients with AF who are treated with warfarin. The fear of hemorrhagic complications may lead some clinicians to favor the use of aspirin over warfarin in the elderly. However, recent data indicate that the risk-to-benefit ratio of warfarin is more favorable than that of aspirin even in patients older than 75 years. A recent randomized clinical trial (the Birmingham Atrial Fibrillation Treatment of the Aged Study) enrolled 973 patients older than 75 years (mean age, 82 years) with AF and randomly assigned them to treatment with 75 mg/day of aspirin or warfarin adjusted to maintain an INR of 2.0 to 3.0.[19] The primary endpoint was the composite of stroke (ischemic or hemorrhagic), intracranial hemorrhage, and arterial embolism, and the mean duration of follow-up was 2.7 years. The annual risk of the composite endpoint was significantly higher in the aspirin group (3.8%) than in the warfarin group (1.8%), even when the analysis was limited to patients older than 85 years. These data suggest that age should not be considered a contraindication to warfarin in patients with AF.

It is well established that genetic factors influence the dose of warfarin required to maintain the INR within therapeutic range. Several single-nucleotide polymorphisms that affect warfarin metabolism have been identified. Algorithms based on pharmacogenetic (see Chap. 10) and clinical factors improve the accuracy of warfarin dose initiation compared with algorithms based only on clinical factors, particularly for outliers who require ≤21 mg/wk or ≥49 mg/wk of warfarin to maintain a therapeutic INR.[20] However, a randomized study demonstrated that warfarin dosing that took into account the results of genotyping for *CYP2C9* (a cytochrome P-450 isoform) and *VKORC1* (a vitamin K epoxide reductase complex subunit) did not improve the time in therapeutic range, which was approximately 70% in both groups.[21] Additional studies are required to determine whether the clinical benefits of genotyping of warfarin candidates justify the cost of genetic testing.

Direct thrombin inhibitors have several advantages over vitamin K antagonists such as warfarin, the most notable being a fixed dosing regimen that is not affected by dietary factors. Dabigatran, an oral direct thrombin inhibitor, at a dose of 110 mg/day, was recently shown in AF patients to produce rates of stroke and systemic embolism similar to those associated with warfarin,[22] but with lower rates of major hemorrhage, and might offer an alternative choice for anticoagulation in the future.

Low-Molecular-Weight Heparin

Low-molecular-weight heparin has a longer half-life than unfractionated heparin and a predictable antithrombotic effect that is attained with a fixed dosage administered subcutaneously twice a day. Because low-molecular-weight heparin can be self-injected by patients outside of the hospital, it has been a practical alternative to unfractionated heparin for initiation of anticoagulation in patients with AF. A randomized study compared low-molecular-weight heparin with the combination of a vitamin K antagonist (phenprocoumon) plus unfractionated heparin until the INR was ≥2.0 in patients undergoing cardioversion of AF who were not already anticoagulated.[23] Both study groups were anticoagulated for 4 weeks after cardioversion. The primary endpoint (a composite of all embolic and hemorrhagic events and all-cause mortality) occurred in 2.8% of patients in the group that received low-molecular-weight heparin compared with 4.8% of patients in the group that received unfractionated heparin plus phenprocoumon. This study demonstrated that low-molecular-weight heparin is noninferior to conventional anticoagulation for prevention of ischemic and thromboembolic events after cardioversion of AF.

Because of its high cost, low-molecular-weight heparin rarely is used in clinical practice as a substitute for long-term conventional anticoagulation. Low-molecular-weight heparin typically is used as a temporary bridge to therapeutic anticoagulation when therapy with warfarin is initiated or in high-risk patients for a few days before and after a medical or dental procedure when anticoagulation with warfarin has been suspended.

Excision or Closure of the Left Atrial Appendage

Approximately 90% of left atrial thrombi form in the appendage, and therefore excision or closure of the left atrial appendage, at least in theory, should markedly reduce the risk of thromboembolic complications in patients with AF. Surgical techniques consist of either excision or closure by suturing or stapling. The efficacy of these techniques is variable and probably both technique and operator dependent. Postoperative transesophageal echocardiography demonstrated that there was successful closure of the appendage in only 40% of 137 patients.[24] The rate of successful closure was higher when the appendage was excised (73%) than when it was closed by suturing (23%). Of note is that complete closure never was achieved by stapling of the appendage. Left atrial appendage thrombus was never present by transesophageal echocardiography after excision of the appendage but was observed in 41% of patients who underwent closure of the appendage. Therefore, transesophageal echocardiography should be performed after surgical closure of the left atrial appendage to confirm successful closure before discontinuation of anticoagulation.

Left atrial appendage closure also can achieved percutaneously with an implanted device intended to seal the appendage. A randomized clinical trial (PROTECT AF)[25] compared the efficacy of a percutaneous closure device versus warfarin for prevention of thromboembolic complications in 707 patients with AF and a $CHADS_2$ score ≥1. The device was found to be noninferior to warfarin for the primary efficacy composite endpoint of stroke, systemic emboli, and cardiovascular death and superior to warfarin for hemorrhagic stroke (91% reduction). The complication rate was approximately four times higher in the device arm, with the most common complication being pericardial effusion. The study demonstrated that percutaneous closure of the left atrial appendage is a safe and effective alternative to warfarin in patients with AF. Final approval of the left atrial appendage closure device by the Food and Drug Administration is pending.

It is likely that the left atrial appendage closure device will have its greatest utility in high-risk patients with AF who cannot tolerate warfarin or who strongly dislike taking warfarin because of the inconveniences associated with its long-term use to improve their quality of life.

Acute Management of Atrial Fibrillation

Patients who present to the emergency department because of AF generally have a rapid ventricular rate, and control of the ventricular rate is most rapidly achieved with intravenous diltiazem or esmolol. If the patient is hemodynamically unstable, immediate transthoracic cardioversion may be appropriate. If the AF has been present for more than 48 hours or if the duration is unclear and the patient is not already anticoagulated, cardioversion ideally should be preceded by transesophageal echocardiography to rule out a left atrial thrombus. However, a delay in cardioversion may not be appropriate in the setting of severe cardiovascular decompensation.

If the patient is hemodynamically stable, the decision to restore sinus rhythm by cardioversion is based on several factors, including symptoms, prior AF episodes, age, left atrial size, and current antiarrhythmic drug therapy. For example, in an elderly patient whose symptoms resolve once the ventricular rate is controlled and who already has had early recurrences of AF despite rhythm-control drug therapy, further attempts at cardioversion usually are not appropriate. On the other hand, cardioversion usually is appropriate for patients with symptomatic AF who present with a first episode of AF or who have had long intervals of sinus rhythm between prior episodes.

If cardioversion is decided on for a hemodynamically stable patient who presents with AF that does not appear to be self-limited, there are two management decisions to be made: early versus delayed cardioversion and pharmacologic versus electrical cardioversion.

The advantages of early cardioversion are rapid relief of symptoms, avoidance of the need for transesophageal echocardiography or therapeutic anticoagulation for 3 to 4 weeks before cardioversion if cardioversion is performed within 48 hours of AF onset, and possibly a lower risk of early AF recurrence because of less atrial remodeling (see Chap. 35). Possible reasons to defer cardioversion include an AF duration longer than 48 hours or duration unclear in a patient who is not anticoagulated and for whom transesophageal echocardiography is not available, a left atrial thrombus by transesophageal echocardiography (see Fig. 15-91), a suspicion (based on prior AF episodes) that AF will convert spontaneously within a few days, and a correctable cause of AF (e.g., hyperthyroidism).

When cardioversion is performed early in the course of an episode of AF, there is the option of either pharmacologic or electrical cardioversion. Pharmacologic cardioversion has the advantage of not requiring general anesthesia or deep sedation. In addition, the probability of an immediate recurrence of AF may be lower with pharmacologic cardioversion than with electrical cardioversion. However, pharmacologic cardioversion is associated with the risk of adverse drug effects and is not as effective as electrical cardioversion. Pharmacologic cardioversion is very unlikely to be effective if the duration of AF is longer than 7 days.

Drugs that can be administered intravenously for cardioversion of AF consist of ibutilide, procainamide, and amiodarone. For AF episodes less than 2 to 3 days in duration, the efficacy of these drugs is approximately 60% to 70% for ibutilide, 40% to 50% for amiodarone, and 30% to 40% for procainamide. To minimize the risk of QT prolongation and polymorphic ventricular tachycardia (torsades de pointes; see Chap. 39), the use of ibutilide should be limited to patients with an ejection fraction >35%. Acute pharmacologic cardioversion of AF also can be attempted with orally administered drugs in patients without structural heart disease. The most commonly used oral agents for acute conversion of AF are propafenone (300 to 600 mg) and flecainide (100 to 200 mg). It is prudent to administer these drugs under surveillance the first time they are used. If no adverse drug effects are observed, the patient may then be an appropriate candidate for episodic, self-administered antiarrhythmic drug therapy on an outpatient basis.

The efficacy of transthoracic cardioversion is approximately 95%. Biphasic waveform shocks convert AF more effectively than monophasic waveform shocks and allow the use of lower energy shocks, resulting in a lower risk of skin irritation. An appropriate first-shock strength using a biphasic waveform is 150 to 200 J followed by higher output shocks if needed. If a 360-J biphasic shock is unsuccessful, ibutilide should be infused before another shock is delivered because it lowers the defibrillation energy requirement and improves the success rate of transthoracic cardioversion.

There are two types of failure of transthoracic cardioversion in patients with AF. The first type is a complete failure to restore sinus rhythm. For this situation, an increase in shock strength or infusion of ibutilide often results in successful cardioversion. The second type of failure is an immediate recurrence of AF within a few seconds of successful conversion to sinus rhythm. The incidence of an immediate recurrence of AF is approximately 25% for episodes less than 24 hours in duration and approximately 10% for episodes more than 24 hours in duration. For this type of failure of cardioversion, an increase in shock strength is of no value. If the patient has not been receiving an oral rhythm-control agent, infusion of ibutilide may be helpful for prevention of an immediate recurrence of AF.

Regardless of whether cardioversion is performed pharmacologically or electrically, therapeutic anticoagulation is necessary for 3 weeks or more before cardioversion to prevent thromboembolic complications if the AF has been ongoing for more than 48 hours. If the time of onset of AF is unclear, for the sake of safety, the AF duration should be assumed to be more than 48 hours. These patients should be therapeutically anticoagulated for 4 weeks after cardioversion to prevent thromboembolic complications that may occur because of atrial stunning. If the duration of AF is known to be less than 48 hours, cardioversion can be performed without anticoagulation. To improve the safety margin, it may be appropriate to use a 24-hour cutoff for the AF duration that allows safe cardioversion without anticoagulation.

When the AF duration is longer than 48 hours or unclear, an alternative to 3 weeks of therapeutic anticoagulation before cardioversion is anticoagulation with heparin and transesophageal echocardiography to check for a left atrial thrombus. If no thrombi are seen, the patient can safely be cardioverted but still requires 4 weeks of therapeutic anticoagulation after cardioversion to prevent thromboembolism related to atrial stunning. The major clinical benefit of the transesophageal echocardiography–guided approach over the conventional approach is that sinus rhythm is restored several weeks sooner. Compared with the conventional approach, the transesophageal echocardiography–guided approach has not been found to reduce the risk of stroke or major bleeding or to affect the proportion of patients still in sinus rhythm at 8 weeks after cardioversion.

Long-Term Management of Atrial Fibrillation

Pharmacologic Rate Control Versus Rhythm Control

Several randomized studies have compared a rate-control strategy with a rhythm-control strategy in patients with AF. The largest study by far was the AFFIRM study, which consisted of 4060 patients with a mean age of 70 years who had AF for 6 hours to 6 months.[26] At 5 years of follow-up, the prevalence of sinus rhythm was 35% in the rate-control arm and 63% in the rhythm-control arm. There was no significant difference between the two study arms in total mortality, stroke rate, or quality of life. The percentage of patients requiring hospitalization was significantly lower in the rate-control arm (73%) than in the rhythm-control arm (80%), and the incidence of adverse drug effects such as torsades de pointes also was significantly lower in the rate-control arm (0.2% versus 0.8%). The authors of the AFFIRM study concluded that there is no survival advantage of a rhythm-control strategy over a rate-control strategy and that a rate-control strategy has advantages such as a lower probability of hospitalization and of adverse drug effects.

In a post hoc analysis of the AFFIRM study, the relationship between sinus rhythm, treatment, and survival was determined by an on-treatment analysis instead of an intention-to-treat analysis used in the original report.[27] Sinus rhythm was found to be independently associated with lower mortality (hazard ratio, 0.53), and antiarrhythmic drug therapy was independently associated with increased mortality (hazard ratio, 1.49). Therefore, the potential benefit of maintaining sinus rhythm with antiarrhythmic drugs was negated by the adverse effects of the antiarrhythmic drug therapy. This suggested that therapies that maintain sinus rhythm without major adverse effects may have a beneficial effect on survival.

The results of the AFFIRM study should not be applied routinely to all patients with AF. The decision to pursue a rhythm-control strategy versus a rate-control strategy should be individualized, with several factors taken into account. These include the nature, frequency, and severity of symptoms; the length of time that AF has been present continuously in patients with persistent AF; left atrial size; comorbidities; the response to prior cardioversions; age; the side effects and efficacy of the antiarrhythmic drugs already used to treat the patient; and the patient's preference.

The AFFIRM study convincingly demonstrated that a rate-control strategy is preferable to a rhythm-control strategy in asymptomatic or minimally symptomatic patients ≥65 years old. In patients with persistent AF, it is reasonable to attempt to restore sinus rhythm with antiarrhythmic drug therapy or transthoracic cardioversion at least once in patients ≤65 years old and in patients ≥65 years old who are symptomatic from the AF despite adequate heart rate control. If the AF has been continuous for more than 1 year or if the left atrial diameter is very large (>5.0 cm), there is a high probability of an early recurrence of AF, and this should be taken into account in deciding on the best strategy. After cardioversion, the decision to maintain the patient on antiarrhythmic drug therapy to delay the next episode of AF is based on the patient's preference, the perceived risk of an early recurrence of AF, and the duration of sinus rhythm between prior cardioversions. Treatment by cardioversion without daily antiarrhythmic drug therapy is acceptable if episodes of AF are separated by at least 6 months. Treatment with a rhythm-control drug usually is appropriate when AF recurs within a few months of cardioversion.

The most realistic goal of antiarrhythmic drug therapy in patients with persistent AF is to delay the onset of the next episode by at least several months, not for several years. It often is appropriate to continue therapy with a particular antiarrhythmic drug if recurrences of AF are limited to approximately one episode per year.

In patients with symptomatic paroxysmal AF, the aggressiveness with which a rhythm-control strategy is pursued should be dictated by the frequency and severity of symptoms and how well antiarrhythmic drug therapy is tolerated. Drug therapy is more likely to be judged successful when patients are reminded that the goal of therapy is not complete suppression of AF but a clinically meaningful reduction in frequency, duration, and severity of episodes.

A pharmacologic rhythm-control strategy need not necessarily consist of daily drug therapy. Episodic drug therapy (the "pill-in-the-pocket" approach) is useful for patients whose episodes of AF are relatively infrequent. Episodic drug therapy is a reasonable option for patients who are clearly aware of the onset and termination of AF episodes and who have lone AF or only minimal structural heart disease. A typical drug regimen consists of a class IC drug (flecainide or propafenone) plus a short-acting beta blocker (e.g., propranolol) or calcium channel blocker (e.g., verapamil) for rate control before cardioversion or if the antiarrhythmic drug converts AF to atrial flutter. Many patients with infrequent episodes prefer this approach because it eliminates the inconvenience, cost, and possible side effects of daily prophylactic therapy. However, patients who are disabled by severe symptoms during AF may prefer daily prophylactic therapy even if episodes are infrequent.

Many patients with symptomatic AF also have asymptomatic episodes. Therefore, daily antithrombotic therapy to prevent thromboembolic events is appropriate for *all* patients being treated for recurrent AF, whether it is persistent or paroxysmal and whether a rhythm-control or rate-control strategy is employed. The choice of aspirin, warfarin, or the combination of aspirin plus clopidogrel should be dictated by an analysis of risk factors and drug tolerance.

Pharmacologic Rate Control

An excessively rapid ventricular rate during AF often results in uncomfortable symptoms and decreased effort tolerance and can cause a tachycardia-induced cardiomyopathy if it is sustained for several weeks to months. Optimal heart rates during AF vary with age and should be similar to the heart rates that a patient would have at a particular degree of exertion during sinus rhythm. Heart rate control must be assessed both at rest and during exertion. At rest, the ideal ventricular rate during AF is in the range of 60 to 75 beats/min. During mild to moderate exertion (e.g., rapid walking), the target rate should be 90 to 115 beats/min; and during strenuous exercise, the ideal rate is in the range of 120 to 160 beats/min. Optimal assessment of the degree of heart rate control is provided by an ambulatory 24-hour Holter recording or an exercise test.

Oral agents available for long-term heart rate control in patients with AF are digitalis, beta blockers, calcium channel antagonists, and amiodarone. The first-line agents for rate control are beta blockers and the calcium channel antagonists verapamil and diltiazem. A combination is often used to improve efficacy or to limit side effects by allowing the use of smaller dosages of the individual drugs. In patients with sinus node dysfunction and tachy-brady syndrome, the use of a beta blocker with intrinsic sympathomimetic activity (pindolol, acebutolol) may provide rate control without aggravating sinus bradycardia.

Digitalis may adequately control the rate at rest but often does not provide adequate rate control during exertion. Its use is appropriate in patients with systolic heart failure, in whom digitalis has been shown to improve outcomes such as heart failure hospitalizations and mortality. However, in patients with the vagotonic form of paroxysmal AF, the vagotonic effect of digitalis may promote AF. Furthermore, in patients without systolic heart failure, the use of a digitalis glycoside may have a deleterious effect on survival. In a large anticoagulation trial comparing warfarin with a direct thrombin inhibitor (SPORTIF III-IV), digitalis was found to be independently associated with a 53% higher risk of all-cause mortality.[28] Although this was demonstrated by post hoc analysis and not by a randomized comparison of digitalis versus a placebo, the results are of enough concern to limit the use of digitalis to patients with heart failure.

Amiodarone is much less frequently used for rate control than the other negative dromotropic agents because of the risk of organ toxicity associated with long-term therapy. Amiodarone may be an appropriate choice for rate control if the other agents are not tolerated or are ineffective. As an example, amiodarone would be an appropriate choice for a patient with persistent AF, heart failure, and reactive airway disease who cannot tolerate either a calcium channel antagonist or a beta blocker and who has a rapid ventricular rate despite treatment with digitalis.

Pharmacologic Rhythm Control

The results of published studies on the efficacy of antiarrhythmic drugs for AF suggest that all of the available drugs except amiodarone have similar efficacy and are associated with a 50% to 60% reduction in the odds of recurrent AF during 1 year of treatment.[29] The one drug that stands out as having higher efficacy than the others is amiodarone. In studies that directly compared amiodarone with sotalol or class I drugs, amiodarone was 60% to 70% more effective in suppressing AF. However, because of the risk of organ toxicity, amiodarone is not appropriate first-line drug therapy for most categories of patients with AF. Because their efficacy is in the same general range, the selection of an antiarrhythmic drug to prevent AF often is dictated by the issues of safety and side effects.

Ventricular proarrhythmia from class IA agents (quinidine, procainamide, disopyramide) and class III agents (sotalol, dofetilide, dronedarone, amiodarone) is manifested as QT prolongation and polymorphic ventricular tachycardia (torsades de pointes). Risk factors for this type of proarrhythmia include female gender, left ventricular dysfunction, and hypokalemia. The risk of torsades de pointes appears to be much lower with dronedarone and amiodarone than with the other class III drugs. The ventricular proarrhythmia from class IC agents (flecainide and propafenone) is manifested as monomorphic ventricular tachycardia, sometimes associated with widening of the QRS complex during sinus rhythm but not QT prolongation. Published studies indicate that the drugs most likely to result in ventricular proarrhythmia are quinidine, flecainide, sotalol, and dofetilide. In controlled studies, these agents increased the risk of ventricular tachycardia by a factor of 2 to 6.[29]

Adverse drug events resulting in discontinuation of drug therapy are fairly common with rhythm-control drugs. Withdrawal due to adverse effects was most common with quinidine, disopyramide, flecainide, sotalol, and amiodarone.[29] A review of studies in which 32 treatment arms received an antiarrhythmic drug for AF found that 10.4% of patients discontinued drug therapy because of an adverse drug event, most commonly gastrointestinal side effects and neuropathy.[30]

The best options for drug therapy to suppress AF depend on the patient's comorbidities. In patients with lone AF or minimal heart disease (e.g., mild left ventricular hypertrophy), flecainide, propafenone, sotalol, and dronedarone are reasonable first-line drugs, and amiodarone and dofetilide can be considered if the first-line agents are ineffective or not tolerated. In patients with substantial left ventricular hypertrophy (left ventricular wall thickness >13 mm), the hypertrophy may heighten the risk of ventricular proarrhythmia, and the safest choice for drug therapy is amiodarone. In patients with coronary artery disease, several of the class I drugs have been found to increase the risk of death, and the safest first-line options are dofetilide, sotalol, and dronedarone, with amiodarone reserved for use as a second-line agent. In patients with heart failure, several antiarrhythmic drugs have been associated with increased mortality, and the only two drugs known to have a neutral effect on survival are amiodarone and dofetilide (see Chap. 37).

Experimental studies indicate that angiotensin-converting enzyme (ACE) inhibitors and angiotensin receptor blockers (ARBs) have favorable effects on electrical and structural remodeling (see Chap. 35). This explains why ACE inhibitors and ARBs have been shown in some studies to prevent AF. In a meta-analysis of 11 trials that included a total of 56,308 patients, ACE inhibitors and ARBs reduced the relative risk of AF by 28%.[31] The effect was limited to patients with left ventricular systolic dysfunction or hypertrophy. However, in a randomized clinical trial of the ARB valsartan versus placebo in 1442 patients with structural heart disease and recurrent AF, the AF recurrence rate was approximately 50% in both study arms, and there was no evidence that valsartan prevented AF.[32] Therefore, whether ACE inhibitors and ARBs prevent AF is unclear, and there is insufficient evidence to support their use for the sole purpose of preventing AF.

There also is some evidence that statins prevent AF, perhaps because of their anti-inflammatory effects. A systematic review of 10 observational studies demonstrated a 23% reduction in the relative risk of AF in patients treated with statins.[33] However, a meta-analysis of six randomized clinical trials concluded that statins do not prevent AF, except after open heart surgery.[33] Therefore, the available data do not support the use of statins solely for the prevention of AF.

Nonpharmacologic Management of Atrial Fibrillation

Pacing to Prevent Atrial Fibrillation

Randomized clinical trials comparing dual-chamber (DDD) pacing with right ventricular pacing concluded that atrial pacing prevents AF.[34] Studies suggest that the higher incidence of AF during ventricular pacing than during DDD pacing may be at least partially due to a proarrhythmic effect of ventricular pacing, not only to a suppressive effect of atrial pacing.

Studies in small numbers of patients suggested that dual-site right atrial pacing or pacing of the interatrial septum in the region of Bachmann bundle prevents AF. Although it is possible that these atrial pacing techniques decrease the propensity for AF, the magnitude of the effect appears to be minimal.

Some antibradycardia pacemakers are designed also to prevent and to terminate AF. Pacing algorithms to prevent AF consist of atrial pacing to overdrive sinus rhythm, suppression of postextrasystolic pauses, and acceleration of the atrial pacing rate when repetitive premature atrial complexes are sensed. When these pacing algorithms have been evaluated in rigorous fashion, they have been found to be ineffective or at best minimally effective in reducing the AF burden.[35] Antitachycardia pacing (ATP) to terminate AF consists of a burst of rapid atrial pacing at the onset of AF. ATP may be useful for termination of atrial flutter or an atrial tachycardia, but it is rarely if ever effective for AF.

Because of insufficient evidence to support its use, atrial pacing is not indicated for prevention of AF in patients without bradycardia. In patients with a bradycardia indication for a pacemaker and paroxysmal AF or recurrent episodes of persistent AF, the available data clearly support the use of atrial-based pacing and programming to minimize the amount of ventricular pacing.

Implanted Atrial Defibrillator

The energy required for atrial defibrillation is much lower when a shock is delivered within the heart than when transthoracic cardioversion is performed. When the shock is delivered between a lead in the superior vena cava plus the generator can and the right ventricular apex, the atrial defibrillation threshold typically is in the range of 3 to 5 J. However, internal shocks >1 J generally are painful. Because even an R wave–synchronized shock can precipitate ventricular fibrillation, there currently is no stand-alone implanted atrial defibrillator available for clinical use. The implanted atrial defibrillators that are available are built into conventional ICDs.

The limitations of atrial defibrillation are painful shocks and the potential for immediate recurrences of AF after cardioversion, and the clinical utility of the atrial defibrillator has been limited. The most appropriate candidates for an implanted atrial defibrillator are patients with relatively infrequent episodes of poorly tolerated AF who do not respond well to pharmacologic therapy, who are not good candidates for catheter ablation, and who qualify for an ICD.

Catheter Ablation of Atrial Fibrillation

CHALLENGES OF ABLATING ATRIAL FIBRILLATION. Catheter ablation reliably and permanently eliminates several types of arrhythmias, such as AV nodal reentrant tachycardia and accessory pathway–mediated tachycardias[36] (see Chaps. 37 and 39). Success rates of more than 95% are attainable when the arrhythmia substrate is well defined, localized, and temporally stable. In contrast, the arrhythmia substrate of AF as yet is not well understood, usually is widespread, is variable between patients, and may be progressive. Furthermore, there are several factors that promote AF that cannot be addressed simply by catheter ablation, such as hypertension and obstructive sleep apnea, structural remodeling of the atria, inflammatory factors, and genetic factors (see Chap. 9). Therefore, whereas late recurrences of AV nodal reentrant tachycardia or accessory pathway conduction are very rare, AF may recur more than 2 or 3 years after an initially successful ablation procedure.

SELECTION OF PATIENTS. Given the limitations of catheter ablation of AF, it usually is appropriate to treat the patient with at least one rhythm-control drug before catheter ablation is considered. This is particularly so if the AF is persistent because the efficacy of catheter ablation is lower for persistent AF than for paroxysmal AF. The most appropriate candidates for catheter ablation have symptomatic AF that is affecting quality of life and that has not adequately responded to drug therapy. The ideal candidate has lone AF or only minimal structural heart disease. The recommendation for catheter ablation should be influenced by the estimated probability of success, and the procedure is least likely to be successful if the left atrium is markedly dilated or if the AF has been persistent for more than 4 years.

Catheter ablation may be appropriate first-line therapy in some patients with AF: patients younger than 35 years with symptomatic AF; patients with sinus node dysfunction in whom antiarrhythmic drug therapy is likely to create the need for a permanent pacemaker; and occasional patients who express a strong aversion to drug therapy.

CONVENTIONAL RADIOFREQUENCY CATHETER ABLATION. The most commonly used technique to eliminate paroxysmal AF in the laboratory is radiofrequency ablation using a 3.5-mm irrigated-tip catheter or an 8-mm tip catheter. Radiofrequency energy is delivered point by point, typically in association with a three-dimensional electroanatomic mapping system as a navigation guide and to indicate the points that already have been ablated. To improve anatomic accuracy, the electroanatomic map of the left atrium can be merged with a computed tomography scan or magnetic resonance image of the left atrium and pulmonary veins (**Fig. 40-6**) or with an ultrasound image generated by intracardiac echocardiography.

Because of their important role in triggering and maintaining episodes of AF, almost all ablation strategies include electrical isolation of the pulmonary veins (**Fig. 40-7**). This can be accomplished by either ostial ablation or wide-area ablation 1 to 2 cm away from the ostia, in the antral regions of the pulmonary veins. Most of the available data indicate that wide-area ablation is more effective than ostial ablation, probably because it also targets drivers that may be in the antrum, outside the pulmonary vein itself.[37] Triggers of AF can also arise from other thoracic veins, such as the superior vena cava, coronary sinus, and vein of Marshall. After the pulmonary veins have been isolated, infusion of isoproterenol is helpful to determine whether any non–pulmonary vein triggers are present.

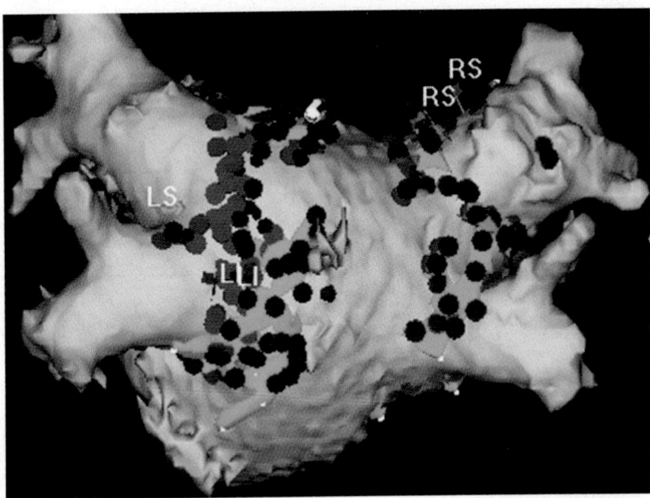

FIGURE 40-6 An electroanatomic map of the left atrium merged with a computed tomography scan of the left atrium and pulmonary veins. The red and gray tags indicate the sites at which radiofrequency energy was delivered in the antrum of the pulmonary veins. LI = left inferior pulmonary vein; LS = left superior pulmonary vein; RS = right superior pulmonary vein.

Pulmonary vein isolation often is sufficient to eliminate paroxysmal AF but rarely is sufficient for persistent AF. A variety of ablation strategies have been used for persistent AF after the pulmonary veins have been isolated: linear ablation across the left atrial roof, mitral isthmus, or cavotricuspid isthmus; ablation of CFAEs in the left atrium, coronary sinus, or right atrium; various combinations of linear and CFAE ablation; and ablation of ganglionated plexi. The endpoint of catheter ablation of persistent AF is either completion of a prespecified lesion set (in which case sinus rhythm is restored by cardioversion) or stepwise ablation until the AF converts to sinus rhythm.

A wide range of success rates for radiofrequency catheter ablation of AF has been reported. A meta-analysis of 63 studies in which radiofrequency catheter ablation of paroxysmal or persistent AF was performed reported an overall single-procedure success rate of 57% at a mean follow-up of 14 months and a multiple-procedure success rate of 71%.[30] In another meta-analysis, four prospective, randomized studies were analyzed, and radiofrequency catheter ablation was found to result in AF-free survival significantly more often than antiarrhythmic drug therapy (76% versus 19%).[38] In a subsequent multicenter study of 112 patients with paroxysmal AF resistant to one or more antiarrhythmic drugs, the patients were randomly assigned to pulmonary vein isolation plus additional ablation at the operator's discretion or antiarrhythmic drug therapy.[39] AF-free survival at 12 months was 89% in the ablation arm after a median of two procedures per patient compared with 23% in the drug arm.[39]

On the basis of published reports and the experience at high-volume centers, it is reasonable to expect a single-procedure 1-year success rate of 70% to 80% in patients with paroxysmal AF and approximately 50% in patients with persistent AF. After a redo procedure, a success rate of approximately 90% appears to be realistic for patients with paroxysmal AF compared with approximately 75% for patients with persistent AF.

The risk of a major complication from radiofrequency catheter ablation of AF is reported to be 5% to 6%.[30,40] In a large international survey, the most common major complications were cardiac tamponade (1.2%), pulmonary vein stenosis (1.3%), and cerebral thromboembolism (0.94%).[40] The risk of vascular injury is reported to be 1% to 2%.[40,41] The risk of atrioesophageal fistula is probably less than 0.1%; however, this complication is of great concern because it often is lethal. Large international surveys have reported the risk of a fatal complication to

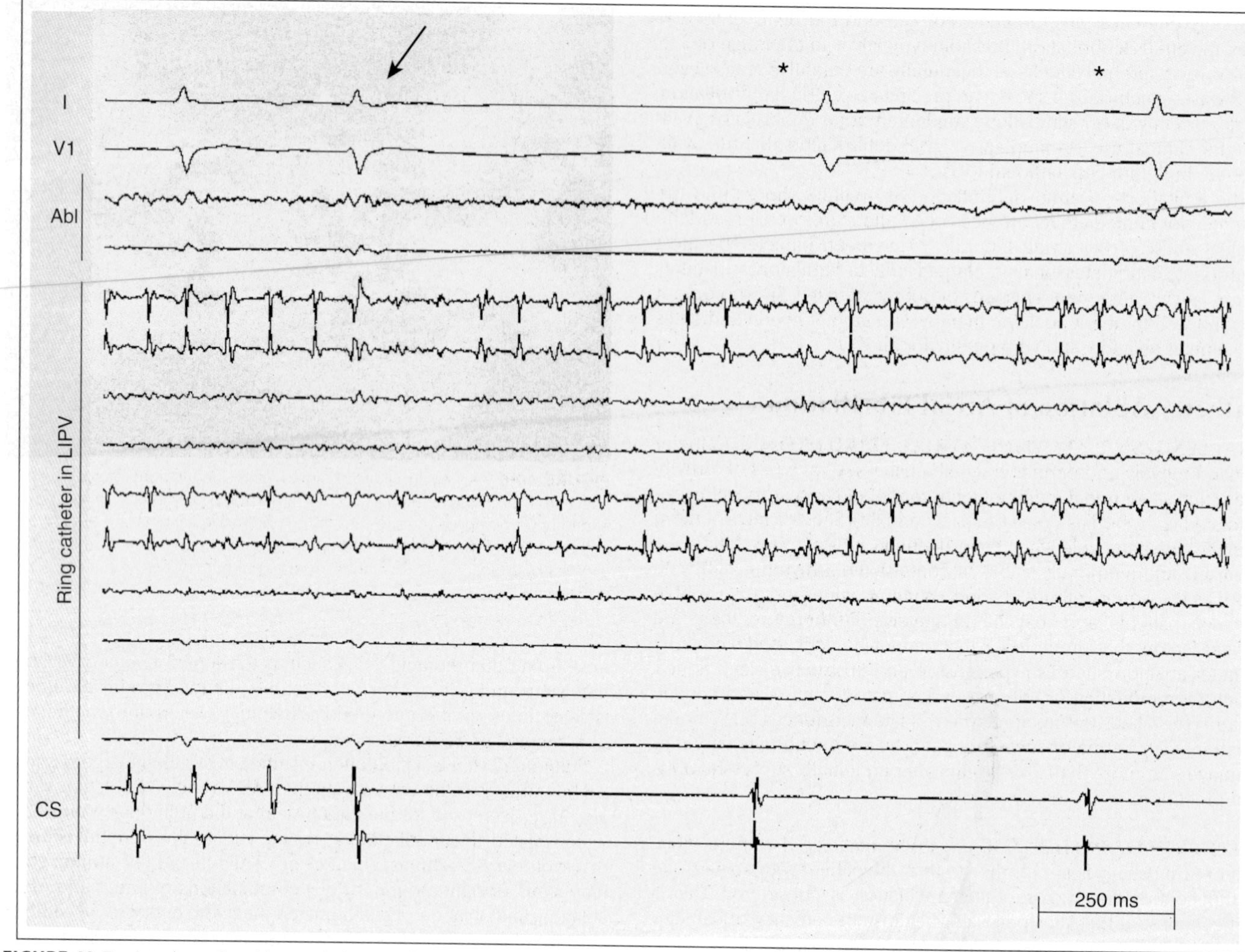

FIGURE 40-7 A tachycardia with a cycle length of 80 milliseconds arising in a left inferior pulmonary vein. This tachycardia was responsible for generating AF. During radiofrequency ablation in the antrum of this pulmonary vein, AF terminated (arrow) and converted to sinus rhythm when the pulmonary vein became electrically isolated. The sinus beats are indicated with an asterisk. The pulmonary vein tachycardia was still present inside the vein. Shown are leads I and V_1, the electrograms recorded by the ablation catheter (Abl) outside the left inferior pulmonary vein (LIPV) and by a ring catheter in the LIPV, and the coronary sinus electrograms (CS).

be in the range of 0.05% to 0.1%.[40,42] In a survey of 32,569 patients who underwent catheter ablation of AF, the mortality rate was 0.1%, and the most common causes of death were cardiac tamponade (25% of deaths), stroke (16%), atrioesophageal fistula (16%), and pneumonia (16%).[42]

NEWER ABLATION TOOLS. Two systems currently are available for remote navigation of a radiofrequency ablation catheter. In one system, large magnets are positioned on each side of the patient, and small magnets embedded in the tip of the ablation catheter allow remote navigation by shifting the magnetic field vectors. With the other system, an ablation catheter is navigated remotely by a robotic steerable sheath system. The advantages of these systems are improved catheter stability, marked reduction in radiation exposure to the operator, and avoidance of the technical challenges of manual catheter manipulation. Preliminary experience with remote magnetic navigation and a robotic steerable sheath system suggests that the efficacy and safety of radiofrequency catheter ablation of AF are comparable to those of conventional radiofrequency catheter ablation.[43,44]

One of the main reasons that radiofrequency catheter ablation of AF often is a lengthy procedure (≥3 hours) is that point-by-point ablation is required at a large number of sites. Ablation catheters that allow the delivery of radiofrequency energy simultaneously at multiple electrodes have resulted in decreased procedure times (<2 hours) without compromising efficacy.[45,46] These catheters are available for clinical use in Europe and parts of Asia but have yet to be approved for clinical use in the United States.

Several new types of ablation catheters have been developed to facilitate isolation of the pulmonary veins, including a cryoballoon catheter, a laser balloon catheter, a high-intensity focused ultrasound balloon catheter, and a high-density mesh ablator. These new ablation tools are designed to fit into the antrum of a pulmonary vein and to create a circumferential ablation lesion with a minimal number of energy applications. None of these catheters is market approved as of yet in the United States. Among these new technologies, the most experience to date has been accumulated with the cryoballoon catheter.

An important advantage of cryoenergy is that it appears to be much less likely than radiofrequency energy to cause pulmonary vein stenosis or esophageal injury. In two studies in which a total of 363 patients with paroxysmal AF underwent pulmonary vein isolation with a cryoballoon catheter, the success rate was 74% at 12 months in one study[47] and 49% at a mean follow-up of 33 months in the other study.[48] A major complication occurred in 4% to 10% of patients,[47,48] with the most common complication being transient phrenic nerve paralysis in 7.5% of patients, with recovery within 1 year.[47]

Definitive assessment of the relative advantages of these new technologies over conventional radiofrequency ablation of AF will have to await more experience with their use and longer follow-up periods. Nevertheless, it seems likely that catheter ablation of AF will be facilitated and probably be made safer by one or more of these new technologies.

Ablation of the Atrioventricular Node

Radiofrequency catheter ablation of the AV node results in complete AV nodal block and substitutes a regular, paced rhythm for an irregular and rapid native rhythm. It is a useful strategy in patients who are symptomatic from AF because of a rapid ventricular rate that cannot be adequately controlled pharmacologically as a result of either inefficacy of or intolerance to rate-control drugs and who either are not good candidates for ablation of the AF or already have undergone an unsuccessful attempt at catheter ablation of the AF. Because of the better success rate with catheter ablation of paroxysmal AF than of persistent AF, AV node ablation is more often performed in patients with persistent than with paroxysmal AF.

In patients with AF and an uncontrolled ventricular rate, AV node ablation improves the left ventricular ejection fraction if there is a tachycardia-induced cardiomyopathy. AV node ablation also has been shown to improve symptoms, quality of life, and functional capacity and to reduce the use of health care resources. However, the studies demonstrating these favorable outcomes were mostly descriptive cohort studies.[49] There is no evidence that AV node ablation is of benefit in patients whose ventricular rate is well controlled by medications.

The disadvantages of AV node ablation are that it creates a lifelong need for ventricular pacing and does not restore AV synchrony. Although symptoms and functional capacity typically improve after AV node ablation in patients with AF and an uncontrolled ventricular rate, some patients may not feel as well as during sinus rhythm.

AV node ablation is a technically simple procedure with a very high acute and long-term success rate (≥98%) and a very low risk of complications. In patients with persistent AF, a ventricular pacemaker is implanted, and a dual-chamber pacemaker is appropriate if the AF is paroxysmal. Most patients have a good clinical outcome with right ventricular pacing; but in patients with left ventricular dysfunction, biventricular pacing for cardiac resynchronization therapy is appropriate. In patients with an ischemic or nonischemic cardiomyopathy and an ejection fraction ≤30% to 35%, an ICD may be appropriate for primary prevention of sudden death. However, a simple pacemaker without the ICD often is adequate for patients with a borderline ejection fraction (30% to 35%) and a rapid ventricular rate because the ejection fraction is likely to improve to >35% after the ventricular rate has been controlled by AV node ablation.

Surgical Approaches to Atrial Fibrillation

The most effective surgical procedure for AF is the "cut-and-sew" maze procedure developed by Cox in 1987.[50] This operation involves 12 atrial incisions to isolate the pulmonary veins and to create lines of block in the left atrium and right atrium. In addition, the left and right atria are excised. Long-term freedom from AF after the Cox maze procedure has been reported to range from 70% to 95%, but 10% to 35% of patients still require antiarrhythmic drug therapy.[51-54] The efficacy of the Cox maze procedure is lower in patients with very large left atria or with persistent AF for many years.[55,56] The Cox maze procedure has not been widely performed because it requires cardiopulmonary bypass, is technically difficult, and is associated with a mortality risk of approximately 1% to 2%.[53]

A large variety of surgical ablation tools have been developed to simplify the classic Cox maze procedure. These tools allow the surgeon to substitute an ablation line for a surgical incision. Several different types of energy have been used for surgical ablation: radiofrequency energy, cryoenergy, microwave, laser, and high-intensity focused ultrasound.[57] The tool that most consistently produces transmural ablation lines is a clamp device intended to isolate the pulmonary veins by use of bipolar radiofrequency energy.[58]

Various surgical ablation strategies have been used, including pulmonary vein isolation, left atrial ablation, and the Cox maze lesion set. In patients who do not require concomitant coronary artery bypass grafting or valve repair or replacement, surgical ablation typically is performed by a nonsternotomy approach. The efficacy of these procedures generally has been reported to range from 70% to 85%.[57] However, because of inadequate monitoring for recurrent AF during follow-up, it is likely that these success rates are overestimates.

At present, surgery for AF most commonly is performed as a concomitant procedure in patients with AF undergoing open heart surgery for coronary artery disease or valvular disease. A stand-alone surgical procedure for AF may be appropriate for patients who have not had a successful outcome from catheter ablation, who are not good candidates for catheter ablation, or who prefer a surgical procedure over catheter ablation.

Specific Clinical Syndromes

Postoperative Atrial Fibrillation (see Chaps. 84 and 85)

AF is common after open heart surgery and is reported to occur in 25% to 40% of patients who undergo coronary artery bypass graft surgery or valve replacement. It is associated with a twofold increase in the risk of postoperative stroke and is the most common reason for prolonged hospitalization. The risk of AF peaks on the second postoperative day. The pathogenesis of postoperative AF is multifactorial and probably involves adrenergic activation, inflammation, atrial ischemia, electrolyte disturbances, and genetic factors. Several risk factors for AF after open heart surgery have been identified, including age older than 70 years, history of prior AF, male gender, left ventricular dysfunction, left atrial enlargement, chronic lung disease, diabetes, and obesity.

The antiarrhythmic drugs that have been shown to decrease the risk of postoperative AF are beta blockers, sotalol, and amiodarone. A meta-analysis of studies that included several thousand patients who underwent open heart surgery concluded that the incidence of AF in the treatment arms of these studies was 17% to 22% compared with 33% to 37% in the control groups of these studies.[59] Amiodarone and sotalol decreased the risk of postoperative AF by 52% to 66%, and beta blockers appeared to be somewhat less effective, decreasing the risk by 31%. Amiodarone was the only one of these three drugs that was associated with a significant decrease in the length of hospitalization (by approximately 1 day) and in the postoperative stroke rate (by 46%). Hypomagnesemia is common after open heart surgery and probably heightens the risk of AF. Magnesium administration immediately preoperatively, perioperatively, or postoperatively decreases the risk of postoperative AF. A meta-analysis of 20 randomized trials that enrolled approximately 2500 patients who underwent open heart surgery found that the administration of magnesium reduced the odds of AF by 46%.[60] However, magnesium reduced the odds of postoperative AF by only approximately 20% in patients also receiving a beta blocker.[59]

Atrial pacing using temporary electrodes attached to the right or left atrium also has been shown to decrease the probability of postoperative AF. A meta-analysis reported that there was a 40% reduction in the risk of postoperative AF attributable to right atrial or biatrial pacing.[59]

Other agents that have been demonstrated in randomized studies to reduce the risk of AF after open heart surgery consist of long-chain polyunsaturated fatty acids (fish oil), which reduced the risk by 54%[61]; atorvastatin, which decreased the risk by 61%[62]; and hydrocortisone, which decreased the risk by 37%.[63] The main mechanism by which these agents prevent AF may be an anti-inflammatory effect. Other factors, such as modulation of autonomic tone or an antioxidant effect, also may play a role.

Wolff-Parkinson-White Syndrome (see Chaps. 37 and 39)

Patients with the Wolff-Parkinson-White syndrome and an accessory pathway with a short refractory period can experience a very rapid ventricular rate during AF. Ventricular rates of more than 250 to 300 beats/min can result in loss of consciousness or precipitate ventricular fibrillation and a cardiac arrest. Patients with Wolff-Parkinson-White syndrome who present in AF with a rapid ventricular rate should undergo transthoracic cardioversion if there is hemodynamic instability. If the patient is hemodynamically stable, intravenous procainamide or ibutilide can be used for pharmacologic cardioversion. Procainamide may be preferable to ibutilide because it blocks accessory pathway conduction and slows the ventricular rate before AF has converted to sinus rhythm. Digitalis and calcium channel antagonists are contraindicated in patients with Wolff-Parkinson-White syndrome and AF. These agents selectively block conduction in the AV node and can result in acceleration of conduction through the accessory pathway.

The preferred therapy for patients with Wolff-Parkinson-White syndrome and AF with a rapid ventricular rate is catheter ablation of the accessory pathway. The efficacy of catheter ablation is more than 95% for most types of accessory pathways, and the risk of a major complication is very low.[36] AF typically no longer recurs after successful accessory pathway ablation, probably because the AF in the Wolff-Parkinson-White syndrome often is tachycardia induced and a result of AV reciprocating tachycardia.

Congestive Heart Failure (see Chap. 28)

AF is a common arrhythmia in patients with heart failure, with a prevalence reported to range from 10% in patients with a New York Heart Association functional class I up to 50% in class IV patients. AF may be the cause of heart failure in patients who present with a nonischemic cardiomyopathy and AF with a rapid ventricular rate. In patients with structural heart disease and preexisting left ventricular dysfunction, AF may be responsible for worsening of heart failure. The deleterious hemodynamic effects of AF are mediated by a rapid rate or irregular ventricular rate and loss of AV synchrony.

The most appropriate rate-control drugs in patients with heart failure are digitalis and beta blockers. If necessary, amiodarone also can be used for rate control. The only rhythm-control drugs safe to use in patients with heart failure are amiodarone and dofetilide. These are the only two rhythm-control drugs that have been demonstrated to not increase the risk of death in patients with heart failure.

As in other patients with AF, the decision to pursue a rate-control strategy or a rhythm-control strategy in patients with heart failure should be individualized. In a multicenter trial, 1376 patients (mean age, 67 years) with AF, congestive heart failure, and mean left ventricular ejection fraction of 27% were randomly assigned to a rate-control strategy (most commonly digitalis and a beta blocker) or a rhythm-control strategy (amiodarone in 82% of patients) and observed for a mean of approximately 3 years.[64] There were no significant differences in all-cause mortality (10%/year), cardiovascular mortality (8%/year), or worsening heart failure (approximately 7% to 8%/year), and the hospitalization rate was higher in the rhythm-control group. Therefore, this study demonstrated no beneficial effect of a rhythm-control strategy on outcomes in patients with heart failure. However, endpoints such as ejection fraction and functional capacity were not examined in this study, and many patients in the rhythm-control arm continued to have AF. Although the study demonstrated that a pharmacologic rhythm-control strategy does not improve survival compared with a rate-control strategy in patients with heart failure and AF, this should not be taken to imply that sinus rhythm has no advantages over AF with a controlled ventricular rate in patients with heart failure.

Another randomized study demonstrated that rhythm control by catheter ablation improves left ventricular ejection fraction, functional capacity, and quality of life compared with a highly effective rate-control strategy, namely, AV node ablation plus a biventricular pacemaker.[65] Eighty-one patients with AF, heart failure, and ejection fraction <40% were randomly assigned to radiofrequency catheter ablation of the AF or AV node ablation and biventricular pacing. Freedom from AF at 6 months in the AF ablation arm was 71% in the absence of antiarrhythmic drug therapy and 88% with antiarrhythmic drug therapy. The mean ejection fraction improved from approximately 27% to 35% in the AF ablation group and remained unchanged in the AV node ablation group. Functional capacity (measured by the 6-minute walk test) and quality of life also improved significantly in the AF ablation group but not in the AV node ablation group. The failure of AV node ablation to improve these parameters is attributable to the fact that these patients already had adequate rate control with drug therapy.

These results suggest that attempts at restoration of sinus rhythm are worthwhile in patients with heart failure and that catheter ablation of the AF should be considered if sinus rhythm is not maintained by amiodarone or dofetilide. A rate-control strategy is appropriate for patients who do not respond adequately to amiodarone or dofetilide and either are not suitable candidates for catheter ablation of the AF or have an unsuccessful outcome from ablation. AV node ablation should be reserved for patients whose ventricular rate during AF is not adequately controlled by drug therapy. Because left ventricular dysfunction and heart failure can be aggravated by right ventricular pacing, biventricular pacing should be performed after AV node ablation. The decision to implant a biventricular pacemaker versus a biventricular ICD is based on clinical judgment. If it seems likely that the ejection fraction will remain <30% to 35% after optimal heart rate control, a biventricular ICD would be appropriate for primary prevention of sudden cardiac death.

Pregnancy

New-onset AF is rare during pregnancy (see Chap. 82), and when it does occur, it is usually in the setting of underlying congenital or valvular heart disease, thyrotoxicosis, or electrolyte abnormalities. In women with paroxysmal AF before pregnancy, the frequency of episodes may or may not increase during pregnancy.[66] Specific recommendations for the management of AF during pregnancy are provided in the Guidelines for Atrial Fibrillation.

Future Perspectives

The ideal antiarrhythmic drug to prevent AF would affect the atrium only, thereby eliminating the potential for ventricular proarrhythmia. Such drugs are under development and may improve the safety and efficacy of pharmacologic therapy for AF. Very likely, drugs that modify a single channel will not be as effective as those with multiple actions, and it is possible that targeting of nonchannel function like the development of fibrosis will prove useful.

For stroke prevention in patients with AF, there is the need for anticoagulation therapy that is more convenient, stable, and safer than vitamin K inhibitors such as warfarin. It seems likely that direct thrombin inhibitors, which provide a stable degree of anticoagulation with the need for monitoring of the INR or frequent dose adjustments, will become available in the near future.

In the past few years, significant progress has been made in the field of catheter ablation of AF, but there still is much room for improvement in efficacy and procedure duration. A better understanding of AF mechanisms and the ability to accurately identify the specific mechanisms at play in a given individual would allow a tailored approach to ablation that could maximize both efficacy and efficiency. In addition, efficacy, safety, and procedure duration most likely will be improved by tools for catheter ablation and surgical ablation of AF that allow the rapid creation of controllable and permanent lesions.

Finally, whereas multiple studies show that maintenance of rate provides no outcome advantage over maintenance of rhythm, those results are probably influenced by the side effects of the drugs used for rhythm control. It is possible that in the future, better drugs to maintain sinus rhythm will show the advantage of rhythm over rate control in AF.

REFERENCES

Epidemiology

1. Lloyd-Jones D, Adams R, Carnethon M, et al: Heart disease and stroke statistics—2009 update: A report from the AHA Statistics Committee and Stroke Statistics Subcommittee. Circulation 119:e21, 2009.

2. Lloyd-Jones DM, Wang TJ, Leip EP, et al: Lifetime risk for development of atrial fibrillation: The Framingham Heart Study. Circulation 110:1042, 2004.
3. Gami AS, Hodge DO, Herges RM, et al: Obstructive sleep apnea, obesity, and the risk of incident atrial fibrillation. J Am Coll Cardiol 49:565, 2007.
4. Wang TJ, Parise H, Levy D, et al: Obesity and the risk of new-onset atrial fibrillation. JAMA 292:2471, 2004.
5. Miyasaka Y, Barnes ME, Gersh BJ, et al: Secular trends in incidence of atrial fibrillation in Olmsted County, Minnesota, 1980 to 2000, and implications on the projections for future prevalence. Circulation 114:119, 2006.

Prevention of Thromboembolic Conditions

6. Lip GY, Edwards SJ: Stroke prevention with aspirin, warfarin and ximelagatran in patients with non-valvular atrial fibrillation: A systematic review and meta-analysis. Thromb Res 118:321, 2006.
7. Fuster V, Ryden LE, Cannom DS, et al: ACC/AHA/ESC 2006 guidelines for the management of patients with atrial fibrillation—executive summary: A report of the ACC/AHA Task Force and the ESC Committee for Practice Guidelines. J Am Coll Cardiol 48:854, 2006.
8. Gage BF, van Walraven C, Pearce L, et al: Selecting patients with atrial fibrillation for anticoagulation: Stroke risk stratification in patients taking aspirin. Circulation 110:2287, 2004.
9. Go AS, Fang MC, Udaltsova N, et al: Impact of proteinuria and glomerular filtration rate on risk of thromboembolism in atrial fibrillation: The anticoagulation and risk factors in atrial fibrillation (ATRIA) study. Circulation 119:1363, 2009.
10. Nieuwlaat R, Dinh T, Olsson SB, et al: Should we abandon the common practice of withholding oral anticoagulation in paroxysmal atrial fibrillation? Eur Heart J 29:915, 2008.
11. Akar JG, Jeske W, Wilber DJ: Acute onset human atrial fibrillation is associated with local cardiac platelet activation and endothelial dysfunction. J Am Coll Cardiol 51:1790, 2008.
12. Mandava A, Mittal S: Clinical significance of pacemaker-detected atrial high-rate episodes. Curr Opin Cardiol 23:60, 2008.
13. Glotzer TV, Daoud EG, Wyse DG, et al: Rationale and design of a prospective study of the clinical significance of atrial arrhythmias detected by implanted device diagnostics: The TRENDS study. J Interv Card Electrophysiol 15:9, 2006.
14. van Walraven C, Hart RG, Wells GA, et al: A clinical prediction rule to identify patients with atrial fibrillation and a low risk for stroke while taking aspirin. Arch Intern Med 163:936, 2003.
15. Singer DE, Chang Y, Fang MC, et al: The net clinical benefit of warfarin anticoagulation in atrial fibrillation. Ann Intern Med 151:297, 2009.
16. Connolly SJ, Pogue J, Hart RG, et al: Effect of clopidogrel added to aspirin in patients with atrial fibrillation. N Engl J Med 360:2066, 2009.
17. Oden A, Fahlen M, Hart RG: Optimal INR for prevention of stroke and death in atrial fibrillation: A critical appraisal. Thromb Res 117:493, 2006.
18. Rose AJ, Ozonoff A, Henault LE, Hylek EM: Warfarin for atrial fibrillation in community-based practise. J Thromb Haemost 6:1647, 2008.
19. Mant J, Hobbs FD, Fletcher K, et al: Warfarin versus aspirin for stroke prevention in an elderly community population with atrial fibrillation (the Birmingham Atrial Fibrillation Treatment of the Aged Study, BAFTA): A randomised controlled trial. Lancet 370:493, 2007.
20. Klein TE, Altman RB, Eriksson N, et al: Estimation of the warfarin dose with clinical and pharmacogenetic data. N Engl J Med 360:753, 2009.
21. Anderson JL, Horne BD, Stevens SM, et al: Randomized trial of genotype-guided versus standard warfarin dosing in patients initiating oral anticoagulation. Circulation 116:2563, 2007.
22. Connolly SJ, Ezekowitz MD, Yusuf S, et al: Dabigatran versus warfarin in patients with atrial fibrillation. N Engl J Med 361:1139, 2009.
23. Stellbrink C, Nixdorff U, Hofmann T, et al: Safety and efficacy of enoxaparin compared with unfractionated heparin and oral anticoagulants for prevention of thromboembolic complications in cardioversion of nonvalvular atrial fibrillation: The Anticoagulation in Cardioversion using Enoxaparin (ACE) trial. Circulation 109:997, 2004.
24. Kanderian AS, Gillinov AM, Pettersson GB, et al: Success of surgical left atrial appendage closure: Assessment by transesophageal echocardiography. J Am Coll Cardiol 52:924, 2008.
25. Holmes DR, Reddy VY, Turi ZG, et al: Percutaneous closure of the left atrial appendage versus warfarin therapy for prevention of stroke in patients with atrial fibrillation: A randomised non-inferiority trial. Lancet 374:534, 2009.

Long-Term Management

26. Wyse DG, Waldo AL, DiMarco JP, et al: A comparison of rate control and rhythm control in patients with atrial fibrillation. N Engl J Med 347:1825, 2002.
27. Corley SD, Epstein AE, DiMarco JP, et al: Relationships between sinus rhythm, treatment, and survival in the Atrial Fibrillation Follow-Up Investigation of Rhythm Management (AFFIRM) Study. Circulation 109:1509, 2004.
28. Gjesdal K, Feyzi J, Olsson SB: Digitalis: A dangerous drug in atrial fibrillation? An analysis of the SPORTIF III and V data. Heart 94:191, 2008.
29. Lafuente-Lafuente C, Mouly S, Longas-Tejero MA, et al: Antiarrhythmic drugs for maintaining sinus rhythm after cardioversion of atrial fibrillation: A systematic review of randomized controlled trials. Arch Intern Med 166:719, 2006.
30. Calkins H, Reynolds MR, Spector P, et al: Treatment of atrial fibrillation with antiarrhythmic drugs or radiofrequency ablation. Two systematic literature reviews and meta-analyses. Circ Arrhythm Electrophysiol 2:349, 2009.
31. Healey JS, Baranchuk A, Crystal E, et al: Prevention of atrial fibrillation with angiotensin-converting enzyme inhibitors and angiotensin receptor blockers: A meta-analysis. J Am Coll Cardiol 45:1832, 2005.
32. Disertori M, Latini R, Barlera S, et al: Valsartan for prevention of recurrent atrial fibrillation. N Engl J Med 360:1606, 2009.
33. Liu T, Li L, Korantzopoulos P, et al: Statin use and development of atrial fibrillation: A systematic review and meta-analysis of randomized clinical trials and observational studies. Int J Cardiol 126:160, 2008.

Nonpharmacologic Management

34. Knight BP, Gersh BJ, Carlson MD, et al: Role of permanent pacing to prevent atrial fibrillation: Science advisory from the American Heart Association Council on Clinical Cardiology (Subcommittee on Electrocardiography and Arrhythmias) and the Quality of Care and Outcomes Research Interdisciplinary Working Group, in collaboration with the Heart Rhythm Society. Circulation 111:240, 2005.
35. Blanc JJ, De Roy L, Mansourati J, et al: Atrial pacing for prevention of atrial fibrillation: Assessment of simultaneously implemented algorithms. Europace 6:371, 2004.
36. Morady F: Catheter ablation of supraventricular arrhythmias: State of the art. J Cardiovasc Electrophysiol 15:124, 2004.
37. Calkins H, Brugada J, Packer DL, et al: HRS/EHRA/ECAS expert Consensus Statement on catheter and surgical ablation of atrial fibrillation: Recommendations for personnel, policy, procedures and follow-up. A report of the Heart Rhythm Society (HRS) Task Force on catheter and surgical ablation of atrial fibrillation. Heart Rhythm 4:816, 2007.
38. Noheria A, Kumar A, Wylie JV Jr, Josephson ME: Catheter ablation vs antiarrhythmic drug therapy for atrial fibrillation: A systematic review. Arch Intern Med 168:581, 2008.
39. Jais P, Cauchemez B, Macle L, et al: Catheter ablation versus antiarrhythmic drugs for atrial fibrillation: The A4 study. Circulation 118:2498, 2008.
40. Cappato R, Calkins H, Chen SA, et al: Worldwide survey on the methods, efficacy, and safety of catheter ablation for human atrial fibrillation. Circulation 111:1100, 2005.
41. Spragg DD, Dalal D, Cheema A, et al: Complications of catheter ablation for atrial fibrillation: Incidence and predictors. J Cardiovasc Electrophysiol 19:627, 2008.
42. Cappato R, Calkins H, Chen SA, et al: Prevalence and causes of fatal outcome in catheter ablation of atrial fibrillation. J Am Coll Cardiol 53:1798, 2009.
43. Katsiyiannis WT, Melby DP, Matelski JL, et al: Feasibility and safety of remote-controlled magnetic navigation for ablation of atrial fibrillation. Am J Cardiol 102:1674, 2008.
44. Saliba W, Reddy VY, Wazni O, et al: Atrial fibrillation ablation using a robotic catheter remote control system: Initial human experience and long-term follow-up results. J Am Coll Cardiol 51:2407, 2008.
45. Boersma LV, Wijffels MC, Oral H, et al: Pulmonary vein isolation by duty-cycled bipolar and unipolar radiofrequency energy with a multielectrode ablation catheter. Heart Rhythm 5:1635, 2008.
46. Fredersdorf S, Weber S, Jilek C, et al: Safe and rapid isolation of pulmonary veins using a novel circular ablation catheter and duty-cycled RF generator. J Cardiovasc Electrophysiol 20:1097, 2009.
47. Neumann T, Vogt J, Schumacher B, et al: Circumferential pulmonary vein isolation with the cryoballoon technique results from a prospective 3-center study. J Am Coll Cardiol 52:273, 2008.
48. Moreira W, Manusama R, Timmermans C, et al: Long-term follow-up after cryothermic ostial pulmonary vein isolation in paroxysmal atrial fibrillation. J Am Coll Cardiol 51:850, 2008.
49. Bradley DJ, Shen WK: Atrioventricular junction ablation combined with either right ventricular pacing or cardiac resynchronization therapy for atrial fibrillation: The need for large-scale randomized trials. Heart Rhythm 4:224, 2007.
50. Cox JL, Boineau JP, Schuessler RB, et al: Electrophysiologic basis, surgical development, and clinical results of the maze procedure for atrial flutter and atrial fibrillation. Adv Card Surg 6:1, 1995.
51. Damiano RJ Jr, Gaynor SL, Bailey M, et al: The long-term outcome of patients with coronary disease and atrial fibrillation undergoing the Cox maze procedure. J Thorac Cardiovasc Surg 126:2016, 2003.
52. Gillinov AM, McCarthy PM: Advances in the surgical treatment of atrial fibrillation. Cardiol Clin 22:147, 2004.
53. Prasad SM, Maniar HS, Camillo CJ, et al: The Cox maze III procedure for atrial fibrillation: Long-term efficacy in patients undergoing lone versus concomitant procedures. J Thorac Cardiovasc Surg 126:1822, 2003.
54. Ballaux PK, Geuzebroek GS, van Hemel NM, et al: Freedom from atrial arrhythmias after classic maze III surgery: A 10-year experience. J Thorac Cardiovasc Surg 132:1433, 2006.
55. Gillinov AM, Sirak J, Blackstone EH, et al: The Cox maze procedure in mitral valve disease: Predictors of recurrent atrial fibrillation. J Thorac Cardiovasc Surg 130:1653, 2005.
56. Gaynor SL, Schuessler RB, Bailey MS, et al: Surgical treatment of atrial fibrillation: Predictors of late recurrence. J Thorac Cardiovasc Surg 129:104, 2005.
57. Khargi K, Hutten BA, Lemke B, Deneke T: Surgical treatment of atrial fibrillation; a systematic review. Eur J Cardiothorac Surg 27:258, 2005.
58. Schneeberger EW, Osterday RM: Lateral placement of bipolar clamp facilitates pulmonary vein isolation. Ann Thorac Surg 84:1412, 2007.

Specific Clinical Syndromes

59. Burgess DC, Kilborn MJ, Keech AC: Interventions for prevention of post-operative atrial fibrillation and its complications after cardiac surgery: A meta-analysis. Eur Heart J 27:2846, 2006.
60. Miller S, Crystal E, Garfinkle M, et al: Effects of magnesium on atrial fibrillation after cardiac surgery: A meta-analysis. Heart 91:618, 2005.
61. Calo L, Bianconi L, Colivicchi F, et al: N-3 Fatty acids for the prevention of atrial fibrillation after coronary artery bypass surgery: A randomized, controlled trial. J Am Coll Cardiol 45:1723, 2005.
62. Patti G, Chello M, Candura D, et al: Randomized trial of atorvastatin for reduction of postoperative atrial fibrillation in patients undergoing cardiac surgery: Results of the ARMYDA-3 (Atorvastatin for Reduction of MYocardial Dysrhythmia After cardiac surgery) study. Circulation 114:1455, 2006.
63. Halonen J, Halonen P, Jarvinen O, et al: Corticosteroids for the prevention of atrial fibrillation after cardiac surgery: A randomized controlled trial. JAMA 297:1562, 2007.
64. Roy D, Talajic M, Nattel S, et al: Rhythm control versus rate control for atrial fibrillation and heart failure. N Engl J Med 358:2667, 2008.
65. Khan MN, Jais P, Cummings J, et al: Pulmonary-vein isolation for atrial fibrillation in patients with heart failure. N Engl J Med 359:1778, 2008.
66. Silversides CK, Harris L, Haberer K, et al: Recurrence rates of arrhythmias during pregnancy in women with previous tachyarrhythmia and impact on fetal and neonatal outcomes. Am J Cardiol 97:1206, 2006.

GUIDELINES FRED MORADY AND DOUGLAS P. ZIPES

Atrial Fibrillation

The most recent and comprehensive guidelines for the management of atrial fibrillation (AF) were published in 2006 by the American College of Cardiology/American Heart Association (ACC/AHA) Task Force on Practice Guidelines and the European Society of Cardiology Committee for Practice Guidelines.[1] The following classification system was used for recommendations and for the level of evidence on which the recommendations are based:

Class I: conditions for which there is evidence and/or general agreement that the test is useful and effective

Class IIa: weight of evidence or opinion is in favor of usefulness/efficacy

Class IIb: usefulness or efficacy is less well established by evidence or opinion

Class III: conditions for which there is evidence and/or general agreement that the test is not useful or effective and in some cases may be harmful

Level A: recommendations are derived from data from multiple randomized clinical trials

Level B: recommendations are derived from a single randomized trial or nonrandomized studies

Level C: recommendations are based on the consensus opinion of experts

The guidelines do not necessarily define the standard of care. Management decisions must be individualized on the basis of the particular circumstances of a patient, and there are situations in which a deviation from the guidelines may be appropriate.

CLASSIFICATION OF ATRIAL FIBRILLATION

The terminology used to classify AF in the guidelines is as follows: paroxysmal AF is defined as episodes of AF that last less than 7 days; persistent AF is defined as AF that lasts more than 7 days; longstanding AF refers to AF that has been persistent for more than 1 year. These designations are not altered by termination of AF by drug therapy or electrical cardioversion. AF that is resistant to electrical cardioversion is referred to as permanent AF. AF is considered recurrent after two or more episodes have occurred.

Some patients with paroxysmal AF occasionally have episodes that are persistent, and vice versa. In this event, the AF should be categorized on the basis of the predominant form. Lone AF refers to AF in patients younger than 60 years who do not have structural heart disease or hypertension. AF that is secondary to acute myocardial infarction, cardiac surgery, pericarditis, myocarditis, hyperthyroidism, or an acute pulmonary process is considered separately because the AF often resolves after treatment of the underlying disorder.

MANAGEMENT OF ATRIAL FIBRILLATION

The guidelines address five aspects of the management of AF: pharmacologic rate control; prevention of thromboembolic complications; cardioversion; maintenance of sinus rhythm; and special considerations, including postoperative AF, myocardial infarction, Wolff-Parkinson-White syndrome, hyperthyroidism, pregnancy, hypertrophic cardiomyopathy, and pulmonary disease.

An important aspect in the management of patients with AF that is not specifically addressed in the guidelines is how to decide on a rate-control strategy versus a rhythm-control strategy. Several clinical trials have demonstrated that pharmacologic rhythm-control and rate-control strategies result in similar outcomes, even in patients with AF who have left ventricular dysfunction and heart failure. On the other hand, a randomized trial of left atrial radiofrequency catheter ablation versus atrioventricular (AV) node ablation and biventricular pacing demonstrated significantly greater improvement in left ventricular function, exercise capacity, and quality of life in patients with heart failure who were treated by ablation. It is possible that the side effects from the drugs used for rhythm control offset the benefits of sinus rhythm. Specific recommendations regarding rhythm-control versus rate-control strategies are difficult to provide because the decision must be individualized on the basis of several factors, including age, symptom severity, functional limitations, preference of the patient, comorbidities, sinus node function, and response to drug therapy.

Pharmacologic Rate Control During Atrial Fibrillation (Table 40G-1)

In addition to specific recommendations on the use of particular drugs for control of the ventricular rate, the guidelines recommend that the effects of drug therapy on the ventricular rate be measured at rest and during exercise to ensure adequate heart rate control. The criteria used for rate control are rates of 60 to 80 beats/min at rest and 90 to 115 beats/min during moderate exercise.

Digitalis is much less effective for control of the ventricular rate during exercise than at rest and is indicated for patients with heart failure or left ventricular dysfunction and for sedentary patients. A combination of digitalis and either a beta blocker or nondihydropyridine calcium channel antagonist is appropriate to control the rate at rest and during exercise. The guidelines recommend that digitalis not be used as the sole agent for rate control in patients with paroxysmal AF. Catheter ablation of the AV node should be reserved for patients whose ventricular rate cannot be adequately controlled by drug therapy because of either inefficacy or drug intolerance.

Prevention of Thromboembolism (Table 40G-2)

The guidelines recommend antithrombotic therapy with either aspirin or a vitamin K antagonist such as warfarin for all patients with AF except those who have lone AF or contraindications. The choice between aspirin and a vitamin K antagonist is based on the patient's risk profile. The factors associated with the highest risk of thromboembolism are a prior thromboembolic event and rheumatic mitral stenosis, and a vitamin K antagonist (e.g., warfarin) is recommended for patients with one of these risk factors. The risk factors associated with a moderate risk of thromboembolism are age ≥75 years, hypertension, heart failure, ejection fraction ≤35%, and diabetes. Aspirin is recommended if none of these risk factors is present, and a vitamin K antagonist is recommended for patients with one or more of these risk factors. In patients with only one of the moderate risk factors, either aspirin or a vitamin K antagonist is reasonable, and the choice should be individualized. Of note is that the guidelines recommend against use of a vitamin K antagonist for stroke prevention in patients with lone AF and in patients without any risk factors. New antithrombin and anti–factor Xa drugs are being investigated.

Cardioversion of Atrial Fibrillation (Table 40G-3)

The first-line drugs recommended for cardioversion are flecainide, dofetilide, propafenone, and ibutilide. Amiodarone is considered a reasonable option. The guidelines state that digoxin and sotalol may be harmful when they are used for cardioversion and recommend against use of these agents for that purpose.

Direct-current cardioversion is recommended when there is a rapid ventricular rate that does not respond quickly to drug therapy in patients with myocardial ischemia, hypotension, or heart failure and in patients with the Wolff-Parkinson-White syndrome and AF with a very rapid rate or hemodynamic instability. If there is an early recurrence of AF after direct-current cardioversion, repeated cardioversion is recommended after treatment with an antiarrhythmic drug.

If AF has been present for >48 hours or if the duration is unknown, anticoagulation with an international normalized ratio (INR) of 2 to 3 is recommended for ≥3 weeks before cardioversion, whether pharmacologic or electrical, and for 4 weeks afterward. When cardioversion is performed within 48 hours of the onset of AF, anticoagulation before and after cardioversion may be based on the patient's risk profile.

In patients with AF >48 hours in duration or in whom the duration is unknown, an alternative to anticoagulation for ≥3 weeks before cardioversion is to perform transesophageal echocardiography, to anticoagulate the patient with heparin, to initiate oral anticoagulation, and to proceed with immediate cardioversion if no thrombi are present in the left atrium or left atrial appendage. Anticoagulation with heparin should be continued until the INR is 2, and oral anticoagulation with an INR of 2 to 3 should be continued for ≥4 weeks.

TABLE 40G-1 ACC/AHA Recommendations for Pharmacologic Rate Control of Atrial Fibrillation

CLASS	INDICATION	LEVEL OF EVIDENCE
Class I (indicated)	Measurement of the heart rate at rest and control of the rate with pharmacologic agents (either a beta blocker or nondihydropyridine calcium channel antagonist, in most cases) are recommended for patients with persistent or permanent AF	B
	In the absence of preexcitation, intravenous administration of beta blockers (esmolol, metoprolol, or propranolol) or nondihydropyridine calcium channel antagonists (verapamil, diltiazem) is recommended to slow the ventricular response to AF in the acute setting, exercising caution in patients with hypotension or heart failure	B
	Intravenous administration of digoxin or amiodarone is recommended to control heart rate in patients with AF and heart failure who do not have an accessory pathway	B
	In patients who experience symptoms related to AF during activity, the adequacy of heart rate control should be assessed during exercise, adjusting pharmacologic treatment as necessary to keep the rate in the physiologic range	C
	Digoxin is effective after oral administration to control the heart rate at rest in patients with AF and is indicated for patients with heart failure or left ventricular dysfunction and for sedentary individuals	C
Class IIa (strong supportive evidence)	A combination of digoxin and either a beta blocker or nondihydropyridine calcium channel antagonist is reasonable to control the heart rate both at rest and during exercise in patients with AF. The choice of medication should be individualized and the dose modulated to avoid bradycardia.	B
	It is reasonable to use ablation of the AV node or accessory pathway to control heart rate when pharmacologic therapy is insufficient or associated with side effects	B
	Intravenous amiodarone can be useful to control heart rate in patients with AF when other measures are unsuccessful or contraindicated	C
	When electrical cardioversion is not necessary in patients with AF and an accessory pathway, intravenous procainamide or ibutilide is a reasonable alternative	C
Class IIb (weak supportive evidence)	When the ventricular rate cannot be adequately controlled both at rest and during exercise in patients with AF by a beta blocker, nondihydropyridine calcium channel antagonist, or digoxin, alone or in combination, oral amiodarone may be administered to control the heart rate	C
	Intravenous procainamide, disopyramide, ibutilide, or amiodarone may be considered for hemodynamically stable patients with AF involving conduction over an accessory pathway	B
	When the rate cannot be controlled with pharmacologic agents or tachycardia-mediated cardiomyopathy is suspected, catheter-directed ablation of the AV node may be considered in patients with AF to control the heart rate	C
Class III (not indicated)	Digitalis should not be used as the sole agent to control the rate of ventricular response in patients with paroxysmal AF	B
	Catheter ablation of the AV node should not be attempted without a prior trial of medication to control the ventricular rate in patients with AF	C
	In patients with decompensated heart failure and AF, intravenous administration of a nondihydropyridine calcium channel antagonist may exacerbate hemodynamic compromise and is not recommended	C
	Intravenous administration of digitalis glycosides or nondihydropyridine calcium channel antagonists to patients with AF and a preexcitation syndrome may paradoxically accelerate the ventricular response and is not recommended	C

Maintenance of Sinus Rhythm (Table 40G-4)

A reasonable outcome of antiarrhythmic drug therapy is infrequent recurrences of well-tolerated AF. Initiation of a rhythm-control medication is reasonable on an outpatient basis in patients without heart disease when the medication is well tolerated. The guidelines consider catheter ablation of symptomatic AF to be a reasonable alternative to rhythm-control medications in patients with little or no left atrial enlargement.

Special Considerations (Table 40G-5)

Postoperative Atrial Fibrillation The guidelines recommend prophylactic treatment with an oral beta blocker to prevent postoperative AF in patients undergoing cardiac surgery. Preoperative amiodarone also is considered to be appropriate prophylactic therapy to prevent postoperative AF. The use of cardioversion, rhythm-control medications, and antithrombotic medication should be based on the same considerations as in nonsurgical patients.

Acute Myocardial Infarction Electrical cardioversion is recommended if there is hemodynamic compromise or ongoing ischemia or when adequate rate control cannot be achieved with drug therapy. The guidelines recommend intravenous amiodarone or digitalis to slow the ventricular rate in patients and to improve left ventricular function in patients with an acute myocardial infarction. If there is no left ventricular dysfunction, bronchospasm, or AV block, an intravenous beta blocker or nondihydropyridine calcium antagonist is recommended for rate control.

Atrial Fibrillation in the Wolff-Parkinson-White Syndrome Catheter ablation of the accessory pathway is recommended in patients with symptomatic AF and the Wolff-Parkinson-White syndrome. Immediate electrical cardioversion is recommended if there is AF with a rapid ventricular rate and hemodynamic instability. If the patient is hemodynamically stable, intravenous procainamide or ibutilide is recommended for pharmacologic conversion of AF. Intravenous digitalis and nondihydropyridine calcium channel antagonists should be avoided in patients with ventricular preexcitation during AF.

Hyperthyroidism The guidelines recommend a beta blocker as first-line therapy for rate control in patients with AF and thyrotoxicosis. If a beta blocker cannot be used, verapamil or diltiazem should be used for rate control. Recommendations for therapy to prevent thromboembolic complications are as for patients without hyperthyroidism.

Atrial Fibrillation during Pregnancy The guidelines recommend digoxin, a beta blocker, or a nondihydropyridine calcium channel antagonist for rate control of AF during pregnancy. Direct-current cardioversion is recommended if there is hemodynamic instability.

Except in patients with a low-risk profile, either aspirin or an anticoagulant is recommended for prevention of thromboembolic complications, depending on the stage of pregnancy (see Chap. 82). Unfractionated or low-molecular-weight heparin can be considered during the first trimester and last month of pregnancy in patients with risk factors for thromboembolism, and an oral anticoagulant can be considered during the second trimester in patients at high risk of thromboembolism.

When AF occurs during pregnancy, quinidine or procainamide can be considered for pharmacologic cardioversion in hemodynamically stable patients.

Hypertrophic Cardiomyopathy The guidelines point out that there are not adequate data on the best rhythm-control medication to use for AF in the setting of hypertrophic cardiomyopathy. The preferred therapy is

TABLE 40G-2 ACC/AHA Recommendations for Prevention of Thromboembolism in Atrial Fibrillation

CLASS	INDICATION	LEVEL OF EVIDENCE
Class I (indicated)	Antithrombotic therapy to prevent thromboembolism is recommended for all patients with AF, except those with lone AF or contraindications	A
	The selection of the antithrombotic agent should be based on the absolute risks of stroke and bleeding and the relative risk and benefit for a given patient	A
	For patients without mechanical heart valves at high risk of stroke, chronic oral anticoagulant therapy with a vitamin K antagonist is recommended in a dose adjusted to achieve the target intensity international normalized ratio (INR) of 2.0 to 3.0 unless contraindicated. Factors associated with highest risk for stroke in patients with AF are prior thromboembolism (stroke, transient ischemic attack, or systemic embolism) and rheumatic mitral stenosis.	A
	Anticoagulation with a vitamin K antagonist is recommended for patients with more than one moderate risk factor. Such factors include age ≥75 years, hypertension, heart failure, impaired left ventricular systolic function (ejection fraction ≤35% or fractional shortening <25%), and diabetes mellitus.	A
	INR should be determined at least weekly during initiation of therapy and monthly when anticoagulation is stable	A
	Aspirin, 81 to 325 mg daily, is recommended as an alternative to vitamin K antagonists in low-risk patients or in those with contraindications to oral anticoagulation	A
	For patients with AF who have mechanical heart valves, the target intensity of anticoagulation should be based on the type of prosthesis, maintaining an INR of at least 2.5	B
	Antithrombotic therapy is recommended for patients with atrial flutter as for those with AF	C
Class IIa (strong supportive evidence)	For primary prevention of thromboembolism in patients with nonvalvular AF who have just one of the following validated risk factors, antithrombotic therapy with either aspirin or a vitamin K antagonist is reasonable, based on an assessment of the risk of bleeding complications, ability to safely sustain adjusted chronic anticoagulation, and the patient's preferences: age ≥75 years (especially in female patients), hypertension, heart failure, impaired left ventricular function, or diabetes mellitus	A
	For patients with nonvalvular AF who have one or more of the following less well validated risk factors, antithrombotic therapy with either aspirin or a vitamin K antagonist is reasonable for prevention of thromboembolism: age 65 to 74 years, female gender, or coronary artery disease. The choice of agent should be based on the risk of bleeding complications, ability to sustain adjusted chronic anticoagulation, and the patient's preferences	B
	It is reasonable to select antithrombotic therapy by the same criteria irrespective of the pattern (i.e., paroxysmal, persistent, or permanent) of AF	B
	In patients with AF who do not have mechanical prosthetic heart valves, it is reasonable to interrupt anticoagulation for up to 1 week without substituting heparin for surgical or diagnostic procedures that carry a risk of bleeding	C
	It is reasonable to reevaluate the need for anticoagulation at regular intervals	C
Class IIb (weak supportive evidence)	In patients ≥75 years at increased risk of bleeding but without frank contraindications to oral anticoagulant therapy, and in other patients with moderate risk factors for thromboembolism who are unable to safely tolerate anticoagulation at the standard intensity of INR 2.0 to 3.0, a lower INR target of 2.0 (range, 1.6 to 2.5) may be considered for prevention of ischemic stroke and systemic embolism	C
	When surgical procedures require interruption of oral anticoagulant therapy for longer than 1 week in high-risk patients, unfractionated heparin may be administered or low-molecular-weight heparin given by subcutaneous injection, although the efficacy of these alternatives in this situation is uncertain	C
	After percutaneous coronary intervention or revascularization surgery in patients with AF, low-dose aspirin (<100 mg/day) and/or clopidogrel (75 mg/day) may be given concurrently with anticoagulation to prevent myocardial ischemic events, but these strategies have not been thoroughly evaluated and are associated with an increased risk of bleeding	C
	In patients undergoing percutaneous coronary intervention, anticoagulation may be interrupted to prevent bleeding at the site of peripheral arterial puncture, but the vitamin K antagonist should be resumed as soon as possible after the procedure and the dose adjusted to achieve an INR in the therapeutic range. Aspirin may be given temporarily during the hiatus, but the maintenance regimen should then consist of the combination of clopidogrel, 75 mg daily, plus warfarin (INR, 2.0 to 3.0). Clopidogrel should be given for a minimum of 1 month after implantation of a bare-metal stent, at least 3 months for a sirolimus-eluting stent, at least 6 months for a paclitaxel-eluting stent, and12 months or longer in selected patients, following which warfarin may be continued as monotherapy in the absence of a subsequent coronary event. When warfarin is given in combination with clopidogrel or low-dose aspirin, the dose intensity must be carefully regulated.	C
	In patients with AF younger than 60 years without heart disease or risk factors for thromboembolism (lone AF), the risk of thromboembolism is low without treatment, and the effectiveness of aspirin for primary prevention of stroke relative to the risk of bleeding has not been established	C
	In patients with AF who sustain ischemic stroke or systemic embolism during treatment with low-intensity anticoagulation (INR, 2.0 to 3.0), rather than add an antiplatelet agent, it may be reasonable to raise the intensity of the anticoagulation to a maximum target INR of 3.0 to 3.5	C
Class III (not indicated)	Long-term anticoagulation with a vitamin K antagonist is not recommended for primary prevention of stroke in patients younger than 60 years without heart disease (lone AF) or any risk factors for thromboembolism	C

TABLE 40G-3 **ACC/AHA Recommendations for Cardioversion of Atrial Fibrillation**

CLASS	INDICATION	LEVEL OF EVIDENCE
Pharmacologic Cardioversion		
Class I (indicated)	Administration of flecainide, dofetilide, propafenone, or ibutilide is recommended for pharmacologic cardioversion of AF	A
Class IIa (strong supportive evidence)	Administration of amiodarone is a reasonable option for pharmacologic cardioversion of AF	A
	A single oral bolus dose of propafenone or flecainide ("pill-in-the-pocket") can be administered to terminate persistent AF outside the hospital once treatment has proved safe in the hospital for selected patients without sinus or AV node dysfunction, bundle branch block, QT interval prolongation, the Brugada syndrome, or structural heart disease. Before antiarrhythmic medication is initiated, a beta blocker or nondihydropyridine calcium channel antagonist should be given to prevent rapid AV conduction in the event atrial flutter occurs.	C
	Administration of amiodarone can be beneficial on an outpatient basis in patients with paroxysmal or persistent AF when rapid restoration of sinus rhythm is not deemed necessary	C
Class IIb (weak supportive evidence)	Administration of quinidine or procainamide might be considered for pharmacologic cardioversion of AF, but the usefulness of these agents is not well established	C
Class III (not indicated)	Digoxin and sotalol may be harmful when used for pharmacologic cardioversion of AF and are not recommended	A
	Quinidine, procainamide, disopyramide, and dofetilide should not be started out of the hospital for conversion of AF to sinus rhythm	B
Direct-Current Cardioversion		
Class I (indicated)	When a rapid ventricular response does not respond promptly to pharmacologic measures for patients with AF with ongoing myocardial ischemia, symptomatic hypotension, angina, or heart failure, immediate R wave–synchronized direct-current cardioversion is recommended	C
	Immediate direct-current cardioversion is recommended for patients with AF involving preexcitation when very rapid tachycardia or hemodynamic instability occurs	B
	Cardioversion is recommended in patients without hemodynamic instability when symptoms of AF are unacceptable to the patient. In case of early relapse of AF after cardioversion, repeated direct-current cardioversion attempts may be made after administration of antiarrhythmic medication.	C
Class IIa (strong supportive evidence)	Direct-current cardioversion can be useful to restore sinus rhythm as part of a long-term management strategy for patients with AF	B
	The patient's preference is a reasonable consideration in the selection of infrequently repeated cardioversions for the management of symptomatic or recurrent AF	C
Class III (not indicated)	Frequent repetition of direct-current cardioversion is not recommended for patients who have relatively short periods of sinus rhythm between relapses of AF after multiple cardioversion procedures despite prophylactic antiarrhythmic drug therapy	C
	Electrical cardioversion is contraindicated in patients with digitalis toxicity or hypokalemia	C
Pharmacologic Enhancement of Direct-Current Cardioversion		
Class IIa (strong supportive evidence)	Pretreatment with amiodarone, flecainide, ibutilide, propafenone, or sotalol can be useful to enhance the success of direct-current cardioversion and to prevent recurrent AF	B
	In patients who relapse to AF after successful cardioversion, it can be useful to repeat the procedure after prophylactic administration of antiarrhythmic medication	C
Class IIb (weak supportive evidence)	For patients with persistent AF, administration of beta blockers, disopyramide, diltiazem, dofetilide, procainamide, or verapamil may be considered, although the efficacy of these agents to enhance the success of direct-current cardioversion or to prevent early recurrence of AF is uncertain	C
	Out-of-hospital initiation of antiarrhythmic medications may be considered in patients without heart disease to enhance the success of cardioversion of AF	C
	Out-of-hospital administration of antiarrhythmic medications may be considered to enhance the success of cardioversion of AF in patients with certain forms of heart disease once the safety of the drug has been verified for the patient	C
Prevention of Thromboembolism in Patients with Atrial Fibrillation Undergoing Cardioversion		
Class I (indicated)	For patients with AF of 48-hour duration or longer, or when the duration of AF is unknown, anticoagulation (INR 2.0 to 3.0) is recommended for at least 3 weeks before and 4 weeks after cardioversion, regardless of the method (electrical or pharmacologic) used to restore sinus rhythm	B
	For patients with AF of more than 48-hour duration requiring immediate cardioversion because of hemodynamic instability, heparin should be administered concurrently (unless contraindicated) by an initial intravenous bolus injection, followed by a continuous infusion in a dose adjusted to prolong the activated partial thromboplastin time to 1.5 to 2 times the reference control value. Thereafter, oral anticoagulation (INR 2.0 to 3.0) should be provided for at least 4 weeks, as for patients undergoing elective cardioversion. Limited data support subcutaneous administration of low-molecular-weight heparin in this indication.	C
	For patients with AF of less than 48-hour duration associated with hemodynamic instability (angina pectoris, myocardial infarction, shock, or pulmonary edema), cardioversion should be performed immediately, without delay, for prior initiation of anticoagulation	C

Continued

TABLE 40G-3 ACC/AHA Recommendations for Cardioversion of Atrial Fibrillation—cont'd

CLASS	INDICATION	LEVEL OF EVIDENCE
Class IIa (strong supportive evidence)	During the 48 hours after onset of AF, the need for anticoagulation before and after cardioversion may be based on the patient's risk of thromboembolism	C
	As an alternative to anticoagulation before cardioversion of AF, it is reasonable to perform transesophageal echocardiography in search of thrombus in the left atrium or left atrial appendage	B
	a. For patients with no identifiable thrombus, cardioversion is reasonable immediately after anticoagulation with unfractionated heparin (e.g., initiated by intravenous bolus injection and an infusion continued at a dose adjusted to prolong the activated partial thromboplastin time to 1.5 to 2 times the control value until oral anticoagulation has been established with an oral vitamin K antagonist [e.g., warfarin] as evidenced by an INR ≥2.0)	B
	Thereafter, continuation of oral anticoagulation (INR 2.0 to 3.0) is reasonable for a total anticoagulation period of at least 4 weeks, as for patients undergoing elective cardioversion	B
	Limited data are available to support the subcutaneous administration of a low-molecular-weight heparin in this indication	C
	b. For patients in whom thrombus is identified by transesophageal echocardiography, oral anticoagulation (INR 2.0 to 3.0) is reasonable for at least 3 weeks before and 4 weeks after restoration of sinus rhythm, and a longer period of anticoagulation may be appropriate even after apparently successful cardioversion because the risk of thromboembolism often remains elevated in such cases	C
	For patients with atrial flutter undergoing cardioversion, anticoagulation can be beneficial according to the recommendations as for patients with AF	C

TABLE 40G-4 ACC/AHA Recommendations for Maintenance of Sinus Rhythm in Patients with Atrial Fibrillation

CLASS	INDICATION	LEVEL OF EVIDENCE
Class I (indicated)	Before initiation of antiarrhythmic drug therapy, treatment of precipitating or reversible causes of AF is recommended	C
Class IIa (strong supportive evidence)	Pharmacologic therapy can be useful in patients with AF to maintain sinus rhythm and to prevent tachycardia-induced cardiomyopathy	C
	Infrequent, well-tolerated recurrence of AF is reasonable as a successful outcome of antiarrhythmic drug therapy	C
	Outpatient initiation of antiarrhythmic drug therapy is reasonable in patients with AF who have no associated heart disease when the agent is well tolerated	C
	In patients with lone AF without structural heart disease, initiation of propafenone or flecainide can be beneficial on an outpatient basis in patients with paroxysmal AF who are in sinus rhythm at the time of drug initiation	B
	Sotalol can be beneficial in outpatients in sinus rhythm with little or no heart disease, prone to paroxysmal AF, if the baseline uncorrected QT interval is shorter than 460 msec, serum electrolyte values are normal, and risk factors associated with class III drug–related proarrhythmia are not present	C
	Catheter ablation is a reasonable alternative to pharmacologic therapy to prevent recurrent AF in symptomatic patients with little or no left atrial enlargement	C
Class III (not indicated)	Antiarrhythmic therapy with a particular drug is not recommended for maintenance of sinus rhythm in patients with AF who have well-defined risk factors for proarrhythmia with that agent	A
	Pharmacologic therapy is not recommended for maintenance of sinus rhythm in patients with advanced sinus node disease or AV node dysfunction unless they have a functioning electronic cardiac pacemaker	C

TABLE 40G-5 ACC/AHA Recommendations for Special Considerations in Atrial Fibrillation

CLASS	INDICATION	LEVEL OF EVIDENCE
Postoperative Atrial Fibrillation		
Class I (indicated)	Unless contraindicated, treatment with an oral beta blocker to prevent postoperative AF is recommended for patients undergoing cardiac surgery	A
	Administration of AV nodal blocking agents is recommended to achieve rate control in patients who develop postoperative AF	B
Class IIa (strong supportive evidence)	Preoperative administration of amiodarone reduces the incidence of AF in patients undergoing cardiac surgery and represents appropriate prophylactic therapy for patients at high risk for postoperative AF	A
	It is reasonable to restore sinus rhythm by pharmacologic cardioversion with ibutilide or direct-current cardioversion in patients who develop postoperative AF, as advised for nonsurgical patients	B
	It is reasonable to administer antiarrhythmic medications in an attempt to maintain sinus rhythm in patients with recurrent or refractory postoperative AF, as recommended for other patients who develop AF	B
	It is reasonable to administer antithrombotic medication in patients who develop postoperative AF, as recommended for nonsurgical patients	B
Class IIb (weak supportive evidence)	Prophylactic administration of sotalol may be considered for patients at risk for development of AF after cardiac surgery	B
Acute Myocardial Infarction		
Class I (indicated)	Direct-current cardioversion is recommended for patients with severe hemodynamic compromise or intractable ischemia, or when adequate rate control cannot be achieved with pharmacologic agents in patients with acute myocardial infarction and AF	C
	Intravenous administration of amiodarone is recommended to slow a rapid ventricular response to AF and to improve left ventricular function in patients with acute myocardial infarction	C
	Intravenous beta blockers and nondihydropyridine calcium antagonists are recommended to slow a rapid ventricular response to AF in patients with acute myocardial infarction who do not display clinical left ventricular dysfunction, bronchospasm, or AV block	C
	For patients with AF and acute myocardial infarction, administration of unfractionated heparin by either continuous intravenous infusion or intermittent subcutaneous injection is recommended in a dose sufficient to prolong the activated partial thromboplastin time to 1.5 to 2 times the control value, unless contraindications to anticoagulation exist	C
Class IIa (strong supportive evidence)	Intravenous administration of digitalis is reasonable to slow a rapid ventricular response and to improve left ventricular function in patients with acute myocardial infarction and AF associated with severe left ventricular dysfunction and heart failure	C
Class III (not indicated)	The administration of class IC antiarrhythmic drugs is not recommended in patients with AF in the setting of acute myocardial infarction	C
Management of Atrial Fibrillation Associated with the Wolff-Parkinson-White (WPW) Preexcitation Syndrome		
Class I (indicated)	Catheter ablation of the accessory pathway is recommended for symptomatic patients with AF who have WPW syndrome, particularly those with syncope due to rapid heart rate or those with a short bypass tract refractory period	B
	Immediate direct-current cardioversion is recommended to prevent ventricular fibrillation in patients with a short anterograde bypass tract refractory period in whom AF occurs with a rapid ventricular response associated with hemodynamic instability	B
	Intravenous procainamide or ibutilide is recommended to restore sinus rhythm in patients with WPW in whom AF occurs without hemodynamic instability in association with a wide QRS complex on the electrocardiogram (≥120-msec duration) or with a rapid preexcited ventricular response	C
Class IIa (strong supportive evidence)	Intravenous flecainide or direct-current cardioversion is reasonable when very rapid ventricular rates occur in patients with AF involving conduction over an accessory pathway	B
Class IIb (weak supportive evidence)	It may be reasonable to administer intravenous quinidine, procainamide, disopyramide, ibutilide, or amiodarone to hemodynamically stable patients with AF involving conduction over an accessory pathway	B
Class III (not indicated)	Intravenous administration of digitalis glycosides or nondihydropyridine calcium channel antagonists is not recommended in patients with WPW syndrome who have preexcited ventricular activation during AF	B
Hyperthyroidism		
Class I (indicated)	Administration of a beta blocker is recommended to control the rate of ventricular response in patients with AF complicating thyrotoxicosis, unless contraindicated	B
	In circumstances when a beta blocker cannot be used, administration of a nondihydropyridine calcium channel antagonist (diltiazem or verapamil) is recommended to control the ventricular rate in patients with AF and thyrotoxicosis	B
	In patients with AF associated with thyrotoxicosis, oral anticoagulation (INR 2.0 to 3.0) is recommended to prevent thromboembolism, as recommended for AF patients with other risk factors for stroke	C
	Once a euthyroid state is restored, recommendations for antithrombotic prophylaxis are the same as for patients without hyperthyroidism	C

Continued

CH 40

TABLE 40G-5 ACC/AHA Recommendations for Special Considerations in Atrial Fibrillation—cont'd

CLASS	INDICATION	LEVEL OF EVIDENCE
Management of Atrial Fibrillation During Pregnancy		
Class I (indicated)	Digoxin, a beta blocker, or a nondihydropyridine calcium channel antagonist is recommended to control the rate of ventricular response in pregnant patients with AF	C
	Direct-current cardioversion is recommended in pregnant patients who become hemodynamically unstable because of AF	C
	Protection against thromboembolism is recommended throughout pregnancy for all patients with AF (except those with lone AF and/or low thromboembolic risk). Therapy (anticoagulant or aspirin) should be chosen according to the stage of pregnancy.	C
Class IIb (weak supportive evidence)	Administration of heparin may be considered during the first trimester and last month of pregnancy for patients with AF and risk factors for thromboembolism. Unfractionated heparin may be administered either by continuous intravenous infusion in a dose sufficient to prolong the activated partial thromboplastin time to 1.5 to 2 times the control value or by intermittent subcutaneous injection in a dose of 10,000 to 20,000 units every 12 hours, adjusted to prolong the mid-interval (6 hours after injection) activated partial thromboplastin time to 1.5 times control	B
	Despite the limited data available, subcutaneous administration of low-molecular-weight heparin may be considered during the first trimester and last month of pregnancy for patients with AF and risk factors for thromboembolism	C
	Administration of an oral anticoagulant may be considered during the second trimester for pregnant patients with AF at high thromboembolic risk	C
	Administration of quinidine or procainamide may be considered to achieve pharmacologic cardioversion in hemodynamically stable patients who develop AF during pregnancy	C
Management of Atrial Fibrillation in Patients with Hypertrophic Cardiomyopathy (HCM)		
Class I (indicated)	Oral anticoagulation (INR 2.0 to 3.0) is recommended in patients with HCM who develop AF, as for other patients at high risk of thromboembolism	B
Class IIa (strong supportive evidence)	Antiarrhythmic medications can be useful to prevent recurrent AF in patients with HCM. Available data are insufficient to recommend one agent over another in this situation, but (a) disopyramide combined with a beta blocker or nondihydropyridine calcium channel antagonist or (b) amiodarone alone is generally preferred.	C
Management of Atrial Fibrillation in Patients with Pulmonary Disease		
Class I (indicated)	Correction of hypoxemia and acidosis is the recommended primary therapeutic measure for patients who develop AF during an acute pulmonary illness or exacerbation of chronic pulmonary disease	C
	A nondihydropyridine calcium channel antagonist (diltiazem or verapamil) is recommended to control the ventricular rate in patients with obstructive pulmonary disease who develop AF	C
	Direct-current cardioversion should be attempted in patients with pulmonary disease who become hemodynamically unstable as a consequence of AF	C
Class III (not indicated)	Theophylline and beta-adrenergic agonist agents are not recommended for patients with bronchospastic lung disease who develop AF	C
	Beta blockers, sotalol, propafenone, and adenosine are not recommended in patients with obstructive lung disease who develop AF	C

either disopyramide plus a beta blocker, verapamil, or diltiazem for rate control or amiodarone by itself.

Pulmonary Disease

The primary therapy for AF in the setting of an acute pulmonary illness or exacerbation of chronic pulmonary disease should be correction of hypoxemia and acidosis. Verapamil or diltiazem is recommended for rate control in patients with obstructive pulmonary disease. Theophylline and beta-adrenergic agonists are not recommended in patients with bronchospastic disease, and beta blockers, sotalol, propafenone, and adenosine are not recommended in patients with obstructive lung disease.

REFERENCES

1. Fuster V, Ryden LE, Cannom DS, et al: ACC/AHA/ESC 2006 guidelines for the management of patients with atrial fibrillation—executive summary: A report of the American College of Cardiology/American Heart Association Task Force on Practice Guidelines and the European Society of Cardiology Committee for Practice Guidelines (Writing Committee to Revise the 2001 Guidelines for the Management of Patients With Atrial Fibrillation). J Am Coll Cardiol 48:854, 2006.

CHAPTER 41 Cardiac Arrest and Sudden Cardiac Death

Robert J. Myerburg and Agustin Castellanos

Perspective

Sudden cardiac death (SCD) persists as a major public health problem, on the basis of numbers and demographics. With average numerical estimates in the range of 300,000 to 350,000 deaths per year in the United States alone, it accounts for half of all cardiovascular deaths. It is commonly an unexpected first cardiac event, often striking during the victim's productive years. Despite recognition of an association between forewarning symptoms of chest pain or syncope and SCD dating to Hippocrates around 400 BCE, the description of coronary artery anatomy in a victim of SCD in the late 1490s by DaVinci, and an epidemiologic survey in Rome by Lancisi at the request of Pope Clement XI in1706, advances in prediction, prevention, and management of unexpected cardiac arrest and SCD did not begin to emerge until 50 years ago. It is anticipated that the major insights into causes, pathophysiology, and preventive and management strategies developed during the past few decades, described in this chapter, will continue to evolve.

Definitions

SCD is natural death from cardiac causes, heralded by abrupt loss of consciousness within 1 hour of the onset of an acute change in cardiovascular status (**Table 41-1**). Preexisting heart disease may or may not have been known to be present, but the time and mode of death are unexpected. This definition incorporates the key elements of natural, rapid, and unexpected. It consolidates previous definitions that have conflicted, mainly because the most useful operational definition of SCD in the past differed for the clinician, the cardiovascular epidemiologist, the pathologist, and the scientist attempting to define pathophysiologic mechanisms. As epidemiology, causes, and mechanisms began to be understood, these differences faded.

To satisfy clinical, scientific, legal, and social considerations, four temporal elements must be considered: (1) prodromes, (2) onset, (3) cardiac arrest, and (4) biologic death (**Fig. 41-1**). Because the proximate cause of SCD is an abrupt disturbance of cardiovascular function, any definition must recognize the brief time interval between the onset of the mechanism directly responsible for cardiac arrest and the consequent loss of consciousness. Therefore, the 1-hour definition, which primarily refers to the duration of the "terminal event," defines the interval between the onset of symptoms signaling the pathophysiologic disturbance leading to cardiac arrest and the onset of the cardiac arrest itself.

Prodromes, occurring weeks or months before an event, are not sensitive or specific predictors of an impending event; but premonitory signs and symptoms, which can occur during the days or weeks before a cardiac arrest, may be more specific for an imminent cardiac arrest when they begin abruptly. Sudden onset of chest pain, dyspnea, or palpitations and other symptoms of arrhythmias often precede the onset of cardiac arrest and define the 1-hour onset of the terminal event that brackets the cardiac arrest. The fourth element, biologic death, was considered an immediate consequence of cardiac arrest in the past, usually occurring within minutes. However, the generally accepted clinical-pathophysiologic definition of up to 1 hour between onset of the terminal event and biologic death requires qualifications for specific circumstances. For example, since the development of community-based interventions and life support systems, patients may now remain biologically alive for a long period after the onset of a pathophysiologic process that has caused irreversible damage and will ultimately lead to death. In this circumstance, the causative pathophysiologic and clinical event is the cardiac arrest itself rather than the factors responsible for the delayed biologic death. Thus, death remains defined biologically, legally, and literally as an absolute and irreversible event timed to cessation of all biologic functions, but most studies link the definition of SCD to the cardiac arrest rather than a biologic death that occurs during hospitalization after cardiac arrest or within 30 days. Finally, the forensic pathologist studying unwitnessed deaths may use the definition of sudden death for a person known to be alive and functioning normally 24 hours before, and this remains appropriate within obvious limits.

TABLE 41-1 Terms Related to Sudden Cardiac Death

TERM	DEFINITION	QUALIFIERS	MECHANISMS
Sudden cardiac death	Sudden, irreversible cessation of all biologic functions	None	—
Cardiac arrest	Abrupt cessation of cardiac mechanical function, which may be reversible by a prompt intervention but will lead to death in its absence	Rare spontaneous reversions; likelihood of successful intervention relates to mechanism of arrest, clinical setting, and prompt return of circulation	Ventricular fibrillation, ventricular tachycardia, asystole, bradycardia, pulseless electrical activity, mechanical factors
Cardiovascular collapse	Sudden loss of effective blood flow due to cardiac and/or peripheral vascular factors that may reverse spontaneously (e.g., neurocardiogenic syncope; vasovagal syncope) or require interventions (e.g., cardiac arrest)	Nonspecific term; includes cardiac arrest and its consequences and transient non–life-threatening conditions that usually revert spontaneously	Same as cardiac arrest, plus vasodepressor syncope or other causes of transient loss of blood flow

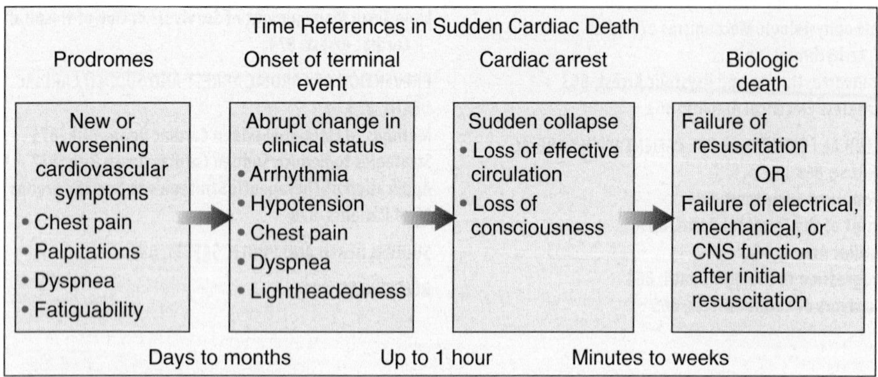

FIGURE 41-1 Sudden cardiac death viewed from four temporal perspectives: (1) prodromes, (2) onset of the terminal event, (3) cardiac arrest, and (4) progression to biologic death. Individual variability of the components influences clinical expression. Some victims experience no prodromes, with onset leading almost instantaneously to cardiac arrest; others may have an onset that lasts up to 1 hour before clinical arrest. Some patients may live days to weeks after the cardiac arrest before biologic death, often because of irreversible brain damage and dependence on life support. These factors influence interpretation of the 1-hour definition. The two most relevant clinical factors are onset of the terminal event and the clinical cardiac arrest itself; legal and social considerations focus on the time of biologic death. CNS = central nervous system.

Epidemiology

Epidemiologic Overview

Epidemiologic studies of SCD are difficult to interpret for both theoretical and practical reasons. There are persisting inconsistencies about definition and challenges in accessing data and adjudicating individual cases in data sets, in determining pathophysiologic mechanisms, and in making distinctions between population risk and individual risk.[1] In addition, the fact that cardiac arrest leading to SCD has short-term dynamics superimposed on a long-term static or dynamic substrate introduces unusual epidemiologic complexities. These include long-term risk prediction based on evolution of atherogenesis, myocardial hypertrophy, and ventricular muscle dysfunction over time and modulation by transient (short-term) variables such as ischemia, hemodynamic shifts, atherosclerotic plaque disruption and thrombosis, and autonomic variations. The differences between chronic disease evolution and transient events call for different forms of epidemiologic modeling. Furthermore, the emerging field of genetic epidemiology adds another dimension for study, and there is a need for focusing on interventional epidemiology, a term coined to define the population dynamics of therapeutic outcomes.

Incidence and the Population Burden of Sudden Cardiac Death

The worldwide incidence of SCD is difficult to estimate because numbers vary as a function of coronary heart disease prevalence in different countries (see Chap. 1).[2] Estimates of the annual number of SCDs in the United States are largely based on retrospective death certificate analyses,[3] American Heart Association statistical updates based on data from the National Center for Health Statistics,[4] and national extrapolations from a large emergency rescue experience in one community[5] and a community-wide multisource data set from another.[6] Death certificate statistics from the same data sources range from fewer than 250,000 SCDs annually when the etiologic definition is limited to coronary heart disease to more than 460,000 SCDs per year when all causes are included.[3,4,7] The extrapolations from two community-based sources set nationwide figures at fewer than 200,000 SCDs per year.[5,6] Because these broad ranges and the reported regional differences in incidence and outcomes of cardiac arrest[8] suggest that an accurate number can be found only by performing a carefully designed prospective epidemiologic study, the most widely cited estimates remain in the range of 300,000 to 350,000 SCDs annually.[9] These figures suggest an overall incidence between one and two deaths per 1000 persons among the general population.

The temporal definition of sudden death strongly influences epidemiologic data. Retrospective death certificate studies have demonstrated that a temporal definition of death less than 2 hours after the onset of symptoms results in 12% to 15% of all natural deaths being defined as "sudden" and nearly 90% of all natural sudden deaths having cardiac causes. In contrast, the application of a 24-hour definition of sudden death increases the fraction of all natural deaths falling into the sudden category to more than 30% but reduces the proportion of all sudden natural deaths resulting from cardiac causes to 75%.

Prospective studies have demonstrated that about 50% of all coronary heart disease deaths are sudden and unexpected, occurring shortly (instantaneous to 1 hour) after the onset of symptoms. Because coronary heart disease is the dominant cause of both sudden and nonsudden cardiac deaths in the United States, the fraction of total cardiac deaths that are sudden is similar to the fraction of deaths from coronary heart disease that are sudden, although there does appear to be a geographic variation in the fraction of coronary deaths that are sudden.[7,9] It is also of interest that the age-adjusted decline in coronary heart disease mortality in the United States during the past half-century has not changed the fraction of coronary deaths that are sudden and unexpected,[10,11] even though there may be a decline in out-of-hospital deaths compared with emergency department deaths. Furthermore, the decreasing age-adjusted mortality does not imply a decrease in absolute numbers of cardiac or sudden deaths because of the growth and aging of the U.S. population and the increasing prevalence of chronic heart disease.[7]

Population Pools and Time Dependence of Risk

Three factors are of primary importance for identification of populations at risk and consideration of strategies for prevention of SCD: (1) the absolute numbers and event rates (incidence) among population subgroups (**Fig. 41-2A**); (2) the clinical subgroups in which SCDs occur (Fig. 41-2B); and (3) the time dependence of risk (**Fig. 41-3**).

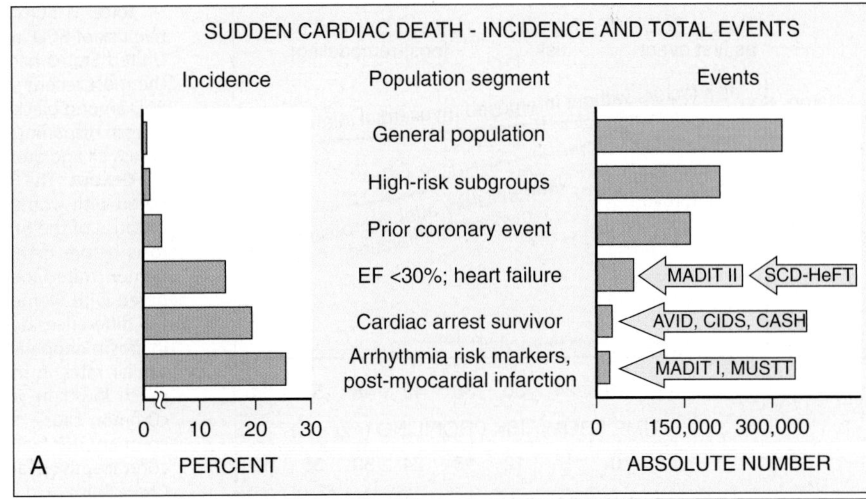

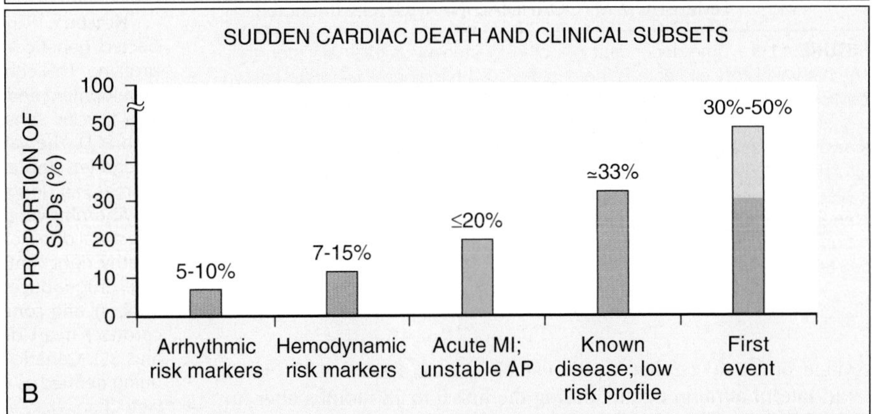

FIGURE 41-2 Impact of population subgroups and time from events on the clinical epidemiology of SCD. **A,** Estimates of incidence (percent/year) and the total number of events per year for the general adult population in the United States and for increasingly high risk subgroups. The overall adult population has an estimated sudden death incidence of 0.1% to 0.2%/year, accounting for a total of more than 300,000 events/year. With the identification of increasingly powerful risk factors, the incidence increases progressively, but this is accompanied by a progressive decrease in the total number of events represented by each group. The inverse relationship between incidence and total number of events occurs because of the progressively smaller denominator pool in the highest subgroup categories. Successful interventions in larger population subgroups require identification of specific markers to increase the ability to identify specific patients who are at particularly high risk for a future event. (Note: The horizontal axis for the incidence figures is not linear and should be interpreted accordingly.) **B,** The distribution of clinical status of victims at the time of SCD. Nearly two thirds of cardiac arrests occur as the first clinically manifested event or in the clinical setting of known disease in the absence of strong risk predictors. Less than 25% of the victims have high-risk markers based on arrhythmic or hemodynamic parameters. AP = angina pectoris; EF = ejection fraction; MI = myocardial infarction. (***A*** *modified from Myerburg RJ, Kessler KM, Castellanos A: Sudden cardiac death: Structure, function, and time-dependence of risk. Circulation 85[Suppl I]:I2, 1992.* ***B*** *modified from Myerburg RJ: Sudden cardiac death: Exploring the limits of our knowledge. J Cardiovasc Electrophysiol 12:369, 2001.)*

POPULATION AND SUBGROUP RISK VERSUS INDIVIDUAL RISK ASSESSMENT. When the more than 300,000 adult SCDs that occur annually in the United States are viewed as a global figure for an unselected adult population 35 years of age and older, the overall incidence is 0.1% to 0.2%/year (1 to 2/1000 population; see Fig. 41-2A). This general population includes the large proportion of SCDs that occur as a first clinical manifestation as well as SCDs that can be predicted with greater accuracy in higher risk subgroups (see Fig. 41-2B). Any intervention designed for the general population must therefore be applied to the 999 per 1000 who do not have an event in order to reach and possibly to influence the 1 per 1000 who does. Thus, despite the large absolute number at risk among the general population and the impact of proven interventions on populations, the practical ability to apply the principles of population risk to targeted individual patients is challenging. The cost and risk-to-benefit uncertainties limit the nature of such broad-based interventions and demand a higher resolution of risk identification. Figure 41-2A highlights this problem by expressing the incidence (percent/year) of SCD among various subgroups and comparing the incidence figures with the total number of events that occur annually in each subgroup.

On moving from the total adult population to a subgroup at higher risk because of the presence of selected coronary risk factors, there may be a 10-fold or greater increase in the annual incidence of events, with the magnitude dependent on the number and types of risk factors operating in specific subgroups. The size of the denominator pool, however, remains very large, and implementation of interventions remains problematic, even at this heightened level of risk. Higher resolution is desirable and can be achieved by identification of more specific subgroups. However, the corresponding absolute number of deaths becomes progressively smaller as the subgroups become more focused (see Fig. 41-2A), limiting the potential benefit of interventions to a much smaller fraction of the total number of patients at risk. Up to half of all SCDs due to coronary heart disease are first clinical events,[8,9] and another 20% to 30% occur among subgroups of patients with known coronary heart disease profiled at relatively low risk for SCD on the basis of current clinically available markers (see Fig. 41-2B). The principle of a high proportion of SCDs occurring as first events or in previously asymptomatic individuals applies to the less common causes as well.[12]

BIOLOGIC AND CLINICAL TIME-DEPENDENT RISK. Temporal elements in risk of SCD have been analyzed in the context of both biologic and clinical chronology. In the former, epidemiologic analyses of SCD risk among populations have identified three patterns: diurnal, weekly, and seasonal. General patterns of heightened risk during the morning hours, on Mondays, and during the winter months have been described.[13] An exception to the diurnal risk pattern is SCD in sleep apnea, in which risk tends to be nocturnal.[14]

Ambient temperature is an environmental factor that associates with risk of SCD. Both excessive cold[15] and excessive heat[16] have been associated with cardiac arrest risk, although the studies do not determine whether temperature extremes link to ventricular tachyarrhythmias versus other mechanisms of cardiac arrest. Another environmental variable, transient ambient air pollution conditions, has been associated with increased incidence of ventricular arrhythmias stored in implantable cardioverter-defibrillator (ICD) memories,[17] but the question of whether these are cardiac arrest equivalents is uncertain.

In the longer term clinical paradigm, the risk of SCD is not linear as a function of time after changes in cardiovascular status.[9,10,18] Survival curves after major cardiovascular events, which identify risk for both

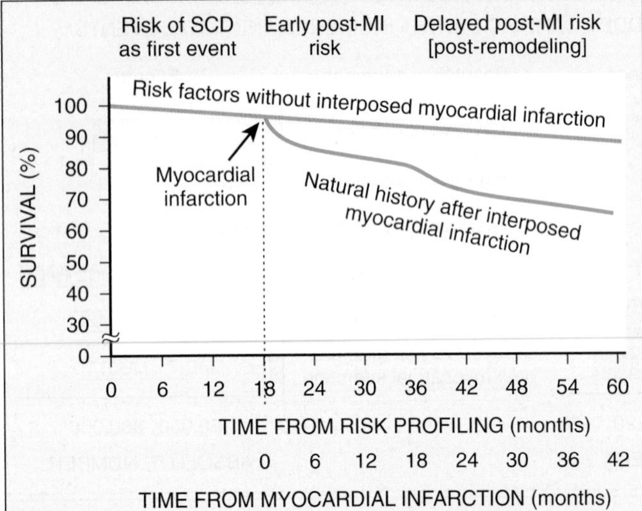

FIGURE 41-3 Time-dependent risk of SCD after myocardial infarction (MI). The natural history of a population of patients with major risk factors or known cardiovascular disease but at low risk because of freedom from major cardiovascular events (top curve) is compared with that of patients who have survived a myocardial infarction (bottom curve). SCD risk is accelerated during the initial 6 to 18 months after the major cardiovascular event, then plateaus, followed by a secondary acceleration during the next 2 to 3 years, probably due to the consequences of remodeling. *(Modified from Myerburg RJ, Kessler KM, Castellanos A: Sudden cardiac death: Structure, function, and time-dependence of risk. Circulation 85[Suppl I]:I2, 1992.)*

sudden and total cardiac death, usually demonstrate that the most rapid rate of attrition occurs during the first 6 to 18 months after an index event (see Fig. 41-3). Thus, there is a time dependence of risk that focuses the potential opportunity for maximum efficacy of an intervention during the early period after a conditioning event. Curves that have these characteristics have been generated from among survivors of out-of-hospital cardiac arrest, new onset of heart failure, and unstable angina and from patients having recent myocardial infarction with low ejection fractions or heart failure. For the latter, however, early nonarrhythmic deaths also contribute a large proportion of the fatal events. Even though the rate of attrition decreases after the early spike in mortality, a secondary delayed increase in risk occurs in post–myocardial infarction patients 2 to 5 years after an index event, probably related to ventricular remodeling and heart failure.

Age, Race, Gender, and Heredity

AGE. There are two ages of peak incidence of sudden death: within the first year of life (including the sudden infant death syndrome; see Chap. 65) and between 45 and 75 years of age. Among the general populations of infants younger than 1 year and middle-aged or older adults, the incidences are surprisingly similar.[19] Among adults older than 35 years, the incidence of SCD is 1/1000 persons per year (**Fig. 41-4A**), with an age-related increase in risk over time as the prevalence of coronary heart disease increases as a function of advancing age.[9] The incidence in infants is 0.73/1000 person-years,[19] and the incidence in adolescents and adults younger than 30 years is approximately 6/100,000 person-years,[19,20] or 1% of the risk in the middle-aged and older adults (Fig. 41-4A). In contrast to incidence, however, the proportion of deaths caused by coronary heart diseases that are sudden and unexpected decreases with advancing age. In the 20- to 39-year age group, approximately 75% of coronary heart disease deaths in men are sudden and unexpected, with the proportion falling to approximately 60% in the 45- to 54-year age group and hovering close to 50% thereafter. Age also influences the proportion of any cardiovascular cause among all causes of natural sudden death in that the proportion of coronary deaths and of all cardiac causes of death that are sudden is highest in the younger age groups, whereas the fraction of total sudden natural deaths that result from any cardiovascular cause is higher in the older age groups. At the other end of the age range, only 19% of sudden natural deaths among children between 1 and 13 years of age have cardiac causes; the proportion increases to 30% in the 14- to 21-year age group.

RACE. A number of studies comparing racial differences in the relative risk of SCD in whites and blacks with coronary heart disease in the United States had yielded conflicting and inconclusive data. However, the most recent studies demonstrate a higher risk of cardiac arrest and SCD among blacks compared with whites (Fig. 41-4B; see Chap. 2).[21] SCD rates in Hispanic populations were smaller. The differences were observed across all age groups.

GENDER. The SCD syndrome has a large preponderance in men compared with women during the young adult and early middle-age years because of the protection that women enjoy from coronary atherosclerosis before menopause (Fig. 41-4B). Various population studies have demonstrated fourfold to sevenfold excesses of SCD among men compared with women before the 65-year and older age groups, in which the differences decrease to 2:1 or less. As coronary event risk increases in postmenopausal women, SCD risk increases proportionately, with similar rates in men and women. Even though the overall SCD risk is much lower in younger women, coronary artery disease is the most common cause of SCD in women older than 40 years, and the classic coronary risk factors, including cigarette smoking, diabetes, use of oral contraceptives, and hyperlipidemia, all influence risk in women (see Chap. 81).[22]

HEREDITY. Familial patterns of SCD risk, resulting from known or suspected genetic variations, are emerging as important factors for risk profiling. This concept is applicable generally in regard to both disease development and SCD expression in the common acquired disorders and in a specific sense to inherited arrhythmogenic conditions associated with SCD. The various genetic associations can be separated into four categories (**Table 41-2**): inherited uncommon primary arrhythmic syndromes (e.g., long-QT syndromes, Brugada syndrome, catecholaminergic polymorphic ventricular tachycardia or fibrillation), inherited uncommon structural diseases associated with SCD risk (e.g., hypertrophic cardiomyopathy, right ventricular dysplasia), "acquired" or induced arrhythmia risk (e.g., drug-induced long-QT interval or proarrhythmia, electrolyte disturbances), and common acquired diseases associated with SCD risk (e.g., coronary heart disease, nonischemic cardiomyopathies) (see Chaps. 9 and 35). Genetic variants mapped to loci on many chromosomes are being defined as the molecular bases for these entities and associations (see Chap. 9).

The multiple specific mutations at gene loci encoding ion channel proteins associated with the various inherited arrhythmia syndromes (see Chap. 9) represent a major advance in the understanding of a genetic and pathophysiologic basis for these causes of sudden death. In addition, the role of modifier genes and mutation specificity in the severity of clinical phenotypes in long-QT interval syndromes[23,24] and structural diseases such as hypertrophic cardiomyopathy[25] are of increasing interest. These observations may provide screening tools for individuals at risk as well as the potential to devise specific therapeutic strategies. In addition, gene loci identified by genome-wide association studies may also serve as candidates for investigation of the role of low-penetrance mutations or polymorphisms in SCD due to more common causes, such as coronary heart disease.[26] At this time, it appears that the hope for common variants linking to common syndromes such as SCD will be superseded by multiple rare variant associations.

To the extent that SCD is an expression of underlying coronary heart disease, hereditary factors that contribute to coronary heart disease risk operate nonspecifically for the SCD syndrome. However, studies have identified mutations and relevant polymorphisms along multiple steps of the cascade, from atherogenesis to plaque destabilization, thrombosis, and arrhythmogenesis, each of which is associated with increased risk of a coronary event (**Fig. 41-5**).[27,28] Integration of these individual markers may provide more powerful individual risk prediction in the future. In addition, several population studies have suggested that SCD, as an expression of coronary heart disease, clusters in specific families.[29-32]

Risk Factors for Sudden Cardiac Death

GENERAL PROFILE OF SUDDEN CARDIAC DEATH RISK (see Chaps. 7 to 9). Risk profiling for coronary artery disease, by means of the conventional risk factors for coronary atherogenesis, is useful to identify levels of population risk and individual risk but cannot be used to distinguish individual patients at risk for SCD from those at risk for other manifestations of coronary heart disease. Multivariate analyses of selected risk factors (e.g., age, diabetes mellitus, systolic blood pressure, heart rate, electrocardiographic abnormalities, vital capacity, relative weight, cigarette consumption, and serum cholesterol level) have determined that approximately 50% of all SCDs occur

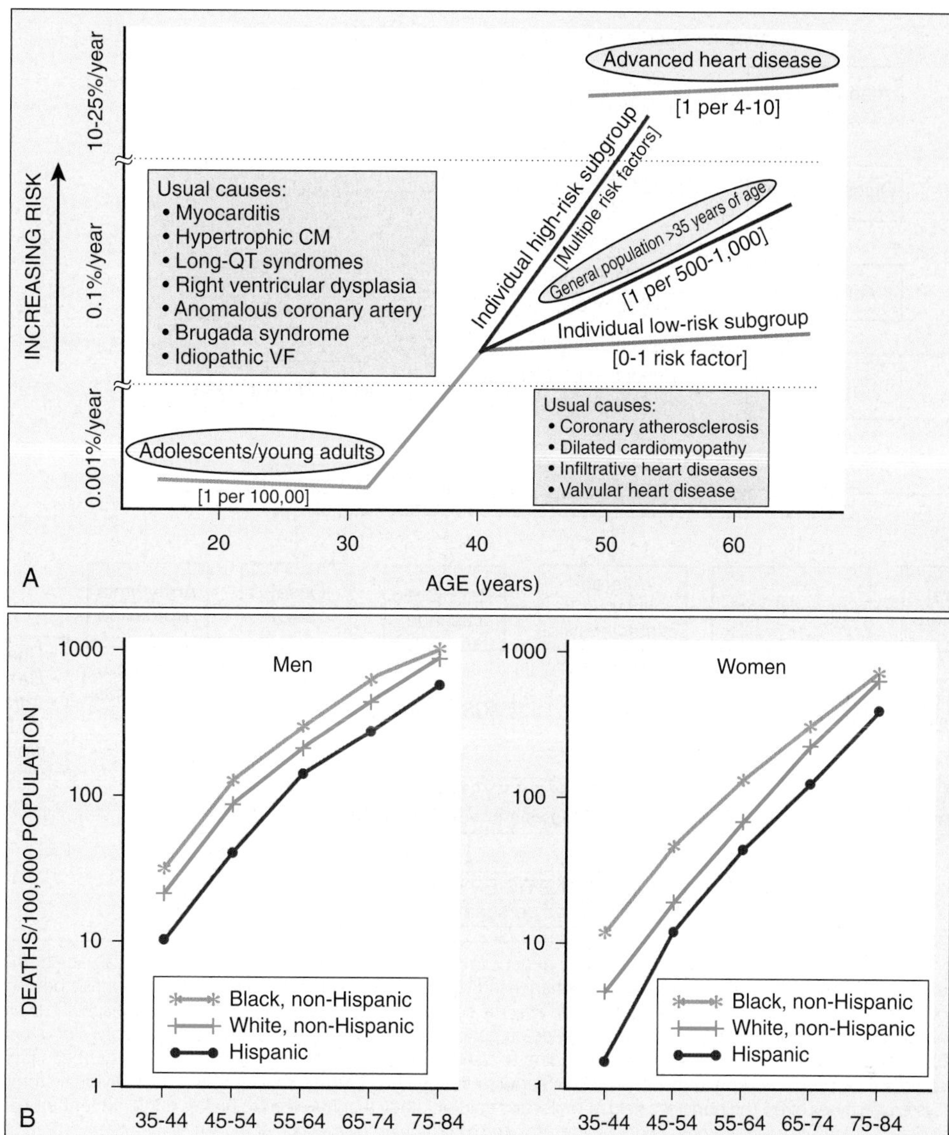

FIGURE 41-4 Age-, gender-, and race-specific risks of SCD. **A,** Age-related and disease-specific risk for SCD. For the general population 35 years of age and older, SCD risk is 0.1% to 0.2%/year (1/500 to 1000 population), with a wide spread in subgroup risk based on number and power of individual risk factors. Among the general population of adolescents and adults younger than 30 years, the overall risk of SCD is 1/100,000 population or 0.001%/year. The risk of SCD increases dramatically beyond the age of 35 years and continues to increase past the age of 70 years. Among patients older than 30 years with advanced structural heart disease and markers of high risk for cardiac arrest, the event rate may exceed 25%/year, and age-related risk is attenuated. Among adolescents and young adults at risk for SCD from specific identified causes, it is difficult to ascertain risk for individual patients because of variable expression of the disease state (see text for details). **B,** SCD risk as a function of age, gender, and race or culture (white, black, and Hispanic). CM = cardiomyopathy; VF = ventricular fibrillation. *(**B,** Data modified from Gillum RF: Sudden cardiac death in Hispanic Americans and African Americans. Am J Public Health 87:1461, 1997.)*

TABLE 41-2 Genetic Contributors to Sudden Cardiac Death Risk

Genetically Based Primary Arrhythmia Disorders
Congenital long-QT interval syndrome, short-QT syndrome
Brugada syndrome
Catecholaminergic polymorphic ("idiopathic") ventricular tachycardia/fibrillation
Inherited Structural Disorders with Arrhythmic SCD Risk
Hypertrophic cardiomyopathy
Right ventricular dysplasia/cardiomyopathy
Genetic Predisposition to Induced Arrhythmias and SCD
Drug-induced "acquired" long-QT interval syndrome (drugs, electrolytes)
Electrolyte and metabolic arrhythmogenic effects
Genetic Modulation of Complex Acquired Diseases
Coronary artery disease, acute coronary syndromes
Congestive heart failure, dilated cardiomyopathies

among the 10% of the population in the highest risk decile on the basis of multiple risk factors (**Fig. 41-6**). Thus, the cumulative risk derived from multiple risk factors exceeds the simple arithmetic sum of the individual risks. The comparison of risk factors in the victims of SCD with those in people who develop any manifestations of coronary artery disease does not provide useful patterns, by either univariate or multivariate analysis, to distinguish victims of SCD from the overall pool. However, a history of diabetes mellitus and a tendency to longer QTc intervals on random electrocardiograms are suggested as potential markers of interest for SCD prediction.[33] Angiographic and hemodynamic patterns discriminate SCD risk from non-SCD risk only under limited conditions. In addition, familial clustering of SCD as a specific manifestation of the disease may lead to identification of specific genetic abnormalities that predispose to SCD.[30-32]

Hypertension is a clearly established risk factor for coronary heart disease and also emerges as a highly significant risk factor for incidence of SCD. However, there is no influence of increasing systolic blood pressure levels on the ratio of sudden deaths to total coronary

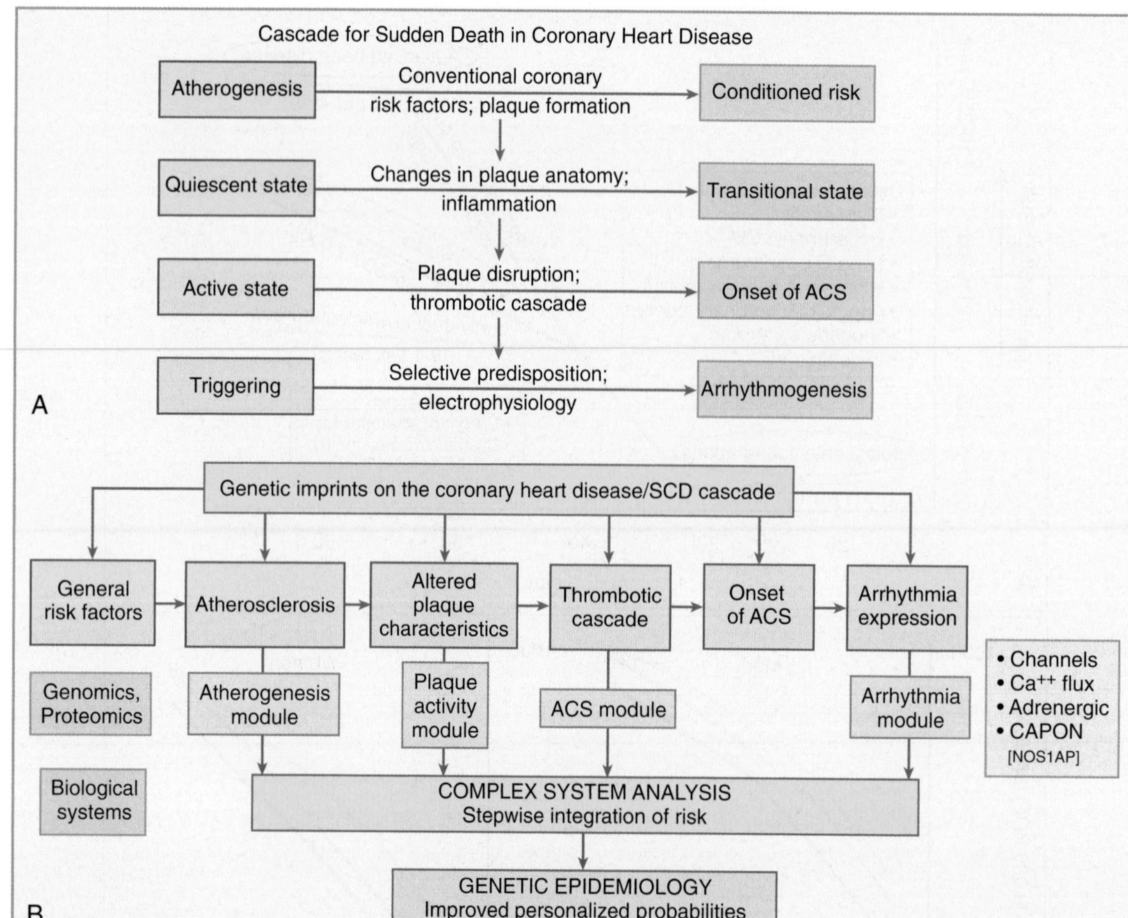

FIGURE 41-5 The coronary atherosclerosis heart disease cascade and genetic imprints on the progression to SCD. **A,** The cascade from conventional risk factors for coronary atherosclerosis to arrhythmogenesis in SCD related to coronary heart disease. The cascade identifies four levels of risk, beginning with lesion initiation and development and progressing to the transition to an active state, then to acute coronary syndromes (ACS), and finally to the specific expression of life-threatening arrhythmias. Multiple factors enter at each level, including specific risk based on genetic profiles of individual patients. **B,** Positions along multiple sites in the cascade from general risk factors for atherosclerosis to arrhythmia expression leading to SCD. Individual risk based on genetic profiles has been identified for atherogenesis, plaque evolution, the thrombotic cascade, and arrhythmia expression. Stepwise integration of these characteristics for individuals through genetics, genomics, proteomics, and biologic system analyses offers the hope of a field of molecular epidemiology that may lead to higher single-patient probabilities for individual SCD risk prediction. See text for details. *(Modified from Myerburg RJ: Scientific gaps in the prediction and prevention of sudden cardiac death. J Cardiovasc Electrophysiol 13:709, 2002.)*

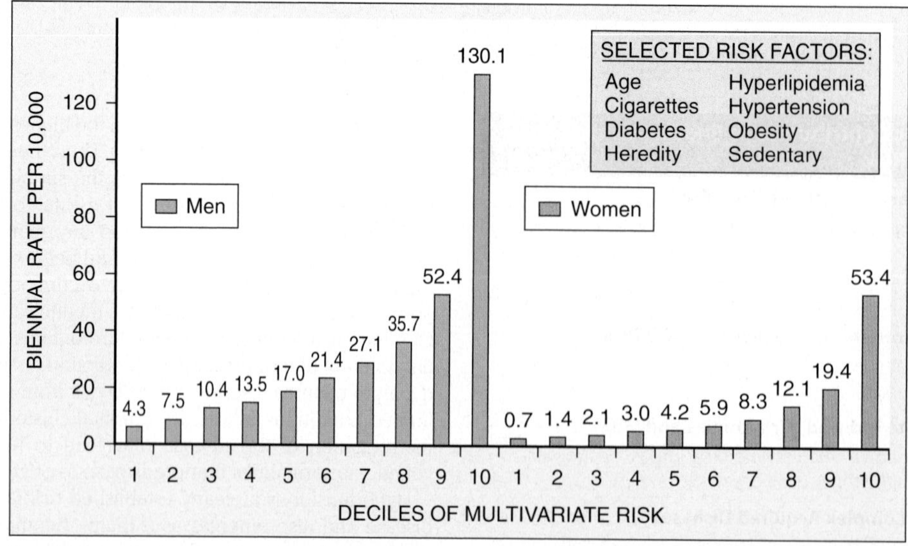

FIGURE 41-6 Risk of sudden death by decile of multivariate risk—the Framingham Study. Selected risk variables are shown. *(Modified from Kannel WB, Shatzkin A: Sudden death: Lessons from subsets in population studies. J Am Coll Cardiol 5[Suppl 6]:141B, 1985. Reprinted by permission of the American College of Cardiology.)*

heart disease deaths. No relationship has been observed between cholesterol concentration and the proportion of coronary deaths that were sudden. Neither the electrocardiographic pattern of left ventricular hypertrophy nor nonspecific ST-T wave abnormalities influence the proportion of total coronary deaths that are sudden and unexpected; only intraventricular conduction abnormalities are suggestive of a disproportionate number of SCDs, an old observation that is reinforced by data from some device trials that suggest the importance of QRS duration as a risk marker. A low vital capacity also suggests a disproportionate risk for sudden versus total coronary deaths. This is of interest because such a relationship was particularly striking in the Framingham Study in the analysis of data from women who had died suddenly.

The conventional risk factors used in early studies of SCD are the risk factors for the evolution of coronary artery disease. The rationale is based on two facts: (1) coronary disease is the structural basis for 80% of SCDs in the United States and (2) the coronary risk factors are easy to identify because they tend to be present continuously over time (see Fig. 41-5A). However, risk factors specific for fatal arrhythmias are dynamic pathophysiologic events and occur transiently.[34] Transient pathophysiologic events are being modeled epidemiologically in an attempt to express and to use them as clinical risk factors for both profiling and intervention.[1] However, data suggest that longitudinal and transient risk predictors may have their power blunted by clinical interventions, such as PCI during acute coronary syndromes and post–myocardial infarction beta blocker therapy.[35]

The identification of specific clinical markers of risk for SCD as a specific expression of both coronary heart disease and other cardiovascular disorders has been a goal for many years.[9,10] Left ventricular ejection fraction has been the most popular of such markers for clinical trials and patient profiling. However, its sensitivity limitations and inability to identify the large subgroup in which SCD is the first expression of heart disease have encouraged investigators to seek additional markers. For example, exercise data from a large cohort of men observed for years after a stress test demonstrated that a profile of higher resting heart rates, smaller increments in rate during exercise, and lower decrement in heart rate during the first minute after exercise predicted higher risk of SCD during follow-up.[36] In addition, a number of electrocardiographic indicators (such as microvolt T wave alternans and indices of QT duration and dispersion), genetic profiles, and other indices of extent of disease are also predictive (see Chap. 37).

FUNCTIONAL CAPACITY AND SUDDEN DEATH. The Framingham Study demonstrated a striking relationship between functional classification and death during a 2-year follow-up period. However, the proportion of deaths that were sudden did not vary with functional classification, ranging from 50% to 57% in all groups and from those free of clinical heart disease to those in functional Class IV. Other studies have also suggested that patients with heart failure with better functional capacity are at lower risk of dying, as expected, but a higher proportion of those deaths are sudden.[37]

LIFESTYLE AND PSYCHOSOCIAL FACTORS

LIFESTYLE. There is a strong association between cigarette smoking and all manifestations of coronary heart disease. The Framingham Study demonstrated that cigarette smokers have a twofold to threefold increase in sudden death risk in each decade of life at entry between 30 and 59 years and that this is one of the few risk factors in which the proportion of coronary heart disease deaths that are sudden increases in association with the risk factor. Excess risk of SCD in current smokers with coronary heart disease was not observed in former smokers, whose risk was similar to that of those who never smoked.[38] In addition, in a study of 310 survivors of out-of-hospital cardiac arrest, the recurrent cardiac arrest rate was 27% at 3 years of follow-up among those who continued to smoke compared with 19% in those who stopped. Conversely, light to moderate alcohol consumption was associated with a reduced risk of SCD among male physicians.[39] Obesity is a second factor that appears to influence the proportion of coronary deaths that occur suddenly. With increasing relative weight, the percentage of coronary heart disease deaths that were sudden in the Framingham Study increased linearly from a low of 39% to a high of 70%. Total coronary heart disease deaths increased with increasing relative weight as well.

Associations between levels of physical activity and SCD have been studied with variable results. Epidemiologic observations have suggested a relationship between low levels of physical activity and increased coronary heart disease death risk. The Framingham Study, however, showed an insignificant relationship between low levels of physical activity and incidence of sudden death but a high proportion of sudden to total cardiac deaths at higher levels of physical activity. An association between acute physical exertion and the onset of myocardial infarction has been suggested, particularly among individuals who are habitually physically inactive. A subsequent case-crossover cohort study confirmed this observation for SCD, demonstrating a 17-fold relative increase in SCD associated with vigorous exercise compared with lower level activity or inactive states.[40] However, the absolute risk for events was very low (1 event/1.5 million exercise sessions). Habitual vigorous exercise markedly attenuated risk. In contrast, SCD among young athletes has a higher incidence than among young nonathletic individuals in the same age range (see Chap. 83). Information about physical activity relationships in various clinical settings, such as overt and silent disease states, is still lacking.

PSYCHOSOCIAL FACTORS (see Chap. 91)**.** The magnitude of recent life changes in the realms of health, work, home and family, and personal and social factors has been related to myocardial infarction and SCD.[41] There is an association with significant elevations of life change scores during the 6 months before a coronary event, and the association is particularly striking in victims of SCD. Among women, those who die suddenly are less often married, had fewer children, and had greater educational discrepancies with their spouses than did age-related control subjects living in the same neighborhood as the victims of sudden death. A history of psychiatric treatment including phobic anxieties,[42] cigarette smoking, and greater quantities of alcohol consumption than in the control subjects also characterized the sudden death group. Controlling for other major prognostic factors, risk of sudden and total deaths and other coronary events is affected by social and economic stresses. Alteration of modifiable lifestyle factors has been proposed as a strategy to reduce risk of SCD in patients with coronary heart disease,[43] although studies of pharmacologic and psychotherapeutic treatment of depression after myocardial infarction failed to demonstrate an effect on event rates,[44] even though symptoms of depressive states improved.[45] Behavioral changes (e.g., inactivity) secondary to depression appeared to relate more closely to event rates than did depression itself. Acute psychosocial stressors have been associated with a higher risk of cardiovascular events, including SCD.[46-48] The risk appears to cluster around the time of the stress and appears to occur among victims at preexisting risk, with the stressor simply advancing the time of an impending event.[48] The possibility of physical stress–induced coronary plaque disruption also has been suggested.

LEFT VENTRICULAR EJECTION FRACTION IN CHRONIC ISCHEMIC HEART DISEASE. A marked reduction of the left ventricular ejection fraction is the most powerful of the known predictors of SCD in patients with chronic ischemic heart disease as well as in those at risk for SCD from other causes (see later). Increased risk, independent of other risk factors, is measurable at ejection fractions higher than 40%, but the greatest rate of change of risk is between 30% and 40%. An ejection fraction ≤30% is the single most powerful independent predictor for SCD but has low sensitivity and specificity.[49] Nonetheless, relying on a low ejection fraction as the sole major predictor limits predictive power because of the large number of SCDs that occur at low incidence rates among the very large subset of patients with normal or moderately reduced ejection fractions with unrecognized disease.[50]

VENTRICULAR ARRHYTHMIAS IN CHRONIC ISCHEMIC HEART DISEASE (see Chaps. 39 and 57)**.** Most forms of ambient ventricular ectopic activity (premature ventricular complexes [PVCs] and short runs of nonsustained ventricular tachycardia [VT]) have a benign prognosis in the absence of structural heart disease. An exception is polymorphic forms of nonsustained VT that occur in patients without structural heart disease but can have a molecular, functional, drug-related, or electrolyte-related basis for high-risk arrhythmias. When they are present in subjects in the coronary-prone age groups, however, PVCs select a subgroup with a higher probability of coronary artery disease and of SCD. Exercise-induced PVCs and short runs of nonsustained VT indicate some level of SCD risk,[51] even in the absence of recognizable structural heart disease. However, the data available to support this hypothesis are conflicting, with the possible exception of polymorphic runs of nonsustained VT. Additional data suggest that PVCs and nonsustained VT during both the exercise and recovery phases of a stress test are predictive of increased risk.[52] Arrhythmias in the recovery phase, previously thought to be benign, appear to predict higher risk than arrhythmias in the exercise phase, and there is a gradient of risk with increasing severity of arrhythmias.

The occurrence of PVCs in survivors of myocardial infarction, particularly if frequent and of complex forms such as repetitive PVCs, predicts an increased risk of SCD and total mortality during long-term follow-up. There are conflicting data on the role of measures of frequency and forms of ventricular ectopic activity as discriminators of risk, but most studies have cited a frequency cutoff of 10 PVCs/hour as a threshold level for increased risk. Several investigators have emphasized that the most powerful predictors among the various forms of PVCs are runs of nonsustained VT, although this relationship is now questioned. Many of the reported studies have been based on a single ambulatory monitor sample recorded 1 week to several months after the onset of acute myocardial infarction, and the duration of the samples has ranged from 1 to 48 hours. Other studies have suggested that ambulatory ventricular arrhythmias in patients with heart failure do not specifically predict an increased risk of death.[53]

The results of the Cardiac Arrhythmia Suppression Trial (CAST; see Chap. 37), designed to test the hypothesis that PVC suppression by antiarrhythmic drugs alters the risk of SCD after myocardial infarction, were surprising for two reasons. First, the death rate in the randomized placebo group was lower than expected; and second, the death rate among patients in the encainide and flecainide arms exceeded control rates by more than three times. Subgroup analysis has demonstrated increased risk in the placebo group for patients with nonsustained VT and an ejection fraction of 30% or less, but excess risk in the treated group was still observed. The excess death rates may be accounted for by the occurrence of ischemic events in the presence of drug. No adverse effect (other than short-term proarrhythmic risk at initiation of therapy) was observed with the other drug in the study (moricizine), but neither did long-term benefit emerge with further study. The Survival with Oral *d*-Sotalol (SWORD) study, a comparison of *d*-sotalol with placebo in a post–myocardial infarction population with a low death rate, also demonstrated excess risk in the drug-treated group. Whether the conclusions from CAST, CAST II, and SWORD extend beyond the drugs studied or to other diseases remains to be learned.

Left ventricular dysfunction is the major modulator of risk implied by chronic PVCs after myocardial infarction. The risk of death predicted by post–myocardial infarction PVCs is enhanced by the presence of left ventricular dysfunction, which appears to exert its influence most strongly in the first 6 months after infarction. Delayed deterioration of LV function, likely consequent to remodeling after myocardial infarction, may increase risk further. Finally, there are data suggesting that the risk associated with postinfarction ventricular arrhythmias is higher in patients who have non–Q-wave infarctions than in those with transmural infarctions.

EMERGING MARKERS OF SCD RISK. Additional risk markers with independent or added predictive power are being studied for risk profiling. Among these are techniques such as microvolt T wave alternans,[54] contrast-enhanced magnetic resonance imaging of the postinfarction border,[55,56] measures of QT variability,[57] derivatives of heart rate variability methods,[58-60] and studies of familial clustering of SCD as an expression of coronary heart disease[30-32] and for the potential of genetic risk profiling.[61] With the possible exception of predictive accuracy of a negative T wave alternans study,[62] these are all in their infancy for clinical application.

Causes of Sudden Cardiac Death

Coronary Artery Abnormalities

Disease of the coronary arteries and its consequences account for at least 80% of SCDs in Western countries, and the nonischemic cardiomyopathies cause another 10% to 15%. Coronary artery disease is also the most common cause in many areas of the world in which the prevalence of atherosclerosis is lower.[63] In regard to the latter, it is anticipated that as third-world countries improve access to heath care for communicable disease in earlier years of life, coronary atherosclerosis and its consequences will emerge as a larger problem.[64]

Despite the established dominant relationship between coronary atherosclerosis and SCD, a complete understanding of SCD requires recognition that less common and often rare coronary vascular disorders (**Table 41-3**) may be identifiable before death and have therapeutic implications.[61,65] Many of these entities are relatively more common causes of SCD in adolescents and young adults, among whom the prevalence of coronary atherosclerosis is much lower (see Fig. 41-4A).

ATHEROSCLEROTIC CORONARY ARTERY DISEASE (see Chaps. 54 to 58). The structural and functional abnormalities of the coronary vasculature due to coronary atherosclerosis interact with electrophysiologic alterations that result from the myocardial impact of an ischemic burden. The relationship between the vascular and myocardial components of this pathophysiologic model, and its modulation by hemodynamic, autonomic, genetic, and other influences, establishes multiple patterns of risk derived from the fundamental disease state (**Fig. 41-7**). Risk is modulated by multiple factors that can be either transient or persistent, and transient modulations may interact with persistent changes. The myocardial component of this pathophysiologic model is not static over time, and the term *persistent* must be viewed with caution because of the gradual effects of remodeling after an initial ischemic event and the effects of recurrent ischemic events. Cardiac arrest and SCD resulting from transient ischemia or acute myocardial infarction differ in physiology and prognosis from the risk of cardiac arrest implied by a prior myocardial infarction with or without a subsequent ischemic cardiomyopathy. In general, short-term risk of life-threatening events associates more closely with acute ischemia or the acute phase of myocardial infarction, and longer term risk associates more with transient ischemia, myocardial scarring, remodeling, ischemic cardiomyopathy, and heart failure.

NONATHEROSCLEROTIC CORONARY ARTERY ABNORMALITIES. Nonatherosclerotic coronary artery abnormalities include congenital lesions, coronary artery embolism, coronary arteritis, and mechanical abnormalities of the coronary arteries. Among the congenital lesions, anomalous origin of a left coronary artery from the pulmonary artery (see Chaps. 65 and 83) is relatively common and associated with a high death rate in infancy and early childhood without surgical treatment. The early risk for SCD is not excessively high, but patients who survive to adulthood without surgical intervention are at risk for SCD. Other forms of coronary arteriovenous fistulas are much less frequent and associated with a low incidence of SCD.

ANOMALOUS ORIGIN OF CORONARY ARTERIES FROM THE WRONG SINUS OF VALSALVA (see Chaps. 21 and 83)**.** These anatomic variants are associated with an increased risk of SCD, particularly during exercise. When the anomalous artery passes between the aortic and the pulmonary artery root, the takeoff angle of the anomalous ostium creates a slitlike opening of the vessel, reducing the effective cross-sectional area for blood flow. Congenitally hypoplastic, stenotic, or atretic left coronary arteries are uncommon abnormalities associated with a risk of myocardial infarction in the young, but not of SCD.

EMBOLISM TO THE CORONARY ARTERIES. Coronary artery emboli occur most commonly in aortic valve endocarditis and from thrombotic material on diseased or prosthetic aortic or mitral valves. Emboli can also originate from left ventricular mural thrombi or as a consequence of surgery or cardiac catheterization. Symptoms and signs of myocardial ischemia or infarction are the most common manifestations. In each of these categories, SCD is a risk resulting from the electrophysiologic consequences of embolic ischemia.

CORONARY ARTERITIS. Mucocutaneous lymph node syndrome (Kawasaki disease; see Chap. 89) carries a risk of SCD in association with coronary arteritis. Polyarteritis nodosa and related vasculitis syndromes can cause SCD, presumably because of coronary arteritis, as can coronary ostial stenosis in syphilitic aortitis. The latter has become a rare manifestation of syphilis.

MECHANICAL OBSTRUCTION TO CORONARY ARTERIES. Several types of mechanical abnormalities are listed among the causes of SCD. Coronary artery dissection, with or without dissection of the aorta, occurs in Marfan syndrome (see Chap. 65) and has also been reported after trauma

TABLE 41-3 Causes of and Contributing Factors in Sudden Cardiac Death

I. Coronary artery abnormalities
  A. Coronary atherosclerosis
    1. Chronic coronary atherosclerosis with acute or transient myocardial ischemia—thrombosis, spasm, physical stress
    2. Acute myocardial infarction, onset and early phase
    3. Chronic atherosclerosis with change in myocardial substrate, including prior myocardial infarction
  B. Congenital abnormalities of coronary arteries
    1. Anomalous origin from pulmonary artery
    2. Other coronary arteriovenous fistula
    3. Origin of a left coronary branch from right or noncoronary sinus of Valsalva
    4. Origin of right coronary artery from left sinus of Valsalva
    5. Hypoplastic or aplastic coronary arteries
    6. Coronary-intracardiac shunt
  C. Coronary artery embolism
    1. Aortic or mitral endocarditis
    2. Prosthetic aortic or mitral valves
    3. Abnormal native valves or left ventricular mural thrombus
    4. Platelet embolism
  D. Coronary arteritis
    1. Polyarteritis nodosa, progressive systemic sclerosis, giant cell arteritis
    2. Mucocutaneous lymph node syndrome (Kawasaki disease)
    3. Syphilitic coronary ostial stenosis
  E. Miscellaneous mechanical obstruction of coronary arteries
    1. Coronary artery dissection in Marfan syndrome
    2. Coronary artery dissection in pregnancy
    3. Prolapse of aortic valve myxomatous polyps into coronary ostia
    4. Dissection or rupture of sinus of Valsalva
  F. Functional obstruction of coronary arteries
    1. Coronary artery spasm with or without atherosclerosis
    2. Myocardial bridges

II. Hypertrophy of ventricular myocardium
  A. Left ventricular hypertrophy associated with coronary heart disease
  B. Hypertensive heart disease without significant coronary atherosclerosis
  C. Hypertrophic myocardium secondary to valvular heart disease
  D. Hypertrophic cardiomyopathy
    1. Obstructive
    2. Nonobstructive
  E. Primary or secondary pulmonary hypertension
    1. Advanced chronic right ventricular overload
    2. Pulmonary hypertension in pregnancy (highest risk peripartum)

III. Myocardial diseases and heart failure
  A. Chronic congestive heart failure
    1. Ischemic cardiomyopathy
    2. Idiopathic dilated cardiomyopathy
      a. Acquired
      b. Hereditary
    3. Alcoholic cardiomyopathy
    4. Hypertensive cardiomyopathy
    5. Postmyocarditis cardiomyopathy
    6. Peripartum cardiomyopathy
  B. Acute and subacute cardiac failure
    1. Massive acute myocardial infarction
    2. Acute myocarditis
    3. Acute alcoholic cardiac dysfunction
    4. Takotsubo syndrome (uncertain sudden death risk)
    5. Ball valve embolism in aortic stenosis or prosthesis
    6. Mechanical disruptions of cardiac structures
      a. Rupture of ventricular free wall
      b. Disruption of mitral apparatus
        (1) Papillary muscle
        (2) Chordae tendineae
        (3) Leaflet
      c. Rupture of interventricular septum
    7. Acute pulmonary edema in noncompliant ventricles

IV. Inflammatory, infiltrative, neoplastic, and degenerative processes
  A. Viral myocarditis, with or without ventricular dysfunction
    1. Acute phase
    2. Postmyocarditis interstitial fibrosis
  B. Myocarditis associated with the vasculitides
  C. Sarcoidosis
  D. Progressive systemic sclerosis
  E. Amyloidosis
  F. Hemochromatosis
  G. Idiopathic giant cell myocarditis
  H. Chagas disease
  I. Cardiac ganglionitis
  J. Arrhythmogenic right ventricular dysplasia; right ventricular cardiomyopathy
  K. Neuromuscular diseases (e.g., muscular dystrophy, Friedreich ataxia, myotonic dystrophy)
  L. Intramural tumors
    1. Primary
    2. Metastatic
  M. Obstructive intracavitary tumors
    1. Neoplastic
    2. Thrombotic

V. Diseases of the cardiac valves
  A. Valvular aortic stenosis/insufficiency
  B. Mitral valve disruption
  C. Mitral valve prolapse
  D. Endocarditis
  E. Prosthetic valve dysfunction

VI. Congenital heart disease
  A. Congenital aortic or pulmonic valve stenosis
  B. Congenital septal defects with Eisenmenger physiology
    1. Advanced disease
    2. During labor and delivery
  C. Late after surgical repair of congenital lesions (e.g., tetralogy of Fallot)

VII. Electrophysiologic abnormalities
  A. Abnormalities of the conducting system
    1. Fibrosis of the His-Purkinje system
      a. Primary degeneration (Lenègre's disease)
      b. Secondary to fibrosis and calcification of the "cardiac skeleton" (Lev disease)
      c. Postviral conducting system fibrosis
      d. Hereditary conducting system disease
    2. Anomalous pathways of conduction (Wolff-Parkinson-White syndrome, short refractory period bypass)
  B. Abnormalities of repolarization
    1. Congenital abnormalities of QT interval duration
      a. Congenital long-QT interval syndromes
        (1) Romano-Ward syndrome (without deafness)
        (2) Jervell and Lange-Nielsen syndrome (with deafness)
      b. Congenital short-QT interval syndrome
    2. Acquired (or provoked) long-QT interval syndromes
      a. Drug effect (with genetic predisposition?)
        (1) Cardiac, antiarrhythmic
        (2) Noncardiac
        (3) Drug interactions
      b. Electrolyte abnormality (response modified by genetic predisposition?)
      c. Toxic substances
      d. Hypothermia
      e. Central nervous system injury; subarachnoid hemorrhage
    3. Brugada syndrome—right bundle branch block and ST-segment elevations in the absence of ischemia
    4. Early repolarization syndrome
  C. Ventricular fibrillation of unknown or uncertain cause
    1. Absence of identifiable structural or functional causes
      a. "Idiopathic" ventricular fibrillation
      b. Short-coupled torsades de pointes, polymorphic ventricular tachycardia
      c. Nonspecific fibrofatty infiltration in previously healthy victim (variation of right ventricular dysplasia?)
    2. Sleep-death in Southeast Asians (see VIIB3, Brugada syndrome)
      a. Bangungut
      b. Pokkuri
      c. Lai-tai

Continued

TABLE 41-3 Causes of and Contributing Factors in Sudden Cardiac Death—cont'd

VIII. Electrical instability related to neurohumoral and central nervous system influences
  A. Catecholaminergic polymorphic ventricular tachycardia
  B. Other catecholamine-dependent arrhythmias
  C. Central nervous system related
    1. Psychic stress, emotional extremes (takotsubo syndrome)
    2. Auditory related
    3. "Voodoo death" in primitive cultures
    4. Diseases of the cardiac nerves
    5. Arrhythmia expression in congenital long-QT interval syndrome

IX. Sudden infant death syndrome and sudden death in children
  A. Sudden infant death syndrome
    1. Immature respiratory control functions
    2. Long-QT interval syndrome
    3. Congenital heart disease
    4. Myocarditis
  B. Sudden death in children
    1. Eisenmenger syndrome, aortic stenosis, hypertrophic cardiomyopathy, pulmonary atresia
    2. After corrective surgery for congenital heart disease
    3. Myocarditis
    4. Genetic disorders of electrical function (e.g., long-QT interval syndrome)
    5. No identified structural or functional cause

X. Miscellaneous
  A. Sudden death during extreme physical activity (seek predisposing causes)
  B. Commotio cordis—blunt chest trauma
  C. Mechanical interference with venous return
    1. Acute cardiac tamponade
    2. Massive pulmonary embolism
    3. Acute intracardiac thrombosis
  D. Dissecting aneurysm of the aorta
  E. Toxic and metabolic disturbances (other than QT interval effects listed above)
    1. Electrolyte disturbances
    2. Metabolic disturbances
    3. Proarrhythmic effects of antiarrhythmic drugs
    4. Proarrhythmic effects of noncardiac drugs
  F. Mimics sudden cardiac death
    1. "Café coronary"
    2. Acute alcoholic states ("holiday heart")
    3. Acute asthmatic attacks
    4. Air or amniotic fluid embolism

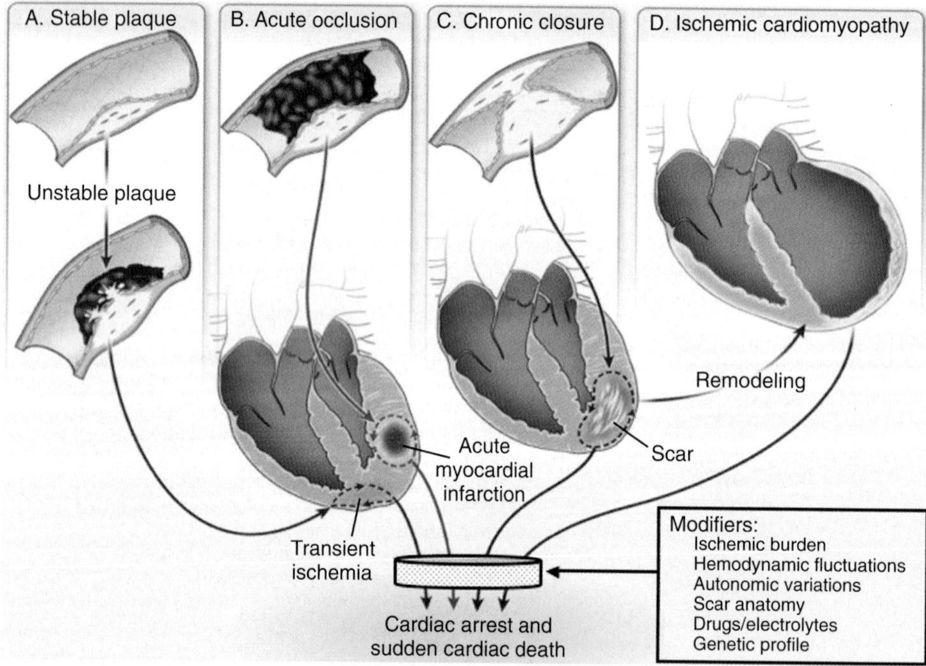

FIGURE 41-7 Pathophysiology of ventricular tachyarrhythmias in coronary heart disease. Short- and long-term risks of generating ventricular tachycardia or fibrillation (VT/VF) and of recurrent events are related to the presence of transient or persistent physiologic factors. VT/VF caused by transient ischemia **(A)** and the acute phase (24 to 48 hours) of myocardial infarction **(B)** are not predictive of recurrent events if recurrent ischemia is preventable. In contrast, VT/VF associated with healed myocardial infarction, with or without acute transient ischemia **(C)**, is associated with risk of recurrence. Longstanding ischemic cardiomyopathy **(D)**, especially when it is accompanied by heart failure, establishes a substrate associated with risk of VT/VF and recurrences over time. A series of modifying influences contribute to individual expression. *(Modified from Myerburg RJ: Implantable cardioverter-defibrillators after myocardial infarction. N Engl J Med 359:2245, 2008.)*

and in the peripartum period of pregnancy. Among the rare mechanical causes of SCD is prolapse of myxomatous polyps from the aortic valve into coronary ostia as well as dissection or rupture of a sinus of Valsalva aneurysm, with involvement of the coronary ostia and proximal coronary arteries. Finally, deep myocardial bridges over coronary arteries (see Chap. 83) have been reported in association with SCD occurring during strenuous exercise, possibly caused by dynamic mechanical obstruction. Scattered fibrosis in the distribution of the affected vessel is commonly seen at postmortem examination, suggesting a chronic or intermittent ischemic burden over time. Deep bridging seems to be more common in association with hypertrophic cardiomyopathy. However, the more common superficial bridges in the absence of other disorders are of less concern, and SCD associated with this anatomy is uncommon.

CORONARY ARTERY SPASM (see Chap. 54**).** Coronary vasospasm may cause serious arrhythmias and SCD. It is usually associated with some degree of concomitant coronary atherosclerotic disease. Painless myocardial ischemia, associated with either spasm or fixed lesions, is now recognized as a mechanism of previously unexplained sudden death.[66] Different patterns of silent ischemia (e.g., totally asymptomatic, post–myocardial infarction, and mixed silent-anginal pattern) may have different prognostic implications. In post–myocardial infarction patients, silent ischemia has been associated with an increased risk of SCD.[67]

Ventricular Hypertrophy and Hypertrophic Cardiomyopathy

(see Chaps. 69 and 83)

Left ventricular hypertrophy is an independent risk factor for SCD, associates with many causes of SCD, and may be a physiologic contributor to mechanisms of potentially lethal arrhythmias. The underlying states resulting in left ventricular hypertrophy include hypertensive heart disease with or without atherosclerosis, valvular heart disease, obstructive and nonobstructive hypertrophic cardiomyopathy, primary pulmonary hypertension with right ventricular hypertrophy, and advanced right ventricular overload secondary to congenital heart disease. Each of these conditions is associated with risk of SCD, and it has been suggested that patients with severely hypertrophic ventricles are particularly susceptible to arrhythmic death.

Risk of SCD in obstructive and nonobstructive hypertrophic cardiomyopathy was identified in the early clinical and hemodynamic descriptions of this entity. Among patients who have the obstructive form, up to 70% of all deaths are sudden. However, survivors of cardiac arrest in this group may have a better long-term outcome than survivors with other causes, and reports have suggested that the risk of primary cardiac arrest and SCD in hypertrophic cardiomyopathy is lower than previously thought.

A substantial proportion of patients with obstructive and nonobstructive hypertrophic cardiomyopathy have a family history of affected relatives or premature SCDs of unknown cause. Genetic studies have confirmed autosomal dominant inheritance patterns, with a great deal of allele and phenotypic heterogeneity. Most of the mutations are at loci that encode elements in the contractile protein complex, the most common being beta-myosin heavy chain and cardiac troponin T, which together account for more than half of identified abnormalities. In the beta-myosin heavy chain form, there is a relationship between severity of left ventricular hypertrophy and risk of SCD; in the troponin T form, left ventricular hypertrophy may be less severe, despite SCD risk. The genetics of hypertrophic cardiomyopathy is characterized by a large number of private mutations with variable expression. Possible interaction with modifier genes, such as variations in ion channel genes, remains to be clarified.

Specific clinical markers have not been especially predictive of SCD in individual patients, although young age at onset, strong family history of SCD, magnitude of left ventricular mass, ventricular arrhythmias, and worsening symptoms (especially syncope) appear to indicate higher risk.[68-70] Early studies suggested that a low resting outflow gradient, with a substantial provocable gradient, identifies a high risk of SCD, but recent data support the predictive power of a high resting gradient.[70] The mechanism of SCD in patients with hypertrophic cardiomyopathy was initially thought to involve outflow tract obstruction, possibly as a consequence of catecholamine stimulation, but later data have focused on lethal arrhythmias as the common mechanism of sudden death in this disease. Risk is also thought to be suggested by nonsustained VT on ambulatory recording or the inducibility of potentially lethal arrhythmias during programmed electrical stimulation. Rapid or polymorphic symptomatic nonsustained tachycardias, or both, have better predictive power.

The question of whether the pathogenesis of the arrhythmias represents an interaction between electrophysiologic and hemodynamic abnormalities or is a consequence of electrophysiologic derangement of hypertrophied muscle is unanswered. The observation that patients with nonobstructive hypertrophic cardiomyopathy are also at risk for SCD suggests that an electrophysiologic mechanism secondary to the hypertrophied muscle itself plays a major role. In athletes younger than 35 years, hypertrophic cardiomyopathy is the most common cause of SCD, in contrast to athletes older than 35 years, among whom ischemic heart disease is the most common cause.

Dilated Cardiomyopathy and Heart Failure

The advent of therapeutic interventions that provide better long-term control of congestive heart failure has improved long-term survival of these patients (see Chaps. 26, 28, and 68). However, the proportion of patients with heart failure who die suddenly is substantial, especially among those who appear clinically stable (i.e., functional Class I or II).[37] The mechanism of SCD (VT or ventricular fibrillation [VF] versus bradyarrhythmia or asystole) appears to be related to cause (i.e., ischemic versus nonischemic). The absolute risk of SCD increases with deteriorating left ventricular function, but the ratio of sudden to nonsudden deaths is related inversely to the extent of functional impairment.[37] Among patients with cardiomyopathy who have good functional capacity (Classes I and II), total mortality risk is considerably lower than for those with poor functional capacity (Classes III and IV), but the probability that a death will be sudden is higher (**Fig. 41-8**). Unexplained syncope has been observed to be a powerful predictor of SCD in patients who have functional Class III or IV symptoms, regardless of the cause of cardiomyopathy. Ambulatory ventricular arrhythmias do not appear to indicate specific SCD risk in such patients.[53]

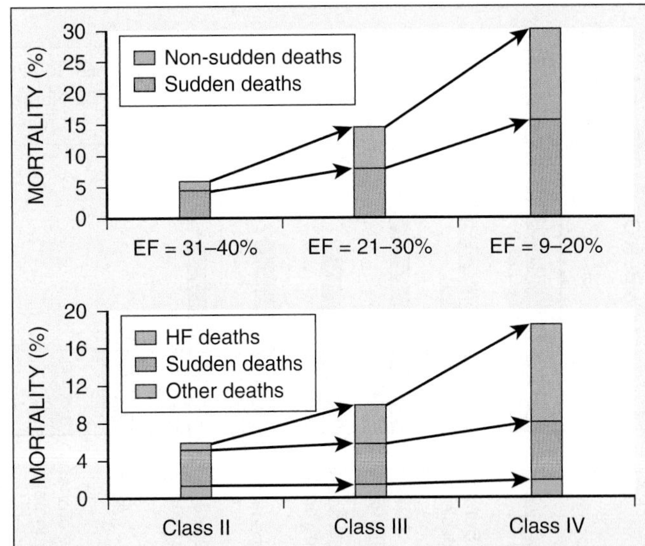

FIGURE 41-8 Risk of sudden cardiac death related to left ventricular ejection fraction (EF) and functional classification in heart failure (HF). The relative probability of death being sudden is higher, and absolute mortality risk is lower, among patients with higher ejection fractions and better functional capacity. *(Modified from Cleland JG, Chattopadhyay S, Khand A, et al: Prevalence and incidence of arrhythmias and sudden death in heart failure. Heart Fail Rev 7:229, 2002, with permission from Springer Science and Business Media.)*

The interaction between post–myocardial infarction ventricular arrhythmia and depressed ejection fraction in determining risk for SCD has been described. The most common etiologic basis for the association between chronic heart failure and SCD is ischemic cardiomyopathy. The prevalence of ischemic cardiomyopathy has been increasing because of better acute myocardial infarction survival statistics coupled with late remodeling. Other causes include idiopathic, alcoholic, and postmyocarditis congestive cardiomyopathies and the familial pattern of dilated cardiomyopathy, many of the latter being associated with a lamin A/C mutation.[71] Other gene loci are also implicated. Peripartum cardiomyopathy (see Chap. 82) may also cause SCD.

Acute Heart Failure

All causes of acute cardiac failure (see Chaps. 25 and 27), in the absence of prompt interventions, can result in SCD caused by the circulatory failure itself or secondary arrhythmias. The electrophysiologic mechanisms involved have been proposed to be caused by acute stretching of ventricular myocardial fibers or the His-Purkinje system on the basis of its experimentally demonstrated arrhythmogenic effects. However, the roles of neurohumoral mechanisms and acute electrolyte shifts have not been fully evaluated. Among the causes of acute cardiac failure associated with SCD are massive acute myocardial infarction, acute myocarditis, acute alcoholic cardiac dysfunction, acute pulmonary edema in any form of advanced heart disease, and a number of mechanical causes of heart failure, such as massive pulmonary embolism, mechanical disruption of intracardiac structures secondary to infarction or infection, and ball valve embolism in aortic or mitral stenosis (see Table 41-3).

INFLAMMATORY, INFILTRATIVE, NEOPLASTIC, AND DEGENERATIVE DISEASES OF THE HEART. Almost all diseases in this category have been associated with SCD, with or without concomitant cardiac failure. Acute viral myocarditis with left ventricular dysfunction (see Chap. 70) is commonly associated with cardiac arrhythmias, including potentially lethal arrhythmias.[72] Serious ventricular arrhythmias or SCD can occur in myocarditis in the absence of clinical evidence of left ventricular dysfunction.[73,74] In a report of 19 SCDs among 1,606,167 previously screened U.S. Air Force recruits, 8 of 19 victims (42%) had evidence of myocarditis (5 nonrheumatic, 3 rheumatic) at postmortem examination, and 15 of 19 (79%) suffered their cardiac arrests during strenuous exertion. Sixty-eight percent of SCDs

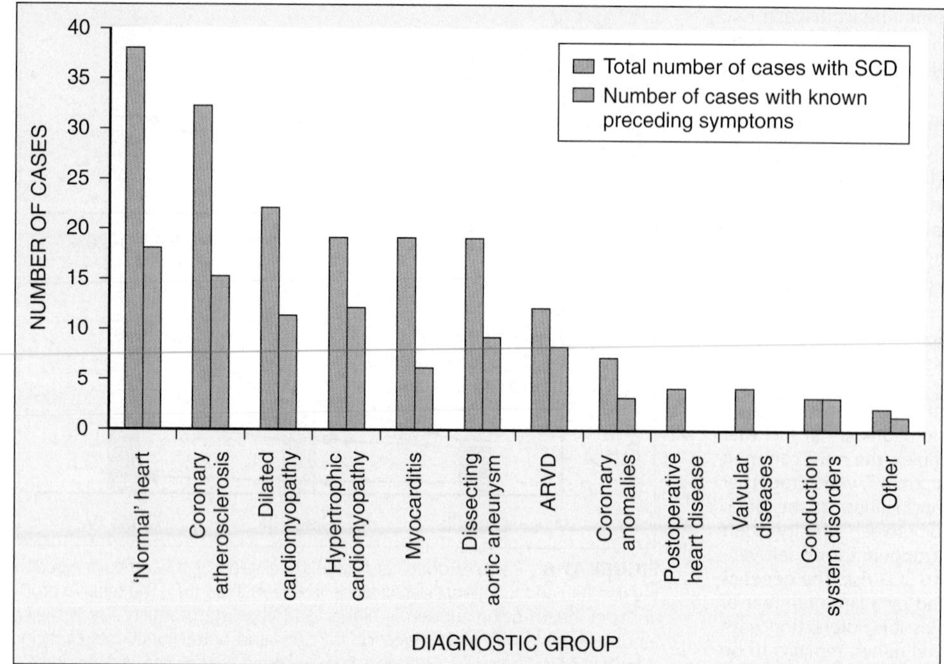

FIGURE 41-9 SCD in adolescents and young adults in Sweden. Frequency of preceding symptoms in 181 cases of sudden cardiac death in persons 15 to 35 years old, by diagnostic group. ARVD = arrhythmogenic right ventricular dysplasia. *(Modified from Wisten A, Forsberg H, Krantz P, Messner T: Sudden cardiac death in 15-35-year olds in Sweden during 1992-99. J Intern Med 252:529, 2002, with permission of the publisher.)*

due to myocarditis in a study from Sweden had no premortem symptoms[11] (**Fig. 41-9**), and most available data suggest a bias toward victims younger than 35 years, both for absolute numbers and for percentages of SCDs due to myocarditis.[10,75] Giant cell myocarditis and acute necrotizing eosinophilic myocarditis are particularly virulent for both myocardial damage and arrhythmias.[72] Viral carditis can also cause damage isolated to the specialized conducting system and result in a propensity to arrhythmias; the rare association of this process with SCD has been reported. Varicella in adults is a rare cause of striking conduction system disorders, but left ventricular function is usually preserved; its relationship to SCD is unclear.

Myocardial involvement in collagen-vascular disorders, tumors, chronic granulomatous diseases, infiltrative disorders, and protozoan infestations varies widely, but SCD can be the initial or terminal manifestation of the disease process in all cases. Among the granulomatous diseases, sarcoidosis (see Chap. 68) stands out because of the frequency of SCD associated with it. It has been reported that SCD was the terminal event in 67% of sarcoid heart disease deaths. The risk of SCD has been related to the extent of cardiac involvement, but ambient arrhythmias, such as nonsustained VT, may indicate risk in such patients with lesser degrees of cardiac involvement. In a report on the pathologic findings in nine patients who died of progressive systemic sclerosis (see Chap. 68), eight who died suddenly had evidence of transient ischemia and reperfusion histologically, suggesting that this might represent Raynaud-like involvement of coronary vessels. Amyloidosis of the heart (see Chap. 68) may also cause sudden death. An incidence of 30% has been reported, and diffuse involvement of ventricular muscle or of the specialized conducting system may be associated with SCD.

Arrhythmogenic Right Ventricular Dysplasia or Right Ventricular Cardiomyopathy (see Chaps. 39 and 68)**.** This condition is associated with a high incidence of ventricular arrhythmias, including polymorphic nonsustained VT and VF and recurrent sustained monomorphic VT.[76] Although symptomatic monomorphic VT has been well recognized in the syndrome for many years, the risk of SCD had been unclear and thought to be relatively low until the risks associated with the disease were clarified by a number of subsequent studies.[77] In a high proportion of victims, perhaps as many as 80%, the first manifestation of the disease is "unexplained" syncope or SCD. SCD is often exercise related, and in some areas of the world where screening for hypertrophic cardiomyopathy has excluded the affected athletes from competition, right ventricular dysplasia has emerged as the most common cause of sports-related SCD. Although it is generally considered a right ventricular abnormality, with possible late involvement of the left ventricle in advanced cases, a left ventricle–dominant pattern has also been described.[78]

The genetic basis for right ventricular dysplasia has been explored because a large proportion of the cases have a familial distribution.[68] The inheritance pattern is autosomal dominant, except in one geographically isolated cluster in which it is autosomal recessive (Naxos disease, plakoglobin locus on chromosome 17). Autosomal dominant mutations have been identified in the ryanodine receptor locus on chromosome 1 [1q42][79] and four loci encoding desmosome structure (plakoglobin, desmoplakin, plakophilin 2, and desmoglein 2).[80-82] The desmosomal loci collectively are the most common known mutations associated with right ventricular dysplasia. Linkage analyses have implicated a heterogeneous distribution of a number of other loci that might contribute to inheritance patterns (see Chap. 9).

Valvular Heart Disease (see Chap. 66)**.** Before the advent of surgery for valvular heart disease, severe aortic stenosis was associated with a high mortality risk. Approximately 70% of deaths were sudden, accounting for an absolute SCD mortality rate of 15% to 20% among all affected patients. A retrospective observational study of 133 asymptomatic patients with normal left ventricular function and severe aortic stenosis, defined as a peak aortic gradient of >60 mm Hg, followed up without surgery, identified 7 SCDs (5%) during a mean follow-up of 3.3 years. Three of the deaths were preceded by a change in status: onset of dyspnea, decreasing left ventricular function, and a coronary event.[83] The advent of safe and effective procedures for aortic valve replacement has reduced the incidence of this cause of sudden death, but patients with prosthetic or heterograft aortic valve replacements remain at some risk for SCD caused by arrhythmias, prosthetic valve dysfunction, or coexistent coronary heart disease. The incidence peaks 3 weeks after operation and then levels off after 8 months. Nonetheless, the risk is still appreciably lower than the historical risk among patients before the advent of valve surgery. A high incidence of ventricular arrhythmia has been observed during follow-up of patients with valve replacement, especially those who had aortic stenosis, multiple valve surgery, or cardiomegaly. Sudden death during follow-up was associated with ventricular arrhythmias and thromboembolism. Hemodynamic variables were less predictive. Stenotic lesions of other valves imply a much lower risk of SCD. Regurgitant lesions, particularly chronic aortic regurgitation and acute mitral regurgitation, may cause SCD, but the risk is also lower than with aortic stenosis.

Mitral Valve Prolapse (see Chap. 66)**.** This entity is prevalent, but probably less than previously thought,[84] and associated with a high incidence of annoying low-risk cardiac arrhythmias. However, a risk of SCD is apparent although low.[85] This uncommon complication appears to correlate best with marked redundancy of mitral leaflets seen on echocardiography, in conjunction with nonspecific ST-T wave changes in the inferior leads on the electrocardiogram. Reported associations between QT interval prolongation or preexcitation and SCD in mitral prolapse syndrome are less consistent.

Endocarditis of the Aortic and Mitral Valves (see Chap. 67)**.** This may be associated with rapid death resulting from acute disruption of the valvular apparatus, coronary embolism, or abscesses of valvular rings or the septum; however, such deaths are rarely true sudden deaths because conventionally defined tachyarrhythmic mechanisms are uncommon. Coronary embolism from valvular vegetations can trigger fatal ischemic arrhythmia on rare occasions.

Congenital Heart Disease. The congenital lesions most commonly associated with SCD are aortic stenosis (see Chap. 65) and communications between the left and right sides of the heart with the Eisenmenger physiology. In the latter, the risk of SCD is a function of the severity of pulmonary vascular disease; also, there is an extraordinarily high risk of maternal mortality during labor and delivery in the pregnant patient with Eisenmenger syndrome (see Chap. 82).[86] Potentially lethal arrhythmias and SCD have been described as late complications after surgical repair of complex congenital lesions, particularly tetralogy of Fallot, transposition of the great arteries, and atrioventricular (AV) canal. These patients should be observed closely and treated aggressively when cardiac arrhythmias are identified, although the late risk of SCD may not be as high as previously thought.

Electrophysiologic Abnormalities

Acquired disease of the AV node and His-Purkinje system and the presence of accessory pathways of conduction (see Chap. 39) are two groups of structural abnormalities of specialized conduction that may be associated with SCD. Clinical surveillance and follow-up studies have suggested that intraventricular conduction disturbances in coronary heart disease are one of the few factors that can increase the proportion of SCD in coronary heart disease. Several studies from the late 1970s and 1980s had demonstrated increased total mortality and SCD risk during the late in-hospital course and first few months after hospital discharge in patients with anterior myocardial infarctions and right bundle branch or bifascicular block. In one study, 47% of patients who had late hospital VF had had the combination of anteroseptal infarction and bundle branch block. This finding corresponded to a VF incidence of 35% in a subgroup that represented only 4.1% of a total of 966 myocardial infarctions. In a later study evaluating the impact of thrombolytic therapy compared with the pre–thrombolytic era experience, the incidence of pure right bundle branch block was higher but that of bifascicular block was lower, as were late complications and mortality. These observations suggest a benefit of thrombolytic therapy, but the principle of increased risk among those who develop advanced conduction abnormalities (probably related to infarct size) is not attenuated by the therapy, and the condition still requires aggressive management.

Primary fibrosis (Lenègre's disease) or injury secondary to other disorders (Lev disease) of the His-Purkinje system is commonly associated with intraventricular conduction abnormalities and symptomatic AV block and less commonly with SCD. The identification of those at risk and the efficacy of pacemakers for prevention of SCD, rather than only amelioration of symptoms, have been subjects of debate. However, survival appears to depend more on the nature and extent of the underlying disease than on the conduction disturbance itself.

Patients with congenital AV block (see Chap. 39) or nonprogressive congenital intraventricular block, in the absence of structural cardiac abnormalities and with stable heart rate and rhythm, have been characterized as being at low risk for SCD in the past. In contrast, progressive congenital intraventricular blocks and the coexistence of structural congenital defects predicted a high risk and were considered pacemaker indications. Later data have suggested that patients with the patterns of congenital AV block previously thought to be benign are at risk for a dilated cardiomyopathy,[87] and routine pacemaker implantation in patients older than 15 years, if not indicated sooner, has been suggested by at least one group. Whether there is mortality benefit from pacemakers or a reduction in the incidence of dilated cardiomyopathy is not yet clear. Hereditary forms of AV heart block have also been reported in association with a familial propensity to SCD. Sodium channel gene mutations have been associated with progressive conduction system disturbances, along with aging, and some are variants of Brugada gene expression.[88,89] External ophthalmoplegia and retinal pigmentation with progressive conduction system disease (Kearns Sayre syndrome), associated with mitochondrial DNA variants, may lead to high-grade heart block and pacemaker dependence.

The anomalous pathways of conduction, bundles of Kent in the Wolff-Parkinson-White syndrome and Mahaim fibers, are commonly associated with nonlethal arrhythmias. However, when the anomalous pathways of conduction have short anterograde refractory periods, the occurrence of atrial fibrillation may allow the initiation of VF during very rapid conduction across the bypass tract (see Chap. 39). The incidence of SCD in patients with short refractory period bypass tracts is unknown because an accurate estimate of its incidence in the general population is not available. Patients who have multiple pathways appear to be at higher risk for SCD, as do patients with a familial pattern of anomalous pathways and premature SCD. Family history is relevant because a genetic predisposition to Wolff-Parkinson-White syndrome has been suggested.[90]

Long-QT Syndromes (see Chaps. 9 and 35 to 39)**.** The congenital long-QT syndrome is a functional abnormality usually caused by inherited mutations affecting molecular structure of ion channel proteins and is associated with environmental or neurogenic triggers that can initiate symptomatic or lethal arrhythmias.[91] Less commonly, but not rarely, such mutations may occur de novo or may be transmitted from an apparently normal mosaic parent,[92] influencing the reliability of family histories. Two hereditary patterns have been described: the much more common autosomal dominant pattern known as the Romano-Ward syndrome; and the rare autosomal recessive inheritance pattern, associated with deafness, the Jervell and Lange-Nielsen syndrome. There is a broad range of phenotypic expression, with syncope being the most common expression among symptomatic patients. SCD is less common, although data are limited by the absence of information about the number of undiagnosed carriers in whom fatal cardiac arrest is the first clinical event. Some patients have prolonged QT intervals throughout life without any manifest arrhythmias, whereas others are highly susceptible to symptomatic and potentially fatal ventricular arrhythmias, particularly the torsades de pointes pattern of VT.[93,94] Moreover, genetic studies have demonstrated that penetrance may be low or variable in some families, making electrocardiographic identification of affected members difficult. The relationship between low penetrance and risk of SCD remains undefined, but such patients are likely to be susceptible to QT-lengthening effects of drugs or serum electrolyte level variations, expressed clinically as acquired long-QT syndrome (see later).

Higher levels of risk are associated with female gender, greater degrees of QT prolongation or QT alternans, unexplained syncope, family history of premature SCD, and documented torsades de pointes or prior VF. Patients with the syndrome require avoidance of drugs that are associated with QT lengthening and careful medical management, which may include implantable defibrillators. Moreover, a potentially important preventive strategy is to identify and to manage relatives medically who carry the mutation (see Chaps. 9 and 35 to 39 for details). A large number of mutations at loci on chromosomes 3, 7, and 11 that encode the K^+ and Na^+ channel alpha subunits (*KCNQ1, KCNH2, SCN5A*) and on chromosome 21 that encode the corresponding beta subunits (*KCNE1, KCNE2, SCN4B*) are implicated in various patterns of the Romano-Ward and Jervell and Lange-Nielsen syndromes. Additional loci are associated with less common genetic variants associated with long QT. Another form of long-QT syndrome, LQT4, is associated with a mutation at a locus on chromosome 4 encoding the cytoskeletal element ankyrin-B[95] (see Chaps. 9 and 35). It has been suggested that ankyrin-B mutations may have arrhythmia implications extending beyond the long-QT syndromes.

From an epidemiologic perspective, there is interest in whether QT interval abnormalities or the propensity thereto, interacting with acquired diseases predisposes to SCD as a specific clinical expression.[1,9,61] In a prospective cohort study of a population having a mean age of 69 years at entry, a prolonged QTc emerged as a powerful risk factor for SCD in the presence of cardiovascular disorders, such as myocardial infarction, hypertension, and heart failure.[96] The hypothesis that common genetic variants may modulate QTc in unselected populations stimulates interest in the relationship to selective risk for SCD in individuals with acquired diseases.[26] However, a number of rare variants may be even more important.

The acquired form of prolonged QT interval syndrome refers to excessive lengthening of the QT interval and the potential for development of torsades de pointes in response to environmental influences. Like congenital long-QT syndrome, it is more common in women. The syndrome may be caused by drug effects or an individual patient's idiosyncrasies (particularly related to class IA or III antiarrhythmic drugs and psychotropic drugs; see Chap. 91), electrolyte abnormalities, hypothermia, toxic substances, bradyarrhythmia-induced QT adjustments, and central nervous system injury (most commonly, subarachnoid hemorrhage). It has also been reported in intensive weight reduction programs that involve the use of liquid protein diets and in anorexia nervosa. Lithium carbonate can prolong the QT interval and has been reported to be associated with an increased incidence of SCD in cancer patients with preexisting heart disease. Drug interactions have been recognized as a mechanism of prolongation of the QT interval and torsades de pointes.[97] A growing body of evidence has suggested that inherited polymorphisms or mutations with low penetrance, involving the same gene loci associated with phenotypically expressed long-QT syndrome, underlie the so-called individual idiosyncrasies to the acquired form in many if not

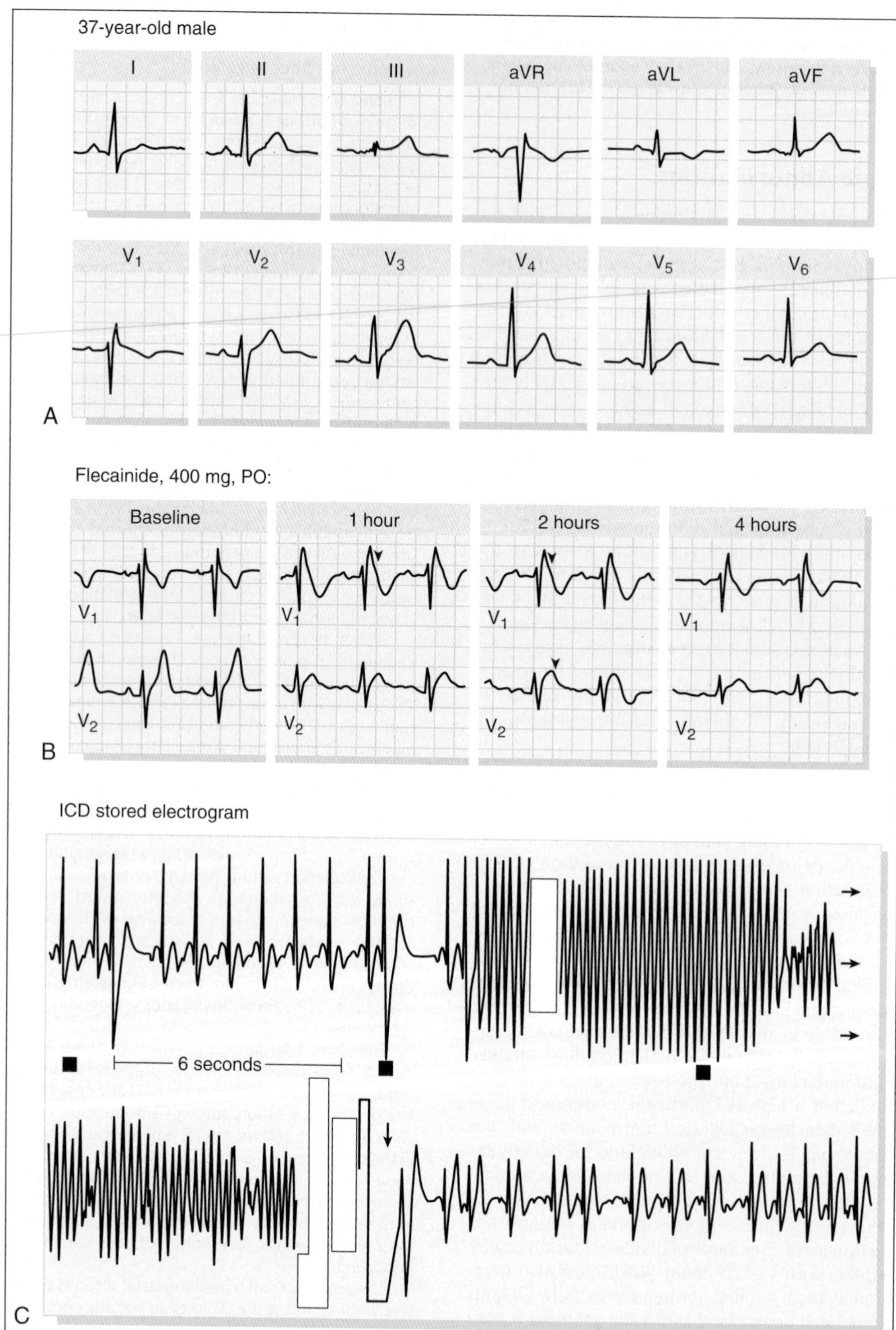

FIGURE 41-10 Electrocardiographic and clinical findings in a 37-year-old man with Brugada syndrome. The patient was resuscitated after out-of-hospital ventricular fibrillation. No structural disease was identified. **A,** The 12-lead electrocardiogram shows an incomplete right bundle branch block pattern, which is not typical for Brugada syndrome. **B,** Typical repolarization changes of Brugada syndrome (arrowheads) were elicited by a single oral dose of flecainide, 400 mg. The patient received an ICD and 6 months later had an appropriate shock (arrow, **C**), as shown on the accompanying electrogram stored in the device.

most cases.[98,99] In acquired prolonged QT syndrome, as in the congenital form, torsades de pointes is commonly the specific arrhythmia that triggers or degenerates into VF.

Short-QT Syndrome (see Chaps. 9 and 39**).** A familial pattern of SCD risk has been associated with abnormally short QT intervals, defined as a QTc <300 milliseconds (QT <280 milliseconds).[100] Short-QT syndrome is much less common than long-QT syndrome, and there is little to guide risk profiling other than documented life-threatening arrhythmias and familial clustering of SCD.[100,101] Several ion channel gene loci variants have been suggested.

Brugada Syndrome (see Chaps. 35 and 39**).** This disorder is characterized by right bundle branch block and an unusual form of nonischemic ST-T wave elevations in the anterior precordial leads (**Fig. 41-10**) associated with risk of SCD. It is a familial disorder and occurs most commonly in young and middle-aged men. A mutation involving the cardiac Na^+ channel gene (*SCN5A*) has been observed in a minority of cases, and there are compelling data suggesting that other ion channel defects may be a cause. The right bundle branch block and ST-T wave changes may be intermittent and evoked or exaggerated by Na^+ channel blockers (e.g., flecainide). Risk of SCD is difficult to predict in individuals. Persistent baseline electrocardiographic changes, syncope, life-threatening arrhythmias, strong family history of SCD, and inducibility of ventricular tachyarrhythmias during electrophysiologic testing, in various combinations, are thought to be the best predictors.[102,103]

Long before the description of Brugada syndrome, a specific pattern of SCD in young men had been observed in Southeast Asia. Syndromes referred to as *bangungut* in the Philippines, *pokkuri* in Japan, and *lai-tai* in Laos were reported. In each, there was a tendency for death to occur unexpectedly during sleep, and a toxic cause was suspected at one time. Documented cases were reported in Laotians who came to the United States after the Vietnam War. The mechanism was identified as VF in some of these cases. The fact that these cases continue to occur in a new cultural setting has suggested that there might be a hereditary predisposition. Further clinical and genetic observations have led to the conclusion that many if not all of the subjects had Brugada syndrome.[104]

Early Repolarization Pattern and SCD (see Chap. 39). An association between the electrocardiographic pattern of early repolarization and risk of idiopathic VF has been described.[105] Early repolarization was observed in 64 (31%) of 206 survivors of sudden cardiac arrest in the absence of identifiable structural or molecular causes compared with 5% among 412 well-matched normal controls. The survivors with early repolarization patterns had a higher rate of recurrence of VF (41% of subjects; median of eight events per subject) than did the 142 without early repolarization (23% of subjects; median of two events per subject). Early repolarization was limited to the inferior and lateral leads, in contrast to anterior leads used for the conventional definition of benign early repolarization. The magnitude of J-point elevation was significantly greater among cardiac arrest survivors than among the controls with early repolarization. Interestingly, a number of the clinical features were similar to the responses seen in patients with Brugada syndrome, leading to speculation whether the reported cases of VF associated with early repolarization might be another expression of the Brugada pathophysiologic process.[106]

Catecholaminergic Polymorphic Ventricular Tachycardia (see Chaps. 9, 35, and 39). Catecholaminergic polymorphic ventricular tachycardia is an inherited syndrome associated with catecholamine-dependent lethal arrhythmias in the absence of forewarning electrocardiographic abnormalities and with at least partial control by beta adrenoceptor blocking agents.[107] An autosomal dominant pattern involving the ryanodine receptor locus (RyR2) was initially described predominantly in younger patients, usually men, with bidirectional or polymorphic VT associated with SCD risk. A pattern not associated with that genotype appeared more likely in older patients (young adults), usually women.[107] More recent data suggest less dominance by male gender for RyR2 variants and another variant involving autosomal recessive inheritance of calsequestrin loci (*CASQ2*) in about 10% of genotyped cases and relatives.[108]

Electrical Instability Resulting from Neurohumoral and Central Nervous System Influences. Several central nervous system–related interactions with cardiac electrical stability have been suggested (see Chaps. 35 and 94). Epidemiologic data have also suggested an association between behavioral abnormalities and the risk of SCD. Psychological stress and emotional extremes have been suggested as triggering mechanisms for advanced arrhythmias and SCD for many years,[109] but there are only limited, largely observational data supporting such associations. Stress-induced arrhythmias are better supported than is stress-induced mortality risk, which requires further study. Data from the 1994 Los Angeles earthquake have identified an increased rate of fatal cardiac events on that day, but the event rate was reduced during the ensuing 2 weeks, suggesting a triggering of events about to happen rather than independent causation.[110] Associations between auditory stimulation and auditory auras and SCD have been reported. Auditory abnormalities in some forms of congenital QT prolongation have also been observed.

A variant of torsades de pointes, characterized by short coupling intervals between a normal impulse and the initiating impulse, has been described (see Fig. 41-e1 on website). It appears to have familial trends and to be related to alterations in autonomic nervous system activity. The 12-lead electrocardiogram demonstrates normal QT intervals, but VF and sudden death are common (see Chaps. 9 and 39).

Acute emotional stress has been reported as a cause of a specific form of reversible left ventricular dysfunction and heart failure, characterized by ballooning of the apex with a narrow neck at the base of the heart (termed *takotsubo* cardiomyopathy, named for the similarity of this shape to a Japanese octopus fishing pot).[111,112] It is suspected to be catecholamine mediated and its long-term prognosis is good, but short-term risk of SCD during the acute phase remains uncertain.

The phenomenon of voodoo death has been studied in underdeveloped countries. There appears to be an association between isolation from the tribe, a sense of hopelessness, severe bradyarrhythmias, and sudden death. With cultural changes in many of these areas, the syndrome has become less amenable to observation and study; however, there remain pockets of cultural isolation in which the syndrome may still exist. Limited clinical observations and experimental data modeling voodoo death have suggested a mechanism related to parasympathetic overactivity, as opposed to the evidence for an adrenergic basis for syndromes related to acute emotional stress.

Sudden Infant Death Syndrome and Sudden Cardiac Death in Children

The sudden infant death syndrome (SIDS) occurs between birth and 6 months of age, is more common in male infants, and had an incidence of 1.2 deaths/1000 live births before widespread publication of appropriate sleep positions in at-risk infants.[113] Between 1992 and 2002, the incidence fell to 0.57 death/1000 live births as attention to sleep position grew, supporting a major role for obstructive sleep apnea as a mechanism. Vulnerability due to various mechanisms of central respiratory control dysfunction, both inherent and prematurity related, is likely to interact with sleep position as a multicomponent mechanism.[114]

Because of its abrupt nature, a primary cardiac mechanism had been suspected as the basis of this syndrome in some victims for many years, and a large study of electrocardiograms of infants has suggested an association of risk of SIDS with prolonged QT intervals. Subsequently, a near-miss survivor was shown to have a de novo mutation of the Na^+ channel gene (*SCN5A;* chromosome 3), validating the concept that long QT may be one mechanism of SIDS.[115] The relative incidence of SIDS among victims with the longer QT intervals and documentation of additional long-QT–related arrhythmias in near-misses have supported the notion that as many as 15% of SIDS deaths may occur by this mechanism. Other cardiac causes have also been reported. Accessory pathways (two cases) and dispersed or immature AV nodal or bundle branch cells in the annulus (four cases) have been described in a group of seven SIDS victims studied by detailed histopathologic examination.

Sudden death in children beyond the SIDS age group and in adolescents and young adults is associated with identifiable heart disease in the majority of cases.[116] Although one earlier study identified cardiac causes in only 25% of victims of sudden natural death between the ages of 1 and 21 years, a later report identified cardiac causes in 65%, with cardiac causes attributed in 80% of older children and adolescents. About 25% of SCDs in children occur in those who have undergone previous surgery for congenital cardiac disease. Of the remaining 75%, more than half occur in children who have one of four lesions: congenital aortic stenosis, Eisenmenger syndrome, pulmonary stenosis or atresia, or obstructive hypertrophic cardiomyopathy. Neuspiel and Kuller have observed 14 cases of myocarditis among 51 SCDs in children (27%). In a more recent autopsy study of victims aged 5 to 35 years, 29% of the deaths were presumed arrhythmias in the absence of structural diseases and 25% were acute myocardial infarctions, primarily in the 30- to 35-year age group.[116] Other common causes included myocarditis, hypertrophic and dilated cardiomyopathies, congenital heart diseases, and aortic dissections.

Other Causes and Circumstances Associated with Sudden Death

SCD can occur during or after extreme physical activity in competing athletes or under special circumstances within the general population. Examples of the latter include intense exercise and basic military training. Among adolescent and young adult competitive athletes, the incidence estimate is in the range of 1/75,000 annually in Italy[117] compared with less than 1/125,000 for the general nonathlete population in the same age group. However, Maron (see Chap. 83) has reported the frequency of sudden unexpected death related to cardiovascular disease during competitive sports to be 1 in 200,000 individual student athletes per academic year and 1 in 70,000 during a 3-year high-school career. Exercise-related incidence figures are more difficult to ascertain in other populations, but one study reported an incidence of one SCD per 1.5 million exercise sessions in health clubs.[38] The incidence of exercise-related cardiac arrest appears to be lower in women.[118] Most athletes and nonathletes have a previously known or unrecognized cardiac abnormality. In middle-aged and older adults, in whom coronary disease dominates as the cause of SCD, exercise-related deaths appear to be associated with acute plaque disruptions.[47] Whether exercise contributed to the initiation of plaque disruption or preexisting disruption simply set the stage for the fatal response during exercise remains unclear. Among athletes, hypertrophic cardiomyopathy with or without obstruction and occult congenital or acquired coronary artery disease are the most common causes identified after death (see Chap. 83),[119] with myocarditis contributing a significant minority. In a report of a large cohort of U.S. Air Force recruits, a surprisingly large fraction of those who died suddenly during exertion had unsuspected myocarditis. Diseases attributed to molecular structural abnormalities, such as long-QT syndrome and right ventricular dysplasia, are being increasingly recognized as causes of SCD in athletes and exercising nonathletes. Blunt chest wall trauma by sports objects, such as baseballs and hockey pucks, can initiate lethal arrhythmias, a syndrome known as commotio cordis (see Chap. 83).[120]

Sudden death from true cardiac causes in athletes should not be confused with precipitous death related to heat stroke or malignant hyperthermia. In the latter, the victim has usually exercised excessively in hot weather, often with athletic gear that impairs heat dissipation and sometimes in association with the use of substances that cause heat production and vasoconstriction impairing heat exchange. This leads to collapse, with markedly elevated core body temperatures and ultimately irreversible organ system damage. Ingestion of exogenous dietary supplements, particularly ephedrine and caffeine-containing preparations, taken in excess quantities, has been proposed to have a role in precipitation of life-threatening arrhythmias, largely on the basis of case report data. As a result, the U.S. Food and Drug Administration (FDA) has banned marketing of these substances for athletic performance enhancement or weight loss.

A small group of victims have neither previously determined functional abnormality nor identifiable structural abnormalities at postmortem examination. Such events or deaths, when they are associated with documented VF, are classified as idiopathic. Although long-term survival after an idiopathic potentially fatal event is still unclear, some degree of risk appears to remain. The idiopathic category is decreasing as the subtle molecular causes become better defined, including recognition by postmortem genetic studies. Limited data suggest that higher risk persists primarily in patients with subtle cardiac structural abnormalities, in contrast to patients who are truly normal. In addition, these events tend to occur in young, otherwise healthy people.

There also are a number of noncardiac conditions that can cause or mimic SCD. Sleep apnea is associated with a risk of nocturnal death, including deaths attributable to cardiac causes. In these circumstances, the risk of death peaks during the night rather than in the early morning hours.[14] Another respiratory system–based cause of sudden death is the so-called café coronary, in which food, usually an unchewed piece of meat, lodges in the oropharynx and causes an abrupt obstruction at the glottis. The classic description of a café coronary is sudden cyanosis and collapse in a restaurant during a meal accompanied by lively conversation. The holiday heart syndrome is characterized by cardiac arrhythmias, most commonly atrial, and other cardiac abnormalities associated with acute alcoholic states. It has not been determined whether potentially lethal arrhythmias occurring in such settings account for reported sudden deaths associated with acute alcoholic states. Massive pulmonary embolism (see Chap. 77) can cause acute cardiovascular collapse and sudden death; sudden death in severe acute asthmatic attacks, without prolonged deterioration of the patient's condition, is well recognized. Air or amniotic fluid embolism at the time of labor and delivery may cause sudden death on rare occasions, with the clinical picture mimicking that of SCD. Peripartum air embolism caused by unusual sexual practices has been reported as a cause of such sudden deaths.

Finally, a number of abnormalities that do not directly involve the heart may cause sudden deaths that mimic SCD. These include aortic dissection (see Chap. 60), acute cardiac tamponade (see Chap. 75), and rapid exsanguination.

Pathology and Pathophysiology

Pathologic studies in SCD victims reflect the epidemiologic and clinical observations that coronary atherosclerosis is the major predisposing cause. In one report, 81% of 220 victims of SCD had significant coronary heart disease at autopsy. At least one vessel with more than 75% stenosis was found in 94% of victims, acute coronary occlusion in 58%, healed myocardial infarction in 44%, and acute myocardial infarction in 27%. These observations are consistent with subsequent studies of the frequency of coronary disease in SCD victims, but the focus has evolved from the simple anatomic presence of coronary lesions to the specific associations with unstable plaques. All other causes of SCD (see Table 41-3) collectively account for no more than 15% to 20% of cases, but they have provided a large base of enlightening pathologic data.

Pathology of Sudden Death Caused by Coronary Artery Abnormalities

Coronary Arteries. Extensive atherosclerosis has long been recognized as the most common pathologic finding in the coronary arteries of victims of SCD. The combined results of a number of studies have suggested a general pattern of at least two coronary arteries with 75% or greater narrowing in more than 75% of the victims. Several studies have demonstrated no specific pattern of distribution of coronary artery lesions that preselect for SCD. In a quantitative analysis comparing coronary artery narrowing at postmortem examination in SCD victims and control subjects, 36% of the 5-mm segments of the coronary arteries from the SCD group had 76% to 100% cross-sectional area reductions compared with 3% in the control group. An additional 34% of sections from the SCD group had 51% to 75% reductions in cross-sectional area. Only 7% of sections from the SCD patients had 0% to 25% reductions in cross-sectional area.

The role of active coronary artery lesions, characterized by plaque fissuring, plaque erosion or rupture, platelet aggregation, and thrombosis, as a major pathophysiologic mechanism of the onset of cardiac arrest has become clarified (see Chap. 54). Among 100 consecutive victims of sudden coronary death, 44% had major (more than 50% luminal occlusion) recent coronary thrombi, 30% had minor occlusive thrombi, and 21% had plaque fissuring. Only 5% had no acute coronary artery changes; 65% of the thrombi occurred at sites of preexisting high-grade stenoses, and an additional 19% were found at sites of more than 50% stenosis. In a subsequent study, 50 (30%) of 168 victims had occlusive intraluminal coronary thrombi, and 73 (44%) had mural intraluminal thrombi. Single-vessel disease, acute infarction at postmortem examination, and prodromal symptoms were associated with the presence of thrombi. In a later study, plaque rupture or erosion was observed in 66% of culprit vessel lesions in victims of SCD related to coronary heart disease.[37] Disruption, platelet aggregation, and thrombosis are associated with markers of inflammation and various conventional risk factors for coronary atherosclerosis, such as cigarette smoking and hyperlipidemia.[121]

Some of the less common, nonatherosclerotic coronary artery abnormalities have specific pathologic features as well. Coronary artery spasm, an established cause of acute ischemia and SCD,[66] is commonly associated with nonobstructive plaques, and spasm itself has been recognized at postmortem examination in rare cases. When deep myocardial bridges are identified in association with SCD, patchy fibrosis in areas subserved by the affected vessel is commonly seen at postmortem examination. Coronary vasculitis in association with various autoimmune disorders may cause diffuse myocardial abnormalities, but asymptomatic cardiac involvement or global myocardial dysfunction is more common than SCD.

Myocardium. Myocardial injury in SCD caused by coronary heart disease reflects the extensive atherosclerosis usually present. Studies of victims of out-of-hospital SCD and from epidemiologic sources have indicated that healed myocardial infarction is a common finding in SCD victims, with most investigators reporting frequencies ranging from 40% to more than 70%. In one study, 72% of men in the 25- to 44-year age group who died suddenly (≤24 hours) with no previous clinical history of coronary heart disease had scars of large (63%) or small (<1-cm cross-sectional area, 9%) areas of healed myocardial necrosis. The incidence of acute myocardial infarction is considerably less, with cytopathologic evidence of recent myocardial infarction averaging about 20%. This estimate corresponds well with results of studies of out-of-hospital cardiac arrest survivors, who were found to have an incidence of new myocardial infarction in the range of 20% to 30%. These pathologic observations do not provide insight into the likely possibility that many SCDs occur by acute coronary syndrome mechanisms and progress from ischemia to fatal arrhythmias without time for structural markers to become visible. Even though there is an association between troponin level elevations during chest pain syndromes and risk of subsequent cardiac death, and troponin level increases are seen in a substantial proportion of cardiac arrest survivors, the question of whether the myocardial injury preceded or resulted from the cardiac arrest is difficult to resolve in individual cases.

Ventricular Hypertrophy. Myocardial hypertrophy can coexist and interact with acute or chronic ischemia but appears to confer an independent mortality risk. There is no close correlation between increased heart weight and severity of coronary heart disease in SCD victims; heart weights are higher in SCD victims than in those whose death is not sudden, despite similar prevalences of history of hypertension before death. Hypertrophy-associated mortality risk is also independent of left ventricular function and extent of coronary artery disease, and left ventricular hypertrophy itself may predispose to SCD. Experimental data have also suggested increased susceptibility to potentially lethal ventricular arrhythmias in left ventricular hypertrophy with ischemia and reperfusion. A study of massively enlarged hearts (i.e., weighing more than 1000 g), however, did not indicate an excess incidence of SCD, but the underlying pathologic process in that study was dominated by lesions that produce volume overload.

Specialized Conducting System in Sudden Cardiac Death. Fibrosis of the specialized conducting system may be observed in SCD victims. Although this process is associated with AV block or intraventricular conduction abnormalities, its role in SCD is uncertain. Lev disease, Lenègre's disease, ischemic injury caused by small-vessel disease, and numerous infiltrative or inflammatory processes can result in such changes. In addition, active inflammatory processes such as myocarditis and infiltrative processes such as amyloidosis, scleroderma, hemochromatosis, and morbid obesity may damage or destroy the AV node, bundle of His, or both and result in AV block.[122]

Focal diseases such as sarcoidosis, Whipple disease, and rheumatoid arthritis and fibrotic or fatty infiltration of the AV node or His-Purkinje system with apparent discontinuities[71] can also involve the conducting system (see Chap. 39). These various categories of conducting system disease have been considered possible pathologic substrates for SCD that might be overlooked because of the difficulty in doing careful postmortem examinations of the conducting system routinely. Focal involvement of conducting tissue by tumors (especially mesothelioma of the AV node but also lymphoma, carcinoma, rhabdomyoma, and fibroma) has also been reported, and rare cases of SCD have been associated with these lesions. It has been suggested that abnormal postnatal morphogenesis of the specialized conducting system may be a significant factor in some SCDs in infants and children.

Cardiac Nerves and Sudden Cardiac Death. Diseases of cardiac nerves have been postulated to have a role in SCD. Neural involvement may be the result of random damage to neural elements within the myocardium (i.e., secondary cardioneuropathy) or may be primary, as in a selective cardiac viral neuropathy. Secondary involvement can be a consequence of ischemic neural injury in coronary heart disease and has been postulated to result in autonomic destabilization, enhancing the propensity to arrhythmias. Nerve sprouting may be important.[123] Some experimental data have supported this hypothesis, and a clinical technique for imaging of cardiac neural fibers suggests a changing pattern over time after myocardial infarction. Viral, neurotoxic, and hereditary causes (e.g., progressive muscular dystrophy and Friedreich ataxia) have been emphasized.

Mechanisms and Pathophysiology

Electrical mechanisms of cardiac arrest are divided into tachyarrhythmic and bradyarrhythmia-asystolic events. The tachyarrhythmias include VF and pulseless or sustained VT, in which adequate blood flow cannot be maintained and perfusion is inadequate to meet the body's needs. Asystolic events include severe bradyarrhythmias—heart rates slow enough to impede adequate tissue perfusion and inability to generate a mechanical event because of complete absence of electrical activity (asystole) or dissociation between abnormal spontaneous electrical activity and mechanical function (pulseless electrical activity). It is likely that VF, or VT deteriorating to VF, is the initiating event in most cardiac arrests. After a variable time, fibrillation may cease and asystole or pulseless electrical activity emerges. In a significant minority of cases, however, the documented initial recording is asystole or pulseless electrical activity, which can continue as such or transform into VF.[124] More commonly, asystolic events or pulseless electrical activity follows an initial tachyarrhythmic event.

The occurrence of potentially lethal tachyarrhythmias, or of severe bradyarrhythmia or asystole, is the end of a cascade of pathophysiologic abnormalities that result from complex interactions between coronary vascular events, myocardial injury, variations in autonomic tone, and the metabolic and electrolyte state of the myocardium (see Fig. 41-5).[10] There is no uniform hypothesis of mechanisms by which these elements interact to lead to the final pathway of lethal arrhythmias. However, Figure 41-7 shows models of the pathophysiologic process of SCD that include vascular, myocardial, and functional components. The risk for cardiac arrest is conditioned by the presence of structural abnormalities and modulated by functional variations.[10,48,49]

Pathophysiologic Mechanisms of Lethal Tachyarrhythmias

Coronary Artery Structure and Function. Among the 80% of SCDs associated with coronary atherosclerosis, an extensive distribution of chronic arterial narrowing has been well defined by pathologic studies. However, the specific mechanisms by which these lesions lead to potentially lethal disturbances of electrical stability are not simply the consequence of steady-state reductions in regional myocardial blood flow in association with variable demands (see Chap. 43).[9,10] A simple increase in myocardial oxygen demand, in the presence of a fixed supply, may be a mechanism of exercise-induced arrhythmias and sudden death during intense physical activity or in others whose heart disease had not previously become clinically manifested. However, the dynamic nature of the pathophysiologic mechanism of coronary events has led to the recognition that superimposed acute lesions create a setting in which alterations in the metabolic or electrolyte state of the myocardium are the common circumstance leading to disturbed electrical stability. Active vascular events, leading to acute or transient reduction in regional myocardial blood flow in the presence of a normal or previously compromised circulation, constitute a common mechanism of ischemia, angina pectoris, arrhythmias, and SCD.[9,65] Coronary artery spasm or modulation of coronary collateral flow, predisposed to by local endothelial dysfunction, exposes the myocardium to the double hazard of transient ischemia and reperfusion (**Fig. 41-11**).[65] Neurogenic influences may play a role but do not appear to be a sine qua non for the production of spasm. Vessel susceptibility and humoral factors, particularly those related to platelet activation and aggregation, also appear to be important mechanisms.

Transition of stable atherosclerotic plaques to an "active" state because of endothelial damage, with plaque fissuring leading to platelet activation and aggregation followed by thrombosis, is a mechanism that appears to be present in most SCDs related to coronary heart disease (see Chap. 54). Inflammatory responses in atherosclerotic plaques are now viewed as the condition leading to lesion progression, including erosion, disruption, platelet activation, and thrombosis. In addition to causing subacute or acute critical reduction in regional blood flow, these mechanisms produce a series of biochemical alterations that may enhance or retard susceptibility to VF by means of vasomotor modulation.

The final step in the role of coronary artery pathophysiology leading to ischemia-induced arrhythmias is platelet aggregation and thrombosis (see Figs. 41-5 and 41-7; see Chap. 43). In 1984, Davies and Thomas noted that 95 of 100 subjects who died suddenly (less than 6 hours after the onset of symptoms) had acute coronary thrombi, plaque fissuring, or both. This incidence was considerably higher than in many previous reports, but it is noteworthy that only 44% of the patients had the largest thrombus occluding 51% or more of the cross-sectional area of the involved vessel and only 18% of the patients had more than 75% occlusion. These findings raised questions about whether mechanical obstruction to flow was dominant or whether the high incidence of nonoccluding thrombi simply reflected the state of activation of the platelets. The discrepancy between the relatively high incidence of acute thrombi in postmortem studies and the low incidence of evolution of new myocardial infarction among survivors of out-of-hospital VF highlights this point. The rapid initiation of lethal arrhythmias, the spontaneous thrombolysis, a dominant role of spasm induced by platelet products, or a combination of these factors may explain this observation.

Acute Ischemia and Initiation of Lethal Arrhythmias. The onset of acute ischemia produces immediate electrical, mechanical, and biochemical dysfunction of cardiac muscle. The specialized conducting tissue is more resistant to acute ischemia than working myocardium is, and therefore the electrophysiologic consequences are less intense and

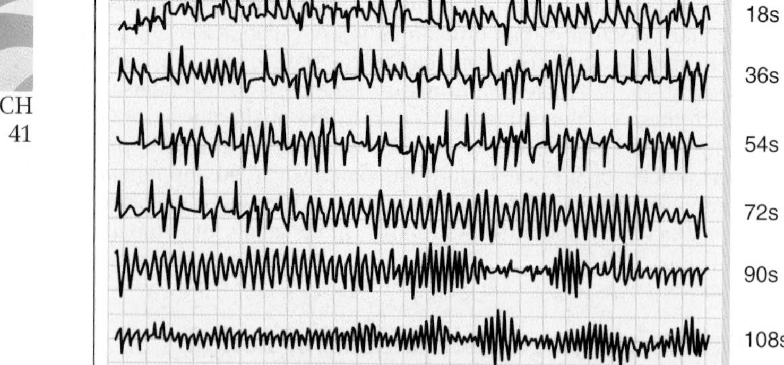

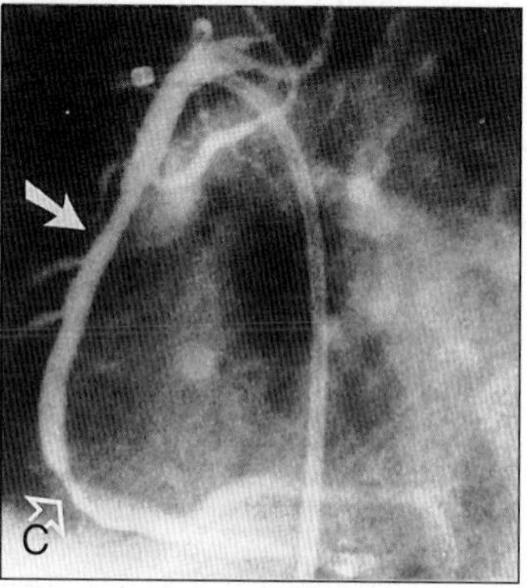

FIGURE 41-11 Life-threatening ventricular arrhythmias associated with acute myocardial ischemia related to coronary artery spasm and with reperfusion. **A,** Continuous lead II electrocardiographic monitor recording during ischemia (time, 0 to 55 seconds) caused by spasm of the right coronary artery **(B).** There is an abrupt transition (time, 56 to 72 seconds) from repetitive ventricular ectopy to a rapid polymorphic, prefibrillatory tachyarrhythmia (time, 80 to 130 seconds) associated with nitroglycerin-induced reversal of the spasm **(C).** Closed arrows indicate site of spasm before and after nitroglycerin; open arrow indicates lower grade distal lesion. *(Modified from Myerburg RJ, Kessler KM, Mallon SM, et al: Life-threatening ventricular arrhythmias in patients with silent myocardial ischemia due to coronary artery spasm. N Engl J Med 326:1451, 1992.)*

delayed in onset in specialized conduction tissue. Experimental studies have also provided data on the long-term consequences of left ventricular hypertrophy and healed experimental myocardial infarction. Tissue exposed to chronic stress produced by long-term left ventricular pressure overload and tissue that has healed after ischemic injury both show lasting cellular electrophysiologic abnormalities, including regional changes in transmembrane action potentials and refractory periods. Moreover, acute ischemic injury or acute myocardial infarction in the presence of healed myocardial infarction is more arrhythmogenic than the same extent of acute ischemia in previously normal tissue. In addition to the direct effect of ischemia on normal or previously abnormal tissue, reperfusion after transient ischemia can cause lethal arrhythmias (see Fig. 41-11). Reperfusion of ischemic areas can occur by three mechanisms: (1) spontaneous thrombolysis, (2) collateral flow from other coronary vascular beds to the ischemic bed, and (3) reversal of vasospasm. Some mechanisms of reperfusion-induced arrhythmogenesis appear to be related to the duration of ischemia before reperfusion. Experimentally, there is a window of vulnerability beginning 5 to 10 minutes after the onset of ischemia and lasting up to 20 to 30 minutes.

Electrophysiologic Effects of Acute Ischemia (see Chap. 35)**.** Within the first minutes after experimental coronary ligation, there is a propensity to ventricular arrhythmias that abates after 30 minutes and reappears after several hours. The initial 30 minutes of arrhythmias is divided into two periods, the first of which lasts for about 10 minutes and is presumably directly related to the initial ischemic injury. The second period (20 to 30 minutes) may be related either to reperfusion of ischemic areas or to the evolution of different injury patterns in the epicardial and endocardial muscle. Multiple mechanisms of reperfusion arrhythmias have been observed experimentally, including slow conduction and reentry and afterdepolarizations and triggered activity.

At the level of the myocyte, the immediate consequences of ischemia, which include alterations of cell membrane physiology, with efflux of K^+, influx of Ca^{2+}, acidosis, reduction of transmembrane resting potentials, and enhanced automaticity in some tissues, are followed by a separate series of changes during reperfusion. Those of particular interest are the possible continued influx of Ca^{2+}, which may produce electrical instability; responses to alpha or beta adrenoceptor stimulation, or both; and afterdepolarizations as triggering responses for Ca^{2+}-dependent arrhythmias. Other possible mechanisms studied experimentally include formation of superoxide radicals in reperfusion arrhythmias and differential responses of endocardial and epicardial muscle activation times and refractory periods during ischemia or reperfusion. The adenosine triphosphate–dependent K^+ current ($I_{K,ATP}$), which is inactive during normal conditions, is activated during ischemia. Its activation results in a strong efflux of K^+ ions from myocytes, markedly shortening the time course of repolarization and leading to slow conduction and ultimately to inexcitability. The fact that this response is more marked in epicardium than in endocardium leads to a prominent dispersion of repolarization across the myocardium during transmural ischemia. At an intercellular level, ischemia alters the distribution of connexin43, the primary gap junction protein between myocytes.[125] This alteration results in uncoupling of myocytes, a factor that is arrhythmogenic because of altered patterns of excitation and regional changes in conduction velocity.[126]

The importance of the myocardial response to the onset of ischemia has been emphasized on the basis of the demonstration of dramatic cellular electrophysiologic changes during the early period after coronary occlusion. However, the state of the myocardium at the time of onset of ischemia is a critical additional factor. Tissue healed after previous injury appears to be more susceptible to the electrical destabilizing effects of acute ischemia, as is chronically hypertrophied muscle. There are data suggesting that remodeling-induced local stretch, regional hypertrophy, or intrinsic cellular alteration may contribute to this vulnerability. Of more direct clinical relevance is the suggestion that potassium depletion by diuretics and clinical hypokalemia may make ventricular myocardium more susceptible to potentially lethal arrhythmias.

The association of metabolic and electrolyte abnormalities, and neurophysiologic and neurohumoral changes, with lethal arrhythmias emphasizes the importance of integrating changes in the myocardial substrate with systemic influences. Most direct among myocardial metabolic changes in response to ischemia are local acute increase in interstitial K^+ levels to values exceeding 15 mM, a decrease in the tissue pH to below 6.0, changes in adrenoceptor activity, and alterations in autonomic nerve traffic, all of which tend to create and to maintain electrical instability, especially if it is regional in distribution. Other metabolic changes, such as cyclic adenosine monophosphate elevation, accumulation of free fatty acids and their metabolites, formation of lysophosphoglycerides, and impaired myocardial glycolysis, have also been suggested as myocardial destabilizing influences.[127] These local myocardial changes integrate with systemic patterns of autonomic fluctuation that can be observed as patterns of altered heart rate variability and fractal dynamics,[128] potentially identifying subsets of patients predetermined to be at higher risk for SCD during an ischemic event.

TRANSITION FROM MYOCARDIAL INSTABILITY TO LETHAL ARRHYTHMIAS. The combination of a triggering event and a susceptible myocardium is a fundamental electrophysiologic concept for the mechanism of initiation of potentially lethal arrhythmias (see Figs.

41-5 and 41-7). The triggering event may be electrophysiologic, ischemic, metabolic, or hemodynamic. The endpoint of their interaction is disorganization of patterns of myocardial activation into multiple uncoordinated reentrant pathways (i.e., VF). Clinical, experimental, and pharmacologic data have suggested that triggering events in the absence of myocardial instability are unlikely to initiate lethal arrhythmias. Therefore, in the absence of myocardial vulnerability, many triggering events, such as frequent and complex PVCs, may be innocuous.

The onset of ischemia is accompanied by abrupt reductions in transmembrane resting potential and amplitude and in duration of the action potentials in the affected area, with little change in remote areas. When ischemic cells depolarize to resting potentials less than −60 mV, they may become inexcitable and of little electrophysiologic importance (see Chap. 35). As they are depolarizing to that range, however, or repolarizing as a consequence of reperfusion, the membranes pass through ranges of reduced excitability, upstroke velocity, and time courses of repolarization. These characteristics result in slow conduction and electrophysiologic heterogeneity. When this occurs in ischemic myocardium that is adjacent to nonischemic tissue, it creates a setting for the key elements of reentry, slow conduction, and unidirectional block, which makes the myocardium vulnerable to reentrant arrhythmias. When premature impulses are generated in this environment, regardless of their electrical mechanism (e.g., reentrant, triggered activity, automaticity), they may further alter the dispersion of recovery between ischemic tissue, chronically abnormal tissue, and normal cells, ultimately leading to complete disorganization and VF.

The dispersion of refractory periods produced by acute ischemia, which provides the substrate for reentrant tachycardias and VF, may be further enhanced by a healed ischemic injury. The time course of repolarization is lengthened after healing of ischemic injury and shortened by acute ischemia. The coexistence of the two appears to make the ventricle more susceptible to sustained arrhythmias in some experimental models.

Bradyarrhythmias and Asystolic Arrest

The basic electrophysiologic mechanism in this form of arrest is failure of normal subordinate automatic activity to assume the pacemaking function of the heart in the absence of normal function of the sinus node, AV junction, or both. Asystolic arrests are more common in severely diseased hearts and with cardiac arrest in patients with a number of end-stage disorders, cardiac and noncardiac. These mechanisms may result, in part, from diffuse involvement of subendocardial Purkinje fibers in advanced heart disease. Systemic influences that increase extracellular K^+ concentration, such as anoxia, acidosis, shock, renal failure, trauma, and hypothermia, can result in partial depolarization of normal or already diseased pacemaker cells in the His-Purkinje system, with a decrease in the slope of spontaneous phase 4 depolarization and ultimate loss of automaticity. These processes can produce global dysfunction of automatic cell activity, in contrast to the regional dysfunction more common in acute ischemia. Functionally depressed automatic cells (e.g., because of increased extracellular K^+ concentration) are more susceptible to overdrive suppression. Under these conditions, brief bursts of tachycardia may be followed by prolonged asystolic periods, with further depression of automaticity by the consequent acidosis and increased local K^+ concentration or by changes in adrenergic tone. The ultimate consequence may be degeneration into VF or persistent asystole.

Pulseless Electrical Activity

Pulseless electrical activity, formerly called electromechanical dissociation, is separated into primary and secondary forms. The common denominator in both is continued electrical rhythmicity of the heart in the absence of effective mechanical function. The secondary form includes the causes that result from an abrupt cessation of cardiac venous return, such as massive pulmonary embolism, acute malfunction of prosthetic valves, exsanguination, and cardiac tamponade from hemopericardium. The primary form is the more familiar; in this form, none of these obvious mechanical factors is present, but ventricular muscle fails to produce an effective contraction despite continued electrical activity (i.e., failure of electromechanical coupling). It usually occurs as an end-stage event in advanced heart disease, but it can occur in patients with acute ischemic events or, more commonly, after electrical resuscitation from a prolonged cardiac arrest. Although it is not thoroughly understood, it appears that diffuse disease, metabolic abnormalities, or global ischemia provides the pathophysiologic substrate. The proximate mechanism for failure of electromechanical coupling may be abnormal intracellular Ca^{2+} metabolism, intracellular acidosis, or perhaps adenosine triphosphate depletion.

Clinical Features of the Patient with Cardiac Arrest

Although the pathologic anatomy associated with SCD caused by coronary artery disease often reflects the changes associated with acute myocardial injury, only one of five survivors of out-of-hospital VF has clinical evidence of a new transmural myocardial infarction. Nonetheless, many have enzyme level elevations, with nonspecific electrocardiographic changes suggesting myocardial damage, which may be caused by transient ischemia as a triggering event or may be a consequence of the loss of myocardial perfusion during the cardiac arrest. The former supports the concept of transient pathophysiologic changes associated with acute coronary syndromes as the trigger for cardiac arrest. The recurrence rate is low among survivors of out-of-hospital cardiac arrest due to documented transmural myocardial infarction. In contrast, early studies have demonstrated a 30% recurrence rate at 1 year and 45% at 2 years in the survivors who did not have a new transmural myocardial infarction. Recurrence rates decreased subsequently, probably in part the result of long-term interventions. However, it is not known whether the decrease resulted from a change in the natural history, changes in preventive strategies for underlying disease, or long-term interventions for control of arrhythmic risk.

Clinical cardiac arrest and SCD can be described in the framework of the same four phases of the event used to establish temporal definitions (see Fig. 41-1): prodromes, onset of the terminal event, the cardiac arrest, and progression to biologic death or survival.

Prodromal Symptoms

Patients at risk for SCD can have prodromes such as chest pain, dyspnea, weakness or fatigue, palpitations, syncope, and a number of nonspecific complaints. Several epidemiologic and clinical studies have demonstrated that such symptoms can presage coronary events, particularly myocardial infarction and SCD, and result in contact with the medical system weeks to months before SCD. Among a group of patients successfully resuscitated after out-of-hospital cardiac arrest, 28% reported retrospectively that they had had new or changing angina pectoris or dyspnea in the 4 weeks before arrest, and 31% had seen a physician during this time, but only 12% because of these symptoms.

Attempts to identify early prodromal symptoms specific for risk of SCD have not been successful. Although several studies have reported that 12% to 46% of fatalities occur in patients who had seen a physician 1 to 6 months before death, such visits are more likely to presage myocardial infarction or nonsudden deaths, and most complaints responsible for those visits are not heart related. However, patients who have chest pain as a prodrome to SCD appear to have a higher probability of intraluminal coronary thrombosis at postmortem examination. Fatigue has been a particularly common symptom in the days or weeks before SCD in a number of studies, but this symptom is nonspecific. The symptoms that occur within the last hours or minutes before cardiac arrest are more specific for heart disease and may include symptoms of arrhythmias, ischemia, and heart failure.

Onset of the Terminal Event

The period of 1 hour or less between acute changes in cardiovascular status and the cardiac arrest itself is defined as the "onset of the terminal event." Ambulatory recordings fortuitously obtained during the onset of an unexpected cardiac arrest have indicated dynamic changes in cardiac electrical activity during the minutes or hours before the event. Increasing heart rate and advancing grades of ventricular ectopy are common antecedents of VF. Alterations in autonomic nervous system activity may also contribute to the onset of the event. Studies of short-term variations of heart rate variability, or related measures, have identified changes that correlate with the occurrence of ventricular arrhythmias. Although these physiologic properties may be associated with transient electrophysiologic destabilization of the myocardium, the extent to which they are paralleled by clinical symptoms or events has been less well documented.[129] SCDs caused by arrhythmias or acute circulatory failure mechanisms correlate with a high incidence of acute myocardial disorders at the onset of the terminal event; such disorders are more likely to be ischemic when the death is caused by arrhythmias and to be associated with low-output states or myocardial anoxia when the deaths are caused by circulatory failure.

Abrupt, unexpected loss of effective circulation can be caused by cardiac arrhythmias or mechanical disturbances, but most such events that terminate in SCD are arrhythmic. Hinkle and Thaler classified cardiac deaths in 142 subjects who died during a follow-up of 5 to 10 years. Class I was labeled arrhythmic death, and class II was death caused by circulatory failure. The distinction between the two classes was based on whether circulatory failure preceded (class II) or followed (class I) the disappearance of the pulse. Among deaths that occurred less than 1 hour after the onset of the terminal illness, 93% were caused by arrhythmias; in addition, 90% of deaths caused by heart disease were initiated by arrhythmic events rather than by circulatory failure. Deaths caused by circulatory failure occurred predominantly among patients who could be identified as having terminal illnesses (95% were comatose), were associated more frequently with bradyarrhythmias than with VF as the terminal arrhythmias, and were dominated by noncardiac events as the terminal illness. In contrast, 98% of the arrhythmic deaths were associated primarily with cardiac disorders.

Cardiac Arrest

Cardiac arrest is characterized by abrupt loss of consciousness caused by lack of adequate cerebral blood flow due to failure of cardiac pump function. It almost always leads to death in the absence of a successful intervention, although spontaneous reversions occur rarely. The most common electrical mechanism is VF, followed by asystole or pulseless electrical activity and pulseless VT. Mechanical mechanisms include rupture of the ventricle, cardiac tamponade, acute mechanical obstruction to flow, and acute disruption of a major blood vessel.

The potential for successful resuscitation is a function of the setting in which cardiac arrest occurs, the mechanism of the arrest, and the underlying clinical status of the victim. Closely related to the potential for successful resuscitation is the decision of whether to attempt to resuscitate.[130]

At present, there are fewer low-risk patients with otherwise uncomplicated myocardial infarctions weighting in-hospital cardiac arrest statistics than occurred previously. In one report, only 14% of patients receiving in-hospital cardiopulmonary resuscitation (CPR) were discharged from the hospital alive, and 20% of these patients died within the ensuing 6 months. Although 41% of the patients had suffered an acute myocardial infarction, 73% had a history of congestive heart failure and 20% had had prior cardiac arrests. The mean age of 70 years may have influenced the outcome statistics, but patients with high-risk complicated myocardial infarction and those with other high-risk markers heavily influenced the population of patients at risk for in-hospital cardiac arrest. Noncardiac clinical diagnoses were dominated by renal failure, pneumonia, sepsis, diabetes, and a history of cancer. The strong male preponderance consistently reported in out-of-hospital cardiac arrest studies is not present in in-hospital patients, but the better prognosis of VT or VF mechanisms, compared with pulseless electrical activity or asystolic mechanisms, persists (27% survival versus 8% survival). However, the proportion of arrests caused by in-hospital VT or VF is considerably less (33%), with the combination of respiratory arrest, asystole, and pulseless electrical activity dominating the statistics (61%). In another report, a 22% survival to hospital discharge was observed. Adverse risks were age older than 70 years, prior stroke or renal failure, and heart failure on admission. Better outcomes were predicted by prior angina pectoris or admission because of ventricular arrhythmias. Strategic factors affecting in-hospital cardiac arrest survival include the location in hospital, the type of hospital, daytime and evening events compared with nights and weekends, and a rapid time to defibrillation.[131]

The important risk factors for death after CPR are listed in **Table 41-4**. The fraction of out-of-hospital cardiac arrest survivors who are discharged from the hospital alive may now equal or exceed the fraction of in-hospital cardiac arrest victims who are discharged alive, and the post-discharge mortality rate for in-hospital cardiac arrest survivors is higher than that for out-of-hospital cardiac arrest survivors; these are telling clinical statistics. They emphasize the success of preventive measures for cardiac arrest in low-risk in-hospital patients, causing those statistics to be dominated by higher risk patients. However, other data demonstrate that in-hospital cardiac arrest survival is lower for events that occur during weeknights and weekends than during the daytime and evening hours during the week[131] and that more rapid times to defibrillation are advantageous.[132] These suggest the need for additional strategies for uniformly rapid in-hospital responses.[133]

Among elderly persons, the outcomes after community-based responses to out-of-hospital cardiac arrest are not as good as for younger victims. In one study comparing persons younger than 80 years (mean age, 64 years) with those in their 80s and 90s, survival to hospital discharge among the younger group was 19.4% compared with 9.4% for octogenarians and 4.4% for nonagenarians.[134] However, when the groups were analyzed according to markers favoring survival (e.g., VF, pulseless VT), the incremental benefit was even better for the elderly than for the younger patients (36%, 24%, and 17%, respectively), but the frequency of ventricular tachyarrhythmias compared with nonshockable rhythms was lower among elderly persons.[134] Overall, age is only a weak predictor of an adverse outcome and should not be used in isolation as a reason not to resuscitate. Long-term neurologic status and length of hospitalization were similar among older and younger surviving patients.

TABLE 41-4 Predictors of Mortality After In-Hospital Cardiopulmonary Resuscitation

Before Arrest
Hypotension (systolic BP < 100 mm Hg)
Pneumonia
Renal failure (BUN > 50 mg/dL)
Cancer
Homebound lifestyle
During Arrest
Arrest duration >15 min
Intubation
Hypotension (systolic BP < 100 mm Hg)
Pneumonia
Homebound lifestyle
After Resuscitation
Coma
Need for pressors
Arrest duration > 15 min

BP = blood pressure; BUN = blood urea nitrogen.
Modified from Bedell SE, Delbanco TL, Cook EF, Epstein FH: Survival after cardiopulmonary resuscitation in the hospital. N Engl J Med 309:569, 1983.

Progression to Biologic Death

The time course for progression from cardiac arrest to biologic death is related to the mechanism of the cardiac arrest, the nature of the underlying disease process, and the delay between onset and resuscitative efforts. The onset of irreversible brain damage usually begins within 4 to

6 minutes after loss of cerebral circulation, and biologic death follows quickly in unattended cardiac arrest. In large series, however, it has been demonstrated that a limited number of victims can remain biologically alive for longer periods and may be resuscitated after delays in excess of 8 minutes before beginning of basic life support and in excess of 16 minutes before advanced life support. Despite these exceptions, it is clear that the probability of a favorable outcome—survival neurologically intact—deteriorates rapidly as a function of time after cardiac arrest. Younger patients with less severe cardiac disease and the absence of coexistent multisystem disease have a higher probability of a favorable outcome after such delays.

Irreversible injury of the central nervous system usually occurs before biologic death, and the interval may extend days to weeks, and occasionally into very prolonged persistent vegetative states, in patients who are resuscitated during the temporal gap between brain damage and biologic death. In-hospital cardiac arrest caused by VF is less likely to have a protracted course between the arrest and biologic death, with patients surviving after a prompt intervention or succumbing rapidly because of inability to stabilize cardiac rhythm or hemodynamics.

The patients whose cardiac arrest is caused by sustained VT with cardiac output inadequate to maintain consciousness can remain in VT for considerably longer periods, with blood flow that is marginally sufficient to maintain viability. Thus, there is a longer interval between the onset of cardiac arrest and the end of the period that allows successful resuscitation. The lives of such patients usually end in VF or an asystolic arrest if the VT is not actively or spontaneously reverted. Once the transition from VT to VF or to a bradyarrhythmia has occurred, the subsequent course to biologic death is similar to that in patients in whom VF or bradyarrhythmias are the initiating event.

The progression in patients with asystole or pulseless electrical activity as the initiating event is more rapid. Such patients, whether in an in-hospital or out-of-hospital environment, have a poor prognosis because of advanced heart disease or coexistent multisystem disease. They tend to respond poorly to interventions, even if the heart is successfully paced. Although a small subgroup of patients with bradyarrhythmias associated with electrolyte or pharmacologic abnormalities may respond well to interventions, most progress rapidly to biologic death. The infrequent cardiac arrests caused by mechanical factors such as tamponade, structural disruption, and impedance to flow by major thromboembolic obstructions to right or left ventricular outflow are reversible only in patients in whom the mechanism is recognized and an intervention is feasible. Most of these events lead to rapid biologic death, although prompt relief of tamponade-induced cardiac arrests will save some lives.

Survivors of Cardiac Arrest

HOSPITAL COURSE. Cardiac arrests during the acute phase of myocardial infarction are classified as *primary* (electrical event not associated with hemodynamic dysfunction) or *secondary* (electrical event linked to hemodynamic dysfunction). Patients who are resuscitated immediately from primary VF associated with acute coronary syndromes usually stabilize promptly, and they require no long-term arrhythmia management based on the early arrhythmia (see Chap. 55). The management after secondary cardiac arrest in myocardial infarction is dominated by the hemodynamic status of the patient.

Survivors of out-of-hospital cardiac arrest may have repetitive ventricular arrhythmias during the initial 24 to 48 hours of hospitalization. These arrhythmias have variable responses to antiarrhythmic therapy, depending on hemodynamic status. The overall rate of recurrent cardiac arrest is low, 10% to 20%, but the mortality rate in patients who have recurrent cardiac arrests is about 50%. Only 5% to 10% of in-hospital deaths after out-of-hospital resuscitation are caused by recurrent cardiac arrhythmias. Patients who have recurrent cardiac arrest have a high incidence of new or preexisting AV or intraventricular conduction abnormalities.

The most common causes of death in hospitalized survivors of out-of-hospital cardiac arrest are noncardiac events related to central nervous system injury.[135] These include anoxic encephalopathy and sepsis related to prolonged intubation and hemodynamic monitoring lines. Fifty-nine percent of deaths during index hospitalization after out-of-hospital resuscitation have been reported to be from these causes. Approximately 40% of those who arrive at the hospital in coma never awaken after admission to the hospital and die after a median survival of 3.5 days. Two thirds of those who regain consciousness have no gross deficits, and an additional 20% have persisting cognitive deficits only. Of the patients who do awaken, 25% do so by admission, 71% by the first hospital day, and 92% by the third day. A small number of patients have awakened after prolonged hospitalization. Among those who die in the hospital, 80% do not awaken before death. Two studies have suggested a potential benefit of therapeutic hypothermia for patients with post–cardiac arrest coma (see later, Clinical Profile of Survivors of Out-of-Hospital Cardiac Arrest).[136,137]

Cardiac causes of delayed death during hospitalization after out-of-hospital cardiac arrest are most commonly related to hemodynamic deterioration, which accounts for about one third of deaths in hospitals. Among all deaths, those that occurred within the first 48 hours of hospitalization were usually caused by hemodynamic deterioration or arrhythmias regardless of the neurologic status; later deaths were related to neurologic complications. Admission characteristics most predictive of subsequent awakening included motor response, pupillary light response, spontaneous eye movement, and blood glucose level below 300 mg/dL.

CLINICAL PROFILE OF SURVIVORS OF OUT-OF-HOSPITAL CARDIAC ARREST. The clinical features of survivors of out-of-hospital cardiac arrest are heavily influenced by the type and extent of the underlying disease associated with the event. Causation is dominated by coronary heart disease, which accounts for approximately 80% of out-of-hospital cardiac arrest in the United States[7] and is commonly extensive. The cardiomyopathies collectively account for another 10% to 15%; all other structural heart diseases plus functional abnormalities and toxic or environmental causes account for the remainder (see Table 41-3).[63,138]

In a study of 63 survivors of cardiac arrest with normal ejection fractions and no obvious heart disease, no cause was identified after intensive studies in 44% of the patients.[139] The remainder were found to have long-QT syndromes (23%), catecholaminergic polymorphic ventricular tachycardia (23%), right ventricular dysplasia (17%), early repolarization (14%), coronary spasm (11%), Brugada syndrome (9%), and myocarditis (3%). The mean age of this group was 43 years, and 46% had had no prior history of presyncope or syncope.

LEFT VENTRICULAR FUNCTION. Left ventricular function is abnormal in most survivors of out-of-hospital cardiac arrest, often severely abnormal, but there is a wide variation, ranging from severe dysfunction to normal or near-normal measurements.[140] The severity of myocardial dysfunction estimated shortly after cardiac arrest is due to a combination of myocardial stunning consequent to the cardiac arrest itself with the extent of preexisting dysfunction. Stunning commonly improves within the first 24 to 48 hours,[141] and the residual is assumed to be due to preexisting disease or the acute injury leading to the cardiac arrest. If the ejection fraction is severely reduced initially, failure to begin improvement within the first 48 hours is an adverse short-term prognostic sign. In a study of resuscitated out-of-hospital cardiac arrest victims admitted to the hospital and subsequently discharged alive and neurologically intact, 47% had acute coronary syndromes identified during workup and had a mean ejection fraction of 42% compared with 32% in nonsurvivors.[142] Among survivors to hospital discharge, a reduced ejection fraction is an adverse long-term prognostic sign.

CORONARY ANGIOGRAPHY. Survivors of out-of-hospital cardiac arrest tend to have extensive coronary disease but no specific pattern of abnormalities. Acute coronary lesions, often multifocal, are present in most survivors.[139] Significant lesions in two or more vessels are present in at least 70% of patients who have any coronary lesion. Among patients who have recurrent cardiac arrests, the incidence of triple-vessel disease is higher than among those who do not. However, the frequency of moderate to severe stenosis of the left main coronary artery does not differ between cardiac arrest survivors and the overall population of patients with symptomatic coronary heart disease.

EXERCISE TESTING. Exercise testing is no longer commonly used to evaluate the need for and response to anti-ischemic therapy in survivors of out-of-hospital cardiac arrest, except when there is a question of transient ischemia as a mechanism for onset. The probability of a positive test result related to ischemia is relatively low, although termination of testing because of fatigue is common. Mortality during follow-up is higher in patients who fail to achieve a normal rise in systolic blood pressure during exercise.

Electrocardiographic Observations. Among survivors of out-of-hospital cardiac arrest, the 12-lead electrocardiogram (see Chap. 13) has proved of value only for discriminating risk of recurrence among those whose cardiac arrest was associated with new transmural myocardial infarction. Patients who develop documented new Q waves in association with a clinical picture that supports the assumption that an ST elevation myocardial infarction began before the cardiac arrest itself are at lower risk for recurrence.[1] In contrast, nonspecific electrocardiographic markers of ischemia, associated with elevations of troponin or creatine kinase MB levels, indicate higher risk of recurrence. A higher incidence of repolarization abnormalities (e.g., ST-segment depression, flat T waves, prolonged QT) occurs in out-of-hospital cardiac arrest survivors than in post–myocardial infarction patients, and these might be markers for increased risk. Prolonged QRS duration in association with a markedly reduced ejection fraction portends increased mortality risk.[143]

Blood Chemistry. Lower serum potassium levels are observed in survivors of cardiac arrest than in patients with acute myocardial infarction or stable coronary heart disease. This finding is often a consequence of resuscitation interventions rather than a preexisting hypokalemic state because of chronic diuretic use or other causes. Low ionized calcium levels, with normal total calcium levels, were also observed during resuscitation from out-of-hospital cardiac arrest. Higher resting lactate levels have been reported in out-of-hospital cardiac arrest survivors than in normal subjects. Lactate levels correlated inversely with ejection fractions and directly with PVC frequency and complexity.

LONG-TERM PROGNOSIS. Studies from the early 1970s had indicated that the risk of recurrent cardiac arrest in the first year after survival of an initial VT/VF event was about 30% and at 2 years was 45%. Total mortality at 2 years was about 60% in both studies. More recent mortality data,[144] including those from the control groups of the secondary prevention ICD trials,[145-147] have demonstrated 2-year mortality rates between 15% and 25%. The apparent improved outcomes, independent of the benefit provided by ICD therapy, are probably attributable to the current interventions used among survivors, such as beta adrenoceptor blockers, anti-ischemic procedures, and heart failure therapies that were not available or in general use at the earlier time. Risk of recurrent cardiac arrest and all-cause mortality is higher during the first 12 to 24 months after the index event and relates best to ejection fraction during the first 6 months.

Management of Cardiac Arrest

The response to a cardiac arrest is driven by two urgent principles: (1) maintenance of continuous artificial cardiopulmonary support until return of spontaneous circulation has been achieved; and (2) restoration of spontaneous circulation as quickly as possible. To achieve these goals, the management strategy is divided into five elements: (1) initial assessment and summoning of an emergency response team; (2) basic life support; (3) early defibrillation by a first responder (if available); (4) advanced life support; and (5) post–cardiac arrest care. If successful, the algorithm is followed by a sixth element, long-term management. The initial elements can be applied by a broad array of responders, which includes physicians and nurses as well as paramedical personnel, emergency rescue technicians, and lay people trained in bystander interventions. The requirements for specialized knowledge and skills increase progressively as the patient is moved through post–cardiac arrest management and into long-term follow-up care.[148] These emergency response principles are intended for both in-hospital application and community-based responses.

Community-Based Interventions

The initial systems responding to out-of-hospital cardiac arrests were integrated into fire departments as primary emergency rescue systems. Paramedical personnel were trained in CPR and in the use of monitoring equipment, defibrillators, and specific intravenous drug therapy. Although the initial out-of-hospital intervention experience in Miami and Seattle, reported in the mid-1970s, yielded only 14% and 11% rates of survival to discharge, respectively, later improvements in the systems saved more lives (**Fig. 41-12A**). Both had increased survival rates to about 25% by the early 1980s and to 30% or more by the late 1980s. Improvements correlated with the addition of emergency medical technicians as another tier of responders to provide CPR and earlier defibrillation. Survival rates have decreased since then, presumably because of the extension of rescue systems into less densely populated regions, in addition to increased traffic congestion and "verticalization" of buildings in urban areas (Fig. 41-12A). In general, rural areas have lower success rates, and the national success rate for the United States is probably 5% or less. Regional variability is highlighted by a 10-community analysis in the United States and Canada demonstrating a range of VF survival rates from 0% to 39.5%.[8]

Reports from different areas in the United States show marked variations in outcomes.[149] Some very densely populated areas (i.e., Chicago and New York City) have provided disturbing outcome data. A study from Chicago has reported that only 9% of out-of-hospital cardiac arrest victims survive to be hospitalized and that only 2% are discharged alive. Moreover, outcomes in blacks are far worse than those in whites (0.8% versus 2.6%). The fact that a large majority had bradyarrhythmias, asystole, or pulseless electrical activity on initial contact with emergency medical services suggests prolonged times between collapse and emergency medical service arrival, absent or ineffective bystander interventions, or both. The New York City report has indicated a survival to hospital discharge rate of only 1.4%. Among those who have bystander CPR, the rate increases to 2.9%, and bystander CPR plus VF as the initial rhythm yields a further increase to 5.3%. Finally, for those whose arrests occurred after the arrival of emergency medical services, the success rate increases further, to 8.5%. These trends support the concept that delays and breaks in the "chain of survival"[130] have a major negative impact on results of emergency medical services in densely populated areas.[149]

There are circumstances in which resuscitative efforts in the out-of-hospital setting are deemed futile. The victim found unconscious after an unwitnessed collapse, reasonably assumed to be found after a prolonged interval (e.g., cool skin, rigor mortis), obviously fulfills this classification. However, studies have provided markers of futility under less stark circumstances. In a study involving trained responders with automated external defibrillators (AEDs), only 0.5% of victims survived if (1) the arrest was not witnessed by emergency medical service personnel, (2) there was no return of spontaneous circulation, and (3) no shocks were delivered per protocol. Adding a response time longer than 8 minutes reduced survival to 0.3%, and events unwitnessed by a bystander yielded no survivors.[150]

IMPACT OF TIERED RESPONSE SYSTEMS. Improvements in both out-of-hospital care and in-hospital technology and practices can contribute to better outcomes, as described in the chain of survival concept.[148] Of these two general factors, the influence of out-of-hospital care has been studied in more detail. The importance of early defibrillation for improving outcome has been supported by a number of studies (see Fig. 41-e2 on website).[148,151-153] These observations have motivated the search for strategies that shorten response times, largely by the development of two-tiered systems (**Fig. 41-13A**) in which nonconventional first responders, such as police, firemen, security guards, and lay people, deploy AEDs in public places.[148,153-155] Preliminary data suggest that this strategy may improve outcome by substantial increments by the rationale of shortening response times (Fig. 41-13B).

In rural communities, earlier defibrillation by ambulance technicians yielded a 19% survival compared with only 3% for standard CPR. In another report, an analysis of the relationship between response delay and survival to hospital discharge revealed a 48% survival for response times of 2 minutes or less compared with less than 10% survival when responses were longer than 10 minutes (Fig. 41-13A).[152] Mean response time was approximately 13 minutes, and overall survival was 5%. It was 9.5% for those in VT or VF on first contact. A second element in out-of-hospital care that contributes to outcome is the role of bystander CPR by lay people awaiting the arrival of emergency rescue personnel.[156,157] It has been reported that although there was no significant difference in the percentage of patients successfully resuscitated and admitted to the hospital alive with (67%) or without (61%) bystander intervention, almost twice as many out-of-hospital

HISTORY OF COMMUNITY-BASED EMERGENCY RESPONSE SYSTEMS

Year	Outcome	Survival
1971–1974	Initial Miami/Seattle outcomes	14%, 11%
1978–1985	Peak Miami/Seattle outcomes	25%–35%
1984	Rural outcomes:	
	• Standard basic life support	3%
	• Ambulance-based expanded access	19%
1991	Estimated cumulative U.S. survival	1%–3%
1992–1994	Major metropolitan population centers	2%
1996	Dade county, Florida, current outcomes	9%
1996–1998	Updated U.S. EMS outcomes, cumulative	<5%
1999	"Optimized" EMS systems [OPALS]	5%
2000–2004	Non-conventional responders; Public access sites [Police, security guards, airline personnel, lay persons; airports and airliners, malls, casinos, stadiums]	17%–>50%

A

AED DEPLOYMENT STRATEGIES

Deployment	Examples	Rescuers	Advantages	Limitations
Emergency vehicles	• Police cars • Fire engines • Ambulances	• Trained emergency personnel	• Experienced users • Broad deployment • Objectivity	• Deployment time • Arrival delays • Community variations
Public access sites	• Public buildings • Stadiums, malls • Airports • Airliners	• Security personnel • Designated rescuers • Random laypersons	• Population density • Shorter delays • Lay and emergency personnel access	• Low event rates • Inexperienced users • Panic and confusion
Multifamily dwellings	• Apartments • Condominiums • Hotels	• Security personnel • Designated rescuers • Family members	• Familiar locations • Defined personnel • Shorter delays	• Infrequent use • Low event rates • Geographic factors
Single-family dwellings	• Private homes • Apartments • Neighborhood "Heart watch"	• Family members	• Immediate access • Familiar setting	• Acceptance • Victim may be alone • One-time user; panic

B

FIGURE 41-12 Out-of-hospital cardiac arrest survival and automated external defibrillator (AED) deployment strategies. **A,** The history of out-of-hospital cardiac arrest survival statistics demonstrates that standard emergency rescue systems are not sufficient to have a meaningful impact on sudden cardiac death in the community. **B,** Various deployment strategies for nonconventional responders with access to AEDs. For each example, the type of rescuer and the advantages and limitations of each strategy are provided. It is unlikely that any single strategy will dominate; rather, there will be a cumulative benefit from the additive effect of multiple approaches. EMS = emergency medical service; OPALS = Ontario Prehospital Advanced Life Support. *(From Myerburg RJ: Sudden cardiac death: Exploring the limits of our knowledge. J Cardiovasc Electrophysiol 12:369, 2001.)*

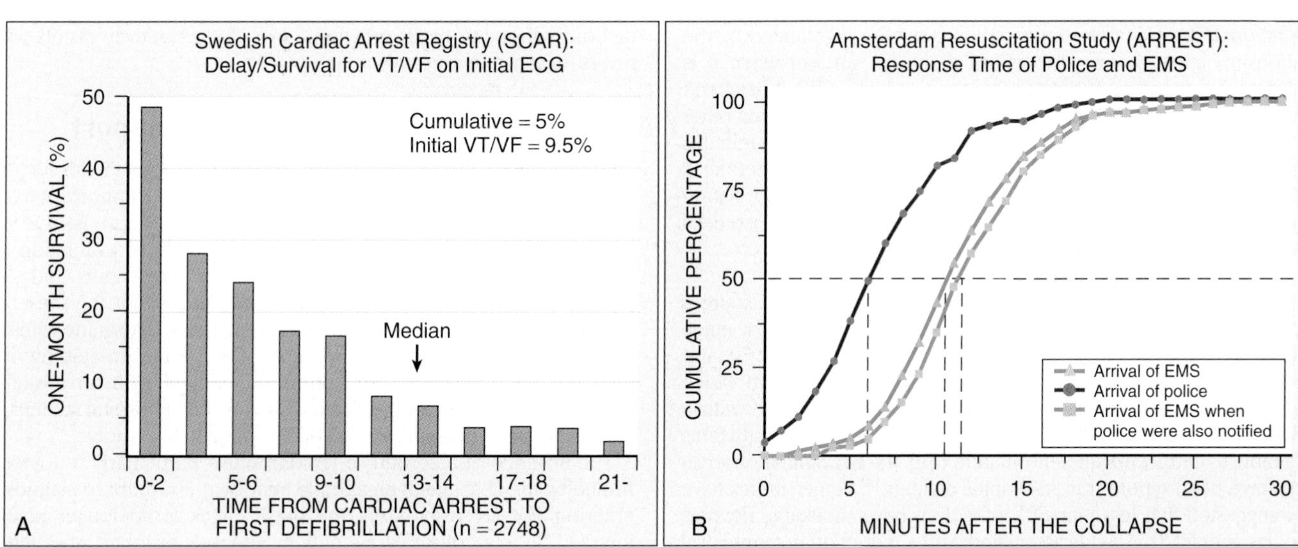

FIGURE 41-13 Influence of response time on survival from out-of-hospital cardiac arrest. **A,** The time from onset of cardiac arrest to initial defibrillation attempt is related to 1-month survival on the basis of data from the Swedish Cardiac Arrest Registry.[173] The cumulative survival rate was 5%, and the survival rate for victims whose initial rhythm was ventricular tachycardia (VT) or ventricular fibrillation (VF) was 9.5%. The median response time was nearly 13 minutes. Thirty-day survival ranged from a maximum of 48% with responses shorter than 2 minutes to less than 5% with response time longer than 15 minutes. *(Modified from Holmberg M, Holmberg S, Herlitz J: The problem of out-of-hospital cardiac arrest: Prevalence of sudden death in Europe today. Am J Cardiol 83:88D, 1999, with permission of the publisher.)* **B,** The potential for faster response systems, based on the Amsterdam Resuscitation Study, is demonstrated, comparing response times of police vehicles with those of conventional emergency medical systems (EMS). At the 50th percentile of response times, police vehicles provided a nearly 5-minute improvement in arrival time (approximately 6 minutes). *(Modified from Waalewijn RA, de Vos R, Koster RW: Out-of-hospital cardiac arrests in Amsterdam and its surrounding areas: Results from the Amsterdam resuscitation study [ARREST] in "Utstein" style. Resuscitation 28:157, 1998.)*

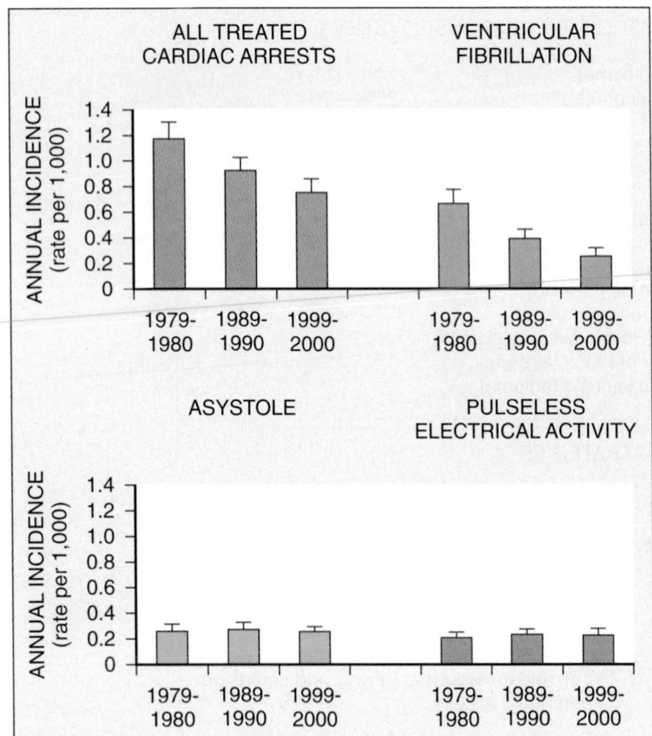

FIGURE 41-14 Changing incidence of ventricular fibrillation in the community. Between 1980 and 2000, there was a progressive decrease in the ventricular fibrillation event rate in the Seattle, Washington, community for unexplained reasons. Of note is the fact that there was no concomitant increase in nonshockable rhythms. The proportion of events with ventricular fibrillation at initial contact is decreasing, as observed in several other studies. *(Modified from Cobb LA, Fahrenbruch CE, Olsufka M, Copass MK: Changing incidence of out-of-hospital ventricular fibrillation, 1980-2000. JAMA 288:3008, 2002.)*

cardiac arrest victims were ultimately discharged alive when they had had bystander CPR (43%) than when such support was not provided (22%). Central nervous system protection, expressed as early regaining of consciousness, is the major protective element of bystander CPR. The rationale for bystander intervention is further highlighted by the relationship between time to defibrillation and survival when it is analyzed as a function of time to initiation of basic CPR. It has been reported that more than 40% of victims whose defibrillation and other advanced life support activities were instituted more than 8 minutes after collapse survived if basic CPR had been initiated less than 2 minutes after onset of the arrest. A period of CPR before defibrillation may also be helpful,[156] particularly if the time to defibrillation exceeds 4 minutes from onset of arrest.[151,158]

IMPORTANCE OF ELECTRICAL MECHANISMS. Several sources have identified a disturbing trend in initial rhythms recorded by emergency rescue personnel.[5,154,159] Compared with data from the 1970s and 1980s, there has been a decrease in the number of events in which ventricular tachyarrhythmias are the initial rhythm recorded, with a consequent reduction in the proportion of victims who have rhythms amenable to cardioversion-defibrillation (**Fig. 41-14**). Similar observations have been reported in in-hospital settings.[160] Some studies have now suggested that less than 50% of victims have shockable rhythms at initial contact. This fact is associated with a reduction in cumulative survival probabilities from community-based interventions,[5] even though data from studies using nonconventional AED strategies have suggested improvement for outcomes in VT or VF victims.[154,159] Because this finding does not appear to be related to time from the 911 summons to arrival, it is likely that pre-911 delays in recognition and reaction to an event may be playing a role, which suggests a need for more extensive public education programs. Thus, response times may not be as close to true downtimes as one would hope, impairing the potential for success. The 4- to 6-minute time for a desirable response is not optimal. By 4 minutes, significant circulatory and ischemic changes have occurred, and conditions worsen rapidly beyond that time.[151]

The electrical mechanism of out-of-hospital cardiac arrest, as defined by the initial rhythm recorded by emergency rescue personnel, has a powerful impact on outcome. The subgroup of patients who are in sustained VT at the time of first contact, although small, has the best outcome. Eighty-eight percent of patients in cardiac arrest related to VT were successfully resuscitated and admitted to the hospital alive, and 67% were ultimately discharged alive. However, this relatively low risk group represents only 7% to 10% of all cardiac arrests. Because of the inherent time lag between collapse and initial recordings, it is likely that many more cardiac arrests begin as rapid sustained VT and degenerate into VF before arrival of rescue personnel.

Patients who have a bradyarrhythmia or asystole, or pulseless electrical activity, at initial contact have the worst prognosis; only 9% of such patients in the Miami study were admitted to the hospital alive, and none was discharged. In a later experience, there was some improvement in outcome, although the improvement was limited to patients in whom the initial bradyarrhythmia recorded was an idioventricular rhythm that responded promptly to chronotropic agents in the field. In a large prospective observational in-hospital study of cardiac arrests in children and adults, children had a higher probability of asystole or pulseless electrical activity as the initial documented rhythm but had a better overall survival rate because they had better outcomes of interventions for these rhythms than adults did.[160]

Bradyarrhythmias also have adverse prognostic implications after defibrillation from VF in the field. Patients who developed a heart rate lower than 60 beats/min after defibrillation regardless of the specific bradyarrhythmic mechanism had a poor prognosis, with 95% of such patients dying before hospitalization or in the hospital. The outcome in the group of patients in whom VF is the initial rhythm recorded is intermediate between the outcomes associated with sustained VT and bradyarrhythmia and asystole. Of such patients, 40% were successfully resuscitated and admitted to the hospital alive, and 23% were ultimately discharged alive. Later data indicate improvement in outcome. The proportion of each of the electrophysiologic mechanisms responsible for cardiac arrest varied among the earlier reports, with VF ranging from 65% to more than 90% of the study populations and bradyarrhythmia and asystole ranging from 10% to 30%. However, in reports from densely populated metropolitan areas, the ratios of tachyarrhythmic to bradyarrhythmic or pulseless activity events were reversed, and outcomes were far worse.[149]

Initial Assessment and Basic Life Support

The activities at initial contact with the unconscious victim include diagnostic maneuvers and basic cardiopulmonary support interventions. The first action must be confirmation that collapse is or is suspected of being a cardiac arrest. A few seconds of evaluation for response to voice, observation for respiratory movements and skin color, and simultaneous palpation of major arteries for the presence or absence of a pulse yield sufficient information to determine whether a life-threatening incident is in progress. Once a life-threatening incident has been suspected or confirmed, contact with an available emergency medical rescue system (911) for out-of-hospital settings, or a "code" team in-hospital, should be an immediate priority.

The absence of a carotid or femoral pulse, particularly if it is confirmed by the absence of an audible heartbeat, is a primary diagnostic criterion. For lay responders, the pulse check is no longer recommended.[130] Skin color may be pale or intensely cyanotic. Absence of respiratory efforts or the presence of only agonal respiratory efforts, in conjunction with an absent pulse, is diagnostic of cardiac arrest; however, respiratory efforts can persist for 1 minute or longer after the onset of the arrest. In contrast, absence of respiratory efforts or severe stridor with persistence of a pulse suggests a primary respiratory arrest that will lead to a cardiac arrest in a short time. In the latter circumstance, initial efforts should include exploration of the oropharynx in search of a foreign body and the Heimlich maneuver, particularly if the incident occurs in a setting in which aspiration is likely (e.g., restaurant death or café coronary).

CHEST THUMP. When the diagnosis of a pulseless collapse is established, a blow to the chest (precordial thump, "thumpversion") may be attempted by a properly trained rescuer. It has been recommended that it be reserved as an advanced life support activity.[130] Its use has been supported on the basis of a prospective study in 5000 patients. Precordial thumps successfully reverted VF in 5 events, VT in 11, asystole in 2, and undefined cardiovascular collapse in 2 others in which the electrical mechanism was unknown. In no case was conversion of VT to VF observed. Because the latter is the only major concern about the precordial thump technique and electrical activity can be initiated by mechanical stimulation in the asystolic heart, the technique is considered optional for responding to a pulseless cardiac arrest in the absence of monitoring when a defibrillator is not immediately available. It should not be used unmonitored for the patient with a rapid tachycardia without complete loss of consciousness. The thumpversion technique employs one or two blows delivered firmly to the junction of the middle and lower thirds of the sternum from a height of 8 to 10 inches. The effort should be abandoned if the patient does not immediately develop a spontaneous pulse and begin breathing. Another mechanical method, which requires that the patient be still conscious, is so-called cough-induced cardiac compression, or cough version. It is a conscious act of forceful coughing by the patient that may support forward flow by cyclic increases in intrathoracic pressure during VF or may cause conversion of sustained VT. Available data supporting its successful use are limited, and it is not considered an alternative to conventional techniques.

BASIC LIFE SUPPORT—THE ABCS OF CARDIOPULMONARY RESUSCITATION. The goal of this activity is to maintain viability of the central nervous system, heart, and other vital organs until definitive intervention can be achieved. Basic life support encompasses both the initial responses outlined earlier and their natural flow into establishing ventilation and perfusion. This range of activities can be carried out not only by professional and paraprofessional personnel but also by trained emergency technicians and lay people. Time is crucial, so there should be minimal delay between the diagnosis and preparatory efforts in the initial response and the institution of basic life support. This principle has measurable impact for out-of-hospital and in-hospital cardiac arrest. Survival to discharge for in-hospital cardiac arrests, considering all causes and mechanisms, was reported to be 33% when CPR was initiated within the first minute compared with 14% when the time was longer than 1 minute (odds ratio, 3.06).[133] When VF was the initial rhythm, the corresponding figures were 50% and 32%, respectively. In the out-of-hospital setting, if only one witness is present, notification of emergency personnel (calling 911) is the only activity that should precede basic life support.

AIRWAY. Clearing of the airway is a critical step in preparing for successful resuscitation. This process includes tilting the head backward and lifting the chin, in addition to exploring the airway for foreign bodies, including dentures, and removing them. The Heimlich maneuver should be performed if there is reason to suspect that a foreign body is lodged in the oropharynx. This maneuver entails wrapping the arms around the victim from the back and delivering a sharp thrust to the upper abdomen with a closed fist. If it is not possible for the person in attendance to carry out the maneuver because of insufficient physical strength, mechanical dislodgment of the foreign body can sometimes be achieved by abdominal thrusts with the unconscious patient in a supine position. The Heimlich maneuver is not entirely benign; ruptured abdominal viscera in the victim have been reported, as has a case in which the rescuer disrupted his own aortic root and died. If there is strong suspicion that respiratory arrest precipitated cardiac arrest, particularly in the presence of a mechanical airway obstruction, a second precordial thump should be delivered after the airway has been cleared.

BREATHING. With the head properly placed and the oropharynx clear, mouth-to-mouth resuscitation can be initiated if no specific rescue equipment is available. To a large extent, the procedure used to establish ventilation depends on the site at which the cardiac arrest occurs. Various devices are available, including plastic oropharyngeal airways, esophageal obturators, the masked Ambu bag, and endotracheal tubes. Intubation is the preferred procedure, but time should not be sacrificed, even in the in-hospital setting, while awaiting an endotracheal tube or a person trained to insert it quickly and properly. Thus, in the in-hospital setting, temporary support with Ambu bag ventilation is the usual method until endotracheal intubation can be carried out, and in the out-of-hospital setting, mouth-to-mouth resuscitation is used while awaiting emergency rescue personnel. The effect of the acquired immunodeficiency syndrome and hepatitis B transmission on attitudes about mouth-to-mouth resuscitation by bystanders and even professional personnel in hospitals is an area of concern, but currently available data assessing risk of infection suggest that it is minimal.[130] The impact of this concern on attitudes toward and outcomes of resuscitative efforts has not been assessed.

CIRCULATION. This element of basic life support is intended to maintain blood flow (i.e., circulation) until definitive steps can be taken. The rationale is based on the hypothesis that chest compression allows the heart to maintain an externally driven pump function by sequential emptying and filling of its chambers, with competent valves favoring the forward direction of flow. In fact, the application of this technique has proved successful when it is used as recommended.[130] The palm of one hand is placed over the lower sternum and the heel of the other rests on the dorsum of the lower hand. The sternum is then depressed, with the resuscitator's arms straight at the elbows to provide a less tiring and more forceful fulcrum at the junction of the shoulders and back (see Fig. 41-e3 on website). By use of this technique, sufficient force is applied to depress the sternum about 4 to 5 cm, with abrupt relaxation, and the cycle is carried out at a rate of about 100 compressions/min.[130]

Techniques of CPR based on the hypothesis that increased intrathoracic pressure is the prime mover of blood, rather than cardiac compression itself, have been evaluated, and the guidelines for conventional CPR ventilatory techniques were modified in 2005. For single responders to victims from infancy (excluding newborns) through adulthood, and for adults responded to by two rescuers, a compression-ventilation ratio of 30 : 2 is now recommended.[130] For two-rescuer CPR for infants and children, the former compression-ventilation ratio of 15 : 2 is retained. A more recent modification intended to encourage more bystander participation in CPR and to allay concerns about mouth-to-mouth ventilation of unknown victims is the "hands-only" (compression-only) technique.[161] This technique is intended for untrained or remotely trained bystanders who are not confident about their ability to perform compression-ventilation sequences. Bystanders familiar with the standard technique should use the 30 : 2 compression-ventilation ratio. The 2005 changes in CPR recommendations, reducing the number of successive shocks and pulse checks during initial responses (see Defibrillation-Cardioversion), are intended in part to increase the cumulative time of circulatory support during CPR, before restoration of a spontaneous pulse.[162]

CONCEPT OF CARDIOCEREBRAL RESUSCITATION. This concept, also referred to as minimally interrupted cardiac resuscitation, is based on the hypothesis that the primary benefit in CPR is pumping action rather than the combination of compression and ventilation. It challenges the general guidelines that assume a benefit of interrupting compression to provide ventilation and that an initial phase of ventilation before initial defibrillation improves outcomes with response times longer than 4 or 5 minutes. Cardiocerebral resuscitation emphasizes continuous chest compressions, interrupted primarily for single shocks and evaluation of responses to shocks, deferring and limiting ventilatory and certain pharmacologic actions. Data from studies in Japan[163] and the United States[164,165] suggest a neurologically intact survival advantage of the cardiocerebral protocol compared with conventional CPR based on the 2000 Guidelines and 2005 Update. For witnessed arrests with documented VF, the study from Japan demonstrated a neurologically intact survival advantage of 22% versus 10%. The two recent reports from the United States demonstrated comparable advantages of 39% versus 15% for neurologically intact survival and 28.4% versus 11.9% for survival, respectively. Despite these interesting data, it remains generally agreed that a randomized trial is needed before the minimal interruption concept can replace the current guidelines.

Despite the fact that conventional techniques produce measurable carotid artery flow and a record of successful resuscitations, the absence of a pressure gradient across the heart in the presence of an extrathoracic arteriovenous pressure gradient has led to the concept that it is not cardiac compression per se but rather a pumping action produced by pressure changes in the entire thoracic cavity that optimizes systemic blood flow during resuscitation. Experimental work in which the chest is compressed during ventilations rather than between

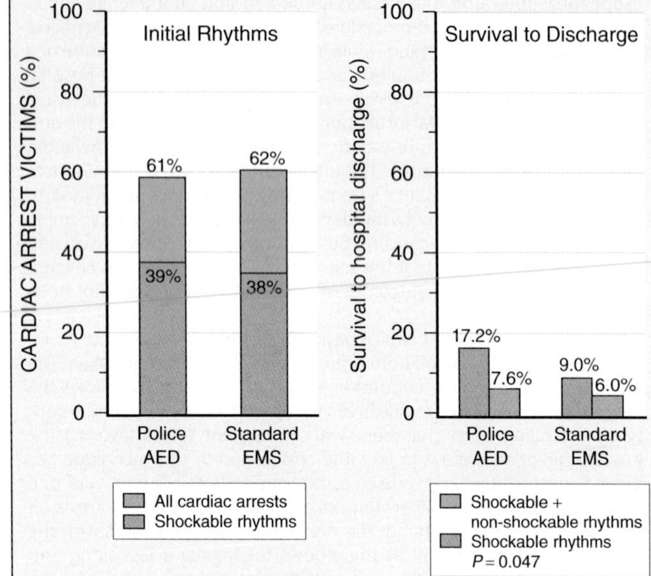

FIGURE 41-15 Rhythms at initial contact and survival statistics from the Miami–Dade County, Florida, police automated external defibrillator (AED) project. Shockable rhythms were observed in just below 40% of cardiac arrest victims in both the police AED program and the standard emergency medical system (EMS) historical control data. Those with shockable rhythms had improved survival to hospital discharge, with only a small improvement when both shockable and nonshockable rhythms were included in the analyzed data. *(Modified from Myerburg RJ, Fenster J, Velez M, et al: Impact of community-wide police car deployment of automated external defibrillators on out-of-hospital cardiac arrest. Circulation 106:1058, 2002.)*

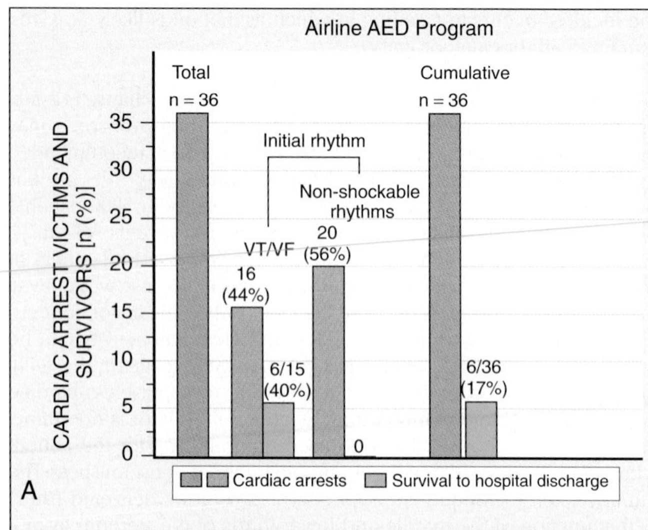

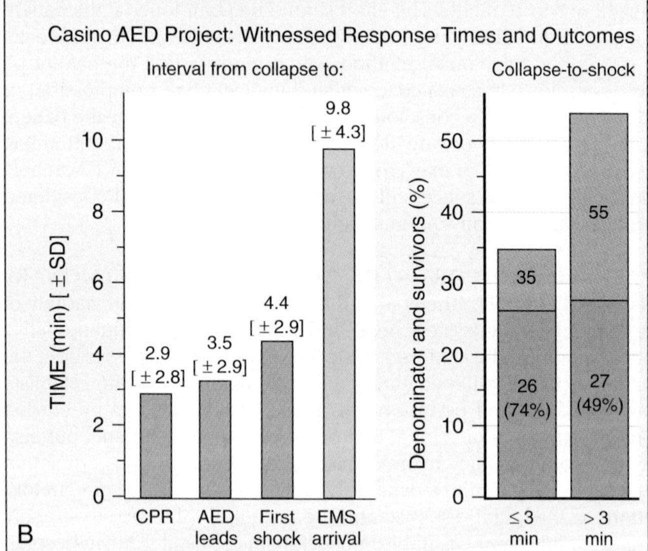

FIGURE 41-16 Outcomes of automated external defibrillator (AED) deployment programs at specific public sites. **A,** The data on outcomes after deployment of AEDs on a major airline demonstrated that approximately 44% of the cardiac arrests were associated with a documented ventricular tachycardia or fibrillation (VT/VF) mechanism and 40% of those victims survived. There were no survivors among the 56% of the victims who had nonshockable rhythms. Cumulative survival for the program was 17%. **B,** The results of AED deployment in the controlled environment of casinos. Because the onset of cardiac arrest can frequently be witnessed, short intervals from onset of collapse to CPR and AED shocks were achieved. Response times were reduced by more than 50% compared with the standard emergency medical system (EMS). For those found in VT/VF, survival was better than expected from other community-based systems and approached 60% for VT/VF with a witnessed onset. When response time was less than 3 minutes, survival for VT/VF was more than 70%. *(**A** modified from Page RL, Joglar JA, Kowal RC, et al: Use of automated external defibrillators by a U.S. airline. N Engl J Med 343:1210, 2000. **B** modified from Valenzuela TD, Roe DJ, Nichol G, et al: Outcomes of rapid defibrillation by security officers after cardiac arrest in casinos. N Engl J Med 343:1206, 2000.)*

them (simultaneous compression-ventilation) has demonstrated better extrathoracic arterial flow. However, increased carotid artery flow does not necessarily equate with improved cerebral perfusion, and the reduction in coronary blood flow caused by elevated intrathoracic pressures with use of certain techniques may be too high a price for the improved peripheral flow. In addition, a high thoracoabdominal gradient has been demonstrated during experimental simultaneous compression-ventilation, which could divert flow from the brain in the absence of concomitant abdominal binding. On the basis of these observations, new mechanically assisted techniques, including an active decompression phase (i.e., active compression-decompression), have been evaluated for improved circulation during CPR.[166] More clinical studies are needed before their general clinical applications are established.

Early Defibrillation by First Responders

The time from onset of cardiac arrest to advanced life support influences outcome statistics. Improvement in both early neurologic status and survival occurs in patients defibrillated by first responders, compared with outcomes associated with awaiting the assistance of more highly trained paramedics. The term *first responder* refers to the person on scene providing the initial resuscitative action and has emerged from minimally trained emergency technicians allowed to carry out defibrillation in conjunction with basic life support to nonconventional responders, such as trained security guards and police, and most recently to laypersons knowledgeable in CPR with access to AEDs. Because the time to defibrillation plays a central role in determining outcome in cardiac arrest caused by VF, the development and deployment of AEDs (see Chap. 38) in the community hold promise for progress in the future. This technology is potentially applicable to a number of different strategic models, each with its own benefits and limitations (see Fig. 41-12B).

Among the strategies that have yielded identifiable survival benefits to date are deployment in police vehicles,[152,154,159] airliners and airports,[167,168] casinos,[169] and more general community-based sites.[159,170] Police AED deployment data have been inconsistent in various studies,[148,152,156] possibly because of appropriateness for various types of communities and specific deployment strategies used, but data suggest that there is benefit in large metropolitan areas (**Fig. 41-15**).[154] Initial airline data were similarly uncertain, but a more recent report on data from a large airline with a well-organized system has suggested benefit (**Fig. 41-16A**).[167] Similar encouraging results have been reported from deployment of AEDs in the Chicago airport system.[168] Finally, the special circumstance of casinos, in which continuous television monitoring alerts security officers to medical problems immediately, has yielded impressive survival rates (Fig. 41-16B).[169] For more general community sites, defined as true public access, a large study has suggested a twofold benefit.[170] However, there appears to be a great deal of variability of efficiency on the basis of expected event rates at different types of community sites, and deployment strategies have been suggested on the basis of projected event rates at various locations.[171] Deployment in schools, accompanied by comprehensive response planning, demonstrates relatively low event rates but good outcomes.[172] A study of the deployment of AEDs in the home for patients who had recent myocardial infarctions and were not candidates for implantable defibrillators did not demonstrate benefit.[173] Because the home is the most common site of cardiac arrest and has lower survival rates than in public sites, additional strategies for both AEDs and other technologies should be tested. A study evaluating the LifeVest in this setting is under way.[174]

As is the case for any medical device,[175] infrequent malfunctions of AEDs may occur, caused by design or manufacturing defects[176] or by failure to adhere to manufacturers' recommendations for replacement of batteries and leads. It is an obligation of those responsible for maintaining AEDs to remain cognizant of FDA safety alerts and recalls and shelf-lives of batteries and leads.

Advanced Life Support

This next step in the resuscitative sequence is designed to achieve a stable return of spontaneous circulation and hemodynamic stabilization.[130] The implementation of advanced life support is not intended to suggest an abrupt cessation of basic life support activities but rather a merging and transition from one level of activity to the next. In the past, advanced life support required judgments and technical skills that removed it from the realm of activity of lay bystanders and even emergency medical technicians, limiting these activities to specifically trained paramedical personnel, nurses, and physicians. With further education of emergency technicians, most community-based CPR programs now permit them to carry out advanced life support activities. However, some studies suggest that addition of advanced life support to an otherwise optimized out-of-hospital response system (i.e., bystander CPR and early defibrillation) does not improve statistics for neurologically intact survival.[177] In this regard, the development and testing of AEDs that have the ability to sense and to analyze cardiac electrical activity and prompt the user to deliver definitive electrical intervention provide a role for less highly trained rescue personnel (i.e., police, ambulance drivers) and even untrained or minimally trained lay bystanders[168,170] for rapid defibrillation.

The general goals of advanced life support are to revert the cardiac rhythm to one that is hemodynamically effective, to optimize ventilation, and to maintain and support the restored circulation. Thus, during advanced life support, the patient's cardiac rhythm is promptly cardioverted or defibrillated as the first priority if appropriate equipment is immediately available. A short period of closed chest cardiac compression immediately before defibrillation enhances the probability of survival, especially if circulation has been absent for ≥4 to 5 minutes.[151,156,158] After the initial attempt to restore a hemodynamically effective rhythm, the patient is intubated and oxygenated, if needed, and the heart is paced if a bradyarrhythmia or asystole occurs. An intravenous line is established to deliver medications. After intubation, the goal of ventilation is to reverse hypoxemia and not merely to achieve a high alveolar oxygen pressure (P_{O_2}). Thus, oxygen rather than room air should be used to ventilate the patient; if possible, the arterial P_{O_2} should be monitored. Respiratory support in the hospital and an Ambu bag by means of an endotracheal tube, or facemasks in the out-of-hospital setting, are generally used.

DEFIBRILLATION-CARDIOVERSION. Rapid conversion to an effective cardiac electrical mechanism is a key step for successful resuscitation (**Fig. 41-17**). Delay should be minimal, even when conditions for CPR are optimal. When VF or VT that is pulseless or accompanied by loss of consciousness is recognized on a monitor or by telemetry, defibrillation should be carried out immediately. An initial shock of 360 J should be delivered by monophasic devices and 120 to 200 J by biphasic devices, with the energy depending on the recommendations for individual biphasic devices. Energies delivered through AEDs are generally preprogrammed and vary among available devices. Failure of

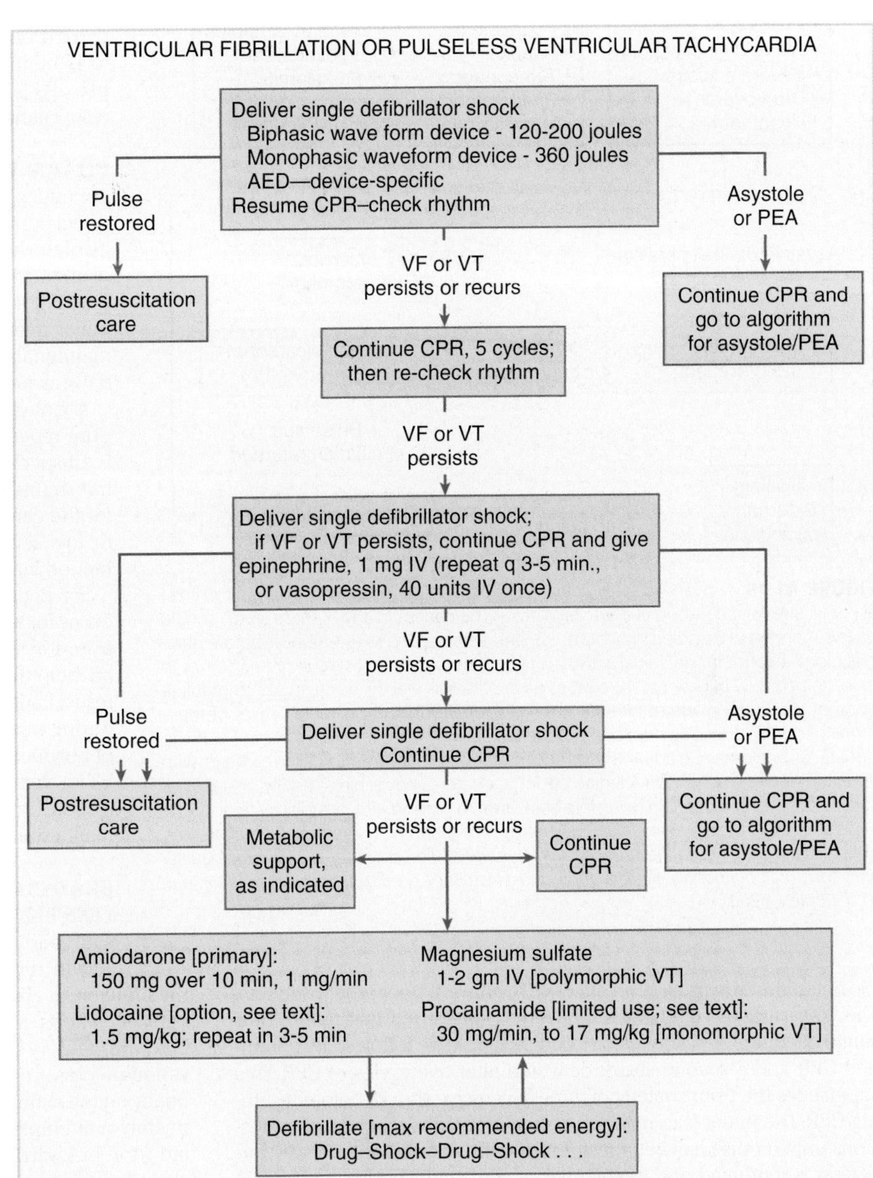

FIGURE 41-17 Advanced life support for ventricular fibrillation (VF) and pulseless ventricular tachycardia (VT). If initial defibrillation fails, the patient should be intubated and intravenous access immediately established while CPR is continued. Epinephrine, 1 mg intravenously, should be administered and may be repeated several times with additional attempts to defibrillate with 360 J. If the conversion is still unsuccessful, epinephrine may be administered again, although it is unlikely that higher doses will provide any further benefit. Sodium bicarbonate should be administered at this time only if the patient is known to be hyperkalemic, but intravenous antiarrhythmic drugs should be tried (see text). Additional attempts to defibrillate should follow the administration of each drug attempted. Concomitant with all steps, continuation of CPR is paramount. PEA = pulseless electrical activity. *(Modified from ECC Committee, Subcommittees and Task Forces of the AHA: 2005 AHA Guidelines for Cardiopulmonary Resuscitation and Emergency Cardiovascular Care. Circulation 112[Suppl]:IV1, 2005.)*

CH 41

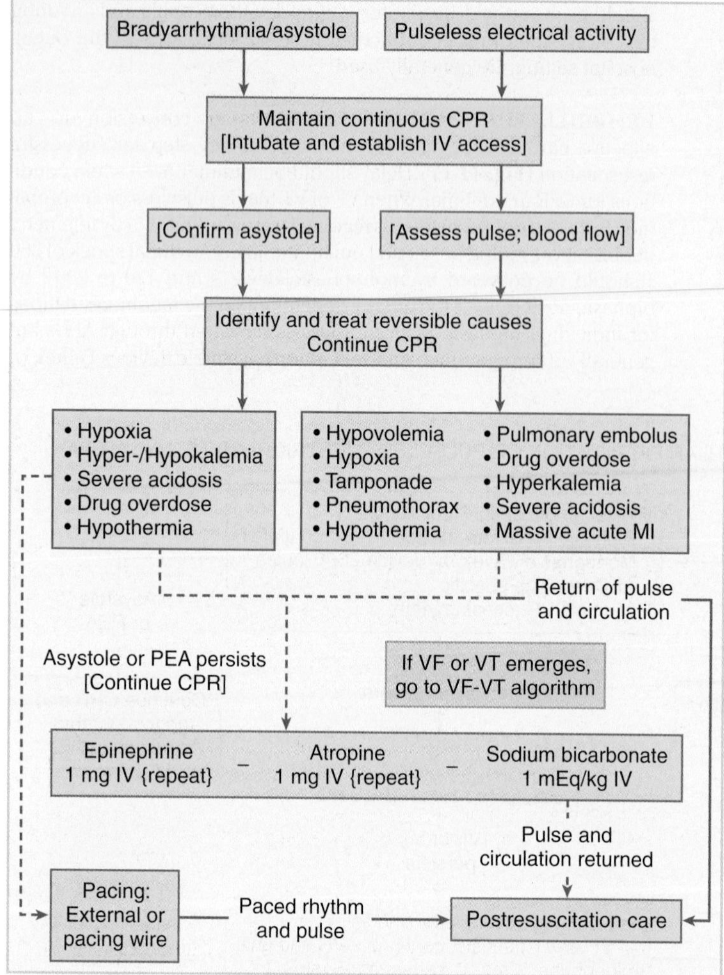

FIGURE 41-18 Advanced cardiac life support for patients with bradyarrhythmic-asystolic arrests and pulseless electrical activity. The patient in any of these states should have continued CPR and be intubated, with intravenous access established, before pharmacologic treatment. The initial activity is to confirm persisting asystole or to attempt to assess blood flow in patients thought to have pulseless electrical activity. An immediate attempt should be made to identify and to treat reversible or treatable causes of these forms of cardiac arrest. Epinephrine is generally administered first, and atropine or bicarbonate, or both, may be administered subsequently. An attempt to pace the heart with an external device or an intracardiac pacing catheter is advisable although usually not successful, except for certain reversible bradyarrhythmias. MI = myocardial infarction; PEA = pulseless electrical activity; VF = ventricular fibrillation; VT = ventricular tachycardia. *(Modified from ECC Committee, Subcommittees and Task Forces of the AHA: 2005 AHA Guidelines for Cardiopulmonary Resuscitation and Emergency Cardiovascular Care. Circulation 112[Suppl]:IV1, 2005.)*

the initial shock to provide an effective rhythm is a poor prognostic sign. The 2005 updated guidelines[130] have recommended that failure of a single adequate shock to restore a pulse should be followed by continued CPR and a second shock delivered after five cycles of CPR. This supersedes the prior strategy of three successive shocks before resuming CPR. The intent is to maximize circulatory time by chest compressions until a pulse has been restored. If cardiac arrest still persists, the patient is intubated and intravenous access achieved. Epinephrine is administered and followed by repeated defibrillation attempts at 360 J (monophasic) or 200 J or more (biphasic). Epinephrine may be repeated at 3- to 5-minute intervals with a defibrillator shock in between,[130] but high-dose epinephrine does not appear to provide added benefit.[178] Vasopressin has been suggested as an alternative to epinephrine.

Simultaneously, the rescuer should focus on ventilation to correct the chemistry of the blood, efforts that render the heart more likely to reestablish a stable rhythm (i.e., improved oxygenation, reversal of acidosis, and improvement of the underlying electrophysiologic condition). Although adequate oxygenation of the blood is crucial in the immediate management of the metabolic acidosis of cardiac arrest, additional correction can be achieved, if necessary, by intravenous administration of sodium bicarbonate. Sodium bicarbonate is recommended for circumstances of known or suspected preexisting bicarbonate-responsive causes of acidosis, certain drug overdoses, and prolonged resuscitation runs.[130] The more general role for bicarbonate during cardiac arrest has been questioned, but in any circumstance, much less sodium bicarbonate than was previously recommended is adequate for treatment of acidosis in this setting. Excessive quantities can be deleterious. Although some investigators have questioned the use of sodium bicarbonate because risks of alkalosis, hypernatremia, and hyperosmolality may outweigh its benefits, the circumstances cited may benefit from administration of sodium bicarbonate while CPR is being carried out. Up to 50% of the dose may be repeated every 10 to 15 minutes during the course of CPR. When possible, arterial pH, P_{O_2}, and P_{CO_2} should be monitored during the resuscitation.

PHARMACOTHERAPY (see Chap. 37). For the patient who continues to have persistent or recurrent VT or VF despite direct-current cardioversion after epinephrine, electrical stability of the heart may be achieved by intravenous administration of antiarrhythmic agents during continued resuscitation efforts (see Fig. 41-17). Intravenous amiodarone has emerged as the initial treatment of choice.[124] Bolus therapy is followed by a maintenance dose during the next 18 hours and for several days, as necessary, depending on the stability of the rhythm.

A bolus of lidocaine may be given intravenously and the dose repeated in 2 minutes for patients in whom amiodarone is unsuccessful and possibly for those who have an acute transmural myocardial infarction as the triggering mechanism for the cardiac arrest. Intravenous procainamide is rarely used in this setting any longer, but it may be tried for persisting, hemodynamically stable arrhythmias.

For patients in whom acute hyperkalemia is the triggering event for resistant VF or who have hypocalcemia or are toxic from Ca^{2+} entry blocking drugs, 10% calcium gluconate may be helpful.[130] Calcium should not be used routinely during resuscitation, even though ionized calcium levels may be low during resuscitation from cardiac arrest. Some resistant forms of polymorphic VT or torsades de pointes, rapid monomorphic VT or ventricular flutter (rate ≥260/min), or resistant VF may respond to intravenous beta blocker therapy or intravenous magnesium sulfate.

BRADYARRHYTHMIC AND ASYSTOLIC ARREST; PULSELESS ELECTRICAL ACTIVITY. The approach to the patient with bradyarrhythmic or asystolic arrest or pulseless electrical activity differs from the approach to the patient with a tachyarrhythmic event (**Fig. 41-18**).[130] When this form of cardiac arrest is recognized, efforts should focus first on establishing control of the cardiorespiratory status (i.e., continue CPR, intubate, and establish intravenous access), reconfirming the rhythm (in two leads if possible), and finally taking actions that favor the emergence of a stable spontaneous rhythm or attempt to pace the heart. Possible reversible causes, particularly for bradyarrhythmia and asystole, should be considered and excluded (or treated) promptly. These include hypovolemia, hypoxia, cardiac tamponade, tension pneumothorax, preexisting acidosis, drug overdose, hypothermia, and hyperkalemia. Epinephrine and atropine are commonly used in an attempt to elicit spontaneous electrical activity or to increase the rate of a bradycardia. These have had only limited success, as have intravenous isoproterenol infusions in doses up to 15 to 20 μg/min. In the absence of an intravenous line, epinephrine, 1 mg (10 mL of a 1:10,000 solution), may be given by the intracardiac route, but there is danger of coronary or myocardial laceration. Sodium bicarbonate, 1 mEq/kg, may be tried for known or strongly suspected preexisting hyperkalemia or bicarbonate-responsive acidosis.

Pacing of the bradyarrhythmic or asystolic heart has been limited in the past by the unavailability of personnel capable of carrying out such procedures at the scene of cardiac arrests. With the development of more effective external pacing systems, the role of pacing and its influence on outcome must now be reevaluated. Unfortunately, all data to date have suggested that the asystolic patient continues to have a very poor prognosis, despite new techniques.

The published standards for CPR and emergency cardiac care[130] include a series of teaching algorithms to be used as guides to appropriate care. Figures 41-17 and 41-18 provide the algorithms for VF and pulseless VT, asystole (or cardiac standstill), and pulseless electrical activity. These general guides are not to be interpreted as inclusive of all possible approaches or contingencies. The special circumstance of CPR in pregnant women requires additional attention to effects of drugs on the gravid uterus and the fetus, mechanical and physiologic influences of pregnancy on the efficacy of CPR, and risk of complications, such as ruptured uterus and lacerated liver.

STABILIZATION. When electrical resuscitation from VT, VF, bradycardia, asystole, or pulseless electrical activity has been achieved, the focus shifts to maintaining a stable electrical, hemodynamic, and central nervous system status. If frequent PVCs and runs of nonsustained VT persist after restoration of a sinus mechanism, a continuous infusion of an effective antiarrhythmic drug is used. Intravenous amiodarone is the preferred agent. Lidocaine is an option for arrhythmias caused by acute ischemic events, and intravenous procainamide may be considered if the others fail. On occasion, a continuous infusion of propranolol or esmolol is used, sometimes in conjunction with magnesium sulfate, especially for recurrent episodes of polymorphic VT or VT storm unresponsive to amiodarone.

Catecholamines are used in cardiac arrest not only in an attempt to achieve better electrical stability (e.g., conversion from fine to coarse VF, or increasing the rate of spontaneous contraction during bradyarrhythmias) but also for their inotropic and peripheral vascular effects. Epinephrine is the first choice among the catecholamines for use in cardiac arrest because it increases myocardial contractility, elevates perfusion pressure, may convert electromechanical dissociation to electromechanical coupling and improves chances for defibrillation. Because of its adverse effects on renal and mesenteric flow, norepinephrine is a less desirable agent, despite its inotropic effects. When the chronotropic effect of epinephrine is undesirable, dopamine or dobutamine is preferable to norepinephrine for inotropic effect. Isoproterenol may be used for the treatment of primary or postdefibrillation bradycardia when heart rate control is the primary goal of therapy intended to improve cardiac output. Calcium chloride is sometimes used in patients with pulseless electrical activity that persists after administration of catecholamines. The efficacy of this intervention is uncertain. Stimulation of alpha adrenoceptors may be important during definitive resuscitative efforts. For example, the alpha adrenoceptor–stimulating effects of epinephrine and higher dosages of dopamine, producing elevation of aortic diastolic pressures by peripheral vasoconstriction with increased cerebral and myocardial flow, have been reemphasized.

Post–Cardiac Arrest Care

For successfully resuscitated cardiac arrest victims, whether the event occurred in or out of the hospital, post–cardiac arrest care includes admission to an intensive care unit and continuous monitoring for a minimum of 48 to 72 hours. Some elements of postarrest management are common to all resuscitated patients, but prognosis and certain details of management are specific for the clinical setting in which the cardiac arrest occurred. The major management categories include (1) primary cardiac arrest in acute myocardial infarction, (2) secondary cardiac arrest in acute myocardial infarction, (3) cardiac arrest associated with noncardiac diseases, drug effects, or electrolyte disorders, and (4) survival after out-of-hospital cardiac arrest.

PRIMARY CARDIAC ARREST IN ACUTE MYOCARDIAL INFARCTION. VF in patients with acute myocardial infarction free of concomitant hemodynamic complications (i.e., primary VF; see Chap. 55) is now less common in hospitalized patients than the 15% to 20% incidence before the availability of cardiac care units. The events that do occur are almost always successfully reverted by prompt interventions in properly equipped emergency departments or cardiac care units. If ventricular arrhythmias persist after successful resuscitation, a lidocaine infusion is used. Antiarrhythmic support is usually discontinued after 24 hours if sustained arrhythmias do not recur (see Chap. 37). The occurrence of VF during the early phase of acute myocardial infarction (i.e., first 24 to 48 hours) does not identify long-term risk and is not an indication for long-term antiarrhythmic or device therapy. Pulseless VT, producing the clinical picture of cardiac arrest in acute myocardial infarction, is treated similarly; its intermediate- and long-term implications are the same as those of VF. Cardiac arrest caused by bradyarrhythmias or asystole in acute *inferior* wall myocardial infarction, in the absence of primary hemodynamic deterioration, is uncommon and may respond to atropine or pacing. The prognosis is good, with no special long-term care required in most cases. Persistent symptomatic bradyarrhythmias, requiring permanent pacemakers, rarely occur in such patients. In contrast, bradyarrhythmic cardiac arrest associated with large *anterior* wall infarctions (and AV or intraventricular block) has a poor prognosis.

SECONDARY CARDIAC ARREST IN ACUTE MYOCARDIAL INFARCTION. This condition is defined as cardiac arrest occurring in association with or as a result of hemodynamic or mechanical dysfunction. The immediate mortality among patients in this setting ranges from 59% to 89%, depending on the severity of the hemodynamic abnormalities and size of the myocardial infarction. Resuscitative efforts commonly fail in such patients, and when they are successful, the post–cardiac arrest management is often difficult. When secondary cardiac arrest occurs by the mechanisms of VT or VF, aggressive hemodynamic or anti-ischemic measures may help achieve rhythm stability. Intravenous amiodarone has emerged as the antiarrhythmic therapy of choice.[124] Lidocaine may also be tried if the mechanism appears to be ischemic but is less likely to be successful in this setting than in primary VF. The success of interventions and prevention of recurrent cardiac arrest are related closely to the success in managing the hemodynamic status. The incidence of cardiac arrest caused by bradyarrhythmias or asystole, or by electromechanical dissociation, is higher in the secondary form of cardiac arrest in acute myocardial infarction. Such patients usually have large myocardial infarctions and major hemodynamic abnormalities and may be acidotic and hypoxemic. Even with aggressive therapy, the prognosis after asystolic arrest in such patients is poor, and patients are resuscitated only rarely from pulseless electrical activity. All patients in circulatory failure at the onset of arrest are in a high-risk category, with only a 2% survival rate among hypotensive patients in one study.

CARDIAC ARREST AMONG IN-HOSPITAL PATIENTS WITH NONCARDIAC ABNORMALITIES. These patients fall into two major categories: (1) those with life-limiting diseases, such as malignant neoplasms, sepsis, organ failure, end-stage pulmonary disease, and advanced central nervous system disease; and (2) those with acute toxic or proarrhythmic states that are potentially reversible. In the former category, the ratio of tachyarrhythmic to bradyarrhythmic cardiac arrest is low and the prognosis for survival of cardiac arrest is poor. Although the data may be somewhat skewed by the practice of assigning "do not resuscitate" orders to patients with end-stage disease, available data for attempted resuscitations show a poor outcome. Only 7% of cancer patients, 3% of renal failure patients, and no patients with sepsis or acute central nervous system disease were successfully resuscitated and discharged from the hospital. For the few successfully resuscitated patients in these categories, postarrest management is dictated by the underlying precipitating factors.

Most antiarrhythmic drugs (see Chap. 37), a number of drugs used for noncardiac purposes, and electrolyte disturbances can precipitate potentially lethal arrhythmias and cardiac arrest. The class IA and class III antiarrhythmic drugs can cause proarrhythmic responses by lengthening the QT interval and generating torsades de pointes. The class IC drugs rarely cause torsades de pointes but cause excess SCD risk in patients with recent myocardial infarction, possibly by interacting with transient ischemia. Among other categories of drugs, the phenothiazines, tricyclic antidepressants, lithium, terfenadine interacting with ketoconazole (or other blockers of enzymes in the hepatic P-450 system), pentamidine, cocaine, erythromycin, and cardiovascular drugs that are not antiarrhythmics (such as lidoflazine) are recognized causes. Beyond these, a broad array of pharmacologic and pathophysiologic-metabolic causes have been reported. Hypokalemia, hypomagnesemia, and perhaps hypocalcemia are the electrolyte disturbances most closely associated with cardiac arrest. Acidosis and hypoxia can potentiate the vulnerability associated with electrolyte disturbances. Proarrhythmic effects are often prewarned by prolongation of the QT interval, although this electrocardiographic change is not always present.

Impending or manifest cardiac arrest caused by torsades de pointes is managed by intravenous administration of magnesium, pacing, or treatment with isoproterenol and removal of the offending agent. When QT prolongation is the basis, magnesium may effectively control the arrhythmia without shortening the QT interval. Class IC drugs may cause a rapid, sinusoidal VT pattern, especially in patients with poor left ventricular function. This VT has a tendency to recur repetitively after cardioversion until the drug has begun to clear and has been controlled by propranolol in some patients. When the patient's condition can be stabilized until the offending factor is removed (e.g., proarrhythmic drugs) or corrected (e.g., electrolyte imbalances, hypothermia), the prognosis is excellent. The recognition of torsades de pointes (see Chap. 39) and the identification of its risk by prolongation of the QT interval in association with the offending agent are helpful in managing these patients.

POST–CARDIAC ARREST CARE IN SURVIVORS OF OUT-OF-HOSPITAL CARDIAC ARREST. The initial management of survivors of out-of-hospital cardiac arrest centers on stabilizing the cardiac electrical status, supporting hemodynamics, and providing supportive care for reversal of organ damage that has occurred as a consequence of the cardiac arrest. The in-hospital risk of recurrent cardiac arrest is relatively low, and arrhythmias account for only 10% of in-hospital deaths after successful out-of-hospital resuscitation. However, the mortality rate during the index hospitalization is 50%, indicating that nonarrhythmic mortality dominates the mechanisms of early postresuscitation deaths (30% hemodynamic, 60% central nervous system related). Antiarrhythmic therapy, usually intravenous amiodarone, is used in an attempt to prevent recurrent cardiac arrest among patients who demonstrate recurrent arrhythmia during the first 48 hours of postarrest hospitalization. Patients who have preexisting or new AV or intraventricular conduction disturbances are at particularly high risk for recurrent cardiac arrest. The routine use of temporary pacemakers has been evaluated in such patients but has not been found to be helpful for prevention of early recurrent cardiac arrest. Invasive techniques for hemodynamic monitoring are used in patients whose condition is unstable but are not used routinely for those whose condition is stable on admission.

Anoxic encephalopathy is a strong predictor of in-hospital death. A suggested addition to the management of this condition is the use of induced mild hypothermia to reduce metabolic demands and cerebral edema.[136,137] When this strategy is applied promptly to the postarrest survivor who remains unconscious on hospital admission, there is a modest but measurable survival benefit. During the later convalescent period, continued attention to central nervous system status, including physical rehabilitation, is of primary importance for an optimal outcome. Respiratory support by conventional methods is used as necessary. Management of other organ system injury (e.g., renal, hepatic) as well as early recognition and treatment of infectious complications also contributes to ultimate survival.

Long-Term Management of Survivors of Out-of-Hospital Cardiac Arrest

When the survivor of an out-of-hospital cardiac arrest has awakened and achieved electrical and hemodynamic stability, usually within a few days if it is to occur at all, decisions must be made about the nature and extent of the workup required to establish a long-term management strategy. The goals of the workup are to identify the specific causative and triggering factors of the cardiac arrest, to clarify the functional status of the patient's cardiovascular system, and to establish long-term therapeutic strategies. The extent of the workup is largely dictated by the degree of central nervous system recovery and the factors already known to have contributed to the cardiac arrest. Patients who have limited return of central nervous system function usually do not undergo extensive workups, and patients whose cardiac arrests were triggered by an acute transmural myocardial infarction have workups similar to those for other patients with acute myocardial infarction (see Chap. 55).

Survivors of out-of-hospital cardiac arrest not associated with acute myocardial infarction who have good return of neurologic function appear to have a long-term survival probability commensurate with their age, gender, and extent of disease when they are treated according to existing guidelines.[142,179,180] These patients should undergo diagnostic workups to define the cause of cardiac arrest and to tailor long-term therapy, the latter targeted to the underlying disease and strategies for prevention of recurrent cardiac arrests or SCD. The workup includes cardiac catheterization with coronary angiography, if coronary atherosclerosis is known or considered to be the possible cause of the event; evaluation of the functional significance of coronary lesions by stress imaging techniques, if indicated; determination of functional and hemodynamic status; and assessment of whether the life-threatening arrhythmic event was caused by a transient risk associated with acute myocardial infarction or there is persisting risk based on clinical characteristics.

GENERAL CARE. The general management of survivors of cardiac arrest is determined by the specific cause and the underlying pathophysiologic process. For patients with ischemic heart disease (see Chaps. 56 and 57), who constitute approximately 80% of cardiac arrest victims, interventions to prevent myocardial ischemia, optimization of therapy for left ventricular dysfunction, and attention to general medical status are all addressed. Although there are limited data suggesting that revascularization procedures may improve the recurrence rate and total mortality rates after survival from out-of-hospital cardiac arrest, no properly controlled prospective studies have validated this impression for bypass surgery or percutaneous interventions. Moreover, a randomized trial of prophylactic implantable defibrillators versus usual therapy in patients with low ejection fractions undergoing coronary bypass surgery in the absence of a history of cardiac arrest or other life-threatening arrhythmia or arrhythmia markers (the Coronary Artery Bypass Graft [CABG] Patch trial) revealed no mortality benefit of implantable defibrillators after revascularization.[181] The indications for revascularization after a cardiac arrest are limited to those who have a generally accepted indication for angioplasty or surgery, including (but not limited to) a documented ischemic mechanism for the cardiac arrest.

Although no data from placebo-controlled trials are available to define a benefit of various anti-ischemic strategies (including beta blockers or other medical anti-ischemic therapy) for long-term management after out-of-hospital cardiac arrest, medical, catheter interventional, or surgical anti-ischemic therapy, rather than antiarrhythmic drug therapy, is generally considered the primary approach to long-term management of the subgroup of prehospital cardiac arrest survivors in whom transient myocardial ischemia was the inciting factor. Moreover, in an uncontrolled observation comparing cardiac arrest survivors who had ever received beta blockers after the index event with those who had not received that class of drug, a significant improvement in long-term outcome was observed among those who had received beta blockers. Further evaluation of the specific role of revascularization procedures and anti-ischemic medical therapy after out-of-hospital cardiac arrest is needed.

The long-term management of the consequences of left ventricular dysfunction by conventional means, such as digitalis preparations and chronic diuretic use, has been evaluated in several studies. Data from the Multiple Risk Factor Intervention Trial (MRFIT) have suggested a higher mortality rate in the special intervention group, presumably related to diuretic use and potassium depletion, and other data regarding the relation between potassium depletion and arrhythmias have focused attention on the routine use of such drugs. Although the facts are currently far from conclusive, it is advisable that diuretic use be accompanied by careful monitoring of electrolyte levels.

The various pharmacologic strategies (e.g., angiotensin-converting enzyme inhibitors, carvedilol and other beta-adrenergic blocking agents, and spironolactone) that have been shown to provide a clinical and mortality benefit in patients with left ventricular dysfunction, with or without heart failure, provide SCD benefit in conjunction with total mortality benefit. The extent to which there is a specific SCD benefit for cardiac arrest survivors is uncertain, although some primary prevention trials have suggested that such benefit occurs.

Prevention of Cardiac Arrest and Sudden Cardiac Death

Prevention of SCD can be classified into five clinical subgroup categories: (1) prevention of recurrent events in survivors of cardiac arrest or pulseless VT (secondary prevention) or other symptomatic tachycardias considered life-threatening (**Table 41-5**); (2) prevention of an initial event among patients at high risk because of advanced heart disease with low ejection fractions and other markers of risk (primary prevention) (**Table 41-6**); (3) primary prevention in patients with less advanced common or uncommon structural heart diseases; (4) primary prevention in patients with structurally normal hearts, subtle or minor structural abnormalities, or genetically based molecular disorders that establish risk for ventricular arrhythmias (**Table 41-7**); and (5) primary prevention among the general population. The last category includes the substantial proportion of SCDs that occur as a first cardiac event among victims previously free of known disease (see earlier).

Four antiarrhythmic strategies, which are not mutually exclusive, may be considered for patients at risk for cardiac arrest: implantable defibrillators, antiarrhythmic drugs, catheter ablation, and antiarrhythmic surgery. In addition to these specific antiarrhythmic strategies, therapies for other medical and cardiovascular conditions are integral to management of SCD risk.

The choice of a therapy, or combinations of therapies, is based on estimation of risk determined by evaluation of the individual patient by various risk-profiling techniques, coupled with available efficacy and safety data.

Methods to Estimate Sudden Cardiac Death Risk

GENERAL MEDICAL AND CARDIOVASCULAR RISK MARKERS. The presence and severity of acquired medical disorders, such as myocardial ischemia, left ventricular dysfunction, and heart failure, and general medical conditions, such as hypertension, diabetes, dyslipidemias, chronic renal failure, and cigarette smoking, are integral to estimation of SCD risk. Although lacking the specificity of individual SCD risk prediction attributable to some of the specific arrhythmia markers, they provide general indicators of risk and data supporting the benefit of therapies, such as beta blockers, angiotensin-converting enzyme inhibitors and receptor blockers, and statins, in appropriate subgroups of patients. Other noninvasive markers of risk are being explored, including measures reflecting autonomic function, QT interval stability, and genetic influences on SCD risk (see Risk Factors for Sudden Cardiac Death). The potential importance of proper timing and combining of risk markers has been explored.[55,120] A study suggests greater predictive power for risk of post–myocardial infarction adverse events when markers are evaluated after 8 weeks, as opposed to closer to the index event.[182]

AMBULATORY MONITORING (see Chap. 36)**.** The development of reliable methods of analysis of ambulatory recordings has led some investigators to study the usefulness of such recordings for profiling risk of sustained tachyarrhythmic events and to measure suppressibility of ambient arrhythmias as a specific and individualized means of evaluating drug therapy for prevention of SCD. The latter is now obsolete as a primary approach in the cardiac arrest survivor, but ambulatory monitoring is still used for profiling the risk for development of life-threatening sustained arrhythmias in individuals with certain forms of structural or electrophysiologic disease who are considered at high risk. For example, the strategies in the Multicenter Automatic Defibrillator Implantation Trial (MADIT)[183] and the Multicenter Unsustained Tachycardia Trial (MUSTT)[184] used identification of nonsustained VT in post–myocardial infarction patients with other risk markers for early mortality. Although the ambient arrhythmias were not a target for therapy in the design of the studies, they have established the usefulness of this technique for identification of risk. Similarly, ambulatory recordings, particularly among patients with symptoms, are used as an aid to risk profiling in disorders such as hypertrophic cardiomyopathy, long-QT syndrome, and right ventricular dysplasia and in patients with dilated cardiomyopathy or heart failure. For patients with possible SCD risk based on low-frequency symptomatic events, such as near-syncope or syncope, with or without a perception of repetitive palpitations or tachycardias, an implantable loop recorder for recording and retrieval of transient events may provide risk profiling benefit.

TABLE 41-5 Secondary Prevention ICD Trials

TRIAL (F/U ANALYSIS) YEAR PUBLISHED	STUDY GROUP, DEFINED ENTRY CRITERIA	TIME FROM DIAGNOSIS OF QUALIFYING CONDITION TO RANDOMIZATION	EJECTION FRACTION, ENROLLED PATIENTS	*ALL-CAUSE MORTALITY*		*BENEFIT*	
				CONTROL	ICD	RelRR	AbsRR
AVID (2-year analysis) 1997	VFib, VT with syncope, VT with EF ≤40%	Entry criterion: undefined Actual: not reported EF: 3 days post–qualifying event (median)	32% (SD = ±13%)	25%	18%	−27%	−7%
CIDS (2-year analysis) 2000	VFib, out-of-hospital cardiac arrest due to VFib or VT, VT with syncope, VT with symptoms and EF ≤35%, unmonitored syncope with subsequent spontaneous or induced VT	Entry criterion: undefined Actual: Time from qualifying event to randomization not reported Median time from randomization to ICD 7 days (>90% in ≤21 days) EF: not reported	34% (SD = ±14%)	21%	15%	−30%	−6%
CASH (9-year analysis) 2000	VFib, VT	Entry criteria: not defined Actual: not reported EF: not reported	46% (SD = ±18%)	44%	36%	−23%	−8%

AbsRR = absolute risk reduction; EF = ejection fraction; F/U = follow-up; RelRR = relative risk reduction; VFib = ventricular fibrillation; VT = ventricular tachycardia.
From Myerburg RJ, Reddy V, Castellanos A: Indications for implantable cardioverter-defibrillators based on evidence and judgment. J Am Coll Cardiol 2009, 54:747-763, with permission of the publisher.

TABLE 41-6 Primary Prevention ICD Trials

TRIAL (F/U ANALYSIS) YEAR PUBLISHED	STUDY GROUP, DEFINED ENTRY CRITERIA	TIME FROM DIAGNOSIS OF QUALIFYING CONDITION TO RANDOMIZATION	EJECTION FRACTION, ENROLLED PATIENTS	ALL-CAUSE MORTALITY		BENEFIT	
				CONTROL	ICD	RelRR	AbsRR
MADIT (2-year analysis) 1996	Prior MI, EF ≤35%, N-S VT, inducible VT, failed IV PA	Entry criterion: ≥3 weeks Actual: 75% ≥6 months Qualifying EF: interval not reported	26% (SD = ±7%)	32%	13%	−59%	19%
CABG Patch (2-year analysis) 1997	Coronary bypass surgery, EF <36%, SAECG (+)	Diagnosis of CAD: interval not reported Qualifying EF: interval not reported SAECG: day of randomization	27% (SD = ±6%)	18%	18%	N/A	N/A
MUSTT (5-year analysis) 1999	CAD (prior MI ~95%), EF ≤40%, N-S VT, inducible VT	Qualifying N-S VT: ≥4 days from MI Time from MI: 17% ≤1 month 50% ≥3 years Qualifying EF: interval not reported	30% (21%, 35%) [median (25th, 75th percentile)]	55% [E-P guided arm: AAD versus ICD at 60 m]	24%	−58%	−31%
MADIT II (2-year analysis) 2002	Prior MI (>1 month), EF ≤30%	Entry criteria: ≥1 month Actual: 88% ≥6 months Qualifying EF: interval not reported	23% (SD = ±5%)	22%	16%	−28%	−6%
DEFINITE (2½-year analysis) 2004	Nonischemic CM, Hx HF, EF ≤35%, ≥10 PVCs/hr or N-S VT	Heart failure onset (mean): Controls = 3.27 years ICD group = 2.39 years	21% (range = 7%-35%)	14%	8%	−44%	−6%
DINAMIT (2½-year analysis) 2004	Recent MI (6-40 days), EF ≤35%, abnormal HRV or mean 24-hr heart rate >80/min	Entry criteria: 6-40 days Actual: mean = 18 days	28% (SD = ±5%)	17%	19%	N/A	N/A
SCD-HeFT (5-year analysis) 2005	Class II-III CHF, EF ≤35%	Entry criteria: interval not reported Qualifying EF: interval not reported	25% (20%, 30%) [median (25th, 75th percentile)]	36%	29%	−23%	−7%

AAD = antiarrhythmic drug; AbsRR = absolute risk reduction; CAD = coronary artery disease; CHF = congestive heart failure; CM = cardiomyopathy; EF = ejection fraction; E-P = electrophysiologically; F/U = follow-up; HRV = heart rate variability; Hx HF = history of heart failure; IV PA = intravenous procainamide; MI = myocardial infarction; N-S = non-sustained; RelRR = relative risk reduction; PVCs = premature ventricular complexes; SAECG (+) = positive signal-averaged electrocardiography; VT = ventricular tachycardia.

From Myerburg RJ, Reddy V, Castellanos A: Indications for implantable cardioverter-defibrillators based on evidence and judgment. J Am Coll Cardiol 54:747-763, 2009, with permission of the publisher.

TABLE 41-7 ICD Indications in Genetic Disorders Associated with Sudden Cardiac Death Risk

DIAGNOSIS	ICD INDICATION	PRIMARY SOURCE OF DATA	RISK INDICATORS	GUIDELINES	
				CLASSIFICATION	EVIDENCE
HCM	Secondary SCA protection	Registries; cohorts	Prior SCA, pulseless VT	Class I	Level B
			Sustained VT, unexplained syncope	Class IIa	Level C
	Primary SCA protection	Registries; cohorts	Left ventricle thickness >30 mm, high left ventricular outflow gradient, family history of SCD, N-S VT, blunted blood pressure response to exercise	Class IIa	Level C
ARVD/RVCM	Secondary SCA protection	Registry; case series	Prior SCA, sustained VT	Class I	Level B, C
			Unexplained syncope	Class IIa	Level C
	Primary SCA protection	Registry; case series	Induced VT, ambient N-S VT, extensive disease	Class IIa	Level C
Congenital LQT	Secondary SCA protection	Registry; cohorts	Prior SCA, symptomatic VT	Class I	Level B
	Primary SCA protection	Registry; cohorts	VT or syncope on beta blocker, QTc >500 msec, family history of premature SCA (?)	Class IIa, IIb	Level B
Familial SQT	Secondary SCA protection	Small case series	Prior SCA, "idiopathic" VF	Class I	Level C
	Primary SCA protection	Small case series	Unknown; family history of SCD (?)	Class IIb, III	Level C
Brugada syndrome	Secondary SCA protection	Case cohorts	Prior SCA, pulseless VT	Class I	Level B
	Primary SCA protection	Case cohorts	Symptomatic VT, unexplained syncope, family history of premature SCA with type I electrocardiographic pattern	Class IIa	Level C
CPVT/F	Secondary SCA protection	Small case series	Prior SCA, pulseless VT	Class I	Level C
	Primary SCA protection	Small case series	Syncope or VT while receiving beta blockers, family history of premature SCA (?)	Class IIa	Level C

ARVD/RVCM = arrhythmogenic right ventricular dysplasia/cardiomyopathy; CPVT/F = catecholaminergic polymorphic ventricular tachycardia/"idiopathic" ventricular fibrillation; HCM = hypertrophic cardiomyopathy; LQT = long-QT syndrome; N-S = non-sustained; PVT = polymorphic ventricular tachycardia; SCA = sudden cardiac arrest; SCD = sudden cardiac death; SQT = short-QT syndrome; VA = ventricular arrhythmias; VF = ventricular fibrillation; VT = ventricular tachycardia; (?) = uncertain.

Guideline classifications and levels of evidence are derived from an amalgamation of narrative and tabular statements in two recent Guidelines documents (references 179 and 180) with variations in the documents adjudicated by the authors. Definitions are the standard usages provided in Guidelines documents.

From Myerburg RJ, Reddy V, Castellanos A: Indications for implantable cardioverter-defibrillators based on evidence and judgment. J Am Coll Cardiol 54:747-763, 2009, with permission of the publisher.

PROGRAMMED ELECTRICAL STIMULATION. Whereas there is a large albeit somewhat conflicting data base on the role of electrophysiologic testing for risk profiling, particularly in patients with advanced heart disease, its use is currently more limited than in the past. In primary prevention trials, such as MADIT[183] and MUSTT,[184] electrophysiologic testing was used to profile risk and demonstrated large benefits. MADIT II,[185] which enrolled patients with lower ejection fractions than MADIT or MUSTT and did not use programmed stimulation or other arrhythmia markers, also demonstrated a survival benefit of ICD therapy. The extent to which MADIT II differs from MADIT and MUSTT and the question of whether the electrophysiologic testing criteria in the latter are necessary have yet to be fully resolved. However, a follow-up study of MADIT II patients suggested that cumulative ICD discharge rates were equivalent in patients who had inducible and noninducible ventricular tachyarrhythmias, although inducibility was associated with a higher incidence of VT and noninducibility with VF.[186]

The secondary prevention trials among cardiac arrest survivors did not seek to determine whether routine electrophysiologic testing offered any predictive value,[145-147] and it is no longer necessary, particularly if ICD therapy is available to the patient. Most prior studies had demonstrated limitations on the basis of the relatively small fraction of cardiac arrest survivors (an average of less than 50% on the basis of multiple studies) who had inducible arrhythmias. Under conditions in which a potentially reversible trigger for cardiac arrest can be identified, and perhaps among some cardiac arrest survivors in whom transient ischemia was the initiating mechanism and the ejection fraction is higher than 40%, there might be a persistent limited role for such testing as a guide to therapy.

For patients with symptomatic arrhythmia or those considered at potentially high risk, programmed stimulation is still used. Inducibility of sustained or hemodynamically unstable arrhythmias, initiated with an appropriate protocol, is considered positive and predictive. However, the implications of induced *nonsustained* forms of VT are more controversial. Although it has been suggested that induction of nonsustained ventricular rhythms may indicate risk, it is generally considered nonspecific in the absence of structural heart disease or when an aggressive protocol is used. The reliability of *non*-inducibility to predict absence of risk is also questioned.[186] In the past, opinions ranged from the conclusion that potentially high-risk patients free of inducible ventricular arrhythmias were electrophysiologically stable and required no long-term antiarrhythmic therapy to the other extreme that such patients remained at risk but did not have an objective endpoint of therapy by this method and therefore must be treated by other techniques. Despite these conflicting opinions, it is generally accepted now that survivors of cardiac arrest without clearly identifiable transient and treatable causes remain at high risk, regardless of inducibility status. Some out-of-hospital cardiac arrests can be clearly demonstrated to result from transient ischemia, and this subgroup appears to achieve benefit from anti-ischemic therapy.[142]

Strategies to Reduce Sudden Cardiac Death Risk

ANTIARRHYTHMIC DRUGS. Historically, the earliest approach to the management of risk of out-of-hospital cardiac arrest and VT with hemodynamic compromise was the use of membrane-active antiarrhythmic agents. This approach was based initially on the assumption that a high frequency of ambient ventricular arrhythmias constituted a triggering mechanism for potentially lethal arrhythmias and that their suppression by antiarrhythmic drugs was protective. It was also assumed that electrophysiologic instability of the myocardium that predisposed to potentially lethal arrhythmias could be modified by these drugs and that suppression of inducibility of VT or VF during programmed electrical stimulation studies reflected this effect. Suppression of ambient arrhythmias was demonstrated by the empiric use of amiodarone, beta-adrenergic blocking agents, or membrane-active antiarrhythmic drugs, but a scientifically valid demonstration of a survival benefit was lacking. The observations that post–cardiac arrest survivors who had been treated with class I antiarrhythmic drugs had a worse outcome than did those who were not treated challenged the concept of benefit. That skepticism was definitively reinforced by the results of CAST, which demonstrated that certain class I antiarrhythmic drugs are neutral or harmful. In contrast, beta blocker therapy might have some benefit in such patients, and amiodarone might also be effective for some patients.[187] Ultimately, affirmative data have defined the superiority of ICD therapy for most survivors of tachyarrhythmic cardiac arrest.

In summary, ambient arrhythmia suppression and empiric antiarrhythmic drug therapy enjoyed a short period of popularity as a strategy for reduction of risk among VT/VF survivors but in time yielded to the apparently greater benefits of amiodarone, and perhaps beta blockers, prescribed empirically. A study of cardiovascular effects of a new amiodarone analogue, dronedarone, suggested an arrhythmic death survival benefit among patients with atrial fibrillation.[188] However, this observation was based on a secondary analysis of a small number of events and should not be considered conclusive absent more data. The combination of amiodarone and beta blocker therapy in the post–myocardial infarction patient has been suggested as a strategy that provides greater benefit than either drug alone from subgroup analysis of the European Myocardial Infarct Amiodarone Trial (EMIAT) and Canadian Amiodarone Myocardial Infarction Trial (CAMIAT), and another study reinforced the benefit of beta blockers for the specific prevention of SCD in unselected post–myocardial infarction patients.[35]

THERAPY GUIDED BY PROGRAMMED ELECTRICAL STIMULATION. The second major antiarrhythmic strategy was based on suppression of inducibility of sustained ventricular arrhythmias, considered to be a marker of risk during electrophysiologic testing. The use of programmed electrical stimulation to identify benefit on the basis of suppression of inducibility by an antiarrhythmic drug gained popularity for evaluation of long-term therapy among survivors of out-of-hospital cardiac arrest. It had evolved as the preferred method of management, despite concerns about the sensitivity and specificity of the various pacing protocols and the extent to which the myocardial status at the time of the programmed electrical stimulation study reflects that present at the time of the clinical cardiac arrest. Nonetheless, most studies have demonstrated limitations based on observations that a relatively small fraction of cardiac arrest survivors (an average of less than 50% on the basis of multiple studies) had inducible arrhythmias.

Drug suppression of inducibility during electrophysiologic testing as an endpoint for secondary prevention of SCD or primary prevention in high-risk post–myocardial infarction patients has yielded to the benefits of ICD therapy in most subgroups, with a few exceptions among primary prevention categories. It still has use, however, for risk profiling in a number of clinical circumstances.[183,184,189] The use of the suppression of nonsustained arrhythmias as an endpoint of therapy is not considered valid.

SURGICAL INTERVENTION STRATEGIES. The previously popular antiarrhythmic surgical techniques now have limited applications. Intraoperative map-guided cryoablation may be used for patients who have inducible, hemodynamically stable sustained monomorphic VT during electrophysiologic testing and have suitable ventricular and coronary artery anatomy amenable to catheter ablation. However, it has little applicability to survivors of out-of-hospital cardiac arrest because the type of arrhythmia favoring this surgical approach is infrequently observed in cardiac arrest survivors. It can be used as adjunctive therapy for ICD recipients whose arrhythmia burden requires frequent shocks. In addition, coronary revascularization procedures have a clearly defined role for cardiac arrest survivors in whom an ischemic mechanism was responsible for the event and suitable surgical anatomy is present.

CATHETER ABLATION THERAPY. The use of catheter ablation techniques to treat ventricular tachyarrhythmias has been most successful for the benign focal tachycardias that originate in the right ventricle or left side of the interventricular septum (see Chap. 37) and for some reentrant VTs. With rare exceptions, catheter ablation techniques are not used for the treatment of higher risk ventricular tachyarrhythmias or for definitive therapy in patients at risk for progression of the arrhythmic substrate. For VT caused by bundle branch reentrant mechanisms, which occur in cardiomyopathies as well as in other structural cardiac disorders, ablation of the right bundle branch to interrupt the reentrant cycle has been successful. However, this has limited applicability to the large number of patients with structural heart disease at risk for SCD or those who have survived a cardiac arrest. Nonetheless, catheter ablation is an appropriate adjunctive treatment strategy for patients with ICDs who are having multiple tachyarrhythmic events. A study has suggested a potential preventive benefit of VT substrate ablation for survivors of cardiac arrest equivalents (VF, hemodynamically limiting VT, or syncope with VT inducibility) with a history of myocardial infarction.[190] Presently, this benefit is limited to reducing the number of patients receiving ICD therapy (33% with ICD alone versus 12% with ICD plus ablation; $HR = 0.35$; $P = 0.007$), and further studies are needed to determine whether there is an expanded role.

Implantable Defibrillators. The development of the ICD added a new dimension to the management of patients at high risk for cardiac arrest (see Chap. 38). After the initial reports of small case series of very high risk patients in the early 1980s, a number of observational studies have confirmed that ICDs can achieve rates of sudden death consistently less than 5% at 1 year and total death rates in the 10% to 20% range in populations who have high mortality risks, as predicted by mortality surrogates such as historical controls or time to first appropriate shock.[101] However, determination of the mortality benefit of ICDs remained uncertain and was debated for many years. More than 16 years elapsed between the first clinical use of an implanted defibrillator and publication of the first major randomized clinical trial comparing implantable defibrillator therapy with antiarrhythmic drug therapy.[183] During that period, reports had documented the ability of ICDs to revert potentially fatal arrhythmias but could not identify a valid relative or absolute mortality benefit because of confounding factors, such as competing risks for sudden and nonsudden death and determination of whether appropriate shocks represented the interruption of an event that would have been fatal. Despite these limitations, ICD therapy continued to increase its relative position among other forms of therapy for survivors of out-of-hospital cardiac arrest and, to a lesser extent, for those considered to be at high risk for a primary cardiac arrest on the basis of specific clinical markers.

With publication of the results of MADIT,[183] information on the relative benefit of defibrillators over antiarrhythmic drug therapy (largely amiodarone) for primary prevention of SCD in a very high risk population, based on controlled randomized trial data, finally became available. The outcome demonstrated a 59% reduction in relative risk of total mortality at 2 years of follow-up (54% cumulative) and a 19% reduction in absolute risk of dying at 2 years of follow-up. It was followed during a period of less than 10 years by a series of randomized trial reports evaluating ICD therapy for primary and secondary prevention of SCD among patients with prior myocardial infarction, prior cardiac arrests, and heart failure.

Whereas the studies cited documented the ability of implantable devices to revert potentially fatal arrhythmias and subsequently showed a relative benefit over amiodarone in some groups of patients, the absence of placebo-controlled trials still prevents quantitation of the true magnitude of any mortality benefit because of the inability of positive-controlled trials to identify the absolute benefit of an intervention.[191] Despite these limitations, the ICD is now the preferred therapy for survivors of cardiac arrest at risk for recurrences and for primary prevention in patients in a number of high-risk categories. Major questions still unanswered include the relative benefit of amiodarone versus defibrillators among lower risk subgroups of survivors of out-of-hospital cardiac arrest, the role of beta blockers, and the role of anti-ischemic surgical and medical therapy as definitive approaches.

A much larger issue, and one that has not yet been defined, is the use of implantable defibrillators for primary prevention of cardiac arrest in patients thought to be at intermediate levels of risk. Studies of cost-effectiveness, in addition to medical efficacy, are needed.

Application of Therapeutic Strategies to Specific Groups of Patients

SECONDARY PREVENTION OF SCD AFTER SURVIVAL OF CARDIAC ARREST. As populations of cardiac arrest survivors began to accumulate from community-based emergency rescue activities, therapeutic strategies intended to improve long-term survival emerged as a mandate for clinical investigators. The problem that affects all long-term strategies for cardiac arrest survivors, however, is the lack of a reliable concurrent natural history denominator against which to compare the results of interventions. This lack is a consequence of ethical concerns about withholding therapy in a placebo-controlled study model for patients at high risk of dying,[191] in conjunction with the confounding influence of general therapies used in such patients that may also improve survival. Early approaches to long-term therapy centered on the use of antiarrhythmic drug therapy, largely guided by the results of electrophysiologic testing or the empiric use of antiarrhythmic drugs, particularly amiodarone. Various observational and positive-controlled studies had suggested that suppression of inducible ventricular arrhythmias yielded a better outcome than failure of suppression and that amiodarone is better than class I antiarrhythmic drugs. The first adequately powered secondary prevention trial of ICDs versus antiarrhythmic drugs was published in 1997. This study, the AVID trial, demonstrated a 27% reduction in relative risk of total mortality at 2 years of follow-up, with an absolute risk reduction of 7% (**Fig. 41-19**).[145] It was followed shortly thereafter by reports of two other studies, the Canadian Implantable Defibrillator Study (CIDS)[146] and the Cardiac Arrest Study Hamburg (CASH),[147] both limited by the power of the enrollment numbers but suggesting trends toward similar benefits (see Table 41-5). As a consequence of the secondary prevention trials, ICDs have emerged as the preferred therapy for survivors of out-of-hospital cardiac arrest or hemodynamically important VT. A subgroup analysis of AVID has suggested that the advantage of ICDs over antiarrhythmic drugs might be limited to patients with ejection fractions <35%.[187] As a retrospective analysis, the observation calls for confirmation in a controlled trial.

Although only one of the secondary prevention trials (AVID) demonstrated a statistically significant survival benefit of the ICD compared with antiarrhythmic therapy, usually using amiodarone, the other two showed trends to a survival benefit, supported by a meta-analysis.[192] Despite this limitation, ICD therapy has emerged as preferred therapy, regardless of ejection fraction, for survivors without identifiable and correctable transient causes of cardiac arrest. It has largely supplanted anatomically based antiarrhythmic surgery and pharmacologic antiarrhythmic approaches for secondary prevention.

AVID: Drug 25%, ICD 18% — 27% relative reduction, 7% absolute reduction, 18% residual risk (2-year analysis)

MADIT II: Usual therapy 22%, ICD 16% — 28% relative reduction, 6% absolute reduction, 16% residual risk (2-year analysis)

SCD-HeFT: Placebo/usual therapy 36%, ICD 29% — 23% relative reduction, 7% absolute reduction, 29% residual risk (5-year analysis)

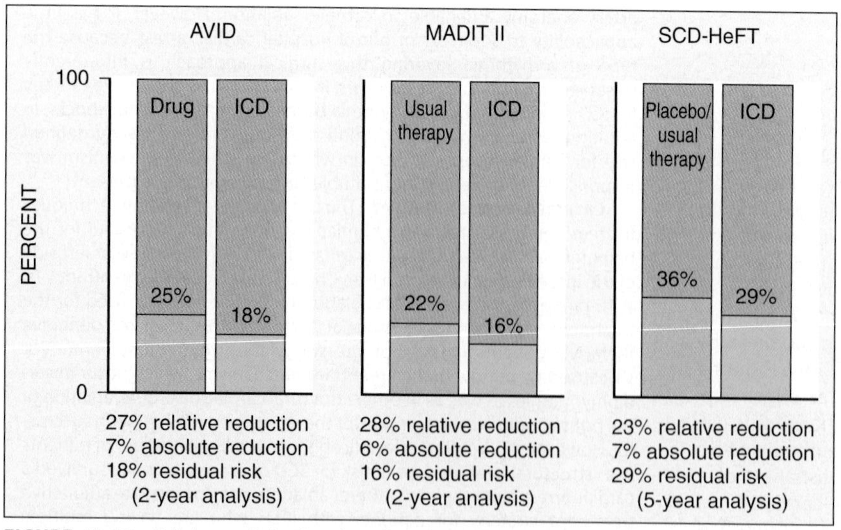

FIGURE 41-19 Relative and absolute benefits of ICDs in three ICD trials: a secondary prevention study (AVID) trial, a primary prevention trial (MADIT II), and a heart failure sudden death trial (SCD-HeFT); see text for definitions and trial descriptions. Relative risk reductions indicate proportional differences in outcomes between test and control populations, absolute reductions indicate proportional benefits for individuals, and residual risks indicate mortality remaining after accounting for ICD benefits. *(Modified from Myerburg RJ, Mitrani R, Interian A Jr, Castellanos A: Interpretation of outcomes of antiarrhythmic clinical trials: Design features and population impact. Circulation 97:1514, 1998.)*

PRIMARY PREVENTION OF SCD IN PATIENTS WITH ADVANCED HEART DISEASE. After the disturbing outcome of CAST and the suggestions of lack of efficacy or adverse effects of the class I antiarrhythmic drugs generally when used for primary or secondary prevention of SCD, interest shifted to the use of amiodarone and implantable defibrillators. Two major trials of amiodarone in post–myocardial infarction patients,[193,194] one of which required ejection fractions <40%, demonstrated no total mortality benefit, even though both trials demonstrated antiarrhythmic benefit, expressed as a reduction in arrhythmic deaths or resuscitated VF. Subgroup analyses have suggested that the concomitant use of beta blockers does confer a mortality benefit.

In parallel with the amiodarone trials, the first randomized controlled trial comparing antiarrhythmic therapy (primarily amiodarone) with ICD therapy (MADIT) was carried out (see Table 41-6).[183] The randomized patients had ejection fractions <35%, nonsustained VT during ambulatory recording, and inducible VT that was not suppressible by procainamide. This very high risk group demonstrated a 54% reduction in total mortality with ICD therapy compared with drug therapy, primarily amiodarone. At the same time, a trial comparing ICD implantation with no specific therapies for arrhythmias among patients with ejection fractions <36% who were undergoing coronary bypass surgery (CABG Patch trial) demonstrated no benefit of defibrillators for total mortality.[181] The only marker for arrhythmic risk required for entry into the study was a positive signal-averaged electrocardiogram. A third trial, MUSTT,[184] was a complex study designed to determine whether electrophysiologically guided therapy would lead to an improved outcome in patients with ambient nonsustained VT, inducible VT, history of prior myocardial infarction, and ejection fractions <40%. The results demonstrated that although a statistically significant beneficial effect on total mortality was achieved by guiding therapy according to the results of electrophysiologic testing, compared with patients with inducible tachycardia who did not receive therapy, the subgroup of patients who received ICDs because they failed to respond to drug therapy accounted for all the benefit. There was 24% mortality among ICD-treated patients at 5 years of follow-up compared with 55% among those receiving electrophysiologically guided drug therapy and 48% among those randomly assigned to no therapy. MADIT II was next among the post–myocardial infarction primary prevention trials reported.[185] In this study, ICD therapy provided a mortality benefit compared with conventional therapy among patients with prior myocardial infarction and ejection fractions <30%, with a relative risk reduction of 28% and an absolute risk reduction of 6% (22% versus 16%) at 2 years (see Fig. 41-19). During long-term follow-up, a constant annualized risk of about 8.5% was estimated among survivors, with the most powerful risk predictors being age >65 years, Class III or IV heart failure, diabetes, non–sinus rhythm, and blood urea nitrogen elevation.[195]

MADIT and MADIT II had set entry requirements of >3 weeks and >1 month after the qualifying infarction, with the actual enrollment into those and MUSTT being considerably longer on average. Because both old and recent[18] data suggested higher risk for SCD early after myocardial infarctions, the Defibrillator in Acute Myocardial Infarction Trial (DINAMIT) was designed to evaluate possible benefit of ICD implantation early after a myocardial infarction in patients with ejection fractions ≤35%[196] and other markers of risk. DINAMIT demonstrated no survival benefit attributable to early implantation of ICDs in patients randomized at 6 to 40 days after myocardial infarction (mean = 18 days), despite a reduced arrhythmic mortality. There was also an unexplained increase in nonarrhythmic mortality compared with conventional therapy that needs to be explored in future studies. The absence of early ICD benefit in light of early SCD risk has led some to call for further studies of this question.

A study designed to determine whether patients with nonischemic cardiomyopathy, accompanied by a history of heart failure, ejection fractions ≤35%, and PVCs or nonsustained VT, benefit from prophylactic ICD therapy, DEFINITE was underpowered to achieve statistical significance (P = 0.08). However, the reported results demonstrated a strong trend for benefit, with a 35% relative risk reduction and a 6% absolute risk reduction during 2 years of follow-up.[197] Subgroups with prolonged QRS durations, ejection fraction >20%, and Class III heart failure performed better than the overall cohort data. Finally, the Sudden Cardiac Death-Heart Failure Trial (SCD-HeFT) was designed to test the potential benefit of ICDs versus amiodarone, compared with placebo, in patients with functional Class II or III congestive heart failure and ejection fractions <35%. Nonischemic and ischemic cardiomyopathy were almost equally represented, with 85% of the ischemic cardiomyopathy patients having a history of prior myocardial infarction. The results of this study demonstrated a 23% reduction in relative risk and an absolute risk reduction of 7% during 5 years[198] (see Fig. 41-19). Amiodarone provided no added benefit to conventional therapy. In contrast to DEFINITE, the Class II patients in SCD-HeFT had better outcomes than Class III patients.

The mortality benefit of ICDs combined with cardiac resynchronization therapy is unclear. Although one study suggested a small mortality benefit in patients with Class III and IV heart failure,[199] another study that enrolled Class I and II heart failure patients (the majority of enrollees being Class II), with prolonged QRS durations, demonstrated a heart failure hospitalization benefit without a mortality benefit.[200]

Primary Prevention in Patients with Less Advanced Common Heart Diseases or Uncommon Diseases. Primary prevention trials have been designed to enroll populations of patients with advanced heart disease who were estimated to be at very high risk for SCD and total mortality as a consequence of the severity of the underlying disease. Most clinical trials testing the question of relative efficacy of antiarrhythmic versus ICD therapy have used the ejection fraction as the marker for advanced disease, with the upper limits of qualifying ejection fractions between 30% and 40%, the majority set at 35%. The mean or median values of those actually enrolled ranged from 21% to 30%[101]; and subgroups with ejection fractions >30%, and particularly those in the range of 35% to 40%, had lower if any benefit (**Fig. 41-20**). Moreover, in the secondary prevention trial AVID, a subgroup analysis suggested that there is no survival advantage of ICD therapy compared with amiodarone for patients with ejection fractions >35%.[187] This observation is important because it raises a question about therapeutic options, for both primary and secondary prevention strategies, when ejection fractions are >35%. However, because of the absence of controls receiving neither therapy, it is unknown whether there is equivalent benefit attributable to both therapies.

Whereas the risk for SCD and total mortality is highest among patients with advanced structural heart disease and low ejection fractions, impaired functional capacity, or both, a substantial portion of the total SCD burden occurs among patients with coronary heart disease or the various nonischemic cardiomyopathies with ejection fractions

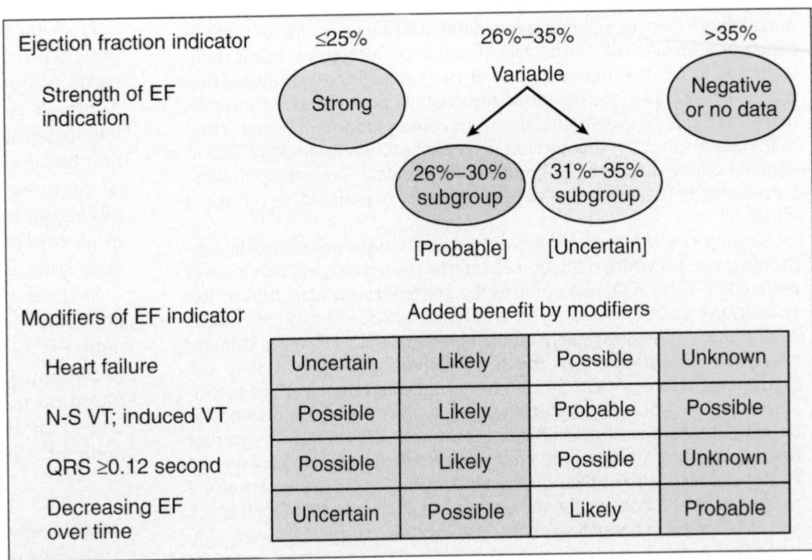

FIGURE 41-20 Modifiers of post–myocardial infarction ejection fraction indicators for ICDs. The strength of ejection fraction (EF) as a primary determinant of ICD indications after myocardial infarction varies and is apparently modulated by a number of clinical modifiers. Although stratified trial data are not available, indications from subgroup analyses suggest general patterns of modification of EF indicators by other influences. In the circumstance when EF alone appears to be a strong indicator (e.g., 20% to 25%), modifiers that have an effect at other levels of EF (e.g., heart failure) may not add further strength of prediction for total mortality. *(Modified from Myerburg RJ: Implantable cardioverter-defibrillators after myocardial infarction. N Engl J Med 359:2245, 2008.)*

between 35% and 40% and higher. In addition, among patients with heart failure related to various forms of cardiomyopathy, whereas the total mortality risk is considerably lower in patients in functional Class I or early Class II than in those with late Class III or Class IV status, the probability of a death's being sudden is higher in the former group[37,201] (see Fig. 41-8). Despite this observation, there are no data available to guide therapy for primary prevention of cardiac arrest in such patients.[10] This limitation is confounded by the fact that patients in these categories generally have low event rates but cumulatively account for large numbers of SCDs (see Fig. 41-2A, B). In addition, certain other structural entities associated with some elevation of risk for SCD in the absence of a severely reduced ejection fraction, such as some patterns of viral myocarditis, hypertrophic cardiomyopathy, right ventricular dysplasia, and sarcoidosis, are managed without the benefit of clinical trials to guide therapeutic decisions (see Table 41-7). Patients with symptomatic ventricular arrhythmias related to structural disorders such as right ventricular dysplasia, in which most of the mortality risk is arrhythmic, are often advised to have an ICD, even in the absence of a prior cardiac arrest or hemodynamically significant VT. Whether antiarrhythmic therapy would be just as effective remains unknown, but the judgment of using defibrillators in patients with a disorder whose fatal expression is primarily arrhythmic carries the strength of logic, often supported by risk profiling based on observational data of clinical markers. Among the entities in which family history is helpful for defining risk, clinical judgment is made easier when there is a strong family history of SCD. Specific support for this approach derives from genetic studies in hypertrophic cardiomyopathy. In addition, clinical observational data have supported the use of ICDs in high-risk subsets of patients with hypertrophic cardiomyopathy.[202]

Primary Prevention in Patients with Structurally Normal Hearts or Molecular Disorders of Cardiac Electrical Activity. Clinically subtle or inapparent structural disorders and entities with pure electrophysiologic expression, such as the congenital long-QT syndromes, Brugada syndrome, and idiopathic VF, are receiving increasing attention in regard to preventive activities. The decision-making process for cardiac arrest or symptomatic VT survivors with the long-QT syndrome is similar to that for other entities, in that those who have survived a potentially fatal arrhythmia are generally treated with ICDs (see Table 41-7). In contrast, individuals who express the electrocardiographic phenotype of long-QT syndrome in the absence of symptomatic arrhythmias are generally treated with beta blocker therapy. Beta blockers are also considered useful for affected family members who have not had an event and subgroups of long-QT patients with syncope of undocumented mechanism.[94] Between these extremes are the asymptomatic affected family members of patients with symptomatic long-QT syndrome. Given the complexity of the pathophysiology of potentially fatal arrhythmias among such patients, the threshold for consideration of ICD therapy is decreasing.[94] Genetic screening may ultimately prove useful for identification of a specific risk, particularly if individual arrhythmic risk is demonstrated to be determined by one or more modifier genes interacting with the defect responsible for an ion channel pore defect.[61] Currently, many such clinical therapeutic decisions remain judgment based rather than data driven.[101] In this context, a family history of premature SCD in affected relatives appears to be useful for the decision-making process for preventive therapy in this general category of patients (see Chaps. 9 and 37).

Among the other molecular arrhythmia syndromes, Brugada syndrome is one for which management strategies remain problematic and debated.[102-103] The ICD is accepted as the preferred secondary prevention strategy in cardiac arrest survivors and symptomatic affected individuals, even though it is based solely on observational data. However, primary prevention approaches for affected relatives, especially if they are asymptomatic, are unclear. Studies have suggested that syncope associated with electrocardiographic changes suggestive of the disorder at baseline is a marker of risk sufficient to warrant ICD therapy[102] and that baseline electrocardiographic changes associated with inducibility of ventricular tachyarrhythmias during electrophysiologic testing are also a marker of risk.[103] Conversely, the absence of right bundle branch block and ST-T wave changes without provocation suggests lower risk. However, a family history of SCD remains an important factor in judgment-based decisions. Similar arguments, but supported by even fewer data, apply to affected family members of patients with right ventricular dysplasia.

PRIMARY PREVENTION AMONG THE GENERAL POPULATION. Because SCD is frequently the first clinical expression of underlying structural heart disease or occurs in identified patients profiled to be at low risk (see Fig. 41-2B), there has been a longstanding interest in therapeutic strategies targeted to primary prevention. To have a major impact on the problem of SCD in the general population, including adolescents and young adults, we need to move beyond the identification of high-risk patients who have specific clinical entities, advanced or subtle, that predict a high risk for SCD. Rather, it is necessary to find small subgroups of patients in the general population at specific risk for SCD as a manifestation of underlying heart disease, if and when that disease becomes manifested. As an example, the studies that have demonstrated familial clustering of SCD as the first expression of underlying coronary artery disease suggesting genetic or behavioral predisposition may provide some help for the future.[31-33] If highly specific markers can be found, related to electrophysiologic properties or along multiple points in the cascade of coronary events (see Fig. 41-5), preventive therapy before the first expression of an underlying disease may have a major effect on the population problem of SCD. Short of that, successes will be limited to community-based intervention and to the subgroups that are easier to identify and in whom it is more justifiable to use prophylactic interventional therapy on the basis of population size and magnitude of risk.[9,10,101]

Adolescents and young adults, including athletes (see Chap. 83), constitute a group for special consideration. The SCD risk in these groups is an order of magnitude of 1% of that of the general adult population older than 35 years (see Fig. 41-4).[9,138] However, most causes of SCD in these populations are not characterized by advanced life-limiting structural heart disease, and therefore surviving cardiac arrest victims can, with appropriate long-term therapy, be expected to have significant extensions of life. Because most deaths are arrhythmic, the ability to identify individuals at risk in advance of a life-threatening arrhythmic event offers more long-term impact than for older populations. For both the general young population and athletes, identification of individuals at risk may lead to prevention of events triggered by physical activity.[203] One study has demonstrated a reduction in SCDs in athletes with the use of widespread electrocardiographic screening.[204] In the United States, strategies for screening of adolescents, young adults, and athletes to identify the entities that create a risk have largely been limited to medical and family histories and a physical examination.[205] The European[206] and the International Olympic Committee recommendations[207] add electrocardiographic screening for athletes, which continues to be debated in the United States,[208,209] despite data indicating both feasibility[210,211] and suggestions of cost-effectiveness.[203] Electrocardiographic screening of the general adolescent population, including athletes, can identify many of those at potential risk because of congenital long-QT syndrome, hypertrophic cardiomyopathy, right ventricular dysplasia, and Brugada syndrome. Although electrocardiographic screening in the adolescent and athletic subgroups is imperfect and usually accompanied by depolarization and repolarization patterns that may be difficult to interpret, this strategy can lead to further testing in appropriate individuals. Echocardiography has also been suggested as a screening method, but it is more expensive and less cost-efficient and does not recognize conditions such as long-QT syndrome and Brugada syndrome.

SCD risk must be evaluated in competitive athletes with previously known cardiovascular disorders or those discovered during preparticipation screening as well as in those with known disorders who wish to participate in recreational sports. Recommendations for the latter, based on intensity of exercise and nature of disease, are available.[212] Issues for competing athletes are more complex, including both medical[213] and legal considerations.[214]

SUDDEN DEATH AND PUBLIC SAFETY

The unexpectedness of SCD has raised questions concerning secondary risk to the public created by people in the throes of a cardiac arrest. There are no data from controlled studies available to guide public policy regarding people at high risk for potentially lethal arrhythmias and for abrupt incapacitation. In a report of observations on 1348 sudden deaths caused by coronary heart disease in people 65 years of age or younger during a 7-year period in Dade County, Florida, 101 (7.5%) of the deaths occurred in people who were engaged in activities at the time of death that were potentially hazardous to the public (e.g., driving a motor vehicle, working at altitude, piloting aircraft), and 122 (9.1%) of the victims had occupations that could create potential hazards to others if an abrupt loss of consciousness had occurred while they were at work. There were no catastrophic events as a result of these cardiac arrests, only minor property damage in 19 and minor injuries in 5.

Other studies have also led to the conclusion that risk to the public is low. In specific reference to private automobile drivers, a study from Seattle identified 33 SCDs/year while driving the estimated 1.32 million vehicles in the community. Available data suggest that unexpected cardiac arrest at the wheel usually involves a prodrome sufficient to allow the driver to get to the roadside before losing consciousness. An analysis of recurrent VT/VF events among cardiac arrest survivors has suggested limitation of driving privileges for the first 8 months after the index event on the basis of the clustering of recurrent event rates early after the index event.[18,215] Therefore, although there are likely to be isolated cases in which cardiac arrest causes public hazards, the risk appears to be small, and because it is difficult to identify specific individuals at risk, sweeping restrictions to avoid such risks appear unwarranted. The exceptions are people with multisystem disease, particularly senility, and individual circumstances that require specific consideration, such as patients with documented or substantial risk for loss of consciousness associated with the onset of arrhythmias and high-risk patients who have special responsibilities—school bus drivers, aircraft pilots, train operators, and truck drivers.[215]

REFERENCES

Epidemiology

1. Myerburg RJ, Castellanos A: Emerging paradigms of the epidemiology and demographics of sudden cardiac arrest. Heart Rhythm 3:235, 2006.
2. Priori SG, Aliot E, Blomstrom-Lundqvist C, et al: Task Force on Sudden Cardiac Death of the European Society of Cardiology. Eur Heart J 22:1374, 2001.
3. Zheng ZJ, Croft JB, Giles WH, Mensah GA: Sudden cardiac death in the United States, 1989 to 1998. Circulation 104:2158, 2001.
4. Rosamond W, Flegal K, Furie K, et al: American Heart Association Statistics Committee and Stroke Statistics Subcommittee: Heart Disease and Stroke Statistics—2008 Update: A Report from the AHA Statistics Committee and Stroke Statistics Subcommittee. Circulation 117:e25, 2008.
5. Cobb LA, Fahrenbruch CE, Olsufka M, Copass MK: Changing incidence of out-of-hospital ventricular fibrillation, 1980-2000. JAMA 288:3008, 2002.
6. Chugh SS, Jui J, Gunson K, et al: Current burden of sudden cardiac death: Multiple source surveillance versus retrospective death certificate–based review in a large U.S. community. J Am Coll Cardiol 44:1268, 2004.
7. Myerburg RJ, Wellens HJJ: Epidemiology of cardiac arrest and sudden cardiac death. *In* Priori S, Zipes D (eds): Sudden Cardiac Death: A Handbook for Clinical Practice. Oxford, UK, Blackwell Publishing, 2006, pp 3-19.
8. Nichol G, Thomas E, Callaway CW, et al: Regional variation in out-of-hospital cardiac arrest incidence and outcome. JAMA 300:1423, 2008.
9. Myerburg RJ: Sudden cardiac death: Exploring the limits of our knowledge. J Cardiovasc Electrophysiol 12:369, 2001.
10. Huikuri H, Castellanos A, Myerburg RJ: Sudden death due to cardiac arrhythmias. N Engl J Med 345:1473, 2001.
11. Fox CS, Evans JC, Larson MG, et al: Temporal trends in coronary heart disease mortality and sudden cardiac death from 1950–1999: The Framingham Heart Study. Circulation 110:522, 2004.
12. Wisten A, Forsberg H, Krantz P, Messner T: Sudden cardiac death in 15-35-year olds in Sweden during 1992-1999. J Intern Med 252:529, 2002.
13. Arntz HR, Willich SN, Schreiber C, et al: Diurnal, weekly and seasonal variation of sudden death. Population-based analysis of 24,061 consecutive cases. Eur Heart J 21:315, 2000.
14. Gami AS, Howard DE, Olson EJ, Somers VK: Day-night pattern of sudden death in obstructive sleep apnea. N Engl J Med 351:1206, 2005.
15. Gerber Y, Jacobsen SJ, Killian JM, et al: Seasonality and daily weather conditions in relation to myocardial infarction and sudden cardiac death in Olmsted County, Minnesota, 1979 to 2002. J Am Coll Cardiol 48:287, 2006.
16. Empana JP, Sauval P, Ducimetiere P, et al: Increase in out-of-hospital cardiac arrest attended by the medical mobile intensive care units, but not myocardial infarction, during the 2003 heat wave in Paris, France. Crit Care Med 37:3079, 2009.
17. Rich DQ, Schwartz J, Mittleman MA, et al: Association of short-term ambient air pollution concentrations and ventricular arrhythmias. Am J Epidemiol 161:1123, 2005.
18. Solomon SD, Zelenkofske S, McMurray JJV, et al: Sudden death in patients with myocardial infarction and left ventricular dysfunction, heart failure or both. N Engl J Med 352:2581, 2005.
19. Atkins DL, Everson-Stewart S, Sears GK, et al: Epidemiology and outcomes from out-of-hospital cardiac arrest in children: The Resuscitation Outcomes Consortium Investigators Epistry—Cardiac Arrest. Circulation 119:1484, 2009.
20. Wren C, O'Sullivan JJ, Wright C: Sudden death in children and adolescents. Heart 83:410, 2000.
21. Gillum RF: Sudden cardiac death in Hispanic Americans and African Americans. Am J Public Health 87:1461, 1997.
22. Albert CM, Chae CU, Grodstein F, et al: Prospective study of sudden cardiac death among women in the United States. Circulation 107:2096, 2003.
23. Crotti L, Lundquist AL, Insolia R, et al: KCNH2-K897T is a genetic modifier of latent congenital long QT syndrome. Circulation 112:1251, 2005.
24. Crotti L, Spazzolini C, Schwartz PJ, et al: The common long-QT syndrome mutation KCNQ1/A341V causes unusually severe clinical manifestations in patients with different ethnic backgrounds: Toward a mutation-specific risk stratification. Circulation 116:2366, 2007.
25. Bos JM, Towbin JA, Ackerman MJ: Diagnostic, prognostic, and therapeutic implications of genetic testing for hypertrophic cardiomyopathy. J Am Coll Cardiol 54:201, 2009.
26. Pfeufer A, Sanna S, Arking DE, et al: Common variants at ten loci modulate the QT interval duration in the QTSCD study. Nat Genet 41:407, 2009.
27. Samani NJ, Erdmann J, Hall AS, et al: Genomewide association analysis of coronary artery disease. N Engl J Med 357:443, 2007.
28. Faber BC, Cleutjens KB, Niessen RL, et al: Identification of genes potentially involved in rupture of human atherosclerotic plaques. Circ Res 89:547, 2001.
29. Friedlander Y, Siscovick DS, Weinmann S, et al: Family history as a risk factor for primary cardiac arrest. Circulation 97:155, 1998.
30. Jouven X, Desnos M, Guerot C, Ducimetiere P: Predicting sudden death in the population: The Paris Prospective Study I. Circulation 99:1978, 1999.
31. Dekker LR, Bezzina CR, Henriques JP, et al: Familial sudden death is an important risk factor for primary ventricular fibrillation: A case-control study in acute myocardial infarction patients. Circulation 114:1140, 2006.
32. Kaikkonen KS, Kortelainen ML, Linna E, Huikuri HV: Family history and the risk of sudden cardiac death as a manifestation of an acute coronary event. Circulation 114:1462, 2006.
33. Chugh SS, Reinier K, Singh T, et al: Determinants of prolonged QT interval and their contribution to sudden death risk in coronary artery disease: The Oregon Sudden Unexpected Death Study. Circulation 119:663, 2009.
34. Taylor AJ, Burke AP, O'Malley PG, et al: A comparison of the Framingham risk index, coronary artery calcification, and culprit plaque morphology in sudden cardiac death. Circulation 101:1243, 2000.
35. Huikuri HV, Tapanainen JM, Lindgran K, et al: Prediction of sudden cardiac death after myocardial infarction in the beta-blocking era. J Am Coll Cardiol 42:652, 2003.
36. Jouven X, Empana JP, Schwartz PJ, et al: Heart-rate profile during exercise as a predictor of sudden death. N Engl J Med 352:1951, 2005.
37. Cleland JG, Chattopadhyay S, Khand A, et al: Prevalence and incidence of arrhythmias and sudden death in heart failure. Heart Fail Rev 7:229, 2002.
38. Goldenberg I, Jonas M, Tenenbaum A, et al: Bezafibrate Infarction Prevention Study Group: Current smoking, smoking cessation, and the risk of sudden cardiac death in patients with coronary artery disease. Arch Intern Med 163:2301, 2003.
39. Albert CM, Manson JE, Cook NR, et al: Moderate alcohol consumption and the risk of sudden cardiac death among US male physicians. Circulation 100:944, 1999.
40. Albert CM, Mittleman MA, Chae CU, et al: Triggering of sudden death from cardiac causes by vigorous exertion. N Engl J Med 343:1355, 2000.
41. Rozanski A, Blumenthal JA, Kaplan J: Impact of psychological factors on the pathogenesis of cardiovascular disease and implications for therapy. Circulation 99:2192, 1999.
42. Albert CM, Chae CU, Rexrode KM, et al: Phobic anxiety and risk of coronary heart disease and sudden cardiac death among women. Circulation 111:480, 2005.
43. de Vreede-Swagemakers JJ, Gorgels AP, Weijenberg MP, et al: Risk indicators for out-of-hospital cardiac arrest in patients with coronary artery disease. J Clin Epidemiol 52:601, 1999.
44. Thombs BD, de Jonge P, Coyne JC, et al: Depression screening and patient outcomes in cardiovascular care: A systematic review. JAMA 300:2161, 2008.
45. Whooley MA, de Jonge P, Vittinghoff E, et al: Depressive symptoms, health behaviors, and risk of cardiovascular events in patients with coronary heart disease. JAMA 300:2379, 2008.
46. Leor J, Poole WK, Kloner RA: Sudden cardiac death triggered by an earthquake. N Engl J Med 334:413, 1996.
47. Lampert R, Joska T, Burg MM, et al: Emotional and physical precipitants of ventricular arrhythmia. Circulation 106:1800, 2002.
48. Kloner RA: Natural and unnatural triggers of myocardial infarction. Prog Cardiovasc Dis 48:285, 2006.
49. Myerburg RJ: Implantable cardioverter-defibrillators after myocardial infarction. N Engl J Med 359:2245, 2008.
50. Stecker EC, Vickers C, Waltz J, et al: Population-based analysis of sudden cardiac death with and without left ventricular systolic dysfunction. J Am Coll Cardiol 47:1161, 2006.
51. Jouven X, Zureik M, Desnos M, et al: Long-term outcome in asymptomatic men with exercise-induced premature ventricular depolarizations. N Engl J Med 343:826, 2000.
52. Frolkis JP, Pothier CE, Blackstone EH, Lauer MS: Frequent ventricular ectopy after exercise as a predictor of death. N Engl J Med 348:781, 2003.
53. Teerlink JR, Jalaluddin M, Anderson S, et al: Ambulatory ventricular arrhythmias in patients with heart failure do not specifically predict an increased risk of sudden death. PROMISE (Prospective Randomized Milrinone Survival Evaluation) Investigators. Circulation 101:40, 2000.
54. Bloomfield DM, Steinman RC, Namerow PB, et al: Microvolt T-wave alternans distinguishes between patients likely and patients not likely to benefit from implanted cardiac defibrillator therapy: A solution to the Multicenter Automatic Defibrillator Implantation Trial (MADIT) II conundrum. Circulation 110:1885, 2004.
55. Yan AT, Shayne AJ, Brown KA, et al: Characterization of the peri-infarct zone by contrast-enhanced cardiac magnetic resonance imaging is a powerful predictor of post–myocardial infarction mortality. Circulation 114:32, 2006.
56. Schmidt A, Azevedo CF, Cheng A, et al: Infarct tissue heterogeneity by magnetic resonance imaging identifies enhanced cardiac arrhythmia susceptibility in patients with left ventricular dysfunction. Circulation 115:2006, 2007.
57. Haigney MC, Zareba W, Gentlesk PJ, et al: QT interval variability and spontaneous ventricular tachycardia or fibrillation in the Multicenter Automatic Defibrillator Implantation Trial (MADIT) II patients. J Am Coll Cardiol 44:1481, 2004.
58. Bauer A, Kantelhardt JW, Barthel P, et al: Deceleration capacity of heart rate as a predictor of mortality after myocardial infarction: Cohort study. Lancet 367:1674, 2006.
59. Barthel P, Schneider R, Bauer A, et al: Risk stratification after acute myocardial infarction by heart rate turbulence. Circulation 108:1221, 2003.
60. Makikallio TH, Barthel P, Schneider R, et al: Prediction of sudden cardiac death after acute myocardial infarction: Role of Holter monitoring in the modern treatment era. Eur Heart J 26:762, 2005.
61. Myerburg RJ: Scientific gaps in the prediction and prevention of sudden cardiac death. J Cardiovasc Electrophysiol 13:709, 2002.
62. Costantini O, Hohnloser SH, Kirk MM, et al: ABCD Trial Investigators: The ABCD (Alternans Before Cardioverter Defibrillator) Trial: Strategies using T-wave alternans to improve efficiency of sudden cardiac death prevention. J Am Coll Cardiol 53:471, 2009.

63. Tunstall-Pedoe H (ed): MONICA Monograph and Multimedia Sourcebook. World's largest study of heart disease, stroke, risk factors and population trends, 1979-2002. Geneva, World Health Organization, 2003.
64. Nabel EG, Stevens S, Smith R: Combating chronic disease in developing countries. Lancet 373:2004, 2009.

Causes of Sudden Cardiac Death

65. Myerburg RJ, Interian A Jr, Mitrani RM, et al: Frequency of sudden cardiac death and profiles of risk. Am J Cardiol 80:10F, 1997.
66. Myerburg RJ, Kessler KM, Mallon SM, et al: Life-threatening ventricular arrhythmias in patients with silent myocardial ischemia due to coronary artery spasm. N Engl J Med 326:1451, 1992.
67. Schoenenberger AW, Kobza R, Jamshidi P, et al: Sudden cardiac death in patients with silent myocardial ischemia after myocardial infarction (from the Swiss Interventional Study on Silent Ischemia Type II [SWISSI II]). Am J Cardiol 104:158, 2009.
68. McKenna WJ, Behr ER: Hypertrophic cardiomyopathy: Management, risk stratification, and prevention of sudden death. Heart 87:169, 2002.
69. Elliott PM, Gimeno Blanes JR, Mahon NG, et al: Relation between severity of left-ventricular hypertrophy and prognosis in patients with hypertrophic cardiomyopathy. Lancet 357:420, 2001.
70. Maron MS, Olivotto I, Betocchi S, et al: Effect of left ventricular outflow tract obstruction on clinical outcome in hypertrophic cardiomyopathy. N Engl J Med 348:295, 2003.
71. Pasotti M, Klersy C, Pilotto A, et al: Long-term outcome and risk stratification in dilated cardiolaminopathies. J Am Coll Cardiol 52:1250, 2008.
72. Cooper LT: Myocarditis. N Engl J Med 360:1526, 2009.
73. Corrado D, Basso C, Thiene G: Sudden cardiac death in young people with apparently normal heart. Cardiovasc Res 50:399, 2001.
74. Theleman KP, Kuiper JJ, Roberts WC: Acute myocarditis (predominately lymphocytic) causing sudden death without heart failure. Am J Cardiol 88:1078, 2001.
75. Diaz FJ, Loewe C, Jackson A: Death caused by myocarditis in Wayne County, Michigan: A 9-year retrospective study. Am J Forensic Med Pathol 27:300, 2006.
76. Corrado D, Basso C, Nava A, Thiene G: Arrhythmogenic right ventricular cardiomyopathy: Current diagnostic and management strategies. Cardiol Rev 9:259, 2001.
77. Thiene G, Nava A, Corrado D, et al: Right ventricular cardiomyopathy and sudden death in young people. N Engl J Med 318:129, 1988.
78. Sen-Chowdhry S, Syrris P, Prasad SK, et al: Left-dominant arrhythmogenic cardiomyopathy: An under-recognized clinical entity. J Am Coll Cardiol 52:2175, 2008.
79. Tiso N, Stephan DA, Nava A, et al: Identification of mutations in the cardiac ryanodine receptor gene in families affected with arrhythmogenic right ventricular cardiomyopathy type 2 (ARVD2). Hum Mol Genet 10:189, 2001.
80. Pilichou K, Nava A, Basso C, et al: Mutations in desmoglein-2 gene are associated with arrhythmogenic right ventricular cardiomyopathy. Circulation 113:1171, 2006.
81. Norman M, Simpson M, Mogensen J, et al: Novel mutation in desmoplakin causes arrhythmogenic left ventricular cardiomyopathy. Circulation 112:636, 2005.
82. Sen-Chowdhry S, Syrris P, McKenna WJ: Genetics of right ventricular cardiomyopathy. J Cardiovasc Electrophysiol 16:927, 2005.
83. Avakian SD, Grinberg M, Ramires JA, Mansur AP: Outcome of adults with asymptomatic severe aortic stenosis. Int J Cardiol 123:322, 2008.
84. Freed LA, Levy D, Levine RA, et al: Prevalence and clinical outcome of mitral valve prolapse. N Engl J Med 341:1, 1999.
85. Chugh SS, Kelly KL, Titus JL: Sudden cardiac death with apparently normal heart. Circulation 102:649, 2000.
86. Weiss BM, Hess OM: Pulmonary vascular disease and pregnancy: Current controversies, management strategies, and perspectives. Eur Heart J 21:104, 2000.
87. Udink ten Cate FE, Breur JM, Cohen MI, et al: Dilated cardiomyopathy in isolated congenital complete atrioventricular block: Early and long-term risk in children. J Am Coll Cardiol 37:1129, 2001.
88. Tan HL, Bink-Boelkens MT, Bezzina CR, et al: A sodium-channel mutation causes isolated cardiac conduction disease. Nature 409:1043, 2001.
89. Probst V, Allouis M, Sacher F, et al: Progressive cardiac conduction defect is the prevailing phenotype in carriers of a Brugada syndrome *SCN5A* mutation. J Cardiovasc Electrophysiol 17:270, 2006.
90. Gollob MH, Green MS, Tang AS, et al: Identification of a gene responsible for familial Wolff-Parkinson-White syndrome. N Engl J Med 344:1823, 2001.
91. Roden DM: Long QT syndrome. N Engl J Med 358:169, 2008.
92. Miller TE, Estrella E, Myerburg RJ, et al: Recurrent third-trimester fetal loss and maternal mosaicism for long-QT syndrome. Circulation 109:3029, 2004.
93. Priori SG, Schwartz PJ, Napolitano C, et al: Risk stratification in the long-QT syndrome. N Engl J Med 348:1866, 2003.
94. Moss AJ, Zareba W, Hall WJ, et al: Effectiveness and limitations of beta-blocker therapy in congenital long-QT syndrome. Circulation 101:616, 2000.
95. Mohler PJ, Schott JJ, Gramolini AO, et al: Ankyrin-B mutation causes type 4 long-QT cardiac arrhythmia and sudden cardiac death. Nature 421:634, 2003.
96. Straus SM, Kors JA, De Bruin ML, et al: Prolonged QTc interval and risk of sudden cardiac death in a population of older adults. J Am Coll Cardiol 47:362, 2006.
97. Ray WA, Murray KT, Meredith S, et al: Oral erythromycin and the risk of sudden death from cardiac causes. N Engl J Med 351:1089, 2004.
98. Roden DM, Viswanathan PC: Genetics of acquired long QT syndrome. J Clin Invest 115:2025, 2005.
99. Makita N, Horie M, Nakamura T, et al: Drug-induced long-QT syndrome associated with a subclinical *SCN5A* mutation. Circulation 106:1269, 2002.
100. Gaita F, Giustetto C, Bianchi F, et al: Short QT syndrome: A familial cause of sudden death. Circulation 108:965, 2003.
101. Myerburg RJ, Reddy V, Castellanos A: Indications for implantable cardioverter-defibrillators based on evidence and judgment. J Am Coll Cardiol 54:747, 2009.
102. Priori SG, Napolitano C, Gasparini M, et al: Natural history of Brugada syndrome: Insights for risk stratification and management. Circulation 105:1342, 2002.
103. Brugada J, Brugada R, Antzelevitch C, et al: Long-term follow-up of individuals with the electrocardiographic pattern of right bundle-branch block and ST-segment elevation in precordial leads V_1 to V_3. Circulation 105:73, 2002.
104. Vatta M, Dumaine R, Varghese G, et al: Genetic and biophysical basis of sudden unexplained nocturnal death syndrome (SUNDS), a disease allelic to Brugada syndrome. Hum Mol Genet 11:337, 2002.
105. Haïssaguerre M, Derval N, Sacher F, et al: Sudden cardiac arrest associated with early repolarization. N Engl J Med 358:2016, 2008.
106. Myerburg RJ, Castellanos A: Early repolarization and sudden cardiac arrest: Theme or variation on a theme? Nat Clin Pract Cardiovasc Med 5:760, 2008.
107. Priori SG, Napolitano C, Memmi M, et al: Clinical and molecular characterization of patients with catecholaminergic polymorphic ventricular tachycardia. Circulation 106:69, 2002.
108. Hayashi M, Denjoy I, Extramiana F, et al: Incidence and risk factors of arrhythmic events in catecholaminergic polymorphic ventricular tachycardia. Circulation 119:2426, 2009.
109. Lampert R, Joska T, Burg MM, et al: Emotional and physical precipitants of ventricular arrhythmia. Circulation 106:1800, 2002.
110. Leor J, Poole WK, Kloner RA: Sudden cardiac death triggered by an earthquake. N Engl J Med 334:413, 1996.
111. Akashi YJ, Nakazawa K, Sakakibara M, et al: The clinical features of takotsubo cardiomyopathy. Q J Med 96:563, 2003.
112. Sharkey SW, Lesser JR, Zenovich AG, et al: Acute and reversible cardiomyopathy provoked by stress in women from the United States. Circulation 111:472, 2005.
113. Task Force on Sudden Infant Death Syndrome: The changing concept of sudden infant death syndrome: Diagnostic coding shifts, controversies regarding the sleeping environment, and new variables to consider in reducing risk. Pediatrics 116:1245, 2005.
114. Kinney HC, Thach BT: The sudden infant death syndrome. N Engl J Med 361:795, 2009.
115. Schwartz P, Priori S, Dumaine R, et al: A molecular link between the sudden infant death syndrome and the long-QT syndrome. N Engl J Med 343:262, 2000.
116. Puranik R, Chow CK, Duflou JA, et al: Sudden death in the young. Heart Rhythm 2:1277, 2005.
117. Corrado D, Basso C, Schiavon M, Thiene G: Screening for hypertrophic cardiomyopathy in young athletes. N Engl J Med 339:364, 1998.
118. Whang W, Manson JE, Hu FB, et al: Physical exertion, exercise, and sudden cardiac death in women. JAMA 295:1399, 2006.
119. Maron BJ, Doerer JJ, Haas TS, et al: Sudden deaths in young competitive athletes: Analysis of 1866 deaths in the United States, 1980-2006. Circulation 119:1085, 2009.
120. Madias C, Maron BJ, Weinstock J, et al: Commotio cordis—sudden cardiac death with chest wall impact. J Cardiovasc Electrophysiol 18:115, 2007.

Pathology and Pathophysiology

121. Burke AP, Farb A, Malcom GT, et al: Coronary risk factors and plaque morphology in men with coronary disease who died suddenly. N Engl J Med 336:1276, 1997.
122. Cohle SD, Suarez-Mier MP, Aguilera B: Sudden death resulting from lesions of the cardiac conduction system. Am J Forensic Med Pathol 23:83, 2002.
123. Liu YB, Wu CC, Lu LS, et al: Sympathetic nerve sprouting, electrical remodeling, and increased vulnerability to ventricular fibrillation in hypercholesterolemic rabbits. Circ Res 92:1145, 2003.
124. Dorian P, Cass D, Schwartz B, et al: Amiodarone as compared with lidocaine for shock-resistant ventricular fibrillation. N Engl J Med 347:368, 2002.
125. Beardslee MA, Lerner DL, Tadros PN, et al: Dephosphorylation and intracellular redistribution of ventricular connexin43 during electrical uncoupling induced by ischemia. Circ Res 87:656, 2000.
126. Yao JA, Hussain W, Patel P, et al: Remodeling of gap junctional channel function in epicardial border zone of healing canine infarcts. Circ Res 92:437, 2003.
127. McLennan PL: Myocardial membrane fatty acids and the antiarrhythmic actions of dietary fish oil in animal models. Lipids 36(Suppl):S111, 2001.
128. Makikallio TH, Koistinen J, Jordaens L, et al: Heart rate dynamics before spontaneous onset of ventricular fibrillation in patients with healed myocardial infarcts. Am J Cardiol 83:880, 1999.

Clinical Characteristics of the Patient with Cardiac Arrest

129. Huikuri HV, Makikallio TH, Raatikainen MJ, et al: Prediction of sudden cardiac death: Appraisal of the studies and methods assessing the risk of sudden arrhythmic death. Circulation 108:110, 2003.
130. ECC Committee, Subcommittees and Task Forces of the American Heart Association: 2005 AHA Guidelines for Cardiopulmonary Resuscitation and Emergency Cardiovascular Care. Circulation 112(Suppl):IV1, 2005.
131. Peberdy MA, Ornato JP, Larkin GK, et al: National Registry of Cardiopulmonary Resuscitation Investigators: Survival from in-hospital cardiac arrest during nights and weekends. JAMA 299:785, 2008.
132. Chan PS, Krumholz HM, Nichol G, Nallamothu BK: American Heart Association National Registry of Cardiopulmonary Resuscitation Investigators: Delayed time to defibrillation after in-hospital cardiac arrest. N Engl J Med 358:9, 2008.
133. Herlitz J, Bang A, Alsen B, Aune S: Characteristics and outcome among patients suffering from in hospital cardiac arrest in relation to the interval between collapse and start of CPR. Resuscitation 53:21, 2002.
134. Kim C, Becker L, Eisenberg MS: Out-of-hospital cardiac arrest in octogenarians and nonagenarians. Arch Intern Med 160:3439, 2000.
135. Kette F, Sbrojavacca R, Rellini G, et al: Epidemiology and survival rate of out-of-hospital cardiac arrest in northeast Italy: The F.A.C.S. study. Friuli Venezia Giulia Cardiac Arrest Cooperative Study. Resuscitation 36:153, 1998.
136. The Hypothermia after Cardiac Arrest Study Group: Mild therapeutic hypothermia to improve the neurologic outcome after cardiac arrest. N Engl J Med 346:549, 2002.
137. Bernard SA, Gray TW, Buist MD, et al: Treatment of comatose survivors of out-of-hospital cardiac arrest with induced hypothermia. N Engl J Med 346:557, 2002.
138. Myerburg RJ: Sudden cardiac death in persons with normal (or near normal) hearts. Am J Cardiol 79(Suppl 6A):3, 1997.

139. Krahn AD, Healey JS, Chauhan V, et al: Systematic assessment of patients with unexplained cardiac arrest: Cardiac Arrest Survivors With Preserved Ejection Fraction Registry (CASPER). Circulation 120:278, 2009.
140. Gorgels AP, Gijsbers C, de Vreede-Swagemakers J, et al: Out-of-hospital cardiac arrest—the relevance of heart failure. The Maastricht Circulatory Arrest Registry. Eur Heart J 24:1204, 2003.
141. Laurent I, Monchi M, Chiche JD, et al: Reversible myocardial dysfunction in survivors of out-of-hospital cardiac arrest. J Am Coll Cardiol 40:2110, 2002.
142. Bunch TJ, White RD, Gersh BJ, et al: Long-term outcomes of out-of-hospital cardiac arrest after successful early defibrillation. N Engl J Med 348:2626, 2003.
143. Iuliano S, Fisher SG, Karasik PE, et al: QRS duration and mortality in patients with congestive heart failure. Am Heart J 143:1085, 2002.
144. Pell JP, Corstorphine M, McConnachie A, et al: Post-discharge survival following pre-hospital cardiopulmonary arrest due to cardiac aetiology: Temporal trends and impact of changes in clinical management. Eur Heart J 27:406, 2006.
145. The Antiarrhythmics versus Implantable Defibrillators (AVID) Investigators: A comparison of antiarrhythmic-drug therapy with implantable defibrillators in patients resuscitated from near-fatal ventricular arrhythmias. N Engl J Med 337:1576, 1997.
146. Connolly SJ, Gent M, Roberts RS, et al: Canadian Implantable Defibrillator Study (CIDS): A randomized trial of the implantable cardioverter defibrillator against amiodarone. Circulation 101:1297, 2000.
147. Kuck KH, Cappato R, Siebels J, Ruppel R: Randomized comparison of antiarrhythmic drug therapy with implantable defibrillators in patients resuscitated from cardiac arrest: The Cardiac Arrest Study Hamburg (CASH). Circulation 102:748, 2000.

Management of Cardiac Arrest

148. Waalewijn RA, de Vos R, Koster RW: Out-of-hospital cardiac arrests in Amsterdam and its surrounding areas: Results from the Amsterdam resuscitation study (ARREST) in "Utstein" style. Resuscitation 28:157, 1998.
149. Eisenberg MS, Psaty BM: Defining and improving survival rates from cardiac arrest in US communities. JAMA 301:860, 2009.
150. Morrison LJ, Visentin LM, Kiss A, et al: Validation of a rule for termination of resuscitation in out-of-hospital cardiac arrest. N Engl J Med 355:478, 2006.
151. Weisfeldt ML, Becker LB: Resuscitation after cardiac arrest: A three-phase time-sensitive model. JAMA 288:3035, 2002.
152. Holmberg M, Holmberg S, Herlitz J: The problem of out-of-hospital cardiac arrest: Prevalence of sudden death in Europe today. Am J Cardiol 83:88D, 1999.
153. White RD, Hankins DG, Bugliosi TF: Seven years' experience with early defibrillation by police and paramedics in an emergency medical services system. Resuscitation 39:145, 1998.
154. Myerburg RJ, Fenster J, Velez M, et al: Impact of community-wide police car deployment of automated external defibrillators on out-of-hospital cardiac arrest. Circulation 106:1058, 2002.
155. Hollenberg J, Riva G, Bohm K, et al: Dual dispatch early defibrillation in out-of-hospital cardiac arrest: The SALSA-pilot. Eur Heart J 30:1781, 2009.
156. Cobb LA, Fahrenbruch CE, Walsh TR, et al: Influence of cardiopulmonary resuscitation prior to defibrillation in patients with out-of-hospital ventricular fibrillation. JAMA 281:1182, 1999.
157. Dowie R, Campbell H, Donohoe R, Clarke P: "Event tree" analysis of out-of-hospital cardiac arrest data: Confirming the importance of bystander CPR. Resuscitation 56:173, 2003.
158. Wik L, Hansen TB, Fylling F, et al: Delaying defibrillation to give basic cardiopulmonary resuscitation to patients with out-of-hospital ventricular fibrillation: A randomized trial. JAMA 289:1389, 2003.
159. Capucci A, Aschiere D, Piepoli MF, et al: Tripling survival from sudden cardiac arrest via early defibrillation without traditional education in cardiopulmonary resuscitation. Circulation 106:1065, 2002.
160. Nadkarni VM, Larkin GL, Peberdy MA, et al: First documented rhythm and clinical outcome from in-hospital cardiac arrest among children and adults. JAMA 295:50, 2006.
161. Sayre MR, Berg RA, Cave DM, et al: Hands-only (compression-only) cardiopulmonary resuscitation: A call to action for bystander response to adults who experience out-of-hospital sudden cardiac arrest: A science advisory for the public from the American Heart Association Emergency Cardiovascular Care Committee. Circulation 117:2162, 2008.
162. Valenzuela TD, Kern KB, Clark LL, et al: Interruptions of chest compressions during emergency medical systems resuscitation. Circulation 112:1259, 2005.
163. SOS-KANTO Study Group: Cardiopulmonary resuscitation by bystanders with chest compression only (SOS-KANTO): An observational study. Lancet 369:920, 2007.
164. Kellum MJ, Kennedy KW, Barney R, et al: Cardiocerebral resuscitation improves neurologically intact survival of patients with out-of-hospital cardiac arrest. Ann Emerg Med 52:244, 2008.
165. Bobrow BJ, Clark LL, Ewy GA, et al: Minimally interrupted cardiac resuscitation by emergency medical services providers for out-of-hospital cardiac arrest. JAMA 229:1158, 2008.
166. Havel C, Berzlanovich A, Sterz F, et al: Safety, feasibility, and hemodynamic and blood flow effects of active compression-decompression of thorax and abdomen in patients with cardiac arrest. Crit Care Med 36:1832, 2008.
167. Page RL, Joglar JA, Kowal RC, et al: Use of automated external defibrillators by a U.S. airline. N Engl J Med 343:1210, 2000.
168. Caffrey SL, Willoughby PJ, Pepe PE, Becker LB: Public use of automated external defibrillators. N Engl J Med 347:1242, 2002.
169. Valenzuela TD, Roe DJ, Nichol G, et al: Outcomes of rapid defibrillation by security officers after cardiac arrest in casinos. N Engl J Med 343:1206, 2000.
170. Hallstrom AP, Ornato JP, Weisfeldt M, et al: Public-access defibrillation and survival after out-of-hospital cardiac arrest. N Engl J Med 351:637, 2004.
171. Folke F, Lippert FK, Nielsen SL, et al: Location of cardiac arrest in a city center: Strategic placement of automated external defibrillators in public locations. Circulation 120:510, 2009.
172. Drezner JA, Rao AL, Heistand J, et al: Effectiveness of emergency response planning for sudden cardiac arrest in United States high schools with automated external defibrillators. Circulation 120:518, 2009.
173. Bardy GH, Lee KL, Mark DB, et al: Home use of automated external defibrillators for sudden cardiac arrest. N Engl J Med 358:1793, 2008.
174. Evaluating the effectiveness of the LifeVest defibrillator and improving methods for determining the use of implantable cardioverter defibrillators (The VEST/PREDICTS Study). Available at: www.clinicaltrials.gov. Accessed August 1, 2009.
175. Myerburg RJ, Feigal DW, Lindsay BD: Life-threatening malfunction of implantable cardiac devices. N Engl J Med 354:2309, 2006.
176. Shah JS, Maisel WH: Recalls and safety alerts affecting automated external defibrillators. JAMA 296:655, 2006.
177. Stiell IG, Wells GA, Field B, et al: Advanced cardiac life support in out-of-hospital cardiac arrest. N Engl J Med 351:647, 2004.
178. Gueugniaud PY, Mols P, Goldstein P, et al: A comparison of repeated high doses and repeated standard doses of epinephrine for cardiac arrest outside the hospital: European Epinephrine Study Group. N Engl J Med 339:1595, 1998.
179. Zipes DP, Camm AJ, Borggrefe M, et al: ACC/AHA/ESC 2006 Guidelines for Management of Patients With Ventricular Arrhythmias and the Prevention of Sudden Cardiac Death—Executive Summary: A Report of the ACC/AHA Task Force and the ESC Committee for Practice Guidelines. J Am Coll Cardiol 48:1064, 2006.
180. Epstein AE, DiMarco JP, Ellenbogen KA, et al: ACC/AHA/HRS 2008 Guidelines for device-based therapy of cardiac rhythm abnormalities: Executive Summary: A Report of the ACC/AHA Task Force on Practice Guidelines. J Am Coll Cardiol 51:2085, 2008.
181. Bigger JT Jr: Prophylactic use of implanted cardiac defibrillators in patients at high risk for ventricular arrhythmias after coronary-artery bypass graft surgery. Coronary Artery Bypass Graft (CABG) Patch Trial Investigators. N Engl J Med 337:1569, 1997.

Prevention of Cardiac Arrest and Sudden Cardiac Death

182. Exner DV, Kavanagh KM, Slawnych MP, et al: Noninvasive risk assessment early after a myocardial infarction: The REFINE study. J Am Coll Cardiol 50:2275, 2007.
183. Moss AJ, Hall WJ, Cannom DS, et al: Improved survival with an implanted defibrillator in patients with coronary disease at high risk for ventricular arrhythmia. N Engl J Med 335:1933, 1996.
184. Buxton AE, Lee KL, Fisher JD, et al: A randomized study of the prevention of sudden death in patients with coronary artery disease. N Engl J Med 341:1882, 1999.
185. Moss AJ, Zareba W, Hall WJ, et al: Prophylactic implantation of a defibrillator in patients with myocardial infarction and reduced ejection fraction. N Engl J Med 346:877, 2002.
186. Daubert JP, Zareba W, Hall WJ, et al: Predictive value of ventricular arrhythmia inducibility for subsequent ventricular tachycardia or ventricular fibrillation in Multicenter Automatic Defibrillator Implantation Trial (MADIT) II patients. J Am Coll Cardiol 47:98, 2006.
187. Domanski MJ, Sakseena S, Epstein AE, et al: Relative effectiveness of the implantable cardioverter-defibrillator and antiarrhythmic drugs in patients with varying degrees of left ventricular dysfunction who have survived malignant ventricular arrhythmias. J Am Coll Cardiol 34:1090, 1999.
188. Hohnloser SH, Crijns HJGM, van Eickels M, et al: Effect of dronedarone on cardiovascular events in atrial fibrillation. N Engl J Med 360:668, 2009.
189. Priori SG, Aliot E, Blomstrom-Lundqvist C, et al: Update of the guidelines on sudden cardiac death of the European Society of Cardiology. Eur Heart J 24:13, 2003.
190. Reddy VY, Reynolds MR, Neuzil P, et al: Prophylactic catheter ablation for the prevention of defibrillator therapy. N Engl J Med 357:2657, 2007.
191. Myerburg RJ, Mitrani R, Interian A Jr, Castellanos A: Interpretation of outcomes of antiarrhythmic clinical trials: Design features and population impact. Circulation 97:1514, 1998.
192. Connolly SJ, Hallstrom AP, Cappato R, et al: Meta-analysis of the implantable cardioverter defibrillator secondary prevention trials. Eur Heart J 21:2071, 2000.
193. Julian DG, Camm AJ, Frangin G, et al: Randomised trial of effect of amiodarone on mortality in patients with left-ventricular dysfunction after recent myocardial infarction: EMIAT. Lancet 349:667, 1997.
194. Cairns JA, Connolly SJ, Roberts R, Gent M: Randomised trial of outcome after myocardial infarction in patients with frequent or repetitive ventricular premature depolarisations: CAMIAT. Lancet 349:675, 1997.
195. Cygankiewicz I, Gillespie J, Zareba W, et al: Predictors of long-term mortality in Multicenter Automatic Defibrillator Implantation Trial II (MADIT II) patients with implantable cardioverter-defibrillators. Heart Rhythm 6:468, 2009.
196. Hohnloser SH, Kuck KH, Dorian P, et al: Prophylactic use of an implantable cardioverter-defibrillator after acute myocardial infarction. N Engl J Med 351:2481, 2004.
197. Kadish A, Dyer A, Daubert JP, et al: Prophylactic defibrillator implantation in patients with nonischemic dilated cardiomyopathy. N Engl J Med 350:2151, 2004.
198. Bardy GH, Lee KL, Mark DB, et al: Amiodarone or an implantable cardioverter-defibrillator for congestive heart failure. N Engl J Med 352:225, 2005.
199. Bristow MR, Saxon LA, Boehmer J, et al: Cardiac-resynchronization therapy with or without an implantable defibrillator in advanced chronic heart failure. N Engl J Med 350:2140, 2004.
200. Moss AJ, Hall WJ, Cannom DS, et al: Cardiac-resynchronization therapy for the prevention of heart-failure events. N Engl J Med 361:1329, 2009.
201. MERIT-HF Study Group: Effect of metoprolol CR/XL in chronic heart failure: Metoprolol CR/XL Randomised Intervention Trial in Congestive Heart Failure (MERIT-HF). Lancet 353:2001, 1999.
202. Maron BJ, Spirito P, Shen WK, et al: Implantable cardioverter-defibrillators and prevention of sudden cardiac death in hypertrophic cardiomyopathy. JAMA 298:405, 2007.
203. Fuller CM: Cost effectiveness analysis of screening of high school athletes for risk of sudden cardiac death. Med Sci Sports Exerc 32:887, 2000.
204. Corrado D, Basso C, Pavei A, et al: Trends in sudden cardiovascular death in young competitive athletes after implementation of a preparticipation screening program. JAMA 296:1593, 2006.
205. Maron BJ, Thompson PD, Ackerman MJ, et al: Recommendations and considerations related to preparticipation screening for cardiovascular abnormalities in competitive athletes: 2007 update: A scientific statement from the American Heart Association Council on Nutrition, Physical Activity, and Metabolism. Circulation 115:1643, 2007.
206. Corrado D, Pelliccia A, Bjornstad HH, et al: Cardiovascular pre-participation screening of young competitive athletes for prevention of sudden death: Proposal for a common European protocol. Consensus Statement of the Study Group of Sport Cardiology of the Working Group of Cardiac Rehabilitation and Exercise Physiology and the Working Group of Myocardial and Pericardial Diseases of the European Society of Cardiology. Eur Heart J 26:516, 2005.

207. International Olympic Committee Medical Commission: Sudden cardiovascular death in sport. Lausanne Recommendations; Preparticipation Cadiovascular Screening: 10 December 2004. Available at: http://multimedia.olympic.org/pdf/en_report_886.pdf. Accessed August 8, 2009.
208. Chaitman BR: An electrocardiogram should not be included in routine preparticipation screening of young athletes. Circulation 116:2610, 2007.
209. Myerburg RJ, Vetter VL: Electrocardiograms should be included in pre-participation screening of athletes. Circulation 116:2616, 2007.
210. Pelliccia A, Di Paolo FM, Corrado D, et al: Evidence for efficacy of the Italian national pre-participation screening programme for identification of hypertrophic cardiomyopathy in competitive athletes. Eur Heart J 27:2196, 2006.
211. Pelliccia A, Culasso F, Di Paolo FM, et al: Prevalence of abnormal electrocardiograms in a large, unselected population undergoing pre-participation cardiovascular screening. Eur Heart J 28:2006, 2007.
212. Maron BJ, Chaitmen BR, Ackerman MJ, et al: Recommendations for physical activities and recreational sports participation for young patients with genetic cardiovascular diseases. Circulation 109:2807, 2004.
213. Douglas PS: Saving athletes' lives a reason to find common ground? J Am Coll Cardiol 52:1997, 2008.
214. Paterick TE, Paterick TJ, Fletcher GF, Maron BJ: Medical and legal issues in the cardiovascular evaluation of competitive athletes. JAMA 294:3011, 2005.

Sudden Death and Public Safety

215. Epstein AE, Miles WM, Benditt DG, et al: Personal and public safety issues related to arrhythmias that may affect consciousness: Implications for regulation and physician recommendations. A medical/scientific statement from the AHA and the NASPE. Circulation 94:1147, 1996.

CHAPTER 42 Hypotension and Syncope

Hugh Calkins and Douglas P. Zipes

Definition

Syncope is a transient loss of consciousness due to transient global cerebral hypoperfusion characterized by rapid onset, short duration, and spontaneous recovery.[1] Loss of consciousness results from a reduction of blood flow to the reticular activating system located in the brainstem and does not require electrical or chemical therapy for reversal. The metabolism of the brain, in contrast to that of many other organs, is exquisitely dependent on perfusion. Consequently, cessation of cerebral blood flow leads to loss of consciousness within approximately 10 seconds. Restoration of appropriate behavior and orientation after a syncopal episode is usually immediate. Retrograde amnesia, although uncommon, can be present in the elderly. Syncope, as defined here, represents a subset of a much wider spectrum of conditions that can result in transient loss of consciousness, including conditions such as stroke and epileptic seizures. Nonsyncopal causes of transient loss of consciousness differ in their mechanism and duration.[1]

Syncope is an important clinical problem because it is common, costly, and often disabling; it may cause injury, and it may be the only warning sign before sudden cardiac death (see Chap. 41)[1-3]. Wisten and colleagues[3] reported that 25% of 162 victims of sudden death 15 to 35 years old initially presented with syncope or presyncope. Patients with syncope account for 1% of hospital admissions and 3% of emergency department visits. Surveys of young adults have revealed that up to 50% report a prior episode of loss of consciousness. Most of these episodes are isolated events that never come to medical attention. There is a particularly high prevalence of a first episode of syncope between the age of 10 and 30 years with a peak around the age of 15 years. The age distribution of syncopal episodes is bimodal, with a second peak ≥65 years and especially ≥70 years. The annual incidence of syncope in the elderly has been reported to be 6% per year. It is therefore not surprising that a study derived from the Medicare data base reported an annual cost of hospitalizations of $2.4 billion for management of patients with syncope.[4] Patients who experience syncope also report a markedly reduced quality of life. In addition, syncope can result in traumatic injury. One study reported that 29% of syncope patients who presented to an emergency department suffered from a minor traumatic injury, and 5% experienced severe traumatic injury including major injury resulting from syncope-induced motor vehicle accidents.[5]

The prognosis of patients with syncope varies greatly with the diagnosis. Patients with syncope in the setting of structural heart disease or primary electrical disease have an increased incidence of sudden death and overall mortality. Syncope due to orthostatic hypotension is associated with a twofold increased mortality, which results largely from the multiple comorbidities in this group of patients. In contrast, young patients with neurally mediated syncope have an excellent prognosis.

Classification

Shown in **Tables 42-1 and 42-2** are the diagnostic considerations in patients with real or apparent transient loss of consciousness (Table 42-1) and those with syncope (Table 42-2). An approach to the differential diagnosis of transient loss of consciousness is outlined in **Figure 42-1**.[1] Syncope can be distinguished from most other causes of transient loss of consciousness by asking whether the loss of consciousness was transient, rapid in onset, of short duration, and followed by spontaneous recovery. If the answer to each of these questions is yes and the transient loss of consciousness did not result from head trauma, the diagnostic considerations include true syncope in which the mechanism of transient loss of consciousness is global cerebral hypoperfusion, epileptic seizures, psychogenic syncope, and other rare causes. In evaluating a patient with transient loss of consciousness, it is important to consider nonsyncopal conditions, such as metabolic disorders, epilepsy, and alcohol, as well as conditions in which consciousness is only apparently lost (i.e., conversion reaction). These psychogenic causes of syncope, being recognized with increased frequency, are typically diagnosed in patients ≤40 years and especially in those with a history of psychiatric disease.

The differential diagnosis of syncope (see Table 42-2) includes vascular causes as most common, followed by cardiac causes, with arrhythmias most common (see Chap. 39). Although knowledge of the common conditions that can cause syncope is essential and allows the clinician to arrive at a probable cause of syncope in the majority of patients, it is equally important to be aware of several less common but potentially lethal causes of syncope, such as the long-QT syndrome, arrhythmogenic right ventricular dysplasia, Brugada syndrome, hypertrophic cardiomyopathy, idiopathic ventricular fibrillation (VF), catecholaminergic polymorphic ventricular tachycardia, short-QT syndrome, and pulmonary emboli.[6-13]

The distribution of causes of syncope varies both with the patient's age and with the clinical setting in which the patient is evaluated.[14,15] Neurally mediated syncope and other causes of reflex-mediated syncope are the most common causes of syncope at any age and in any setting. Cardiac causes of syncope, especially cardiac tachyarrhythmias and bradyarrhythmias, are the second most common causes of syncope. The incidence of cardiac causes of syncope is higher in the elderly and in patients who present to emergency departments for evaluation. Orthostatic hypotension is extremely uncommon in patients younger than 40 years but is common in the very elderly (see Chap. 80).

CH 42

TABLE 42-1 Causes of Real or Apparent Transient Loss of Consciousness

Syncope (see Table 42-2)
Neurologic or cerebrovascular disease
- Epilepsy
- Vertebrobasilar transient ischemic attack

Metabolic syndromes and coma
- Hyperventilation with hypocapnia
- Hypoglycemia
- Hypoxemia
- Intoxication with drugs or alcohol
- Coma

Psychogenic syncope
- Anxiety, panic disorder
- Somatization disorders

Vascular Causes of Syncope

Vascular causes of syncope, particularly reflex-mediated syncope and orthostatic hypotension, are by far the most common causes, accounting for at least one third of all syncopal episodes.[1,2,16-18] In contrast, vascular steal syndromes are exceedingly uncommon causes of syncope.

Orthostatic Hypotension

Standing displaces 500 to 800 mL of blood to the abdomen and lower extremities, resulting in an abrupt drop in venous return to the heart. This drop leads to a decrease in cardiac output and stimulation of aortic, carotid, and cardiopulmonary baroreceptors that trigger a reflex increase in sympathetic outflow. As a result, heart rate, cardiac contractility, and vascular resistance increase to maintain a stable systemic blood pressure on standing. Orthostatic intolerance is a term used to refer to the signs and symptoms of an abnormality in any portion of this blood pressure control system. Symptoms of orthostatic intolerance include syncope, lightheadedness or presyncope, tremulousness, weakness, fatigue, palpitations, diaphoresis, and blurred or tunnel vision. Orthostatic hypotension is defined as a drop of 20 mm Hg in systolic blood pressure or a drop of 10 mm Hg in diastolic blood pressure within 3 minutes of standing. Orthostatic hypotension can be asymptomatic or associated with the symptoms of orthostatic intolerance listed before. These symptoms are often worse immediately on arising in the morning or after meals or exercise. Initial orthostatic hypotension is defined as a decrease of >40 mm Hg in blood pressure immediately on standing with rapid return to normal (<30 seconds).[19] In contrast, delayed progressive orthostatic hypotension is characterized by a slow progressive decrease in systolic blood pressure on standing.[20] Syncope that occurs after meals, particularly in elderly people, can result from a redistribution of blood to the gut. A decline in systolic blood pressure of about 20 mm Hg approximately 1 hour after eating has been reported in up to one third of elderly nursing home residents. Although usually asymptomatic, it can result in lightheadedness or syncope.

Drugs that either cause volume depletion or result in vasodilation are the most common cause of orthostatic hypotension (**Table 42-3**). Elderly patients are particularly susceptible to the hypotensive effects of drugs because of reduced baroreceptor sensitivity, decreased cerebral blood flow, renal sodium wasting, and impaired thirst mechanism that develops with aging. Orthostatic hypotension can also result from neurogenic causes, which can be subclassified into primary and secondary autonomic failure (see Chap. 94). Primary causes are generally idiopathic, whereas secondary causes are associated with a known biochemical or structural anomaly or are seen as part of a particular disease or syndrome. There are three types of primary autonomic failure. Pure autonomic failure (Bradbury-Eggleston syndrome) is an idiopathic sporadic disorder characterized by orthostatic hypotension, usually in conjunction with evidence of more widespread autonomic failure, such as disturbances in bowel, bladder, thermoregulatory, and sexual function. Patients with pure autonomic failure have

TABLE 42-2 Causes of Syncope

Vascular
- Anatomic
  - Vascular steal syndromes (subclavian steal syndrome)
- Orthostatic
  - Autonomic insufficiency
  - Idiopathic
  - Volume depletion
  - Drug and alcohol induced
- Reflex mediated
  - Carotid sinus hypersensitivity
  - Neurally mediated syncope (common faint, vasodepressor, neurocardiogenic, vasovagal)
  - Glossopharyngeal syncope
  - Situational (acute hemorrhage, cough, defecation, laugh, micturition, sneeze, swallow, postprandial)

Cardiac
- Anatomic
  - Obstructive cardiac valve disease
  - Aortic dissection
  - Atrial myxoma
  - Pericardial disease, tamponade
  - Hypertrophic obstructive cardiomyopathy
  - Myocardial ischemia, infarction
  - Pulmonary embolism
  - Pulmonary hypertension
- Arrhythmias
  - Bradyarrhythmias
    - Atrioventricular block
    - Sinus node dysfunction, bradycardia
  - Tachyarrhythmias
    - Supraventricular tachycardia
      - Atrial fibrillation
        - Paroxysmal supraventricular tachycardia (AVNRT, WPW)
        - Other
      - Ventricular tachycardia
        - Structural heart disease
        - Inherited syndromes (ARVD, HCM, Brugada syndrome, long-QT syndrome)
        - Drug-induced proarrhythmia
      - Implanted pacemaker or ICD malfunction

Syncope of Unknown Origin

AVNRT = AV nodal reentrant tachycardia; ARVD = arrhythmogenic right ventricular dysplasia; HCM = hypertrophic cardiomyopathy; ICD = implantable cardioverter-defibrillator; WPW = Wolff-Parkinson-White syndrome.

reduced supine plasma norepinephrine levels. Multiple system atrophy (Shy-Drager syndrome) is a sporadic, progressive, adult-onset disorder characterized by autonomic dysfunction, parkinsonism, and ataxia in any combination. The third type of primary autonomic failure is Parkinson disease with autonomic failure. A small subset of patients with Parkinson disease may also experience autonomic failure, including orthostatic hypotension. In addition to these forms of chronic autonomic failure there is a rare acute panautonomic neuropathy. This neuropathy generally occurs in young people and results in widespread severe sympathetic and parasympathetic failure with orthostatic hypotension, loss of sweating, disruption of bladder and bowel function, fixed heart rate, and fixed dilated pupils.

Postural orthostatic tachycardia syndrome (POTS) is a milder form of chronic autonomic failure and orthostatic intolerance characterized by symptoms of orthostatic intolerance, increase of 28 beats/min or more in heart rate, and absence of a significant change in blood pressure within 5 minutes of standing or upright tilt.[1,2,17] The precise pathophysiologic basis for POTS syndrome has not been well defined. Some patients have both POTS and neurally mediated syncope.

Reflex-Mediated Syncope

The reflex-mediated causes of syncope are listed in Table 42-2. These are a group of conditions in which cardiovascular reflexes that control circulation become inappropriate in response to a trigger that results in vasodilation with or without bradycardia and a drop in blood pressure and global cerebral hypoperfusion. In each case, the reflex is composed of a trigger (the afferent limb) and a response (the efferent limb). This group of reflex-mediated syncopal syndromes has in common the response limb of the reflex, which consists of increased vagal tone and a withdrawal of peripheral sympathetic tone that leads to bradycardia, vasodilation, and, ultimately, hypotension, presyncope, or syncope. If hypotension due to peripheral vasodilation predominates, it is classified as a vasodepressor-type reflex response; if bradycardia or asystole predominates, it is classified as a cardioinhibitory response; and when both vasodilation and bradycardia play a role, it is classified as a mixed response. The specific triggers are what distinguish these causes of syncope. For example, micturition syncope results from activation of mechanoreceptors in the bladder; defecation syncope results from neural inputs from gut wall tension receptors; and swallowing syncope results from afferent neural impulses arising from the upper gastrointestinal tract. The two most common types of reflex-mediated syncope, carotid sinus hypersensitivity and neurally mediated hypotension, are discussed later. Identification of the trigger is of importance because of its therapeutic implications as avoidance of the trigger may prevent further syncopal episodes.

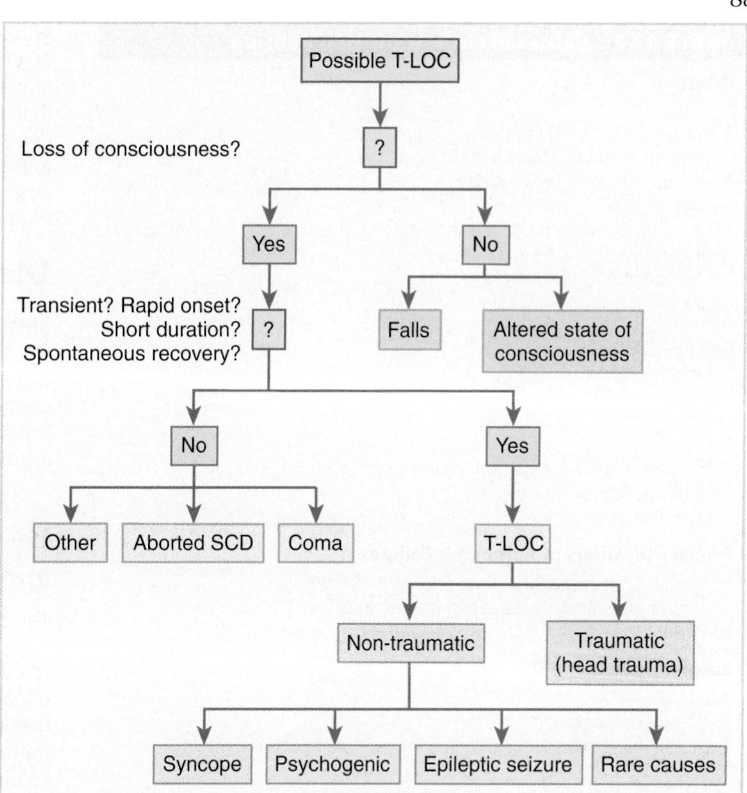

FIGURE 42-1 Approach to the evaluation of patients with transient loss of consciousness (T-LOC). SCD = sudden cardiac death. *(Modified from Moya A, Sutton R, Ammirati F, et al: Guidelines for the diagnosis and management of syncope (version 2009): The Task Force for the Diagnosis and Management of Syncope of the European Society of Cardiology [ESC]. Eur Heart J 30:2631, 2009.)*

Neurally Mediated Hypotension or Syncope (Vasovagal Syncope)

The term *neurally mediated hypotension* or *syncope* (also known as neurocardiogenic, vasodepressor, and vasovagal syncope and "fainting") has been used to describe a common abnormality of blood pressure regulation characterized by the abrupt onset of hypotension with or without bradycardia. Triggers associated with the development of neurally mediated syncope include orthostatic stress, such as can occur with prolonged standing or a hot shower, and emotional stress, such as can result from the sight of blood.[1,2,16] It has recently been recognized that a large proportion of patients with neurally mediated syncope have minor psychiatric disorders.[21,22] It has been proposed that neurally mediated syncope results from a paradoxical reflex that is initiated when ventricular preload is reduced by venous pooling. This reduction leads to a reduction in cardiac output and blood pressure, which is sensed by arterial baroreceptors. The resultant increased catecholamine levels, combined with reduced venous filling, lead to a vigorously contracting volume-depleted ventricle. The heart itself is involved in this reflex by virtue of the presence of mechanoreceptors, or C fibers, consisting of nonmyelinated fibers found in the atria, ventricles, and pulmonary artery. It has been proposed that vigorous contraction of a volume-depleted ventricle leads to activation of these receptors in susceptible individuals. These afferent C fibers project centrally to the dorsal vagal nucleus of the medulla, leading to a "paradoxical" withdrawal of peripheral sympathetic tone and an increase in vagal tone, which in turn causes vasodilation and bradycardia. The ultimate clinical consequence is syncope or presyncope. Not all neurally mediated syncope results from activation of mechanoreceptors. In humans, the sight of blood or extreme emotion can trigger syncope, suggesting that higher neural centers can also participate in the pathophysiologic process of vasovagal syncope. In addition, central mechanisms can contribute to the production of neurally mediated syncope.

Carotid Sinus Hypersensitivity

Syncope caused by carotid sinus hypersensitivity results from stimulation of carotid sinus baroreceptors located in the internal carotid artery above the bifurcation of the common carotid artery. Carotid sinus hypersensitivity is detected in approximately one third of elderly patients who present with either syncope or falls.[1,2,23] However, carotid sinus hypersensitivity is also commonly observed in asymptomatic elderly patients.[24] Thus, the diagnosis of carotid sinus hypersensitivity should be approached cautiously after exclusion of alternative causes of syncope. Once it is diagnosed, dual-chamber pacemaker implantation is recommended for patients with recurrent syncope or falls resulting from carotid sinus hypersensitivity[25] on the basis of a large number of both nonrandomized and randomized clinical trials.[26,27] The AHA/ACC/HRS Guidelines for device implantation have given this a Class I indication for pacemaker implantation.[25] If the diagnosis of carotid sinus hypersensitivity is based on a >3-second pause with carotid sinus massage without clear, provocative events, pacemaker implantation is less strongly recommended (Class IIa).

Cardiac Causes of Syncope

Cardiac causes of syncope, particularly tachyarrhythmias and bradyarrhythmias, are the second most common cause of syncope, accounting for 10% to 20% of syncopal episodes (see Table 42-2; see Chap. 39). Ventricular tachycardia (VT) is the most common tachyarrhythmia that can cause syncope. Supraventricular tachycardia (SVT) can also cause syncope, although most patients with supraventricular arrhythmias present with less severe symptoms, such as palpitations, dyspnea, and lightheadedness. Bradyarrhythmias that can result in syncope include sick sinus syndrome and atrioventricular (AV) block. Anatomic causes of syncope include obstruction to blood flow, such as a massive pulmonary embolus (see Chap. 77), atrial myxoma (see Chap. 74), and aortic stenosis (see Chap. 66).

TABLE 42-3 Causes of Orthostatic Hypotension

Drugs
Diuretics
Alpha-adrenergic blocking drugs
Terazosin (Hytrin), labetalol
Adrenergic neuron blocking drugs
Guanethidine
Angiotensin-converting enzyme inhibitors
Antidepressants
Monoamine oxidase inhibitors
Alcohol
Diuretics
Ganglion-blocking drugs
Hexamethonium, mecamylamine
Tranquilizers
Phenothiazines, barbiturates
Vasodilators
Prazosin, hydralazine, calcium channel blockers
Centrally acting hypotensive drugs
Methyldopa, clonidine
Primary Disorders of Autonomic Failures
Pure autonomic failure (Bradbury-Eggleston syndrome)
Multiple system atrophy (Shy-Drager syndrome)
Parkinson disease with autonomic failure
Secondary Neurogenic
Aging
Autoimmune disease
Guillain-Barré syndrome, mixed connective tissue disease, rheumatoid arthritis
Eaton-Lambert syndrome, systemic lupus erythematosus
Carcinomatosis autonomic neuropathy
Central brain lesions
Multiple sclerosis, Wernicke encephalopathy
Vascular lesions or tumors involving the hypothalamus and midbrain
Dopamine beta-hydroxylase deficiency
Familial hyperbradykinism
General medical disorders
Diabetes, amyloid, alcoholism, renal failure
Hereditary sensory neuropathies, dominant or recessive
Infections of the nervous system
Human immunodeficiency virus infection, Chagas disease, botulism, syphilis
Metabolic disease
Vitamin B_{12} deficiency, porphyria, Fabry disease, Tangier disease
Spinal cord lesions

Modified from Bannister SR (ed): Autonomic Failure. 2nd ed. Oxford, Oxford University Press, 1988, p 8.

Neurologic Causes of Transient Loss of Consciousness (see Chaps. 62 and 92)

Neurologic causes of transient loss of consciousness, including migraines, seizures, Arnold-Chiari malformations, and transient ischemic attacks, are surprisingly uncommon, accounting for less than 10% of all cases of syncope. The majority of patients in whom a "neurologic" cause of transient loss of consciousness is established are found in fact to have had a seizure rather than true syncope.

Metabolic Causes of Transient Loss of Consciousness

Metabolic causes of transient loss of consciousness are rare, accounting for less than 5% of syncopal episodes. The most common metabolic causes of syncope are hypoglycemia (see Chap. 64), hypoxia, and hyperventilation. Establishment of hypoglycemia as the cause of an apparent loss of consciousness requires demonstration of hypoglycemia during the syncopal episode. Although hyperventilation-induced syncope has been generally considered to be due to a reduction in cerebral blood flow, one study demonstrated that hyperventilation alone was not sufficient to cause syncope. This observation suggests that hyperventilation-induced syncope may also have a psychological component. Psychiatric disorders can also cause syncope. Up to one fourth of patients with syncope of unknown origin may have psychiatric disorders for which apparent syncope is one of the presenting symptoms[1,2] (see Chap. 91).

Diagnostic Tests

Identification of the precise cause of syncope is often challenging. Because syncope usually occurs sporadically and infrequently, it is extremely difficult either to examine a patient or to obtain an electrocardiogram (ECG) during an episode of syncope. For this reason, the primary goal in the evaluation of a patient with syncope is to arrive at a presumptive determination of the cause of syncope.

History, Physical Examination, and Carotid Sinus Massage

The history and physical examination are by far the most important components of the evaluation of a patient with transient loss of consciousness and syncope and can identify the cause in more than 25% of patients.[1,2,15] Maximal information can be obtained from the clinical history when it is approached in a systematic and detailed fashion. Initial evaluation should begin by determining whether the patient did, in fact, experience a syncopal episode by asking these questions: (1) Did the patient experience a complete loss of consciousness? (2) Was the loss of consciousness transient with rapid onset and short duration? (3) Did the patient recover spontaneously, completely, and without sequelae? (4) Did the patient lose postural tone? If the answer to one or more of these questions is negative, other nonsyncopal causes of transient loss of consciousness should be suspected. Although falls can be differentiated from syncope by the absence of loss of consciousness, an overlap between symptoms of falls and syncope has been reported[1,2] because elderly individuals may experience amnesia for the episode of loss of consciousness. In evaluating a patient with syncope, particular attention should then be focused on (1) determining whether the patient has a history of cardiac disease, metabolic disease (i.e., diabetes), or a family history of cardiac disease, syncope, or sudden death; (2) identifying medications that may have played a role in syncope, especially those that may cause hypotension, bradycardia or heart block, or a proarrhythmic response (antiarrhythmic medications); (3) quantifying the number and chronicity of prior syncopal and presyncopal episodes; (4) identifying precipitating factors, including body position and activity immediately before syncope; and (5) quantifying the type and duration of prodromal and recovery symptoms. It is also useful to obtain careful accounts from witnesses to provide a detailed account of the episode, including how the patient collapsed, the patient's skin color and breathing pattern, the duration of unconsciousness, and the movements during the episode of unconsciousness. The features of the clinical history most helpful in differentiating neurally mediated hypotension, arrhythmia, seizure, or psychogenic syncope are summarized in **Table 42-4**.

The clinical histories obtained from patients with syncope related to AV block and VT are similar. In each case, syncope typically occurs with less than 5 seconds of warning and few if any prodromal and recovery symptoms. Demographic features suggesting that syncope results from an arrhythmia such as VT or AV block include male gender, fewer than three prior episodes of syncope, and increased age. Features of the clinical history that point toward a diagnosis of neurally mediated syncope include palpitations, blurred vision, nausea, warmth, diaphoresis, or lightheadedness before syncope and nausea, warmth, diaphoresis, or fatigue after syncope.

Features of the clinical history useful in distinguishing seizures from syncope include orientation after an event, a blue face or not becoming pale during the event, frothing at the mouth, aching muscles,

TABLE 42-4 Differentiation of Syncope Caused by Neurally Mediated Hypotension, Arrhythmias, Seizures, and Psychogenic Causes

	NEURALLY MEDIATED HYPOTENSION	ARRHYTHMIAS	SEIZURE	PSYCHOGENIC
Demographics and clinical setting	Female > male gender Younger age (<55 yr) More episodes (>2) Standing, warm room, emotional upset	Male > female gender Older age (>54 yr) Fewer episodes (<3) During exertion or supine Family history of sudden death	Younger age (<45 yr) Any setting	Female > male gender Occurs in the presence of others Younger age (<40 yr) Many episodes (often many episodes in a day) No identifiable trigger
Premonitory symptoms	Longer duration (>5 sec) Palpitations Blurred vision Nausea Warmth Diaphoresis Lightheadedness	Shorter duration (<6 sec) Palpitations less common	Sudden onset or brief aura (déjà vu, olfactory, gustatory, visual)	Usually absent
Observations during the event	Pallor Diaphoretic Dilated pupils Slow pulse, low blood pressure Incontinence may occur Brief clonic movements may occur	Blue, not pale Incontinence can occur Brief clonic movements can occur	Blue face, no pallor Frothing at the mouth Prolonged syncope (duration >5 minutes) Tongue biting Horizontal eye deviation Elevated pulse and blood pressure Incontinence more likely* Tonic-clonic movements if grand mal	Normal color Not diaphoretic Eyes closed Normal pulse and blood pressure No incontinence Prolonged duration (minutes) is common
Residual symptoms	Residual symptoms common Prolonged fatigue common (>90%) Oriented	Residual symptoms uncommon (unless prolonged unconsciousness) Oriented	Residual symptoms common Aching muscles Disoriented Fatigue Headache Slow recovery	Residual symptoms uncommon Oriented

*May be observed with any of these causes of syncope but more common with seizures.

feeling sleepy after the event, and a duration of unconsciousness of more than 5 minutes. Tongue biting strongly points toward a seizure rather than syncope as the cause of loss of consciousness. Other findings suggestive of a seizure as a cause of the syncopal episode include (1) an aura before the episode, (2) horizontal eye deviation during the episode, (3) an elevated blood pressure and pulse during the episode, and (4) a headache after the event. Urinary or fecal incontinence can be observed with either a seizure or a syncopal episode but occurs more commonly with a seizure. Grand mal seizures are usually associated with tonic-clonic movements. Syncope caused by cerebral ischemia can result in decorticate rigidity with clonic movements of the arms. Akinetic or petit mal seizures can be recognized by the patient's lack of responsiveness in the absence of a loss of postural tone. Temporal lobe seizures last several minutes and are characterized by confusion, changes in the level of consciousness, and autonomic signs such as flushing. Vertebral basilar insufficiency should be considered the cause of syncope if syncope occurs in association with other symptoms of brainstem ischemia (i.e., diplopia, tinnitus, focal weakness or sensory loss, vertigo, or dysarthria). Migraine-mediated syncope is often associated with a throbbing unilateral headache, scintillating scotomata, and nausea.

PHYSICAL EXAMINATION. In addition to a complete cardiac examination, particular attention should focus on determining whether structural heart disease is present, defining the patient's level of hydration, and detecting significant neurologic abnormalities suggestive of a dysautonomia or a cerebrovascular accident. Orthostatic vital signs are a critical component of the evaluation. The patient's blood pressure and heart rate should be obtained supine and then each minute for approximately 3 minutes while standing. The two abnormalities that should be searched for are (1) early orthostatic hypotension, defined as a drop of 20 mm Hg in systolic blood pressure or a drop of 10 mm Hg in diastolic blood pressure within 3 minutes of standing, and (2) POTS, which is defined as an increase of 28 beats/min or more within 5 minutes of standing with symptoms of orthostatic intolerance. The significance of POTS lies in its close overlap with neurally mediated syncope.

CAROTID SINUS MASSAGE. Carotid sinus massage should be performed after checking for bruits in patients with syncope older than 40 years by applying gentle pressure over the carotid pulsation just below the angle of the jaw, where the carotid bifurcation is located. Pressure should be applied for 5 to 10 seconds in both supine and upright positions because an abnormal response to carotid sinus massage is present only in the upright position in up to one third of patients. Because the main complications associated with carotid sinus massage are neurologic, carotid sinus massage should be avoided in patients with prior transient ischemic attacks, strokes within the past 3 months, and carotid bruits, except if significant stenosis has been excluded by carotid Doppler studies. A normal response to carotid sinus massage is a transient decrease in the sinus rate or prolongation of AV conduction, or both. Carotid sinus hypersensitivity is defined as a sinus pause of more than 3 seconds in duration or a fall in systolic blood pressure of 50 mm Hg or more. The response to carotid sinus massage can be classified as cardioinhibitory (asystole), vasodepressive (fall in systolic blood pressure), or mixed. Diagnosis of carotid sinus hypersensitivity as the cause of syncope requires the reproduction of the patient's symptoms during carotid sinus massage.

Laboratory Tests

BLOOD TESTS. The routine use of blood tests, such as serum electrolyte, cardiac enzyme, glucose, and hematocrit levels, is of low diagnostic value in syncopal patients and therefore is not recommended routinely.

Tilt-Table Testing

The tilt-table test is a valuable diagnostic test for evaluation of patients with syncope[1,2,16,26]; a positive response indicates susceptibility to neurally mediated syncope. Upright tilt testing is generally performed for 30 to 45 minutes after a 20-minute horizontal pre-tilt stabilization phase, at an angle between 60 and 80 degrees (with 70 degrees the most common). The sensitivity of the test can be increased, with an associated fall in specificity, by the use of longer tilt durations, steeper tilt angles, and provocative agents such as isoproterenol and nitroglycerin. When isoproterenol is employed as a provocative agent, it is recommended that the infusion rate be increased incrementally from 1 to 3 μg/min to increase the heart rate 25% greater than baseline. When nitroglycerin is employed, a fixed dose of 300 to 400 μg nitroglycerin spray should be administered sublingually after a 20-minute unmedicated phase with the patient in the upright position. These two provocative approaches are equivalent in diagnostic accuracy. In the absence of pharmacologic provocation, the specificity of the test has been estimated to be 90%, decreasing significantly when provocative agents are used.

The main indication for upright tilt testing is to confirm a diagnosis of neurally mediated syncope when the initial evaluation is insufficient to establish this diagnosis. In patients without structural heart disease, the induction of reflex hypotension or bradycardia with reproduction of syncope is considered diagnostic of neurally mediated syncope.[1,2,26] Upright tilt testing is generally not recommended in patients in whom the diagnosis can be established by the initial history and physical examination. However, for some patients, confirmation of the diagnosis with a positive response to upright tilt testing is reassuring. The induction of reflex hypotension or bradycardia without reproduction of syncope points toward a diagnosis of neurally mediated syncope but is a less specific response. If a patient has structural heart disease, other cardiovascular causes of syncope should be excluded before a positive response to upright tilt testing is considered to be diagnostic of neurally mediated syncope. Upright tilt testing is also indicated in the evaluation of patients for whom the cause of syncope has been determined (i.e., asystole) but the presence of neurally mediated syncope on upright tilt would influence treatment. Upright tilt testing has also been shown to be of value in patients with psychogenic causes of syncope as it may trigger a loss of consciousness in association with a normal blood pressure and heart rate. The induction of loss of consciousness with no change in vital signs points strongly toward a diagnosis of psychogenic pseudosyncope. Upright tilt testing has no value in assessing the efficacy of treatment of neurally mediated syncope.

Echocardiography

Echocardiography is commonly used to evaluate patients with syncope, but current guidelines suggest that echocardiography be performed only in patients suspected of having structural heart disease (see Chap. 15).[1,2,15] For example, an echocardiogram should be obtained in patients who have clinical features suggestive of a cardiac cause of syncope, such as syncope with exertion or while supine, family history of sudden death, or syncope of abrupt onset. Echocardiographic findings considered diagnostic of the cause of syncope include severe aortic stenosis, pericardial tamponade, aortic dissection, congenital abnormalities of the coronary arteries, and obstructive atrial myxomas or thrombi. Findings of impaired right or left ventricular function, evidence of right ventricular overload or pulmonary hypertension (pulmonary emboli), and hypertrophic cardiomyopathy (see Chap. 69) are of prognostic importance and justify additional diagnostic testing.

Stress Tests and Cardiac Catheterizations

Myocardial ischemia is an unlikely cause of syncope and, when present, is usually accompanied by angina (see Chap. 52). The use of stress tests (see Chap. 14) is best reserved for patients in whom syncope or presyncope occurred during or immediately after exertion, in association with chest pain, and for patients at high risk for coronary artery disease.[1,2,15] Syncope occurring during exercise is suggestive of a cardiac cause. In contrast, syncope that follows exercise usually is caused by neurally mediated syncope. Even among patients with syncope during exertion, exercise stress testing is highly unlikely to trigger another event. Coronary angiography is recommended in patients with syncope thought to be due, directly or indirectly, to myocardial ischemia.

Electrocardiography

The 12-lead ECG is another important component in the workup of a patient with syncope (see Chap. 13). The initial ECG results in establishment of a diagnosis in approximately 5% of patients and suggests a diagnosis in another 5% of patients. Specific findings that can identify the probable cause of syncope include QT prolongation (long-QT syndrome), short PR interval and delta wave (Wolff-Parkinson-White syndrome), right bundle branch block pattern with ST-segment elevation (Brugada syndrome), and evidence of an acute myocardial infarction, high-grade AV block, or T wave inversion in the right precordial leads (arrhythmogenic right ventricular dysplasia). Any abnormality of the baseline ECG is an independent predictor of cardiac syncope or increased mortality and suggests the need to pursue an evaluation of cardiac causes of syncope.[1,2] Most patients with syncope have a normal ECG. This finding is useful as it suggests a low likelihood of a cardiac cause of syncope and is associated with an excellent prognosis, particularly in a young patient with syncope. Despite the low diagnostic yield of electrocardiography, the test is inexpensive and risk free and is considered a standard part of the evaluation of virtually all patients with syncope.[1,2,15]

SIGNAL-AVERAGED ELECTROCARDIOGRAPHY. A noninvasive technique, signal-averaged electrocardiography (SAECG; see Chap. 36) is used to detect low-amplitude signals in the terminal portion of the QRS complex (late potentials), which are a substrate for ventricular arrhythmias. In contrast to standard electrocardiography, the role of SAECG in the evaluation of patients with syncope is not well established, and it is not recommended as a standard part of the evaluation of patients with syncope.[1,2,15] One of the few situations in which SAECG is of diagnostic value is when a diagnosis of arrhythmogenic right ventricular dysplasia is being considered.[7]

HOLTER RECORDING AND TELEMETRY. Continuous electrocardiographic monitoring by telemetry or Holter monitoring (see Chap. 36) is commonly performed in patients with syncope but is unlikely to identify the cause of syncope. The information provided by electrocardiographic monitoring at the time of syncope is extremely valuable because it allows an arrhythmic cause of syncope to be established or excluded. However, because of the infrequent and sporadic nature of syncope, the diagnostic yield of Holter monitoring in the evaluation of patients with syncope and presyncope is extremely low. Another clinically useful finding is the detection of symptoms in the absence of an arrhythmia. This finding is observed in up to 15% of patients undergoing continuous electrocardiographic monitoring. The absence of an arrhythmia and symptoms during continuous electrocardiographic monitoring may not exclude an arrhythmia as the cause of syncope. In patients suspected of having an arrhythmia as the cause of syncope, additional evaluation, such as electrophysiologic (EP) testing or event monitoring, should be considered. In-patient telemetry monitoring or Holter monitoring is recommended for patients who have the clinical or electrocardiographic features suggestive of an arrhythmic syncope or a history of recurrent syncope with injury. Holter monitoring and in-patient telemetry monitoring are most likely to be diagnostic in the occasional patient with frequent (i.e., daily) episodes of syncope or presyncope.

EVENT RECORDERS. Some transtelephonic event monitors (see Chap. 36) are worn continuously to capture both retrospective and prospective ECG recordings, whereas other types record only when they are activated by the patient. Continuous-loop event monitors are preferred, often programmed with 5 to 15 minutes of preactivation memory stored by the device that can be retrieved for analysis. Prospective event monitors not worn continuously by the patient are of value to investigate palpitations but play no role in the evaluation of patients with syncope. Event monitors are indicated in patients with infrequent but recurrent episodes of presyncope or syncope, particularly when potentially malignant causes of syncope have been excluded.[1,2,15] When they are used in selected populations of patients, a diagnostic yield as high as 25% can be observed. However, a much lower diagnostic yield can be expected in less selected populations. Compared with standard Holter monitors, event monitors have an increased diagnostic yield.[27]

During the past 5 years, external and implantable devices for real-time outpatient telemetry monitoring have been developed with wireless cell phone–like technology to transmit real-time ECG recordings to a service center. Studies have demonstrated that these devices result in a higher diagnostic yield in patients with syncope or presyncope than with the conventional event monitors described before.[28]

IMPLANTABLE EVENT RECORDERS. In patients with extremely infrequent episodes of syncope (e.g., once or twice a year), a traditional event monitor is unlikely to record an event. Implantable event monitors (see Chap. 36) address this problem by triggering automatically on the basis of programmed detection criteria as well as with a hand-held activator and storing of the ECG signal in a circular buffer. Some of these devices can transmit the signals transtelephonically. These devices allow a longer monitoring period (12 to 36 months) and have a higher diagnostic yield but have the disadvantage of requiring surgical implantation and increased cost.

Current guidelines recommend that when the mechanism of syncope remains unclear after a full evaluation, an implantable event recorder is indicated in patients who have clinical or electrocardiographic features suggestive of arrhythmic syncope or a history of recurrent syncope with injury.[1,2] There is no consensus whether a standard 30-day event monitor should be ordered before placement of an implantable event monitor. One study reported that early application of an implantable event monitor in patients with recurrent severe syncopal episodes thought to be due to neurally mediated hypotension identified a subset of patients in whom specific therapy was instituted (i.e., pacemaker for asystole, catheter ablation for paroxysmal SVT) and resulted in a very low 1-year recurrence of syncope.[29] As a result of this and other studies, current guidelines also recognize that an implantable event recorder may be appropriate in the initial phase of a syncope workup instead of at completion of conventional investigations in patients with preserved cardiac function who have the clinical or electrocardiographic features suggestive of an arrhythmic syncope. An implantable event recorder can also be used to assess the contribution of bradycardia before implantation of a permanent pacemaker in patients with suspected or certain neurally mediated syncope who present with frequent or traumatic syncopal episodes.

Electrophysiologic Testing

EP testing (see Chap. 36) can provide important diagnostic information in patients presenting with syncope by establishing a diagnosis of sick sinus syndrome, carotid sinus hypersensitivity, heart block, SVT, and VT. The indications for EP testing and diagnostic findings in the evaluation of patients with syncope are shown in **Table 42-5**.[1] There is general agreement that EP testing should be performed in patients when the initial evaluation suggests an arrhythmic cause of syncope,[1,2,15] such as in those with an abnormal ECG or structural heart disease, those whose clinical history suggests an arrhythmic cause of syncope, and those with a family history of sudden death. EP testing should not be performed in patients with a normal ECG and no heart disease and in whom the clinical history does not suggest an arrhythmic cause of syncope. The Class II indications for performance of an EP study are shown in Table 42-5, indicating that EP testing is appropriate when the results may have an impact on treatment and also in patients with "high-risk" occupations, in whom every effort should be

TABLE 42-5 Indications for and Diagnostic Findings of Electrophysiologic Testing in the Evaluation of Patients with Syncope

	CLASS	LEVEL OF EVIDENCE
Indications		
In patients with ischemic heart disease when the initial evaluation suggests an arrhythmic cause and there is no established indication for an ICD	I	B
In patients with BBB, EPS should be considered when noninvasive tests do not establish a diagnosis	IIa	B
In patients with syncope of abrupt onset or preceded by palpitations when noninvasive tests do not establish a diagnosis	IIb	B
In patients with syncope and Brugada syndrome, ARVD, and hypertrophic cardiomyopathy, EPS is appropriate in selected cases	IIb	C
In patients with high-risk occupations, in whom every effort to exclude a cardiovascular cause of syncope is warranted	IIb	C
EPS is not recommended in syncope patients with a normal ECG, with no heart disease, and in whom the clinical history does not suggest an arrhythmic cause of syncope	III	B
Diagnostic Criteria		
EPS is diagnostic and no additional tests are required in the following situations:		
Sinus bradycardia and a prolonged CSNRT (>525 msec)	I	B
BBB and either a baseline H-V >100 msec or second- or third-degree His-Purkinje block during incremental atrial pacing or with pharmacologic challenge	I	B
Induction of sustained monomorphic VT in patients with a prior myocardial infarction	I	B
Induction of SVT that causes hypotension or hypotensive symptoms	I	B
H-V interval between 70 and 100 msec should be considered diagnostic	IIa	B
The induction of polymorphic VT or VF in patients with Brugada syndrome, patients with ARVD, and patients resuscitated from cardiac arrest	IIb	B
The induction of polymorphic VT or VF in patients with ischemic disease or DCM should not be considered a diagnostic finding	III	B

ARVD = arrhythmogenic right ventricular dysplasia; BBB = bundle branch block; CSNRT = corrected sinus node recovery time; DCM = dilated cardiomyopathy; EPS = electrophysiologic study; H-V = His-ventricle; ICD = implantable cardioverter-defibrillator; SVT = supraventricular tachycardia; VF = ventricular fibrillation; VT = ventricular tachycardia.

Modified from Moya A, Sutton R, Ammirati F, et al: Guidelines for the diagnosis and management of syncope (version 2009): The Task Force for the Diagnosis and Management of Syncope of the European Society of Cardiology (ESC). Eur Heart J 30:2631, 2009.

expended to determine the probable cause of syncope. EP testing is no longer indicated in patients with a severely depressed ejection fraction because in this setting, an implantable cardioverter-defibrillator (ICD) is indicated regardless of the presence or mechanism of syncope.[1]

ELECTROPHYSIOLOGIC TESTING PROTOCOL. A comprehensive EP evaluation should be performed in a patient with syncope, including an evaluation of sinus node function by measurement of the sinus node recovery time (SNRT) and an evaluation of AV conduction by measurement of the H-V interval at baseline, with atrial pacing and after pharmacologic challenge with intravenous procainamide. In addition, programmed electrical stimulation by standard techniques should be performed to evaluate the inducibility of ventricular and supraventricular arrhythmias. Although the minimal suggested EP protocol includes only double extrastimuli and two basic drive train cycle lengths, it is common practice in the United States to include triple extrastimuli and three basic drive train cycle lengths. It is also common practice to limit the shortest coupling interval to 200 milliseconds. In select patients in whom suspicion of a ventricular arrhythmia is high, EP testing with atrial and ventricular programmed stimulation may be repeated after an infusion of isoproterenol, which is of particular importance when a supraventricular arrhythmia such as AV nodal reentrant tachycardia or orthodromic AV reciprocating tachycardia is suspected as the cause of syncope.

Sinus node function is evaluated during EP testing primarily by determination of the SNRT. Identification of sinus node dysfunction as the cause of syncope is uncommon during EP tests (<5%). The sensitivity of an abnormal SNRT or corrected SNRT (CSNRT) is approximately 50% to 80%. The specificity of an abnormal SNRT or CSNRT is >95%.[2] The absence of evidence of sinus node dysfunction during EP testing does not exclude a bradyarrhythmia as the cause of syncope.

During EP testing, AV conduction is assessed by measurement of the AV nodal to His bundle conduction time (A-H interval) and the His bundle to ventricular conduction time (H-V interval) and also by determination of the response of AV conduction to incremental atrial pacing and atrial premature stimuli. If the results of an initial assessment of AV conduction in the baseline state are inconclusive, procainamide (10 mg/kg) can be administered intravenously and atrial pacing and programmed stimulation repeated. According to the 2004 European Guidelines on Management of Syncope,[1] the findings at EP study that allow heart block to be established as the probable cause of syncope are bundle branch block and a baseline H-V interval ≥100 milliseconds or demonstration of second- or third-degree His-Purkinje block during incremental atrial pacing or provoked by an infusion of procainamide (see Table 42-5). These guidelines indicate that finding of an H-V interval between 70 and 100 milliseconds is of less certain diagnostic value. Among studies on EP testing in evaluation of patients with syncope, AV block was identified as the probable cause of syncope in approximately 10% to 15% of patients.

Although it is uncommon for SVT to result in syncope, this is an important diagnosis to establish as most types of supraventricular arrhythmias can be cured with catheter ablation (see Chap. 37). The usual setting in which SVT causes syncope is in a patient with underlying heart disease or limited cardiovascular reserve, SVT of abrupt onset and with an extremely rapid rate, or in a patient who has a propensity for the development of neurally mediated syncope. The typical pattern is the development of syncope or near-syncope at the onset of the SVT because of an initial drop in blood pressure. The patient often regains consciousness despite the continuation of the arrhythmia owing to the activation of a compensatory mechanism. Completion of a standard EP test allows accurate identification of most types of supraventricular arrhythmias that may have caused syncope, repeated during an isoproterenol infusion to increase the sensitivity of the study, particularly for detection of AV nodal reentrant tachycardia in a patient with dual AV node physiology or catecholamine-sensitive atrial fibrillation. According to the 2004 European Guidelines on Management of Syncope, an EP study is considered diagnostic of SVT as the cause of syncope when there is induction of a rapid supraventricular arrhythmia that reproduces hypotensive or spontaneous symptoms (see Table 42-5).[1] A supraventricular arrhythmia is diagnosed as the probable cause of syncope in less than 5% of patients who undergo EP testing for evaluation of syncope of unknown origin, but the probability is increased in patients who report a history of palpitations or heart racing before syncope.

VT is the most common abnormality uncovered during EP testing in patients with syncope and is identified as the probable cause in approximately 20% of patients. In general, an EP test result is interpreted as positive for VT when sustained monomorphic VT is induced. The induction of polymorphic VT and VF may represent a nonspecific response to EP testing. The diagnostic and prognostic importance of the induction of polymorphic VT or VF remains uncertain. According to the 2004 European Guidelines on Management of Syncope, an EP study is considered diagnostic of VT as the cause of syncope when there is induction of sustained monomorphic VT (see Table 42-5),[1] with less certain diagnostic value with the induction of polymorphic VT or VF in patients with Brugada syndrome, patients with arrhythmogenic right ventricular dysplasia, and patients resuscitated from a cardiac arrest. The role of EP testing and pharmacologic challenge with procainamide in syncope patients with suspected Brugada syndrome is controversial. A recent meta-analysis reported that 54% of 1036 such patients had VT or VF induced at EP testing. No difference in outcome was observed regardless of the results of EP testing at 3 years of follow-up.[30] These guidelines also state that the induction of polymorphic VT or VF in patients with ischemic or dilated cardiomyopathy has low predictive value.

Overall, approximately one third of patients with syncope referred for diagnostic EP testing have a presumptive diagnosis established.

Tests to Screen for Neurologic Causes of Syncope

Syncope as an isolated symptom rarely has a neurologic cause. As a result, widespread use of tests to screen for neurologic conditions is rarely diagnostic.[1,2,15,31] In many institutions, computed tomography scans, electroencephalograms, and carotid duplex scans are overused, being obtained for more than 50% of patients with syncope. A diagnosis is almost never uncovered that was not first suspected on the basis of a careful history and neurologic examination. Transient ischemic attacks that result from carotid disease are not accompanied by loss of consciousness. No studies have suggested that carotid Doppler ultrasonography is beneficial in patients with syncope. Electroencephalograms should be obtained only when there is a relatively high likelihood of epilepsy. Computed tomography and magnetic resonance imaging (see Chaps. 18 and 19) should be avoided in patients with uncomplicated syncope. Although the low diagnostic yield of screening "neurologic tests" has been recognized for more than a decade, studies demonstrate that they continue to be overused, resulting in a dramatic increase in costs.[31]

Approach to the Evaluation of Patients with Syncope

Figure 42-2 outlines the approach to the diagnostic evaluation of a patient presenting with a transient loss of consciousness proposed by the European Society of Cardiology Task Force on Syncope.[1] The initial evaluation begins with a careful history, physical examination, supine and upright blood pressure evaluation, and 12-lead ECG, followed by additional testing in selected subgroups, including carotid sinus massage, echocardiography, electrocardiographic monitoring, and tilt-table testing as explained earlier. The various types of neurologic testing are generally of little or no value except in the case of head trauma and when nonsyncopal causes of transient loss of consciousness, such as epilepsy, are suspected.

On the basis of this initial evaluation, patients can be classified into those with true syncope and those with nonsyncopal transient loss of consciousness. Those patients with syncope can be further divided into two groups: those in whom a certain diagnosis has been

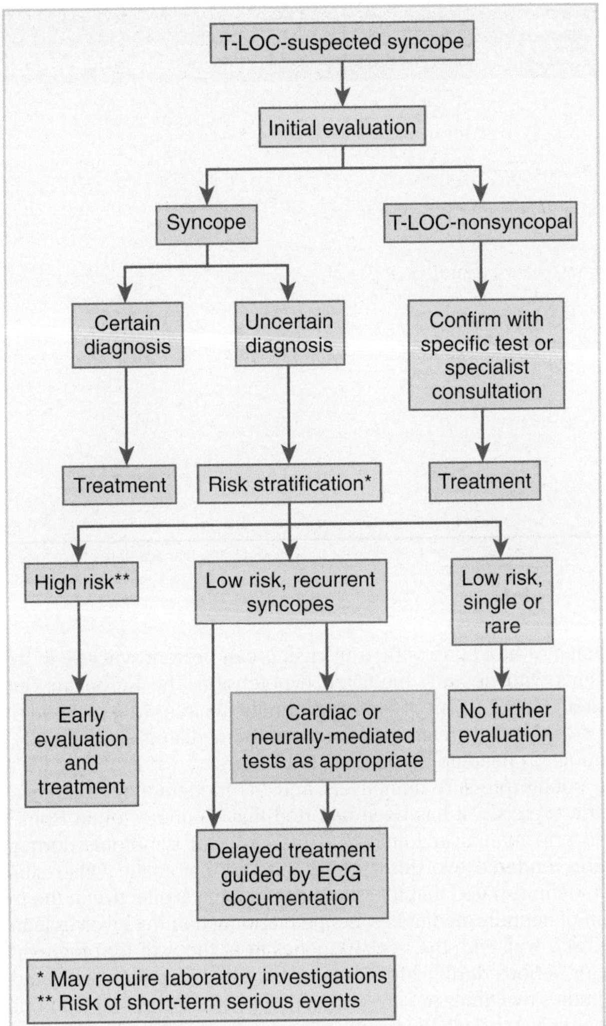

FIGURE 42-2 Diagnostic approach to the evaluation of patients with transient loss of consciousness (T-LOC) and syncope.

established and in whom treatment can be initiated, and those with an uncertain diagnosis. For the latter, attention should focus on determination of whether the patient is at increased risk of a cardiovascular event or death. These patients should be hospitalized or undergo an intensive timely outpatient cardiovascular evaluation that may include exercise stress testing, cardiac catheterization, and EP testing (**Table 42-6**). Conversely, patients who have experienced only a single episode of syncope and are determined to be at low risk of a cardiovascular event or death may require no further evaluation. Patients who fall between these two extremes can undergo further testing selected on the basis of the results of their initial evaluation (see Fig. 42-2). When this diagnostic approach has been completed, a probable cause of syncope can be determined in more than three fourths of patients.

The European Guidelines on Management of Syncope have recently called attention to the importance of a structured care pathway in the evaluation of patients with syncope.[1] Other studies have reported favorable outcomes when a syncope evaluation unit or standardized approach to the evaluation of syncope is used.[31-33] Brignole and coworkers,[32] for example, employed decision-based software to standardize the evaluation of syncope in the emergency departments of 11 general hospitals. A diagnostic workup consistent with the guidelines was accomplished in 86% of patients and resulted in a presumptive diagnosis in nearly 100% of patients. Hospitalization was deemed appropriate for evaluation of syncope in 25% of patients. Another study randomized patients to a syncope evaluation unit or a standard

TABLE 42-6 Clinical Variables for Identification of High-Risk Syncope Patients Who May Benefit from Hospitalization or an Accelerated Outpatient Evaluation

Severe structural heart disease (low ejection fraction, prior myocardial infarction, heart failure)
Clinical or electrocardiographic features suggesting arrhythmic syncope
Syncope during exertion or while supine
Palpitations at the time of syncope
Family history of sudden death
Nonsustained VT
Bifascicular block or QRS >120 msec
Severe sinus bradycardia (<50 beats/min) in absence of medications or physical training
Preexcitation
Prolonged or very short QT interval
Brugada electrocardiographic pattern (right bundle branch block with ST elevation in leads V_1-V_3)
Arrhythmogenic right ventricular dysplasia electrocardiographic pattern (T wave inversion in leads V_1-V_3 with or without epsilon waves)
Electrocardiogram suggestive of hypertrophic dilated cardiomyopathy
Clinical evidence or suspicion of a pulmonary embolus (clinical setting, sinus tachycardia, shortness of breath)
Severe anemia
Important comorbidities
Significant electrolyte abnormalities
Severe anemia

evaluation. The syncope evaluation unit resulted in a diagnosis of 67% of patients versus 10% of patients who underwent a standard evaluation.[33]

Management of Patients

There are three goals of treatment in a patient with syncope: (1) prolong survival, (2) prevent traumatic injuries, and (3) prevent recurrences of syncope. The approach to treatment of a patient with syncope depends largely on the cause and mechanism of syncope. For example, the appropriate treatment of a patient with syncope related to AV block would be a pacemaker in most situations.[34] However, a patient with syncope due to heart block in the setting of an inferior wall myocardial infarction will usually not require a permanent pacemaker as the heart block usually resolves spontaneously. Similarly, heart block resulting from neurally mediated syncope generally does not require pacemaker implantation. Treatment of a patient with syncope related to the Wolff-Parkinson-White syndrome typically involves catheter ablation, and treatment of a patient with syncope related to VT or in the setting of an ischemic or nonischemic cardiomyopathy would probably involve placement of an implantable defibrillator[34] (see Chap. 38). However, ICD implantation may not be required for patients with VT/VF occurring within 48 hours of an acute myocardial infarction. For other types of syncope, optimal management may involve discontinuation of an offending pharmacologic agent, an increase in salt intake, or education of the patient.

Other issues that need to be considered include the indication for hospitalization of a patient with syncope and duration of driving restrictions. Current guidelines recommend that patients with syncope be hospitalized when there is known or suspected heart disease, electrocardiographic abnormalities suggestive of arrhythmic syncope, syncope with severe injury or during exercise, and syncope when there is a family history of sudden death (see Table 42-6).[1]

Physicians who care for patients with syncope are often asked to address the issue of driving risk. Patients who experience syncope while driving pose a risk both to themselves and to others. Although some would argue that all patients with syncope should never drive again because of the theoretical possibility of a recurrence, this is an impractical solution that would be ignored by many patients. Factors that should be considered in making a recommendation for a particular patient include (1) the potential for recurrent syncope, (2) the

TABLE 42-7 Treatment of Neurally Mediated and Reflex-Mediated Syncope

TREATMENT	CLASS	LEVEL OF EVIDENCE
Reassurance and education	I	C
Isometric physical counterpressure maneuvers with prodrome	I	B
Cardiac pacing should be considered in patients with dominant cardioinhibitory carotid sinus hyposensitivity	IIa	B
Cardiac pacing should be considered with frequent recurrent reflex syncope, age >40 yr, and documented spontaneous cardioinhibitory response during monitoring of recurrent syncope	IIb	B
Midodrine may be indicated in patients with neurally mediated syncope refractory to conservative treatment approaches	IIb	B
Tilt training may be useful for education of patients, but long-term benefit depends on compliance	IIb	B
Cardiac pacing may be indicated in patients with tilt-induced cardioinhibitory response with recurrent, frequent, unpredictable syncope and age >40 yr after alternative treatment has failed	IIb	C
Triggers of situations inducing syncope must be avoided as much as possible	III	C
Hypotensive drugs should be discontinued or modified	III	C
Cardiac pacing is not indicated in the absence of a documented cardioinhibitory reflex	III	C
Beta blockers are not indicated	III	A

Modified from Moya A, Sutton R, Ammirati F, et al: Guidelines for the diagnosis and management of syncope (version 2009): The Task Force for the Diagnosis and Management of Syncope of the European Society of Cardiology (ESC). Eur Heart J 30:2631, 2009.

presence and duration of warning symptoms, (3) whether syncope occurs while seated or only when standing, (4) how often and in what capacity the patient drives, and (5) whether any state laws may be applicable. When considering these issues, physicians should note that acute illnesses, including syncope, are unlikely to cause a motor vehicle accident. A study among 3877 patients with syncope reported that syncope occurred while driving in 380 (9.8%).[35] The most common cause was reflex syncope (see Table 42-2) in more than one third. Recurrence of syncope during driving occurred in only 10 patients. During 8 years of follow-up, the cumulative probability of recurrence while driving was 7%. Importantly, no difference in the total recurrence rate was observed in syncope patients regardless of whether syncope occurred while driving. The American Heart Association and the Canadian Cardiovascular Society have published guidelines concerning this issue. For noncommercial drivers, it is generally recommended that driving be restricted for several months. If the patient remains asymptomatic for several months, driving can then be resumed.

Neurally Mediated Syncope

Because neurally mediated syncope and reflex syncope are so common, treatment options are reviewed (**Table 42-7**).[1] Treatment of syncope due to neurally mediated hypotension begins with a careful history. Particular attention is focused on identification of precipitating factors; quantification of the degree of salt intake and current medication use; and determination of whether the patient has a prior history of peripheral edema, hypertension, asthma, or other conditions that may alter the approach used for treatment. For most patients with neurally mediated syncope, particularly those with infrequent episodes associated with an identifiable precipitant, education and reassurance are sufficient.[36] Patients should be educated about common precipitating factors, such as dehydration, prolonged standing, alcohol, and medications such as diuretics and vasodilators. Patients should also be taught to sit or to lie down at the onset of symptoms and to initiate physical counterpressure maneuvers. Volume expansion by salt supplementation is also commonly recommended. Ingestion of approximately 500 mL of water acutely improves orthostatic tolerance to tilt in healthy subjects and may be of value as prophylaxis for syncope in blood donors. The effectiveness of water ingestion in the management of patients with recurrent neurally mediated syncope has not been well studied.

A recent important shift in the approach used for treatment of neurally mediated syncope results from the effectiveness of "physical" measures and maneuvers in the treatment of patients with this condition.[12] Isometric physical counterpressure maneuvers, such as leg crossing or hand grip with arm tensing, can prevent syncope in many patients with neurally mediated hypotension. The European Guidelines on Management of Syncope identify the following physical measures as Class II treatments for neurally mediated syncope: (1) tilt training, (2) head-up tilt sleeping (>10 degrees), (3) isometric leg and arm counterpressure maneuvers, and (4) moderate aerobic and isometric exercise.[1] It has been reported that 2 minutes of an isometric hand grip maneuver initiated at the onset of symptoms during tilt testing rendered two thirds of patients asymptomatic. Other studies have demonstrated that tilt (standing) training is effective in the treatment of neurally mediated syncope. Standing training involves leaning against a wall with the heel 10 inches from the wall for progressively longer periods during 2 to 3 months. Standing time initially should be 5 minutes two times per day with a progressive increase to 40 minutes twice daily. Although the results of nonrandomized studies of standing training have been positive, the results of randomized trials suggest that standing training may have only limited effectiveness.[37]

In contrast to these effective physical maneuvers, the value of pharmacologic agents is less certain. The medications that are generally relied on to treat neurally mediated syncope include beta blockers, fludrocortisone, serotonin reuptake inhibitors, and midodrine. Despite the widespread use of these agents, none of these pharmacologic agents has been demonstrated to be effective in multiple large prospective randomized clinical trials. Although beta blockers were previously considered first-line therapy by many, studies have reported that the beta blockers metoprolol, propranolol, and nadolol are no more effective than placebo.[38,39]

Although pacemakers have also been found to be valuable in the treatment of some patients with neurally mediated syncope in nonrandomized or nonblinded clinical trials, two blinded randomized clinical trials have shown that pacemakers have no benefit.[36,40,41] Additional trials are under way, but the results will not be available for several years. At present, pacemaker implantation has been given a Class IIb indication for treatment of patients with highly symptomatic neurally mediated syncope associated with bradycardia documented spontaneously or at the time of tilt-table testing.[25] The European Guidelines on Management of Syncope provide a somewhat more restrictive recommendation concerning the indications for pacemaker implantation in this setting (see Table 42-7).

Future Perspectives

As the U.S. population ages and the prevalence of cardiac disease increases, it is inevitable that syncope will remain an important clinical problem with which physicians of all types will need to be familiar. We anticipate that during the next 5 years, additional studies will confirm the clinical and economic value of syncope evaluation units. This will lead to more widespread use of syncope evaluation units, much like chest pain emergency units now routinely employed to evaluate patients with chest pain. It also seems likely that genetic testing will grow in diagnostic importance in the evaluation of patients with syncope. It is notable that genetic testing is now available on a routine clinical basis for many of the inherited cardiac conditions that may present with syncope, including the long-QT syndrome, arrhythmogenic right ventricular dysplasia, and hypertrophic cardiomyopathy. We are also hopeful that new pharmacologic or nonpharmacologic treatments will be developed for treatment of patients with severe disabling orthostatic hypotension, postural orthostatic tachycardia syndrome, and neurally mediated syncope.

REFERENCES

1. Moya A, Sutton R, Ammirati F, et al: Guidelines for the diagnosis and management of syncope (version 2009): The Task Force for the Diagnosis and Management of Syncope of the European Society of Cardiology (ESC). Eur Heart J 30:2631, 2009.
2. Brignole M, Alboni P, Benditt DG, et al: Guidelines on management (diagnosis and treatment) of syncope—Update 2004. Eur Heart J 25:2054, 2004.
3. Wisten A, Forsberg H, Krantz P, Messner T: Sudden cardiac death in 15-35-year olds in Sweden during 1992-1999. J Intern Med 252:529, 2002.
4. Sun B, Emond J, Comargo D Jr: Direct medical costs of syncope-related hospitalizations in the United States. Am J Cardiol 95:668, 2005.
5. Bartoletti A, Fabiani P, Bagnoli L, et al: Physical injuries caused by a transient loss of consciousness: Main clinical characteristics of patients and diagnostic contribution of carotid sinus massage. Eur Heart J 29:618, 2008.
6. Spirito P, Autore C, Rapezzi C, et al: Syncope and risk of sudden death in hypertrophic cardiomyopathy. Circulation 119:1703, 2009.
7. Dalal D, Nasir K, Bomma C, et al: Arrhythmogenic right ventricular dysplasia: A United States experience. Circulation 25:3823, 2005.
8. Antzelevitch C, Brugada P, Borggrefe M, et al: Brugada syndrome: Report of the second consensus conference. Heart Rhythm 4:429, 2005.
9. Roden DM: Long-QT syndrome. N Engl J Med 358:169, 2008.
10. Hayashi M, Denjoy I, Extramiana F, et al: Incidence and risk factors of arrhythmic events in catecholaminergic polymorphic ventricular tachycardia. Circulation 119:2426, 2009.
11. Calder Kirsten K, Berbert M, Henderson SO: The mortality of untreated pulmonary embolism in emergency department patients. Ann Emerg Med 45:302, 2005.
12. Noda T, Shimizu W, Taguchi A, et al: Malignant entity of idiopathic ventricular fibrillation and polymorphic ventricular tachycardia initiated by premature extrasystoles originating from the right ventricular outflow tract. J Am Coll Cardiol 4:1288, 2005.
13. Bjerregaard P, Gussak I: Short QT syndrome: Mechanisms, diagnosis and treatment. Nat Clin Pract Cardiovasc Med 2:84, 2005.
14. Del Rosso A, Alboni P, Brignole M, et al: Relation of clinical presentation of syncope to the age of patients. Am J Cardiol 96:1431, 2005.
15. Strickberger SA, Benson DW, Biaggioni I, et al: AHA/ACCF Scientific Statement on the evaluation of syncope. Circulation 113:316, 2006.
16. Grubb BP: Neurocardiogenic syncope and related disorders of orthostatic intolerance. Circulation 111:2997, 2005.
17. Grubb BP, Kanjwal Y, Kosinski D: The postural tachycardia syndrome: A concise guide to diagnosis and management. J Cardiovasc Electrophysiol 17:108, 2006.
18. Grubb BP: Neurocardiogenic syncope. N Engl J Med 352:1004, 2005.
19. Wieling W, Krediet P, van Dijk N, et al: Initial orthostatic hypotension: Review of a forgotten condition. Clin Sci (Lond) 112:157, 2007.
20. Gibbons CH, Freeman R: Delayed orthostatic hypotension: A frequent cause of orthostatic intolerance. Neurology 67:28, 2006.
21. Giada F, Silvestri I, Rossillo A, et al: Psychiatric profile, quality of life and risk of syncopal recurrence in patients with tilt-induced vasovagal syncope. Europace 7:465, 2005.
22. Leftheriotis D, Michopoulou I, Flevari P, et al: Minor psychiatric disorders and syncope: The role of psychopathology in the expression of vasovagal reflex. Psychother Psychosom 77:372, 2008.
23. Parry SW, Steen IN, Baptist M, Kenny RA: Amnesia for loss of consciousness in carotid sinus syndrome. J Am Coll Cardiol 45:1840, 2005.
24. Kerr SR, Pearce MS, Brayne C, et al: Carotid sinus hypersensitivity in asymptomatic older persons. Arch Intern Med 166:515, 2006.
25. Epstein AE, DiMarco JP, Ellenbogen KA, et al: ACC/AHA/HRS 2008 Guidelines for Device-Based Therapy of Cardiac Rhythm Abnormalities: A report of the ACC/AHA Task Force on Practice Guidelines. Circulation 117:e350, 2008.
26. Benditt DG, Sutton R: Tilt-table testing in the evaluation of syncope. J Cardiovasc Electrophysiol 16:356, 2005.
27. Rockx MA: Is ambulatory monitoring for "community-acquired" syncope economically attractive? A cost-effectiveness analysis of a randomized trial of external loop recorders versus Holter monitoring. Am Heart J 150:1065, 2005.
28. Rothman SA, Laughlin JC, Seltzer J, et al: The diagnosis of cardiac arrhythmias: A prospective multi-center randomized study comparing mobile cardiac outpatient telemetry versus standard loop event monitoring. J Cardiovasc Electrophysiol 18:241, 2007.
29. Brignole M, Sutton R, Menozzi C, et al: Early application of an implantable loop recorder allows effective specific therapy in patients with recurrent suspected neurally mediated syncope. Eur Heart J 27:1085, 2006.
30. Paul M, Gerss J, Schulze-Bahr E, et al: Role of programmed ventricular stimulation in patients with Brugada syndrome: A meta-analysis of worldwide published data. Eur Heart J 28:2126, 2007.
31. Bartoletti A, Fabiani P, Adriani P, et al: Hospital admission of patients referred to the emergency department for syncope: A single-hospital prospective study based on the application of the European Society of Cardiology Guidelines on syncope. Eur Heart J 27:83, 2006.
32. Brignole M, Menozzi C, Bartoletti A, et al: A new management of syncope: Prospective systematic guideline-based evaluation of patients referred urgently to general hospitals. Eur Heart J 27:76, 2006.
33. Shen WK, Decker WW, Smars PA, et al: Syncope evaluation in the emergency department study (SEEDS). A multidisciplinary approach to syncope management. Circulation 110:3636, 2004.
34. Epstein AE, DiMarco JP, Ellenbogen KA, et al: ACC/AHA/HRS Guidelines for device-based therapy of cardiac rhythm disorders. Heart Rhythm 5:934, 2008.
35. Sorajja D, Newbitt G, Hodge D, et al: Syncope while driving: Clinical characteristics, causes and prognosis. Circulation 120:928, 2009.
36. Kuriachan V, Sheldon RS, Platonov M: Evidence-based treatment for vasovagal syncope. Heart Rhythm 5:1609, 2008.
37. van Dijk, N, Quartieri F, Blanc JJ, et al: Effectiveness of physical counterpressure maneuvers in preventing vasovagal syncope. J Am Coll Cardiol 48:1652, 2008.
38. Gurevitz O, Barsheshet A, Bar-Lev D, et al: Tilt training: Does it have a role in preventing vasovagal syncope? Pacing Clin Electrophysiol 30:1499, 2007.
39. Sheldon R, Connolly S, Rose S, et al: Prevention of syncope trial (POST): A randomized, placebo-controlled study of metoprolol in the prevention of vasovagal syncope. Circulation 113:1164, 2006.
40. Flevari P, Livanis EG, Theodorakis GN, et al: Vasovagal syncope. A prospective, randomized, crossover evaluation of the effect of propranolol, nadolol and placebo on syncope recurrence and patients' well-being. J Am Coll Cardiol 40:499, 2002.
41. Raviele A, Giada F, Menozzi D, et al: A randomized, double-blind, placebo-controlled study of permanent cardiac pacing for the treatment of recurrent tilt-induced vasovagal syncope. The Vasovagal Syncope and Pacing Trial (SYNPACE). Eur Heart J 25:1741, 2004.

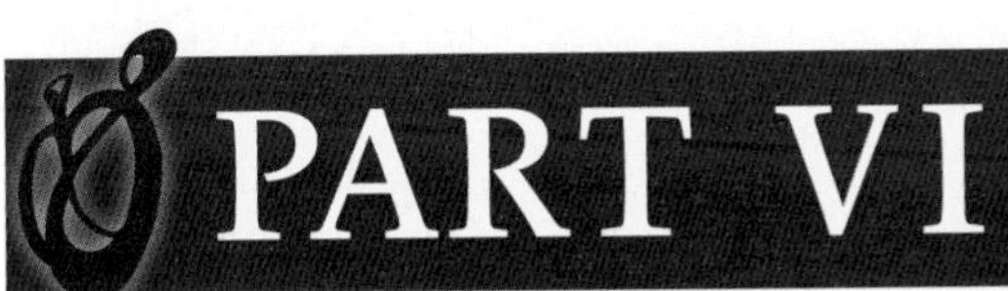

PREVENTIVE CARDIOLOGY

CHAPTER 43 The Vascular Biology of Atherosclerosis

Peter Libby

The 20th century witnessed a remarkable evolution in concepts concerning the pathogenesis of atherosclerosis. This disease has a venerable history, having left traces in the arteries of Egyptian mummies. Apparently uncommon in antiquity, atherosclerosis became epidemic as populations increasingly survived early mortality caused by communicable diseases and malnutrition. Economic development and urbanization promoted habits of poor diet (e.g., a surfeit of saturated fats) and diminished physical activity, which can favor atherogenesis (see Chaps. 1, 44, and 48). These environmental factors have spread steadily, such that we face an epidemic of atherosclerosis that reaches far beyond Western societies.

We no longer view arteries as inanimate tubes. In the mid-19th century, Rudolf Virchow recognized the participation of cells in atherogenesis. A controversy raged between Virchow, who viewed atherosclerosis as a proliferative disease, and Karl Rokitansky, who believed that atheroma derived from healing and resorption of thrombi. Experiments performed in the early part of the 20th century used dietary modulation to produce fatty lesions in the arteries of rabbits and ultimately identified cholesterol as the culprit.[1] These observations, followed by the characterization of human lipoprotein particles in the mid-20th century, promoted the insudation of lipids as a cause for atherosclerosis. We now recognize that elements of all these mechanisms contribute to atherogenesis. This chapter summarizes evidence from human studies, animal experimentation, and in vitro work and presents a synoptic view of atherogenesis from the biologic perspective.

Acquaintance with the vascular biology of atherosclerosis should prove useful to the practitioner. Our daily contact with this common disease lulls us into a complacent belief that we understand it better than we actually do. For example, we are just beginning to learn why atherosclerosis affects certain regions of the arterial tree preferentially and why its clinical manifestations occur only at certain times. Atherosclerosis can involve both large and mid-size arteries diffusely. Postmortem and intravascular ultrasound studies have revealed widespread intimal thickening in patients with atherosclerosis. Many asymptomatic individuals have intimal lesions in their coronary or carotid arteries even in the early decades of life. At the same time, atherosclerosis produces focal stenoses in certain areas of affected vessels much more than in others. An understanding of the biologic basis of the predilection of certain sites to develop atherosclerotic lesions has begun to emerge.

Atherosclerosis also displays heterogeneity in time; this disease has both chronic and acute manifestations. Few human diseases have a longer "incubation" period than atherosclerosis, which begins to affect the arteries of many North Americans in the second and third decades of life (**Fig. 43-1**). Indeed, many young Americans have abnormal thickening of the coronary arterial intima; yet typically, symptoms of atherosclerosis occur after several decades of delay, characteristically occurring even later in women. Despite this indolent time course and prolonged period of clinical inactivity, the dreaded complications of atheroma—such as myocardial infarction, unstable angina, and stroke—typically occur suddenly.

Another poorly understood issue regarding atherogenesis is its role in the narrowing, or stenosis, of some vessels and in the dilation, or ectasia, of others. Typically, we fear stenoses in coronary atherosclerosis, but aneurysm is a common manifestation of this disease in other vessels, including the aorta. Even in the life history of a single atherosclerotic lesion, a phase of ectasia known as positive remodeling, or compensatory enlargement, precedes the formation of stenotic lesions. Contemporary vascular biology has begun to shed light on some of these puzzling aspects of atherosclerosis.

Structure of the Normal Artery

Cell Types Composing the Normal Artery

ENDOTHELIAL CELLS. The endothelial cell of the arterial intima constitutes the crucial contact surface with blood. Arterial endothelial cells possess many highly regulated mechanisms of capital importance in vascular homeostasis that often go awry during the

Abdominal Aorta

Age, 15-19 y (n = 559) Age, 15-19 y (n = 559)

Age, 20-24 y (n = 692) Age, 20-24 y (n = 692)

Age, 25-29 y (n = 790) Age, 25-29 y (n = 790)

Age, 30-34 y (n = 610) Age, 30-34 y (n = 610)

0-10 10-20 20-30 30-40 40-50 50+

Prevalence of Fatty Streaks, %

0-2 2-4 4-6 6-8 8-10 10+

Prevalence of Raised Lesions, %

A

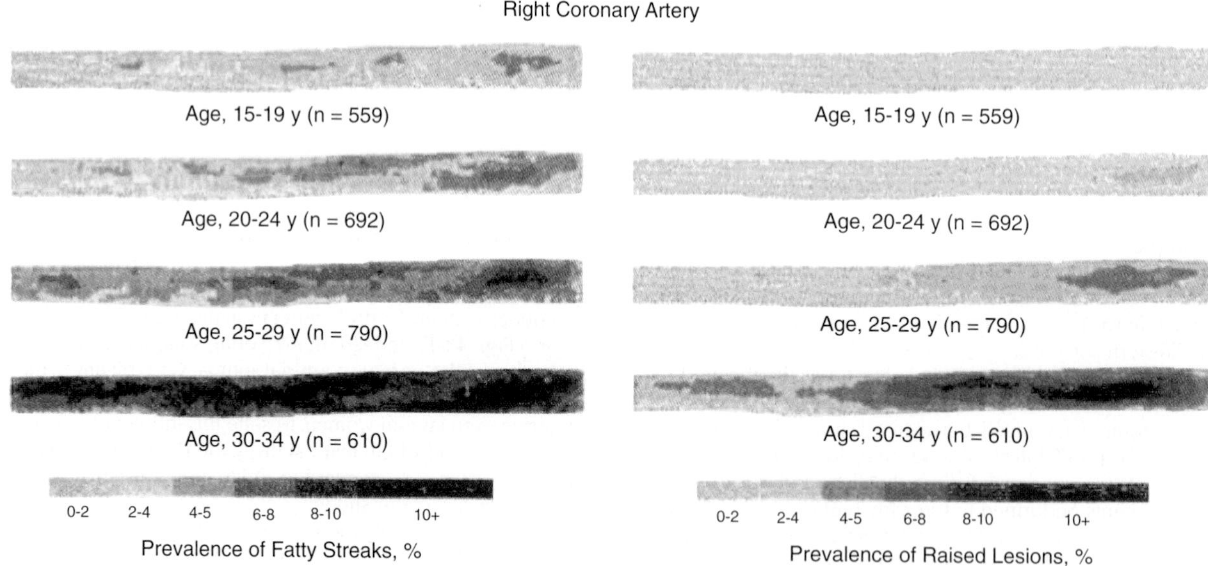

FIGURE 43-1 Prevalence maps of fatty streaks and raised lesions in the abdominal aorta. Composite data from the Pathobiological Determinants of Atherosclerosis in Youth (PDAY) study show a pseudocolored representation of morphometric analysis of more than 2800 aortas from Americans younger than 35 years who succumbed for noncardiac reasons. **A,** Note the early involvement of the dorsal surface of the infrarenal abdominal aorta by fatty streaks, followed by raised lesions. **B,** A similar but slightly slower progression of lesions affects the right coronary artery. The scales at the bottom of the panels show the coding of the pseudocoloring. *(From Strong JP, Malcolm GJ, McMahan CA, et al: Prevalence and extent of atherosclerosis in adolescents and young adults. JAMA 281:727, 1999.)*

pathogenesis of arterial diseases. For example, the endothelial cell provides one of the only surfaces, either natural or synthetic, that can maintain blood in a liquid state during protracted contact (**Fig. 43-2**). This remarkable blood compatibility derives in part from the expression of heparan sulfate proteoglycan molecules on the surface of the endothelial cell. These molecules, like heparin, serve as a cofactor for antithrombin III, causing a conformational change that allows this inhibitor to bind to and inactivate thrombin. The surface of the endothelial cell also contains thrombomodulin, which binds thrombin molecules and can exert antithrombotic properties by activating proteins S and C. Should a thrombus begin to form, the normal endothelial cell possesses potent fibrinolytic mechanisms associated with its surface. The endothelial cell can produce both tissue and urokinase-type plasminogen activators. These enzymes catalyze the activation of

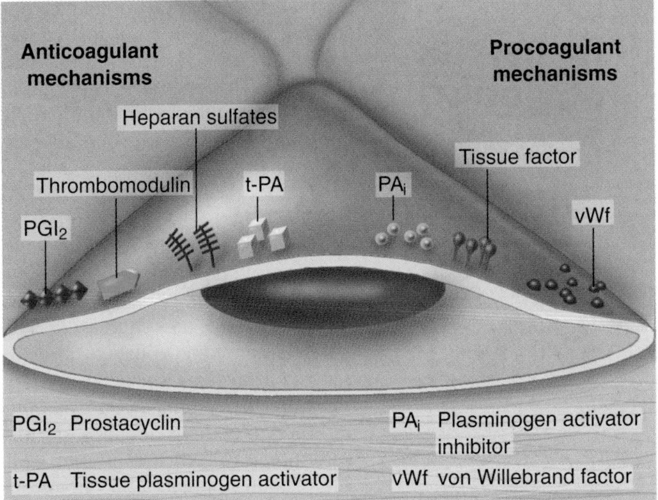

FIGURE 43-2 The endothelial thrombotic balance. This diagram depicts the anticoagulant profibrinolytic functions of the endothelial cell **(left)** and certain procoagulant and antifibrinolytic functions **(right)**.

plasminogen to form plasmin, a fibrinolytic enzyme. (For a complete discussion of the role of endothelium in hemostasis and fibrinolysis, see Chap. 87.)

Endothelial cells have a common origin but acquire bed-specific characteristics during development. The endothelial cells that form the inner lining of all blood vessels arise during embryogenesis from regions known as the blood islands, located on the embryo's periphery. Angioblasts, the predecessors of endothelial cells, share this site with the precursors of blood cells. Despite arising from the same site, cells display considerable heterogeneity even during embryologic and early postnatal development. Although endothelial cells presumably derive from a common precursor, the signals they encounter during vessel development differ. As rudimentary blood vessels begin to form, endothelial precursors interact with surrounding cells. The interchange permits spatial and temporal gradients of various stimuli and their receptors on the endothelial cells, leading to this cell type's heterogeneity in the adult. Endothelial cell heterogeneity depends on both environmental stimuli and epigenetic features acquired during development.

Some recent evidence has indicated that the cells that make up various compartments of the arterial wall can originate from bone marrow during postnatal life as well as from their traditional embryologic sources. In particular, peripheral blood appears to contain endothelial precursor cells that may help repair areas of endothelial desquamation.[2,3] Moreover, in injured or transplanted arteries, smooth muscle cells (SMCs) of apparent bone marrow origin can take up residence in the intima or media (see sections later in this chapter). The endothelial progenitor cells (EPCs) bear characteristic markers such as CD133, CD34, and vascular endothelial growth factor receptor 2 (VEGFR-2). Circulating numbers of EPCs, as assayed in vitro, vary among individuals. Those with a higher burden of risk factors for atherosclerosis have fewer EPCs. EPC number may correlate with prognosis in atherosclerotic patients. Older individuals may have impaired EPC numbers and hence less ability to repair breaches in intimal integrity.[4] Recent experimental evidence has challenged the notion that EPCs populate murine atherosclerotic plaques.[5]

Differential expression of endothelial genes in various types of blood vessels depends on transcriptional regulation by the local environment.[6] For example, the promoter region of the gene that encodes von Willebrand factor directs expression in the endothelium of brain and heart microvessels but not in larger arteries. Co-culture of endothelial cells with cardiac myocytes, but not other cell types, could selectively activate a von Willebrand factor gene promoter construct. Likewise, endothelial nitric oxide synthase gene activity in the heart shows bed-specific regulation. Members of the EPH family of tyrosine kinase receptors and their ligands, known as ephrins, display heterogeneous expressions in arterial versus venous endothelial cells during development. In the adult, arterial endothelial cells and SMCs, but not venous vascular cells, express ephrin-B2. This finding supports a stable lineage difference between cells that make up arteries and veins. Phage display and proteomic techniques have begun to substantiate the in vivo significance of vascular cell heterogeneity in atherogenesis.

ARTERIAL SMOOTH MUSCLE CELLS. The second major cell type of the normal artery wall, the SMC, has many important functions in normal vascular homeostasis, as a target of therapies in cardiovascular medicine, and in the pathogenesis of arterial diseases. These cells contract and relax and thus control blood flow through the various arterial beds, generally at the level of the muscular arterioles. In the larger types of arteries involved in atherosclerosis, however, abnormal smooth muscle contraction may cause vasospasm, a complication of atherosclerosis that may aggravate the embarrassment of blood flow. SMCs synthesize the bulk of the complex arterial extracellular matrix that plays a key role in normal vascular homeostasis and in the formation and complication of atherosclerotic lesions. These cells also can migrate and proliferate, contributing to the formation of intimal hyperplastic lesions, including atherosclerosis and restenosis; stent stenosis after percutaneous intervention; or anastomotic hyperplasia, complicating vein grafts. Death of SMCs may promote destabilization of atheromatous plaques or favor ectatic remodeling and ultimately aneurysm formation.

In contrast to endothelial cells, thought to derive from a common precursor, SMCs can arise from many sources (**Fig. 43-3**).[7] After endothelial cells form tubes, the rudimentary precursor of blood vessels, they recruit the cells that will become smooth muscle, or pericytes (smooth muscle–like cells associated with microvessels). In the descending aorta and arteries of the lower body, the regional mesoderm serves as the source of smooth muscle precursors. The mesodermal cells in somites give rise to the SMCs that invest much of the distal aorta and its branches. In arteries of the upper body, however, SMCs can actually derive from a completely different germ layer—neurectoderm, rather than mesoderm. Before the neural tube closes, neuroectodermal cells migrate and become the precursors of SMCs in the ascending aorta and some of its branches, including the carotid arteries. SMCs in the coronary arteries derive from mesoderm, but in a special way. The precursors of coronary artery SMCs arise from yet another embryologic source, a structure known as the proepicardial organ.

The transcription factor serum response factor (SRF) binds to sequences in the promoters of many genes selectively expressed by SMCs, known as CArG elements. SRF appears to act in conjunction with multiple accessory factors that may differ in SMCs derived from different lineages. In vitro evidence suggests that developmental origin modulates responses to mediators implicated in arterial disease, such as transforming growth factor-β (TGF-β) and plasminogen activator inhibitor 1 (PAI-1), both involved in hemostasis and extracellular matrix macromolecule regulation and in healing of injured vessels. Lineage analyses indicate that large patches of SMCs in arteries arise as expansions of small clones established early in development.[7] Thus, the heterogeneity of SMCs may have direct clinical implications for understanding several common observations, such as the propensity of certain arteries or regions of arteries to develop atherosclerosis or heightened responses to injury (e.g., the proximal left anterior descending coronary artery), and medial degeneration (e.g., the proximal aorta in Marfan disease). Differential responses of SMCs to regulators of extracellular matrix production help explain why the clinical manifestations of systemic defects in fibrillin and elastin characteristically occur locally in the ascending aorta (see Chap. 60).[8]

INTIMA. Understanding of the pathogenesis of atherosclerosis first requires knowledge of the structure and biology of the normal artery and its indigenous cell types. Normal arteries have a well-developed trilaminar structure (**Fig. 43-4**). The innermost layer, the tunica intima, is thin at birth in humans and many nonhuman species. Although it is often depicted as a monolayer of endothelial cells abutting directly on a basal lamina, the structure of the adult human intima is actually much more complex and heterogeneous. The endothelial monolayer resides on a basement membrane containing nonfibrillar collagen types, such as type IV collagen, laminin, fibronectin, and other extracellular matrix molecules. With aging, human arteries develop a more complex intima containing arterial SMCs and fibrillar forms of interstitial collagen (types I and III). SMCs produce these extracellular matrix constituents of the arterial intima. The presence of a more

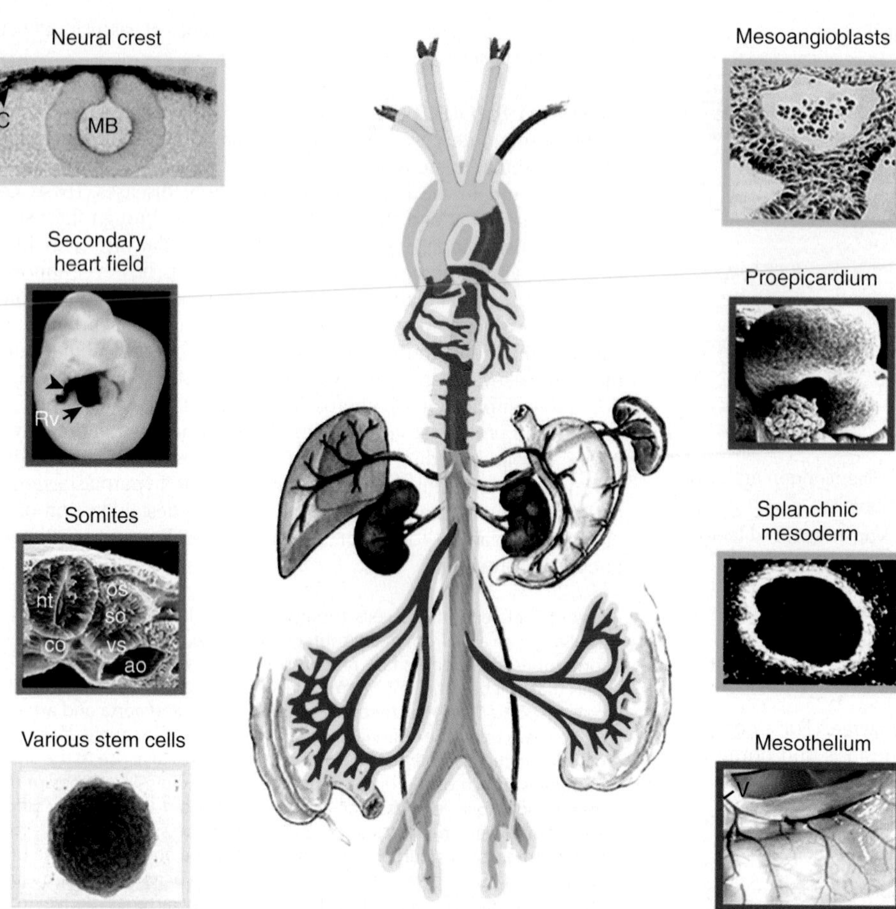

FIGURE 43-3 Diversity of the embryologic origin of vascular SMCs. Different colors represent different embryonic sources for SMCs, as indicated in the boxed images on the sides of the figure. The yellow outline indicates local and systemic contributions by various sources of vascular stem cells. The fate map shows a diverse distribution of SMCs derived from different sources in the aorta and its major branch arteries. With few exceptions, the exact boundaries of SMCs from various sources within the arteries shown are uncertain, and thus the figure depicts approximate boundaries. In the left boxed image labeled Somites, note the close proximity of the developing dorsal aorta (ao) to the ventral sclerotome (vs) of the somite (so). The lineage-specific boundaries shown may shift during growth and aging of vessels. *(Reproduced from Majesky MW: Developmental basis of vascular smooth muscle diversity. Arterioscler Thromb Vasc Biol 27:1248, 2007.)*

complex intima, known by pathologists as diffuse intimal thickening, characterizes most adult human arteries. Some locales in the arterial tree tend to develop a thicker intima than other regions, even in the absence of atherosclerosis (**Fig. 43-5**). For example, the proximal left anterior descending coronary artery often contains an intimal cushion of SMCs more fully developed than that in typical arteries. The diffuse intimal thickening process does not necessarily go hand in hand with lipid accumulation and may occur in individuals without substantial burden of atheroma. The internal elastic membrane bounds the tunica intima abluminally and serves as the border between the intimal layer and the underlying tunica media.

TUNICA MEDIA. The tunica media lies under the intima and internal elastic lamina. The media of elastic arteries such as the aorta has well-developed concentric layers of SMCs, interleaved with layers of elastin-rich extracellular matrix (see Fig. 43-4A). This structure appears well adapted to the storage of the kinetic energy of left ventricular systole by the walls of great arteries. The lamellar structure also certainly contributes to the structural integrity of the arterial trunks. The media of smaller muscular arteries usually has a less stereotyped organization (see Fig. 43-4B). SMCs in these smaller arteries generally embed in the surrounding matrix in a more continuous than lamellar array. The SMCs in normal arteries seldom proliferate. Indeed, rates of both cell division and cell death are low under usual circumstances. In the normal artery, a state of homeostasis of extracellular matrix also typically prevails. Because extracellular matrix neither accumulates nor atrophies, rates of arterial matrix synthesis and dissolution usually balance each other. The external elastic lamina bounds the tunica media abluminally, forming the border with the adventitial layer.

ADVENTITIA. The adventitia of arteries has typically received little attention, although appreciation of its potential roles in arterial homeostasis and pathology has increased. The adventitia contains collagen fibrils in a looser array than is usually encountered in the intima. Vasa vasorum and nerve endings localize in this outermost layer of the arterial wall. The cellular population in the adventitia is sparser than in other arterial layers. Cells encountered in this layer include fibroblasts and mast cells (see Fig. 43-4). Emerging evidence suggests a role for mast cells in atheroma and aneurysm formation in animal models, but their importance in humans remains speculative.[9]

Atherosclerosis Initiation

Extracellular Lipid Accumulation

The first steps in human atherogenesis remain largely conjectural, but the integration of observations of tissues obtained from young humans with the results of experimental studies of atherogenesis in animals provides hints in this regard. On initiation of an atherogenic diet, typically rich in cholesterol and saturated fat, small lipoprotein particles accumulate in the intima (**Fig. 43-6**, steps 1 and 2). These lipoprotein particles appear to decorate the proteoglycan of the arterial intima and tend to coalesce into aggregates (**Fig. 43-7**).[10] Detailed kinetic studies of labeled lipoprotein particles indicate that a prolonged residence time characterizes sites of early lesion formation in rabbits. The binding of lipoproteins to proteoglycan in the intima captures and retains these particles, accounting for their prolonged residence time. Lipoprotein particles bound to proteoglycan have increased susceptibility to oxidative or other chemical modifications, considered by many to contribute to the pathogenesis of early atherosclerosis (Fig. 43-6, step 2). Other studies suggest that permeability of the endothelial monolayer increases at sites of lesion predilection to low-density lipoprotein (LDL). Contributors to oxidative stress in the nascent atheroma could include NADH/NADPH oxidases expressed by vascular cells, lipoxygenases expressed by infiltrating leukocytes, or the enzyme myeloperoxidase.

Leukocyte Recruitment

Another hallmark of atherogenesis, leukocyte recruitment and accumulation, also occurs early in lesion generation (Fig. 43-6, step 4; **Fig. 43-8**). The normal endothelial cell generally resists adhesive interactions with leukocytes. Even in inflamed tissues, most recruitment and trafficking of leukocytes occur in postcapillary venules and not in

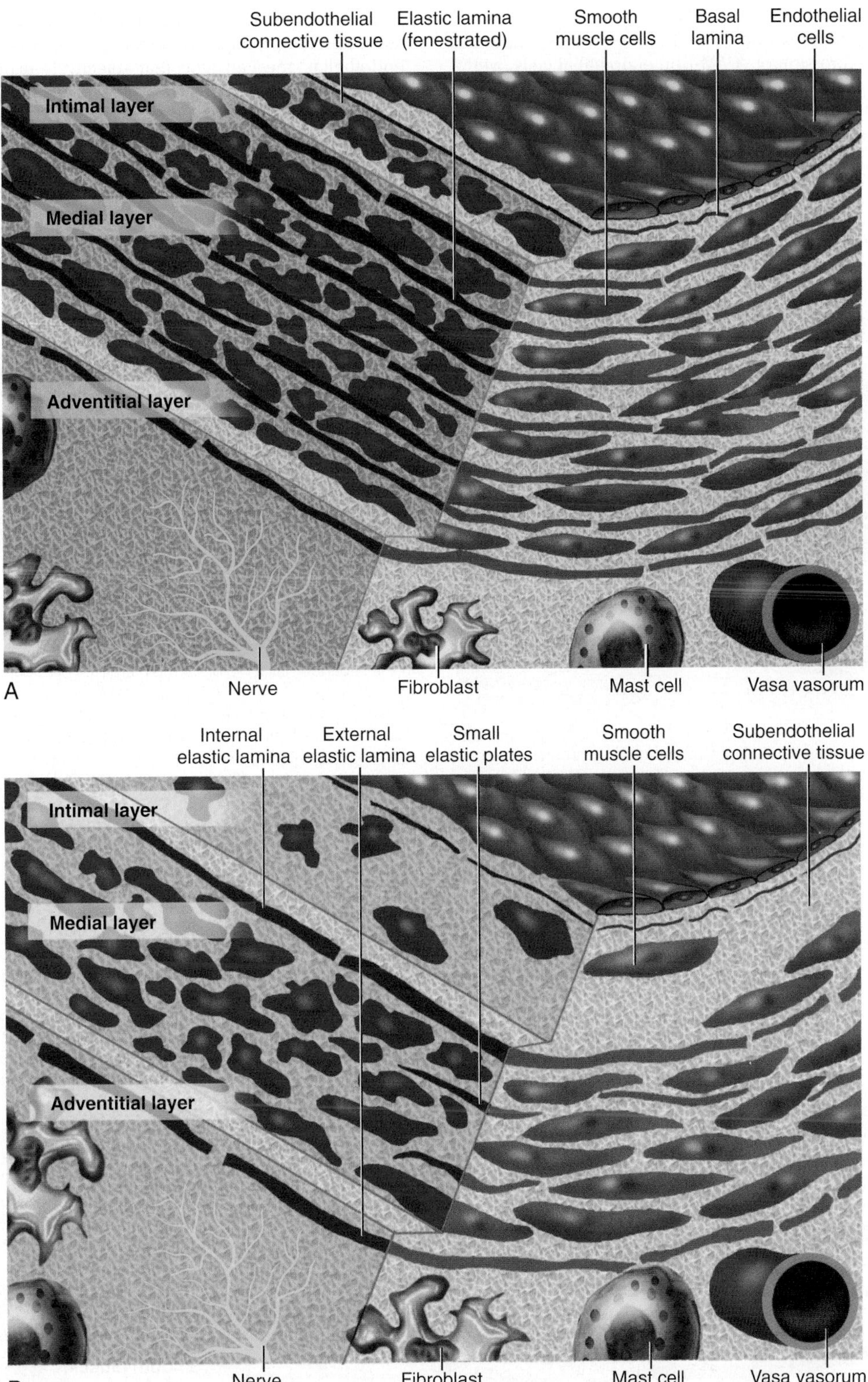

FIGURE 43-4 The structures of normal arteries. **A,** Elastic artery. Note the concentric laminae of elastic tissue that form sandwiches with successive layers of SMCs. Each level of the elastic arterial tree has a characteristic number of elastic laminae. **B,** Muscular artery. In the muscular artery, the SMCs are surrounded by a collagenous matrix but lack the concentric rings of the well-organized elastic tissue characteristic of larger arteries.

arteries. But very soon after initiation of hypercholesterolemia, leukocytes adhere to the endothelium and move between endothelial cell junctions, or even penetrate though endothelial cells (transcytosis) to enter the intima, where they begin to accumulate lipids and become foam cells (Fig. 43-6, step 5; Fig. 43-8).[11] In addition to the monocyte, T lymphocytes also tend to accumulate in early human and animal atherosclerotic lesions. The expression of certain leukocyte adhesion molecules on the surface of the endothelial cell regulates the adherence of monocytes and T cells to the endothelium.[12] Two broad categories of leukocyte adhesion molecules exist. Members of the immunoglobulin superfamily include structures such as vascular cell adhesion molecule 1 (VCAM-1) or CD106. This adhesion molecule has particular interest in the context of early atherogenesis because it interacts with an integrin (very late antigen 4, VLA-4) characteristically expressed by only those classes of leukocytes that accumulate in nascent atheroma—monocytes and T cells. Moreover, experimental studies have shown expression of VCAM-1 on endothelial cells overlying very early atheromatous lesions. Other members of the immunoglobulin superfamily of leukocyte adhesion molecules include intercellular adhesion molecule 1 (ICAM-1). This molecule is more promiscuous, both in the types of leukocytes it binds and because of its wide and constitutive expression at low levels by endothelial cells in many parts of the circulation.

Selectins constitute the other broad category of leukocyte adhesion molecules. The prototypical selectin, E-selectin or CD62E (E stands for "endothelial," the cell type that selectively expresses this particular family member), probably has little to do with early atherogenesis. E-selectin preferentially recruits polymorphonuclear leukocytes, a cell type seldom found in early atheroma (but an essential protagonist in acute inflammation and host defenses against bacterial pathogens).

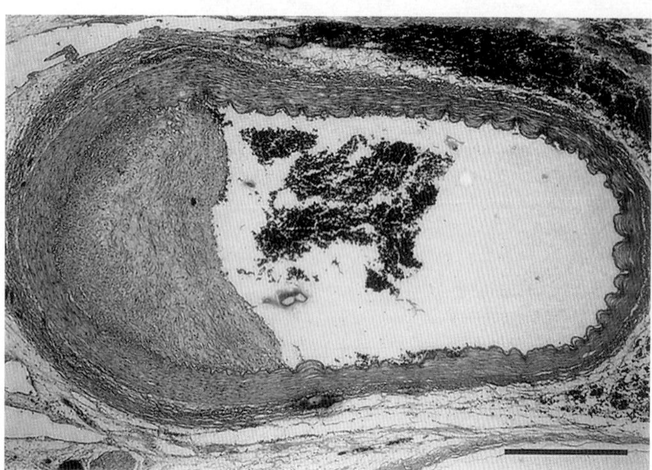

FIGURE 43-5 An intimal cushion shown in a cross section through the internal carotid artery of a 10-week-old male infant. Areas where intimal cushions form in early life tend to develop atheromas more commonly in later years. Bar = 0.5 mm. *(From Weniger WJ, Muller GB, Reiter C, et al: Intimal hyperplasia of the infant parasellar carotid artery: A potential developmental factor in atherosclerosis and SIDS. Circ Res 85:970, 1999.)*

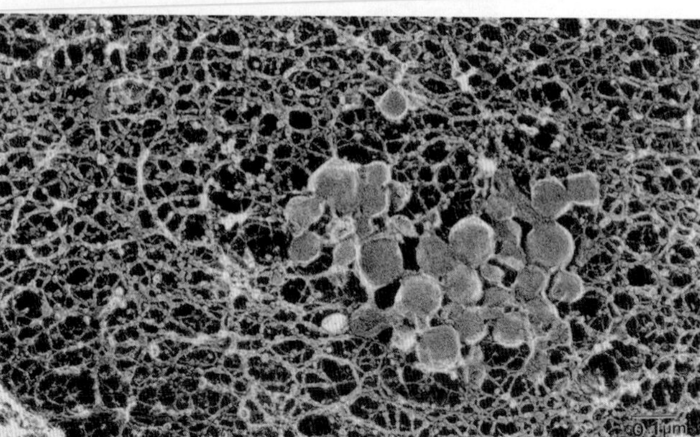

FIGURE 43-7 Scanning electron micrograph of a freeze-etch preparation of rabbit aorta that received an intravenous injection of human low-density lipoprotein (LDL). Round LDL particles decorate the strands of proteoglycan found in the subendothelial region of the intima. By binding LDL particles, proteoglycan molecules can retard their traversal of the intima and promote their accumulation. Proteoglycan-associated LDL appears particularly susceptible to oxidative modification. Accumulation of extracellular lipoprotein particles is one of the first morphologic changes noted after initiation of an atherogenic diet in experimental animals. *(Reproduced from Nievelstein PF, Fogelman AM, Mottino G, Frank JS: Lipid accumulation in rabbit aortic intima 2 hours after bolus infusion of low density lipoprotein. A deep-etch and immunolocalization study of ultrarapidly frozen tissue. Arterioscler Thromb 11:1795, 1991.)*

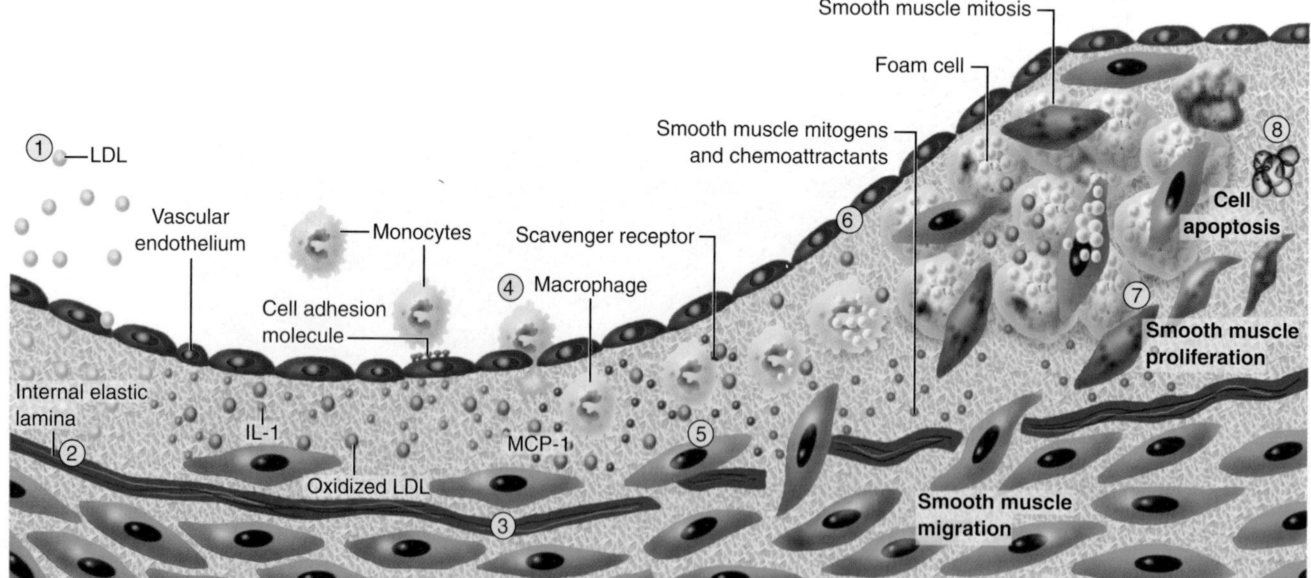

FIGURE 43-6 Schematic of the evolution of the atherosclerotic plaque. **1,** Accumulation of lipoprotein particles in the intima. The modification of these lipoproteins is depicted by the darker color. Modifications include oxidation and glycation. **2,** Oxidative stress, including products found in modified lipoproteins, can induce local cytokine elaboration. **3,** The cytokines, thus induced, increase expression of adhesion molecules for leukocytes that cause their attachment and chemoattractant molecules that direct their migration into the intima. **4,** Blood monocytes, on entering the artery wall in response to chemoattractant cytokines such as monocyte chemoattractant protein 1 (MCP-1), encounter stimuli such as macrophage colony-stimulating factor that can augment their expression of scavenger receptors. **5,** Scavenger receptors mediate the uptake of modified lipoprotein particles and promote the development of foam cells. Macrophage foam cells are a source of mediators, such as further cytokines and effector molecules like hypochlorous acid, superoxide anion (O_2^-), and matrix metalloproteinases. **6,** SMCs migrate into the intima from the media. **7,** SMCs can then divide and elaborate extracellular matrix, promoting extracellular matrix accumulation in the growing atherosclerotic plaque. In this manner, the fatty streak can evolve into a fibrofatty lesion. **8,** In later stages, calcification can occur (not depicted) and fibrosis continues, sometimes accompanied by SMC death (including programmed cell death or apoptosis), yielding a relatively acellular fibrous capsule surrounding a lipid-rich core that may also contain dying or dead cells and their detritus.

Moreover, endothelial cells overlying atheroma do not express high levels of this adhesion molecule. Other members of this family, including P-selectin or CD62P (P stands for "platelet," the original source of this adhesion molecule), may play a greater role in leukocyte recruitment in atheroma as endothelial cells overlying human atheroma do express this adhesion molecule. Selectins tend to promote saltatory or rolling locomotion of leukocytes over the endothelium. Adhesion molecules belonging to the immunoglobulin superfamily tend to promote tighter adhesive interactions and immobilization of leukocytes. Studies in genetically altered mice have proven roles for VCAM-1 and P-selectin (including both platelet- and endothelium-derived P-selectin) in experimental atherosclerosis. Increasing evidence supports the accumulation in atheromas of distinct subtypes of mononuclear phagocytes.[13] The functional consequences of this heterogeneity of macrophage populations in plaques require further study, especially in humans.[14]

Once adherent to the endothelium, leukocytes must receive a signal to penetrate the endothelial monolayer and enter the arterial wall (Fig. 43-6, step 4). The current concept of directed migration of leukocytes involves the action of protein molecules known as chemoattractant cytokines or chemokines.[15,16] Among the many chemokines implicated in atherogenesis, two have particular interest in recruiting the mononuclear cells characteristic of the early atheroma. One such molecule, known as monocyte chemoattractant protein 1 (MCP-1) or CCL2, is produced by the endothelium in response to oxidized lipoprotein and other stimuli. Cells intrinsic to the normal artery, including endothelial cells and SMCs, can produce this chemokine when they are stimulated by inflammatory mediators, as do many other cell types. MCP-1 selectively promotes the directed migration, or chemotaxis, of monocytes. Genetically modified mice lacking MCP-1 or its receptor CCR2 have delayed and attenuated atheroma formation when placed on an atherosclerosis-prone hyperlipidemic genetic background. Human atherosclerotic lesions express increased levels of MCP-1 compared with uninvolved vessels. Thus, several chemokines appear causally to contribute to monocyte recruitment during atherogenesis in vivo. Interleukin-8 (CXCL8), a chemokine that binds to CXCR2 on leukocytes, also participates in experimental atherosclerosis. Fractalkine, a unique cell surface–bound chemokine, also appears to contribute to atherogenesis. Another group of chemoattractant cytokines may heighten lymphocyte accumulation in plaques as well. Atheromas express a trio of lymphocyte-selective chemokines (IP-10 or CXCL10, I-TAC or CXCL11, and MIG or CXCL9). Interferon-γ, a cytokine known to be present in atheromatous plaques, induces the genes encoding this family of T-cell chemoattractants.[17]

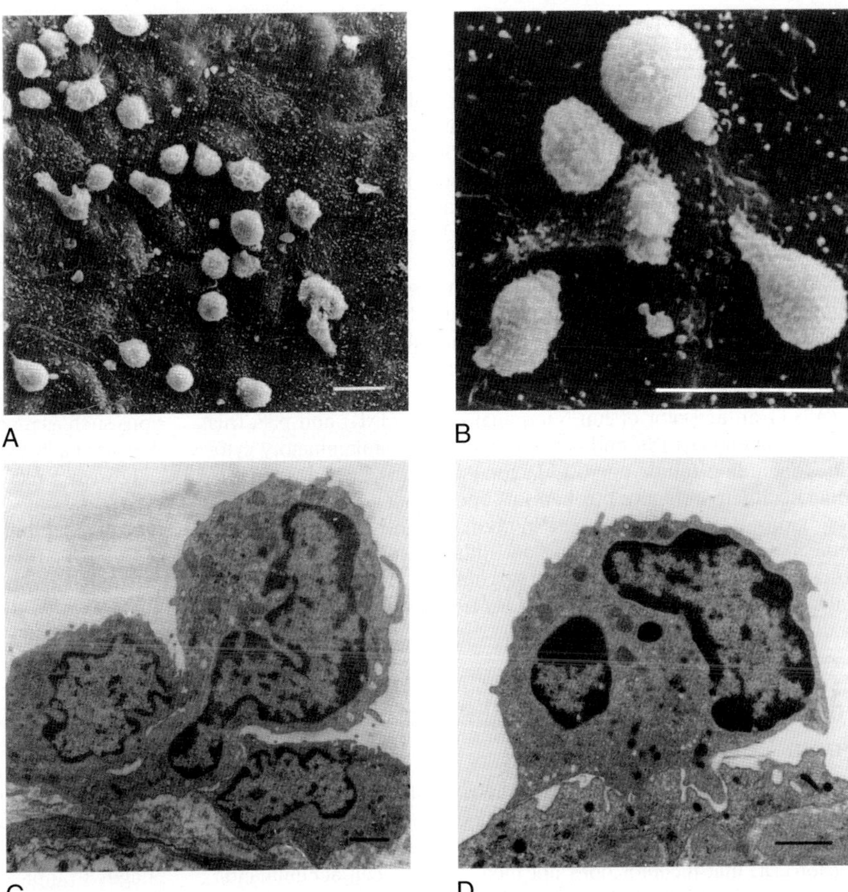

FIGURE 43-8 Electron microscopy of leukocyte interactions with the artery wall in hypercholesterolemic nonhuman primates. **A, B,** Scanning electron micrographs demonstrate the adhesion of mononuclear phagocytes to the intact endothelium 12 days after initiation of a hypercholesterolemic diet in rabbits. **C, D,** Transmission electron micrographs. Note the abundant interdigitations and intimate association of the monocyte with the endothelium in **C**. In **D,** a monocyte appears to come between two endothelial cells to enter the intima. *(Reproduced from Faggiotto A, Ross R, Harker L: Studies of hypercholesterolemia in the nonhuman primate. I. Changes that lead to fatty streak formation. Arteriosclerosis 4:323, 1984.)*

Focality of Lesion Formation

The spatial heterogeneity of atherosclerosis is challenging to explain in mechanistic terms. Equal concentrations of blood-borne risk factors such as lipoproteins bathe the endothelium throughout the vasculature. It is difficult to envisage how injury due to inhalation of cigarette smoke could produce any local rather than global effect on arteries, yet stenoses due to atheromas typically form focally. Some have invoked a multicentric origin hypothesis of atherogenesis, positing that atheromas arise as benign leiomyomas of the artery wall. The monotypia of various molecular markers in individual atheromas supports this monoclonal hypothesis of atherogenesis.[7] The location of sites of lesion predilection at proximal portions of arteries after branch points or bifurcations at flow dividers, however, suggests a hydrodynamic basis for early lesion development. Arteries without many branches (e.g., the internal mammary and radial arteries) tend not to develop atherosclerosis.

Two concepts can aid in understanding how local flow disturbances might render certain foci sites of lesion predilection. Locally disturbed flow could induce alterations that promote the steps of early atherogenesis. Alternatively, the laminar flow that usually prevails at sites that do not tend to develop early lesions may elicit antiatherogenic homeostatic mechanisms (atheroprotective functions). The endothelial cell experiences the laminar shear stress of normal flow and the disturbed flow (usually yielding decreased shear stress) at sites of predilection. In vitro data suggest that laminar shear stress can augment the expression of genes that may protect against atherosclerosis, including forms of the enzymes superoxide dismutase and nitric oxide synthase. Superoxide dismutase can reduce oxidative stress by catabolizing the reactive and injurious superoxide anion. Endothelial nitric oxide synthase produces the well-known endogenous vasodilator nitric oxide. Beyond its vasodilating actions, though, nitric oxide can resist inflammatory activation of endothelial functions, such as expression of the adhesion molecule VCAM-1. Nitric oxide appears to exert this anti-inflammatory action at the level of gene expression by interfering with the transcriptional regulator nuclear factor kappa B (NF-κB). Nitric oxide increases the production of IκBα, an intracellular inhibitor of this important transcription factor. NF-κB regulates numerous genes involved in inflammatory responses in general and in atherogenesis in particular.

Studies also implicate a transcription factor (Krüppel-like factor 2, KLF2) as an important regulator of endothelial anti-inflammatory properties.[18] KLF2 can induce endothelial nitric oxide synthase expression, and KLF2 inhibits NF-κB function by sequestering cofactors needed to boost NF-κB transcriptional activity, resulting in inhibition of the expression of the cassette of NF-κB–dependent genes involved in the inflammatory pathways that operate during atherogenesis (**Fig. 43-9**). Mice with partial disruption of KLF2 signaling have increased atherosclerosis.[19] Laminar shear stress can also limit expression of another regulator of endothelial function, thioredoxin-interacting protein (Txnip).[20] Txnip inhibits the action of thioredoxin. Augmented thioredoxin in regions of laminar shear stress due to decreased Txnip levels in turn attenuates activity of apoptosis signal-regulating kinase 1 (ASK1), an activator of Jun N-terminal kinase (JNK) and p38. This pathway attenuates JNK and p38 activation by proinflammatory cytokines including tumor necrosis factor (see Fig. 43-9). Thus, several separate atheroprotective mechanisms operate such that under usual conditions of laminar shear stress in normal arteries, the endothelium tonically expresses locally acting anti-inflammatory function. Future study of the molecular regulation of vascular cell function by mechanical stimuli should clarify the mechanisms of lesion formation at particular sites in the circulation.

Intracellular Lipid Accumulation: Foam Cell Formation

The monocyte, once recruited to the arterial intima, can there imbibe lipid and become a foam cell or lipid-laden macrophage (Fig. 43-6, step 5). Whereas most cells can express the classic cell surface receptor for LDL, that receptor does not mediate foam cell accumulation (see Chap. 47). This is evident clinically, as patients lacking functional LDL receptors (familial hypercholesterolemia homozygotes) still develop tendinous xanthomas filled with foamy macrophages. The LDL receptor does not mediate foam cell formation because of its exquisite regulation by cholesterol. As soon as a cell collects enough cholesterol for its metabolic needs from LDL capture, an elegant transcriptional control mechanism quenches expression of the receptor (see Chap. 47).

Instead of the classic LDL receptor, various molecules known as scavenger receptors appear to mediate the excessive lipid uptake characteristic of foam cell formation. These surface molecules, which belong to several families, bind modified rather than native lipoproteins and participate in their internalization.[21,22] Atherosclerosis-prone mice with mutations that delete functional scavenger receptor-A have less exuberant fatty lesion formation than do mice with functional scavenger receptor-A molecules. As scavenger receptors have functions such as recognition of apoptotic cells and modified lipoproteins, they are likely to have complex roles during different stages of atherosclerosis.[21,22] Other receptors that bind modified lipoprotein and that may participate in foam cell formation include CD36 and macrosialin, the latter exhibiting preferential binding specificity for oxidized forms of LDL. (See Chap. 47 for a table of scavenger receptors.)

Once macrophages have taken up residence in the intima and become foam cells, they can replicate. The factors that trigger macrophage cell division in the atherosclerotic plaque probably include macrophage colony-stimulating factor (M-CSF). This co-mitogen and survival factor for mononuclear phagocytes exists in human and experimental atheromatous lesions. Atherosclerosis-prone mice lacking functional M-CSF have retarded fatty lesion development as well. Other candidates for macrophage mitogens or co-mitogens include interleukin-3 and granulocyte-macrophage colony-stimulatory factor (GM-CSF). Up to this point in the development of the nascent atheroma, the lesion consists primarily of lipid-engorged macrophages. Complex features such as fibrosis, thrombosis, and calcification do not characterize the fatty streak, the precursor lesion of the complex atheroma. Several lines of evidence suggest that such fatty streaks can regress, at least to some extent.

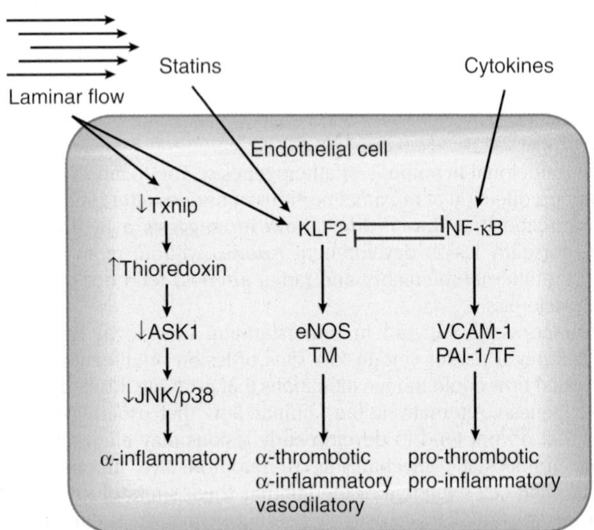

FIGURE 43-9 Novel transcriptional mechanisms that link shear stress to altered expression of genes that influence thrombosis and inflammation. Laminar shear stress can activate Krüppel-like factor 2 (KLF2), a transcription factor that activates endothelial nitric oxide synthase (eNOS), which generates nitric oxide as well as thrombomodulin (TM), yielding downstream anti-inflammatory and antithrombotic effects. By competing for coactivators of nuclear factor kappa B (NF-κB), KLF2 activation attenuates its downstream proinflammatory, prothrombotic, and antifibrinolytic effects, mediated by adhesion molecules such as vascular cell adhesion molecule 1 (VCAM-1), plasminogen activator inhibitor 1 (PAI-1), and tissue factor (TF) procoagulant. Laminar flow also limits Txnip (thioredoxin-interacting protein), which in turn augments thioredoxin function, attenuating apoptosis signal-regulating kinase 1 (ASK1) and hence suppressing Jun N-terminal kinase (JNK) and the kinase p38, ultimately leading to reduced inflammation.

Evolution of Atheroma

Innate and Adaptive Immunity: Mechanisms of Inflammation in Atherogenesis

During the last decade, the convergence of basic and clinical evidence has demonstrated a fundamental role for inflammation in atherogenesis (see Chap. 44).[23,24] The macrophage foam cells recruited to the artery wall early in this process serve not only as a reservoir for excess lipid; in the established atherosclerotic lesion, these cells are a rich source of proinflammatory mediators, including proteins such as cytokines and chemokines and various eicosanoids and lipids such as platelet-activating factor. These phagocytic cells also can elaborate large quantities of oxidant species, such as superoxide anion, in the milieu of the atherosclerotic plaque. This ensemble of inflammatory mediators can promote inflammation in the plaque and thus contribute to the progression of lesions. The term *innate immunity* describes this type of amplification of the inflammatory response that does not depend on antigenic stimulation (**Fig. 43-10**).

In addition to innate immunity, mounting evidence supports a prominent role for antigen-specific or adaptive immunity in plaque progression.[25] In addition to the mononuclear phagocytes, dendritic cells in atherosclerotic lesions can present antigens to the T cells that constitute an important minority of the leukocytes in atherosclerotic lesions. Candidate antigens for stimulation of this adaptive immune response include modified lipoproteins, heat shock proteins, beta$_2$-glycoprotein Ib, and infectious agents.[26,27] The antigen-presenting cells (macrophages, dendritic cells, or endothelial cells) allow the antigen to interact with T cells in a manner that triggers their activation. The activated T cells then can secrete copious quantities of cytokines that can modulate atherogenesis.

The helper T cells (bearing CD4) fall into two general categories. Cells of the T helper 1 subtype elaborate proinflammatory cytokines such as interferon-γ, lymphotoxin, CD40 ligand, and tumor necrosis factor-α. This panel of Th1 cytokines can in turn activate vascular wall cells and orchestrate alterations in plaque biology that can lead to plaque destabilization and heightened thrombogenicity. On the other hand, helper T cells slanted toward the production of Th2 cytokines, such as interleukin-10, can inhibit inflammation in the context of atherogenesis.[28] Cytolytic T cells (bearing CD8) can express Fas ligand and other cytotoxic factors that can promote cytolysis and apoptosis of target cells, including SMCs, endothelial cells, and macrophages. The death of all three of these cell types can occur in the atherosclerotic lesion and may contribute to plaque progression and complication. Regulatory T cells (Treg) can elaborate TGF-β and interleukin-10. Treg lymphocytes bear the markers CD4 and CD25. Both TGF-β and interleukin-10 can exert anti-inflammatory effects. Several experimental preparations suggest an antiatherosclerotic function of Treg cells in vivo.[25,29] The role of B cells and antibody in atherosclerosis remains incompletely explored. Humoral immunity may have either atheroprotective or atherogenic properties, depending on the circumstances.[30] Antibodies that recognize oxidatively modified LDL can protect against experimental atherosclerosis. This observation has incited interest in vaccination with modified LDL to mitigate atherosclerosis.

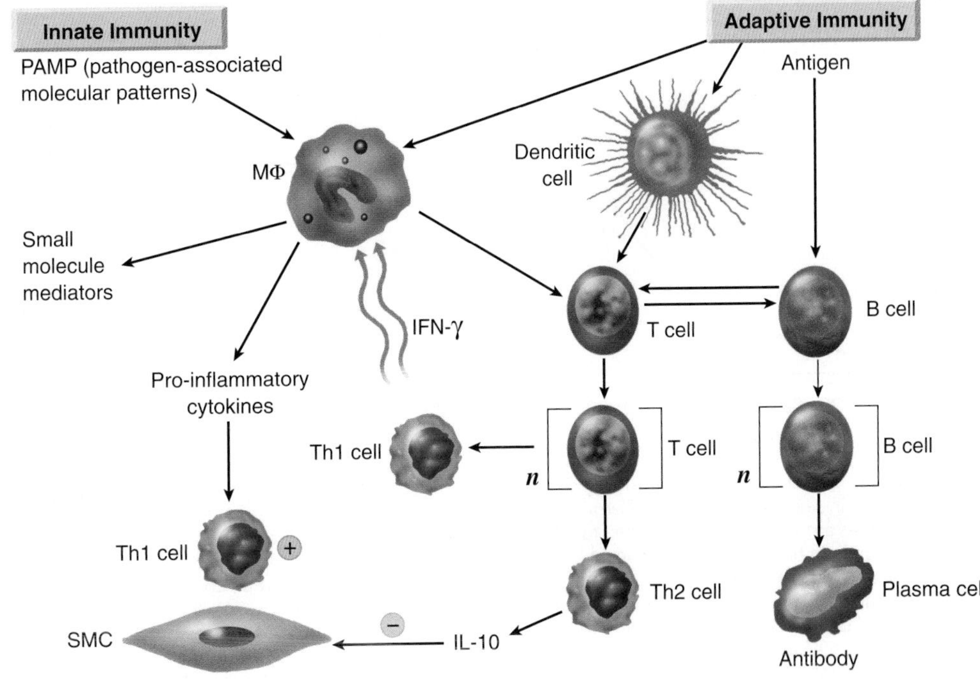

FIGURE 43-10 Innate and adaptive immunity in atherosclerosis. A diagram of the pathways of innate **(left)** and adaptive **(right)** immunity operating during atherogenesis. IFN-γ = interferon-γ; MΦ = macrophage; Th = T helper cell. *(After Hansson G, Libby P, Schoenbeck U, Yan Z-Q: Innate and adaptive immunity in the pathogenesis of atherosclerosis. Review. Circ Res 91:281, 2002.)*

Smooth Muscle Cell Migration and Proliferation

Whereas the early events in atheroma initiation involve primarily altered endothelial function and recruitment and accumulation of leukocytes, the subsequent evolution of atheroma into more complex plaques also involves SMCs (Fig. 43-6, steps 6 and 7). SMCs in the normal arterial tunica media differ considerably from those in the intima of an evolving atheroma.[31,32] Whereas some SMCs probably arrive in the arterial intima early in life, others accumulate in advancing atheroma after recruitment from the underlying media into the intima or arise from blood-borne precursors. Recent experimental evidence in mice has challenged the concept of recruitment of blood-borne SMCs into plaques.[33,34] The chemoattractants for SMCs likely include molecules such as platelet-derived growth factor (PDGF), a potent SMC chemoattractant secreted by activated macrophages and overexpressed in human atherosclerosis. SMCs in the atherosclerotic intima can also multiply by cell division. Estimated rates of division of SMCs in human atherosclerotic lesions are on the order of less than 1%, but even such indolent replication might yield considerable SMC accumulation during the decades of lesion evolution.

SMCs in the atherosclerotic intima appear to exhibit a less mature phenotype than the quiescent SMCs in the normal arterial medial layer. Instead of expressing primarily isoforms of smooth muscle myosin characteristic of adult SMCs, those in the intima have higher levels of the embryonic isoform of smooth muscle myosin. Thus, SMCs in the intima seem to recapitulate an embryonic phenotype. These intimal SMCs in atheroma appear morphologically distinct as well. They contain more rough endoplasmic reticulum and fewer contractile fibers than do normal medial SMCs.

Although replication of SMCs in the steady state appears infrequent in mature human atheroma, bursts of SMC replication may occur during the life history of a given atheromatous lesion. For example, and as discussed in considerable detail later in this chapter, episodes of plaque disruption with thrombosis may expose SMCs to potent mitogens, including the coagulation factor thrombin itself. Thus, accumulation of SMCs during atherosclerosis and growth of the intima may not occur in a continuous and linear fashion. Rather, "crises" may punctuate the history of an atheroma, during which bursts of smooth muscle replication or migration may occur (**Fig. 43-11**).

Smooth Muscle Cell Death During Atherogenesis

In addition to SMC replication, death of these cells may also participate in complication of the atherosclerotic plaque (Fig. 43-6, step 8).[35] Some SMCs in advanced human atheroma exhibit fragmentation of their nuclear DNA that is characteristic of programmed cell death or apoptosis. Apoptosis may occur in response to inflammatory cytokines present in the evolving atheroma. In addition to soluble cytokines that may trigger programmed cell death, T cells in atheroma may participate in eliminating some SMCs. In particular, certain T-cell populations known to accumulate in plaques can express Fas ligand on their surface. Fas ligand can engage Fas on the surface of SMCs and in conjunction with soluble proinflammatory cytokines lead to SMC death.[36]

Thus, SMC accumulation in the growing atherosclerotic plaque probably results from a tug-of-war between cell replication and cell death.[37] Contemporary cell and molecular biologic research has identified candidates for mediation of both the replication and the attrition of SMCs, a concept that originated from Virchow's careful morphologic observations almost 150 years ago. Referring to the SMCs in the intima, Virchow noted that early atherogenesis involves a "multiplication of their nuclei" but noted that cells in lesions can "hurry on to their own destruction."

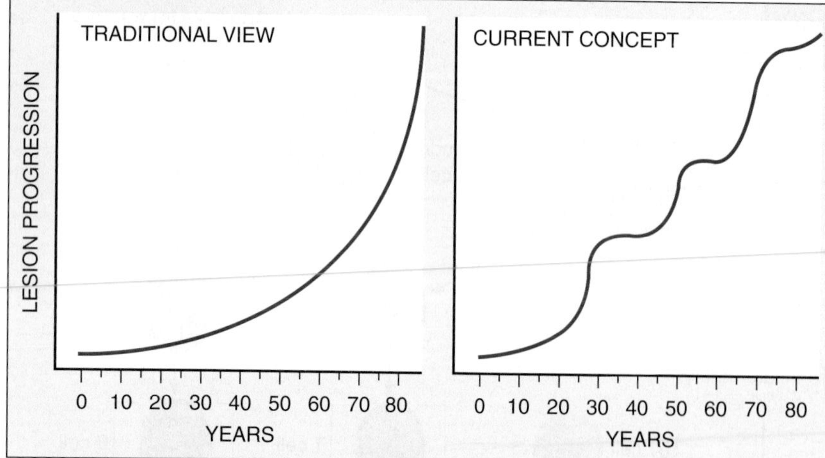

FIGURE 43-11 The time course of atherosclerosis. Traditional teaching held that atheroma formation followed an inexorably progressive course with age, as depicted in the left-hand curve. Current thinking suggests an alternative model, a step function rather than a monotonically upward course of lesion evolution in time (right-hand curve). According to this latter model, "crises" can punctuate periods of relative quiescence during the life history of a lesion. Such crises might follow an episode of plaque disruption, with mural thrombosis, and healing, yielding a spurt in smooth muscle proliferation and matrix deposition. Intraplaque hemorrhage due to rupture of a friable microvessel might produce a similar scenario. Such episodes are usually clinically inapparent. Extravascular events, such as an intercurrent infection with systemic cytokinemia or endotoxemia, could elicit an "echo" at the level of the artery wall, evoking a round of local cytokine gene expression by "professional" inflammatory leukocytes resident in the lesion. The episodic model of plaque progression, shown on the right, fits better with human angiographic data than does the continuous function depicted on the left.

Arterial Extracellular Matrix

Extracellular matrix, rather than cells themselves, makes up much of the volume of an advanced atherosclerotic plaque. Thus, extracellular constituents of plaque also require consideration. The major extracellular matrix macromolecules that accumulate in atheroma include interstitial collagens (types I and III) and proteoglycans such as versican, biglycan, aggrecan, and decorin. Elastin fibers may also accumulate in atherosclerotic plaques. Arterial SMCs produce these matrix molecules in disease, just as they do during development and maintenance of the normal artery (Fig. 43-6, step 7). Stimuli for excessive collagen production by SMCs include PDGF and TGF-β, a constituent of platelet granules, and a product of many cell types found in lesions, including Treg.

Much like the accumulation of SMCs, extracellular matrix secretion also depends on a balance, as noted earlier. In this case, the counterpoise to biosynthesis of the extracellular matrix molecules is breakdown catalyzed in part by catabolic enzymes known as matrix metalloproteinases (MMPs). Dissolution of extracellular matrix macromolecules undoubtedly plays a role in the migration of SMCs as they penetrate into the intima from the media through a dense extracellular matrix, traversing the elastin-rich internal elastic lamina. In injured arteries, overexpression of such proteinase inhibitors (known as tissue inhibitors of metalloproteinases, or TIMPs) can delay smooth muscle accumulation in the intima of injured arteries.[38]

Extracellular matrix breakdown also is likely to play a role in arterial remodeling that accompanies lesion growth. During the early life of an atheromatous lesion, plaques grow outwardly, in an abluminal direction, rather than inwardly, in a way that would lead to luminal stenosis. This outward growth of the intima leads to an increase in the caliber of the entire artery. This so-called positive remodeling or compensatory enlargement must involve turnover of extracellular matrix molecules to accommodate the circumferential growth of the artery. Luminal stenosis tends to occur only after the plaque burden exceeds some 40% of the cross-sectional area of the artery.

Angiogenesis in Plaques

Atherosclerotic plaques develop their own microcirculation as they grow because of endothelial migration and replication. Histologic examination with appropriate markers for endothelial cells reveals a rich neovascularization in evolving plaques. These microvessels probably form in response to angiogenic peptides overexpressed in atheroma. These angiogenesis factors include vascular endothelial growth factor (VEGF) forms of fibroblast growth factors, placental growth factor (PlGF), and oncostatin M.

These microvessels within plaques probably have considerable functional significance. For example, the abundant microvessels in plaques provide a relatively large surface area for the trafficking of leukocytes, which could include both entry and exit of leukocytes. Indeed, in the advanced human atherosclerotic plaque, microvascular endothelium displays mononuclear-selective adhesion molecules such as VCAM-1 much more prominently than does the macrovascular endothelium overlying the plaque. The microvascularization of plaques may also allow growth of the plaque, overcoming diffusion limitations on oxygen and nutrient supply, in analogy with the concept of tumor angiogenic factors and growth of malignant lesions.[39] Consistent with this view, administration of inhibitors of angiogenesis to mice with experimentally induced atherosclerosis limits lesion expansion. Finally, the plaque microvessels may be friable and prone to rupture like the neovessels in the diabetic retina. Hemorrhage and thrombosis in situ could promote a local round of SMC proliferation and matrix accumulation in the area immediately adjacent to the microvascular disruption (**Fig. 43-12**). This scenario illustrates a special case of one of the crises described earlier in the evolution of the atheromatous plaque (see Fig. 43-11). Attempts to augment myocardial perfusion by enhancing new vessel growth through the transfer of angiogenic proteins or their genes might have adverse effects on lesion growth or clinical complications of atheroma by these mechanisms.

Plaque Mineralization

Plaques often develop areas of calcification as they evolve. Indeed, Virchow recognized morphologic features of bone formation in atherosclerotic plaques in early microscopic descriptions of atherosclerosis. Understanding of the mechanism of mineralization during evolution of atherosclerotic plaques has advanced. Some subpopulations of SMCs may foster calcification by enhanced secretion of cytokines such as bone morphogenetic proteins, homologues of TGF-β. Atheroma calcification shares many mechanisms with bone formation. Receptor activator of NF-κB ligand (RANKL), a member of the tumor necrosis factor family, appears to promote SMC mineral formation through a bone morphogenetic protein 4 (BNP4)–dependent pathway. Osteoprotegerin can antagonize plaque mineralization by inhibiting RANKL signaling. Genetic absence of osteoprotegerin augments calcification of mouse atheromas, and administration of exogenous osteoprotegerin limits it.[40,41] The transcription factor Runx-2, activated by inflammatory mediators and oxidative stress among other stimuli, can promote SMC mineral formation by activating AKT.[42,43]

Complication of Atherosclerosis

Arterial Stenoses and Their Clinical Implications

The previous sections have discussed the initiation and evolution of the atherosclerotic plaque. These phases of the atherosclerotic process generally last many years, during which the affected individual often has no symptoms. After the plaque burden exceeds the capacity of the artery to remodel outward, encroachment on the arterial lumen begins.

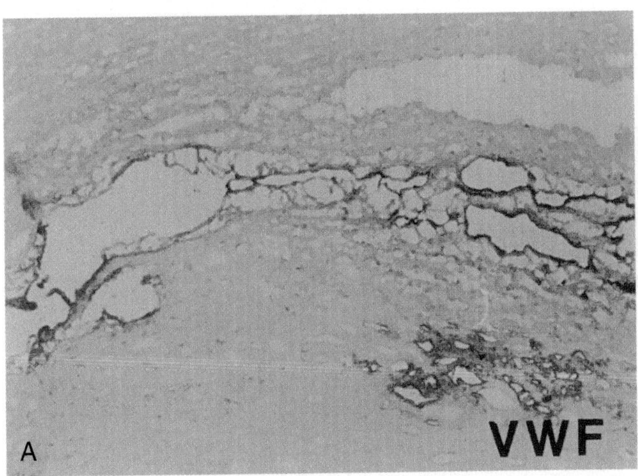

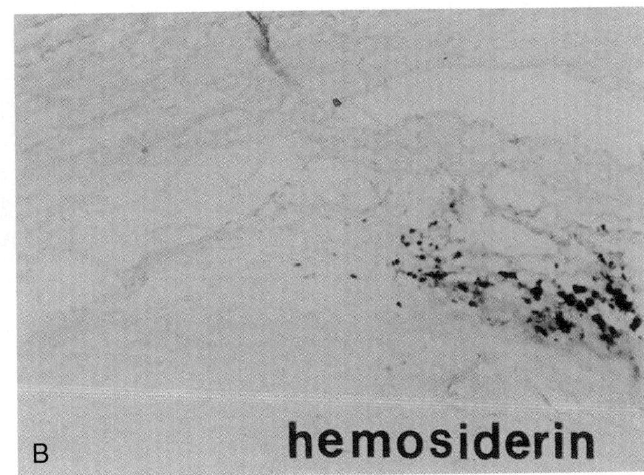

FIGURE 43-12 Intraplaque hemorrhage surrounding neovessels in an atheroma. A typical human atherosclerotic plaque, stained for von Willebrand factor **(A)** and iron by Prussian blue **(B)**. The von Willebrand factor stains the endothelial cells that line the microvascular channels and lakes. Note the extravasated von Willebrand factor that colocalizes with iron deposition, indicating hemosiderin deposition consistent with an intraplaque hemorrhage. *(After Brogi E, Winkles JA, Underwood R, et al: Distinct patterns of expression of fibroblast growth factors and their receptors in human atheroma and non-atherosclerotic arteries: Association of acidic FGF with plaque microvessels and macrophages. J Clin Invest 92:2408, 1993.)*

During the chronic asymptomatic or stable phase of lesion evolution, growth probably occurs discontinuously, with periods of relative quiescence punctuated by episodes of rapid progression (see Fig. 43-11). Human angiographic studies support this discontinuous growth of coronary artery stenoses. Eventually, the stenoses may progress to a degree that impedes blood flow through the artery. Lesions that produce stenoses of greater than 60% can cause flow limitations under conditions of increased demand. This type of athero-occlusive disease commonly produces chronic stable angina pectoris or intermittent claudication on increased demand. Thus, the symptomatic phase of atherosclerosis usually occurs many decades after lesion initiation.

In many cases of myocardial infarction, however, no history of prior stable angina heralds the acute event. Several kinds of clinical observation suggest that many myocardial infarctions result not from high-grade stenoses but from lesions that do not limit flow. For example, in individuals who have undergone coronary arteriography in the months preceding myocardial infarction, the culprit lesion most often shows less than 50% stenosis. In a compilation of four such serial angiographic studies, only approximately 15% of acute myocardial infarctions arose from lesions with degrees of stenosis greater than 60% on an antecedent angiogram.

Instead of progressive growth of the intimal lesion to a critical stenosis, we now recognize that thrombosis, complicating a not necessarily occlusive plaque, most often causes episodes of unstable angina or acute myocardial infarction.[44] Angiographic studies performed in individuals undergoing thrombolysis support this view. In one such study, almost half of patients undergoing thrombolysis for a first myocardial infarction had an underlying stenosis of less than 50% once the acute thrombus was lysed.

These findings do not imply that small atheromas cause most myocardial infarctions. Indeed, culprit lesions of acute myocardial infarction may be sizeable; but they may not produce a critical luminal narrowing because of compensatory enlargement. Of course, critical stenoses do cause myocardial infarctions, and high-grade stenoses more likely cause acute myocardial infarction than do nonocclusive lesions; yet because the noncritical stenoses by far outnumber the tight focal lesions in a given coronary tree, the lesser stenoses cause more infarctions even though high-grade stenoses have a greater individual probability of causing myocardial infarctions.

Thrombosis and Atheroma Complication

This evolution in our view of the pathogenesis of the acute coronary syndromes places new emphasis on thrombosis as the critical mechanism of transition from chronic to acute atherosclerosis. Understanding of the mechanisms of coronary thrombosis has advanced considerably. We now appreciate that a physical disruption of the atherosclerotic plaque commonly causes acute thrombosis.[45] Several major modes of plaque disruption provoke most coronary thrombi. The first mechanism, accounting for some two thirds of acute myocardial infarctions, involves a fracture of the plaque's fibrous cap (**Fig. 43-13**). Another mode involves a superficial erosion of the intima (**Fig. 43-14**), accounting for up to a quarter of acute myocardial infarctions in selected referral cases of individuals who have succumbed to sudden cardiac death. Superficial erosion appears more frequently in women than in men as a mechanism of coronary sudden death.[46]

Plaque Rupture and Thrombosis

The rupture of the plaque's fibrous cap probably reflects an imbalance between the forces that impinge on the plaque's cap and the mechanical strength of the fibrous cap. Interstitial forms of collagen provide most of the biomechanical resistance to disruption of the fibrous cap. Hence, the metabolism of collagen probably participates in regulating the propensity of a plaque to rupture (**Fig. 43-15**). Factors that decrease collagen synthesis by SMCs can impair their ability to repair and to maintain the plaque's fibrous cap. For example, the T cell–derived cytokine interferon-γ potently inhibits SMC collagen synthesis. On the other hand, as already noted, certain mediators released from platelet granules during activation (including TGF-β and PDGF) can increase SMC collagen synthesis, tending to reinforce the plaque's fibrous structure.

In addition to reduced de novo collagen synthesis by SMCs, increased catabolism of the extracellular matrix macromolecules that compose the fibrous cap can also contribute to weakening of this structure and render it susceptible to rupture and hence thrombosis. The same matrix-degrading enzymes thought to contribute to smooth muscle migration and arterial remodeling also may contribute to weakening of the fibrous cap (see Fig. 43-15). Macrophages in advanced human atheroma overexpress matrix metalloproteinases and elastolytic cathepsins that can break down the collagen and elastin of the arterial extracellular matrix.[38,47] Thus, the strength of the plaque's fibrous cap undergoes dynamic regulation, linking the inflammatory response in the intima with the molecular determinants of plaque stability and hence thrombotic complications of atheroma. The thinning of the plaque's fibrous cap, a result of reduced collagen synthesis and increased degradation, probably explains why histologic study has shown that thin fibrous caps characterize atherosclerotic plaques that have ruptured and caused fatal myocardial infarction.

CH 43

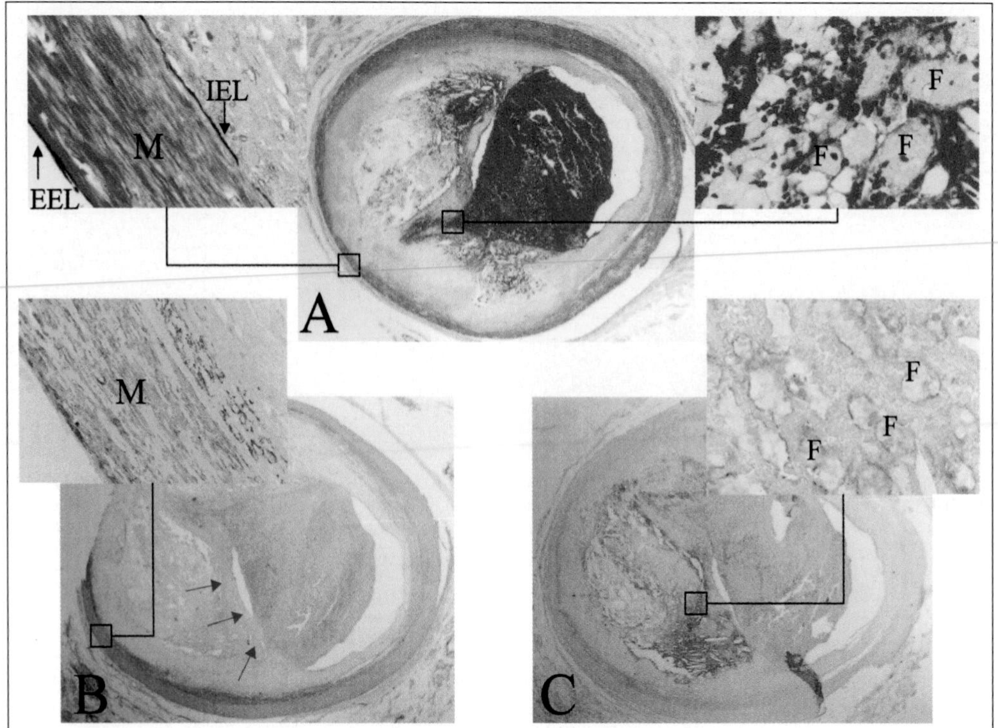

FIGURE 43-13 An example of a ruptured plaque that caused a fatal thrombosis. **A,** Movat stain. **B,** Immunostaining with HHF-38 discloses SMCs. Note the paucity of SMCs in the fibrous cap (red arrows), in contrast with the abundant SMCs in the medial layer (inset; M denotes the tunica media). **C,** Macrophage staining (CD68) shows accumulation of the inflammatory cells near the fibrous cap (inset; F denotes foam cell). EEL = external elastic lamina; IEL = internal elastic lamina. *(Reproduced from Bezerra HG, Higuchi ML, Gutierrez PS, et al: Atheromas that cause fatal thrombosis are usually large and frequently accompanied by vessel enlargement. Cardiovasc Pathol 10:189, 2001.)*

Another feature of the so-called vulnerable atherosclerotic plaque defined by pathologic analysis is a relative lack of SMCs (see Fig. 43-13B). As explained earlier, inflammatory mediators, both soluble and associated with the surface of T lymphocytes, can provoke programmed death of SMCs. Dropout of SMCs from regions of local inflammation within plaques probably contributes to the relative lack of SMCs at places where plaques rupture. Because these cells produce new collagen needed to repair and to maintain the matrix of the fibrous cap, the lack of SMCs may contribute to weakening of the fibrous cap and hence the propensity of that plaque to rupture.[48]

A prominent accumulation of macrophages and a large lipid pool is a third microanatomic feature of the so-called vulnerable atherosclerotic plaque. From a strictly biomechanical viewpoint, a large lipid pool can serve to concentrate biomechanical forces on the shoulder regions of plaques, which are common sites of rupture of the fibrous cap. From a metabolic standpoint, the activated macrophage characteristic of the plaque's core region produces the cytokines and the matrix-degrading enzymes thought to regulate aspects of matrix catabolism and SMC apoptosis in turn. Apoptotic macrophages and SMCs can generate particulate tissue factor, a potential instigator of microvascular thrombosis after spontaneous or iatrogenic plaque disruption. The success of lipid-lowering therapy in reducing the incidence of acute myocardial infarction or unstable angina in patients at risk may result from a reduced accumulation of lipid and a decrease in inflammation and plaque thrombogenicity. Animal studies and monitoring of peripheral markers of inflammation in humans support this concept.[49]

Thrombosis due to Superficial Erosion of Plaques

The preceding section discusses the pathophysiology of rupture of the plaque's fibrous cap. The pathobiology of superficial erosion is much less well understood. In experimental atherosclerosis in the nonhuman primate, areas of endothelial loss and platelet deposition occur in the more advanced plaques (see Fig. 43-14). In humans, superficial erosion appears more likely to cause fatal acute myocardial infarction in women and in individuals with hypertriglyceridemia and diabetes mellitus, but the underlying molecular mechanisms remain obscure. Apoptosis of endothelial cells could contribute to desquamation of endothelial cells in areas of superficial erosion. Likewise, matrix metalloproteinases, such as certain gelatinases specialized in degrading the nonfibrillar collagen found in the basement membrane (e.g., collagen type IV), might also sever the tetherings of the endothelial cell to the subjacent basal lamina and promote their desquamation.

Most plaque disruptions do not give rise to clinically apparent coronary events. Careful pathoanatomic examination of hearts obtained from individuals who have succumbed to noncardiac death has shown a surprisingly high incidence of focal plaque disruptions with limited mural thrombi. Moreover, hearts fixed immediately after explantation from individuals with severe but chronic stable coronary atherosclerosis who had undergone transplantation for ischemic cardiomyopathy show similar evidence for ongoing but asymptomatic plaque disruption. Experimentally, in atherosclerotic nonhuman primates, mural platelet thrombi can complicate plaque erosions without causing arterial occlusion. Therefore, repetitive cycles of plaque disruption, thrombosis in situ, and healing probably contribute to lesion evolution and plaque growth. Such episodes of thrombosis and healing constitute one type of crisis in the history of a plaque that may cause a burst of SMC proliferation, migration, and matrix synthesis (see Fig. 43-11). Recent observations suggest that plaque disruptions with healing underlie many thrombi that cause sudden death, indicating that nonocclusive thrombosis may precede the mortal event more frequently than previously recognized.[46] TGF-β and PDGF released from platelet granules may promote healing at the site of thrombosis by stimulating migration and collagen synthesis by SMCs, as noted earlier. Thrombin, generated at sites of mural thrombosis, potently stimulates SMC proliferation. The "burnt-out" fibrous and calcific atheroma may represent a late stage of a plaque that was previously lipid rich and vulnerable but now is rendered fibrous and hypocellular

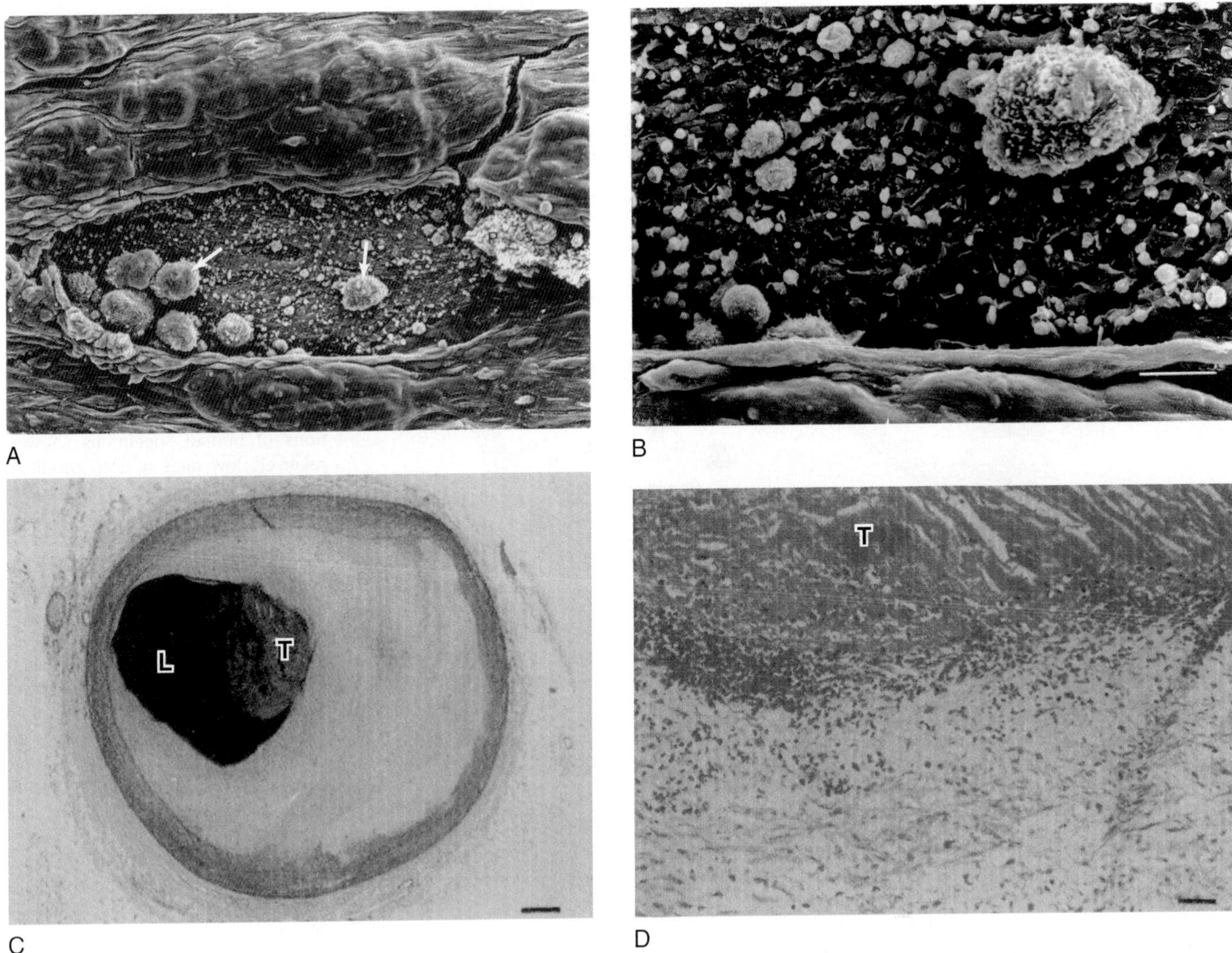

FIGURE 43-14 Superficial erosion of experimental atherosclerotic lesions, shown by scanning electron microscopy. Advanced atherosclerotic plaques can promote thrombosis by superficial erosion of the endothelial layer, exposing the blood and platelets to the subendothelial basement membrane containing collagen platelet activation and thrombosis. **A,** In the low-power view, the rent in endothelium is evident. Leukocytes (arrows) have adhered to the subendothelium, which is beginning to be covered with a carpet of platelets. **B,** The high-power view shows a field selected from the center of **A** that shows the leukocytes and platelets adherent to the subendothelium. *(Reproduced from Faggiotto A, Ross R: Studies of hypercholesterolemia in the nonhuman primate. II. Fatty streak conversion to fibrous plaque. Arteriosclerosis 4:341, 1984.)* **C,** A low-power histologic section through a coronary artery, thrombosed as a result of superficial erosion. L = lumen; T = thrombus. **D,** A high-power histologic section through a coronary artery, thrombosed as a result of superficial erosion. T = thrombus. *(Reproduced from Farb A, Burke AP, Tang AL, et al: Coronary plaque erosion without rupture into a lipid core. A frequent cause of coronary thrombosis in sudden coronary death. Circulation 93:1354, 1996.)*

because of a wound healing response mediated by the products of thrombosis.

Diffuse and Systemic Nature of Plaque Vulnerability and Inflammation in Atherogenesis

Studies at autopsy of atherosclerotic plaques that caused fatal thrombosis brought the notion of the vulnerable high-risk plaque to the fore. This observation stimulated many to seek ways of identifying and treating such high-risk atherosclerotic lesions. Current evidence, however, suggests that more than one such high-risk plaque often resides in a given coronary tree.[50,51] Moreover, the inflammation thought to characterize the so-called vulnerable plaque appears widespread. Studies using various imaging modalities have underscored the multiplicity of such high-risk plaques (see Chap. 23). Careful analysis of angiograms of individuals with acute coronary syndromes has demonstrated evidence for plaque ulceration or thrombosis in more than one lesion in many cases. Individuals with multiple unstable lesions by angiographic criteria tend to have worse outcomes during follow-up. Angioscopic studies have also shown multiple sites of intracoronary thrombosis in patients with acute coronary syndromes. Intravascular ultrasound, optical coherence tomography, magnetic resonance imaging, and computed tomographic angiography (among other technologies) have served to understand better the morphology of plaques that cause acute coronary syndromes.[52] These various modalities have generally found an association of lesions that cause acute manifestations ("culprit lesions") with positive remodeling or compensatory enlargement of arteries.[53]

Several concordant lines of evidence support the systemic and diffuse nature of inflammation in individuals with acute coronary syndromes.[54] Moreover, multiple studies have shown that various systemic markers of inflammation, such as C-reactive protein, increase in patients at risk for acute coronary syndromes. Inflammation precedes the acute coronary syndrome, as revealed by profiling of the platelet transcriptome, providing a window on gene transcription many days before the acute event. Two of the most elevated transcripts comparing mRNA from platelets of patients with ST-segment elevation to that from patients with stable coronary artery disease encode proteins implicated in inflammation.[55] Thus, a combination of imaging studies and investigations using inflammatory markers supports the diffuse and systemic nature of instability of atheromas in individuals with or at risk for acute coronary syndromes. This recognition has

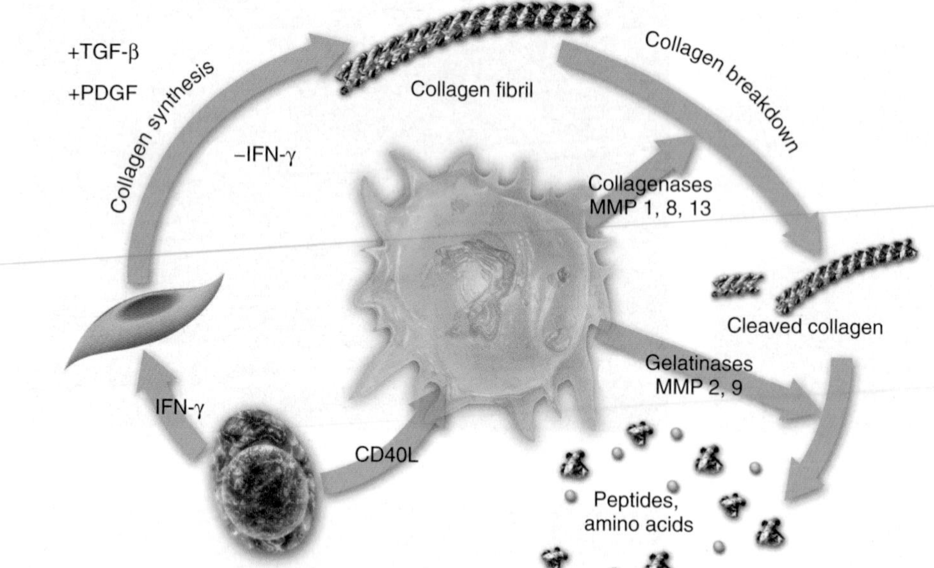

FIGURE 43-15 Inflammation regulates metabolism of fibrillar collagen, which may influence atherosclerotic plaque disruption. The T lymphocyte releases proinflammatory cytokines such as IFN-γ (lower left) that inhibit smooth muscle cells from producing the new collagen required to lay down the collagenous matrix of the plaque's fibrous cap, which protects the plaque from rupture. The T cell–derived cytokine CD40L stimulates mononuclear phagocytes (center) to elaborate interstitial collagenases including MMP-1, MMP-8, and MMP-13, which catalyze the initial proteolytic cleavage of the intact collagen fibril. The cleaved collagen can then undergo additional degradation by gelatinases such as MMP-9. In this way, inflammation can threaten the stability of atherosclerotic plaques, increase their tendency to rupture, and hence cause thromboses that trigger most acute coronary syndromes. *(Reproduced from Libby P: The molecular mechanisms of the thrombotic complications of atherosclerosis. J Intern Med 263:517, 2008.)*

important therapeutic implications. In addition to appropriately deployed local revascularization strategies, such individuals should also receive systemic therapy aimed at stabilizing the usually multiple high-risk lesions that may cause recurrent events.

Thrombosis depends not only on the "solid state" of the plaque that may rupture or erode to trigger thrombosis but also on the "fluid phase" of blood that determines the consequences of a given plaque disruption (**Fig. 43-16**).[44] The amount of tissue factor in the lipid core of a plaque (the solid state) can control the degree of clot formation that will ensue after disruption. The level of fibrinogen in the fluid phase of blood can influence whether a plaque disruption will cause an occlusive thrombus that can precipitate an acute ST-segment elevation myocardial infarction or merely a small mural thrombus. Likewise, levels of inhibitors of fibrinolysis, such as PAI-1, will impede the ability of endogenous plasminogen activator to limit thrombus growth or persistence. Inflammation regulates both the fluid-phase and solid-state factors delineated earlier, including tissue factor, fibrinogen, and PAI-1. This model helps explain the links between inflammation and thrombotic complications of atherosclerosis that have emerged from laboratory and clinical investigations.

Special Cases of Arteriosclerosis

Restenosis After Arterial Intervention (See Chap. 58.)

The problems of restenosis and in-stent stenosis after percutaneous arterial intervention represent special cases of arterial hyperplastic disease. After balloon angioplasty, luminal narrowing recurs in approximately one third of cases within 6 months. Initially, work on the pathophysiology of restenosis after angioplasty focused on smooth muscle proliferation. Much of the thinking regarding the pathobiology of restenosis or in-stent stenosis depended on extension to the human situation of the results of withdrawal of an overinflated balloon or overexpanded stents in previously normal animal arteries. Study of balloon-injured rat carotid arteries permitted precise understanding of the kinetics of intimal thickening after this type of injury, but the attempts to transfer this information to human restenosis met with considerable frustration. This disparity between experimental injury of animal arteries and human restenosis is not surprising. The substrate of the animal studies was usually a normal artery rather than an atherosclerotic one, with all the attendant cellular and molecular differences highlighted earlier.

Although SMC proliferation appears prominent in the simple experimental models of intimal thickening, observations of human specimens showed relatively low rates of SMC proliferation and called into question the therapeutic targeting of this process. Moreover, intravascular ultrasound studies in humans and considerable evidence from animal experimentation suggested that a substantial proportion of the loss of luminal caliber after balloon angioplasty resulted from a constriction of the vessel from the adventitial side (negative remodeling). These observations renewed interest in adventitial inflammation, with scar formation and wound contraction as a mechanism of arterial constriction after balloon angioplasty.

The widespread use of stents has changed the face of the restenosis problem. The process of in-stent stenosis, in contrast with restenosis after balloon angioplasty, depends uniquely on intimal thickening as opposed to negative remodeling. The stent provides a firm scaffold that prevents constriction from the adventitia. Histologic analyses reveal that a great deal of the volume of the in-stent stenotic lesion is made up of "myxomatous" tissue, comprising occasional stellate SMCs embedded in a loose and highly hydrated extracellular matrix. The introduction of stents has reduced the clinical impact of restenosis because of the technique's efficacy in increasing luminal diameter. Even if a considerable degree of lumen loss occurs as a result of intimal thickening, the luminal caliber remains sufficient to alleviate the patient's symptoms because of the excellent dilation achieved. Currently, stents that elute antiproliferative and anti-inflammatory substances have shown great benefit in terms of preventing in-stent stenosis, albeit with a potential for augmenting late stent thrombosis (see Chap. 58). The risk of late thrombosis after radiation brachytherapy or in stents that contain antiproliferative agents may relate to impaired endothelial healing, with the attendant loss of the anticoagulant and profibrinolytic properties of the normal intimal lining (see Fig. 43-2).

Accelerated Arteriosclerosis After Transplantation

Since the advent of effective immunosuppressive therapy such as cyclosporin, the major limitation to long-term survival of cardiac allografts is the development of an accelerated form of arterial hyperplastic disease (see Chap. 31). We favor the term *arteriosclerosis* (hardening of the arteries) rather than atherosclerosis (gruel-hardening) to describe this process because of the inconstant association with lipids (the "gruel" in atherosclerosis). This form of arterial disease often presents a diagnostic challenge. The patient may not experience typical anginal symptoms because of post-transplantation cardiac denervation. In addition, graft coronary disease is concentric and diffuse, not only affecting the proximal epicardial coronary vessels but also penetrating smaller intramyocardial branches (**Fig. 43-17**). For this reason, the angiogram, well suited to visualize focal and eccentric stenoses, consistently underestimates the degree of transplantation arteriosclerosis.

In most centers, a majority of patients undergoing transplantation have atherosclerotic disease and ischemic cardiomyopathy. However, a sizeable minority undergo heart transplantation for idiopathic dilated cardiomyopathy and may have few (if any) risk factors for atherosclerosis. Even in the absence of traditional risk factors, this latter group of individuals shares the risk for development of accelerated arteriosclerosis. This observation suggests that the pathophysiology of this form of accelerated arteriosclerosis differs from that of typical atherosclerosis.

The selective involvement of the engrafted vessels, with sparing of the host's native arteries, suggests that accelerated arteriopathy does not merely result from immunosuppressive therapy or other systemic factors in the transplantation recipient. Rather, these observations suggest that the immunologic differences between the host and recipient vessels might contribute to the pathogenesis of this disease. Considerable evidence from both human and experimental studies currently supports this viewpoint.[56] Endothelial cells in the transplanted coronary arteries express histocompatibility antigens that can engender an allogeneic immune response from host T cells. The activated T cells can secrete cytokines (e.g., interferon-γ) that can augment histocompatibility gene expression, recruit leukocytes by induction of adhesion molecules, and activate macrophages to produce SMC chemoattractants and growth factors. Interruption of interferon-γ signaling can prevent experimental graft coronary disease in mice. This disease appears to occur despite cyclosporin therapy, as this immunosuppressant is relatively ineffective as a suppressor of the endothelial allogeneic response. Indeed, immunosuppressive agents that more effectively suppress the endothelial allogeneic response appear better able to retard graft arteriosclerosis.

These considerations suggest that graft arteriosclerosis represents an extreme case of immunologically driven arterial hyperplasia (**Fig. 43-18**) that can happen in the absence of other risk factors. At the other extreme, patients with homozygous familial hypercholesterolemia can develop fatal atherosclerosis in the first decade of life solely as a result of an elevation in LDL. Most patients with atherosclerosis fall somewhere between these two extremes. Analysis of usual atherosclerotic lesions shows evidence for a chronic immune response and lipid accumulation. Therefore, by studying the extreme cases, such as transplantation arteriopathy and familial hypercholesterolemia, one can gain insight into elements of the pathophysiology that contribute to the multifactorial form of atherosclerosis that affects the majority of patients.

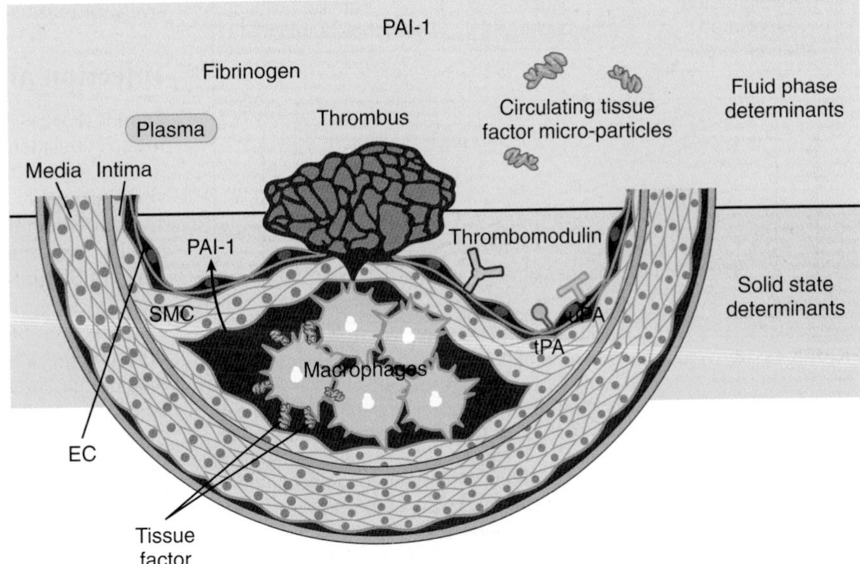

FIGURE 43-16 A two-state model of atherothrombosis. The high-risk atheroma has a thin fibrous cap overlying a large lipid core that contains tissue factor–bearing macrophages. When the fibrous cap fractures, coagulation proteins in the fluid phase of blood gain access to tissue factor–associated macrophages and tissue factor–bearing microparticles derived from apoptotic cells in the solid state of the plaque. These events trigger thrombus formation on the ruptured plaque. The clinical consequences depend on the amount of tissue factor and apoptosis in the plaque's core and on the levels of fibrinogen and PAI-1 in the fluid phase of blood. The interaction of the fluid phase with the solid state will determine whether a given plaque disruption provokes a partial or transient coronary artery occlusion (that can be clinically silent or less commonly cause an episode of unstable angina) or a devastating persistent and occlusive thrombus that can precipitate an acute myocardial infarction. Inflammation regulates the thrombotic/fibrinolytic balance in both the solid state and the fluid phase as PAI-1 and fibrinogen are both acute-phase reactants and because the inflammatory mediator CD40 ligand (CD154) induces tissue factor expression. EC = endothelial cell; PAI-1 = plasminogen activator inhibitor 1; SMC = smooth muscle cell; tPA = tissue plasminogen activator; uPA = urokinase-type plasminogen activator. *(Reproduced from Libby P, Theroux P: Pathophysiology of coronary artery disease. Circulation 111:3481, 2005.)*

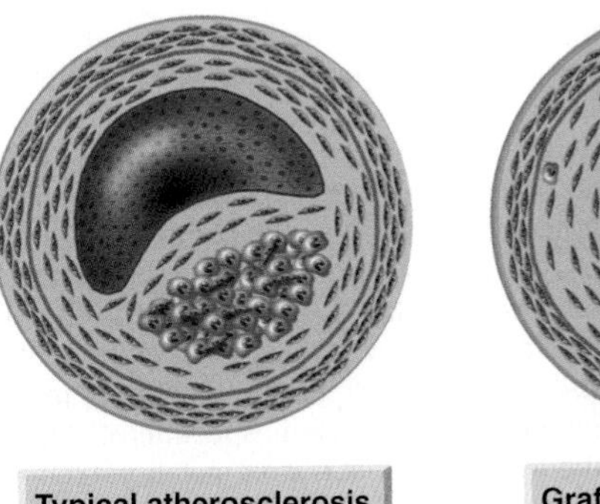

FIGURE 43-17 Comparison of typical atherosclerosis and transplantation arteriosclerosis. Typical atherosclerosis **(left)** characteristically forms an eccentric lesion with a lipid core and fibrous capsule. In contrast, the lesion of transplantation-associated accelerated arteriosclerosis **(right)** characteristically has a concentric intimal expansion without a clear central lipid core.

Aneurysmal Disease

Atherosclerosis also produces aneurysmal disease (see Chap. 60). Why is a single disease process manifested in directionally opposite manners, for example, most commonly producing stenoses in the coronary arteries but also causing ectasia of the abdominal aorta? In particular, aneurysmal disease characteristically affects the infrarenal abdominal aorta. This region is highly prone to the development of atherosclerosis. Data from the Pathobiological Determinants of Atherosclerosis in Youth (PDAY) study show that the dorsal surface of the infrarenal abdominal aorta has a particular predilection for the development of fatty streaks and raised lesions in Americans younger than 35 years who succumbed for noncardiac reasons (see Fig. 43-1). Because of the absence of vasa vasorum, the relative lack of blood supply to the tunica media in this portion of the abdominal aorta might explain the regional susceptibility of this portion of the arterial tree to aneurysm formation. In addition, the lumbar lordosis of the biped human may alter the hydrodynamics of blood flow in the distal aorta, yielding flow disturbances that may promote lesion formation.

CH 43

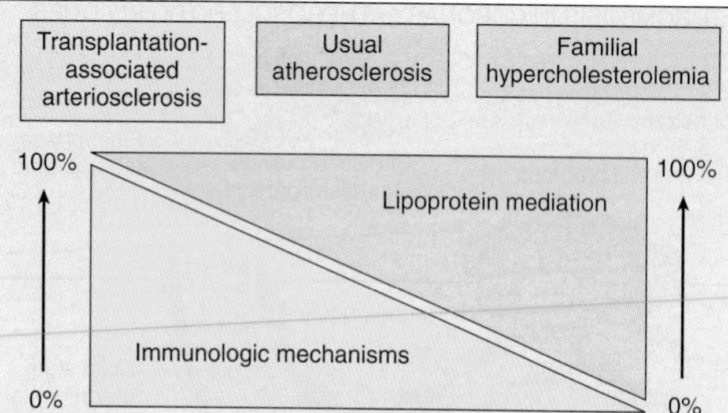

FIGURE 43-18 A multifactorial view of the pathogenesis of atherosclerosis. This diagram depicts two extreme cases of atherosclerosis. One (far left side) represents accelerated arteriosclerosis that can occur in the transplanted heart in the absence of traditional coronary risk factors. This disease probably represents primarily immune-mediated arterial intimal disease. The other extreme (far right side) depicts the case of a child who may succumb to rampant atherosclerosis in the first decade of life solely because of an elevated LDL level due to a mutation in the LDL receptor (homozygous familial hypercholesterolemia). Between these two extremes lie most patients with atherosclerosis, probably involving various mixtures of immune and inflammatory or lipoprotein-mediated disease. One can further consider that this diagram extends to a third dimension that would involve other candidate risk factors, such as homocysteine, lipoprotein(a), infection, and tobacco abuse.

Histologic examination shows considerable distinction between occlusive atherosclerotic disease and aneurysmal disease. In typical coronary artery atherosclerosis, expansion of the intimal lesion produces stenotic lesions. The tunica media underlying the expanded intima is often thinned, but its general structure remains relatively well preserved. In contrast, transmural destruction of the arterial architecture occurs in aneurysmal disease. In particular, the usually well-defined laminar structure of the normal tunica media disappears with obliteration of the elastic laminae. The medial SMCs, usually well preserved in typical stenotic lesions, are notable for their paucity in the media of advanced aortic aneurysms.

Study of the pathophysiology that underlies these anatomic pathologic findings has proven frustrating. Experimental aneurysm formation in animals has uncertain relevance to the clinical disease. The human specimens obtainable for analysis generally represent the late stages of this disease. Nonetheless, recent work has identified several mechanisms that may underlie the peculiar pathology of aneurysmal disease. Widespread destruction of the elastic laminae suggests a role for degradation of elastin, collagen, and other constituents of the arterial extracellular matrix. Many studies have documented overexpression of matrix-degrading proteinases, including matrix metalloproteinases in human aortic aneurysm specimens. Current clinical trials are testing the hypothesis that matrix metalloproteinase inhibitors can reduce the expansion of aneurysms. Recent experimental work has implicated angiotensin II as a potentiator of aneurysm formation in mice. Alterations in TGF-β signaling can predispose to aneurysm formation. Mutations in TGF-β receptors can cause arterial ectasia.[8]

Thus, heightened elastolysis may explain the breakdown of the usually ordered structure of the tunica media in this disease. A slant toward T helper cell Th2 populations in aneurysmal versus occlusive disease may contribute to the overexpression of certain elastolytic enzymes.[57,58] Thoracic aortic aneurysms may, in contrast, harbor a predominantly Th1 response.[59] In addition, aortic aneurysms show evidence for considerable inflammation, particularly in the adventitia. The lymphocytes that characteristically abound on the adventitial side of aneurysmal tissue suggest that apoptosis of SMCs triggered by inflammatory mediators including soluble cytokines and Fas ligand, elaborated by these inflammatory cells, may contribute to SMC destruction and promote aneurysm formation. Although extracellular matrix degradation and SMC death also occur in sites where atherosclerosis causes stenosis, they appear to predominate in regions of aneurysm formation and to affect the tunica media much more extensively, for reasons that remain obscure.

Infection and Atherosclerosis

Interest persists in the possibility that infections may cause atherosclerosis. A considerable body of seroepidemiologic evidence supports a role for certain bacteria, notably *Chlamydia pneumoniae*, and certain viruses, notably cytomegalovirus, in the etiology of atherosclerosis. The seroepidemiologic studies have spurred a number of in vivo and in vitro experiments that lend varying degrees of support to this concept. Several caveats apply in the evaluation of the seroepidemiologic evidence. First, confounding factors should be carefully considered. For example, smokers may have a higher incidence of bronchitis due to *C. pneumoniae*. Therefore, evidence for infection with *C. pneumoniae* may merely serve as a marker for tobacco use, a known risk factor for atherosclerotic events. In addition, a strong bias favors the publication of positive studies as opposed to negative studies. Thus, meta-analyses of seroepidemiologic studies may be slanted toward the positive merely because of underreporting of negative studies. Finally, atherosclerosis is a common and virtually ubiquitous disease in developed countries. In most societies, many adults have serologic evidence of prior infections with Herpesviridae, such as cytomegalovirus, and respiratory pathogens, such as *C. pneumoniae*. It is difficult to sort out coincidence from causality when the majority of the population studied has evidence of both infection and atherosclerosis.

Whereas proof that bacteria or viruses can cause atherosclerosis remains elusive, it is quite plausible that infections may potentiate the action of traditional risk factors, such as hypercholesterolemia. Based on the vascular biology of atherosclerosis discussed in this chapter, a number of scenarios might apply. First, cells within the plaque itself may harbor infection. For example, macrophages existing in an established atherosclerotic lesion might become infected with *C. pneumoniae*, which could spur their activation and accelerate the inflammatory pathways that we currently believe operate within the atherosclerotic intima. Specific microbial products, such as lipopolysaccharides, heat shock proteins, or other virulence factors, might act locally at the level of the artery wall to potentiate atherosclerosis in infected lesions.

Extravascular infection might also influence the development of atheromatous lesions and provoke their complication. For example, circulating endotoxin or cytokines produced in response to a remote infection can act locally at the level of the artery wall to promote the activation of vascular cells and of leukocytes in preexisting lesions, producing an "echo" at the level of the artery wall of a remote infection. Also, the acute-phase response to an infection in a nonvascular site might affect the incidence of thrombotic complications of atherosclerosis by increasing fibrinogen or plasminogen activator inhibitor or otherwise altering the balance between coagulation and fibrinolysis. Such disturbance in the prevailing prothrombotic, fibrinolytic balance may critically influence whether a given plaque disruption will produce a clinically inapparent transient or nonocclusive thrombus or sustained and occlusive thrombi that could cause an acute coronary event.

Acute infections might also produce hemodynamic alterations that could trigger coronary events. For example, the tachycardia and increased metabolic demands of fever could augment the oxygen requirements of the heart, precipitating ischemia in an otherwise compensated individual. These various scenarios illustrate how infectious processes, either local in the atheroma or extravascular, might aggravate atherogenesis, particularly in preexisting lesions or in concert with traditional risk factors. Sufficiently powered clinical trials, however, have not shown that treatment with macrolide or fluoroquinolone antibiotics can reduce recurrent coronary events in survivors of myocardial infarction. Even if such studies had been positive, they would not establish a role for a particular infectious agent, nor could they prove that the antibiotic effect of the agents tested, rather than some other action not related to their antimicrobial effect, could produce benefit. However plausible, current clinical evidence does not support a role for bacterial infection in recurrent coronary events.[60,61]

REFERENCES

Mechanisms of Atherogenesis

1. Steinberg D: The Cholesterol Wars: The Skeptics vs. the Preponderance of Evidence. San Diego, Elsevier Academic Press, 2007.
2. Shantsila E, Watson T, Lip GY: Endothelial progenitor cells in cardiovascular disorders. J Am Coll Cardiol 49:741, 2007.
3. Reed MJ, Karres N, Eyman D, Edelberg J: Endothelial precursor cells. Stem Cell Rev 3:218, 2007.
4. Dong C, Crawford LE, Goldschmidt-Clermont PJ: Endothelial progenitor obsolescence and atherosclerotic inflammation. J Am Coll Cardiol 45:1458, 2005.
5. Hagensen MK, Shim J, Thim T, et al: Circulating endothelial progenitor cells do not contribute to plaque endothelium in murine atherosclerosis. Circulation 121:898, 2010.
6. Aird WC: Mechanisms of endothelial cell heterogeneity in health and disease. Circ Res 98:159, 2006.
7. Majesky MW: Developmental basis of vascular smooth muscle diversity. Arterioscler Thromb Vasc Biol 27:1248, 2007.
8. Loeys BL, Schwarze U, Holm T, et al: Aneurysm syndromes caused by mutations in the TGF-beta receptor. N Engl J Med 355:788, 2006.
9. Libby P, Shi GP: Mast cells as mediators and modulators of atherogenesis. Circulation 115:2471, 2007.
10. Kruth HS: Sequestration of aggregated low-density lipoproteins by macrophages. Curr Opin Lipidol 13:483, 2002.
11. Muller WA: Mechanisms of transendothelial migration of leukocytes. Circ Res 105:223, 2009.
12. Galkina E, Ley K: Vascular adhesion molecules in atherosclerosis. Arterioscler Thromb Vasc Biol 27:2292, 2007.
13. Woollard KJ, Geissmann F: Monocytes in atherosclerosis: Subsets and functions. Nat Rev Cardiol 7:77, 2010.
14. Libby P, Nahrendorf M, Pittet MJ, Swirski FK: Diversity of denizens of the atherosclerotic plaque: Not all monocytes are created equal. Circulation 117:3168, 2008.
15. Charo IF, Ransohoff RM: The many roles of chemokines and chemokine receptors in inflammation. N Engl J Med 354:610, 2006.
16. Gleissner CA, von Hundelshausen P, Ley K: Platelet chemokines in vascular disease. Arterioscler Thromb Vasc Biol 28:1920, 2008.
17. Libby P: Inflammation in atherosclerosis. Nature 420:868, 2002.
18. Parmar KM, Larman HB, Dai G, et al: Integration of flow-dependent endothelial phenotypes by Kruppel-like factor 2. J Clin Invest 116:49, 2006.
19. Atkins GB, Wang Y, Mahabeleshwar GH, et al: Hemizygous deficiency of Kruppel-like factor 2 augments experimental atherosclerosis. Circ Res 103:690, 2008.
20. Yamawaki H, Pan S, Lee RT, Berk BC: Fluid shear stress inhibits vascular inflammation by decreasing thioredoxin-interacting protein in endothelial cells. J Clin Invest 115:733, 2005.
21. Moore KJ, Freeman MW: Scavenger receptors in atherosclerosis: Beyond lipid uptake. Arterioscler Thromb Vasc Biol 26:1702, 2006.
22. van Berkel TJ, Out R, Hoekstra M, et al: Scavenger receptors: Friend or foe in atherosclerosis? Curr Opin Lipidol 16:525, 2005.

Inflammation and Immunity in Atherogenesis

23. Hartvigsen K, Chou MY, Hansen LF, et al: The role of innate immunity in atherogenesis. J Lipid Res 50(Suppl):S388, 2009.
24. Libby P, Ridker PM, Hansson GK: Inflammation in atherosclerosis: From pathophysiology to practice. J Am Coll Cardiol 54:2129, 2009.
25. Andersson J, Libby P, Hansson GK: Adaptive immunity and atherosclerosis. Clin Immunol 134:33, 2010.
26. Tsimikas S, Brilakis ES, Miller ER, et al: Oxidized phospholipids, Lp(a) lipoprotein, and coronary artery disease. N Engl J Med 353:46, 2005.
27. Chou MY, Hartvigsen K, Hansen LF, et al: Oxidation-specific epitopes are important targets of innate immunity. J Intern Med 263:479, 2008.
28. Ait-Oufella H, Taleb S, Mallat Z, Tedgui A: Cytokine network and T cell immunity in atherosclerosis. Semin Immunopathol 31:23, 2009.
29. Taleb S, Tedgui A, Mallat Z: Regulatory T-cell immunity and its relevance to atherosclerosis. J Intern Med 263:489, 2008.
30. Binder CJ, Chou MY, Fogelstrand L, et al: Natural antibodies in murine atherosclerosis. Curr Drug Targets 9:190, 2008.
31. Manabe I, Nagai R: Regulation of smooth muscle phenotype. Curr Atheroscler Rep 5:214, 2003.
32. Mulvihill ER, Jaeger J, Sengupta R, et al: Atherosclerotic plaque smooth muscle cells have a distinct phenotype. Arterioscler Thromb Vasc Biol 24:1283, 2004.
33. Bentzon JF, Weile C, Sondergaard CS, et al: Smooth muscle cells in atherosclerosis originate from the local vessel wall and not circulating progenitor cells in ApoE knockout mice. Arterioscler Thromb Vasc Biol 26:2696, 2006.
34. Bentzon JF, Sondergaard CS, Kassem M, Falk E: Smooth muscle cells healing atherosclerotic plaque disruptions are of local, not blood, origin in apolipoprotein E knockout mice. Circulation 116:2053, 2007.

Apoptosis in Atherosclerosis

35. Clarke MC, Figg N, Maguire JJ, et al: Apoptosis of vascular smooth muscle cells induces features of plaque vulnerability in atherosclerosis. Nat Med 12:1075, 2006.
36. Kavurma MM, Tan NY, Bennett MR: Death receptors and their ligands in atherosclerosis. Arterioscler Thromb Vasc Biol 28:1694, 2008.
37. Geng YJ, Libby P: Progression of atheroma: A struggle between death and procreation. Arterioscler Thromb Vasc Biol 22:1370, 2002.

Mechanisms of Plaque Complication

38. Dollery CM, Libby P: Atherosclerosis and proteinase activation. Cardiovasc Res 69:625, 2006.
39. Moulton KS: Angiogenesis in atherosclerosis: Gathering evidence beyond speculation. Curr Opin Lipidol 17:548, 2006.
40. Bennett BJ, Scatena M, Kirk EA, et al: Osteoprotegerin inactivation accelerates advanced atherosclerotic lesion progression and calcification in older ApoE$^{-/-}$ mice. Arterioscler Thromb Vasc Biol 26:2117, 2006.
41. Morony S, Tintut Y, Zhang Z, et al: Osteoprotegerin inhibits vascular calcification without affecting atherosclerosis in ldlr$^{-/-}$ mice. Circulation 117:411, 2008.
42. Aikawa E, Nahrendorf M, Figueiredo JL, et al: Osteogenesis associates with inflammation in early-stage atherosclerosis evaluated by molecular imaging in vivo. Circulation 116:2841, 2007.
43. Byon CH, Javed A, Dai Q, et al: Oxidative stress induces vascular calcification through modulation of the osteogenic transcription factor Runx2 by AKT signaling. J Biol Chem 283:15319, 2008.
44. Libby P, Theroux P: Pathophysiology of coronary artery disease. Circulation 111:3481, 2005.
45. Virmani R, Burke AP, Farb A, Kolodgie FD: Pathology of the vulnerable plaque. J Am Coll Cardiol 47(Suppl):C13, 2006.
46. Kramer MC, Rittersma SZ, de Winter RJ, et al: Relationship of thrombus healing to underlying plaque morphology in sudden coronary death. J Am Coll Cardiol 55:122, 2010.
47. Libby P: The molecular mechanisms of the thrombotic complications of atherosclerosis. J Intern Med 263:517, 2008.
48. Clarke MC, Littlewood TD, Figg N, et al: Chronic apoptosis of vascular smooth muscle cells accelerates atherosclerosis and promotes calcification and medial degeneration. Circ Res 102:1529, 2008.
49. Libby P: Molecular and cellular mechanisms of the thrombotic complication of atherosclerosis. J Lipid Res 50:S352, 2009.
50. Libby P: Act local, act global: Inflammation and the multiplicity of "vulnerable" coronary plaques. J Am Coll Cardiol 45:1600, 2005.
51. Lombardo A, Rizzello V, Natale L, et al: Magnetic resonance imaging of carotid plaque inflammation in acute coronary syndromes: A sign of multisite plaque activation. Int J Cardiol 136:103, 2009.
52. Choi SH, Chae A, Chen CH, et al: Emerging approaches for imaging vulnerable plaques in patients. Curr Opin Biotechnol 18:73, 2007.
53. Motoyama S, Sarai M, Harigaya H, et al: Computed tomographic angiography characteristics of atherosclerotic plaques subsequently resulting in acute coronary syndrome. J Am Coll Cardiol 54:49, 2009.
54. Abbate A, Bussani R, Liuzzo G, et al: Sudden coronary death, fatal acute myocardial infarction and widespread coronary and myocardial inflammation. Heart 94:737, 2008.
55. Healy AM, Pickard MD, Pradhan AD, et al: Platelet expression profiling and clinical validation of myeloid-related protein-14 as a novel determinant of cardiovascular events. Circulation 113:2278, 2006.

The Vascular Biology of Allograft Arterial Disease

56. Mitchell RN, Libby P: Vascular remodeling in transplant vasculopathy. Circ Res 100:967, 2007.

Mechanisms of Aneurysm Formation

57. Shimizu K, Libby P, Mitchell RN: Local cytokine environments drive aneurysm formation in allografted aortas. Trends Cardiovasc Med 15:142, 2005.
58. Shimizu K, Mitchell RN, Libby P: Inflammation and cellular immune responses in abdominal aortic aneurysms. Arterioscler Thromb Vasc Biol 26:987, 2006.
59. Tang PC, Yakimov AO, Teesdale MA, et al: Transmural inflammation by interferon-gamma–producing T cells correlates with outward vascular remodeling and intimal expansion of ascending thoracic aortic aneurysms. FASEB J 19:1528, 2005.

Infection in Atherosclerosis

60. Anderson JL: Infection, antibiotics, and atherothrombosis—end of the road or new beginnings? N Engl J Med 352:1706, 2005.
61. Andraws R, Berger JS, Brown DL: Effects of antibiotic therapy on outcomes of patients with coronary artery disease: A meta-analysis of randomized controlled trials. JAMA 293:2641, 2005.

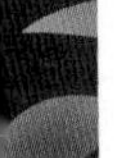

CHAPTER 44 Risk Markers for Atherothrombotic Disease

Paul M Ridker and Peter Libby

Atherothrombosis can no longer be considered a disease of the developed world, because myocardial infarction and stroke are increasingly prevalent worldwide, across all socioeconomic strata (see Chap. 1). By 2025, cardiovascular mortality on a worldwide scale will likely surpass that of every major disease group, including infection, cancer, and trauma.[1,2]

From our current perspective, it is perhaps surprising that the formal conceptual basis for considering specific cardiovascular risk factors and risk markers emerged as recently as the 1960s, when the findings of the Framingham Heart Study began to appear. From an epidemiologic perspective, a risk marker is a characteristic or feature of an individual or population that presents early in life and associates with an increased risk of developing future disease. The risk marker of interest may be an acquired behavior (e.g., smoking), an inherited trait (e.g., familial hyperlipidemia), or a laboratory value (e.g., cholesterol, C-reactive protein). For a risk marker to have clinical usefulness, it typically must predate the onset of clinical disease. Most risk markers used in daily practice have demonstrated a consistent graded response effect in large prospective epidemiologic studies. Several risk markers, such as hyperlipidemia and hypertension, are modifiable, and trials have demonstrated that lowering these factors reduces vascular risk. For other risk factors such as smoking, the attributable risk and assumed pathways of effect make trials unethical, but a biomarker need not be proved causal for it to have substantial clinical usefulness. For example, although controversy persists regarding whether markers of inflammation are directly or indirectly associated with atherothrombosis, several inflammatory biomarkers have proved effective in clinical practice for evaluating vascular risk and selecting individuals at risk who benefit from specific interventions.

This chapter reviews the epidemiologic evidence underlying risk markers for atherothrombosis in three parts. The first section describes the conventional risk factors of smoking, hypertension, hyperlipidemia, insulin resistance and diabetes, physical activity, and obesity, as well as general strategies for reducing risk related to these disorders. This section will explore some of the issues and controversy surrounding the concept of the metabolic syndrome. It also briefly reviews evidence on how mental stress and depression affect traditional measures of vascular risk.

Not all coronary events occur in individuals with multiple traditional risk factors, however, and in some individuals, abnormalities of inflammation, hemostasis, and/or thrombosis appear to contribute decisively. In particular, almost half of all myocardial infarctions and strokes occur in individuals without hyperlipidemia. Thus, the second section of this chapter reviews atherothrombotic risk markers, including high-sensitivity C-reactive protein (hsCRP) and other markers of inflammation, as well as homocysteine and lipoprotein(a). We evaluate evidence that describes whether these novel risk indicators add to risk prediction beyond conventional factors. The third section presents brief overviews of imaging techniques and emerging genetic approaches that may contribute to risk evaluation in the future. The chapter concludes with a discussion of a novel approach to overall risk prediction that can be applied immediately and that encompasses emerging concepts of inflammatory and heritable risk.[3] The need for future clinical guidelines to incorporate biologic changes in our understanding of atherosclerosis is also discussed.

With the exception of glucose intolerance and obesity, the prevalence of most cardiovascular risk factors has declined in the United States over the past 40 years. These favorable U.S. trends indicate that interventions to lower risk can reduce not only coronary disease but also stroke. Adherence to a healthy lifestyle may prevent many cases of coronary heart disease (CHD). Therefore, targeting risk reduction by lifestyle modification for those who have clusters of risk factors seems a sensible primary goal for preventive cardiovascular practice globally.

Conventional Risk Factors

Smoking

Other than advanced age, smoking is the single most important risk factor for coronary artery disease. Cigarette consumption is the leading preventable cause of death in the United States, where it accounts for more than 400,000 deaths annually.[4] Ischemic heart disease causes 35% to 40% of all smoking-related deaths, with an additional 8% attributable to second-hand smoke exposure. Despite the relative stability in prevalence of current smokers in the United States, rates of tobacco use are increasing among adolescents, young adults, and women.[5] Although increased recognition of the hazards of smoking might be hoped to slow these trends, almost 1 billion individuals now smoke worldwide. Smoking has a particularly large impact in the developing world (see Chap. 1). In China alone, more than 670,000 deaths annually are already attributable to smoking[6] and, by the end of 2010, 930,000 adult deaths may occur from smoking-related causes in India.[7] Even among nonsmokers, inhaled smoke—whether from passive exposure or cigar or pipe consumption—increases coronary risk. Passive smoking exposure can impair coronary vasodilatory capacity and increase bronchial responsiveness and concomitant pulmonary dysfunction.

An exceptionally consistent series of prospective studies has documented the effects of smoking on coronary risk. Compared with nonsmokers, persons who consume 20 or more cigarettes daily have a two- to threefold increase in total CHD. Moreover, these effects depend on dose; consumption of as few as one to four cigarettes daily increases coronary artery disease risk. Such light levels of smoking have a major impact on myocardial infarction and all-cause mortality, even among smokers who do not report inhalation. In addition to myocardial infarction, cigarette consumption relates directly to increased rates of sudden death, aortic aneurysm formation, symptomatic peripheral vascular disease, and ischemic stroke. Risk of coronary disease directly increases with the number of cigarettes consumed. Prospective evidence links cigarette consumption to an elevated risk of hemorrhagic stroke, including intracranial hemorrhage and subarachnoid hemorrhage, again in a dose-response manner. Continued smoking is also a major risk factor for recurrent myocardial infarction.

Historically, cigarette consumption was prevalent in men before women and, at least in the United States, smoking prevalence remains lower in women than men. However, this gap has markedly narrowed, with overall consumption rates in women now in excess of 20%. Native Americans and those with less education have higher rates, whereas black and Hispanic women appear to smoke less than white women (**Fig. 44-1**). Because of adverse synergy with oral contraceptives, young female smokers who take oral contraceptives have particularly elevated risks of premature coronary disease and stroke. Smoking has special hazards for women with diabetes.

Beyond acute unfavorable effects on blood pressure and sympathetic tone, and a reduction in myocardial oxygen supply, smoking affects atherothrombosis through several other mechanisms. In addition to accelerating atherosclerotic progression, long-term smoking may enhance the oxidation of low-density lipoprotein (LDL) cholesterol and impair endothelium-dependent coronary artery vasodilation. In addition, smoking has adverse hemostatic and inflammatory effects, including increased levels of CRP, soluble intercellular adhesion molecule-1 (ICAM-1), fibrinogen, and homocysteine. Smoking may provoke spontaneous platelet aggregation, increased monocyte adhesion to endothelial cells, and adverse alterations in endothelial-derived fibrinolytic and antithrombotic factors, including tissue-type plasminogen activator and tissue pathway factor inhibitor (see Chap. 87). Compared with nonsmokers, smokers have an increased prevalence of coronary spasm and reduced thresholds for ventricular arrhythmia. Accruing evidence suggests that insulin resistance represents an additional mechanistic link between smoking and premature atherosclerosis.

Cessation of cigarette consumption overwhelmingly remains the single most important intervention in preventive cardiology. In a major overview, smoking cessation was found to reduce CHD mortality by 36% as compared with mortality in subjects who continued smoking, an effect that did not vary by age, sex, or country of origin.[8] The observed 35% to 40% risk reductions equal or exceed other secondary prevention interventions that have received more attention from physicians and the pharmaceutical industry, including the use of aspirin, statins, beta-adrenergic blocking agents, and angiotensin-converting enzyme inhibitors.

Reductions in smoking from any mechanism improve health outcomes, particularly when linked to lifestyle changes, including exercise and dietary control. Trials of nicotine replacement therapy using transdermal nicotine or nicotine chewing gum increase abstention rates after cessation. Such pharmacologic programs, as well as physician-guided counseling, are cost-effective and should be provided as standard prevention services. Low-yield cigarettes do not appear to reduce the risks of myocardial infarction. Although the elevated cardiovascular risks associated with smoking decrease significantly after cessation, the risks of cancer of the lungs, pancreas, and stomach persist for more than a decade, as do the risks of developing chronic obstructive pulmonary disease. Smoking cessation has clear benefit, but smoking reduction alone appears to have only a marginal effect.[9]

Poor patient understanding of the importance of smoking cessation continues, particularly in the developing world. The observation that smoking predicts better outcome following various reperfusion strategies (the so-called smoker's paradox) is not because of any benefit of smoking but simply because smokers are likely to undergo such procedures at a younger age and hence generally have lower comorbidity on average. Despite public health legislation, the tobacco industry continues its aggressive targeting of young adults, who are most susceptible to new addiction. Recent agreements to regulate tobacco by the U.S. Food and Drug Administration provide an opportunity to re-address smoking prevention efforts on a national scale.[10] Studies of social networking indicate that smoking cessation by a spouse decreases a person's chance of smoking by 67%, whereas smoking cessation by a sibling, friend, or coworker decreases a person's chance of smoking by 25% to 36%.[11] Although novel smoking cessation programs that include direct financial incentives have been evaluated and found effective,[12] community education and physician-based primary prevention remain the most important components of any smoking reduction strategy.

Hypertension

High blood pressure often confers silent cardiovascular risk, and its prevalence is steadily increasing (see Chap. 45). Of the estimated 50 million Americans with high blood pressure, almost one third evade diagnosis and only one fourth receive effective treatment.[13] In the National Health and Nutrition Examination Survey (NHANES), 28.7% of subjects evaluated had a measured blood pressure higher than 140/90 mm Hg or reported use of antihypertensive medications, an increase of almost 4% from similar survey data a decade earlier.[14] Hypertension prevalence was highest in non-Hispanic blacks (33.5%), increased with age (reaching more than 65% after the age of 60 years), and tended to be more prevalent in women than in men. Although 68% of the study participants were aware of their hypertension, only 58% received therapy, and only 31% had their hypertension controlled (**Fig. 44-2**). Thus, in contrast to hyperlipidemia, hypertension prevalence is increasing and treatment rates remain poor, highlighting the need for programs targeting prevention. In Europe, the prevalence of hypertension exceeds that in the United States and Canada by 60%. Worldwide, almost 1 billion adults have hypertension, 333 million in developed countries and 639 million in developing countries; by 2025,

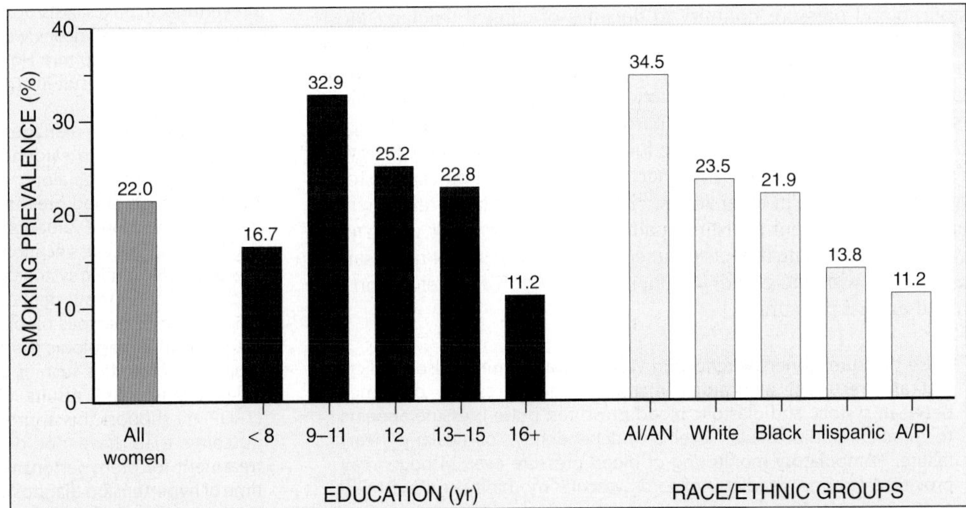

FIGURE 44-1 Prevalence of current smoking among American women 18 years of age and older by education and by race and ethnicity. AI/AN = American Indian/Alaska Native; A/PI = Asian/Pacific Islander. *(From Lucas JW, Schiller JS, Benson V: Summary health statistics for U.S. adults: National Health Interview Survey, 2001. Vital Health Stat 10:1, 2004.)*

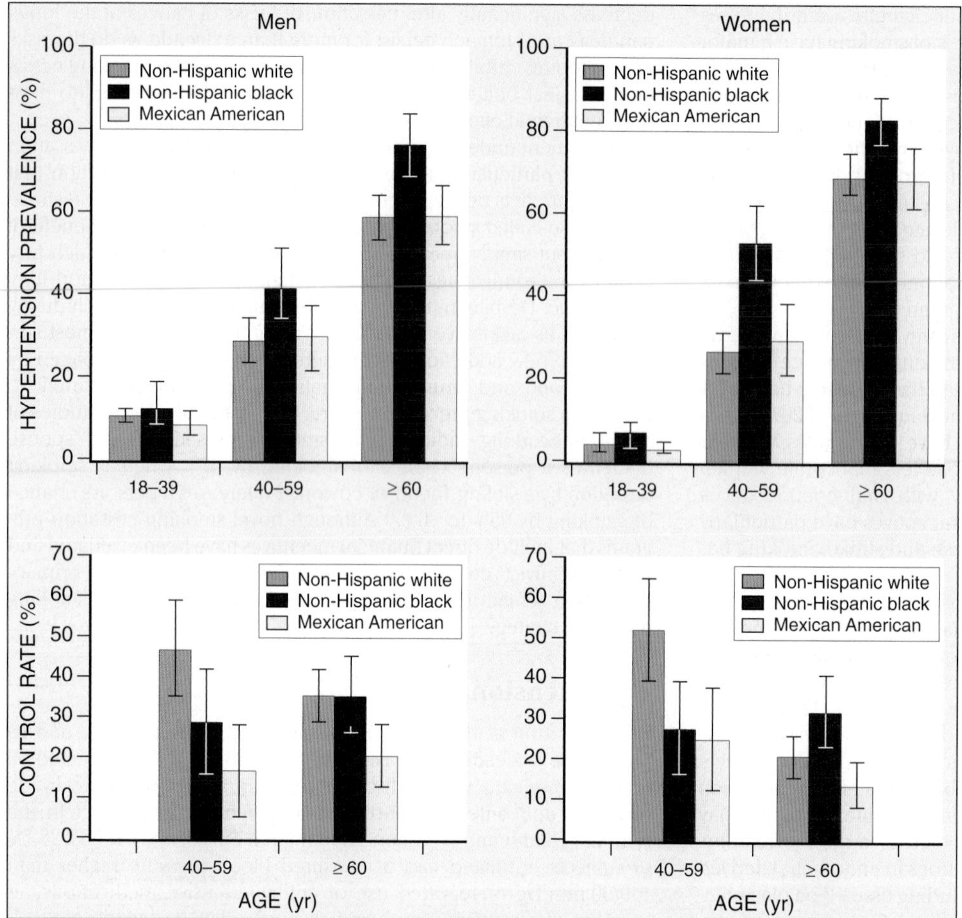

FIGURE 44-2 Hypertension prevalence (top) and hypertension control rates (bottom) by age and ethnicity among American men and women. *(From Hajjar I, Kotchen TA: Trends in prevalence, awareness, treatment, and control of hypertension in the United States, 1988-2000. JAMA 290:199, 2003.)*

the total number of adults with hypertension is anticipated to exceed 1.5 billion (**Fig. 44-3**).[15] Worldwide, hypertension causes 7.6 million premature deaths annually, with 80% of this burden occurring in low- and middle-income countries (see Chap. 1).[16]

Part of the complexity of hypertension as a risk factor relates to changing definitions of risk and an understanding that systolic blood pressure and pulse pressure may have greater importance than diastolic blood pressure, contrary to decades of clinical teaching. Most epidemiologic studies now recognize the joint contributions of systolic and diastolic blood pressure to the development of cardiovascular risk, an issue that has influenced strategies for risk detection. Isolated systolic hypertension, in particular, has at least as much importance as diastolic blood pressure for the outcomes of total cardiovascular mortality and stroke. Evidence supports the treatment of systolic hypertension, even in older adults.[17] Isolated systolic hypertension thus appears to represent a distinct pathophysiologic state in which elevated blood pressure reflects reduced arterial elasticity not necessarily associated with increased peripheral resistance or an elevation in mean arterial pressure.

Pulse pressure, generally reflecting vascular wall stiffness, also predicts first and recurrent myocardial infarction. Defined as the difference between systolic and diastolic blood pressures, pulse pressure appears to predict cardiovascular events independently, particularly heart failure.[18] Ambulatory monitoring of blood pressure over 24 hours may provide a stronger predictor of cardiovascular morbidity and mortality compared with office-based measures.

Studies of home blood pressure evaluation have yielded mixed results. In one older cohort, self-measurement of blood pressure had better prognostic accuracy for vascular events than office-based evaluation,[19] whereas another study has determined that nocturnal hypertension diagnosed by continuous monitoring is associated with an increased risk of congestive heart failure.[20] By contrast, in a randomized trial comparing office with home blood pressure measurement, self-measurement allowed identification of those with white coat hypertension but did not greatly improve overall management nor alter objective measures of compliance, such as left ventricular mass.[21] A more recent trial has indicated that home monitoring and consequent blood pressure control improve when an Internet-based pharmacist is available for consultation.[22]

The importance of these changing definitions of hypertension has received support from intervention trials specifically targeting isolated systolic hypertension that have generally shown benefit. Blood pressure reductions as small as 4 to 5 mm Hg result in large and clinically significant reductions in risk for stroke, vascular mortality, congestive heart failure, and total CHD in middle-aged subjects, older adults, and high-risk groups, such as those with diabetes and peripheral arterial disease.[23] Among compliant patients, sodium reduction and weight loss can lower blood pressure, but not all patients respond to such measures, and the long-term success of nonpharmacologic approaches to hypertension control has often proven disappointing. By contrast, relatively simple therapies such as low-dose diuretics can have a major public health benefit. In an overview of 42 clinical trials that included 192,000 patients, low-dose diuretics compared with placebo yielded reductions of 21% in total CHD, 49% in congestive heart failure, 29% in stroke, and 19% in cardiovascular mortality.[24] In this meta-analysis, although combined therapy was often superior, none of the other first-line therapies for hypertension, including beta-adrenergic blocking agents, angiotensin-converting enzyme inhibitors, angiotensin receptor blockers, or calcium channel blockers yielded benefits beyond those of low-dose diuretics. Combined low-dose therapies, however, have considerable efficacy in both blood pressure reduction and event prevention. In an analysis of 354 randomized trials, regimens of multiple drugs given at low doses were estimated capable of reducing systolic blood pressure by 20 mm Hg and diastolic blood pressure by 11 mm Hg, effects that could result in stroke reductions of 63% and CHD risk reductions of 46%.[25]

Diet and lifestyle management remain the cornerstone of prevention of hypertension, and evidence continues to accrue that adopting low-risk dietary measures along with weight reduction greatly reduces the burden of high blood pressure.[26] The Joint National Committee on Prevention, Detection, Evaluation and Treatment of High Blood Pressure has suggested a new classification of blood pressure, with normal defined as less than 120 mm Hg systolic and less than 80 mm Hg diastolic for adults, and prehypertension defined as systolic blood pressure of 120 to 139 mm Hg or diastolic blood pressure of 80 to 89 mm Hg. In this latter category, pharmacologic therapy is suggested in the presence of other major comorbidities such as diabetes, renal dysfunction, or known vascular disease. The results of the Trial of Preventing Hypertension (TROPHY) support this approach and the feasibility of treatment,[27] but outcome trials have not demonstrated the superiority of initiating treatment for prehypertensive patients over initiating treatment at the time of hypertension diagnosis, or the cost-effectiveness of this approach. By contrast, pharmacologic therapy is mandated for those with stage 1 hypertension (systolic blood pressure 140 to 159 mm Hg, or diastolic blood pressure 90 to 99 mm Hg) or stage 2 hypertension (systolic blood pressure higher than 160 mm Hg, or diastolic blood pressure higher than

100 mm Hg). The recent Action to Control Cardiovascular Risk in Diabetes (ACCORD) trial found that targeting a systolic blood pressure of less than 120 mm Hg, as compared to less than 140 mm Hg, did not reduce the rate of cardiovascular events among diabetic patients.[28]

Patients with chronic kidney disease (estimated glomerular filtration rate < 60 mL/m^2) also merit blood pressure reduction, both for the prevention of cardiovascular disease and to slow progression to end-stage renal disease. Genetic variants associated with atrial natriuretic polypeptides may modify the effect of antihypertensive therapy, indicating that pharmacogenetics could play a role in future care.[29] As also recently demonstrated among diabetic patients, good blood pressure control must continue long term to maintain clinical benefits.[30]

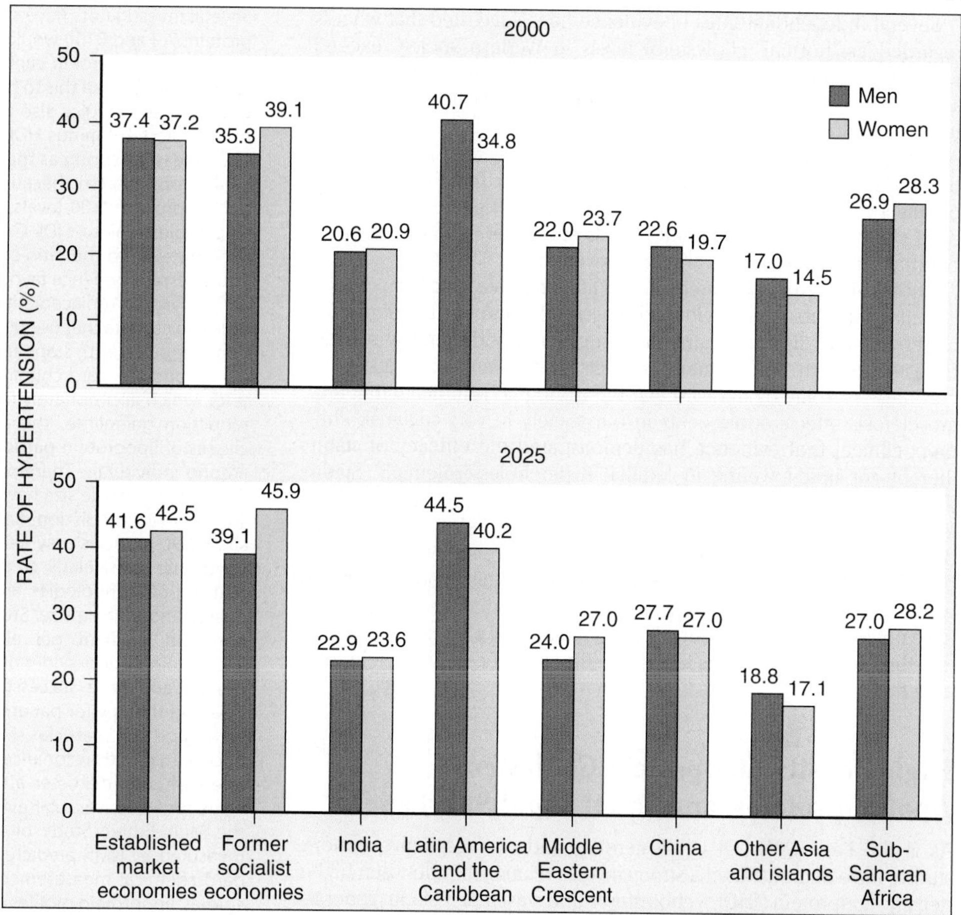

FIGURE 44-3 Hypertension prevalence rates by geographic region, 2000 and 2025. *(From Kearney PM, Whelton M, Reynolds K, et al: Global burden of hypertension: Analysis of worldwide data. Lancet 365:217, 2005.)*

Hyperlipidemia and Elevated Low-Density Lipoprotein Cholesterol

(see Chap. 47)

Cross-sectional population studies have consistently revealed a relationship between serum cholesterol levels and CHD death. Confounding factors, however, limit the validity of such studies. The emergence of data from prospective cohort studies, such as that begun in Framingham in the 1950s, bolstered the relationship between cholesterol and CHD. This study, as well as others performed with different populations around the world, established the concept of cholesterol more firmly as a culprit in CHD. The Atherosclerosis Risk in Communities (ARIC) study has particular relevance to current clinical practice in the United States because it included substantial numbers of women and members of racial minority groups.

Although based on more than a century of experimental and clinical observation, doubt lingered regarding the role of cholesterol in atherosclerosis until surprisingly recently. Through the beginning of the 1990s, controversy enveloped the role of cholesterol-lowering therapy in CHD risk reduction. Despite evidence that high cholesterol levels correlated with coronary death, the proposition that cholesterol-lowering therapy could reduce CHD morbidity remained unproven. Critics pointed to the J-shaped curve, which apparently described the relationship of serum cholesterol to mortality. Advocates of the cholesterol hypothesis countered that the heightened risk for all-cause death in individuals with low levels of cholesterol might reflect comorbidities such as cancer, inanition, or liver disease. The goal of reducing CHD mortality by drug therapy eluded convincing proof for decades. Some cholesterol-lowering medications appeared to cause an increase in the incidence of some events, including noncoronary death. In the pioneering coronary drug project, estrogen treatment led to excess mortality in the cohort of men studied. The World Health Organization study of clofibrate showed excess noncoronary death. Dietary interventions to lower cholesterol often proved ineffective and, together, such results seemed to challenge the validity of cholesterol as a therapeutic target.

Conclusive evidence regarding the cholesterol hypothesis awaited clinical trials of cholesterol lowering using the hydroxymethylglutaryl coenzyme A (HMG-CoA) reductase inhibitors (statins), agents that lowered LDL cholesterol much more efficiently than previously available drugs. Unassailable clinical trial evidence now shows that lowering LDL cholesterol levels reduces coronary events in broad segments of the population. The ensemble of large clinical trials of statins has substantiated a decrease in total mortality in almost all major study populations. As a group, placebo-controlled trials of statins lowered LDL cholesterol levels by 20% to 60% and reduced coronary events by up to one third over a 5-year period, with no evidence of an increase in nonvascular mortality.

The Heart Protection Study showed that statins can reduce stroke and coronary events in those with preexisting vascular disease.[31] Several head to head trials comparing different statin regimens have shown that even more aggressive LDL reduction is associated with greater clinical improvements (see Chap. 47).

The case for LDL cholesterol as a CHD risk factor thus meets most of the criteria established by Robert Koch in the 19th century to establish a causative agent in a disease. High cholesterol levels consistently predict risk of future cardiovascular events in human populations. Animal studies in multiple species have shown a causal relationship between hypercholesterolemia and atherosclerosis. Knowledge of the LDL receptor pathway plus emerging understanding of the vascular biology of atherosclerosis provides biologic plausibility for the involvement of LDL in atherogenesis. The human mutations in the LDL receptor produce hypercholesterolemia on a monogenic basis that causes accelerated atherosclerosis as early as the first decade of life in individuals with homozygous familial hypercholesterolemia. Finally, interventions in large clinical trials to lower LDL cholesterol levels by various approaches (e.g., bile acid–binding resins, intestinal bypass surgery, statins) have shown a reduction in cardiovascular events. Thus, LDL cholesterol fulfills the criteria of modified Koch's postulates as one causative agent in atherosclerosis.

Several independent lines of evidence have suggested that what is regarded as "normal" cholesterol levels in Western society exceed levels that good health requires.[32] In particular, certain rural agrarian societies with very low rates of atherothrombosis have total cholesterol levels well below those accepted as normal in Western societies. Another line of evidence derives from phylogeny. Contemporary humans have much higher total cholesterol levels than those of many other species of higher organisms that thrive nonetheless. Clinical trials have shown that LDL cholesterol levels as low as 50 mg/dL provide optimal outcomes, even in primary prevention.

Cholesterol levels measured early in life influence long-term cardiovascular risk. Substantial evidence suggests that the burden of risk for cardiovascular disease begins in young adulthood. Autopsy studies from the Korean and Vietnam conflicts, and recent explorations of coronary anatomy by intravascular ultrasonography, indicate that atherosclerosis affects adolescents in our society. In very high-risk children, clinical trial evidence has demonstrated the efficacy of statin therapy for lipid-lowering in familial hypercholesterolemia.[33] Statin trials have now demonstrated convincing benefits on hard clinical endpoints, even among those without established cardiovascular disease.[34] Not all patient subgroups, however, have shown such clear benefits with statin therapy. As described later in this chapter, in those with severe congestive heart failure or on hemodialysis, recent trials have not found lowered event rates in statin-treated patients, suggesting that the use of these agents late in the disease process may yield less benefit.

High-Density Lipoprotein Cholesterol, Apolipoproteins, and Other Lipid Subclasses

As is the case with LDL cholesterol, abundant prospective cohort studies have demonstrated a strong inverse relationship between high-density lipoprotein (HDL) cholesterol and vascular risk. In general, each increase of HDL cholesterol by 1 mg/dL is associated with a 2% to 3% decrease in risk of total cardiovascular disease. Patients with angiographically proven coronary artery disease more often have low levels of HDL than high levels of LDL, as defined by current criteria. The process of reverse cholesterol transport may explain in part the apparent protective role of HDL against coronary death. According to this concept, HDL could ferry cholesterol from the vessel wall, augmenting peripheral catabolism of cholesterol (see Chap. 47). HDL can also carry antioxidant enzymes that may reduce the levels of oxidized phospholipids in atheromatous lesions, which could enhance atherogenesis. Furthermore, overexpressing the apolipoprotein A-I gene in transgenic mice and infusing complexes of apolipoprotein A-I and phospholipids into hyperlipidemic rabbits not only increases HDL cholesterol levels (HDL-C) but also decreases atherosclerotic development. Evidence is also accruing of anti-inflammatory properties for HDL-C.

In contrast to LDL, however, we currently lack evidence that increasing HDL-C levels reduces risk. The Investigation of Lipid Level Management to Understand Its Impact in Atherosclerotic Events (ILLUMINATE) trial, in which the cholesteryl ester transfer protein inhibitor torcetrapib was given to patients at high vascular risk, showed an unanticipated increase in all-cause mortality,[35] findings that have led to considerable controversy as to whether HDL-C remains a viable therapeutic target.[36]

Nonetheless, the consistency of the observational data, both cross-sectional and prospective, strongly supports the HDL level as a negative risk factor, as incorporated in the Adult Treatment Panel (ATP-III) guidelines, and supports the continued careful evaluation of agents that can directly increase HDL levels. This recognition by the ATP-III—that a biomarker can be useful without fulfilling Koch's postulates—has importance for clinical practice and has implications for several other emerging risk factors (see later). Optimism that HDL-C remains in the causal pathway for atherosclerotic events also comes from recent genetic studies evaluating the relationships of polymorphisms in HDL-related loci as predictors of incident vascular events.[37,38]

Several investigators have suggested that the measurement of apolipoproteins A-I and B100 would predict cardiovascular risk better than HDL and LDL cholesterol in clinical practice. Two recent prospective cohort studies have shown this to be the case for men[39] and women.[40] However, both of these studies also found that non-HDL cholesterol (defined as total cholesterol minus HDL cholesterol) provided clinical risk information at least as strong as that of apolipoprotein B100; this was an unsurprising observation, because non–HDL-C correlates very closely with apolipoprotein B100 levels. Furthermore, these studies found that the total cholesterol–to–HDL-C ratio remained a very strong predictor of risk, superior even to the ratio of apolipoprotein B100 to apolipoprotein A-I. Thus, despite evidence favoring apolipoproteins A-I and B100 in univariate analyses as replacements for HDL and LDL cholesterol, there remain little clinical data that use of these measures improves overall risk prediction compared with standard lipid testing.

Beyond standard chemical measures of total, LDL, and HDL cholesterol, which appropriately form the basis of current lipid screening and reduction guidelines, the amount of cholesterol carried by different classes of lipoprotein particles may influence function and vary widely among individuals. Therefore, measures of core lipid composition and lipoprotein particle size have been hypothesized to provide better measures for risk prediction. Several lines of evidence have indicated that small LDL particles may be more atherogenic than large particles and contribute particularly to the dyslipidemia of diabetes. Currently, a number of technologies are available for the evaluation of LDL subclasses and particle size. Studies using density gradient ultracentrifugation and gradient gel electrophoresis have generally found that lipoprotein subclass identifies individuals at higher risk for coronary disease and have successfully shown a preferential benefit of lipid-lowering therapy for patients with small, dense LDL particles compared with large LDL particles. LDL particle concentration, as measured by nuclear magnetic resonance (NMR) studies, correlates well with coronary arterial lumen diameter after statin therapy and may offer predictive value for future vascular events. In both the Women's Health Study and the Multi-Ethnic Study of Atherosclerosis, LDL particle concentration measured by NMR predicted incident vascular events better than standard chemical measurement of LDL cholesterol.[41,42] However, in these studies, lipoprotein profiles evaluated by NMR were not superior to those of other standard measures, such as the total cholesterol–to–HDL-C ratio or non–HDL-C. Thus, although intriguing pathophysiologic information regarding lipid reduction with statins and gemfibrozil has come from NMR studies, as well as density gradient studies,[43,44] it remains unclear whether these novel methods of lipid evaluation add importantly to standard lipid screening in routine practice or should remain specialized tools for research and lipid clinics.

Triglyceride-Rich Lipoproteins and Cardiovascular Risk

In contrast to compelling evidence favoring a causal role for LDL-C in atherogenesis, the role of triglycerides remains controversial. Part of this controversy reflects the inverse correlation of triglyceride levels with HDL-C. Adjustment for HDL-C attenuates the relationship between triglycerides and cardiovascular disease. A recent meta-analysis has suggested that the adjusted risk ratio for coronary disease among those in the top third of triglyceride levels, compared with the bottom third, decreases from approximately 2.0 to 1.5 after accounting for HDL-C.[45] A second controversy reflects the continued recommendation in guidelines that triglycerides be measured in the fasting state, whereas much of the prognostic value of plasma triglyceride levels depends on postprandial levels. Two major cohort studies have recently reported that nonfasting triglycerides predict vascular events, independent of traditional risk factors, but that fasting triglyceride levels show little independent relationship.[46,47] On this basis, prediction of vascular risk may need to be based on an oral triglyceride tolerance test, analogous to a glucose tolerance test used to diagnose diabetes.[48] Nonfasting triglycerides have also recently been found to predict incident stroke, again in contrast to fasting levels.[49]

For these reasons, among others, current guidelines do not establish a target value of triglycerides. However, in view of the tight link of triglyceride levels with known risk factors for atherosclerosis (e.g., low HDL-C level, uncontrolled diabetes, hypothyroidism), the finding of marked and persistently elevated triglyceride levels should enter into overall risk assessment for an individual and stimulate consideration of the reason for triglyceride level elevation, including careful exclusion of secondary causes (see Chap. 47). A cautious approach to triglyceride reduction seems prudent, because randomized trials using fenofibrate in diabetic patients have not shown significant reductions in risk when added to statin therapy.[50,51]

Metabolic Syndrome, Insulin Resistance, and Diabetes

Insulin resistance and diabetes (see Chap. 64) rank among the major cardiovascular risk factors; in one major survey, the presence of diabetes conferred an equivalent risk to aging 15 years, an impact higher than that of smoking.[52] Almost 35 million Americans have some degree of abnormal glucose tolerance, a condition along with obesity that markedly increases the risk for type 2 diabetes and premature atherothrombosis. Patients with diabetes have two- to eightfold higher rates of future cardiovascular events as compared with age- and ethnicity-matched nondiabetic individuals, and 75% of all deaths in diabetic patients result from CHD. Compared with unaffected individuals, diabetic patients have a greater atherosclerotic burden, both in the major arteries and in microvascular tone. Not surprisingly, diabetic patients have substantially increased rates of atherosclerotic complications in the settings of primary prevention and after coronary intervention procedures. Insulin resistance alone confers an elevated risk of heart failure and probably explains the association of obesity with this diagnosis.[53] Moreover, the risk of cardiovascular disease starts to increase long before the onset of clinical diabetes. In the Nurses Health Study, women who eventually developed type 2 diabetes had a threefold elevated relative risk of myocardial infarction before the diagnosis of diabetes, a cardiovascular event rate almost as high as that in patients with overt diabetes at study entry.[54] These effects are magnified in ethnic minority populations and in patients with other concomitant risk factors.

Although hyperglycemia associates with microvascular disease, insulin resistance itself promotes atherosclerosis even before it produces frank diabetes, and available data corroborate the role of insulin resistance as an independent risk factor for atherothrombosis. This finding has prompted recommendations for increased surveillance for the metabolic syndrome, a cluster of glucose intolerance and hyperinsulinemia accompanied by hypertriglyceridemia, low HDL levels, hypofibrinolysis, hypertension, microalbuminuria, a predominance of small, dense LDL particles, and central obesity. Although several formal definitions of the metabolic syndrome have been proposed, the definition adopted by the National Cholesterol Education Program Adult Treatment Panel requires at least three of the following five criteria: (1) waist circumference larger than 102 cm in men and 88 cm in women; (2) serum triglyceride levels of at least 150 mg/dL; (3) HDL cholesterol less than 40 mg/dL in men and less than 50 mg/dL in women; (4) blood pressure of at least 130/85 mm Hg; and (5) serum glucose concentration of at least 110 mg/dL. Using these criteria, the prevalence of metabolic syndrome in the United States is almost 25%, or almost 50 million persons.

Some have raised concerns regarding the concept of metabolic syndrome[55] (**Table 44-1**). The definition of metabolic syndrome differs among various national guidelines and statements. Some of these criteria require measurement of insulin resistance, whereas others, including the ATP-III criteria, use variables readily available from a standard clinical evaluation. The disparity in these definitions underscores the arbitrary nature of including or excluding various risk factors in the definition of metabolic syndrome. Moreover, disagreement persists regarding insulin resistance as a unifying pathophysiologic pathway that accounts for all the features of the metabolic syndrome, rendering it a true syndrome. In addition, the question of whether coalescence of risk factors incorporated in the concept of metabolic syndrome augment risk beyond the sum of risk attributable to the individual components remains controversial. Several studies have documented that individuals with the metabolic syndrome have elevated vascular event rates. In the Kuopio Ischaemic Heart Disease Risk Factor Study, patients with metabolic syndrome showed markedly increased rates of coronary, cardiovascular, and all-cause mortality (**Fig. 44-4**).[56] However, not all those with metabolic syndrome have similar risk. One compilation of two studies suggested minimal contribution of the ATP-III definition of metabolic syndrome to the prediction of cardiovascular events[57]—data regarded by one editorialist as "another nail in the coffin of the metabolic syndrome."[58] However, both of the studies included in this analysis focused on older individuals, in the seventh decade of life or older. Currently, this constellation of risk factors affects many younger individuals, and the issue of additive risk over time in this population remains unanswered.[59,60]

TABLE 44-1 Controversy Regarding the Metabolic Syndrome Concept

CONCERNS*	COUNTERPOINTS
Criteria are ambiguous or incomplete; rationale for thresholds is ill-defined.	Practical concerns would favor a definition that does not involve measurements of insulin resistance or imaging.
Value of including diabetes in definition is questionable.	Metabolic syndrome concept may not help predict diabetes, but may have value in cardiovascular risk assessment.
Insulin resistance as unifying cause is uncertain.	Current criteria do not include an index of inflammation that may contribute mechanistically to some of the risk.
No clear basis for including or excluding other cardiovascular risk factors.	Concerns regarding clinical practicality may influence the choice of criteria.
Cardiovascular risk value is variable and depends on specific risk factors present.	Inflammatory status (e.g., hsCRP) may add to risk captured by individual components of the metabolic syndrome.
Cardiovascular risk associated with the syndrome may be no higher than sum of its parts.	Sufficient outcome data in younger populations to assess the added value of clustered components of the metabolic syndrome to risk prediction are lacking.
Treatment of syndrome is no different from treatment for each of its components.	We lack rigorous prospective intervention trials predicated on metabolic syndrome criteria.
Medical value of diagnosing the syndrome is unclear.	May help motivate patients and physicians to seek associated risk factors and advocate and adhere to preventive measures.

*Modified from Kahn R: Metabolic syndrome—what is the clinical usefulness? Lancet 371:1892, 2008.

Although most definitions of the metabolic syndrome include a measurement of central obesity, none of the current criteria includes a direct measurement of visceral fat deposition. Much evidence supports the visceral adipose depot as a driver of dysmetabolism, including many components of the metabolic syndrome.[61] Traditional risk algorithms and definitions of the metabolic syndrome alike do not explicitly include biomarkers of inflammation. One of the pathobiologic hypotheses regarding mechanisms whereby visceral adipose tissue may contribute to cardiovascular risk invokes inflammatory stimuli arising from the visceral fat depot. Multiple experimental and clinical studies have implicated an inflammatory response operating in visceral adipose tissue. Therefore, inflammation may furnish a pathophysiologic link between the features of the metabolic syndrome and cardiovascular risk.

The most recent definition of metabolic syndrome from the National Heart, Lung, and Blood Institute includes a proinflammatory state.[62] Thus, inflammatory biomarkers such as hsCRP may help further stratify clinical risk and improve the prognostic value of metabolic

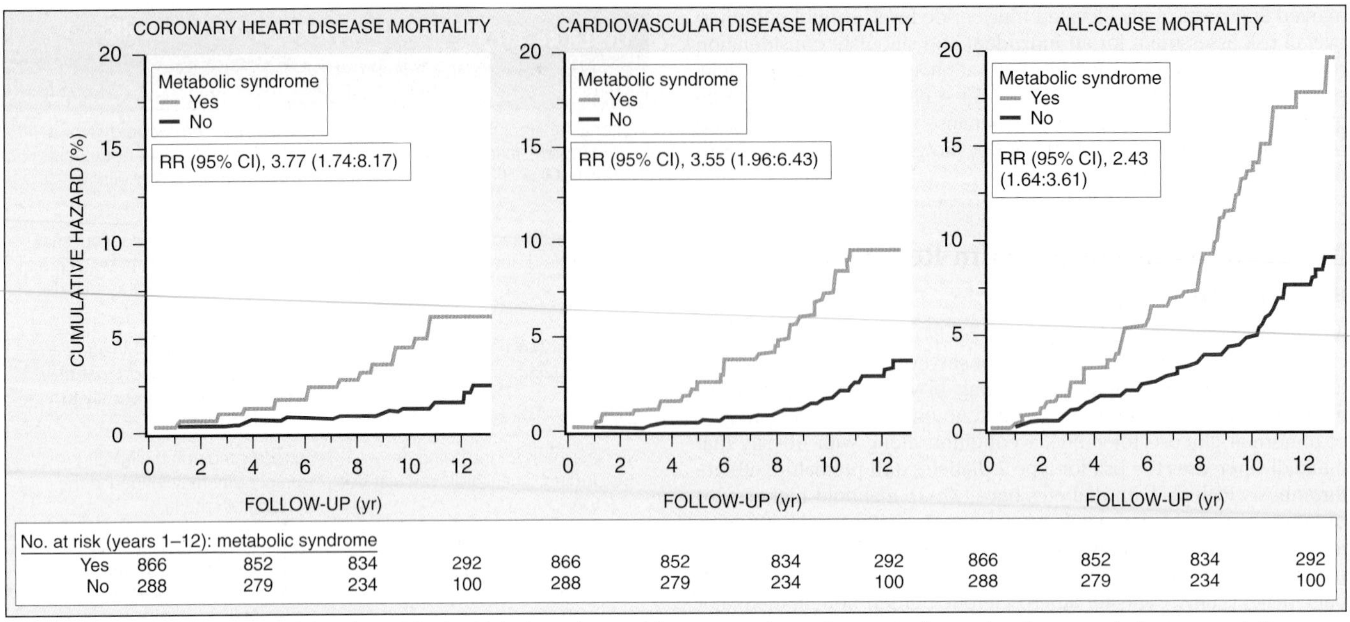

CORONARY HEART DISEASE MORTALITY — RR (95% CI), 3.77 (1.74:8.17)

CARDIOVASCULAR DISEASE MORTALITY — RR (95% CI), 3.55 (1.96:6.43)

ALL-CAUSE MORTALITY — RR (95% CI), 2.43 (1.64:3.61)

No. at risk (years 1–12): metabolic syndrome												
Yes	866	852	834	292	866	852	834	292	866	852	834	292
No	288	279	234	100	288	279	234	100	288	279	234	100

FIGURE 44-4 Cumulative hazard (unadjusted Kaplan-Meier hazard curves) for coronary heart disease, cardiovascular disease, and all-cause mortality among individuals with and without metabolic syndrome. *(From Lakka H, Laaksonen DE, Lakka TA, et al: The metabolic syndrome and total and cardiovascular disease mortality in middle-aged men. JAMA 288:2709, 2002.)*

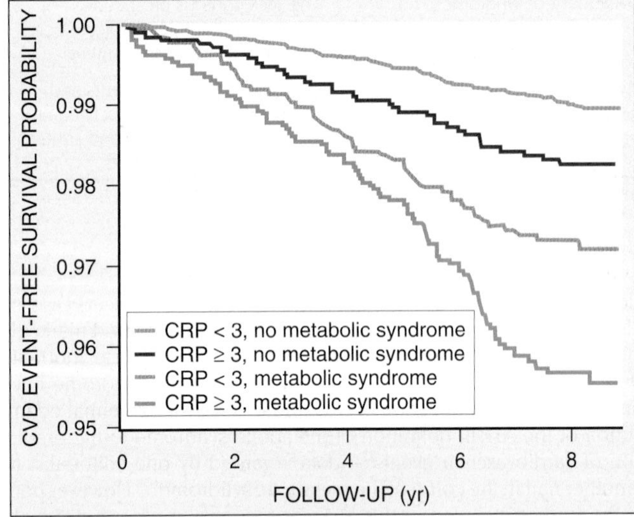

FIGURE 44-5 High-sensitivity C-reactive protein (hsCRP) adds prognostic information on risk for individuals with and without the metabolic syndrome. CVD = cardiovascular disease. *(From Ridker PM, Buring JE, Cook NR, Rifai N: C-reactive protein, the metabolic syndrome, and risk of incident cardiovascular events: An 8-year follow-up of 14,719 initially healthy American women. Circulation 107:441, 2003.)*

syndrome. For example, data from the Women's Health Study have indicated that an hsCRP level higher than 3 mg/liter adds important prognostic information about cardiovascular risk at all levels of the metabolic syndrome, whereas those with levels lower than 1 mg/liter are at substantially lower risk (**Fig. 44-5**).[63] This observation is important, because levels of hsCRP also predict incident type 2 diabetes.[64,65] Almost identical data regarding the additive value of hsCRP to the metabolic syndrome in terms of future vascular risk prediction have arisen from the West of Scotland Coronary Prevention Study.[66] Because hsCRP levels correlate with impaired fibrinolysis and with basal insulin levels, hsCRP evaluation may well become a routine part of the definition of metabolic syndrome. As reviewed later in this chapter in sections describing inflammatory markers, this conclusion has emerged in part from observations that atherosclerosis and type 2 diabetes share a common inflammatory basis.[67]

Because traditional risk algorithms and metabolic syndrome definitions do not capture inflammation explicitly, integrating features of the metabolic syndrome may explain part of the usefulness of adding hsCRP to traditional cardiovascular risk prediction instruments such as the Framingham algorithm. Obesity and intra-abdominal fat, which require imaging studies for rigorous definition, account for much, but not all, of hsCRP's ability to refine cardiovascular risk prediction. Obesity itself does not necessarily raise cardiovascular risk. Individuals with predominantly subcutaneous fat, in the gynoid or "pear" distribution, have less cardiovascular risk for a given body mass index (BMI) than those with the centripetal android or "apple" pattern associated with visceral adiposity. Some obese individuals do not develop insulin resistance or other cardiovascular risk factors related to the metabolic syndrome. This observation has given rise to the concept of the so-called "fit fat". For this reason, BMI itself may not predict incremental cardiovascular risk as well as hsCRP does.

Many clinicians find the concept of metabolic syndrome useful, because it fits the profile of many patients presenting in contemporary primary care practice. Some argue that the concept of metabolic syndrome can encourage physicians to engage in tighter control of risk factors and lifestyle modification, and encourage patients to adhere to lifestyle modification or therapy designed to address the individual components of metabolic syndrome as mandated by prevailing guidelines. Skeptics argue that evidence is lacking that the construct of the metabolic syndrome can influence physicians or the public to adopt or maintain a healthy lifestyle or preventive therapies.

In the end, the current controversy regarding the concept of the metabolic syndrome, its validity, and its clinical usefulness may present a false dichotomy. Given the growing epidemic of obesity and the foreseen burden of cardiovascular risk that it entails, professionals should reach beyond pedantic arguments regarding the nosology of the metabolic syndrome and combine forces to address the risk factors that comprise this cluster. In particular, there is not enough evidence to reject the notion that the sum of the risk factors outweighs the parts in younger populations, in whom concern regarding obesity and cardiovascular risk has become urgent. All individuals with components of the metabolic syndrome should adopt and adhere to a healthy lifestyle and appropriate treatment of individual risk factors.

For therapeutic interventions for patients with diabetes, see Chaps. 49 and 64. Unfortunately, poor control of concomitant risk factors in diabetic patients represents a major challenge; in NHANES, only 31% of participants achieved the target goal of hemoglobin A1c (HbA1c) less than 7.0%, only 36% achieved the target blood pressure goals of less than 130/80 mm Hg, and more than half had total cholesterol levels in excess of 200 mg/dL. Moreover, only 7% of all adults with diabetes in NHANES achieved all three of these crucial target goals. This situation also concerns European general practices, where diet-only treatment remains common and complication rates are very high.

Exercise, Weight Loss, and Obesity

Most epidemiologic studies have demonstrated a strong graded association between levels of physical activity and reduced rates of cardiovascular morbidity and all-cause mortality (see Chap. 83). Observational studies have cast doubt on the long-held belief that exercise must be vigorous to be beneficial. In both men and women, exercise levels achieved with as little as 30 minutes of walking daily provide major cardiovascular benefits[68] (**Fig. 44-6**). Accumulated episodes of exercise, even if brief, have further demonstrated benefit, suggesting that risk reduction does not require prolonged vigorous work. Smaller but consistent benefits of modest exercise have been observed for incident stroke, independent of hypertension. A regular exercise program also reduces the transient increase in risk of sudden death that, although extremely rare, can occur during vigorous exercise.[69] Thus, a "no pain, no gain" approach to the prescription of physical activity to reduce vascular risk now appears passé.

Regular exercise affects a number of risk factors for atherosclerosis. Aerobic exercise is associated with a mean reduction of systolic blood pressure of 5 mm Hg in hypertensive participants, a level comparable with that of many drug interventions. Although traditionally considered to have only modest effects on total and LDL-C levels, exercise consistently improves HDL-C and reduces triglyceride levels. More recent data have indicated that physical activity can increase the average size of LDL particles without a change in plasma LDL concentration. These effects occur even in the absence of clinically significant weight loss and relate more strongly to amount than intensity of exercise. In children, physical activity levels need to exceed 1 hour daily considerably to prevent clustering of cardiovascular risk factors at an early age.[70]

Exercise further improves insulin sensitivity and glycemic control, with major benefits for diabetic patients, including reductions in glycated hemoglobin and reduced requirements for therapy. These data agree with prospective epidemiologic observations that moderate-intensity activity is associated with a reduced incidence of diabetes and with randomized intervention studies. Regular exercise lowers CRP levels, improves coronary endothelial function, and appears to benefit hemostatic variables, including tissue-type plasminogen activator, fibrinogen, von Willebrand factor, fibrin D-dimer, and plasma viscosity.

Controversy remains as to whether obesity itself is a true risk factor for cardiovascular disease, or whether its impact on vascular risk derives solely from interrelations with glucose intolerance, insulin resistance, hypertension, physical inactivity, and dyslipidemia.[71] Midlife obesity, however, strongly presages hospitalization and future complications of coronary heart disease, even among those with few or no other major risk factors.[72] From an epidemiologic perspective, obesity alone is associated with elevated vascular risk regardless of activity levels, and the waist-to-hip ratio, a biomarker of centripetal or abdominal obesity, independently predicts vascular risk in women and older men. Among U.S. adults, the prevalence of obesity (defined as a BMI of 30 kg/m^2 or higher) has doubled over the past decade, now reaching more than 30% across the population. Even among children, particularly girls, obesity is a major problem, with rates in excess of 10% for white girls and 20% for black girls. Thus, weight control must play a fundamental role in all preventive cardiology practices, preferably in

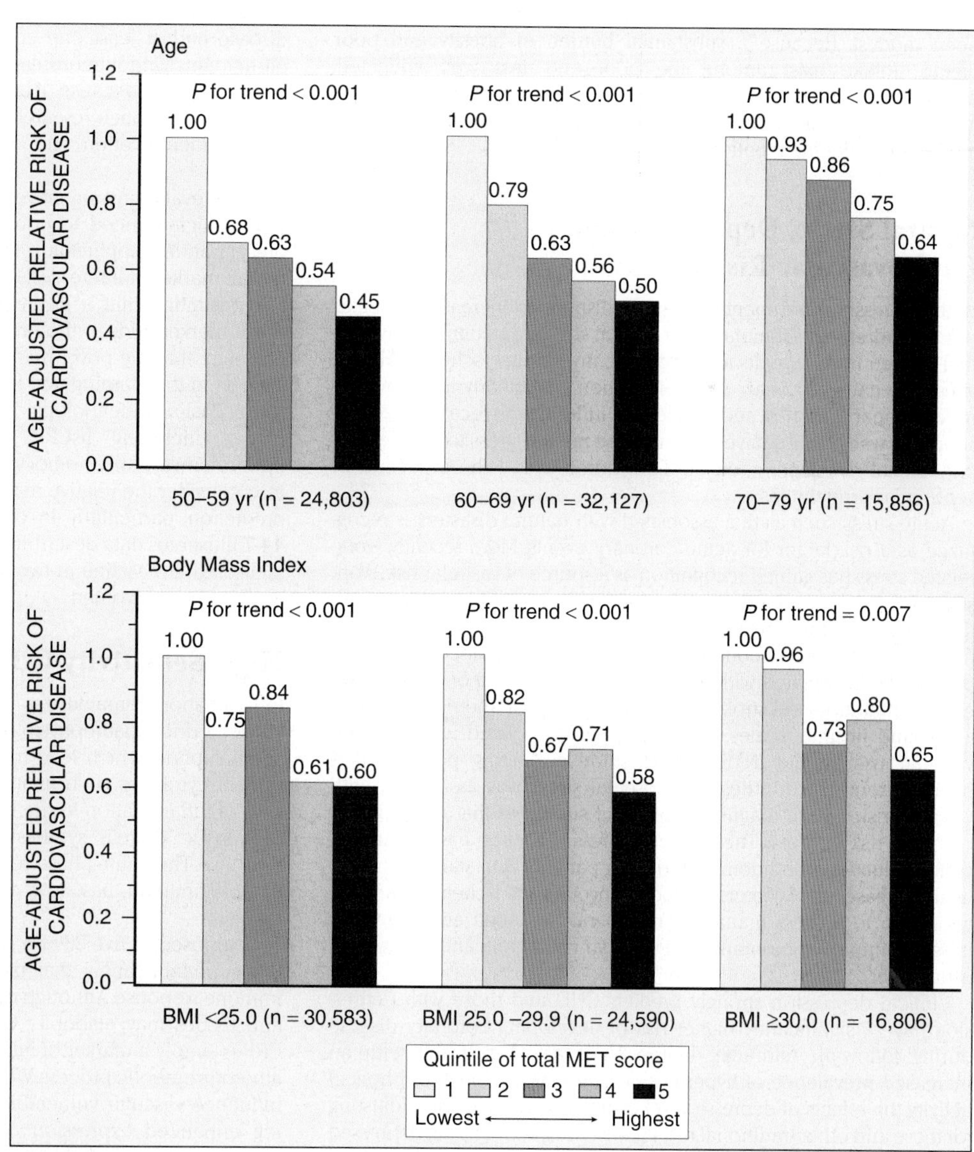

FIGURE 44-6 Relative risks of cardiovascular disease according to quintile of energy expenditure (metabolic equivalent [MET] score) from recreational activities stratified by age (top) and body mass index (bottom). *(From Manson JE, Greenland P, LaCroix AZ, et al: Walking compared with vigorous exercise for the prevention of cardiovascular events in women. N Engl J Med 347:716, 2002.)*

conjunction with advice regarding diet and exercise. Both fitness and fatness have implications for vascular risk. In the Women's Health Study, a high BMI was more strongly associated with adverse cardiovascular biomarkers than physical activity; however, within BMI categories, physical activity directly influenced overall levels of risk.[73] As also made clear from randomized trial data, lifestyle modification, including physical activity, is a crucial adjunct to any pharmacologic weight loss program.[74]

Despite consistent data from cohort studies,[75] randomized diet intervention trials have provided mixed results. In the Women's Health Initiative Dietary Modification trial, interventions that reduced total fat intake and increased intake of vegetables, fruits, and grains did not significantly reduce event rates in postmenopausal women and achieved only modest effects on traditional risk factors.[76] In a comparison of four popular diet regimens,[77] as well as in a study of carbohydrate substitution,[78] modest weight reductions and beneficial effects were observed with all interventions, but long-term adherence levels were low. In one of the few trials to attempt follow-up beyond 1 year, reduced caloric intake resulted in clinically meaningful weight loss, regardless of which macronutrients were emphasized, suggesting that caloric intake is more important than any specific dietary plan.[79] This recent trial, along with others,[80,81] also emphasizes the importance of counseling, behavioral factors, and motivation. Nonetheless, even in trials limited to motivated participants, long-term weight reduction has been modest. Because a substantial burden of obesity and poor dietary intake exist among the poor and less well educated, community-based efforts such as the total community approach being implemented in many European towns may provide an alternative model for social intervention.[82]

Mental Stress, Depression, and Cardiovascular Risk

Both depression and mental stress predispose to increased vascular risk. The adrenergic stimulation of mental stress can augment myocardial oxygen requirements and aggravate myocardial ischemia. Mental stress can cause coronary vasoconstriction, particularly in atherosclerotic coronary arteries, and hence can influence myocardial oxygen supply as well. Studies have further linked mental stress to platelet and endothelial dysfunction, metabolic syndrome, and the induction of ventricular arrhythmias.

Acute stress, such as that associated with natural disasters, is recognized as a risk factor for acute coronary events. More recently, work-related stress has gained recognition as a source of vascular risk. Work stress has two components—job strain, which combines high work demands and low job control, and effort-reward imbalance, which more closely reflects economic factors in the workplace. Both components are associated with an approximate doubling of risk for myocardial infarction and stroke.[83] Other psychological metrics, including anger and hostility scales, have also been associated with elevated vascular risk. In the INTERHEART study evaluating postinfarction patients from 52 countries, psychosocial stress was associated with vascular risk, with a magnitude of effect similar to that of the major coronary risk factors.[84] The impact of stress reduction has also undergone evaluation in randomized trials. In patients with stable ischemic heart disease and exercise-induced myocardial ischemia, random allocation to a stress management program reduced emotional distress and improved biomarkers of vascular risk significantly more than usual care.[85]

Clinical depression strongly predicts CHD, and those with depression have a significantly higher risk of developing coronary disease during follow-up. Although depression is also associated with an increased prevalence of hypertension, smoking, and lack of physical activity, the effects of depression on overall risk remain after adjusting for these and other traditional risk factors. Thus, findings that depressed individuals also have increased platelet activation, elevated levels of hsCRP, and decreased heart rate variability support depression as an independent predictor of events. Depression occurs in one of five outpatients with coronary artery disease and in one of three patients with heart failure,[86] but this component of patient care is often ignored in cardiovascular practices. Whether therapy for postinfarction depression reduces recurrent event rates remains controversial (see Chap. 49).

Novel Atherosclerotic Risk Markers

Despite the importance of blood lipids, 50% of all myocardial infarctions occur in individuals without overt hyperlipidemia. In a major prospective study of healthy American women, 77% of all future cardiovascular events occurred in patients with LDL-C levels less than 160 mg/dL and 46% occurred in those with LDL-C levels less than 130 mg/dL.[87] Although the use of global prediction models such as those developed in Framingham greatly improves the detection of heart disease risk, as many as 20% of all events occur in the absence of any of the major classic vascular risk factors.

This fact challenges several basic issues related to current screening programs for risk detection and disease prevention, but clinical data continue to accrue that demonstrate the hazard of relying solely on classic risk factors. In one analysis of more than 120,000 patients with CHD, 15% of the women and 19% of the men had no evidence of hyperlipidemia, hypertension, diabetes, or smoking, and more than 50% had only one of these general risk factors.[88] In another large analysis, between 85% and 95% of participants with coronary disease had at least one conventional risk factor, but so did those participants without coronary disease, despite follow-up for as long as 30 years.[89] Thus, because of the considerable need to improve vascular risk detection, much research over the past 10 or 15 years has focused on the identification and evaluation of novel atherosclerotic risk factors.

When evaluating any novel risk factor as a potential new screening tool, clinicians need to consider whether any of the following are present and/or applicable: (1) a standardized and reproducible assay for the marker of interest; (2) a consistent series of prospective studies demonstrating that a given parameter predicts future risk; (3) the novel marker adds to the predictive value of lipid screening; and (4) evidence that the novel marker adds to global risk prediction scores, such as in the Framingham Heart Study. The following section applies these basic epidemiologic requirements to a series of novel risk factors, including hsCRP and other markers of inflammation, lipoprotein(a), and homocysteine (**Table 44-2**). Physicians should also consider the relative magnitude of novel markers in terms of risk prediction, particularly in comparison with lipid screening. **Figure 44-7** illustrates data describing the relative efficacy of several variables measured at baseline in two large cohorts of initially healthy middle-aged men and women.

High-Sensitivity C-Reactive Protein

Inflammation characterizes all phases of atherothrombosis and provides a critical pathophysiologic link between plaque formation and acute rupture, which lead to occlusion and infarction.[90] The expression of cytokines such as interleukin-6, which can travel from local sites of inflammation to the liver and trigger a change in the program of hepatic protein synthesis, is characteristic of the acute-phase response. The acute-phase reactant CRP, a simple downstream marker of inflammation, has now emerged as a major cardiovascular risk marker.[91]

Composed of five 23-kDa subunits, CRP is a circulating member of the pentraxin family that plays a major role in the human innate immune response. Although derived primarily from the liver, other cells and tissues may elaborate CRP. Controversy remains as to whether CRP is simply a marker of inflammatory risk or has a direct role in the atherothrombotic process. With regard to the latter possibility, CRP may influence vascular vulnerability through several mechanisms, including enhanced expression of local adhesion molecules, increased expression of endothelial plasminogen activator inhibitor type 1 (PAI-1), reduced endothelial nitric oxide bioactivity, altered LDL uptake by macrophages, and colocalization with complement within atherosclerotic lesions.

TABLE 44-2 Clinical Epidemiology of Proposed Plasma-Based Biomarkers for Prediction of Future Cardiovascular Events

BIOMARKER	PROSPECTIVE STUDIES CONVINCING?	STANDARDIZED COMMERCIAL ASSAY?	ADDITIVE TO LIPID SCREENING?	ADDITIVE TO FRAMINGHAM RISK SCORE?
Inflammation				
hsCRP	++++	+++	+++	+++
Lp-PLA$_2$	++	++/−	++	+/−
sICAM-1	++	±	+	−
SAA	++	−	+	−
IL-6, IL-18	++	−	+	−
Myeloperoxidase	+	−	±	−
sCD40L	+	−	−	−
Altered thrombosis				−
t-PA, PAI-1	++	±	−	−
Fibrinogen	+++	±	++	−
Homocysteine	++++	+++	±	−
D-dimer	++	+	−	−
Oxidative stress-oxidized LDL	±	−	−	−
Altered lipids				−
Lipoprotein(a)	+++	±	±	−
LDL particle size	++	±	±	−

IL = interleukin; PAI-1 = plasminogen activator inhibitor-1; SAA = serum amyloid A; sCD40L = soluble CD40 ligand; t-PA = tissue plasminogen activator. Plus signs indicate increasing strength of evidence.

Modified from Ridker PM, Brown NJ, Vaughan DE, et al: Established and emerging plasma biomarkers in the prediction of first atherothrombotic events. Circulation 109(Suppl 1):IV6, 2004.

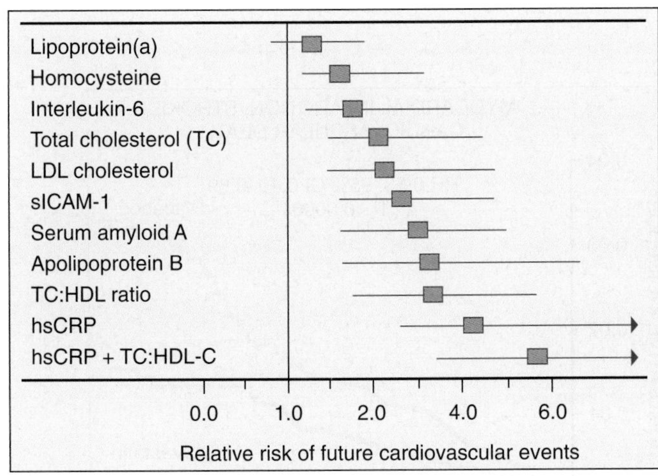

FIGURE 44-7 Relative risks of future myocardial infarction among apparently healthy women according to baseline levels of Lp(a), homocysteine, interleukin-6, total cholesterol, low-LDL-C, sICAM-1, serum amyloid A, apolipoprotein B, ratio of total cholesterol to high-density lipoprotein cholesterol (TC:HDL-C), high-sensitivity C-reactive protein (hsCRP), and the combination of hsCRP with the TC:HDL-C. *(From Ridker PM: Clinical application of C-reactive protein for cardiovascular disease detection and prevention. Circulation 107:363, 2003.)*

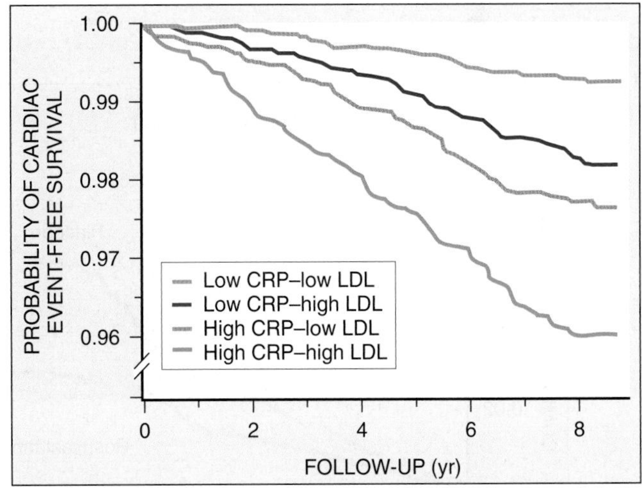

FIGURE 44-8 Cardiovascular event–free survival among apparently healthy individuals according to baseline levels of high-sensitivity CRP and LDL-C. *(From Ridker PM, Rifai N, Rose L, et al: Comparison of C-reactive protein and low-density lipoprotein cholesterol levels in the prediction of first cardiovascular events. N Engl J Med 347:1557, 2002.)*

Regardless of whether CRP is a marker or mediator, a large series of prospective epidemiologic studies has demonstrated that CRP, when measured with high-sensitivity assays (hsCRP), strongly and independently predicts risk of myocardial infarction, stroke, peripheral arterial disease, and sudden cardiac death in apparently healthy individuals, even when LDL-C plasminogen activator inhibitor-1 levels are low.[92] In recent comprehensive meta-analyses, the multivariable hazard associated with hsCRP was, if anything, larger than that associated with either blood pressure or cholesterol.[93] These data apply to women and men across all age levels and have been consistent in diverse populations. Most importantly, hsCRP adds prognostic information at all LDL-C levels and at all levels of risk, as determined by the Framingham Risk Score.[87] In other major studies from the United States and Europe, hsCRP levels predicted subsequent risk better than LDL-C levels.[94] Because hsCRP levels reflect a component of vascular risk different from that of cholesterol, the addition of hsCRP to lipid evaluation provides a major opportunity to improve global risk prediction. In clinical terms, absolute vascular risk is higher in individuals with elevated hsCRP levels and low LDL-C levels than in those with elevated LDL-C levels but low levels of hsCRP, but current guidelines consider only the latter group to be at high risk (**Fig. 44-8**). Even in studies that have reported the effect of hsCRP as modest, the magnitude of the effect was at least as large as that of hypertension and smoking, data demonstrating the importance of inflammation in atherogenesis.[95]

The American Heart Association and the Centers for Disease Control and Prevention issued a statement in 2003 regarding the use of hsCRP in clinical practice.[96] Briefly, hsCRP levels less than 1, 1 to 3, and higher than 3 mg/liter should be interpreted as lower, moderate, and higher relative vascular risk, respectively, when considered along with traditional markers of risk, a finding recently corroborated within the Framingham Heart Study itself.[97] Screening for hsCRP should be done at the discretion of the physician as part of global risk evaluation, not as a replacement for LDL and HDL testing. Although hsCRP predicts risk across the entire population spectrum, it likely has greatest usefulness for those at intermediate risk—that is, those with anticipated 10-year event rates between 5% and 20%. Current guidelines from the Canadian Cardiovascular Society strongly endorse evaluation of hsCRP in these intermediate-risk individuals and suggest that statin therapy be considered for those with levels higher than 2 mg/liter.[98] Values of hsCRP higher than 8 mg/liter may represent an acute-phase response caused by an underlying inflammatory disease or intercurrent major infection and should lead to repeat testing in approximately 2 to 3 weeks. Consistently high values, however, represent very high risk of future cardiovascular disease, because risk appears to be linear across the full range of hsCRP levels.[99] Because hsCRP levels are stable over long periods, have no circadian variation, and do not depend on prandial state, screening can easily be done on an outpatient basis at the time of cholesterol evaluation.

In clinical practice, many physicians routinely use both hsCRP and family history as part of the global risk prediction process. This is easily accomplished using the Reynolds Risk Scores (available at www.reynoldsriskscore.com).[3,100] Levels of hsCRP higher than 3 mg/liter also predict recurrent coronary events, thrombotic complications after angioplasty, poor outcome in the setting of unstable angina, and vascular complications after bypass surgery. All these data support a critical role for inflammation throughout atherothrombosis. Additionally, hsCRP has prognostic usefulness in cases of acute ischemia, even without troponin level elevation, suggesting that an enhanced inflammatory response at the time of hospital admission can determine subsequent plaque rupture.[101] These findings help explain why those with elevated hsCRP levels are also more likely to benefit from aggressive interventions compared with those with low hsCRP levels.

Elevated levels of hsCRP predict not only cardiovascular events but also the onset of type 2 diabetes, perhaps because hsCRP levels correlate with several components of the metabolic syndrome—including those not easily measured in clinical practice, such as insulin sensitivity, endothelial dysfunction, and hypofibrinolysis, as noted earlier.

The use of statin therapy to reduce vascular risk in individuals with elevated hsCRP, even when LDL-C levels are low, represents a fundamental change in treatment strategies for the prevention of cardiovascular disease. Most importantly, in the recent JUPITER trial[102] of apparently healthy men and women with LDL-C levels lower than 130 mg/dL who were at increased risk because of hsCRP levels of 2 mg/liter or higher, the use of rosuvastatin resulted in a 44% reduction in the trial primary endpoint of all vascular events ($P < 0.000001$), a 54% reduction in myocardial infarction ($P = 0.0002$), a 48% reduction in stroke ($P = 0.002$), a 46% reduction in the need for arterial revascularization ($P < 0.001$), and a 20% reduction in all-cause mortality ($P = 0.02$; **Fig. 44-9**). All prespecified subgroups within JUPITER significantly benefited from statin therapy, including those previously considered to be at low risk, such as women, nonsmokers, those without metabolic syndrome, and those with a Framingham score less than 10%. From a public policy perspective, the 5-year number needed to treat (NNT) within JUPITER was only 25, a value smaller

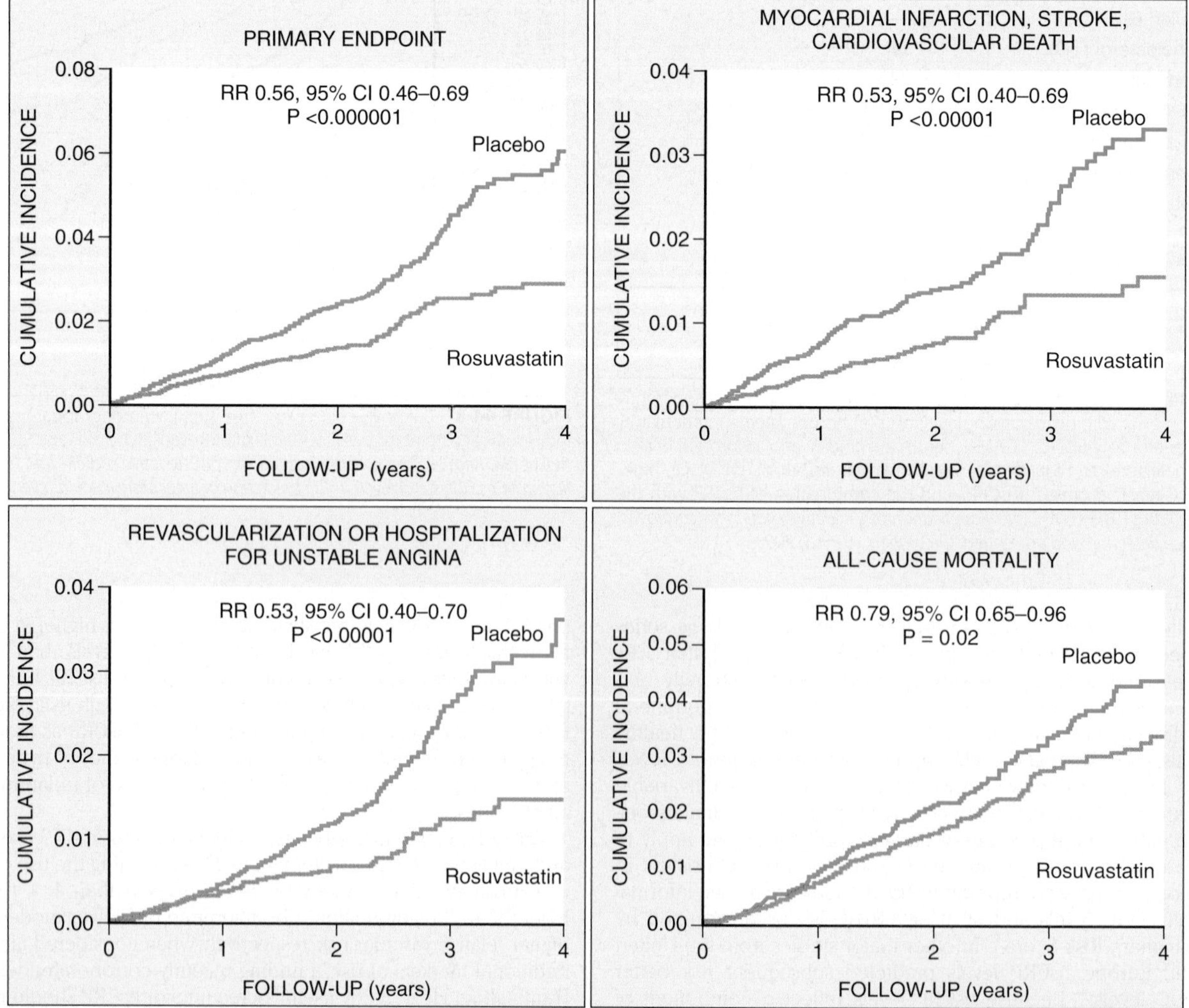

FIGURE 44-9 Primary results of the JUPITER trial of rosuvastatin therapy among apparently healthy men and women with LDL-C < 130 mg/dL and hsCRP > 2 mg/L. *(From Ridker PM, Danielson E, Fonseca FA, et al: Rosuvastatin to prevent vascular events in men and women with elevated C-reactive protein. N Engl J Med 359:2195, 2008.)*

than the comparable 5-year NNT associated with the treatment of hyperlipidemia or hypertension in primary prevention. In an additional prespecified analysis, rosuvastatin reduced incident venous thromboembolism by 43%, a result with clinical relevance and an important observation regarding the pleiotropic effects of statin therapy.[103]

The JUPITER trial also demonstrated that achieving low levels of both LDL-C and hsCRP after the initiation of statin therapy are critical goals for maximizing preventive efforts, at least with statin therapy. Within the JUPITER cohort, an 80% risk reduction was observed among those who not only reduced LDL-C to less than 70 mg/dL, but who also reduced hsCRP to below 1 mg/liter (**Fig. 44-10**).[104] This observation, made in a primary prevention setting, confirms prior work in high-risk secondary prevention demonstrating the importance of achieving dual goals for LDL-C and hsCRP. For example, in the PROVE IT-TIMI 22 trial of patients with acute coronary syndromes treated with statin therapy, achieving levels of hsCRP lower than 2 mg/liter was as important for long-term event-free survival as was achieving LDL-C levels lower than 70 mg/dL; in fact, the best long-term outcomes were found in those who achieved both these goals (**Fig. 44-11**).[105]

The concept of dual goals for statin therapy, which includes CRP and LDL-C level reduction, has been corroborated in the A-to-Z clinical trial,[106] as well as in studies using intravascular ultrasound to monitor disease progression. In this latter setting, only those with CRP reduction had coronary regression with statin therapy, whereas those who achieved both CRP and LDL-C level reduction had the greatest regression overall.[107] The JUPITER trial also provides data demonstrating the efficacy of statin therapy in women,[108] older patients,[109] and those with moderate renal insufficiency,[110] as well as in the prevention of stroke.[111]

hsCRP levels correlate only modestly with underlying atherosclerotic disease, as measured by carotid intimal medial thickness or by coronary calcification. This observation suggests that hsCRP does not simply reflect the presence of subclinical disease but indicates an increased propensity for plaque disruption and/or thrombosis. Autopsy data support this hypothesis: elevated hsCRP levels occur more often in patients with frankly ruptured plaques than in those with erosive disease or those who died of nonvascular causes. hsCRP levels predict incident hypertension and add prognostic information on vascular risk at all levels of blood pressure.[112] Finally, in patients with

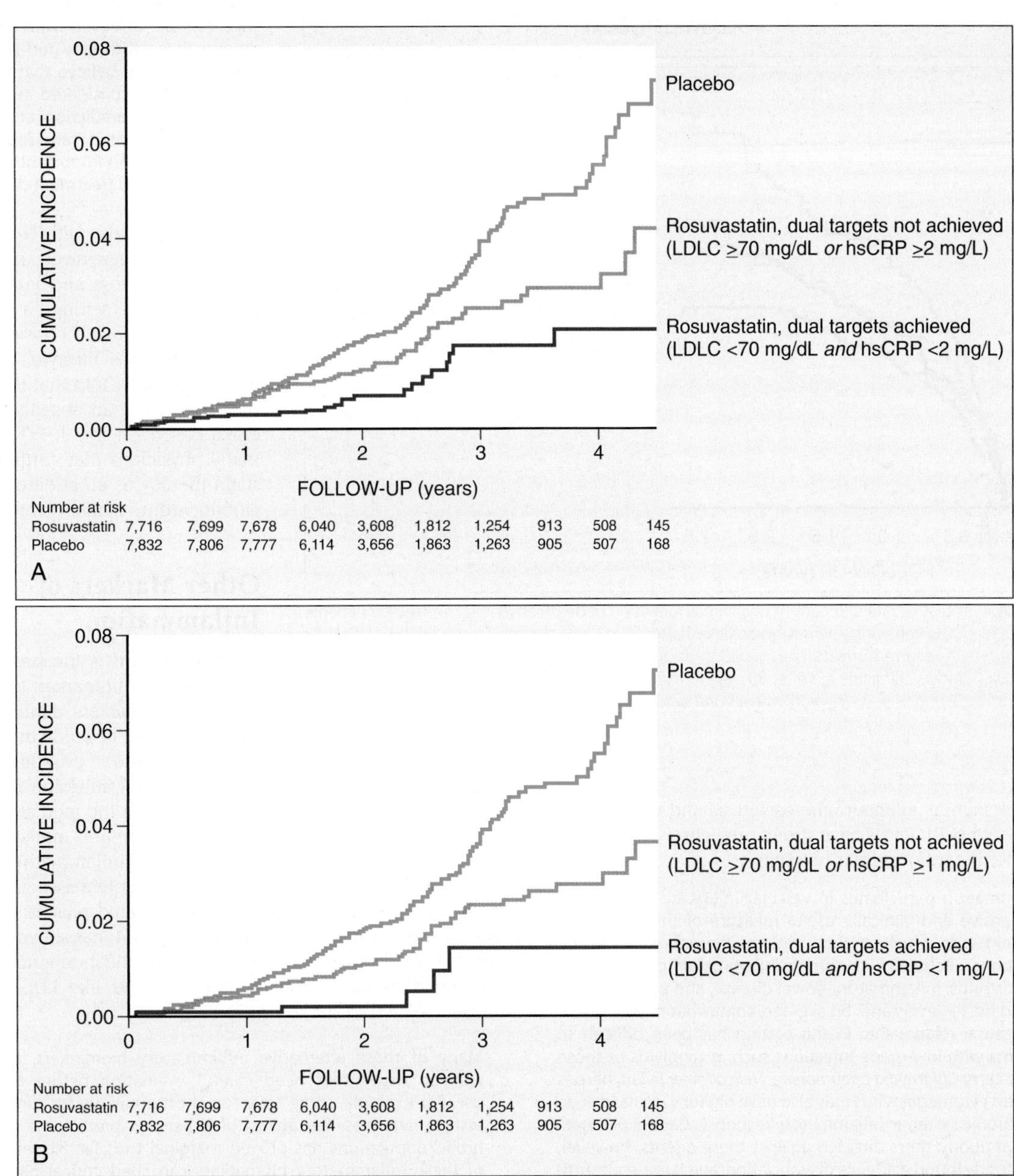

FIGURE 44-10 Incident cardiovascular events in the JUPITER trial according to achieved concentrations of LDL cholesterol and hsCRP after initiation of rosuvastatin. **A,** Analysis using targets of LDL cholesterol less than 70 mg/dL and hsCRP less than 2 mg/liter. **B,** Analysis using targets of LDL cholesterol less than 70 mg/dL and hsCRP less than 1 mg/liter. *(From Ridker PM, Danielson E, Fonseca FA, et al; JUPITER Trial Study Group: Reduction in C-reactive protein and LDL cholesterol and cardiovascular event rates after initiation of rosuvastatin: A prospective study of the JUPITER trial. Lancet 373:1175, 2009.)*

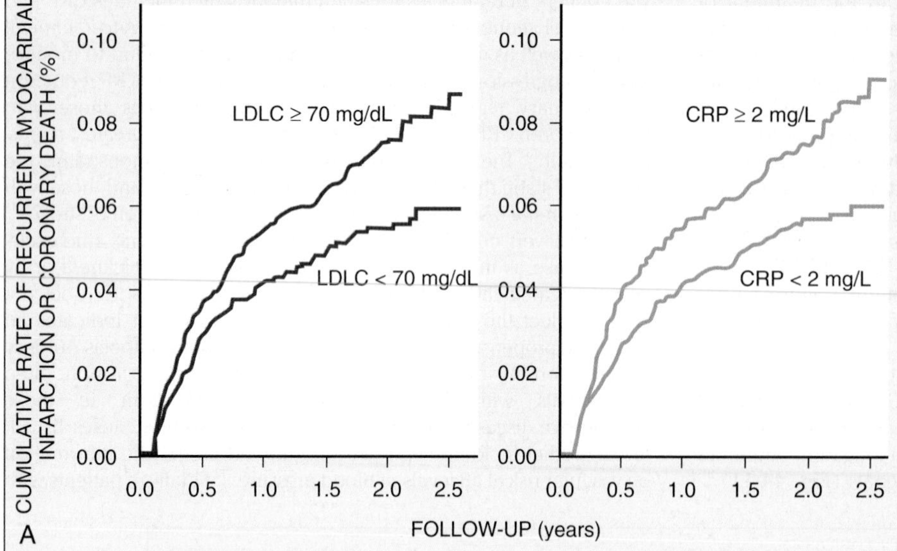

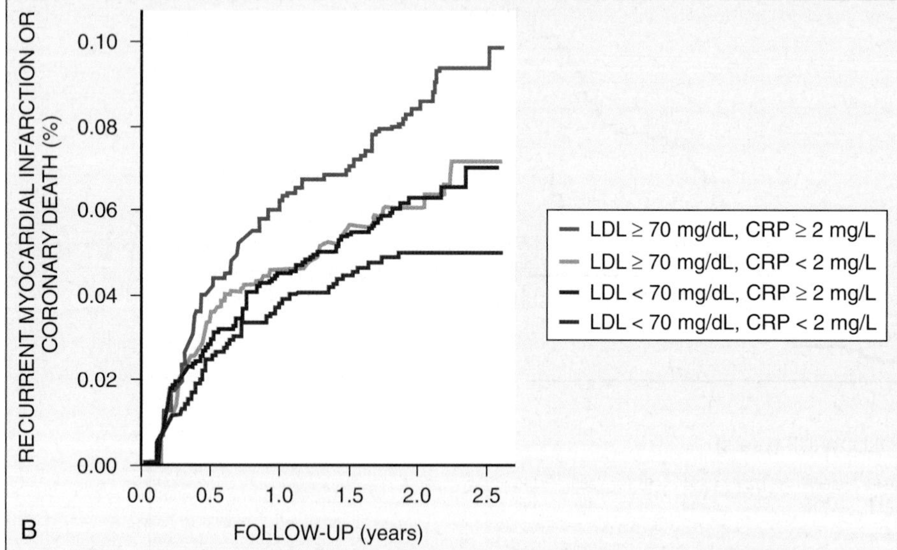

FIGURE 44-11 **A,** Cumulative rate of recurrent myocardial infarction or death among statin-treated patients according to levels of LDL-C (left) or hsCRP (right) achieved after 30 days of therapy in the PROVE IT-TIMI 22 trial. **B,** Cumulative rate of recurrent myocardial infarction or death among statin-treated patients according to both levels of LDL-C and hsCRP achieved after 30 days of therapy in the PROVE IT-TIMI 22 trial. *(From Ridker PM, Cannon CP, Morrow D, et al: C-reactive protein levels and outcomes after statin therapy. N Engl J Med 352:20, 2005.)*

other conditions, such as allograft atherosclerosis and chronic renal failure and dialysis, hsCRP levels have strong predictive value for poor short- and long-term cardiovascular outcomes.

Although inflammation participates in vascular injury and hsCRP provides an inexpensive and clinically useful measure of this process, it remains uncertain as to which stimulus initiates the underlying proinflammatory response. Patients with chronic inflammatory diseases such as rheumatoid arthritis, inflammatory bowel disease, and psoriasis tend to have elevated hsCRP levels and, on average, somewhat higher vascular risk, but a causal relationship in this setting has been difficult to establish. Patients with low-grade infections such as gingivitis or those who chronically carry *Chlamydia pneumoniae*, *Helicobacter pylori*, herpes simplex virus, and cytomegalovirus may also have higher vascular risk on the basis of a chronic systemic inflammatory response. Careful prospective studies of antibody titers directed against these agents, however, have not consistently found evidence of association, and large-scale antibiotic trials have not shown reduced event rates. Whether novel targeted anti-inflammatory therapies, including specific cytokine inhibitors or agents commonly used to treat arthritis, such as very low-dose methotrexate, can improve coronary outcomes is an active area of research.[113]

Some have suggested that measurement of hsCRP has only a marginal clinical effect, a conclusion largely based on the observation that the addition of hsCRP to risk prediction models minimally increases the C-statistic, a traditional measure of model fit.[114] Once age and smoking are accounted for, neither blood pressure, LDL-C, nor HDL-C increase the C-statistic, suggesting that this statistical tool lacks sensitivity to major pathophysiologic effects.[115] Other investigators have noted that mendelian randomization analyses have not supported a direct causal role for CRP in atherothrombosis.[116] Such studies, however, cannot exclude the possibility of effect for CRP and, more importantly, do not address the broader issue of inflammation as a determinant of vascular damage. Thus, even if hsCRP is a biomarker of risk rather than a causal risk factor, given the robustness of laboratory and epidemiologic data, the low cost of testing, and the definitive results that can be achieved with statin therapy among those with elevated hsCRP and low LDL-C levels, we believe that hsCRP evaluation should be considered as a routine part of coronary risk prediction, at a minimum for those with estimated Framingham risks of 5% or more for whom important reclassification of risk occurs and treatment decisions can be altered.

All individuals with elevated hsCRP levels should aggressively undergo physical activity, weight loss, and smoking cessation programs. In this setting, an elevated hsCRP level should provide considerable motivation to improve lifestyle, particularly for those previously told that they were not at risk because of an absence of hyperlipidemia. Based on the JUPITER trial results, many physicians may further elect to use statin therapy as an additional method for global cardiovascular risk reduction.[117]

Other Markers of Inflammation

Although hsCRP is the best-characterized inflammatory biomarker for clinical use, several other markers of inflammation have shown promise in predicting vascular risk. These include cytokines such as interleukin-6, soluble forms of certain cell adhesion molecules such as soluble ICAM-1 (sICAM-1), P-selectin, or the mediator CD40 ligand, as well as the total white blood cell count and markers of leukocyte activation such as myeloperoxidase. Other inflammatory markers associated with lipid oxidation, such as lipoprotein-associated phospholipase A_2 (Lp-PLA$_2$) and pregnancy-associated plasma protein A, have also shown promise.[118,119] Like hsCRP, Lp-PLA$_2$ has shown efficacy in the prediction of stroke, demonstrating again the independence of inflammatory biomarkers from lipid parameters like LDL-C that are not closely related to stroke risk.[120]

Many of these alternative inflammatory biomarkers, however, have analytic issues that need careful evaluation before routine clinical use. For example, some have too short a half-life for clinical diagnostic testing, whereas the ability of others to predict risk in settings of broad populations has proved marginal thus far. Nonetheless, several of these inflammatory biomarkers can shed critical pathophysiologic light on the atherothrombotic process, particularly at the time of plaque rupture. Similarly, myeloperoxidase may provide prognostic information in cases of acute ischemia beyond that associated with troponin or CRP.[121]

Although also an acute-phase reactant and thus often considered an inflammatory biomarker, plasma fibrinogen additionally influences platelet aggregation and blood viscosity, interacts with plasminogen binding and, in combination with thrombin, mediates the final step in clot formation and the response to vascular injury.[122] In addition, fibrinogen associates positively with age, obesity, smoking, diabetes, and LDL-C level, and inversely with HDL-C level, alcohol use, and physical activity/exercise level.

Given these relationships, it is not surprising that fibrinogen was among the first novel risk factors evaluated. Early reports from the Gothenburg, Northwick Park, and Framingham heart studies all found significant positive associations between fibrinogen levels and future risk of cardiovascular events. Since then, a number of other prospective studies have confirmed these findings and, in a meta-analysis, there was an approximately linear logarithmic association between usual fibrinogen level and risk of CHD and stroke.[123] In more recent studies, hsCRP and fibrinogen levels appeared to be additive in their ability to predict risk, although the absolute effect of hsCRP appeared larger. Other studies have suggested that the predictive usefulness of fibrinogen is highest in those with other concomitant elevations of lipoprotein(a) or homocysteine.

Despite the consistency of these data, fibrinogen evaluation has found limited use in clinical practice because of suboptimal assay standardization, and consistency across reference laboratories remains poor. Fibrates and niacin lower fibrinogen levels but statin therapy does not, an effect also different than that observed for hsCRP. Three clinical trials have evaluated the potential benefits of fibrinogen reduction, and all have found disappointing results. The Bezafibrate Infarction Prevention Trial showed no reduction in event rates with active therapy, despite a significant reduction in fibrinogen levels and despite evidence that within the study population, baseline fibrinogen levels predicted vascular risk.[124] In the MRC General Practice Research Framework trial of more than 1500 patients with peripheral vascular disease, bezafibrate reduced fibrinogen levels by 13% but again had no significant effect on clinical outcomes.[125] Finally, in the Heart and Estrogen/Progestin Replacement Study (HERS) and in the Women's Health Initiative, hormone replacement therapy lowered fibrinogen levels but did not benefit outcomes.

Given these results, continued evaluation of novel inflammatory biomarkers may provide targets for or monitors of therapy, particularly in the setting of acute coronary ischemia. However, in a comprehensive overview conducted by the National Academy of Clinical Biochemists that included multiple inflammatory biomarkers, only hsCRP met all the stated clinical criteria for acceptance as a biomarker for risk assessment in primary prevention.[126]

Homocysteine

Homocysteine is a sulfhydryl-containing amino acid derived from the demethylation of dietary methionine. Patients with rare inherited defects of methionine metabolism can develop severe hyperhomocysteinemia (plasma levels higher than 100 mmol/liter) and have a markedly elevated risk of premature atherothrombosis and venous thromboembolism. In contrast to severe hyperhomocysteinemia, mild to moderate elevations of homocysteine (plasma levels higher than 15 mmol/liter) are more common in the general population, primarily because of insufficient dietary intake of folic acid. Other patient groups who tend to have elevated levels of homocysteine include those receiving folate antagonists such as methotrexate and carbamazepine, and those with impaired homocysteine metabolism caused by hypothyroidism or renal insufficiency.

A common polymorphism in the methylene tetrahydrofolate reductase gene (*MTHFR*) that encodes a thermolabile protein has also been linked to elevated homocysteine levels and to increased vascular risk, at least among individuals homozygous for the variant. Familial association studies have reported higher homocysteine levels in offspring of parents with premature coronary artery disease. However, the clinical importance of the *MTHFR* polymorphism appears modest, and heterozygous individuals display little evidence of elevated homocysteine levels, even in those with low folate intake. In a meta-analysis of 40 observational studies, individuals homozygous for the *MTHFR* 677 TT variant had a 16% increase in relative risk (odds ratio [OR], 1.16; 95% confidence interval [CI], 1.05 to 1.28), and this observation was evident only in studies originating in Europe.[127] In populations in whom folate fortification exists, such as in North America, no compelling evidence supports the genetic evaluation of *MTHFR* to predict vascular risk. For example, in the large-scale Women's Health Study, *MTHFR* variants were associated with plasma homocysteine levels, which in turn were associated with modest elevation of risk, but there was no independent effect of the gene variants on clinical outcomes.[128]

Reliable immunoassays for total plasma homocysteine (the combination of free homocysteine, bound homocysteine, and mixed disulfides), now widely available, have largely replaced the use of high-performance liquid chromatography. Despite the availability of newer assays, measurement of homocysteine remains controversial, and recent guidelines have not advocated their use. This lack of enthusiasm reflects modest overall effects in prospective cohort studies and the results of several large trials of homocysteine reduction. With regard to epidemiologic evidence, although there is some heterogeneity among prospective studies, on average a 25% lower homocysteine level appears to be associated with an approximate 11% lower risk of CHD. However, at least in the United States, fortification of the food supply has greatly reduced the frequency of low folate and elevated homocysteine levels, particularly for those initially in the moderately elevated range. Thus, the number of individuals potentially identifiable by screening for homocysteine has decreased considerably.

With regard to clinical trials of homocysteine reduction, several major studies have shown no substantive benefit. In the Vitamin Intervention for Stroke Prevention (VISP) trial conducted in 3680 patients with prior stroke allocated to high-dose or low-dose vitamin regimens containing folate and pyridoxine, there was no evidence of differential benefit in the high-dose group, despite greater homocysteine level reduction.[129] In a second trial, of 636 postangioplasty patients treated with folate, vitamin B_6, and vitamin B_{12}, rates of in-stent stenosis were actually higher in most intervention groups compared with those allocated to placebo.[130] This negative trial is clinically important, because it conflicts with prior work that had suggested benefit in this setting. A net harmful effect associated with combined vitamin B supplementation was also observed in the Norwegian Vitamin Trial (NORVIT) involving 3749 participants with recent myocardial infarction. In that trial, mean total homocysteine was lowered by 27% in the intervention group, but there was no significant effect on the primary endpoint (hazard ratio [HR], 1.08; 95% CI, 0.93 to 1.25), whereas a trend toward increased risk was observed in those allocated to folate, vitamin B_6, and vitamin B_{12} (HR, 1.22; 95% CI, 1.00 to 1.50).[131] Similarly, in the Heart Outcomes Prevention Evaluation (HOPE-2) trial of 5522 patients with vascular disease or diabetes, 5 years of therapy with folate, vitamin B_6, and vitamin B_{12} resulted in no benefit compared with placebo for total vascular events (HR, 0.95; 95% CI, 0.84 to 1.07), cardiovascular mortality (HR, 0.96; 95% CI, 0.81 to 1.13), or any of several prespecified secondary endpoints.[132] Finally, in a major Veterans Administration trial including 2056 patients with advanced renal disease, treatment with high doses of folic acid and B vitamins did not improve survival nor reduce incidence of vascular events.[133] As a group, these sharply negative trial results conflict with the supposition made from studies of mendelian randomization that had previously argued for a clear causal role between homocysteine concentration and vascular events.[134]

Despite reduced enthusiasm and lack of evidence that homocysteine reduction lowers risk, there remain specific patient populations for whom homocysteine evaluation may prove appropriate, including those lacking traditional risk factors, those with renal failure, or those with markedly premature atherosclerosis or a family history of myocardial infarction and stroke at a young age.[135] It is also crucial to continue folate supplementation in the general population to reduce the risk of neural tube defects, an inexpensive practice that has been in place in the United States for over a decade, yet remains a public health challenge for much of Europe and the developing world.[136]

Lipoprotein(a)

Lipoprotein(a) (Lp[a]) consists of an LDL particle with its apolipoprotein B-100 (apo B100) component linked by a disulfide bridge to apolipoprotein(a) (apo[a]), a variable-length protein that has sequence homology to plasminogen. The apo(a) component of Lp(a) is a complex molecule composed in part of varying numbers of cysteine-rich kringle IV repeats that result in great heterogeneity. As such, plasma Lp(a) concentrations vary inversely with apo(a) isoform size but may also vary even in isoform size, based on differential levels of production. Underlying its molecular complexity, more than 25 heritable forms of Lp(a) exist, demonstrating the importance of the genome in determining plasma levels, an important issue for risk prediction across different population groups. The close homology between Lp(a) and plasminogen has raised the possibility that this lipoprotein may inhibit endogenous fibrinolysis by competing with plasminogen binding on the endothelium. More recent studies have suggested that Lp(a) binds and inactivates tissue factor pathway inhibitor and may increase the expression of plasminogen activator inhibitor, further linking lipoproteins and thrombosis. Lp(a) also colocalizes within atherosclerotic lesions and may have local actions through oxidized phospholipids pathways.[137] Thus, several mechanisms may contribute to a role of Lp(a) in atherothrombosis.

Many prospective cohort studies have supported a role for Lp(a) as a determinant of vascular risk. In an updated meta-analysis of 36 prospective studies that included more than 12,000 cardiovascular endpoints, the adjusted risk ratios for each standard deviation increase in plasma Lp(a) level were 1.13 for CHD and 1.10 for ischemic stroke.[138] Adjustment for classic cardiovascular risk factors only modestly attenuated these effects, in part because there is little correlation between Lp(a) and other markers of risk. Whether the assessment of Lp(a) truly adds prognostic information to overall risk in primary prevention remains uncertain, however, because in most studies, Lp(a) has typically predictive value for those already known to be at high risk as a result of the presence of other risk factors, in particular elevated LDL-C levels.

Several prospective evaluations have shown that Lp(a) predicts risk in a nonlinear manner, so that risk increases are very small until Lp(a) levels within the top 5% to 10% are reached.[139] Some investigators have advocated Lp(a) assessment in certain patient groups, such as those with established coronary disease or renal failure, although data remain controversial. Evidence that children with recurrent ischemic stroke have elevated Lp(a) levels also supports the potential use of this biomarker in unusual high-risk settings.

Standardization of commercial Lp(a) assays remains problematic; the inaccuracy of commercial Lp(a) assays has resulted from the use of techniques sensitive to apo(a) size. However, commercial assays that measure Lp(a) in a manner independent of apo(a) isoform size are now available in some reference laboratories.[140] Using one such assay, investigators in the Women's Health Study have found that extremely high levels of Lp(a)—higher than the 90th percentile or higher than 65.6 mg/liter—are associated with increased cardiovascular risk, independent of other traditional risk factors.[141] This risk increase was nonlinear, however, and was limited almost entirely to those with concomitant elevations of LDL-C levels, confirming earlier work. Thus, the presence of threshold effects and interactions with LDL-C limit the routine measurement of Lp(a) for cardiovascular risk stratification in the general population.

With the exception of high-dose niacin, few interventions lower Lp(a) level, and no study has shown that Lp(a) reduction lowers vascular risk. This limitation, as well as the observation that LDL-C reduction markedly reduces any hazard associated with Lp(a), has also dampened enthusiasm for screening. Genetic investigations have suggested important insights into Lp(a) regulation and suggest a causal relationship between Lp(a) and increased risk.[142,143] Thus, continued development of therapies that inhibit Lp(a) merit consideration and direct testing in clinical trials. In one recent pharmacogenetic study, the benefit of prophylactic aspirin was closely linked to specific genetic polymorphisms associated with Lp(a) expression.[144]

Future Directions in Cardiovascular Risk Assessment

Some 40% of the U.S. adult population is at intermediate risk, but these individuals do not currently qualify for intensive risk factor intervention, despite the presence of one or more traditional risk factors. Current evidence suggests that the readiest tool to improve risk stratification among these individuals is the inflammatory biomarker hsCRP as an adjunct to global risk prediction. Strong evidence, as reviewed earlier, has shown that hsCRP adds prognostic information at all LDL-C levels of the Framingham risk score and of the metabolic syndrome. Thus, hsCRP evaluation, along with standard lipid screening and knowledge of family history, may become common practice in the near future. The pathophysiologic implications that follow from the inflammatory hypothesis of atherothrombosis should lead to novel interventions for primary prevention as well as for the treatment of acute ischemia.

Direct Plaque Imaging

In addition to the use of inflammatory markers and family history, strategies to detect vascular disease will likely take several forms. One approach eschews risk factor measurement, but identifies preclinical disease through the noninvasive detection of atherosclerotic plaque (see Chaps. 18, 19, 22, and 23). Such an approach can never truly prevent disease; it can only lead to early detection. However, because many therapies can delay clinical expression of disease once existing lesions are diagnosed, this approach merits consideration.

Several studies indicate that coronary calcification, as detected by computed tomography (CT), can detect preclinical atherosclerosis (see Chap. 19).[144a] Much controversy remains, however, as to whether this approach is cost-effective or has an acceptable false-negative rate.[145] Enrollment in some of these studies may be biased by referral patterns or self-selection by patients. Part of the difficulty with coronary calcification as a clinical biomarker that CT imaging probably detects the plaques least likely to rupture and does not detect the less calcified lesions that appear to cause most clinical events. Thus, although coronary calcium provides a noninvasive measure of atherosclerotic burden, patients with low calcium scores cannot be dismissed as being at low risk. Furthermore, the clinical determinants of calcification are largely unknown and may not reflect propensity to plaque rupture. Studies indicating that hsCRP elevation corresponds to an approximate doubling of the risk of plaque rupture at all levels of coronary calcium have demonstrated the complexity of this approach.[146] Although advocates of CT imaging have noted that sensitivity for the presence of angiographic coronary disease is comparable with that of noninvasive stress testing, such as perfusion scintigraphy or dobutamine echocardiography, the specificity of CT imaging in this setting is low.[147]

Considerable public health concern has also arisen regarding the consequences of overinterpreting the positive and negative predictive values of findings from imaging techniques, such as coronary calcium scores. For example, in one study of initially asymptomatic individuals, 41% of all future vascular events occurred in those with a coronary artery calcium score (CACS) lower than 100, and 17% occurred in those with a CACS of 0.[148] Thus, a low CACS does not preclude the risk of coronary events. Moreover, in the same study, those with high Framingham risk scores but low coronary calcium scores remained at high risk.

Relative to simple blood-based biomarkers, imaging tests currently incur considerable expense and thus may not be cost-effective. One study has shown that the provision of calcium scores does not effectively motivate patients' adherence to risk reduction regimens.[149] In other cases, whole-body scans obtained for vascular screening have led to expensive and unnecessary workups and biopsies of incidental findings, often requiring repeat imaging at substantial radiation doses. Even when the costs of these false-positive findings are ignored, the quality-adjusted life-year cost estimates for CT screening have been found to be unfavorable.[150] Several other modalities for the noninvasive assessment of atherosclerosis exist, ranging from those that are well documented and inexpensive (e.g., ankle-brachial index) to those that are exploratory (e.g., magnetic resonance imaging). Perhaps the best-studied noninvasive approach is the ultrasonic measurement of carotid intimal medial thickness. This technique has proved to have strong predictive value in general population studies and minimal additional expense is required, because most centers already have the required sonographic tools in place.[151]

Whether any imaging technique will prove cost-effective as a screening tool is currently under study in the Multiethnic Study of Atherosclerosis (MESA) funded by the National Heart, Lung, and Blood Institute. In the Rotterdam Heart Study, in which simultaneous measures of atherosclerotic burden were obtained, the ankle-brachial index performed as well as carotid intimal medial thickness (IMT) and x-ray evidence of abdominal aortic calcification, but can be performed at no cost at the bedside.[152] Finally, unlike plasma-based biomarkers, there has been little evidence in randomized trial settings that information obtained through imaging improves outcomes. The importance of performing such trials has been underscored by the recent Detection of Ischemia in Asymptomatic Diabetics (DIAD) trial, in which random allocation to ischemia screening with myocardial perfusion imaging failed to reduce incident myocardial infarction, vascular death, or episodes of ischemia during follow-up.[153] Thus, given issues of cost (and, in some cases, radiation exposure), substantive work is needed before any broad recommendations can be made for the expanded use of imaging as a screening tool for vascular risk detection.[154]

Genetic Determinants of Atherothrombosis

Venous thromboembolism has a major genetic component, and advances in genetic diagnosis (factor V Leiden and the G20210A prothrombin mutation), as well as pharmacogenetic management of warfarin, have already been implemented in many clinical practices (see Chaps. 8 and 9). Similarly, genetic evaluation has found an important role in several well-described heritable disorders that affect cardiac morphology (e.g., those associated with hypertrophic cardiomyopathy) or that cause myocardial conduction defects (e.g., long-QT syndrome). By contrast, although clinicians understand that myocardial infarction, stroke, and other forms of arterial disease also have a major heritable component, no genetic screening test for atherothrombosis has yet found a substantive role in routine clinical practice. Nonetheless, with heritability estimates approaching 50% in several studies, this situation may well change in the future and has stimulated intensive ongoing investigation.

Deciphering the genetic underpinnings of atherothrombosis presents considerable challenges because of major gene-environment interactions. Also, atherothrombosis represents a prototypic complex disease in which multiple small effects accumulate and have a substantial population-attributable risk.[155] Some genetic determinants of atherothrombotic cardiovascular disease were initially described on a candidate gene basis and have been replicated in multiple cohorts. Perhaps the best known of these is the relationship between polymorphisms in the apolipoprotein E (apo E) gene that codes for three common isoforms (E2, E3, and E4), which in turn are associated with differential risks of coronary heart disease. In a meta-analysis of 48 studies incorporating information from over 15,000 affected patients and 33,000 controls, carriers of the apo E e4 allele had a 42% higher risk for coronary heart disease (OR, 1.42; 95% CI, 1.26 to 1.61) compared with those with the more common e3/3 genotype, whereas carriers of the e4 allele had no significant increase in risk.[156]

By contrast, the advent of the genome-wide association study (GWAS) has made it possible to discover gene loci that previously were not anticipated as determinants of vascular risk.[157] For example, a common polymorphism on chromosome 9p21 has repeatedly been found to be associated with coronary artery disease that is not strongly related to any known intermediate phenotype, such as cholesterol or blood pressure.[158,159]

Yet, despite clear replication in more than a dozen cohorts to date, no study has shown that measurement of 9p21 alters global risk prediction.[160] In fact, in one major study, knowledge of single-nucleotide polymorphisms (SNPs) within the chromosome 9 loci lead, if anything, to a worsening of risk prediction as compared with usual risk factors and a simple question regarding parental history.[161] These data underscore the complexity of genetic biomarkers with risk and greatly reduce enthusiasm for screening.

Multiple recent GWASs have reported novel associations of genes with lipid levels and with incident cardiovascular disease.[162-164] Other potential genetic determinants of myocardial infarction reported in the cardiovascular literature include polymorphisms in the arachidonate 5-lipooxygenase–activating protein gene and its related pathways,[165] in the cyclooxygenase-2 gene,[166] in the proprotein convertase subtilisin-kexin type 9 (*PCSK9*) gene,[167] in the *OX40* ligand gene,[168] and in the *ROS1* gene encoding for tyrosine kinase. Similarly, variation in the beta$_2$-adrenergic receptor gene has been found in two study populations to be associated with an increased risk of sudden death.[169] Other observations that ultimately may relate to atherothrombotic risk include the finding of a common genetic variant associated with adult and childhood obesity,[170] polymorphisms associated with an increased risk of diabetes and impaired glucose tolerance,[171] and replicable genetic determinants of CRP.[172] Much of this ongoing work will require careful replication before attaining wide scientific or clinical acceptance.

Although clinically effective genetic screens are not yet available, in daily practice the simple ascertainment of a parental history of early-onset atherosclerosis has proved to be an important predictor of future cardiovascular events. In the Framingham Offspring Study, when compared with those with no parental history of cardiovascular disease, men with at least one parent with premature atherothrombosis (onset younger than age 55 for fathers and younger than age 65 for mothers) had an age-adjusted odds ratio of 2.6 (95% CI, 1.7 to 4.1), whereas the similar odds ratio for women was 2.3 (95% CI, 1.2 to 3.1).[173] These effects compare in magnitude with those of smoking, hypertension, and hyperlipidemia in the Framingham cohort itself. As noted subsequently, analysis of data from the Women's Health Study has also found that a parental history of myocardial infarction before 60 years of age, along with knowledge of CRP levels, can reclassify large numbers of patients as being at higher or lower risk than would have been anticipated on the basis of traditional risk factors alone.

Improved genetic understanding of cardiovascular risk should facilitate the deployment of interventions so that the right patient gets the right therapy at the right time—the concept of personalized medicine. Pharmacogenetic evaluation also has the potential to allow physicians to predict unwanted actions of drugs in advance and thus avoid a particular environmental exposure that might adversely interact with a common genetic variant. For example, polymorphism in the HMG-CoA reductase gene is associated with differential effects of statin therapy,[174] and one report has suggested that mean leukocyte telomere length both predicts incident vascular events and may identify individuals who would most benefit from statin treatment.[175] By contrast, the SEARCH investigators have reported a common variant in SLCO1B1 that relates strongly to an increased risk of statin-induced myopathy.[176]

Although evaluations of single genetic markers have not been of much clinical usefulness to date, the concept of using multimarker approaches has generated somewhat greater optimism. For example, in the Malmo Diet and Cancer Study, a genotype score based on nine validated SNPs known to be associated with modulation of LDL-C or HDL-C levels was found to be an independent risk factor for incident cardiovascular disease[177] (**Fig. 44-12**). In that study, however, the genetic risk score did not improve discrimination and only modestly improved reclassification. Little clinical efficacy was also seen in a very recent analysis of the Women's Genome Health Study in which more than 100 previously validated SNPS from earlier GWASs were used to generate a second-generation genetic risk score.[178] Thus, although considerable biologic insight into mechanisms and pathogenesis have already come from large-scale genomic studies of vascular disease, currently available data do not support the use of genetic biomarkers as clinical tools in the prediction or prevention of cardiovascular disease.

Novel Approaches to Global Risk Detection

In the half century since the identification of the major coronary risk factors of age, hypertension, smoking, and hyperlipidemia, our understanding of atherothrombosis has expanded to include the biology of hemostasis, thrombosis, inflammation, and endothelial function. Despite this more ample view of pathophysiology, the variables in current risk assessment algorithms remain largely unchanged from those evaluated a half-century ago.

An expanded and updated approach to vascular risk detection is needed so that primary care physicians can be guided by the most modern biologic constructs. New risk prediction algorithms must involve rigorous evaluation, with particular care given not only to the concepts of discrimination but also to calibration and reclassification.[179] This change in focus for prevention must include an understanding that reliance on the C-statistic as a traditional method for selecting variables for inclusion in risk prediction models is outmoded and subject to considerable error.[115] Careful investigation has shown that inappropriate reliance on the C-statistic would actually eliminate LDL-C, HDL-C, and blood pressure from most global prediction models. Furthermore, continued reliance on 10-year risk estimates rather than estimates of lifetime risk may actually restrain more effective prevention efforts.[180]

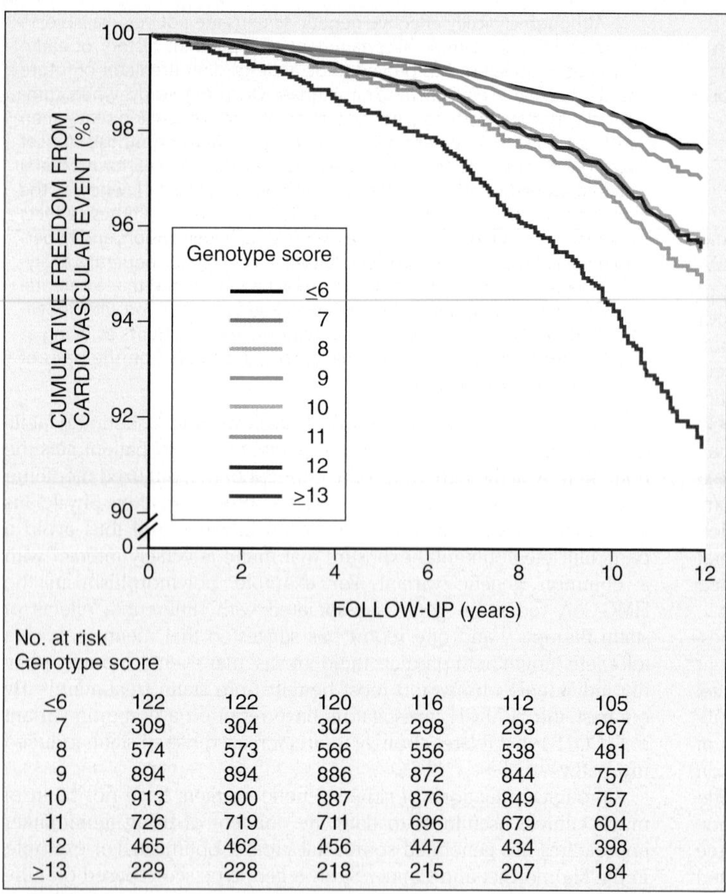

FIGURE 44-12 Predicted cumulative freedom from myocardial infarction, stroke, or cardiovascular death according to genotype score in the Malmo Diet and Cancer Study. *(From Kathiresan S, Melander O, Anevski D, et al: Polymorphisms associated with cholesterol and risk of cardiovascular events. N Engl J Med 358:1240, 2008.)*

TABLE 44-3 Estimated 10-Year Risk of Atherothrombotic Disease for a 50-Year-Old Nondiabetic Female Smoker*,†

hsCRP (MG/LITER)	PARENTAL HISTORY?	ATP-III (%)	RRS (%)
0.1	No	11.5	4.9
0.5	No	11.5	6.5
1.0	No	11.5	7.4
3.0	No	11.5	8.9
5.0	No	11.5	9.7
8.0	No	11.5	10.5
10.0	No	11.5	10.9
0.1	Yes	11.5	7.5
0.5	Yes	11.5	9.9
1.0	Yes	11.5	11.2
3.0	Yes	11.5	13.4
5.0	Yes	11.5	14.6
8.0	Yes	11.5	15.8
10.0	Yes	11.5	16.4

*Blood pressure = 155/85 mm Hg; high-density lipoprotein = 35 mg/dL; TC = 240 mg/dL.

†Based on traditional Framingham variables as used in Adult Treatment Panel III (ATP-III) that additionally takes into account hsCRP and parental history of myocardial infarction before 60 years of age.

Modified from Ridker PM, Buring JE, Rifai N, Cook N: Development and validation of improved algorithms for the assessment of global cardiovascular risk in women: The Reynolds Risk Score. JAMA 297:611, 2007.

In an effort to move beyond traditional risk variables, a few recent investigations have ascertained wide panels of biomarkers in large cohorts of initially healthy individuals who were then followed prospectively for incident vascular events. For example, using such data in the Women's Health Study, nine variables—age, current smoking, systolic blood pressure, HbA1c among diabetics, hsCRP, apo B100, apo A-I, Lp(a), and a parental history of premature atherosclerosis—were found to improve risk prediction substantially when compared with traditional Framingham covariates.[3] Importantly, use of this novel algorithm reclassified almost 50% of those otherwise considered to be at intermediate risk on the basis of usual risk factors, an effect that was also seen for a simplified prediction model that substituted non–HDL-C for apo B100 and HDL-C for apo A-I. Moreover, this reclassification was correct in over 90% of cases. For a hypothetical nondiabetic woman with a calculated 10-year Framingham risk of 10.8% , the estimated risks calculated by this updated approach range from a low of 4.7% to a high of 16.0% (**Table 44-3**). This new algorithm, the Reynolds Risk Score (www.reynoldsriskscore.org), mentioned earlier,[3] has recently been prospectively validated in the Physicians Health Study of men.[100] Both hsCRP and parental history of premature atherothrombosis, the two novel parameters included in the Reynolds Risk Score, have also been shown to improve risk reclassification within the Framingham Heart Study.[97] Other major epidemiologic investigations,[181-183] but not all,[184] have reported similar results, underscoring continued controversy in this arena. As a general rule, those studies that have not found novel biomarkers to add risk information have been conducted in very low-risk cohorts with only small numbers of individuals at intermediate risk for whom reclassification is possible.

The effective practice of preventive cardiology also requires a careful reevaluation of the core purposes of screening, evaluations of cost-effectiveness, and appropriate use of imaging tests. **Figure 44-13** provides a conceptual basis for such an approach. At the bottom of the population pyramid, of those at unknown risk, a generalized evaluation for smoking status and blood pressure, along with blood measurements of total and HDL cholesterol, hsCRP, and glucose levels, provides a broad basis for ascertaining lifetime risk while simultaneously providing an index of risk for developing incident type 2 diabetes. With this information, most individuals can be categorized as lower, moderate, or higher vascular risk, thus greatly reducing the need for screening in imaging tests that can increase cost and radiation exposure. For those at the top of the risk pyramid who have indications for statin therapy, monitoring of LDL-C levels is needed for application of current guidelines. In this setting, particularly for postinfarction patients, data from several studies have also indicated that achieving a low level of hsCRP, along with a low level of LDL-C, can aid in the assessment of long-term prognosis. As noted, the concept that reducing both inflammation and cholesterol is important for clinical outcomes has now been extended to the primary prevention setting.[104] Use of such modified methods for global risk prediction holds considerable promise, even if only to heighten interest in prevention. Several studies continue to find wide underuse of proven preventive interventions, an education gap that will require new and more aggressive approaches to primary and secondary prevention.

Moving Toward Evidence-Based Guidelines

Whereas this chapter has thus far focused on risk markers for atherothrombotic disease, a controversy exists regarding how to put data on biomarkers of risk into clinical practice. In a recent scientific statement from the American Heart Association, initial proof of concept, prospective validation in independent populations, documentation of incremental information when added to standard risk factors, assessment of effects on patient management and outcomes, and ultimately cost-effectiveness are all appropriately highlighted.[185] The translation of evidence into practice guidelines remains equally controversial. In a comprehensive analysis of guidelines issued by the American Heart Association and the American College of Cardiology through September 2008, less than half were based on firm evidence from randomized trials.[186]

The use of statin therapy for the prevention of vascular disease provides an example of this complexity. In current clinical guidelines, statin therapy is typically recommended for use in those with levels of absolute risk exceeding certain thresholds—typically, a 20% estimated 10-year risk using global risk assessment tools such as those pioneered by the Framingham Heart Study. At first glance, this approach would seem to be intuitive and effective; multiple randomized trials of patients with high absolute risk caused by prior myocardial infarction or stroke clearly benefit from statin therapy. Furthermore, on the assumption that the relative risk reductions associated with statin therapy are independent of absolute risk, using absolute risk thresholds should allow for cost-effective targeting of therapy. If this core assumption were incorrect, however, then continuing to use absolute risk as a method of determining whom to treat with statin therapy would result in overuse in some groups and underuse in others.

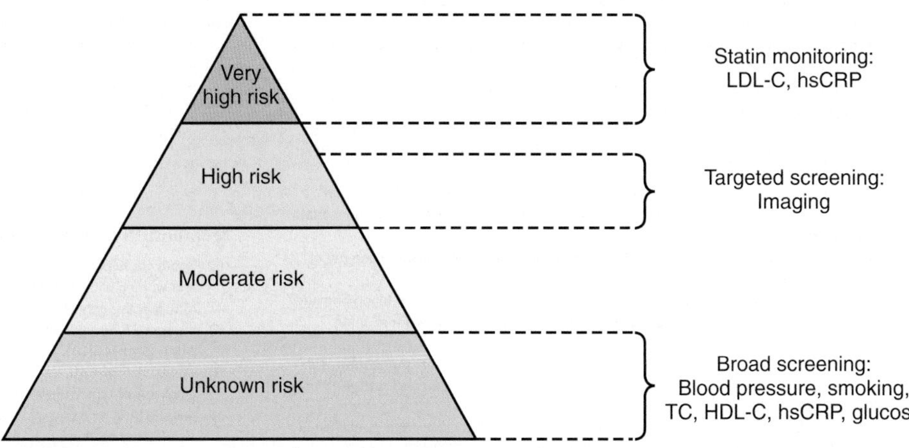

FIGURE 44-13 A cost-effective approach to cardiovascular risk screening. TC = total cholesterol.

The results of six recent randomized clinical trials of statin therapy compared with placebo suggest that reexamining the assumption that absolute risk should dictate statin prescription may be warranted. Two of these trials dealt with individuals suffering from congestive heart failure, a group with exceptionally high absolute risk. In the first of these trials, the CORONA investigators randomly allocated 5011 systolic heart failure patients 60 years of age or older to rosuvastatin, 10 mg, or placebo; after 36 months, almost one third of the trial participants had suffered myocardial infarction, stroke, or cardiovascular death, confirming the very high absolute risk among such patients.[187] Yet, despite a 45% reduction in LDL-C and good compliance with the study medication, there was no significant benefit associated with statin therapy (HR, 0.92; 95% CI, 0.83 to 1.02; $P = 0.12$). An almost identical finding was observed in the GISSI-HF trial, in which 4574 patients with chronic heart failure were allocated to rosuvastatin, 10 mg daily, or to placebo and followed over a 4-year period.[188] During follow-up, 57% were hospitalized for cardiovascular reasons and 29% died from any cause, again demonstrating the very high absolute risk among such individuals. However, as in CORONA, there was no benefit associated with statin therapy on either cardiac events (HR, 1.01; 95% CI, 0.91 to 1.11; $P = 0.9$) or all-cause mortality (HR, 1.00; 95% CI, 0.90 to 1.12; $P = 0.9$).

The disconnect between absolute risk and statin efficacy observed in CORONA and GISSI is not unique, as demonstrated in two other trials of individuals on hemodialysis. In the German Diabetes and Dialysis Study, 1255 patients with type 2 diabetes receiving maintenance hemodialysis were allocated to 20 mg, atorvastatin, or to placebo[189]; after 4 years, the cumulative incidence of myocardial infarction, stroke, or cardiovascular death approached 50%, indicating exceptionally high risk, yet allocation to atorvastatin had no significant effect on clinical outcomes (HR, 0.92; 95% CI, 0.77 to 1.10; $P = 0.37$). Similarly, in a recent study of 2776 patients undergoing maintenance hemodialysis in the AURORA trial, rosuvastatin had no benefit on vascular event rates (HR, 0.96; 95% CI, 0.84 to 1.11; $P = 0.59$), despite a 5-year cumulative incidence of myocardial infarction, stroke, or cardiovascular death exceeding 35%.[190]

These four trials documented a lack of efficacy for statin therapy in at least some high-risk and very high-risk individuals. However, the JUPITER trial of rosuvastatin discussed earlier, and the MEGA trial of pravastatin conducted in 7832 apparently healthy Japanese men and women,[191] have demonstrated the efficacy of statin therapy in groups considered to be at too low a risk according to traditional global risk algorithms to merit intervention. For example, in JUPITER, all participants had LDL-C levels below treatment targets in primary prevention and more than half had Framingham scores below 10%; nonetheless, the absolute event rates in JUPITER and consequent NNT calculations were comparable to those of prior primary prevention trials that selected patients on the basis of overt hyperlipidemia.[102]

Given trial evidence that some low-global-risk patients benefit markedly from statin therapy whereas some high-global-risk patients do not, it may be necessary to reconsider methods for selecting populations to treat with statin therapy. Although the Framingham investigators have proposed an updated risk score that incorporates more clinical endpoints such as stroke, intermittent claudication, peripheral arterial disease, and congestive heart failure,[192] this score does not incorporate novel biomarkers or parental history and improves overall risk evaluation only modestly.[193] By contrast, a recent European evaluation has confirmed that screening for hsCRP levels higher than 2 mg/L defines a population in whom statin therapy is highly effective.[183] Thus, evolving guidelines that better match recommendations to trial outcomes will help the primary care community implement optimal methods for risk factor assessment and improve targeting of preventive interventions. Finally, as the costs of pharmaceutical interventions for prevention continue to decline, novel approaches to broad population usage of proven therapies as adjuncts to diet, exercise, and smoking cessation will be needed.[194] This represents a crucial shift in policy toward primary prevention; approximately 50% of the decline in U.S. deaths from CHD over the past 20 years is attributable to reductions in major risk factors and the rest to the use of evidence-based therapies.[195]

REFERENCES

1. Bhatt DL, Steg PG, Ohman EM, et al: International prevalence, recognition, and treatment of cardiovascular risk factors in outpatients with atherothrombosis. JAMA 95:180, 2006.
2. He J, Gu D, Wu X, et al: Major causes of death among men and women in China. N Engl J Med 353:1124, 2005.

Smoking

3. Ridker PM, Buring JE, Rifai N, Cook NR: Development and validation of improved algorithms for the assessment of global cardiovascular risk in women: The Reynolds Risk Score. JAMA 97:611, 2007.
4. Centers for Disease Control and Prevention (CDC): Smoking-attributable mortality, years of potential life lost, and productivity losses—United States. JAMA 301:593, 2009.
5. Centers for Disease Control and Prevention (CDC): Cigarette smoking among adults—United States. JAMA 301:373, 2009.
6. Gu D, Kelly TN, Wu X, et al: Mortality attributable to smoking in China. N Engl J Med 360:150, 2009.
7. Jha P, Jacob B, Gajalakshmi V, et al: A nationally representative case-control study of smoking and death in India. N Engl J Med 358:1137, 2008.
8. Critchley JA, Capewell S: Mortality risk reduction associated with smoking cessation in patients with coronary heart disease: A systematic review. JAMA 2003:290:86, 2003.
9. Kenfield SA, Stampfer MJ, Rosner BA, Colditz GA: Smoking and smoking cessation in relation to mortality in women. JAMA 299:2037, 2008.
10. Brandt AM: FDA regulation of tobacco—pitfalls and possibilities. N Engl J Med 359:445, 2008.
11. Christakis NA, Fowler JH. The collective dynamics of smoking in a large social network. N Engl J Med 358:2249, 2008.

Hypertension

12. Volpp KG, Troxel AB, Pauly MV, et al: A randomized, controlled trial of financial incentives for smoking cessation. N Engl J Med 360:699, 2009.
13. Chobanian AV, Bakris GL, Black HR, et al: The Seventh Report of the Joint National Committee on Prevention, Detection, Evaluation, and Treatment of High Blood Pressure: The JNC 7 report. JAMA 289:2560, 2003.

14. Hajjar I, Kotchen TA: Trends in prevalence, awareness, treatment, and control of hypertension in the United States. JAMA 90:199, 2003.
15. Kearney PM, Whelton M, Reynolds K, et al: Global burden of hypertension: Analysis of worldwide data. Lancet 365:217, 2005.
16. Lawes CMM, VanderHoorn S, Rodgers A: Global burden of blood-pressure related disease. Lancet 371:1513, 2008.
17. Beckett NS, Peters R, Fletcher AE, et al: Treatment of hypertension in patients 80 years of age or older. N Engl J Med 358:1887, 2008.
18. Haider AW, Larson MG, Franklin SS, Levy D: Systolic blood pressure, diastolic blood pressure, and pulse pressure as predictors of risk for congestive heart failure in the Framingham Heart Study. Ann Intern Med 38:10, 2003.
19. Bobrie G, Chatellier G, Genes N, et al: Cardiovascular prognosis of "masked hypertension" detected by blood pressure self-measurement in elderly treated hypertensive patients. JAMA 291:1342, 2004.
20. Ingelsson E, Bjorklund-Bodegard K, Lind L, et al: Diurnal blood pressure pattern and risk of congestive heart failure. JAMA 295:2859, 2006.
21. Staessen JA, Den Hond E, Celis H, et al: Antihypertensive treatment based on blood pressure measurement at home or in the physician's office: A randomized controlled trial. JAMA 291:955, 2004.
22. Green BB, Cook AJ, Ralston JD, et al: Effectiveness of home blood pressure monitoring, Web communication, and pharmacist care on hypertension control: A randomized controlled trial. JAMA 299:2857, 2008.
23. Nissen SE, Tuzcu EM, Libby P, et al: Effect of antihypertensive agents on cardiovascular events in patients with coronary disease and normal blood pressure: The CAMELOT study: A randomized controlled trial. JAMA 292:2217, 2004.
24. Psaty BM, Lumley T, Furberg CD, et al: Health outcomes associated with various antihypertensive therapies used as first-line agents: a network meta-analysis. JAMA 289:2534, 2003.
25. Law MR, Wald NJ, Morris JK, Jordan RE: Value of low dose combination treatment with blood pressure lowering drugs: Analysis of 354 randomised trials. BMJ 26:1427, 2003.
26. Forman JP, Stampfer MJ, Curhan GC: Diet and lifestyle risk factors associated with incident hypertension in women. JAMA 302:401, 2009.
27. Julius S, Nesbitt SD, Egan BM, et al: Feasibility of treating prehypertension with an angiotensin-receptor blocker. N Engl J Med 354:1685, 2006.
28. The ACCORD Study Group; Cushman WC, Evans GW, Byington RP, et al: Effects of intensive blood-pressure control in type 2 diabetes mellitus. N Engl J Med 362:1575, 2010.
29. Lynch AI, Boerwinkle E, Davis BR, et al: Pharmacogenetic association of the NPPA T2238C genetic variant with cardiovascular disease outcomes in patients with hypertension. JAMA 299:296, 2008.
30. Holman RR, Paul SK, Bethel MA, et al: Long-term follow-up after tight control of blood pressure in type 2 diabetes. N Engl J Med 359:1565, 2008.

Lipid Disorders

31. Collins R, Armitage J, Parish S, et al: Effects of cholesterol-lowering with simvastatin on stroke and other major vascular events in 20,536 people with cerebrovascular disease or other high-risk conditions. Lancet 363:757, 2004.
32. Libby P: The forgotten majority: Unfinished business in cardiovascular risk reduction. J Am Coll Cardiol 46:1225, 2005.
33. Wiegman A, Hutten BA, de Groot E, et al: Efficacy and safety of statin therapy in children with familial hypercholesterolemia: A randomized controlled trial. JAMA 292:331, 2004.
34. Brugts JJ, Yetgin T, Hoeks SE, et al: The benefits of statins in people without established cardiovascular disease but with cardiovascular risk factors: Meta-analysis of randomised controlled trials. BMJ 338:b2376, 2009.
35. Barter PJ, Caulfield M, Eriksson M, et al: Effects of torcetrapib in patients at high risk for coronary events. N Engl J Med 357:2109, 2007.
36. Rader DJ: Illuminating HDL—is it still a viable therapeutic target? N Engl J Med 357:2180, 2007.
37. Thompson A, Di Angelantonio E, Sarwar N, et al: Association of cholesteryl ester transfer protein genotypes with CETP mass and activity, lipid levels, and coronary risk. JAMA 299:2777, 2008.
38. Ridker PM, Pare G, Parker AN, et al: Polymorphism in the CETP gene region, HDL cholesterol, and risk of future myocardial infarction: Genomewide analysis among 18,245 initially healthy women from the Women's Genome Health Study. Circ Cardiovasc Genet 2:26, 2009.
39. Pischon T, Girman CJ, Sacks FM, et al: Non-high-density lipoprotein cholesterol and apolipoprotein B in the prediction of coronary heart disease in men. Circulation 112:3375, 2005.
40. Ridker PM, Rifai N, Cook NR, et al: Non-HDL cholesterol, apolipoproteins A-I and B100, standard lipid measures, lipid ratios, and CRP as risk factors for cardiovascular disease in women. JAMA 294:326, 2005.
41. Mora S, Szklo M, Otvos JD, et al: LDL particle subclasses, LDL particle size, and carotid atherosclerosis in the Multi-Ethnic Study of Atherosclerosis (MESA). Atherosclerosis 192:211, 2007.
42. Mora S, Otvos JD, Rifai N, et al: Lipoprotein particle profiles by nuclear magnetic resonance compared with standard lipids and apolipoproteins in predicting incident cardiovascular disease in women. Circulation 119:931, 2009.
43. Otvos JD, Collins D, Freedman DS, et al: Low-density lipoprotein and high-density lipoprotein particle subclasses predict coronary events and are favorably changed by gemfibrozil therapy in the Veterans Affairs High-Density Lipoprotein Intervention Trial. Circulation 113:1556, 2006.
44. Kathiresan S, Otvos JD, Sullivan LM, et al: Increased small low-density lipoprotein particle number: A prominent feature of the metabolic syndrome in the Framingham Heart Study. Circulation 113:20, 2006.
45. Sarwar N, Danesh J, Eiriksdottir G, et al: Triglycerides and the risk of coronary heart disease: 10,158 incident cases among 262,525 participants in 29 Western prospective studies. Circulation 115:450, 2007.
46. Bansal S, Buring JE, Rifai N, et al: Fasting compared with nonfasting triglycerides and risk of cardiovascular events in women. JAMA 298:309, 2007.
47. Nordestgaard BG, Benn M, Schnohr P, Tybjaerg-Hansen A: Nonfasting triglycerides and risk of myocardial infarction, ischemic heart disease, and death in men and women. JAMA 298:299, 2007.
48. Ridker PM: Fasting versus nonfasting triglycerides and the prediction of cardiovascular risk: Do we need to revisit the oral triglyceride tolerance test? Clin Chem 54:11, 2008.
49. Freiberg JJ, Tybjaerg-Hansen A, Jensen JS, Nordestgaard BG: Nonfasting triglycerides and risk of ischemic stroke in the general population. JAMA 300:2142, 2008.
50. Keech A, Simes RJ, Barter P, et al: Effects of long-term fenofibrate therapy on cardiovascular events in 9795 people with type 2 diabetes mellitus (the FIELD study): Randomised controlled trial. Lancet 366:1849, 2005.
51. The ACCORD Study Group: Effects of combination lipid therapy in type 2 diabetes mellitus. N Engl J Med 362:1563, 2010.

Metabolic Syndrome, Insulin Resistance, and Diabetes

52. Booth GL, Kapral MK, Fung K, Tu JV: Relation between age and cardiovascular disease in men and women with diabetes compared with non-diabetic people: A population-based retrospective cohort study. Lancet 368:29, 2006.
53. Ingelsson E, Sundstrom J, Arnlov J, et al: Insulin resistance and risk of congestive heart failure. JAMA 294:334, 2005.
54. Hu FB, Stampfer MJ, Haffner SM, et al: Elevated risk of cardiovascular disease prior to clinical diagnosis of type 2 diabetes. Diabetes Care 25:1129, 2002.
55. Kahn R, Buse J, Ferrannini E, Stern M: The metabolic syndrome: Time for a critical appraisal: Joint statement from the American Diabetes Association and the European Association for the Study of Diabetes. Diabetes Care 28:2289, 2005.
56. Lakka HM, Laaksonen DE, Lakka TA, et al: The metabolic syndrome and total and cardiovascular disease mortality in middle-aged men. JAMA 288:2709, 2002.
57. Sattar N, McConnachie A, Shaper AG, et al: Can metabolic syndrome usefully predict cardiovascular disease and diabetes? Outcome data from two prospective studies. Lancet 371:1927, 2008.
58. Kahn R: Metabolic syndrome—what is the clinical usefulness? Lancet 371:1892, 2008.
59. Wang J, Ruotsalainen S, Moilanen L, et al: The metabolic syndrome predicts cardiovascular mortality: A 13-year follow-up study in elderly non-diabetic Finns. Eur Heart J 28:857, 2007.
60. Jeppesen J, Hansen TW, Rasmussen S, et al: Insulin resistance, the metabolic syndrome, and risk of incident cardiovascular disease: a population-based study. J Am Coll Cardiol 49:2112, 2007.
61. Mathieu P, Lemieux I, Despres JP: Obesity, inflammation, and cardiovascular risk. Clin Pharmacol Ther 87:407, 2010.
62. Grundy SM, Brewer HB Jr, Cleeman JI, et al: Definition of metabolic syndrome: Report of the National Heart, Lung, and Blood Institute/American Heart Association conference on scientific issues related to definition. Circulation 109:433, 2004.
63. Ridker PM, Buring JE, Cook NR, Rifai N: C-reactive protein, the metabolic syndrome, and risk of incident cardiovascular events: An 8-year follow-up of 14,719 initially healthy American women. Circulation 107:391, 2003.
64. Pradhan AD, Manson JE, Rifai N, et al: C-reactive protein, interleukin 6, and risk of developing type 2 diabetes mellitus. JAMA 286:327, 2001.
65. Hu FB, Meigs JB, Li TY, et al: Inflammatory markers and risk of developing type 2 diabetes in women. Diabetes 53:693, 2004.
66. Sattar N, Gaw A, Scherbakova O, et al: Metabolic syndrome with and without C-reactive protein as a predictor of coronary heart disease and diabetes in the West of Scotland Coronary Prevention Study. Circulation 108:414, 2003.
67. Eckel RH, Grundy SM, Zimmet PZ: The metabolic syndrome. Lancet 365:1415, 2005.

Exercise, Weight Loss, and Obesity

68. Manson JE, Greenland P, LaCroix AZ, et al: Walking compared with vigorous exercise for the prevention of cardiovascular events in women. N Engl J Med 347:716, 2002.
69. Whang W, Manson JE, Hu FB, et al: Physical exertion, exercise, and sudden cardiac death in women. JAMA 295:1399, 2006.
70. Andersen LB, Harro M, Sardinha LB, et al: Physical activity and clustered cardiovascular risk in children: A cross-sectional study (The European Youth Heart Study). Lancet 368:299, 2006.
71. Poirier P, Giles TD, Bray GA, et al: Obesity and cardiovascular disease: Pathophysiology, evaluation, and effect of weight loss: An update of the 1997 American Heart Association Scientific Statement on Obesity and Heart Disease from the Obesity Committee of the Council on Nutrition, Physical Activity, and Metabolism. Circulation 113:898, 2006.
72. Yan LL, Daviglus ML, Liu K, et al: Midlife body mass index and hospitalization and mortality in older age. JAMA 295:190, 2006.
73. Mora S, Lee IM, Buring JE, Ridker PM: Association of physical activity and body mass index with novel and traditional cardiovascular biomarkers in women. JAMA 295:1412, 2006.
74. Wadden TA, Berkowitz RI, Womble LG, et al: Randomized trial of life style modification and pharmacotherapy for obesity. N Engl J Med 353:2111, 2005.
75. He FJ, Nowson CA, MacGregor GA: Fruit and vegetable consumption and stroke: Meta-analysis of cohort studies. Lancet 367:320, 2006.
76. Howard BV, Van Horn L, Hsia J, et al: Low-fat dietary pattern and risk of cardiovascular disease: The Women's Health Initiative Randomized Controlled Dietary Modification Trial. JAMA 295:655, 2006.
77. Dansinger ML, Gleason JA, Griffith JL, et al: Comparison of the Atkins, Ornish, Weight Watchers, and Zone diets for weight loss and heart disease risk reduction: A randomized trial. JAMA 293:43, 2005.
78. Appel LJ, Sacks FM, Carey VJ, et al: Effects of protein, monounsaturated fat, and carbohydrate intake on blood pressure and serum lipids: Results of the OmniHeart randomized trial. JAMA 294:2455, 2005.
79. Sacks FM, Bray GA, Carey VJ, et al: Comparison of weight-loss diets with different compositions of fat, protein, and carbohydrates. N Engl J Med 360:859, 2009.
80. Wing RR, Tate DF, Gorin AA, et al: A self-regulation program for maintenance of weight loss. N Engl J Med 355:1563, 2006.
81. Svetkey LP, Stevens VJ, Brantley PJ, et al: Comparison of strategies for sustaining weight loss: The weight loss maintenance randomized controlled trial. JAMA 299:1139, 2008.

The complex regulation of BP has thwarted the genetic dissection of primary human hypertension.[9] Whereas mutations in 20 salt-handling genes cause ultrarare monogenic forms of severe early-onset hypotension (salt-wasting syndromes) and hypertension (all inherited as mendelian traits), the applicability to common primary hypertension has been difficult to show. The first genome-wide associations for hypertension were recently reported, with small affect sizes for each loci.[10,10a] New data from the Framingham Heart Study indicate that gene mutations underlying the pediatric salt-wasting syndromes (Bartter and Gitelman) are carried by 1% to 2% of the general adult population and confer resistance against primary hypertension (**Fig. 45-3**).[10b]

Mechanisms of Primary (Essential) Hypertension

Hemodynamic Subtypes

Primary hypertension can be divided into three distinctly different hemodynamic subtypes that vary sharply by age.

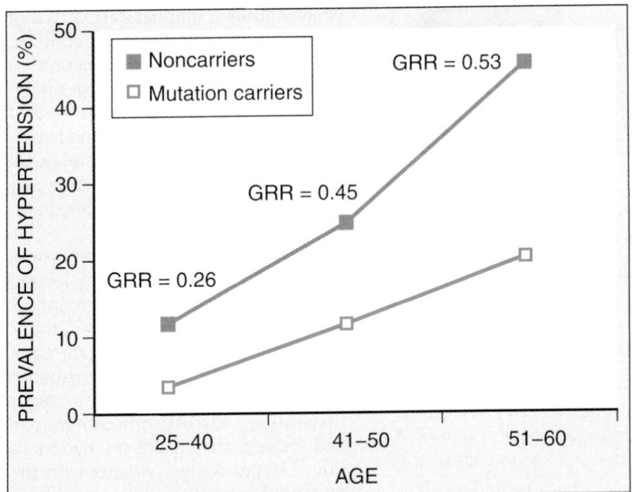

FIGURE 45-3 Reduced prevalence of hypertension among mutation carriers. Prevalence of hypertension at the last examination within ages 25-40, 41-50, and 51-60 years, for mutation carriers and noncarriers of genes causing Bartter and Gitelman syndromes. The genotype relative risk (GRR) for mutation carriers is shown. *(From Ji W, Foo JN, O'Roak BJ, et al: Rare independent mutations in renal salt handling genes contribute to blood pressure variation. Nat Genet 40:592, 2008.)*

SYSTOLIC HYPERTENSION IN YOUNG ADULTS. At one end of the age spectrum is isolated systolic hypertension (ISH) in young adults (typically 17 to 25 years of age). The key hemodynamic abnormalities are increased cardiac output and a stiff aorta, both presumably reflecting an overactive sympathetic nervous system.[11] The prevalence is estimated to be as high as 25% in young men but only 2% in young women. These figures may be too high because brachial artery BP overestimates central aortic pressure by approximately 20 mm Hg in young adults from peripheral pulse wave amplification. However, in the largest study to date, central aortic pressures were 20 mm Hg higher than normal in young adults with ISH.[11] A hyperdynamic circulation in youth may precede diastolic hypertension in middle age.

DIASTOLIC HYPERTENSION IN MIDDLE AGE. When hypertension is diagnosed in middle age (typically, 30 to 50 years of age), the most common BP pattern is elevated diastolic pressure, with systolic pressure being normal (isolated diastolic hypertension) or elevated (combined systolic-diastolic hypertension). This pattern constitutes classic "essential hypertension." Isolated diastolic hypertension is more common in men and is often associated with middle-age weight gain.[12] Without treatment, isolated diastolic hypertension often progresses to combined systolic-diastolic hypertension. The fundamental hemodynamic fault is an elevated systemic vascular resistance coupled with an inappropriately normal cardiac output. Vasoconstriction at the level of the resistance arterioles results from increased neurohormonal drive and an autoregulatory reaction of vascular smooth muscle to an expanded plasma volume, the latter because of impairment in the kidneys' ability to excrete sodium.

ISOLATED SYSTOLIC HYPERTENSION IN OLDER ADULTS. After the age of 55 years, ISH (systolic BP >140 mm Hg and diastolic BP <90 mm Hg) is the most common form.[13] In developed countries, systolic pressure rises steadily with age; in contrast, diastolic pressure rises until about 55 years of age, then falls progressively thereafter (**Fig. 45-4**). The resultant widening of pulse pressure indicates stiffening of the central aorta and a more rapid return of reflected pulse waves from the periphery, causing an augmentation of systolic aortic pressure (see Fig. 45-4; also see Figs. 45-e1, 45-e2, and 45-e3 on website).[14] Accumulation of collagen (which is poorly distensible) adversely affects its ratio to elastin in the aortic wall.

ISH may represent an exaggeration of this age-dependent stiffening process, although systolic BP and pulse pressure do not rise with age in the absence of urbanization (e.g., cloistered nuns). ISH is more

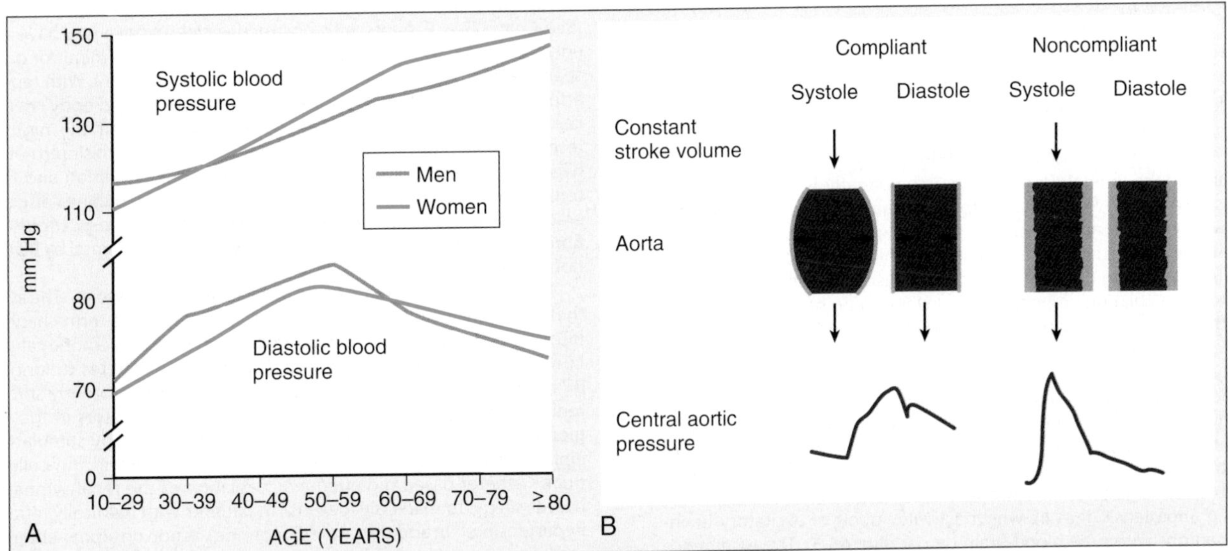

FIGURE 45-4 **A,** Age-dependent changes in systolic and diastolic blood pressure in the United States. **B,** Schematic representation of the relationship between aortic compliance and pulse pressure. *(**A** from Burt V, Whelton P, Rocella EJ, et al: Prevalence of hypertension in the U.S. adult population. Results from the Third National Health and Nutrition Examination Survey, 1988-1991. Hypertension 25:305, 1995. **B** from Dr. Stanley Franklin, University of California at Irvine, with permission.)*

CH 45

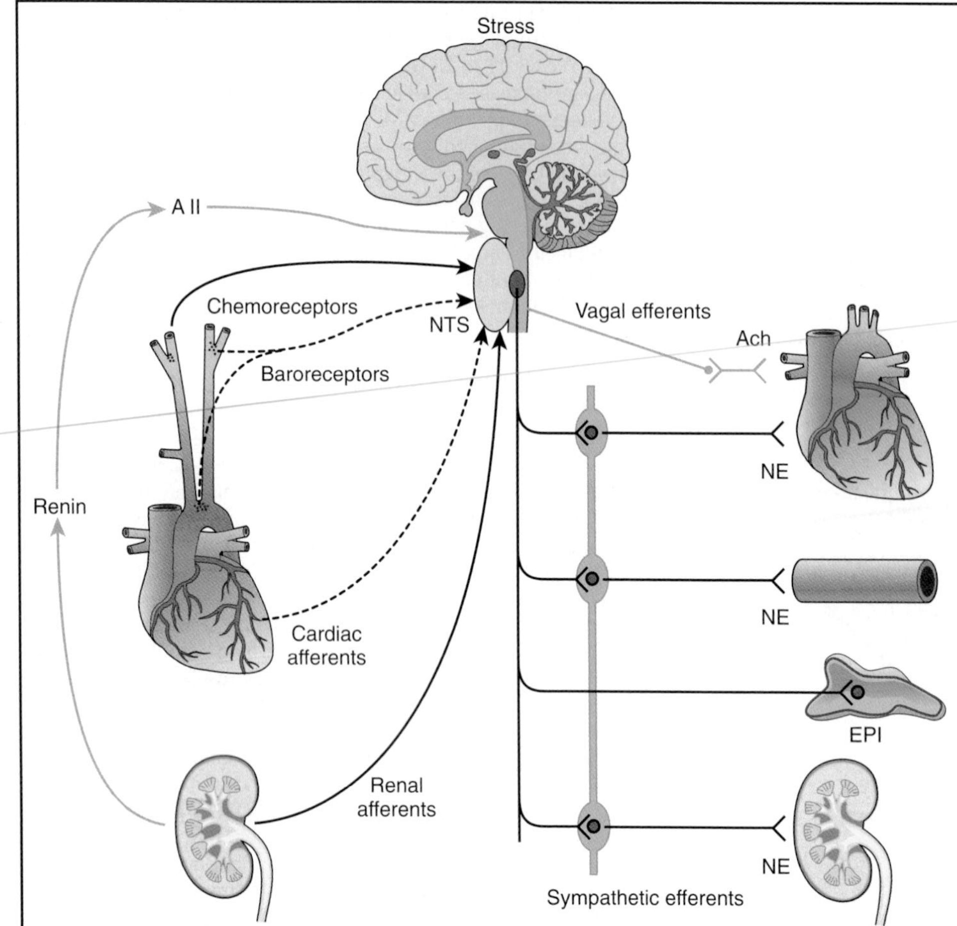

FIGURE 45-5 Sympathetic nervous system. Dotted arrows represent inhibitory neural influences and solid arrows represent excitatory neural influences on sympathetic outflow to the heart, peripheral vasculature, and kidneys. A II = angiotensin II; Ach = acetylcholine; EPI = epinephrine; NE = norepinephrine; NTS = nucleus tractus solitarius.

common in women and is a major risk factor for diastolic heart failure, which also is more common in women (see Chaps. 30, 80, and 81). Most cases of ISH arise de novo after the age of 55 years and are not "burned-out" middle-age diastolic hypertension.[12] Compared with young or middle-aged adults with optimal BP, those with BP in the high-normal range (prehypertension) are more likely to develop ISH after 55 years of age.[12]

A multitude of neurohormonal, renal, and vascular mechanisms interact to varying degrees in contributing to these different hemodynamic forms of hypertension.

Neural Mechanisms

In young adults, primary hypertension consistently is associated with increased heart rate and cardiac output, plasma and urinary norepinephrine levels, regional norepinephrine spillover, peripheral postganglionic sympathetic nerve firing (determined by microelectrode recordings), and alpha-adrenergic receptor–mediated vasoconstrictor tone in the peripheral circulation.[15] Sympathetic overactivity has been demonstrated in early primary hypertension and in several other forms of established human hypertension, including hypertension associated with obesity, sleep apnea, early type 2 diabetes mellitus and prediabetes, chronic kidney disease (CKD), heart failure, and immunosuppressive therapy with calcineurin inhibitors such as cyclosporine. In these conditions, central sympathetic outflow can be driven by deactivation of inhibitory neural inputs (e.g., baroreceptors), activation of excitatory neural inputs (e.g., carotid body chemoreceptors, renal afferents), or circulating angiotensin II (A II), which activates pools of excitatory brainstem neurons without a blood-brain barrier (**Fig. 45-5**). The emergence of new invasive procedures for lowering of sympathetic activity and BP in patients with refractory hypertension—an implantable carotid baroreceptor pacemaker[16] and catheter-based radiofrequency ablation of the renal sympathetic nerves[17]—has rekindled excitement about neural mechanisms, even before the procedures have approval by the Food and Drug Administration.

Baroreceptors and Hypertension. In hypertension, the baroreceptors reset to defend a higher level of BP. Baroreflex control of sinus node function is abnormal even in mild hypertension, but baroreflex control of systemic vascular resistance and BP is well preserved until diastolic function is impaired.[18] The surgically implanted carotid baroreceptor pacemaker produces sustained BP reductions in dog models of hypertension and is being evaluated in patients with medically refractory hypertension.[16] Complete baroreflex failure (see Chap. 94) rarely causes labile hypertension, most often seen in throat cancer survivors as a late complication of radiation therapy, which causes a gradual destruction of the baroreceptor nerves. In contrast, partial baroreceptor dysfunction is common in elderly hypertensives and typically is manifested with a triad of orthostatic hypotension, supine hypertension, and symptomatic postprandial hypotension, the last initiated by splanchnic pooling after carbohydrate-rich meals.

Obesity-Related Hypertension. Neural mechanisms of obesity-related hypertension deserve special mention. With weight gain, reflex sympathetic activation may be an important compensation to burn fat but at the expense of sympathetic overactivity in target tissues (i.e., vascular smooth muscle and kidney) that produces hypertension.[19] Hypertensive patients with the metabolic syndrome with or without new-onset type 2 diabetes have near-maximal rates of sympathetic firing. Although the sympathetic activation associates with insulin resistance, the precise stimulus to sympathetic outflow is unknown; candidates include leptin, other adipokines, and A II. Why weight loss causes much less improvement in hypertension than in diabetes remains unknown.[20]

Obstructive Sleep Apnea as a Cause of Neurogenic Hypertension (See Chap. 79.)**.** Patients with obstructive sleep apnea can have markedly elevated plasma and urine catecholamine levels, mimicking those seen in patients with pheochromocytoma (see Chap. 86). With repeated arterial desaturation during apneas, activation of carotid body chemoreceptors causes dramatic pressor episodes throughout the night and resets the chemoreceptor reflex; daytime normoxia is misinterpreted as hypoxia, producing sustained reflex sympathetic activation and hypertension even during waking hours.[21] Obstructive sleep apnea also accelerates the risk of several hypertensive complications (e.g., stroke, atrial fibrillation, and cardiovascular death) beyond that explained by BP elevation alone.

Long-Term Sympathetic Regulation of Blood Pressure. The sympathetic nervous system is well known to regulate short-term changes in BP, such as transient surges in BP during physical and emotional stress. In addition, sustained sympathetic activation contributes to long-term BP regulation because the renal sympathetic nerves potently stimulate renin release by stimulation of beta$_1$-adrenergic receptors in the juxtaglomerular apparatus and renal sodium reabsorption by stimulation of alpha$_1$-adrenergic receptors regulating Na^+,K^+-ATPase in the collecting duct. Catheter-based radiofrequency ablation of the renal sympathetic nerves seems to markedly lower BP in patients with medically refractory hypertension.[17] In addition, norepinephrine's action on alpha$_1$-adrenergic receptors stimulates cardiac and vascular smooth muscle hypertrophy. In patients with hypertension and left ventricular hypertrophy (LVH), cardiac norepinephrine spillover increases and may predispose to sudden cardiac death.

Renal Mechanisms

In many forms of experimental and human hypertension, the fundamental abnormality is an acquired or inherited defect in the kidneys' ability to excrete the excessive sodium load imposed by a modern diet high in salt.[22] As humans evolved in a low-sodium/high-potassium environment, the human kidney is ill-equipped to handle the current exposure to high sodium and low potassium.[8] Renal sodium retention expands the plasma volume, increasing cardiac output and triggering autoregulatory responses that increase systemic vascular resistance. Salt retention also augments the smooth muscle contraction produced by endogenous vasoconstrictors. Beyond raising BP, a high-salt diet also accelerates hypertensive target organ damage. A successful 30-year campaign in Finland to lower salt intake by one third was associated with a population-level fall in systolic and diastolic BP of 10 mm Hg and a 75% reduction in the incidence of CAD and stroke deaths.

Resetting of Pressure-Natriuresis. In normotensive individuals, BP elevation invokes an immediate increase in renal sodium excretion to shrink plasma volume and to return BP to normal. In almost all forms of hypertension, the pressure-natriuresis curve is shifted to the right, and in salt-sensitive hypertension, the slope is reduced. Resetting of the pressure-natriuresis curve prevents the return of BP to normal so that fluid balance is maintained but at the expense of high BP. It also leads to nocturia, one of the most common and bothersome symptoms in patients with uncontrolled hypertension. Hypertensive individuals excrete the same amount of a given dietary sodium load as normotensive individuals do, but at a higher BP, and require many more hours to excrete the sodium load and to achieve sodium balance. Renal inflammation is both the cause and consequence of renal medullary ischemia, the hallmark of both the initiation and progression of salt-dependent hypertension in rodent models.[23]

Low Birth Weight. Because of fetal undernutrition, low birth weight with reduced nephrogenesis increases the risk for development of adult salt-dependent hypertension. This association is independent of shared genes, shared postnatal environment, and adult risk factors for hypertension.[24] Adult hypertensives have fewer glomeruli per kidney but very few obsolescent glomeruli, suggesting that nephron dropout with decreased total filtration surface area is the cause and not the consequence of the hypertension. When they are exposed to a fast-food diet, low-birth-weight children are susceptible to rapid postnatal weight gain, leading to adolescent obesity and hypertension.

Genetic Contributions. Animal and human studies have implicated an important genetic contribution to salt-sensitive hypertension. Rats with inbred defects in the kidneys' ability to excrete sodium remain relatively normotensive on a sodium-restricted diet but become severely hypertensive when fed a high-sodium diet, a model of salt-sensitive hypertension that can be cured by interstrain renal transplantation. A similar gene-environment interaction has been postulated to explain why persons of sub-Saharan African ancestry remain normotensive on a sodium-restricted diet but are predisposed to hypertension when they are exposed to a high-sodium Western diet. Ancestral gene analysis has not defined the molecular basis for salt-dependent human hypertension but has identified a common genetic predisposition of African-origin populations to all nondiabetic forms of CKD, including focal glomerulosclerosis, AIDS, and hypertensive nephropathy. Sequence variations in the *MYH9* gene encoding nonmuscle myosin found in podocytes associate strongly with African ancestry and confer a twofold to fourfold increased risk of end-stage renal disease, independent of BP.[25] As the kidneys fail, BP becomes increasingly salt dependent.

Vascular Mechanisms

Alterations in the structure and function of small and large arteries play a pivotal role in the pathogenesis and progression of hypertension.

ENDOTHELIAL CELL DYSFUNCTION. The endothelial lining of blood vessels is critical to vascular health and constitutes a major defense against hypertension. Dysfunctional endothelium is characterized by impaired release of endothelium-derived relaxing factors (e.g., nitric oxide, endothelium-derived hyperpolarizing factor) and enhanced release of endothelium-derived constricting, proinflammatory, prothrombotic, and growth factors (**Fig. 45-6**).[26]

The endothelium of all blood vessels expresses the enzyme nitric oxide synthase, which can be activated by bradykinin, acetylcholine, or cyclic laminar shear stress. Nitric oxide synthase generates nitric oxide, a volatile gas that diffuses to the adjacent vascular smooth muscle and activates a series of G kinases that culminate in vasodilation (see Fig. 45-6).

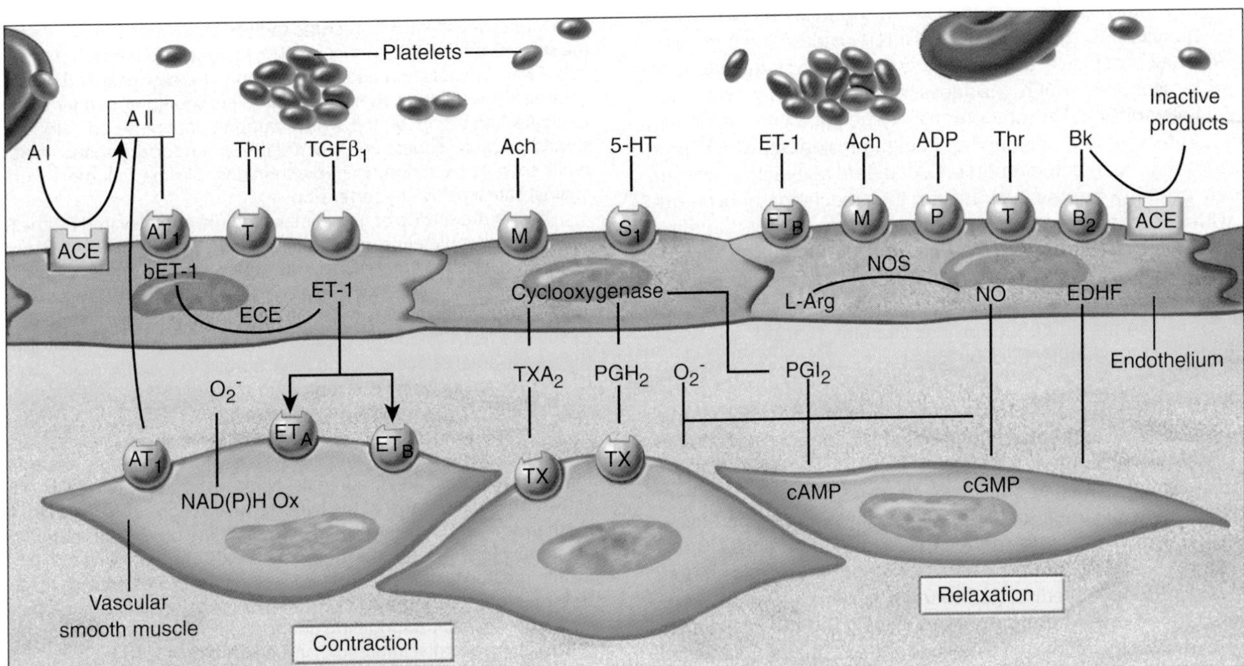

FIGURE 45-6 Endothelium-derived relaxing and constricting factors. Various blood- and platelet-derived substances can activate specific receptors (orange circles) on the endothelial membrane to release relaxing factors such as nitric oxide (NO), prostacyclin (PGI_2), and an endothelium-derived hyperpolarizing factor (EDHF). Contracting factors also are released, such as endothelin (ET-1), angiotensin (A II), and thromboxane A_2 (TXA_2), as well as prostaglandin H_2 (PGH_2). ACE = angiotensin-converting enzyme; 5-HT = serotonin; Bk = bradykinin; ECE = endothelin-converting enzyme; L-Arg = L-arginine; NOS = nitric oxide synthase; O_2^- = superoxide; $TGF\beta_1$ = transforming growth factor β1; Thr = thrombin. *(From Ruschitzka F, Corti R, Noll G, et al: A rationale for treatment of endothelial dysfunction in hypertension. J Hypertens 17[Suppl 1]:25, 1999.)*

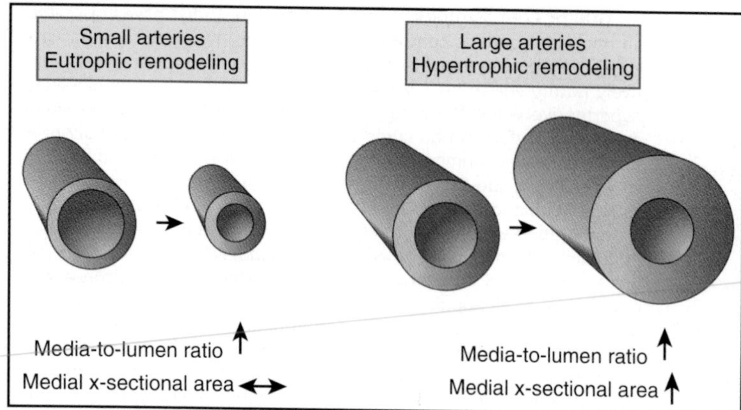

FIGURE 45-7 Vascular remodeling of small and large arteries in hypertension. Diagrams represent arteries in cross section showing the tunica adventitia, tunica media, and tunica intima. *(Modified from Duprez DA: Role of renin-angiotensin-aldosterone system in vascular remodeling and inflammation: A clinical review. J Hypertens 24:983, 2006.)*

In humans, endothelium-dependent vasodilation can be assessed by measuring increases in the large artery (forearm or coronary) diameter after intra-arterial infusion of acetylcholine or release of ischemia (e.g., arrested forearm circulation) or a sudden elevation in BP (cold pressor test; see Chaps. 52 and 61).

Mounting evidence indicates that smoldering vascular inflammation plays a central role in the genesis and complications of high BP. C-reactive protein (CRP; see Chap. 44), an easily measured serum biomarker, reports on inflammation.[27] Cross-sectional studies show strong correlations between elevated CRP and arterial stiffness and elevated pulse pressure. Longitudinal studies implicate elevated CRP levels as a risk marker (or risk factor) for new onset of hypertension and accelerated progression of hypertensive target organ disease, possibly beyond that explained by BP elevation alone.

Oxidative stress also contributes to endothelial cell vasodilator dysfunction in hypertension. Superoxide anion and other reactive oxygen species quench nitric oxide, thereby reducing its bioavailability.[28] Several pathways produce superoxide in arteries: nicotinamide adenine dinucleotide phosphate (NADPH) oxidases, which are expressed in all vascular cell types and activated by circulating A II; nitric oxide synthase, which produces superoxide only when an important cofactor (tetrahydrobiopterin) is deficient, a process known as nitric oxide synthase uncoupling; xanthine oxidase, which produces uric acid; and mitochondria. Generation of reactive oxygen species by xanthine oxidase accounts for the association of hyperuricemia with endothelial dysfunction and hypertension. The xanthine oxidase inhibitor allopurinol can normalize BP in two thirds of adolescents with hyperuricemia and recently diagnosed hypertension,[29] but allopurinol cannot be recommended as a routine antioxidant because of its serious side effect profile. Vitamins C and E are weak antioxidants that have little effect on BP.

VASCULAR REMODELING. Over time, endothelial cell dysfunction, neurohormonal activation, and elevated BP cause remodeling of blood vessels, which further perpetuates hypertension (**Fig. 45-7**).[30] An increase in the medial thickness relative to lumen diameter (increased media-to-lumen ratio) is the hallmark of hypertensive remodeling in small and large arteries. Vasoconstriction initiates small artery remodeling, which normalizes wall stress. Normal smooth muscle cells rearrange themselves around a smaller lumen diameter, a process termed inward eutrophic remodeling. The media-to-lumen ratio increases, but the medial cross-sectional area remains unchanged. By decreasing lumen diameter in the peripheral circulation, inward eutrophic remodeling increases systemic vascular resistance, the hemodynamic hallmark of diastolic hypertension.

In contrast, large artery remodeling is characterized by the expression of hypertrophic genes, triggering increases in medial thickness and in the media-to-lumen ratio. Such hypertrophic remodeling involves an increase in the size of vascular smooth muscle cells and an accumulation of extracellular matrix proteins, such as collagen, because of activation of transforming growth factor-β (TGF-β). The resultant large artery stiffness is the hemodynamic hallmark of ISH.

Antihypertensive therapy may not provide optimal cardiovascular protection unless it prevents or reverses vascular remodeling by normalizing hemodynamic load, restoring normal endothelial cell function, and eliminating the underlying neurohormonal activation.[30]

Hormonal Mechanisms: Renin-Angiotensin-Aldosterone System (See Fig. 25-3.)

Activation of the renin-angiotensin-aldosterone system (RAAS) is one of the most important mechanisms contributing to endothelial cell dysfunction, vascular remodeling, and hypertension (**Fig. 45-8**). Renin, a protease produced solely by the renal juxtaglomerular cells, cleaves angiotensinogen (renin substrate produced by the liver) to A I, which is converted by angiotensin-converting enzyme (ACE) to A II (see Chap. 93). ACE is most abundant in the lungs but is also present in the heart and systemic vasculature (tissue ACE). Chymase, a serine protease in the heart and systemic arteries, provides an alternative pathway for conversion of A I to A II. The interaction of A II with G protein–coupled AT_1 receptors activates numerous cellular processes that contribute to hypertension and accelerate hypertensive end-organ damage (see Fig. 45-8), including vasoconstriction, generation of reactive oxygen species, vascular inflammation, vascular and cardiac remodeling, and production of aldosterone, the principal mineralocorticoid. There is increasing evidence that aldosterone, A II, and even renin and prorenin activate multiple signaling pathways that can damage vascular health and cause hypertension.

ALDOSTERONE AND EPITHELIAL SODIUM CHANNEL REGULATION. RAAS activation is a major homeostatic mechanism to counter hypovolemic hypotension (as with hemorrhage or salt and water deprivation). Interaction of aldosterone with cytosolic mineralocorticoid receptors in the renal collecting duct cells recruits sodium channels from the cytosol to the surface of the renal epithelium. The recruited epithelial sodium channels (ENaCs) increase sodium reabsorption, thereby reexpanding plasma volume. Conversely, modern high-salt diets should engender continual feedback inhibition of the RAAS. Suppression of serum aldosterone should trigger sequestration of ENaCs by endocytosis and increased renal sodium excretion, thereby shrinking plasma volume to protect against salt-sensitive hypertension.

Thus, in the setting of high dietary sodium and elevated BP, the RAAS should be completely suppressed, and any degree of RAAS activity is inappropriate. In normotensive individuals, the risk for development of hypertension increases with increasing levels of serum aldosterone that are well within the normal range. By stimulating mineralocorticoid receptors in the heart and kidney, circulating aldosterone may contribute to the development of cardiac and renal fibrosis in hypertension.[31] By stimulating mineralocorticoid receptors in the brainstem, aldosterone also may contribute to sympathetic overactivity.

RECEPTOR-MEDIATED ACTIONS OF ANGIOTENSIN II. Two main angiotensin receptor types (AT) are known. AT_1 receptors are widely expressed in the vasculature, kidneys, adrenals, heart, liver, and brain. A I receptor activation explains most of the hypertensive actions of A II (see Fig. 45-8). Furthermore, enhanced AT_1-mediated signaling provides a central mechanistic explanation for the frequent coexistence of elevated BP with insulin resistance and atherosclerosis and constitutes a major therapeutic target for interruption of every step in cardiovascular disease progression, from vascular remodeling and formation of atherosclerotic plaque to stroke, myocardial infarction, and death (**Fig. 45-9**).

In contrast, AT_2 receptors distribute widely in the fetus, but in adults they localize only in the adrenal medulla, uterus, ovaries, vascular endothelium, and distinct brain regions. In rodents, AT_2 receptor activation opposes some of the deleterious effects of AT_1 receptors by promoting endothelium-dependent vasodilation by bradykinin and nitric oxide pathways. Animal studies have suggested that AT_2 receptors can be profibrotic, but their role in human hypertension remains speculative. The

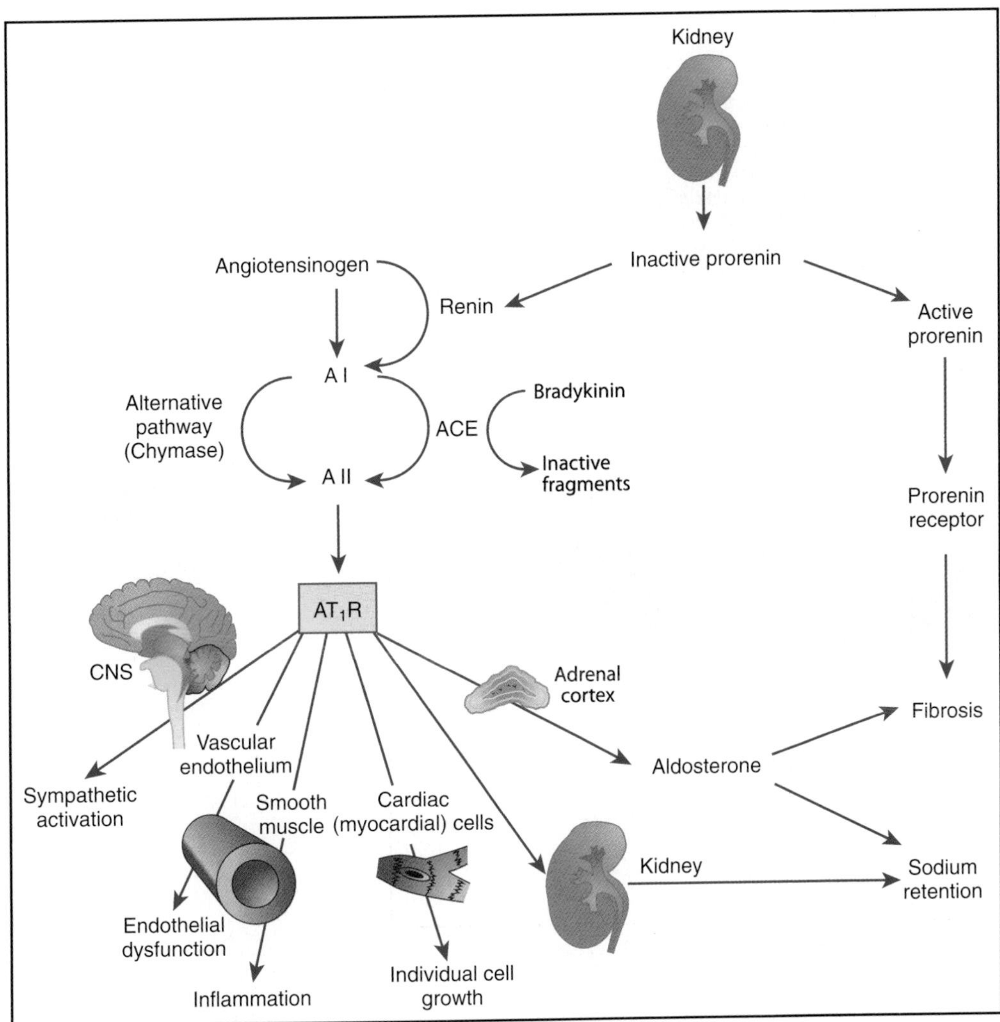

FIGURE 45-8 The renin-angiotensin-aldosterone system. A I = angiotensin I; A II = angiotensin II; ACE = angiotensin-converting enzyme; AT_1R = angiotensin I receptor.

finding of several angiotensin metabolites also has added to the complexity of the RAAS (see Fig. 45-e4 on website).

Receptor-Mediated Actions of Renin and Prorenin. Traditionally, prorenin was considered the inactive precursor of renin, an enzyme that functions solely to generate A I by enzymatic cleavage of angiotensinogen. These concepts are rapidly evolving as newer studies implicate prorenin and renin as direct cardiac and renal toxins. Prorenin is inactive because a 43–amino acid hinge is closed and prevents it from binding to angiotensinogen. The kidneys convert inactive prorenin to active renin by enzymatic cleavage of this inhibitory hinge region. When circulating prorenin binds to a newly discovered (pro)renin receptor in the heart and kidneys, the hinge is opened (but not cleaved), and this nonenzymatic process fully activates prorenin (see Fig. 45-e5 on website).[32] Activation of the (pro)renin receptor increases TGF-β production, leading to collagen deposition and fibrosis. This receptor-mediated process does not depend on A II generation, ACE inhibitors (ACEIs), or angiotensin receptor blockers (ARBs). Although these are excellent antihypertensives (see Chap. 46), they trigger large reactive increases in prorenin and renin production that may counter some of the cardiovascular protection afforded by reduced AT_1 receptor activation. The reactive increases are even greater with the new direct renin inhibitor aliskiren, which reduces renin's ability to cleave angiotensinogen and to generate A I but nevertheless does not inhibit profibrotic signaling by the (pro)renin receptor.[33] As prorenin blood levels normally exceed those of renin by 100-fold, (pro) renin receptor activation may turn out to be an important factor in human hypertension.

T Cells and Angiotensin II–Induced Hypertension. T cells, which express AT_1 receptors and NADPH oxidase, may play an important role in the genesis of A II–dependent hypertension, particularly obesity-related hypertension, as the activated T cells are selectively sequestered in adipose tissue.[34] Homing of activated T cells to perivascular fat promotes vasoconstriction and vascular remodeling. Homing of activated T cells to perinephric fat promotes renal dysfunction and sodium retention (**Fig. 45-10**) (see also Fig. 93-2).

Pathogenesis of Hypertensive Heart Disease

Hypertension is a major risk factor not only for CAD but also for LVH and heart failure.

Pressure Overload Hypertrophy

In hypertensive patients, LVH powerfully and independently predicts morbidity and mortality, predisposing to heart failure, ventricular tachyarrhythmia, ischemic stroke, atrial fibrillation, and embolic stroke. Major advances have increased our understanding of the molecular signal transduction pathways underlying pressure overload cardiomyocyte hypertrophy.[35] Moreover, the structural abnormalities in the hypertensive heart extend beyond myocyte hypertrophy; they also include medial hypertrophy of the intramyocardial coronary arteries and collagen deposition leading to cardiac fibrosis.[36] These changes result from pressure overload and the neurohormonal activation that contributes to hypertension. In animal models, A II, aldosterone, norepinephrine, and prorenin accelerate pressure overload cardiomyocyte hypertrophy and promote cardiac fibrosis, the hallmarks of pathologic LVH (in contrast to the physiologic hypertrophy of exercise training, which does not involve fibrosis).

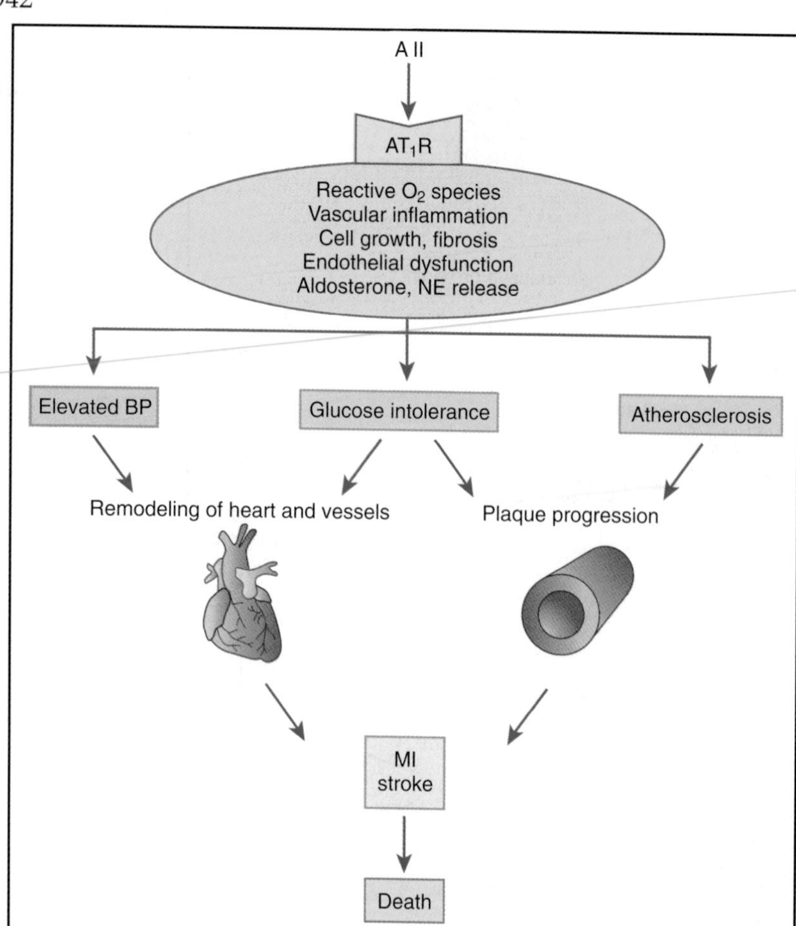

FIGURE 45-9 Schematic representation of the central role of angiotensin 1 receptor (AT_1R)–mediated signaling in cardiovascular disease progression. A II = angiotensin II; MI = myocardial infarction; NE = norepinephrine.

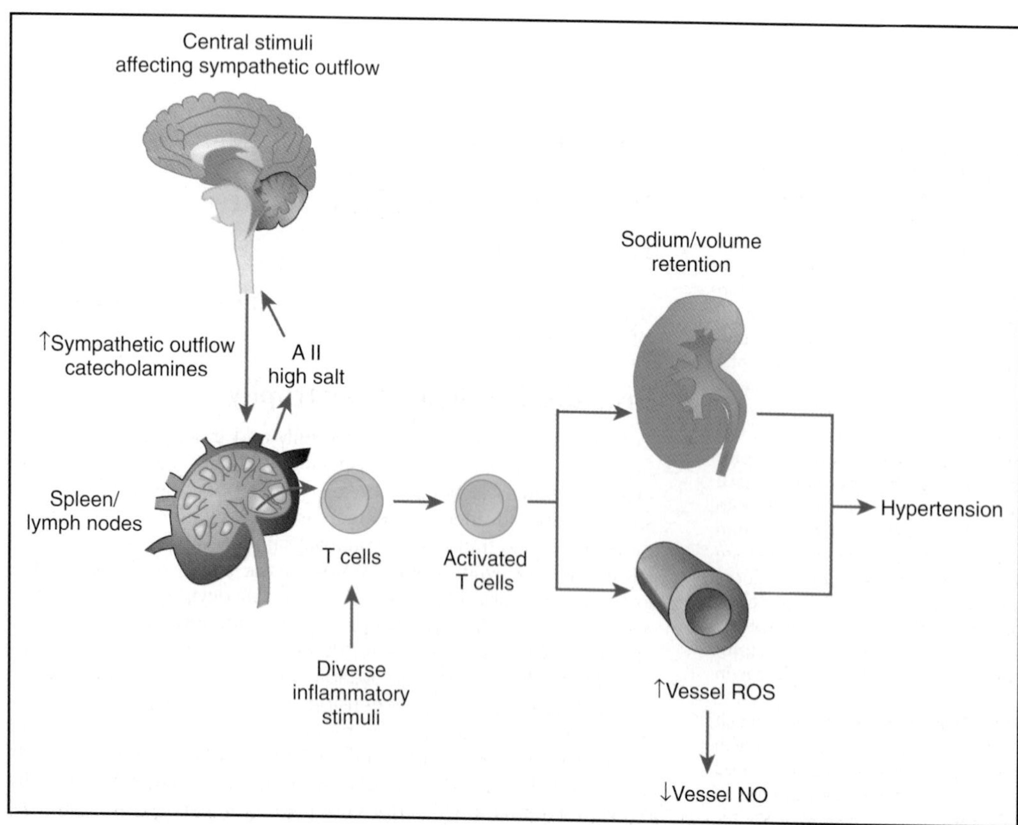

FIGURE 45-10 Proposed mechanism for the role of adaptive immunity in hypertension. Hypertensive stimuli such as angiotensin II (A II) can participate in T-cell activation by directly acting on T cells and via central nervous system activation. Central nervous system activation leads to increased sympathetic outflow, which also promotes T-cell activation and enhances chemokine production in perivascular fat and perinephric adipose tissue, promoting T-cell accumulation at these sites. Diverse inflammatory stimuli also promote hypertension by activating T cells. Activated T cells enter the perivascular fat, activating the vascular production of reactive oxygen species (ROS) and reducing nitric oxide (NO) production, thus causing vasoconstriction. T cells also affect renal sodium and volume handling. These actions on the kidney and vasculature lead to hypertension. *(From Harrison DG, Guzik TJ, Goronzy J, Weyand C: Is hypertension an immunologic disease? Curr Cardiol Rep 10:464, 2008.)*

IMPAIRED CORONARY VASODILATOR RESERVE. The hypertrophied hypertensive heart has normal resting coronary blood flow, but vasodilator reserve becomes impaired when myocyte mass outstrips the blood supply. Even in the absence of atherosclerosis, the hypertensive heart has blunted or absent coronary vasodilator reserve, leading to subendocardial ischemia under conditions of increased myocardial oxygen demand. The combination of subendocardial ischemia and cardiac fibrosis impairs diastolic relaxation, leading to exertional dyspnea and diastolic heart failure.

Heart Failure (see Chaps. 26 and 30)

Before the advent of effective drug therapy for hypertension in the late 1950s, heart failure caused most deaths from hypertension. Better management has substantially reduced hypertension-related deaths from heart failure and significantly delayed its onset, but hypertension remains the most common cause of heart failure with preserved systolic function. In addition, hypertension indirectly leads to systolic heart failure as a major risk factor for myocardial infarction. It is unclear whether mild or moderate hypertension alone, without myocardial infarction, leads to systolic heart failure.[36]

Diagnosis and Initial Evaluation of Hypertension

Hypertension has been termed the silent killer, an asymptomatic chronic disorder that, undetected and untreated, silently damages the blood vessels, heart, brain, and kidneys. However, it may not be entirely asymptomatic; in double-blind placebo-controlled trials, patients' quality of life ratings were often found to improve with successful drug treatment of hypertension. Control of hypertension can improve exertional dyspnea caused by diastolic dysfunction, nocturia caused by resetting of pressure-natriuresis, and possibly even erectile dysfunction caused by endothelial dysfunction.

Initial Evaluation of the Hypertensive Patient

The initial evaluation for hypertension should accomplish three goals: the accurate measurement of BP; the assessment of the patient's overall cardiovascular risk; and the detection of secondary (i.e., identifiable and potentially curable) forms of hypertension.

MEASUREMENT OF BLOOD PRESSURE

Staging of Office Blood Pressure

According to the 2003 guidelines of the Seventh Report of the Joint National Committee on Prevention, Detection, Evaluation, and Treatment of High Blood Pressure (JNC 7),[3] which are still in effect until the publication of JNC 8, BP is staged as normal, prehypertension, or hypertension by the average of two or more readings taken at two or more office visits (**Table 45-1**; see Table 49-5).

MEASUREMENT TECHNIQUE (see Chap. 12). In the office, BP should be measured at least twice after 5 minutes of rest, with the patient seated in a chair, the back supported, and the arm bare and at heart level. A large adult-sized cuff should be used to measure BP in overweight adults because the standard-sized cuff can spuriously elevate readings. Tobacco and caffeine should be avoided for at least 30 minutes. BP should be measured in both arms and after 5 minutes of standing, the latter to exclude a significant postural fall in BP, particularly in older persons and in those with diabetes or other conditions (e.g., Parkinson's disease) that predispose to autonomic insufficiency.

TABLE 45-1 Staging of Office Blood Pressure*

BP STAGE	SYSTOLIC BP (MM HG)	DIASTOLIC BP (MM HG)
Normal	<120	<80
Prehypertension	120-139	80-89
Stage 1 hypertension	140-159	90-99
Stage 2 hypertension	≥160	≥100

*Calculation of seated BP is based on the mean of two or more readings on two separate office visits.

From Chobanian AV, Bakris GL, Black HR, et al: The Seventh Report of the Joint National Committee on Prevention, Detection, Evaluation, and Treatment of High Blood Pressure: The JNC 7 report. JAMA 289:2560, 2003.

Home and Ambulatory Monitoring

An individual's BP varies widely throughout a 24-hour period and is therefore impossible to characterize accurately, except by repeated measurements under various conditions (see Fig. 45-e6 on website). Out-of-office readings provide a clear picture of usual BP for accurate diagnosis and management. These readings predict cardiovascular events better than office readings do, and they overcome many of the pitfalls of office measurement, including physician errors and alerting (i.e., "white coat") reactions. Home BP monitoring also improves medication adherence by actively involving patients in their own medical care.

For these reasons, new position papers on home BP monitoring from both the United States and Europe make the following recommendations: that home BP monitoring should become a routine part of the clinical management of patients with known or suspected hypertension the same way that home blood glucose monitoring is essential to the management of diabetes; that two (or three) readings should be taken in the morning and at night for 1 week, with a total of at least 12 readings being averaged to make clinical decisions; and that the target treatment goal is an average home BP <135/85 mm Hg for most patients and <130/80 mm Hg for high-risk patients, such as those with CAD, heart failure, diabetes, or CKD.[37,38]

A validated electronic oscillometric monitor with an arm cuff should be chosen from the Dabl educational website (*dableducational.com*). Each patient's monitor needs to be checked in the office for accuracy and cuff size because many manufacturers provide only a standard adult cuff. Patients need to be taught correct measurement technique and how to avoid reporting bias. Wrist monitors are inaccurate and thus not recommended. The oscillometric method may not work well in patients with atrial fibrillation or frequent extrasystoles. Some patients become obsessed about taking their BP and need to limit measurement.

Ambulatory monitoring provides automated measurements of BP during a 24-hour period while patients are engaged in their usual activities, including sleep. Prospective outcome studies in both treated and untreated patients have shown that ambulatory BP measurement predicts fatal and nonfatal myocardial infarction and stroke better than standard office measurement does (**Fig. 45-11**).[39] Recommended normal values include an average daytime BP <135/85 mm Hg, nighttime BP <120/70 mm Hg, and 24-hour BP <130/80 mm Hg. Some experts have recommended a lower cutoff value of 130/80 mm Hg as a more stringent definition of normal daytime BP.

WHITE COAT HYPERTENSION. About 20% of patients with elevated office BPs have normal home or ambulatory BPs. If the daytime BP is <135/85 mm Hg (or preferably <130/80 mm Hg) and there is no target organ damage despite consistently elevated office readings, the patient has "office-only" or white coat hypertension, caused by a transient adrenergic response to the measurement of BP only in the physician's office. The prognostic importance of white coat hypertension remains unresolved. The cardiovascular risk seems intermediate between that in persons with consistently normal BP and that in persons with consistently high BP.

Many patients do not have pure white coat hypertension but rather "white coat aggravation," a white coat reaction superimposed on a milder level of out-of-office hypertension that nevertheless needs treatment (see Fig. 45-e6 on website). Currently, Medicare reimburses ambulatory BP monitoring for suspected white coat hypertension if the following criteria are met: office BP >140/90 mm Hg on at least three separate office visits with two measurements made at each visit; at least two out-of-office BPs <140/90 mm Hg; and no evidence of target organ damage. The indications for ambulatory monitoring

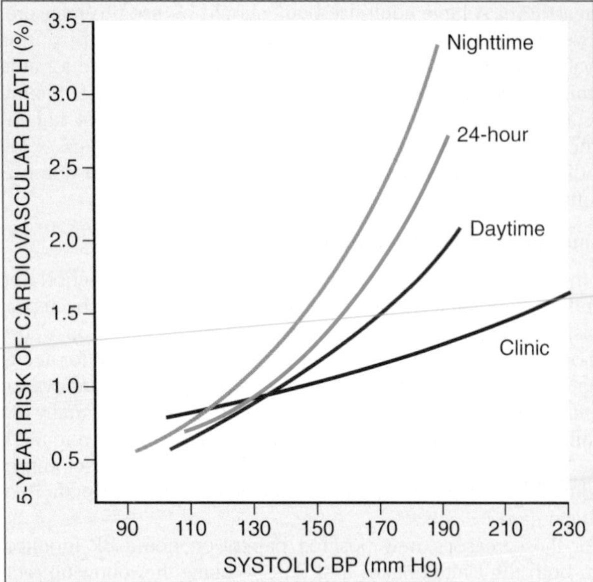

FIGURE 45-11 Superiority of ambulatory over office BP measurement as a measure of cardiovascular risk. Shown is the adjusted 5-year risk of cardiovascular death (number of deaths per 100 subjects) in the study cohort of 5292 patients for office BP and ambulatory BP. *(From Dolan E, Santon A, Thijs L, et al: Superiority of ambulatory over clinic BP measurement in predicting mortality: The Dublin outcome study. Hypertension 46:156, 2005.)*

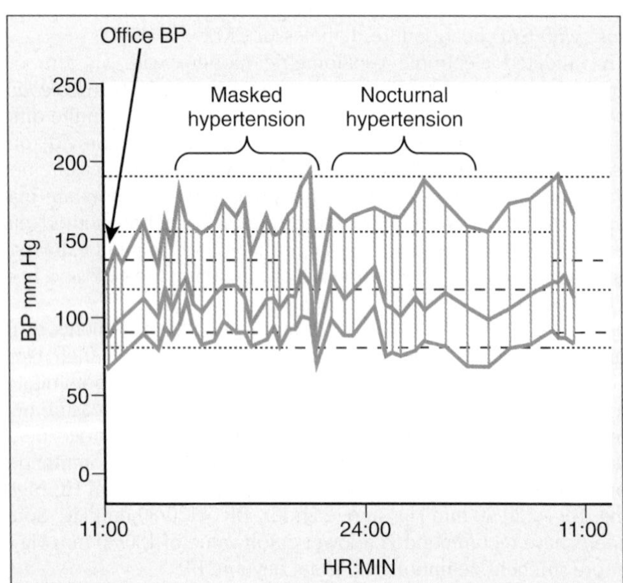

FIGURE 45-12 A 24-hour ambulatory BP recording in a patient with apparently normal office BP but with masked hypertension and nocturnal hypertension. *(From Dr. R. G. Victor, Cedars-Sinai Medical Center, Los Angeles, California.)*

should be expanded. In up to 30% of treated patients with persistently elevated office BP, for example, ambulatory monitoring documents adequate or excessive control of hypertension, eliminating overtreatment.

MASKED HYPERTENSION. Another example of the importance of ambulatory monitoring is in patients in whom office readings underestimate out-of-office BP, presumably because of sympathetic overactivity in daily life caused by job or home stress, tobacco abuse, or other adrenergic stimulation that dissipates when they come to the office (**Fig. 45-12**). Such documentation prevents undertreatment of this masked hypertension, which can affect more than 10% of patients and clearly increases cardiovascular risk, despite normal office BP readings.

TABLE 45-2 Risks Influencing Prognosis in Patients with Hypertension

Risk Factors for Cardiovascular Disease
Systolic and diastolic BP levels
Levels of pulse pressure (in the elderly)
Age: men >55 years; women >65 years
Smoking
Dyslipidemia (LDL-C >115 mg/dL)
Impaired fasting glucose (102-125 mg/dL) or abnormal glucose tolerance test result
Family history of premature cardiovascular disease
Abdominal obesity
Diabetes mellitus
Subclinical Target Organ Damage
Left ventricular hypertrophy
Carotid wall thickening or plaque
Low estimated glomerular filtration rate ≤60 mL/min/1.73 m^2
Microalbuminuria
Ankle-brachial BP index <0.9
Established Target Organ Damage
Cerebrovascular disease: ischemic stroke, cerebral hemorrhage, transient ischemic attack
Heart disease: myocardial infarction, angina, coronary revascularization, heart failure
Renal disease: diabetic nephropathy, renal impairment
Peripheral arterial disease
Advanced retinopathy: hemorrhages or exudates, papilledema

Modified from Mancia G, De Backer G, Dominiczak A, et al: 2007 Guidelines for the Management of Arterial Hypertension: The Task Force for the Management of Arterial Hypertension of the European Society of Hypertension (ESH) and of the European Society of Cardiology (ESC). Eur Heart J 28:1462, 2007.

OTHER USES OF AMBULATORY MONITORING. Ambulatory monitoring is the only way to detect hypertension during sleep (see Fig. 45-12). BP normally dips during sleep and increases sharply when a person awakens and becomes active (see Fig. 45-e6 on website). Nocturnal hypertension increases the aggregate hemodynamic load on the cardiovascular system and predicts cardiovascular outcomes better than either daytime ambulatory BP or standard office measurements (see Fig. 45-11).[39] Nocturnal hypertension is particularly common in patients with CKD, presumably because of increased cardiac output (centralization of an expanded plasma volume while supine) and increased systemic vascular resistance (failure of sympathetic vasoconstrictor drive to suppress normally during sleep because of persistent activation of an excitatory reflex in the diseased kidneys). In addition, ambulatory BP monitoring is particularly useful in diagnosis of baroreflex impairment.

CARDIOVASCULAR RISK STRATIFICATION (see Chap. 44). In hypertensive individuals, cardiovascular risk increases sharply with BP stage (see Table 45-1; see Table 49-5), but this is not the only factor to consider. The gradient between increasing levels of BP and cardiovascular risk becomes progressively steeper as additional risk factors are added. Cardiovascular risk also increases dramatically with hypertensive target organ damage and with additional cardiovascular risk factors often present in patients with hypertension or prehypertension (**Table 45-2**).[40] In particular, more than 75% of hypertensive patients meet current criteria for initiation of lipid-lowering medication (low-density lipoprotein cholesterol level >130 mg/dL), and 25% have diabetes.[41] Thus, the minimal laboratory testing required for the initial evaluation of hypertension includes determination of blood electrolyte values, fasting glucose concentration, and serum creatinine level with calculated glomerular filtration rate (GFR); fasting lipid panel; hematocrit; spot urinalysis, including urine albumin-to-creatinine ratio; and resting 12-lead electrocardiogram.

Definition of High Risk

Whereas hypertension is present in 25% of adults in the general population, it is present in 75% of adults with diabetes and in more than

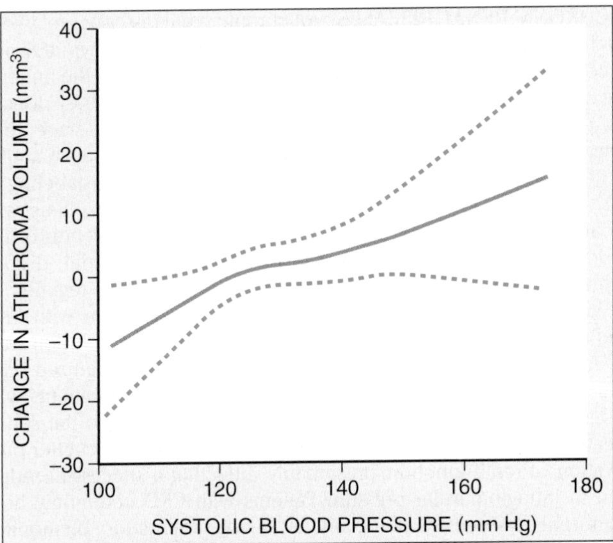

FIGURE 45-13 Relationship between systolic blood pressure and the rate of progression of coronary atheroma in 274 patients who completed the intravascular ultrasound substudy of the CAMELOT (Comparison of Amlodipine Versus Enalapril to Limit Occurrences of Thrombosis) trial. A systolic blood pressure in the range of 120 to 140 mm Hg corresponded to no net progression or regression of coronary disease. Values above this range were associated with progression and those below were associated with regression of disease. *(From Sipahi I, Tuzcu EM, Schoenhagen P, et al: Effects of normal, pre-hypertensive, and hypertensive blood pressure levels on progression of coronary atherosclerosis. J Am Coll Cardiol 48:833, 2006.)*

90% of those with CKD. Either of these two comorbidities dramatically increases the cardiovascular risk associated with hypertension, and the presence of hypertension greatly accelerates the progression to end-stage renal disease. Therefore, the 2003 JNC 7 guidelines recommend a usual BP of 140/90 mm Hg as the threshold for initiation of antihypertensive medication in most patients, with a lower threshold of 130/80 mm Hg for high-risk patients with diabetes or CKD.[3] On the basis of more recent data, the operational definition of high-risk patients now includes most cardiology patients—those with established CAD, CAD risk equivalents, carotid artery disease (carotid bruit or abnormal carotid ultrasound study), peripheral artery disease, abdominal aortic aneurysm, heart failure, or high risk for CAD (10-year Framingham risk score of >10%) (see Chaps. 44 and 49).[5] In particular, in patients with established CAD, a continuous relationship exists between systolic BP and the rate of progression of coronary atherosclerosis (determined by intravascular ultrasound) over a wide range of systolic pressures, beginning as low as 100 mm Hg (**Fig. 45-13**).[42]

Evaluation of Target Organ Disease

Traditionally, the complications of hypertension are viewed as hypertensive, caused by the increased level of BP per se, or atherosclerotic, caused by concomitant atherosclerosis, with BP elevation playing a variable role. This view is oversimplified, however, because both types of complications frequently coexist, as exemplified by hypertensive retinopathy (see Fig. 45-e7 on website)[43] or hypertensive heart disease.

HYPERTENSIVE HEART DISEASE. Hypertension may contribute to CAD more than is commonly realized because hypertensives have more silent ischemia and unrecognized myocardial infarctions, and patients with acute myocardial infarction often have preexisting hypertension that evaded detection or treatment. Assessment of BP is inaccurate during an acute coronary syndrome because of pain-induced BP rise or dysautonomia or pump failure decreasing BP. Preexisting hypertension increases the case-fatality rate associated with an acute myocardial infarction and substantially increases the risk of hemorrhagic stroke during thrombolytic therapy, especially when systolic BP exceeds 175 mm Hg.

On the electrocardiogram, LVH with strain is a serious harbinger of new-onset heart failure and heart failure death.[44] Echocardiography detects LVH more sensitively than electrocardiography does. Whereas electrocardiographic LVH is present in 5% to 10% of hypertensives, echocardiographic LVH is present in nearly 30% of unselected hypertensive adults and in up to 90% of patients with severe uncontrolled hypertension. Cardiac magnetic resonance imaging (MRI) is even more sensitive, detecting LVH in 28% of white hypertensives but in 62% of black hypertensives.[45]

LARGE-VESSEL DISEASE (see Chaps. 60 and 61). Hypertension also constitutes a major risk factor for and is present in the overwhelming majority of patients with aortic dissection (distal more than proximal dissection), abdominal aortic aneurysm, and peripheral arterial disease. One-time abdominal ultrasound screening for abdominal aortic aneurysm is recommended after the age of 65 years in smokers and in those with severe systolic hypertension, and it should be performed if aortic pulsations are detected below the umbilicus because most abdominal aortic aneurysms occur below the origin of the renal arteries. Hypertension is present in 50% of patients with Takayasu arteritis, a large-cell arteritis common in Asia and India.

CEREBROVASCULAR DISEASE (see Chap. 62). Hypertension is a major risk factor for stroke and dementia, often the two most dreaded complications of aging. Hypertension accounts for 50% of strokes. In hypertensives, 80% of strokes are ischemic (thrombotic or embolic) and 20% are hemorrhagic. The onset of ischemic stroke markedly increases on wakening, corresponding to the morning surge in BP. Hypertensive patients with asymptomatic carotid bruits should undergo Doppler ultrasonography. The risk of stroke is greatest in older patients with ISH. In middle-aged and elderly hypertensives, asymptomatic cerebral white matter lesions on MRI are remarkably common and likely accelerate the brain atrophy and vascular dementia that occur with aging.

CHRONIC KIDNEY DISEASE (see Chap. 93). Hypertension follows only diabetes as a risk factor for CKD. Traditionally, the typical pathologic change of small scarred kidneys (termed hypertensive nephrosclerosis) was assumed to result from chronic exposure of the renal parenchyma to excessive pressure and flow and to be the most common cause of end-stage renal disease among blacks. However, recent work on the *MYH9* gene locus suggests that many cases of presumed hypertensive nephrosclerosis in blacks may result primarily from an abnormal gene product: nonmuscle myosin, a protein that regulates podocyte function.[46]

Quantitative estimates of urinary albumin excretion and GFR (the latter from *www.kdoqi.org*) should be obtained from a spot urine collection. Microalbuminuria (defined as a urine albumin–to–urine creatinine ratio of 30 to 300 mg/mg) is a sensitive early marker of kidney damage and a powerful independent predictor of cardiovascular complications from hypertension, presumably because it reflects systemic vascular disease (see Chaps. 44 and 93). In patients with hypertension, the presence of renal damage dramatically increases the risk of a cardiovascular event. Most patients with hypertension-associated CKD die of heart attack or stroke before renal function deteriorates sufficiently to require chronic hemodialysis.

IDENTIFIABLE (SECONDARY) FORMS OF HYPERTENSION. The third goal of the initial evaluation is to detect identifiable causes of hypertension, thereby offering the possibility of cure to some patients, particularly those with severe or refractory hypertension (**Table 45-3**).

Renal Parenchymal Disease (see Chap. 93)

Renal parenchymal disease is the most common cause of secondary hypertension, responsible for 2% to 5% of cases. As chronic glomerulonephritis has become less common, diabetes and hypertension are the most common risk factors for CKD. The prevalence of chronic renal disease, defined by a reduction in the GFR to less than 60 mL/min/1.73 m² or persistent albuminuria of more than 300 mg/day, affects some 11% (19.2 million) of the adult U.S. population.[47]

As previously noted, microalbuminuria of 30 to 300 mg/day relates closely to target organ damage and should be determined in every

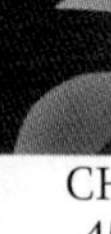

CH 45

TABLE 45-3 Overall Guide to Workup for Identifiable Causes of Hypertension

	DIAGNOSTIC PROCEDURE	
DIAGNOSIS	INITIAL	ADDITIONAL
Chronic renal disease	Urinalysis, serum creatinine, renal sonography	Isotopic renography, renal biopsy
Renovascular disease	Renal sonography (atrophic kidney)	Magnetic resonance or computed tomography (CT) angiography, Duplex Doppler sonography, digital subtraction renal angiography
Coarctation	Blood pressure in legs	Echocardiography, magnetic resonance imaging, aortography
Primary aldosteronism	Plasma renin, serum aldosterone	Salt loading, adrenal vein sampling
Cushing syndrome	1-mg dexamethasone suppression test	Urinary cortisol after variable doses of dexamethasone, adrenal CT, scintiscans
Pheochromocytoma	Plasma-free metanephrines	24-hr urinary metanephrines and catecholamines, adrenal CT

new hypertensive patient by testing of a single voided urine specimen. Measurement of the serum creatinine level by itself is an inadequate screening test for significant renal damage, particularly in elderly patients. Therefore, creatinine clearance should be calculated with the Cockcroft-Gault equation or the Modification of Diet in Renal Disease (MDRD) equation, taking age, sex, and body weight into account.[47] However, the MDRD equation does not account for other factors that affect creatinine generation by muscle, such as diet and physical conditioning. Serum cystatin C, an endogenous 13-kDa protein filtered by the glomeruli and reabsorbed and metabolized by the proximal tubular epithelium, with very little being excreted in the urine, is being evaluated as a potential replacement for serum creatinine because it is less affected by muscle mass.[48] Once renal disease begins, it usually progresses, following the concept that a loss of filtration surface leads to both glomerular and systemic hypertension, which engenders more glomerular sclerosis, setting up a cycle of progressive disease. Therefore, it is critical to identify renal damage early, because removal of causal or aggravating factors can prevent the otherwise inexorable progress of renal damage. These factors include obstruction of the urinary tract, depletion of effective circulating volume, nephrotoxic agents, and most important, uncontrolled hypertension.

ACUTE RENAL DISEASES. Hypertension may appear with any sudden, severe insult to the kidneys that markedly impairs excretion of salt and water, which leads to volume expansion, or reduces renal blood flow (e.g., sudden bilateral renal ischemia because of cholesterol emboli), which activates the RAAS (e.g., bilateral ureteral obstruction). Reversal of hypertension has been particularly striking in men with high-pressure chronic retention of urine, who may manifest renal failure and severe hypertension, both of which may be ameliorated by relief of the obstruction. Some vasculitides also produce rapidly progressive renal damage.

Two commonly used classes of drugs, nonsteroidal anti-inflammatory drugs (NSAIDs) and inhibitors of the renin-angiotensin system, may suddenly worsen renal function in patients with preexisting renal diseases. NSAIDs block the synthesis of prostaglandins, which act as vasodilators within the kidney. Renin-angiotensin inhibitors, both ACEIs and ARBs, may precipitate acute renal failure in patients with bilateral renovascular disease whose renal perfusion depends on high levels of A II.

CHRONIC RENAL DISEASES. All chronic renal diseases are associated with a higher prevalence of hypertension, and hypertension accelerates the progression of renal damage, regardless of the underlying cause of the renal disease. In patients with chronic kidney disease, the control of hypertension slows the progression to end-stage renal disease.[49] However, uncertainty remains about the BP goal of antihypertensive therapy in patients with CKD. Perhaps the mislabeling of *MYH9* nephropathy as hypertensive nephrosclerosis explains why renal function continued to decline 5 years after completion of the African American Study of Kidney Disease (AASK) trial, despite achievement of a BP of 133/78 mm Hg on an ACEI-based regimen.[46]

With whatever drugs are chosen to treat hypertension with CKD, and particularly with ACEIs and ARBs, caution is needed in lowering BP too rapidly and in the presence of previously unrecognized bilateral renovascular disease, found in as many as 20% of patients with progressive renal damage. However, a modest increase in the serum creatinine level, averaging 30% above baseline, predicts a better preservation of renal function, presumably reflecting a successful reduction in intraglomerular pressure. Patients with CKD commonly have nocturnal hypertension detectable by 24-hour ambulatory BP monitoring (see Figs. 45-11 and 45-12).[50]

Patients with diabetic nephropathy (see Chaps. 64 and 93) show particular protection against progressive renal damage by reduction of elevated BP with an ARB- or ACEI-based regimen. The role of the direct renin inhibitors has yet to be established; CKD patients should be monitored often for hyperkalemia. Most CKD patients require the addition of at least two more drugs in addition to ACEI or ARB, typically a loop diuretic and a calcium channel blocker, to control their hypertension.

Hemodialysis Patients

In patients on dialysis, hypertension is a risk factor for mortality. Beyond the primary influence of excess fluid volume, hypertension can be accentuated by the accumulation of endogenous inhibitors of nitric oxide synthase and sympathetic overactivity. With neither the vasoconstrictor effects of renal renin nor the vasodepressor actions of various renal hormones, BP may be particularly labile and sensitive to changes in fluid volume. In patients receiving maintenance hemodialysis every 48 hours, elevated BPs tend to fall progressively after dialysis is completed, remain depressed during the first 24 hours, and rise again during the second day as a result of excessive fluid retention. Only gradually achieving and maintaining dry weight, as with 8-hour nocturnal hemodialysis, can control BP.

Renal Transplantation

Although successful renal transplantation may cure primary hypertension, various problems can result, with about 50% of recipients becoming hypertensive within 1 year. These problems include stenosis of the renal artery at the site of anastomosis, rejection reactions, high doses of glucocorticoids and cyclosporine or tacrolimus, and excess renin derived from the retained diseased kidneys. ACEI or ARB therapy may obviate the need to remove the native diseased kidneys to relieve hypertension caused by their persistent secretion of renin. The source of the donor kidney may also play a role in the subsequent development of hypertension in the recipient. Hypertension occurs more frequently when donors have had a family history of hypertension or when the donors have died of subarachnoid hemorrhage and had probably had high BP.

Renovascular Hypertension

The prevalence of proven renovascular hypertension in the overall hypertensive population is unknown, but significant renal artery stenosis has been found in 14% of hypertensive patients undergoing coronary angiography followed by renal angiography. Such "drive-by" renal angiography is discouraged. Renal artery stenosis is rather easy to find but difficult to prove as the cause of reversible hypertension. Moreover, the risks of revascularization often outweigh the benefits (see Chap. 63).[51]

Screening should focus on those hypertensive patients who have multiple features known to be associated with renovascular

TABLE 45-4 Clinical Clues for Renovascular Hypertension

History
Onset of hypertension before 30 years or after 50 years of age
Abrupt onset of hypertension
Severe or resistant hypertension
Symptoms of atherosclerotic disease elsewhere
Negative family history of hypertension
Smoker
Worsening renal function after renin-angiotensin inhibition
Recurrent "flash" pulmonary edema

Examination
Abdominal bruits
Other bruits
Advanced fundal changes

Laboratory Findings
Secondary aldosteronism
Higher plasma renin level
Low serum potassium level
Low serum sodium level
Proteinuria, usually moderate
Elevated serum creatinine level
Unilateral small (atrophic) kidney size by ultrasound examination

hypertension. The greater the number of clues, the more extensive the search should be (**Table 45-4**).

CLASSIFICATION. In adults, the two major types of renovascular disease tend to appear at different times and to affect men and women differently. Atherosclerotic disease affecting mainly the proximal third of the main renal artery is seen mostly in older men. Fibroplastic disease involving mainly the distal two thirds and branches of the renal arteries appears most commonly in younger women. As the population grows older, 90% of cases are caused by atherosclerotic disease and only 10% by fibroplastic disease. Although the nonatherosclerotic stenoses may involve all layers of the renal artery, the most common is fibromuscular dysplasia.

A number of other intrinsic and extrinsic causes of renovascular hypertension are known, including cholesterol emboli in the renal artery or compression of this vessel by nearby tumors. Most renovascular hypertension develops from partial obstruction of one main renal artery, but only a branch need be involved; segmental disease has been found in about 10% of cases. On the other hand, if apparent complete occlusion of the renal artery is slow to develop, enough collateral flow will become available to preserve the viability of the kidney. Such seemingly nonfunctioning kidneys may secrete renin and cause hypertension. If recognized, such totally occluded vessels can sometimes be repaired, resulting in return of renal function and relief of hypertension. Renovascular stenosis is often bilateral, although usually one side is predominant. Bilateral disease should be suspected in those with renal insufficiency, particularly if rapidly progressive oliguric renal failure develops without evidence of obstructive uropathy, and even more so if it develops after the start of ACEI or ARB therapy.

MECHANISMS. The sequence of changes in patients with renovascular hypertension starts with the release of increased amounts of renin when sufficient ischemia is induced to diminish pulse pressure against the juxtaglomerular cells in the renal afferent arterioles. A reduction in renal perfusion pressure by 50% leads to an immediate and persistent increase in renin secretion from the ischemic kidney, along with suppression of secretion from the contralateral one. With time, an expanded body fluid volume causes renin levels to fall but not to the low level expected from the elevated BP.

DIAGNOSIS. The presence of the clinical features listed in Table 45-4, found in perhaps 5% to 10% of all hypertensive persons, indicates the need for a screening test for renovascular hypertension. A positive screening test result or very strong clinical features call for more definitive confirmatory tests. The initial diagnostic study in most patients should be noninvasive and, if abnormal, followed by a study of renal perfusion to ensure that any renovascular lesion is pathogenic and to decide whether revascularization is indicated (**Fig. 45-14**) (see Fig. 63-11).[51]

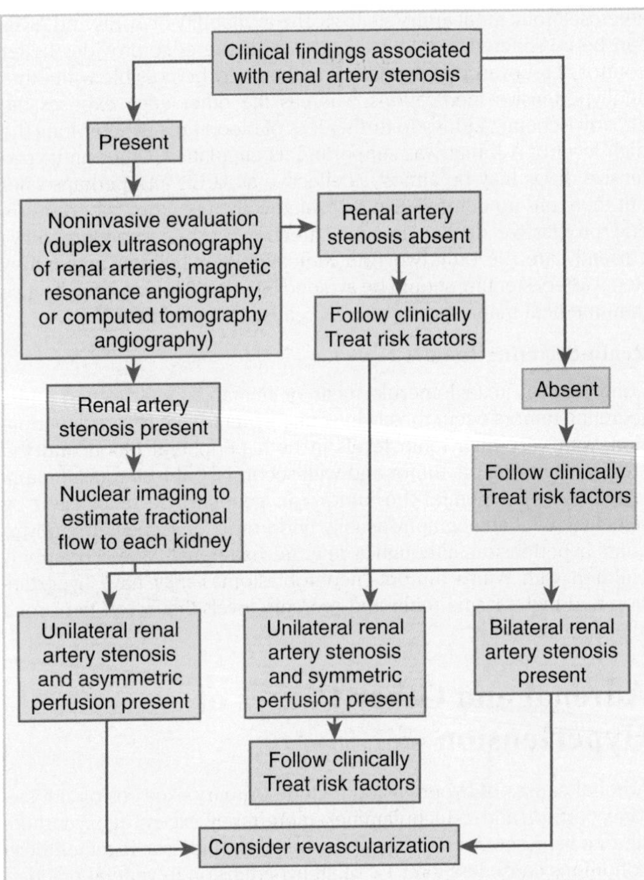

FIGURE 45-14 Algorithm for evaluation of patients in whom renal artery stenosis is suspected. Clinical follow-up includes periodic reassessment with duplex ultrasonography, magnetic resonance angiography, and nuclear imaging to estimate fractional blood flow to each kidney. The treatment of risk factors includes smoking cessation and the use of aspirin, lipid-lowering agents, and antihypertensive therapy. *(Modified from Safian RD, Textor SC: Renal-artery stenosis. N Engl J Med 344:431, 2001.)*

All screening tests have limitations. Considerable asymmetry of renal blood flow, 25% or more, was found in 148 hypertensive patients whose renal arteries were patent on prior angiography. Such normal asymmetry is likely to account for the low sensitivity and specificity of captopril-enhanced renal scans. Similarly, the sensitivity of renal duplex sonography for the detection of hemodynamically significant renovascular disease is only about 50%. The accuracy of ultrasonography is operator dependent, but the outcome of revascularization associates with the use of a resistance index to assess flow in renal arteries. Patients with high resistance index values (above 80), reflecting marked intrarenal vascular disease, had generally poor outcomes. Those with lower values had generally good outcomes.

During the past decade, contrast-enhanced computed tomography (CT) and magnetic resonance angiography have become the preferred screening tests for renal artery stenosis because initial studies suggested better sensitivity and specificity (see Fig. 45-e8 on website). However, more recent data indicate that even in experienced centers, these imaging modalities cannot reliably exclude renal artery stenosis. Gadolinium-enhanced MRI is contraindicated in patients with advanced CKD to avoid causing nephrogenic systemic fibrosis, a potentially fatal complication seen mainly in patients with low GFR.[52]

MANAGEMENT. Balloon angioplasty (without stenting) is the treatment of choice for fibromuscular dysplasia of the renal arteries (see also Chap. 63). Pending better outcomes data, however, a conservative approach based on medical management of cardiovascular risk factors—with antihypertensive medication, statins, and antiplatelet therapy—is the cornerstone for the treatment of patients with atherosclerotic renal artery stenosis. The availability of ACEIs and ARBs can be considered a double-edged sword; one edge provides better control of renovascular hypertension than may be possible with other antihypertensive medications, whereas the other edge exposes the already ischemic kidney to further loss of blood flow by inhibiting the high level of A II that was supporting its circulation. Other antihypertensive drugs may be almost as effective as ACEIs and perhaps safer, but there are no comparative data. Medically refractory hypertension and progressive decline in renal function (ischemic nephropathy) currently are the only two firm indications for balloon angioplasty. Renal artery stenting should be avoided because it is no more effective than medical management and can cause complications.[53]

Renin-Secreting Tumors

Composed of juxtaglomerular cells or hemangiopericytomas, renin-secreting tumors occur mostly in young patients with severe hypertension, with very high renin levels in both peripheral blood and the kidney harboring the tumor, and with secondary aldosteronism manifested by hypokalemia. The tumor can generally be recognized by selective renal angiography, usually performed for suspected renovascular hypertension, although a few are extrarenal. More commonly, children with Wilms tumors (nephroblastoma) may have hypertension and high plasma renin and prorenin levels that revert to normal after nephrectomy.

Adrenal and Other Causes of Hypertension (see Chap. 86)

Adrenal causes of hypertension include primary excesses of aldosterone, cortisol, and catecholamines; more rarely, excess deoxycorticosterone is present with congenital adrenal hyperplasia. Together, these conditions cause less than 1% of all hypertension in general practice, although primary aldosteronism accounts for 10% to 20% of patients referred to specialists for the evaluation of refractory hypertension. Each of these adrenal disorders can be recognized with relative ease, but they are easily overlooked because they are rare.

More problematic than the diagnosis of these adrenal disorders is the need to exclude their presence because of the increasing identification of an incidental solitary adrenal mass on abdominal imaging with CT or MRI.[54] An adrenal "incidentaloma" is found on about 5% of abdominal CT scans obtained for nonadrenal indications. Some advocate that these findings require screening for hormonal excess (see Table 45-3). Most of these incidentalomas appear to be nonfunctional on the basis of normal basal adrenal hormone levels. When more detailed studies are done, however, a significant number show incomplete suppression of cortisol by dexamethasone, that is, subclinical Cushing disease that does not appear to progress to overt hypercortisolism but may be associated with insulin resistance and osteopenia.

The probability of adrenal cancer varies by the imaging phenotype. The risk of cancer is low if a non–contrast-enhanced CT scan shows a tumor density of less than 10 HU, consistent with low-density lipid; if an MRI scan confirms a high lipid content by loss of signal on out-of-phase images; and if the tumor is smaller than 4 cm. Tumors 4 cm or larger should be resected because many are malignant.

Primary Aldosteronism and Other Forms of Mineralocorticoid-Induced Hypertension

A number of syndromes with mineralocorticoid excess have been recognized (**Table 45-5**); primary aldosteronism is the most common. Debate continues about the prevalence of primary aldosteronism in an unselected hypertensive population, but most experts agree that the condition is common in patients with resistant hypertension.[55] Moreover, in keeping with the profibrotic effects of aldosterone, many more cardiovascular events are seen in patients with primary aldosteronism than in patients with primary hypertension matched for age, gender, and BP levels.

TABLE 45-5 Syndromes of Mineralocorticoid Excess

Adrenal origin
Aldosterone excess (primary)
Aldosterone-producing adenoma
Bilateral hyperplasia
Primary unilateral adrenal hyperplasia
Glucocorticoid-remediable aldosteronism (familial hyperaldosteronism, type I)
Adrenal carcinoma
Extra-adrenal tumors
Deoxycorticosterone excess
Deoxycorticosterone-secreting tumors
Congenital adrenal hyperplasia
11β-Hydroxylase deficiency
17α-Hydroxylase deficiency
Cortisol excess
Cushing syndrome from ACTH-producing tumor
Glucocorticoid receptor resistance
Renal origin
Activating mutation of mineralocorticoid receptor
Pseudohypoaldosteronism, type II (Gordon)
11β-Hydroxysteroid dehydrogenase deficiency
Congenital: apparent mineralocorticoid excess
Acquired: licorice, carbenoxolone

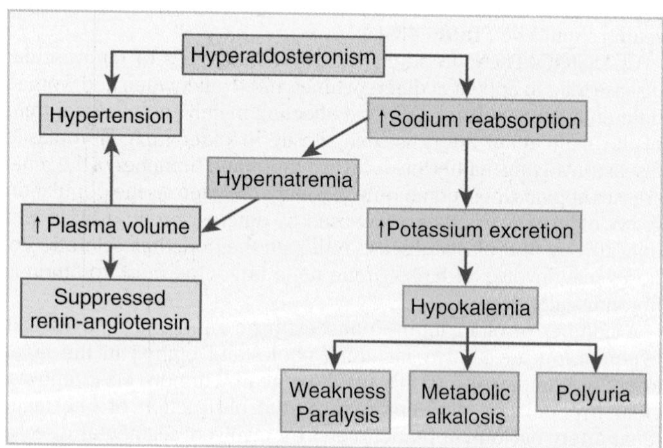

FIGURE 45-15 Pathophysiology of primary hyperaldosteronism.

Pathophysiology of Mineralocorticoid Excess

Until recently, the most frequently found source of hyperaldosteronism was a solitary aldosterone-producing adenoma. Recently, measurements of plasma renin and aldosterone have identified milder forms of hyperaldosteronism, usually associated with bilateral adrenal hyperplasia (BAH).

Aldosterone excess from any source causes hypertension and renal potassium wastage, which should induce hypokalemia (**Fig. 45-15**), but most patients with aldosteronism caused by BAH are normokalemic. The lack of overt hypokalemia could exist because potassium wastage has lowered the serum potassium level, but not yet to hypokalemic levels; because with milder degrees of aldosteronism, as are typical with BAH, the excess of aldosterone induces hypertension without causing potassium wastage, a scenario that has never been experimentally or clinically recognized; or because the BAH is related to the typical progressive increase in adrenal nodular hyperplasia with age that has no relationship to hypertension. The third explanation would fit with the long-held belief that BAH is simply a form of low-renin hypertension, that is, primary hypertension with plasma renin levels that fall progressively with age while plasma aldosterone levels remain stable.

This explanation could account for the common findings of an increased aldosterone-to-renin ratio, caused not by increased aldosterone but by decreased renin, and by the presence of BAH in most normokalemic hypertensive patients.

Diagnosis. The three steps to the recommended evaluation of primary aldosteronism are screening, salt loading for biochemical confirmation, and adrenal vein sampling for localization.[56] Screening involves measurement of plasma renin and serum aldosterone. Despite the recommendation by a few experts that virtually all hypertensive patients be screened by an aldosterone-to-renin ratio measurement, only 1% will have a surgically correctable adenoma.[55] Moreover, if screening is done, rather than using a ratio that could be high only because of a low renin level, a positive result should be based on both an elevated plasma aldosterone level (above 15 ng/dL) and a suppressed low renin level.

Screening is recommended only for hypertensive subjects who have a higher likelihood of aldosterone-producing adenoma, including those with unprovoked hypokalemia or excessive hypokalemia on diuretic therapy, a family history of aldosteronism, resistant hypertension, or an adrenal incidentaloma. Hyperaldosteronism has been found in as many as 20% of patients with resistant hypertension, with half of these being unilateral and thus surgical candidates.[55]

If the screening plasma aldosterone and renin levels are suggestive, the next step is an oral salt-loading suppression to document the autonomy of hyperaldosteronism. If the suppression test result is abnormal, adrenal vein sampling by an experienced tertiary center is strongly recommended to differentiate unilateral adenoma from bilateral hyperplasia and to confirm exactly which gland should be removed by laparoscopic surgery (see Fig. 45-e9 on website). Because detection of microscopic adenomas may be below the resolution of CT scanning and because minor adrenal nodularity and nonfunctioning adrenal incidentalomas are common, CT findings alone may lead to the wrong conclusion almost half of the time.[57]

Differential Diagnosis: Mendelian Forms of Hypertension. In patients presenting with severe hypertension and hypokalemia, primary aldosteronism needs to be distinguished from rare forms of mineralocorticoid-induced hypertension that are inherited as mendelian traits. Clinical clues of syndromic hypertension are the premature onset (often before the age of 30 years), the severity of the hypertension (which is frequently dramatic), and a compelling family history indicative of mendelian inheritance. All these familial syndromes involve excessive activation of ENaC as a final common mechanism, caused either by gain-of-function mutations of ENaC or of the mineralocorticoid receptor, or by increased production or decreased clearance of the mineralocorticoid receptor ligands—aldosterone, as well as deoxycorticosterone and cortisol (**Fig. 45-16**).

One type, familial glucocorticoid-remediable aldosteronism, is caused by recombination of genes encoding the aldosterone synthase enzyme (CYP11B2), normally found only in the outer zona glomerulosa, and the 11β-hydroxylase enzyme (CYP11B1) in the zona fasciculata. The chimeric gene induces an enzyme that catalyzes the synthesis of 18-hydroxylated cortisol in the zona fasciculata. Because this zone is under the control of adrenocorticotropic hormone (ACTH), the glucocorticoid suppressibility of the syndrome is explained. The diagnosis should be made by genetic testing for the chimeric gene, and treatment should be provided with glucocorticoid suppression.

Another rare form is apparent mineralocorticoid excess caused by deficiency of the enzyme 11β-hydroxysteroid dehydrogenase type 2 (11β-OHSD2) in the renal tubule, where it normally converts cortisol, which has the ability to act on the mineralocorticoid receptor, to cortisone, which does not. Persistence of high levels of cortisol induces all the features of mineralocorticoid excess. The 11β-OHSD2 enzyme may be congenitally absent (the syndrome of apparent mineralocorticoid excess) or inhibited by the glycyrrhizic acid contained in licorice. Another unusual syndrome with hypertension and hypokalemia but suppressed mineralocorticoid secretion is Liddle syndrome, in which the kidney reabsorbs excess sodium and wastes potassium because of a mutation in the beta or gamma subunits of the epithelial sodium channel.

In most of these cases, volume expansion and severe hypertension cause feedback suppression of plasma renin, and mineralocorticoid receptor activation leads to renal potassium wasting and hypokalemia. One exception is pseudohypoaldosteronism type II, in which the disease-causing mutation produces both low-renin and salt-sensitive hypertension caused by overactivity of the thiazide-sensitive Na-Cl cotransporter in the distal collecting duct and hyperkalemia caused by underactivity of the renal outer medullary potassium channel.

THERAPY. Once the diagnosis of primary aldosteronism is made and the type of adrenal disorder has been established, the choice of therapy is relatively simple. Patients with a solitary adenoma should have the tumor resected by laparoscopic surgery, and those with bilateral hyperplasia should be treated with an aldosterone antagonist (spironolactone or eplerenone) and other antihypertensive drugs as needed. Laparoscopic adrenalectomy eliminates the need for antihypertensive medication in up to 50% of patients and reduces

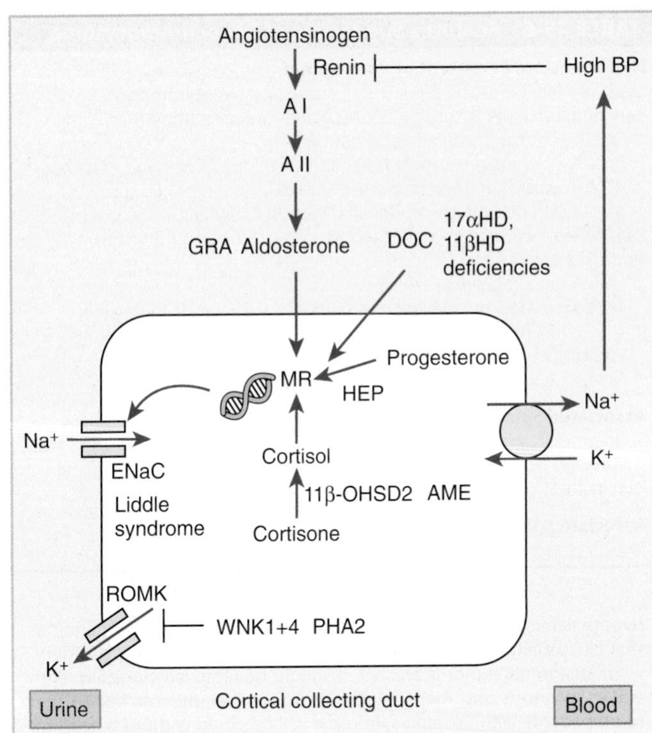

FIGURE 45-16 Mendelian forms of hypertension that cause mineralocorticoid-induced hypertension. AME = apparent mineralocorticoid excess; A I = angiotensin I; A II = angiotensin II; BP = blood pressure; GRA = glucocorticoid-remediable aldosteronism; 11β-OHSD2 = 11β-hydroxysteroid dehydrogenase type 2; DOC = deoxycorticosterone; ENaC = epithelial sodium channel; MR = mineralocorticoid receptor; PHA2 = pseudohypoaldosteronism type II; ROMK = rectifying outer medullary potassium channel; WNK = with no lysine kinases; HEP = hypertension exacerbated by pregnancy; 11βHD = 11β-hydroxylase; 17αHD = 17α-hydroxylase. The effect of PHA2 on the activity of the thiazide-sensitive Na-Cl cotransporter in the distal collecting duct is not shown. See text for explanation. *(Modified from Lifton RP, Gharavi AG, Geller DS: Molecular mechanisms of human hypertension. Cell 104:545, 2001.)*

medication requirements in patients who may have coexisting primary hypertension or renal damage from prolonged exposure to elevated BP and undiagnosed hyperaldosteronism.

Cushing Syndrome (see Chap. 86)

Hypertension occurs in about 80% of patients with Cushing syndrome. If left untreated, it can cause marked LVH and congestive heart failure. As with hypertension of other endocrine causes, the longer it is present, the less likely it is to disappear when the underlying cause is relieved.

Mechanism of Hypertension. BP can increase for a number of reasons. The secretion of mineralocorticoids can increase along with cortisol, which itself is a potent activator of the mineralocorticoid receptor. The excess cortisol can overwhelm the ability of renal 11β-OHSD2 to convert it to cortisone, which is not a mineralocorticoid receptor ligand; the excess cortisol overstimulates renal mineralocorticoid receptors to retain sodium and expand plasma volume. Cortisol stimulates the synthesis of renin substrate and the expression of A I receptors, which may be responsible for enhanced pressor effects.

Diagnosis. The syndrome should be suspected in patients with truncal obesity, wide purple striae, thin skin, muscle weakness, and osteoporosis. If clinical features are suggestive, the diagnosis often can be either ruled out or virtually ensured by the measurement of free cortisol in a 24-hour urine sample, the simple overnight dexamethasone suppression test, or the determination of late-night salivary cortisol. Some cases of metabolic syndrome may be caused by subclinical Cushing syndrome.

Therapy. In about two thirds of patients with Cushing syndrome, the process begins with overproduction of ACTH by the pituitary, which leads to BAH. Although pituitary hyperfunction may reflect a

CH 45

TABLE 45-6 Features Suggestive of Pheochromocytoma

Hypertension, Persistent or Paroxysmal
Markedly variable blood pressures (± orthostatic hypotension)
Sudden paroxysms (± subsequent hypertension) in relation to
Stress: anesthesia, angiography, parturition
Pharmacologic provocation: histamine, nicotine, caffeine, beta blockers, glucocorticoids, tricyclic antidepressants
Manipulation of tumors: abdominal palpation, urination
Rare patients persistently normotensive
Unusual settings
Childhood, pregnancy, familial
Multiple endocrine adenomas: medullary carcinoma of the thyroid (MEN-2), mucosal neuromas (MEN-2B)
Von Hippel–Lindau syndrome
Neurocutaneous lesions: neurofibromatosis
Associated Symptoms
Sudden spells with headache, sweating, palpitations, nervousness, nausea, vomiting
Pain in chest or abdomen
Associated Signs
Sweating, tachycardia, arrhythmia, pallor, weight loss

hypothalamic disorder, most patients have discrete pituitary adenomas that can usually be resected by selective transsphenoidal microsurgery.

If an adrenal tumor is present, it should be removed surgically. With earlier diagnosis and more selective surgical therapy, it is hoped that more patients with Cushing syndrome will be cured without a need for lifelong glucocorticoid replacement therapy and with permanent relief of their hypertension. Therapy may require one of a number of drugs temporarily, but rarely permanently.

Congenital Adrenal Hyperplasia. Enzymatic defects may induce hypertension by interfering with cortisol biosynthesis. Low levels of cortisol lead to increased ACTH levels; this increases the accumulation of precursors proximal to the enzymatic block, specifically deoxycorticosterone, which induces mineralocorticoid hypertension. The more common of these is 11-hydroxylase deficiency, which has been attributed to various mutations in the gene and leads to virilization (from excessive androgens) and hypertension with hypokalemia (from excessive deoxycorticosterone). The other is 17-hydroxylase deficiency, which also causes hypertension from excess deoxycorticosterone, in addition to failure of secondary sexual development because sex hormones are also deficient. Affected children are hypertensive, but the defect in sex hormone synthesis may not become obvious until pubertal failure is recognized in adolescence.

Pheochromocytoma and Paraganglioma (see Chaps. 86 and 94)

Pheochromocytomas are rare catecholamine-secreting tumors of the adrenal chromaffin cells. Paragangliomas are even rarer extra-adrenal tumors of the sympathetic or vagal ganglion cells. For clinical purposes, the term *pheo* generally refers to any catecholamine-secreting tumor, whether a true adrenal pheochromocytoma or a functional extra-adrenal paraganglioma. The wild fluctuations in BP and dramatic symptoms of pheo usually alert both the patient and physician to the possibility of this diagnosis (**Table 45-6**). However, such fluctuations may be missed or, as occurs in 50% of patients, the hypertension may be persistent. On one hand, the spells typical of a pheochromocytoma (with headache, sweating, palpitations, and pallor) may be incorrectly attributed to migraine, menopause, or panic attacks. On the other hand, most patients with severe paroxysmal hypertension do not have a pheochromocytoma but rather marked anxiety. When they are correctly diagnosed and treated, most pheos are curable. When they are undiagnosed or improperly treated, they can be fatal.[58] See Chap. 86 for details regarding the pathophysiology, diagnosis, and treatment of pheochromocytoma.

Other Causes of Hypertension

A host of other causes of hypertension are known. One that is probably becoming more common is the ingestion of various drugs—prescribed (e.g., cyclosporine, tacrolimus, erythropoietin), purchased over the counter (e.g., ephedra), and illicit (e.g., cocaine, methamphetamine). As previously noted, obstructive sleep apnea commonly causes substantial, and often reversible, hypertension.

TABLE 45-7 Hypertension Associated with Cardiac Surgery

Preoperative
Anxiety, angina, other manifestations
Discontinuation of antihypertensive therapy
Rebound from beta blockers in patients with coronary artery disease
Intraoperative
Induction of anesthesia: tracheal intubation
Nasopharyngeal, urethral, or rectal manipulation
Before, during, or after cardiopulmonary bypass
Postoperative
Obvious cause: hypoxia, hypercarbia, ventilatory difficulties, hypothermia, shivering, arousal from anesthesia
With no obvious cause: after myocardial revascularization; less frequently after valve replacement; after resection of aortic coarctation

COARCTATION OF THE AORTA (see Chap. 65). Congenital narrowing of the aorta can occur at any level of the thoracic or abdominal aorta, but is typically found just beyond the origin of the left subclavian artery or distal to the insertion of the ligamentum arteriosum. With less severe postductal lesions, symptoms may not appear until the teenage years or later, particularly during pregnancy. Hypertension in the arms, weak or absent femoral pulses, and a loud murmur heard over the back are the classic features of coarctation. The pathogenesis of the hypertension can involve more than simple mechanical obstruction and probably involves a generalized vasoconstrictor mechanism. The lesion can be detected by echocardiography, and MRI or contrast aortography proves the diagnosis. Once it is repaired, patients may continue to have hypertension that requires careful monitoring and treatment.

HORMONAL DISTURBANCES (see Chap. 86). Hypertension is seen in as many as half of patients with various hormonal disturbances, including acromegaly, hypothyroidism, and hyperparathyroidism. Diagnosis of the last two conditions has been made easier by readily available blood tests, and affected hypertensive patients can be relieved of their high BP by correction of the hormonal disturbance. Such relief occurs more frequently in patients with hypothyroidism than in those with hyperparathyroidism.

PERIOPERATIVE HYPERTENSION (see Chap. 85). Preexisting hypertension should be well controlled before elective surgery, with particular attention to correction of diuretic-induced hypokalemia. Antihypertensive agents should not be discontinued perioperatively, in particular to avoid rebound from beta blockers or clonidine. Fortunately, intravenous formulations of most classes are available if oral intake is not possible. Hypertension may appear or worsen in the perioperative period, perhaps more commonly with cardiac than with noncardiac surgery (**Table 45-7**). Hypertension is of particular concern after heart transplantation, appearing for a number of reasons, including immunosuppression with calcineurin inhibitors (cyclosporine and tacrolimus) and possibly cardiac denervation; treatment includes dihydropyridine calcium channel blockers, diuretics, and central sympatholytics.

Special Considerations for Hypertensive Diseases in Women (see Chap. 81)

Oral Contraceptive Use

The use of estrogen-containing oral contraceptive (OC) pills can cause secondary hypertension in young women. Most women who take them experience a slight rise in BP. Moreover, newer progestins such as drospirenone contain a spironolactone-like moiety with mild mineralocorticoid antagonist action; as a result, drospirenone-estrogen combinations generally cause a small decrease in BP.[59]

CLINICAL FEATURES. In most women, the hypertension is mild, but in some it may accelerate rapidly and cause severe renal damage. When use of the OC is discontinued, BP falls to normal within 3 to 6 months in about 50% of patients. Whether the OC causes permanent hypertension in the other half or just uncovers primary hypertension at an earlier time is not clear.

MECHANISMS. OC use probably causes hypertension by volume expansion because estrogens and some synthetic progestogens used in OC pills cause sodium retention. Although plasma renin levels rise in response to increased levels of angiotensinogen, ACEIs do not alter BP any more in women with OC-induced hypertension than in women with primary hypertension. Drospirenone-containing OC pills may cause a reactive rise in serum aldosterone.

MANAGEMENT. The use of estrogen-containing OCs should be restricted in women older than 35 years, particularly if they also smoke or are hypertensive or obese. Drospirenone-containing OC pills are a better alternative. Women given OCs should be monitored as follows: the initial supply should be limited; they should be asked to return for a BP check before an additional supply is provided; and if BP has risen, an alternative contraceptive method should be offered. If OC remains the only acceptable contraceptive method, the elevated BP can be reduced with appropriate therapy. In women who stop taking OCs, evaluation for secondary hypertensive diseases should be postponed for at least 3 months to allow changes in the RAAS to remit. If the hypertension does not recede, additional workup and therapy may be needed.

Postmenopausal Sex Hormone Therapy

Estrogen therapy does not appear to induce hypertension, although it does induce the various changes in the RAAS seen with oral contraceptive use. In fact, most controlled trials have found a decrease in daytime ambulatory BP and a greater dipping of nocturnal BP in users of estrogen replacement therapy. Such lower BPs may reflect a number of effects, including improved endothelium-dependent vasodilation and reduced muscle sympathetic nerve activity.

Hypertension During Pregnancy (see Chap. 82)

In about 12% of first pregnancies in previously normotensive women, hypertension appears after 20 weeks (gestational hypertension). In about half of cases, this hypertension will progress to preeclampsia when it is complicated by proteinuria, edema, or hematologic or hepatic abnormalities, which in turn increase the risk of progress to eclampsia, defined by the occurrence of convulsions.[60] Women with hypertension predating pregnancy have an even higher incidence of preeclampsia and a greater likelihood of early delivery of small-for-gestational-age babies. Additional predisposing factors include young or older age, multiple gestations, concomitant heart or renal disease, and chronic hypertension.[60] The diagnosis is usually based on a rise in pressure of 30/15 mm Hg or more to a level above 140/90 mm Hg. As with other forms of hypertension, ambulatory BP monitoring makes the diagnosis most precisely.

CLINICAL FEATURES. The features shown in **Table 45-8** should help distinguish gestational hypertension and preeclampsia from chronic primary hypertension; the distinction should be made because management and prognosis are different. Gestational hypertension is self-limited and less commonly recurs in subsequent pregnancies, whereas chronic hypertension progresses and usually complicates subsequent pregnancies. Differentiation may be difficult because of a lack of knowledge of the pre-pregnancy BP and because of the usual tendency for BP to fall considerably during the middle trimester, so that hypertension present before pregnancy may not be recognized.

TABLE 45-8 Differences Between Preeclampsia and Chronic Hypertension

FEATURE	PREECLAMPSIA	CHRONIC HYPERTENSION
Age	Young (<20 years)	Older (>30 years)
Parity	Primigravida	Multigravida
Onset	After 20 weeks of pregnancy	Before 20 weeks of pregnancy
Weight gain and edema	Sudden	Gradual
Systolic blood pressure	<160 mm Hg	>160 mm Hg
Funduscopic findings	Spasm, edema	Arteriovenous nicking, exudates
Left ventricular hypertrophy	Rare	More common
Proteinuria	Present	Absent
Plasma uric acid level	Increased	Normal
Blood pressure after delivery	Normal	Elevated

MECHANISMS. The hemodynamic features of gestational hypertension are a further rise in cardiac output than is usually seen in normal pregnancy, accompanied by profound vasoconstriction that reduces intravascular capacity even more than blood volume, which may reflect increased central and peripheral sympathetic activity. Increasingly strong evidence has indicated that preeclampsia starts from immune maladaptation leading to inadequate placentation; this results in reduced angiogenic growth factors and increased placental debris entering the maternal circulation, where it provokes a maternal inflammatory response with hypertension.[60] The mother may be particularly vulnerable to encephalopathy because of her previously normal BP. As described in more detail later (see Hypertensive Crisis), cerebral blood flow is normally maintained constant over a fairly narrow range of mean arterial pressure, roughly between 60 and 100 mm Hg in normotensive individuals. In a previously normotensive young woman, an acute rise in BP to 150/100 mm Hg can exceed the upper limit of autoregulation and result in a breakthrough of cerebral blood flow (acute dilation) that leads to cerebral edema and convulsions.

PREVENTION AND TREATMENT. Beyond delay of pregnancy until after the teenage years and better prenatal care, the only other effective strategy to prevent preeclampsia is the use of low doses of aspirin. The only cure for preeclampsia is delivery, which removes the diseased placenta. To achieve this apparently simple end, the clinician must detect the often-symptomless prodromal condition by screening all pregnant women, admitting those with advanced preeclampsia to the hospital so as to keep track of an unpredictable situation, and timing preemptive delivery to maximize the safety of mother and baby. Caution is advised in the use of drugs for gestational hypertension; it is traditionally limited to methyldopa in the United States, but other drugs are used elsewhere. Drug treatment of maternal BP does not improve perinatal outcome and may be associated with fetal growth retardation. Most authorities recommend antihypertensive drugs only if diastolic pressures remain above 100 mm Hg. The only drugs contraindicated are ACEIs and ARBs because of their propensity to induce neonatal renal failure.

CHRONIC HYPERTENSION. If pregnancy begins while a woman is receiving antihypertensive drug therapy, medications including diuretics but excluding ACEIs and ARBs are usually continued, in the belief that the mother should be protected and that the fetus will not suffer from any sudden hemodynamic shifts that occur when therapy is first begun. However, despite currently available treatment, the

CH 45

TABLE 45-9 Circumstances Requiring Rapid Treatment of Hypertension

Accelerated-malignant hypertension with papilledema
Cerebrovascular
Hypertensive encephalopathy
Atherothrombotic brain infarction with severe hypertension
Intracerebral hemorrhage
Subarachnoid hemorrhage
Cardiac
Acute aortic dissection
Acute left ventricular failure
Acute or impending myocardial infarction
After coronary bypass surgery
Renal
Acute glomerulonephritis
Renal crises from collagen-vascular diseases
Severe hypertension after kidney transplantation
Excessive circulating catecholamines
Pheochromocytoma crisis
Food or drug interactions with monoamine oxidase inhibitors
Sympathomimetic drug use (cocaine)
Rebound hypertension after sudden cessation of antihypertensive drugs
Eclampsia
Surgical
Severe hypertension in patients requiring immediate surgery
Postoperative hypertension
Postoperative bleeding from vascular suture lines
Severe body burns
Severe epistaxis
Thrombotic thrombocytopenic purpura

incidence of perinatal mortality and fetal growth restriction remains higher in patients with chronic hypertension.

MANAGEMENT OF ECLAMPSIA. With appropriate care of gestational hypertension, eclampsia hardly ever supervenes; when it does, however, maternal and fetal mortality increase markedly. Excellent results have been reported with the use of magnesium sulfate to prevent and to treat convulsions.[60] Caution is needed to avoid volume overload because pulmonary edema is the most common cause of maternal mortality. Compared with women who were normotensive, the overall prognosis for women who had hypertension during pregnancy is not as good, probably because of causes other than preeclampsia, including unrecognized chronic primary hypertension. After delivery, transient or persistent hypertension can develop in the mother. In many cases, early primary hypertension may have been masked by the hemodynamic changes of pregnancy.

Hypertensive Crisis

Definitions

A number of clinical circumstances require prompt reduction of BP (**Table 45-9**). These circumstances can be separated into emergencies, which require immediate (but controlled) reduction of BP (within 1 hour), and urgencies, which can be treated more slowly. A persistent diastolic pressure exceeding 130 mm Hg is often associated with acute vascular damage; some patients may suffer vascular damage from lower levels of pressure, whereas others are able to withstand even higher levels without apparent harm. The rapidity of the rise may be more important than the absolute level in producing acute vascular damage, as explained later. Therefore, in practice, all patients with diastolic BP above 130 mm Hg should be treated, some more rapidly with parenteral drugs and others more slowly with oral agents. When the rise in pressure causes retinal hemorrhages, exudates, or papilledema, the term *accelerated-malignant hypertension* is used. Hypertensive encephalopathy is characterized by headache, irritability, alterations in consciousness, and other manifestations of central nervous dysfunction with sudden and marked elevations in BP.

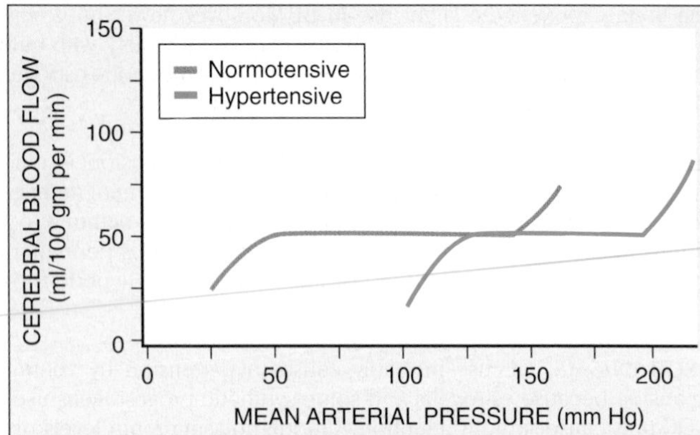

FIGURE 45-17 Idealized curves of cerebral blood flow at varying levels of systemic blood pressure in normotensive and hypertensive subjects. A rightward shift in autoregulation is shown with chronic hypertension. *(Modified from Strandgaard S, Olesen J, Skinhtoi E, Lassen NA: Autoregulation of brain circulation in severe arterial hypertension. Br Med J 1:507, 1973.)*

Incidence

Less than 1% of patients with primary hypertension progress to an accelerated-malignant phase. The incidence probably has receded because of more widespread treatment of hypertension. Any hypertensive disease can be manifested as a crisis. Some, including pheochromocytoma and renovascular hypertension, do so at a higher rate than that seen with primary hypertension. However, because hypertension is of unknown cause in more than 90% of all patients, most hypertensive crises appear in the setting of preexisting primary hypertension.

Pathophysiology

Whenever BP rises and remains above a critical level, various processes set off a series of local and systemic effects that cause further rises in pressure and vascular damage, eventually resulting in accelerated-malignant hypertension. Classic studies in animals and humans elucidated the mechanism of hypertensive encephalopathy. The caliber of pial arterioles over the cerebral cortex was measured in normotensive cats whose BP was varied over a wide range of infusion by vasodilators or A II. As the pressure fell, the arterioles became dilated; as the pressure rose, they became constricted. Thus, constant cerebral blood flow was maintained by means of autoregulation, which depends on the cerebral sympathetic nerves. However, when mean arterial pressure rose above 180 mm Hg (i.e., 220/110), the tightly constricted vessels could no longer withstand the pressure and suddenly dilated. The dilation began in an irregular manner, first in areas with less muscle tone and then diffusely, with production of generalized vasodilation. This breakthrough of cerebral blood flow hyperperfuses the brain under high pressure and causes leakage of fluid into the perivascular tissue, resulting in cerebral edema and the syndrome of hypertensive encephalopathy.

In humans, cerebral blood flow has been measured repetitively by an isotopic technique while BP was lowered or raised with vasodilators or vasoconstrictors in a manner similar to that used in animal studies. Curves depicting cerebral blood flow as a function of arterial pressure demonstrated autoregulation, with a constancy of flow over mean pressures in normotensive persons from about 60 to 120 mm Hg and in hypertensive patients from about 110 to 180 mm Hg (**Fig. 45-17**). This shift to the right in hypertensive patients results from structural thickening of the arterioles as an adaptation to the chronically elevated pressure. When pressure was raised beyond the upper limit of autoregulation, the same breakthrough with hyperperfusion occurred as was seen in the animal studies. In previously normotensive persons whose vessels have not been altered by prior exposure to high pressure, breakthrough occurred at a mean arterial pressure

TABLE 45-10 Clinical Characteristics of Hypertensive Crisis

Blood pressure: usually >140 mm Hg diastolic
Funduscopic findings: hemorrhages, exudates, papilledema
Cardiac findings: prominent apical impulse, cardiac enlargement, congestive heart failure
Renal findings: oliguria, azotemia
Gastrointestinal findings: nausea, vomiting
Hematologic findings: microangiopathic hemolysis

of about 120 mm Hg (i.e., 140/80 mm Hg); in hypertensive patients, the breakthrough occurred at about 180 mm Hg (i.e.,220/110 mm Hg).

These studies have confirmed clinical observations. In previously normotensive persons, severe encephalopathy occurs with relatively little hypertension. In children with acute glomerulonephritis and in women with eclampsia, convulsions can occur as a result of hypertensive encephalopathy, with BP readings as low as 150/100 mm Hg. Obviously, chronically hypertensive patients withstand such pressures without difficulty, but when pressure increases significantly, encephalopathy can develop even in these patients.

Manifestations and Course

The symptoms and signs of hypertensive crises are usually dramatic (**Table 45-10**), probably reflecting acute damage to endothelium and platelet activation. However, some patients may be relatively asymptomatic, despite markedly elevated pressure and extensive organ damage. Young black men are particularly prone to hypertensive crisis, with severe renal insufficiency. Even in elderly persons, however, hypertension can initially present in an accelerated-malignant phase. If left untreated, patients die quickly of brain damage or more gradually of renal damage. Before effective therapy was available, less than 25% of patients with malignant hypertension survived 1 year and only 1% survived 5 years. With therapy, including renal dialysis, more than 90% survive 1 year and about 80% survive 5 years.

Differential Diagnosis

The presence of hypertensive encephalopathy or accelerated-malignant hypertension demands immediate aggressive therapy to lower BP effectively, often before the specific cause is known. However, certain serious diseases and psychological problems can mimic a hypertensive crisis, and management of these conditions usually requires different diagnostic and therapeutic approaches. In particular, BP should not be lowered too abruptly, if at all, in a patient with a stroke.[61] See Chap. 46 for specific therapy for hypertensive crises.

Future Perspectives

The measurement of BP will become more accurate for diagnosis and cardiovascular risk stratification with the greater use of out-of-office measurements and assessments of vascular health by measures of vascular compliance, central aortic pressure, and inflammatory biomarkers. Future research on underlying mechanisms of primary hypertension should aim to make treatment less empiric and more effective than current practice.

REFERENCES

Epidemiology of Hypertension

1. Lawes CM, Vander HS, Rodgers A: Global burden of blood-pressure-related disease, 2001. Lancet 371:1513, 2008.
2. Victor RG, Leonard D, Hess P, et al: Factors associated with hypertension awareness, treatment, and control in Dallas County, Texas. Arch Intern Med 168:1285, 2008.
3. Chobanian AV, Bakris GL, Black HR, et al: The Seventh Report of the Joint National Committee on Prevention, Detection, Evaluation, and Treatment of High Blood Pressure: The JNC 7 report. JAMA 289:2560, 2003.
4. Lewington S, Clarke R, Qizilbash N, et al: Age-specific relevance of usual blood pressure to vascular mortality: A meta-analysis of individual data for one million adults in 61 prospective studies. Lancet 360:1903, 2002.
5. Rosendorff C, Black HR, Cannon CP, et al: Treatment of hypertension in the prevention and management of ischemic heart disease: A scientific statement from the American Heart Association Council for High Blood Pressure Research and the Councils on Clinical Cardiology and Epidemiology and Prevention. Circulation 115:2761, 2007.
6. Cooper RS, Wolf-Maier K, Luke A, et al: An international comparative study of blood pressure in populations of European vs. African descent. BMC Med 3:2, 2005.
7. Chen L, Davey SG, Harbord RM, Lewis SJ: Alcohol intake and blood pressure: A systematic review implementing a Mendelian randomization approach. PLoS Med 5:e52, 2008.
8. Adrogue HJ, Madias NE: Sodium and potassium in the pathogenesis of hypertension. N Engl J Med 356:1966, 2007.
9. Ehret GB, Morrison AC, O'Connor AA, et al: Replication of the Wellcome Trust genome-wide association study of essential hypertension: The Family Blood Pressure Program. Eur J Hum Genet 16:1507, 2008.
10. Levy D, Ehret GB, Rice K, et al: Genome-wide association study of blood pressure and hypertension. Nat Genet 41:677, 2009.
10a. Newton-Cheh C, Johnson T, Gateva V, et al: Genome-wide association study identifies eight loci associated with blood pressure. Nat Genet 41:666, 2009.
10b. Ji W, Foo JN, O'Roak BJ, et al: Rare independent mutations in renal salt handling genes contribute to blood pressure variation. Nat Genet 40:592, 2008.
11. McEniery CM, Yasmin, Wallace S, et al: Increased stroke volume and aortic stiffness contribute to isolated systolic hypertension in young adults. Hypertension 46:221, 2005.
12. Franklin SS, Pio JR, Wong ND, et al: Predictors of new-onset diastolic and systolic hypertension: The Framingham Heart Study. Circulation 111:1121, 2005.
13. Franklin SS: Hypertension in older people: Part 1: J Clin Hypertens (Greenwich) 8:444, 2006.
14. Agabiti-Rosei E, Mancia G, O'Rourke MF, et al: Central blood pressure measurements and antihypertensive therapy: A consensus document. Hypertension 50:154, 2007.

Pathophysiology of Hypertension

15. Victor RG, Shafiq MM: Sympathetic neural mechanisms in human hypertension. Curr Hypertens Rep 10:241, 2008.
16. Mohaupt MG, Schmidli J, Luft FC: Management of uncontrollable hypertension with a carotid sinus stimulation device. Hypertension 50:825, 2007.
17. Krum H, Schlaich M, Whitbourn R, et al: Catheter-based renal sympathetic denervation for resistant hypertension: A multicentre safety and proof-of-principle cohort study. Lancet 373:1275, 2009.
18. Grassi G, Seravalle G, Quarti-Trevano F, et al: Sympathetic and baroreflex cardiovascular control in hypertension-related left ventricular dysfunction. Hypertension 53:205, 2009.
19. Landsberg L: A teleological view of obesity, diabetes and hypertension. Clin Exp Pharmacol Physiol 33:863, 2006.
20. Mark AL; Dietary therapy for obesity: An emperor with no clothes. Hypertension 51:1426, 2008.
21. Butt M, Dwivedi G, Khair O, Lip GY: Obstructive sleep apnea and cardiovascular disease. Int J Cardiol 139:7, 2010. Epub 2009 Jun 7.
22. He FJ, MacGregor GA: Salt, blood pressure and cardiovascular disease. Curr Opin Cardiol 22:298, 2007.
23. Rodriguez-Iturbe B, Romero F, Johnson RJ: Pathophysiological mechanisms of salt-dependent hypertension. Am J Kidney Dis 50:655, 2007.
24. Bergvall N, Iliadou A, Johansson S, et al: Genetic and shared environmental factors do not confound the association between birth weight and hypertension: A study among Swedish twins. Circulation 115:2931, 2007.
25. Kao WH, Klag MJ, Meoni LA, et al: MYH9 is associated with nondiabetic end-stage renal disease in African Americans. Nat Genet 40:1185, 2008.
26. Munzel T, Sinning C, Post F, et al: Pathophysiology, diagnosis and prognostic implications of endothelial dysfunction. Ann Med 40:180, 2008.
27. Ridker PM, Silvertown JD: Inflammation, C-reactive protein, and atherothrombosis. J Periodontol 79(Suppl):1544, 2008.
28. Harrison DG, Gongora MC: Oxidative stress and hypertension. Med Clin North Am 93:621, 2009.
29. Feig DI, Soletsky B, Johnson RJ: Effect of allopurinol on blood pressure of adolescents with newly diagnosed essential hypertension: A randomized trial. JAMA 300:924, 2008.
30. Duprez DA: Role of the renin-angiotensin-aldosterone system in vascular remodeling and inflammation: A clinical review. J Hypertens 24:983, 2006.
31. Schiffrin EL: Effects of aldosterone on the vasculature: Hypertension 47:312, 2006.
32. Danser AH: Prorenin: Back into the arena. Hypertension 47:824, 2006.
33. Feldt S, Batenburg WW, Mazak I, et al: Prorenin and renin-induced extracellular signal-regulated kinase 1/2 activation in monocytes is not blocked by aliskiren or the handle-region peptide. Hypertension 51:682, 2008.
34. Harrison DG, Guzik TJ, Goronzy J, Weyand C: Is hypertension an immunologic disease? Curr Cardiol Rep 10:464, 2008.
35. Hill JA, Olson EN: Cardiac plasticity. N Engl J Med 358:1370, 2008.
36. Gradman AH, Alfayoumi F: From left ventricular hypertrophy to congestive heart failure: Management of hypertensive heart disease. Prog Cardiovasc Dis 48:326, 2006.
37. Parati G, Stergiou GS, Asmar R, et al: European Society of Hypertension guidelines for blood pressure monitoring at home: A summary report of the Second International Consensus Conference on Home Blood Pressure Monitoring. J Hypertens 26:1505, 2008.
38. Pickering TG, Miller NH, Ogedegbe G, et al: Call to action on use and reimbursement for home blood pressure monitoring: A joint scientific statement from the American Heart Association, American Society of Hypertension, and Preventive Cardiovascular Nurses Association. J Cardiovasc Nurs 23:299, 2008.
39. Dolan E, Stanton A, Thijs L, et al: Superiority of ambulatory over clinic blood pressure measurement in predicting mortality: The Dublin outcome study. Hypertension 46:156, 2005.
40. Messerli FH, Williams B, Ritz E: Essential hypertension. Lancet 370:591, 2007.
41. Mancia G, De Backer G, Dominiczak A, et al: 2007 Guidelines for the Management of Arterial Hypertension: The Task Force for the Management of Arterial Hypertension of the European Society of Hypertension (ESH) and of the European Society of Cardiology (ESC). Eur Heart J 28:1462, 2007.

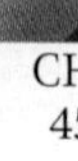

42. Sipahi I, Tuzcu EM, Schoenhagen P, et al: Effects of normal, pre-hypertensive, and hypertensive blood pressure levels on progression of coronary atherosclerosis. J Am Coll Cardiol 48:833, 2006.
43. Wong TY, Mitchell P: The eye in hypertension. Lancet 369:425, 2007.
44. Okin PM, Devereux RB, Nieminen MS, et al: Electrocardiographic strain pattern and prediction of new-onset congestive heart failure in hypertensive patients: The Losartan Intervention for Endpoint Reduction in Hypertension (LIFE) study. Circulation 113:67, 2006.
45. Drazner MH, Dries DL, Peshock RM, et al: Left ventricular hypertrophy is more prevalent in blacks than whites in the general population: The Dallas Heart Study. Hypertension 46:124, 2005.
46. Freedman BI, Hicks PJ, Bostrom MA, et al: Polymorphisms in the non-muscle myosin heavy chain 9 gene (MYH9) are strongly associated with end-stage renal disease historically attributed to hypertension in African Americans. Kidney Int 75:736, 2009.
47. Stevens LA, Coresh J, Greene T, Levey AS: Assessing kidney function—measured and estimated glomerular filtration rate. N Engl J Med 354:2473, 2006.
48. Stevens LA, Schmid CH, Greene T, et al: Factors other than glomerular filtration rate affect serum cystatin C levels. Kidney Int 75:652, 2009.
49. Casas JP, Chua W, Loukogeorgakis S, et al: Effect of inhibitors of the renin-angiotensin system and other antihypertensive drugs on renal outcomes: Systematic review and meta-analysis. Lancet 366:2026, 2005.
50. Pogue V, Rahman M, Lipkowitz M, et al: Disparate estimates of hypertension control from ambulatory and clinic blood pressure measurements in hypertensive kidney disease. Hypertension 53:20, 2009.
51. Levin A, Linas S, Luft FC, et al: Controversies in renal artery stenosis: A review by the American Society of Nephrology Advisory Group on Hypertension. Am J Nephrol 27:212, 2007.
52. Kallen AJ, Jhung MA, Cheng S, et al: Gadolinium-containing magnetic resonance imaging contrast and nephrogenic systemic fibrosis: A case-control study. Am J Kidney Dis 5:966, 2008.
53. Bax L, Woittiez AJ, Kouwenberg HJ, et al: Stent placement in patients with atherosclerotic renal artery stenosis and impaired renal function: A randomized trial. Ann Intern Med 150:840, 2009.
54. Young WF Jr: Clinical practice. The incidentally discovered adrenal mass. N Engl J Med 356:601, 2007.
55. Douma S, Petidis K, Doumas M, et al: Prevalence of primary hyperaldosteronism in resistant hypertension: A retrospective observational study. Lancet 371:1921, 2008.
56. Funder JW, Carey RM, Fardella C, et al: Case detection, diagnosis, and treatment of patients with primary aldosteronism: An endocrine society clinical practice guideline. J Clin Endocrinol Metab 93:3266, 2008.
57. Nwariaku FE, Miller BS, Auchus R, et al: Primary hyperaldosteronism: Effect of adrenal vein sampling on surgical outcome. Arch Surg 141:497, 2006.
58. Yu R, Nissen NN, Chopra P, et al: Diagnosis and treatment of pheochromocytoma in an academic hospital from 1997 to 2007. Am J Med 122:85, 2009.
59. Shufelt CL, Bairey Merz CN: Contraceptive hormone use and cardiovascular disease. J Am Coll Cardiol 53:221, 2009.
60. Sibai B, Dekker G, Kupferminc M: Pre-eclampsia. Lancet 365:785, 2005.
61. Adams HP Jr, del Zoppo G, Alberts MJ, et al: Guidelines for the early management of adults with ischemic stroke: A guideline from the American Heart Association/American Stroke Association Stroke Council, Clinical Cardiology Council, Cardiovascular Radiology and Intervention Council, and the Atherosclerotic Peripheral Vascular Disease and Quality of Care Outcomes in Research Interdisciplinary Working Groups. Circulation 115:e478, 2007.

CHAPTER 46 Systemic Hypertension: Therapy

Norman M. Kaplan

Hypertension is the most common modifiable risk factor for cardiovascular diseases in the United States and other developed countries.[1] Its prevalence will continue to increase, both among the young because of increasing obesity and in older adults because of longer life expectancy. Despite it continuing to be the most common indication for nonpregnant adults to visit a physician, hypertension remains inadequately treated.[2] There are many reasons for this, especially physician inertia and the cost of medications. The main fault, however, resides in the inherent nature of the disease—genetically determined, induced by a common but unhealthy lifestyle, asymptomatic, and persistent, with overt consequences delayed by 10 to 30 years—so that the cost of therapy, both in money and in adverse effects, appears to outweigh benefits to be derived from adherence to the regimen. Furthermore, behind the inherent nature of the disease lurks another disquieting feature of the therapy of most hypertension; it may not benefit the majority of patients who adhere faithfully to their treatment. Even among older patients, such as those enrolled in the Systolic Hypertension in the Older Program (SHEP) trial, 111 patients would need to be treated for 5 years to prevent one cardiovascular death and 19 treated to prevent one cardiovascular event.[1,2a] This relatively small benefit and the cost and side effects of drug therapy have raised questions regarding the use of medication for the prevention of hypertension.

The situation may change for at least three reasons. First, significant increases in cardiovascular morbidity and mortality have now been amply documented, even in those with levels of blood pressure below 140/90 mm Hg.[3] Second, blood pressure levels above the assumed normal (i.e., 120/80 mm Hg) interact with other cardiovascular risk factors, calling for the need to address not only blood pressure but the patient's multiple risk factors.[4] Third, and perhaps most importantly, treatment with drugs that have almost no side effects can delay, if not prevent, the progression of prehypertension into overt hypertension.[5] Beyond these reasons, the potential for an inexpensive polypill with antilipemic, antihypertensive, and antithrombotic components may soon be realized.[6] All these reasons are amplified by the realization that the prevalence of hypertension, as noted in Chaps. 1 and 44, continues to increase as the population grows fatter and older.

Benefits of Therapy

For the largest group of hypertensive patients—those older than 65 years of age—the benefits of antihypertensive therapy are even greater than in younger patients, simply because older adults start at a much greater risk[7] (**Fig. 46-1**). Such benefit has now been shown to apply to those older than 80 years of age.[8] Despite claims that one or another therapy provides additional benefit for certain patients, the benefits of therapy are likely derived from the extent of blood pressure reduction rather than from the manner in which it was reduced[9] (**Fig. 46-2**).

The difficulty in showing clear benefits of treatment in much of the hypertensive population, either for younger individuals with blood pressures below 140/90 mm Hg or older adults with systolic pressures below 160 mm Hg, requires consideration. Even though their individual risk is relatively low, their sheer number causes them to make the major contribution to the overall population at risk for hypertension. This has given rise to two important guidelines for clinical practice: (1) the critical need for prevention of hypertension by population-wide lifestyle modifications; and (2) the rationale for considering blood pressure in the larger context of overall cardiovascular risk.

Threshold of Therapy

With any blood pressure above 120/80 mm Hg, lifestyle changes should be strongly emphasized and practical guidance should be provided for achieving the desired changes (see later). Other risk factors for cardiovascular disease also require attention (see Chap. 44). Some physicians use the presence of an overall risk of greater than 10% over the next 10 years, based on the Framingham risk score, to begin active drug therapy. The use of such overall risk estimates indicates the need for antihypertensive drug therapy more accurately than blood pressure criteria alone.

The algorithm shown in **Figure 46-3** closely follows recommendations in various national guidelines. Even lower thresholds for beginning drug therapy may be advised if the principle proven by the TROPHY trial in upper-range prehypertensives[5] is upheld in larger and longer trials with cardiovascular endpoints. Such trials are now ongoing but likely will require 3 to 5 years to complete. If drug therapy is not given, close surveillance must still be provided, because 10% to 17% of placebo-treated patients with initial blood pressure (BP) from 140/90 to 160/95 mm Hg in various randomized controlled trials (RCTs) had progression of their BP to a level above 170/100 mm Hg. All patients should be strongly advised to follow appropriate lifestyle modifications (see later, "Lifestyle Modifications").

Systolic Pressure in Older Patients

Current guidelines recommend that therapy be given to older patients with isolated systolic hypertension (ISH) because they generally have a higher absolute risk of cardiovascular disease and therefore derive greater benefit from treatment. Regardless of age, as long as the patient appears to have a reasonable life expectancy, active therapy is appropriate for all those who have a systolic level above 160 mm Hg, with or without an elevated diastolic pressure. No published RCTs have involved older patients with systolic BPs between 140 and 160 mm Hg, so the decision to treat should be based on overall risk. Those at high risk (e.g., diabetics, smokers) should be started on therapy at systolic levels above 140 mm Hg. Moreover, in one double-blinded parallel group study, a significant slowing of loss of cognitive function was noted in the 600 patients older than 80 years of age whose BP was reduced by an angiotensin II receptor blocker.[10]

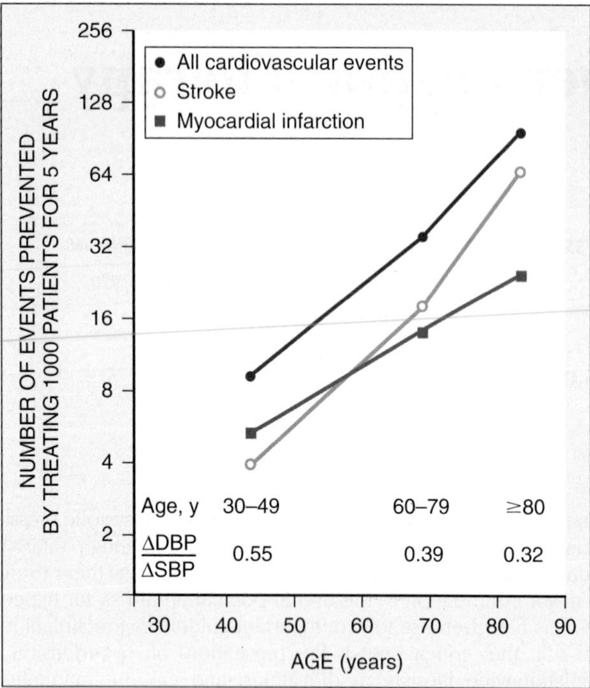

FIGURE 46-1 Absolute benefits in the prevention of fatal and nonfatal cardiovascular events, stroke, and myocardial infarction in three age groups. Symbols represent the number of events that can be prevented by treating 1000 patients for 5 years (y). *(Modified from Wang J-G, Staessen JA, Franklin SS, et al: Systolic and diastolic blood pressure lowering as determinants of cardiovascular outcome. Hypertension 45:907, 2005.)*

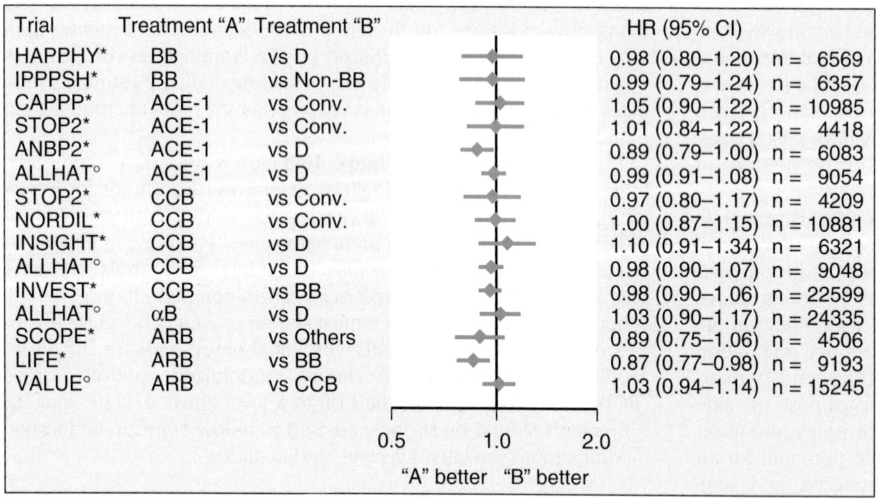

Trial	Treatment "A"	Treatment "B"	HR (95% CI)	n
HAPPHY*	BB	vs D	0.98 (0.80–1.20)	n = 6569
IPPPSH*	BB	vs Non-BB	0.99 (0.79–1.24)	n = 6357
CAPPP*	ACE-1	vs Conv.	1.05 (0.90–1.22)	n = 10985
STOP2*	ACE-1	vs Conv.	1.01 (0.84–1.22)	n = 4418
ANBP2*	ACE-1	vs D	0.89 (0.79–1.00)	n = 6083
ALLHAT°	ACE-1	vs D	0.99 (0.91–1.08)	n = 9054
STOP2*	CCB	vs Conv.	0.97 (0.80–1.17)	n = 4209
NORDIL*	CCB	vs Conv.	1.00 (0.87–1.15)	n = 10881
INSIGHT*	CCB	vs D	1.10 (0.91–1.34)	n = 6321
ALLHAT°	CCB	vs D	0.98 (0.90–1.07)	n = 9048
INVEST*	CCB	vs BB	0.98 (0.90–1.06)	n = 22599
ALLHAT°	αB	vs D	1.03 (0.90–1.17)	n = 24335
SCOPE*	ARB	vs Others	0.89 (0.75–1.06)	n = 4506
LIFE*	ARB	vs BB	0.87 (0.77–0.98)	n = 9193
VALUE°	ARB	vs CCB	1.03 (0.94–1.14)	n = 15245

0.5 1.0 2.0
"A" better "B" better

FIGURE 46-2 Trials comparing the effect on primary endpoint of treatments based on different antihypertensive drugs. Primary endpoint was cardiovascular (*) or cardiac (°) morbidity and mortality. Data are shown as differences in hazard ratio (HR) and a 95% confidence interval (CI). αB = α blocker; ACE-1 = angiotensin-converting enzyme inhibitor; Conv. = conventional treatment (based on diuretic, beta blocker, or both); D = diuretic. *(Modified from Mancia G: Role of outcome trials in providing information on antihypertensive treatment: Importance and limitations. Am J Hypertens 19:2, 2006.)*

Goal of Therapy

When the decision has been made to treat, the clinician must consider the goal of therapy. In the past, most physicians assumed that the effects of blood pressure reduction on cardiovascular risk would fit a straight line downward (**Fig. 46-4**, line A), justifying the belief that "the lower, the better." However, data from a number of large trials have indicated a more gradual decline in risk when pressures were reduced to moderate levels (see Fig. 46-4, line B). Subsequently, evidence has been presented suggesting a J curve—that is, a fall in risk until some critical level of pressure is reached, below which the risk goes back up (see Fig. 46-4, line B). The J curve has been found to apply for coronary events with falls in diastolic pressure below 80 mm Hg in patients with diastolic hypertension,[11] and for strokes with falls of systolic pressure to below 120 mm Hg in patients with chronic kidney disease.[12]

Rather than danger from drug-induced falls in BP below some critical level needed for tissue perfusion, poor general health may cause low BP and increase the risk for death. Nonetheless, excessive antihypertensive treatment may increase cardiovascular morbidity and mortality. The problem may be even more ominous in older patients with ISH, whose diastolic pressures are often low before therapy is started. Regardless, the major clinical problem is not overtreatment but undertreatment. Even in carefully conducted clinical trials, in which good control should be at a maximum, systolic BPs usually remain above 140 mm Hg, even though diastolic levels can usually be brought down to below 90 mm Hg.

The current consensus is that the optimal goal of antihypertensive therapy in most patients with combined systolic and diastolic hypertension who are not at high risk is a BP below 140/90 mm Hg. The greatest benefit is probably derived from lowering the diastolic pressure to 80 to 85 mm Hg. Not only is there no proven benefit with more intensive control, but also added cost and probable increased side effects are associated with more intensive antihypertensive therapy.

In older patients with ISH, the goal should be a systolic blood pressure of 150 mm Hg, because that was the level reached in the RCTs that showed benefit.[8] Caution is advised if, inadvertently, diastolic pressures fall below 65 mm Hg. In this case, less than ideal reductions in systolic levels need to be balanced against the potential for harm if diastolic levels fall below that level.[1]

Although the evidence is scant, more intensive therapy to attain a diastolic pressure of 80 mm Hg or lower may be desirable in some groups, including the following:

- Black patients, who are at greater risk for hypertensive complications and who may continue to have progressive renal damage despite a diastolic pressure of 85 to 90 mm Hg.
- Patients with diabetes mellitus, in whom a blood pressure of less than 130/80 mm Hg reduces the incidence of cardiovascular events.
- Patients with slowly progressive chronic renal disease who excrete more than 1 to 2 g of protein/day, in whom reducing the blood pressure to 125/75 mm Hg or lower may slow the rate of loss of renal function.[13] However, in the African American Study of Kidney Disease (AASK) trial of 759 blacks with nondiabetic hypertensive renal disease, most of those given enough therapy to reach a level of 133/78 mm Hg continued to have progressive renal damage.[14]
- Patients with significant coronary disease, if more evidence supports the finding that additional benefit is seen when the systolic BP (SBP) is reduced from 129 to 125 mm Hg, as seen in the CAMELOT trial.[15]

Despite the difficulties in achieving the appropriate goal of therapy, good control can be achieved in most patients if they are given enough antihypertensive medication in a progressive manner. Ready access to health care, frequent contact with the same physician, and surveillance of physician performance enhances control.

Lifestyle Modifications

Lifestyle modifications are indicated for almost all hypertensive individuals (**Table 46-1**). Adverse lifestyle habits are ubiquitous in those with hypertension and may play a major role in the development of the disease. Multiple modifications of lifestyle can lower blood pressure and reduce the incidence and mortality from heart attacks and strokes.[16]

Observational and trial data support the importance of simultaneous modifications of lifestyle to accomplish the greatest benefits. Although success in modifying lifestyle may be as difficult or even more difficult to achieve than having patients continue long-term antihypertensive drug therapy, even a small persistent reduction in blood pressure can have a major protective effect regarding the development of cardiovascular (CV) disease. With obesity rapidly increasing in children, attention must be directed at improving their nutrition.[17]

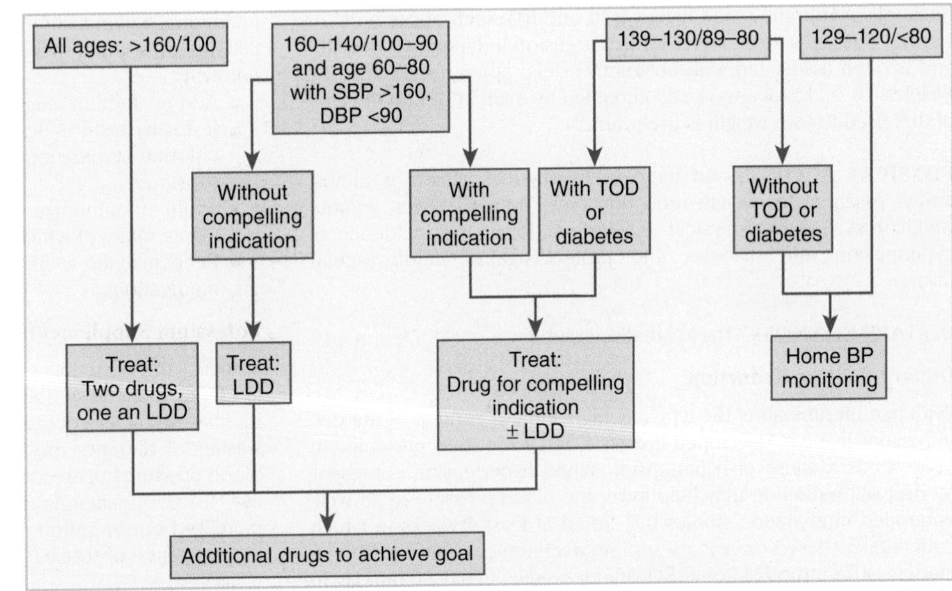

FIGURE 46-3 Algorithm for the decision to manage patients with different average blood pressure levels, determined by repeated office readings or, preferably, out of office readings, with specific attention to those aged 60 to 80 years. The recommended initial drug choices are indicated. DBP = diastolic blood pressure; LDD = low-dose diuretic; SBP = systolic blood pressure; TOD = target organ damage.

AVOIDANCE OF TOBACCO. Smoking cigarettes has long been known to be a major risk factor for CV disease, yet 21% of U.S. adults continue to smoke (see Chap. 44). Part of their risk comes from the major pressor effect of tobacco, which is easily missed because patients are not allowed to smoke in places where blood pressures are recorded. With automatic monitoring, the effect is easy to demonstrate, and blood pressure usually falls immediately when smokers quit.

Tolerance does not develop to the pressor effect of nicotine, and sympathetic outflow increases with each cigarette, leading to an increase in arterial stiffness. The noxious effects of smoking include an increase in insulin resistance, visceral obesity, and a particularly detrimental effect on the progression of nephropathy. Those who smoke must be told to stop on every contact with a health practitioner. Nicotine replacement therapies are effective and have minimal pressor effects.

WEIGHT REDUCTION. Even small increases in weight have impressive consequences on blood pressure. Over 18 years, women with an initial body mass index (BMI) of 24 were five times more likely to have diabetes and twice as likely to have hypertension as women with a BMI of 21 or lower. In many people, most of this increased weight is deposited in the upper body, constituting a major component of the

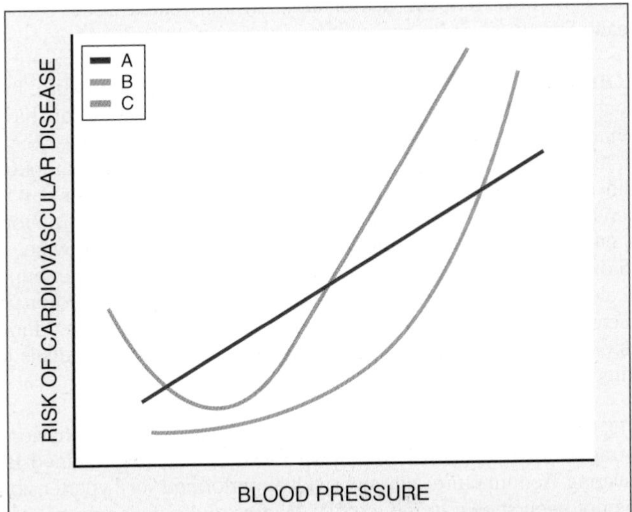

FIGURE 46-4 Three models representing hypothetical relationships between levels of blood pressure and risk of cardiovascular disease. See text for details.

TABLE 46-1 Lifestyle Modifications to Manage Hypertension

MODIFICATION	RECOMMENDATION	APPROXIMATE SYSTOLIC BLOOD PRESSURE REDUCTION (RANGE)
Weight reduction	Maintain normal body weight (body mass index, 18.5-24.9 kg/m²).	5-20 mm Hg/10 kg
Adoption of DASH eating plan	Consume a diet rich in fruits, vegetables, low-fat dairy products, with reduced content of saturated and total fat.	8-14 mm Hg
Dietary sodium reduction	Reduce dietary sodium intake to no more than 100 mmol/day (2.4 g sodium or 6 g sodium chloride).	2-8 mm Hg
Physical activity	Engage in regular aerobic physical activity such as brisk walking (at least 30 min/day, most days of the week).	4-9 mm Hg
Moderation of alcohol consumption	Limit daily consumption to no more than two drinks (1 oz [30 mL] ethanol—24 oz beer, 10 oz wine, or 3 oz 80-proof whiskey) for most men and to no more than one drink for women and lighter weight persons.	2.5-4 mm Hg

DASH = Dietary Approaches to Stop Hypertension.
From Chobanian AV, Bakris GL, Black HR, et al: The Seventh Report of the Joint National Committee on Prevention, Detection, Evaluation, and Treatment of High Blood Pressure: The JNC 7 report. JAMA 289:2560, 2003.

metabolic syndrome (see Chaps. 44, 49, and 64). Such upper body or visceral obesity is a risk factor for hypertension independent of BMI[18] and is often associated with obstructive sleep apnea (see Chap. 79). Weight loss is almost always accompanied by a fall in BP, and the type of diet used to lose weight is irrelevant.[19]

PHYSICAL ACTIVITY. An increase in physical activity is almost always essential for weight reduction (see Chap. 83). Even without weight loss, however, physical activity can lower the incidence of hypertension and diabetes and protect against cardiovascular disease.[20]

DIETARY CHANGES. These are discussed in Chaps. 45, 48, and 49.

Dietary Sodium Reduction

Evidence incriminating the typically high sodium content of the diet of persons living in developed industrialized societies is presented in Chap. 45 as a cause of hypertension. When hypertension is present, modest salt reduction may help lower the blood pressure. In 28 well-controlled intervention studies that lasted at least 4 weeks in which daily intake (based on urinary sodium excretion) was reduced by a median of 78 mmol/24 hours, BPs fell an average of 5.0/2.0 mm Hg in 734 hypertensive subjects and 2.0/1.0 mm Hg in 2220 normotensive subjects in a dose-dependent manner (**Fig. 46-5**).[21] Not all hypertensive persons respond to a moderate degree of sodium reduction to the recommended level of 100 mmol sodium or 2.4 g/day. Nevertheless, even if the BP does not fall with moderate degrees of sodium restriction, patients may still benefit. Lower sodium intake associates with multiple CV and non-CV benefits.[22] Components of the metabolic syndrome are associated with increasing BP sensitivity to dietary sodium.[23]

Rigid degrees of sodium restriction, however, are not only difficult for patients to achieve but also may be counterproductive. The marked stimulation of renin-aldosterone and sympathetic nervous activity that accompanies rigid sodium restriction may prevent the BP from falling and increase the amount of potassium wastage if diuretics are used concurrently. Sodium reduction is useful for everyone—as a preventive measure in those who are normotensive and, more certainly, as partial therapy in those who are hypertensive. The easiest way to accomplish moderate sodium reduction is to substitute natural foods for processed foods because natural foods are low in sodium and high in potassium, whereas most processed foods have had sodium added and potassium removed. It is hoped that those who process food will gradually reduce the large amounts of salt that are often added, as is being done in the United Kingdom.[21] In the meantime, patients should be asked to avoid foods with more than 300 mg of sodium per serving. Additional guidelines include the following:

- Add no sodium chloride to food during cooking or at the table.
- If a salty taste is desired, use a half-sodium and half-potassium chloride preparation (e.g., Lite-Salt) or a pure potassium chloride substitute.
- Avoid or minimize consumption of fast foods and processed meats, many of which have high sodium content.
- Recognize the sodium content of some antacids and proprietary medications.

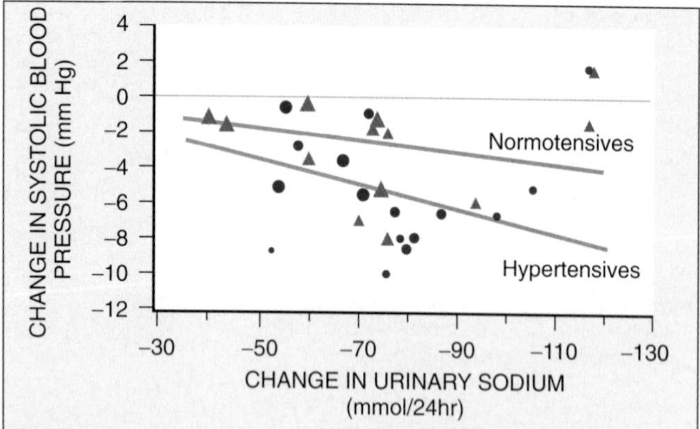

FIGURE 46-5 Relationship between the net change in urinary sodium excretion and systolic blood pressure. The blue triangles represent normotensive subjects and the magenta circles represent hypertensive subjects. The slope is weighted by the inverse of the variance of the net change in systolic blood pressure. The size of the circle is proportional to the weight of the trial. *(Modified from He J, MacGregor GA: A comprehensive review on salt and health and current experience of worldwide salt reduction programmes. J Hum Hypertens 23:363, 2009.)*

Potassium Supplementation

Some of the advantages of a lower sodium intake may relate to its tendency to increase body potassium content, both by a coincidental increase in dietary potassium intake and by a decrease in potassium wastage if diuretics are being used. Potassium supplements reduce blood pressure but are too costly and potentially hazardous for routine use in normokalemic hypertensive persons. The best source is increased consumption of fruits and vegetables, which also reduces the incidence of stroke.[24]

Calcium Supplements

Additional calcium, either in the diet or from supplements, may have a small antihypertensive effect. However, in one recent study, the 732 healthy women who took 1 g of elemental calcium/day had significantly more CV events over 5 years than those who took a placebo.[25]

Magnesium Supplements

Magnesium supplements reduce blood pressure only in patients with low serum magnesium levels.[26]

Other Dietary Constituents

Under tightly controlled conditions, the DASH diet—providing less sodium and saturated fat and more potassium, calcium, and fiber—was found to lower BP significantly. However, these results may not realistically apply because they were obtained in a short study that was tightly controlled. A more realistic view of what can be expected comes from the PREMIER trial, in which 810 adults with a mean initial blood pressure of 135/85 mm Hg were allocated to three groups; one third had minimal contact, one third was given intensive advice and close follow-up, and the rest were given the same advice and follow-up plus instruction to prepare their own DASH diet.[27] After 6 months, the latter two groups had identical reductions in coronary heart disease risks, with no additional benefit from the DASH diet. Caffeine acutely but transiently raises blood pressure, but no association between habitual coffee consumption and the incidence of hypertension has emerged. Moreover, increased coffee consumption was associated with a modestly reduced risk of stroke in the women in the Nurses Health Study.[28]

MODERATION OF ALCOHOL. Alcohol is a two-edged sword. Too much, particularly in a binge, raises blood pressure and can have lethal effects; too little may deny a number of CV benefits (see Chaps. 44, 49, and 73). The so-called safe level of regular alcohol consumption with regard to hypertension is no more than two drinks per day in men and one drink per day in women. One drink is defined as about 12 mL of alcohol—the equivalent of 12 oz of beer, 4 oz of wine, or 1.5 oz of liquor. Although regular consumption of moderate amounts of alcohol is associated with a reduction in the risk of coronary disease, heart failure, ischemic stroke, diabetes, and dementia,[29] most experts do not recommend encouraging hypertensive individuals to drink.

OTHER MODALITIES. Most studies of various cognitive-behavioral therapies for relaxation have shown transient but not sustained BP lowering. Acupuncture, although widely performed for hypertension, has not been shown to reduce BP.[30] Microvascular decompression of the brainstem may have a transient but not persistent antihypertensive effect.[31] Statin drugs may lower BP.[32] Despite the attraction that lifestyle

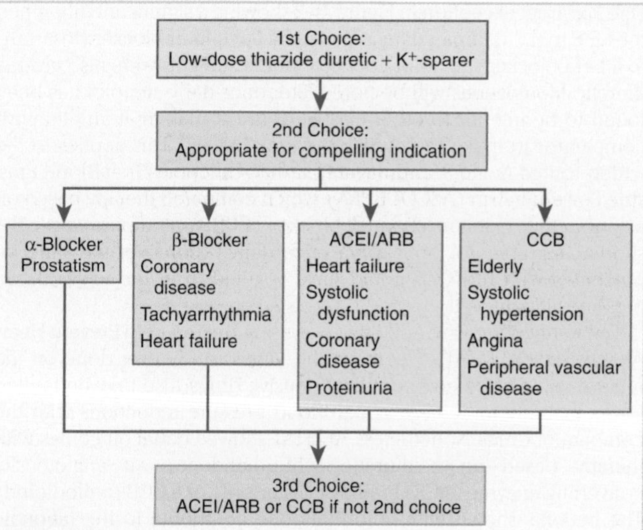

FIGURE 46-6 Algorithm for therapy of hypertension. Increasing evidence favors an aldosterone blocker as the fourth choice and perhaps as the third choice for many patients.

modifications may prevent hypertension and help manage the disease once it has developed, there is limited success of achieving significant lifestyle changes in clinical practice. Therefore, although lifestyle changes should be pursued, patients must not be denied the proven benefits of antihypertensive drug therapy.

Antihypertensive Drug Therapy

If the lifestyle modifications described are not adequate to bring the blood pressure to goal (<140/90 mm Hg for most individuals; <130/80 mm Hg for those with diabetes or renal insufficiency), or if the level of hypertension at the onset is so high that immediate drug therapy is deemed necessary (>160/100 mm Hg), an overall algorithm for treatment should be followed (**Fig. 46-6**).

General Guidelines

When drug therapy is decided on, the guidelines listed in **Table 46-2** should be followed to provide effective 24-hour control of hypertension in a manner that encourages adherence to the regimen. The approach is based on known pharmacologic principles and proven ways to improve adherence.

For most patients who do not require more intensive immediate therapy following the selection of the most appropriate agent for initial therapy (see later), a relatively low dose of a single drug should be started, aiming for a reduction of 5 to 10 mm Hg in blood pressure at each step. Many physicians, by nature and training, wish to control a patient's hypertension rapidly and completely. Regardless of which drugs are used, this approach often leads to undue fatigue, weakness, and postural dizziness, which many patients find intolerable, particularly when they felt well before therapy was begun.

Although hypokalemia and other electrolyte abnormalities may be responsible for some of these symptoms, a more likely explanation has been provided by the studies of Strandgaard and Haunsø.[33] They demonstrated the constancy of cerebral blood flow by autoregulation over a range of mean arterial pressures from about 60 to 120 mm Hg in normal subjects and from 110 to 180 mm Hg in patients with hypertension (**Fig. 46-7**; also see Fig. 45-17). This shift to the right protects hypertensive patients from a surge of blood flow, which could cause cerebral edema. However, the shift also predisposes hypertensive patients to cerebral ischemia when blood pressure is lowered to a normal level. The lower limit of autoregulation necessary to preserve a constant cerebral blood flow in hypertensive patients is a mean BP of approximately 110 mm Hg. Thus, acutely lowering the pressure from 160/110 mm Hg (mean = 127 mm Hg) to 140/85 mm Hg (mean = 102 mm Hg) may induce cerebral hypoperfusion, despite not producing hypotension in the accepted sense.

Thus, a graded approach to antihypertensive therapy for most patients should help avoid symptoms related to overly intensive

TABLE 46-2 Guidelines to Improve Maintenance of Antihypertensive Therapy

Be aware of the problem and be alert to signs of inadequate intake of medications:
- Recognize and manage depression.

Articulate the goal of therapy, which is to reduce blood pressure to near-normotension with few or no side effects.

Educate the patient about the disease and its treatment:
- Provide individual assessments of current risks and potential benefits of control.
- Involve the patient in decision making.
- Provide written instructions.
- Encourage family support.

Maintain contact with the patient:
- Encourage visits and calls to allied health personnel.
- Allow the pharmacist to monitor therapy.
- Give feedback to the patient through home blood pressure readings.
- Make contact with patients who do not return.

Keep care inexpensive and simple:
- Do the least workup needed to rule out secondary causes.
- Only obtain follow-up laboratory data yearly unless indicated more often.
- Use home blood pressure readings.
- Use nondrug low-cost therapies.
- Use once-daily doses of long-acting drugs.
- Use generic drugs and break larger doses of tablets in half.
- If appropriate, use combination tablets.
- Use calendar blister packs.
- Tailor medication to daily routines.
- Use detailed clinical protocols monitored by nurses and assistants.

Prescribe according to pharmacologic principles:
- Add one drug at a time.
- Start with small doses, aiming for reductions of 5 to 10 mm Hg at each step.
- Have medication taken immediately on awakening in the morning or after 4 am if patient awakens to void.

Be willing to stop unsuccessful therapy and try a different approach.

Anticipate and address side effects:
- Adjust therapy to ameliorate side effects that do not disappear spontaneously.

Continue to add effective and tolerated drugs stepwise in sufficient doses to achieve the goal of therapy.

Provide feedback and validation of success.

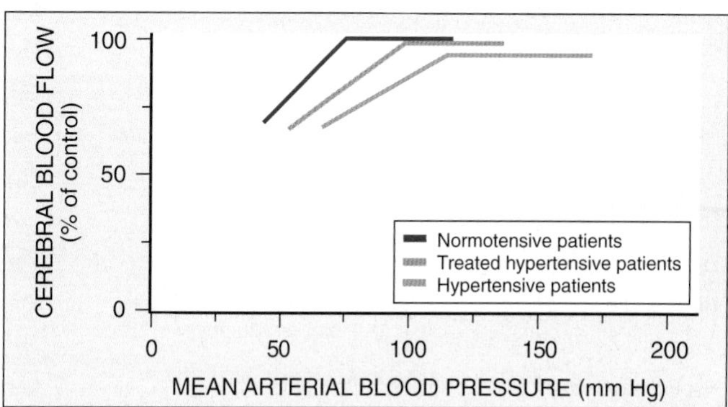

FIGURE 46-7 Mean cerebral blood flow autoregulation curves from normotensive, hypertensive, and effectively treated hypertensive patients. *(Modified from Strandgaard S: Autoregulation of cerebral blood flow in hypertensive patients. The modifying influence of prolonged antihypertensive treatment of the tolerance to acute, drug-induced hypotension. Circulation 53:720, 1976; and Strandgaard S, Haunso S: Why does antihypertensive treatment prevent stroke but not myocardial infarction? Lancet 2:658, 1987.)*

blood pressure reduction. Fortunately, if therapy is continued for a period, the curve of cerebral autoregulation shifts back toward normal, allowing patients to tolerate greater reductions in blood pressure without experiencing adverse symptoms (see Fig. 46-7, middle curve).[33]

STARTING DOSAGES. The need to start with a fairly small dose also reflects a greater responsiveness of some patients to doses of medication that may be appropriate for most patients. All drugs exert increasing effect with increasing dose up to a threshold, but the response to a given dose varies from patient to patient; some are very sensitive to that dose and some very resistant, with most having a moderate response. Without knowing how individual patients will respond, the safest and easiest approach is to start at a dose that may not be enough for most patients.

CHOICE OF INITIAL DRUG. In the past, the choice of initial drug was largely based on perceived differences in the efficacy of lowering blood pressure and the likelihood of side effects. Although comparative trials have shown some differences, largely determined by age and race,[34] most have found that moderate doses of all classes of drugs provide similar efficacy. This conclusion is hardly surprising because the formulations of almost all antihypertensive drugs are designed for the same purpose—to lower the BP by at least 10% in most hypertensive patients. More than that would probably be unacceptable to patients; less would be unacceptable to physicians.

Recommendations for the choice of initial therapy increasingly depend on the ability of drugs to have favorable effects on other conditions that frequently coexist with hypertension while avoiding those that may have unfavorable effects (**Table 46-3**).[35] Yet overall, data clearly show that with equal reductions in achieved BP, most drugs are equally effective in the hypertensive population[9] (see Fig. 46-2). One apparent exception in Figure 46-2 showing a significant difference, the LIFE trial,[36] compared an angiotensin II receptor blocker (losartan) to a beta blocker (atenolol), but 80% of the subjects were also given a diuretic. Moreover, as will be noted later, once-daily atenolol has been found to be inferior to other classes of drugs, making it an attractive comparator to make the other drug look better.[37] This applies to the widely touted Anglo-Scandinavian Cardiac Outcomes Trial-Blood Pressure Lowering Arm (ASCOT-BPLA), which compared therapy based on a long-acting calcium channel blocker (CCB; amlodipine) with the short-acting atenolol, both given once daily.[36] Moreover, the superior outcomes with the CCB could have resulted from the lower blood pressures it achieved.

The Antihypertensive and Lipid Lowering Treatment to Prevent Heart Attack Trial (ALLHAT),[38] perhaps the largest study ever done on the relative value of different antihypertensive drugs, also may be faulted for its inability to achieve equal blood pressure reductions with the comparator drugs. Nonetheless, ALLHAT showed equal outcomes with therapy based on a diuretic (chlorthalidone), an angiotensin-converting enzyme (ACE) inhibitor (lisinopril), or a CCB (amlodipine). The benefits shown with chlorthalidone contribute to the rationale for the choice of this agent over hydrochlorothiazide (see later, "Diuretics").

Even some of the favorable indications in Table 46-3 do not hold up when large data bases are carefully examined. ACE inhibitors (ACEIs) and angiotensin receptor blockers (ARBs) are widely thought to be especially renoprotective and are listed as "favorable" for diabetic or other nephropathy in Table 46-3. However, in a systemic review and meta-analysis of all currently available trials, it was concluded that "in patients with diabetes, additional renoprotective actions of [ACEIs and ARBs] beyond blood pressure remain unproven, and there is uncertainty about the greater renoprotection seen in nondiabetic renal disease."[39]

TABLE 46-3 Considerations for Individualizing Antihypertensive Drug Therapy*

May Have Favorable Effects On Comorbid Conditions		*May Have Unfavorable Effects on Comorbid Conditions*†	
CONDITION	**DRUG**	**CONDITION**	**DRUG**
Angina	Beta blocker, CCB	Bronchospastic disease	Beta blocker
Atrial tachycardia and fibrillation	Beta blocker CCB (non-DHP)	Second- or third-degree heart block	Beta blocker, CCB (non-DHP)
Cough from ACE inhibitor	ARB	Depression	Central alpha-adrenergic agonist, reserpine‡
Cyclosporine-induced hypertension	CCB	Dyslipidemia	Beta blocker (non-ISA), diuretic (high-dose)
		Gout	Diuretic
Diabetes mellitus, particularly with proteinuria	ACEI, ARB, low-dose diuretic, CCB, beta blocker	Heart failure	CCB†
		Hyperkalemia	ACEI, ARB, DRI, aldo blocker
Dyslipidemia	Alpha blocker	Liver disease	Labetalol, methyldopa‡
Essential tremor	Beta blocker (non-CS)	Peripheral vascular disease	Beta blocker†
Heart failure	ACEI, ARB, carvedilol, beta blocker, diuretic	Pregnancy	ACEI,‡ ARB,‡ DRI‡
		Renal insufficiency	Potassium-sparing agent, aldo blocker†
Hyperthyroidism	Beta blocker	Renovascular disease, bilateral	ACEI, ARB, DRI
Migraine	Beta blocker (non-CS), CCB	Types 1 and 2 diabetes	Beta blocker, high-dose diuretic
Osteoporosis	Thiazide		
Preoperative hypertension	Beta blocker		
Previous MI	Beta blocker, ACEI, ARB		
Prostatism	Alpha blocker		
Renal insufficiency	ACEI, ARB, loop diuretic		
Systolic hypertension in older persons	Diuretic, CCB		

*Conditions and drugs are listed in alphabetical order.
†These drugs may be used with special monitoring, unless contraindicated.
‡Contraindicated.
aldo = aldosterone; MI = myocardial infarction; non-CS = noncardioselective; non-ISA = non–intrinsic sympathomimetic activity.

Overall, the achieved BP reduction seems to account for clinical benefit. In one likely important regard, however, both ACEIs and ARBs may be better than diuretics and beta blockers for protection against the onset of diabetes, even during the relatively short duration of most trials.[40] Experimental data support the results of multiple clinical trials in this regard.

It should be noted that drugs in a given class may not provide the same long-term cardiovascular or renal protection as other members of the same class, even if they provide equal short-term BP reduction. There have been few direct comparative studies of drugs in the same class, so caution is advised. The duration of antihypertensive action may be the major determinant, as appears to be true of the failure of once-daily atenolol compared with other drugs (see later).[37]

OVERALL ALGORITHM. On the basis of these data, the algorithm shown in Figure 46-6 provides an appropriate approach to the treatment of stage 1 hypertension—BP below 160/100 mm Hg. A low-dose thiazide diuretic should be the foundation but is likely to be adequate by itself in only about 30% of patients. The remainder should be given whatever choice seems appropriate for their coexisting conditions (see Table 46-3). On the basis of these short-term efficacy trials, those with only hypertension could logically be given an ACEI or ARB if they are younger or nonblack, or given a diuretic or CCB if they are older or black.[41] Because concomitant diuretic therapy largely obviates differential responses in BP, there seems to be little reason to favor any drug class in the absence of a specific indication or contraindication.

COMBINATION THERAPY. Because a low dose of a thiazide diuretic potentiates the effect of all other drug classes, and because most patients require two or more drugs for adequate control, a combination of a low-dose diuretic and an appropriate second choice has been widely advocated and used. However, the results of the Avoiding Cardiovascular Events through Combination Therapy in Patients Living with Systolic Hypertension (ACCOMPLISH) trial question this practice.[42] In the ACCOMPLISH trial, the combination of an ACEI (benazepril) and CCB (amlodipine) provided a 20% greater reduction in the relative rates of cardiovascular morbidity and mortality than the combination of the same ACEI and a diuretic (hydrochlorothiazide), despite equal reductions in BP with the two combinations. Especially if these results are replicated, the initial and second drug would be either an ACEI (or ARB) or a CCB, and a diuretic would be the third choice. A number of combination tablets with the CCB amlodipine plus an ACEI or an ARB have become available. A tablet with three components—diuretic, ARB, and CCB—is also available,[43] so the polypill will likely soon become a reality,[6] although its composition remains in question (see Chap. 1).

COMPLETE COVERAGE WITH ONCE-DAILY DOSING. A number of choices within each of the six major classes of antihypertensive drugs now available provide full 24-hour efficacy (e.g., the beta blocker metoprolol-XL, the alpha blocker doxazosin, the CCB amlodipine, the ACEI trandolapril, and the ARB telmisartan). Therefore, once-daily dosing should be feasible for almost all patients, resulting in improved adherence to therapy. The use of longer-acting agents avoids the potential for inducing too great a peak effect to provide an adequate effect at the end of the dosing interval (the trough). Moreover, because many patients occasionally skip a dose of their drugs, there is an additional value in using an agent with an inherently long duration of action that also covers the skipped dose.

Because patients differ not only in terms of degree of response but also in terms of the duration of effect, the prudent course is to document the patient's response at the end of the dosing interval, usually in the early morning before that day's dosing. With this approach, the abrupt surge in blood pressure that occurs on awakening is blunted, and patients may receive better protection against the increased incidence of CV catastrophes at this critical time. The assessment of adequate 24-hour control requires home BP monitoring, an approach that all patients should use. BP management is almost always better because it is based on frequent home readings rather than occasional office readings. These general principles of therapy provide a basis for the following discussion of the various classes of available drugs.

Diuretics

Diuretics fall into four major groups by their primary site of action within the tubule, starting in the proximal portion and moving to the collecting duct: (1) agents acting on the proximal tubule, such as carbonic anhydrase inhibitors, which have limited antihypertensive efficacy; (2) loop diuretics; (3) thiazides and related sulfonamide compounds; and (4) potassium-sparing diuretics (**Table 46-4**). A thiazide is the usual choice, often in combination with a potassium-sparing agent. An aldosterone blocker is the more logical choice among potassium sparers. Loop diuretics should be reserved for patients with renal insufficiency or resistant hypertension.

MECHANISM OF ACTION. All diuretics initially lower BP by increasing urinary sodium excretion and by reducing plasma volume, extracellular fluid volume, and cardiac output. Within 6 to 8 weeks, the lowered plasma, extracellular fluid volume, and cardiac output return toward normal, but not completely back to normal. At this point and beyond, the lower BP is related to a decline in peripheral resistance, thereby improving the underlying hemodynamic defect of hypertension. However, initial diuresis is needed because diuretics fail to lower the BP when the excreted sodium is returned or when given to patients who have nonfunctioning kidneys. With the shrinkage in blood volume and lower BP, increased secretion of renin and aldosterone retards the continued sodium diuresis. Both renin-induced vasoconstriction and aldosterone-induced sodium retention prevent continued diminution of body fluids and progressive reduction in BP during continuous diuretic therapy.

CLINICAL EFFECTS. With daily diuretic therapy, systolic pressure usually falls about 10 mm Hg, although the degree depends on various factors, including the initial height of the pressure, the quantity of sodium ingested, the adequacy of renal function, and the intensity of the counterregulatory renin-aldosterone response. Those with initially lower renin or aldosterone levels, including many older or black hypertensive individuals, tend to have a greater antihypertensive effect. The antihypertensive effect of the diuretic persists indefinitely, although excessive dietary sodium intake may overwhelm it. If other antihypertensive drugs are used without diuretic, those that do not block the

TABLE 46-4 Representative Diuretics and Potassium-Sparing Agents

AGENT	DAILY DOSE (MG)	DURATION OF ACTION (HR)
Thiazides		
Bendroflumethiazide	1.25-5.0	>18
Hydrochlorothiazide	6.25-50	12-18
Methyclothiazide	2.5-5.0	>24
Trichlormethiazide	1-4	>34
Related Sulfonamide Compounds		
Chlorthalidone	12.5-50	24-72
Indapamide	1.25-2.5	24
Metolazone	0.5-10	24
Loop Diuretics		
Bumetanide	0.5-5	4-6
Ethacrynic acid	25-100	12
Furosemide	40-480	4-6
Torsemide	5-40	12
Potassium-Sparing Agents		
Amiloride	5-10	24
Eplerenone	50-200	24
Spironolactone	25-100	8-12
Triamterene	50-100	12

renin-aldosterone mechanism may have their efficacy blunted by sodium retention. This mechanism probably reflects the success of the drugs in initially lowering the BP and involve the abnormal renal pressure-natriuresis relationship that is present in primary hypertension. Just as more pressure is needed to excrete a given load of sodium in a hypertensive individual, so does a lowering of pressure toward normal lead to sodium retention. Drugs that inhibit the renin-aldosterone mechanism, such as ACEIs, ARBs, and direct renin inhibitors (DRIs), or drugs that induce some natriuresis themselves, such as CCBs, may continue to work without the need for concomitant diuretics. However, a diuretic enhances the effectiveness of all other types of drugs, including calcium channel blockers.

DOSAGE AND CHOICE OF AGENT. Most patients with mild to moderate hypertension and a serum creatinine concentration less than 1.5 mg/dL respond to the lower doses of the various diuretics (thiazides and related compounds) listed in Table 46-4. Until now, hydrochlorothiazide (HCTZ) in doses of 12.5 to 25 mg has been the overwhelming choice and is the diuretic combined with various beta blockers, ACEIs, ARBs, and DRIs that are now available, with the exception of three other drugs—atenolol, clonidine, and captopril—which are combined with chlorthalidone. However, HCTZ in these doses has not been shown to reduce morbidity or mortality. Conversely, chlorthalidone, 12.5 to 25 mg, has shown benefit in National Institutes of Health (NIH)–sponsored trials (HDFP, MRFIT, SHEP, ALLHAT). After many years of not being prescribed, chlorthalidone is now being recommended as an appropriate diuretic.[44,45] With renal damage, manifested by a serum creatinine level higher than 1.5 mg/dL or estimated glomerular filtration rate (GFR) below 30 mL/min, thiazides are usually not effective; such patients usually require two or three daily doses of furosemide, one or two doses of torsemide, or a single dose of metolazone. The combination of a thiazide with a loop diuretic may provide even better efficacy by countering the distal nephron hypertrophy seen with loop diuretics alone.

SIDE EFFECTS. Many biochemical changes often accompany successful diuresis, including a decrease in plasma potassium level and increases in glucose, insulin, and uric acid levels (**Fig. 46-8**). The use of low doses of diuretic minimizes or obviates most of these undesired effects.

Hypokalemia

The degree of potassium wastage and hypokalemia is directly related to the dose of diuretic; the serum potassium level falls an average of 0.7 mmol/liter with 50 mg of hydrochlorothiazide, 0.4 mmol/liter with 25 mg, and little if any decrease with 12.5 mg of HCTZ. Hypokalemia related to high doses of diuretic may precipitate potentially hazardous ventricular arrhythmia and increase the risk of primary cardiac arrest, particularly in patients known to be susceptible because of concomitant digitalis therapy or myocardial irritability.

The following maneuvers should help prevent diuretic-induced hypokalemia:

- Use the smallest dose of diuretic needed.
- Restrict dietary sodium intake to less than 100 mmol/day.
- Increase dietary potassium intake.
- Use a combination of a thiazide with a potassium-sparing agent, preferably an aldosterone blocker, with caution in patients with renal insufficiency.
- Use a concomitant beta blocker, ACEI, ARB, or DRI, which diminishes potassium loss by blunting the diuretic-induced rise in renin and aldosterone.

Hypomagnesemia

In some patients, concomitant diuretic-induced magnesium deficiency prevents restoration of intracellular deficits of potassium, so hypomagnesemia should be corrected.

Hyperuricemia

The serum uric acid level is elevated in as many as one third of untreated hypertensive patients. With long-term high-dose diuretic therapy, hyperuricemia appears in another third of patients as a consequence of increased proximal tubule reabsorption accompanying volume contraction and may precipitate acute gout. Hyperuricemia may also potentiate atherosclerosis and hypertension.[46]

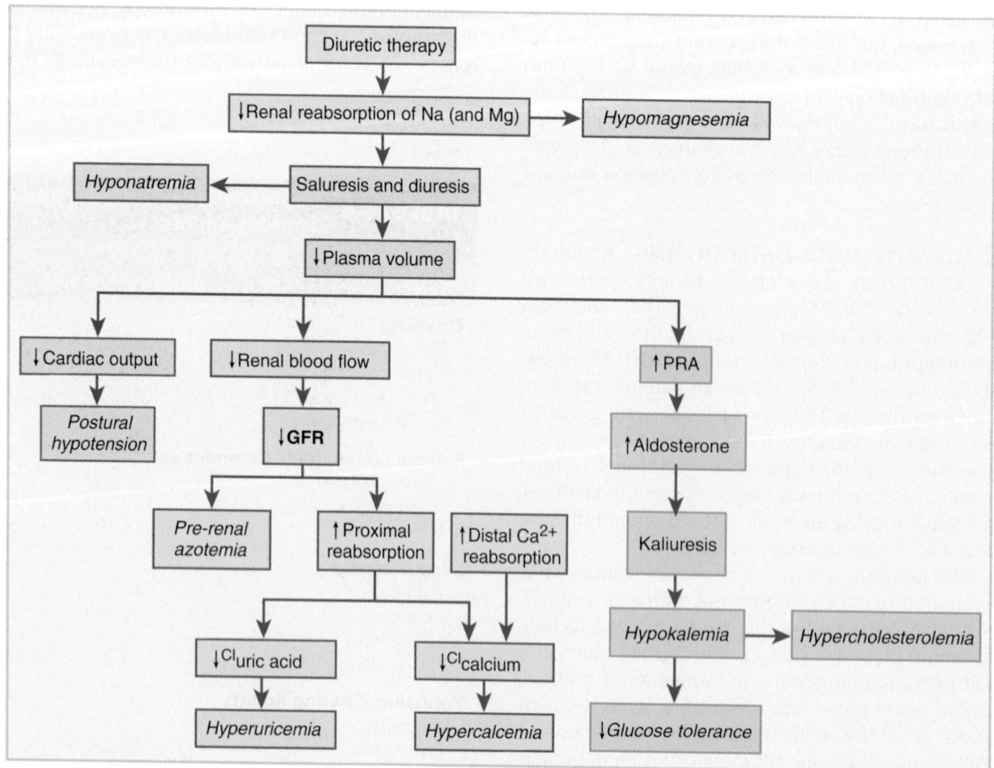

FIGURE 46-8 Mechanisms whereby chronic diuretic therapy may lead to various complications. The mechanism for hypercholesterolemia remains in question, although it is shown as arising from hypokalemia. Cl = clearance; PRA = plasma renin activity.

Hyperglycemia and Insulin Resistance

High doses of diuretics may impair glucose tolerance and precipitate diabetes mellitus, probably because they increase insulin resistance and hyperinsulinemia.

Hypercalcemia

Thiazide diuretic therapy frequently causes a slight rise in serum calcium levels, less than 0.5 mg/dL, in conjunction with a 40% to 50% decrease in urinary calcium excretion. Thiazide therapy thereby protects against renal stones and osteoporosis.

Hyponatremia

Thiazides may cause insidious hyponatremia, usually in older women.

Erectile Dysfunction

An increase in the incidence of impotence was noted among men who took 15 mg of chlorthalidone, with the diuretic being the only one of five classes of agents accompanied by this effect.[47]

Sulfa Sensitivity

Ethacrynic acid is the only diuretic that does not have a sulfonamide structure. A slow rechallenge with a sulfonamide diuretic may be successful in overcoming sulfa sensitivity.

LOOP DIURETICS. Loop diuretics are usually needed in the treatment of hypertensive patients with renal insufficiency, defined here as a serum creatinine level exceeding 1.5 mg/dL or estimated GFR below 30 mL/min. Furosemide has had the widest use, although metolazone may be as effective and requires only a single daily dose. Furosemide in uncomplicated hypertension provides less antihypertensive action than longer-acting diuretics when given once or twice daily, which better maintains the slight volume contraction required for the antihypertensive diuretic effect.

POTASSIUM-SPARING AGENTS. These drugs are normally used in combination with thiazide diuretics. Of the four currently available, two (eplerenone and spironolactone) are aldosterone blockers; the other two (triamterene and amiloride) directly inhibit potassium secretion. In combination with a thiazide diuretic, these agents diminish the amount of potassium wasting. Moreover, low doses of spironolactone may prevent myocardial fibrosis, reduce mortality in patients with heart failure, and lower blood pressure significantly in patients with resistant hypertension.[48]

Eplerenone more selectively antagonizes aldosterone than it does spironolactone,[49] thereby avoiding the gynecomastia and menstrual irregularities sometimes seen with spironolactone. In view of the increasing evidence that even normal levels of aldosterone promote fibrosis of various tissues, such a selective aldosterone blocker may find much wider use as a potassium sparer.

OVERVIEW OF DIURETICS IN HYPERTENSION. Until publication of the results of the ACCOMPLISH trial,[42] a low dose of a thiazide diuretic, preferably chlorthalidone, was recommended as the initial choice of drug therapy for most hypertensive individuals. If not the first choice, conventional wisdom has certainly favored a diuretic as the second drug used. In those with more severe hypertension or renal damage, larger doses of a thiazide or a loop-acting agent are needed. The potential for adverse effects associated with diuretics requires appropriate surveillance, particularly in patients with systolic or diastolic dysfunction who may have borderline renal perfusion. Overall, diuretics remain the least expensive choice that may also provide other benefits, such as protection against osteoporosis.

Adrenergic Inhibitors

A number of drugs that inhibit the adrenergic nervous system are available, including some that act centrally on vasomotor center activity, peripherally on neuronal catecholamine discharge, or by blocking alpha- or beta-adrenergic receptors, or both (**Table 46-5**); some act at numerous sites.

TABLE 46-5 Adrenergic Inhibitors Used in Treatment of Hypertension

Peripheral Neuronal Inhibitors
Reserpine
Guanethidine
Guanadrel
Central Adrenergic Inhibitors
Methyldopa
Clonidine
Guanabenz
Guanfacine
Alpha-Adrenergic Receptor Blockers
$Alpha_1$ and $alpha_2$ receptors
Phenoxybenzamine
$Alpha_1$ receptors
Doxazosin
Prazosin
Terazosin
Beta-Adrenergic Receptor Blockers
Acebutolol
Atenolol
Betaxolol
Bisoprolol
Carteolol
Metoprolol
Nadolol
Penbutolol
Pindolol
Propranolol
Timolol
Vasodilating Beta Blockers
Carvedilol
Labetalol
Nebivolol

An important aspect of sympathetic activity involves the feedback of norepinephrine to alpha- and beta-adrenergic receptors located on the neuronal surface (i.e., presynaptic receptors). Presynaptic alpha-adrenergic receptor activation inhibits release, whereas presynaptic beta-adrenergic receptor activation stimulates further norepinephrine release.

DRUGS THAT ACT ON THE NEURON. Reserpine, guanethidine, and related compounds act in different ways to inhibit the release of norepinephrine from peripheral adrenergic neurons.

Reserpine. Reserpine, the most active and widely used of the derivatives of the rauwolfia alkaloids, depletes the postganglionic adrenergic neurons of norepinephrine by inhibiting its uptake into storage vesicles, exposing it to degradation by cytoplasmic monoamine oxidase. The peripheral effect is predominant, although the drug enters the brain and depletes central catecholamine stores as well. This effect probably accounts for the sedation and depression accompanying reserpine use. The drug has certain advantages: only one daily dose is needed, in combination with a diuretic; the antihypertensive effect is significant; little postural hypotension is noted; and many patients experience no side effects. The drug has a relatively flat dose-response curve, so that a dose of only 0.05 mg/day gives almost as much antihypertensive effect as 0.125 or 0.25 mg/day, but with fewer side effects. Although it remains popular in some areas and is recommended as an inexpensive choice where resources are limited, the use of reserpine has progressively declined because it has no commercial sponsor.

Guanethidine. This agent and a series of related guanidine compounds, including guanadrel, bethanidine, and debrisoquine, act by inhibiting the release of norepinephrine from the adrenergic neurons. These drugs reduce BP mainly when the patient is upright as a result of gravitational pooling of blood in the legs, because compensatory sympathetic nervous system–mediated vasoconstriction is blocked. This effect results in the most common side effect, postural hypotension. As less bothersome other drugs have become available, guanethidine and

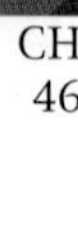
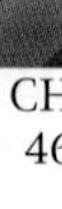

related compounds have been relegated mainly to the treatment of severe hypertension unresponsive to all other agents.

DRUGS THAT ACT ON RECEPTORS

PREDOMINANTLY CENTRAL ALPHA AGONISTS. Of these, only clonidine has much current use, although methyldopa remains one of the few drugs approved for treatment of pregnancy-induced hypertension (see Chap. 82).

METHYLDOPA. Methyldopa acts primarily within the central nervous system, where alpha-methylnorepinephrine, derived from methyldopa, is released from adrenergic neurons and stimulates central alpha-adrenergic receptors, reducing the sympathetic outflow from the central nervous system. The blood pressure falls mainly as a result of a decrease in peripheral resistance, with little effect on cardiac output. Renal blood flow is well maintained, and significant postural hypotension is unusual. Methyldopa needs to be given no more than twice daily, in doses ranging from 250 to 3000 mg/day.

Side effects include some that are common to centrally acting drugs that reduce sympathetic outflow—sedation, dry mouth, impotence, and galactorrhea. However, methyldopa causes some unique side effects that are probably of an autoimmune nature because a positive antinuclear antibody test result is obtained in about 10% of patients who take the drug, and red cell autoantibodies occur in about 20%. Inflammatory disorders in various organs have been reported, most commonly involving the liver, with diffuse parenchymal injury similar to that in viral hepatitis.

CLONIDINE. Although of a different structure, clonidine shares many features with methyldopa. It acts at the same central sites, has similar antihypertensive efficacy, and causes many of the same bothersome but less serious side effects (e.g., sedation, dry mouth). It does not, however, induce the autoimmune and inflammatory side effects.

The drug has a fairly short biologic half-life so that when it is discontinued, the inhibition of norepinephrine release disappears within about 12 to 18 hours and plasma catecholamine levels rise. This effect is responsible for the rapid rebound of BP to pretreatment levels and the occasional appearance of withdrawal symptoms, including tachycardia, restlessness, and sweating. If the rebound requires treatment, clonidine may be reintroduced or alpha-adrenergic receptor antagonists may be given. Clonidine is available in a transdermal preparation, which may provide smoother BP control for as long as 7 days with fewer side effects. Bothersome skin rashes preclude its use in perhaps 25% of patients, however.

GUANABENZ. This drug differs in structure from but shares many characteristics with both methyldopa and clonidine, acting primarily as a central alpha agonist.

GUANFACINE. This drug also resembles clonidine but is longer acting, which enables once-daily dosing and minimizes rebound hypertension. This agent, although used less than clonidine, is the preferred choice of a central alpha agonist.

ALPHA-ADRENERGIC RECEPTOR BLOCKERS. These agents may have many attractive features, but their use has been limited, initially because of the potential for postural hypotension and more recently because of a greater likelihood of fluid retention that could provoke congestive heart failure.[38] The first of this class was prazosin, but the two agents now used—doxazosin and terazosin—have slower onset and longer duration of action so that they may be given once daily, with less propensity for first-dose hypotension.

Selective alpha blockers are as effective as other antihypertensives. The favorable hemodynamic changes—a fall in peripheral resistance, with maintenance of cardiac output—make them an attractive choice for patients who wish to remain physically active. In addition, these agents do not adversely alter blood lipids and insulin sensitivity, risk factors that may actually improve with alpha blockers, unlike the adverse effects observed with diuretics and beta blockers.

The ALLHAT data[38] clearly indicate the need to use a diuretic with an alpha blocker, particularly in those with left ventricular hypertrophy (LVH) or other risk factors for congestive heart failure. Alpha blockers are now being used primarily for the relief of prostatism. By decreasing the tone of the smooth muscle at the bladder neck and prostate, they relieve the obstructive symptoms of prostatic hypertrophy. Tamsulosin has a greater effect on the bladder and less of an antihypertensive effect, but its use is associated with a serious complication after cataract surgery.[50]

BETA-ADRENERGIC RECEPTOR BLOCKERS. In the 1980s, beta-adrenergic receptor blockers (beta blockers) became the most popular form of antihypertensive therapy after diuretics, reflecting their relative effectiveness and freedom from many bothersome side effects. Because beta blockers reduce mortality in patients post–myocardial infarction or heart failure (i.e., secondary prevention), it was assumed they would also provide special protection against initial cardiac events (i.e., primary prevention). In multiple large RCTs, however, the use of a beta blocker (particularly atenolol) provided no more protection against the first myocardial infarction (MI) than other drugs and was associated with a statistically significant 16% increase in the incidence of stroke. The rationale for this has long been known but only recently appreciated—beta blockers lower brachial systolic BP equally but do not lower aortic pressure as well as other drugs. They reduce heart rate and increase peripheral resistance, so that the arterial wave reflection from the periphery returns during systole rather than during diastole.[51] Therefore, Lindholm and coworkers have concluded that "beta blockers should not remain [as] first choice in the treatment of primary hypertension."[37]

Types of Beta Blockers

Various beta blockers are now available in the United States (**Fig. 46-9**). Pharmacologically, these agents differ considerably with respect to degree of absorption, protein binding, and bioavailability. However, the three most important differences affecting their clinical use are cardioselectivity, intrinsic sympathomimetic activity, and lipid solubility. Despite these differences, they all seem to be about as effective as antihypertensives.

Cardioselectivity

Cardioselectivity refers to the relative blocking effect on the $beta_1$-adrenergic receptors in the heart compared with that on the $beta_2$ receptors in the bronchi, peripheral blood vessels, and elsewhere. Such cardioselectivity can easily be shown using small doses in acute studies; with the rather high doses used to treat hypertension, much of this selectivity is lost.

Intrinsic Sympathomimetic Activity

Some of these drugs, such as pindolol, have intrinsic sympathomimetic activity and interact with beta receptors to cause a measurable agonist response while blocking the greater agonist effects of endogenous catecholamines at the same time.

Lipid Solubility

Atenolol and nadolol are among the least lipid-soluble of the beta blockers, so they escape hepatic metabolism and are excreted unchanged. Lipid-soluble agents, such as metoprolol and propranolol, are taken up and metabolized in the liver and are consequently more bioavailable after intravenous than oral administration.

Mechanism of Action

Despite these and other differences, the various beta blockers now available are approximately as effective as antihypertensive agents. A

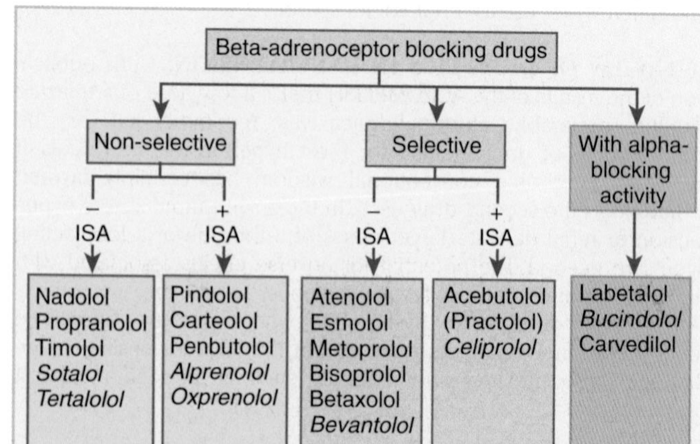

FIGURE 46-9 Classification of beta-adrenergic receptor blockers on the basis of cardioselectivity and intrinsic sympathomimetic activity. Drugs not approved for use in the United States for the treatment of hypertension are in italics. ISA = intrinsic sympathomimetic activity.

number of possible mechanisms likely contribute to their antihypertensive action. For those without intrinsic sympathomimetic activity, cardiac output falls 15% to 20% and renin release drops about 60%. At the same time that beta blockers lower BP through various means, their blockade of peripheral beta-adrenergic receptors inhibits vasodilation, leaving alpha receptors open to catecholamine-mediated vasoconstriction. Over time, however, vascular resistance tends to return to normal, which presumably preserves the antihypertensive effect of a reduced cardiac output.

Clinical Effects

Even in small doses, beta blockers begin to lower BP within a few hours. Although progressively higher doses have usually been given, careful study has shown a near-maximal effect from smaller doses. Even though beta blockers are less protective than other antihypertensive drugs for primary prevention, they remain important for the secondary protection that they provide to hypertensive patients with coexisting coronary disease or heart failure. Because beta blockers inhibit sympathetic activity, they have been widely used to reduce the somatic manifestations of stress in people as divergent as violin players or race car drivers. However, their value in younger, hyperkinetic, hypertensive individuals has never been documented.

Side Effects

Most of the side effects of beta blockers are related to their major pharmacologic action, the blockade of beta-adrenergic receptors. Certain concomitant problems may worsen when beta-adrenergic receptors are blocked, including peripheral vascular disease and bronchospasm. The most common side effect is fatigue, probably a consequence of decreased cardiac output. Sexual dysfunction may be increased by beta blockers, but depression likely is not.

Beta blockers increase the incidence of diabetes, presumably through a decrease in insulin sensitivity secondary to reduced skeletal muscle perfusion from peripheral vasoconstriction. Diabetic patients may have additional problems with beta blockers, even more with nonselective ones. The responses to hypoglycemia—both the symptoms (except sweating) and counterregulatory hormonal changes that raise blood glucose levels—depend partially on sympathetic nervous activity. Diabetic patients who are susceptible to hypoglycemia may not be aware of the usual warning signals (except sweating) and may not rebound as quickly.

Perturbations of lipoprotein metabolism accompany the use of beta blockers. Nonselective agents cause rises in triglyceride levels and reductions in cardioprotective high-density lipoprotein cholesterol levels. When a beta blocker is suddenly discontinued, angina pectoris and MI may occur because the increased number of beta receptors that appear after beta blockade are suddenly exposed to sympathetic nervous activity. Because patients with hypertension are more susceptible to coronary disease, they should be weaned gradually and given appropriate coronary vasodilator therapy.

Caution is advised in the use of beta blockers for patients suspected of harboring a pheochromocytoma (see Chaps. 45 and 86), because unopposed alpha-adrenergic agonist action may precipitate a serious hypertensive crisis if this disorder is present. The use of beta blockers during pregnancy has been clouded by scattered case reports of various fetal problems.

Overview of Beta Blockers in Hypertension

Beta blockers are specifically recommended for hypertensive patients with concomitant coronary disease, particularly after a myocardial infarction, congestive heart failure, or tachyarrhythmias (see Table 46-3). If a beta blocker is chosen, the agents that are more cardioselective offer the likelihood of fewer perturbations of lipid and carbohydrate metabolism and, because of fewer side effects (except for bradycardia), better adherence to therapy. Long-acting formulations are available for once-daily dosing.

VASODILATING BETA BLOCKERS. The combination of an alpha and a beta blocker in a single molecule is available in the forms of labetalol and carvedilol, with the latter agent also approved for the treatment of heart failure. The fall in pressure results mainly from a decrease in peripheral resistance, with little or no decline in cardiac output. The most bothersome side effects are related to postural hypotension. Labetalol should be given twice daily, but a longer acting preparation of carvedilol is available. Intravenous labetalol is used to treat hypertensive emergencies.

Nebivolol, the most selective $beta_1$-blocker of this family of drugs, exerts its effect by generating and releasing NO while having a complimentary antioxidant effect.[52] It may be particularly effective in the treatment of older patients with isolated systolic hypertension. In addition to reducing aortic stiffness, as do other beta blockers, it also reduces the amplification of central systolic pressure by reducing wave reflection from the periphery.[53]

Direct Vasodilators

Three agents differ from drugs that produce vasodilation indirectly, such as ACEIs and ARBs, which inhibit a vasoconstricting hormone. Hydralazine is the most widely used of this type. Minoxidil is more potent, but it is usually reserved for patients with severe refractory hypertension associated with renal failure. Nitroprusside, nitroglycerin, and some CCBs may be given intravenously for hypertensive crises (see later, "Therapy for Hypertensive Crises").

HYDRALAZINE. Hydralazine, in combination with a diuretic and a beta blocker, has been used frequently to treat severe hypertension. It acts directly to relax the smooth muscle in precapillary resistance vessels, with little or no effect on postcapillary venous capacitance vessels. As a result, blood pressure falls by a reduction in peripheral resistance, but meanwhile a number of compensatory processes, which are activated by the arterial baroreceptor arc, blunt the decrease in pressure and cause side effects. With the concomitant use of a diuretic to overcome the tendency for fluid retention and an adrenergic inhibitor to prevent the reflex increase in sympathetic activity and increase in renin level, the vasodilator is more effective and causes few, if any, side effects. Hydralazine needs be given only twice daily. Its daily dosage should be kept below 400 mg to prevent the lupus-like syndrome that appears in 10% to 20% of patients who receive more. This reaction, although uncomfortable to the patient, is almost always reversible. The reaction is uncommon with daily doses of 200 mg or less and is more common in slow acetylators of the drug.

MINOXIDIL. This drug vasodilates by opening potassium channels in vascular smooth muscle. Its hemodynamic effects are similar to those of hydralazine, but minoxidil is even more effective and may be used once daily. It is particularly useful for patients with severe hypertension and renal failure. Even more than with hydralazine, diuretics and adrenergic receptor blockers must be used with minoxidil to prevent the reflex increase in cardiac output and fluid retention. Pericardial effusion has appeared in about 3% of those given minoxidil, even in some without renal or cardiac failure. The drug also causes hair to grow profusely, and the facial hirsutism precludes use of the drug in most women.

CALCIUM CHANNEL BLOCKERS. These drugs are among the most popular classes of agents used in the treatment of hypertension. Claims of multiple serious side effects of their use, mostly based on biased observational studies, have been repudiated by data from multiple RCTs, including ALLHAT, in which coronary events were the same for the CCB as for the diuretic or ACEI, and mortality from non-CV causes was significantly lower in the CCB group than in the diuretic or ACEI group.[38]

Mechanisms of Action

All currently available CCBs interact with the same L-type voltage-gated plasma membrane channel, but at different sites and with different consequences. Dihydropyridines (DHPs) have the greatest peripheral vasodilatory action, with little effect on cardiac automaticity, conduction, or contractility. But comparative trials have shown that the non-DHP CCBs verapamil and diltiazem, which do affect these

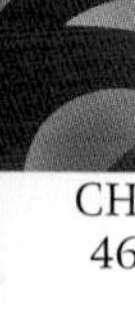

TABLE 46-6 Comparative Randomized Controlled Trials for Hypertension—Hazard Rate (95% CI)*

THERAPY	STROKE	CORONARY DISEASE	HEART FAILURE	CV EVENTS	CV DEATH	TOTAL MORTALITY
ACEI versus placebo	0.84 (0.72-0.97)	0.79 (0.71-0.88)	0.82 (0.69-0.96)	0.78 (0.71-0.85)	0.80 (0.68-0.93)	0.88 (0.81-0.96)
CCB versus placebo	0.65 (0.55-0.78)	0.83 (0.67-1.03)	0.99 (0.53-1.86)	0.81 (0.70-0.94)	0.75 (0.59-0.96)	0.88 (0.74-1.04)
ACEI versus D/βB	1.09 (0.96-1.24)	0.97 (0 90-1.05)	0.94 (0.55-1 59)	1.02 (0.97-1.08)	1.03 (0.95-1.11)	0.94 (0.80-1.11)
CCB versus D/βB	0.92 (0.85-0.99)	1.02 (0.96-1.09)	1.27 (1.01-1.61)	1.04 (0.97-1.08)	1.05 (0.97-1.15)	0.95 (0.87-1.03)
ACEI versus CCB	1.08 (0.91-1.28)	0.83 (0.65-1.05)	0.84 (0.75-0.95)	0.95 (0.86-1.04)	1.03 (0.83-1.27)	1.04 (0.94-1.15)

*The trials included in these two meta-analyses differed somewhat. In the report from Turnbull and colleagues, 27 trials from 1985 to 2003, which included congestive heart failure and mortality endpoints, were included; in the report from Verdecchia and associates, 29 trials comparing ACEIs and CCBs for the prevention only of coronary heart disease and stroke from 1996 through 2004 were included.

CI = confidence interval; D/βB = diuretic/beta blocker.

Data from Turnbull F, Neal B, Algert C, et al: Effects of different blood pressure-lowering regimens on major cardiovascular events in individuals with and without diabetes mellitus. Results of prospectively designed overviews of randomized trials. Arch Intern Med 165:1410, 2005; and Verdecchia P, Reboldi G, Angeli F, et al: Angiotensin-converting enzyme inhibitors and calcium channel blockers for coronary heart disease and stroke prevention. Hypertension 46:386, 2005.

properties, are also effective antihypertensives and may cause fewer side effects related to vasodilation, such as flushing and ankle edema. They induce slight bradycardia and should be used cautiously with a beta blocker or for patients with a conduction defect.

Clinical Use

CCBs are effective in hypertensive patients of all ages and races. Against placebo in RCTs, DHP CCBs reduced cardiovascular events and deaths (**Table 46-6**). Compared with other classes of drugs, they may protect better against stroke but less well against heart failure.[54]

CCBs have been found to be particularly effective in the prevention of stroke in older hypertensive individuals, perhaps because they tend to have a greater antihypertensive effect than that seen in younger patients. They also appear to lower BP in blacks better than in others[9]; however, with equal degrees of BP reduction, they are no better as a cardioprotective than a diuretic or ACEI (see Table 46-6). CCBs may cause at least an initial natriuresis, probably by producing renal afferent vasodilation, which may lessen the need for concurrent diuretic therapy. Unlike all other antihypertensive agents, their effectiveness may lessen rather than improve with concomitant dietary sodium restriction; most careful studies have shown an enhancement of their effect by concomitant diuretic therapy.

The use of CCBs has been questioned in two important groups of hypertensives: those with diabetes and those with nephropathy. Concerning the use of CCBs in patients with type 2 diabetes, a DHP CCB, nitrendipine, provided excellent protection in those enrolled in the Systolic Hypertension in Europe (Syst-Eur) trial, even better than that provided by a diuretic in the SHEP trial. Therapy based on the DHP CCB felodipine provided a 51% reduction in major CV events in the 1501 patients with diabetes enrolled in the HOT trial.[54a] Among the almost 12,000 diabetic patients in the ALLHAT trial, the CCB amlodipine was as protective as the ACEI or diuretic.[38]

Concerning the use of CCBs in patients with nephropathy, experts agree that an ACEI or ARB should be the first drug used. To provide the degree of BP reduction required to protect such patients maximally almost always necessitates the administration of additional drugs. A CCB is an appropriate choice as the third drug, with a diuretic as the second. On the basis of greater reduction in proteinuria seen with non–DHP CCBs, some believe a non–DHP CCB should be used.[55] However, the addition of a DHP CCB does not interfere with the renoprotective effects of ACEIs or ARBs.[56] Moreover, renal function, assessed by the estimated GFR, was better preserved by the DHP CCB than by the diuretic or the ACEI in ALLHAT.[38]

Side Effects

Side effects preclude the use of these drugs in perhaps 10% of patients. Most side effects—headaches, flushing, local ankle edema—are related to the vasodilation that these drugs produce. Slow-release and longer acting formulations reduce vasodilative side effects. In a few patients, the antihypertensive effect of the short-acting agents, particularly liquid nifedipine, may be so marked as to reduce blood flow and induce ischemia of vital organs, which requires their use to be discontinued. The decrease in coronary events in large RCTs with long-acting DHPs is the best proof of the safety of these agents.[54] CCBs may be unique in not having their antihypertensive efficacy blunted by nonsteroidal anti-inflammatory drugs (NSAIDs).

Overview of Calcium Channel Blockers

Compared with other classes of agents, CCBs reduce the risk of coronary disease equally, stroke more but heart failure less, and have similar effects on overall mortality.[54a] They work well and are usually well tolerated across the entire spectrum of hypertensives. They have some particular niches—coexisting angina and cyclosporine or NSAID use. If chosen, an inherently long-acting, second-generation DHP such as amlodipine seems to be the best choice, because it maintains better BP control in the critical early morning hours and throughout the next day if the patient misses a dose. Rate-slowing CCBs, such as verapamil or diltiazem, may be preferable in certain cases.

Inhibitors of the Renin-Angiotensin-Aldosterone System

ANGIOTENSIN-CONVERTING ENZYME INHIBITORS. Activity of the renin-angiotensin system may be inhibited in four ways, all of which can be applied clinically (**Fig. 46-10**). The first, use of beta-adrenergic receptor blockers to inhibit the release of renin, was discussed earlier. The second, an agent that directly inhibits renin activity, is now available.[57] The third, inhibition of the enzyme that converts the inactive decapeptide angiotensin I (A I) to the active octapeptide angiotensin II (A II), is being widely used with orally effective ACEIs. The fourth, blockade of angiotensin's actions by a competitive receptor blocker, is the basis for the fastest growing class of antihypertensive agents, the ARBs. ARBs may offer additional benefits, in particular the absence of cough that often accompanies ACEIs, as well as less angioedema. ARBs and DRIs are considered after the ACEIs.

Mechanism of Action

The first of the ACEIs, captopril, was synthesized as a specific inhibitor of the ACE that in the classic pathway breaks the peptidyl dipeptide bond in A I. The enzyme is thereby prevented from attaching to and splitting the A I structure. Because A II cannot be formed and A I is inactive, the ACEI paralyzes the classic renin-angiotensin system, thereby removing the effects of most endogenous A II as both a vasoconstrictor and a stimulant to aldosterone synthesis. Interestingly, with long-term use of ACEIs, the plasma A II levels actually return to previous values while the blood pressure remains lowered,[58] which suggests that the antihypertensive effect may involve other mechanisms. The same ACE that converts A I to A II is also responsible for inactivation of the vasodilating hormone bradykinin. By inhibiting the breakdown of bradykinin, ACEIs increase the concentration of a vasodilating hormone while decreasing the concentration of a vasoconstrictor hormone. The increased plasma kinin levels may contribute to the vasodilation and other beneficial effects of ACEIs, but they are also probably responsible for the most common and bothersome side effects of their use—a dry hacking cough and, less frequently, angioedema. Regardless of their mechanism of action, ACEIs lower blood pressure mainly by reducing peripheral resistance with little if any effect on heart rate, cardiac output, or body fluid volumes, probably reflecting preservation of baroreceptor reflexes. As they restore endothelium-dependent relaxation, resistance arteries become less thickened and more responsive.

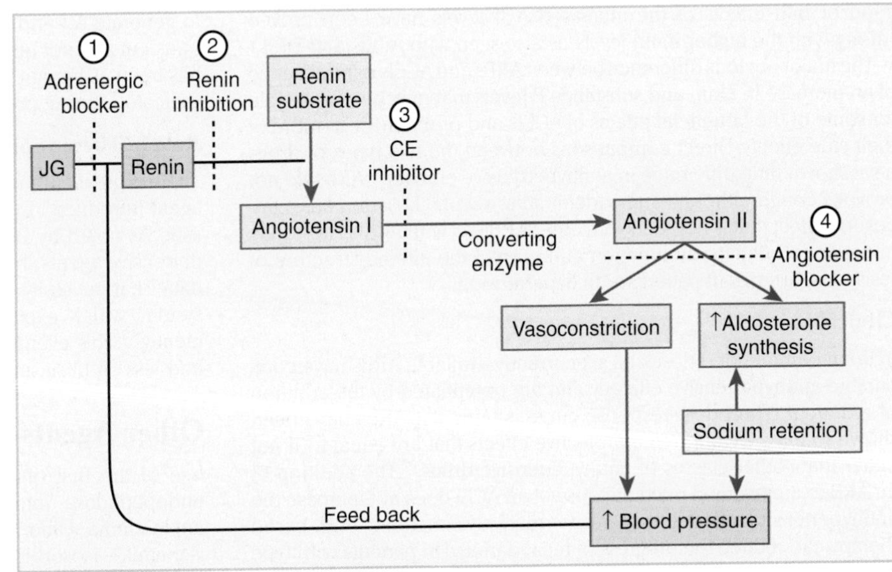

FIGURE 46-10 Renin-angiotensin-aldosterone system and four sites where its activity can be inhibited. CE = converting enzyme; JG = juxtaglomerular cells.

Clinical Use

In patients with uncomplicated primary hypertension, ACEIs as monotherapy provide antihypertensive effects equal to those obtained with other classes, but are somewhat less effective in blacks and older people because of their lower renin levels. Addition of a diuretic enhances the efficacy of an ACEI. More importantly, ACEI-based therapy has provided significant protection against CV disease and death when compared with placebo, and comparable if not better protection than other classes of drugs (see Table 46-6). In the ALLHAT trial involving predominantly older, high-risk hypertensive individuals, ACEI-based therapy was generally equal to diuretic- or CCB-based therapies except against strokes in the black enrollees, probably because of less antihypertensive efficacy.[38]

ACEIs have proven impressively effective in the treatment of hypertensives (and nonhypertensives) with coronary disease or congestive heart failure (see Chaps. 55 and 28). Another area in which they have become the drug of choice is chronic renal disease, whether diabetic or nondiabetic in origin. The high levels of renin, arising in the juxtaglomerular cells within the renal afferent arterioles, flood the glomeruli and renal efferent arterioles, providing ACEIs (and ARBs and DRIs) with the opportunity to dilate these vessels selectively and lower intraglomerular pressure more effectively than other classes of drugs. These hemodynamic effects may lower renal perfusion and glomerular filtration. However, because acute increases of serum creatinine levels up to 30% that stabilize within the first 2 months of ACEI therapy are associated with better long-term renoprotection, such increases should not prompt withdrawal of the drug.[59] On the other hand, a retrospective observational study has reported renal failure after prolonged use of an ACEI in diabetic patients.[60] Whether ACEIs (and ARBs and DRIs) provide renal (and cardiac) protection beyond their antihypertensive effects remains in question. The issue has been most intensively studied in patients with proteinuria because it is easy to measure. Controlled trials have suggested that the antiproteinuric effect of an ACEI is directly related to its antihypertensive effect, but data are inadequate. These drugs have been a mixed blessing for patients with renovascular hypertension. On the one hand, they usually control the blood pressure effectively. On the other hand, the removal of the high levels of A II that follow their use may deprive the stenotic kidney of the hormonal drive to its blood flow, thereby causing a marked decline in renal perfusion, so that patients with only one kidney or bilateral disease may develop acute and sometimes persistent renal failure.

Side Effects

Most patients who take an ACEI experience neither the side effects nor the biochemical changes that often accompany other drugs; this may be of even more concern, albeit less obvious, such as rises in lipid, glucose, or uric acid levels or reductions in potassium levels. ACEIs may have specific and nonspecific adverse effects. Specific side effects include rare rashes, loss of taste, and leukopenia. In addition, they may cause a hypersensitivity reaction with angioneurotic edema, most frequently in blacks, or a cough, most frequently in Asians.[61] The cough is infrequently associated with pulmonary dysfunction but may not disappear for 3 weeks after the ACEI is discontinued. If a cough appears in a patient who needs an ACEI, an ARB or DRI should be substituted. Angioedema occurs more frequently in diabetics who take both a glitazone and an ACEI. Each drug inhibits an enzyme responsible for the degradation of substance P, dipeptidyl peptidase-4, and an ACE respectively. Higher levels of substance P have been blamed for the increase in angioedema.[62]

Another serious problem with ACEIs and ARBs is their effect on the fetuses of women who take them during pregnancy. The interference with renal development has long been recognized with their use in the second and third trimesters. Even more threatening is the possibility that their use during the first trimester may cause major cardiac and central nervous system malformations.[63] If further documented, this would limit use of these drugs in almost all women with childbearing potential.

The antihypertensive efficacy of ACEIs may be blunted by large (300-mg) doses of aspirin and most NSAIDs. Patients with renal insufficiency or those taking potassium supplements or potassium-sparing agents may not be able to excrete potassium loads and may thus develop hyperkalemia.

Overview of Angiotensin-Converting Enzyme Inhibitors

The rationale for the use of ACEIs in the treatment of hypertension has steadily expanded beyond their proven efficacy as antihypertensive agents. In particular, they provide special advantages in three large groups of patients—those with heart failure, coronary ischemia, or nephropathy. They are the drugs of choice for these patients (see Table 46-3). Moreover, the evidence from the Heart Outcomes Prevention Evaluation (HOPE) trial has led to the recommendation that an ACEI be given to all patients at high risk for coronary disease, whether hypertensive or not.[64] Although an ACEI-based therapy did not outperform a diuretic or a CCB in the ALLHAT trial,[38] their proven special benefits ensure their continued growth. Even as ACEIs have become increasingly popular and less expensive, their position has been threatened by the aggressive marketing of ARBs, agents acting at a more distal site of the renin-angiotensin system.

ANGIOTENSIN II RECEPTOR BLOCKERS

Mechanisms of Action

ARBs displace A II from its specific A II type 1 (AT_1) receptor, antagonizing all its known effects and resulting in a dose-dependent fall in peripheral resistance and little change in heart rate or cardiac output. As a consequence of the competitive displacement, circulating levels of A II increase but, at the same time, the blockade of the renin-angiotensin mechanism is more complete, including any A II that is generated through pathways that do not involve the ACE. No obvious good or bad effects of the increased A II levels have been proved (along with the higher renin levels, as also seen with ACEIs and DRIs).

The major obvious difference between ARBs and ACEIs is the absence of an increase in kinin and substance P levels that may be responsible for some of the beneficial effects of ACEIs and probably even more of their side effects. Direct comparisons between the two types of drugs have shown little difference in antihypertensive efficacy.[65] ARBs do not provoke cough, although angioedema may occur.[66] Losartan has a uricosuric effect that is not seen with other ARBs. As with ACEIs, ARBs may improve endothelial dysfunction and correct the altered structure of resistance arteries in patients with hypertension.

Clinical Use

In the recommended doses, all six currently available ARBs have comparable antihypertensive efficacy and are potentiated by the addition of a diuretic. Their dose-response curve is fairly flat. ARBs have been shown to have CV and renal protective effects that are equal to, if not better than, other classes of antihypertensive drugs.[67] The addition of an ARB to a presumed maximal dose of an ACEI does not increase the antihypertensive effect but increases renal dysfunction.[68] ARB-based therapy can reduce the progress of renal damage in patients with type 2 diabetes with nephropathy (Chap. 28 describes their use in heart failure).

Side Effects

Whether or not they are more effective than ACEIs, ARBs are easier to take. In various clinical trials, side effects were generally no greater than with placebo, and the agent was better tolerated than other antihypertensive agents. Fetal toxicity, hyperkalemia, hypotension, and renal impairment are almost certain to be noted occasionally because they are expected consequences of the blockade of the renin-angiotensin mechanism. However, no major surprises have surfaced to date. Their superior side effect profile prompted the use of one, candesartan, in the TROPHY trial of treating prehypertension.[5]

Overview of Angiotensin II Receptor Blockers

As reflected by the fast growth of the use of ARBs, it appears that they are being prescribed for many more patients than the 10% or so who are intolerant of an ACEI.

DIRECT RENIN INHIBITORS. A DRI, aliskerin, is now approved for the treatment of hypertension. Despite its limited absorption and bioavailability (3%), aliskerin works because of its high aqueous solubility, high specificity for the enzymatically active site of human renin, and long half-life (40 hours), and because it is minimally metabolized.[69] Other orally effective DRIs are likely to follow aliskerin (see Chap. 45).

Mechanism of Action

The renal juxtaglomerular apparatus secretes prorenin, which is enzymatically converted to the active renin, largely in the kidney. Renin cleaves the 10–amino acid A I from the protein substrate angiotensinogen. Aliskerin blocks renin's catalytic site, reducing the formation of A I and its generation of A II, resulting in a fall of BP. The lower levels of angiotensin I and II remove inhibition of prorenin secretion from the juxtaglomerular apparatus so that levels of prorenin and renin are markedly increased. It is believed that as long as aliskerin blocks the catalytic action of prorenin and renin, BP will fall. Experimentally, however, prorenin can bind to a cognate receptor in various tissues where it exerts profibrotic effects, without interference from aliskerin.[70] Moreover, in transgenic mice with markedly elevated prorenin levels, no increase in tissue fibrosis occurred, even though hypertension developed.[71] Therefore, the eventual benefits and potential dangers of a DRI remain uncertain.

Antihypertensive Efficacy

Aliskerin lowers BP and reduces left ventricular hypertrophy. Its combination with an ARB appears to provide additional antihypertensive effect and end-organ protection.[72] The rationale for the combination is the potential of nonrenin enzymes, such as cathepsin D and chymase, to generate A I and A II that will not be inhibited by DRIs. Except for transient and not unexpected rises in serum potassium levels, aliskerin has been as benign as ARBs. As with ACEIs and ARBs, DRIs are contraindicated during pregnancy.

Role in Therapy of Hypertension

There is great enthusiasm over aliskerin, the only new antihypertensive agent introduced in more than a decade,[72] but some are less enthusiastic. As noted by Birkenhager and Staessen, "No new class of antihypertensive agents should make it to routine use without hard outcome data. That necessity applies even more to dual inhibition of the renin system, which exposes patients to hyperkalemia and renal insufficiency."[73] This eventually may be found to be true, but more caution and less enthusiasm may be appropriate at this point.

Other Agents

Use of the first of the most promising new class of drugs, neutral endopeptidase inhibitors, was curtailed by a high incidence of angioedema. Older vasodilators now used extensively for coronary ischemia—isosorbide dinitrate and transdermal glyceryl trinitrate—can effectively lower BP, but they probably have not undergone rigorous trials because of the lack of commercial sponsors. Statins have a small but significantly antihypertensive effect.[32] Glitazones, sildenafil, progestins with antimineralocorticoid activity, uricosurics, and other agents may have beneficial antihypertensive effects. Others now in development will likely be added.

Special Therapeutic Considerations

WITHDRAWAL OF DRUGS. As many as 20% of treated patients with well-controlled hypertension are able to maintain normotension for as long as 1 year after withdrawal of their drugs. Considering how difficult it may be to achieve adequate control, withdrawal seems inappropriate if the therapy is causing no adverse effects.

RESISTANT HYPERTENSION. There are numerous causes of resistance to therapy, usually defined as the failure of diastolic blood pressure to fall below 90 mm Hg despite the use of three or more drugs, including a diuretic (**Table 46-7**).[74] Patients often do not respond well because they do not take their medications. Often overlooked is physician inertia to modify therapy, a problem that can be overcome particularly within an integrated health care delivery system with appropriate surveillance.

What appears to be a poor response on the basis of office readings of blood pressure may be found to be an adequate response by ambulatory or home readings. Several factors—such as obstructive sleep apnea[75] or, most commonly, volume overload caused by inadequate diuretic or excessive dietary sodium intake—may account for a poor response even if the medication is taken regularly. Larger doses, more potent diuretics, or small doses of an aldosterone blocker often bring resistant hypertension under control.

HYPERTENSIVE CHILDREN. Almost nothing is known about the effects of various antihypertensive medications given to children over long periods. In the absence of adequate data, an approach similar to that advocated for adults is advised.[76] Emphasis should be placed on weight reduction in hypertensive children who are obese in the hope of controlling hypertension without the need for drug therapy.

HYPERTENSION DURING PREGNANCY. (see Chap. 82)

HYPERTENSION IN OLDER PERSONS. A few older persons may have high blood pressure when measured by the sphygmomanometer, but they may have less or no hypertension when direct intra-arterial readings are made—that is, pseudohypertension related to rigid arteries that do not collapse under the cuff. If the systolic pressure is above 160 mm Hg alone or with diastolic levels above 90 mm Hg, careful lowering of BP with a diuretic plus an ACEI (if needed to reach the goal of 150 mm Hg systolic) can reduce CV events in patients up to

TABLE 46-7 Causes of Inadequate Response to Therapy

Pseudoresistance
"White coat syndrome" or office elevations
Pseudohypertension in older persons

Nonadherence to Therapy
Side effects of medication
Cost of medication
Lack of consistent and continuous primary care
Inconvenient and chaotic dosing schedules
Instructions not understood
Inadequate education of patients
Dementia (e.g., memory deficit)

Drug-Related Causes
Doses too low
Inappropriate combinations (e.g., two centrally acting adrenergic inhibitors)
Rapid inactivation (e.g., hydralazine)
Drug interactions

Nonsteroidal anti-inflammatory drugs	Oral contraceptives
Sympathomimetics	Adrenal steroids
Nasal decongestants	Licorice (chewing tobacco)
Appetite suppressants	Cyclosporine
Cocaine	Erythropoietin
Caffeine	Cholestyramine
Antidepressants	Monoamine oxidase inhibitors

Excessive volume contraction with stimulation of renin and aldosterone
Hypokalemia (usually diuretic-induced)
Rebound after clonidine withdrawal

Associated Conditions
Smoking
Increasing obesity
Sleep apnea
Insulin resistance or hyperinsulinemia
Ethanol intake more than 1 oz/day (more than three drinks)
Anxiety-induced hyperventilation or panic attacks
Chronic pain
Intense vasoconstriction (Raynaud phenomenon, arteritis)

Secondary Hypertension
Renal insufficiency
Renovascular hypertension
Pheochromocytoma
Primary aldosteronism

Volume Overload
Excessive sodium intake
Progressive renal damage (nephrosclerosis)
Fluid retention related to reduction of blood pressure
Inadequate diuretic therapy

TABLE 46-8 RCTs on Treatment of Hypertensives under Age 65 versus over Age 65

DRUG	DIFFERENCE IN SBP/DBP (MM HG)	RELATIVE RISK (95% CI)
ACEI vs Placebo		
Age < 65 yr	−4.6/−2.1	0.76 (0.66-0.88)
Age > 65 yr	−4.2/−2.0	0.83 (0.74-0.94)
CCB vs Placebo		
Age < 65 yr	−7.2/−2.9	0.84 (0.54-1.31)
Age > 65 yr	−9.3/−3.8	0.74 (0.59-0.92)

DBP = diastolic blood pressure; SBP = systolic blood pressure.
Data from Blood Pressure Lowering Treatment Trialists' Collaboration; Turnbull F, Neal B, Ninomiya T, et al: Effects of different regimens to lower blood pressure on major cardiovascular events in older and younger adults: meta-analysis of randomised trials. BMJ 336:1121, 2008.

TABLE 46-9 Possible Causes of Increased Risk of Pharmacologic Treatment of Hypertension in Older Adults

CAUSE	POTENTIAL COMPLICATIONS
Diminished baroreceptor activity	Orthostatic hypotension
Decreased intravascular volume	Orthostatic hypotension, dehydration
Sensitivity of hypokalemia	Arrhythmia, muscle weakness
Decreased renal and hepatic function	Drug accumulation
Polypharmacy	Drug interaction
Central nervous system changes	Depression, confusion

and older than 80 years of age.[8] Overall, CCBs reduce BP and risks of stroke more effectively than ACEIs[54] (**Table 46-8**).

Care is needed because older adults may have a number of problems with the medications (**Table 46-9**). In view of the reduced effectiveness of the baroreceptor reflex and the failure of peripheral resistance to rise appropriately with standing, postural hypotension should be carefully sought and, if present, addressed before starting antihypertensive therapy.[77] All drugs should be given in slowly increasing doses to prevent excessive lowering of BP.

HYPERTENSION IN BLACKS. Blacks have more hypertension and suffer more target organ damage from it, particularly stroke and renal damage. Therapy may need to be started earlier and pursued more vigorously. Blacks, similar to older individuals, tend to respond better to diuretics or CCBs as monotherapy, because both groups tend to have lower renin levels and therefore respond less to renin-inhibiting drugs. They also have more angioedema with ACEIs but no more cough than nonblacks. (See also Fig. 2-3 and Table 2-1.)[61]

PATIENTS WITH HYPERTENSION AND DIABETES. Special attention should be given to diabetic patients with hypertension (see Chap. 64). The two commonly coexist and multiply the cardiovascular risks of each alone. Fortunately, evidence from several trials has now documented the protection provided by intensive control of hypertension, in concert with management of the diabetes and the dyslipidemia that commonly accompanies the two. Most diabetic hypertensive patients need two or more antihypertensive drugs to bring their BP to below the goal of 130/80 mm Hg.[78] The benefits of such intensive management were clearly documented in a 13.3-year follow-up of 160 patients with type 2 diabetes and hypertension with microalbuminuria.[79] Half of these patients were given more intensive management, and the risks of having a CV event, nephropathy, retinopathy, or autonomic neuropathy decreased by 50% or more. An ACEI and/or ARB should be included if proteinuria is present. A diuretic and long-acting DHP are likely to be required. Keep in mind the effects of the combination of an ACEI and glitazone, which increase levels of substance P.[62]

HYPERTENSIVE PATIENTS WITH IMPOTENCE. Erectile dysfunction is common in hypertensive patients, and more so in those who are also diabetic. The problem may be exacerbated by diuretic therapy, even in appropriately low doses. Fortunately, 5-phosphodiesterase inhibitors often return erectile ability, even in the presence of various antihypertensive drugs, with no greater likelihood of adverse events than in those not receiving antihypertensive therapy (with the exception of nitrates).

HYPERTENSION WITH CARDIAC DISEASE. Any drug that reduces BP will regress LVH, except for naked direct vasodilators. Better and equally efficacious results have been seen with ACEIs, ARBs, and CCBs, whereas less regression has been seen with diuretics and beta blockers.

Coronary Artery Disease

Guidelines from an expert committee of the American Heart Association have recommended these targets for BP: less than 140/90 mm Hg for general coronary artery disease (CAD) prevention, less than 130/80 mm Hg for high CAD risk, including stable angina, and less than 120/80 mm Hg for left ventricular systolic or diastolic dysfunction.[80]

Heart Failure

Older hypertensive individuals have a high prevalence of left ventricular (LV) diastolic dysfunction, present in 25.8% of 2545 patients studied in Italy.[81] There are inadequate data on the benefits of treating LV diastolic dysfunction, but the evidence for treatment of systolic dysfunction is unequivocal. Aldosterone blockade is particularly indicated for post-MI patients with LV dysfunction.

Atrial Fibrillation

The most common cardiac arrhythmia, atrial fibrillation (AF), is even more common in hypertensive patients. After conducting a literature search, Novo and colleagues[82] stated that "Although many studies and meta-analyses have supported the advantage of RAS [renin-angiotensin system] blockade in preventing AF recurrence, it is premature to recommend the use of ACEIs and ARBs specifically for the prevention of AF."

HYPERTENSION WITH CEREBROVASCULAR DISEASE. As the most direct cause of strokes, hypertension causes even more strokes than heart attacks as people grow older (see Chap. 62). Reduction of elevated blood pressure protects against stroke even more than heart attack.[7] However, if a thrombotic stroke occurs and BP is high, as it usually is, there has been uncertainty about whether to lower it or not because lowering BP could extend cerebral ischemia by lowering cerebral blood flow and perfusion. Patients eligible for intravenous thrombolysis must have a BP below 185 mm Hg systolic or 110 mm Hg diastolic; if BP is higher, antihypertensive therapy should be given to reach these levels.[83] After stroke, reduction of hypertension unquestionably reduces recurrence.

ANESTHESIA IN HYPERTENSIVE PATIENTS. In the absence of significant cardiac dysfunction or other target organ damage, hypertension adds little to the cardiovascular risks of surgery. If possible, however, hypertension should be well controlled by means of medications before anesthesia (see Chap. 85) and surgery to reduce the risk of myocardial ischemia. Therefore, patients taking antihypertensive medications should continue these drugs, if necessary using dermal or intravenous formulations, as long as the anesthesiologist is aware of their use and takes reasonable precautions to prevent wide swings in BP. Use of a beta blocker just before surgery to reduce cardiac events in high-risk patients has been found to increase strokes and mortality[84]; if started 7 days before surgery and slowly titrated, however, a beta blocker may be protective.[85]

Therapy for Hypertensive Crises

When diastolic blood pressure exceeds 140 mm Hg, rapidly progressive damage to the arterial vasculature is demonstrable experimentally, and a surge of cerebral blood flow may rapidly lead to encephalopathy (see Chap. 45). If such high pressure persists or if there are any signs of encephalopathy, the pressure should be lowered using parenteral agents in patients considered to be in immediate danger or using oral agents in those who are alert and in no other acute distress.

Several drugs for this purpose are currently available (**Table 46-10**). If diastolic pressure exceeds 140 mm Hg and the patient has any complications, such as an aortic dissection, a constant infusion of nitroprusside is most effective and almost always lowers the pressure to the desired level. Constant monitoring with an intra-arterial line is mandatory because a slightly excessive dose may lower BP abruptly to levels that induce shock. The potency and rapidity of action of nitroprusside have made it the treatment of choice for life-threatening hypertension. However, because nitroprusside acts as a venous and arteriolar dilator, venous return and cardiac output are lowered and intracranial pressures may increase. Therefore, other parenteral agents are more widely used, including labetalol and the rapidly acting CCBs, nicardipine and clevidipine.[86] With any of these agents, intravenous furosemide is often needed to lower BP further and prevent retention of sodium and water.

For patients in less immediate danger, oral therapy may be used. Almost every drug has been used and most, with repeated doses, reduce high pressures. Oral doses of short-acting formulations include furosemide, propranolol, captopril, or felodipine, but clonidine is a

TABLE 46-10 Parenteral Drugs for Treatment of Hypertensive Emergency

DRUG*	DOSE	ONSET OF ACTION	DURATION OF ACTION	ADVERSE EFFECTS†	SPECIAL INDICATIONS
Vasodilators					
Nitroprusside	0.25-10.00 μg/kg/min IV	Immediate	1-2 min	Nausea, vomiting, muscle twitching, thiocyanate and cyanide toxicity	Not preferred for most hypertensive emergencies
Nitroglycerin	5-100 μg/min	2-5 min	5-10 min	Headache, vomiting, methemoglobinemia, tolerance with prolonged use	Not preferred but may be useful for coronary ischemia
Fenoldopam (Corlopam)	0.1-0.6 μg/kg/min IV	4-5 min	10-15 min	Tachycardia, increased intraocular pressure	May be indicated for renal insufficiency
Nicardipine‡ (Cardene IV)	5-15 mg/h	5-10 min	1-4 hr	Headache, nausea, flushing, tachycardia	Most hypertensive emergencies
Clevidipine (Cleviprex)	1-2 mg IV, rapidly increasing dose to 16 mg max	2-4 min	5-15 min		Most hypertensive emergencies
Hydralazine	5-20 mg IV 10-40 mg IM	10-20 min 20-30 min	1-4 hr 4-6 hr	Tachycardia, flushing, headache, vomiting, aggravation of angina	Eclampsia; not for aortic dissection
Adrenergic Inhibitors					
Phentolamine	5-15 mg IV	1-2 min	3-10 min	Tachycardia, flushing, headache	Catecholamine excess
Esmolol (Brevibloc)	250-500 μg/kg/min for 4 min, then 50-300 μg/kg/min IV	1-2 min	1-20 min	Hypotension, nausea	Aortic dissection after surgery
Labetalol (Normodyne, Trandate)	20-80 mg IV bolus every 10 min, 2-mg/min IV infusion	5-10 min	3-6 hr	Vomiting, scalp tingling, burning in throat, dizziness, nausea, heart block, orthostatic hypotension	Most hypertensive emergencies, except acute heart failure

*In order of rapidity of action.
†Hypotension may occur with any of these.
‡Intravenous formulations of other calcium channel blockers are also available.

poor choice because of the difficulty of maintaining it for long-term therapy. A safer course for many patients, particularly if their current high pressures simply reflect stopping previously effective oral medication and they are asymptomatic, is simply to restart the previous medication and monitor their response closely. If their nonadherence to therapy was caused by side effects, appropriate changes should be made.

Future Perspectives

The treatment of hypertension will continue to improve. However, because the genetic foundations will likely never be correctable and the environmental precipitants will likely never be controllable, the management of hypertension will continue to require considerable resources and work.

Treatment may become easier with more long-acting, easier to take medications, but there will not likely be a magic bullet to cure the disease. The greatest need is to prevent young people from developing the bad habits that many of their parents have—in particular, leading to obesity. Prevention may only be possible with pills. Perhaps, as in spontaneously hypertensive rats, therapy may need to begin in early life. Without reliable markers to identify those who will become hypertensive, even that possibility seems unlikely. Finally, the number of older people will continue to increase, and without the ability to prevent atherosclerotic stiffening of their arteries, they will be the neediest and least manageable of those with hypertension.

REFERENCES

General Considerations

1. Kaplan NM, Victor R: Hypertension in the population at large. *In* Kaplan NM, Victor RG (eds): Kaplan's Clinical Hypertension. 10th ed. Philadelphia, Lippincott Williams & Wilkins, 2010, pp 1-19.
2. Lloyd-Jones D, Adams R, Carnethon M, et al: Heart disease and stroke statistics—2009 update: A report from the American Heart Association Statistics Committee and Stroke Statistics Subcommittee. Circulation 119:480, 2009.

2a. SHEP Cooperative Research Group: Prevention of stroke by antihypertensive-drug treatment in older persons with isolated systolic hypertension. JAMA 265:3255, 1991.

3. Bo S, Gambino R, Gentile L, et al: High-normal blood pressure is associated with a cluster of cardiovascular and metabolic risk factors: A population-based study. J Hypertens 27:102, 2009.
4. Asayama K, Ohkubo T, Yoshida S, et al: Stroke risk and antihypertensive drug treatment in the general population: The Japan Arteriosclerosis Longitudinal Study. J Hypertens 27:357, 2009.
5. Julius S, Nesbitt SD, Egan BM, et al: Feasibility of treating prehypertension with an angiotensin-receptor blocker. N Engl J Med 354:1685, 2006.
6. Yusuf S, Pais P, Afzal R, et al: Effects of a polypill (polycap) on risk factors in middle-aged individuals without cardiovascular disease (TIPS): A phase II, double-blind, randomised trial. Lancet 373:1341, 2009.

Benefits and Targets of Therapy

7. Wang JG, Staessen JA, Franklin SS, et al: Systolic and diastolic blood pressure lowering as determinants of cardiovascular outcome. Hypertension 45:907, 2005.
8. Beckett NS, Peters R, Fletcher AE, et al: Treatment of hypertension in patients 80 years of age or older. N Engl J Med 358:1887, 2008.
9. Mancia G: Role of outcome trials in providing information on antihypertensive treatment: Importance and limitations. Am J Hypertens 19:1, 2006.
10. Skoog I, Lithell H, Hansson L, et al: Effect of baseline cognitive function and antihypertensive treatment on cognitive and cardiovascular outcomes: Study on COgnition and Prognosis in the Elderly (SCOPE). Am J Hypertens 18:1052, 2005.
11. Messerli FH, Mancia G, Conti CR, et al: Dogma disputed: Can aggressively lowering blood pressure in hypertensive patients with coronary artery disease be dangerous? Ann Intern Med 144:884, 2006.
12. Weiner DE, Tighiouart H, Levey AS, et al: Lowest systolic blood pressure is associated with stroke in stages 3 to 4 chronic kidney disease. J Am Soc Nephrol 18:960, 2007.
13. De Galan BE, Perkovic V, Ninomiya T, et al: Lowering blood pressure reduces renal events in type 2 diabetes. J Am Soc Nephrol 20:883, 2009.
14. Appel LJ, Wright JT Jr, Greene T, et al: Long-term effects of renin-angiotensin system-blocking therapy and a low blood pressure goal on progression of hypertensive chronic kidney disease in African Americans. Arch Intern Med 168:832, 2008.
15. Nissen SE, Tuzcu EM, Libby P, et al: Effect of antihypertensive agents on cardiovascular events in patients with coronary disease and normal blood pressure: The CAMELOT study: A randomized controlled trial. JAMA 292:2217, 2004.

Lifestyle Modifications

16. Kotseva K, Wood D, De BG, et al: Cardiovascular prevention guidelines in daily practice: A comparison Of EUROASPIRE I, II, and III surveys in eight European countries. Lancet 373:929, 2009.
17. Gidding SS, Lichtenstein AH, Faith MS, et al: Implementing American Heart Association pediatric and adult nutrition guidelines: A scientific statement from the American Heart Association Nutrition Committee of the Council on Nutrition, Physical Activity and Metabolism, Council on Cardiovascular Disease in the Young, Council on Arteriosclerosis, Thrombosis and Vascular Biology, Council on Cardiovascular Nursing, Council on Epidemiology and Prevention, and Council for High Blood Pressure Research. Circulation 119:1161, 2009.
18. Mathieu P, Poirier P, Pibarot P, et al: Visceral obesity: The link among inflammation, hypertension, and cardiovascular disease. Hypertension 53:577, 2009.
19. Sacks FM, Bray GA, Carey VJ, et al: Comparison of weight-loss diets with different compositions of fat, protein, and carbohydrates. N Engl J Med 360:859, 2009.
20. Kokkinos P, Manolis A, Pittaras A, et al: Exercise capacity and mortality in hypertensive men with and without additional risk factors. Hypertension 53:494, 2009.
21. He FJ, Macgregor GA: A comprehensive review on salt and health and current experience of worldwide salt reduction programmes. J Hum Hypertens 23:363, 2009.
22. Dickinson KM, Keogh JB, Clifton PM: Effects of a low-salt diet on flow-mediated dilatation in humans. Am J Clin Nutr 89:485, 2009.
23. Chen J, Gu D, Kelly TN, et al: Metabolic syndrome and blood pressure response to sodium—authors' reply. Lancet 373:1946, 2009.
24. Cook NR, Obarzanek E, Cutler JA, et al: Joint effects of sodium and potassium intake on subsequent cardiovascular disease: The Trials of Hypertension Prevention follow-up study. Arch Intern Med 169:32, 2009.
25. Bolland MJ, Barber PA, Doughty RN, et al: Vascular events in healthy older women receiving calcium supplementation: Randomised controlled trial. BMJ 336:262, 2008.
26. Guerrero-Romero F, Rodriguez-Moran M: The effect of lowering blood pressure by magnesium supplementation in diabetic hypertensive adults with low serum magnesium levels: A randomized, double-blind, placebo-controlled clinical trial. J Hum Hypertens 23:245, 2009.
27. Maruthur NM, Wang NY, Appel LJ: Lifestyle interventions reduce coronary heart disease risk: Results From the PREMIER trial. Circulation 119:2026, 2009.
28. Lopez-Garcia E, Rodriguez-Artalejo F, Rexrode KM, et al: Coffee consumption and risk of stroke in women. Circulation 119:1116, 2009.
29. Fillmore KM, Kerr WC, Stockwell T, et al: Moderate alcohol use and reduced mortality risk: Systematic error in prospective studies. Addict Res Theory 14:101, 2006.
30. Lee H, Kim SY, Park J, et al: Acupunture for lowering blood pressure: Systemic review and meta-analysis. Am J Hypertens 22:122, 2009.
31. Frank H, Heusser K, Geiger H, et al: Temporary reduction of blood pressure and sympathetic nerve activity in hypertensive patients after microvascular decompression. Stroke 40:47, 2009.
32. Bautista LE: Blood pressure-lowering effects of statins: Who benefits? J Hypertens 27:1478, 2009.

Pharmacologic Therapy

33. Strandgaard S, Haunso S: Why does antihypertensive treatment prevent stroke but not myocardial infarction? Lancet 2:658, 1987.
34. Brown MJ: Hypertension and ethnic group. BMJ 332:833, 2006.
35. Mancia G, De Backer G, Dominiczak A, et al: 2007 ESH-ESC Practice Guidelines for the Management of Arterial Hypertension: ESH-ESC Task Force on the Management of Arterial Hypertension. J Hypertens 25:1751, 2007.
36. Dahlof B, Devereux RB, Kjeldsen SE, et al: Cardiovascular morbidity and mortality in the Losartan Intervention for Endpoint Reduction in Hypertension Study (LIFE): A randomised trial against atenolol. Lancet 359:995, 2002.
37. Lindholm LH, Carlberg B, Samuelsson O: Should beta blockers remain first choice in the treatment of primary hypertension? A meta-analysis. Lancet 366:1545, 2005.
38. Wright JT, Jr, Probstfield JL, Cushman WC, et al: ALLHAT findings revisited in the context of subsequent analyses, other trials, and meta-analyses. Arch Intern Med 169:832, 2009.
39. Casas JP, Chua W, Loukogeorgakis S, et al: Effect of inhibitors of the renin-angiotensin system and other antihypertensive drugs on renal outcomes: Systematic review and meta-analysis. Lancet 366:2026, 2005.
40. Messerli FH, Bangalore S, Julius S: Should β-blockers and diuretics remain as first-line therapy for hypertension? Circulation 117:2706, 2008.
41. Williams B, Poulter NR, Brown MJ, et al: Guidelines for management of hypertension: Report of the Fourth Working Party of the British Hypertension Society, 2004-BHS IV. J Hum Hypertens 18:139, 2004.
42. Jamerson K, Weber MA, Bakris GL, et al: Benazepril plus amlodipine or hydrochlorothiazide for hypertension in high-risk patients. N Engl J Med 359:2417, 2008.
43. Calhoun DA, Lacourciere Y, Chiang YT, et al: Triple antihypertensive therapy with amlodipine, valsartan, and hydrochlorothiazide: A randomized clinical trial. Hypertension 54:32, 2009.
44. Ernst ME, Carter BL, Basile JN: All thiazide-like diuretics are not chlorthalidone: Putting the ACCOMPLISH study into perspective. J Clin Hypertens 11:5, 2009.
45. Messerli FH, Bangalore S: Antihypertensive efficacy of aliskerin: Is hydrochlorothiazide an appropriate benchmark? Circulation 119:371, 2009.
46. Feig DI, Kang D-H, Johnson RJ: Uric acid and cardiovascular risk. N Engl J Med 359:1811, 2008.
47. Grimm RH, Jr., Grandits GA, Prineas RJ, et al: Long-term effects on sexual function of five antihypertensive drugs and nutritional hygienic treatment in hypertensive men and women. Treatment of Mild Hypertension Study (TOMHS). Hypertension 29:8, 1997.
48. Sowers JR, Whaley-Connell A, Epstein M: Narrative review: The emerging clinical implications of the role of aldosterone in the metabolic syndrome and resistant hypertension. Ann Intern Med 150:776, 2009.
49. Takeda Y: Effects of eplerenone, a selective mineralocorticoid receptor antagonist, on clinical and experimental salt-sensitive hypertension. Hypertens Res 32:321, 2009.
50. Bell CM, Hatch WV, Fischer HD, et al: Association between tamsulosin and serious ophthalmic adverse events in older men following cataract surgery. JAMA 301:1991, 2009.
51. Williams B, Lacy PS, Thom SM, et al: Differential impact of blood pressure-lowering drugs on central aortic pressure and clinical outcomes: Principal results of the Conduit Artery Function Evaluation (CAFE) study. Circulation 113:1213, 2006.
52. Hillebrand U, Lang D, Telgmann RG, et al: Nebivolol decreases endothelial cell stiffness via the estrogen receptor beta: A nano-imaging study. J Hypertens 27:517, 2009.
53. Dhakam Z, Yasmin, Mceniery CM, et al: A comparison of atenolol and nebivolol in isolated systolic hypertension. J Hypertens 26:351, 2008.
54. Costanzo P, Perrone-Filardi P, Petretta M, et al: Calcium channel blockers and cardiovascular outcomes: A meta-analysis of 175,634 patients. J Hypertens 27:1136, 2009.

54a. Zanchetti A, Hansson L, Clement D, et al: Benefits and risks of more intensive blood pressure lowering in hypertensive patients in the HOT study with different risk profiles: Does a J-shaped curve exist in smokers? J Hypertens 21:797, 2003.

55. Hart P, Bakris GL: Calcium antagonists: Do they equally protect against kidney injury? Kidney Int 73:795, 2008.
56. Bakris GL, Weir MR, Shanifar S, et al: Effects of blood pressure level on progression of diabetic nephropathy: Results from the RENAAL study. Arch Intern Med 163:1555, 2003.
57. Schmieder RE, Philipp T, Guerediaga J, et al: Long-term antihypertensive efficacy and safety of the oral direct renin inhibitor aliskiren: A 12-month randomized, double-blind comparator trial with hydrochlorothiazide. Circulation 119:417, 2009.
58. Azizi M, Menard J: Combined blockade of the renin-angiotensin system with angiotensin-converting enzyme inhibitors and angiotensin II type 1 receptor antagonists. Circulation 109:2492, 2004.
59. Bakris GL, Weir MR: Angiotensin-converting enzyme inhibitor-associated elevations in serum creatinine: Is this a cause for concern? Arch Intern Med 160:685, 2000.
60. Suissa S, Hutchinson T, Brophy JM, et al: ACE-inhibitor use and the long-term risk of renal failure in diabetes. Kidney Int 69:913, 2006.
61. Mcdowell SE, Coleman JJ, Ferner RE: Systematic review and meta-analysis of ethnic differences in risks of adverse reactions to drugs used in cardiovascular medicine. BMJ 332:1177, 2006.
62. Brown NJ, Byiers S, Maldonado M, et al: Dipeptidyl peptidase-IV inhibitor use associated with increased risk of ACE inhibitor-associated angioedema. Hypertension 54:516, 2009.
63. Cooper WO, Hernandez-Diaz S, Arbogast PG, et al: Major congenital malformations after first-trimester exposure to ACE inhibitors. N Engl J Med 354:2443, 2006.
64. Danchin N, Cucherat M, Thuillez C, et al: Angiotensin-converting enzyme inhibitors in patients with coronary artery disease and absence of heart failure or left ventricular systolic dysfunction: An overview of long-term randomized controlled trials. Arch Intern Med 66:787, 2006.
65. Matchar DB, Mccrory DC, Orlando LA, et al: Systematic review: Comparative effectiveness of angiotensin-converting enzyme inhibitors and angiotensin II receptor blockers for treating essential hypertension. Ann Intern Med 148:16, 2009.
66. Sica DA, Black HR: Current concepts of pharmacotherapy in hypertension. ACE inhibitor-related angioedema: Can angiotensin-receptor blockers be safely used? J Clin Hypertens 4:375, 2002.
67. Volpe M, Tocci G, Sciarretta S, et al: Angiotensin II receptor blockers and myocardial infarction: An updated analysis of randomized clinical trials. J Hypertens 27:941, 2009.
68. Mann JF: What's new in hypertension 2008? Nephrol Dial Transplant 24:38, 2009.
69. Brown MJ: Aliskiren. Circulation 118:773, 2008.
70. Feldt S, Batenburg WW, Mazak I, et al: Prorenin and renin-induced extracellular signal-regulated kinase 1/2 activation in monocytes is not blocked by aliskiren or the handle-region peptide. Hypertension 51:682, 2008.
71. Mercure C, Prescott G, Lacombe MJ, et al: Chronic increases in circulating prorenin are not associated with renal or cardiac pathologies. Hypertension 53:1062, 2009.
72. Oparil S, Yarows SA, Patel S, et al: Efficacy and safety of combined use of aliskiren and valsartan in patients with hypertension: A randomised, double-blind trial. Lancet 370:221, 2007.
73. Birkenhager WH, Staessen JA: Dual inhibition of the renin system by aliskiren and valsartan. Lancet 370:195, 2007.
74. Calhoun DA, Jones D, Textor S, et al: Resistant hypertension: Diagnosis, evaluation, and treatment. A scientific statement from the American Heart Association Professional Education Committee of the Council for High Blood Pressure Research. Hypertension 51:1403, 2008.
75. Ruttanaumpawan P, Nopmaneejumruslers C, Logan AG, et al: Association between refractory hypertension and obstructive sleep apnea. J Hypertens 27:1439, 2009.
76. Flynn J: Hypertension in childhood and adolescence. *In* Kaplan NM, Victor R (eds): Kaplan's Clinical Hypertension. 10th ed. Philadelphia, Lippincott Williams & Wilkins, Press, 2010, pp 430-454.
77. Freeman R: Clinical practice. Neurogenic orthostatic hypotension. N Engl J Med 358:615, 2008.
78. Bakris GL, Sowers JR: Treatment of hypertension in patients with diabetes—an update. J Am Soc Hypertens 3:150, 2009.
79. Gaede P, Lund-Andersen H, Parving HH, et al: Effect of a multifactorial intervention on mortality in type 2 diabetes. N Engl J Med 358:5801, 2008.
80. Rosendorff C, Black HR, Cannon CP, et al: Treatment of hypertension in the prevention and managment of ischemic heart disease. Hypertension 50:E28, 2007.
81. Zanchetti A, Cuspidi C, Comarella L, et al: Left ventricular diastolic dysfunction in older hypertensives: Results of the APROS-diadys study. J Hypertens 25:2158, 2007.
82. Novo G, Guttilla D, Fazio G, et al: The role of the renin-angiotensin system in atrial fibrillation and the therapeutic effects of ACE-Is And ARBS. Br J Clin Pharmacol 66:345, 2008.
83. Aiyagari V, Gorelick PB: Management of blood pressure for acute and recurrent stroke. Stroke 40:2251, 2009.
84. Devereaux PJ, Yang H, Yusuf S, et al: Effects of extended-release metoprolol succinate in patients undergoing non-cardiac surgery (POISE Trial): A randomised controlled trial. Lancet 371:1839, 2008.
85. Fleisher LA, Poldermans D: Perioperative beta blockade: Where do we go from here? Lancet 371:1813, 2008.
86. Varon J: Treatment of acute severe hypertension: current and newer agents. Drugs 68:283, 2008.

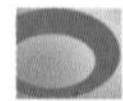

GUIDELINES Norman M. Kaplan

Treatment of Hypertension

The major U.S. guidelines for the management of hypertension are issued by the Joint National Committee on Prevention, Detection, Evaluation, and Treatment of High Blood Pressure, a group coordinated by the National Heart Lung and Blood Institute (NHLBI). Its seventh and most recent guidelines were published in 2003, and are known as JNC-7.[1] Other recent recommendations have been published in other countries, such as guidelines from the British Hypertension Society in 2004[2] and the Canadian Hypertension Education Program in 2006.[3,4] In 2003, recommendations for blood pressure control in patients with diabetes were issued by the American College of Physicians[5] and for blacks by the International Society on Hypertension in Blacks.[6]

INITIAL EVALUATION

JNC-7 updated NHLBI recommendations from prior guidelines issued in 1997[7] in several important ways. First, JNC-7 introduced the concept of "prehypertension," which is a systolic blood pressure of 120 to 139 mm Hg or a diastolic blood pressure of 80 to 89 mm Hg. JNC-7 recommended a more aggressive approach to patients with blood pressures in this range, with an emphasis on lifestyle modifications to prevent cardiovascular disease. JNC-7 describes normal blood pressure as a systolic pressure below 120 mm Hg and a diastolic blood pressure below 80 mm Hg. Stage 1 hypertension is a systolic blood pressure of 140 to 159 mm Hg or a diastolic blood pressure of 90 to 99 mm Hg. Patients with higher blood pressures have stage 2 hypertension.

Health care providers rarely follow established procedures for measuring blood pressure. In addition, there is increasing evidence that clinical blood pressure measurements made by a trained professional using a mercury sphygmomanometer and the Korotkoff sound technique may lead to the misclassification of many individuals. Guidelines from the American Heart Association[8] define proper procedures for measuring blood pressure. These include the following:

- Allow the patient to sit quietly for 5 minutes before measuring blood pressure.
- The patient should be seated comfortably with the back supported and the upper arm bared without constrictive clothing. The legs should not be crossed.
- The arm should be supported at heart level, and the bladder of the cuff should encircle at least 80% of the arm circumference. Larger or smaller cuffs must be used as needed.
- The mercury column should be deflated at 2 to 3 mm/sec, and the first and last audible sounds should be taken as systolic and diastolic pressure. The column should be read to the nearest 2 mm Hg.
- Neither the patient nor the observer should talk during the measurement.

These measurement guidelines recommend a mercury sphygmomanometer as the standard for measurement, but recognize that these devices are being replaced by newer technologies. The guidelines recommend ambulatory monitoring for the evaluation of white coat hypertension, and home monitoring in select patients may be useful for predicting cardiovascular events and monitoring the effects of treatment.

TABLE 46G-1 Joint National Committee (JNC)-7 Guidelines for Follow-up Based on Initial Blood Pressure Measurements for Adults

Initial Blood Pressure (mm Hg)*		
SYSTOLIC	DIASTOLIC	FOLLOW-UP RECOMMENDATION
<130	<85	Recheck in 2 yr.
130-139	85-89	Recheck in 1 yr (provide information about lifestyle modifications).
140-159	90-99	Confirm within 2 mo (provide information about lifestyle modifications).
160-179	100-109	Evaluate or refer to source of care within 1 mo.
≥180	≥110	Evaluate or refer to source of care immediately or within 1 wk, depending on clinical situation.

*If systolic and diastolic categories are different, follow recommendations for shorter time follow-up.

JNC-7 provides recommendations for follow-up of patients after the initial measurement of blood pressure (**Table 46G-1**). These should be guided by the blood pressure and other clinical data, including past blood pressure measurements, other cardiovascular risk factors, or target organ disease. JNC-7 recommends routine laboratory tests before the initiation of therapy that include 12-lead electrocardiography, urinalysis, determination of blood glucose, hematocrit, lipid profile, and serum potassium, creatinine, and calcium levels. More extensive testing for identifiable causes of hypertension is not routinely indicated.

INITIAL MANAGEMENT STRATEGY

The goal of treatment according to JNC-7 is to reduce blood pressure to below 140 mm Hg systolic and 90 mm Hg diastolic; in patients with concomitant diabetes or renal disease, the goal is blood pressure below 130/80 mm Hg.

These guidelines recommend that initial management be based on the patient's blood pressure stage and other medical issues (**Table 46G-2**). Lifestyle modifications should be encouraged for all patients, including those with normal blood pressure, and should be used as the sole therapy for patients with prehypertension unless they have clinical evidence of compelling indications. These indications include heart failure, post-myocardial infarction, high coronary artery disease risk, diabetes, chronic kidney disease, and need for recurrent stroke prevention.

Recommended lifestyle modifications include the following:

- Weight reduction to maintain normal body weight (body mass index, 18.5 to 24.9 kg/m^2)
- Adoption of the Dietary Approaches to Stop Hypertension (DASH) eating plan[9]
- Dietary sodium reduction to no more than 100 mmol/day (2.4 g sodium or 6 g sodium chloride)
- Physical activity—at least 30 minutes per day, most days of the week
- Limit daily alcohol intake to no more than two drinks (1 oz [30 mL] ethanol— beer, 24 oz; wine, 10 oz; or 80-proof whiskey, 3 oz) in most men and to no more than one drink in women and lighter weight persons.

DRUG THERAPY

JNC-7 guidelines recommend thiazide-type diuretics as the initial therapy for most patients with hypertension, either alone or in combination with one of the other classes. **Table 46G-3** describes JNC-7's list of "compelling indications" and recommended therapies. The guidelines note that most patients who are hypertensive will require two or more antihypertensive agents to achieve their blood pressure goals. When blood pressure is more than 20/10 mm Hg above goal, the guidelines recommend that clinicians consider initiating therapy with two drugs.

Guidelines from other organizations vary slightly in thresholds for initiating therapy. For example, the British Hypertension Society's guidelines support initiation of drug therapy for all patients with systolic blood pressure of 160 mm Hg or sustained diastolic blood pressure of 100 mm Hg, despite nonpharmacologic measures. Drug treatment is also indicated for patients with sustained systolic blood pressure of 140 to 159 mm Hg or diastolic blood pressure of 90 to 99 mm Hg if target organ damage is present, there is evidence of established cardiovascular disease or diabetes, or the 10-year coronary heart disease risk is higher than 15%. For most patients, these guidelines recommend a target of reducing systolic pressure below 140 mm Hg and diastolic pressure below 85 mm Hg. For patients with diabetes, a lower target is recommended. These guidelines recommend initiation of therapy with a diuretic unless there is a contraindication or a compelling indication for another drug class.

For patients with hypertension and diabetes, the 2003 recommendations from the American College of Physicians include a target blood pressure of no more than 135/80 mm Hg.[5] These guidelines recommend thiazide diuretics or angiotensin-converting enzyme (ACE) inhibitors as first-line agents for blood pressure control in most patients.

Guidelines developed for the treatment of blacks recommend lower thresholds for drug therapy and more aggressive treatment strategies.[6]

TABLE 46G-2 Joint National Committee (JNC)-7 Guidelines for Classification and Management of Hypertension in Adults

BLOOD PRESSURE CLASSIFICATION	SYSTOLIC BLOOD PRESSURE (mm Hg)	DIASTOLIC BLOOD PRESSURE (mm Hg)	LIFESTYLE MODIFICATION	Initial Drug Therapy	
				WITHOUT COMPELLING INDICATIONS	WITH COMPELLING INDICATIONS*
Normal	<120	And <80	Encourage	No antihypertensive drug indicated	Drug(s) for compelling indications†
Prehypertension	120-139	Or 80-89	Yes	No antihypertensive drug indicated	Drug(s) for compelling indications†
Stage 1 hypertension	140-159	Or 90-99	Yes	Thiazide-type diuretics for most	Drug(s) for compelling indications†
Stage 2 hypertension	≥160	Or ≥100	Yes	Two-drug combination for most (usually thiazide-type diuretic plus ACEI, ARB, BB, or CCB)	Other antihypertensive drugs (diuretics, ACEI, ARB, BB, CCB) as needed

*Heart failure, post-myocardial infarction, high coronary artery disease risk, diabetes, chronic kidney disease, recurrent stroke prevention.
†Treat patients with chronic kidney disease or diabetes to blood pressure goal of <130/80 mm Hg.
ACEI = angiotensin-converting enzyme inhibitor; ARB = angiotensin receptor blocker; BB = beta blocker; CCB = calcium channel blocker.

TABLE 46G-3 Joint National Committee (JNC)-7 Guidelines for Recommended Drugs for Patients with Compelling Indications

	DIURETIC	BETA BLOCKER	ACE INHIBITOR	ANGIOTENSIN RECEPTOR BLOCKER	CALCIUM CHANNEL BLOCKER	ALDOSTERONE ANTAGONIST
Heart failure	+	+	+	+		+
Post-myocardial infarction		+	+			+
High coronary disease risk	+	+	+		+	
Diabetes	+	+	+	+	+	
Chronic kidney disease			+	+		
Recurrent stroke prevention	+		+			

ACE = angiotensin-converting enzyme.

These guidelines recommend a lower blood pressure target (130/80 mm Hg) for blacks with hypertension who also have conditions such as heart disease, kidney disease, or diabetes. This statement notes that physicians should have a low threshold for using more than one drug for the treatment of hypertension in blacks.

FOLLOW-UP AND REFERRAL TO SPECIALISTS

In follow-up, the JNC-7 guidelines recommend that most patients should be seen at approximately monthly intervals until the blood pressure goal is reached. More frequent visits are recommended for patients with stage 2 hypertension or with complicating comorbid conditions. Serum potassium and creatinine levels should be monitored at least once or twice annually. After blood pressure is at goal and stable, follow-up visits can be scheduled at 3- to 6-month intervals. Low-dose aspirin therapy should be considered only after blood pressure is controlled because of the risk of hemorrhagic stroke in patients with uncontrolled hypertension.

REFERENCES

1. Chobanian AV, Bakris GL, Black HR, et al: The Seventh Report of the Joint National Committee on Prevention, Detection, Evaluation, and Treatment of High Blood Pressure: The JNC 7 report. JAMA 289:2560, 2003.
2. Williams B, Poulter NR, Brown MJ, et al: Guidelines for management of hypertension: Report of the fourth working party of the British Hypertension Society, 2004-BHS IV. J Hum Hypertens 18:139, 2004.
3. Khan NA, McAlister FA, Rabkin SW, et al: The 2006 Canadian Hypertension Education Program recommendations for the management of hypertension: Part II—therapy. Can J Cardiol 22:583, 2006.
4. Hemmelgarn BR, McAlister FA, Grover S, et al: The 2006 Canadian Hypertension Education Program recommendations for the management of hypertension: Part I—blood pressure measurement, diagnosis and assessment of risk. Can J Cardiol 22:573, 2006.
5. Snow V, Weiss KB, Mottur-Pilson C: The evidence base for tight blood pressure control in the management of type 2 diabetes mellitus. Ann Intern Med 138:587, 2003.
6. Douglas JG, Bakris GL, Epstein M, et al: Management of high blood pressure in African Americans: Consensus statement of the Hypertension in African Americans Working Group of the International Society on Hypertension in Blacks. Arch Intern Med 163:525, 2003.
7. The sixth report of the Joint National Committee on prevention, detection, evaluation, and treatment of high blood pressure. Arch Intern Med 157:2413, 1997.
8. Pickering TG, Hall JE, Appel LJ, et al: Recommendations for blood pressure measurement in humans and experimental animals: Part 1: Blood pressure measurement in humans: A statement for professionals from the Subcommittee of Professional and Public Education of the American Heart Association Council on High Blood Pressure Research. Hypertension 45:142, 2005.
9. Sacks FM, Svetkey LP, Vollmer WM, et al: Effects on blood pressure of reduced dietary sodium and the Dietary Approaches to Stop Hypertension (DASH) diet. DASH-Sodium Collaborative Research Group. N Engl J Med 344:3, 2001.

CHAPTER 47 Lipoprotein Disorders and Cardiovascular Disease

Jacques Genest and Peter Libby

Serum levels of lipids and lipoprotein lipids have proven among the most potent and best substantiated risk factors for atherosclerosis in general and coronary heart disease (CHD) in particular. The uptake of oxidized low-density lipoprotein (LDL)–derived cholesterol by subintimal macrophages characterizes the formation of the atherosclerotic plaque, initiating and promulgating a local inflammatory reaction and leading to foam cell formation. Cholesterol accumulation in macrophages leads to apoptosis and favors the formation of the necrotic core in complex atherosclerotic plaques. Chap. 43 discusses the biological basis of atherosclerosis, and Chap. 44 presents the epidemiologic observational data on serum (or plasma) lipids and lipoprotein lipids as a key component of cardiovascular risk factors. This chapter discusses the fundamentals of lipid metabolism, therapeutic approaches to treatment of lipid disorders, and the evidence base regarding their clinical use.

The term *hyperlipidemia* has long been used in clinical practice. However, the term *dyslipoproteinemia* more appropriately reflects the disorders of the lipid and lipoprotein transport pathways associated with arterial diseases. *Dyslipidemia* encompasses disorders increasingly encountered in clinical practice, such as low high-density lipoprotein (HDL) cholesterol and elevated triglyceride levels, but an average total plasma cholesterol level. Certain rare lipoprotein disorders can cause overt clinical manifestations, but most common dyslipoproteinemias themselves only rarely cause symptoms or produce clinical signs that are evident on physical examination. Rather, they require laboratory tests for detection. Dyslipoproteinemias constitute a major risk factor for atherosclerosis and coronary artery disease (CAD), and their proper recognition and management can reduce cardiovascular and total mortality rates. Thus, the fundamentals of lipidology presented here have importance for the daily practice of cardiovascular medicine.

Lipoprotein Transport System

Biochemistry of Lipids

The lipid transport system has evolved in animals to carry hydrophobic molecules (fat) from their sites of origin (the gastrointestinal system and liver) to their sites of uptake (muscles and hormone-producing tissues) through the aqueous environment of plasma. The proteins (apolipoproteins) that mediate this process have shown high conservation throughout evolution in organisms with a circulatory system. Most apolipoproteins derive from an ancestral gene and contain both hydrophilic and hydrophobic domains. This amphipathic structure enables these proteins to bridge the interface between the aqueous environment of plasma and the phospholipid constituents of the lipoprotein. The major types of lipids that circulate in plasma include cholesterol and cholesteryl esters, phospholipids, and triglycerides (**Fig. 47-1**).

Cholesterol constitutes an essential component of mammalian cell membranes and furnishes substrate for steroid hormones and bile acids. Many cell functions depend critically upon membrane cholesterol, and cells tightly regulate cholesterol content. Most of the cholesterol in plasma circulates in the form of cholesteryl esters, in the core of lipoprotein particles. The enzyme lecithin-cholesterol acyltransferase (LCAT) forms cholesteryl esters in the blood compartment by transferring a fatty acyl moiety from phosphatidyl choline to cholesterol.

Triglycerides consist of a three-carbon glycerol backbone covalently linked to three fatty acid chains (designated R_1, R_2, and R_3). The fatty acid composition varies in terms of chain length and presence of double bonds (degree of saturation). Triglyceride molecules, nonpolar and hydrophobic, travel packaged in the core of the lipoprotein. Hydrolysis of triglycerides by lipases generates free fatty acids (FFAs) used for energy.

Phospholipids, constituents of all cellular membranes, consist of a glycerol molecule linked to two fatty acids (R_1 and R_2; see Fig. 47-1). The fatty acids differ in length and degree of saturation (double bonds). The third carbon of the glycerol moiety carries a phosphate group that links in turn to one of four molecules—choline (phosphatidyl choline, also called lecithin), ethanolamine (phosphatidylethanolamine), serine (phosphatidyl serine), or inositol (phosphatidylinositol). A related phospholipid, sphingomyelin, has special functions in the plasma membrane in the formation of membrane microdomains, such as rafts and caveolae. The structure of sphingomyelin resembles that of phosphatidylcholine. The backbone of sphingolipids uses the amino acid serine rather than glycerol. Phospholipids are polar molecules, more water-soluble than triglycerides or cholesterol or its esters. Phospholipids participate in signal transduction pathways; hydrolysis by membrane-associated phospholipases generates second messengers such as diacyl glycerols, lysophospholipids, phosphatidic acids, and FFAs such as arachidonate that regulate many cell functions.

Lipoproteins, Apolipoproteins, Receptors, and Processing Enzymes

Lipoproteins have complex macromolecular structures, comprising a core of more hydrophobic cholesteryl esters and triglycerides

CH 47

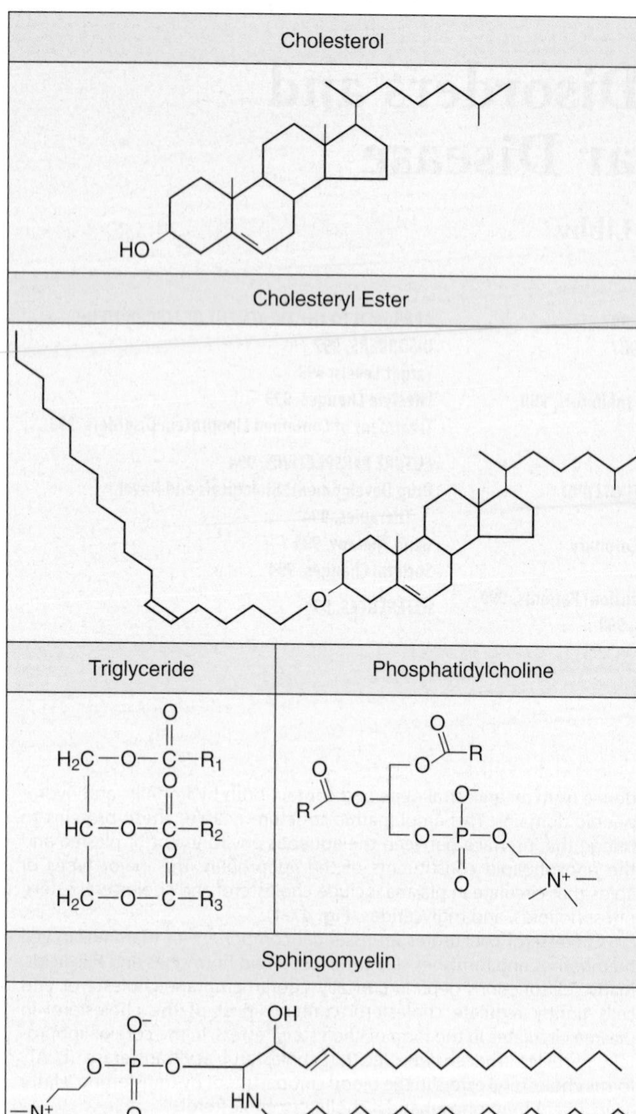

FIGURE 47-1 Structures of the major lipid molecules—cholesterol, cholesteryl esters, triglycerides, and phospholipids (phosphatidylcholine and sphingomyelin). R indicates a fatty acyl chain.

enveloped by hydrophilic phospholipids and free cholesterol. The apolipoproteins furnish the protein moiety of lipoproteins (**Fig. 47-2**). Lipoproteins vary in size, in density in the aqueous environment of plasma, and in lipid and apolipoprotein content (**Fig. 47-3**; **Table 47-1**). The classification of lipoproteins reflects their density in plasma (the density of plasma is 1.006 g/mL), as gauged by flotation in the ultracentrifuge. The triglyceride-rich lipoproteins, consisting of chylomicrons, chylomicron remnants, and very low-density lipoprotein (VLDL), have a density lower than 1.006 g/mL. The rest (bottom fraction) of the ultracentrifuged plasma consists of LDL, HDL, and lipoprotein(a) [(Lp(a)].

Apolipoproteins (apo) have four major roles: (1) assembly and secretion of the lipoprotein (apo A-I, apo B100, apo B48); (2) structural integrity of the lipoprotein (apo B, apo E, apo A-I, apo A-II); (3) coactivator or inhibitor of enzymes (apo A-I, A-V, C-I, C-II, C-III); and (4) binding or docking to specific receptors and proteins for cellular uptake of the entire particle or selective uptake of a lipid component (apo A-I, apo B100, apo E; **Table 47-2**). The roles of several

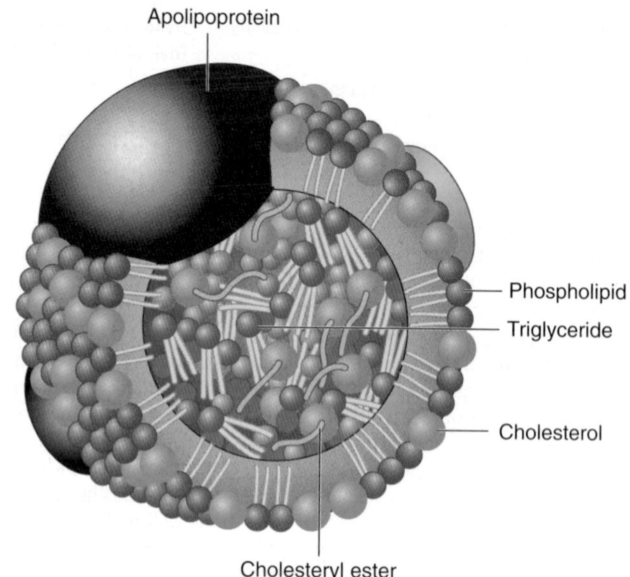

FIGURE 47-2 Structure of lipoproteins. Phospholipids are oriented with their polar group toward the aqueous environment of plasma. Free cholesterol is inserted within the phospholipid layer. The core of the lipoprotein is made up of cholesteryl esters and triglycerides. Apolipoproteins are involved in the secretion of the lipoprotein, provide structural integrity, and act as cofactors for enzymes or as ligands for various receptors.

TABLE 47-1 Plasma Lipoprotein Composition

COMPONENT	ORIGIN	DENSITY (G/ML)	SIZE (NM)	PROTEIN (%)	CHOLESTEROL IN PLASMA (MMOL/L)†	TRIGLYCERIDE IN FASTING PLASMA (MMOL/L)‡	APOPROTEIN MAJOR	APOPROTEIN OTHER
Chylomicron*	Intestine	<0.95	100-1000	1-2	0.0	0.0	B48	A-I, Cs
Chylomicron remnants*	Chylomicron metabolism	0.95-1.006	30-80	3-5	0.0	0.0	B48, E	A-I, A-IV, Cs
VLDL	Liver	<1.006	40-50	10	0.1-0.4	0.2-1.2	B100	AI, Cs
IDL	VLDL	1.006-1.019	25-30	18	0.1-0.3	0.1-0.3	B100, E	
LDL	IDL	1.019-1.063	20-25	25	1.5-3.5	0.2-0.4	B100*	
HDL	Liver, intestine	1.063-1.210	6-10	40-55	0.9-1.6	0.1-0.2	A-I, A-II	A-IV
Lipoprotein(a)	Liver	1.051-1.082	25	30-50			B100, (a)	

*In the fasted state, serum (or plasma) should not contain chylomicrons or their remnants.
†In mmol/L. For mg/dL, multiply by 38.67.
‡In mmol/L. For mg/dL, multiply by 88.5.

apolipoproteins (apo A-IV, apo A-V, apo D, apo H, apo J, apo L, apo M) remain incompletely understood.

Many proteins regulate the synthesis, secretion, and metabolic fate of lipoproteins. Their characterization has provided insights into molecular cellular physiology and elucidated targets for drug development (**Table 47-3**). The discovery of the LDL receptor (LDL-R) furnished a landmark in understanding cholesterol metabolism and receptor-mediated endocytosis.[1] The LDL-R regulates the entry of cholesterol into cells; tight control mechanisms alter its expression on the cell surface, depending on need. Other receptors for lipoproteins include several that bind VLDL but not LDL. The LDL receptor–related peptide (LRP), which mediates the uptake of chylomicron remnants and VLDL, preferentially recognizes apo E. The LRP interacts with hepatic lipase. A specific VLDL receptor exists. Hepatocytes and the various lipoproteins containing apo E have complex interactions involving cell surface proteoglycans that provide scaffolding for lipolytic enzymes (lipoprotein lipase and hepatic lipase) involved in remnant lipoprotein recognition. Macrophages express receptors that bind modified (especially oxidized) lipoproteins. These scavenger lipoprotein receptors mediate the uptake of oxidized LDL into

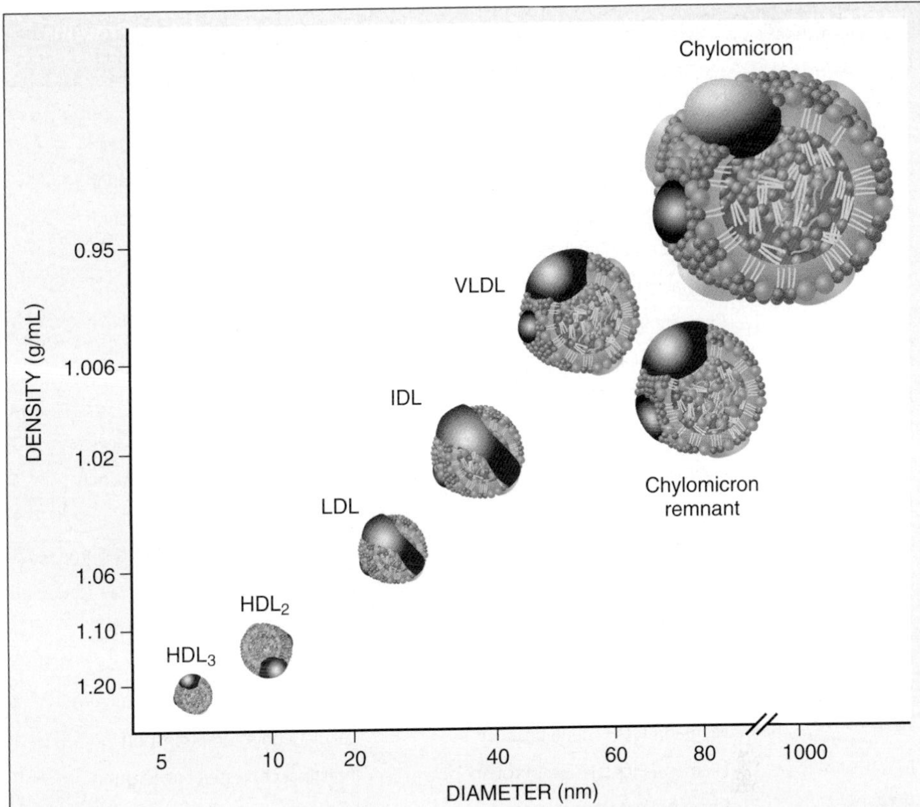

FIGURE 47-3 Relative size of plasma lipoproteins according to their hydrated density. The density of plasma is 1.006 g/mL.

TABLE 47-2 Roles and Functions of Apolipoproteins

APOLIPOPROTEIN	PREDOMINANT LIPOPROTEIN	MOLECULAR WEIGHT (KDA)	PLASMA CONCENTRATION (MG/DL)	CHROMOSOME	ROLE	DISEASE
A-I	HDL	28.3	90-160	11q23	ACAT activation, structural	HDL deficiency
A-II	HDL	17	25-45	1q21-23	Structural	
A-IV	HDL	45	10-20	11q23	Structural, absorption	
A-V	VLDL, HDL			11q23	TRL metabolism	Hypertriglyceridemia
B100	LDL, VLDL	512	50-150	2q23-24	Structural, LDL-R binding	Hypobetalipoproteinemia
B48	Chylomicrons	241	0-100	2q23-24	Structural	
C-I	Chylomicrons	6.63	5-6	19q13.2	TRL metabolism	
C-II	Chylomicrons, VLDL	8.84	3-5	19q13.2	LPL activation	Hyperchylomicronemia
C-III	Chylomicrons, VLDL	8.76	10-14	11q23	LPL inhibition	Hypertriglyceridemia
D	HDL	33	4-7	3q26.2	LCAT	
E	Chylomicron remnants, IDL	34	2-8	19q13.2	LDL-R, apo E-R binding	Type III
H	Chylomicrons, VLDL, LDL, HDL	—	—	17q23-ter	B_2 glycoprotein	Cofactor for anionic phospholipid binding by antiphospholipid autoantibodies
J	HDL	70	10	18p21	Complement system	
L1-6	HDL	43.9	—	22q12.3	Unknown	Anti-trypansomial
M	HDL	25	1 uM	66p21.3	Unknown	
(a)	Lipoprotein(a)	250-800	0-200	6q27	Tissue injury (?)	

Apo E-R = apolipoprotein E receptor.

CH 47

TABLE 47-3 Lipoprotein Processing Enzymes, Receptors, and Modulating Proteins

ABBREVIATION	NAME	ROLE	CHROMOSOME	DISEASE
ABCA1	ATP binding cassette A1	Cellular phospholipid efflux	9q31	Tangier disease
ABCG5/G8	ATP binding cassette G5 and G8	Intestinal sitosterol transporter	21	Sitosterolemia
ACAT1	Acetyl-CoA acetyltransferase 1	Cellular cholesterol esterification	1q22.3	
ACAT2	Acetyl-CoA acetyltransferase 2	Cellular cholesterol esterification	6q25.3	
Apo E-R	Apo E–containing lipoprotein receptor	TRL uptake	1p34	
CD36	Fatty acid translocase	Fatty acid transport	7q11.2	
CETP	Cholesteryl ester transfer protein	Lipid exchange in plasma	16q21	Elevated HDL cholesterol
EL (LIPG)	Endothelial lipase	Phospholipid hydrolysis	18q21.1	
HL (LIPC)	Hepatic lipase	Triglyceride hydrolysis	15q21	Remnant accumulation
HSL (LIPE)	Hormone-sensitive lipase	Fatty acid release from adipocytes	19q13.2	
LCAT	Lecithin cholesterol acyltransferase	Cholesterol esterification (Plasma)	16q22.1	LCAT deficiency, low HDL
LDL-R	Low-density lipoprotein receptor	LDL uptake	19p13	Familial hypercholesterolemia
Lox1	Scavenger receptor	Oxidized LDL uptake, endothelium	12p12-13	Oxidized lipoprotein uptake
LPL	Lipoprotein lipase	Triglyceride hydrolysis	8p22	Hyperchylomicronemia
LRP1	LDL-R–related protein	Protease uptake, many ligands	19q12	
LRP2	LDL-R–related protein 2 (megalin)	Protease uptake, apo J	2q24-31	
MTP	Microsomal triglyceride transfer protein	Apo B assembly	4q22-24	Abetalipoproteinemia
NPC1	Niemann-Pick C gene product	Cellular cholesterol transport	18q11-12	Niemann-Pick type C
NPC1L1	Niemann-Pick C1–like 1 protein	Intestinal cholesterol absorption	7p13	
PLTP	Phospholipid transfer protein	Lipid exchange in plasma	20q12	
PCSK9	Proprotein convertase, subtilisin/kexin-9	Protein cleavage	1p34.1	Hypercholesterolemia
SMPD1	Sphingomyelinase phosphodiesterase	Sphingomyelin hydrolysis	11p15.4	Niemann-Pick types A and B
SRA	Scavenger receptor A	Oxidized LDL uptake, macrophages	8p21	
SR-B1	Scavenger receptor B1	HDL CE uptake	12	
VLDL-R	Very low-density lipoprotein receptor	VLDL uptake	9q24	

CE = Cholesteryl ester.

macrophages. In contrast to the exquisitely regulated LDL receptor, high cellular cholesterol content does not suppress scavenger receptors, enabling the subintimal macrophages to accumulate abundant cholesterol, become foam cells, and form fatty streaks. Sterol accumulation in the endoplasmic reticulum may lead to cell apoptosis via the unfolded protein response.[2] Endothelial cells can also take up modified lipoproteins through receptors such as Lox-1. To reach lipid-laden macrophages, HDL particles traverse vascular endothelial cells by transcytosis; cholesterol uptake from macrophages by HDL depends in part on the scavenger receptor class B (SR-B1) and adenosine triphosphate–binding cassette transporter G1 (ABCG1) transporter.[3]

At least three physiologically relevant receptors bind HDL particles—SR-B1 (also named CLA-1 in humans), the adenosine triphosphate–binding cassette transporter A1 (ABCA1), and ABCG1. SR-B1 binds not only HDL but also LDL and VLDL, albeit with lower affinity. SR-B1 mediates the selective uptake of HDL cholesteryl esters in steroidogenic tissues, hepatocytes, and endothelium. ABCA1 mediates cellular phospholipid (and possibly cholesterol) efflux and functions critically in HDL biogenesis. The ABCG1 transporter transfers cellular cholesterol to more mature, spherical HDL particles.[4]

Lipoprotein Metabolism and Transport

The lipoprotein transport system has two major roles; the efficient transport of triglycerides from the intestine and the liver to sites of uptake (fat tissue or muscle) and the transport of cholesterol to peripheral tissues for membrane synthesis and steroid hormone production or to the liver for bile acid synthesis.

INTESTINAL PATHWAY (CHYLOMICRONS TO CHYLOMICRON REMNANTS). Life requires fats. The human body derives essential fatty acids that it cannot make from the diet. Fat typically furnishes 20% to 40% of daily calories. Triglycerides comprise the major portion of ingested fats. For an individual consuming 2000 kcal/day, with 30% in the form of fat, this represents approximately 66 g of triglycerides/day and approximately 250 mg (0.250 g) of cholesterol. The intestine has highly efficient fat absorption mechanisms. This property likely reflects the evolutionary value of providing the organism with nutrients when food availability was not regular.

On ingestion, pancreatic lipases hydrolyze triglycerides into free fatty acids and monoglycerides or diglycerides. Emulsification by bile salts leads to the formation of intestinal micelles. Micelles resemble lipoproteins in that they consist of phospholipids, free cholesterol, bile acids, diglycerides and monoglycerides, free fatty acids, and glycerol.

The mechanism of micelle uptake by the intestinal brush border cells still engenders debate. The Niemann-Pick C1–like 1 (NPC1-L1) protein is part of an intestinal cholesterol transporter complex and is the target for the selective cholesterol absorption inhibitor ezetimibe[5] (see later). After uptake into intestinal cells, fatty acids undergo reesterification to form triglycerides and packaging into chylomicrons inside the intestinal cell and enter the portal circulation (**Fig. 47-4**, part 1). Chylomicrons contain apo B48, the amino-terminal component of apo B100. In the intestine, the apo B gene is modified during transcription into mRNA, with a substitution of a uracil for a cytosine by an apo B48–editing enzyme complex (ApoBec).[6] This mechanism involves a cytosine deaminase and leads to a termination codon at residue 2153 and a truncated form of apo B. Only intestinal cells express ApoBec. These cells also absorb plant sterols (e.g., sitosterol, campesterol), which undergo intracellular sorting and resecretion into the intestinal lumen via the ABCG5/8 heterodimeric transporter. Mutations of the ABCG5/8 genes cause the rare disorder sitosterolemia.[7]

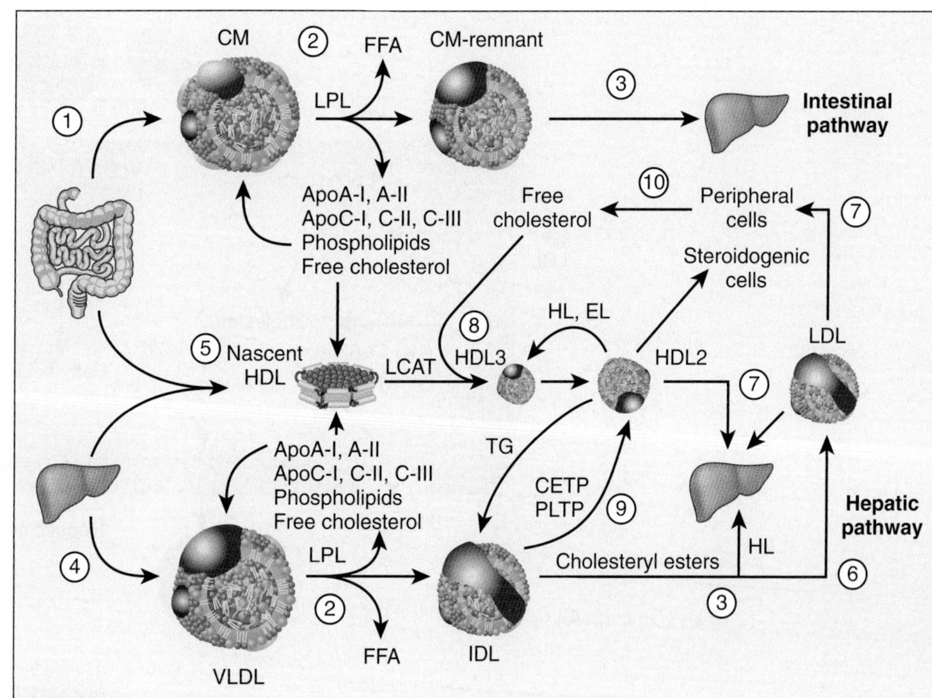

FIGURE 47-4 Schematic diagram of the lipid transport system. Numbers in circles refer to explanation in the text. EL = endothelial lipase; HL = hepatic lipase.

Chylomicrons rapidly enter the plasma compartment after meals. In capillaries of adipose tissue or muscle cells in the peripheral circulation, chylomicrons encounter lipoprotein lipase (LPL), an enzyme attached to heparan sulfate proteoglycans present on the luminal side of endothelial cells (see Fig. 47-4, part 2). Apolipoproteins regulate LPL activity—apo C-II and apo AV activate and apo C-III inhibits LPL. LPL has broad specificity for triglycerides; it cleaves all fatty acyl residues attached to glycerol, generating three molecules of FFA for each molecule of glycerol. Muscle cells take up fatty acids rapidly. Adipose cells can store triglycerides made from fatty acids for energy utilization, a process that requires insulin. Fatty acids can also bind to fatty acid–binding proteins and travel to the liver, where they are repackaged in VLDL. Peripheral resistance to insulin (in diabetes or the metabolic syndrome) can thus increase the delivery of FFAs to the liver, with a consequent increase in VLDL secretion and increased apo B particles in plasma (see Chap. 64).[8] The remnant particles, derived from chylomicrons following LPL action, contain apo E and enter the liver for degradation and reuptake of their core constituents (see Fig. 47-4, part 3).

HEPATIC PATHWAY (VERY-LOW-DENSITY LIPOPROTEIN TO INTERMEDIATE-DENSITY LIPOPROTEIN). Food supply varies, as does dietary fat content. The body must ensure readily available triglyceride to meet energy demands. Hepatic secretion of VLDL particles serves this function (see Fig. 47-4, part 4). VLDLs are triglyceride-rich lipoproteins smaller than chylomicrons (see Table 47-1 and Fig. 47-3). They contain apo B100 as their main lipoprotein. As opposed to apo B48, apo B100 contains a domain recognized by the LDL receptor (the apo B/E receptor). VLDL particles follow the same catabolic pathway through lipoprotein lipase as chylomicrons (see Fig. 47-4, part 2). During hydrolysis of triglyceride-rich lipoproteins by LPL, an exchange of proteins and lipids takes place; VLDL particles (and chylomicrons) acquire apo Cs and apo E, in part from HDL particles. VLDLs also exchange triglycerides for cholesteryl esters from HDL (mediated by cholesteryl ester transfer protein [CETP]) (see Fig. 47-4, part 9). Such bidirectional transfer of constituents between lipoproteins serves several purposes, allowing lipoproteins to do the following: acquire specific apolipoproteins that will dictate their metabolic fate; transfer phospholipids onto nascent HDL particles mediated by phospholipid transfer protein (PLTP); and transfer cholesterol from HDL to VLDL remnants so it can be metabolized in the liver. During the loss of core triglycerides, the phospholipid envelope becomes redundant and sheds phospholipids, which can then associate with apo A-I to form new HDL particles. Such exchanges contribute importantly to the reverse cholesterol transport pathway.

After hydrolysis of triglycerides partly depletes VLDL of triglycerides, VLDL particles have relatively more cholesterol, shed several apolipoproteins (especially the C apolipoproteins), and acquire apo E. The VLDL remnant lipoprotein, called intermediate-density lipoprotein (IDL), binds to hepatic LDL receptors via its apo E moiety (see Fig. 47-4, part 3) or undergoes further delipidation by hepatic lipase to form an LDL particle (see Fig. 47-4, part 6). At least four receptors bind triglyceride-rich lipoproteins (TRLs), TRL remnants, and apo B–containing lipoproteins—the VLDL receptor, remnant receptor, LDL receptor (also called the apo B/E receptor), and LDL receptor–related peptide. Most hepatic lipoprotein receptors share an ability to bind apo E, an engagement that mediates uptake of several classes of lipoproteins, including VLDL and IDL.[9] The interactions between apo E and its receptors are complex, often involving the docking of TRL on heparan sulfate proteoglycans before presentation of the ligand to its receptor.

LOW-DENSITY LIPOPROTEINS. LDL particles contain predominantly cholesteryl esters packaged with the protein moiety apo B100. Normally, triglycerides constitute only 4% to 8% of the LDL mass (see Table 47-1). In the presence of elevated plasma triglyceride levels, LDL particles can become enriched in triglycerides and depleted in core cholesteryl esters. LDL particle size variation results from changes in core constituents, with an increase in triglycerides and a relative decrease in cholesteryl esters leading to smaller, denser LDL particles.

LDL particles serve as the main serum carriers of cholesterol, typical in humans and in nonhuman primates fed a cholesterol-enriched diet. In other mammals, such as rodents or rabbits, VLDL and HDL particles transport most of the cholesterol. Cells can either make cholesterol from acetate through enzymatic reactions requiring at least 33 steps or obtain it as cholesteryl esters from LDL particles. Cells internalize LDL via the LDL-R (**Fig. 47-5A**). LDL particles contain one molecule of apo B. Although several domains of apo B are highly lipophilic and associate with phospholipids, a region surrounding residue 3500 binds with saturability and high affinity to the LDL-R. The LDL-R localizes in a region of the plasma membrane rich in the protein clathrin (see Fig. 47-4, part 7, and Fig. 47-5A). Once bound to the receptor, clathrin polymerizes and forms an endosome that contains LDL bound to its receptor, a portion of the plasma membrane, and clathrin. This internalized particle then fuses with lysosomes whose catalytic enzymes (cholesteryl ester hydrolase, cathepsins) release free cholesterol and degrade apo B. The LDL-R will detach itself from its ligand and recycle to the plasma membrane.

Cells tightly regulate cholesterol content by the following: (1) cholesterol synthesis in the smooth endoplasmic reticulum (via the rate-limiting step with hydroxymethylglutaryl coenzyme A [HMG-CoA]

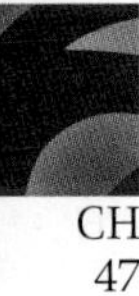

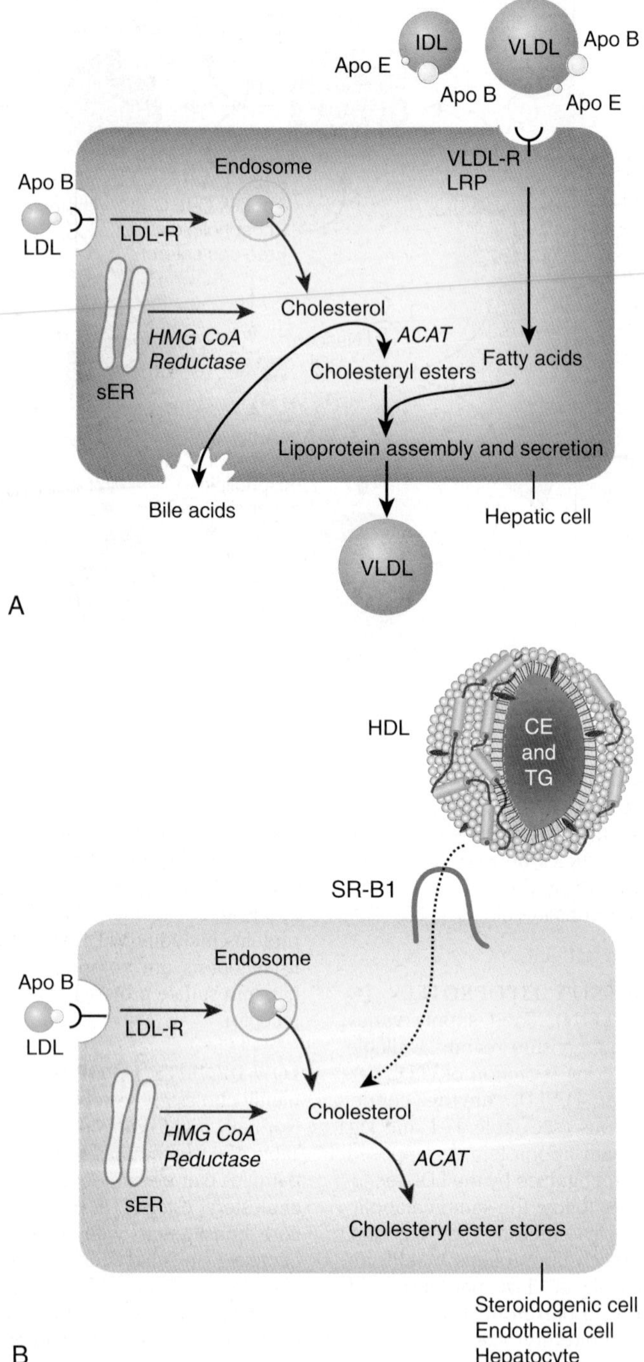

FIGURE 47-5 Cellular cholesterol homeostasis in various tissues. **A,** Cholesterol homeostasis (hepatocytes). **B,** Selective uptake of cholesterol (adrenal cells, hepatocytes, endothelial cells).

reductase); (2) receptor-mediated endocytosis of LDL (two mechanisms under the control of the steroid-responsive element binding protein [SREBP]); (3) cholesterol efflux from plasma membrane to cholesterol acceptor particles (predominantly apo A-I and HDL) via the ABCA1 and ABCG1 transporters; and (4) intracellular cholesterol esterification via the enzyme acyl CoA–cholesteryl acyltransferase (ACAT; see Fig. 47-5A, B, and C). The SREBP regulates the first two pathways at the level of gene transcription in a coordinated fashion. Cellular cholesterol binds to a protein called SCAP (SREPB cholesterol-activated protein) residing on the endoplasmic reticulum. Cholesterol inhibits the interaction of SCAP with SREPB. In the absence of cholesterol, SCAP mediates the cleavage of SREBP at two sites by specific proteases and release an amino-terminal (NH_2) fragment of SREBP.The SREBP NH_2 fragment migrates to the nucleus and increases the transcriptional activity of genes involved in cellular cholesterol and fatty acid homeostasis. Cleavage of SREBP depends on a proprotein convertase related to the subtilisin/kexin family of convertases. Another member of the convertase superfamily, proprotein convertase subtilisin/kexin 9 (PCSK9), functions in the internalization and cellular processing of the LDL-R. Gain-of-function mutations in PCSK9 cause dominant familial hypercholesterolemia, whereas loss of function increases LDL-R and lowers LDL cholesterol (LDL-C), and cardiovascular event rates, significantly.[10] The ACAT pathway regulates cholesterol content in membranes. Humans express two separate forms of ACAT. ACAT1 and ACAT2 are derived from different genes and mediate cholesterol esterification in cytoplasm and in the

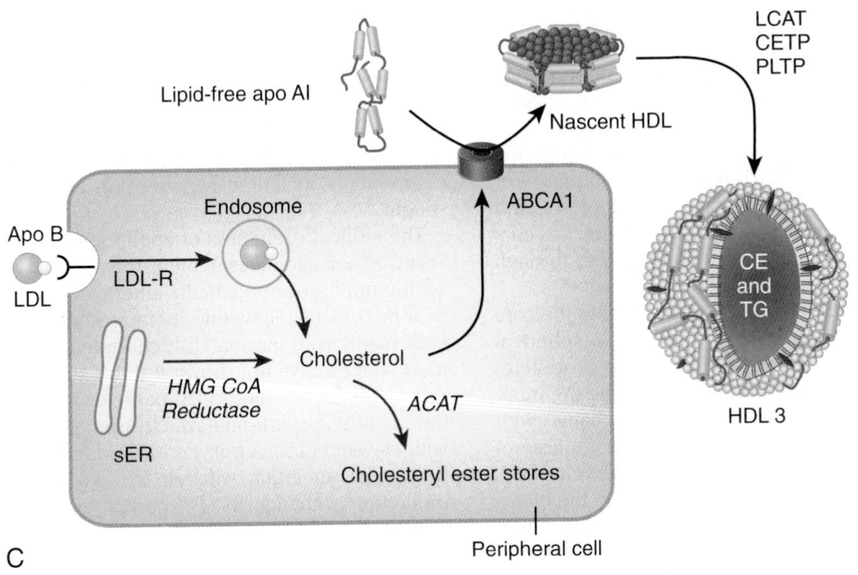

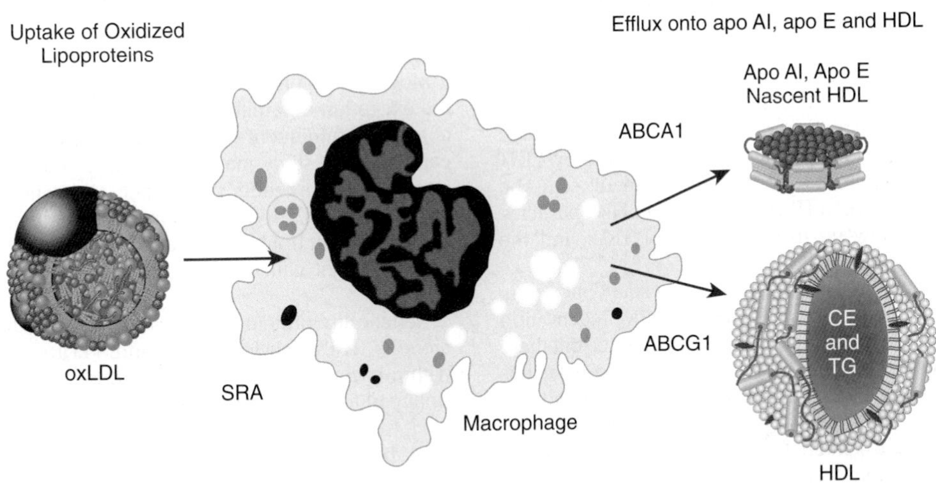

FIGURE 47-5, cont'd **C,** Cellular cholesterol efflux (peripheral cells). **D,** Macrophage. CE = cholesterol esters; LRP = low-density lipoprotein receptor– related peptide; sER = smooth endoplasmic reticulum; TG = triglycerides; VLDL-R = very-low-density lipoprotein receptor.

endoplasmic reticulum lumen for lipoprotein assembly and secretion.

Regulation of cholesterol efflux depends in part on the ABCA1 pathway, controlled in turn by hydroxysterols (especially 24-hydroxycholesterol and 27-hydroxycholesterol, which act as ligands for the liver-specific receptor [LxR] family of transcriptional regulatory factors). In conditions of cholesterol sufficiency, the cell can decrease its input of cholesterol by decreasing the de novo synthesis of cholesterol. The cell can also decrease the amount of cholesterol that enters via the LDL-R, increase the amount stored as cholesteryl esters, and promote the removal of cholesterol by increasing its movement to the plasma membrane for efflux.

HIGH-DENSITY LIPOPROTEIN AND REVERSE CHOLESTEROL TRANSPORT. Epidemiologic studies consistently have shown an inverse relationship between plasma levels of HDL cholesterol and CAD events. HDL promotes reverse cholesterol transport and can prevent lipoprotein oxidation, exert anti-inflammatory actions in vitro, and promote cell proliferation and survival.[11]

HDL particles have complex and incompletely understood metabolism. The complexity arises because the particles acquire their components from several sources and these components undergo metabolism at different sites. Apolipoprotein A-I, the main protein of HDL, is synthesized in the intestine and liver. Approximately 80% of HDL originates from the liver and 20% from the intestine (see Fig. 47-4, part 5). Lipid-free apo A-I acquires phospholipids from cell membranes and from redundant phospholipids shed during hydrolysis of triglyceride-rich lipoproteins. Lipid-free apo A-I binds to ABCA1 and promotes its phosphorylation via cyclic adenosine monophosphate (cAMP), which increases the net efflux of phospholipids and cholesterol onto apo A-I to form a nascent HDL particle (see Fig. 47-4, part 10). This particle contains apo A-I, phospholipids, and some free cholesterol; its structure is currently a matter of scientific debate (see Fig. 47-5C). These nascent HDL particles will mediate further cellular cholesterol efflux. Currently, standard laboratory tests do not measure these HDL precursors because they contain little or no cholesterol.

On reaching a cell membrane, the nascent HDL particles capture membrane-associated cholesterol and promote the efflux of free cholesterol onto other HDL particles (see Fig. 47-4, part 10). Conceptually, the formation of HDL particles appears to involve two steps. The first step involves ABCA1-dependent cellular phospholipid and cholesterol efflux, and the second step probably does not require ABCA1. The efflux of cellular cholesterol from cells such as macrophages does not contribute importantly to overall HDL-C mass but may have a critical effect on the export of cholesterol from atheromas. Macrophages can efflux cholesterol onto apo A-I and apo E, onto nascent discoidal HDL particles via the ABCA1 transporter, or onto spherical HDL particles via the ABCG1 transporter (see Fig. 47-5D). ABCG1 transporter does not promote cellular cholesterol efflux to lipid-free or lipid-poor apo A-I but to mature HDL particles. The plasma enzyme LCAT, an enzyme activated by apo A-I, then esterifies the free cholesterol (see Figs. 47-4, part 8, and 47-5C). LCAT transfers an acyl chain (a fatty acid) from the R2 position of a phospholipid to the 3′-hydroxy residue of cholesterol, resulting in the formation of a cholesteryl ester (see Fig. 47-1). In a process called selective uptake of cholesterol, HDL also provides cholesterol to steroid hormone–producing tissues and the liver through the scavenger SR-B1 receptor (see Fig. 47-5B).

Because of their hydrophobicity, cholesteryl esters move to the core of the lipoprotein, and the HDL particle now assumes a spherical configuration (a particle denoted as HDL3). With further cholesterol esterification, the HDL particle increases in size to become the more buoyant HDL2. Cholesterol within HDL particles can exchange with TRLs via CETP, which mediates an equimolar exchange of cholesterol from HDL to TRLs and triglyceride movement from TRLs onto HDL (see Fig. 47-4, part 9). Inhibition of CETP increases HDL-C in the blood and represents a therapeutic target for cardiovascular disease (CVD) prevention. PLTP mediates the transfer of phospholipids between TRLs and HDL particles. Triglyceride-enriched HDLs are denoted HDL2b. Hepatic lipase can hydrolyze triglycerides and endothelial lipase can hydrolyze phospholipids within these particles, converting them back to HDL3 particles.

One mechanism of reverse cholesterol transport includes the uptake of cellular cholesterol from extrahepatic tissues, such as lipid-laden macrophages,[12] and its esterification by LCAT, transport by large HDL particles, and exchange for one triglyceride molecule by CETP. Originally, on an HDL particle, the cholesterol molecule can be taken up by hepatic receptors on a TRL or LDL particle. HDL particles, therefore, act as shuttles between tissue cholesterol, TRLs, and the liver.

Reverse cholesterol transport by HDL constitutes a small but potentially important portion of the plasma HDL mass. Selective inactivation of macrophage ABCA1 does not change HDL-C levels in mice but there is an increase in atherosclerosis. The catabolism of HDL particles has engendered debate among lipoprotein researchers. The protein component of HDL particles is exchangeable with lipoproteins of other classes. The kidneys appear to eliminate apolipoprotein A-I and other HDL apolipoproteins. The lipid components of HDL particles also follow a different metabolic route (see Fig. 47-5B, C, and D).

Lipoprotein Disorders

Definitions

Time and new information have stimulated changes to the classification of lipoprotein disorders. The original classification of lipoprotein disorders by Donald Fredrickson and colleagues in 1967 used the measurement of total plasma cholesterol and triglycerides and lipoprotein patterns analyzed by electrophoresis. This classification recognized elevations of chylomicrons (type I), VLDL or prebeta lipoproteins (type IV), broad beta disease (or type III hyperlipoproteinemia), beta lipoproteins (LDL; type II), and elevations of both chylomicrons and VLDL (type V). In addition, the combined elevation of prebeta (VLDL) and beta (LDL) lipoproteins was denoted type IIb hyperlipoproteinemia. Although providing a useful conceptual framework, this classification has some drawbacks; it does not include HDL cholesterol and it does not differentiate severe monogenic lipoprotein disorders from the more common polygenic disorders. Subsequently, the World Health Organization, the European Atherosclerosis Society, and more recently, the National Cholesterol Education Program, have classified lipoprotein disorders on the basis of arbitrary cut points.

A practical clinical approach describes a lipoprotein disorder by the absolute plasma levels of lipids (cholesterol and triglycerides) and lipoprotein cholesterol (LDL and HDL cholesterol), and considers clinical manifestations of hyperlipoproteinemia in the context of biochemical characterization. For example, a young patient presenting with eruptive xanthomas and a plasma triglyceride level of 11.3 mmol/L (1000 mg/dL) likely has familial hyperchylomicronemia caused by LPL deficiency. An obese, hypertensive middle-aged man with a cholesterol level of 6.4 mmol/L (247 mg/dL), triglyceride level of 3.1 mmol/L (274 mg/dL), HDL cholesterol level of 0.8 mmol/L (31 mg/dL), and calculated LDL cholesterol level of 4.2 mmol/L (162 mg/dL) likely has the metabolic syndrome, and the identification of its other components, including hypertension and hyperglycemia, should be sought.

The clinical usefulness of apolipoprotein levels has stirred debate. Taken as a single measurement, the apo B level provides information on the number of potentially atherogenic particles and can be used as a goal of lipid-lowering therapy. Similarly, LDL particle size correlates highly with plasma HDL cholesterol and triglyceride levels, and most studies have not shown it to be an independent cardiovascular risk factor. Small, dense LDL particles tend to track with features of the metabolic syndrome, which usually involves dyslipoproteinemia with elevated plasma triglyceride and reduced HDL cholesterol levels. It remains uncertain whether in addition to LDL particle number reduction, a change in LDL particle size will bring further clinical benefit.

Genetic Lipoprotein Disorders

Understanding of the genetics of lipoprotein metabolism has expanded rapidly. Classification of genetic lipoprotein disorders usually requires a biochemical phenotype in addition to a clinical phenotype. With the exception of familial hypercholesterolemia, monogenic disorders tend to be infrequent or very rare. Disorders considered heritable on careful family study may be difficult to characterize unambiguously because of age, gender, penetrance, and gene-gene and environmental interactions. Most common lipoprotein disorders encountered clinically result from the interaction of increasing age, lack of physical activity, weight gain, and a suboptimal diet with individual genetic makeup.

Genetic lipoprotein disorders can affect LDL, Lp(a), remnant lipoproteins, TRLs (chylomicrons and VLDL), or HDL (**Table 47-4**). Within each of these, genetic disorders can cause an excess or deficiency of a specific class of lipoprotein.

LOW-DENSITY LIPOPROTEINS (TYPE II HYPERLIPIDEMIA)

Familial Hypercholesterolemia

Familial hypercholesterolemia is the most thoroughly studied lipoprotein disorder. The elucidation of the pathway whereby complex molecules enter the cell by receptor-mediated endocytosis and the discovery of the LDL-R represent landmarks in cell biology and clinical investigation. Affected subjects have an elevated LDL cholesterol level higher than the 95th percentile for age and sex. In adulthood, clinical manifestations include corneal arcus, tendinous xanthomas over the extensor tendons (metacarpophalangeal joints, patellar, triceps, and Achilles tendons), and xanthelasmas. Transmission is autosomal codominant. Familial hypercholesterolemia affects approximately 1 in 500, although this prevalence is higher in populations with a founder effect. Patients with familial hypercholesterolemia have a high risk of developing CAD by the third to fourth decade in men and approximately 8 to 10 years later in women. Diagnosis is based on an elevated plasma LDL cholesterol level, family history of premature CAD, and presence of xanthomas.[13]

LOW-DENSITY LIPOPROTEIN RECEPTOR GENE. Defects of the *LDL-R* gene cause an accumulation of LDL particles in plasma, thus altering the function of the LDL-R protein and causing familial hypercholesterolemia (see Fig. 47-4, part 7). To date, there are over 1000 identified mutations of the *LDL-R* gene (see http://www.umd.necker.fr). LDL-R mutations are the most frequent cause of familial hypercholesterolemia.

FAMILIAL DEFECTIVE APO B. Mutations within the apo B gene that lead to an abnormal ligand-receptor interaction can cause a form of familial hypercholesterolemia clinically indistinguishable from the primary form. Several mutations at the postulated binding site to the LDL-R cause familial defective apo B100 (see Fig. 47-4, part 7). These

TABLE 47-4 Genetic Lipoprotein Disorders

DISORDER	GENE	FIGURE 47-4 PART
LDL Particles		
Familial hypercholesterolemia	*LDL-R*	7
Familial defective apo B100	*Apo B*	7
Autosomal dominant hypercholesterolemia	*PCSK9*	7
Autosomal recessive hypercholesterolemia	*ARH*	7
Abetalipoproteinemia	*MTP*	
Hypobetalipoproteinemia	*Apo B*	
Familial sitosterolemia	*ABCG5/ABCG8*	
Familial lipoprotein(a) hyperlipoproteinemia	*Apo (a)*	
Remnant Lipoproteins		
Dysbetalipoproteinemia type III	*Apo E*	3
Hepatic lipase deficiency	*HL*	6
Triglyceride-rich Lipoproteins		
Lipoprotein lipase deficiency	*LPL*	2
Apo C-II deficiency	*Apo C-II*	2
Apo A-V deficiency	*Apo A-V*	
Familial hypertriglyceridemia	*Polygenic*	
Familial combined hyperlipidemia	*Polygenic*	
HDL Particles		
Apo A-I deficiency	*Apo A-I*	
Tangier disease, familial HDL deficiency	*ABCA1*	10
Familial LCAT deficiency syndromes	*LCAT*	8
CETP deficiency	*CETP*	9
Niemann-Pick disease types A and B	*SMPD1*	
Niemann-Pick disease type C	*NPC1*	

consist of apo $B_{Arg3500Gln}$, apo $B_{Arg3500Trp}$, and apo $B_{Arg3531Cys}$.[13] The apo $B_{Arg3500Gln}$ results from a G → A substitution at nucleotide 3500 within exon 26 of the apo B gene. The defective apo B has a reduced affinity (20% to 30% of control) for the LDL-R. LDL particles with defective apo B have a plasma half-life three- to fourfold longer than the half-life of normal LDL. Because of their increased persistence, these LDL particles can undergo oxidative modifications that can enhance their atherogenicity more readily. Affected subjects usually have elevated LDL cholesterol levels up to 400 mg/dL (10.4 mmol/L) but may also have normal levels. Familial defective apo B 100 has a prevalence similar to that of familial hypercholesterolemia (1 in 500). In subjects with the classic presentation of familial hypercholesterolemia, the prevalence of familial defective apo B 100 is reported to be 1 in 50 to 1 in 20. The reasons for the variability of plasma LDL cholesterol levels remain unexplained.

PROPROTEIN CONVERTASE, SUBTILISIN/KEXIN TYPE 9 (PCSK9) GENE. An autosomal dominant form of hypercholesterolemia that maps to chromosome 1p34.1 involves a mutation in the *PCSK9* gene. *PCSK9* codes for a protein identified as neural apoptosis-regulated convertase 1 (NARC1), a novel proprotein convertase belonging to the subtilase family of convertases. It is related to subtilisin/kexin isoenzyme-1 (site-1 protease) required for cleavage of SREBP. Subjects with loss-of-function mutation of *PCSK9* have a markedly lower LDL-C level than subjects without the mutation. Black Americans have a higher prevalence of this protective mutation than white Americans. In the Atherosclerosis Risk in Communities study, subjects with lifelong low LDL-C levels because of a mutation at the *PCSK9* gene locus had a marked reduction in coronary events,[14] confirming that genetic low LDL-C states confer a cardioprotective advantage.

AUTOSOMAL RECESSIVE HYPERCHOLESTEROLEMIA (ARH). An autosomal recessive form of familial hypercholesterolemia, known as autosomal recessive hypercholesterolemia (ARH), has been identified in kindred from Sardinia. It is caused by mutations in the *ARH* gene that encode a protein involved in the recycling of the LDL-R.

HYPOBETALIPOPROTEINEMIA AND ABETALIPOPROTEINEMIA. Mutations within the apo B gene can lead to truncations of the mature apo B100 peptide. Many such mutations cause a syndrome characterized by reduced LDL and VLDL cholesterol levels but little or no clinical manifestations and no known risk of CVD—a condition called hypobetalipoproteinemia. Apo B truncated close to its amino terminus loses the ability to bind lipids, producing a syndrome similar to abetalipoproteinemia, a rare recessive lipoprotein disorder of infancy that causes mental retardation and growth abnormalities. Abetalipoproteinemia is caused by a mutation in gene coding for the microsomal triglyceride transfer protein (MTP) required for the assembly of apo B–containing lipoproteins in the liver and intestine. The resulting lack of apo B–containing lipoproteins in plasma causes a marked deficiency of fat-soluble vitamins (A, D, E, and K) that circulate in lipoproteins. In turn, this deficiency results in mental and developmental retardation in affected children.

SITOSTEROLEMIA. A rare condition of increased intestinal absorption and decreased excretion of plant sterols (sitosterol and campesterol) can mimic severe familial hypercholesterolemia, with extensive xanthoma formation. Premature atherosclerosis, often apparent clinically well before adulthood, occurs in patients with sitosterolemia. Diagnosis requires specialized analysis of plasma sterols, demonstrating an elevation in sitosterol, campesterol, cholestanol, sitostanol, and campestanol levels. Interestingly, the level of plasma cholesterol is normal or reduced, and triglycerides are normal. Mutations in the adenosine triphosphate binding cassette G5 and G8 genes (*ABCG5* and *ABCG8*) associate with sitosterolemia.[5] The gene products of *ABCG5* and *ABCG8* are half-ABC transporters thought to form a heterodimer characteristic of the full ABC transporters. The complex is located in the villous border of intestinal cells and actively pumps plant sterols back into the intestinal lumen. A defect in either of the genes renders the complex inactive, and absorption of plant sterols (rather than their elimination) ensues. *ABCG5* and *ABCG8* mutations leading to sitosterolemia are very rare.

LIPOPROTEIN (A). Lp(a), pronounced "lipoprotein little a," consists of an LDL particle linked covalently with one molecule of apo (a). The apo (a) moiety consists of a protein with a high degree of homology with plasminogen. The apo (a) gene appears to have arisen from the plasminogen gene by nonhomologous recombination. The apo (a) gene has multiple repeats of one of the kringle motifs (kringle IV), varying in number from 12 to more than 40 in each individual. Plasma Lp(a) levels depend almost entirely on genetics and correlate inversely with the number of kringle repeats and, therefore, with the molecular weight of apo (a). Using mendelian randomization, data from the Copenhagen Heart study have indicated that Lp(a) is a genetically determined cardiovascular risk factor; genome-wide association analysis also supports a causal role for Lp(a) in CVD.[15,15a] Few environmental factors or medications modulate plasma Lp(a) levels. The pathogenesis of Lp(a) may result from an antifibrinolytic potential and/or ability to bind oxidized lipoproteins. Prospective epidemiologic studies have shown a positive association between Lp(a) and CAD (see Chap. 44).

Triglyceride-Rich Lipoproteins

In subjects with the metabolic syndrome and in diabetic patients (see Chap. 64), elevation of plasma triglyceride levels occurs most often in the presence of visceral (abdominal) obesity and a diet rich in calories, carbohydrates, and saturated fats. Severe elevation of plasma triglyceride levels can result from genetic disorders of the processing enzymes or apolipoproteins and from poorly controlled diabetes.

FAMILIAL HYPERTRIGLYCERIDEMIA (TYPE IV HYPERLIPOPROTEINEMIA). Familial hypertriglyceridemia is not associated with clinical signs such as corneal arcus, xanthoma, and xanthelasmas. Plasma triglyceride, VLDL cholesterol, and VLDL triglyceride levels are moderately to markedly elevated; LDL and HDL cholesterol levels are usually low. Total cholesterol is normal or elevated, depending on VLDL cholesterol levels. Fasting plasma concentrations of triglycerides range from approximately 2.3 to 5.7 mmol/L (200 to 500 mg/dL). After a meal, plasma triglyceride levels may exceed 11.3 mmol/L (1,000 mg/dL). The disorder clusters in first-degree relatives, but phenotypic variability is related to sex, age, hormone use (especially estrogens), and diet. Alcohol intake potently stimulates hypertriglyceridemia in these subjects, as does caloric or carbohydrate intake. The relationship with CAD is not as strong as with familial combined hyperlipidemia and has not been seen in all studies. Depending on the criteria used, the prevalence of familial hypertriglyceridemia ranges from 1 in 100 to 1 in 50. The disorder is highly heterogeneous and likely results from several genes, with a strong environmental influence. An unrelated disorder, familial glycerolemia, a chromosome X-linked genetic disorder, may mimic familial hypertriglyceridemia because most measurement techniques for triglycerides determine glycerol after the enzymatic hydrolysis of triglycerides. The diagnosis of familial hyperglycerolemia requires the ultracentrifugation of plasma and analysis of glycerol.

Hepatic overproduction of VLDL is one cause of familial hypertriglyceridemia (see Fig. 47-4, part 4); the catabolism (uptake) of VLDL particles can be normal or reduced. Lipolysis by LPL appears not to be a limiting factor, although the triglyceride load, especially in the postprandial state, may limit processing of VLDL particles. The genetic basis of familial hypertriglyceridemia is unknown, and the candidate approach to find the gene(s) involved has not yielded fruit thus far. Treatment is based first on lifestyle modifications, including withdrawal of hormones (estrogens and progesterone), limiting alcohol intake, reducing caloric intake, and increasing physical activity. The decision to treat this disorder with medications (see later) depends on the global cardiovascular risk.

Type V hyperlipidemia, an infrequent disorder characterized by severe elevation in plasma triglyceride levels (both VLDL and chylomicrons), associates with a fat-rich diet, obesity, and poorly controlled diabetes. Its pathogenesis is multifactorial and results from the overproduction of VLDL and chylomicrons and from decreased catabolism of these particles.

FAMILIAL HYPERCHYLOMICRONEMIA (TYPE I HYPERLIPIDEMIA). This rare disorder of severe hypertriglyceridemia associates with elevations in fasting plasma triglyceride levels higher than 11.3 mmol/L (>1000 mg/dL). These patients have recurrent bouts of pancreatitis and eruptive xanthomas. Interestingly, severe hypertriglyceridemia can also be associated with xerostomia, xerophthalmia, and behavioral abnormalities. The hypertriglyceridemia results from a markedly reduced or absent LPL activity or, more rarely, the absence of its activator, apo CII (see Fig. 47-4, part 2). These defects lead to a lack of hydrolysis of chylomicrons and VLDL and their accumulation in plasma, especially after meals. Extreme elevations of plasma triglyceride levels (>113 mmol/L; >10,000 mg/dL) can result.

Patients with very high triglyceride levels have milky white plasma, and a visible band of chylomicrons forms on top of the plasma after it stands overnight in a refrigerator. Populations with a founder effect can have high prevalence of LPL mutations. At least 60 LPL mutations can cause LPL deficiency. LPL188, LPLasn291ser, and LPL207 frequently associate with hyperchylomicronemia. Heterozygotes for the disorder tend to have an increase in fasting plasma triglyceride levels and smaller, denser LDL particles. Many patients with complete LPL deficiency present in childhood fail to thrive and have recurrent bouts of pancreatitis. To underscore the importance of the role of LPL, mice deficient in LPL die soon after birth. The treatment of acute pancreatitis includes intravenous hydration and avoidance of fat in the diet (including in parenteral nutrition). Plasma filtration is required only rarely. Chronic treatment includes avoidance of alcohol and dietary fats. To make the diet more palatable, short-chain fatty acids, which are not incorporated in chylomicrons, can be used to supplement the diet.

TYPE III HYPERLIPOPROTEINEMIA. Type III hyperlipoproteinemia, also referred to as dysbetalipoproteinemia or broad beta disease, is a rare genetic lipoprotein disorder characterized by an accumulation in plasma of remnant lipoprotein particles. On lipoprotein agarose gel electrophoresis, a typical pattern of a broad band between the prebeta (VLDL) and beta (LDL) lipoproteins is observed—hence the name, broad beta disease. Patients with this disease clearly have increased cardiovascular risk. The clinical presentation consists of pathognomonic tuberous xanthomas and striated palmar xanthomas. The lipoprotein profile shows increased cholesterol and triglyceride levels and reduced HDL cholesterol levels. Remnant lipoproteins (partly catabolized chylomicrons and VLDL) accumulate in plasma and accumulate cholesterol esters. The defect results from abnormal apo E, which does not bind to hepatic receptors that recognize apo E as a ligand (see Fig. 47-4, part 3). The ratio of VLDL cholesterol to triglycerides, normally less than 0.7 (when measured in mmol/L; <0.30 in mg/dL), is elevated in patients with type III hyperlipoproteinemia because of cholesteryl ester enrichment of remnant particles. Thus, the calculation of LDL-C in such patients is unreliable, and direct LDL-C measurement may be required for clinical purposes. The diagnosis includes plasma ultracentrifugation for lipoprotein separation, lipoprotein electrophoresis, and apo E phenotyping or genotyping. Patients with type III hyperlipoproteinemia have the apo E2/2 phenotype or genotype. There are three common alleles for apo E: apo E2, E3, and E4. The apo E2 allele has markedly decreased binding to the apo B/E receptor.

In a normal population, the prevalence of the apo E2/2 phenotype is approximately 0.7% to 1.0%. Type III hyperlipoproteinemia occurs in approximately 1% of subjects bearing the apo E2/2 phenotype. The reasons for the relative rarity of type III dyslipoproteinemia are not fully understood. As discussed, a second "hit" may impart the full expression of the disorder. Other rare mutations of the apo E gene can cause type III hyperlipoproteinemia. In general, type III dyslipoproteinemia responds well to dietary therapy, correction of other metabolic abnormalities (e.g., diabetes, obesity, hypothyroidism) and, in cases requiring drug therapy, fibric acid derivatives or statins. The importance of the apo E gene and protein is underscored by the widespread use of the apo E–deficient mouse, which develops experimental atherosclerosis.

FAMILIAL COMBINED HYPERLIPIDEMIA. One of the most common familial lipoprotein disorders is familial combined hyperlipoproteinemia (FCH). Described initially in survivors of myocardial infarction (MI), its definition has undergone several refinements. It is characterized by the presence of elevated total cholesterol and/or triglyceride levels based on arbitrary cut points in several members of the same family. Advances in analytic techniques have added the measurement of LDL cholesterol and, in some cases, apo B levels. Because of the lack of a clear-cut clinical or biochemical marker, considerable overlap exists among FCH, familial dyslipidemic hypertension, the metabolic syndrome, and hyperapobetalipoproteinemia. Genetic heterogeneity probably underlies FCH, which has a prevalence of approximately 1 in 50 and accounts for 10% to 20% of patients with premature CAD. The condition has few clinical signs; corneal arcus, xanthomas, and xanthelasmas occur infrequently. The biochemical abnormalities include elevation of plasma total and LDL cholesterol levels (>90th to 95th percentile) and/or an elevation of plasma triglyceride levels (>90th to 95th percentile)—a type IIb lipoprotein phenotype, often in correlation with low HDL cholesterol and elevated apo B levels; small, dense LDL particles occur frequently. For a diagnosis of FCH, the disorder must affect at least one first-degree relative. The underlying metabolic disorder appears to be hepatic overproduction of apo B–containing lipoproteins, delayed postprandial TRL clearance, and increased flux of FFAs to the liver.

Experimental data have shown that substrate levels drive hepatic apo B secretion, with the most important substrates being FFA and cholesteryl esters. Increased delivery of FFA to the liver, as in states of insulin resistance, leads to increased hepatic apo B secretion. FCH has complex genetics. It was initially considered an autosomal codominant trait; modifying factors include sex, age of onset, and comorbid states such as obesity, lack of exercise, and diet. Novel loci in the upstream transcription factor 1 (USF1) and stearoyl-CoA desaturase 1 genes are promising candidate genes related to FCH.[16,17]

High-Density Lipoproteins

Reduced plasma levels of HDL cholesterol consistently correlate with the development or presence of CAD. Most cases of reduced HDL cholesterol result from elevated plasma triglyceride or apo B levels and often accompany other features of the metabolic syndrome. Primary forms of reduced HDL cholesterol levels, which occur in cases of premature CAD, have helped shed light on the complex metabolism of HDL particles. Genetic disorders of HDL can result from decreased production or abnormal maturation and increased catabolism.[18] While HDL-C is a strong and graded cardiovascular risk factor in epidemiological studies, recent trials using statins show that with aggressive LDL-C lowering (to <80 mg/dL or 2.0 mmol/L), HDL-C level no longer predicts residual cardiovascular risk.[18a] Combined with Mendelian randomization data[19] on genetic HDL deficiency states, these data cast doubt on the validity of HDL-C as a therapeutic target. Genetic lipoprotein disorders leading to moderate to severe elevations in plasma triglyceride levels cause a reduction in HDL cholesterol levels. Familial hyperchylomicronemia, familial hypertriglyceridemia, and FCH are all associated with reduced HDL cholesterol levels. In complex disorders of lipoprotein metabolism, such as FCH, the metabolic syndrome, and common forms of hypertriglyceridemia, several factors most likely correlate with low HDL cholesterol levels. Plasma triglyceride and HDL cholesterol levels vary inversely. There are several reasons for this association: (1) decreased lipolysis of TRLs lowers substrate (phospholipid) availability for HDL maturation; (2) triglyceride enrichment of HDL increases their catabolic rate and hence reduces their plasma concentration; and (3) reduced exchange of lipids between HDL and TRLs leads to a more rapid disappearance of HDL from plasma.

APO A-I GENE DEFECTS. Primary defects affecting the production of HDL particles may be caused by mutations at the apo A-I–C-III–A-IV gene complex. More than 46 mutations affect the structure of apo A-I, leading to a marked reduction in HDL cholesterol levels. Not all these defects are associated with premature CVD. Clinical presentations can vary from extensive atypical xanthomatosis and corneal infiltration of lipids to no manifestations at all. Treatment of these apo A-I gene defects generally fails to raise HDL cholesterol levels. Other mutations of apo A-I lead to an increased catabolic rate of apo A-I and may not be associated with CVD. One such mutation, apo $A\text{-}I_{Milano}$ (apo $A\text{-}I_{Arg173Cys}$), appears to confer longevity, despite very low HDL levels.

LECITHIN-CHOLESTEROL ACYLTRANSFERASE DEFICIENCY. Genetic defects in the HDL-processing enzymes give rise to interesting phenotypes. Deficiencies of LCAT, the enzyme that catalyzes the formation of cholesteryl esters in plasma, cause corneal infiltration of neutral lipids and hematologic abnormalities caused by abnormal constitution of red blood cell membranes. LCAT deficiency can lead to an entity called fish eye disease because of the characteristic pattern of corneal infiltration observed in affected individuals. Despite very low HDL-C levels, CAD risk does not appear increased in LCAT deficiency.

CHOLESTERYL ESTER TRANSFER PROTEIN DEFICIENCY. Patients without CETP have very elevated HDL cholesterol levels, enriched in cholesteryl esters. Because CETP facilitates the transfer of HDL cholesteryl esters into TRLs, a deficiency of this enzyme causes accumulation of cholesteryl esters in HDL particles. CETP deficiency is not associated with premature CAD, but may not afford protection against CAD.

TANGIER DISEASE AND FAMILIAL HIGH-DENSITY LIPOPROTEIN DEFICIENCY. A rare disorder of HDL deficiency was identified in a proband from the Chesapeake Bay island of Tangier in the United States. The proband, whose sister was also affected, had markedly enlarged yellow tonsils and almost absent HDL cholesterol, an entity now called Tangier disease. The cellular defect in Tangier disease consists of a reduced cellular cholesterol efflux in skin fibroblasts and macrophages from affected subjects. A more common entity, familial HDL deficiency, was also found to result from decreased cellular cholesterol. Tangier disease and familial HDL deficiency result from mutations at the ATP-binding cassette A1 gene (*ABCA1*) that encodes the ABCA1 transporter (see Fig. 47-5C). Over 100 mutations in the *ABCA1* gene can cause Tangier disease (homozygous or compound heterozygous mutations) or familial HDL deficiency (heterozygous mutations). Although subjects with Tangier disease and familial HDL deficiency may have increased risk for CAD, their very low levels of LDL cholesterol appear to have a protective effect. Using mendelian randomization principles, mutations of the ABCA1 gene were not associated with CAD in the Copenhagen Heart Study.[19] ABCA1 appears to shuttle from the late endosomal compartment to the plasma membrane and act as a membrane-bound transporter of phospholipids (and cholesterol) onto acceptor proteins such as apo A-I and apo E. Hydroxysterols regulate ABCA1 via the LXR/RXR nuclear receptor pathway. ABCA1 undergoes phosphorylation via protein kinase A and acts as a receptor for apo AI.

OTHER CHOLESTEROL TRANSPORT DEFECTS. Niemann-Pick type C disease is a disorder of lysosomal cholesterol transport. In patients with Niemann-Pick type C disease, mental retardation and neurologic manifestations occur frequently. The cellular phenotype involves markedly decreased cholesterol esterification and a cellular cholesterol transport defect to the Golgi apparatus (see Chap. 7). Unlike Tangier disease and familial HDL deficiency, the cellular defect in Niemann-Pick type C disease appears proximal to the transport of cholesterol to the plasma membrane. The gene for Niemann-Pick type C disease (*NPC1*) has been mapped to 18q21; the gene codes for a 1278–amino acid protein, which appears to function in cholesterol shuttling between the late endosomal pathway and the plasma membrane. The *NPC1* gene product shares homology with the morphogen receptor *patched* and with SCAP. Niemann-Pick type C cells lack NPC1 protein, and cholesterol sequestration in the late endosome compartment prevents increased expression of ABCA1; these patients thus have impaired cellular cholesterol efflux and HDL assembly. Niemann-Pick type I disease (subtypes A and B), caused by mutations at the sphingomyelin phosphodiesterase-1 (*SMPD-1*) gene, associates with a low HDL cholesterol level. The *SMPD-1* gene encodes a lysosomal (acidic) and secretory sphingomyelinase. The low HDL cholesterol level in Niemann-Pick A and B patients appears to result from a decrease in LCAT reaction because of abnormal HDL constituents.

Secondary Causes of Hyperlipidemia and the Metabolic Syndrome

Several clinical disorders lead to alterations in lipoprotein status (**Table 47-5**). See Chap. 44.

HORMONAL CAUSES. Hypothyroidism, a not infrequent cause of secondary lipoprotein disorders, often manifests with elevated levels of LDL cholesterol, triglycerides, or both. An elevated level of thyroid-stimulating hormone is key to the diagnosis (see Chap. 86), and the lipoprotein abnormalities often revert to normal after correction of the thyroid status. Rarely, hypothyroidism may uncover a genetic lipoprotein disorder such as type III hyperlipidemia. Estrogens can elevate plasma triglyceride and HDL cholesterol levels, probably because of increases in hepatic VLDL and apo A-I production. In postmenopausal women, estrogens may reduce LDL cholesterol levels by up to 15%. The use of estrogens for the treatment of lipoprotein disorders is no longer recommended because of the slight increase in cardiovascular risk with prolonged use of estrogens in the postmenopausal period (see Chap. 81). Rarely, pregnancy causes severe increases in plasma triglyceride levels on a background of lipoprotein lipase deficiency or unidentified genetic defects. Such cases present a serious threat to mother and child and require referral to specialized centers. Male sex hormones and anabolic steroids can increase hepatic lipase activity and have been used in the treatment of hypertriglyceridemia in men. Growth hormone can reduce LDL cholesterol and augment HDL cholesterol levels but is not recommended in the treatment of lipoprotein disorders.

METABOLIC CAUSES. Most secondary dyslipoproteinemia results from the constellation of metabolic abnormalities seen in patients with

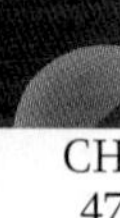

TABLE 47-5 Secondary Causes of Dyslipoproteinemias

CAUSE	DISORDER
Metabolic	Diabetes Lipodystrophy Glycogen storage disorders
Renal	Chronic renal failure Glomerulonephritis with nephritic syndrome
Hepatic	Cirrhosis Biliary obstruction Porphyria
Hormonal	Estrogens Progesterones Growth hormone Thyroid disorders (hypothyroidism) Corticosteroids
Lifestyle	Physical inactivity Obesity Diet rich in fats, saturated fats Alcohol intake Smoking
Medications	Retinoic acid derivatives Glucocorticoids Exogenous estrogens Thiazide diuretics Beta-adrenergic blockers (non-selective) Testosterone and other anabolic steroids Immunosuppressive medications (cyclosporine) Antiviral medications (human immunodeficiency virus protease inhibitors) Antischizophrenic agents

the metabolic syndrome (see Chap. 44). The findings of increased visceral fat (abdominal obesity), elevated blood pressure, and impaired glucose tolerance often cluster with increased plasma triglyceride and reduced HDL cholesterol levels and comprises the major components of the metabolic syndrome. Internationally recognized uniform criteria for the metabolic syndrome have now been established,[19a] but recent data from the INTERHEART study cast doubt on its validity as an independent risk factor (see Chap. 44).[19b] Overt diabetes, especially type 2 diabetes, frequently elevates plasma triglyceride and reduces HDL cholesterol levels (see Chap. 64). These abnormalities have prognostic implications for patients with type 2 diabetes. Poor control of diabetes, obesity, and moderate to severe hyperglycemia can yield severe hypertriglyceridemia, with chylomicronemia and increased VLDL cholesterol levels. Subjects with type 1 diabetes can also have severe hypertriglyceridemia when poorly controlled. Familial lipodystrophy (complete or partial) may be associated with increased VLDL secretion. Dunnigan lipodystrophy, a genetic disorder with features of the metabolic syndrome, is caused by mutations within the lamin A/C gene and is associated with limb-girdle fat atrophy. Excess plasma triglyceride levels often accompany glycogen storage disorders.

RENAL DISORDERS. In subjects with glomerulonephritis and protein-losing nephropathies, a marked increase in the secretion of hepatic lipoproteins can raise LDL cholesterol levels, which may approach those seen in subjects with FH. By contrast, patients with chronic renal failure have a pattern of hypertriglyceridemia with reduced HDL cholesterol levels (see Chap. 93). Patients with end-stage renal disease, including those on hemodialysis or chronic ambulatory peritoneal dialysis, have a poor prognosis and accelerated atherosclerosis. Recent trials have challenged the use of statins in end-stage renal disease and dialysis; diabetic patients on dialysis had no reduction in cardiovascular endpoints when treated with statins.[20,21] After organ transplantation, the immunosuppressive regimen (glucocorticoids and cyclosporine) typically elevates triglyceride and reduces HDL cholesterol levels. Because transplant patients generally have an increase in cardiovascular risk, a secondary hyperlipidemia may warrant treatment. Patients receiving the combination of statin plus cyclosporine merit careful dose titrations and monitoring for myopathy.

LIVER DISEASE. Obstructive liver disease, especially primary biliary cirrhosis, may lead to the formation of an abnormal lipoprotein termed *lipoprotein-x*. This type of lipoprotein is found in cases of LCAT deficiency; it consists of an LDL-like particle but with a marked reduction in cholesteryl esters. Extensive xanthoma formation on the face and palmar areas can be the result of accumulation of lipoprotein-x.

LIFESTYLE. Factors contributing to obesity, such as an imbalance between caloric intake and energy expenditure, lack of physical activity, and a diet rich in saturated fats and refined sugars, contribute in large part to the lipid and lipoprotein lipid levels in a population (see Chaps. 48 and 49).

MEDICATION. Several medications can alter lipoproteins. Thiazide diuretics can increase plasma triglyceride levels. Beta-adrenergic receptor blockers (beta blockers), especially non-beta$_1$ selective beta blockers, increase triglyceride and lower HDL cholesterol levels. Retinoic acid and estrogens can increase triglyceride levels, sometimes dramatically. Corticosteroids and immunosuppressive agents can increase plasma triglyceride and lower HDL cholesterol levels. Estrogens can increase plasma HDL cholesterol levels substantially and often also increase triglyceride concentrations. Anabolic steroids, often used by endurance or body-building athletes, can cause hypertriglyceridemia and very low HDL-C levels. The exact composition, dosage, and frequency of use of anabolic steroids are often impossible to determine from the patient. The use of second-generation antipsychotic medications may lead to metabolic disorders, weight gain, and lipoprotein abnormalities.[22] The use of highly active antiretroviral therapy (HAART) may cause severe lipoprotein disorders and an increase in the prevalence of CAD among patients with chronic HIV infection treated with such agents (see Chap. 72).[23,24]

In clinical practice, many dyslipoproteinemias, other than the genetic forms mentioned earlier, share an important environmental cause. Lifestyle changes (e.g., diet, exercise, reduction of abdominal obesity) should be the foundation for the treatment of most dyslipidemias. The effects of marked alterations in lifestyle, reduction in dietary fats (especially saturated fats), and exercise can improve the cardiovascular prognosis. Translating these findings into practice, however, has proven difficult.

Drugs That Affect Lipid Metabolism

See **Table 47-6**.

After the initiation of medical therapy, the response should be checked within the first 3 months, along with transaminase and creatinine kinase levels. Thereafter, clinical judgment should dictate the interval between follow-up visits. Although frequent visits are probably not useful for the detection of serious side effects, they serve to encourage compliance and adherence to diet and lifestyle changes.

Bile Acid–Binding Resins

Bile acid–binding resins interrupt the enterohepatic circulation of bile acids by inhibiting their reabsorption in the intestine; more than 90% of bile acids usually undergo reabsorption. Currently, their main use is as adjunctive therapy for patients with severe hypercholesterolemia caused by increased LDL-C levels. Because bile acid–binding resins are not absorbed systemically—they remain in the intestine and are eliminated in the stool—they are considered safe in children. Cholestyramine (Questran) is used in 4-g unit doses as powder, and colestipol (Colestid) is used in 5-g unit doses; a 1-g tablet of colestipol is available. Effective doses range from 2 to 6 unit doses/day, always taken with meals. The most important side effects are predominantly gastrointestinal, with constipation, a sensation of fullness, and gastrointestinal discomfort. Hypertriglyceridemia can result from the use of these drugs. Decreased drug absorption dictates careful scheduling of medications 1 hour before or 3 hours after the patient takes

TABLE 47-6 Current Lipid-Lowering Medications

GENERIC NAME	BRAND NAME	RECOMMENDED DOSAGE RANGE
Statins		
Atorvastatin	Lipitor	10-80 mg
Fluvastatin	Lescol	20-80 mg
Lovastatin	Mevacor	20-80 mg
Pravastatin	Pravachol	10-40 mg
Rosuvastatin	Crestor	15-40 mg
Simvastatin	Zocor	10-80 mg
Pitavastatin	Levacol	2-4 mg
Bile Acid Absorption Inhibitors		
Cholestyramine	Questran	2-24 g
Colestipol	Colestid	5-30 g
Colesevelam	WelChol	3.8-4.5 g
Cholesterol Absorption Inhibitor		
Ezetimibe	Zetia (Ezetrol)	10 mg
Fibrates*		
Bezafibrate	Bezalip	400 mg
Fenofibrate	Tricor, Trilipix, Lipidil Micro, Lipidil EZ	40-200 mg
Gemfibrozil†	Lopid	600-1200 mg
Niacin‡	Niacin	1-3 g
Nicotinic acid	Niaspan	1-2 g

*Avoid in patients with renal insufficiency.
†Not recommended in combination with statins.
‡Use with caution in patients with diabetes or glucose intolerance.

a bile acid–binding resin. Bile acid–binding resins can be used in combination with statins and/or cholesterol absorption inhibitors in cases of severe hypercholesterolemia.

Hydroxymethylglutaryl–Coenzyme A Reductase Inhibitors (Statins)

Statins inhibit HMG-CoA reductase and prevent the formation of mevalonate, the rate-limiting step of sterol synthesis. To maintain cellular cholesterol homeostasis, expression of the LDL-R increases and the rate of cholesteryl ester formation declines. These homeostatic adjustments to HMG-CoA reductase inhibition increase LDL cholesterol clearance from plasma and decrease hepatic production of VLDL and LDL. In addition to blocking the synthesis of cholesterol, statins also interfere with the synthesis of lipid intermediates, with important biologic effects. In the cholesterol synthetic pathway, intermediate molecules of dimethylallyl pyrophosphate are metabolized by prenyltransferase into geranyl pyrophosphate and subsequently into farnesyl pyrophosphate. This step occurs before the formation of squalenes. These intermediates, geranylgeranyl and farnesyl pyrophosphates, prenylate proteins—a mechanism whereby a lipid moiety attaches covalently to a protein, allowing anchoring into cell membranes and enhancing its biologic activity. The guanosine triphosphate (GTP)–binding proteins Rho A, Rac, and Ras undergo prenylation. Statins may increase HDL cholesterol levels in part by preventing the geranylgeranylation of Rho A and phosphorylation of peroxisome proliferator–activated receptor alpha (PPARα), a factor that regulates apo A-I transcription. Altered protein prenylation may also mediate some of the putative effects of statins not related to a reduction in LDL cholesterol levels.

Atherosclerosis is an inflammatory disease (see Chap. 43). Statins decrease C-reactive protein levels, induce apoptosis in smooth-muscle cells, augment collagen content of atherosclerotic plaques, alter endothelial function, and decrease the inflammatory component of plaques. Some investigators have argued that statins possess effects independent of their inhibition of HMG-CoA reductase. The clinical importance of these possible LDL-independent actions, and the differences in efficacy between statins for a given percentage reduction in LDL cholesterol levels, remain speculative.

Statins are generally well tolerated; side effects include reversible elevation in transaminase levels and myositis, which causes discontinuation of the drug in less than 1% of patients. The currently available drugs (**Table 47-7**) are as follows: fluvastatin (Lescol), 20 to 80 mg/day; lovastatin (Mevacor), 10 to 80 mg/day; pravastatin (Pravachol), 20 to 40 mg/day; simvastatin (Zocor), 10 to 80 mg/day; atorvastatin (Lipitor), 10 to 80 mg/day; and rosuvastatin (Crestor), 5 to 40 mg/day. Pitavastatin, 2 to 4 mg/day, is currently available in Asia. Concomitant drugs that interfere with the metabolism of statins by inhibiting the cytochrome P-450 3A4 and 2C9 systems (see Chap. 10) can increase plasma concentrations of statins. These include antibiotics, antifungal medications, certain antiviral drugs, grapefruit juice, cyclosporine, and amiodarone.

Cholesterol Absorption Inhibitors

The development of selective inhibitors of intestinal sterol absorption has added to the treatment of lipoprotein disorders. Ezetimibe is the first such compound. Ezetimibe limits the selective uptake of cholesterol and other sterols by intestinal epithelial cells, by interfering with the NPC1-L1 protein. It can help patients achieve targeted LDL cholesterol levels who do not do so on maximally tolerated statin doses. Ezetimibe lowers LDL cholesterol levels by about 18% and adds to the effect of statins. Because ezetimibe also prevents the intestinal absorption of sitosterol, it might be the drug of choice in cases of sitosterolemia. The current dosage of ezetimibe is 10 mg/day. Studies evaluating the effects of ezetimibe on cardiovascular endpoints are ongoing.

Fibric Acid Derivatives (Fibrates)

Two derivatives of fibric acid are currently available in the United States. Gemfibrozil (Lopid) is used at a dosage of 600 mg twice daily and is indicated in cases of hypertriglyceridemia and in the secondary prevention of CVDs in patients with low HDL cholesterol levels. These latter recommendations are based on the Veterans Administration HDL Intervention Trial (VA-HIT). Fenofibrate (Tricor, Trilipix, Lipidil Micro, Lipidil EZ) is used to treat hypertriglyceridemia and combined hyperlipoproteinemia. The dosage is 200 mg/day; a new formulation is available to vary the dosage from 40 (especially in cases of renal failure) to 267 mg/day. Ciprofibrate (Lipanthyl, Lipanor), clofibrate (Atromid), and bezafibrate (Bezalip) are more widely used in Europe. The main indications for the use of fibrates are the treatment of hypertriglyceridemia when diet and lifestyle changes are not sufficient. Another potential indication is in the prevention of CVD in patients with elevated plasma triglyceride and low HDL cholesterol levels, although the data supporting their use are weaker than those for statins (**Table 47-8**). A meta-analysis of fibrate studies has shown a decrease in MIs, but no effect on mortality (see later, Fig. 47-7).[24a,24b] The mechanism of action of fibrates involves interaction with the nuclear transcription factor PPARα, which regulates the transcription of the LPL, apo C-III, and apo A-I genes. The side effects of fibrates include cutaneous manifestations, gastrointestinal effects (abdominal discomfort, increased bile lithogenicity), erectile dysfunction, elevated transaminase levels, interaction with oral anticoagulants, and elevated plasma homocysteine levels, especially with fenofibrate and, to a lesser extent, with bezafibrate. Because fibrates increase LPL activity, LDL cholesterol levels may rise in patients with hypertriglyceridemia treated with this class of medications. Fibrates, especially gemfibrozil, can inhibit the glucuronidation of statins and thus retard their elimination. For this reason, combination of gemfibrozil with statins may increase the risk of myotoxicity and is therefore contraindicated.

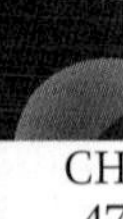

TABLE 47-7 Review of Statin Trials

TRIAL (YEAR)	DURATION (YR)	MEDICATION USED	COMPARATOR	NO. OF PATIENTS IN STUDY	AGE (YR)	NO. OF WOMEN (%)	POPULATION	ΔLDL-C (MG/DL)	RELATIVE RISK MCE	RELATIVE RISK CHD, DEATH
4S (1994)	5.2	Simva 20-40	Placebo	4,444	35-70	19	Sec	−68	0.657	0.658
WOSCOP (1995)	4.8	Prava 40	Placebo	6,596	45-64	0	Prim	−41	0.685	0.683
CARE (1996)	4.8	Prava 40	Placebo	4,159	21-75	14	Sec	−40	0.773	0.847
Post-CABG (1997)	4.2	Lova 40-80	Placebo	1,351	21-74	8	Sec	−41	0.874	1.498
AFCAPS (1998)	5.3	Lova 20-40	Placebo	6,605	45-73	15	Prim	−36	0.629	0.679
LIPID (1998)	5.6	Prava 40	Placebo	9,014	31-75	17	Sec	−40	0.778	0.763
GISSI (2000)	1.9	Prava 20	Placebo	4,271	19-90	14	Sec	−14	0.841	0.769
HPS (2002)	5.0	Simva 40	Placebo	20,536	40-80	25	Prim/Sec	−50	0.740	0.833
ALLHAT LLT (2002)	4.8	Prava 40	Placebo	10,355	>55	49	Prim	−20	0.905	0.986
GREACE (2002)	3.0	Atorva 10-80	UC	1,600	58 (mean)	22	Sec	−73	0.461	0.526
LIPS (2002)	3.1	Fluva 80	Placebo	1,677	18-80	16	Sec	−36	0.808	0.535
PROSPER (2002)	3.2	Prava 40	Placebo	5,804	70-82	52	Prim	−40	0.826	0.866
ALERT (2003)	5.1	Fluva 40	Placebo	2,102	30-75	34	Prim	−32	0.754	0.906
ASCOT LLA (2003)	3.2	Atorva 10	Placebo	10,305	40-79	19	Prim	−41	0.646	0.898
CARDS (2004)	3.9	Atorva 10	Placebo	2,838	40-75	32	DM	−44	0.687	0.667
ALLIANCE (2004)	4.3	Atorva 10-80	UC	2,442	31-78	18	Prim	−15	0.617	0.710
A-to-Z (2004)	2.0	Simva 80	Simva 20	4,497	52-69 IQR	24	Sec (ACS)	−14	0.862	0.757
PROVE-IT (2004)	2.0	Atorva 80	Prava 40	4,162	58 (mean)	22	Sec (ACS)	−31	0.843	0.774
4D (2005)	4.0	Atorva 20	Placebo	1,255	66 (mean)	46	DM, ESKD	−42	0.881	0.939
TNT (2005)	4.9	Atorva 80	Atorva 10	10,001	29-76	19	Sec	−25	0.790	0.781
IDEAL (2005)	4.0	Atorva 80	Simva 20-40	8,888	30-80	19	Sec	−23	0.882	0.972
ASPEN (2006)	4.0	Atorva 10	Placebo	2,410	61 (mean)	34	DM	−41	0.834	1.017
SPARCL (2006)	4.9	Atorva 80	Placebo	4,731	63 (mean)	40	Sec (CVA)	−61	0.675	0.800
MEGA (2006)	5.3	Prava 10-20	Placebo	3,966	58 (mean)	68	Prim	−27	0.539	0.627
CORONA (2007)	2.7	Rosuva 10	Placebo	5,013	>60	24	HF	−63	0.936	0.995
JUPITER (2008)	1.9	Rosuva 20	Placebo	17,802	66 (mean)	38	Prim	−47	0.538	0.838
GISSI-HF (2008)	3.9	Rosuva 10	Placebo	4,574	>18		HF			
SEARCH (2008)	6.7	Simva 80	Simva 20	12,064	18-80	18	Sec	14	0.860	1.013

Atorva = atorvastatin; CVA = cerebrovascular accident; DM = diabetes mellitus; ESKD = end-stage kidney disease; Fluva = fluvastatin; HF = heart failure; IQR = interquartile range; Lova = lovastatin; MCE = major cardiac event; Prava = pravastatin; Prim = primary; Rosuva = rosuvastatin; Sec = secondary; Simva = simvastatin; UC = usual care.

Modified from Delahoy PJ, Magliano DJ, Webb K, et al: The relationship between reduction in low-density lipoprotein cholesterol by statins and reduction in risk of cardiovascular outcomes: An updated meta-analysis. Clin Ther 31:236, 2009.

Nicotinic Acid (Niacin)

Niacin can substantially increase HDL cholesterol and lower triglyceride levels, but has a more modest effect on LDL cholesterol levels. Effective doses of niacin are approximately 2000 to 3000 mg/day, in three separate doses. An escalating dose schedule to reach the full dose in 2 to 3 weeks rather than starting with the full dose can improve tolerability. Slow-release forms of niacin, including Niaspan (1 to 2 g/day) decrease the side effect profile of the drug. Skin flushing can be attenuated by taking a daily aspirin. Niacin decreases the hepatic secretion of VLDL from the liver and decreased FFA mobilization for the periphery. In the long-term follow-up of the Coronary Drug Project, niacin decreased mortality at 15 years. Significant and common minor side effects, and much less frequent serious adverse actions, hamper its more widespread adoption. Side effects of niacin include flushing, hyperuricemia, hyperglycemia, hepatotoxicity, acanthosis nigricans, and gastritis. Close laboratory monitoring of side effects is warranted. Long-acting niacin has the advantage of a once- or twice-daily dosing schedule, but older preparations of slow-release niacin were potentially more hepatotoxic. Niacin effectively raises HDL cholesterol levels and, in combination with a low-dose statin, can retard the angiographic progression of CAD and decrease adverse cardiac events. Recent studies have identified cell surface receptors for nicotinic acid that belong to the G protein–coupled heptahelical superfamily. This discovery may speed the elucidation of the molecular mechanism of nicotinic acid's effects on lipid metabolism.

Cholesteryl Ester Transfer Protein Inhibitors

The inhibition of cholesteryl ester transfer protein (CETP) by pharmacologic agents mimics the genetic heterozygous CETP deficiency state (see Fig. 47-4, part 9). Of several agents tested in humans, torcetrapib proved toxic and increased mortality, an effect attributed to off-target effects. Two CETP inhibitors, anacetrapib and dalcetrapib, are undergoing clinical trials. A marked increase in larger, more buoyant HDL particles occurred in patients on torcetrapib; these particles appear to promote cellular cholesterol efflux efficiently. Reported side effects include elevation in hepatic transaminase levels, an increase in blood pressure (with torcetrapib), and abdominal symptoms.

TABLE 47-8 Trials of Fibrate Therapy

STUDY (YEAR)	STUDY SIZE (N)	FIBRATE	FOLLOW-UP (WK)	TOTAL CHOLESTEROL (MG/DL)			TRIGLYCERIDES (MG/DL)			LDL (MG/DL)			HDL (MG/DL)		
				BASELINE*	FOLLOW-UP TX	FOLLOW-UP PCBO	BASELINE*	FOLLOW-UP TX	FOLLOW-UP PCBO	BASELINE*	FOLLOW-UP TX	FOLLOW-UP PCBO	BASELINE*	FOLLOW-UP TX	FOLLOW-UP PCBO
BIP (2000)	3090	Beza 400	322	212.5	207.5	213.2	145.0	124.2	149.6	148.5	141.5	147.7	34.6	52.5	38.1
Frick (1993)	628	Gem 1200	260	270.1	249.2	281.3	183.2	125.7	201.3	188.1	180.3	201.7	46.3	50.4	45.7
HHS (1987)	4081	Gem 1200	262	269.8	246.9	272.6	176.0	114.8	177.7	188.7	173.5	191.4	47.3	51.2	47.0
VA-HIT (1999)	2531	Gem 1200	52	175.0	170.0	177.0	160.5	115.0	166.0	111.5	113.0	113.0	32.0	34.0	32.0
FIELD (2005)	9795	Feno 200	260	194.4	163.3	176.1	153.5	130.1	165.5	118.5	93.8	100.4	42.5	43.6	43.2
ACCORD (2010)	5518	Feno 200	360	174.7	151.1	153.7	189.0	147.0	170.0	100.0	81.1	80.0	38.0	41.2	40.5

Beza = bezafibrate; Feno: fenofibrate; Gem = gemfibrozil; Pcbo = placebo; Tx = treatment.
Modified from Abourbih S, Filion KB, Joseph L, et al: Effect of fibrates on lipid profiles and cardiovascular outcomes: A systematic review of randomized controlled trials. Am J Med 122:962.e1, 2009.

Fish Oils

Fish oils contain polyunsaturated fatty acids,such as eicosapentaenoic acid or docosahexaenoic acid, with the first double on the omega-3 position (see Chap. 48). These fatty acids lower plasma triglyceride levels and have antithrombotic properties, and have a place in the treatment of hypertriglyceridemia. Fish oils decrease VLDL synthesis and decrease VLDL apo B. The response to fish oils depends on dose, requiring a daily intake of up 10 g of eicosapentaenoic acid or docosahexaenoic acid for a maximal benefit on plasma triglyceride levels. A prescription form of omega-3 fatty acids has become available in the United States for use in cases of extreme hypertriglyceridemia (>500 mg/dL, or 5.6 mmol/L).

Phytosterols

Phytosterols are derivatives of cholesterol from plants and trees. They interfere with the formation of micelles in the intestine and prevent intestinal cholesterol absorption. They can be obtained as neutraceuticals or incorporated into soft margarines. Phytosterols may prove useful for the adjunctive management of lipoprotein disorders. Current guidelines include their use as part of the therapeutic lifestyle change regimen.

Clinical Trials of Drugs Affecting Lipoprotein Metabolism

Numerous pathologic, epidemiologic, genetic, and interventional trials have validated the central tenet of the lipid hypothesis, which proposes a causal relationship between dyslipidemia and atherogenesis and identifies lipid modification as a risk-reducing strategy for CHD (see Chap. 49). Small trials using dietary or drug therapies have demonstrated the angiographic benefit of managing elevated total cholesterol and LDL cholesterol levels. Early clinical trials using bile acid sequestrants, fibrates, or nicotinic acid have reported modest reductions in coronary risk with modest reductions in LDL-C levels.

The advent of the HMG-CoA reductase inhibitors, or statins, in the mid-1980s made more aggressive reduction of LDL cholesterol levels possible. By the late 1990s, several large-scale, prospective randomized trials with these drugs had reported robust reductions in relative cardiovascular risks compared with placebo. This section discusses clinical trials in high-risk patients and those with acute coronary syndromes, and in high-risk primary prevention. There are 27 trials with statins reporting cardiovascular outcomes, each with more than 1000 subjects randomized to a statin versus placebo[25] (or a statin comparator; see the review by Delahoy and associates[26] and http://www.ctsu.ox.ac.uk/~search). Subgroup meta-analysis has explored effects of statins in women, nonwhites, older patients, and diabetics. The focus on statin trials reflects the widespread clinical success of this category of drugs.

Secondary Prevention and Acute Coronary Syndromes

Secondary prevention trials have undergone extensive review inthe past two editions of this chapter. Using a strategy of lower LDL is better, five trials have compared moderate with more robust LDL-C reduction, using maximum doses of atorvastatin or simvastatin (see Table 47-7). The Aggrastat-to-Zocor (A-to-Z), Pravastatin or Atorvastatin Evaluation and Infection Therapy (PROVE-IT), Treating to New Targets (TNT), Incremental Decrease in End Points Through Aggressive Lipid Lowering (IDEAL), and Study of the Effectiveness of Additional Reductions in Cholesterol and Homocysteine (SEARCH) trials have shown that more intensive reduction of LDL-C in patients at high or very high risk of recurrent CAD events reduces risk further compared with more modest LDL-C lowering. These data were analyzed as part of a new meta-analysis of statin trials (**Fig. 47-6**; also see http://www.ctsu.ox.ac.uk/~search/results/results.htm).

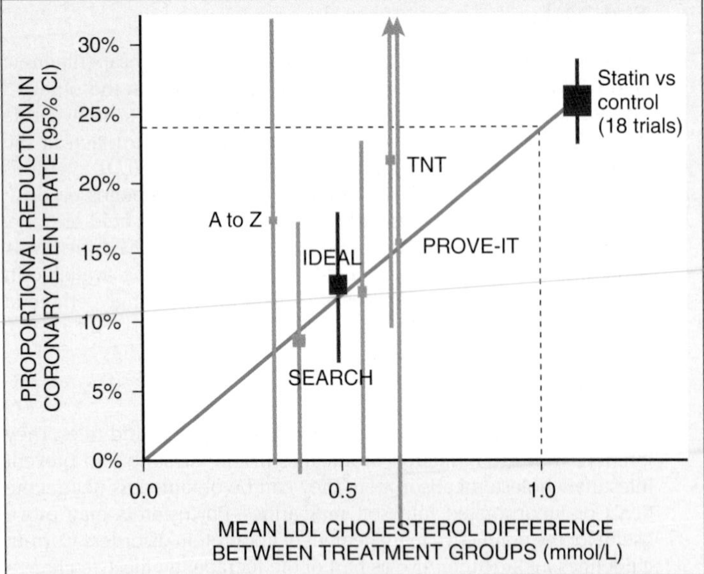

FIGURE 47-6 Meta-analysis of clinical trials of statin therapy. This graphic illustration shows the proportional reduction in nonfatal MI or CHD death versus absolute LDL-C reduction. The red boxes indicate the meta-analysis of statin trials compared with placebo and the results of the five trials of maximal doses of statin are indicated in yellow (see http://searchinfo.org).

Treating High-Risk (Primary Prevention) Patients

As the interaction of multiple coronary risk factors has received greater clinical importance, recommendations for clinical practice have increasingly embraced the concept of global risk management. This global risk is calculated using an algorithm that considers not only total cholesterol but also HDL cholesterol, smoking, age, hypertension, and sex (see Chaps. 44 and 49). The Reynolds risk score (http//www.reynoldsriskscore.org) now includes the conventional cardiovascular risk factors, as presented in the Framingham risk score,[27] with family history and high-sensitivity C-reactive protein (hsCRP) level. Adult diabetic subjects are considered to be at high cardiovascular risk (see Chap. 64), with few exceptions. Cardiovascular risk is determined as cardiovascular death or nonfatal MI in the next 10 years, based on the Framingham Heart Study risk score, and determines the intensity of lipid intervention. Based on the evidence from clinical trials, the 2004 U.S. Adult Treatment Panel (ATP III) has modified its guidelines, recommending a more aggressive LDL-C target in very high-risk subjects to an LDL-C of less than 70 mg/dL (1.8 mmol/L). Similar risk stratification and targets exist in Europe.[28]

Because global risk assessment shifts emphasis away from abnormal lipids alone to the patient's overall risk profile, it raises an important issue for the future of lipid management. That is, should the decision to initiate lipid modification for cardiovascular risk reduction be based on high risk or high cholesterol? This question has been evaluated in recent reviews, which have analyzed large trials of statin therapy in the secondary prevention of CAD, acute coronary syndromes, high-risk primary prevention, and selective primary prevention. Table 47-7 summarizes 28 randomized clinical trials of statins. There is some overlap among studies in terms of entry criteria, especially as they pertain to secondary and high-risk prevention. Some studies included diabetic subjects and others used diabetes as an entry criterion. The cumulative data indicate the following:

1. Statin therapy reduces the relative risk of major cardiovascular events in relation to the absolute magnitude of LDL-C (or apo B) reduction.
2. Statins are well tolerated and the benefits, for the vast majority of patients, far outweigh the potential risks.
3. The absolute benefits correlate with baseline risk—from a purely economical point of view, the higher the cardiovascular risk, the greater the benefit.
4. Also, paradoxically, the large-scale impact of LDL-C reduction on a lower-risk population is likely to confer societal benefits in terms of CVD reduction, albeit at a high monetary cost.

Over the past decade, several issues have been addressed.

DIABETIC SUBJECTS. Patients with diabetes should receive a statin (see Chap. 64). Multiple observational studies have documented a markedly increased risk of CHD in adult diabetics over the long term. Data from the Cholesterol Treatment Trialists (CTT) meta-analysis of statin trials in subjects with diabetes have shown a 21% CVD event reduction and 9% all-cause mortality benefit in favor of statins.[29-31] Tight diabetes control is not necessarily cardio-protective.[30,31]

OLDER PATIENTS. A recent meta-analysis of statin trials using data on patients older than 75 years has shown a 22% relative reduction in all-cause mortality (see Chap. 80).[32] These data provide no valid reasons to withdraw statins from older patients if clinically indicated. Physicians must nevertheless exercise caution in implementing preventive strategies in older patients who are already on multiple medications.

WOMEN. Controversy arose on the basis of selective analysis of data showing a lack of benefit for statins in women, especially in the primary prevention setting.[32a] Most studies were not powered statistically to show an effect on women (see Table 47-7). The results of the JUPITER study,[33] which randomized 6801 women (3426 to rosuvastatin and 3375 to placebo), showed a statistically significant reduction in the primary endpoint of acute MI, stroke, CVD death, arterial revascularization, and hospitalization for unstable angina in favor of the rosuvastatin arm. These results, together with those of a meta-analysis of statin treatment in high-risk women, should eliminate the notion that statins do not confer cardiovascular protection for women.

NONWHITES. The INTERHEART study has shown the universality of cardiovascular risk factors in a study of almost 15,000 acute MIs compared with healthy controls.[34] The number of nonwhites and various ethnic groups are underrepresented in most studies, but there is presently no reason to believe that lipid-lowering therapy will not reduce cardiovascular risk in various ethnic groups. The MEGA study showed statin efficacy in a Japanese population.[35] JUPITER included more than 4,400 black or Hispanic individuals randomized to placebo or rosuvastatin, 20 mg/day, and found no heterogeneity in the response to therapy compared with whites.[33]

ACUTE CORONARY SYNDROMES. Earlier secondary prevention statin studies generally selected patients who were at least 3 to 6 months post–coronary event and stabilized. Substantial interest has turned to the question of statin treatment in the period immediately following an acute coronary syndrome.

The Aggrastat-to-Zocor (A-to-Z) study randomized patients with acute coronary syndromes (randomized to tirofiban or heparin) to receive either simvastatin, 40 to 80 mg/day, versus diet plus simvastatin, 20 mg/day. Overall, the results of this trial were neutral (i.e., the observed reduction in events did not reach statistical significance). The Pravastatin or Atorvastatin Evaluation and Infection Therapy (PROVE-IT) trial compared pravastatin, 40 mg/day, with atorvastatin, 80 mg/day, in 4162 post–acute coronary event patients. PROVE-IT showed that in patients who have recently survived an acute coronary syndrome, an intensive statin regimen that yielded a median LDL cholesterol level of 62 mg/dL (1.60 mmol/L) provided greater protection against death or major cardiovascular events than less aggressive therapy that lowered LDL cholesterol to a median of 95 mg/dL (2.5 mmol/L). Taken together, these data suggest that statin therapy should be initiated promptly in patients with acute coronary syndromes and that a robust reduction in LDL-C levels is warranted.

Starting statins in hospital may also improve compliance on discharge.[36]

MEDICAL THERAPY VERSUS REVASCULARIZATION. The multicenter, randomized Clinical Outcomes Utilizing Revascularization and Aggressive Drug Evaluation (COURAGE) trial studied 3260 patients in the United States and Canada (see Chap. 57).[37] The protocol targeted global risk reduction, emphasizing the following: (1) lifestyle modification; (2) maximal use of drugs to lower blood pressure to Joint National Committee on Prevention, Detection, and Treatment of High Blood Pressure (JNC-VI) goals; (3) maximal use of statin (simvastatin to 80 mg) to lower the cholesterol level to below current U.S. goals for secondary prevention (with a primary goal of LDL = 1.55 to 2.2 mmol/L and secondary goals of HDL > 1.04 mmol/L and triglycerides < 1.7 mmol/L); (4) maximal use of a drug to alleviate anginal symptoms. Patients were randomized to a strategy of medical therapy or the best interventional devices to conduct percutaneous coronary intervention (PCI). The COURAGE study tested the hypothesis that revascularization plus maximal medical therapy would be superior to maximal therapy alone. Men and women (15%) with angiographically documented one-, two-, or three-vessel disease (>70% visual stenosis of proximal coronary segment), with objective evidence of ischemia at baseline and American College of Cardiology/American Heart Association (ACC/AHA) class I or II indications for PCI, were randomized. The outcomes were death, MI, or stroke, hospitalization for biomarker-negative acute coronary syndrome (ACS), cost and resource use, quality of life, including angina, and cost-effectiveness.

After 5 years, there were no significant differences in any of the prespecified outcomes. The early benefit of freedom from angina disappeared within 3 years of the trial. Costs were significantly lower in the medical management group compared with the revascularization group. It was concluded that "as an initial management strategy in patients with stable CAD, PCI did not reduce the risk of death, MI, or other major cardiovascular events when added to optimal medical therapy."[37]

REGRESSION STUDIES. The Reversal of Atherosclerosis with Lipitor (REVERSAL) trial used intravascular ultrasonography (IVUS) to examine the effect of differing degrees of lipid lowering on plaque volume.[37a] Over 18 months, patients treated with pravastatin (40 mg/day) had a 25% drop in LDL cholesterol levels, and those randomized to atorvastatin (80 mg/day) had a 46% decrease, to an average LDL cholesterol level of 79 mg/dL (2.6 mmol/L). The more aggressive lipid-lowering regimen reduced lesion volume. The primary endpoint was a reduction in the total atheroma volume, which increased by 0.4% on pravastatin but decreased by 2.7% ($P = 0.02$) on atorvastatin. The ASTEROID study[38] evaluated whether 24-month treatment with rosuvastatin, 40 mg/day, would result in regression of coronary atherosclerosis, as measured by intravascular ultrasound (IVUS), in 507 patients. During treatment with rosuvastatin, the LDL-C level decreased from 130 to 61 mg/dL (from 3.4 to1.6 mmol/L); HDL-C increased by 14.7%. After 2 years, 349 patients underwent follow-up IVUS. Several efficacy parameters were used; the median change in atheroma volume decreased by 0.79%, and the median change in most diseased subsegments decreased by 5.6% (both, $P < 0.001$). No control or comparator group was used. The ASTEROID study showed that rosuvastatin, 40 mg/day, promotes coronary atherosclerosis regression.

RISKS ASSOCIATED WITH LOW LOW-DENSITY LIPOPROTEIN CHOLESTEROL. Combined with the cumulative evidence from large-scale clinical outcomes data, reaching a low total and LDL cholesterol is associated with decreased cardiovascular risk. Some have expressed concern that a low LDL-C level may be detrimental for health, but there are several arguments against this:

1. Most animal species have little or no LDL-C, and produce LDL particles only when dietary cholesterol and saturated fats increase.
2. Because of its importance in cellular functions, most (if not all) cell types have the cellular machinery to make cholesterol endogenously.
3. The HDL transport system, via the SR-B1 receptor, appears to be a major delivery system of cholesterol from hepatic sources to organs.
4. LDL deficiency states in humans, hypobetalipoproteinemia caused by mutations in the apo B gene, and loss of function mutations in the PCSK9 gene are associated with normal health but with a marked reduction in lifelong cardiovascular events.[14]

The Cholesterol Treatment Trialists meta-analysis of more than 90,000 patients treated with statins has not shown an increase in cancers[25]; the JUPITER trial[33] did not show increases in cancers, renal or hepatic diseases, or hemorrhagic strokes, despite 25% of patients having reached an LDL-C less than 44 mg/dL (1.2 mmol/L) for up to 5 years.

END-STAGE HEART FAILURE. Recent studies (CORONA[39] and GISSI-HF[40]) have addressed statin treatment in end-stage heart failure (left ventricular ejection fraction < 30%). These studies suggest that statin therapy does not reduce CVD morbidity or mortality in advanced heart failure of ischemic or nonischemic cause.

END-STAGE RENAL FAILURE. Two studies of atorvastatin or rosuvaststin (4D and AURORA) performed in subjects with diabetes and end-stage renal failure on dialysis failed to show improved cardiovascular outcomes.[20,21] Patients enrolled in these two trials had a baseline LDL-C of approximately 130 mg/dL.

RISKS ASSOCIATED WITH LONG-TERM STATINS. The JUPITER trial showed a slight but statistically significant increase in physician-reported diabetes.[33] Pravastatin, atorvastatin, and simvastatin can produce similar findings. Careful analysis of the data has shown that most patients who became diabetic during the course of the trial have features of the metabolic syndrome and insulin resistance. Although this finding cannot be ignored, its clinical significance is uncertain, given the importance of statins in the treatment of diabetes. However, it should spur more basic research on the effects of statins on insulin signaling and glucose homeostasis.

Trials of Drugs Other Than Statins

FIBRATES. See Table 47-8 and **Figure 47-7**.[24b] The FIELD trial was carried out for 5 years in Australia, New Zealand, and Finland and examined the effect of fenofibrate, 200 mg/day, on the development of CHD in 9795 patients with diabetes, aged 50 to 75 years. The primary composite endpoint of CHD death or nonfatal MI was not significantly lower in the fenofibrate group compared with the placebo group (5.2% versus 5.8%; $P = 0.16$).

The Veteran's Affairs Cooperative Studies Program High-Density Lipoprotein Cholesterol Intervention Trial (VA-HIT; see Table 47-8) was a multicenter randomized study that assessed the effects of gemfibrozil, 1200 mg/day, versus dietary therapy on the incidence of cardiovascular events in 2531 men with known CHD and low baseline HDL cholesterol levels. The primary endpoint of the VA-HIT study was the combination of CHD death and nonfatal MI. Patients randomized to receive placebo accounted for 275 events, compared with 219 events in the gemfibrozil group. The decline in coronary events represented a 22% risk reduction that was statistically significant ($P = 0.006$).

The Bezafibrate Infarction Prevention (BIP) study (see Table 47-8) reported no reduction in fatal and nonfatal MI and CHD death in a cohort of 3090 men and women with CHD, total cholesterol of 180 to 250 mg/dL, HDL cholesterol less than 45 mg/dL (1.2 mmol/L), triglycerides less than 300 mg/dL (3.4 mmol/L), and LDL cholesterol less than 180 mg/dL (4.7 mmol/L), who were treated with bezafibrate, 400 mg/day, or placebo.

The Action to Control Cardiovascular Risk in Diabetes (ACCORD) trial examined the effect of fenofibrate added to statin therapy (simvastatin) in the prevention of cardiovascular events in diabetic patients. With a target LDL-C of 80 mg/dL (2.0 mmol/L) reached in study participants, patients were further randomized to fenofibrate 200 mg/day or placebo. After up to 7 years of follow-up, the combination of fenofibrate and simvastatin did not reduce the rate of fatal cardiovascular events, nonfatal MI, or nonfatal stroke, as compared with simvastatin alone.[24a]

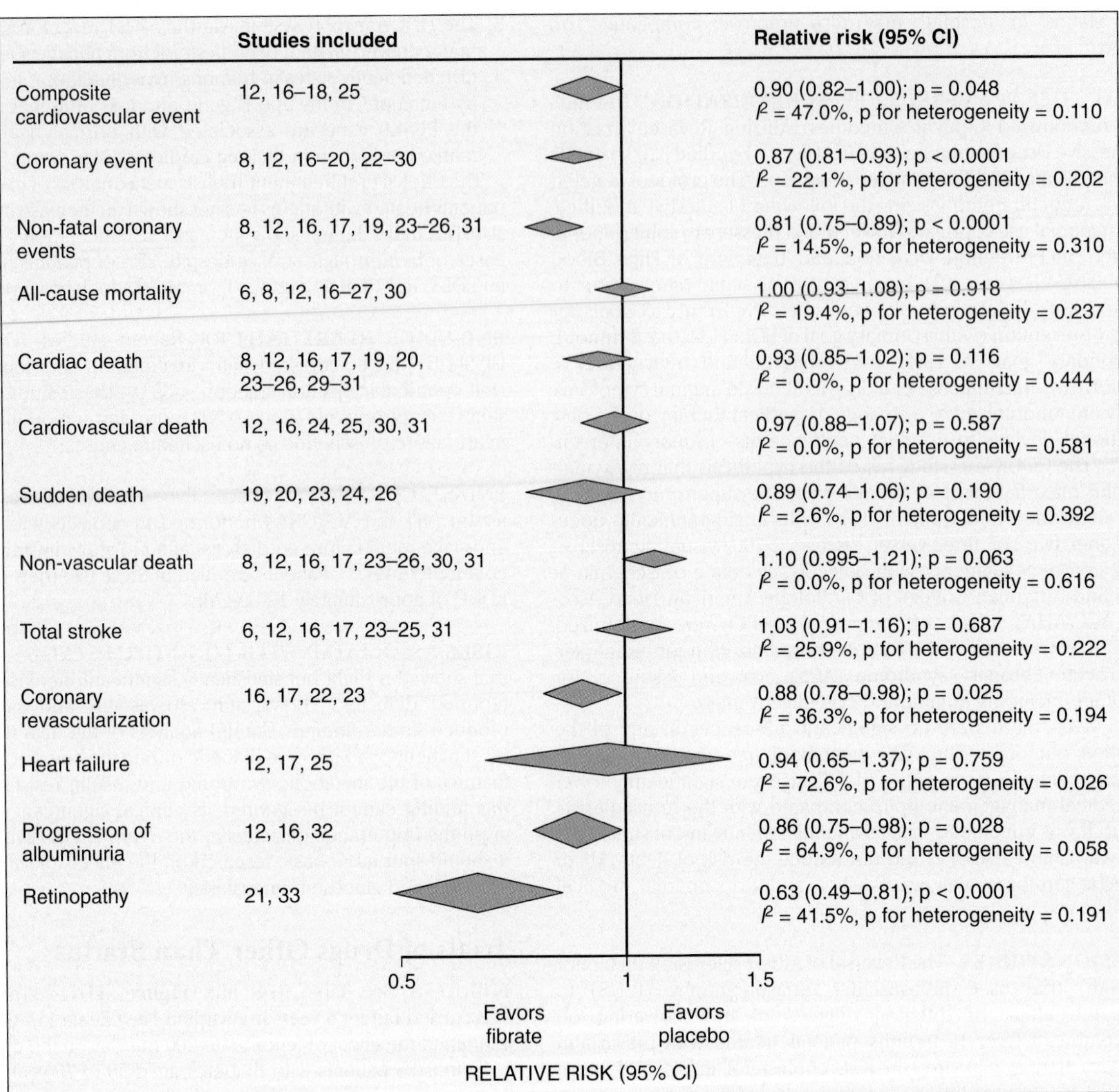

FIGURE 47-7 Meta-analysis of trials of fibrates. *(From Jun M, Foote C, Lv J, et al: Effects of fibrates on cardiovascular outcomes: a systematic review and meta-analysis. Lancet 375:1875, 2010.)*

NIACIN. Niacin is a naturally occurring vitamin with a daily requirement of 25 to 50 mg/day.[41] Early trials performed in the 1970s showed a benefit of niacin in the coronary drug project, although this was during an era without the current therapies of aspirin, beta blockers, revascularization, and the more potent statins. Almost all the trials using niacin that are discussed here included relatively small numbers of subjects, used combination medications, and often used biomarkers such as luminal angiography, rather than hard cardiovascular events. Niacin lowers levels of LDL-C by 15% to 25%, can increase HDL-C by 20% to 30%, and lowers triglycerides.

The combination of a statin with niacin improves the lipid profile in patients with combined dyslipidemia and low HDL-C levels. Niacin increases serum HDL-C levels more effectively than fibrates alone. The results of the AIM-HIGH and HPS-THRIVE trials,[42] using combined statin and niacin in high-risk patients and powered for CVD endpoints, will provide important guidance regarding the clinical effectiveness of niacin in contemporary practice.

Approach to the Treatment of Lipoprotein Disorders

Patients with lipoprotein disorders should undergo comprehensive evaluation and management in the context of a global risk reduction program. Most patients with dyslipoproteinemias lack symptoms, except for those with severe hypertriglyceridemia who can present with acute pancreatitis and those with familial lipoprotein disorders who have cutaneous manifestations (e.g., xanthomas, xanthelasmas). In the evaluation of patients with dyslipidemia, secondary causes should be sought and treated. The clinical evaluation should include a thorough history, including a complete family history, which may reveal clues about the genetic cause and also the genetic susceptibility to CVD. The physician should seek and address other risk factors (e.g., cigarette smoking, obesity, diabetes, hypertension, lack of exercise) and institute measures to improve lifestyle (e.g., diet, physical activity, alcohol intake). Such interventions should make use of nonphysician health professionals (e.g., those with training in diet and nutrition, physical therapy, and smoking cessation). The ATP III Therapeutic Lifestyle Change program offers one such approach. Achievement of current guideline goals will often require concomitant medication in addition to lifestyle changes (see Chap. 49).

The physical examination should include a search for xanthomas (in extensor tendons, including hands, elbows, knees, Achilles tendons, and palmar xanthomas), and the presence of xanthelasmas, corneal arcus, and corneal opacifications. The blood pressure, waist circumference, weight, and height should be recorded and signs of arterial compromise sought; a complete cardiovascular examination must be performed. The evaluation of peripheral pulses and the determination of the ankle-brachial index may reveal important clues for the presence of peripheral vascular disease.

TABLE 47-9 Laboratory Tests for the Diagnosis of Lipoprotein Disorders

LIPID PROFILE	MAY HELP IN DIAGNOSIS	TEST PERFORMED IN SPECIALIZED CENTERS	RESEARCH TOOLS
Cholesterol	LDL particle size (NMR, PAGE)	Lipoprotein separation by UTC	Molecular diagnosis
Triglycerides	Apo B	Specific enzyme assays (LCAT, LPL)	Cell-based assays
	Direct LDL-C measurement	Apo E levels	—
LDL cholesterol*	Apo A-I	Apolipoprotein separation by PAGE, apo C-II, apo C-III	—
	Apo E genotype, phenotype	HDL size (NMR), LDL-R assay	—
	Lipoprotein(a)	Sterol analysis by gas chromatography	—

NMR = nuclear magnetic resonance; PAGE = polyacrylamide gel electrophoresis; UTC = ultracentrifugation.

*Calculated as follows:

LDL-C total cholesterol + −[(triglycerides 2.2) −HDL-C)

in mmol/liter, or triglycerides divided by 5, in mg/dL. This is valid for triglycerides < 4.5 mmol/liter (<400 mg/dL). LDL cholesterol can also be directly measured in plasma.

The diagnosis of lipoprotein disorders depends on laboratory measurements (**Table 47-9**). The fasting lipid profile generally suffices for most lipoprotein disorders, and specialized laboratories can refine the diagnosis and provide expertise for extreme cases. Additional tests often involve considerable expense and may not increase the predictive value beyond that of the lipid profile, although they can help in refining the diagnosis. To assess baseline risk in individuals on lipid-lowering therapy, the medication should be stopped for 1 month before a lipid profile is determined. Many advanced lipid tests can be done in specialized centers, but they seldom add to the clinical assessment specified earlier.

After diagnosis of a lipid disorder, based on at least two lipid profiles, secondary causes should be evaluated by measurement of thyroid-stimulating hormone and glucose levels. Patients who are to receive medications should have their liver function evaluated (alanine aminotransferase [ALT]) and creatinine kinase levels). A decision to treat high-risk subjects (e.g., ACS patients, post-MI or coronary revascularization) should be made immediately, and therapy should commence concomitantly with lifestyle changes.[43]

Target Levels

The National Cholesterol Education Program Adult Treatment Panel III (NCEP ATP III) has made recommendations for the treatment of hypercholesterolemia.[43] Target levels (see Chap. 49) depend on the overall risk of cardiovascular death or nonfatal MI. Patients with CAD or atherosclerosis of other vascular beds (carotid arteries, peripheral vascular disease), adult patients with diabetes, and patients with an estimated 10-year risk of more than 20% of developing CAD fall into a high-risk category and merit aggressive treatment. This includes medications and lifestyle modifications, exercise, and diet to achieve a primary target of an LDL-C level lower than 2.6 mmol/L (100 mg/dL). In subjects with triglyceride levels higher than 200 mg/dL, ATP III presents a secondary target of a non–HDL-C level less than 3.4 mmol/L (130 mg/dL). Many of these individuals have the metabolic syndrome. A stricter LDL-C target for ACS patients to lower than 80 mg/dL (1.8 mmol/L) is supported by clinical studies, such as the PROVE-IT and A-to-Z trials.

Once the LDL-C target has been reached, patients still remain at increased cardiovascular risk. Age is still the most important determinant of risk. Secondary targets include the non–HDL-C level, total cholesterol–to–HDL-C ratio, apo B/apo A-I ratio, and triglyceride and hsCRP levels[44,45] Although each of these potential targets has been shown in post hoc analysis of outcome studies or as part of a prespecified data analysis, there are no clinical studies specifically addressing the issue of reaching these targets. Physicians must thus exercise judgment when considering a combination of statins with other lipid-lowering agents.

Lifestyle Changes (see Chaps. 48 and 49)

TREATMENT. The therapeutic options consist of lifestyle modifications, treatment of secondary causes and, if possible, diet and medications.

DIET. Individuals with dyslipoproteinemias should always adopt dietary therapy. High-risk subjects should have medications started concomitantly with a diet because, in many cases, diet may not suffice to reach target levels. The diet should have three objectives: (1) it should allow the patient to reach and maintain ideal body weight; (2) it should be well balanced, with fruits, vegetables, and whole grains; and (3) it should be restricted in sodium, saturated fats, and refined carbohydrates. Dietary counseling should involve a professional dietitian. Often, the help of dietitians, weight loss programs, and/or diabetic outpatient centers can aid in sustaining weight loss. Currently, the ATP III and AHA recommend a diet in which protein intake is 15% to 20% of calories, fats less than 35% (with only 7% from saturated fats) and the remaining calories derived from carbohydrates. Cholesterol intake should be less than 300 mg/day.

Treatment of Combined Lipoprotein Disorders

Combined lipoprotein disorders, characterized by an increase in plasma total cholesterol and triglyceride levels, frequently occur in clinical practice and present difficult challenges. Patients with combined lipoprotein disorders have an increase in LDL cholesterol levels and particle numbers (as reflected by an increase in total or LDL apo B), small dense LDL particles, increased VLDL cholesterol and VLDL triglyceride levels, and reduced HDL cholesterol levels. Patients with this pattern of combined dyslipidemia often have obesity and the metabolic syndrome. Treatment should begin with lifestyle modifications, with a diet reduced in total calories and saturated fats, weight reduction, and increased physical activity.

Drug treatment, when warranted, aims to correct the predominant lipoprotein abnormality. Statins can reduce plasma triglyceride levels, particularly in those with high baseline triglyceride levels. Fibrates reduce triglyceride levels and may change the composition of LDL to larger and less dense particles. The results of the FIELD trial do not support the use of fibric acid derivatives in the prevention of CVD in diabetic subjects with low HDL cholesterol levels, although greater drop-in statin use in the placebo arm may have confounded the results (see Table 47-7). Fibrates can paradoxically increase LDL cholesterol levels because of increased lipoprotein lipase activity. Plasma creatinine and homocysteine levels may increase with fibrates. In view of the effects of gemfibrozil on the glucuronidation of statins, we advise against gemfibrozil use in combination with a statin. The combination of a statin with a fibrate is effective in correcting combined lipoprotein disorders. Sub-group analysis of fibrate trials suggest that this approach may be of some benefit in the prevention of cardiovascular events in patients with elevated triglycerides and a low HDL-C.[24a] Patients taking a fibrate plus a statin merit close medical follow-up for evidence of hepatotoxicity or myositis within the first 6 weeks of therapy and every 6 months thereafter. The combined use of a statin and ezetimibe for the treatment of severe hypercholesterolemia or to reach recommended target levels when monotherapy with a statin is insufficient or causes unwanted side effects has a good rationale, although unsubstantiated by clinical endpoint trials.

Other combinations, including fibric acid derivatives with bile acid–binding resins and niacin with bile acid–binding resins, have also proven useful in specific cases. The combination of fibrates or statins with niacin requires careful monitoring because of the risk of hepatotoxicity and myositis. The search for correctable causes (e.g., uncontrolled diabetes, obesity, hypothyroidism, alcohol use) of combined dyslipidemia and the benefit of lifestyle modifications require reemphasis. As noted earlier, the help of dietitians, weight loss programs, and/or diabetic outpatient centers may be of considerable benefit.

EXTRACORPOREAL LOW-DENSITY LIPOPROTEIN FILTRATION. Patients with severe hypercholesterolemia, especially those with homozygous familial hypercholesterolemia or severe heterozygous familial hypercholesterolemia, may warrant treatment with extracorporeal LDL elimination modalities. These techniques use selective filtration, adsorption, or precipitation of LDL (or apo B–containing particles) after plasma separation. Specialized centers have LDL-pheresis available. This approach can dramatically reduce the risk of developing CVD and improve survival.

Future Perspectives

Drug Development: Biologicals and Novel Therapies

The development of novel pharmaceutical agents for the treatment of lipoprotein disorders will likely continue because CVD caused by atherosclerosis represents the largest burden of disease in most countries in the near future. Better targeting of high-risk individuals will allow optimization of expensive therapies. The finding that subjects previously considered at relatively low risk of CAD on the basis of their LDL cholesterol levels but who have an elevated CRP level benefit from a statin in the primary prevention of CAD may radically alter the concept of cardiovascular risk stratification (JUPITER study[33,45]; see Chaps. 44 and 49). Markers of inflammation (especially hsCRP), in addition to conventional risk factors, can help in cardiovascular risk stratification.

Targeting LDL has withstood the test of time and clinical trials. Molecular targets, other than HMG CoA reductase, will likely include inhibition of PCSK9[46]; encouraging results already have been seen in animals. Novel biologicals, such as antisense RNA directed against apo B synthesis in the liver, have shown great promise in patients with severe familial hypercholesterolemia.[47] More refined techniques, using small interfering RNA (siRNA) or short hairpin RNA (shRNA) silencing techniques, may advance the treatment of lipoprotein disorders. Cost considerations will likely restrict these novel agents to severely ill and drug-refractory patients.

Novel therapies to raise HDL-C levels have received some support in a proof of concept clinical trial in which ACS patients were given weekly injections of apo A-I_{Milano}–reconstituted proteoliposomes, in effect nascent HDL particles. Although a reduction in atheroma volume was found, the widespread application of such techniques remains confined to the experimental setting. Other therapeutic modalities in the treatment of atherosclerosis by modulating lipoprotein metabolism include the development of new inhibitors of CETP to increase HDL cholesterol levels. The first compound, torcetrapib, increased HDL-C by 70% and further decreased LDL-C by 25%. However, it proved to have off-target effects, leading to an increase in mortality in the ILLUMINATE trial. Two new CETP inhibitors, anacetrapib and dalcetrapib,[48] are currently undergoing clinical trials. Pharmacologic modulation of HDL-C levels, other than by niacin, has not led to results proportional to those achieved for LDL-C. Potential modulators of HDL-C levels include SR-B1, ABCA1, and ABCG1 pathways and apo A-I and its homologues and mimetics.

The burgeoning field of pharmacogenomics might, in the near future, allow treatment of patients on the basis of their genetic makeup. Resistance to statins has been shown to be associated with genetic variability at the organic anion-transporting polypeptide *OATP1B1* gene[49] and likely to genes associated with muscular dystrophies. Genetic screening may become a useful clinical tool as technology improves and rapid genotyping for diagnostic and prognostic purposes becomes available to clinicians. Other than cost issues, the ethics of screening for genetic predisposition to disease and access to information represent daunting challenges. The discovery that the apo E4 allele carries the risk of early-onset Alzheimer disease, one of the familial forms of the disorder, illustrates the ethical complexities of genetic testing in the realm of lipoprotein disorders.

Gene Therapy

Severe, homozygous, monogenic disorders may eventually be treated by gene therapy. The initial trials of gene therapy in cases of homozygous familial hypercholesterolemia have not led to a major improvement and have largely been abandoned. However, the lifelong burden of these rare disorders and the potential for cure makes this approach appealing. Other diseases, such as abetalipoproteinemia, LPL deficiency,[50] Niemann-Pick type C disease, sitosterolemia, and Tangier disease may become targets for gene therapy. If the approach to correct these disorders is successful, the more widespread applications of gene-based therapies for the purpose of reducing potential cardiovascular risk will become a daunting medical, social, and ethical problem.

Societal Changes

Drug therapy alone will likely not suffice to stem the current worldwide epidemic of atherosclerosis. In the 19th century, societal changes aimed at preserving the benefits of hygiene and public health measures and infrastructure greatly reduced human suffering and pestilence as a cause of death. Today, public health measures to reduce cigarette smoking have already lowered the incidence of MI. Because more than 50% of the population worldwide resides in cities, urban planning should encourage physical activity (e.g., by construction of sidewalks and bicycle lanes). Shifts in patterns of food consumption in the past 50 years have doubtless contributed to the epidemic of obesity and increased prevalence of lipoprotein disorders, hypertension, and diabetes, with consequent cardiovascular diseases. Personal changes with respect to food consumption, caloric intake, and physical activity will remain a major challenge requiring societal intervention.

REFERENCES

Lipoprotein Transport System and Lipoprotein Disorders

1. Goldstein JL, Brown MS: The LDL receptor. Arterioscler Thromb Vasc Biol 29:431, 2009.
2. Seimon T, Tabas I: Mechanisms and consequences of macrophage apoptosis in atherosclerosis. J Lipid Res 50:S382, 2009.
3. Rohrer L, Ohnsorg PM, Lehner M, et al: High-density lipoprotein transport through aortic endothelial cells involves scavenger receptor BI and ATP-binding cassette transporter G1. Circ Res 104:1142, 2009.
4. Rader DJ, Alexander ET, Weibel GL, et al: The role of reverse cholesterol transport in animals and humans and relationship to atherosclerosis. J Lipid Res 50:S189, 2009.
5. Davis HR Jr, Altmann SW: Niemann-Pick C1 Like 1 (NPC1L1), an intestinal sterol transporter. Biochim Biophys Acta 1791:679, 2009.
6. Bransteitter R, Prochnow C, Chen XS: The current structural and functional understanding of APOBEC deaminases. Cell Mol Life Sci 66:3137, 2009.
7. Tang W, Ma Y, Jia L, et al: Genetic inactivation of NPC1L1 protects against sitosterolemia in mice lacking ABCG5/ABCG8. J Lipid Res 50:293, 2009.
8. Su Q, Tsai J, Xu E, et al: Apolipoprotein B100 acts as a molecular link between lipid-induced endoplasmic reticulum stress and hepatic insulin resistance. Hepatology 50:77, 2009.
9. Hu L, van der Hoogt CC, Espirito Santo SM, et al: The hepatic uptake of VLDL in lrp-ldlr-/-vldlr-/- mice is regulated by LPL activity and involves proteoglycans and SR-BI. J Lipid Res 49:1553, 2008.
10. Poirier S, Mayer G, Benjannet S, et al: The proprotein convertase PCSK9 induces the degradation of low-density lipoprotein receptor (LDLR) and its closest family members VLDLR and ApoER2. J Biol Chem 283:2363, 2008.
11. Rader DJ: Mechanisms of disease: HDL metabolism as a target for novel therapies. Nat Clin Pract Cardiovasc Med 4:102, 2007.
12. Wang X, Rader DJ: Molecular regulation of macrophage reverse cholesterol transport. Curr Opin Cardiol 22:368, 2007.
13. Minhas R, Humphries SE, Qureshi N, Neil HA: Controversies in familial hypercholesterolaemia: Recommendations of the NICE Guideline Development Group for the identification and management of familial hypercholesterolaemia. Heart 95:584, 2009.
14. Cohen JC, Boerwinkle E, Mosley TH Jr, Hobbs HH: Sequence variations in PCSK9, low LDL, and protection against coronary heart disease. N Engl J Med 354:1264, 2006.
15. Kamstrup PR, Tybjaerg-Hansen A, Steffensen R, Nordestgaard BG: Genetically elevated lipoprotein(a) and increased risk of myocardial infarction. JAMA 301:2331, 2009.

15a. Clarke R, Peden JF, Hopewell JC, et al: Genetic variants associated with Lp(a) lipoprotein level and coronary disease. N Engl J Med 361:2518, 2009.
16. Mar-Heyming R, Miyazaki M, Weissglas-Volkov D, et al: Association of stearoyl-CoA desaturase 1 activity with familial combined hyperlipidemia. Arterioscler Thromb Vasc Biol 28:1193, 2008.
17. Lee JC, Weissglas-Volkov D, Kyttälä M, et al: USF1 contributes to high serum lipid levels in Dutch FCHL families and U.S. whites with coronary artery disease. Arterioscler Thromb Vasc Biol 27:2222, 2007.
18. Genest J, Dastani Z, Engert J, Marcil M: Genetics of high-density lipoproteins. *In* Fielding CJ, (ed): High-Density Lipoproteins: From Basic Biology to Clinical Aspects. Weinheim, Germany, Wiley-VCH, 2007, pp 465-490.
18a. Ridker PM, Genest J, Boekholdt SM, et al: HDL cholesterol and residual risk of first cardiovascular events after treatment with potent statin therapy: an analysis from the JUPITER trial. Lancet 376:333, 2010.
19. Frikke-Schmidt R, Nordestgaard BG, Stene MC, et al: Association of loss-of-function mutations in the ABCA1 gene with high-density lipoprotein cholesterol levels and risk of ischemic heart disease. JAMA 299:2524, 2008.
19a. Alberti KG, Eckel RH, Grundy SM, et al: Harmonizing the metabolic syndrome. A joint interim statement of the International Diabetes Federation Task Force on Epidemiology and Prevention; National Heart, Lung, and Blood Institute; American Heart Association; World Heart Federation; International Atherosclerosis Society; and International Association for the Study of Obesity. Circulation 120:1640, 2009.
19b. Mente A, Yusuf S, Islam S, et al: Metabolic syndrome and risk of acute myocardial infarction: A case-control study of 26,903 subjects from 52 countries. J Am Coll Cardiol 55:2390, 2010.
20. Wanner C, Krane V, März W, et al: Atorvastatin in patients with type 2 diabetes mellitus undergoing hemodialysis. N Engl J Med 353:238, 2005.
21. Fellstrom BC, Jardine AG, Schmieder RE, et al: Rosuvastatin and cardiovascular events in patients undergoing hemodialysis. N Engl J Med 360:1395, 2009.

Drugs That Affect Lipoprotein Metabolism

22. Krakowski M, Czobor P, Citrome L: Weight gain, metabolic parameters, and the impact of race in aggressive inpatients randomized to double-blind clozapine, olanzapine or haloperidol. Schizophr Res 110:95, 2009.
23. DAD Study Group; Friis-Møller N, Reiss P, Sabin CA, et al: Class of antiretroviral drugs and the risk of myocardial infarction. N Engl J Med 356:1723, 2007.
24. Barbaro G, Iacobellis G: Metabolic syndrome associated with HIV and highly active antiretroviral therapy. Curr Diab Rep 9:37, 2009.

Clinical Trials of Drugs Affecting Lipid Metabolism and Approach to the Treatment of Lipid Disorders

24a. The ACCORD Study Group: Effects of combination lipid therapy in type 2 diabetes mellitus. N Engl J Med 362:1563, 2010.
24b. Jun M, Foote C, Lv J, et al: Effects of fibrates on cardiovascular outcomes: a systematic review and meta-analysis. Lancet 375:1875, 2010.
25. Baigent C, Keech A, Kearney P, et al: Efficacy and safety of cholesterol-lowering treatment: Prospective meta-analysis of data from 90,056 participants in 14 randomised trials of statins. Lancet 366:1267, 2005.
26. Delahoy PJ, Magliano DJ, Webb K, et al: The relationship between reduction in low-density lipoprotein cholesterol by statins and reduction in risk of cardiovascular outcomes: An updated meta-analysis. Clin Ther 31:236, 2009.
27. D'Agostino RB, Ramachandran SV, Pencina MJ, et al: General cardiovascular risk profile for use in primary care. The Framingham Heart Study. Circulation 117:743, 2008.
28. Graham I, Atar D, Borch-Johnsen K, Boysen G, et al: European guidelines on cardiovascular disease prevention in clinical practice. Eur J Cardiovasc Prev Rehabil 14:S1, 2007.
29. Cholesterol Treatment Trialists' (CTT) Collaborators: Efficacy of cholesterol-lowering therapy in 18,686 people with diabetes in 14 randomised trials of statins: A meta-analysis. Lancet 371:117, 2008.
30. Skyler JS, Bergenstal R, Bonow RO, et al: Intensive glycemic control and the prevention of cardiovascular events: implications of the ACCORD, ADVANCE, and VA Diabetes Trials: A position statement of the American Diabetes Association and a Scientific Statement of the American College of Cardiology Foundation and the American Heart Association. Circulation 119:351, 2009.
31. Holman RR, Paul SK, Bethel MA, et al: 10-year follow-up of intensive glucose control in type 2 diabetes. N Engl J Med 359:1577, 2008.
32. Afilalo J, Duque G, Steele R, et al: Statins for secondary prevention in elderly patients: A hierarchical bayesian meta-analysis. J Am Coll Cardiol 51:37, 2008.
32a. Mora S, Glynn RJ, Hsia J, et al: Statins for the primary prevention of cardiovascular events in women with elevated high-sensitivity C-reactive protein or dyslipidemia: results from the Justification for the Use of Statins in Prevention: An Intervention Trial Evaluating Rosuvastatin (JUPITER) and meta-analysis of women from primary prevention trials. Circulation 9;121:1069, 2010.
33. Ridker PM, Danielson E, Fonseca FA, et al: Rosuvastatin to prevent vascular events in men and women with elevated C-reactive protein. N Engl J Med 359:2195, 2008.
34. Yusuf S, Hawken S, Ounpuu S, et al: Effect of potentially modifiable risk factors associated with myocardial infarction in 52 countries (the INTERHEART study): Case-control study. Lancet 364:937, 2004.
35. Mizuno K, Nakaya N, Ohashi Y, et al: Usefulness of pravastatin in primary prevention of cardiovascular events in women: Analysis of the Management of Elevated Cholesterol in the Primary Prevention Group of Adult Japanese (MEGA study). Circulation 117:494, 2008.
36. Wiviott SD, de Lemos JA, Cannon CP, et al: A tale of two trials: A comparison of the post-acute coronary syndrome lipid-lowering trials A to Z and PROVE IT-TIMI 22. Circulation 113:1406, 2006.
37. Boden WE, O'Rourke RA, Teo KK, et al; COURAGE Trial Research Group: Optimal medical therapy with or without PCI for stable coronary disease. N Engl J Med 356:1503, 2007.
37a. REVERSAL Investigators: Effect of intensive compared with moderate lipid-lowering therapy on progression of coronary atherosclerosis: a randomized controlled trial. JAMA 291:1071, 2004.
38. Nissen SE, Nicholls SJ, Sipahi I, et al: Effect of very high-intensity statin therapy on regression of coronary atherosclerosis: The ASTEROID trial. JAMA 295:1556, 2006.
39. Kjekshus J, Apetrei E, Barrios V, et al; CORONA Group: Rosuvastatin in older patients with systolic heart failure. N Engl J Med 357:2248, 2007.
40. Gissi-HF Investigators; Tavazzi L, Maggioni AP, Marchioli R, et al: Effect of rosuvastatin in patients with chronic heart failure (the GISSI-HF trial): A randomised, double-blind, placebo-controlled trial. Lancet 372:1231, 2008.
41. Carlson LA: Nicotinic acid: The broad-spectrum lipid drug. A 50th anniversary review. J Intern Med 258:94, 2005.
42. Brown BG, Zhao XQ: Nicotinic acid, alone and in combinations, for reduction of cardiovascular risk. Am J Cardiol 101:58B, 2008.
43. Smith SC Jr, Allen J, Blair SN, et al: AHA/ACC guidelines for secondary prevention for patients with coronary and other atherosclerotic vascular disease: 2006 update: Endorsed by the National Heart, Lung, and Blood Institute. Circulation 113:2363, 2006.
44. Fruchart JC, Sacks F, Hermans MP, et al: The Residual Risk Reduction Initiative: A call to action to reduce residual vascular risk in patients with dyslipidemia. Am J Cardiol 102:1K, 2008.
45. Ridker PM, Danielson E, Fonseca FA, et al: Reduction in C-reactive protein and LDL cholesterol and cardiovascular event rates after initiation of rosuvastatin: A prospective study of the JUPITER trial. Lancet 373:1175, 2009.

Future Perspectives

46. Chan JC, Piper DE, Cao Q, et al: A proprotein convertase subtilisin/kexin type 9 neutralizing antibody reduces serum cholesterol in mice and nonhuman primates. Proc Natl Acad Sci U S A 106:9820, 2009.
47. Kastelein JJ, Wedel MK, Baker BF, et al: Potent reduction of apolipoprotein B and low-density lipoprotein cholesterol by short-term administration of an antisense inhibitor of apolipoprotein B. Circulation 114:1729, 2006.
48. Joy T, Hegele RA: The end of the road for CETP inhibitors after torcetrapib? Curr Opin Cardiol 24:364, 2009.
49. SEARCH Collaborative Group: SLCO1B1 variants and statin-induced myopathy—a genomewide study. N Engl J Med 359:789, 2008.
50. Stroes ES, Nierman MC, Meulenberg JJ, et al: Intramuscular administration of AAV1-lipoprotein lipase S447X lowers triglycerides in lipoprotein lipase-deficient patients. Arterioscler Thromb Vasc Biol 28:2303, 2008.

CHAPTER 48 Nutrition and Cardiovascular Disease

Dariush Mozaffarian

Together with smoking and physical activity, dietary habits form the foundation for the causation, prevention, and treatment of most cardiovascular and metabolic diseases, including coronary heart disease (CHD), stroke, and type 2 diabetes mellitus (DM), as well as sudden cardiac death, atrial fibrillation, heart failure, and cognitive decline. In developed countries such as the United States, higher intake of dietary salt and industrial trans fat, and lower intake of omega-3 fatty acids, fruits, and vegetables, are some of the major modifiable causes of both total deaths and deaths from cardiovascular disease (CVD).[1] In developing countries, the burgeoning epidemics of obesity, DM, and CVD result directly from rapid social and environmental changes transmitted primarily through changes in diet and other lifestyle behaviors.[2] Familiarity with the beneficial and harmful effects of various nutritional factors is essential to mitigate and eventually reverse the substantial disease burdens caused by suboptimal dietary habits in individuals and in populations.

Knowledge of how diet affects CVD has rapidly progressed in recent years. Limited past inferences from ecologic studies and short-term experiments have given way to more robust and consistent evidence from randomized trials and prospective cohort studies of disease endpoints (e.g., myocardial infarction [MI], CHD death) that provide more direct evidence for total causal effects, supported by well-conducted trials of multiple risk markers and pathways (e.g., blood pressure [BP], glucose and insulin levels, lipids). Conclusions are most robust when studies across these different designs provide concordant findings, with supporting evidence from in vitro and animal work, retrospective studies, and ecologic studies. Dietary factors exert acute and chronic effects on a complex set of established and novel risk factors, mechanistic pathways, and disease conditions (**Fig. 48-1**).

Translation of this knowledge into action at the public health, policy, practitioner, and health care system levels is essential. Strong drug-, device-, and procedure-driven research and profits have often minimized direct financial incentives to focus on diet and other lifestyle habits to prevent and treat cardiometabolic diseases. However, the global pandemics of obesity, DM, and CVD highlight the tremendous direct and indirect costs of undesirable diet, and the financial imperatives of placing clinical and policy emphasis on nutrition have now become fully evident. Translation of knowledge to action has also been limited by evolving messages and confusion about which dietary factors are most relevant; by uncertainty regarding effective methods for behavior change; and by the need for tools to monitor diets efficiently. Fortunately, substantial research advances have addressed these challenges to provide a more clear and consistent picture of the most relevant dietary factors for cardiometabolic health, to inform evidence-based strategies for effective individual- and population-based dietary change, and to show that simple targeted assessments are acceptable and practical for monitoring dietary change. Increased emphasis on nutrition by the public, health care providers, and policy makers should facilitate informed formulation and translation of dietary recommendations for improving cardiovascular health.

Macronutrients

Carbohydrates

Total carbohydrate quantity consumed does not associate strongly with CHD risk (**Fig. 48-2**), but the types and quantity of carbohydrate consumed are important determinants of health effects. Traditionally, carbohydrates have been grouped as simple (e.g., glucose, fructose, galactose, sucrose, lactose, lactulose) or complex (e.g., starch, cellulose, hemicellulose, glycogen). Recent evidence indicates that this classification scheme has little relevance to health effects. Specific factors that determine quality and health effects of high-carbohydrate foods include dietary fiber content, glycemic index (GI) and glycemic load (GL), and the extent of processing (i.e., refined grains versus whole grains). Dietary fiber, lower GI and GL, and whole-grain content tend to cluster together in certain foods, and differentiating their independent effects is challenging. Nonetheless, it is clear that carbohydrate quality, as characterized by one or more of these measures, influences a variety of cardiometabolic pathways, including glucose-insulin homeostasis and triglyceride (TG) levels and related endothelial and inflammatory responses. Effects may be especially relevant in the immediate postprandial period and in those predisposed to insulin resistance.[3-6]

DIETARY FIBER. Dietary fiber is comprised of nondigestible polysaccharides, resistant starch and oligosaccharides, and lignins in plants. Trials have demonstrated consistent benefits of dietary fiber on multiple CVD risk factors, including serum TG, low-density lipoprotein cholesterol (LDL-C), blood glucose, and BP.[7,8] In hypertensive patients, for example, higher fiber intake reduces systolic (S) BP and diastolic (D) BP by 6.0 and 4.2 mm Hg, respectively. Unfortunately, few long-term trials have been performed. In the Diet and Reinfarction Trial in men with prior MI, advice to consume cereal fiber had no significant effect on CHD endpoints, but follow-up was limited to 2 years. In contrast, in long-term prospective cohorts, fiber from grains, cereals, and fruits is associated with a lower incidence of CHD, and fiber from

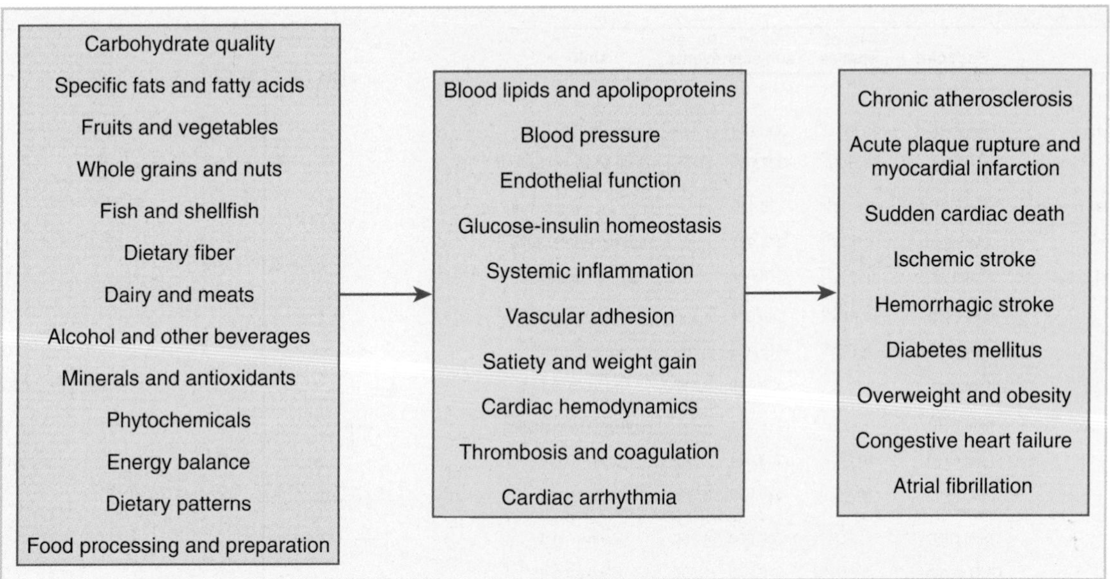

FIGURE 48-1 Pathways of effects of diet on cardiometabolic diseases.

grains and cereals with a lower incidence of DM (see Fig. 48-2).[9,10] Cereal fiber intake may also reduce risk via a substitution effect, replacing more refined carbohydrates that may have detrimental effects.

GLYCEMIC INDEX AND GLYCEMIC LOAD. GI is an empiric measure of effects on postprandial glucose-insulin homeostasis, calculated as the relative increase over time (area under the curve) of the blood glucose level after ingestion of a carbohydrate of interest versus a standard (e.g., glucose, GI = 100). Less refined, higher fiber foods tend to have a lower GI; starchy, refined, lower fiber foods tend to have a higher GI. High GI foods include corn flakes (GI = 81), potatoes (GI = 78), white bread (GI = 75), and white rice (GI = 73); low GI foods include milk (GI = 39), apples (GI = 36), lentils (GI = 32), and nuts (GI = 24).[11] To account for both carbohydrate quality and quantity, GL is calculated as GI × g/serving of carbohydrate. This distinction is important when comparing foods that contain very different absolute amounts of carbohydrate, such as potatoes, cereals, or grains versus fruits or nonstarchy vegetables. For example, watermelon and white rice have a similar GI (76 and 73, respectively), but the GL of watermelon is far lower (4.5 versus 29). Compared to higher GI and GL foods, lower GI and GL foods improve blood glucose, TG, and LDL-C levels, and perhaps also inflammation, endothelial function, and fibrinolysis.[3-6] In short-term trials, lower GI meals increase satiety,[12] but long-term effects on weight or adiposity have not been confirmed. Higher average dietary GI and GL are associated with a higher risk of CHD and DM in prospective studies (see Fig. 48-2).[13,14] Long-term trials have not tested the independent effects of GI and GL on cardiometabolic events. Cardiovascular effects of whole versus refined grains are discussed later in this chapter.

Fats

TOTAL FAT. In the 1960s and 1970s, ecologic (cross-national) studies and short-term feeding trials evaluating single risk factors (e.g., total cholesterol levels) suggested that higher fat consumption, as a percentage of total energy (%E), increased CHD risk. However, subsequent evidence has demonstrated convincingly that the proportion of energy consumed from total fat has no appreciable effect on CHD. Lower total fat intake reduces serum total cholesterol and LDL-C, but also reduces high-density lipoprotein cholesterol (HDL-C) and increases TG levels, with little overall net change in the total cholesterol–to–HDL-C (TC/HDL-C) ratio in men, and no change or slight worsening of the TC/HDL-C ratio in women.[15,16] Lower %E from total fat is also typically accompanied by increased %E from carbohydrates that, if they are largely refined and lower fiber, may adversely affect postprandial glucose-insulin homeostasis and related responses (see earlier, "Carbohydrates"). Evidence from prospective cohorts and trials confirms negligible effects of total fat consumption on CHD events (see Fig. 48-2).[13] In the Women's Health Initiative (WHI) clinical trial (N = 48,835), lowering total fat intake from 37.8 to 24.3 %E (at 1 year) and to 28.8 %E (at 6 years) had no effect on incident CHD (relative risk [RR], 0.98; 95% confidence interval [CI], 0.88 to 1.09), stroke (RR, 1.02; 95% CI, 0.90 to 1.15), or total CVD (RR, 0.98; 95% CI, 0.92 to 1.05).[17] Based on these multiple lines of evidence for no effect, both the U.S. Department of Agriculture (USDA) and the American Heart Association (AHA) have dropped prior recommendations to maintain total fat intake less than 30%E,[18,19] and a 2003 report from the World Health Organization (WHO) concluded that "there is no evidence to directly link the quantity of daily fat intake to increased risk of CVD."[20]

Evidence for the effects of total fat intake on stroke is more mixed, with several long-term observational studies finding null or inverse (protective) associations.[21] Whether the protective associations seen in some studies are related to total fat per se, or to other associated nutritional factors (e.g., animal protein or saturated fat, that have been hypothesized to reduce stroke risk), is unclear. The WHI results provide good evidence that at least within the range of 24% to 38%E, total fat intake has little impact on incident stroke in women. There is also little evidence that low-fat diets either prevent DM or improve glycemic control. Prospective cohorts generally find no relationship between total fat intake and incident DM.[22] In the WHI trial, a diet low in total fat had no effect on homeostasis model assessment of insulin resistance (HOMA-IR) or DM incidence over 8.1 years (RR, 0.96, 95% CI, 0.90 to 1.03), even with 1.9 kg lower weight in the intervention group.[23] Post hoc analyses have suggested slightly lower DM incidence in highly compliant women (P = 0.04), but other factors determining compliance would bias such results. Growing evidence also suggests that %E from total fat has little effect on weight loss or overweight or obesity (see later, "Energy Balance").

TYPES OF FAT. In contrast to the relatively limited health effects of the proportion of energy consumed from total fat, substantial health effects can occur from increases or decreases in specific types of fats consumed, either as a replacement for other fats or for carbohydrates. Nomenclature schemes and dietary recommendations for fats traditionally follow broad chemical classifications defined by the degree of unsaturation (e.g., saturated, monounsaturated, polyunsaturated) or the type of double bond (e.g., omega[n]-3 or omega[n]-6; see

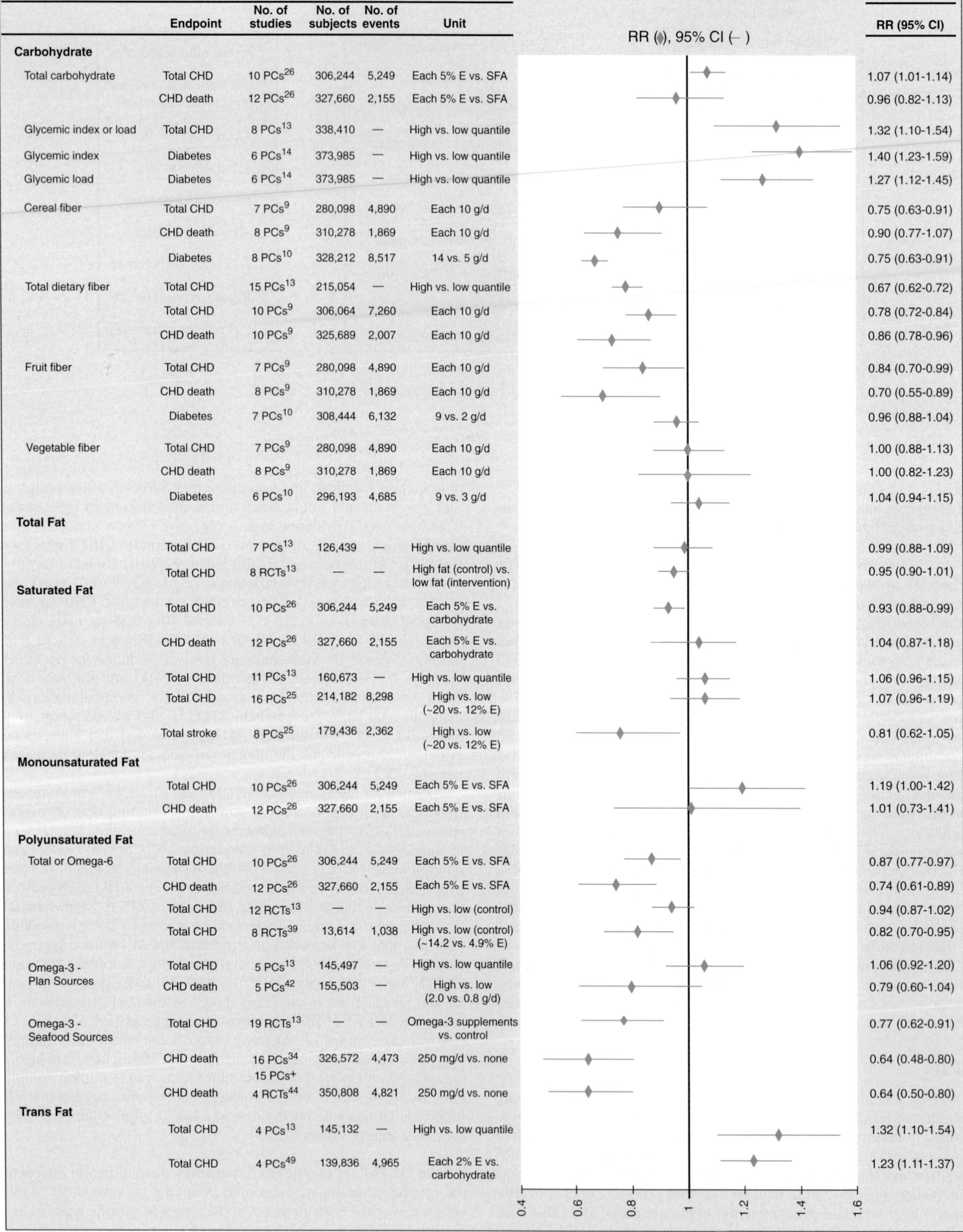

	Endpoint	No. of studies	No. of subjects	No. of events	Unit	RR (95% CI)
Carbohydrate						
Total carbohydrate	Total CHD	10 PCs[26]	306,244	5,249	Each 5% E vs. SFA	1.07 (1.01-1.14)
	CHD death	12 PCs[26]	327,660	2,155	Each 5% E vs. SFA	0.96 (0.82-1.13)
Glycemic index or load	Total CHD	8 PCs[13]	338,410	—	High vs. low quantile	1.32 (1.10-1.54)
Glycemic index	Diabetes	6 PCs[14]	373,985	—	High vs. low quantile	1.40 (1.23-1.59)
Glycemic load	Diabetes	6 PCs[14]	373,985	—	High vs. low quantile	1.27 (1.12-1.45)
Cereal fiber	Total CHD	7 PCs[9]	280,098	4,890	Each 10 g/d	0.75 (0.63-0.91)
	CHD death	8 PCs[9]	310,278	1,869	Each 10 g/d	0.90 (0.77-1.07)
	Diabetes	8 PCs[10]	328,212	8,517	14 vs. 5 g/d	0.75 (0.63-0.91)
Total dietary fiber	Total CHD	15 PCs[13]	215,054	—	High vs. low quantile	0.67 (0.62-0.72)
	Total CHD	10 PCs[9]	306,064	7,260	Each 10 g/d	0.78 (0.72-0.84)
	CHD death	10 PCs[9]	325,689	2,007	Each 10 g/d	0.86 (0.78-0.96)
Fruit fiber	Total CHD	7 PCs[9]	280,098	4,890	Each 10 g/d	0.84 (0.70-0.99)
	CHD death	8 PCs[9]	310,278	1,869	Each 10 g/d	0.70 (0.55-0.89)
	Diabetes	7 PCs[10]	308,444	6,132	9 vs. 2 g/d	0.96 (0.88-1.04)
Vegetable fiber	Total CHD	7 PCs[9]	280,098	4,890	Each 10 g/d	1.00 (0.88-1.13)
	CHD death	8 PCs[9]	310,278	1,869	Each 10 g/d	1.00 (0.82-1.23)
	Diabetes	6 PCs[10]	296,193	4,685	9 vs. 3 g/d	1.04 (0.94-1.15)
Total Fat						
	Total CHD	7 PCs[13]	126,439	—	High vs. low quantile	0.99 (0.88-1.09)
	Total CHD	8 RCTs[13]	—	—	High fat (control) vs. low fat (intervention)	0.95 (0.90-1.01)
Saturated Fat						
	Total CHD	10 PCs[26]	306,244	5,249	Each 5% E vs. carbohydrate	0.93 (0.88-0.99)
	CHD death	12 PCs[26]	327,660	2,155	Each 5% E vs. carbohydrate	1.04 (0.87-1.18)
	Total CHD	11 PCs[13]	160,673	—	High vs. low quantile	1.06 (0.96-1.15)
	Total CHD	16 PCs[25]	214,182	8,298	High vs. low (~20 vs. 12% E)	1.07 (0.96-1.19)
	Total stroke	8 PCs[25]	179,436	2,362	High vs. low (~20 vs. 12% E)	0.81 (0.62-1.05)
Monounsaturated Fat						
	Total CHD	10 PCs[26]	306,244	5,249	Each 5% E vs. SFA	1.19 (1.00-1.42)
	CHD death	12 PCs[26]	327,660	2,155	Each 5% E vs. SFA	1.01 (0.73-1.41)
Polyunsaturated Fat						
Total or Omega-6	Total CHD	10 PCs[26]	306,244	5,249	Each 5% E vs. SFA	0.87 (0.77-0.97)
	CHD death	12 PCs[26]	327,660	2,155	Each 5% E vs. SFA	0.74 (0.61-0.89)
	Total CHD	12 RCTs[13]	—	—	High vs. low (control)	0.94 (0.87-1.02)
	Total CHD	8 RCTs[39]	13,614	1,038	High vs. low (control) (~14.2 vs. 4.9% E)	0.82 (0.70-0.95)
Omega-3 - Plan Sources	Total CHD	5 PCs[13]	145,497	—	High vs. low quantile	1.06 (0.92-1.20)
	CHD death	5 PCs[42]	155,503	—	High vs. low (2.0 vs. 0.8 g/d)	0.79 (0.60-1.04)
Omega-3 - Seafood Sources	Total CHD	19 RCTs[13]	—	—	Omega-3 supplements vs. control	0.77 (0.62-0.91)
	CHD death	16 PCs[34]	326,572	4,473	250 mg/d vs. none	0.64 (0.48-0.80)
	CHD death	15 PCs+ 4 RCTs[44]	350,808	4,821	250 mg/d vs. none	0.64 (0.50-0.80)
Trans Fat						
	Total CHD	4 PCs[13]	145,132	—	High vs. low quantile	1.32 (1.10-1.54)
	Total CHD	4 PCs[49]	139,836	4,965	Each 2% E vs. carbohydrate	1.23 (1.11-1.37)

FIGURE 48-2 Meta-analyses of dietary nutrients and incidence of coronary heart disease (CHD), stroke, and diabetes. PC = prospective cohort. RCT = randomized controlled trial. — = not reported.

Chap. 47). Such broad groupings obscure substantial differences in the dietary sources and biologic effects of individual fatty acids within each class that can have very specific effects on gene transcription, cell membrane fluidity and function, and metabolites generated. As these distinct biologic properties are elucidated, clinical and public health focus should focus on the types and amounts of individual fatty acids. This chapter follows the conventional groupings, but also highlights some effects of individual fatty acids.

Saturated Fatty Acids

Meats, dairy products, and tropical oils (e.g., palm, coconut) are major sources of saturated fatty acids (SFAs). Based on ecologic comparisons, effects on LDL-C, and animal experiments, SFA intake would be expected to increase CHD risk. When replacing equivalent calories from carbohydrates, for example, each 1%E greater intake of SFA increases LDL-C by 0.032 mmol/liter.[15] But growing evidence indicates that the SFA story is not as simple as it appears. First, lauric acid (12:0), myristic acid (14:0), and palmitic acid (16:0) raise LDL-C compared with carbohydrates, but stearic acid (18:0) does not. More importantly, because dietary factors affect chronic disease via multiple pathways (see Fig. 48-1), effects on any single risk marker cannot be assumed to translate directly into changes in disease incidence. For example, the 12-, 14-, and 16-carbon SFAs raise LDL-C compared with carbohydrates, but they also lower TG, raise HDL-C, and raise apolipoprotein A-I (apo A-I) levels.[15] SFAs also lower lipoprotein(a) when consumed in place of monounsaturated fatty acids (MUFAs) or carbohydrates.[24] In the setting of multiple complex lipid and lipoprotein changes, effects on a more global lipid risk marker may be most informative. For each 1%E substituted for carbohydrates, the TC/HDL-C ratio is not affected by myristic acid (−0.003; $P = 0.83$) or palmitic acid (0.005; $P = 0.43$), is nonsignificantly decreased by stearic acid (−0.013; $P = 0.12$), and is significantly decreased by lauric acid (−0.037; $P < 0.001$). These changes suggest minimal effects or even small CHD benefits of SFAs compared with carbohydrates.

Faced with conflicting evidence from risk markers, prospective cohorts and trials of disease endpoints may provide better evidence for total clinical effects. In the large WHI trial, SFA intake was reduced from approximately 12.5% to 9%E—largely replaced with carbohydrates—without effects on incident CHD (RR, 0.98), stroke (RR, 1.02), total CVD (RR, 0.98), or diabetes (RR, 0.96).[17,23] Similarly, two systematic reviews and meta-analyses of prospective cohort studies found no significant association between SFA intake and incident CHD (see Fig. 48-2).[13,25] These three large studies indicate no overall effect of SFA consumption on CHD events. Evidence from a pooled analysis of individual-level data, including 344,696 men and women in 11 prospective cohorts in the United States, Europe, and Israel, suggests that the effects of SFAs on CHD may depend on the nutrient replaced.[26] Consuming SFAs in place of carbohydrates was associated with lower CHD risk (for each 5 %E, RR = 0.93, 95% CI = 0.88 to 0.99), whereas consuming SFAs in place of polyunsaturated fatty acids (PUFAs) was associated with higher risk,[26] consistent with some clinical trials (see later). Observational analysis of replacing SFAs with MUFAs is limited by their common dietary sources,[26] and no clinical trials of CHD events have tested the effects of replacing SFAs with MUFAs.

These lines of evidence, together with the favorable effects of PUFAs on CVD risk factors, suggest that PUFA intake is beneficial in place of SFA or carbohydrates (see later), but that replacing SFAs with carbohydrates may cause little benefit or even slight harm. Data on effects of carbohydrate (see above) would suggest that carbohydrate quality or individual susceptibility to insulin resistance would modify this latter effect; indeed, a recent cohort demonstrated that SFA consumption was associated with significantly lower CHD risk compared with high-GI (highly refined) carbohydrates, similar risk compared with medium-GI carbohydrates, and a trend toward higher risk compared with low-GI carbohydrates.[26a] Evidence for CVD effects of replacing SFAs with MUFAs is mixed (see later). Thus, a focus on decreasing SFAs alone may not result in substantial intended CHD benefits, compared with a focus on increasing PUFAs or improving overall diet quality (see later, "Dietary Patterns").

Six controlled trials have evaluated the effects of SFA versus various replacement nutrients on glucose-insulin homeostasis among individuals predisposed to insulin resistance.[27] Three of five trials found improvements in some glucose-insulin biomarkers when SFAs were replaced with MUFAs; one of three trials, with PUFAs; one trial, with carbohydrate; and zero of two trials, with trans fatty acids (TFAs). Four controlled trials have evaluated similar questions among generally healthy individuals.[27] Only one of four trials found improvements when SFAs were replaced with MUFAs; one of two trials, with carbohydrate; and zero of one trial, with PUFAs or TFAs. These mixed findings do not allow robust conclusions on the effects of dietary fats on glucose-insulin metabolism; the most promising evidence is for potential benefits when SFAs are replaced with MUFAs among those predisposed to insulin resistance. In observational studies, circulating or tissue SFA biomarkers are often associated with insulin resistance, but endogenous SFA levels are increased by both SFA and carbohydrate consumption and also altered by lipolysis, lipogenesis, and beta oxidation. SFA intake was lowered in the WHI trial without effects on HOMA-IR or incident DM.[23] Among four large prospective cohorts evaluating dietary fats and incident DM, none found independent associations between SFA or MUFA intake and DM.[27] In contrast, all four cohorts found protective associations of PUFAs, vegetable oils, and/or the ratio of PUFA to SFA intake with incident DM. These results point to PUFAs as protective against DM, consistent with findings for CHD.

Evidence for the effects of SFAs on other CVD risk factors or endpoints, such as BP or stroke, is limited.[27] Several cohorts have observed a lower risk of stroke—total, ischemic, or hemorrhagic—with higher SFA intake.[25,27] Causal mechanisms and independence from other nutrients in animal fats and proteins require further study.

Monounsaturated Fatty Acids

Animal fats and vegetable oils (e.g., olive and canola) are each major sources of MUFAs, largely oleic acid (18:1n-9). Compared with carbohydrates, MUFA intake lowers LDL-C and TG, raises HDL-C, and lowers BP.[15,28,29] Compared with SFAs, MUFA intake lowers LDL-C and raises lipoprotein(a), without substantial change in TG or HDL-C.[15,24] Fewer studies have compared MUFAs and PUFAs; as a replacement for carbohydrates, MUFAs may raise HDL-C slightly more and lower LDL-C and TG slightly less than PUFAs, with a similar overall improved TC/HDL-C ratio. Trials testing the effects of MUFAs on glucose-insulin homeostasis have shown mixed results compared with SFA or carbohydrates.[27,30,31] Four large prospective cohorts have found no relationship between MUFA intake and incident DM.[31]

Relatively few individual prospective studies have reported on the relationship between MUFA consumption and CHD events, with inconsistent results.[13,16] In a pooled analysis from 11 cohorts, higher MUFA intake, as an isocaloric replacement for SFA, was associated with a trend toward higher CHD risk (for each 5%E, RR = 1.19, 95% CI = 1.00 to 1.42).[26] In nonhuman primates, SFA and MUFA intake were both similarly proatherogenic.[32] No randomized controlled trials have tested whether MUFA intake reduces CHD events compared with carbohydrates, SFAs, or PUFAs.

Animal experiments have suggested that MUFAs alter LDL-C particle composition, increasing cholesteryl oleate content, a change that may increase atherogenicity.[32] This could explain why MUFAs lower LDL-C concentrations and improve the TC/HDL-C ratio but might not reduce CHD risk. In contrast, observational studies and randomized trials have consistently shown that overall dietary patterns that have included MUFAs, typically from olive oil as part of an overall Mediterranean-type diet, improve CHD risk factors and lower CHD events.[13] It is unclear whether these benefits derive from protective effects of MUFAs per se, other related components in olive oil (in particular polyphenols in extra virgin olive oil), or other factors in the Mediterranean-type dietary pattern.

Polyunsaturated Fatty Acids

Dietary PUFAs can be classified broadly into n-6 PUFAs, largely linoleic acid (LA; 18:2n-6) from vegetable oils, and n-3 PUFAs, including

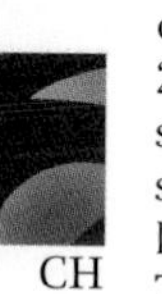

CH 48

alpha-linoleic acid (ALA; 18:3n-3) from plant sources (e.g., flaxseed, canola, walnuts, soybeans), and eicosapentaenoic acid (EPA, 20:5n-3) and docosahexaenoic acid (DHA; 22:6n-3) from fish and shellfish. LA and ALA are essential fatty acids that cannot be synthesized by humans. Humans synthesize relatively little EPA and even less DHA,[33] so that seafood consumption provides the major source. The ratio of n-6 to n-3 fatty acids is not a useful metric of health effects compared with absolute consumption levels of these dietary fats.[34-36]

LINOLEIC ACID. LA typically comprises more than 90% of dietary PUFAs. Compared with carbohydrates, LA lowers LDL-C and TG, raises HDL-C, and improves TC/HDL-C ratio.[15] Effects on other CHD risk markers are less established; some trials have suggested that LA may be anti-inflammatory or improve insulin resistance, but findings have been mixed.[30,31,36] In a pooled analysis from 11 cohorts, greater PUFA intake in place of SFAs was associated with a significantly lower incidence of CHD (for each 5%E, RR = 0.87, 95% CI = 0.77 to 0.97).[26] PUFA intake was also associated with lower CHD risk when replacing carbohydrates.[37] Consistent with observational studies, a meta-analysis of randomized trials that increased total PUFAs or LA in place of SFAs demonstrated reduction in CHD events (see Fig. 48-2).[38] No clinical trials have tested whether consuming PUFAs in place of carbohydrates or MUFAs reduces CHD events. Overall, the evidence suggests that total PUFA or LA intake reduces CHD risk, whether in place of SFAs or carbohydrates. Relationships between PUFA intake and DM were discussed earlier ("Saturated Fatty Acids").

ALPHA-LINOLEIC ACID. In some controlled trials, ALA intake has favorably affected some CVD risk markers related to platelet function, inflammation, endothelial function, and arterial compliance[34]; a meta-analysis of 14 trials found improvements in fibrinogen and fasting glucose levels.[39] Whether such effects are caused directly by ALA or by its longer-chain metabolites (e.g., EPA) is unclear. Ecologic studies have suggested benefits of increasing ALA consumption in populations with low overall n-3 PUFA intake.[40] Prospective cohorts have shown mixed results, with overall no significant relationships seen between ALA intake and CHD events (see Fig. 48-2).[13,34,41,42] One trial in the 1960s demonstrated no significant change in CHD events with ALA supplementation, but follow-up was limited to 1 year.[34] No other trials have tested the effects of ALA intake on CHD events, although several trials are planned or ongoing. Because ALA is an accessible and inexpensive source of n-3 PUFAs, better understanding of its effects is essential.

EICOSAPENTAENOIC ACID AND DOCOSAHEXAENOIC ACID. Controlled trials have demonstrated clear benefits of marine n-3 PUFAs on heart rate, BP, and TG levels, and potential benefits on cardiac relaxation and efficiency, inflammatory responses, endothelial function, autonomic tone, and urine proteinuria.[43-45] Small trials of prevention of recurrent ventricular tachyarrhythmias in patients with implantable cardioverter-defibrillators (ICDs) have yielded inconsistent results.[46] Meta-analyses of observational and clinical trial data have consistently indicated that longer-chain n-3 PUFAs reduce CHD events, especially fatal CHD or arrhythmic death (see Fig. 48-2),[13,33,42,43] in agreement with evidence from dog and primate models for the prevention of ischemia-induced ventricular fibrillation. Four of five large randomized controlled trials of fish or fish oil intake have demonstrated significant reductions in CHD events.[33,47] In a meta-analysis of randomized trials, fish oil supplementation reduced total mortality by 17% (RR, 0.83; 95% CI, 0.68 to 1.00; $P = 0.046$); these populations were generally higher risk, and effects on total mortality should be more modest in populations at lower risk of ischemia-induced arrhythmic death.[43] The dose-response relationship for preventing CHD death appears to be nonlinear, with substantial benefits up to approximately 250 mg/day of EPA plus DHA and then decreasing benefits thereafter.[43] Observational studies have suggested benefits for other endpoints, such as nonfatal MI, ischemic stroke, and atrial fibrillation, but intervention trials have not established these benefits.[33,42,43] In a randomized open-label trial in 18,645 Japanese subjects with statin-treated hypercholesterolemia, the addition of EPA (1.8 g/day for 4.6 years) reduced nonfatal coronary events by 19% ($P = 0.01$). Most studies have assessed combined intakes of EPA plus DHA; insufficient evidence exists to make recommendations about EPA versus DHA separately.

Trans Fatty Acids

TFA are unsaturated fats with at least one double bond in a trans configuration. Major dietary sources are foods made with partially hydrogenated oils, such as baked goods, deep-fried foods, packaged snacks, and shortening used for home cooking. Ruminant (e.g., cow, sheep, goat) meats and milk contain small amounts of TFAs, formed by gut microorganisms. Compared with TFAs from partially hydrogenated oils, the low levels of ruminant TFAs consumed (<0.5%E) do not appear to increase CVD risk appreciably.[48] Higher amounts of TFA intake have clear adverse lipid effects, including raising LDL-C, TG, and lipoprotein(a), lowering HDL-C, and increasing TC/HDL-C and apo B–to–apo-A-I ratios.[49] In contrast to other macronutrients, many of these adverse effects occur regardless of the type of nutrient replaced. In controlled feeding trials, consuming 1%E from TFAs in place of SFAs, MUFAs, or PUFAs raised the TC/HDL-C ratio by 0.031, 0.054, and 0.67, raised apo B by 3.5, 10.0, and 10.9 mg/liter, raised lipoprotein(a) by 3.8, 1.4, and 1.1 mg/liter, and decreased apo A-I by 7.0, 5.3, and 5.3 mg/liter, respectively.[49] Based on controlled trials, observational studies, and animal experiments, TFAs may also promote inflammation, endothelial dysfunction, insulin resistance, visceral adiposity, and arrhythmia.[50,51] The strength of the evidence for these nonlipid effects varies, but the implicated pathways suggest an unusual constellation of effects on adipocyte dysfunction and insulin resistance. In prospective cohorts, small amounts of TFA intake (e.g., 2 %E) were associated with a substantially higher risk of CHD and sudden death (see Fig. 48-2).[13,48] Numerous TFAs exist, each with varying dietary sources and biologic and physiologic effects. Emerging evidence suggests that 18-carbon TFAs, especially trans-18:2 isomers, may be most adverse.

Dietary Cholesterol

Dietary cholesterol raises both LDL-C and HDL-C, with a net increase in total cholesterol–to–HDL-C ratio of 0.02 units/100 mg dietary intake.[52] In animal experiments, dietary cholesterol is proatherogenic. Long-term prospective studies generally have shown no significant associations of dietary cholesterol or selected dietary sources (e.g., eggs, shellfish) with incident CVD.[13,53-55] Conversely, higher cholesterol, egg, or shellfish consumption is associated with a higher incidence of DM in five cohorts[56,57] and with higher CVD risk in patients with established DM in three cohorts,[53,58] suggesting potential interactions between dietary cholesterol, DM susceptibility, and CVD that require further study.

Protein

CVD effects of dietary protein have been relatively understudied. In short-term trials, protein intake in place of carbohydrates improves BP, TG and LDL-C levels, and possibly glycemic control.[59-61] In the setting of stable weight, higher protein diets lower HDL-C when replacing unsaturated fats. Few prospective cohorts have reported on total protein intake and CHD events, with generally null results.[62-65] In some studies, plant but not animal protein sources in diet associate with lower CHD risk,[63] suggesting that types of foods consumed or overall diet patterns may be more relevant than protein per se. Four cohorts have observed protective associations between animal protein intake and risk of hemorrhagic stroke[21]; this emerging relationship requires further study.

Foods

Controlled trials of cardiometabolic risk factors and prospective cohorts of disease endpoints have provided evidence for CVD effects of specific foods. Such effects often reflect the summed influence of a complex assortment of fatty acids, proteins, carbohydrate quality, micronutrients, and phytochemicals, making it difficult to pinpoint individual active constituents. Conversely, such summed effects have particular relevance for understanding effects of the whole food and for making dietary recommendations.

Fruits and Vegetables

Higher fruit and vegetable intake associates consistently with lower CHD incidence (**Fig. 48-3**).[66] Fruit intake is also associated with lower stroke risk[67] and dietary fiber from fruits with lower onset of DM (see Fig. 48-2). In controlled trials lasting up to 2 years, diets with an emphasis on consuming fruits and vegetables substantially improved multiple cardiometabolic risk factors, including BP, lipid levels, insulin resistance, inflammation, adiposity, and endothelial function.[28,61,68-72] In trials, the benefits of fruit and vegetable intake have not been reproduced with equivalent amounts of potassium, magnesium, and fiber supplements[73] and do not depend on the macronutrient (fat, protein, or carbohydrate) content of the diet.[28] This suggests that benefits are derived from a more complex set of micronutrients, phytochemicals, and fiber in fruits and vegetables, as well as from the replacement of less healthful foods. These studies provide convincing evidence that fruit and vegetable consumption lowers CVD risk. The benefits of specific types of fruits and vegetables, as well as of 100% juice, require further study.

Whole Versus Refined Grains

Whole grains contain endosperm, bran, and germ from the natural cereal; their refined counterparts are largely starchy endosperm (complex carbohydrate) with bran and germ removed. Bran contains fiber, B vitamins, minerals, flavonoids, and tocopherols; germ contains numerous antioxidants and phytochemicals. Intake of whole grains associates consistently with lower risk of CHD, DM, and possibly stroke (see Fig. 48-3). Whole-grain intake has been found to improve glucose-insulin homeostasis, endothelial function, and possibly weight loss and inflammation.[74-76] Whole-grain oats reduce LDL-C.[77] As with fruits and vegetables, it is not clear that any single micronutrient accounts for these benefits; the benefits may result from the synergistic effects of multiple constituents. Refined grain foods (e.g., carbohydrates in packaged foods, white bread, rice) have not associated consistently with incident CVD.[75] But such foods, together with starchy vegetables such as potatoes, are major contributors to dietary GI and GL, which in turn associate with higher CHD and DM risk (see Fig. 48-2). Whether this higher risk relates to replacement (e.g., relative absence of whole grains, fruits, vegetables), or to direct adverse effects on postprandial glucose-insulin, endothelial, and inflammatory responses, is unclear. Based on at best neutral effects, it seems prudent to limit frequency and portion sizes of refined grains, replacing them with whole grains, fruits, and vegetables.

Nuts

In prospective cohorts, modest nut consumption associates with lower CHD incidence (see Fig. 48-3).[13,78] Potentially bioactive constituents include unsaturated fats, vegetable protein, fiber, folate, minerals, tocopherols, and phenolic compounds.[79] In cross-sectional observational studies and controlled trials, nut intake lowers total and LDL-C and variably improves oxidative, inflammatory, and endothelial biomarkers.[79-83] Nut intake associates with lower body mass index (BMI) in observational studies and similar or greater weight loss in intervention trials.[84] Effects of different types of nuts require further study, but benefits in short-term trials and the magnitude and consistency of lower risk in observational studies support the importance of modest nut consumption for lowering CHD risk.

Legumes

CVD effects of legumes (beans) are not well established. Trials of soy foods have demonstrated nonsignificant trends toward lowering of SBP and DBP (−5.8 and −4.0 mm Hg, respectively).[85] Isolated soy protein or isoflavones (phytoestrogens) have smaller effects, with modest reductions in LDL-C (−3%) and DBP (−2 mm Hg).[85,86] Legumes provide an overall package of micronutrients, phytochemicals, and fiber that could reduce CVD and DM; this hypothesis requires further evaluation in controlled interventions and long-term cohorts.

Fish

More prospective cohorts have reported on fish intake and CHD events than any other dietary factor (see Fig. 48-3). Benefits appear strongest for CHD mortality, with observed lower risk of 15% for intake once weekly, 23% for two to four times weekly, and 38% for five or more times weekly.[87] Nutrients include unsaturated fats, selenium, and vitamin D, but prevention of CHD death appears mainly related to n-3 PUFAs in fish (see earlier, "Eicosapentaenoic Acid and Docosahexaenoic Acid"). In a pooled analysis of 16 prospective cohorts from the United States, Europe, China, and Japan, consumption of 250 mg/day of EPA plus DHA from fish associated with 36% lower CHD mortality, and four of five large randomized controlled trials demonstrated reductions in CHD events with fish or fish oil intake.[33] Consumption of fish also associates with a lower risk of nonfatal MI, ischemic stroke, and possibly atrial fibrillation,[43,88] but controlled trials have not yet established these benefits. Fish intake was recently linked to more frequently diagnosed DM (comparing five times/week or more with less than once/month, 22% higher risk)[89]; n-3 PUFAs regulate hepatic genes (e.g., *PPAR-α, SREBP-1*) and may modestly raise glucose production and reduce hyperinsulinemia without causing peripheral insulin resistance or metabolic dysfunction.[90,91] Fish and n-3 PUFAs improve other metabolic risks (e.g., TG, BP, inflammation).[33,43] Types of fish consumed and preparation methods may influence blood EPA and DHA levels and CVD effects, with greatest benefits from nonfried oily (dark meat) fish that contain up to 10-fold more n-3 PUFAs than other species.[43,57,92-94] Evidence for possible CVD effects of methylmercury found in a few fish species is limited and conflicting; if modest adverse effects occur, these may reduce net CVD benefits of some fish consumed.[43]

Meats

Based on SFA and cholesterol content, meat consumption has been thought to increase CVD risk. Relationships of total meat intake with incident CHD and DM are mixed, with overall nonsignificant trends toward higher risk (see Fig. 48-3).[13,95,96] When types of meat are evaluated separately, the intake of processed meats, but not unprocessed red meats, associates more consistently with higher risk of CHD and DM. These findings suggest that different types of meat may have different cardiometabolic effects that may relate to wide variations in preservatives (e.g., sodium, nitrites) or preparation methods (e.g., frying, commercial cooking), or to smaller variations in the contents of specific fatty acids or heme iron. Few studies have reported on meat intake and incident stroke,[96] limiting conclusions for this endpoint.

Dairy Products

Biologic effects of dairy foods are still being elucidated. Milk or dairy intake increases fecal fat excretion but inconsistently affects satiety and weight loss.[97,98] DASH (Dietary Approaches to Stop Hypertension)–type diet patterns that include low-fat dairy products improve BP, lipid levels, insulin resistance, and endothelial function,[28,69,70,73] but these trials cannot confirm isolated effects of dairy products. Long-term observational studies have suggested that dairy consumption associates with lower risk of CHD, stroke, and DM (see Fig. 48-3), as well as lower risk of metabolic syndrome or its components.[99] Overall, these studies suggest potential benefits of dairy intake for cardiometabolic risk, but active constituents have not been established. Calcium and linoleic acid have been proposed as potential mediators, but experimental studies of each have shown small or no effects on risk factors. Potentially different effects of low-fat versus whole-fat dairy products are also unclear. Low-fat dairy is currently recommended, given its lower SFA and calories, but if benefits are partly related to bioactive fatty acids, whole-fat dairy could have similar or even greater benefits.

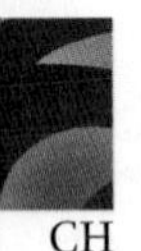

	Endpoint	No. of studies	No. of subjects	No. of events	Unit	RR (95% CI)
Fruits						
	Total CHD	10 PCs[13]	222,706	—	High vs. low quantile	0.80 (0.66-0.93)
	Total CHD	6 PCs[67]	184,412	3,346	Each serving/d	0.93 (0.89-0.96)
	Total stroke	5 PCs[68]	210,601	1,853	Each serving/d	0.89 (0.85-0.93)
	Ischemic stroke	4 PCs[68]	209,769	1,756	Each serving/d	0.88 (0.85-0.92)
Vegetables						
	Total CHD	9 PCs[13]	220,564	—	High vs. low quantile	0.77 (0.68-0.87)
	Total CHD	7 PCs[67]	199,632	3,833	Each serving/d	0.89 (0.83-0.95)
	Total stroke	4 PCs[68]	172,164	933	Each serving/d	0.97 (0.92-1.04)
	Ischemic stroke	3 PCs[68]	171,332	836	Each serving/d	0.99 (0.93-1.04)
Whole Grains						
	Total CHD	11 PCs[13]	356,070	—	High vs. low quantile	0.81 (0.75-0.86)
	Total CHD	6 PCs[76]	284,841	4,385	2.5 vs. 0.2 servings/d	0.76 (0.69-0.83)
	Total stroke	4 PCs[76]	208,143	933	2.5 vs. 0.2 servings/d	0.83 (0.68-1.02)
	Total CVD	7 PCs[76]	285,376	6,504	2.5 vs. 0.2 servings/d	0.79 (0.73-0.85)
	Diabetes	6 PCs[75]	286,125	10,944	Each 2 servings/d	0.79 (0.72-0.87)
Nuts						
	Total CHD	6 PCs[13]	184,194	—	High vs. low quantile	0.70 (0.57-0.82)
	CHD death	4 PCs[79]	153,604	1,597	4 servings/wk vs. never	0.63 (0.51-0.83)
Fish						
	Total CHD	29 PCs[13]	363,228	—	High vs. low quantile	0.81 (0.70-0.92)
	CHD death	13 PCs[88]	222,364	3,032	5+/wk vs. <1/mo	0.62 (0.46-0.82)
	Nonfatal MI	5 PCs[88]	181,151	2,216	5+/wk vs. <1/mo	0.79 (0.64-0.99)
	Total stroke	8 PCs[89]	200,575	3,491	5+/wk vs. <1/mo	0.69 (0.54-0.88)
	Ischemic stroke	3 PCs[89]	154,337	1,138	5+/wk vs. <1/mo	0.65 (0.46-0.93)
	Hemorrhagic stroke	3 PCs[89]	154,337	548	5+/wk vs. <1/mo	0.80 (0.44-1.47)
Meats						
Total meats	Total CHD	12 PCs[13]	236,414	—	High vs. low quantile	1.23 (0.98-1.49)
	Diabetes	4 PCs[96]	180,205	5,579	Each serving/d (120 g)	1.26 (0.84-1.88)
Unprocessed red meats	Total CHD	4 PCs[97]	56,311	1,252	Each serving/d (100 g)	1.00 (0.81-1.23)
	Diabetes	5 PCs[97]	298,982	7,582	Each serving/d (100 g)	1.16 (0.92-1.46)
Processed meats	Total CHD	6 PCs[97]	614,062	21,336	Each serving/d (50 g)	1.42 (1.07-1.89)
	Diabetes	8 PCs[96]	372,205	9,456	Each serving/d (50 g)	1.57 (1.28-1.93)
	Diabetes	7 PCs[97]	302,725	8,331	Each serving/d (50 g)	1.19 (1.11-1.27)
Milk/Dairy						
	Total CHD	11 PCs[101]	263,346	7,434	High vs. low quantile	0.91 (0.82-1.00)
	Total CHD	8 PCs[13]	216,820	—	High vs. low quantile	0.94 (0.75-1.13)
	Total stroke	7 PCs[101]	414,097	14,358	High vs. low quantile	0.79 (0.75-0.82)
	Diabetes	4 PCs[101]	120,263	4,851	High vs. low quantile	0.92 (0.86-0.97)
Eggs						
	Total CHD	6 PCs[13]	258,221	—	High vs. low quantile	1.06 (0.89-1.23)

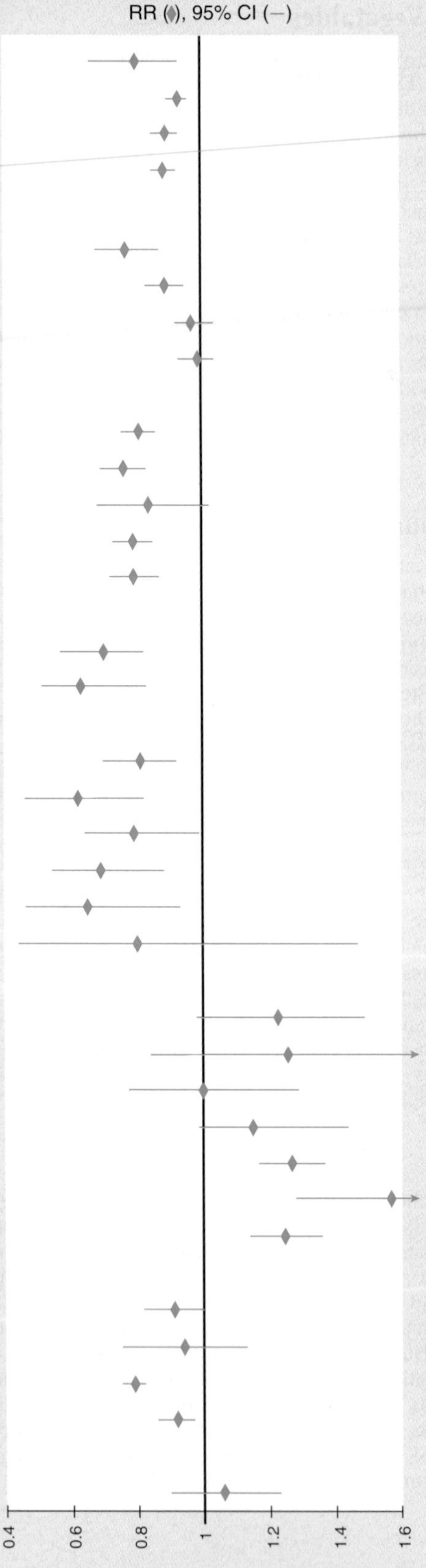

FIGURE 48-3 Meta-analyses of foods and incidence of coronary heart disease (CHD), stroke, and diabetes. PC = prospective cohort. RCT = randomized controlled trial. — = not reported.

Among observational studies of CHD, DM, or metabolic syndrome, three suggested greater benefits of low-fat dairy, three suggested similar effects of low-fat and whole-fat dairy, and one suggested greater benefits of whole-fat dairy.[100] Few controlled trials have directly compared low-fat and whole-fat products. In a trial of 45 young healthy volunteers provided 3.5 daily servings of low-fat or whole-fat dairy (milk and yogurt) for 8 weeks, similar effects on BP were seen, but consumption of whole-fat dairy led to 1.2 kg greater weight gain.[101] The effects of specific dairy products (e.g., milk, cheese, butter) also require further investigation; for example, in three controlled trials, cheese raised total cholesterol and LDL-C less than an equivalent intake of butter.[102-104]

Beverages

Alcohol

Habitual heavy alcohol consumption (see Chap. 73) causes up to one third of nonischemic dilated cardiomyopathy in many countries.[105] Ventricular dysfunction is often irreversible, even when alcohol use is stopped; continued drinking associates with high mortality. Higher habitual intake and acute binges may increase the risk of atrial fibrillation, sometimes termed *holiday heart*.[106] Compared with nondrinkers, regular moderate consumption, up to two drinks per day for men and one drink per day for women, is associated with lower incidence of CHD and DM.[13,107] Benefits may be overstated in these observational analyses because of inclusion among the nondrinkers of former drinkers who had quit because of poor health.[108] Nevertheless, the magnitude and consistency of the observed lower risks, together with the favorable effects of alcohol on HDL-C and insulin resistance in controlled trials,[109,110] provide convincing evidence for at least modest cardiometabolic benefit of moderate alcohol intake. Meaningful differences have not been seen among types of drinks (e.g., wine, beer, liquor), but drinking patterns appear important, with the greatest benefits seen in those who drink moderate amounts regularly (i.e., over several days per week), rather than irregular or binge drinking.[111] Because of high rates of alcohol-related accidents, homicides, and suicides, especially in young adults, alcohol use has net adverse effects on population mortality.[1] Thus, it is not advisable as a means to reduce CVD risk, but adults who already drink alcohol can continue to consume it moderately from a cardiovascular risk perspective.

Coffee and Tea

Caffeine supplements raise BP and acutely worsen insulin sensitivity and glucose tolerance; similar amounts of caffeine consumed from coffee may have smaller effects, suggesting other partly offsetting factors.[112,113] Results from 21 prospective cohorts have suggested no significant relationship between coffee use and CHD risk.[114] Very frequent coffee use (four or more cups daily) associates with lower DM incidence,[115] but a biologic basis for this observation is not yet established. Short-term trials have suggested that green tea intake may augment weight loss and weight maintenance[116]; however, consistent effects are not seen on endothelial function, BP, or cholesterol levels.[85] Observational studies of tea drinking and CHD endpoints are inconsistent; very frequent use (three or more cups daily) associates with a modestly lower risk of stroke and DM.[117,118] Mixed results of observational studies and a lack of clear physiologic benefits in trials currently do not allow definitive conclusions about the CVD effects of coffee or tea (see chapter on website for more details).

Sugar-Sweetened Beverages

Ecologic and cohort data suggest causal effects of sugar-sweetened beverage (SSB) intake on adiposity. Calories from beverages increased from 11.8% to 21.0% of all calories consumed in the United States from 1965 to 2002, an increase of 222 kcal/person/day.[119] SSBs (largely sodas and colas, but also sweetened fruit drinks) comprised 60% of this increase; alcohol comprised 32%; and 100% fruit juices comprised 9%. The average American teenage boy or girl consumes 22 and 15 8-oz servings, respectively, of SSBs each week[120]; most of this consumption occurs at home.[121] Observational studies generally find positive associations between SSB intake and adiposity or weight gain; controlled trials of SSB reduction have shown mixed results, possibly because of variable intervention efficacy.[122] Short-term trials have suggested that calories in liquid form may be less satiating and thus increase the total quantity of calories consumed, compared with solid foods.[123,124] In post hoc analyses of an 18-month diet trial, reduction in liquid calories were related most strongly to weight loss; each daily serving of reduced SSBs associated with 0.65 kg greater weight loss.[125] In prospective cohort studies, higher SSB intake predicted higher incidence of DM and metabolic syndrome.[126-129a] SSB intake has also been linked to incident CHD in cohort studies.[130,130a]

Milk

See earlier, "Dairy Products."

Micronutrients

Sodium

Dietary sources of sodium (see Chaps. 1 and 45) vary worldwide.[131] In North America and Europe, 75% comes from packaged foods, with the minority naturally occurring or added at home. In contrast, in Asian countries, most sodium is added at home or from soy sauce. In a meta-analysis of 28 trials lasting 4 weeks or longer, reducing sodium by approximately 1800 mg/day lowered SBP and DBP by 5.0 and 2.7 mm Hg in hypertensive individuals, and by 2.0 and 1.0 mm Hg in normotensive individuals.[132] Effects are larger in blacks than in whites[133] and also larger when overall dietary quality is suboptimal (see later, "Dietary Patterns"). In two large Japanese cohorts, higher dietary sodium was associated with CVD mortality, largely due to a twofold higher risk of ischemic stroke.[134,135] In contrast, higher dietary sodium associated with trends toward *lower* CVD mortality in the National Health and Nutrition Examination Survey (NHANES),[136] although earlier studies suggested a positive relationship between dietary sodium and CVD death and incident heart failure when restricted to overweight adults. Two cohorts evaluating 24-hour urine sodium, a more accurate measure of dietary intake, observed positive associations with CVD events, including a 42% higher risk per approximately 2700 mg/day of dietary sodium[137]; a third cohort found no significant association between 24-hour urine sodium and CVD events.[138] Mixed results of these studies may be the result of varying measurement error or differing sensitivity of the underlying population to the effects of sodium—for example, differences in hypertensive status, ethnicity, or background diet. In post hoc analyses of two completed sodium reduction trials, dietary sodium reductions of approximately 965 mg/day during interventions lasting up to 4 years reduced CVD events by 25% (95% CI, 1 to 43%, $P = 0.04$) after 10 to 15 years of follow-up.[139] Relatively few prospective studies have reported on the relationship between dietary sodium and CVD events, raising concerns about publication bias and many unreported null findings. Nonetheless, sodium intake convincingly alters BP and, based on these relatively few studies of disease events, has probable causal relationships with CVD, especially stroke.

Other Minerals

Vegetables, fruits, whole grains, legumes, nuts, and dairy are major sources of minerals. In observational studies, dietary sources of potassium, calcium, and magnesium are linked to lower BP and, in some studies, to a lower risk of CVD events. A meta-analysis of 33 potassium supplement trials demonstrated modest reductions in SBP and DBP (−3.1 and −2.0 mm Hg), with effects appearing strongest when dietary sodium intake was high. In six trials limited to hypertensive patients, potassium supplements produced larger reductions in SBP and DBP

(−11.2 and −5.0 mm Hg), but these effects did not achieve statistical significance.[140] Trials of calcium supplements that often included vitamin D found small reductions in SBP and DBP (−1.9 and −1.0 mm Hg).[141] Thirteen trials using calcium alone in hypertensive patients demonstrated similar small reductions in SBP and DBP (−2.5 and −0.8 mm Hg); heterogeneity suggested potential overestimation of effects.[140] Twelve trials of magnesium supplements in hypertensive patients showed modestly lower DBP (−2.2 mm Hg), but again with significant heterogeneity.[140] Overall, the evidence indicates that potassium modestly lowers BP, more so in hypertensive patients or when dietary sodium is high; evidence for calcium and magnesium is mixed, and BP effects may be smaller.

Antioxidants and Vitamins

B vitamins (e.g., thiamin) are diet-derived, water-soluble, and renally excreted. B vitamin deficiency is a known cause of cardiomyopathy (beriberi) in developing countries, and emerging evidence suggests that patients with chronic heart failure may commonly have lower B vitamin levels.[142,143] Whether this latter deficiency relates to poor nutritional status, diuretic-induced urinary loss, or other metabolic causes—or whether replacement improves clinical outcomes—remains unknown.

Several dietary vitamins and nutrients are associated with lower CVD risk in observational studies, but multiple trials of supplements, including folate, B vitamins, beta-carotene, vitamin C, vitamin E, and selenium, have shown no significant effects on atherosclerosis progression or CVD events (see Chap. 49).[13,144-146] Many of these trials, for reasons of power, evaluated individuals with established CVD or clinical risk factors, whereas most observational studies evaluated generally healthy individuals. Thus, discrepancies in findings could partly be related to different time periods of biologic sensitivity (i.e., some vitamins and nutrients could be important only early in the disease course). Such explanations should be considered speculative until confirmed in prospective studies and trials. Discrepancies between observational studies and supplement trials more likely relate to residual bias in observational studies from other lifestyle behaviors (i.e., observed benefits are not caused by diet) or because of other nutritional factors (i.e., observed benefits are caused by diet but not by the specifically identified vitamins or nutrients). Diets higher in beta-carotene and other vitamins, for example, are often rich in fruits and vegetables that contain a number of other beneficial factors, including other antioxidants, minerals, phytochemicals, and dietary fiber, as well as having replacement effects for less healthy foods. Thus, isolating one or even several components would unlikely produce similar effects as from consuming the whole food, as seen in short-term trials of fruits and vegetables versus supplements.

Two cohorts have found that plasma vitamin D levels, largely driven by sun exposure, are inversely associated with CVD events.[147,148] Trials of vitamin D supplements show inconclusive effects on BP,[149] and the WHI trial in 36,282 postmenopausal women showed no effects on incident CHD (RR, 1.04; 95% CI, 0.92 to 1.18), stroke (RR, 0.95; 95% CI, 0.82 to 1.10), or DM (RR, 1.01; 95% CI, 0.94 to 1.10).[150,151] A meta-analysis of 18 vitamin D trials (mean dose, 528 IU/day) in 57,311 participants suggested a modest benefit for total mortality (RR, 0.93; 95% CI, 0.87 to 0.99),[152] but whether this result was related to fewer deaths from CVD or cancers, which might be prevented by vitamin D, was not evaluated. High plasma vitamin D levels may be needed for CVD benefits; if so, brief sun exposure can provide high levels efficiently compared with dietary intake.

Marine n-3 PUFAs are a notable exception to discordance between observational studies and supplement trials. Observational studies of habitual fish intake and controlled trials of fish oil supplements have shown similar effects on CVD risk factors; numerous prospective cohorts of generally healthy individuals have demonstrated lower risk of CHD death with fish intake; four of five randomized controlled trials in individuals with and without established CHD have demonstrated significant reductions in CVD events with fish or fish oil intake; and, in a meta-analysis of controlled trials, fish oil supplementation lowered total mortality (see earlier, "Eicosapentaenoic Acid and Docosahexaenoic Acid," "Fish").

Flavonoids

Flavonoids are bioactive polyphenols that include flavonols (in onions, broccoli, tea, and various fruits), flavones (in parsley, celery, and chamomile tea), flavanones (in citrus fruits), flavanols such as catechins and procyanidins (in cocoa, apples, grapes, red wine, and tea), anthocyanidins (in colored berries), and isoflavones (in soy).[85,153] In laboratory experiments and short-term trials, flavonoids lower BP and exhibit antioxidant, antiplatelet, and anti-inflammatory effects.[153] In trials, intake of cocoa or dark chocolate improves endothelial function and reduces SBP and DBP (−5.9 and −3.3 mm Hg).[85] BP lowering occurs with as little as 6.3 g (30 kcal)/day of dark chocolate, increases over time, and is related to increased endothelial nitric oxide production.[154] This restorative mechanism suggests important benefits beyond lowering of BP, because nitric oxide–related endothelial dysfunction is fundamental to atherosclerotic and metabolic diseases. A few short-term trials of other dietary sources (e.g., tea, red wine or grapes) or of specific flavonoid extracts have not consistently found improved endothelial function, BP, or lipid levels.[85] In prospective cohorts evaluating total or selected dietary flavonoids and risk of CVD, 9 of 12 cohorts observed lower CHD death (pooled RR, 0.81 across tertiles; 95% CI, 0.71 to 0.92).[153,155,156] Heterogeneity of specific flavonoids and their dietary sources limits inference for class effects, but observed lower risk of CHD death plus endothelial and BP benefits of cocoa or dark chocolate provide strong impetus for further study.

Further Considerations

Energy Balance

Energy balance, or calories expended versus calories consumed, is the principal determinant of weight gain and adiposity (see website for references for this section). Calorie expenditure is influenced by physical activity, body size, muscle mass, age, and sex that together with goals for weight loss, gain, or stability, determine the need for dietary calories. Some individuals may consume more calories but have neutral or negative energy balance (because of high calories expended), whereas others may consume fewer calories but have positive energy balance (because of low calories expended). Thus, metrics of weight or adiposity provide the most practical tools to assess energy balance.

A number of factors influence energy balance. Societal and environmental determinants include education, income, and race or ethnicity; the presence of fast food restaurants, grocery stores, safety considerations related to crime, parks or open spaces, and walking or biking paths; and advertising, social norms, and work and home dynamics. Ultimately, these influences act through changes in diet and/or physical activity to influence adiposity. Where sufficient data are available, the recent obesity epidemic appears temporally related to increased energy intake in developed nations, and to increased intake and decreased expenditure in some developing nations (see Chap. 1). Both diet quantity and quality influence energy intake. Dietary factors linked to excess consumption include larger portion sizes, higher intake of SSBs, processed snacks, energy-dense foods, fast-food meals, and trans fat, and lower intake of fruits, vegetables, and whole grains. More time watching television and lower average sleep duration also are associated with energy imbalance and adiposity, with evidence that their effects may be related more closely to changes in energy intake than expenditure.

Habitual excess energy intakes as small as approximately 50 kcal/day are sufficient to explain the gradual weight gain seen in most individuals. This makes unintended weight gain very easy, but also means that modest lifestyle and environmental changes can mitigate or reverse such energy gaps and adiposity.

Compared with types and quality of foods consumed, dietary macronutrient composition (i.e., %E from fat, protein, or carbohydrates) has little effect on energy balance. Ad libitum diet trials through 2000 and the recent WHI trial have observed that low-fat diet interventions associate with initial weight loss, but many of these trials were not randomized and all were confounded by intervention intensity: low-fat groups had active dietary advice with multiple counseling visits, group sessions, and follow-up contacts, whereas control groups had no intervention. In contrast, multiple randomized trials with equal intensity intervention in each diet arm have provided convincing evidence that macronutrient composition has little effect on weight loss.

Dietary Patterns

The study of individual nutrients and foods provides important information about biologic pathways and health effects, but growing evidence indicates that overall dietary quality is equally relevant. Several diet patterns, including the Prudent, DASH-type, and Mediterranean-type diets, significantly reduce CVD risk factors in controlled trials and are consistently linked to lower onset of CHD, stroke, and DM in prospective cohorts.[13,19,59,68,157] A Mediterranean-type diet also reduced CVD events, compared with a low total fat and low-SFA diet, in a randomized trial in patients with recent MI.[158] Rather than targeting single risk factors, overall diet patterns improve multiple pathways of risk, including BP, glucose-insulin homeostasis, blood lipids, inflammation, endothelial function, arrhythmic risk, and possibly coagulation and thrombosis.

These dietary patterns share several characteristics that highlight key features of a cardiometabolically healthy diet (**Table 48-1**).[19] These characteristies include a diet rich in whole foods such as fruits, vegetables, whole grains, and nuts, including fish, modest dairy intake, and vegetable oils, and with lower intakes of SSBs and processed, energy-dense, and deep-fried foods. Moderate intake of unprocessed meats, poultry, and alcohol can also be part of a healthier food–based dietary pattern. Such diets are naturally higher in fiber, antioxidants, minerals, phytochemicals, and unsaturated fats, and lower in salt, TFAs, and SFAs. Appropriate caloric intake and physical activity are also critical for preventing adiposity and DM, supported by the diet pattern described and by modest portion sizes, limited television watching, and adequate sleep. Focus on the overall diet pattern, rather than on individual foods or nutrients, can be effective for both individual counseling and population recommendations by facilitating communication, allowing individual flexibility and preferences in diet choices, and increasing health impact because of the combined benefits of multiple modest changes.

Individual Susceptibility

See website for details.

Changing Behavior (see Chap. 49)

Current evidence permits recommendation of many specific dietary habits to prevent and treat cardiometabolic risk factors and conditions (**Table 48-2**; see Table 48-1). Translation of this knowledge into behaviors is critical (see website for references for this section). Cigarette and food industries have mastered the science of behavioral change; clinical and public health expertise lag behind. Nevertheless, a growing knowledge base now highlights several effective individual- and population-based strategies. By combining such methods, many developed countries have dramatically reduced tobacco use since the 1950s, and the promotion of seatbelt, bike helmet, and sunscreen use has also had success. These efforts provide a roadmap for combined strategies to improve diet. Because modest dietary differences can substantially alter disease risk at the population level, large changes are frequently unnecessary. Also, relative to most drugs, devices, and procedures, changes in diet are low risk, low cost, and broadly available—advantages that are highly germane to disease prevention and treatment.

INDIVIDUAL-BASED STRATEGIES. Several features of the health care system can facilitate behavior change at the individual patient level, including provider familiarity with key dietary factors for improving CVD health, practical tools for assessing and following dietary habits, evidence-based strategies for behavior change and monitoring, and prevention-oriented care systems. Some evidence suggests that

TABLE 48-1 Food-Based Components of Dietary Patterns that Improve Cardiometabolic Health*

RECOMMENDATION	GOAL†	SERVING SIZE
Consume More		
Fruits	Four to five servings/day	One medium-sized fruit; ½ cup of fresh, frozen, or canned fruit; ¼ cup of dried fruit; ½ cup of 100% juice; goals should not be met with juice alone
Vegetables	Four to five servings/day	1 cup of raw leafy vegetable; ½ cup of cut-up raw vegetables, cooked vegetables, or 100% juice; limit starchy vegetables such as potatoes to ½ cup or less/day
Whole grains‡	Three or more servings/day, in place of refined grains	One slice of whole-grain bread; 1 cup of high-fiber whole-grain cereal; ½ cup cooked whole-grain rice, pasta, or cereal
Nuts	Four to five servings/wk	50 g (1.75 oz)
Fish and shellfish	Two or more servings/wk, preferably oily	100 g (3.5 oz); goals should not be met with commercially prepared deep-fried or breaded fish
Dairy products§	Two to three servings/day	1 cup of milk or yogurt; 1.5 oz of cheese
Vegetable oils	Two to six servings/day	1 teaspoon oil (e.g., in cooking or salad dressing); 1 tablespoon vegetable spread
Consume Less		
Foods containing partially hydrogenated vegetable oils (trans fat)	Avoid intake	
Processed meats (e.g., bacon, sausage, hot dogs, processed deli meats)	Limit intake (e.g., up to two servings/wk)	100 g (3.5 oz)
Sugar-sweetened beverages, sweets, and bakery foods	Limit intake (e.g., up to five servings/wk)	8 oz of soda; one small cookie, doughnut, or muffin; one slice of cake or pie
Alcohol	Up to two drinks daily for men, one drink daily for women	5 oz wine; 12 oz beer; 1.5 oz other alcoholic beverage
Energy balance	Reduce portion sizes, increase physical activity, limit TV watching, ensure adequate sleep	

*Adapted from the evidence described in this chapter, together with USDA and AHA guidelines.[18,19] Food-based recommendations can facilitate communication and translation to individual patients and populations. Dietary patterns containing these components are naturally higher in fiber, antioxidants, minerals, and phytochemicals and lower in salt, saturated fat, and trans fat.

†Based on a 2000 kcal/day diet. Servings should be adjusted accordingly for higher or lower energy consumption.

‡Or potentially whole legumes (beans), although evidence for equivalent effects is limited. Characterization of whole-grain content in packaged foods is challenging; pragmatically, sufficient whole-grain content could be defined by the fiber content of whole wheat (i.e., at least 1.1 g of naturally occurring dietary fiber per 10 g of carbohydrate).

§Based on indirect lines of evidence, most guidelines recommend low-fat dairy products.

CH 48

TABLE 48-2 Effects of Food and Nutrients on Specific Cardiometabolic Risk Factors and Disease Endpoints

RISK FACTOR OR DISEASE	*Strength of Evidence for Benefits** CONVINCING	PROBABLE	POSSIBLE	INSUFFICIENT EVIDENCE FOR EFFECTS
Hypertension	Higher intakes of Mediterranean- or DASH-type dietary pattern, dietary fiber, fruits and vegetables, fish or fish oil, cocoa or dark chocolate, potassium; lower intake of sodium	Higher intakes of calcium, soy foods; lower intake of caffeine	Higher intakes of whole grains, magnesium, vitamin D, soy protein; MUFAs in place of SFAs	Isoflavones; coffee or tea; PUFAs or carbohydrates in place of SFAs
High LDL-C	Higher intakes of MUFAs or PUFAs, dietary fiber, fruits and vegetables, green tea, soy protein; lower intakes of trans fat, SFAs (12:0-16:0), dietary cholesterol	Higher intakes of dairy, whole grains; lower intake of unfiltered coffee		
Atherogenic dyslipidemia (low HDL-C, high triglycerides)	Higher intakes of Mediterranean- or DASH-type dietary pattern, MUFAs or PUFAs, fish or fish oil; lower intakes of simple or complex refined carbohydrates (high GI or GL), trans fat	Higher intake of dairy products	Higher intakes of fruits and vegetables	
Insulin-resistant type 2 diabetes	Higher intake of whole grains; lower intake of processed meats; moderate alcohol use	Higher intakes of PUFAs or vegetable oils, dairy products; lower intake of simple or complex refined carbohydrates (high GI or GL)	Higher intakes of fruits and vegetables, MUFAs or PUFAs in place of SFAs, coffee; lower intake of dietary cholesterol, trans fats	Carbohydrates in place of SFAs; unprocessed meats; fish or fish oil; tea
Obesity	Higher intakes of whole unprocessed foods (e.g., whole grains, vegetables, nuts, fruits); lower intake of sugar-sweetened beverages	Higher intake of dietary fiber; lower intakes of large portion sizes, simple or complex refined carbohydrates (high GI or GL), energy-dense foods (high carbohydrate–low fiber or high fat); less TV watching	Higher intakes of green tea; lower intakes of deep-fried foods, meals from fast food restaurants, trans fat; longer sleep duration	Total fat (%E); SFAs, MUFAs, or PUFAs
Systemic inflammation	Higher intakes of fruits and vegetables	Higher intakes of Mediterranean- or DASH-type diet pattern, whole grains, fish oil (supplements); lower intakes of TFAs	Higher intakes of fish, fish oil (diet), ALA, PUFAs, nuts; lower intakes of simple or complex refined carbohydrates (high GI, GL)	SFAs or MUFAs
Coronary heart disease	Higher intakes of fish or fish oil (CHD mortality), PUFAs in place of SFAs, Mediterranean- or DASH-type dietary pattern, fruits and vegetables, whole grains, nuts, dietary fiber; lower intakes of trans fat, processed meats; moderate alcohol use	Lower intakes of simple or complex refined carbohydrates (high GI or GL), dietary cholesterol in patients with diabetes	Higher intakes of fish or fish oil (nonfatal CHD); dairy, legumes, ALA, MUFAs in place of SFAs, vitamin D; lower intakes of sodium, unprocessed meats, dietary cholesterol in patients without diabetes	Total fat (% E); carbohydrates in place of SFAs; antioxidant or vitamin supplements; coffee or tea
Ischemic stroke	Higher intakes of Mediterranean- or DASH-type dietary pattern, fruits, whole grains	Higher intake of fish; lower intake of sodium	Higher intakes of vegetables, SFAs, fish oil, tea; lower intakes of processed meats	ALA; antioxidant or vitamin supplements
Hemorrhagic stroke		Higher intakes of whole grains, Mediterranean- or DASH-type dietary pattern; lower intake of sodium	Higher intakes of SFAs, animal protein, tea	Fish or fish oil
Heart failure†	Lower intake of heavy alcohol use		Higher intakes of Mediterranean- or DASH-type dietary pattern, whole grains, fish; moderate alcohol use	
Atrial fibrillation		Lower intake of heavy alcohol use	Higher intake of fish or fish oil	

*Strength of evidence defined by World Health Organization criteria.[20] For most dietary factors, evidence is derived from controlled trials of risk factors plus long-term prospective cohorts of disease endpoints. For fish, EPA + DHA, omega-6 PUFAs, and total fat intake, evidence is also derived from randomized trials of CHD endpoints.

†Incidence; limited data on dietary treatment for secondary prevention, except for one large randomized trial of EPA + DHA supplementation that reduced total mortality and clinical experience with sodium restriction to prevent fluid overload.

practitioners recognize the importance of nutrition but inconsistently use tailored guidance or monitoring. Variable knowledge barriers have been identified, including inadequate relevant training in medical school and residency. For practicing providers, education and live and media presentations can improve provider knowledge and performance. Providers and patients also benefit from consultation and assistance from allied professionals for dietary counseling and intervention. Emphasizing foods to be consumed for good health, rather than just foods to be avoided, may also improve success. Familiarity with selected evidence-based foods and dietary patterns (see Tables 48-1 and 48-2), rather than comprehensive nutritional expertise, is an effective goal for providers.

Accessible tools for dietary evaluation are important to facilitate clinical assessment and monitoring of progress. Brief self-administered diet questionnaires could be completed at home or in the waiting room, but lack of systematic evaluation or consensus about the best tool has limited their widespread use. Validated biomarkers are available for some nutrients and fatty acids, but their roles in clinical practice require further study. Until standardized questionnaires and/or biomarker panels are developed and evaluated, practitioners can perform simple office-based assessments by asking patients about selected modifiable dietary habits. Because targeted goals are also most effective, physicians should focus on those dietary factors with the strongest evidence base, individualizing as necessary based on the risk factor or disease condition of greatest interest (see Table 48-2).

Randomized trials have demonstrated that dietary advice alone improves dietary habits, including changes in the intakes of fruits, vegetables, dietary fiber, sodium, and fats, as well as corresponding improvements in BP and lipid levels. Several evidence-based strategies are effective, including the following: individual sessions to assess readiness for behavior change, collaboratively identify goals, and develop plans to achieve these goals; a focus on specific proximal goals for targeted behaviors; self-monitoring with oral, written, or electronic feedback; group sessions for peer support, problem solving, and skill development for behavior change; and trained motivational interviewing when individuals are ambivalent about change. Supplementary strategies include long-term support from family, peers, or community programs, especially after several months, when adherence often wanes, and electronic feedback or e-counseling. Imperfect success should not dissuade efforts. Compliance with both behavioral and drug treatments is incomplete but such strategies, even imperfectly implemented, can improve clinical outcomes.

Many health care systems are structured toward the detection and treatment of acute illness, rather than the prevention and management of chronic disease. These limitations can be improved by using planned visits for individual or group education and medical care, and by adding methods for sustained in-person, telephone, or electronic follow-up. Such efforts are complemented by changes in quality and reimbursement guidelines that support behavior change efforts, now being developed and implemented by some private and public payers.

POPULATION-BASED STRATEGIES. Whereas individual-based approaches can effectively improve diet, population-based strategies at national, state, community, school, or workplace levels can have a larger and more sustained impact. Overlapping approaches include policy and legislation, media and other educational campaigns, environmental change, and social and community supports. Population-based interventions have most success when multiple stakeholders, including policy makers, community members, and local organizations, are involved throughout planning, implementation, and sustainability stages.

Policy and legislation can substantially alter—either improving or worsening—behaviors and risk factors by altering knowledge, access, and environments related to food. Simple policy approaches have proven effective at targeting specific nutrients, such as trans fat and sodium, for population-wide reduction. Subsidies, taxation, and point-of-purchase prompts can influence food selection, especially when price differences are larger or among price-sensitive groups (e.g., children and adolescents, lower socioeconomic groups). Compared with other policy strategies, media or other educational campaigns alone are often less successful at improving diet; intensive campaigns with a simple message or "healthy choice" logos are often most effective. It is unclear whether posting ingredients or calories on food labels and menu boards alters consumer behavior, but such labeling at least partly alters industry behavior in terms of what is offered. Regulation of advertising has been important for antismoking efforts; similar strategies have been proposed for children's television programs, which largely advertise processed foods, fast foods, and SSBs.

Social and physical environments, together with family and community supports, also influence behavior. Schools and workplaces are important settings for monitoring risk and implementing behavioral and policy approaches to improving diet. Multipronged interventions, including educational curricula, supportive environmental policies, a parental or family component, and healthier food options at schools, have been most successful. Similar multicomponent interventions are effective in workplaces, complemented by employee participation in planning and implementation, individual behavior change strategies, and self-monitoring. Multicomponent approaches that target specific high-risk groups in the community are also effective, as are multicomponent approaches planned and implemented in religious settings. Evidence for the independent effects of food environments, availability, and pricing is at an early stage. Increasing the availability of healthier foods (e.g., in cafeterias, grocery stores, or neighborhoods) and point-of-purchase prompts each appear to be effective.

Combining various population level strategies has proven particularly successful—for example, integrated approaches including upstream policy measures, midstream media campaigns, and downstream community approaches. Such population-based strategies also complement individual-based approaches and are effective in tandem. Because of clustering of suboptimal diet habits, local environments, and disease risk factors, population-based behavioral change strategies are also relevant for reducing social and racial inequities.

REFERENCES

1. Danaei G, Ding EL, Mozaffarian D, et al: The preventable causes of death in the United States: comparative risk assessment of dietary, lifestyle, and metabolic risk factors. PLoS Med 6:2028, 2009.
2. Popkin BM: Global nutrition dynamics: The world is shifting rapidly toward a diet linked with noncommunicable diseases. Am J Clin Nutr 84:289, 2006.

Macronutrients

3. Riccardi G, Rivellese AA, Giacco R: Role of glycemic index and glycemic load in the healthy state, in prediabetes, and in diabetes. Am J Clin Nutr 87:269S, 2008.
4. Livesey G, Taylor R, Hulshof T, et al: Glycemic response and health—a systematic review and meta-analysis: relations between dietary glycemic properties and health outcomes. Am J Clin Nutr 87:258S, 2008.
5. O'Keefe JH, Gheewala NM, O'Keefe JO: Dietary strategies for improving post-prandial glucose, lipids, inflammation, and cardiovascular health. J Am Coll Cardiol 51:249, 2008.
6. Thomas D, Elliott EJ: Low glycaemic index, or low glycaemic load, diets for diabetes mellitus. Cochrane Database Syst Rev (1):CD006296, 2009.
7. Anderson JW, Randles KM, Kendall CW, et al: Carbohydrate and fiber recommendations for individuals with diabetes: A quantitative assessment and meta-analysis of the evidence. J Am Coll Nutr 23:5, 2004.
8. Whelton SP, Hyre AD, Pedersen B, et al: Effect of dietary fiber intake on blood pressure: A meta-analysis of randomized, controlled clinical trials. J Hypertens 23:475, 2005.
9. Pereira MA, O'Reilly E, Augustsson K, et al: Dietary fiber and risk of coronary heart disease: A pooled analysis of cohort studies. Arch Intern Med 164:370-376, 2004.
10. Schulze MB, Schulz M, Heidemann C, et al: Fiber and magnesium intake and incidence of type 2 diabetes: A prospective study and meta-analysis. Arch Intern Med 167:956, 2007.
11. Atkinson FS, Foster-Powell K, Brand-Miller JC. International tables of glycemic index and glycemic load values: 2008. Diabetes Care 31:2281, 2008.
12. Bornet FR, Jardy-Gennetier AE, Jacquet N, et al: Glycaemic response to foods: Impact on satiety and long-term weight regulation. Appetite 49:535, 2007.
13. Mente A, de Koning L, Shannon HS, et al: A systematic review of the evidence supporting a causal link between dietary factors and coronary heart disease. Arch Intern Med 169:659, 2009.
14. Barclay AW, Petocz P, McMillan-Price J, et al: Glycemic index, glycemic load, and chronic disease risk—a meta-analysis of observational studies. Am J Clin Nutr 87:627, 2008.
15. Mensink RP, Zock PL, Kester AD, et al: Effects of dietary fatty acids and carbohydrates on the ratio of serum total to HDL cholesterol and on serum lipids and apolipoproteins: A meta-analysis of 60 controlled trials. Am J Clin Nutr 77:1146, 2003.
16. Mozaffarian D: Effects of dietary fats versus carbohydrates on coronary heart disease: A review of the evidence. Curr Atheroscler Rep 7:435, 2005.
17. Howard BV, Van Horn L, Hsia J, et al: Low-fat dietary pattern and risk of cardiovascular disease: The Women's Health Initiative Randomized Controlled Dietary Modification Trial. JAMA 295:655, 2006.

18. Dietary Guidelines Advisory Committee: 2005 Dietary Guidelines Advisory Committee Report (http://www.health.gov/dietaryguidelines/dga2005/report).
19. Lichtenstein AH, Appel LJ, Brands M, et al: Diet and lifestyle recommendations revision 2006: A scientific statement from the American Heart Association Nutrition Committee. Circulation 114:82, 2006.
20. World Health Organization, Food and Agriculture Organization of the United Nations: Diet, Nutrition and the Prevention of Chronic Diseases: Report of a Joint WHO/FAO Expert Consultation (WHO Technical Report Series 916). Geneva, World Health Organization, 2003.
21. Ding EL, Mozaffarian D: Optimal dietary habits for the prevention of stroke. Semin Neurol 26:11, 2006.
22. Halton TL, Liu S, Manson JE, et al: Low-carbohydrate-diet score and risk of type 2 diabetes in women. Am J Clin Nutr 87:339, 2008.
23. Tinker LF, Bonds DE, Margolis KL, et al: Low-fat dietary pattern and risk of treated diabetes mellitus in postmenopausal women: The Women's Health Initiative randomized controlled dietary modification trial. Arch Intern Med 168:1500, 2008.
24. Berglund L, Lefevre M, Ginsberg HN, et al: Comparison of monounsaturated fat with carbohydrates as a replacement for saturated fat in subjects with a high metabolic risk profile: Studies in the fasting and postprandial states. Am J Clin Nutr 86:1611, 2007.
25. Siri-Tarino PW, Sun Q, Hu FB, et al: Meta-analysis of prospective cohort studies evaluating the association of saturated fat with cardiovascular disease. Am J Clin Nutr 91:535, 2010.
26. Jakobsen MU, O'Reilly EJ, Heitmann BL, et al: Major types of dietary fat and risk of coronary heart disease: a pooled analysis of 11 cohort studies. Am J Clin Nutr 89:1425, 2009.
26a. Jakobsen MU, Dethlefsen C, Joensen AM, et al: Intake of carbohydrates compared with intake of saturated fatty acids and risk of myocardial infarction: Importance of the glycemic index. Am J Clin Nutr 91:1764, 2010.
27. Micha R, Mozaffarian D: Saturated fat and cardiometabolic risk factors, coronary heart disease, stroke, and diabetes: A fresh look at the evidence. Lipids 45:893, 2010.
28. Miller ER, 3rd, Erlinger TP, Appel LJ: The effects of macronutrients on blood pressure and lipids: an overview of the DASH and OmniHeart trials. Curr Atheroscler Rep 8:460, 2006.
29. Shah M, Adams-Huet B, Garg A: Effect of high-carbohydrate or high-cis-monounsaturated fat diets on blood pressure: A meta-analysis of intervention trials. Am J Clin Nutr 85:1251, 2007.
30. Galgani JE, Uauy RD, Aguirre CA, et al: Effect of the dietary fat quality on insulin sensitivity. Br J Nutr 100:471, 2008.
31. Riserus U, Willett WC, Hu FB: Dietary fats and prevention of type 2 diabetes. Prog Lipid Res 48:44, 2009.
32. Degirolamo C, Shelness GS, Rudel LL: LDL cholesteryl oleate as a predictor for atherosclerosis: evidence from human and animal studies on dietary fat. J Lipid Res 50(Suppl):S434, 2009.
33. Harris WS, Mozaffarian D, Lefevre M, et al: Towards establishing dietary reference intakes for eicosapentaenoic and docosahexaenoic acids. J Nutr 139:804S, 2009.
34. Mozaffarian D: Does alpha-linolenic acid intake reduce the risk of coronary heart disease? A review of the evidence. Altern Ther Health Med 11:24, 2005.
35. Griffin BA: How relevant is the ratio of dietary n-6 to n-3 polyunsaturated fatty acids to cardiovascular disease risk? Evidence from the OPTILIP study. Curr Opin Lipidol 19:57, 2008.
36. Harris WS, Mozaffarian D, Rimm E, et al: Omega-6 fatty acids and risk for cardiovascular disease: A science advisory from the American Heart Association Nutrition Subcommittee of the Council on Nutrition, Physical Activity, and Metabolism; Council on Cardiovascular Nursing; and Council on Epidemiology and Prevention. Circulation 119:902, 2009.
37. Oh K, Hu FB, Manson JE, et al: Dietary fat intake and risk of coronary heart disease in women: 20 years of follow-up of the nurses' health study. Am J Epidemiol 161:672, 2005.
38. Mozaffarian D, Wallace S, Micha R: Effects on coronary heart disease of increasing polyunsaturated fat in place of saturated fat: A systematic review and meta-analysis of randomized controlled trials. PLoS Med 7:e1000252, 2010.
39. Wendland E, Farmer A, Glasziou P, et al: Effect of alpha linolenic acid on cardiovascular risk markers: A systematic review. Heart 92:166, 2006.
40. Zatonski W, Campos H, Willett W: Rapid declines in coronary heart disease mortality in Eastern Europe are associated with increased consumption of oils rich in alpha-linolenic acid. Eur J Epidemiol 23:3, 2008.
41. Brouwer IA, Katan MB, Zock PL: Dietary alpha-linolenic acid is associated with reduced risk of fatal coronary heart disease, but increased prostate cancer risk: a meta-analysis. J Nutr 134:919, 2004.
42. Wang C, Harris WS, Chung M, et al: n-3 Fatty acids from fish or fish-oil supplements, but not alpha-linolenic acid, benefit cardiovascular disease outcomes in primary- and secondary-prevention studies: A systematic review. Am J Clin Nutr 84:5, 2006.
43. Mozaffarian D, Rimm EB. Fish intake, contaminants, and human health: Evaluating the risks and the benefits. JAMA 296:1885, 2006.
44. Mozaffarian D: Fish, n-3 fatty acids, and cardiovascular haemodynamics. J Cardiovasc Electrophysiol 8:S23, 2007.
45. Peoples GE, McLennan PL, Howe PR, et al: Fish oil reduces heart rate and oxygen consumption during exercise. J Cardiovasc Pharmacol 52:540, 2008.
46. Brouwer IA, Raitt MH, Dullemeijer C, et al: Effect of fish oil on ventricular tachyarrhythmia in three studies in patients with implantable cardioverter defibrillators. Eur Heart J 30:820, 2009.
47. GISSI-Heart Failure Investigators: Effect of n-3 polyunsaturated fatty acids in patients with chronic heart failure (the GISSI-HF trial): A randomised, double-blind, placebo-controlled trial. Lancet 372:1223, 2008.
48. Mozaffarian D, Katan MB, Ascherio A, et al: Trans fatty acids and cardiovascular disease. N Engl J Med 354:1601, 2006.
49. Mozaffarian D, Clarke R: Quantitative effects on cardiovascular risk factors and coronary heart disease risk of replacing partially hydrogenated vegetable oils with other fats and oils. Eur J Clin Nutr 63(Suppl 2):S22, 2009.
50. Micha R, Mozaffarian D: Trans fatty acids: effects on metabolic syndrome, heart disease and diabetes. Nat Rev Endocrinol 5:335, 2009.
51. Wallace SK, Mozaffarian D: Trans fatty acids and nonlipid risk factors. Curr Atheroscler Rep 11:423, 2009.
52. Weggemans RM, Zock PL, Katan MB: Dietary cholesterol from eggs increases the ratio of total cholesterol to high-density lipoprotein cholesterol in humans: A meta-analysis. Am J Clin Nutr 73:885, 2001.
53. Djousse L, Gaziano JM: Egg consumption in relation to cardiovascular disease and mortality: The Physicians' Health Study. Am J Clin Nutr 87:964, 2008.
54. Matheson EM, Mainous AG 3rd, Hill EG, et al: Shellfish consumption and risk of coronary heart disease. J Am Diet Assoc 109:1422, 2009.
55. Kratz M: Dietary cholesterol, atherosclerosis and coronary heart disease. Handb Exp Pharmacol (170):195, 2005.
56. Djousse L, Gaziano JM, Buring JE, et al: Egg consumption and risk of type 2 diabetes in men and women. Diabetes Care 32:295, 2009.
57. Patel PS, Sharp SJ, Luben RN, et al: The association between type of dietary fish and seafood intake and the risk of incident type 2 diabetes: The EPIC-Norfolk cohort study. Diabetes Care 32:1857, 2009.
58. Tanasescu M, Cho E, Manson JE, et al: Dietary fat and cholesterol and the risk of cardiovascular disease among women with type 2 diabetes. Am J Clin Nutr 79:999, 2004.
59. Appel LJ, Sacks FM, Carey VJ, et al: Effects of protein, monounsaturated fat, and carbohydrate intake on blood pressure and serum lipids: Results of the OmniHeart randomized trial. JAMA 294:2455, 2005.
60. Layman DK, Clifton P, Gannon MC, et al: Protein in optimal health: heart disease and type 2 diabetes. Am J Clin Nutr 87:1571S-1575S, 2008.
61. Jenkins DJ, Wong JM, Kendall CW, et al: The effect of a plant-based low-carbohydrate ("Eco-Atkins") diet on body weight and blood lipid concentrations in hyperlipidemic subjects. Arch Intern Med 169:1046, 2009.
62. Kelemen LE, Kushi LH, Jacobs DR Jr, et al: Associations of dietary protein with disease and mortality in a prospective study of postmenopausal women. Am J Epidemiol 161:239, 2005.
63. Halton TL, Willett WC, Liu S, et al: Low-carbohydrate-diet score and the risk of coronary heart disease in women. N Engl J Med 355:1991, 2006.
64. Trichopoulou A, Psaltopoulou T, Orfanos P, et al: Low-carbohydrate-high-protein diet and long-term survival in a general population cohort. Eur J Clin Nutr 61:575, 2007.
65. Lagiou P, Sandin S, Weiderpass E, et al: Low carbohydrate-high protein diet and mortality in a cohort of Swedish women. J Intern Med 261:366, 2007.

Foods

66. Dauchet L, Amouyel P, Hercberg S, et al: Fruit and vegetable consumption and risk of coronary heart disease: A meta-analysis of cohort studies. J Nutr 136:2588, 2006.
67. Dauchet L, Amouyel P, Dallongeville J: Fruit and vegetable consumption and risk of stroke: A meta-analysis of cohort studies. Neurology 65:1193, 2005.
68. Esposito K, Marfella R, Ciotola M, et al: Effect of a mediterranean-style diet on endothelial dysfunction and markers of vascular inflammation in the metabolic syndrome: A randomized trial. JAMA 292:1440, 2004.
69. Ard JD, Grambow SC, Liu D, et al: The effect of the PREMIER interventions on insulin sensitivity. Diabetes Care 27:340, 2004.
70. Elmer PJ, Obarzanek E, Vollmer WM, et al: Effects of comprehensive lifestyle modification on diet, weight, physical fitness, and blood pressure control: 18-month results of a randomized trial. Ann Intern Med 144:485, 2006.
71. Svendsen M, Blomhoff R, Holme I, et al: The effect of an increased intake of vegetables and fruit on weight loss, blood pressure and antioxidant defense in subjects with sleep-related breathing disorders. Eur J Clin Nutr 61:1301, 2007.
72. McCall DO, McGartland CP, McKinley MC, et al: Dietary intake of fruits and vegetables improves microvascular function in hypertensive subjects in a dose-dependent manner. Circulation 119:2153, 2009.
73. Al-Solaiman Y, Jesri A, Mountford WK, et al: DASH lowers blood pressure in obese hypertensives beyond potassium, magnesium and fibre. J Hum Hypertens 24:237, 2010.
74. de Munter JS, Hu FB, Spiegelman D, et al: Whole grain, bran, and germ intake and risk of type 2 diabetes: A prospective cohort study and systematic review. PLoS Med 4:e261, 2007.
75. Mellen PB, Walsh TF, Herrington DM: Whole grain intake and cardiovascular disease: A meta-analysis. Nutr Metab Cardiovasc Dis 18:283, 2008.
76. Katcher HI, Legro RS, Kunselman AR, et al: The effects of a whole grain-enriched hypocaloric diet on cardiovascular disease risk factors in men and women with metabolic syndrome. Am J Clin Nutr 87:79, 2008.
77. Kelly SA, Summerbell CD, Brynes A, et al: Wholegrain cereals for coronary heart disease. Cochrane Database Syst Rev (2):CD005051, 2007.
78. Kelly JH Jr, Sabate J: Nuts and coronary heart disease: An epidemiological perspective. Br J Nutr 96 Suppl 2:S61, 2006.
79. Ros E: Nuts and novel biomarkers of cardiovascular disease. Am J Clin Nutr 89:1649S, 2009.
80. Kris-Etherton PM, Hu FB, Ros E, et al: The role of tree nuts and peanuts in the prevention of coronary heart disease: multiple potential mechanisms. J Nutr 138:1746S, 2008.
81. Banel DK, Hu FB: Effects of walnut consumption on blood lipids and other cardiovascular risk factors: a meta-analysis and systematic review. Am J Clin Nutr 90:56, 2009.
82. Mena MP, Sacanella E, Vazquez-Agell M, et al: Inhibition of circulating immune cell activation: a molecular antiinflammatory effect of the Mediterranean diet. Am J Clin Nutr 89:248, 2009.
83. Llorente-Cortés V, Estruch R, Mena MP, et al: Effect of Mediterranean diet on the expression of pro-atherogenic genes in a population at high cardiovascular risk. Atherosclerosis 208:44, 2010.
84. Mattes RD, Kris-Etherton PM, Foster GD: Impact of peanuts and tree nuts on body weight and healthy weight loss in adults. J Nutr 138:1741S, 2008.
85. Hooper L, Kroon PA, Rimm EB, et al: Flavonoids, flavonoid-rich foods, and cardiovascular risk: a meta-analysis of randomized controlled trials. Am J Clin Nutr 88:38, 2008.
86. Sacks FM, Lichtenstein A, Van Horn L, et al: Soy protein, isoflavones, and cardiovascular health: an American Heart Association Science Advisory for professionals from the Nutrition Committee. Circulation 113:1034, 2006.
87. He K, Song Y, Daviglus ML, et al: Accumulated evidence on fish consumption and coronary heart disease mortality: a meta-analysis of cohort studies. Circulation 109:2705, 2004.
88. He K, Song Y, Daviglus ML, et al: Fish consumption and incidence of stroke: a meta-analysis of cohort studies. Stroke 35:1538, 2004.
89. Kaushik M, Mozaffarian D, Spiegelman D, et al: Long-chain omega-3 fatty acids, fish intake, and the risk of type 2 diabetes mellitus. Am J Clin Nutr 90:613-620, 2009.
90. Jump DB: N-3 polyunsaturated fatty acid regulation of hepatic gene transcription. Curr Opin Lipidol 19:242-247, 2008.

91. Giacco R, Cuomo V, Vessby B, et al: Fish oil, insulin sensitivity, insulin secretion and glucose tolerance in healthy people: Is there any effect of fish oil supplementation in relation to the type of background diet and habitual dietary intake of n-6 and n-3 fatty acids? Nutr Metab Cardiovasc Dis 17:572, 2007.
92. Mozaffarian D, Gottdiener JS, Siscovick DS: Intake of tuna or other broiled or baked fish versus fried fish and cardiac structure, function, and hemodynamics. Am J Cardiol 97:216, 2006.
93. Chung H, Nettleton JA, Lemaitre RN, et al: Frequency and type of seafood consumed influence plasma (n-3) fatty acid concentrations. J Nutr 138:2422, 2008.
94. He K, Liu K, Daviglus ML, et al: Intakes of long-chain n-3 polyunsaturated fatty acids and fish in relation to measurements of subclinical atherosclerosis. Am J Clin Nutr 88:1111, 2008.
95. Aune D, Ursin G, Veierod MB: Meat consumption and the risk of type 2 diabetes: A systematic review and meta-analysis of cohort studies. Diabetologia 52:2277, 2009.
96. Micha R, Wallace S, Mozaffarian D: Red and processed meat consumption and risk of incident coronary heart disease, stroke, and diabetes: A systematic review and meta-analysis. Circulation 121:2271, 2010.
97. Lanou AJ, Barnard ND: Dairy and weight loss hypothesis: an evaluation of the clinical trials. Nutr Rev 66:272, 2008.
98. Christensen R, Lorenzen JK, Svith CR, et al: Effect of calcium from dairy and dietary supplements on faecal fat excretion: A meta-analysis of randomized controlled trials. Obes Rev 10:475, 2009.
99. Tremblay A, Gilbert JA: Milk products, insulin resistance syndrome and type 2 diabetes. J Am Coll Nutr 28 Suppl 1:91S, 2009.
100. Elwood PC, Givens DI, Beswick AD, et al: The survival advantage of milk and dairy consumption: An overview of evidence from cohort studies of vascular diseases, diabetes and cancer. J Am Coll Nutr 27:723S, 2008.
101. Alonso A, Zozaya C, Vazquez Z, et al: The effect of low-fat versus whole-fat dairy product intake on blood pressure and weight in young normotensive adults. J Hum Nutr Diet 22:336, 2009.
102. Tholstrup T, Hoy CE, Andersen LN, et al: Does fat in milk, butter and cheese affect blood lipids and cholesterol differently? J Am Coll Nutr 23:169, 2004.
103. Biong AS, Muller H, Seljeflot I, et al: A comparison of the effects of cheese and butter on serum lipids, haemostatic variables and homocysteine. Br J Nutr 92:791, 2004.
104. Nestel PJ, Chronopulos A, Cehun M: Dairy fat in cheese raises LDL cholesterol less than that in butter in mildly hypercholesterolaemic subjects. Eur J Clin Nutr 59:1059, 2005.

Beverages

105. Laonigro I, Correale M, et al: Alcohol abuse and heart failure. Eur J Heart Fail 11:453, 2009.
106. Conen D, Tedrow UB, Cook NR, et al: Alcohol consumption and risk of incident atrial fibrillation in women. JAMA 300:2489, 2008.
107. Koppes LL, Dekker JM, et al: Moderate alcohol consumption lowers the risk of type 2 diabetes: A meta-analysis of prospective observational studies. Diabetes Care 28:719, 2005.
108. Fillmore KM, Stockwell T, Chikritzhs T, et al: Moderate alcohol use and reduced mortality risk: Systematic error in prospective studies and new hypotheses. Ann Epidemiol 17:S16, 2007.
109. Shai I, Wainstein J, Harman-Boehm I, et al: Glycemic effects of moderate alcohol intake among patients with type 2 diabetes: A multicenter, randomized, clinical intervention trial. Diabetes Care 30:3011, 2007.
110. Joosten MM, Beulens JW, Kersten S, et al: Moderate alcohol consumption increases insulin sensitivity and ADIPOQ expression in postmenopausal women: A randomised, crossover trial. Diabetologia 51:1375, 2008.
111. Bagnardi V, Zatonski W, Scotti L, et al: Does drinking pattern modify the effect of alcohol on the risk of coronary heart disease? Evidence from a meta-analysis. J Epidemiol Community Health 62:615, 2008.
112. Noordzij M, Uiterwaal CS, Arends LR, et al: Blood pressure response to chronic intake of coffee and caffeine: A meta-analysis of randomized controlled trials. J Hypertens 23:921, 2005.
113. van Dam RM: Coffee consumption and risk of type 2 diabetes, cardiovascular diseases, and cancer. Appl Physiol Nutr Metab 33:1269, 2008.
114. Wu JN, Ho SC, Zhou C, et al: Coffee consumption and risk of coronary heart diseases: A meta-analysis of 21 prospective cohort studies. Int J Cardiol 137:216, 2009.
115. van Dam RM, Hu FB: Coffee consumption and risk of type 2 diabetes: A systematic review. JAMA 294:97, 2005.
116. Hursel R, Viechtbauer W, Westerterp-Plantenga MS: The effects of green tea on weight loss and weight maintenance: A meta-analysis. Int J Obes (Lond) 33:956, 2009.
117. Arab L, Liu W, Elashoff D: Green and black tea consumption and risk of stroke: A meta-analysis. Stroke 40:1786, 2009.
118. Jing Y, Han G, Hu Y, et al: Tea consumption and risk of type 2 diabetes: A meta-analysis of cohort studies. J Gen Intern Med 24:557, 2009.
119. Duffey KJ, Popkin BM: Shifts in patterns and consumption of beverages between 1965 and 2002. Obesity (Silver Spring) 15:2739, 2007.
120. Lloyd-Jones D, Adams R, Carnethon M, et al: Heart disease and stroke statistics—2009 update: A report from the American Heart Association Statistics Committee and Stroke Statistics Subcommittee. Circulation 119:e21, 2009.
121. Wang YC, Bleich SN, Gortmaker SL: Increasing caloric contribution from sugar-sweetened beverages and 100% fruit juices among US children and adolescents, 1988-2004. Pediatrics 121:e1604, 2008.
122. Wolff E, Dansinger ML: Soft drinks and weight gain: How strong is the link? Medscape J Med 10:189, 2008.
123. Stull AJ, Apolzan JW, Thalacker-Mercer AE, et al: Liquid and solid meal replacement products differentially affect postprandial appetite and food intake in older adults. J Am Diet Assoc 108:1226, 2008.
124. Zijlstra N, Mars M, de Wijk RA, et al: The effect of viscosity on ad libitum food intake. Int J Obes (Lond) 32:676, 2008.
125. Chen L, Appel LJ, Loria C, et al: Reduction in consumption of sugar-sweetened beverages is associated with weight loss: The PREMIER trial. Am J Clin Nutr 89:1299, 2009.
126. Schulze MB, Manson JE, Ludwig DS, et al: Sugar-sweetened beverages, weight gain, and incidence of type 2 diabetes in young and middle-aged women. JAMA 292:927, 2004.
127. Paynter NP, Yeh HC, et al: Coffee and sweetened beverage consumption and the risk of type 2 diabetes mellitus: the atherosclerosis risk in communities study. Am J Epidemiol 164:1075, 2006.
128. Dhingra R, Sullivan L, Jacques PF, et al: Soft drink consumption and risk of developing cardiometabolic risk factors and the metabolic syndrome in middle-aged adults in the community. Circulation 116:480, 2007.
129. Palmer JR, Boggs DA, Krishnan S, et al: Sugar-sweetened beverages and incidence of type 2 diabetes mellitus in African American women. Arch Intern Med 168:1487, 2008.
129a. Malik VS, Popkin BM, Bray GA, et al: Sugar-sweetened beverages, obesity, type 2 diabetes mellitus, and cardiovascular disease risk. Circulation 121:1356, 2010.
130. Fung TT, Malik V, Rexrode KM, et al: Sweetened beverage consumption and risk of coronary heart disease in women. Am J Clin Nutr 89:1037, 2009.
130a. Malik VS, Popkin BM, Bray GA, et al: Sugar-sweetened beverages and risk of metabolic syndrome and type 2 diabetes: A meta-analysis. Diabetes Care 33:2477, 2010.

Micronutrients

131. Brown IJ, Tzoulaki I, Candeias V, et al: Salt intakes around the world: Implications for public health. Int J Epidemiol 38:791, 2009.
132. He FJ, MacGregor GA: Effect of longer-term modest salt reduction on blood pressure. Cochrane Database Syst Rev (3):CD004937, 2004.
133. Jurgens G, Graudal NA: Effects of low sodium diet versus high sodium diet on blood pressure, renin, aldosterone, catecholamines, cholesterols, and triglyceride. Cochrane Database Syst Rev (1):CD004022, 2004.
134. Nagata C, Takatsuka N, Shimizu N, et al: Sodium intake and risk of death from stroke in Japanese men and women. Stroke 35:1543, 2004.
135. Umesawa M, Iso H, Date C, et al: Relations between dietary sodium and potassium intakes and mortality from cardiovascular disease: The Japan Collaborative Cohort Study for Evaluation of Cancer Risks. Am J Clin Nutr 88:195, 2008.
136. Cohen HW, Hailpern SM, Alderman MH: Sodium intake and mortality follow-up in the Third National Health and Nutrition Examination Survey (NHANES III). J Gen Intern Med 23:1297, 2008.
137. Cook NR, Obarzanek E, Cutler JA, et al: Joint effects of sodium and potassium intake on subsequent cardiovascular disease: The Trials of Hypertension Prevention follow-up study. Arch Intern Med 169:32, 2009.
138. Geleijnse JM, Witteman JC, Stijnen T, et al: Sodium and potassium intake and risk of cardio-vascular events and all-cause mortality: The Rotterdam Study. Eur J Epidemiol 22:763, 2007.
139. Cook NR, Cutler JA, Obarzanek E, et al: Long term effects of dietary sodium reduction on cardiovascular disease outcomes: Observational follow-up of the trials of hypertension prevention (TOHP). BMJ 334:885, 2007.
140. Dickinson HO, Mason JM, Nicolson DJ, et al: Lifestyle interventions to reduce raised blood pressure: A systematic review of randomized controlled trials. J Hypertens 24:215, 2006.
141. van Mierlo LA, Arends LR, Streppel MT, et al: Blood pressure response to calcium supplementation: A meta-analysis of randomized controlled trials. J Hum Hypertens 20:571-580, 2006.
142. Wooley JA: Characteristics of thiamin and its relevance to the management of heart failure. Nutr Clin Pract 23:487, 2008.
143. Keith ME, Walsh NA, Darling PB, et al: B-vitamin deficiency in hospitalized patients with heart failure. J Am Diet Assoc 109:1406, 2009.
144. Bleys J, Miller ER 3rd, Pastor-Barriuso R, et al: Vitamin-mineral supplementation and the progression of atherosclerosis: A meta-analysis of randomized controlled trials. Am J Clin Nutr 84:880, 2006.
145. Flores-Mateo G, Navas-Acien A, Pastor-Barriuso R, et al: Selenium and coronary heart disease: A meta-analysis. Am J Clin Nutr 84:762, 2006.
146. Bjelakovic G, Nikolova D, Gluud LL, et al: Antioxidant supplements for prevention of mortality in healthy participants and patients with various diseases. Cochrane Database Syst Rev (2):CD007176, 2008.
147. Giovannucci E, Liu Y, Hollis BW, et al: 25-hydroxyvitamin D and risk of myocardial infarction in men: A prospective study. Arch Intern Med 168:1174, 2008.
148. Dobnig H, Pilz S, Scharnagl H, et al: Independent association of low serum 25-hydroxyvitamin D and 1,25-dihydroxyvitamin D levels with all-cause and cardiovascular mortality. Arch Intern Med 168:1340, 2008.
149. Witham MD, Nadir MA, Struthers AD: Effect of vitamin D on blood pressure: a systematic review and meta-analysis. J Hypertens 27:1948, 2009.
150. Hsia J, Heiss G, Ren H, et al: Calcium/vitamin D supplementation and cardiovascular events. Circulation 115:846, 2007.
151. de Boer IH, Tinker LF, Connelly S, et al: Calcium plus vitamin D supplementation and the risk of incident diabetes in the Women's Health Initiative. Diabetes Care 31:701, 2008.
152. Autier P, Gandini S: Vitamin D supplementation and total mortality: A meta-analysis of randomized controlled trials. Arch Intern Med 167:1730, 2007.
153. Ding EL, Hutfless SM, Ding X, et al: Chocolate and prevention of cardiovascular disease: A systematic review. Nutr Metab (Lond) 3:2, 2006.
154. Taubert D, Roesen R, Lehmann C, et al: Effects of low habitual cocoa intake on blood pressure and bioactive nitric oxide: a randomized controlled trial. JAMA 298:49, 2007.
155. Mink PJ, Scrafford CG, Barraj LM, et al: Flavonoid intake and cardiovascular disease mortality: A prospective study in postmenopausal women. Am J Clin Nutr 85:895-909, 2007.
156. Mursu J, Voutilainen S, Nurmi T, et al: Flavonoid intake and the risk of ischaemic stroke and CVD mortality in middle-aged Finnish men: The Kuopio Ischaemic Heart Disease Risk Factor Study. Br J Nutr 100:890-895, 2008.

Further Considerations

157. Mozaffarian D, Marfisi R, Levantesi G, et al: Incidence of new-onset diabetes and impaired fasting glucose in patients with recent myocardial infarction and the effect of clinical and lifestyle risk factors. Lancet 370:667, 2007.
158. de Lorgeril M, Salen P: The Mediterranean-style diet for the prevention of cardiovascular diseases. Public Health Nutr 9:118, 2006.

CHAPTER 49 Primary and Secondary Prevention of Coronary Heart Disease

J. Michael Gaziano, Paul M Ridker, and Peter Libby

Both the primary prevention and secondary prevention of coronary heart disease (CHD) have indisputable public health importance. Given the prevalence of CHD, prevention of even a small proportion of events saves thousands of lives, avoids inestimable suffering, and conserves billions of health care dollars. In addition, measures preventing CHD may also mitigate other manifestations of atherosclerosis, such as stroke and peripheral artery disease, and may have an impact on hypertension, diabetes, cognitive function, cancer, depression, and other chronic conditions. Because cardiovascular disease (CVD) has become the number-one killer worldwide, both developed and developing countries should highly prioritize the widespread deployment of affordable preventive strategies.

Our ever-increasing knowledge about the pathogenesis of atherosclerosis and about the interrelationship between lifestyle, biochemical factors, genetic risk factors, and heart disease has yielded substantial declines in age-adjusted cardiovascular mortality (**Fig. 49-1**). Beyond prediction of an individual's risk of future cardiovascular events (see Chap. 44), disease prevention must identify and apply interventions that reduce this risk. Trials must weigh the benefits of given interventions against their risks and costs to aid in the formulation of guidelines.

Single risk factor guidelines have achieved some success in the screening and treatment of several major risk factors, such as smoking, dyslipidemia, and hypertension. Implementation of these guidelines, however, remains difficult. The number and complexity of the guidelines impede their implementation. Lack of time for physicians to act on guidelines presents an additional hurdle; clinicians need a minimum of 1.5 hours per day to deliver only those cardiovascular-related preventive services recommended by the U.S. Preventive Services Task Force (USPSTF).[1] Lack of payment for preventive care further limits its delivery.

This chapter classifies preventive interventions into three categories based on the strength of the evidence that supports the efficacy of intervention. We examine potentially modifiable risk factor domains and interventions, with information on prevalence, associated risk, benefit of treatment, cost-efficacy, and recommendations and guidelines for each; a discussion of multiple risk factor intervention strategies follows. We conclude with a summary of the approach to the individual.

Using Risk Factor Information

When CVD first emerged as the dominant chronic disease in high-income countries, it was considered a natural consequence of aging. We currently view CVD as a "human-made" disease, heavily influenced by the choices humans make. The past 50 years have witnessed great progress in the identification of many "lifestyle factors" (as well as biochemical and genetic factors) associated with CVD and in the dissemination of this information to the public. "Risk factor" has become an integral part of the language of epidemiology, cardiology, and a host of other disciplines (see Chap. 44).

Types of Evidence About Risk Factors

Autopsy studies have shown that atherosclerosis can begin at an early age if risk factors—the same risk factors that lead to CVD in adults—are present (see Chap. 43). The establishment of cause and effect, a crucial step in the identification of predictors and development of preventive intervention, requires data from several types of research (**Table 49-1**). Basic research and human physiologic studies reveal the mechanisms underlying atherogenesis and help elucidate the biologic plausibility of potential interventions to modify these effects. Human observational studies, such as case-control studies and prospective cohorts, help establish the risk attributable to a single factor. Randomized trials can support causation and establish interventions to modify risk.

Each of these strategies has strengths and weaknesses. Descriptive studies (case reports, case series, cross-sectional surveys, cross-cultural studies, and studies of population-based temporal trends) have considerable value in their ability to generate hypotheses, but their design prevents adequate control for factors that may confound apparent associations. Observational studies (case-control and prospective cohort studies) give researchers greater control over potential confounders. Such studies can help estimate the risk attributable to a single factor, particularly when the effect of a given factor is large, as is the case for smoking and lung cancer. Yet, in searching for small to moderate effects, the amount of uncontrolled confounding in observational studies may be as large as the probable risk itself. Such instances require randomized trials to confirm causation.

For factors associated with diseases for which causality remains uncertain, the factor may still have clinical utility for identification of groups at high risk that might benefit from specific interventions. Even when causality is not in question, trials help quantify the magnitude of the effect of an intervention that targets a risk factor. When the intervention involves competing risks and benefits, randomized trials can assess the net clinical effect of the intervention. This consideration has critical importance, because the magnitude of associated risk does not relate necessarily to the magnitude of benefit derived from the

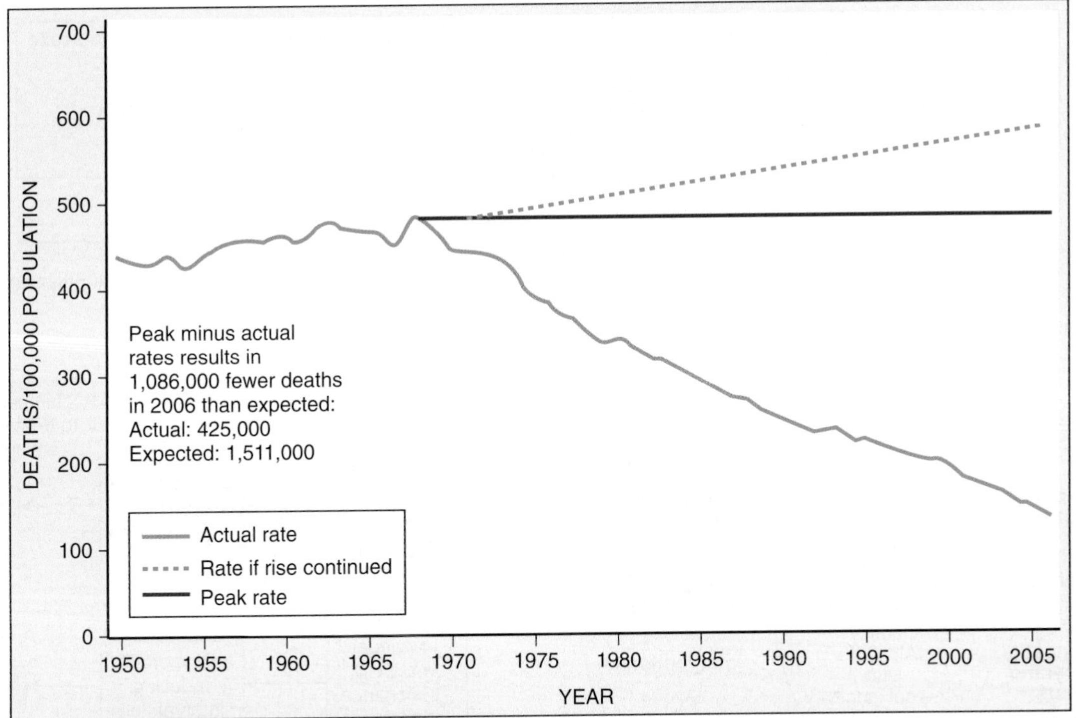

FIGURE 49-1 Actual and expected change in age-adjusted mortality from coronary heart disease in the United States, 1950 to 2006. *(From Morbidity and Mortality: 2009 Chart Book on Cardiovascular, Lung, and Blood Diseases. Bethesda, Md, National Heart, Lung and Blood Institute, 2009, p 32.)*

TABLE 49-1 Types of Studies Used in Establishing Preventive Strategies

Basic research
- In vitro studies
- Animal studies

Human physiologic studies

Epidemiologic studies
- Descriptive studies
  - Case reports
  - Cross-sectional surveys
  - Cross-cultural comparison studies
  - Temporal trend studies
- Analytical studies
  - Observational
  - Case-control studies
  - Cohort studies
  - Intervention (randomized trials)

Cost-efficacy studies

Meta-analyses

intervention. Such lack of correlation may result from the inability of the intervention to achieve the necessary change, or a change in the variable may not yield a proportional change in risk. For example, the observed risk associated with a rise of 1 mm Hg in blood pressure exceeds the benefit on CHD derived from reducing blood pressure by this amount.[2] Similarly, although elevated levels of homocysteine may elevate CHD risk and folic acid can reduce homocysteine levels, evidence from randomized trials indicates that reduction of homocysteine levels with folic acid does not reduce vascular risk (see Chap. 44). In contrast, although C-reactive protein (CRP) may or may not contribute causally to atherosclerosis, randomized trial evidence has demonstrated that those indentified as being at high risk because of increased CRP can benefit from specific therapies, such as statins.

Meta-analyses can provide better estimates of risk associated with a given factor or of the benefits of a given intervention. For example, the best estimate of the benefit of aspirin in secondary prevention has come from a large meta-analysis of nearly 300 trials demonstrating that aspirin reduces the risk of a major CVD event by 25% among those with vascular disease. Once reasonable estimates of benefit and risk have been established for a given intervention, cost-effectiveness should be analyzed, although this step can be quite difficult with heart disease because the benefit often accrues decades after the intervention.

Cost-effectiveness estimates are calculated as the ratio of net cost to gain in life expectancy, and the common currency used to compare interventions is the quality-adjusted life-year (QALY) or disability-adjusted life-year (DALY). Interventions with an incremental cost-effectiveness ratio of less than $40,000 per QALY, such as those for hypertension management and hemodialysis, are typically accepted by most insurers, whereas those exceeding $40,000 per QALY are not. The economic impact of ineffective primary prevention among persons with two or more modifiable risk factors has been estimated at $13.2 billion annually.[3]

Coronary Heart Disease as a Multifactorial Disease (see Chaps. 43, 44, 45, and 47)

Our knowledge of the biology of atherosclerosis has led to a working model for the progression of this disease and its many causative factors. CHD generally results from the convergence of a number of features. Most people with CVD have small, concurrent adverse changes in multiple risk factors rather than extreme deviations in any single risk factor. Left unchecked, atherosclerosis will progress through stages (**Fig. 49-2**). Predisposing factors, such as heredity, interact with behavioral factors, such as diet, alcohol consumption, and exercise. This combination of predisposing factors and behaviors can lead to metabolic abnormalities such as dyslipidemia, hypertension, obesity, and diabetes, which may eventually result in quiescent disease. Various diagnostic tests can yield clues (see Chap. 44) to this underlying quiescent disease.

Risk Predictors and Risk Reducers

Regardless of where risk factors fit in the progression of the disease, they fall into two broad categories based on how we use them in clinical practice: those that are useful for predicting risk, denoted risk

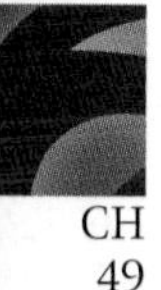

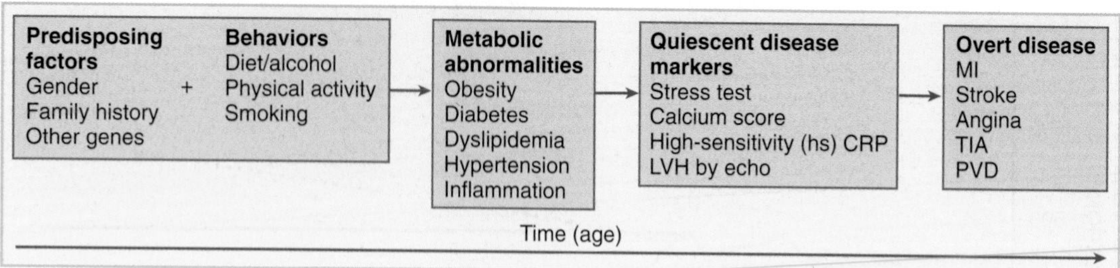

FIGURE 49-2 Progression of atherosclerosis. CRP = C-reactive protein; LVH = left ventricular hypertrophy; MI = myocardial infarction; TIA = transient ischemic attack; PVD = peripheral vascular disease.

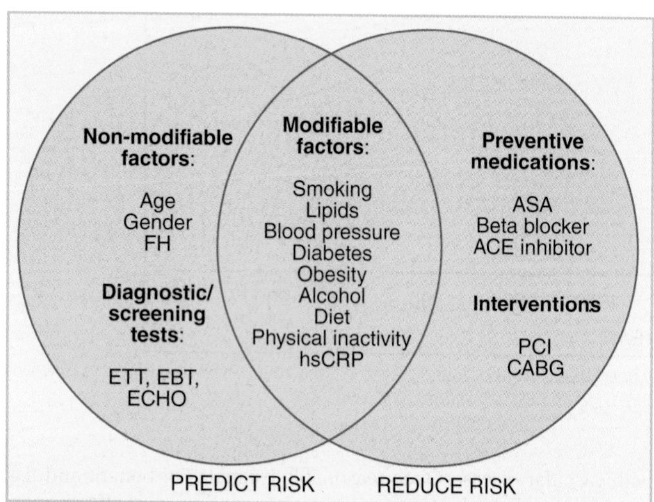

FIGURE 49-3 Risk factors can be divided into those that are useful in predicting risk and those that are useful targets for lowering risk. ACE = angiotensin-converting enzyme; ASA = acetylsalicylic acid; CABG = coronary artery bypass graft; EBT = electron beam tomography; ECHO = echocardiography; ETT = exercise tolerance test; FH = family history; hsCRP = high-sensitivity C-reactive protein; PCI = percutaneous coronary intervention.

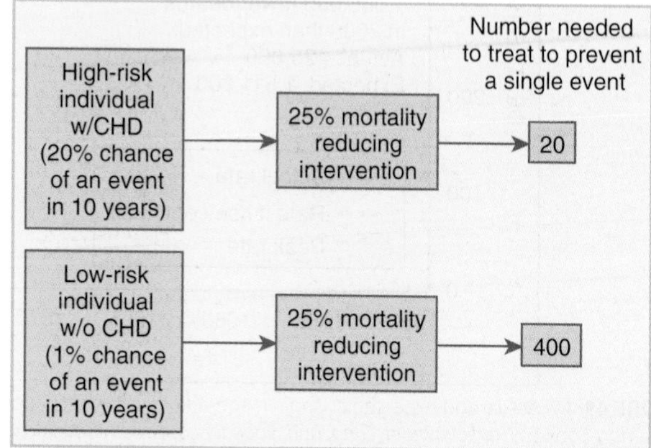

FIGURE 49-4 The cost-efficacy of an intervention that reduces risk by 25% among those who are high risk and those who are low risk varies by baseline level of risk. In a population with a 20% risk of an event in 10 years, only 20 patients need to be treated to prevent a single event, compared with 400 low-risk individuals.

predictors, and those that are targets for risk reduction or potential risk-reducing interventions, called risk reducers (**Fig. 49-3**). Some factors, such as cigarette smoking and blood pressure, fall into both categories. How do we decide which factors to use for risk prediction and which to use as targets to lower risk? In the following sections, we define an approach to the use of risk factors for prediction; this chapter later discusses using them for risk reduction. This chapter considers only those factors that modify intermediate or long-term risk. For discussion of interventions used acutely to modify short-term risk, such as aspirin or thrombolysis in the setting of an acute myocardial infarction (MI), see Chaps. 55 and 56.

Predicting and Assessing Risk

Risk prediction can apply to a population or to an individual. Population information can be gathered on a representative sample to estimate the rates of various risk factors for the purposes of planning public health messages and allocating resources for screening programs. Assessment of individual risk can help target subsegments of the population with more intensive programs for risk reduction. This section describes briefly the assessment of risk factors and event rates in the overall population and discusses in detail the assessment of risk in the individual.

ASSESSING RISK AT A POPULATION LEVEL: INCIDENCE, PREVALENCE, AND POPULATION ATTRIBUTABLE RISK. Sound public policy requires evaluation of the impact of different factors on the population. Population risk depends on the strength of the risk factor–disease association, on the benefit of intervention, and on how common the factor is in the general population. Incidence, prevalence, and population-attributable risk capture these concepts. Although incidence rates reflect the frequency of new cases of disease or a risk factor during a given period, prevalence reflects the proportion of individuals with a given condition or factor at a single point. Population-attributable risk—how much of the population's risk of disease a given factor accounts for—depends on the proportion of the public with a given risk factor and the magnitude of the associated risk.

Population-attributable risk also reflects the shape of the relation between the exposure and the disease. Many factors increase risk in a linear fashion, so population-attributable risk can be computed against an ideal standard or a low-risk individual. For example, hypertension has a linear relationship with heart disease and stroke; thus, lowering of blood pressure at any level above normal reduces risk. In contrast, the risk curve for obesity appears nonlinear, with risk increasing logarithmically, so each incremental pound gained is associated with much more risk in the already overweight. Population-attributable risk is an important concept for determining resource allocation between various preventive interventions and in establishing priorities for public health messages such as antismoking campaigns.

ASSESSING INDIVIDUAL RISK. A fundamental step in targeting individual preventive strategies involves assessing the risk for development of a clinically relevant outcome, because the cost-efficacy of many interventions varies according to overall risk in a given individual or population. For example, fewer high-risk individuals require treatment to save one life or to prevent one event in comparison to those at lower risk, even if relative risk reductions are identical in both groups.

To illustrate this concept, assume that an intervention reduces mortality by 25% in both primary and secondary prevention (**Fig. 49-4**). Furthermore, assume that a high-risk individual with CHD has a 20%

chance of death from CVD during the next 10 years, whereas a low-risk individual has a 1% chance of death during the same period. To save a life among those at high risk, one would have to treat only 20 patients (4 of whom are destined to die) for 10 years, so that a 25% relative risk reduction would result in one life saved (3 deaths instead of 4); but one would have to treat 400 low-risk patients (4 of whom are also destined to die) so that the same 25% relative risk reduction would yield 3 deaths instead of 4. Thus, the total cost per life saved is considerably lower (1/20 the cost) among individuals at higher absolute risk. High-cost interventions are generally cost-effective only in high-risk individuals, but if the cost of intervention is low, then treatment of even low-risk subgroups can prove cost-beneficial.

A "perfect" risk predictor is prevalent in the population, can be easily and safely measured, and has good predictive value. It must also be inexpensive to measure, a major limitation for imaging techniques such as screening with computed tomography or magnetic resonance imaging. Further, the false-positive rate associated with screening must be low to avoid unnecessary and potentially hazardous consequences. Age and sex are nonmodifiable risk factors that meet these criteria; similarly, blood pressure and smoking status exemplify readily assessable modifiable factors.

GLOBAL AND INDIVIDUAL RISK SCORES. (see Chap. 44) Because many risk predictors are correlated, risk often can be predicted with information on just a few factors. In most initial screenings, a handful of easily measured risk factors suffice to determine an individual's overall risk of CHD. For those who clearly have very low or very high risk after initial screening, measurement and evaluation of numerous additional risk factors will provide very little, if any, incremental information helpful in managing the patient. Those at intermediate risk (see later) will derive the most value from additional screening. Assessment of an individual's absolute risk enables cost-effective targeting of interventions; the National Cholesterol Education Program (NCEP) Adult Treatment Panel (ATP) III, the Seventh Joint National Committee on Prevention, Detection, Evaluation, and Treatment of High Blood Pressure (JNC 7), and the USPSTF all suggest a tiered approach to management based on absolute risk.

An initial categorization of an individual's risk depends on the presence or absence of established CVD. Those with known CVD, including coronary, cerebrovascular, or peripheral disease, have on average a much higher risk than those without known disease. Approximately 80% of those with known CVD will die of some form of the disease, whereas those without known CVD have approximately half that mortality rate from CVD. Thus, men and women with CVD generally warrant aggressive preventive interventions. Risk reduction in these individuals is referred to as secondary prevention, as opposed to primary prevention among those without overt CVD.

Individuals with diabetes compose a second high-risk group. Rates of CVD events and mortality among diabetic patients considerably exceed those in the general population; thus, patients with diabetes warrant aggressive preventive interventions. Similarly, patients with chronic renal failure (many of whom have diabetes) have exceedingly high risk for CVD events and death.

For those who do not have known CVD or diabetes, several risk prediction strategies have been developed with use of some of the predictive risk factors outlined in Figure 49-3 (as discussed extensively in Chap. 44). The National Heart, Lung and Blood Institute has made available an online version of the 10-year risk calculator based on the Framingham algorithm (*hin.nhlbi.nih.gov/atpiii/calculator.asp*) as well as versions that can be downloaded to a computer or handheld device (*hin.nhlbi.nih.gov/atpiii/riskcalc.htm*).

There are a number of alternatives to the Framingham Risk Score. The Reynolds Risk Score, a variation on the Framingham score, incorporates two additional pieces of information, the high-sensitivity (hs) CRP level and whether a parent suffered an MI before the age of 60 years.[4,5] The Reynolds score is on par with the Framingham score in estimating risk among individuals at high or low risk but seems to be a better predictor for those in the middle. In both the Women's Health Study and the Physicians' Health Study, use of the Reynolds score showed that approximately 20% of those considered to be at "intermediate" risk can be correctly reclassified to higher or lower risk groups, a potentially important issue in considering which patients should receive aggressive preventive therapies. To date, the Reynolds score has not been evaluated in nonwhite populations.

The Systematic Coronary Risk Evaluation project, or SCORE, was assembled by a European joint task force using data from cohort studies in 12 European countries involving 250,000 individuals. SCORE replaces earlier risk stratification models promulgated by the European Society of Cardiology (ESC) and shifts the emphasis from the prevention of CHD to the prevention of CVD.[6] Using age, sex, systolic blood pressure, total cholesterol or the HDL–total cholesterol ratio, and smoking status, SCORE calculates the 10-year risk of CVD death rather than any cardiovascular event. Diabetes was not included because it was not reliably measured in the cohorts used to develop the scores. When the ESC updated its guidelines in 2007, it created two SCORE charts, one for high-risk European countries and another for low-risk European countries (e.g., Belgium, France, Greece, Italy, Luxembourg, and Portugal).[7] Drug treatment is recommended if the SCORE risk exceeds 5%, and particularly as it approaches 10%. SCORE charts are available for download at *http://www.escardio.org/communties/EACPR/toolbox/health-professionals/Pages/SCORE-Risk-Charts.aspx.*

The New Zealand Guidelines Group has assembled tables, updated in 2009, assessing absolute cardiovascular risk during 5 years instead of 10 years (**Fig. 49-5**). This model predicts the 5-year total CVD risk based on age, sex, ethnicity (e.g., Maori, Pacific peoples, or people from the Indian subcontinent), smoking history, lipid and glucose levels, and systolic blood pressure. Risk assessment for asymptomatic patients without known risk factors should begin at 45 years of age for men and at 55 years of age for women. Patients are categorized as being at very high, high, moderate, or mild risk. Those with known CVD, genetic lipid disorders, or diabetes and renal disease constitute the very-high-risk category because most have a greater than 20% chance of a CVD event during 5 years. Drug therapy is recommended for those whose total CVD risk is 15% or greater.

All of these scores predict 5- or 10-year risk, but atherosclerosis is a lifelong disease, and lifetime risk is another important way to express risk—particularly for young individuals in whom early institution of lifestyle change is crucial.[8]

Lowering Risk: Interventions at an Individual and Population Level

Three complementary approaches may reduce the population burden of CVD: (1) therapeutic interventions for secondary prevention in patients with known CVD; (2) identification and targeting of high-risk individuals for primary prevention through mass screening or case finding; and (3) general recommendations disseminated throughout the population. Each of these approaches has merit in different situations, depending on the cost-effectiveness of the intervention and on the overall benefit-to-risk ratio. Targeted interventions such as specialized cardiac rehabilitation and lifestyle programs show the greatest efficacy among motivated individuals who hope to avoid a recurrent MI (secondary prevention), whereas mass screening programs for high blood pressure and hyperlipidemia are cost-effective (primary prevention). Population-wide campaigns against cigarette smoking offer an example of an effective public health approach. Implementation of the first two strategies requires risk assessment at the individual level; the third strategy requires knowledge of risk at the population level.

If individuals can reduce their risk factor burden before 50 years of age, they may substantially lower their lifetime risk for development of CVD. Framingham Heart Study participants who were free of CVD at 50 years of age and free of any major risk factors had substantially lower lifetime risks (5.2% versus 68.9% for men; 8.2% versus 50.2% for women) and markedly longer median survival (>39 years versus 28 years for men; >39 years versus 31 years for women) than participants who had two or more major risk factors at 50 years of age.[8]

Classification of Interventions for Modifiable Risk Factors

Because of the multiplicity of targets for CVD risk modification, implementation of a preventive strategy for a given patient requires a

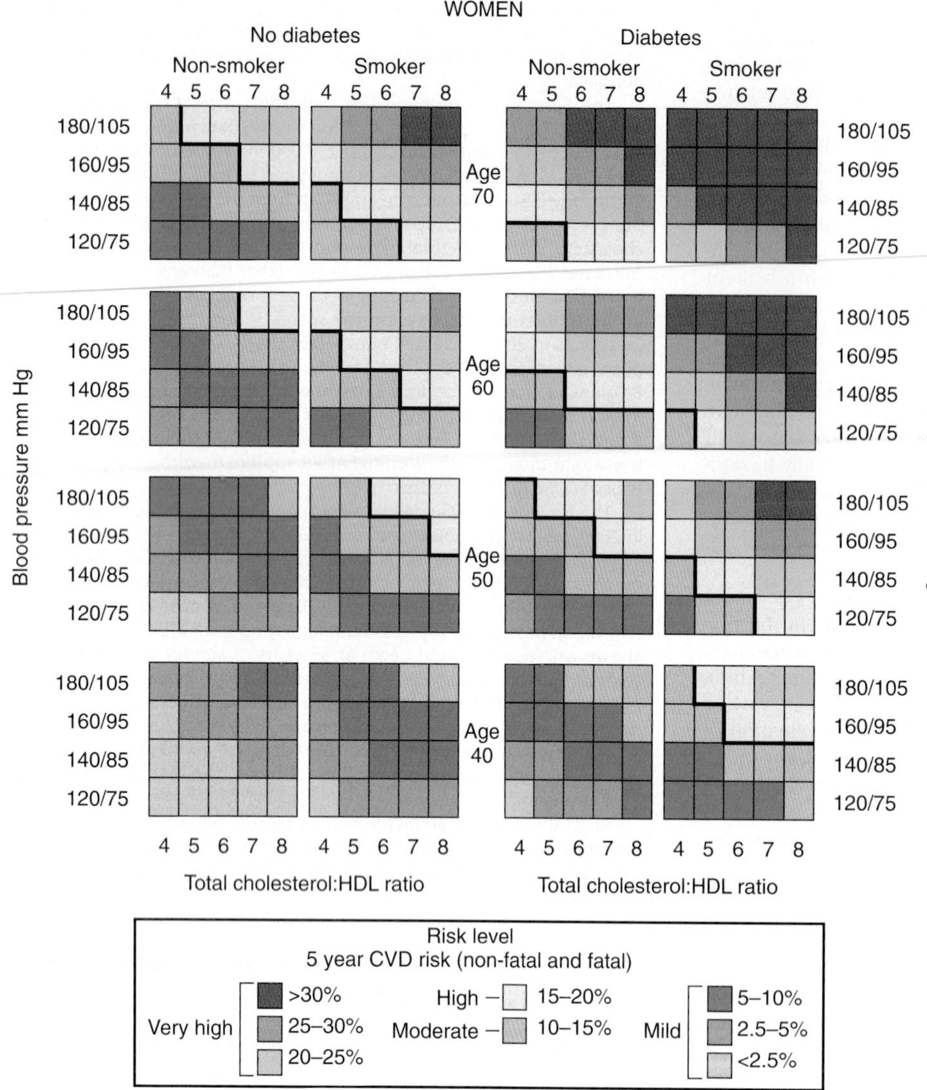

How to use the table:

- Within the table choose the cell nearest to the person's age, blood pressure and TC:HDL ratio. When the systolic and diastolic values fall in different risk levels, the higher category applies.
- For example, the lower left cell contains all non-smokers without diabetes who are less than 45 years and have a TC:HDL ratio less than 4.5 and a blood pressure less than 130/80 mm Hg. People who fall exactly on a threshold between cells are placed in the cell indicating higher risk.

FIGURE 49-5 Risk assessment tool devised by a New Zealand task force to determine 5-year total cardiovascular disease (CVD) risk based on age, sex, smoking history, lipid and glucose levels, and blood pressure. This chart shows the risk level for women; a similar chart exists to assess risk in men. HDL = high-density lipoprotein; TC = total cholesterol. *(From New Zealand Guidelines Group: New Zealand Cardiovascular Guidelines Handbook: A Summary Resource for Primary Care Practitioners. 2nd ed. Wellington, New Zealand, 2009. http://www.nzgg.org.nz/guidelines/0154/CVD_handbook_june_2009_update.pdf.)*

practical, systematic approach to ranking of interventions and allocation of resources. Risk factors fall into four categories according to the likelihood that modification of the factor will lower risk: factors for which interventions have been proved to reduce risk; factors for which interventions are likely to lower the incidence of events; factors clearly associated with CHD risk that, if modified, might lower the incidence of coronary events; and factors associated with CHD risk that cannot be modified or, if modified, are not likely to decrease risk. Adapting this classification scheme to clinical practice requires consideration of feasibility and cost-efficacy. We present a modified classification scheme of interventions for major modifiable risk factors based not only on the strength of the association and evidence of the benefit of intervention, but also on cost-efficacy (**Table 49-2**).

CLASS 1. Class 1 interventions have a clear causal relationship with heart disease (**Table 49-3**). Reliable data, generally from randomized clinical trials, demonstrate the magnitude of the intervention's benefit as well as its risks and cost. Cigarette smoking, hypertension, and dyslipidemias relate causally to CHD, and the corresponding interventions—smoking cessation, blood pressure management, and lipid profile management—all are cost-effective in both primary and secondary prevention. For management of hypertension and dyslipidemia, extensive trial and cost-efficacy data enable a tiered approach based on absolute risk at baseline. Other beneficial and cost-effective pharmacologic approaches include aspirin, beta-adrenergic receptor blockers (beta blockers), and angiotensin-converting enzyme (ACE) inhibitors in specific situations in secondary prevention, and aspirin in higher-risk primary prevention.

CLASS 2. Class 2 includes interventions for which the available data (largely basic research and human observational studies) strongly indicate a causal relationship and suggest that intervention will probably reduce the incidence of events, but with less abundant data on the benefits, risks, and costs of intervention. For example, data from large-scale, long-term randomized trials on weight management and physical activity with CHD outcomes will likely remain limited.

CLASS 3. Class 3 interventions are currently under active investigation. Incomplete data support many factors in this class, restricting conclusions about an independent causal relationship with CHD. Examples include various strategies to raise HDL level. Thus, although these factors may have utility for risk assessment, their role as targets for the prevention of CHD remains uncertain. For these reasons, hormone replacement therapy, dietary practices such as the consumption of nutritional supplements, psychological factors, and interventions that target several novel biochemical and genetic markers currently fall into class 3.

The sections that follow provide a summary of the data on the given interventions, followed by a summary of how to implement the specific strategies. The subsequent sections summarize the approach to intervention for each category of factors.

Class 1 Interventions

This category includes the "big three" interventions—smoking cessation, management of dyslipidemia, and management of blood pressure—as well as prophylactic pharmacologic interventions in selected patients. Each of these interventions should be seriously considered in those with CVD and diabetes, and in primary prevention patients when appropriate, and this consideration should be documented. A population-level comparative risk assessment for 12 major modifiable dietary, lifestyle, and metabolic risks recently found that

TABLE 49-2 Classification Scheme for Modifiable Risk Factors

CLASS	DEFINITION
1	Basic research and human observational studies identify targets with strong potential for risk reduction. Intervention data (typically from randomized trials) demonstrate the magnitude of the benefit and risk. Interventions are cost-effective.
2	Basic research and human observational studies identify targets with potential for risk reduction. Intervention data from large-scale trials are limited. Lack of adequate intervention data precludes determination of cost-effectiveness.
3	Basic research and human observational studies demonstrate associations, but the nature of the relationship is not yet clear. Interventions are not yet available or have not been adequately tested.

TABLE 49-3 Risk Factors and Interventions for Coronary Heart Disease

CLASS	RISK FACTOR	INTERVENTION
1	Smoking Dyslipidemia High blood pressure Preventive medications	Smoking cessation Lipid management Blood pressure management Aspirin, angiotensin-converting enzyme inhibitor, beta blocker
2	Diabetes, prediabetes Physical inactivity Overweight, obesity Unhealthy diet, alcohol Inflammation	Diabetes management Activity management Weight management Improved diet Various interventions
3	Menopause, hormone replacement therapy Micronutrients Psychological factors Novel biochemical and genetic markers	

smoking and high blood pressure, both of which have effective interventions, cause the largest number of deaths in the United States.[9]

Cigarette Smoking and Cessation (see Chap. 44)

PREVALENCE. In the United States, per capita cigarette consumption rose dramatically in the first half of the 20th century. More than 65% of men born between 1911 and 1920 were smoking by 1945. Annual per capita consumption of cigarettes hit an astonishing 4286 (more than 200 packs per year) in 1963. The prevalence of smoking among men peaked in 1955, when more than half were smokers; among women, that point came 10 years later, with more than one third smoking. Smoking rates have declined substantially since then, with 21% of adults smoking. Slightly more men than women—approximately 23% of men aged 18 years and older, compared with 18% of women aged 18 years and older—are smokers.[10] Smoking rates among high-school seniors rose from 30% in the mid-1980s (with higher rates among girls) to approximately 36.5% by 1997,[11] but now appear to be on a steady downward trend. Smoking rates tend to be higher among those with lower socioeconomic status and those with a high-school education or less. According to data from the 2008 National Health Interview Survey, 41% of adults aged 25 years or older with GED certificates smoke, and 32% of individuals living below the federal poverty level are smokers.

ASSOCIATED RISK. Smoking increases the risk of CHD (see Chap. 44). Seminal studies linking smoking and heart disease appeared by the middle of the 20th century. The 1964 Surgeon General's report reaffirmed the epidemiologic relation, and by 1983 the Surgeon General had firmly established cigarette smoking as the leading avoidable cause of CVD. Based largely on studies among men, the 1989 Surgeon General's report showed that smoking doubles the incidence of CHD and increases CHD mortality by 50%, and that these risks increase with age and the number of cigarettes smoked. Women incur similar increases in the relative risk for CHD.

In the United States, cigarette smoking is the leading preventable cause of death and accounts for an estimated 443,000 deaths each year and more than 5 million years of potential life lost.[12] Among smokers 35 years of age or older who die of smoking-related causes, 33% die of CVD. Smoking rates continue to rise worldwide, with the greatest increases in the developing world; 1 million more deaths were attributable to tobacco in 2000 than in 1990.[13] Tobacco use causes an estimated 5 million deaths annually.[14]

BENEFIT OF INTERVENTION. Although data from large-scale, randomized trials concerning the risk reduction associated with smoking cessation are limited, observational studies demonstrate clear benefits of smoking cessation. Smokers who quit reduce their excess risk of a coronary event by 50% within the first 2 years after cessation, with much of this gain in the first few months. This period is followed by a more gradual decline, with the risk of former smokers approaching that of never smokers after 3 to 5 years.

COST-EFFICACY. Smoking cessation is highly cost-effective in both primary and secondary prevention. The intervention is usually short term and thus low cost. In fact, smoking cessation programs generally cost less than continued smoking. The gains in life expectancy are large, and the earlier in life an individual stops smoking, the larger the potential gain; a 35-year-old male smoker, for example, may add 3 years to his life expectancy on cessation. Costs vary, depending on the intensity of intervention and the use of pharmacologic agents. A Swedish study found that during a 20-year period, the incremental costs per QALY saved were relatively low for bupropion in comparison to nicotine patches: approximately $660 per QALY gained for men and about $490 per QALY gained for women.[15] Several nonpharmacologic approaches also have been effective.

GUIDELINES AND RECOMMENDATIONS. Clinical practice guidelines from the U.S. Public Health Service recognize that tobacco dependence is a chronic condition that generally requires repeated intervention. Although there has been some improvement, according to the National Committee for Quality Assurance's State of Health Care Quality Report, clinicians do not always capitalize on opportunities to intervene with smokers. In 2005, 71.2% of commercially insured smokers received cessation advice, up slightly from 69.6% in 2004; and 75.5% of smokers receiving Medicare were given advice to quit, up 11 percentage points from 2004. In another report, only 25% of Medicaid patients said that they had any practical assistance with quitting or any follow-up regarding their progress.[16] The Public Health Service guidelines support a combination of counseling and medication and stress the importance of multiple counseling sessions to increase the success rate. Seven first-line pharmacotherapies that reliably increase long-term smoking abstinence were also identified: sustained-release bupropion hydrochloride, five nicotine replacement therapies (gum, patch, inhaler, nasal spray, and lozenges), and varenicline. Prescription-only varenicline, approved by the U.S. Food and Drug Administration (FDA) in 2006, works in two ways; by imitating the effects of nicotine, it reduces cravings and withdrawal symptoms, and it partially blocks the effects of nicotine, providing the smoker with less of a reward. Varenicline is typically taken for 12 weeks, and although it is not intended to be used with nicotine replacement products, some studies show that they might be safely combined. A 2008 Cochrane review found no overall difference in the effectiveness of the various forms of nicotine replacement therapy.[17] For people smoking more than 15 cigarettes per day, use of any form increased the chances of quitting long term by 50% to 70%. Another approach, an antismoking vaccine, is under development; antibodies would bind nicotine to prevent it from leaving the blood and entering the brain, eliminating the enjoyable sensation.

In view of the addictive nature of smoking and the tendency to increase smoking over time, smoking reduction—as opposed to cessation—is not an acceptable strategy. Although it is important to counsel patients at all stages about the hazards of smoking and the benefits of quitting, the period soon after a cardiac event is an opportune time to encourage a patient to stop smoking.

FUTURE CHALLENGES. In the United States, the recently enacted Family Smoking Prevention and Tobacco Control Act bans the use in cigarettes of flavorings, such as strawberry and grape, and gives the FDA broad authority to regulate labeling, packaging, and advertising of tobacco products, all of which should make smoking less appealing to minors. Intense public health efforts are needed worldwide to reverse the alarming rise in smoking rates occurring in many developing countries; nearly 60% of men in China now smoke. Approximately 82% of the 1.1 billion people who smoke worldwide reside in low- and middle-income countries.[14] The low success rates in cessation efforts offer a challenge to clinicians, and greater emphasis must be placed on preventing smoking in the first place.

Dyslipidemia and Its Management (see Chaps. 44 and 47)

PREVALENCE. Mean cholesterol levels have declined modestly in the United States since the early 1960s. Even with this decline, about 45% of all American adults have cholesterol levels greater than 200 mg/dL, and 16% have levels higher than 240 mg/dL (National Health and Nutrition Examination Survey 2005-2006). Low HDL-cholesterol levels and high triglyceride levels tend to coincide and often result from metabolic phenomena distinct from those leading to high levels of LDL-cholesterol. Thus, low HDL and high triglyceride levels can occur alone or in combination with high LDL levels.

ASSOCIATED RISK. Several lipid variables causally associate with increased risk of CHD. A 1-mg/dL increase in serum LDL-cholesterol associates with a 2% to 3% increase in risk for CHD, and elevations earlier in life may be associated with higher increases in risk. HDL-cholesterol independently predicts CHD; every 1-mg/dL decrease in HDL-cholesterol causes a 3% to 4% increase. Furthermore, the ratio of total cholesterol or LDL-cholesterol to HDL-cholesterol may predict CHD risk better than LDL alone. A 1-unit decrease in this ratio (easily achievable with statins) reduces the risk of MI by more than 50%. See Chaps. 44 and 47 for discussion of hypertriglyceridemia.

BENEFIT OF INTERVENTION. Dietary and pharmacologic treatments that lower serum cholesterol have clear benefits (see Chap. 47). A 2005 meta-analysis of 14 randomized trials with 90,056 participants showed that statin therapy safely reduces the 5-year incidence of major coronary events, coronary revascularization, and stroke by about one fifth per 1 mmol/liter reduction in LDL level, irrespective of pretreatment cholesterol level, age, sex, or preexisting disease and without any increases in cancer.[18] This reduction in risk is linear, resulting in comparable risk reductions across the spectrum of lipid levels (see Fig. 47-6).

Long-term daily compliance appears to be far more important in determining outcome efficacy than any demonstrated differences between statins in terms of potency. A recent meta-analysis of four large randomized trials among those with existing disease found that intensive therapy with high-dose statins had clear benefits over standard-dose therapy in reducing the risk of MI, stroke, or any cardiovascular event.[19] Trial data support the early initiation of statin therapy after MI or coronary artery bypass grafting.

For a discussion of fibrates and nicotinic acid, consult Chap. 47.

COST-EFFICACY. The cost-efficacy of nonpharmacologic interventions to lower LDL-cholesterol is unclear. Pharmacologic intervention, however, is clearly cost-effective under certain conditions, and available data permit tailoring of recommendations to the level of baseline CHD risk. Early analyses of cholesterol reduction for secondary prevention (which used data from cholestyramine trials) resulted in very costly interventions, largely because the available drugs were relatively ineffective. In contrast, data for statin therapy are remarkably consistent, and with the availability of generic statins, analyses indicate that they may prove cost-effective for a larger number of individuals.

Statins are highly cost-effective. QALY evaluations are highly sensitive to drug cost and will decline substantially as more statins transition into generic drugs. Simvastatin and pravastatin both became available as generics in 2006, joining lovastatin, which has been prescribed in generic form since 1999. An analysis found that a daily dose of 40 mg of generic simvastatin would cost less than $1350 per life year gained for those with an annual risk of major vascular events of 1% or more, regardless of their age at the start of treatment.[20]

GUIDELINES AND TREATMENT. All patients with CVD should be screened for serum cholesterol levels, but in primary prevention, some controversy remains. Physicians can choose from several sets of guidelines, but each has become increasingly complex, with multiple steps to determine who should be treated and demanding procedures to evaluate the success of treatment. The NCEP recommends routine screening of all adults older than 20 years of age,[21] and the USPSTF recommends screening of all men 35 years of age and older and women 45 years of age and older if they are at increased risk for CHD.[22] Screening of patients with CVD should include a full fasting lipid profile that measures total cholesterol, HDL, and triglycerides. For patients without CVD, screening for HDL remains controversial. Because HDL and the ratio of total cholesterol to HDL-cholesterol powerfully predict risk and aid in the detection of individuals who have elevated LDL despite moderate levels of total cholesterol, it seems prudent to check HDL along with total cholesterol. Similarly, measuring hsCRP also may be useful.

Since the NCEP issued its first Adult Treatment Panel (ATP) report in 1988, the guidelines have been revised twice; a new version is slated for release in 2011. Under the current guidelines, 65 million U.S. adults are eligible for therapeutic lifestyle changes, and 36 million meet the criteria for drug therapy. The ATP III guidelines rely on assessment of a risk score (Framingham Risk Score, consideration of other markers of risk such as elevated triglycerides and hsCRP, and family history) and the LDL level. Once they are receiving lipid-lowering therapy, patients are observed for the attainment of one of three or four fixed LDL targets. Patients with existing CHD (or a CHD risk equivalent such as diabetes or peripheral arterial disease) are at the highest risk for a cardiovascular event and thus have the lowest LDL target (<100 mg/dL), with the option of setting the goal at <70 mg/dL for those who have had a recent acute coronary event or who have CVD combined with either diabetes or severe or poorly controlled risk factors (**Table 49-4**).

In 2006, the American Heart Association (AHA) and American College of Cardiology (ACC) updated their secondary prevention guidelines for lipid management, echoing the recommendations made by the NCEP 2 years earlier but strengthening some of them as

TABLE 49-4 Low-Density Lipoprotein Goals for Three Risk Levels

RISK LEVEL	LDL GOAL (MG/DL)
CHD and CHD risk equivalent*	<100
Multiple (2+) risk factors	<130†
0-1 risk factor	<160

*Diabetes, chronic kidney disease.

†LDL goal for individuals with multiple risk factors and a 10-year overall risk >20% is <100 mg/dL.

From Third Report of the National Cholesterol Education Program (NCEP) Expert Panel on Detection, Evaluation, and Treatment of High Blood Cholesterol in Adults (Adult Treatment Panel III) final report. Circulation 106:3143, 2002.

well. As with the NCEP guidelines, the LDL goal remains at <100 mg/dL, and <70 mg/dL has been added as an optional goal. The AHA/ACC update extends the <70 mg/dL option to all patients with coronary artery disease (CAD), not just to those at very high risk, a view that remains controversial.[23] Patients with a triglyceride level of 200 to 499 mg/dL should have a non-HDL cholesterol level <130 mg/dL, with further reduction to <100 mg/dL considered reasonable.

According to the NCEP guidelines for primary prevention, patients at moderately high risk for development of CHD (two or more risk factors and a 10-year overall risk of 10% to 20%) should be treated to an LDL target of less than 130 mg/dL or, optionally, to 100 mg/dL. This is also the target for patients with moderate risk (two or more risk factors and a <10% risk for heart attack in the next 10 years). Those at even lower risk should be treated to a target LDL level of less than 160 mg/dL.

An important question regarding the NCEP guidelines is whether both risk levels and LDL levels are necessary, especially if the LDL level is used in the risk assessment tool. The linear association between cholesterol levels and CVD risk provides no biologic justification for current threshold levels. Even within an ATP risk category, use of the LDL thresholds may mean favoring treatment of a patient whose LDL level is above a certain threshold but who has a relatively low overall risk, while forgoing treatment of a patient who is at higher overall risk but whose LDL level is just below the arbitrary threshold.

Guidelines from the European Society of Cardiology (ESC) also have tiers. Although the target is identical for all patients (total cholesterol <190 mg/dL [5 mmol/liter] and LDL cholesterol <115 mg/dL [3 mmol/liter]), the timing and intensity of drug therapy are different.[7] In primary prevention, using the ESC's SCORE scale, if the 10-year risk of cardiovascular death is 5% or greater, or if the projected risk at the age of 60 years is 5% or greater, lifestyle modifications are recommended and lipids should be checked in 3 months. If the total cholesterol or LDL-cholesterol level is above target at this checkup, drug therapy may be instituted. For high-risk asymptomatic individuals whose total cholesterol and LDL-cholesterol levels are already close to the target levels (<5 mmol/liter and <3 mmol/liter, respectively), the treatment goals are total cholesterol <4.5 mmol/liter (175 mg/dL) and LDL <2.5 mmol/liter (100 mg/dL), or lower if feasible. These are the same goals for those with established CVD or diabetes.

New Canadian guidelines published in 2009 specify more aggressive lipid control and have redefined LDL targets. For high-risk patients, the guidelines recommend a 50% reduction in LDL. The previous target for this group was <2 mmol/liter, so for some patients, the new goal would be a level significantly below this. However, much of the focus is on primary prevention and those at intermediate risk, defined as a 10% to 19% estimated likelihood of a thrombotic event during the next 10 years. With use of the new guidelines, some patients in this group would be subject to the same intensive lipid-lowering treatment as previously recommended for individuals at high risk; this includes individuals who have an LDL level of >3.5 mmol/liter or a total cholesterol–HDL ratio >5.0, as well as men older than 50 years of age or women older than 60 years of age with hsCRP >2.0 mg/liter.[24]

In secondary prevention, individuals with a high LDL level who also have a low HDL or high triglyceride level should be treated aggressively (see Chap. 47). In primary prevention, individuals who have a normal LDL level but a low HDL or high triglyceride level warrant nonpharmacologic interventions, pending further trial data regarding drug therapy in such cases. Intervention data for patients with isolated elevated triglyceride levels are also needed.

FUTURE CHALLENGES. Whereas the last 20 years have witnessed much progress in identifying and treating patients with dyslipidemia, current guidelines are overly complicated. Current data support a simplified, risk-based approach. New research shows that among Americans with high LDL levels, one third have not been screened, and one third of those at high risk are not receiving medication that would likely benefit them.[25] The absolute CVD risk, rather than the LDL level, should trigger initiation of treatment. Given the linear relation between cholesterol level and risk and the similar linear relation between lowering of risk and change in total or LDL cholesterol, the new Canadian guidelines focusing on change in LDL-cholesterol rather than on fixed targets have merit. A simple risk assessment would classify individuals into only two strata: those for whom lipid-lowering therapy should be considered, and those for whom it is not warranted. Additional randomized trial data are needed to clarify the role of cholesterol screening. Although cholesterol levels are falling or stable in industrialized countries, they are rising in developing countries as Western diets increasingly become adopted. Developing countries need low-cost strategies for screening and intervention (see Chap. 1).

Hypertension and Blood Pressure Control (see Chap. 46)

PREVALENCE. One in three American adults is hypertensive, and another 25% fall into the prehypertensive category (**Table 49-5**; see Table 45-1).[26,27] High blood pressure is more common among blacks than whites and among men than women until 45 years of age, when it equally affects both sexes. After 65 years of age, however, a higher percentage of women are hypertensive. Data from the Framingham

TABLE 49-5 Classification and Management of Blood Pressure for Adults

				Management	
				INITIAL DRUG THERAPY	
BP CLASSIFICATION	SYSTOLIC BP (MM HG)	DIASTOLIC BP (MM HG)	LIFESTYLE MODIFICATION	*WITHOUT COMPELLING INDICATION*	*WITH COMPELLING INDICATION*
Normal	<120	*and* <80	Encourage		
Prehypertension	120-139	*or* 80-89	Yes	None indicated	Drugs for compelling indications* (treat to BP target <130/80)
Stage 1 hypertension	140-159	*or* 90-99	Yes	Thiazide-type diuretics for most May consider ACEI, ARB, BB, CCB, or combination	Drugs for compelling indications* Other antihypertensive drugs (diuretics, ACEI, ARB, BB, CCB) as needed
Stage 2 hypertension	≥160	*or* ≥100	Yes	Two-drug combination for most (usually thiazide-type diuretic and ACEI or ARB or BB or CCB)	

*Patients with chronic kidney disease or diabetes.

ACEI = angiotensin-converting enzyme inhibitor; ARB = angiotensin receptor blocker; BB = beta blocker; BP = blood pressure; CCB = calcium channel blocker.

From Chobanian AV, Bakris GL, Black HR, et al: The Seventh Report of the Joint National Committee on Prevention, Detection, Evaluation, and Treatment of High Blood Pressure: The JNC 7 Report. JAMA 289:2560, 2003.

Heart Study suggest that normotensive individuals at 55 years of age have a 90% lifetime risk for the development of hypertension. A recently published long-term study of nurses suggests that women adopting healthy practices such as maintaining normal weight, eating a healthful diet, exercising daily, drinking a moderate amount of alcohol, and limiting use of over-the-counter analgesics could greatly reduce the risk of hypertension in young women.[28] In the United States, hypertension prevalence appears to be increasing. Although control of hypertension improved throughout the 1990s, particularly among older patients, control rates remain low (30%).[29]

ASSOCIATED RISK. Elevated systolic or diastolic blood pressure associates with an increased risk of CVD (see Chaps. 44 to 46).[2,30] A collaborative meta-analysis of individual participant data from 61 prospective, observational studies with 1 million participants showed a linear risk relation between blood pressure and the risk of vascular mortality down to a pressure of at least 115/75 mm Hg throughout middle and old age.[30] Hypertension also associates with increased risk of heart failure, stroke, and kidney disease. The CVD risk curve is linear; for individuals 40 to 70 years of age, each increment of 20 mm Hg in systolic blood pressure or 10 mm Hg in diastolic blood pressure doubles the risk of CVD across a blood pressure range of 115/75 to 185/115 mm Hg. Systolic blood pressure remains the most useful clinical predictor of risk.

BENEFIT OF INTERVENTION. Randomized trials have demonstrated the protective effect of treating mild to moderate hypertension. Precise estimates of risk reduction have come from meta-analyses reporting that lowering of diastolic blood pressure by 5 to 6 mm Hg results in a 42% reduction in the risk of stroke and a 15% reduction in the risk of CHD events.[31] The Antihypertensive and Lipid-Lowering Treatment to Prevent Heart Attack Trial (ALLHAT) demonstrated the efficacy of thiazide diuretics compared with other antihypertensive agents.[32] Some of the benefit of the diuretics may have resulted from slightly better reduction in blood pressure.[33] ALLHAT was one of 29 randomized trials included in a 2003 meta-analysis that examined the effects of various blood pressure–lowering regimens on major CVD events. No significant differences were observed between treatment approaches based on ACE inhibitors, calcium antagonists, diuretics, or beta blockers, although ACE inhibitor–based regimens reduced blood pressure less. In addition, this study demonstrated a linear relation such that larger reductions in blood pressure produced larger reductions in risk.[34] Two antihypertensive agents will be needed for initial therapy for many patients, in particular those with stage 2 hypertension.

Until recently, treatment rates among those older than 80 years of age were low because of concern that treatment might lead to kidney and other problems. Yet, the Hypertension in the Very Elderly Trial (HYVET)[35] found that treatment of this growing patient population with a diuretic and an ACE inhibitor if needed was both safe and effective, reducing not only the risk of heart failure and death from stroke, but also the risk of death from any cause.

COST-EFFICACY. Detection and management of hypertension are highly cost-effective in both primary and secondary prevention. More aggressive management in those at high risk, based on the existence of CVD or diabetes, is warranted on the basis of greater cost-efficacy. In secondary prevention, for agents such as diuretics and beta blockers, the cost is below $10,000 per QALY for patients with established CHD, even when blood pressure is only mildly elevated.[36] In primary prevention, cost ranges from $10,000 to $20,000 per QALY among individuals with moderate to severe elevations in blood pressure, but the cost approaches an unacceptable $100,000 per QALY for higher priced medications. Cost-efficacy decreases with increasing age. Careful cost-efficacy evaluation is needed for recommendations from JNC 7, as this guideline suggests the use of multiple agents and favors intervention for a wider group of individuals, including those with slight elevations of blood pressure.

GUIDELINES AND TREATMENT. Several guidelines exist for the management of hypertension, often characterized by complexity. The USPSTF recommends routine blood pressure testing of all adults.[37,38] The JNC 7 (to be superseded by the JNC 8 in 2010) defines four levels of blood pressure according to the risk imparted (see Table 49-5; see Table 45-1).

Recommendations for intervention from the JNC 7 are based on the level of blood pressure and the level of absolute risk. The absolute risk strata are defined according to the presence or absence of target organ disease, clinical CVD, diabetes, and cardiovascular risk factors (such as smoking, hyperlipidemia, age older than 60 years, sex, and family history of early-onset CVD). The JNC 7 sets a blood pressure goal of 140/90 mm Hg for lower-risk patients and 130/80 mm Hg for those with CVD, diabetes, or chronic kidney disease. Because the relation of blood pressure to CVD risk is linear, a significant portion of the population-attributable risk occurs among those with blood pressure in the JNC 7 category of prehypertension—a systolic blood pressure of 120 to 139 mm Hg or a diastolic pressure of 80 to 89 mm Hg.

For all individuals with blood pressure of 120/80 mm Hg or greater, JNC 7 recommends lifestyle modifications including smoking cessation, weight reduction if needed, increased physical activity, limited alcohol intake, limited sodium intake, adequate potassium and calcium intake, and adoption of the Dietary Approaches to Stop Hypertension (DASH) eating plan—a diet with a reduced content of saturated and total fat that is also rich in fruits, vegetables, and low-fat dairy products (see Chaps. 46 and 48).[39]

Initiation of drug therapy depends on blood pressure and the absolute level of risk. For example, among individuals with stage 1 hypertension but no evidence of end-organ damage, vascular disease, or diabetes and one CVD risk factor, lifestyle modification and drug therapy are recommended. For individuals with stage 2 hypertension, combination therapy including a thiazide-type diuretic is usually the starting point. The guidelines also recommend initiation of therapy with two drugs (one being a diuretic) when blood pressure is more than 20/10 mm Hg above the target level. For specific therapeutic agents recommended by JNC 7, see Chap. 46. Most patients require more than one agent to achieve their blood pressure goal.

Guidelines from the European Society of Hypertension/European Society of Cardiology (ESH/ESC) stratify initial therapy somewhat differently. High-normal is defined as systolic pressure between 130 and 139 mm Hg or diastolic pressure of 85 to 89 mm Hg, and drug therapy is recommended only for individuals at very high risk because of prior MI, diabetes, or a similar clinical condition.[40] Among patients with grade 1 hypertension (systolic pressure of 140 to 159 mm Hg or diastolic pressure of 90 to 99 mm Hg) or grade 2 hypertension (systolic pressure of 160 to 179 mm Hg or diastolic pressure of 100 to 109 mm Hg), drug treatment should be started promptly in those at high risk (three or more risk factors, target organ damage, or diabetes) or very high risk (obvious clinical disease). For patients in these two categories who are at moderate risk, the guidelines call for lifestyle modification for several weeks, then drug treatment if blood pressure is uncontrolled. This is a change from earlier ESH/ESC guidelines, which recommended monitoring for "extended periods" (at least 3 months) before initiation of drug therapy. Low-risk individuals with grade 2 hypertension should also be advised to try lifestyle changes for several weeks before medication is introduced, but low-risk patients with grade 1 hypertension can try lifestyle changes for several months before drug treatment is considered. As with the JNC 7 recommendations, lifestyle modifications should always accompany drug therapy. Updated ESH/ESC guidelines were released in late 2009, and the guidelines now include a recommendation for a lower threshold level of about 120 mm Hg systolic and 70 mm Hg diastolic for high-risk patients, reflecting the J-curve phenomenon and the possible danger of going lower.

Data from ALLHAT also have indicated that a thiazide-type diuretic may be a good choice for first-line antihypertensive therapy.[32] The available evidence no longer supports the use of beta blockers as a first-line therapy for primary prevention. The Anglo-Scandinavian Cardiac Outcomes Trial–Blood Pressure Lowering Arm (ASCOT-BPLA) trial assigned 19,257 hypertensive patients at moderate risk for development of CVD events to one of two regimens: a beta blocker, plus a thiazide diuretic if needed; or a long-acting calcium channel blocker, plus an ACE inhibitor when needed.[41] The trial was halted early, as subjects receiving beta blockers became increasingly disadvantaged. A meta-analysis of 20 trials and a 2007 Cochrane review concluded that beta blockers should not remain the first choice in treatment of primary hypertension.[42,43]

In 2006, the British Hypertension Society updated pharmacologic treatment guidelines ahead of schedule to revise its previous recommendation concerning beta blockers as the preferred first-line therapy for hypertension.[44] The working group cited evidence that beta blockers produce less benefit than other drugs, particularly in the elderly, and increasing evidence that the most frequently used beta blockers at usual doses carry an unacceptable risk of provoking type 2 diabetes. According to the new guidelines, for all patients 55 years of age and older and for black patients of any age, a calcium channel blocker or a thiazide-type diuretic is the first choice. If a second drug is required, an ACE inhibitor (or an angiotensin receptor blocker [ARB] if an ACE inhibitor is not tolerated) is preferred. In patients younger than 55 years of age, the first-choice therapy should be an ACE inhibitor or an ARB. A calcium channel blocker or a thiazide-type diuretic should be added if another drug is required. Regardless of age, if three drugs are needed, the guidelines recommend a combination of an ACE inhibitor, a calcium channel blocker, and a thiazide-type diuretic. The revised ESH/ESC guidelines do not emphasize which antihypertensive should be used as a first-line or second-line drug, instead advising physicians to tailor therapy to individual patients.

FUTURE CHALLENGES. The relations between risk and increasing levels of blood pressure and between risk reduction and degree of blood pressure lowering are linear. Thus, more attention should be focused on changing blood pressure rather than on treating to a specific target. In the developed world, the prevalence of hypertension is increasing as populations age. Approximately 40% of those with hypertension do not know they have it and are not being treated, and only one third of patients treated for hypertension have their blood pressure under control.[45] In developing countries, hypertension rates are rising rapidly with urbanization and lifestyle changes. A new estimate of the attributable global burden of nonoptimal blood pressure (>115 mm Hg) shows that approximately two thirds of the disease burden occurs in the developing world, and that roughly two thirds of the worldwide burden occurs in those 45 to 69 years of age.[46]

Cardiac Protection with Aspirin and Other Pharmacologic Agents

Several pharmacologic interventions are highly effective in the prevention of CVD events, including aspirin, beta blockers, and ACE inhibitors. Each of these agents has proven efficacy in intermediate and longer-term secondary prevention among various subgroups of patients. Aspirin also has benefit in primary prevention for some groups.

ANTIPLATELET THERAPY: SECONDARY PREVENTION. Aspirin therapy in patients with existing CVD (see Chaps. 55 to 57 and 87) reduces the risk of subsequent events by 25%. Meta-analyses demonstrate clear reductions in mortality and nonfatal CVD events among those with prior MI, stroke, bypass surgery, angioplasty, peripheral vascular surgery, or angina.[47] In these meta-analyses, doses above 75 mg/day showed clear benefit, with no trend toward increasing benefit at higher doses. In contrast, below 75 mg/day, there was a nonsignificant attenuated risk reduction of only 15%. The AHA/ACC recently lowered the recommended prophylactic dose from 75 to 325 mg/day to 75 to 162 mg/day, on the basis of antiplatelet trials that show no difference in benefit but a reduced risk of bleeding with a lower dose.[23] Other antiplatelet agents do not offer much benefit over aspirin. In the Antiplatelet Trialists' Collaboration analysis, other agents did not offer superiority. Whether there is a modest benefit of clopidogrel over aspirin is not clear, despite randomized trials including thousands of patients, and data on comparative cost-efficacy are unclear. A recent trial comparing clopidogrel and aspirin versus aspirin alone in high-risk patients found that clopidogrel plus aspirin was not significantly more effective than aspirin alone in reducing the rate of MI, stroke, or death from CVD, but that dual antiplatelet therapy did increase the risk of moderate to severe bleeding.[48] Whereas data support the addition of clopidogrel to aspirin in certain high-risk patients, such as those with acute ischemia or after stent placement, the increased bleeding risk makes this strategy unacceptable for primary prevention.

Unless it is contraindicated, most patients with known CVD should use aspirin. Other antiplatelet agents with demonstrated efficacy, such as clopidogrel, should be limited to patients with aspirin allergy or intolerance. Clopidogrel has a much less favorable cost-efficacy than aspirin (and associates with increased hemorrhage), so it should not be used instead of aspirin in primary prevention. Data from the Coronary Heart Disease Policy Model suggest that extending the use of aspirin therapy for secondary prevention from current levels to all eligible patients for 25 years would have an estimated cost-effectiveness ratio of about $11,000 per QALY gained. Clopidogrel alone in all patients or in routine combination with aspirin had an incremental cost of more than $130,000 per QALY gained.[49]

ASPIRIN IN PRIMARY PREVENTION. Six large-scale trials have assessed the benefits of low-dose aspirin in the prevention of CVD. Three of the trials were limited to men, and one was limited to women. Taken together, these studies suggest a benefit of prophylactic aspirin in primary prevention of MI and ischemic stroke (**Fig. 49-6**).[50] The Women's Health Study addressed the benefit-to-risk ratio of aspirin therapy for primary prevention of CVD specifically in women. In that study, a 100-mg dose of aspirin every other day lowered the risk of stroke but did not affect the risk of MI or death from other cardiovascular causes in a group of initially healthy women who were 45 years of age or older.[51] Among study participants 65 years of age or older, however, the 100-mg alternate-day aspirin dose reduced the risk of major cardiovascular events by 26%. The Women's Health Study also examined primary prevention using an aspirin dose below 75 mg, which produced a suboptimal effect. The nonsignificant 9% reduction in CVD events was consistent with the nonsignificant reduction of 13% in the secondary meta-analysis for doses below 75 mg.[47]

These six trials were included in a 2009 collaborative meta-analysis of aspirin use for primary prevention, which found that the risk of bleeding was comparable to the potential benefit associated with routine use of aspirin in healthy individuals at lower risk for CHD. Conducted by the Antithrombotic Trialists' Collaboration, the analysis also included 16 secondary prevention trials that compared long-term aspirin with controls.[52] Ongoing trials are assessing the risk of bleeding in high-risk individuals.

The USPSTF [22] and the AHA have concluded that aspirin decreases the incidence of CHD in adults at increased risk for heart disease. In 2007, the AHA updated its guidelines for women, recommending aspirin for high-risk women whose 10-year risk of a first coronary event exceeds 20%, and for all women 65 years of age or older if blood pressure is controlled and the potential benefit for prevention of ischemic stroke or MI outweighs the risk of bleeding or hemorrhagic stroke. In 2009, the USPSTF updated its guidelines, recommending aspirin for men 45 to 79 years of age and women 55 to 79 years of age if the potential benefit—a reduction in risk of MI in men and risk of ischemic stroke in women—outweighs the increased risk of gastrointestinal bleeding.[53] The agency did not specify an optimum dose, noting that this is currently unknown. The ESC had recommended aspirin in primary prevention only for men at particularly high risk of CHD, but it has now changed that recommendation to anyone who has a SCORE risk of greater than 10%.[7] Ongoing trials among higher-risk individuals will help to refine these recommendations.

BETA-ADRENERGIC RECEPTOR BLOCKERS. Several trials have demonstrated the long-term efficacy of beta-adrenergic receptor blocking agents (beta blockers) in reducing mortality after MI, and meta-analyses suggest a 23% mortality reduction with long-term use (see Chaps. 55 and 56). Long-term use of beta blockers also lowers the risk of recurrent cardiovascular events. Cross-trial comparisons suggest that the higher the level of beta blockade, as measured by heart rate reduction relative to the control group, the greater the

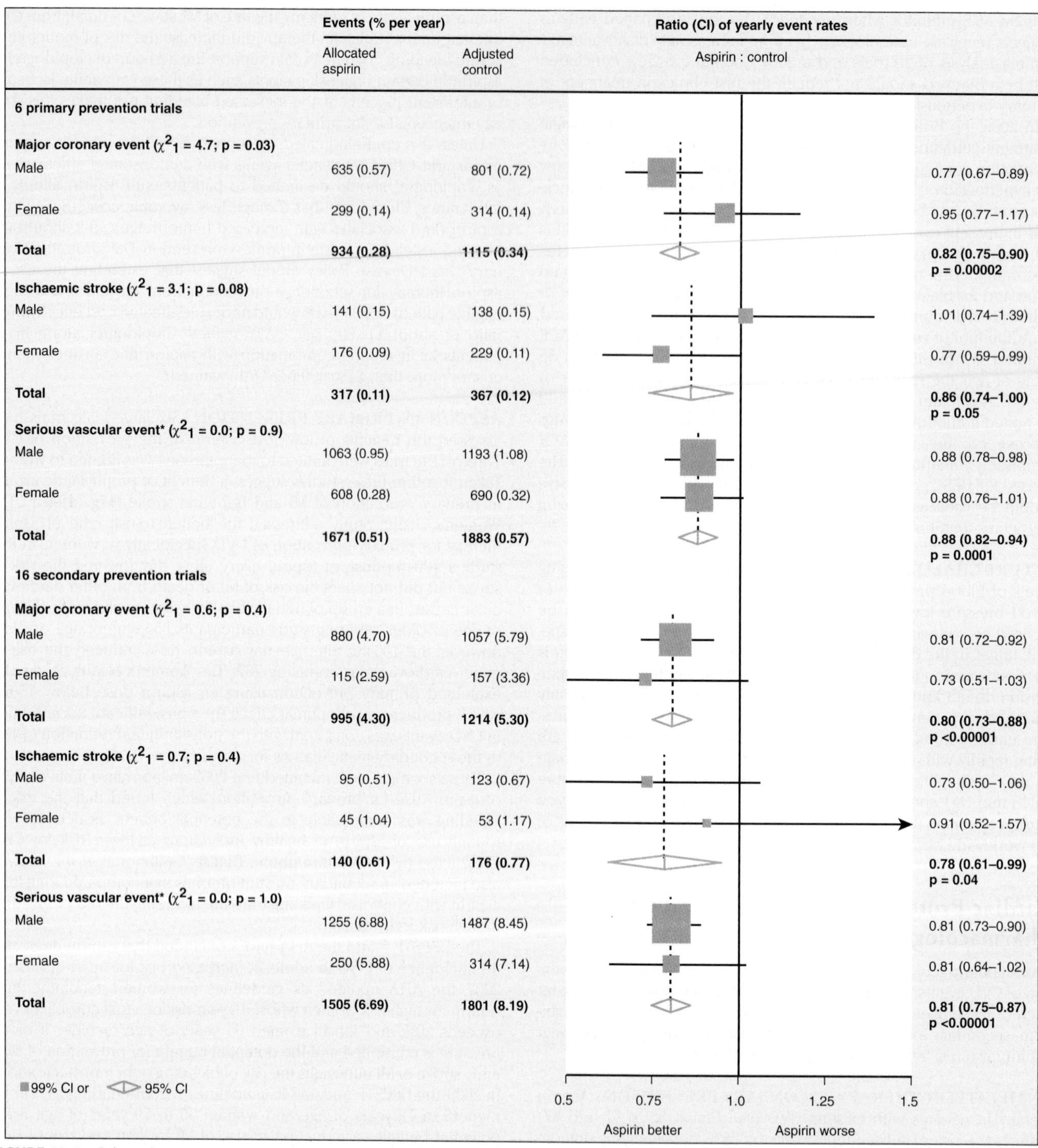

FIGURE 49-6 Selected outcomes in primary and secondary prevention trials of aspirin, by sex. Actual numbers for aspirin-allocated trial participants and adjusted numbers for control-allocated trial participants are presented together with the corresponding mean yearly event rate (in parentheses). Rate ratios for all trials are indicated by squares, and their 99% confidence intervals (CIs) by horizontal lines. Subtotals and their 95% CIs are represented by diamonds. Squares or diamonds to the left of the solid line indicate benefit. *Myocardial infarction, stroke (hemorrhagic or other), or vascular death. *(From Antithrombotic Trialists' [ATT] Collaboration; Baigent C, Blackwell L, Collins R, et al: Aspirin in the primary and secondary prevention of vascular disease: Collaborative meta-analysis of individual participant data from randomised trials. Lancet 373:1849, 2009.)*

benefit. Beta blockade after MI and in the setting of congestive heart failure is also extremely cost-effective. Data from the Coronary Heart Disease Policy Model suggest that implementing beta blocker therapy in all first-MI survivors annually during 20 years would prevent 62,000 MIs and result in 72,000 fewer CHD deaths; the cost-effectiveness of beta blocker therapy would be less than $11,000 per QALY gained, even under unfavorable assumptions.[54]

ANGIOTENSIN-CONVERTING ENZYME INHIBITORS. ACE inhibitors provide substantial benefit to individuals at high risk for CHD events. After MI, the use of an ACE inhibitor is associated with a 7% reduction in mortality at 30 days.[55] Among individuals with a low ejection fraction after MI, total mortality is reduced by 26% (see Chap. 55). A meta-analysis of six randomized, controlled trials suggests that long-term ACE inhibitor therapy reduces the risk of major clinical outcomes by 22%. The benefits of ACE inhibitors extend to those with clinical CHD and diabetes, even in the absence of left ventricular dysfunction.[56]

ORAL ANTICOAGULANTS. (see Chaps. 55, 56, and 87) Oral anticoagulants prevent embolic events in patients with prosthetic heart valves and atrial fibrillation. Their role in the secondary prevention of events in those with CHD, either alone or in combination with aspirin, is less certain. The results of randomized, controlled trials are inconsistent, a troubling issue because oral anticoagulants can cause serious bleeding.

A meta-analysis including the results from newer trials (CHAMP, LoWASA, WARIS-II, and ASPECT-2) concluded that moderate- to high-intensity anticoagulants should not be used routinely as an alternative or supplement to aspirin in high-risk acute coronary syndrome patients because of the increased risk of bleeding.[57] Clinical trials are needed to compare anticoagulants with clopidogrel alone or in combination with clopidogrel in acute coronary syndrome patients.

In 2009, a panel of international experts published a white paper on the topic of "triple" antithrombotic therapy; dual antiplatelet therapy plus an anticoagulant is likely to become more common as the population ages and the number of patients with CAD plus atrial fibrillation or deep venous thrombosis grows.[58] To reduce the possibility of bleeding complications, the panel stressed the importance of frequently reevaluating the need for all three drugs and also recommended that patients taking warfarin who must undergo angioplasty consider a bare-metal stent rather than a drug-eluting stent to limit the amount of time they would be required to take aspirin and clopidogrel after the procedure.

RECOMMENDATIONS. Aspirin should be used for any patient with any form of known ischemic disease. Aspirin in combination with a second antiplatelet agent such as clopidogrel is used in acute settings and should be reserved for the highest-risk patients. Beta blockers should be considered after MI and in those with heart failure. ACE inhibitors are cost-effective and should be considered standard therapy in patients with low ejection fraction and other high-risk patients. All three agents are recommended for secondary prevention by the AHA, the ACC, and the ESC. The USPSTF recommends aspirin in primary prevention if the potential benefit—a reduction in risk of MI in men and risk of ischemic stroke in women—outweighs the increased risk of gastrointestinal bleeding. According to the USPSTF, men 45 to 79 years of age and women 55 to 79 years of age should take aspirin. In light of the 2009 Antithrombotic Trialists' Collaboration meta-analysis, however, some of these recommendations may be revised in the near future.[52] Oral anticoagulants, although offering clear benefit in appropriate patients with atrial fibrillation and certain prosthetic valves, are not recommended in general prevention of CHD events.

Class 2 Interventions

Class 2 interventions relate to risk factors with strong causal associations with CHD risk and for which intervention might reduce risk, although data are limited (see Table 49-3). Factors in this category include diabetes, obesity, physical inactivity, and alcohol intake. Inflammation is another potential target for which there are several interventions (discussed elsewhere), such as not smoking, aggressive lipid lowering, and weight management. In general, cost-efficacy analyses are not available because of a lack of adequate intervention studies.

Diabetes and Its Control (see Chaps. 44 and 64)

PREVALENCE. In the United States, nearly 24 million people—about 8% of the population—have diabetes mellitus. Approximately 90% to 95% of adult cases are type 2 diabetes.[59] About 25% of people with diabetes are not aware they have it. The prevalence of diabetes appears to have increased during the last decade, which may reflect increasing body mass index (BMI). Another alarming trend is the recent increase in type 2 diabetes (formerly called adult-onset diabetes) among children. Current projections foresee almost 50 million people in the United States with diagnosed diabetes by 2050, with the largest increase in minority groups.[60]

ASSOCIATED RISK. Diabetes is a powerful risk factor for atherosclerotic disease, its complications, and cardiovascular-related mortality. CHD is the leading cause of death in diabetic men and women; surveys show heart disease listed on 68% of death certificates among people with diabetes 65 years of age or older. Diabetes affects the risk of CHD and death in both women and men, and indeed, diabetic women may face a greater risk of CHD mortality.[61,62] The increased CHD risk associated with diabetes affects individuals with normal weight but rises with increasing adiposity.[63]

Some data have indicated that individuals with diabetes but without established CHD have as high a risk for fatal CHD as do those with established CHD but without diabetes; but at least one study concluded that established CHD signifies a higher risk than diabetes for CHD mortality in men, whereas diabetes is associated with greater risk for CHD mortality in women.[61] In the end, individuals with diabetes must be considered at high risk for CHD, whether or not they have other risk factors.

BENEFITS OF TREATMENT. Maintaining normoglycemia may reduce the risk of microvascular (renal and eye) disease. However, in reducing the risk of macrovascular disease, the "more is better" hypothesis was not borne out by the 2008 results from three trials that employed intensive glycemic control in those with type 2 diabetes, or in earlier trials of patients with type 1 diabetes. In the Veterans Affairs Diabetes Trial (VADT) of 1791 participants with poorly controlled diabetes, intensive glucose control was defined as an HbA1c level of <7%, and although intensive control did suggest some benefits, it did not affect CVD risk.[64] Recent subanalyses of the VADT results, however, found that intensive glucose control initiated within 15 years after diagnosis of type 2 diabetes reduced the risk of cardiovascular events, including death, by 40%; initiation of intensive control 20 years or more after diagnosis was associated with increased risk of cardiovascular events and death.[64] The initial VADT results concur with the Action in Diabetes and Vascular Disease (ADVANCE) study, in which participants achieved an HbA1c mean level of 6.5% after 5 years of treatment. The ADVANCE trial showed a reduction in the progression of albuminuria with intensive glucose control but no effect on cardiovascular event rates.[65] The third study, ACCORD (Action to Control Cardiovascular Risk in Diabetes), enrolled more than 10,000 patients with type 2 diabetes at especially high risk for CVD; in the intensive treatment group, the target was an HbA1c level of <6%.[66] The aggressive treatment wing of the trial was stopped when patients assigned to intensive glucose lowering had a 22% higher relative risk for death compared with patients assigned to standard glucose control (HbA1c 7% to 7.9%).

ACCORD, ADVANCE, and VADT were included in a meta-analysis of five major trials, which found that intensive glycemic control decreased nonfatal MIs by 17% and CHD events by 15%, with no increase in the risk of all-cause mortality.[67] Intensive treatment did, however, double the rate of severe hypoglycemic episodes. The combined United Kingdom Prospective Diabetes Studies (UKPDS) and the Prospective Pioglitazone Clinical Trial in Macrovascular Events (PROACTIVE) were also part of the analysis.

Among patients with type 1 diabetes assigned to intensive therapy in the Diabetes Complications and Control Trial (DCCT), an apparent reduction in CVD events achieved statistical significance in an updated analysis despite a relatively small number of events in a younger cohort.[68]

The 10-year follow-up of the UKPDS found that a period of intensive glycemic control decreased MI (by 21%; $P = 0.01$).[69] As in DCCT in type 1 diabetes, this recent analysis of UKPDS in type 2 diabetes patients suggests a "legacy" effect yielding macrovascular benefit during a longer time span than is usually encompassed by clinical trials.[70]

Whereas several trials have suggested that ACE inhibitor therapy reduces the onset of diabetes, the prospective DREAM trial, which was designed to address this question directly, did not confirm this concept.[71] DREAM found that rosiglitazone, commonly used to treat type 2 diabetes, may delay the onset of frank diabetes, although the long-term benefits of this approach are unknown.[72]

Aggressive multifactorial intervention among diabetic patients does appear to reduce CHD events. In a trial of 160 patients with type 2 diabetes and microalbuminuria allocated to conventional care or intensive therapy (lifestyle and pharmacologic interventions intended to maintain glycated hemoglobin below 6.5%, total cholesterol below 175 mg/dL, triglycerides below 150 mg/dL, and blood pressure below 130/80 mm Hg), rates of incident cardiovascular events were decreased by more than half during an 8-year follow-up period (hazard ratio, 0.47; 95% CI, 0.24 to 0.73).[73] The cardiovascular benefits of blood pressure control in diabetic patients require sustained treatment.[74] Recent data suggest that aiming for a blood pressure target of 120 mm Hg does not confer clinical benefit over a target of less than 140 mm Hg in diabetic patients.[75]

Diabetic patients enrolled in cardiovascular event reduction trials of statins, aspirin, ACE inhibitors, and lifestyle management derive considerable event reduction. Subgroup analyses of large placebo-controlled trials of cholesterol- and triglyceride-lowering therapy indicate that individuals with diabetes benefit as much from these therapies as do nondiabetics.[45] Improved screening would help ensure that the diabetic population benefits from these advances.

GUIDELINES AND RECOMMENDATIONS. Diet and exercise are integral components of the treatment strategy for patients with diabetes. In many patients with type 2 diabetes, glycemic control can be achieved by modest weight loss through diet and exercise. A Cochrane data base meta-analysis of 14 trials with 377 participants with type 2 diabetes showed significant improvement in glycemia, visceral adiposity, and triglycerides, even without weight loss.[76] Lifestyle risk factors associate with new-onset diabetes even in older adults.[77]

In contrast to patients with type 1 diabetes, those with type 2 diabetes are much more likely than the general population to have multiple coronary risk factors. Thus, aggressive modification of associated risk factors, including treatment of hypertension, LDL reduction, weight reduction, and increased physical activity, is of paramount importance in reducing the risk of CHD among people with diabetes.

In 2007, the American Diabetes Association (ADA) and the AHA issued joint guidelines on the primary prevention of CVD in patients with diabetes, calling for treatment of these patients to a target blood pressure lower than 130/80 mm Hg.[78] Individuals with borderline readings up to 139 mm Hg systolic or 89 mm Hg diastolic should receive lifestyle and behavioral therapy for 3 months. If the follow-up pressures reach 140 mm Hg systolic or 90 mm Hg diastolic, or higher, pharmacotherapy is recommended, with one of the medications being an ACE inhibitor or ARB. Updates may revise these goals on the basis of the data from ACCORD.[75] The LDL-cholesterol goal is below 100 mg/dL for adults older than 40 years of age who have diabetes and at least one major CVD risk factor (but not overt CVD). Drug therapy should aim for an LDL reduction of at least 30% to 40%. Guidelines from the NCEP consider diabetes to be a CHD equivalent and advocate an LDL-cholesterol goal lower than 100 mg/dL. Lifestyle changes should be attempted first and supplemented with a statin when necessary, or if starting LDL levels are higher than 130 mg/dL. The ACCORD lipid arm did not show benefit on outcomes of adding a fibrate to a statin in diabetic patients.[79] For management of diabetic dyslipidemia (high triglycerides, low HDL, and excessive small dense LDL), see Chap. 47. The key measures are weight control, physical activity, and diabetes control. For hypertriglyceridemia that persists despite these measures, omega-3 fatty acids may be useful, although clinical trial evidence for benefit on outcomes in diabetic patients is lacking. Nicotinic acid can raise HDL concentration but can worsen glycemic control in some individuals, and we await clinical trial evidence regarding efficacy in this population. The AHA/ADA guidelines also recommend daily low-dose aspirin therapy (75 to 162 mg) for all adults with diabetes older than 40 years of age and for younger adults who are 21 years of age or older and who smoke or are hypertensive or who have other additional risk factors.

In light of the findings from the ACCORD, ADVANCE, and VADT studies, the ACC, ADA, and AHA issued a joint statement in 2008 revising the glycemic target recommendations for some patients. The consensus was that most patients should continue with the target goal of A1c level of less than 7%.[80]

Prediabetes and Metabolic Syndrome

ASSOCIATED RISK. The metabolic syndrome concept comprises a cluster of metabolic abnormalities that includes insulin resistance, dyslipidemia, hypertension, a proinflammatory state, and excess weight, particularly abdominal adiposity (see Chaps. 44 and 64). It is quite common; approximately 27% of U.S. adults[81] and 10% of adolescents aged 12 to 19 years[82] meet the criteria for metabolic syndrome. Individuals classified as having metabolic syndrome have increased risk for diabetes and CVD and increased risk of mortality from CVD. Not all patients with metabolic syndrome have equal risk for development of type 2 diabetes or vascular events, and several studies suggest that other factors, such as inflammation, can identify a subgroup of high-risk individuals (see Fig. 44-5). An Australian study that followed up more than 10,000 participants for a median of 5.2 years to examine the impact of impaired fasting glucose (prediabetes) on the risk of cardiovascular and all-cause mortality found that these individuals were twice as likely as the controls to die of CVD.[83]

BENEFITS OF TREATMENT. Two randomized clinical trials have demonstrated that patients with metabolic syndrome or impaired glucose tolerance benefit markedly from lifestyle interventions. In the Finnish Diabetes Prevention Study, 522 overweight individuals with impaired glucose tolerance received no intervention or individualized counseling with regard to reducing weight, total fat intake, and increasing physical activity. During a 3.2-year follow-up period, weight loss was significantly greater in the active intervention group, and the incidence of type 2 diabetes was reduced from 23% to 11%, a risk reduction of almost 60% ($P < 0.001$).[84] By use of this simple intervention, five subjects with impaired glucose tolerance treated for 5 years would prevent one case of incident type 2 diabetes. Further support for this hypothesis derives from the Diabetes Prevention Program, which randomly assigned 3234 nondiabetic American patients with abnormal glucose metabolism to placebo, metformin, or a lifestyle intervention program targeting weight loss and exercise.[85] The lifestyle intervention reduced the incidence of type 2 diabetes by 58% compared with placebo, whereas metformin reduced risk by 31%. The lifestyle-induced reduction exceeded that achieved with pharmacologic therapy. A Cochrane review incorporating eight trials supports the ability of exercise and diet to decrease the incidence of type 2 diabetes.[86]

Taken together, trials demonstrate that type 2 diabetes can be prevented or delayed, an effect that in turn will likely reduce atherosclerotic complications in this high-risk group. In the absence of precise estimates for risk reduction in CVD events, however, cost-efficacy cannot be assessed. Lifestyle intervention can have a large population impact. In a prospective study of women, more than 90% of all incident cases of diabetes occurred among those who failed to exercise, had a BMI greater than 25, smoked, or had poor dietary habits.[87]

RECOMMENDATIONS. Both the ATP III[21] and JNC 7[45] guidelines address the metabolic syndrome, although some challenge the concept (see Table 44-1). The safest and most effective strategies to reduce risk factors associated with the metabolic syndrome include weight reduction in overweight and obese patients and increased physical activity. Although drugs that can improve insulin resistance are available, there is no clear evidence that they reduce CHD risk in patients with metabolic syndrome.

Overweight, Obesity, and Weight Management

(see Chaps. 44 and 48)

PREVALENCE. During the past four decades, the proportion of the U.S. population considered to be overweight (BMI ≥25.0) and obese

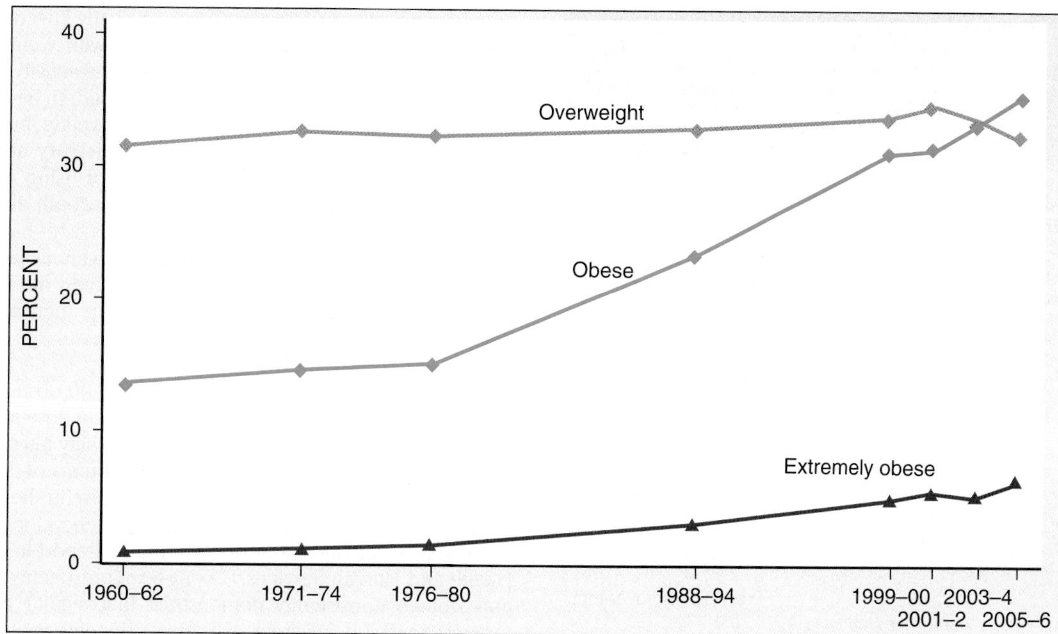

FIGURE 49-7 Trends in overweight, obesity, and extreme obesity, ages 20 to 74 years. Age-adjusted by the direct method to the year 2000 U.S. Bureau of the Census by age groups 20-39, 40-59, and 60-74 years. Pregnant women excluded. Overweight defined as 25 ≤ BMI < 30; obesity defined as BMI ≥ 30; extreme obesity defined as BMI ≥ 40.

(BMI ≥30.0) has risen steadily (**Fig. 49-7**). Recent data establish that more than one third of Americans are obese, although the rise of obesity has slowed recently, and some two thirds are overweight.[88]

The prevalence of overweight and obesity in children and adolescents has risen in parallel with that in adults. More than a quarter of American youth have obesity, defined as a BMI at or above the 95th percentile for age.[89] An estimated 17% of those aged 2 to 19 years are considered overweight or obese—an alarming trend, as early obesity strongly predicts later CVD. A large Swedish study found that being overweight in late adolescence was on par with light smoking (fewer than 11 cigarettes per day) in increasing the risk of premature death.[90] Being obese in late adolescence was as hazardous as heavy smoking in increasing the risk of death during a 38-year period. Excess weight may explain the dramatic increases in type 2 diabetes among children.

ASSOCIATED RISK. Obesity and overweight strongly associate with risks of CHD and stroke. Differences in definitions of overweight and obesity account for inconsistency in reports on the magnitude of their association with CHD. Whether excess weight is an independent risk factor for CHD is disputed because its impact on CHD risk may depend at least in part on other coronary risk factors such as hypertension, dyslipidemia, glucose intolerance, and inflammatory and hemostatic factors. However, given its strong association with CVD, obesity, especially abdominal obesity, is an important and easily assessed marker of risk.[91]

Data from numerous cohort and metabolic studies provide consistent evidence linking excess weight and inactivity with impaired health. A long-term study of women looked at the relative importance of obesity and physical activity as predictors of CHD risk. Whereas BMI, waist-to-hip ratio, and physical inactivity all independently contributed to CHD, the study found that obesity confers a greater level of risk than physical inactivity during a 20-year period.[92] Excess weight increases the risk of metabolic disorders such as hypertension, dyslipidemia, insulin resistance, and glucose intolerance. In the Multi-Ethnic Study of Atherosclerosis, obesity independently associated with biomarkers of subclinical disease.[93] A collaborative analysis of 57 prospective studies including almost 900,000 individuals showed a strong relationship between BMI and CHD and stroke risk.[94] In adults and children, excess weight associates with increases in inflammatory markers such as CRP and fibrinogen, which in turn associate with elevated risk of CVD. Excess weight is also strongly linked to increased risk of CHD, ischemic stroke, type 2 diabetes mellitus, and other chronic conditions. The distribution of body fat also assists the development of CHD, with abdominal adiposity posing a substantially greater risk in both women and men. A waist circumference greater than 35 inches in women and greater than 40 inches in men is an easily measured marker of increased CHD risk.[91] Whereas distribution of weight assessed by waist circumference, waist-to-hip ratio, or even computed tomography or magnetic resonance imaging adds marginal predictive value, BMI remains the most practical and readily obtained measurement for assessment of this metabolic variable.[95]

Excess weight has enormous personal and economic burdens. Women with markers of abdominal obesity have excess cardiovascular and all-cause mortality.[96] Medical spending for weight-related conditions accounted for an estimated 9% of the total annual U.S. medical expenses in 1998, or $78 billion,[97] an amount that rivals expenditures on smoking-related conditions. A study that examined the impact of weight gain per se in initially overweight men and women 35 to 65 years of age found that the 3-year increase in health care costs was $561 greater for individuals who gained 20 pounds or more during this period than for their weight-stable counterparts.[98]

BENEFIT OF INTERVENTION. Lack of large-scale randomized trials of weight reduction as an isolated intervention limit the estimation of the benefits of weight loss in lowering risk of CHD; but information from numerous observational studies and small or short-term randomized clinical trials supports the substantial health benefits of weight loss (**Table 49-6**). Modest weight loss of 5% to 10% associates with a significant improvement in blood pressure among individuals with and without hypertension. Modest weight loss improves the lipoprotein profile, yielding lower levels of serum triglycerides, higher levels of HDL-cholesterol, and small reductions in total cholesterol and LDL-cholesterol as well as improvements in glucose tolerance and insulin resistance. Weight loss also improves sleep apnea (see Chap. 79).

There is little consensus, however, on the ideal approach to weight reduction. Promotion of lifestyle changes to encourage weight reduction has been disappointing. Although 25% of American men and 43% of American women may attempt to lose weight in any given year, failure rates are exceedingly high. One reason may be that most individuals who are trying to lose weight are not following

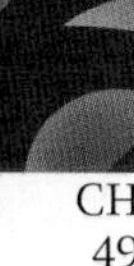

TABLE 49-6 Weight Loss and Physical Activity Benefits for Those Overweight or Obese (or with Insufficient Daily Activity)

DISEASE/RISK FACTOR	WEIGHT LOSS	PHYSICAL ACTIVITY
Hypertension	↓↓↓	↓↓↓
Type 2 diabetes mellitus	↓↓↓	↓↓
Lipid profile	Definite improvement	Definite improvement
Coronary heart disease	↓↓	↓↓↓
Stroke	↓	↓↓
Colorectal cancer	↓	↓↓
Breast cancer	↓	↓
Osteoarthritis	↓↓	↓
Osteoporosis	→	↓↓↓
Gallbladder disease	↓	↓
Sleep apnea	↓↓	Unknown
Mental health	Probable improvement	Probable improvement

↓↓↓ = strong decrease in risk; ↓↓ = moderate decrease in risk; ↓ = slight decrease in risk; → = no benefit.

From Manson JE, Skerrett PJ, Greenland P, VanItallie TB: The escalating pandemics of obesity and sedentary lifestyle: A call to action for clinicians. Arch Intern Med 164:249, 2004.

recommendations to reduce calorie intake and to engage in at least 150 minutes of leisure-time physical activity per week. Effective treatment strategies generally involve a multifaceted approach, including dietary counseling, behavioral modification, increased physical activity, and psychosocial support. Observational studies and clinical trials suggest that pharmacotherapy and bariatric surgery hold some promise in promoting weight loss, but long-term success, long-term risks, and cost-effectiveness have not been fully evaluated.[99] Pharmacologic blockers of endocannabinoids promote weight loss and improve metabolic profiles, but concern about depression has forestalled their clinical use.

COST-EFFICACY. The lack of precise estimates of benefit and the substantial variability in the intervention strategy render impossible the calculation of the cost-to-benefit ratio of weight loss programs or interventions.

RECOMMENDATIONS AND GUIDELINES. Numerous options are available to help patients lose weight. Guidelines produced by the National Heart, Lung and Blood Institute (currently being updated), the North American Association for the Study of Obesity, and the Centers for Disease Control and Prevention (CDC)[100,101] emphasize a three-part strategy for weight loss that includes calorie restriction, structured physical activity, and behavior therapy for all patients with a BMI greater than 30 kg/m^2 and those with a BMI of 25.0 to 29.9 kg/m^2 and a history of CHD or two or more disease risk factors. The CDC recently released a practical compendium of community strategies for obesity prevention.[101] See the following sections for discussions of interventions for specific physical activity and diet recommendations. Pharmacotherapy may be appropriate for some individuals, and bariatric surgery can prove effective for morbidly obese patients.

Physical Inactivity and Exercise (see Chaps. 44, 50, and 83)

PREVALENCE. Physical inactivity is one of the most common modifiable risk factors for CHD. Data from the National Health Interview Survey indicate that 70% of adult Americans do not meet the current recommendation of 30 minutes of light to moderate physical activity at least 5 days per week or vigorous activity for at least 20 minutes on 3 days or more per week.[102] Nearly 25% do not engage in any leisure-time physical activity at all,[102] with women being more sedentary than men. Lack of sufficient physical activity is also endemic among children. Only a minority of schoolchildren have daily physical education classes,[103] and walking and bicycling by children have declined. In contrast, the time spent in sedentary activities such as watching television, playing video games, or using a computer has increased dramatically.[103] Physical activity in youth declines between the ages of 9 and 15 years. Older individuals, who have elevated risk for CVD, are less likely than younger individuals to be physically active, and women tend to be less active than men. Each of these demographic changes has contributed to the increase in childhood diabetes.

ASSOCIATED RISK. Data from more than 40 observational studies demonstrate clear evidence of an inverse linear dose-response relation between physical activity and all-cause mortality rates in younger and older men and women. For detailed descriptions of this abundant literature, consult the AHA statement on exercise in the prevention and treatment of atherosclerotic CVD[104] and the encyclopedic 2008 Physical Activity Guidelines Advisory Committee Report to the Secretary of Health and Human Services.[105] Long-term prospective studies of men and women consistently demonstrate that regular physical activity protects against death from CHD. These benefits apply to activities as simple as brisk walking, which reduces the risk of CHD in women and men and reduces the risk of type 2 diabetes. Shifting even late in life from a sedentary lifestyle to a more active one confers a reduction in mortality from CHD. Physical activity also associates with a decreased risk of stroke in men and women, primarily because of its beneficial effects on body weight, blood pressure, serum cholesterol, and glucose tolerance.

Although no large-scale, randomized trials of physical activity are available, numerous studies of moderate size and duration have included healthy individuals, those at high risk for CVD, and those with existing CVD. Despite differences in design, these trials generally demonstrate a cardiovascular benefit. The ideal intensity, frequency, and duration of physical activity, however, remain uncertain.

BENEFIT OF INTERVENTION. Whereas cessation of activity appears to result in increased risk of CHD, the lack of large-scale, randomized, primary prevention trials makes it difficult to determine the precise magnitude of the benefit of exercise for CHD. Physical activity does, however, benefit cardiovascular risk factors. Exercise increases HDL, reduces LDL and triglycerides, increases insulin sensitivity, and reduces blood pressure in both hypertensive and normotensive individuals. It also improves endothelial function and reduces CRP levels.

In secondary prevention, cardiac rehabilitation programs with an exercise component tend to report benefit in reducing subsequent events. Pooled data suggest reductions in total and cardiovascular mortality of about 25%.[106]

GUIDELINES AND TREATMENT. The AHA issued diet and lifestyle recommendations in 2006 that offer guidance for anyone older than 2 years of age, with or without CVD.[107] The recommendations call for 30 minutes or more of physical activity most days of the week, even if it is broken up into smaller increments. Ten-minute increments of moderate-intensity aerobic activity can be accumulated toward the 30-minute minimum as long as heart rate is noticeably accelerated (a brisk walk or pushing a lawn mower, for example), according to updated recommendations from the AHA and the American College of Sports Medicine.[108] Described as the first comprehensive guidelines ever to be issued by the federal government, the 2008 Physical Activity Guidelines for Americans are the exercise equivalent of the government's Dietary Guidelines for Americans. According to the exercise guidelines, every adult should accumulate 30 minutes of moderately intense physical activity most days of the week and more activity if weight loss is desired, which echoes earlier recommendations from the U.S. Surgeon General. The new recommendations go a step further by advocating that adults add muscle-strengthening activities on 2 days or more a week. Strength training may offer additional cardiovascular and other benefits, making these recommendations an excellent starting point for primary prevention.

In addition, the AHA has said that Americans need to focus on reducing sedentary activities, such as watching television and surfing the Web, and instead make "daily choices to move rather than be moved" (e.g., taking the stairs instead of the elevator). Previously issued guidelines from the AHA/ACC for secondary prevention also encouraged patients to be physically active. An "exercise prescription" might include walking, jogging, cycling, swimming, or other aerobic activity for 30 to 60 minutes on most days of the week, supplemented with an increase in daily lifestyle activities such as walking up stairs when possible. Structured exercise programs may enhance long-term compliance. From a practical standpoint, advice on physical activity should begin with an assessment of a patient's current activities, including physical activity at work and during leisure time. If the assessment indicates that activity is less than optimal, an evaluation of the barriers preventing increased activity should be performed. Common potential barriers include lack of time, energy, desire, or a safe and convenient place to exercise. Other barriers include medical conditions such as osteoarthritis and prior stroke. Physicians should empower patients to overcome these barriers and advise them to add calorie expenditure to everyday activities, such as taking stairs instead of the elevator or walking instead of driving. Advice from a physician should include gradual increase in leisure-time physical activity to 30 minutes or more per day. Intensity of exercise should be discussed with those who have made a commitment to the recommended 30 minutes or more per day.

Diet and Moderate Alcohol Consumption

DIET (see Chaps. 44 and 48). Diet has an important impact on CHD risk. Cross-cultural studies suggest that diet plays a role in CHD as well as in other chronic diseases. For example, the Ni-Hon-San study demonstrated that Japanese immigrants who moved to Hawaii and California developed CHD and ischemic stroke at rates comparable to those of lifetime residents of the United States. Understanding of the specific components of the Western diet that impart this risk has proven challenging; dietary research is hampered by the difficulty of measuring dietary components. Nonetheless, several dietary factors have been well studied. This section discusses macronutrients (fats, carbohydrates, and protein sources) and alcohol. Supplements, nutraceuticals, and specific foods are discussed later in class 3 interventions.

Observational Studies

Observational studies suggest a number of dietary factors that may influence the risk of CHD. Excess calorie intake relative to calorie expenditure characterizes the contemporary Western lifestyle. Observational dietary research consistently finds that individuals who consume higher amounts of fruits and vegetables have lower rates of heart disease and stroke, as documented in detail in Chap. 48. Other components of the Western diet that may increase the risk of CHD include saturated and trans fats, simple carbohydrates that represent a higher glycemic load, and lack of fiber. Recent data highlight the adverse cardiovascular and metabolic consequences of sugar-sweetened beverages.[109]

METABOLIC TRIALS. Metabolic trials suggest that diet is an important component of any prevention program. Diet can have a profound effect on weight reduction, which can improve dyslipidemia, hypertension, and diabetes. Even without weight loss, a healthy diet can improve the lipid profile and deliver nutrients with salutary effects on the cardiovascular system. In the DASH trial, 459 adults with systolic blood pressure lower than 160 mm Hg and diastolic pressure lower than 80 to 95 mm Hg were randomized to a control diet low in fruits, vegetables, and dairy products, with a fat content of 37%; a diet rich in fruits and vegetables; or a combination diet rich in fruits, vegetables, and low-fat dairy products. Both of the intervention diets substantially reduced systolic and diastolic blood pressure in individuals with and without hypertension.[39]

A review of data from 147 metabolic studies, prospective cohort studies, and clinical trials suggests that at least three dietary strategies are effective in preventing CHD.[110] These include substitution of nonhydrogenated unsaturated fats for saturated and trans fats; increase in the consumption of omega-3 fatty acids from fish, fish oil supplements, or plant sources; and adherence to a diet high in fruits, vegetables, nuts, and whole grains and low in refined grain products.

DIET TRIALS WITH CHD ENDPOINTS. Trial data exploring the impact of dietary changes alone on CHD events are limited. The Lyon Diet Heart Study randomized 605 survivors of a first MI to a Mediterranean-type diet or a "prudent Western-type diet." After a mean follow-up of 46 months, the risk of cardiac death or acute MI was 65% lower for those consuming the Mediterranean diet.[111] However, the results of a more recent study, the Women's Health Initiative randomized controlled dietary modification trial, which included postmenopausal women 50 to 79 years of age, confounded conventional wisdom.[112] Intensive behavioral modification designed to reduce dietary fat intake and to increase consumption of fruits, vegetables, and grains during more than 8 years did not significantly reduce the risk of CHD, stroke, or total CVD. Critiques of the trial included the design, which did not distinguish saturated and trans fat that increases the risk of CVD from unsaturated fat that is thought to be protective. In addition, as all of the participants were postmenopausal women, these findings may not apply to all women.

Dietary Recommendations

With limited trial data, it is difficult to answer when patients ask what they should eat to prevent heart disease. When it comes to overweight patients, a 2009 study found that what they eat may be less important than how much they eat. All four of the diets compared in this trial produced weight loss to the same extent, and those who lost weight reduced their risk of heart disease and diabetes and improved their blood pressure.[113] On the basis of observational studies, all patients should be advised of some general principles that consistently emerge from other data. To help patients understand these general recommendations, a simple set of rules can be the basis for improved diet:

- Total calorie intake must be balanced with energy expenditure. If weight reduction is desired, the balance must be fewer calories in than out.
- Simple carbohydrates (sugars and starches) that have a high glycemic load should be avoided in favor of high-fiber carbohydrate sources (whole-wheat products, beans) to delay the absorption of sugars and to reduce the insulin response. Sugar-sweetened beverages should be minimized.
- Maximize fruit and vegetable intake. The U.S. Department of Agriculture recommends 1 to 2.5 cups of fruit and 1 to 4 cups of vegetables per day.
- Minimize intake of saturated and trans fats. Instead, select monounsaturated and polyunsaturated fats and whole grains. Adequate intake of omega-3 fatty acids also appears to be beneficial in primary prevention and especially in secondary prevention of CVD.[114] The AHA recommends two servings of oily fish per week (equivalent to about 500 mg/day of combined EPA and DHA) for primary prevention; consider a dose of approximately 1000 mg/day of combined EPA and DHA for individuals with CHD.
- Protein sources that are low in saturated or trans fats should replace those that are high in these harmful fats.
- Added salt should be limited, particularly for those whose blood pressure seems to be more responsive to salt restriction.

ALCOHOL. Alcohol consumption has complex effects on CVD. Observational studies demonstrate that heavy alcohol intake increases total mortality and CVD mortality. In contrast, more than 100 prospective studies show an inverse association between light to moderate drinking and risk of heart attack, ischemic stroke, peripheral vascular disease, sudden cardiac death, and death from all cardiovascular causes.[115] The effect is relatively consistent, corresponding to a 20% to 45% reduction in risk. Moderate alcohol consumption associates with decreased cardiovascular risk in both primary and secondary prevention and among men and women. Mechanisms underlying the effect of moderate alcohol consumption, defined as one or two drinks daily, include raising of HDL levels, improvement in fibrinolytic capacity, and reduction of platelet aggregation and hsCRP.[116] Trials demonstrate that alcohol raises HDL levels. Whereas some have suggested unique cardioprotective properties associated with red wine consumption, most studies have found equal benefits for all forms of alcohol when it is consumed in moderation.

Recommendations.

Any individual or public health recommendation must consider the complexity of alcohol's metabolic, physiologic, and psychological effects. With alcohol, the difference between daily intake of small to moderate quantities and large quantities may be the difference between preventing and causing disease. All individuals should avoid excessive alcohol consumption. One or two drinks per day generally are safe for men. Lower levels may be prudent for women because of their generally smaller lean body mass and potential differences in liver metabolism. Counseling must be individualized. Discussions of alcohol consumption should take into account other medical problems, including other coronary risk factors (particularly hypertension and diabetes), liver disease, tendency toward excess use, family history of alcoholism, and possibly a family history of breast and colon cancer.

Class 3 Interventions

Class 3 interventions relate to risk factors that are currently under investigation (see Table 49-3) but not ready for clinical practice. For some, limited data preclude demonstration of a causal relationship with CHD. For others with apparent causal relationships, interventions are not yet available or tested. Clinicians need to be prepared to discuss these factors with their patients; they often come up in conversation, as they are areas of active research and often the subject of media attention.

Menopause and Postmenopausal Estrogen Therapy (see Chap. 81)

RISK ASSOCIATED WITH MENOPAUSE. CVD afflicts relatively few women younger than 45 years of age in the United States and other developed countries. By 60 years of age, however, it is the leading cause of death among women.[102] Although men exhibit a higher incidence of CHD at every age as well as higher CHD mortality rates, the gap narrows substantially after both natural menopause and bilateral oophorectomy.

A wide range of factors may explain the increased risk of CHD after menopause. These include adverse changes in lipid and glucose metabolism that result in an increase in LDL-cholesterol and a decrease in HDL-cholesterol, an increase in glucose intolerance, and changes in hemostatic factors and vascular function. These changes have long been attributed to the decline in endogenous estrogen that accompanies menopause, but results from a longitudinal study that followed more than 900 premenopausal women for 9 years suggest that the hormonal shift toward androgen dominance as estradiol levels fall contributes to the increase in CVD after menopause.[117] This study was designed specifically to evaluate further the previously identified association between menopause and the metabolic syndrome; the incidence increased progressively from 6 years before to 6 years after the final period, independent of aging and known CVD risk factors. The dip in estrogen levels was a weak and nonsignificant predictor of metabolic syndrome risk.

Abundant observational studies suggested that postmenopausal hormone therapy reduced the risk of CHD. Such data, together with the known favorable effects of oral estrogen on the lipid profile, provided the foundation for widespread use of postmenopausal hormone therapy to prevent CVD.[118]

EFFECTS OF HORMONE REPLACEMENT. Physiologic effects of exogenous estrogen are compatible with cardioprotection effect. Estrogen reduces LDL and increases HDL levels; reduces lipoprotein(a), plasminogen activator inhibitor type 1, and insulin levels; inhibits oxidation of LDL; and improves endothelial vascular function. The effects of estrogen on inflammation are complex, as levels of fibrinogen decrease while levels of hsCRP increase. Many of these effects are prominent with oral estrogen and minimal when estrogen is given transdermally, suggesting a first-pass effect at the level of the liver. Estrogen may also improve glucose tolerance.

Despite observational data and physiologic data suggesting benefits of hormone replacement therapy, data from at least seven randomized trials (five on secondary prevention and two on primary prevention) not only failed to support a possible benefit of hormone therapy on CHD, but also indicated that combined estrogen and progestin may actually increase CHD risk (**Fig. 49-8**).[118,119] This abrupt about-face with regard to the possible benefits of hormone therapy illustrates the problem of uncontrolled confounding in observational cohort studies and the importance of randomized, controlled trials. Emerging evidence indicates that age and time since menopause may also modulate the effect of estrogen on cardiovascular risk.

The first secondary prevention trial, the Heart and Estrogen/Progestin Replacement Study (HERS), found no cardiovascular benefit of estrogen-progestin supplementation even with extended follow-up.[118] Subsequent trials found no beneficial effect of hormone therapy or an increased risk of CHD events.[118]

One arm of the large-scale Women's Health Initiative evaluated the relative benefits and risks of estrogen plus progestin among 16,608 postmenopausal women 50 to 79 years of age with an intact uterus at baseline during a planned 8.5-year period. After a mean of 5.2 years of follow-up, however, the trial's data and safety monitoring board recommended stopping the trial because the test statistic for invasive breast cancer exceeded the stopping boundary for this adverse effect, and the global index statistic indicated that risks exceeded benefits. At that time, the estimated hazard ratios were 1.29 (95% CI, 1.02 to 1.63) for CHD, 1.41 (95% CI, 1.07 to 1.85) for stroke, and 2.13 (95% CI, 1.39 to 3.25) for pulmonary embolism. The hazard ratio for total CVD was 1.22 (95% CI, 1.09 to 1.36). The absolute excess cardiovascular risks per 10,000 person-years attributable to estrogen plus progestin were seven more CHD events, eight more strokes, and eight more pulmonary emboli. Benefits included a reduced risk of fracture and colorectal cancer.[120]

The unopposed estrogen arm of the Women's Health Initiative, which included 10,739 generally healthy postmenopausal women 50 to 79 years of age without a uterus, was also halted early because of a slightly increased risk of stroke, particularly in women 60 years of age or older.[121] After 6.8 years of follow-up, the use of estrogen associated with a 39% increase in incidence of stroke, a 9% reduction in CHD, and a 30% to 39% reduction in fracture rate. A closer examination suggested that younger and more recently menopausal women had a reduced risk of CHD (MI and coronary revascularization) and a more favorable global index with estrogen than with placebo.[120]

Whereas menopause increases the risk of CVD, trial data indicate that estrogen and progestin replacement does not confer cardiovascular protection, especially among older women. Whether other hormone treatment regimens or agents provide CVD protection is being addressed in other trials.

RECOMMENDATIONS. Hormone therapy is no longer recommended as an approach to the prevention of CVD by the USPSTF, the North American Menopause Society, the AHA, or other scientific organizations.[119] Furthermore, the FDA revised the labeling for all postmenopausal hormone therapies containing estrogen alone or estrogen plus a progestogen to include a boxed warning that highlights the increased risk for heart disease, MI, stroke, and breast cancer.[122] Hormone therapy continues to have a role in clinical practice for the treatment of moderate to severe menopausal symptoms. In a 2008 position statement, the North American Menopause Society supported the initiation of hormone therapy "around the time of menopause" to treat menopause-related symptoms or disorders such as osteoporosis in select postmenopausal women.[123] Current-generation oral contraceptive hormone preparations do not appear to increase risk of MI, but they do heighten risk for venous thromboembolism.[124]

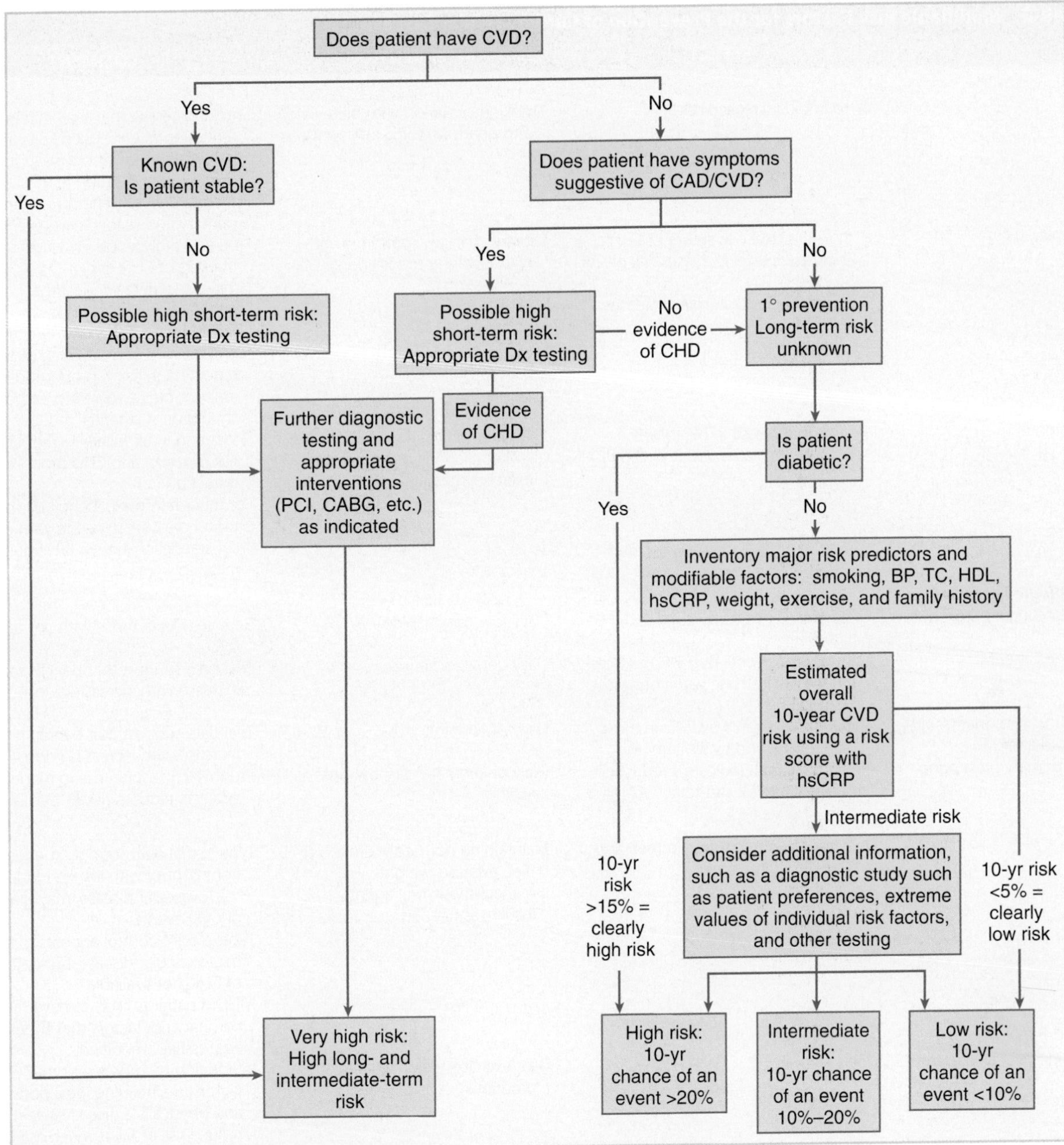

FIGURE 49-10 Cardiovascular disease risk assessment algorithm. By asking a few simple questions, clinicians can determine a patient's long-term risk of a coronary event. BP = blood pressure; CABG = coronary artery bypass graft; CAD = coronary artery disease; CVD = cardiovascular disease; HDL = high-density lipoprotein; hsCRP = high-sensitivity C-reactive protein; PCI = percutaneous coronary intervention; TC = total cholesterol.

in five physicians were aware that more women than men die of CVD each year.[142] The AHA recently published the guidelines for CVD prevention in women,[119] consisting of a set of clinical recommendations tailored to a woman's individual level of risk. The elderly also represent a special population. Interventions described earlier generally apply to healthy elderly individuals. As is the case with any pharmacologic intervention, starting dose may be lower in elderly individuals than in younger individuals, and comorbid conditions and medication interactions must be taken into account; but beneficial interventions should not be withheld on the basis of age alone. Special attention must be given to improving education to enhance adherence to preventive advice for those with low socioeconomic status (see Chap. 2).

Future Challenges

Primary prevention and secondary prevention have contributed substantially to the reduction in CHD mortality rates, yet challenges remain.[143] First, as the population ages, the number of individuals with factors putting them at risk for CVD will increase. Similarly, the number of people living with CVD will increase, thus necessitating greater secondary preventive efforts.

Second, trends of several modifiable risk factors are troubling. Obesity and physical inactivity are epidemic in all sectors of the population, including children. These factors will increase rates of diabetes and hypertension and slow the favorable trends in mean lipid levels. These shifts may lead to slowing of the decline in age-adjusted CHD and stroke rates, or even to reversal of these positive trends (see Chap. 1).[144]

Third, in addition to developing a better understanding of the mechanistic and epidemiologic determinants of atherosclerotic disease, we must find more effective strategies to establish priorities for interventions in prevention programs, to implement existing guidelines for risk factor modification, and to develop low-cost interventions for factors for which guidelines are not yet available. Many lifestyle changes are

CH 49

TABLE 49-8 Modifiable Risk Factors for the Prevention of Cardiovascular Disease

FACTOR	EFFECT	INTERVENTION	COMMENT
Class 1			
Smoking	2- to 3-fold increased risk	Smoking cessation with behavioral and pharmacologic interventions	Smoking cessation results in 60% reduction of CHD risk by 3 years; about half of that benefit occurs in first 3-6 months after quitting Interventions cost-effective in both primary and secondary prevention
Dyslipidemias	1-mg/dL increase in serum LDL-cholesterol level increases risk of CVD by 2%-3% 1-mg/dL decrease in HDL increases CHD risk by 3%-4%	Dietary changes combined with lipid-lowering medications	HDL and triglyceride measures useful markers of CHD risk Limited trial data suggest that intervention reduces risk Lipid-lowering drugs cost-effective in any patient with 10-year CHD risk >10%; reduction in risk is proportional to amount of LDL lowering, so goal should be substantial reduction in LDL
Hypertension	7-mm Hg increase in BP above baseline increases risk of CVD by 27%	Lifestyle modifications, weight loss, limited alcohol intake, aerobic exercise, medications	Reduction in BP results in reduction in risk of stroke and CHD proportional to reduction in BP For moderate-risk patient, pharmacologic blood pressure lowering with goal of substantial change in BP should be initiated
Pharmacologic Therapies			
Aspirin in secondary prevention	Reduce CVD events by 23%	Daily low-dose aspirin	Reduces risk in those with any form of CVD
Beta blockers after MI	Reduce CVD events by 18% and clearly reduce risk in those with congestive heart failure	Daily beta blocker use	Trial data suggest that benefit may increase with increasing dose
ACE inhibitors for patients with low EF and after MI	Reduce CVD events by 22% in those with low EF and by 7% after MI	Daily ACE inhibitor use	Trial data suggest that benefit may increase with increasing dose
Aspirin in primary prevention	Pooled trial data indicate a reduction in risk of first MI and total CVD	Daily or alternate-day low-dose aspirin	Prophylactic aspirin use in higher risk subjects reduces risk of CVD events
Class 2			
Diabetes	Increases risk 2- to 4-fold in men and 3- to 7-fold in women	Maintaining normoglycemia with diet, exercise, weight management, oral agents, insulin, as needed	Type 1: trial data strongly suggest that tight control with insulin reduces risk of microvascular disease, may reduce risk of CVD events Type 2: tight control appears to reduce microvascular disease, but data on risk of CHD not available NIDDM patients likely to have multiple coronary risk factors that should be aggressively modified
Obesity and physical inactivity	Increase risk	Diet, exercise, weight management programs	In addition to improving other CVD risk factors, maintaining ideal body weight and physically active lifestyle may reduce risk of MI as much as 50%, but trial data limited
Dietary factors	Fruit and vegetable intake, type and amount of fat, type and amount of carbohydrate, fiber, trans fatty acids affect CHD rates		USDA and AHA recommend a diet rich in fruits and vegetables; reduction in saturated and trans fatty acid intake, increase in whole grains also appear to be helpful
Moderate alcohol intake (one drink per day)	Decreases risk of MI by 30%-50%	Discussion of alcohol intake with all patients	Risk-to-benefit ratio for moderate alcohol consumption may vary widely by gender, also based on underlying risk of CHD Recommendations must be made individually, with careful regard for conditions such as hypertension, diabetes, liver disease, history of alcohol abuse, risk of breast cancer
Class 3			
Menopause	Increases CVD risk Large randomized controlled trial results suggest that hormone replacement therapy does not confer cardioprotection, may increase risk of stroke Long-term use associated with increased risk of breast cancer; unopposed estrogen increases risk of endometrial cancer		Neither estrogen alone nor combination of estrogen and progestin recommended as strategy for decreasing CVD risk in postmenopausal women
Dietary supplements	Examples include multivitamins, antioxidant supplements, folate, vitamins B_{12} and B_6, fish oils		Randomized trial results of antioxidant supplements, folic acid, B vitamins have been disappointing

TABLE 49-8 Modifiable Risk Factors for the Prevention of Cardiovascular Disease—cont'd

SPECIFIC FACTORS	COMMENT	
Psychological factors	Examples include depression, lack of social support, stress, type A personality	Trials of antidepressants for secondary prevention have not demonstrated clear reduction in risk of CHD
Novel biochemical and genetic markers	Examples include fibrinogen, homocysteine, Lp(a), $LpPLA_2$, t-PA, von Willebrand factor, factor VII, C-reactive protein, soluble adhesion molecules (sICAM, sVCAM), antibodies to various infectious agents, measures of oxidative stress	Additional observational data needed to clarify role of these factors in clinical practice; potential genetic markers, therapies emerging at rapid rate

ACE = angiotensin-converting enzyme; BP = blood pressure; CHD = coronary heart disease; CVD = cardiovascular disease; EF = ejection fraction; HDL = high-density lipoprotein; LDL = low-density lipoprotein; Lp(a) = lipoprotein (a); LpPLA2 = lipoprotein-associated phospholipase A_2; MI = myocardial infarction; NIDDM = non–insulin-dependent diabetes mellitus; RCTs = randomized controlled trials; sICAM = soluble intercellular adhesion molecule; sVCAM = soluble vascular cell adhesion molecule; t-PA = tissue plasminogen activator; USDA = U.S. Department of Agriculture.

difficult to achieve and even more difficult to maintain during the long term. Effective interventions need to involve not only the affected individuals but also families, workplaces, schools, and even whole communities. Translating evidence into practice presents considerable challenges, as exemplified in a recent advisory regarding stroke.[145]

Fourth, for clinicians, it is of critical importance to identify a successful strategy for each patient. Further research on cost-benefit and risk-benefit ratios will enable better targeting of interventions for maximal individual and societal benefit. More widespread use of multifaceted self-help and health professional–directed prevention programs should help sustain the decline in CVD mortality rates.

Finally, a unified single set of guidelines for primary and secondary CVD prevention would likely improve the ease of implementation. Both primary and secondary prevention merit increased attention worldwide, especially in low- and moderate-income countries (see Chap. 1). We must strive to reinforce the scientific data base and rigor of the information used for guideline generation.[146] The development of country-specific prevention guidelines that take into account the prevalence of various risk factors, cultural beliefs, and health care resources, such as those developed by New Zealand, should be encouraged.

REFERENCES

General

1. Yarnall KS, Pollak KI, Ostbye T, et al: Primary care: Is there enough time for prevention? Am J Public Health 93:635, 2003.
2. MacMahon S, Peto R, Cutler J, et al: Blood pressure, stroke, and coronary heart disease. Part 1, Prolonged differences in blood pressure: Prospective observational studies corrected for the regression dilution bias. Lancet 335:765, 1990.
3. Qureshi AI, Suri MF, Kirmani JF, Divani AA: The relative impact of inadequate primary and secondary prevention on cardiovascular mortality in the United States. Stroke 35:2346, 2004.

Risk Estimation

4. Ridker PM, Buring JE, Rifai N, Cook NR: Development and validation of improved algorithms for the assessment of global cardiovascular risk in women: The Reynolds Risk Score. JAMA 297:611, 2007.
5. Ridker PM, Paynter NP, Rifai N, et al: C-reactive protein and parental history improve global cardiovascular risk prediction: The Reynolds Risk Score for men. Circulation 118:2243, 2008.
6. Conroy RM, Pyorala K, Fitzgerald AP, et al: Estimation of ten-year risk of fatal cardiovascular disease in Europe: The SCORE project. Eur Heart J 24:987, 2003.
7. Graham I, Atar D, Borch-Johnsen K, et al: European guidelines on cardiovascular disease prevention in clinical practice: Executive summary. Eur Heart J 28:2375, 2007.
8. Lloyd-Jones DM, Leip EP, Larson MG, et al: Prediction of lifetime risk for cardiovascular disease by risk factor burden at 50 years of age. Circulation 113:791, 2006.
9. Danaei G, Ding EL, Mozaffarian D, et al: The preventable causes of death in the United States: Comparative risk assessment of dietary, lifestyle, and metabolic risk factors. PLoS Med 6:e1000058, 2009.

Smoking Cessation

10. Cigarette smoking among adults and trends in smoking cessation—United States, 2008. MMWR Morb Mortal Wkly Rep 58:1227, 2009.
11. Johnston LD, O'Malley PM, Bachman JG: Monitoring the Future: National Survey Results on Drug Use, 1975-2005. Vol I: Secondary School Students. Rockville, Md, National Institutes of Health, National Institute on Drug Abuse, 2005. NIH publication no. 99-4660.
12. Annual smoking-attributable mortality, years of potential life lost, and productivity losses—United States, 1997-2001. MMWR Morb Mortal Wkly Rep 54:625, 2005.
13. Reducing Risks, Promoting Healthy Life: World Health Report 2002. Geneva, World Health Organization, 2002.
14. Jha P, Chaloupka FJ, Moore J, et al (eds): Disease Control Priorities in Developing Countries. 2nd ed. New York, Oxford University Press, 2006, pp 869-885.
15. Bolin K, Lindgren B, Willers S: The cost utility of bupropion in smoking cessation health programs: Simulation model results for Sweden. Chest 129:651, 2006.
16. Chase EC, McMenamin SB, Halpin HA: Medicaid provider delivery of the 5A's for smoking cessation counseling. Nicotine Tob Res 9:1095, 2007.
17. Stead LF, Perera R, Bullen C, et al: Nicotine replacement therapy for smoking cessation. Cochrane Database Syst Rev (1):CD000146, 2008.

Lipid Lowering

18. Baigent C, Keech A, Kearney PM, et al: Efficacy and safety of cholesterol-lowering treatment: Prospective meta-analysis of data from 90,056 participants in 14 randomised trials of statins. Lancet 366:1267, 2005.
19. Cannon CP, Steinberg BA, Murphy SA, et al: Meta-analysis of cardiovascular outcomes trials comparing intensive versus moderate statin therapy. J Am Coll Cardiol 48:438, 2006.
20. Mihaylova B, Briggs A, Armitage J, et al: Lifetime cost effectiveness of simvastatin in a range of risk groups and age groups derived from a randomised trial of 20,536 people. BMJ 333:1145, 2006.
21. Third Report of the National Cholesterol Education Program (NCEP) Expert Panel on Detection, Evaluation, and Treatment of High Blood Cholesterol in Adults (Adult Treatment Panel III) final report. Circulation 106:3143, 2002.
22. U.S. Preventive Services Task Force: Guide to Clinical Preventive Services 2009. Rockville, Md, Agency for Healthcare Research and Quality, 2000-2003.
23. Smith SC Jr, Allen J, Blair SN, et al: AHA/ACC guidelines for secondary prevention for patients with coronary and other atherosclerotic vascular disease: 2006 update endorsed by the National Heart, Lung, and Blood Institute. J Am Coll Cardiol 47:2130, 2006.
24. Genest J, McPherson R, Frohlich J, et al: 2009 Canadian Cardiovascular Society/Canadian guidelines for the diagnosis and treatment of dyslipidemia and prevention of cardiovascular disease in the adult—2009 recommendations. Can J Cardiol 25:567, 2009.
25. Kuklina EV, Yoon PW, Keenan NL: Trends in high levels of low-density lipoprotein cholesterol in the United States, 1999-2006. JAMA 302:2104, 2009.
26. Lloyd-Jones D, Adams R, Carnethon M, et al: Heart disease and stroke statistics—2009 update: A report from the American Heart Association Statistics Committee and Stroke Statistics Subcommittee. Circulation 119:e21, 2009.
27. Lloyd-Jones D, Adams R, Carnethon M, et al: Heart disease and stroke statistics—2009 update: A report from the American Heart Association Statistics Committee and Stroke Statistics Subcommittee. Circulation 119:480-486, 2009.

Blood Pressure Control

28. Forman JP, Stampfer MJ, Curhan GC: Diet and lifestyle risk factors associated with incident hypertension in women. JAMA 302:401, 2009.
29. Sawicki PT, McGauran N: Have ALLHAT, ANBP2, ASCOT-BPLA, and so forth improved our knowledge about better hypertension care? Hypertension 48:1, 2006.
30. Lewington S, Clarke R, Qizilbash N, et al: Age-specific relevance of usual blood pressure to vascular mortality: A meta-analysis of individual data for one million adults in 61 prospective studies. Lancet 360:1903, 2002.
31. Collins R, Peto R, MacMahon S, et al: Blood pressure, stroke, and coronary heart disease. Part 2, Short-term reductions in blood pressure: Overview of randomised drug trials in their epidemiological context. Lancet 335(8693):827-838, 1990.
32. ALLHAT Officers and Coordinators for the ALLHAT Collaborative Research Group: Major outcomes in high-risk hypertensive patients randomized to angiotensin-converting enzyme inhibitor or calcium channel blocker vs diuretic: The Antihypertensive and Lipid-Lowering Treatment to Prevent Heart Attack Trial (ALLHAT). JAMA 288:2981, 2002.
33. Webster M: New results and analysis expand and modify key interpretations of the ALLHAT trial. Rev Cardiovasc Med 5:164, 2004.
34. Turnbull F: Effects of different blood-pressure-lowering regimens on major cardiovascular events: Results of prospectively-designed overviews of randomised trials. Lancet 362:1527, 2003.
35. Beckett NS, Peters R, Fletcher AE, et al: Treatment of hypertension in patients 80 years of age or older. N Engl J Med 358:1887, 2008.
36. Pearce KA, Furberg CD, Psaty BM, Kirk J: Cost-minimization and the number needed to treat in uncomplicated hypertension. Am J Hypertens 11:618, 1998.
37. Guide to Clinical Preventive Services, 2005. Rockville, Md, Agency for Healthcare Research and Quality, 2005.
38. Screening for high blood pressure: U.S. Preventive Services Task Force reaffirmation recommendation statement. Ann Intern Med 147:783, 2007.

39. Appel LJ, Moore TJ, Obarzanek E, et al: A clinical trial of the effects of dietary patterns on blood pressure. DASH Collaborative Research Group. N Engl J Med 336:1117, 1997.
40. Mancia G, De Backer G, Dominiczak A, et al: 2007 Guidelines for the Management of Arterial Hypertension: The Task Force for the Management of Arterial Hypertension of the European Society of Hypertension (ESH) and of the European Society of Cardiology (ESC). J Hypertens 25:1105, 2007.
41. Dahlof B, Sever PS, Poulter NR, et al: Prevention of cardiovascular events with an antihypertensive regimen of amlodipine adding perindopril as required versus atenolol adding bendroflumethiazide as required, in the Anglo-Scandinavian Cardiac Outcomes Trial–Blood Pressure Lowering Arm (ASCOT-BPLA): A multicentre randomised controlled trial. Lancet 366:895, 2005.
42. Lindholm LH, Carlberg B, Samuelsson O: Should beta blockers remain first choice in the treatment of primary hypertension? A meta-analysis. Lancet 366:1545, 2005.
43. Wiysonge CS, Bradley H, Mayosi BM, et al: Beta-blockers for hypertension. Cochrane Database Syst Rev (1):CD002003, 2007.
44. Hypertension: Management of Hypertension in Adults in Primary Care. NICE Clinical Guideline 34. National Institute for Health and Clinical Excellence, London, 2006.
45. Chobanian AV, Bakris GL, Black HR, et al: The Seventh Report of the Joint National Committee on Prevention, Detection, Evaluation, and Treatment of High Blood Pressure: The JNC 7 report. JAMA 289:2560, 2003.
46. Lawes CM, Vander Hoorn S, Law MR, et al: Blood pressure and the global burden of disease 2000. Part II: Estimates of attributable burden. J Hypertens 24:423, 2006.

Antiplatelet Therapy

47. Antithrombotic Trialists' Collaboration: Collaborative meta-analysis of randomised trials of antiplatelet therapy for prevention of death, myocardial infarction, and stroke in high risk patients. BMJ 324:71, 2002.
48. Bhatt DL, Fox KA, Hacke W, et al: Clopidogrel and aspirin versus aspirin alone for the prevention of atherothrombotic events. N Engl J Med 354:1706, 2006.
49. Gaspoz JM, Coxson PG, Goldman PA, et al: Cost effectiveness of aspirin, clopidogrel, or both for secondary prevention of coronary heart disease. N Engl J Med 346:1800, 2002.
50. Berger JS, Roncaglioni MC, Avanzini F, et al: Aspirin for the primary prevention of cardiovascular events in women and men: A sex-specific meta-analysis of randomized controlled trials. JAMA 295:306, 2006.
51. Ridker PM, Cook NR, Lee IM, et al: A randomized trial of low-dose aspirin in the primary prevention of cardiovascular disease in women. N Engl J Med 352:1293, 2005.
52. Baigent C, Blackwell L, Collins R, et al: Aspirin in the primary and secondary prevention of vascular disease: Collaborative meta-analysis of individual participant data from randomised trials. Lancet 373:1849, 2009.
53. Wolff T, Miller T, Ko S: Aspirin for the primary prevention of cardiovascular events: An update of the evidence for the U.S. Preventive Services Task Force. Ann Intern Med 150:405, 2009.
54. Phillips KA, Shlipak MG, Coxson P, et al: Health and economic benefits of increased beta-blocker use following myocardial infarction. JAMA 284:2748, 2000.
55. Tokmakova M, Solomon SD: Inhibiting the renin-angiotensin system in myocardial infarction and heart failure: Lessons from SAVE, VALIANT and CHARM, and other clinical trials. Curr Opin Cardiol 21:268, 2006.
56. Baker WL, Coleman CI, Kluger J, et al: Systematic review: Comparative effectiveness of angiotensin-converting enzyme inhibitors or angiotensin II–receptor blockers for ischemic heart disease. Ann Intern Med 151:861, 2009.
57. Husted SE, Ziegler BK, Kher A: Long-term anticoagulant therapy in patients with coronary artery disease. Eur Heart J 27:913, 2006.
58. Holmes DR Jr, Kereiakes DJ, Kleiman NS, et al: Combining antiplatelet and anticoagulant therapies. J Am Coll Cardiol 54:95, 2009.

Diabetes Control

59. National Diabetes Fact Sheet: General Information and National Estimates on Diabetes in the United States, 2007. Atlanta, Ga, U.S. Department of Health and Human Services, Centers for Disease Control and Prevention, 2007.
60. Narayan KM, Boyle JP, Geiss LS, et al: Impact of recent increase in incidence on future diabetes burden: U.S., 2005-2050. Diabetes Care 29:2114, 2006.
61. Natarajan S, Liao Y, Cao G, et al: Sex differences in risk for coronary heart disease mortality associated with diabetes and established coronary heart disease. Arch Intern Med 163:1735, 2003.
62. Franco OH, Steyerberg EW, Hu FB, et al: Associations of diabetes mellitus with total life expectancy and life expectancy with and without cardiovascular disease. Arch Intern Med 167:1145, 2007.
63. Fox CS, Pencina MJ, Wilson PW, et al: Lifetime risk of cardiovascular disease among individuals with and without diabetes stratified by obesity status in the Framingham heart study. Diabetes Care 31:1582, 2008.
64. Duckworth W, Abraira C, Moritz T, et al: Glucose control and vascular complications in veterans with type 2 diabetes. N Engl J Med 360:129, 2009.
65. Patel A, MacMahon S, Chalmers J, et al: Intensive blood glucose control and vascular outcomes in patients with type 2 diabetes. N Engl J Med 358:2560, 2008.
66. Gerstein HC, Miller ME, Byington RP, et al: Effects of intensive glucose lowering in type 2 diabetes. N Engl J Med 358:2545, 2008.
67. Ray KK, Seshasai SR, Wijesuriya S, et al: Effect of intensive control of glucose on cardiovascular outcomes and death in patients with diabetes mellitus: A meta-analysis of randomised controlled trials. Lancet 373:1765, 2009.
68. Nathan DM, Cleary PA, Backlund JY, et al: Intensive diabetes treatment and cardiovascular disease in patients with type 1 diabetes. N Engl J Med 353:2643, 2005.
69. Holman RR, Paul SK, Bethel MA, et al: 10-year follow-up of intensive glucose control in type 2 diabetes. N Engl J Med 359:1577, 2008.
70. Chalmers J, Cooper ME: UKPDS and the legacy effect. N Engl J Med 359:1618, 2008.
71. Bosch J, Yusuf S, Gerstein HC, et al: Effect of ramipril on the incidence of diabetes. N Engl J Med 355:1551, 2006.
72. Gerstein HC, Yusuf S, Bosch J, et al: Effect of rosiglitazone on the frequency of diabetes in patients with impaired glucose tolerance or impaired fasting glucose: A randomised controlled trial. Lancet 368:1096, 2006.
73. Gaede P, Vedel P, Larsen N, et al: Multifactorial intervention and cardiovascular disease in patients with type 2 diabetes. N Engl J Med 348:383, 2003.
74. Holman RR, Paul SK, Bethel MA, et al: Long-term follow-up after tight control of blood pressure in type 2 diabetes. N Engl J Med 359:1565, 2008.
75. Cushman WC, Evans GW, Byington RP, et al: Effects of intensive blood-pressure control in type 2 diabetes mellitus. N Engl J Med 362:1575, 2010.
76. Thomas DE, Elliott EJ, Naughton GA: Exercise for type 2 diabetes mellitus. Cochrane Database Syst Rev (3):CD002968, 2006.
77. Mozaffarian D, Kamineni A, Carnethon M, et al: Lifestyle risk factors and new-onset diabetes mellitus in older adults: The cardiovascular health study. Arch Intern Med 169:798, 2009.
78. Buse JB, Ginsberg HN, Bakris GL, et al: Primary prevention of cardiovascular diseases in people with diabetes mellitus: A scientific statement from the American Heart Association and the American Diabetes Association. Circulation 115:114, 2007.
79. Ginsberg HN, Elam MB, Lovato LC, et al: Effects of combination lipid therapy in type 2 diabetes mellitus. N Engl J Med 362:1563, 2010.
80. Skyler JS, Bergenstal R, Bonow RO, et al: Intensive glycemic control and the prevention of cardiovascular events: Implications of the ACCORD, ADVANCE, and VA diabetes trials: A position statement of the American Diabetes Association and a scientific statement of the American College of Cardiology Foundation and the American Heart Association. Circulation 119:351, 2009.
81. Ford ES, Giles WH, Mokdad AH: Increasing prevalence of the metabolic syndrome among U.S. adults. Diabetes Care 27:2444, 2004.
82. de Ferranti SD, Gauvreau K, Ludwig DS, et al: Prevalence of the metabolic syndrome in American adolescents: Findings from the Third National Health and Nutrition Examination Survey. Circulation 110:2494, 2004.
83. Barr EL, Zimmet PZ, Welborn TA, et al: Risk of cardiovascular and all-cause mortality in individuals with diabetes mellitus, impaired fasting glucose, and impaired glucose tolerance: The Australian Diabetes, Obesity, and Lifestyle Study (AusDiab). Circulation 116:151, 2007.
84. Tuomilehto J, Lindstrom J, Eriksson JG, et al: Prevention of type 2 diabetes mellitus by changes in lifestyle among subjects with impaired glucose tolerance. N Engl J Med 344:1343, 2001.
85. Knowler WC, Barrett-Connor E, Fowler SE, et al: Reduction in the incidence of type 2 diabetes with lifestyle intervention or metformin. N Engl J Med 346:393, 2002.
86. Orozco LJ, Buchleitner AM, Gimenez-Perez G, et al: Exercise or exercise and diet for preventing type 2 diabetes mellitus. Cochrane Database Syst Rev (3):CD003054, 2008.
87. Hu FB, Stampfer MJ, Solomon CG, et al: The impact of diabetes mellitus on mortality from all causes and coronary heart disease in women: 20 years of follow-up. Arch Intern Med 161:1717, 2001.

Obesity Management

88. Flegal KM, Carroll MD, Ogden CL, Curtin LR: Prevalence and trends in obesity among US adults, 1999-2008. JAMA 303:235, 2010.
89. Van Cleave J, Gortmaker SL, Perrin JM: Dynamics of obesity and chronic health conditions among children and youth. JAMA 303:623, 2010.
90. Neovius M, Sundstrom J, Rasmussen F: Combined effects of overweight and smoking in late adolescence on subsequent mortality: Nationwide cohort study. BMJ 338:b496, 2009.
91. Mathieu P, Lemieux I, Despres JP: Obesity, inflammation, and cardiovascular risk. Clin Pharmacol Ther 87:407, 2010.
92. Li TY, Rana JS, Manson JE, et al: Obesity as compared with physical activity in predicting risk of coronary heart disease in women. Circulation 113:499, 2006.
93. Burke GL, Bertoni AG, Shea S, et al: The impact of obesity on cardiovascular disease risk factors and subclinical vascular disease: The Multi-Ethnic Study of Atherosclerosis. Arch Intern Med 168:928, 2008.
94. Whitlock G, Lewington S, Sherliker P, et al: Body-mass index and cause-specific mortality in 900,000 adults: Collaborative analyses of 57 prospective studies. Lancet 373:1083, 2009.
95. Flegal KM, Graubard BI: Estimates of excess deaths associated with body mass index and other anthropometric variables. Am J Clin Nutr 89:1213, 2009.
96. Zhang C, Rexrode KM, van Dam RM, et al: Abdominal obesity and the risk of all-cause, cardiovascular, and cancer mortality: Sixteen years of follow-up in US women. Circulation 117:1658, 2008.
97. Finkelstein EA, Fiebelkorn IC, Wang G: National medical spending attributable to overweight and obesity: How much, and who's paying? Health Aff (Millwood) Suppl Web Exclusives :W3-219, 2003.
98. Elmer PJ, Brown JB, Nichols GA, Oster G: Effects of weight gain on medical care costs. Int J Obes Relat Metab Disord 28:1365, 2004.
99. Manson JE, Skerrett PJ, Greenland P, VanItallie TB: The escalating pandemics of obesity and sedentary lifestyle. A call to action for clinicians. Arch Intern Med 164:249, 2004.
100. The Practical Guide: Identification, Evaluation, and Treatment of Overweight and Obesity in Adults. Washington, DC, National Heart, Lung and Blood Institute, North American Association for the Study of Obesity, 2000.
101. Khan LK, Sobush K, Keener D, et al: Recommended community strategies and measurements to prevent obesity in the United States. MMWR Recomm Rep 58:1, 2009.
102. Lloyd-Jones D, Adams RJ, Brown TM, et al: Heart disease and stroke statistics—2010 update: A report from the American Heart Association. Circulation 121:e46, 2010.

Physical Activity

103. Nader PR, Bradley RH, Houts RM, et al: Moderate-to-vigorous physical activity from ages 9 to 15 years. JAMA 300:295, 2008.
104. Thompson PD, Buchner D, Pina IL, et al: Exercise and physical activity in the prevention and treatment of atherosclerotic cardiovascular disease: A statement from the Council on Clinical Cardiology (Subcommittee on Exercise, Rehabilitation, and Prevention) and the Council on Nutrition, Physical Activity, and Metabolism (Subcommittee on Physical Activity). Circulation 107:3109, 2003.

105. Physical Activity Guidelines Advisory Committee Report, 2008. Washington, DC, U.S. Department of Health and Human Services, 2008.
106. Jolliffe JA, Rees K, Taylor RS, et al: Exercise-based rehabilitation for coronary heart disease. Cochrane Database Syst Rev (3):CD001800, 2003.
107. Lichtenstein AH, Appel LJ, Brands M, et al: Diet and lifestyle recommendations revision 2006: A scientific statement from the American Heart Association Nutrition Committee. Circulation 114:82, 2006.
108. Haskell WL, Lee IM, Pate RR, et al: Physical activity and public health: Updated recommendation for adults from the American College of Sports Medicine and the American Heart Association. Med Sci Sports Exerc 39:1423, 2007.

Dietary Intervention

109. Malik VS, Popkin BM, Bray GA, et al: Sugar-sweetened beverages, obesity, type 2 diabetes mellitus, and cardiovascular disease risk. Circulation 121:1356, 2010.
110. Hu FB, Willett WC: Optimal diets for prevention of coronary heart disease. JAMA 288:2569, 2002.
111. de Lorgeril M, Salen P, Martin JL, et al: Mediterranean diet, traditional risk factors, and the rate of cardiovascular complications after myocardial infarction: Final report of the Lyon Diet Heart Study. Circulation 99:779, 1999.
112. Howard BV, Van Horn L, Hsia J, et al: Low-fat dietary pattern and risk of cardiovascular disease: The Women's Health Initiative Randomized Controlled Dietary Modification Trial. JAMA 295:655, 2006.
113. Sacks FM, Bray GA, Carey VJ, et al: Comparison of weight-loss diets with different compositions of fat, protein, and carbohydrates. N Engl J Med 360:859, 2009.
114. Lavie CJ, Milani RV, Mehra MR, Ventura HO: Omega-3 polyunsaturated fatty acids and cardiovascular diseases. J Am Coll Cardiol 54:585, 2009.
115. Goldberg IJ, Mosca L, Piano MR, Fisher EA: AHA Science Advisory: Wine and your heart: A science advisory for healthcare professionals from the Nutrition Committee, Council on Epidemiology and Prevention, and Council on Cardiovascular Nursing of the American Heart Association. Circulation 103:472, 2001.
116. Lindberg ML, Amsterdam EA: Alcohol, wine, and cardiovascular health. Clin Cardiol 31:347, 2008.

Hormone Therapy

117. Janssen I, Powell LH, Crawford S, et al: Menopause and the metabolic syndrome: The Study of Women's Health Across the Nation. Arch Intern Med 168:1568, 2008.
118. Magliano DJ, Rogers SL, Abramson MJ, Tonkin AM: Hormone therapy and cardiovascular disease: A systematic review and meta-analysis. BJOG 113:5, 2006.
119. Mosca L, Banka CL, Benjamin EJ, et al: Evidence-based guidelines for cardiovascular disease prevention in women: 2007 update. Circulation 115:1481, 2007.
120. Hsia J, Langer RD, Manson JE, et al: Conjugated equine estrogens and coronary heart disease: The Women's Health Initiative. Arch Intern Med 166:357, 2006.
121. Anderson GL, Limacher M, Assaf AR, et al: Effects of conjugated equine estrogen in postmenopausal women with hysterectomy: The Women's Health Initiative randomized controlled trial. JAMA 291:1701, 2004.
122. FDA approves new labels for estrogen and estrogen with progestin therapies for postmenopausal women following review of Women's Health Initiative data. U.S. Food and Drug Administration. Available at: http://www.fda.gov/bbs/topics/NEWS/2003/NEW00863.html.
123. Utian WH, Archer DF, Bachmann GA, et al: Estrogen and progestogen use in postmenopausal women: July 2008 position statement of The North American Menopause Society. Menopause 15(pt 1):584, 2008.
124. Shufelt CL, Bairey Merz CN: Contraceptive hormone use and cardiovascular disease. J Am Coll Cardiol 53:221, 2009.

Vitamin Use

125. Gaziano JM: Vitamin E and cardiovascular disease: Observational studies. Ann N Y Acad Sci 1031:280, 2004.
126. Lee IM, Cook NR, Gaziano JM, et al: Vitamin E in the primary prevention of cardiovascular disease and cancer: The Women's Health Study: A randomized controlled trial. JAMA 294:56, 2005.
127. Hercberg S, Galan P, Preziosi P, et al: The SU.VI.MAX Study: A randomized, placebo-controlled trial of the health effects of antioxidant vitamins and minerals. Arch Intern Med 164:2335, 2004.
128. Sesso HD, Buring JE, Christen WG, et al: Vitamins E and C in the prevention of cardiovascular disease in men: The Physicians' Health Study II randomized controlled trial. JAMA 300:2123, 2008.
129. GISI-Prevenzione Investigators (Gruppo Italiano per lo Studio della Sopravvivenza nell'Infarto miocardico): Dietary supplementation with n-3 polyunsaturated fatty acids and vitamin E after myocardial infarction: Results of the GISSI-Prevenzione trial. Lancet 354:447, 1999.
130. Yokoyama M, Origasa H, Matsuzaki M, et al: Effects of eicosapentaenoic acid on major coronary events in hypercholesterolaemic patients (JELIS): A randomised open-label, blinded endpoint analysis. Lancet 369:1090, 2007.
131. Toole JF, Malinow MR, Chambless LE, et al: Lowering homocysteine in patients with ischemic stroke to prevent recurrent stroke, myocardial infarction, and death: The Vitamin Intervention for Stroke Prevention (VISP) randomized controlled trial. JAMA 291:565, 2004.
132. Bonaa KH, Njolstad I, Ueland PM, et al: Homocysteine lowering and cardiovascular events after acute myocardial infarction. N Engl J Med 354:1578, 2006.
133. Lonn E, Yusuf S, Arnold MJ, et al: Homocysteine lowering with folic acid and B vitamins in vascular disease. N Engl J Med 354:1567, 2006.
134. NIH State of the Science Panel: National Institutes of Health State-of-the-Science Conference Statement: Multivitamin/mineral supplements and chronic disease prevention. Ann Intern Med 145:364, 2006.
135. Sacks FM, Lichtenstein A, Van Horn L, et al: Soy protein, isoflavones, and cardiovascular health: An American Heart Association Science Advisory for professionals from the Nutrition Committee. Circulation 113:1034, 2006.

Behavioral Factors and Depression

136. De Vogli R, Chandola T, Marmot MG: Negative aspects of close relationships and heart disease. Arch Intern Med 167:1951, 2007.
137. Whang W, Kubzansky LD, Kawachi I, et al: Depression and risk of sudden cardiac death and coronary heart disease in women: Results from the Nurses' Health Study. J Am Coll Cardiol 53:950, 2009.
138. Glassman AH, O'Connor CM, Califf RM, et al: Sertraline treatment of major depression in patients with acute MI or unstable angina. JAMA 288:701, 2002.
139. Berkman LF, Blumenthal J, Burg M, et al: Effects of treating depression and low perceived social support on clinical events after myocardial infarction: The Enhancing Recovery in Coronary Heart Disease Patients (ENRICHD) Randomized Trial. JAMA 289:3106, 2003.
140. Lichtman JH, Bigger JT Jr, Blumenthal JA, et al: Depression and coronary heart disease: Recommendations for screening, referral, and treatment: A science advisory from the American Heart Association Prevention Committee of the Council on Cardiovascular Nursing, Council on Clinical Cardiology, Council on Epidemiology and Prevention, and Interdisciplinary Council on Quality of Care and Outcomes Research: Endorsed by the American Psychiatric Association. Circulation 118:1768, 2008.
141. Thombs BD, de Jonge P, Coyne JC, et al: Depression screening and patient outcomes in cardiovascular care: A systematic review. JAMA 300:2161, 2008.

Implementation of Preventive Interventions

142. Mosca L, Linfante AH, Benjamin EJ, et al: National study of physician awareness and adherence to cardiovascular disease prevention guidelines. Circulation 111:499, 2005.
143. Ford ES, Ajani UA, Croft JB, et al: Explaining the decrease in U.S. deaths from coronary disease, 1980-2000. N Engl J Med 356:2388, 2007.
144. Franks PW, Hanson RL, Knowler WC, et al: Childhood obesity, other cardiovascular risk factors, and premature death. N Engl J Med 362:485, 2010.
145. Schwamm L, Fayad P, Acker JE 3rd, et al: Translating evidence into practice: A decade of efforts by the American Heart Association/American Stroke Association to reduce death and disability due to stroke: A presidential advisory from the American Heart Association/American Stroke Association. Stroke 41:1051, 2010.
146. Tricoci P, Allen JM, Kramer JM, et al: Scientific evidence underlying the ACC/AHA clinical practice guidelines. JAMA 301:831, 2009.

CHAPTER 50 Exercise-Based, Comprehensive Cardiac Rehabilitation

Paul D. Thompson

Historical Perspective

Prolonged hospitalizations lasting several weeks, followed by months of restricted physical activity, were the standard treatment of myocardial infarction (MI) until the early 1950s. Indeed, as recently as the early 1970s, patients were routinely hospitalized for 3 weeks after MI. Exercise-based cardiac rehabilitation programs were begun in the 1950s to reverse the physical deconditioning and reduced exercise capacity produced by such hospitalizations and attendant, restricted physical activity. Exercise training was central to reversal of this deconditioning process. It was also central to cardiac rehabilitation efforts, because exercise was one of the few interventions documented to delay the onset of classic angina pectoris before the availability of beta-adrenergic blocking agents (beta blockers), calcium channel blockers, coronary artery bypass graft surgery (CABG), and percutaneous coronary intervention (PCI).[1,2]

Abbreviated hospital stays, as well as effective medicines and procedures to treat myocardial ischemia, have changed the purpose and design of cardiac rehabilitation programs. Exercise training remains the cornerstone of cardiac rehabilitation efforts, but education and counseling to improve psychological well-being, to reduce cigarette smoking, and to increase adherence to medicines and diet are now key components of the comprehensive rehabilitation effort.[3] New Medicare guidelines reflect these changes and stipulate that "cardiac rehabilitation programs must be comprehensive and... must include a medical evaluation, a program to modify cardiac risk factors..., prescribed exercise, education, and counseling." Counseling includes dietary counseling, psychosocial intervention, lipid treatment, and stress management.[4]

Nevertheless, exercise training remains a critical key component of cardiac rehabilitation programs because of its ability to increase exercise capacity, to reduce exercise-induced cardiac ischemia and angina, and to reduce cardiac risk factors such as serum lipids, blood pressure, and endothelial dysfunction.[5] Consequently, this chapter addresses the totality of the cardiac rehabilitation effort but emphasizes the use of exercise training in this process.

Basic Principles of Exercise Physiology and of Exercise Training (see Chaps. 14 and 83)

Maximal Oxygen Uptake

Only small amounts of energy are immediately available in skeletal muscle. Consequently, both aerobic exercise and resistance exercise (**Table 50-1**) increase the body's oxygen requirements to supply energy to the exercising muscle. The amount of energy used during exercise is measured indirectly as the amount of oxygen consumed. This is referred to as the ventilatory oxygen consumption, or $\dot{V}O_2$. Rearrangement of the Fick equation, cardiac output (Q) = $\dot{V}O_2$/arterial-venous O_2 difference (A-V $O_2\Delta$), demonstrates that $\dot{V}O_2$ is the product of Q and A-V $O_2\Delta$. Thus, the metabolic demands of exercise are met by increasing oxygen delivery by increases in Q, which in turn is the product of heart rate (HR) and cardiac stroke volume (SV), as well as by increases in the A-V $O_2\Delta$. The A-V $O_2\Delta$ increases during exercise by blood flow redistribution from nonexercising tissue (such as the kidney and splanchnic bed) to exercising muscle, by increased oxygen extraction in the exercising muscle, and by hemoconcentration due to plasma fluid losses into the exercising muscle interstitial space. The increase in Q during exercise is tightly coupled to the increase in $\dot{V}O_2$ so that a 1-liter increase in $\dot{V}O_2$ elicits an ≅6-liter increase in Q. Maximal exercise capacity is measured as $\dot{V}O_2$max, or the maximal amount of oxygen that the individual can transport during exercise before being limited by fatigue or dyspnea. $\dot{V}O_2$max in an individual is a highly stable and reproducible measure of exercise capacity. It is expressed as either an absolute value in liters per minute, or relative to body weight as milliliters per kilogram of body weight per minute. The maximal increase in the A-V $O_2\Delta$ is fixed at approximately 15 to 17 volumes percentage. Because the exercise work rate determines $\dot{V}O_2$, which is the product of Q and the A-V $O_2\Delta$, and because the maximal A-V $O_2\Delta$ is relatively fixed, maximal exercise capacity or $\dot{V}O_2$max is an indirect measure of maximal cardiac pump capacity or maximal Q and SV.

Myocardial Oxygen Uptake

Myocardial oxygen demand (MO_2) can be estimated as the product of HR and systolic blood pressure (SBP) or the so-called double product. Although the absolute exercise work rate determines $\dot{V}O_2$ and Q, the increase in HR and SBP are determined by the exercise $\dot{V}O_2$ requirement as a percentage of $\dot{V}O_2$max. Consequently, for any absolute exercise level, an individual with a larger $\dot{V}O_2$max uses less of his or her maximal capacity and demonstrates a lower HR and SBP exercise response. The key point is that MO_2 is determined not solely by the external exercise work rate, but by the exercise work rate relative to maximal exercise capacity.

Ventilatory Threshold

Expired carbon dioxide ($\dot{V}CO_2$) also increases as the exercise work rate increases. Increases in $\dot{V}O_2$ and $\dot{V}CO_2$ are parallel early during exercise, but the rate of carbon dioxide expiration increases more rapidly and the coupling of $\dot{V}O_2$ and $\dot{V}CO_2$ diverges at what is termed the ventilatory threshold (VT). This divergence is due to the production of lactic acid, buffering of the lactic acid H^+ ions by bicarbonate, and the subsequent exhalation of additional carbon dioxide. The VT has also been known as the anaerobic threshold and as OBLA for "onset of blood lactate accumulation." Because carbon dioxide stimulates respiratory drive, the VT is also associated with a nonlinear increase in the respiratory rate and mild

TABLE 50-1 Terms to Describe Exercise

Physical activity: any body movement
Exercise: physical activity to stress and train
Aerobic exercise: exercise that primarily stresses the oxygen transport system and includes activities such as walking, jogging, swimming, and cycling
Resistance exercise: exercise that primarily stresses the muscular skeletal system and includes weightlifting
Exercise training: exercise performed repetitively to increase the performance capacity of the cardiovascular (aerobic exercise training) or muscular skeletal (resistance exercise training) systems

From Thompson PD: Exercise prescription and proscription for patients with coronary artery disease. Circulation 112:2354, 2005.

dyspnea. The VT generally occurs at approximately 50% of $\dot{V}O_2$max in exercise-untrained individuals, but at higher levels of percentage $\dot{V}O_2$max in exercise-trained subjects. VT is an important measurement of exercise tolerance because it represents the maximal steady work rate that can be maintained during submaximal exercise.

Effect of Cardiac Disease on Exercise Performance

Exercise performance may be normal for age and sex in individuals with cardiac disease. Alternatively, exercise capacity in cardiac patients may be limited by diseases that limit maximal SV, impair the HR response, or produce myocardial ischemia that causes limiting symptoms or a diminished increase in SV. Medications that limit the HR response to exercise (such as beta blockers) or physical activity restrictions that produce a detraining effect may also contribute to reduced exercise tolerance in cardiac patients.

Effect of Exercise Training on Exercise Performance

The primary effect of exercise training, either aerobic or strength training, is to increase exercise capacity. With strength training, the primary adaptation is to increase muscle strength and muscle endurance in the exercise-trained muscle. The principal effect of primarily aerobic exercise training is to increase $\dot{V}O_2$max. This increase in maximal exercise capacity means that any submaximal work rate requires a lower percentage of $\dot{V}O_2$max, thereby reducing the HR and SBP response and the MO_2 requirements. Endurance exercise training also increases both the absolute VT and the VT as a percentage of $\dot{V}O_2$max. Multiple adaptations contribute to the improvement in exercise tolerance after exercise training, including increases in SV and a widening of the A-V $O_2\Delta$, although the magnitude of the latter has obvious physiologic limits.

The magnitude of the increase in exercise $\dot{V}O_2$max with endurance exercise training depends on multiple factors, including the age of the subject, the intensity and duration of the training regimen, genetic factors, underlying disease states, and whether testing and training are done by use of similar exercises. In general, the magnitude of the improvement in exercise tolerance is greater in young subjects trained intensely. For cardiac rehabilitation patients, reported increases in $\dot{V}O_2$max average 11% to 36%,[6] although the response varies with the severity of the underlying disease. For example, individuals with markedly reduced ventricular function may achieve much of their increase in exercise capacity by widening the A-V $O_2\Delta$, whereas increases in cardiac output have been documented with 12 months of exercise training in some cardiac patients.[5] In addition to increasing maximal exercise capacity, endurance exercise training increases endurance capacity by virtue of its effects on VT. This is extremely important, because increased submaximal exercise endurance capacity reduces dyspnea at submaximal work rates and facilitates performance of most daily tasks, virtually none of which require maximal effort.

Effects of Cardiac Rehabilitation and Exercise Training on Morbidity and Mortality in Cardiac Patients

Angina Pectoris

Most patients with angina pectoris control or eliminate their symptoms with medication, PCI, or CABG. Consequently, and with rare exceptions,[7] much of the evidence that exercise training improves effort tolerance in patients with angina pectoris was obtained before 1990. Exercise training increases the exercise time to the onset of angina or even eliminates angina entirely by at least two mechanisms.

First, exercise training reduces the MO_2 requirements during submaximal exercise.[5] Endurance exercise training increases $\dot{V}O_2$max. Because the HR and SBP response to exercise is more closely related to the percentage $\dot{V}O_2$max elicited by an exercise task and not to the absolute exercise work rate, the increase in $\dot{V}O_2$max with exercise training reduces the HR and SBP response to submaximal exercise. This reduction in double product reduces the MO_2 requirements and delays the onset of angina.

Second, exercise training improves endothelial vasodilator function.[8-10] Normal coronary arteries dilate with exercise, whereas atherosclerotic coronary arteries often demonstrate endothelial dysfunction evidenced by failure to dilate or even exercise-induced vasoconstriction. Exercise training reduces endothelial dysfunction as measured by quantitative coronary angiography during infusions of the endothelial agonist acetylcholine.[8] Some patients also demonstrate increases in the rate-pressure product at the onset of exercise after only a short period of exercise training,[5] also supporting the concept of improved endothelial function (**Fig. 50-1**).

Exercise training in patients with angina, at least in the United States, is primarily relegated to use in patients who are not amenable to coronary interventions, but recent clinical trial evidence challenges this approach. Hambrecht and colleagues[7] evaluated changes in exercise performance, coronary artery anatomy, and clinical outcomes in 101 men aged ≤70 years with stable angina pectoris. Subjects were randomized to either a year of exercise training or PCI. Subjects were excluded if the coronary lesion was not suitable for PCI or if they had high-grade stenosis of the left anterior descending artery, >25% left main stenosis, valvular disease, ejection fraction <40%, MI within 2 months, or PCI or CABG within 12 months. The exercise training consisted of 2 weeks of six 10-minute sessions daily at 70% of

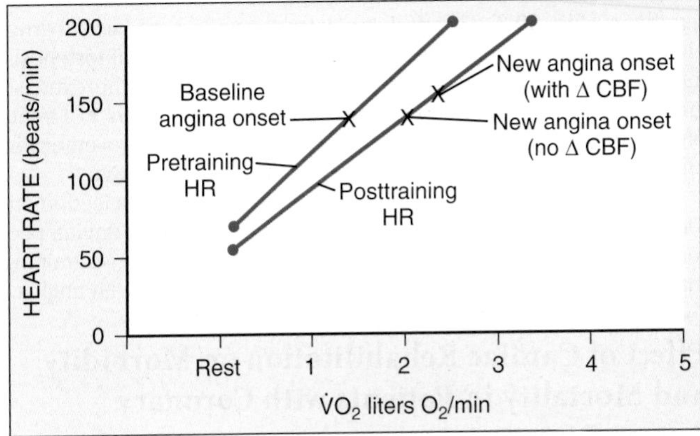

FIGURE 50-1 Changes in exercise tolerance and the onset of angina with exercise training. The heart rate (HR) versus $\dot{V}O_2$ slope is shifted so that any work rate ($\dot{V}O_2$) elicits a slower HR response. Angina is delayed to the same HR if there is no change in coronary blood flow (new angina onset [no Δ CBF]) or delayed to a higher HR if coronary blood flow is increased by improved endothelial function (new angina onset [with Δ CBF]). *(From Thompson PD: Exercise prescription and proscription for patients with coronary artery disease. Circulation 112:2354, 2005.)*

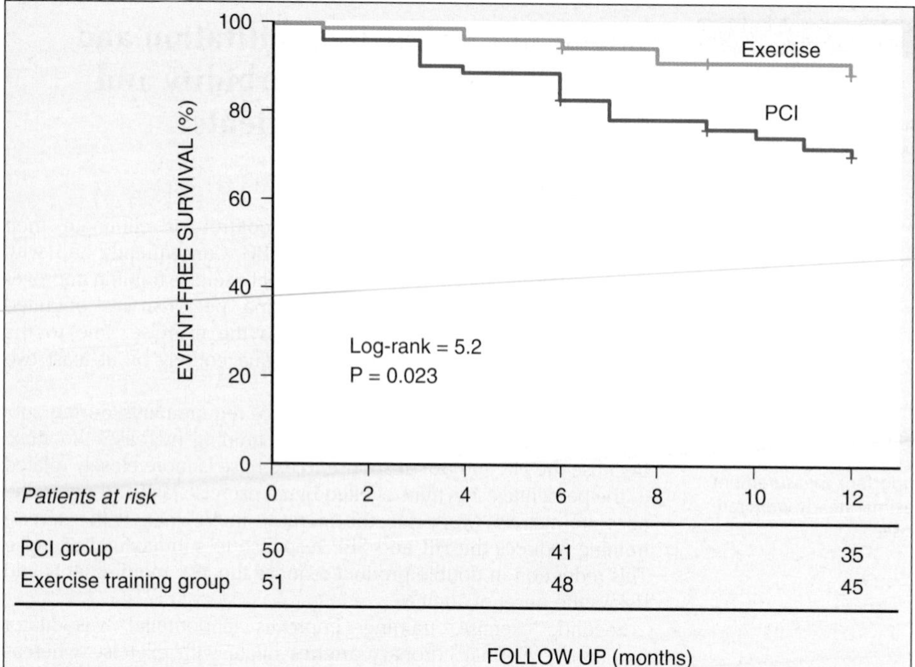

FIGURE 50-2 Event-free survival in 101 carefully selected patients with stable angina randomly assigned to percutaneous coronary intervention (balloon angioplasty or stent) or to a year of exercise training. Numbers at the bottom of the figure indicate patients free of events. Event-free survival was significantly better in the exercise training group (88% versus 70%; $P = 0.02$ by log-rank test). *(Reproduced from Hambrecht R, Walther C, Mobius-Winkler S, et al: Percutaneous coronary angioplasty compared with exercise training in patients with stable coronary artery disease: A randomized trial. Circulation 109:1371, 2004.)*

maximal tolerated HR, followed by daily 20-minute home exercise sessions, plus a weekly 60-minute supervised session.

Forty-seven subjects in each group completed the trial. The exercise level at the onset of ischemia increased 30% in the exercise-trained subjects and 20% in the PCI subjects. These differences were not significant, but increases in maximal exercise capacity (20% versus 0%) and $\dot{V}O_2$ max (16% versus 2%) were significantly greater in the exercise-trained subjects. The potential target lesion did not change in the exercise subjects, and only 15% of the PCI subjects demonstrated restenosis defined as >50% luminal narrowing at the PCI site. Total coronary artery disease (CAD) progression measured by angiographic scoring was less in the exercise-trained group, however, and 88% of the PCI versus only 70% of the exercise-trained subjects experienced a major cardiovascular event including MI, stroke, revascularization procedure, or hospitalization for angina. This difference was statistically significant (**Fig. 50-2**). This study predated the widespread use of drug-eluting stents (see Chap. 58), but even assuming no in-stent restenosis, the event-free survival would still have been greater in the exercise group (88% versus 72%; $P = 0.039$). As noted by the authors, PCI treats one culprit lesion, whereas exercise training, by its improvement in endothelial dysfunction, addresses the entire vascular system.

These results require confirmation, and because of the selection criteria, they cannot be generalized to all subjects with stable angina pectoris. Nevertheless, these findings do document that exercise training may be suitable for the management of selected patients with angina.

Effect of Cardiac Rehabilitation on Morbidity and Mortality in Patients with Coronary Artery Disease

At least four meta-analyses have examined the effect of exercise-based cardiac rehabilitation on clinical outcomes.[5] All provide essentially identical results because they include many of the same studies. The most recent analysis examined 48 trials and included 8940 patients randomized to either cardiac rehabilitation or usual care.[11] Total mortality and cardiac mortality were 20% and 26% lower, respectively, in the cardiac rehabilitation participants ($P < 0.05$ for both). Recurrent MIs were also 20% lower, but this change was not statistically significant.

The majority of the trials in this meta-analysis were performed before modern revascularization strategies were available, so it is possible that many of the subjects in these early studies had residual coronary stenoses and inducible ischemia. Such patients are now routinely revascularized by PCI or CABG. Given the beneficial effects of exercise training on cardiac ischemia and the widespread use of revascularization strategies, it is not certain that similar reductions in cardiac mortality would accrue with present-day cardiac rehabilitation patients. The most recent meta-analysis found no differences in results from studies before and after 1995, suggesting that the benefits of cardiac rehabilitation do apply to the modern practice of cardiology. There was also no difference between exercise-only and more comprehensive rehabilitation programs, supporting the importance of exercise training in reducing cardiac mortality.

These meta-analyses support the benefits of cardiac rehabilitation, but no single trial was of sufficient size to evaluate cardiac mortality on its own.[5] Meta-analyses are plagued by the propensity for positive results to be published—the "positive paper bias." On the other hand, the inclusion of so many exercise-only trials may underestimate the real benefit of more comprehensive cardiac rehabilitation.

GOSPEL (GlObal Secondary Prevention strategiEs to Limit events after myocardial infarction study) enrolled 3241 patients in 78 Italian centers.[12] Subjects underwent 3 months of standard cardiac rehabilitation and were then randomized to 3 years of an intensive rehabilitation effort or to the care of their primary physicians. Participants in the intensive rehabilitation arm participated in exercise, lifestyle and risk factor counseling, and clinical assessments monthly for 6 months, and then biannually for the duration of the study. The primary endpoint was a combination of cardiovascular mortality, nonfatal MI, nonfatal stroke, and hospitalization for angina, heart failure (HF), or revascularization. Endpoint events occurred in 16.1% of the intensive rehabilitation group versus 18.2% of the usual care group (−12%), but this decrease was not significant ($P = 0.12$). Nonfatal MI was the only individual endpoint that decreased significantly (−48%; $P = 0.01$).

GOSPEL did not compare a postevent cardiac rehabilitation program with usual care, because all participants in GOSPEL underwent a standard 3-month rehabilitation program. Furthermore, it is not possible to judge the quality of the usual care provided to the nonrehabilitation participants. Nevertheless, the overall effect of GOSPEL on cardiovascular outcomes was small, given the intensity of the effort required for such prolonged care. Specifically, there were only 34 fewer cardiovascular endpoint events in the intensively treated group, and only 21 fewer nonfatal MIs. Such results do not negate the possible benefits of standard exercise rehabilitation, but they do question the additional benefit of prolonged cardiac rehabilitation, at least in a population of patients willing to volunteer for such a study.

Cardiac Rehabilitation in Patients After PCI

Few large trials have examined the effects of exercise-based cardiac rehabilitation in patients after PCI. The ETICA (Exercise Training Intervention after Coronary Angioplasty) trial examined exercise and clinical outcomes in 118 patients who had undergone one-vessel (n = 81) or two-vessel (n = 37) PCI.[13] Subjects were assigned to either exercise training or a usual-care control group. Exercise subjects participated in a 6-month exercise training program consisting of 30 minutes of stationary cycling and 15 minutes of calisthenics thrice weekly. Exercise testing before and after the study used fatigue, a target HR, or ≥1 mm ST depression as the endpoint.

$\dot{V}O_2$ max and quality of life measures each improved ≈26% ($P <$ 0.001), and only in the exercise-trained subjects. Angiographic restenosis, defined as >50% luminal narrowing at the angioplasty site, was not different at 6 months between the two groups (29% versus 33%), but luminal diameter at the angioplasty site was ≈30% greater in the exercise-trained patients ($P < 0.05$). Disease progression and new lesions in major coronary arteries, both defined as >20% decrease in coronary diameter, were significantly less frequent in the exercise subjects. Cardiac ischemia, measured as thallium uptake, also improved only in the exercise-trained subjects. Subjects were observed for 33 ± 7 months after the end of the protocol. During this time, there were no deaths in either group, but there were 20% ($P < 0.008$) fewer PCIs (4 versus 11), MIs (1 versus 3), and CABGs (2 versus 5) in the exercise-trained subjects.

This study preceded the frequent use of stents during PCI and the use of drug-eluting stents. Specifically, only 19 of the exercise-trained subjects and 18 of the control subjects received a stent. Also, lipid-lowering therapy was prohibited because a secondary study examined the effect of exercise on lipid levels. Consequently, it is not clear if exercise training would produce similar reductions in atherosclerotic progression and cardiac events in patients treated with contemporary therapies. Nevertheless, more current therapies should not alter the differences in exercise performance or quality of life measures observed in this trial. Also, it is not clear how much of the improvement in the angiographic appearance of the coronary tree was due to structural change in the atherosclerotic plaque versus functional changes in coronary artery tone due to improved endothelial function.

Cardiac Rehabilitation in Heart Failure

Until 2009, only meta-analyses supported an exercise benefit in HF patients. For example, Smart and Marwick[14] collected 81 studies that included 2387 patients with HF. $\dot{V}O_2$ max increased 16% with exercise training. Outcome data were available for 622 exercise patients and 575 control patients. There was no difference in total adverse events between the exercise and control groups during a mean follow-up of 5.9 months. On the other hand, there was a 29% decrease in deaths in the exercise training subjects ($P = 0.06$). Such results suggest that exercise training not only increases exercise capacity, but also reduces cardiac mortality in patients with systolic HF (see Chap. 28).

HF-ACTION (Heart Failure: A Controlled Trial Investigating Outcomes of Exercise Training) was the first large-scale, adequately powered trial to examine the effect of exercise training on cardiovascular outcomes in patients with stable HF.[15] HF-ACTION randomized 2331 patients with left ventricular ejection fraction (LVEF) of ≤35% to an exercise training or control group. Exercise training subjects were encouraged to participate in 36 supervised exercise sessions during 3 months, similar to standard cardiac rehabilitation, and were transitioned to home exercise with the goal of exercising five times weekly for 40 minutes. The training target HR was 60% to 70% of maximum HR reserve, calculated as maximal HR minus resting HR.

The mean duration of follow-up was 3.1 years, ranging from 1 to 4 years. There were decreases in total mortality (−4%; $P = 0.7$), cardiovascular mortality or cardiovascular hospitalization (−8%; $P = 0.14$), and cardiovascular mortality or HF hospitalization (−13%; $P = 0.06$) in the exercise-trained versus the control group, but these differences were not statistically significant. These results were adjusted for baseline exercise duration, LVEF, psychological depression index, and history of atrial fibrillation or flutter (**Fig. 50-3**). After this adjustment, total mortality or hospitalization (−11%; $P = 0.03$), cardiovascular mortality or hospitalization (−9%; $P = 0.09$), and cardiovascular mortality or cardiovascular hospitalization (−15%; $P = 0.03$) decreased, suggesting that exercise training has some beneficial effects in patients with HF.

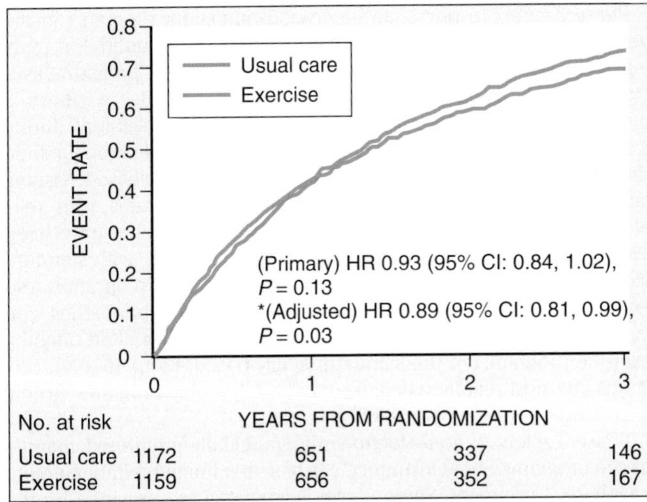

FIGURE 50-3 All-cause mortality or all-cause hospitalization in HF-ACTION. The hazard ratio (HR) was not reduced in the unadjusted data but was statistically significant with adjustment for baseline exercise duration, left ventricular ejection fraction, Beck Depression Inventory II score, history of atrial fibrillation or flutter, and heart failure etiology. *(From O'Connor CM, Whellan DJ, Lee KL, et al: Efficacy and safety of exercise training in patients with chronic heart failure: HF-ACTION randomized controlled trial. JAMA 301:1439, 2009.)*

These are not overwhelming results, but they probably underestimate the potential benefits of exercise training in HF patients. Results were examined on an intention-to-treat basis, as is appropriate for such studies. Unfortunately, exercise compliance in the exercise group was not ideal. Only 736 subjects completed the 36 supervised exercise sessions. The investigators attempted to enhance long-term exercise compliance by providing home treadmills or exercise cycles and HR monitors. They also employed various adherence optimization strategies. Despite such efforts, peak $\dot{V}O_2$ increased only 4% in the exercise group. This was short of the 10% increase projected by study investigators, and well below the 18% increase reported in HF patients exercising in supervised sessions.[16] Consequently, these results probably do not reflect the improvements that can occur with motivated subjects who adhere to an exercise regimen. On the other hand, these results may overestimate the potential benefits of exercise for the general HF population. All participants in HF-ACTION volunteered for exercise training and were provided with exercise equipment, but many still could not adhere to an exercise regimen. Clinicians should probably use these results to recommend exercise training for HF patients and to encourage such patients to participate in supervised programs to maximize adherence and benefit.

Practical Aspects of Cardiac Rehabilitation Programs

Program Structure

Cardiac rehabilitation programs are divided into three phases based on the patient's clinical status. Phase 1 refers to inpatient programs started soon after the acute cardiac event or intervention. Phase 1 programs currently are less common because of the brevity of most hospital stays, although some European countries still have inpatient rehabilitation programs that may last several weeks. Even with the short duration of many cardiac hospital admissions, phase 1 programs remain useful in mobilizing elderly patients after complicated cardiac events and in many patients after cardiac surgery. Phase 1 programs in the United States are often directed by physical therapy departments or a dedicated cardiac rehabilitation staff. Phase 1 is also an excellent way to introduce patients to the concept of cardiac rehabilitation and to solicit appropriate referrals. Separate reimbursement for phase 1 programs in the United States is not available because this service, if it is provided, is included in the charges for the acute event.[4]

Phase 2 refers to physician-supervised outpatient programs in the postdischarge period.[4] Physician supervision is required for reimbursement by most U.S. insurance carriers for phase 2 programs, as is electrocardiographic monitoring. Historically, patients in phase 2 programs exercise three times weekly for a total of 36 sessions during 3 to 4 months. Other approaches to cardiac rehabilitation include simple home-based, self-supervised programs; home-based, visiting nurse–supervised programs; and home-based programs with telephone electrocardiographic monitoring. Such approaches have been examined in research settings and compare favorably with standard facility-based programs.[17] Other approaches to program duration also examined one session weekly for a year.[18] Such approaches can increase exercise capacity and may facilitate adoption of an ongoing exercise program, but the standard facility-based, 12- to 16-week programs are most readily recognized and are the only programs (to my knowledge) covered by insurance carriers.

Phase 3 refers to non–electrocardiographically monitored, maintenance programs. Some insurance carriers offer limited reimbursement for phase 3 programs. Some phase 3 programs are provided by the same facilities providing phase 2 programs, but because these do not usually provide medical supervision, phase 3 programs may also be provided by health clubs and fitness facilities. Phase 3 programs are not covered by medical insurance in the United States.[4]

Staff Coverage

The standard cardiac rehabilitation program has a physician medical director, a staff nurse, and other nurses or individuals with training in exercise physiology to design the exercise and educational programs and to supervise the exercise sessions. To qualify for Medicare reimbursement in the United States, phase 2 cardiac rehabilitation programs must have the supervising physician immediately available during the rehabilitation sessions. Definition of the term *immediately available* is open to interpretation, but has generally referred to being in the facility and available within moments for any emergency. Also for reimbursement, patients must have an electrocardiogram strip recorded, interpreted, and mounted in the chart for each session. All cardiac rehabilitation staff must be trained in advanced cardiac life support. A nurse must be available during the exercise rehabilitation sessions to handle emergencies and to administer medications. Staffing levels are recommended at 1 staff member per 5 participants during phase 2 and 1 staff member per 10 to 15 participants during phase 3 sessions.

Design and Administration of the Exercise Training Program

Patients referred to cardiac rehabilitation should undergo a symptom-limited exercise test before entering the program. The exercise test serves to exclude important symptoms, ischemia, or arrhythmias that might require other interventions before exercise training. The exercise test is also useful in establishing baseline exercise capacity and for determination of maximum HR for use in preparing an exercise prescription. These tests are usually done with the patient taking the usual medications to mimic the HR response likely to occur during exercise training.

Typical exercise training sessions for cardiac rehabilitation patients consist of 5 minutes of warm-up followed by at least 20 minutes of aerobic exercise training and 5 to 15 minutes of cool-down. The warm-up session consists of stretching and light calisthenics. Some resistance exercise training with light weights or exercise machines should also be performed, often after the aerobic session and as part of an extended cool-down. Such exercises as biceps curls, triceps extensions, military presses (for patients without shoulder problems), shoulder shrugs, bent-knee pushups, bent-knee "crunches," and quarter squats address most of the major muscle groups and increase the patient's ability to perform the tasks of work and daily living, which often require lifting and carrying activities.

The aerobic exercise training component is generally performed at 60% to 70% of $\dot{V}O_2\,max$, which corresponds to ≈70% to 80% of maximum HR. Some patients require lower training intensities. Although 20 minutes of exercise training is standard, shorter periods of exercise training are beneficial, and longer sessions almost certainly provide additional benefit. Most cardiac rehabilitation programs recommend other activities, such as yard work and walking, on days when patients do not attend supervised sessions.

Exercise testing is useful before cardiac rehabilitation is started, but not all patients, especially those after recent MI, undergo such testing. Patients who did not undergo exercise testing before the program can exercise at a heart rate 20 beats faster than their resting value. Another approach is to exercise patients at their resting HR plus a specified additional percentage of the resting rate. For example, during month 1, the patient might exercise at rest HR + 20% to 30% rest HR; month 2, rest HR + 20% to 40% rest HR; and month 3, rest HR + 20% to 50% rest HR. Alternatively, such patients can exercise to the point of mild dyspnea and maintain that level during the training session. As discussed before, the onset of dyspnea approximates the VT and is an adequate intensity for a training stimulus. Finally, patients can exercise to a "somewhat hard" level using number scales designed to estimate the intensity of exertion, such as the modified Borg scale.

Unsupervised Exercise Training

Many patients cannot attend supervised exercise training sessions because a cardiac rehabilitation program is not available, because it is not convenient to attend supervised sessions, or because of costs not covered by insurance. Nevertheless, all CAD patients should be advised to exercise for its cardiovascular benefits.

Patients without lower limb orthopedic problems should be encouraged to use brisk walking as their exercise training modality. Patients in unsupervised programs should generally be encouraged to exercise to the onset of mild dyspnea for the reasons mentioned earlier. Such an approach obviates the need for pulse monitoring. Many patients either cannot accurately monitor their heart rate or become unduly concerned about pulse irregularities caused by premature atrial or ventricular contractions. Patients exercising on their own can also be encouraged to judge their exercise intensity with the "talk test" or by exercising at the fastest walking rate that still permits comfortable conversation. This work rate corresponds to the exercise training range recommended for cardiac patients.[5]

Other Components of Comprehensive Cardiac Rehabilitation

The American Heart Association recommended in 1994 that cardiac rehabilitation programs expand to include other strategies designed to reduce cardiovascular risk (see Chap. 49).[6] These measures included nutritional, psychological, and vocational counseling, as well as serum lipid, blood pressure, and smoking risk factor management—components required by Medicare.[4] There is no doubt about the critical importance of these components of secondary CAD prevention. Addressing such issues as blood pressure and lipid management and smoking cessation often requires a balancing of the roles of the cardiac rehabilitation staff and those of the primary care physician. The cardiac rehabilitation personnel generally focus on counseling aspects of risk factor management. They can also serve as a knowledgeable source to interpret laboratory results and the physician's instructions and as patient advocates with the primary health care provider. With lipid management, for example, the rehabilitation staff may evaluate the results from the patient's physician and suggest that the patient request a more aggressive treatment approach to achieve cholesterol goals.

Programs differ as to how they deliver counseling and education components. Evaluation of the patient's learning style may help maximize the program's education potential. Many programs use the aerobic exercise time to visit with and educate the patient while he or she is on the exercise apparatus. Some programs simply make printed material available to patients. Other programs use television monitors and either commercially available or locally prepared video programs to deliver the counseling and risk-reduction messages. Some programs have replaced exercise sessions with educational programs—an approach that I oppose, given the physiologic benefits of exercise training. Classroom activities can be creatively scheduled along with exercise sessions, allowing participants to choose which education programs best meet their needs. Ideally, educational programs on nutrition, lipid management, smoking cessation, and psychological issues should be delivered by experts in the field, but such experts are often not available, requiring the rehabilitation staff to provide these sessions or to purchase commercially available programs.

Insurance Coverage

Insurance coverage of cardiac rehabilitation activities is critically important for patients to be able to receive these services. Medicare in the United States[19] provides reimbursement for patients who have stable angina pectoris, or who have within the prior 12 months suffered an acute MI, undergone CABG, undergone a cardiac valve repair or replacement, had PCI, or received a heart or heart-lung transplant. Medicare coverage is critically important in the United States because most private insurers follow the Medicare reimbursement procedures. Routine coverage is for a total of 36 exercise sessions. Cardiac rehabilitation is not covered by Medicare for HF, but it is covered by some insurance carriers. It is not clear how HF-ACTION will affect this policy. Insurance coverage in other countries varies greatly.

Current Problems with Cardiac Rehabilitation

The major current problem with exercise-based cardiac rehabilitation is its underuse. Only ≈25% to 30% of men and ≈11% to 20% of women eligible for cardiac rehabilitation participate in such programs.[20] Physician endorsement of cardiac rehabilitation is one of the most important predictors of participation.[20] It is unclear why physicians do not routinely refer patients, although underestimation by physicians of the benefits of exercise, lack of knowledge of health professionals about exercise training, and absence of exercise advocates similar to pharmaceutical representatives may contribute. Absence of a conclusive, appropriately powered clinical trial may also contribute to underuse. Nevertheless, the bulk of the evidence strongly supports the use of standard cardiac rehabilitation. Consequently, all physicians should be encouraged to refer most patients to cardiac rehabilitation. Even when the physician is not convinced of the benefit, the patient often finds the experience rewarding and reassuring. One of the most effective ways to combat the lack of referral is to include cardiac rehabilitation in standardized order sets for appropriate cardiac patients.

The Future of Cardiac Rehabilitation

Cardiac rehabilitation has an uncertain future. Efforts to control medical care costs will place increased scrutiny on any programs that add cost without documented efficacy. Excellent meta-analysis evidence indicates that cardiac rehabilitation reduces cardiac events, but as discussed, most of the studies analyzed predate present aggressive medical and interventional therapy for cardiac disease. Consequently, insurance companies may limit cardiac rehabilitation coverage or increase the copayment required for these services. These changes, if they occur, will force the development of a different form of cardiac rehabilitation. Programs will need to shift from the thrice-weekly supervised format to programs that use less frequent staff interaction.

Alternatively, the more distant future may actually see more use of exercise-based cardiac rehabilitation if it is supported by appropriate trials. This subject would seem highly appropriate for comparative efficacy study. Exercise training and risk factor reduction are inexpensive compared with invasive therapies for ischemic disease. Exercise training and risk reduction also treat the entire vascular tree, rather than a specific lesion. Exercise-based cardiac rehabilitation could be more widely used in the future to improve endothelial dysfunction and to manage angina pectoris and stable CAD, thereby reducing such costly interventions as PCI and CABG. Such a shift will require much more documentation of the benefits of such programs. As noted before, evidence from a small controlled clinical trial suggested that exercise training decreases cardiovascular events compared with PCI in selected patients with angina pectoris (see Fig. 50-2).[7] This trial requires confirmation in a larger study that uses optimum medical therapy and contemporary percutaneous coronary intervention. Additional trials should be initiated to compare intensive rehabilitation and risk factor reduction with PCI or CABG in CAD patients. The evidence that CABG is superior to medical therapy in selected CAD patients is decades old and may no longer be valid in the era of statins and other highly effective pharmacologic interventions. Appropriately designed trials may document that comprehensive cardiac rehabilitation, including exercise training and aggressive lifestyle and medication management of risk factors, may obviate the need for surgical intervention and assist in controlling medical care costs.

Acknowledgments

The author thanks the staff of the Hartford Hospital Cardiac Rehabilitation Program for the years of education they have provided to the author and Lucie Bohannon, MS, PT, and Donna Polk, MD, MPH, for advice on the practical aspects of rehabilitation.

REFERENCES

1. Redwood DR, Rosing DR, Epstein SE: Circulatory and symptomatic effects of physical training in patients with coronary-artery disease and angina pectoris. N Engl J Med 286:959, 1972.
2. Detry JM, Rousseau M, Vandenbroucke G, et al: Increased arteriovenous oxygen difference after physical training in coronary heart disease. Circulation 44:109, 1971.
3. Ades PA: Cardiac rehabilitation and secondary prevention of coronary heart disease. N Engl J Med 345:892, 2001.
4. National Government Services. Available at: http://www.ngsmedicare.com/ngsmedicare/PartA/Coverage/CoverageArticles/files/CardiacRehabilitationProgramA45888archive07172008.htm. Accessed June 10, 2009.
5. Thompson PD: Exercise prescription and proscription for patients with coronary artery disease. Circulation 112:2354, 2005.
6. Leon AS, Franklin BA, Costa F, et al: Cardiac rehabilitation and secondary prevention of coronary heart disease: An American Heart Association scientific statement from the Council on Clinical Cardiology (Subcommittee on Exercise, Cardiac Rehabilitation, and Prevention) and the Council on Nutrition, Physical Activity, and Metabolism (Subcommittee on Physical Activity), in collaboration with the American Association of Cardiovascular and Pulmonary Rehabilitation. Circulation 111:369, 2005.
7. Hambrecht R, Walther C, Mobius-Winkler S, et al: Percutaneous coronary angioplasty compared with exercise training in patients with stable coronary artery disease: A randomized trial. Circulation 109:1371, 2004.
8. Hambrecht R, Wolf A, Gielen S, et al: Effect of exercise on coronary endothelial function in patients with coronary artery disease. N Engl J Med 342:454, 2000.
9. Moyna NM, Thompson PD: The effect of physical activity on endothelial function in man. Acta Physiol Scand 180:113, 2004.
10. Hambrecht R, Adams V, Erbs S, et al: Regular physical activity improves endothelial function in patients with coronary artery disease by increasing phosphorylation of endothelial nitric oxide synthase. Circulation 107:3152, 2003.
11. Taylor RS, Brown A, Ebrahim S, et al: Exercise-based rehabilitation for patients with coronary heart disease: Systematic review and meta-analysis of randomized controlled trials. Am J Med 116:682, 2004.
12. Giannuzzi P, Temporelli PL, Maggioni AP, et al: GlObal Secondary Prevention strategiEs to Limit event recurrence after myocardial infarction: The GOSPEL study. A trial from the Italian Cardiac Rehabilitation Network: Rationale and design. Eur J Cardiovasc Prev Rehabil 12:555, 2005.
13. Belardinelli R, Paolini I, Cianci G, et al: Exercise training intervention after coronary angioplasty: The ETICA trial. J Am Coll Cardiol 37:1891, 2001.
14. Smart N, Marwick TH: Exercise training for patients with heart failure: A systematic review of factors that improve mortality and morbidity. Am J Med 116:693, 2004.
15. O'Connor CM, Whellan DJ, Lee KL, et al: Efficacy and safety of exercise training in patients with chronic heart failure: HF-ACTION randomized controlled trial. JAMA 301:1439, 2009.
16. Belardinelli R, Georgiou D, Cianci G, Purcaro A: Randomized, controlled trial of long-term moderate exercise training in chronic heart failure: Effects on functional capacity, quality of life, and clinical outcome. Circulation 99:1173, 1999.
17. Jolly K, Taylor RS, Lip GY, Stevens A: Home-based cardiac rehabilitation compared with centre-based rehabilitation and usual care: A systematic review and meta-analysis. Int J Cardiol 111:343, 2006.
18. Hamm LF, Kavanagh T, Campbell RB, et al: Timeline for peak improvements during 52 weeks of outpatient cardiac rehabilitation. J Cardiopulm Rehabil 24:374, 2004.
19. Decision Memo for Cardiac Rehabilitation Programs. Available at: https://www.cms.hhs.gov/mcd/viewdecisionmemo.asp?id=164. March 22, 2006.
20. Jackson L, Leclerc J, Erskine Y, Linden W: Getting the most out of cardiac rehabilitation: A review of referral and adherence predictors. Heart 91:10, 2005.

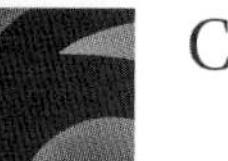

CHAPTER 51 Complementary and Alternative Approaches to Management of Patients with Heart Disease

Edzard Ernst

Complementary and Alternative Medicine: Definitions, Prevalence, and Reasons for Use

Complementary and alternative medicine (CAM) includes a range of therapeutic approaches that have little in common with each other. Thus, CAM is far from easy to define. For the purpose of this chapter, the following definition is used: "CAM is diagnosis, treatment and/or prevention which complements mainstream medicine by contributing to a common whole, by satisfying a demand not met by orthodoxy or by diversifying the conceptual frameworks of medicine."[1] **Table 51-1** provides short definitions of the most important modalities in the context of this chapter.

The 1-year prevalence of CAM use in the general population varies considerably from country to country. In the United States, the figure has been increasing during the last decades and is currently around 60%.[2] In specific populations of patients, it may be even higher. Many patients who use CAM fail to tell their physicians; therefore, physicians are likely to have a wrong impression about CAM use by their patients unless they ask specific questions. Most who try CAM would use it as an adjunct to rather than as a replacement of mainstream health care.

The reasons for use of CAM are diverse and depend, amongst a myriad of other factors, on whether CAM is employed in the hope of staying healthy, to improve well-being, or for treatment of a specific medical condition. Prominent "pull factors" are philosophical congruence with the world view of CAM, wanting control over one's own health, and a good therapeutic relationship with a CAM practitioner. Important "push factors" are dissatisfaction with conventional health care, rejection of science, desperation (when seriously ill), and the high cost of private orthodox medicine.[3]

This chapter provides a brief summary of the evidence base as it pertains to CAM for heart disease. For more detailed and fully referenced discussions, the reader is referred elsewhere.[3,4]

Complementary and Alternative Medicine for Congestive Heart Failure

(see Chaps. 26 and 27)

According to the results of rigorous clinical trials, the CAM approach that seems most promising for congestive heart failure is hawthorn (*Crataegus* spp). Extracts of this plant contain cardiac glycosides and thus have pharmacologic effects similar to those of digitalis (digitalis itself was, of course, plant based originally, but pure, single, and synthetically produced constituents are used today, which by definition is *not* herbal medicine). The main constituents of hawthorn extracts are catechin, epicatechin, flavonoids, and procyanidins. Their pharmacologic actions include dilation of the coronary arteries, positive inotropic effects, decrease of atrioventricular conduction time, and increase of the refractory period. In addition, cardioprotective, antiarrhythmic, hypotensive, beta-blocking, and angiotensin-converting enzyme–inhibiting properties have been documented.[3]

A meta-analysis of eight double-blind, placebo-controlled, randomized clinical trials (RCTs) with patients suffering from congestive heart failure in New York Heart Association (NYHA) Class I to III is available.[5] All RCTs used a monoextract of hawthorn leaves and flowers. Effects in favor of hawthorn extract were found for maximal workload and pressure–heart rate product. Symptoms such as dyspnea and fatigue also improved better than with placebo.

Since the publication of this meta-analysis, new, important findings have emerged from an RCT including 1442 patients with congestive heart failure in NYHA Class II or III.[6] They received 900 mg/day of a standardized hawthorn extract or placebo for 24 months. The primary outcome measure, time to first cardiac event, showed a nonsignificant trend in favor of the herbal medicine (620 versus 606 days). In a subgroup analysis of severely ill patients (left ventricular ejection fraction 25% or lower), hawthorn intake was associated with a 40% reduction in sudden cardiac deaths.

Adverse effects of hawthorn extracts are rare, usually mild, and reversible: nausea, dizziness, vertigo, fatigue, sweating, palpitations, tachycardia, and gastrointestinal complaints. Additive effects with antihypertensive drugs, nitrates, other cardiac glycosides, and central nervous system depressants are conceivable. The correct dose of hawthorn depends on the nature of the extract; for a standardized extract, it is 900 mg/day.

Other natural remedies supported by some but less conclusive evidence include goldenseal *(Hydrastis canadensis)*, horsetail (*Equisetum* spp), and rutin.[7]

Coronary Heart Disease (see Chaps. 53-57)

Treatment

ACUPUNCTURE. A fundamental concept of traditional acupuncture is *qi*, often translated as "energy." *Qi* is thought to flow through the body in 12 "meridians" where acupuncture points are located. There is no reliable evidence for the existence of *qi* or meridians. Modern concepts try to explain acupuncture's mode of action through neurophysiologic phenomena. For instance, acupuncture has been found to release neurotransmitters such as opioid peptides and serotonin.

Several clinical trials have tested whether acupuncture is an effective adjunctive treatment of coronary heart disease. An overview has been provided elsewhere.[4] The results of clinical trials tend to be encouraging in terms of symptom control or nitroglycerin consumption. However, the studies available to date are small and frequently not rigorous. Therefore, the currently available evidence is far from conclusive.

TABLE 51-1 Examples of Complementary and Alternative Treatment Modalities That Are Important Through Their Popularity

NAME OF THERAPY	BRIEF DESCRIPTION
Acupuncture	Stimulation of acupuncture points by insertion of a needle, electrical current (electroacupuncture), heat (moxibustion), laser (laser acupuncture), or pressure (acupressure)
Aromatherapy	Application of "essential" oils from plants, usually through gentle massage
Autogenic training	Form of self-hypnosis that can be taught and subsequently self-applied, usually to control stress
Bach flower remedies	A therapeutic system of plant infusions aimed at balancing physical and emotional disturbances
Biofeedback	Use of information (e.g., audible or visible) on physiologic responses so that a patient can learn to control these responses
Body-mind medicine	A healing approach emphasizing the connections between the physician, mental and emotional aspects of disease
Chelation therapy	Intravenous infusion of EDTA, vitamins, and minerals used in CAM predominantly to treat vascular diseases
Chiropractic	School of predominantly manipulative techniques aimed at correcting malalignment of the spine with the aim of restoring function and health
Herbalism	Treatment or prevention of disease using plant-based medicines; various medical cultures have produced their own type of herbalism, e.g., Ayurveda (India), Kampo (Japan), traditional Chinese medicine
Hypnotherapy	Form of cognitive information processing using suspension of peripheral awareness aimed at apparently involuntary changes in perception, memory, mood, and physiology
Imagery	Use of imagery to correct unhealthy attitudes aimed at helping to restore health
Massage	Manual techniques of rubbing, stroking, tapping, or kneading of the body with a view to treating physical or emotional conditions
Music therapy	The use of a music-accredited professional to achieve individualized therapeutic goals
Osteopathy	System of health care using manual spinal mobilization and manipulation to restore function and health
Qigong	Branch of traditional Chinese medicine aimed at restoring balance and flow of "life energy"
Relaxation	Techniques for eliciting a "relaxation response" of the autonomic nervous system
Supplements	Umbrella term for dietary supplements ranging from herbal remedies to vitamins
Yoga	Indian philosophy used therapeutically by way of gentle physical exercises, breathing control, and meditation

The risks of acupuncture are mostly minor; for example, pain during needling and minor bleeding occur in about 10% of all patients. Serious complications, such as pneumothorax, cardiac tamponade, infections, and even deaths, are also on record. Perhaps the greatest risk would be to use acupuncture as an alternative to conventional treatment of coronary heart disease.

CHELATION THERAPY. Chelation therapists claim that the infusion of EDTA, usually combined with vitamins and minerals, can reduce a stenosis in a coronary artery. This concept is biologically implausible, however, and the trial data fail to show that this treatment is clinically effective.[8]

RELAXATION. Several CAM approaches can produce a "relaxation response" via the autonomic nervous system (e.g., autogenic training, biofeedback, hypnotherapy, imagery, or meditation). One of the best-researched relaxation techniques is progressive muscle relaxation. This technique has been shown to decrease oxygen consumption, heart rate, respiration, and skeletal muscle activity and to increase skin resistance and alpha brain wave activity. Relaxation therapies can be clinically useful for treatment of anxiety, hypertension, and coronary syndrome X as well as for prevention of complications after myocardial infarction.[3]

No significant risks are associated with relaxation techniques as long as they are used wisely. They can serve only as an adjunct to therapy and not as an alternative therapy for coronary heart disease.

OTHERS. Several other CAM approaches have been tested in clinical trials, such as Ayurvedic herbal mixtures, Chinese herbal medicines,[9] homeopathic remedies, pomegranate *(Punica granatum)*, and *Terminalia arjuna*. The evidence is insufficient for any of them.[10]

Prevention and Risk Factor Normalization

HYPERTENSION (see Chap. 46). The use of CAM seems higher in hypertensive people compared with people without hypertension.[11] Numerous CAM approaches have been tested for their potential to decrease elevated blood pressure. A fully referenced overview has been published elsewhere.[3]

Acupuncture

The current trial data are scarce and contradictory. Even if the totality of the evidence would suggest an antihypertensive effect, this might not be clinically relevant. The effect sizes of the positive studies are small, and the practicality of regular treatment for lowering of blood pressure seems doubtful.

Autogenic Training

A systematic review of five clinical trials found encouraging evidence to support the notion that this autohypnotic technique generates hypotensive effects. However, because of methodologic limitations of these data, firm conclusions cannot be drawn.

Biofeedback

Several RCTs have shown that biofeedback lowers both systolic and diastolic blood pressure to a clinically relevant extent. A meta-analysis of these data concluded that feedback is effective in lowering blood pressure.[12]

Chiropractic

A systematic review of four RCTs of mostly poor methodologic quality found no convincing evidence to suggest that chiropractic is an effective treatment of hypertension.[13] As this treatment is by no means free of risks,[3] its risk-benefit balance fails to be positive.

Herbal Medicine

Many herbal medicines have been tested for possible antihypertensive effects. Encouraging results emerged for the following[3]:

- *Achillea wilhelmsii*, a popular folk remedy from Iran
- *Adenia cissampeloides* lowered elevated systolic but not diastolic blood pressure.

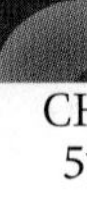

- Various Chinese herbal medicines have been tested, invariably with positive results (several groups have shown that Chinese studies of Chinese herbal medicines never report negative findings).
- Garlic *(Allium sativum)*: a meta-analysis found a small pooled effect size.
- Ginseng *(Panax ginseng)*: findings are contradictory.
- Hawthorn *(Crataegus)* has produced mixed results regarding blood pressure.
- *Hibiscus sabdariffa*: too few trial data.[14]
- Maritime pine bark extract *(Pinus pinaster)*: too few data.
- Pomegranate *(Punica granatum)*: too few trial data.

Clinical trials of *Gingko biloba, Punica granatum,* and *Trifolium subterraneum* have failed to demonstrate significant effects on blood pressure.[3]

Hypnotherapy

Two small clinical trials suggested that hypnotherapy may have hypotensive effects in patients suffering from elevated blood pressure. However, the practicality of using this approach on a regular basis seems doubtful.[3]

Meditation

A systematic review of six RCTs of transcendental meditation failed to generate convincing evidence that meditation is an effective treatment of hypertension.[15]

Music Therapy

A systematic review of 12 RCTs has provided encouraging preliminary evidence to suggest that music therapy might be a useful adjunct to standard antihypertensive treatments.[16]

Relaxation

A meta-analysis of nine RCTs found small effects of various stress reduction programs on both systolic and diastolic blood pressure. However, the effects are probably too small to be clinically relevant.

Qigong

The regular practice of *qigong*, a Chinese meditative practice using slow graceful movements and controlled breathing techniques, for 8 to 10 weeks has been shown to normalize elevated systolic and diastolic blood pressure. A meta-analysis of 12 RCTs concluded that there is encouraging but limited evidence for an antihypertensive effect.[17]

Supplements (Nonherbal)

A systematic review of four relatively small RCTs found that 100 to 200 mg of coenzyme Q10 per day for 8 to 12 weeks decreased systolic blood pressure by 6 to 12 mm Hg and systolic blood pressure by 2 to 16 mm Hg. Further, large-scale studies seem warranted.

Fish oil (omega-3 fatty acids) has produced contradictory results in clinical trials testing its potential for lowering of elevated blood pressure.

Other studies have demonstrated encouraging but small effects for the following nonherbal supplements:

- Green algae *(Chlorella)*
- L-Arginine
- Melatonin
- *Ganoderma lucidum*
- Vitamin C
- Vitamin E

Yoga

A systematic review suggested that regular adherence to a yoga regimen has modest, positive effects on a range of cardiovascular risk factors, including hypertension.[18] More recent trial data seem to confirm this notion.[19]

HYPERCHOLESTEROLEMIA (see Chaps. 47 and 48). Several herbal and other supplements have been tested for their potential to decrease elevated cholesterol levels. A fully referenced overview has been published elsewhere.[3]

Herbal Medicine

For the following herbal medicines, encouraging trial data exist.[3]

- Aloe vera juice *(Aloe vera)*
- Artichoke *(Cynara scolymus)*
- Dai-saiko-to, a Kampo medicine
- Fenugreek *(Trigonella foenum-graecum)*
- Garlic *(Allium sativum)*
- Ginseng *(Panax ginseng)*
- Green tea *(Camellia sinensis)*
- Guar gum *(Cyamopsis tetragonolobus)*
- Guggul *(Commiphora mukul)*
- Oat and other fiber products
- Psyllium *(Plantago ovata)*
- Saiko-ka-ryukotsu-borei-to, a Kampo medicine
- Yerba maté *(Ilex paraguariensis)*[20]

Unfortunately, the effect sizes are usually small or modest, and the clinical relevance of the effect is therefore debatable.

Supplements (Nonherbal)

A Cochrane review of the cholesterol-lowering properties of chitosan identified nine RCTs.[21] On average, there was a small but significant (–0.2 mmol/liter) reduction. Because of methodologic limitations of several of the primary studies, no firm conclusions can be drawn.

Another Cochrane review assessed the effects of fish oil on blood lipid levels in patients with type 2 diabetes mellitus. A reduction in triglyceride levels was noted, but there was no effect on total cholesterol or HDL-cholesterol levels and a slight increase in LDL-cholesterol levels.

Limited evidence from clinical trials exists furthermore for the following nonherbal supplements:

- Konjac glucomannan
- Milk products fermented by the probiotic *Bifidobacterium longum* strain BL1
- Red yeast rice
- Soy protein

SMOKING. A large percentage of smokers trying to quit employ CAM for that purpose,[22] and many forms of CAM are being advocated to facilitate nicotine withdrawal. However, relatively few of them have been tested in clinical trials. A fully referenced review has been published elsewhere.[3]

Acupuncture

A Cochrane review included 24 RCTs of acupuncture as a means to aid smoking cessation.[23] The overall long-term result achieved with acupuncture shows no difference from that obtained with sham-acupuncture.

Hypnotherapy

Another Cochrane review of nine RCTs evaluated various hypnotherapeutic techniques for smoking cessation. The results were far from uniform, but the overall conclusion was negative. There is no good evidence for the superiority of hypnotherapy compared with other therapeutic options.

Other Treatments

Encouraging evidence has emerged for massage therapy and relaxation techniques for alleviation of nicotine withdrawal symptoms. Independent replications of these studies are required before recommendations can be issued.

OBESITY (see Chap. 48). Many CAM approaches have been tested for body weight reduction. For a fully referenced overview, see elsewhere.[24]

Acupuncture and Acupressure

A systematic review included four sham-controlled RCTs. Overall, the evidence was contradictory and not convincing.

Herbal Medicine

Compared with placebo, *Ephedra sinica* and ephedrine generate a small weight loss of about 0.9 kg per month. However, the use of such stimulants is associated with an increased risk of psychiatric, autonomic, and gastrointestinal symptoms and cardiovascular problems (e.g., hypertension, myocardial infarction, arrhythmias, and stroke). They should therefore not be recommended and have been removed from the U.S. market.

Garcinia cambogia has been shown to suppress fatty acid synthesis and to reduce food intake. Four double-blind RCTs are available. Overall, the evidence is encouraging but not convincing. Further independent studies are needed.

Small effects on body weight have also been shown for the following botanical supplements:

- Glucomannan, a component of konjac root, derived from *Amorphophallus konjac*
- Guar gum, a dietary fiber derived from *Cyamopsis tetragonolobus*
- Maté extract
- Psyllium *(Plantago ovata)*

No effect was shown in clinical trials of *Citrus aurantium* extracts.

Hypnotherapy

A meta-analysis of six RCTs suggested that the addition of hypnotherapy to cognitive-behavioral therapy leads to a small reduction in body weight. However, the effect seems to be too small to be clinically relevant.

Supplements (Nonherbal)

Small effects on body weight have been suggested for the following supplements[3]:

- Beta-hydroxy-beta-methylbutyrate, a metabolite of leucine
- Chitosan, a product made of the shells of shellfish[21]
- Chromium, a cofactor to insulin
- Conjugated linoleic acid

No clear effects have been demonstrated in clinical studies of oral capsaicin or yohimbine.[3]

STRESS. Several forms of CAM have a reputation for being "de-stressing." Some of the evidence from clinical trials seems to confirm this. A fully referenced overview was published elsewhere.[3]

Acupuncture

Several RCTs suggested that needle acupuncture induces a more pronounced relaxation response than sham-acupuncture does. Unfortunately, most of these studies are methodologically weak, and their findings are therefore less than compelling.

Aromatherapy

A systematic review concluded that aromatherapy has anxiolytic effects. However, these are short term and too small to have clinical relevance.

Autogenic Training

A systematic review including six clinical trials suggested that autogenic training generates anxiolytic effects that might be clinically relevant.[25]

Biofeedback

Various forms of biofeedback can generate anxiolytic effects in a range of clinical situations. However, the trial data are not entirely uniform and therefore not compelling.

Flower Remedies

A systematic review found no evidence that Bach flower remedies reduce stress.[26]

Herbal Medicine

A Cochrane review of 11 RCTs concluded that kava *(Piper methysticum)* appears to be effective for the symptomatic treatment of anxiety.[27] Unfortunately, kava is thought to cause liver damage. Therefore, its use cannot be recommended.

Less convincing trial data exist for the following herbal medicines:

- *Crataegus oxyacantha*
- *Eschscholzia californica*
- German chamomile *(Matricaria recutita)*
- Lemon balm *(Melissa officinalis)*
- Passion flower *(Passiflora incarnata)*

One RCT tested the anxiolytic effects of valerian *(Valeriana officinalis)*, but its results were negative.

Hypnotherapy

Anxiety was reduced more effectively by hypnotherapy in patients before painful and stressful diagnostic procedures than by a nonhypnotic behavioral technique.

Imagery

A systematic review of six RCTs of imagery as an adjuvant therapy found encouraging evidence to suggest that this approach alleviates anxiety.[28]

Massage

An overview of 10 studies showed that massage therapy decreases anxiety in a variety of settings.[29]

Meditation

Meditation can reduce anxiety levels and neuroendocrine responses to stress more effectively than attention control in volunteers placed in stressful conditions. A meta-analysis of controlled and uncontrolled studies of mindfulness-based stress reduction concluded that this approach has anxiolytic effects, but the primary data were methodologically weak.

Music Therapy

A systematic review of 29 RCTs showed that music therapy reduces anxiety in hospitalized patients.[30]

Relaxation

Various relaxation techniques have been used to manage the anxiety associated with a range of medical conditions.[3] For instance, audiotapes with relaxation instructions were superior to music tapes or blank tapes at reducing both anxiety and pain during femoral angiography. Relaxation before a magnetic resonance imaging scan reduced the anxiety associated with the procedure more than no intervention.

DIABETES (see Chap. 86). Herbal and other dietary supplements have repeatedly been tested for their antiglycemic effects. A fully referenced overview is available elsewhere.[3]

Herbal Medicine

A systematic review assessed the effectiveness of various Ayurvedic preparations for diabetes.[31] According to its findings, holy basil, fenugreek, and the herbal formulas Ayush-82 and D-400 may have a glucose-lowering effect, but more and better quality studies are required to be sure.

A Cochrane review assessed the effects of 69 different Chinese herbal medicines.[32] It concluded that some of them may have beneficial effects on glucose metabolism in type 2 diabetes mellitus. Unfortunately, the majority of the trials had low methodologic quality, and it is therefore not possible to recommend any of these preparations.

Other herbal medicines supported by tentative evidence from RCTs are *Camellia sinensis*, cinnamon *(Cinnamomum zeylanicum)*, and ginseng *(Panax ginseng* and *Panax quinquefolius)* as well as guar gum *(Cyamopsis tetragonolobus)*, white sweet potatoes *(Ipomoea batatas)*, mulberry *(Morus indica)*, psyllium *(Plantago ovata)*, and the French maritime pine *(Pinus pinaster)*.[3]

TABLE 51-2 The Most Promising Complementary and Alternative Medicine (CAM) Approaches for Heart Disease or Risk Factors

CONDITION	CAM	COMMENT
Congestive heart failure	Hawthorn	Recent data were not convincing
Coronary heart disease	Acupuncture	Practicality is debatable
	Relaxation	Potentially useful self-treatments
Hypertension	Acupuncture	Practicality is debatable
	Autogenic training	Potentially useful self-treatments
	Biofeedback	Potentially useful self-treatments
	Herbal medicines	More research required
	Hypnotherapy	Practicality is debatable
	Music therapy	Practicality is debatable
	Relaxation	Potentially useful self-treatments
	Qigong	Potentially useful self-treatments
	Coenzyme Q10	More research required
Hypercholesterolemia	Various herbs	More research required
Stress	Aromatherapy	Pleasant experience, popular treatment
	Autogenic training	Potentially useful self-treatments
	Biofeedback	Potentially useful self-treatments
	Various herbal medicines	More research required
	Hypnotherapy	Practicality is debatable
	Imagery	Potentially useful self-treatments
	Massage	Pleasant experience, popular treatment
	Music therapy	Practicality is debatable
	Relaxation	Potentially useful self-treatments

Supplements (Nonherbal)

A meta-analysis of 20 RCTs assessing the effect of chromium on blood glucose levels, insulin, or glycated hemoglobin HbA1c concluded that the data are inconclusive. No effect on glucose or insulin concentrations was noted in nondiabetic subjects.[33]

Other nonherbal supplements supported by encouraging albeit preliminary data are the following[3,7]:

- Beta-glucan
- Coenzyme Q10
- Ginseng (*Panax* spp)
- *Gymnema sylvestre*
- Soy
- *Stevia rebaudiana*

No effects on glucose metabolism were reported for fish oil and magnesium.

Other Types of Heart Disease

The field of CAM is plagued by proponents who advocate CAM even for serious conditions without having good evidence in support. Patients can thus easily find positive recommendations for CAM options as treatments for a range of other types of heart disease. In the absence of sound evidence, such advice seems irresponsible. Cardiologists should be aware that many of their patients are tempted by such claims to try CAM. They should discuss these issues openly with their patients and provide advice that is firmly based on evidence.

Conclusions

This overview shows that several forms of CAM have the potential to become useful adjuncts to conventional treatments or preventative measures of various types of heart disease (**Table 51-2**). In the majority of cases, however, this evidence is limited by the paucity or the low quality of the primary studies. The most promising treatments are those that seem to induce a relaxation response, which might be particularly useful to manage stress and hypertension (see Table 51-2).

The CAM research community has a most unfortunate tendency to draw misleading conclusions from investigations into CAM; when a treatment fails to emerge as effective, it is often not the treatment but the trial methodology that is deemed to be at fault. Moreover, there are hardly any equivalence studies comparing the effects of conventional with CAM options. Overall, one does not get the impression that CAM therapies would be more effective in treating any type of heart disease than the currently available conventional treatments.

It follows, in my view, that the most promising CAM options should be submitted to more extensive testing in rigorous clinical trials. Only when this has been done will we be able to define with certainty which forms of CAM generate more good than harm and which do not.

REFERENCES

Complementary and Alternative Medicine: Definitions, Prevalence, and Reasons for Use

1. Ernst E, Resch KL, Mills S, et al: Complementary medicine—a definition. Br J Gen Pract 45:506, 1995.
2. Barnes PM, Powell-Griner E, McFann K, Nahin RL: Complementary and alternative medicine use among adults: United States, 2002. Adv Data 343:1, 2004.
3. Ernst E, Pittler MH, Wider B, Boddy K: The Desktop Guide to Complementary and Alternative Medicine. 2nd ed. Edinburgh, Elsevier Mosby, 2006.
4. Ernst E, Pittler MH, Wider B, Boddy K: Complementary Therapies for Pain Management. An Evidence-Based Approach. London, Elsevier, 2007.
5. Pittler MH, Schmidt K, Ernst E: Hawthorn extract for treating chronic heart failure: Meta-analysis of randomized trials. Am J Med 114:665, 2003.
6. Holubarsch CJ, Colucci WS, Meinertz T, et al: The efficacy and safety of *Crataegus* extract WS 1442 in patients with heart failure: The SPICE trial. Eur J Heart Fail 10:1255, 2008.
7. Ulbricht C, Seaman E: Natural Standard Herbal Pharmacotherapy. An Evidence-Based Approach. St. Louis, Mosby, 2010.

Coronary Heart Disease

8. Villarruz MV, Dans A, Tan F: Chelation therapy for atherosclerotic cardiovascular disease. Cochrane Database Syst Rev (4):CD002785, 2002.
9. Tam WY, Chook P, Qiao M, et al: The efficacy and tolerability of adjunctive alternative herbal medicine (*Salvia miltiorrhiza* and *Pueraria lobata*) on vascular function and structure in coronary patients. J Altern Complement Med 15:415, 2009.
10. Ernst E, Pittler M, Wider B, Boddy K: Oxford Handbook of Complementary Medicine. Oxford, Oxford University Press, 2008.

Hypertension

11. Bell RA, Suerken CK, Grzywacz JG, et al: CAM use among older adults age 65 or older with hypertension in the United States: General use and disease treatment. J Altern Complement Med 12:903, 2006.
12. Nakao M, Yano E, Nomura S, Kuboki T: Blood pressure–lowering effects of biofeedback treatment in hypertension: A meta-analysis of randomized controlled trials. Hypertens Res 26:37, 2003.
13. Ernst E: Chiropractic spinal manipulation as a treatment of hypertension? A systematic review of randomised clinical trials. Perfusion 21:188, 2008.
14. Wahabi HA, Alansary LA, Al-Sabban AH, Glasziuo P: The effectiveness of *Hibiscus sabdariffa* in the treatment of hypertension: A systematic review. Phytomedicine 17:83, 2010. Epub 2009 Oct 3.
15. Canter PH, Ernst E: Insufficient evidence to conclude whether or not Transcendental Meditation decreases blood pressure: Results of a systematic review of randomized clinical trials. J Hypertens 22:2049, 2004.
16. Schmidt K, Ernst E: Music therapy for patients with cardiovascular diseases—a systematic review. Perfusion 17:136, 2004.
17. Lee MS, Pittler MH, Guo R, Ernst E: Qigong for hypertension: A systematic review of randomized clinical trials. J Hypertens 25:1525, 2007.
18. Hutchinson S, Ernst E: Yoga therapy for coronary heart disease: A systematic review. Perfusion 17:44, 2004.
19. Cohen DL, Bloedon LT, Rothman RL, et al: Iyengar yoga versus enhanced usual care on blood pressure in patients with prehypertension to stage I hypertension: A randomized controlled trial. Evid Based Complement Alternat Med 2009 Sep 4. [Epub ahead of print].

Hypercholesterolemia

20. de Morais EC, Stefanuto A, Klein GA, et al: Consumption of yerba mate *(Ilex paraguariensis)* improves serum lipid parameters in healthy dyslipidemic subjects and provides an additional LDL-cholesterol reduction in individuals on statin therapy. J Agric Food Chem 57:8316, 2009.
21. Jull AB, Ni Mhurchu C, Bennett DA, et al: Chitosan for overweight or obesity. Cochrane Database Syst Rev (3):CD003892, 2008. DOI: 10.1002/14651858.CD003892.pub3.

Smoking

22. Sood A, Ebbert JO, Sood R, Stevens SR: Complementary treatments for tobacco cessation: A survey. Nicotine Tobacco Res 8:767, 2006.
23. White AR, Rampes H, Campbell JL: Acupuncture and related interventions for smoking cessation. Cochrane Database Syst Rev (1):CD000009, 2006.

Obesity

24. Pittler MH, Ernst E: Complementary therapies for reducing body weight: A systematic review. Int J Obes (Lond) 29:1030, 2005.

Stress

25. Kanji N, Ernst E: Autogenic training for stress and anxiety: A systematic review. Complement Ther Med 8:106, 2000.
26. Ernst E: "Flower remedies": A systematic review of the clinical evidence. Wien Klin Wochenschr 114:963, 2002.
27. Pittler MH, Ernst E: Kava extract for treating anxiety. Cochrane Database Syst Rev (1):CD003383, 2003.
28. Roffe L, Schmidt K, Ernst E: A systematic review of guided imagery as an adjuvant cancer therapy. Psychooncology 14:607, 2005.
29. Richards KC, Gibson R, Overton-McCoy AL: Effects of massage in acute and critical care. AACN Clin Issues 11:76, 2000.
30. Evans D: The effectiveness of music as an intervention for hospital patients: A systematic review. J Adv Nurs 37:8, 2002.

Diabetes

31. Hardy ML, Coulter I, Venuturupalli S, et al: Ayurvedic interventions for diabetes mellitus. Evid Rep Technol Assess (Summ) 41:2, 2001.
32. Liu JP, Zhang M, Wang WY, Grimsgaard S: Chinese herbal medicines for type 2 diabetes mellitus. Cochrane Database Syst Rev (3):CD003642, 2002.
33. Althuis MD, Jordan NE, Ludington EA, Wittes JT: Glucose and insulin responses to dietary chromium supplements: A meta-analysis. Am J Clin Nutr 76:148, 2002.

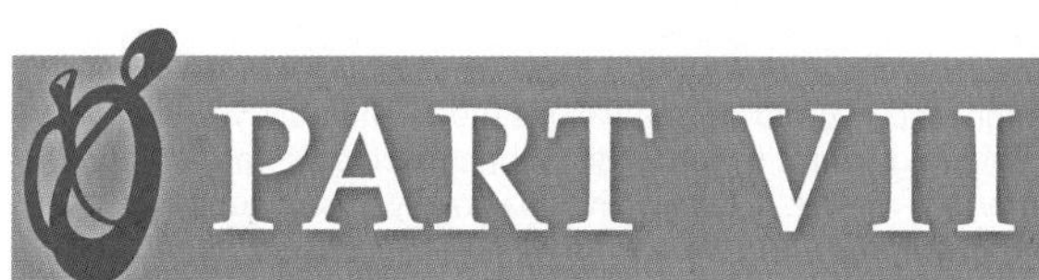

ATHEROSCLEROTIC CARDIOVASCULAR DISEASE

CHAPTER 52 Coronary Blood Flow and Myocardial Ischemia

John M. Canty, Jr.

The coronary circulation is unique in that it is responsible for generating the arterial pressure that is required to perfuse the systemic circulation and yet, at the same time, has its own perfusion impeded during the systolic portion of the cardiac cycle. Because myocardial contraction is closely connected to coronary flow and oxygen delivery, the balance between oxygen supply and demand is a critical determinant of the normal beat-to-beat function of the heart. When this relationship is acutely disrupted by diseases affecting coronary blood flow, the resulting imbalance can immediately precipitate a vicious cycle, whereby ischemia-induced contractile dysfunction precipitates hypotension and further myocardial ischemia. Thus, a knowledge of the regulation of coronary blood flow, determinants of myocardial oxygen consumption, and relationship between ischemia and contraction is essential for understanding the pathophysiologic basis and management of many cardiovascular disorders.[1]

Control of Coronary Blood Flow

There are pronounced systolic and diastolic coronary flow variations throughout the cardiac cycle, with coronary arterial inflow out of phase with venous outflow (**Fig. 52-1**).[2] Systolic contraction increases tissue pressure, redistributes perfusion from the subendocardial to the subepicardial layers of the heart, and impedes coronary arterial inflow, which reaches a nadir. At the same time, systolic compression reduces the diameter of intramyocardial microcirculatory vessels (arterioles, capillaries, and venules) and increases coronary venous outflow, which peaks during systole. During diastole, coronary arterial inflow increases with a transmural gradient that favors perfusion to the subendocardial vessels. At this time, coronary venous outflow falls.

Determinants of Myocardial Oxygen Consumption

In contrast to most other vascular beds, myocardial oxygen extraction is near-maximal at rest, averaging approximately 75% of arterial oxygen content.[3] The ability to increase oxygen extraction as a means to increase oxygen delivery is limited to circumstances associated with sympathetic activation and acute subendocardial ischemia. Nevertheless, coronary venous oxygen tension (Pv_{O_2}) can only decrease from 25 to approximately 15 torr. Because of the high resting oxygen extraction, increases in myocardial oxygen consumption are primarily met by proportional increases in coronary flow and oxygen delivery (**Fig. 52-2**). In addition to coronary flow, oxygen delivery is directly determined by arterial oxygen content (Pa_{O_2}). This is equal to the product of hemoglobin concentration and arterial oxygen saturation plus a small amount of oxygen dissolved in plasma that is directly related to Pa_{O_2}. Thus, for any given flow level, anemia results in proportional reductions in oxygen delivery, whereas the nonlinear oxygen dissociation curve results in relatively small reductions in oxygen content until Pa_{O_2} falls to the steep portion of the oxygen dissociation curve (below 50 torr).

The major determinants of myocardial oxygen consumption are heart rate, systolic pressure (or myocardial wall stress), and left ventricular (LV) contractility. A twofold increase in any of these individual determinants of oxygen consumption requires an approximately 50% increase in coronary flow. Experimentally, the systolic pressure-volume area is proportional to myocardial work and linearly related to myocardial oxygen consumption. The basal myocardial oxygen requirements needed to maintain critical membrane function are low (approximately 15% of resting oxygen consumption) and the cost of electrical activation is trivial when mechanical contraction ceases during diastolic arrest (as with cardioplegia) and diminishes during ischemia.

Coronary Autoregulation. Regional coronary blood flow remains constant as coronary artery pressure is reduced below aortic pressure over a wide range when the determinants of myocardial oxygen consumption are kept constant.[4] This phenomenon is termed *autoregulation* (**Fig. 52-3**). When pressure falls to the lower limit of autoregulation, coronary resistance arteries are maximally vasodilated to intrinsic stimuli and flow becomes pressure-dependent, resulting in the onset of subendocardial ischemia. Resting coronary blood flow under normal

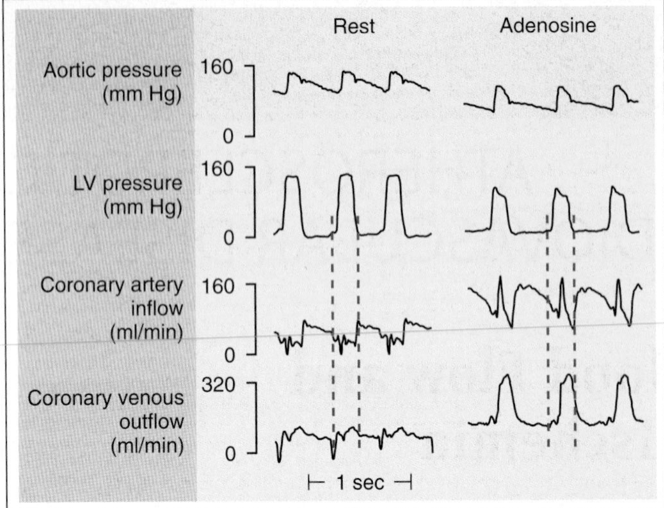

FIGURE 52-1 Phasic coronary arterial inflow and venous outflow at rest and adenosine vasodilation. Arterial inflow primarily occurs during diastole. During systole (dotted vertical lines), arterial inflow declines as venous outflow peaks, reflecting the compression of microcirculatory vessels during systole. After adenosine administration, the phasic variations in venous outflow are more pronounced. *(Modified from Canty JM Jr, Brooks A: Phasic volumetric coronary venous outflow patterns in conscious dogs. Am J Physiol 258:H1457, 1990.)*

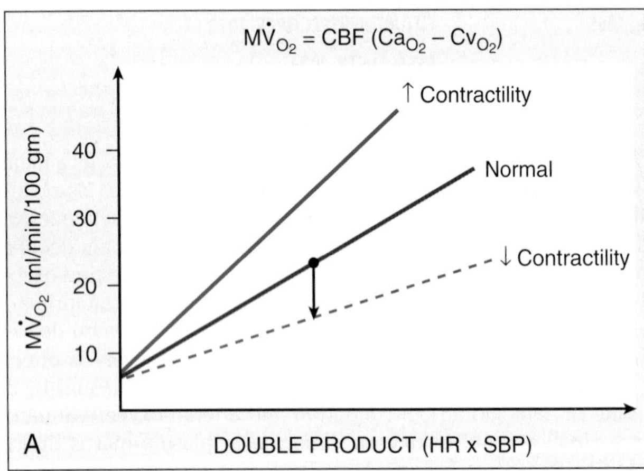

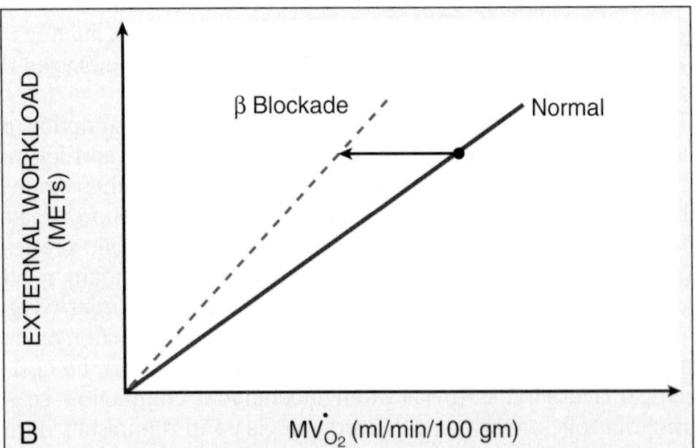

FIGURE 52-2 Fick equation and the relationship between heart rate (HR)–systolic pressure (SBP) double product and myocardial oxygen consumption ($M\dot{V}O_2$). **A,** Increases in $M\dot{V}O_2$ are primarily met by increases in coronary flow and linearly related to the double product. Twofold increases in HR, SBP, or contractility each result in approximately 50% increases in myocardial oxygen consumption. **B,** Beta blockade allows the same external workload to be accomplished at a lower cardiac workload ($M\dot{V}O_2$) by reducing the double product and myocardial contractility. CaO_2 = coronary arterial oxygen content; CBF = coronary blood flow; CvO_2 = coronary venous oxygen content.

hemodynamic conditions averages 0.7 to 1.0 mL/min/g and can increase between four- and fivefold during vasodilation.[5] The ability to increase flow above resting values in response to pharmacologic vasodilation is termed *coronary reserve.* Flow in the maximally vasodilated heart is dependent on coronary arterial pressure. Maximum perfusion and coronary reserve are reduced when the diastolic time available for subendocardial perfusion is decreased (tachycardia) or the compressive determinants of diastolic perfusion (preload) are increased. Coronary reserve is also diminished by anything that increases resting flow, including increases in the hemodynamic determinants of oxygen consumption (systolic pressure, heart rate, contractility) and reductions in arterial oxygen supply (anemia, hypoxia). Thus, circumstances can develop that precipitate subendocardial ischemia in the presence of normal coronary arteries.[1] Although initial studies have suggested that the lower pressure limit of autoregulation is 70 mm Hg, studies in conscious dogs in the basal state have shown that coronary flow can be autoregulated to mean coronary pressures as low as 40 mm Hg (diastolic pressures of 30 mm Hg).[4] These coronary pressure levels are similar to those recorded in humans without symptoms of ischemia, distal to chronic coronary occlusions, using pressure wire micromanometers. The lower autoregulatory pressure limit increases during tachycardia because of an increase in flow requirements, as well as a reduction in the time available for perfusion.[6]

Figure 52-4 illustrates important transmural variations in the lower autoregulatory pressure limit, which result in increased vulnerability of the subendocardium to ischemia.[1] Subendocardial flow primarily occurs in diastole and begins to decrease below a mean coronary pressure of 40 mm Hg.[4] In contrast, subepicardial flow occurs throughout the cardiac cycle and is maintained until coronary pressure falls below 25 mm Hg. This difference arises from increased oxygen consumption in the subendocardium, requiring a higher resting flow level, as well as the more pronounced effects of systolic contraction on subendocardial vasodilator reserve. The transmural difference in the lower autoregulatory pressure limit results in vulnerability of the subendocardium to ischemia in the presence of a coronary stenosis. Although there is no pharmacologically recruitable flow reserve during ischemia in the normal coronary circulation,[7] reductions in coronary flow below the lower limit of autoregulation can occur in the presence of pharmacologically recruitable coronary flow reserve under certain circumstances.[8]

ENDOTHELIUM-DEPENDENT MODULATION OF CORONARY TONE. Epicardial arteries do not normally contribute significantly to coronary vascular resistance, yet arterial diameter is modulated by a wide variety of paracrine factors that can be released from platelets, as well as circulating neurohormonal agonists, neural tone, and local control through vascular shear stress.[9] The most common factors related to cardiovascular disease are summarized in **Table 52-1** (see Fig. 52-e1 on website). The net effect of many of these agonists is critically dependent on whether a functional endothelium is present. Furchgott and Zawadzki[10] originally demonstrated that acetylcholine normally dilates arteries via an endothelium-dependent relaxing factor (EDRF) that was later identified to be nitric oxide (NO). This binds to guanylyl cyclase and increases cyclic guanosine monophosphate (cGMP), resulting in vascular smooth muscle relaxation. When the endothelium is removed, the dilation to acetylcholine is converted to vasoconstriction, reflecting the effect of muscarinic vascular smooth muscle contraction. Subsequent studies have demonstrated that coronary artery resistance arteries also exhibit endothelial modulation of diameter and that the response to physical forces such as shear stress, as well as paracrine mediators, vary with resistance vessel size.[11] The major endothelium-dependent biochemical pathways involved in regulating coronary epicardial and resistance artery diameter are as follows.

Nitric Oxide (Endothelium-Derived Relaxing Factor)

NO (EDRF) is produced in endothelial cells by the enzymatic conversion of L-arginine to citrulline via type III NO synthase (NOS). This reaction is controlled by calcium and calmodulin and is dependent on molecular oxygen, nicotinamide adenine dinucleotide phosphate, reduced form (NADPH), tetrahydrobiopterin, adenosine diphosphate (ADP), flavin adenine dinucleotide, and flavin mononucleotide. Endothelial NO diffuses abluminally into vascular smooth muscle, where it binds to guanylate cyclase, increasing cGMP production and causing relaxation through a reduction in intracellular calcium. NO-mediated vasodilation is enhanced by cyclical or pulsatile changes

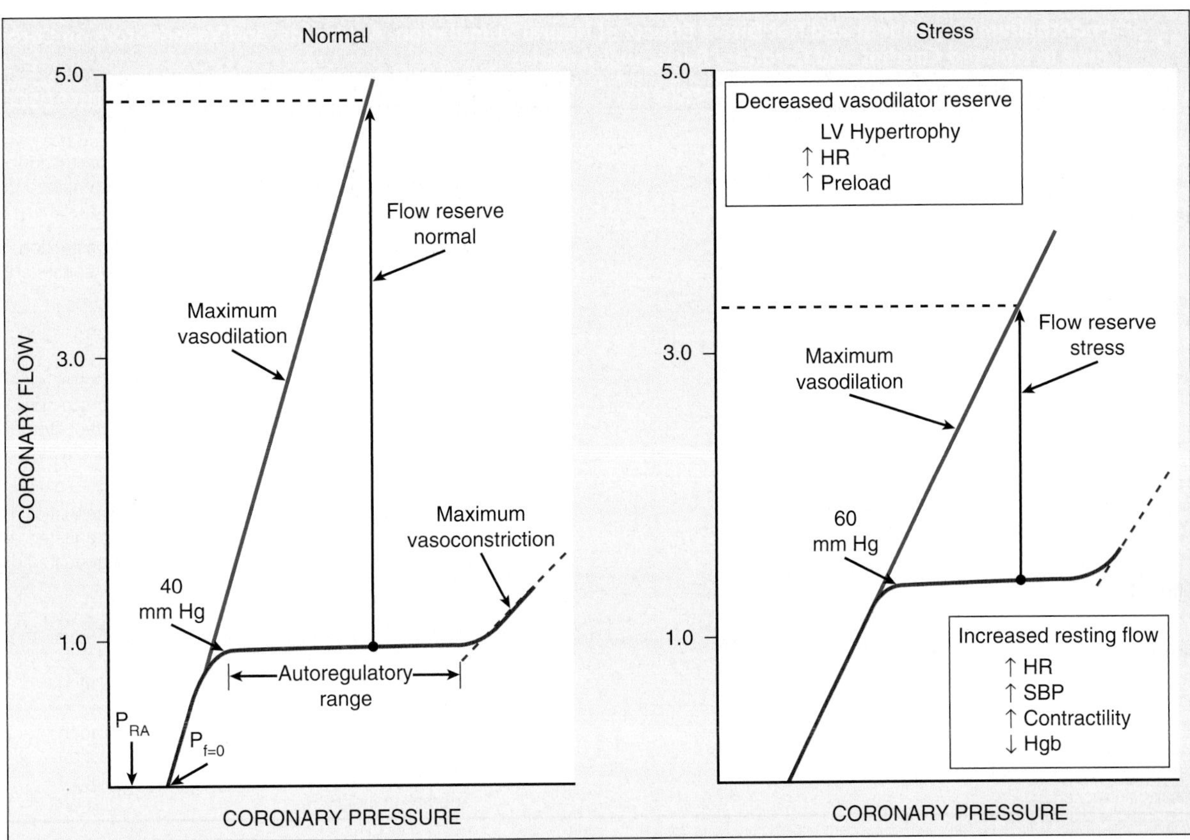

FIGURE 52-3 Autoregulatory relationship under basal conditions and following metabolic stress (e.g., tachycardia). The normal heart maintains coronary blood flow constant **(left panel)** as regional coronary pressure is varied over a wide range when the global determinants of oxygen consumption are kept constant (red lines). Below the lower autoregulatory pressure limit (approximately 40 mm Hg), subendocardial vessels are maximally vasodilated and myocardial ischemia develops. During vasodilation (blue lines), flow increases four to five times above resting values at a normal arterial pressure. Coronary flow ceases at a pressure higher than right atrial pressure (P_{RA}), called zero flow pressure ($P_{f=0}$), which is the effective backpressure to flow in the absence of coronary collaterals. Following stress **(right panel)**, tachycardia increases the compressive determinants of coronary resistance by decreasing the time available for diastolic perfusion and thus reduces maximum vasodilated flow. In addition, increases in myocardial oxygen demand or reductions in arterial oxygen content increase resting flow. These changes reduce coronary flow reserve, the ratio between dilated and resting coronary flow, and cause ischemia to develop at higher coronary pressures. Hgb = hemoglobin.

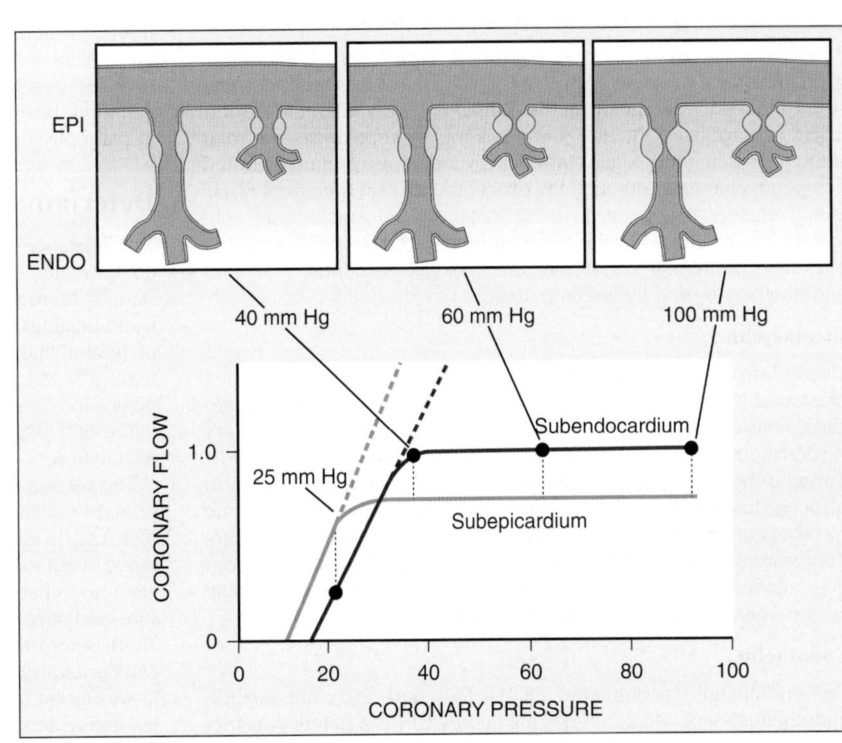

FIGURE 52-4 Transmural variations in coronary autoregulation and myocardial metabolism. Increased vulnerability of the subendocardium (ENDO; red) versus subepicardium (EPI; gold) to ischemia reflects the fact that autoregulation is exhausted at a higher coronary pressure (40 versus 25 mm Hg). This is the result of increased resting flow and oxygen consumption in the subendocardium and an increased sensitivity to systolic compressive effects, because subendocardial flow only occurs during diastole. Subendocardial vessels become maximally vasodilated before those in the subepicardium as coronary artery pressure is reduced. These transmural differences can be increased further during tachycardia or during conditions with elevated preload, which reduce maximum subendocardial perfusion.

TABLE 52-1 Endothelium-Dependent and Net Direct Effects of Neural Stimulation, Autacoids, and Vasodilators on Coronary Tone in Isolated Conduit and Coronary Resistance Arteries

SUBSTANCE	ENDOTHELIUM-DEPENDENT	NORMAL RESPONSE	ATHEROSCLEROSIS
Acetylcholine			
Conduit	Nitric oxide	Net dilation	Constriction
Resistance	Nitric oxide, EDHF	Dilation	Attenuated dilation
Norepinephrine			
Alpha$_1$		Constriction	Constriction
Beta$_2$	Nitric oxide	Dilation	Attenuated dilation
Platelets			
Thrombin	Nitric oxide	Dilation	Constriction
Serotonin			
Conduit	Nitric oxide	Constriction	Constriction
Resistance	Nitric oxide	Dilation	Constriction
ADP	Nitric oxide	Dilation	Attenuated dilation
Thromboxane	Endothelin	Constriction	Constriction
Paracrine Agonists			
Bradykinin	Nitric oxide, EDHF	Dilation	Attenuated dilation
Histamine	Nitric oxide	Dilation	Attenuated dilation
Substance P	Nitric oxide	Dilation	Attenuated dilation
Endothelin (ET)			
ET-1	Nitric oxide	Net constriction	Increased constriction
Vasodilators			
Adenosine		Dilation	Dilation
Regadenoson		Dilation	Dilation
Dipyridamole		Dilation	Dilation
Papaverine		Dilation	Dilation
Nitroglycerin		Dilation	Dilation
Calcium channel blockers		Submaximal dilation	Dilation

ADP = adenosine diphosphate; EDHF = endothelium-dependent hyperpolarizing factor.

in coronary shear stress. Chronic upregulation of NO synthase occurs in response to episodic increases in coronary flow, such as during exercise training, which also potentiates the relaxation to various endothelium-dependent vasodilators. NO-mediated vasodilation is impaired in many disease states and in patients with one or more risk factors for coronary artery disease (CAD). This occurs via inactivation of NO by superoxide anion generated in response to oxidative stress. Such inactivation is the hallmark of impaired NO-mediated vasodilation in atherosclerosis, hypertension, and diabetes.

Endothelium-Dependent Hyperpolarizing Factor

Endothelium-dependent hyperpolarization (EDHF) is an additional mechanism for selected agonists (e.g., bradykinin), as well as shear stress–induced vasodilation, in the human coronary microcirculation. EDHF is produced by the endothelium, hyperpolarizes vascular smooth muscle, and dilates arteries by opening calcium-activated potassium channels. Although the exact biochemical species of EDHF is still unclear, it appears to be a metabolite of arachidonic acid metabolism produced by the cytochrome P-450 epoxygenase pathway. The most prominent candidates are epoxyeicosatrienoic acid and endothelium-derived hydrogen peroxide.

Prostacyclin

Metabolism of arachidonic acid via cyclooxygenase can also produce prostacyclin, which is a coronary vasodilator when administered exogenously. Although prostacyclin contributes to tonic coronary vasodilation in humans, inhibitors of cyclooxygenase fail to alter flow during ischemia distal to a stenosis or limit oxygen consumption in response to increases in metabolism. This suggests that it is overcome by other compensatory vasodilator pathways.[9] In contrast to the coronary resistance vasculature, vasodilator prostaglandins are important determinants of coronary collateral vessel resistance, and inhibiting cyclooxygenase reduces collateral perfusion in dogs.

Endothelin

The endothelins (endothelin-1 [ET-1], ET-2, and ET-3) are peptide endothelium-dependent constricting factors. ET-1 is a potent constrictor derived from the enzymatic cleavage of a larger precursor molecule (pre-proendothelin) via endothelin-converting enzyme. In contrast to the rapid vascular smooth muscle relaxation and recovery characteristic of endothelium-derived vasodilators (NO, EDHF, and prostacyclin), the constriction to ET is prolonged. Changes in ET levels are largely mediated through transcriptional control and produce longer term changes in coronary vasomotor tone. The effects of ET are mediated by binding to both ET-A and ET-B receptors. ET-A–mediated constriction is caused by the activation of protein kinase C in vascular smooth muscle. ET-B–mediated constriction is less pronounced and is counterbalanced by prominent ET-B–mediated endothelium-dependent NO production and vasodilation. ET is not involved in regulating coronary blood flow in the normal heart but can modulate vascular tone when circulating concentrations increase in pathophysiologic states, such as heart failure.

Determinants of Coronary Vascular Resistance

The resistance to coronary blood flow can be divided into three major components, as summarized in **Figure 52-5**.[5] Under normal circumstances, there is no measurable pressure drop in the epicardial arteries, indicating negligible conduit resistance (R_1). With the development of hemodynamically significant epicardial artery narrowing (more than 50% diameter reduction), the fixed conduit artery resistance begins to contribute an increasing component to total coronary resistance and, when severely narrowed (more than 90%), may reduce resting flow.

The second component of coronary resistance (R_2) is dynamic and primarily arises from microcirculatory resistance arteries and arterioles. This is distributed throughout the myocardium across a broad range of microcirculatory resistance vessel size (20 to 200 μm in diameter) and changes in response to physical forces (intraluminal pressure and shear stress), as well as the metabolic needs of the tissue. There is normally little resistance contributed by coronary venules and capillaries and their resistance remains fairly constant during changes in vasomotor tone. Even in the maximally vasodilated heart, capillary resistance accounts for no more than 20% of the microvascular resistance.[12] Thus, a twofold increase in capillary density would only increase maximal myocardial perfusion by approximately 10%. Minimal coronary vascular resistance of the microcirculation is primarily determined by the size and density of arterial resistance vessels and results in substantial coronary flow reserve in the normal heart.

The third component, or compressive resistance (R_3), varies with time throughout the cardiac cycle and is related to cardiac contraction and systolic pressure development within the left ventricle. In heart failure, compressive effects from elevated ventricular diastolic pressure also impede perfusion via passive compression of microcirculatory vessels by elevated extravascular tissue pressure during diastole. Increases in preload effectively raise the normal back pressure to coronary flow above coronary venous pressure levels.[8] Compressive effects are most prominent in the subendocardium and are discussed in greater detail later.

EXTRAVASCULAR COMPRESSIVE RESISTANCE (R_3). During systole, cardiac contraction raises extravascular tissue pressure to values equal to LV pressure at the subendocardium. This declines to values near pleural pressure at the subepicardium.[3] The increased effective backpressure during systole produces a time-varying reduction in the driving pressure for coronary flow that impedes perfusion to the subendocardium. Although this paradigm can explain variations in systolic coronary inflow, it is not able to account for the increase in coronary venous systolic outflow. To explain both impaired inflow and accelerated venous outflow, some investigators have proposed the concept of the intramyocardial pump.[8] In this model, microcirculatory vessels are compressed during systole and produce a capacitive discharge of blood that accelerates flow from the microcirculation to the coronary venous system (**Fig. 52-6**). At the same time, the upstream capacitive discharge impedes systolic coronary arterial inflow. Although this explains the phasic variations in coronary arterial inflow and venous outflow, as well as its transmural distribution in systole, vascular capacitance cannot explain compressive effects related to elevated tissue pressure during diastole. Thus, components of intramyocardial capacitance, compressive changes in resistance, and time-varying driving pressure all contribute to the compressive determinants of phasic coronary blood flow.

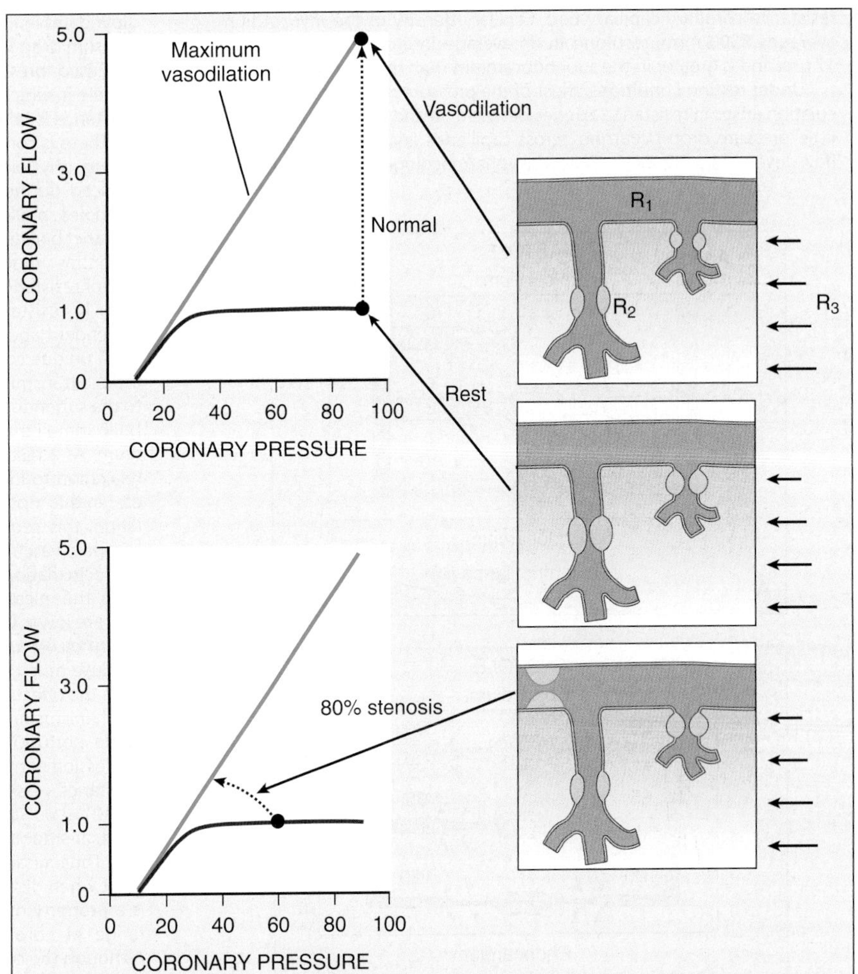

FIGURE 52-5 Schematic of components of coronary vascular resistance with and without a coronary stenosis. R_1 is epicardial conduit artery resistance, which is normally insignificant; R_2 is resistance secondary to metabolic and autoregulatory adjustments in flow and occurs in arterioles and resistance arteries; and R_3 is the time-varying compressive resistance that is higher in subendocardial than subepicardial layers. In the normal heart, $R_2 > R_3 >> R_1$. The development of a proximal stenosis or pharmacologic vasodilation reduces arteriolar resistance (R_2). In the presence of a severe epicardial stenosis, $R_1 > R_3 > R_2$.

TRANSMURAL VARIATIONS IN MINIMUM CORONARY RESISTANCE (R_2) AND DIASTOLIC DRIVING PRESSURE. The subendocardial vulnerability to compressive determinants of vascular resistance[1] is partially compensated for by a reduced minimal resistance from an increased arteriolar and capillary density. Because of this vascular gradient, transmural flow during maximal pharmacologic vasodilation of the beating heart is uniform at rest. Coronary vascular resistance in the maximally vasodilated heart is also pressure-dependent, reflecting passive distention of arterial resistance vessels. Thus, the instantaneous vasodilated value of coronary resistance obtained at a normal coronary distending pressure will be lower than that at a reduced pressure.

The precise determinants of the effective driving pressure for diastolic perfusion continue to be controversial.[8] Most experimental studies have demonstrated that the effective backpressure to flow in the heart is higher than right atrial pressure. This has been termed *zero flow pressure* ($P_{f=0}$) and its minimum value is approximately 10 mm Hg in the maximally vasodilated heart. This increases to values close to LV diastolic filling pressure when preload is elevated above 20 mm Hg. Elevated preload reduces coronary driving pressure and diminishes subendocardial perfusion. It is particularly important in determining flow when coronary pressure is reduced by a stenosis, as well as in the failing heart.

STRUCTURE AND FUNCTION OF THE CORONARY MICROCIRCULATION. The schematics in Figures 52-4 and 52-5 suggest a fairly localized site for the control of coronary vascular resistance that is useful for conceptualizing the major determinants of coronary vascular resistance. Individual coronary resistance arteries are a longitudinally distributed network and in vivo studies of the coronary microcirculation have demonstrated considerable spatial heterogeneity of specific resistance vessel control mechanisms (**Fig. 52-7**).[9,11] Each resistance vessel needs to dilate in an orchestrated fashion to meet the needs of the downstream vascular bed, which is frequently removed from the site of resistance artery control. This can be accomplished independently of metabolic signals by sensing physical forces such as intraluminal flow (shear stress–mediated control) or intraluminal pressure changes (myogenic control). Epicardial arteries (>400 μm in diameter) serve a conduit artery function, with diameter primarily regulated by shear stress, and contribute little pressure drop (<5%) over a wide range of coronary flow. Coronary resistance vessels can be divided into resistance arteries (100 to 400 μm), which regulate their tone in response to local shear stress and luminal pressure changes (myogenic response), and arterioles (>100 μm), which are sensitive to changes in local tissue metabolism and directly control perfusion of the low-resistance coronary capillary bed. Capillary density of the myocardium averages 3500/mm^2, resulting in an average intercapillary distance of 17 μm, and is greater in the subendocardium than the subepicardium.

Under resting conditions, most of the pressure drop in the microcirculation arises in resistance arteries between 50 and 200 μm in size, with little pressure drop occurring across capillaries and venules at normal flow levels (**Fig. 52-8A**).[12] Following pharmacologic vasodilation with dipyridamole, resistance artery vasodilation minimizes the precapillary pressure drop in arterial resistance vessels. At the same time, there is an increased pressure drop and redistribution of resistance to venular vessels, in which smooth muscle relaxation is limited and the already low resistance is fairly fixed.

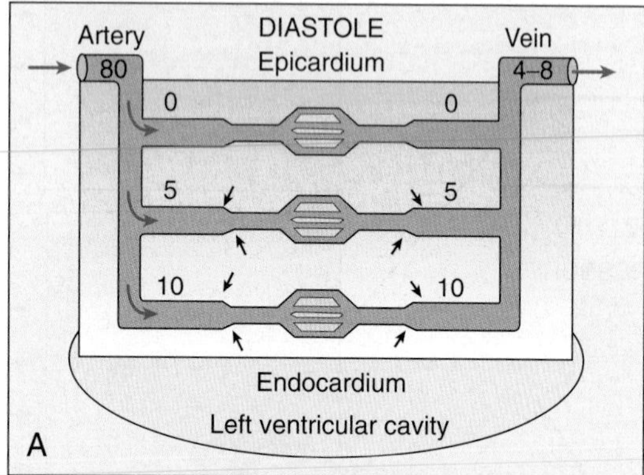

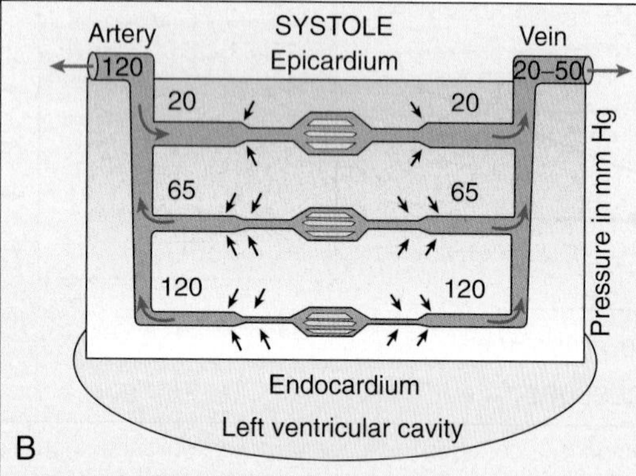

FIGURE 52-6 Effects of extravascular tissue pressure on transmural perfusion. **A,** Compressive effects during diastole are related to tissue pressures that decrease from the subendocardium to subepicardium. At diastolic LV pressures greater than 20 mm Hg, preload determines the effective backpressure to coronary diastolic perfusion. **B,** During systole, cardiac contraction increases intramyocardial tissue pressure surrounding compliant arterioles and venules. This produces a concealed arterial "backflow" that reduces systolic epicardial artery inflow, as depicted in Figure 52-1. Compression of venules accelerates venous outflow. *(Modified from Hoffman JIE, Baer RW, Hanley FL, et al: Regulation of transmural myocardial blood flow. J Biomech Eng 107:2, 1985.)*

There is considerable heterogeneity in microcirculatory vasodilation during physiologic adjustments in flow. For example, as pressure is reduced during autoregulation, dilation is primarily accomplished by arterioles smaller than 100 μm, whereas larger resistance arteries tend to constrict because of the reduction in perfusion pressure (see Fig. 52-8B).[13] In contrast, metabolic vasodilation results from a more uniform vasodilation of resistance vessels of all sizes (see Fig. 52-8C).[14] Similar inhomogeneity in resistance vessel dilation occurs in response to endothelium-dependent agonists and pharmacologic vasodilators.

A unique component of subendocardial coronary resistance vessels are the transmural penetrating arteries that course from the epicardium to the subendocardial plexus.[9] These vessels are removed from the metabolic stimuli that develop when ischemia is confined to the subendocardium. As a result, local control from altered shear stress and myogenic relaxation to local pressure become very critical determinants of diameter in this "upstream" resistance segment. Even during maximal vasodilation, this segment creates an additional longitudinal component of coronary vascular resistance that must be traversed before the arteriolar microcirculation is reached. Because of this greater longitudinal pressure drop, the microcirculatory pressures in subendocardial coronary arterioles are lower than in the subepicardial arterioles.

INTRALUMINAL PHYSICAL FORCES REGULATING CORONARY RESISTANCE. Because much of the coronary resistance vasculature can be upstream from the effects of metabolic mediators of control, local vascular control mechanisms are critically important in orchestrating adequate regional tissue perfusion to the distal microcirculation. There is a differential expression of mechanisms among different sizes and classes of coronary resistance vessels, which coincides with their function.

MYOGENIC REGULATION. The myogenic response refers to the ability of vascular smooth muscle to oppose changes in coronary arteriolar diameter. Thus, vessels relax when distending pressure is decreased and constrict when distending pressure is elevated (**Fig. 52-9A**). Myogenic tone is a property of vascular smooth muscle and occurs across a large size range of coronary resistance arteries in animals and in humans.[15] Although the cellular mechanism is uncertain, it is dependent on vascular smooth muscle calcium entry, perhaps through stretch-activated L-type Ca^{2+} channels, eliciting cross-bridge activation. The resistance changes arising from the myogenic response tend to bring local coronary flow back to the original level. Myogenic regulation has been postulated to be one of the important mechanisms of the coronary autoregulatory response and, in vivo, appears to occur primarily in arterioles smaller than 100 μm (e.g., during autoregulation; see Fig. 52-8B).[13]

FLOW-MEDIATED RESISTANCE ARTERY CONTROL. Coronary resistance arteries and arterioles also regulate their diameter in response to changes in local shear stress (see Fig. 52-9B). Flow-induced dilation in isolated coronary arterioles was originally demonstrated by Kuo and colleagues.[11,16] They found this to be endothelium-dependent and mediated by NO, because it could be abolished with an L-arginine analogue. In contrast, isolated

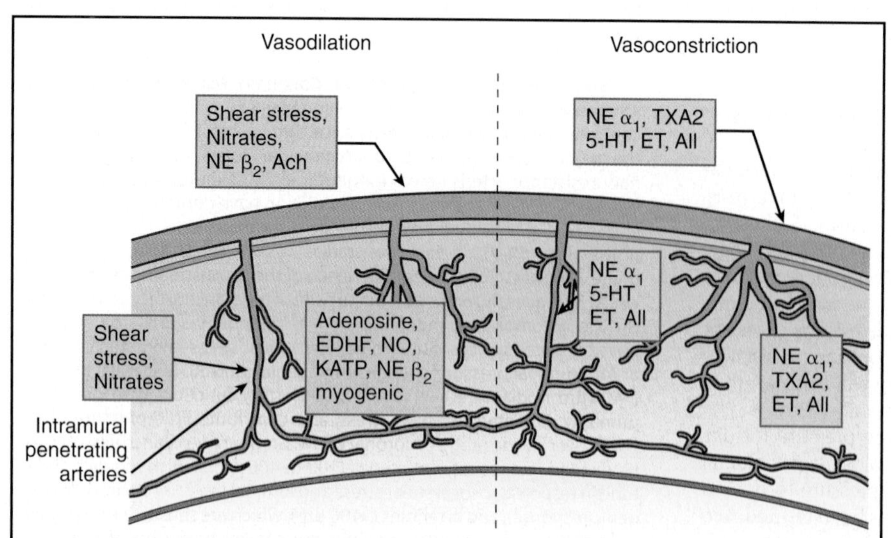

FIGURE 52-7 Transmural distribution of coronary resistance vessels—major vasodilatory and vasoconstrictor mechanisms in epicardial conduit arteries and different sites of the microcirculation. The epicardial conduit arteries arborize into subepicardial and subendocardial resistance arteries. Intramural penetrating resistance arteries are unique in that they are removed from subendocardial metabolic stimuli and theoretically are more dependent on regulating their tone in response to shear stress and luminal pressure as mechanisms to produce dilation in response to changes in metabolism of the distal subendocardial arteriolar plexus. See text for further discussion. Ach = acetylcholine; EDHF = endothelium-dependent hyperpolarizing factor; ET = endothelin; 5-HT = serotonin; KATP = ATP-dependent potassium channel; NE β_2 = norepinephrine beta$_2$ adrenergic; NE α_1 = norepinephrine alpha$_1$ adrenergic; TXA2 = thromboxane A_2. *(Modified from Duncker DJ, Bache RJ: Regulation of coronary vasomotor tone under normal conditions and during acute myocardial hypoperfusion. Pharmacol Ther 86:87, 2000.)*

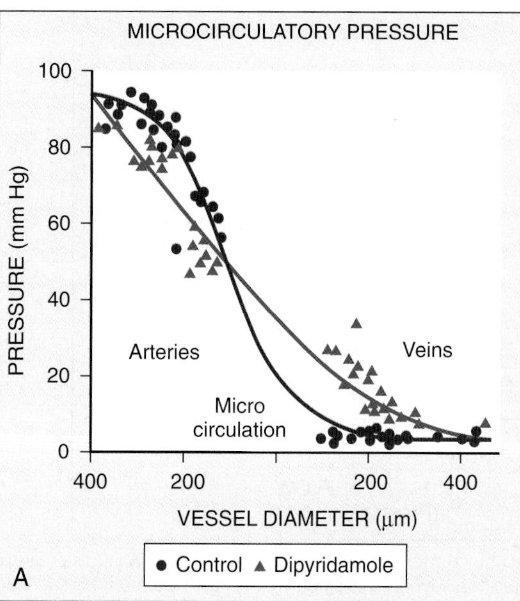

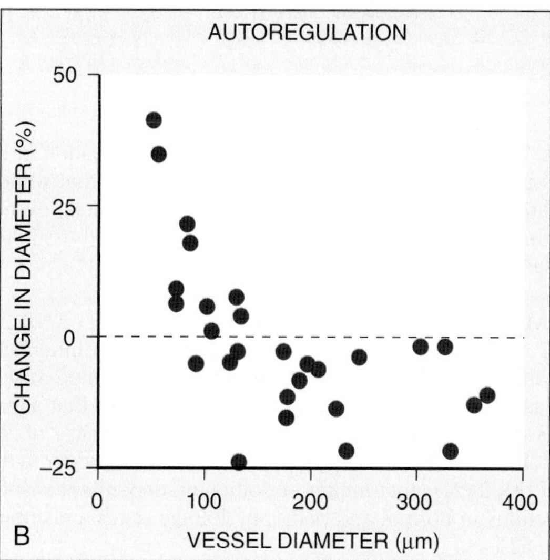

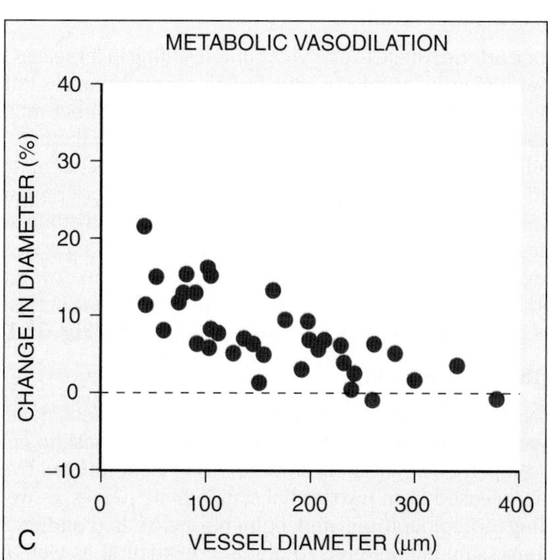

FIGURE 52-8 Microcirculatory pressure profile and local resistance changes to physiologic stimuli in subepicardial vessels. **A,** Under resting conditions, most of the pressure drop to flow arises from resistance arteries and arterioles. Following dipyridamole vasodilation, there is a redistribution of microcirculatory resistance. with a greater pressure drop occurring across postcapillary venules that do not alter their resistance. **B,** Heterogeneous arterial microvessel response during autoregulation. A reduction in pressure to 38 mm Hg elicited dilation in arterioles smaller than 100 μm, whereas larger arteries tended to constrict passively from the reduction in distending pressure. **C,** Homogeneous vasodilation of resistance arteries during increases in myocardial oxygen consumption. There is dilation in all microvascular resistance arteries that is greatest in vessels smaller than 100 μm. *(**A** modified from Chilian WM, Layne SM, Klausner EC, et al: Redistribution of coronary microvascular resistance produced by dipyridamole. Am J Physiol 256:H383, 1989; **B** modified from Kanatsuka H, Lamping KG, Eastham CL, et al: Heterogeneous changes in epimyocardial microvascular size during graded coronary stenosis. Evidence of the microvascular site for autoregulation. Circ Res 66:389, 1990; **C** modified from Kanatsuka H, Lamping KG, Eastham CL, et al: Comparison of the effects of increased myocardial oxygen consumption and adenosine on the coronary microvascular resistance. Circ Res 65:1296, 1989.)*

atrial vessels from patients undergoing cardiac surgery exhibit flow-mediated vasodilation that is mediated by EDHF.[17,18] The disparity with animal studies may reflect age or species variability in the relative importance of EDHF versus NO in the coronary circulation. The mechanisms also appear to vary as a function of vessel size, with studies in pigs demonstrating that hyperpolarization regulates epicardial conduit arteries[19] and NO predominates in the resistance vasculature.[16] Finally, EDHF may represent a compensatory pathway that is normally inhibited by NO and becomes upregulated in acquired disease states, in which NO-mediated vasodilation is impaired. Despite the variability in isolated vessels, blocking NO synthase with an L-arginine analogue in the coronary circulation of humans reduces vasodilation to pharmacologic endothelium-dependent agonists and attenuates flow increases during metabolic vasodilation, demonstrating that NO-mediated vasodilatation plays a role in determining physiologic vascular tone in some segments of the coronary resistance vasculature.[20]

METABOLIC MEDIATORS OF CORONARY RESISTANCE. Despite increasing knowledge regarding the distribution of coronary microvascular resistance, there is still no consensus regarding specific mediators of metabolic vasodilation. Coronary resistance in any segment of the microcirculation represents the integration of local physical factors (e.g., pressure and flow), vasodilator metabolites (e.g., adenosine, PO_2, pH), autacoids, and neural modulation. Each of these mechanisms contributes to net coronary vascular smooth muscle tone, which may ultimately be controlled by opening and closing vascular smooth muscle adenosine triphosphate (ATP)–sensitive K^+ (K^+-ATP) channels. There is considerable redundancy in the available local control mechanisms.[9] Because of this, blocking single mechanisms fails to alter coronary autoregulation or metabolic flow regulation at normal coronary pressures. This redundancy can, however, be unmasked by stressing the heart and evaluating flow regulation at reduced pressures distal to a coronary stenosis at rest or during exercise.[9] Some of the proposed candidates and their role in metabolic resistance control and ischemia-induced vasodilation are summarized here.[3]

Adenosine

There has been a longstanding interest in the role of adenosine as a metabolic mediator of resistance artery control. It is released from cardiac myocytes when the rate of ATP hydrolysis exceeds its synthesis during ischemia. Its production and release also increase with myocardial metabolism. Adenosine has an extremely short half-life (<10 seconds) caused by its rapid inactivation by adenosine deaminase. It binds to A2 receptors on vascular smooth muscle, increases cyclic adenosine monophosphate (cAMP), and opens intermediate calcium-activated potassium channels.[21] Adenosine has a differential effect on coronary resistance arteries, primarily dilating vessels smaller than 100 μm.[14] Although adenosine has no direct effect on larger resistance arteries and conduit arteries, these dilate through endothelium-dependent vasodilation from the concomitant increases

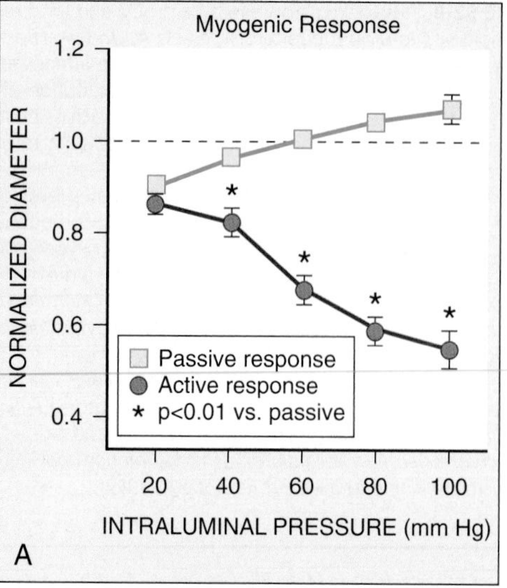

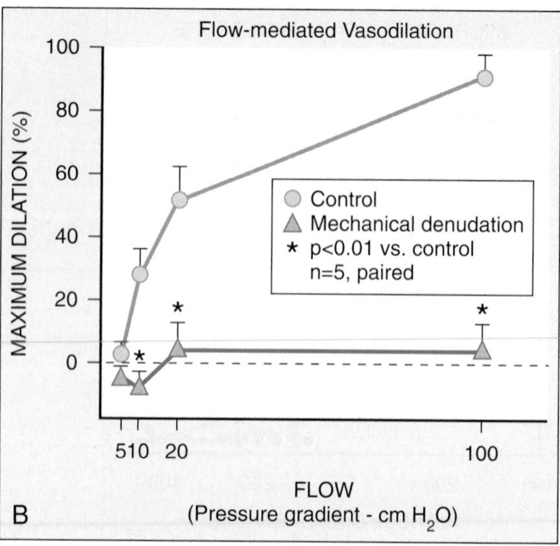

FIGURE 52-9 Effects of physical forces on coronary diameter in isolated human coronary resistance arteries (nominal diameter, 100 μm). **A**, As distending pressure is reduced from 100 mm Hg, there is progressive vasodilation consistent with myogenic regulation. Myogenic dilation reaches the maximum passive diameter of the vessel at 20 mm Hg. **B**, Flow-mediated vasodilation in cannulated human resistance arteries. As the pressure gradient across the isolated vessel is increased, intraluminal flow rises and causes progressive dilation that is abolished by removing the endothelium. Similar flow-mediated dilation occurs in most arterial vessels, including the coronary conduit arteries. *(**A** modified from Miller FJ, Dellsperger KC, Gutterman DD: Myogenic constriction of human coronary arterioles. Am J Physiol 273:H257, 1997; **B** modified from Miura H, Wachtel RE, Liu Y, et al: Flow-induced dilation of human coronary arterioles: Important role of Ca^{2}+-activated K+ channels. Circulation 103:1992, 2001.)*

in local shear stress as arteriolar resistance falls.[22] Despite the attractiveness of adenosine as a local metabolic control mechanism, there is now substantial in vivo experimental data to demonstrate convincingly that it is not required for adjusting coronary flow to increases in metabolism or autoregulation.[23] It may, however, contribute to vasodilation during hypoxia and during acute exercise-induced myocardial ischemia distal to a stenosis.[9]

ATP-Sensitive K^+ Channels

Coronary vascular smooth muscle K^+-ATP channels are tonically active, contributing to coronary vascular tone under resting conditions. Preventing K^+-ATP channel opening with glibenclamide causes constriction of arterioles smaller than 100 μm, reduces coronary flow, and accentuates myocardial ischemia distal to a coronary stenosis by overcoming intrinsic vasodilatory mechanisms.[9] The K^+-ATP channels can modulate the coronary metabolic and autoregulatory responses. It is a potentially attractive mechanism, because many of the other candidates for metabolic flow regulation (e.g., adenosine, NO, $beta_2$ adrenoreceptors, and prostacyclin) are ultimately affected by blocking this pathway. It is likely that K^+-ATP channel opening is a common effector rather than sensor of metabolic activity or of autoregulatory adjustments in flow. It is also possible that the reductions in coronary flow observed after blocking K^+-ATP channel vasodilation are pharmacologic, caused by vasoconstriction of the microcirculation that overcomes intrinsic vasodilatory stimuli, as seen when other potent vasoconstrictors (e.g., endothelin or vasopressin) are administered at pharmacologic doses.

Hypoxia

Although a potent coronary vasodilatory stimulus, the role of local PO_2 in the regulation of arteriolar tone remains unresolved. Coronary flow increases in proportion to reductions in arterial oxygen content (reduced PO_2 or anemia) and there is a twofold increase in perfused capillary density in response to hypoxia.[3] Nevertheless, studies demonstrating a direct effect of oxygen on metabolic or autoregulatory adjustments are lacking and the vasodilatory response to reduced arterial oxygen delivery may simply reflect the close coupling between myocardial metabolism and flow.

Acidosis

Arterial hypercapnea and acidosis (PCO_2) are potent stimuli that have been demonstrated to produce coronary vasodilation independent of hypoxia. Whereas their precise role in the local regulation of myocardial perfusion remains unclear, it seems reasonable that some of the vasodilation occurring with increased myocardial metabolism could arise from increased myocardial CO_2 production and tissue acidosis in the setting of acute ischemia.[3]

NEURAL CONTROL OF CORONARY CONDUIT AND RESISTANCE ARTERIES. Sympathetic and vagal nerves innervate coronary conduit arteries and segments of the resistance vasculature. Neural stimulation affects tone through mechanisms that alter vascular smooth muscle as well as by stimulating the release of NO from the endothelium. Diametrically opposite effects can occur in the presence of risk factors that impair endothelium-dependent vasodilation. Their actions in normal and pathophysiologic states are summarized in Table 52-1.

Cholinergic Innervation

Resistance arteries dilate to acetylcholine, resulting in increases in coronary flow. In conduit arteries, acetylcholine normally causes mild coronary vasodilation. This reflects the net action of a direct muscarinic constriction of vascular smooth muscle counterbalanced by an endothelium-dependent vasodilation caused by direct stimulation of NOS and an increased flow-mediated dilation from concomitant resistance vessel vasodilation. The response in humans with atherosclerosis or risk factors for CAD is distinctly different. The resistance vessel dilation to acetylcholine is attenuated and the reduction in flow-mediated NO production leads to net epicardial conduit artery vasoconstriction, which is particularly prominent in stenotic segments (**Fig. 52-10A**).

Sympathetic Innervation

Under basal conditions, there is no resting sympathetic tone in the heart and thus there is no effect of denervation on resting perfusion. During sympathetic activation, coronary tone is modulated by norepinephrine released from myocardial sympathetic nerves, as well as by circulating norepinephrine and epinephrine.[3,24] In conduit arteries, sympathetic stimulation leads to $alpha_1$ constriction as well as $beta_2$-mediated vasodilation. The net effect is to dilate epicardial coronary arteries. This dilation is potentiated by concomitant flow-mediated vasodilation from metabolic vasodilation of coronary resistance vessels. When NO-mediated vasodilation is impaired, $alpha_1$ constriction predominates and can dynamically increase stenosis severity in asymmetrical lesions in which the stenosis is compliant. This is one of the mechanisms that can provoke ischemia during cold pressor testing (see Fig. 52-10B).

The effects of sympathetic activation on myocardial perfusion and coronary resistance vessel tone are complex and dependent on the net actions of beta$_1$-mediated increases in myocardial oxygen consumption (resulting from increases in the determinants of myocardial oxygen consumption), direct beta$_2$-mediated coronary vasodilation, and alpha$_1$-mediated coronary constriction. Under normal conditions, exercise-induced beta$_2$-adrenergic feed-forward dilation predominates, resulting in a higher flow relative to the level of myocardial oxygen consumption.[23] This neural control mechanism produces transient vasodilation before the buildup of local metabolites during exercise and prevents the development of subendocardial ischemia during abrupt changes in demand. After nonselective beta blockade, sympathetic activation unmasks alpha$_1$-mediated coronary artery constriction. Although flow is mildly decreased, oxygen delivery is maintained by increased oxygen extraction and a reduction in coronary venous Po_2 at similar levels of cardiac workload. Intense alpha$_1$-adrenergic constriction can overcome intrinsic stimuli for metabolic vasodilation and result in ischemia in the presence of pharmacologic vasodilator reserve.[24] The role of pre- and postsynaptic alpha$_2$ responses is controversial. They appear to have a less significant role in controlling flow. This partly reflects the competing effects of presynaptic alpha$_2$ receptor stimulation, leading to reduced vasoconstriction by inhibiting norepinephrine release.

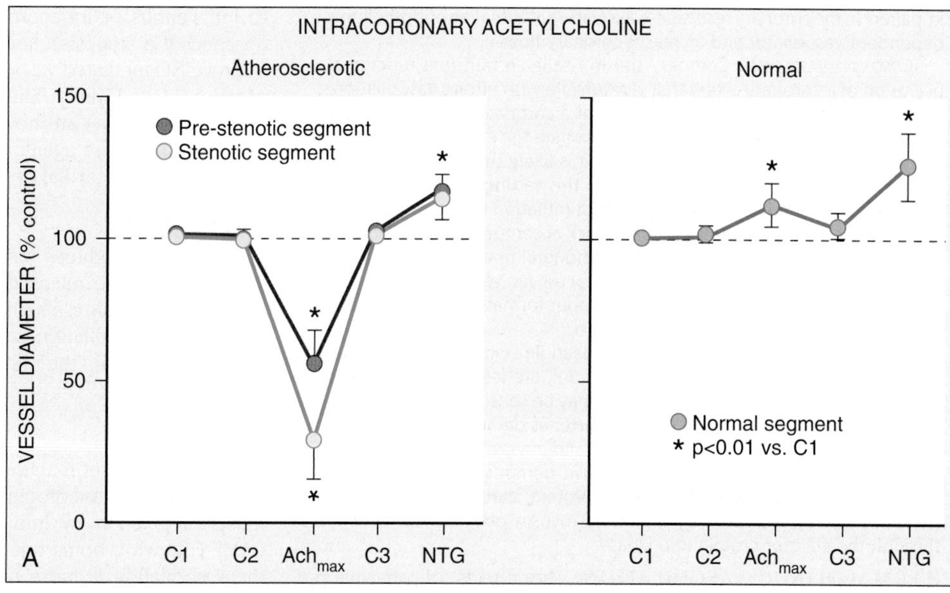

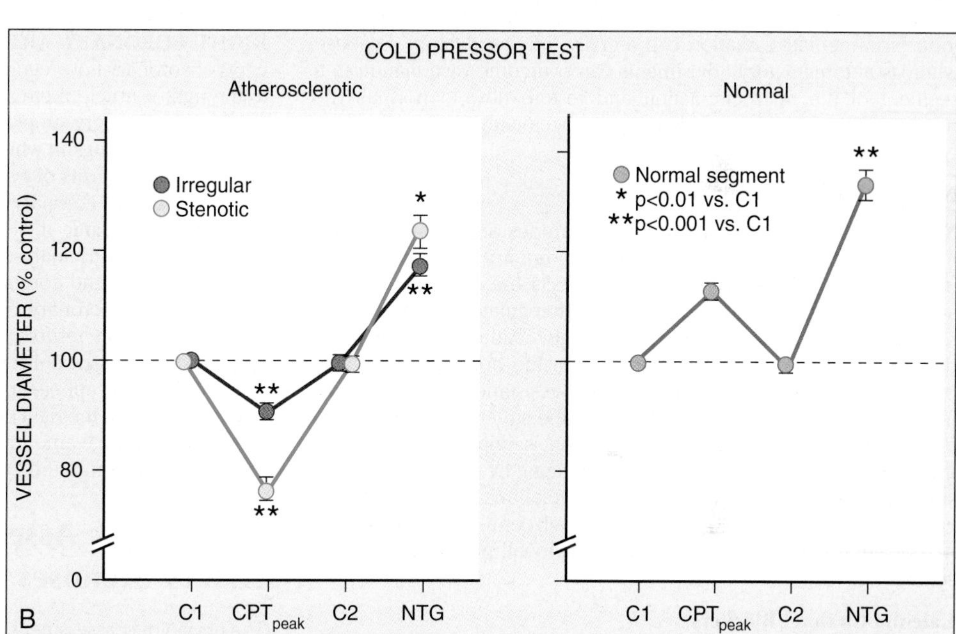

FIGURE 52-10 Differential conduit artery diameter responses in normal and atherosclerotic epicardial arteries. **A,** Acetylcholine. In normal arteries, acetylcholine elicits vasodilation but there is vasoconstriction in the atherosclerotic artery, which is particularly pronounced in the stenosis. **B,** Cold pressor testing. Activation of sympathetic tone normally leads to net epicardial dilation but there is vasoconstriction in irregular and stenotic coronary segments in patients with atherosclerosis. Ach = acetylcholine; C = control; CPT = cold pressor test; NTG = nitroglycerin. *(**A** modified from Ludmer PL, Selwyn AP, Shook TL, et al: Paradoxical vasoconstriction induced by acetylcholine in atherosclerotic coronary arteries. N Engl J Med 315:1046, 1986; **B** modified from Nabel EG, Ganz P, Gordon JB, et al: Dilation of normal and constriction of atherosclerotic coronary arteries caused by the cold pressor test. Circulation 77:43, 1988.)*

PARACRINE VASOACTIVE MEDIATORS AND CORONARY VASOSPASM. There are a large number of paracrine factors that can affect coronary tone in normal and pathophysiologic states that are unrelated to normal coronary circulatory control. The most important of these are summarized in Table 52-1 (see Fig. 52-e1 on website). Paracrine factors are released from epicardial artery thrombi after activation of the thrombotic cascade initiated by plaque rupture. They can modulate epicardial tone in regions near eccentric ulcerated plaques that are still responsive to stimuli that alter smooth muscle relaxation and constriction, leading to dynamic changes in the physiologic significance of a stenosis. Paracrine mediators can also have differential effects on downstream vessel vasomotion that are dependent on vessel size (conduit arteries versus resistance arteries) as well as on the presence of a functionally normal endothelium, because many also stimulate the release of NO and EDHF.

Serotonin released from activated platelets causes vasoconstriction in normal and atherosclerotic conduit arteries and can increase the functional severity of a dynamic coronary stenosis through superimposed vasospasm. In contrast, it dilates coronary resistance vessels (<100 μm) and increases coronary flow through the endothelium-dependent release of NO. In atherosclerosis or circumstances in which NO production is impaired, the direct effects on smooth muscle predominate and the response of the microcirculation is converted to vasoconstriction. As a result, serotonin release generally exacerbates ischemia in CAD.

Thromboxane A_2 is a potent vasoconstrictor that is a product of endoperoxide metabolism and is released during platelet aggregation. It produces vasoconstriction of conduit arteries and isolated coronary resistance vessels and can accentuate acute myocardial ischemia.

ADP is another platelet-derived vasodilator that relaxes coronary microvessels and conduit arteries. It is mediated by NO and abolished by removing the endothelium.

Thrombin normally leads to vasodilation in vitro that is endothelium-dependent and mediated by the release of prostacyclin as well as NO. In vivo, it also releases thromboxane A_2, leading to vasoconstriction in epicardial stenoses in which endothelium-dependent vasodilation is impaired. In the coronary resistance vasculature, it acts as an endothelium-dependent vasodilator and increases coronary flow.

Coronary Vasospasm. Coronary spasm results in transient functional occlusion of a coronary artery that is reversible with nitrate vasodilation. It most commonly occurs in the setting of a coronary stenosis, leading to dynamic stenosis behavior, and can dissociate the effects on perfusion from anatomic stenosis severity. In CAD, it is likely that endothelial disruption plays a role in focal vasospasm. In this setting, the normal vasodilation from autacoids and sympathetic stimulation is converted into a vasoconstrictor response because of the lack of competing endothelium-dependent vasodilation. Nevertheless, although impaired endothelium-dependent vasodilation is a permissive factor for vasospasm, it is not causal, and a trigger is required (e.g., thrombus formation or sympathetic activation).

The mechanisms responsible for variant angina with normal coronary arteries, or Prinzmetal angina (see Chap. 56), are less clear. Data from animal models have indicated that there may be sensitization of intrinsic vasoconstrictor mechanisms.[25] Coronary arteries demonstrate supersensitivity to vasoconstrictor agonists in vivo and in vitro as well as reduced vasodilatory responses. Some studies have demonstrated that Rho, a guanosine triphosphate (GTP)–binding protein, can sensitize vascular smooth muscle to calcium by inhibiting myosin phosphatase activity through the effector protein Rho kinase.

PHARMACOLOGIC VASODILATION. The effects of pharmacologic vasodilators on coronary flow reflect direct actions on vascular smooth muscle as well as secondary adjustments in resistance artery tone. Flow-mediated dilation can amplify the vasodilatory response, whereas autoregulatory adjustments can overcome vasodilation in a segment of the microcirculation and restore flow to normal. The potent resistance vessel vasodilators are specifically used in assessing coronary stenosis severity.[26]

Nitroglycerin

Nitroglycerin dilates epicardial conduit arteries and small coronary resistance arteries but does not increase coronary blood flow in the normal heart. This latter observation reflects the fact that transient arteriolar vasodilation is overcome by autoregulatory escape, which returns coronary resistance to control levels.[27] Although nitroglycerin does not increase coronary blood flow in the normal heart, it can produce vasodilation of large coronary resistance arteries, which improves the distribution of perfusion to the subendocardium when flow-mediated[9] NO-dependent vasodilation is impaired. It can also improve subendocardial perfusion by reducing LV end-diastolic pressure through systemic venodilation in heart failure. Similarly, coronary collateral vessels dilate in response to nitroglycerin, and the reduction in collateral resistance can improve regional perfusion in some settings.

Calcium Channel Blockers

All calcium channel blockers lead to vascular smooth muscle relaxation and are, to various degrees, pharmacologic coronary vasodilators. In epicardial arteries, the vasodilation is similar to that of nitroglycerin and is effective in preventing coronary vasospasm superimposed on a coronary stenosis as well as in normal arteries of patients with variant angina. They also submaximally vasodilate coronary resistance vessels. In this regard, dihydropyridine derivatives such as nifedipine are particularly potent and can sometimes precipitate subendocardial ischemia in the face of a critical stenosis. This arises from a transmural redistribution of blood flow as well and the tachycardia and hypotension that transiently occur with short half-life formulations of nifedipine.

Adenosine and A_2 Receptor Agonists

Adenosine dilates coronary arteries through activation of A2 receptors on vascular smooth muscle and is independent of the endothelium in coronary arterioles isolated from humans with heart disease.[21] Experimentally, there is a differential sensitivity of the microcirculation to adenosine, with the direct effects related to resistance vessel size and primarily restricted to vessels smaller than 100 μm.[14] Larger upstream resistance arteries dilate via an NO-dependent mechanism from the increase in shear stress. Thus, in states in which endothelium-dependent vasodilation is impaired, maximal coronary flow responses to intravenous or intracoronary adenosine may be reduced in the absence of a stenosis[22] and can be increased by interventions that improve NO-mediated vasodilation, such as lowering low-density lipoprotein (LDL) levels.[28] Single-dose adenosine A_2 receptor agonists (e.g., regadenoson) are now clinically available and are as effective as adenosine. These agents circumvent the need for continuous infusions during myocardial perfusion imaging (see Chap. 17).[26]

Dipyridamole

Dipyridamole produces vasodilation by inhibiting the myocyte reuptake of adenosine released from cardiac myocytes. It therefore has actions and mechanisms similar to those of adenosine, with the exception that the vasodilation is more prolonged. It can be reversed via the administration of the nonspecific adenosine receptor blocker aminophylline.

Papaverine

Papaverine is a short-acting coronary vasodilator that was the first agent used for intracoronary vasodilation. It causes vascular smooth muscle relaxation by inhibiting phosphodiesterase and increasing cAMP. Following bolus injection, it has a rapid onset of action, but the vasodilation is more prolonged than after adenosine (approximately 2 minutes). Its actions are independent of the endothelium.

RIGHT CORONARY ARTERY FLOW. Although the general concepts of coronary flow regulation developed for the left ventricle apply to the right ventricle, there are differences related to the extent of the right coronary artery supply to the right ventricular free wall. This has been studied in dogs, in which the right coronary artery is a nondominant vessel.[29] In terms of coronary flow reserve, arterial pressure supplying the right coronary substantially exceeds right ventricular pressure, minimizing the compressive determinants of coronary reserve. Right ventricular oxygen consumption is lower than that in the left ventricle, and coronary venous oxygen saturations are higher than in the left coronary circulation. Because there is considerable oxygen extraction reserve, coronary flow decreases as pressure is reduced and oxygen delivery is maintained by increased extraction. These differences appear specific to the right ventricular free wall. In humans, in whom the right coronary artery is dominant (see Chap. 21) and supplies a large amount of the inferior left ventricle, factors affecting flow regulation to the LV myocardium are likely to predominate.

Physiologic Assessment of Coronary Artery Stenoses

The physiologic assessment of stenosis severity is a critical component of the management of patients with obstructive epicardial CAD.[30] Epicardial artery stenoses arising from atherosclerosis increase coronary resistance and reduce maximal myocardial perfusion. Abnormalities in coronary microcirculatory control can also contribute to causing myocardial ischemia in many patients. Separating the role of a stenosis from coronary resistance vessels can be accomplished by simultaneously assessing coronary flow and distal coronary pressure using intracoronary transducers that are currently available for clinical care.[31]

Stenosis Pressure-Flow Relationship

The angiographically visible epicardial coronary arteries are normally able to accommodate large increases in coronary flow without producing any significant pressure drop and thus serve a conduit function to the coronary resistance vasculature. This changes dramatically in CAD, in which the epicardial artery resistance becomes dominant. This fixed component of resistance increases with stenosis severity and limits maximal myocardial perfusion.

As a starting point, it is helpful to consider the idealized relationship between stenosis severity, pressure drop, and flow that has been validated in animals as well as humans studied in circumstances in which diffuse atherosclerosis and risk factors that can impair microcirculatory resistance vessel control are minimized. **Figure 52-11** summarizes the major determinants of stenosis energy losses. The relationship between pressure drop across a stenosis and coronary flow for stenoses between

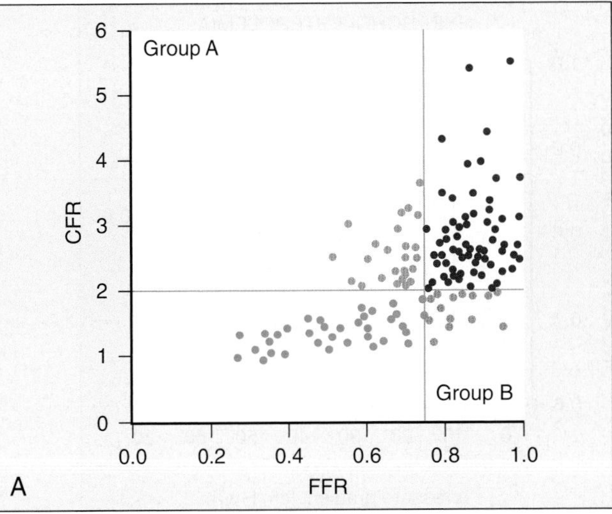

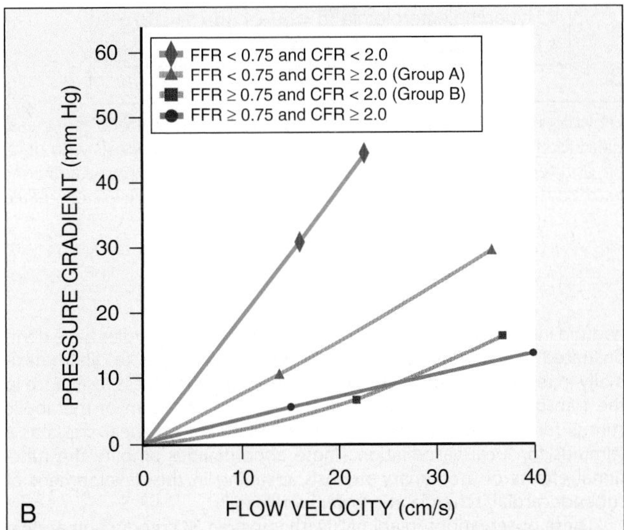

FIGURE 52-17 Characterization of coronary stenosis severity with simultaneous measurements of intracoronary pressure and flow. **A,** Vertical line represents a threshold fractional flow reserve (FFR) of 0.75 and the horizontal line predicts a threshold coronary flow reserve (CFR) of 2. Group A depicts patients with significant stenoses by FFR who have relatively preserved microvascular function and a CFR higher than 2. Group B depicts patients with microcirculatory impairment or submaximal vasodilation in whom CFR is limited but FFR is not reduced. **B,** Instantaneous stenosis pressure-flow relationships corresponding to the four groups depicted in **A**. *(Modified from Meuwissen M, Chamuleau S, Siebes M, et al: Role of variability in microvascular resistance on fractional flow reserve and coronary blood flow velocity reserve in intermediate coronary lesions. Circulation 103:184, 2001.)*

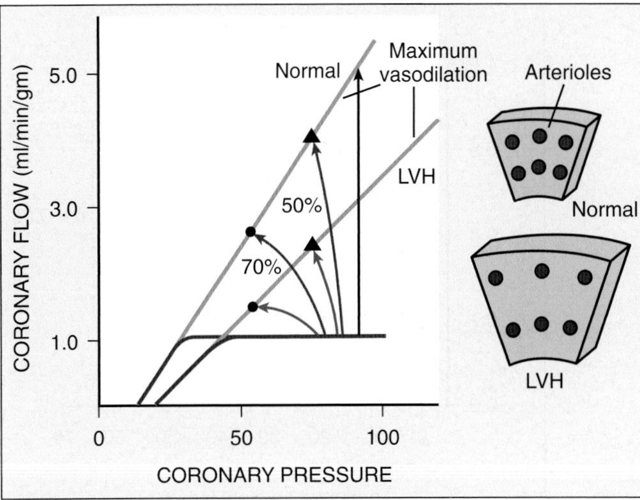

FIGURE 52-18 Effects of left ventricular hypertrophy (LVH) on maximal coronary flow. With acquired LVH, myocardial mass increases without proliferation of the microcirculatory resistance arteries (right side). Because the maximal absolute flow per minute during vasodilation remains unchanged, the maximum flow per gram of tissue falls inversely with the change in LV mass. In contrast, whereas the resting flow per gram of myocardium remains constant with hypertrophy, the increase in LV mass requires a higher absolute resting flow. The net effect of these opposing actions is to decrease coronary flow reserve at any coronary pressure. As a result of the reduction in microcirculatory reserve in the absence of a coronary stenosis, the functional significance of a 50% stenosis (triangles) in the hypertrophied heart could approach a more severe stenosis (in the example, 70%, circles) in normal myocardium. This can even result in ischemia with normal coronary arteries during stress.

The major assumption common to all flow reserve measurements is that the pharmacologic vasodilator used consistently achieves maximal vasodilation of the resistance vasculature in normals as well as in patients with atherosclerotic disease and impaired endothelial function. The reductions in absolute flow reserve in people with angiographically insignificant stenoses (see Fig. 52-16B), as well as variability in quantitative perfusion measurements with normal epicardial arteries and coronary risk factors, indicate that this may not always be the case. The extent to which this is related to a structural abnormality in the microcirculation (e.g., caused by regional hypertrophy or vascular remodeling) versus a functional abnormality in the microcirculation (altered microcirculatory vasodilatory response versus impaired endothelium-dependent vasodilation) remains unclear. A second limitation is that currently available approaches can only measure coronary flow reserve averaged across the entire wall of the heart. This is because they are based on invasive epicardial coronary measurements or, in the case of imaging (SPECT and PET), have insufficient spatial resolution to assess transmural variations in flow (see Chap. 17). An imaging technique that could assess the physiologic significance of a stenosis in the subendocardial layers would be a major advance, because this region is the most severely affected by an epicardial stenosis. This is feasible with CMR (see Chap. 18).[35a]

Pathophysiologic States Affecting Microcirculatory Coronary Flow Reserve

Various pathophysiologic states can accentuate the effects of a fixed-diameter coronary stenosis as well as precipitate subendocardial ischemia during stress in the presence of normal coronary arteries. Thus, it is important to incorporate measurements of stenosis severity with abnormalities of coronary resistance vessel control. In the former case, treatment will be directed at the epicardial stenosis, whereas in the latter, medical therapies designed to improve abnormalities in resistance vessel control will be required. The prognostic importance of abnormalities in coronary resistance vessel control is underscored by emerging data in women evaluated for chest pain thought to be of ischemic origin. Abnormalities in coronary flow reserve and endothelium-dependent vasodilation are common in women with insignificant coronary disease and can be accompanied by metabolic ischemia, assessed by magnetic resonance spectroscopy (see Chap. 18), and they negatively affect prognosis.[36] The two most common factors affecting microcirculatory resistance control independently of coronary stenosis severity in patients are LV hypertrophy and impaired NO-mediated resistance vessel vasodilation.

LEFT VENTRICULAR HYPERTROPHY. The effects of hypertrophy on coronary flow reserve are complex and need to be thought of in terms of the absolute flow level (e.g., measured with an intracoronary Doppler probe) as well as the flow per gram of myocardium. With acquired hypertrophy, resting flow per gram of myocardium remains constant, but the increase in LV mass necessitates an increase in the absolute level of resting flow (mL/min) through the coronary artery.[37] In terms of maximal perfusion, acquired hypertrophy does not result in vascular proliferation and coronary resistance vessels remain unchanged (**Fig. 52-18**). Because

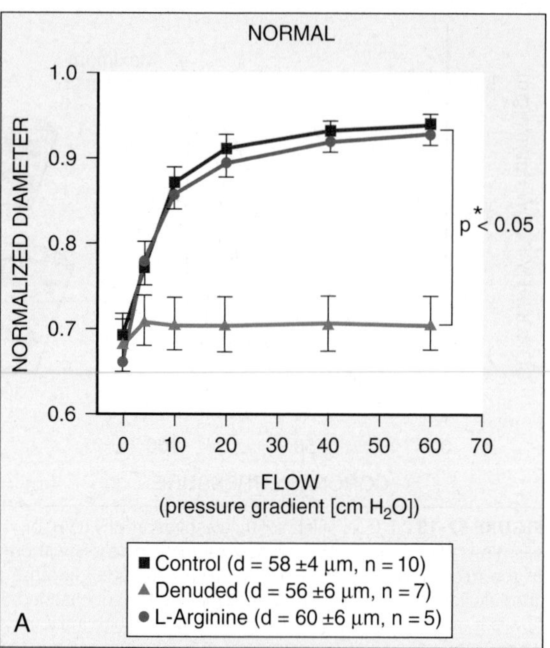

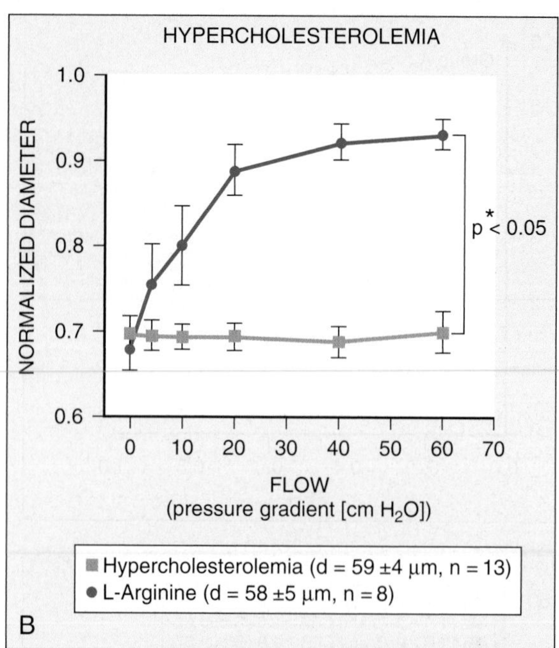

FIGURE 52-19 Flow-mediated vasodilation in coronary resistance arteries is abolished by dietary hypercholesterolemia in swine. **A,** In normal arterioles, increased flow (pressure gradient) elicits vasodilation that is abolished by removing the endothelium (denuded), similar to that in human vessels. **B,** In animals with dietary hypercholesterolemia but no significant epicardial stenosis, flow-mediated vasodilation of arterioles is abolished. It was restored by administering L-arginine to increase NO production. *(Modified from Kuo L, Davis MJ, Cannon MS, et al: Pathophysiological consequences of atherosclerosis extend into the coronary microcirculation: Restoration of endothelium-dependent responses by L-arginine. Circ Res 70:465, 1992.)*

maximum absolute flow (mL/min) remains unchanged, maximum perfusion per gram of myocardium falls. The net effect is that coronary flow reserve at any given coronary arterial pressure is reduced and inversely related to the change in LV mass. For example, in the absence of a change in mean aortic pressure, a twofold increase in LV mass, as is associated with severe LV hypertrophy, can reduce coronary flow reserve in a nonstenotic artery from 4 to 2 mL/min/g. This will increase the functional severity of any anatomic degree of coronary artery narrowing and can even precipitate subendocardial ischemia with normal coronary arteries.

Some degree of LV hypertrophy is common in patients with CAD and it likely contributes to reductions in coronary flow reserve that are independent of stenosis severity. The actual coronary flow reserve in hypertrophy will be critically dependent on the underlying cause of hypertrophy and its effects on coronary driving pressure. A similar degree of hypertrophy caused by untreated systemic hypertension will have a higher coronary flow reserve than in aortic stenosis, in which mean arterial pressure remains normal. Similarly, when hypertrophy is from systolic hypertension and increased pulse pressure caused by reduced aortic compliance, the accompanying reduction in diastolic pressure can lower coronary reserve.

Impaired Endothelium-Dependent Vasodilation. Measurements of coronary flow reserve in humans with risk factors for atherosclerosis are systematically lower than normals without coronary risk factors and underscore the importance of abnormalities in microvascular control in determining coronary flow reserve. Much of this may reflect abnormal local resistance vessel control via impaired endothelial-dependent vasodilation arising from NO inactivation associated with risk factors for CAD. Kuo and colleagues have demonstrated that experimental hypercholesterolemia markedly attenuates the dilation of coronary arterioles in response to shear stress and pharmacologic agonists that stimulate NOS in the absence of epicardial stenoses (**Fig. 52-19**).[38] This was reversed with L-arginine, suggesting that it reflects impaired NO synthesis or availability.

Abnormalities in NO-mediated vasodilation in vivo are functionally significant and impair the ability of the heart to autoregulate coronary blood flow. **Figure 52-20** shows the effects of inhibiting NO on the coronary autoregulatory relationship in normal dogs.[39] Although resting blood flow is not altered, there is a marked increase in the coronary pressure at which intrinsic autoregulatory adjustments become exhausted, with flow beginning to decrease at a distal coronary pressure of 60 versus 45 mm Hg, approximately similar to the shift occurring in response to a twofold increase in heart rate. In vivo microcirculatory studies have demonstrated that there is an inability of resistance arteries to dilate maximally in response to shear stress.[22] This likely reflects excess resistance in the transmural penetrating arteries, which are upstream of metabolic stimuli for vasodilation and extremely dependent on shear stress as a stimulus for local vasodilation. These abnormalities amplify the functional effects of a coronary stenosis, resulting in the development of subendocardial ischemia at a lower workload.[40]

These observations in animals with impaired NO production appear to be relevant to pathophysiologic states associated with impaired endothelium-dependent vasodilation in humans. For example, coronary flow reserve is markedly reduced in the absence of a coronary stenosis in familial hypercholesterolemia,[33] and improving endothelial function by lowering elevated LDL levels with statins produces a delayed improvement in coronary flow reserve in normal and stenotic arteries and also ameliorates clinical signs of myocardial ischemia.[28] Impaired NO-mediated vasodilation likely affects the regulation of myocardial perfusion in other disease states in which endothelium-dependent vasodilation is impaired.

Coronary Collateral Circulation

Following a total coronary occlusion, residual perfusion to the myocardium persists through native coronary collateral channels that open when an intercoronary pressure gradient between the source and recipient vessel develops. In animals, the native collateral flow during occlusion is less than 10% of the resting flow levels and is insufficient to maintain tissue viability for longer than 20 minutes. There is tremendous individual variability in the function of coronary collaterals among patients with chronic stenoses. In people without coronary collaterals, coronary pressure during balloon angioplasty occlusion falls to approximately 10 mm Hg. In other patients, collaterals proliferate to the point where they are sufficient not only to maintain normal resting perfusion but also to prevent stress-induced ischemia at submaximal cardiac workloads. Ischemia does not develop during PCI balloon occlusion when fractional flow reserve (based on coronary wedge pressure during occlusion minus venous pressure) is greater than 0.25.[31] A large observational cross-sectional study has demonstrated that patients with elevated distal coronary pressure arising

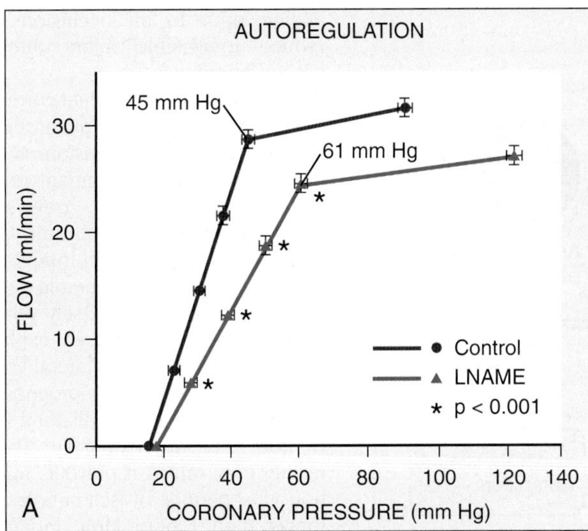

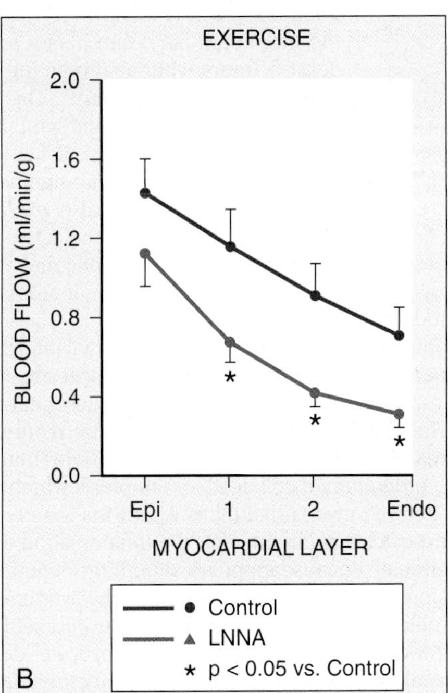

FIGURE 52-20 Impaired microcirculatory control with abnormal NO-mediated endothelium-dependent resistance artery dilation. **A,** Effects of blocking nitric oxide synthase (NOS) with the L-arginine analogue LNAME in chronically instrumented dogs. There is an increase in the lower autoregulatory pressure limit, resulting in the onset of ischemia at a coronary pressure of 61 mm Hg versus 45 mm Hg under normal conditions that occurred without a change in heart rate. **B,** Transmural perfusion before and after blocking NO-mediated dilation with LNNA in exercising dogs subjected to a coronary stenosis. Although coronary pressure and hemodynamics were similar, blood flow was lower in each layer of the heart after blocking NOS and not overcome by metabolic dilator mechanisms during ischemia. Collectively, these experimental data support the notion that abnormalities in endothelium-dependent vasodilation can amplify the functional effects of a coronary stenosis. Endo = endocardium; Epi = epicardium; LNAME = NG-nitro-L-arginine methyl ester; LNNA = NG-nitro-L-arginine. *(**A** modified from Smith TP Jr, Canty JM Jr: Modulation of coronary autoregulatory responses by nitric oxide: Evidence for flow-dependent resistance adjustments in conscious dogs. Circ Res 73:232, 1993; **B** modified from Duncker DJ, Bache RJ: Inhibition of nitric oxide production aggravates myocardial hypoperfusion during exercise in the presence of a coronary artery stenosis. Circ Res 74:629, 1994.)*

from recruitable collaterals during transient total balloon occlusion (fractional flow reserve > 0.25) have a lower cardiovascular event rate and improved survival (see Fig. 52-e3 on website).[41]

Arteriogenesis and Angiogenesis

Proliferation of coronary collaterals (see Chap. 21) occurs in response to repetitive stress-induced ischemia as well as the development of transient interarterial pressure gradients between the source and recipient vessel through a process termed *arteriogenesis.*[42] Resting distal coronary pressure consistently falls as stenosis severity exceeds 70% and the resultant interarterial pressure gradient increases endothelial shear stress in preexisting collaterals smaller than 200 μm in diameter. This causes progressive enlargement of collaterals through a process dependent on physical forces and growth factors, particularly vascular endothelial growth factor (VEGF) that is mediated via NO synthase. Thus, patients with impaired NO-mediated vasodilation resulting from coronary risk factors may have a limited ability to develop coronary collaterals in response to a chronic coronary stenosis.

Most functional collateral flow arises from arteriogenesis in existing epicardial anastomoses that enlarge into mature vessels that can reach 1 to 2 mm in diameter. Collateral perfusion can also originate from de novo vessel growth, or angiogenesis, which refers to the sprouting of smaller, capillary-like structures from preexisting blood vessels. These vessels may provide nutritive collateral flow when they develop in the border between ischemic and nonischemic regions. Capillary angiogenesis may also occur within the ischemic region and can reduce the intercapillary distance for oxygen exchange. Nevertheless, because capillary resistance is already a small component of microcirculatory resistance, increases in capillary density in the absence of changes in arteriolar resistance will not significantly increase myocardial perfusion.

There is currently great interest in experimental interventions to improve collateral flow (e.g., recombinant growth factors, in vivo gene transfer, and endothelial progenitor cells; see Chap. 11). Although many interventions have been shown to cause favorable angiogenesis of capillaries and improve myocardial function, few interventions have increased arteriogenesis in mature collaterals, and randomized human clinical trials have been disappointing.[43] Part of this may arise from the fact that no intervention has resulted in measurable increases in maximum vasodilated myocardial perfusion or coronary flow reserve indices, the sine qua non of functional collateral formation. Improvements in myocardial function have been used as an endpoint, but these may occur independently of increased perfusion and arise from mechanisms that alter cardiac myocyte growth and repair rather than angiogenesis.[44]

Regulation of Collateral Resistance

The control of blood flow to collateral-dependent myocardium is governed by a series resistance arising from interarterial collateral anastomoses, largely epicardial, as well as the native downstream microcirculation. Collateral resistance is therefore the major determinant of perfusion and coronary pressure distal to a chronic occlusion is already near the lower autoregulatory pressure limit. Because of this, subendocardial perfusion is critically dependent on mean aortic pressure and LV preload with ischemia easily provoked by systemic hypotension, increases in LV end-diastolic pressure, and tachycardia. Like the distal resistance vessels, collaterals constrict when NO synthesis is blocked, which aggravates myocardial ischemia and can be overcome by nitroglycerin.[9] In contrast to the native coronary circulation, experimental studies have shown that coronary collaterals are under tonic dilation from vasodilator prostaglandins, and blocking cyclooxygenase with aspirin exacerbates myocardial ischemia in dogs. The role of prostanoids in human coronary collateral resistance regulation is unknown.

The distal microcirculatory resistance vasculature in collateral-dependent myocardium appears to be regulated by mechanisms similar to those present in the normal circulation but is characterized by impaired endothelium-dependent vasodilation as compared with

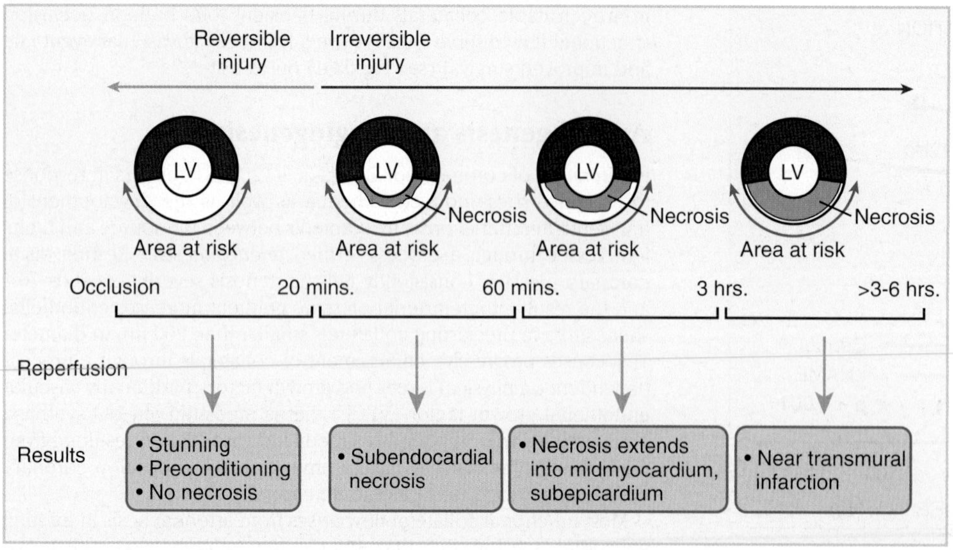

FIGURE 52-21 Wave front of necrosis in infarction in the absence of collaterals. Total occlusions shorter than 20 minutes do not cause irreversible injury but can cause myocardial stunning as well as precondition the heart and protect it against recurrent ischemic injury. Irreversible injury begins after 20 minutes and progresses as a wave front from endocardium to epicardium. After 60 minutes, the inner third of the LV wall is irreversibly injured. After 3 hours, there is a subepicardial rim of tissue remaining, with the transmural extent of infarction completed between 3 and 6 hours after occlusion. The most important factor delaying the progression of irreversible injury is the magnitude of collateral flow, which is primarily directed to the outer layers of the heart. *(Modified from Kloner RA, Jennings RB: Consequences of brief ischemia: Stunning, preconditioning, and their clinical implications: Part 1. Circulation 104:2981, 2001.)*

normal vessels. The extent to which these microcirculatory abnormalities alter the normal metabolic and coronary autoregulatory responses in collateral dependent myocardium is unknown.

Metabolic and Functional Consequences of Ischemia

Because oxygen delivery to the heart is closely coupled to coronary blood flow, a sudden cessation of regional perfusion following a thrombotic coronary occlusion quickly leads to the cessation of aerobic metabolism, depletion of creatine phosphate, and onset of anaerobic glycolysis. This is followed by the accumulation of tissue lactate, a progressive reduction in tissue ATP levels, and an accumulation of catabolites, including those of the adenine nucleotide pool. As ischemia continues, tissue acidosis develops and there is an efflux of potassium into the extracellular space. Subsequently, ATP levels fall below those required to maintain critical membrane function, resulting in the onset of myocyte death.

Irreversible Injury and Myocyte Death

The temporal evolution and extent of irreversible tissue injury after coronary occlusion are variable and dependent on transmural location, residual coronary flow, and the hemodynamic determinants of oxygen consumption. Irreversible myocardial injury begins after 20 minutes of coronary occlusion in the absence of significant collaterals.[45] Irreversible injury begins in the subendocardium and progresses as a wave front over time, from the subendocardial layers to the subepicardial layers (**Fig. 52-21**). This reflects the higher oxygen consumption in the subendocardium and the redistribution of collateral flow to the outer layers of the heart by the compressive determinants of flow at reduced coronary pressure. In experimental infarction, the entire subendocardium is irreversibly injured within 1 hour of occlusion and the transmural progression of infarction is largely completed within 4 to 6 hours after coronary occlusion. Factors that increase myocardial oxygen consumption (e.g., tachycardia) or reduce oxygen delivery (e.g., anemia, arterial hypotension) accelerate the progression of irreversible injury. In contrast, repetitive reversible ischemia or angina prior to an occlusion can reduce irreversible injury through preconditioning.[46]

The magnitude of residual coronary flow through collaterals or through a subtotal coronary occlusion is the most important determinant of the actual time course of irreversible injury in patients with chronic CAD. The relationship between infarct size and the area at risk of ischemia during a total occlusion is inversely related to collateral flow and likely explains the important role of collateral vessel function in determining prognosis.[41] When subendocardial collateral flow is more than approximately 30% of resting flow values, it prevents infarction after periods of ischemia lasting longer than 1 hour. More moderate subendocardial ischemia from a subtotal occlusion (e.g., flow reduced by no more than 50%) can persist for at least 5 hours without producing significant irreversible injury.[47] This explains the fact that signs and symptoms of ischemia can be present for long periods without producing significant myocardial necrosis. It also explains the clinical observation that late coronary reperfusion with ongoing ischemia can salvage myocardium beyond the 6-hour time limit predicted from experimental models of infarction.

Cell death arises from multiple mechanisms in myocardial infarction (see Chap. 54).[48] Reperfusion immediately causes myocyte necrosis and sarcolemmal disruption, with the leakage of cell contents into the extracellular space. The injury is further amplified by the reentry of leukocytes into the area of injury. At later time points, myocytes initially salvaged can undergo programmed cell death or apoptosis, which can contribute to further delayed myocardial injury. Apoptosis is a coordinated involution of myocytes that circumvents the inflammation associated with necrotic cell death. Because apoptosis is an energy-dependent process, cells can be forced to switch to a necrotic pathway if energy levels are depleted below critical levels. In more chronic settings, autophagy can contribute to the mechanisms of myocyte death. Because of the temporal complexity of irreversible injury, the relative importance of each mechanism in myocardial infarction continues to be controversial. Nevertheless, modulating mechanisms contributing to late cell death could prevent deleterious LV remodeling.

Reversible Ischemia and Perfusion-Contraction Matching

Reversible ischemia is considerably more frequent than irreversible injury. Supply-induced ischemia can arise from transient coronary occlusion resulting from coronary vasospasm or transient thrombosis in a critically stenosed coronary artery, producing transmural ischemia similar to that present at the onset of infarction. Demand-induced ischemia arises from an inability to increase flow in response to increases in myocardial oxygen consumption in which ischemia predominantly affects the subendocardium. These have fundamentally different effects on myocardial diastolic relaxation, with supply-induced ischemia increasing LV compliance and demand-induced ischemia reducing it. There is a fairly stereotypical sequence of physiologic changes that develop during an episode of spontaneous transmural ischemia (**Fig. 52-22**). Coronary occlusion results in an immediate fall in coronary venous oxygen saturation, with a reduction in ATP production. This causes a decline in regional contraction within several beats, reaching dyskinesis within 1 minute. As regional contraction ceases, there is a reduction in global LV contractility (dP/dt), a progressive rise in LV end-diastolic pressure, and a fall in systolic pressure. The magnitude of the systemic hemodynamic changes varies with the severity of ischemia as well as the amount of the left ventricle subjected to ischemia. Significant electrocardiographic ST-segment changes develop within 2 minutes as efflux of potassium into the extra-

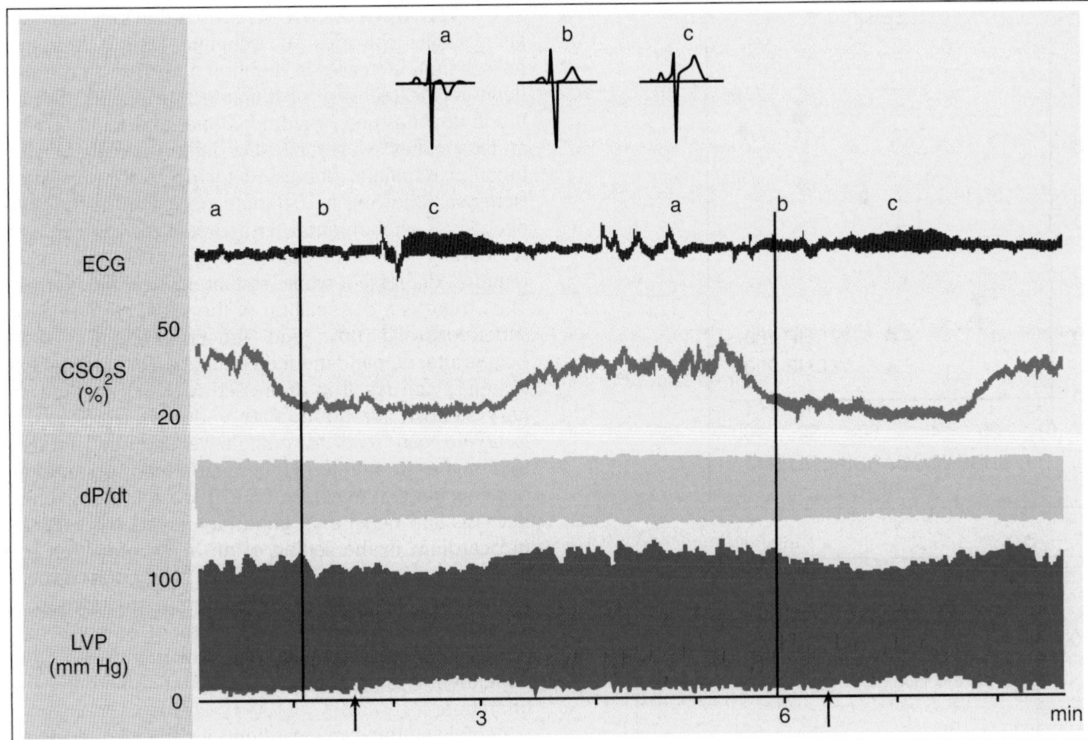

FIGURE 52-22 Physiologic changes during two episodes of spontaneous asymptomatic ischemia in a patient with acute coronary syndrome. High-speed electrocardiographic tracings depict the baseline ECG (a), pseudonormalization of T waves in early ischemia (b), and ST-segment elevation with late ischemia (c). A primary reduction in coronary flow is depicted by the sudden fall in coronary venous oxygen saturation (CSO_2S). Shortly thereafter, LV dP/dt falls, reflecting regional contractile dysfunction (solid vertical lines). Within 1 minute, LV end-diastolic pressure begins to rise (arrows) and is associated with a reduction in systolic pressure. Significant ST-segment elevation begins after the rise in LV end-diastolic pressure (c). On spontaneous resolution of ischemia (rise in CSO_2S), the changes resolve. Each episode lasted 2 minutes and was not associated with chest pain. LVP = left ventricular pressure. *(Modified from Chierchia S, Brunelli C, Simonetti I, et al: Sequence of events in angina at rest: Primary reduction in coronary flow. Circulation 61:759, 1980.)*

cellular space reaches a critical level. Symptoms of chest pain are variable and usually the last event to occur in the evolution of ischemia. On restoring perfusion, the sequence is reversed with resolution of chest pain occurring before hemodynamic changes resolve, but regional contraction can remain depressed, reflecting the development of stunned myocardium. A similar temporal sequence of events occurs during exercise-induced ischemia, although the time frame of evolution can be more protracted because ischemia primarily occurs in the subendocardium. Because of the temporal delay in the development of angina and other factors, many episodes of ST depression are symptomatically silent. It is also likely that very brief episodes of ischemia, as reflected by more sensitive indices, such as reduced regional contraction or elevations in end-diastolic pressure, can be electrocardiographically silent.

Acute Perfusion-Contraction Matching During Subendocardial Ischemia. When coronary pressure distal to a stenosis falls below the lower limit of autoregulation, flow reserve is exhausted, resulting in the onset of subendocardial ischemia. In this case, reductions in subendocardial flow are closely coupled to reductions in regional contractile function of the heart as measured by sensitive approaches, such as regional wall thickening. There is an approximately linear relationship between relative reductions in subendocardial blood flow and relative reductions in regional wall thickening at rest,[4] during tachycardia,[6] and during exercise-induced dysfunction distal to a critical stenosis (**Fig. 52-23**).[49,50] This forms the basis for using regional myocardial function as an index of the severity of subendocardial ischemia during stress imaging (see Chap. 15).

Short-Term Hibernation. In steady-state ischemia, the close matching between perfusion and contraction leads to reduced regional oxygen consumption and energy utilization, a phenomenon termed *short-term hibernation*.[47] This reestablishes a balance between supply and demand, as reflected by regeneration of creatine phosphate and ATP with the resolution of lactate production, despite persistent hypoperfusion. Short-term hibernation is an extremely tenuous state and small increases in the determinants of myocardial oxygen demand precipitate further ischemia and a rapid deterioration in function and metabolism. Thus, the ability of short-term hibernation to prevent necrosis is limited by the severity and duration of ischemia, with irreversible injury developing frequently after periods of more than 12 to 24 hours.[51]

Functional Consequences of Reversible Ischemia

There are various late consequences of ischemia after normal myocardial perfusion is reestablished (see Fig. 17-28). These reflect acute and delayed effects on regional function, as well as protection of the heart from subsequent ischemic episodes. In the most chronic state, they result in hibernating myocardium, characterized by chronic contractile dysfunction and regional cellular mechanisms that downregulate contractile and metabolic function of the heart to protect it from irreversible injury. The complex interplay among these entities is summarized in **Figure 52-24**. Clinically, it is difficult to separate all the various mechanisms involved in contributing to ischemia-induced viable dysfunctional myocardium because they may all coexist to some extent in the same heart. They can, however, be separated experimentally, and the important features and mechanisms from basic studies are summarized here.

MYOCARDIAL PRECONDITIONING AND POSTCONDITIONING. Brief reversible ischemia preceding a prolonged coronary occlusion reduces myocyte necrosis, a phenomenon termed *acute preconditioning*.[46,52] Because acute infarction is frequently preceded by angina, preconditioning is an endogenous mechanism that can delay the evolution of irreversible myocardial injury. Acute preconditioning can be induced pharmacologically using adenosine A1 receptor stimulation as well as various pharmacologic agonists that stimulate protein kinase C or open K^+-ATP channels. It has been demonstrated in humans during angioplasty with reduced subjective and objective ischemia during successive coronary occlusions as an endpoint. Preconditioning also develops on a chronic basis (termed *delayed preconditioning*) and, once induced, persists for up to 4 days.[53] It reduces myocardial infarct size and protects the heart from ischemia-induced stunning. The mechanisms of chronic preconditioning involve protein

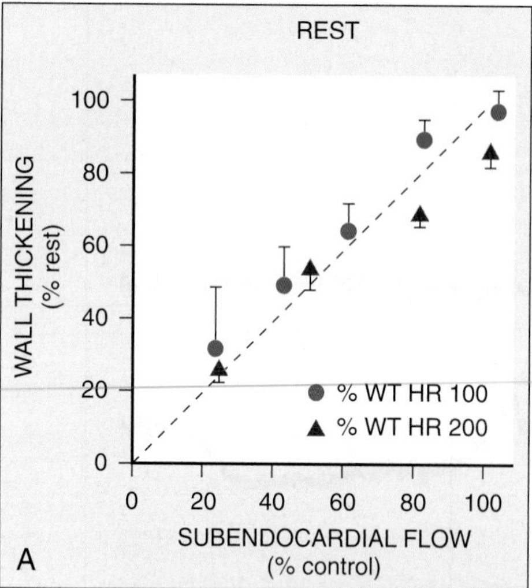

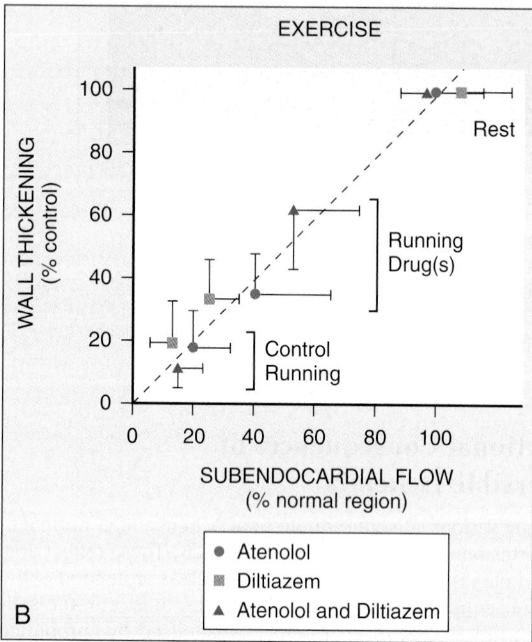

FIGURE 52-23 Perfusion contraction matching during acute ischemia. Relative reductions in function (regional wall thickening) are proportional to the relative reduction in subendocardial flow measured with microspheres in conscious dogs. This relationship is maintained over a wide range of heart rates during autoregulation **(A)** as well as during exercise with a fixed coronary stenosis **(B).** In the latter case, medical interventions that ameliorate ischemia improve both subendocardial flow and wall thickening during exercise. HR = heart rate; WT = wall thickening. *(**A** modified from Canty JM Jr: Coronary pressure-function and steady-state pressure-flow relations during autoregulation in the unanesthetized dog. Circ Res 63:821, 1988; and Canty JM Jr, Giglia J, Kandath D: Effect of tachycardia on regional function and transmural myocardial perfusion during graded coronary pressure reduction in conscious dogs. Circulation 82:1815,1990; **B** modified from Matsuzaki M, Gallagher KB, Kemper WS, et al: Sustained regional dysfunction produced by prolonged coronary stenosis: Gradual recovery after reperfusion. Circulation 68:170, 1983.)*

synthesis, with upregulation of the inducible form of NO synthase (iNOS), cyclooxygenase 2 (COX-2), and opening of the mitochondrial K^+-ATP channel. A final protective mechanism, myocardial postconditioning,[54] refers to the ability to cause cardiac protection by producing intermittent ischemia or administering pharmacologic agonists at the time of reperfusion. It is a relatively new observation and, although less extensively studied, has a greater potential to affect irreversible injury because it can be induced after myocardial ischemia is established rather than requiring pretreatment.[46]

STUNNED MYOCARDIUM. Myocardial function normalizes rapidly after single episodes of ischemia lasting less than 2 minutes. As ischemia increases in duration and/or severity, there is a temporal delay in the recovery of function that occurs, despite the fact that blood flow has been restored. Kloner and Jennings[52] and Heyndrickx and associates[55] were the first to demonstrate that regional myocardial function remained depressed for up to 6 hours after resolution of ischemia following a 15-minute occlusion in the absence of tissue necrosis, a phenomenon termed *stunned myocardium* (**Fig. 52-25**). A defining feature of isolated myocardial stunning is that function remains depressed while resting myocardial perfusion is normal. Thus, there is a dissociation of the usual close relationship between subendocardial flow and function. Stunned myocardium also occurs after demand-induced ischemia. For example, exercise-induced ischemia can result in depressed regional function distal to a coronary stenosis for hours after perfusion is restored, and repetitive ischemia can lead to cumulative stunning. Prolonged sublethal ischemia, as in short-term hibernation, leads to stunning on restoration of perfusion that may take up to 1 week to resolve in the absence of necrosis and may be an important cause of reversibly dysfunctional myocardium in the setting of an acute reduction in flow, as in an acute coronary syndrome (ACS).[56] Stunned myocardium is also responsible for postoperative pump dysfunction following cardiopulmonary bypass. Finally, areas of stunned myocardium can coexist with irreversibly injured myocardium and contribute to time-dependent improvements in function following myocardial infarction.

Acutely stunned myocardium is clinically important to recognize because contractile function normalizes during stimulation with various inotropic agents, including beta-adrenergic agonists. In contrast to other dysfunctional states, function will spontaneously normalize within 1 week, provided that there is no recurrent ischemia. If repetitive episodes of reversible ischemia develop before function normalizes, they can cause a state of persistent dysfunction or chronic stunning. The cellular mechanism of stunning likely involves free radical–mediated myocardial injury and reduced myofilament calcium sensitivity.[57]

CHRONIC HIBERNATING MYOCARDIUM. Viable dysfunctional myocardium is defined as any myocardial region where contractile function improves after coronary revascularization.[58,59] This broad definition of reversible dyssynergy includes three distinct categories with fairly diverse pathophysiologic mechanisms, summarized in **Table 52-2**. Complete normalization of function is the rule after acute ischemia but the exception in chronically dysfunctional myocardium. Brief occlusions or prolonged moderate ischemia (short-term hibernation) result in postischemic stunning in the absence of infarction, with complete functional recovery occurring rapidly (within 1 week after reperfusion).[56,57] The time course of improvement is roughly dependent on the duration and severity of the ischemic episode. Reversible dyssynergy with delayed functional improvement can also arise from structural remodeling of the heart that is independent of ischemia or a coronary stenosis (e.g., remote myocardial remodeling in heart failure or the reduced infarct volume that occurs over the initial weeks following coronary reperfusion). The latter conditions can be readily identified when the clinical setting, coronary anatomy, and assessment of myocardial perfusion are taken into account. Many clinical studies have evaluated the presence of contractile reserve during dobutamine administration as a predictor of functional recovery. Although this identifies the likelihood of functional recovery (see Chap. 15), it cannot distinguish the diverse pathophysiologic states underlying reversible dyssynergy. Understanding the cause may be important to the extent that this affects the time course and magnitude of functional recovery after revascularization in patients undergoing revascularization to treat ischemic heart failure.[59]

Chronic segmental dysfunction arising from repetitive episodes of ischemia (frequently clinically silent) is common and present in at least one coronary distribution in over 60% of patients with ischemic cardiomyopathy (**Fig. 52-26**).[60] When resting flow relative to a remote

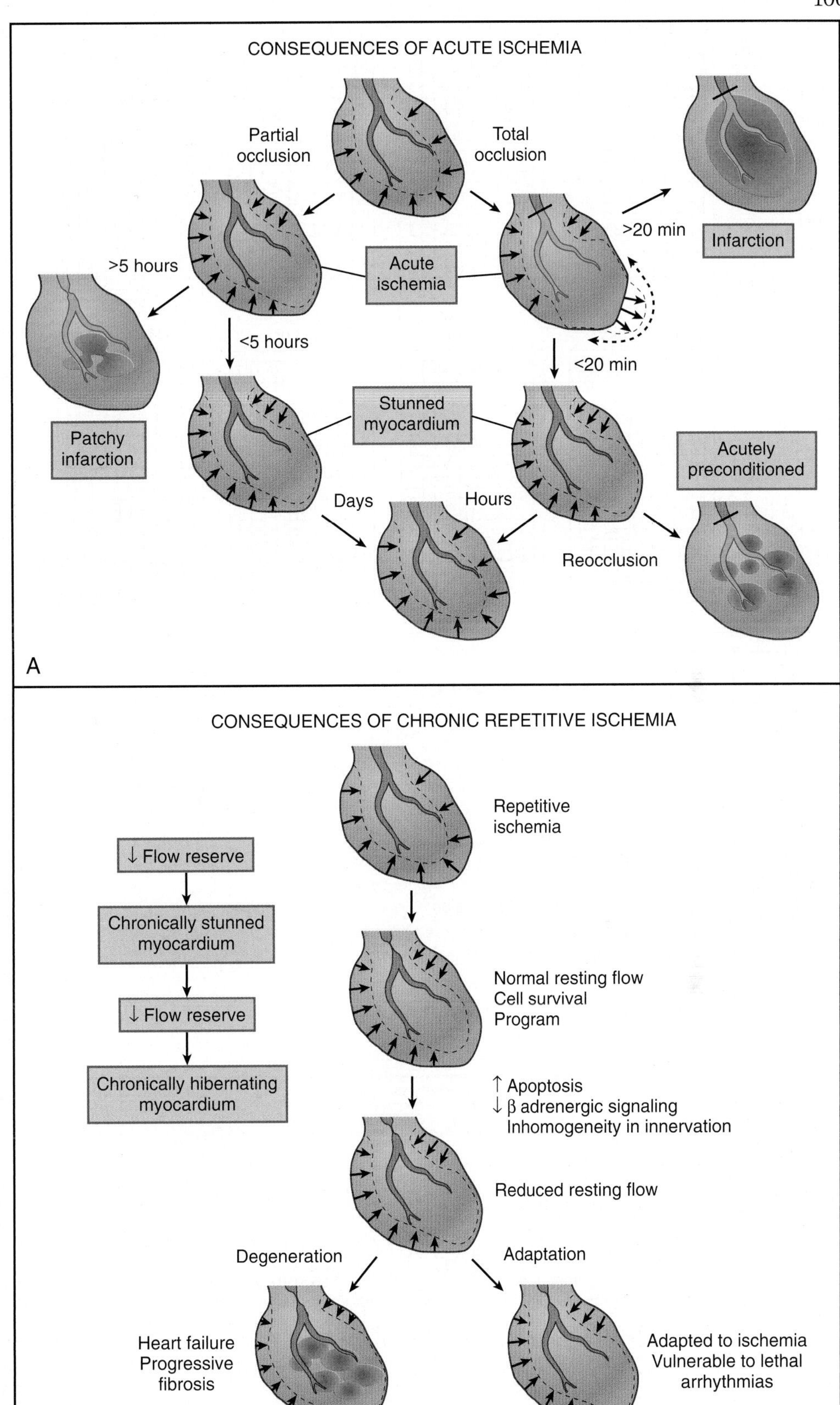

FIGURE 52-24 Effects of ischemia on LV function and irreversible injury. The ventriculograms illustrate contractile dysfunction (dashed lines and arrows). **A,** Consequences of acute ischemia. A brief total occlusion (right) or a prolonged partial occlusion (caused by an acute high-grade stenosis, left) leads to acute contractile dysfunction proportional to the reduction in blood flow. Irreversible injury begins after 20 minutes following a total occlusion but is delayed for up to 5 hours following a partial occlusion (or with significant collaterals) caused by short-term hibernation. When reperfusion is established before the onset of irreversible injury, stunned myocardium develops and the time required for recovery of function is proportional to the duration and severity of ischemia. With prolonged ischemia, stunning in viable myocardium coexists with subendocardial infarction and accounts for reversible dysfunction. Brief episodes of ischemia preceding prolonged ischemia elicit protection against infarction (acute preconditioning). **B,** Effects of chronic repetitive ischemia on function distal to a stenosis. As stenosis severity increases, coronary flow reserve decreases and the frequency of reversible ischemia increases. Reversible repetitive ischemia initially leads to chronic preconditioning against infarction and stunning (not shown). Subsequently, there is a gradual progression from contractile dysfunction with normal resting flow (chronically stunned myocardium) to contractile dysfunction with depressed resting flow (hibernating myocardium). This transition is related to the physiologic significance of a coronary stenosis and can occur in a time period as short as 1 week or develop chronically in the absence of severe angina. The cellular response during the progression to chronic hibernating myocardium is variable, with some patients exhibiting successful adaptation with little cell death and fibrosis and others developing degenerative changes difficult to distinguish from subendocardial infarction. See text for further discussion.

region is normal in dysfunctional myocardium distal to a stenosis, the region is chronically stunned. In contrast, when relative resting flow is reduced in the absence of symptoms or signs of ischemia, hibernating myocardium is present. Although there has previously been controversy over whether flow is normal or reduced at rest, both entities exist in patients and represent extremes in the spectrum of adaptive and maladaptive responses to chronic reversible ischemia. Viability studies are primarily required to distinguish infarction from hibernating myocardium because the myocardium is always viable when the resting flow is normal.[51]

CH 52

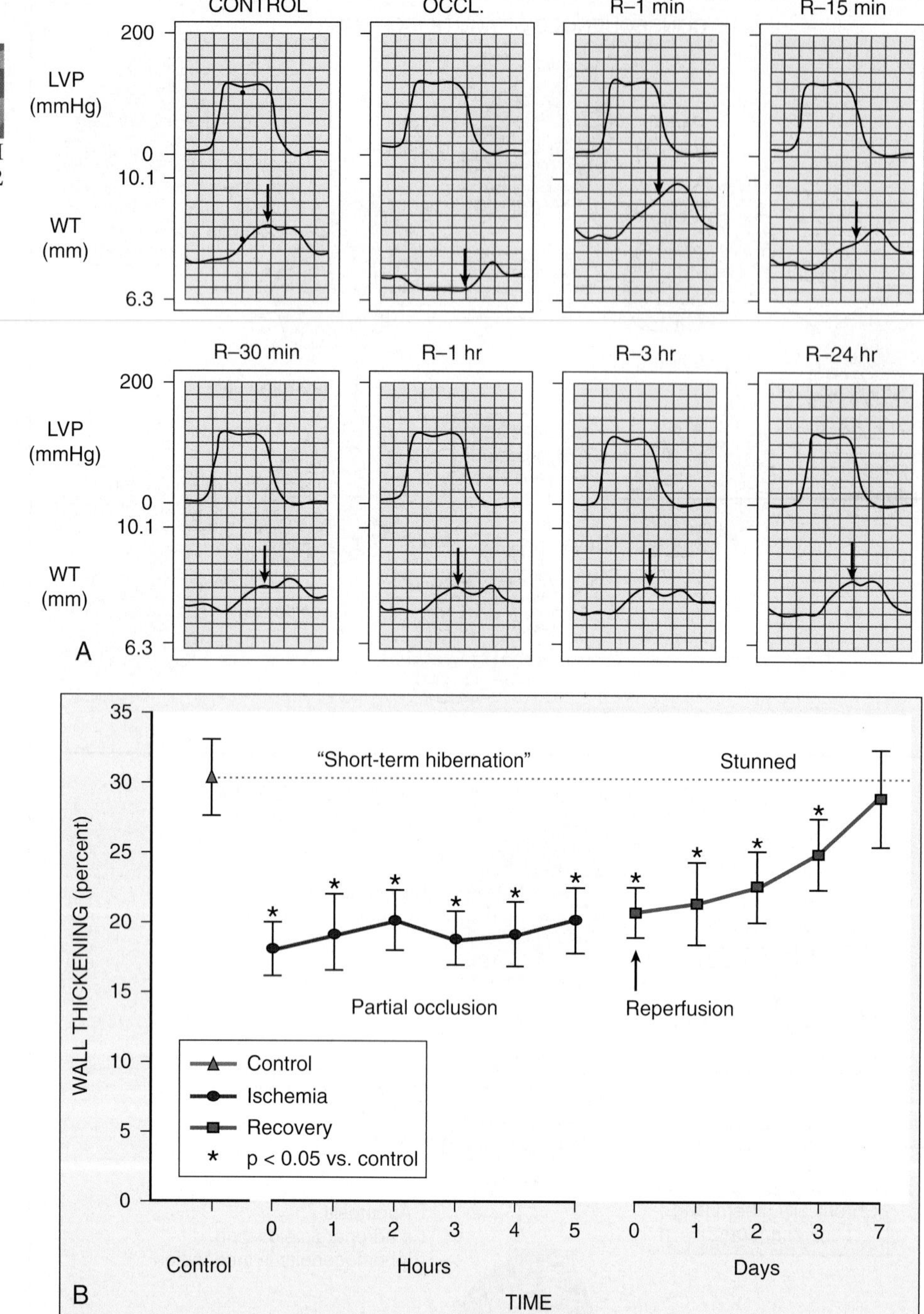

FIGURE 52-25 Stunned myocardium. **A,** Myocardial stunning following a brief total occlusion (OCCL.). Wall thickening (WT) measured by ultrasonic crystals is dyskinetic, with systolic thinning during occlusion. After reperfusion (R), function is completely normal after 24 hours. **B,** Myocardial stunning following a prolonged partial occlusion. During acute ischemia (red circles), there is short-term hibernation reflecting an acute match between reduced flow, wall thickening, and metabolism. With reperfusion (blue squares), wall thickening remains depressed and gradually returns to normal after 1 week. LVP = left ventricular pressure. (***A*** *modified from Heyndrickx GR, Baig H, Nellens P, et al: Depression of regional blood flow and wall thickening after brief coronary occlusions. Am J Physiol 234:H653, 1978;* ***B*** *modified from Matsuzaki M, Gallagher KP, Kemper WS, et al: Sustained regional dysfunction produced by prolonged coronary stenosis: Gradual recovery after reperfusion. Circulation 68:170, 1983.)*

It was originally thought that hibernating myocardium arises from a primary reduction in flow similar to experimental models of prolonged moderate ischemia and short-term hibernation. Whereas this is a plausible mechanism for the development of hibernating myocardium in association with an ACS, experimental studies have subsequently demonstrated that delayed subendocardial infarction is the rule rather than the exception when moderate flow reductions are maintained for more than 24 hours.[51] Many patients with hibernating myocardium present with LV dysfunction rather than symptomatic ischemia. Serial studies in animals have now demonstrated that the reductions in relative resting flow are a consequence rather than a cause of the contractile dysfunction.[61,62] This paradigm, relevant to chronic coronary disease, was proposed after experimental studies with a slowly progressive left anterior descending artery (LAD) stenosis demonstrated that dysfunction with normal resting flow consistent with chronic stunning precedes the development of hibernating myocardium after 3 months (**Fig. 52-27**).[63] The progression from chronically stunned myocardium (with normal resting flow) to hibernating myocardium (with reduced flow) is related to the functional significance of the chronic stenosis supplying the region and is probably a reflection of its propensity to develop repetitive supply or demand-induced ischemia. This progression can develop in as little as 1 week after placement of a critical stenosis that exhausts coronary flow reserve.[64] As regional dysfunction progresses from chronically stunned to hibernating myocardium, the myocyte takes on regional characteristics similar to those from an explanted heart with advanced failure. Normally perfused remote zone cardiac myocytes can be normal or take on structural alterations similar to those in the dysfunctional region. Some of the major cellular responses are summarized here.

Apoptosis, Myocyte Loss, and Myofibrillar Loss. The frequency of focal myocyte death from apoptosis varies during the development of viable dysfunctional myocardium and thus is probably responsible for the variability in the frequency of apoptosis when analyzing biopsies from patients.[65,66] Experimentally, apoptosis is particularly prominent during the transition from chronically stunned to hibernating myocardium, at which time there is a loss of approximately 30% of the regional myocytes (**Fig. 52-28**).[67] The myocyte loss results in compensatory regional myocyte hypertrophy to maintain approximately normal wall thickness. Vanoverschelde and coworkers[68] have previously described light microscopic and ultrastructural characteristics of hibernating myocardium from transmural biopsies, which are characterized by small increases in interstitial connective tissue, myofibrillar loss (myolysis), increased glycogen deposition, and minimitochondria. Experimental animal models of hibernating myocardium also develop these structural changes in as little as 2 weeks but they are also present in remote, normally perfused regions of the heart.[51,69] Global cellular changes have also been reported in patients in the absence of a stenosis, suggesting that the structural changes are probably the result of chronically elevated preload. Thus, although cellular dedifferentiation had been emphasized as a mechanism of adaptation, the global ultrastructural changes are probably not causally related to the regional responses to ischemia in hibernating myocardium.[59]

Cell Survival and Antiapoptotic Program in Response to Repetitive Ischemia. There is variability in the regulation of cell survival pathways in response to repetitive ischemia. Some studies have demonstrated

TABLE 52-2 Viable Dysfunctional Myocardium: Patterns of Contractile Reserve, Resting Perfusion, and Temporal Recovery of Function after Revascularization

PARAMETER	CONTRACTILE RESERVE	RESTING FLOW	EXTENT OF FUNCTIONAL RECOVERY	TIME COURSE OF RECOVERY
Transient Reversible Ischemia				
Postischemic stunning	Present	Normal	Normalizes	<24 hr
Short-term hibernation	Present	Normal	Normalizes	<7 days
Chronic Repetitive Ischemia				
Chronic hibernating myocardium	Variable	Reduced	Improves	Up to 12 mo
Chronic stunning	Present	Normal	Improves	Days to weeks
Structural Remodeling				
Subendocardial infarction	Variable	Reduced	Variable	Weeks
Remodeled, tethered myocardium	Present	Normal	Improves	Months

upregulation of cardioprotective mechanisms in response to repetitive reversible ischemia, which may be operative in minimizing myocyte cell death and fibrosis in the chronic setting.[70] An interesting mechanism potentially linking altered metabolism and protection is the regional downregulation of glycogen synthase kinase-3β, which can ameliorate cell death and also explains the increased tissue glycogen in hibernating myocardium.[71] In experimental studies in animals without heart failure, antiapoptotic and stress proteins such as HSP-70 have been found to be upregulated,[72] whereas increased proapoptotic proteins and a profile of progressive cell death and fibrosis have been reported in human biopsies of patients with hibernating myocardium and heart failure.[66] It is likely that the variability among studies reflects the frequency and severity of ischemia, modulation by neurohormonal activation in heart failure, and the complexity of the temporal expression of adaptive and maladaptive responses in myocardium subjected to chronic repetitive ischemia.

Metabolism and Energetics in Hibernating Myocardium. Once adapted, the metabolic and contractile response of hibernating myocardium appears to be dissociated from external determinants of workload. As a result, submaximal increases in oxygen consumption can occur without immediately leading to subendocardial ischemia.[73] Experimentally, the hibernating myocardial region appears to operate over a lower range of the normal myocardial supply-demand relationship in a fashion similar to that of the nonischemic failing heart. Although glycogen content is increased, maximum rates of glucose uptake during insulin stimulation are not altered. In addition, creatine phosphate and ATP levels are not regionally altered, contrasting with the depressed ATP levels in stunning. Recently, studies of isolated mitochondria from swine with hibernating myocardium have demonstrated a downregulation of energy uptake and oxygen consumption.[74] This slows ATP uptake and presumably maintains cell viability during superimposed acute ischemia. Proteomic analysis has demonstrated a reduction in multiple proteins involved in oxidative metabolism and electron transport.[72]

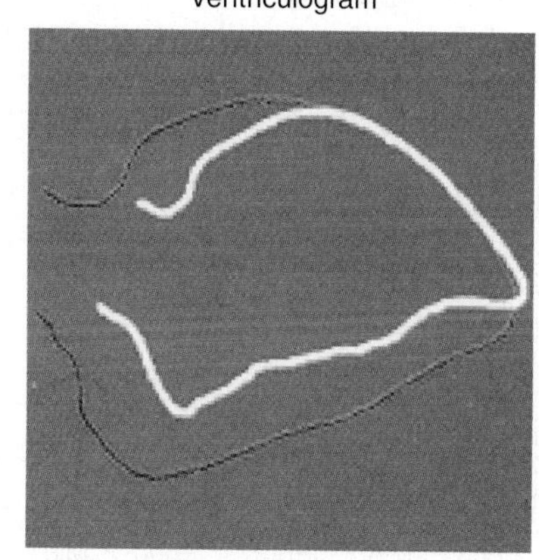

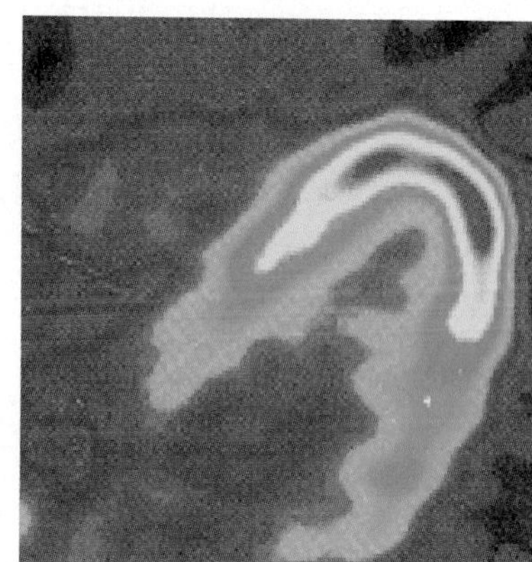

Resting flow

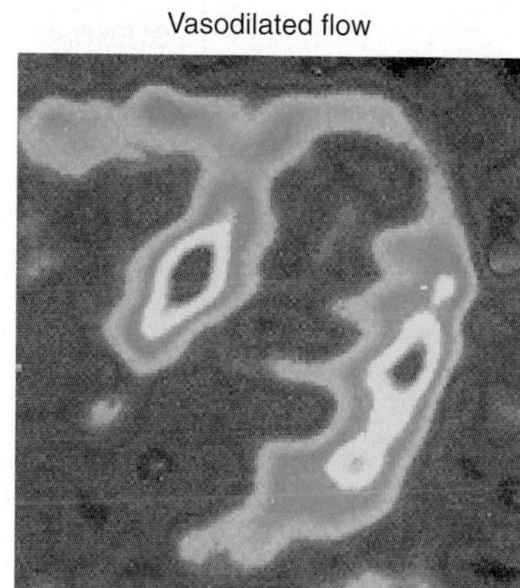

FIGURE 52-26 Hibernating myocardium in humans with a chronic LAD occlusion and collateral dependent myocardium. The RAO tracings of the left ventriculogram show anterior akinesis (upper left). Transaxial PET scans (see Chap. 17) illustrate $^{13}NH_3$ flow measurements at rest (lower left) and following pharmacologic vasodilation with dipyridamole (lower right). Quantitative perfusion measurements showed LAD flow to be critically impaired. Viability (following an oral glucose load) is identified by increased ^{18}F-fluorodeoxyglucose (FDG) uptake in the anterior wall (upper right). RAO = right anterior oblique. *(Modified from Vanoverschelde J-LJ, Wijns W, Depre C, et al: Mechanisms of chronic regional postischemic dysfunction in humans: New insights from the study of noninfarcted collateral-dependent myocardium. Circulation 87:1513, 1993.)*

Inhomogeneity in Sympathetic Innervation, Beta-Adrenergic Responses, and Sudden Death. The contractile response of hibernating myocardium is blunted and partially related to a regional downregulation in beta-adrenergic adenylyl cyclase coupling, similar to that found globally in advanced heart failure.[75] This may be related to local norepinephrine overflow because the presynaptic uptake of norepinephrine is reduced when assessed using nuclear tracers such as ^{11}C-hydroxyephedrine.[76] The resultant inhomogeneity in myocardial sympathetic nerve function may be one of the reasons responsible for the vulnerability of experimental hibernating myocardium to develop lethal ventricular arrhythmias and ventricular fibrillation.[77] Thus, normalizing electrical instability and improving contractile dysfunction may account for the profound impact of revascularization on survival when hibernating myocardium is present.[59]

Successful Adaptation Versus Degeneration in Hibernating Myocardium. There is considerable divergence among studies regarding the pathology of reversibly dyssynergic hibernating myocardium. At one extreme, some investigators believe that it is destined to undergo irreversible myocyte death, which is supported by data showing large amounts of fibrosis (more than 30% of the tissue), markedly abnormal high-energy phosphate metabolism, and retrospective analysis suggesting that the degree of fibrosis is related to the duration of hibernating myocardium.[66] At the other extreme, there are circumstances in which fibrosis is not a prominent feature with normal myocardial energetics at

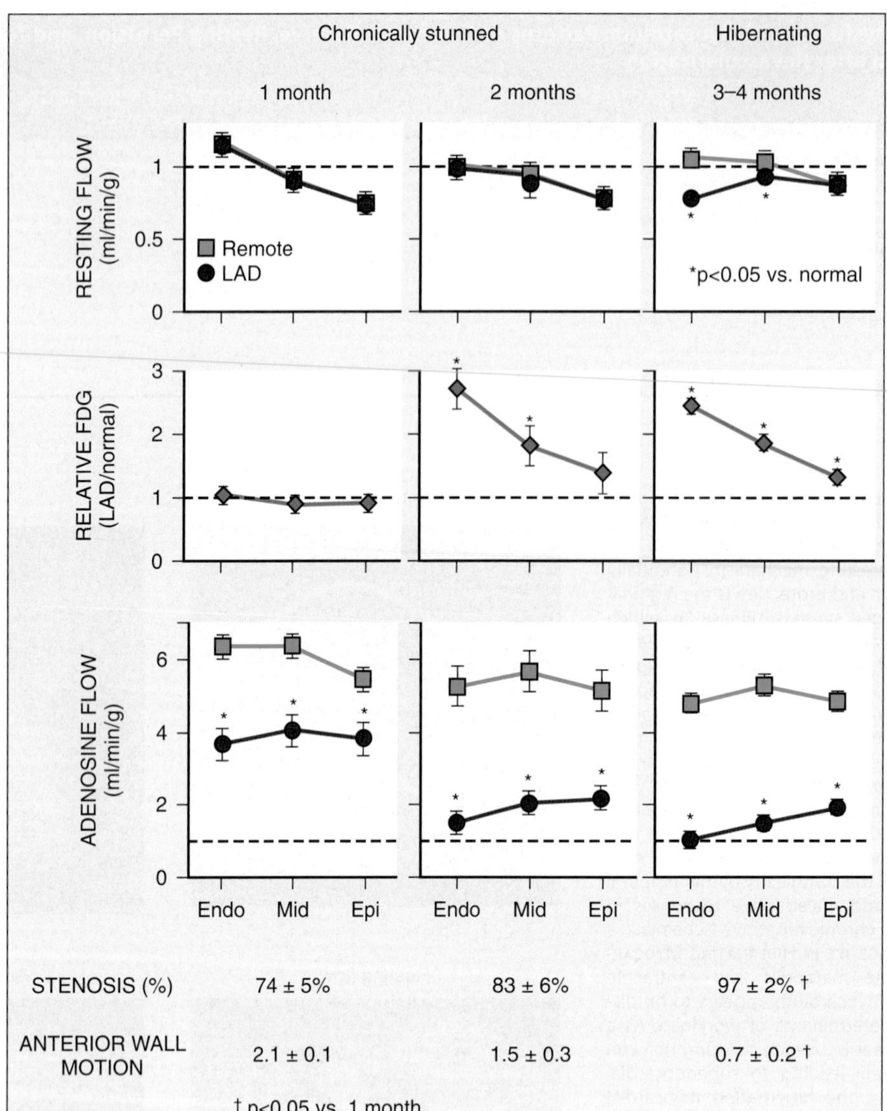

FIGURE 52-27 Progression from chronically stunned to hibernating myocardium as stenosis severity increases in swine with viable dysfunctional myocardium from a chronic LAD stenosis. Transmural flow measurements (microspheres) at rest and adenosine vasodilation are shown, along with regional FDG uptake (fasting conditions). Below are the angiographic stenosis severity and anterior wall motion score (3, normal; 2, mild hypokinesis; 1, severe hypokinesis). As stenosis severity increases over time, there is a reduction in vasodilated flow (adenosine) to the LAD region. Initially, there is anterior hypokinesis, with normal resting flow consistent with chronically stunned myocardium. After 3 months, the stenosis progresses to occlusion with collateral dependent myocardium. Subendocardial flow is critically reduced and there is a reduction in resting flow to the inner two thirds of the LAD myocardium. At this time, hibernating myocardium is present and there is no evidence of infarction. The temporal progression of abnormalities demonstrate that chronic stunning precedes the development of hibernating myocardium. In contrast to short-term hibernation resulting from acute ischemia, the reduction in resting flow is a consequence, rather than a cause, of the contractile dysfunction. Endo = endocardium; Epi = epicardium; FDG = ^{18}F-fluorodeoxyglucose. *(Modified from Fallavollita JA, Canty JM Jr: Differential ^{18}F-2-deoxyglucose uptake in viable dysfunctional myocardium with normal resting perfusion: Evidence for chronic stunning in pigs. Circulation 99:2798, 1999.)*

rest, suggesting that hibernating myocardium can be sustained for long periods without progressive degeneration.[77,78] The factors that determine the path to progressive structural degeneration versus adaptation are currently unknown but may be modulated by the superimposed neurohormonal activation, elevation in cytokine levels associated with advanced clinical heart failure, and structural degeneration that arises from small reductions in coronary flow reserve below the threshold required to maintain myocyte viability.

Future Perspectives

There has been considerable progress in advancing the mechanistic understanding of the coronary circulation and myocardial ischemia in health and disease, yet important gaps remain in basic knowledge and in its translation to clinical care. The major factors determining myocardial perfusion and oxygen delivery were established over 30 years ago, have been incorporated into how angina is managed, and have stood the test of time. The basic understanding of the fluid mechanical behavior of coronary stenoses has only recently been translated to the cardiac catheterization laboratory, where it can facilitate routine clinical decision making. Here, measurements of coronary pressure distal to a stenosis and flow have been demonstrated to provide a physiologic approach to guiding interventional procedures (see Chap. 58). This ischemia-guided physiologic approach results in reduced major adverse cardiovascular events in comparison to an anatomically guided strategy based on the angiographic severity of potential lesions, and is likely to be increasingly used in future clinical decisions.

Basic research has led to the discovery of many new signaling pathways involved in the control of coronary blood flow, extended the understanding of flow regulation in microcirculatory vessels, and identified the importance of physical factors such as shear stress and local

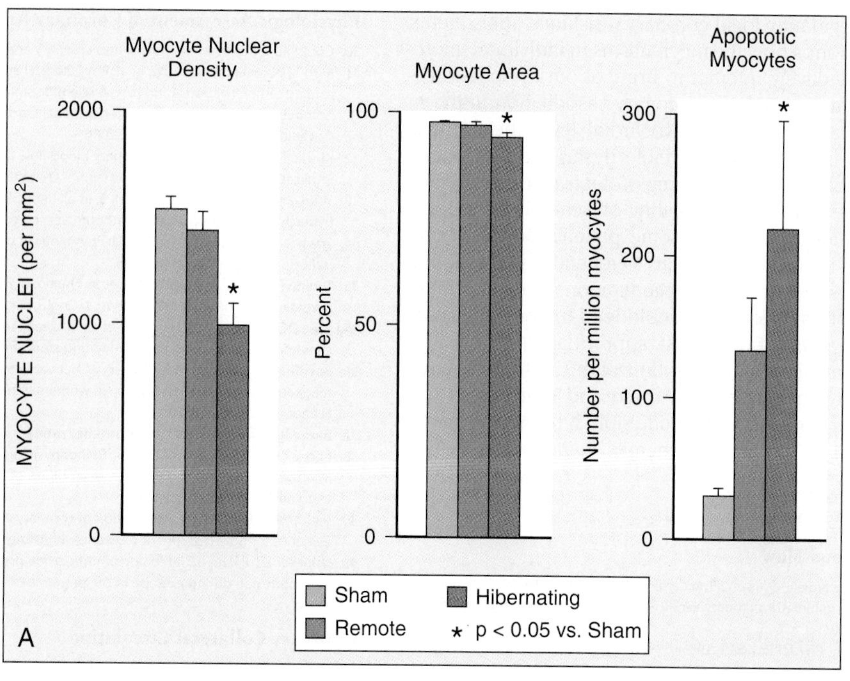

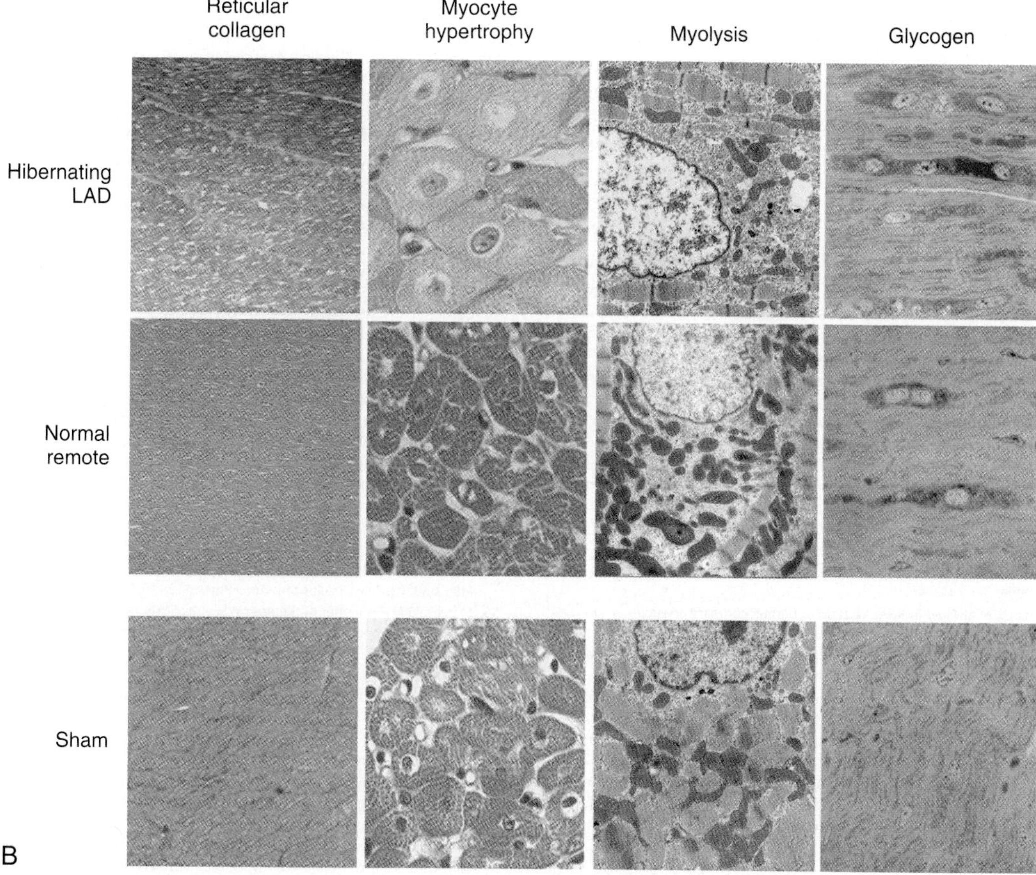

FIGURE 52-28 Apoptosis, hypertrophy, and myocyte cellular morphology in hibernating myocardium. Data in hibernating LAD regions are compared with remote regions as well as with LAD regions from normal animals. **A,** The progression from chronically stunned to hibernating myocardium is accompanied by regional apoptosis-induced myocyte loss. There is about a 30% reduction in myocyte nuclear number without significant fibrosis, because the myocyte area is almost normal. **B,** Myocyte cellular changes in hibernating myocardium. The increased myocyte loss results in compensatory myocyte cellular hypertrophy in hibernating myocardium. Whereas reticular collagen is regionally increased (about 2%), there is no evidence of infarction. The electron microscopic characteristics of hibernating myocardium demonstrate myofibrillar loss, an increased number of small mitochondria, and increased glycogen content. Although these are markedly different from normal myocardium (sham), biopsies of normal remote, nonischemic segments show similar morphologic changes, indicating that these structural abnormalities are not directly related to ischemia nor are they the cause of regional contractile dysfunction. (***A** from Lim H, Fallavollita JA, Hard R, et al: Profound apoptosis-mediated regional myocyte loss and compensatory hypertrophy in pigs with hibernating myocardium. Circulation 100:2380, 1999; **B** from Canty JM, Fallavollita JA: Hibernating myocardium. J Nucl Cardiol 12:104, 2005.*)

coronary pressure in regulating local coronary resistance adjustments. Nevertheless, the question of how the mechanisms in individual microcirculatory vessels collectively interact to bring about the phenomenon of autoregulation and metabolic coronary vasodilation in the in vivo heart remains unanswered. At a myocardial level, the intrinsic mechanisms involved in patients with viable dysfunctional myocardium appear to be diverse, with some being protective and beneficial in maintaining myocyte viability in the setting of ischemia and others being detrimental. Understanding why some patients develop coronary collaterals and/or intrinsic adaptations to repetitive ischemia but others undergo progressive structural degeneration is an important gap in our knowledge. This information could lead to novel therapies and a better identification of the most appropriate patients and approach for high-risk myocardial revascularization. Continued bench to bedside translational investigation in these and other areas will allow us to expand our understanding and apply it to improving the management of patients with chronic ischemic heart disease.

REFERENCES

Control of Coronary Blood Flow

1. Hoffman JIE: Transmural myocardial perfusion. Prog Cardiovasc Dis 29:429, 1987.
2. Canty JM Jr, Brooks A: Phasic volumetric coronary venous outflow patterns in conscious dogs. Am J Physiol 258:H1457, 1990.
3. Feigl EO: Coronary physiology. Physiol Rev 63:1, 1983.
4. Canty JM Jr: Coronary pressure-function and steady-state pressure-flow relations during autoregulation in the unanesthetized dog. Circ Res 63:821, 1988.
5. Klocke FJ: Coronary blood flow in man. Prog Cardiovasc Dis XIX:117, 1976.
6. Canty JM Jr, Giglia J, Kandath D: Effect of tachycardia on regional function and transmural myocardial perfusion during graded coronary pressure reduction in conscious dogs. Circulation 82:1815, 1990.
7. Canty JM Jr, Smith TP Jr: Adenosine-recruitable flow reserve is absent during myocardial ischemia in unanesthetized dogs studied in the basal state. Circ Res 76:1079, 1995.
8. Hoffman JIE, Spaan JAE: Pressure-flow relations in coronary circulation. Physiol Rev 70:331, 1990.
9. Duncker DJ, Bache RJ: Regulation of coronary vasomotor tone under normal conditions and during acute myocardial hypoperfusion. Pharmacol Ther 86:87, 2000.

Coronary Microcirculation

10. Furchgott RF, Zawadzki JV: The obligatory role of endothelial cells in the relaxation of arterial smooth muscle by acetylcholine. Nature 288:373, 1980.
11. Kuo L, Davis MJ, Chilian WM: Longitudinal gradients for endothelium-dependent and -independent vascular responses in the coronary microcirculation. Circulation 92:518, 1995.
12. Chilian WM, Layne SM, Klausner EC, et al: Redistribution of coronary microvascular resistance produced by dipyridamole. Am J Physiol 256:H383, 1989.
13. Kanatsuka H, Lamping KG, Eastham CL, et al: Heterogeneous changes in epimyocardial microvascular size during graded coronary stenosis. Evidence of the microvascular site for autoregulation. Circ Res 66:389, 1990.
14. Kanatsuka H, Lamping KG, Eastham CL, et al: Comparison of the effects of increased myocardial oxygen consumption and adenosine on the coronary microvascular resistance. Circ Res 65:1296, 1989.
15. Miller FJ, Dellsperger KC, Gutterman DD: Myogenic constriction of human coronary arterioles. Am J Physiol Heart Circ Physiol 273:H257, 1997.
16. Kuo L, Davis MJ, Chilian WM: Endothelium-dependent, flow-induced dilation of isolated coronary arterioles. Am J Physiol 259:H1063, 1990.
17. Liu Y, Gutterman DD: Vascular control in humans: Focus on the coronary microcirculation. Basic Res Cardiol 104:211, 2009.
18. Miura H, Wachtel RE, Liu Y, et al: Flow-induced dilation of human coronary arterioles: Important role of Ca^{2+}-activated K^+ channels. Circulation 103:1992, 2001.
19. Dube S, Canty JM Jr: Shear-stress induced vasodilation in porcine coronary conduit arteries is independent of nitric oxide release. Am J Physiol 280:H2581, 2001.
20. Quyyumi AA, Dakak N, Andrews NP, et al: Contribution of nitric oxide to metabolic coronary vasodilation in the human heart. Circulation 92:320, 1995.
21. Sato A, Terata K, Miura H, et al: Mechanism of vasodilation to adenosine in coronary arterioles from patients with heart disease. Am J Physiol Heart Circ Physiol 288:H1633, 2005.
22. Jones CJ, Kuo L, Davis MJ, et al: Role of nitric oxide in the coronary microvascular responses to adenosine and increased metabolic demand. Circulation 91:1807, 1995.
23. Duncker DJ, Bache RJ: Regulation of coronary blood flow during exercise. Physiol Rev 88:1009, 2008.

Coronary Vasoconstriction, Vasospasm, and Pharmacologic Vasodilation

24. Heusch G, Baumgart D, Camici P, et al: α-Adrenergic coronary vasoconstriction and myocardial ischemia in humans. Circulation 101:689, 2000.
25. Konidala S, Gutterman DD: Coronary vasospasm and the regulation of coronary blood flow. Prog Cardiovasc Dis 46:349, 2004.
26. Druz RS: Current advances in vasodilator pharmacological stress perfusion imaging. Semin Nucl Med 39:204, 2009.
27. Jones CJH, Kuo L, Davis MJ, et al: In vivo and in vitro vasoactive reactions of coronary arteriolar microvessels to nitroglycerin. Am J Physiol 271:H461, 1996.
28. Guethlin M, Kasel AM, Coppenrath K, et al: Delayed response of myocardial flow reserve to lipid-lowering therapy with fluvastatin. Circulation 99:475, 1999.
29. Zong P, Tune JD, Downey HF: Mechanisms of oxygen demand/supply balance in the right ventricle. Exp Biol Med (Maywood) 230:507, 2005.

Physiologic Assessment of Coronary Artery Stenosis

30. Gould KL: Does coronary flow trump coronary anatomy? J Am Coll Cardiol Img 2:1009, 2009.
31. Kern MJ, Lerman A, Bech JW, et al: Physiological assessment of coronary artery disease in the cardiac catheterization laboratory. A scientific statement from the American Heart Association Committee on Diagnostic and Interventional Cardiac Catheterization, Council on Clinical Cardiology. Circulation 114:1321, 2006.
32. Klocke FJ: Measurements of coronary blood flow and degree of stenosis: Current clinical implications and continuing uncertainties. J Am Coll Cardiol 1:31, 1983.
33. Yokoyama I, Ohtake T, Momomura S, et al: Reduced coronary flow reserve in hypercholesterolemic patients without overt coronary stenosis. Circulation 94:3232, 1996.
34. Spaan JA, Piek JJ, Hoffman JI, et al: Physiological basis of clinically used coronary hemodynamic indices. Circulation 113:446, 2006.
35. Tonino PA, De Bruyne B, Pijls NH, et al: Fractional flow reserve versus angiography for guiding percutaneous coronary intervention. N Engl J Med 360:213, 2009.
35a. Lee DC, Simonetti OP, Harris KR, et al: Magnetic resonance versus radionuclide pharmacologic stress perfusion imaging for flow-limiting stenoses of varying severity. Circulation 110:58, 2004.
36. Buchthal SD, den Hollander JA, Merz CN, et al: Abnormal myocardial phosphorus-31 nuclear magnetic resonance spectroscopy in women with chest pain but normal coronary angiograms. N Engl J Med 342:829, 2000.
37. Bache RJ: Effects of hypertrophy on the coronary circulation. Prog Cardiovasc Dis 31:403, 1988.
38. Kuo L, Davis MJ, Cannon MS, et al: Pathophysiological consequences of atherosclerosis extend into the coronary microcirculation: Restoration of endothelium-dependent responses by L-arginine. Circ Res 70:465, 1992.
39. Smith TP Jr, Canty JM Jr: Modulation of coronary autoregulatory responses by nitric oxide: Evidence for flow-dependent resistance adjustments in conscious dogs. Circ Res 73:232, 1993.
40. Duncker DJ, Bache RJ: Inhibition of nitric oxide production aggravates myocardial hypoperfusion during exercise in the presence of a coronary artery stenosis. Circ Res 74:629, 1994.

Coronary Collateral Circulation

41. Meier P, Gloekler S, Zbinden R, et al: Beneficial effect of recruitable collaterals: A 10-year follow-up study in patients with stable coronary artery disease undergoing quantitative collateral measurements. Circulation 116:975, 2007.
42. Schaper W: Collateral circulation: past and present. Basic Res Cardiol 104:5, 2009.
43. Simons M: Angiogenesis: Where do we stand now? Circulation 111:1556, 2005.
44. Suzuki G, Lee TC, Fallavollita JA, et al: Adenoviral gene transfer of FGF-5 to hibernating myocardium improves function and stimulates myocytes to hypertrophy and reenter the cell cycle. Circ Res 96:767, 2005.

Metabolic and Functional Consequence of Ischemia

45. Kloner RA, Jennings RB: Consequences of brief ischemia: Stunning, preconditioning, and their clinical implications: part 1. Circulation 104:2981, 2001.
46. Downey JM, Cohen MV: Reducing infarct size in the setting of acute myocardial infarction. Prog Cardiovasc Dis 48:363, 2006.
47. Heusch G: Hibernating myocardium. Physiol Rev 78:1055, 1998.
48. Dorn GW 2nd, Diwan A: The rationale for cardiomyocyte resuscitation in myocardial salvage. J Mol Med 86:1085, 2008.
49. Gallagher KP, Matsuzaki M, Osakada G, et al: Effect of exercise on the relationship between myocardial blood flow and systolic wall thickening in dogs with acute coronary stenosis. Circ Res 52:716, 1983.
50. Matsuzaki M, Guth B, Tajimi T, et al: Effect of the combination of diltiazem and atenolol on exercise-induced regional myocardial ischemia in conscious dogs. Circulation 72:233, 1985.
51. Heusch G, Schulz R, Rahimtoola SH: Myocardial hibernation: A delicate balance. Am J Physiol Heart Circ Physiol 288:H984, 2005.
52. Kloner RA, Jennings RB: Consequences of brief ischemia: Stunning, preconditioning, and their clinical implications: part 2. Circulation 104:3158, 2001.
53. Bolli R: The late phase of preconditioning. Circ Res 87:972, 2000.
54. Vinten-Johansen J, Zhao ZQ, Jiang R, et al: Preconditioning and postconditioning: Innate cardioprotection from ischemia-reperfusion injury. J Appl Physiol 103:1441, 2007.
55. Heyndrickx GR, Baig H, Nellens P, et al: Depression of regional blood flow and wall thickening after brief coronary occlusions. Am J Physiol 234:H653, 1978.
56. Matsuzaki M, Gallagher KP, Kemper WS, et al: Sustained regional dysfunction produced by prolonged coronary stenosis: Gradual recovery after reperfusion. Circulation 68:170, 1983.
57. Bolli R, Marban E: Molecular and cellular mechanisms of myocardial stunning. Physiol Rev 79:609, 1999.
58. Rahimtoola SH, Dilsizian V, Kramer CM, et al: Chronic ischemic left ventricular dysfunction: From pathophysiology to imaging and its integration into clinical practice. J Am Coll Cardiol Img 1:536, 2008.
59. Canty JM Jr, Fallavollita JA: Hibernating myocardium. J Nucl Cardiol 12:104, 2005.
60. Vanoverschelde J-LJ, Wijns W, Depre C, et al: Mechanisms of chronic regional postischemic dysfunction in humans: New insights from the study of noninfarcted collateral-dependent myocardium. Circulation 87:1513, 1993.
61. Fallavollita JA, Perry BJ, Canty JM Jr: ^{18}F-2-deoxyglucose deposition and regional flow in pigs with chronically dysfunctional myocardium: Evidence for transmural variations in chronic hibernating myocardium. Circulation 95:1900, 1997.
62. Fallavollita JA, Canty JM Jr: Differential ^{18}F-2-deoxyglucose uptake in viable dysfunctional myocardium with normal resting perfusion: Evidence for chronic stunning in pigs. Circulation 99:2798, 1999.
63. Canty JM Jr, Fallavollita JA: Chronic hibernation and chronic stunning: A continuum. J Nucl Cardiol 7:509, 2000.
64. Thomas SA, Fallavollita JA, Borgers M, et al: Dissociation of regional adaptations to ischemia and global myolysis in an accelerated swine model of chronic hibernating myocardium. Circ Res 91:970, 2002.
65. Dispersyn GD, Borgers M, Flameng W: Apoptosis in chronic hibernating myocardium: Sleeping to death? Cardiovasc Res 45:696, 2000.
66. Elsasser A, Vogt AM, Nef H, et al: Human hibernating myocardium is jeopardized by apoptotic and autophagic cell death. J Am Coll Cardiol 43:2191, 2004.

67. Lim H, Fallavollita JA, Hard R, et al: Profound apoptosis-mediated regional myocyte loss and compensatory hypertrophy in pigs with hibernating myocardium. Circulation 100:2380, 1999.
68. Vanoverschelde J-L, Wijns W, Borgers M, et al: Chronic myocardial hibernation in humans. From bedside to bench. Circulation 95:1961, 1997.
69. Thijssen VL, Borgers M, Lenders M-H, et al: Temporal and spatial variations in structural protein expression during the progression from stunned to hibernating myocardium. Circulation 110:3313, 2004.
70. Depre C, Vatner SF: Mechanisms of cell survival in myocardial hibernation. Trends Cardiovasc Med 15:101, 2005.
71. Kim SJ, Peppas A, Hong SK, et al: Persistent stunning induces myocardial hibernation and protection: Flow/function and metabolic mechanisms. Circ Res 92:1233, 2003.
72. Page B, Young R, Iyer V, et al: Persistent regional downregulation in mitochondrial enzymes and upregulation of stress proteins in swine with chronic hibernating myocardium. Circ Res 102:103, 2008.
73. Fallavollita JA, Malm BJ, Canty JM Jr: Hibernating myocardium retains metabolic and contractile reserve despite regional reductions in flow, function, and oxygen consumption at rest. Circ Res 92:48, 2003.
74. Hu Q, Suzuki G, Young RF, et al: Reductions in mitochondrial O_2 consumption and preservation of high-energy phosphate levels after simulated ischemia in chronic hibernating myocardium. Am J Physiol Heart Circ Physiol 297:H223, 2009.
75. Iyer V, Canty JM Jr: Regional desensitization of β-adrenergic receptor signaling in swine with chronic hibernating myocardium. Circ Res 97:789, 2005.
76. Luisi AJ Jr, Suzuki G, deKemp R, et al: Regional ^{11}C-hydroxyephedrine retention in hibernating myocardium: Chronic inhomogeneity of sympathetic innervation in the absence of infarction. J Nucl Med 46:1368, 2005.
77. Canty JM Jr, Suzuki G, Banas MD, et al: Hibernating myocardium: Chronically adapted to ischemia but vulnerable to sudden death. Circ Res 94:1142, 2004.
78. Dispersyn GD, Ramaekers FCS and Borgers M: Clinical pathophysiology of hibernating myocardium. Coron Artery Dis 12:381, 2001.

CHAPTER 53 Approach to the Patient with Chest Pain

Marc S. Sabatine and Christopher P. Cannon

Acute chest pain is one of the most common reasons for presentation to the emergency department (ED), accounting for approximately 7 million ED visits annually in the United States. This presentation suggests acute coronary syndrome (ACS), but after diagnostic evaluation, only 15% to 25% of patients with acute chest pain actually have ACS.[1,2] The difficulty lies in discriminating patients with ACS or other life-threatening conditions from patients with noncardiovascular, non–life-threatening chest pain. The diagnosis of ACS is missed in approximately 2% of patients, leading to substantial consequences—for example, the short-term mortality for patients with acute myocardial infarction (MI) who are mistakenly discharged from the ED increases twofold over that expected for patients who are admitted to the hospital. For patients with a low risk of complications, however, these concerns must be balanced against the costs and inconvenience of admission and against the risk of complications from tests and procedures with a low probability of improving patient outcomes.

Several recent advances have enhanced the accuracy and efficiency of the evaluation of patients with acute chest pain, including better blood markers for myocardial injury,[3] decision aids to stratify patients according to their risk of complications, early and even immediate exercise testing[4] and radionuclide scanning for lower risk patient subsets (see Chap. 17),[5] multislice computed tomography for the anatomic evaluation of coronary artery disease, pulmonary embolism, and aortic dissection (see Chap. 19),[6] and the use of chest pain units[7] and critical pathways for efficient and rapid evaluation of lower-risk patients.[8]

Causes of Acute Chest Pain

In a typical population of patients presenting for the evaluation of acute chest pain in EDs, about 15% to 25% have acute MI or unstable angina.[2] A small percentage have other life-threatening problems, such as pulmonary embolism or acute aortic dissection, but most are discharged without a diagnosis or with a diagnosis of a noncardiac condition. These noncardiac conditions include musculoskeletal syndromes, disorders of the abdominal viscera (including gastroesophageal reflux disease), and psychological conditions (**Table 53-1**).

Myocardial Ischemia or Infarction

The most common serious cause of acute chest discomfort is myocardial ischemia or infarction (see Chaps. 54 to 56), which occurs when the supply of myocardial oxygen is inadequate compared with the demand. Myocardial ischemia usually occurs in the setting of coronary atherosclerosis, but it may also reflect dynamic components of coronary vascular resistance. Coronary spasm can occur in normal coronary arteries or, in patients with coronary disease, near atherosclerotic plaques and in smaller coronary arteries (see Chap. 52). Other less common causes of impaired coronary blood flow include syndromes that compromise the orifices or lumina of the coronary arteries, such as coronary arteritis, proximal aortitis, spontaneous coronary dissection, proximal aortic dissection, coronary emboli from infectious or noninfectious endocarditis or thrombus in the left atrium or left ventricle, myocardial bridge, or a congenital abnormality of the coronary arteries (see Chap. 21).

The classic manifestation of ischemia is angina, which is usually described as a heavy chest pressure or squeezing, a burning feeling, or difficulty breathing (see Chap. 12). The discomfort often radiates to the left shoulder, neck, or arm. It typically builds in intensity over a period of a few minutes. The pain may begin with exercise or psychological stress, but ACS most commonly occurs without obvious precipitating factors.

Atypical descriptions of chest pain reduce the likelihood that the symptoms represent myocardial ischemia or injury. The American College of Cardiology (ACC) and American Heart Association (AHA) guidelines list the following as pain descriptions that are not characteristic of myocardial ischemia[8]:

- Pleuritic pain (i.e., sharp or knifelike pain brought on by respiratory movements or cough)
- Primary or sole location of discomfort in the middle or lower abdominal region
- Pain that may be localized at the tip of one finger, particularly over the left ventricular apex
- Pain reproduced with movement or palpation of the chest wall or arms
- Constant pain that persists for many hours
- Very brief episodes of pain that last a few seconds or less
- Pain that radiates into the lower extremities

Data from large populations of patients with acute chest pain indicate that ACS occurs in patients with atypical symptoms with sufficient frequency that no single factor should be used to exclude the diagnosis of acute ischemic heart disease. In particular, women, older persons, and individuals with diabetes may be more likely to report atypical symptoms of myocardial ischemia or infarction (see Chap. 81).

Pericardial Disease

The visceral surface of the pericardium is insensitive to pain, as is most of the parietal surface. Therefore, noninfectious causes of pericarditis (e.g., uremia; see Chap. 75) usually cause little or no pain. In contrast, infectious pericarditis almost always involves surrounding pleura, so that patients typically experience pleuritic pain with breathing, coughing, and changes in position. Swallowing may induce the pain because of the proximity of the esophagus to the posterior heart. Because the central diaphragm receives its sensory supply from the phrenic nerve, and the phrenic nerve arises from the third to fifth cervical segments of the spinal cord, pain from infectious pericarditis is frequently felt in the shoulders and neck. Involvement of the more lateral diaphragm can lead to symptoms in the upper abdomen and

TABLE 53-1 Common Causes of Acute Chest Pain

SYSTEM	SYNDROME	CLINICAL DESCRIPTION	KEY DISTINGUISHING FEATURES
Cardiac	Angina	Retrosternal chest pressure, burning, or heaviness; radiating occasionally to neck, jaw, epigastrium, shoulders, left arm	Precipitated by exercise, cold weather, or emotional stress; duration 2-10 min
	Rest or unstable angina	Same as angina, but may be more severe	Typically <20 min; lower tolerance for exertion; crescendo pattern
	Acute myocardial infarction	Same as angina, but may be more severe	Sudden onset, usually lasting ≥30 min; often associated with shortness of breath, weakness, nausea, vomiting
	Pericarditis	Sharp, pleuritic pain aggravated by changes in position; highly variable duration	Pericardial friction rub
Vascular	Aortic dissection	Excruciating, ripping pain of sudden onset in anterior of chest, often radiating to back	Marked severity of unrelenting pain; usually occurs in setting of hypertension or underlying connective tissue disorder such as Marfan syndrome
	Pulmonary embolism	Sudden onset of dyspnea and pain, usually pleuritic with pulmonary infarction	Dyspnea, tachypnea, tachycardia, signs of right heart failure
	Pulmonary hypertension	Substernal chest pressure, exacerbated by exertion	Pain associated with dyspnea and signs of pulmonary hypertension
Pulmonary	Pleuritis and/or pneumonia	Pleuritic pain, usually brief, over involved area	Pain pleuritic and lateral to midline, associated with dyspnea
	Tracheobronchitis	Burning discomfort in midline	Midline location, associated with coughing
	Spontaneous pneumothorax	Sudden onset of unilateral pleuritic pain, with dyspnea	Abrupt onset of dyspnea and pain
Gastrointestinal	Esophageal reflux	Burning substernal and epigastric discomfort, 10-60 min in duration	Aggravated by large meal and postprandial recumbency; relieved by antacid
	Peptic ulcer	Prolonged epigastric or substernal burning	Relieved by antacid or food
	Gallbladder disease	Prolonged epigastric or right upper quadrant pain	Unprovoked or following meal
	Pancreatitis	Prolonged, intense epigastric and substernal pain	Risk factors including alcohol, hypertriglyceridemia, medications
Musculoskeletal	Costochondritis	Sudden onset of intense fleeting pain	May be reproduced by pressure over affected joint; occasionally, swelling and inflammation over costochondral joint
	Cervical disc disease	Sudden onset of fleeting pain	May be reproduced with movement of neck
	Trauma or strain	Constant pain	Reproduced by palpation or movement of chest wall or arms
Infectious	Herpes zoster	Prolonged burning pain in dermatomal distribution	Vesicular rash, dermatomal distribution
Psychological	Panic disorder	Chest tightness or aching, often accompanied by dyspnea and lasting 30 minutes or more, unrelated to exertion or movement	Patient may have other evidence of emotional disorder

back, creating confusion with pancreatitis or cholecystitis. Pericarditis occasionally causes a steady, crushing substernal pain that resembles that of acute myocardial infarction.[9]

Vascular Disease

Acute aortic dissection (see Chap. 60) usually causes the sudden onset of excruciating ripping pain, the location of which reflects the site and progression of the dissection. Ascending aortic dissections tend to manifest with pain in the midline of the anterior chest, and posterior descending aortic dissections tend to manifest with pain in the back of the chest. Aortic dissections are rare, with an estimated annual incidence of 3/100,000, and usually occur in the presence of risk factors including Marfan and Ehlers-Danlos syndromes, bicuspid aortic valve, pregnancy (for proximal dissections), and hypertension (for distal dissections).

Pulmonary emboli (see Chap. 77) often cause the sudden onset of dyspnea and pleuritic chest pain, although they may be asymptomatic. The annual incidence is approximately 1 per 1000, though this number is likely an underestimate. Massive pulmonary emboli tend to cause severe and persistent substernal pain, attributed to distention of the pulmonary artery. Smaller emboli that lead to pulmonary infarction can cause lateral pleuritic chest pain. Hemodynamically significant pulmonary emboli may cause hypotension, syncope, and signs of right heart failure. Pulmonary hypertension (see Chap. 78) can cause chest pain similar to that of angina pectoris, presumably because of right heart hypertrophy and ischemia.

Pulmonary Conditions

Pulmonary conditions that cause chest pain usually produce dyspnea and pleuritic symptoms, the location of which reflects the site of pulmonary disease. Tracheobronchitis tends to be associated with a burning midline pain, whereas pneumonia can produce pain over the involved lung. The pain of a pneumothorax is sudden in onset and is usually accompanied by dyspnea. Primary pneumothorax typically occurs in tall, thin young men; secondary pneumothorax occurs in the setting of pulmonary disease such as chronic obstructive pulmonary disease, asthma, or cystic fibrosis. Asthma exacerbations can present with chest discomfort, typically characterized as tightness.

Gastrointestinal Conditions

Irritation of the esophagus by acid reflux can produce a burning discomfort that is exacerbated by alcohol, aspirin, and some foods. Symptoms often are worsened by a recumbent position and relieved by sitting upright and by acid-reducing therapies. Esophageal spasm can produce a squeezing chest discomfort similar to that of angina.[10] Mallory-Weiss tears of the esophagus can occur in patients who have had prolonged vomiting episodes. Severe vomiting can also cause esophageal rupture (Boerhaave syndrome) with mediastinitis. Chest pain caused by peptic ulcer disease usually occurs 60 to 90 minutes after meals and is typically relieved rapidly by acid-reducing therapies. This pain is usually epigastric in location but can radiate into the chest and shoulders. Cholecystitis produces a wide range of pain syndromes and usually causes right upper quadrant abdominal pain, but chest and back pain caused by this disorder is not unusual. The pain is often described as aching or colicky. Pancreatitis typically causes an intense, aching epigastric pain that may radiate to the back. Relief through acid-reducing therapies is limited.

Musculoskeletal and Other Causes

Chest pain can arise from musculoskeletal disorders involving the chest wall, such as costochondritis, by conditions affecting the nerves of the chest wall, such as cervical disc disease, by herpes zoster, or following heavy exercise. Musculoskeletal syndromes causing chest pain are often elicited by direct pressure over the affected area or by movement of the patient's neck. The pain itself can be fleeting, or can be a dull ache that lasts for hours. Panic syndrome is a major cause of chest discomfort in ED patients. The symptoms typically include chest tightness, often accompanied by shortness of breath and a sense of anxiety, and generally last 30 minutes or longer.

Diagnostic Considerations

Clinical Evaluation

When evaluating patients with acute chest pain, the clinician must address a series of issues related to prognosis and immediate management. Even before trying to arrive at a definite diagnosis, high-priority questions include the following:

- *Clinical stability:* Does the patient need immediate treatment for actual or impending circulatory collapse or respiratory insufficiency?
- *Immediate prognosis:* If the patient is currently clinically stable, what is the risk that he or she has a life-threatening condition such as an ACS, pulmonary embolism, or aortic dissection?
- *Safety of triage options:* If the risk of a life-threatening condition is low, is it safe to discharge the patient for outpatient management, or should he or she undergo further testing or observation to guide management?

Initial Assessment

Evaluation of the patient with acute chest pain can begin before the physician sees the patient, and thus effectiveness may depend on the actions of the office staff and other nonphysician personnel. Guidelines from the ACC and AHA[8] (see Chaps. 55 and 56, Guidelines sections) emphasize that patients with symptoms consistent with ACS should not be evaluated solely over the telephone but should be referred to facilities that allow evaluation by a physician and the recording of a 12-lead electrocardiogram (ECG).[11] These guidelines also recommend strong consideration of immediate referral to an ED or a specialized chest pain unit for patients with suspected ACS who experience chest discomfort at rest for longer than 20 minutes, hemodynamic instability, or recent syncope or near-syncope. Transport as a passenger in a private vehicle is considered an acceptable alternative to an emergency vehicle only if the wait would lead to a delay longer than 20 to 30 minutes.

The National Heart Attack Alert Program guidelines[12] recommend that patients with the following chief complaints should undergo immediate assessment by triage nurses and be referred for further evaluation:

- Chest pain, pressure, tightness, or heaviness; pain that radiates to neck, jaw, shoulders, back, or one or both arms
- Indigestion or heartburn; nausea and/or vomiting associated with chest discomfort
- Persistent shortness of breath
- Weakness, dizziness, lightheadedness, loss of consciousness

For such patients, the initial assessment involves taking a history, performing a physical examination, obtaining an ECG and chest radiograph, and measuring biomarkers of myocardial injury.

HISTORY. If the patient does not need immediate intervention because of impending or actual circulatory collapse or respiratory insufficiency, the physician's assessment should begin with a clinical history that captures the characteristics of the patient's pain, including its quality, location, and radiation, the time and tempo (abrupt or gradual) of onset, the duration of symptoms, provoking or palliating activities, and any associated symptoms, particularly those that are pulmonary or gastrointestinal. ACS is typically described as a diffuse substernal chest pressure that starts gradually, radiates to the jaw or arms, and is worsened by exertion and relieved by rest or nitroglycerin. Studies have suggested that response to nitroglycerin may not reliably discriminate cardiac chest pain from noncardiac chest pain.[13] In contrast to the tempo of the chest pain in ACS, pulmonary embolism, aortic dissection, and pneumothorax all present with chest pain that is sudden and severe in onset. Moreover, pain that is pleuritic or positional in nature suggests pulmonary embolism, pericarditis, pneumonia, or a musculoskeletal condition.

In addition to the characteristics of the acute episode, the presence of risk factors for atherosclerosis (e.g., advanced age, male sex, diabetes) increases the likelihood that the chest pain is caused by myocardial ischemia. A history of MI is associated not only with a high risk of obstructive coronary disease but also with an increased likelihood of multivessel disease. Younger patients have a lower risk of ACS but should be screened with greater care for histories of recent cocaine use (see Chap. 73).[14]

PHYSICAL EXAMINATION (see Chap. 12). The initial examination of patients with acute chest pain should aim to identify potential precipitating causes of myocardial ischemia (e.g., uncontrolled hypertension), important comorbid conditions (e.g., chronic obstructive pulmonary disease), and evidence of hemodynamic complications (e.g., congestive heart failure, new mitral regurgitation, hypotension).[8] In addition to vital signs, examination of the peripheral vessels should include assessment of the presence of bruits or absent pulses that suggest extracardiac vascular disease.

For patients whose clinical presentations do not suggest myocardial ischemia, the search for noncoronary causes of chest pain should focus first on potentially life-threatening issues (e.g., aortic dissection, pulmonary embolism), and then turn to the possibility of other cardiac diagnoses (e.g., pericarditis) and noncardiac diagnoses (e.g., esophageal discomfort). Aortic dissection is suggested by blood pressure or pulse disparities or by a new murmur of aortic regurgitation accompanied by back or midline anterior chest pain. Differences in breath sounds in the presence of acute dyspnea and pleuritic chest pain raise the possibility of pneumothorax. Tachycardia, tachypnea, and an accentuated pulmonic component of the second heart sound (P_2) may be the major manifestations of pulmonary embolism on physical examination.

ELECTROCARDIOGRAPHY (see Chap. 13). A critical source of data, the ECG, should be obtained within 10 minutes after presentation in patients with ongoing chest discomfort and as rapidly as possible in patients who have a history of chest discomfort consistent with ACS but whose discomfort has resolved by the time of evaluation, to identify patients who might benefit from immediate reperfusion therapy (mechanical or pharmacologic).[11]

The ECG provides critical information for both diagnosis and prognosis. New persistent or transient ST-segment abnormalities (≥0.05 mV) that develop during a symptomatic episode at rest and resolve when the symptoms resolve strongly suggest acute ischemia and severe coronary disease. Nonspecific ST-segment and T wave abnormalities are usually defined as lesser amounts of ST-segment deviation or T wave inversion of 0.2 mV or less, and are less helpful for risk stratification. A completely normal ECG does not exclude the possibility of ACS; the risk of acute MI is about 4% among patients with a history of coronary artery disease and 2% among patients with no such history.[15] However, patients with a normal or near-normal ECG have a better prognosis than patients with clearly abnormal ECGs at presentation. Moreover, a normal ECG has a negative predictive value of 80% to 90%, regardless of whether the patient was experiencing chest pain at the time the ECG was obtained.[16] Diffuse ST-segment elevation and PR-segment depression suggest pericarditis. Right axis deviation, right bundle branch block, T wave inversions in leads V_1 to V_4, and an S wave in lead I and Q wave and T wave inversion in lead III suggest pulmonary embolism.

The availability of a prior ECG improves diagnostic accuracy and reduces the rate of admission for patients with abnormal baseline tracings. Serial electrocardiographic tracings improve the clinician's ability to diagnose acute MI, particularly if combined with serial measurement of cardiac biomarkers. Continuous electrocardiographic monitoring to detect ST-segment shifts is technically feasible but makes an uncertain contribution to patient management. Posterior leads can be useful for identifying ischemia in the territory supplied by the left circumflex coronary artery, which is otherwise relatively silent electrocardiographically.

CHEST RADIOGRAPHY. A chest radiograph is typically obtained in all patients presenting with chest pain. It is usually nondiagnostic in patients with ACS, but can show pulmonary edema caused by ischemia-induced diastolic or systolic dysfunction. It is more useful for diagnosing or suggesting other disorders; for example, it may show a widened mediastinum or aortic knob in aortic dissection. The chest radiograph is usually normal in pulmonary embolism, but can show atelectasis, an elevated hemidiaphragm, a pleural effusion or, more rarely, Hampton's hump or Westermark's sign. The chest radiograph can reveal pneumonia or pneumothorax.

BIOMARKERS. Patients presenting with chest discomfort possibly consistent with ACS should have biomarkers of myocardial injury measured (see Chaps. 55 and 56). The preferred biomarker is a cardiac troponin (T or I; cTnT or cTnI); creatine kinase MB isoenzyme (CK-MB) is less sensitive.[8]

Diagnostic Performance

Studies of the diagnostic performance of cTnI, cTnT, or CK-MB indicate that when any of these test findings are abnormal, the patient has a high likelihood of having an ACS. It should be acknowledged, however, that it is inherently challenging to define the diagnostic performance of biomarkers for MI because part of the definition of MI includes the rise and fall of a cardiac biomarker of necrosis. Nevertheless, these assays are indispensible in the diagnosis of MI, and using the totality of clinical evidence as the reference standard for diagnosis, they have excellent sensitivity and specificity.

TROPONINS. Different genes encode troponins I and T in cardiac muscle, slow skeletal muscle, and fast skeletal muscle; hence, the assays for cardiac troponins are more specific than the assay for CK-MB for myocardial injury, and cardiac troponin is the preferred diagnostic biomarker.[17] The high specificity of cardiac troponins for myocardium make false-positive elevations (i.e., an elevated cardiac troponin in the absence of myocardial injury) exceedingly rare. Rather, elevations in the absence of other clinical data consistent with an ACS usually represent true myocardial damage from causes other than atherosclerotic coronary artery disease. Such damage may occur with other forms of myocardial injury, such as in the setting of myocarditis, myocardial contusion, or cardioversion or defibrillation, left ventricular strain from congestive heart failure,[18] hypertensive crisis, or extreme exercise, right ventricular strain from pulmonary embolus,[19] or other causes of acute pulmonary hypertension. Elevated levels of cardiac troponins have been reported in patients with renal disease.[20] The exact mechanism remains unclear, but in patients with a clinical history suggestive of ACS, an elevated cardiac troponin level conveys a similarly increased risk of ischemic complications in patients across a broad range of renal function.[21] Elevated cardiac troponin levels can also occur in patients with severe sepsis[22]; again, the mechanism remains unclear.

With serial sampling up to 12 hours after presentation, cardiac troponins offer a sensitivity higher than 95% and a specificity of 90%. When using only a single sample at presentation, performance has been substantially worse, with a sensitivity of only 70% to 75%. Recently, however, sensitive assays have been developed that offer a lower limit of detection, (approximately 0.001 to 0.01 ng/mL, depending on the specific assay) and acceptable imprecision at low levels that, importantly, are now below the 99th percentile in a normal reference population (typically 0.01 to 0.07 ng/mL), thereby improving the ability to detect myocardial injury. Using such assays, the sensitivity for detecting myocardial infarction using a single sample at presentation is approximately 90%, the specificity approximately 90%, and the negative predictive value approximately 97% to 99%.[3,23,24] Moreover, among patients presenting within 3 hours of the onset of chest pain, the superior performance of high-sensitivity assays is even more striking, a sensitivity of 80% to 85%, compared with approximately 55% for older assays. The area under the receiver operator characteristic curve is as high as 0.98 using serial samples for high-sensitivity assays.

Ultrasensitive assays with even lower limits of detection (e.g., <0.001 ng/mL or <1 pg/mL) are also being developed, allowing almost all individuals (including healthy persons) to have a quantifiable troponin result. Using such assays, in patients with non–ST-elevation MI, 72% had circulating troponin levels at baseline above the 99th percentile and another 28% had levels above the limit of detection. Moreover, in patients with unstable angina (defined as lack of elevation of troponin level using a current-generation commercial assay), 44% had circulating troponin levels above the 99th percentile and another 52% had levels above the limit of detection at baseline; 6 to 8 hours later, these values were 82% and 18%, respectively.[25] Similarly, ultrasensitive assays can detect increases in circulating troponin in proportion to the amount of ischemia experienced during exercise stress testing.[26] Thus, in the future, troponin may move from a semiquantitative assay (negative in most individuals, quantified in a subset) to quantifiable in all. The clinical implications of very low level values reported from ultrasensitive assays will need to be defined.

CREATINE KINASE MB ISOENZYME. Until the advent of cardiac troponin assays, CK-MB was the biomarker of choice for the diagnosis of MI. The major limitation to CK-MB as a diagnostic biomarker is its relative lack of specificity, because it can be found in skeletal muscle, tongue, diaphragm, small intestine, uterus, and prostate. Use of the CK-MB relative index (the ratio of CK-MB to total CK) partially addresses this limitation for skeletal muscle as a source. However, the amount of CK-MB is increased in skeletal muscle in patients with conditions that cause chronic muscle destruction and regeneration, such as muscular dystrophy, high-performance athletics (e.g., marathon running), or rhabdomyolysis.[27] CK-MB elevations are particularly common in ED patients because they have higher rates of histories of alcohol abuse or trauma. One advantage of CK-MB is a shorter half-life in the circulation, which makes it useful for gauging the timing of an MI (a normal CK-MB with an elevated troponin level could represent a small MI or an MI that occurred several days ago) and for diagnosing reinfarction in a patient who has had an MI in the past week.

OTHER MARKERS. Serum myoglobin and heart-type fatty acid binding protein (H-FABP) are smaller molecules and diffuse through interstitial fluids more rapidly after cell death than the larger CK and troponin molecules; they become abnormal as early as 30 minutes after myocardial injury.[28] Because neither is specific to myocardial tissue, however, false-positive rates in ED populations are high.[29]

Many patients presenting with ACS, including those without evidence of myocyte necrosis, have elevated concentrations of inflammatory biomarkers such as C-reactive protein,[30] serum amyloid A, myeloperoxidase,[31] or interleukin-6 (IL-6). To date, no study has identified exact decision cut points or shown an incremental benefit on an admission or treatment strategy based on these new markers, so the clinical usefulness of these observations remains uncertain.

Ischemia-modified albumin (IMA) has been approved by the U.S. Food and Drug Administration for clinical use. The albumin cobalt binding test for the detection of IMA is based on the observation that the affinity of the N-terminus of human albumin for cobalt is reduced in patients with myocardial ischemia.[32] As with the other markers, however, the clinical specificity of IMA in the broad population of patients with chest pain and suspected ACS remains an area for further investigation.[33]

D-dimer testing is useful for patients with chest pain to help rule out pulmonary embolism, because a negative enzyme-linked immunosorbent assay (ELISA) test has a negative predictive value of more than 99% in patients with a low clinical probability (patients with a higher clinical probability should undergo an imaging study).[34]

B-type natriuretic peptides (BNP and N-terminal pro-BNP [NT-proBNP]) arise in the setting of increased ventricular wall stress. Natriuretic peptides are most commonly used to aid in the diagnosis of heart failure.[35] BNP levels can be elevated in the setting of transient myocardial ischemia,[36] and the magnitude of elevation in ACS is correlated with prognosis.[37] However, the lack of specificity of natriuretic peptide elevation for ACS limits its use as a diagnostic marker.

PROGNOSTIC IMPLICATIONS OF TEST RESULTS. Abnormal levels of CK-MB, cTnI, and cTnT predict an increased risk of complications.[8] Even if patients do not have CK-MB elevations, cTnI and cTnT are helpful for early risk stratification in patients with acute chest pain. The notion that a patient who has a slight elevation in troponin has an "infarctlet" of questionable prognostic significance should be abandoned.[38] The prognostic value of cTnI seems to be comparable to that of cTnT.

Testing Strategy

The 2007 National Academy of Clinical Biochemistry (NACB) practice guidelines recommend the measurement of biomarkers of cardiac injury in patients with symptoms that suggest ACS (**Table 53-2**). Furthermore, patients with a very low probability of ACS should not undergo measurement of biomarkers because false-positive results could lead to unnecessary hospitalizations, tests, procedures, and complications.

The ACC, AHA, and NACB guidelines recommend cTnI or cTnT as the preferred first-line markers, but CK-MB (by mass assay) is an acceptable alternative. The preference for cardiac troponins reflects the greater specificity of these markers compared with CK-MB and the prognostic value of troponin elevations in the presence of normal CK-MB levels. If the initial set of markers is negative in patients who have presented within the first 6 hours of the onset of pain, the guidelines recommend that another sample be drawn in the time frame of 8 to 12 hours after symptom onset.

Decision Aids

An algorithm for the diagnostic evaluation of chest pain is shown in **Figure 53-1**. The history, physical examination, ECG, and biomarkers of myocardial injury can be integrated to allow the clinician to assess the likelihood of ACS and the risk of complications (**Tables 53-3 and 53-4**). Furthermore, in terms of prognosis, multivariable algorithms have been developed and prospectively validated, with the goal of improving risk stratification in patients with acute chest pain. These algorithms can be used to estimate the probability of acute myocardial infarction, acute ischemic heart disease, or the risk of major cardiac complications in individual patients.[15] They serve mainly to identify patients who are at low risk for complications and who therefore do not require admission to the hospital or coronary care unit.

A prospectively validated algorithm for the prediction of the risk of complications requiring intensive care is presented as a flow chart in **Figure 53-2**.[39] In this algorithm, patients with suspected myocardial infarction on their ECGs are immediately classified as having a high risk (approximately 16%) of major complications within the next 72 hours. Patients whose ECGs are consistent with ischemia but not infarction are then classified as having an intermediate (approximately 8%) or high risk for complications, depending on the presence or absence of clinical risk factors, including systolic blood pressure below 110 mm Hg, bilateral rales heard above the bases, and known unstable ischemic heart disease (defined as worsening of previously stable angina, a new onset of angina after infarction or after a coronary revascularization procedure, or pain that was the same as that associated with a prior MI). These same risk factors help stratify patients without ischemic changes on their ECGs.

TABLE 53-2 National Academy of Clinical Biochemistry Recommendations for Use of Biochemical Markers for Risk Stratification in Acute Coronary Syndrome

Class I

1. Patients with suspected ACS should undergo early risk stratification based on an integrated assessment of symptoms, physical examination findings, electrocardiographic findings, and biomarkers (level of evidence: C).
2. A cardiac troponin is the preferred marker for risk stratification and, if available, should be measured in all patients with suspected ACS. In patients with a clinical syndrome consistent with ACS, a maximal (peak) concentration exceeding the 99th percentile of values for a reference control group should be considered indicative of increased risk of death and recurrent ischemic events (level of evidence: A).
3. Blood should be obtained for testing on hospital presentation followed by serial sampling, with timing of sampling based on the clinical circumstances. For most patients, blood should be obtained for testing at hospital presentation, and at 6 to 9 hours (level of evidence: B).

Class IIa

4. Measurement of hs-CRP may be useful, in addition to a cardiac troponin, for risk assessment in patients with a clinical syndrome consistent with ACS. The benefits of therapy based on this strategy remain uncertain (level of evidence: A).
5. Measurement of B-type natriuretic peptide (BNP) or N-terminal pro-BNP (NT-proBNP) may be useful, in addition to a cardiac troponin, for risk assessment in patients with a clinical syndrome consistent with ACS. The benefits of therapy based on this strategy remain uncertain (level of evidence: A).

Class IIb

6. Measurement of markers of myocardial ischemia, in addition to cardiac troponin and ECG, may aid in excluding ACS in patients with a low clinical probability of myocardial ischemia (level of evidence: C).
7. A multimarker strategy that includes measurement of two or more pathobiologically diverse biomarkers, in addition to a cardiac troponin, may aid in enhancing risk stratification in patients with a clinical syndrome consistent with ACS. BNP and high-sensitivity C-reactive protein (hsCRP) are the biomarkers best studied using this approach. The benefits of therapy based on this strategy remain uncertain (level of evidence: C).
8. Early repeat sampling of cardiac troponin (e.g., 2-4 hours after presentation) may be appropriate if tied to therapeutic strategies (level of evidence: C).

Class III

Biomarkers of necrosis should not be used for routine screening of patients with low clinical probability of ACS (level of evidence: C).

From Morrow DA, Cannon CP, Jesse RL, et al: National Academy of Clinical Biochemistry Laboratory medicine practice guidelines: Clinical characteristics and utilization of biochemical markers in acute coronary syndromes. Circulation 115:e356, 2007.

Immediate Management

The ACC and AHA guidelines suggest an approach to the immediate management of patients with possible ACS that integrates information from the history, physical examination, 12-lead ECG, and initial cardiac marker tests to assign patients to four categories—noncardiac diagnosis, chronic stable angina, possible ACS, and definite ACS (**Fig. 53-3**).[8] In this algorithm, patients with ST-segment elevations are triaged immediately for reperfusion therapy, in accordance with the ACC and AHA guidelines for acute MI. Patients with ACS who have ST wave or T wave changes, ongoing pain, positive cardiac markers, or hemodynamic abnormalities should be admitted to the hospital for the management of acute ischemia. Cost-effectiveness analyses support triage of such patients to the coronary care unit for their initial care. For patients with possible or definite ACS who do not have diagnostic ECGs and whose initial serum cardiac markers are within normal limits, observation in a chest pain unit or other nonintensive care facility is appropriate, with subsequent additional testing (see later).

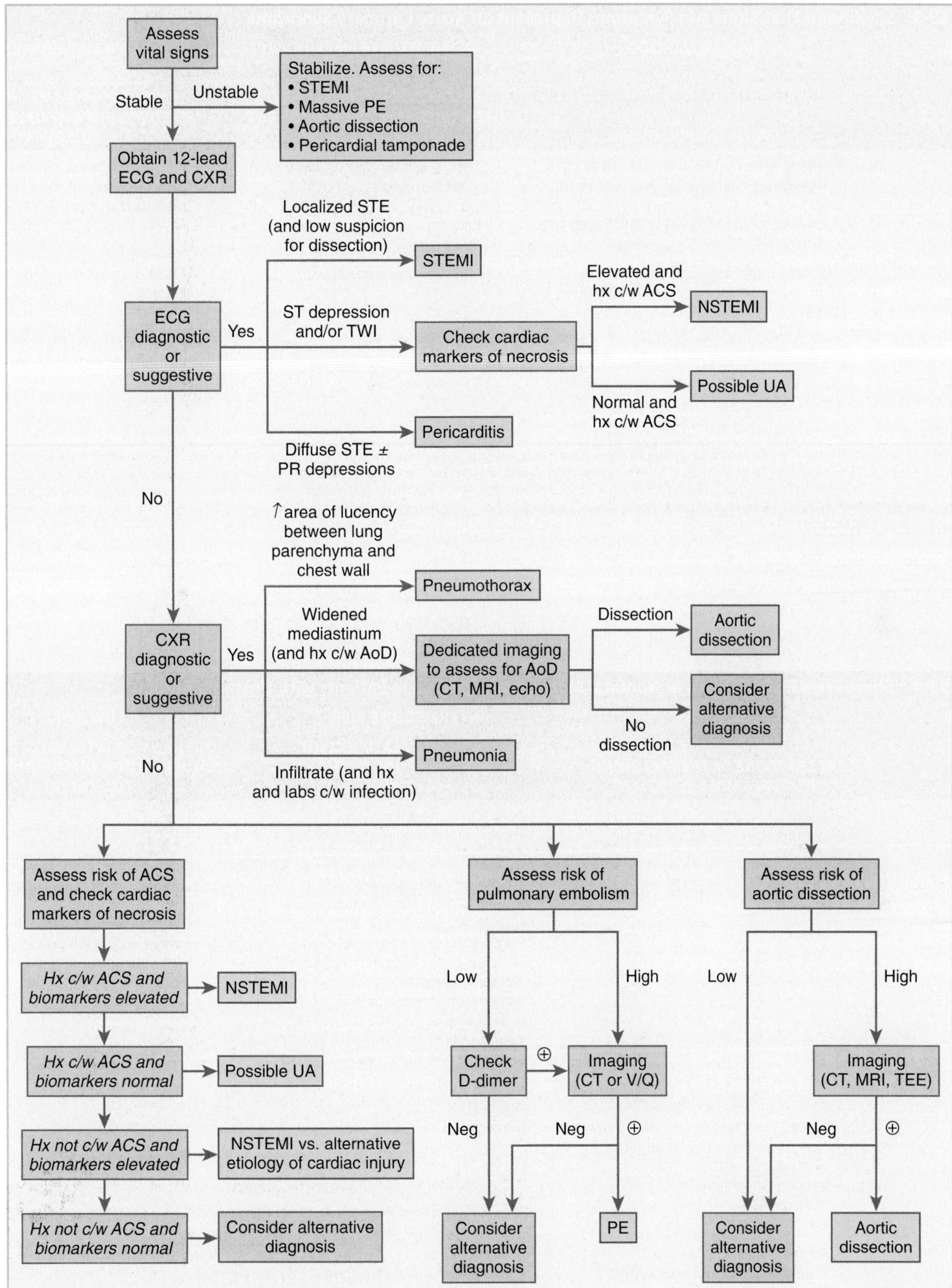

FIGURE 53-1 Algorithm for the initial diagnostic approach to a patient with chest pain. AoD = aortic dissection; c/w = consistent with; CXR = chest x-ray; hx = history; NSTEMI = non–ST-segment myocardial infarction; PE = pulmonary embolism; STE = ST elevation; STEMI = ST-segment myocardial infarction; TEE = transesophageal echocardiography; UA = unstable angina; V/Q = ventilation-perfusion scan.

CH 53

TABLE 53-3 Likelihood That Signs and Symptoms Represent an Acute Coronary Syndrome

FEATURE	HIGH LIKELIHOOD *ANY OF THE FOLLOWING*	INTERMEDIATE LIKELIHOOD *ABSENCE OF HIGH-LIKELIHOOD FEATURES AND PRESENCE OF ANY OF THE FOLLOWING*	LOW LIKELIHOOD *ABSENCE OF HIGH- OR INTERMEDIATE-LIKELIHOOD FEATURES, BUT MAY HAVE ANY OF THE FOLLOWING*
History	• Chest or left arm pain or discomfort as chief symptom reproducing documented angina prior • Known history of coronary artery disease, including MI	• Chest or left arm pain or discomfort as chief symptom • Age > 70 yr • Male sex • Diabetes mellitus	• Probable ischemic symptoms in absence of any of the intermediate-likelihood characteristics • Recent cocaine use
Examination	• Transient mitral regurgitation murmur, hypotension, diaphoresis, pulmonary edema, or rales	• Extracardiac vascular disease	• Chest discomfort reproduced by palpation
Electrocardiogram	• New, or presumably new, transient ST-segment deviation (≥0.1 mV) or T wave inversion (≥0.2 mV) in multiple precordial leads	• Fixed Q waves • ST-segment depression 0.05-0.1 mV or T wave inversion > 0.1 mV	• T wave flattening or inversion < 0.1 mV in leads with dominant R waves • Normal ECG
Cardiac markers	• Elevated cardiac TnI, TnT, or CK-MB	• Normal	• Normal

From Anderson JL, Adams CD, Antman EM, et al: ACC/AHA 2007 guidelines for the management of patients with unstable angina/non ST-elevation myocardial infarction: A report of the American College of Cardiology/American Heart Association Task Force on Practice Guidelines (Writing Committee to Revise the 2002 Guidelines for the Management of Patients With Unstable Angina/Non ST-Elevation Myocardial Infarction): Developed in collaboration with the American College of Emergency Physicians, the Society for Cardiovascular Angiography and Interventions, and the Society of Thoracic Surgeons: Endorsed by the American Association of Cardiovascular and Pulmonary Rehabilitation and the Society for Academic Emergency Medicine. Circulation 116:e148, 2007.

TABLE 53-4 Short-Term Risk of Death or Nonfatal Myocardial Ischemia in Patients with Unstable Angina

FEATURE	HIGH RISK *AT LEAST ONE OF THE FOLLOWING FEATURES MUST BE PRESENT*	INTERMEDIATE RISK *NO HIGH-RISK FEATURES, BUT MUST HAVE ONE OF THE FOLLOWING*	LOW RISK *NO HIGH- OR INTERMEDIATE-RISK FEATURES, BUT MAY HAVE ANY OF THE FOLLOWING*
History	• Accelerating tempo of ischemic symptoms in preceding 48 hours	• Prior MI, peripheral or cerebrovascular disease, or CABG; prior ASA use	
Character of pain	• Prolonged ongoing (>20 min) pain at rest	• Prolonged (>20 min) rest angina, now resolved, with intermediate or high likelihood of CAD • Rest angina (>20 min) or relieved with rest or sublingual nitroglycerin • Nocturnal angina • New-onset or progressive CCS class III or IV angina in past 2 wk without prolonged (20 min) rest pain, but with intermediate or high likelihood of CAD	• Increased angina frequency, severity, or duration • Angina provoked at a lower threshold • New-onset angina with onset 2 wk-2 mo prior to presentation
Clinical findings	• Pulmonary edema, most likely caused by ischemia • New or worsening MR murmur • S_3 or new or worsening rales • Hypotension, bradycardia, tachycardia • Age >75 yr	• Age > 70 yr	
Electrocardiogram	• Angina at rest with transient ST-segment changes > 0.05 mV • Bundle branch block, new or presumed new • Sustained ventricular tachycardia	• T wave changes • Pathologic Q waves or resting ST-segment depression < 0.1 mV in multiple lead groups (anterior, inferior, lateral)	• Normal or unchanged ECG
Cardiac markers	• Elevated cardiac TnI, TnT, or CK-MB	• Slightly elevated cardiac TnI, TnT, or CK-MB	• Normal

ASA = acetylsalicylic acid; CABG = coronary artery bypass grafting; CCS = *Canadian Cardiovascular Society;* MR = mitral regurgitation; NTG = nitroglycerin.

From Anderson JL, Adams CD, Antman EM, et al: ACC/AHA 2007 guidelines for the management of patients with unstable angina/non ST-elevation myocardial infarction: A report of the American College of Cardiology/American Heart Association Task Force on Practice Guidelines (Writing Committee to Revise the 2002 Guidelines for the Management of Patients With Unstable Angina/Non ST-Elevation Myocardial Infarction): Developed in collaboration with the American College of Emergency Physicians, the Society for Cardiovascular Angiography and Interventions, and the Society of Thoracic Surgeons: Endorsed by the American Association of Cardiovascular and Pulmonary Rehabilitation and the Society for Academic Emergency Medicine. Circulation 116:e148, 2007.

Suspected myocardial infarction on electrocardiogram
Suspected ischemia on electrocardiogram
No
Yes
No risk factors
One risk factor
Two or more risk factors
One risk factor or none
Two or more risk factors
Very low risk (< 1%)
Low risk (approximately 4%)
Intermediate risk (approximately 8%)
High risk (> 16%)

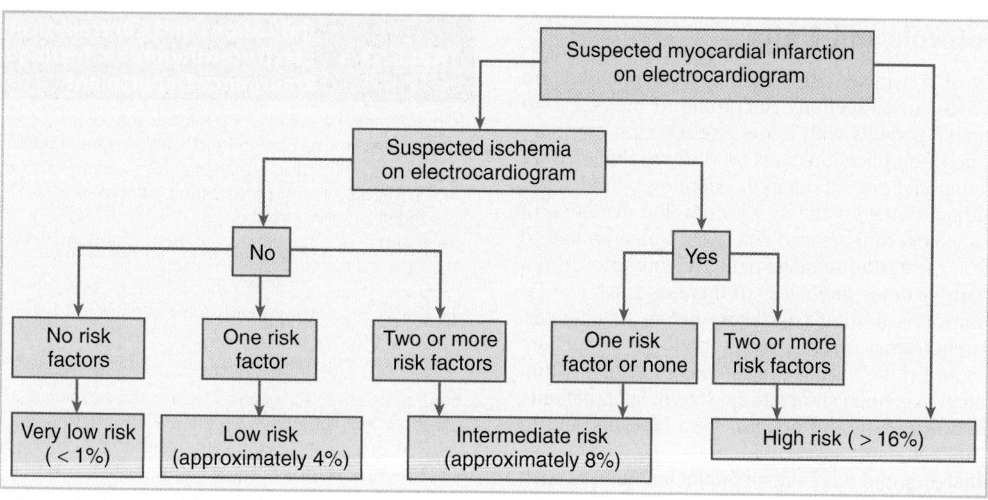

FIGURE 53-2 Derivation and validation of four groups into which patients can be categorized, according to the risk of major cardiac events within 72 hours after admission. Risk factors include: systolic blood pressure below 110 mm Hg, bilateral rales heard above the bases, and known unstable ischemic heart disease (see text for details). *(From Goldman L, Cook EF, Johnson PA, et al: Prediction of the need for intensive care in patients who come to emergency departments with acute chest pain. N Engl J Med 334:1498, 1996.)*

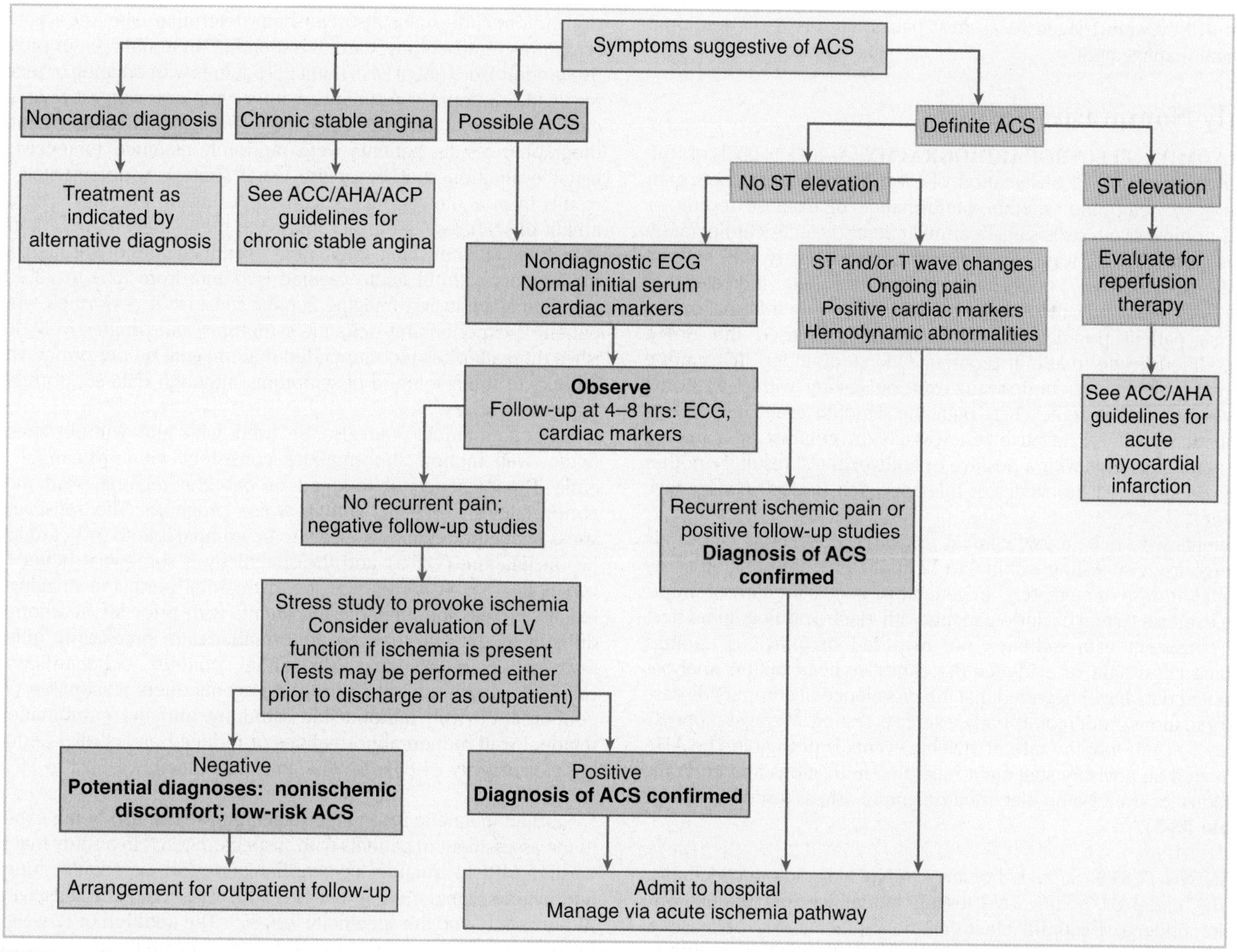

Symptoms suggestive of ACS
Noncardiac diagnosis
Chronic stable angina
Possible ACS
Definite ACS
Treatment as indicated by alternative diagnosis
See ACC/AHA/ACP guidelines for chronic stable angina
No ST elevation
ST elevation
Nondiagnostic ECG Normal initial serum cardiac markers
ST and/or T wave changes Ongoing pain Positive cardiac markers Hemodynamic abnormalities
Evaluate for reperfusion therapy
Observe Follow-up at 4–8 hrs: ECG, cardiac markers
See ACC/AHA guidelines for acute myocardial infarction
No recurrent pain; negative follow-up studies
Recurrent ischemic pain or positive follow-up studies Diagnosis of ACS confirmed
Stress study to provoke ischemia Consider evaluation of LV function if ischemia is present (Tests may be performed either prior to discharge or as outpatient)
Negative Potential diagnoses: nonischemic discomfort; low-risk ACS
Positive Diagnosis of ACS confirmed
Arrangement for outpatient follow-up
Admit to hospital Manage via acute ischemia pathway

FIGURE 53-3 Algorithm for the evaluation and management of patients suspected of having ACS. ACP = American College of Physicians. *(From Anderson JL, Adams CD, Antman EM, et al: ACC/AHA 2007 guidelines for the management of patients with unstable angina/non ST-elevation myocardial infarction: A report of the American College of Cardiology/American Heart Association Task Force on Practice Guidelines [Writing Committee to Revise the 2002 Guidelines for the Management of Patients With Unstable Angina/Non ST-Elevation Myocardial Infarction]: Developed in collaboration with the American College of Emergency Physicians, the Society for Cardiovascular Angiography and Interventions, and the Society of Thoracic Surgeons: Endorsed by the American Association of Cardiovascular and Pulmonary Rehabilitation and the Society for Academic Emergency Medicine. Circulation 116:e148, 2007.)*

Chest Pain Protocols and Units

The main elements of a typical chest pain critical pathway are included in Figure 53-3 (lower section). According to the ACC and AHA recommendations,[8] patients with a low risk of acute coronary syndrome or associated complications can be observed for 6 to 12 hours while undergoing electrocardiographic monitoring and serial measurement of cardiac markers. Patients who develop evidence of ischemia or other indicators of increased risk should be admitted to the coronary care unit for further management. Patients who do not develop recurrent pain or other predictors of increased risk can be triaged for early noninvasive testing (see later) before or after discharge. Outpatient stress testing is a reasonable option if the patient is at low risk for ACS and if the testing can be accomplished within 72 hours; such a strategy has been shown to be safe. In such patients, it is prudent to prescribe aspirin and possibly beta blockers, and to provide them with sublingual nitroglycerin.

To enhance the efficiency and reliability of implementation of such chest pain protocols, many hospitals triage low-risk patients with chest pain to special chest pain units.[40] These units often are located adjacent to or within EDs, but sometimes are located elsewhere in the hospital. In most of these units, the rate of MI has been about 1% to 2%, and they have proven to be safe and cost-saving sites of care for low-risk patients. Chest pain units are also sometimes used for intermediate-risk patients, such as those with a prior history of coronary disease but no other high-risk predictors. In one community-based randomized trial, patients with unstable angina and an overall intermediate risk of complications had similar outcomes and lower costs if they were triaged to a chest pain unit versus conventional hospital management.

Early Noninvasive Testing

TREADMILL ELECTROCARDIOGRAPHY. A major goal of the initial short period of observation of low-risk patients in chest pain units is to determine whether performance of exercise testing or other noninvasive tests is safe. Treadmill exercise electrocardiography is inexpensive and available at many hospitals every day, beyond traditional laboratory hours, and prospective data indicate that early exercise test results provide reliable prognostic information for low-risk patient populations. Most studies have used the Bruce or modified Bruce treadmill protocol. One study found that among low-risk patients who underwent exercise testing within 48 hours of presentation for acute chest pain, the 6-month event rate among 195 patients with a negative test was 2%, in contrast to a rate of 15% among patients with a positive or equivocal test result.[41] Another study documented the safety of this approach in 3000 consecutive patients.[4]

Patients who have a low clinical risk of complications can safely undergo exercise testing within 6 to 12 hours after presentation at the hospital or even immediately.[4] In general, protocols for early or immediate exercise testing exclude patients with electrocardiographic findings consistent with ischemia not recorded on previous tracings, ongoing chest pain, or evidence of congestive heart failure. Analyses of pooled data have suggested that the prevalence of coronary disease in populations undergoing early exercise testing averages approximately 5%, and that the rate of adverse events is negligible. The AHA has issued an advisory statement regarding indications and contraindications for exercise on electrocardiographic stress testing in the ED (**Table 53-5**).[4,42]

TABLE 53-5 Indications and Contraindications for Exercise Electrocardiographic Testing in the Emergency Department

Requirements before exercise electrocardiographic testing that should be considered in the Emergency Department setting:

- Two sets of cardiac enzymes at 4-hr intervals should be normal.
- ECG at the time of presentation and preexercise 12-lead ECG shows no significant abnormality.
- Absence of rest electrocardiographic abnormalities that would preclude accurate assessment of the exercise ECG
- From admission to time that results are available from the second set of cardiac enzymes: patient asymptomatic, lessening chest pain symptoms, or persistent atypical symptoms
- Absence of ischemic chest pain at the time of exercise testing

Contraindications to exercise electrocardiographic testing in the Emergency Department setting:

- New or evolving electrocardiographic abnormalities on the rest tracing
- Abnormal cardiac enzyme levels
- Inability to perform exercise
- Worsening or persistent ischemic chest pain symptoms from admission to the time of exercise testing
- Clinical risk profiling indicating that imminent coronary angiography is likely

IMAGING TESTS. Stress echocardiography and radionuclide scans are the preferred noninvasive testing modalities for patients who cannot undergo treadmill electrocardiographic testing because of physical disability or who have resting ECGs that confound interpretation. Imaging studies are less readily available and more expensive than exercise electrocardiography, but have increased sensitivity for the detection of coronary disease and the ability to quantify the extent of, and localize, jeopardized myocardium. High-risk rest perfusion scans are associated with an increased risk of major cardiac complications, whereas patients with low-risk scans have low 30-day cardiac event rates (<2%).[43-45]

In addition to stress imaging studies to detect provocable ischemia, rest radionuclide scans also can help determine whether a patient's symptoms represent myocardial ischemia.[46] In a multicenter prospective randomized trial of 2475 adult ED patients with ongoing or recently resolved (<3 hours) chest pain or other symptoms suggestive of acute cardiac ischemia, and with normal or nondiagnostic initial electrocardiographic results, patients were randomly assigned to receive the usual evaluation strategy or the usual strategy supplemented with results from acute resting myocardial perfusion imaging.[47] The availability of scan results did not influence the management of patients with acute MI or unstable angina, but it reduced rates of hospitalization for patients without acute cardiac ischemia from 52% to 42%. Rest myocardial perfusion imaging is most sensitive if performed when a patient is experiencing ischemic symptoms, and progressively diminishes thereafter. It is recommended that imaging be performed within 2 hours of the resolution of symptoms, although data support its use for up to 4 hours.[48]

Echocardiography can also be used, with and without stress, to detect wall motion abnormalities consistent with myocardial ischemia. The presence of induced or baseline regional wall motion abnormalities correlates with a worse prognosis. The sensitivity of stress echocardiography appears to be comparable to myocardial perfusion imaging (~85%), and the specificity is somewhat better (95% versus 90%).[49] As is the case for myocardial perfusion imaging, the results are less interpretable in patients with prior MI, in whom it is difficult to exclude that the abnormalities are preexisting unless a prior study is available. Myocardial contrast echocardiography (MCE)[50] using microbubble imaging agents offers reasonable (77%) concordance with radionuclide scanning, and the combination of regional wall motion abnormalities or reduced myocardial perfusion has a sensitivity of 80% to 90% and a specificity of 60% to 90% for ACS.[51,52]

Cardiac magnetic resonance imaging (MRI) is also being explored in the assessment of patients with suspected ACS.[53] In a study that used cardiac MRI to quantify myocardial perfusion, ventricular function, and hyperenhancement in patients with chest pain, the sensitivity for ACS was 84% and the specificity was 85%. The addition of T2-weighted imaging, which can detect myocardial edema and thus help differentiate acute from chronic perfusion defects, improves the specificity to 96% without sacrificing sensitivity.[54] Integration of MRI coronary angiography is being studied.[55] Stress MRI using adenosine, although more labor intensive, has also been studied and shows excellent sensitivity and specificity.[56]

In contrast to the functional imaging data from stress testing, coronary computed tomography angiography (CTA) offers noninvasive anatomic data. Using multidetector computed tomography (MDCT), coronary CTA has a sensitivity of approximately 90% and a specificity of 65% to 90% for coronary stenosis greater than 50%. Coronary CTA has been evaluated in a single-center study of chest pain patients presenting to the ED.[6] Of 368 patients with a nondiagnostic ECG and negative initial biomarker of necrosis, 31 were ultimately diagnosed with ACS. Approximately half of the patients were free of coronary artery disease (CAD) on coronary CTA and 0% had an ACS, yielding a negative predictive value of 100%. The remaining 50% had evidence of atherosclerosis, with 32% having minor plaque and 18% having a stenosis greater than 50%. A final diagnosis of ACS was made in 6% of those with only minor plaque and in 35% with a significant stenosis. The negative predictive value of coronary stenosis by coronary CTA for ACS was 98%. Thus, given the anatomic rather than the functional data provided, coronary CTA may be best suited to rule out rather than rule in ACS. Of the patients who underwent CTA in a randomized comparison of myocardial perfusion imaging versus coronary CTA, 68% had a normal test and were discharged home. Another 24% had an intermediate or nondiagnostic test and underwent myocardial perfusion imaging; most of the results were negative. In total, 89% were discharged from the ED. Among patients who underwent myocardial perfusion imaging, 97% were discharged from the ED. The patients randomized to coronary CTA had a time to diagnosis that was 8 hours shorter, and consequently incurred lower hospital costs. Higher rates of cardiac catheterization and coronary revascularization occurred in the coronary CTA group (11% versus 3% and 5% versus 1%, respectively).[57] The most recent ACC and AHA guidelines acknowledge that coronary CTA is a reasonable alternative to stress testing in patients with low to intermediate probability of CAD.[8]

For both MRI and coronary CTA, additional multicenter studies and considerations related to radiation exposure are needed before such approaches are widely adopted clinically.

REFERENCES

Causes of Acute Chest Pain

1. Pope JH, Aufderheide TP, Ruthazer R, et al: Missed diagnoses of acute cardiac ischemia in the emergency department. N Engl J Med 342:1163, 2000.
2. Lindsell CJ, Anantharaman V, Diercks D, et al: The Internet Tracking Registry of Acute Coronary Syndromes (i*trACS): A multicenter registry of patients with suspicion of acute coronary syndromes reported using the standardized reporting guidelines for emergency department chest pain studies. Ann Emerg Med 48:666, 2006.
3. Morrow DA: Clinical application of sensitive troponin assays. N Engl J Med 361:913, 2009.
4. Amsterdam EA, Kirk JD, Diercks DB, et al: Exercise testing in chest pain units: Rationale, implementation, and results. Cardiol Clin 23:503, 2005.
5. Ekelund U, Forberg JL: New methods for improved evaluation of patients with suspected acute coronary syndrome in the emergency department. Emerg Med J 24:811, 2007.
6. Hoffmann U, Bamberg F, Chae CU, et al: Coronary computed tomography angiography for early triage of patients with acute chest pain: The ROMICAT (Rule Out Myocardial Infarction using Computer Assisted Tomography) trial. J Am Coll Cardiol 53:1642, 2009.
7. Blomkalns AL, Gibler WB: Chest pain unit concept: rationale and diagnostic strategies. Cardiol Clin 23:411, 2005.
8. Anderson JL, Adams CD, Antman EM, et al: ACC/AHA 2007 guidelines for the management of patients with unstable angina/non ST-elevation myocardial infarction: A report of the American College of Cardiology/American Heart Association Task Force on Practice Guidelines (Writing Committee to Revise the 2002 Guidelines for the Management of Patients With Unstable Angina/Non ST-Elevation Myocardial Infarction): Developed in collaboration with the American College of Emergency Physicians, the Society for Cardiovascular Angiography and Interventions, and the Society of Thoracic Surgeons: Endorsed by the American Association of Cardiovascular and Pulmonary Rehabilitation and the Society for Academic Emergency Medicine. Circulation 116:e148, 2007.
9. Lange RA, Hillis LD: Clinical practice. Acute pericarditis. N Engl J Med 351:2195, 2004.
10. Eslick GD: Noncardiac chest pain: Epidemiology, natural history, health care seeking, and quality of life. Gastroenterol Clin North Am 33:1, 2004.

Initial Assessment

11. Antman EM, Anbe DT, Armstrong PW, et al: ACC/AHA guidelines for the management of patients with ST-elevation myocardial infarction: A report of the American College of Cardiology/American Heart Association Task Force on Practice Guidelines (Committee to Revise the 1999 Guidelines for the Management of Patients with Acute Myocardial Infarction). Circulation 110:e82, 2004.
12. National Heart Attack Alert Program Coordinating Committee, 60 Minutes to Treatment Working Group: Emergency department: rapid identification and treatment of patients with acute myocardial infarction. Ann Emerg Med 23:311, 1994.
13. Diercks DB, Boghos E, Guzman H, et al: Changes in the numeric descriptive scale for pain after sublingual nitroglycerin do not predict cardiac etiology of chest pain. Ann Emerg Med 45:581, 2005.
14. McCord J, Jneid H, Hollander JE, et al: Management of cocaine-associated chest pain and myocardial infarction: A scientific statement from the American Heart Association Acute Cardiac Care Committee of the Council on Clinical Cardiology. Circulation 117:1897, 2008.
15. Lee TH, Goldman L: Evaluation of the patient with acute chest pain. N Engl J Med 342:1187, 2000.
16. Turnipseed SD, Trythall WS, Diercks DB, et al: Frequency of acute coronary syndrome in patients with normal electrocardiogram performed during presence or absence of chest pain. Acad Emerg Med 16:495, 2009.

Biomarkers

17. Thygesen K, Alpert JS, White HD: Universal definition of myocardial infarction. J Am Coll Cardiol 50:2173, 2007.
18. Peacock WF 4th, De Marco T, Fonarow GC, et al: Cardiac troponin and outcome in acute heart failure. N Engl J Med 358:2117, 2008.
19. Becattini C, Vedovati MC, Agnelli G: Prognostic value of troponins in acute pulmonary embolism: A meta-analysis. Circulation 116:427, 2007.
20. Khan NA, Hemmelgarn BR, Tonelli M, et al: Prognostic value of troponin T and I among asymptomatic patients with end-stage renal disease: A meta-analysis. Circulation 112:3088, 2005.
21. Wu AH, Jaffe AS, Apple FS, et al: National Academy of Clinical Biochemistry laboratory medicine practice guidelines: Use of cardiac troponin and B-type natriuretic peptide or N-terminal proB-type natriuretic peptide for etiologies other than acute coronary syndromes and heart failure. Clin Chem 53:2086, 2007.
22. Favory R, Neviere R: Significance and interpretation of elevated troponin in septic patients. Crit Care 10:224, 2006.
23. Reichlin T, Hochholzer W, Bassetti S, et al: Early diagnosis of myocardial infarction with sensitive cardiac troponin assays. N Engl J Med 361:858, 2009.
24. Keller T, Zeller T, Peetz D, et al: Sensitive troponin I assay in early diagnosis of acute myocardial infarction. N Engl J Med 61:868, 2009.
25. Wilson SR, Sabatine MS, Braunwald E, et al: Detection of myocardial injury in patients with unstable angina using a novel nanoparticle cardiac troponin I assay: Observations from the PROTECT-TIMI 30 Trial. Am Heart J 158:386, 2009.
26. Sabatine MS, Morrow DA, de Lemos JA, et al: Detection of acute changes in circulating troponin in the setting of transient stress test-induced myocardial ischaemia using an ultrasensitive assay: results from TIMI 35. Eur Heart J 30:162, 2009.
27. Leers MP, Schepers R, Baumgarten R: Effects of a long-distance run on cardiac markers in healthy athletes. Clin Chem Lab Med 44:999, 2006.
28. O'Donoghue M, de Lemos JA, Morrow DA, et al: Prognostic utility of heart-type fatty acid binding protein in patients with acute coronary syndromes. Circulation 2114:550, 2006.
29. Morrow DA, Cannon CP, Jesse RL, et al: National Academy of Clinical Biochemistry Laboratory Medicine Practice Guidelines: Clinical characteristics and utilization of biochemical markers in acute coronary syndromes. Circulation 115:e356, 2007.
30. Scirica BM, Morrow DA, Cannon CP, et al: Clinical application of C-reactive protein across the spectrum of acute coronary syndromes. Clin Chem 53:1800, 2007.
31. Schindhelm RK, van der Zwan LP, Teerlink T, Scheffer PG: Myeloperoxidase: A useful biomarker for cardiovascular disease risk stratification? Clin Chem 55:1462, 2009.
32. Peacock F, Morris DL, Anwaruddin S, et al: Meta-analysis of ischemia-modified albumin to rule out acute coronary syndromes in the emergency department. Am Heart J 152:253, 2006.
33. Sabatine MS: When prognosis precedes diagnosis: Putting the cart before the horse. CMAJ 172:1697, 2005.
34. van Belle A, Buller HR, Huisman MV, et al: Effectiveness of managing suspected pulmonary embolism using an algorithm combining clinical probability, D-dimer testing, and computed tomography. JAMA 295:172, 2006.
35. Braunwald E: Biomarkers in heart failure. N Engl J Med 358:2148, 2008.
36. Sabatine MS, Morrow DA, de Lemos JA, et al: Acute changes in circulating natriuretic peptide levels in relation to myocardial ischemia. J Am Coll Cardiol 44:1988, 2004.
37. Morrow DA, de Lemos JA, Blazing MA, et al: Prognostic value of serial B-type natriuretic peptide testing during follow-up of patients with unstable coronary artery disease. JAMA 294:2866, 2005.
38. Bonaca MP, Morrow DA: Defining a role for novel biomarkers in acute coronary syndromes. Clin Chem 54:1424, 2008.
39. Goldman L, Cook EF, Johnson PA, et al: Prediction of the need for intensive care in patients who come to the emergency departments with acute chest pain. N Engl J Med 334:1498, 1996.

Immediate Management

40. Farkouh ME, Smars PA, Reeder GS, et al: A clinical trial of a chest-pain observation unit for patients with unstable angina. N Engl J Med 339:1882, 1998.
41. Polanczyk CA, Johnson PA, Hartley LH, et al: Clinical correlates and prognostic significance of early negative exercise tolerance test in patients with acute chest pain seen in the hospital emergency department. Am J Cardiol 81:288, 1998.
42. Gibbons RJ, Balady GJ, Bricker JT, et al: ACC/AHA 2002 guideline update for exercise testing: summary article: A report of the American College of Cardiology/American Heart Association Task Force on Practice Guidelines (Committee to Update the 1997 Exercise Testing Guidelines). Circulation 106:1883, 2002.
43. Kontos MC, Tatum JL: Imaging in the evaluation of the patient with suspected acute coronary syndrome. Cardiol Clin 23:517, 2005.
44. Marcassa C, Bax JJ, Bengel F, et al: Clinical value, cost-effectiveness, and safety of myocardial perfusion scintigraphy: a position statement. Eur Heart J 29:557, 2008.
45. Wyrick JJ, Kalvaitis S, McConnell KJ, et al: Cost-efficiency of myocardial contrast echocardiography in patients presenting to the emergency department with chest pain of suspected cardiac origin and a nondiagnostic electrocardiogram. Am J Cardiol 102:649, 2008.
46. Klocke FJ, Baird MG, Lorell BH, et al: ACC/AHA/ASNC guidelines for the clinical use of cardiac radionuclide imaging—executive summary: A report of the American College of Cardiology/American Heart Association Task Force on Practice Guidelines (ACC/AHA/ASNC Committee to Revise the 1995 Guidelines for the Clinical Use of Cardiac Radionuclide Imaging). Circulation 108:1404, 2003.

47. Udelson JE, Beshansky JR, Ballin DS, et al: Myocardial perfusion imaging for evaluation and triage of patients with suspected acute cardiac ischemia: A randomized controlled trial. JAMA 288:2693, 2002.
48. Schaeffer MW, Brennan TD, Hughes JA, et al: Resting radionuclide myocardial perfusion imaging in a chest pain center including an overnight delayed image acquisition protocol. J Nucl Med Technol 35:242, 2007.
49. Conti A, Sammicheli L, Gallini C, et al: Assessment of patients with low-risk chest pain in the emergency department: Head-to-head comparison of exercise stress echocardiography and exercise myocardial SPECT. Am Heart J 149:894, 2005.
50. Kaul S: Myocardial contrast echocardiography: A 25-year retrospective. Circulation 118:291, 2008.
51. Kaul S, Senior R, Firschke C, et al: Incremental value of cardiac imaging in patients presenting to the emergency department with chest pain and without ST-segment elevation: A multicenter study. Am Heart J 148:129, 2004.
52. Korosoglou G, Labadze N, Hansen A, et al: Usefulness of real-time myocardial perfusion imaging in the evaluation of patients with first time chest pain. Am J Cardiol 94:1225, 2004.
53. Lockie T, Nagel E, Redwood S, Plein S: Use of cardiovascular magnetic resonance imaging in acute coronary syndromes. Circulation 119:1671, 2009.
54. Cury RC, Shash K, Nagurney JT, et al: Cardiac magnetic resonance with T2-weighted imaging improves detection of patients with acute coronary syndrome in the emergency department. Circulation 2118:837, 2008.
55. Yang Q, Li K, Liu X, et al: Contrast-enhanced whole-heart coronary magnetic resonance angiography at 3.0-T: A comparative study with X-ray angiography in a single center. J Am Coll Cardiol 54:69, 2009.
56. Ingkanisorn WP, Kwong RY, Bohme NS, et al: Prognosis of negative adenosine stress magnetic resonance in patients presenting to an emergency department with chest pain. J Am Coll Cardiol 47:1427, 2006.
57. Goldstein JA, Gallagher MJ, O'Neill WW, et al: A randomized controlled trial of multi-slice coronary computed tomography for evaluation of acute chest pain. J Am Coll Cardiol 49:863, 2007.

CHAPTER 54 ST-Segment Elevation Myocardial Infarction: Pathology, Pathophysiology, and Clinical Features

Elliott M. Antman

The pathologic diagnosis of myocardial infarction (MI) requires evidence of myocyte cell death caused by prolonged ischemia. Characteristic findings include coagulation necrosis and contraction band necrosis, often with patchy areas of myocytolysis at the periphery of the infarct. During the acute phase of MI, most myocyte loss in the infarct zone occurs via coagulation necrosis and proceeds to inflammation, phagocytosis of necrotic myocytes, and repair eventuating in scar formation.

The clinical diagnosis of MI requires an integrated assessment of the history with some combination of indirect evidence of myocardial necrosis using biochemical, electrocardiographic, and imaging modalities (**Table 54-1**). The sensitivity and specificity of the clinical tools for diagnosing MI vary considerably, depending on the time after onset of the infarction (**Table 54-2**).

The World Heath Organization and American Heart Association previously required the presence of at least two of the following for the diagnosis of myocardial infarction: characteristic symptoms, electrocardiographic changes, and a typical rise and fall in biochemical markers. Advances in the techniques for diagnosing MI led to a consensus document published jointly by several prominent cardiac societies[1] (see Table 54-2). In addition to codifying the criteria for the diagnosis of MI, the revised definition classifies MI into five types, depending on the circumstances in which the MI occurs (**Table 54-3**). The revised definition of MI (see Table 54-2) has important implications not only for the clinical care of patients, but also for epidemiologic studies, public policy, and clinical trials.[2,3] The shift to cardiac-specific troponins as the markers of choice for the diagnosis of MI requires new cutoff values for cardiac injury. The term *normal range* has been replaced by the term *upper reference limit*, defined as the 99th percentile of a normal reference control group.[1]

The contemporary approach to patients presenting with ischemic discomfort is to consider them as experiencing an acute coronary syndrome. The 12-lead electrocardiogram (ECG) defines those presenting with ST-segment elevation, the subject of Chaps. 54 and 55, and those without ST-segment elevation, the subject of Chap. 56. Although the revised definition of MI has greater impact on the non–ST-segment elevation end of the acute coronary syndrome spectrum (i.e., distinction between unstable angina and non–ST-segment elevation MI), the issues also pertain to discussion of ST-segment elevation myocardial infarction (STEMI).

Changing Patterns in Clinical Care

Despite advances in diagnosis and management, STEMI continues to be a major public health problem in the industrialized world and is rising in developing countries (see Chap. 1).[4] In the United States, almost 1 million patients per year suffer from an acute MI, and more than 1 million patients with suspected acute MI yearly enter coronary care units in the United States.[5] The rate of MI rises for both men and women sharply with increasing age, and racial differences exist, with MI occurring more frequently in black men and women, regardless of age (**Fig. 54-1**). Of particular concern from a global perspective, the burden of MI in developing countries may approach those now afflicting developed countries. Limitations in available resources to treat STEMI in developing countries mandate major efforts on an international level to strengthen primary prevention programs.[6]

Improvements in Outcome

Mortality from STEMI has declined steadily.[7-9] This drop in mortality appears to result from a fall in the incidence of STEMI (replaced in part by an increase in the rate of unstable angina/non–ST-segment elevation MI [NSTEMI][10]) and a fall in the case fatality rate once STEMI has occurred.[5]

Several phases in the management of patients have contributed to the decline in mortality from STEMI.[11] The "clinical observation phase" of coronary care consumed the first half of the 20th century and focused on a detailed recording of physical and laboratory findings, with little active treatment for the infarction. The "coronary care unit phase" began in the mid-1960s and was notable for detailed analysis and vigorous management of cardiac arrhythmias. The "high-technology phase" heralded by the introduction of the pulmonary artery balloon flotation catheter set the stage for bedside hemodynamic monitoring and more precise hemodynamic management. The modern "reperfusion era" of coronary care was introduced by intracoronary and then intravenous fibrinolysis, increased use of aspirin, and the development of primary percutaneous coronary intervention (PCI; see Chap. 58).

Contemporary care of patients with STEMI has entered an evidence-based coronary care phase and is increasingly influenced by guidelines and performance measures for clinical practice.[12-14] Government websites now benchmark mortality rates for patients with MI who are treated at various hospitals (www.hospitalcompare.hhs.gov).

Limitations of Current Therapy

The short-term mortality rate of patients with STEMI who receive aggressive pharmacologic reperfusion therapy as part of a randomized trial is in the range of 6.5% to 7.5%,[15] whereas observational data bases suggest that the mortality rate in STEMI patients in the community is

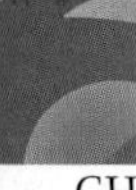

CH 54

TABLE 54-1 Aspects of Diagnosis of Myocardial Infarction by Different Techniques

TECHNIQUE	FEATURES
Pathology	Myocardial cell death
Biochemistry	Markers of myocardial cell death recovered from blood samples
Electrocardiography	Evidence of myocardial ischemia (ST and T wave abnormalities); evidence of loss of electrically functioning cardiac tissue (Q waves)
Imaging	Reduction or loss of tissue perfusion; cardiac wall motion abnormalities

Modified from Thygesen K, Alpert JS, White HD, et al: Universal definition of myocardial infarction. Circulation 116:2634, 2007.

TABLE 54-2 Revised Definition of Myocardial Infarction

Criteria for Acute, Evolving, or Recent MI

Either of the following criteria satisfies the diagnosis for acute, evolving, or recent MI:

1. Typical rise and/or fall of biochemical markers of myocardial necrosis with at least one of the following:
   a. Ischemic symptoms
   b. Development of pathologic Q waves in the ECG
   c. Electrocardiographic changes indicative of ischemia (ST-segment elevation or depression)
   d. Imaging evidence of new loss of viable myocardium or new regional wall motion abnormality
2. Pathologic findings of an acute myocardial infarction

Criteria for Healing or Healed Myocardial Infarction

Any one of the following criteria satisfies the diagnosis for healing or healed myocardial infarction:

1. Development of new pathologic Q waves in serial ECGs. The patient may or may not remember previous symptoms. Biochemical markers of myocardial necrosis may have normalized, depending on the length of time that has passed since the infarction developed.
2. Pathologic findings of a healed or healing infarction

From Thygesen K, Alpert JS, White HD, et al: Universal definition of myocardial infarction. Circulation 116:2634, 2007.

TABLE 54-3 Classification of Myocardial Infarction

TYPE	FEATURES
1	Spontaneous myocardial infarction related to ischemia caused by a primary coronary event such as plaque erosion and/or rupture, fissuring, or dissection
2	Myocardial infarction secondary to ischemia caused by increased oxygen demand or decreased supply (e.g., coronary artery spasm, coronary embolism, anemia, arrhythmias, hypertension, hypotension)
3	Sudden unexpected cardiac death, including cardiac arrest, often with symptoms suggestive of myocardial ischemia, accompanied by presumably new ST-segment elevation, or new LBBB, or presumably new major obstruction in a coronary artery by angiography and/or pathology, but death occurring before blood samples could be obtained, or before the appearance of cardiac biomarkers in the blood
4a	Myocardial infarction associated with PCI
4b	Myocardial infarction associated with stent thrombosis, as documented by angiography or autopsy
5	Myocardial infarction associated with CABG

CABG = coronary artery bypass grafting; LBBB = left bundle branch block.
From Thygesen K, Alpert JS, White HD, et al: Universal definition of myocardial infarction. Circulation 2007;116(22):2634-2653.

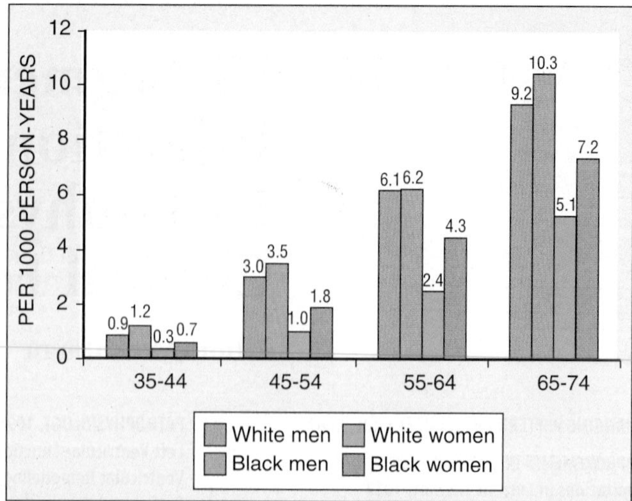

FIGURE 54-1 Annual rate of first heart attacks by age, sex, and race (data, Atherosclerosis Risk in Communities [ARIC] surveillance, 1987-2004). *(From Lloyd-Jones D, Adams R, Carnethon M, et al: Heart disease and stroke statistics—2009 update: A report from the American Heart Association Statistics Committee and Stroke Statistics Subcommittee. Circulation 119:e21, 2009.)*

15% to 20%.[16] About 30% of patients with STEMI who are eligible to receive reperfusion therapy do not receive that lifesaving treatment.[17] In part, this difference relates to the selection of patients without serious comorbidities for clinical trials.

Advanced age consistently emerges as one of the principal determinants of mortality in patients with STEMI.[18] Cardiac catheterization and other invasive procedures are being performed more commonly at some point during hospitalization in older patients with STEMI. Nevertheless, evidence suggests that the greatest reductions in mortality for older patients derive from those strategies used during the first 24 hours, a time frame during which prompt and appropriate use of lifesaving reperfusion therapy has paramount importance, emphasizing the need to extend advances in drug therapy for STEMI to older patients.[5]

Considerable variation exists in the management and outcomes of patients with STEMI.[19,20] Mortality rates for STEMI are lower in hospitals with a high clinical volume, a high rate of invasive procedures, and a top ranking in quality reports. Conversely, mortality rates are higher in STEMI patients not cared for by a cardiovascular specialist.[21] Variation also occurs in the treatment patterns of certain population subgroups with STEMI, notably women and blacks.[22] Evidence exists that much of the regional variation in outcomes derives from the characteristics of the patient and treatments received as opposed to the location where those treatments were delivered.

Pathology

Almost all MIs result from coronary atherosclerosis, generally with superimposed coronary thrombosis. Nonatherogenic forms of coronary artery disease are discussed later in this chapter, and causes of STEMI without coronary atherosclerosis are shown in **Table 54-4**.

Before the fibrinolytic era, clinicians typically divided patients with MI into those suffering a Q wave and those suffering a non–Q-wave infarction on the basis of evolution of the pattern on the ECG over several days. The term *Q-wave infarction* was frequently considered to be virtually synonymous with transmural infarction, whereas non–Q-wave infarctions were often referred to as subendocardial infarctions. Contemporary studies using cardiac magnetic resonance imaging indicate that the development of a Q wave on the ECG is determined more by the size of the infarct than the depth of mural involvement.[23,24] A more suitable framework that puts STEMI in perspective, along with unstable angina–NSTEMI (UA/NSTEMI) based on pathophysiology, is referred to as *acute coronary syndromes* (**Fig. 54-2**).

TABLE 54-4 Causes of Myocardial Infarction Without Coronary Atherosclerosis

Coronary Artery Disease Other Than Atherosclerosis
Arteritis
 Luetic
 Granulomatous (Takayasu disease)
 Polyarteritis nodosa
 Mucocutaneous lymph node (Kawasaki) syndrome
 Disseminated lupus erythematosus
 Rheumatoid spondylitis
 Ankylosing spondylitis
Trauma to coronary arteries
 Laceration
 Thrombosis
 Iatrogenic
 Radiation (radiation therapy for neoplasia)
Coronary mural thickening with metabolic disease or intimal proliferative disease
 Mucopolysaccharidoses (Hurler disease)
 Homocystinuria
 Fabry disease
 Amyloidosis
 Juvenile intimal sclerosis (idiopathic arterial calcification of infancy)
 Intimal hyperplasia associated with contraceptive steroids or with the postpartum period
 Pseudoxanthoma elasticum
 Coronary fibrosis caused by radiation therapy
Luminal narrowing by other mechanisms
 Spasm of coronary arteries (Prinzmetal angina with normal coronary arteries)
 Spasm after nitroglycerin withdrawal
 Dissection of the aorta
 Dissection of the coronary artery

Emboli to Coronary Arteries
Infective endocarditis
Nonbacterial thrombotic endocarditis
Prolapse of mitral valve
Mural thrombus from left atrium, left ventricle, or pulmonary veins
Prosthetic valve emboli
Cardiac myxoma
Associated with cardiopulmonary bypass surgery and coronary arteriography
Paradoxical emboli
Papillary fibroelastoma of the aortic valve (fixed embolus)
Thrombi from intracardiac catheters or guidewires

Congenital Coronary Artery Anomalies
Anomalous origin of left coronary from pulmonary artery
Left coronary artery from anterior sinus of Valsalva
Coronary arteriovenous and arteriocameral fistulas
Coronary artery aneurysms

Myocardial Oxygen Demand-Supply Disproportion
Aortic stenosis, all forms
Incomplete differentiation of the aortic valve
Aortic insufficiency
Carbon monoxide poisoning
Thyrotoxicosis
Prolonged hypotension
Takotsubo cardiomyopathy

Hematologic (In Situ Thrombosis)
Polycythemia vera
Thrombocytosis
Disseminated intravascular coagulation
Hypercoagulability, thrombosis, thrombocytopenic purpura

Miscellaneous
Cocaine abuse
Myocardial contusion
Myocardial infarction with normal coronary arteries
Complication of cardiac catheterization

Modified from Cheitlin MD, McAllister HA, de Castro CM: Myocardial infarction without atherosclerosis. JAMA 231:951, 1975.

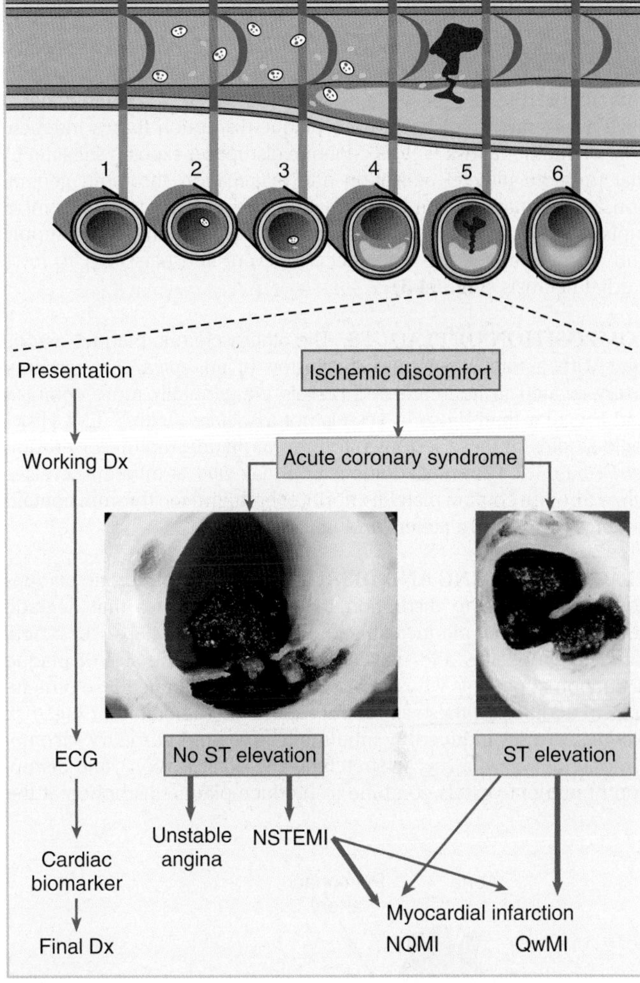

FIGURE 54-2 Acute coronary syndromes. The longitudinal section of an artery depicts the time line of atherogenesis from a normal artery (1), to lesion initiation and accumulation of extracellular lipid in the intima (2), to the evolution to the fibrofatty stage (3), and to lesion progression with procoagulant expression and weakening of the fibrous cap (4). An ACS develops when the vulnerable or high-risk plaque undergoes disruption of the fibrous cap (5); disruption of the plaque is the stimulus for thrombogenesis. Thrombus resorption may be followed by collagen accumulation and smooth muscle cell growth (6). Following disruption of a vulnerable or high-risk plaque, patients experience ischemic discomfort resulting from a reduction of flow through the affected epicardial coronary artery. The flow reduction may be caused by a completely occlusive thrombus (bottom half, right) or subtotally occlusive thrombus (bottom half, left). Patients with ischemic discomfort may present with or without ST-segment elevation on the ECG. Of patients with ST-segment elevation, most ultimately develop a Q-wave MI (QwMI), whereas a few develop a non–Q-wave MI (NQMI). Patients who present without ST-segment elevation are suffering from unstable angina or NSTEMI, a distinction that is ultimately made on the presence or absence of a serum cardiac marker such as CK-MB or a cardiac troponin detected in the blood. Most patients presenting with NSTEMI ultimately develop an NQMI on the ECG; a few may develop a QwMI. The spectrum of clinical presentations ranging from unstable angina through NSTEMI and STEMI are referred to as the acute coronary syndromes. Dx = diagnosis. *(Modified from Libby P: Circulation 104:365, 2001; Hamm CW, Bertrand M, Braunwald E: Lancet 358:1533, 2001; Davies MJ: Heart 83:361, 2000; and Antman EM, Anbe DT, Armstrong PW, et al: ACC/AHA guidelines for the management of patients with ST-elevation myocardial infarction: A report of the American College of Cardiology/American Heart Association Task Force on Practice Guidelines [Committee to Revise the 1999 Guidelines for the Management of Patients with Acute Myocardial Infarction]. Circulation 110:e82, 2004.)*

Plaque

During the natural evolution of atherosclerotic plaques, especially lipid-laden plaques, an abrupt and catastrophic transition can occur, characterized by plaque disruption (see Chap. 43).[25,26] Some patients have a systemic predisposition to plaque disruption that is independent of traditional risk factors.[27] Plaque disruption exposes substances that promote platelet activation and aggregation, thrombin generation, and ultimately thrombus formation. The resultant thrombus interrupts blood flow and leads to an imbalance between oxygen supply and demand and, if this imbalance is severe and persistent, to myocardial necrosis (**Fig. 54-3**).

COMPOSITION OF PLAQUES. The atherosclerotic plaques associated with a total thrombotic occlusion of an epicardial coronary artery, located in infarct-related vessels, are generally more complex and irregular than those in vessels not associated with STEMI. Histologic studies of these lesions often reveal plaque rupture or erosion (see Chap. 43). Thrombus composition may vary at different levels—white thrombi contain platelets, fibrin, or both, and red thrombi contain erythrocytes, fibrin, platelets, and leukocytes.

PLAQUE FISSURING AND DISRUPTION. Atherosclerotic plaques considered prone to disruption overexpress enzymes that degrade components of the plaque extracellular matrix (see Chap. 43).[28,29] Activated macrophages and mast cells abundant at the site of plaque disruption in patients who died of STEMI can elaborate these proteinases. In addition to these structural aspects of vulnerable or high-risk plaques, stresses induced by intraluminal pressure, coronary vasomotor tone, tachycardia (cyclic stretching and compression), and disruption of nutrient vessels combine to produce plaque disruption at the margin of the fibrous cap near an adjacent, less involved segment of the coronary artery wall (shoulder region of plaque).[30] A number of key physiologic variables such as systolic blood pressure, heart rate, blood viscosity, endogenous tissue plasminogen activator (t-PA) activity, plasminogen activator inhibitor type 1 (PAI-1) levels, plasma cortisol levels, and plasma epinephrine levels exhibit circadian and seasonal variations and increase at times of stress. These factors act in concert to heighten propensity to plaque disruption and coronary thrombosis, yielding the clustering of STEMI in the early morning hours, especially in the winter and after natural disasters.[31]

ACUTE CORONARY SYNDROMES. Plaque disruption exposes thrombogenic substances that may produce an extensive thrombus in the infarct-related artery (see Fig. 54-2). An adequate collateral network that prevents necrosis from occurring can result in clinically silent episodes of coronary occlusion. Characteristically, completely occlusive thrombi lead to transmural injury of the ventricular wall in the myocardial bed subtended by the affected coronary artery and typically produce ST-segment elevation on the ECG (see Figs. 54-2 to 54-4). Infarction alters the sequence of depolarization, ultimately reflected as changes in the QRS.[32] The most characteristic change in the QRS that develops in most patients initially presenting with ST-segment elevation is the evolution of Q waves in the leads overlying the infarct zone, leading to the term *Q-wave infarction* (see Fig. 54-2).[32] In the minority of patients presenting with ST-segment elevation, no Q waves develop, but other abnormalities of the QRS complex are frequently seen, such as diminution in R wave height and notching or splintering of the QRS. Patients presenting without ST-segment elevation are initially diagnosed as suffering from unstable angina or NSTEMI (see Fig. 54-2 and Chap. 56).

The acute coronary syndrome (ACS) spectrum concept, organized around a common pathophysiologic substrate, furnishes a useful framework for developing therapeutic strategies.[33] Patients presenting with persistent ST-segment elevation are candidates for reperfusion therapy (either pharmacologic or catheter-based) to restore flow in the occluded epicardial infarct-related artery. ACS patients presenting without ST-segment elevation are not candidates for pharmacologic reperfusion but should receive anti-ischemic therapy, followed by PCI. All patients with ACS should receive anticoagulant therapy and antiplatelet therapy, regardless of the presence or absence of ST-segment elevation. Thus, the 12-lead ECG remains at the center of the decision pathway for the management of patients with ACS to distinguish between presentations with ST-segment elevation and without ST-segment elevation (**Fig. 54-4**; see Fig. 54-2).[10] Prognostic considerations must take into account other important factors, such as whether the electrocardiographic abnormality is caused by a first infarct versus subsequent infarct, the location of infarction (anterior versus inferior [see Fig. 54-4]), infarct size, and demographic factors such as patient age.[32,33]

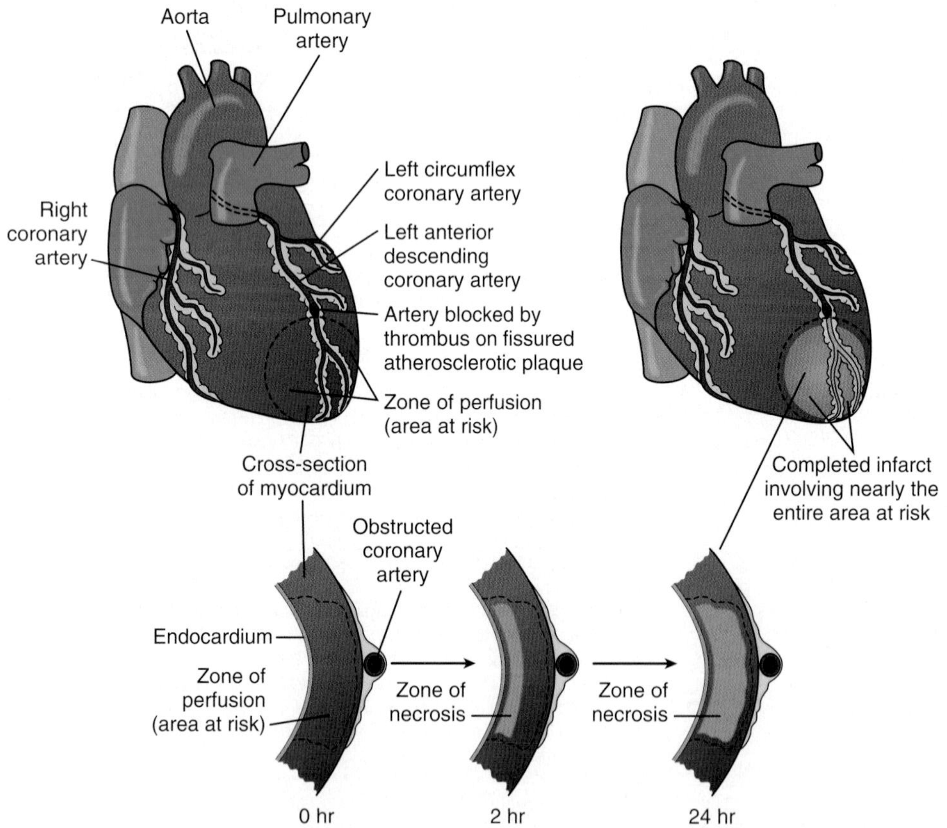

FIGURE 54-3 Schematic representation of the progression of myocardial necrosis after coronary artery occlusion. Necrosis begins in a small zone of the myocardium beneath the endocardial surface in the center of the ischemic zone. This entire region of myocardium (dashed outline) depends on the occluded vessel for perfusion and is the area at risk. A narrow zone of myocardium immediately beneath the endocardium is spared from necrosis because it can be oxygenated by diffusion from the ventricle. *(From Schoen FJ: The heart. In Kumar V, Abbas AK, Fausto N, Aster J [eds]: Robbins and Cotran Pathologic Basis of Disease. 8th ed. Philadelphia, WB Saunders, 2010, pp 529-587.)*

Heart Muscle

GROSS PATHOLOGY. On gross inspection, MI can be divided into two major types: transmural infarcts, in which myocardial necrosis involves the full thickness (or nearly full

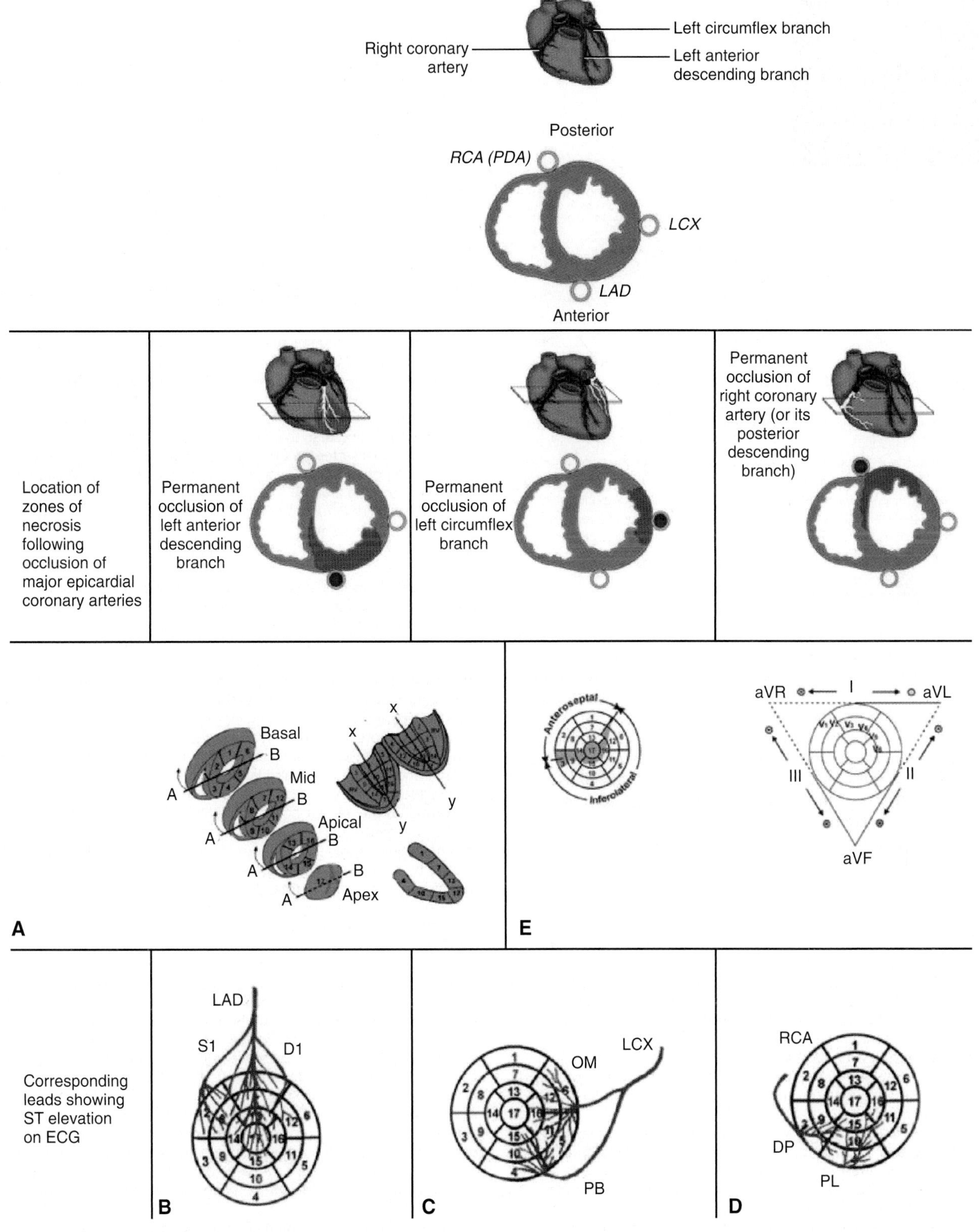

FIGURE 54-4 Correlation of sites of coronary occlusion, zones of necrosis, and electrocardiographic abnormalities. **Top,** Schematic diagram of the heart with the location of the major epicardial coronary arteries. Immediately below is another schematic diagram depicting a short-axis view of the left and right ventricles (LV, RV) and approximate location of the left anterior descending (LAD), left circumflex (LCX), and right coronary artery (RCA); the latter gives rise to the posterior descending artery (PDA) in most patients. **Middle,** Location of the zones of necrosis following occlusion of a major epicardial coronary artery. **Bottom,** Identification of the infarct artery from the 12-lead ECG. **A,** The 17 myocardial segments in a polar map format with superimposition of the arterial supply provided by the LAD **(B)**, LCX **(C)**, and RCA **(D)**. **E,** Position of the standard electrocardiographic leads relative to the polar map. The infarct artery can be deduced by identifying the leads that show ST-segment elevation and referencing that information to panels **A** through **D**. For example, ST-segment elevation seen most prominently in the leads overlying segments 1, 2, 7, 8, 13, 14, and 17 indicates that the LAD is the infarct artery. D_1 = first diagonal; DP = posterior descending; OM = obtuse marginal; PB = posterobasal; PL = posterolateral; S_1 = first septal. *(From Bayes de Luna A, Wagner G, Birnbaum Y, et al: A new terminology for the left ventricular walls and location of myocardial infarcts that present Q wave based on the standard of cardiac magnetic resonance imaging. Circulation 114:1755, 2006.)*

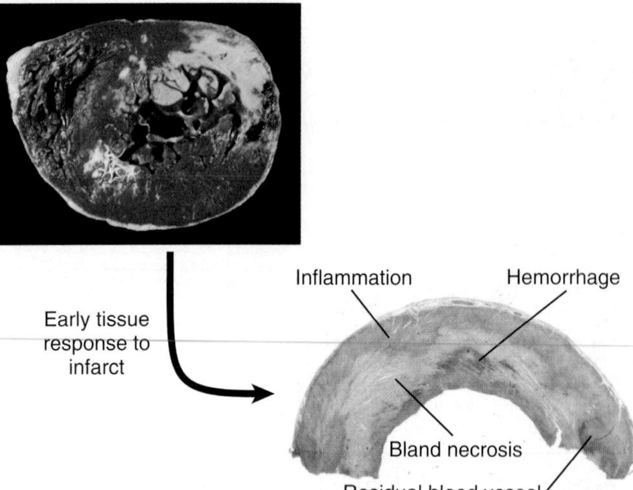

FIGURE 54-5 Top, Acute MI, predominantly of the posterolateral left ventricle, demonstrated histochemically by a lack of staining by the triphenyltetrazolium chloride stain in areas of necrosis. The staining defect is caused by the enzyme leakage that follows cell death. The myocardial hemorrhage at one edge of the infarct was associated with cardiac rupture, and the anterior scar (lower left) was indicative of old infarct (specimen oriented with posterior wall at top). **Bottom,** The early tissue response to the infarction process involves a mixture of bland necrosis, inflammation, and hemorrhage. *(From Schoen FJ: The heart. In Kumar V, Abbas AK, Fausto N, Aster J [eds]: Robbins and Cotran Pathologic Basis of Disease. 8th ed. Philadelphia, WB Saunders, 2010, pp 529-587.)*

thickness) of the ventricular wall, and subendocardial (nontransmural) infarcts, in which the necrosis involves the subendocardium, the intramural myocardium, or both without extending all the way through the ventricular wall to the epicardium (**Fig. 54-5A**).

An occlusive coronary thrombosis appears to be far more common when the infarction is transmural and localized to the distribution of a single coronary artery (see Fig. 54-4). Nontransmural infarctions, however, frequently occur in the presence of severely narrowed but still patent coronary arteries. Patchy nontransmural infarction may arise from fibrinolysis or PCI of an originally occlusive thrombus with restoration of blood flow before the wave front of necrosis has extended from the subendocardium across the full thickness of the ventricular wall (see Fig. 54-3).

Gross alterations of the myocardium are difficult to identify until at least 6 to 12 hours have elapsed following the onset of necrosis (**Fig. 54-6**). However, a variety of histochemical stains can be used to identify zones of necrosis that can be discerned after only 2 to 3 hours (see Fig. 54-5A).[34] Subsequently, the infarcted myocardium undergoes a sequence of gross pathologic changes summarized in Figures 54-5 and 54-6.[35]

HISTOLOGIC AND ULTRASTRUCTURAL CHANGES

LIGHT MICROSCOPY: PATTERNS OF MYOCARDIAL NECROSIS. Histologic evaluation of MI reveals various stages of the healing process (**Fig. 54-7**; see Figs. 54-5B, and 54-6).

COAGULATION NECROSIS. Coagulation necrosis results from severe persistent ischemia and is usually present in the central region of infarcts, which results in the arrest of muscle cells in the relaxed state and the passive stretching of ischemic muscle cells. The myofibrils are stretched, many with nuclear pyknosis, vascular congestion, and healing by phagocytosis of necrotic muscle cells (see Fig. 54-6). Mitochondrial damage with prominent amorphous (flocculent) densities but no calcification is evident.

NECROSIS WITH CONTRACTION BANDS. This form of myocardial necrosis, also termed *contraction band necrosis* or *coagulative myocytolysis*, results primarily from severe ischemia followed by reflow.[35] It is characterized by hypercontracted myofibrils with contraction bands and mitochondrial damage, frequently with calcification, marked vascular congestion, and healing by lysis of muscle cells. Necrosis with contraction bands is caused by increased Ca^{2+} influx into dying cells, resulting in the arrest of cells in the contracted state, which occurs in the periphery of large infarcts and to a greater extent in nontransmural than in transmural infarcts. The entire infarct may show this form of necrosis after reperfusion (see Fig. 54-7F).[36]

MYOCYTOLYSIS. Ischemia without necrosis generally causes no acute changes visible by light microscopy. However, severe prolonged ischemia can cause myocyte vacuolization, often termed *myocytolysis*. Prolonged severe ischemia, which is potentially reversible, causes cloudy swelling, as well as hydropic, vascular, and fatty degeneration.

ELECTRON MICROSCOPY. In experimental infarction, the earliest ultrastructural changes in cardiac muscle following ligation of a coronary artery, noted within 20 minutes, consist of reduction in the size and number of glycogen granules, intracellular edema, and swelling and distortion of the transverse tubular system, sarcoplasmic reticulum, and mitochondria (see Fig. 54-6).[37] These early changes are reversible. Changes after 60 minutes of occlusion include myocyte swelling, swelling and internal disruption of mitochondria, development of amorphous, flocculent aggregation and margination of nuclear chromatin, and relaxation of myofibrils. After 20 minutes to 2 hours of ischemia, changes in some cells become irreversible and there is progression of these alterations.[35]

APOPTOSIS. An additional pathway of myocyte death involves apoptosis, or programmed cell death. In contrast to coagulation necrosis, myocytes undergoing apoptosis exhibit shrinkage of cells, fragmentation of DNA, and phagocytosis, but without the usual cellular infiltrate indicative of inflammation (**Fig. 54-8**).[34] The role of apoptosis in the setting of MI is less well understood than that of classic coagulation necrosis. Apoptosis may occur shortly after the onset of myocardial ischemia. However, the major impact of apoptosis appears to be on late myocyte loss and ventricular remodeling after MI.[38]

MODIFICATION OF PATHOLOGIC CHANGES BY REPERFUSION. When reperfusion of myocardium undergoing the evolutionary changes from ischemia to infarction occurs sufficiently early (i.e., within 15 to 20 minutes), it can successfully prevent necrosis from developing. Beyond this early stage, the number of salvaged myocytes and therefore the amount of salvaged myocardial tissue (area of necrosis/area at risk) relates directly to the length of time of total coronary artery occlusion, level of myocardial oxygen consumption, and collateral blood flow (**Fig. 54-9**).[37] Typically, reperfused infarcts show a mixture of necrosis, hemorrhage within zones of irreversibly injured myocytes, coagulative necrosis with contraction bands, and distorted architecture of the cells in the reperfused zone (**Fig. 54-10**). Reperfusion of infarcted myocardium accelerates the washout of intracellular proteins, producing an exaggerated and early peak value of substances such as creatine kinase-MB (CK-MB) and cardiac-specific troponin T and I (see Fig. 54-6 and later).[39]

CORONARY ANATOMY AND LOCATION OF INFARCTION. Angiographic studies performed in the earliest hours of STEMI have revealed approximately a 90% incidence of total occlusion of the infarct-related vessel.[40] Recanalization from spontaneous fibrinolysis, as well as attrition caused by some mortality among those patients with total occlusion, diminishes angiographic total occlusion in the period following the onset of MI. Pharmacologic fibrinolysis and PCI markedly increase the proportion of patients with a patent infarct-related artery early after STEMI.

A STEMI with transmural necrosis typically occurs distal to an acutely totally occluded coronary artery, with thrombus superimposed on a ruptured plaque (see Fig. 54-4). The converse is not the case, however, in that chronic total occlusion of a coronary artery does not always cause MI. Collateral blood flow and other factors such as the level of myocardial metabolism, presence and location of stenoses in other coronary arteries, rate of development of the obstruction, and quantity of myocardium supplied by the obstructed vessel all influence the viability of myocardial cells distal to the occlusion. In many series of patients studied at necropsy or by coronary arteriography, a small number (5%) of patients with STEMI have normal coronary vessels. In these patients, an embolus that has lysed, a transiently occlusive platelet aggregate, or a prolonged episode of severe coronary spasm may have caused the infarct.

Studies of patients who ultimately develop STEMI after having undergone coronary angiography at some time before its occurrence have helped clarify coronary anatomy before infarction. Although high-grade stenoses, when present, more frequently lead to STEMI than less severe lesions, most occlusions actually occur in vessels with a previously identified stenosis of less than 50% on angiograms performed months to years earlier. This finding supports the concept that STEMI occurs as a result of sudden thrombotic occlusion at the site of rupture of previously nonobstructive but lipid-rich plaques. When collateral vessels perfuse an area of the ventricle, an infarct may occur at a distance from a coronary occlusion. For example, following the gradual obliteration of the lumen of the right coronary artery, the inferior wall of the left ventricle can be kept

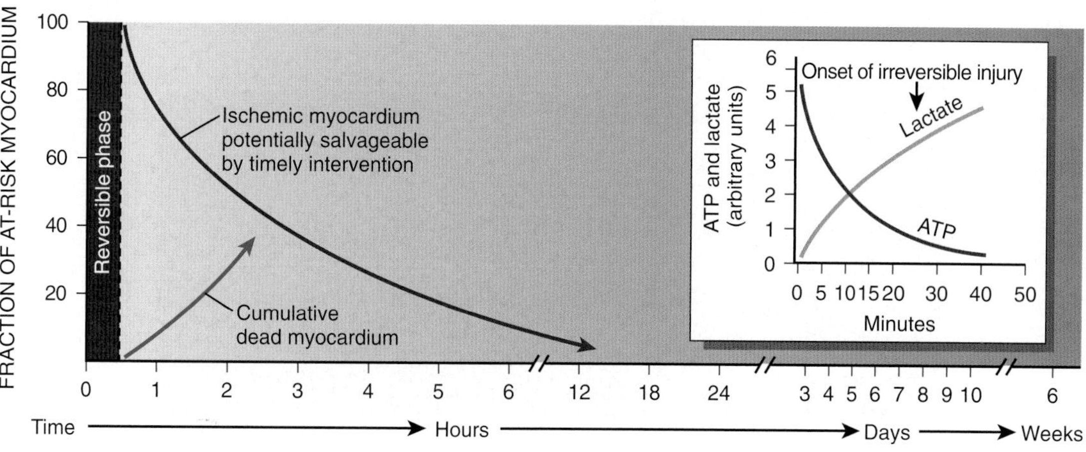

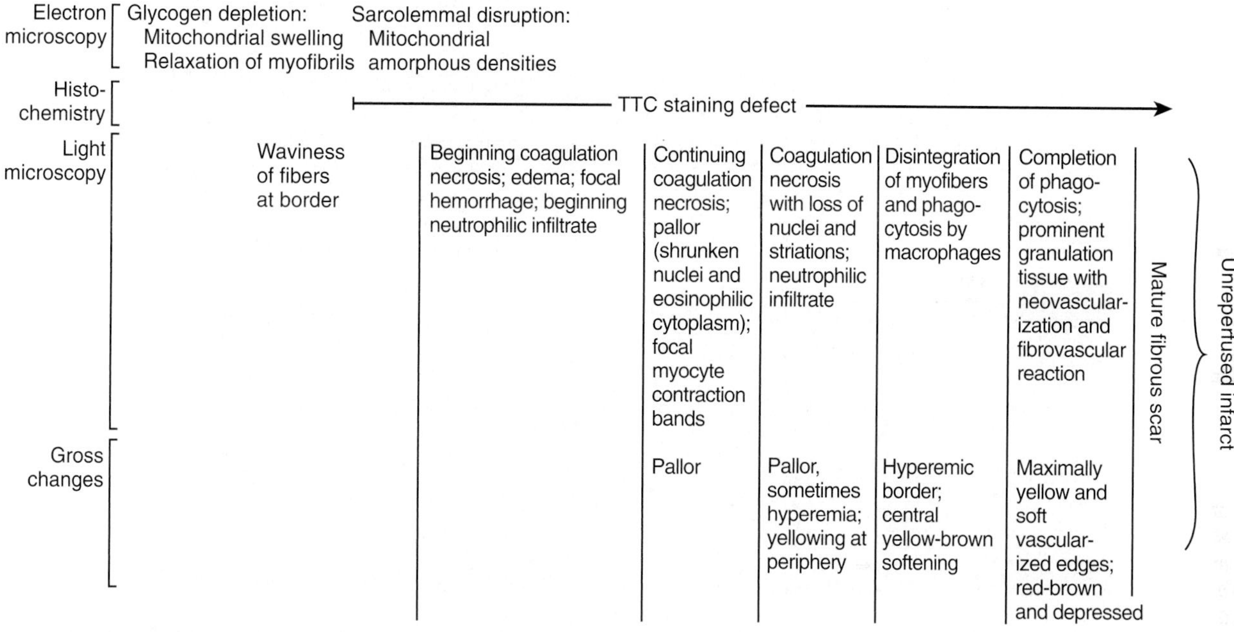

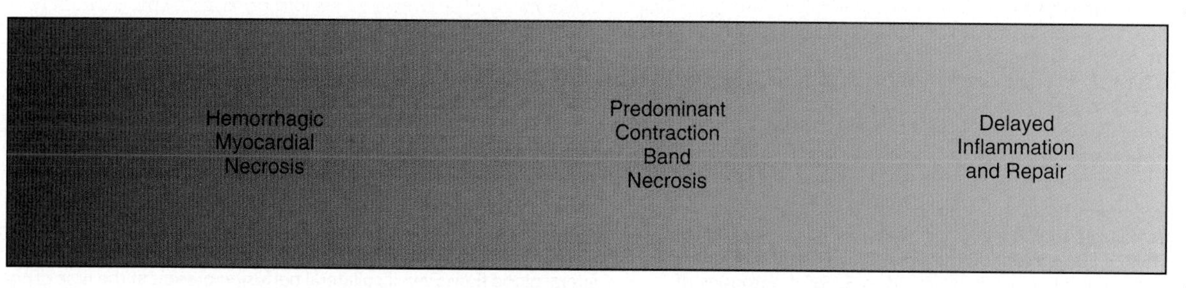

FIGURE 54-6 Temporal sequence of early biochemical, ultrastructural, histochemical, and histological findings after onset of myocardial infarction. **Top,** Schematics of the time frames for early and late reperfusion of the myocardium supplied by an occluded coronary artery. For approximately 30 minutes after the onset of even the most severe ischemia, myocardial injury is potentially reversible; after that, there is progressive loss of viability that is complete by 6 to 12 hours. The benefits of reperfusion (both early and late) are greatest when it is achieved early, with progressively smaller benefits occurring as reperfusion is delayed. Note the alterations in the temporal sequence in the reperfused infarct. The pattern of pathologic findings following reperfusion is variable, depending on the timing of reperfusion, prior infarction, and collateral flow. TTC = triphenyltetrazolium chloride. *(From Schoen FJ: The heart. In Kumar V, Abbas AK, Fausto N, Aster J [eds]: Robbins and Cotran Pathologic Basis of Disease. 8th ed. Philadelphia, WB Saunders, 2010, pp 529-587.)*

viable by collateral vessels arising from the left anterior descending coronary artery. Later, an occlusion of the left anterior descending artery may cause an infarct of the diaphragmatic wall.

Right Ventricular Infarction. Approximately 50% of patients with inferior infarction have some involvement of the right ventricle.[41] Among these patients, right ventricular infarction occurs exclusively in those with transmural infarction of the inferoposterior wall and posterior portion of the septum. Right ventricular infarction almost invariably develops in association with infarction of the adjacent septum and inferior left ventricular walls, but isolated infarction of the right ventricle is seen in 3% to 5% of autopsy-proven cases of MI (**Fig. 54-11**). Right ventricular infarction occurs less commonly than would be anticipated from the frequency of atherosclerotic lesions involving the right coronary artery. The right ventricle can sustain long periods of ischemia but still demonstrate excellent recovery of contractile function after reperfusion.[42]

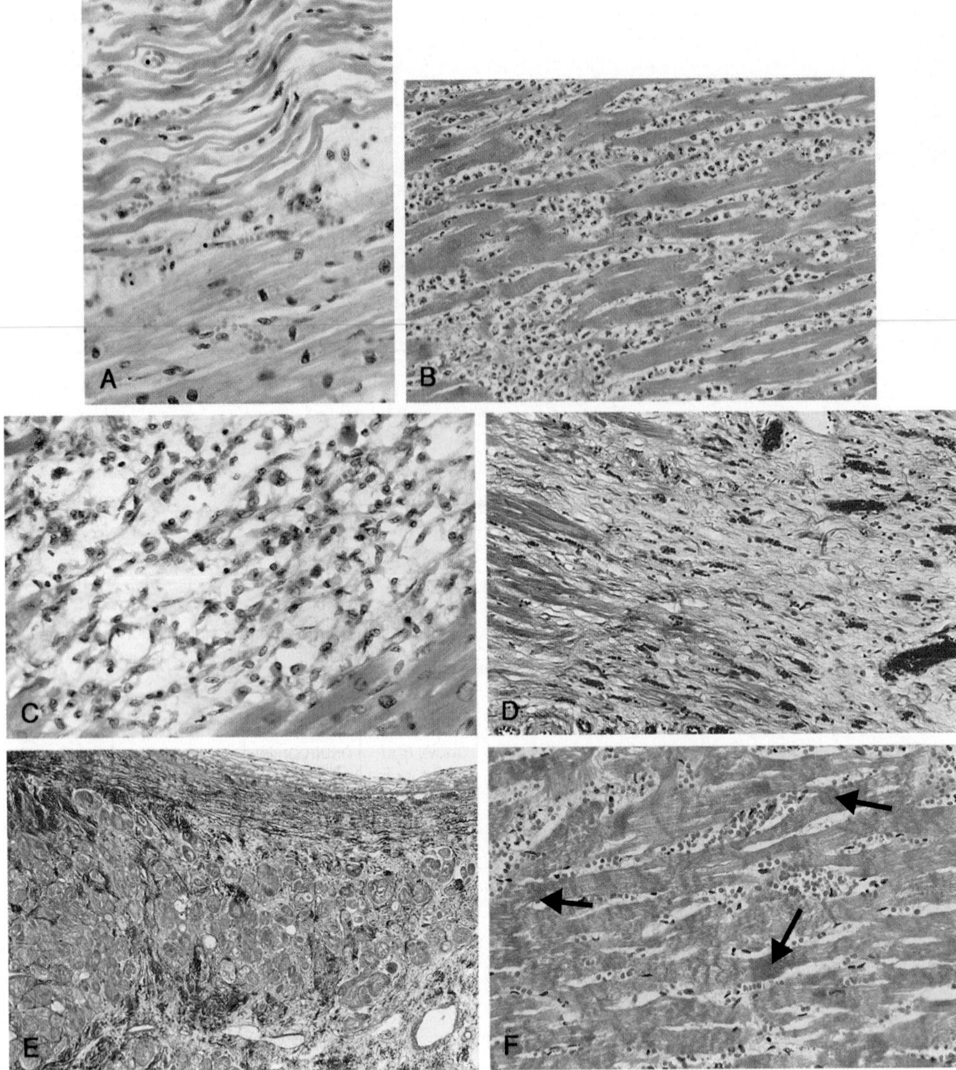

FIGURE 54-7 Microscopic features of myocardial infarction. **A,** 1-day-old infarct showing coagulative necrosis, wavy fibers with elongation, and narrowing compared with adjacent normal fibers (lower right). Widened spaces between the dead fibers contain edema fluid and scattered neutrophils. **B,** Dense polymorphonuclear leukocytic infiltrate in an area of acute myocardial MI of 3 to 4 days' duration. **C,** Almost complete removal of necrotic myocytes by phagocytosis (≈7 to 10 days). **D,** Granulation tissue with a rich vascular network and early collagen deposition, approximately 3 weeks after infarction. **E,** Well-healed myocardial infarct with replacement of the necrotic fibers by dense collagenous scar. A few residual cardiac muscle cells are present. (In **D** and **E**, collagen is highlighted as blue in this Masson trichrome stain.) **F,** Myocardial necrosis with hemorrhage and contraction bands, visible as dark bands spanning some myofibers (arrows). This is the characteristic appearance of markedly ischemic myocardium that has been reperfused. *(From Schoen FJ: The heart. In Kumar V, Abbas AK, Fausto N, Aster J [eds]: Robbins and Cotran Pathologic Basis of Disease. 8th ed. Philadelphia, WB Saunders, 2010, pp 529-587.)*

Atrial Infarction. Atrial infarction can be seen in up to 10% of patients with STEMI if PR-segment displacement is used as the criterion. Although isolated atrial infarction is observed in 3.5% of autopsies of patients with STEMI, it often occurs in conjunction with ventricular infarction and can cause rupture of the atrial wall.[43] This type of infarct is more common on the right side than on the left side, occurs more frequently in the atrial appendages than in the lateral or posterior walls of the atrium, and can result in thrombus formation. Atrial infarction is frequently accompanied by atrial arrhythmias.[44] It has also been linked to inadequate secretion of atrial natriuretic peptide and a low cardiac output syndrome when right ventricular infarction coexists.

Collateral Circulation in Acute Myocardial Infarction. The coronary collateral circulation (see Chap. 52) is particularly well developed in patients with the following: (1) coronary occlusive disease, especially with reduction of the luminal cross-sectional area by more than 75% in one or more major vessels; (2) chronic hypoxia, as in cases of severe anemia, chronic obstructive pulmonary disease, and cyanotic congenital heart disease; and (3) left ventricular hypertrophy.

The magnitude of coronary collateral flow is one of the principal determinants of infarct size. Indeed, patients with abundant collaterals commonly can have totally occluded coronary arteries without evidence of infarction in the distribution of that artery; thus, the survival of the myocardium distal to such occlusions depends in large measure on collateral blood flow. Even if collateral perfusion present at the time of coronary occlusion does not prevent infarction, it may still exert a beneficial effect by preventing the formation of a left ventricular aneurysm. It is likely that the presence of a high-grade stenosis (90%), possibly with periods of intermittent total occlusion, permits the development of collaterals that remain only as potential conduits until a total occlusion occurs or recurs. Total occlusion then brings these channels into full operation.

Nonatherosclerotic Causes of Acute Myocardial Infarction. Numerous pathologic processes other than atherosclerosis can involve the coronary arteries and result in STEMI (see Table 54-4). For example, coronary arterial occlusions can result from embolization of a coronary artery. The causes of coronary embolism are numerous and include infective endocarditis and nonbacterial thrombotic endocarditis (see Chap. 67), mural thrombi, prosthetic valves, neoplasms, air introduced at the time of cardiac surgery, and calcium deposits from manipulation of calcified valves at operation. In situ thrombosis of coronary arteries can occur secondary to chest wall trauma (see Chap. 76).

A variety of inflammatory processes can be responsible for coronary artery abnormalities, some of which mimic atherosclerotic disease and

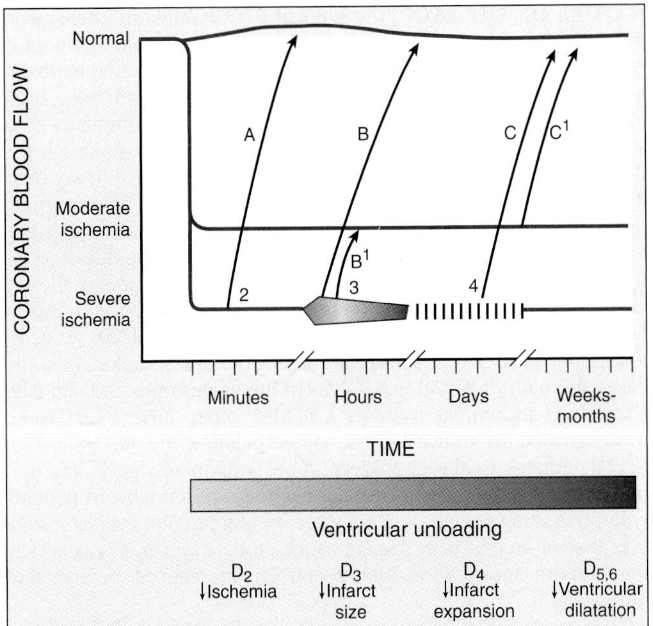

FIGURE 54-13 Therapeutic maneuvers in various stages of ischemia and infarction. Severely ischemic tissue (2) may be reperfused, thereby averting myocardial infarction (A). Infarcting tissue (3) may be reperfused, leading to sparing of myocardial tissue (B). If blood flow is restored only in part B, the myocardium may remain noncontractile, although viable (i.e., hibernating). After completion of the infarct (4), late reperfusion (C) may still be useful. Mechanical reperfusion of moderately ischemic myocardium (C^1) may restore contractility of hibernating myocardium to normal. Ventricular unloading may be useful throughout the preinfarct and postinfarct periods. Unloading may reduce ischemia (D_2), infarct size (D_3), infarct expansion (D_4), and ventricular dilatation ($D_{5,6}$). *(From Braunwald E, Pfeffer MA: Ventricular enlargement and remodeling following acute myocardial infarction: Mechanisms and management. Am J Cardiol 68:4D, 1991.)*

The increase in P50 results from increased levels of erythrocyte 2,3-diphosphoglycerate (2,3-DPG), which constitutes an important compensatory mechanism, responsible for an estimated 18% increase in oxygen release from oxyhemoglobin in patients with cardiogenic shock.

ENDOCRINE FUNCTION

PANCREAS. Although the absolute levels of blood insulin are often in the normal range, they are usually inappropriately low for the level of blood sugar, and there may be relative insulin resistance as well. Patients with cardiogenic shock often demonstrate marked hyperglycemia and depressed levels of circulating insulin. Abnormalities in insulin secretion and the resultant impaired glucose tolerance appear to be caused by a reduction in pancreatic blood flow as a consequence of splanchnic vasoconstriction accompanying severe LV failure. In addition, increased activity of the sympathetic nervous system with augmented circulating catecholamines inhibits insulin secretion and augments glycogenolysis, also contributing to the elevation of blood sugar.

Glucose appears to be a more favorable energy source than free fatty acids for the ischemic myocardium by permitting adenosine triphosphate (ATP) generation by anaerobic glycolysis.[54] Because hypoxic heart muscle derives a considerable portion of its energy from the metabolism of glucose (see Chap. 24) and because insulin is essential for the uptake of glucose by the myocardium, insulin deficiency has clear deleterious effects. These metabolic considerations, combined with epidemiologic observations that diabetic patients have a markedly worse prognosis, have served as the foundation for efforts to administer insulin-glucose infusions to diabetic patients with STEMI.[55]

ADRENAL MEDULLA. The plasma and urinary catecholamine levels peak during the first 24 hours after the onset of chest pain, with the greatest rise in plasma catecholamine secretion occurring during the first hour after the onset of STEMI. These high levels of circulating catecholamines in patients with STEMI correlate with the occurrence of serious arrhythmias and result in an increase in myocardial oxygen consumption, directly and indirectly, as a consequence of catecholamine-induced elevation of circulating free fatty acids. The concentration of circulating catecholamines correlates with the extent of myocardial damage and incidence of cardiogenic shock, as well as with early and late mortality rates.

Circulating catecholamines enhance platelet aggregation; when this occurs in the coronary microcirculation, the release of the potent local vasoconstrictor thromboxane A_2 may further impair cardiac perfusion. The marked increase in sympathetic activity associated with STEMI serves as the foundation for beta-adrenergic receptor blocker regimens in the acute phase.

ACTIVATION OF THE RENIN-ANGIOTENSIN-ALDOSTERONE SYSTEM. Noninfarcted regions of the myocardium appear to exhibit activation of the tissue RAAS with increased angiotensin II production. Both locally generated and systemically generated angiotensin II can stimulate the production of various growth factors, such as platelet-derived growth factor and transforming growth factor-β, that promote compensatory hypertrophy in the noninfarcted myocardium, as well as control the structure and tone of the infarct-related coronary and other myocardial vessels. Additional potential actions of angiotensin II that have a more negative impact on the infarction process include the release of endothelin, PAI-1, and aldosterone, which may cause vasoconstriction, impaired fibrinolysis, and increased sodium retention, respectively.

NATRIURETIC PEPTIDES. The peptides atrial natriuretic factor (ANF) and N-terminal pro-ANF are released from cardiac atria in response to elevation of atrial pressure. B-type natriuretic peptide (BNP) and its precursor, N-terminal pro-BNP (NT-proBNP), are secreted by human atrial and ventricular myocardium. Given the larger mass of ventricular rather than atrial myocardium, the total amount of mRNA for BNP is higher in the ventricles than in the atria. Natriuretic peptides are released early after STEMI, peaking at about 16 hours. Evidence has shown that natriuretic peptides released from the left ventricle during STEMI originate from the infarcted myocardium and from viable noninfarcted myocardium. The rise in BNP and NT-proBNP levels after STEMI correlates with infarct size and regional wall motion abnormalities. Measurement of natriuretic peptides can provide useful information early and late in the course of STEMI.[56]

ADRENAL CORTEX. Levels of plasma and urinary 17-hydroxycorticosteroids and ketosteroids, as well as aldosterone, rise markedly in patients with STEMI. Their concentrations correlate directly with the peak level of serum CK, implying an association between the stress imposed by larger infarcts and greater secretion of adrenal steroids. The magnitude of the elevation of cortisol correlates with infarct size and mortality. Glucocorticosteroids also contribute to impaired glucose tolerance.

THYROID GLAND. Although patients with STEMI are generally clinically euthyroid, there is evidence of a transient decrease in serum triiodothyronine (T_3) levels, a fall that is most marked on approximately the third day after the infarct. This fall in T_3 is usually accompanied by a rise in reverse T_3, with variable changes or no change in thyroxine (T_4) and thyroid-stimulating hormone (TSH) levels. The alteration in peripheral T_4 metabolism appears to correlate with infarct size and may be mediated by the rise in endogenous levels of cortisol that accompanies STEMI.

RENAL FUNCTION. Both prerenal azotemia and acute renal failure can complicate the marked reduction of cardiac output that occurs in cardiogenic shock. On the other hand, an increase in circulating atrial natriuretic peptide occurs following STEMI, which is correlated with the severity of LV failure. An increase in BNP is also found when right ventricular infarction accompanies inferior wall infarction, suggesting that this hormone may play a role in the hypotension that accompanies right ventricular infarction.

HEMATOLOGIC ALTERATIONS

PLATELETS. STEMI generally occurs in the presence of extensive coronary and systemic atherosclerotic plaques, which may serve as the site for the formation of platelet aggregates, a sequence that has been suggested as the initial step in the process of coronary thrombosis, coronary occlusion, and subsequent MI. Circulating platelets are hyperaggregable in patients with STEMI. Platelets from STEMI patients have an increased propensity for aggregation locally in the area of a disrupted plaque and also release vasoactive substances.[57]

HEMOSTATIC MARKERS. Elevated levels of serum fibrinogen degradation products, an end product of thrombosis, as well as the release of distinctive proteins when platelets are activated, such as platelet factor 4 and beta-thromboglobulin, have been reported in some patients with STEMI. Fibrinopeptide A (FPA), a protein released from fibrin by thrombin, is a marker of ongoing thrombosis and is increased during the early hours of STEMI. Marked elevations of hemostatic markers such as FPA, thrombin-antithrombin complex (TAT), and prothrombin fragment 1+2 (F1+2) are associated with an increased risk of mortality in STEMI patients. The interpretation of the coagulation tests in patients with STEMI may be complicated by elevated blood levels of catecholamines, concomitant shock, and/or pulmonary embolism—conditions that all may alter various tests of platelet and coagulation function. Additional factors that affect coagulation tests in STEMI include the type and dosage of antithrombotic agents and reperfusion of the infarct artery.

Leukocytes. Leukocytosis usually accompanies STEMI in proportion to the magnitude of the necrotic process, elevated glucocorticoid levels, and possibly inflammation in the coronary arteries. The magnitude of elevation of the leukocyte count is associated with in-hospital mortality after STEMI.[58]

Blood Viscosity. Clinical and epidemiologic studies have suggested that several hemostatic and hemorheologic factors (e.g., fibrinogen, factor VII, plasma viscosity, hematocrit, red blood cell aggregation, total white blood cell count) participate in the pathophysiology of atherosclerosis and also play an integral role in acute thrombotic events. An increase in blood viscosity also occurs in patients with STEMI attributable to hemoconcentration during the first few days and later to elevated serum concentrations of alpha$_2$-globulin and fibrinogen, components of the acute-phase response to tissue necrosis, which is also responsible for the elevated sedimentation rate characteristic of STEMI.

Clinical Features

Predisposing Factors

In up to half of patients with STEMI, a precipitating factor or prodromal symptoms can be identified (see Chap. 44). Evidence suggests that unusually heavy exercise, particularly in fatigued or habitually inactive patients, and emotional stress can precipitate STEMI.[59] Such infarctions could result from marked increases in myocardial oxygen consumption in the presence of severe coronary arterial narrowing.

Accelerating angina and rest angina, two patterns of unstable angina, may culminate in STEMI (see Fig. 54-2). Noncardiac surgical procedures have also been noted as precursors of STEMI. Perioperative risk stratification may reduce the likelihood of STEMI and cardiac-related mortality (see Chap. 85).[60] Reduced myocardial perfusion secondary to hypotension (e.g., hemorrhagic or septic shock) and increased myocardial oxygen demands caused by aortic stenosis, fever, tachycardia, and agitation can also contribute to myocardial necrosis. Other factors reported as predisposing to STEMI include respiratory infections, hypoxemia of any cause, pulmonary embolism, hypoglycemia, administration of ergot preparations, use of cocaine, sympathomimetics, serum sickness, allergy, and on rare occasion, wasp stings. In patients with Prinzmetal angina (see Chap. 57), STEMI may develop in the territory of the coronary artery that repeatedly undergoes spasm. Rarely, munitions workers exposed to high concentrations of nitroglycerin develop MI when they are withdrawn from this exposure, suggesting that it is caused by vasospasm.

CIRCADIAN PERIODICITY. The time of onset of STEMI has a pronounced circadian periodicity, with a peak incidence of events between 6 AM and noon.[61] Circadian rhythms affect many physiologic and biochemical variables; the early morning hours are associated with rises in levels of plasma catecholamines and cortisol and increases in platelet aggregability. Interestingly, the characteristic circadian peak was absent in patients receiving a beta blocker or aspirin before their presentation with STEMI. The concept of triggering a STEMI is a complex one and likely involves the superimposition of multiple factors such as time of day, season, and the stress of natural disasters.[62]

History (see Chaps. 12 and 53)

PRODROMAL SYMPTOMS. The patient's history remains crucial to establishing a diagnosis. The prodrome is usually characterized by chest discomfort, resembling classic angina pectoris, but it occurs at rest or with less activity than usual and can therefore be classified as unstable angina. However, it is often not disturbing enough to induce patients to seek medical attention and, if they do, they may not be hospitalized. A feeling of general malaise or frank exhaustion often accompanies other symptoms preceding STEMI.

NATURE OF THE PAIN. The pain of STEMI varies in intensity; in most patients, it is severe and, in some cases, intolerable. The pain is prolonged, usually lasting for more than 30 minutes and frequently for a number of hours. The discomfort is described as constricting, crushing, oppressing, or compressing; often, the patient complains of a sensation of a heavy weight or squeezing in the chest. Although the discomfort is typically described as a choking, viselike, or heavy pain, it can also be characterized as a stabbing, knifelike, boring, or burning discomfort. The pain is usually retrosternal in location, spreading frequently to both sides of the anterior chest, with a predilection for the left side. Often, the pain radiates down the ulnar aspect of the left arm, producing a tingling sensation in the left wrist, hand, and fingers. Some patients note only a dull ache or numbness of the wrists in association with severe substernal or precordial discomfort. In some cases, the pain of STEMI may begin in the epigastrium and simulate a variety of abdominal disorders, a fact that often causes STEMI to be misdiagnosed as indigestion. In other patients, the discomfort of STEMI radiates to the shoulders, upper extremities, neck, jaw, and interscapular region, again usually favoring the left side. In patients with preexisting angina pectoris, the pain of infarction usually resembles that of angina with respect to location. However, it is generally much more severe, lasts longer, and is not relieved by rest and nitroglycerin.

The pain of STEMI may have subsided by the time the physician first encounters the patient (or the patient reaches the hospital), or it may persist for many hours. Opiates, in particular morphine, usually relieve the pain. Both angina pectoris and the pain of STEMI are thought to arise from nerve endings in ischemic or injured, but not necrotic, myocardium. Thus, in cases of STEMI, stimulation of nerve fibers in an ischemic zone of myocardium surrounding the necrotic central area of infarction probably gives rise to the pain.

The pain often disappears suddenly and completely when blood flow to the infarct territory is restored. In patients in whom reocclusion occurs after fibrinolysis, pain recurs if the initial reperfusion has left viable myocardium. Thus, what has previously been thought of as the pain of infarction, sometimes lasting for many hours, probably represents pain caused by ongoing ischemia. The recognition that pain implies ischemia and not infarction heightens the importance of seeking ways to relieve the ischemia, for which the pain is a marker. This finding suggests that the clinician should not be complacent about ongoing cardiac pain under any circumstances. In some patients, particularly older patients, diabetic patients, and heart transplantation recipients, STEMI manifests clinically not by chest pain, but rather by symptoms of acute LV failure and chest tightness or by marked weakness or frank syncope. Diaphoresis, nausea, and vomiting may accompany these symptoms.

OTHER SYMPTOMS. Nausea and vomiting may occur, presumably because of activation of the vagal reflex or stimulation of LV receptors as part of the Bezold-Jarisch reflex. These symptoms occur more commonly in patients with inferior STEMI than in those with anterior STEMI. Moreover, nausea and vomiting are common side effects of opiates. When the pain of STEMI is epigastric in location and is associated with nausea and vomiting, the clinical picture can easily be confused with that of acute cholecystitis, gastritis, or peptic ulcer. Occasionally, a patient complains of diarrhea or a violent urge to defecate during the acute phase of STEMI. Other symptoms include feelings of profound weakness, dizziness, palpitations, cold perspiration, and a sense of impending doom. On occasion, symptoms arising from an episode of cerebral embolism or other systemic arterial embolism herald a STEMI. Chest discomfort may not accompany these symptoms.

DIFFERENTIAL DIAGNOSIS. The pain of STEMI may simulate that of acute pericarditis (see Chap. 75), which usually associates with some pleuritic features. Pericardial discomfort is aggravated by respiratory movements and coughing and often involves the shoulder, the ridge of the trapezius, and the neck. An important feature that distinguishes pericardial pain from ischemic discomfort is that ischemic discomfort does not radiate to the trapezius ridge, a characteristic site of radiation of pericardial pain. Pleural pain is usually sharp, knifelike, and aggravated in a cyclical fashion by each breath, which distinguishes it from the deep, dull, steady pain of STEMI. Pulmonary embolism (see Chap. 77) generally produces pain laterally in the chest, is often pleuritic in nature, and may be associated with hemoptysis. The pain caused by acute aortic dissection (see Chap. 60) is usually localized to the center of the chest, is extremely severe and described by the patient as a "ripping" or "tearing" sensation, is at its maximal intensity shortly after onset, persists for many hours, and often radiates to the back or lower extremities. Often, one or more major arterial pulses are absent. Pain arising from the costochondral and chondrosternal articulations may be associated with localized swelling and redness; it is usually sharp and "darting" and is characterized by marked localized tenderness. Episodes of retrosternal discomfort induced by peristalsis in patients with increased esophageal stiffness and episodes of sustained esophageal contraction can mimic the pain of STEMI.

Silent STEMI and Atypical Presentation

Nonfatal STEMI can be unrecognized by the patient and discovered only on subsequent routine electrocardiographic or postmortem examinations. Of these unrecognized infarctions, approximately half are truly silent, with patients unable to recall any symptoms whatsoever. The other half of patients with so-called *silent infarction* can recall an event characterized by symptoms compatible with acute infarction when leading questions are posed after the electrocardiographic abnormalities are discovered. Unrecognized or silent infarction occurs more commonly in patients without antecedent angina pectoris and in patients with diabetes and hypertension.[63] Silent STEMI is often followed by silent ischemia (see Chap. 57). The prognoses of patients with silent and symptomatic presentations of STEMI appear to be similar.

Atypical presentations of STEMI include the following: (1) heart failure (i.e., dyspnea without pain beginning de novo or worsening of established failure); (2) classic angina pectoris without a particularly severe or prolonged episode; (3) atypical location of the pain; (4) central nervous system manifestations, resembling those of stroke, secondary to a sharp reduction in cardiac output in a patient with cerebral arteriosclerosis; (5) apprehension and nervousness; (6) sudden mania or psychosis; (7) syncope; (8) overwhelming weakness; (9) acute indigestion; and (10) peripheral embolization.

Physical Examination (see Chaps. 12 and 53)

GENERAL APPEARANCE. Patients suffering STEMI often appear anxious and in considerable distress. An anguished facial expression is common and—in contrast to patients with severe angina pectoris, who often lie, sit, or stand still, recognizing that all forms of activity increase the discomfort—some patients suffering STEMI may be restless and move about in an effort to find a comfortable position. They often massage or clutch their chests and frequently describe their pain with a clenched fist held against the sternum (the Levine sign). In patients with LV failure and sympathetic stimulation, cold perspiration and skin pallor may be evident; they typically sit or are propped up in bed, gasping for breath. Between breaths, they may complain of chest discomfort or a feeling of suffocation. Cough productive of frothy, pink, or blood-streaked sputum is common.

Patients in cardiogenic shock often lie listlessly, making few, if any, spontaneous movements. The skin is cool and clammy, with a bluish or mottled color over the extremities, with marked facial pallor and severe cyanosis of the lips and nail beds. Depending on the degree of cerebral perfusion, the patient in shock may converse normally or may evidence confusion and disorientation.

HEART RATE. The heart rate can vary from a marked bradycardia to a rapid regular or irregular tachycardia, depending on the underlying rhythm and degree of LV failure. Most commonly, the pulse is rapid and regular initially (sinus tachycardia at 100 to 110 beats/min), slowing as the patient's pain and anxiety are relieved; premature ventricular beats are common.

BLOOD PRESSURE. Most patients with uncomplicated STEMI are normotensive, although the reduced stroke volume accompanying the tachycardia can cause declines in systolic and pulse pressures and elevation of diastolic pressure. Among previously normotensive patients, a hypertensive response is occasionally seen during the first few hours, with the arterial pressure exceeding 160/90 mm Hg, presumably as a consequence of adrenergic discharge secondary to pain, anxiety, and agitation. Previously hypertensive patients often become normotensive without treatment after STEMI, although many of these previously hypertensive patients eventually regain their elevated levels of blood pressure, generally 3 to 6 months after infarction. In patients with massive infarction, arterial pressure falls acutely because of LV dysfunction and venous pooling secondary to administration of morphine and/or nitrates. As recovery occurs, the arterial pressure tends to return to preinfarction levels.

Patients in cardiogenic shock by definition have systolic pressures below 90 mm Hg and evidence of end-organ hypoperfusion. Hypotension alone does not necessarily signify cardiogenic shock, however, because some patients with inferior infarction with Bezold-Jarisch reflex activation may also have a transient systolic blood pressure below 90 mm Hg. Their hypotension eventually resolves spontaneously, although the process can be accelerated by intravenous atropine (0.5 to 1 mg) and assumption of the Trendelenburg position. Other patients who are initially only slightly hypotensive may demonstrate gradually falling blood pressures with progressive reduction in cardiac output over several hours or days as they develop cardiogenic shock as a consequence of increasing ischemia and extension of infarction (see Fig. 54-12). Evidence of autonomic hyperactivity is common, varying in type with the location of the infarction. At some time during their initial presentation, more than half of patients with inferior STEMI have evidence of excess parasympathetic stimulation, with hypotension, bradycardia, or both, whereas about half of patients with anterior STEMI show signs of sympathetic excess, with hypertension, tachycardia, or both.

TEMPERATURE AND RESPIRATION. Most patients with extensive STEMI develop fever, a nonspecific response to tissue necrosis, within 24 to 48 hours of the onset of infarction. Body temperature often begins to rise within 4 to 8 hours after the onset of infarction, and rectal temperature may reach 38.3° to 38.9°C (101° to 102°F). Fever usually resolves by the fourth or fifth day after infarction.

The respiratory rate may be slightly elevated soon after the development of STEMI; in patients without heart failure, it results from anxiety and pain because it returns to normal with treatment of physical and psychological discomfort. In patients with LV failure, the respiratory rate correlates with the severity of failure; patients with pulmonary edema may have respiratory rates exceeding 40/min. But the respiratory rate is not necessarily elevated in patients with cardiogenic shock. Cheyne-Stokes (periodic) respiration may occur in older patients with cardiogenic shock or heart failure, particularly after opiate therapy or in the presence of cerebrovascular disease.

JUGULAR VENOUS PULSE. The jugular venous pulse usually fails to show any abnormalities. The *a* wave may be prominent in patients with pulmonary hypertension secondary to LV failure or reduced compliance. In contrast, right ventricular infarction (whether or not it accompanies LV infarction) often results in marked jugular venous distention and, when complicated by necrosis or ischemia of the right ventricular papillary muscles, tall *c-v* waves of tricuspid regurgitation are evident. Patients with STEMI and cardiogenic shock usually have elevated jugular venous pressure. In patients with STEMI, hypotension, and hypoperfusion (findings that may resemble those of patients with cardiogenic shock) but who have flat neck veins, it is likely that the depression of LV performance may relate, at least in part, to hypovolemia. The differentiation can be made only by assessing LV performance using echocardiography or by measuring LV filling pressure with a pulmonary artery flotation catheter.

CAROTID PULSE. Palpation of the carotid arterial pulse provides a clue to the LV stroke volume; a small pulse suggests a reduced stroke volume, whereas a sharp brief upstroke is often observed in patients with mitral regurgitation or ruptured ventricular septum with a left-to-right shunt. Pulsus alternans reflects severe LV dysfunction.

CHEST. Moist rales are audible in patients who develop LV failure and/or a reduction of LV compliance with STEMI. Diffuse wheezing can present in patients with severe LV failure. Cough with hemoptysis, suggesting pulmonary embolism with infarction, can also occur. In 1967, Killip and Kimball[64] proposed a prognostic classification scheme on the basis of the presence and severity of rales detected in patients presenting with STEMI. Class I patients are free of rales and a third heart sound. Class II patients have rales but only to a mild to moderate degree (<50% of lung fields), and they may or may not have an S_3. Patients in Class III have rales in more than half of each lung field and frequently have pulmonary edema. Finally, Class IV patients are in cardiogenic shock. Despite overall improvement in mortality rate in each class, compared with data observed during the original development of the classification scheme, the classification scheme remains useful today, as evidenced by data from large MI trials of STEMI patients.[65]

CARDIAC EXAMINATION

Palpation

Palpation of the precordium may yield normal findings, but in patients with transmural STEMI, it more commonly reveals a presystolic pulsation, synchronous with an audible fourth heart sound, which reflects a vigorous left atrial contraction filling a ventricle with reduced compliance. In the presence of LV systolic dysfunction, an outward movement of the left ventricle can be palpated in early diastole, coincident with a third heart sound.

Auscultation

HEART SOUNDS. The heart sounds, particularly the first sound, are frequently muffled and occasionally inaudible immediately after the infarct, and their intensity increases during convalescence. A soft first heart sound may also reflect prolongation of the P-R interval. Patients with marked ventricular dysfunction and/or left bundle branch block may have paradoxical splitting of the second heart sound.

A fourth heart sound is almost universally present in patients in sinus rhythm with STEMI. However, it has limited diagnostic value because it is commonly audible in most patients with chronic ischemic heart disease and is recordable, although not often audible, in many normal subjects older than 45 years of age.

A third heart sound in patients with STEMI usually reflects severe LV dysfunction with elevated ventricular filling pressure. It is caused by rapid deceleration of transmitral blood flow during protodiastolic filling of the left ventricle and is usually heard in patients with large infarctions. This sound is detected best at the apex, with the patient in the left lateral recumbent position. A third heart sound may be caused not only by LV failure but also by increased inflow into the left ventricle, as occurs when mitral regurgitation or ventricular septal defect complicates STEMI. Third and fourth heart sounds emanating from the left ventricle are heard best at the apex; in patients with right ventricular infarcts, these sounds can be heard along the left sternal border and increase on inspiration.

MURMURS. Transient or persistent systolic murmurs are commonly audible in patients with STEMI and generally result from mitral regurgitation secondary to dysfunction of the mitral valve apparatus (e.g., papillary muscle dysfunction, LV dilation). A new, prominent, apical holosystolic murmur, accompanied by a thrill, may represent rupture of a head of a papillary muscle (see Chap. 55). The findings in cases of rupture of the interventricular septum are similar, although the murmur and thrill are usually most prominent along the left sternal border and may be audible at the right sternal border as well. The systolic murmur of tricuspid regurgitation (caused by right ventricular failure because of pulmonary hypertension and/or right ventricular infarction or by infarction of a right ventricular papillary muscle) is also heard along the left sternal border. It is characteristically intensified by inspiration and is accompanied by a prominent *c-v* wave in the jugular venous pulse and a right ventricular fourth sound.

FRICTION RUBS. Pericardial friction rubs may be heard in patients with STEMI, especially those sustaining large transmural infarctions.[66] Rubs are notorious for their evanescence and hence are probably even more common than reported. Although friction rubs can be heard within 24 hours or as late as 2 weeks after the onset of infarction, most commonly they are noted on the second or third day. Occasionally, in patients with extensive infarction, a loud rub can be heard for many days. Patients with STEMI and a pericardial friction rub may have a pericardial effusion on echocardiographic study, but only rarely does this cause the classic electrocardiographic changes of pericarditis. Delayed onset of the rub and the associated discomfort of pericarditis (as late as 3 months postinfarction) are characteristic of the now rare postmyocardial infarction syndrome (Dressler syndrome).

Pericardial rubs are most readily audible along the left sternal border or just inside the apical impulse. Loud rubs may be audible over the entire precordium and even over the back. Occasionally, only the systolic portion of a rub is heard; it can be confused with a systolic murmur, and the diagnosis of rupture of the ventricular septum or mitral regurgitation may be incorrectly considered.

OTHER FINDINGS

FUNDI. Hypertension, diabetes, and generalized atherosclerosis commonly accompany STEMI, and because these conditions can produce characteristic changes in the fundus, a funduscopic examination may provide information concerning the underlying vascular status. This is particularly useful for patients unable to provide a detailed history.

ABDOMEN. Pain in the abdomen associated with nausea, vomiting, restlessness, and even abdominal distention is often interpreted by patients as a sign of "indigestion," resulting in self-medication with antacids, and it can suggest an acute abdominal process to the physician. Right heart failure, characterized by hepatomegaly and a positive abdominojugular reflux, is unusual in patients with acute LV infarction, but does occur in patients with severe and prolonged LV failure or right ventricular infarction.

EXTREMITIES. Coronary atherosclerosis is often associated with systemic atherosclerosis, and therefore patients with STEMI may have a history of intermittent claudication and demonstrate physical findings of peripheral vascular disease (see Chap. 61). Thus, diminished peripheral arterial pulses, loss of hair, and atrophic skin in the lower extremities may be noted in patients with coronary artery disease. Peripheral edema is a manifestation of right ventricular failure and, like congestive hepatomegaly, is unusual in patients with acute LV infarction. Cyanosis of the nail beds is common in patients with severe LV failure and is particularly striking in patients with cardiogenic shock.

NEUROPSYCHIATRIC FINDINGS. Except for the altered mental status that occurs in patients with STEMI who have a markedly reduced cardiac output and cerebral hypoperfusion, neurologic findings are normal unless the patient has suffered cerebral embolism secondary to a mural thrombus. The coincidence between these two conditions can be explained by systemic hypotension caused by STEMI precipitating a cerebral infarction and the converse, as well as by mural emboli from the left ventricle causing cerebral emboli.

Patients with STEMI often exhibit alterations of the emotional state including intense anxiety, denial, and depression. Medical staff caring for STEMI patients must be sensitive to changes in the patient's emotional state; a calm, professional atmosphere, with thorough explanations of equipment and prognosis, can help alleviate the distress associated with STEMI.

Laboratory Findings

SERUM MARKERS OF CARDIAC DAMAGE. The availability of serum cardiac markers with markedly enhanced sensitivity for myocardial damage enables clinicians to diagnose MI in approximately an additional one third of patients who would not have fulfilled criteria for MI in the past.[67] The increased use of more sensitive biomarkers of MI, combined with more precise imaging techniques, has necessitated the establishment of new criteria for MI (see Table 54-2). As a consequence of the enhanced sensitivity for detection of smaller infarcts using cardiac-specific troponins, clinicians now face a new set of issues. More patients are discharged with a diagnosis of MI rather than UA, lifestyle and insurance implications need to be considered, and epidemiologic studies tracking the incidence of MI over time must account for the improved ability to diagnose MI in more contemporary patient cohorts.[1]

Although these considerations apply directly to patients on the UA/NSTEMI end of the ACS spectrum (see Chap. 56), a general discussion of cardiac biomarkers is presented here because the scientific aspects of the pathophysiologic concepts and assay methodology overlap when biomarkers are used to evaluate STEMI patients. It should be emphasized that clinicians should *not* wait for the results of biomarker assays to initiate treatment for the STEMI patient. Because there is a time urgency for reperfusion in STEMI, the 12-lead ECG should serve to initiate such strategies.

Necrosis compromises the integrity of the sarcolemmal membrane; intracellular macromolecules (serum cardiac markers) begin to diffuse into the cardiac interstitium, and ultimately into the microvasculature and lymphatics in the region of the infarct (**Fig. 54-14**; **Table 54-5**).[68,69] The rate of appearance of these macromolecules in the peripheral circulation depends on several factors, including intracellular location, molecular weight, local blood and lymphatic flow, and rate of elimination from the blood.[69,70]

Creatine Kinase

Serum CK activity exceeds the normal range within 4 to 8 hours after the onset of STEMI and declines to normal within 2 to 3 days (see Fig. 54-14). Although the peak CK level occurs on average at about 24 hours, peak levels occur earlier in patients who have had reperfusion as a result of the administration of fibrinolytic therapy or mechanical recanalization, as well as in patients with early spontaneous fibrinolysis (**Fig. 54-15**).

Although elevation of the serum CK concentration is a sensitive enzymatic detector of STEMI that is routinely available in most hospitals, important drawbacks include false-positive results in patients with muscle disease, alcohol intoxication, diabetes mellitus, skeletal muscle trauma, after vigorous exercise, convulsions, intramuscular injections, thoracic outlet syndrome, and pulmonary embolism.[71]

CREATINE KINASE ISOENZYMES. Three isoenzymes of CK exist (MM, BB, and MB). Extracts of brain and kidney contain predominantly the BB isoenzyme; skeletal muscle contains principally MM, but also contains some MB (1% to 3%), and cardiac muscle contains both MM and MB isoenzymes. The MB isoenzymes of CK can also be present in small quantities in the small intestine, tongue, diaphragm, uterus, and prostate. Strenuous exercise, particularly in trained long-distance runners or professional athletes, can cause elevation of both total CK and CK-MB.[72] Because CK-MB can be detected in the blood of healthy subjects, the cutoff value for abnormal elevation of CK-MB is usually set a few units above the upper reference limit for a given laboratory (see Fig. 54-14).[71] Although small quantities of CK-MB isoenzyme occur in tissues other than the heart, elevated levels of CK-MB may be considered, for practical purposes, to be the result of MI, except in the case of trauma or surgery on the organs noted.

Creatine kinase MB is analyzed in most laboratories by highly sensitive and specific enzyme immunoassays that use monoclonal antibodies directed against CK-MB.[71] It has been proposed that a ratio (relative index) of CK-MB mass to CK activity of approximately 2.5 indicates a myocardial rather than a skeletal source of the CK-MB elevation. Although this ratio may be satisfied by many patients with STEMI, it is inaccurate in several circumstances: (1) when high levels of total CK are present because of skeletal muscle injury (a large quantity of CK-MB must be released from the myocardium to satisfy criteria); (2) when chronic skeletal muscle injury releases large amounts of CK-MB; and (3) when total CK measurements are within the normal reference range for the laboratory and CK-MB is elevated, possibly indicating that a microinfarction has occurred. Clinicians should not rely on measurements of CK and CK-MB at a single time, but instead should evaluate the temporal rise and fall of serial values (see Fig. 54-14). Of note, because cardiac-specific troponins I and T (cTnI and cTnT; see Figs. 54-14 and 54-15 and Tables 54-2 and 54-5) accurately distinguish skeletal from cardiac muscle damage, the troponins are now considered the preferred biomarker for diagnosing MI.[69]

In addition to STEMI secondary to coronary obstruction, other forms of injury to cardiac muscle, such as those resulting from myocarditis, trauma, cardiac catheterization, shock, and cardiac surgery, may also produce elevated serum CK-MB levels.[71] These latter causes of elevation of serum CK-MB values can usually be readily distinguished from STEMI by the clinical setting.

OTHER BIOMARKERS. Isoforms of the MM and MB isoenzymes have been identified,[73] but with the increased availability of assays for the cardiac-specific troponins, measurement of CK isoforms has little, if any, important clinical role (see Table 54-5 and Fig. 54-14).[69] Myoglobin has now given way to more cardiac-specific markers, such as cTnI or cTnT.[74]

Cardiac-Specific Troponins

The troponin complex consists of three subunits that regulate the calcium-mediated contractile process of striated muscle. These include troponin C, which binds Ca^{2+}, troponin I (TnI), which binds to actin and inhibits actin-myosin interactions, and troponin T (TnT), which binds to tropomyosin, thereby attaching the troponin complex to the thin filament. Although the majority of TnT is incorporated into the troponin complex, approximately 6% is dissolved in the cytosol; about 2% to 3% of TnI is found in a cytosolic pool. Following myocyte injury, the initial release of cTnT and cTnI is from the cytosolic pool, followed subsequently by release from the structural (myofilament-bound) pool (see Fig. 54-14).[1]

Different genes encode TnT and TnI in cardiac and skeletal muscle, thus permitting the production of specific antibodies for the cardiac form (cTnT and cTnI) that enable their quantitative assay (see Fig. 54-14 and Table 54-4).[68] The measurement of cTnT or cTnI is now at the center of the new diagnostic criteria for MI.[1]

When interpreting the results of assays for cTnT or cTnI, clinicians must be cognizant of several analytic issues.[75] The cTnT assays are produced by a single manufacturer, leading to relative uniformity of cutoffs, whereas several manufacturers produce cTnI assays. There is evidence that the release pattern of troponin complexes and degradation into various troponin fragments may affect the results of various commercial assays, especially for cTnI, and may be useful in the future to gain insight into pathophysiologic events (e.g., ischemia, reperfusion).[76]

CUTOFF VALUES. Variations in the cutoff concentration for abnormal levels of cTnI in the immunoassays clinically available may be caused in part by different specificities of the antibodies used for detecting free and complexed cTnI. Thus, when using the measurement of cTnI for diagnosing STEMI, clinicians should apply the cutoff values for the particular assay used in their laboratory.[74] For both cTnT and cTnI, the definition of an abnormally increased level is a value exceeding that of 99% of a reference control group.[1]

Furthermore, whereas CK-MB usually increases 10- to 20-fold above the upper limit of the reference range, cTnT and cTnI typically increase more than 20 times above the reference range (see Fig. 54-14). These features of the cardiac-specific troponin assays provide an improved signal-to-noise ratio, enabling the detection of even minor degrees of myocardial necrosis. In patients with MI, cTnT and cTnI levels first begin to rise above the upper reference limit by 3 hours from the onset of chest pain. Because of a continuous release from a degenerating contractile apparatus in necrotic myocytes, elevations of cTnI may persist for 7 to 10 days after MI; elevations of cTnT may persist for up to 10 to 14 days. The prolonged time course of elevation of cTnT and cTnI is advantageous for the late diagnosis of MI. Patients with STEMI who undergo successful recanalization of the infarct-related artery have a rapid release of cardiac troponins, which can indicate reperfusion (see Fig. 54-15).[33]

TROPONIN VERSUS CK-MB. When comparing the diagnostic efficiency of the cardiac troponins versus CK-MB for MI, it is important to remember that the troponin assays can probably detect episodes of myocardial necrosis that are below the detection limit of the current CK-MB assays. This can lead to false-positive cases of troponin elevations if CK-MB is used as the reference standard or, conversely, to false-negative cases of CK-MB elevation if troponin is used as the reference standard. From a clinical perspective, it is desirable to have diagnostic

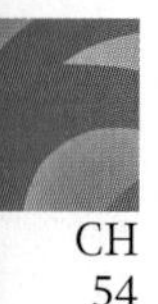

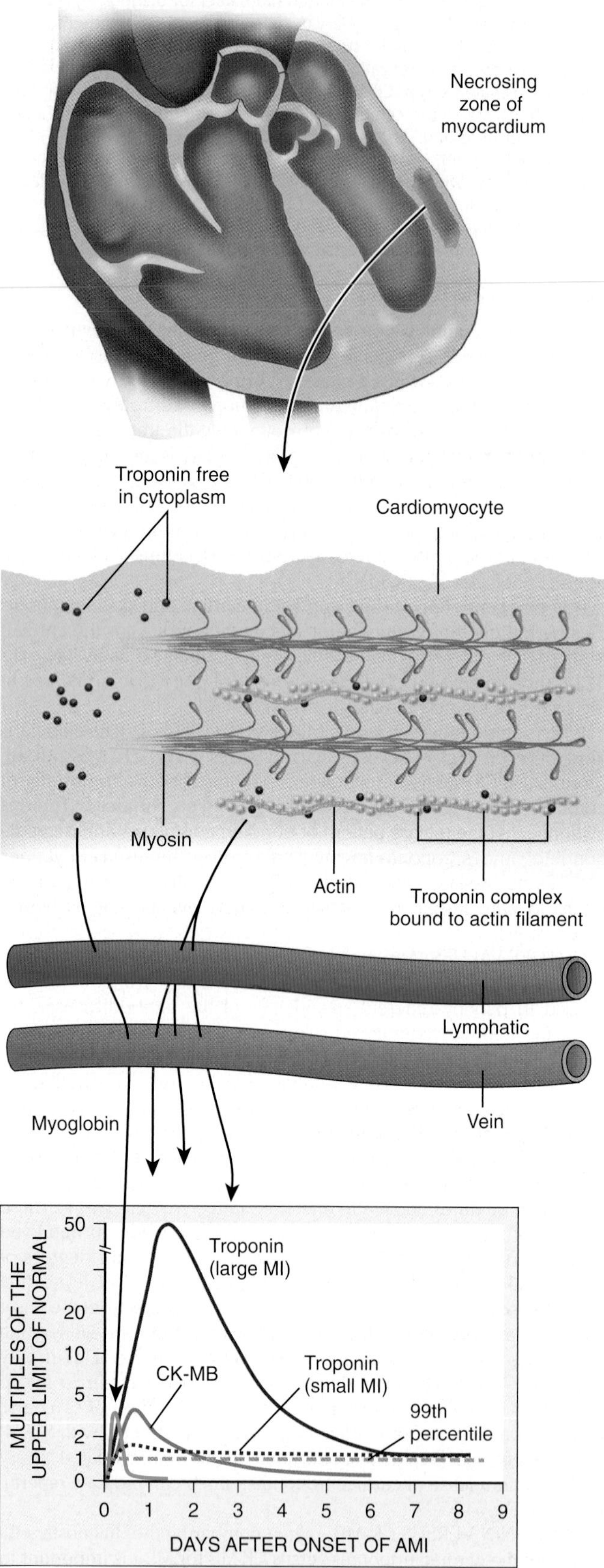

FIGURE 54-14 Top, Zone of necrosing myocardium, followed by a diagram of a cardiomyocyte that is in the process of releasing biomarkers **(middle)**. **Bottom,** After disruption of the sarcolemmal membrane of the cardiomyocyte, the cytoplasmic pool of biomarkers is released first (leftmost arrow). Markers such as myoglobin and CK isoforms are rapidly released, and blood levels rise quickly above the cutoff limit. This is then followed by a more protracted release of biomarkers from the disintegrating myofilaments that may continue for several days (three-headed arrow). Cardiac troponin levels rise to about 20 to 50 times the upper reference limit (the 99th percentile of values in a reference control group) in patients who have a classic acute MI and sustain sufficient myocardial necrosis to result in abnormally elevated levels of the MB fraction of creatine kinase (CK-MB). Clinicians can now diagnose episodes of microinfarction by sensitive assays that detect cardiac troponin elevations above the upper reference limit, even though CK-MB levels may still be in the normal reference range (not shown). CV = coefficient of variation. *(Modified from Antman EM: Decision making with cardiac troponin tests. N Engl J Med 346:2079, 2002; and Jaffe AS, Babiun L, Apple FS: Biomarkers in acute cardiac disease: The present and the future. J Am Coll Cardiol 48:1, 2006.)*

TABLE 54-5 Biomarkers for Evaluation of Patients with ST-Segment Elevation Myocardial Infarction

BIOMARKER	MOLECULAR WEIGHT (DA)	RANGE OF TIME TO INITIAL ELEVATION (HR)	MEAN TIME TO PEAK ELEVATIONS (NONREPERFUSED)	TIME TO RETURN TO NORMAL RANGE
Frequently Used in Clinical Practice				
MB-CK*	86,000	3-12	24 hr	48-72 hr
cTnI†	23,500	3-12	24 hr	5-10 days
cTnT	33,000	3-12	12 hr-2 days	5-14 days
Infrequently Used in Clinical Practice				
Myoglobin	17,800	1-4	6-7 hr	24 hr
MB-CK tissue isoform	86,000	2-6	18 hr	Unknown
MM-CK tissue isoform	86,000	1-6	12 hr	38 hr

*Increased sensitivity can be achieved with sampling every 6 or 8 hr.
†Multiple assays available for clinical use; clinicians should be familiar with the cutoff value used in their institution.
Modified from Antman EM, Anbe DT, Armstrong PW, et al: ACC/AHA guidelines for the management of patients with ST-elevation myocardial infarction: A report of the American College of Cardiology/American Heart Association Task Force on Practice Guidelines (Committee to Revise the 1999 Guidelines for the Management of Patients with Acute Myocardial Infarction). Circulation 110:e82, 2004.

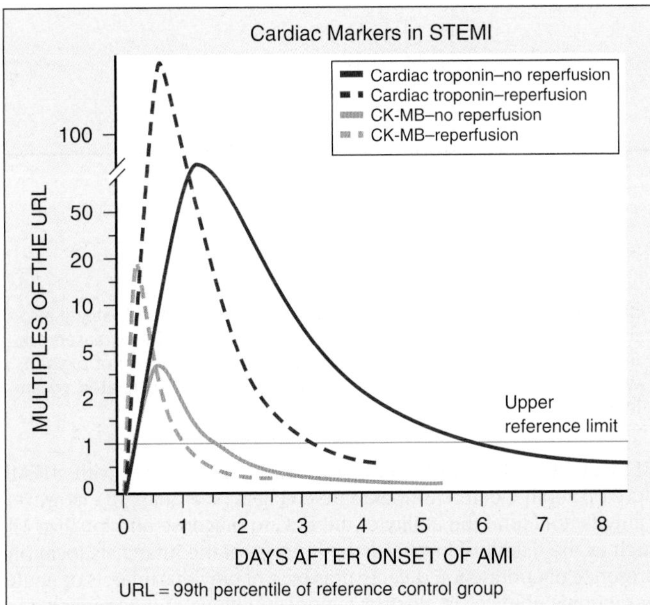

FIGURE 54-15 The kinetics of release of CK-MB and cardiac troponin in patients who do not undergo reperfusion are shown in the solid blue and pink curves as multiples of the upper reference limit (URL). When patients with STEMI undergo reperfusion (dashed blue and pink curves), the cardiac biomarkers are detected sooner and rise to a higher peak value, but decline more rapidly, resulting in a smaller area under the curve and limitation of infarct size. AMI = acute MI. *(Modified from Antman EM, Anbe DT, Armstrong PW, et al: ACC/AHA guidelines for the management of patients with ST-elevation myocardial infarction: A report of the American College of Cardiology/American Heart Association Task Force on Practice Guidelines [Committee to Revise the 1999 Guidelines for the Management of Patients with Acute Myocardial Infarction]. Circulation 110:e82, 2004.)*

tests for MI with increased sensitivity to increase the number of MI cases identified, and with increased specificity to reduce the number of cases incorrectly diagnosed and treated for MI. The prognostic value of the troponins is independent of other risk factors such as age and electrocardiographic abnormalities, as well as the measurement of older biomarkers such as CK-MB.[68]

Recommendations for Measurement of Serum Markers

It seems reasonable for clinicians to measure cTnT or cTnI in all patients with suspected MI. From a cost-effectiveness perspective, it is unnecessary to measure both a cardiac-specific troponin and CK-MB. Routine diagnosis of MI can be accomplished within 12 hours using CK-MB, cTnT, or cTnI by obtaining measurements approximately every 8 to 12 hours (see Tables 54-2 and 54-4). Retrospective diagnosis or diagnosis of MI in the presence of skeletal muscle injury is more readily accomplished with cTnT or cTnI. Assays for the cardiac-specific troponins should supersede assays for CK-MB, not only for the diagnosis of MI but also for the assessment of reperfusion, reinfarction, and estimation of infarct size.[1]

The universal definition of MI not only recommends classifying infarctions into five types (see Table 54-3), but also recommends assessing the magnitude of the infarction by tabulating the fold elevation of cardiac biomarkers above the 99th percentile of a normal reference group. A suggested grid for reporting the results is shown in **Table 54-6**. An example from a clinical trial comparing prasugrel with clopidogrel as supportive antiplatelet therapy for moderate-high risk ACS patients undergoing PCI is shown in **Figure 54-16**.[3]

Clinicians should measure a cardiac biomarker reflective of muscle death in a patient with suspected MI. **Figure 54-17** illustrates the temporal rise and fall of such biomarkers of muscle death along the chronology of the disease process, which begins with the development of a vulnerable plaque and ends with the release of biomarkers of muscle overload.[29] Markers such as pregnancy-associated plasma protein (PAPP) and ischemia-modified albumin (IMA) are not routinely measured in patients with MI. Measurement of BNP and related compounds may be useful for the assessment of the hemodynamic impact of the MI, although no clear guidance is available as to how to structure specific therapeutic maneuvers in the setting of STEMI in response to BNP measurements.

OTHER LABORATORY MEASUREMENTS

SERUM LIPIDS. During the first 24 to 48 hours after admission, total cholesterol and high-density lipoprotein (HDL) cholesterol remain at or near baseline values but generally fall precipitously after that (see Chap. 47). The fall in HDL cholesterol after STEMI is greater than the fall in total cholesterol; thus, the ratio of total cholesterol to HDL cholesterol is no longer useful for risk assessment unless measured early after MI. A lipid profile should be obtained on all STEMI patients who are admitted within 24 to 48 hours of symptoms. The success of lipid-lowering therapy in primary and secondary prevention studies and evidence that hypolipidemic therapy improves endothelial function and inhibits thrombus formation[77] indicate that early management of serum lipids in patients hospitalized for STEMI is advisable.[78] For patients admitted beyond 24 to 48 hours, more accurate determinations of serum lipid levels are obtained approximately 8 weeks after the infarction has occurred.

HEMATOLOGIC FINDINGS. The elevation of the white blood cell count usually develops within 2 hours after the onset of chest pain, reaches a peak 2 to 4 days after infarction, and returns to normal in 1 week. The peak white blood cell count usually ranges from 12 to 15×10^3/mL but occasionally rises to as high as 20×10^3/mL in patients with large STEMI. Often, there is an increase in the percentage of polymorphonuclear leukocytes and a shift of the differential count to band forms. An epidemiologic association has been reported, indicating a worse angiographic appearance of culprit lesions and increased risk of adverse clinical outcomes the higher the white blood cell count is at presentation with an ACS.[79]

The erythrocyte sedimentation rate (ESR) is usually normal during the first day or two after infarction, even though fever and leukocytosis may

TABLE 54-6 Classification of Different Types of Myocardial Infarction: Suggested Grid for Reporting Results*

	MI Type					
MULTIPLES X 99%	1 (SPONTANEOUS)	2 (SECONDARY)	3† (SUDDEN DEATH)	4‡ (PCI)	5‡ (CABG)	TOTAL NO.
1-2×						
2-3×						
3-5×						
5-10×						
>10×						
Total no.						

TYPES OF MI	TREATMENT A NO. OF PATIENTS	TREATMENT B NO. OF PATIENTS
MI type 1		
MI type 2		
MI type 3		
MI type 4		
MI type 5		
Total no.		

*According to multiples of the 99th percentile of a control group of the applied cardiac biomarker.
†Biomarkers are not available for this type of myocardial infarction because the patients expired before biomarker determination could be performed.
‡For the sake of completeness, the total distribution of biomarker values should be reported. The shaded areas represent biomarker elevations below the decision limit used for these types of myocardial infarction.
From Thygesen K, Alpert JS, White HD, et al: Universal definition of myocardial infarction. Circulation 116:2634, 2007.

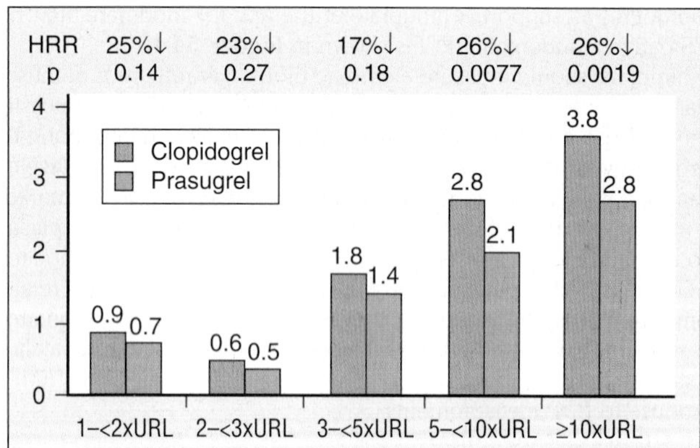

FIGURE 54-16 Effect of prasugrel compared with clopidogrel with respect to the total number of new or recurrent MIs classified using the biomarker categories recommended by the universal definition of MI (see Table 54-6). The biomarker categories are groupings of fold elevations above the upper reference limit (URL) of normal. The data shown for each bar are from Kaplan-Meier estimates for the incidence of MI; the percentage reductions represent the relative reductions in the hazard rate ratio (HRR) for the development of an MI in the prasugrel versus clopidogrel groups. *(From Morrow DA, Wiviott SD, White HD, et al: Effect of the novel thienopyridine prasugrel compared with clopidogrel on spontaneous and procedural myocardial infarction in the Trial to Assess Improvement in Therapeutic Outcomes by Optimizing Platelet Inhibition with Prasugrel-Thrombolysis in Myocardial Infarction 38: An application of the classification system from the universal definition of myocardial infarction. Circulation 119:2758, 2009.)*

be present. It then rises to a peak on the fourth or fifth day and may remain elevated for several weeks. The increase in the ESR does not correlate well with the size of the infarction or with the prognosis. The hematocrit often increases during the first few days after infarction as a consequence of hemoconcentration. An elevated C-reactive protein (CRP) level appears to identify patients presenting with STEMI, with worse angiographic appearance of the infarct artery and a greater likelihood of developing heart failure.[80]

The hemoglobin value at presentation with STEMI predicts major cardiovascular events powerfully and independently.[81] Of note is a J-shaped relationship between baseline hemoglobin values and clinical events. Cardiovascular mortality increases progressively as the presenting hemoglobin level falls below 14 to 15 g/dL; conversely, it also rises as the hemoglobin level increases above 17 g/dL. The increased risk from anemia probably relates to diminished tissue delivery of oxygen, whereas the increased risk with polycythemia may be related to an increase in blood viscosity.

ELECTROCARDIOGRAPHY. The majority of patients with STEMI develop serial electrocardiographic changes (see Chap. 13). However, many factors limit the ability of the ECG to diagnose and localize MI, such as the extent of myocardial injury, age of the infarct, its location, presence of conduction defects, presence of previous infarcts or acute pericarditis, changes in electrolyte concentrations, and administration of cardioactive drugs. Changes in the ST segment and T wave are nonspecific and may occur in a variety of conditions, including stable and unstable angina pectoris, ventricular hypertrophy, acute and chronic pericarditis, myocarditis, early repolarization, electrolyte imbalance, shock, and metabolic disorders, and following the administration of digitalis. Serial ECGs help differentiate these conditions from STEMI. Transient changes favor angina or electrolyte disturbances, whereas persistent changes argue for infarction if other causes such as shock, administration of digitalis, and persistent metabolic disorders can be eliminated. Nevertheless, serial standard 12-lead ECGs remain a potent and extremely useful method for the detection and localization of MI.[32] Analysis of the constellation of electrocardiographic leads showing ST-segment elevation may also be useful for identifying the site of occlusion in the infarct artery (see Fig. 54-4).[82] The extent of ST-segment deviation on the ECG, location of infarction, and QRS duration correlate with risk of adverse outcomes. Even when left bundle branch block is present on the ECG, MI can be diagnosed when striking ST-segment deviation is present beyond that which can be explained by the conduction defect. In addition to the diagnostic and prognostic information contained within the 12-lead ECG, it also provides valuable noninvasive information about the success of reperfusion for STEMI (see Chap. 55).[83]

Although general agreement exists on electrocardiographic and vectorcardiographic criteria for the recognition of infarction of the anterior and inferior myocardial walls, less agreement pertains to criteria for lateral and posterior infarcts; in this area, even the terminology can be confusing. A consensus group has recommended elimination of the term *posterior* and suggests using the term *lateral* to be consistent with current understanding of the segmental anatomy of the heart as it sits in the thorax.[84] Patients with an abnormal R wave in V_1 (0.04 second in duration and/or R/S ratio ≥ 1 in the absence of preexcitation or right ventricular hypertrophy), with inferior or lateral Q waves, have an increased incidence of isolated occlusion of a dominant left circumflex coronary artery without collateral circulation. These patients have a lower ejection fraction, increased end-systolic volume, and higher complication rate than patients with inferior infarction caused by isolated occlusion of the right coronary artery.

Although most patients bear the electrocardiographic changes from an infarction for the rest of their lives, particularly if they evolve Q waves, in a substantial minority the typical changes disappear, Q waves regress, and the ECG can even return to normal after a number of years. Under many circumstances, Q-wave patterns simulate MI. Conditions that may mimic the electrocardiographic features of MI by producing a pattern of "pseudoinfarction" include ventricular hypertrophy, conduction disturbances, preexcitation, primary myocardial disease, pneumothorax, pulmonary embolus, amyloid heart disease, primary and metastatic tumors of the heart, traumatic heart disease, intracranial hemorrhage, hyperkalemia, pericarditis, early repolarization, and cardiac sarcoidosis.

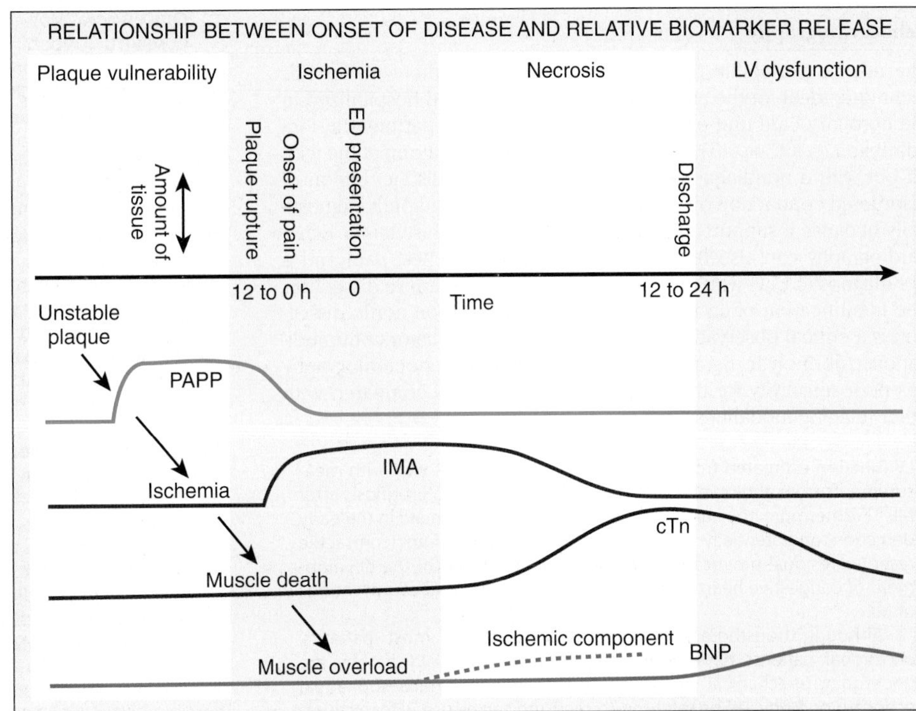

FIGURE 54-17 Coronary artery plaques vulnerable to rupture are caused by infiltration of inflammatory elements that release cytokines and enzymes, resulting in degradation of the fibrous cap. PAPP-A is a metalloproteinase that is released into blood during the stage of plaque vulnerability. Once a plaque has ruptured, myocardial ischemia is the initial consequence. This can be detected by the IMA test. Prolonged ischemia leads to myocardial necrosis and the release of cTn. After 12 to 24 hours, there can be LV dysfunction and myocardial muscle overloading, causing the release of BNP. There may also be release of BNP because of myocardial ischemia (dotted line). IMA = ischemia-modified albumin. *(From Wu AHB: Early detection of acute coronary syndromes and risk stratification by multimarker analysis. Biomarkers Med 1:52, 2007.)*

Q-Wave and Non–Q-Wave Infarction

The presence or absence of Q waves on the surface ECG does not reliably distinguish between transmural and nontransmural (subendocardial) MI.[85] Q waves on the ECG signify abnormal electrical activity but are not synonymous with irreversible myocardial damage. Also, the absence of Q waves may simply reflect the insensitivity of the standard 12-lead ECG, especially in zones of the left ventricle supplied by the left circumflex artery (see Fig. 54-4). Angiographic studies in MI patients without ST-segment elevation show a higher incidence of subtotal occlusion of the culprit coronary vessel and greater collateral flow to the infarct zone. Observational data suggest that MI without ST-segment elevation occurs more commonly in older patients and in patients with a prior MI.

Ischemia at a Distance

Patients with new Q waves and ST-segment elevation diagnostic for STEMI in one territory often have ST-segment depression in other territories. These additional ST-segment changes, which imply a poor prognosis, are caused by ischemia in a territory other than the area of infarction, termed *ischemia at a distance*, or by reciprocal electrical phenomena. A good deal of attention has been directed to associated ST-segment depression in the anterior leads when it occurs in patients with acute inferior STEMI. However, despite the clinical importance of differentiation among causes of anterior ST-segment depression in such patients, including anterior ischemia, inferolateral wall infarction, and true reciprocal changes, such a differentiation cannot be made reliably by electrocardiographic or even vectorcardiographic techniques. Although precordial ST-segment depression is associated more commonly with extensive infarction of the lateral or inferior septal segments, rather than anterior wall subendocardial ischemia, imaging techniques such as echocardiography are necessary to ascertain whether an anterior wall motion abnormality is present.[86]

Right Ventricular Infarction

ST-segment elevation in the right precordial leads (V_1, V_3R to V_6R) is a relatively sensitive and specific sign of right ventricular infarction.[82,87] Occasionally, ST-segment elevation in leads V_2 and V_3 results from acute right ventricular infarction; this appears to occur only when the injury to the left inferior wall is minimal (see Fig. 54-11).[88] Usually, the concurrent inferior wall injury suppresses this anterior ST-segment elevation resulting from right ventricular injury. Similarly, right ventricular infarction appears to reduce the anterior ST-segment depression often observed with inferior wall myocardial infarction. A QS or QR pattern in leads V_3R and/or V_4R also suggests right ventricular myocardial necrosis but has less predictive accuracy than ST-segment elevation in these leads.

IMAGING

Roentgenography

The initial chest roentgenogram (see Chap. 16) in patients with STEMI is almost invariably a portable film obtained in the emergency department or coronary care unit. When present, prominent pulmonary vascular markings on the roentgenogram reflect elevated LV end-diastolic pressure, but significant temporal discrepancies can occur because of what have been termed *diagnostic lags* and *post-therapeutic lags*. Up to 12 hours can elapse before pulmonary edema accumulates after ventricular filling pressure has become elevated. The post-therapeutic phase lag represents a longer time interval; up to 2 days are required for pulmonary edema to resorb and the radiographic signs of pulmonary congestion to clear after ventricular filling pressure has returned toward normal. The degree of congestion and size of the left side of the heart on the chest film are useful for defining groups of patients with STEMI who are at increased risk of dying after the acute event.

Echocardiography

The relative portability of echocardiographic equipment makes this technique ideal for the assessment of patients with MI hospitalized in the coronary care unit or even in the emergency department before admission (see Chap. 15).[86] In patients with chest pain compatible with MI but with a nondiagnostic ECG, the finding of a distinct region of disordered contraction on echocardiography can be helpful diagnostically because it supports the diagnosis of myocardial ischemia. Echocardiography can also help evaluate patients with chest pain and a nondiagnostic ECG who are suspected of having an aortic dissection. The identification of an intimal flap consistent with an aortic dissection is a critical observation because it represents a major contraindication to fibrinolytic therapy (see Chap. 60). However, echocardiography has poor sensitivity for detection of the intimal flaps compared with other imaging modalities, such as CT angiography.

LV function estimated from echocardiograms correlates well with measurements from angiograms and is useful in establishing prognosis after MI.[86] Furthermore, the early use of echocardiography can aid in the early detection of potentially viable but stunned myocardium (contractile reserve), residual provocable ischemia, patients at risk for the development of congestive heart failure after MI, and mechanical complications of MI.

Although transthoracic imaging is adequate in most patients, occasional patients have poor echo windows, especially if they are undergoing mechanical ventilation. In such patients, transesophageal echocardiography can be safely performed and can be useful for evaluating ventricular septal defects and papillary muscle dysfunction.[33]

Doppler techniques allow the assessment of blood flow in the cardiac chambers and across cardiac valves. Used in conjunction with echocardiography, it can help detect and assess the severity of mitral or tricuspid regurgitation after STEMI. Identification of the site of acute ventricular septal rupture, quantification of shunt flow across the resulting defect, and assessment of acute cardiac tamponade are also possible.[33]

Other Imaging Modalities

Computed Tomography. This technique (see Chap. 19) can provide useful cross-sectional information in patients with MI. In addition to the assessment of cavity dimensions and wall thickness, LV aneurysms can be detected and, of particular importance in patients with STEMI, intracardiac thrombi can be identified. Although cardiac computed tomography is a less convenient technique, it probably is more sensitive than echocardiography for thrombus detection.

Cardiac Magnetic Resonance Imaging. In addition to localizing and sizing the area of infarction, cardiac magnetic resonance (CMR) techniques (see Chap. 18) permit early recognition of MI and can provide an assessment of the severity of the ischemic insult (see Fig. 56-5). This modality is attractive because it can assess perfusion of infarcted and noninfarcted tissue, as well as of reperfused myocardium; identify areas of jeopardized but not infarcted myocardium; identify myocardial edema, fibrosis, wall thinning, and hypertrophy; assess ventricular chamber size and segmental wall motion; and identify the temporal transition between ischemia and infarction (**Fig. 54-18**).[89] It has limited application during the acute phase because of the need to transport patients with MI to the MRI facility, but as discussed later, it is an extremely useful imaging technique during the subacute and chronic phases of MI.

Contrast-enhanced CMR can detect myocardial infarction accurately. The transmural extent of late gadolinium enhancement in regions of dysfunctional myocardium accurately predicts the likelihood of contractile recovery after successful restoration of coronary flow from mechanical revascularization.[90] Numerous clinical studies have also demonstrated high sensitivity of late gadolinium enhancement (delayed hyperenhancement) of CMR in detecting small amounts of myonecrosis. In patients with a prior MI, estimation of the size of the peri-infarct zone by CMR using the delayed enhancement technique provides incremental prognostic value beyond LV volumes and ejection fraction.[91] Beyond detecting infarction, this imaging technique can characterize the presence and size of microvascular obstruction from infarction, which portends an adverse clinical outcome postinfarction (see Fig. 18-4).[92] Clinically unrecognized myocardial scar detected by late gadolinium enhancement imaging is associated with a high risk of adverse cardiac events in patients with signs and symptoms of coronary artery disease but without a history of infarction.[93]

Nuclear Imaging. Radionuclide angiography, perfusion imaging, infarct-avid scintigraphy, and positron emission tomography have been used to evaluate patients with STEMI (see Chap. 17).[94] Nuclear cardiac imaging techniques can be useful for detecting MI, assessing infarct size, collateral flow, and jeopardized myocardium, determining the effects of the infarct on ventricular function, and establishing a prognosis of patients with STEMI. However, the necessity of moving a critically ill patient from the coronary care unit to the nuclear medicine department limits practical application unless a portable gamma camera is available. Cardiac radionuclide imaging for the diagnosis of MI should be restricted to special limited situations in which the triad of clinical history, electrocardiographic findings, and serum marker measurements is unavailable or unreliable.

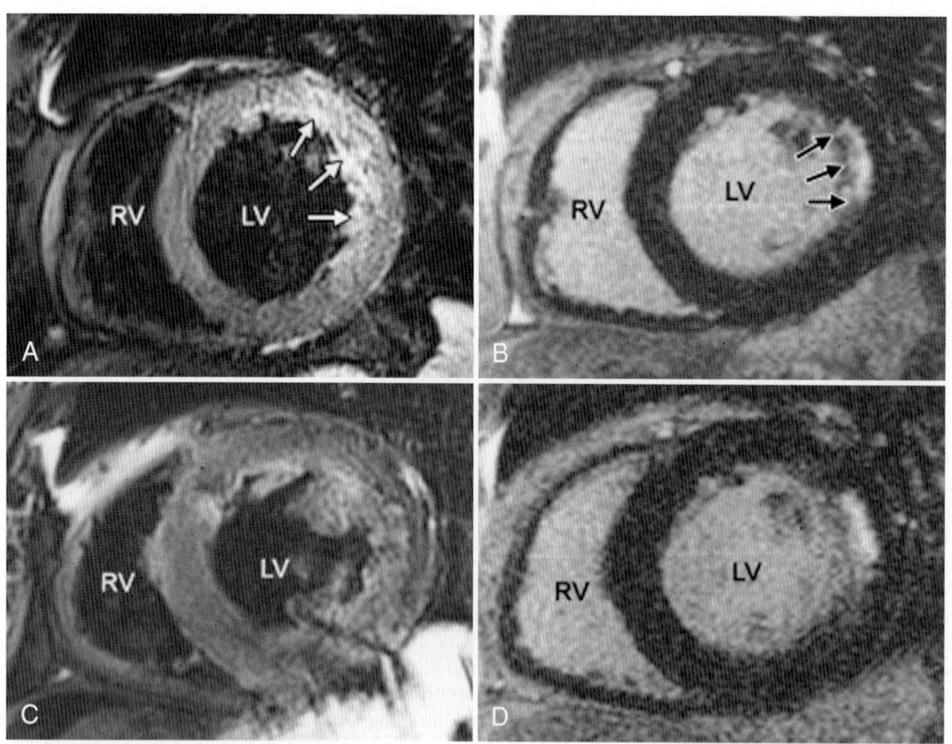

FIGURE 54-18 **A,** T2-weighted edema imaging showing acute transmural myocardial edema surrounding a subendocardial infarction *(arrows)* **(B)**. The patient suffered from an acute MI 2 days before the CMR, secondary to acute plaque rupture and thrombus formation in the proximal diagonal territory *(arrows)*. **C,** CMR was repeated 3 weeks after the initial presentation, showing marked resolution of the T2-weighted transmural myocardial edema. **D,** Infarct size is relatively unchanged compared with the first CMR study. *(Courtesy of Dr. Raymond Kwong, Brigham and Women's Hospital, Boston.)*

Estimation of Infarct Size

ELECTROCARDIOGRAPHY. Interest in limiting infarct size, in large part because of the recognition that the quantity of myocardium infarcted has important prognostic implications, has focused attention on the accurate determination of MI size. The sum of ST-segment elevations measured from multiple precordial leads correlates with the extent of myocardial injury in patients with anterior MI.[32] However, there is a relationship between the number of electrocardiographic leads showing ST-segment elevation and mortality rate. Patients with 8 or 9 of 12 leads with ST-segment elevation have 3 to 4 times the mortality of those with only 2 or 3 leads with ST-segment elevation. The duration of ischemia time, as estimated from continuous ST-segment monitoring, correlates with infarct size, ratio of infarct size to the area at risk, and extent of regional wall motion abnormality observed subsequently.[95]

SERUM CARDIAC MARKERS. Estimation of infarct size by the analysis of serum cardiac markers requires accounting for the quantity of the marker lost from the myocardium, its volume of distribution, and its release ratio. Serial measurements of proteins released by necrotic myocardium help determine MI size. Clinically, the peak CK or CK-MB value provides an approximate estimate of infarct size and is widely used prognostically. Coronary artery reperfusion dramatically changes the washout kinetics of CK and other markers from myocardium, resulting in early and exaggerated peak levels and limiting the usefulness of such curves as a measure of infarct size. Measuring a cardiac-specific troponin level several days after STEMI, even in cases of successful reperfusion, may provide a reliable estimate of infarct size, because such late troponin measurements reflect delayed release from the myofilament-bound pool in damaged myocytes.[96]

NONINVASIVE IMAGING TECHNIQUES. These imaging modalities can aid in the experimental and clinical assessment of infarct size.[94] Contrast-enhanced CMR can demonstrate regional heterogeneity of infarction patterns in patients with persistently occluded infarct arteries, compared with those with successfully reperfused vessels.[97]

REFERENCES

Changing Patterns in Clinical Care

1. Thygesen K, Alpert JS, White HD, et al: Universal definition of myocardial infarction. Circulation 116:2634, 2007.
2. Hochholzer W, Buettner HJ, Trenk D, et al: New definition of myocardial infarction: Impact on long-term mortality. Am J Med 121:399, 2008.
3. Morrow DA, Wiviott SD, White HD, et al: Effect of the novel thienopyridine prasugrel compared with clopidogrel on spontaneous and procedural myocardial infarction in the Trial to Assess Improvement in Therapeutic Outcomes by Optimizing Platelet Inhibition with Prasugrel-Thrombolysis in Myocardial Infarction 38: An application of the classification system from the universal definition of myocardial infarction. Circulation 119:2758, 2009.
4. Gaziano TA: Reducing the growing burden of cardiovascular disease in the developing world. Health Aff (Millwood) 26:13, 2007.
5. Lloyd-Jones D, Adams R, Carnethon M, et al: Heart disease and stroke statistics—2009 update: A report from the American Heart Association Statistics Committee and Stroke Statistics Subcommittee. Circulation 119:e21, 2009.
6. Napoli C, Cacciatore F: Novel pathogenic insights in the primary prevention of cardiovascular disease. Prog Cardiovasc Dis 51:503, 2009.
7. Goldberg RJ, Glatfelter K, Burbank-Schmidt E, et al: Trends in community mortality due to coronary heart disease. Am Heart J 151:501, 2006.
8. Kamalesh M, Subramanian U, Ariana A, et al: Similar decline in post-myocardial infarction mortality among subjects with and without diabetes. Am J Med Sci 329:228, 2005.
9. Myerson M, Coady S, Taylor H, et al: Declining severity of myocardial infarction from 1987 to 2002: The Atherosclerosis Risk in Communities (ARIC) Study. Circulation 119:503, 2009.
10. Anderson JL, Adams CD, Antman EM, et al: ACC/AHA 2007 guidelines for the management of patients with unstable angina/non ST-elevation myocardial infarction: A report of the American College of Cardiology/American Heart Association Task Force on Practice Guidelines (Writing Committee to Revise the 2002 Guidelines for the Management of Patients With Unstable Angina/Non ST-Elevation Myocardial Infarction): Developed in collaboration with the American College of Emergency Physicians, the Society for Cardiovascular Angiography and Interventions, and the Society of Thoracic Surgeons: Endorsed by the American Association of Cardiovascular and Pulmonary Rehabilitation and the Society for Academic Emergency Medicine. Circulation 116:e148, 2007.
11. Braunwald E, Antman EM: Evidence-based coronary care. Ann Intern Med 126:551, 1997.
12. Antman EM, Peterson ED: Tools for guiding clinical practice from the American Heart Association and the American College of Cardiology: What are they and how should clinicians use them? Circulation 119:1180, 2009.
13. Krumholz HM, Anderson JL, Bachelder BL, et al: ACC/AHA 2008 performance measures for adults with ST-elevation and non-ST-elevation myocardial infarction: A report of the American College of Cardiology/American Heart Association Task Force on Performance Measures (Writing Committee to develop performance measures for ST-elevation and non-ST-elevation myocardial infarction): Developed in collaboration with the American Academy of Family Physicians and the American College of Emergency Physicians: Endorsed by the American Association of Cardiovascular and Pulmonary Rehabilitation, Society for Cardiovascular Angiography and Interventions, and Society of Hospital Medicine. Circulation 118:2596, 2008.
14. Kushner FG, Hand M, Smith SC Jr, et al: 2009 focused updates of the ACC/AHA guidelines for the management of patients with ST-elevation myocardial infarction (updating the 2004 guideline and 2007 focused update) and the ACC/AHA/SCAI guidelines on percutaneous coronary intervention (updating the 2005 guideline and 2007 focused update): A report of the American College of Cardiology Foundation/American Heart Association Task Force on Practice Guidelines. Circulation 120:2271, 2009.
15. Antman EM, Morrow DA, McCabe CH, et al: Enoxaparin versus unfractionated heparin with fibrinolysis for ST-elevation myocardial infarction. N Engl J Med 354:1477, 2006.
16. Canto JG, Rogers WJ, Chandra NC, et al: The association of sex and payer status on management and subsequent survival in acute myocardial infarction. Arch Intern Med 162:587, 2002.
17. Fox KA, Steg PG, Eagle KA, et al: Decline in rates of death and heart failure in acute coronary syndromes, 1999-2006. JAMA 297:1892, 2007.
18. Ahmed S, Antman EM, Murphy SA, et al: Poor outcomes after fibrinolytic therapy for ST-segment elevation myocardial infarction: Impact of age (a meta-analysis of a decade of trials). J Thromb Thrombolysis 21:119, 2006.
19. Orlandini A, Diaz R, Wojdyla D, et al: Outcomes of patients in clinical trials with ST-segment elevation myocardial infarction among countries with different gross national incomes. Eur Heart J 27:527, 2006.
20. Steinberg BA, Moghbeli N, Buros J, et al: Global outcomes of ST-elevation myocardial infarction: Comparisons of the Enoxaparin and Thrombolysis Reperfusion for Acute Myocardial Infarction Treatment-Thrombolysis In Myocardial Infarction study 25 (ExTRACT-TIMI 25) registry and trial. Am Heart J 154:54, 2007.
21. Birkhead JS, Weston C, Lowe D. Impact of specialty of admitting physician and type of hospital on care and outcome for myocardial infarction in England and Wales during 2004-5: Observational study. BMJ 332:1306, 2006.
22. Jani SM, Montoye C, Mehta R, et al: Sex differences in the application of evidence-based therapies for the treatment of acute myocardial infarction: The American College of Cardiology's Guidelines Applied in Practice projects in Michigan. Arch Intern Med 166:1164, 2006.

Pathology

23. Bayes de Luna A: Location of Q-wave myocardial infarction in the era of cardiac magnetic resonance imaging techniques: An update. J Electrocardiol 40:69, 2007.
24. Engblom H, Carlsson MB, Hedstrom E, et al: The endocardial extent of reperfused first-time myocardial infarction is more predictive of pathologic Q waves than is infarct transmurality: A magnetic resonance imaging study. Clin Physiol Funct Imaging 27:101, 2007.
25. Achenbach S: Can CT detect the vulnerable coronary plaque? Int J Cardiovasc Imaging 24:311, 2008.
26. Fox JJ, Strauss HW: One step closer to imaging vulnerable plaque in the coronary arteries. J Nucl Med 50:497, 2009.
27. Wasserman EJ, Shipley NM: Atherothrombosis in acute coronary syndromes: mechanisms, markers, and mediators of vulnerability. Mt Sinai J Med 73:431, 2006.
28. Katritsis DG, Pantos J, Efstathopoulos E: Hemodynamic factors and atheromatic plaque rupture in the coronary arteries: From vulnerable plaque to vulnerable coronary segment. Coron Artery Dis 18:229, 2007.
29. Wu AHB: Early detection of acute coronary syndromes and risk stratification by multimarker analysis. Biomarkers Med 1:45, 2007.
30. Barlis P, Serruys PW, Devries A, Regar E: Optical coherence tomography assessment of vulnerable plaque rupture: Predilection for the plaque 'shoulder'. Eur Heart J 29:2023, 2008.
31. Manfredini R, Boari B, Salmi R, et al: Circadian rhythms and reperfusion in patients with acute ST-segment elevation myocardial infarction. JAMA 294:2846, 2005.
32. Wagner GS, Macfarlane P, Wellens H, et al: AHA/ACCF/HRS recommendations for the standardization and interpretation of the electrocardiogram: Part VI: Acute ischemia/infarction: A scientific statement from the American Heart Association Electrocardiography and Arrhythmias Committee, Council on Clinical Cardiology; the American College of Cardiology Foundation; and the Heart Rhythm Society: Endorsed by the International Society for Computerized Electrocardiology. Circulation 119:e262, 2009.
33. Antman EM, Anbe DT, Armstrong PW, et al: ACC/AHA guidelines for the management of patients with ST-elevation myocardial infarction: A report of the American College of Cardiology/American Heart Association Task Force on Practice Guidelines (Committee to Revise the 1999 Guidelines for the Management of Patients with Acute Myocardial Infarction). Circulation 110:e82, 2004.
34. Chua S, Chang LT, Sun CK, et al: Time courses of subcellular signal transduction and cellular apoptosis in remote viable myocardium of rat left ventricles following acute myocardial infarction: Role of pharmacomodulation. J Cardiovasc Pharmacol Ther 14:104, 2009.
35. Schoen FJ: The heart. *In* Kumar V, Abbas AK, Fausto N (eds): Robbins & Cotran Pathologic Basis of Disease. 8th ed. Philadelphia, WB Saunders, 2010, pp 529-587.
36. Pasotti M, Prati F, Arbustini E: The pathology of myocardial infarction in the pre- and post-interventional era. Heart 92:1552, 2006.
37. Vargas SO, Sampson BA, Schoen FJ: Pathologic detection of early myocardial infarction: A critical review of the evolution and usefulness of modern techniques. Mod Pathol 12:635, 1999.
38. Abbate A, Bussani R, Sinagra G, et al: Right ventricular cardiomyocyte apoptosis in patients with acute myocardial infarction of the left ventricular wall. Am J Cardiol 102:658, 2008.
39. Noel TE, Kontos MC: Troponin and other markers of necrosis for risk stratification in patients with acute coronary syndromes. *In* de Lemos JA (ed): Biomarkers in Heart Disease. Oxford, Blackwell Publishing, 2008, pp 22-39.
40. DeWood MA, Spores J, Notske R, et al: Prevalence of total coronary occlusion during the early hours of transmural myocardial infarction. N Engl J Med 303:897, 1980.
41. Hamon M, Agostini D, Le Page O, Riddell JW: Prognostic impact of right ventricular involvement in patients with acute myocardial infarction: Meta-analysis. Crit Care Med 36:2023, 2008.
42. Popescu BA, Antonini-Canterin F, Temporelli PL, et al: Right ventricular functional recovery after acute myocardial infarction: Relation with left ventricular function and interventricular septum motion. GISSI-3 echo substudy. Heart 91:484, 2005.
43. Neven K, Crijns H, Gorgels A: Atrial infarction: A neglected electrocardiographic sign with important clinical implications. J Cardiovasc Electrophysiol 14:306, 2003.
44. Tjandrawidjaja MC, Fu Y, Kim DH, et al: Compromised atrial coronary anatomy is associated with atrial arrhythmias and atrioventricular block complicating acute myocardial infarction. J Electrocardiol 38:271, 2005.
45. Park SM, Prasad A, Rihal C, et al: Left ventricular systolic and diastolic function in patients with apical ballooning syndrome compared with patients with acute anterior ST-segment elevation myocardial infarction: A functional paradox. Mayo Clin Proc 84:514, 2009.

Pathophysiology

46. Schuster EH, Bulkley BH: Ischemia at a distance after acute myocardial infarction: A cause of early postinfarction angina. Circulation 62:509, 1980.

47. Forrester JS, Wyatt HL, Da Luz PL, et al: Functional significance of regional ischemic contraction abnormalities. Circulation 54:64, 1976.
48. Funaro S, La Torre G, Madonna M, et al: Incidence, determinants, and prognostic value of reverse left ventricular remodelling after primary percutaneous coronary intervention: results of the Acute Myocardial Infarction Contrast Imaging (AMICI) multicenter study. Eur Heart J 30:566, 2009.
49. McMurray J, Solomon S, Pieper K, et al: The effect of valsartan, captopril, or both on atherosclerotic events after acute myocardial infarction: An analysis of the Valsartan in Acute Myocardial Infarction Trial (VALIANT). J Am Coll Cardiol 47:726, 2006.
50. Hochman JS: Cardiogenic shock complicating acute myocardial infarction: Expanding the paradigm. Circulation 107:2998, 2003.
51. Ruan W, Lu L, Zhang Q, et al: Serial assessment of left ventricular remodeling and function by echo-tissue Doppler imaging after myocardial infarction in streptozotocin-induced diabetic swing. J Am Soc Echocardiogr 22:530, 2009.
52. Weisman HF, Bush DE, Mannisi JA, et al: Cellular mechanisms of myocardial infarct expansion. Circulation 78:186, 1988.
53. Konstam MA: Patterns of ventricular remodeling after myocardial infarction: Clues toward linkage between mechanism and morbidity. JACC Cardiovasc Imaging 1:592, 2008.
54. Kosiborod M, Inzucchi SE, Krumholz HM, et al: Glucose normalization and outcomes in patients with acute myocardial infarction. Arch Intern Med 169:438, 2009.
55. Hofsten DE, Logstrup BB, Moller JE, et al: Abnormal glucose metabolism in acute myocardial infarction: Influence on LV function and prognosis. JACC Cardiovasc Imaging 2:592, 2009.
56. Lorgis L, Zeller M, Dentan G, et al: Prognostic value of N-terminal pro-brain natriuretic peptide in elderly people with acute myocardial infarction: Prospective observational study. BMJ 338:b1605, 2009.
57. White HD, Chew DP: Acute myocardial infarction. Lancet 372:570, 2008.
58. Smit JJ, Ottervanger JP, Kolkman JJ, et al: Change of white blood cell count more prognostic important than baseline values after primary percutaneous coronary intervention for ST-segment elevation myocardial infarction. Thromb Res 122:185, 2008.

Clinical Features

59. Bodis J, Boncz I, Kriszbacher I: Permanent stress may be the trigger of an acute myocardial infarction on the first work-day of the week. Int J Cardiol 2009.
60. Fleischmann KE, Beckman JA, Buller CE, et al: ACCF/AHA 2009 focused update on perioperative beta blockade: A report of the American College of Cardiology Foundation/American Heart Association Task Force on Practice Guidelines. Circulation 120:2123, 2009.
61. Assali AR, Brosh D, Vaknin-Assa H, et al: The impact of circadian variation on outcomes in emergency acute anterior myocardial infarction percutaneous coronary intervention. Catheter Cardiovasc Interv 67:221, 2006.
62. Leiza JR, de Llano JM, Messa JB, et al: New insights into the circadian rhythm of acute myocardial infarction in subgroups. Chronobiol Int 24:129, 2007.
63. Feringa HH, Karagiannis SE, Vidakovic R, et al: The prevalence and prognosis of unrecognized myocardial infarction and silent myocardial ischemia in patients undergoing major vascular surgery. Coron Artery Dis 18:571, 2007.
64. Killip T 3rd, Kimball JT: Treatment of myocardial infarction in a coronary care unit. A two-year experience with 250 patients. Am J Cardiol 20:457, 1967.
65. Montalescot G, Wiviott SD, Braunwald E, et al: Prasugrel compared with clopidogrel in patients undergoing percutaneous coronary intervention for ST-elevation myocardial infarction (TRITON-TIMI 38): Double-blind, randomised controlled trial. Lancet 373:723, 2009.
66. Dorfman TA, Aqel R: Regional pericarditis: A review of the pericardial manifestations of acute myocardial infarction. Clin Cardiol 32:115, 2009.
67. Ravkilde J, Horder M, Gerhardt W, et al: Diagnostic performance and prognostic value of serum troponin T in suspected acute myocardial infarction. Scand J Clin Lab Invest 53:677, 1993.
68. Antman EM: Decision making with cardiac troponin tests. N Engl J Med 346:2079, 2002.
69. Jaffe AS, Babuin L, Apple FS: Biomarkers in acute cardiac disease: The present and the future. J Am Coll Cardiol 48:1, 2006.
70. Penttila K, Koukkunen H, Halinen M, et al: Myoglobin, creatine kinase MB isoforms and creatine kinase MB mass in early diagnosis of myocardial infarction in patients with acute chest pain. Clin Biochem 35:647, 2002.
71. Apple FS, Quist HE, Doyle PJ, et al: Plasma 99th percentile reference limits for cardiac troponin and creatine kinase MB mass for use with European Society of Cardiology/American College of Cardiology consensus recommendations. Clin Chem 49:1331, 2003.
72. Apple FS: Tissue specificity of cardiac troponin I, cardiac troponin T and creatine kinase-MB. Clin Chim Acta 284:151, 1999.
73. Roberts R, Kleiman NS: Earlier diagnosis and treatment of acute myocardial infarction necessitates the need for a 'new diagnostic mind-set.' Circulation 89:872, 1994.
74. Morrow DA, Cannon CP, Jesse RL, et al: National Academy of Clinical Biochemistry Laboratory Medicine Practice Guidelines: Clinical characteristics and utilization of biochemical markers in acute coronary syndromes. Circulation 115:e356, 2007.
75. Aviles RJ, Askari AT, Lindahl B, et al: Troponin T levels in patients with acute coronary syndromes, with or without renal dysfunction. N Engl J Med 346:2047, 2002.
76. Jaffe AS, Van Eyk JE: Degradation of cardiac troponins: implications for clinical practice. *In* Morrow DA (ed): Cardiovascular Biomarkers: Pathophysiology and Disease Management. Totowa, NJ, Humana Press, 2006, pp 161-174.
77. Wolfrum S, Jensen KS, Liao JK: Endothelium-dependent effects of statins. Arterioscler Thromb Vasc Biol 23:729, 2003.
78. Smith SC Jr, Allen J, Blair SN, et al: AHA/ACC guidelines for secondary prevention for patients with coronary and other atherosclerotic vascular disease: 2006 update: Endorsed by the National Heart, Lung and Blood Institute. Circulation 113:2363, 2006.
79. Barron HV, Cannon CP, Murphy SA, et al: Association between white blood cell count, epicardial blood flow, myocardial perfusion, and clinical outcomes in the setting of acute myocardial infarction: A thrombolysis in myocardial infarction 10 substudy. Circulation 102:2329, 2000.
80. Ziakas A, Gavrilidis S, Giannoglou G, et al: In-hospital and long-term prognostic value of fibrinogen, CRP, and IL-6 levels in patients with acute myocardial infarction treated with thrombolysis. Angiology 57:283, 2006.
81. Sabatine MS, Morrow DA, Giugliano RP, et al: Association of hemoglobin levels with clinical outcomes in acute coronary syndromes. Circulation 111:2042, 2005.
82. Zimetbaum PJ, Josephson ME: Use of the electrocardiogram in acute myocardial infarction. N Engl J Med 348:933, 2003.
83. Scirica BM, Morrow DA, Sadowski Z, et al: A strategy of using enoxaparin as adjunctive antithrombin therapy reduces death and recurrent myocardial infarction in patients who achieve early ST-segment resolution after fibrinolytic therapy: The ExTRACT-TIMI 25 ECG study. Eur Heart J 28:2070, 2007.
84. Bayes de Luna A, Wagner G, Birnbaum Y, et al: A new terminology for left ventricular walls and location of myocardial infarcts that present Q wave based on the standard of cardiac magnetic resonance imaging: A statement for health care professionals from a committee appointed by the International Society for Holter and Noninvasive Electrocardiography. Circulation 114:1755, 2006.
85. Moon JC, De Arenaza DP, Elkington AG, et al: The pathologic basis of Q-wave and non-Q-wave myocardial infarction: A cardiovascular magnetic resonance study. J Am Coll Cardiol 44:554, 2004.
86. Cheitlin MD, Armstrong WF, Aurigemma GP, et al: ACC/AHA/ASE 2003 Guideline Update for the Clinical Application of Echocardiography: Summary article. A report of the American College of Cardiology/American Heart Association Task Force on Practice Guidelines (ACC/AHA/ASE Committee to Update the 1997 Guidelines for the Clinical Application of Echocardiography). J Am Soc Echocardiogr 16:1091, 2003.
87. Lopez-Sendon J, Coma-Canella I, Alcasena S, et al: Electrocardiographic findings in acute right ventricular infarction: Sensitivity and specificity of electrocardiographic alterations in right precordial leads V4R, V3R, V1, V2, and V3. J Am Coll Cardiol 6:1273, 1985.
88. Finn AV, Antman EM: Images in clinical medicine. Isolated right ventricular infarction. N Engl J Med 349:1636, 2003.
89. Ibrahim T, Makowski MR, Jankauskas A, et al: Serial contrast-enhanced cardiac magnetic resonance imaging demonstrates regression of hyperenhancement within the coronary artery wall in patients after acute myocardial infarction. JACC Cardiovasc Imaging 2:580, 2009.
90. Silva C, Cacciavillani L, Corbetti F, et al: Natural time course of myocardial infarction at delayed enhancement magnetic resonance. Int J Cardiol 2009.
91. Yan AT, Shayne AJ, Brown KA, et al: Characterization of the peri-infarct zone by contrast-enhanced cardiac magnetic resonance imaging is a powerful predictor of post-myocardial infarction mortality. Circulation 114:32, 2006.
92. Habis M, Capderou A, Sigal-Cinqualbre A, et al: Comparison of delayed enhancement patterns on multislice computed tomography immediately after coronary angiography and cardiac magnetic resonance imaging in acute myocardial infarction. Heart 95:624, 2009.
93. Kwong RY, Chan AK, Brown KA, et al: Impact of unrecognized myocardial scar detected by cardiac magnetic resonance imaging on event-free survival in patients presenting with signs or symptoms of coronary artery disease. Circulation 113:2733, 2006.
94. Klocke FJ, Baird MG, Lorell BH, et al: ACC/AHA/ASNC guidelines for the clinical use of cardiac radionuclide imaging: A report of the American College of Cardiology/American Heart Association Task Force on Practice Guidelines (ACC/AHA/ASNC Committee to Revise the 1995 Guidelines for the Clinical Use of Radionuclide Imaging). Circulation 108:1404, 2003.
95. Krucoff MW, Johanson P, Baeza R, et al: Clinical utility of serial and continuous ST-segment recovery assessment in patients with acute ST-elevation myocardial infarction: assessing the dynamics of epicardial and myocardial reperfusion. Circulation 110:e533, 2004.
96. Giannitsis E, Katus HA: Biomarkers of necrosis for risk assessment and management of ST-elevation myocardial infarction. *In* Morrow DA (ed): Cardiovascular Biomarkers: Pathophysiology and Disease Management. Totowa, NJ, Humana Press, 2006, pp 119-128.
97. Baur LH: Magnetic resonance imaging of persistent myocardial obstruction after myocardial infarction. A tool becoming increasingly important in clinical cardiology? Int J Cardiovasc Imaging 25:549, 2009.

CHAPTER 55 ST-Segment Elevation Myocardial Infarction: Management

Elliott M. Antman and David A. Morrow

Despite considerable advances in the care for patients with ST-segment elevation myocardial infarction (STEMI),[1-4] room for improvement exists, especially in special populations such as older adults, women, members of ethnic minority groups, and those with a low education level and low socioeconomic status.[5-7] A discussion of the phases of management of STEMI can follow the chronology of the interface of clinicians with the patient. Chap. 49 deals with the primary and secondary prevention of coronary artery disease. This chapter deals with the treatment at the time of onset of STEMI (prehospital issues, initial recognition and management in the emergency department, and reperfusion), hospital management (medications, arrhythmias, complications, and preparation for discharge), and secondary prevention after STEMI. Chap. 58 discusses percutaneous coronary intervention (PCI) in patients with STEMI.

Prehospital and Initial Management

Given the progressive loss of functioning myocytes with persistent occlusion of the infarct-related artery in STEMI (see Chap. 54), the initial management aims to restore blood flow to the infarct zone. Despite some deficiencies in the evidence base for selection of a reperfusion strategy, it is generally accepted that primary PCI is the preferred option, provided it can be delivered in a timely fashion by an experienced operator (>75 PCI procedures/year) and team (at least 200 PCI procedures/year, including at least 36 primary PCI procedures/year).[1,8] Missed opportunities for improvement of care for STEMI include failure to deliver any form of reperfusion therapy in about 30% of patients and failure to minimize delays in reperfusion because of perpetuation of inefficient systems of care.[2,9,10] The chain of survival for STEMI involves a highly integrated strategy, beginning with patient education about the symptoms of STEMI (see Chap. 54) and early contact with the medical system, coordination of destination protocols in emergency medical services (EMS) systems, efficient practices in emergency departments to shorten door-to-reperfusion time, and expeditious implementation of the reperfusion strategy by a trained team.[11-14] The next major breakthrough in the care of patients with STEMI will more likely come from the implementation of systems that shorten total ischemic time than from modifying adjunctive therapies that complement a reperfusion strategy or deal with the consequences of the infarction.[15-17] Much like the clinical research enterprise has been reorganized around translational steps, we must now follow a road map for the transformation of reperfusion therapy for STEMI (**Table 55-1**). The American Heart Association has launched a national initiative to engineer improved health care delivery for STEMI and proposed the criteria for an ideal STEMI system (**Table 55-2**). When considering such initiatives to streamline timely delivery of reperfusion therapies, it is also important to focus on overall quality of care measures for STEMI.[18]

PREHOSPITAL CARE. The prehospital care of patients with suspected STEMI is a crucial element bearing directly on the likelihood of survival. Most deaths associated with STEMI occur within the first hour of its onset and are usually caused by ventricular fibrillation (see Chap. 41). Hence, the immediate implementation of definitive resuscitative efforts and of rapidly transporting the patient to a hospital is of prime importance. Major components of the delay from the onset of symptoms consistent with acute myocardial infarction (MI) to reperfusion include the following[1]: (1) the time for the patient to recognize the seriousness of the problem and seek medical attention; (2) prehospital evaluation, treatment, and transportation; (3) the time for diagnostic measures and initiation of treatment in the hospital (e.g., door-to-needle time for patients receiving a fibrinolytic agent and door-to-balloon time for patients undergoing a catheter-based reperfusion strategy); and (4) the time from initiation of treatment to restoration of flow (**Fig. 55-1**).

Patient-related factors that correlate with a longer time to the decision to seek medical attention include the following: older age; female sex; black race; low socioeconomic status; low emotional or somatic awareness; history of angina, diabetes, or both; consulting a spouse or other relative; and consulting a physician.[19,20] Health care professionals should heighten the level of awareness of patients at risk for STEMI (e.g., those with hypertension, diabetes, history of angina pectoris).[1,14] They should use each patient encounter as a teachable moment to review and reinforce with patients and their families the need to seek urgent medical attention for a pattern of symptoms, including chest discomfort, extreme fatigue, and dyspnea, especially if accompanied by diaphoresis, lightheadedness, palpitations, or a sense of impending doom. Although many patients shun such discussions and tend to minimize the likelihood of ever needing emergency cardiac treatment, emphasis should be placed on the prevention and treatment of potentially fatal arrhythmias, as well as salvage of the jeopardized myocardium by reperfusion, for which time is crucial.[21] Patients should also be instructed in the proper use of sublingual nitroglycerin and to call 911 emergency services if the ischemic-type discomfort persists for longer than 5 minutes.[22]

EMERGENCY MEDICAL SERVICES SYSTEMS. These systems have three major components—emergency medical dispatch, first

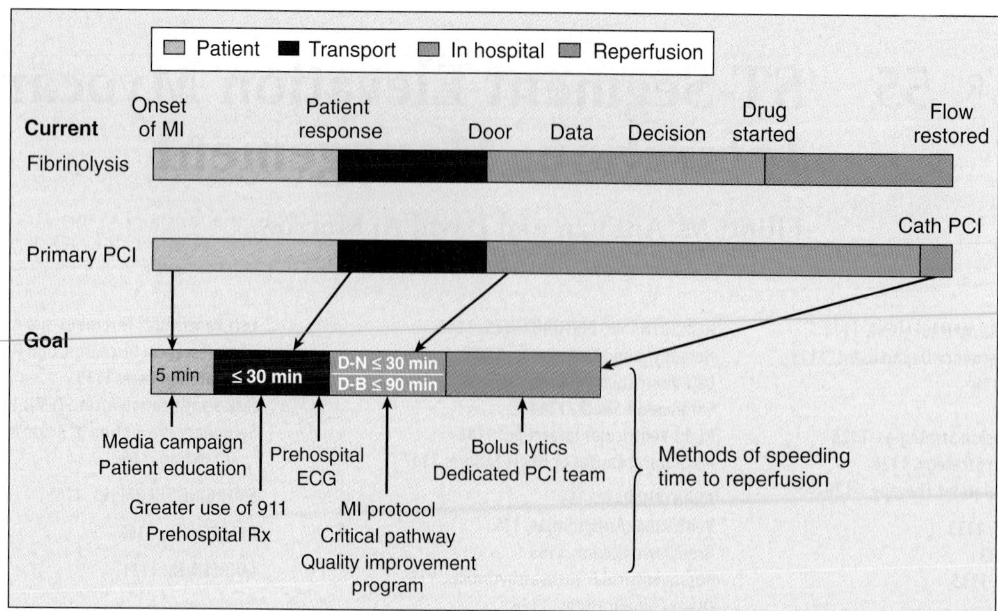

FIGURE 55-1 Major components of time delay between onset of infarction and restoration of flow in the infarct-related artery. Plotted sequentially from left to right are the time for patients to recognize symptoms and seek medical attention, transportation to the hospital, in-hospital decision making and implementing reperfusion strategy, and time for restoration of flow once the reperfusion strategy has been initiated. The time to initiate fibrinolytic therapy is the door-to-needle (D-N) time; this is followed by the period of time required for pharmacological restoration of flow. More time is required to move the patient to the catheterization laboratory for a PCI procedure, referred to as the door-to-balloon (D-B) time, but restoration of flow in the epicardial infarct-related artery occurs promptly after PCI. **Bottom,** Various methods for speeding the time to reperfusion are shown, along with the goals for the time intervals for the various components of the time delay. *(Modified from Antman EM, Anbe DT, Armstrong PW, et al: ACC/AHA guidelines for the management of patients with ST-elevation myocardial infarction: A report of the American College of Cardiology/American Heart Association Task Force on Practice Guidelines [Committee to Revise the 1999 Guidelines for the Management of Patients with Acute Myocardial Infarction]. Circulation 110:e82, 2004.)*

TABLE 55-1 Translational Approach to Systems of Care for STEMI

TRANSLATIONAL STEP	KEY ASPECTS OF TRANSLATIONAL STEP	REPERFUSION FOR STEMI
1	Activity to test what care works: • Clinical efficacy research	Randomized clinical trials of fibrinolysis and catheter-based therapies
2	Activities to test who benefits from providing care: • Outcomes research • Comparative effectiveness research • Health services research	Registries such as the joint ACC/AHA ACTION-GWTG Registry
3	Activities to test how to deliver high-quality care reliably and in all settings: • Measurement and accountability of health care quality and cost • Implementation of interventions and health care system redesign • Scaling and spread of effective interventions • Research in above domains	ACC D2B Alliance; AHA Mission: Lifeline

ACC = American College of Cardiology; ACTION = Acute Coronary Treatment and Intervention Outcomes Network; AHA = American Heart Association; D2B = door-to-balloon; GWTG = Get With the Guidelines.

Modified from Dougherty D, Conway PH: The "3T's" road map to transform US health care: the "how" of high-quality care. JAMA 299:2319, 2008; and Antman EM: Time is muscle: translation into practice. J Am Coll Cardiol 52:1216, 2008.

response, and EMS ambulance response. A major advance in the contribution of EMS systems is the expansion of the capability to record a prehospital 12-lead electrocardiogram (ECG).[23] The ability to transmit such ECGs and to activate the STEMI care team prior to hospital

TABLE 55-2 Criteria for a STEMI System of Care

1. The system should be registered with Mission: Lifeline.
2. There should be ongoing multidisciplinary team meetings that include EMS, non-PCI hospitals and STEMI referral centers, and PCI hospitals and STEMI receiving centers to evaluate outcomes and quality improvement data. Operational issues should be reviewed, problems identified, and solutions implemented.
3. Each STEMI system should include a process for prehospital identification and activation, destination protocols to STEMI receiving centers, and transfer for patients who arrive at STEMI referral centers and are primary PCI candidates and/or are fibrinolytic-ineligible and/or in cardiogenic shock.
4. Each system should have a recognized system coordinator, physician champion, and EMS medical director.
5. Each system component (EMS, STEMI referral centers and STEMI receiving centers) should meet the appropriate criteria.[13]

Modified from American Heart Association, Mission: Lifeline, 2010 (http://www.heart.org/HEARTORG/HealthcareProfessional/Mission-Lifeline-Home-Page_UCM_305495_SubHomePage.jsp).

arrival places EMS efforts at the center of the early response to STEMI.[24,25] Ongoing efforts to shorten the time to treatment of patients with STEMI include improvement in the medical dispatch component by expanding 911 coverage, providing automated external defibrillators to first responders, placing automated external defibrillators in critical public locations, and greater coordination of EMS ambulance response.[26,27] Well-equipped ambulances and helicopters staffed by personnel trained in the acute care of the STEMI patient allow definitive therapy to commence while the patient is being transported to the hospital (**Table 55-3**). To serve effectively, EMS units must be placed strategically within a community and have excellent radio communication systems. These units should be equipped with battery-operated monitoring equipment, a DC defibrillator, oxygen, endotracheal tubes and suction apparatus, and commonly used cardiovascular drugs. Radiotelemetry systems that allow transmission of the electrocardiographic signal to a medical control officer are highly desirable to facilitate triage of STEMI patients and are becoming increasingly

TABLE 55-3 Reperfusion Checklist for Evaluation of the STEMI Patient

Step 1: Has patient experienced chest discomfort for >15 min and <12 hr?

→ YES → Step 2

→ NO → STOP

Step 2: Are there contraindications to fibrinolysis?
If *ANY* of the following are checked, fibrinolysis *may* be contraindicated.

Systolic blood pressure >180 mm Hg	☐ YES	☐ NO
Diastolic blood pressure >110 mm Hg	☐ YES	☐ NO
Right versus left arm systolic blood pressure difference >15 mm Hg	☐ YES	☐ NO
History of structural central nervous system disease	☐ YES	☐ NO
Significant closed head/facial trauma within the previous 3 mo	☐ YES	☐ NO
Recent (within 6 wk) major trauma, surgery (including laser eye surgery), gastrointestinal or genitourinary bleed	☐ YES	☐ NO
Bleeding or clotting problem on blood thinners	☐ YES	☐ NO
CPR more than 10 min	☐ YES	☐ NO
Pregnant female	☐ YES	☐ NO
Serious systemic disease (e.g., advanced/terminal cancer, severe liver or kidney disease)	☐ YES	☐ NO

Step 3: Does the patient have severe heart failure or cardiogenic shock such that percutaneous coronary intervention is preferable?

Pulmonary edema (rales more than halfway up)	☐ YES	☐ NO
Systemic hypoperfusion (cold, clammy)	☐ YES	☐ NO

CPR = cardiopulmonary resuscitation.

From Antman EM, Anbe DT, Armstrong PW, et al: ACC/AHA guidelines for the management of patients with ST-elevation myocardial infarction: A report of the American College of Cardiology/American Heart Association Task Force on Practice Guidelines (Committee to Revise the 1999 Guidelines for the Management of Patients with Acute Myocardial Infarction) Circulation 110:e82, 2004.

available in many communities (**Fig. 55-2**). Observations of simple variables such as age, heart rate, and blood pressure permit initial classification of patients into high- or low-risk subgroups.[28]

In addition to prompt defibrillation, the efficacy of prehospital care appears to depend on several factors, including early relief of pain with its deleterious physiologic sequelae, reduction of excessive activity of the autonomic nervous system, and abolition of prelethal arrhythmias such as ventricular tachycardia. Such efforts must not, however, impede rapid transfer to the hospital (see Fig. 55-2).

PREHOSPITAL FIBRINOLYSIS. Several randomized trials have evaluated the potential benefits of prehospital versus in-hospital fibrinolysis. Although none of the individual trials showed a significant reduction in mortality with prehospital-initiated fibrinolytic therapy, earlier treatment generally provides greater benefit; a meta-analysis of all the available trials demonstrated a 17% reduction in mortality. The CAPTIM trial reported a trend toward a lower rate of mortality among STEMI patients receiving prehospital fibrinolysis as compared with primary PCI, especially if patients were treated within 2 hours of the onset of symptoms.[1] Several registry reports have provided additional support for the benefit of prehospital lysis.[29-31]

Several factors enter consideration of whether ambulances and emergency transport vehicles should initiate fibrinolytic therapy. The greatest reduction in mortality is observed when reperfusion can be initiated within 60 to 90 minutes of the onset of symptoms.[1] Streamlining of emergency department triage practices so that treatment can be started within 30 minutes, when coupled with the 15- to 30-minute transport time that is common in most urban centers, may be more cost-effective than equipping all ambulances to administer prehospital fibrinolytic therapy (see Fig. 55-2).[19,20] The latter would require extensive training of personnel (see Table 55-3), installation of computer-assisted electrocardiography or systems for radio transmission of the electrocardiographic signal to a central station, and stocking of medicine kits with the necessary drug supplies. In some communities, in which transport delays may be 60 to 90 minutes or longer and experienced personnel are available on ambulances, prehospital fibrinolytic therapy is beneficial. Therefore, prehospital fibrinolysis is reasonable in settings in which physicians are present in the ambulance or there is a well-organized EMS system with full-time paramedics, capability for obtaining and transmitting 12-lead electrocardiographic readings from the field, and online medical command to authorize prehospital fibrinolysis.[32,33]

Management in the Emergency Department

When evaluating patients in the emergency department, physicians must confront the difficult task of rapidly identifying patients who require urgent reperfusion therapy, triaging lower-risk patients to the appropriate facility within the hospital, and not discharging patients inappropriately, while avoiding unnecessary admissions. A history of ischemic-type discomfort and the initial 12-lead ECG are the primary tools for screening patients with acute coronary syndromes in the emergency department.[34] More extensive use of prehospital 12-lead electrocardiographic recordings facilitate triage of STEMI patients in

Hospital fibrinolysis:
Door-needle ≤ 30 min

Not PCI capable

Call 911, call fast

Patient symptom onset of STEMI

911 EMS dispatch

EMS on-scene
Encourage 12-lead ECGs
Consider prehospital fibrinolytic if capable and EMS-needle ≤ 30 min

EMS triage plan

Interhospital transfer

PCI capable

Goals†

Patient — 5 min after symptom onset

Dispatch — 1 min

EMS on scene — ≤ 8 min

EMS transport — Prehospital fibrinolysis: EMS-needle ≤ 30 min

EMS transport: EMS-balloon ≤ 90 min

Patient self-transport: hospital door-balloon ≤ 90 min

Total ischemic time: <120 min*

*Golden hour=first 60 minutes

A

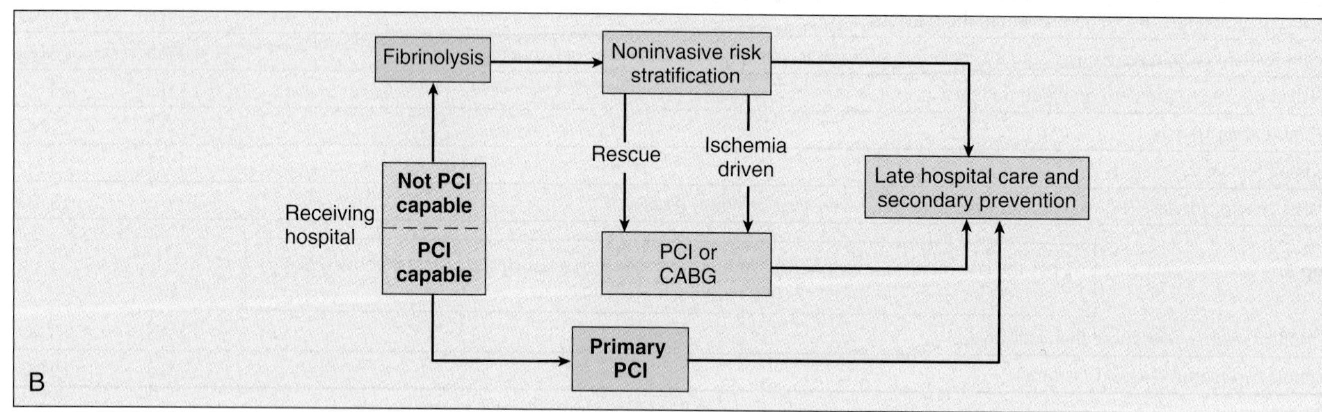

FIGURE 55-2 Options for transporting STEMI patients and initial reperfusion treatment. Reperfusion in patients with STEMI can be accomplished by the pharmacologic (fibrinolysis) or catheter-based (PCI) approach. Implementation of these strategies varies based on the mode of transportation of the patient and capabilities at the receiving hospital. **A,** Patient transported by EMS after calling 911. Transport time to the hospital varies from case to case, but the goal is to keep total ischemic time <120 minutes. There are three options: (1) If EMS has fibrinolytic capability and the patient qualifies for therapy, prehospital fibrinolysis should be started within 30 minutes of EMS arrival on scene. (2) If EMS is not capable of administering prehospital fibrinolysis and the patient is transported to a non–PCI-capable hospital, the hospital door-to-needle time should be ≤30 minutes for patients in whom fibrinolysis is indicated. (3) If EMS cannot administer prehospital fibrinolysis and the patient is transported to a PCI-capable hospital, the hospital door-to-balloon time should be ≤90 minutes. *Interhospital transfer:* It is also appropriate to consider emergency interhospital transfer of the patient to a PCI-capable hospital for mechanical revascularization if (1) there is a contraindication to fibrinolysis, (2) PCI can be initiated promptly (≤90 minutes after the patient presents to the initial receiving hospital or ≤60 minutes compared to when fibrinolysis could be initiated at the initial receiving hospital), or (3) fibrinolysis is administered and is unsuccessful (i.e., rescue PCI). Secondary nonemergency interhospital transfer can be considered for recurrent ischemia **(B).** *Patient self-transport:* Patient self-transportation is discouraged. If the patient arrives at a non–PCI-capable hospital, the door-to-needle time should be ≤30 minutes. If the patient arrives at a PCI-capable hospital, the door-to-balloon time should be ≤90 minutes. The treatment options and time recommendations after first hospital arrival are the same. **B,** For patients who receive fibrinolysis, noninvasive risk stratification is recommended to identify the need for rescue PCI (failed fibrinolysis) or ischemia-driven PCI. Regardless of the initial method of reperfusion treatment, all patients should receive late hospital care and secondary prevention of STEMI. †The medical system goal is to facilitate rapid recognition and treatment of patients with STEMI so that door-to-needle (or EMS-to-needle) for initiation of fibrinolytic therapy can be achieved within 30 minutes, or that door-to-balloon (or EMS-to-balloon) or PCI can be achieved within 90 minutes. These goals should not be understood as ideal times, but rather the longest times that should be considered acceptable for a given system. Systems that can achieve even more rapid times for treatment of patients with STEMI should be encouraged. *(Modified from Armstrong PW, Collen D, Antman E: Fibrinolysis for acute myocardial infarction: The future is here and now. Circulation 107:2533, 2003; and Antman EM, Anbe DT, Armstrong PW, et al: ACC/AHA guidelines for the management of patients with ST-elevation myocardial infarction: A report of the American College of Cardiology/American Heart Association Task Force on Practice Guidelines [Committee to Revise the 1999 Guidelines for the Management of Patients with Acute Myocardial Infarction]. Circulation 110:e82, 2004.)*

the emergency department.[23] ST-segment elevation on the ECG of a patient with ischemic discomfort highly suggests thrombotic occlusion of an epicardial coronary artery, and its presence should serve as the trigger for a well-rehearsed sequence of rapid assessment of the patient for contraindications to fibrinolysis and initiation of a reperfusion strategy (**Tables 55-4** and **55-5**).[1] Because the 12-lead ECG is at the center of the decision pathway for initiation of reperfusion therapy, it should be obtained promptly (≤10 minutes) in patients presenting with ischemic discomfort.

Because lethal arrhythmias can occur suddenly in patients with STEMI, all patients should be attached to a bedside electrocardiographic monitor and intravenous access should be obtained. If the initial reading shows ST-segment elevation of 1 mm or more in at least two contiguous leads or a new or presumably new left bundle branch block, the patient should be evaluated immediately for a reperfusion strategy. Critical factors that weigh into the selection of a reperfusion strategy include the following: (1) the time elapsed since the onset of symptoms; (2) the risk associated with STEMI; (3) the risk of

TABLE 55-4 Assessment of Reperfusion Options for STEMI Patients

Step 1: Assess time and risk.
- Time since onset of symptoms
- Risk of STEMI
- Risk of fibrinolysis
- Time required for transport to a skilled PCI laboratory

Step 2: Determine if fibrinolysis or invasive strategy is preferred.
- *If presentation is <3 hr and there is no delay to an invasive strategy, there is no preference for either strategy.*

Fibrinolysis is generally preferred if:
- Early presentation (≤3 hr from symptom onset and delay to invasive strategy; see below)
- Invasive strategy is not an option:
  - Catheterization laboratory occupied or not available
  - Vascular access difficulties
  - Lack of access to a skilled PCI laboratory*†
- Delay to invasive strategy:
  - Prolonged transport
  - (Door-to-balloon)–(door-to-needle) more than 1 hr‡§
  - Medical contact-to-balloon or door-to-balloon more than 90 min

An invasive strategy is generally preferred if:
- Skilled PCI laboratory is available with surgical backup
  - Skilled PCI laboratory is available, defined by†‡
  - Medical contact-to-balloon or door-to-balloon less than 90 min
  - (Door-to-balloon)–(door-to-needle) less than 1 hr‡
- High risk from STEMI
  - Cardiogenic shock
  - Killip class ≥ 3
- Contraindications to fibrinolysis, including increased risk of bleeding and ICH
- Late presentation
  - Symptom onset was more than 3 hr ago
- Diagnosis of STEMI is in doubt

*Operator experience > a total of 75 primary PCI cases/yr.
†Team experience > a total of 36 primary PCI cases/yr.
‡Applies to fibrin-specific agents.
§This calculation implies that the estimated delay to the implementation of the invasive strategy is >1 hr versus immediate initiation of fibrinolytic therapy.
ICH = intracranial hemorrhage.
From Antman EM, Anbe DT, Armstrong PW, et al: ACC/AHA guidelines for the management of patients with ST-elevation myocardial infarction: A report of the American College of Cardiology/American Heart Association Task Force on Practice Guidelines (Committee to Revise the 1999 Guidelines for the Management of Patients with Acute Myocardial Infarction) Circulation 110:e82, 2004.

administering a fibrinolytic; and (4) the time required to initiate an invasive strategy (see Table 55-4).

Given the importance of time to reperfusion,[8] the concept of medical system goals has arisen.[13] Benchmarks for medical systems to use when assessing the quality of their performance are a door-to-needle time of less than or equal to 30 minutes for initiation of fibrinolytic therapy and a door-to-balloon time of less than or equal to 90 minutes for percutaneous coronary perfusion (see Fig. 55-2).[35-37] Increasing sophistication of EMS systems facilitates initiating the process of evaluation and implementation of a reperfusion strategy even before the patient arrives in the emergency department.[23] For those patients transported by ambulance, the medical system goals can be restated as an EMS-to-needle time of less than or equal to 30 minutes for initiation of fibrinolysis and an EMS-to-balloon time of less than or equal to 90 minutes for initiation of PCI (see Fig. 55-2).[1,38]

Patients with an initial electrocardiographic reading that reveals new or presumably new ST-segment depression and/or T wave inversion, although not considered candidates for fibrinolytic therapy, should be treated as though they are suffering from MI without ST-segment elevation or unstable angina (a distinction to be made subsequently after scrutiny of serial ECGs and cardiac biomarker measurements; see Chap. 56).

In patients with a clinical history suggestive of STEMI (see Chap. 54) and an initial nondiagnostic electrocardiographic reading (i.e., no ST-segment deviation or T wave inversion), serial tracings should be

TABLE 55-5 Contraindications and Cautions for Fibrinolytic Use in STEMI*

Absolute Contraindications
- Any prior intracranial hemorrhage
- Known structural cerebral vascular lesion (e.g., arteriovenous malformation)
- Known malignant intracranial neoplasm (primary or metastatic)
- Ischemic stroke within 3 mo *except* acute ischemic stroke within 3 hr
- Suspected aortic dissection
- Active bleeding or bleeding diathesis (excluding menses)
- Significant closed head or facial trauma within 3 mo

Relative Contraindications
- History of chronic severe poorly controlled hypertension
- Severe uncontrolled hypertension on presentation (SBP >180 mm Hg or DBP >110 mm Hg)†
- History of prior ischemic stroke > 3 mo, dementia, or known intracranial pathology not covered in contraindications
- Traumatic or prolonged (>10 min) CPR or major surgery (<3 wk)
- Recent (within 2-4 wk) internal bleeding
- Noncompressible vascular punctures
- For streptokinase, anistreplase: Prior exposure (>5 days ago) or prior allergic reaction to these agents
- Pregnancy
- Active peptic ulcer
- Current use of anticoagulants: the higher the INR, the higher the risk of bleeding

*Viewed as advisory for clinical decision-making and may not be all-inclusive or definitive.
†Could be an absolute contraindication in low-risk patients with myocardial infarction.
CPR = cardiopulmonary resuscitation; DBP = diastolic blood pressure; INR = international normalized ratio; SBP = systolic blood pressure.
From Antman EM, Anbe DT, Armstrong PW, et al: ACC/AHA guidelines for the management of patients with ST-elevation myocardial infarction: A report of the American College of Cardiology/American Heart Association Task Force on Practice Guidelines (Committee to Revise the 1999 Guidelines for the Management of Patients with Acute Myocardial Infarction). Circulation 110:e82, 2004.

obtained while the patients are being evaluated in the emergency department. Emergency department staff can be alerted to the sudden development of ST-segment elevation by periodic visual inspection of the bedside electrocardiographic monitor, by continuous ST-segment recording, or by auditory alarms when the ST-segment deviation exceeds programmed limits. Decision aids such as computer-based diagnostic algorithms, identification of high-risk clinical indicators, rapid determination of cardiac biomarkers, echocardiographic screening for regional wall motion abnormalities, and myocardial perfusion imaging have greatest clinical usefulness when the electrocardiographic reading is nondiagnostic. In an effort to improve the cost-effectiveness of care of patients with a chest pain syndrome, nondiagnostic electrocardiographic reading, and low suspicion of MI, but in whom the diagnosis has not been entirely excluded, many medical centers have developed critical pathways that involve a coronary observation unit with a goal of ruling out MI in less than 12 hours.[39,40]

GENERAL TREATMENT MEASURES

Aspirin

Aspirin is useful not only for the primary prevention of vascular events (see Chap. 49) but is also effective across the entire spectrum of acute coronary syndromes and forms part of the initial management strategy for patients with suspected STEMI (see Chap. 87). Because low doses (40 to 80 mg) take several days to achieve full antiplatelet effect, at least 162 to 325 mg should be administered acutely in the emergency department.[1] To achieve therapeutic blood levels rapidly, the patient should chew the tablet to promote buccal absorption rather than absorption through the gastric mucosa.[41]

Control of Cardiac Pain

Management of STEMI patients in the emergency department should aim to relieve pain. A tendency to underdose the patient for fear of obscuring response to antiischemic or reperfusion therapy should be avoided because pain heightens sympathetic activity during the early phase of STEMI. Control of cardiac pain typically uses a combination of nitrates, analgesics (e.g., morphine), oxygen, and in appropriately selected patients, beta-adrenergic blocking agents (referred to hereafter as beta blockers).[35] Similar pharmacologic principles apply in the coronary care unit, where many of the therapies discussed herein should continue after initial dosing in the emergency department. Because the pain associated with STEMI is related to ongoing ischemia, many interventions that improve the oxygen supply-demand relationship (by increasing supply or decreasing demand) can alleviate the cause of pain.

ANALGESICS. Although a wide variety of analgesic agents has been used to treat the pain associated with STEMI, including meperidine, pentazocine, and morphine, morphine remains the drug of choice, except in patients with well-documented morphine hypersensitivity. A dose of 4 to 8 mg should be administered intravenously, and doses of 2 to 8 mg should be repeated at intervals of 5 to 15 minutes until the pain is relieved or there is evident toxicity—hypotension, depression of respiration, or severe vomiting—which should preclude further administration of the drug.

The reduction of anxiety resulting from morphine diminishes the patient's restlessness and activity of the autonomic nervous system, with a consequent reduction of the heart's metabolic demands. Morphine has unequivocal beneficial effects in patients with pulmonary edema because of peripheral arterial and venous dilation (particularly among patients with excessive sympathoadrenal activity), reduction of the work of breathing, and slowing of heart rate secondary to combined withdrawal of sympathetic tone and augmentation of vagal tone.

Hypotension following the administration of nitroglycerin and morphine can be minimized by maintaining the patient in a supine position and elevating the lower extremities if systolic arterial pressure declines below 100 mm Hg. Such positioning is undesirable in the presence of pulmonary edema, but morphine rarely produces hypotension under these circumstances. The concomitant administration of atropine in doses of 0.5 to 1.5 mg intravenously may be helpful in treating eventual excessive vagomimetic effects of morphine, particularly when hypotension and bradycardia are present before it is administered.[1] Respiratory depression is an unusual complication of morphine in the presence of severe pain or pulmonary edema, but as the patient's cardiovascular status improves, impairment of ventilation may supervene. It can be treated with naloxone, in doses of 0.1 to 0.2 mg intravenous initially, repeated after 15 minutes if necessary. Nausea and vomiting may be troublesome side effects of large doses of morphine and can be treated with a phenothiazine.

NITRATES. Because of their ability to enhance coronary blood flow by coronary vasodilation and to decrease ventricular preload by increasing venous capacitance, sublingual nitrates are indicated for most patients with an acute coronary syndrome. At present, the only groups of patients with STEMI in whom sublingual nitroglycerin should *not* be given are those with inferior MI and suspected right ventricular infarction[42] or marked hypotension (systolic pressure <90 mm Hg), especially if accompanied by bradycardia.

Once hypotension is excluded, a sublingual nitroglycerin tablet should be administered and the patient observed for improvement in symptoms or change in hemodynamics. If an initial dose is well tolerated and appears to be of benefit, further nitrates should be administered, with monitoring of the vital signs. Even small doses can produce sudden hypotension and bradycardia, a reaction that can be life-threatening but is usually easily reversed with intravenous atropine if recognized quickly. Long-acting oral nitrate preparations should be avoided in the early course of STEMI because of the frequently changing hemodynamic status of the patient. In patients with a prolonged period of waxing and waning chest pain, intravenous nitroglycerin may help to control symptoms and correct ischemia, but requires frequent monitoring of blood pressure.

BETA BLOCKERS. Beta blockers relieve ischemic pain, reduce the need for analgesics in many patients, and reduce infarct size and life-threatening arrhythmias. Avoiding early intravenous beta blockade in patients presenting in Killip class II or higher is important, however, because of the risk of precipitating cardiogenic shock.[1,43,44] A popular and relatively safe protocol for the use of a beta blocker in this situation is as follows:

1. Patients with heart failure (rales > 10 cm up from diaphragm), hypotension (blood pressure < 90 mm Hg), bradycardia (heart rate < 60 beats/min), or first-degree atrioventricular (AV) block (PR interval > 0.24 second) are first excluded.
2. Metoprolol is given in three 5-mg intravenous boluses.
3. Patients are observed for 2 to 5 minutes after each bolus and, if the heart rate falls below 60 beats/min or systolic blood pressure falls below 100 mm Hg, no further drug is given.
4. If hemodynamic stability continues 15 minutes after the last intravenous dose, the patient is begun on oral metoprolol, 50 mg every 6 hours for 2 days, and then switched to 100 mg twice daily.

An infusion of an extremely short-acting beta blocker, esmolol (50 to 250 μg/kg/min), may be useful for patients with relative contraindications to beta blocker administration in whom heart rate slowing is considered highly desirable.

OXYGEN. Hypoxemia can occur in patients with STEMI and usually results from ventilation-perfusion abnormalities that are sequelae of left ventricular failure; pneumonia and intrinsic pulmonary disease are additional causes of hypoxemia. Treating all patients hospitalized with STEMI with oxygen for at least 24 to 48 hours is common practice on the basis of the empiric assumption of hypoxia and evidence that increased oxygen in the inspired air may protect ischemic myocardium. But this practice may not be cost-effective. Augmentation of the fraction of oxygen in the inspired air does not elevate oxygen delivery significantly in patients who are not hypoxemic. Furthermore, it may increase systemic vascular resistance and arterial pressure and thereby lower cardiac output slightly.

In view of these considerations, arterial oxygen saturation can be estimated by pulse oximetry, and oxygen therapy can be omitted if it is normal. On the other hand, oxygen should be administered to patients with STEMI when arterial hypoxemia is clinically evident or can be documented by measurement (e.g., SaO_2 < 90%).[1] In these patients, serial arterial blood gas measurements can be employed to follow the efficacy of oxygen therapy. The delivery of 2 to 4 liters/min of 100% oxygen by mask or nasal prongs for 6 to 12 hours is satisfactory for most patients with mild hypoxemia. If arterial oxygenation is still depressed on this regimen, the flow rate may have to be increased, and other causes for hypoxemia should be sought. In patients with pulmonary edema, endotracheal intubation and positive-pressure controlled ventilation may be necessary.

LIMITATION OF INFARCT SIZE. Infarct size is an important determinant of prognosis in patients with STEMI. Patients who succumb from cardiogenic shock generally exhibit a single massive infarct or a small to moderate-sized infarct superimposed on multiple prior infarctions.[45] Survivors with large infarcts frequently exhibit late impairment of ventricular function, and the long-term mortality rate is higher than for survivors with small infarcts, who tend not to develop cardiac decompensation.[46]

In view of the prognostic importance of infarct size, the possibility of modification of infarct size has attracted a great deal of experimental and clinical attention (see Fig. 54-9).[8,12,47] Efforts to limit infarct size have been divided among several different (sometimes overlapping) approaches: (1) early reperfusion; (2) reduction of myocardial energy demands; (3) manipulation of sources of energy production in the myocardium; and (4) prevention of reperfusion injury. Despite the many advances in reperfusion therapy for STEMI, practical clinical decision making for individual patients is complex. Persistent uncertainties about the risk (bleeding)-benefit balance in older patients and those arriving late after the onset of symptoms appear to be the major factors explaining the underuse of reperfusion for STEMI in routine practice.[48]

Dynamic Nature of Infarction

STEMI is a dynamic process that does not occur instantaneously but evolves over hours. The fate of jeopardized ischemic tissue can be affected favorably by interventions that restore myocardial perfusion, reduce microvascular damage in the infarct zone, reduce myocardial oxygen requirements, inhibit accumulation of or facilitate washout of noxious metabolites, augment the availability of substrate for anaerobic metabolism, or blunt the effects of mediators of injury that compromise the structure and function of intracellular organelles and constituents of cell membranes. Strong evidence in experimental animals and suggestive evidence in patients have indicated that ischemic preconditioning, a form of endogenous protection against STEMI (see Chap. 24), before sustained coronary occlusion decreases infarct size and is associated with a more favorable outcome, with decreased risk of extension of infarction and recurrent ischemic events. Brief episodes of ischemia in one coronary vascular bed may precondition myocardium in a remote zone, attenuating the size of infarction in the latter when sustained coronary occlusion occurs.[49]

The perfusion of the myocardium in the infarct zone appears to be reduced maximally immediately following coronary occlusion. Up to one third of patients develop spontaneous recanalization of an occluded infarct-related artery beginning at 12 to 24 hours. This delayed spontaneous reperfusion may improve left ventricular function because it improves healing of infarcted tissue, prevents ventricular remodeling, and reperfuses hibernating myocardium. To maximize the amount of salvaged myocardium by accelerating the process of reperfusion and also implementing it in those patients who would otherwise have an occluded infarct-related artery, the strategies of pharmacologically induced and catheter-based reperfusion of the infarct vessel have been developed (**Fig. 55-3**; see Chap. 58). An overarching concept that applies to all methods of reperfusion is the critical importance of time. Mortality reduction from STEMI is highest the earlier the infarct artery is reperfused (**Fig. 55-4**).[47]

Additional factors that may contribute to limitation of infarct size in association with reperfusion include relief of coronary spasm, prevention of damage to the microvasculature, improved systemic hemodynamics (augmentation of coronary perfusion pressure and reduced left ventricular end-diastolic pressure), and development of collateral circulation. The prompt implementation of measures designed to protect ischemic myocardium and support myocardial perfusion may provide sufficient time for the development of anatomic and physiologic compensatory mechanisms that limit the ultimate extent of infarction (see Chap. 54). Interventions designed to protect ischemic myocardium during the initial event may also reduce the incidence of extension of infarction or early reinfarction.

Routine Measures for Infarct Size Limitation

Although timely reperfusion of ischemic myocardium is the most important technique for limiting infarct size, several routine measures to accomplish this goal apply to all patients with STEMI, whether or not they receive reperfusion therapy. The treatment strategies discussed in this section can be initiated in the emergency department and then continued in the coronary care unit.

It is important to maintain an optimal balance between myocardial oxygen supply and demand so that as much as possible of the jeopardized zone of the myocardium surrounding the most profoundly ischemic zones of the infarct can be salvaged. During the period before irreversible injury has occurred, myocardial oxygen consumption should be minimized by maintaining the patient at rest, physically and emotionally, and by using mild sedation and a quiet atmosphere that may lower heart rate, a major determinant of myocardial oxygen consumption. If the patient was receiving a beta blocker when the clinical manifestations of the infarction commenced, the drug should be continued unless a specific contraindication is noted, such as left ventricular systolic failure or bradyarrhythmia.[35] Marked sinus bradycardia (heart rate ≤ 50 beats/min) and the frequently coexisting hypotension should be treated with postural maneuvers (the Trendelenburg position) to increase central blood volume and with atropine and electrical pacing, but not with isoproterenol. On the other hand, the routine administration of atropine, with the resultant increase in heart rate, to patients without serious bradycardia is contraindicated. All forms of tachyarrhythmias require prompt treatment because they increase myocardial oxygen needs.[1]

Congestive heart failure should be treated promptly. Given their multiple beneficial actions in STEMI patients, inhibitors of the

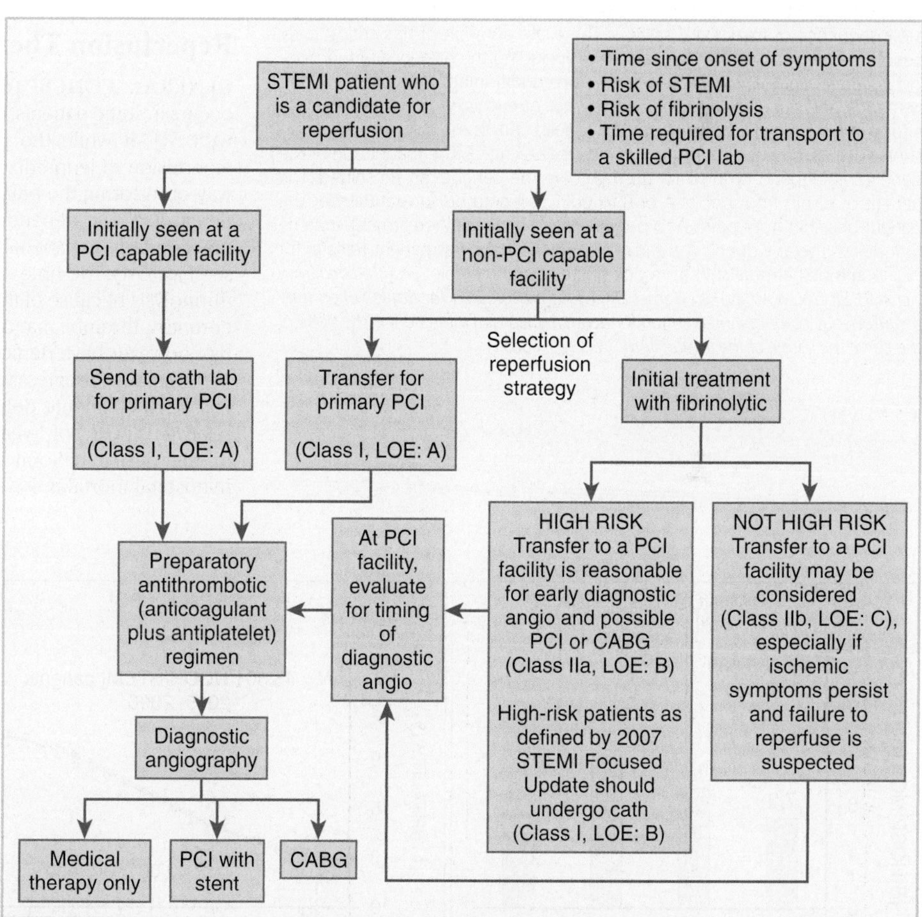

FIGURE 55-3 Each community, and each facility in that community, should have an agreed-on plan for how STEMI patients are to be treated. This plan should include which hospitals should do the following: (1) receive STEMI patients from EMS units capable of obtaining diagnostic ECGs, management at the initial receiving hospital, and written criteria and agreement for expeditious transfer of patients from non–PCI-capable to PCI-capable facilities; and (2) consider initiating a preparatory pharmacologic regimen as soon as possible in preparation for and during patient transfer to a catheterization laboratory. The optimal regimen is not yet established, although published studies (see text for details) have used various combinations of anticoagulants, oral antiplatelet agents, and IV antiplatelets. LOE = level of evidence. *(From Kushner FG, Hand M, Smith SC Jr, et al: 2009 Focused Updates: ACC/AHA Guidelines for the Management of Patients With ST-Elevation Myocardial Infarction (updating the 2004 Guideline and 2007 Focused Update) and ACC/AHA/SCAI Guidelines on Percutaneous Coronary Intervention [updating the 2005 Guideline and 2007 Focused Update]: A report of the American College of Cardiology Foundation/American Heart Association Task Force on Practice Guidelines. Circulation 120:2271, 2009.)*

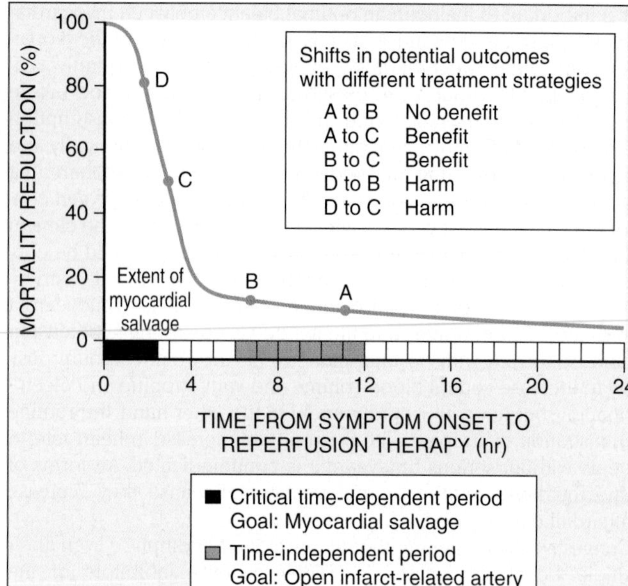

FIGURE 55-4 Mortality reduction as a benefit of reperfusion therapy is greatest in the first 2 to 3 hours after the onset of symptoms of acute MI, most likely a consequence of myocardial salvage. The exact duration of this critical early period may be modified by several factors, including the presence of functioning collateral coronary arteries, ischemic preconditioning, myocardial oxygen demands, and duration of sustained ischemia. After this early period, the magnitude of the mortality benefit is much reduced and, as the mortality reduction curve flattens, time to reperfusion therapy is less critical. The magnitude of the benefit will depend on how far up the curve the patient can be shifted. The benefit of a shift from points A or B to point C would be substantial, but the benefit of a shift from point A to point B would be small. A treatment strategy that delays therapy during the early critical period, such as patient transfer for PCI, would be harmful (shift from point D to point C or point B). *(Modified from Gersh BJ, Stone GW, White HD, Homes DR Jr: Pharmacological facilitation of primary percutaneous coronary intervention for acute myocardial infarction: Is the slope of the curve the shape of the future? JAMA 293:979, 2005.)*

renin-angiotensin-aldosterone system (RAAS) are indicated for the treatment of congestive heart failure associated with STEMI unless the patient is hypotensive. Inotropic agents that increase myocardial oxygen consumption (e.g., isoproterenol) should be avoided.

Arterial oxygenation should be restored to normal in patients with hypoxemia, such as occurs in patients with chronic pulmonary disease, pneumonia, or left ventricular failure. Oxygen-enriched air should be administered to patients with hypoxemia, and bronchodilators and expectorants should be used when indicated. Severe anemia, which also can extend the area of ischemic injury, should be corrected by the cautious administration of packed red blood cells, accompanied by a diuretic if there is any evidence of left ventricular failure. Associated conditions, particularly infections and the accompanying tachycardia, fever, and elevated myocardial oxygen needs, require immediate attention.

Systolic arterial pressure should not be allowed to deviate by more than approximately 25 to 30 mm Hg from the patient's usual level unless marked hypertension had been present before the onset of STEMI. It is likely that each patient has an optimal range of arterial pressure; as coronary perfusion pressure deviates from this level, the unfavorable balance that ensues between oxygen supply (which is related to coronary perfusion pressure) and myocardial oxygen demand (which is related to ventricular wall tension) increases the extent of ischemic injury.

Reperfusion Therapy

GENERAL CONCEPTS. Although late spontaneous reperfusion occurs in some patients, thrombotic occlusion persists in most patients with STEMI while the myocardium is undergoing necrosis. Timely reperfusion of jeopardized myocardium represents the most effective way of restoring the balance between myocardial oxygen supply and demand.[2,47] The dependence of myocardial salvage on time to treatment pertains to patients treated with fibrinolysis or PCI[1,12,50] (**Fig. 55-5**; see Fig. 55-4). The time dependence may be particularly critical with fibrinolysis because of the decreasing efficacy of fibrinolytic agents as coronary thrombi mature over time. Analyses adjusting for baseline risk, however, have demonstrated a statistically significant increase in mortality with progressive delays between the onset of symptoms and PCI. Each 30-minute delay from symptom onset to PCI increases the relative risk (RR) of 1-year mortality by 8%. Similarly, progressive delays in the door-to-balloon time have a significant adverse effect on in-hospital mortality.

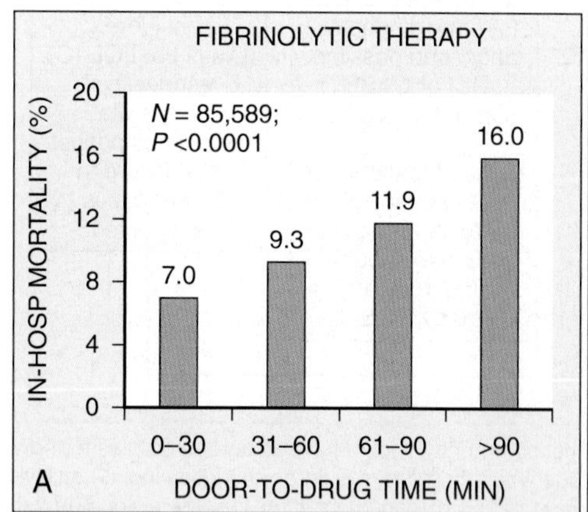

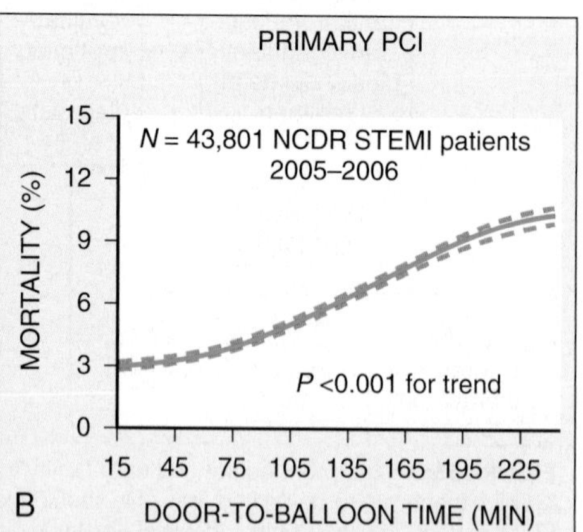

FIGURE 55-5 Importance of time to reperfusion in patients undergoing fibrinolysis **(A)** or primary PCI **(B)** for STEMI. **A,** Graph based on data from 85,589 patients treated with fibrinolysis. For every 30-minute delay, there is a progressive increase in the in-hospital mortality rate. **B,** Based on data from 43,801 patients, this depicts the adjusted in-hospital mortality rate as a function of door-to-balloon time. Estimated mortality ranged from 3% with a door-to-balloon time of 30 minutes to 10.3% for patients with a door-to-balloon time of 240 minutes. NCDR = National Cardiovascular Data Registry. *(Data from Cannon CP, Gibson CM, Lambrew CT, et al: Relationship of symptom-onset-to-balloon time and door-to-balloon time with mortality in patients undergoing angioplasty for acute myocardial infarction. JAMA 283:2941, 2000; and Rathore SS, Curtis J, Chen J, et al: Association of door-to-balloon time and mortality in patients admitted to hospital with ST elevation myocardial infarction: National cohort study. BMJ 338:b1807, 2009.)*

In some patients, particularly those with cardiogenic shock, tissue damage occurs in a stuttering manner rather than abruptly, a condition that might more properly be termed *subacute infarction*. This concept of the nature of the infarction process, as well as the observation that the incidence of complications of STEMI in the early and late postinfarction periods is a function of infarct size, underscores the need for careful history taking to ascertain whether the patient appears to have had repetitive cycles of spontaneous reperfusion and reocclusion. Determining the time of onset of the infarction process in such patients can be difficult. In such patients, with waxing and waning ischemic discomfort, a rigid time interval from the first episode of pain should not be used when determining whether a patient is outside the window for benefit from acute reperfusion therapy.

PATHOPHYSIOLOGY OF MYOCARDIAL REPERFUSION. Prevention of cell death by the restoration of blood flow depends on the severity and duration of preexisting ischemia. Substantial experimental and clinical evidence has indicated that the earlier blood flow is restored, the more favorably influenced are recovery of left ventricular systolic function, improvement in diastolic function, and reduction in overall mortality.[12,51] Collateral coronary vessels also appear to influence left ventricular function following reperfusion.[52] They provide sufficient perfusion of myocardium to retard cell death and are probably of greater importance in patients having reperfusion later rather than 1 to 2 hours after coronary occlusion. Even after successful reperfusion and despite the absence of irreversible myocardial damage, a period of postischemic contractile dysfunction can occur, a phenomenon termed *myocardial stunning*.[53] Periods of myocardial stunning have been well described in experimental animals but also apply to STEMI patients who undergo PCI.

REPERFUSION INJURY. The process of reperfusion, although beneficial in terms of myocardial salvage, may come at a cost because of a process known as reperfusion injury.[54] Several types of reperfusion injury have been observed in experimental animals.[55] These consist of the following: (1) lethal reperfusion injury—reperfusion-induced death of cells that were still viable at the time of restoration of coronary blood flow; (2) vascular reperfusion injury—progressive damage to the microvasculature so that there is an expanding area of no reflow and loss of coronary vasodilatory reserve; (3) stunned myocardium—salvaged myocytes display a prolonged period of contractile dysfunction following restoration of blood flow because of abnormalities of intracellular metabolism leading to reduced energy production; and (4) reperfusion arrhythmias—bursts of ventricular tachycardia and, on occasion, ventricular fibrillation—that occur within seconds of reperfusion.[56] The available evidence suggests that vascular reperfusion injury, stunning, and reperfusion arrhythmias can all occur in patients with STEMI. The concept of lethal reperfusion injury of potentially salvageable myocardium remains controversial in experimental animals and in patients.[57]

Reperfusion increases the cell swelling that occurs with ischemia. Reperfusion of the myocardium in which the microvasculature is damaged leads to the creation of a hemorrhagic infarct (see Chap. 54). Fibrinolytic therapy appears more likely to produce hemorrhagic infarction than catheter-based reperfusion. Although concern has been raised that this hemorrhage may lead to extension of the infarct, this does not appear to be the case. Histologic study of patients not surviving in spite of successful reperfusion has revealed hemorrhagic infarcts, but this hemorrhage usually does not extend beyond the area of necrosis.

Protection Against Reperfusion Injury

A variety of adjunctive approaches may protect the myocardium against injury that occurs after reperfusion: (1) preservation of microvascular integrity by using antiplatelet agents and antithrombins to minimize embolization of atheroembolic debris; (2) prevention of inflammatory damage; and (3) metabolic support of the ischemic myocardium.[58] The effectiveness of agents directed against reperfusion injury rapidly declines the later they are administered after reperfusion[59]; eventually, no beneficial effect is detectable in animal models after 45 to 60 minutes of reperfusion has elapsed.

An alternative experimental approach to protection against reperfusion injury is called postconditioning, which involves introducing brief repetitive episodes of ischemia alternating with reperfusion.[60] This appears to activate a number of cellular protective mechanisms centering around prosurvival kinases.[61] Many of these protective kinases are also activated during ischemic preconditioning. Clinical studies in STEMI patients undergoing PCI have provided evidence that postconditioning protects the human heart and is associated with a reduction in infarct size and improvement in myocardial perfusion.[62]

REPERFUSION ARRHYTHMIAS. Transient sinus bradycardia occurs in many patients with inferior infarcts at the time of acute reperfusion; it is most often accompanied by some degree of hypotension. This combination of hypotension and bradycardia with a sudden increase in coronary flow may involve activation of the Bezold-Jarisch reflex.[63] Premature ventricular contractions, accelerated idioventricular rhythm, and nonsustained ventricular tachycardia also commonly follow successful reperfusion. Although some investigators have postulated that early afterdepolarizations participate in the genesis of reperfusion ventricular arrhythmias, early afterdepolarizations are present during ischemia and reperfusion and are therefore unlikely to be involved in the development of reperfusion ventricular tachycardia or fibrillation.

When present, rhythm disturbances may actually indicate successful restoration of coronary flow. While reperfusion arrhythmias have a high sensitivity for detecting successful reperfusion, the high incidence of identical rhythm disturbances in patients without successful coronary artery reperfusion limits their specificity for detection of restoration of coronary blood flow. In general, clinical features are poor markers of reperfusion, with no single clinical finding or constellation of findings being reliably predictive of angiographically demonstrated coronary artery patency.[1]

Although reperfusion arrhythmias may show a temporal clustering at the time of restoration of coronary blood flow in patients with successful fibrinolysis, the overall incidence of such arrhythmias appears to be similar in patients not receiving a fibrinolytic agent who may develop these arrhythmias as a consequence of spontaneous coronary artery reperfusion or the evolution of the infarct process itself. These considerations, as well as the fact that the brief electrical storm occurring at the time of reperfusion is generally innocuous, indicate that no prophylactic antiarrhythmic therapy is necessary when fibrinolytics are prescribed.

LATE ESTABLISHMENT OF PATENCY OF THE INFARCT VESSEL. Improved survival and ventricular function after successful reperfusion may not result entirely from limitation of infarct size.[64] Poorly contracting or noncontracting myocardium in a zone that is supplied by a stenosed infarct-related artery with slow antegrade perfusion may still contain viable myocytes. This situation is referred to as hibernating myocardium,[65] and its function can be improved by PCI to augment flow in the infarct-related artery.

SUMMARY OF EFFECTS OF MYOCARDIAL REPERFUSION. Plaque disruption in the culprit vessel produces complete occlusion of the infarct-related coronary artery. STEMI occurs with the ensuing development of left ventricular dilation and ultimate death through a combination of pump failure and electrical instability (**Fig. 55-6**; see Chap. 54). Early reperfusion shortens the duration of coronary occlusion, minimizes the degree of ultimate left ventricular dysfunction and dilation, and reduces the probability that the STEMI patient will develop pump failure or malignant ventricular tachyarrhythmias. Late reperfusion of stenosed infarct arteries may restore contractile function in hibernating myocardium.[65]

Fibrinolysis

Fibrinolysis recanalizes thrombotic occlusion associated with STEMI, and restoration of coronary flow reduces infarct size and improves myocardial function and survival over the short and the long term.[66,67] Most of the mortality benefit seen at 10-year follow-up in the GISSI trial

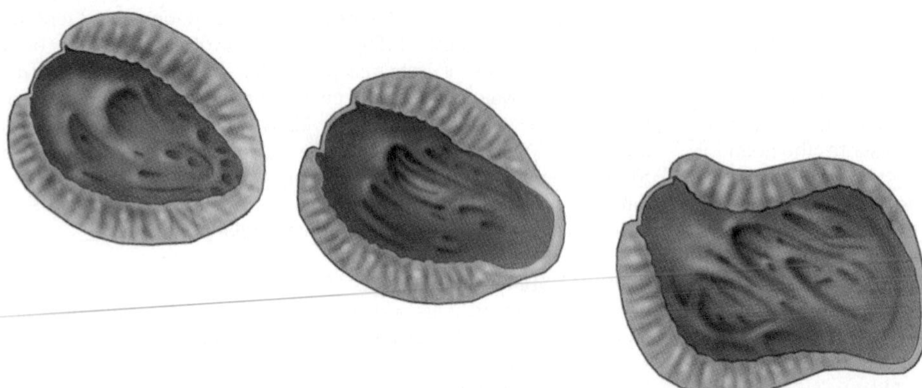

FIGURE 55-6 Remodeling of left ventricle after STEMI. **Left,** Apical STEMI (white zone of left ventricle). Over time, the infarct zone elongates and thins. Progressive remodeling of the left ventricle occurs **(center and right),** ultimately converting the left ventricle from an oval shape to a spherical shape. Pharmacologic and catheter-based reperfusion strategies for STEMI have a favorable impact on this process by minimizing the extent of myocardial necrosis **(left)** through prompt restoration of flow in the epicardial infarct vessel. *(Modified from McMurray JJV, Pfeffer MA [eds]: Heart Failure Updates. London, Martin Dunitz, 2003.)*

was obtained before hospital discharge because no survival difference was seen in fibrinolysed and control patients discharged alive except for those treated within the first hour after onset of symptoms.[1]

INTRACORONARY FIBRINOLYSIS. In current practice, patients are more likely to be treated by PCI. This has reopened the concept of delivering fibrinolytic agents via the intracoronary route, but such efforts at present are largely restricted to adjunctive use during complicated PCI procedures.[68]

INTRAVENOUS FIBRINOLYSIS

Thrombolysis in Myocardial Infarction Flow Grade

To provide a level of standardization for comparison of the various regimens, most investigators describe the flow in the infarct vessel according to the Thrombolysis in Myocardial Infarction (TIMI) trial grading system: grade 0, complete occlusion of the infarct-related artery; grade 1, some penetration of the contrast material beyond the point of obstruction but without perfusion of the distal coronary bed; grade 2, perfusion of the entire infarct vessel into the distal bed but with delayed flow compared with a normal artery; and grade 3, full perfusion of the infarct vessel with normal flow.[69] When evaluating reports of angiographic studies of fibrinolytic agents, it must be noted that only in studies in which a pretreatment coronary arteriogram documents occlusion of the culprit vessel can the term *recanalization* be applied if flow is restored. If the status of the culprit vessel is not known before treatment, one can only ascertain the patency rate of the vessel at the moment that the contrast material is injected. This snapshot in time does not reflect the fluctuating status of flow in the infarct vessel that characteristically undergoes repeated cycles of patency and reocclusion, as has been documented angiographically and by continuous ST-segment monitoring.

Issues of the fluctuating nature of patency of the infarct-related artery notwithstanding, most angiographic studies of reperfusion regimens for STEMI have used an assessment of the TIMI flow grade at 90 or preferably 60 minutes after the start of fibrinolytic therapy.[2,66] TIMI grade 3 flow is far superior to grade 2 in terms of infarct size reduction and short- and long-term mortality benefit. Therefore, TIMI grade 3 flow should be the goal when assessing flow in the epicardial infarct artery (**Fig. 55-7**).

TIMI Frame Count

To provide a more quantitative statement of the briskness of coronary blood flow in the infarct artery and to account for differences in the size and length of vessels (e.g., left anterior descending versus right coronary artery) and interobserver variability, Gibson and colleagues[70] have developed the TIMI frame count, a simple count of the number of angiographic frames elapsed until the contrast material arrives in the distal bed of the vessel of interest. This objective and quantitative index of coronary blood flow independently predicts in-hospital mortality from STEMI and also discriminates patients with TIMI grade 3 flow into low-risk and high-risk groups. Using the TIMI frame count, they determined that the following are univariate predictors of delayed coronary blood flow after fibrinolytic administration: greater percentage diameter stenosis; decreased minimum lumen diameter; greater percentage of the culprit artery distal to stenosis; and presence of delayed achievement of patency, a culprit artery location in the left coronary circulation, pulsatile flow (i.e., reversible flow in systole), or intraluminal thrombus. The TIMI frame count can also be used to quantitate coronary blood flow (mL/second), as calculated by the following:

$$(21 \div \text{observed TIMI frame count}) \times 1.7$$

This is based on Doppler velocity wire data showing that normal flow equals 1.7 cm^3/second, which is proportional to 21 frames. Calculated coronary perfusion relates to mortality for patients treated with

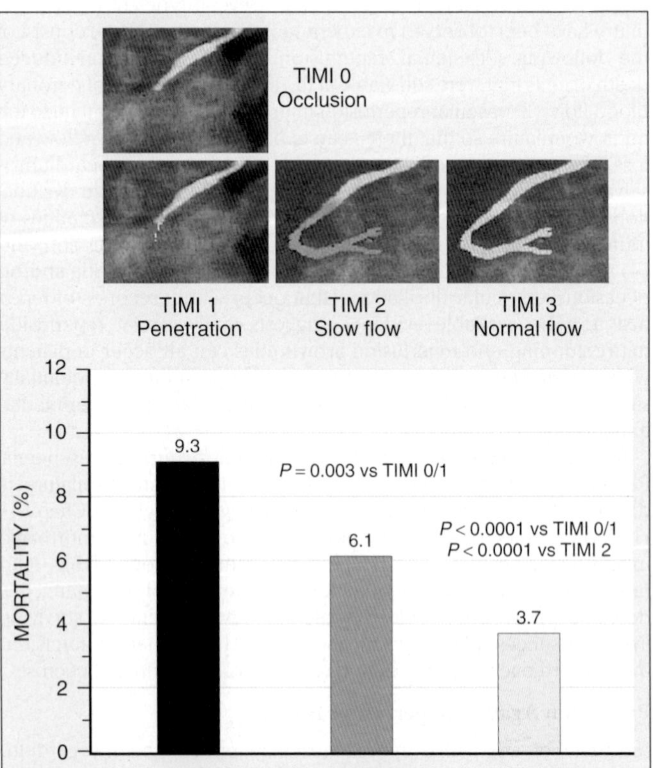

FIGURE 55-7 Correlation of TIMI flow grade and mortality. A pooled analysis of data from 5498 patients in several angiographic trials of reperfusion for STEMI showed a gradient of mortality when the angiographic findings were stratified by TIMI flow grade. Patients with TIMI 0 or TIMI 1 flow had the highest rate of mortality, TIMI 2 flow was associated with an intermediate rate of mortality, and the lowest rate of mortality was observed in patients with TIMI 3 flow. TIMI = Thrombolysis in Myocardial Infarction. *(Dr. Michael Gibson, personal communication, 2008.)*

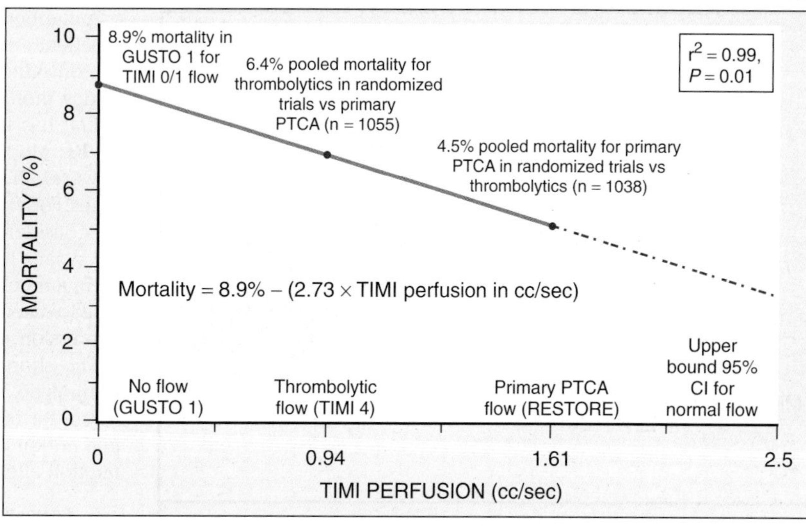

FIGURE 55-8 Relationship between coronary blood flow and mortality rate in patients with acute myocardial infarction. PTCA = percutaneous transluminal coronary angioplasty. *(From Gibson CM: Primary angioplasty, rescue angioplasty, and new devices.* In *Hennekens CH [ed]: Clinical Trials in Cardiovascular Disease: A Companion to Braunwald's Heart Disease. Philadelphia, WB Saunders, 1999, p 194.)*

fibrinolytics or primary PCI and serves to assess various modalities for reperfusion in STEMI (**Fig. 55-8**).

Myocardial Perfusion

Despite intense interest in the development of reperfusion regimens that normalize flow in the epicardial infarct-related artery, reperfusion in patients with STEMI aims to improve actual myocardial perfusion in the infarct zone. Myocardial perfusion cannot be improved adequately without restoration of flow in the occluded infarct-related artery. Yet, even patients with TIMI grade 3 flow may not achieve adequate myocardial perfusion, especially if there is a great delay between the onset of symptoms and restoration of epicardial flow.[71] The term *myocardial no-reflow* has been used to describe the state in which there is reduced myocardial perfusion after opening of an epicardial infarct artery.[72] The two major impediments to normalization of myocardial perfusion are microvascular damage (**Fig. 55-9**) and reperfusion injury. Obstruction of the distal microvasculature in the downstream bed of the infarct-related artery is caused by platelet microemboli and thrombi.[73] Fibrinolysis may actually exacerbate microembolization of platelet aggregates because of the exposure of clot-bound thrombin, an extremely potent platelet agonist. Spasm can also occur in the microvasculature because of the release of substances from activated platelets. Reperfusion injury results in cellular edema, formation of reactive oxygen species, and calcium overload. In addition, cytokine activation leads to neutrophil accumulation and inflammatory mediators that contribute to tissue injury.

Several techniques can evaluate the adequacy of myocardial perfusion. Electrocardiographic ST-segment resolution strongly predicts outcome in STEMI patients but is a better predictor of an occluded artery than of a patent infarct-related artery.[74,75] The absence of early ST-segment resolution after angiographically successful primary PCI identifies patients with a higher risk of left ventricular dysfunction and mortality, presumably because of microvascular damage in the infarct zone. Thus, the 12-lead ECG is a marker of the biologic integrity of myocytes in the infarct zone and can reflect inadequate myocardial perfusion, even in the presence of TIMI grade 3 flow.[71] ST-segment resolution in combination with cardiac biomarkers (e.g., troponins, natriuretic peptides) provides powerful prognostic information early in the management of STEMI patients.[76] Given the dynamic nature of coronary occlusion, continuous ST-segment monitoring may prove more informative than static 12-lead electrocardiographic recordings, but practical limitations have prevented continuous ST-segment monitoring in widespread clinical application.[77] Defects in perfusion patterns seen with myocardial contrast echocardiography correlate with regional wall motion abnormalities and lack of myocardial viability on dobutamine stress echocardiography. A practical limitation to myocardial contrast echocardiography is the need for intracoronary injection of echo contrast, although this can be circumvented by the availability of new echo contrast agents that can be injected intravenously. Doppler flow wire studies, cardiac magnetic resonance (CMR), and nuclear imaging with positron emission tomography can also define abnormalities of myocardial perfusion.

An angiographic method for assessing myocardial perfusion has been developed by Gibson and coworkers,[71] the TIMI myocardial perfusion (TMP) grade (**Fig. 55-10**). Abnormalities of increasing myocardial perfusion as assessed by the TMP grade correlate with mortality risk even after adjusting for the presence of TIMI grade 3 flow or a normal TIMI frame count.

EFFECT OF FIBRINOLYTIC THERAPY ON MORTALITY. Early intravenous fibrinolysis undoubtedly improves survival in patients with STEMI.[1] Mortality varies considerably, depending on the patients included for study and the adjunctive therapies used. The benefit of fibrinolytic therapy appears to be greatest when agents are administered as early as possible, with the most dramatic results obtained when the drug is given less than 2 hours after symptoms begin.[2]

A comprehensive overview of nine trials of thrombolytic therapy has been performed, and each trial enrolled more than 1,000 patients; the absolute mortality rates for the control and fibrinolytic groups stratified by presenting features are shown in **Figure 55-11**. The overall results indicated an 18% reduction in short-term mortality, but as much as a 25% reduction in mortality for the subset of 45,000 patients with ST-segment elevation or bundle branch block. Two trials, LATE and EMERAS, viewed together have provided evidence that a mortality reduction may still be observed in patients treated with thrombolytic agents between 6 and 12 hours from the onset of ischemic symptoms. The data from LATE and EMERAS and the FTT overview form the basis for extending the window of treatment with fibrinolytics up to 12 hours from the onset of symptoms. Boersma and colleagues have pooled the trials in the FTT overview, two smaller studies with data on time to randomization, and 11 additional trials of more than 100 patients.[1] Patients were divided into six time categories from symptom onset to randomization. A nonlinear relationship of treatment benefit to time was observed, with the greatest benefit occurring in the first 1 to 2 hours from the onset of symptoms (**Fig. 55-12**).

The mortality effect of fibrinolytic therapy in older patients is of considerable interest and controversy. Although patients older than 75 years of age were initially excluded from randomized trials of fibrinolytic therapy, they now constitute about 15% of the patients studied in megatrials of fibrinolysis and about 35% of patients analyzed in

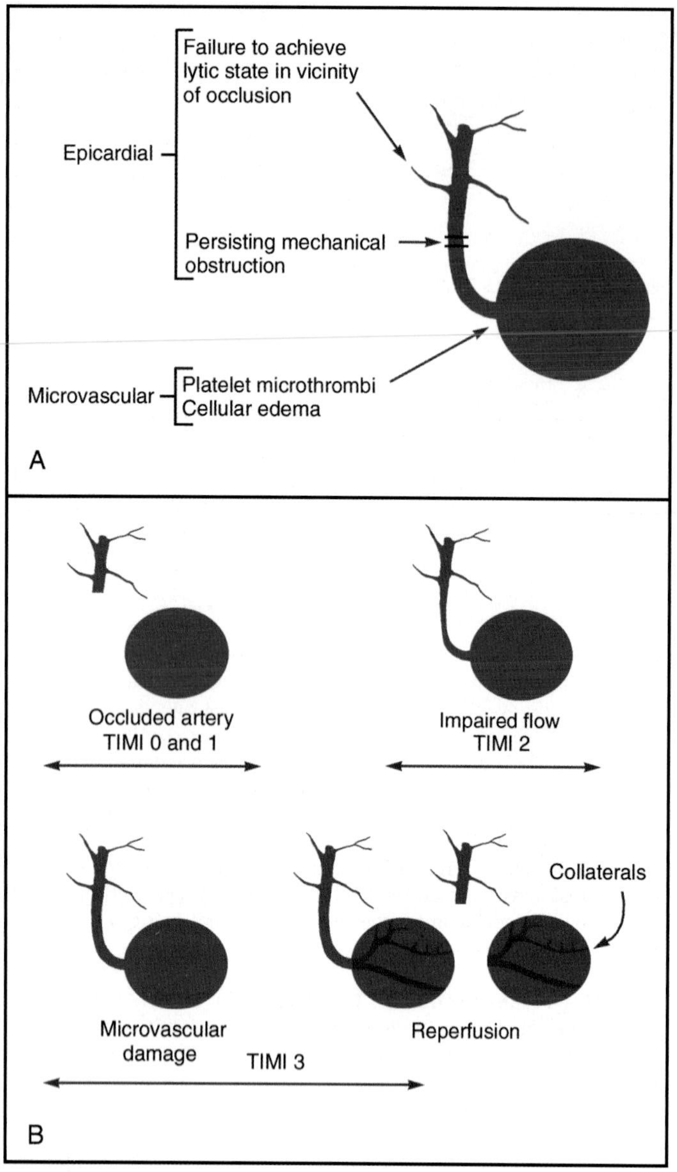

FIGURE 55-9 Patterns of response to fibrinolysis. **A,** Failure of epicardial reperfusion can occur because of failure to induce a lytic state or because of mechanical factors at the site of occlusion. Failure of microvascular reperfusion is caused by a combination of platelet microthrombi followed by endothelial swelling and myocardial edema (no reflow). **B,** Fibrinolysis may fail because of persistent occlusion of the epicardial infarct-related artery (TIMI grades 0 and 1), patency of an epicardial artery in the presence of impaired (TIMI grade 2) flow, or microvascular occlusion in the presence of angiographically normal (TIMI grade 3) flow. Successful reperfusion requires a patent artery with an intact microvascular network. Conversely, reperfusion may occur despite an occluded epicardial artery because of the presence of collateral arteries. *(From Davies CH, Ormerod OJ: Failed coronary thrombolysis. Lancet 351:1191, 1998.)*

registries of STEMI patients.[78] Barriers to the initiation of therapy in older patients with STEMI include a protracted period of delay in seeking medical care, a lower incidence of ischemic discomfort and greater incidence of atypical symptoms and concomitant illnesses, and an increased incidence of nondiagnostic electrocardiographic readings. Younger patients with STEMI achieve a slightly greater relative reduction in mortality compared with older patients, but the higher absolute mortality in older adults results in similar absolute mortality reductions.[79] Other important baseline characteristics that have an impact on the mortality effect of fibrinolytic therapy include the vital signs at presentation and presence of diabetes mellitus (see Fig. 55-11).

A number of models integrate the many clinical variables that affect a patient's mortality risk before administration of fibrinolytic therapy. A convenient, simple, bedside risk-scoring system for predicting 30-day mortality at presentation for fibrinolytic-eligible patients with STEMI has been developed using the InTIME-II trial database (**Fig. 55-13**). Modeling of mortality risk cannot cover all clinical scenarios, however, and should not substitute for clinical judgment in individual cases. For example, patients with inferior STEMI who might otherwise be considered to have a low risk of mortality, and for whom many physicians have questioned the benefits of fibrinolytic therapy, might be in a much higher mortality risk subgroup if their inferior infarction is associated with right ventricular infarction, precordial ST-segment depression, or ST-segment elevation in the lateral precordial leads.

The short-term survival benefit enjoyed by patients who receive fibrinolytic therapy is maintained over the 1- to 10-year follow-up. Room for improvement remains. Advances in adjunctive antiplatelet and antithrombin therapies have led to reductions in the rate of reinfarction after fibrinolysis for STEMI.[2,66]

Comparison of Fibrinolytic Agents. Approved fibrinolytic agents for intravenous therapy have distinct features (**Table 55-6**; see Chap. 87). The tissue plasminogen activator (t-PA) molecule contains the following five domains: finger, epidermal growth factor, kringle 1 and kringle 2, and serine protease (**Fig. 55-14**).[66] In the absence of fibrin, t-PA is a weak plasminogen activator; fibrin provides a scaffold on which t-PA and plasminogen are held in such a way that the catalytic efficiency for plasminogen activation of t-PA is increased many-fold. Plasma clearance of t-PA is mediated to a varying degree by residues in each of the domains except the serine protease domain, which is responsible for the enzymatic activity of t-PA. The accelerated dose regimen of t-PA over 90 minutes produces more rapid thrombolysis than the standard 3-hour infusion of t-PA. The recommended dosage regimen for t-PA is a 15-mg intravenous bolus followed by an infusion of 0.75 mg/kg (maximum 50 mg) over 30 minutes, followed by an infusion of 0.5 mg/kg (maximum 35 mg) over 60 minutes.

Modifications of the native t-PA structure yielded a group of third-generation fibrinolytics (see Fig. 55-14 and Table 55-6). A common feature among these is prolonged plasma clearance, allowing them to be administered as a bolus rather than the bolus and double-infusion technique whereby an accelerated-dose t-PA is administered.[66]

Reteplase. Reteplase is a recombinant deletion mutant form of t-PA lacking the finger, epidermal growth factor, and kringle 1 domains, as well as the carbohydrate side chains (see Fig. 55-14 and Table 55-6).

The GUSTO III trial compared the 10 + 10 unit regimen of reteplase with accelerated t-PA in 15,059 patients.[1] The 30-day mortality rate was 7.47% in the reteplase group and 7.24% in the t-PA group, corresponding to an absolute difference of 0.23%, with a 95% confidence interval (CI) of −0.66 to +1.1%. The results of GUSTO III did not demonstrate superiority of reteplase over t-PA and, using a 1% absolute difference as a boundary for noninferiority, the mortality results also do not formally demonstrate noninferiority. The intracranial hemorrhage rate was 0.91% with reteplase and 0.87% with t-PA. The secondary composite endpoint of net clinical benefit (death or disabling stroke) was 7.89% with reteplase and 7.91% with accelerated t-PA. Although GUSTO III did not fulfill formal criteria for noninferiority of reteplase and t-PA, many clinicians consider the two agents to be therapeutically similar and consider the double-bolus method of administration of reteplase to be an advantage over t-PA.

Tenecteplase. Tenecteplase is a mutant form of t-PA with specific amino acid substitutions in the kringle 1 domain and protease domain introduced to decrease plasma clearance, increase fibrin specificity, and reduce sensitivity to plasminogen activator inhibitor-1 (see Fig. 55-14 and Table 55-6). ASSENT 2 was a randomized, double-blind, phase III equivalence trial comparing single-bolus tenecteplase with accelerated dose t-PA in 16,949 patients.[1] The 30-day mortality rate with tenecteplase was 6.179% and with t-PA it was 6.151% ($P = 0.0059$ for equivalence). The rate of intracranial hemorrhage was 0.93% with tenecteplase and 0.94% with t-PA. Major bleeding occurred in 4.66% of tenecteplase-treated patients compared with 5.94% of t-PA–treated patients ($P = 0.0002$). There was no specific subgroup of patients for whom tenecteplase or t-PA was significantly better, with the exception of patients treated after 4 hours from the onset of symptoms, among whom the mortality rate was 7.0% with tenecteplase and 9.2% with t-PA ($P = 0.018$).

Other Fibrinolytic Agents. Urokinase is used on rare occasions as an intracoronary infusion (6000 IU/min) to an average cumulative dose of 5,000,000 IU to lyse intracoronary thrombi that are believed to be

TMP Grade 0
No or
minimal blush.
TMP Grade 1
Stain present.
Blush persists on
next injection.
TMP Grade 2
Contrast strongly
persistent at end
of washout. Gone
by next injection.
TMP Grade 3
Normal ground
glass appearance
of blush. Contrast
mildly persistent
at end of washout.
Mortality (%)
8
6
4
2
0
6.2
5.1
4.4
2.0

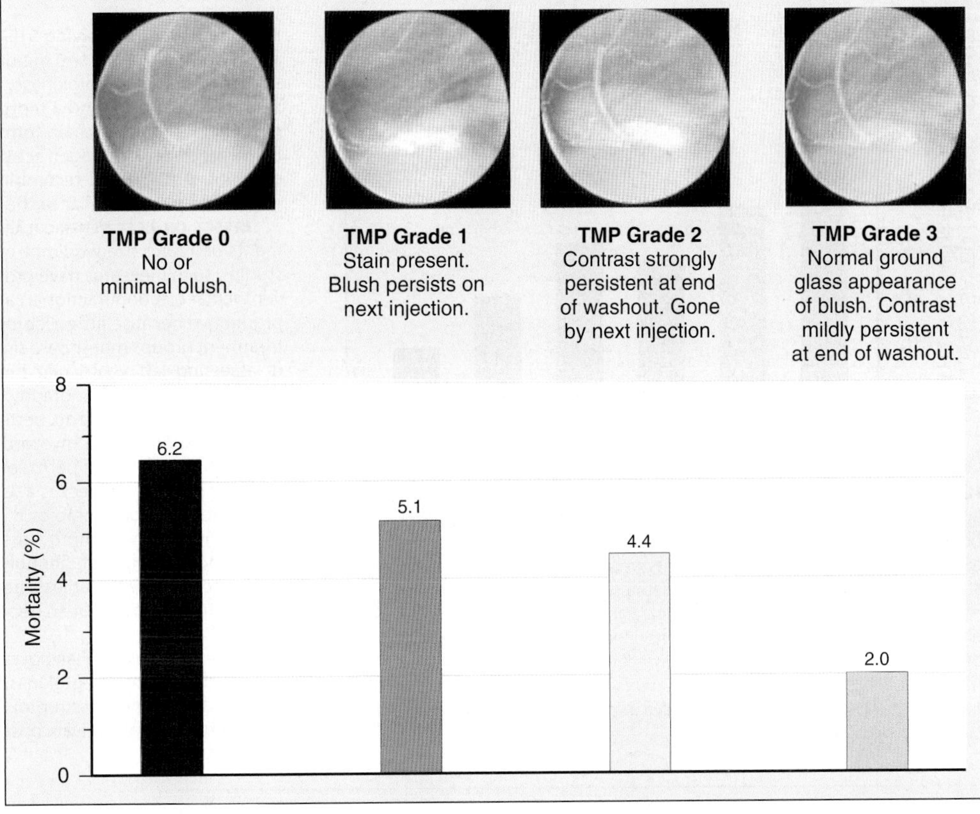

FIGURE 55-10 Relationship between TIMI myocardial perfusion (TMP) grade and mortality. TMP grade 0 or no perfusion of the myocardium is associated with the highest rate of mortality. If the stain of the myocardium is present (grade 1), mortality is also high. A reduction in mortality is seen if the contrast enters the microvasculature but is still persistent at the end of the washout phase (grade 2). The lowest mortality rate is observed in those patients with normal perfusion (grade 3) in whom the contrast is minimally persistent at the end of the washout phase. *(From Gibson CM, Cannon CP, Murphy SA, et al: Relationship of TIMI myocardial perfusion grade to mortality after administration of thrombolytic drugs. Circulation 101:125, 2000.)*

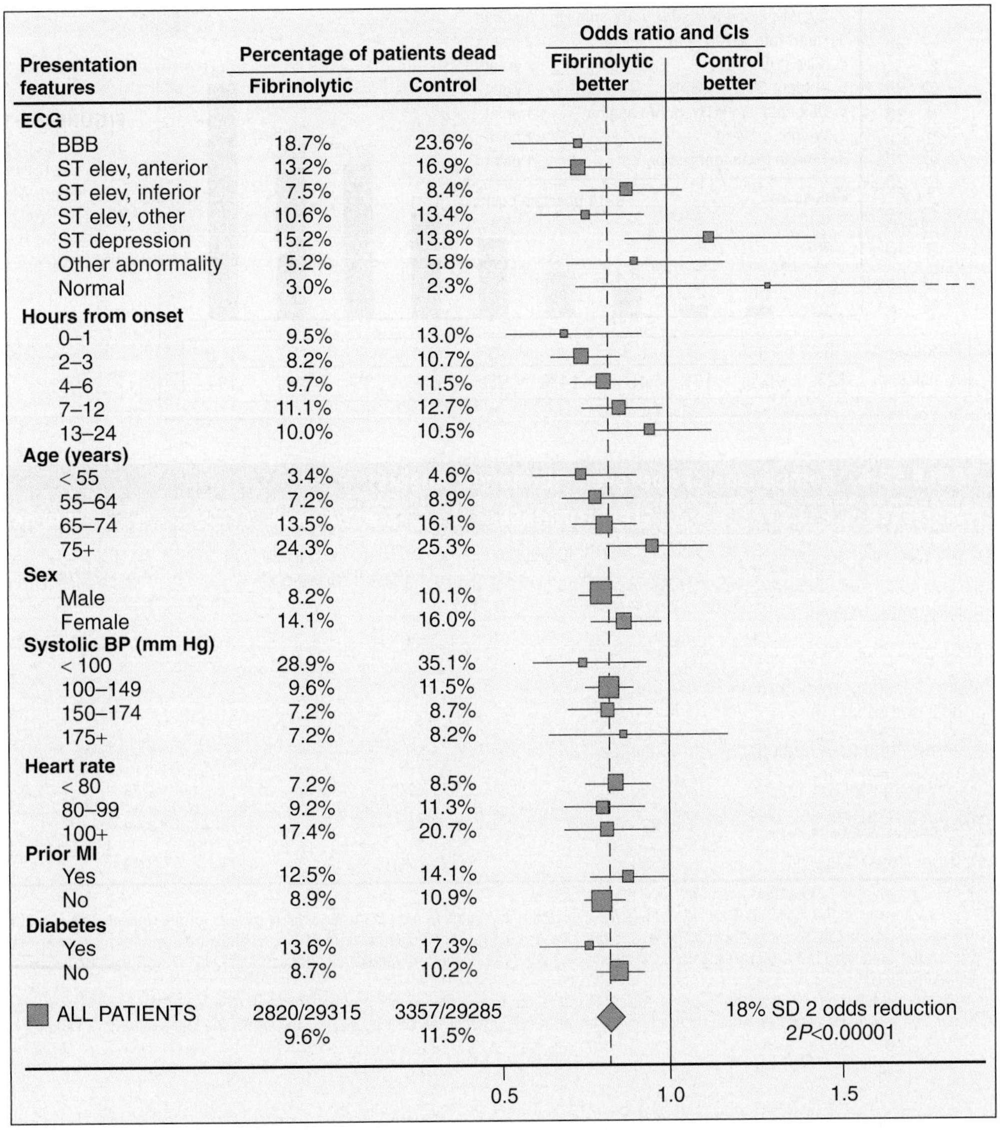

Presentation features
Percentage of patients dead
Fibrinolytic
Control
Odds ratio and CIs
Fibrinolytic better
Control better
ECG
BBB 18.7% 23.6%
ST elev, anterior 13.2% 16.9%
ST elev, inferior 7.5% 8.4%
ST elev, other 10.6% 13.4%
ST depression 15.2% 13.8%
Other abnormality 5.2% 5.8%
Normal 3.0% 2.3%
Hours from onset
0–1 9.5% 13.0%
2–3 8.2% 10.7%
4–6 9.7% 11.5%
7–12 11.1% 12.7%
13–24 10.0% 10.5%
Age (years)
< 55 3.4% 4.6%
55–64 7.2% 8.9%
65–74 13.5% 16.1%
75+ 24.3% 25.3%
Sex
Male 8.2% 10.1%
Female 14.1% 16.0%
Systolic BP (mm Hg)
< 100 28.9% 35.1%
100–149 9.6% 11.5%
150–174 7.2% 8.7%
175+ 7.2% 8.2%
Heart rate
< 80 7.2% 8.5%
80–99 9.2% 11.3%
100+ 17.4% 20.7%
Prior MI
Yes 12.5% 14.1%
No 8.9% 10.9%
Diabetes
Yes 13.6% 17.3%
No 8.7% 10.2%
ALL PATIENTS 2820/29315 9.6% 3357/29285 11.5%
18% SD 2 odds reduction
2P<0.00001
0.5
1.0
1.5

FIGURE 55-11 Mortality differences during days 0 to 35 subdivided by presentation features in a collaborative overview of results from nine trials of thrombolytic therapy. The absolute mortality rates are shown for fibrinolytic and control groups in the center portion of the figure for each of the clinical features at presentation listed on the left side of the figure. The ratio of the odds of death in the fibrinolytic group to that in the control group is shown for each subdivision (magenta squares), along with its 99% confidence interval (horizontal line). The summary OR at the bottom of the figure corresponds to an 18% proportional reduction in 35-day mortality and is highly statistically significant. This translates to a reduction of 18 deaths/1000 patients treated with thrombolytic agents. BBB = bundle branch block; BP = blood pressure; SD = standard deviation. *(From Fibrinolytic Therapy Trialists' [FTT] Collaborative Group: Indications for fibrinolytic therapy in suspected acute myocardial infarction: Collaborative overview of mortality and major morbidity results from all randomized trials of more than 1000 patients. Lancet 343:311, 1994.)*

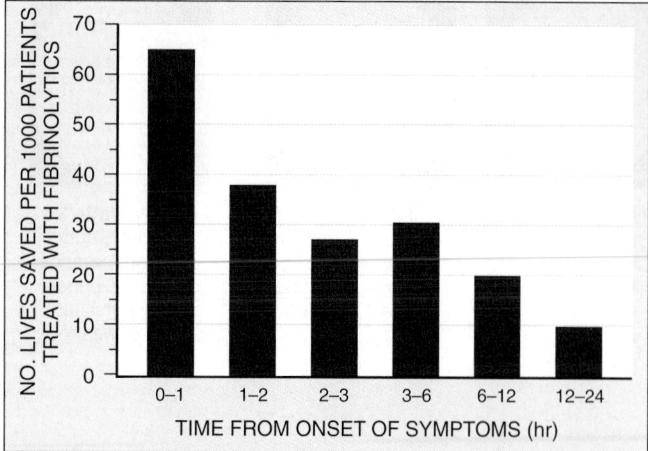

FIGURE 55-12 Importance of time to reperfusion in patients receiving fibrinolytic therapy for STEMI. The data from 22 trials of fibrinolytic therapy were pooled and the findings stratified by the six time categories shown in the figure. The number of lives saved/1000 patients treated with fibrinolytics compared with placebo is greatest the earlier treatment is initiated after the onset of symptoms, and this decreases in a nonlinear fashion with incremental time delays. Because the lifesaving effect of fibrinolysis is maximal in the first hour from onset of symptoms, this has been referred to as the "golden hour" for pharmacologic reperfusion. *(From Boersma E, Maas AC, Deckers JW, et al: Early thrombolytic treatment in acute myocardial infarction: Reappraisal of the golden hour. Lancet 348:771, 1996.)*

responsible for an evolving STEMI. Anistreplase, usually administered in a dose of 30 mg over 2 to 5 minutes intravenously, has a side effect profile similar to that of streptokinase, a patency profile similar to that of conventional dose t-PA, and a mortality benefit similar to that of streptokinase or t-PA (double-chain form, duteplase). Staphylokinase is a highly fibrin-specific plasminogen activator that requires priming on the surface of a clot. A pegylated recombinant form of staphylokinase yields TIMI grade 3 flow rates similar to those obtained with t-PA.[66]

EFFECT ON LEFT VENTRICULAR FUNCTION. Although precise measurements of infarct size would be an ideal endpoint for clinical reperfusion studies, such measures have proven impractical. Attempts to use the left ventricular ejection fraction as a surrogate for infarct size have not been productive because little difference is seen in ejection fraction between treatment groups that show a significant difference in mortality. Methods of assessing left ventricular function, such as end-systolic volume or quantitative echocardiography, are more revealing because patients with smaller volumes and better preserved ventricular shape have an improved survival. The myocardial salvage index, defined as the difference between an initial perfusion defect (e.g., by sestamibi scintigraphy) and final perfusion defect, is a useful means for comparing the effectiveness of reperfusion therapies.[80]

As with survival, improvement in global left ventricular function is related to the time of fibrinolytic treatment, with greatest improvement occurring with earliest therapy.[2] Greater improvement in left ventricular function has been reported with anterior than with inferior infarcts.[81]

COMPLICATIONS OF FIBRINOLYTIC THERAPY. Recent (<1 year) exposure to streptococci or streptokinase produces some degree of antibody-mediated resistance to streptokinase and anistreplase in most patients. Although this is of clinical consequence only rarely, it is recommended

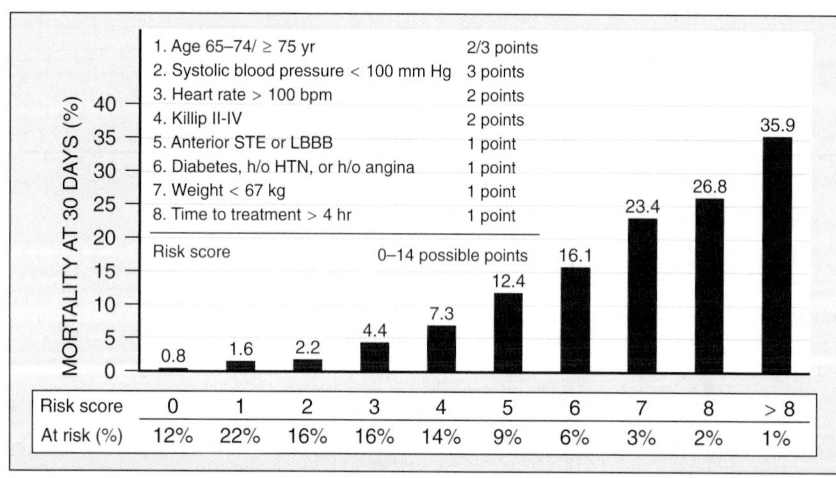

FIGURE 55-13 TIMI risk score for STEMI predicting 30-day mortality. h/o = history of; HTN = hypertension; LBBB = left bundle branch block; STE = ST-segment elevation. *(From Morrow DA, Antman EM, Charlesworth A, et al: The TIMI risk score for ST elevation myocardial infarction: A convenient, bedside, clinical score for risk assessment at presentation: An InTIME II substudy. Circulation 102:2031, 2000.)*

TABLE 55-6 Comparison of Approved Fibrinolytic Agents*

PARAMETER	STREPTOKINASE	ALTEPLASE	RETEPLASE	TNK T-PA
Dose	1.5 MU in 30-60 min	Up to 100 mg in 90 min (based on weight)	10 U × 2 (30 min apart) each over 2 min	30-50 mg based on weight
Bolus administration	No	No	Yes	Yes
Antigenic				
Allergic reactions (hypotension most common)	Yes	No	No	No
Systemic fibrinogen depletion	Marked	Mild	Moderate	Minimal
90-min patency rates (%)	≈50	≈75	≈75	≈75†
TIMI grade 3 flow (%)	32	54	60	63
Cost per dose (U.S. $)‡	568	2750	2750	2750 for 50 mg

TIMI = Thrombolysis in Myocardial Infarction; TNK = tenecteplase.

*Data from Armstrong PW, Collen D: Fibrinolysis for acute myocardial infarction: Current status and new horizons for pharmacological reperfusion, part 1. Circulation 103:2862, 2001. †Data from Cannon CP, Gibson CM, McCabe CH, et al: TNK-tissue plasminogen activator compared with front-loaded alteplase in acute myocardial infarction: results of the TIMI 10B trial. Thrombolysis in Myocardial Infarction (TIMI) 10B Investigators. Circulation 98:2805, 1998. ‡Data from Medical Economics Staff: 2001 Drug Topics Red Book. 105th ed. Montvale, NJ, Medical Economics Company, 2001.

From Antman EM, Anbe DT, Armstrong PW, et al: ACC/AHA guidelines for the management of patients with ST-elevation myocardial infarction: A report of the American College of Cardiology/American Heart Association Task Force on Practice Guidelines (Committee to Revise the 1999 Guidelines for the Management of Patients with Acute Myocardial Infarction). Circulation 110:e82, 2004.

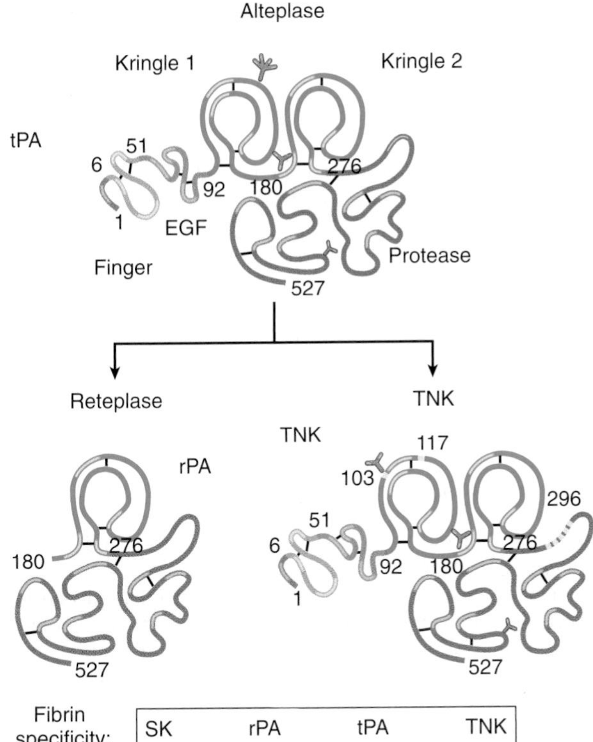

FIGURE 55-14 Molecular structure of alteplase (tPA), reteplase (rPA), and tenecteplase (TNK). Streptokinase (SK) is the least fibrin-specific thrombolytic agent in clinical use; the progressive increase in relative fibrin specificity for the various thrombolytics is shown at the bottom. *(Modified from Brener SJ, Topol EJ: Third-generation thrombolytic agents for acute myocardial infarction.* In *Topol EJ [ed]: Acute Coronary Syndromes. New York, Marcel Dekker, 1998, p 169.)*

that patients not receive streptokinase for STEMI if they have been treated with a streptokinase product within the past year. Bleeding complications are most common and potentially the most serious. Most bleeding is relatively minor with all agents, with more serious episodes occurring in patients requiring invasive procedures.[82] Intracranial hemorrhage is the most serious complication of fibrinolytic therapy; its frequency varies with the clinical characteristics of the patient and the fibrinolytic agent prescribed (**Fig. 55-15**).[1]

There have been reports of an early hazard with fibrinolytic therapy—that is, an excess of deaths in the first 24 hours in fibrinolytic-treated patients compared with control subjects, especially in older patients treated more than 12 hours.[51] However, this excess early mortality is more than offset by the deaths prevented beyond the first day, culminating in an 18% (range, 13% to 23%) reduction in mortality by 35 days. The mechanisms responsible for this early hazard are not clear but are probably multiple, including an increased risk of myocardial rupture (particularly in older patients), fatal intracranial hemorrhage, inadequate myocardial reperfusion resulting in pump failure and cardiogenic shock, and possible reperfusion injury of reperfused myocardium. Reports of more unusual complications such as splenic rupture, aortic dissection, and cholesterol embolization have also appeared.

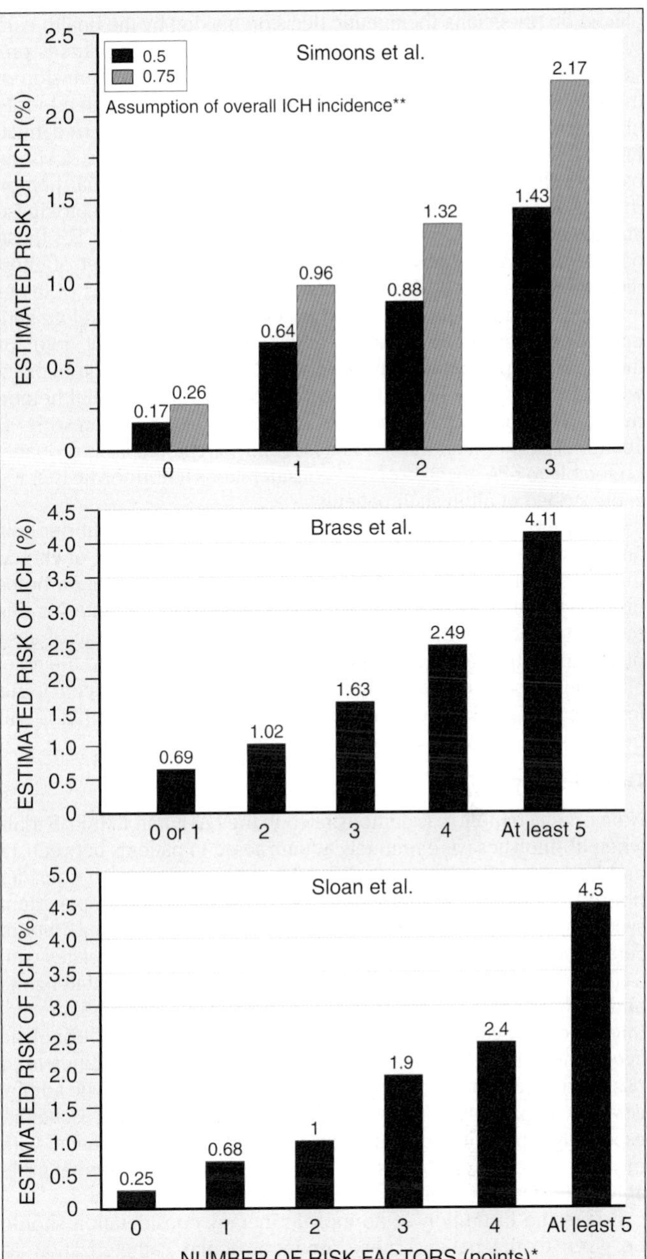

FIGURE 55-15 Estimation of risk of intracranial hemorrhage (ICH) with fibrinolysis. The number of risk factors is the sum of the points based on criteria established in the studies shown. *Although the exact risk factors varied among the studies, common risk factors across all the studies included increased age, low body weight, and hypertension on admission. **If the overall incidence of ICH is assumed to be 0.75%, patients without risk factors who receive streptokinase have a 0.26% probability of ICH. The risk is 0.96%, 1.32%, and 2.17% in patients with one, two, or three risk factors, respectively. See references for further discussion. *(Data from Simoons ML, Maggioni AP, Knatterud G, et al: Individual risk assessment for intracranial haemorrhage during thrombolytic therapy. Lancet 342:1523, 1993; Brass LM, Lichtman JH, Wang Y, et al: Intracranial hemorrhage associated with thrombolytic therapy for elderly patients with acute myocardial infarction: results from the Cooperative Cardiovascular Project. Stroke 31:1802, 2000; Sloan et al: J Am Coll Cardiol 37(Suppl A):372A, 2001.)*

RECOMMENDATIONS FOR FIBRINOLYTIC THERAPY

Net Clinical Outcome with Fibrinolysis

Hesitancy in prescribing a fibrinolytic agent is often the result of uncertainty about the risk of bleeding. Patients with a higher baseline risk of mortality are more likely to benefit from fibrinolytic therapy. The mortality benefit associated with fibrinolytic therapy must be weighed against the excess risk of stroke. A useful concept that incorporates the benefits and risks of fibrinolytic therapy in a single composite endpoint is net clinical outcome. Thus, composite endpoints such as death or nonfatal stroke and death, nonfatal MI, or nonfatal major bleed may be used to compare various pharmacologic reperfusion regimens.[83]

Choice of Agent

Analysis of the net clinical outcome and cost-effectiveness of one agent versus another does not easily yield recommendations for treatment because clinicians must weigh the risk of mortality and the risk of intracranial hemorrhage when confronting a fibrinolytic-eligible patient with STEMI. Additional considerations may be the constraints placed on physicians' therapeutic decision making by the health care system in which they are practicing. In the subgroup of patients presenting within 4 hours of symptom onset, the speed of reperfusion of the infarct vessel is of paramount importance and a high-intensity fibrinolytic regimen such as accelerated t-PA is the preferred treatment, except in those for whom the risk of death is low (e.g., a young patient with a small inferior MI) and the risk of intracranial hemorrhage is increased (e.g., acute hypertension), in whom streptokinase and accelerated t-PA are approximately equivalent choices. For those patients presenting between 4 and 12 hours after the onset of chest discomfort, the speed of reperfusion of the infarct vessel is of lesser importance, and streptokinase and accelerated t-PA are therefore generally equivalent options, given the difference in costs. Of note, for those patients presenting between 4 and 12 hours from symptom onset with a low mortality risk but an increased risk of intracranial hemorrhage (e.g., older patients with inferior MI, systolic pressure > 100 mm Hg, and heart rate < 100 beats/min), streptokinase is probably preferable to t-PA because of cost considerations if fibrinolytic therapy is prescribed at all in such patients.

In those patients considered appropriate candidates for fibrinolysis and for whom t-PA would have been selected as the agent of choice in the past, we believe clinicians should now consider using a bolus fibrinolytic such as reteplase or tenecteplase. The rationale for this recommendation is that bolus fibrinolysis has the advantage of ease of administration, a lower chance of medication errors (and the associated increase in mortality when such medication errors occur), and less noncerebral bleeding, and also offers the potential for prehospital treatment.[66]

Late Therapy

No mortality benefit was demonstrated in the LATE and EMERAS trials when fibrinolytics were routinely administered to patients between 12 and 24 hours, although we believe it is still reasonable to consider fibrinolytic therapy in appropriately selected patients with persistent symptoms and ST-segment elevation on the ECG beyond 12 hours. Persistent chest pain late after the onset of symptoms correlates with a higher incidence of collateral or antegrade flow in the infarct zone and is therefore a marker for patients with viable myocardium that might be salvaged. Because older patients treated with fibrinolytic agents more than 12 hours after the onset of symptoms are at increased risk of cardiac rupture, it is preferable to restrict late fibrinolytic administration to patients younger than 65 years with ongoing ischemia, especially those with large anterior infarctions. The older patient with ongoing ischemic symptoms but presenting late (>12 hours) is probably better managed with PCI than with fibrinolytic therapy.

Before the institution of fibrinolytic therapy, consideration should be given to the patient's need for intravascular catheterization, as would be required for the placement of an arterial pressure monitoring line, pulmonary artery catheter for hemodynamic monitoring, or temporary transvenous pacemaker. If any of these are required, ideally they should be placed as expeditiously as possible before infusion of the fibrinolytic agent. If such procedures require an additional delay of more than 30 minutes, they should be deferred as long as possible after fibrinolytic therapy is begun. In the early hours after institution of fibrinolytic therapy, such catheterization should be performed only if crucial to the patient's survival, and then sites where excessive bleeding can be controlled should be chosen (e.g., subclavian vein catheterization should be avoided).

As noted, all patients with suspected STEMI should receive aspirin (160 to 325 mg) regardless of the fibrinolytic agent prescribed. Aspirin should be continued indefinitely. The issues surrounding antithrombin therapy as an adjunct to thrombolysis are complex and are discussed in detail later.

Catheter-Based Reperfusion Strategies

The infarct artery can also be reperfused by a catheter-based strategy (see Chap. 58). This approach has now evolved from passage of a balloon catheter over a guidewire to include potent antiplatelet therapy (intravenous glycoprotein [GP] IIb/IIIa inhibitors and P2Y12 adenosine diphosphate [ADP] antagonists), coronary stents, and thrombectomy.[35] When PCI is used in lieu of fibrinolytic therapy, it is referred to as direct or primary PCI (see Fig. 55-3). When fibrinolysis has failed to reperfuse the infarct vessel or a severe stenosis is present in the infarct vessel, a rescue PCI can be performed. A strategy of routine delayed angiography and PCI after successful fibrinolytic therapy may also be considered for patients who are not at high risk.[84,85] Lastly, a conservative approach of elective PCI only when spontaneous or exercise-provoked ischemia occurs can be used to manage STEMI patients, whether or not they have received a previous course of fibrinolytic therapy.

SURGICAL REPERFUSION. Despite the extensive improvement in intraoperative preservation with cardioplegia and hypothermia and numerous surgical techniques (see Chap. 84), it is not logistically possible to provide surgical reperfusion in a timely fashion. Therefore, patients with STEMI who are candidates for reperfusion routinely receive fibrinolysis or PCI. However, STEMI patients are currently referred for coronary artery bypass grafting (CABG) for one of the following indications: persistent or recurrent chest pain despite fibrinolysis or PCI, high-risk coronary anatomy (e.g., left main stenosis) discovered at catheterization, or a complication of STEMI such as ventricular septal rupture or severe mitral regurgitation caused by papillary muscle dysfunction. Patients with STEMI with continued severe ischemic and hemodynamic instability are likely to benefit from emergency revascularization. PCI with stenting as needed is the preferable technique when revascularization is required in the first 48 to 72 hours following STEMI; surgery should be reserved for patients in whom PCI has been unsuccessful or whose anatomy dictates the need for CABG, such as patients with left main or extensive multivessel coronary artery disease.

Patients undergoing successful fibrinolysis but with important residual stenoses, who on anatomic grounds are more suitable for surgical revascularization than for PCI, have undergone CABG with low rates of mortality (about 4%) and morbidity, provided that they are operated on more than 24 hours from STEMI. Those patients requiring urgent or emergency CABG within 24 to 48 hours of STEMI have mortality rates between 12% and 15%.[1] When surgery is performed under urgent conditions with active and ongoing ischemia or cardiogenic shock, the operative mortality rate rises steeply.

Selection of Reperfusion Strategy

Despite strong evidence in the literature that prompt use of reperfusion therapy improves survival of STEMI patients, reperfusion therapy remains underused and is too often tardy.[35] When performed rapidly after presentation in an experienced center, primary PCI is superior to pharmacologic reperfusion therapy.[86] Nevertheless, controversy exists about the optimum form of reperfusion therapy when there is an anticipated delay to PCI, such as in centers without 24-hour availability of primary PCI.[35] This controversy has been difficult to resolve in the context of a dynamic and rapidly changing evidence base regarding the best approach to reperfusion for patients with STEMI when immediate primary PCI is not an option. With respect to pharmacologic reperfusion, newer fibrinolytic agents and combinations of adjunctive treatments have improved medical measures to restore and maintain flow in the infarct artery (**Fig. 55-16**). From the perspective of PCI, improvements in catheterization laboratory facilities, new stents, evolution of adjunctive antithrombotic therapy, and thrombus aspiration devices have improved the efficacy and safety of PCI for patients with STEMI (see Chap. 58).[87] Importantly, the outcomes in patients treated with primary PCI also vary with the experience of the operator and the center. High-volume operators and centers can consistently achieve better outcomes in STEMI patients.[88] Selection of the optimal form of reperfusion therapy therefore involves judgment regarding system resources and individual patient characteristics.

Several issues should be considered in choosing the type of reperfusion therapy (see Fig. 55-3):

1. *Time from the onset of symptoms to initiation of reperfusion therapy.* This important variable predicts infarct size and patient outcome.

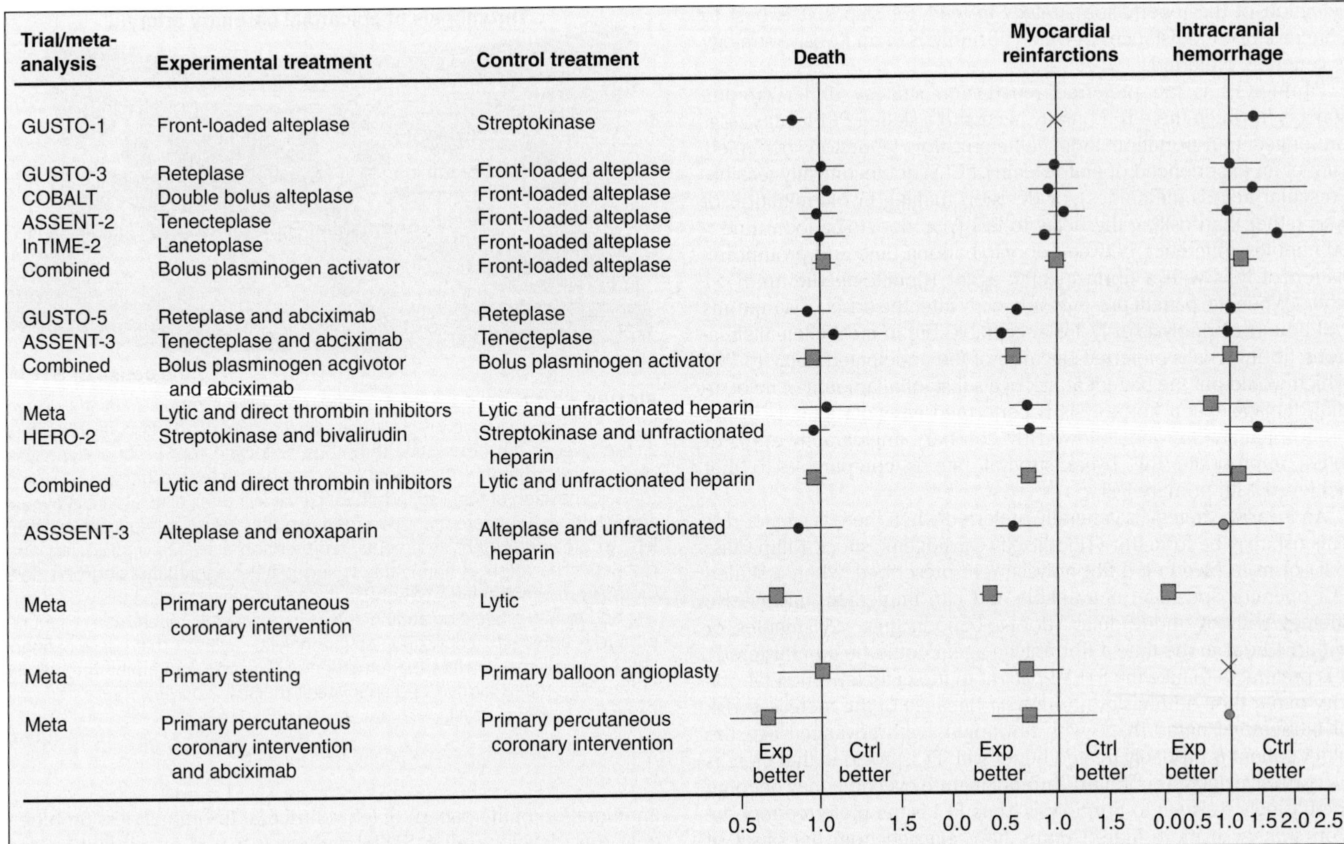

FIGURE 55-16 Relative treatment effect associated with several acute reperfusion modalities in patients presenting with STEMI. Data are odds ratios and 95% confidence intervals. Ctrl = control; Exp = experimental. *(Modified from Boersma E, Mercado N, Poldermans D, et al: Acute myocardial infarction. Lancet 361:851, 2003.)*

Although infarct size is one factor that affects patient outcomes, others include the coexistence of obstructions in non–infarct-related coronary arteries, level of electrical stability of the myocardium, extent of left ventricular remodeling, and appropriate use of evidence-based medical therapies following STEMI. Thus, for patients treated by fibrinolysis or PCI, time from the onset of symptoms predicts mortality, underscoring the need for prompt reperfusion, whichever strategy is selected (see Figs. 55-1 and 55-2).[35]

2. *Risk of death after STEMI.* Patients presenting with cardiogenic shock have an improved 1-year survival chance if they are treated with an early revascularization strategy (PCI and/or CABG, as indicated).[89] Patients at highest risk of mortality from STEMI account for the most deaths from STEMI (see Fig. 55-13). Accordingly, the mortality benefit associated with PCI is highest in patients who are at highest risk of mortality; the mortality benefit of PCI decreases progressively as the patient's risk of mortality from STEMI decreases, so that the mortality advantage of PCI is no longer evident among patients whose 30-day mortality rate is estimated to be between 2% and 3% if treated with fibrinolytic therapy.
3. *Risk of bleeding.* In patients with an increased risk of bleeding, particularly intracranial hemorrhage, therapeutic decision making strongly favors a PCI-based reperfusion strategy (see Fig. 55-15).[90] If PCI is unavailable, the benefit of pharmacologic reperfusion should be balanced against the risk of bleeding. A decision analysis has suggested that when PCI is not available, fibrinolytic therapy should still be favored over no reperfusion treatment until the risk of a life-threatening bleed exceeds 4%. For patients who are not candidates for acute reperfusion because of lack of availability of PCI and contraindications to fibrinolysis, aspirin and antithrombin therapy can be prescribed.

Thus, every effort should be made to provide reperfusion therapy, even in clinical circumstances in which there is a perceived increase in the risk of bleeding. Arrangements for urgent primary PCI should be made for patients with a constellation of advanced age, low body weight, and hypertension on presentation because of the substantially increased risk of intracranial hemorrhage with fibrinolytic therapy. When the estimated delay to implementation of primary PCI is substantial (>90 minutes), fibrinolysis (with a fibrin-specific agent) may be preferable to no reperfusion therapy in such patients when the risk from the STEMI is high (e.g., anterior infarction with hemodynamic compromise).[91] In the setting of absolute contraindications to fibrinolysis (see Table 55-5) and lack of access to PCI facilities, antithrombotic therapy should be prescribed because of the small but finite chance (10%) of restoration of TIMI grade 3 flow in the infarct vessel and decreasing the chance of thrombotic complications of STEMI.[1]

4. *Time required for transportation to a skilled PCI center.* The greatest operational impediment to routine implementation of a PCI reperfusion strategy is the delay required for transportation to a skilled PCI center (see Figs. 55-1 and 55-2).[92] Although several studies have reported that referral to a PCI center is superior to fibrinolysis administered in a local hospital, such studies were conducted in dedicated health care systems with extremely short transportation and door-to-balloon times at the PCI centers.[93] Some evidence has suggested that if the delay to implementation of primary PCI is longer than 1 hour, the mortality advantage compared with administration of a fibrin-specific agent is lost.[35]

Circumstances in which fibrinolysis or PCI is the preferred reperfusion strategy are summarized in Table 55-4. The assessment of reperfusion options for STEMI is a two-step process. Step 1 involves the integrated assessment of the time since onset of symptoms (see Figs. 55-1 to 55-4), risk of death after STEMI (see Fig. 55-13), risk of bleeding if fibrinolysis were to be administered (see Fig. 55-15), and time required for transportation to a skilled PCI center (see Fig. 55-5).[91] The complexities of clinical medicine do not permit decision making to be reduced to a simple equation or one-size-fits-all approach to selection of the reperfusion strategy. Instead, for step 2, it is best to conceive of circumstances in which fibrinolysis or an invasive strategy is generally preferred.

Fibrinolysis is the preferred reperfusion strategy under circumstances in which there is no ready access to a skilled PCI facility (e.g., prolonged transportation time, catheterization laboratory occupied, lack of an experienced operator/team), PCI is not technically feasible (vascular access difficulties), or decision making favors initiation of lysis rather than risking the delay to PCI (e.g., door-to-balloon time > 90 minutes; difference between door-to-balloon time and prompt initiation of lysis with a fibrin-specific agent [door-to-needle time] >1 hour). When the patient presents very early after the onset of symptoms (<3 hours), fibrinolysis or PCI is acceptable, but in most clinical situations, fibrinolysis is preferred because of the anticipated delay to PCI, which would put the patient at risk of a substantial amount of myocardial damage. When fibrinolysis is performed early, particularly in the prehospital setting, and followed by coronary angiography and PCI when appropriate, the 1-year survival rate is comparable to that achieved with primary PCI.[29]

An invasive strategy is generally preferred when there is greater risk. This risk may be from the STEMI itself (cardiogenic shock, Killip Class ≥ II) or from bleeding if fibrinolysis were prescribed. When a skilled PCI operator and team is available and can implement an invasive strategy without undue delay (door-to-balloon time <90 minutes, or within 1 hour of the time a fibrinolytic agent could be administered), it is preferable to take the STEMI patient to the catheterization laboratory rather than administer fibrinolysis. Because of the increased risk of intracranial hemorrhage with fibrinolysis with advanced age, the older patient is probably treated better with PCI, provided that there is no excessive delay. As coronary thrombi mature over time, they become increasingly resistant to fibrinolysis. Thus, PCI is the preferred reperfusion strategy if more than 3 hours have elapsed from the onset of symptoms, again assuming that there is no significant delay in the anticipated time to balloon inflation (see Fig. 55-2). Finally, when the diagnosis is in doubt, an invasive strategy is clearly the preferred strategy because it not only provides key diagnostic information regarding the patient's symptoms, but does so without the risk of intracranial hemorrhage associated with fibrinolysis.

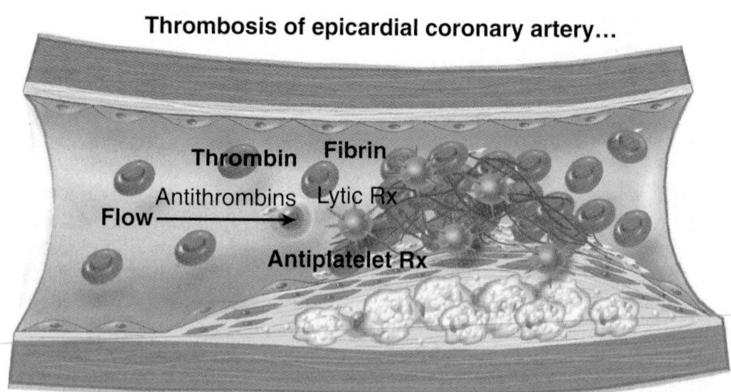

FIGURE 55-17 Pharmacologic dissolution of thrombus in infarct-related artery. This schematic view is of a longitudinal section of an infarct-related artery at the level of the obstructive thrombus. Following rupture of a vulnerable plaque (bottom center), the coagulation cascade is activated, ultimately leading to the deposition of fibrin strands (blue curvilinear arcs); platelets are activated and begin to aggregate (transition from flat discs, representing inactive platelets, to green spiked-ball elements, representing activated and aggregating platelets). The mesh of fibrin strands and platelet aggregates obstructs flow (normally moving from left to right) in the infarct-related artery; this would correspond to TIMI grade 0 on angiography. Pharmacologic reperfusion is a multipronged approach consisting of fibrinolytic agents that digest fibrin, antithrombins that prevent the formation of thrombin and inhibit the activity of thrombin that is formed, and antiplatelet therapy. *(Courtesy of Luke Wells, the Exeter Group, New York, NY.)*

Anticoagulant and Antiplatelet Therapy

ANTICOAGULANT THERAPY. The rationale for administering anticoagulant therapy acutely in STEMI patients includes prevention of deep venous thrombosis, pulmonary embolism, ventricular thrombus formation, and cerebral embolization. In addition, establishing and maintaining patency of the infarct-related artery, whether or not a patient receives fibrinolytic therapy, provides another rationale for anticoagulant therapy in cases of STEMI (**Fig. 55-17**).

EFFECT OF HEPARIN ON MORTALITY. Randomized trials in STEMI patients conducted in the prefibrinolytic era showed lower risks of pulmonary embolism, stroke, and reinfarction in patients who received intravenous heparin, supporting the administration of heparin to STEMI patients not treated with fibrinolytic therapy. With the introduction of the fibrinolytic era and, importantly, after the publication of the ISIS-2 trial, the situation became more complicated because of strong evidence of a substantial mortality reduction with aspirin alone and confusing and conflicting data regarding the risk-benefit ratio of heparin used as an adjunct to aspirin or in combination with aspirin and a fibrinolytic agent.[1] For every 1000 patients treated with heparin compared with aspirin alone, there are five fewer deaths ($P = 0.03$) and three fewer recurrent infarctions ($P = 0.04$), at the expense of three more major bleeds ($P = 0.001$).[94]

OTHER EFFECTS OF HEPARIN. A number of angiographic studies have examined the role of heparin therapy in establishing and maintaining patency of the infarct-related artery in patients with STEMI. The evidence favoring the use of heparin for enhancing patency of the infarct artery when a fibrin-specific fibrinolytic agent is prescribed is not conclusive. However, the suggestion of a mortality benefit and amelioration of the pattern of left ventricular thrombus (less protuberant) that develops after STEMI indicates that it is prudent to use heparin for at least 48 hours after fibrinolysis and to maintain an activated partial thromboplastin time (aPTT) target of 1.5 to 2 times that of control.[35]

Although heparin may induce thrombocytopenia through an immunologic mechanism, this effect occurs only rarely, probably occurring in only 2% to 3% of patients (see Chap. 87).[95] The most serious complication of antithrombotic therapy is bleeding, especially intracranial hemorrhage, when fibrinolytic agents are prescribed.[96] Major hemorrhagic events occur more frequently in patients of low body weight, advanced age, and female sex, with marked prolongation of the aPTT (>90 to 100 seconds), and with the performance of invasive procedures. Frequent monitoring of the aPTT (facilitated by the use of a bedside testing device) reduces the risk of major hemorrhagic complications in patients treated with heparin. It should be noted, however, that during the first 12 hours following fibrinolytic therapy, the aPTT may be elevated from the fibrinolytic agent alone (particularly if streptokinase is administered), making it difficult to interpret accurately the effects of a heparin infusion on the patient's coagulation status.

NEWER ANTITHROMBOTIC AGENTS. Potential disadvantages of unfractionated heparin (UFH) include dependency on antithrombin III for inhibition of thrombin activity, sensitivity to platelet factor 4, inability to inhibit clot-bound thrombin, marked interpatient variability in therapeutic response, and the need for frequent aPTT monitoring. Even with standardized weight-based dosing nomograms, less than 35% of initial aPTT measurements are within the therapeutic range.[97] An effort to circumvent these disadvantages of UFH has stimulated interest in the development of alternative anticoagulants (see Chap. 87).

Hirudin and Bivalirudin

In patients undergoing fibrinolysis, direct thrombin inhibitors such as hirudin or bivalirudin reduce the incidence of recurrent MI by 25% to 30% compared with heparin but have not reduced mortality.[98] In addition, both hirudin and bivalirudin result in higher rates of major bleeding versus heparin when used with fibrinolytic agents. In contrast, when administered for a short period as an adjunct to primary PCI in an open-label trial, bivalirudin significantly reduced major bleeding by

40% compared with heparin and a GPIIb/IIIa receptor blocker and was associated with a significant reduction in mortality at 30 days and at 1 year (**Fig. 55-18**).[99] Bivalirudin was associated with an increased early risk of stent thrombosis, demonstrating an early trade-off of bleeding and antithrombotic efficacy.[100]

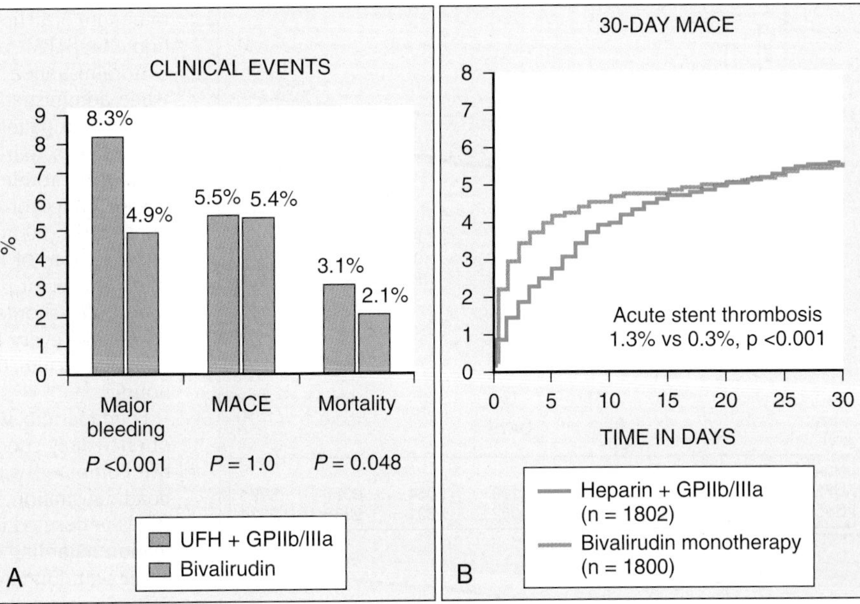

FIGURE 55-18 Results of an open-label randomized clinical trial comparing bivalirudin with unfractionated heparin (UFH) and a glycoprotein IIb/IIIa receptor antagonist (GPIIb/IIIa) as adjunctive medical therapy to support primary percutaneous coronary intervention in patients with ST-elevation STEMI. **A,** Treatment with bivalirudin was associated with a significantly lower rate of major bleeding and mortality at 30 days. **B,** Kaplan-Meier curves of the cumulative incidence of major adverse cardiac events (MACE), which did not differ between the two strategies at 30 days. Acute stent thrombosis during the first 24 hours was higher in patients treated with bivalirudin alone. *(From Stone GW, Witzenbichler B, Guagliumi G et al: Bivalirudin during primary PCI in acute myocardial infarction. N Eng J Med 358:2218, 2008.)*

Low-Molecular-Weight Heparins

Advantages of low-molecular-weight heparins include a stable, reliable anticoagulant effect, high bioavailability, permitting administration via the subcutaneous route, and a high anti-Xa–to–anti-IIa ratio, producing blockade of the coagulation cascade in an upstream location, resulting in a marked decrement in thrombin generation. Compared with UFH, the rate of early (60 to 90 minutes) reperfusion of the infarct artery, either assessed angiographically or by noninvasive means, is not enhanced by the administration of a low-molecular-weight heparin.[94] However, the rates of reocclusion of the infarct artery, reinfarction, or recurrent ischemic events appear to be reduced by low-molecular-weight heparins.[101] This effect may underlie a significant reduction in recurrent MI with a strategy of extended anticoagulation with low-molecular-weight heparins or a factor Xa antagonist compared with standard therapy in patients with STEMI undergoing fibrinolysis.

The CREATE investigators have studied the effects of the low-molecular-weight heparin reviparin compared with placebo in 15,570 patients with STEMI, 73% of whom received a fibrinolytic (predominantly a non–fibrin-specific agent).[102] The primary composite outcome of death, recurrent MI, or stroke was reduced by 13% both at 7 days (P = 0.005) and at 30 days (P = 0.001) with reviparin. The AMI-SK investigators reported that ST-segment resolution at 90 and 180 minutes, as well as angiographic patency, was improved in streptokinase-treated STEMI patients who received enoxaparin compared with placebo. These observations support the hypotheses that antithrombin therapy is a useful adjunct to a pharmacologic reperfusion regimen and that low-molecular-weight heparins are clinically effective in STEMI.[94,95]

The ASSENT-3 trial compared UFH with enoxaparin (30 mg intravenous bolus followed by subcutaneous injections of 1 mg/kg every 12 hours until hospital discharge).[103] The composite endpoint of 30-day mortality, in-hospital reinfarction, or in-hospital refractory ischemia was reduced from 15.4% with UFH to 11.4% with enoxaparin (RR, 0.74; 95% CI, 0.63 to 0.87). The rate of intracranial hemorrhage was similar with UFH versus enoxaparin (0.93% versus 0.88%; P = 0.98). The ASSENT-3 PLUS study compared the same UFH and enoxaparin regimens but initiated therapy in the prehospital setting.[94,95] The composite endpoint of 30-day mortality, in-hospital reinfarction, or in-hospital refractory ischemia was reduced from 17.4% with UFH to 14.2% with enoxaparin (P = 0.08). Of concern, however, was the increased rate of intracranial hemorrhage observed in ASSENT-3 PLUS—1% with UFH versus 2.2% with enoxaparin (P = 0.05). The increase in intracranial hemorrhage in ASSENT-3 PLUS was seen predominantly in patients older than 75 years of age—0.8% with UFH versus 6.7% with enoxaparin (P = 0.01).

The ExTRACT-TIMI 25 trial, in a double-blind, double-dummy design, tested the hypothesis that a strategy of enoxaparin administered for the duration of the index hospitalization is superior to the conventional antithrombin strategy of UFH for 48 hours after fibrinolysis.[104] The enoxaparin dosing strategy was adjusted according to the patient's age and renal function. For patients younger than 75 years of age, enoxaparin (or matching placebo) was to be given as a fixed, 30-mg intravenous bolus followed 15 minutes later by a subcutaneous injection of 1 mg/kg, with injections administered every 12 hours. For patients 75 years of age and older, the intravenous bolus was eliminated and the subcutaneous dose was reduced to 0.75 mg/kg every 12 hours. The primary endpoint of death or recurrent nonfatal MI through 30 days occurred in 12% of patients in the UFH group and 9.9% of those in the enoxaparin group (17% reduction in RR; P = 0.001). Nonfatal reinfarction occurred in 4.5% of the patients receiving UFH and 3% of those receiving enoxaparin (33% reduction in RR; P = 0.001); 7.5% of patients given UFH died, as did 6.9% of those given enoxaparin (P = 0.11). The composite of death, nonfatal reinfarction, or urgent revascularization occurred in 14.5% of patients given UFH and 11.7% of those given enoxaparin (P = 0.001); major bleeding occurred in 1.4% and 2.1%, respectively (P = 0.001) (**Fig. 55-19**). The composite of death, nonfatal reinfarction, or nonfatal intracranial hemorrhage (a measure of net clinical benefit) occurred in 12.2% of patients given UFH and 10.1% of those given enoxaparin (P = 0.001).

FACTOR XA ANTAGONISTS. The OASIS-6 trial evaluated the specific factor Xa antagonist fondaparinux (2.5 mg subcutaneously) in 12,092 patients with STEMI.[105] The trial design compared fondaparinux given for 8 days versus placebo in patients when the treating physician thought that UFH was not indicated (stratum I) and versus UFH for 48 hours when the treating physician thought that heparin was indicated (stratum II). The primary endpoint, death or reinfarction, occurred in 14% of placebo patients and 11.2% of fondaparinux patients in stratum I (HR 0.79; 95% CI, 0.68 to 0.92), and in 8.7% of UFH patients and 8.3% of fondaparinux patients in stratum II (HR 0.96; 95% CI, 0.81 to 1.13). Thus, fondaparinux was superior to placebo (stratum I) but yielded similar results to those achieved with UFH (stratum II). The outcome of patients in stratum II who underwent PCI tended to be worse when fondaparinux was used compared with UFH, probably because of an increased risk of catheter thrombosis when fondaparinux is administered without coadministration of another antithrombin that has anti-IIa activity. Severe hemorrhage occurred in 1.3% of control patients and 1% of fondaparinux patients through 9 days (P = 0.13).

Recommendations for Anticoagulant Therapy

ANTICOAGULATION WITH FIBRINOLYSIS. Given the pivotal role of thrombin in the pathogenesis of STEMI, antithrombotic therapy remains an important intervention (see Fig. 55-17). A regimen of intravenous unfractionated heparin bolus at 60 U/kg to a maximum of 4000 U, followed by an initial infusion of 12 U/kg/hr to a maximum of 1000 U/hr given for 48 hours, has established efficacy in patients receiving fibrinolytic therapy. However, infusions of unfractionated

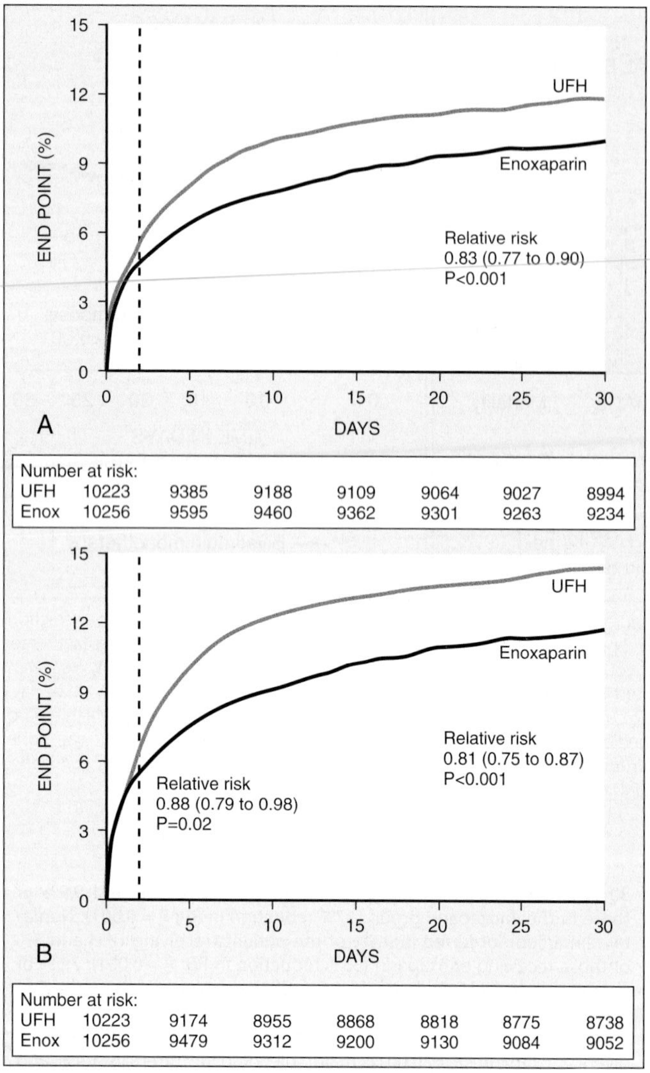

A

Number at risk:

UFH	10223	9385	9188	9109	9064	9027	8994
Enox	10256	9595	9460	9362	9301	9263	9234

B

Number at risk:

UFH	10223	9174	8955	8868	8818	8775	8738
Enox	10256	9479	9312	9200	9130	9084	9052

FIGURE 55-19 Comparison of enoxaparin with unfractionated heparin as adjunctive therapy in STEMI patients receiving fibrinolysis. **A,** The rate of the primary endpoint (death or nonfatal MI) at 30 days was significantly lower in the enoxaparin (Enox) group than in the unfractionated heparin (UFH) group (9.9% versus 12%; $P < 0.001$ by the log-rank test). The dashed vertical line indicates the comparison at day 2 (direct pharmacologic comparison), at which time a trend in favor of enoxaparin was seen. **B,** The rate of the main secondary endpoint (death, nonfatal MI, or urgent revascularization) at 30 days was significantly lower in the Enox group than in the UFH group (11.7% versus 14.5%; $P < 0.001$ by the log-rank test). The difference was already significant at 48 hours (6.1% in the UFH group versus 5.3% in the Emox group; $P = 0.02$ by the log-rank test). The interval shown is the time (in 24-hour intervals) from randomization to an event or the last follow-up visit. *(From Antman EM, Morrow DA, McCabe CH, et al: Enoxaparin versus unfractionated heparin with fibrinolysis for ST-elevation myocardial Infarction. N Engl J Med 354: 1477, 2006.)*

heparin are cumbersome to administer and provide unreliable levels of anticoagulation, requiring frequent measurements of aPTT to adjust the infusion rate.[106] In addition, because of the risk of heparin-induced thrombocytopenia with prolonged administration of unfractionated heparin, alternative anticoagulant regimens are preferred if administered for longer than 48 hours.[35]

Both ExTRACT-TIMI 25 and OASIS 6 have indicated that more prolonged administration of an antithrombin for the duration of hospitalization is beneficial compared with the prior practice of administering UFH only for 48 hours, unless clear-cut indications for continued anticoagulation were present. As such, patients managed with pharmacologic reperfusion therapy should receive anticoagulant therapy for a minimum of 48 hours and preferably for the duration of the hospitalization after STEMI, up to 8 days.[35]

Administration of enoxaparin or fondaparinux is preferred when administration of an anticoagulant for longer than 48 hours is planned for patients with STEMI treated with a fibrinolytic.[35] The benefits of enoxaparin over UFH are evident regardless of the type of fibrinolytic administered (streptokinase or fibrin-specific) and across a wide range of patient subgroups. An initial intravenous bolus of enoxaparin (30 mg) should be administered, followed by subcutaneous injections of 1 mg/kg every 12 hours for patients younger than 75 years of age; for patients 75 years of age and older, the initial intravenous bolus should be omitted and the maintenance dose should be 0.75 mg/kg every 12 hours. If the estimated creatinine clearance is less than 30 mL/min, the maintenance dose should be 1 mg/kg every 24 hours.

Fondaparinux was superior to placebo in OASIS 6. The convenience of once-daily subcutaneous injections of fondaparinux is also attractive compared with UFH, but its use is complicated by the need for coadministration of an additional antithrombin with anti-IIa activity if PCI is performed in a patient treated with fondaparinux. Further information regarding the appropriate dosing of additional antithrombins along with fondaparinux in the catheterization laboratory is needed.

In patients with a known history of heparin-induced thrombocytopenia, it is reasonable to consider bivalirudin as a useful alternative to heparin to be used in conjunction with streptokinase. Dosing according to the HERO 2 regimen (a bolus of 0.25 mg/kg followed by an intravenous infusion of 0.5 mg/kg/hr for the first 12 hours, and 0.25 mg/kg/hr for the subsequent 36 hours) is recommended but with a reduction in the infusion rate if the aPTT is longer than 75 seconds within the first 12 hours.[1]

For patients who are referred for CABG, the preferred antithrombin is UFH. When an alternative antithrombin has been used, it should be discontinued prior to surgery, with a sufficiently long interval to avoid double anticoagulation when the patient enters the operating room and receives UFH.

ADJUNCTIVE ANTICOAGULATION FOR PRIMARY PERCUTANEOUS INTERVENTION. Based on expert consensus, UFH is recommended for patients undergoing primary PCI (see Chap. 58). On the basis of the results of the HORIZONS-AMI trial,[99] bivalirudin is an alternative for adjunctive anticoagulation during primary PCI. Fondaparinux is not recommended as the sole anticoagulant in this setting.[35] A large randomized trial of fondaparinux in patients with STEMI, including 3789 patients undergoing primary PCI, revealed a possible hazard related to catheter thrombosis. Low-molecular-weight heparins have not had sufficient evaluation in primary PCI to formulate recommendations for treatment. Some investigators who have used enoxaparin to support primary PCI for STEMI administered 0.5 mg/kg intravenously at the time of the procedure.

PATIENTS TREATED WITHOUT REPERFUSION THERAPY. In STEMI patients not receiving reperfusion therapy, fondaparinux reduces the composite of death or recurrent MI without an increase in severe bleeding as compared with placebo or UFH.[107]

ANTIPLATELET THERAPY. Platelets play a major role in the response to disruption of a coronary artery plaque, especially in the early phase of thrombus formation (**Fig. 55-20**).[108] Platelets are also activated in response to fibrinolysis, and platelet-rich thrombi are more resistant to fibrinolysis than fibrin and erythrocyte-rich thrombi (see Fig. 55-17). Thus, there is a sound scientific basis for inhibiting platelet aggregation in all STEMI patients, regardless of the reperfusion management strategy. Comprehensive overviews of randomized trials of antiplatelet therapy have summarized the overwhelming evidence of benefit of antiplatelet therapy for a wide range of vascular disorders.[109] In patients at risk for STEMI, patients with a documented prior STEMI, and patients in the acute phase of STEMI, there is a 22% reduction in the odds of the composite endpoint of death, nonfatal recurrent infarction, and nonfatal stroke with antiplatelet therapy (**Fig. 55-21**). Not unexpectedly, the absolute benefits are greatest in those patients at highest baseline risk. Although several antiplatelet regimens have been evaluated, the agent most extensively tested has been aspirin.

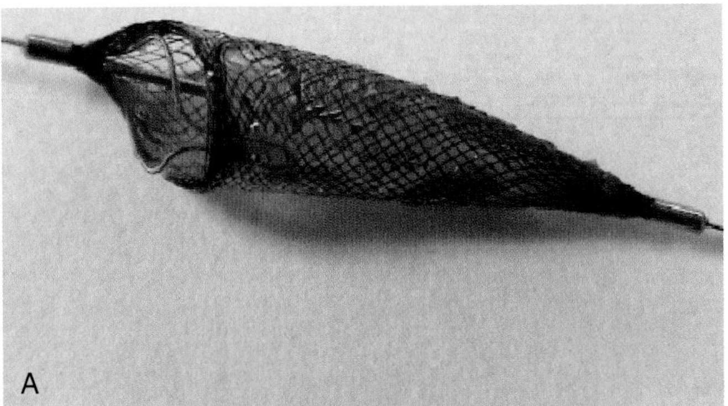

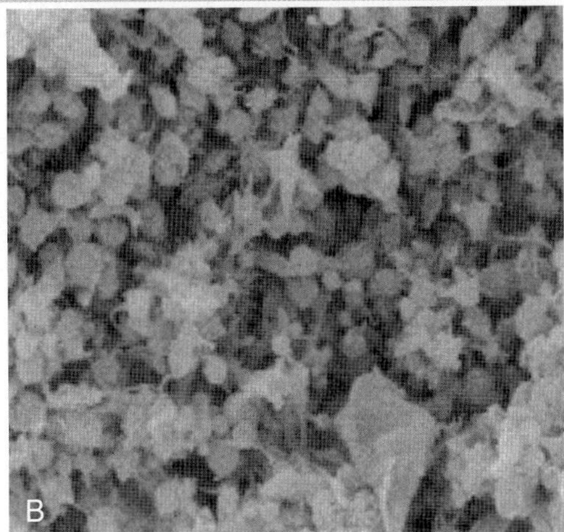

FIGURE 55-20 Importance of platelet aggregation early in STEMI. A 46-year-old man presented with STEMI resulting from occlusion of the right coronary artery. At the time of primary percutaneous PCI, which was performed within 90 minutes of the onset of symptoms, a nonocclusive distal protection filter was placed downstream from the obstruction in the infarct artery. **A,** Macroscopically, the obstructing thrombus was white. **B,** Scanning electron microscopy at high magnification (×2000) showed a platelet-rich thrombus without fibrin or erythrocytes. This case emphasizes the important role of platelet activation and aggregation early after the onset of disruption of a coronary artery plaque and underscores the necessity for antiplatelet therapy in STEMI patients. *(Modified from Beygui F, Collet JP, Nagaswami C, et al: Images in cardiovascular medicine. Architecture of intracoronary thrombi in ST-elevation acute myocardial infarction: Time makes the difference. Circulation 113:e21, 2006.)*

Antiplatelet Therapy with Fibrinolysis

The ISIS-2 study was the largest trial of aspirin in STEMI patients[1]; it provides the single strongest piece of evidence that aspirin reduces mortality in STEMI patients. In contrast to the observations of a time-dependent mortality effect of fibrinolytic therapy, the mortality reduction with aspirin was similar in patients treated within 4 hours (25% reduction in mortality), between 5 and 12 hours (21% reduction), and between 13 and 24 hours (21% reduction). There was an overall 23% reduction in mortality from aspirin in ISIS-2 that was largely additive to the 25% reduction in mortality from streptokinase, so patients receiving both therapies experienced a 42% reduction in mortality. The mortality reduction was as high as 53% in patients who received both aspirin and streptokinase within 6 hours of symptoms. Of particular interest was the finding that the combination of streptokinase and aspirin reduced mortality without increasing the risk of stroke or hemorrhage.

Obstructive platelet-rich arterial thrombi resist fibrinolysis and have an increased tendency to produce reocclusion after initial successful reperfusion in patients with STEMI. Despite the inhibition of cyclooxygenase by aspirin, platelet activation continues to occur through thromboxane A_2–independent pathways, leading to platelet aggregation and increased thrombin formation.[41] The addition of other antiplatelet agents to aspirin has been proven to benefit patients with STEMI. Inhibitors of the P2Y12 ADP receptor help prevent activation and aggregation of platelets. In the CLARITY-TIMI 28 trial, the addition of the P2Y12 inhibitor clopidogrel to background treatment with aspirin to STEMI patients younger than 75 years of age who received fibrinolytic therapy reduced the risk of clinical events (death, reinfarction, stroke) and reocclusion of a successfully reperfused infarct artery (**Fig. 55-22**).[110] An ST Resolution (STRes) electrocardiographic substudy from the CLARITY-TIMI 28 trial has provided insight into the mechanism of the benefit of clopidogrel in STEMI.[111] There was no difference in the rate of complete STRes between the clopidogrel and placebo groups at 90 minutes (38.4% versus 36.6% at 90 minutes). When patients were stratified by STRes category, treatment with clopidogrel resulted in greater benefit among those with evidence of early STRes, with greater odds of an open artery at late angiography in patients with partial (odds ratio [OR], 1.4; $P = 0.04$) or complete (OR, 2; $P = 0.001$) STRes, but no improvement in those with no STRes at 90 minutes (OR, 0.89; $P = 0.48$) (P for interaction, 0.003). Clopidogrel was also associated with a significant reduction in the odds of in-hospital death or MI in patients who achieved partial (OR, 0.30; $P = 0.003$) or complete STRes at 90 minutes (OR, 0.49; $P = 0.056$), whereas clinical benefit was not apparent in patients who had no STRes (OR, 0.98; $P = 0.95$) (P for interaction, 0.027). Thus it appears that clopidogrel did not increase the rate of complete opening of occluded infarct arteries when fibrinolysis was administered but was highly effective in preventing reocclusion of an initially reperfused infarct artery.

In the COMMIT trial, 45,852 patients with suspected MI were randomized to clopidogrel, 75 mg/day (without a loading dose), or placebo in addition to aspirin, 162 mg/day (see Fig. 55-22).[43] The patients in the clopidogrel group had a lower rate of the composite endpoint of death, reinfarction, or stroke (9.2% versus 10.1%; $P = 0.002$). They also had a significantly lower rate of death (7.5% versus 8.1%; $P = 0.03$). No excess of bleeding with clopidogrel occurred in this trial.

Combination Pharmacologic Reperfusion

Several studies have evaluated the combination of GP IIb/IIIa inhibitors and fibrinolytics.[1] The first series of trials combined full doses of thrombolytic agents with IIb/IIIa inhibitors. Although these initial trials provided proof of the hypothesis that the addition of an intravenous GP IIb/IIIa inhibitor enhanced the efficacy of a full dose of a fibrinolytic agent, unacceptably high rates of major bleeding were observed.

The combination of a reduced dose of a fibrinolytic agent and IIb/IIIa inhibitor was tested in a subsequent series of trials. The rates of TIMI grade 3 flow at 60 and 90 minutes were only slightly higher with combination reperfusion compared with full-dose fibrinolytic monotherapy. These trials generally showed improved myocardial perfusion, reflected in enhanced ST-segment resolution and faster angiographic frame counts.

The GUSTO V trial tested half-dose reteplase (5 U and 5 U) and full-dose abciximab compared with full-dose reteplase (10 U and 10 U) in 16,588 patients in the first 6 hours of STEMI. Thirty-day mortality rates were similar in the two treatment groups (5.9% versus 5.6%) but nonfatal reinfarction and other complications of MI were reduced in the group receiving combination reperfusion therapy. Although the rates of intracranial hemorrhage were the same in the two treatment groups (0.6%), moderate to severe bleeding was significantly increased from 2.3% to 4.6% with combination reperfusion therapy ($P = 0.001$). This excess bleeding risk appeared to be limited to patients older than 75 years of age. The greatest mortality benefit was observed in those patients who presented with anterior MI.

The ASSENT-3 trial randomized 6095 patients with STEMI to full-dose tenecteplase with UFH versus full-dose tenecteplase with enoxaparin or half-dose tenecteplase plus abciximab (with weight-adjusted reduced-dose UFH).[103] Similar to the GUSTO V trial, combination reperfusion therapy with half-dose tenecteplase and abciximab was not associated with a reduction in 30-day mortality; however, in-hospital reinfarction and refractory ischemia were reduced with combination reperfusion therapy. Of note, the major bleeding rate other than intracranial hemorrhage was increased from 2.2% to 4.3% with combination reperfusion therapy ($P = 0.0005$). Older patients were at greatest risk for excess bleeding, experiencing a threefold increase in the rate of that complication.

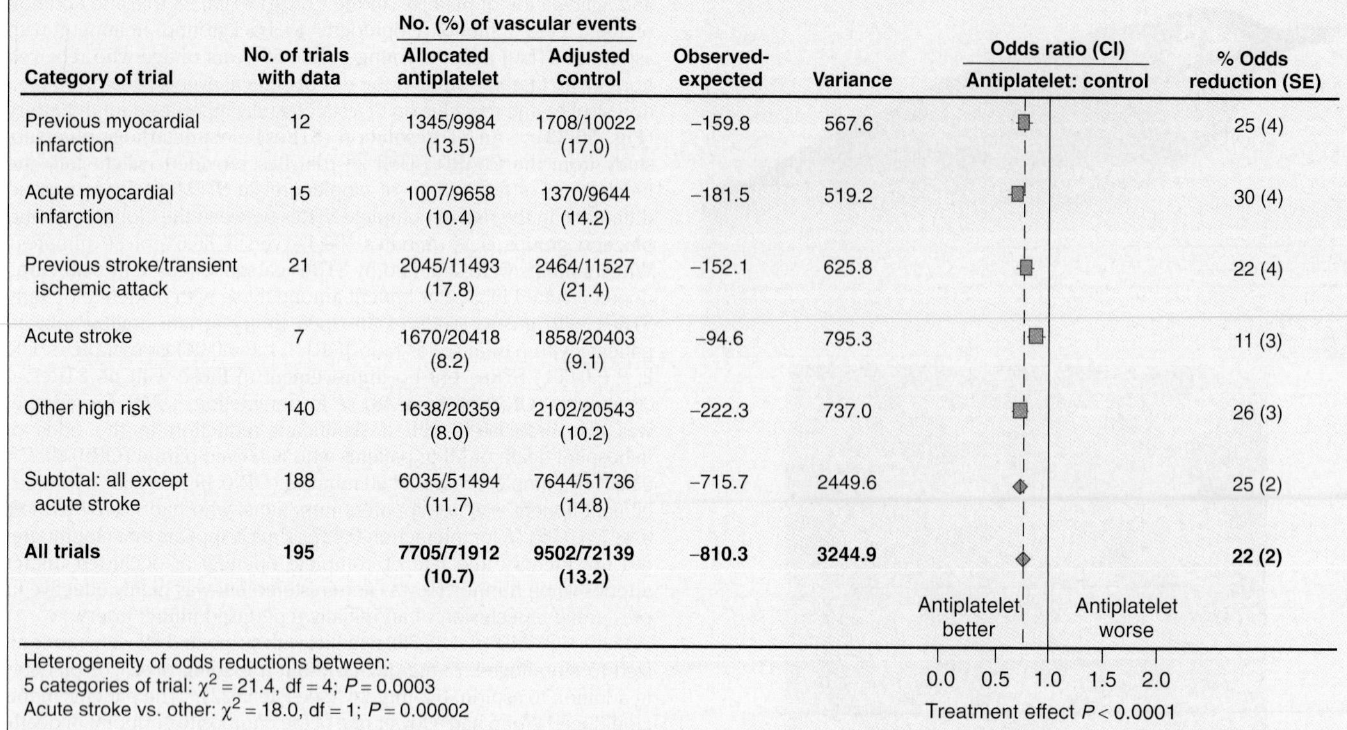

Category of trial	No. of trials with data	No. (%) of vascular events: Allocated antiplatelet	No. (%) of vascular events: Adjusted control	Observed-expected	Variance	Odds ratio (CI) Antiplatelet: control	% Odds reduction (SE)
Previous myocardial infarction	12	1345/9984 (13.5)	1708/10022 (17.0)	−159.8	567.6		25 (4)
Acute myocardial infarction	15	1007/9658 (10.4)	1370/9644 (14.2)	−181.5	519.2		30 (4)
Previous stroke/transient ischemic attack	21	2045/11493 (17.8)	2464/11527 (21.4)	−152.1	625.8		22 (4)
Acute stroke	7	1670/20418 (8.2)	1858/20403 (9.1)	−94.6	795.3		11 (3)
Other high risk	140	1638/20359 (8.0)	2102/20543 (10.2)	−222.3	737.0		26 (3)
Subtotal: all except acute stroke	188	6035/51494 (11.7)	7644/51736 (14.8)	−715.7	2449.6		25 (2)
All trials	**195**	**7705/71912 (10.7)**	**9502/72139 (13.2)**	**−810.3**	**3244.9**		**22 (2)**

FIGURE 55-21 Proportional effects of antiplatelet therapy on vascular events (MI, stroke, or vascular death) in the main high-risk categories. The stratified ratio of odds of an event in treatment groups to that in control groups is plotted for each group of trials (square) along with its 99% CI (horizontal line). Meta-analysis of results for all trials (95% CI) is represented by a diamond; SE = standard error. *(From Antithrombotic Trialists' Collaboration: Collaborative meta-analysis of randomised trials of antiplatelet therapy for prevention of death, myocardial infarction, and stroke in high-risk patients. BMJ 324:71, 2002.)*

Given the increased bleeding risk with combination reperfusion therapy, it cannot be recommended for routine clinical use. However, the combination of an intravenous GP IIb/IIIa inhibitor with a reduced dose of a fibrinolytic agent might be considered in high-risk patients (e.g., anterior STEMI) when long transfer delays for primary PCI are anticipated.[1]

Antiplatelet Therapy for Primary Percutaneous Intervention in STEMI

All patients with STEMI should receive aspirin as soon as possible after presentation, in the absence of contraindications. The addition of the P2Y12 inhibitor clopidogrel to aspirin appears to offer additional benefit in patients undergoing PCI after STEMI. An analysis of the subgroup of patients who underwent PCI in the CLARITY-TIMI 28 trial showed that pretreatment with clopidogrel significantly reduces the incidence of cardiovascular death, MI, or stroke following PCI (3.6% versus 6.2%; adjusted OR, 0.54 [95% CI, 0.35 to 0.85]; P = 0.008).[112] Pretreatment with clopidogrel also reduces the incidence of MI or stroke prior to PCI (4% versus 6.2%; OR, 0.62 [95% CI, 0.40 to 0.95]; P = 0.03). There was no significant excess in the rates of TIMI major or minor bleeding (2% versus 1.9%; P = 0.99).

Moreover, in patients undergoing primary or delayed PCI after initial therapy for STEMI, the more potent P2Y12 inhibitor prasugrel has been found to be superior to clopidogrel for reducing the risk of cardiovascular death, MI, or stroke.[113] In the subgroup of patients with STEMI enrolled in the TRITON-TIMI 38 trial (N = 3534), this endpoint was lowered by 32% at 30 days with prasugrel compared with aspirin (6.5% versus 9.5%; P = 0.0017) and by 21% at 15 months (10.0% versus 12.4%; P = 0.022) (**Fig. 55-23**).[114] Prasugrel reduced stent thrombosis by 42% compared with clopidogrel. This reduction in recurrent ischemic events with prasugrel was associated with a similar increase in major bleeding as seen in the overall trial population. Analogously, in the PLATO trial, compared with clopidogrel, treatment with the reversible P2Y12 inhibitor ticagrelor in patients with STEMI undergoing primary PCI reduced the primary endpoint of cardiovascular death, recurrent MI, or stroke by 16%, a magnitude similar to that for the overall trial population.[114a] A discussion of the use of GP IIb/IIIa inhibitors as part of adjunctive therapy for patients with STEMI undergoing PCI is presented in Chap. 58.

Recommendations for Antiplatelet Therapy

Nonenteric-coated aspirin should be chewed by patients who have not taken aspirin prior to presentation with STEMI. The initial dose should be 162 to 325 mg. During the maintenance phase of antiplatelet therapy following STEMI, the dose of aspirin should be reduced to 75 to 162 mg to minimize bleeding risk.[115] If true aspirin allergy is present, other antiplatelet agents such as clopidogrel (loading dose, 300 to 600 mg; maintenance dose, 75 mg/day) or ticlopidine (loading dose, 500 mg; maintenance dose, 250 mg twice daily) can be substituted.

The addition of a P2Y12 inhibitor to aspirin is warranted for most patients with STEMI.[35] Based on the results of the COMMIT[116] and CLARITY-TIMI 28[110] trials, clopidogrel at 75 mg/day orally is an alternative for all patients with STEMI, regardless of whether they receive fibrinolytic therapy, undergo primary PCI, or do not receive reperfusion therapy.[35] The available data suggest that a loading dose of 300 mg of clopidogrel should be given to patients younger than 75 years of age who receive fibrinolytic therapy. There is insufficient data to recommend a loading dose in patients 75 years of age and older who receive a fibrinolytic. When primary PCI is the mode of reperfusion therapy, an oral loading dose of 300 to 600 mg of clopidogrel before stent implantation is an established alternative.[117] In addition, on the basis of the results of the TRITON-TIMI 38 trial, prasugrel administered with an oral loading dose of 60 mg and 10 mg orally daily thereafter is a superior alternative to clopidogrel, 300 mg, for patients not at particularly high risk of life-threatening bleeding, such as those with a history of cerebrovascular disease.[113,114] Similarly, ticagrelor administered with a loading dose of 180 mg and 90 mg twice daily thereafter is superior to clopidogrel.[114a]

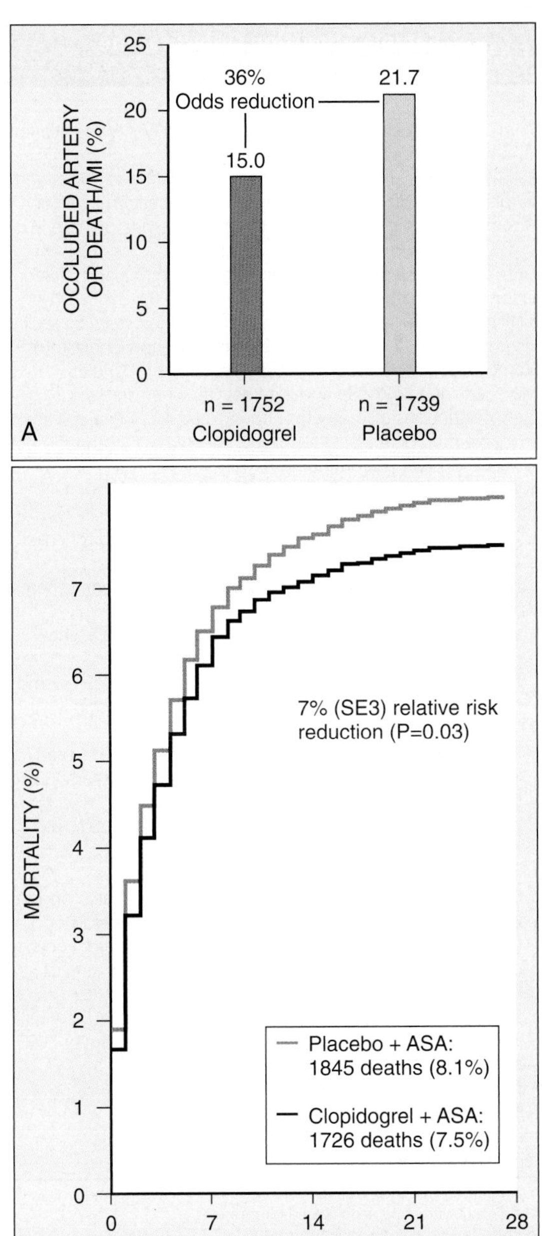

FIGURE 55-22 Impact of addition of clopidogrel to aspirin (ASA) in STEMI patients. **A,** Effects of the addition of clopidogrel in patients receiving fibrinolysis for STEMI. Patients in the clopidogrel group (n = 1752) had a 36% reduction in the odds of dying, sustaining a recurrent infarction, or having an occluded infarct artery compared with the placebo group (n = 1739) in the CLARITY-TIMI 28 trial. **B,** Effect of the addition of clopidogrel on in-hospital mortality after STEMI. These time-to-event curves show a 0.6% reduction in mortality in the group receiving clopidogrel plus aspirin (n = 22,961) compared with placebo plus aspirin (n = 22,891) in the COMMIT trial. *(**A** modified from Sabatine MS, Cannon CP, Gibson, CM, et al: Addition of clopidogrel to aspirin and fibrinolytic therapy for myocardial infarction with ST-segment elevation. N Engl J Med 352:1179, 2005; **B** modified from Chen ZM, Jiang LX, Chen YP, et al: Addition of clopidogrel to aspirin in 45,852 patients with acute myocardial infarction: Randomised placebo-controlled trial. Lancet 366:1607, 2005.)*

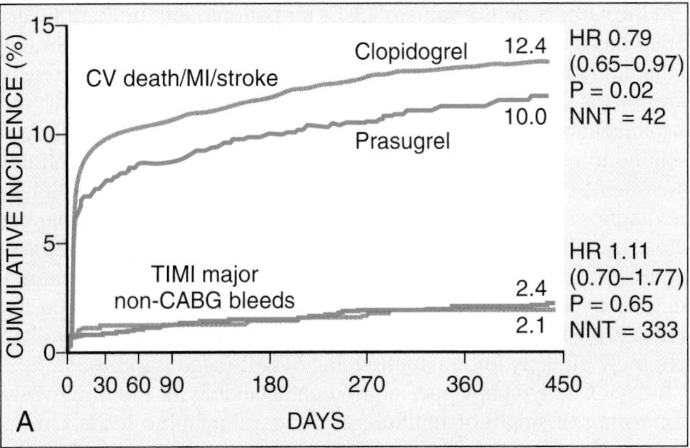

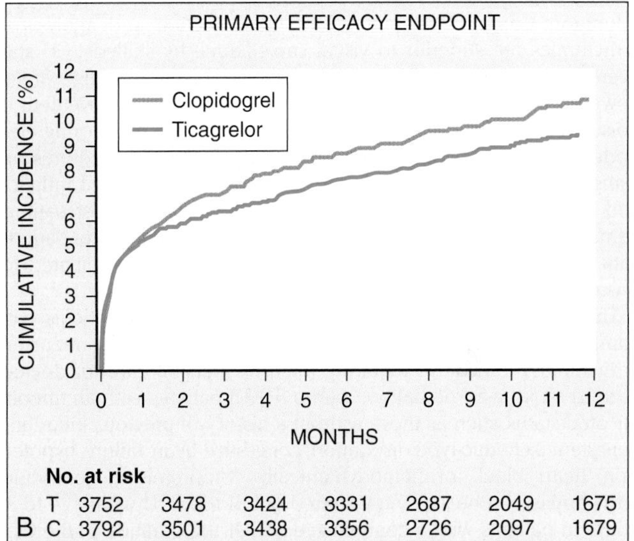

FIGURE 55-23 **A,** Efficacy and safety of prasugrel among the subgroup of patients with STEMI enrolled in a randomized clinical trial of prasugrel compared with clopidogrel in patients undergoing PCI after presentation with acute coronary syndrome. Treatment with prasugrel was associated with a 21% relative reduction in the risk cardiovascular death, myocardial infarction, or stroke during 15 months of follow-up. Major bleeding was increased with prasugrel in the trial overall, but not among patients with ST-elevation myocardial infarction. **B,** Efficacy results for ticagrelor (versus clopidogrel) in patients with STEMI enrolled in the PLATO trial. Ticagrelor reduced the primary endpoint (incidence of MI, stroke, or vascular death) versus clopidogrel, from 11.0% to 9.3% (hazard ratio [HR] 0.85; 95% CI, 0.74 to 0.97; P = 0.02). CV = cardiovascular; NNT = number needed to treat. *(**A** from Montalescot G, Wiviott SD, Braunwald E, et al: Prasugrel compared with clopidogrel in patients undergoing percutaneous coronary intervention for ST-segment elevation myocardial infarction [TRITON-TIMI 38]: Double-blind, randomised controlled trial. Lancet 373:723, 2009; **B** from Steg G, et al: Circulation [in press].)*

Hospital Management

Coronary Care Units

Deaths from primary ventricular fibrillation in patients with STEMI have been prevented because the coronary care unit (CCU) allows continuous monitoring of cardiac rhythm by highly trained nurses with the authority to initiate immediate treatment of arrhythmias in the absence of physicians, and because of the specialized equipment (e.g., defibrillators, pacemakers) and drugs available. Although all these benefits can be achieved for patients scattered throughout the hospital, the clustering of patients with STEMI in the CCU has greatly improved the efficient use of trained personnel, facilities, and equipment. With increasing emphasis on hemodynamic monitoring and treatment of the serious complications of STEMI with such modalities as pharmacologic or catheter-based reperfusion therapy, afterload reduction, and intra-aortic balloon counterpulsation, and other advanced hemodynamic support, the presence of a CCU and experienced teams of physicians has assumed even greater importance. As reperfusion strategies, including fibrinolytic therapy and PCI, are used more routinely for STEMI patients, facilities in which patients can undergo diagnostic and therapeutic angiographic procedures are being integrated into an expanded structure of a coronary care team.[11]

At the same time, the value of CCUs for patients with uncomplicated STEMI has undergone reevaluation. With increasing attention directed to the limitations of resources and to the economic impact of intensive care, efforts have been made to select patients likely to benefit from hospitalization in a CCU. The ECG, on presentation, particularly in conjunction with previous tracings and an immediate general clinical assessment, can be useful both for predicting which patients will have the diagnosis of STEMI confirmed and for identifying low-risk patients who may require less intensive care. Analysis of the quality of pain can help identify low-risk patients. Patients without a history of angina pectoris or MI who present with pain that is sharp or stabbing and pleuritic, positional, or reproduced by palpation of the chest wall are extremely unlikely to be experiencing STEMI (see Chap. 53).[118]

Today, CCUs typically have equipment available for the noninvasive monitoring of single or multiple electrocardiographic leads, cardiac rhythm, ST-segment deviation, arterial pressure, and arterial oxygen saturation. Computer algorithms for the detection and analysis of arrhythmias are superior to visual surveillance by skilled CCU staff. Even the most sophisticated electrocardiographic monitoring systems, however, are susceptible to artifacts because of patient movement or noise on the signal from poor skin preparation when monitoring electrodes are applied. Noninvasive monitoring of arterial blood pressure using a sphygmomanometric cuff that undergoes cycles of inflation and deflation at programmed intervals is suitable for most patients admitted to a CCU. Invasive arterial monitoring is preferred for patients with a low output syndrome when inotropic therapy is initiated for severe left ventricular failure.

The CCU remains the appropriate hospital unit for patients with complicated infarctions (e.g., hemodynamic instability, recurrent arrhythmias) and those requiring intensive nursing care for devices such as an intra-aortic balloon pump. STEMI patients with an uncomplicated status, such as those without a history of previous infarction, persistent ischemic-type discomfort, congestive heart failure, hypotension, heart block, or hemodynamically compromising ventricular arrhythmias, can be safely transferred out of the CCU within 24 to 36 hours. In patients with a complicated STEMI, the duration of the CCU stay should be dictated by the need for intensive care—that is, hemodynamic monitoring, close nursing supervision, intravenous vasoactive drugs, and frequent changes in the medical regimen.

For patients with a low risk of mortality from STEMI, the clinician should consider admission to an intermediate care facility (see later) equipped with simple electrocardiographic monitoring and resuscitation equipment.[1] This strategy has proven cost-effective and may reduce CCU use by one third, shorten hospital stays, and have no deleterious effect on a patient's recovery. Intermediate care units for low-risk STEMI patients can also be appealing to patients who stand to gain little benefit from the high staffing, intense activity, and elaborate technology available in current CCUs (but with their attendant high costs) and who may be disturbed by that activity and equipment.

TABLE 55-7 Sample Admitting Orders for the STEMI Patient

1. Condition: Serious
2. IV: NS on D_5W to keep vein open. Start a second IV if IV medication is being given. This may be saline lock.
3. Vital signs: Every 1.5 hr until stable, then every 4 hr and as needed. Notify physician if HR is <60 beats/min or >100 beats/min, BP is <100 mm Hg systolic or >150 mm Hg systolic, respiratory rate is <8 or >22.
4. Monitor: Continuous ECG monitoring for dysrhythmia and ST-segment deviation.
5. Diet: NPO except for sips of water until stable. Then start 2 g sodium/day, low saturated fat (<7% of total calories/day), low cholesterol (<200 mg/day) diet, such as total lifestyle change (TLC) diet.
6. Activity: Bedside commode and light activity when stable.
7. Oxygen: Continuous oximetry monitoring. Nasal cannula at 2 liters/min when stable for 6 hr, reassess for oxygen need (i.e., O_2 saturation of <90%) and consider discontinuing oxygen.
8. Medications:
   a. Nitroglycerin (NTG)
      1. Use sublingual NTG 0.4 mg every 5 min as needed for chest discomfort.
      2. Intravenous NTG for CHF, hypertension, or persistent ischemia.
   b. Aspirin (ASA; acetylsalicylic acid)
      1. If ASA not given in the emergency department (ED), chew nonenteric-coated ASA* 162-325 mg.
      2. If ASA has been given, start daily maintenance of 75-162 mg daily; may use enteric coated for gastrointestinal protection.
   c. Beta blocker
      1. If not given in the ED, assess for contraindication (i.e., bradycardia and hypotension); continue daily assessment to ascertain eligibility for beta blocker.
      2. If given in the ED, continue daily dose and optimize as dictated by heart rate and blood pressure.
   d. Angiotensin-converting enzyme (ACE) inhibitor
      1. Start ACE inhibitor orally in patients with pulmonary congestion or LVEF <40% if the following are absent: hypotension (SBP <100 mm Hg or <30 mm Hg below baseline) or known contraindications to this class of medications.
   e. Angiotensin receptor blocker (ARB)
      1. Start ARB orally in patients who are intolerant of ACE inhibitors and with either clinical or radiologic signs of heart failure or LVEF <40%.
   f. Pain medications
      1. IV morphine sulfate 2-4 mg with increments of 2-8 mg IV at 5- to 15-min intervals as needed to control pain.
   g. Anxiolytics (based on a nursing assessment)
   h. Daily stool softener

*Although some trials have used enteric-coated ASA for initial dosing, more rapid buccal absorption occurs with nonenteric-coated formulations.

BP = blood pressure; CHF = congestive heart failure; HR = heart rate; IV = intravenous; NS = normal saline; NPO = nothing by mouth.

Modified from Antman EM, Anbe DT, Armstrong PW, et al: ACC/AHA guidelines for the management of patients with ST-elevation myocardial infarction: A report of the American College of Cardiology/American Heart Association Task Force on Practice Guidelines (Committee to Revise the 1999 Guidelines for the Management of Patients with Acute Myocardial Infarction). Circulation 110:e82, 2004.

GENERAL MEASURES. The CCU staff must be sensitive to patient concerns about mortality, prognosis, and future productivity. A calm, quiet atmosphere and the laying on of hands with a gentle but confident touch help allay anxiety and reduce sympathetic tone, ultimately leading to a reduction in hypertension, tachycardia, and arrhythmias.[1] To reduce the risk of nausea and vomiting early after infarction and to reduce the risk of aspiration, during the first 4 to 12 hours after admission patients should receive nothing by mouth or a clear liquid diet (**Table 55-7**). Subsequently, a diet with 50% to 55% of calories from complex carbohydrates and up to 30% from monounsaturated and unsaturated fats should be given. The diet should be enriched in foods that are high in potassium, magnesium, and fiber but low in sodium.

The results of laboratory tests obtained in the CCU should be scrutinized for any derangements potentially contributing to arrhythmias, such as hypoxemia, hypovolemia, disturbances of acid-base balance or of electrolytes, and drug toxicity. Oxazepam, 15 to 30 mg orally four times a day, is useful to allay the anxiety that is common in the first 24 to 48 hours (see Table 55-7). Delirium can be provoked by medications frequently used in the CCU, including antiarrhythmic drugs, H_2 blockers, narcotics, and beta blockers. Potentially offending agents should be discontinued in patients with an abnormal mental status. Haloperidol, a butyrophenone, can be used safely in patients with STEMI, beginning with a dose of 2 mg intravenously for mildly agitated patients and 5 to 10 mg for progressively more agitated patients. Hypnotics, such as temazepam, 15 to 30 mg, or an equivalent, should be provided as needed for sleep. Docusate, 200 mg daily, or another stool softener should be used to prevent constipation and straining.

Coronary precautions that do not appear to be supported by evidence from clinical research include the avoidance of iced fluids, hot beverages, caffeinated beverages, rectal examinations, and back rubs.[1]

Physical Activity

In the absence of complications, patients with STEMI need not be confined to bed for more than 12 hours and, unless they are hemodynamically compromised, they may use a bedside commode shortly after admission (see Table 55-7). Progression of activity should be individualized depending on the patient's clinical status, age, and physical capacity.

In patients without hemodynamic compromise, early mobilization, including dangling the feet on the side of the bed, sitting in a chair, standing, and walking around the bed, does not cause important changes in heart rate, blood pressure, or pulmonary wedge pressure. Although heart rate increases slightly (usually by less than 10%), pulmonary wedge pressures fall slightly as the patient assumes the upright posture for activities. Early ambulatory activities are rarely associated with any symptoms, and when symptoms do occur, they generally are related to hypotension. Thus, when Levine and Lown proposed the armchair treatment of STEMI in the 1950s, they were undoubtedly correct that stress to the myocardium is less in the upright position. As long as blood pressure and heart rate are monitored, early mobilization offers considerable psychological and physical benefit, without any clear medical risk.

INTERMEDIATE CORONARY CARE UNIT. Patients with STEMI are at risk for late in-hospital mortality from recurrent ischemia or infarction, hemodynamically significant ventricular arrhythmias, and severe congestive heart failure after discharge from the CCU. Therefore, continued surveillance in intermediate CCUs (also called step-down units) is justifiable. Risk factors for mortality in the hospital after discharge from the CCU include significant congestive heart failure evidenced by persistent sinus tachycardia for more than 2 days and rales in more than one third of the lung fields, recurrent ventricular tachycardia and ventricular fibrillation, atrial fibrillation or flutter while in the CCU, intraventricular conduction delays or heart block, anterior location of infarction, and recurrent episodes of angina with marked electrocardiographic ST-segment abnormalities at low activity levels.

The availability of intermediate care units may also be helpful for identifying those patients who remain free of complications and are suitable candidates for early discharge from the hospital. Aggressive reperfusion protocols with angioplasty or fibrinolytics can reduce the length of hospital stay without compromising mortality after discharge.[119] In patients who are thought to have undergone successful reperfusion, the absence of early sustained ventricular tachyarrhythmias, hypotension, or heart failure, coupled with a well-preserved left ventricular ejection fraction, predicts a low risk of in-hospital late complications. Such patients are suitable candidates for discharge from the hospital in less than 5 days from the onset of symptoms.

Following STEMI, patients are often eager for information, in need of reassurance, confused by misinformation and prior impressions, capable of counterproductive denial, and simply frightened. Intermediate care facilities provide ideal settings and ample opportunity to begin the rehabilitation process. The capacity for the early detection of problems following STEMI and the social and educational benefits of grouping such patients together strongly argue for continued use of intermediate CCUs. Furthermore, the economic advantage of grouping such patients together for the sharing of skilled personnel and resources outweighs any questions raised by the lack of a clear consensus regarding reduced mortality. An additional potential advantage is the facilitation of patient education in a group setting, with lectures and audiovisual programs.

Pharmacologic Therapy

BETA BLOCKERS. The effects of beta blockers for the treatment of patients with STEMI can be divided into those that are immediate (when the drug is given early in the course of infarction) and those that are long term (secondary prevention). The immediate intravenous administration of beta blockers reduces cardiac index, heart rate, and blood pressure.[120] The net effect is a reduction in myocardial oxygen consumption per minute and per beat. Favorable effects of acute intravenous administration of beta blockers on the balance of myocardial oxygen supply and demand are reflected in reductions in chest pain, in the proportion of patients with threatened infarction who actually evolve STEMI, and in the development of ventricular arrhythmias.[121] Because beta-adrenergic blockade diminishes circulating levels of free fatty acids by antagonizing the lipolytic effects of catecholamines, and because elevated levels of fatty acids augment myocardial oxygen consumption and probably increase the incidence of arrhythmias, these metabolic actions of beta-blocking agents may also benefit the ischemic heart. Despite these favorable effects of early administration of intravenous beta blockers, there are potentially detrimental effects for some patients,[43] which have led to the modification of guidelines for early administration of intravenous beta blockers.[35]

More than 52,000 patients have been randomized in clinical trials studying beta-adrenergic blockade in acute MI. These trials cover a range of beta blockers and timing of administration and were largely conducted in the era before reperfusion strategies were developed for STEMI. The available data in the prereperfusion era have suggested there were favorable trends toward a reduction in mortality, reinfarction, and cardiac arrest. However, in the reperfusion era, the addition of an intravenous beta blocker to fibrinolytic therapy was not associated with a reduction in mortality but was helpful in reducing the rate of recurrent ischemic events.[122] Concern arose regarding the potential risk of provoking cardiogenic shock if early intravenous followed by oral beta-adrenergic blockade was routinely administered to all patients with STEMI.[121] The largest trial testing beta blockade in patients with acute MI was COMMIT, which randomized 45,852 patients within 24 hours of MI to metoprolol given as sequential intravenous boluses of 5 mg, up to 15 mg, followed by 200 mg/day orally or placebo.[43] There was no difference in the rate of the composite endpoint of death, reinfarction, or cardiac arrest in the metoprolol group (9.4%) compared with the placebo group (9.9%). But significant reductions occurred in reinfarction and episodes of ventricular fibrillation in the metoprolol group, translating into five fewer events for each of these endpoints per 1000 patients treated. However, there were 11 more episodes of cardiogenic shock in the metoprolol group per 1000 patients treated. The risk of developing cardiogenic shock, which was recorded as part of the COMMIT protocol in contrast to earlier studies, was greatest in those patients presenting with moderate to severe left ventricular dysfunction (Killip Class II or higher).

Combining the results of the low-risk patients from COMMIT with the data from earlier trials, an overview of the effects of early intravenous therapy followed by oral beta blocker therapy can be seen (**Fig. 55-24**). There is a 13% reduction in all-cause mortality (7 lives saved/1000 patients treated), 22% reduction in reinfarction (5 fewer events/1000 patients treated), and 15% reduction in ventricular fibrillation or cardiac arrest (5 fewer events/1000 patients treated).[43] To achieve these benefits safely, it is important to avoid the early administration of beta blockers to patients with relative contraindications, as outlined in **Table 55-8**.

Recommendations

Given the evidence of the benefits of early beta blocker administration in STEMI, patients without a contraindication (see Table 55-8), irrespective of administration of concomitant fibrinolytic therapy or performance of primary PCI, should promptly receive *oral* beta blockers. It is also reasonable to administer intravenously beta blockers promptly to STEMI patients, especially if a tachyarrhythmia or hypertension is present, in the absence of signs of heart failure or low output, increased risk of developing shock, indicators of high risk of developing shock, or other relative contraindications to beta blockers.[35] We use metoprolol 5 mg intravenously every 2 to 5 minutes for three doses, provided the heart rate does not fall below 60 beats/min and the systolic blood pressure does not drop below 100 mm Hg. Oral maintenance dosing

TABLE 55-8 Contraindications to Early Intravenous Beta Blocker Therapy in STEMI

Signs of heart failure
Evidence of a low-output state
Increased risk for cardiogenic shock*

*The more risk factors present, the higher the risk of developing cardiogenic shock: age older than 70 years, systolic blood pressure <120 mm Hg, sinus tachycardia >110 beats/min or heart rate <60 beats/min, and increased time since onset of symptom of STEMI.

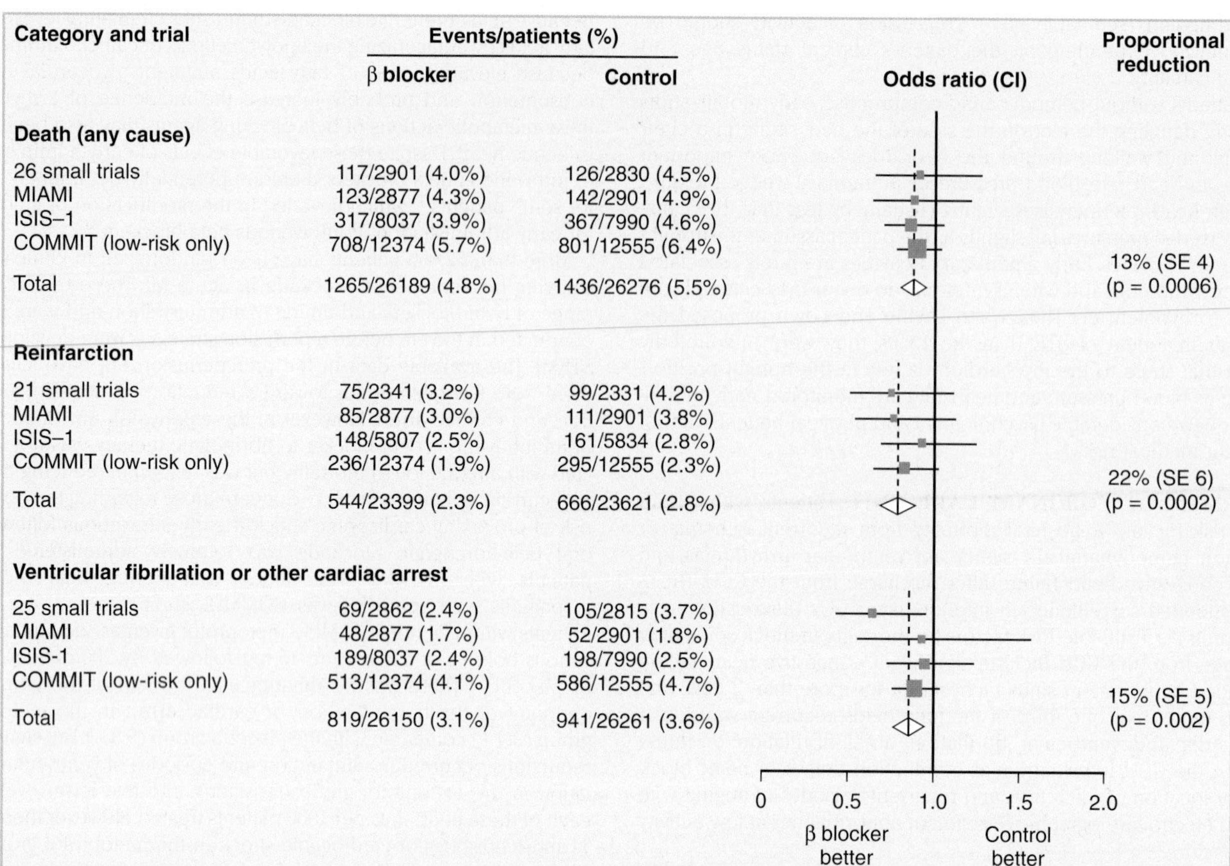

FIGURE 55-24 Meta-analysis of effects of intravenous and then oral beta blocker therapy on death, reinfarction, and cardiac arrest during the scheduled treatment periods in 26 small randomized trials, MIAMI, ISIS-1, and the low-risk subset of COMMIT. For COMMIT, data are included only for patients who presented with systolic blood pressure > 105 mm Hg, heart rate > 65 beats/min, and Killip Class I (as in MIAMI7). Five small trials included in the ISIS-1 report did not have any data on reinfarction. In the ISIS-1 trial, data on reinfarction in hospital were available for the last three quarters of the study, involving 11,641 patients. Odds ratios (ORs) in each (blue squares with area proportional to number of events) comparing outcome in patients allocated beta blockers to that in patients allocated controls, along with 99% CIs (horizontal line). Overall OR and 95% CI are indicated by diamonds. *(From Chen ZM, Pan HC, Chen YP, et al: Early intravenous then oral metoprolol in 45,852 patients with acute myocardial infarction: Randomised placebo-controlled trial. Lancet 366:1622, 2005.)*

is initiated with metoprolol, 50 mg every 6 hours for 2 days, and then 100 mg twice daily.

Beta blockers are especially helpful for patients in whom STEMI is complicated by persistent or recurrent ischemic pain, progressive or repetitive serum enzyme level elevations suggestive of infarct extension, or tachyarrhythmias early after the onset of infarction.[123] If adverse effects of beta blockers develop or if patients present with complications of infarction that are contraindications to beta blockade, such as heart failure or heart block, the beta blocker should be withheld. Unless there are contraindications (see Table 55-8), beta blockade probably should be continued in patients who develop STEMI.[35] Moreover, patients who initially have contraindications to a beta blocker, such as heart failure, should be reevaluated with respect to their candidacy for such therapy after 24 hours.

Selection of Beta Blocker

Favorable effects have been reported with metoprolol, atenolol, carvedilol, timolol, and alprenolol; these benefits probably occur with propranolol and with esmolol, an ultrashort-acting agent, as well. In the absence of any favorable evidence supporting the benefit of agents with intrinsic sympathomimetic activity, such as pindolol and oxprenolol, and with some unfavorable evidence for these agents in secondary prevention, beta blockers with intrinsic sympathomimetic activity probably should not be chosen for treatment of STEMI. The CAPRICORN trial randomized 1959 patients with MI and systolic dysfunction (ejection fraction < 40%) to carvedilol or placebo in addition to current pharmacotherapeutic agents, including angiotensin-converting enzyme (ACE) inhibitors in 98% of patients. All-cause mortality was reduced over a mean follow-up of 1.3 years from 15.3% in the placebo group to 11.9% in the carvedilol group (23% RR reduction; $P = 0.031$), with a similar pattern during the first 30 days.[124] Thus, CAPRICORN confirms the benefit of beta blocker administration in addition to ACE inhibitor therapy for patients with transient or sustained left ventricular dysfunction after MI. An algorithm for the use of beta blockers in STEMI patients is shown in **Figure 55-25**.

Occasionally, the clinician may wish to proceed with beta blocker therapy even in the presence of relative contraindications, such as a history of mild asthma, mild bradycardia, mild heart failure, or first-degree heart block. In this situation, a trial of esmolol may help determine whether the patient can tolerate beta-adrenergic blockade. Because the hemodynamic effects of this drug, with a half-life of 9 minutes, disappear in less than 30 minutes, it offers considerable advantage over longer acting agents when the risk of a beta blocker complication is relatively high.

INHIBITORS OF THE RENIN-ANGIOTENSIN-ALDOSTERONE SYSTEM (RAAS). The rationale for inhibition of the RAAS includes experimental and clinical evidence of a favorable impact on ventricular remodeling, improvement in hemodynamics, and reductions in congestive heart failure. Unequivocal evidence from randomized, placebo-controlled trials has shown that ACE inhibitors reduce the rate of mortality from STEMI.[1] These trials can be grouped into two categories. The first group consisted of selected MI patients for randomization on the basis of features indicative of increased mortality, such as left ventricular ejection fraction less than 40%, clinical signs and symptoms of congestive heart failure, anterior location of infarction, and

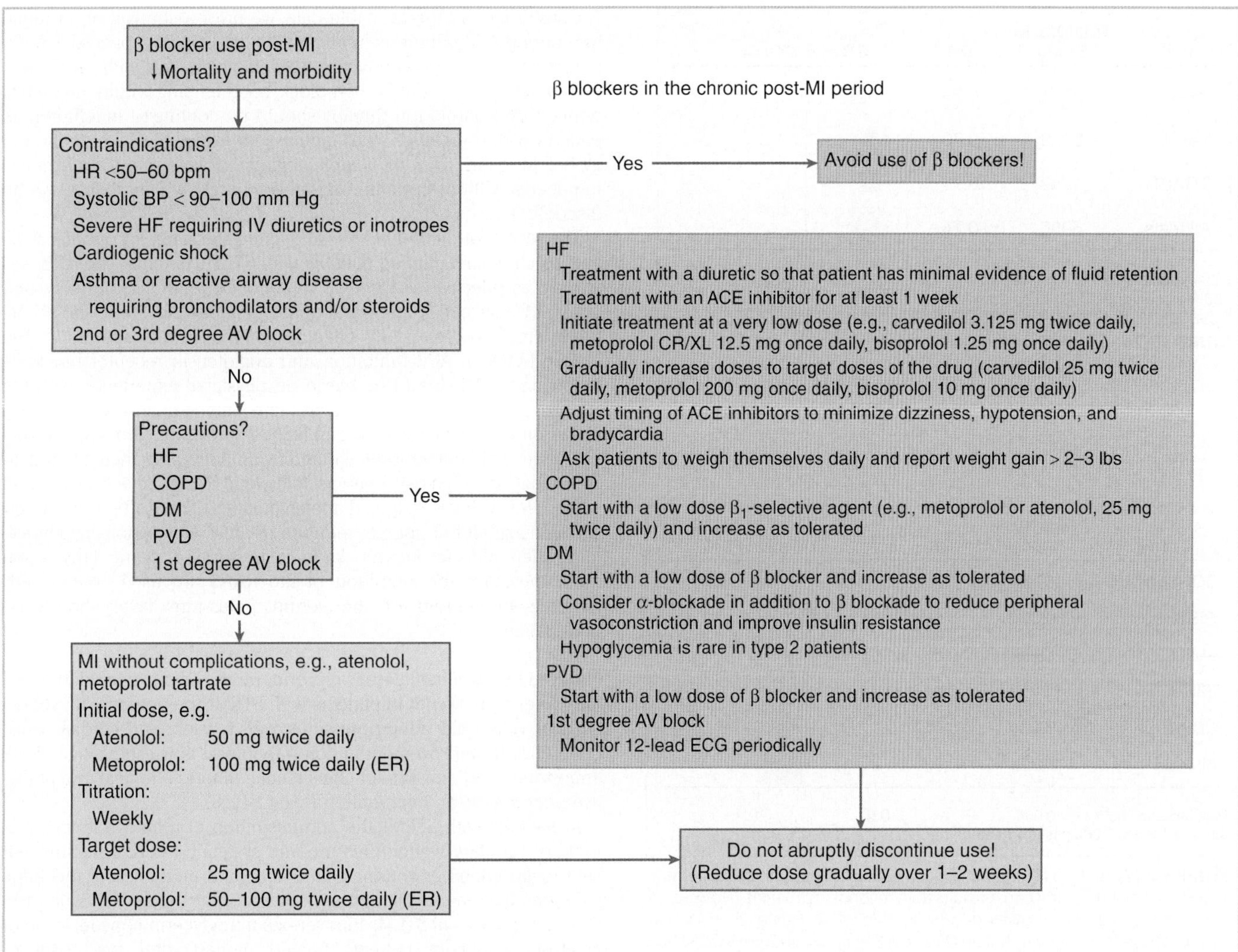

FIGURE 55-25 Algorithm for use of beta blockers in the treatment of patients with STEMI. COPD = chronic obstructive pulmonary disease; DM = diabetes mellitus; ER = extended release; HF = heart failure; PVD = peripheral vascular disease. *(From Gheorghiade M, Goldstein S: Beta-blockers in the post-myocardial infarction patient. Circulation 106:394, 2002.)*

abnormal wall motion score index (**Fig. 55-26**). Trials in the second group were unselective and randomized all patients with MI, provided they had a minimum systolic pressure of approximately 100 mm Hg (ISIS-4, GISSI-3, CONSENSUS II, and Chinese Captopril Study); (**Fig. 55-27**). With the exception of the SMILE trial, all the selective trials initiated ACE inhibitor therapy between 3 and 16 days after MI and maintained it for 1 to 4 years, whereas the unselective trials all initiated treatment within the first 24 to 36 hours and maintained it for only 4 to 6 weeks.

A consistent survival benefit was observed in all the trials already noted, except for CONSENSUS II, the one study that used an intravenous preparation early in the course of MI. An estimate of the mortality benefit of ACE inhibitors in the unselective, short duration trials was 5/1000 patients treated. Analysis of these unselective short-term trials indicates that approximately one third of lives was saved within the first 1 to 2 days. Certain subgroups, such as patients with anterior infarction, showed proportionately greater benefit from early administration (11 lives saved/1000) of ACE inhibitors. Not unexpectedly, greater survival benefits of 42 to 76 lives saved/1000 patients treated were obtained in the selective long-duration therapy trials. Of note, there was generally a 20% reduction in the risk of death attributable to ACE inhibitor treatment in the selective trials. The mortality reduction with ACE inhibitors is accompanied by significant reductions in the development of congestive heart failure, supporting the underlying pathophysiologic rationale for administering this class of drugs in patients with STEMI. In addition, some data have suggested that chronic administration of ACE inhibitors after a STEMI reduces ischemic events, including recurrent infarction and the need for coronary revascularization.[125]

The mortality benefits of ACE inhibitors add to those achieved with aspirin and beta blockers. Thus, ACE inhibitors should not be considered a substitute for these other therapies with proven benefit in STEMI patients. The benefits of ACE inhibition appear to be a class effect, because mortality and morbidity have been reduced by several agents. To replicate these benefits in clinical practice, however, physicians should select a specific agent and prescribe the drug according to the protocols used in the successful clinical trials reported to date.[126]

The major contraindications to the use of ACE inhibitors in patients with STEMI include hypotension in the setting of adequate preload, known hypersensitivity, and pregnancy. Adverse reactions include hypotension, especially after the first dose, and intolerable cough with chronic dosing; much less commonly, angioedema can occur.

An alternative method of pharmacologic inhibition of the RAAS is by administration of angiotensin II receptor blockers (ARBs). The VALIANT trial compared the effects of the ARB valsartan versus captopril alone and in combination with captopril on mortality in patients with acute MI complicated by left ventricular systolic dysfunction and/or heart failure.[127] Patients were randomized within 10 days of MI to valsartan (20 mg initially, titrated to 160 mg twice daily), valsartan added to captopril (20 mg and 6.25 mg initially, titrated to 80 mg twice

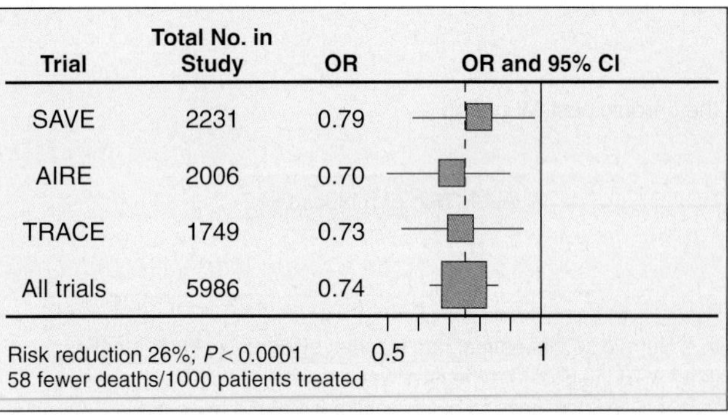

FIGURE 55-26 Effect of angiotensin-converting enzyme inhibitors on mortality after myocardial infarction—results from the long-term trials. *(From Gornik H, O'Gara PT: Adjunctive medical therapy.* In *Manson JE, Buring JE, Ridker PM, Gaziano JM [eds]: Clinical Trials in Heart Disease: A Companion to Braunwald's Heart Disease. Philadelphia, Elsevier Saunders, 2004, p 114.)*

Trial	Total No. in Study	OR	OR and 95% CI
CONSENSUS-II	6090	1.1	
GISSI-3	19394	0.88	
SMILE	1556	0.67	
ISIS-4	58050	0.94	
CCS-1	13634	0.94	
All trials	98724	0.93	

Risk reduction 6.7%; $P < 0.006$
4.9 fewer deaths/1000 patients treated
0.5 1

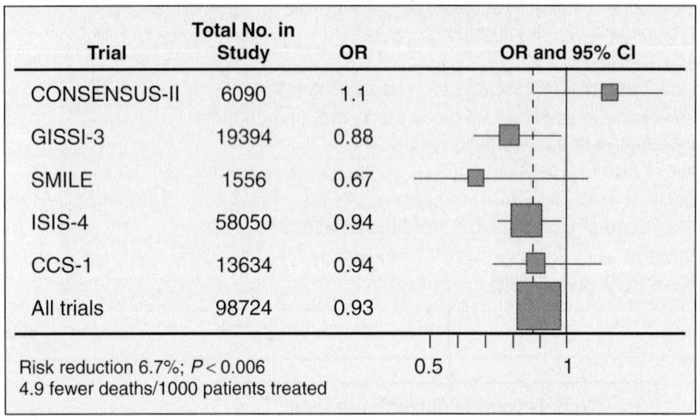

FIGURE 55-27 Effects of angiotensin-converting enzyme inhibitors on mortality after myocardial infarction—results from the short-term trials. *(From Gornik H, O'Gara PT: Adjunctive medical therapy.* In *Manson JE, Buring JE, Ridker PM, Gaziano JM [eds]: Clinical Trials in Heart Disease: A Companion to Braunwald's Heart Disease. Philadelphia, Elsevier Saunders, 2004, p 114.)*

daily and 50 mg three times daily), or captopril (6.25 mg initially, titrated to 50 mg three times daily) added to conventional therapy. Rates of mortality were similar in the three treatment groups—19.9% in the valsartan group, 19.3% in the valsartan plus captopril group, and 19.5% in the captopril alone group (**Fig. 55-28**).

Aldosterone blockade is another pharmacologic strategy for inhibition of the RAAS. The EPHESUS trial randomized 6642 patients with acute MI complicated by left ventricular dysfunction and heart failure to the selective aldosterone blocker eplerenone or placebo in conjunction with current postinfarction pharmacotherapy.[128] During a mean follow-up period of 16 months, there was a 15% reduction in the RR of mortality favoring eplerenone (**Fig. 55-29**). Cardiovascular mortality or hospitalization for cardiovascular events was also reduced by eplerenone. Serious hyperkalemia (serum potassium concentration ≥6 mmol/liter) occurred in 5.5% of patients in the eplerenone group compared with 3.9% of patients in the placebo group ($P = 0.002$).

Recommendations

After administration of aspirin and initiation of reperfusion strategies and, where appropriate, beta blockers, all STEMI patients should be considered for inhibition of the RAAS. Although there is little disagreement that high-risk STEMI patients (older, anterior infarction, prior infarction, Killip Class II or higher, and asymptomatic patients with evidence of depressed global ventricular function on an imaging study) should receive lifelong treatment with ACE inhibitors, short-term (4 to 6 weeks) therapy to a broader group of patients has also been proposed on the basis of the pooled results of the unselective mortality trials.[35,126]

Considering all the available data, we favor a strategy of an initial trial of oral ACE inhibitors in all STEMI patients with congestive heart failure, as well as in hemodynamically stable patients with ST-segment elevation or left bundle branch block, commencing within the first 24 hours.[129] ACE inhibition therapy should be continued indefinitely in patients with congestive heart failure, with evidence of a reduction in global function, or with a large regional wall motion abnormality. In patients without these findings at discharge, ACE inhibitors can be discontinued.

The results of the VALIANT trial expand the range of options available to clinicians treating patients with STEMI. Because the ARB was at least as effective as the ACE inhibitor in reducing mortality and other adverse cardiovascular outcomes following MI, it should be considered as a clinically effective alternative to captopril.[130] The choice between ACE inhibition and angiotensin receptor blockade following STEMI should be based on physician experience with the agents, patient tolerability, safety, convenience, and cost. Finally, based on experience from the EPHESUS study, long-term aldosterone blockade with eplerenone, 25 mg/day initially and then titrated to 50 mg/day for high-risk patients following STEMI (ejection fraction ≤40%, clinical heart failure, diabetes mellitus), should be considered. Given the small but definite increase in the risk of serious hyperkalemia when aldosterone blockade is prescribed, particularly when other measures for inhibition of the RAAS are used concurrently, periodic monitoring of the serum potassium level should be undertaken.[131]

NITRATES. Sublingual nitroglycerin rarely opens occluded coronary arteries. However, in patients with STEMI, the potential for reductions in ventricular filling pressures, wall tension, and cardiac work, coupled with improvement in coronary blood flow, especially in ischemic zones, and antiplatelet effects make nitrates a logical and attractive pharmacologic intervention (see Chap. 57).[35]

In patients with STEMI, the administration of nitrates reduces pulmonary capillary wedge pressure and systemic arterial pressure, left ventricular chamber volume, infarct size, and incidence of mechanical complications. As with other interventions to spare ischemic myocardium in cases of STEMI, intravenous nitroglycerin appears to be of greatest benefit in patients treated earliest after the onset of symptoms.

Clinical Trial Results

In the prefibrinolytic era, 10 randomized trials of acute administration of intravenous nitroglycerin (or nitroprusside, another nitric oxide donor) collectively enrolled 2042 patients. A meta-analysis of these trial results showed a reduction in mortality of 35% associated with nitrate therapy.[132]

In the fibrinolytic era, two megatrials of nitrate therapy have been conducted, GISSI-3 and ISIS-4.[1] In GISSI-3, there was no independent effect of nitrates on short-term mortality. Similarly, in ISIS-4, no effect of a mononitrate on 35-day mortality was observed. A pooled analysis of more than 80,000 patients treated with nitrate-like preparations intravenously or orally in 22 trials revealed a mortality rate of 7.7% in the control group, which was reduced to 7.4% in the nitrate group. These data suggest a small treatment effect of nitrates on mortality such that three to four fewer patients would die for every 1000 patients treated.

Nitrate Preparations and Mode of Administration

Intravenous nitroglycerin can be administered safely to patients with evolving STEMI as long as the dose is titrated to avoid induction of reflex tachycardia or systemic arterial hypotension. Patients with inferior wall infarction are particularly sensitive to an excessive fall in preload, particularly with concurrent right ventricular infarction.[35] In such cases, nitrate-induced venodilation could impair cardiac output and reduce coronary blood flow, thus worsening rather than improving myocardial oxygenation. A reasonable regimen begins with an initial infusion rate of 5 to 10 µg/min, with increases of 5 to 20 µg/min, until the mean arterial blood pressure is reduced by 10% of its baseline level in normotensive patients and by 30% for hypertensive patients, avoiding a systolic pressure lower than 90 mm Hg.

Adverse Effects

Clinically significant methemoglobinemia has been reported to occur during the administration of intravenous nitroglycerin. Although uncommon, this problem is seen when unusually large doses of nitrates are administered. It is important not only for its potential to cause symptoms of lethargy and headache, but also because elevated methemoglobin levels can impair the oxygen-carrying capacity of blood, potentially exacerbating ischemia. Dilation of the pulmonary vasculature supplying poorly ventilated lung segments may produce a ventilation-perfusion mismatch. Tolerance to intravenous nitroglycerin, as manifested by increasing nitrate requirements, develops in many patients, often as soon as 12 hours after the infusion is started. Despite the theoretical and demonstrated benefit of sulfhydryl agents in diminishing tolerance, their use has not become widespread.

Recommendations for Nitrates in Patients with STEMI

Nitroglycerin is indicated for the relief of persistent pain and as a vasodilator in patients with infarction associated with left ventricular failure. In the absence of recurrent angina or congestive heart failure, we do not routinely prescribe nitrates for STEMI patients. Higher-risk patients such as those with large infarctions, especially of the anterior wall, have the most to gain from nitrates in terms of reduction of ventricular remodeling, and therefore it is reasonable to consider using intravenous nitrates for 24 to 48 hours in such patients. There is no clear benefit to empirical long-term cutaneous or oral nitrates in the asymptomatic patient, and we therefore do not prescribe nitrates beyond the first 48 hours unless angina or ventricular failure is present.

CALCIUM CHANNEL ANTAGONISTS. Despite sound experimental and clinical evidence of an antiischemic effect, calcium antagonists have not been helpful in the acute phase of STEMI, and concern has been raised in several systematic overviews about an increased risk of mortality when they are prescribed on a routine basis. A distinction should be made between the dihydropyridine type of calcium channel antagonists (e.g., nifedipine) and the nondihydropyridine agents (e.g., verapamil and diltiazem).

Nifedipine

In multiple trials involving more than 5000 patients, the immediate-release preparation of nifedipine has not resulted in any reduction in infarct size, prevention of progression to infarction, control of recurrent ischemia, or lowering of mortality rate. When trials of the immediate-release form of nifedipine are pooled in a meta-analysis, evidence suggests a dose-related increased risk of in-hospital mortality (especially at a dose of >80 mg of nifedipine), although posthospital mortality does not appear to be increased in nifedipine-treated patients. Nifedipine does not appear to be helpful in conjunction with fibrinolytic therapy or beta blockade. Thus, we do not recommend the use of immediate-release nifedipine early in the treatment of STEMI. No trials of the sustained-release preparations of nifedipine in patients with STEMI have been reported to date.

Verapamil and Diltiazem

When administered during the acute phase of STEMI, these drugs have not had any demonstrated favorable effect on infarct size or other important endpoints in patients with STEMI, with the exception of control of supraventricular arrhythmias.[1] The INTERCEPT trial compared 300 mg of diltiazem with placebo in patients who received fibrinolytic therapy for STEMI. Diltiazem did not reduce the cumulative occurrence of cardiac death, nonfatal reinfarction, or refractory ischemia during a 6-month follow-up.

Based on the available data, we do not recommend the routine use of verapamil or diltiazem for patients with STEMI. Verapamil and diltiazem can be given for relief of ongoing ischemia or slowing of a rapid ventricular response in atrial fibrillation in patients for whom beta blockers are ineffective or contraindicated.[1] Their use should be avoided in patients with Killip Class II or greater hemodynamic findings.

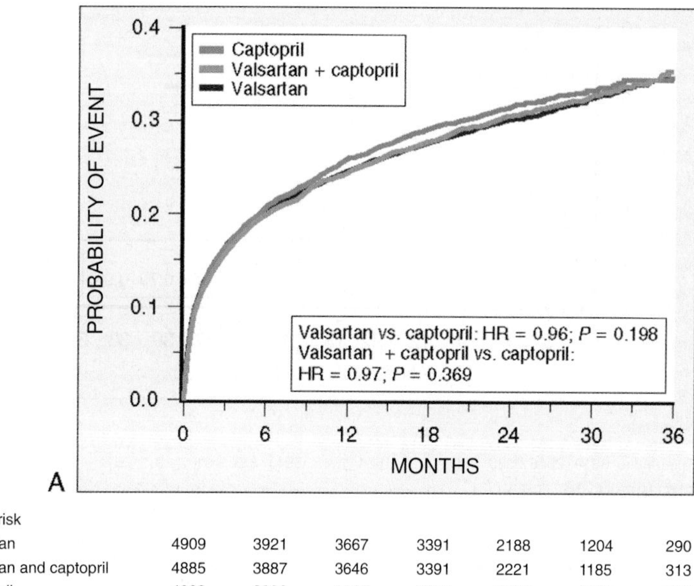

No. at risk							
Valsartan	4909	3921	3667	3391	2188	1204	290
Valsartan and captopril	4885	3887	3646	3391	2221	1185	313
Captopril	4909	3896	3610	3355	2155	1148	295

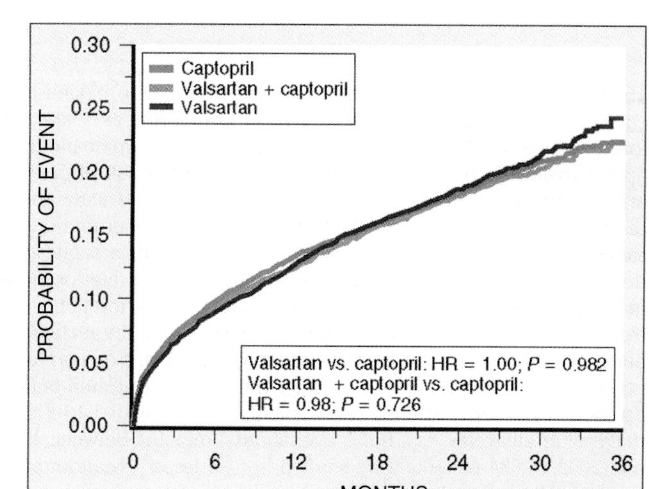

No. at risk							
Valsartan	4909	4464	4272	4007	2648	1437	357
Valsartan and captopril	4885	4414	4265	3994	2648	1435	382
Captopril	4909	4428	4241	4018	2635	1432	364

FIGURE 55-28 Effects of an ACE inhibitor (captopril), ARB (valsartan), or combination after myocardial infarction. The Kaplan-Meier estimates of **(A)** mortality and **(B)** cardiovascular death, reinfarction, or hospitalization for heart failure by treatment in the VALIANT trial are depicted. HR = hazard ratio. *(From Pfeffer M, McMurray JJ, Velasquez EJ, et al: Valsartan, captopril, or both in myocardial infarction complicated by heart failure, left ventricular dysfunction, or both. N Engl J Med 349:1893, 2003.)*

OTHER THERAPIES

Magnesium

Patients with STEMI may have a total body deficit of magnesium because of a low dietary intake, advanced age, or prior diuretic use.

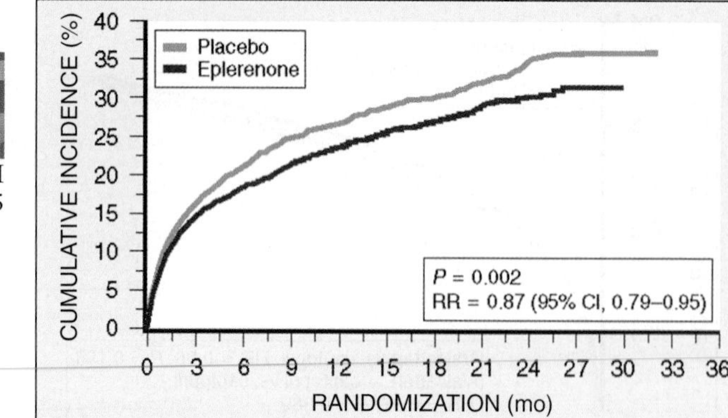

No. at risk

Placebo	3313	2754	2580	2388	2013	1494	995	558	247	77	2	0	0
Eplerenone	3319	2816	2680	2504	2096	1564	1061	594	273	91	0	0	0

FIGURE 55-29 Effect of a selective aldosterone receptor blocker (eplerenone) after myocardial infarction. The Kaplan-Meier estimates of the rate of death from cardiovascular causes or hospitalization for cardiovascular events in the EPHESUS trial are depicted. *(From Pitt B, Remme W, Zannad F, et al: Eplerenone, a selective aldosterone blocker, in patients with left ventricular dysfunction after myocardial infarction [abstract]. N Engl J Med 348:14, 2003.)*

They may also acquire a functional deficit of available magnesium caused by trapping of free magnesium in adipocytes, as soaps are formed when free fatty acids are released by catecholamine-induced lipolysis with the onset of infarction. Because of the risk of cardiac arrhythmias when electrolyte deficits are present in the early phase of infarction, all patients with STEMI should have their serum magnesium level measured on admission. We advocate repleting magnesium deficits to maintain a serum magnesium level of 2 mEq/liter or more. In the presence of hypokalemia (<4 mEq/liter) during the course of treatment of STEMI, the serum magnesium level should be rechecked and repleted if necessary because it is often difficult to correct a potassium deficit in the presence of a concurrent magnesium deficit. Episodes of torsades de pointes should be treated with 1 to 2 g of magnesium delivered as a bolus over about 5 minutes. Between 1980 and 2002, 68,684 patients were studied in a series of 14 randomized trials. On the basis of the totality of available evidence and current coronary care practice, there is no indication for the routine administration of intravenous magnesium to patients with STEMI at any level of risk.[133]

Glucose Control During STEMI

During the acute phase of STEMI, there is an increase in catecholamine levels in both the blood and ischemic myocardium. Insulin levels remain low, whereas cortisol, glucagon, and free fatty acid levels increase. These factors may contribute to an elevation of the blood glucose level, which should be measured routinely on admission to the coronary care unit (see Chap. 64). An infusion of insulin is recommended to treat persistent hyperglycemia in STEMI patients with a complicated course.[134] Given the evidence supporting glucose control in critically ill patients, it is also reasonable to administer an insulin infusion to hyperglycemic STEMI patients, even if they have an uncomplicated course. However, intensive treatment of hyperglycemia to a target less than 110 mg/dL in the critical care setting is not recommended.

It was proposed that routine administration of infusions of glucose-insulin-potassium (GIK) to STEMI patients would reduce mortality. A series of small trials, most of which were performed in the prereperfusion era, along with some in the setting of fibrinolysis or PCI, has suggested that GIK infusions are of benefit. However, the CREATE-ECLA investigators randomized 20,201 STEMI patients (83% of whom received reperfusion therapy) to GIK or placebo and found no evidence of a mortality benefit (30-day mortality, 9.7% in control patients and 10% in GIK patients).[135] Thus, in the current era of STEMI management, in which other effective therapies (e.g., reperfusion, aspirin, ACE inhibitors) are administered, there appears to be no benefit to the routine use of GIK infusions.

Other Agents

Several adjunctive pharmacotherapies have been investigated to prevent inflammatory damage in the infarct zone but have not been shown to provide a clinical benefit. For example, pexelizumab, a monoclonal antibody against the C5 component of complement, had no effect on infarct size in STEMI patients treated with fibrinolytics or PCI.[136,137] It also had no effect on mortality in STEMI patients treated with primary PCI.[138] The AMISTAD II trial was a dose-ranging study of adenosine in patients with anterior STEMI.[81] Although high-dose adenosine (70 μg/kg/min infusion for 3 hours) was associated with a reduction in infarct size, neither high- nor low-dose adenosine reduced the primary composite clinical endpoint of death or the development of heart failure at 6 months compared with placebo.[59]

Hemodynamic Disturbances

Hemodynamic Assessment

Patients with clinically uncomplicated STEMI do not require invasive hemodynamic monitoring because clinical evaluation can assess the status of the circulation. This approach ordinarily consists of monitoring of heart rate and rhythm, repeated measurement of systemic arterial pressure by cuff, obtaining chest radiographs to detect heart failure, repeated auscultation of the lung fields for pulmonary congestion, measurement of urine flow, examination of the skin and mucous membranes for evidence of the adequacy of perfusion, and arterial sampling for pO_2, pCO_2, and pH when hypoxemia or metabolic acidosis is suspected.

In contrast, in patients with STEMI whose ventricular contractile performance is abnormal, as evidenced by clinical signs and symptoms of heart failure, it is important to assess the degree of hemodynamic compromise to initiate therapy with drugs such as vasodilators and diuretics. In the past, central venous or right atrial pressure was used to gauge the degree of left ventricular failure in patients with STEMI. However, this technique is limited because central venous pressure reflects right rather than left ventricular function. Right ventricular function and therefore systemic venous pressure may be normal or almost normal in patients with significant left ventricular failure. Conversely, patients with right ventricular failure caused by right ventricular infarction or pulmonary embolism may exhibit elevated right atrial and central venous pressures, despite normal left ventricular function. Low values for right atrial and central venous pressures imply hypovolemia, whereas elevated right atrial pressures usually result from right ventricular failure secondary to left ventricular failure, pulmonary hypertension, or right ventricular infarction or, less commonly, from tricuspid regurgitation or pericardial tamponade.

Major advances in the management of complicated STEMI have resulted from the hemodynamic monitoring that has become widespread in CCUs (**Table 55-9**). This approach often uses both an intra-arterial catheter and pulmonary artery catheter for the measurement of pulmonary artery, pulmonary artery occlusive (equivalent to pulmonary wedge), and right atrial pressures, and cardiac output by thermodilution. In patients with hypotension, a Foley catheter provides accurate and continuous measurement of urine output.

NEED FOR INVASIVE MONITORING. The use of invasive hemodynamic monitoring is based on the following needs and challenges:

1. Difficulty in interpreting clinical and radiographic findings of pulmonary congestion, even after a review of noninvasive studies such as an echocardiogram.
2. Need for identifying noncardiac causes of arterial hypotension, particularly hypovolemia.
3. Possible contribution of reduced ventricular compliance to impaired hemodynamics, requiring judicious adjustment of intravascular volume to optimize left ventricular filling pressure.

TABLE 55-9 Indications for Hemodynamic Monitoring in Patients with STEMI

Management of complicated acute myocardial infarction
- Hypovolemia versus cardiogenic shock
- Ventricular septal rupture versus acute mitral regurgitation
- Severe left ventricular failure
- Right ventricular failure

Refractory ventricular tachycardia
Differentiating severe pulmonary disease from left ventricular failure
Assessment of cardiac tamponade
Assessment of therapy in *selected* individuals
- Afterload reduction in patients with severe left ventricular failure
- Inotropic agent therapy
- Beta blocker therapy
- Temporary pacing (ventricular versus atrioventricular)
- Intra-aortic balloon counterpulsation
- Mechanical ventilation

From Gore JM, Zwernet PL: Hemodynamic monitoring of acute myocardial infarction. *In* Francis GS, Alpert JS (eds): Modern Coronary Care. Boston, Little, Brown, 1990, p 138.

TABLE 55-10 Hemodynamic Classifications of Patients with Acute Myocardial Infarction

*Based on Clinical Examination**		*Based on Invasive Monitoring*†	
CLASS	**DEFINITION**	**SUBSET**	**DEFINITION**
I	Rales and S_3 absent	I	Normal hemodynamics; PCWP < 18 mm Hg, CI > 2.2
II	Crackles, S_3 gallop, elevated jugular venous pressure	II	Pulmonary congestion; PCWP > 18 mm Hg, CI > 2.2
III	Frank pulmonary edema	III	Peripheral hypoperfusion; PCWP < 18 mm Hg, CI < 2.2
IV	Shock	IV	Pulmonary congestion and peripheral hypoperfusion; PCWP > 18 mm Hg, CI < 2.2

CI = cardiac index; PCWP = pulmonary capillary wedge pressure.
*Modified from Killip T, Kimball J: Treatment of myocardial infarction in a coronary care unit. A two year experience with 250 patients. Am J Cardiol 20:457, 1967.
†Modified from Forrester J, Diamond G, Chatterjee K, et al: Medical therapy of acute myocardial infarction by the application of hemodynamic subsets. N Engl J Med 295:1356, 1976.

4. Difficulty in assessing the severity and sometimes the presence of complications such as mitral regurgitation and ventricular septal defect when the cardiac output or systemic pressures is (are) depressed.
5. Establishing a baseline of hemodynamic measurements and guiding therapy in patients with clinically apparent pulmonary edema or cardiogenic shock.
6. Underestimation of systemic arterial pressure by the cuff method in patients with intense vasoconstriction.

The prognosis and clinical status of patients with STEMI relate to the cardiac output and pulmonary artery wedge pressure. Patients with normal cardiac output after STEMI have a low expected mortality rate; prognosis worsens as cardiac output declines. Patients with intraventricular conduction defects, AV block, or both after anterior infarction have lower cardiac indices and higher pulmonary capillary wedge pressures than patients without these conduction disturbances. Conversely, patients with these conduction defects and inferior STEMI usually do not demonstrate such hemodynamic abnormalities.

PULMONARY ARTERY PRESSURE MONITORING. Patients most likely to benefit from pulmonary artery catheter monitoring include those whose STEMI is complicated by the following: (1) hypotension that is not easily corrected by fluid administration; (2) hypotension in the presence of congestive heart failure; (3) hemodynamic compromise severe enough to require intravenous vasopressors or vasodilators or intra-aortic balloon counterpulsation; (4) mechanical lesions (or suspected lesions) such as cardiac tamponade, severe mitral regurgitation, and a ruptured ventricular septum; and (5) right ventricular infarction.[139] Other indications for hemodynamic monitoring include assessment of the effects of mechanical ventilation, differentiating pulmonary disease from left ventricular failure as the cause of hypoxemia, and management of septic shock (see Table 55-9).[35] Before inserting a pulmonary artery catheter into a patient with STEMI, the physician must consider that the potential benefit of the information to be obtained outweighs any potential risks. Accumulating evidence from settings other than STEMI suggest that invasive hemodynamic monitoring does not improve outcomes.[140]

Major complications from pulmonary artery catheters are not common (about 3% to 5% of cases), but severe problems can occur, including sepsis, pulmonary infarction, and pulmonary artery rupture.[141] Minimized duration of catheterization and strict adherence to aseptic techniques can diminish risk. Catheter-related bloodstream infections can also be reduced by using antiseptic-impregnated dressings.[142] Noninvasive methods of determining cardiac output, such as pulse contour analysis and thoracic electrical bioimpedance, are under investigation.[143]

Accurate determination of hemodynamics by clinical assessment is difficult in critically ill patients. Consequently, the use of a pulmonary artery catheter often leads to important changes in therapy. Of note, it has been reported that rates of complications and mortality may be higher in patients who undergo pulmonary artery catheterization, although such patients are often at higher risk initially. These observations emphasize the importance of patient selection, meticulous technique, and correct interpretation of the data obtained.[141]

HEMODYNAMIC ABNORMALITIES. In 1976, Swan and coworkers measured the cardiac output and wedge pressure simultaneously in a large series of patients with acute MI and identified four major hemodynamic subsets of patients (**Table 55-10**): (1) patients with normal systemic perfusion and without pulmonary congestion (normal cardiac output and normal wedge pressure); (2) patients with normal perfusion and pulmonary congestion (normal cardiac output and elevated wedge pressure); (3) patients with decreased perfusion but without pulmonary congestion (reduced cardiac output and normal wedge pressure); and (4) patients with decreased perfusion and pulmonary congestion (reduced cardiac output and elevated wedge pressure). This classification, which overlaps with a crude clinical classification proposed earlier by Killip and Kimball (see Table 55-10), has proved to be useful, but it should be noted that patients frequently pass from one category to another with therapy and sometimes apparently even spontaneously.

Hemodynamic Subsets

The patient's clinical status generally reflects these subsets. Hypoperfusion usually becomes evident clinically when the cardiac index falls below approximately 2.2 liters/min/m^2, whereas pulmonary congestion is noted when the wedge pressure exceeds approximately 20 mm Hg. However, approximately 25% of patients with cardiac indices lower than 2.2 liters/min/m^2 and 15% of patients with elevated pulmonary capillary wedge pressures are not recognized clinically. Discrepancies in hemodynamic and clinical classification of patients with STEMI arise for a variety of reasons. Patients may exhibit phase lags as clinical pulmonary congestion develops or resolves, symptoms secondary to chronic obstructive pulmonary disease may be confused with those resulting from pulmonary congestion, or long-standing left ventricular dysfunction may mask signs of hypoperfusion because of compensatory vasoconstriction.

The hemodynamic findings shown in **Table 55-11** allow for rational approaches to therapy (see Table 55-10). The goals of hemodynamic therapy include maintenance of ventricular performance, blood pressure support, and protection of jeopardized myocardium. Because these goals occasionally may be at cross purposes, recognition of the

TABLE 55-11 Hemodynamic Patterns for Common Clinical Conditions

CARDIAC CONDITION	CHAMBER PRESSURE (MG HG)				
	RA	RV	PA	PCW	CI
Normal	0-6	25/0-6	25/0-12	6-12	≥2.5
AMI without LVF	0-6	25/0-6	30/12-18	≤18	≥2.5
AMI with LVF	0-6	30-40/0-6	30-40/18-25	>18	>2.0
Biventricular failure	>6	50-60/>6	50-60/25	18-25	>2.0
RVMI	12-20	30/12-20	30/12	≤12	<2.0
Cardiac tamponade	12-16	25/12-16	25/12-16	12-16	<2.0
Pulmonary embolism	12-20	50-60/12-20	50-60/12	<12	<2.0

AMI = acute myocardial infarction; CI = cardiac index; LVF = left ventricular failure; PA = pulmonary artery; PCW = pulmonary capillary wedge; RA = right atrium; RV = right ventricle; RVMI = right ventricular myocardial infarction.

From Gore JM, Zwernet PL: Hemodynamic monitoring of acute myocardial infarction. *In* Francis GS, Alpert JS (eds): Modern Coronary Care. Boston, Little, Brown, 1990, pp 139-164.

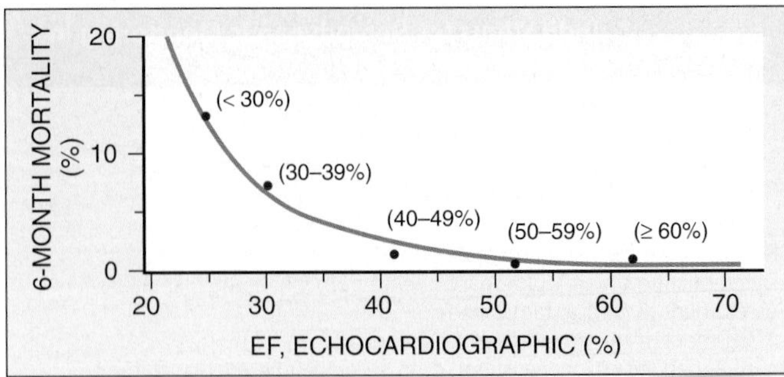

FIGURE 55-30 Impact of left ventricular function on survival following MI. The curvilinear relationship between left ventricular ejection fraction (EF) for patients treated in the fibrinolytic era is shown. Among patients with a left ventricular EF below 40%, the rate of mortality is markedly increased at 6 months. Thus, interventions such as thrombolysis, aspirin, and ACE inhibitors should be of considerable benefit in patients with acute MI to minimize the amount of left ventricular damage and interrupt the neurohumoral activation seen with congestive heart failure. *(Modified from Volpi A, De Vita C, Franzosi MG, et al: Determinants of 6-month mortality in survivors of myocardial infarction after thrombolysis. Results of the GISSI-2 data base. The Ad Hoc Working Group of the Gruppo Italiano per lo Studio della Sopravvivenza nell'Infarto Miocardico [GISSI]-2 Data Base. Circulation 88:416, 1993.)*

hemodynamic profile, as assessed clinically or as determined from hemodynamic monitoring, is required to design an optimal therapeutic management strategy.

Hypotension in the Prehospital Phase

During the prehospital phase of STEMI, invasive hemodynamic monitoring is not feasible and therapy should be guided by frequent clinical assessment and measurement of arterial pressure by cuff, recognizing that intense vasoconstriction can provide a falsely low pressure measured by this method. Hypotension associated with bradycardia often reflects excessive vagotonia. Relative or absolute hypovolemia is often present when hypotension occurs with a normal or rapid heart rate, particularly among patients receiving diuretics just before the infarction. Marked diaphoresis, reduction of fluid intake, or vomiting during the period preceding and accompanying the onset of STEMI may all contribute to the development of hypovolemia. Even if the effective vascular volume is normal, relative hypovolemia may be present because ventricular compliance is reduced in cases of STEMI, and a left ventricular filling pressure as high as 20 mm Hg may be necessary to provide an optimal preload.

MANAGEMENT. In the absence of rales involving more than one third of the lung fields, patients should be put in the reverse Trendelenburg position and, in patients with sinus bradycardia and hypotension, atropine should be administered (0.3 to 0.6 mg IV repeated at 3- to 10-minute intervals, up to 2 mg). If these measures do not correct the hypotension, normal saline should be administered intravenously, beginning with a bolus of 100 mL followed by 50-mL increments every 5 minutes. The patient should be observed and the infusion stopped when the systolic pressure returns to approximately 100 mm Hg, if the patient becomes dyspneic, or if pulmonary rales develop or increase. Because of the poor correlation between left ventricular filling pressure and mean right atrial pressure, assessment of systemic (even central) venous pressure is of limited value as a guide to fluid therapy. Administration of positive inotropic agents is indicated during the prehospital phase if systemic hypotension persists despite correction of hypovolemia and excessive vagotonia.

Hypovolemic Hypotension

Recognition of hypovolemia is of particular importance in hypotensive patients with STEMI because of the hazard it poses and because of the improvement in circulatory dynamics that can be achieved so readily and safely by augmentation of vascular volume. Because hypovolemia is often occult, it is frequently overlooked in the absence of invasive hemodynamic monitoring. Hypovolemia may be absolute, with low left ventricular filling pressure (8 mm Hg), or relative, with normal (8 to 12 mm Hg) or even modestly increased (13 to 18 mm Hg) left ventricular filling pressures.

Exclusion of hypovolemia as the cause of hypotension requires the documentation of a reduced cardiac output despite the left ventricular filling pressure exceeding 18 mm Hg. If, in a hypotensive patient, the pulmonary capillary wedge pressure (ordinarily measured as the pulmonary artery occlusive pressure) is below this level, fluid challenge should be carried out as noted. Hypotension caused by right ventricular infarction may be confused with that caused by hypovolemia because both are associated with a low, normal, or minimally elevated left ventricular filling pressure. The findings and management of right ventricular infarction are discussed elsewhere in this chapter.

Hyperdynamic State

When infarction is not complicated by hemodynamic impairment, no therapy other than general supportive measures and treatment of arrhythmias is necessary. However, if the hemodynamic profile is of the hyperdynamic state—that is, elevation of sinus rate, arterial pressure, and cardiac index, occurring singly or together in the presence of a normal or low left ventricular filling pressure—and if other causes of tachycardia such as fever, infection, and pericarditis can be excluded, treatment with beta blockers is indicated. Presumably, the increased heart rate and blood pressure result from inappropriate activation of the sympathetic nervous system, possibly because of the augmented release of catecholamines triggered by pain and/or anxiety.

Left Ventricular Failure

Left ventricular dysfunction is the single most important predictor of mortality following STEMI (**Fig. 55-30**).[144,145] In patients with STEMI, systolic dysfunction alone or both systolic and diastolic dysfunction can occur. Left ventricular diastolic dysfunction leads to pulmonary venous hypertension and pulmonary congestion. Clinical manifestations of left ventricular failure become more common as the extent of the injury to the left ventricle increases. In addition to infarct size, other important predictors of the development of symptomatic left ventricular dysfunction include advanced age and diabetes.[146,147] Mortality increases are related to the severity of the hemodynamic deficit.

THERAPEUTIC IMPLICATIONS. Classification of patients with STEMI by hemodynamic subsets has therapeutic relevance. As noted, patients with normal wedge pressures and hypoperfusion often benefit from the infusion of fluids because the peak value of stroke volume is usually not attained until left ventricular filling pressure reaches 18 to 24 mm Hg. However, a low level of left ventricular filling pressure does not necessarily imply that left ventricular damage is slight. Such patients may be relatively hypovolemic and/or may have suffered a right ventricular infarct, with or without severe left ventricular damage.

When preload is increased by fluid infusion, the relationship between ventricular filling pressure and cardiac index can provide valuable hemodynamic information in addition to that obtained from baseline measurements. For example, the ventricular function curve rises steeply (marked increase in cardiac index, small increase in filling pressure) in patients with normal left ventricular function and hypovolemia, whereas the curve rises gradually or remains flat in those patients with a combination of hypovolemia and depressed cardiac function. Invasive hemodynamic monitoring is essential to guide therapy of patients with severe left ventricular failure (pulmonary capillary wedge pressure > 18 mm Hg and cardiac index < 2.5 liters/min/m^2). Although positive inotropic agents can be useful, they do not represent the initial therapy of choice in patients with STEMI. Instead, heart failure is managed most effectively first by reduction of ventricular preload and then, if possible, by lowering of afterload. Arrhythmias can contribute to hemodynamic compromise and should be treated promptly in patients with left ventricular failure.

HYPOXEMIA. Patients with STEMI complicated by congestive heart failure characteristically develop hypoxemia caused by a combination of pulmonary vascular engorgement and, in some cases, pulmonary interstitial edema, diminished vital capacity, and respiratory depression from narcotic analgesics. Hypoxemia can impair the function of ischemic tissue at the margin of the infarct and thereby contribute to establishing or perpetuating the vicious cycle (see Chap. 54). The ventilation-perfusion mismatch that results in hypoxemia requires careful attention to ventilatory support. Increasing fractions of inspired oxygen (FiO_2) via face mask should be used initially, but if the oxygen saturation of the patient's blood cannot be maintained above 85% to 90% on 100% FiO_2, strong consideration should be given to endotracheal intubation with positive-pressure ventilation. The improvement of arterial oxygenation and hence myocardial oxygen supply may help restore ventricular performance. Positive end-expiratory pressure may diminish systemic venous return and reduce effective left ventricular filling pressure. This may require reduction in the amount of positive end-expiratory pressure, normal saline infusions to maintain left ventricular filling pressure, adjustment of the rate of infusion of vasodilators such as nitroglycerin, or some combination of these. Because myocardial ischemia frequently occurs during the return to unsupported spontaneous breathing, weaning should be accompanied by observation for signs of ischemia and is potentially facilitated by a period of intermittent mandatory ventilation or pressure support ventilation before extubation.

DIURETICS. Mild heart failure in patients with STEMI frequently responds well to diuretics such as furosemide, administered intravenously in doses of 10 to 40 mg and repeated at 3- to 4-hour intervals if necessary. The resultant reduction of pulmonary capillary pressure reduces dyspnea, and the lowering of left ventricular wall tension that accompanies the reduction of left ventricular diastolic volume diminishes myocardial oxygen requirements and may lead to improvement of contractility and augmentation of the ejection fraction, stroke volume, and cardiac output. The reduction of elevated left ventricular filling pressure may also enhance myocardial oxygen delivery by diminishing the impedance to coronary perfusion attributable to elevated ventricular wall tension. It may also improve arterial oxygenation by reducing pulmonary vascular congestion.

The intravenous administration of furosemide reduces pulmonary vascular congestion and pulmonary venous pressure within 15 minutes, before renal excretion of sodium and water has occurred; presumably, this action results from a direct dilating effect of this drug on the systemic arterial bed. It is important not to reduce left ventricular filling pressure much below 18 mm Hg, the lower range associated with optimal left ventricular performance in STEMI, because this could reduce cardiac output further and cause arterial hypotension. Excessive diuresis may also result in hypokalemia.

AFTERLOAD REDUCTION. Myocardial oxygen requirements depend on left ventricular wall stress, which in turn is proportional to the product of peak developed left ventricular pressure, volume, and wall thickness. Vasodilator therapy is recommended in patients with STEMI complicated by the following: (1) heart failure unresponsive to treatment with diuretics; (2) hypertension; (3) mitral regurgitation; or (4) ventricular septal defect. In these patients, treatment with vasodilator agents increases stroke volume and may reduce myocardial oxygen requirements and thereby lessen ischemia. Hemodynamic monitoring of systemic arterial and, in many cases, pulmonary capillary wedge (or at least pulmonary artery) pressure and cardiac output in patients treated with these agents is important. Improvement of cardiac performance and energetics requires three simultaneous effects: (1) reduction of left ventricular afterload; (2) avoidance of excessive systemic arterial hypotension to maintain effective coronary perfusion pressure; and (3) avoidance of excessive reduction of ventricular filling pressure with consequent diminution of cardiac output. In general, pulmonary capillary wedge pressure should be maintained at approximately 20 mm Hg and arterial pressure above 90/60 mm Hg in patients who were normotensive before developing STEMI.

Vasodilator therapy is particularly useful when STEMI is complicated by mitral regurgitation or rupture of the ventricular septum. In such patients, vasodilators alone or in combination with intra-aortic balloon counterpulsation can sometimes serve as a temporary measure and provide hemodynamic stabilization to permit definitive catheterization and angiographic studies and prepare the patient for early surgical intervention. Because of the precarious state of patients with complicated infarction and the need for meticulous adjustment of dosage, therapy is best initiated with agents that can be administered intravenously and that have a short duration of action (e.g., nitroprusside, nitroglycerin, isosorbide dinitrate). After initial stabilization, the medication of choice is generally an ACE inhibitor, but long-acting nitrates given by mouth, sublingually, or by ointment can also be useful.

Nitroglycerin

This drug has been shown in animal experiments to be less likely than nitroprusside to produce a coronary steal (i.e., to divert blood flow from the ischemic to the nonischemic zone). Therefore, apart from consideration of its routine use in STEMI patients discussed earlier, it may be a particularly useful vasodilator in patients with STEMI complicated by left ventricular failure. Ten to 15 mg/min is infused and the dose is increased by 10 mg/min every 5 minutes until the desired effect (improvement of hemodynamics or relief of ischemic chest pain) is achieved or a decline in systolic arterial pressure to 90 mm Hg, or by more than 15 mm Hg, has occurred. Although both nitroglycerin and nitroprusside lower systemic arterial pressure, systemic vascular resistance, and the heart rate–systolic blood pressure product, the reduction of left ventricular filling pressure is more prominent with nitroglycerin because of its relatively greater effect than nitroprusside on venous capacitance vessels. Nevertheless, in patients with severe left ventricular failure, cardiac output often increases, despite the reduction in left ventricular filling pressure produced by nitroglycerin.

Oral Vasodilators

The use of oral vasodilators in the treatment of chronic congestive heart failure is discussed in Chap. 28. Patients with STEMI and persistent heart failure should receive long-term inhibition of the RAAS.[35] Reduced ventricular load decreases the remodeling of the left ventricle that occurs commonly in the period after STEMI and thereby reduces the development of heart failure and risk of death.[148,149]

DIGITALIS. Although digitalis increases the contractility and oxygen consumption of normal hearts, when heart failure is present, the diminution of heart size and wall tension frequently results in a net reduction of myocardial oxygen requirements (see Chap. 28). In animal experiments, it fails to improve ventricular performance immediately following experimental coronary occlusion, but salutary effects are elicited when it is administered several days later. The absence of early beneficial effects may be caused by the inability of ischemic tissue to respond to digitalis or the already maximal stimulation of contractility of the normal heart by circulating and neuronally released catecholamines.

Although the issue is still controversial, arrhythmias can be increased by digitalis glycosides when they are given to patients in the first few hours after the onset of STEMI, particularly in the presence of hypokalemia. Also, undesirable peripheral systemic and coronary vasoconstriction can result from the rapid intravenous administration of rapidly acting glycosides such as ouabain.

Administration of digitalis to patients with STEMI in the hospital phase should generally be reserved for the management of supraventricular tachyarrhythmias, such as atrial flutter and fibrillation, and of heart failure that persists despite treatment with diuretics, vasodilators, and beta blockers. There is no indication for its use as an inotropic agent in patients without clinical evidence of left ventricular dysfunction, and it is too weak an inotropic agent to be relied on as the principal cardiac stimulant in patients with overt pulmonary edema or cardiogenic shock.

BETA-ADRENERGIC AGONISTS. When left ventricular failure is severe, as manifested by marked reduction of the cardiac index (<2 liters/min/m^2), and pulmonary capillary wedge pressure is at optimal (18 to 24 mm Hg) or excessive (>24 mm Hg) levels, despite therapy with diuretics, beta-adrenergic agonists are indicated.[150] Although isoproterenol is a potent cardiac stimulant and improves ventricular performance, it should be avoided in STEMI patients. It also causes tachycardia and augments myocardial oxygen consumption and lactate production; in addition, it reduces coronary perfusion pressure by causing systemic vasodilation, and in animal experiments it increases the extent of experimentally induced infarction. Norepinephrine also increases myocardial oxygen consumption because of its peripheral vasoconstrictor and positive inotropic actions. Nevertheless, in a randomized trial of norepinephrine as a first-line vasopressor in patients with shock, norepinephrine associated with similar survival to dopamine as the comparator, with fewer arrhythmias.[150a] Subgroup analysis suggested that use of norepinephrine associated with lower mortality in patients with cardiogenic shock.

Dopamine and dobutamine can be particularly useful for patients with STEMI and reduced cardiac output, increased left ventricular filling pressure, pulmonary vascular congestion, and hypotension. Fortunately, the potentially deleterious alpha-adrenergic vasoconstrictor effects exerted by dopamine occur only at higher doses than those required to increase contractility. The vasodilating actions of dopamine on renal and splanchnic vessels and its positive inotropic effects generally improve hemodynamics and renal function. In patients with STEMI and severe left ventricular failure, this drug should be administered at a dose of 3 μg/kg/min while pulmonary capillary wedge and systemic arterial pressures and cardiac output are monitored. The dose can be increased stepwise to 20 μg/kg/min to reduce pulmonary capillary wedge pressure to approximately 20 mm Hg and elevate the cardiac index to exceed 2 liters/min/m^2. Dopamine doses exceeding 5 μg/kg/min can, however, activate peripheral alpha receptors and cause vasoconstriction.

Dobutamine has a positive inotropic action comparable to that of dopamine but a slightly less positive chronotropic effect and less vasoconstrictor activity.[150] In patients with STEMI, dobutamine improves left ventricular performance without augmenting enzymatically estimated infarct size. It can be administered in a starting dose of 2.5 μg/kg/min and increased stepwise to a maximum of 30 μg/kg/min. Both dopamine and dobutamine must be given carefully and with constant monitoring of the ECG, systemic arterial pressure, pulmonary artery or pulmonary artery occlusive pressure and, if possible, frequent measurements of cardiac output. The dose must be reduced if the heart rate exceeds 100 to 110 beats/min, if supraventricular or ventricular tachyarrhythmias occur, or if ST-segment deviations increase.

OTHER POSITIVE INOTROPIC AGENTS. Milrinone is a noncatecholamine, nonglycoside, phosphodiesterase inhibitor with inotropic and vasodilating actions.[150] It is useful for selected patients whose heart failure persists despite treatment with diuretics, who are not hypotensive, and who are likely to benefit from both an enhancement in contractility and afterload reduction. Milrinone should be given as a loading dose of 0.5 μg/kg/min over 10 minutes, followed by a maintenance infusion of 0.375 to 0.75 μg/kg/min. The loading dose may be reduced or omitted if the patient has borderline hypotension.

Cardiogenic Shock

Cardiogenic shock is the most severe clinical expression of left ventricular failure and is associated with extensive damage to the left ventricular myocardium in more than 80% of STEMI patients in whom it occurs; the remainder have a mechanical defect such as ventricular septal or papillary muscle rupture or predominant right ventricular infarction. In the past, cardiogenic shock was reported to occur in up to 20% of patients with STEMI, but estimates from recent large trials and observational databases report an incidence in the range of 5% to 8%.[145] This low-output state is characterized by elevated ventricular filling pressures, low cardiac output, systemic hypotension, and evidence of vital organ hypoperfusion (e.g., clouded sensorium, cool extremities, oliguria, acidosis). Patients with cardiogenic shock caused by STEMI are more likely to be older, to have a history of diabetes mellitus, a prior MI or congestive heart failure, and to have sustained an anterior infarction at the time of development of shock. Mechanical complications should be strongly considered in patients with nonanterior MI who develop shock. Of note, although the incidence of cardiogenic shock in patients with STEMI has been relatively stable since the mid-1970s, the short-term mortality rate has decreased from 70% to 80% in the 1970s to 50% to 60% in the 1990s. Moreover, it is possible to stratify risk among patients with shock to identify those with a mortality rate lower than 50% with intensive therapy, including revascularization. Cardiogenic shock is the cause of death in about 60% of patients dying after fibrinolysis for STEMI.[89,151]

PATHOLOGIC FINDINGS. At autopsy, more than two thirds of patients with cardiogenic shock demonstrate stenosis of 75% or more of the luminal diameter of all three major coronary vessels, usually including the left anterior descending coronary artery. Almost all patients with cardiogenic shock are found to have thrombotic occlusion of the artery supplying the major region of recent infarction, with loss of about 40% of the left ventricular mass.[145] Patients who die as a consequence of cardiogenic shock often have piecemeal necrosis—that is, progressive myocardial necrosis from marginal extension of their infarct into an ischemic zone bordering on the infarction. This finding generally is associated with persistent elevation of cardiac biomarker levels. Such extensions and focal lesions are probably in part the result of the shock state itself. Early deterioration in left ventricular function secondary to apparent extension of infarction may, in some cases, result from expansion of the necrotic zone of myocardium without actual extension of the necrotic process. Hydrodynamic forces that develop during ventricular systole can disrupt necrotic myocardial muscle bundles, with resultant expansion and thinning of the akinetic zone of myocardium; this in turn results in the deterioration of overall left ventricular function.

Other causes of cardiogenic shock in patients with STEMI include mechanical defects such as rupture of the ventricular septum, a papillary muscle, or free wall with tamponade, right ventricular infarction, or a marked reduction of preload caused by conditions such as hypovolemia.[145]

PATHOPHYSIOLOGY. The shock state in patients with STEMI appears to be the result of a vicious cycle (see Chap. 54, Fig. 54-12).

DIAGNOSIS. Cardiogenic shock is characterized by marked and persistent (longer than 30 minutes) hypotension, with systolic arterial pressure lower than 80 mm Hg and a marked reduction of cardiac index (generally, <1.8 liters/min/m^2) in the face of elevated left ventricular filling pressure (pulmonary capillary wedge pressure

>18 mm Hg). Spurious estimates of left ventricular filling pressure based on measurements of the pulmonary artery wedge pressure can occur in the presence of marked mitral regurgitation, in which the tall *v* wave in the left atrial (and pulmonary artery wedge) pressure tracing elevates the mean pressure above the left ventricular end-diastolic pressure. Accordingly, mitral regurgitation and other mechanical lesions such as ventricular septal defect, ventricular aneurysm, and pseudoaneurysm must be excluded before the diagnosis of cardiogenic shock caused by impairment of left ventricular function can be established. Mechanical complications should be suspected in any patient with STEMI in whom circulatory collapse occurs. Immediate hemodynamic, angiographic, and echocardiographic evaluations are necessary in patients with cardiogenic shock. It is important to exclude mechanical complications because primary therapy of such lesions usually requires immediate operative treatment, with intervening support of the circulation by intra-aortic balloon counterpulsation.

MEDICAL MANAGEMENT. When the mechanical complications noted are absent, cardiogenic shock is caused by impairment of left ventricular function. Inotropic and vasopressor agents may be given as pharmacologic support and should be used in the lowest possible doses. Although dopamine or dobutamine usually improves the hemodynamics in these patients, unfortunately neither appears to improve hospital survival significantly. Similarly, vasodilators have been used to elevate cardiac output and reduce left ventricular filling pressure, but by lowering the already markedly reduced coronary perfusion pressure, myocardial perfusion can be compromised further, accelerating the vicious cycle illustrated in Figure 54-12. Vasodilators may nonetheless be used in conjunction with intra-aortic balloon counterpulsation and inotropic agents to increase cardiac output while sustaining or elevating coronary perfusion pressure.

The systemic vascular resistance is usually elevated in patients with cardiogenic shock, but occasionally resistance is normal and, in a few cases, vasodilation actually predominates.[152] When systemic vascular resistance is not elevated (i.e., <1800 dynes/sec/cm^5) in patients with cardiogenic shock, norepinephrine, which has both alpha- and beta-adrenergic agonist properties, can be used to increase diastolic arterial pressure, maintain coronary perfusion, and improve contractility, in doses ranging from 2 to 10 μg/min. The use of alpha-adrenergic agents such as phenylephrine and methoxamine is contraindicated in patients with cardiogenic shock unless systemic vascular resistance is inordinately low. Calcium sensitizing agents, such as levosimendan, have been studied but have shown little incremental value in randomized trials.[153]

MECHANICAL SUPPORT (see Chap. 32).

Intra-Aortic Balloon Counterpulsation

Intra-aortic balloon counterpulsation is used in the treatment of STEMI in three groups of patients: (1) those whose conditions are hemodynamically unstable and for whom support of the circulation is required for the performance of cardiac catheterization and angiography to assess lesions that are potentially correctable surgically or by angioplasty; (2) those with cardiogenic shock that is unresponsive to medical management; and (3) rarely, those with refractory ischemia that is unresponsive to other treatments. In experimental animals, intra-aortic balloon counterpulsation decreases preload, increases coronary blood flow, and improves cardiac performance. Unfortunately, among patients with cardiogenic shock, improvement is often only temporary. Although a response to intra-aortic balloon counterpulsation correlates with better outcomes, counterpulsation alone does not improve overall survival in patients with or without a surgically remediable mechanical lesion.

Percutaneous Left Ventricular Assist Devices

Temporary mechanical support with left ventricular assist devices may allow time for recovery of stunned or hibernating myocardium.[154] A percutaneous left ventricular assist device may be placed by cannulation of the left femoral vein and advancement to the left atrium via transseptal puncture.[155] Blood from the left atrium is then returned via a nonpulsatile motor into the femoral artery. This system may provide up to 5 liters/min of flow. Small randomized trials have not revealed any outcomes advantage compared with intraaortic balloon counterpulsation,[145] but hemodynamic improvement is greater with the percutaneous left ventricular assist device. Another percutaneous alternative is a motorized device that is placed across the aortic valve and provides continuous flow of blood from the left ventricle into the aorta; it has been shown to provide superior hemodynamic support to intra-aortic balloon pump in patients with MI.[156] External surgically placed left ventricular devices as a bridge to transplantation or as a destination therapy are discussed in Chap. 32.

Complications

Complications of intra-aortic balloon counterpulsation include damage to or perforation of the aortic wall, ischemia distal to the site of insertion of the balloon in the femoral artery, thrombocytopenia, hemolysis, atheroemboli, infection, and mechanical failure, such as rupture of the balloon. Patients at highest risk include those with peripheral vascular disease, older patients, and women, particularly if they are small. These risk indicators should be taken into consideration before the institution of intra-aortic balloon counterpulsation. Because of the potential for vascular bleeding complications, there has been a reluctance to use intra-aortic pumps in patients who have undergone fibrinolytic therapy. But despite the increased bleeding risk, because of the poor outcome among patients with shock following thrombolysis (usually ineffective thrombolysis), this modality should be considered for selected patients who are candidates for an aggressive approach to revascularization. In addition to vascular complications, and complications associated with transseptal puncture, percutaneous left ventricular assist devices are also associated with the development of a systemic inflammatory response syndrome (SIRS) in some cases.[154]

REVASCULARIZATION. Of the five therapeutic modalities frequently used to treat patients with cardiogenic shock (vasopressors, mechanical support, fibrinolysis, PCI, and CABG), the first two are useful temporizing maneuvers. Revascularization, however, is associated with an improvement in survival.

The SHOCK study evaluated early revascularization for the treatment of patients with MI complicated by cardiogenic shock. Patients with shock caused by left ventricular failure complicating STEMI were randomized to emergency revascularization (n = 152), accomplished by CABG or angioplasty, or initial medical stabilization (n = 150). In 86% of patients in both groups, intra-aortic balloon counterpulsation was performed. The primary endpoint was all-cause mortality at 30 days; a secondary endpoint was mortality at 6 months. At 30 days, the overall mortality rate was 46.7% in the revascularization group, not significantly different from the 56% mortality rate observed in the medical therapy group (P = 0.11). Subgroups of patients in the SHOCK trial that showed particular benefit from the early revascularization strategy (i.e., reduced 6-month mortality) were those who were younger than 75 years of age, had a prior MI, and were randomized less than 6 hours from onset of infarction. Long-term survival improved significantly in patients with cardiogenic shock who underwent early revascularization (**Fig. 55-31**).[89] A subsequent observational study of patients with MI complicated by shock indicated that well-selected older patients undergoing PCI had similar 1-year survival to younger patients undergoing early revascularization.[157]

RECOMMENDATIONS. We recommend assessment of patients on an individualized basis to determine their desire for aggressive care and overall candidacy for further treatment (e.g., age, mental status, comorbidities). Patients with shock who are potential candidates for revascularization receive intra-aortic balloon counterpulsation and undergo coronary arteriography as soon as possible. Those with suitable anatomy should be revascularized as completely as possible with PCI and/or CABG.[35,89,145] There appears to be a benefit of revascularization with respect to survival as long as 48 hours after MI and 18 hours after the onset of shock. Left ventricular assist devices

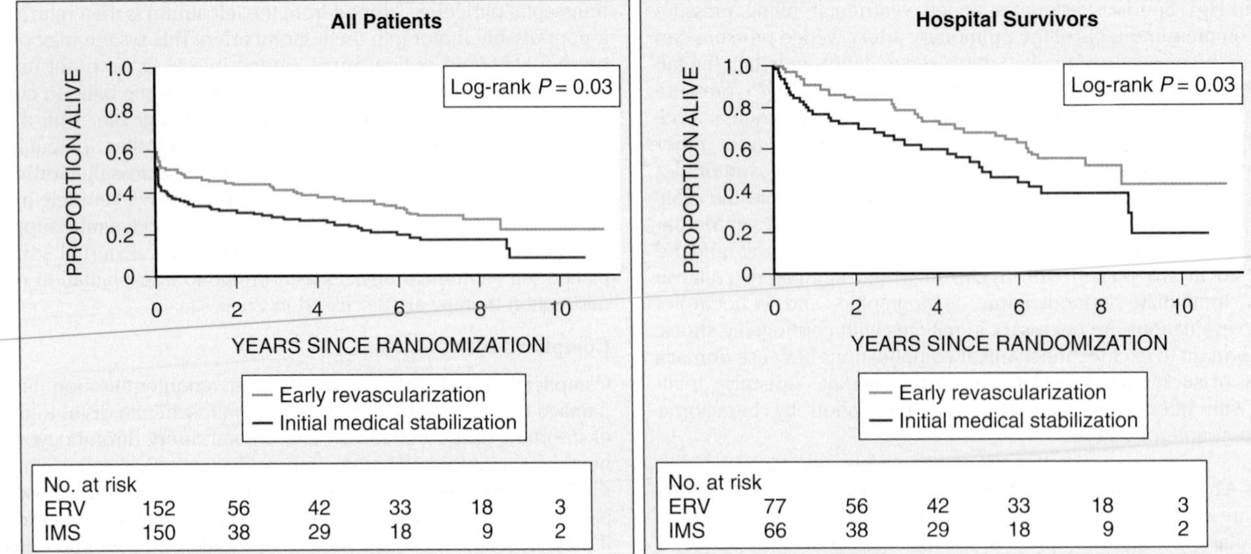

FIGURE 55-31 Impact of revascularization in patients in the SHOCK trial. Among all patients, the survival rates in the early revascularization (ERV) and initial medical stabilization (IMS) groups, respectively, were 41.4% versus 28.3% at 3 years and 32.8% versus 19.6% at 6 years. With the exclusion of eight patients with aortic dissection, tamponade, or severe mitral regurgitation identified shortly after randomization, the survival curves remained significantly different ($P = 0.02$), with a 14% absolute difference at 6 years. Among hospital survivors, the survival rates in the ERV and IMS groups, respectively, were 78.8% versus 64.3% at 3 years and 62.4% versus 44.4% at 6 years. *(From Hochman JS, Sleeper LA, Webb JG, Dzavik V, et al: Early revascularization and long-term survival in cardiogenic shock complicating acute myocardial infarction. JAMA 295:2511, 2006.)*

may be considered for patients with refractory shock after revascularization.

Right Ventricular Infarction

Right ventricular infarction can have a range of clinical presentations, from mild right ventricular dysfunction through cardiogenic shock. A characteristic hemodynamic pattern (**Fig. 55-32**) has been observed in patients with clinically significant right ventricular infarction, which frequently accompanies inferior left ventricular infarction or rarely occurs in isolated form. Right heart filling pressures (central venous, right atrial, and right ventricular end-diastolic pressures) are elevated, whereas left ventricular filling pressure is normal or only slightly raised, right ventricular systolic and pulse pressures are decreased, and cardiac output is often markedly depressed. Rarely, this disproportionate elevation of right-sided filling pressure causes right-to-left shunting through a patent foramen ovale. This possibility should be considered in patients with right ventricular infarction who have unexplained systemic hypoxemia. The finding of an elevation in the atrial natriuretic factor level in patients with this condition has led to the suggestion that abnormally high levels of this peptide might be partly responsible for the hypotension seen in patients with right ventricular infarction.

DIAGNOSIS. Many patients with the combination of normal left ventricular filling pressure and depressed cardiac index have right ventricular infarcts, with accompanying inferior left ventricular infarcts. The hemodynamic picture may superficially resemble that seen in patients with pericardial disease (see Chap. 75). It includes elevated right ventricular filling pressure, steep, right atrial *y* descent, and an early diastolic drop and plateau (resembling the square root sign) in the right ventricular pressure tracing. Moreover, patients with right ventricular infarction may display the Kussmaul sign (an increase in jugular venous pressure with inspiration) and pulsus paradoxus (a fall in systolic pressure of more than 10 mm Hg with inspiration; see Fig. 55-32).[158] The Kussmaul sign in the setting of inferior STEMI strongly predicts right ventricular involvement.

The ECG can provide the first clue that right ventricular involvement is present in the patient with inferior STEMI (see Fig. 55-32). Most patients with right ventricular infarction have ST-segment elevation in lead V_4R (right precordial lead in the V_4 position).[159] Transient elevation of the ST segment in any of the right precordial leads can occur with right ventricular MI, and the presence of ST-segment elevation of 0.1 mV or more in any one or a combination of leads V_4R, V_5R, and V_6R in patients with the clinical picture of acute MI indicates the diagnosis of right ventricular MI. Wellens[160] has emphasized that in addition to noting the presence or absence of convex upward ST-segment elevation in V_4R, clinicians should determine whether the T wave is positive or negative; such distinctions help distinguish proximal versus distal occlusion of the right coronary artery versus occlusion of the left circumflex artery (see Fig. 55-32). Elevation of the ST segments in leads V_1 through V_4 caused by right ventricular infarction can be confused with elevation caused by anteroseptal infarction. Although the elevated ST segments are oriented anteriorly in both cases, the frontal plane can provide important clues; the ST segments are oriented to the right in right ventricular infarction (e.g., +120 degrees), whereas they are oriented to the left in anteroseptal infarction (e.g., −30 degrees).

Noninvasive Assessment

Echocardiography is helpful in the differential diagnosis because in right ventricular infarction, in contrast to pericardial tamponade, little or no pericardial fluid accumulates. The echocardiogram shows abnormal wall motion of the right ventricle, as well as right ventricular dilation and depression of right ventricular ejection fraction.[161] CMR can also aid in the recognition of right ventricular infarction.[162] Serial studies have shown that some degree of recovery of an initially depressed right ventricular ejection fraction is the rule with right ventricular infarction, to a greater degree than with the left ventricular ejection fraction.[158]

Hemodynamics

Impaired left atrial filling in patients with right ventricular infarction can result in marked reductions in stroke volume and arterial blood pressure. Disproportionate elevation of the right-sided filling pressure is the hemodynamic hallmark of right ventricular infarction. Therefore, ventricular pacing may fail to increase cardiac output and atrioventricular sequential pacing may be required.

TREATMENT. Because of their ability to reduce preload, medications routinely prescribed for left ventricular infarction may produce profound hypotension in patients with right ventricular infarction. In

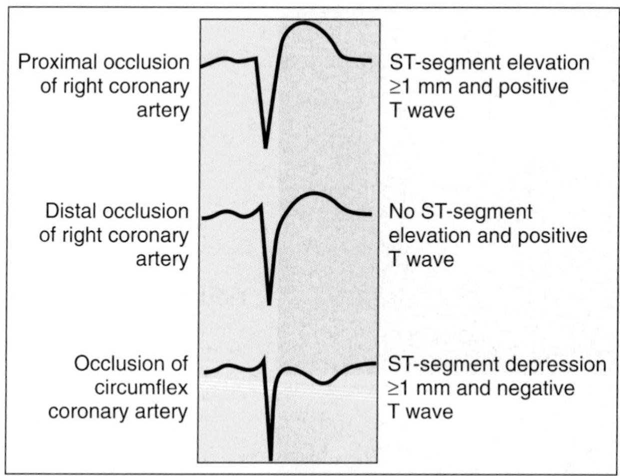

Clinical findings:
Shock with clear lungs, elevated JVP
Kussmaul sign

Hemodynamics:
Increased RA pressure (*y* descent)
Square root sign in RV tracing

ECG:
ST elevation in right-sided leads

Echo:
Depressed RV function

Management:
Maintain RV preload
Lower RV afterload (PA---PCW)
Restore AV synchrony
Inotropic support
Reperfusion

FIGURE 55-32 Right ventricular infarction, clinical features and management. Patients with hemodynamically significant right ventricular infarction present with shock but clear lungs and elevated JVP. ST-segment elevation exists in right-sided electrocardiographic leads with variation in the repolarization pattern depending on the infarct artery and the location of the occlusion. Management recommendations are shown at the bottom, right. Echo = echocardiogram; JVP = jugular venous pressure; PA = pulmonary artery; PCW = pulmonary capillary wedge; RA = right atrial; RV = right ventricular. *(Modified from Wellens HJ: The value of the right precordial leads of the electrocardiogram. N Engl J Med 340:381, 1999; and Antman EM, Anbe DT, Armstrong PW, et al: ACC/AHA guidelines for the management of patients with ST-elevation myocardial infarction: A report of the American College of Cardiology/American Heart Association Task Force on Practice Guidelines [Committee to Revise the 1999 Guidelines for the Management of Patients with Acute Myocardial Infarction]. Circulation 110:e82, 2004.)*

patients with hypotension caused by right ventricular MI, hemodynamics can be improved by a combination of expanding plasma volume to augment right ventricular preload and cardiac output and, when left ventricular failure is present, arterial vasodilators.[1] The initial therapy for hypotension in patients with right ventricular infarction should almost always be volume expansion. If hypotension has not been corrected after brisk administration of 1 liter or more of fluid, however, consideration should be given to hemodynamic monitoring with a pulmonary artery catheter, because further volume infusion may be of little use and may produce pulmonary congestion. Vasodilators reduce the impedance to left ventricular outflow and in turn left ventricular diastolic, left atrial, and pulmonary (arterial) pressures, thereby lowering the impedance to right ventricular outflow and enhancing right ventricular output.

Right ventricular infarction is common among patients with inferior left ventricular infarction. Therefore, otherwise unexplained systemic arterial hypotension or diminished cardiac output, or marked hypotension in response to small doses of nitroglycerin in patients with inferior infarction, should lead to the prompt consideration of this diagnosis. Patients requiring pacing should have atrial or atrioventricular sequential pacing. Successful reperfusion of the right coronary artery significantly improves right ventricular mechanical function and lowers in-hospital mortality in patients with right ventricular infarction. Replacement of the tricuspid valve and repair of the valve with annuloplasty rings have been carried out in the treatment of severe tricuspid regurgitation caused by right ventricular infarction.

Mechanical Causes of Heart Failure

FREE WALL RUPTURE. The most dramatic complications of STEMI are those that involve tearing or rupture of acutely infarcted tissue (**Fig. 55-33**). The clinical characteristics of these lesions vary considerably and depend on the site of rupture, which may involve the papillary muscles, interventricular septum, or free wall of either ventricle. The overall incidence of these complications is hard to assess because clinical and autopsy series differ considerably, but the incidence appears to be decreasing with the increasing use of reperfusion therapy.[163,164] **Table 55-12** shows the comparative clinical profile of these complications, as gathered from different studies. Rupture of the free wall of the infarcted ventricle (see Fig. 55-33) occurs in up to 10% of patients dying in the hospital of STEMI. Thinness of the apical wall, marked intensity of necrosis at the terminal end of the blood supply, poor collateral flow, the shearing effect of muscular contraction against an inert and stiffened necrotic area, and aging of the myocardium with laceration of the myocardial microstructure may all promote rupture.

Clinical Characteristics

The following are some features that characterize this serious complication of STEMI[164]:

1. Occurs more frequently in older patients, and possibly more frequently in women than in men with infarction.
2. Appears to be more common in hypertensive than in normotensive patients.
3. Occurs more frequently in the left than in the right ventricle and seldom occurs in the atria.
4. Usually involves the anterior or lateral walls of the ventricle in the area of the terminal distribution of the left anterior descending coronary artery.
5. Is usually associated with a relatively large transmural infarction involving at least 20% of the left ventricle.
6. Occurs between 1 day and 3 weeks, but most commonly 1 to 4 days, after infarction.
7. Is usually preceded by infarct expansion—that is, thinning and a disproportionate dilation within the softened necrotic zone.
8. Most commonly results from a distinct tear in the myocardial wall or a dissecting hematoma that perforates a necrotic area of myocardium (see Fig. 55-33).
9. Usually occurs near the junction of the infarct and the normal muscle.
10. Occurs less frequently in the center of the infarct, but when rupture occurs here, is usually during the second rather than the first week after the infarct.
11. Rarely occurs in a greatly thickened ventricle or in an area of extensive collateral vessels.
12. Most often occurs in patients without previous infarction.
13. No evidence that the intensity of anticoagulation influences the occurrence of rupture.
14. Occurs more commonly in patients who have received reperfusion therapy with a fibrinolytic versus PCI.[1]

Rupture of the free wall of the left ventricle usually leads to hemopericardium and death from cardiac tamponade. Occasionally, rupture

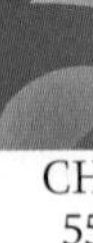

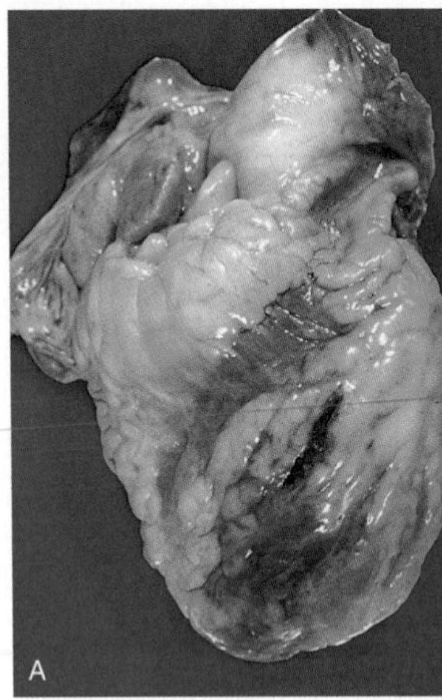

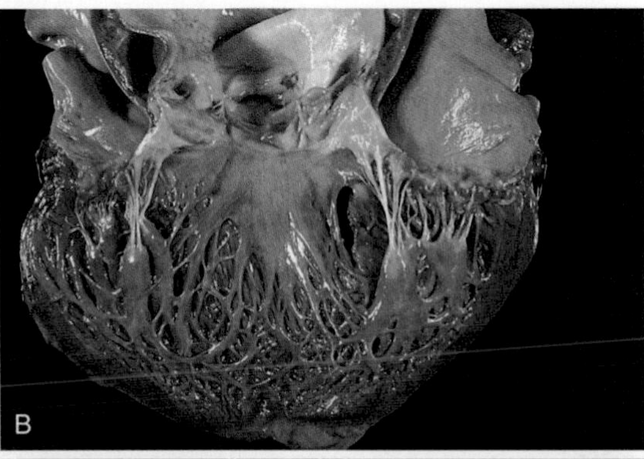

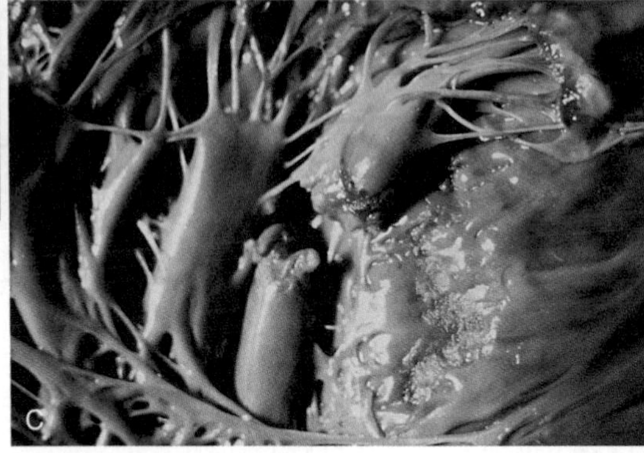

FIGURE 55-33 Cardiac rupture syndromes complicating STEMI. **A,** Anterior myocardial rupture in an acute infarct. **B,** Rupture of the ventricular septum. **C,** Complete rupture of a necrotic papillary muscle. *(From Schoen FJ: The heart. In Kumar V, Abbas AK, Fausto N [eds]: Robbins & Cotran Pathologic Basis of Disease. 8th ed. Philadelphia, Saunders, 2010, pp 529-587.)*

TABLE 55-12 Features of Ventricular Septal Rupture (VSR), Rupture of Ventricular Free Wall, and Papillary Muscle Rupture

FEATURE	VSR	RUPTURE OF VENTRICULAR FREE WALL	PAPILLARY MUSCLE RUPTURE
Incidence	1%-3% without reperfusion therapy, 0.2%-0.34% with fibrinolytic therapy, 3.9% among patients with cardiogenic shock	0.8%-6.2%; fibrinolytic therapy does not reduce risk; primary PTCA seems to reduce risk	About 1% (posteromedial more frequent than anterolateral papillary muscle)
Time course	Bimodal peak; within 24 hr and 3-5 days; range, 1-14 days	Bimodal peak; within 24 hr and 3-5 days; range, 1-14 days	Bimodal peak; within 24 hr and 3-5 days; range, 1-14 days
Clinical manifestations	Chest pain, shortness of breath, hypotension	Anginal, pleuritic, or pericardial chest pain, syncope, hypotension, arrhythmia, nausea, restlessness, sudden death	Abrupt onset of shortness of breath and pulmonary edema; hypotension
Physical findings	Harsh holosystolic murmur, thrill (+), S_3, accentuated second heart sound, pulmonary edema, RV and LV failure, cardiogenic shock	Jugular venous distention (29% of patients), pulsus paradoxus (47%), electromechanical dissociation, cardiogenic shock	A soft murmur in some cases, no thrill, variable signs of RV overload, severe pulmonary edema, cardiogenic shock
Echocardiographic findings	VSR, left-to-right shunt on color flow Doppler echocardiography through the ventricular septum, pattern of RV overload	>5 mm pericardial effusion not visualized in all cases; layered, high-acoustic echoes within the pericardium (blood clot); direct visualization of tear; signs of tamponade	Hypercontractile LV, torn papillary muscle or chordae tendineae, flail leaflet, severe MR on color flow Doppler echocardiography
Right-heart catheterization	Increase in oxygen saturation from the RA to RV, large *v* waves	Ventriculography insensitive, classic signs of tamponade not always present (equalization of diastolic pressures among the cardiac chambers)	No increase in oxygen saturation from the RA to RV, large *v* waves,* very high pulmonary-capillary wedge pressures

*Large *v* waves are from the pulmonary capillary wedge pressure.

LV = left ventricle or left ventricular; MR = mitral regurgitation; PTCA = percutaneous transluminal coronary angioplasty; RA = right atrium; RV = right ventricle or right ventricular.

From Antman EM, Anbe DT, Armstrong PW et al: ACC/AHA guidelines for the management of patients with ST-elevation myocardial infarction: A report of the American College of Cardiology/American Heart Association Task Force on Practice Guidelines (Committee to Revise the 1999 Guidelines for the Management of Patients with Acute Myocardial Infarction). Circulation 110:e82, 2004.

of the free wall of the ventricle occurs as the first clinical manifestation in patients with undetected or silent MI, and then it may be considered a form of sudden cardiac death (see Chap. 41).

The course of rupture varies from catastrophic, with an acute tear leading to immediate death, to subacute, with nausea, hypotension, and pericardial type of discomfort being the major clinical clues to its presence. Survival depends on the recognition of this complication, on hemodynamic stabilization of the patient—usually with inotropic agents and/or intra-aortic balloon pump—and, most importantly, on prompt surgical repair.[1] Initial percutaneous treatment of small or medium-sized ventricular septal defects with an occluder device offers a promising alternative to surgical closure or as an approach to initial medical stabilization facilitating delayed, definitive, surgical correction.[154,165]

Pseudoaneurysm

Incomplete rupture of the heart may occur when organizing thrombus and hematoma, together with pericardium, seal a rupture of the left ventricle and thus prevent the development of hemopericardium (**Fig. 55-34**). With time, this area of organized thrombus and pericardium can become a pseudoaneurysm (false aneurysm) that maintains communication with the cavity of the left ventricle. In contrast to true aneurysms, which always contain some myocardial elements in their walls, the walls of pseudoaneurysms are composed of organized hematoma and pericardium and lack any elements of the original myocardial wall. Pseudoaneurysms can become large, even equaling the true ventricular cavity in size, and communicate with the left ventricular cavity through a narrow neck. Frequently, pseudoaneurysms contain significant quantities of old and recent thrombi, superficial portions of which can cause arterial emboli. Pseudoaneurysms can drain off a portion of each ventricular stroke volume in the same manner as true aneurysms. The diagnosis of pseudoaneurysm can usually be made by echocardiography and contrast angiography, although at times, differentiation between true aneurysm and pseudoaneurysm can be difficult by any imaging technique.[166]

Diagnosis

The rupture usually presents with sudden profound shock, often rapidly leading to pulseless electrical activity caused by pericardial tamponade. Immediate pericardiocentesis confirms the diagnosis and relieves the pericardial tamponade, at least momentarily. If the patient's condition is relatively stable, echocardiography may help in establishing the diagnosis of tamponade.[1] Under the most favorable conditions, cardiac catheterization can be carried out, not necessarily to confirm the diagnosis of rupture but to delineate the coronary anatomy. This information helps guide CABG in patients with high-grade obstructive lesions during ventricular repair. In patients with critically compromised hemodynamics, establishment of the diagnosis should be followed immediately by surgical resection of the necrotic and ruptured myocardium with primary reconstruction. When rupture is subacute and a pseudoaneurysm is suspected or present, prompt elective surgery is indicated because rupture of the pseudoaneurysm occurs relatively frequently.[167]

RUPTURE OF THE INTERVENTRICULAR SEPTUM. Clinical features associated with an increased risk of rupture of the interventricular septum (see Table 55-12) include lack of development of a collateral network, advanced age, hypertension, anterior location of infarction, and possibly fibrinolysis.[168] Rupture of the interventricular septum after STEMI confers a high 30-day mortality.[164] The perforation can range in length from 1 cm to several centimeters (see Fig. 55-33). It can be a direct through-and-through opening or more irregular and serpiginous. The size of the defect determines the magnitude of the left-to-right shunt and the extent of hemodynamic deterioration, which in turn affects the likelihood of survival. As in rupture of the free wall of the ventricle, transmural infarction underlies rupture of the ventricular septum. Rupture of the septum with an anterior infarction tends to be apical in location, whereas inferior infarctions are associated with perforation of the basal septum and have a worse prognosis than those in an anterior location. In contrast with rupture of the free wall, rupture of the ventricular septum is more often associated with complete heart block, right bundle branch block, or atrial fibrillation. Almost all patients have multivessel coronary artery disease, with most exhibiting lesions in all the major vessels. The likelihood of survival depends on the degree of impairment of ventricular function and the size of the defect.

A ruptured interventricular septum is characterized by the appearance of a new harsh, loud holosystolic murmur that is heard best at the lower left sternal border and that is usually accompanied by a thrill.[1] Biventricular failure generally ensues within hours to days. The defect can also be recognized by echocardiography with color flow Doppler imaging (**Fig. 55-35**; see Fig. 15-31) or insertion of a pulmonary artery balloon catheter to document the left-to-right shunt. Catheter placement of an umbrella-shaped device within the ruptured septum may stabilize the condition of critically ill patients with acute septal rupture after STEMI.

RUPTURE OF A PAPILLARY MUSCLE. Partial or total rupture of a papillary muscle is a rare but often fatal complication of transmural MI (see Fig. 55-33).[169,170] Inferior wall infarction can lead to rupture of

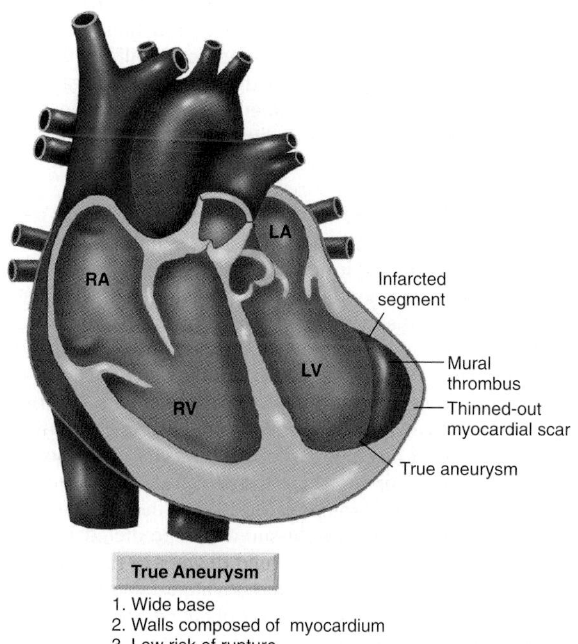

FIGURE 55-34 Differences between a pseudoaneurysm and a true aneurysm. LA = left atrium; LV = left ventricle; RA = right atrium; RV = right ventricle. *(From Shah PK: Complications of acute myocardial infarction.* In *Parmley W, Chatterjee K [eds]: Cardiology. Philadelphia, JB Lippincott, 1987.)*

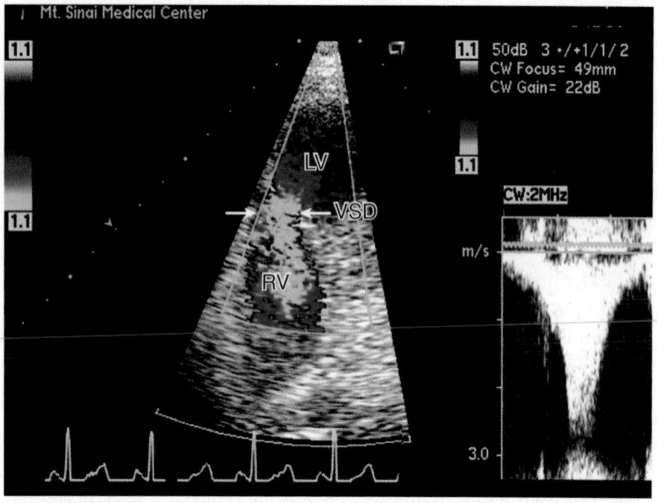

FIGURE 55-35 Two-dimensional echocardiography in an older female patient with a ventricular septal defect (VSD) that developed after a STEMI caused by occlusion of the left anterior descending coronary artery. Close-up of ventricular septum in apical four-chamber view **(left)** demonstrates turbulent systolic color flow Doppler across large VSD. Continuous wave Doppler **(right)** demonstrates systolic flow across VSD. LV = left ventricle; RV = right ventricle. *(From Kamran M, Attari M, Webber G: Images in cardiovascular medicine. Ventricular septal defect complicating an acute myocardial infarction. Circulation 112:e337, 2005.)*

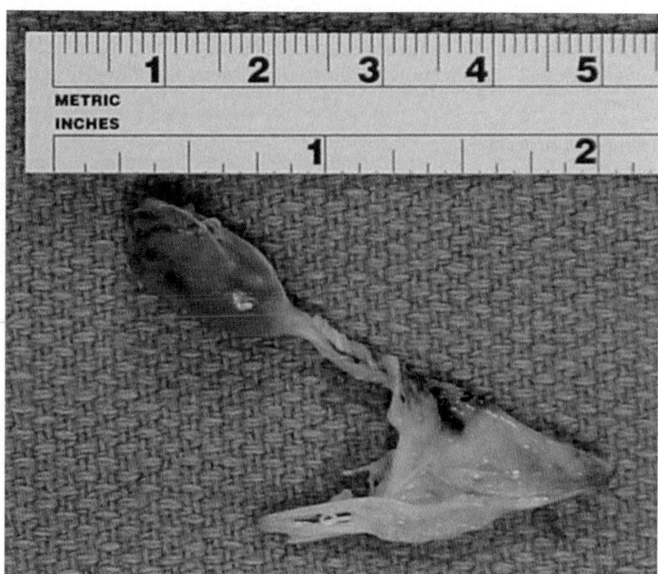

FIGURE 55-36 Surgical specimen showing papillary muscle **(top left),** chordae, and anterior mitral leaflet **(bottom right)** from a patient who had partial rupture of the papillary muscle and underwent mitral valve replacement for severe mitral regurgitation after STEMI. *(Courtesy of Dr. John Byrne.)*

the posteromedial papillary muscle, which occurs more commonly than rupture of the anterolateral muscle, a consequence of anterolateral MI. Rupture of a right ventricular papillary muscle is unusual but can cause massive tricuspid regurgitation and right ventricular failure. Complete transection of a left ventricular papillary muscle is incompatible with life because the sudden massive mitral regurgitation that develops cannot be tolerated. Rupture of a portion of a papillary muscle, usually the tip or head of the muscle, resulting in severe, although not necessarily overwhelming, mitral regurgitation, is much more frequent and is not immediately fatal (**Fig. 55-36**). Unlike rupture of the ventricular septum, which occurs with large infarcts, papillary muscle rupture occurs with a relatively small infarction in approximately half of the cases seen. The extent of coronary artery disease in these patients sometimes is modest as well. In a small number of patients, rupture of more than one cardiac structure is noted clinically or at postmortem examination; all possible combinations of rupture of the free left ventricular wall, interventricular septum, and papillary muscles can occur.[171]

As with patients who have a ruptured ventricular septal defect, those with papillary muscle rupture manifest a new holosystolic murmur and develop increasingly severe heart failure.[170] In both conditions, the murmur may become softer or disappear as arterial pressure falls. Mitral regurgitation caused by partial or complete rupture of a papillary muscle can be promptly recognized echocardiographically. Color flow Doppler imaging is particularly helpful in distinguishing acute mitral regurgitation from a ventricular septal defect in the setting of STEMI (see Table 55-12).[1] Therefore, an echocardiogram should be obtained immediately on any patient in whom the diagnosis is suspected because hemodynamic deterioration can ensue rapidly. Echocardiography also often permits differentiation of papillary muscle rupture from other, generally less severe forms of mitral regurgitation that occur with STEMI.

DIFFERENTIATION BETWEEN VENTRICULAR SEPTAL RUPTURE AND MITRAL REGURGITATION. It may be difficult, on clinical grounds, to distinguish between acute mitral regurgitation and rupture of the ventricular septum in patients with STEMI who suddenly develop a loud systolic murmur.[170] This differentiation can be made most readily by color flow Doppler echocardiography. In addition, a right-heart catheterization with a balloon-tipped catheter can readily distinguish between these two complications. Patients with ventricular septal rupture demonstrate a "step-up" in oxygen saturation in blood samples from the right ventricle and pulmonary artery compared with those from the right atrium. Patients with acute mitral regurgitation lack this step-up. They also may demonstrate tall *c-v* waves in both the pulmonary capillary and pulmonary arterial pressure tracings.

Invasive monitoring, which is essential in these patients, also allows for the critically important assessment of ventricular function.[1] Right and left ventricular filling pressures (right atrial and pulmonary capillary wedge pressures) guide fluid administration or the use of diuretics, whereas measurements of cardiac output and mean arterial pressure permit the calculation of systemic vascular resistance to direct vasodilator therapy. Unless systolic pressure is below 90 mm Hg, this therapy, generally using nitroglycerin or nitroprusside, should be instituted as soon as possible once hemodynamic monitoring is available. This may be critically important for stabilizing the patient's condition in preparation for further diagnostic studies and surgical repair. If vasodilator therapy is not tolerated or if it fails to achieve hemodynamic stability, intra-aortic balloon counterpulsation should be instituted rapidly.

SURGICAL TREATMENT. Operative intervention is most successful in patients with STEMI and circulatory collapse when a surgically correctable mechanical lesion such as ventricular septal defect or mitral regurgitation can be identified and repaired. In such patients, the circulation should at first be supported by intra-aortic balloon pulsation and a positive inotropic agent such as dopamine or dobutamine in combination with a vasodilator, unless the patient is hypotensive. Surgery should not be delayed in patients with a correctable lesion who agree to an aggressive management strategy and require pharmacologic and/or mechanical (counterpulsation) support. Such patients frequently develop a serious complication (e.g., infection, adult respiratory distress syndrome, extension of the infarct, renal failure) if surgery is delayed. Surgical survival is predicted by early operation, short duration of shock, and mild degrees of right and left ventricular impairment.[164,172] When the hemodynamic status of a patient with one of these mechanical lesions complicating STEMI remains stable after the patient has been weaned from pharmacologic and/or mechanical support, it may be possible to postpone the operation for 2 to 4 weeks to allow some healing of the infarct to occur).[1] Surgical repair involves correction of mitral regurgitation, insertion of a prosthetic mitral valve

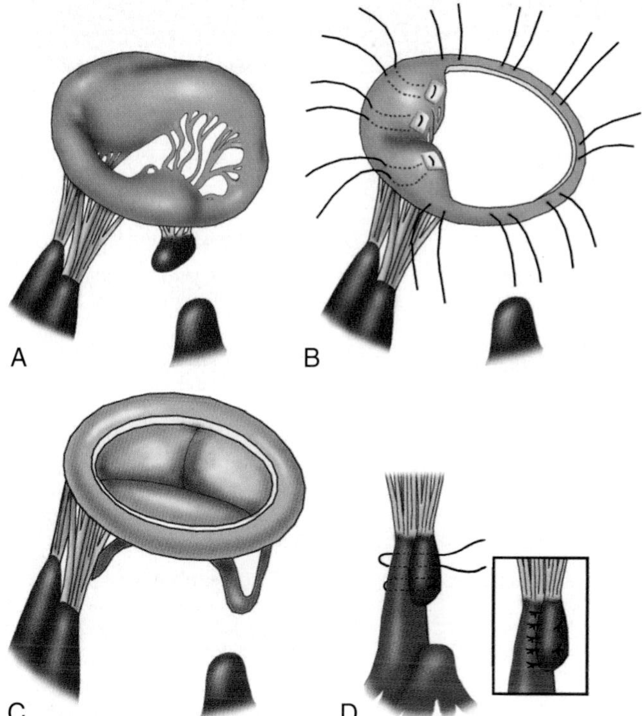

FIGURE 55-37 Surgical management of mitral regurgitation caused by ruptured papillary muscle. **A,** Acute papillary muscle rupture results in severe mitral regurgitation caused by leaflet and commissural prolapse. Mitral valve replacement is usually necessary. **B,** Mitral débridement with retention of the unruptured commissural and leaflet segment is performed to preserve partial annular papillary continuity. **C,** Mitral valve replacement is then performed. **D,** Occasionally, mitral valve repair can be performed by transfer of a papillary head to a nonruptured segment. *(Courtesy of Dr. David Adams, Division of Cardiac Surgery, Mount Sinai Hospital, New York.)*

repair, or closure of a ventricular septal defect, usually accompanied by coronary revascularization (**Figs. 55-37** and **55-38**).

Arrhythmias

Arrhythmias that can complicate the course of patients with STEMI and their prevention and treatment in this setting are discussed here and summarized in **Table 55-13**.

The incidence of arrhythmias is higher in patients the earlier they are seen after the onset of symptoms. Many serious arrhythmias develop before hospitalization, even before the patient is monitored. Some abnormality of cardiac rhythm also occurs in most patients with STEMI treated in CCUs. Patients seen very early during the course of STEMI almost invariably exhibit evidence of increased activity of the autonomic nervous system. Thus, sinus bradycardia, sometimes associated with AV block, and hypotension reflect augmented vagal activity.

MECHANISM OF ARRHYTHMIAS. A leading hypothesis for a major mechanism of arrhythmias in the acute phase of coronary occlusion is reentry caused by inhomogeneity of the electrical characteristics of ischemic myocardium.[173,174] The cellular electrophysiologic mechanisms for reperfusion arrhythmias appear to include washout of various ions, such as lactate and potassium, and toxic metabolic substances that have accumulated in the ischemic zone.

HEMODYNAMIC CONSEQUENCES. Patients with significant left ventricular dysfunction have a relatively fixed stroke volume and depend on changes in heart rate to alter cardiac output. However, there is a narrow range of heart rate over which the cardiac output is maximal, with significant reductions occurring at faster and slower

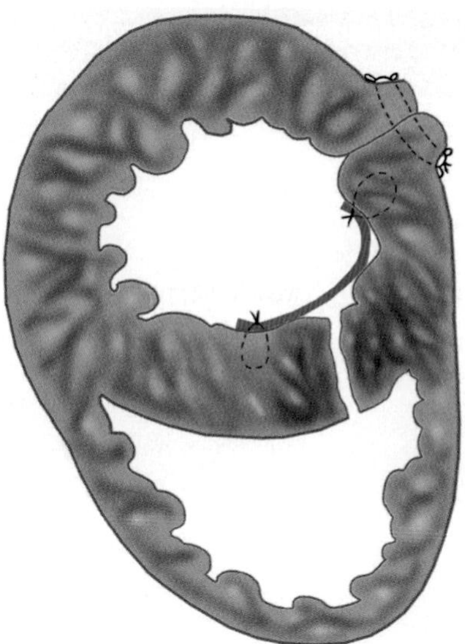

FIGURE 55-38 Repair of ischemic ventricular septal defect. The infarct typically involves a free wall and septum. Repair of the defect is performed through an incision in the ventricular wall infarct. The septal defect is closed with a prosthetic patch and a second patch is used to close the incision in the free wall. *(Courtesy of Dr. David Adams, Division of Cardiac Surgery, Mount Sinai Hospital, New York.)*

rates. Thus, all forms of bradycardia and tachycardia can depress cardiac output in patients with STEMI. Although the optimal rate insofar as cardiac output is concerned may exceed 100 beats/min, it is important to consider that heart rate is one of the major determinants of myocardial oxygen consumption and that at more rapid heart rates, myocardial energy needs can be elevated to levels that adversely affect the ischemic myocardium. Therefore, in patients with STEMI, the optimal rate is usually lower, in the range of 60 to 80 beats/min.

A second factor to consider in assessing the hemodynamic consequences of a particular arrhythmia is the loss of the atrial contribution to ventricular preload. In patients without STEMI, loss of atrial transport decreases left ventricular output by 15% to 20%. In patients with reduced diastolic left ventricular compliance of any cause (including STEMI), however, atrial systole is of greater importance for left ventricular filling. In patients with STEMI, atrial systole boosts end-diastolic volume by 15%, end-diastolic pressure by 29%, and stroke volume by 35%.

Ventricular Arrhythmias (see Chap. 39)

VENTRICULAR PREMATURE DEPOLARIZATIONS. Before the widespread use of reperfusion therapy, aspirin, beta blockers, and intravenous nitrates in the management of STEMI, it was believed that frequent ventricular premature complexes (VPCs; more than five/min), VPCs with multiform configuration, early coupling (the R-on-T phenomenon), and repetitive patterns in the form of couplets or salvos presaged ventricular fibrillation. It is now clear, however, that such warning arrhythmias are present in as many patients who do not develop fibrillation as in those who do. Several reports have shown that primary ventricular fibrillation (see later) occurs without antecedent warning arrhythmias and may even develop in spite of suppression of warning arrhythmias.[1] Both primary ventricular fibrillation and VPCs, especially R-on-T beats, occur during the early phase of STEMI, when considerable heterogeneity of electrical activity is present. Although R-on-T beats expose this heterogeneity and can precipitate ventricular fibrillation in a small minority of patients, the ubiquitous nature of VPCs in patients with STEMI and the extremely infrequent nature of ventricular fibrillation in the current era of STEMI management produce unacceptably low sensitivity and specificity of electrocardiographic patterns observed on monitoring systems for identifying patients at risk of ventricular fibrillation.

TABLE 55-13 Management of Cardiac Arrhythmias During Acute Myocardial Infarction

CATEGORY	ARRHYTHMIA	OBJECTIVE OF TREATMENT	THERAPEUTIC OPTIONS
Electrical instability	Ventricular premature beats	Correction of electrolyte deficits and increased sympathetic tone	Potassium and magnesium solutions, beta blocker
	Ventricular tachycardia	Prophylaxis against ventricular fibrillation, restoration of hemodynamic stability	Antiarrhythmic agents; cardioversion/defibrillation
	Ventricular fibrillation	Urgent reversion to sinus rhythm	Defibrillation; bretylium tosylate
	Accelerated idioventricular rhythm	Observation unless hemodynamic function is compromised	Increase sinus rate (atropine, atrial pacing); antiarrhythmic agents
	Nonparoxysmal atrioventricular junctional tachycardia	Search for precipitating causes (e.g., digitalis intoxication); suppress arrhythmia only if hemodynamic function is compromised	Atrial overdrive pacing; antiarrhythmic agents; cardioversion relatively contraindicated if digitalis intoxication present
Pump failure, excessive sympathetic stimulation	Sinus tachycardia	Reduce heart rate to diminish myocardial oxygen demands	Antipyretics; analgesics; consider beta blocker unless congestive heart failure present; treat latter if present with anticongestive measures (diuretics, afterload reduction)
	Atrial fibrillation and/or atrial flutter	Reduce ventricular rate; restore sinus rhythm	Verapamil, digitalis glycosides; anticongestive measures (diuretics, afterload reduction); cardioversion; rapid atrial pacing (for atrial flutter)
	Paroxysmal supraventricular tachycardia	Reduce ventricular rate; restore sinus rhythm	Vagal maneuvers; verapamil, cardiac glycosides, beta-adrenergic blockers; cardioversion; rapid atrial pacing
Bradyarrhythmias and conduction disturbances	Sinus bradycardia	Acceleration of heart rate only if hemodynamic function is compromised	Atropine; atrial pacing
	Junctional escape rhythm	Acceleration of sinus rate only if loss of atrial "kick" causes hemodynamic compromise	Atropine; atrial pacing
	Atrioventricular block and intraventricular block		Insertion of pacemaker

Modified from Antman EM, Rutherford JD (eds): Coronary Care Medicine: A Practical Approach. Boston, Martinus Nijhoff, 1986, p 78.

Management

Because the incidence of ventricular fibrillation in patients with STEMI seen in CCUs over the past three or four decades appears to be declining, the prior practice of prophylactic suppression of ventricular premature beats with antiarrhythmic drugs no longer is necessary, and its use may actually increase the risk of fatal bradycardic and asystolic events.[175] Therefore, we pursue a conservative course when VPCs are observed in STEMI patients and do not routinely prescribe antiarrhythmic drugs, but instead determine whether recurrent ischemia or electrolyte or metabolic disturbances are present.[1] When, at the inception of an infarction, VPCs accompany sinus tachycardia, augmented sympathoadrenal stimulation is often a contributing factor and can be treated by beta-adrenergic blockade. In fact, the early administration of an intravenous beta blocker is effective in reducing the incidence of ventricular fibrillation in cases of evolving MI.

ACCELERATED IDIOVENTRICULAR RHYTHM. This arrhythmia is seen in up to 20% of patients with STEMI. It occurs frequently during the first 2 days, with about equal frequency in anterior and inferior infarctions. Most episodes are of short duration. Accelerated idioventricular rhythm is often observed shortly after successful reperfusion has been established. However, the frequent occurrence of this rhythm in patients without reperfusion limits their reliability as markers of restoration of patency of the infarct-related coronary artery.[1] In contrast to rapid ventricular tachycardia, accelerated idioventricular rhythm is thought not to affect prognosis, and we do not routinely treat accelerated idioventricular rhythms.

VENTRICULAR TACHYCARDIA. Nonsustained runs of ventricular tachycardia early after presentation do not appear to be associated with an increased mortality risk, either during hospitalization or over the first year. Ventricular tachycardia occurring late in the course of STEMI is more common in patients with transmural infarction and left ventricular dysfunction, is likely to be sustained, usually induces marked hemodynamic deterioration, and is associated with increased rates of hospital and long-term mortality.

Management

Because hypokalemia can increase the risk of developing ventricular tachycardia, low serum potassium levels should be identified quickly after a patient's admission for STEMI and should be treated promptly. We strive to maintain the serum potassium level above 4.5 mEq/liter and serum magnesium level above 2 mEq/liter. Rapid abolition of sustained ventricular tachycardia in patients with STEMI is mandatory because of its deleterious effect on pump function and because it frequently deteriorates into ventricular fibrillation. After reversion to sinus rhythm, every effort should be made to correct underlying abnormalities, such as hypoxia, hypotension, acid-base or electrolyte disturbances, and digitalis excess. Although no definitive data are available, it is a common clinical practice to continue maintenance infusions of antiarrhythmic drugs for several days after an index episode of ventricular tachycardia, discontinue the drug, and either observe the patient for recurrence or perform a diagnostic electrophysiology study. Patients with recurrent or refractory ventricular tachycardia should be considered for specialized procedures, such as implantation of antitachycardia devices or surgery. Occasionally, urgent attempts at revascularization with angioplasty or CABG can help control refractory ventricular tachycardia.

VENTRICULAR FIBRILLATION. Ventricular fibrillation can occur in three settings in hospitalized patients with STEMI. (Its occurrence as a mechanism of sudden death is discussed in Chap. 41.) Primary ventricular fibrillation occurs suddenly and unexpectedly in patients with no or few signs or symptoms of left ventricular failure. Although primary ventricular fibrillation occurred in up to 10% of patients hospitalized with STEMI several decades ago, analyses have suggested that its incidence has declined. Secondary ventricular fibrillation is often the final event of a progressive downhill course with left ventricular failure and cardiogenic shock. So-called late ventricular fibrillation develops more than 48 hours after STEMI and frequently but not exclusively occurs in patients with large infarcts and ventricular dysfunction. Patients with intraventricular conduction defects and anterior wall infarction, with persistent sinus tachycardia, atrial flutter, or fibrillation early in the clinical course, and with right ventricular infarction who require ventricular pacing are at higher risk for suffering late in-hospital ventricular fibrillation than are patients without these features.

Prognosis

Debate continues on the effect of primary ventricular fibrillation on prognosis.[176] Now, with the availability of amiodarone and implantable cardioverter-defibrillators (ICDs), the prognosis of late ventricular fibrillation is improving and is probably driven more by residual ventricular function and recurrent ischemia than by the arrhythmic risk per se.

Prophylaxis

Lidocaine prophylaxis to prevent primary ventricular fibrillation is no longer advised. Hypokalemia is associated with the risk of ventricular fibrillation in the CCU.[1] Although it has not been conclusively shown that correction of hypokalemia to a level of 4.5 mEq/liter actually reduces the incidence of ventricular fibrillation, our experience suggests that this probably is protective and of little risk. Despite the lack of a consistent relationship between hypomagnesemia and ventricular fibrillation, magnesium deficits may still be linked to the risk of ventricular fibrillation because intracellular magnesium levels are reduced in patients with STEMI and are not adequately reflected by serum measurements. For these reasons, and because it is often difficult to repair a potassium deficit without administering supplemental magnesium, we routinely replete magnesium to a level of 2 mEq/liter. The only situation in which we might consider prophylactic lidocaine (bolus of 1.5 mg/kg, followed by 20 to 50 μg/kg/min) would be the unusual circumstance in which a patient within the first 12 hours of a STEMI must be managed in a facility in which cardiac monitoring is not available and equipment for prompt defibrillation is not readily accessible.

Management

Treatment for ventricular fibrillation (see Chaps. 37 and 39) consists of an unsynchronized electrical countershock with at least 200 to 300 J, implemented as rapidly as possible.[1] When ventricular fibrillation occurs outside an intensive care unit, resuscitative efforts are much less likely to be successful, primarily because the time interval between the onset of the episode and institution of definitive therapy tends to be prolonged. Failure of electrical countershock to restore an effective cardiac rhythm is almost always caused by rapidly recurrent ventricular tachycardia or ventricular fibrillation, electromechanical dissociation, or, rarely, electrical asystole.

Successful interruption of ventricular fibrillation or prevention of refractory recurrent episodes can also be facilitated by administration of intravenous amiodarone. When synchronous cardiac electrical activity is restored by countershock but contraction is ineffective (i.e., pulseless electrical activity), the usual underlying cause is extensive myocardial ischemia or necrosis or rupture of the ventricular free wall or septum. If rupture has not occurred, intracardiac administration of calcium gluconate or epinephrine may promote restoration of an effective heartbeat. We do not usually administer bicarbonate injections to correct acidosis because of the high osmotic load they impose and the fact that hyperventilation of the patient is probably a more suitable means of clearing the acidosis.

Bradyarrhythmias (see Chap. 39)

SINUS BRADYCARDIA. Sinus bradycardia occurs commonly during the early phases of STEMI, particularly in patients with inferior and posterior infarction.[1] On the basis of data obtained in experimental infarction studies and from some clinical observations, the increased vagal tone that produces sinus bradycardia during the early phase of STEMI may actually be protective, perhaps because it reduces myocardial oxygen demands. Thus, the acute mortality rate appears similar in patients with sinus bradycardia to the rate in those without this arrhythmia.

Management

Isolated sinus bradycardia, unaccompanied by hypotension or ventricular ectopy, should be observed rather than treated initially. In the first 4 to 6 hours after infarction, if the sinus rate is extremely slow (<40 to 50 beats/min) and associated with hypotension, intravenous atropine in doses of 0.3 to 0.6 mg every 3 to 10 minutes (with a total dose not exceeding 2 mg) can be administered to bring the heart rate up to approximately 60 beats/min.

ATRIOVENTRICULAR AND INTRAVENTRICULAR BLOCK. Ischemic injury can produce conduction block at any level of the AV or intraventricular conduction system. Such blocks can occur in the AV node and the bundle of His, producing various grades of AV block, in either main bundle branch, producing right or left bundle branch block, and in the anterior and posterior divisions of the left bundle, producing left anterior or left posterior (fascicular) divisional blocks. Disturbances of conduction can occur in various combinations. Clinical features of proximal and distal AV conduction disturbances in patients with STEMI are summarized in **Table 55-14.**

First-Degree Atrioventricular Block

First-degree AV block generally does not require specific treatment. Beta blockers and calcium antagonists (other than nifedipine) prolong AV conduction and may be responsible for first-degree AV block as well. However, discontinuation of these drugs in the setting of STEMI has the potential of increasing ischemia and ischemic injury. Therefore, it is our practice not to decrease the dosage of these drugs unless the PR interval is longer than 0.24 second. Only if higher degree block or hemodynamic impairment occurs should these agents be stopped. If the block is a manifestation of excessive vagotonia and is associated with sinus bradycardia and hypotension, administration of atropine, as already outlined, may be helpful. Continued electrocardiographic monitoring is important in such patients in view of the possibility of progression to higher degrees of block.

Second-Degree Atrioventricular Block

First-degree and type I second-degree AV blocks do not appear to affect survival, are most commonly associated with occlusion of the right coronary artery, and are caused by ischemia of the AV node (see Table 55-14). Specific therapy is not required in patients with second-degree type I AV block when the ventricular rate exceeds 50 beats/min and premature ventricular contractions, heart failure, and bundle branch block are absent. However, if these complications develop or if the heart rate falls below approximately 50 beats/min and the patient is symptomatic, immediate treatment with atropine (0.3 to 0.6 mg) is indicated; temporary pacing systems are almost never needed in the management of this arrhythmia.

Type II second-degree block usually originates from a lesion in the conduction system below the His bundle (see Table 55-14). Because of its potential for progression to complete heart block, type II second-degree AV block should be treated with a temporary external or transvenous demand pacemaker, with the rate set at approximately 60 beats/min.[1]

TABLE 55-14 Atrioventricular Conduction Disturbances in Acute Myocardial Infarction

	Location of Disturbance	
PARAMETER	**PROXIMAL**	**DISTAL**
Site of block	Intranodal	Infranodal
Site of infarction	Inferoposterior	Anteroseptal
Compromised arterial supply	RCA (90%), LCX (10%)	Septal perforators of LAD
Pathogenesis	Ischemia, necrosis, hydropic cell swelling, excess parasympathetic activity	Ischemia, necrosis, hydropic cell swelling
Predominant type of AV nodal block	(a) First-degree (PR > 200 msec) Mobitz type I, second-degree	(a) Mobitz type II, second-degree Third-degree
Common premonitory features of third-degree AV block	(a) First- or second-degree AV block (b) Mobitz I pattern	(a) Intraventricular conduction block (b) Mobitz II pattern
Features of escape rhythm following third-degree block (a) Location (b) QRS width (c) Rate (d) Stability of escape rhythm	(a) Proximal conduction system (His bundle) (b) <0.12/sec* (c) 45-60/min but may be as low as 30/min (d) Rate usually stable; asystole uncommon	(a) Distal conduction system (bundle branches) (b) >0.12/sec (c) Often <30/min (d) Rate often unstable with moderate to high risk of ventricular asystole
Duration of high-grade AV block	Usually transient (2-3 days)	Usually transient, but some form of AV conduction disturbance and/or intraventricular defect may persist
Associated mortality rate	Low unless associated with hypotension and/or congestive heart failure	High because of extensive infarction associated with power failure or ventricular arrhythmias
Pacemaker therapy (a) Temporary (b) Permanent	(a) Rarely required; may be considered for bradycardia associated with left ventricular power failure, syncope, or angina (b) Almost never indicated because conduction defect is usually transient	(a) Should be considered in patients with anteroseptal infarction and acute bifascicular block (b) Indicated for patients with high-grade AV block with block in His-Purkinje system and those with transient advanced AV block and associated bundle branch block

*Some studies have suggested that a wide QRS escape rhythm (>0.12 second) following high-grade AV block in inferior infarction is associated with a worse prognosis.
LAD = left anterior descending coronary artery; LCX = left circumflex coronary artery; RCA = right coronary artery.
Modified from Antman EM, Rutherford JD: Coronary Care Medicine: A Practical Approach. Boston, Martinus Nijhoff, 1986; and Dreifus LS, Fisch C, Griffin JC, et al: Guidelines for implantation of cardiac pacemakers and antiarrhythmia devices. J Am Coll Cardiol 18:1, 1991.

Complete (Third-Degree) Atrioventricular Block

Complete AV block can occur in patients with anterior or inferior infarction. Complete heart block in patients with inferior infarction usually results from an intranodal or supranodal lesion and develops gradually, often progressing from first-degree or type I second-degree block.[177] The escape rhythm is usually stable, without asystole and often junctional, with a rate exceeding 40 beats/min and a narrow QRS complex in 70% of cases and a slower rate and wide QRS in the others. This form of complete AV block is often transient, may be responsive to pharmacologic antagonism of adenosine with methylxanthines,[178] and resolves in most patients within a few days (see Table 55-14).

In patients with anterior infarction, third-degree AV block often occurs suddenly, 12 to 24 hours after the onset of infarction, although it is usually preceded by intraventricular block and often type II (not first-degree or type I) AV block. Such patients have unstable escape rhythms with wide QRS complexes and rates less than 40 beats/min; ventricular asystole may occur suddenly. In patients with anterior infarction, AV block usually develops as a result of extensive septal necrosis that involves the bundle branches. The high rate of mortality in this group of patients with slow idioventricular rhythm and wide QRS complexes is the consequence of extensive myocardial necrosis, which results in severe left ventricular failure and often shock (see Table 55-14).

Patients with inferior infarction often have concomitant ischemia or infarction of the AV node secondary to hypoperfusion of the AV node artery. However, the His-Purkinje system usually escapes injury in such individuals. Patients with inferior STEMI who develop AV block generally have lesions in both right and left anterior descending coronary arteries. Similarly, patients with inferior STEMI and AV block have larger infarcts and more depressed right ventricular and left ventricular function than patients with inferior infarct and no AV block. As noted, junctional escape rhythms with narrow QRS complexes occur commonly in this setting.

Although data suggest that complete AV block is not an independent risk factor for mortality, whether temporary transvenous pacing per se improves survival of patients with anterior STEMI remains controversial. Some investigators have contended that ventricular pacing is of no value when used to correct complete AV block in patients with anterior infarction in view of the poor prognosis in this group, regardless of therapy. However, pacing may protect against transient hypotension, with its attendant risks of extending infarction and precipitating malignant ventricular tachyarrhythmias. Also, pacing protects against asystole, a particular hazard in patients with anterior infarction and infranodal block. Improved survival with pacing probably occurs in only a small fraction of patients with complete AV block and anterior wall infarcts, because the extensive destruction of the myocardium that almost invariably accompanies this condition results in a high mortality rate, even in paced patients. Given these considerations, an extremely large series of patients would be required to demonstrate the small reduction of mortality that might be achieved by pacing. The absence of data supporting such an effect, however, by no means excludes the possibility that it may be present.

Pacing is not usually necessary in patients with inferior wall infarction and complete AV block that is often transient in nature, but it is indicated if the ventricular rate is slow (<40 to 50 beats/min), if ventricular arrhythmias or hypotension is present, or if pump failure develops; atropine is only rarely of value in these patients. Only when complete heart block develops in less than 6 hours after the onset of symptoms is atropine likely to abolish the AV block or cause acceleration of the escape rhythm. In such cases, the AV block is more likely to be transient and related to increases in vagal tone, rather than the more persistent block seen later in the course of STEMI, which generally requires cardiac pacing.

INTRAVENTRICULAR BLOCK. The right bundle branch and left posterior division have a dual blood supply from the left anterior descending and right coronary arteries, whereas the left anterior division is supplied by septal perforators originating from the left anterior descending coronary artery. Not all conduction blocks observed in patients with STEMI can be considered to be complications of infarcts because almost half are already present when the first ECG is recorded, and they may represent antecedent disease of the conduction system.[179] Compared with patients without conduction defects, STEMI patients with bundle branch blocks have more comorbid conditions, are less likely to receive therapies such as thrombolytics, aspirin, and beta blockers, and have an increased in-hospital mortality rate.[180] In the prefibrinolytic era, studies of intraventricular conduction disturbances (i.e., block within one or more of the three subdivisions [fascicles] of the His-Purkinje system [the anterior and posterior divisions of the left bundle and the right bundle]) had been reported to occur in 5% to 10% of patients with STEMI. More recent series in the reperfusion era have suggested that intraventricular blocks occur in about 2% to 5% of patients with MI.[181] Investigators performing primary PCI for STEMI have reported an association between new-onset bundle branch block and abnormal myocardial perfusion, even if flow through epicardial arteries is restored.[182]

Isolated Fascicular Block

Isolated left anterior divisional block is unlikely to progress to complete AV block. Mortality is increased in these patients, although not as much as in patients with other forms of conduction block. The posterior fascicle is larger than the anterior fascicle and, in general, a larger infarct is required to block it. As a consequence, mortality is markedly increased. Complete AV block is not a frequent complication of either form of isolated divisional block.

Right Bundle Branch Block

This conduction defect alone can lead to AV block because it is often a new lesion, associated with anteroseptal infarction. Isolated right bundle branch block is associated with an increased mortality risk in patients with anterior STEMI, even if complete AV block does not occur, but this appears to be the case only if it is accompanied by congestive heart failure.

Bifascicular Block

The combination of right bundle branch block with left anterior or posterior divisional block, or the combination of left anterior and posterior divisional blocks (i.e., left bundle branch block), is known as bidivisional or bifascicular block. If new block occurs in two of the three divisions of the conduction system, the risk of developing complete AV block is high. Mortality is also high because of the occurrence of severe pump failure secondary to the extensive myocardial necrosis required to produce such an extensive intraventricular block.[183] Patients with intraventricular conduction defects, particularly right bundle branch block, account for the majority of patients who develop ventricular fibrillation late in their hospital stay. However, the high rate of mortality in these patients occurs even in the absence of high-grade AV block and appears to be related to cardiac failure and massive infarction, rather than to the conduction disturbance.

Preexisting bundle branch block or divisional block is less often associated with the development of complete heart block in patients with STEMI than are conduction defects acquired during the course of the infarct. Bidivisional block in the presence of prolongation of the P-R interval (first-degree AV block) may indicate disease of the third subdivision rather than of the AV node; it is associated with a greater risk of complete heart block than if first-degree AV block is absent.

Complete bundle branch block (left or right), the combination of right bundle branch block and left anterior divisional (fascicular) block, and any of the various forms of trifascicular block are all more often associated with anterior than with inferoposterior infarction. All these forms are more frequent with large infarcts and in older patients, and have a higher incidence of other accompanying arrhythmias than that seen in patients without bundle branch block.

USE OF PACEMAKERS IN PATIENTS WITH ACUTE MYOCARDIAL INFARCTION (see Chap. 38)

Temporary Pacing

Just as is the case for complete AV block, transvenous ventricular pacing has not resulted in a statistically demonstrable improvement in prognosis in patients with STEMI who develop intraventricular conduction defects. However, temporary pacing is advisable in some of these patients because of the high risk of developing complete AV block. This includes patients with new bilateral (bifascicular) bundle branch block (i.e., right bundle branch block with left anterior or posterior divisional block and alternating right and left bundle branch block); first-degree AV block adds to this risk. Isolated new block in only one of the three fascicles, even with P-R prolongation and preexisting bifascicular block and a normal P-R interval, poses somewhat less risk; these patients should be monitored closely, with insertion of a temporary pacemaker deferred unless higher degree AV block occurs.

Noninvasive external temporary cardiac pacing is possible routinely in conscious patients and is acceptable to many patients, despite the discomfort. Used in a standby mode, it is almost free of complications and contraindications and provides an important alternative to transvenous endocardial pacing.[1] Once it is clinically evident that continuous pacing is required, external pacing, which is generally not well tolerated for more than minutes to hours, should be replaced by a temporary transvenous pacemaker.

Asystole

The presence of apparent ventricular asystole on monitor displays of continuously recorded ECGs may be misleading because the rhythm may actually be fine ventricular fibrillation. Because of the predominance of ventricular fibrillation as the cause of cardiac arrest in this setting, initial therapy should include electrical countershock, even if definitive electrocardiographic documentation of this arrhythmia is not available. In the rare case in which asystole can be documented as the responsible electrophysiologic disturbance, immediate transcutaneous pacing, or stimulation with a transvenous pacemaker if one is already in place, is indicated.[1]

Permanent Pacing

The question of the advisability of permanent pacemaker insertion is complicated because not all sudden deaths in STEMI patients with conduction defects are caused by high-grade AV block. A high incidence of late ventricular fibrillation occurs in CCU survivors with anterior STEMI complicated by right or left bundle branch block. Therefore, ventricular fibrillation, rather than asystole caused by failure of AV conduction and infranodal pacemakers, could be responsible for late sudden death.

Long-term pacing is often helpful when complete heart block persists throughout the hospital phase in a patient with STEMI, when sinus node function is markedly impaired, or when type II second- or third-degree block occurs intermittently.[1] When high-grade AV block is associated with newly acquired bundle branch block or other criteria of impairment of conduction system function, prophylactic long-term pacing may also be justified. Additional considerations that drive a decision to insert a permanent pacemaker include whether the patient is a candidate for an ICD or has severe heart failure that might be improved with biventricular pacing (see Chap. 28).

Supraventricular Tachyarrhythmias (see Chaps. 39 and 40)

SINUS TACHYCARDIA. This arrhythmia is typically associated with augmented sympathetic activity and may provoke transient hypertension or hypotension. Common causes are anxiety, persistent pain, left ventricular failure, fever, pericarditis, hypovolemia, pulmonary embolism, and the administration of cardioaccelerator drugs such as atropine, epinephrine, or dopamine; rarely, it occurs in patients with atrial infarction. Sinus tachycardia is particularly common in patients with anterior infarction, especially if there is significant accompanying left ventricular dysfunction. It is an undesirable rhythm in patients with STEMI because it results in an augmentation of myocardial oxygen consumption, as well as a reduction in the time available for coronary perfusion, thereby intensifying myocardial ischemia and/or external myocardial necrosis. Persistent sinus tachycardia can signify persistent heart failure and, under these circumstances, connotes poor prognosis and excess mortality. An underlying cause should be sought and appropriate treatment instituted, such as analgesics for pain, diuretics for heart failure, oxygen, beta blockers, and nitroglycerin for ischemia, and aspirin for fever or pericarditis.

Administration of beta blockers, in the dosage and manner described elsewhere in this chapter, may be helpful in the treatment of sinus tachycardia, particularly when this arrhythmia is a manifestation of a hyperdynamic circulation, which is seen particularly in young patients with an initial STEMI without extensive cardiac damage. Beta blocker administration is contraindicated, however, in patients in whom the sinus tachycardia is a manifestation of hypovolemia or of pump failure; the latter is indicated by a systolic arterial pressure below 100 mm Hg, rales involving more than one third of the lung fields, a pulmonary capillary wedge pressure exceeding 20 to 25 mm Hg, or a cardiac index below approximately 2.2 liters/min/m^2. A possible exception to this is a patient in whom persistent ischemia is believed to be the cause or the result of tachycardia—cautious administration of an ultrashort-acting beta blocker such as esmolol (25 to 200 µg/kg/min) can evaluate the patient's response to slowing of the heart rate.

ATRIAL FLUTTER AND FIBRILLATION. Atrial flutter is usually transient and, in patients with STEMI, is typically a consequence of augmented sympathetic stimulation of the atria, often occurring in patients with left ventricular failure, pulmonary emboli in whom the arrhythmia intensifies hemodynamic deterioration, or atrial infarction (see Table 55-13).

As with atrial premature complexes and atrial flutter, fibrillation is usually transient and tends to occur in patients with left ventricular failure but also occurs in those with pericarditis and ischemic injury to the atria and right ventricular infarction.[184] The increased ventricular rate and loss of the atrial contribution to left ventricular filling result in a significant reduction in cardiac output. Atrial fibrillation during STEMI is associated with increased mortality and stroke, particularly in patients with anterior wall infarction.[185] However, because it is more common in patients with clinical and hemodynamic manifestations of extensive infarction and a poor prognosis, atrial fibrillation is probably a marker of poor prognosis, with only a small independent contribution to increased mortality.

Management

Atrial flutter and fibrillation in patients with STEMI are treated in a manner similar to that in other settings (see Chap. 40). Patients with recurrent episodes of atrial fibrillation should be treated with oral anticoagulants to reduce the risk of stroke, even if sinus rhythm is present at the time of hospital discharge, because no antiarrhythmic regimen can be relied on to be completely effective in suppressing atrial fibrillation. In the absence of contraindications, patients should receive a beta blocker after STEMI; in addition to their several other beneficial effects, these agents are helpful in slowing the ventricular rate if atrial fibrillation recurs. Digitalis may also be helpful in slowing the ventricular rate and managing ventricular dysfunction when atrial fibrillation develops after STEMI.[186]

Other Complications

RECURRENT CHEST DISCOMFORT. Evaluation of postinfarction chest discomfort is sometimes complicated by previous abnormalities on the ECG and a vague description of the discomfort by the patient, who may be exquisitely sensitive to fleeting discomfort or may deny a potential recrudescence of symptoms. The critical task for clinicians is to distinguish recurrent angina or infarction from nonischemic causes of discomfort that might be caused by infarct expansion, pericarditis, pulmonary embolism, and noncardiac conditions. Important diagnostic maneuvers include a repeat physical examination, repeat reading of the ECG, and assessment of the response to sublingual nitroglycerin, 0.4 mg. (The use of noninvasive diagnostic evaluation for recurrent ischemia in patients whose symptoms appear only with moderate levels of exertion is discussed elsewhere in this chapter.)

Recurrent Ischemia and Infarction

The incidence of postinfarction angina without reinfarction is reduced in patients undergoing primary PCI for STEMI compared with fibrinolysis.[187] More effective antiplatelet and antithrombin therapies significantly reduce the rate of recurrent ischemic events after fibrinolysis to a range similar to that reported for primary PCI.[104,110,113] When accompanied by ST and T wave changes in the same leads where Q waves have appeared, it may be caused by occlusion of an initially patent vessel, reocclusion of an initially recanalized or stented vessel, or coronary spasm.

Diagnosis

Extension of the original zone of necrosis or reinfarction in a separate myocardial zone can be a difficult diagnosis, especially within the first 24 hours after the index event. It is more convenient to refer to extension and reinfarction collectively under the more general term *recurrent infarction.* Serum cardiac marker levels may remain elevated from the initial infarction, and it may not be possible to distinguish the electrocardiographic changes that are part of the normal evolution after the index infarction from those caused by recurrent infarction. Within the first 18 to 24 hours following the initial infarction, when serum cardiac marker levels may not have returned to the normal range, recurrent infarction should be strongly considered when there is repeat ST-segment elevation on the ECG. Although pericarditis remains a possibility in such patients, the two can usually be distinguished by the presence of a rub and lack of responsiveness to nitroglycerin in patients with pericardial discomfort. Beyond the first 24 hours, recurrent infarction can be diagnosed either by re-elevation of the cardiac markers or the appearance of new Q waves on the ECG.[1] Reinfarction is more common in patients with diabetes mellitus and those with a previous MI. The predominant angiographic predictors of reinfarction in patients undergoing primary PCI include a final coronary stenosis larger than 30%, post-PCI coronary dissection, and post-PCI intracoronary thrombus. Diabetic patients and those with advanced Killip class are more likely to experience reinfarction.[188]

Prognosis

Regardless of whether postinfarction angina is persistent or limited, its presence is important because the short-term morbidity rate is higher among such patients; mortality is increased if the recurrent ischemia is accompanied by electrocardiographic changes and hemodynamic compromise.[1] Recurrent infarction, often caused by reocclusion of the infarct-related coronary artery, carries serious adverse prognostic information because it is associated with higher rates of in-hospital complications (e.g., congestive heart failure, heart block) and early and long-term mortality.[189] Presumably, the higher mortality rate is related to the larger mass of myocardium whose function becomes compromised.

Management

As with the acute phase of treatment of STEMI, algorithms for the management of patients with recurrent ischemic discomfort at rest center on the 12-lead ECG (**Fig. 55-39**). Patients with ST-segment re-elevation should be referred for urgent catheterization and PCI; repeat fibrinolysis can be considered if PCI is not available. Insertion of an intra-aortic balloon pump may help stabilize the patient while other procedures are being arranged. For patients who are thought to have recurrent ischemia but no evidence of hemodynamic compromise, an attempt should be made to control symptoms

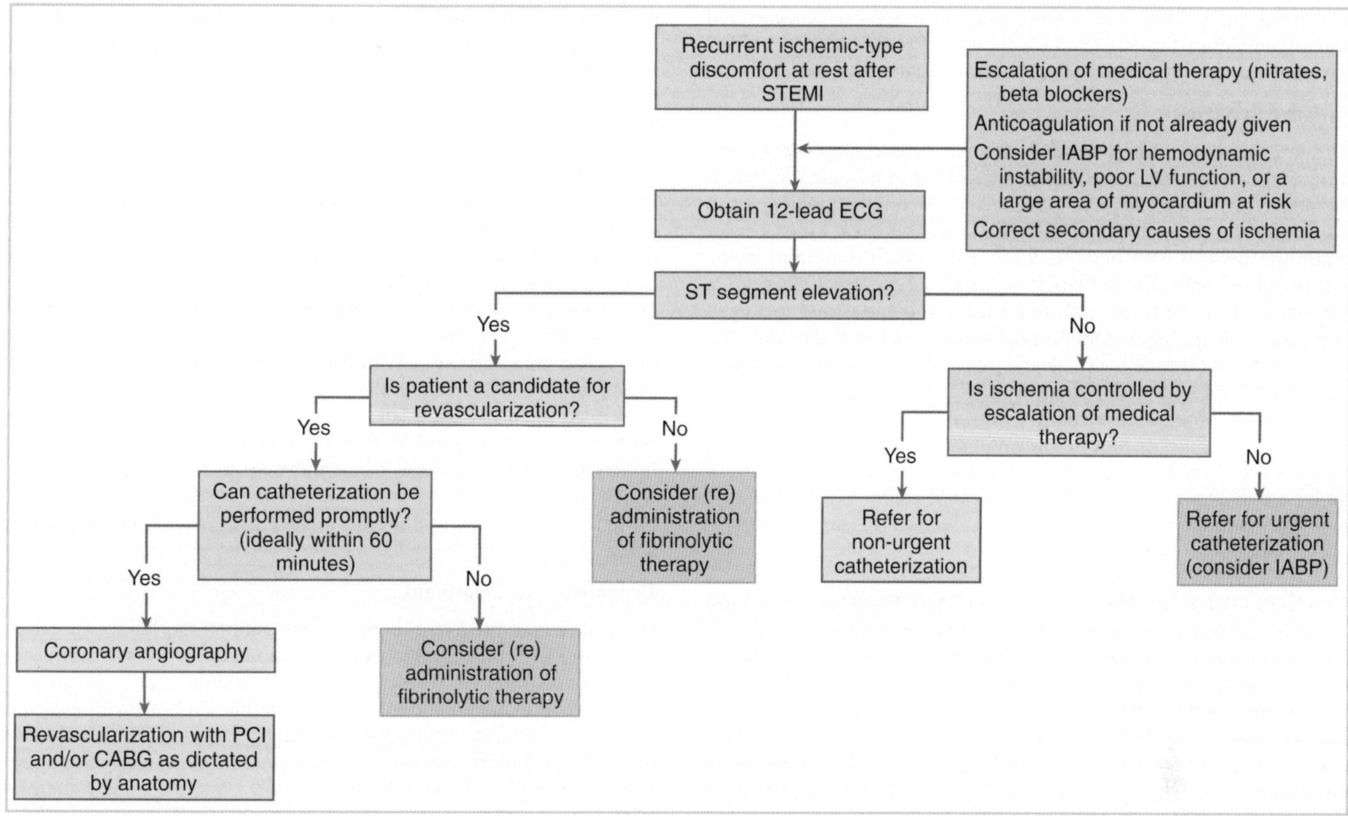

FIGURE 55-39 Algorithm for management of ischemia/infarction after STEMI. IABP = intra-aortic balloon pump; LV = left ventricular. *(Modified from Antman EM, Anbe DT, Armstrong PW, et al: ACC/AHA guidelines for the management of patients with ST-elevation myocardial infarction: A report of the American College of Cardiology/American Heart Association Task Force on Practice Guidelines [Committee to Revise the 1999 Guidelines for the Management of Patients with Acute Myocardial Infarction]. Circulation 110:e82, 2004.)*

with sublingual or intravenous nitroglycerin and intravenous beta blockade to slow the heart rate to 60 beats/min. When hypotension, congestive heart failure, or ventricular arrhythmias develop during recurrent ischemia, urgent catheterization and revascularization are indicated.

High-risk patients with STEMI who receive fibrinolysis benefit from a strategy of routine referral for catheterization and revascularization (<24 hours).[85] However, current trials that compared primary PCI with PCI performed as soon as possible after a preparatory pharmacologic regimen had been administered have not shown such a facilitated PCI approach to be more effective than primary PCI; there are even suggestions of increased mortality because of excess bleeding in the facilitated PCI group.[35]

Finally, with increasing use of PCI in the management of patients with STEMI, clinicians should be alert to the problem of stent thrombosis as a cause of recurrent ischemia. Stent thrombosis can occur acutely (hours to days after deployment of a stent) or in a more subacute fashion (many months after deployment of a stent; see Chap. 58).

PERICARDIAL EFFUSION AND PERICARDITIS (see Chap. 75)

Pericardial Effusion

Effusions are generally detected echocardiographically and their incidence varies with technique, criteria, and laboratory expertise.[190] Effusions are more common in patients with anterior STEMI and with larger infarcts and when congestive failure is present. Most pericardial effusions that occur following STEMI do not cause hemodynamic compromise; when tamponade occurs, it is usually caused by ventricular rupture or hemorrhagic pericarditis. The reabsorption rate of a postinfarction pericardial effusion is slow, with resolution often taking several months. The presence of an effusion does not indicate that pericarditis is present; although they may occur together, most effusions occur without other evidence of pericarditis.

Pericarditis

Pericarditis can produce pain as early as the first day and as late as 6 weeks after STEMI. The pain of pericarditis may be confused with that resulting from postinfarction angina, recurrent infarction, or both. An important distinguishing feature is the radiation of the pain to either trapezius ridge, a finding that is almost pathognomonic of pericarditis and is rarely seen with ischemic discomfort. Transmural MI, by definition, extends to the epicardial surface and is responsible for local pericardial inflammation. An acute fibrinous pericarditis (pericarditis epistenocardiaca) occurs commonly after transmural infarction, but most patients do not report any symptoms from this process. Although transient pericardial friction rubs are relatively common in patients with transmural infarction within the first 48 hours, pain or electrocardiographic changes occur much less often. However, the development of a pericardial rub appears to be correlated with a larger infarct and greater hemodynamic compromise. The discomfort of pericarditis usually becomes worse during a deep inspiration, but it can be relieved or diminished when the patient sits up and leans forward.

Although anticoagulation clearly increases the risk for hemorrhagic pericarditis early after STEMI, this complication does not occur with sufficient frequency during heparinization or following fibrinolytic therapy to warrant absolute prohibition of such agents when a rub is present. Nevertheless, the detection of a pericardial effusion on echo is usually an indication for discontinuation of anticoagulation. In patients for whom continuation or initiation of anticoagulant therapy is strongly indicated (e.g., during cardiac catheterization or following coronary angioplasty), heightened monitoring of clotting parameters and observation for clinical signs of possible tamponade are necessary. Late pericardial constriction caused by anticoagulant-induced hemopericardium has been reported.

Treatment of pericardial discomfort consists of aspirin, but usually in higher doses than prescribed routinely following infarction; doses of 650 mg orally every 4 to 6 hours may be necessary. Nonsteroidal anti-inflammatory drugs (NSAIDs) and steroids should be avoided because they may interfere with myocardial scar formation.[1,191]

Dressler Syndrome

Also known as the postmyocardial infarction syndrome, Dressler syndrome usually occurs 1 to 8 weeks after infarction. Dressler cited an incidence of 3% to 4% of all MI patients in 1957, but the incidence has decreased dramatically since then. Clinically, patients with Dressler syndrome present with malaise, fever, pericardial discomfort, leukocytosis, an elevated sedimentation rate, and a pericardial effusion. At autopsy, patients with this syndrome usually demonstrate localized fibrinous pericarditis containing polymorphonuclear leukocytes. The cause of this syndrome is not clearly established, although the detection of antibodies to cardiac tissue has raised the notion of an immunopathologic process. Treatment is with aspirin, 650 mg, as often as every 4 hours. Glucocorticosteroids and NSAIDs are best avoided in patients with Dressler syndrome within 4 weeks of STEMI because of their potential to impair infarct healing, cause ventricular rupture, and increase coronary vascular resistance. Aspirin in large doses is effective.[192]

VENOUS THROMBOSIS AND PULMONARY EMBOLISM. Almost all peri-MI pulmonary emboli originate from thrombi in the veins of the lower extremities; much less commonly, they originate from mural thrombi overlying an area of right ventricular infarction. Bed rest and heart failure predispose to venous thrombosis and subsequent pulmonary embolism, and both these factors occur commonly in patients with STEMI, particularly those with large infarcts. At a time when patients with STEMI were routinely subjected to prolonged periods of bed rest, significant pulmonary embolism was found in more than 20% of patients with STEMI coming to autopsy, and massive pulmonary embolism accounted for 10% of deaths from MI. In current practice, with early mobilization and the widespread use of low-dose anticoagulant prophylaxis, especially using low-molecular-weight heparins, pulmonary embolism has become an uncommon cause of death in patients with STEMI. When pulmonary embolism does occur in patients with STEMI, management is generally similar to that described for noninfarction patients (see Chap. 77).

LEFT VENTRICULAR ANEURYSM. The term *left ventricular aneurysm* (often termed *true aneurysm*) is generally reserved for a discrete dyskinetic area of the left ventricular wall with a broad neck to differentiate it from pseudoaneurysm caused by a contained myocardial rupture. Dyskinetic or akinetic areas of the left ventricle are far more common than true aneurysms after STEMI; such poorly contracting segments are termed *regional wall motion abnormalities*. True left ventricular aneurysms probably develop in less than 5% of all patients with STEMI and perhaps somewhat more frequently in patients with transmural infarction (especially anterior).[193] The wall of the true aneurysm is thinner than the wall of the rest of the left ventricle (see Fig. 55-34); it is usually composed of fibrous tissue and necrotic muscle, occasionally mixed with viable myocardium.

Pathogenesis

Aneurysm formation presumably occurs when intraventricular tension stretches the noncontracting infarcted heart muscle, thus producing infarct expansion, a relatively weak thin layer of necrotic muscle, and fibrous tissue that bulges with each cardiac contraction. With the passage of time, the wall of the aneurysm becomes more densely fibrotic, but it continues to bulge with systole, causing some of the left ventricular stroke volume during each systole to be ineffective.

When an aneurysm is present after anterior STEMI, there is generally a total occlusion of a poorly collateralized left anterior descending coronary artery. An aneurysm rarely occurs with multivessel disease when there are extensive collaterals or a nonoccluded left anterior descending artery. Aneurysms usually range from 1 to 8 cm in diameter. They occur approximately four times more often at the apex and in the anterior wall than in the inferoposterior wall. The overlying pericardium is usually densely adherent to the wall of the aneurysm, which may even become partially calcified after several years. True left ventricular aneurysms, in contrast to pseudoaneurysms, rarely rupture soon after development. Late rupture, when the true aneurysm has become stabilized by the formation of dense fibrous tissue in its wall, almost never occurs.

Diagnosis

The presence of persistent ST-segment elevation in an electrocardiographic area of infarction, classically thought to suggest aneurysm formation, actually indicates a large infarct with a regional wall motion abnormality but does not necessarily imply an aneurysm. The diagnosis of aneurysm is best made noninvasively by an echocardiographic study, by CMR, or by left ventriculography at the time of cardiac catheterization. With the loss of shortening from the area of the aneurysm, the remainder of the ventricle may become hyperkinetic to compensate. With relatively large aneurysms, complete compensation is impossible. The stroke volume falls or, if it is maintained, it is at the expense of an increase in end-diastolic volume, which in turn leads to increased wall tension and myocardial oxygen demand. Heart failure may ensue, and angina may appear or worsen.

Prognosis and Treatment

Left ventricular aneurysm increases the risk of a mortality, even when compared with that in patients with comparable left ventricular ejection fraction. Death in these patients is often sudden and presumably related to the high incidence of ventricular tachyarrhythmias that occur with aneurysms.[194] Aggressive management of STEMI, including prompt reperfusion, may diminish the incidence of ventricular aneurysms. Surgical aneurysmectomy generally only succeeds if there is relative preservation of contractile performance in the nonaneurysmal portion of the left ventricle. In such a case, when the operation is performed for worsening heart failure or angina, operative mortality is relatively low and clinical improvement can be expected. Because of the importance of maintaining as normal a left ventricular shape as possible, several surgical techniques for ventricular reconstruction have been developed; these may be combined with the general approach shown in **Figure 55-40**.[195] Because of the risk of mural thrombosis and systemic embolization, we favor long-term oral anticoagulation with warfarin in patients with a left ventricular aneurysm after STEMI.

Left Ventricular Thrombus and Arterial Embolism

Endocardial inflammation during the acute phase of infarction probably provides a thrombogenic surface for clots to form in the left ventricle. With extensive transmural infarction of the septum, however, mural thrombi may overlie infarcted myocardium in both ventricles. The incidence of left ventricular thrombus formation after STEMI appears to have dropped from about 20% to 5% with more aggressive use of antithrombotic strategies.[196] Prospective studies have suggested that patients who develop a mural thrombus early, within 48 to 72 hours of infarction, have an extremely poor early prognosis, with a high rate of mortality from the complications of a large infarction (e.g., shock, reinfarction, rupture, ventricular tachyarrhythmia), rather than emboli from the left ventricular thrombus.

Although a mural thrombus adheres to the endocardium overlying the infarcted myocardium, superficial portions of it can become detached and produce systemic arterial emboli. Although estimates vary on the basis of patient selection, about 10% of mural thrombi result in systemic embolization. Echocardiographically detectable features that suggest a given thrombus is more likely to embolize include increased mobility and protrusion into the ventricular chamber, visualization in multiple views, and contiguous zones of akinesis and hyperkinesis.

MANAGEMENT. Data from previous trials with limited sample size have suggested that anticoagulation (intravenous heparin or high-dose

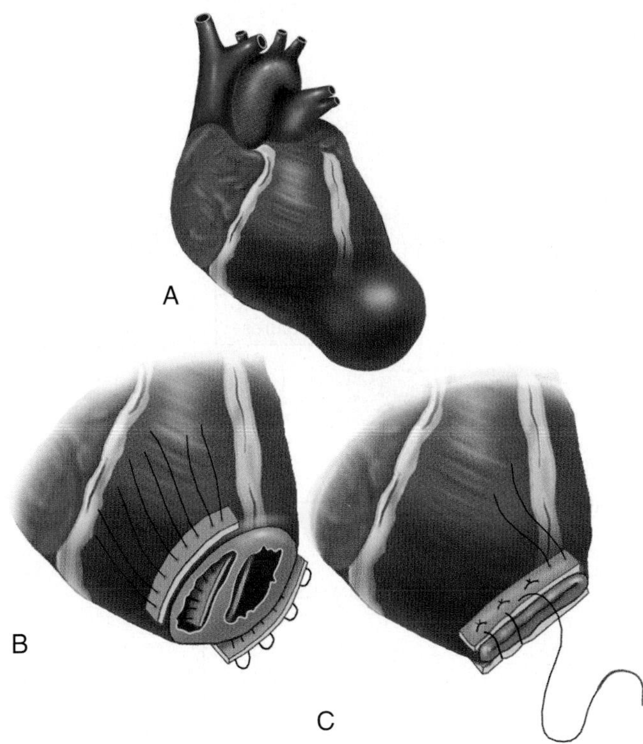

FIGURE 55-40 Surgical management of ventricular aneurysm. **A,** In this case, the aneurysm is located at the apex. **B,** The aneurysmal segment is resected and felt pledget strips are used to reinforce interrupted suture closure of the apex. **C,** Completed repair partially restores apical geometry. *(Courtesy of Dr. David Adams, Division of Cardiac Surgery, Mount Sinai Hospital, New York.)*

subcutaneous heparin) reduce the development of left ventricular thrombi by 50% but, because of the low event rate, it is not possible to demonstrate a reduction in the incidence of systemic embolism. Fibrinolysis reduces the rate of thrombus formation and the character of the thrombi so that they are less protuberant. However, the data from fibrinolytic trials are difficult to interpret because of the confounding effect of antithrombotic therapy with heparin. Recommendations for anticoagulation vary considerably, and fibrinolysis has precipitated fatal embolization. Nevertheless, anticoagulation for 3 to 6 months with warfarin is advocated for many patients with demonstrable mural thrombi.[1,197]

On the basis of the available data, it is our practice to recommend anticoagulation (intravenous heparin to elevate the aPTT to 1.5 to 2 times that of control, followed by a minimum of 3 to 6 months of warfarin) in the following clinical situations: (1) an embolic event has already occurred or (2) the patient has a large anterior infarction whether or not a thrombus is visualized echocardiographically. We are also inclined to follow the same anticoagulation practice in patients with infarctions other than in the anterior distribution if a thrombus or large wall motion abnormality is detected. Aspirin, although probably not able to affect thrombus size in most patients, may prevent further platelet deposition on existing thrombi and also protects against recurrent ischemic events. Aspirin should be prescribed in conjunction with warfarin to patients who are candidates for long-term anticoagulation therapy on the basis of the indications discussed earlier.

Convalescence, Discharge, and Post–Myocardial Infarction Care

TIMING OF HOSPITAL DISCHARGE. The timing of discharge from the hospital is variable. As noted, patients who have undergone aggressive reperfusion protocols and have no significant ventricular arrhythmias, recurrent ischemia, or congestive heart failure have been safely discharged in less than 5 days. More commonly, discharge occurs 5 or 6 days after admission for patients who experience no complications, who can be followed readily at home, and whose family setting is conducive to convalescence. Most complications that would preclude early discharge occur within the first day or two of admission; therefore, patients suitable for early discharge can be identified early during their hospitalization.[1] Several controlled trials and many uncontrolled trials of early discharge after STEMI have failed to show any increase in risk in patients appropriately selected for early discharge. The decision regarding timing of discharge in the patients with uncomplicated STEMI should take into account the patient's psychological state after STEMI, the adequacy of the dose titration for essential drugs such as beta blockers and inhibitors of the RAAS, and the availability and timing of follow-up with visiting nurses and the patient's primary care physician. For patients who have experienced a complication, discharge is deferred until their condition has been stable for several days and it is clear that they are responding appropriately to necessary medications such as antiarrhythmic agents, vasodilators, or positive inotropic agents or that they have undergone the appropriate workup for recurrent ischemia.

COUNSELING. Before discharge from the hospital, all patients should receive detailed instruction concerning physical activity. Initially, this should consist of walking at home with avoidance of isometric exercise such as lifting; several rest periods should be taken daily. In addition, the patient should be given fresh nitroglycerin tablets and instructed in their use (see Chap. 57) and should receive careful instructions about the use of any other medications prescribed. As convalescence progresses, graded resumption of activity should be encouraged (see Chaps. 50 and 83). Many approaches have been used, ranging from formal rigid guidelines to general advice advocating moderation and avoidance of any activity that evokes symptoms. Sexual counseling is often overlooked during recovery from STEMI and should be included as part of the educational process. Such counseling should begin early after STEMI and include the recommendation that sexual activity be resumed after successful completion of early submaximal or later symptom-limited exercise stress testing.[1]

Some evidence indicates that behavioral alteration is possible after recovery from STEMI and that this may improve prognosis. A cardiac rehabilitation program with supervised physical exercise and an educational component has been recommended for most STEMI patients after discharge. Although the overall clinical benefit of such programs continues to be debated, there is little question that most people derive considerable information and psychological security from such interventions, and they continue to be endorsed by experienced clinicians.[1] Meta-analyses of randomized trials of medically supervised rehabilitation programs versus usual care that were conducted in an era before widespread use of beta blockers and aggressive reperfusion strategies have shown a reduction in cardiovascular death but no change in the incidence of nonfatal reinfarction. Given the relationship between depression and STEMI, interest has arisen in psychosocial intervention programs during the convalescent phase of STEMI (see Chaps. 50 and 91).[198,199] Psychosocial intervention programs can decrease symptoms of depression and are a useful adjunct to standard cardiac rehabilitation programs after STEMI; however, they do not have a significant impact on the risk of mortality or recurrent MI after STEMI.[200]

Risk Stratification After STEMI

The process of risk stratification following STEMI occurs in several stages—initial presentation, in-hospital course (CCU, intermediate care unit), and at the time of hospital discharge. The tools used to form an integrated and dynamic assessment of the patient consist of baseline demographic information, serial ECGs and serum and plasma cardiac biomarker measurements, hemodynamic monitoring data, noninvasive tests and, if performed, the findings at cardiac catheterization (**Fig. 55-41**).[1] These are integrated with the occurrence of in-hospital complications to provide information regarding survival.

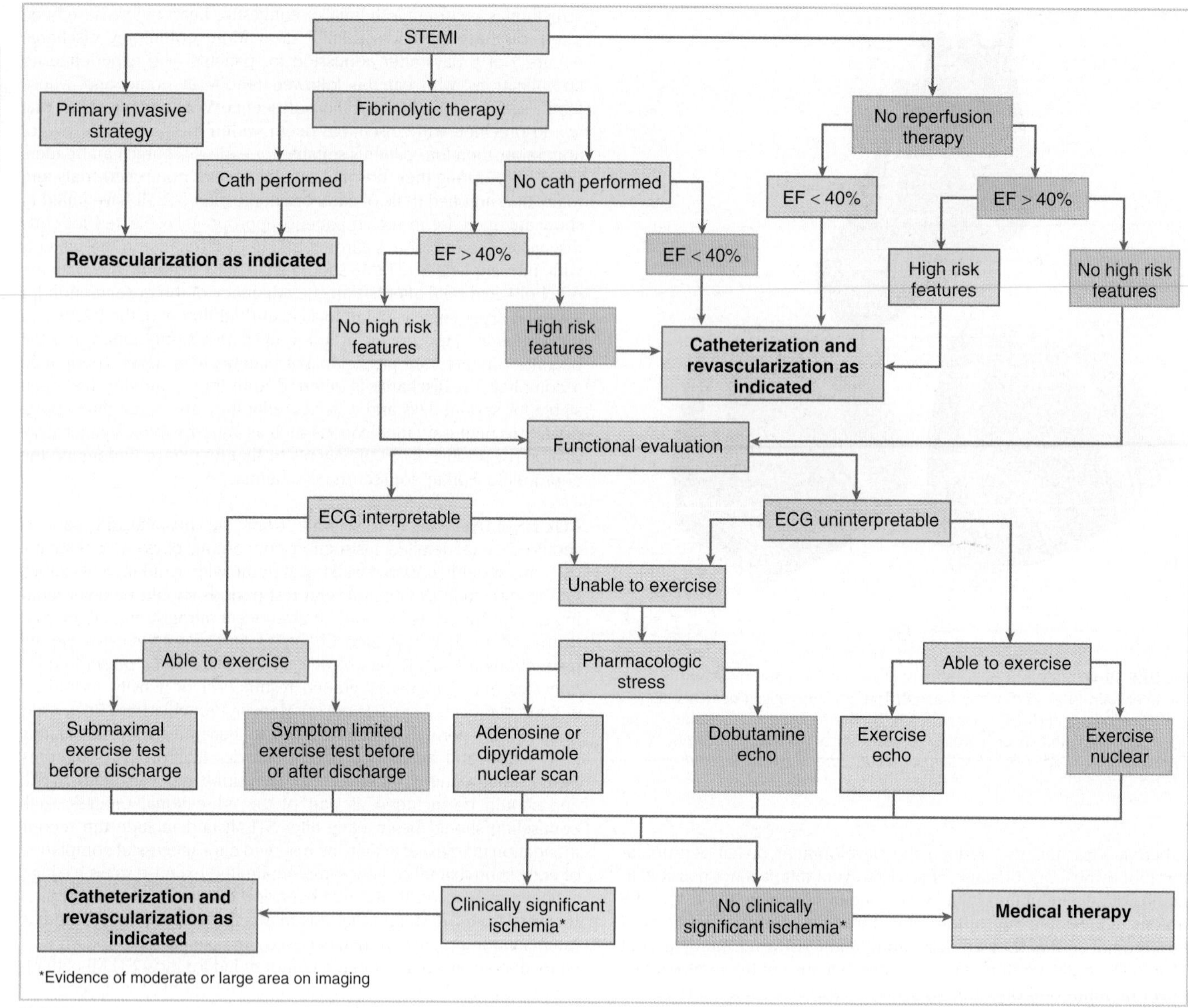

FIGURE 55-41 Algorithm for catheterization and revascularization after STEMI. The algorithm shows the treatment paths for patients who initially undergo a primary invasive strategy, receive fibrinolytic therapy, or do not undergo reperfusion therapy for STEMI. Patients who have not undergone a primary invasive strategy and have no high-risk features should undergo functional evaluation using one of the noninvasive tests shown. When clinically significant ischemia (evidence of moderate or large area of ischemia by imaging) is detected, patients should undergo catheterization and revascularization as indicated; if no clinically significant ischemia is detected, medical therapy is prescribed post-STEMI. cath = catheterization; echo = echocardiography; EF = ejection fraction. *(From Antman EM, Anbe DT, Armstrong PW, et al: ACC/AHA guidelines for the management of patients with ST-elevation myocardial infarction: A report of the American College of Cardiology/American Heart Association Task Force on Practice Guidelines [Committee to Revise the 1999 Guidelines for the Management of Patients with Acute Myocardial Infarction]. Circulation 110:e82, 2004.)*

INITIAL PRESENTATION. Certain demographic and historical factors portend a worse prognosis in patients with STEMI, including female gender, age older than 65 years, a history of diabetes mellitus, prior angina pectoris, and previous MI (see Fig. 55-13). Diabetes mellitus, in particular, appears to confer a more than 40% increase in adjusted risk of death by 30 days (see Chap. 64).[201] Surviving diabetic patients also experience a more complicated post-MI course, including a greater incidence of postinfarction angina, infarct extension, and heart failure.[1] These higher rates of complications likely relate to the extensive accelerated atherosclerosis and higher risk of thrombosis and heart failure associated with diabetes mellitus.

In addition to playing a central role in the decision pathway for the management of patients with STEMI based on the presence or absence of ST-segment elevation, the 12-lead ECG carries important prognostic information.[202] Mortality is higher in patients experiencing anterior wall STEMI than after inferior STEMI, even when corrected for infarct size. Patients with right ventricular infarction complicating inferior infarction, as suggested by ST-segment elevation in V_4R, have a higher mortality rate than patients sustaining an inferior infarction without right ventricular involvement.[158] Patients with multiple leads showing ST-segment elevation and a high sum of ST-segment elevation have an increased mortality rate, especially if their infarct is anterior in location. Patients whose ECG demonstrates persistent advanced heart block (e.g., type II, second-degree, or third-degree AV block) or new intraventricular conduction abnormalities (bifascicular or trifascicular) in the course of STEMI have a worse prognosis than patients without these abnormalities. The influence of a high degree of heart block is particularly important in patients with right ventricular infarction because such patients have a markedly increased mortality risk. Other electrocardiographic findings that augur poorly are persistent horizontal or downsloping ST-segment depression, Q waves in multiple leads,[203] evidence of right ventricular infarction accompanying inferior infarction, ST-segment depressions in anterior leads in patients with inferior infarction, and atrial arrhythmias, especially atrial fibrillation.

Several validated clinical risk stratification tools may be used at presentation to assess the short- and long-term risk of death after MI.[204] In addition to the patient's age and historical factors such as diabetes and prior MI, clinical signs of heart failure, including tachycardia and hypotension, are common to many of these clinical scores for risk assessment.

HOSPITAL COURSE. Soon after CCUs were instituted, it became apparent that left ventricular function is an important early determinant of survival. Hospital mortality from STEMI depends directly on the severity of left ventricular dysfunction. Risk stratification via physical findings, estimation of infarct size and, in appropriate patients, invasive hemodynamic monitoring in the CCU, provide an assessment of the likelihood of a complicated hospital course and may also identify important abnormalities, such as hemodynamically significant mitral regurgitation, that convey an adverse long-term prognosis (see Table 55-10). In particular, the development of heart failure after MI entails a higher risk of sudden cardiac death.[205]

Recurrent ischemia and infarction following STEMI, in the same location as the index infarction or at a distance, influence prognosis adversely.[206] Poor prognosis comes from the loss of viable myocardium, with the resulting larger area of infarction creating a greater compromise in ventricular function. Postinfarction angina generally connotes a less favorable prognosis because it indicates the presence of jeopardized myocardium. In the current era of aggressive revascularization, early postinfarction angina often leads to early interventions that tend to improve outcome, diminishing the long-term impact and significance of angina soon after STEMI.[205,207]

ASSESSMENT AT HOSPITAL DISCHARGE. Both short- and long-term survival after STEMI depend on three factors—resting left ventricular function, residual potentially ischemic myocardium, and susceptibility to serious ventricular arrhythmias. The most important of these factors is the state of left ventricular function (see Fig. 55-30).[1] The second most important factor is how the severity and extent of the obstructive lesions in the coronary vascular bed perfusing residual viable myocardium affect the risk of recurrent infarction, additional myocardial damage, and serious ventricular arrhythmias. Thus, survival relates to the quantity of myocardium that has become necrotic and the quantity at risk of becoming necrotic. At one end of the spectrum, the prognosis is best for the patient with normal intrinsic coronary vessels whose completed infarction constitutes a small fraction (5%) of the left ventricle as a consequence of a coronary embolus and who has no jeopardized myocardium. At the other extreme is the patient with a massive infarct with left ventricular failure whose residual viable myocardium is perfused by markedly obstructed vessels. Progression of atherosclerosis or lowering of perfusion pressure in these vessels impairs the function and viability of the residual myocardium on which left ventricular function depends. Revascularization may reduce the threat to the jeopardized myocardium, even in such a patient. The third risk factor, the susceptibility to serious arrhythmias, is reflected in ventricular ectopic activity and other indicators of electrical instability, such as reduced heart rate variability or baroreflex sensitivity and an abnormal signal-averaged ECG.[204] All these identify patients at increased risk of death.

Left Ventricular Function

Left ventricular ejection fraction may be the most easily assessed measurement of left ventricular function and is extremely useful for risk stratification (see Fig. 55-30). However, imaging of the left ventricle at rest may not distinguish adequately among infarcted, irreversibly damaged, and stunned or hibernating myocardium. To circumvent this difficulty, various techniques have been investigated to assess the extent of residual viable myocardium including exercise and pharmacologic stress echocardiography, stress radionuclide ventricular angiography, perfusion imaging in conjunction with pharmacological stress, positron emission tomography, and gadolinium-enhanced CMR.[208,209] All these techniques can be performed safely in postinfarction patients. Because no study has clearly shown one imaging modality to be superior to others, clinicians should be guided in their selection of ventricular imaging technique by the availability and level of expertise with a given modality at their institution.[210] Because of the dynamic nature of LV function recovery after STEMI, clinicians should consider the timing of the imaging study relative to the index event when assessing LV function.[1]

In patients with low left ventricular ejection fraction, the measurement of exercise capacity is useful for further identifying those patients at particularly high risk and also for establishing safe exercise limits after discharge.[1] Patients with a good exercise capacity despite a reduced ejection fraction have a better long-term outcome than those with exercise impairment (see Chaps. 50 and 83).

Myocardial Ischemia

Because of the potent adverse consequences of recurrent MI after STEMI, it is important to assess a patient's risk for future ischemia and infarction. Given the increasing array of pharmacologic, interventional, and surgical options available to modify the likelihood of developing recurrent episodes of myocardial ischemia, most clinicians find it helpful to identify patients at risk for provocable myocardial ischemia before discharge. A predischarge evaluation for ischemia allows clinicians to select patients who might benefit from catheterization and revascularization following fibrinolysis for STEMI and to assess the adequacy of medical therapy for those patients who are suitable for a more conservative management strategy (see Fig. 55-41).

EXERCISE TESTING. An exercise test also offers the clinician an opportunity to formulate a more precise exercise prescription and is helpful for boosting patients' confidence in their ability to conduct their daily activities after discharge. Patients who are unable to exercise can be evaluated by the use of a pharmacologic stress protocol, such as an infusion of dobutamine or dipyridamole with echocardiography or perfusion imaging (see Fig. 55-41).

Treadmill exercise testing after STEMI has traditionally used a submaximal protocol that requires the patient to exercise until symptoms of angina appear, electrocardiographic evidence of ischemia is seen, or a target workload (≈5 metabolic equivalents) has been reached (see Chap. 50). Symptom-limited exercise tests can be performed safely before discharge in patients with an uncomplicated in-hospital postinfarction course. Variables derived from exercise tests after STEMI that have been evaluated for their ability to predict the occurrence of death or recurrent nonfatal infarction include the development and magnitude of ST-segment depression, development of angina, exercise capacity, and systolic blood pressure response during exercise.[204]

Electrical Instability

After STEMI, patients are at greatest risk for the development of sudden cardiac death caused by malignant ventricular arrhythmias over the course of the first 1 to 2 years.[1,211] Several techniques have been proposed to stratify patients into those who are at increased risk of sudden death following STEMI, including the following: measurement of Q-T dispersion (variability of Q-T intervals between electrocardiographic leads); ambulatory electrocardiographic recordings for detection of ventricular arrhythmias (Holter monitoring); invasive electrophysiologic testing; recording a signal-averaged ECG (a measure of delayed, fragmented conduction in the infarct zone); and measuring heart rate variability (beat to beat variability in R-R intervals) or baroreflex sensitivity (slope of a line relating beat to beat change in sinus rate in response to alteration of blood pressure). However, these have not proved sufficiently useful to recommend their use in routine practice.[204]

Despite the increased risk of arrhythmic events following STEMI in patients who are found to have abnormal results on one or more of the noninvasive tests described earlier, several points should be emphasized. The low positive predictive value (<30%) for the noninvasive screening tests limits their usefulness when viewed in isolation. Although the predictive value of screening tests can be improved by combining several of them together, the therapeutic implications of an increased risk profile for arrhythmic events have not been established. The mortality reductions achievable with the general use of beta blockers, ACE inhibitors, aspirin, and revascularization when appropriate after infarction, coupled with concerns about the efficacy and safety of antiarrhythmic drugs and the cost of implanted defibrillators, leave considerable uncertainty about the therapeutic implications of an abnormal noninvasive test for electrical instability in an asymptomatic patient. Additional data on patient outcomes when clinicians act on the results of an abnormal finding are required before definitive recommendations can be made for asymptomatic patients.[1] The management of patients with sustained, hemodynamically compromising arrhythmias is discussed in Chaps. 37 to 39.

PROPHYLACTIC ANTIARRHYTHMIC THERAPY. Although it has been recognized for decades that antiarrhythmic therapy can control atrial and ventricular arrhythmias effectively in many patients, reviews of clinical trials following STEMI have reported an increased risk of mortality with type I drugs. The most notable postinfarction trial in this area was the Cardiac Arrhythmia Suppression Trial (CAST), which tested whether encainide, flecainide, or moricizine for suppression of ventricular arrhythmias detected on ambulatory electrocardiographic monitoring would reduce the risk of cardiac arrest and death over the long term. Both the first phase of the trial (encainide or flecainide versus placebo) and the second phase of the trial (moricizine versus placebo) were stopped prematurely because of increased mortality in the active treatment groups. The mechanism of the increased risk after STEMI remains a subject of investigation. One hypothesis that has been proposed is an adverse interaction between recurrent ischemia and the presence of an antiarrhythmic drug because the risk of death or cardiac arrest was greater in patients with a non–Q-wave acute MI than with Q-wave MI. Sodium channel blockade by antiarrhythmics may exacerbate electrophysiologic differences between subepicardial and subendocardial zones of myocardium, rendering the latter more susceptible to ischemic injury.

Subsequent to CAST, another postinfarction, prophylactic, antiarrhythmic drug trial was undertaken with oral D-sotalol (Survival With ORal D-sotalol, or SWORD). SWORD also was stopped prematurely after enrollment of only 3121 of a planned 6400 patients because statistical evidence of increased mortality emerged in the active treatment group. The Canadian Amiodarone Myocardial Infarction Trial (CAMIAT) showed that amiodarone reduces the frequency of ventricular premature depolarization in patients with recent MI; this is correlated with a reduction in arrhythmic death or resuscitation from ventricular fibrillation. However, 42% of patients discontinued amiodarone during maintenance therapy in CAMIAT because of intolerable side effects. The European Amiodarone Myocardial Infarction Trial (EMIAT) showed a reduction in arrhythmic death after MI in patients with depressed left ventricular function, but there was no reduction in total mortality or other cardiovascular-related mortality.

The routine use of antiarrhythmic agents (including amiodarone) cannot be recommended. Given the data cited earlier on the protective effects of beta blockers against sudden death and the ability of aspirin to reduce the risk of reinfarction, it is unclear that additional mortality reductions would be achieved by the empirical addition of amiodarone in the patient who is convalescing from a STEMI and is free of symptomatic sustained ventricular arrhythmias.

Several trials that included post-STEMI patients in the study population have shown significant mortality reductions in patients randomized to ICD implantation versus conventional medical therapy (see Chap. 38). However, early implantation of an ICD in the first few weeks after MI has not been shown to be beneficial; at present, there is insufficient evidence to support routine risk stratification to guide ICD placement soon after STEMI.[212] At present, the selection of STEMI patients who are candidates for ICD implantation is based on the algorithm in **Figure 55-42**.

Secondary Prevention of Acute Myocardial Infarction

Patients who survive the initial course of STEMI still have considerable risk of recurrent events rendering imperative efforts to reduce this risk (see Chap. 49).

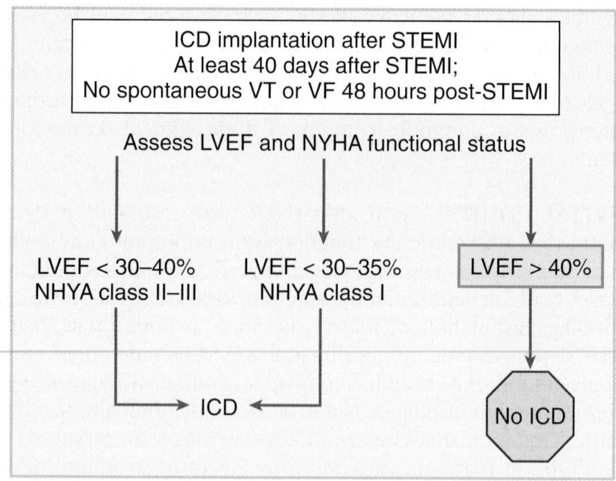

FIGURE 55-42 Algorithm for implantation of an ICD in STEMI patients without ventricular fibrillation (VF) or sustained ventricular tachycardia (VT) more than 48 hours after STEMI. The appropriate management path is based on measurement of the left ventricular ejection fraction (LVEF); measurements obtained 3 days or less after STEMI should be repeated before proceeding with the algorithm. Patients with an LVEF < 30% to 40% at least 40 days post-STEMI are referred for insertion of an ICD if they are in New York Heart Association (NYHA) Class II or III. Patients with a more depressed LVEF < 30% to 35% are referred for ICD implantation even if they are NYHA Class I because of their increased risk of sudden cardiac death. Patients with preserved left ventricular function (LVEF > 40%) do not receive an ICD and are treated with medical therapy post-STEMI. *(Modified from Zipes DP, Camm AJ, Borggrefe M, et al: ACC/AHA/ESC 2006 guidelines for management of patients with ventricular arrhythmias and the prevention of sudden cardiac death: A report of the American College of Cardiology/American Heart Association Task Force and the European Society of Cardiology Committee for Practice Guidelines [Writing Committee to Develop Guidelines for Management of Patients with Ventricular Arrhythmias and the Prevention of Sudden Cardiac Death]. Developed in collaboration with the European Rhythm Association and the Heart Rhythm Society. Circulation 114:e385, 2006.)*

LIFESTYLE MODIFICATION. Efforts to improve survival and quality of life after MI that relate to lifestyle modification of known risk factors are considered in Chap. 49. Of these, cessation of smoking and control of hypertension are probably most important. Within 2 years of quitting smoking, the risk of a nonfatal MI in former smokers falls to a level similar to that in patients who never smoked. Being hospitalized for STEMI is a powerful motivation for patients to cease cigarette smoking, and this is an ideal time to encourage that clearly beneficial and highly cost-effective lifestyle change. Use of hospital-based smoking cessation programs and referral to cardiac rehabilitation programs have been associated with successful smoking cessation.[213] Smoking cessation intervention should therefore be a routine part of the discharge planning post-STEMI for all smokers. It is also an ideal time to begin to treat hypertension, counsel patients to achieve optimal body weight, and consider various strategies to improve the patient's lipid profile.[1]

TREATING DEPRESSION. Physicians caring for patients following a STEMI need to be sensitive to the prevalence of major depression after infarction (see Chap. 91).[214] This problem is associated independently with a higher risk of death. In addition, lack of an emotionally supportive network in the patient's environment after discharge is associated with an increased risk of recurrent cardiac events.[1] The precise mechanisms relating depression and lack of social support to a worse prognosis after STEMI are not clear, but one possibility is lack of adherence to prescribed treatments, a behavior that has been shown to be associated with increased risk of mortality after infarction. Evidence exists that a comprehensive rehabilitation program using primary health care personnel who counsel patients and make home visits favorably affects the clinical course of patients after infarction and reduces the rate of rehospitalization for recurrent ischemia and infarction.[215] A supportive physician attitude can also have a positive impact on the rate of return to work after STEMI.

MODIFICATION OF LIPID PROFILE. Increased cholesterol level, and most importantly an increased low-density lipoprotein (LDL) cholesterol level, is associated with an increased risk of coronary heart disease and is a modifiable risk factor for recurrent events (see Chaps. 47 and 49). A target LDL cholesterol level lower than 100 mg/dL with an optimal target lower than 70 mg/dL has been recommended for patients with clinically evident coronary heart disease.[216] This recommendation clearly applies to patients with STEMI, and it is therefore important to obtain a lipid profile on admission in all patients admitted with acute infarction. (It should be recalled that cholesterol levels may fall 24 to 48 hours after infarction.) In addition to lowering LDL cholesterol, therapy with statins reduces levels of C-reactive protein, suggesting an anti-inflammatory effect.[217] Surveys of physician practice in the past have revealed a disappointingly low rate of treatment of hypercholesterolemia to recommended targets in patients with proven coronary artery disease, indicating considerable room for improvement in this aspect of secondary prevention.[218]

Recommendations

The dietary prescription after STEMI should be low saturated fat (<7% of total calories) and low cholesterol (<200 mg/day).[219] Patients with an LDL cholesterol level higher than 100 mg/dL should be discharged on statin therapy with the goal of reducing the LDL level to less than 70 mg/dL (see Chaps. 47 and 49). It is also reasonable to prescribe statin therapy to patients recovering from STEMI whose LDL cholesterol level is unknown or is lower than 100 mg/dL.[1] For many patients recovering from an acute MI, a low high-density lipoprotein cholesterol level is their primary lipid abnormality.

ANTIPLATELET AGENTS. On the basis of the compelling data from the Antiplatelet Trialists' Collaboration of a 22% reduction in the risk of recurrent infarction, stroke, or vascular death in high-risk vascular patients receiving prolonged antiplatelet therapy (see Chap. 87) in the absence of a true aspirin allergy, all STEMI patients should receive 75 to 162 mg of aspirin daily indefinitely.[109,216] Additional benefits of long-term aspirin that can accrue in the STEMI patient are an increased likelihood of patency of the infarct artery and smaller infarcts if recurrent MI does take place. Patients with true aspirin allergy can be treated with clopidogrel (75 mg once daily) on the basis of experience from patients with unstable angina/non–ST-segment elevation MI (UA/NSTEMI). Given the results of the CLARITY-TIMI 28[110] and COMMIT[116] trials, as well as experience with clopidogrel in UA/NSTEMI, clopidogrel (75 mg/day) should be added to aspirin in patients discharged after a STEMI.[35] Prasugrel (10 mg/day) may be considered for patients with STEMI who have undergone PCI for STEMI.[113] The optimum duration of treatment with dual antiplatelet therapy needs further study, but benefit has been shown to continue after 30 days and it seems reasonable to continue a thienopyridine for at least 1 year after STEMI and maintain aspirin treatment indefinitely.[220,221] In addition, there is accumulating evidence that more potent antiplatelet therapy than aspirin and clopidogrel is beneficial for the patient treated for an acute coronary syndrome with a drug-eluting stent, at least for a period of 30 days.[222]

INHIBITION OF THE RENIN-ANGIOTENSIN-ALDOSTERONE SYSTEM. The rationale for inhibition of this neurohormonal axis after STEMI was discussed earlier. To prevent late remodeling of the left ventricle and also to decrease the likelihood of recurrent ischemic events, we advocate indefinite therapy with an ACE inhibitor to all patients with clinically evident congestive heart failure, a moderate decrease in global ejection fraction, or a large regional wall-motion abnormality, even in the presence of a normal global ejection fraction. Once the STEMI patient is discharged from the hospital, the evidence based on long-term management of patients with chronic coronary artery disease is the most relevant for long-term decision making. Based on the results of the HOPE and EUROPA trials, we advocate indefinite treatment with an ACE inhibitor for all STEMI patients with an ejection fraction less than 40%, renal dysfunction, or diabetes regardless of ejection fraction, provided no contraindications exist.[216] As discussed earlier, the VALIANT trial results suggest that valsartan may be used as an alternative to an ACE inhibitor for the long-term management of patients with left ventricular dysfunction after STEMI.

BETA BLOCKERS. Meta-analyses of trials from the prethrombolytic era involving more than 24,000 patients who received beta blockers in the convalescent phase of STEMI have shown a 23% reduction in long-term mortality.[1] When beta blockers are administered early (6 hours) in the acute phase of infarction and continued in the chronic phase of treatment, some of the benefit may result from a reduction in infarct size. In most patients who have beta blockade initiated during the convalescent phase of STEMI, however, reduction in long-term mortality is probably the result of a combination of an antiarrhythmic effect (prevention of sudden death) and prevention of reinfarction.

Given the well-documented benefits of beta blocker therapy, it is disturbing that this form of therapy continues to be underused, especially in high-risk groups such as older adults.[1] Patients with a relative contraindication to beta blockers (moderate heart failure, bradyarrhythmias) should undergo a monitored trial of therapy in the hospital. The dosage should be sufficient to blunt the heart rate response to stress or exercise. Much of the impact of beta blockers in preventing mortality occurs in the first weeks; treatment should commence as soon as possible. Evidence exists that programs providing physician feedback improve adherence to guidelines such as those noted earlier for prescription of beta adrenoceptor blockers after acute MI.[223]

Some controversy exists as to how long patients should be treated. The collective data from five trials providing information on long-term follow-up of beta blockers after infarction have suggested that therapy be continued for at least 2 to 3 years.[1] At that time, if the beta blocker is well tolerated and if there is no reason to discontinue therapy, such therapy probably should be continued in most patients.

Not all patients derive the same benefit from beta blocker therapy. The cost-effectiveness of treatment in medium- or high-risk persons compares favorably with that of many other accepted interventions, such as CABG, angioplasty, and lipid-lowering therapy. In patients with an extremely good prognosis (first acute MI, good ventricular function, no angina, negative stress test result, and no complex ventricular ectopy) among whom a mortality rate of approximately 1%/year can be anticipated, beta blockers would have a smaller impact on survival. However, it is our preference to prescribe beta blockers to such patients for whatever postinfarction benefit is achieved and also to include them as part of the patient's usual regimen should MI recur at an unpredictable time in the future.

NITRATES. Although nitrates are suitable for the management of specific conditions after STEMI, such as recurrent angina or as part of a treatment regimen for congestive heart failure, little evidence indicates that they reduce mortality over the long term when prescribed on a routine basis to all patients with infarction.[1]

ANTICOAGULANTS. After several decades of evaluation, the weight of evidence now suggests that anticoagulants have a favorable effect on late mortality, stroke, and reinfarction in patients hospitalized with STEMI (**Table 55-15**). Given the complexities of combining long-term therapy with warfarin alone with antiplatelet therapy, clinicians must weigh the need for warfarin based on established indications for anticoagulation and the risk of bleeding.[96] An algorithm to guide decision making with respect to warfarin is shown in **Figure 55-43**.

There are at least three hypothetical reasons for anticipating that anticoagulants might be beneficial in the long-term management of patients after STEMI:

1. Because the coronary occlusion responsible for the STEMI is often caused by a thrombus, anticoagulants might be expected to halt progression, slow progression, or prevent the development of new thrombi elsewhere in the coronary arterial tree.
2. Anticoagulants might be expected to diminish the formation of mural thrombi and resultant systemic embolization.
3. Anticoagulants might be expected to reduce the incidence of venous thrombosis and pulmonary embolization.

TABLE 55-15 Aspirin Versus Warfarin Therapy after ST-Elevation Myocardial Infarction (STEMI)

STUDY	STUDY DESIGN	DRUGS USED	ASA	SECOND ARM	THIRD ARM	PATIENTS	ENDPOINTS	Results (%) ASA ALONE	WARFARIN ALONE	ASA + WARFARIN
STEMI-Specific Trials										
WARIS II*	Randomized Open label $N = 3630$ FU = 4 yr (mean)	ASA monotherapy vs. warfarin monotherapy vs. warfarin + ASA	160 mg daily	Dosed to target INR 2.8-4.2	Dosed to target INR 2.0-2.5 + ASA 75 mg daily	Age <75 yr Hospitalized for acute MI % STEMI = 71.8	Death, nonfatal reinfarction, or thromboembolic stroke Major, nonfatal bleeding (P <0.001)	20 0.17	16.7 (P = 0.03 vs. ASA) 0.68	15 (P = 0.001 vs. ASA) 0.57
APRICOT II[†]	Randomized Open label $N = 308$ FU = 3 mo	ASA monotherapy vs. warfarin + ASA	If TIMI grade 3, post-48 hr UFH, then 160 mg initially and then 80 mg daily	Dosed to target INR 2-3 if TIMI 3 post–48 hr, UFH + 160 mg initially and then 80 mg daily	N/A	Age ≤76 yr Acute STEMI ≤6 yr prior to thrombolytic Tx % STEMI = 100	Reocclusion (TIMI ≤ 2) (P <0.02) Total occlusion (TIMI 0-1) (P <0.02) Revascularization (P < 0.01) Reinfarction (P <0.05) Event-free survival rate* (P <0.01) Bleeding (TIMI major and minor (P = NS)	28 20 31 8 66 3	N/A	15 9 13 2 86 5
Trials Not Specific to STEMI										
ASPECT II[‡]	Randomized Open label $N = 999$ FU = 26 mo	ASA monotherapy vs. warfarin monotherapy vs. warfarin + ASA	80 mg daily	Dosed to target INR 3-4	Dosed to target INR 2-2.5 + ASA 80 mg daily	Acute MI or UA within preceding 8 wk	Death, MI, or stroke (P = 0.02479 Major bleeding Minor bleeding (P <0.0001) Almost 20% of warfarin and combined group discontinued therapy; 40% in therapeutic range	9 1 5	5 1 8	5 2 15
CHAMP[§]	Randomized Open label $N = 5059$ FU = median 2.7 yr	ASA monotherapy vs. warfarin + ASA	162 mg daily	Dosed to target INR 1.5-2.5 + 81 mg ASA daily	N/A	Acute MI within preceding 14 days prior to enrollment	Death (P = 0.76) Recurrent MI (P = 0.78) Stroke (P = 0.52) Major bleeding (P = 0.001)	17.3 13.1 3.5 0.72**	N/A	17.6 13.3 3.1 1.2**
CARS[¶]	Randomized Blinded $N = 8803$ FU = 33 mo Median = 14 mo	ASA monotherapy vs. warfarin 1 mg + ASA	160 mg daily (avg INR @ wk 4 = 1.02)	1 mg + 80 mg ASA (avg INR @ wk 4 = 1.05)	N/A	Age 21-85 yr (82% < 70 yr) MI 3-21 days (mean, 9.6 days) prior to enrollment	Ischemic stroke (P = 0.0534)	0.6	N/A	1.1

*Hurlen M, Abdelnoor M, Smith P, et al: Warfarin, aspirin, or both after myocardial infarction. N Engl J Med 347:969, 2002.
[†]Brouwer MA, van den Bergh PJ, Aengevaeren WR, et al: Aspirin plus coumarin versus aspirin alone in the prevention of reocclusion after fibrinolysis for acute myocardial infarction: Results of the Antithrombotics in the Prevention of Reocclusion In Coronary Thrombolysis (APRICOT)-2 Trial. Circulation 106:659, 2002.
[‡]Van Es RF, Jonker JJ, Verheugt FW, et al: Aspirin and coumadin after acute coronary syndromes (the ASPECT-2 study): A randomised controlled trial. Lancet 360:109, 2002.
[§]Fiore LD, Ezekowitz MD, Brophy MT, et al: Department of Veterans Affairs Cooperative Studies Program Clinical Trial comparing combined warfarin and aspirin with aspirin alone in survivors of acute myocardial infarction: Primary results of the CHAMP study. Circulation 105:557, 2002.
[¶]O'Connor CM, Gattis WA, Hellkamp AS, et al: Comparison of two aspirin doses on ischemic stroke in post-myocardial infarction patients in the warfarin (Coumadin) Aspirin Reinfarction Study (CARS). Am J Cardiol 88:541, 2001.
** Reported as number of events per 100 person-years of follow-up.
ASA = acetylsalicylic acid (aspirin); FU = follow-up; INR = international normalized ratio; MI = myocardial infarction; N/A = not applicable; STEMI = ST-segment myocardial infarction ; TIMI = Thrombosis In Myocardial Infarction; Tx = treatment; UA = unstable angina; UFH = unfractionated heparin; vs. = versus.
Modified from Antman EM, Anbe DT, Armstrong PW, et al: ACC/AHA Guidelines for the Management of Patients with ST-Elevation Myocardial Infarction: A report of the American College of Cardiology/American Heart Association Task Force on Practice Guidelines (Committee to Revise the 1999 Guidelines for the Management of Patients with Acute Myocardial Infarction). Circulation 110:e82, 2004.

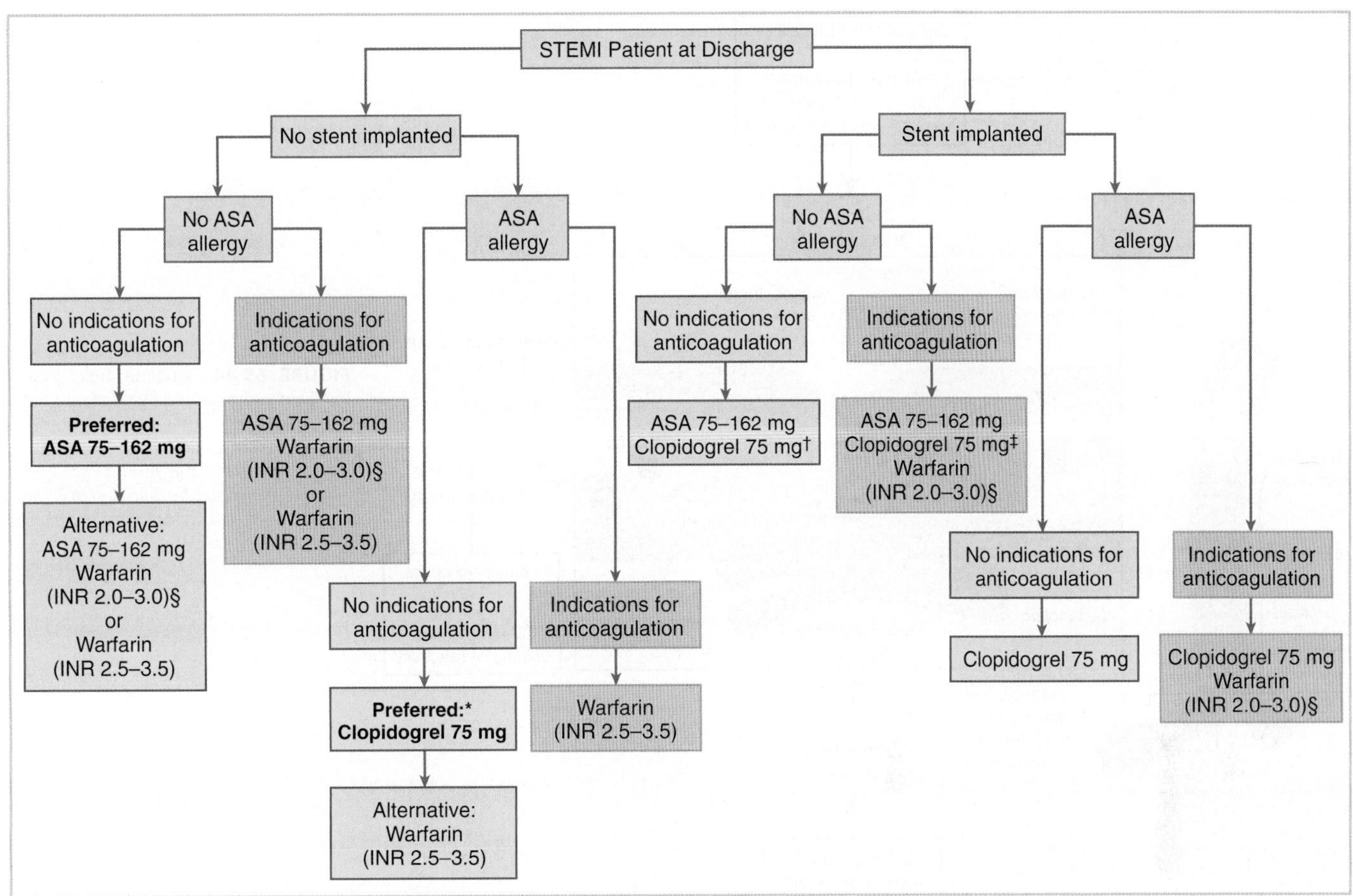

FIGURE 55-43 Algorithm for antithrombotic therapy at hospital discharge after STEMI. *Clopidogrel is preferred over warfarin because of an increased risk of bleeding and low patient compliance in warfarin trials. †For 12 months. ‡Discontinue clopidogrel 1 month after implantation of a bare metal stent or several months after implantation of a drug-eluting stent (3 months after sirolimus and 6 months after paclitaxel) because of the potential increased risk of bleeding with warfarin and two antiplatelet agents. Continue ASA and warfarin long term if warfarin is indicated for other reasons such as atrial fibrillation, LV thrombus, cerebral emboli, or extensive regional wall motion abnormality. §An INR of 2 to 3 is acceptable with tight control, but the lower end of this range (2.0-2.5) is preferable. The combination of antiplatelet therapy and warfarin may be considered in patients younger than 75 years, with low bleeding risk, who can be monitored reliably. ASA = acetylsalicylic acid; INR = international normalized ratio; LV = left ventricular. *(Modified from Antman EM, Anbe DT, Armstrong PW, et al: ACC/AHA guidelines for the management of patients with ST-elevation myocardial infarction: A report of the American College of Cardiology/American Heart Association Task Force on Practice Guidelines [Committee to Revise the 1999 Guidelines for the Management of Patients with Acute Myocardial Infarction]). Circulation 110:e82, 2004.)*

Alternative oral anticoagulants, such as the oral factor Xa inhibitors, that have the advantage of more predictable anticoagulation without stable oral dosing, have undergone initial evaluation in patients with acute coronary syndrome, including STEMI, and are being evaluated in larger trials.[224,225]

CALCIUM CHANNEL ANTAGONISTS. At present, we do not recommend the routine use of calcium antagonists for secondary prevention of infarction. A possible exception is a patient who cannot tolerate a beta blocker because of adverse effects on bronchospastic lung disease but who has well-preserved left ventricular function; such patients may be candidates for a rate-slowing calcium antagonist such as diltiazem or verapamil.

HORMONE THERAPY. The decision to prescribe hormone therapy (see Chap. 81) is often a complex one that involves the desire to suppress postmenopausal symptoms versus the risks of breast and endometrial cancer and vascular events. Despite improvement in lipid profiles, hormone therapy with estrogen plus progestin in postmenopausal women with established coronary heart disease does not prevent recurrent coronary events and is associated with a significantly increased risk of coronary and venous thromboembolic events.[1] At present, we recommend not starting hormone therapy with estrogen plus progestin after STEMI and discontinuing it in postmenopausal women after STEMI.

ANTIOXIDANTS. Dietary supplementation with omega-3 polyunsaturated fatty acids has been associated with a reduction in coronary heart disease death and nonfatal reinfarction in patients within 3 months of a MI (see Chap. 48). Vitamin E (300 mg/day) does not confer any significant clinical benefit, however.[1]

NONSTEROIDAL ANTI-INFLAMMATORY DRUGS. Evidence has emerged that cyclooxygenase-2 (COX-2) selective drugs and NSAIDs that have varying COX-1:COX-2 inhibitory ratios promote a prothrombotic state, and their use is associated with an increased risk of atherothrombotic events.[226,227] Given the increased risk of atherothrombosis related to the index STEMI event, the desire not to interfere with the beneficial pharmacologic actions of low-dose aspirin post-STEMI, and reports of increased mortality and reinfarction when they are used after MI, clinicians should avoid prescribing NSAIDs to patients recovering from STEMI.[35] If NSAIDs must be prescribed for pain relief, the lowest dose required to control symptoms should be administered for the shortest period of time required.[228]

Emerging Therapies

Although there has been a substantial increase in the number of patients with STEMI who receive primary PCI, there remains considerable room for improvement. Although PCI usually restores flow through epicardial arteries, many patients do not achieve adequate nutrient

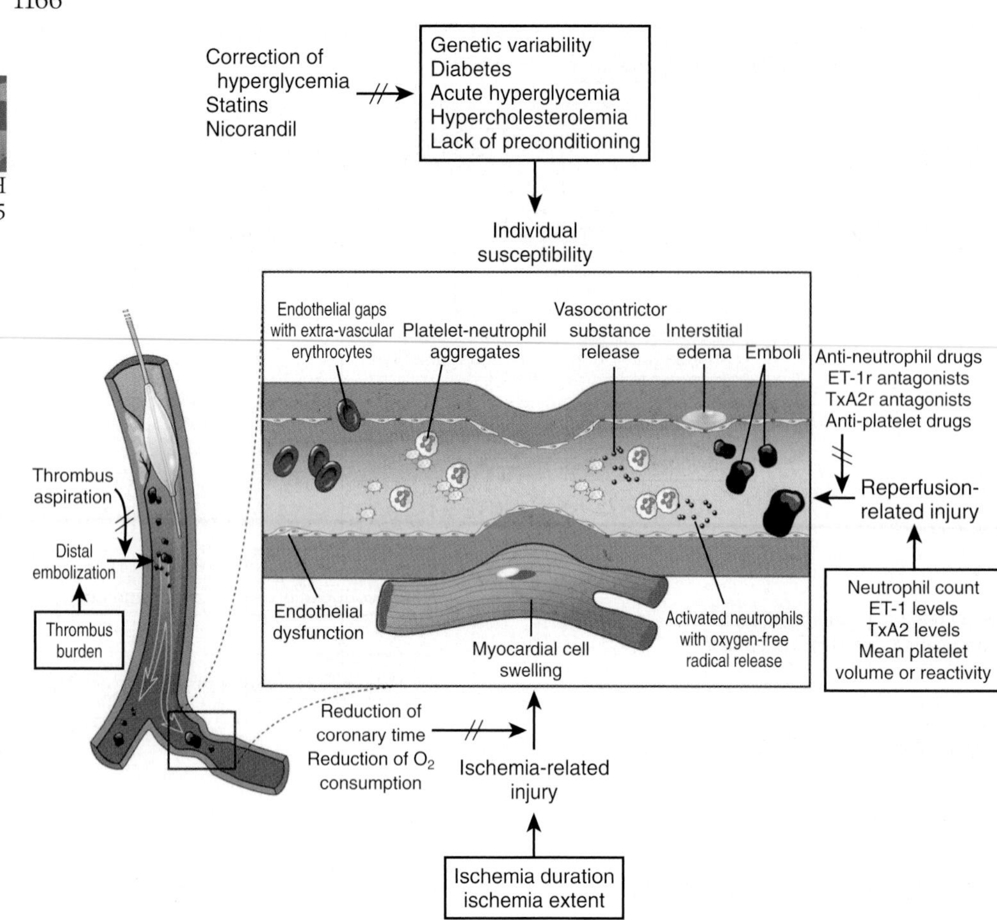

FIGURE 55-44 Multiple mechanisms involved in the pathogenesis of no-reflow that might be targeted by appropriate therapy. ET = endothelin; r = receptor; TxA2 = thromboxane A2. *(Modified from Niccoli G, Burzotta F, Galiuto L, Crea F: Myocardial no-reflow in humans. J Am Coll Cardiol 54:281, 2009.)*

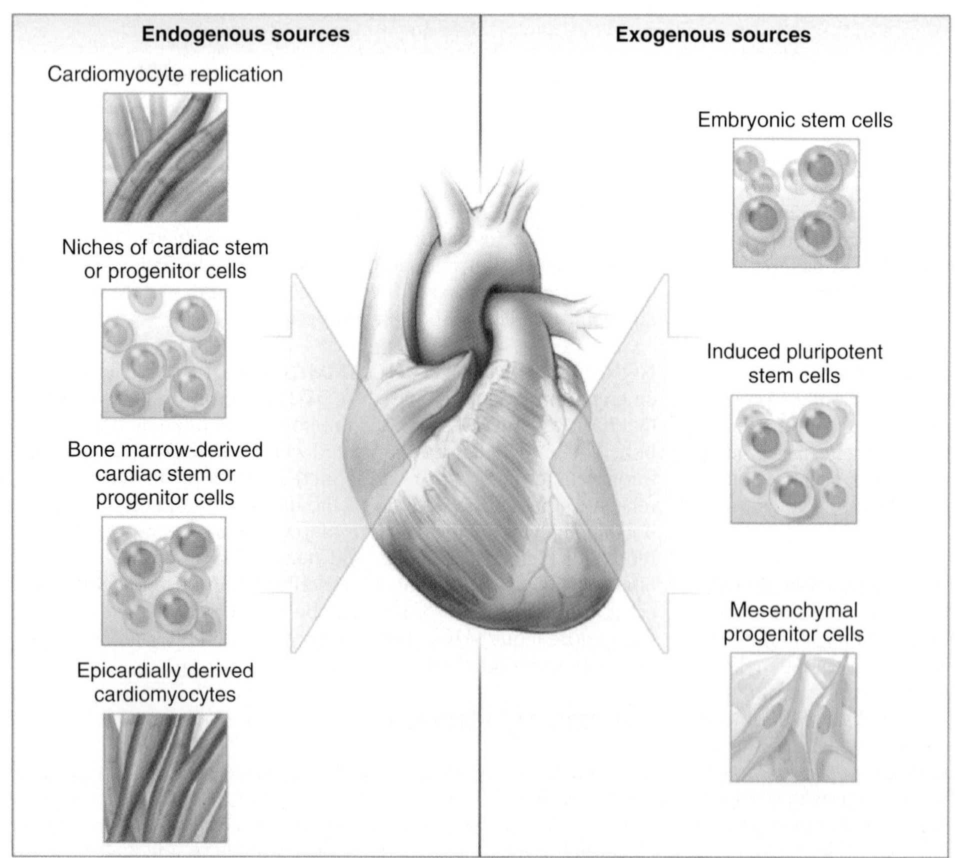

FIGURE 55-45 The demonstration that some cardiomyocytes are regenerated after birth highlights the promise and challenges of future regenerative cardiac therapies. Autologous and allogeneic sources of cells that may give rise to cardiomyocytes are under investigation. See Chap. 11. *(From Parmacek MS, Epstein JA: Cardiomyocyte renewal. N Engl J Med 361:86, 2009.)*

flow at the myocardial level in the infarct zone because of a process referred to as no-reflow.[72] The no-reflow phenomenon occurs more frequently when there is a large thrombus burden, high platelet count, increased platelet reactivity, presence of hyperglycemia, and lack of preconditioning. The duration and extent of myocardial ischemia also bear directly on the likelihood of the occurrence of the no-reflow phenomenon. Potential therapies designed to address the pathogenetic mechanisms underlying the no-reflow phenomenon are summarized in **Figure 55-44**.

Even if reperfusion is achieved in a timely fashion and no-reflow is minimized, there is an inevitable loss of a finite number of myocytes in a patient with STEMI. The secondary damage to the left ventricle after STEMI occurs through a process of postinfarction ventricular remodeling. Treatments to minimize ventricular remodeling include the standard approaches to disruption of the RAAS and potential new therapies, such as renin inhibition, reducing the amount of central nervous system generation of aldosterone, enhancing the synthesis of endothelial nitric oxide synthase, modulating beta-adrenergic signaling, and minimizing the processes that lead to cardiac apoptosis.[229]

Finally, in contradistinction to the traditional teaching that the heart is a terminally differentiated organ, it is now clear that myocytes are capable of entering the cell cycle and dividing (see Chaps. 11 and 33).[230] The burgeoning field of cardiac regenerative medicine is now focusing on several approaches using endogenous and exogenous sources of cells that may give rise to myocytes (**Fig. 55-45**).[231]

REFERENCES

General

1. Antman EM, Anbe DT, Armstrong PW, et al: ACC/AHA guidelines for the management of patients with ST-elevation myocardial infarction: A report of the American College of Cardiology/American Heart Association Task Force on Practice Guidelines (Committee to Revise the 1999 Guidelines for the Management of Patients with Acute Myocardial Infarction). Circulation 110:e82, 2004.
2. White HD, Chew DP: Acute myocardial infarction. Lancet 372:570, 2008.
3. Kuch B, von Scheidt W, Ehmann A, et al: Extent of the decrease of 28-day case fatality of hospitalized patients with acute myocardial infarction over 22 years: Epidemiological versus clinical view: The MONICA/KORA Augsburg Infarction Registry. Circ Cardiovasc Qual Outcomes 2:313, 2009.
4. Krumholz HM, Wang Y, Chen J, et al: Reduction in acute myocardial infarction mortality in the United States: Risk-standardized mortality rates from 1995-2006. JAMA 302:767, 2009.
5. Lloyd-Jones D, Adams R, Carnethon M, et al: Heart disease and stroke statistics—2009 update: A report from the American Heart Association Statistics Committee and Stroke Statistics Subcommittee. Circulation 119:e21, 2009.
6. Ting HH, Bradley EH, Wang Y, et al: Factors associated with longer time from symptom onset to hospital presentation for patients with ST-elevation myocardial infarction. Arch Intern Med 168:959, 2008.
7. Floyd KC, Yarzebski J, Spencer FA, et al: A 30-year perspective (1975-2005) into the changing landscape of patients hospitalized with initial acute myocardial infarction: Worcester Heart Attack Study. Circ Cardiovasc Qual Outcomes 2:88, 2009.
8. Antman EM: Time is muscle: translation into practice. J Am Coll Cardiol 52:1216, 2008.
9. Fox KA, Steg PG, Eagle KA, et al: Decline in rates of death and heart failure in acute coronary syndromes, 1999-2006. JAMA 297:1892, 2007.

Emergency Department Management

10. Tricomi AJ, Magid DJ, Rumsfeld JS, et al: Missed opportunities for reperfusion therapy for ST-segment elevation myocardial infarction: Results of the Emergency Department Quality in Myocardial Infarction (EDQMI) study. Am Heart J 155:471, 2008.
11. Jacobs AK, Antman EM, Faxon DP, et al: Development of systems of care for ST-elevation myocardial infarction patients: Executive summary. Circulation 116:217, 2007.
12. Rathore SS, Curtis JP, Chen J, et al: Association of door-to-balloon time and mortality in patients admitted to hospital with ST elevation myocardial infarction: National cohort study. BMJ 338:b1807, 2009.
13. American Heart Associaton, Mission: Lifeline, 2010 (http://www.heart.org/HEARTORG/HealthcareProfessional/Mission-Lifeline-Home-Page_UCM_305495_SubHomePage.jsp).
14. Jones DW, Peterson ED, Bonow RO, et al: Partnering to reduce risks and improve cardiovascular outcomes: American Heart Association initiatives in action for consumers and patients. Circulation 119:340, 2009.
15. Le May MR, So DY, Dionne R, et al: A citywide protocol for primary PCI in ST-segment elevation myocardial infarction. N Engl J Med 358:231, 2008.
16. Peterson ED, Roe MT, Mulgund J, et al: Association between hospital process performance and outcomes among patients with acute coronary syndromes. JAMA 295:1912, 2006.
17. Frendl DM, Palmeri ST, Clapp JR Jr, et al: Overcoming barriers to developing seamless ST-segment elevation myocardial infarction care systems in the United States: Recommendations from a comprehensive Prehospital 12-lead Electrocardiogram Working Group. J Electrocardiol 42:426, 2009.
18. Wang TY, Fonarow GC, Hernandez AF, et al: The dissociation between door-to-balloon time improvement and improvements in other acute myocardial infarction care processes and patient outcomes. Arch Intern Med 169:1411, 2009.
19. Mensah GA, Hand MM, Antman EM, et al: Development of systems of care for ST-elevation myocardial infarction patients: the patient and public perspective. Circulation 116:e33, 2007.
20. Moser DK, Kimble LP, Alberts MJ, et al: Reducing delay in seeking treatment by patients with acute coronary syndrome and stroke: A scientific statement from the American Heart Association Council on cardiovascular nursing and stroke council. Circulation 114:168, 2006.
21. Ting HH, Bradley EH, Wang Y, et al: Delay in presentation and reperfusion therapy in ST-elevation myocardial infarction. Am J Med 121:316, 2008.
22. National Heart Lung and Blood Institute: Act in Time to Heart Attack Signs (http://www.nhlbi.nih.gov/actintime).
23. Rokos IC, French WJ, Koenig WJ, et al: Integration of pre-hospital electrocardiograms and ST-elevation myocardial infarction receiving center (SRC) networks: Impact on door-to-balloon times across 10 independent regions. JACC Cardiovasc Interv 2:339, 2009.
24. Granger CB: Accelerating ST-segment elevation myocardial infarction care: Emergency medical services take center stage. JACC Cardiovasc Interv 2:347, 2009.
25. Sivagangabalan G, Ong AT, Narayan A, et al: Effect of prehospital triage on revascularization times, left ventricular function, and survival in patients with ST-elevation myocardial infarction. Am J Cardiol 103:907, 2009.
26. Jacobs AK, Antman EM, Ellrodt G, et al: Recommendation to develop strategies to increase the number of ST-segment-elevation myocardial infarction patients with timely access to primary percutaneous coronary intervention. Circulation 113:2152, 2006.
27. Millin MG, Brooks SC, Travers A, et al: Emergency medical services management of ST-elevation myocardial infarction. Prehosp Emerg Care 12:395, 2008.
28. Wiviott SD, Morrow DA, Frederick PD, et al: Performance of the thrombolysis in myocardial infarction risk index in the National Registry of Myocardial Infarction-3 and -4: A simple index that predicts mortality in ST-segment elevation myocardial infarction. J Am Coll Cardiol 44:783, 2004.
29. Danchin N, Coste P, Ferrieres J, et al: Comparison of thrombolysis followed by broad use of percutaneous coronary intervention with primary percutaneous coronary intervention for ST-segment-elevation acute myocardial infarction: Data from the French registry on acute ST-elevation myocardial infarction (FAST-MI). Circulation 118:268, 2008.
30. Bjorklund E, Stenestrand U, Lindback J, et al: Pre-hospital thrombolysis delivered by paramedics is associated with reduced time delay and mortality in ambulance-transported real-life patients with ST-elevation myocardial infarction. Eur Heart J 27:1146, 2006.
31. Zeymer U, Arntz HR, Dirks B, et al: Reperfusion rate and inhospital mortality of patients with ST-segment elevation myocardial infarction diagnosed already in the prehospital phase: Results of the German Prehospital Myocardial Infarction Registry (PREMIR). Resuscitation 80:402, 2009.
32. Morrison LJ, Brooks S, Sawadsky B, et al: Prehospital 12-lead electrocardiography impact on acute myocardial infarction treatment times and mortality: A systematic review. Acad Emerg Med 13:84, 2006.
33. Goldstein P, Lapostolle F, Steg G, et al: Lowering mortality in ST-elevation myocardial infarction and non-ST-elevation myocardial infarction: Key prehospital and emergency room treatment strategies. Eur J Emerg Med 16:244, 2009.
34. Atzema CL, Austin PC, Tu JV, Schull MJ: Emergency department triage of acute myocardial infarction patients and the effect on outcomes. Ann Emerg Med 53:736, 2009.
35. Antman EM, Hand M, Armstrong PW, et al: 2007 focused update of the ACC/AHA 2004 guidelines for the management of patients with ST-elevation myocardial infarction: A report of the American College of Cardiology/American Heart Association Task Force on Practice Guidelines: Developed in collaboration With the Canadian Cardiovascular Society: Endorsed by the American Academy of Family Physicians: 2007 Writing Group to Review New Evidence and Update the ACC/AHA 2004 Guidelines for the Management of Patients With ST-Elevation Myocardial Infarction, Writing on Behalf of the 2004 Writing Committee. Circulation 117:296, 2008.
36. Bradley EH, Herrin J, Wang Y, et al: Strategies for reducing the door-to-balloon time in acute myocardial infarction. N Engl J Med 355:2308, 2006.
37. Wang OJ, Wang Y, Lichtman JH, et al: "America's Best Hospitals" in the treatment of acute myocardial infarction. Arch Intern Med 167:1345, 2007.
38. Van de Werf F, Bax J, Betriu A, et al: Management of acute myocardial infarction in patients presenting with persistent ST-segment elevation: The Task Force on the Management of ST-Segment Elevation Acute Myocardial Infarction of the European Society of Cardiology. Eur Heart J 29:2909, 2008.
39. Cannon CP: Updated Strategies and Therapies for Reducing Ischemic and Vascular Events (STRIVE) unstable angina/non-ST elevation myocardial infarction critical pathway toolkit. Crit Pathw Cardiol 7:43, 2008.
40. Ross MA, Amsterdam E, Peacock WF, et al: Chest pain center accreditation is associated with better performance of centers for Medicare and Medicaid services core measures for acute myocardial infarction. Am J Cardiol 102:120, 2008.
41. Sweeny JM, Gorog DA, Fuster V: Antiplatelet drug 'resistance'. Part 1: Mechanisms and clinical measurements. Nat Rev Cardiol 6:273, 2009.
42. Hamon M, Agostini D, Le Page O, Riddell JW: Prognostic impact of right ventricular involvement in patients with acute myocardial infarction: meta-analysis. Crit Care Med 36:2023, 2008.
43. Chen ZM, Pan HC, Chen YP, et al: Early intravenous then oral metoprolol in 45,852 patients with acute myocardial infarction: randomised placebo-controlled trial. Lancet 366:1622, 2005.
44. Sabatine MS: Something old, something new: Beta blockers and clopidogrel in acute myocardial infarction. Lancet 366:1587, 2005.
45. Goldberg RJ, Spencer FA, Gore JM, et al: Thirty-year trends (1975 to 2005) in the magnitude of, management of, and hospital death rates associated with cardiogenic shock in patients with acute myocardial infarction: a population-based perspective. Circulation 119:1211, 2009.
46. Roik M, Opolski G: Long-term outcome among patients with ST-segment elevation myocardial infarction complicated by shock. J Am Coll Cardiol 52:315, 2008.

47. Gersh BJ, Stone GW, White HD, Holmes DR Jr: Pharmacological facilitation of primary percutaneous coronary intervention for acute myocardial infarction: Is the slope of the curve the shape of the future? JAMA 293:979, 2005.
48. Alter DA, Ko DT, Newman A, Tu JV: Factors explaining the under-use of reperfusion therapy among ideal patients with ST-segment elevation myocardial infarction. Eur Heart J 27:1539, 2006.
49. Gross ER, Gross GJ: Ischemic preconditioning and myocardial infarction: An update and perspective. Drug Discov Today Dis Mech 4:165, 2007.
50. De Luca G, Suryapranata H, Ottervanger JP, Antman EM: Time delay to treatment and mortality in primary angioplasty for acute myocardial infarction: Every minute of delay counts. Circulation 109:1223, 2004.
51. Fibrinolytic Therapy Trialists' (FTT) Collaborative Group: Indications for fibrinolytic therapy in suspected acute myocardial infarction: Collaborative overview of early mortality and major morbidity results from all randomised trials of more than 1000 patients. Lancet 343:311, 1994.
52. Park HJ, Chang K, Park CS, et al: Coronary collaterals: The role of MCP-1 during the early phase of acute myocardial infarction. Int J Cardiol 130:409, 2008.
53. Depre C, Vatner SF: Cardioprotection in stunned and hibernating myocardium. Heart Fail Rev 12:307, 2007.
54. Wu KC: Fighting the "fire" of myocardial reperfusion injury: How to define success? J Am Coll Cardiol 53:730, 2009.
55. Piper HM, Garcia-Dorado D: Cardiac protection takes off. Cardiovasc Res 83:163, 2009.
56. Majidi M, Kosinski AS, Al-Khatib SM, et al: Reperfusion ventricular arrhythmia 'bursts' in TIMI 3 flow restoration with primary angioplasty for anterior ST-elevation myocardial infarction: A more precise definition of reperfusion arrhythmias. Europace 10:988, 2008.
57. Garcia-Dorado D, Ruiz-Meana M, Piper HM: Lethal reperfusion injury in acute myocardial infarction: facts and unresolved issues. Cardiovasc Res 83:165, 2009.
58. Cannon RO 3rd: Mechanisms, management and future directions for reperfusion injury after acute myocardial infarction. Nat Clin Pract Cardiovasc Med 2:88, 2005.
59. Kloner RA, Forman MB, Gibbons RJ, et al: Impact of time to therapy and reperfusion modality on the efficacy of adenosine in acute myocardial infarction: The AMISTAD-2 trial. Eur Heart J 27:2400, 2006.
60. Laskey WK, Yoon S, Calzada N, Ricciardi MJ: Concordant improvements in coronary flow reserve and ST-segment resolution during percutaneous coronary intervention for acute myocardial infarction: A benefit of postconditioning. Catheter Cardiovasc Interv 72:212, 2008.
61. Granfeldt A, Lefer DJ, Vinten-Johansen J: Protective ischaemia in patients: Preconditioning and postconditioning. Cardiovasc Res 83:234, 2009.
62. Thibault H, Piot C, Staat P, et al: Long-term benefit of postconditioning. Circulation 117:1037, 2008.
63. Kawasaki T, Akakabe Y, Yamano M, et al: Vagal enhancement as evidence of residual ischemia after inferior myocardial infarction. Pacing Clin Electrophysiol 32:52, 2009.
64. Takemura G, Nakagawa M, Kanamori H, et al: Benefits of reperfusion beyond infarct size limitation. Cardiovasc Res 83:269, 2009.
65. Kelly RF, Sluiter W, McFalls EO: Hibernating myocardium: Is the program to survive a pathway to failure? Circ Res 102:3, 2008.
66. Van de Werf FJ, Topol EJ, Sobel BE: The impact of fibrinolytic therapy for ST-segment-elevation acute myocardial infarction. J Thromb Haemost 7:14, 2009.
67. Kiernan TJ, Gersh BJ: Thrombolysis in acute myocardial infarction: Current status. Med Clin North Am. 91:617, 2007.
68. Kelly RV, Crouch E, Krumnacher H, et al: Safety of adjunctive intracoronary thrombolytic therapy during complex percutaneous coronary intervention: Initial experience with intracoronary tenecteplase. Catheter Cardiovasc Interv. 66:327, 2005.
69. TIMI Study Group: The Thrombolysis in Myocardial Infarction (TIMI) trial. Phase I findings. N Engl J Med 312:932, 1985.
70. Gibson CM, Murphy S, Menown IB, et al: Determinants of coronary blood flow after thrombolytic administration. TIMI Study Group. Thrombolysis in Myocardial Infarction. J Am Coll Cardiol 34:1403, 1999.
71. Appelbaum E, Kirtane AJ, Clark A, et al: Association of TIMI myocardial perfusion grade and ST-segment resolution with cardiovascular magnetic resonance measures of microvascular obstruction and infarct size following ST-segment elevation myocardial infarction. J Thromb Thrombolysis 27:123, 2009.
72. Niccoli G, Burzotta F, Galiuto L, Crea F: Myocardial no-reflow in humans. J Am Coll Cardiol 54:281, 2009.
73. Kirtane AJ, Vafai JJ, Murphy SA, et al: Angiographically evident thrombus following fibrinolytic therapy is associated with impaired myocardial perfusion in STEMI: A CLARITY-TIMI 28 substudy. Eur Heart J 27:2040, 2006.
74. Rakowski T, Dziewierz A, Siudak Z, et al: ST-segment resolution assessed immediately after primary percutaneous coronary intervention correlates with infarct size and left ventricular function in cardiac magnetic resonance at 1-year follow-up. J Electrocardiol 42:152, 2009.
75. Rekik S, Mnif S, Sahnoun M, et al: Total absence of ST-segment resolution after failed thrombolysis is correlated with unfavorable short- and long-term outcomes despite successful rescue angioplasty. J Electrocardiol 42:73, 2009.
76. Bjorklund E, Jernberg T, Johanson P, et al: Admission N-terminal pro-brain natriuretic peptide and its interaction with admission troponin T and ST-segment resolution for early risk stratification in ST elevation myocardial infarction. Heart 92:735, 2006.
77. Terkelsen CJ, Norgaard BL, Lassen JF, et al: Potential significance of spontaneous and interventional ST-changes in patients transferred for primary percutaneous coronary intervention: Observations from the ST-MONitoring in Acute Myocardial Infarction study (the MONAMI study). Eur Heart J 27:267, 2006.
78. Gershlick AH: Managing myocardial infarction in the elderly: Time to bury inappropriate concerns instead. Eur Heart J 30:887, 2009.
79. Schiele F, Meneveau N, Seronde MF, et al: Changes in management of elderly patients with myocardial infarction. Eur Heart J 30:987, 2009.
80. Acikel S, Akdemir R, Cagirci G, et al: The treatment of clopidogrel resistance: Triple antiplatelet therapy and future directions. Int J Cardiol 144:79, 2009.
81. Ross AM, Gibbons RJ, Stone GW, et al: A randomized, double-blinded, placebo-controlled multicenter trial of adenosine as an adjunct to reperfusion in the treatment of acute myocardial infarction (AMISTAD-II). J Am Coll Cardiol 45:1775, 2005.
82. Assessment of the Safety and Efficacy of a New Treatment Strategy with Percutaneous Coronary Intervention (ASSENT-4 PCI) investigators: Primary versus tenecteplase-facilitated percutaneous coronary intervention in patients with ST-segment elevation acute myocardial infarction (ASSENT-4 PCI): Randomised trial. Lancet 367:569, 2006.
83. Carter NJ, McCormack PL, Plosker GL: Enoxaparin: A review of its use in ST-segment elevation myocardial infarction. Drugs 68:691, 2008.
84. Fernandez-Aviles F, Alonso JJ, Castro-Beiras A, et al: Routine invasive strategy within 24 hours of thrombolysis versus ischaemia-guided conservative approach for acute myocardial infarction with ST-segment elevation (GRACIA-1): a randomised controlled trial. Lancet 364:1045, 2004.
85. Cantor WJ, Fitchett D, Borgundvaag B, et al: Routine early angioplasty after fibrinolysis for acute myocardial infarction. N Engl J Med 360:2705, 2009.
86. Huynh T, Perron S, O'Loughlin J, et al: Comparison of primary percutaneous coronary intervention and fibrinolytic therapy in ST-segment-elevation myocardial infarction: bayesian hierarchical meta-analyses of randomized controlled trials and observational studies. Circulation 119:3101, 2009.
87. Stone GW: Angioplasty strategies in ST-segment-elevation myocardial infarction: part I: primary percutaneous coronary intervention. Circulation 118:538, 2008.
88. Srinivas VS, Hailpern SM, Koss E, et al: Effect of physician volume on the relationship between hospital volume and mortality during primary angioplasty. J Am Coll Cardiol 53:574, 2009.
89. Hochman JS, Sleeper LA, Webb JG, et al: Early revascularization and long-term survival in cardiogenic shock complicating acute myocardial infarction. JAMA 295:2511, 2006.
90. Grzybowski M, Clements EA, Parsons L, et al: Mortality benefit of immediate revascularization of acute ST-segment elevation myocardial infarction in patients with contraindications to thrombolytic therapy: A propensity analysis. JAMA 290:1891, 2003.
91. Pinto DS, Kirtane AJ, Nallamothu BK, et al: Hospital delays in reperfusion for ST-elevation myocardial infarction: Implications when selecting a reperfusion strategy. Circulation 114:2019, 2006.
92. Chakrabarti A, Krumholz HM, Wang Y, et al: Time to reperfusion in patients undergoing interhospital transfer for primary percutaneous coronary intervention in the U.S: An analysis of 2005 and 2006 data from the National Cardiovascular Data Registry. J Am Coll Cardiol 51:2442, 2008.
93. Busk M, Maeng M, Rasmussen K, et al: The Danish multicentre randomized study of fibrinolytic therapy vs. primary angioplasty in acute myocardial infarction (the DANAMI-2 trial): Outcome after 3 years follow-up. Eur Heart J 29:1259, 2008.
94. Morrow DA: Heparin and low-molecular-weight heparin. *In* Manson JE, Buring JE, Ridker PM, Gaziano JM (eds): Clinical Trials in Heart Disease: A Companion to Braunwald's Heart Disease. 2nd ed. Philadelphia, Elsevier Saunders, 2004, pp 45-65.
95. Crespo EM, Oliveira GB, Honeycutt EF, et al: Evaluation and management of thrombocytopenia and suspected heparin-induced thrombocytopenia in hospitalized patients: The Complications After Thrombocytopenia Caused by Heparin (CATCH) registry. Am Heart J 157:651, 2009.
96. Holmes DR Jr, Kereiakes DJ, Kleiman NS, et al: Combining antiplatelet and anticoagulant therapies. J Am Coll Cardiol 54:95, 2009.
97. Cheng S, Morrow DA, Sloan S, et al: Predictors of initial nontherapeutic anticoagulation with unfractionated heparin in ST-segment elevation myocardial infarction. Circulation 119:1195, 2009.
98. Bittl JA, White HD, Antman EM: Direct thrombin inhibitors. *In* Manson JE, Buring JE, Ridker PM, Gaziano JM (eds): Clinical Trials in Heart Disease: A Companion to Braunwald's Heart Disease. 2d ed. Philadelphia, Elsevier Saunders; 2004, pp 83-96.
99. Stone GW, Witzenbichler B, Guagliumi G, et al: Bivalirudin during primary PCI in acute myocardial infarction. N Engl J Med 358:2218, 2008.
100. Morrow DA: Antithrombotic therapy to support primary PCI. N Engl J Med 358:2280, 2008.
101. Singh S, Bahekar A, Molnar J, et al: Adjunctive low molecular weight heparin during fibrinolytic therapy in acute ST-segment elevation myocardial infarction: A meta-analysis of randomized control trials. Clin Cardiol 32:358, 2009.
102. Yusuf S, Mehta SR, Xie C, et al: Effects of reviparin, a low-molecular-weight heparin, on mortality, reinfarction, and strokes in patients with acute myocardial infarction presenting with ST-segment elevation. JAMA 293:427, 2005.
103. Assessment of the Safety and Efficacy of a New Thrombolytic Regimen (ASSENT)-3 Investigators: Efficacy and safety of tenecteplase in combination with enoxaparin, abciximab, or unfractionated heparin: the ASSENT-3 randomised trial in acute myocardial infarction. Lancet 358:605, 2001.
104. Antman EM, Morrow DA, McCabe CH, et al: Enoxaparin versus unfractionated heparin with fibrinolysis for ST-elevation myocardial infarction. N Engl J Med 354:1477, 2006.
105. Yusuf S, Mehta SR, Chrolavicius S, et al: Effects of fondaparinux on mortality and reinfarction in patients with acute ST-segment elevation myocardial infarction: The OASIS-6 randomized trial. JAMA 295:1519, 2009.
106. Eikelboom JW, Weitz JI: Anticoagulation for ST-segment elevation myocardial infarction. Circulation 119:1186, 2009.
107. Oldgren J, Wallentin L, Afzal R, et al: Effects of fondaparinux in patients with ST-segment elevation acute myocardial infarction not receiving reperfusion treatment. Eur Heart J 29:315, 2008.
108. Beygui F, Collet JP, Nagaswami C, et al: Images in cardiovascular medicine. Architecture of intracoronary thrombi in ST-elevation acute myocardial infarction: Time makes the difference. Circulation 113:e21, 2006.
109. Antithrombotic Trialists' Collaboration: Collaborative meta-analysis of randomised trials of antiplatelet therapy for prevention of death, myocardial infarction, and stroke in high risk patients. BMJ 324:71, 2002.
110. Sabatine MS, Cannon CP, Gibson CM, et al: Addition of clopidogrel to aspirin and fibrinolytic therapy for myocardial infarction with ST-segment elevation. N Engl J Med 352:1179, 2005.
111. Scirica BM, Sabatine MS, Morrow DA, et al: The role of clopidogrel in early and sustained arterial patency after fibrinolysis for ST-segment elevation myocardial infarction: The ECG CLARITY-TIMI 28 Study. J Am Coll Cardiol 48:37, 2006.

112. Sabatine MS, Cannon CP, Gibson CM, et al: Effect of clopidogrel pretreatment before percutaneous coronary intervention in patients with ST-elevation myocardial infarction treated with fibrinolytics: The PCI-CLARITY study. JAMA 294:1224, 2005.

Hospital Management

113. Wiviott SD, Braunwald E, McCabe CH, et al: Prasugrel versus clopidogrel in patients with acute coronary syndromes. N Engl J Med 357:2001, 2007.
114. Montalescot G, Wiviott SD, Braunwald E, et al: Prasugrel compared with clopidogrel in patients undergoing percutaneous coronary intervention for ST-elevation myocardial infarction (TRITON-TIMI 38): Double-blind, randomised controlled trial. Lancet 373:723, 2009.
114a. Wallentin L, Becker RC, Budaj A, et al: Ticagrelor versus clopidogrel in patients with acute coronary syndromes. N Engl J Med 361:1045, 2009.
115. Peters RJ, Mehta SR, Fox KA, et al: Effects of aspirin dose when used alone or in combination with clopidogrel in patients with acute coronary syndromes: Observations from the Clopidogrel in Unstable angina to prevent Recurrent Events (CURE) study. Circulation 108:1682, 2003.
116. Chen ZM, Jiang LX, Chen YP, et al: Addition of clopidogrel to aspirin in 45,852 patients with acute myocardial infarction: Randomised placebo-controlled trial. Lancet 366:1607, 2005.
117. King SB 3rd, Smith SC Jr, Hirshfeld JW Jr, et al: 2007 focused update of the ACC/AHA/SCAI 2005 guideline update for percutaneous coronary intervention: A report of the American College of Cardiology/American Heart Association Task Force on Practice Guidelines: 2007 Writing Group to Review New Evidence and Update the ACC/AHA/SCAI 2005 Guideline Update for Percutaneous Coronary Intervention, Writing on Behalf of the 2005 Writing Committee. Circulation 117:261, 2008.
118. Anderson JL, Adams CD, Antman EM, et al: ACC/AHA 2007 guidelines for the management of patients with unstable angina/non ST-elevation myocardial infarction: A report of the American College of Cardiology/American Heart Association Task Force on Practice Guidelines (Writing Committee to Revise the 2002 Guidelines for the Management of Patients With Unstable Angina/Non ST-Elevation Myocardial Infarction): Developed in collaboration with the American College of Emergency Physicians, the Society for Cardiovascular Angiography and Interventions, and the Society of Thoracic Surgeons: Endorsed by the American Association of Cardiovascular and Pulmonary Rehabilitation and the Society for Academic Emergency Medicine. Circulation 116:e148, 2007.
119. Berger AK, Duval S, Jacobs DR Jr, et al: Relation of length of hospital stay in acute myocardial infarction to postdischarge mortality. Am J Cardiol 101:428, 2008.
120. Bates ER: Role of intravenous beta-blockers in the treatment of ST-elevation myocardial infarction: Of mice (dogs, pigs) and men. Circulation 115:2904, 2007.
121. Freemantle N, Cleland J, Young P, et al: Beta blockade after myocardial infarction: Systematic review and meta regression analysis. BMJ 318:1730, 1999.
122. The TIMI Study Group: Comparison of invasive and conservative strategies after treatment with intravenous tissue plasminogen activator in acute myocardial infarction. Results of the thrombolysis in myocardial infarction (TIMI) phase II trial. N Engl J Med 320:618, 1989.
123. Piccini JP, Hranitzky PM, Kilaru R, et al: Relation of mortality to failure to prescribe beta blockers acutely in patients with sustained ventricular tachycardia and ventricular fibrillation following acute myocardial infarction (from the VALsartan In Acute myocardial iNfarcTion trial [VALIANT] Registry). Am J Cardiol 102:1427, 2008.
124. Fonarow GC, Lukas MA, Robertson M, et al: Effects of carvedilol early after myocardial infarction: Analysis of the first 30 days in Carvedilol Post-Infarct Survival Control in Left Ventricular Dysfunction (CAPRICORN). Am Heart J 154:637, 2007.
125. Rutherford JD, Pfeffer MA, Moye LA, et al: Effects of captopril on ischemic events after myocardial infarction. Results of the Survival and Ventricular Enlargement trial. SAVE Investigators. Circulation 90:1731, 1994.
126. Schocken DD, Benjamin EJ, Fonarow GC, et al: Prevention of heart failure: A scientific statement from the American Heart Association Councils on Epidemiology and Prevention, Clinical Cardiology, Cardiovascular Nursing, and High Blood Pressure Research; Quality of Care and Outcomes Research Interdisciplinary Working Group; and Functional Genomics and Translational Biology Interdisciplinary Working Group. Circulation 117:2544, 2008.
127. Pfeffer MA, McMurray JJ, Velazquez EJ, et al: Valsartan, captopril, or both in myocardial infarction complicated by heart failure, left ventricular dysfunction, or both. N Engl J Med 349:1893, 2003.
128. Pitt B, Remme W, Zannad F, et al: Eplerenone, a selective aldosterone blocker, in patients with left ventricular dysfunction after myocardial infarction. N Engl J Med 348:1309, 2003.
129. Pedrazzini G, Santoro E, Latini R, et al: Causes of death in patients with acute myocardial infarction treated with angiotensin-converting enzyme inhibitors: Findings from the Gruppo Italiano per lo Studio della Sopravvivenza nell'Infarto (GISSI)-3 trial. Am Heart J 155:388, 2008.
130. Tokmakova M, Solomon SD: Inhibiting the renin-angiotensin system in myocardial infarction and heart failure: lessons from SAVE, VALIANT and CHARM, and other clinical trials. Curr Opin Cardiol 21:268, 2006.
131. Phillips CO, Kashani A, Ko DK, et al: Adverse effects of combination angiotensin II receptor blockers plus angiotensin-converting enzyme inhibitors for left ventricular dysfunction: A quantitative review of data from randomized clinical trials. Arch Intern Med 167:1930, 2007.
132. Gornik H, O'Gara PT: Adjunctive medical therapy. *In* Manson JE, Buring JE, Ridker PM, Gaziano JM (eds): Clinical Trials in Heart Disease: A Companion to Braunwald's Heart Disease. Philadelphia, Elsevier Saunders, 2004, pp 109-128.
133. MAGIC Investigators: Early administration of intravenous magnesium to high-risk patients with acute myocardial infarction in the Magnesium in Coronaries (MAGIC) Trial: A randomised controlled trial. Lancet 360:1189, 2002.
134. Moghissi ES, Korytkowski MT, DiNardo M, et al: American Association of Clinical Endocrinologists and American Diabetes Association consensus statement on inpatient glycemic control. Endocr Pract 15:353, 2009.
135. Mehta SR, Yusuf S, Diaz R, et al: Effect of glucose-insulin-potassium infusion on mortality in patients with acute ST-segment elevation myocardial infarction: The CREATE-ECLA randomized controlled trial. JAMA 293:437, 2005.
136. Granger CB, Mahaffey KW, Weaver WD, et al: Pexelizumab, an anti-C5 complement antibody, as adjunctive therapy to primary percutaneous coronary intervention in acute myocardial infarction: The COMplement inhibition in Myocardial infarction treated with Angioplasty (COMMA) trial. Circulation 108:1184, 2003.
137. Mahaffey KW, Granger CB, Nicolau JC, et al: Effect of pexelizumab, an anti-C5 complement antibody, as adjunctive therapy to fibrinolysis in acute myocardial infarction: The COMPlement inhibition in myocardial infarction treated with thromboLYtics (COMPLY) trial. Circulation 108:1176, 2003.
138. Armstrong PW, Granger CB, Adams PX, et al: Pexelizumab for acute ST-elevation myocardial infarction in patients undergoing primary percutaneous coronary intervention: A randomized controlled trial. JAMA 297:43, 2007.

Hemodynamic Disturbances

139. Chatterjee K: The Swan-Ganz catheters: Past, present, and future. A viewpoint. Circulation 119:147, 2009.
140. Stewart RM, Park PK, Hunt JP, et al: Less is more: Improved outcomes in surgical patients with conservative fluid administration and central venous catheter monitoring. J Am Coll Surg. 208:725, 2009.
141. Finfer S, Delaney A: Pulmonary artery catheters. BMJ 333:930, 2006.
142. Timsit JF, Schwebel C, Bouadma L, et al: Chlorhexidine-impregnated sponges and less frequent dressing changes for prevention of catheter-related infections in critically ill adults: A randomized controlled trial. JAMA 301:1231, 2009.
143. Funk DJ, Moretti EW, Gan TJ: Minimally invasive cardiac output monitoring in the perioperative setting. Anesth Analg 108:887, 2009.
144. Frisch DR, Giedrimas E, Mohanavelu S, et al: Predicting irreversible left ventricular dysfunction after acute myocardial infarction. Am J Cardiol 103:1206, 2009.
145. Reynolds HR, Hochman JS: Cardiogenic shock: Current concepts and improving outcomes. Circulation 117:686, 2008.
146. Harinstein ME, Flaherty JD, Fonarow GC, Gheorghiade M: Directions for research in the post-myocardial infarction patient with left ventricular dysfunction. Am J Cardiol 102:57G, 2008.
147. Lewis EF, Velazquez EJ, Solomon SD, et al: Predictors of the first heart failure hospitalization in patients who are stable survivors of myocardial infarction complicated by pulmonary congestion and/or left ventricular dysfunction: A VALIANT study. Eur Heart J 29:748, 2008.
148. Flaherty JD, Udelson JE, Gheorghiade M, et al: Assessment and key targets for therapy in the post-myocardial infarction patient with left ventricular dysfunction. Am J Cardiol 102:5G, 2008.
149. Ishii H, Amano T, Matsubara T, Murohara T: Pharmacological intervention for prevention of left ventricular remodeling and improving prognosis in myocardial infarction. Circulation 118:2710, 2008.
150. Overgaard CB, Dzavik V: Inotropes and vasopressors: Review of physiology and clinical use in cardiovascular disease. Circulation 118:1047, 2008.
150a. De Backer D, Biston P, Devriendt J, et al: Comparison of dopamine and norepinephrine in the treatment of shock. N Engl J Med 362:779, 2010.
151. Babaev A, Frederick PD, Pasta DJ, et al: Trends in management and outcomes of patients with acute myocardial infarction complicated by cardiogenic shock. JAMA 294:448, 2005.
152. Hochman JS: Cardiogenic shock complicating acute myocardial infarction: Expanding the paradigm. Circulation 107:2998, 2003.
153. Mebazaa A, Nieminen MS, Packer M, et al: Levosimendan vs dobutamine for patients with acute decompensated heart failure: The SURVIVE Randomized Trial. JAMA 297:1883, 2007.
154. Thiele H, Smalling RW, Schuler GC: Percutaneous left ventricular assist devices in acute myocardial infarction complicated by cardiogenic shock. Eur Heart J 28:2057, 2007.
155. Al-Husami W, Yturralde F, Mohanty G, et al: Single-center experience with the TandemHeart percutaneous ventricular assist device to support patients undergoing high-risk percutaneous coronary intervention. J Invasive Cardiol 20:319, 2008.
156. Seyfarth M, Sibbing D, Bauer I, et al: A randomized clinical trial to evaluate the safety and efficacy of a percutaneous left ventricular assist device versus intra-aortic balloon pumping for treatment of cardiogenic shock caused by myocardial infarction. J Am Coll Cardiol 52:1584, 2008.
157. Lim HS, Farouque O, Andrianopoulos N, et al: Survival of elderly patients undergoing percutaneous coronary intervention for acute myocardial infarction complicated by cardiogenic shock. JACC Cardiovasc Interv 2:146, 2009.
158. Pfisterer M: Right ventricular involvement in myocardial infarction and cardiogenic shock. Lancet 362:392, 2003.
159. Zimetbaum PJ, Josephson ME: Use of the electrocardiogram in acute myocardial infarction. N Engl J Med 348:933, 2003.
160. Wellens HJ: The value of the right precordial leads of the electrocardiogram. N Engl J Med 340:381, 1999.
161. Anavekar NS, Skali H, Bourgoun M, et al: Usefulness of right ventricular fractional area change to predict death, heart failure, and stroke following myocardial infarction (from the VALIANT ECHO Study). Am J Cardiol 101:607, 2008.
162. Larose E, Ganz P, Reynolds HG, et al: Right ventricular dysfunction assessed by cardiovascular magnetic resonance imaging predicts poor prognosis late after myocardial infarction. J Am Coll Cardiol 49:855, 2007.
163. Figueras J, Alcalde O, Barrabes JA, et al: Changes in hospital mortality rates in 425 patients with acute ST-elevation myocardial infarction and cardiac rupture over a 30-year period. Circulation 118:2783, 2008.
164. Poulsen SH, Praestholm M, Munk K, et al: Ventricular septal rupture complicating acute myocardial infarction: Clinical characteristics and contemporary outcome. Ann Thorac Surg. 85:1591, 2008.
165. Maltais S, Ibrahim R, Basmadjian AJ, et al: Postinfarction ventricular septal defects: Towards a new treatment algorithm? Ann Thorac Surg 87:687, 2009.
166. Freixa X, Sitges M, Pare C: Images in cardiology. Left ventricular pseudoaneurysm complicating acute myocardial infarction: Improved diagnosis by real-time three-dimensional echocardiography. Heart 92:154, 2006.
167. Atik FA, Navia JL, Vega PR, et al: Surgical treatment of postinfarction left ventricular pseudoaneurysm. Ann Thorac Surg 83:526, 2007.
168. Birnbaum Y, Fishbein MC, Blanche C, Siegel RJ: Ventricular septal rupture after acute myocardial infarction. N Engl J Med 347:1426, 2002.
169. Bursi F, Enriquez-Sarano M, Jacobsen SJ, Roger VL: Mitral regurgitation after myocardial infarction: A review. Am J Med 119:103, 2006.

170. Stout KK, Verrier ED: Acute valvular regurgitation. Circulation 119:3232, 2009.
171. Liuzzo JP, Shin YT, Choi C, et al: Simultaneous papillary muscle avulsion and free wall rupture during acute myocardial infarction. Intra-aortic balloon pump: A bridge to survival. J Invasive Cardiol 18:135, 2006.
172. Russo A, Suri RM, Grigioni F, et al: Clinical outcome after surgical correction of mitral regurgitation due to papillary muscle rupture. Circulation 118:1528, 2008.
173. Carmeliet E: Cardiac ionic currents and acute ischemia: From channels to arrhythmias. Physiol Rev 79:917, 1999.
174. Tang L, Deng C, Long M, et al: Thrombin receptor and ventricular arrhythmias after acute myocardial infarction. Mol Med. 14:131, 2008.
175. Yadav AV, Zipes DP: Prophylactic lidocaine in acute myocardial infarction: Resurface or reburial? Am J Cardiol 94:606, 2004.
176. Piccini JP, Berger JS, Brown DL: Early sustained ventricular arrhythmias complicating acute myocardial infarction. Am J Med 121:797, 2008.
177. Hreybe H, Saba S: Location of acute myocardial infarction and associated arrhythmias and outcome. Clin Cardiol 32:274, 2009.
178. Altun A, Kirdar C, Ozbay G. Effect of aminophylline in patients with atropine-resistant late advanced atrioventricular block during acute inferior myocardial infarction. Clin Cardiol 21:759, 1998.
179. Di Chiara A: Right bundle branch block during the acute phase of myocardial infarction: Modern redefinitions of old concepts. Eur Heart J 27:1, 2006.
180. Wong CK, Stewart RA, Gao W, et al: Prognostic differences between different types of bundle branch block during the early phase of acute myocardial infarction: insights from the Hirulog and Early Reperfusion or Occlusion (HERO)-2 trial. Eur Heart J 27:21, 2006.
181. Kleemann T, Juenger C, Gitt AK, et al: Incidence and clinical impact of right bundle branch block in patients with acute myocardial infarction: ST elevation myocardial infarction versus non-ST elevation myocardial infarction. Am Heart J 156:256, 2008.
182. Suzuki M, Sakaue T, Tanaka M, et al: Association between right bundle branch block and impaired myocardial tissue-level reperfusion in patients with acute myocardial infarction. J Am Coll Cardiol 47:2122, 2006.
183. Bogale N, Orn S, James M, et al: Usefulness of either or both left and right bundle branch block at baseline or during follow-up for predicting death in patients following acute myocardial infarction. Am J Cardiol 99:647, 2007.
184. Køber L, Swedberg K, McMurray JJ, et al: Previously known and newly diagnosed atrial fibrillation: A major risk indicator after a myocardial infarction complicated by heart failure or left ventricular dysfunction. Eur J Heart Fail 8:591, 2006.
185. Saczynski JS, McManus D, Zhou Z, et al: Trends in atrial fibrillation complicating acute myocardial infarction. Am J Cardiol 104:169, 2009.
186. Berton G, Cordiano R, Cucchini F, et al: Atrial fibrillation during acute myocardial infarction: Association with all-cause mortality and sudden death after 7-year of follow-up. Int J Clin Pract. 63:712, 2009.
187. Keeley EC, Boura JA, Grines CL: Primary angioplasty versus intravenous thrombolytic therapy for acute myocardial infarction: A quantitative review of 23 randomised trials. Lancet 361:13, 2003.
188. Kruk M, Kadziela J, Reynolds HR, et al: Predictors of outcome and the lack of effect of percutaneous coronary intervention across the risk strata in patients with persistent total occlusion after myocardial infarction: Results from the OAT (Occluded Artery Trial) study. JACC Cardiovasc Interv 1:511, 2008.
189. Fokkema ML, van der Vleuten PA, Vlaar PJ, et al: Incidence, predictors, and outcome of reinfarction and stent thrombosis within one year after primary percutaneous coronary intervention for ST-elevation myocardial infarction. Catheter Cardiovasc Interv 73:627, 2009.
190. Gueret P, Khalife K, Jobic Y, et al: Echocardiographic assessment of the incidence of mechanical complications during the early phase of myocardial infarction in the reperfusion era: A French multicentre prospective registry. Arch Cardiovasc Dis 101:41, 2008.
191. Jugdutt BI: Cyclooxygenase inhibition and adverse remodeling during healing after myocardial infarction. Circulation 115:288, 2007.
192. Imazio M, Negro A, Belli R, et al: Frequency and prognostic significance of pericarditis following acute myocardial infarction treated by primary percutaneous coronary intervention. Am J Cardiol 103:1525, 2009.
193. Napodano M, Tarantini G, Ramondo A, et al: Myocardial abnormalities underlying persistent ST-segment elevation after anterior myocardial infarction. J Cardiovasc Med (Hagerstown) 10:44, 2009.
194. Abildstrom SZ, Ottesen MM, Rask-Madsen C, et al: Sudden cardiovascular death following myocardial infarction: The importance of left ventricular systolic dysfunction and congestive heart failure. Int J Cardiol 104:184, 2005.
195. Marchenko AV, Cherniavsky AM, Volokitina TL, et al: Left ventricular dimension and shape after postinfarction aneurysm repair. Eur J Cardiothorac Surg 27:475, 2005.
196. Rehan A, Kanwar M, Rosman H, et al: Incidence of post myocardial infarction left ventricular thrombus formation in the era of primary percutaneous intervention and glycoprotein IIb/IIIa inhibitors. A prospective observational study. Cardiovasc Ultrasound 4:20, 2006.
197. Hirsh J, Fuster V, Ansell J, Halperin JL: American Heart Association/American College of Cardiology Foundation guide to warfarin therapy. Circulation 107:1692, 2003.
198. Jaffe AS, Krumholz HM, Catellier DJ, et al: Prediction of medical morbidity and mortality after acute myocardial infarction in patients at increased psychosocial risk in the Enhancing Recovery in Coronary Heart Disease Patients (ENRICHD) study. Am Heart J 152:126, 2006.
199. Alter DA, Chong A, Austin PC, et al: Socioeconomic status and mortality after acute myocardial infarction. Ann Intern Med 144:82, 2006.
200. Mendes de Leon CF, Czajkowski SM, Freedland KE, et al: The effect of a psychosocial intervention and quality of life after acute myocardial infarction: The Enhancing Recovery in Coronary Heart Disease (ENRICHD) clinical trial. J Cardiopulm Rehabil 26:9, 2006.
201. Donahoe SM, Stewart GC, McCabe CH, et al: Diabetes and mortality following acute coronary syndromes. JAMA 298:765, 2007.
202. Petrina M, Goodman SG, Eagle KA: The 12-lead electrocardiogram as a predictive tool of mortality after acute myocardial infarction: current status in an era of revascularization and reperfusion. Am Heart J 152:11, 2006.
203. Wong CK, Gao W, Raffel OC, et al: Initial Q waves accompanying ST-segment elevation at presentation of acute myocardial infarction and 30-day mortality in patients given streptokinase therapy: An analysis from HERO-2. Lancet 367:2061, 2006.
204. Morrow DA: Cardiovascular risk prediction in patients with stable and unstable coronary heart disease. Circulation 121:2681, 2010.
205. Adabag AS, Therneau TM, Gersh BJ, et al: Sudden death after myocardial infarction. JAMA 300:2022, 2008.
206. Gibson CM, Karha J, Murphy SA, et al: Early and long-term clinical outcomes associated with reinfarction following fibrinolytic administration in the Thrombolysis in Myocardial Infarction trials. J Am Coll Cardiol 42:7, 2003.
207. De Luca G, Ernst N, van 't Hof AW, et al: Predictors and clinical implications of early reinfarction after primary angioplasty for ST-segment elevation myocardial infarction. Am Heart J 151:1256, 2006.
208. Bodi V, Sanchis J, Nunez J, et al: Prognostic value of a comprehensive cardiac magnetic resonance assessment soon after a first ST-segment elevation myocardial infarction. JACC Cardiovasc Imaging 2:835, 2009.
209. Wright J, Adriaenssens T, Dymarkowski S, et al: Quantification of myocardial area at risk with T2-weighted CMR: Comparison with contrast-enhanced CMR and coronary angiography. JACC Cardiovasc Imaging 2:825, 2009.
210. Di Carli MF, Hachamovitch R: New technology for noninvasive evaluation of coronary artery disease. Circulation 115:1464, 2007.

Arrhythmias

211. Zipes DP, Camm AJ, Borggrefe M, et al: ACC/AHA/ESC 2006 Guidelines for Management of Patients With Ventricular Arrhythmias and the Prevention of Sudden Cardiac Death: A report of the American College of Cardiology/American Heart Association Task Force and the European Society of Cardiology Committee for Practice Guidelines (writing committee to develop Guidelines for Management of Patients With Ventricular Arrhythmias and the Prevention of Sudden Cardiac Death): Developed in collaboration with the European Heart Rhythm Association and the Heart Rhythm Society. Circulation 114:e385, 2006.
212. Estes NA 3rd: The challenge of predicting and preventing sudden cardiac death immediately after myocardial infarction. Circulation 120:185, 2009.

Other Complications

213. Dawood N, Vaccarino V, Reid KJ, et al: Predictors of smoking cessation after a myocardial infarction: The role of institutional smoking cessation programs in improving success. Arch Intern Med 168:1961, 2008.
214. Thombs BD, de Jonge P, Coyne JC, et al: Depression screening and patient outcomes in cardiovascular care: A systematic review. JAMA 300:2161, 2008.
215. Milani RV, Lavie CJ: Impact of cardiac rehabilitation on depression and its associated mortality. Am J Med 120:799, 2007.
216. Smith SC Jr, Allen J, Blair SN, et al: AHA/ACC guidelines for secondary prevention for patients with coronary and other atherosclerotic vascular disease: 2006 update: Endorsed by the National Heart, Lung, and Blood Institute. Circulation 113:2363, 2006.
217. Morrow DA, de Lemos JA, Sabatine MS, et al: Clinical relevance of C-reactive protein during follow-up of patients with acute coronary syndromes in the Aggrastat-to-Zocor Trial. Circulation 114:281, 2006.
218. Waters DD, Brotons C, Chiang CW, et al: Lipid treatment assessment project 2: A multinational survey to evaluate the proportion of patients achieving low-density lipoprotein cholesterol goals. Circulation 120:28, 2009.
219. Lichtenstein AH, Appel LJ, Brands M, et al: Diet and lifestyle recommendations revision 2006: A scientific statement from the American Heart Association Nutrition Committee. Circulation 114:82, 2006.
220. Morrow DA, Wiviott SD, White HD, et al: Effect of the novel thienopyridine prasugrel compared with clopidogrel on spontaneous and procedural myocardial infarction in the Trial to Assess Improvement in Therapeutic Outcomes by Optimizing Platelet Inhibition with Prasugrel-Thrombolysis in Myocardial Infarction 38: An application of the classification system from the universal definition of myocardial infarction. Circulation 119:2758, 2009.
221. Antman EM, Wiviott SD, Murphy SA, et al: Early and late benefits of prasugrel in patients with acute coronary syndromes undergoing percutaneous coronary intervention: A TRITON-TIMI 38 (TRial to Assess Improvement in Therapeutic Outcomes by Optimizing Platelet InhibitioN with Prasugrel-Thrombolysis In Myocardial Infarction) analysis. J Am Coll Cardiol 51:2028, 2008.
222. Abdel-Latif A, Moliterno DJ: Antiplatelet polypharmacy in primary percutaneous coronary intervention: Trying to understand when more is better. Circulation 119:3168, 2009.
223. Fonarow GC: Beta-blockers for the post-myocardial infarction patient: Current clinical evidence and practical considerations. Rev Cardiovasc Med 7:1, 2006.
224. Mega JL, Braunwald E, Mohanavelu S, et al: Rivaroxaban versus placebo in patients with acute coronary syndromes (ATLAS ACS-TIMI 46): A randomised, double-blind, phase II trial. Lancet 374:29, 2009.
225. Alexander JH, Becker RC, Bhatt DL, et al: Apixaban, an oral, direct, selective factor Xa inhibitor, in combination with antiplatelet therapy after acute coronary syndrome: Results of the Apixaban for Prevention of Acute Ischemic and Safety Events (APPRAISE) trial. Circulation 119:2877, 2009.
226. Antman EM, Bennett JS, Daugherty A, et al: Use of nonsteroidal antiinflammatory drugs: An update for clinicians: A scientific statement from the American Heart Association. Circulation 115:1634, 2007.
227. Gibson CM, Pride YB, Aylward PE, et al: Association of non-steroidal anti-inflammatory drugs with outcomes in patients with ST-segment elevation myocardial infarction treated with fibrinolytic therapy: An ExTRACT-TIMI 25 analysis. J Thromb Thrombolysis 27:11, 2009.
228. Garcia Rodriguez LA, Tacconelli S, Patrignani P: Role of dose potency in the prediction of risk of myocardial infarction associated with nonsteroidal anti-inflammatory drugs in the general population. J Am Coll Cardiol 52:1628, 2008.
229. Dorn GW 2nd: Novel pharmacotherapies to abrogate postinfarction ventricular remodeling. Nat Rev Cardiol 6:283, 2009.
230. Bergmann O, Bhardwaj RD, Bernard S, et al: Evidence for cardiomyocyte renewal in humans. Science 324:98, 2009.
231. Parmacek MS, Epstein JA: Cardiomyocyte renewal. N Engl J Med 361:86, 2009.

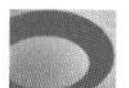

GUIDELINES Stephen D. Wiviott and Elliott M. Antman

Management of Patients with ST-Segment Elevation Myocardial Infarction

The American College of Cardiology and American Heart Association (ACC/AHA) comprehensive recommendations for the management of ST-segment elevation myocardial infarction (STEMI) were initially published in 2004,[1] followed by focused updates.[2,3]

PRE-STEMI GOALS, EARLY RISK STRATIFICATION, AND MANAGEMENT

The ACC/AHA guidelines on pre-STEMI management aim to identify patients at risk for STEMI and to provide therapies to prevent STEMI and promote patient education to identify symptoms and signs of STEMI to allow for early activation of emergency medical systems (EMS) rather than self-transport. The early risk stratification and management guidelines for STEMI aim to provide early access to known therapies that improve outcomes.

Prehospital, EMS providers should administer aspirin (162 to 325 mg) to all patients not already taking aspirin (Class I; level of evidence [LOE], C), obtain a 12-lead electrocardiogram (ECG) in patients suspected of having STEMI (Class IIa; LOE, B), review a reperfusion checklist, and relay this information to a medical facility (Class IIa; LOE, C; see Fig. 55-2). Patients with STEMI who have cardiogenic shock, those with contraindications to lytics (Class I; LOE, A), and those at high-risk of dying because of heart failure (Class IIa; LOE, B) should be channeled immediately to a facility capable of cardiac catheterization.

INITIAL RECOGNITION AND EVALUATION IN THE EMERGENCY DEPARTMENT

Initial evaluation in the emergency department focuses on identification of STEMI, early therapy, and reperfusion strategy. Selection of reperfusion strategy depends on hospital and patient characteristics (**Fig. 55G-1**; see Table 55-4). Time to reperfusion therapy strongly influences outcomes in STEMI. Patients presenting to a hospital with percutaneous coronary intervention (PCI) capability should undergo PCI within 90 minutes of first medical contact as a systems goal. Patients with STEMI presenting to a non-PCI–capable hospital should be considered for transfer to a PCI-capable hospital based on patient characteristics, time from symptom onset, and time to available PCI therapy. STEMI patients presenting to a hospital without PCI capability and who cannot be transferred to a PCI center and undergo PCI within 90 minutes of first medical contact should receive fibrinolytic therapy within 30 minutes of hospital presentation as a systems goal in the absence of contraindications (Class I; LOE, B). Communities should have well-developed plans for transfer of patients with STEMI to PCI-capable hospitals (Class I; LOE, C).

Achieving these goals requires rapid and focused evaluation (Class I; LOE, C), including the following:

- History of coronary artery disease (CAD), cerebrovascular disease (CVD), and risk factors associated with fibrinolytic therapy, including prior stroke, bleeding risk, or signs and symptoms of stroke
- Physical examination to assess the extent and complications of STEMI and to identify evidence of prior stroke or cognitive deficits
- 12-lead ECG interpreted by an experienced physician within 10 minutes of hospital arrival at the emergency department in patients with suggestive symptoms
- Laboratory examinations, including cardiac-specific troponin levels should be performed—but not delay reperfusion
- Patients with STEMI should have portable chest X-ray, when possible, without delaying reperfusion (unless a potential contraindication, such as aortic dissection, is suspected)—if the distinction between STEMI and aortic dissection remains unclear, imaging should be used.

Initial medical therapies in the emergency department should include the following:

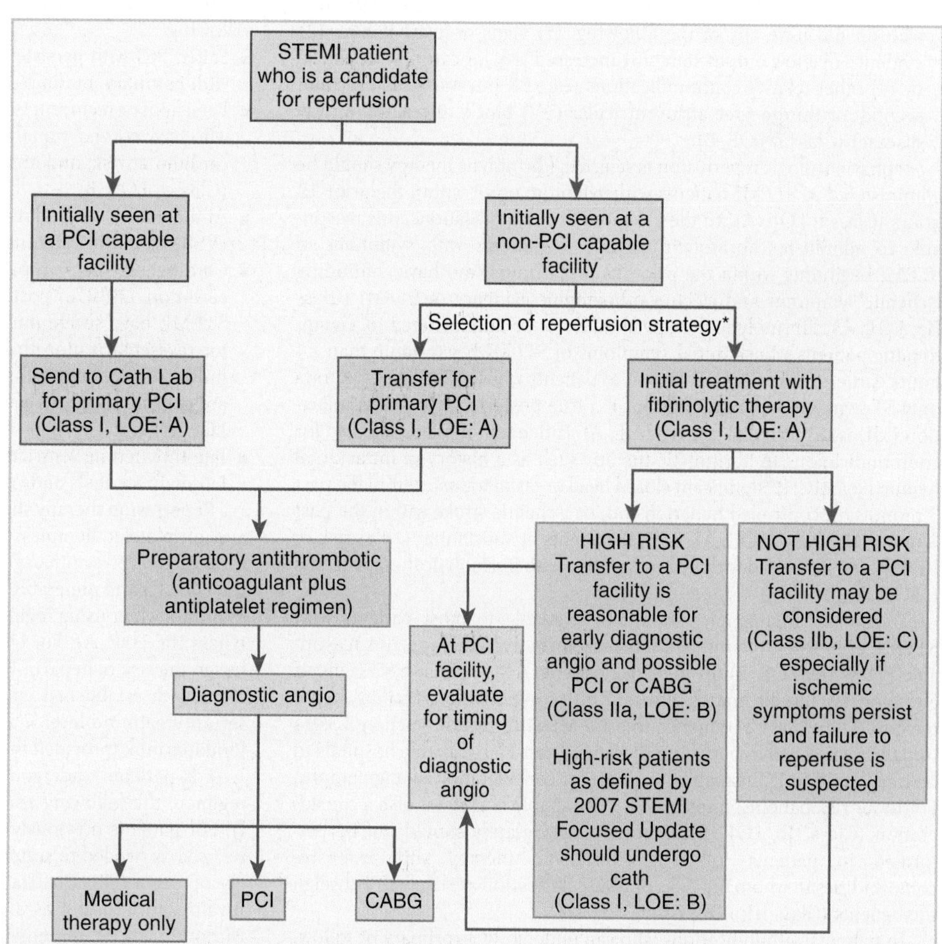

FIGURE 55G-1 Each community and each facility in that community should have an agreed-on plan for how STEMI patients are to be treated. It should include which hospitals should receive STEMI patients from emergency medical services units capable of obtaining diagnostic ECGs, management at the initial receiving hospital, and written criteria and agreements for expeditious transfer of patients from non-PCI–capable to PCI-capable facilities. Consideration should be given to initiating a preparatory pharmacologic regimen as soon as possible in preparation for and during patient transfer to the catheterization laboratory. The optimal regimen has not yet been established, although published studies have used various combinations for the following: anticoagulant, oral antiplatelet agents, intravenous antiplatelet. *Time since onset of symptoms, risk of STEMI, risks associated with fibrinolytic therapy; time required for transport to a skilled PCI laboratory. Angio, angiography; Cath Lab, catheterization laboratory. *(Modified from Kushner FG, Hand M, Smith SC Jr, et al: 2009 Focused Updates: ACC/AHA Guidelines for the Management of Patients With ST-Elevation Myocardial Infarction (updating the 2004 Guideline and 2007 Focused Update) and ACC/AHA/SCAI Guidelines on Percutaneous Coronary Intervention (updating the 2005 Guideline and 2007 Focused Update): a report of the American College of Cardiology Foundation/American Heart Association Task Force on Practice Guidelines. Circulation 120:2271, 2009.)*

- *Supplemental oxygen:* Supplemental oxygen should be administered to patients with arterial oxygen desaturation (i.e., $SaO_2 < 90\%$) (Class I; LOE, B), but it is reasonable to administer supplemental oxygen to all patients with uncomplicated STEMI during the first 6 hours (Class IIa; LOE, C).
- *Nitroglycerin:* Sublingual nitroglycerin should be given to patients with ongoing ischemic discomfort, 0.4 mg every 5 minutes, for a total of three doses. Intravenous (IV) nitroglycerin is then indicated for relief of ongoing ischemic discomfort, control of hypertension, or management of pulmonary congestion (Class I; LOE, C). Nitrates should not be administered to patients with systolic blood pressure (SBP) < 90 mm Hg or SBP ≥ 30 mm Hg below baseline, severe bradycardia (<50 beats/min), tachycardia (>100 beats/min), or suspected right ventricular (RV) infarction (Class III; LOE, C).
- *Analgesia:* Morphine sulfate (2 to 4 mg IV, with increments of 2 to 8 mg IV repeated at 5- to 15-minute intervals) is the analgesic of choice for management of pain associated with STEMI (Class I; LOE, C).
- *Aspirin:* Aspirin should be chewed by patients who have not taken aspirin before presentation with STEMI (Class I). The initial dose should be 162 mg (LOE, A) to 325 mg (LOE, C). Nonenteric-coated aspirin provides more rapid buccal absorption.
- *Beta blockers:* Oral beta blocker therapy should be initiated for patients who do not have any of the following: (1) signs of heart failure; (2) evidence of a low output state; (3) increased risk for cardiogenic shock; or (4) other relative contraindications (e.g., PR interval > 0.24 second, second- or third-degree atrioventricular (AV) block, or reactive airway disease) (Class I; LOE, B).

If pharmacologic reperfusion is selected, fibrinolytic therapy should be administered to STEMI patients with symptom onset within the prior 12 hours (Class I; LOE, A). In the absence of contraindications, it is reasonable to administer fibrinolytic therapy to patients with symptoms of STEMI beginning within the prior 12 to 24 hours who have continuing ischemic symptoms and electrocardiographic evidence of STEMI (Class IIa; LOE, C). Fibrinolytic therapy should not be administered to asymptomatic patients whose initial symptoms of STEMI began more than 24 hours earlier (Class III; LOE, C) nor to patients whose 12-lead ECG shows only ST-segment depression, except if a true posterior myocardial infarction (MI) is suspected (Class III; LOE, A). Patients should be evaluated for contraindications to fibrinolytic therapy such as a history of intracranial hemorrhage (ICH), significant closed head or facial trauma within the past 3 months, uncontrolled hypertension, or ischemic stroke within the past 3 months (Class I; LOE, A). STEMI patients at substantial (≥4%) risk of ICH should be treated with PCI rather than with fibrinolytic therapy (Class I; LOE, A).

Diagnostic angiography should be available to most patients with STEMI, even when the initial strategy is fibrinolytic therapy. It is reasonable (Class IIa; LOE, B) for high-risk patients (e.g., extensive ST-segment elevation, left bundle branch block [LBBB], congestive heart failure, hypotension, Killip Class 2 or higher, inferior MI with ejection fraction ≤ 35%) initially treated with reperfusion therapy at non-PCI—capable hospitals to be transferred to PCI-capable hospitals for consideration of angiography. For lower risk patients, transfer to a PCI-capable hospital is also a consideration (Class IIb; LOE, B). Coronary angiography should not be performed in patients following fibrinolytic therapy with extensive comorbidities in whom the risks of revascularization are likely to outweigh the benefits (Class III; LOE, C).

In patients with indications who can undergo PCI (primary or following fibrinolytics), the procedure should be performed by skilled personnel. PCI should not be performed in a noninfarct artery at the time of primary PCI in patients without hemodynamic compromise (Class III; LOE, C). Primary PCI should not be performed in asymptomatic patients more than 12 hours after the onset of STEMI if they are hemodynamically and electrically stable (Class III; LOE, C).

A strategy of coronary angiography with intent to perform PCI (or emergency coronary artery bypass grafting [CABG]) is recommended for patients who have received fibrinolytic therapy and have any of the following: (1) cardiogenic shock, younger than 75 years, and are suitable candidates for revascularization; (2) severe congestive heart failure and/or pulmonary edema (Killip Class III); or (3) hemodynamically compromising ventricular arrhythmias (Class I; LOE, C). It is reasonable to perform rescue PCI for patients with one or more of the following: hemodynamic or electrical instability, persistent ischemic symptoms or fibrinolytic therapy has failed (ST-segment elevation < 50%, resolved after 90 minutes following initiation of fibrinolytic therapy in the lead showing the worst initial elevation), and a moderate or large area of myocardium at risk (Class II; LOE, B).

Indications for PCI following STEMI depend on clinical considerations and coronary anatomy. In patients whose anatomy is suitable, PCI should be performed in the following situations: (1) when there is objective evidence of recurrent MI (Class I; LOE, C); (2) for moderate or severe spontaneous or provocable myocardial ischemia during recovery from STEMI (Class I; LOE, B); or (3) for cardiogenic shock or hemodynamic instability (Class I; LOE, B).

Emergency CABG can be useful as the primary reperfusion strategy in patients who have suitable anatomy, are not candidates for fibrinolysis or PCI, and are within 6 to 12 hours of an evolving STEMI, especially with severe multivessel or left main disease (Class IIa; LOE, B). Emergency CABG should not be performed in patients with persistent angina and a small area of myocardium at risk if they are hemodynamically stable or after successful reperfusion with PCI but persistent ischemia on the basis of microvascular obstruction (Class III; LOE, C). Additionally, emergency or urgent CABG in patients with STEMI should be considered for the following:

- Failed PCI with persistent pain or hemodynamic instability in patients with coronary anatomy suitable for surgery (Class I; LOE, B)
- Persistent or recurrent ischemia refractory to medical therapy in patients who have coronary anatomy suitable for surgery, have substantial myocardium at risk, and are not candidates for PCI or fibrinolytic therapy (Class I; LOE, B)
- At the time of surgical repair of postinfarction ventricular septal rupture (VSR) or mitral valve insufficiency (Class I; LOE, B)
- Cardiogenic shock in patients younger than 75 years with ST-segment elevation, LBBB, or posterior MI who develop shock within 36 hours of STEMI, have severe multivessel or left main disease, and are suitable for revascularization that can be performed within 18 hours of shock, unless further support is futile because of the patient's wishes or there are contraindications or unsuitability for further invasive care (Class I; LOE, A)
- Life-threatening ventricular arrhythmias in the presence of 50% or more left main stenosis and/or triple-vessel disease (Class I; LOE, B)

Reperfusion therapy should be supported with ancillary anticoagulants and antiplatelet therapies. Patients undergoing reperfusion with fibrinolytics should receive anticoagulant therapy for a minimum of 48 hours (Class IIa; LOE, C) and preferably for the duration of the index hospitalization, up to 8 days when using regimens other than unfractionated heparin (UFH) (Class IIa; LOE, A). For UFH, therapy is generally limited to 48 hours to lessen the risk of heparin-induced thrombocytopenia. Anticoagulant regimens with established efficacy include UFH, enoxaparin (provided the serum creatinine level < 2.5 mg/dL in men and 2.0 mg/dL in women), fondaparinux (provided the creatinine level < 3.0 mg/dL).

For patients undergoing PCI after having received an anticoagulant regimen, the following additional therapies should be considered (Class I). For patients previously receiving UFH additional boluses of UFH can be used as needed to support the procedure, taking into account whether glycoprotein (GP) IIb/IIIa antagonists have been administered (LOE, C). Bivalirudin is useful as a supportive measure for primary PCI, with or without prior treatment with UFH (Class I; LOE, B), and is a reasonable consideration in patients at high risk for bleeding. For patients with prior treatment with enoxaparin, if the last subcutaneous dose was administered at least 8 to 12 hours earlier, an additional intravenous dose should be given (Class I; LOE, B). Because of the risk of catheter thrombosis, fondaparinux should not be used as the sole anticoagulant to support PCI. An additional anticoagulant with anti-IIa activity should be administered (Class III; LOE, C).

Adjunctive antiplatelet therapies play a key role in the management of STEMI. A daily dose of aspirin (initial dose, 162 to 325 mg orally; maintenance dose, 75 to 162 mg) should be given indefinitely after STEMI to all patients without a true aspirin allergy (Class I; LOE, A). Clopidogrel, 75 mg/day orally, should be added to aspirin in patients with STEMI if fibrinolytic therapy or no reperfusion therapy is administered (Class I;

LOE, A). Treatment with clopidogrel in these settings should continue for at least 14 days (Class I; LOE, B).

A loading dose of a thienopyridine is recommended for STEMI patients for whom PCI is planned. The regimen should be one of the following:

- At least 300 to 600 mg of clopidogrel should be given as early as possible before or at the time of primary or nonprimary PCI (Class I; LOE, C).
- Prasugrel, 60 mg, should be given as soon as possible for primary PCI (Class I; LOE, B)

For STEMI patients undergoing nonprimary PCI, the following regimens are recommended:

- If the patient has received fibrinolytic therapy and has been given clopidogrel, clopidogrel should be continued as the thienopyridine of choice (Class I; LOE, C).
- If the patient has received fibrinolytic therapy without a thienopyridine, a loading dose of 300 to 600 mg of clopidogrel should be given as the thienopyridine of choice (Class I; LOE, C).
- If the patient did not receive fibrinolytic therapy, either a loading dose of 300 to 600 mg of clopidogrel should be given (Class I; LOE, C) or, once the coronary anatomy is known and PCI is planned, a loading dose of 60 mg of prasugrel should be given promptly, no later than 1 hour after the PCI (Class I; LOE, B).
- In STEMI patients with a history of prior stroke or transient ischemic attack for whom primary PCI is planned, prasugrel is not recommended (Class III; LOE, C).

The duration of thienopyridine therapy should be as follows:

- In patients receiving a stent (bare metal stent [BMS] or drug-eluting stent [DES]) during PCI for acute coronary syndrome (ACS), clopidogrel, 75 mg daily, or prasugrel, 10 mg daily, should be given for at least 12 months (Class I; LOE, B).
- If the risk of morbidity because of bleeding outweighs the anticipated benefit afforded by thienopyridine therapy, earlier discontinuation should be considered (Class I; LOE, C).
- In patients with DES, consideration of continuation of clopidogrel or prasugrel beyond 15 months may be considered (Class IIb; LOE, C).

Beyond these recommendations, consideration of long-term maintenance therapy (e.g., 1 year) with clopidogrel (75 mg/day, orally) is reasonable in STEMI patients whether they undergo reperfusion with fibrinolytic therapy or do not receive reperfusion therapy (Class IIa; LOE, C). In patients taking a thienopyridine for whom CABG is planned and can be delayed, it is recommended that the drug be discontinued to allow dissipation of the antiplatelet effect. The period of withdrawal should be at least 5 days in patients receiving clopidogrel and at least 7 days in patients receiving prasugrel, unless the need for revascularization and/or the net benefit of the thienopyridine outweighs the potential risks of excess bleeding (Class I; LOE, C) .

It is reasonable to start treatment with GP IIb/IIIa antagonists at the time of primary PCI (with or without stenting) in selected patients with STEMI (Class IIa; LOE, A, abciximab; LOE, B, tirofiban or eptifibatide). GP IIb/IIIa antagonists, as part of a preparatory pharmacologic strategy for patients with STEMI before their arrival in the cardiac catheterization laboratory for angiography and PCI, have uncertain usefulness (Class IIb; LOE, B).

HOSPITAL MANAGEMENT

After initial patient evaluation and management in the emergency department and selection of reperfusion therapy, STEMI guidelines focus on the in-hospital management on monitoring for and treating secondary complications of STEMI, initiation of secondary preventive measures and transition to long-term management of STEMI. Care should be structured around protocols that promote guideline-based management. Critical pathways, protocols, and other quality improvement tools (e.g., ACC, "Guidelines Applied in Practice,"[4] and AHA, "Mission: Lifeline"[5]) can aid in the application of evidence-based treatments for patients with STEMI by caregivers and institutions (Class I; LOE, C). A standard set of admitting orders summarizes the key features of care (see Table 55-7).

STEMI patients should be admitted to a coronary care unit (CCU) or step-down unit (for low-risk patients) (Class I; LOE, C). Nursing care should be provided by individuals certified in critical care (Class I; LOE, C). STEMI patients originally admitted to the CCU who are stable after 12 to 24 hours should be transferred to the step-down unit (Class I; LOE, C). Additional general measures include limiting bed rest to less than 12 to 24 hours for stable patients.

A medical assessment to determine the appropriateness of adjunctive medical therapies should include the following:

1. Beta-adrenergic blocking agents (beta blockers)
   - Patients receiving beta-blockers within the first 24 hours of STEMI without adverse effects should continue their use during the early convalescent phase of STEMI (Class I; LOE, A).
   - Patients without contraindications to beta blockers who did not receive them within the first 24 hours after STEMI should have them started in the early convalescent phase (Class I; LOE, A).
   - Patients with early contraindications within the first 24 hours of STEMI should be reevaluated for candidacy for beta blocker therapy (Class I; LOE, X).
2. Nitroglycerin
   - Intravenous nitroglycerin is indicated in the first 48 hours after STEMI for the treatment of persistent ischemia, congestive heart failure (CHF), or hypertension. The decision to administer intravenous nitroglycerin and the dose used should not preclude therapy with other proven mortality-reducing interventions, such as beta blockers or angiotensin-converting enzyme (ACE) inhibitors (Class I; LOE, B).
   - Intravenous, oral, or topical nitrates are useful beyond the first 48 hours after STEMI for treatment of recurrent angina or persistent CHF if their use does not preclude therapy with beta blockers or ACE inhibitors (Class I; LOE, B).
   - Nitrates should not be administered to patients with systolic pressure lower than 90 mm Hg or 30 mm Hg or more below baseline, severe bradycardia (less than 50 beats/min), tachycardia (more than 100 beats/min), or RV infarction (Class III; LOE, C).
3. Inhibition of the renin-angiotensin-aldosterone system
   - An ACE inhibitor should be administered orally during convalescence from STEMI in patients who tolerate this class of medication (Class I; LOE, A).
   - An angiotensin receptor blocker (ARB) should be administered to STEMI patients who cannot tolerate ACE inhibitors and have clinical or radiologic signs of heart failure or left ventricular ejection fraction (LVEF) less than 0.40 (Class I; LOE, B).
   - Long-term aldosterone blockade should be prescribed for post-STEMI patients without significant renal dysfunction (creatinine level ≤2.5 mg/dL in men and ≤ 2.0 mg/dL in women) or without hyperkalemia (potassium level ≤ 5.0 mEq/L) who are already receiving therapeutic doses of an ACE inhibitor, have an LVEF ≤0.40, and have either symptomatic heart failure or diabetes (Class I; LOE, A).
   - In STEMI patients who tolerate ACE inhibitors, an ARB can be useful as an alternative to ACE inhibitors provided there are clinical or radiologic signs of heart failure or LVEF <0.40 (Class IIa; LOE, B).

COMPLICATIONS FOLLOWING STEMI

The management of patients with hypotension, pulmonary edema, arrhythmias, or shock depends on the most likely underlying disorder (**Fig. 55G-2**). For most conditions, LV function and the presence of a mechanical complication should be assessed by echocardiography if not previously evaluated invasively. Recommended treatments for low-output states include inotropic support, intra-aortic counterpulsation (IABP), mechanical reperfusion with PCI or CABG, and surgical correction of mechanical complications (Class I; LOE, B). Beta blockers or calcium channel antagonists should not be administered to patients in a low-output state because of pump failure (Class III; LOE, B).

For patients with cardiogenic shock not quickly reversed with pharmacologic therapy, the IABP is a stabilizing measure for angiography and prompt revascularization (Class I; LOE, B). Early revascularization, either PCI or CABG, is recommended for patients younger than 75 years with ST-segment elevation or LBBB who develop shock within 36 hours of MI and are suitable for revascularization that can be performed within 18 hours of shock, unless further support is futile because of the patient's

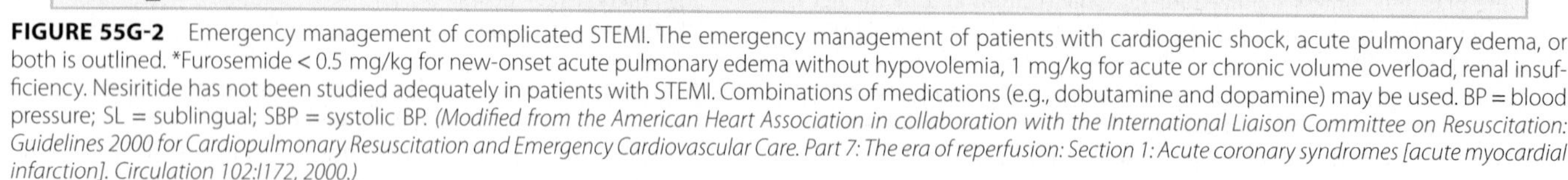

FIGURE 55G-2 Emergency management of complicated STEMI. The emergency management of patients with cardiogenic shock, acute pulmonary edema, or both is outlined. *Furosemide < 0.5 mg/kg for new-onset acute pulmonary edema without hypovolemia, 1 mg/kg for acute or chronic volume overload, renal insufficiency. Nesiritide has not been studied adequately in patients with STEMI. Combinations of medications (e.g., dobutamine and dopamine) may be used. BP = blood pressure; SL = sublingual; SBP = systolic BP. *(Modified from the American Heart Association in collaboration with the International Liaison Committee on Resuscitation: Guidelines 2000 for Cardiopulmonary Resuscitation and Emergency Cardiovascular Care. Part 7: The era of reperfusion: Section 1: Acute coronary syndromes [acute myocardial infarction]. Circulation 102:I172, 2000.)*

wishes or contraindications or unsuitability for further invasive care (Class I; LOE, A).

RV infarction should be considered for patients with inferior STEMI and hemodynamic compromise and should be assessed with a right precordial V_4R lead to detect ST-segment elevation and an echocardiogram to screen for RV infarction (Class I; LOE, B). For such patients, early reperfusion should be achieved, if possible, AV synchrony should be achieved, and bradycardia should be corrected. RV preload should be optimized (intravenous volume challenge), RV afterload should be optimized (therapy of concomitant LV dysfunction), and inotropic support should be used for hemodynamic instability not responsive to volume challenge (Class I; LOE, C).

Mechanical causes of heart failure or low-output syndrome, including mitral valve regurgitation, ventricular septal rupture, and left-ventricular free wall rupture, should prompt consideration for urgent cardiac surgical repair unless further support is considered futile because of the patient's wishes or contraindications or unsuitability for further invasive care (Class I; LOE, B or C). CABG should generally be undertaken at the same time as repair of these defects when coronary anatomy is appropriate (Class I; LOE, C).

Tachyarrhythmias after STEMI include ventricular fibrillation, ventricular tachycardia, and atrial fibrillation or flutter. In general, ventricular and atrial arrhythmias in the setting of STEMI are treated according to advanced cardiac life support (ACLS) guidelines that include electrical and pharmacologic therapies. Beyond standard measures, it is reasonable to manage refractory arrhythmias in the setting of recent STEMI, particularly polymorphic ventricular tachycardia (VT), by aggressive attempts to reduce myocardial ischemia and adrenergic stimulation, including therapies such as beta-adrenergic blockade, IABP use, consideration of emergency PCI-CABG surgery (Class IIa; LOE, B), and normalization of serum potassium and magnesium levels (Class IIa; LOE, B). The routine use of prophylactic antiarrhythmic drugs is not indicated for suppression of isolated ventricular premature beats, couplets, runs of accelerated idioventricular rhythm, or nonsustained VT (Class III). The use of implantable cardioverter-defibrillator (ICD) implantation post-STEMI is summarized in Figure 55-42. For episodes of sustained atrial fibrillation or flutter without hemodynamic compromise or ischemia, rate control is indicated (Class I; LOE, C). In addition, patients with sustained atrial fibrillation or flutter should be given anticoagulant therapy unless contraindications exist (Class I; LOE, C). Consideration should be given to cardioversion to sinus rhythm for patients with a history of atrial fibrillation or flutter prior to STEMI (Class I; LOE, C).

The guidelines provide an approach to the management of bradyarrhythmias and AV block (**Table 55G-1**). There are four possible actions for bradycardias: observation, medical therapy with atropine, transcutaneous pads with standby pacing, or temporary venous pacing. Actions depend on the severity of bradycardia, type of STEMI, and likely anatomic site of block. Permanent ventricular pacing is indicated for persistent second-degree AV block in the His-Purkinje system with bilateral bundle branch block or third-degree AV block within or below the His-Purkinje system after STEMI, transient advanced second- or third-degree infranodal AV block, and associated bundle-branch block. Uncertainty regarding the site of the block may warrant an electrophysiologic study for persistent and symptomatic second- or third-degree AV block. Permanent ventricular pacing may be considered for persistent second- or third-degree AV block at the AV node level. Permanent ventricular pacing is not recommended for transient AV block in the absence of intraventricular conduction defects, in the presence of isolated left anterior fascicular block, for acquired left anterior fascicular block in the absence of AV block, or first-degree AV block in the presence of bundle branch block that predated STEMI or is of indeterminate age.

Recurrent chest pain after STEMI may indicate pericarditis or recurrent ischemia. Aspirin is recommended for treatment of pericarditis after STEMI. Doses as high as 650 mg orally (enteric) every 4 to 6 hours may be needed, and anticoagulation should be immediately discontinued if pericardial effusion develops or increases (Class I; LOE, B). Nonsteroidal anti-inflammatory drugs (NSAIDs) may be considered for pain relief; however, they should not be used for extended periods because of their continuous effect on platelet function, an increased risk of myocardial scar thinning, and infarct expansion (Class IIb; LOE, B). Corticosteroids might be considered only as a last resort in patients with pericarditis refractory to aspirin or NSAIDs (Class IIb; LOE, C).

The guidelines recommend an approach to management of recurrent ischemic discomfort (**Fig. 55G-3**). Initial assessment is based on the presence or absence of recurrent ST-elevation. Patients with recurrent ischemic chest discomfort after initial reperfusion therapy for STEMI should undergo escalation of medical therapy with nitrates and beta blockers. Intravenous anticoagulation should be initiated if not already started (Class I; LOE, B). In addition to intensified medical therapy, patients with recurrent ischemic chest discomfort with recurrent ST-segment elevation, hemodynamic instability, poor LV function, or a large area of myocardium at risk should be referred urgently for cardiac catheterization and revascularization as needed. Insertion of an IABP should also be considered (Class I; LOE, C). Patients with recurrent ischemic-type chest discomfort who are considered candidates for revascularization should undergo coronary arteriography and PCI or CABG, as dictated by coronary anatomy (Class I; LOE, B).

CONVALESCENCE, DISCHARGE, AND POST–MYOCARDIAL INFARCTION CARE

After the acute phase of STEMI management, assessment of ventricular function, exercise testing, and further invasive assessment merit consideration. Echocardiography should be used for patients with STEMI not undergoing LV angiography to assess baseline LV function, especially if the patient is hemodynamically unstable (Class I; LOE, C). Echocardiography should also be used to evaluate suspected mechanical complications, shock, intracardiac thrombus, and pericardial effusion (Class I; LOE, B).

The guidelines offer an approach to exercise testing and repeat catheterization (see Fig. 55-41). Exercise testing is not recommended routinely for patients who have undergone successful revascularization. Functional

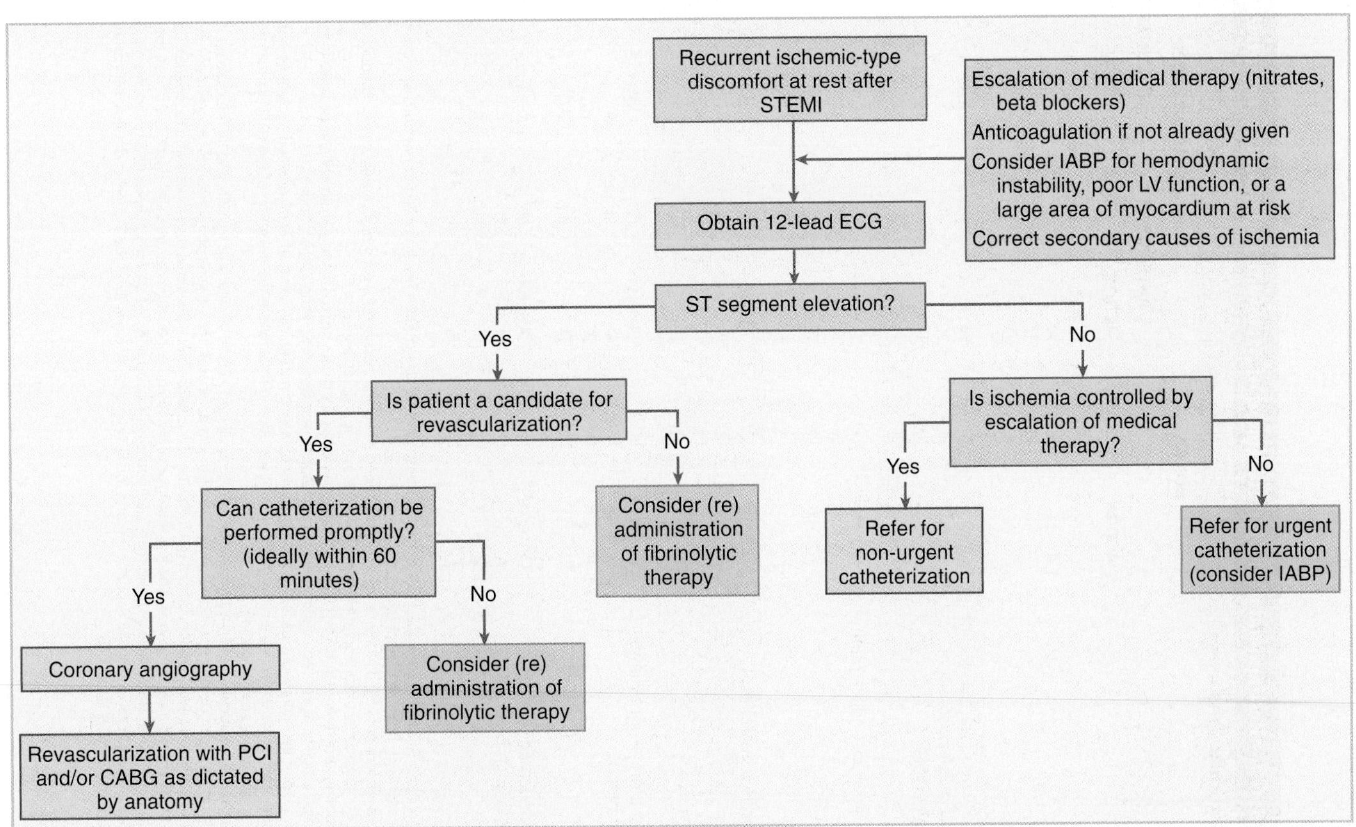

FIGURE 55G-3 Algorithm for the management of ischemia or infarction after STEMI. *(Modified from Antman EM, Anbe DT, Armstrong PW, et al: ACC/AHA guidelines for the management of patients with ST-elevation myocardial infarction: A report of the American College of Cardiology/American Heart Association Task Force on Practice Guidelines [Committee to Revise the 1999 Guidelines for the Management of Patients with Acute Myocardial Infarction]. Circulation 110:e82, 2004.)*

TABLE 55G-1 Recommendations for Treatment of Atrioventricular and Intraventricular Conduction Disturbances during STEMI

Intraventricular Conduction	Atrioventricular Conduction													
	NORMAL		FIRST-DEGREE AV BLOCK				MOBITZ I SECOND-DEGREE AV BLOCK				MOBITZ II SECOND-DEGREE AV BLOCK			
			ANTERIOR MI		NONANTERIOR MI		ANTERIOR MI		NONANTERIOR MI		ANTERIOR MI		NONANTERIOR MI	
	ACTION	*CLASS*	*ACTION*	*CLASS*	*ACTION*	*CLASS*	*ACTION*	*CLASS*	*ACTION*	*CLASS*	*ACTION*	*CLASS*	*ACTION*	*CLASS*
	Observe	I	Observe	I	Observe	I	Observe	IIb	Observe	IIa	Observe	III	Observe	III
	A	III	A	III	A	III	A*	III	A	III	A	III	A	III
	TC	III	TC	IIb	TC	IIb	TC	I	TC	I	TC	I	TC	I
	TV	III	TV	III	TV	III	TV	III	TV	III	TV	IIa	TV	IIa
Old or new fascicular block (left anterior or left posterior or fascicular block)	Observe	I	Observe	IIb	Observe	IIb	Observe	IIb	Observe	IIb	Observe	III	Observe	III
	A	III	A	III	A	III	A*	III	A	III	A	III	A	III
	TC	IIb	TC	I	TC	IIa	TC	I	TC	I	TC	I	TC	I
	TV	III	TV	III	TV	III	TV	III	TV	III	TV	IIa	TV	IIb
Old bundle branch block (BBB)	Observe	I	Observe	III	Observe	III	Observe	III	Observe	III	Observe	III	Observe	III
	A	III	A	III	A	III	A*	III	A	III	A	III	A	III
	TC	IIb	TC	I	TC	I	TC	I	TC	I	TC	I	TC	I
	TV	III	TV	IIb	TV	IIb	TV	IIb	TV	IIb	TV	IIa	TV	IIa
New bundle branch block	Observe	III	Observe	III	Observe	III	Observe	III	Observe	III	Observe	III	Observe	III
	A	III	A	III	A	III	A*	III	A	III	A	III	A	III
	TC	I	TC	I	TC	I	TC	I	TC	I	TC	IIb	TC	IIb
	TV	IIb	TV	IIa	TV	IIa	TV	IIa	TV	IIa	TV	I	TV	I
Fascicular block + right bundle branch block	Observe	III	Observe	III	Observe	III	Observe	III	Observe	III	Observe	III	Observe	III
	A	III	A	III	A	III	A*	III	A	III	A	III	A	III
	TC	I	TC	I	TC	I	TC	I	TC	I	TC	IIb	TC	IIb
	TV	IIb	TV	IIa	TV	IIa	TV	IIa	TV	IIa	TV	I	TV	I
Alternating left and right bundle branch block	Observe	III	Observe	III	Observe	III	Observe	III	Observe	III	Observe	III	Observe	III
	A	III	A	III	A	III	A*	III	A	III	A	III	A	III
	TC	IIb	TC	IIb	TC	IIb	TC	IIb	TC	IIb	TC	IIb	TC	IIb
	TV	I	TV	I	TV	I	TV	I	TV	I	TV	I	TV	I

Explanation of table: This table is designed to summarize the atrioventricular (column headings) and intraventricular (row headings) conduction disturbances that may occur during acute anterior or nonanterior STEMI, the possible treatment options, and the indications for each possible therapeutic option.

Actions: There are four possible actions, or therapeutic options, listed and classified for each bradyarrhythmia or conduction problem:

1. Observe: Continued electrocardiographic monitoring, no further action planned.
2. A, A*: Atropine administered at 0.6 to 1.0 mg intravenously every 5 minutes, up to 0.04 mg/kg. In general, because the increase in sinus rate with atropine is unpredictable, this is to be avoided unless there is symptomatic bradycardia that will likely respond to a vagolytic agent (e.g., sinus bradycardia or Mobitz I), as denoted by the asterisk, above.
3. TC: Application of transcutaneous pads and standby transcutaneous pacing, with no further progression to transvenous pacing imminently planned.
4. TV: Temporary transvenous pacing. It is assumed, but not specified in the table, at the discretion of the clinician, that transcutaneous pads will be applied and standby transcutaneous pacing will be in effect as the patient is transferred to the fluoroscopy unit for temporary transvenous pacing.

Class: Each possible therapeutic option is further classified according to ACC/AHA criteria as I, IIa, IIb, and III. There are no randomized trials available that address or compare specific treatment options. Moreover, the data for this table and recommendations are largely derived from observational data of prefibrinolytic era databases. Thus, the recommendations above must be taken as recommendations and tempered by the clinical circumstances.

Level of evidence: This table was developed from the following:: (1) published observational case reports and case series; (2) published summaries, not meta-analyses, of these data; and (3) expert opinion, largely from the prereperfusion era. There are no published randomized trials comparing different strategies of managing conduction disturbances post-STEMI. Thus, the level of evidence for the recommendations in the table is C.

How to use the table: For example, a 54-year-old man is admitted with an anterior STEMI and a narrow QRS on admission. On day 1, he develops a right bundle branch block (RBBB), with a PR interval of 0.28 second. RBBB is an intraventricular conduction disturbance, so look at row "New BBB." Find the column for "First-Degree AV Block." Find the "Action" and "Class" cells at the convergence. Note that "Observe" and "Atropine" are Class III, not indicated; transcutaneous pacing (TC) is Class I. Temporary transvenous pacing (TV) is Class IIb.

testing should be performed in the hospital or early after discharge in STEMI patients not selected for cardiac catheterization, and without high-risk features, to assess the presence and extent of inducible ischemia (Class I; LOE, B). In patients judged to be unable to exercise, pharmacologic stress nuclear scintigraphy or dobutamine echocardiography before or early after discharge should be used for patients with STEMI who are not undergoing cardiac catheterization to assess for inducible ischemia (Class I; LOE, B).

Coronary arteriography should be performed in patients with spontaneous episodes of myocardial ischemia or episodes of myocardial ischemia provoked by minimal exertion during recovery from STEMI (Class I; LOE, A). Coronary arteriography should be performed for intermediate- or high-risk findings on noninvasive testing after STEMI or in survivors of STEMI who had clinical heart failure during the acute episode but subsequently demonstrated well-preserved LV function (Class I; LOE, B or C). It is reasonable to perform coronary arteriography when STEMI is suspected to have occurred by a mechanism other than thrombotic occlusion (Class IIa; LOE, C). These circumstances would include coronary embolism, certain metabolic or hematologic diseases, or coronary artery spasm. Coronary arteriography is also considered reasonable for STEMI patients with any of the following: diabetes mellitus, LVEF < 0.40, CHF, prior revascularization, or life-threatening ventricular arrhythmias, without the above features (Class I; LOE, C).

SECONDARY PREVENTION AND LONG-TERM MANAGEMENT

Patients who survive the acute phase of STEMI should have plans initiated for secondary prevention therapies (Class I; LOE, A). Contemporary recommendations for secondary prevention after STEMI include the following:

- Complete smoking cessation
- Blood pressure at goal < 140/90 mm Hg unless diabetes or chronic kidney disease is present (blood pressure < 130/90 mm Hg)
- Physical activity 30 minutes, 3 to 4 days/week, optimally daily
- Hemoglobin A1c (HbA1c) < 7%
- Body mass index (BMI), 18.5 to 24.9

In addition, cardiac rehabilitation and secondary prevention programs are recommended for patients with STEMI, particularly those with a number of modifiable risk factors and/or those moderate- to high-risk patients for whom supervised exercise training is warranted. Before discharge, follow-up therapy with a medical provider should be arranged to evaluate functional recovery, assess medication use and titrate doses as needed, and address physical activity, return to work, sexual activity, and travel in detail (Class I; LOE, C).

REFERENCES

1. Antman EM, Anbe DT, Armstrong PW, et al: ACC/AHA guidelines for the management of patients with ST-elevation myocardial infarction: A report of the American College of Cardiology/American Heart Association Task Force on Practice Guidelines (Committee to Revise the 1999 Guidelines for the Management of Patients with Acute Myocardial Infarction). Circulation 110:e82, 2004.
2. Antman EM, Hand M, Armstrong PW, et al: 2007 Focused Update of the ACC/AHA 2004 Guidelines for the Management of Patients with ST-Elevation Myocardial Infarction: A report of the American College of Cardiology/American Heart Association Task Force on Practice Guidelines: Developed in collaboration with the Canadian Cardiovascular Society endorsed by the American Academy of Family Physicians: 2007 Writing Group to Review New Evidence and Update the ACC/AHA 2004 Guidelines for the Management of Patients With ST-Elevation Myocardial Infarction, Writing on Behalf of the 2004 Writing Committee. Circulation 117:296, 2008.
3. Kushner FG, Hand M, Smith SC Jr, et al: 2009 Focused Updates: ACC/AHA Guidelines for the Management of Patients With ST-Elevation Myocardial Infarction (updating the 2004 Guideline and 2007 Focused Update) and ACC/AHA/SCAI Guidelines on Percutaneous Coronary Intervention (updating the 2005 Guideline and 2007 Focused Update): A report of the American College of Cardiology Foundation/American Heart Association Task Force on Practice Guidelines. Circulation 120:2271, 2009.
4. Montoye CK, Eagle KA; Michigan ACC-GAP Investigators; ACC-GAP Steering Committee; American College of Cardiology: An Organizational Framework for the AMI ACC-GAP Project. J Am Coll Cardiol 46 (10 Suppl):1, 2005.
5. American Heart Associaton, Mission: Lifeline, 2010 (http://www.heart.org/HEARTORG/HealthcareProfessional/Mission-Lifeline-Home-Page_UCM_305495_SubHomePage.jsp).

CHAPTER 56 Unstable Angina and Non–ST Elevation Myocardial Infarction

Christopher P. Cannon and Eugene Braunwald

Each year, approximately one million patients in the United States are hospitalized for unstable angina or non–ST elevation myocardial infarction (UA/NSTEMI), a condition also referred to as non–ST elevation acute coronary syndrome (NSTE-ACS).[1,2] Acute total occlusion of a coronary artery usually causes STEMI (see Chap. 54), whereas UA/NSTEMI most commonly results from severe obstruction, but not total occlusion, of the culprit coronary artery. The incidence of NSTE-ACS, both absolute and relative to STEMI, is increasing, probably as a result of demographic changes in the population, including progressively increasing numbers of older persons and higher rates of diabetes.[3]

Definition

Stable angina pectoris typically manifests as a deep, poorly localized chest or arm discomfort (rarely described as pain), reproducibly precipitated by physical exertion or emotional stress, and relieved within 5 to 10 minutes by rest or sublingual nitroglycerin (see Chaps. 53 and 54). In contrast, *unstable* angina is defined as angina pectoris (or equivalent type of ischemic discomfort) with at least one of three features: (1) occurring at rest (or minimal exertion) and usually lasting >20 minutes (if not interrupted by the administration of a nitrate or an analgesic); (2) being severe and usually described as frank pain; or (3) occurring with a crescendo pattern (i.e., pain that awakens the patient from sleep or that is more severe, prolonged, or frequent than previously). Approximately two thirds of patients with unstable angina have evidence of myocardial necrosis on the basis of elevated cardiac serum markers, such as cardiac-specific troponin T or I and creatine kinase isoenzyme (CK)–MB, and thus have a diagnosis of NSTEMI. As troponin measurements become progressively more sensitive, an increasing fraction of patients with NSTE-ACS exhibit some release of troponin, and therefore these should be considered cases of NSTEMI with a reciprocal reduction in the fraction with unstable angina.

Pathophysiology

Five pathophysiologic processes may contribute to the development of UA/NSTEMI (**Fig. 56-1A**)[4]:

1. plaque rupture or erosion with superimposed nonocclusive thrombus (this causes by far the most UA/NSTEMI);
2. dynamic obstruction due to
   a. spasm of an epicardial coronary artery, as in Prinzmetal variant angina;
   b. constriction of the small, intramural muscular coronary arteries, that is, the coronary resistance vessels[5];
   c. local vasoconstrictors, such as thromboxane A_2, released from platelets;
   d. dysfunction of the coronary endothelium; and
   e. adrenergic stimuli including cold and cocaine;
3. severe coronary luminal narrowing caused by progressive coronary atherosclerosis or post–percutaneous coronary intervention restenosis;
4. inflammation; and
5. secondary unstable angina, that is, severe myocardial ischemia related to increased myocardial oxygen demand or decreased oxygen supply (e.g., tachycardia, fever, hypotension, or anemia).

Individual patients may have several of these processes coexisting as the cause of UA/NSTEMI. Several serum markers can serve as effective tools in identifying these pathophysiologic processes. As noted later, these serum markers form the foundation of a "multimarker strategy" for evaluation and risk stratification (**Fig. 56-1B**).

Thrombosis

Six sets of observations support the central role of coronary artery thrombosis in the pathogenesis of UA/NSTEMI: (1) the findings, at autopsy, of thrombi in the coronary arteries, usually localized to the site of a ruptured or eroded coronary plaque[6]; (2) the demonstration in coronary atherectomy specimens from patients with UA/NSTEMI of a high incidence of thrombotic lesions compared with those obtained from patients with stable angina; (3) the frequent finding of thrombus at coronary angioscopy; (4) the demonstration at coronary angiography (**Fig. 56-2**), intravascular ultrasound, optical coherence tomography, and computed tomography angiography of plaque ulceration or irregularities suggesting a ruptured plaque or thrombus; (5) the elevation of several serum markers of platelet activity and fibrin formation; and (6) the improvement in clinical outcome by antiplatelet and antithrombotic therapy.

Platelet Activation and Aggregation

Platelets play a key role in the transformation of a stable atherosclerotic plaque to an unstable lesion (**Fig. 56-3**). Rupture or ulceration of an atherosclerotic plaque often exposes the subendothelial matrix (e.g., collagen and tissue factor) to circulating blood. The first step in

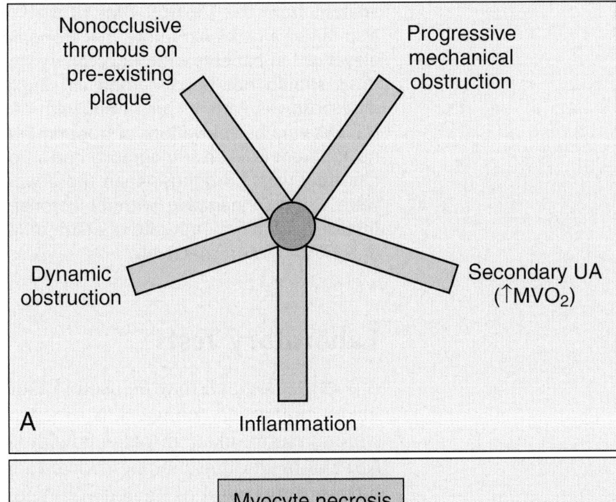

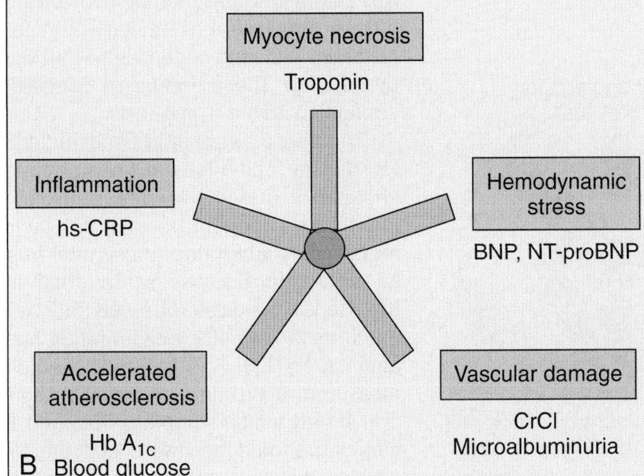

FIGURE 56-1 **A,** Schematic representation of the causes of unstable angina (UA). MVO_2 = myocardial O_2 consumption. *(Reproduced from Braunwald E: Unstable angina: An etiologic approach to management. Circulation 98:2219, 1998.)* **B,** A multimarker strategy for evaluation of the etiology and prognosis of UA/NSTEMI. In addition, these now have been seen to be independent markers of an adverse prognosis. BNP = B-type natriuretic peptide; CrCl = creatinine clearance; Hb A_{1c} = hemoglobin A_{1c}; hs-CRP = high-sensitivity C-reactive protein; NT-proBNP = N-terminal pro-BNP; UA/NSTEMI = unstable angina or non–ST elevation myocardial infarction. *(Modified with permission from Morrow DA, Braunwald E: Future of biomarkers in acute coronary syndromes: Moving toward a multimarker strategy. Circulation 108:250, 2003.)*

thrombus formation is platelet *adhesion* via platelet glycoprotein (GP) Ib binding to von Willebrand factor and GP VI binding to collagen. The ensuing platelet *activation* leads to (1) a shape change in the platelet (from a smooth discoid shape to a spiculated form, which increases the surface area on which thrombin generation can occur); (2) degranulation of the platelet alpha and dense granules, releasing thromboxane A_2, serotonin, and other platelet aggregatory and chemoattractant agents; (3) increased expression of the GP IIb/IIIa receptor on the platelet surface followed by a conformational change of the receptor that enhances its affinity for fibrinogen; and (4) platelet *aggregation,* in which fibrinogen binds to the activated platelet fibrinogen inhibitor GP IIb/IIIa, causing a growing platelet plug.

SECONDARY HEMOSTASIS. Simultaneous with the formation of the platelet plug, the plasma coagulation system is activated. Tissue factor triggers most coronary artery thrombosis (see Chaps. 43 and 87). Ultimately, factor X is activated (to factor Xa), which leads to the generation of thrombin (factor IIa, which plays a central role in arterial thrombosis). Thrombin, which converts fibrinogen to fibrin, is also a powerful stimulant of platelet aggregation and activates factor XIII, which leads to cross-linking of fibrin and stabilization of the clot.

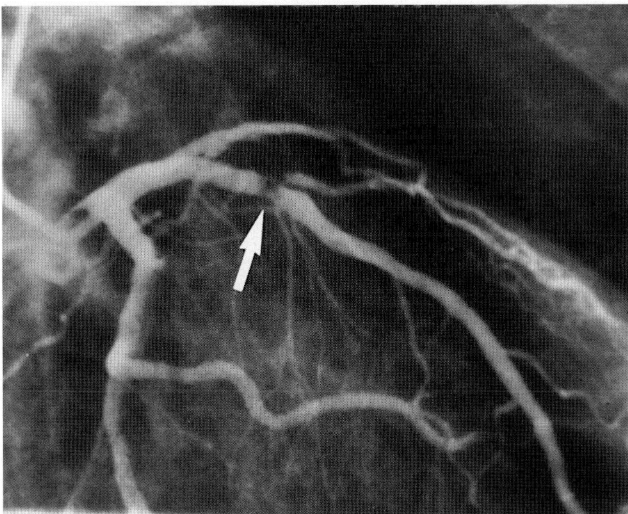

FIGURE 56-2 Coronary artery thrombus in a 60-year-old patient with unstable angina. Coronary angiography shows an irregular hazy filling defect in the left anterior descending artery at the level of the second diagonal branch (arrow). Contrast medium surrounds the globular thrombus, which extends into the diagonal branch.

Thrombin molecules are incorporated into coronary thrombi and can form the nidus of rethrombosis.

Clinical Presentation

Among patients with ACS, women present more often with unstable angina, representing 30% to 45% of patients with this condition, compared with 25% to 30% of patients with NSTEMI and only 20% of patients with STEMI.[7] In comparison to the latter, patients with UA/NSTEMI are older and have higher rates of prior MI, stable angina, diabetes, previous coronary revascularization, and extracardiac vascular disease than do patients with STEMI.[7] Indeed, approximately 80% of patients with UA/NSTEMI have a history of coronary artery disease (CAD) before the acute event.[8]

Clinical Examination

The physical examination may be unremarkable or may support the diagnosis of cardiac ischemia. Signs suggesting that ischemia involves a large fraction of the left ventricle include diaphoresis, pale cool skin, sinus tachycardia, a third or fourth heart sound, and basilar rales on lung examination. In some patients, ischemia of a large area of myocardium reduces left ventricular dysfunction and causes hypotension.

Electrocardiography

ST depression (or transient ST elevation) and T wave changes occur in up to 50% of patients with UA/NSTEMI[9] (see Chap. 13). New (or presumably new) ST-segment deviation (≥0.1 mV) is a useful measure of ischemia and prognosis. When electrocardiograms preceding the acute event are available, further ST depression of only 0.05 mV is a sensitive although nonspecific finding of UA/NSTEMI.[9] Transient (i.e., <20 minutes) ST elevation, which occurs in approximately 10% of patients with UA/NSTEMI, portends a high risk of future cardiac events. T wave changes are sensitive but not specific for acute ischemia unless they are marked (>0.3 mV) (**Fig. 56-4**).

CONTINUOUS ELECTROCARDIOGRAPHIC MONITORING. Continuous electrocardiographic monitoring serves two purposes in UA/NSTEMI: (1) to identify arrhythmias and (2) to identify recurrent ST-segment deviation indicative of ischemia. Recurrent ST-segment deviation is a strong *independent* marker of adverse outcome,[10] even in the presence of troponin release.

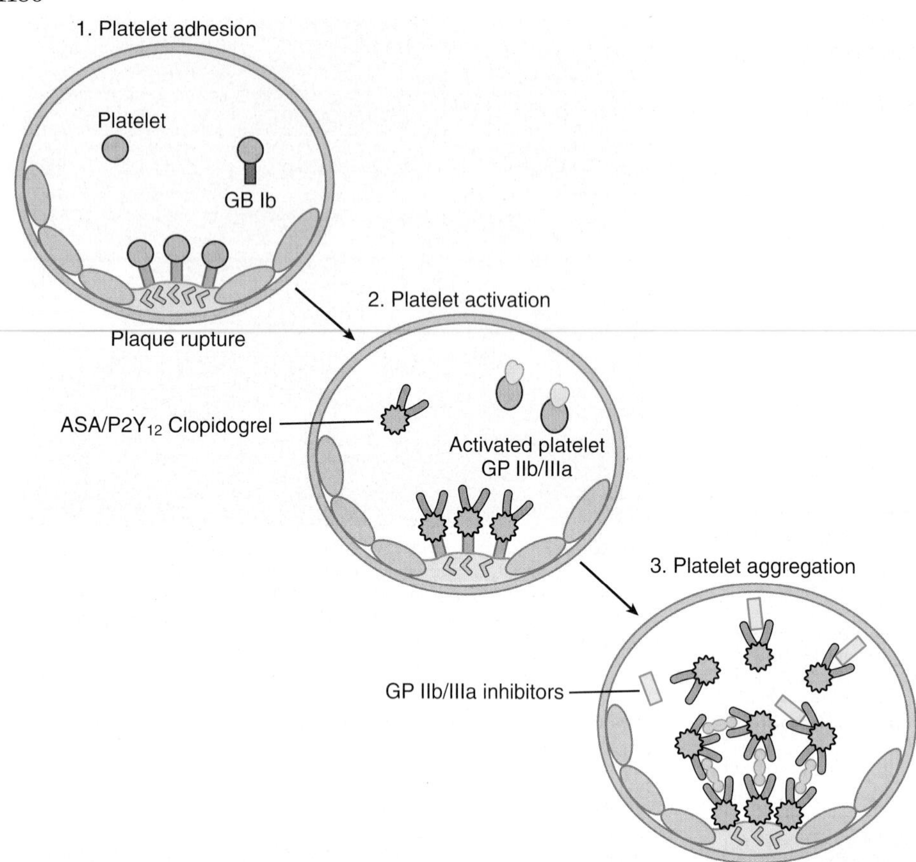

FIGURE 56-3 Platelet adhesion (1), activation (2), and aggregation (3). Platelets initiate thrombosis at the site of a ruptured or eroded plaque: the first step is platelet adhesion (1) via the GP Ib receptor in conjunction with von Willebrand factor. This is followed by platelet activation (2), which leads to a shape change in the platelet, degranulation of the alpha and dense granules, and expression of GP IIb/IIIa receptors on the platelet surface with activation of the receptor, such that it can bind fibrinogen. The final step is platelet aggregation (3), in which fibrinogen (yellow) binds to the activated GP IIb/IIIa receptors of two platelets. Aspirin (ASA) and clopidogrel act to decrease platelet activation (see text for details), whereas the GP IIb/IIIa inhibitors inhibit the final step of platelet aggregation. GP = glycoprotein. (See Fig. 87-3.)

Markers of Cardiac Necrosis

Among patients presenting with symptoms consistent with UA/NSTEMI, elevations of markers of myocardial necrosis (i.e., CK-MB, troponin T or I) identify patients with the diagnosis of NSTEMI. With the use of troponins, which are more sensitive than CK-MB, a greater percentage of patients are classified as having NSTEMI, which is associated with a worse prognosis.[11] Persistent elevation of troponin after an acute event also associates with worse clinical outcomes.[12]

Although the appropriate cut point to define an elevation of troponin I has engendered controversy, growing consensus has focused on use of the 99th percentile of a normal population (approximately 0.10 ng/mL) with a coefficient of variation (a measure of reproducibility of the assay) not greater than 10% and a sensitivity (lower level of detection) of as low as 0.02 ng/mL. As more sensitive assays for troponin are being developed, revision of these characteristics will be required. Even slight elevations of cardiac troponin presage a higher risk of death or recurrent ischemic events.[11,12]

Because assays differ, each hospital needs to review the specific cut points defined by the assay used. Most point-of-care tests for troponins provide a binary (positive or negative) result, whereas some provide a quantitative result, although the sensitivity and diagnostic accuracy of some of these tests have only recently matched the accuracy of current-generation laboratory-based assays.

Despite increasingly accurate assays, apparent false-positive troponin elevations have been found in patients later found at coronary angiography not to have epicardial stenoses.[13] These elevations result from an alternative diagnosis, such as congestive heart failure, in which troponin elevations in the absence of CAD portend an adverse prognosis. An analysis from the TACTICS–TIMI 18 trial[14,15] also raised a cautionary note that troponin elevations in patients without coronary stenosis should not be discarded as simply false-positives. Patients presenting with UA/NSTEMI who had elevations of troponin but no apparent CAD on angiography had a significantly worse prognosis than those who were troponin negative without coronary disease, with a 6-month rate of death or MI of 5.3% and 0%, respectively.[14]

Laboratory Tests

A chest radiograph may be useful in identifying pulmonary congestion or edema, which is more likely in patients with UA/NSTEMI in whom ischemia involves a significant proportion of the left ventricle or in those with antecedent left ventricular dysfunction. The presence of congestion confers an adverse prognosis.

Obtaining a serum lipid panel including low-density and high-density lipoprotein cholesterol and triglyceride is useful in identifying important, treatable risk factors for coronary atherothrombosis after hospital discharge. Because serum total and high-density cholesterol levels fall by as much as 30% to 40% beginning 24 hours after UA/NSTEMI or STEMI, they should be measured at the time of initial presentation. If only a later sample is obtained, the clinician should be aware that the total and low-density cholesterol values may be as much as 30% to 40% lower than the patient's actual baseline concentration (see Chap. 47). Other circulating markers of increased risk are discussed subsequently. Evaluation for other secondary causes of UA/NSTEMI[16] may also be appropriate in selected patients (e.g., assessing thyroid function in patients who present with UA/NSTEMI and persistent tachycardia).

Noninvasive Testing

In the management of UA/NSTEMI, noninvasive testing is employed for several purposes: (1) at presentation, usually in the emergency department, to diagnose the presence or absence of CAD (see Chap. 53); (2) to evaluate the extent of residual ischemia after medical therapy has been initiated and to guide further therapy as part of an "early conservative" strategy; (3) to evaluate left ventricular function; and (4) in risk stratification. The markers of high risk include evidence of severe ischemia or ventricular tachyarrhythmia on continuous electrocardiography or stress testing and the development of left ventricular dysfunction, either at rest or stress induced.

The safety of early stress testing in patients with UA/NSTEMI has been debated, but observations made in several trials have suggested that pharmacologic or symptom-limited stress testing is safe after a period of at least 24 hours of stabilization.[17] Contraindications to stress testing are a recent (less than 24 hours) occurrence of rest pain, especially if it is associated with electrocardiographic changes or other signs of hemodynamic instability or arrhythmia.

The merits of various modalities of stress testing have been compared. Stress myocardial perfusion imaging with sestamibi or stress echocardiography is slightly more sensitive than electrocardiographic stress testing alone and has greater prognostic value, but myocardial perfusion has been proven cost-effective only in higher-risk patients. A useful approach is to individualize the choice on the basis of patient characteristics, local availability, and expertise in interpretation. For most patients, electrocardiographic stress testing is recommended if the

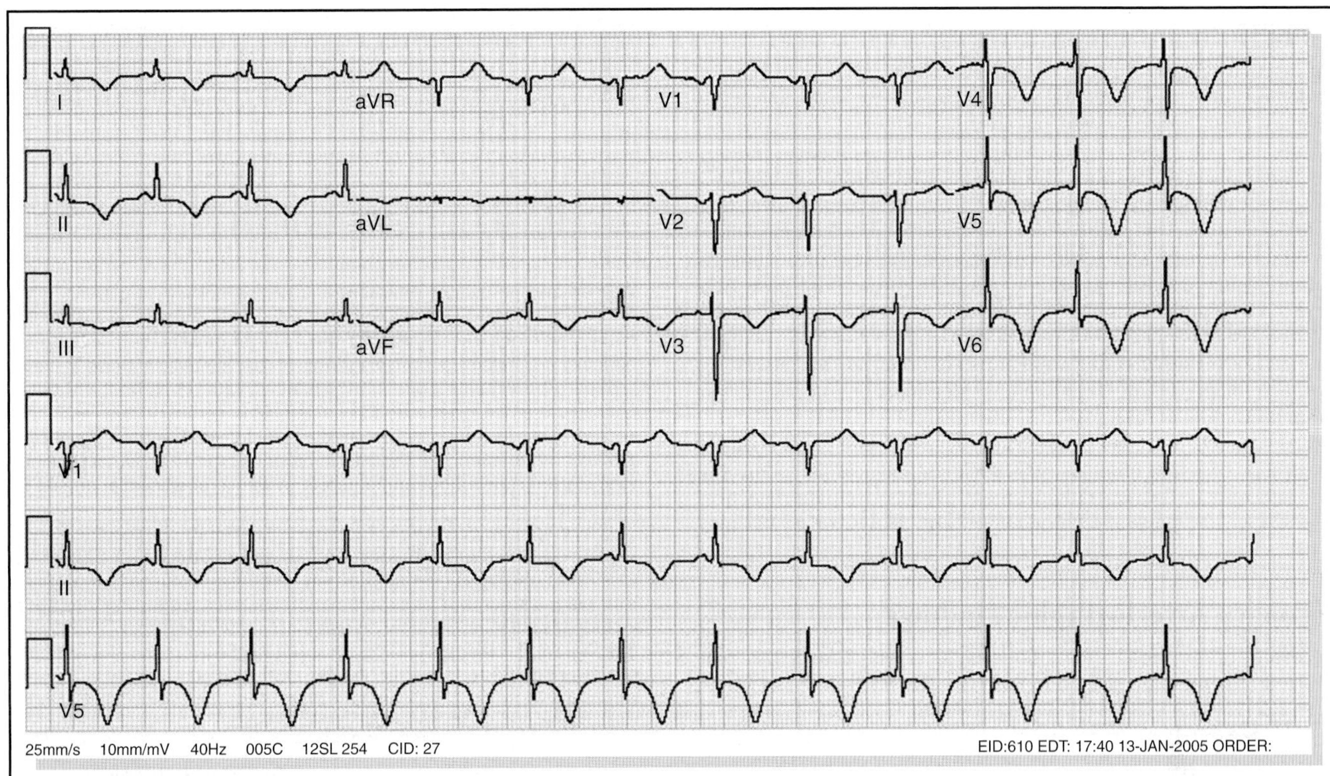

FIGURE 56-4 Electrocardiogram showing deep symmetric inferolateral T wave inversion with 1-mm ST-segment deviation. Such electrocardiographic findings are frequently associated with critical stenosis of a coronary artery (although localization of which artery is often difficult). These findings are also a useful marker of patients at high risk of subsequent death or myocardial infarction.

TABLE 56-1 Braunwald Clinical Classification of UA/NSTEMI

CLASS	DEFINITION	DEATH OR MI TO ONE YEAR* (%)
Severity		
Class I	New onset of severe angina or accelerated angina; no rest pain	7.3
Class II	Angina at rest within past month but not within preceding 48 hr (angina at rest, subacute)	10.3
Class III	Angina at rest within 48 hr (angina at rest)	10.8†
Clinical Circumstances		
A. Secondary angina	Develops in the presence of extracardiac condition that intensifies myocardial ischemia	14.1
B. Primary angina	Develops in the absence of extracardiac condition	8.5
C. Postinfarction angina	Develops within 2 wk after acute myocardial infarction	18.5‡
Intensity of treatment	Patients with unstable angina may also be divided into three groups according to whether unstable angina occurs: (1) in the absence of treatment for chronic stable angina, (2) during treatment for chronic stable angina, or (3) despite maximal anti-ischemic drug therapy. The three groups may be designated by subscripts 1, 2, and 3, respectively.	
Electrocardiographic changes	Patients with unstable angina may be further divided into those with or without transient ST-T wave changes during pain.	

*Data from TIMI III Registry: Scirica BM, Cannon CP, McCabe CH, et al: Prognosis in the thrombolysis in myocardial ischemia III registry according to the Braunwald unstable angina pectoris classification. Am J Cardiol 90:821, 2002.

†$P = 0.057$.

‡$P = 0.001$.

UA/NSTEMI = unstable angina/non–ST elevation myocardial infarction.

From Braunwald E: Unstable angina: A classification. Circulation 80:410, 1989.

electrocardiogram at rest lacks significant ST-segment abnormalities. If ST abnormalities at rest exist, then perfusion or echocardiographic imaging is recommended. Exercise testing is generally recommended unless the patient cannot walk sufficiently to achieve a significant workload, in which case pharmacologic stress testing provides an alternative (see Chaps. 14 and 50).

Clinical Classification

Because UA/NSTEMI comprises such a heterogeneous group of patients, classification schemes based on clinical features are useful. A clinical classification of UA/NSTEMI (**Table 56-1**)[16] provides a useful means to stratify risk. Patients fall into three groups according to the clinical circumstances of the acute ischemic episode: (1) primary unstable angina caused by reductions of myocardial perfusion; (2) secondary unstable angina (e.g., with ischemia related to precipitating factors such as anemia or an acute MI); and (3) post-MI unstable angina. Patients are classified simultaneously according to the severity of the ischemia. This classification provides valuable prognostic information (with postinfarction angina at rest having the worst prognosis).

Imaging

Intravascular ultrasound (IVUS) was the first imaging technique to demonstrate that patients who had recently had an acute coronary event had disrupted plaques that exhibited more positive remodeling (i.e., less encroachment on the coronary lumen) and larger plaque areas than did patients with chronic stable CAD. Computed tomography angiography (CTA) has also shown that ruptured plaques were characterized by positive vascular remodeling, low plaque density, and spotty calcification. Patients presenting to the emergency department without these features could have ACS ruled out with great reliability.[18,19] Motoyama and colleagues[20] showed that contrast-enhanced CTA could also identify vulnerable plaques that had not yet ruptured but were at risk of doing so. This interesting approach might, in the future, allow identification of patients in whom prevention of rupture by invasive means might be considered.[21] Cardiac magnetic resonance (CMR) imaging with T2-weighted imaging, assessment of left ventricular wall thickness, myocardial perfusion, and detection of delayed enhancement permits accurate detection of ACS as well as acute and chronic MI[22] (**Fig. 56-5**; see Figs. 18-4 and 54-18).

Coronary Arteriographic Findings

The extent of epicardial CAD among patients with UA/NSTEMI randomized to the invasive arm of the TACTICS–TIMI 18 trial, who systematically underwent angiography, was as follows: 34% had significant obstruction (>50% luminal diameter stenosis) of three vessels; 28% had two-vessel disease; 26% had single-vessel disease; and 13% had no coronary stenosis >50%. Approximately 10% had left main stem stenosis >50%.[16] Registries of unselected UA/NSTEMI patients have reported similar findings. Women and nonwhites with UA/NSTEMI have less extensive coronary disease than their counterparts do,[7] whereas patients with NSTEMI have more extensive disease on coronary angiography than do those who present with unstable angina alone.

Women and nonwhites represent a larger proportion of patients with symptoms of UA/NSTEMI without epicardial CAD, suggesting a different pathophysiologic mechanism for their clinical presentation, leading to difficulty in making a firm diagnosis of UA/NSTEMI in these patient groups.[7] Approximately one third of patients with UA/NSTEMI without a critical epicardial obstruction have impaired coronary flow assessed angiographically, suggesting a pathophysiologic role for coronary microvascular dysfunction. The short-term prognosis in this group of patients with UA/NSTEMI without angiographic evidence of epicardial disease is excellent.[23]

The culprit lesion in UA/NSTEMI typically exhibits an eccentric stenosis with scalloped or overhanging edges and a narrow neck (see Chap. 21). These angiographic findings may represent disrupted atherosclerotic plaque, thrombus, or a combination. Features suggesting thrombus include globular intraluminal masses with a rounded or polypoid shape (see Fig. 56-2). "Haziness" of a lesion suggests the presence of thrombus, but this finding is not specific. Patients with angiographically visualized thrombus have impaired coronary blood flow and worse clinical outcomes compared with those without thrombus.

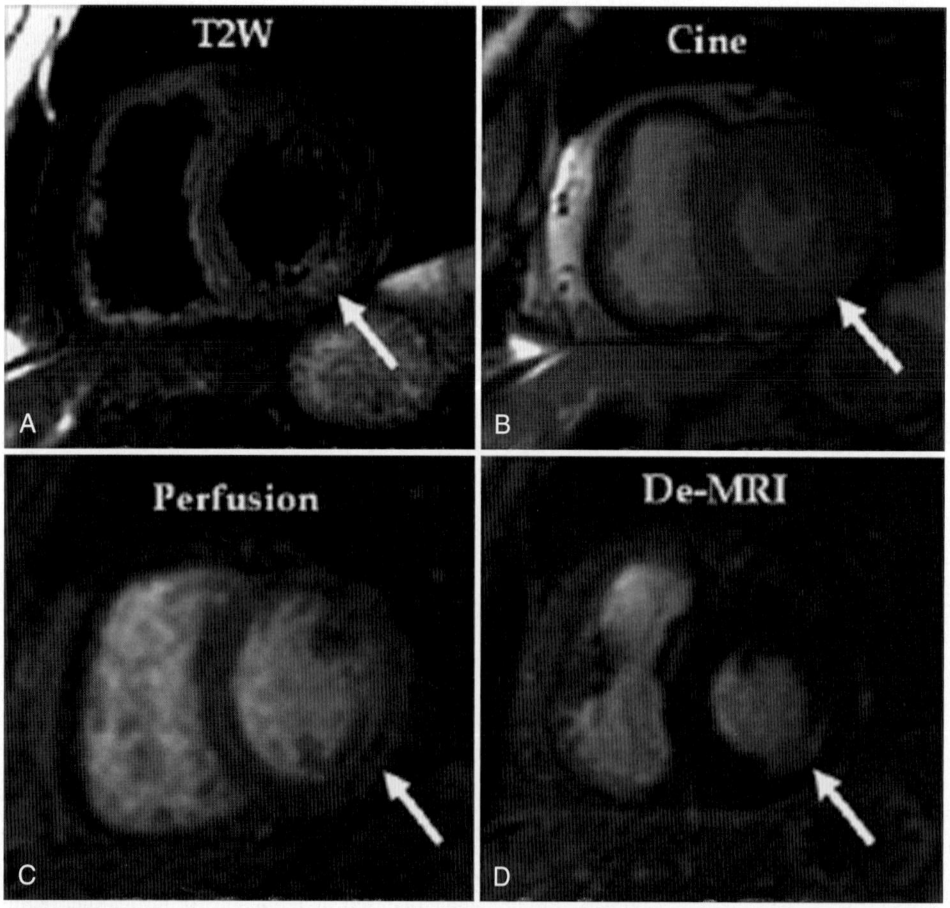

FIGURE 56-5 Example of a patient with NSTEMI. CMR imaging was performed in a 63-year-old man 1 hour after his arrival at the emergency department with initially normal cardiac enzymes; it revealed a small area of T2 hyperintensity **(A)** in the inferolateral wall (myocardial edema) with associated subtle hypokinesis **(B)**, a resting perfusion defect **(C)**, and delayed hyperenhancement **(D)**; (myocardial necrosis) in the same area (arrows). Troponin level was elevated 7 hours after CMR imaging. Invasive angiography revealed triple-vessel disease with a 95% stenosis in the posterolateral branch. *(From Cury RC, Shash K, Nagurney JT, et al: Cardiac magnetic resonance with T2-weighted imaging improves detection of patients with acute coronary syndrome in the emergency department. Circulation 118:837, 2008.)*

RISK STRATIFICATION

Risk After Acute Coronary Syndrome. An important emerging concept is that the risk of recurrent ischemic events is more dependent on the presence of multifocal lesions other than the culprit lesion responsible for the ACS event. Studies of coronary anatomy by angiography, IVUS, or angioscopy have shown multiple active plaques in addition to the culprit lesion. Thus, as aggressive interventional approaches are used increasingly successfully to treat the culprit lesion, the remaining plaques often provoke recurrent events. The percentage of patients with more than one active plaque on angiography relates to an increasing baseline level of C-reactive protein (CRP),[23] a marker of inflammation. These findings provide an important pathophysiologic link between inflammation, more diffuse active CAD, and recurrent cardiac events in the months to years after a clinical ACS event.

Natural History. Patients with unstable angina have lower *short-term* mortality (1.5% to 2.0% from first presentation to 30 days) than do those with NSTEMI or STEMI; the early mortality risk of the two types of MI is similar and between 3% and 5%. The *early* mortality risk in UA/NSTEMI relates to the extent of myocardial damage and resulting hemodynamic compromise and is less than in patients with STEMI. In contrast, *long-term* outcome—for both mortality and nonfatal events—is actually *worse* for patients with UA/NSTEMI compared with STEMI. This finding probably results from the greater likelihood of recurrence of ACS in patients with UA/NSTEMI as well as their older age, greater extent of coronary disease, prior MI, and comorbidities such as diabetes and impaired renal function.

Methods of Risk Stratification

CLINICAL VARIABLES

High-Risk Clinical Subgroups

The aforementioned classification of unstable angina (see Table 56-1) has proved clinically useful in several studies for the identification of high-risk patients, notably those with ongoing or recurrent rest pain, post-MI unstable angina, or secondary unstable angina.[15] Increasing age associates with a significant increase in adverse outcomes.[24] Patients with UA/NSTEMI and diabetes mellitus or extracardiac vascular disease (i.e., cerebrovascular disease or peripheral arterial vascular disease) are at approximately 50% higher risk than those without these comorbidities even after controlling for other differences in baseline characteristics (**Table 56-2**). As with STEMI, patients with UA/NSTEMI who present with evidence of congestive heart failure (Killip class ≥II) also have an increased risk of death.

RISK ASSESSMENT BY ELECTROCARDIOGRAPHY. In the TIMI III registry of patients with UA/NSTEMI, independent predictors of 1-year death or MI included left bundle branch block (risk ratio, 2.8); and ST-segment deviation >0.05 mV (risk ratio, 2.45); both $P < 0.001$.[9] There appears to be a gradient of risk based on the degree of ST-segment deviation.[25]

RISK ASSESSMENT BY CARDIAC MARKERS (Table 56-3)

Markers of Myocyte Necrosis

Patients with NSTEMI, defined as associated with an elevated biomarker of necrosis (CK-MB or troponin), have a worse long-term prognosis than do those with unstable angina.[26] Beyond just a positive versus negative test result, there is a linear relation between the level of circulating troponin T or I and subsequent risk of death.[27] However, in several studies, a higher risk of MI (or recurrent MI) was observed even with small elevations of positive troponins.[11,28]

C-Reactive Protein and Other Markers of Inflammation (see Chaps. 44 and 49)

Elevated levels of CRP relate to increased risk of death, MI, and the need for urgent revascularization. Because CRP is an acute-phase reactant, it is elevated by MI, with or without ST-segment elevation. Thus, the level of CRP in patients with very recent ACS is approximately five times that of stable patients.[25] Among patients with negative troponin I, CRP can discriminate between high- and low-risk groups. When both CRP and troponin T are used, mortality can be stratified from 0.4% for patients with both markers negative, to 4.7% if either CRP or troponin is positive, to 9.1% if both are positive.[29] CRP measured after stabilization post-ACS strongly predicts outcome after 3 to 12 months.[30]

Study of other inflammatory markers has offered consistent evidence of an association between systemic inflammation and recurrent adverse events, including serum amyloid A, monocyte chemoattractant protein

TABLE 56-2 Clinical Indicators of Increased Risk in UA/NSTEMI

History
Advanced age (>70 yr)
Diabetes mellitus
Post–myocardial infarction angina
Prior peripheral vascular disease
Prior cerebrovascular disease

Clinical Presentation
Braunwald class II or III (acute or subacute rest pain)
Braunwald class B (secondary unstable angina)
Heart failure or hypotension
Multiple episodes of pain within 24 hr

Electrocardiogram
ST-segment deviation ≥0.05 mV
T wave inversion ≥0.3 mV
Left bundle branch block

Cardiac Markers
Increased troponin T or I or creatine kinase–MB
Increased C-reactive protein or white blood cell count
Increased B-type natriuretic peptide
Elevated creatinine
Elevated glucose or hemoglobin A_{1c}

Angiogram
Thrombus
Multivessel disease
Left ventricular dysfunction

UA/NSTEMI = unstable angina/non–ST elevation myocardial infarction.

TABLE 56-3 Emerging Biomarkers in Acute Coronary Syndrome

	POSSIBLE MECHANISM	MAJOR FINDINGS
Markers Predicting the Development of ACS		
von Willebrand factor[1]	Mediates platelet adhesion, aggregation (at high shear stress), and stabilizes factor VIIIc	OR = 3.0 for the 4th quartile compared with 1st quartile in patients developing ACS
Erythrocyte membrane–bound interleukin-8[2]	Increases inflammatory response on release from erythrocyte membrane during intraplaque hemorrhage	1 SD increase was associated with 5.1-fold higher odds of having ACS (compared with chronic stable angina), adjusted for baseline characteristics and other markers
Platelet collagen receptor glycoprotein (GP) VI[3]	Enhances platelet aggregability	Mean fluorescence intensity above the cutoff of >18.6 (i.e., an elevated level of surface expression of GP VI) had a 1.4-fold relative risk for ACS
Platelet-bound stromal cell–derived factor 1[4]	May play a role in vascular and myocardial remodeling or regeneration	1.4-fold higher level in patients with ACS compared with stable angina
Linoleic acid[5]	Varies inversely with low-density lipoprotein Other undefined mechanism	1 SD decrease was associated with a >3-fold increase in the odds of being a case (ACS) compared with controls
Trans isomer of oleic acid[6]	Unfavorable effects on lipid profile, endothelial function, and inflammatory markers	1 SD increase was associated with an OR of 1.2 of being a case (ACS) compared with controls
Markers Predicting Prognosis in Patients with ACS		
Thrombus precursor protein[7]	Reflects enhanced systemic activation of the coagulation system	Elevated levels independently associated with increased risk of death, reMI, or recurrent ischemia (HR, 1.5) and death or MI (HR, 1.6), adjusted for baseline characteristics and other biomarkers
Chromogranin A[8]	Negative inotropy, induction of apoptosis, inhibition of catecholamine secretion, vasodilation	1 SD increase associated with increases in mortality (1.3-fold), CHF hospitalizations (1.2-fold) after adjustment for conventional cardiovascular risk markers
Free plasma homocysteine[9]	Causes endothelial damage and dysfunction	Level >4.11 μmol/liter (highest quintile) was independently associated with increased risk of cardiovascular death, MI, or stroke (HR, 2.3) after a median follow-up of 2.7 years

ACS = acute coronary syndrome; CHF = congestive heart failure; HR = hazard ratio; OR = odds ratio; reMI = recurrent infarction; SD = standard deviation.
From Giugliano RP, Braunwald E: The year in non–ST-segment elevation acute coronary syndrome. J Am Coll Cardiol 54:1544, 2009. See this paper for references in the table.

1,[30a] and interleukin-6. Neopterin, a marker of monocyte activation, has been reported to be an independent predictor of long-term adverse outcomes.[31] Elevated levels of this inflammatory biomarker (as well as of CRP) can be reduced by high doses of potent statins (e.g., 80 mg/daily of atorvastatin or 40 mg/daily of rosuvastatin). These studies, taken together, indicate that inflammation relates to patient instability and to an increased risk of recurrent cardiac events.

White Blood Cell Count. This is an even simpler, universally available but nonspecific marker of inflammation. Several studies of patients with UA/NSTEMI[32] have reported that patients with elevated white cell counts have a higher risk of mortality and recurrent MI. This association was independent of CRP, suggesting that no one marker, such as CRP, captures all of the information about the influence of inflammation on outcomes.

Myeloperoxidase. Myeloperoxidase (MPO) is a heme protein released during degranulation of neutrophils and some monocytes that generates hypochlorous acid, a potent pro-oxidant. Elevated concentrations in patients presenting with a significantly higher risk of recurrent ACS have associated with increased short-term risk of recurrent ischemic events.[33] Elevations of MPO occur even in coronary arteries remote from the culprit lesion of a UA/NSTEMI episode.[33,34] Thus, leukocyte activation appears to extend beyond a single coronary artery lesion in patients with ACS.

Natriuretic Peptides (BNP and NT-proBNP). B-type natriuretic peptide (BNP) is a neurohormone that is synthesized in ventricular myocardium and is released in response to increased wall stress (see Chap. 25). Its actions include natriuresis, vasodilation, inhibition of sympathetic nerve activity, and inhibition of the renin-angiotensin-aldosterone system. BNP is a useful diagnostic and prognostic marker among patients with heart failure. BNP has prognostic value across the full spectrum of patients with ACS, including those with UA/NSTEMI. In OPUS–TIMI 16, patients with elevated levels of BNP (>80 pg/mL) or NT-proBNP had a twofold to threefold higher risk of death by 10 months,[35] a finding that has been confirmed.[36,37] Together, these data suggest that measurement of natriuretic peptides in patients presenting with UA/NSTEMI adds importantly to current tools for risk stratification.

Creatinine. Another simple tool for risk stratification is the use of creatinine or calculation of creatinine clearance.[38] The risk of impaired renal function appears to be independent of other standard risk factors, such as troponin elevation. Reduced renal function may also play a role in reduced drug clearance, indicating the need for downward adjustment of doses of medications frequently used in the treatment of ACS, such as low-molecular-weight heparin (LMWH) or the small molecule GP IIb/IIIa blockers eptifibatide and tirofiban.

Glucose. Elevated admission values of glucose or hemoglobin A1c predict adverse outcomes among diabetic and nondiabetic patients with acute UA/NSTEMI compared with those without hyperglycemia (see Chap. 64).[39] A synergistic relationship between hyperglycemia and inflammation has also been described.[40] The risk associated with hyperglycemia was amplified in patients with an elevated CRP level compared with a normal one.

Thrombus Precursor Protein. This soluble fibrin polymer is a precursor to the formation of insoluble fibrin that may be increased in patients with acute MI. A significant correlation between thrombus precursor protein levels and the incidence of adverse clinical outcomes in ACS has been reported.[41]

Combined Risk Assessment Scores

Integrating all of these factors, several groups have developed comprehensive risk scores that use clinical variables and findings from the electrocardiogram or from serum cardiac markers.[42,43] The TIMI risk score identified seven independent risk factors: age >65 years, >3 risk factors for CAD, documented CAD at catheterization, ST deviation >0.5 mm, >2 episodes of angina in last 24 hours, ASA within prior week, and elevated cardiac markers. Use of this scoring system allowed risk stratification of patients across an almost 10-fold gradient of risk, from 4.7% to 40.9% ($P < 0.001$) (**Fig. 56-6A**). More important, this risk score predicts the response to several of the therapies in UA/NSTEMI. Patients with higher TIMI risk scores had significant reductions in events when treated with enoxaparin compared with unfractionated heparin,[43] with a GP IIb/IIIa inhibitor compared with placebo, and with an invasive versus conservative strategy (Fig. 56-6B).

The Global Registry of Acute Coronary Events (GRACE) has also identified factors that were associated independently with increased mortality; the most important baseline determinants of higher mortality were increased age, Killip class, increased heart rate, ST-segment depression, signs of heart failure, lower systolic pressure, cardiac arrest at presentation, and elevated serum creatinine or cardiac marker enzymes.[44]

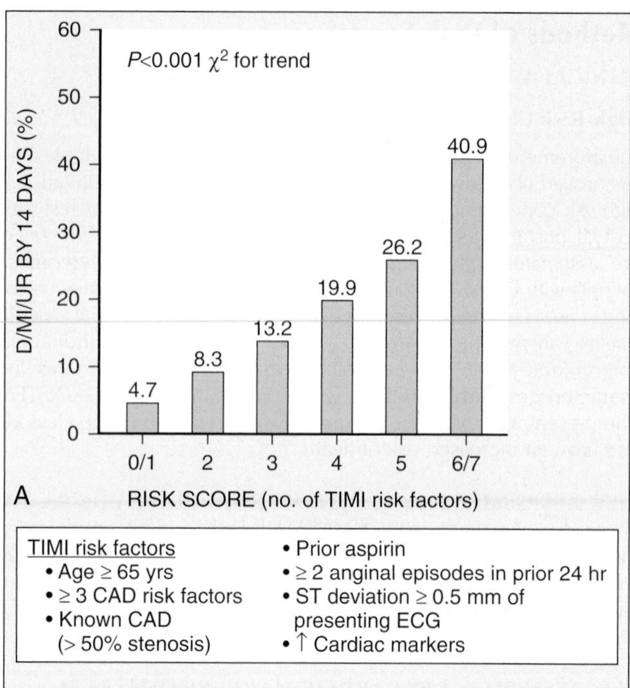

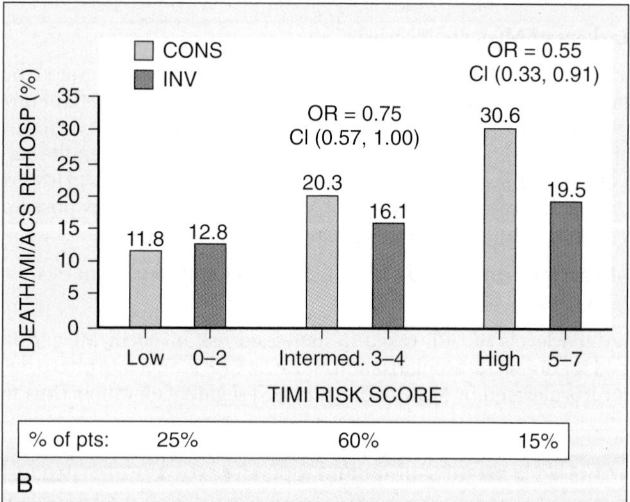

FIGURE 56-6 **A,** Thrombolysis In Myocardial Ischemia (TIMI) risk score for unstable angina or non–ST elevation myocardial infarction (UA/NSTEMI). The risk factors are shown at the bottom, and the risk of death (D), myocardial infarction (MI), or urgent revascularization (UR) is shown along the vertical axis. **B,** Use of the TIMI risk score for UA/NSTEMI to predict the benefit of an early invasive strategy. In a prospectively defined analysis, the TIMI risk score was applied in the Treat Angina with Aggrastat and determine Cost of Therapy with an Invasive or Conservative Strategy (TACTICS)–TIMI 18 trial. As shown, 75% of patients had a risk score of 3 or higher, and a significant benefit of an invasive strategy was observed in these patients. ACS = acute coronary syndrome; CAD = coronary artery disease; CI = confidence interval; CONS = conservative; ECG = electrocardiogram; INV = invasive; OR = odds ratio. *(**A,** modified from Antman EM, Cohen M, Bernink PJLM, et al: The TIMI risk score for unstable angina/non–ST elevation MI: A method for prognostication and therapeutic decision-making. JAMA 284:835, 2000. **B,** data from Cannon CP, Weintraub WS, Demopoulos LA, et al: Comparison of early invasive and conservative strategies in patients with unstable coronary syndromes treated with the glycoprotein IIb/IIIa inhibitor tirofiban. N Engl J Med 344:1879, 2001.)*

With the ever-growing number of new cardiac markers, comprehensive risk scores will likely include these new markers as they become more widely available in clinical practice, as shown in several studies using three markers in a "multimarker strategy" evaluation for prediction of mortality[45] or of nonfatal events.[46]

A risk score to predict major bleeding has also been developed from the CRUSADE registry. Patients with worsening creatinine clearance, women, diabetics, patients with lower blood pressure, and patients with higher heart rates had higher rates of bleeding.[47] In addition, when antithrombotic agents were not dose-adjusted for renal function or weight, rates of bleeding were two to three times higher.[48]

Medical Therapy

General Measures

Patients with UA/NSTEMI at medium or high risk should be admitted to an intensive (cardiac) or intermediate care unit; patients at low risk should be admitted to a monitored bed, preferably in a cardiac step-down unit.[2] In these settings, continuous electrocardiographic monitoring (i.e., telemetry) is used to detect tachyarrhythmias, alterations in atrioventricular and intraventricular conduction, and changes in ST-segment deviation. Bed rest should be prescribed initially. Ambulation, as tolerated, is permitted if the patient has been stable without recurrent chest discomfort for at least 12 to 24 hours. It is advisable to provide supplemental oxygen to patients with cyanosis or extensive rales and when arterial oxygen saturation, measured by oximetry, declines below 90%.

Relief of chest pain is an initial goal of treatment. In patients with persistent pain despite therapy with nitrates and beta blockers (see later), morphine sulfate by intravenous bolus in doses of 2 to 5 mg may be administered. Contraindications to morphine include allergy for this drug, for which meperidine can be substituted, and hypotension. With careful blood pressure monitoring, repeated doses can be administered every 5 to 30 minutes. Morphine may act as both an analgesic and an anxiolytic, but its venodilatory effects may produce beneficial hemodynamic effects by reducing ventricular preload, which is especially useful in the presence of pulmonary congestion. However, morphine may also cause hypotension, and if that occurs, supine positioning and intravenous saline should restore blood pressure; pressors are rarely needed. If respiratory depression develops, naloxone (0.4 to 2.0 mg) may be given.

NITRATES. Nitrates are endothelium-independent vasodilators that both increase myocardial blood flow by coronary vasodilation and reduce myocardial oxygen demand. The latter effect results from arteriolar and venous dilation leading to reduced myocardial afterload, preload, and ventricular wall stress. If the patient is experiencing ischemic pain, nitrates should initially be given sublingually or by buccal spray (0.3 to 0.6 mg). If pain persists after three sublingual tablets (or buccal sprays) administered at 5-minute intervals, intravenous nitroglycerin by use of nonabsorbing tubing (5 to 10 μg/min) is recommended. The rate of the nitroglycerin infusion may be increased by 10 μg/min every 3 to 5 minutes until relief of symptoms occurs or systolic blood pressure falls to below 100 mm Hg.[2] Although there is no absolute maximum dose, a dose of 200 μg/min is generally used as a ceiling.

Contraindications to the use of nitrates are hypotension and the use of sildenafil or related phosphodiesterase type 5 inhibitors within the previous 24 to 48 hours. Topical or long-acting oral nitrates can be used if the patient has been pain free for 12 to 24 hours. Dosing of nitrates depends on the formulation, but an attempt should be made to have an 8- to 10-hour nitrate-free interval to avoid the development of tolerance. Chronic nitrate therapy can frequently be tapered in the long-term management of patients unless they develop chronic, stable angina (see Chap. 57).

The effect of nitrates on mortality was evaluated in ISIS-4, a large randomized trial for patients with suspected MI (both STEMI and NSTEMI).[49] No effect on mortality was observed in the overall population or in the subgroup of patients with NSTEMI.

BETA BLOCKERS. Early placebo-controlled trials in UA/NSTEMI demonstrated the benefit of beta blockers in reducing subsequent MI or recurrent ischemia.[46] In patients with acute MI (both STEMI and NSTEMI), beta blockers have also been shown to reduce reinfarction and ventricular fibrillation (see Chap. 57).[50] A reduction in mortality achieved by beta blockers in more recent times (i.e., the 21st century) is less clear.[51]

Oral beta blockers in doses used in chronic stable angina (see Chap. 57) should be begun 24 hours after presentation and should be continued at discharge in patients with UA/NSTEMI who do not have contraindications. Oral beta blocker therapy should be initiated within the first 24 hours for patients who do not have one or more of the following: (1) signs of heart failure, (2) evidence of a low-output state, (3) increased risk for cardiogenic shock, or (4) other relative contraindications to beta blockade (PR interval >0.24 second, second- or third-degree heart block, active asthma, or reactive airway disease). Beta blockers can be administered at low doses to patients with heart failure once they are stabilized. If ischemia and chest pain are ongoing despite intravenous nitrate therapy, intravenous beta blockers may be used cautiously, followed by oral administration. The choice of beta blocker can be individualized on the basis of the drug's pharmacokinetics, cost, and physician familiarity. However, those with intrinsic sympathomimetic activity, such as pindolol, should not be selected.

CALCIUM CHANNEL BLOCKERS. Calcium channel blockers have vasodilatory effects and reduce blood pressure. Some, such as verapamil and diltiazem, also slow heart rate and reduce myocardial contractility. Early studies suggested that they reduce recurrent MI.[52] Calcium antagonists may be used in patients with persistent ischemia despite treatment with full-dose nitrates and beta blockers, in patients with contraindications to beta blockers (see earlier), and in those with hypertension. Such patients should be treated with heart rate–slowing calcium channel blockers (e.g., diltiazem or verapamil). Oral doses of diltiazem and verapamil range from 30 to 90 mg four times daily to 360 mg once daily of the long-acting preparation. Nifedipine (short acting), which accelerates heart rate, has been shown to be harmful in patients with acute MI when it is not coadministered with a beta blocker. No harm with long-term treatment with the long-acting drugs (amlodipine and felodipine) was observed in patients with documented left ventricular dysfunction and CAD,[53] indicating that these agents may be safely used in patients with UA/NSTEMI with left ventricular dysfunction. In addition, two recent trials documented the benefit of amlodipine in patients with hypertension and stable CAD.[54,55]

Antithrombotic Therapy (see Chap. 87)

ANTIPLATELET AGENTS. The importance of platelets in the pathogenesis of UA/NSTEMI was discussed earlier. Accordingly, antiplatelet therapy plays a central role in management.

Aspirin (ASA)

This drug acetylates platelet cyclooxygenase 1 (COX-1), thereby blocking the synthesis and release of thromboxane A_2, a platelet activator (**Fig. 56-7**). ASA thereby decreases overall platelet aggregation and arterial thrombus formation. Because this inhibition of COX-1 is irreversible, the antiplatelet effects last for the lifetime of the platelets, approximately 7 to 10 days. Several trials have demonstrated clear beneficial effects of ASA in patients with UA/NSTEMI[56] (**Fig. 56-8**). In addition to reducing adverse clinical events early in the course of treatment of UA/NSTEMI, ASA also prevents recurrence of ischemic events in secondary prevention.

In the randomized trials of ASA versus placebo, the dose of aspirin ranged from 75 mg/day to 1300 mg/day, and each trial showed an approximately 25% reduction in death or MI.[56] Thus, there does not appear to be a dose-response in the efficacy of aspirin.[57] In the case of patients with UA/NSTEMI, after an initial loading dose of 162 to 325 mg, doses of 75 or 81 mg daily appear to be efficacious and cause less gastrointestinal irritation or bleeding than higher doses. The OASIS-7 trial randomized 25,087 ACS patients (UA/NSTEMI, 70.8%; STEMI, 29.2%) to receive high-dose (300 to 325 mg/day) versus low-dose (75 to 100 mg/day) aspirin for 30 days (and to high-dose versus regular-dose clopidogrel; see later). Preliminary results found no difference in the risk of cardiovascular death, MI, or stroke, and no difference in the overall rate of major bleeding—2.3% in each group. More complete analysis of this short-term comparison of aspirin dosing will be needed.

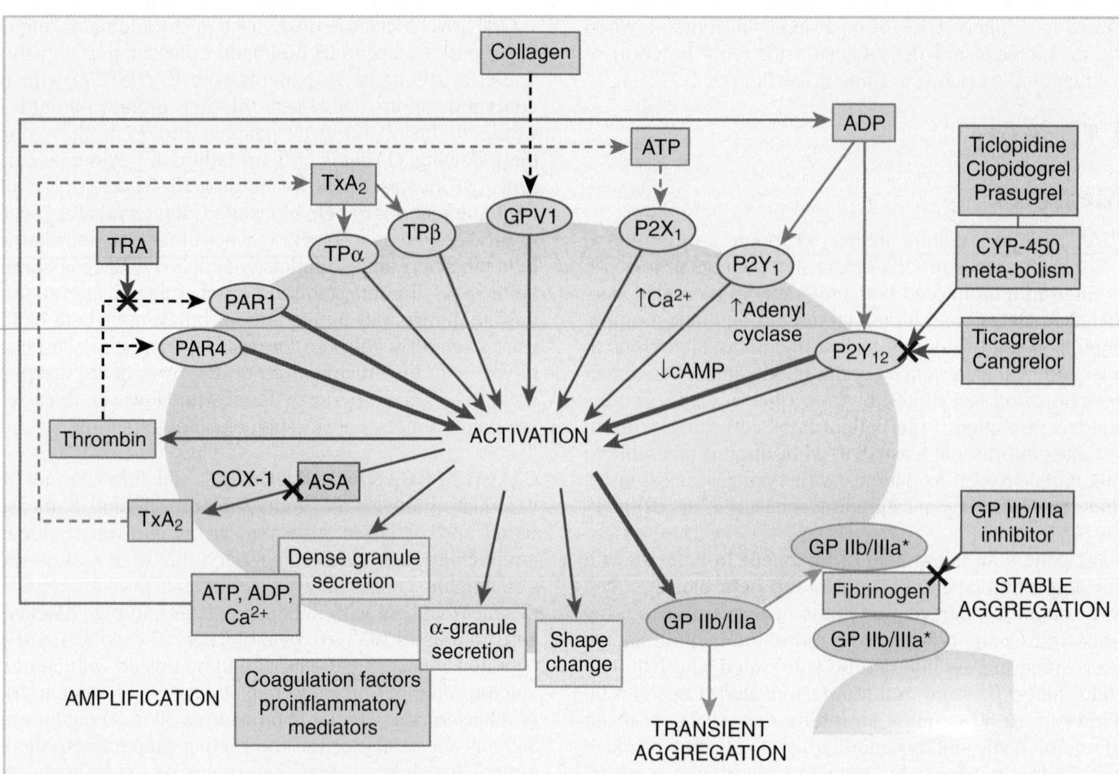

FIGURE 56-7 Platelet activation mechanisms and sites of blockade of antiplatelet therapies. Platelet activation is initiated by soluble agonists, such as thrombin, thromboxane A_2, 5HT, ADP (via $P2Y_1$), and ATP, and by adhesive ligands, such as collagen and von Willebrand factor. Consequently, dense granule secretion of platelet agonists and secretion of thromboxane A_2 (as a result of phospholipase A_2 activation) lead to amplification of platelet activation and the associated responses. The $P2Y_{12}$ receptor plays a major role in the amplification of platelet activation, supported also by outside-in signaling via the $\alpha_{IIb}\beta_3$ (GP IIb/IIIa) receptor. Combined $P2Y_{12}$ and $\alpha_{IIb}\beta_3$ blockade, therefore, has additive effects on platelet activation and the associated platelet responses. See text for details. ADP = adenosine; cAMP = cyclic adenosine monophosphate; COX = cyclooxygenase diphosphate; GP = glycoprotein; TxA_2 = thromboxane A_2. *(Modified after Storey RF: Biology and pharmacology of the platelet $P2Y_{12}$ receptor. Curr Pharm Des 12:1255, 2006. From Wallentin L: $P2Y_{12}$ inhibitors: Differences in properties and mechanisms of action and potential consequences for clinical use. Eur Heart J 30:1964, 2009, with permission.)*

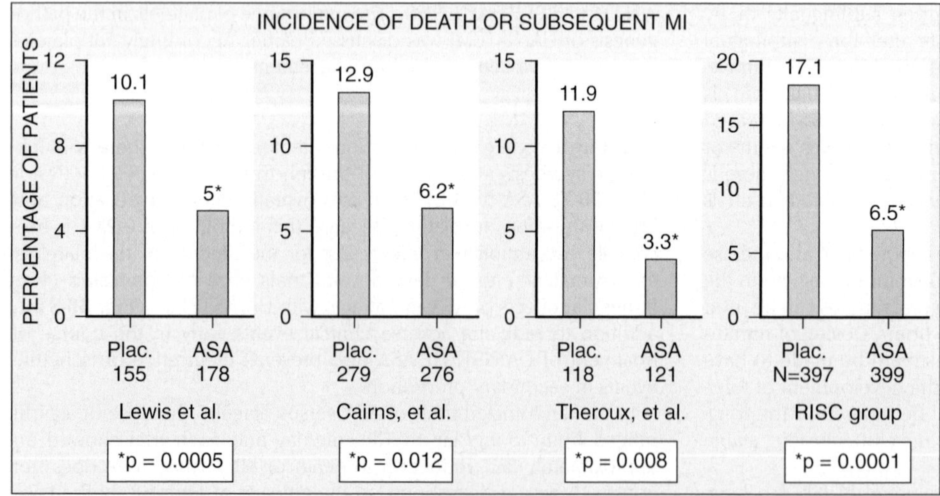

FIGURE 56-8 Four randomized trials showing the benefit of aspirin in UA/NSTEMI, in which the incidence of death or MI was reduced by more than 50% in each of the four trials. The doses of aspirin in the four trials were 325 mg, 1300 mg, 650 mg, and 75 mg daily, indicating no difference in efficacy for aspirin across these doses. ASA = aspirin; Plac. = placebo. *(Data from Lewis HD, et al: N Engl J Med 309:396, 1983; Cairns JA, et al: N Engl J Med 313:1369, 1985; Theroux P, et al: N Engl J Med 319:1105, 1988; RISC Group: Lancet 349:827, 1990.)*

In patients who have an allergy or who cannot tolerate aspirin, clopidogrel is recommended.[2]

"Aspirin resistance" may occur during chronic therapy.[58,59] Small studies have identified 2% to 8% of patients in whom treatment with ASA appears to have a limited antiplatelet effect (i.e., minimal change in the degree of platelet aggregation). These patients tend to have a greater risk of recurrent cardiac events.[60] There is increasing evidence that so-called aspirin resistance is often related to poor compliance. Other causes include poor absorption, interaction with ibuprofen, and overexpression of COX-2 mRNA. Whether routine monitoring of antiplatelet effects by light transmission aggregometry or point-of-care devices with adjustment of dose is an effective strategy has not been evaluated in large trials or registries, but such monitoring would seem to be a potentially useful approach.

Contraindications to ASA therapy include documented allergy (e.g., asthma), active bleeding, and a known platelet disorder. Dyspepsia and other gastrointestinal symptoms with long-term ASA therapy (i.e., aspirin intolerance) do not usually preclude therapy in the short term.

ADP ANTAGONISTS

Thienopyridines

These agents (ticlopidine, clopidogrel, and prasugrel) are prodrugs that are converted to active metabolites through oxidation by the

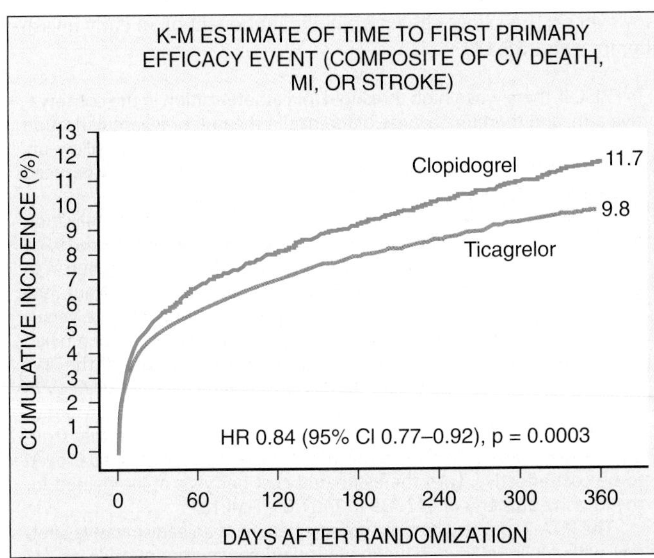

FIGURE 56-13 The primary endpoint of the PLATO trial—a composite of death from cardiovascular (CV) causes, myocardial infarction (MI), or stroke—occurred significantly less often in the ticagrelor group than in the clopidogrel group (9.8% versus 11.7% at 12 months; HR, 0.84; 95% CI, 0.77 to 0.92; $P < 0.001$). K-M = Kaplan-Meier; HR = hazard ratio; CI = confidence interval. *(From Wallentin L, Becker R, Budaj A, et al: Ticagrelor versus clopidogrel in patients with acute coronary syndromes. N Engl J Med 361:1045, 2009.)*

TABLE 56-4 Standardized Nomogram for Titration of Heparin*

APTT (SEC)†	CHANGE	IV INFUSION (UNITS/KG/HR)
<35	70 units/kg bolus	+3
35-49	35 units/kg bolus	+2
50-70	0	0
71-90	0	−2
>100	Hold infusion for 30 min	−3

*Initial dose: 60 units/kg bolus and 12 units/kg/hr infusion.

†Activated partial thromboplastin time (APTT) should be checked and infusion adjusted at 6, 12, and 24 hours after initiation of heparin, daily thereafter, and 4 to 6 hours after any adjustment in dose.

From Becker RC, Ball SP, Eisenberg P, et al: A randomized, multicenter trial of weight-adjusted intravenous heparin dose titration and point-of-care coagulation monitoring in hospitalized patients with active thromboembolic disease. Am Heart J 137:59, 1999.

LMWH, when added to ASA, has proved to be effective compared with ASA alone, leading to a 66% reduction in the odds of death or MI.[98] Early trials with enoxaparin showed a 20% reduction in death, MI, or recurrent ischemia compared with UFH.[102] In two more recent trials, enoxaparin was found to be noninferior to UFH.[103,104] In a meta-analysis of all trials in ACS, enoxaparin yielded a statistically significant 16% reduction in the odds of death or MI at 30 days.[102] Enoxaparin provides significant benefit over UFH in patients with UA/NSTEMI who are managed conservatively and who typically receive UFH or LMWH for at least 48 hours, but not in patients managed invasively who are taken to the catheterization laboratory within 24 hours.[105] Treatment with enoxaparin was associated with an excess of major bleeding compared with UFH.[102] Although several LMWHs have been approved, the weight of evidence supports the choice of enoxaparin.[2]

FONDAPARINUX. Fondaparinux, a synthetic pentasaccharide, is an *indirect* factor Xa inhibitor and requires the presence of antithrombin for its action. The OASIS-5 trial compared fondaparinux, administered at a relatively low dose (2.5 mg subcutaneously once daily) with standard-dose enoxaparin in 20,078 patients with high-risk UA/NSTEMI. The rates of death, MI, or refractory ischemia throughout the first 9 days were similar.[106] Of importance, however, the rate of major bleeding was reduced significantly—almost by half—in the fondaparinux arm (2.2% versus 4.1%). By 30 days, mortality was significantly lower in the fondaparinux arm (2.9% versus 3.5%). However, in patients undergoing PCI, fondaparinux has associated with more than a threefold increased risk of catheter-related thrombi, a complication also observed in STEMI patients treated with fondaparinux.[107] Supplemental UFH at the time of catheterization appeared to minimize the risk of this problem with fondaparinux. Thus, fondaparinux is an alternative for patients with UA/NSTEMI. It is associated with a lower risk of bleeding and is recommended, in particular, in patients at a higher risk of bleeding.[2]

Direct Thrombin Inhibitors. Direct thrombin inhibitors have a potential advantage over indirect thrombin inhibitors, such as UFH, LMWH, and fondaparinux, in that they do not require antithrombin and can inhibit clot-bound thrombin. They do not interact with plasma proteins, provide a stable level of anticoagulation, and do not cause thrombocytopenia. A meta-analysis of all direct thrombin inhibitors, including hirudin, bivalirudin, argatroban, efegatran, or inogatran, showed a modest 9% reduction in death or MI at 30 days, favoring the direct thrombin inhibitor over unfractionated heparin.[108] The only current indication approved by the Food and Drug Administration for lepirudin and argatroban is for anticoagulation in patients with heparin-induced thrombocytopenia and associated thromboembolic disease.

Bivalirudin binds reversibly to thrombin. The open-label ACUITY trial randomized 13,819 patients with UA/NSTEMI managed with an early invasive strategy to one of three treatments: (1) UFH or enoxaparin with or without a GP IIb/IIIa inhibitor, (2) bivalirudin with a GP IIb/IIIa inhibitor, and (3) bivalirudin alone. The primary endpoint was the composite of death, MI, unplanned revascularization for ischemia, and major bleeding at 30 days.[109] No differences were observed for efficacy or major bleeding in the direct comparison of the anticoagulants, that is, between UFH or enoxaparin plus a GP IIb/IIIa inhibitor and bivalirudin plus a GP IIb/IIIa inhibitor. For the bivalirudin-alone group, compared with the group receiving UFH or enoxaparin plus a GP IIb/IIIa inhibitor, there were no differences in efficacy but a significantly lower rate of bleeding (3.0% versus 5.7%).[109] Thus, the substitution of bivalirudin for UFH or enoxaparin as the anticoagulant among patients receiving supplemental GP IIb/IIIa inhibitors did not change efficacy or safety outcomes, but the strategy of bivalirudin alone (i.e., without a GP IIb/IIIa inhibitor) was associated with less bleeding than the combination of a GP IIb/IIIa inhibitor with either UFH or enoxaparin. The ISAR–REACT 3[110] trial compared UFH and bivalirudin in patients who had received 600 mg of clopidogrel. The reduced rate of major bleeding with bivalirudin was largely offset by an increase in ischemic events.

Oral Anticoagulation. Several trials have examined oral anticoagulation with warfarin after ACS, with the rationale that prolonged treatment might extend the benefit of early anticoagulation with a parenteral antithrombin agent. They have suggested that if a sufficient degree of anticoagulation were achieved, a benefit accrued from the combination of ASA plus warfarin.[111,112] In the WARIS trial, patients with ACS within the prior 8 weeks were randomized to warfarin alone (target international normalized ratio [INR] of 2.8 to 4.2), ASA alone (160 mg daily), or aspirin (80 mg daily) combined with warfarin (target INR of 2.0).[111] During a follow-up of 4 years, the rate of death, MI, or thromboembolic stroke occurred in 20% of patients receiving ASA alone, 16.7% of patients receiving warfarin alone ($P = 0.03$), and 15% of patients receiving warfarin and ASA ($P = 0.001$). Rates of major bleeding were 0.62% per treatment-year in both groups receiving warfarin and 0.17% in patients receiving ASA ($P < 0.001$). Thus, the combination of ASA plus warfarin was more effective than aspirin alone for long-term secondary prevention but was associated with increased serious bleeding.

However, given the similar benefits seen with clopidogrel and warfarin added to ASA, the lack of need for monitoring of the INR, and the frequent use of PCI and stenting in the patient population in whom the need for clopidogrel is well established, the clinical use of ASA and warfarin has been limited. Among patients *without a coronary stent* but with another indication for warfarin, such as chronic atrial fibrillation or severe left ventricular dysfunction, who are at high risk of systemic embolization, the combination of ASA and warfarin would be preferable as the long-term antithrombotic strategy. The combination of all three agents (ASA, clopidogrel, and warfarin) has not been tested prospectively to date, but it may be associated with a high bleeding risk during long-term therapy. Use of this combination is sometimes required in UA/NSTEMI patients after stenting with atrial fibrillation or other strong indications for warfarin. In such patients, it is recommended to use low-dose aspirin (75 to 81 mg daily), warfarin (titrated meticulously to an INR of 2.0 to 2.5), and clopidogrel for as short a time as recommended for the type of stent placed.[2]

FACTOR XA INHIBITORS. Two potent oral direct factor Xa inhibitors with a high bioavailability are undergoing phase III testing. In the ATLAS ACS–TIMI 46 trial, a phase II dose-finding study with rivaroxaban, the addition of this drug to ASA in patients with recent ACS[113] was associated with a significant 31% reduction of the hard endpoints of death, MI, and stroke, but a significant increase in bleeding. In the APPRAISE trial, carried out with apixaban (a factor Xa inhibitor with properties similar to those of rivaroxaban), a dose-related increase in bleeding and a trend to a reduction in ischemic events were observed.[114] In both trials, the reduction of ischemic events trended to be greater with the ASA plus a factor Xa inhibitor combination, whereas bleeding was higher in the group receiving triple therapy (ASA, clopidogrel, and factor Xa inhibitor).

Ongoing phase III trials will help in the elucidation of the clinical role of this therapeutic class.

PROTEASE-ACTIVATED RECEPTOR (PAR-1) ANTAGONISTS. Thrombin potently stimulates platelets by activating PAR-1. The thrombin receptor blocker Vorapaxar blocks this interaction.[115-117] This thrombin receptor antagonist was tested in a phase II trial of patients undergoing PCI, in whom it was associated with a trend toward a lower incidence of death or MI but without an increase in bleeding.[118] It is now undergoing testing in two large phase III trials. One trial, Thrombin Receptor Antagonist for Clinical Events Reduction (TRACER), is in patients who recently experienced an ACS; the other trial is in patients with chronic CAD.[119]

Treatment Strategies and Interventions

There are two general approaches to the use of cardiac catheterization and revascularization in UA/NSTEMI: (1) an early *invasive* strategy, involving routine early cardiac catheterization followed by PCI, CABG, or continuing medical therapy, depending on the coronary anatomy; and (2) a more *conservative* approach, with initial medical management and catheterization reserved for patients with recurrent ischemia either at rest or on a noninvasive stress test and, if the anatomy is suitable, revascularization. To date, the relative merits of these two strategies have been studied in 10 randomized trials. The first three and the most recent trial did not demonstrate a significant difference; however, six trials have shown a significant benefit of an early invasive therapy (**Fig. 56-14**).[119-121]

In FRISC II, there was a high threshold for catheterization in the conservative arm, and therefore a large difference in the rate of revascularization between the invasive and conservative strategies. In a 5-year follow-up, overall death or MI was lower, while mortality was significantly reduced in patients at high risk at baseline but not in those at low risk.[122]

In the TACTICS–TIMI 18 trial, the rate of death, MI, or rehospitalization for ACS at 6 months (the primary endpoint) fell significantly, from 19.4% in the conservative group to 15.9% in the early invasive group.[15] In patients with a troponin I level >0.1 ng/mL, there was a significant 39% relative risk reduction in the primary endpoint with the invasive versus the conservative strategy, whereas patients with a negative troponin had similar outcomes with either strategy (**Fig. 56-15**). With use of the TIMI risk score, there was significant benefit of the early invasive strategy in intermediate-risk (score, 3 to 4) patients and high-risk (5 to 7) patients, whereas low-risk (0 to 2) patients had similar outcomes with either strategy[15] (see Fig. 56-6B). Interestingly, the invasive strategy has also proved to be cost-effective, with the estimated cost per year of life gained for the invasive strategy of $12,739 in TACTICS–TIMI 18.[123]

The RITA-3 trial also demonstrated a benefit of an early invasive strategy, with a 34% relative reduction in the primary endpoint of death, MI, or refractory angina at 4 months; this benefit was driven primarily by a reduction in refractory angina. By 5 years, there was a significantly lower cardiovascular mortality rate in the early invasive arm.[124] In the most recent trial (ICTUS) that examined an invasive versus a conservative approach, all patients received ASA, enoxaparin, and abciximab for PCI, followed by intensive statin therapy. At 1 year, there was no significant difference in the rate of the primary endpoint—death, MI, or rehospitalization for angina.[125] In this trial, a very low threshold was used in the definition of periprocedural MI, and thus there was a much higher periprocedural MI rate compared with earlier trials, explaining, at least in part, the disparate results of this trial. However, even in ICTUS, the risk of rehospitalization was significantly lower in the invasive arm.

A meta-analysis of the more recent trials has confirmed an overall significant reduction in death, MI, or rehospitalization and of mortality during follow-up (see Fig. 56-14).[121] A sex-specific collaborative meta-analysis demonstrated benefit of an invasive strategy in all men and in high-risk women, but not in low-risk women, consistent with the 2007 Guidelines[120] (**Fig. 56-16**; see Fig. 81-6). Subgroup analyses of registries and clinical trials have shown a benefit of an early invasive strategy among women,[120] the elderly,[126] and patients with chronic

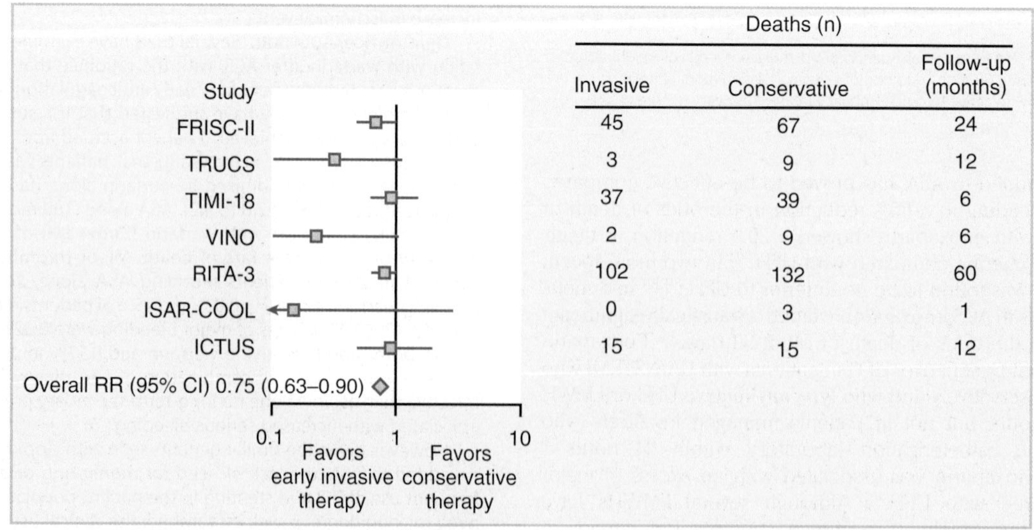

Study	Invasive	Conservative	Follow-up (months)
FRISC-II	45	67	24
TRUCS	3	9	12
TIMI-18	37	39	6
VINO	2	9	6
RITA-3	102	132	60
ISAR-COOL	0	3	1
ICTUS	15	15	12

FIGURE 56-14 Meta-analysis of the benefit of a routine invasive versus "selective" invasive (i.e., conservative) strategy for patients with unstable angina or NSTEMI on the rate of death, myocardial infarction, or rehospitalization through follow-up. FRISC-II = Fragmin and Fast Revascularization During Instability in Coronary Artery Disease; ICTUS = Invasive Versus Conservative Treatment in Unstable Coronary Syndromes; ISAR-COOL = Intracoronary Stenting With Antithrombotic Regimen Cooling-Off; RITA-3 = Randomized Intervention Trial of Unstable Angina; RR = risk ratio; TACTICS–TIMI 18 = Treat Angina With Aggrastat and Determine the Cost of Therapy With an Invasive or Conservative Strategy–Thrombolysis in Myocardial Infarction; TRUCS = Treatment of Refractory Unstable Angina in Geographically Isolated Areas Without Cardiac Surgery; VINO = Value of First Day Coronary Angiography/Angioplasty in Evolving Non–ST-Segment Elevation Myocardial Infarction. *(Reproduced with permission from Bavry AA, Kumbhani DJ, Rassi AN, et al: Benefit of early invasive therapy in acute coronary syndromes: A meta-analysis of contemporary randomized clinical trials. J Am Coll Cardiol 48:1319, 2006.)*

kidney disease[127]—groups that are less likely to undergo early coronary arteriography.

Indications for Invasive Versus Conservative Management Strategies

On the basis of several recent randomized trials and meta-analyses, an early invasive strategy is now recommended in patients with UA/NSTEMI who have ST-segment changes or positive troponin on admission or who evolve these high-risk features during the subsequent 24 hours. Other high-risk indicators, such as recurrent ischemia and evidence of congestive heart failure, are also indications for an early invasive strategy. An early invasive strategy is also advised in patients who present with UA/NSTEMI within 6 months of a prior PCI and in whom restenosis may be the cause. An early invasive approach is also indicated in patients with UA/NSTEMI with prior CABG.[2]

The Intracoronary Stenting with Antithrombotic Regimen Cooling-Off (ISAR-COOL) trial found a benefit of an immediate invasive strategy with an average time of only 2 hours from randomization to catheterization, compared with a delayed invasive strategy, in which the average time to catheterization was 4 days.[128] The TIMACS trial compared early (median = 14 hours after randomization) with later (median = 50 hours) angiography.[129] It showed a trend for reduction of the primary endpoint (death, MI, and stroke) in the group as a whole but a significant reduction in the primary endpoint in patients with a high GRACE risk score. There was also a significant 28% reduction of the secondary endpoint of death, MI, and refractory ischemia with earlier angiography. Both of these trials lend support to a very early invasive strategy, especially in high-risk patients.

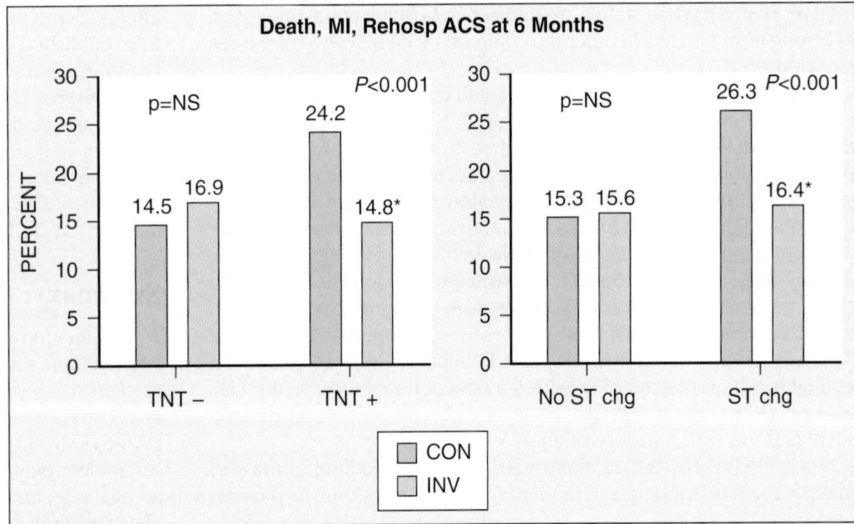

FIGURE 56-15 Risk stratification with troponin T (TnT) or ST-segment changes to determine the benefit of an early invasive (INV) versus conservative (CON) strategy in the TACTICS–TIMI 18 trial. *(Data from Cannon CP, Weintraub WS, Demopoulos LA, et al: Comparison of early invasive and conservative strategies in patients with unstable coronary syndromes treated with the glycoprotein IIb/IIIa inhibitor tirofiban. N Engl J Med 344:1879, 2001.)*

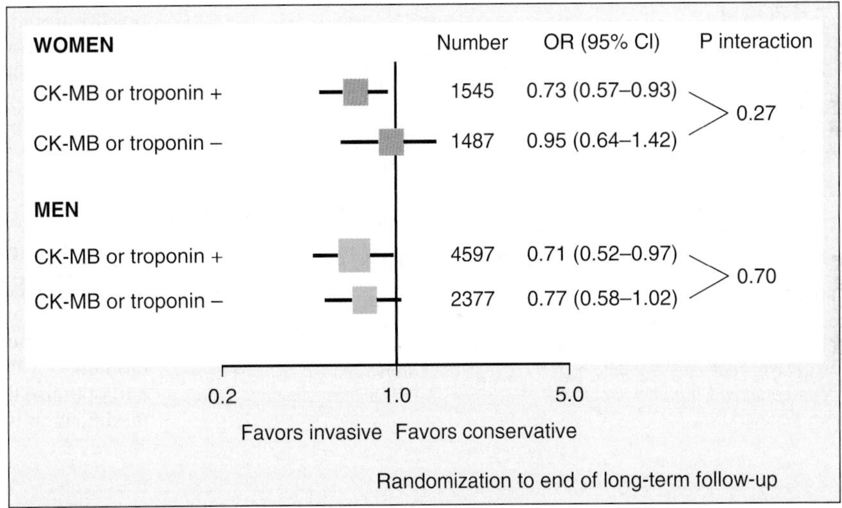

FIGURE 56-16 Meta-analysis, by sex, of the benefit of a routine invasive versus "selective" invasive (i.e., conservative) strategy for patients with unstable angina or NSTEMI on the rate of death, myocardial infarction, or rehospitalization through follow-up. *(From O'Donoghue M, Boden WE, Braunwald E, et al: Early invasive vs. conservative treatment strategies in women and men with unstable angina and non–ST-segment elevation myocardial infarction. A meta-analysis. JAMA 300:71, 2008.)*

Percutaneous Coronary Intervention. (See Chap. 58.) Current angiographic success rates of PCI are high, generally >95%, although the presence of UA/NSTEMI or visualized thrombus can increase the risk of acute complications, such as abrupt closure and MI. Thus, use of GP IIb/IIIa inhibitors or a thienopyridine (clopidogrel or prasugrel) in such patients improves both acute and long-term outcomes after PCI. Implantation of drug-eluting stents reduces the risk of restenosis. There is a risk of late stent thrombosis after drug-eluting stent implantation, especially when clopidogrel is stopped. This serious complication can be reduced by long-term (at least 1 year or perhaps longer) dual antiplatelet therapy (i.e., ASA and a thienopyridine) in patients treated in this manner.

Percutaneous Coronary Intervention versus Coronary Artery Bypass Grafting. Several trials have compared PCI and CABG in patients with ischemic heart disease, many of whom had UA/NSTEMI (see Chap. 58). On the basis of the results, CABG is recommended for patients with disease of the left main coronary artery as well as for those with multivessel disease and impaired left ventricular function or diabetes mellitus. For other patients treated invasively, PCI is ordinarily employed if the coronary anatomy is suitable. If it is not, CABG is the treatment of choice. PCI associates with a slightly lower initial morbidity and mortality than CABG, but there is a higher need of repeated PCI.

Other Therapies

ANGIOTENSIN-CONVERTING ENZYME INHIBITORS AND ANGIOTENSIN RECEPTOR BLOCKERS. Large trials have shown a 0.5% absolute mortality benefit of early (initiated within 24 hours) angiotensin-converting enzyme (ACE) inhibitor therapy in patients with acute MI. However, the ISIS-4 trial did not show a benefit in patients without ST elevation.[49] Long-term use of ACE inhibition prevents recurrent ischemic events and mortality (see Chap. 55). Angiotensin receptor blockers (ARBs) may be substituted for ACE inhibitors on the basis of the Valsartan in Acute Myocardial Infarction Trial (VALIANT), which showed equivalent outcomes in post-MI patients treated with the ACE inhibitors captopril and the ARB valsartan.[130] ARBs are certainly indicated in patients who cannot tolerate ACE inhibitors.

LIPID-LOWERING THERAPY. Long-term treatment with lipid-lowering therapy, especially with statins, has shown benefit in patients after acute MI and UA/NSTEMI (see Chaps. 47 and 55).[131] In a prespecified subgroup of more than 3200 patients with unstable angina, in the Long-Term Intervention with Pravastatin in Ischemic Disease (LIPID) trial, pravastatin therapy led to a significant 26% reduction in total mortality.[132] When statins are initiated in-hospital at the time of an ACS, long-term benefits in outcome compared with placebo have been reported.[133]

In the PROVE IT–TIMI 22 trial, conducted in 4162 patients who were enrolled an average of 10 days after an ACS, intensive lipid-lowering therapy with atorvastatin 80 mg resulted in a 16% reduction in the primary endpoint and a 25% reduction in death, MI, or urgent revascularization, compared with moderate lipid-lowering therapy with pravastatin (40 mg).[134] A benefit emerged only 30 days after randomization,[135] highlighting the importance of early initiation of intensive statin therapy after ACS (**Fig. 56-17**). The average low-density lipoprotein (LDL) levels achieved in the two arms were 62 mg/dL and 95 mg/dL, respectively. In part on the basis of these results, the Adult Treatment Panel III of the National Cholesterol Education Program issued an update in which they recommended a new optional therapeutic LDL goal of <70 mg/dL in high-risk patients with coronary heart disease, such as those with a history of an ACS.[136]

Since PROVE IT–TIMI 22, there have been four additional trials of intensive versus moderate (standard) statin therapy, one in patients after ACS and three in patients with stable CAD. A meta-analysis of the four published trials showed a highly significant 16% reduction in coronary death or MI with intensive versus standard statin therapy (**Fig. 56-18**).[137]

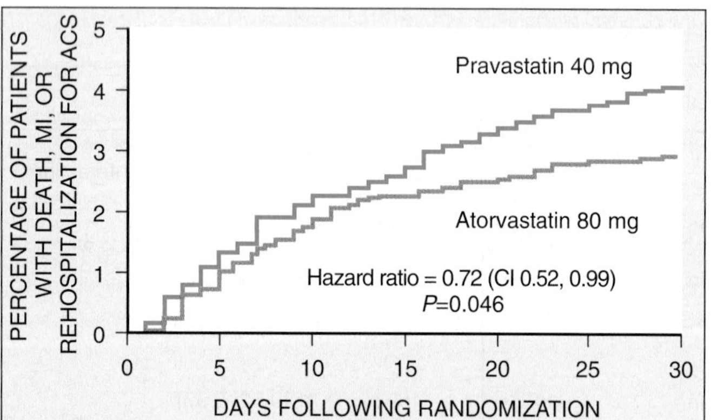

FIGURE 56-17 The benefit of intensive statin therapy initiated early after acute coronary syndrome (ACS) in the PROVE IT–TIMI 22 trial. A significant reduction in events is seen in the first 30 days. *(Modified from Ray KK, Cannon CP, McCabe C, et al: Early and late benefits of high-dose atorvastatin in patients with acute coronary syndromes: Results from the PROVE IT–TIMI 22 Trial. J Am Coll Cardiol 46:1405, 2005.)*

Intensive statin therapy should start at least at the time of hospital discharge, according to the ACC/AHA guidelines. However, benefit of intensive statin therapy before PCI has been seen in five small- to moderately-sized randomized trials,[138] suggesting that high-dose statin therapy should be started at the time of admission.

Summary: Acute Management of UA/NSTEMI

The evaluation of patients with UA/NSTEMI begins with the clinical examination, electrocardiography, and measurement of cardiac biomarkers to assess (1) the likelihood of CAD and (2) the risk of death or recurrent cardiac events. Patients with a low likelihood of having UA/NSTEMI should undergo a "diagnostic pathway" evaluation via serial electrocardiograms, cardiac biomarkers, and early stress testing to evaluate for CAD. This can be accomplished frequently in an observation/chest pain unit or in association with a hospital emergency department. Patients with a clinical history strongly consistent with UA/NSTEMI should undergo risk stratification by a clinical scoring system, such as the TIMI or GRACE risk scores,[43,44] as well as troponin measurement. Those at low risk should be treated with antiplatelet therapy with aspirin and clopidogrel as well as an anticoagulant, nitrates, and beta blockers. An early conservative strategy is adequate in low-risk patients. For moderate- to high-risk patients (e.g., those with positive troponin, ST-segment changes, TIMI risk score >3), the aforementioned medications should be used, and an early invasive strategy is preferred. GP IIb/IIIa inhibition should be added for patients who are unstable or at the time of PCI. Clopidogrel should be begun on admission. For patients in whom prasugrel is intended, omitting a loading dose of clopidogrel at the time of presentation would be warranted.

Long-Term Secondary Prevention After UA/NSTEMI (see Chap. 49)

The time of hospital discharge after UA/NSTEMI affords a "teachable moment" for the patient,[139] when the physician and staff can review and optimize the medical regimen for long-term treatment. Risk factor modification is critical and includes discussions with the patient (as appropriate to the risk factors) on the importance of smoking cessation, achieving optimal weight, exercise, following appropriate diet, good blood pressure control, control of hyperglycemia in diabetic patients, and intensive statin therapy (**Table 56-5**).

	Odds ratio (95% CI)	Odds reduction	Event rates No./Total (%) High dose	Event rates No./Total (%) Std dose
PROVE IT-TIMI 22		−17%	147/2099 (7.0)	172/2063 (8.3)
A-to-Z		−15%	205/2265 (9.1)	235/2232 (10.5)
TNT		−21%	334/4995 (6.7)	418/5006 (8.3)
IDEAL		−12%	411/4439 (9.3)	463/4449 (10.4)
Total	OR, 0.84; 95% CI, 0.77–0.91; P=0.00003	−16%	1097/13798 (8.0)	1288/13750 (9.4)

.66 1 1.5
High-dose better High-dose worse

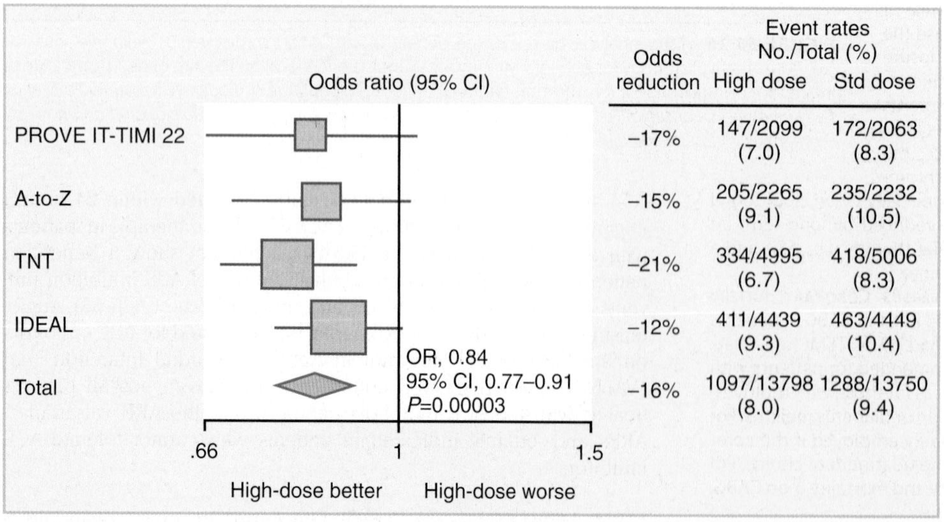

FIGURE 56-18 Meta-analysis of trials of intensive versus standard statin therapy, showing a highly significant 16% reduction in the risk of coronary death or myocardial infarction ($P < 0.0001$). A-to-Z = Aggrastat-to-Zocor trial; IDEAL = Incremental Decrease in End Points Through Aggressive Lipid-Lowering trial; PROVE IT–TIMI 22 = Pravastatin or Atorvastatin Evaluation and Infection Therapy–Thrombolysis In Myocardial Infarction 22 trial; TNT = Treating to New Targets trial. *(Reproduced from Cannon CP, Steinberg BA, Murphy SA, et al: Meta-analysis of cardiovascular outcomes trials comparing intensive versus moderate statin therapy. J Am Coll Cardiol 48:438, 2006.)*

Six classes of therapies that have improved outcomes after UA/NSTEMI in large randomized trials should be instituted for long-term treatment. Each may contribute to long-term clinical stability in different ways:

1. Intensive LDL-C reduction with high-dose statins.[134,137,140]
2. ACE inhibitors or ARBs are recommended for long-term treatment that may facilitate plaque stabilization or retard progression of atherosclerosis.
3. Beta blockers are indicated for anti-ischemic therapy and may help decrease triggers for MI during follow-up.
4. For antiplatelet therapy, the combination of low-dose aspirin and a $P2Y_{12}$ inhibitor for at least a year confers clinical benefit

TABLE 56-5 Cardiac Checklist for UA/NSTEMI*

CARDIAC CHECKLIST—ADMISSION		CARDIAC CHECKLIST—DISCHARGE	
Admit Date: ________		**Admit Date:** ________	
Patient Name: ________ (First Name) (Middle Initial) (Last Name)		**Patient Name:** ________ (First Name) (Middle Initial) (Last Name)	
Brief History: ________		**Brief History:** ________	
Medications:		**Medications:**	
1. Aspirin	□	1. Aspirin (low dose)	□
2. Clopidogrel or ticagrelor	□	2. Clopidogrel/prasugrel/ticagrelor	□
3. Heparin, LMWH, or other anticoagulant	□	3. Statin (high dose)	□
4. GP IIb/IIIa inhibitor	□	4. ACE inhibitor	□
5. Beta blocker	□	5. Beta blocker	□
6. Nitrate	□	**Interventions:**	
7. ACE inhibitor	□	6. LDL controlled to goal	□
Interventions:		7. Blood pressure controlled	□
8. Cath/revascularization for recurrent ischemia or in intermediate- and high-risk patients	□	8. Diabetes controlled	□
Risk Factor Modification:		9. Smoking cessation counseling (if applicable)	□
9. Cholesterol—check and treat as needed	□	10. Cardiac rehabilitation/lifestyle change	□
10. Treat other risk factors (e.g., smoking)	□		

*These simple lists serve as reminders of guideline-recommended therapies, such as aspirin, clopidogrel, heparin, or LMWH. This "cardiac checklist" could be used in two ways: the physician could keep a copy on a small index card in a pocket or in a personal digital assistant (PDA) and run down the list when writing admission orders for patients, or it could be used in developing standard orders for UA/NSTEMI—either printed order sheets or computerized orders. See text for details of specific indications and contraindications for medications.
ACE = angiotensin-converting enzyme; cath = catheterization; GP = glycoprotein; LDL = low-density lipoprotein; LMWH = low-molecular-weight heparin.

by preventing or decreasing the severity of any thrombosis that occurs if a plaque ruptures and reducing thrombosis if a stent has been implanted. Longer duration of dual antiplatelet therapy may be appropriate in patients at high risk of recurrent ischemic events and is generally recommended in patients with drug-eluting stents.

5. Smoking cessation programs involving counseling, the use of nicotine patches or gum, the anxiolytic agent bupropion, or the acetylcholine partial agonist varenicline should be strongly encouraged.[141]
6. Exercise-based cardiac rehabilitation programs coupled with education on weight control, diet, and drug adherence are also advisable.

Thus, a multifactorial approach to long-term medical therapy can address the various components of atherothrombosis.

REGISTRY EXPERIENCE. A major problem identified in clinical practice is that a large proportion of patients fail to receive guideline-recommended therapies after UA/NSTEMI. Many large registries, in the United States and worldwide, have documented that 10% to 15% of patients do not receive any antithrombotic therapy and 40% to 50% of medically managed patients do not receive clopidogrel, despite Class I recommendations for their use.[142,143] These data suggest that in addition to guideline development and education, there is a need for specific tools to improve implementation of guideline recommendations on a patient-by-patient basis. Most important, lack of adherence to the guidelines has associated with adverse outcomes.[144] Paradoxically, patients at high risk for recurrent events (the elderly and patients with diabetes mellitus, renal dysfunction, and heart failure) were less likely than lower-risk patients to receive guideline-recommended therapies.[145]

CRITICAL PATHWAYS AND QUALITY IMPROVEMENT. Critical pathways and the process of Continuous Quality Improvement (CQI) are means of trying to improve care[146,147] (see Chap. 5). Critical pathways are standardized protocols for the management of specific diseases (e.g., ACS) that aim to optimize and streamline patient care.[148] In general, these pathways involve standardized or computerized order sets or simple pocket cards, reminders, or checklists of the appropriate therapies. The process of pathway implementation generally involves physician and nursing education, including presentations at grand rounds, "in-services," and other educational meetings throughout the institution to the relevant caregivers. Another key part of an overall CQI effort is to monitor performance—that is, actual use of guideline-recommended therapies.[148]

CRITICAL PATHWAYS IMPROVE OUTCOMES. There are now several well-conducted studies showing that the use of critical pathways can improve the quality of care. The American Heart Association's Get With The Guidelines (GWTG) program aims to support and facilitate improvement in the quality of care of patients with cardiovascular disease. The GWTG-CAD program includes learning sessions, didactic sessions, best-practice sharing, interactive workshops, post-meeting follow-up, and a web-based Patient Management Tool, which provides the opportunity for concurrent data collection, ongoing real-time feedback of hospital data, and clinical decision support to enable rapid cycle improvement. GWTG-CAD also has a performance recognition program.[147] Participation in GWTG-CAD improves the use of therapies such as ASA, beta blockers, ACE inhibitors, and statins at the time of hospital discharge.

The American College of Cardiology–sponsored Guidelines Applied in Practice (GAP) program has also provided important multicenter data supporting the efficacy of critical pathways.[149] Better compliance with the use of guideline-recommended therapies is associated with lower mortality (**Fig. 56-19**). In the GAP program, patients in whom the clinical records showed that the pathways and tools had been used had the highest rates of treatment with the recommended therapies and better outcomes.[149]

Prinzmetal Variant Angina

In 1959, Prinzmetal and colleagues described a syndrome of ischemic pain that occurred at rest, accompanied by ST-segment elevation.[150] This syndrome, known as Prinzmetal variant angina (PVA), may be associated with acute MI, ventricular tachycardia or fibrillation, and sudden cardiac death. The incidence of PVA has always been greater in Japan than in Western countries, but across the world, the incidence appears to have fallen markedly during the past three decades; this

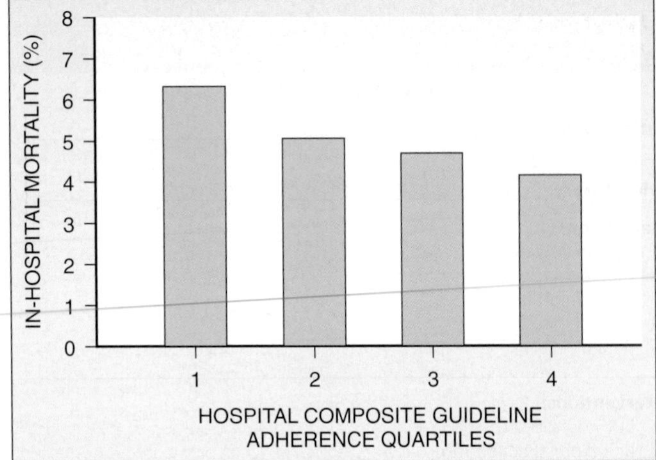

FIGURE 56-19 Association between hospital guideline adherence and in-hospital mortality. Hospitals in quartile 1 had the poorest adherence. *(Modified with permission from Peterson ED, Roe MT, Mulgund J, et al: Association between hospital process performance and outcomes among patients with acute coronary syndromes. JAMA 295:1912, 2006.)*

decline may be related, in part, to the more aggressive use of calcium antagonists for hypertension.[151]

Mechanisms

The original hypothesis of Prinzmetal and colleagues was that variant angina results from transient increases in coronary vasomotor tone or vasospasm. The focal vasospasm in PVA should not be confused with the generalized vasoconstriction of both the large and small coronary vessels, a normal response to stimuli such as cold exposure; the latter response, although widespread in the coronary vascular bed, is much less intense.

The precise mechanisms responsible for PVA have not been established, but a reduction in nitric oxide production by the coronary arterial endothelium or an imbalance between endothelium-derived relaxing and contracting factors may prevail.[152] Enhanced phospholipase C (PLC) activity has also been documented. Because PLC (through activation of the inositol triphosphate pathway) mobilizes Ca^{2+} from intracellular stores, it may enhance contraction of smooth muscle cells.[153] An inflammatory cause is supported by the finding of elevated levels of serum hs-CRP in many patients.[154] Polymorphisms of the $alpha_2$ presynaptic and the postsynaptic $beta_2$ receptor may also associate with PVA.[155]

Histologic findings in patients with PVA who underwent coronary atherectomy suggest that repetitive coronary vasospasm may provoke vascular injury and lead to the formation of neointimal hyperplasia at the initial site of spasm, which in turn caused rapid progression of coronary stenosis in some patients. Imaging with iodine-123–labeled metaiodobenzylguanidine (^{123}I-MIBG) has demonstrated regional myocardial sympathetic denervation in the area of distribution of the vessel in which vasospasm developed.[156]

Clinical and Laboratory Findings

Patients with PVA tend to be younger than patients with chronic stable angina or unstable angina secondary to coronary atherosclerosis, and many do not exhibit classic coronary risk factors, except that they are often heavy cigarette smokers. The anginal pain is often extremely severe and may be accompanied by syncope related to atrioventricular block, asystole, or ventricular tachyarrhythmias.[156]

Attacks of PVA tend to cluster between midnight and 8 AM,[157] and they sometimes occur in clusters of two or three within 30 to 60 minutes. Although exercise capacity is generally well preserved in patients with PVA, some patients experience typical pain and ST-segment elevations not only at rest but also during or after exertion. Patients with the combination of PVA and severe fixed coronary obstruction may have a combination of exertion-induced angina with ST-segment depression and episodes of angina at rest with ST-segment elevation. Some patients appear to have a distinct relation between emotional distress and episodes of coronary vasospasm, in agreement with studies suggesting that sympathovagal imbalance may precipitate spasm in patients with PVA. In rare cases, PVA develops after coronary artery bypass surgery and may occur adjacent to a drug-eluting stent[158]; on occasion, PVA appears to be a manifestation of a generalized vasospastic disorder associated with migraine or Raynaud phenomenon. PVA can also occur in association with ASA-induced asthma and administration of 5-fluorouracil and cyclophosphamide.

ELECTROCARDIOGRAPHY. The key to the diagnosis of PVA lies in the detection of episodic ST-segment elevation often accompanied by severe chest pain, usually occurring at rest (**Fig. 56-20**). Many patients also exhibit multiple episodes of asymptomatic (silent) ST-segment elevation. ST-segment deviations may be present in any leads, depending on the artery involved. Serious arrhythmias can sometimes be precipitated by the cold pressor test. Transient conduction disturbances may occur during episodes of ischemia. Myocardial cell damage may occur in the absence of persistent electrocardiographic changes in patients with prolonged attacks of PVA. STEMI caused by coronary artery spasm in the absence of angiographically demonstrable obstructive CAD has been well documented.[159]

Exercise testing in patients with PVA can yield variable responses. Approximately equal numbers of patients show ST-segment depression, no change, or ST-segment elevation. These changes reflect the presence of underlying fixed CAD in some patients, the absence of significant lesions in others, and the provocation of spasm by exercise in the remainder. Ambulatory electrocardiographic monitoring or the use of a telephone transmitter may be helpful in capturing ST-segment elevations during symptomatic episodes.

Serious arrhythmias including sinus node dysfunction causing asystole and syncope, complete atrioventricular block, ventricular tachycardia, ventricular fibrillation, and sudden cardiac death have been reported.[160,161] Implantation of a pacemaker or an implanted automatic defibrillator may be required.[162]

CORONARY ARTERIOGRAPHY. (see Chap. 21) Spasm of a proximal coronary artery with resultant transmural ischemia and abnormalities in left ventricular function are the diagnostic hallmarks of PVA (see Fig. 56-20). Patients with no or mild fixed coronary obstruction tend to experience a more benign course than patients with PVA and associated severe obstructive lesions.[163] The vasospastic process almost always involves large segments of the epicardial vessels at a single site, but other sites may be involved at different times. The right coronary artery is the most frequent site, followed by the left anterior descending coronary artery. Simultaneous spasm of all three major coronary arteries may mimic three-vessel atherosclerotic disease.[164]

PROVOCATIVE TESTS

ERGONOVINE. Several provocative tests for coronary spasm have been developed. Of these, the ergonovine test is the most sensitive. Ergonovine maleate, an ergot alkaloid, stimulates both alpha-adrenergic and serotonergic receptors, and therefore exerts a direct constrictor effect on vascular smooth muscle and can induce coronary artery spasm.

When it is administered intravenously in bolus doses rising from 0.05 to 0.20 mg, ergonovine provides a sensitive and specific test for provocation of coronary artery spasm. The majority of patients who have a response to ergonovine do so at a dose of less than 0.20 mg. In low doses, and in carefully controlled clinical situations, ergonovine is a relatively safe drug, but prolonged coronary artery spasm precipitated by ergonovine may cause MI. On occasion, conduction disturbances (heart block) or severe tachyarrhythmias develop. Because of these hazards, it is recommended that ergonovine be administered only to patients in whom coronary arteriography has demonstrated normal or nearly normal coronary arteries and in gradually increasing doses, beginning with a very low dose. Intracoronary nitrates and calcium antagonists are usually effective in providing prompt relief from drug-induced spasm. Absolute contraindications to ergonovine testing include pregnancy, severe hypertension, severe left ventricular dysfunction, moderate to severe aortic stenosis, and high-grade left main coronary artery stenosis.

ACETYLCHOLINE. Stimulation of acetylcholine receptors produces a uniform endothelium-dependent dilation of normal coronary arteries but leads to vasoconstriction when endothelial function is impaired. In patients with PVA, intracoronary injections of acetylcholine can induce severe coronary spasm and reproduce the clinical syndrome.[165] This focal spasm should not be confused with the mild diffuse constriction that acetylcholine induces in patients with abnormal coronary endothelium. Acetylcholine is infused during a 1-minute period into a coronary artery in incremental doses of 10, 25, 50, and 100 μg, and doses should be separated by 5-minute intervals.

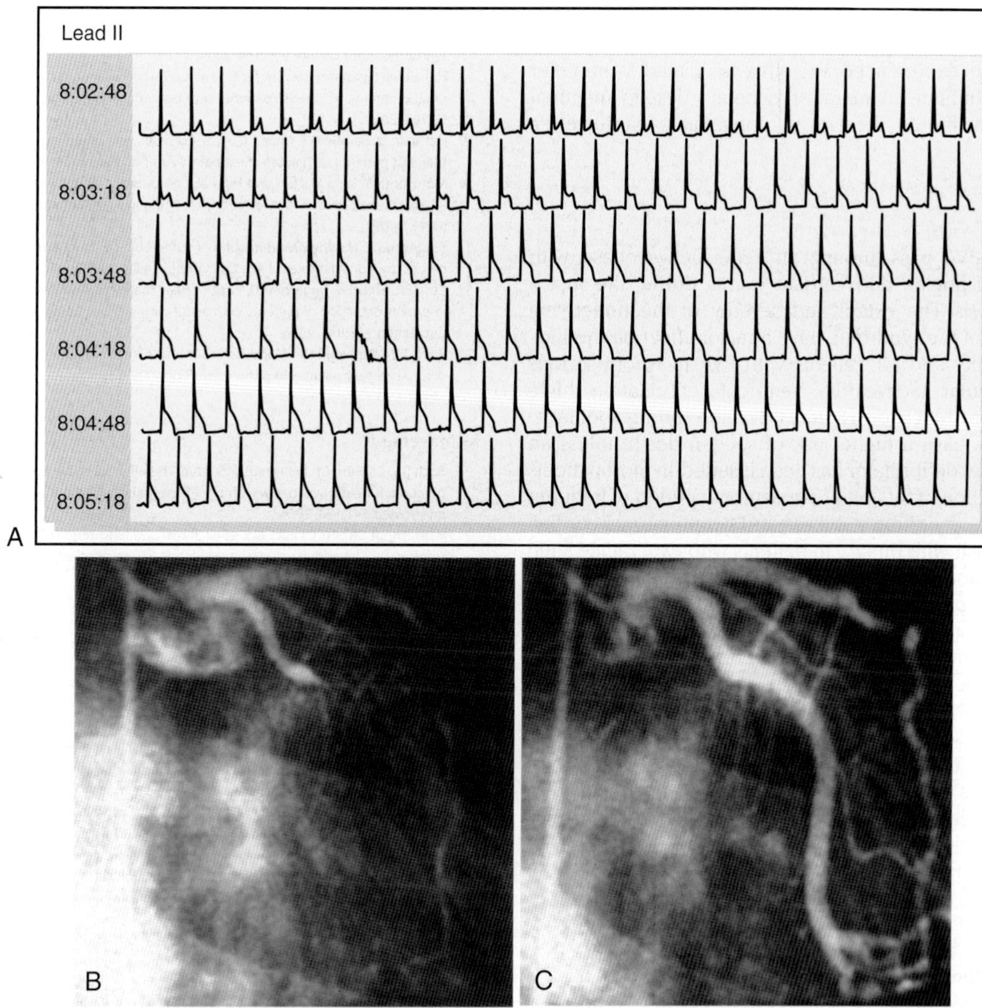

FIGURE 56-20 Continuous electrocardiography in a 39-year-old man with Prinzmetal angina. **A,** During an episode of angina, transient ST-segment elevation (in lead II) was noted on continuous telemetry. **B,** Hyperventilation-induced total occlusion of the proximal left circumflex artery (visible on angiography from the right anterior oblique caudal view). **C,** Spasm that resolved with the administration of intracoronary nitroglycerin and diltiazem. The patient's symptoms were controlled with oral nitrates and calcium channel blockade during a follow-up of 2 years. *(From Chen HSV, Pinto DS: Prinzmetal angina. N Engl J Med 349:e1, 2003.)*

Histamine, dopamine, and serotonin can also induce coronary artery spasm. Exercise, the cold pressor test, and alkalosis induced by hyperventilation[166] can all cause coronary spasm in patients with PVA, but none of these tests is as sensitive as ergonovine or acetylcholine.

Management

Patients with PVA should be urged strongly to discontinue smoking. The mainstay of therapy is a calcium antagonist alone or in combination with a long-acting nitrate. There are several similarities and differences between the optimal management of PVA and that of classic (stable and unstable) angina.

1. Patients with both PVA and classic angina usually respond well to nitrates; sublingual or intravenous nitroglycerin often abolishes attacks of PVA promptly, and long-acting nitrates are useful in preventing attacks. Calcium antagonists have proved extremely effective in preventing the coronary artery spasm of PVA,[167] and they should ordinarily be prescribed in maximally tolerated doses on a long-term basis. Because calcium antagonists act through a mechanism different from that of nitrates, these two classes of drugs may exert additive vasodilatory effects. All first- and second-generation calcium antagonists have similar (approximately 90%) efficacy in producing relief of symptoms, and they also suppress asymptomatic ischemia.
2. Response to beta blockade in patients with PVA is variable.[168,169] Some, particularly those with associated fixed lesions, exhibit a reduction in the frequency of exertion-induced angina caused primarily by augmentation of myocardial oxygen requirements. In others, however, nonselective beta blockers may actually be detrimental because blockade of $beta_2$ receptors, which mediate coronary dilation, allows unopposed alpha receptor–mediated coronary vasoconstriction to occur; in these patients, the duration of episodes of vasospastic angina may be prolonged by beta blockers.
3. Prazosin, a selective alpha-adrenergic receptor blocker, may also have value in the treatment of patients with PVA.[170] Nicorandil, a coronary vasodilator that acts by activating the potassium channel, also appears to be effective.[171] This agent has been approved in Europe but not in the United States.
4. ASA, helpful in unstable angina, may theoretically increase the severity of ischemic episodes in patients with PVA because it inhibits biosynthesis of the naturally occurring coronary vasodilator prostacyclin.
5. PCI and occasionally CABG may be helpful in patients with PVA and discrete, proximal fixed obstructive lesions. However, spasm may develop at a site different from the initial stenosis; therefore, calcium antagonists should be continued for at least 6 months after successful revascularization in patients with PVA. PCI and CABG

are contraindicated in patients with isolated coronary artery spasm without accompanying fixed obstructive disease.

6. Patients who have experienced ischemia-associated ventricular fibrillation who continue to manifest ischemia despite maximal medical treatment should receive an implantable cardioverter-defibrillator.[162,172]

Prognosis

Many patients with PVA pass through an acute, active phase, with frequent episodes of angina and cardiac events during the first 6 months after diagnosis. The extent and severity of the underlying CAD and the tempo of the syndrome have a major effect on the incidence of late mortality and MI. Patients with PVA in whom serious arrhythmias (ventricular tachycardia, ventricular fibrillation, high-degree atrioventricular block, or asystole) develop during spontaneous episodes of pain have a higher risk of sudden death unless an implanted cardioverter-defibrillator has been inserted. In most patients who survive an infarction or the initial 3- to 6-month period of frequent ischemic episodes, the condition stabilizes, and symptoms and cardiac events tend to diminish with time.[173] In patients who experience such remissions, cautious tapering of calcium antagonists may be attempted. In one series, 16% of patients had spontaneous remission 3 months after withdrawal of therapy, 44% continued to have symptoms despite treatment with calcium antagonists and nitrates, and the other 40% were free of angina but receiving treatment. Remission occurred more frequently in patients without significant coronary artery stenoses and in those who stopped smoking.[174]

For reasons that are not clear, some patients, after a relatively quiescent period of months or even years, experience a recrudescence of vasospastic activity with frequent and severe episodes of ischemia. Fortunately, these patients usually respond to re-treatment with calcium antagonists and nitrates.

REFERENCES

Epidemiology and Pathophysiology

1. Lloyd-Jones D, Adams R, Carnethon M, et al: Heart disease and stroke statistics—2009 update: A report from the American Heart Association Statistics Committee and Stroke Statistics Subcommittee. Circulation 119:480, 2009.
2. Anderson JL, Adams CD, Antman EM, et al: ACC/AHA 2007 guidelines for the management of patients with unstable angina/non–ST-elevation myocardial infarction: Executive summary. A report of the American College of Cardiology/American Heart Association Task Force on Practice Guidelines. Circulation 116:803, 2007.
3. Giugliano RP, Braunwald E: The year in non–ST-segment elevation acute coronary syndrome. J Am Coll Cardiol 54:1544, 2009.
4. Braunwald E: Unstable angina: An etiologic approach to management. Circulation 98:2219, 1998.
5. Ong P, Athanasiadis A, Hill S, et al: Coronary artery spasm as a frequent cause of acute coronary syndrome: The CASPAR (Coronary Artery Spasm in Patients with Acute Coronary Syndrome) study. J Am Coll Cardiol 52:523, 2008.
6. Davies MJ: The composition of coronary-artery plaques. N Engl J Med 336:1312, 1997.
7. Hochman JS, Tamis JE, Thompson TD, et al: Sex, clinical presentation, and outcome in patients with acute coronary syndromes. N Engl J Med 341:226, 1999.
8. Khot UN, Khot MB, Bajzer CT, et al: Prevalence of conventional risk factors in patients with coronary heart disease. JAMA 290:898, 2003.
9. Cannon CP, McCabe CH, Stone PH, et al: The electrocardiogram predicts one-year outcome of patients with unstable angina and non–Q wave myocardial infarction: Results of the TIMI III Registry ECG Ancillary Study. J Am Coll Cardiol 30:133, 1997.
10. Scirica BM, Morrow DA, Budaj A, et al: Ischemia detected on continuous electrocardiography following acute coronary syndrome: Observations from the MERLIN-TIMI 36 trial. J Am Coll Cardiol 53:1411, 2009.

Biomarkers

11. Morrow DA, Cannon CP, Rifai N, et al: Ability of minor elevations of troponin I and T to predict benefit from an early invasive strategy in patients with unstable angina and non–ST elevation myocardial infarction: Results from a randomized trial. JAMA 286:2405, 2001.
12. Eggers KM, Lagerqvist B, Venge P, et al: Persistent cardiac troponin I elevation in stabilized patients after an episode of ACS predicts long-term mortality. Circulation 116:1907, 2007.
13. Fleming SM, O'Byrne L, Finn J, et al: False-positive cardiac troponin I in a routine clinical population. Am J Cardiol 89:1212, 2002.
14. Dokainish H, Pillai M, Murphy S, et al: Prognostic implications of elevated troponin in patients with suspected acute coronary syndromes but no epicardial coronary disease. J Am Coll Cardiol 45:19, 2005.
15. Cannon CP, Weintraub WS, Demopoulos LA, et al: Comparison of early invasive and conservative strategies in patients with unstable coronary syndromes treated with the glycoprotein IIb/IIIa inhibitor tirofiban. N Engl J Med 344:1879, 2001.
16. Braunwald E: Unstable angina: A classification. Circulation 80:410, 1989.
17. Karha J, Cannon CP, Murphy S, et al: Safety of stress testing following an acute coronary syndrome. Am J Cardiol 94:1534, 2004.
18. Hollander JE, Chang AM, Shofer F, et al: Coronary computed tomographic angiography for rapid discharge of low-risk patients with potential acute coronary syndromes. Ann Emerg Med 53:295, 2009.
19. Hoffman U, Bamberg F, Chae CU, et al: Coronary computed tomography angiography for early triage of patients with acute chest pain. J Am Coll Cardiol 53:1642, 2009.
20. Motoyama S, Sarai M, Harigaya H, et al: Computed tomographic angiography characteristics of atherosclerotic plaques subsequently resulting in acute coronary syndrome. J Am Coll Cardiol 54:49, 2009.
21. Braunwald E: Noninvasive detection of vulnerable coronary plaques: Locking the barn door before the horse is stolen. J Am Coll Cardiol 54:58, 2009.
22. Cury RC, Shash K, Nagurney JT, et al: Cardiac magnetic resonance with T2-weighted imaging improves detection of patients with acute coronary syndrome in the emergency department. Circulation 118:837, 2008.
23. Zairis MN, Papadaki OA, Manousakis SJ, et al: C-reactive protein and multiple complex coronary artery plaques in patients with primary unstable angina. Atherosclerosis 164:355, 2002.

Management

24. Bach RG, Cannon CP, Weintraub WS, et al: The effect of routine, early invasive management on outcome for elderly patients with non–ST segment elevation acute coronary syndromes. Ann Intern Med 141:186, 2004.
25. Westerhout CM, Fu Y, Lauer MS, et al: Short- and long-term risk stratification in acute coronary syndromes: The added value of quantitative ST-segment depression and multiple biomarkers. J Am Coll Cardiol 48:939, 2006.
26. Kleiman N, Lakkis N, Cannon C, et al: Prospective analysis of creatine kinase muscle-brain fraction and comparison with troponin T to predict cardiac risk and benefit of an invasive strategy in patients with non–ST elevation acute coronary syndromes. J Am Coll Cardiol 40:1044, 2002.
27. Antman EM, Tanasijevic MJ, Thompson B, et al: Cardiac-specific troponin I levels to predict the risk of mortality in patients with acute coronary syndromes. N Engl J Med 335:1342, 1996.
28. Kastrati A, Mehilli J, Neumann FJ, et al: Abciximab in patients with acute coronary syndromes undergoing percutaneous coronary intervention after clopidogrel pretreatment: The ISAR-REACT 2 randomized trial. JAMA 295:1531, 2006.
29. Morrow DA, Rifai N, Antman EM, et al: C-reactive protein is a potent predictor of mortality independently and in combination with troponin T in acute coronary syndromes: A TIMI 11A substudy. J Am Coll Cardiol 31:1460, 1998.
30. Morrow DA, de Lemos JA, Sabatine MS, et al: Clinical relevance of C-reactive protein during follow-up of patients with acute coronary syndromes in the Aggrastat-to-Zocor Trial. Circulation 114:281, 2006.
30a de Lemos JA, Morrow DA, Sabatine MS, et al: Association between plasma levels of monocyte chemoattractant protein-1 and long-term clinical outcomes in patients with acute coronary syndromes. Circulation 107:690, 2003.
31. Ray KK, Morrow DA, Sabatine MS, et al: Long-term prognostic value of neopterin: A novel marker of monocyte activation in patients with acute coronary syndrome. Circulation 115:3071, 2007.
32. Sabatine MS, Morrow DA, Cannon CP, et al: Relationship between baseline white blood cell count and degree of coronary artery disease and mortality in patients with acute coronary syndromes: A TACTICS-TIMI 18 substudy. J Am Coll Cardiol 40:1761, 2002.
33. Baldus S, Heeschen C, Meinertz T, et al: Myeloperoxidase serum levels predict risk in patients with acute coronary syndromes. Circulation 108:1440, 2003.
34. Buffon A, Biasucci LM, Liuzzo G, et al: Widespread coronary inflammation in unstable angina. N Engl J Med 347:5, 2002.
35. de Lemos JA, Morrow DA, Bentley JH, et al: The prognostic value of B-type natriuretic peptide in patients with acute coronary syndromes. N Engl J Med 345:1014, 2001.
36. Omland T, de Lemos JA, Morrow DA, et al: Prognostic value of N-terminal pro-atrial and pro-brain natriuretic peptide in patients with acute coronary syndromes. Am J Cardiol 89:463, 2002.
37. Morrow DA, de Lemos JA, Sabatine MS, et al: Evaluation of B-type natriuretic peptide for risk assessment in unstable angina/non–ST-elevation myocardial infarction: B-type natriuretic peptide and prognosis in TACTICS-TIMI 18. J Am Coll Cardiol 41:1264, 2003.
38. Gibson CM, Pinto DS, Murphy SA, et al: Association of creatinine and creatinine clearance on presentation in acute myocardial infarction with subsequent mortality. J Am Coll Cardiol 42:1535, 2003.
39. Bhadriraju S, Ray KK, DeFranco AC, et al: Association between blood glucose and long-term mortality in patients with acute coronary syndromes in the OPUS-TIMI 16 trial. Am J Cardiol 97:1573, 2006.
40. Ray KK, Cannon CP, Morrow DA, et al: Synergistic relationship between hyperglycemia and inflammation with respect to clinical outcomes in non–ST elevation acute coronary syndromes: Analyses from OPUS-TIMI 16 and TACTICS-TIMI 18. Eur Heart J 28:806, 2007.
41. Mega JL, Morrow DA, de Lemos JA, et al: Thrombus precursor protein and clinical outcomes in patients with acute coronary syndromes. J Am Coll Cardiol 51:2422, 2008.
42. Boersma E, Pieper KS, Steyerberg EW, et al: Predictors of outcome in patients with acute coronary syndromes without persistent ST-segment elevation. Results from an international trial of 9461 patients. Circulation 101:2557, 2000.
43. Antman EM, Cohen M, Bernink PJ, et al: The TIMI risk score for unstable angina/non–ST elevation MI: A method for prognostication and therapeutic decision making. JAMA 284:835, 2000.
44. Granger CB, Goldberg RJ, Dabbous O, et al: Predictors of hospital mortality in the global registry of acute coronary events. Arch Intern Med 163:2345, 2003.
45. Sabatine MS, Morrow DA, de Lemos J, et al: Multimarker approach to risk stratification in non–ST elevation acute coronary syndromes: Simultaneous assessment of troponin I, C-reactive protein, and B-type natriuretic peptide. Circulation 105:1760, 2002.

46. Gottlieb SO, Weisfeldt ML, Ouyang P, et al: Effect of the addition of propranolol to therapy with nifedipine for unstable angina: A randomized, double-blind, placebo-controlled trial. Circulation 73:331, 1986.
47. Subherwal S, Bach RG, Chen AY, et al: Baseline risk of major bleeding in non–ST-segment elevation myocardial infarction: The CRUSADE bleeding score. Circulation 119:1873, 2009.
48. Alexander KP, Chen AY, Roe MT, et al: Excess dosing of antiplatelet and antithrombin agents in the treatment of non–ST-segment elevation acute coronary syndromes. JAMA 294:3108, 2009.
49. ISIS-4 (Fourth International Study of Infarct Survival) Collaborative Group): Randomized factorial trial assessing early oral captopril, oral mononitrate, and intravenous magnesium sulphate in 58,050 patients with suspected acute myocardial infarction. Lancet 345:669, 1995.
50. Yusuf S, Peto R, Lewis J, et al: Beta-blockade during and after myocardial infarction: An overview of the randomized trials. Prog Cardiovasc Dis 27:335, 1985.
51. Chen ZM, Pan HC, Chen YP, et al: Early intravenous then oral metoprolol in 45,852 patients with acute myocardial infarction: Randomised placebo-controlled trial. Lancet 366:1622, 2005.
52. The Multicenter Diltiazem Postinfarction Trial Research Group: The effect of diltiazem on mortality and reinfarction after myocardial infarction. N Engl J Med 319:385, 1998.
53. Cohn JN, Ziesche S, Smith R, et al: Effect of the calcium antagonist felodipine as supplementary vasodilator therapy in patients with chronic heart failure treated with enalapril: V-HeFT III. Circulation 96:856, 1997.
54. Jamerson K, Weber MA, Bakris GL, et al: Benazepril plus amlodipine or hydrochlorothiazide for hypertension in high-risk patients. N Engl J Med 359:2417, 2008.
55. Nissen SE, Tuzcu EM, Libby P, et al: Effect of antihypertensive agents on cardiovascular events in patients with coronary disease and normal blood pressure: The CAMELOT study: A randomized controlled trial. JAMA 292:2217, 2004.
56. Antithrombotic Trialists' Collaboration: Collaborative meta-analysis of randomised trials of antiplatelet therapy for prevention of death, myocardial infarction, and stroke in high risk patients. BMJ 324:71, 2002.
57. Bhatt DL, Bertrand ME, Berger PB, et al: Meta-analysis of randomized and registry comparisons of ticlopidine with clopidogrel after stenting. J Am Coll Cardiol 39:9, 2002.
58. Patrono C, Rocca B: Aspirin, 110 years later. J Thromb Haemost 7(Suppl 1):258, 2009.
59. Frelinger AL 3rd, Furman MI, Linden MD, et al: Residual arachidonic acid–induced platelet activation via an adenosine diphosphate–dependent but cyclooxygenase-1– and cyclooxygenase-2–independent pathway: A 700-patient study of aspirin resistance. Circulation 113:2888, 2006.
60. Eikelboom JW, Hirsh J, Weitz JI, et al: Aspirin-resistant thromboxane biosynthesis and the risk of myocardial infarction, stroke, or cardiovascular death in patients at high risk for cardiovascular events. Circulation 105:1650, 2002.
61. Cattaneo M: New $P2Y_{12}$ blockers. J Thromb Haemost 7(Suppl 1):262, 2009.
62. Clopidogrel in Unstable Angina to Prevent Recurrent Events Trial Investigators: Effects of clopidogrel in addition to aspirin in patients with acute coronary syndromes without ST-segment elevation. N Engl J Med 345:494, 2001.
63. Yusuf S, Mehta SR, Zhao F, et al: Early and late effects of clopidogrel in patients with acute coronary syndromes. Circulation 107:966, 2003.
64. Mehta SR, Yusuf S, Peters RJ, et al: Effects of pretreatment with clopidogrel and aspirin followed by long-term therapy in patients undergoing percutaneous coronary intervention: The PCI-CURE study. Lancet 358:527, 2001.
65. Sabatine MS, Cannon CP, Gibson CM, et al: Effect of clopidogrel pretreatment before percutaneous coronary intervention in patients with ST-elevation myocardial infarction treated with fibrinolytics: The PCI-CLARITY study. JAMA 294:1224, 2005.
66. Smith SC Jr, Feldman TE, Hirshfeld JW Jr, et al: ACC/AHA/SCAI 2005 Guideline Update for Percutaneous Coronary Intervention—Summary Article: A Report of the American College of Cardiology/American Heart Association Task Force on Practice Guidelines (ACC/AHA/SCAI Writing Committee to Update the 2001 Guidelines for Percutaneous Coronary Intervention). J Am Coll Cardiol 47:216, 2006.
67. Fox KAA, Mehta SR, Peters R, et al: Benefits and risks of the combination of clopidogrel and aspirin in patients undergoing surgical revascularization for non–ST-elevation acute coronary syndrome: The Clopidogrel in Unstable angina to prevent Recurrent ischemic Events (CURE) trial. Circulation 110:1202, 2004.
68. Berger JS, Frye CB, Harshaw Q, et al: Impact of clopidogrel in patients with acute coronary syndromes requiring coronary artery bypass surgery: A multicenter analysis. J Am Coll Cardiol 52:1693, 2008.
69. Montalescot G, Sideris G, Meuleman C, et al: A randomized comparison of high clopidogrel loading doses in patients with non–ST-segment elevation acute coronary syndromes: The ALBION (Assessment of the Best Loading Dose of Clopidogrel to Blunt Platelet Activation, Inflammation, and Ongoing Necrosis) trial. J Am Coll Cardiol 48:931, 2006.
70. Patti G, Colonna G, Pasceri V, et al: Randomized trial of high loading dose of clopidogrel for reduction of periprocedural myocardial infarction in patients undergoing coronary intervention: Results from the ARMYDA-2 (Antiplatelet therapy for Reduction of MYocardial Damage during Angioplasty) study. Circulation 111:2099, 2005.
71. OASIS 7. Mehta S, presented at the European Society of Cardiology, Barcelona, 2009.
72. Gurbel PA, Bliden KP, Hayes KM, et al: The relation of dosing to clopidogrel responsiveness and the incidence of high post-treatment platelet aggregation in patients undergoing coronary stenting. J Am Coll Cardiol 45:1392, 2005.
73. Erlinge D, Varenhorst C, Braun OO, et al: Patients with poor responsiveness to thienopyridine treatment or with diabetes have lower levels of circulating active metabolite, but their platelets respond normally to active metabolite added ex vivo. J Am Coll Cardiol 52:1968, 2008.
74. Wiviott SD, Trenk D, Frelinger AL, et al: Prasugrel compared with high loading- and maintenance-dose clopidogrel in patients with planned percutaneous coronary intervention. The Prasugrel in Comparison to Clopidogrel for Inhibition of Platelet Activation and Aggregation–Thrombolysis in Myocardial Infarction 44 trial. Circulation 116:2923, 2007.
75. Cuisset T, Frere C, Quilici J, et al: Relationship between aspirin and clopidogrel responses in acute coronary syndrome and clinical predictors of non response. Thromb Res 123:597, 2009.
76. Matetzky S, Shenkman B, Guetta V, et al: Clopidogrel resistance is associated with increased risk of recurrent atherothrombotic events in patients with acute myocardial infarction. Circulation 109:3171, 2004.
77. Marcucci R, Gori AM, Paniccia R, et al: Cardiovascular death and nonfatal myocardial infarction in acute coronary syndrome patients receiving coronary stenting are predicted by residual platelet reactivity to ADP detected by a point-of-care assay: A 12-month follow-up. Circulation 119:237, 2009.
78. van Werkum JW, Heestermans AA, Zomer AC, et al: Predictors of coronary stent thrombosis: The Dutch Stent Thrombosis Registry. J Am Coll Cardiol 53:1399, 2009.
79. Wiviott SD, Braunwald E, McCabe CH, et al: Prasugrel versus clopidogrel in patients with acute coronary syndromes. N Engl J Med 357:2001, 2007.
80. Han Y, Li Y, Wang S, et al: Cilostazol in addition to aspirin and clopidogrel improves long-term outcomes after percutaneous coronary intervention in patients with acute coronary syndromes: A randomized, controlled study. Am Heart J 157:733, 2009.
81. Mega JL, Close SL, Wiviott SD, et al: Cytochrome p-450 polymorphisms and response to clopidogrel. N Engl J Med 360:354, 2009.
82. Simon T, Verstuyft C, Mary-Krause M et al: Genetic determinants of response to clopidogrel and cardiovascular events. N Engl J Med 360:363, 2009.
83. Collet J-P, Hulot J-S, Pena A, et al: Cytochrome P450 2C19 polymorphism in young patients treated with clopidogrel after myocardial infarction: A cohort study. Lancet 373:309, 2009.
84. Sibbing D, Stegherr J, Latz W, et al: Cytochrome P450 2C19 loss-of-function polymorphism and stent thrombosis following percutaneous coronary intervention. Eur Heart J 30:916, 2009.
85. Trenk D, Hochholzer W, Fromm MF, et al: Cytochrome P450 2C19 681G>A polymorphism and high on-clopidogrel platelet reactivity associated with adverse 1-year clinical outcome of elective percutaneous coronary intervention with drug-eluting or bare-metal stents. J Am Coll Cardiol 51:1925, 2008.
86. Mega JL, Close SL, Wiviott SD, et al: Cytochrome P450 genetic polymorphisms and the response to prasugrel. Relationship to pharmacokinetic, pharmacodynamic, and clinical outcomes. Circulation 119:2553, 2009.
87. Montalescot MM, Wiviott SD, Braunwald E, et al: Prasugrel compared with clopidogrel in patients undergoing percutaneous coronary intervention for ST-elevation myocardial infarction (TRITON-TIMI 38): Double-blind, randomized controlled trial. Lancet 373:723, 2009.
88. Husted S, Emanuelsson H, Heptinstall S, et al: Pharmacodynamics, pharmacokinetics, and safety of the oral reversible $P2Y_{12}$ antagonist AZD6140 with aspirin in patients with atherosclerosis: A double-blind comparison to clopidogrel with aspirin. Eur Heart J 27:1038, 2006.
89. Wallentin L: $P2Y_{12}$ inhibitors: Differences in properties and mechanisms of action and potential consequences for clinical use. Eur Heart J 30:1964, 2009.
90. Storey RF, Husted S, Harrington RA, et al: Inhibition of platelet aggregation by AZD6140, a reversible oral $P2Y_{12}$ receptor antagonist, compared with clopidogrel in patients with acute coronary syndromes. J Am Coll Cardiol 50:1852, 2007.
91. Wallentin L, Becker R, Budaj A, et al: Ticagrelor versus clopidogrel in patients with acute coronary syndromes. N Engl J Med 361:1045, 2009.
92. Boersma E, Harrington RA, Moliterno DJ, et al: Platelet glycoprotein IIb/IIIa inhibitors in acute coronary syndromes: A meta-analysis of all major randomised clinical trials. Lancet 359:189, 2002.
93. Kastrati A, Mehilli J, Neumann FJ, et al: Abciximab in patients with acute coronary syndromes undergoing percutaneous coronary intervention after clopidogrel pretreatment: The ISAR-REACT 2 randomized trial. JAMA 295:1531, 2006.
94. Giugliano RP, White JA, Bode C, et al: Early versus delayed, provisional eptifibatide in acute coronary syndromes. N Engl J Med 360:2176, 2009.
95. Stone GW, Bertrand ME, Moses JW, et al: Routine upstream initiation vs deferred selective use of glycoprotein IIb/IIIa inhibitors in acute coronary syndromes: The ACUITY Timing trial. JAMA 297:591, 2007.
96. Fung AY, Saw J, Starovoytov A, et al: Abbreviated infusion of eptifibatide after successful coronary intervention: The BRIEF-PCI (Brief Infusion of Eptifibatide Following Percutaneous Coronary Intervention) randomized trial. J Am Coll Cardiol 53:837, 2009.
97. Theroux P, Ouimet H, McCans J, et al: Aspirin, heparin or both to treat unstable angina. N Engl J Med 319:1105, 1988.
98. Eikelboom JW, Anand SS, Malmberg K, et al: Unfractionated heparin and low-molecular-weight heparin in acute coronary syndrome without ST elevation: A meta-analysis. Lancet 355:1936, 2000.
99. Rich JD, Maraganore JM, Young E, et al: Heparin resistance in acute coronary syndromes. J Thromb Thrombolysis 23:93, 2007.
100. Warkentin TE, Kelton JG: Temporal aspects of heparin-induced thrombocytopenia. N Engl J Med 344:1286, 2001.
101. Hirsh J, Warkentin TE, Shaughnessy SG, et al: Heparin and low-molecular-weight heparin: Mechanisms of action, pharmacokinetics, dosing, monitoring, efficacy, and safety. Chest 119:64S, 2001.
102. Murphy SA, Gibson CM, Morrow DA, et al: Efficacy and safety of the low-molecular weight heparin enoxaparin compared with unfractionated heparin across the acute coronary syndrome spectrum: A meta-analysis. Eur Heart J 28:2077, 2007.
103. Blazing MA, de Lemos JA, White HD, et al: Safety and efficacy of enoxaparin vs unfractionated heparin in patients with non–ST-segment elevation acute coronary syndromes who receive tirofiban and aspirin: A randomized controlled trial. JAMA 292:55, 2004.
104. Ferguson JJ, Califf RM, Antman EM, et al: Enoxaparin vs unfractionated heparin in high-risk patients with non–ST-segment elevation acute coronary syndromes managed with an intended early invasive strategy: Primary results of the SYNERGY randomized trial. JAMA 292:45, 2004.
105. de Lemos JA, Blazing MA, Wiviott SD, et al: Enoxaparin versus unfractionated heparin in patients treated with tirofiban, aspirin and an early conservative initial management strategy: Results from the A phase of the A-to-Z trial. Eur Heart J 25:1688, 2004.

106. Yusuf S, Mehta SR, Chrolavicius S, et al: Comparison of fondaparinux and enoxaparin in acute coronary syndromes. N Engl J Med 354:1464, 2006.
107. Yusuf S, Mehta SR, Chrolavicius S, et al: Effects of fondaparinux on mortality and reinfarction in patients with acute ST-segment elevation myocardial infarction: The OASIS-6 randomized trial. JAMA 295:1519, 2006.
108. Direct Thrombin Inhibitor Trialists' Collaborative Group: Direct thrombin inhibitors in acute coronary syndromes: Principal results of a meta-analysis based on individual patients' data. Lancet 359:294, 2002.
109. Stone GW, McLaurin BT, Cox DA, et al: Bivalirudin for patients with acute coronary syndromes. N Engl J Med 355:2203, 2006.
110. Kastrati A, Neumann F-J, Mehilli J, et al: Bivalirudin versus unfractionated heparin during percutaneous coronary intervention. N Engl J Med 359:688, 2008.
111. Hurlen M, Abdelnoor M, Smith P, et al: Warfarin, aspirin, or both after myocardial infarction. N Engl J Med 347:969, 2002.
112. van Es RF, Jonker JJC, Verheugt FWA, et al: Aspirin and coumadin after acute coronary syndromes (the ASPECT-2 study): A randomised controlled trial. Lancet 360:109, 2002.
113. Mega J, Braunwald E, Mohanavelu S, et al: Rivaroxaban versus placebo in patients with acute coronary syndromes (ATLAS ACS–TIMI 46): A randomized, double blind, phase II trial. Lancet 374:29, 2009.
114. APPRAISE Steering Committee and Investigators: Apixaban, an oral, direct, selective factor Xa inhibitor, in combination with antiplatelet therapy after acute coronary syndrome: Results of the Apixaban for Prevention of Acute Ischemic and Safety Events (APPRAISE) trial. Circulation 119:2877, 2009.
115. Becker RC, Smyth S: The evolution of platelet-directed pharmacotherapy. J Thromb Haemost 7:266, 2009.
116. Chakalamannil S, Wang Y, Greenlee WJ, et al: Discovery of a novel, orally active himbacine-based thrombin receptor antagonist (SCH 530348) with potent antiplatelet activity. J Med Chem 51:3061, 2008.
117. Smuth SS, Woulfe DS, Weitz CG, et al: G-protein coupled receptors as signaling targets for antiplatelet therapy. Arterioscler Thromb Vasc Biol 29:449, 2009.
118. Becker RC, Moliterno DJ, Jennings LK, et al: Safety and tolerability of SCH 530348 in patients undergoing non-urgent percutaneous coronary intervention: A randomised, double-blind, placebo-controlled phase II study. Lancet 373:919, 2009.
119. Morrow DA, Scirica BM, Fox KA, et al: Evaluation of a novel antiplatelet agent for secondary prevention in patients with a history of atherosclerotic disease: Design and rationale for the Thrombin-Receptor Antagonist in Secondary Prevention of Atherothrombotic Ischemic Events (TRA 2 P)–TIMI 50 trial. Am Heart J 158:335, 2009.
120. O'Donoghue M, Boden WE, Braunwald E, et al: Early invasive vs. conservative treatment strategies in women and men with unstable angina and non–ST-segment elevation myocardial infarction. A meta-analysis. JAMA 300:71, 2008.
121. Bavry AA, Kumbhani DJ, Rassi AN, et al: Benefit of early invasive therapy in acute coronary syndromes: A meta-analysis of contemporary randomized clinical trials. J Am Coll Cardiol 48:1319, 2006.
122. Lagerqvist B, Husted S, Kontny F, et al: 5-Year outcomes in the FRISC-II randomised trial of an invasive versus a non-invasive strategy in non–ST-elevation acute coronary syndrome: A follow-up study. Lancet 368:998, 2006.
123. Mahoney EM, Jurkovitz CT, Chu H, et al: Cost and cost-effectiveness of an early invasive versus conservative strategy for the treatment of unstable angina and non–ST elevation myocardial infarction. JAMA 288:1851, 2002.
124. Fox KA, Poole-Wilson P, Clayton TC, et al: 5-Year outcome of an interventional strategy in non–ST-elevation acute coronary syndrome: The British Heart Foundation RITA 3 randomised trial. Lancet 366:914, 2005.
125. de Winter RJ, Windhausen F, Cornel JH, et al: Early invasive versus selectively invasive management for acute coronary syndromes. N Engl J Med 353:1095, 2005.
126. Bauer T, Koeth O, Junger C, et al: Effect of an invasive strategy on in-hospital outcome in elderly patients with non–ST-elevation myocardial infarction. Eur Heart J 28:2873, 2007.
127. Charytan DM, Wallentin L, Lagerqvist B, et al: Early angiography in patients with chronic kidney disease: A collaborative systematic review. Clin J Am Soc Nephrol 4:1032, 2009.
128. Neumann FJ, Kastrati A, Pogatsa-Murray G, et al: Evaluation of prolonged antithrombotic pretreatment ("cooling-off" strategy) before intervention in patients with unstable coronary syndromes: A randomized controlled trial. JAMA 290:1593, 2003.
129. Mehta SR, Granger CB, Boden WE, et al: Early versus delayed invasive intervention in acute coronary syndromes. N Engl J Med 360:2165, 2009.
130. Pfeffer MA, McMurray JJ, Velazquez EJ, et al: Valsartan, captopril, or both in myocardial infarction complicated by heart failure, left ventricular dysfunction, or both. N Engl J Med 349:1893, 2003.
131. Heart Protection Study Collaborative Group: MRC/BHF Heart Protection Study of cholesterol lowering with simvastatin in 20,536 high-risk individuals: A randomised placebo controlled trial. Lancet 360:7, 2002.
132. Tonkin AM, Colquhoun D, Emberson J, et al: Effects of pravastatin in 3260 patients with unstable angina: Results from the LIPID study. Lancet 356:1871, 2000.
133. Hulten E, Jackson JL, Douglas K, et al: The effect of early, intensive statin therapy on acute coronary syndrome: A meta-analysis of randomized controlled trials. Arch Intern Med 166:1814, 2006.
134. Cannon CP, Braunwald E, McCabe CH, et al: Intensive versus moderate lipid lowering with statins after acute coronary syndromes. N Engl J Med 350:1495, 2004.
135. Ray KK, Cannon CP, McCabe C, et al: Early and late benefits of high-dose atorvastatin in patients with acute coronary syndromes: Results from the PROVE IT–TIMI 22 Trial. J Am Coll Cardiol 46:1405, 2005.
136. Grundy SM, Cleeman JI, Merz CNB, et al: Implications of recent clinical trials for the National Cholesterol Education Program Adult Treatment Panel III Guidelines. Circulation 110:227, 2004.
137. Cannon CP, Steinberg BA, Murphy SA, et al: Meta-analysis of cardiovascular outcomes trials comparing intensive versus moderate statin therapy. J Am Coll Cardiol 48:438, 2006.
138. Di Sciascio G, Patti G, Pasceri V, et al: Efficacy of atorvastatin reload in patients on chronic statin therapy undergoing percutaneous coronary intervention: Results of the ARMYDA-RECAPTURE (Atorvastatin for Reduction of Myocardial Damage During Angioplasty) randomized trial. J Am Coll Cardiol 54:558, 2009.
139. Fonarow GC: In-hospital initiation of statins: Taking advantage of the "teachable moment." Cleve Clin J Med 70:502, 504, 2003.
140. Baigent C, Keech A, Kearney PM, et al: Efficacy and safety of cholesterol-lowering treatment: Prospective meta-analysis of data from 90,056 participants in 14 randomised trials of statins. Lancet 366:1267, 2005.
141. Tonstad S, Tonnesen P, Hajek P, et al: Effect of maintenance therapy with varenicline on smoking cessation: A randomized controlled trial. JAMA 296:64, 2006.
142. Fox KA, Steg PG, Eagle KA, et al: Decline in rates of death and heart failure in acute coronary syndromes, 1999-2006. JAMA 297:1892, 2007.
143. Tricoci P, Roe MT, Mulgund J, et al: Clopidogrel to treat patients with non–ST-segment elevation acute coronary syndromes after hospital discharge. Arch Intern Med 166:806, 2006.
144. Peterson ED, Roe MT, Mulgund J, et al: Association between hospital process performance and outcomes among patients with acute coronary syndromes. JAMA 295:1912, 2006.
145. Roe MT, Peterson ED, Newby LK, et al: The influence of risk status on guideline adherence for patients with non–ST-segment elevation acute coronary syndromes. Am Heart J 151:1205, 2006.
146. Cannon CP, O'Gara PT: Goals, design and implementation of critical pathways in cardiology. In Cannon CP, O'Gara PT (eds): Critical Pathways in Cardiology. Philadelphia, Lippincott Williams & Wilkins, 2001, pp 3-6.
147. Califf RM, Peterson ED, Gibbons RJ, et al: Integrating quality into the cycle of therapeutic development. J Am Coll Cardiol 40:1895, 2002.
148. Cannon CP, Hand MH, Bahr R, et al: Critical pathways for management of patients with acute coronary syndromes: An assessment by the National Heart Attack Alert Program. Am Heart J 143:777, 2002.
149. Eagle KA, Montoye CK, Riba AL, et al: Guideline-based standardized care is associated with substantially lower mortality in Medicare patients with acute myocardial infarction: The American College of Cardiology's Guidelines Applied in Practice (GAP) Projects in Michigan. J Am Coll Cardiol 46:1242, 2005.

Prinzmetal Variant Angina

150. Prinzmetal M, Kennamer R, Merliss R, et al: A variant form of angina pectoris. Am J Med 27:375, 1959.
151. Sueda S, Kohno H, Fukuda H, Uraoka T: Did the widespread use of long-acting calcium antagonists decrease the occurrence of variant angina? Chest 124:2074, 2003.
152. Mayer S, Hillis LD: Prinzmetal's variant angina. Clin Cardiol 21:243, 1998.
153. Okumura K, Osanai T, Kosugi T, et al: Enhanced phospholipase C activity in the cultured skin fibroblast obtained from patients with coronary spastic angina: Possible role for enhanced vasoconstrictor response. J Am Coll Cardiol 36:1847, 2000.
154. Hung MJ, Cherng WJ, Yang NI, et al: Relation of high-sensitivity C-reactive protein level with coronary vasospastic angina pectoris in patients without hemodynamically significant coronary artery disease. Am J Cardiol 96:1484, 2005.
155. Park JS, Zhang SY, Jo SH, et al: Common adrenergic receptor polymorphisms as novel risk factors for vasospastic angina. Am Heart J 151:864, 2006.
156. Sakata K, Miura F, Sugino H, et al: Assessment of regional sympathetic nerve activity in vasospastic angina: Analysis of iodine 123–labeled metaiodobenzylguanidine scintigraphy. Am Heart J 133:484, 1997.
157. Kawano H, Motoyama T, Yasue H, et al: Endothelial function fluctuates with diurnal variation in the frequency of ischemic episodes in patients with variant angina. J Am Coll Cardiol 40:266, 2002.
158. Abe M, Yoshida A, Otsuka Y: Intractable Prinzmetal's angina three months after implantation of sirolimus-eluting stent. J Invasive Cardiol 20:E306, 2008.
159. Lip GY, Gupta J, Khan MM, Singh SP: Recurrent myocardial infarction with angina and normal coronary arteries. Int J Cardiol 51:65, 1995.
160. Ledakowicz-Polak A, Ptaszynski P, Polak L, Zielinska M: Prinzmetal's variant angina associated with severe heart rhythm disturbances and syncope: A therapeutic dilemma. Cardiol J 16:269, 2009.
161. Hung M-J, Cheng CW, Yang NI, et al: Coronary vasospasm–induced acute coronary syndrome complicated by life-threatening cardia arrhythmias in patients without hemodynamically significant coronary artery disease. Int J Cardiol 117:37, 2007.
162. Meisel SR, Mazur A, Chetboun I, et al: Usefulness of implantable cardioverter-defibrillators in refractory variant angina pectoris complicated by ventricular fibrillation in patients with angiographically normal coronary arteries. Am J Cardiol 89:1114, 2002.
163. Crea F: Variant angina in patients without obstructive coronary atherosclerosis: A benign form of spasm. Eur Heart J 17:980, 1996.
164. Ahooja V, Thetai D: Multivessel coronary vasospasm mimicking triple-vessel obstructive coronary artery disease. J Invasive Cardiol 19:E178, 2007.
165. Hirano Y, Uehara H, Nakamura H, et al: Diagnosis of vasospastic angina: Comparison of hyperventilation and cold-pressor stress echocardiography, hyperventilation and cold-pressor stress coronary angiography, and coronary angiography with intracoronary injection of acetylcholine. Int J Cardiol 116:331, 2007.
166. Nakao K, Ohgushi M, Yoshimura M, et al: Hyperventilation as a specific test for diagnosis of coronary artery spasm. Am J Cardiol 80:545, 1997.
167. Antman E, Muller J, Goldberg S, et al: Nifedipine therapy for coronary artery spasm. Experience in 127 patients. N Engl J Med 302:1269, 1980.
168. De Cesare N, Cozzi S, Apostolo A, et al: Facilitation of coronary spasm by propranolol in Prinzmetal's angina: Fact or unproven extrapolation? Coron Artery Dis 5:323, 1994.
169. Petrov D, Sardowski S, Gesheva M: "Silent" Prinzmetal's ST elevation related to atenolol overdose. J Emerg Med 33:123, 2007.
170. Tzivoni D, Keren A, Benhorin J, et al: Prazosin therapy for refractory variant angina. Am Heart J 105:262, 1983.

171. Kaski JC: Management of vasospastic angina—role of nicorandil. Cardiovasc Drugs Ther 9(Suppl 2):221, 1995.
172. Al-Sayegh A, Shukkur AM, Akbar M: Automatic implantable cardioverter defibrillator for the treatment of ventricular fibrillation following coronary artery spasm: A case report. Angiology 58:122, 2007.
173. Tashiro H, Shimokawa H, Koyanagi S, Takeshita A: Clinical characteristics of patients with spontaneous remission of variant angina. Jpn Circ J 57:117, 1993.
174. Bory M, Pierron F, Panagides D, et al: Coronary artery spasm in patients with normal or near normal coronary arteries. Long-term follow-up of 277 patients. Eur Heart J 17:1015, 1996.

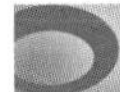

GUIDELINES Christopher P. Cannon and Eugene Braunwald

Unstable Angina and Non–ST Elevation Myocardial Infarction

American College of Cardiology/American Heart Association (ACC/AHA) guidelines for the management of unstable angina and non–ST elevation myocardial infarction (UA/NSTEMI) were published in 2007,[1] presenting updates from prior versions.

Recommendations made in these guidelines pertaining to the initial evaluation of the patient with acute chest pain are included in the text of Chap. 53. For other recommendations relevant to this topic in guidelines for the use of percutaneous coronary interventions (PCI), see Chap. 58.

Like other ACC/AHA guidelines, these use the standard ACC/AHA classification system for indications:

Class I: conditions for which there is evidence and/or general agreement that the treatment is useful and effective.

Class II: conditions for which there is conflicting evidence and/or a divergence of opinion about the usefulness or efficacy of performing the treatment.

Class IIa: weight of evidence or opinion is in favor of usefulness or efficacy.

Class IIb: usefulness or efficacy is less well established by evidence or opinion.

Class III: conditions for which there is evidence and/or general agreement that the treatment is not useful or effective, and in some cases may be harmful.

Three levels are used to rate the evidence on which recommendations have been based. Level A recommendations are derived from data from multiple randomized clinical trials; level B recommendations are derived from a single randomized trial or nonrandomized studies; and level C recommendations are based on the consensus opinion of experts.

EARLY RISK STRATIFICATION AND MANAGEMENT

The initial evaluation of patients with UA/NSTEMI involves risk stratification, which the guidelines term an "integral prerequisite to decision making." This process involves two related but actually separate decision trees. The first, a diagnostic evaluation, estimates the likelihood that obstructive coronary artery disease is the cause of the presenting symptoms and asks, Does this patient have symptoms due to acute ischemia from obstructive coronary artery disease? For this process, the guidelines offer a table of characteristics that portend a high, intermediate, or low likelihood that the patient's presentation is due to ischemia (**Table 56G-1**). For patients of low and sometimes intermediate probability, a diagnostic pathway is provided to determine rapidly if the patient does or does not have an acute coronary syndrome (**Fig. 56G-1**).

The second part of stratification assesses the risk that a patient with UA/NSTEMI has for myocardial infarction or death during the next few weeks. Factors associated with an increased risk are listed in **Table 56G-2**. The guideline notes that risk stratification is useful in (1) selection of the site of care (coronary care unit, monitored step-down unit, or outpatient setting) and (2) selection of therapy, including platelet glycoprotein (GP) IIb/IIIa inhibitors and an invasive versus conservative management strategy.

HOSPITAL CARE

The guidelines recommend that patients admitted for acute coronary syndromes with continuing discomfort or hemodynamic instability, or both, be hospitalized for at least 24 hours in a coronary care unit characterized by a nurse-to-patient ratio sufficient to provide continuous rhythm monitoring and rapid resuscitation and defibrillation should it be necessary. Patients who do not have continuing discomfort or hemodynamic instability can be admitted to a step-down unit.

The 2007 guidelines recommend that the second step after risk stratification is to choose a management strategy (**Table 56G-3**), and then to proceed to the choice of antithrombotic therapy, because choices differ slightly on the basis of which strategy is followed.

TABLE 56G-1 Likelihood That Signs and Symptoms Represent an Acute Coronary Syndrome Secondary to Coronary Artery Disease

FEATURE	HIGH LIKELIHOOD	INTERMEDIATE LIKELIHOOD	LOW LIKELIHOOD
	Any of the Following:	***Absence of High-Likelihood Features and Presence of Any of the Following:***	***Absence of High- or Intermediate-Likelihood Features But May Have:***
History	Chest or left arm pain or discomfort as chief symptom reproducing prior documented angina Known history of CAD, including MI	Chest or left arm pain or discomfort as chief symptom Age >70 years Male sex Diabetes mellitus	Probable ischemic symptoms in absence of any of the intermediate-likelihood characteristics Recent cocaine use
Examination	Transient MR murmur, hypotension, diaphoresis, pulmonary edema, or rales	Extracardiac vascular disease	Chest discomfort reproduced by palpation
ECG	New, or presumably new, transient ST-segment deviation (1 mm or greater) or T wave inversion in multiple precordial leads	Fixed Q waves ST depression 0.5 to 1 mm or T wave inversion greater than 1 mm	T wave flattening or inversion less than 1 mm in leads with dominant R waves Normal ECG
Cardiac markers	Elevated cardiac TnI, TnT, or CK-MB	Normal	Normal

CAD = coronary artery disease; CK-MB = MB fraction of creatine kinase; ECG = electrocardiogram; MI = myocardial infarction; MR = mitral regurgitation; TnI = troponin I; TnT = troponin T.
From Anderson JL, Adams CD, Antman EM, et al: ACC/AHA 2007 guidelines for the management of patients with unstable angina/non–ST-elevation myocardial infarction: A report of the American College of Cardiology/American Heart Association Task Force on Practice Guidelines (Writing Committee to Revise the 2002 Guidelines for the Management of Patients With Unstable Angina/Non–ST-Elevation Myocardial Infarction) developed in collaboration with the American College of Emergency Physicians, the Society for Cardiovascular Angiography and Interventions, and the Society of Thoracic Surgeons endorsed by the American Association of Cardiovascular and Pulmonary Rehabilitation and the Society for Academic Emergency Medicine. J Am Coll Cardiol 50:e1, 2007.

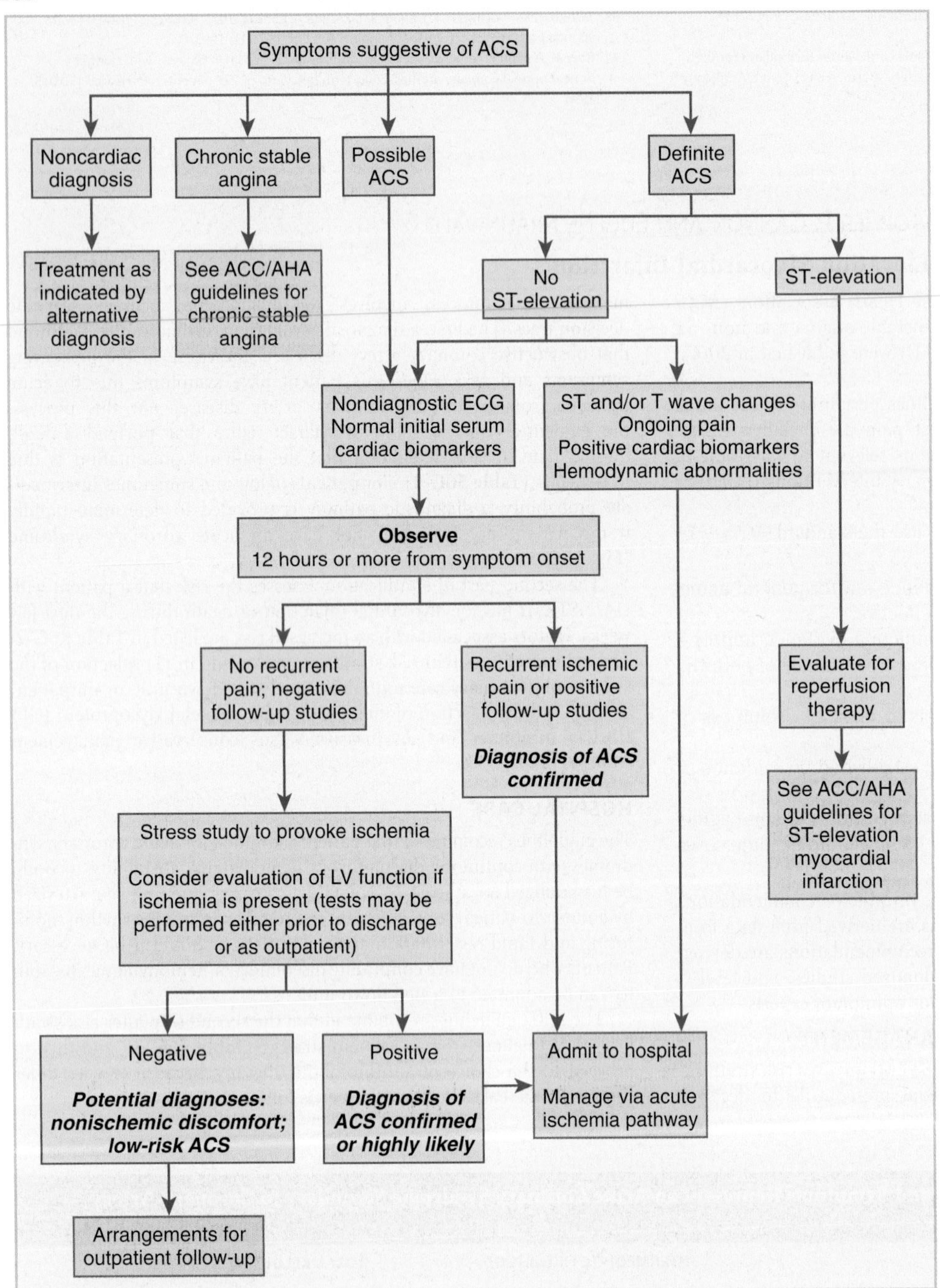

FIGURE 56G-1 ACC/AHA guideline algorithm for acute coronary syndrome (ACS).

An early invasive strategy involves prompt coronary angiography (within approximately 48 hours) followed by revascularization if the anatomy is appropriate. This strategy is recommended for patients with high-risk features as outlined in Tables 56G-2 and 56G-3 and **Figure 56G-2**. In contrast, an early conservative strategy, in which patients are stabilized with medical therapy and angiography is performed only if patients have recurrent symptoms or ischemia, heart failure, or serious arrhythmias, is generally recommended for low-risk patients. As noted in **Figure 56G-3**, patients managed according to the early conservative strategy should undergo an assessment of left ventricular function and a stress test; they should also undergo angiography if they have an ejection fraction below 40% or if they have an intermediate- or high-risk exercise test result. For low-risk women, the 2007 guidelines give a Class I recommendation for an early conservative approach.

Anti-ischemic medical therapy should include nitrates and, in the absence of contraindications, beta blockers (**Table 56G-4**). The 2007 ACC/AHA guidelines emphasize, however, that oral (not intravenous) beta blocker therapy should be initiated within the first 24 hours in patients who do not have one or more of the following: signs of heart failure, evidence of a low-output state, increased risk for cardiogenic shock, or other relative contraindications to beta blockade (PR interval greater than 0.24 second, second- or third-degree heart block, active asthma, or reactive airway disease). If a contraindication to beta blocker therapy exists, patients with recurrent ischemia can be treated with a nondihydropyridine calcium antagonist (e.g., verapamil or diltiazem). Morphine sulfate should be used for patients whose condition is not controlled with nitrates or for patients who have pulmonary congestion, severe agitation, or both. An angiotensin-converting enzyme (ACE) inhibitor should be started if hypertension persists despite anti-ischemic therapy or if patients have left ventricular systolic dysfunction or diabetes. A new recommendation in the 2007 guidelines is that because of the increased risks of mortality, reinfarction, hypertension, heart failure, and myocardial rupture associated with their use, nonsteroidal anti-inflammatory drugs, except for aspirin, whether nonselective or cyclooxygenase 2–selective agents, should be discontinued at the time a patient presents with UA/NSTEMI.

For both treatment strategies, aspirin is indicated, at an initial dose of 160 to 325 mg daily. In addition, the guidelines note that all patients should receive anticoagulants. In the invasive approach, there are four choices: unfractionated heparin (UFH), enoxaparin (Lovenox), bivalirudin (Angiomax), or fondaparinux (Arixtra). Regarding additional antiplatelet therapy, the 2007 guidelines recommend that before diagnostic angiography, at least one of clopidogrel (Plavix) or an intravenous GP IIb/IIIa inhibitor should be initiated. Use of both agents is listed as reasonable; factors favoring administration of both include a delay to the time of angiography, high-risk features, and early recurrent ischemic discomfort.

For patients managed with an initial conservative strategy (see Fig. 56G-3), in addition to aspirin, the ACC/AHA guidelines recommend anticoagulant therapy but have only three options—enoxaparin, fondaparinux, or UFH—with the subcutaneously administered drugs enoxaparin and fondaparinux preferred to UFH as a Class IIa recommendation. In patients with an increased risk of bleeding, fondaparinux is preferable on the basis of lower bleeding risk. Clopidogrel should be started at the time of presentation in conservatively managed patients.

The 2007 ACC/AHA guidelines emphasize reevaluation of medications after angiography (**Fig. 56G-4**). If a patient is selected for coronary artery bypass grafting (CABG), aspirin and UFH should be continued; clopidogrel, GP IIb/IIIa inhibitors, and anticoagulants other than UFH should be stopped. For medically managed patients, reevaluation for the need of clopidogrel is encouraged—so that if it had not been given before angiography (if the physician wished to define the coronary anatomy

TABLE 56G-2 ACC/AHA System for Risk Stratification of Patients with Unstable Angina

FEATURE	HIGH RISK	INTERMEDIATE RISK	LOW RISK
	At Least One of the Following Features:	***No High-Risk Feature But Must Have One of the Following:***	***No High- or Intermediate-Risk Feature But May Have Any of the Following Features:***
History	Accelerating tempo of ischemic symptoms in preceding 48 hr	Prior MI, peripheral or cerebrovascular disease, or CABG; prior aspirin use	
Character of pain	Prolonged ongoing (>20 min) rest pain	Prolonged rest angina, now resolved, with moderate or high likelihood of CAD Rest angina <20 min or relieved with rest or sublingual NTG	New-onset or progressive CCS class III or IV angina the past 2 wk without prolonged rest pain but with moderate or high likelihood of CAD
Clinical findings	Pulmonary edema, most likely caused by ischemia New or worsening MR murmur S_3 or new worsening rales Hypotension, bradycardia, tachycardia Age >75 yr	Age >70 yr	
ECG	Angina at rest with transient ST-segment changes >0.05 mV Bundle branch block, new or presumed new Sustained ventricular tachycardia	T wave inversions >0.2 mV Pathologic Q waves	Normal or unchanged ECG during an episode of chest discomfort
Cardiac markers	Elevated	Slightly elevated	Normal

CABG = coronary artery bypass graft; CAD = coronary artery disease; CCS = Canadian Cardiovascular Society; ECG = electrocardiogram; MI = myocardial infarction; MR = mitral regurgitation; NTG = nitroglycerin.

From Anderson JL, Adams CD, Antman EM, et al: ACC/AHA 2007 guidelines for the management of patients with unstable angina/non–ST-elevation myocardial infarction: A report of the American College of Cardiology/American Heart Association Task Force on Practice Guidelines (Writing Committee to Revise the 2002 Guidelines for the Management of Patients With Unstable Angina/Non–ST-Elevation Myocardial Infarction) developed in collaboration with the American College of Emergency Physicians, the Society for Cardiovascular Angiography and Interventions, and the Society of Thoracic Surgeons endorsed by the American Association of Cardiovascular and Pulmonary Rehabilitation and the Society for Academic Emergency Medicine. J Am Coll Cardiol 50:e1, 2007.

TABLE 56G-3 ACC/AHA Guideline Recommendations for Selection of Initial Treatment Strategy: Invasive Versus Conservative Strategy

PREFERRED STRATEGY	PATIENT CHARACTERISTICS
Invasive	Recurrent angina or ischemia at rest or with low-level activities, despite intensive medical therapy Elevated cardiac biomarkers (TnT or TnI) New or presumably new ST-segment depression Signs or symptoms of HF or new or worsening mitral regurgitation High-risk findings from noninvasive testing Hemodynamic instability Sustained ventricular tachycardia PCI within 6 months Prior CABG High-risk score (e.g., TIMI, GRACE) Reduced left ventricular function (LVEF <40%)
Conservative	Low-risk score (e.g., TIMI, GRACE) Patient or physician preference in the absence of high-risk features

CABG = coronary artery bypass graft surgery; GRACE = Global Registry of Acute Coronary Events; HF = heart failure; LVEF = left ventricular ejection fraction; PCI = percutaneous coronary intervention; TIMI = Thrombolysis In Myocardial Infarction; TnI = troponin I; TnT = troponin T.

From Anderson JL, Adams CD, Antman EM, et al: ACC/AHA 2007 guidelines for the management of patients with unstable angina/non–ST-elevation myocardial infarction: A report of the American College of Cardiology/American Heart Association Task Force on Practice Guidelines (Writing Committee to Revise the 2002 Guidelines for the Management of Patients With Unstable Angina/Non–ST-Elevation Myocardial Infarction) developed in collaboration with the American College of Emergency Physicians, the Society for Cardiovascular Angiography and Interventions, and the Society of Thoracic Surgeons endorsed by the American Association of Cardiovascular and Pulmonary Rehabilitation and the Society for Academic Emergency Medicine. J Am Coll Cardiol 50:e1, 2007.

before starting this agent), it should be given if coronary artery disease is confirmed at angiography. Indeed, use of clopidogrel in medically managed patients is listed as a "test" performance measure in the 2008 ACC/AHA myocardial infarction performance measures.[2]

LATER RISK STRATIFICATION AND MANAGEMENT

Table 56G-5 lists the ACC/AHA guidelines recommendations for risk stratification before discharge. As shown in Figure 56G-1, early stress testing is performed in low-risk patients (see Table 56G-2 for risk category definition); for intermediate-risk patients managed with an early conservative strategy, stress testing can be performed after they have been free of ischemia and heart failure for a minimum of 2 to 3 days. The first choice in noninvasive tests is exercise electrocardiography; imaging technologies and pharmacologic stress tests should be used for subsets of patients for whom exercise electrocardiography would be expected to have a high likelihood of providing inadequate data. Data from noninvasive tests can restratify patients into high-, intermediate-, and low-risk groups (**Table 56G-6**).

For patients who require coronary revascularization, the principles for choosing between CABG and PCI are similar to those used for patients with chronic stable angina (see Chap. 57). The guidelines recommend CABG over PCI for patients with significant left main coronary artery disease and for patients with multivessel disease and diminished ejection fraction or diabetes (**Fig. 56G-5**). Either CABG or PCI is considered appropriate for patients with two-vessel disease (**Table 56G-7**).[3] The UA/NSTEMI guidelines and the 2009 ACC/AHA appropriate use criteria provide some support for revascularization with CABG or PCI for patients with proximal left anterior descending coronary artery disease alone.

HOSPITAL DISCHARGE AND POSTHOSPITAL DISCHARGE CARE

The ACC/AHA guidelines emphasize the importance of aggressive risk factor modification and of teaching patients about management of ischemic episodes (**Table 56G-8**). Five classes of drugs are indicated: aspirin,

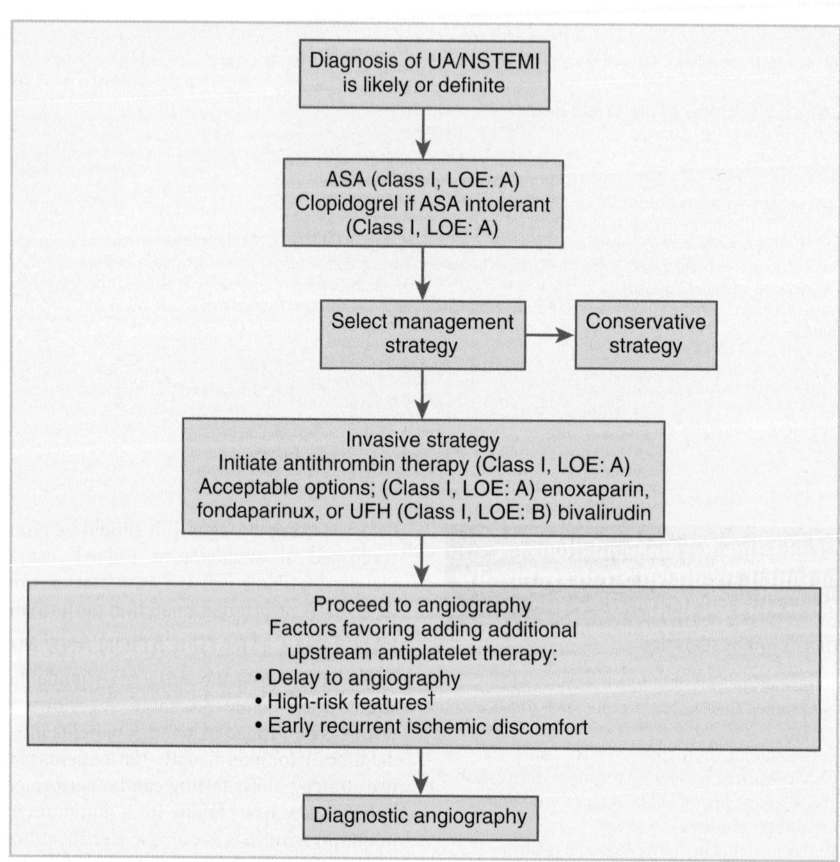

FIGURE 56G-2 ACC/AHA guideline algorithm for patients with UA/NSTEMI managed by an initial invasive strategy. ASA = aspirin; LOE = level of evidence; UFH = unfractionated heparin.

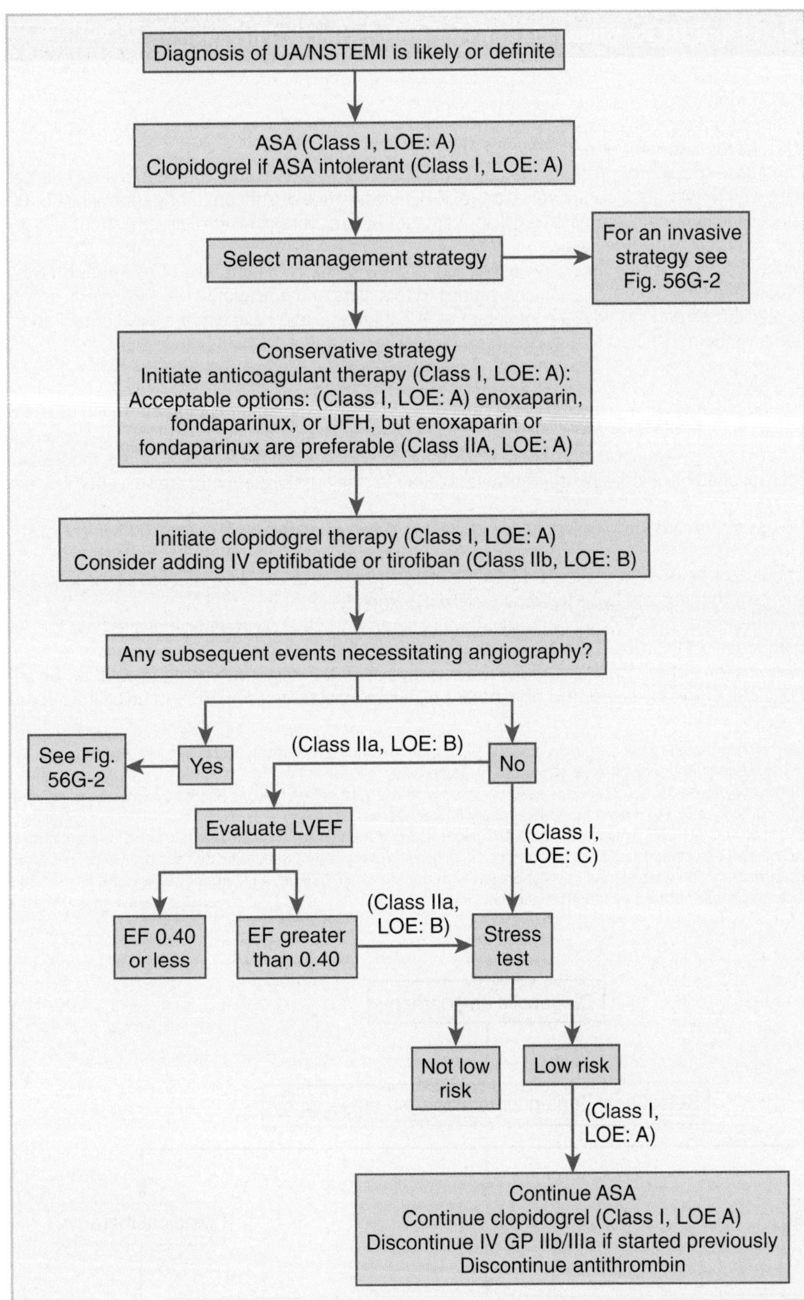

FIGURE 56G-3 ACC/AHA guideline algorithm for patients with UA/NSTEMI managed by an initial conservative strategy. ASA = aspirin; EF = ejection fraction; GP = glycoprotein; IV = intravenous; LOE = level of evidence; LVEF = left ventricular ejection fraction; UFH = unfractionated heparin.

TABLE 56G-4 ACC/AHA Class I and III Recommendations for Anti-Ischemic Therapy

Class I

1. Bed/chair rest with continuous ECG monitoring
2. NTG 0.4 mg sublingually every 5 min for a total of 3 doses; afterward, assess need for IV NTG
3. NTG IV for first 48 hr after UA/NSTEMI for treatment of persistent ischemia, HF, or hypertension
4. Decision to administer NTG IV and dose should not preclude therapy with other mortality-reducing interventions such as beta blockers or ACE inhibitors
5. Beta blockers (via oral route) within 24 hr without a contraindication (e.g., HF) irrespective of concomitant performance of PCI
6. When beta blockers are contraindicated, a nondihydropyridine calcium antagonist (e.g., verapamil or diltiazem) should be given as initial therapy in the absence of severe LV dysfunction or other contraindications
7. ACE inhibitor (via oral route) within first 24 hr with pulmonary congestion, or LVEF ≤0.40, in the absence of hypotension (systolic blood pressure <100 mm Hg or <30 mm Hg below baseline) or known contraindications to that class of medications
8. ARB should be administered to UA/NSTEMI patients who are intolerant of ACE inhibitors and have either clinical or radiologic signs of heart failure or LVEF ≤0.40. Valsartan and candesartan have demonstrated efficacy for this indication.

Class III

1. Nitrates should not be administered to UA/NSTEMI patients with systolic blood pressure <90 mm Hg or ≥30 mm Hg below baseline, severe bradycardia (<50 beats/min), tachycardia (>100 beats/min) in the absence of symptomatic HF, or right ventricular infarction. *(Level of Evidence: C)*
2. Nitroglycerin or other nitrates should not be administered to patients with UA/NSTEMI who have received a phosphodiesterase inhibitor for erectile dysfunction within 24 hr of sildenafil or 48 hr of tadalafil use. The suitable time for the administration of nitrates after vardenafil has not been determined. *(Level of Evidence: C)*
3. Immediate-release dihydropyridine calcium antagonists should not be administered to patients with UA/NSTEMI in the absence of a beta blocker. *(Level of Evidence: A)*
4. An intravenous ACE inhibitor should not be given to patients within the first 24 hours of UA/NSTEMI because of the increased risk of hypotension. (A possible exception may be patients with refractory hypertension.) *(Level of Evidence: B)*
5. It may be harmful to administer intravenous beta blockers to UA/NSTEMI patients who have contraindications to beta blockade, signs of HF or low-output state, or other risk factors* for cardiogenic shock. *(Level of Evidence: A)*
6. Nonsteroidal anti-inflammatory drugs (except for aspirin), whether nonselective or COX-2–selective agents, should not be administered during hospitalization for UA/NSTEMI because of the increased risks of mortality, reinfarction, hypertension, HF, and myocardial rupture associated with their use. *(Level of Evidence: C)*

*Risk factors for cardiogenic shock (the greater the number of risk factors present, the higher the risk of developing cardiogenic shock): age >70 years, systolic blood pressure <120 mm Hg, sinus tachycardia >110 or heart rate <60, increased time since onset of symptoms of UA/NSTEMI.

ACE = angiotensin-converting enzyme; ARB = angiotensin receptor blocker; COX-2 = cyclooxygenase 2; HF = heart failure; IV = intravenous; LV = left ventricular; LVEF = left ventricular ejection fraction; MI = myocardial infarction; NTG = nitroglycerin; PCI = percutaneous coronary intervention.

From Anderson JL, Adams CD, Antman EM, et al: ACC/AHA 2007 guidelines for the management of patients with unstable angina/non–ST-elevation myocardial infarction: A report of the American College of Cardiology/American Heart Association Task Force on Practice Guidelines (Writing Committee to Revise the 2002 Guidelines for the Management of Patients With Unstable Angina/Non–ST-Elevation Myocardial Infarction) developed in collaboration with the American College of Emergency Physicians, the Society for Cardiovascular Angiography and Interventions, and the Society of Thoracic Surgeons endorsed by the American Association of Cardiovascular and Pulmonary Rehabilitation and the Society for Academic Emergency Medicine. J Am Coll Cardiol 50:e1, 2007.

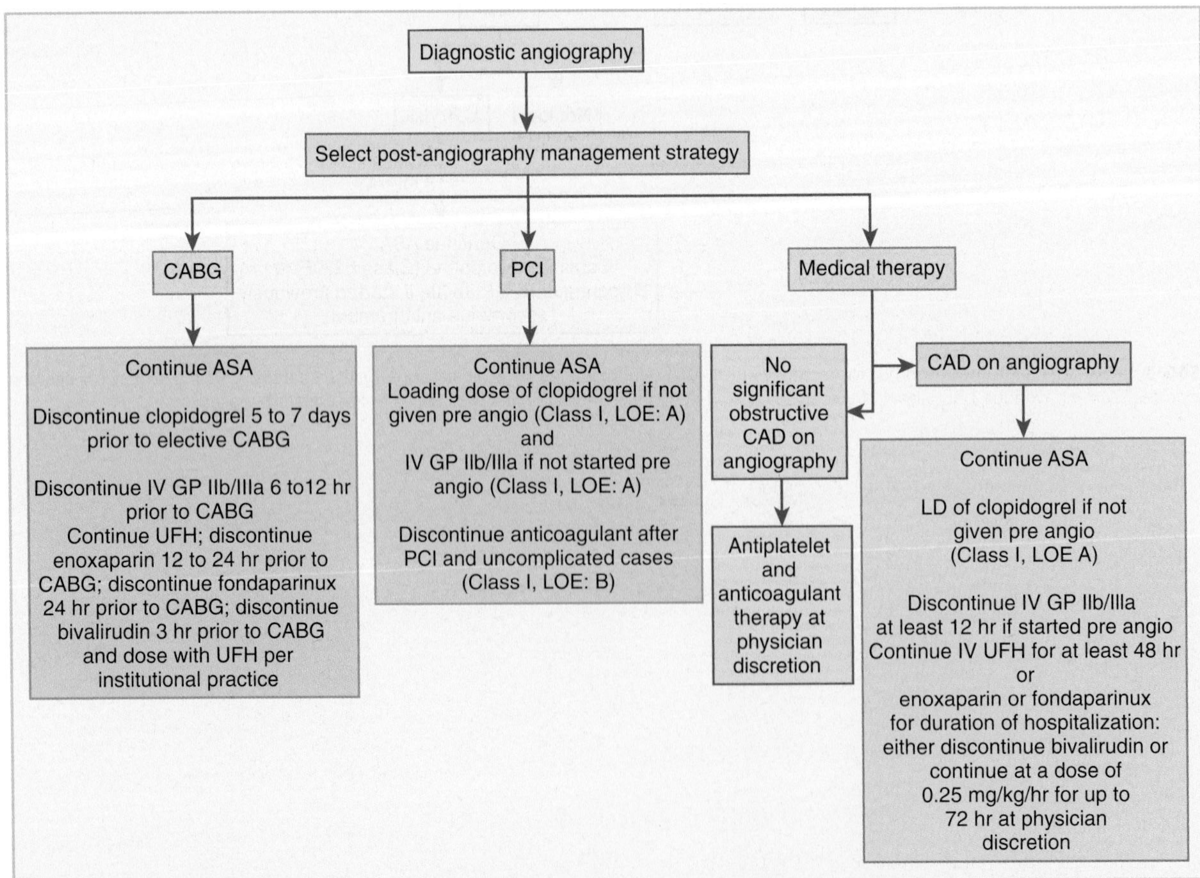

FIGURE 56G-4 ACC/AHA guideline for management after diagnostic angiography in patients with UA/NSTEMI. ASA = aspirin; CABG = coronary artery bypass graft; CAD = coronary artery disease; GP = glycoprotein; IV = intravenous; LD = loading dose; LOE = level of evidence; PCI = percutaneous coronary intervention; pre angio = before angiography; UFH = unfractionated heparin.

TABLE 56G-5 ACC/AHA Guidelines for Risk Stratification Before Discharge in Patients with Acute Coronary Syndromes

Class I

1. Noninvasive stress testing is recommended in low-risk patients who have been free of ischemia at rest or with low-level activity and of HF for a minimum of 12 to 24 hr. *(Level of Evidence: C)*
2. Noninvasive stress testing is recommended in patients at intermediate risk who have been free of ischemia at rest or with low-level activity and of HF for a minimum of 12 to 24 hr. *(Level of Evidence: C)*
3. Choice of stress test is based on the resting ECG, ability to perform exercise, local expertise, and technologies available. Treadmill exercise is useful in patients able to exercise whose ECG lacks baseline ST-segment abnormalities, bundle branch block, LV hypertrophy, intraventricular conduction defect, paced rhythm, preexcitation, or digoxin effect. *(Level of Evidence: C)*
4. An imaging modality should be added in patients with resting ST-segment depression (≥0.1 mV), LV hypertrophy, bundle branch block, intraventricular conduction defect, preexcitation, or digoxin. In patients undergoing a low-level exercise test, an imaging modality can add sensitivity. *(Level of Evidence: B)*
5. Pharmacologic stress testing with imaging is recommended when physical limitations (e.g., arthritis, amputation, severe peripheral vascular disease, severe chronic obstructive pulmonary disease, or general debility) preclude adequate exercise stress. *(Level of Evidence: B)*
6. Prompt angiography without noninvasive risk stratification should be performed for failure of stabilization with intensive medical treatment. *(Level of Evidence: B)*
7. A noninvasive test (echocardiogram or radionuclide angiogram) is recommended to evaluate LV function in patients with definite ACS who are not scheduled for coronary angiography and left ventriculography. *(Level of Evidence: B)*

ACS = acute coronary syndrome; ECG = electrocardiogram; HF = heart failure; LV = left ventricular.

From Anderson JL, Adams CD, Antman EM, et al: ACC/AHA 2007 guidelines for the management of patients with unstable angina/non–ST-elevation myocardial infarction: A report of the American College of Cardiology/American Heart Association Task Force on Practice Guidelines (Writing Committee to Revise the 2002 Guidelines for the Management of Patients With Unstable Angina/Non–ST-Elevation Myocardial Infarction) developed in collaboration with the American College of Emergency Physicians, the Society for Cardiovascular Angiography and Interventions, and the Society of Thoracic Surgeons endorsed by the American Association of Cardiovascular and Pulmonary Rehabilitation and the Society for Academic Emergency Medicine. J Am Coll Cardiol 50:e1, 2007.

TABLE 56G-6 ACC/AHA Noninvasive Risk Stratification

High Risk (>3% Annual Mortality Rate)

1. Severe resting LV dysfunction (LVEF <0.35)
2. High-risk treadmill score (score ≤ −11)
3. Severe exercise LV dysfunction (exercise LVEF <0.35)
4. Stress-induced large perfusion defect (particularly if anterior)
5. Stress-induced multiple perfusion defects of moderate size
6. Large, fixed perfusion defect with LV dilation or increased lung uptake (thallium-201)
7. Stress-induced moderate perfusion defect with LV dilation or increased lung uptake (thallium-201)
8. Echocardiographic wall motion abnormality (involving > two segments) developing at a low dose of dobutamine (≤10 mg/kg/min) or at a low heart rate (<120 beats/min)
9. Stress echocardiographic evidence of extensive ischemia

Intermediate Risk (1%-3% Annual Mortality Rate)

1. Mild/moderate resting LV dysfunction (LVEF 0.35-0.49)
2. Intermediate-risk treadmill score (−11 < score < 5)
3. Stress-induced moderate perfusion defect without LV dilation or increased lung intake (thallium-201)
4. Limited stress echocardiographic ischemia with a wall motion abnormality only at higher doses of dobutamine involving two segments or less

Low Risk (<1% Annual Mortality Rate)

1. Low-risk treadmill score (score ≥5)
2. Normal or small myocardial perfusion defect at rest or with stress
3. Normal stress echocardiographic wall motion or no change of limited resting wall motion abnormalities during stress

LV = left ventricular; LVEF = left ventricular ejection fraction.

From Gibbons RJ, Chatterjee K, Daley J, et al: ACC/AHA/ACP-ASIM guidelines for the management of patients with chronic stable angina. J Am Coll Cardiol 33:2092, 1999.

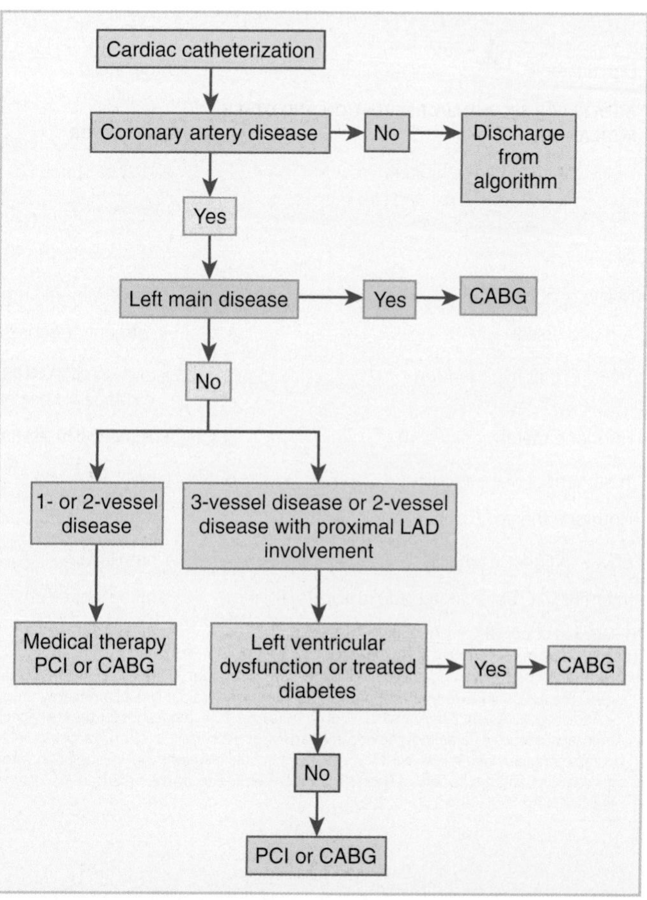

FIGURE 56G-5 ACC/AHA guideline for revascularization strategy in UA/NSTEMI. CABG = coronary artery bypass graft; LAD = left anterior descending coronary artery; PCI = percutaneous coronary intervention.

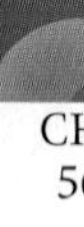

TABLE 56G-7 ACC/AHA Appropriateness Ratings for Type of Revascularization

	CABG			PCI		
	NO DIABETES AND NORMAL LVEF	DIABETES	DEPRESSED LVEF	NO DIABETES AND NORMAL LVEF	DIABETES	DEPRESSED LVEF
Two-vessel coronary artery disease with proximal LAD stenosis	A	A	A	A	A	A
Three-vessel coronary artery disease	A	A	A	U	U	U
Isolated left main stenosis	A	A	A	I	I	I
Left main stenosis and additional coronary artery disease	A	A	A	I	I	I

A = appropriate; I = inappropriate; U = uncertain; CABG = coronary artery bypass graft; LAD = left anterior descending coronary artery; LVEF = left ventricular ejection fraction; PCI = percutaneous coronary intervention.

From Patel MR, Dehmer GJ, Hirshfeld JW, et al: ACCF/SCAI/STS/AATS/AHA/ASNC 2009 Appropriateness Criteria for Coronary Revascularization: A report by the American College of Cardiology Foundation Appropriateness Criteria Task Force, Society for Cardiovascular Angiography and Interventions, Society of Thoracic Surgeons, American Association for Thoracic Surgery, American Heart Association, and the American Society of Nuclear Cardiology Endorsed by the American Society of Echocardiography, the Heart Failure Society of America, and the Society of Cardiovascular Computed Tomography. J Am Coll Cardiol 53:530, 2009.

TABLE 56G-8 Medications Used for Stabilized UA/NSTEMI Patients

ANTI-ISCHEMIC AND ANTITHROMBOTIC/ ANTIPLATELET AGENTS	DRUG ACTION	CLASS/LEVEL OF EVIDENCE
Aspirin	Antiplatelet	I/A
Clopidogrel* or ticlopidine	Antiplatelet when aspirin is contraindicated	I/A
Beta blockers	Anti-ischemic	I/B
ACEI	EF <0.40 or HF EF >0.40	I/A, IIa/A
Nitrates	Antianginal	I/C for ischemic symptoms
Calcium channel blockers (short-acting dihydropyridine antagonists should be avoided)	Antianginal	I for ischemic symptoms; when beta blockers are not successful (B) or contraindicated, or cause unacceptable side effects (C)
Dipyridamole	Antiplatelet	III/A
AGENTS FOR SECONDARY PREVENTION AND OTHER INDICATIONS	**RISK FACTOR**	**CLASS/LEVEL OF EVIDENCE**
HMG-CoA reductase inhibitors	LDL cholesterol >70 mg/dL	Ia
Fibrates	HDL cholesterol <40 mg/dL	IIa/B
Niacin	HDL cholesterol <40 mg/dL	IIa/B
Niacin or fibrate	Triglycerides 200 mg/dL	IIa/B
Antidepressant	Treatment of depression	IIb/B
Treatment of hypertension	Blood pressure >140/90 mm Hg or >130/80 mm Hg if kidney disease or diabetes present	I/A
Hormone therapy (initiation)†	Postmenopausal state	III/A
Treatment of diabetes	HbA1c >7%	I/B
Hormone therapy (continuation)†	Postmenopausal state	III/B
COX-2 inhibitor or NSAID	Chronic pain	IIa/C, IIb/C, or III/C
Vitamins C, E, beta-carotene; folic acid, B_6, B_{12}	Antioxidant effect; homocysteine lowering	III/A

*Preferred to ticlopidine.

†For risk reduction of coronary artery disease.

ACEI = angiotensin-converting enzyme inhibitor; COX-2 = cyclooxygenase 2; EF = ejection fraction; HDL = high-density lipoprotein; HF = heart failure; HMG-CoA = hydroxymethylglutaryl coenzyme A; LDL = low-density lipoprotein; NSAID = nonsteroidal anti-inflammatory drug.

From Anderson JL, Adams CD, Antman EM, et al: ACC/AHA 2007 guidelines for the management of patients with unstable angina/non–ST-elevation myocardial infarction: a report of the American College of Cardiology/American Heart Association Task Force on Practice Guidelines (Writing Committee to Revise the 2002 Guidelines for the Management of Patients With Unstable Angina/Non–ST-Elevation Myocardial Infarction) developed in collaboration with the American College of Emergency Physicians, the Society for Cardiovascular Angiography and Interventions, and the Society of Thoracic Surgeons endorsed by the American Association of Cardiovascular and Pulmonary Rehabilitation and the Society for Academic Emergency Medicine. J Am Coll Cardiol 50:e1, 2007.

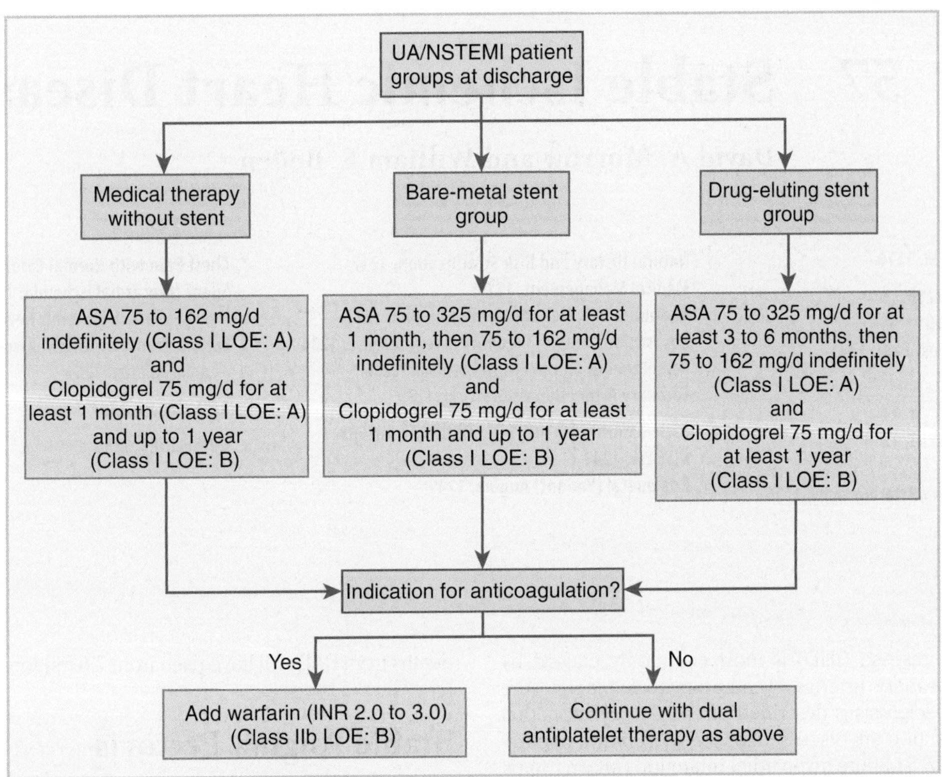

FIGURE 56G-6 ACC/AHA guideline for long-term antithrombotic therapy at hospital discharge after UA/NSTEMI. ASA = aspirin; INR = international normalized ratio; LOE = level of evidence.

clopidogrel, beta blockers, ACE inhibitors, and statins. The 2007 guidelines recommend that statins be given at the time of discharge, regardless of low-density lipoprotein level. Recommendations for antithrombotic therapy are given in **Figure 56G-6**. The dose of aspirin is recommended to be 81 to 162 mg for medically managed patients; after PCI, a slightly higher dose is recommended (162 to 325 mg) for a period of 1, 3, or 6 months, depending on the type of stent, followed by the lower dose. If a patient has an indication for warfarin, it should be added but titrated to an international normalized ratio of 2.0 to 2.5, and aspirin 81 mg daily is recommended.

REFERENCES

1. Anderson JL, Adams CD, Antman EM, et al: ACC/AHA 2007 guidelines for the management of patients with unstable angina/non–ST-elevation myocardial infarction: A report of the American College of Cardiology/American Heart Association Task Force on Practice Guidelines (Writing Committee to Revise the 2002 Guidelines for the Management of Patients With Unstable Angina/Non–ST-Elevation Myocardial Infarction) developed in collaboration with the American College of Emergency Physicians, the Society for Cardiovascular Angiography and Interventions, and the Society of Thoracic Surgeons endorsed by the American Association of Cardiovascular and Pulmonary Rehabilitation and the Society for Academic Emergency Medicine. J Am Coll Cardiol 50:e1, 2007.
2. Masoudi FA, Bonow RO, Brindis RG, et al: ACC/AHA 2008 statement on Performance Measurement and Reperfusion Therapy: A report of the ACC/AHA Task Force on Performance Measures (Work Group to address the challenges of Performance Measurement and Reperfusion Therapy). J Am Coll Cardiol 52:2100, 2008.
3. Patel MR, Dehmer GJ, Hirshfeld JW, et al: ACCF/SCAI/STS/AATS/AHA/ASNC 2009 Appropriateness Criteria for Coronary Revascularization: A report by the American College of Cardiology Foundation Appropriateness Criteria Task Force, Society for Cardiovascular Angiography and Interventions, Society of Thoracic Surgeons, American Association for Thoracic Surgery, American Heart Association, and the American Society of Nuclear Cardiology Endorsed by the American Society of Echocardiography, the Heart Failure Society of America, and the Society of Cardiovascular Computed Tomography. J Am Coll Cardiol 53:530, 2009.

CHAPTER 57 Stable Ischemic Heart Disease

David A. Morrow and William E. Boden

Stable ischemic heart disease (IHD) is most commonly caused by obstruction of the coronary arteries by atheromatous plaque (the pathogenesis of atherosclerosis is described in Chap. 43). Factors that predispose to this condition are discussed in Chap. 44, control of coronary blood flow in Chap. 52, acute myocardial infarction (MI) in Chaps. 54 and 55, and unstable angina in Chap. 56; sudden cardiac death, another significant consequence of coronary artery disease (CAD), is presented in Chap. 41.

The clinical presentations of IHD are highly variable. Chest discomfort is usually the predominant symptom in chronic (stable) angina, unstable angina, Prinzmetal (variant) angina, microvascular angina, and acute myocardial infarction (MI). However, presentations of IHD also occur in which chest discomfort is absent or not prominent, such as asymptomatic (silent) myocardial ischemia, heart failure, cardiac arrhythmias, and sudden death. Obstructive CAD also has nonatherosclerotic causes, including congenital abnormalities of the coronary vessels, myocardial bridging, coronary arteritis in association with the systemic vasculitides, and radiation-induced coronary disease. Myocardial ischemia and angina pectoris may also occur in the absence of obstructive CAD, as in the case of aortic valve disease (see Chap. 66), hypertrophic cardiomyopathy (see Chap. 69), and idiopathic dilated cardiomyopathy (see Chap. 68). Moreover, CAD may coexist with these other forms of heart disease.

Magnitude of the Problem

The importance of IHD in contemporary society is attested to by the almost epidemic number of persons afflicted (see Chap. 1). It is estimated that 17,600,000 Americans have IHD, of whom 10,200,00 have angina pectoris and 8,500,000 have had an MI.[1] Based on data from the Framingham Heart Study, the lifetime risk of developing symptomatic CAD after age 40 is 49% for men and 32% for women. In 2006, IHD accounted for 52% of all deaths caused by cardiovascular disease and was the single most frequent cause of death in American men and women, resulting in more than one in six deaths in the United States. The economic cost of IHD in the United States in 2010 has been estimated at $177.1 billion. Despite a steady decline in age-specific mortality from CAD over the past several decades,[2] ischemic heart disease is now the leading cause of death worldwide, and it is expected that the rate of CAD will only accelerate in the next decade with the burden shifting progressively to lower socioeconomic groups. Contributory factors include aging of the population, alarming increases in the worldwide prevalence of obesity, type 2 diabetes, and a rise in cardiovascular risk factors in younger people. The World Health Organization has estimated that by 2020, the global number of deaths from CAD will have risen from 7.6 million in 2005 to 11.1 million (see Chap. 1).[3]

Stable Angina Pectoris

Clinical Manifestations

CHARACTERISTICS OF ANGINA. Angina pectoris (see Chap. 12) is a discomfort in the chest or adjacent areas caused by myocardial ischemia. It is usually brought on by exertion and is associated with a disturbance in myocardial function. Acute MI, which is usually associated with prolonged severe pain occurring at rest (see Chap. 54), and unstable angina, which is characterized by an accelerated pattern and/or occurrence at rest (see Chap. 56), are discussed separately. Heberden's initial description of angina as conveying a sense of "strangling and anxiety" is still remarkably pertinent. Other adjectives frequently used to describe this distress include tight, constricting, suffocating, crushing, heavy, and squeezing. In other patients, the quality of the sensation is more vague and described as a mild pressure-like discomfort, an uncomfortable numb sensation, or a burning sensation. The site of the discomfort is usually retrosternal, but radiation is common and usually occurs down the ulnar surface of the left arm; the right arm and the outer surfaces of both arms may also be involved (**Fig. 57-1**). Epigastric discomfort alone or in association with chest pressure may occur. Anginal discomfort above the mandible or below the epigastrium is rare. Anginal equivalents (i.e., symptoms of myocardial ischemia other than angina), such as dyspnea, faintness, fatigue, and eructations, are common, particularly in older patients. A history of abnormal exertional dyspnea may be an early indicator of IHD, even when angina is absent or no evidence of CAD can be found on the electrocardiogram (ECG). Dyspnea at rest or with exertion may be a manifestation of severe ischemia, leading to increases in left ventricular (LV) filling pressure.[4] Nocturnal angina should raise the suspicion of sleep apnea (see Chap. 79). Postprandial angina, presumably caused by redistribution of coronary blood flow away from the territory supplied by severely stenosed vessels, may be a marker of severe CAD.

The typical episode of angina pectoris usually begins gradually and reaches its maximum intensity over a period of minutes before dissipating. It is unusual for angina pectoris to reach its maximum severity within seconds, and it is characteristic that patients with angina usually prefer to rest, sit, or stop walking during episodes. Chest discomfort while walking in the cold or uphill is suggestive of angina. Features suggesting the absence of angina pectoris include pleuritic pain, pain localized to the tip of one finger, pain reproduced by movement or palpation of the chest wall or arms, and constant pain lasting

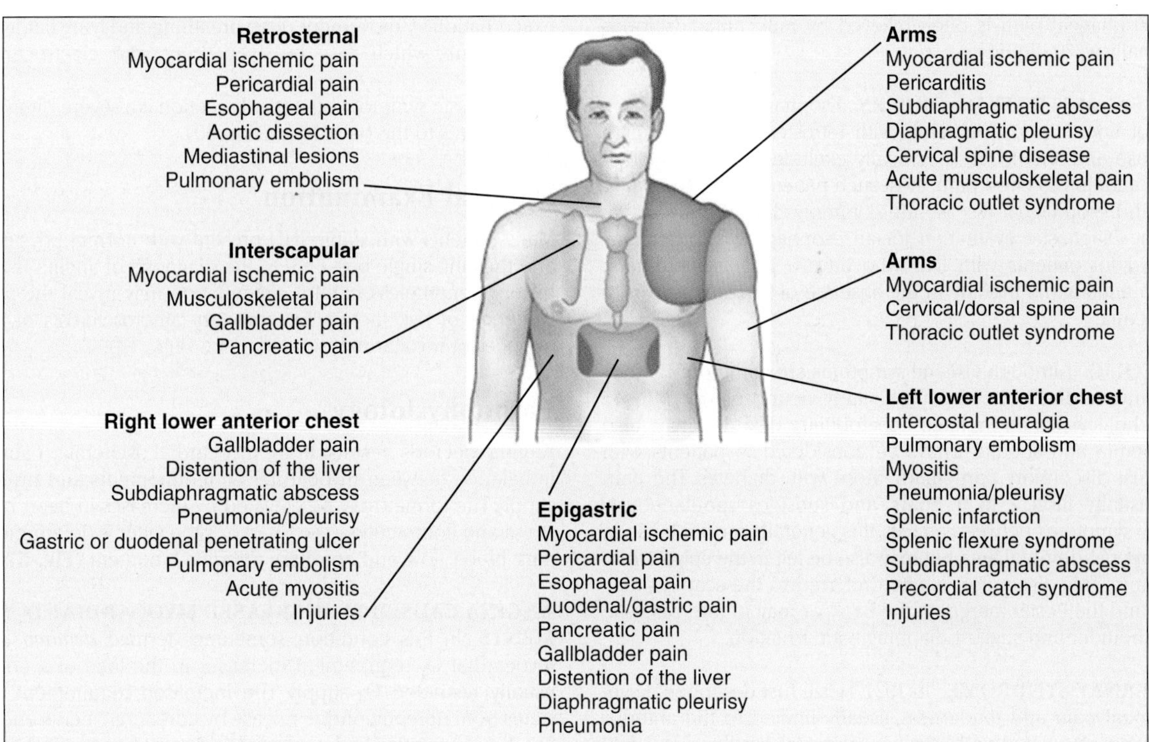

FIGURE 57-1 Location of discomfort and cause of chest symptoms. The location of angina is usually retrosternal but radiation is common. An epigastric location of angina may also occur. *(Modified from Braunwald E: The history. In Zipes D, Libby P, Bonow RO, Braunwald E [eds]: Braunwald's Heart Disease. 7th ed. Philadelphia, WB Saunders, 2005, p 68.)*

many hours or, alternatively, very brief episodes of pain lasting seconds. Pain radiating into the lower extremities is also a highly unusual manifestation of angina pectoris.

Typical angina pectoris is relieved within minutes by rest or the use of nitroglycerin. The response to the latter is often a useful diagnostic tool, although it should be remembered that esophageal pain and other syndromes may also respond to nitroglycerin. A delay of more than 5 to 10 minutes before relief is obtained by rest and nitroglycerin suggests that the symptoms are either not caused by ischemia or are caused by severe ischemia, as with acute MI or unstable angina. The phenomenon of first-effort or warm-up angina is used to describe the ability of some patients in whom angina develops with exertion to continue subsequently at the same or even greater level of exertion without symptoms after an intervening period of rest. This attenuation of myocardial ischemia observed with repeated exertion has been postulated to be caused by ischemic preconditioning and appears to require preceding ischemia of at least moderate intensity to induce the warm-up phenomenon.

GRADING OF ANGINA PECTORIS. A system of grading the severity of angina pectoris proposed by the Canadian Cardiovascular Society (CCS) has gained widespread acceptance (see Table 12-1).[5] The system is a modification of the New York Heart Association (NYHA) functional classification but allows patients to be categorized in more specific terms. Other grading systems[6] include a specific activity scale developed by Goldman and associates and an anginal score developed by Califf and colleagues. The Goldman scale is based on the metabolic cost of specific activities and appears to be valid when used by physicians and nonphysicians. The anginal score of Califf and coworkers integrates the clinical features and tempo of angina together with ST and T wave changes on the ECG and offers independent prognostic information beyond that provided by age, gender, LV function, and coronary angiographic anatomy. A limitation of all these grading systems is their dependence on accurate patient observation and patients' widely varying tolerance for symptoms. Functional estimates based on the CCS criteria have shown a reproducibility of only 73% and do not correlate well with objective measures of exercise performance.

MECHANISMS. The mechanisms of cardiac pain and the neural pathways involved are poorly understood. It is presumed that angina pectoris results from ischemic episodes that excite chemosensitive and mechanosensitive receptors in the heart.[7] Stimulation of these receptors results in the release of adenosine, bradykinin, and other substances that excite the sensory ends of the sympathetic and vagal afferent fibers.[8] The afferent fibers traverse the nerves that connect to the upper five thoracic sympathetic ganglia and upper five distal thoracic roots of the spinal cord. Impulses are transmitted by the spinal cord to the thalamus and hence to the neocortex. Data from animal studies have identified the vanilloid receptor-1 (VR_1), an important sensor for somatic nociception, as present on the sensory nerve endings of the heart and have suggested that VR_1 functions as a transducer of myocardial tissue ischemia.[9] In a murine VR_1 gene knockout model, ischemia-induced activation of VR_1 appeared to play a role in ischemic preconditioning.[10]

Within the spinal cord, cardiac sympathetic afferent impulses may converge with impulses from somatic thoracic structures, which may be the basis for referred cardiac pain—for example, to the chest. In comparison, cardiac vagal afferent fibers synapse in the nucleus tractus solitarius of the medulla and then descend to excite the upper cervical spinothalamic tract cells, which may contribute to the anginal pain experienced in the neck and jaw. Positron emission tomography (PET) imaging of the brain in subjects with silent ischemia has suggested that failed transmission of signals from the thalamus to the frontal cortex may contribute to this phenomenon, along with impaired afferent signaling, such as that caused by autonomic neuropathy. Silent ischemia in diabetic patients, for example, has been proposed to relate to failed development of the cardiac sensory system due to reduced nerve growth factor.[11]

Differential Diagnosis of Chest Pain

ESOPHAGEAL DISORDERS. Common disorders that may simulate or coexist with angina pectoris are gastroesophageal reflux and disorders of esophageal motility, including diffuse spasm and nutcracker esophagus. To compound the difficulty in distinguishing between angina and esophageal pain, both may be relieved by nitroglycerin.

However, esophageal pain is often relieved by milk, antacids, foods or, occasionally, warm liquids.

ESOPHAGEAL MOTILITY DISORDERS. Esophageal motility disorders are not uncommon in patients with retrosternal chest pain of unclear cause and should be specifically excluded or confirmed, if possible. In addition to chest pain, most such patients have dysphagia. Both IHD and esophageal disease are common clinical entities that may coexist. Diagnostic evaluation for an esophageal disorder may be indicated for patients with IHD who have a poor symptomatic response to antianginal therapy in the absence of documentation of severe ischemia.

BILIARY COLIC. Although visceral symptoms are commonly associated with myocardial ischemia (particularly acute inferior MI; see Chap. 54), cholecystitis and related hepatobiliary disorders may also mimic ischemia and should always be considered in patients with atypical chest discomfort, particularly those with diabetes. The pain is steady, usually lasts 2 to 4 hours, and subsides spontaneously, without any symptoms between attacks. It is generally most intense in the right upper abdominal area but may also be felt in the epigastrium or precordium. This discomfort is often referred to the scapula, may radiate around the costal margin to the back, or may in rare cases be felt in the shoulder and suggest diaphragmatic irritation.

COSTOSTERNAL SYNDROME. In 1921, Tietze first described a syndrome of local pain and tenderness, usually limited to the anterior chest wall and associated with swelling of costal cartilage. The full-blown Tietze syndrome—pain associated with tender swelling of the costochondral junctions—is uncommon, whereas costochondritis causing tenderness of the costochondral junctions (without swelling) is relatively common. Pain on palpation of these joints is usually well localized and is a useful clinical sign. Local pressure should be applied routinely to the anterior chest wall during examination of a patient with suspected angina pectoris. Although palpation of the chest wall often reproduces pain in patients with various musculoskeletal conditions, it should be appreciated that chest wall tenderness may also be associated with and does not exclude symptomatic CAD.

OTHER MUSCULOSKELETAL DISORDERS. Cervical radiculitis may be confused with angina. This condition may occur as a constant ache, sometimes resulting in a sensory deficit. The pain may be related to motion of the neck, just as motion of the shoulder triggers attacks of pain from bursitis. Occasionally, pain mimicking angina can be caused by compression of the brachial plexus by the cervical ribs, and tendinitis or bursitis involving the left shoulder may also cause angina-like pain. Physical examination may also detect pain brought about by movement of an arthritic shoulder or a calcified shoulder tendon.

OTHER CAUSES OF ANGINA-LIKE PAIN. Severe pulmonary hypertension may be associated with exertional chest pain with the characteristics of angina pectoris and, indeed, this pain is thought to be caused by right ventricular ischemia that develops during exertion (see Chap. 78). Other associated symptoms include exertional dyspnea, dizziness, and syncope. Associated findings on physical examination, such as parasternal lift, a palpable and loud pulmonary component of the second sound, and right ventricular hypertrophy on the ECG, are usually readily recognized.

Pulmonary embolism is initially characterized by dyspnea as the cardinal symptom, but chest pain may also be present (see Chap. 77). Pleuritic pain suggests pulmonary infarction and a history of exacerbation of the pain with inspiration, along with a pleural friction rub, usually helps distinguish it from angina pectoris. Pleuritic discomfort also may be caused by pneumonia or other causes of pleuritis.

The pain of acute pericarditis (see Chap. 75) may at times be difficult to distinguish from angina pectoris. However, pericarditis tends to occur in younger patients and the diagnosis depends on the combination of chest pain not relieved by rest or nitroglycerin, exacerbation by movement, deep breathing, and lying flat, a pericardial friction rub, which may be evanescent, and electrocardiographic changes.

The classic symptom of aortic dissection is a severe, often sharp pain that radiates to the back (see Chap. 60).

Physical Examination

Many patients with stable IHD present with normal physical findings and thus the single best clue to the diagnosis of angina is the clinical history. Nonetheless, careful examination may reveal the presence or evidence of risk factors for coronary atherosclerosis or the consequences of myocardial ischemia (see Chap. 12).

Pathophysiology

Angina pectoris results from myocardial ischemia, caused by an imbalance between myocardial O_2 requirements and myocardial O_2 supply. The former may be elevated by increases in heart rate, LV wall stress, and contractility (see Chap. 52); the latter is determined by coronary blood flow and coronary arterial O_2 content (**Fig. 57-2**).

ANGINA CAUSED BY INCREASED MYOCARDIAL O_2 REQUIREMENTS. In this condition, sometimes termed *demand angina*, the myocardial O_2 requirement increases in the face of a constant and usually restricted O_2 supply. The increased requirement commonly stems from norepinephrine release by adrenergic nerve endings in the heart and vascular bed, a physiologic response to exertion, emotion, or mental stress. Of great importance to the myocardial O_2 requirement is the rate at which any task is carried out. Hurrying is particularly likely to precipitate angina, as are efforts involving motion of the hands over the head. Mental and emotional stress may also precipitate angina, presumably by increased hemodynamic and catecholamine responses to stress, increased adrenergic tone, and reduced vagal activity. The combination of physical exertion and emotion in association with sexual activity may precipitate angina pectoris. Anger may produce constriction of coronary arteries with pre-existing narrowing, without necessarily affecting O_2 demand. Other precipitants of angina include physical exertion after a heavy meal and the excessive metabolic demands imposed by fever, thyrotoxicosis, tachycardia from any cause, and hypoglycemia.

ANGINA CAUSED BY TRANSIENTLY DECREASED O_2 SUPPLY. Evidence has suggested that not only unstable angina but also chronic stable angina may be caused by transient reductions in O_2 supply, a condition sometimes termed *supply angina*, as a consequence of coronary vasoconstriction that results in dynamic stenosis. In the presence of organic stenoses, platelet thrombi and leukocytes may elaborate vasoconstrictor substances, such as serotonin and thromboxane A_2. Also, endothelial damage in atherosclerotic coronary arteries decreases production of vasodilator substances and may result in an abnormal vasoconstrictor response to exercise and other stimuli. A variable threshold of myocardial ischemia in patients with chronic stable angina may be caused by dynamic changes in peristenotic smooth muscle tone and also by constriction of arteries distal to the stenosis.

In rare patients without organic obstructing lesions, severe dynamic obstruction alone can cause myocardial ischemia and result in angina at rest (see Prinzmetal [variant] angina and Chaps. 52 and 56). On the other hand, in patients with severe fixed obstruction to coronary blood flow, only a minor increase in dynamic obstruction is necessary for blood flow to fall below a critical level and cause myocardial ischemia.

FIXED-THRESHOLD COMPARED WITH VARIABLE-THRESHOLD ANGINA. In patients with fixed-threshold angina precipitated by increased O_2 demands with few if any dynamic (vasoconstrictor) components, the level of physical activity required to precipitate angina is relatively constant. Characteristically, these patients can predict the amount of physical activity that will precipitate angina—for example, walking up exactly two flights of stairs at a customary pace. When tested on a treadmill or

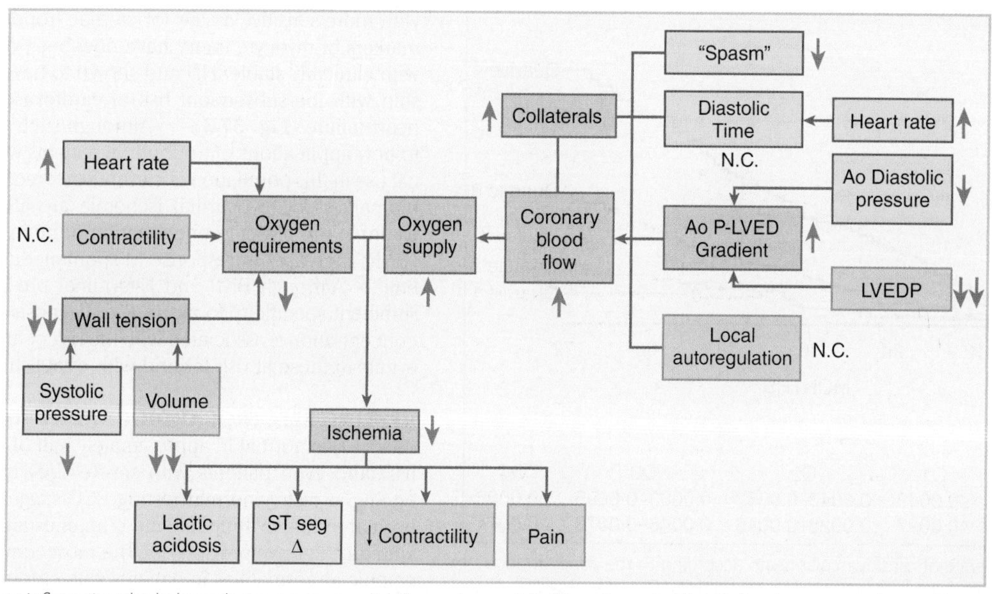

FIGURE 57-2 Factors influencing the balance between myocardial O_2 requirement **(left)** and supply **(right)**. Purple arrows indicate effects of nitrates. In relieving angina pectoris, nitrates exert favorable effects by reducing O_2 requirements and increasing supply. Although a reflex increase in heart rate would tend to reduce the time for coronary flow, dilation of collaterals and enhancement of the pressure gradient for flow to occur as the left ventricular end-diastolic pressure (LVEDP) decreases tend to increase coronary flow. Ao P-LVED = aortic pressure–left ventricular end-diastolic; N.C. = no change. *(From Frishman WH: Pharmacology of the nitrates in angina pectoris. Am J Cardiol 56:8I, 1985.)*

bicycle, the pressure-rate product (the so-called double product, a correlate of the myocardial O_2 requirement) that elicits angina and/or electrocardiographic evidence of ischemia is relatively constant.

Most patients with variable-threshold angina have atherosclerotic coronary arterial narrowing, but dynamic obstruction caused by vasoconstriction plays an important role in causing myocardial ischemia. These patients typically have good days, when they are capable of substantial physical activity, as well as bad days, when even minimal activity can cause clinical and/or electrocardiographic evidence of myocardial ischemia or angina at rest. They often complain of a circadian variation in angina that is more common in the morning. Angina on exertion and sometimes even at rest may be precipitated by cold temperature, emotion, and mental stress.

Mixed Angina. The term *mixed angina* has been proposed by Maseri and colleagues to describe the many patients who fall between the two extremes of fixed-threshold and variable-threshold angina.

The pathophysiologic and clinical correlations of ischemia in patients with stable IHD may have important implications for the selection of anti-ischemic agents, as well as for their timing. The greater the contribution from increased myocardial O_2 requirements to the imbalance between supply and demand, the greater the likelihood that beta-blocking agents will be effective, whereas nitrates and calcium channel blocking agents, at least hypothetically, are likely to be especially effective in episodes caused primarily by coronary vasoconstriction. The finding that in most patients with chronic stable angina, an increase in myocardial O_2 requirement precedes episodes of ischemia—that is, that they have demand angina—argues in favor of controlling heart rate and blood pressure as a primary therapeutic approach.

Evaluation and Management

Testing modalities include noninvasive and invasive procedures.

Noninvasive Testing

BIOCHEMICAL TESTS. In patients with stable IHD, including those with chronic angina, metabolic abnormalities that are risk factors for the development of CAD are frequently detected. These abnormalities include hypercholesterolemia and other dyslipidemias (see Chap. 47), carbohydrate intolerance, and insulin resistance. Moreover, chronic kidney disease is strongly associated with the risk of atherosclerotic vascular disease (see Chap. 93).[12] All patients with established or suspected CAD warrant biochemical evaluation of total cholesterol, low-density lipoprotein (LDL) cholesterol, high-density lipoprotein (HDL) cholesterol, triglyceride, serum creatinine (estimated glomerular filtration), and fasting blood glucose levels.

Other biochemical markers have also been shown to be associated with higher risk of future cardiovascular events (see Chap. 44). Measurement of lipoprotein(a) and other lipid elements that are particularly atherogenic, such as apoprotein B and small dense LDLs, appears to add prognostic information to the measurement of total cholesterol and LDL, and may be considered as a secondary target for therapy in patients who have achieved therapeutic targets for LDL.[13] However, no consensus has been reached regarding routine measurement and a simple approach based on calculation of non-HDL cholesterol may capture the information available from measurement of specific apolipoproteins.[14] Similarly, lipoprotein-associated phospholipase A_2 (Lp-PLA2) is associated with the risk of coronary heart disease as well as recurrent events independent of traditional risk factors.[15] An assay for Lp-PLA2 is available for clinical use but has not been incorporated into guidelines for routine risk assessment.[16] Inhibitors of Lp-PLA2 are under investigation for treatment of IHD and, if proven useful for clinical practice, may stimulate new applications for Lp-PLA2 as a biomarker.[17] Homocysteine has also been linked to atherogenesis and correlates with the risk of CAD; however, in aggregate, prospective studies have supported, at most, a modest increase in risk associated with elevated homocysteine levels and have not consistently demonstrated a relationship independent of traditional risk factors or other biochemical markers. Therefore, general screening for elevated homocysteine levels is not recommended.[18]

Advances in understanding regarding the pathobiology of atherothrombosis (see Chap. 43) have generated interest in inflammatory biomarkers as noninvasive indicators of underlying atherosclerosis and cardiovascular risk. The serum concentration of high-sensitivity C-reactive protein (hsCRP) has shown a consistent relationship to the risk of incident cardiovascular events. The prognostic value of hsCRP is additive to traditional risk factors, including lipids[19]; however, the incremental clinical value for screening continues to be debated.[20] Measurement of hsCRP in patients judged at intermediate risk by global risk assessment (10% to 20% risk of coronary heart disease [CHD]/10 years) may help direct further evaluation and therapy in the primary prevention of CHD (see Chap. 44) and may be useful as an

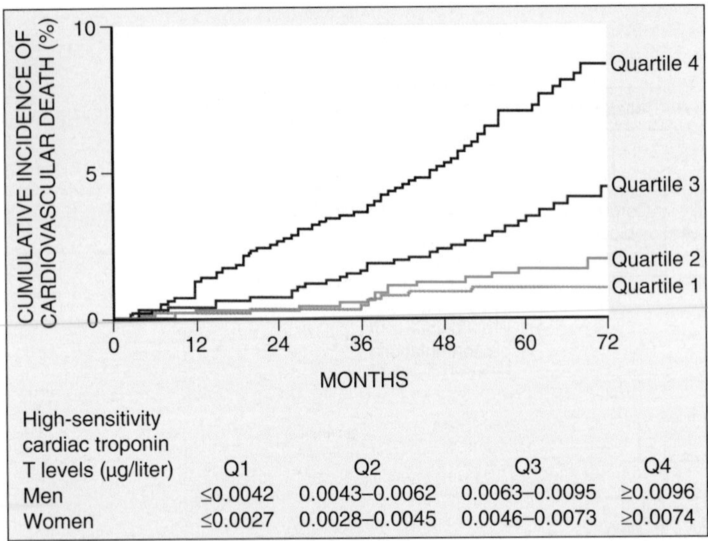

FIGURE 57-3 Incidence of cardiovascular death according to the concentration of high-sensitivity troponin T (hs-TnT) in patients with stable CAD, subgrouped by quartiles of hs-TnT concentration. In a cohort of patients with stable CAD, 97.7% of individuals had detectable circulating cardiac troponin using a sensitive assay, with 11.1% having a concentration that exceeded the 99th percentile reference limit. During a median follow-up of 5.2 years, the incidence of cardiovascular death was associated with the baseline concentration of hs-TnT. This relationship was apparent at concentrations of hs-TnT below the 99th percentile reference limit (0.013 μg/L). *(From Omland T, de Lemos JA, Sabatine MS, et al: A sensitive cardiac troponin T assay in stable coronary artery disease. N Engl J Med 361:2538, 2009.)*

TABLE 57-1 Pretest Likelihood of Coronary Artery Disease in Symptomatic Patients According to Age and Gender*

	Nonanginal Chest Pain		*Atypical Angina*		*Typical Angina*	
AGE (YR)	**MEN**	**WOMEN**	**MEN**	**WOMEN**	**MEN**	**WOMEN**
30-39	4	2	34	12	76	26
40-49	13	3	51	22	87	55
50-59	20	7	65	31	93	73
60-69	27	14	72	51	94	86

*Each value represents the percentage with significant coronary artery disease at coronary angiography.

From Gibbons RJ, Abrams J, Chatterjee K, et al: ACC/AHA 2002 guideline update for the management of patients with chronic stable angina: A report of the American College of Cardiology/American Heart Association Task Force on Practice Guidelines (Committee to update the 1999 guidelines for the management of patients with chronic stable angina) (http://www.acc.org/clinical/guidelines/stable/stable.pdf).

independent marker of prognosis in patients with established CAD. In a randomized double-blind trial in patients free of known atherosclerosis with LDL lower than 130 mg/dL who were identified at higher vascular risk by an elevated hsCRP level (>2 mg/L), treatment with a 3-hydroxy-3-methylglutaryl coenzyme A (HMG-CoA) reductase inhibitor (rosuvastatin) compared with placebo significantly reduced the risk of cardiovascular death and incident atherosclerotic vascular events.[21] On the basis of this finding, some professional society guidelines recommend the use of hsCRP as a risk indicator to support statin therapy in candidates for prevention who are at moderate global risk.[22] Other biomarkers of inflammation, such as myeloperoxidase, growth factors, and metalloproteinases, remain under study as markers of underlying athersclerosis.[23]

Blood levels of cardiac markers of necrosis are typically used to differentiate patients with acute MI from those with stable IHD. However, with more sensitive assays for cardiac troponin, circulating biomarkers of myocyte injury have now been detected in patients with clinically stable IHD and shown to have a graded relationship with the subsequent risk of cardiovascular mortality and heart failure (**Fig. 57-3**).[24,25] Although such evidence may lead to new applications of troponin in patients with stable IHD, clinical use in this population is currently not recommended.[26] Novel biomarkers of myocardial ischemia are also under study. For example, the plasma concentration of brain natriuretic peptide (BNP) increases in response to spontaneous or provoked ischemia.[27] Although BNP and N-terminal pro-BNP may not have sufficient specificity to aid in the diagnosis of stable IHD, their concentration is associated with the risk of future cardiovascular events in those at risk for and with established CAD.[28]

RESTING ELECTROCARDIOGRAPHY. The resting ECG (see Chap. 13) is normal in approximately half of patients with stable IHD, and even patients with severe CAD may have a normal tracing at rest. A normal resting ECG suggests the presence of normal resting LV function and is an unusual finding in a patient with an extensive previous MI. The most common electrocardiographic abnormalities in patients with chronic CAD are nonspecific ST-T wave changes, with or without abnormal Q waves. In addition to myocardial ischemia, other conditions that can produce ST-T wave abnormalities include LV hypertrophy and dilation, electrolyte abnormalities, neurogenic effects, and antiarrhythmic drugs. In patients with known CAD, however, the occurrence of ST-T wave abnormalities on the resting ECG can correlate with the severity of the underlying heart disease. In contrast, a normal resting ECG is a favorable long-term prognostic sign in patients with suspected or definite CAD.

Interval ECGs may reveal the development of Q wave MIs that have gone unrecognized clinically. Various conduction disturbances, most frequently left bundle branch block and left anterior fascicular block, may occur in patients with stable IHD and are often associated with impairment of LV function and reflect multivessel CAD and previous myocardial damage. Hence, such conduction disturbances are an indicator of a relatively poor prognosis. Abnormal Q waves are relatively specific but insensitive indicators of previous MI. Various arrhythmias, especially ventricular premature beats, may be present on the ECG, but they too have low sensitivity and specificity for CAD. LV hypertrophy on the ECG is an indicator of worse prognosis in patients with chronic stable angina. This finding suggests the presence of underlying hypertension, aortic stenosis, hypertrophic cardiomyopathy, or prior MI with remodeling and warrants further evaluation, such as echocardiography to assess LV size, wall thickness, and function.

During an episode of angina pectoris, the ECG becomes abnormal in 50% or more of patients with normal resting ECGs. The most common finding is ST-segment depression, although ST-segment elevation and normalization of resting ST-T wave depression or inversion (pseudonormalization) may develop. Ambulatory electrocardiographic monitoring has shown that many patients with symptomatic myocardial ischemia also have episodes of silent ischemia that would otherwise go unrecognized during normal daily activities. Although this form of electrocardiographic testing provides a quantitative estimate of the frequency and duration of ischemic episodes during routine activities, its sensitivity for detecting CAD is less than that of exercise electrocardiography.

NONINVASIVE STRESS TESTING. Noninvasive stress testing (see Chaps. 14, 15, and 17) can provide useful and often indispensable information to establish the diagnosis and estimate the prognosis in patients with chronic stable angina. However, the indiscriminate use of such tests provides limited incremental information beyond that provided by the physician's detailed and thoughtful clinical assessment. Appropriate application of noninvasive tests requires consideration of Bayesian principles, which state that the reliability and predictive accuracy of any test are defined not only by its sensitivity and specificity but also by the prevalence of disease (or pretest probability) in the population under study. A reasonable estimate of the pretest probability of CAD may be made on clinical grounds (**Table 57-1**).

Noninvasive testing should be performed only if the incremental information provided by a test is likely to alter the planned management strategy. The value of noninvasive stress testing is greatest when the pretest likelihood is intermediate because the test result is likely to have the greatest effect on the post-test probability of CAD and, hence, on clinical decision making.

EXERCISE ELECTROCARDIOGRAPHY

DIAGNOSIS OF CORONARY ARTERY DISEASE. The exercise ECG (see Chap. 14) is particularly helpful for patients with chest pain syndromes who are considered to have a moderate probability of CAD and in whom the resting ECG is normal, provided that they are capable of achieving an adequate workload. Although the incremental diagnostic value of exercise testing is limited in patients in whom the estimated prevalence of CAD is high or low, the test provides useful additional information about the degree of functional limitation in both groups of patients and about the severity of ischemia and prognosis in patients with a high pretest probability of CAD.[29] Interpretation of the exercise test should include consideration of the exercise capacity (duration and metabolic equivalents) and clinical, hemodynamic, and electrocardiographic responses.

INFLUENCE OF ANTIANGINAL THERAPY. Antianginal pharmacologic therapy reduces the sensitivity of exercise testing as a screening tool. Therefore, if the purpose of the exercise test is to diagnose ischemia, it should be performed, if possible, in the absence of antianginal medications. Two or 3 days of interruption is required for patients receiving long-acting beta blockers. For long-acting nitrates, calcium antagonists, and short-acting beta blockers, discontinuing use of the medications the day before testing usually suffices if the purpose of the exercise test is to identify safe levels of daily activity or the extent of functional disability.

NUCLEAR CARDIOLOGY TECHNIQUES (See Chap. 17.)

STRESS MYOCARDIAL PERFUSION IMAGING. Exercise perfusion imaging with simultaneous electrocardiographic testing is superior to exercise electrocardiography alone in detecting CAD, identifying multivessel CAD, localizing diseased vessels, and determining the magnitude of ischemic and infarcted myocardium. Exercise single-photon emission computed tomography (SPECT) yields an average sensitivity and specificity of 88% and 72%, respectively (ranges, 71% to 98% and 36% to 92%, respectively) compared with 68% sensitivity and 77% specificity for exercise electrocardiography alone (**Table 57-2**).[30] Referral bias may account, in part, for the low specificity of many studies, and the few studies that have adjusted for referral bias report a specificity higher than 90%. Perfusion imaging is also valuable for detecting myocardial viability in patients with regional or global LV dysfunction, with or without Q waves, and provides important information in regard to prognosis in all patients.

Stress myocardial scintigraphy is particularly helpful in the diagnosis of CAD in patients with abnormal resting ECGs and in those in whom ST-segment responses cannot be interpreted accurately, such as patients with repolarization abnormalities caused by LV hypertrophy, those with left bundle branch block, and those receiving digitalis. Because stress myocardial perfusion imaging is a relatively expensive test (three to four times the cost of an exercise ECG), stress myocardial perfusion scintigraphy should not be used as a screening test in patients in whom the prevalence of CAD is low, because most abnormal tests will yield false-positive results, and a regular exercise ECG should always be considered first in patients with chest pain and a normal resting ECG for screening and detection of CAD.[30]

PHARMACOLOGIC NUCLEAR STRESS TESTING. For patients unable to exercise adequately, especially older patients and patients with peripheral vascular disease, pulmonary disease, arthritis, other orthopedic limitations, obesity, or a previous stroke, pharmacologic vasodilator stress with dipyridamole or adenosine derivatives may be used.[31] In most nuclear cardiology laboratories, such patients account for approximately 40% of those referred for perfusion imaging. Although the diagnostic accuracy of pharmacologic vasodilator stress perfusion imaging is comparable to that achieved with exercise perfusion imaging (see Table 57-2), treadmill testing is preferred for patients who are capable of exercising because the exercise component of the test provides additional diagnostic and prognostic information, including ST-segment changes, effort tolerance and symptomatic response, and heart rate and blood pressure response. Vasodilator stress agents are also used with PET to diagnose CAD and determine its severity (see Chap. 17).

STRESS ECHOCARDIOGRAPHY. Two-dimensional echocardiography is useful for the evaluation of patients with chronic CAD because it can assess global and regional LV function under basal conditions and during ischemia, as well as detect LV hypertrophy and associated valve disease.[32] Stress echocardiography (see Chap. 15) may be performed using exercise or pharmacologic stress and allows for the detection of regional ischemia by identifying new areas of wall motion disorders. Adequate images can be obtained in more than 85% of patients, and the test is highly reproducible. Numerous studies have shown that exercise echocardiography can detect the presence of CAD with an accuracy similar to that of stress myocardial perfusion imaging and superior to exercise electrocardiography alone (see Table 57-2). Stress echocardiography is also valuable in localizing and quantifying ischemic myocardium (see Fig. 15-25). As with perfusion imaging, stress echocardiography also provides important prognostic information about patients with known or suspected CAD. Pharmacologic stress, such as with dobutamine, should be used for patients unable to exercise, those unable to achieve adequate heart rates with exercise, and those in whom the quality of the echocardiographic images during or immediately after exercise is poor.

Stress echocardiography is an excellent alternative to nuclear cardiology procedures. Limitations imposed by poor visualization of endocardial borders in a sizable subset of patients have been reduced by newer contrast-assisted and imaging technologic modalities (see Chap. 15).[32] Although less expensive than nuclear perfusion imaging, stress echocardiography is more expensive than and not as widely available as exercise electrocardiography.

STRESS CARDIAC MAGNETIC RESONANCE IMAGING. Pharmacologic stress perfusion imaging with cardiac magnetic resonance (CMR) imaging also compares favorably with other methods and is being used clinically in some centers, particularly for individuals who present limitations for the use of other imaging modalities (see Chap. 18).[33,34]

CLINICAL APPLICATIONS OF NONINVASIVE TESTING

GENDER DIFFERENCES IN THE DIAGNOSIS OF CAD. On the basis of earlier studies that indicated a much higher frequency of false-positive stress test results in women than in men, it is generally accepted that electrocardiographic stress testing is not as reliable in women (see Chap. 81). However, the prevalence of CAD in women in the patient populations under study was low, and the lower positive predictive value of exercise electrocardiography in women can be accounted for, in large part, on the basis of Bayesian principles (see Table 57-1).[35] Once men and women are stratified appropriately according to the pretest prevalence of disease, the results of stress testing are similar, although the specificity is probably slightly less in women. Exercise imaging modalities have greater diagnostic accuracy than exercise electrocardiography in men and women.

IDENTIFICATION OF PATIENTS AT HIGH RISK. When applying noninvasive tests to the diagnosis and management of CAD, it is useful to grade the results as negative, indeterminate, positive, not high risk, and positive,

TABLE 57-2 Sensitivity and Specificity of Stress Testing*

MODALITY	TOTAL NO. OF PATIENTS	SENSITIVITY†	SPECIFICITY†
Exercise ECG	24,047	0.68	0.77
Exercise SPECT	5,272	0.88	0.72
Adenosine SPECT	2,137	0.90	0.82
Exercise echocardiography	2,788	0.85	0.81
Dobutamine echocardiography	2,582	0.81	0.79

*Without correction for referral bias.

†Weighted average pooled across individual trials.

Data from Gibbons RJ, Abrams J, Chatterjee K, et al: ACC/AHA 2002 guideline update for the management of patients with chronic stable angina: A report of the American College of Cardiology/American Heart Association Task Force on Practice Guidelines (Committee to update the 1999 guidelines for the management of patients with chronic stable angina) (http://www.acc.org/clinical/guidelines/stable/stable.pdf).

high risk. The criteria for high-risk findings on stress electrocardiography, myocardial perfusion imaging, and stress echocardiography are listed in **Table 57-3**.

Regardless of the severity of symptoms, patients with high-risk noninvasive test results have a high likelihood of CAD and, if they have no obvious contraindications to revascularization, should undergo coronary arteriography. Such patients, even if asymptomatic, are at risk for left main or triple-vessel CAD, and many have impaired LV function. In contrast, patients with clearly negative exercise test results, regardless of symptoms, have an excellent prognosis that cannot usually be improved by revascularization. If they do not have other high risk features or refractory symptoms, coronary arteriography is generally not indicated.

Asymptomatic Persons. Exercise testing in asymptomatic individuals without known CAD is generally not recommended.[36] Exercise testing may be appropriate for asymptomatic individuals with diabetes mellitus who plan to begin vigorous exercise,[37] for those with evidence of myocardial ischemia on ambulatory ECG monitoring, or for those with severe coronary calcifications on cardiac computed tomography (CT; see Chap. 19).

CHEST ROENTGENOGRAPHY. The chest roentgenogram (see Chap. 16) is usually within normal limits in patients with stable IHD, particularly if they have a normal resting ECG and have not experienced an MI. If cardiomegaly is present, it is indicative of severe CAD with previous MI, preexisting hypertension, or an associated nonischemic condition, such as concomitant valvular heart disease, pericardial effusion, or cardiomyopathy.

COMPUTED TOMOGRAPHY. Cardiac multidetector CT (MDCT) has made substantial advances as a noninvasive approach to imaging atherosclerosis (see Chap. 19).[38] In addition to providing a highly sensitive method for detecting coronary calcification which is diagnostic of coronary atherosclerosis, MDCT can also provide an angiogram of the coronary arterial tree.[39]

TABLE 57-3 Risk Stratification Based on Noninvasive Testing

High Risk (>3% Annual Mortality Rate)

1. Severe resting left ventricular dysfunction (LVEF < 0.35)
2. High-risk treadmill score (score ≤ −11)
3. Severe exercise left ventricular dysfunction (exercise LVEF < 0.35)
4. Stress-induced large perfusion defect (particularly if anterior)
5. Stress-induced multiple perfusion defects of moderate size
6. Large, fixed perfusion defect with LV dilation or increased lung uptake (thallium-201)
7. Stress-induced moderate perfusion defect with LV dilation or increased lung uptake (thallium-201)
8. Echocardiographic wall motion abnormality (involving more than two segments) developing at low dose of dobutamine (≤10 μg/kg/min) or at low heart rate (<120 beats/min)
9. Stress echocardiographic evidence of extensive ischemia

Intermediate Risk (1%-3% Annual Mortality Rate)

1. Mild or moderate resting LV dysfunction (LVEF = 0.35-0.49)
2. Intermediate-risk treadmill score (−11 < score < 5)
3. Stress-induced moderate perfusion defect without LV dilation or increased lung intake (thallium-201)
4. Limited stress echocardiographic ischemia with a wall motion abnormality only at higher doses of dobutamine involving two segments or less

Low Risk (<1% Annual Mortality Rate)

1. Low-risk treadmill score (score ≥ 5)
2. Normal or small myocardial perfusion defect at rest or with stress*
3. Normal stress echocardiographic wall motion or no change of limited resting wall motion abnormalities during stress*

*Although the published data are limited, patients with these findings will probably not be at low risk in the presence of a high-risk treadmill score or severe resting LV dysfunction (LVEF < 0.35).

From Gibbons RJ, Abrams J, Chatterjee K, et al: ACC/AHA 2002 guideline update for the management of patients with chronic stable angina: A report of the American College of Cardiology/American Heart Association Task Force on Practice Guidelines (Committee to update the 1999 guidelines for the management of patients with chronic stable angina). (http://www.acc.org/clinical/guidelines/stable/stable.pdf).

The calcium score is a quantitative index of total coronary artery calcium detected by CT, and this score has been shown to be a good marker of the total coronary atherosclerotic burden.[40] Although coronary calcification is a highly sensitive (approximately 90%) finding in patients who have CAD, the specificity for identifying patients with obstructive CAD is low (approximately 50%).[41] In view of this limitation and the potential consequences of unnecessary testing as the result of false-positive results, CT is currently not recommended as a routine approach for screening for obstructive CAD in individuals at low risk for IHD (<10% 10-year estimated risk of coronary events). Moreover, in patients with known or suspected CAD, functional testing is preferable to CT imaging for determining the extent of CAD, the presence of ischemia, and indications for coronary angiography. However, selective screening of individuals at intermediate risk of CAD events may be reasonable to consider because a high calcium score may reclassify an individual at higher risk and thereby lead to more intense risk factor modification. This information should be weighed against the risk of exposure to inonizing radiation.[41a]

CT technology has progressed such that in selected individuals, high-quality images of the coronary arteries may be obtained. As such, CT angiography may be reasonable for symptomatic patients at intermediate risk for coronary disease after initial evaluation—in particular, those with indeterminate results of stress testing.[39] In experienced centers with advanced technology, CT has also been used to characterize plaque composition and, when paired with imaging with PET in a hybrid PET-CT scanner, can offer an assessment of coronary anatomy concurrent with information regarding myocardial blood flow and metabolism.[38] Nevertheless, despite these advances, at present, in most individuals, the temporal resolution of coronary CT angiography is lower than optimal for accurate, complete coronary artery depiction because of nonevaluable segments and limited accuracy in estimating the degree of luminal stenosis. The ability of CT for determination of plaque composition is also currently not sufficient for routine application. The results of ongoing investigation and new technologic innovations will guide evolution of the role of cardiac CT in the assessment and management of IHD.

CARDIAC MAGNETIC RESONANCE IMAGING. Cardiac magnetic resonance imaging (CMR; see Chap. 18) is established as a valuable clinical tool for imaging the aorta and cerebral and peripheral arterial vasculature and is evolving as a versatile noninvasive cardiac imaging modality that has multiple applications for patients with IHD.[39] The clinical use of CMR for myocardial viability assessment has grown based on evidence demonstrating its ability to predict functional recovery after percutaneous or surgical revascularization and its excellent correlation with PET. Pharmacologic stress perfusion imaging with CMR compares favorably with SPECT imaging and also offers accurate characterization of LV function, as well as delineating patterns of myocardial disease that are often useful in discriminating ischemic from nonischemic myocardial dysfunction.

Because of its ability to visualize arteries in three dimensions and differentiate tissue constituents, CMR has received interest as a method to characterize arterial atheroma and assess vulnerability to rupture on the basis of compositional analysis.[42] Arterial plaque has been characterized in the aorta and carotid arteries in humans and has been shown to be predictive of subsequent vascular events.[39] Moreover, CMR coronary angiography in humans is established as a modality to characterize congenital coronary anomalies (see Chaps. 21 and 65), and has shown promise as a method to detect stenoses in the proximal and middle segments of major epicardial vessels or surgical bypass grafts. As such, CMR is continuing to develop as a single approach to assessment of cardiac function, structure, blood flow, and viability without exposing the patient to ionizing radiation.

Catheterization and Coronary Arteriography

The clinical examination and noninvasive techniques described are extremely valuable for establishing the diagnosis of CAD and are indispensable to an overall assessment of patients with this condition.

Currently, however, definitive diagnosis of CAD and precise assessment of its anatomic severity still require cardiac catheterization and coronary arteriography (see Chaps. 20 and 21). In patients with chronic stable angina referred for coronary arteriography, approximately 25% each have single-, double-, or triple-vessel CAD (i.e., more than 70% luminal diameter narrowing); 5% to 10% have obstruction of the left main coronary artery and, in approximately 15%, no flow-limiting obstruction is detectable. Advanced invasive imaging techniques such as intravascular ultrasonography (IVUS) provide a cross-sectional view of the coronary artery and have substantially enhanced the detection and quantification of coronary atherosclerosis, as well as the potential to characterize the vulnerability of coronary atheroma (see Chap. 22).[43] Studies incorporating both coronary angiography and IVUS have demonstrated that the severity of CAD may be underestimated by angiography alone. Intravascular optical coherence tomography, angioscopy, and thermography are evolving as additional tools for more complete characterization of coronary atheroma.[44,45]

Coronary angiographic findings differ between patients presenting with acute MI and those with chronic stable angina. Patients with unheralded MI have fewer diseased vessels, fewer stenoses and chronic occlusions, and less diffuse disease than patients with chronic stable angina, suggesting that the pathophysiologic substrate and propensity for thrombosis differ between these two groups. In patients with chronic angina who have a history of prior MI, total occlusion of at least one major coronary artery is more common than in those without such a history.

CORONARY ARTERY ECTASIA AND ANEURYSMS. Patulous aneurysmal dilation involving most of the length of a major epicardial coronary artery is present in approximately 1% to 3% of patients with obstructive CAD at autopsy or angiography. This angiographic lesion does not appear to affect symptoms, survival, or incidence of MI. Most coronary artery ectasia and/or aneurysms are caused by coronary atherosclerosis (50%), and the rest are caused by congenital anomalies and inflammatory diseases, such as Kawasaki disease.[46] Despite the absence of overt obstruction, 70% of patients with multivessel fusiform coronary artery ectasia or aneurysms have demonstrated evidence of cardiac ischemia based on cardiac lactate levels during ergometry and atrial pacing.

Coronary ectasia should be distinguished from discrete coronary artery aneurysms, which are almost never found in arteries without severe stenosis, are most common in the left anterior descending (LAD) coronary artery, and are usually associated with extensive CAD. These discrete atherosclerotic coronary artery aneurysms do not appear to rupture and their resection is not warranted.

CORONARY COLLATERAL VESSELS. Provided that they are of adequate size, collaterals (see Chap. 21) may protect against MI when total occlusion occurs. In patients with abundant collateral vessels, myocardial infarct size is smaller than in patients without collaterals, and total occlusion of a major epicardial artery may not lead to LV dysfunction. In patients with chronic occlusion of a major coronary artery but without MI, collateral-dependent myocardial segments show almost normal baseline blood flow and O_2 consumption, but severely limited flow reserve. This finding helps explain the ability of collaterals to protect against resting ischemia but not against exercise-induced angina.

MYOCARDIAL BRIDGING. Bridging of coronary arteries (see Chap. 21) is observed by coronary angiography at a rate of less than 5% in otherwise angiographically normal coronary arteries and ordinarily does not constitute a hazard. Occasionally, compression of a portion of a coronary artery by a myocardial bridge can be associated with clinical manifestations of myocardial ischemia during strenuous physical activity and may even result in MI or initiate malignant ventricular arrhythmias. In an autopsy study, increased myocardial bridge thickness and length, as well as proximal vessel location, correlated with an increased risk of MI, proposed to be caused by promotion of proximal atherosclerosis.[47] The functional consequences of myocardial bridging may be characterized with intracoronary Doppler measurements.

LEFT VENTRICULAR FUNCTION. LV function can be assessed by biplane contrast ventriculography (see Chaps. 20 and 21). Global abnormalities of LV systolic function are reflected by elevations in LV end-diastolic and end-systolic volumes and depre[...] fraction. These changes are, however, nonspecif[...] many forms of heart disease. Abnormalities of [...] (e.g., hypokinesis, akinesia, dyskinesia) are more [...] LV relaxation, as reflected in the early diastolic [...] may be impaired at rest in patients with stab[...] becomes even more abnormal (slowed) dur[...] emia intensifies. In patients with stable IHD, the frequen[...] LV end-diastolic pressure and reduced cardiac output at rest, generally attributed to abnormal LV dynamics, increases with the number of vessels exhibiting critical narrowing and with the number of prior MIs. LV end-diastolic pressure may be elevated secondary to reduced LV compliance, LV systolic failure, or a combination of these two processes.

CORONARY BLOOD FLOW AND MYOCARDIAL METABOLISM. Cardiac catheterization can also document abnormal myocardial metabolism in patients with stable IHD. With a catheter in the coronary sinus, arterial and coronary venous lactate measurements are obtained at rest and after suitable stress, such as the infusion of isoproterenol or pacing-induced tachycardia. Because lactate is a byproduct of anaerobic glycolysis, its production by the heart and subsequent appearance in coronary sinus blood is a reliable sign of myocardial ischemia.

Studies of coronary flow reserve (maximum flow divided by resting flow) and endothelial function are frequently abnormal in patients with CAD and may play an important role in determining the functional significance of a stenosis[48] or detecting microvascular dysfunction in those without obstructive epicardial disease. These techniques are discussed in Chap. 52.

Natural History and Risk Stratification

In a registry of patients with a history of stable angina followed in general practices, 29% of patients experienced angina one or more times per week, with associated greater physical limitation and worse quality of life. The frequency of reported angina varied substantially between clinics, suggesting significant heterogeneity in the success of identifying and managing angina.[49] Women have a similar incidence of stable angina to men, and angina in both genders is associated with a higher risk of mortality compared with the general population.[50] Data from the Framingham Study, obtained before the widespread use of aspirin, beta blockers, and aggressive modification of risk factors, revealed an average annual mortality rate of patients with stable IHD of 4%. The combination of these treatments has improved prognosis with an annual mortality rate of 1% to 3% and a rate of major ischemic events of 1% to 2%. For example, among 38,602 outpatients with stable IHD enrolled in 2003 to 2004, the 1-year rate of cardiovascular death was 1.9% (95% confidence interval [CI], 1.7 to 2.1), all-cause mortality was 2.9% (95% CI 2.6 to 3.2), and cardiovascular death, MI, or stroke was 4.5% (95% CI, 4.2 to 4.8).[51] Clinical, noninvasive, and invasive tools are useful for refining the estimate of risk for the individual patient with stable IHD. Moreover, noninvasively acquired information is valuable in identifying patients who are candidates for invasive evaluation with cardiac catheterization.

CLINICAL CRITERIA. Clinical characteristics that include age, male gender, diabetes mellitus, previous MI, and the presence of symptoms typical of angina are predictive of the presence of CAD.[6] A number of studies have attested to the adverse prognostic implications of heart failure in patients with stable IHD. The severity of angina, especially the tempo of intensification, and the presence of dyspnea are also important predictors of outcome.[6]

NONINVASIVE TESTS (see Chaps. 14, 15, and 17)

Exercise Electrocardiography

The prognostic importance of the treadmill exercise test was determined by observational studies in the 1980s and early 1990s. One of the most important and consistent predictors is the maximal exercise capacity, regardless of whether it is measured by exercise duration or workload achieved or whether the test was terminated because of

, fatigue, or angina.[4] After adjustment for age, the peak exercise ity measured in metabolic equivalents (METs) is among the ngest predictors of mortality in men with cardiovascular disease.[29] her factors associated with a poor prognosis identified in patients with chronic stable angina are delineated in Table 57-3.[52]

Stress Nuclear Myocardial Perfusion Imaging

The prognostic value of myocardial perfusion imaging is now well established (see Chap. 17). In particular, the ability of myocardial perfusion SPECT to identify patients at low (less than 1%), intermediate (1% to 5%), or high (more than 5%) risk for future cardiac events is valuable for patient management decisions. The prognostic data obtained from myocardial perfusion SPECT are incremental over clinical and treadmill exercise data for predicting future cardiac events.[38] In patients with normal SPECT imaging findings, the annual risk of death or MI is less than 1%.

Echocardiography

Echocardiographic assessment of LV function is one of the most valuable aspects of noninvasive imaging. Such testing is not necessary for all patients with angina pectoris and, in patients with a normal ECG and no previous history of MI, the likelihood of preserved LV systolic function is high. In contrast, in patients with a history of MI, ST-T wave changes, or conduction defects or Q waves on the ECG, LV function should be measured with echocardiography or an equivalent technique. The presence or absence of inducible regional wall motion abnormalities and the response of the ejection fraction to exercise or pharmacologic stress appear to provide incremental prognostic information to the data provided by the resting echocardiogram. Moreover, a negative stress test portends a low risk for future events (less than 1%/person-year).

Angiographic Criteria. The independent impact of multivessel CAD and LV dysfunction and their interaction with the prognosis of patients with CAD are well established (**Fig. 57-4**). The adverse effects of impaired LV function on prognosis are more pronounced as the number of stenotic vessels increases. Although several indices have been used to quantify the extent of severity of CAD, the simple classification of disease into single-, double-, or triple-vessel or left main CAD is the most widely used and is effective. Additional prognostic information is provided by the severity of obstruction and its location, whether proximal or distal. The concept of the gradient of risk is illustrated in **Figure 57-5**. The importance to survival of the quantity of myocardium that is jeopardized is reflected in the observation that an obstructive lesion proximal to the first septal perforating branch of the LAD coronary artery is associated with a 5-year survival rate of 90% in comparison with 98% for patients with more distal lesions.

High-grade lesions of the left main coronary artery or its equivalent, as defined by severe proximal LAD artery and proximal left circumflex CAD, are particularly life-threatening. Mortality in medically treated patients has been reported to be 29% at 18 months and 43% at 5 years. Survival is better for patients with 50% to 70% stenosis (1- and 3-year survival rates of 91% and 66%, respectively) than for patients with a left main coronary artery stenosis more than 70% (1- and 3-year survival rates of 72% and 41%, respectively).

Limitations of Angiography. The pathophysiologic significance of coronary stenoses lies in their impact on resting and exercise-induced blood flow and in their potential for plaque rupture, with superimposed thrombotic occlusion. It is generally accepted that a stenosis of more than 60% of the luminal diameter is hemodynamically significant in that it may be responsible for a reduction in exercise-induced myocardial blood flow that causes ischemia. The immediate functional significance of obstruction of intermediate severity (approximately 50% diameter stenosis) is less well established. Coronary angiography is not a reliable indicator of the functional significance of stenosis. Moreover, the coronary angiographic determinants of the severity of stenosis are based on a decrease in the caliber of the lumen at the site of the lesion relative to adjacent reference segments, which are considered, often erroneously, to be relatively free of disease. This approach may lead to significant underestimation of the severity and extent of atherosclerosis.

The most serious limitation to the routine use of coronary angiography for prognosis in patients with stable IHD is its inability to identify which coronary lesions can be considered to be at high risk, or vulnerable, for future events, such as MI or sudden death. Although it is widely accepted that MI is the result of thrombotic occlusion at the site of plaque rupture or erosion (see Chaps. 43 and 54), it is clear that it is not necessarily the plaque causing the most severe stenosis that subsequently ruptures. Lesions causing mild obstructions can rupture, thrombose, and occlude, thereby leading to MI and sudden death. Approaches to quantifying the extent of coronary disease, inclusive of nonobstructive lesions, appear to offer additional prognostic information. In contrast, arteries with severe pre-existing stenoses may proceed to clinically silent

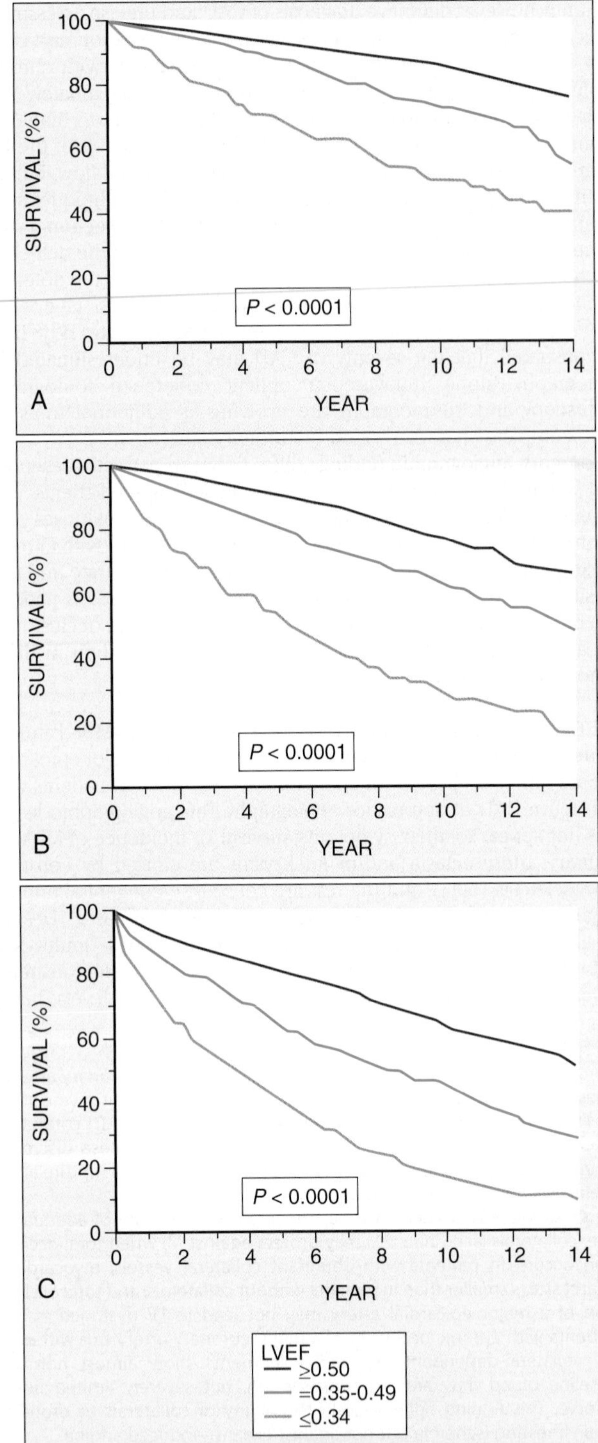

FIGURE 57-4 **A,** Patients with single-vessel coronary disease stratified by normal, moderately, or severely reduced left ventricular ejection fraction (LVEF). **B,** Patients with double-vessel coronary disease stratified by normal, moderately, or severely reduced LVEF. **C,** Patients with triple-vessel coronary disease stratified by normal, moderately, or severely reduced left ventricular LVEF. *(Modified from Emond M, Mock MB, Davis KB, et al: Long-term survival of medically treated patients in the Coronary Artery Surgery Study [CASS] Registry. Circulation 90:2651, 1994.)*

complete occlusion, often without MI, presumably because of the formation of collaterals as the ischemia gradually becomes more severe.

In summary, angiographic documentation of the extent of CAD provides useful information toward assessment of the patient's risk of death and future ischemic events and is an indispensable step in the selection of patients for coronary revascularization, particularly if the interaction between the anatomic extent of disease, LV function, and the severity of ischemia is taken into account. However, angiography is not helpful for predicting the site of subsequent plaque rupture or erosion that can precipitate MI or sudden cardiac death. Additional tools that improve the imaging of coronary atheroma (e.g., IVUS; see Chap. 22) or the functional assessment of a stenosis (e.g., Doppler determination of coronary flow reserve; see Chap. 52) may be helpful in deciding on the flow-limiting significance of a specific lesion and the need for coronary revascularization.[48] Characterization of the atheroma using CT or CMR remains under evaluation but is not yet a routine clinical tool.

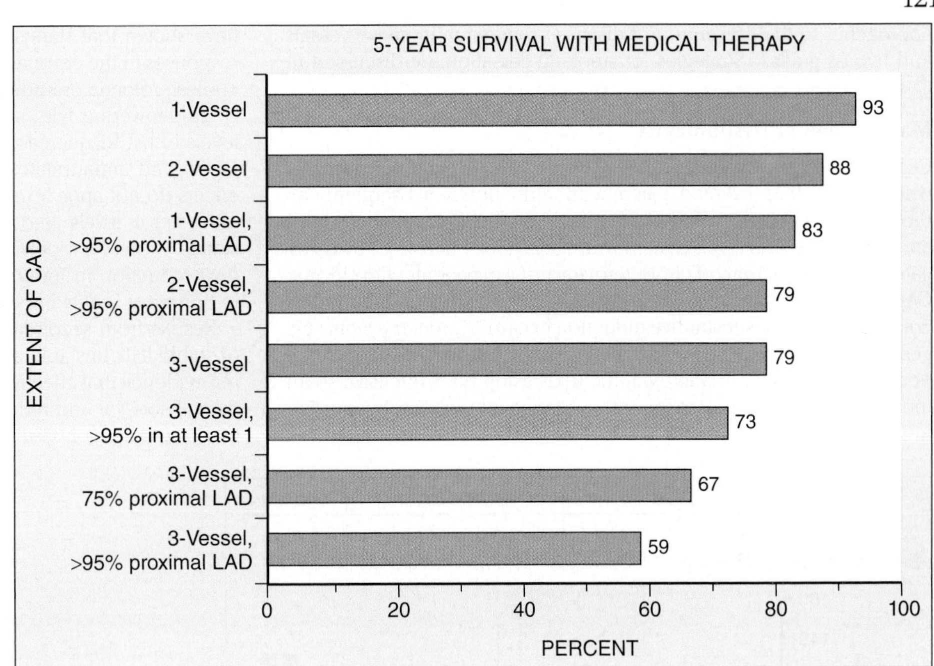

FIGURE 57-5 Angiographic extent of CAD and subsequent survival with medical therapy. A gradient of mortality risk is established based on the number of diseased vessels and the presence and severity of disease of the proximal LAD artery. *(Data from Califf RM, Armstrong PW, Carver JR, et al: Task Force 5: Stratification of patients into high-, medium-, and low-risk subgroups for purposes of risk factor management. J Am Coll Cardiol 27:964, 1996.)*

Medical Management

Comprehensive management of stable IHD has five aspects: (1) identification and treatment of associated diseases that can precipitate or worsen angina and ischemia; (2) reduction of coronary risk factors; (3) application of pharmacologic and nonpharmacologic interventions for secondary prevention, with particular attention to adjustments in lifestyle; (4) pharmacologic management of angina; and (5) revascularization by catheter-based percutaneous coronary intervention (PCI) or by coronary artery bypass grafting (CABG), when indicated. Although discussed individually in this chapter, all five of these approaches must be considered, often simultaneously, in each patient. Of the medical therapies, three (aspirin, angiotensin-converting enzyme [ACE] inhibition, and effective lipid lowering) have been shown to reduce mortality and morbidity in patients with stable IHD and preserved LV function. Other therapies such as nitrates, beta blockers, calcium antagonists, and ranolazine have been shown to improve symptomatology and exercise performance but their effect, if any, on survival in patients with stable IHD has not been demonstrated.

In stable patients with LV dysfunction following MI, evidence has consistently indicated that ACE inhibitors and beta blockers reduce both mortality and the risk of repeat MI, and these agents are recommended for such patients, with or without chronic angina, along with aspirin and lipid-lowering drugs.

TREATMENT OF ASSOCIATED DISEASES. Several common medical conditions that can increase myocardial O_2 demand or reduce O_2 delivery may contribute to the onset of new angina pectoris or the exacerbation of previously stable angina. These conditions include anemia, marked weight gain, occult thyrotoxicosis, fever, infections, and tachycardia. Cocaine, which can cause acute coronary spasm and MI, is discussed in Chap. 73. In patients with CAD, heart failure, by causing cardiac dilation, mitral regurgitation, or tachyarrhythmias (including sinus tachycardia), can increase myocardial O_2 need, along with an increase in the frequency and severity of angina. Identification and treatment of these conditions are critical to the management of stable IHD.

REDUCTION OF CORONARY RISK FACTORS

Hypertension

Epidemiologic links between increased blood pressure (see Chaps. 45, 46, and 49) and CAD severity and mortality are well established. For individuals aged 40 to 70 years, the risk of IHD doubles for each 20-mm Hg increment in systolic blood pressure across the entire range of 115 to 185 mm Hg.[53] Hypertension predisposes to vascular injury, accelerates the development of atherosclerosis, increases myocardial O_2 demand, and intensifies ischemia in patients with preexisting obstructive coronary vascular disease. Although the relationship between hypertension and CAD is linear, LV hypertrophy is a stronger predictor of MI and CAD death than the actual degree of increase in blood pressure.[53] A meta-analysis of clinical trials of treatment of mild to moderate hypertension has shown a statistically significant 16% reduction in CAD events and mortality in patients receiving antihypertensive therapy.[54] This treatment effect is almost twice as great in older compared with younger persons. It is logical to extend these observations about the benefits of antihypertensive therapy to patients with established CAD. Moreover, the number of individuals treated to avoid one death is lower in subjects with established cardiovascular disease. Therefore, blood pressure control is an essential aspect of the management of patients with stable IHD. Although professional society recommendations have advocated a goal of less than 130/80 mm Hg,[53] the results of the Action to Control Cardiovascular Risk in Diabetes (ACCORD) trial, in which 34% of the study population had established cardiovascular disease, did not reveal a significant benefit of targeting a systolic blood pressure below 120 mm Hg versus a level below 140 mm Hg; however, serious adverse events were more frequent in the intensive-therapy group.[54a]

Cigarette Smoking

This remains one of the most powerful risk factors for the development of CAD in all age groups (see Chap. 44). In patients with angiographically documented CAD, cigarette smokers have a higher 5-year risk of sudden death, MI, and all-cause mortality than those who have stopped smoking. Moreover, smoking cessation lessens the risk of adverse coronary events in patients with established CAD. Cigarette smoking may be responsible for aggravating angina other than through the progression of atherosclerosis. It may increase myocardial O_2 demand and reduce coronary blood flow by an alpha-adrenergically mediated increase in coronary artery tone and thereby cause acute ischemia. Moreover, passive exposure to smoke has adverse cardiovascular effects that are almost as great as those of active smoking.[55] Smoking cessation is one of the most effective and cost-effective approaches to the prevention of disease progression in native vessels and bypass grafts.[56] Strategies for smoking cessation are discussed in Chap. 50.

Management of Dyslipidemia

Clinical trials in patients with established atherosclerotic vascular disease have demonstrated a significant reduction in subsequent cardiovascular events in patients with a wide range of serum cholesterol and LDL cholesterol levels treated with statins (see Chap. 47).[57] In aggregate, angiographic trials of cholesterol lowering in patients with chronic CAD have shown that the effects on coronary obstruction are modest compared with the substantive reduction in cardiovascular events, suggesting that atherosclerosis regression is not the primary mechanism of benefit. Nonetheless, in angiographic trials using IVUS, intensive statin therapy has led to regression of coronary atherosclerotic burden in patients with angiographic CAD.[58,59] Also, several, but not all, studies have shown that statins significantly improve endothelium-mediated responses in the coronary and systemic arteries of patients with hypercholesterolemia or known atherosclerosis.

Lipid-lowering with statins has been shown to reduce circulating levels of hsCRP, decrease thrombogenicity, and favorably alter the collagen and inflammatory components of arterial atheroma; these effects do not appear to correlate well with the change in serum LDL cholesterol levels and suggest antiatherothrombotic properties of statins.[60] These properties may contribute to improvement in blood flow, reduction in inducible myocardial ischemia, and the reduction in coronary events in patients treated with statins.

Results from secondary prevention trials of patients with a history of stable IHD, unstable angina, or previous MI have provided convincing evidence that effective lipid-lowering therapy significantly improves overall survival and reduces cardiovascular mortality in patients with CAD, regardless of baseline cholesterol. The National Cholesterol Education Program Guidelines (see Chaps. 47 and 49) advocate cholesterol-lowering therapy for all patients with CAD or extracardiac atherosclerosis to LDL levels below 100 mg/dL, and these guidelines have been adopted in recommendations from the American College of Cardiology/American Heart Association (ACC/AHA).[57] Moreover, results from trials of intensive versus moderate dose statin therapy in patients with recent acute coronary syndrome (ACS) and in patients with stable IHD have provided evidence for a reduction in major cardiovascular events with more aggressive lipid lowering therapy to an LDL concentration lower than 100 mg/dL (**Fig. 57-6**).[61-63] These findings have led to the recommendation that it is reasonable to treat all patients with CAD to an achieved LDL concentration of less than 70 mg/dL (see Chap. 49).

LOW LEVEL OF HDL CHOLESTEROL. Patients with established CAD and low levels of HDL cholesterol represent a subgroup at considerable risk for future coronary events, even when LDL cholesterol is low.[64,65] Low HDL levels are often associated with obesity, hypertriglyceridemia, and insulin resistance and often signify the presence of small lipoprotein remnants and small, dense, LDL particles that are thought to be particularly atherogenic (see Chap. 47). Therapy has focused on diet and exercise, as well as on LDL cholesterol reduction, in patients with a concomitant increase in HDL cholesterol levels. The Veterans Affairs High-Density Lipoprotein Cholesterol Intervention Trial (VA-HIT) Study Group has demonstrated the efficacy of gemfibrozil treatment in men with low HDL cholesterol (40 mg/dL or lower) without elevations in LDL cholesterol (140 mg/dL or lower) or triglyceride levels (mean, 160 mg/dL). Gemfibrozil resulted in a 6% increase in HDL cholesterol and a 31% decrease in triglyceride levels, and these changes were associated with a 24% reduction in death, nonfatal MI, and stroke. Emerging therapies aimed at promoting reverse cholesterol transport and/or interfering

Patients	ACS		Stable CAD		Pooled
n	4162	4497	10001	8888	27548
Prior statin use	25.2%	0%	0%	75.5%	28.2%

LDL-C (mg/dl)

	PROVE IT–TIMI 22	A-to-Z	TNT	IDEAL	Pooled*
Baseline	108	113	152	122	130
Standard	97	101	101	104	101
Intensive	65	69	77	81	75

■ Baseline
● Standard
▲ Intensive

A

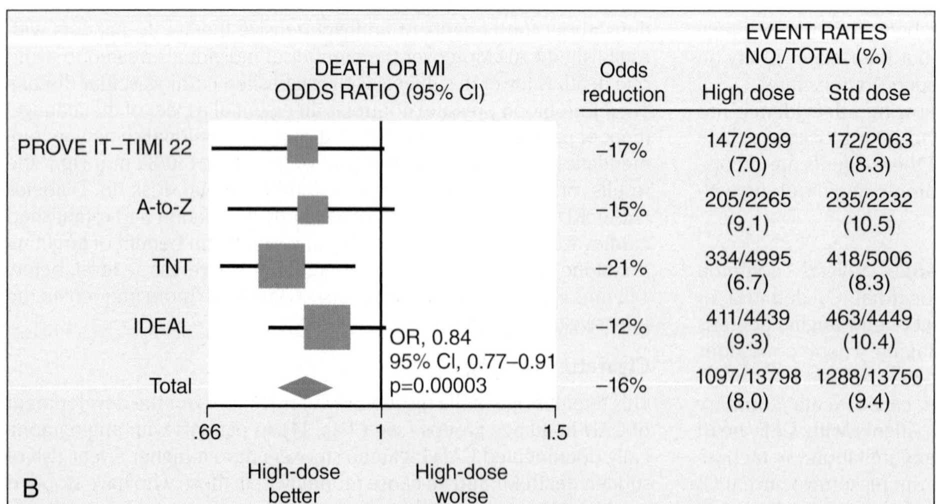

FIGURE 57-6 Pooled evaluation of intensive versus standard statin therapy for patients with established coronary artery disease in the Pravastatin or Atorvastatin Evaluation and Infection Therapy Trial (PROVE-IT-TIMI 22; atorvastatin, 80 mg daily, versus pravastatin, 40 mg daily), Aggrastat-to-Zocor Trial (A-to-Z; simvastatin, 40 mg daily, for 30 days followed by 80 mg daily, versus placebo for 4 months, followed by simvastatin, 20 mg daily), Treat to New Targets Trial (TNT; atorvastatin, 80 mg daily, versus atorvastatin, 10 mg daily), and Incremental Decrease in Endpoints Through Aggressive Lipid-Lowering Trial (IDEAL; atorvastatin, 80 mg daily versus simvastatin, 20 mg daily). Intensive statin therapy was associated with significantly lower achieved levels of low-density lipoprotein cholesterol, LDL-C **(A)** and a 16% lowering of the risk of death or myocardial infarction, MI **(B)**. OR = odds ratio. *(From Cannon CP, Steinberg BA, Murphy SA, et al: Meta-analysis of cardiovascular outcomes trials comparing intensive versus moderate statin therapy. J Am Coll Cardiol 48:438, 2006.)*

with HDL metabolism to raise the concentration of HDL or the related apolipoprotein A-I (the main protein in HDL) are under investigation.[66] In two large randomized trials, torcetrapib, a cholesteryl ester transfer protein (CETP) inhibitor, increased HDL cholesterol by 61% and reduced LDL cholesterol by 20%, but did not decrease progression of atherosclerosis[67] and was associated with an increase in ischemic events, which may be explained by an increase in blood pressure with torcetrapib.[68] It is not known whether there are other unexpected adverse effects specific to this molecule or its drug class.

Management of Diabetes Mellitus. Patients with diabetes mellitus (see Chaps. 49 and 64) are at significantly higher risk of atherosclerotic vascular disease. Although a favorable impact of control of glycemia on microvascular complications of diabetes is established, the effect on macrovascular complications (including CAD) is unclear. During a mean follow-up of 17 years in participants in the Diabetes Control and Complications Trial, patients with type 1 diabetes assigned to intensive glycemic therapy were at lower risk of cardiovascular complications.[69] In an analysis of a secondary endpoint of the Prospective Pioglitazone Clinical Trial in Macrovascular Events Trial (PROACTIVE), treatment of patients with type 2 diabetes with the oral hypoglycemic agent pioglitazone reduced the risk of death, nonfatal MI, or stroke.[70] Caution is raised regarding interpretation of this finding from PROACTIVE on controlling hyperglycemia given the neutral result of the trial with respect to its primary endpoint and effects of pioglitazone on metabolic elements other than blood glucose level. Several large trials evaluating the effects of oral hypoglycemic agents on cardiovascular outcomes are ongoing. Management of hypercholesterolemia and hypertension are particularly important in patients with type 2 diabetes.[57,69]

Estrogen Replacement. In view of the collective data from randomized clinical trials, it is not advised that hormone replacement therapy be initiated or continued for secondary cardiovascular prevention in women with CAD (see Chap. 81).[57]

Exercise

The conditioning effect of exercise (see Chap. 50) on skeletal muscles allows a greater workload at any level of total body O_2 consumption. By decreasing the heart rate at any level of exertion, a higher cardiac output can be achieved at any level of myocardial O_2 consumption. The combination of these two effects of exercise conditioning permits patients with chronic stable angina to increase physical performance substantially following the institution of a continuing exercise program.[71,72]

Most information about the physiologic effects of exercise and their effect on prognosis in patients with CAD has come from studies on patients entered into cardiac rehabilitation programs, many of whom previously sustained a MI. Less information is available on the benefits of exercise in patients with stable IHD without a prior MI., Collectively, small randomized trials evaluating exercise training in patients with stable IHD have indicated improved effort tolerance, O_2 consumption, quality of life, and reduced evidence of ischemia with myocardial perfusion imaging.[71] One randomized trial of exercise training compared with angioplasty in 101 patients with stable angina showed fewer hospitalizations and revascularization procedures in those allocated to regular exercise.[73] Others have demonstrated a striking and direct relationship between the intensity of exercise and favorable changes in inflammatory and hemostatic mediators of cardiovascular risk,[74] the morphology of obstructive lesions on angiography, and vascular endothelial function, thought to be mediated through the expression and phosphorylation of endothelial nitric oxide synthase. Whether exercise accelerates the development of collateral vessels in patients with chronic CAD is unclear.

Exercise is safe if begun under supervision and increased gradually[75] and, if survivors of MI can be used as a yardstick, is probably cost-effective. The psychological benefits of exercise are difficult to evaluate. However, a single nonrandomized study has demonstrated significant improvement in well-being scores and positive affect scores, as well as a reduction in disability scores, in patients in a structured exercise program. Patients who are involved in exercise programs are also more likely to be health conscious, pay attention to diet and weight, and discontinue cigarette smoking. For all these reasons, patients should be urged to participate in regular exercise programs, usually walking, in conjunction with their drug therapy.[72]

Inflammation

Atherothrombosis has been recognized as an inflammatory disease (see Chaps. 43, 44, and 49).[76] Moreover, markers of systemic inflammation, of which hsCRP is the most extensively studied, identify patients with established vascular disease who are at higher risk for death and future ischemic events. Therefore, inflammation has been identified as a potential target for therapeutic intervention in patients with IHD. For example, in a number of studies, treatment with statins has lowered the serum concentration of hsCRP. In addition, lower levels of hsCRP achieved with statin therapy in patients 1 month after an ACS are associated with better long-term prognosis.[77,78] Also, in a large randomized, placebo-controlled trial in individuals with average LDL levels and no known atherosclerosis but an increased risk of atherothrombosis identified with elevated hsCRP, statin therapy reduced the risk of first major cardiovascular events.[21] Although it is challenging to dissect the potential benefit of anti-inflammatory effects of statins from those derived from lowering LDL cholesterol, these findings lend support to the hypothesis that statins are effective in modifying the risk associated with evidence of systemic inflammation and that inflammatory markers may complement LDL measurement in guiding statin therapy.[22] Other established preventive interventions, as well as novel therapeutic strategies, may also have anti-inflammatory effects that could target inflammation. Aspirin, ACE inhibitors, thiazolidinediones, thienopyridines, and fibric acid derivatives are among those agents that have been shown to exert anti-inflammatory or immunoregulatory actions.[76] Additional research is needed to clarify whether inflammation should be a target for routine strategies for risk reduction or novel therapeutic agents in patients with stable IHD.

Obesity

Obesity (see Chaps. 44 and 64) is an independent contributor to the risk for IHD and is associated with a constellation of other risk factors, including hypertension, dyslipidemia, and abnormal glucose metabolism. Weight loss can improve or prevent many of the cardiovascular consequences of obesity.[79]

Additional Disease-Modifying Pharmacotherapy for Secondary Prevention

Aspirin. A meta-analysis of 140,000 patients in 300 studies has confirmed the prophylactic benefit of aspirin (see Chaps. 49 and 87) in men and women with angina pectoris, previous MI, or stroke and after CABG. In a Swedish trial of men and women with chronic stable angina, 75 mg of aspirin in conjunction with the beta blocker sotalol conferred a 34% reduction in acute MI and sudden death. In a smaller study confined to men with chronic stable angina but without a history of MI, 325 mg of aspirin on alternate days reduced the risk of MI by 87% during 5 years of follow-up. Therefore, administration of aspirin daily is advisable for patients with stable IHD without contraindications to this drug.[57,80] Dosing at 75 to 162 mg daily appears to have comparable effects for secondary prevention with dosing at 160 to 325 mg daily and appears to be associated with lower bleeding risk. Aspirin 75 to 162 mg daily is thus preferred for secondary prevention in the absence of recent intracoronary stenting. Although warfarin has proved beneficial in patients after MI, no evidence supports the use of chronic anticoagulation in patients with stable angina.

Clopidogrel. Other orally acting antiplatelet agents have been studied in patients with stable IHD. Clopidogrel, a thienopyridine derivative, may be substituted for aspirin in patients with aspirin hypersensitivity or those who cannot tolerate aspirin (see Chap. 87).[57] In a randomized comparison between clopidogrel and aspirin in patients with established atherosclerotic vascular disease (the Clopidogrel versus Aspirin in Patients at Risk of Ischaemic Events [CAPRIE] trial), treatment with clopidogrel resulted in a modest 8.7% relative reduction in the risk of vascular death, ischemic stroke, or MI ($P = 0.043$) over 2 years. Studies evaluating the addition of clopidogrel to aspirin in patients with non–ST-segment elevation ACS or after PCI have demonstrated robust risk reductions. However, the Clopidogrel for High Atherothrombotic Risk and Ischemic Stabilization Management and Avoidance (CHARISMA) trial showed no overall benefit of the addition of clopidogrel to aspirin with respect to the primary endpoint of cardiovascular death, MI, or stroke over a median of 28 months (6.8%% versus 7.3%; $P = 0.22$) in patients with clinically evident cardiovascular disease (N = 12,153) or multiple risk factors (N = 3,284).[81] In the subgroup of those with established vascular disease, the addition of clopidogrel was associated with a 1% lower risk of these events (6.9 versus

7.9%; $P = 0.046$), supporting a hypothesis of a potential modest benefit from clopidogrel in patients with stable IHD taking aspirin.[82] Ongoing studies are testing the hypothesis that more potent antiplatelet therapy than aspirin alone is useful for patients with stable IHD.[83]

Beta Blockers. The value of beta blockers in reducing death and recurrent MI in patients who have experienced a MI is well established (see Chaps. 49 and 55), as is their usefulness in the treatment of angina. Moreover, patients receiving beta blockers for hypertension are more likely to present with stable angina rather than MI as their first manifestation of CAD.[84] Whether these drugs are also of value in preventing MI and sudden death in patients with stable IHD without previous MI is uncertain and, despite at least one observational study suggesting lower mortality in the patients who were taking beta blockers,[85] there have been no controlled trials against placebo. However, there is no reason to assume that the favorable effects of beta blockers on ischemia and perhaps on arrhythmias should not apply to patients with stable IHD. In addition, observational data have raised the possibility that beta blockers may reduce the progression of coronary atherosclerosis, in part through reduced turbulence and reduced intramural arterial wall stress.[86] Therefore, although the use of beta blockers as first-line agents for uncomplicated hypertension has been questioned, it is sensible to use these drugs when angina, hypertension, or both are present in patients with stable IHD and when these drugs are well tolerated.[87] Emerging evidence also has identified genetic polymorphisms of the $beta_2$-adrenergic receptor gene (*ADRB1* and *ADRB2*) that may influence beta blocker responsiveness.[88]

Angiotensin-Converting Enzyme Inhibitors and Angiotensin Receptor Blockers. Although inhibitors of the renin-angiotensin-aldosterone system are not indicated for the treatment of angina, these drugs appear to have important benefits in reducing the risk of future ischemic events in some patients with cardiovascular disease.[89] An unexpected finding from randomized trials of ACE inhibitors in postinfarction and other patients with ischemic and nonischemic causes of LV dysfunction was a significant reduction in the incidence of subsequent coronary ischemic events. The potentially beneficial effects of ACE inhibitors include reductions in LV hypertrophy, vascular hypertrophy, progression of atherosclerosis, plaque rupture, and thrombosis, in addition to a potentially favorable influence on myocardial O_2 supply and demand relationships, cardiac hemodynamics, sympathetic activity, and coronary endothelial vasomotor function. In addition, in vitro experiments have shown that angiotensin II induces inflammatory changes in human vascular smooth muscle cells, and treatment with ACE inhibitors can reduce signs of inflammation in animal models of atherosclerosis.

Two trials have provided strong evidence supporting the therapeutic benefit of ACE inhibitors in patients with normal LV function and absence of heart failure (**Fig. 57-7**). In the Heart Outcomes Protection Evaluation (HOPE) study, ramipril significantly decreased the risk of the primary

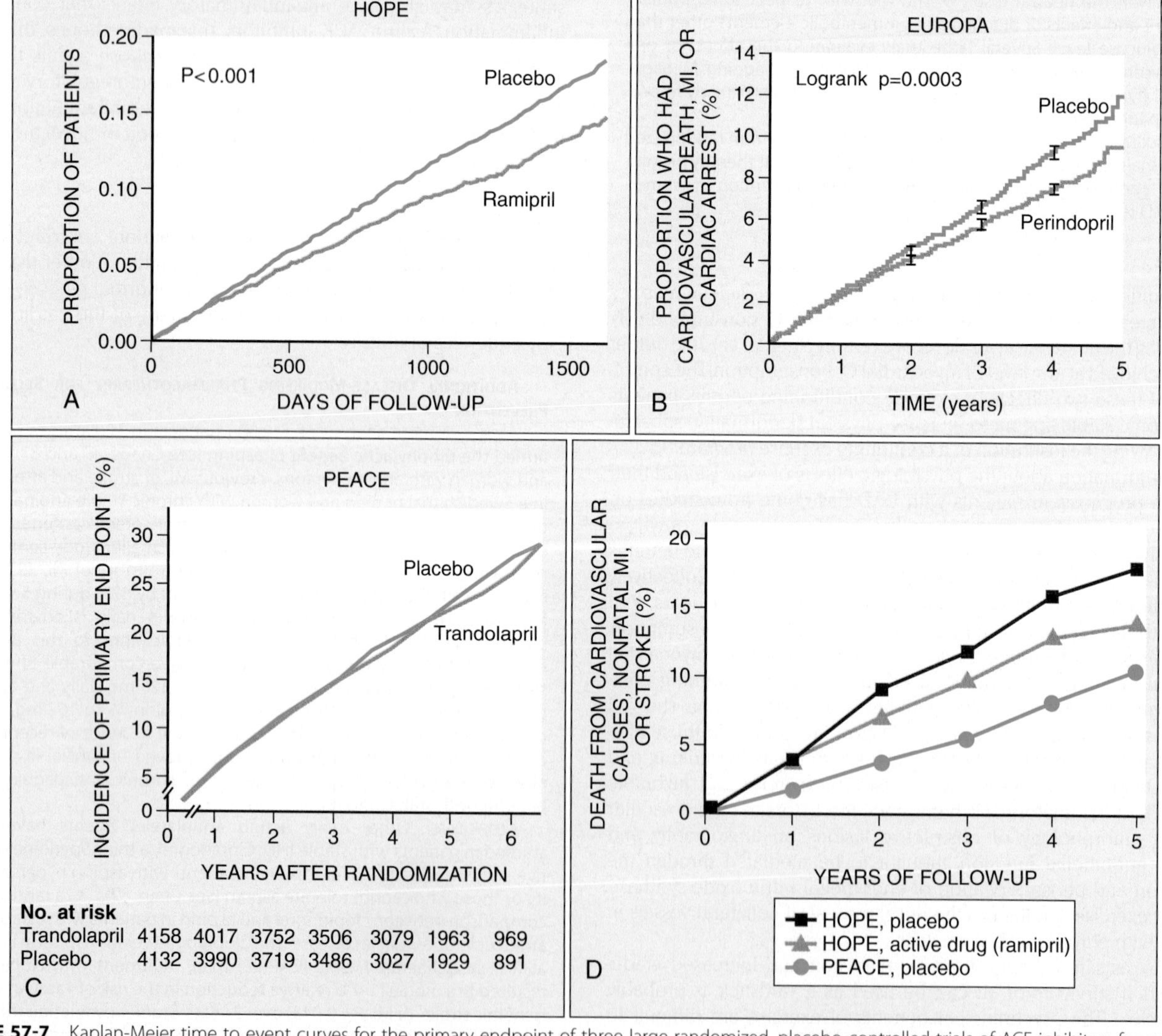

FIGURE 57-7 Kaplan-Meier time to event curves for the primary endpoint of three large randomized, placebo-controlled trials of ACE inhibitors for patients at high risk for or with established cardiovascular disease without heart failure. **A,** Cumulative incidence of cardiovascular death, MI, or stroke with ramipril versus placebo among patients in the HOPE trial. **B,** Cumulative incidence of cardiovascular death, MI, or cardiac arrest with perindopril or placebo in the European Trial on the EUROPA trial. **C,** Cumulative incidence of cardiovascular death, MI, or coronary revascularization in the PEACE trial. **D,** Comparison of cardiovascular death, MI, or stroke in the HOPE and PEACE trials. The cumulative incidence of major cardiovascular events was lower in patients treated with placebo in PEACE than in the patients treated with ramipril in HOPE. (***A,*** *from HOPE Study Investigators: Effects of an angiotensin-converting enzyme inhibitor, ramipril, on cardiovascular events in high risk patients. N Engl J Med 342:145, 2000;* ***B,*** *from EUROPA Investigators: Efficacy of perindopril in reduction of cardiovascular events among patients with stable coronary artery disease: Randomized double-blind, placebo-controlled, multicenter trial [the EUROPA study]. Lancet 363:782, 2003;* ***C,*** *from PEACE Trial Investigators: Angiotensin-converting enzyme inhibition in stable coronary artery disease. N Engl J Med 351:2058, 2004.)*

preparations are available in sublingual, buccal, oral, spray, and ointment forms (see Table 57-5). An oral nitroglycerin spray that dispenses metered, aerosolized doses of 0.4 mg may be better absorbed than the sublingual form by patients with dry mucosal membranes. It can also be quickly sprayed onto or under the tongue. For prophylaxis, the spray should be used 5 to 10 minutes before angina-provoking activities.

Isosorbide Dinitrate

This drug is an effective antianginal agent but has low bioavailability after oral administration. It undergoes hepatic metabolism rapidly, and marked variation in plasma concentrations may be seen after oral administration. It has two metabolites, one with potent vasodilator action, which are cleared less rapidly than the parent drug and excreted unchanged in the urine. It is available in tablets for sublingual use, in chewable form, in tablets for oral use, and in sustained-release capsules.

Partial or complete nitrate tolerance (see later) develops with regimens of isosorbide dinitrate when administered as 30 mg three or four times daily. A dosage schedule should be adopted that allows a 10- to 12-hour nitrate-free interval. If the drug is administered on a three times daily schedule (e.g., at 8 AM, 1 PM, and 6 PM), the antianginal benefit lasts for approximately 6 hours, and the magnitude of the antianginal benefit decreases with each successive dose.

Isosorbide 5-Mononitrate

This active metabolite of the dinitrate is completely bioavailable with oral administration because it does not undergo first-pass hepatic metabolism; it is efficacious in the treatment of chronic stable angina. Plasma levels of isosorbide 5-mononitrate reach their peak between 30 minutes and 2 hours after ingestion, and the drug has a plasma half-life of 4 to 6 hours. A single 20-mg tablet still exhibits activity 8 hours after administration. Tolerance has not been demonstrated with once-daily or eccentric dosing intervals but does occur with a twice-daily dosing regimen at 12-hour intervals. The sustained-release preparation of isosorbide 5-mononitrate may be given once daily in a dosage of 30 to 240 mg. Presumably, this preparation avoids tolerance by providing a sufficiently low nitrate level or a duration of action of 12 hours or less. Once-daily dosing of oral nitrates improves compliance and may offer better efficacy in reducing angina.[109,110]

Topical Nitroglycerin

1. *Ointment.* Nitroglycerin ointment (15 mg/inch) is efficacious when applied (most commonly to the chest) in strips of 0.5 to 2.0 inches. The delay in onset of action is approximately 30 minutes. Because this form of the drug is effective for 4 to 6 hours, it is particularly useful for patients with severe angina or unstable angina who are confined to bed and chair. Nitroglycerin ointment may also be used prophylactically after retiring by patients with nocturnal angina. Skin permeability increases with increased hydration, and absorption is also enhanced if the paste is covered with plastic, with the edges taped to the skin.
2. *Transdermal Patches.* Application of silicone gel or polymer matrix impregnated with nitroglycerin results in absorption for 24 to 48 hours at a rate determined by various methods of preparation of the patch, including a semipermeable membrane placed between the drug reservoir and the skin. The release rate of the patches varies from 0.1 to 0.8 mg/hr. Relatively low doses (0.1 to 0.2 mg/hr) may not produce sufficient plasma and tissue concentrations to sustain consistent, effective antianginal effects. Transdermal nitroglycerin therapy has been shown to increase exercise duration and maintain anti-ischemic effects for 12 hours after patch application throughout 30 days of therapy, without significant evidence of nitrate tolerance or rebound phenomena, provided that the patch is not applied for more than 12 out of 24 hours.

Nitrate Tolerance. A major problem with the use of nitrates is the development of nitrate tolerance, which has been demonstrated with all forms of nitrate administration delivering continuous, relatively stable blood levels of the drug. Although nitrate tolerance is rapid in onset, renewed responsiveness is easily established after a short nitrate-free interval. The problem of tolerance applies to all nitrate preparations; it is particularly important in patients with chronic angina, as opposed to those receiving short-acting courses of nitrates (e.g., with unstable angina and MI). Nitrate tolerance appears to be limited to the capacitance and resistance vessels and has not been noted in the large conductance vessels, including the epicardial coronary arteries and radial arteries, despite continuous administration of nitroglycerin for 48 hours.

Mechanisms. Several mechanisms of nitrate tolerance have been proposed. Evidence has supported the hypothesis that increased generation of vascular superoxide anion ($\cdot O_2^-$) is central to the process.[111] There are various possible contributors to generation of oxygen free radicals, including the effects of nitroglycerin on endothelial nitric oxide synthase (NOS) uncoupling and counterregulatory neurohormonal activation. There are a number of consequences of increased superoxide anion formation; these include plausible links to many of the proposed mechanisms of nitrate tolerance: (1) plasma volume expansion and neurohormonal activation; (2) impaired biotransformation of nitrates to NO; and (3) decreased end-organ responsiveness to NO.

Management. The primary strategy to manage nitrate tolerance is to prevent it by providing a nitrate-free interval. The optimal interval is unknown, but with patches or ointment of nitroglycerin or preparations of isosorbide dinitrate or isosorbide 5-mononitrate, a 12-hour off-period is recommended.

Nitrate Withdrawal. A common form of nitrate withdrawal (rebound) is observed in patients whose angina is intensified after discontinuation of large doses of long-acting nitrates. In this situation, patients may also have heightened sensitivity to constrictor stimuli. The potential for rebound can be modified by adjusting the dose and timing of administration in addition to the use of other antianginal drugs.

Interaction with PDE5 Inhibitors. The combination of nitrates and PDE5 inhibitors, such as sildenafil, may cause serious, prolonged, and potentially life-threatening hypotension.[112] Nitrate therapy is an absolute contraindication to the use of PDE5 inhibitors, and vice versa. Patients who wish to take this class of medications should be aware of the serious nature of this adverse drug interaction and be warned about taking a PDE5 inhibitor within 24 hours of any nitrate preparation, including short-acting sublingual nitroglycerin tablets.

BETA-ADRENERGIC BLOCKING AGENTS. Beta-adrenergic blocking drugs (beta blockers) constitute a cornerstone of therapy for angina.[113] In addition to their antiischemic properties, beta blockers are effective antihypertensives (see Chap. 46) and antiarrhythmics (see Chap. 37). They have also been shown to reduce mortality and reinfarction in patients after MI (see Chap. 55) and to reduce mortality in patients with heart failure (see Chap. 28). This combination of actions makes them extremely useful in the management of stable IHD. A number of studies have shown that beta blockers, in doses that are generally well tolerated, reduce the frequency of anginal episodes and raise the anginal threshold when given alone and when added to other antianginal agents.

The beneficial actions of these drugs depend on their ability to cause competitive inhibition of the effects of neuronally released and circulating catecholamines on beta adrenoceptors (**Table 57-6**). Beta blockade reduces myocardial O_2 requirements, primarily by slowing the heart rate; the slower heart rate in turn increases the fraction of the cardiac cycle occupied by diastole, with a corresponding increase in the time available for coronary perfusion (**Fig. 57-8**; see Table 57-4). These drugs also reduce exercise-induced increases in blood pressure and limit exercise-induced increases in contractility. Thus, beta blockers reduce myocardial O_2 demand primarily during activity or excitement, when surges of increased sympathetic activity occur. In the face of impaired myocardial perfusion, the effects of beta blockers on myocardial O_2 demand may critically and favorably alter the imbalance between supply and demand, thereby resulting in the elimination of ischemia.

Beta blockers may reduce blood flow to most organs by means of the combination of $beta_2$ receptor blockade and unopposed alpha-adrenergic vasoconstriction and (**Table 57-7**). Complications are relatively minor but, in patients with peripheral vascular disease, the reduction in blood flow to skeletal muscles with the use of nonselective beta blockers may reduce maximal exercise capacity. In patients with preexisting LV dysfunction, beta blockade may increase LV volume and thereby increase O_2 demand.

TABLE 57-6 Physiologic Actions of Beta-Adrenergic Receptors

ORGAN	RECEPTOR TYPE	RESPONSE TO STIMULUS
Heart		
SA node	Beta$_1$	Increased heart rate
Atria	Beta$_1$	Increased contractility and conduction velocity
AV node	Beta$_1$	Increased automaticity and conduction velocity
His-Purkinje system	Beta$_1$	Increased automaticity and system conduction velocity
Ventricles	Beta$_1$	Increased automaticity, contractility, and conduction velocity
Arteries		
Peripheral	Beta$_2$	Dilation
Coronary	Beta$_2$	Dilation
Carotid	Beta$_2$	Dilation
Other	Beta$_2$	Increased insulin release; increased liver and muscle glycogenolysis
Lungs	Beta$_2$	Dilation of bronchi
Uterus	Beta$_2$	Smooth muscle relaxation

AV = atrioventricular; SA = sinoatrial.

From Abrams J: Medical therapy of stable angina pectoris. *In* Beller G, Braunwald E (eds): Chronic Ischemic Heart Disease. Atlas of Heart Disease. Vol 5. Philadelphia, WB Saunders 1995, p 7.19.

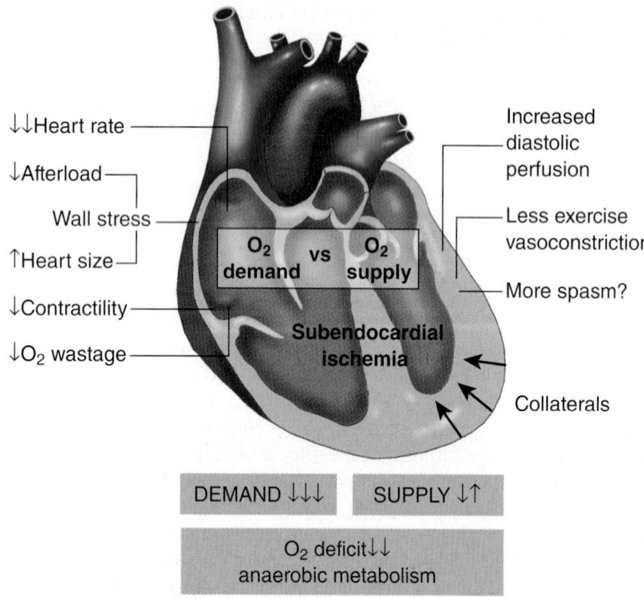

FIGURE 57-8 Effects of beta blockade on the ischemic heart. Beta blockade has a beneficial effect on ischemic myocardium unless (1) the preload rises substantially, as in left-sided heart failure, or (2) vasospastic angina is present, in which case spasm may be promoted in some patients. Note the suggestion that beta blockade diminishes exercise-induced vasoconstriction. *(Modified from Opie LH: Drugs for the Heart. 4th ed. Philadelphia, WB Saunders, 1995, p 6.)*

CHARACTERISTICS OF DIFFERENT BETA BLOCKERS

SELECTIVITY. Two major subtypes of beta receptors, designated beta$_1$ and beta$_2$, are present in different proportions in different tissues. Beta$_1$ receptors predominate in the heart, and stimulation of these receptors leads to an increase in heart rate, atrioventricular (AV) conduction, and contractility, release of renin from juxtaglomerular cells in the kidneys, and lipolysis in adipocytes. Beta$_2$ stimulation causes bronchodilation, vasodilation, and glycogenolysis. Nonselective beta-blocking drugs (e.g., propranolol, nadolol, penbutolol, pindolol, sotalol, timolol, carteolol) block both beta$_1$ and beta$_2$ receptors, whereas cardioselective beta blockers (e.g., acebutolol, atenolol, betaxolol, bisoprolol, esmolol, metoprolol, nebivolol) block beta$_1$ receptors while having less effect on beta$_2$ receptors. Thus, cardioselective beta blockers reduce myocardial O_2 requirements while tending not to block bronchodilation, vasodilation, or glycogenolysis. However, as the doses of these drugs are increased, this cardioselectivity diminishes. Because cardioselectivity is only relative, the use of cardioselective beta blockers in doses sufficient to control angina may still cause bronchoconstriction in some susceptible patients. Nevertheless, beta blockers are relatively well tolerated in most patients with obstructive pulmonary disease.[114]

Some beta blockers also cause vasodilation. Such drugs include labetalol (an alpha-adrenergic blocking agent and beta$_2$ agonist; see Chap. 46), carvedilol (with alpha- and beta$_1$-blocking activity), bucindolol (a nonselective beta blocker that causes direct [non–alpha-adrenergic mediated] vasodilation), and nebivolol (a cardioselective beta blocker with a direct stimulatory effect on endothelial nitric oxide synthase, eNOS).[115]

ANTIARRHYTHMIC ACTIONS. Beta blockers have antiarrhythmic properties as a direct effect of their ability to block sympathoadrenal myocardial stimulation, which in certain situations may be arrhythmogenic (see Chap. 37).

INTRINSIC SYMPATHOMIMETIC ACTIVITY. Beta blockers with intrinsic sympathomimetic activity (ISA), such as acebutolol, bucindolol, carteolol, celiprolol, penbutolol, and pindolol, are partial beta agonists that also produce blockade by shielding beta receptors from more potent beta agonists. Pindolol and acebutolol produce low-grade beta stimulation when sympathetic activity is low (at rest), whereas these partial agonists behave more like conventional beta blockers when sympathetic activity is high. Agents with ISA may not be as effective as those without this property in reducing the heart rate or frequency, duration, and magnitude of ambulatory ST-segment changes or increasing the duration of exercise in patients with severe angina.

POTENCY. Potency can be measured by the ability of beta blockers to inhibit the tachycardia produced by isoproterenol. All drugs are considered in reference to propranolol, which is given a value of 1.0 (see Table 57-7). Timolol and pindolol are the most potent agents, and acebutolol and labetalol are the least potent.

LIPID SOLUBILITY. The hydrophilicity or lipid solubility of beta blockers is a major determinant of their absorption and metabolism. The lipid-soluble (lipophilic) beta blockers propranolol, metoprolol, and pindolol are readily absorbed from the gastrointestinal tract, are metabolized predominantly by the liver, have a relatively short half-life, and usually require administration twice or more daily to achieve continuing pharmacologic effects. If metoprolol or propranolol is administered intravenously, a much higher concentration reaches the bloodstream, and therefore intravenous dosing has much greater potency than oral dosing. The water-soluble (hydrophilic) beta blockers (e.g., atenolol, sotalol, nadolol) are not as readily absorbed from the gastrointestinal tract, are not as extensively metabolized, have relatively long plasma half-lives, and can be administered once daily. Water-soluble beta blockers are usually eliminated unchanged by the kidneys. Lipid-soluble agents are often preferable for patients with significant renal dysfunction for whom clearance of water-soluble agents is reduced. Greater lipid solubility is associated with greater penetration to the central nervous system and may contribute to side effects (e.g., lethargy, depression, hallucinations) that are not clearly related to beta-blocking activity.

ALPHA-ADRENERGIC BLOCKING ACTIVITY. The alpha-blocking potency of labetalol (approximately 10% that of phentolamine) is approximately 20% of its beta-blocking potency (see Table 57-7). Labetalol's combined alpha- and beta-blocking effects make it a particularly useful antihypertensive agent (see Chap. 46), especially in patients with hypertension and angina. The major side effects of labetalol are postural hypotension and retrograde ejaculation. Carvedilol also possesses alpha-adrenergic blocking activity with an alpha$_1$-to-beta-blocking ratio of approximately 1:10.

GENETIC POLYMORPHISMS. The metabolism of metoprolol, carvedilol, and propranolol may be influenced by genetic polymorphisms or other medications that influence hepatic metabolism.[116] The oxidative metabolism of metoprolol occurs primarily through the cytochrome P-450 enzyme CYP2D6 and exhibits the debrisoquin type of genetic polymorphism; poor hydroxylators or metabolizers (10% of whites or less) have significant prolongation of the elimination half-life of the drug in comparison to extensive hydroxylators or metabolizers. Thus, angina might be controlled by a single daily dose of metoprolol in poor metabolizers, whereas extensive metabolizers require the same dose two or three times daily. If a patient exhibits an exaggerated clinical response (e.g., extreme bradycardia) following the administration of metoprolol, propranolol, or other lipid-soluble beta blockers, it may be the result of prolongation of the elimination half-life because of slow oxidative metabolism. Metabolism of metoprolol may also be altered by drugs that interact with CYP2D6. Preliminary evidence has raised the possibility of differences in survival in patients with unstable IHD and provoked ischemia in stable IHD treated with beta blockers based on polymorphisms of the $beta_2$-adrenergic receptor (*ADRB1* and *ADRB2*).[117,118] Moreover, polymorphisms of the beta-adrenergic receptor may lead to variability in response to beta blockers in patients with heart failure.[119]

EFFECTS ON SERUM LIPID LEVELS. Beta blocker therapy (with agents lacking ISA) usually causes no significant changes in total or LDL cholesterol levels but increases triglyceride and reduces HDL cholesterol levels. The most commonly studied drug has been propranolol, which can increase plasma triglyceride concentrations by 20% to 50% and reduce HDL cholesterol levels by 10% to 20%. Increasing $beta_1$ selectivity is associated with lesser effects on lipid levels. Adverse effects on the lipid profile may be more frequent with nonselective than with $beta_1$-selective blockers. The effects of these changes in serum lipid levels by long-term administration of beta blockers must be considered when this therapy is begun or maintained for hypertension or angina.

Dosage

For optimal results, the dosage of a beta blocker should be carefully adjusted. In the case of atenolol, it is useful to start with a dosage of 50 mg once daily. The usual effective dosage is 50 to 100 mg daily; however, some patients benefit from up to 200 mg daily. In the case of metoprolol, it is often preferable from a perspective of the patient's compliance to use an extended-release formulation, which may be started at a dose of 100 mg once daily. Other beta blockers should be started at comparable doses.

Efficacy is determined by the effect on heart rate and symptoms and, when these are unclear, the effect on exercise performance can be evaluated by treadmill exercise testing. The resting heart rate should be reduced to between 50 and 60 beats/min, and an increase of less than 20 beats/min should occur with modest exercise (e.g., climbing one flight of stairs). Therapy with beta blockers needs to be individualized and requires repeated clinical evaluation during the initial period of drug administration.

Adverse Effects and Contraindications

Most of the adverse effects of beta blockers occur as a consequence of the known properties of these drugs and include cardiac effects (e.g., severe sinus bradycardia, sinus arrest, AV block, reduced LV contractility), bronchoconstriction, fatigue, mental depression, nightmares, gastrointestinal upset, sexual dysfunction, intensification of insulin-induced hypoglycemia, and cutaneous reactions (**Table 57-8**; see Table 57-6). Lethargy, weakness, and fatigue may be caused by reduced cardiac output or may arise from a direct effect on the central nervous system. Bronchoconstriction results from blockade of $beta_2$ receptors in the tracheobronchial tree. As a consequence, asthma and chronic obstructive lung disease may be considered as relative contraindications to beta blockers, even to $beta_1$-selective agents.[114]

In patients who already have impaired LV function, heart failure may be intensified, an effect that can be counteracted in part by the use of digitalis or diuretics. Beginning therapy with a very low dose (e.g., metoprolol succinate extended release, 25 mg daily, for 2 weeks in patients with NYHA functional Class II) and then gradually increasing the dose over the course of several weeks has been shown to be well tolerated and beneficial in patients with idiopathic dilated cardiomyopathy and those with heart failure caused by IHD (see Chap. 28). This approach is recommended when using beta blockers for patients with angina and heart failure.[120,121]

Beta blockers should be prescribed with caution for patients with cardiac conduction disease involving the sinus node or AV conduction system. In patients with symptomatic conduction disease, beta blockers are contraindicated unless a pacemaker is in place. In patients with asymptomatic sinus node dysfunction or first-degree AV block, beta blockers may be tolerated, but their administration requires careful observation. Pindolol, because of its ISA activity, may be preferable in this situation. Blockade of noncardiac $beta_2$ receptors inhibits catecholamine-induced glycogenolysis, so noncardioselective beta blockers can mask the premonitory signs of insulin-induced hypoglycemia. Nevertheless, beta blockers are generally well tolerated by patients with diabetes mellitus. Moreover, carvedilol has been shown to exhibit modest insulin-sensitizing properties and can relieve some manifestations of the metabolic syndrome.[122,123] Blockade of $beta_2$ receptors also inhibits the vasodilating effects of catecholamines in peripheral blood vessels and leaves the constrictor (alpha-adrenergic) receptors unopposed, thereby enhancing vasoconstriction. Noncardioselective beta blockers may precipitate episodes of Raynaud phenomenon in patients with this condition and may cause uncomfortable coldness in the distal extremities. Reduced flow to the limbs may occur in patients with peripheral vascular disease.

Abrupt withdrawal of beta-adrenergic blocking agents after prolonged administration can result in increased total ischemic activity in patients with chronic stable angina. This increased ischemia may be caused by a return to the previously high levels of myocardial O_2 demand while the underlying atherosclerotic process has progressed, but a rebound phenomenon resulting in increased beta-adrenergic sensitivity probably occurs in some patients. Occasionally, such withdrawal can precipitate unstable angina and may, in rare cases, even provoke MI. Chronic beta blocker therapy can be safely discontinued by slowly withdrawing the drug in a stepwise manner over the course of 2 to 3 weeks. If abrupt withdrawal of beta blockers is required, patients should be instructed to reduce exertion and manage angina episodes with sublingual nitroglycerin and/or substitute a calcium antagonist.

CALCIUM ANTAGONISTS. The critical role of calcium ions in the normal contraction of cardiac and vascular smooth muscle is discussed in Chaps. 24 and 52. The calcium antagonists (see Chap. 46) are a heterogeneous group of compounds that inhibit calcium ion movement through slow channels in cardiac and smooth muscle membranes by noncompetitive blockade of voltage-sensitive L-type calcium channels.[124] The three major classes of calcium antagonists are the dihydropyridines (nifedipine is the prototype), the phenylalkylamines (verapamil is the prototype), and the modified benzothiazepines (diltiazem is the prototype). Amlodipine and felodipine are additional dihydropyridines that are among the most commonly used calcium antagonists in the United States. The two predominant effects of calcium antagonists result from blocking the entry of calcium ions and slowing recovery of the channel. Phenylalkylamines have a marked effect on recovery of the channel and thereby exert depressant effects on cardiac pacemakers and conduction, whereas dihydropyridines, which do not impair channel recovery, have little effect on the conduction system.

MECHANISM OF ACTION. The efficacy of calcium antagonists in patients with angina pectoris is related to the reduction in myocardial O_2 demand and the increase in O_2 supply that they induce (see Table 57-4). The latter effect is particularly important in patients with conditions in which a prominent vasospastic or vasoconstrictor component may be present, such as Prinzmetal (variant) angina (see Chaps. 52 and 56), variable-threshold angina, and angina related to impaired vasodilator reserve of small coronary arteries. Calcium antagonists may be effective on their own or in combination with beta-adrenergic blockers and nitrates in patients with chronic stable angina. Several calcium antagonists are effective for the treatment of angina pectoris (**Table 57-9**). Each relaxes vascular smooth muscle in the systemic arterial and coronary arterial beds. In addition, blockade of the entry of calcium into myocytes results in a negative inotropic effect, which is counteracted to some extent by peripheral vascular dilation and by activation of the sympathetic nervous system in response to drug-induced hypotension.[124] However, the negative inotropic effect must be taken into consideration in patients with significant LV dysfunction.

With a rapid onset of action and metabolism by the liver, calcium antagonists have a limited bioavailability of between 13% and 52% and a half-life of between 3 and 12 hours. Amlodipine and felodipine are exceptions in that both drugs have long half-lives and may be administered once daily. In the case of some of the other calcium antagonists (e.g., nifedipine and diltiazem), sustained-release preparations have been shown to be effective.

ANTIATHEROGENIC ACTION. Hyperlipidemia-induced changes in the permeability of smooth muscle cells to calcium may play a role in atherogenesis; thus, the hypothesis that calcium antagonists might inhibit

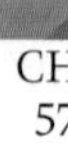

TABLE 57-7 Pharmacokinetics and Pharmacology of Some Beta-Adrenoceptor Blockers

CHARACTERISTIC	ATENOLOL	METOPROLOL/ METOPROLOL XL	NADOLOL	PINDOLOL	PROPRANOLOL/ PROPRANOLOL LA	TIMOLOL	ACEBUTOLOL
Extent of absorption (%)	~50	>95	~30	>90	>90	>90	~70
Extent of bioavailability (% of dose)	~40	~50/77	~30	~90	~30/20	75	~50
Beta-blocking plasma concentration	0.2-0.5 μg/mL	50-100 ng/mL	50-100 ng/mL	50-100 ng/mL	50-100 ng/mL	50-100 ng/mL	0.2-2.0 μg/mL
Protein binding (%)	<5	12	~30	57	93	~10	30-40
Lipophilicity*	Low	Moderate	Low	Moderate	High	Low	Low
Elimination half-life (hr)	6-9	3-7	14-25	3-4	3.5-6/8-11	3-4	3-4†
Drug accumulation in renal disease	Yes	No	Yes	No	No	No	Yes‡
Route of elimination	RE (mostly unchanged)	HM	RE	RE (40% unchanged and HM)	HM	RE (20% unchanged and HM)	HM‡
Beta blocker potency ratio (propranolol = 1)	1.0	1	1.0	6.0	1	6.0	0.3
Adrenergic-receptor blocking activity	β_1¶	β_1¶	β_1/β_2	β_1/β_2	β_1/β_2	β_1/β_2	β_1¶
Intrinsic sympathetic activity	0	0	0	+	0	0	+
Membrane-stabilizing activity	0	0	0	+	++	0	+
Usual maintenance dose	50-100 mg/day	50-100 mg bid-qid/50-400 mg/day	40-80 mg/day	10-40 mg/day (bid-tid)	80-320 mg/day (bid-tid)/ 80-160 mg/day	10-30 mg bid	200-600 mg bid
FDA-approved indications:							
Hypertension	Yes	Yes/yes	Yes	Yes	Yes/yes	Yes	Yes
Angina	Yes	Yes/yes	Yes	No	Yes/yes	No	No
Post-MI	Yes	Yes/no	No	No	Yes/no	Yes	No
Heart failure	No	Yes/yes	No	No	No/no	No	No

*Determined by the distribution ratio between octanol and water.
†Half-life of the active metabolite, diacetolol, is 12 to 15 hours.
‡Acebutolol is mainly eliminated by the liver, but its major metabolite, diacetolol, is excreted by the kidney.

TABLE 57-8 Candidates for Use of Beta-Blocking Agents for Angina

Ideal Candidates
Prominent relationship of physical activity to attacks of angina
Coexistent hypertension
History of supraventricular or ventricular arrhythmias
Previous myocardial infarction
Left ventricular systolic dysfunction
Mild to moderate heart failure symptoms (NYHA functional Classes II, III)
Prominent anxiety state

Poor Candidates
Asthma or reversible airway component in chronic lung disease patients
Severe left ventricular dysfunction with severe heart failure symptoms (NYHA functional Class IV)
History of severe depression
Raynaud phenomenon
Symptomatic peripheral vascular disease
Severe bradycardia or heart block
Brittle diabetes

Modified from Abrams JA: Medical therapy of stable angina pectoris. *In* Beller G, Braunwald E (eds): Chronic Ischemic Heart Disease. Atlas of Heart Disease. Vol. 5. Philadelphia, WB Saunders, 1995. p 7.22.

atherogenesis has been explored since the 1970s but has not yet achieved consensus. Experimental work with calcium channel blockers, in particular with more lipophilic second-generation agents such as amlodipine, have demonstrated improved endothelial function, inhibition of smooth muscle cell proliferation, migration, and ameliorated unfavorable membrane alterations.[125] In a randomized trial in patients with established CAD without hypertension, treatment with amlodipine, compared with placebo, reduced coronary atherosclerosis progression.[126] In a similar trial, nifedipine, compared with placebo, improved coronary endothelial function but did not reduce plaque volume.[125] In summary, although the evidence remains mixed, calcium antagonists may have some role in atheroprotection.

First-Generation Calcium Antagonists

NIFEDIPINE. Nifedipine, a dihydropyridine, is a particularly effective dilator of vascular smooth muscle and is a more potent vasodilator than diltiazem or verapamil. Although its in vitro actions on myocardium and specialized cardiac tissue are similar to those of other agents, the concentration required to reproduce effects on these tissues is not reached in vivo because of the early appearance of its powerful vasodilating effects. Thus, in clinical practice, the potential negative chronotropic, inotropic, and dromotropic (on AV conduction) effects of nifedipine are seldom a problem, with the exception that nifedipine has been reported to worsen heart failure in patients with pre-existing chronic heart failure.

The beneficial effects of nifedipine in the treatment of angina result from its ability to reduce myocardial O_2 requirements because of its afterload-reducing effect and to increase myocardial O_2 delivery as a result of its dilating action on the coronary vascular bed (see Table 57-4). Oral nifedipine in capsule form exerts hypotensive effects within 20 minutes of administration. This immediate-release formulation is no longer recommended because of concerns regarding adverse

LABETALOL	BISOPROLOL	BETAXOLOL	CARTEOLOL	PENBUTOLOL	CARVEDILOL/ CARVEDILOL CR	ESMOLOL (IV)	SOTALOL
>90	>90	>90	>90	100	ND	ND	ND
~25	80	90	85	100	~30/~25	100	>90
0.7-3.0 μg/mL	0.01-0.1 μg/mL	20-50 ng/mL	40-160 ng/mL	ND	ND	0.15-2.0 μg/mL	ND
~50	30	50-60	23-30	80-98	95-98	55	0
Low	Moderate	Moderate	Low	High	High	Low	Low
~6	7-15	12-22	5-7	17-26	6-10/11	4.5 min	12
No	Yes	Yes	Yes	Yes	No	No	Yes
HM	HM 50%; RE 50%	HM	RE	HM	HM	§	RE
0.3	10	4	10	1	10	0.02	0.3
$\beta_1/\beta_2/\alpha_1$	β_1¶	β_1^{∂}	β_1/β_2	β_1/β_2	$\beta_1/\beta_2/\alpha_1$	β_1¶	β_1/β_2
0	0	0	+	+	0	0	0
0	0	0	0	0	+	0	0
100-400 mg bid	5-20 mg/day	5-20 mg/day	2.5-10 mg/day	10-40 mg/day	3.125-50 mg bid 10-18 mg/day	Bolus of 500 μg/kg; infusion at 50-200 μg/kg/min	80-160 mg
Yes No No No	Yes No No No	Yes No No No	Yes No No No	Yes No No No	Yes/Yes No/No No/No Yes/Yes	Yes No Yes No	No No No No

§Rapid metabolism by esterases in the cytosol of red blood cells.

¶Beta$_1$ selectivity is maintained at lower doses, but beta$_2$ receptors are inhibited at higher doses.

FDA = U.S. Food and Drug Administration; HM = hepatic metabolism; MI = myocardial infarction; ND = no data; RE = renal excretion.

events. An extended-release formulation using the gastrointestinal therapeutic system of drug delivery (see Table 57-9) is designed to deliver 30, 60, or 90 mg of nifedipine in a single daily dose at a relatively constant rate over a 24-hour period and is useful for the treatment of chronic stable angina, Prinzmetal angina, and hypertension. Steady-state plasma levels are typically achieved within 48 hours of initiation. The efficacy of the extended-release preparation, either alone or in conjunction with beta blockers, in reducing episodes of angina and ischemia on ambulatory monitoring has been documented.

Adverse Effects

These occur in 15% to 20% of patients and require discontinuation of medication in about 5%. Most adverse effects are related to systemic vasodilation and include headache, dizziness, palpitations, flushing, hypotension, and leg edema (unrelated to heart failure). Gastrointestinal side effects, including nausea, epigastric pressure, and vomiting, are noted in approximately 5% of patients. In rare cases, in patients with extremely severe fixed coronary obstructions, nifedipine aggravates angina, presumably by lowering arterial pressure excessively, with subsequent reflex tachycardia. For this reason, combined treatment of angina with nifedipine and a beta blocker is particularly effective and superior to nifedipine alone. Most adverse effects are reduced by the use of extended-release preparations.

Several clinical case-control studies of hypertension and associated reviews have suggested that short-acting nifedipine may cause an increase in mortality. However, a meta-analysis of 15 studies of long-acting calcium channel antagonists, including nifedipine, in patients with CAD demonstrated a significant reduction in angina, stroke, and heart failure with similar rates of other cardiovascular outcomes.[127] Long-acting nifedipine should be considered as an effective and safe antianginal drug for the treatment of symptomatic patients with chronic CAD who are already receiving beta blockers, with or without nitrates. Short-acting nifedipine should ordinarily be avoided.

Because of its potent vasodilator effects, nifedipine is contraindicated for patients who are hypotensive or have severe aortic valve stenosis and for patients with unstable angina who are not simultaneously receiving a beta blocker in whom reflex-mediated increases in the heart rate may be harmful. Nifedipine (or a second-generation dihydropyridine) is the calcium antagonist of choice in patients with sinus bradycardia, sick sinus syndrome, or AV block, particularly if a beta-adrenergic blocking agent is administered concurrently and additional drug therapy for angina is indicated. This recommendation is based on the observation that in doses used clinically, nifedipine has fewer negative effects on myocardial contractility, heart rate, and AV conduction than verapamil or diltiazem.

Nifedipine interacts significantly with cimetidine and phenytoin (resulting in increased bioavailability of nifedipine). In patients with Prinzmetal angina, abrupt cessation of nifedipine therapy may result in a rebound increase in the frequency and duration of attacks.

VERAPAMIL. Verapamil dilates systemic and coronary resistance vessels and large coronary conductance vessels. It slows the heart rate

TABLE 57-9 Pharmacokinetics of Some Calcium Antagonists Used for Angina Pectoris

CHARACTERISTIC	DILTIAZEM/ DILTIAZEM SR		NICARDIPINE	NIFEDIPINE/ NIFEDIPINE SR		VERAPAMIL/ VERAPAMIL SR		AMLODIPINE	FELODIPINE	ISRADIPINE	NISOLDIPINE
Usual adult dose	IV: 0.25 mg/kg bolus, then 5-15 mg/hr Oral: 30-90 mg tid-qid SR: 60-180 mg bid CD: 120-480 mg/day		IV: 3-15 mg/hr Oral: 20-40 mg tid SR: 30-60 mg bid	Oral: 10-30 mg tid SR: 90 mg/d		IV: 0.075-0.15 mg/kg Oral: 80-120 mg tid-qid SR: 180-480 mg/day		Oral: 2.5-10 mg/day	Oral SR: 2.5-10 mg/day	Oral CR: 2.5-10 mg bid	Oral SR: 10-40 mg/day
Extent of absorption (%)	80-90		100	90		90		>90	>90	>90	ND
Extent of bioavailability (%)	40-70		30	65-75/86		20-35		60-90	20	25	5
Onset of action	IV: 3 min Oral: 30-60 min		IV: 1 min Oral: 20 min	20 min		IV: 2-5 min Oral: 30 min		0.5-1.0 hr	2 hr	20 min	1-3 hr
Time to peak serum concentration (hr)	2-3/6-11		0.5-2.0	0.5/6		IV: 3-5 min Oral: 1-2; SR: 7-9		6-12	2-5	1.5	6-12
Therapeutic serum levels (ng/mL)	50-200		30-50	25-100		80-300		5-20	1-5	2-10	ND
Elimination half-life (hr)	3.5/5-7		2.0-4.0	2.0-5.0		3.0-7.0*		30-50	11-16	8	7-12
Elimination	60% metabolized by liver; remainder excreted by kidneys		High first-pass hepatic metabolism	High first-pass hepatic metabolism		85% eliminated by first-pass hepatic metabolism		Hepatic	High first-pass hepatic metabolism	High first-pass hepatic metabolism	Hepatic
Heart rate	↓		↑	↑↑		↓		0	↑	0	0
Peripheral vascular resistance	↓		↓↓↓	↓↓↓		↓↓		↓↓↓	↓↓↓	↓↓↓	↓↓↓
FDA-approved indications	IR	SR		IR	SR	IR	SR				
Hypertension	No	Yes	Yes[†]	No	Yes	Yes	Yes	Yes	Yes	Yes	Yes
Angina	Yes	Yes	Yes	Yes	Yes	Yes	No	Yes	No	No	Yes
Coronary spasm	Yes	No	No	Yes	Yes	Yes	No	Yes	No	No	No

*Half-life of 4.5 to 12 hr with multiple dosing; may be prolonged in older patients.
[†]The sustained-release formulation may be preferred for hypertension.
CD = combination drug; CR = controlled release; IR = immediate release; ND = no data; SR = sustained release.

and reduces myocardial contractility. This combination of actions results in a reduction in myocardial O_2 requirement, which is the basis for the drug's efficacy in the management of chronic stable angina.

Verapamil reduces the frequency of angina and prolongs exercise tolerance in patients with symptomatic chronic CAD, and the combination of verapamil and a beta blocker provides clinical benefit that is additive. When evaluated in the International Verapamil-Trandolapril Study (INVEST), a strategy combining sustained-release verapamil and trandolapril compared with atenolol and a diuretic for the treatment of patients with hypertension and CAD showed equivalent outcomes with respect to death, MI, or stroke, including patients with prior MI.[128] Despite the marked negative inotropic effects of verapamil in isolated cardiac muscle preparations, changes in contractility are modest in patients with normal cardiac function. However, in patients with cardiac dysfunction, verapamil may reduce cardiac output, increase LV filling pressure, and cause clinical heart failure. In clinically useful doses, verapamil inhibits calcium influx into specialized cardiac cells, sometimes causing slowing of the heart rate and AV conduction. Therefore, it is contraindicated for patients with pre-existing AV nodal disease or sick sinus syndrome, heart failure, and suspected digitalis or quinidine toxicity.

The usual starting dose of verapamil for oral administration is 40 to 80 mg three times daily to a maximal dose of 480 mg daily (see Table 57-9). Sustained-release preparations of verapamil are available, and starting doses are 120 to 240 mg twice daily, with a usual optimal dosage range of 240 to 360 mg daily.

Verapamil interacts significantly with several other drugs. Intravenous verapamil should generally not be used together with a beta blocker (given intravenously or orally), nor should a beta blocker be administered intravenously in patients receiving oral verapamil. Both drugs can be administered orally but with caution in view of the potential for the development of bradyarrhythmias and negative inotropic effects. The bioavailability of verapamil is increased by cimetidine and carbamazepine, whereas verapamil may increase plasma levels of cyclosporine and digoxin and may be associated with excessive hypotension in patients receiving quinidine or prazosin. Hepatic enzyme inducers such as phenobarbital may reduce the effects of verapamil. Verapamil should not be administered in conjunction with the antiarrhythmic drug dofetilide.

Adverse effects of verapamil are noted in approximately 10% of patients and relate to systemic vasodilation (hypotension and facial flushing), gastrointestinal symptoms (constipation and nausea), and central nervous system reactions, such as headache and dizziness. A rare side effect is gingival hyperplasia, which appears after 1 to 9 months of therapy.

DILTIAZEM. Diltiazem's actions are intermediate between those of nifedipine and verapamil. In clinically useful doses, its vasodilator effects are less profound than those of nifedipine, and its cardiac depressant action, on the sinoatrial and AV nodes and myocardium, is less than that of verapamil. This profile may explain the remarkably low incidence of adverse effects of diltiazem. Diltiazem is a systemic vasodilator that lowers arterial pressure at rest and during exertion and increases the workload required to produce myocardial ischemia, but it may also increase myocardial O_2 delivery. Although this drug causes little vasodilation of epicardial coronary arteries under basal conditions, it may enhance perfusion of the subendocardium distal to a flow-limiting coronary stenosis; it also blocks exercise-induced coronary vasoconstriction. In patients with chronic stable angina receiving maximally tolerated doses of diltiazem, the heart rate is significantly reduced at rest, but no effect on peak blood pressure is achieved during exercise, and the duration of symptom-limited treadmill exercise is prolonged.

Several sustained-release formulations of diltiazem are available for once-daily treatment of systemic hypertension and angina pectoris. The usual starting dosage of sustained-release formulations is 120 mg once daily up to a typical maintenance dosage of 180 to 360 mg once daily. The maximum effect on blood pressure may not be observed until 14 days after starting therapy.

Diltiazem is a highly effective antianginal agent. Atenolol and diltiazem have similar efficacy in increasing nonischemic exercise duration in patients with variable-threshold angina and act primarily by slowing the resting heart rate. High doses (mean dose, 340 mg) have been shown to be a relatively safe addition to maximally tolerated doses of isosorbide dinitrate and a beta blocker and cause increases in exercise tolerance and resting and exercise LV ejection fractions. Major side effects are similar to those of the other calcium channel blockers and are related to vasodilation, but they are relatively infrequent, particularly if the dosage does not exceed 240 mg daily. As is the case with verapamil, diltiazem should be prescribed with caution for patients with sick sinus syndrome or AV block. In patients with pre-existing LV dysfunction, diltiazem may exacerbate or precipitate heart failure.

Diltiazem interacts with other drugs, including beta-adrenergic blocking agents (causing enhanced negative inotropic, chronotropic, and dromotropic effects), flecainide, and cimetidine (which increases the bioavailability of diltiazem). It has been associated with increased plasma levels of cyclosporine, carbamazepine, and lithium carbonate. Diltiazem may cause excessive sinus node depression if administered with disopyramide and may reduce digoxin clearance, especially in patients with renal failure.

Second-Generation Calcium Antagonists

The second-generation calcium antagonists (e.g., nicardipine, isradipine, amlodipine, felodipine) are mainly dihydropyridine derivatives, with nifedipine being the prototypical agent. Considerable experience has also accumulated with nimodipine, nisoldipine, and nitrendipine. These agents differ in potency, tissue specificity, and pharmacokinetics and, in general, are potent vasodilators because of greater vascular selectivity than that seen with the first-generation antagonists (e.g., verapamil, nifedipine, diltiazem).

AMLODIPINE. This agent, which is less lipid-soluble than nifedipine, has a slow smooth onset and ultralong duration of action (plasma half-life of 36 hours). It causes marked coronary and peripheral dilation and may be useful in the treatment of patients with angina accompanied by hypertension. It may be used as a once-daily hypotensive or antianginal agent. In a series of randomized placebo-controlled studies in patients with stable exercise-induced angina pectoris, amlodipine was shown to be effective and well tolerated. In two trials in patients with established CAD, amlodipine reduced the risk of major cardiovascular events. Amlodipine has little, if any, negative inotropic action and may be especially useful for patients with chronic angina and LV dysfunction.

The usual dosage of amlodipine is 5 to 10 mg once daily. Downward adjustment of the starting dose is appropriate for patients with liver disease and older patients. Significant changes in blood pressure are typically not evident until 24 to 48 hours after initiation. Steady-state serum levels are achieved at 7 to 8 days.

NICARDIPINE. This drug has a half-life similar to that of nifedipine (2 to 4 hours), but appears to have greater vascular selectivity. Nicardipine may be used as an antianginal and antihypertensive agent and requires administration three times daily, although a sustained-release formulation is available for twice-daily dosing in hypertension. For chronic stable angina pectoris, it appears to be as effective as verapamil or diltiazem, and its efficacy is enhanced when combined with a beta blocker.

FELODIPINE AND ISRADIPINE. In the United States, both drugs are approved by the U.S. Food and Drug Administration for the treatment of hypertension but not for angina pectoris. One study has documented similar efficacy between felodipine and nifedipine in patients with chronic stable angina. Felodipine has also been reported to be more vascular-selective than nifedipine and to have a mild positive inotropic effect as a result of calcium channel agonist properties. Isradipine has a longer half-life than nifedipine and demonstrates greater vascular sensitivity.

Other Pharmacologic Agents

Ranolazine. Ranolazine is a piperazine derivative that was approved in 2006 in the United States for use in patients with chronic stable angina.[129] Ranolazine is unique among currently approved antianginals in that its anti-ischemic effects are achieved without a clinically meaningful change in heart rate or blood pressure.[130] The mechanism of action of this agent remains under investigation. When studied at high

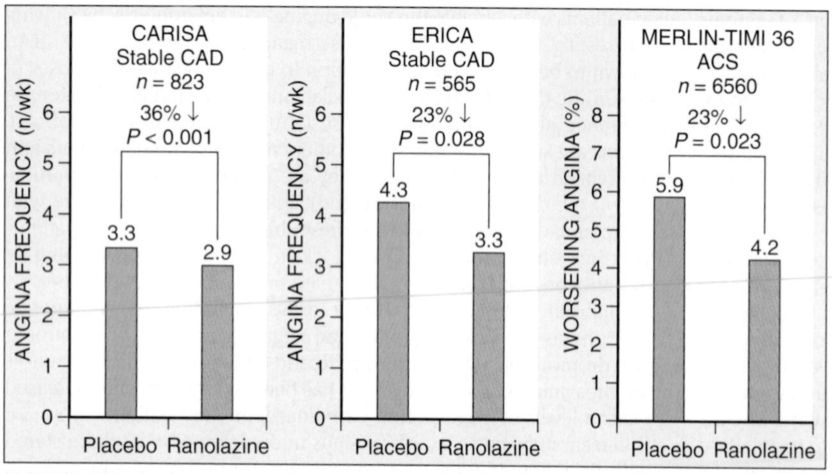

FIGURE 57-9 Reduction in the frequency of angina in three randomized, double-blind, placebo-controlled trials of ranolazine in patients with established CAD. Patients with stable CAD with early positive stress testing treated with standard doses of atenolol, amlodipine, or diltiazem were studied in the Combination Assessment of Ranolazine In Stable Angina (CARISA) trial. Patients with stable CAD and at least three episodes of angina weekly, despite amlodipine, 10 mg daily, were studied in the Efficacy of Ranolazine in Chronic Angina (ERICA) trial. Patients after presentation with non–ST-segment elevation ACS were studied for an average of 12 months in the Metabolic Efficiency With Ranolazine for Less Ischemia in Non-ST-Elevation Acute Coronary Syndromes (MERLIN) trial. In each trial, ranolazine reduced the frequency of angina. *(Data from Chaitman BR, Pepine CJ, Parker JO, et al: Effects of ranolazine with atenolol, amlodipine, or diltiazem on exercise tolerance and angina frequency in patients with severe chronic angina: A randomized controlled trial. JAMA 291:309, 2004; Stone PS, Gratsiansky NA, Blokhin A, et al: Antianginal efficacy of ranolazine when added to treatment with amlodipine. J Am Coll Cardiol 48:566, 2006; and Morrow DA, Scirica BM, Karwatowska-Prokopczuk E, et al: Effects of ranolazine on recurrent cardiovascular events in patients with non-ST-elevation acute coronary syndromes: The MERLIN-TIMI 36 Randomized Trial. JAMA 297:1775, 2007.)*

concentrations in in vitro experiments, ranolazine was shown to shift myocardial substrate utilization from fatty acid to glucose and thus was considered to be a potential metabolic agent. However, subsequent studies at concentrations of ranolazine consistent with doses tested in clinical trials have suggested that ranolazine exerts favorable effects on ischemia through a reduction in calcium overload in the ischemic myocyte via inhibition of the late sodium current (I_{Na}). In animal models of ischemia and reperfusion, ranolazine preserves tissue levels of adenosine triphosphate, improves myocardial contractile function, and reduces the extent of irreversible myocardial injury measured by biomarkers of necrosis and by electron microscopy.

A sustained-release formulation of ranolazine has been studied in three randomized, placebo-controlled clinical trials in patients with stable IHD and has improved exercise performance and increased the time to ischemia during exercise treadmill testing when used as monotherapy or when used in combination with the most frequently used doses of atenolol, amlodipine, or diltiazem.[131] Ranolazine also decreases angina frequency and nitroglycerin use when used in combination with a beta blocker or calcium channel blocker.

When studied in a randomized, blinded, placebo-controlled trial of 6560 patients with non–ST-segment elevation ACS, ranolazine, administered for an average of approximately 1 year, did not add to standard therapy for the secondary prevention of major cardiovascular events.[132] However, ranolazine reduced the incidence of recurrent ischemia, in particular worsening angina, in a significantly more diverse population with established CAD than studied previously with ranolazine (**Fig. 57-9**).[132] Consistent with prior studies, the reduction in angina and improvement in exercise performance were evident only in patients with a history of chronic angina.[133]

The half-life of the sustained-release formulation of ranolazine is approximately 7 hours. A steady state is generally achieved within 3 days of dosing twice daily. Ranolazine is metabolized primarily through the cytochrome P-450 (CYP3A4) pathway and thus the plasma concentration is increased if administered in combination with moderate (e.g., diltiazem) or strong (e.g., ketoconazole and macrolide antibiotic) inhibitors of this system. Verapamil increases the absorption of ranolazine by inhibition of P-glycoprotein. Plasma concentrations of simvastatin are increased approximately twofold after administration of ranolazine.

Ranolazine should be started as 500 mg twice daily and may be increased to a maximum of 1000 mg twice daily in patients with persistent angina. The most commonly reported adverse effects in clinical studies are nausea, generalized weakness, and constipation. Dizziness has also been reported, as has a small dose-related increase in the corrected QT interval, an average of 2 to 5 milliseconds in the dosage range of 500 to 1000 mg twice daily.[129] The electrophysiologic effects of ranolazine include inhibition of the delayed rectifier current and inhibition of I_{Na}; the net effect is to shorten action potential duration and suppress early afterdepolarizations.[134] Thus, ranolazine does not have the electrophysiologic profile that has been observed with QT-prolonging drugs associated with torsades de pointes. Ranolazine should be used with caution in patients receiving other QT-prolonging medications and is contraindicated in patients with clinically significant hepatic impairment, which has been associated with a steeper relationship between ranolazine and the QTc.

There was no adverse trend in the incidence of symptomatic documented arrhythmias, all-cause mortality, or sudden cardiac death with ranolazine in a randomized trial of 6560 patients with recent ACS. A significant reduction in the incidence of arrhythmias detected by 7 days of Holter monitoring with ranolazine compared with placebo in this study suggests possible antiarrhythmic actions of the agent that may warrant additional investigation.[135] In addition to these electrophysiologic effects, ranolazine also appears to have glycometabolic effects, including a reduction in hemoglobin A1c.[136]

*IVABRADINE**. Ivabradine is a specific and selective inhibitor of the I_f ion channel, the principal determinant of the sinoatrial node pacemaker current.[137] Ivabradine reduces the spontaneous firing rate of sinoatrial pacemaker cells and thus slows heart rate through a mechanism that is not associated with negative inotropic effects. Ivabradine reduces peak heart rate during exercise, increases the time to limiting angina compared with placebo, and is equivalent to atenolol with respect to exercise performance and time to ischemia (ST-segment depression) in patients with stable angina undergoing exercise treadmill testing.[138] In a randomized trial of 10,917 patients with CAD and reduced LV function, ivabradine did not reduce the primary endpoint of cardiovascular death, hospitalization for MI, or hospitalization for heart failure.[139] Fewer hospitalizations for MI were observed in the subgroup of patients with a baseline heart rate higher than 70 beats/min who were randomized to ivabradine compared with placebo and in patients with a history of limiting angina.[140]

Investigational Agents

*NICORANDIL**. Nicorandil is a nicotinamide ester that dilates peripheral and coronary resistance vessels via action on ATP-sensitive potassium channels and possesses a nitrate moiety that promotes systemic venous and coronary vasodilation.[141] As a result of these dual actions, nicorandil reduces preload and afterload and results in an increase in coronary blood flow. In addition to these effects, nicorandil may have cardioprotective actions mediated through the activation of potassium channels. Nicorandil has been associated with ulcerations of the gastrointestinal tract.[142]

Nicorandil has antianginal efficacy similar to those of beta blockers, nitrates, and calcium channel blockers. In a recent randomized clinical trial ($N = 5126$), nicorandil reduced the risk of cardiac death, MI, or hospital admission for angina (hazard ratio, 0.83; $P = 0.014$) compared with placebo when added to standard antianginal therapy.[143]

*FASUDIL**. Fasudil is an orally available inhibitor of rho kinase, an intracellular signaling molecule that participates in vascular smooth muscle contraction. Fasudil was shown to increase the time to ischemia in a study of 84 patients with CAD undergoing exercise treadmill testing.[144]

*METABOLIC AGENTS**. Agents aimed at increasing the metabolic efficiency of cardiac myocytes have also been studied in patients with chronic stable angina. Partial inhibitors of fatty acid oxidation appear to shift myocardial metabolism to more oxygen-efficient pathways. Trimetazidine and perhexiline are agents that have been shown to inhibit fatty acid metabolism and to reduce the frequency of angina without hemodynamic effects in patients with chronic stable angina.[145]

---

*Has not been approved by the U.S. Food and Drug Administration at the time of this writing.

OTHER CONSIDERATIONS OF MEDICAL MANAGEMENT OF ANGINA PECTORIS

Relative Advantages of Beta Blockers and Calcium Antagonists

The choice between a beta blocker and calcium channel antagonist as initial therapy in patients with chronic stable angina is controversial because both classes of agents are effective in relieving symptoms and reducing ischemia (**Table 57-10**).[80] Trials comparing beta blockers and calcium antagonists have not shown any difference in the rate of death or MI, although in some studies beta blockers appeared to have greater clinical efficacy and less frequent discontinuation because of side effects. Because long-term administration of beta blockers has been demonstrated to prolong life in patients after acute MI, it is reasonable to consider beta blockers over calcium antagonists as the agents of choice in treating patients with stable IHD. However, it must be recognized that beta blockers (without ISA) increase serum triglyceride levels and decrease HDL cholesterol levels, with uncertain long-term consequences. In addition, these drugs may produce fatigue, depression, and sexual dysfunction. In contrast, although calcium antagonists do not show these adverse effects, their long-term administration has not been shown to improve long-term survival after acute MI. However, diltiazem is apparently effective in preventing severe angina and early reinfarction after non–Q-wave MI. Verapamil reduces reinfarction rates in patients post-MI and, when combined with trandolapril, achieves similar outcomes to atenolol together with a diuretic for the treatment of patients with hypertension and CAD.

The choice of drug with which to initiate therapy is influenced by a number of clinical factors (see Table 57-10)[80]:

1. Calcium antagonists are the preferred agents in patients with a history of asthma or chronic obstructive lung disease with wheezing on clinical examination, in whom beta blockers, even relatively selective agents, are contraindicated. Consideration to a trial of beta blockers should be given if the patient has a history of prior MI.
2. Nifedipine (long-acting), amlodipine, and nicardipine are the calcium antagonists of choice in patients with chronic stable angina and sick sinus syndrome, sinus bradycardia, or significant AV conduction disturbances, whereas beta blockers and verapamil should be used only with great caution in such patients. In patients with symptomatic conduction disease, neither a beta blocker nor a calcium channel blocker should be used unless a pacemaker is in place. If a beta blocker is required in patients with asymptomatic evidence of conduction disease, pindolol, which has the greatest ISA, is useful. In the case of calcium channel blockers in patients with conduction system disease a dihydropyridine is preferable to verapamil and diltiazem, but careful observation for deterioration of conduction is mandatory.
3. Calcium antagonists are clearly preferred for patients with suspected Prinzmetal (variant) angina (see Chap. 56); beta blockers may even aggravate angina under these circumstances.
4. Calcium antagonists may be preferred over beta blockers in patients with significant, symptomatic peripheral arterial disease because the latter may cause peripheral vasoconstriction.
5. Beta blockers should usually be avoided in patients with a history of significant depressive illness and should be prescribed cautiously for patients with sexual dysfunction, sleep disturbance, nightmares, fatigue, or lethargy.
6. The presence of moderate to severe LV dysfunction in patients with angina limits the therapeutic options. The beneficial effects of beta blockers on survival in patients with LV dysfunction after MI, coupled with their beneficial effects on survival and LV performance in patients with heart failure,[121] have established beta blockers as the drug class of choice for the treatment of angina in patients with LV dysfunction, with or without symptoms of heart failure, together with ACE inhibitors, diuretics, and digitalis. If a beta blocker is not tolerated or angina persists despite beta blockade and nitrates, amlodipine can be administered. Ranolazine is also an option for such patients. Verapamil, nifedipine, and diltiazem should be avoided.
7. Short-acting nifedipine should not be used because the reflex-mediated tachycardia may aggravate ischemia.
8. Hypertensive patients with angina pectoris do well with beta blockers or calcium antagonists because both agents have antihypertensive effects. However, beta blockers are the preferred initial agent for treating angina in such patients, as noted earlier, and an ACE inhibitor should be strongly considered for all patients with CAD with hypertension.

TABLE 57-10 Recommended Use of Beta Blockers or Calcium Antagonists for Patients Who Have Angina in Conjunction with Other Medical Conditions

CLINICAL CONDITION	RECOMMENDED DRUG*
Cardiac Arrhythmia or Conduction Disturbance	
Sinus bradycardia	Nifedipine, amlodipine
Sinus tachycardia (not caused by cardiac failure)	Beta blocker
Supraventricular tachycardia	Beta blocker (verapamil)
Atrioventricular block	Nifedipine or amlodipine
Rapid atrial fibrillation	Verapamil or beta blocker
Ventricular arrhythmia	Beta blocker
Left Ventricular Dysfunction	
Heart failure	Beta blocker
Miscellaneous Medical Conditions	
Systemic hypertension	Beta blocker (calcium antagonist)
Severe preexisting headaches	Beta blocker (verapamil or diltiazem)
COPD with bronchospasm or asthma	Nifedipine, amlodipine, verapamil, or diltiazem
Hyperthyroidism	Beta blocker
Raynaud syndrome	Nifedipine or amlodipine
Claudication	Calcium antagonist
Severe depression	Calcium antagonist

*Alternatives in parentheses.
COPD = chronic obstructive pulmonary disease.

Combination Therapy

The combination of multiple agents is widely used in the management of chronic stable angina with options that include a beta blocker, calcium antagonist, long-acting nitrate, or newer agents such as ranolazine, which may be particularly useful when heart rate, blood pressure, or LV dysfunction limit escalation or initiation of other therapy. When adrenergic blockers and calcium antagonists are used together in the treatment of angina pectoris, several issues should be considered:

1. The addition of a beta blocker enhances the clinical effect of nifedipine and other dihydropyridines.
2. In patients with moderate or severe LV dysfunction, sinus bradycardia, or AV conduction disturbances, combination therapy with calcium antagonists and beta blockers should be avoided or initiated with caution. In patients with AV conduction system disease, the preferred combination is a long-acting dihydropyridine and a beta blocker. The negative inotropic effects of calcium antagonists are not usually a problem in combined therapy with low doses of beta blockers but can become significant with higher doses. With such doses, amlodipine is the calcium antagonist of choice, but it should be used cautiously. Ranolazine may be useful for patients who do not tolerate the combination of a beta blocker and calcium channel antagonist.
3. The combination of a dihydropyridine and a long-acting nitrate (without a beta blocker) is not an optimal combination because both are vasodilators.

APPROACH TO PATIENTS WITH CHRONIC STABLE ANGINA. This approach is as follows:

1. Identify and treat precipitating factors such as anemia, uncontrolled hypertension, thyrotoxicosis, tachyarrhythmias, uncontrolled heart failure, and concomitant valvular heart disease.

2. Initiate risk factor modification, physical exercise, diet, and lifestyle counseling. Initiate therapy with a statin, as needed, to reduce the LDL cholesterol level to at least below 100 mg/dL.
3. Initiate pharmacotherapy with aspirin and a beta blocker. Initiate an ACE inhibitor in all patients with an LV ejection fraction of 40% or lower and in those with hypertension, diabetes, or chronic kidney disease. In addition, an ACE inhibitor should be considered for all other patients.
4. Use sublingual nitroglycerin for alleviation of symptoms and for prophylaxis.
5. If angina persists, the next step is usually the addition of a calcium antagonist or long-acting nitrate via dosing schedules to prevent nitrate tolerance. The decision to add a calcium antagonist or long-acting nitrate is not based entirely on the frequency and severity of symptoms. The need to treat concomitant hypertension or the presence of LV dysfunction and symptoms of heart failure may be an indication for the use of one of these agents, even in patients in whom episodes of symptomatic angina are infrequent.
6. If angina persists despite two antianginal agents (a beta blocker with a long-acting nitrate preparation or calcium antagonist), add a third antianginal agent. The selection of the agent will be guided by potential side effects and the presence or absence of concomitant hypertension, relative hypotension, conduction system disease, tachyarrhythmias, or LV dysfunction.
7. Coronary angiography, with a view to considering coronary revascularization, is indicated for patients with refractory symptoms or ischemia despite optimal medical therapy. It should also be carried out in patients with high-risk noninvasive test results (see Table 57-3) and in those with occupations or lifestyles that require a more aggressive approach.

Other Therapies

Spinal Cord Stimulation. An option for patients with refractory angina who are not candidates for coronary revascularization is spinal cord stimulation using a specially designed electrode inserted into the epidural space.[146] The beneficial effects of neuromodulation on pain via this technique are based on the gate theory, in which stimulation of axons in the spinal cord that do not transmit pain to the brain will reduce input to the brain from axons that do transmit pain. Irrespective of the mechanism, several observational studies have reported success rates of up to 80% in terms of reducing the frequency and severity of angina. One small, randomized, sham-controlled study has demonstrated an improvement in symptoms and functional status.[147] What is less easily explained is an apparent anti-ischemic effect of this technique. In a small randomized trial in patients with angina and CAD not amenable to PCI, spinal cord stimulation was associated with similar symptom relief and long-term quality of life compared with CABG. This approach should be reserved for patients in whom all other treatment options have been exhausted.

Enhanced External Counterpulsation. The use of enhanced external counterpulsation (EECP) is another alternative treatment of refractory angina.[148] EECP is generally administered as 35 1-hour treatments over 7 weeks. Observational data have suggested that EECP reduces the frequency of angina and the use of nitroglycerin and improves exercise tolerance and quality of life, and that the responses can last for up to 2 years.[149] In a randomized, double-blind, sham-controlled study of EECP for patients with chronic stable angina, active counterpulsation was associated with an increase in time to ST-segment depression during exercise testing and a reduction in angina, as well as an improvement in health-related quality of life that extended to at least 1 year. There are no definitive data that EECP reduces the extent of ischemia determined by myocardial perfusion imaging.

The mechanisms underlying the effects of EECP are poorly understood. Possible mechanisms include the following: (1) durable hemodynamic changes that reduce myocardial O_2 demand; (2) improvement in myocardial perfusion caused by the ability of increased transmyocardial pressure to open collaterals; and (3) the elaboration of various substances that improve endothelial function and vascular remodeling caused by augmented flow through the arterial vascular bed.[148,150] Finally, the possibility of placebo effects should be recognized; most of the evidence demonstrating favorable effects of EECP is from uncontrolled studies, and data from sham-controlled studies are few.

Chelation. Randomized trials have shown no benefit, and these agents may be harmful.

Revascularization of Coronary Artery Disease

(see Chap. 58)

APPROACH TO DECISIONS REGARDING REVASCULARIZATION. IHD manifests as a continuum of disease with a variable natural history that may, over decades, encompass many phases of clinical expression, ranging from asymptomatic periods, the development of chronic exertional angina, subsequent quiescent periods, progression to accelerating angina, and culmination in unstable angina or acute MI (see Chaps. 54 and 56). Therefore, the approach to treatment should be tailored to the individual's clinical status. Moreover, atherosclerosis is typically a diffuse or multifocal process in which non–flow-limiting coronary stenoses are the principal progenitors of most "hard" clinical events[76] and require a comprehensive systemic approach to management. In general, the principles guiding patient management are predicated on addressing two simultaneous goals, if possible: (1) use of disease-modifying therapies or approaches to prolong life and reduce major cardiovascular events such as acute MI, hospitalization for ACS, or heart failure; (2) optimization of the patient's health status, quality of life, and functional capacity such that angina or ischemia do not adversely affect the activities of daily living.[80]

It is widely accepted that the benefits of revascularization are proportional to the patient's underlying risk, which makes it essential to quantify the patient's prognosis as accurately as possible (see Table 57-3). In addition to the patient's risk for major cardiovascular events, sociodemographic factors, such as age, physical capacity, and ability to adhere to prescribed treatments and lifestyle interventions, overall quality of life, other medical conditions, and patient preferences should be considered. Each of these aspects should be integrated in considering how best to achieve these two fundamental goals of therapy for patients with stable IHD. Revascularization approaches are an integral component of an overall management strategy to improve outcomes and are used when needed in addition to optimal medical therapy. The success of catheter-based or surgical treatment is predicated on the overall success of guideline-directed secondary prevention and lifestyle intervention as a platform for management of all patients with stable IHD.

PATIENT SELECTION. Each of the following considerations may be used to guide decisions regarding the indications for and approach to revascularization: (1) presence and severity of symptoms; (2) physiologic significance of coronary lesions and other anatomic considerations; (3) extent of myocardial ischemia and the presence of LV dysfunction; and (4) other medical conditions that influence the risks of percutaneous or surgical revascularization.

Presence and Severity of Symptoms

A goal of therapy is the complete elimination of angina and resumption of full physical function to the greatest extent possible.[80] Mechanical revascularization (surgical or catheter-based) should be considered if ischemic symptoms persist after intensification of medical therapy, including stringent risk factor modification, or if unacceptable side effects limit antianginal therapy.

Significance of Coronary Lesions and Other Anatomic Considerations

The presence of a 70% or greater stenosis of an epicardial coronary artery is considered to be significant (50% or greater for left main coronary stenosis). Thus, professional guidelines that have informed clinical practice regarding revascularization have been framed principally around these anatomic criteria (number of diseased vessels, extent and severity of anatomic disease), integrating functional considerations (magnitude and distribution of ischemia, and amount of threatened myocardium subtending coronary stenosis).[80,151] However, clinicians also quite often face clinical uncertainty regarding the potential significance of borderline visual coronary stenoses, nominally defined as those lesions in the 50% to 70% range.[152] It is widely acknowledged that angiographic stenosis severity (as a percentage) is often an inaccurate measure of a lesion's functional significance.[45] Whereas cardiac surgeons have used a 50% or greater stenosis as the criterion for significant,[153] many factors other than visual stenosis severity (e.g., lesion eccentricity, tortuousity, presence of plaque rupture or asymmetric luminal filling defects, presence of additional serial lesions) can potentially render a 50% to 70% stenosis functionally or hemodynamically significant. In a study of 325 patients with intermediate stenosis scheduled for PCI, patients with a fractional flow reserve (FFR) more than 0.75 (56%) were randomized to PCI or medical therapy. Patients managed medically had a risk of cardiac death or MI of less than 1%/year that was not increased compared with the group that was stented.[154] Optimally stress testing can be used to determine whether a borderline visual coronary stenosis subtends a segment (or segments) of ischemic myocardium. However, an invasive physiologic tool such as FFR (see Chap. 52) can be used to guide appropriate decisions regarding revascularization of the intermediate stenosis. Judgments regarding the need for revascularization should incorporate angiographic (anatomic) and physiologic (functional) data, including that obtained by intravascular ultrasonography (see Chap. 22).

Other anatomic features, in addition to lesion severity, influence the approach to revascularization for a given patient. These features include vessel size, extent of calcification, tortuosity, and relationships to side branches (see Chap. 58). Each of these characteristics may influence the likelihood of successful catheter-based or, in some cases, surgical revascularization. For example, a patient with single-vessel CAD with a long, complex, and calcified bifurcation lesion of the proximal LAD artery and first diagonal branch may in some cases be a candidate for surgical revascularization. Patients with diffuse severe disease of the distal coronary arteries may be poor candidates for any revascularization procedure.

Extent of Ischemia and Presence of Left Ventricular Dysfunction

The four major determinants of risk in CAD are the extent of ischemia, number of vessels diseased, LV function, and electrical substrate. The extent of ischemia on noninvasive testing is an important predictor for subsequent adverse outcomes and identifies patients for whom revascularization may provide clinical benefit compared with medical therapy beyond the relief of symptoms (**Fig. 57-10**).[155,156] The major effect of coronary revascularization is on ischemia, and the magnitude of the benefit compared with that of medical therapy is enhanced with LV dysfunction, particularly in the presence of reversibly ischemic jeopardized myocardium. Moreover, the greatest survival benefits of CABG, as well as symptomatic and functional improvements, are evident in patients with impaired LV function (generally defined as an ejection fraction of less than 40%; **Tables 57-11** and **57-12**).

Risks of the Procedure

Patients with stable IHD more often than not have other medical conditions, such as renal dysfunction, peripheral atherosclerosis, or pulmonary disease, which may influence the patient's suitability for surgical or percutaneous revascularization. For example, in a patient with peptic ulcer disease and history of GI bleeding, the potential need for long-term dual antiplatelet therapy after a procedure should be considered. Moreover, a patient with three-vessel CAD and impaired LV function who might derive a more durable survival benefit from CABG may be too high risk clinically to undergo surgery and might be a better candidate for multivessel PCI.

In addition, some general principles regarding the choice of treatment in patients with stable IHD should be considered:

1. For most patients with chronic angina, revascularization should not constitute the initial management strategy before evidence-based medical therapy (e.g., pharmacologic antianginal therapy, disease-modifying treatments, therapeutic lifestyle intervention) is initiated and optimized.
2. When improvement in survival is not a relevant consideration, the severity of angina or impairment in health status should play a significant role in determining whether revascularization is appropriate (i.e., limiting angina on optimal medical therapy is a more compelling indication than episodic exertional angina on minimal medical therapy) .
3. The patient's treatment preferences and sociodemographic and/or clinical circumstances should always be a consideration in choosing which treatment strategy to use.

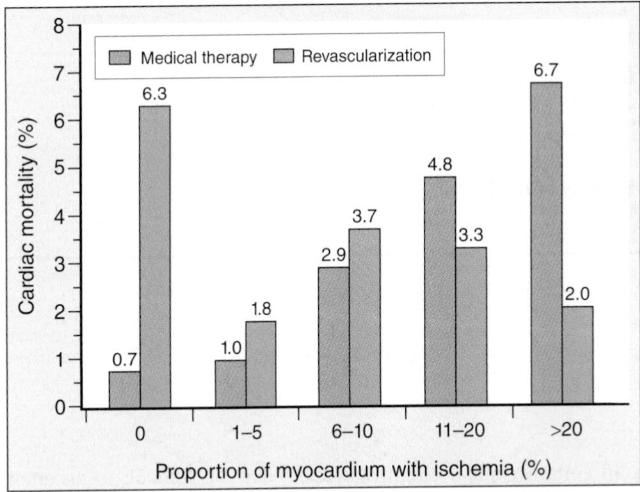

FIGURE 57-10 Rate of cardiac death in patients treated with medical therapy versus revascularization, stratified by the proportion of ischemic myocardium on stress nuclear imaging. A total of 10,627 consecutive patients without prior MI or revascularization were followed for a mean of 1.6 years after exercise or adenosine myocardial perfusion imaging. Patients with moderate to severe ischemia who underwent percutaneous or surgical coronary revascularization within 60 days of stress imaging had lower mortality than those treated with medical therapy ($P < 0.0001$). However, those patients with no or mild ischemia had no survival advantage with revascularization. *(From Hachamovitch R, Hayes SW, Friedman JD, et al: Comparison of the short-term survival benefit associated with revascularization compared with medical therapy in patients with no prior coronary artery disease undergoing stress myocardial perfusion single photon emission computed tomography. Circulation 107:2900, 2003.)*

TABLE 57-11 Impact of Coronary Bypass Surgery on Survival*

CATEGORY OF RISK	NUMBER OF DISEASED VESSELS	SEVERITY OF ISCHEMIA	EJECTION FRACTION	RESULTS OF SURGERY ON SURVIVAL
Mild	2	Mild	>0.50	Unchanged†
	3	Mild	>0.50	Unchanged†
Moderate	2	Moderate to severe	>0.50	Unchanged†
	3	Moderate to severe	>0.50	Improved†
	2	Mild	<0.50	Unchanged†
	3	Mild	<0.50	Improved‡
Severe	2	Moderate to severe	<0.50	Improved‡
	3	Moderate to severe	<0.50	Improved‡

*In subsets of patients studied in the CASS randomized trial and registry studies.
†Randomized trial.
‡Survival improved with surgery versus medicine. In the European Coronary Surgery Trial, patients with double-vessel disease and involvement of the proximal left anterior descending coronary artery had improved survival with surgery, irrespective of left ventricular function.

TABLE 57-12 Effects of Coronary Artery Bypass Grafting on Survival*

SUBGROUP	MEDICAL TREATMENT MORTALITY RATE (%)	P VALUE FOR CABG VERSUS MEDICAL TREATMENT
Vessel Disease		
One vessel	9.9	0.18
Two vessels	11.7	0.45
Three vessels	17.6	<0.001
Left main artery	36.5	0.004
No LAD Disease		
One or two vessels	8.3	0.88
Three vessels	14.5	0.02
Left main artery	45.8	0.03
Overall	12.3	0.05
LAD Disease Present		
One or two vessels	14.6	0.05
Three vessels	19.1	0.009
Left main artery	32.7	0.02
Overall	18.3	0.001
LV Function		
Normal	13.3	<0.001
Abnormal	25.2	0.02
Exercise Test Status		
Missing	17.4	0.10
Normal	11.6	0.38
Abnormal	16.8	<0.001
Severity of Angina		
Class 0, I, II	12.5	0.005
Class III, IV	22.4	0.001

*Systematic overview of the effect of CABG versus medical therapy on survival based on data from seven randomized trials comparing a strategy of initial CABG with one of initial medical therapy. Subgroup results at 5 years are shown.

From Yusuf S, Zucker D, Peduzzi P, et al: Effect of coronary artery bypass surgery on survival: Overview of 10-year results from randomized trials by the Coronary Artery Bypass Surgery Trialists Collaboration. Lancet 344:563, 1994.

4. In certain clinical circumstances, it may be difficult to ascertain reliably whether anginal symptoms or anginal equivalents such as exertional dyspnea or fatigue are a direct manifestation of underlying CAD, especially in patients with significant obesity, those who are sedentary, or those who may have coexisting chronic obstructive pulmonary disease. In such settings, symptoms that are atypical or nondiagnostic for obstructive CAD may not necessarily improve with revascularization, even when such symptoms coexist with physiologically significant coronary disease.
5. The decision to proceed with myocardial revascularization must be individualized according to the specific clinical features and personal preferences of a given patient, often in collaboration with family members and the patient's referring physician, with informed discussion about the potential risks and benefits of all three therapeutic options.

Percutaneous Coronary Intervention

PCI, which includes percutaneous transluminal coronary angioplasty (PTCA), stenting, and related techniques, has continued to evolve significantly over the past three decades (see Chap. 58).[157] PTCA has been largely replaced since the advent of bare metal stents (BMS) in the mid-1990s, with continued evolution over the past 15 years, particularly with the introduction of drug-eluting stents (DES) in 2003. First-generation DES have subsequently been modified through evolutionary design to include thinner struts and improved drug-eluting platforms and delivery systems to minimize restenosis and acute and subacute stent thrombosis. Moreover, the practice of interventional cardiology has changed radically with increased operator experience, improved adjunctive pharmacotherapy, and advances in technology other than stenting, such as distal protection devices and devices directed at specific technical issues (e.g., thrombectomy and atherectomy catheters). As such, PCI is an important treatment modality for patients with stable IHD, particularly those patients with chronic angina who remain symptomatic despite medial therapy.

OUTCOMES

Early Outcome

Continued improvement in the technical aspects of PCI (predominantly coronary stenting), as well as increasing operator experience, has had a favorable impact on the rate of primary success and the rate of reductions in complications.[158] Among the many desirable features of PCI is the fact that it can be performed during the same clinical encounter as the diagnostic angiography. Stable patients can often be discharged on the same or next day and clinical recovery is usually complete within a week or less. In many cases, symptomatic relief can be immediate and dramatic. Such attributes may motivate some patients to elect to undergo PCI, even when optimal medical therapy alone may lower overall risk with equivalent long-term outcomes. A recent examination of data on over 2.6 million patients undergoing PCI between 2005 and 2007 at 968 U.S. sites in the American College of Cardiology National Cardiovascular Data Registry (ACC-NCDR) revealed that among elective PCIs, 58% were performed in patients with stable IHD, of whom 35% had diabetes mellitus.[159] The ACC-NCDR reported an angiographic success rate of 96% and a procedural success rate (angiographic success without death, heart attack, or emergency revascularization) of 93% in patients undergoing PCI. The incidence of death prior to hospital discharge was less than 1% and emergency CABG was required in 0.3% of patients. The ACC-NCDR reported a periprocedural MI rate of 1%, but studies using routine assessments of cardiac biomarkers reported higher rates, although the significance of these periprocedural biomarker increases has been debated.[160,161] Finally, the rate of restenosis with DES is reported to be less than 10%, with a corresponding approximately 20% decrease in the need for repeat revascularization procedures compared with the era of BMS.[162] Outcomes in specific challenging subgroups of patients, such as those with chronic total occlusions or left main coronary stenosis, are discussed in Chap. 58.

Long-Term Outcome

Long-term outcome after PCI is well characterized, with LV function, extent of coronary disease, diabetes, renal function, and the patient's age being the major determinants of mortality risk, and restenosis at the site of intervention being a major contributor to recurrent ischemia and the need for subsequent procedures. The introduction of BMS and DES has dramatically reduced the incidence of restenosis compared with balloon angioplasty. The evolution of stent technology, comparisons of long-term outcomes, and decision-making regarding device selection are discussed in Chap. 58.

Restenosis and Late Stent Thrombosis

(See Chap. 58.)

COMPARISONS BETWEEN PERCUTANEOUS CORONARY INTERVENTION AND MEDICAL THERAPY. Studies comparing balloon angioplasty with medical therapy are of uncertain clinical relevance today because both PCI and medical treatments have undergone profound changes over the last one or two decades. Moreover, randomized clinical trials comparing PCI with medical therapy are few in number and have involved less than 5000 patients (in total). Most have enrolled patients with predominantly single-vessel disease and were completed prior to the routine use of coronary stenting and enhanced adjunctive pharmacotherapy. In aggregate, the results of these 11 trials have supported superior control of angina, improved exercise capacity, and improved quality of life in patients treated with angioplasty compared with medical therapy (**Fig. 57-11**).[163] In 1997, the second Randomized Intervention Treatment of Angina (RITA-2) investigators reported that balloon angioplasty improved angina compared with medical therapy, although this was followed by a higher incidence of ischemic events (combined death and MI) as compared

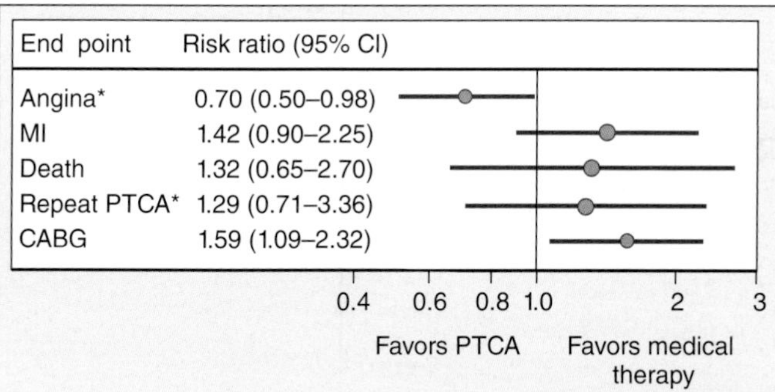

FIGURE 57-11 Relative risk of recurrent cardiac events with PTCA versus medical therapy from a meta-analysis of six randomized trials ($N = 1904$). Compared with medical therapy, angioplasty reduced the relative risk of recurrent angina by 30%. Randomized trials have not included sufficient numbers of patients for informative estimates of the effect of angioplasty on MI, death, or subsequent revascularization; however, trends in the available data do not favor angioplasty. These trials do not reflect the widespread use of coronary stenting. *Test for heterogeneity, $P < 0.0001$. *(From Bucher HC, Hengstler P, Schindler C, et al: Percutaneous transluminal coronary angioplasty versus medical therapy for treatment of non-acute coronary heart disease: A meta-analysis of randomised controlled trials. BMJ 321:73, 2000.)*

with medical therapy, which consisted principally of aspirin, beta blockers, and anti-ischemic therapy. The authors observed an excess of death and periprocedural MI with angioplasty compared with medical therapy (6.3 versus 3.3%; $P < 0.02$). After 7 years, there was no difference in the composite of death or MI, whereas the initial improvement in angina and exercise times with balloon angioplasty versus medical therapy narrowed, mainly because one third of medical patients eventually required PCI because of severe angina.

Meta-analyses of trials of routine stenting compared with balloon angioplasty have not demonstrated differences in the incidence of death, MI, or emergency CABG. In an analysis of 23 trials of 10,347 patients, bare metal stenting compared with balloon angioplasty produced similar rates of mortality (odds ratio, 0.92; $P = 0.60$), and similar rates of a combined endpoint of death or MI (odds ratio, 0.86; $P = 0.2$).[164] However, stenting led to significantly fewer major adverse cardiac events (odds ratio, 0.59; $P < 0.001$), driven exclusively by reduced revascularization. Brophy and coworkers[164a] have analyzed 27 trials with 9918 patients and found that stenting compared with balloon angioplasty produces similar mortality (odds ratio, 0.65; $P =$ NS), death or MI (odds ratio, 0.90; P = not significant [NS]), and need for subsequent CABG surgery (odds ratio, 1.01; $P =$ NS), but less frequent restenosis (odds ratio, 0.52; 95% CI, 0.37 to 0.69). The Medicine, Angioplasty, or Surgery Study (MASS) II study enrolled 651 patients between 1995 and 2000 who were randomized to PCI, CABG, or medical therapy. After 5 years, patients who had undergone PCI were more likely to be free of angina than were medical therapy patients (77% versus 55%; $P < 0.001$), but equally likely to have experienced death, MI, or revascularization for refractory angina and to have undergone subsequent elective revascularization procedures.[165] Currently, no randomized trial or meta-analysis to date has demonstrated a reduction in death or MI with PCI compared with medical therapy for patients with chronic stable angina, although all these comparative studies, by design, assessed PCI in apposition to, not in combination with, medical therapy; no study incorporated guideline-driven disease-modifying medical therapies such as statins or inhibitors of the renin-angiotensin system.

Between 1999 and 2004, the Clinical Outcomes Utilization Revascularization and Aggressive DruG Evaluation (COURAGE) Trial Research Group randomized 2287 patients with objective evidence of ischemia and proximal angiographic CAD (70% visual stenosis) to optimal medical therapy (OMT) with or without PCI.[166] Importantly, the aim and design of COURAGE was to test a strategy of routine, anatomically driven PCI plus OMT versus a strategy of selective, ischemia-driven PCI, if needed, for a failure of initial OMT. Follow-up from 2.5 to 7 years (median, 4.6 years) demonstrated that the combination of death or MI occurred with similar frequency in both arms. The 4.6-year cumulative primary event rates were 19.0% and 18.5% in the PCI + OMT and OMT groups, respectively (hazard ratio [HR] in the PCI + OMT group compared with the OMT group, 1.05; 95% CI, 0.87 to 1.27; $P = 0.62$; **Fig. 57-12**). Comparing PCI and medical therapy groups, there were no differences in death, MI, or stroke (20.0% versus 19.5%; HR, 1.05; 95% CI, 0.87 to 1.27; $P = 0.62$); hospitalization for ACS (12.4% versus 11.8%; HR, 1.07; 95% CI, 0.84 to 1.37; $P = 0.56$); or MI (13.2% versus 12.3%; HR, 1.13; 95% CI, 0.89 to 1.43; $P = 0.33$). Thus, the main study findings indicated that as an initial management strategy in patients with stable CAD, PCI does not reduce death, MI, or other major cardiovascular events when added to OMT. Patients initially treated with PCI had less angina at 1 and 3 years, but not at 5 years, compared with patients initially treated without PCI. As expected, patients who received initial OMT had more frequent subsequent PCIs compared with patients initially treated with PCI, although only 16.5% of OMT patients required revascularization during the first year of follow-up; the remaining 16.5% of patients crossed over to revascularization between year 1 and 7. Subgroup analyses of COURAGE have suggested that there is no difference in the combined endpoint of death and MI in patients with multivessel CAD (compared with those who had single-vessel disease), low ejection fraction (compared with those with ejection fraction > 50%), Class II or III angina (compared with those with Class 0 or I angina), or diabetes (compared with no diabetes; see Fig. 57-12).[166]

Review of the baseline characteristics from COURAGE[167] has revealed that the population was not low risk—34% were diabetic, 71% were dyslipidemic, 67% were hypertensive, 29% were current smokers, 39% had prior MI, and 26% had undergone previous revascularization. Most patients (58%) were in CCS Class II or III and 30% were in Class I (12% had asymptomatic myocardial ischemia); the average number of anginal episodes was six/week, whereas the median was three/week. A total of 95% of patients had ischemia testing and, of those who underwent myocardial perfusion scintigraphy, two thirds had multiple reversible perfusion defects and the remaining third had a single reversible perfusion defect. Almost 70% of patients had multivessel CAD (70% diameter stenosis estimated visually), and LAD coronary disease was common (68%), being significantly more prevalent in the OMT group (37%) than in the PCI group (31%). In the aggregate, these findings indicate that the enrolled patients were highly symptomatic at baseline, had appreciable clinical comorbidity, high prevalence of objective evidence of myocardial ischemia, and extensive angiographic CAD, and thus fall into the population in which a clinical benefit of PCI is expected.[166]

A separately published substudy from COURAGE has demonstrated that patients randomized to receive PCI in addition to OMT had greater reduction in high-grade ischemia on stress nuclear imaging compared with patients who received OMT alone, although such findings were observed in only 20% of the 314 patients in this subgroup.[168] Thus, data support the premise that severe ischemia may identify an important subset of patients with stable IHD who might derive clinical benefit from PCI, but prospective studies in a larger cohort of such patients will be required to evaluate this possibility.

In summary, based on the best available data from randomized trials, it appears reasonable to pursue a strategy of initial medical therapy for most patients with stable IHD and CCS class I or II symptoms and to reserve revascularization for those with persistent and/or more severe symptoms, despite optimal medical therapy, or those with high-risk criteria on noninvasive testing, such as inducible ischemia involving a moderate or large territory of myocardium.[80] The results from the COURAGE trial also underscore the favorable impact that intensive medical therapy and lifestyle interventions have on mitigating clinical events in patients treated with and without PCI. OMT as an initial management strategy in patients with stable IHD is safe and effective.

PATIENT SELECTION. In addition to general considerations regarding the indications and approach to revascularization (see "Approach to Decisions Regarding Revascularization"), additional factors that need to be weighed in patient selection for PCI include the following:

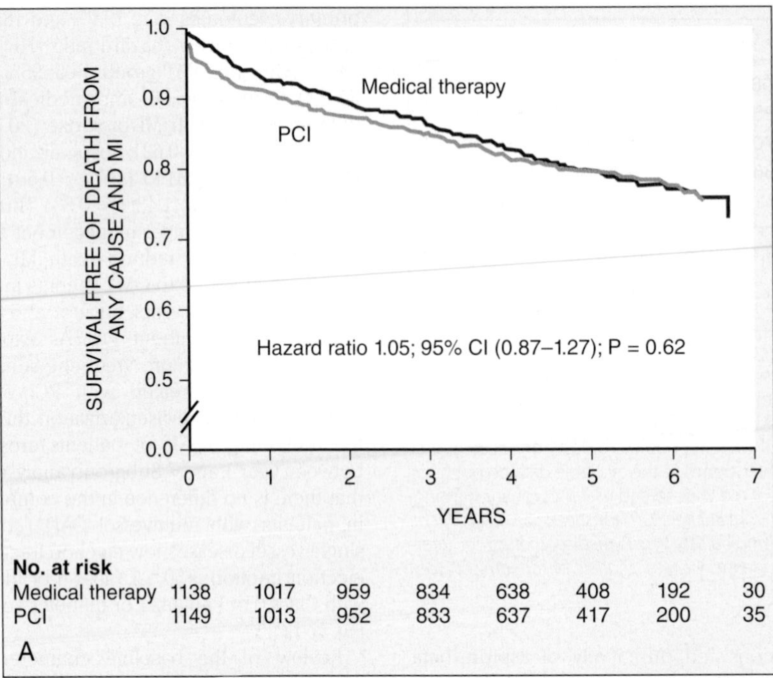

Baseline characteristics	No. of patients	Hazard ratio (95% CI)	Event rate for the primary outcome PCI	Medical therapy	P value*
Overall	2287	1.05 (0.87-1.27)	0.19	0.19	
Sex					
Male	1947	1.15 (0.93-1.42)	0.19	0.18	0.03
Female	338	0.65 (0.40-1.06)	0.18	0.26	
Myocardial infarction					
Yes	876	0.91 (0.69-1.21)	0.23	0.25	0.15
No	1371	1.22 (0.93-1.60)	0.17	0.14	
Extent of CAD					
Multi-vessel disease	1581	1.04 (0.84-1.30)	0.21	0.21	0.65
Single-vessel disease	700	1.17 (0.76-1.80)	0.15	0.12	
Smoking					
Current	653	1.00 (0.71-1.41)	0.20	0.21	0.71
Not current	1631	1.06 (0.86-1.36)	0.19	0.18	
Diabetes					
Yes	766	0.99 (0.73-1.32)	0.25	0.24	0.33
No	1468	1.20 (0.92-1.56)	0.17	0.15	
CCS angina class					
0 or I	964	1.01 (0.75-1.38)	0.17	0.20	0.73
II or III	1371	1.09 (0.85-1.40)	0.20	0.18	
Ejection fraction					
≤50%	406	1.14 (0.77-1.70)	0.28	0.26	0.72
>50%	1848	1.05 (0.84-1.32)	0.17	0.16	
Age					
>65yr	904	1.10 (0.83-1.46)	0.24	0.22	0.62
≤65 yr	1381	1.00 (0.77-1.32)	0.16	0.16	
Previous CABG					
Yes	2039	1.04 (0.84-1.29)	0.17	0.17	0.81
No	248	0.98 (0.52-1.82)	0.34	0.29	
Race					
White	1963	1.08 (0.87-1.34)	0.19	0.18	0.43
Nonwhite	322	0.87 (0.54-1.42)	0.19	0.24	
Health care system					
Canadian	932	1.27 (0.90-1.78)	0.17	0.34	0.17
U.S. non-VA	387	0.71 (0.44-1.14)	0.15	0.21	
U.S. VA	968	1.06 (0.80-1.38)	0.22	0.22	

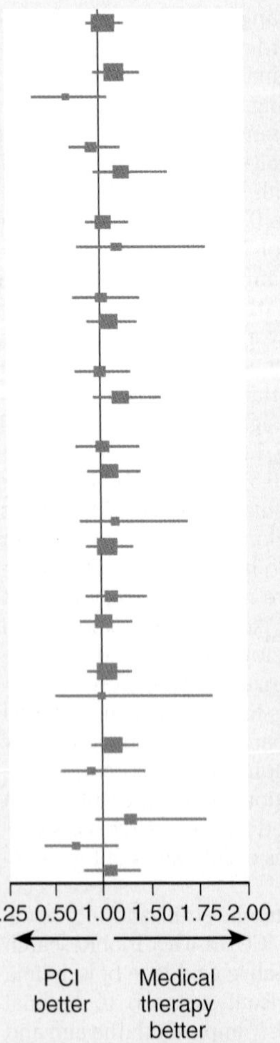

0.25 0.50 1.00 1.50 1.75 2.00

PCI better ← → Medical therapy better

B

FIGURE 57-12 Outcome in 2287 patients with objective evidence of myocardial ischemia and significant coronary artery disease enrolled in the COURAGE trial and randomized to PCI and optimal medical therapy or optimal medical therapy alone (Medical therapy). **A,** No difference in the primary endpoint of death from any cause or MI was observed between the two treatment groups. **B,** The finding of no difference between the two treatment groups was consistent across multiple subgroups, including patients with multivessel disease, diabetes, severe angina, and prior revascularization. *Interaction p-value. *(From Boden WE, O'Rourke RA, Teo KK, et al: Optimal medical therapy with or without PCI for stable coronary disease. N Engl J Med 356:1503, 2007.)*

1. The likelihood of successful catheter-based revascularization based on the angiographic characteristics of the lesion
2. The risk and potential consequences of acute failure of PCI, which are a function, in part, of the coronary artery anatomy (multivessel and/or diffuse disease), percentage of viable myocardium at risk, presence of heart failure, and underlying LV function
3. The likelihood of restenosis, which has been associated with clinical (e.g., diabetes, prior restenosis) and angiographic factors (e.g., small vessel diameter, long lesion length, total occlusion, saphenous vein graft disease; see Chap. 58)
4. The need for complete revascularization based on the extent of CAD, volume of myocardium, and severity of ischemia in the distribution of the artery(ies) amenable to PCI

Percutaneous Coronary Intervention in Subgroups of Patients with Stable Ischemic Heart Disease

Diabetes Mellitus. Patients with diabetes are at substantially higher risk for complications after PCI (see Chap. 64). Possible explanations for the higher rate of adverse outcomes include an altered vascular biologic response in diabetic patients to balloon injury and rapid progression of disease in nondilated segments. The diabetic atherosclerotic milieu is characterized by a procoagulant state, decreased fibrinolytic activity, increased proliferation, and inflammation. Restenosis is more frequent in diabetic patients, as is disease progression. For this reason, CABG, which bypasses most of the vessel instead of a specific lesion, may offer a better intermediate- to long-term outcome.[169] The optimal strategy for revascularization in patients with diabetes is discussed later in this chapter. A strategy of initial optimal medical therapy appears reasonable for most patients with diabetes with stable IHD.[170]

Left Ventricular Dysfunction. Despite advances in interventional cardiology, LV dysfunction remains independently associated with higher in-hospital and long-term mortality after PCI. Specifically, in patients with stable CAD and estimated ejection fractions of 40% or less, 41 to 49, and 50% or higher in the National Heart, Lung, and Blood Institute (NHLBI) Dynamic Registry, mortality at 1 year after PCI was 11.0, 4.5, and 1.9%, respectively. Contemporary trials of PCI versus medical therapy have included too few patients with impaired LV function to guide therapeutic decision-making in this important subset of patients.

Women and Older Patients. Specific issues related to PCI in women and older adults are discussed in Chaps. 80 and 81.

Previous Coronary Bypass Grafting. CABG and PCI are often considered competitive procedures, but it is more appropriate to view them as complementary. An increasing number of patients who have had CABG and later have recurrent ischemia undergo revascularization with PCI. Technical aspects and procedural outcomes of PCI in venous bypass grafts are discussed in Chap. 58.

Coronary Artery Bypass Grafting

In 1964, Garrett and colleagues first used CABG as a "bailout" procedure. Widespread use of the technique by Favoloro and Johnson and their respective collaborators followed in the late 1960s. Use of the internal mammary artery (IMA) graft was pioneered by Kolessov in 1967 and by Green and associates in 1970. Since then, CABG has evolved progressively over the past four decades, and today remains an important treatment modality for many patients with stable IHD. Most bypass operations continue to be performed through a median sternotomy, using cardiopulmonary bypass (CPB) and cardioplegic myocardial arrest or without bypass on a beating heart. Less invasive approaches have become increasingly commonplace in select patients who may be appropriate candidates for more limited coronary revascularization, and include anterior and lateral thoracotomies, partial sternotomies, and epigastric incisions.[171] The technical goal of bypass surgery is to obtain, whenever possible, complete revascularization by grafting all coronary arteries of sufficient caliber that have physiologically significant proximal stenoses. CABG has been documented to prolong survival, relieve angina, and improve quality of life in specific subgroups of patients with CAD.[172]

The annual number of CABG operations in the United States rose steadily over its first three decades, peaking in the late 1990s. Since then, however, rates of CABG have steadily declined, which likely relates to the sustained growth of the use of PCI, particularly in patients with multivessel CAD.[1] CABG provides excellent short- and intermediate-term results in the management of stable IHD; its long-term results are affected by failure of venous grafts. Long-term data with totally arterial surgical revascularization (i.e., using bilateral internal mammary artery [IMA] grafts) are few.

Minimally Invasive Coronary Artery Bypass Grafting. Less invasive or minimally invasive approaches may be divided into four major categories based on the approach and use of CPB (see Chap. 84). Port access CABG is performed using limited incisions with femoral-femoral CPB and cardioplegic arrest. Port access technology has also now enabled totally endoscopic robotically assisted CABG (TECAB) to be performed on the arrested heart.[173] Off-pump CABG is performed using a standard median sternotomy, with generally small skin incisions, and stabilization devices to reduce motion of the target vessels while anastomoses are performed without CPB. Finally, minimally invasive direct coronary artery bypass (MIDCAB) is performed through a left anterior thoracotomy without CPB. Thus, off-pump approaches to CABG include off-pump CAB (OPCAB) and MIDCAB techniques (see Fig. 57-e2 on website).

The potential advantages of the minimally invasive approaches include reduced postoperative patient discomfort, minimized risk of wound infection, and shorter recovery times.[174] The avoidance of CPB may mitigate the risk of bleeding, systemic thromboembolism, renal insufficiency, myocardial stunning, stroke, and the damaging neurologic effects of CABG that could result in cognitive impairment, particularly in older patients and patients with heavily calcified aortas.[175] Amelioration of the systemic inflammatory response that occurs after CABG using CPB is viewed as an additional advantage that might affect these clinical outcomes. The learning curve of minimally invasive CABG has led to some reports of early graft failure. It should be emphasized that with conventional surgical techniques, the early patency rates of an IMA graft are excellent (98.7% in one large series).

Short-term clinical and angiographic outcomes have suggested that the less invasive techniques can be used to achieve results comparable to those of traditional CABG. However, in 2009, a comparative trial of OPCAB versus CABG using CPB in 2203 patients revealed that there was no difference in death or complications at 30 days (7.0% versus 5.6%, respectively; $P = 0.19$) but a significantly worse 1-year composite outcome of all-cause mortality, nonfatal MI, need for repeat revascularization in off-pump versus on-pump procedures (9.9% versus 7.4%, respectively; $P = 0.04$).[176] Additionally, in those patients undergoing follow-up angiography, there was a significantly lower graft patency rate in OPCAB recipients, and no treatment-based differences in neuropsychological outcomes or short-term resource use. Additional data regarding long-term graft patency and more prospective randomized trials of these two approaches will permit the comparative effectiveness of these two approaches on clinical outcomes to be assessed critically.

Novel approaches to coronary revascularization may also include CABG with PCI by combining a minimally invasive surgical CABG procedure on the LAD coronary artery (i.e., a left IMA implant to the proximal LAD artery using OPCAB) with PCI on the remaining vessels. Further experience with these so-called hybrid revascularization procedures is needed to clarify appropriate selection criteria further and to determine whether this strategy offers important advantages over multivessel CABG alone.[177]

Outcomes in Minimally Invasive Coronary Artery Bypass Grafting. Meta-analyses of observational and randomized trials of OPCAB versus CPB[178] have failed to demonstrate clear superiority of OPCAB over CPB with respect to mortality or major morbidity. Intraoperative conversion from OPCAB to CPB appears to be approximately 8%.[179] Early postoperative complications appear to be reduced with OPCAB, along with nonsignificant trends toward lower rates of death, MI, or stroke (see Chap. 84). Generally consistent findings across randomized and observational data sets have revealed comparable completeness of revascularization, reductions in blood loss and/or transfusion requirements, fewer wound infections, less postoperative atrial fibrillation, lower indices of myocardial injury, shorter duration of mechanical ventilation, and earlier hospital discharge with OPCAB. However, the largest randomized trial raises concern regarding possible long-term worse outcomes than with traditional CABG with CPB.[176]

ARTERIAL AND VENOUS CONDUITS. The current standard for bypass grafting advocates routine use of the left IMA for grafting the LAD artery, with supplemental saphenous vein grafts to other vessels. Although the benefits of a single IMA graft over a saphenous vein graft alone are not in dispute, the superiority of bilateral IMA grafts over a single IMA graft and one saphenous vein graft is less well accepted.[180] Initial enthusiasm for the use of bilateral IMA grafts was tempered by a higher rate of postoperative complications, including bleeding, wound infection, and prolonged ventilatory support.[181] Wound infection, most notably, deep sternal wound infection, has been of particular concern, but remains modest in frequency, <3%, except in patients who are obese or diabetic or those who require prolonged ventilatory support. Subsequent series have shown that bilateral versus single IMA grafting is associated with lower rates of recurrent angina pectoris, reoperation, and MI, improved survival in nonrandomized studies and, in some series, the risk of wound infection does not differ substantially from that with single IMA grafts. The increased technical demands and longer operative times of bilateral IMA grafting have also been a barrier to more widespread adoption but may be overcome if evidence supporting a survival advantage continues to accumulate.[182]

Patency of Venous and Arterial Grafts

Early occlusion (before hospital discharge) occurs in 8% to 12% of venous grafts and, by 1 year, 15% to 30% of vein grafts have become occluded. After the first year, the annual occlusion rate is 2% and rises to approximately 4% annually between years 6 and 10. Patency rates with IMA grafts are superior.

DISTAL VASCULATURE. The state of the distal coronary vasculature is important for the fate of bypass grafts. Late patency of grafts is related to coronary arterial runoff as determined by the diameter of the coronary artery into which the graft is inserted, size of the distal vascular bed, and severity of coronary atherosclerosis distal to the site of insertion of the graft. The highest graft patency rates are found when the lumina of the vessels distal to the graft insertion are larger than 1.5 mm in diameter, perfuse a large vascular bed, and are free of atheroma obstructing more than 25% of the vessel lumen. For saphenous veins, optimal patency rates are achieved with a lumen of 2.0 mm or larger.

PROGRESSION OF DISEASE IN NATIVE ARTERIES. The rate of disease progression appears highest in arterial segments already showing evidence of disease, and is between three and six times higher in grafted native coronary arteries than in nongrafted native vessels. These data have suggested that bypassing an artery with minimal disease, even if initially successful, may ultimately be harmful to patients, who incur both the risk of graft closure and the increased risk of accelerated obstruction of native vessels. Lesions in the native vessel that are long (more than 10 mm) and more than 70% in diameter are at increased risk of progressing to total occlusion.

EFFECTS OF THERAPY ON VEIN GRAFT OCCLUSION AND NATIVE VESSEL PROGRESSION. Measures aimed at enhancing long-term patency are generally directed at delaying the overall process of atherosclerosis, and thus may have several additional benefits. Secondary preventive therapy, in particular lipid-lowering treatment, is important to reducing the risk of failure of venous grafts. Chronic anticoagulant therapy has not been shown to alter outcomes convincingly. Other novel approaches, such as pretreatment of venous grafts to increase resistance to atherothrombosis, have not been definitively evaluated.

ANTIPLATELET THERAPY. Several trials have demonstrated the efficacy of aspirin therapy when started 1, 7, or 24 hours preoperatively, but the benefit is lost when aspirin is started more than 48 hours postoperatively. Aspirin, 80 to 325 mg daily, should be continued indefinitely. The addition of dipyridamole or warfarin in conventional doses has not been shown definitively to provide added benefit.[183] Although the effects of clopidogrel on graft patency have not been studied specifically, it is likely to be at least as effective as aspirin and is recommended for those who have an allergy to aspirin or who have had a recent ACS.[184]

LIPID-LOWERING THERAPY. Three randomized trials of lipid-lowering therapy have shown a favorable impact on the development of graft disease.[57] The rationale for lowering LDL cholesterol concentration to less than 100 mg/dL in patients with CAD was extended to postoperative patients in the Post-Coronary Artery Bypass Graft Trial.

PATIENT SELECTION. Indications for CABG are centered on the need for improvement in the quality and/or duration of life.[153] The decision to perform revascularization with PCI or CABG is based largely on coronary anatomy, LV function, other medical comorbidities that may affect the patient's risk for either revascularization procedure, and patient preference (see "Approach to Decisions Regarding Revascularization" and "Choosing Among Percutaneous Coronary Intervention, Coronary Artery Bypass Grafting, and Medical Therapy").[169] CABG is indicated, regardless of symptoms, for patients with CAD in whom survival is likely to be prolonged and for patients with multivessel CAD in whom noninvasive testing suggests high risk (see Table 57-11). Patients with more extensive and severe CAD have an increasing magnitude of benefit from CABG over medical therapy (**Fig. 57-13**; see Fig. 57-10 and Table 57-12). Other factors that must

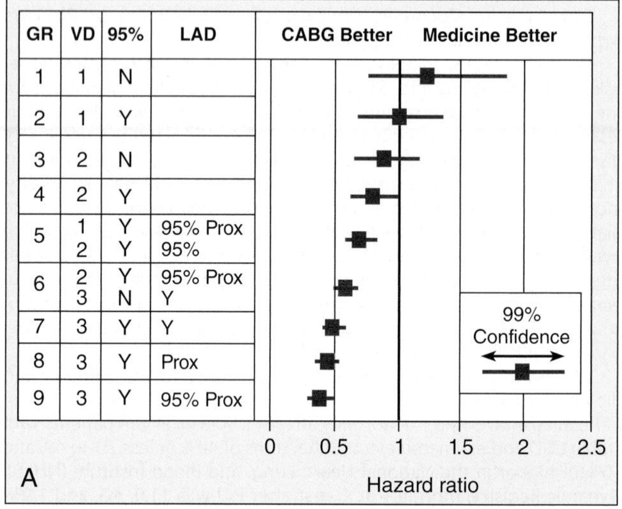

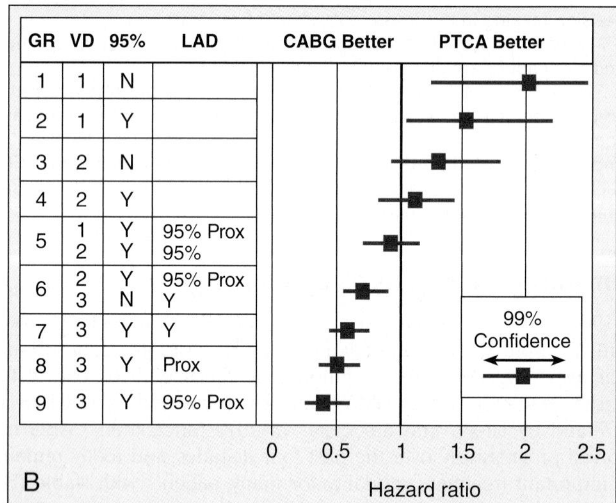

FIGURE 57-13 **A,** Adjusted hazard (mortality) ratios comparing CABG and medical therapy for nine coronary anatomy severity groups (GR) according to the number of vessels diseased (VD), presence or absence of a 95% proximal stenosis (95%), and involvement of the LAD artery. **B,** Adjusted hazard (mortality) ratios comparing CABG and PTCA for nine coronary anatomy groups according to the number of vessels diseased, presence or absence of a 95% proximal stenosis, and LAD artery involvement. In patients with the least severe categories of disease, 5-year survival appears to be better with PTCA (single-vessel disease without proximal stenosis and without LAD artery involvement), whereas for patients with triple-vessel disease and higher grade, more complex, double-vessel disease, a survival benefit is noted with surgery. For other subsets of patients with double-vessel disease, no difference in survival was seen in those treated with CABG or PTCA, and many of these patients are probably similar to those included in the randomized trials. *(Data from the Duke University data base;* ***A*** *and* ***B,*** *from Jones RH, Kesler K, Phillips HR III, et al: Long-term survival benefits of coronary artery bypass grafting and percutaneous transluminal angioplasty in patients with coronary artery disease. J Thorac Cardiovasc Surg 111:1013, 1996.)*

always be considered in the decision are general health and noncoronary comorbid conditions.

SURGICAL OUTCOMES AND LONG-TERM RESULTS. The patient population undergoing CABG has been changing over time, particularly with the wider use of PCI. In comparison with the 1970s, patients undergoing CABG today are older, include a higher percentage of women, and are sicker, in that a greater proportion have unstable angina, triple-vessel CAD, previous coronary revascularization with CABG or PCI, LV dysfunction, and comorbid conditions, including hypertension, diabetes, and peripheral vascular disease. Despite the increasing risk profile of this population, outcomes with CABG have generally remained stable or have improved.

Operative Mortality

Risk factors for death following CABG may be separated into five categories: (1) preoperative factors related to CAD, including recent acute MI, hemodynamic instability, LV dysfunction, extensive CAD, presence of left main CAD, and severe or unstable angina; (2) preoperative factors related to the aggressiveness of the arteriosclerotic process, as reflected in associated carotid or peripheral vascular disease; (3) preoperative biologic factors (older age at surgery, diabetes mellitus, other comorbidities, including pulmonary and renal disease, and perhaps female gender); (4) intraoperative factors (intraoperative ischemic damage, failure to use IMA grafts); and (5) environmental or institutional factors, including the specific surgeon and treatment protocols used.[185] Of these factors, several variables have consistently emerged as the most potent predictors of mortality after CABG: (1) age; (2) urgency of operation; (3) prior cardiac surgery; (4) LV function; (5) percentage stenosis of the left main coronary artery; and (6) number of epicardial vessels with significant disease.

In-hospital mortality after isolated CABG has continued to decline over the last several decades. Despite a shift toward higher risk demographics, increasing age, and clinical comorbidity, early mortality continued to decline in the 1990s. The cumulative mortality for CABG-only operations among more than 1.4 million CABG-only operations recorded in the Society of Thoracic Surgeons (STS) data base declined from 3.05% between 1997 and 1999 to approximately 2% in 2009.[186] Operative mortality rates for isolated CABG surgery now range from approximately 1.5% to 2.0%. Several models have been developed and refined, with the objective of predicting perioperative mortality.[187] Application of such models have demonstrated even greater declines in CABG mortality over the past decade when adjusted for changes in clinical risk profile.

PERIOPERATIVE COMPLICATIONS. Perioperative morbidity (see Chap. 84) has increased because of a larger fraction of higher risk patients. Major morbidity (e.g., death, stroke, renal failure, reoperation, prolonged ventilation, sternal infection) occurred in 13.4% through 30 days among the 503,478 CABG-only operations recorded in the STS data base between 1997 and 1999.[186]

MYOCARDIAL INFARCTION. Perioperative MI, particularly if associated with hemodynamic or arrhythmic complications or pre-existing LV dysfunction, has a major adverse effect on early and late prognosis. The reported incidence varies widely (0% to more than 10%), in large part because of heterogeneous diagnostic criteria, with an average of 3.9% (median, 2.9%). Elevation of the myocardial creatine kinase-MB (CK-MB) isoenzyme level more than five times the upper limit of normal is commonly considered diagnostic of MI in this setting. Data from a prospectively performed study of routine monitoring of CK-MB postoperatively has shown CK-MB to be independently associated with mortality.[188] Predictors of perioperative MI in the Coronary Artery Surgery Study (CASS) were female gender, severe perioperative angina pectoris, severe stenosis of the left main coronary artery, and triple-vessel CAD. It is possible that mortality associated with perioperative MI may be reduced with acadesine, an experimental agent that increases the concentration of adenosine in ischemic tissue.[189]

CEREBROVASCULAR COMPLICATIONS. Neurologic abnormalities following cardiac surgery are dreaded complications and are associated with higher long-term mortality (see Chap. 84).[190] Postulated mechanisms include emboli from atherosclerosis of the aorta or other large arteries, emboli possibly from the CPB machine circuit and its tubing, and intraoperative hypotension, particularly in patients with pre-existing hypertension.[191] Type I injury is associated with major neurologic deficits, stupor, and coma, and type II injury is characterized by a deterioration in intellectual function and memory. The incidence of neurologic abnormalities is variably estimated, depending on how the deficits are defined. The incidence of stroke reported in the Northern New England Cardiovascular Disease Study Group data base between 1992 to 2001 was 1.6% and has been documented as higher in prospective studies (1.5% to 5%).[190] Studies aimed at careful evaluation of neurologic deficits report more frequent neurologic sequelae; type I deficits have been documented in 6% of patients early after CABG, with short-term cognitive decline in 33% to 83%. A prospective long-term study using sophisticated neurocognitive testing revealed cognitive decline in 53% of patients at the time of hospital discharge, 36% at 6 weeks, and 24% at 6 months.[175] In regard to the neurologic sequelae of CPB (including stroke, delirium, and neurocognitive dysfunction), older age, in addition to other comorbid conditions (particularly diabetes), and intraoperative manipulation of the aorta are the more powerful predictors. In most, but not all, studies, atherosclerosis of the proximal aorta has also been a strong predictor of stroke, as has the use of an intra-aortic balloon pump.[192] Mild hypothermia in the intra- and perioperative periods may improve neurocognitive function after CABG.

ATRIAL FIBRILLATION. This arrhythmia is one of the most frequent complications of CABG.[193] It occurs in up to 40% of patients, primarily within 2 to 3 days. In the early postoperative period, rapid ventricular rates and loss of atrial transport may compromise systemic hemodynamics, increase the risk of embolization, and lead to a significant increase in the duration and cost of the hospital stay; it is associated with a twofold to threefold increase in postoperative stroke. Older age, hypertension, prior atrial fibrillation, and heart failure are associated with higher risk of developing atrial fibrillation after cardiac surgery.[194] Prior statin therapy may be associated with less frequent postoperative atrial fibrillation.[195]

Prophylactic use of beta blockers reduces the frequency of postoperative atrial fibrillation; these should be administered routinely before and after CABG to patients without contraindications. Amiodarone is also effective in prophylaxis against postoperative atrial fibrillation and may be considered for patients at high risk for developing this dysrhythmia (see Chap. 84). Off-pump techniques may be associated with less frequent postoperative atrial fibrillation.[175,179] Up to 80% of patients spontaneously revert to sinus rhythm within 24 hours without treatment other than digoxin or other agents used for controlling the ventricular rate. In a randomized trial of patients with postoperative atrial fibrillation that had resolved prior to discharge, there was no detectable benefit of extended antiarrhythmic therapy beyond a short course of 1 week.[193] Most patients return to sinus rhythm by 6 weeks after surgery.

RENAL DYSFUNCTION. The incidence of renal failure requiring dialysis after CABG remains low (0.5% to 1.0%) but is associated with significantly greater morbidity and mortality (see Chap. 84). A decline in renal function defined by a postoperative serum creatinine level higher than 2.0 mg/dL or an increase of more than 0.7 mg/dL is more frequent (7% to 8%). Predictors of postoperative renal dysfunction include advanced age, diabetes, pre-existing renal dysfunction, and heart failure. Patients with preoperative renal dysfunction and a serum creatinine level higher than 2.5 mg/dL appear to be at increased risk of the need for hemodialysis and may be candidates for alternative approaches to revascularization or prophylactic dialysis. A randomized trial of *N*-acetylcysteine for the prevention of development of renal dysfunction in 295 patients undergoing CABG showed no difference compared with placebo.[196]

Relief of Angina

Trials in which the contemporary practice of using one or more arterial grafts was prevalent have demonstrated similar or superior rates of freedom from angina during short- and mid-term follow-up. The major randomized trials all have demonstrated greater relief of angina, better exercise performance, and a lower requirement for antianginal medications for surgically compared with medically treated patients 5 years postoperatively. Independent predictors of recurrence of angina are female gender, obesity, preoperative hypertension, and lack of use of the IMA as a conduit. In patients with triple-vessel CAD undergoing CABG surgery, the completeness of revascularization is a significant determinant of the relief of symptoms at 1 year and over a 5-year period.

In summary, after 5 years, approximately 75% of surgically treated patients can be predicted to be free of an ischemic event, sudden death, occurrence of MI, or recurrence of angina; about 50% remain free for approximately 10 years and about 15% for 15 years or

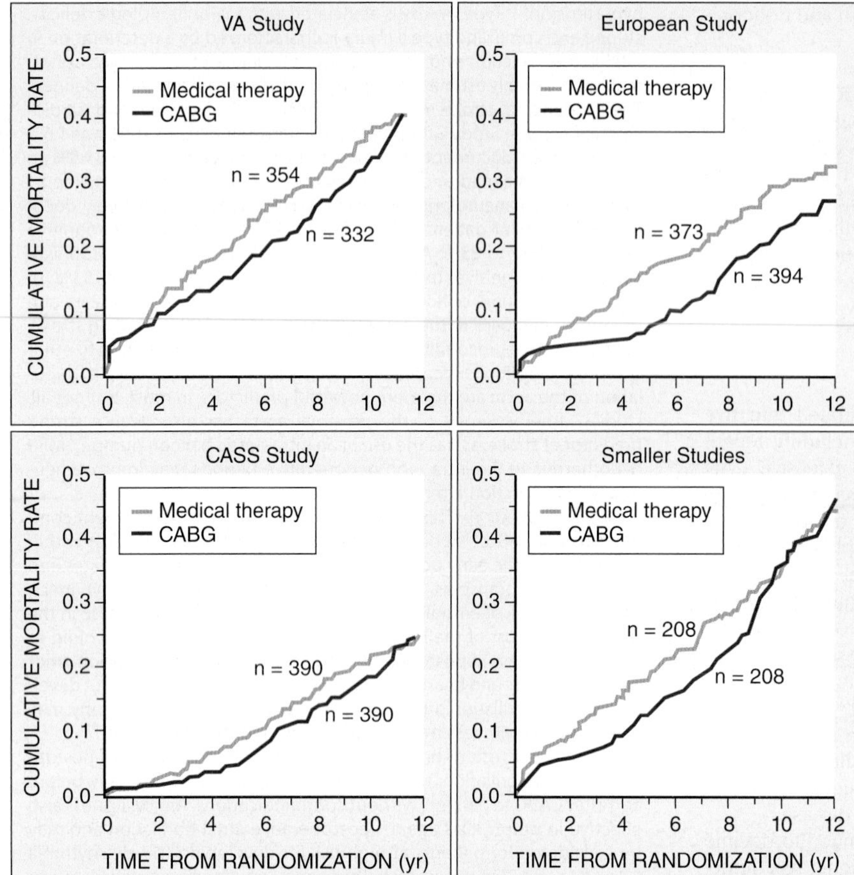

FIGURE 57-14 Survival curves of three large randomized trials and four smaller studies combined. *(From Eagle KA, Guyton RA, Davidoff R, et al: ACC/AHA guidelines for coronary artery bypass graft surgery: A report of the American College of Cardiology/American Heart Association Task Force on Practice Guidelines [Committee to Revise the 1991 Guidelines for Coronary Artery Bypass Graft Surgery]. American College of Cardiology/American Heart Association. J Am Coll Cardiol 34:1262, 1999.)*

more. Symptomatic improvement is best maintained in patients with the most complete revascularization.

Effects on Survival

Current clinical practice has been shaped by three major randomized trials of CABG compared with medical therapy that enrolled patients between 1972 and 1984—the Veterans Affairs (VA) Trial, the European Cardiac Society Study (ECSS), and the National Institutes of Health–supported CASS (**Fig. 57-14**).[153] The evidence base comprises data from 2649 patients participating in these and several smaller trials and has several important limitations with respect to application to current practice because the risk profile of patients referred for surgery, as well as the available surgical and medical interventions, have evolved substantially since these trials were conducted. In particular, these trials antedated the widespread use of one or two IMAs and the disease-modifying therapies (e.g., aspirin, statins, inhibitors of the renin-angiotensin system) that are currently used as guideline-driven intensive medical therapy.

The results of the trials of surgical versus medical therapy have generally been highly consistent, and thus the major points guiding clinical practice may still be drawn from a meta-analysis of the results. In each of the trials, a survival benefit of CABG emerged during mid-term follow-up (2 to 6 years), but this advantage eroded during long-term follow-up and remained statistically significant only in the ECSS. Considered together, the results of these trials support a 4.1% absolute reduction in long-term mortality (10 years) with CABG ($P = 0.03$). Subgroup analyses have revealed several high-risk criteria that identify patients likely to sustain a more substantial survival benefit: (1) left main CAD; (2) single- or double-vessel CAD with proximal LAD artery disease; (3) LV systolic dysfunction; and (4) a composite evaluation that indicates high risk, including severity of symptoms, high-risk exercise tolerance test, history of prior MI, and the presence of ST-segment depression on the resting ECG.

Taken together, the results of all the trials and registries indicate that the sicker the patient—based on the severity of symptoms or ischemia, age, number of diseased vessels, and presence of LV dysfunction—the greater the benefit of surgical over medical therapy on survival (see Figs. 57-10 and 57-13 and Table 57-12). CABG prolongs survival in patients with significant left main CAD irrespective of symptoms, in those with multivessel CAD and impaired LV function, and in patients with triple-vessel CAD that includes the proximal LAD artery, irrespective of LV function. Surgical therapy has also been demonstrated to prolong life in patients with double-vessel CAD and LV dysfunction, particularly those with proximal narrowing of one or more coronary arteries and in the presence of severe angina. Although no study has documented a survival benefit with surgical treatment in patients with single-vessel disease, some evidence has indicated that such patients, who have impaired LV function, have a poor long-term survival with medical therapy.

PATIENTS WITH DEPRESSED LEFT VENTRICULAR FUNCTION. Depressed LV function (see Chap. 52) is one of the most powerful predictors of perioperative and late mortality. In the New York State CABG registry, an ejection fraction of 25% or less was associated with 6.5% in-hospital mortality compared with 1.4% in those with an ejection fraction greater than 40%.[197] In the STS data base, the mean ejection fraction in approximately 136,330 patients undergoing initial CABG in 1999 was 0.51, and approximately 25% had an ejection fraction of less than 0.45. Moreover, as the population ages and the proportion undergoing reoperation increases, the number of patients with preoperative LV dysfunction and clinical heart failure will increase. In the CABG Patch trial confined to patients with an ejection fraction of 0.35 or less, perioperative mortality was 3.5% for patients without clinical signs of heart failure versus 7.7% for those with NYHA Classes I to IV heart failure.

Although the effect of a reduced ejection fraction on operative mortality cannot be eliminated, careful attention to intraoperative metabolic, inotropic, and mechanical support, including preoperative intra-aortic balloon counterpulsation in some patients, may decrease perioperative mortality in comparison with the mortality rates expected from prediction models. In addition to advances in myocardial protection for those undergoing CABG with CPB, off-pump approaches to CABG may also lead to improved surgical outcomes in this high-risk population. Thus, in experienced centers, the in-hospital mortality for patients with severe LV dysfunction is less than 4%.

The powerful effect of the preoperative ejection fraction on late survival currently emphasizes that the presence of LV dysfunction, in association with viable myocardium, has changed from a relative contraindication to CABG to a strong indication. This shift in focus has been caused by the realization that viable dysfunctional myocardium may improve after coronary revascularization.[198] The most striking survival benefits of CABG, as well as symptomatic and functional improvements, are shown by patients with seriously impaired LV function in whom the prognosis of medical therapy is poor. In patients with a history of heart failure and multivessel (particularly triple-vessel) disease, CABG may also reduce the incidence of sudden cardiac death. Although preoperative LV dysfunction creates the potential for significant benefit, the perioperative risk should not be underestimated, particularly in the setting of clinical congestive heart failure.[199] Selection of patients with viable myocardium supplied by a reasonable target vessel(s) for grafting appears critical when considering CABG for patients with severe LV dysfunction.

TABLE 57-13 Markers of Viable Myocardium

CLINICAL INDICATOR	DIAGNOSTIC TEST	ALTERNATIVE TEST
Diastolic wall thickness	Echo	CT, CMR
Systolic wall thickening	Echo	CT, CMR, gated SPECT
Regional wall motion	Echo	CT, CMR, gated SPECT
Regional blood flow	SPECT	PET, CMR
Myocardial metabolism	PET	SPECT
Cell membrane integrity	SPECT	PET
Contractile reserve	Dobutamine echocardiography	Angiography, CT, CMR
Myocardial fibrosis	CMR	CT

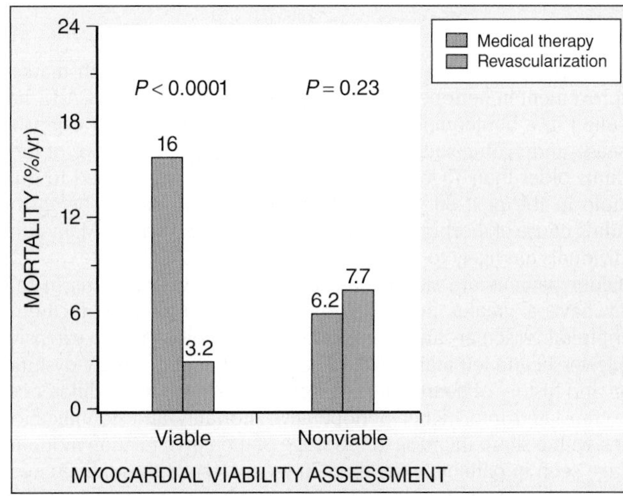

FIGURE 57-15 Meta-analysis of observational studies examining late survival with revascularization versus medical therapy for patients with CAD and LV dysfunction. Analysis of results from 24 studies (N = 3088) demonstrated that revascularization is associated with a significant reduction in annual mortality compared with medical therapy in patients with myocardial viability. No advantage of revascularization was detected in patients without myocardial viability. *(Modified from Allman KC, Shaw LJ, Hachamovitch R, et al: Myocardial viability testing and impact of revascularization on prognosis in patients with coronary artery disease and left-ventricular dysfunction: A meta-analysis. J Am Coll Cardiol 39:1151, 2002.)*

Myocardial Hibernation. Improvement in survival and LV function following CABG depends on the successful reperfusion of viable but noncontractile or poorly contracting myocardium (see Chap. 52). Two related pathophysiologic conditions have been described to explain reversible ischemic contractile dysfunction: (1) myocardial stunning (prolonged but temporary postischemic LV dysfunction without myocardial necrosis); and (2) myocardial hibernation (persistent LV dysfunction when myocardial perfusion is chronically reduced or repetitively stunned but sufficient to maintain the viability of tissue).[200] The reduction in myocardial contractility in hibernating myocardium conserves metabolic demands and may be protective, but more prolonged and severe hibernation may lead to severe ultrastructural abnormalities, irreversible loss of contractile units, and apoptosis.

Hibernating myocardium can cause abnormal systolic or diastolic LV function, or both. The predominant clinical feature of myocardial ischemia in these patients may not be angina but dyspnea secondary to increased LV diastolic pressure. Symptoms of heart failure resulting from chronic LV dysfunction may be inappropriately ascribed to myocardial necrosis and scarring when the symptoms may, in fact, be reversed after the chronic ischemia is relieved by coronary revascularization.

Detection of Hibernating Myocardium. Several clinical markers may be used to determine the likelihood that a dysfunctional myocardial segment is viable or nonviable (**Table 57-13**). The presence of angina and the absence of Q waves on the ECG or a history of prior MI are useful clues. A severe reduction in the diastolic wall thickness of dysfunctional LV segments is indicative of scarring. On the other hand, akinetic or dyskinetic segments with preserved diastolic wall thickness may represent a mixture of scarred and viable myocardium. Although a number of imaging tools may be used for this assessment, the most readily available in most settings is low-dose dobutamine echocardiography[201] (see Chap. 15). PET (see Chap. 17) has emerged as an excellent method for demonstrating viable myocardium in patients with impaired LV function.[156] In comparative studies, PET has yielded the highest predictive accuracy of all imaging modalities for detecting dysfunctional myocardium that will improve after revascularization. However, the high cost, technical difficulty, and need for a cyclotron continue to limit this technique's widespread applicability. Contrast-enhanced CMR is emerging as a valuable alternative technique for the assessment of myocardial viability (see Chap. 18)[202] and thallium-201 rest-redistribution imaging continues to be an alternative (see Chap. 17).

Prognostic Implications of Identifying Viable Myocardium. A growing body of evidence has indicated that the detection of viable myocardium in patients with CAD and LV dysfunction not only identifies those for whom improvement in cardiac function is likely after revascularization, but also identifies a group of high-risk patients for whom revascularization improves survival (**Fig. 57-15**).[156] Studies with PET, thallium-201, and dobutamine echocardiography have uniformly demonstrated that patients with LV dysfunction and evidence of hibernating myocardium have a high mortality rate during medical therapy and appear to have a better outcome with revascularization.[203] All these studies have limitations, including a small number of patients, the retrospective nature of the analysis, and lack of a randomized control group.[198] However, the consistency of the findings has been striking. Viability assessment is also helpful in the selection of patients for revascularization because patients selected for revascularization on the basis of an imaging study demonstrating myocardial viability have lower operative mortality and a higher long-term survival rate than those with no evidence of important myocardial viability, or those in whom a viability assessment is not performed.

The mechanisms for improved survival after revascularization in patients with hibernating myocardium in these retrospective studies may be related to improvement in LV function. However, it is likely that other factors are also operative, including reductions in LV remodeling, propensity for serious arrhythmias, and likelihood of a future fatal acute ischemic event. Prospective trials are needed to provide definitive evidence about whether myocardial viability testing identifies patients with LV dysfunction for whom revascularization improves survival and quality of life. The ongoing follow-up of the revascularization hypothesis treatment groups in the Surgical Treatment of Ischemic Heart Failure (STICH) trial is designed to address this issue.[204]

SURGICAL TREATMENT IN SPECIAL GROUPS

Women

Women are less likely than men to be referred for coronary angiography and subsequent revascularization (see Chap. 81). In some studies, gender-based differences in referral for revascularization are fully explained by clinical factors. Moreover, it has not been established whether gender-based differences represent systematically less consideration of referrals for women, inappropriately more consideration of referrals for men, or both. In comparison with men, women who undergo CABG are sicker, as defined by age, comorbid conditions, severity of angina, and history of heart failure.[205] In-hospital mortality and perioperative morbidity after CABG have remained, on average, two times higher in women compared with men.[206] However, when adjusted for the greater risk profile of women referred for CABG, short-term mortality rates and long-term outcomes are similar to those for men in most, but not all, studies. The independent predictors of long-term prognosis in women are similar to those in men and include older age, previous CABG surgery, previous MI, and diabetes.

With generally similar long-term outcomes after surgical revascularization, gender should not be a significant factor in decisions regarding whether to offer CABG.[205]

CH 57

Older Patients

An evolving change in demographics, in combination with marked improvement in perioperative care and in the outcomes of CABG, has resulted in a burgeoning population of older patients with extensive disease undergoing such surgery (see Chap. 80). The number of individuals older than 75 years in the United States is expected to quadruple in the next 50 years, with cardiovascular disease being the leading cause of morbidity and mortality in this population. Many such individuals are likely to become candidates for CABG.

Older patients are sicker than their younger counterparts in that they have a greater frequency of comorbid conditions, including peripheral vascular and cerebrovascular disease, more extensive triple-vessel and left main CAD, and a higher frequency of LV dysfunction and history of heart failure.[153] Not unexpectedly, these differences are translated into higher perioperative mortality and complication rates, with a sharp increase in the slope of the curve relating mortality to age seen in patients older than 70 years. Despite these differences, in-hospital mortality for older patients has declined over time to 7% to 9% in those undergoing CABG only and has been reported to be as low as 3% to 4% in the subgroup of octogenarians without significant medical comorbidities.[153] Given marked variation in the outcomes in older patients undergoing revascularization, decisions should be based on individual risk and needs assessment.[207]

Renal Disease

Cardiovascular disease is the major cause of mortality in patients with end-stage renal disease (ESRD) and accounts for 54% of deaths (see Chap. 93). Patients with ESRD, as well as those with less severe renal insufficiency, have numerous risk factors that not only accelerate the development of CAD but also complicate its medical management. These risk factors include diabetes, hypertension with LV hypertrophy, systolic and diastolic dysfunction, abnormal lipid metabolism, anemia, and increased homocysteine levels. Therefore, mild or more severe renal dysfunction is prevalent in as many as 50% of patients presenting for CABG.[208] Coronary revascularization with PCI or CABG is feasible and well documented in patients with ESRD, but mortality and complication rates are increased. Patients with milder degrees of renal insufficiency who are not dependent on dialysis are also at higher risk of major perioperative complications, longer recovery times, and lower rates of short- and mid-term survival.[209] Observational data have suggested that in patients on chronic dialysis, CABG is the preferred strategy for revascularization over PCI. However, randomized data are few, and 30-day mortality in patients with ESRD undergoing CABG ranges from 9% to as high as 20%.

Patients with Diabetes

In comparison with age-matched nondiabetic patients, diabetic patients (see Chap. 64) with angiographically proven CAD are more likely to be women with evidence of peripheral vascular disease and a higher number of coronary occlusions. Diabetes is an important independent predictor of mortality among patients undergoing surgical revascularization.[210] Patients with diabetes have smaller distal vessels, which are judged to be poorer targets for bypass grafting. Nevertheless, the patency of arterial and venous grafts appears similar in diabetics and nondiabetic patients. Despite these higher risks with operative intervention, because of the potential long-term benefits of CABG in patients with diabetes and severe CAD, such patients should be considered as candidates for CABG (see "Comparisons Between Percutaneous Coronary Intervention and Coronary Artery Bypass Grafting" and "Choosing Among Percutaneous Coronary Intervention, Coronary Artery Bypass Grafting, and Medical Therapy").

Coronary Bypass Surgery in Patients with Associated Vascular Disease. Management of patients with combined CAD and peripheral vascular disease involving the carotid arteries, the abdominal aorta, or the vessels of the lower extremities presents many challenges (see Chaps. 60 and 61). Polyvascular disease is becoming increasingly frequent as the population of patients under consideration for CABG ages and as technical improvements allow the application of coronary revascularization to ever more complex cases.

Impact of Combined Coronary Artery Disease and Peripheral Vascular Disease. Clinically apparent CAD occurs frequently in patients with peripheral vascular disease. In patients undergoing peripheral vascular surgery, late outcomes are dominated by cardiac causes of morbidity and mortality. Conversely, in patients with CAD, the presence of peripheral vascular disease, even if asymptomatic, is associated with an adverse prognosis, presumably because of the greater total atherosclerotic burden borne by these patients.

Because patients with CAD and peripheral atherosclerosis tend to be older and have more widespread vascular disease and end-organ damage than patients without peripheral atherosclerosis, the perioperative mortality and morbidity consequent to CABG are high and the late outcome is not as favorable.[211] In the Northern New England Cardiovascular data base, in-hospital mortality after CABG was 2.4-fold greater in patients with peripheral vascular disease than in those without it, particularly for patients with lower extremity disease. Diffuse atheroembolism is a particularly serious complication of CABG in patients with peripheral vascular disease and aortic atherosclerosis. It is a major cause of perioperative death, stroke, neurocognitive dysfunction, and multiorgan dysfunction after CABG.

Peripheral vascular disease is also a strong marker of an adverse long-term outcome. For example, in the Northern New England Cardiovascular data base, the 5-year mortality was approximately twofold greater in patients with peripheral vascular disease than in those without it, even after adjusting for other comorbid conditions, which are more frequent in patients with peripheral vascular disease. Nevertheless, given the diffuse nature of coronary disease in patients with peripheral vascular disease, there may be advantages to surgical coronary revascularization rather than PCI in many of these patients.[212]

Carotid Artery Disease. In patients with stable CAD and carotid artery disease for whom carotid endarterectomy is planned, exercise stress testing and consideration of coronary revascularization can ordinarily be performed after the carotid surgery. The prevalence of significant carotid disease in an increasingly older population being considered for CABG is high; approximately 20% have a stenosis of 50% or greater, 6% to 12% have a stenosis of 80% or greater, and the percentage is higher in patients with left main CAD. In patients for whom surgical treatment is considered for both carotid artery disease and CAD, the merits of a combined versus a staged approach have been debated. Neither strategy has been demonstrated to be unequivocally superior to the other, and an individualized approach, depending on the patient's initial condition, severity of symptoms, anatomy of the coronary and carotid vessels, and individual institutional experience, is most appropriate. Preoperative or simultaneous carotid stenting is under investigation as an alternative approach to combined carotid endarterectomy and CABG.

Management of Patients with Associated Vascular Disease. Patients with severe or unstable CAD requiring revascularization can be categorized into two groups according to the severity and instability of the accompanying vascular disease (see Chap. 61). When the noncoronary vascular procedures are elective, they can generally be postponed until the cardiac symptoms have stabilized, either by intensive medical therapy or by revascularization. A combined procedure is necessary in patients with unstable CAD and an unstable vascular condition, such as frequent recurrent transient ischemic attacks or a rapidly expanding abdominal aortic aneurysm. In some patients in this category, PCI offers the potential for stabilizing the patient's cardiac condition before proceeding with a definitive vascular repair. A problem is posed by the use of a thienopyridine after stenting; this will increase bleeding unless surgery is performed at least 5 days after discontinuation of the thienopyridine.

PATIENTS REQUIRING REOPERATION. Currently, approximately 12% of coronary artery procedures are reoperations and, in some centers, particularly tertiary care centers, the proportion is increasing rapidly and accounts for 20% of all CABG operations. The major indication for reoperation is late disease of saphenous vein grafts. An additional factor underlying recurrent symptoms is progression of disease in native vessels between the first and second operations. Several series have emphasized the sicker preoperative status of patients undergoing reoperation, including older age, more serious comorbidity, associated valvular heart disease, and a greater prevalence of LV dysfunction and greater extent of ischemic jeopardized myocardium.[213]

Not unexpectedly, the mortality associated with reoperation is significantly higher than that of initial CABG procedures. For patients undergoing first operations, mortality was 2.6% for urgent and 6% for emergency procedures in comparison with 7.4% and 13.5%, respectively, in patients undergoing repeat CABG.

COMPARISONS BETWEEN PERCUTANEOUS CORONARY INTERVENTION AND CORONARY ARTERY BYPASS GRAFTING

Observational Studies

Catheter-based revascularizations in most comparative studies have been limited mainly to PTCA, and the findings were largely consistent.[153] Over a period of 1 to 5 years, the rates of mortality and nonfatal MI were not significantly different between patients revascularized with CABG versus PTCA, but recurrent events, including angina pectoris and the need for repeat revascularization procedures, were significantly more frequent in the PTCA than the CABG group, largely as a consequence of incomplete revascularization and restenosis. However, several subgroups of patients who may derive a survival benefit from CABG compared with PTCA have been identified. These include patients with LV dysfunction, probably because of the ability to achieve more complete revascularization with CABG. In addition, CABG provides a survival benefit compared with PTCA when proximal LAD artery stenosis (>70%) is present.

More recent studies have included patients undergoing stenting. In an analysis of approximately 60,000 patients with multivessel CAD treated with coronary stenting or CABG and recorded in the New York State Registry between 1997 and 2000, CABG was found to be associated with higher survival after adjustment for medical comorbidities in patients with two or more diseased vessels, with or without involvement of the LAD artery.[214] Nevertheless, the similarity of the unadjusted rates of survival highlights the role of clinical judgment in selecting the optimal therapy for the individual patient and the ability to achieve good outcomes for appropriately selected patients with two-vessel CAD, particularly without involvement of the proximal LAD artery.[169]

Randomized Trials

Overall, the findings from randomized trials indicate that in selected patients with multivessel CAD and preserved ejection fraction, compared with multivessel PCI, CABG results in fewer repeat revascularizations and fewer symptoms, without a significant difference in survival.

Percutaneous Coronary Intervention Versus Coronary Artery Bypass Grafting in Patients with Single-Vessel Disease. Both the Lausanne and the MASS trials were limited to patients with isolated disease of the proximal LAD coronary artery.[153] The results of these small trials were consistent in that over 2 to 3 years, the rates of mortality and MI were similar in the two treatment arms, as was improvement in symptoms, but at the cost of more frequent reintervention in patients treated with PCI. In a trial comparing minimally invasive direct CABG to stenting for patients with isolated stenosis in the proximal LAD artery ($N = 220$), patients treated with CABG were less likely to have recurrent symptoms or undergo repeat revascularization, but showed no detectable difference in the risk of death or MI with PCI.

Multivessel Disease. At least 10 published studies have compared PCI with CABG in patients with multivessel CAD. Despite the heterogeneity of the trials in regard to design, methods, and patient population enrolled, the results are generally comparable and provide a consistent perspective of CABG and PCI in selected patients with multivessel CAD. Nevertheless, there are limitations that should be recognized. Conducted over several decades, the trials evolved substantially with respect to the technology used for both procedures and disease-modifying preventive therapy. Moreover, most patients entered into the trials had well-preserved LV function. Therefore, patients enrolled in these trials were at relatively low risk, with predominantly double-vessel CAD and normal LV ejection fraction—that is, a high proportion of patients in whom CABG surgery had not been previously shown to be superior to medical therapy in regard to survival. Thus, one would not expect a significant mortality difference between PCI and CABG.[80]

As an example, between 1988 and 1991, the Bypass Angioplasty Revascularization Investigation (BARI) trial enrolled 1829 patients with multivessel CAD in the United States and Canada. At 5 years, overall survival rates were not different between the two groups (89.3% with CABG and 86.3% with PTCA; $P = 0.19$), nor was any difference noted in the incidence of MI. CABG was initially associated with greater improvement in angina. Moreover, as anticipated from the observational data, repeat revascularization procedures were more frequent after PCI. This absolute difference was less in subsequent trials in which progressive improvements in stent technology were made. In the Synergy between PCI with Taxus and Cardiac Surgery (SYNTAX) trial, between 2005 and 2007, 1800 patients with three-vessel or left main CAD were randomly assigned to undergo CABG or PCI, for which a multidisciplinary team consisting of a local cardiac surgeon and interventional cardiologist determined that equivalent anatomic revascularization could be achieved with either treatment.[215] The primary outcome measure was the noninferiority comparison of the two groups for major adverse cardiac or cerebrovascular events (i.e., death from any cause, stroke, MI, or repeat revascularization) during the 12-month period after randomization. Rates of major adverse cardiac or cerebrovascular events at 12 months were significantly higher in the PCI group (17.8% versus 12.4% for CABG; $P = 0.002$; **Fig. 57-16**), in large part because of an increased rate of repeat revascularization (13.5% versus 5.9%; $P < 0.001$); thus, the criterion for noninferiority was not met. At 12 months, the rates of death and MI were similar between the two groups. However, stroke was significantly more likely to occur with CABG (2.2% versus 0.6% with PCI; $P = 0.003$).

In-hospital costs are lower for patients undergoing PCI. However, the need for recurrent hospitalization and repeat revascularization procedures over the long term contribute to an increase in postdischarge cost in patients treated with PCI, resulting in similar overall cost over 3 to 5 years.

Patients with Diabetes. An initially unexpected finding in the BARI trial was that patients with previously treated diabetes who underwent PTCA had a 5-year mortality of 34.5% versus 19.4% for those who underwent CABG ($P = 0.003$; see Chap. 64). This advantage of CABG over PTCA for patients with diabetes became more robust by 10 years of follow-up in BARI and was supported in other studies.[216] More rapid progression of atherosclerosis and high rates of restenosis in patients undergoing PCI were plausibly major contributors to this difference. However, subsequent analyses of smaller randomized trials and large clinical registries with mixed results and the introduction of BMS and DES have led to the reevaluation of the relevance of the findings from BARI.[217] Nevertheless, in a collaborative meta-analysis of individual patient data from 7812 patients in ten trials of PCI versus CABG, there was a significant 30% reduction in total mortality with CABG in the subset of 1233 diabetic patients, findings that persisted even after exclusion of the BARI trial (**Fig. 57-17**).[218]

The findings of the Bypass Angioplasty Revascularization Investigation 2 Diabetes (BARI 2D) trial did not directly compare PCI and CABG but provide additional information with respect to revascularization in patients with diabetes mellitus.[170] In the BARI 2D trial, 2368 patients with established diabetes and CAD were randomized to prompt revascularization (PCI or CABG) versus delayed or no revascularization and optimal medical therapy. A notable feature of the prompt revascularization strategy was prespecification to PCI or CABG before randomization, with patients with more severe CAD being allocated to CABG. At 5 years, all-cause mortality did not differ between these two treatment groups (**Fig. 57-18**), However, two prespecified analyses of a secondary composite endpoint (death, MI, or stroke) provide important scientific and clinical insights: (1) compared with optimal medical therapy without revascularization, the CABG cohort had a significantly lower rate of death, MI, or stroke driven mainly by a reduction in nonfatal MI, but accompanied also by a nonsignificant 16% relative decrease in mortality; (2) in contrast to CABG, there was absolutely no difference in the primary survival or secondary composite endpoints in PCI patients versus optimal medical therapy.

In BARI 2D, only 35% of patients received DES; the ongoing Future REvascularization Evaluation in patients with Diabetes mellitus: Optimal management of Multivessel disease (FREEDOM) trial of patients with multivessel CAD who are randomized to either DES or CABG will provide additional information to guide clinical practice.[219]

CHOOSING AMONG PERCUTANEOUS CORONARY INTERVENTION, CORONARY ARTERY BYPASS GRAFTING, AND MEDICAL THERAPY. Optimal medical therapy of stable IHD involves a reduction in reversible risk factors, counseling in lifestyle alteration, treatment of conditions that intensify angina, and pharmacologic management of ischemia. Unlike in ACS patients,[220] revascularization has not been shown to reduce death or MI when used

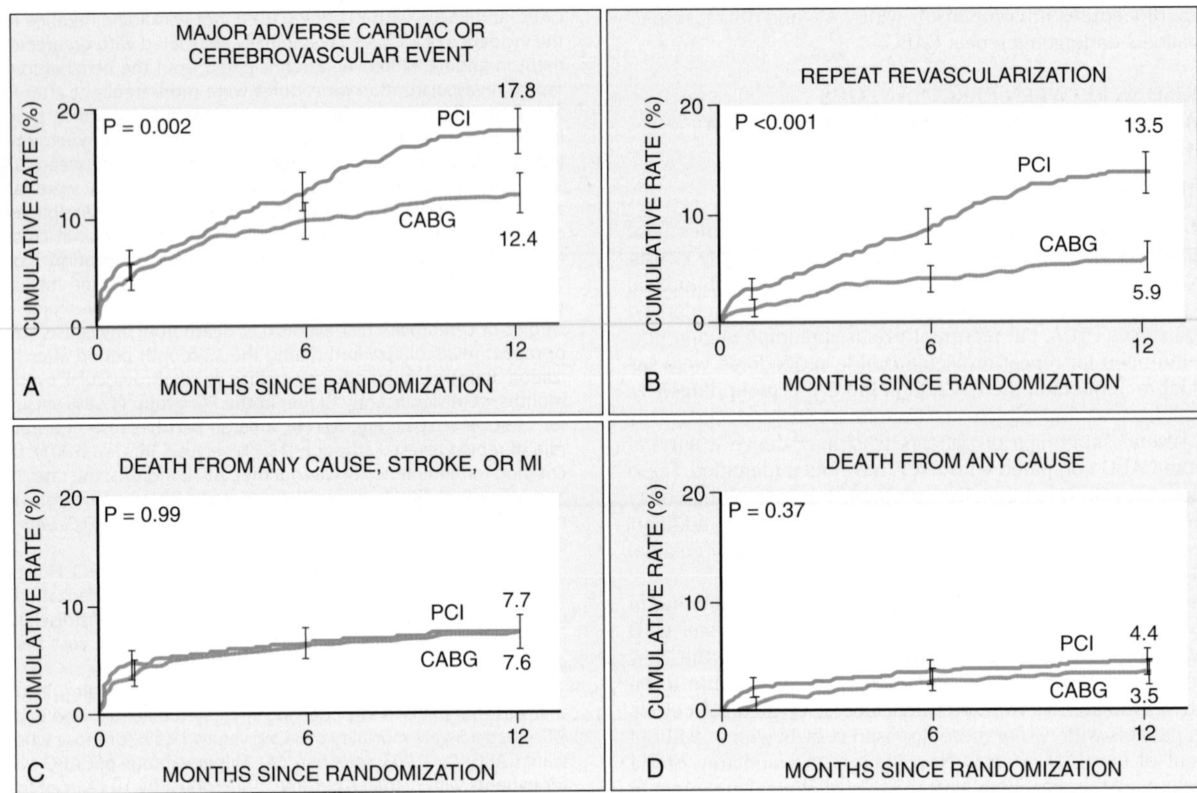

FIGURE 57-16 Outcomes in 1800 patients with stable ischemic heart disease and multivessel coronary artery disease randomized to CABG or PCI. **A,** CABG was superior to PCI at 1 year with respect to the primary outcome measure of death from any cause, MI, stroke, or repeat revascularization. **B,** This result was driven by the need for repeat revascularization, which was reduced significantly in the CABG group. **C, D,** There was no difference in the rate of death, MI, or stroke or death from any cause in the two treatment groups. *(Modified from Serruys PW, Morice MC, Kappetein AP, et al: Percutaneous coronary intervention versus coronary-artery bypass grafting for severe coronary artery disease. N Engl J Med 360:961, 2009.)*

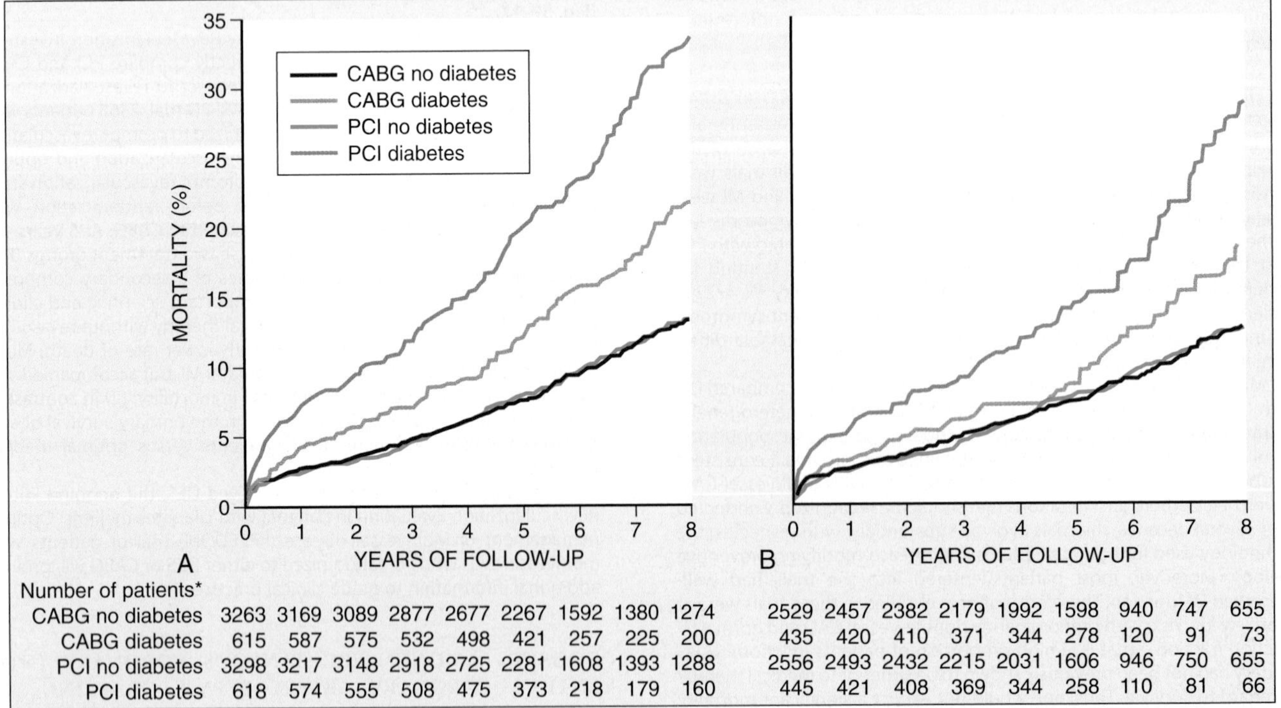

FIGURE 57-17 Kaplan-Meier estimates of death from any cause in a collaborative analysis of individual patient data from 10 randomized trials in patients with stable CAD with and without diabetes mellitus assigned to multivessel PCI or CABG. Patients with diabetes had a significant reduction in mortality with CABG compared with PCI. **A,** Cumulative incidence among patients from all 10 trials. **B,** Cumulative incidence among all trials, excluding the BARI trial. *(Modified from Hlatky MA, Boothroyd DB, Bravata DM, et al: Coronary artery bypass surgery compared with percutaneous coronary interventions for multivessel disease: A collaborative analysis of individual patient data from ten randomised trials. Lancet 373:1190, 2009.)*

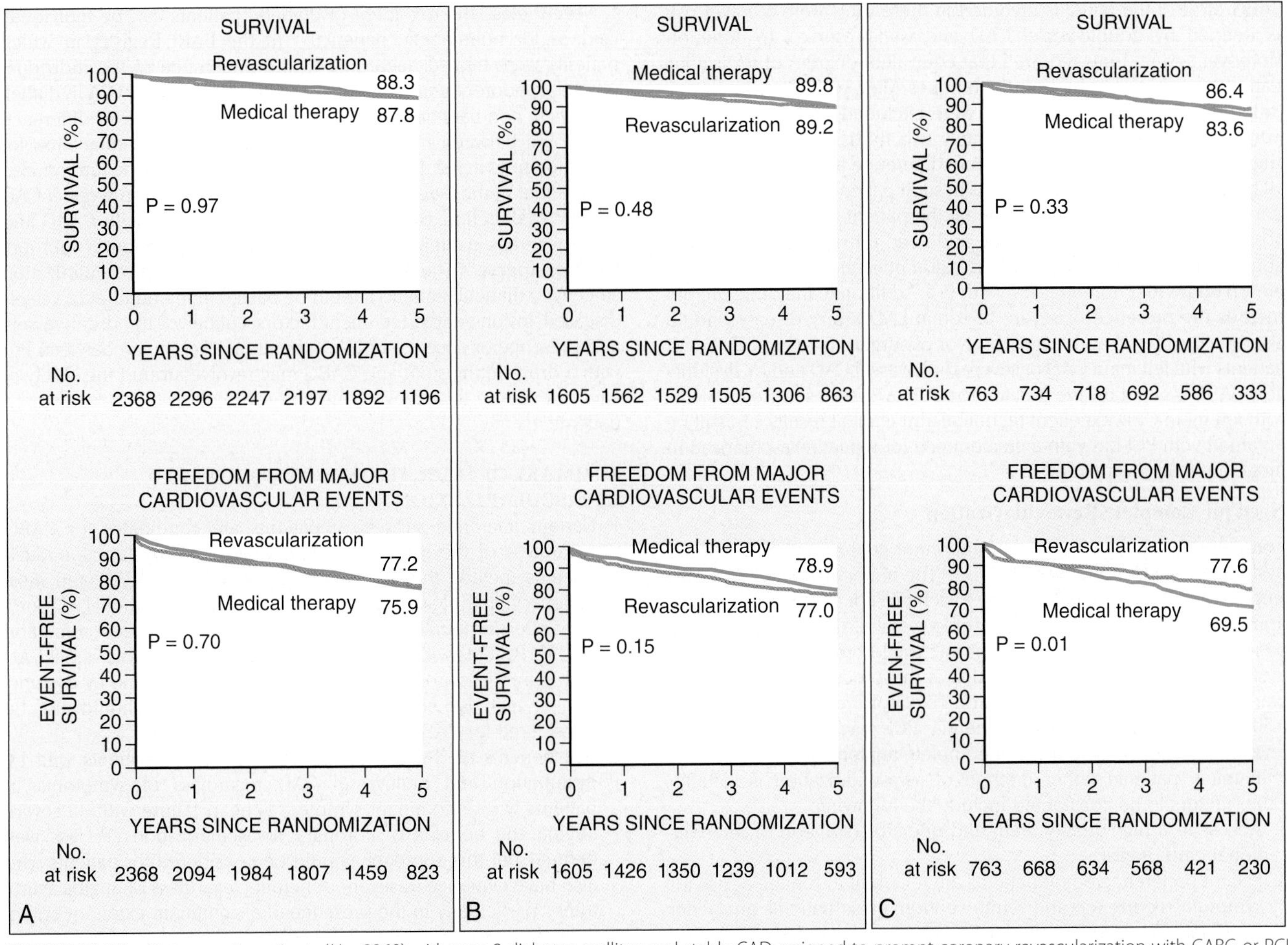

FIGURE 57-18 Outcomes in patients ($N = 2368$) with type 2 diabetes mellitus and stable CAD assigned to prompt coronary revascularization with CABG or PCI versus intensive medical therapy alone in the BARI-2D trial. Intent to revascularize with PCI or CABG was recorded at the time of randomization. **A,** There was no significant difference in the rates of survival (top) or major cardiovascular events (death, myocardial infarction, or stroke; bottom) by treatment group in the overall cohort. **B,** In the PCI stratum, there was no difference between treatment groups with respect to either endpoint. **C,** In patients selected by the investigator to undergo CABG, the rate of major cardiovascular events was significantly lower in patients who underwent prompt revascularization compared with medical therapy alone. *(Modified from Frye RL, August P, Brooks MM, et al: A randomized trial of therapies for type 2 diabetes and coronary artery disease. N Engl J Med 360:2503, 2009.)*

in patients with stable IHD (with the exception of surgery in patients meeting specific anatomic criteria). Recommendations for PCI or CABG should be based both on the extent and severity of ischemia by noninvasive stress testing or invasive assessment of the hemodynamic significance of anatomic stenosis and the severity of anginal symptoms or functional impairment. When an unacceptable level of angina persists despite medical management, the patient has troubling side effects from the anti-ischemic drugs, and/or exhibits a high-risk result on noninvasive testing, the coronary anatomy should be defined to allow selection of the appropriate technique for revascularization.[153] Accordingly, based on these data, and after elucidation of the coronary anatomy, selection of the technique of revascularization should be made as described here (**Table 57-14**; see Figs. 57-16 and 57-18).

Single-Vessel Disease

In patients with single-vessel disease in whom revascularization is deemed necessary and the lesion is anatomically suitable, PCI is almost always preferred over CABG.

Multivessel Disease

The first step is to decide whether a patient falls into the category of those who were included in randomized trials comparing PCI and

TABLE 57-14 Comparison of Revascularization Strategies in Multivessel Disease

ADVANTAGES	DISADVANTAGES
Percutaneous Coronary Intervention	
Less invasive	Restenosis
Shorter hospital stay	High incidence of incomplete revascularization
Lower initial cost	Relative inefficacy in patients with severe left ventricular dysfunction
Easily repeated	Less favorable outcome in diabetics
Effective in relieving symptoms	Limited to specific anatomic subsets
Coronary Artery Bypass Grafting	
Effective in relieving symptoms	Cost
Improved survival in certain subsets	Morbidity
Ability to achieve complete revascularization	
Wider applicability (anatomic subsets)	

Modified from Faxon DP: Coronary angioplasty for stable angina pectoris. *In* Beller G, Braunwald E (eds): Chronic Ischemic Heart Disease. Atlas of Heart Disease. Vol 5. Philadelphia, WB Saunders, 1995, p 9.15.

CABG. Most of the patients included in these trials were at lower risk, as defined by double-vessel CAD and well-preserved LV function. Moreover, several trials required that equivalent degrees of revascularization be achievable by both techniques. Most patients with chronically occluded coronary arteries were excluded and, of those who were clinically eligible, approximately two thirds were excluded for angiographic reasons. The lack of any difference in late mortality and MI between the two treatment arms in such patients indicates that PCI is a reasonable strategy, provided that the patient accepts the distinct possibility of symptom recurrence and need for repeat revascularization. Patients with a single localized lesion in each affected vessel and preserved LV function fare best with PCI. Additional anatomic factors, such as the presence of severe proximal LAD artery disease, should also be considered and weigh in favor of surgery (see Fig. 57-13). For patients with left main CAD or severe triple-vessel CAD and LV dysfunction, CABG is generally the best approach. However, in selected patients with left main CAD, excellent technical and clinical results can still be obtained with PCI but with a greater need for repeat revascularization procedures than with CABG.[215,220]

Need for Complete Revascularization

Complete revascularization is an important goal for patients with LV dysfunction and/or multivessel CAD.[221] The major advantage of CABG surgery over PCI is its greater ability to achieve complete revascularization, particularly in patients with triple-vessel CAD. In most of these patients, particularly those with chronic total coronary occlusion, LV dysfunction, or left main CAD, CABG is the procedure of choice. In patients with borderline LV function (ejection fraction from 0.40 to 0.50) and milder degrees of ischemia, PCI may provide adequate revascularization, even if it is not complete anatomically.

In many patients, either method of revascularization is suitable. Other factors to be considered include the following:

1. Access to a high-quality team and operator (surgeon or interventional cardiologist).
2. Patient preference. Some patients are reluctant to remain at risk for symptom recurrence and reintervention; these patients are better candidates for surgical treatment. Other patients are attracted by the less invasive nature and more rapid recovery from PCI; they prefer to have PCI as their initial revascularization, with the possibility of undergoing CABG if symptoms persist and/or an excellent revascularization has not been achieved.
3. Advanced patient age and comorbidity. Much older patients and those with comorbid conditions are often better candidates for PCI.
4. Younger patient age. PCI is also often preferable for younger patients (<50 years), with the expectation that they may require CABG at some time in the future and that PCI will postpone the need for surgery; this sequence may be preferable to two operations. Patient preference is a pivotal aspect of the decision to perform PCI or CABG in these patient groups.

Patients with Diabetes

The poorer outcomes after PCI than after CABG in treated diabetic patients in the BARI trial, together with similar findings in the ARTS trial, had raised concern whether all diabetic patients with multivessel CAD should be treated surgically (see Chap. 64). The BARI-2D trial results reinforce the principal finding of the COURAGE trial[166] that an initial strategy of PCI provides no incremental clinical benefit over optimal medical therapy, even in patients with diabetes. However, in those patients who remain symptomatic despite medical therapy, or where there is demonstration of significant ischemia or extensive CAD, then a revascularization strategy is warranted. Either PCI or CABG may be reasonable choices, depending on the anatomic complexity of disease. In patients with severe disease, as selected for CABG in the BARI 2D, current evidence supports CABG as the preferred revascularization strategy. A potential advantage is that bypass grafts to the midcoronary vessel both treat the culprit lesion (regardless of anatomic complexity) and may afford prophylaxis against new proximal disease progression, whereas stents only treat suitable stenotic segment(s), with no benefit against the development of new disease.[172]

Nevertheless, the treatment of diabetic patients can be individualized, as for nondiabetic patients.[210] In the BARI Registry, in which patients were treated according to the preference of the individual physician, poorer outcomes were noted for CABG and PTCA in diabetics versus nondiabetics but, among diabetics, no survival difference was noted between PTCA and CABG.[169] A plausible explanation for the differences in results in the registry compared with the randomized trials is that in the latter, sicker diabetic patients with triple-vessel CAD and LV dysfunction, by design, were treated equally with CABG and PTCA, whereas in clinical practice, such patients are referred appropriately for surgery.[169] Therefore, it is reasonable that the revascularization strategy in diabetic patients should be based on the number of vessels diseased, lesion-related technical factors, caliber of the distal vessels, and presence or absence of LV dysfunction. The choice between PCI with a drug-eluting stent and CABG may revolve around the ability of each procedure to achieve complete revascularization in any given patient.[210,219,222]

SUMMARY OF INDICATIONS FOR CORONARY REVASCULARIZATION

1. Certain anatomic subsets of patients are candidates for CABG, regardless of the severity of symptoms or LV dysfunction. Such patients include those with significant left main CAD and most patients with triple-vessel CAD that includes the proximal LAD coronary artery, especially those with LV dysfunction (ejection fraction < 50%). Patients with chronic stable angina and double-vessel CAD with significant proximal disease of the LAD artery and LV dysfunction or high-risk findings on noninvasive testing should also be considered for CABG.[80]
2. The benefits of CABG are well documented in patients with LV dysfunction and multivessel CAD, regardless of symptoms. In patients whose dominant symptom is heart failure without severe angina, the benefits of coronary revascularization are less well defined, but this approach should be considered for patients who also have evidence of severe ischemia (regardless of angina symptoms), particularly in the presence of a significant extent of potentially viable dysfunctional (hibernating) myocardium.[153]
3. The primary objective of coronary revascularization in patients with single-vessel disease is relief of significant symptoms or objective evidence of severe ischemia. For most of these patients, PCI is the revascularization modality of choice.
4. In patients with angina who are not considered to be at high risk, survival is similar for surgery, PCI, and medical management.
5. All the indications discussed earlier relate to the potential benefits of surgery over medical therapy on survival. Coronary revascularization with PCI or CABG is highly efficacious in relieving symptoms and may be considered for patients with moderate to severe ischemic symptoms who are not controlled by and/or who are dissatisfied with medical therapy, even if they are not in a high-risk subset. For such patients, the optimal method of revascularization is selected on the basis of LV function and arteriographic findings and the likelihood of technical success.

OTHER SURGICAL PROCEDURES FOR ISCHEMIC HEART DISEASE. CABG may be combined with surgical procedures aimed at correction of atherosclerotic disease elsewhere in the cardiovascular system, correction of mechanical complications of MI (mitral regurgitation or ventricular septal defect), LV aneurysms, and concomitant valvular heart disease. Not unexpectedly, morbidity and mortality are correspondingly increased because of the added complexity of the procedure and, in many patients who require these other procedures, the presence of underlying LV dysfunction (see later).

Transmyocardial Laser Revascularization

Transmyocardial laser revascularization (TMLR) is performed by placing a laser on the epicardial surface of the left ventricle, exposed through a lateral thoracotomy, and creating small channels from the epicardial to endocardial surfaces. TMLR has been reported to improve symptoms in patients with refractory angina; however, the mechanism and magnitude of benefit remain uncertain. The initial assumption was that laser-mediated channels would provide a network of functional connections between the LV cavity and ischemic myocardium. Subsequent observations demonstrating closure of the channels within hours or days, despite apparent relief of symptoms, have led to other explanations for the apparent clinical success of the procedure. These explanations include improved perfusion by stimulation of angiogenesis, a placebo effect, and an anesthetic effect mediated by the destruction of sympathetic nerves carrying pain-sensitive afferent fibers or periprocedural MI. The failure of two sham-controlled trials of percutaneous laser myocardial revascularization to show any benefit has highlighted the impact of the placebo effect in response to laser myocardial revascularization. On the basis of data from the randomized trials, it would appear that the widespread use of TMLR as a stand-alone method cannot be justified. Because of the perioperative morbidity associated with surgical TMLR, careful selection of patients is necessary.[223]

Other Manifestations of Coronary Artery Disease

Prinzmetal (Variant) Angina

(See Chaps. 52 and 56.)

Chest Pain with Normal Coronary Arteriogram

The syndrome of angina or angina-like chest pain with a normal coronary arteriogram, often termed *syndrome X* (to be differentiated from metabolic syndrome X, characterized by abdominal obesity, hypertriglyceridemia, low HDL cholesterol, insulin resistance, hyperinsulinemia, and hypertension), is an important clinical entity that should be distinguished from classic ischemic heart disease caused by obstructive CAD. Patients with chest pain and normal coronary arteriograms may represent as many as 10% to 20% of those undergoing coronary arteriography because of clinical suspicion of angina. The cause(s) of the syndrome is not conclusively defined and is likely not homogeneous. However, vascular dysfunction and myocardial metabolic abnormalities have been implicated.[224] True myocardial ischemia, reflected in the production of lactate by the myocardium during exercise or pacing, is present in some of these patients; however, others have no metabolic evidence for ischemia as the cause of their discomfort. The incidence of coronary calcification on multislice CT scanning is significantly higher than that of normal controls (53% versus 20%) but lower than that in patients with angina secondary to obstructive CAD (96%). The prognosis of patients with angina and normal or near-normal coronary angiograms is generally more favorable than that for those with angina caused by obstructive atherosclerosis involving the epicardial coronary arteries. However, observational data have indicated that their outcome is not as uniformly excellent as suggested by early cohort studies.[225,226]

It has been postulated that the syndrome of angina pectoris with normal coronary angiograms reflects a number of conditions. Included in syndrome X are patients with endothelial dysfunction or microvascular dysfunction or spasm in whom angina may be the result of ischemia.[224] This condition is frequently termed *microvascular angina*. In others, chest discomfort without ischemia may be caused by abnormal pain perception or sensitivity.[227] Also, IVUS studies have demonstrated anatomic and physiologic heterogeneity of syndrome X, with a spectrum ranging from normal coronary arteries to vessels with intimal thickening and atheromatous plaque but without critical obstructions. It is likely that some patients with syndrome X have a combination of pathobiologic contributors. In addition, it is difficult to distinguish patients with syndrome X in whom chest pain is caused by ischemia from patients with noncardiac pain. Behavioral or psychiatric disorders may be evident.

Microvascular Dysfunction (Inadequate Vasodilator Reserve). Patients with chest pain, angiographically normal coronary arteries, and no evidence of large-vessel spasm, even after an acetylcholine challenge, may demonstrate an abnormally decreased capacity to reduce coronary resistance and increase coronary flow in response to stimuli such as exercise, adenosine, dipyridamole, and atrial pacing.[228] These patients also have an exaggerated response of small coronary vessels to vasoconstrictor stimuli and an impaired response to intracoronary papaverine. Abnormal endothelium-dependent vasoreactivity has been associated with regional myocardial perfusion defects on SPECT and PET imaging. It has been reported that patients with syndrome X also have impaired vasodilator reserve in forearm vessels and airway hyperresponsiveness, which suggests that the smooth muscle of systemic arteries and other organs may be affected, in addition to that of the coronary circulation.

Endothelial dysfunction and endothelial cell activation, reported in patients with syndrome X, may participate in the release of cellular adhesion molecules, proinflammatory cytokines, and constricting mediators that induce changes in the arterial wall, resulting in microvascular dysfunction and higher risk for future development of obstructive CAD. Patients with syndrome X have been observed to have higher levels of circulating intercellular adhesion molecule-1, vasoconstrictor endothelin-1, and the inflammatory marker hsCRP; moreover, the level of hsCRP appears to correlate with the severity of symptoms and burden of ischemic electrocardiographic changes.

Evidence for Ischemia. Despite general acceptance that microvascular and/or endothelial dysfunction is present in many patients with syndrome X, whether ischemia is in fact the putative cause of the symptoms in these patients is not clear. Studies of transmyocardial production of lactate have generated mixed results.[224] The development of LV dysfunction and electrocardiographic or scintigraphic abnormalities during exercise in some of these patients supports an ischemic cause. However, stress echocardiography with dobutamine detects regional contraction abnormalities consistent with ischemia in a subset of patients. More sensitive techniques, such as perfusion analysis with CMR, have demonstrated that subendocardial perfusion abnormalities, in particular, may be associated with syndrome X.

Abnormal Pain Perception. The lack of definitive evidence of ischemia in some patients with syndrome X has focused attention on alternative nonischemic causes of cardiac-related pain, including a decreased threshold for pain perception—the so-called sensitive heart syndrome.[227] This hypersensitivity may result in an awareness of chest pain in response to stimuli such as arterial stretch or changes in heart rate, rhythm, or contractility. A sympathovagal imbalance with sympathetic predominance in some of these patients has also been postulated. At the time of cardiac catheterization, some patients with syndrome X are unusually sensitive to intracardiac instrumentation, with typical chest pain being consistently produced by direct right atrial stimulation and saline infusion. Measurements of regional cerebral blood flow at rest and during chest pain have suggested differential handling of afferent stimuli between patients with syndrome X and those with obstructive CAD.

Clinical Features. The syndrome of angina or angina-like chest pain with normal epicardial arteries occurs more frequently in women (see Chap. 81), many of whom are premenopausal, whereas obstructive CAD is found more commonly in men and postmenopausal women.[224] Fewer than half of patients with syndrome X have typical angina pectoris; most have various forms of atypical chest pain. Although the features are frequently atypical, the chest pain may nonetheless be severe and disabling. The condition may have markedly adverse effects on the quality of life, employment, and use of health care resources.

In some patients with minimal or no CAD, an exaggerated preoccupation with personal health is associated with the chest pain, and panic disorder may be responsible in a portion of such patients. Up to two thirds of patients with chest pain and normal coronary arteries have been observed to have psychiatric disorders. Others have reported that the incidence of obstructive CAD is extremely low in patients with atypical chest pain who are anxious and/or depressed. The association between syndrome X and insulin resistance warrants further study.

Physical and Laboratory Examination. Abnormal physical findings reflecting ischemia, such as a precordial bulge, gallop sound, and the murmur of mitral regurgitation, are uncommon in syndrome X. The resting ECG may be normal, but nonspecific ST-T wave abnormalities are often observed, sometimes occurring in association with the chest pain. Approximately 20% of patients with chest pain and normal coronary arteriograms have positive exercise tests. However, many patients with this syndrome do not complete the exercise test because of fatigue or mild chest discomfort. LV function is usually normal at rest and during stress, unlike the situation in obstructive CAD, in which function often becomes impaired during stress.

Prognosis. Important prognostic information on patients with angina and normal or near-normal coronary arteriograms has been obtained from the CASS Registry. In patients with an ejection fraction of 0.50 or more, the 7-year survival rate was 96% for patients with a normal arteriogram and 92% for those whose arteriogram revealed mild CAD (50% luminal stenosis). Thus, long-term survival of patients with anginal chest pain and normal coronary angiograms is generally excellent, markedly better than in patients with obstructive CAD. Clinical indicators of worse prognosis may be evident. Some but not all studies have indicated that an ischemic response to exercise is associated with increased mortality.[225] Moreover, in women with angina and no obstructive CAD enrolled in the Women's Ischemic Syndrome Evaluation (WISE), persistence of symptoms was associated with a more than twofold higher risk of cardiovascular events.[229] Such patients may be appropriate candidates for formal studies of vascular function and aggressive risk factor modification[224] (see Chap. 81).

MANAGEMENT. In patients with angina-like chest pain syndrome and normal epicardial coronary arteries, noncardiac causes, such as esophageal abnormalities, should be considered. In patients with syndrome X in whom ischemia can be demonstrated by noninvasive stress testing, a trial of anti-ischemic therapy with nitrates, calcium channel blockers, and beta blockers is logical, but the response to this therapy is variable. Perhaps because of the heterogeneity of this population, studies testing these antianginal therapies have produced conflicting results.[224] For example, beta blockers may be most effective in patients with syndrome X who also have evidence of a hyperadrenergic state characterized by increased sympathetic nervous activity (e.g., hypertension, tachycardia, reduced heart rate variability). Sublingual nitroglycerin has shown paradoxical effects on blood flow and exercise tolerance in some studies and beneficial effects in others. Alpha blockers have been demonstrated to be ineffective. Observational studies of calcium antagonists have in general shown disappointing results with respect to amelioration of symptoms.

ACE inhibitors have favorable effects on endothelial function, vascular remodeling, and sympathetic tone that may be relevant to the pathophysiology of syndrome X. Preliminary data studying ACE inhibitors in this population are promising. Similarly, estrogen has been shown to attenuate normal coronary vasomotor responses to acetylcholine, increase coronary blood flow, and potentiate endothelium-dependent vasodilation in postmenopausal women. Studies of estrogen replacement in postmenopausal women with syndrome X have shown improvement in symptoms and/or exercise performance; however, the role of exogenous estrogen in treatment of this group remains in question. Aimed at the altered somatic and visceral pain perception in many patients with syndrome X, imipramine (50 mg) and structured psychological intervention have been reported to be helpful for some patients.[224]

Silent Myocardial Ischemia

The prognostic importance and the mechanisms of silent ischemia have been the subject of considerable interest for almost 30 years. Patients with silent ischemia have been stratified into three categories by Cohn and associates. The first and least common form, type I silent ischemia, occurs in totally asymptomatic patients with obstructive CAD, which may be severe. These patients do not experience angina at any time; some type I patients do not even experience pain in the course of MI. Epidemiologic studies of sudden death (see Chap. 41), as well as clinical and postmortem studies of patients with silent MI and studies of patients with chronic angina pectoris, have suggested that many patients with extensive coronary artery obstruction never experience angina pectoris in any of its recognized forms (stable, unstable, or variant). These patients with type I silent ischemia may be considered to have a defective anginal warning system. Type II silent ischemia is the form that occurs in patients with documented previous MI.

The third and much more frequent form, designated type III silent ischemia, occurs in patients with the usual forms of chronic stable angina, unstable angina, and Prinzmetal angina. When monitored, patients with this form of silent ischemia exhibit some episodes of ischemia associated with chest discomfort and other episodes that are not—that is, episodes of silent (asymptomatic) ischemia. The total ischemic burden in these patients refers to the total period of ischemia, both symptomatic and asymptomatic.

AMBULATORY ELECTROCARDIOGRAPHY. The use of ambulatory electrocardiographic monitoring has led to a greater appreciation of the high frequency of type III silent ischemia, occurring in up to one third of patients with stable angina treated with appropriate therapy. It has become apparent that anginal pain underestimates the frequency of significant cardiac ischemia.[230]

The role of myocardial O_2 demand in the genesis of myocardial ischemia has been evaluated by measuring the heart rate and blood pressure changes preceding silent ischemic events during ambulatory studies. In one series, 92% of all episodes were silent, and 60% to 70% were preceded by significant increases in heart rate or blood pressure. The circadian variations in heart rate and blood pressure also paralleled the increase in silent ischemic events. This and other studies have suggested that increases in myocardial O_2 demand have a significant role in the genesis of silent ischemia, but in other patients reductions in myocardial O_2 supply may make an important contribution to the initiation of symptomatic and asymptomatic episodes. The mechanisms underlying the development of ischemia, as detected by ambulatory electrocardiographic and exercise testing, may be different and, in patients in the ACIP study, concordance between the ambulatory ECG and SPECT was only 50%. For identification of silent ischemia, the two techniques probably complement each other.

Transient ST-segment depression of 0.1 mV or more that lasts longer than 30 seconds is a rare finding in normal subjects. Patients with known CAD show a strong correlation between such transient ST-segment depression and independent measurements of impaired regional myocardial perfusion and ischemia, determined by rubidium-82 uptake as measured by PET. In patients with type III silent ischemia, perfusion defects occur in the same myocardial regions during symptomatic and asymptomatic episodes of ST-segment depression.

Type III silent ischemia is extremely common. Analysis of ambulatory electrocardiographic recordings of patients with CAD who had symptomatic and silent myocardial ischemia has shown that 85% of ambulant ischemic episodes occur without chest pain and 66% of angina reports are unaccompanied by ST-segment depression. Their frequency is such that it has been suggested that overt angina pectoris is merely the "tip of the ischemic iceberg." In patients with stable CAD enrolled 1 to 6 months after hospitalization for an acute ischemic event, only 15% had angina with exercise, but 28% had ST-segment depression and 41% had reversible myocardial perfusion defects on thallium scintigraphy. Episodes of silent ischemia have been estimated to be present in approximately one third of all treated patients with angina, although a higher prevalence has been reported in diabetics (see Chap. 64).[231] Episodes of ST-segment depression, symptomatic and asymptomatic, exhibit a circadian rhythm and are more common in the morning. Asymptomatic nocturnal ST-segment changes are almost invariably an indicator of double- or triple-vessel CAD or left main coronary artery stenosis.

Pharmacologic agents that reduce or abolish episodes of symptomatic ischemia (e.g., nitrates, beta blockers, calcium antagonists) also reduce or abolish episodes of silent ischemia.

MECHANISMS OF SILENT ISCHEMIA. It is not clear why some patients with unequivocal evidence of ischemia do not experience chest pain, whereas others are symptomatic. Differences in peripheral and central neural processing of pain have been proposed as important factors underlying silent ischemia. PET imaging of cerebral blood flow during painful versus silent ischemia has pointed toward differences in handling of afferent signals by the central nervous system. Specifically, overactive gating of afferent signals in the thalamus may reduce the cortical activation necessary for perception of pain from the heart. Autonomic neuropathy has also been implicated as a reason for reduced sensation of pain during ischemia. Although increased release of endorphins may play a role in some patients with silent ischemia, the results of clinical studies are mixed. Some researchers have suggested that anti-inflammatory cytokines are at play in reducing inflammatory processes that may participate in the genesis of cardiac pain.

PROGNOSIS. Although some controversy remains, ample evidence has supported the view that episodes of myocardial ischemia, regardless of whether they are symptomatic or asymptomatic, are of prognostic importance for patients with CAD.[232] In asymptomatic patients (type I), the presence of exercise-induced ST-segment depression has been shown to predict a fourfold to fivefold increase in cardiac mortality in comparison with patients without this finding. Similarly, in patients with stable angina or prior MI, the presence of inducible ischemia evident by ST-segment depression or perfusion abnormalities during exercise testing is associated with unfavorable outcomes, regardless of whether symptoms are present. The strength of this association is greatest when the ischemia is found to occur at a low workload. Several studies evaluating the prognostic implications of silent ischemia on ambulatory monitoring in patients with stable angina (type III) have demonstrated that the presence of myocardial ischemia on the ambulatory ECG, whether silent or symptomatic, is also associated with an adverse cardiac outcome. Moreover, in the ACIP study, in patients treated medically, myocardial ischemia detected by the ambulatory ECG and by an abnormal exercise treadmill test result were each independently associated with adverse cardiac outcomes. However, other studies have not detected a relationship between silent ischemia on ambulatory monitoring and subsequent hard outcomes.

Nevertheless, when the subgroup of patients with ischemia on stress testing is considered, silent ischemia on Holter monitoring is also a significant predictor of subsequent death or MI. In addition, patients with ischemia on the ambulatory ECG are more likely to have multivessel CAD, severe proximal stenoses, and a greater frequency of complex lesion morphology, including intracoronary thrombus, ulceration, and eccentric lesions, than patients without evidence of ischemia on ambulatory monitoring. The presence of severe and complex CAD may partly explain the apparently independent effect of silent ischemia during ambulatory monitoring on prognosis.

Substantial improvements in technology have made long-term ambulatory monitoring for ischemia more convenient and reliable with respect to data quality.[233] Nevertheless, whether the incremental prognostic information provided by adding an ambulatory ECG to a standard stress test justifies the cost of using this modality as a tool for widespread screening remains to be determined, but it is unlikely. The exercise ECG can identify most patients likely to have significant ischemia during their daily activities and remains the most important screening test for significant CAD (see Chap. 14). Many patients with type I silent ischemia have been identified because of an asymptomatic positive exercise ECG obtained following MI. In such patients, with a defective anginal warning system, it is reasonable to assume that asymptomatic ischemia has a significance similar to that of symptomatic ischemia and that their management with respect to disease-modifying preventive therapy, coronary angiography, and revascularization should be similar.

MANAGEMENT. Drugs that are effective for preventing episodes of symptomatic ischemia (e.g., nitrates, calcium antagonists, beta blockers) are also effective for reducing or eliminating episodes of silent ischemia. A number of studies have shown that beta blockers reduce the frequency, duration, and severity of silent ischemia in a dose-dependent fashion. For example, in the Atenolol Silent Ischemia Study Trial (ASIST), 4 weeks of atenolol therapy decreased the number of ischemic episodes detected on ambulatory ECG (from 3.6 to 1.7; $P < 0.001$) and also the average duration (from 30 to 16.4 minutes/48 hours; $P < 0.001$). Coronary revascularization is also effective in reducing the rate of angina and ambulatory ischemia. In the ACIP pilot study, 57% of patients treated with revascularization were free of ischemia at 1 year, compared with 31% and 36% in the ischemia- and angina-guided strategies, respectively ($P < 0.0001$). In the Swiss Interventional Study on Silent Ischemia Type II (SWISSI-II) trial in 201 patients with silent myocardial ischemia who were recovering from acute MI (>2 months), PCI was associated with a significant reduction in late (up to 10-year) mortality as compared with medical therapy,[234] but the medical therapy as used in this study was not as intensive as in the COURAGE and BARI 2D trials, thus making the results of this fairly small study somewhat difficult to interpret. In addition, aggressive secondary prevention with lipid-lowering therapy has also been shown to reduce ischemia on ambulatory monitoring.

Although suppression of ischemia in patients with asymptomatic ischemia appears to be a worthwhile objective, whether treatment should be guided by symptoms or by ischemia as reflected by the ambulatory ECG has not been established. In a study of bisoprolol, nifedipine, and a combination of the two, patients achieving complete eradication of ischemia, symptomatic and asymptomatic, were less likely to suffer death, MI, or angina requiring revascularization. Similarly, amelioration of all symptomatic and asymptomatic ischemia in the ASIST trial conferred an advantage with respect to the primary endpoint of death, resuscitated ventricular tachycardia or ventricular fibrillation, MI, unstable angina, revascularization, or worsening angina. However, in the ACIP trial, no differences in outcome were detected between the groups allocated to ischemia- versus angina-guided therapy. In contrast, the early benefits of revascularization on ischemia were associated with improved clinical outcomes. Specifically, the rate of death or MI was 12.1% in the angina-guided strategy, 8.8% in the ischemia-guided strategy, and 4.7% in the revascularization strategy, and a strong reduction was also seen in recurrent hospitalizations and the revascularization strategies. Patients who continue to suffer silent ischemia after revascularization may be at increased risk for recurrent cardiac events compared with those who are free of any ischemia.

Heart Failure in Ischemic Heart Disease

Currently, the leading cause of heart failure in developed countries is CAD.[235] In the United States, CAD and its complications account for two thirds to three fourths of all cases of heart failure. In many patients, the progressive nature of heart failure reflects the progressive nature of the underlying CAD. The term *ischemic cardiomyopathy* is used for the clinical syndrome in which one or more of the pathophysiologic features just discussed result in LV dysfunction and heart failure symptoms.[236] This condition is the predominant form of heart failure related to CAD. Additional complications of CAD that may become superimposed on ischemic cardiomyopathy and precipitate heart failure are the development of LV aneurysm and mitral regurgitation caused by papillary muscle dysfunction.

ISCHEMIC CARDIOMYOPATHY. In 1970, Burch and associates first used the term *ischemic cardiomyopathy* to describe the condition in which CAD results in severe myocardial dysfunction, with clinical manifestations often indistinguishable from those of primary dilated cardiomyopathy (see Chap. 68). Symptoms of heart failure caused by ischemic myocardial dysfunction and hibernation, diffuse fibrosis, or multiple MIs, alone or in combination, may dominate the clinical picture of CAD. In some patients with chronic CAD, angina may be the principal clinical manifestation at one time, but later this symptom diminishes or even disappears as heart failure becomes more prominent. Other patients with ischemic cardiomyopathy have no history of angina or MI (type I silent ischemia), and it is in this subgroup that ischemic cardiomyopathy is most often confused with dilated cardiomyopathy.

It is important to recognize hibernating myocardium in patients with ischemic cardiomyopathy because symptoms resulting from chronic LV dysfunction may be incorrectly thought to result from necrotic and scarred myocardium rather than from a reversible ischemic process.[237] Hibernating myocardium may be present in patients with known or suspected CAD with a degree of cardiac dysfunction or heart failure not readily accounted for by previous MIs.

The outlook for patients with ischemic cardiomyopathy treated medically is poor, and revascularization or cardiac transplantation may be considered.[198] The prognosis is particularly poor for patients in whom ischemic cardiomyopathy is caused by multiple MIs, those with associated ventricular arrhythmias, and those with extensive amounts of hibernating myocardium. However, this last group of patients, whose heart failure, even if severe, is caused by large segments of reversibly dysfunctional but viable myocardium, appears to have a significantly better prognosis after revascularization. Revascularization in this group also significantly relieves heart failure symptoms. Thus, the key to management of patients with ischemic cardiomyopathy is to assess the extent of residual viable myocardium with a view to coronary revascularization of viable myocardium. Patients with little or no viable myocardium in whom heart failure is secondary to extensive MI and/or fibrosis should be managed in a manner similar to those with dilated cardiomyopathy (see Chaps. 28 and 68) because their prognosis is poor. By contrast, patients with ischemic cardiomyopathy with extensive multivessel CAD and viable myocardium may derive a survival advantage with CABG surgery, particularly the subset of patients with diabetes.

Additional, more rigorous, adequately sized observational studies and randomized controlled trials are needed to determine the efficacy of revascularization versus medical therapy and to define the role of viability testing. Three such studies are underway—the STICH trial,[204] the Heart Failure Revascularization Trial (HEART), and the PET and Recovery Following Revascularization-2 (PARR-2) study.[198]

Left Ventricular Aneurysm. LV aneurysm is usually defined as a segment of the ventricular wall that exhibits paradoxical (dyskinetic) systolic expansion. Chronic fibrous aneurysms interfere with LV performance principally through loss of contractile tissue. Aneurysms made up largely of a mixture of scar tissue and viable myocardium or of thin scar tissue also impair LV function by a combination of paradoxical expansion and loss of effective contraction.[238] False aneurysms (pseudoaneurysms) represent localized myocardial rupture in which the hemorrhage is limited by pericardial adhesions, and have a mouth that is considerably smaller than the maximal diameter (**Fig. 57-19**). True and false aneurysms may coexist, although the combination is extremely rare.

The frequency of LV aneurysms depends on the incidence of transmural MI and heart failure in the population studied. LV aneurysms and the need for aneurysmectomy have declined dramatically during the last 5 to 10 years in concert with the expanded use of acute reperfusion therapy in evolving MI. More than 80% of LV aneurysms are located anterolaterally near the apex. They are often associated with total occlusion of the LAD coronary artery and a poor collateral blood supply. Approximately 5% to 10% of aneurysms are located posteriorly. Three fourths of patients with aneurysms have multivessel CAD.

Almost 50% of patients with moderate or large aneurysms have symptoms of heart failure, with or without associated angina, approximately 33% have severe angina alone, and approximately 15% have symptomatic ventricular arrhythmias that may be intractable and life-threatening. Mural thrombi are found in almost half of patients with chronic LV aneurysms and can be detected by angiography and two-dimensional echocardiography (see Chap. 15). Systemic embolic events in patients with thrombi and LV aneurysm tend to occur early after MI. In patients with chronic LV aneurysm (documented at least 1 month after MI), subsequent systemic emboli were extremely uncommon (0.35/100 patient-years in patients not receiving anticoagulants).

Detection. Clues to the presence of aneurysm include persistent ST-segment elevations on the resting ECG (in the absence of chest pain) and a characteristic bulge of the silhouette of the left ventricle on a chest roentgenogram. Marked calcification of the LV silhouette may be present. These findings, when clear-cut, are relatively specific, but they have limited sensitivity. Radionuclide ventriculography and two-dimensional echocardiography can demonstrate LV aneurysm more readily; the latter is also helpful in distinguishing between true and false aneurysms based on the demonstration of a narrow neck in relation to cavity size in the latter. Color-flow echocardiographic imaging is useful for establishing the diagnosis because flow in and out of the aneurysm, as well as abnormal flow within the aneurysm, can be detected, and subsequent pulsed Doppler imaging can reveal a to-and-fro pattern with characteristic respiratory variation in the peak systolic velocity. CMR may be emerging as the preferred noninvasive technique for the preoperative assessment of LV shape, thinning, and resectability.[238]

Left Ventricular Aneurysmectomy. True LV aneurysms do not rupture, and operative excision is carried out to improve the clinical manifestations, most often heart failure but sometimes also angina, embolization, and life-threatening tachyarrhythmias.[238] Coronary revascularization is frequently performed along with aneurysmectomy, especially for patients in whom angina accompanies heart failure.

A large LV aneurysm in a patient with symptoms of heart failure, particularly if angina pectoris is also present, is an indication for surgery. The operative mortality rate for LV aneurysmectomy is approximately 8% (ranging from 2% to 19%), with rates as low as 3% reported in more recent series. Risk factors for early death include poor LV function, triple-vessel CAD, recent MI, presence of mitral regurgitation, and intractable ventricular arrhythmias. The presence of angina pectoris instead of dyspnea as the dominant preoperative symptom is associated with lower operative mortality. Surgery carries a particularly high risk in patients with severe heart failure, a low-output state, and akinesis of the interventricular septum, as assessed by echocardiography. Akinesis or dyskinesia of the posterior basal segment of the left ventricle and significant right coronary artery stenoses are additional risk factors.

Risk factors for late mortality following survival from surgery include incomplete revascularization, impaired systolic function of the basal segments of the ventricle and septum not involved by the aneurysm, the presence of a large aneurysm with a small quantity of residual viable myocardium, and the presence of severe cardiac failure as the initial feature.

Improvement in LV function has been reported in survivors of resection of LV aneurysms. Anterior ventricular restoration has the potential to reverse adverse remodeling, realign contractile fibers, and decrease LV

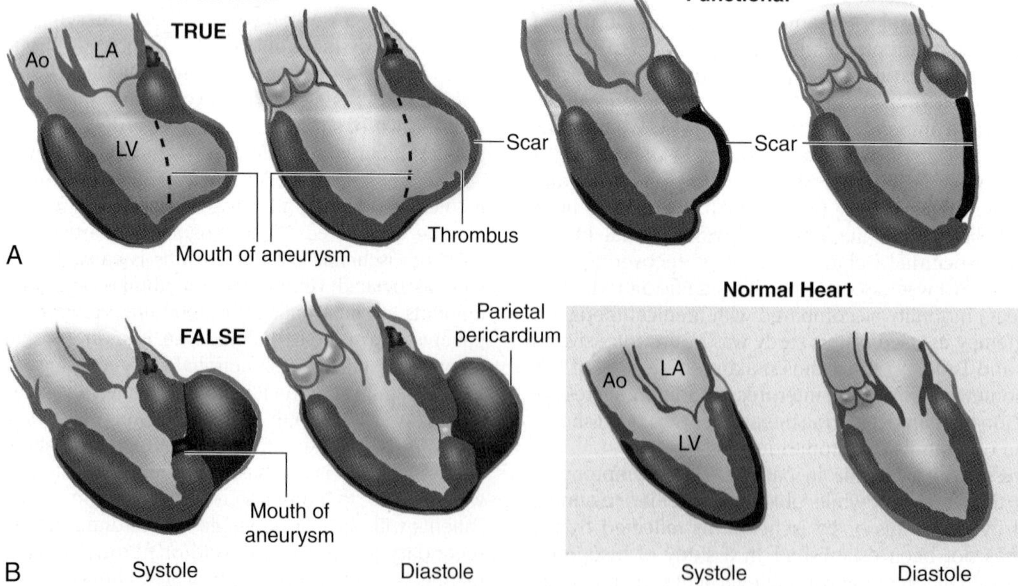

FIGURE 57-19 Hearts in systole and diastole with true and false anatomic and functional LV aneurysms and healed MI. A normal heart in systole and diastole is shown for comparison **(inset)**. **A,** A true anatomic LV aneurysm protrudes during both systole and diastole, has a mouth that is as wide as or wider than the maximal diameter, has a wall that was formerly the wall of the left ventricle, and is composed of fibrous tissue with or without residual myocardial fibers. A true aneurysm may or may not contain thrombus and almost never ruptures once the wall is healed. **B,** A false anatomic LV aneurysm protrudes during both systole and diastole, has a mouth that is considerably smaller than the maximal diameter of the aneurysm and represents a myocardial rupture site, has a wall made up of parietal pericardium, almost always contains thrombus, and often ruptures. A functional LV aneurysm protrudes during ventricular systole but not during diastole and consists of fibrous tissue with or without myocardial fibers. Ao = aorta; LA = left atrium; LV = left ventricle. *(From Cabin HS, Roberts WC: Left ventricular aneurysm, intraaneurysmal thrombus, and systemic embolus in coronary heart disease. Chest 77:586, 1980.)*

wall stress. By removing the abnormal mechanical burden, LV aneurysmectomy has been associated with late improvement in overall systolic function and improvement in the performance of regional nonischemic myocardium in zones remote from the LV aneurysm, in addition to improvement in measures of LV relaxation and cardiovascular neuroregulatory mechanisms. A concomitant improvement in exercise performance and clinical symptoms may also occur, particularly in patients who have undergone complete revascularization. In one series of 285 patients, 67% of patients undergoing ventricular reconstruction had an improvement in symptoms, with a survival of 82% at 5 years.[238]

Newer surgical approaches to the repair of LV aneurysms are designed to restore normal LV geometry by using an alternative method of epicardial closure and/or an endocardial patch to divide the area of the aneurysm from the remainder of the LV cavity (see Fig. 57-e3 on website). Favorable clinical and hemodynamic results following the use of these newer techniques have been reported, with 5-year survival rates ranging from 73% to 87.5% and a corresponding improvement in hemodynamics and clinical symptoms.[239] In one series, 88% of patients treated with the endoaneurysmorrhaphy technique were in NYHA Class I or II after a mean follow-up of approximately 3.5 years.

The value of surgical therapy, including surgical ventricular restoration (SVR), for patients with ischemic cardiomyopathy who do not have frank LV aneurysms was tested in the SVR hypothesis evaluation within the STICH trial. In the first report from this study, SVR failed to confer any benefit when added to CABG in patients with heart failure, dilated left ventricles, and severe regional wall motion abnormalities.[240] In this initial analysis, 1000 patients were recruited at 96 clinical sites in 23 countries. To be included, patients had to have an ejection fraction less than 35%, CAD amenable to CABG, and an area of severe regional dysfunction in the LV anterior wall. Patients were randomized to receive CABG alone (n = 499) or CABG plus SVR (n = 501). All participants received intensive evidence-based medical therapy for heart failure. Both surgical interventions improved symptoms of heart failure and exercise capacity, and SVR reduced end-systolic volume index by 20% versus 3% with CABG, at a median follow-up of 4 years; however, no difference was observed between the two groups for combined rates of death or cardiac hospitalization—56% for CABG and 57% for CABG plus SVR. There were no significant differences between surgical treatments for death, cardiac hospitalization, all-cause hospitalization, acute MI, and stroke.

MITRAL REGURGITATION SECONDARY TO CORONARY ARTERY DISEASE. Mitral regurgitation is an important cause of heart failure in some patients with CAD. Rupture of a papillary muscle or the head of a papillary muscle usually causes severe acute mitral regurgitation in the course of acute MI (see Chaps. 54 and 66). The cause of chronic mitral regurgitation in patients with CAD is multifactorial and the geometric determinants are complex; these include papillary muscle dysfunction from ischemia and fibrosis in conjunction with a wall motion abnormality and changes in LV shape in the region of the papillary muscle and/or dilation of the mitral annulus.[241] Enlargement of the mitral annulus at end-systole is asymmetric, with lengthening primarily involving the posterior annular segments and leading to prolapse of leaflet tissue tethered by the posterior papillary muscle and restriction of leaflet tissue attached to the anterior leaflet. Most patients with chronic CAD and mitral regurgitation have suffered a previous MI. Clinical features that help identify mitral regurgitation secondary to papillary muscle dysfunction as the cause of acute pulmonary edema or of milder symptoms of left-sided failure include a loud systolic murmur and demonstration of a flail mitral valve leaflet on echocardiography.

In some patients with severe mitral regurgitation into a small, noncompliant left atrium, the murmur may be unimpressive or inaudible. Doppler echocardiography is helpful for assessing the severity of the regurgitation (see Chap. 15). As in mitral regurgitation of other causes, the left atrium is not usually greatly enlarged unless mitral regurgitation has been present for more than 6 months. The ECG is nonspecific, and most patients have angiographic evidence of multivessel CAD.

Management

In patients with severe mitral regurgitation, the indications for surgical correction, usually in association with CABG, are fairly clear-cut. Mitral valve repair, as opposed to mitral replacement, is the procedure of choice, but the decision is based on the anatomic characteristics of the structures forming the mitral valve apparatus, urgency of the need for surgery, and severity of LV dysfunction. A more complex and frequently encountered problem involves the indications for mitral valve surgery in patients undergoing CABG in whom the severity of mitral regurgitation is moderate.[241] The decision is based partly on the presence or absence of structural abnormalities of the mitral apparatus and amenability of the valve to repair. Intraoperative transesophageal echocardiography is invaluable for assessing the severity of regurgitation, reparability of the valve, and success of the integrity of the repair after discontinuation of CPB.

The mortality associated with combined CABG and mitral valve placement in the 2005 Society of Thoracic Surgeons data base was approximately 10%. For bypass surgery and mitral valve repair, mortality from 1995 to 2005 was 7% overall, including emergency and reoperative procedures.[186] Predictors of early mortality include the need for replacement versus repair (in some but not all series) but, in addition, may include other variables such as age, comorbid conditions, urgency of surgery, and LV function. Late results are strongly influenced by the pathophysiologic mechanisms underlying mitral regurgitation and are poorer in patients with regurgitation resulting from annular dilation or restrictive leaflet motion than in patients with chordal or papillary muscle rupture. It is encouraging that despite the relatively high operative mortality, late survival of hospital survivors is excellent. In patients with very poor LV function and dilation of the mitral annulus, mitral regurgitation can intensify the severity of LV failure. In such patients, the risk of surgery is high and the long-term benefit is not established,[242] and a trial of intensive medical therapy, including afterload reduction, beta blockade, and biventricular pacing (see Chaps. 28 and 29) may be worthwhile, because favorable remodeling may reduce the severity of mitral regurgitation. For those patients undergoing CABG, the procedural risks associated with combined CABG and mitral valve repair may outweigh the benefit of reduced mitral regurgitation in those at highest perioperative risk.[243] The Cardiothoracic Surgical Trials Network of the National Heart, Lung, and Blood Institute has developed two prospective randomized clinical trials to identify the role of surgery in patients with ischemic mitral regurgitation.[243a]

Cardiac Arrhythmias

In some patients with CAD, cardiac arrhythmias are the dominant clinical manifestation of the disease. Various degrees and forms of ventricular ectopic activity are the most common arrhythmias in patients with CAD, but serious ventricular arrhythmias may be a major component of the clinical findings in other subgroups. The clinical presentation of arrhythmias and their management in patients with CAD are discussed in Chaps. 36 and 37.

Nonatheromatous Coronary Artery Disease

Although atherosclerosis is the most important cause of CAD, other conditions may also be responsible. The most common causes of nonatheromatous CAD resulting in myocardial ischemia are the syndrome of angina-like pain with normal coronary arteriograms (i.e., so-called syndrome X) and Prinzmetal angina (see Chaps. 52 and 56).

Nonatheromatous CAD may result from other diverse abnormalities, including congenital abnormalities in the origin or distribution of the coronary arteries (see Chaps. 21 and 65). The most important of these abnormalities are anomalous origin of a coronary artery (usually the left) from the pulmonary artery, origin of both coronary arteries from either the right or left sinus of Valsalva, and coronary arteriovenous fistula.[244] An anomalous origin of the left main coronary artery or right coronary artery from the aorta, with subsequent coursing between the aorta and pulmonary trunk, is a rare and sometimes fatal coronary arterial anomaly. Coronary anomalies are reported to cause between 12% and 19% of sports-related deaths in U.S. high school and college athletes and account for one third of cardiac anomalies in military recruits with nontraumatic sudden death.[245]

MYOCARDIAL BRIDGING. This cause of systolic compression of the LAD coronary artery is a well-recognized angiographic phenomenon of questionable clinical significance.[246]

CONNECTIVE TISSUE DISORDERS. Several inherited connective tissue disorders are associated with myocardial ischemia (see Chap. 8), including Marfan syndrome (causing aortic and coronary artery dissection),

Hurler syndrome (causing coronary obstruction), homocystinuria (causing coronary artery thrombosis), Ehlers-Danlos syndrome (causing coronary artery dissection), and pseudoxanthoma elasticum (causing accelerated CAD). Kawasaki disease, the mucocutaneous lymph node syndrome, may cause coronary artery aneurysms and ischemic heart disease in children.

Spontaneous Coronary Dissection. This is a rare cause of MI and sudden cardiac death.[247] Chronic dissection manifested as heart failure has been described. In one series, approximately 75% of cases were diagnosed at autopsy and 75% occurred in women, half of which were associated with a postpartum state. Some cases are associated with atherosclerosis. Hypertension has been postulated as a cause of multivessel spontaneous coronary dissection in some patients but, in others, no obvious cause has been identified. In the acute phase, thrombolytic therapy may be dangerous, but early angiography may identify patients who could benefit from stenting or CABG. In survivors of spontaneous coronary artery dissection, the subsequent 3-year mortality was 20%, but complete healing as defined angiographically may lead to a favorable outcome without intervention.

Coronary Vasculitis. This condition, resulting from connective tissue diseases or autoimmune forms of vasculitis, including polyarteritis nodosa, giant cell (temporal) arteritis, and scleroderma, has been well described (see Chap. 89). Coronary arteritis is seen at autopsy in about 20% of patients with rheumatoid arthritis but is rarely associated with clinical manifestations. The incidence of CAD is increased in women with systemic lupus erythematosus (SLE). In SLE patients, CAD has been attributed to a vasculitis, immune complex–mediated endothelial damage, and coronary thrombosis from antiphospholipid antibodies, as well as accelerated atherosclerosis. Giant coronary artery aneurysm associated with SLE is an unusual manifestation that has been associated with the development of acute MI, despite therapy. The antiphospholipid syndrome, characterized by arterial and venous thrombosis and associated with the presence of antiphospholipid antibodies, may be associated with MI, angina, and diffuse LV dysfunction.

Takayasu Arteritis. In rare cases (see Chap. 89), this condition is associated with angina, MI, and cardiac failure in patients younger than 40 years. Coronary blood flow may be decreased by involvement of the ostia or proximal segments of the coronary arteries, but disease in distal coronary segments is rare. The average age at onset of symptoms is 24 years, and the event-free survival rate 10 years after diagnosis is approximately 60%. Luetic aortitis may also produce myocardial ischemia by causing coronary ostial obstruction.

Postmediastinal Irradiation. The occurrence of CAD and morbid cardiac events in young persons after mediastinal irradiation is highly suggestive of a cause-and-effect relationship. Pathologic changes include adventitial scarring and medial hypertrophy with severe intimal atherosclerotic disease. Radiation injury may be latent and may not be manifested clinically for many years after therapy. Contributory factors include higher doses than those currently administered and the presence of cardiac risk factors. Among patients without risk factors who receive an intermediate total dose of 30 and 40 Gy, the risk of cardiac death and MI is low.

Cocaine. Because of its widespread use, cocaine has become a well-documented cause of chest pain, MI, and sudden cardiac death (see Chap. 73).[248] In a population-based study of sudden death in persons 20 to 40 years old in Olmsted County over a 30-year period, a high prevalence of cocaine abuse was observed in the more recent cohort of young adults who died suddenly. The principal effects of cocaine are mediated by alpha-adrenergic stimulation, which causes an increase in myocardial O_2 demand and a reduction in O_2 supply because of coronary vasoconstriction (see Chap. 52).

Other Causes of Myocardial Ischemia. Myocardial ischemia not caused by coronary atherosclerosis can also result from embolism from infective endocarditis (see Chap. 67), implanted prosthetic cardiac valves (see Chap. 66), calcified aortic valves, mural thrombi, and primary cardiac tumors (see Chap. 74).

Cardiac Transplantation–Associated Coronary Arteriopathy

(See Chaps. 31 and 43.)

REFERENCES

1. Lloyd-Jones D, Adams RJ, Brown TM, et al: Heart disease and stroke statistics—2010 update: A report from the American Heart Association. Circulation 121:e46, 2010.
2. Ford ES, Capewell S: Coronary heart disease mortality among young adults in the U.S. from 1980 through 2002: Concealed leveling of mortality rates. J Am Coll Cardiol 50:2128, 2007.
3. American Heart Association: International Cardiovascular Disease Statistics. Dallas, American Heart Association, 2009.
4. Abidov A, Rozanski A, Hachamovitch R, et al: Prognostic significance of dyspnea in patients referred for cardiac stress testing. N Engl J Med 353:1889, 2005.
5. Kaul P, Naylor CD, Armstrong PW, et al: Assessment of activity status and survival according to the Canadian Cardiovascular Society angina classification. Can J Cardiol 25:e225, 2009.
6. Morrow DA: Cardiovascular risk prediction in patients with stable and unstable coronary heart disease. Circulation 121:2681, 2010.
7. Camici PG, Pagani M: Cardiac nociception. Circulation 114:2309, 2006.
8. Qin C, Du JQ, Tang JS, et al: Bradykinin is involved in the mediation of cardiac nociception during ischemia through upper thoracic spinal neurons. Curr Neurovasc Res 6:89, 2009.
9. Wu ZZ, Pan HL: Role of TRPV1 and intracellular Ca^{2+} in excitation of cardiac sensory neurons by bradykinin. Am J Physiol Regul Integr Comp Physiol 293:R276, 2007.
10. Wang L, Wang DH: TRPV1 gene knockout impairs postischemic recovery in isolated perfused heart in mice. Circulation 112:3617, 2005.
11. Ieda M, Kanazawa H, Ieda Y, et al: Nerve growth factor is critical for cardiac sensory innervation and rescues neuropathy in diabetic hearts. Circulation 114:2351, 2006.
12. Brosius FC 3rd, Hostetter TH, Kelepouris E, et al: Detection of chronic kidney disease in patients with or at increased risk of cardiovascular disease: A science advisory from the American Heart Association Kidney and Cardiovascular Disease Council; the Councils on High Blood Pressure Research, Cardiovascular Disease in the Young, and Epidemiology and Prevention; and the Quality of Care and Outcomes Research Interdisciplinary Working Group: developed in collaboration with the National Kidney Foundation. Circulation 114:1083, 2006.
13. Brunzell JD, Davidson M, Furberg CD, et al: Lipoprotein management in patients with cardiometabolic risk: Consensus conference report from the American Diabetes Association and the American College of Cardiology Foundation. J Am Coll Cardiol 51:1512, 2008.
14. Di Angelantonio E, Sarwar N, Perry P, et al: Major lipids, apolipoproteins, and risk of vascular disease. JAMA 302:1993, 2009.
15. O'Donoghue M, Morrow DA, Sabatine MS, et al: Lipoprotein-associated phospholipase A2 and its association with cardiovascular outcomes in patients with acute coronary syndromes in the PROVE IT-TIMI 22 (PRavastatin Or atorVastatin Evaluation and Infection Therapy-Thrombolysis In Myocardial Infarction) trial. Circulation 113:1745, 2006.
16. Davidson MH, Corson MA, Alberts MJ, et al: Consensus panel recommendation for incorporating lipoprotein-associated phospholipase A2 testing into cardiovascular disease risk assessment guidelines. Am J Cardiol 101:51F, 2008.
17. Serruys PW, Garcia-Garcia HM, Buszman P, et al: Effects of the direct lipoprotein-associated phospholipase A(2) inhibitor darapladib on human coronary atherosclerotic plaque. Circulation 118:1172, 2008.
18. Smith SC Jr, Milani RV, Arnett DK, et al: Atherosclerotic Vascular Disease Conference: Writing Group II: Risk factors. Circulation 109:2613, 2004.
19. Buckley DI, Fu R, Freeman M, et al: C-reactive protein as a risk factor for coronary heart disease: a systematic review and meta-analyses for the U.S. Preventive Services Task Force. Ann Intern Med 151:483, 2009.
20. Greenland P, Lloyd-Jones D: Defining a rational approach to screening for cardiovascular risk in asymptomatic patients. J Am Coll Cardiol 52:330, 2008.
21. Ridker PM, Danielson E, Fonseca FA, et al: Rosuvastatin to prevent vascular events in men and women with elevated C-reactive protein. N Engl J Med 359:2195, 2008.
22. Genest J, McPherson R, Frohlich J, et al: 2009 Canadian Cardiovascular Society/Canadian guidelines for the diagnosis and treatment of dyslipidemia and prevention of cardiovascular disease in the adult—2009 recommendations. Can J Cardiol 25:567, 2009.
23. Morrow DA, Cannon CP, Jesse RL, et al: National Academy of Clinical Biochemistry Laboratory Medicine Practice Guidelines: Clinical characteristics and utilization of biochemical markers in acute coronary syndromes. Clin Chem 53:552, 2007.
24. Daniels LB, Laughlin GA, Clopton P, et al: Minimally elevated cardiac troponin T and elevated N-terminal pro-B-type natriuretic peptide predict mortality in older adults: Results from the Rancho Bernardo Study. J Am Coll Cardiol 52:450, 2008.
25. Omland T, de Lemos JA, Sabatine MS, et al: A sensitive cardiac troponin T assay in stable coronary artery disease. N Engl J Med 361:2538, 2009.
26. Morrow DA, Antman EM: Evaluation of high-sensitivity assays for cardiac troponin. Clin Chem 55:5, 2009.
27. Sabatine MS, Morrow DA, de Lemos JA, et al: Acute changes in circulating natriuretic peptide levels in response to myocardial ischemia. J Am Coll Cardiol 44:1988, 2004.
28. Omland T, Sabatine MS, Jablonski KA, et al: Prognostic value of B-Type natriuretic peptides in patients with stable coronary artery disease: The PEACE Trial. J Am Coll Cardiol 50:205, 2007.
29. Arena R, Myers J, Williams MA, et al: Assessment of functional capacity in clinical and research settings: A scientific statement from the American Heart Association Committee on Exercise, Rehabilitation, and Prevention of the Council on Clinical Cardiology and the Council on Cardiovascular Nursing. Circulation 116:329, 2007.
30. Gibbons RJ: Noninvasive diagnosis and prognosis assessment in chronic coronary artery disease: Stress testing with and without imaging perspective. Circ Cardiovasc Imaging 1:257, 2008.
31. Marcassa C, Bax JJ, Bengel F, et al: Clinical value, cost-effectiveness, and safety of myocardial perfusion scintigraphy: A position statement. Eur Heart J 29:557, 2008.
32. Sicari R, Nihoyannopoulos P, Evangelista A, et al: Stress echocardiography expert consensus statement—Executive Summary: European Association of Echocardiography (EAE) (a registered branch of the ESC). Eur Heart J 30:278, 2009.
33. Lee DC, Johnson NP: Quantification of absolute myocardial blood flow by magnetic resonance perfusion imaging. JACC Cardiovasc Imaging 2:761, 2009.
34. Schwitter J, Wacker CM, van Rossum AC, et al: MR-IMPACT: Comparison of perfusion-cardiac magnetic resonance with single-photon emission computed tomography for the detection of coronary artery disease in a multicentre, multivendor, randomized trial. Eur Heart J 29:480, 2008.
35. Gibbons RJ, Balady GJ, Bricker JT, et al: ACC/AHA 2002 guideline update for exercise testing: Summary article: A report of the American College of Cardiology/American Heart Association Task Force on Practice Guidelines (Committee to Update the 1997 Exercise Testing Guidelines). Circulation 106:1883, 2002.

36. Lauer M, Froelicher ES, Williams M, et al: Exercise testing in asymptomatic adults: A statement for professionals from the American Heart Association Council on Clinical Cardiology, Subcommittee on Exercise, Cardiac Rehabilitation, and Prevention. Circulation 112:771, 2005.
37. Albers AR, Krichaversusky MZ, Balady GJ: Stress testing in patients with diabetes mellitus: Diagnostic and prognostic value. Circulation 113:583, 2006.
38. Di Carli MF, Hachamovitch R: New technology for noninvasive evaluation of coronary artery disease. Circulation 115:1464, 2007.
39. Bluemke DA, Achenbach S, Budoff M, et al: Noninvasive coronary artery imaging: Magnetic resonance angiography and multidetector computed tomography angiography: A scientific statement from the american heart association committee on cardiovascular imaging and intervention of the council on cardiovascular radiology and intervention, and the councils on clinical cardiology and cardiovascular disease in the young. Circulation 118:586, 2008.
40. Greenland P, Bonow RO, Brundage BH, et al: ACCF/AHA 2007 clinical expert consensus document on coronary artery calcium scoring by computed tomography in global cardiovascular risk assessment and in evaluation of patients with chest pain: A report of the American College of Cardiology Foundation Clinical Expert Consensus Task Force (ACCF/AHA Writing Committee to Update the 2000 Expert Consensus Document on Electron Beam Computed Tomography). Circulation 115:402, 2007.
41. Chen J, Krumholz HM: How useful is computed tomography for screening for coronary artery disease? Screening for coronary artery disease with electron-beam computed tomography is not useful. Circulation 113:125, 2006.
41a. Gerber TC, Gibbons RJ: Weighing the risks and benefits of cardiac imaging with ionizing radiation. J Am Coll Cardiol Img 3:528, 2010.
42. Fuster V, Kim RJ: Frontiers in cardiovascular magnetic resonance. Circulation 112:135, 2005.
43. Nicholls SJ, Tuzcu EM, Sipahi I, et al: Intravascular ultrasound in cardiovascular medicine. Circulation 114:e55, 2006.
44. Raffel OC, Merchant FM, Tearney GJ, et al: In vivo association between positive coronary artery remodelling and coronary plaque characteristics assessed by intravascular optical coherence tomography. Eur Heart J 29:1721, 2008.
45. Honda Y, Fitzgerald PJ: Frontiers in intravascular imaging technologies. Circulation 117:2024, 2008.
46. Nichols L, Lagana S, Parwani A: Coronary artery aneurysm: A review and hypothesis regarding etiology. Arch Pathol Lab Med 132:823, 2008.
47. Ishikawa Y, Akasaka Y, Suzuki K, et al: Anatomic properties of myocardial bridge predisposing to myocardial infarction. Circulation 120:376, 2009.
48. Tonino PA, De Bruyne B, Pijls NH, et al: Fractional flow reserve versus angiography for guiding percutaneous coronary intervention. N Engl J Med 360:213, 2009.
49. Beltrame JF, Weekes AJ, Morgan C, et al: The prevalence of weekly angina among patients with chronic stable angina in primary care practices: The Coronary Artery Disease in General Practice (CADENCE) Study. Arch Intern Med 169:1491, 2009.
50. Hemingway H, McCallum A, Shipley M, et al: Incidence and prognostic implications of stable angina pectoris among women and men. JAMA 295:1404, 2006.
51. Steg PG, Bhatt DL, Wilson PW, et al: One-year cardiovascular event rates in outpatients with atherothrombosis. JAMA 297:1197, 2007.
52. Kligfield P, Lauer MS: Exercise electrocardiogram testing: Beyond the ST segment. Circulation 114:2070, 2006.
53. Rosendorff C, Black HR, Cannon CP, et al: Treatment of hypertension in the prevention and management of ischemic heart disease: A scientific statement from the American Heart Association Council for High Blood Pressure Research and the Councils on Clinical Cardiology and Epidemiology and Prevention. Circulation 115:2761, 2007.
54. Chobanian AV: Shattuck Lecture. The hypertension paradox—more uncontrolled disease despite improved therapy. N Engl J Med 361:878, 2009.
54a. The ACCORD Study Group: Effects of intensive blood-pressure control in type 2 diabetes mellitus. N Engl J Med 362:1575, 2010.
55. Schane RE, Glantz SA: Education on the dangers of passive smoking: A cessation strategy past due. Circulation 118:1521, 2008.
56. Kahn R, Robertson RM, Smith R, et al: The impact of prevention on reducing the burden of cardiovascular disease. Circulation 118:576, 2008.
57. Smith SC Jr, Allen J, Blair SN, et al: AHA/ACC guidelines for secondary prevention for patients with coronary and other atherosclerotic vascular disease: 2006 update: Endorsed by the National Heart, Lung, and Blood Institute. Circulation 113:2363, 2006.
58. Nissen SE, Nicholls SJ, Sipahi I, et al: Effect of very high-intensity statin therapy on regression of coronary atherosclerosis: The ASTEROID trial. JAMA 295:1556, 2006.
59. Ballantyne CM, Raichlen JS, Nicholls SJ, et al: Effect of rosuvastatin therapy on coronary artery stenoses assessed by quantitative coronary angiography: A study to evaluate the effect of rosuvastatin on intravascular ultrasound-derived coronary atheroma burden. Circulation 117:2458, 2008.
60. Ray KK, Cannon CP: The potential relevance of the multiple lipid-independent (pleiotropic) effects of statins in the management of acute coronary syndromes. J Am Coll Cardiol 46:1425, 2005.
61. LaRosa JC, Grundy SM, Waters DD, et al: Intensive lipid lowering with atorvastatin in patients with stable coronary disease. N Engl J Med 352:1425, 2005.
62. Pedersen TR, Faergeman O, Kastelein JJ, et al: High-dose atorvastatin versus usual-dose simvastatin for secondary prevention after myocardial infarction: The IDEAL study: A randomized controlled trial. JAMA 294:2437, 2005.
63. Cannon CP, Steinberg BA, Murphy SA, et al: Meta-analysis of cardiovascular outcomes trials comparing intensive versus moderate statin therapy. J Am Coll Cardiol 48:438, 2006.
64. Barter P, Gotto AM, LaRosa JC, et al: HDL cholesterol, very low levels of LDL cholesterol, and cardiovascular events. N Engl J Med 357:1301, 2007.
65. Briel M, Ferreira-Gonzalez I, You JJ, et al: Association between change in high density lipoprotein cholesterol and cardiovascular disease morbidity and mortality: Systematic review and meta-regression analysis. BMJ 338:b92, 2009.
66. deGoma EM, deGoma RL, Rader DJ: Beyond high-density lipoprotein cholesterol levels evaluating high-density lipoprotein function as influenced by novel therapeutic approaches. J Am Coll Cardiol 51:2199, 2008.
67. Nissen SE, Tardif JC, Nicholls SJ, et al: Effect of torcetrapib on the progression of coronary atherosclerosis. N Engl J Med 356:1304, 2007.
68. Tall AR: CETP inhibitors to increase HDL cholesterol levels. N Engl J Med 356:1364, 2007.
69. Nathan DM, Cleary PA, Backlund JY, et al: Intensive diabetes treatment and cardiovascular disease in patients with type 1 diabetes. N Engl J Med 353:2643, 2005.
70. Dormandy JA, Charbonnel B, Eckland DJ, et al: Secondary prevention of macrovascular events in patients with type 2 diabetes in the PROactive Study (PROspective pioglitAzone Clinical Trial In macroVascular Events): A randomised controlled trial. Lancet 366:1279, 2005.
71. Marcus BH, Williams DM, Dubbert PM, et al: Physical activity intervention studies: What we know and what we need to know: A scientific statement from the American Heart Association Council on Nutrition, Physical Activity, and Metabolism (Subcommittee on Physical Activity); Council on Cardiovascular Disease in the Young; and the Interdisciplinary Working Group on Quality of Care and Outcomes Research. Circulation 114:2739, 2006.
72. Wenger NK: Current status of cardiac rehabilitation. J Am Coll Cardiol 51:1619, 2008.
73. Hambrecht R, Walther C, Mobius-Winkler S, et al: Percutaneous coronary angioplasty compared with exercise training in patients with stable coronary artery disease: A randomized trial. Circulation 109:1371, 2004.
74. Mora S, Cook N, Buring JE, et al: Physical activity and reduced risk of cardiovascular events: Potential mediating mechanisms. Circulation 116:2110, 2007.
75. Thompson PD, Franklin BA, Balady GJ, et al: Exercise and acute cardiovascular events placing the risks into perspective: A scientific statement from the American Heart Association Council on Nutrition, Physical Activity, and Metabolism and the Council on Clinical Cardiology. Circulation 115:2358, 2007.
76. Libby P, Ridker PM, Hansson GK, et al: Inflammation in atherosclerosis: From pathophysiology to practice. J Am Coll Cardiol 54:2129, 2009.
77. Ridker PM, Cannon CP, Morrow D, et al: C-reactive protein levels and outcomes after statin therapy. N Engl J Med 352:20, 2005.
78. Morrow DA, de Lemos JA, Sabatine MS, et al: Clinical relevance of C-reactive protein during follow-up of patients with acute coronary syndromes in the Aggrastat-to-Zocor Trial. Circulation 114:281, 2006.
79. Poirier P, Giles TD, Bray GA, et al: Obesity and cardiovascular disease: Pathophysiology, evaluation, and effect of weight loss: An update of the 1997 American Heart Association Scientific Statement on Obesity and Heart Disease from the Obesity Committee of the Council on Nutrition, Physical Activity, and Metabolism. Circulation 113:898, 2006.
80. Gibbons RJ, Abrams J, Chatterjee K, et al: ACC/AHA 2002 guideline update for the management of patients with chronic stable angina—summary article: A report of the American College of Cardiology/American Heart Association Task Force on practice guidelines (Committee on the Management of Patients With Chronic Stable Angina). J Am Coll Cardiol 41:159, 2003.
81. Bhatt DL, Fox KA, Hacke W, et al: Clopidogrel and aspirin versus aspirin alone for the prevention of atherothrombotic events. N Engl J Med 354:1706, 2006.
82. Bhatt DL, Flather MD, Hacke W, et al: Patients with prior myocardial infarction, stroke, or symptomatic peripheral arterial disease in the CHARISMA trial. J Am Coll Cardiol 49:1982, 2007.
83. Morrow DA, Scirica BM, Fox KA, et al: Evaluation of a novel antiplatelet agent for secondary prevention in patients with a history of atherosclerotic disease: Design and rationale for the Thrombin-Receptor Antagonist in Secondary Prevention of Atherothrombotic Ischemic Events (TRA 2 degrees P)-TIMI 50 trial. Am Heart J 158:335, 2009.
84. Go AS, Iribarren C, Chandra M, et al: Statin and beta-blocker therapy and the initial presentation of coronary heart disease. Ann Intern Med 144:229, 2006.
85. Bunch TJ, Muhlestein JB, Bair TL, et al: Effect of beta-blocker therapy on mortality rates and future myocardial infarction rates in patients with coronary artery disease but no history of myocardial infarction or congestive heart failure. Am J Cardiol 95:827, 2005.
86. Sipahi I, Tuzcu EM, Wolski KE, et al: Beta-blockers and progression of coronary atherosclerosis: Pooled analysis of 4 intravascular ultrasonography trials. Ann Intern Med 147:10, 2007.
87. Bangalore S, Messerli FH, Kostis JB, et al: Cardiovascular protection using beta-blockers: A critical review of the evidence. J Am Coll Cardiol 50:563, 2007.
88. Pacanowski MA, Gong Y, Cooper-Dehoff RM, et al: Beta-adrenergic receptor gene polymorphisms and beta-blocker treatment outcomes in hypertension. Clin Pharmacol Ther 84:715, 2008.
89. Al-Mallah MH, Tleyjeh IM, Abdel-Latif AA, et al: Angiotensin-converting enzyme inhibitors in coronary artery disease and preserved left ventricular systolic function: A systematic review and meta-analysis of randomized controlled trials. J Am Coll Cardiol 47:1576, 2006.
90. Braunwald E, Domanski MJ, Fowler SE, et al: Angiotensin-converting enzyme inhibition in stable coronary artery disease. N Engl J Med 351:2058, 2004.
91. Solomon SD, Rice MM, Jablonski KA, et al: Renal function and effectiveness of angiotensin-converting enzyme inhibitor therapy in patients with chronic stable coronary disease in the Prevention of Events with ACE inhibition (PEACE) trial. Circulation 114:26, 2006.
92. Yusuf S, Teo KK, Pogue J, et al: Telmisartan, ramipril, or both in patients at high risk for vascular events. N Engl J Med 358:1547, 2008.
93. Yusuf S, Teo K, Anderson C, et al: Effects of the angiotensin-receptor blocker telmisartan on cardiovascular events in high-risk patients intolerant to angiotensin-converting enzyme inhibitors: A randomised controlled trial. Lancet 372:1174, 2008.
94. Lonn E, Yusuf S, Arnold MJ, et al: Homocysteine lowering with folic acid and B vitamins in vascular disease. N Engl J Med 354:1567, 2006.
95. Bonaa KH, Njolstad I, Ueland PM, et al: Homocysteine lowering and cardiovascular events after acute myocardial infarction. N Engl J Med 354:1578, 2006.
96. Levonen A-L, Vahakangas E, Koponen JK, et al: Antioxidant gene therapy for cardiovascular disease: Current status and future perspectives. Circulation 117:2142, 2008.
97. Rutledge T, Vaccarino V, Johnson BD, et al: Depression and cardiovascular health care costs among women with suspected myocardial ischemia: Prospective results from the WISE (Women's Ischemia Syndrome Evaluation) Study. J Am Coll Cardiol 53:176, 2009.
98. Vaccarino V, Johnson BD, Sheps DS, et al: Depression, inflammation, and incident cardiovascular disease in women with suspected coronary ischemia: The National Heart, Lung, and Blood Institute-sponsored WISE study. J Am Coll Cardiol 50:2044, 2007.
99. Lesperance F, Frasure-Smith N, Koszycki D, et al: Effects of citalopram and interpersonal psychotherapy on depression in patients with coronary artery disease: the Canadian Cardiac Randomized Evaluation of Antidepressant and Psychotherapy Efficacy (CREATE) trial. JAMA 297:367, 2007.
100. Dimsdale JE: Psychological stress and cardiovascular disease. J Am Coll Cardiol 51:1237, 2008.

101. Lichtenstein AH, Appel LJ, Brands M, et al: Diet and lifestyle recommendations revision 2006: A scientific statement from the American Heart Association Nutrition Committee. Circulation 114:82, 2006.
102. Mozaffarian D, Wilson PW, Kannel WB: Beyond established and novel risk factors: Lifestyle risk factors for cardiovascular disease. Circulation 117:3031, 2008.
103. Kostis JB, Jackson G, Rosen R, et al: Sexual dysfunction and cardiac risk (the Second Princeton Consensus Conference). Am J Cardiol 96:85M, 2005.
104. Yang MF, Keng F, He ZX: Nitrate-augmented myocardial perfusion imaging for assessment of myocardial viability: Recent advances. Nucl Med Commun 30:415, 2009.
105. Wenzel P, Schulz E, Gori T, et al: Monitoring white blood cell mitochondrial aldehyde dehydrogenase activity: Implications for nitrate therapy in humans. J Pharmacol Exp Ther 330:63, 2009.
106. Gori T, Parker JD: Nitrate-induced toxicity and preconditioning: A rationale for reconsidering the use of these drugs. J Am Coll Cardiol 52:251, 2008.
107. Thomas GR, DiFabio JM, Gori T, et al: Once daily therapy with isosorbide-5-mononitrate causes endothelial dysfunction in humans: Evidence of a free-radical-mediated mechanism. J Am Coll Cardiol 49:1289, 2007.
108. Munzel T, Wenzel P, Daiber A: Do we still need organic nitrates? J Am Coll Cardiol 49:1296, 2007.
109. Kardas P: Comparison of once daily versus twice daily oral nitrates in stable angina pectoris. Am J Cardiol 94:213, 2004.
110. Jansen R, Cleophas TJ, Zwinderman AH, et al: Chronic nitrate therapy in patients with angina with comorbidity. Am J Ther 13:188, 2006.
111. Munzel T, Daiber A, Mulsch A: Explaining the phenomenon of nitrate tolerance. Circ Res 97:618, 2005.
112. Vlachopoulos C, Ioakeimidis N, Rokkas K, et al: Cardiovascular effects of phosphodiesterase type 5 inhibitors. J Sex Med 6:658, 2009.
113. Frishman WH: Fifty years of beta-adrenergic blockade: A golden era in clinical medicine and molecular pharmacology. Am J Med 121:933, 2008.
114. Egred M, Shaw S, Mohammad B, et al: Under-use of beta-blockers in patients with ischaemic heart disease and concomitant chronic obstructive pulmonary disease. QJM 98:493, 2005.
115. Munzel T, Gori T: Nebivolol: The somewhat-different beta-adrenergic receptor blocker. J Am Coll Cardiol 54:1491, 2009.
116. Cheng JW, Frishman WH, Aronow WS: Updates on cytochrome P450-mediated cardiovascular drug interactions. Am J Ther 16:155, 2009.
117. Lanfear DE, Jones PG, Marsh S, et al: Beta2-adrenergic receptor genotype and survival among patients receiving beta-blocker therapy after an acute coronary syndrome. JAMA 294:1526, 2005.
118. Hassan M, York KM, Li H, et al: Association of beta1-adrenergic receptor genetic polymorphism with mental stress-induced myocardial ischemia in patients with coronary artery disease. Arch Intern Med 168:763, 2008.
119. Liggett SB, Mialet-Perez J, Thaneemit-Chen S, et al: A polymorphism within a conserved beta-1-adrenergic receptor motif alters cardiac function and beta-blocker response in human heart failure. Proc Natl Acad Sci U S A 103:11288, 2006.
120. Ko DT, Hebert PR, Coffey CS, et al: Adverse effects of beta-blocker therapy for patients with heart failure: A quantitative overview of randomized trials. Arch Intern Med 164:1389, 2004.
121. Klapholz M: Beta-blocker use for the stages of heart failure. Mayo Clin Proc 84:718, 2009.
122. Bakris GL, Fonseca V, Katholi RE, et al: Metabolic effects of carvedilol versus metoprolol in patients with type 2 diabetes mellitus and hypertension: A randomized controlled trial. JAMA 292:2227, 2004.
123. Torp-Pedersen C, Metra M, Charlesworth A, et al: Effects of metoprolol and carvedilol on pre-existing and new onset diabetes in patients with chronic heart failure: Data from the Carvedilol Or Metoprolol European Trial (COMET). Heart 93:968, 2007.
124. Frishman WH: Calcium channel blockers: Differences between subclasses. Am J Cardiovasc Drugs 7(Suppl 1):17, 2007.
125. Luscher TF, Pieper M, Tendera M, et al: A randomized placebo-controlled study on the effect of nifedipine on coronary endothelial function and plaque formation in patients with coronary artery disease: The ENCORE II study. Eur Heart J 30:1590, 2009.
126. Nissen SE, Tuzcu EM, Libby P, et al: Effect of antihypertensive agents on cardiovascular events in patients with coronary disease and normal blood pressure: The CAMELOT study: A randomized controlled trial. JAMA 292:2217, 2004.
127. Bangalore S, Parkar S, Messerli FH: Long-acting calcium antagonists in patients with coronary artery disease: A meta-analysis. Am J Med 122:356, 2009.
128. Bangalore S, Messerli FH, Cohen JD, et al: Verapamil-sustained release-based treatment strategy is equivalent to atenolol-based treatment strategy at reducing cardiovascular events in patients with prior myocardial infarction: An INternational VErapamil SR-Trandolapril (INVEST) substudy. Am Heart J 156:241, 2008.
129. Chaitman BR: Ranolazine for the treatment of chronic angina and potential use in other cardiovascular conditions. Circulation 113:2462, 2006.
130. Rousseau MF, Pouleur H, Cocco G, et al: Comparative efficacy of ranolazine versus atenolol for chronic angina pectoris. Am J Cardiol 95:311, 2005.
131. Chaitman BR, Pepine CJ, Parker JO, et al: Effects of ranolazine with atenolol, amlodipine, or diltiazem on exercise tolerance and angina frequency in patients with severe chronic angina: A randomized controlled trial. JAMA 291:309, 2004.
132. Morrow DA, Scirica BM, Karwatowska-Prokopczuk E, et al: Effects of ranolazine on recurrent cardiovascular events in patients with non-ST-elevation acute coronary syndromes: The MERLIN-TIMI 36 randomized trial. JAMA 297:1775, 2007.
133. Wilson SR, Scirica BM, Braunwald E, et al: Efficacy of ranolazine in patients with chronic angina observations from the randomized, double-blind, placebo-controlled MERLIN-TIMI (Metabolic Efficiency With Ranolazine for Less Ischemia in Non-ST-Segment Elevation Acute Coronary Syndromes) 36 Trial. J Am Coll Cardiol 53:1510, 2009.
134. Antzelevitch C, Belardinelli L, Zygmunt AC, et al: Electrophysiological effects of ranolazine, a novel antianginal agent with antiarrhythmic properties. Circulation 110:904, 2004.
135. Scirica BM, Morrow DA, Hod H, et al: Effect of ranolazine, an antianginal agent with novel electrophysiological properties, on the incidence of arrhythmias in patients with non ST-segment elevation acute coronary syndrome: Results from the Metabolic Efficiency With Ranolazine for Less Ischemia in Non ST-Elevation Acute Coronary Syndrome Thrombolysis in Myocardial Infarction 36 (MERLIN-TIMI 36) randomized controlled trial. Circulation 116:1647, 2007.
136. Morrow DA, Scirica BM, Chaitman BR, et al: Evaluation of the glycometabolic effects of ranolazine in patients with and without diabetes mellitus in the MERLIN-TIMI 36 randomized controlled trial. Circulation 119:2032, 2009.
137. Tardif JC, Ponikowski P, Kahan T: Efficacy of the I(f) current inhibitor ivabradine in patients with chronic stable angina receiving beta-blocker therapy: A 4-month, randomized, placebo-controlled trial. Eur Heart J 30:540, 2009.
138. Tardif JC, Ford I, Tendera M, et al: Efficacy of ivabradine, a new selective I(f) inhibitor, compared with atenolol in patients with chronic stable angina. Eur Heart J 26:2529, 2005.
139. Fox K, Ford I, Steg PG, et al: Ivabradine for patients with stable coronary artery disease and left-ventricular systolic dysfunction (BEAUTIFUL): A randomised, double-blind, placebo-controlled trial. Lancet 372:807, 2008.
140. Fox K, Ford I, Steg PG, et al: Relationship between ivabradine treatment and cardiovascular outcomes in patients with stable coronary artery disease and left ventricular systolic dysfunction with limiting angina: A subgroup analysis of the randomized, controlled BEAUTIFUL trial. Eur Heart J 30:2337, 2009.
141. Simpson D, Wellington K: Nicorandil: A review of its use in the management of stable angina pectoris, including high-risk patients. Drugs 64:1941, 2004.
142. Brown R, Lee A, Welfare M: Nicorandil-induced colonic ulceration. Heart 94:678, 2008.
143. Walker A, McMurray J, Stewart S, et al: Economic evaluation of the impact of nicorandil in angina (IONA) trial. Heart 92:619, 2006.
144. Vicari RM, Chaitman B, Keefe D, et al: Efficacy and safety of fasudil in patients with stable angina: A double-blind, placebo-controlled, phase 2 trial. J Am Coll Cardiol 46:1803, 2005.
145. Morrow DA, Givertz MM: Modulation of myocardial energetics: Emerging evidence for a therapeutic target in cardiovascular disease. Circulation 112:3218, 2005.
146. Eckert S, Horstkotte D: Management of angina pectoris: The role of spinal cord stimulation. Am J Cardiovasc Drugs 9:17, 2009.
147. Eddicks S, Maier-Hauff K, Schenk M, et al: Thoracic spinal cord stimulation improves functional status and relieves symptoms in patients with refractory angina pectoris: The first placebo-controlled randomised study. Heart 93:585, 2007.
148. Manchanda A, Soran O: Enhanced external counterpulsation and future directions: step beyond medical management for patients with angina and heart failure. J Am Coll Cardiol 50:1523, 2007.
149. Soran O, Kennard ED, Kfoury AG, et al: Two-year clinical outcomes after enhanced external counterpulsation (EECP) therapy in patients with refractory angina pectoris and left ventricular dysfunction (report from The International EECP Patient Registry). Am J Cardiol 97:17, 2006.
150. Akhtar M, Wu GF, Du ZM, et al: Effect of external counterpulsation on plasma nitric oxide and endothelin-1 levels. Am J Cardiol 98:28, 2006.
151. Fox K, Garcia MA, Ardissino D, et al: Guidelines on the management of stable angina pectoris: Executive summary: The Task Force on the Management of Stable Angina Pectoris of the European Society of Cardiology. Eur Heart J 27:1341, 2006.
152. Silber S, Albertsson P, Aviles FF, et al: Guidelines for percutaneous coronary interventions. The Task Force for Percutaneous Coronary Interventions of the European Society of Cardiology. Eur Heart J 26:804, 2005.
153. Eagle KA, Guyton RA, Davidoff R, et al: ACC/AHA 2004 guideline update for coronary artery bypass graft surgery: A report of the American College of Cardiology/American Heart Association Task Force on Practice Guidelines (Committee to Update the 1999 Guidelines for Coronary Artery Bypass Graft Surgery). Circulation 110:e340, 2004.
154. Pijls NH, van Schaardenburgh P, Manoharan G, et al: Percutaneous coronary intervention of functionally nonsignificant stenosis: 5-year follow-up of the DEFER Study. J Am Coll Cardiol 49:2105, 2007.
155. Phillips HR, O'Connor CM, Rogers J: Revascularization for heart failure. Am Heart J 153:65, 2007.
156. Tarakji KG, Brunken R, McCarthy PM, et al: Myocardial viability testing and the effect of early intervention in patients with advanced left ventricular systolic dysfunction. Circulation 113:230, 2006.
157. Dixon SR, Grines CL, O'Neill WW: The year in interventional cardiology. J Am Coll Cardiol 53:2080, 2009.
158. Wu C, Hannan EL, Walford G, et al: A risk score to predict in-hospital mortality for percutaneous coronary interventions. J Am Coll Cardiol 47:654, 2006.
159. Boden WE, Taggart DP: Diabetes with coronary disease—a moving target amid evolving therapies? N Engl J Med 360:2570, 2009.
160. Jeremias A, Kleiman NS, Nassif D, et al: Prevalence and prognostic significance of preprocedural cardiac troponin elevation among patients with stable coronary artery disease undergoing percutaneous coronary intervention: Results from the evaluation of drug eluting stents and ischemic events registry. Circulation 118:632, 2008.
161. Pinto Slottow TL, Waksman R: Overview of the 2007 Food and Drug Administration Circulatory System Devices Panel meeting on the endeavor zotarolimus-eluting coronary stent. Circulation 117:1603, 2008.
162. Malenka DJ, Kaplan AV, Lucas FL, et al: Outcomes following coronary stenting in the era of bare-metal versus the era of drug-eluting stents. JAMA 299:2868, 2008.
163. Katritsis DG, Ioannidis JP: Percutaneous coronary intervention versus conservative therapy in nonacute coronary artery disease: A meta-analysis. Circulation 111:2906, 2005.
164. Al Suwaidi J, Holmes DR Jr, Salam AM, et al: Impact of coronary artery stents on mortality and nonfatal myocardial infarction: Meta-analysis of randomized trials comparing a strategy of routine stenting with that of balloon angioplasty. Am Heart J 147:815, 2004.
164a. Brophy JM, Belisle P, Joseph L: Evidence for use of coronary stents: a hierarchical bayesian meta-analysis. Ann Int Med 138:777, 2003.
165. Hueb W, Lopes NH, Gersh BJ, et al: Five-year follow-up of the Medicine, Angioplasty, or Surgery Study (MASS II): A randomized controlled clinical trial of 3 therapeutic strategies for multivessel coronary artery disease. Circulation 115:1082, 2007.
166. Boden WE, O'Rourke RA, Teo KK, et al: Optimal medical therapy with or without PCI for stable coronary disease. N Engl J Med 356:1503, 2007.
167. Boden WE, O'Rourke RA, Teo KK, et al: The evolving pattern of symptomatic coronary artery disease in the United States and Canada: Baseline characteristics of the Clinical Outcomes Utilizing Revascularization and Aggressive DruG Evaluation (COURAGE) trial. Am J Cardiol 99:208, 2007.

168. Shaw LJ, Berman DS, Maron DJ, et al: Optimal medical therapy with or without percutaneous coronary intervention to reduce ischemic burden: Results from the Clinical Outcomes Utilizing Revascularization and Aggressive Drug Evaluation (COURAGE) trial nuclear substudy. Circulation 117:1283, 2008.
169. Gersh BJ, Frye RL: Methods of coronary revascularization—things may not be as they seem. N Engl J Med 352:2235, 2005.
170. Frye RL, August P, Brooks MM, et al: A randomized trial of therapies for type 2 diabetes and coronary artery disease. N Engl J Med 360:2503, 2009.
171. Keenan TD, Abu-Omar Y, Taggart DP: Bypassing the pump: Changing practices in coronary artery surgery. Chest 128:363, 2005.
172. Taggart DP: PCI or CABG in coronary artery disease? Lancet 373:1150, 2009.
173. Argenziano M, Katz M, Bonatti J, et al: Results of the prospective multicenter trial of robotically assisted totally endoscopic coronary artery bypass grafting. Ann Thorac Surg 81:1666, 2006.
174. Verma S, Fedak PW, Weisel RD, et al: Off-pump coronary artery bypass surgery: Fundamentals for the clinical cardiologist. Circulation 109:1206, 2004.
175. Sellke FW, DiMaio JM, Caplan LR, et al: Comparing on-pump and off-pump coronary artery bypass grafting: Numerous studies but few conclusions: A scientific statement from the American Heart Association council on cardiovascular surgery and anesthesia in collaboration with the interdisciplinary working group on quality of care and outcomes research. Circulation 111:2858, 2005.
176. Shroyer AL, Grover FL, Hattler B, et al: On-pump versus off-pump coronary-artery bypass surgery. N Engl J Med 361:1827, 2009.
177. Vassiliades TA Jr, Douglas JS, Morris DC, et al: Integrated coronary revascularization with drug-eluting stents: Immediate and seven-month outcome. J Thorac Cardiovasc Surg 131:956, 2006.
178. Wijeysundera DN, Beattie WS, Djaiani G, et al: Off-pump coronary artery surgery for reducing mortality and morbidity: meta-analysis of randomized and observational studies. J Am Coll Cardiol 46:872, 2005.
179. Jones RH: The year in cardiovascular surgery. J Am Coll Cardiol 47:2094, 2006.
180. Nishida H, Tomizawa Y, Endo M, et al: Survival benefit of exclusive use of in situ arterial conduits over combined use of arterial and vein grafts for multiple coronary artery bypass grafting. Circulation 112:I299, 2005.
181. Baskett RJ, Cafferty FH, Powell SJ, et al: Total arterial revascularization is safe: Multicenter ten-year analysis of 71,470 coronary procedures. Ann Thorac Surg 81:1243, 2006.
182. Lytle BW, Blackstone EH, Sabik JF, et al: The effect of bilateral internal thoracic artery grafting on survival during 20 postoperative years. Ann Thorac Surg 78:2005, 2004.
183. Okrainec K, Platt R, Pilote L, et al: Cardiac medical therapy in patients after undergoing coronary artery bypass graft surgery: A review of randomized controlled trials. J Am Coll Cardiol 45:177, 2005.
184. Stein PD, Schunemann HJ, Dalen JE, et al: Antithrombotic therapy in patients with saphenous vein and internal mammary artery bypass grafts: The Seventh ACCP Conference on Antithrombotic and Thrombolytic Therapy. Chest 126:600S, 2004.
185. Cram P, Rosenthal GE, Vaughan-Sarrazin MS: Cardiac revascularization in specialty and general hospitals. N Engl J Med 352:1454, 2005.
186. Society of Thoracic Surgeons: STS adult cardiac surgery database—Executive Summary. (http://www.sts.org).
187. Shahian DM, Blackstone EH, Edwards FH, et al: Cardiac surgery risk models: A position article. Ann Thorac Surg 78:1868, 2004.
188. Ramsay J, Shernan S, Fitch J, et al: Increased creatine kinase MB level predicts postoperative mortality after cardiac surgery independent of new Q waves. J Thorac Cardiovasc Surg 129:300, 2005.
189. Mangano DT, Miao Y, Tudor IC, et al: Post-reperfusion myocardial infarction: Long-term survival improvement using adenosine regulation with acadesine. J Am Coll Cardiol 48:206, 2006.
190. Dacey LJ, Likosky DS, Leavitt BJ, et al: Perioperative stroke and long-term survival after coronary bypass graft surgery. Ann Thorac Surg 79:532, 2005.
191. Samuels MA: Can cognition survive heart surgery? Circulation 113:2784, 2006.
192. Bar-Yosef S, Anders M, Mackensen GB, et al: Aortic atheroma burden and cognitive dysfunction after coronary artery bypass graft surgery. Ann Thorac Surg 78:1556, 2004.
193. Izhar U, Ad N, Rudis E, et al: When should we discontinue antiarrhythmic therapy for atrial fibrillation after coronary artery bypass grafting? A prospective randomized study. J Thorac Cardiovasc Surg 129:401, 2005.
194. Sedrakyan A, Zhang H, Treasure T, et al: Recursive partitioning-based preoperative risk stratification for atrial fibrillation after coronary artery bypass surgery. Am Heart J 151:720, 2006.
195. Marin F, Pascual DA, Roldan V, et al: Statins and postoperative risk of atrial fibrillation following coronary artery bypass grafting. Am J Cardiol 97:55, 2006.
196. Burns KE, Chu MW, Novick RJ, et al: Perioperative N-acetylcysteine to prevent renal dysfunction in high-risk patients undergoing CABG surgery: A randomized controlled trial. JAMA 294:342, 2005.
197. Topkara VK, Cheema FH, Kesavaramanujam S, et al: Coronary artery bypass grafting in patients with low ejection fraction. Circulation 112:I344, 2005.
198. Chareonthaitawee P, Gersh BJ, Araoz PA, et al: Revascularization in severe left ventricular dysfunction: the role of viability testing. J Am Coll Cardiol 46:567, 2005.
199. Gibbons RJ, Chareonthaitawee P, Bailey KR: Revascularization in systolic heart failure: A difficult decision. Circulation 113:180, 2006.
200. Klocke FJ. Resting blood flow in hypocontractile myocardium: Resolving the controversy. Circulation 112:3222, 2005.
201. Zaglavara T, Pillay T, Karvounis H, et al: Detection of myocardial viability by dobutamine stress echocardiography: Incremental value of diastolic wall thickness measurement. Heart 91:613, 2005.
202. Selvanayagam JB, Kardos A, Francis JM, et al: Value of delayed-enhancement cardiovascular magnetic resonance imaging in predicting myocardial viability after surgical revascularization. Circulation 110:1535, 2004.
203. Rizzello V, Poldermans D, Schinkel AF, et al: Long-term prognostic value of myocardial viability and ischaemia during dobutamine stress echocardiography in patients with ischaemic cardiomyopathy undergoing coronary revascularisation. Heart 92:239, 2006.
204. Velazquez EJ, Lee KL, O'Connor CM, et al: The rationale and design of the Surgical Treatment for Ischemic Heart Failure (STICH) trial. J Thorac Cardiovasc Surg 134:1540, 2007.
205. Jacobs AK: Women, ischemic heart disease, revascularization, and the gender gap: What are we missing? J Am Coll Cardiol 47:S63, 2006.
206. Blankstein R, Ward RP, Arnsdorf M, et al: Female gender is an independent predictor of operative mortality after coronary artery bypass graft surgery: Contemporary analysis of 31 Midwestern hospitals. Circulation 112:I323, 2005.
207. Peterson ED, Alexander KP, Malenka DJ, et al: Multicenter experience in revascularization of very elderly patients. Am Heart J 148:486, 2004.
208. Cooper WA, O'Brien SM, Thourani VH, et al: Impact of renal dysfunction on outcomes of coronary artery bypass surgery: Results from the Society of Thoracic Surgeons National Adult Cardiac Database. Circulation 113:1063, 2006.
209. Hillis GS, Croal BL, Buchan KG, et al: Renal function and outcome from coronary artery bypass grafting: Impact on mortality after a 2.3-year follow-up. Circulation 113:1056, 2006.
210. Flaherty JD, Davidson CJ: Diabetes and coronary revascularization. JAMA 293:1501, 2005.
211. Hannan EL, Wu C, Bennett EV, et al: Risk stratification of in-hospital mortality for coronary artery bypass graft surgery. J Am Coll Cardiol 47:661, 2006.
212. O'Rourke DJ, Quinton HB, Piper W, et al: Survival in patients with peripheral vascular disease after percutaneous coronary intervention and coronary artery bypass graft surgery. Ann Thorac Surg 78:466, 2004.
213. Sabik JF 3rd, Blackstone EH, Gillinov AM, et al: Occurrence and risk factors for reintervention after coronary artery bypass grafting. Circulation 114:I454, 2006.
214. Hannan EL, Racz MJ, Walford G, et al: Long-term outcomes of coronary-artery bypass grafting versus stent implantation. N Engl J Med 352:2174, 2005.
215. Serruys PW, Morice MC, Kappetein AP, et al: Percutaneous coronary intervention versus coronary-artery bypass grafting for severe coronary artery disease. N Engl J Med 360:961, 2009.
216. BARI Investigators: The final 10-year follow-up results from the BARI randomized trial. J Am Coll Cardiol 49:1600, 2007.
217. Barsness GW, Gersh BJ, Brooks MM, et al: Rationale for the revascularization arm of the Bypass Angioplasty Revascularization Investigation 2 Diabetes (BARI 2D) Trial. Am J Cardiol 97:31G, 2006.
218. Hlatky MA, Boothroyd DB, Bravata DM, et al: Coronary artery bypass surgery compared with percutaneous coronary interventions for multivessel disease: A collaborative analysis of individual patient data from ten randomised trials. Lancet 373:1190, 2009.
219. Farkouh ME, Dangas G, Leon MB, et al: Design of the Future REvascularization Evaluation in patients with Diabetes mellitus: Optimal management of Multivessel disease (FREEDOM) Trial. Am Heart J 155:215, 2008.
220. Kushner FG, Hand M, Smith SC Jr, et al: 2009 Focused Updates: ACC/AHA Guidelines for the Management of Patients With ST-Elevation Myocardial Infarction (updating the 2004 Guideline and 2007 Focused Update) and ACC/AHA/SCAI Guidelines on Percutaneous Coronary Intervention (updating the 2005 Guideline and 2007 Focused Update): A report of the American College of Cardiology Foundation/American Heart Association Task Force on Practice Guidelines. Circulation 120:2271, 2009.
221. Hannan EL, Racz M, Holmes DR, et al: Impact of completeness of percutaneous coronary intervention revascularization on long-term outcomes in the stent era. Circulation 113:2406, 2006.
222. Ong AT, Serruys PW, Mohr FW, et al: The SYNergy between percutaneous coronary intervention with TAXus and cardiac surgery (SYNTAX) study: Design, rationale, and run-in phase. Am Heart J 151:1194, 2006.
223. Bridges CR, Horvath KA, Nugent WC, et al: The Society of Thoracic Surgeons practice guideline series: Transmyocardial laser revascularization. Ann Thorac Surg 77:1494, 2004.
224. Bugiardini R, Bairey Merz CN: Angina with "normal" coronary arteries: A changing philosophy. JAMA 293:477, 2005.
225. Johnson BD, Shaw LJ, Buchthal SD, et al: Prognosis in women with myocardial ischemia in the absence of obstructive coronary disease: Results from the National Institutes of Health-National Heart, Lung, and Blood Institute-Sponsored Women's Ischemia Syndrome Evaluation (WISE). Circulation 109:2993, 2004.
226. Bugiardini R: Women, 'non-specific' chest pain, and normal or near-normal coronary angiograms are not synonymous with favourable outcome. Eur Heart J 27:1387, 2006.
227. Valeriani M, Sestito A, Le Pera D, et al: Abnormal cortical pain processing in patients with cardiac syndrome X. Eur Heart J 26:975, 2005.
228. Handberg E, Johnson BD, Arant CB, et al: Impaired coronary vascular reactivity and functional capacity in women: Results from the NHLBI Women's Ischemia Syndrome Evaluation (WISE) Study. J Am Coll Cardiol 47:S44, 2006.
229. Johnson BD, Shaw LJ, Pepine CJ, et al: Persistent chest pain predicts cardiovascular events in women without obstructive coronary artery disease: Results from the NIH-NHLBI-sponsored Women's Ischaemia Syndrome Evaluation (WISE) study. Eur Heart J 27:1408, 2006.
230. Stern S: Symptoms other than chest pain may be important in the diagnosis of "silent ischemia," or "the sounds of silence." Circulation 111:e435, 2005.
231. Gazzaruso C, Solerte SB, De Amici E, et al: Association of the metabolic syndrome and insulin resistance with silent myocardial ischemia in patients with type 2 diabetes mellitus. Am J Cardiol 97:236, 2006.
232. Sajadieh A, Nielsen OW, Rasmussen V, et al: Prevalence and prognostic significance of daily-life silent myocardial ischaemia in middle-aged and elderly subjects with no apparent heart disease. Eur Heart J 26:1402, 2005.
233. Enseleit F, Duru F: Long-term continuous external electrocardiographic recording: A review. Europace 8:255, 2006.
234. Erne P, Schoenenberger AW, Burckhardt D, et al: Effects of percutaneous coronary interventions in silent ischemia after myocardial infarction: The SWISSI II randomized controlled trial. JAMA 297:1985, 2007.
235. Flaherty JD, Bax JJ, De Luca L, et al: Acute heart failure syndromes in patients with coronary artery disease early assessment and treatment. J Am Coll Cardiol 53:254, 2009.
236. Dickstein K, Cohen-Solal A, Filippatos G, et al: ESC guidelines for the diagnosis and treatment of acute and chronic heart failure 2008: The Task Force for the diagnosis and treatment of acute and chronic heart failure 2008 of the European Society of Cardiology. Developed in collaboration with the Heart Failure Association of the ESC (HFA) and endorsed by the European Society of Intensive Care Medicine (ESICM). Eur J Heart Fail 10:933, 2008.

237. Carluccio E, Biagioli P, Alunni G, et al: Patients with hibernating myocardium show altered left ventricular volumes and shape, which revert after revascularization: Evidence that dyssynergy might directly induce cardiac remodeling. J Am Coll Cardiol 47:969, 2006.
238. Mickleborough LL, Merchant N, Ivanov J, et al: Left ventricular reconstruction: Early and late results. J Thorac Cardiovasc Surg 128:27, 2004.
239. Lundblad R, Abdelnoor M, Geiran OR, et al: Surgical repair of postinfarction ventricular septal rupture: Risk factors of early and late death. J Thorac Cardiovasc Surg 137:862, 2009.
240. Jones RH, Velazquez EJ, Michler RE, et al: Coronary bypass surgery with or without surgical ventricular reconstruction. N Engl J Med 360:1705, 2009.
241. Borger MA, Alam A, Murphy PM, et al: Chronic ischemic mitral regurgitation: Repair, replace or rethink? Ann Thorac Surg 81:1153, 2006.
242. Wu AH, Aaronson KD, Bolling SF, et al: Impact of mitral valve annuloplasty on mortality risk in patients with mitral regurgitation and left ventricular systolic dysfunction. J Am Coll Cardiol 45:381, 2005.
243. Kang DH, Kim MJ, Kang SJ, et al: Mitral valve repair versus revascularization alone in the treatment of ischemic mitral regurgitation. Circulation 114:I499, 2006.
243a. Gardner TJ, O'Gara PT. The cardiothoracic surgery network: Randomized clinical trials in the operating room. J Thorac Cardiovasc Surg 139:830, 2010.
244. Rigatelli G, Docali G, Rossi P, et al: Validation of a clinical-significance-based classification of coronary artery anomalies. Angiology 56:25, 2005.
245. Eckart RE, Scoville SL, Campbell CL, et al: Sudden death in young adults: A 25-year review of autopsies in military recruits. Ann Intern Med 141:829, 2004.
246. Alegria JR, Herrmann J, Holmes DR Jr, et al: Myocardial bridging. Eur Heart J 26:1159, 2005.
247. Egred M, Viswanathan G, Davis GK: Myocardial infarction in young adults. Postgrad Med J 81:741, 2005.
248. Jones JH, Weir WB: Cocaine-associated chest pain. Med Clin North Am 89:1323, 2005.

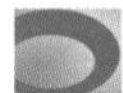

GUIDELINES David A. Morrow and William E. Boden

Chronic Stable Angina

The American College of Cardiology and the American Heart Association (ACC/AHA) updated guidelines for the management of patients with stable chest pain syndromes and known or suspected ischemic heart disease in 2002.[1] Populations addressed by these guidelines include patients with "ischemic equivalents" such as dyspnea or arm pain with exertion and patients with ischemic heart disease who have become asymptomatic, including those who have undergone revascularization procedures. Patients with unstable ischemic syndromes are not included in these guidelines but are instead addressed in guidelines summarized in Chap. 53 Guidelines. As with other ACC/AHA guidelines, indications for interventions are classified into the following four groups:

Class I—for generally accepted indications
Class IIa—when indications are controversial, but the weight of evidence is supportive
Class IIb—when usefulness or efficacy is less well established
Class III—when there is consensus against the usefulness of the intervention

The guidelines use a convention for rating levels of evidence on which recommendations have been based, as follows:

Level A—derived from data from multiple randomized clinical trials
Level B—derived from a single randomized trial or nonrandomized studies
Level C—based on the consensus opinion of experts

OVERVIEW

The ACC/AHA guidelines emphasize the importance of detailed symptom history, focused physical examination, and directed risk factor assessment for patients presenting with chest pain. These data are to be used by the clinician to estimate the probability of significant coronary artery disease (CAD) as low, intermediate, or high. For patients with a low probability of coronary disease (e.g., ≤5%), cardiovascular interventions should be limited, whereas noncardiac causes of chest pain should be evaluated (**Fig. 57G-1**). Recommended initial tests are summarized in **Table 57G-1**. The routine use of chest radiographs or multidetector computed tomography (CT) is not recommended.[2]

For patients with an intermediate or high probability of coronary disease, the clinician should exclude unstable ischemic syndromes and conditions that might exacerbate or cause angina. If these are not present, noninvasive testing should be considered to refine the diagnostic assessment of patients with an intermediate probability of coronary disease and to perform risk stratification for patients with a high probability of coronary disease (**Fig. 57G-2**).

The ACC/AHA guidelines do not mandate exercise testing in all such patients. Pharmacologic imaging studies are recommended for patients who are unable to exercise. Exercise imaging studies are recommended for patients who have had previous coronary revascularization or whose resting electrocardiograms (ECGs) are uninterpretable. Imaging studies are also supported when the clinical evaluation and exercise ECGs have not provided sufficient information to guide management. If the results of noninvasive studies suggest a high risk for complications of coronary heart disease, coronary angiography and revascularization should be considered.

The treatment algorithm recommended by the ACC/AHA guidelines emphasizes the importance of patient education about coronary disease, prevention of ischemia through use of nitrates, beta blockers, and calcium blockers, and prevention of progression of atherosclerosis through risk factor management (**Fig. 57G-3**).

The ACC/AHA guidelines require clarity from the clinician in defining the critical issues for the individual patient. For patients with a chest pain complaint of uncertain cause, the dominant question may be whether coronary artery disease is present or absent (diagnosis). For patients with known or strongly suspected coronary disease, the focus is likely to be on the patient's risk. In these guidelines a specific test may be considered an appropriate option for addressing one or the other of these issues.

The guidelines clearly differentiate between indications for the same tests for the purpose of diagnosis and risk stratification. For example, exercise ECGs are discouraged for establishing diagnosis in patients with a high clinical probability of coronary artery disease on the basis of age, gender, and symptoms (Class IIb indication). However, exercise ECGs are strongly supported as a Class I indication when used to assess prognosis in this same patient population. Thus, interpretation of these guidelines demands rigorous definition of the clinical question at hand.

DIAGNOSIS

Noninvasive Studies

Exercise Electrocardiography

Exercise testing is considered most valuable for diagnosis when the patient's other clinical data suggest an intermediate probability of coronary disease. The ACC/AHA guidelines support the use of exercise ECGs for such patients unless their baseline ECGs show abnormalities likely to render the exercise tracing uninterpretable (**Table 57G-2**). However, exercise ECGs were considered appropriate for patients with complete right bundle branch block or less than 1 mm of ST depression at rest. Use of the exercise test was considered of uncertain value (Class IIb) for patients with high or low pretest probability of coronary disease or those who had less than 1 mm of ST depression and were either using digoxin or had ECG evidence of left ventricular hypertrophy.

Echocardiography

The ACC/AHA guidelines state that "most patients undergoing a diagnostic evaluation for angina do not need an echocardiogram." Echocardiograms are supported to evaluate systolic murmurs suggestive of aortic stenosis or hypertrophic cardiomyopathy and for evaluation of the extent of ischemia when the study can be obtained within 30 minutes after the end of an ischemic episode (**Table 57G-3**). However, routine use of echocardiography for patients with a normal ECG, no history of myocardial infarction, and no evidence of structural heart disease is considered inappropriate (Class III).

Stress Imaging Studies

The ACC/AHA guidelines recommend stress imaging as opposed to exercise ECG in the following: (1) patients who have complete left bundle branch block, electronically paced ventricular rhythm, preexcitation (Wolff-Parkinson-White) syndrome, and other electrocardiographic conduction abnormalities; (2) patients who have more than 1 mm of ST-segment depression at rest including those with left ventricular

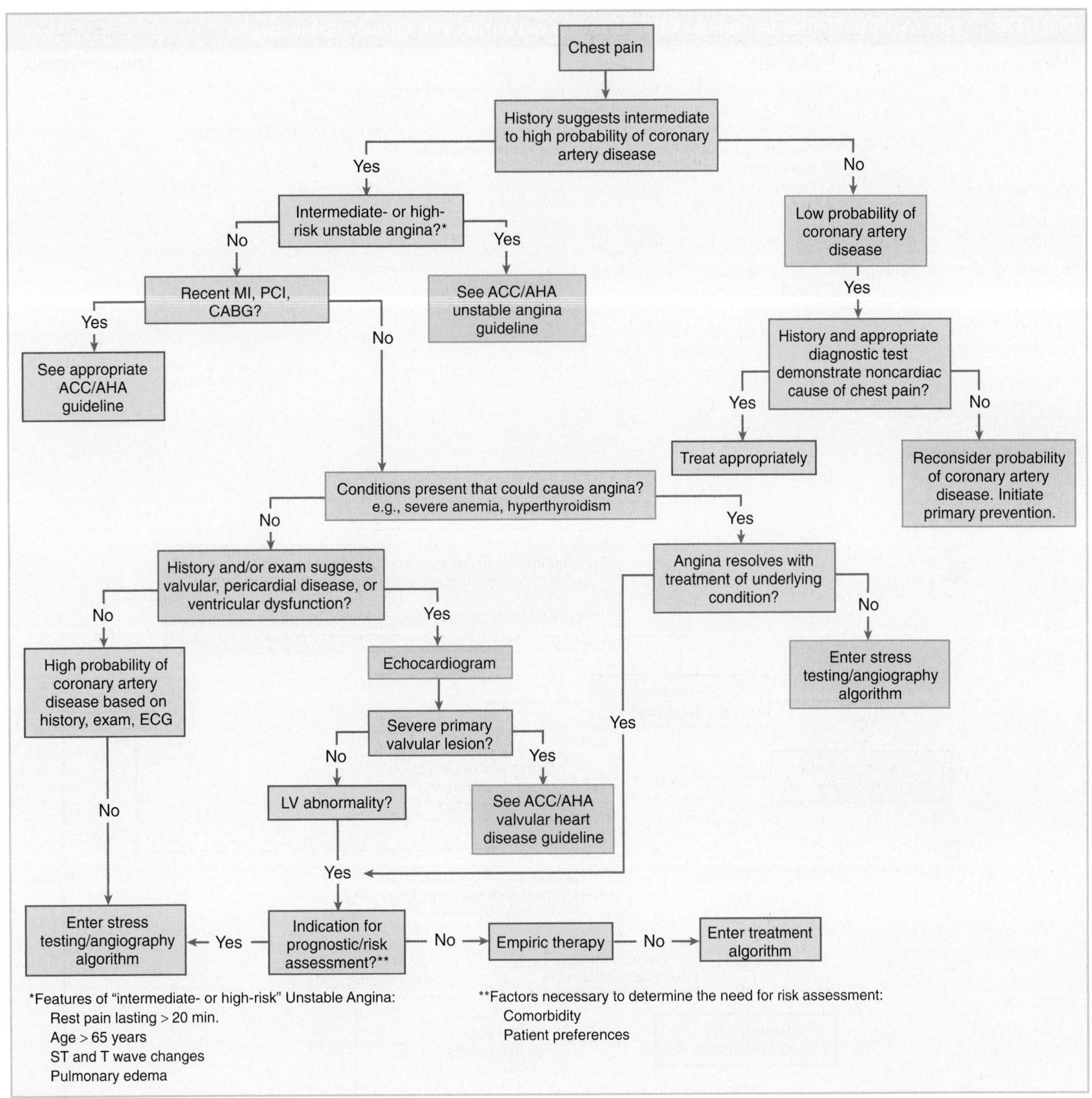

FIGURE 57G-1 Approach to the clinical assessment of chest pain. *(From ACC/AHA 2002 guideline update for the management of patients with chronic stable angina: A report of the American College of Cardiology/American Heart Association Task Force on Practice Guidelines [Committee to Update the 1999 Guidelines for the Management of Patients with Chronic Stable Angina], p 8.) (http://www.acc.org/qualityandscience/clinical/guidelines/stable/stable_clean.pdf.)*

hypertrophy or taking drugs such as digitalis; (3) patients who are unable to exercise to a level high enough to give meaningful results on exercise ECGs; and (4) patients with coronary disease who have undergone prior revascularization, for whom localization of ischemia and establishing the significance of lesions is important.

The guidelines specify that exercise stress testing is preferable to pharmacologic stress testing when the patient can exercise to develop an appropriate level of cardiovascular stress (e.g., 6 to 12 minutes). **Tables 57G-4** and **57G-5** summarize the appropriate indications for stress imaging in patients who are and who are not able to exercise, respectively. As is the case with exercise ECGs, these tests are considered most useful for diagnosis in patients with an intermediate probability of disease.

The guidelines comment on the choice among stress imaging technologies. They conclude that dobutamine perfusion imaging has significant limitations compared with dipyridamole or adenosine perfusion imaging because it does not provoke as great an increase in coronary flow. Therefore, the guidelines recommend that dobutamine be used to provoke ischemia for perfusion imaging only when patients have contraindications to the other agents. In contrast, dobutamine is the agent of choice for pharmacologic stress echocardiography because it enhances myocardial contractile performance and wall motion, which can be observed directly by echocardiography.

Specific Patient Subsets

Although treadmill electrocardiographic testing is less accurate for diagnosis in women than in men, the guidelines note that the diagnostic performance of imaging technologies is also compromised by technical issues (e.g., breast tissue) in women. Therefore, the guidelines conclude

TABLE 57G-1 ACC/AHA Guidelines for Routine Clinical Testing in Patients with Chronic Stable Angina

CLASS	INDICATION	LEVEL OF EVIDENCE*
I (indicated)	1. Rest ECG in patients without obvious noncardiac cause of chest pain	B
	2. Rest ECG during an episode of chest pain	B
	3. Chest radiograph in patients with signs or symptoms of congestive heart failure, valvular heart disease, pericardial disease, or aortic dissection or aneurysm	B
	4. Hemoglobin	C
	5. Fasting glucose	C
	6. Fasting lipid panel	C
IIa (good supportive evidence)	Chest radiograph in patients with signs or symptoms of pulmonary disease	B
IIb (weak supportive evidence)	1. Chest radiograph in other patients	C
	2. Electron beam CT	B
III (not indicated)	None	

*See guidelines text for definitions of level of evidence.

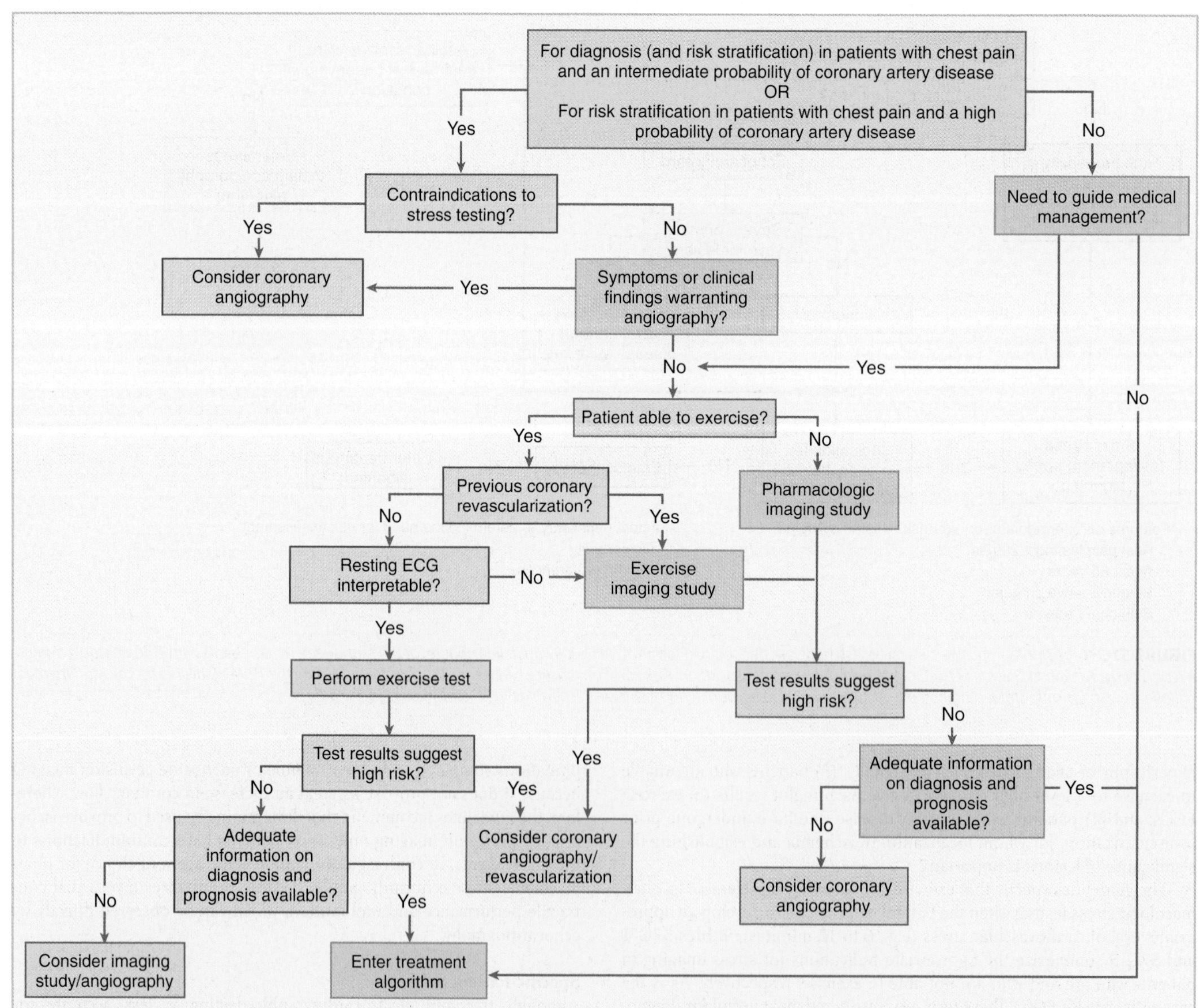

FIGURE 57G-2 Stress testing and angiography in patients with chest pain. *(From ACC/AHA 2002 guideline update for the management of patients with chronic stable angina: A report of the American College of Cardiology/American Heart Association Task Force on Practice Guidelines [Committee to Update the 1999 Guidelines for the Management of Patients with Chronic Stable Angina], p 9.) (http://www.acc.org/qualityandscience/clinical/guidelines/stable/stable_clean.pdf.)*

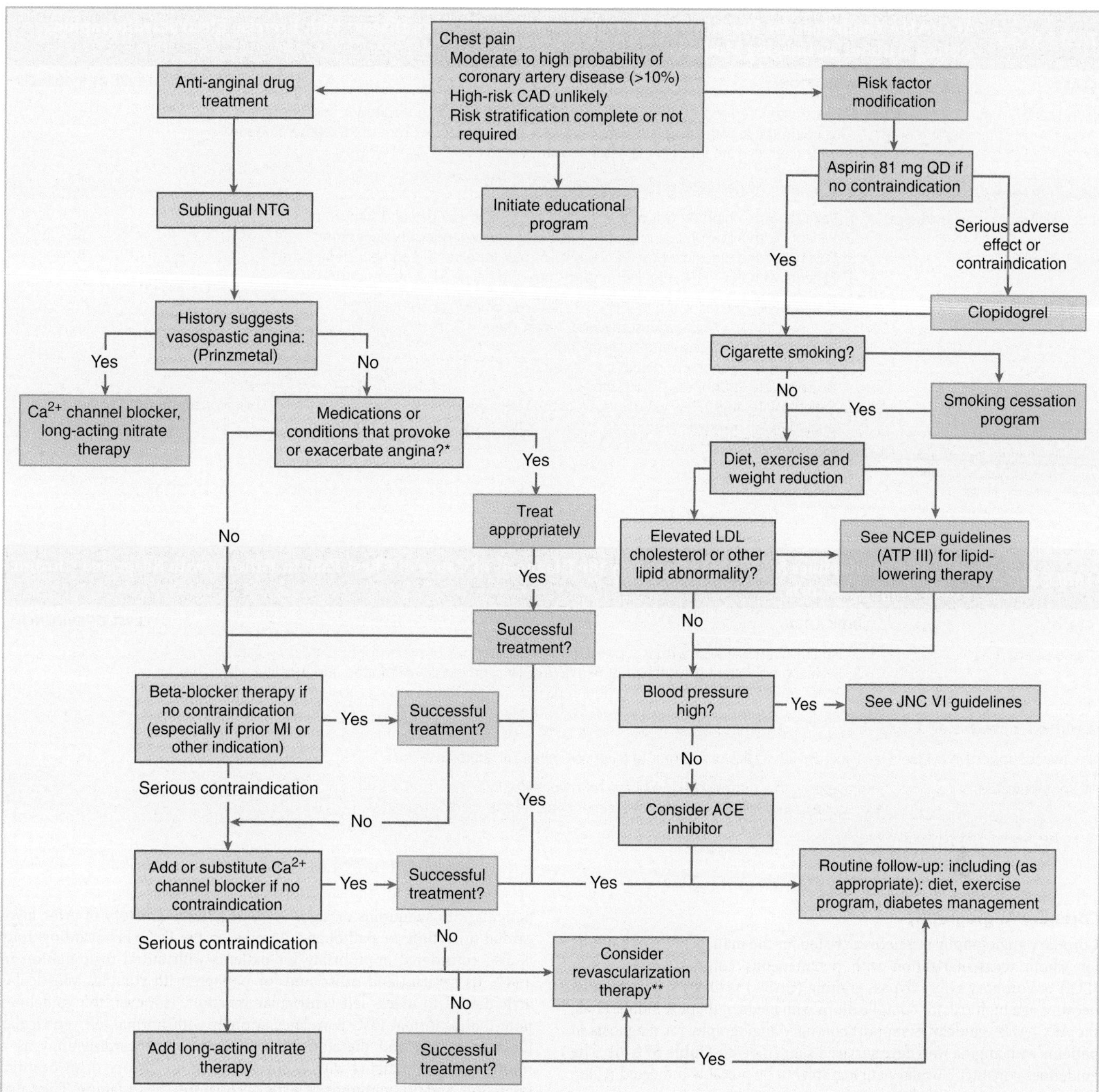

FIGURE 57G-3 Approach to the treatment of chest pain. CAD = coronary artery disease; JNC = Joint National Committee; NCEP = National Cholesterol Education Program; NTG = nitroglycerin. *Conditions that exacerbate or provoke angina are medications (e.g., vasodilators, excessive thyroid replacement, and vasoconstrictors), other cardiac problems (e.g., tachyarrhythmias, bradyarrhythmias, valvular heart disease, especially aortic stenosis), and other medical problems (e.g., hypertrophic cardiomyopathy, profound anemia, uncontrolled hypertension, hyperthyroidism, hypoxemia). **At any point in this process, based on coronary anatomy, severity of anginal symptoms, and patient preferences, it is reasonable to consider evaluation for coronary revascularization. Unless a patient is documented to have left main, triple-vessel, or double-vessel coronary artery disease with significant stenosis of the proximal left anterior descending coronary artery, there is no demonstrated survival advantage associated with revascularization in low-risk patients with chronic stable angina; thus, medical therapy should be attempted in most patients before considering percutaneous coronary intervention or coronary artery bypass grafting. *(From ACC/AHA 2002 guideline update for the management of patients with chronic stable angina: A report of the American College of Cardiology/American Heart Association Task Force on Practice Guidelines [Committee to Update the 1999 Guidelines for the Management of Patients with Chronic Stable Angina], p 10.) (http://www.acc.org/qualityandscience/clinical/guidelines/stable/stable_clean.pdf.)*

that "there currently are insufficient data to justify replacing standard exercise testing with stress imaging in the initial evaluation of women."

The ACC/AHA guidelines discourage the use of noninvasive testing for coronary disease with and without imaging for asymptomatic patients. No Class I and Class IIa indications exist for exercise testing of asymptomatic patients, and there is just one Class IIb indication (weak support): asymptomatic patients with possible myocardial ischemia on ambulatory ECG monitoring or with severe coronary calcification on electron beam CT scanning. Myocardial perfusion imaging testing also receives only weak support (Class IIb) for asymptomatic patients who, despite the recommendations of guidelines, had undergone exercise ECGs and who had an intermediate-risk or high-risk Duke treadmill score or an inadequate exercise ECG.

TABLE 57G-2 ACC/AHA Guidelines for Diagnosis of Obstructive Coronary Artery Disease with Exercise Electrocardiographic Testing Without an Imaging Modality

CLASS	INDICATION	LEVEL OF EVIDENCE*
I (indicated)	Patients with intermediate pretest probability of CAD based on age, gender, and symptoms, including those with complete right bundle branch block or <1 mm of ST-segment depression at rest (exceptions are listed in Classes II and III)	B
IIa (good supportive evidence)	Patients with suspected vasospastic angina	C
IIb (weak supportive evidence)	1. Patients with a high pretest probability of CAD by age, gender, and symptoms	B
	2. Patients with a low pretest probability of CAD by age, gender, and symptoms	B
	3. Patients taking digoxin whose ECG has <1 mm of baseline ST-segment depression	B
	4. Patients with ECG criteria for LVH and <1 mm of baseline ST-segment depression	B
III (not indicated)	1. Patients with the following baseline electrocardiographic abnormalities:	
	a. Preexcitation (Wolff-Parkinson-White) syndrome	B
	b. Electronically paced ventricular rhythm	B
	c. >1 mm of ST-segment depression at rest	B
	d. Complete left bundle branch block	B
	2. Patients with an established diagnosis of CAD because of prior myocardial infarction or coronary angiography; however, testing can assess functional capacity and prognosis	

*See guidelines text for definitions of level of evidence.
LVH = left ventricular hypertrophy.

TABLE 57G-3 ACC/AHA Guidelines for Echocardiography for Diagnosis of Cause of Chest Pain in Patients with Suspected Chronic Stable Angina Pectoris

CLASS	INDICATION	LEVEL OF EVIDENCE*
I (indicated)	1. Patients with systolic murmur suggestive of aortic stenosis or hypertrophic cardiomyopathy	C
	2. Evaluation of extent (severity) of ischemia (e.g., LV segmental wall motion abnormality) when the echocardiogram can be obtained during pain or within 30 min after its abatement	C
IIa (good supportive evidence)		
IIb (weak supportive evidence)	Patients with a click or murmur to diagnose mitral valve prolapse	C
III (not indicated)	Patients with a normal ECG, no history of myocardial infarction, and no signs or symptoms suggestive of heart failure, valvular heart disease, or hypertrophic cardiomyopathy	C

*See guidelines text for definitions of level of evidence.

Coronary Angiography

Coronary angiography is a necessary step for the management of patients for whom revascularization with percutaneous coronary intervention (PCI) or coronary artery bypass grafting (CABG) is likely to be beneficial because of a high risk for complications with medical therapy alone. Thus, the ACC/AHA guidelines support coronary angiography for diagnosis in patients with angina who have survived sudden death (**Table 57G-6**). The guidelines consider coronary angiography to be possibly indicated (Class IIa) when patients with chest pain have contraindications to noninvasive testing or such testing is inadequate or likely to be inadequate to guide management.

The committee thought that noninvasive and clinical data are usually sufficient to establish or exclude the diagnosis of coronary disease and that coronary angiography should rarely be used for this purpose. The guidelines assert that coronary angiography is "generally not indicated" for diagnosis in asymptomatic patients. They offer only weak support (Class IIb) for coronary angiography to establish a definitive diagnosis for patients with recurrent hospitalization for chest pain.

RISK STRATIFICATION

The ACC/AHA guidelines emphasize the following four factors that predict survival for patients with coronary artery disease: (1) left ventricular function; (2) anatomic extent and severity of coronary atherosclerosis; (3) presence of recent plaque rupture; and (4) the patient's general health and noncoronary comorbidity.

Assessment of Left Ventricular Function

The guidelines consider assessment of left ventricular function with either echocardiography or radionuclide angiography appropriate (Class I) in patients with symptoms or signs of heart failure, a history of prior myocardial infarction, or pathologic Q waves on the ECG. Echocardiography is also considered appropriate for patients with mitral regurgitation to assess its severity and cause and for patients with complex ventricular arrhythmias to assess left ventricular function. However, the guidelines note that a normal ECG correlates strongly with normal left ventricular function at rest and therefore do not endorse echocardiography as a routine test for patients with a normal ECG, no history of myocardial infarction, and no symptoms or signs of congestive heart failure. They also do not support routine periodic echocardiography for stable patients in whom no new change in therapy is contemplated.

Noninvasive Tests for Ischemia

Exercise testing is recommended for assessment of prognosis for all patients with an intermediate or high probability of coronary artery disease, except those with electrocardiographic abnormalities that compromise interpretation of the exercise tracing and those for which the information is unlikely to alter management (**Table 57G-7**). The committee directly addressed the issue of whether the additional information provided by imaging technologies might make them preferable tests for risk stratification but concluded that the greater costs of these tests could not be justified for most patients. Therefore, the guidelines endorse a stepwise approach in which the exercise ECG is used as the initial test in patients who are not taking digoxin, have a normal rest ECG, and are able to exercise.

The ACC/AHA guidelines support the use of stress testing with echocardiographic or radionuclide imaging to identify the severity of ischemia in patients who have electrocardiographic abnormalities precluding interpretation of the exercise tracing and for patients in whom the functional

TABLE 57G-4 ACC/AHA Guidelines for Cardiac Stress Imaging as Initial Diagnostic Test for Patients with Chronic Stable Angina Who Are Able to Exercise

CLASS	INDICATION	LEVEL OF EVIDENCE*
I (indicated)	1. Exercise myocardial perfusion imaging or exercise echocardiography in patients with intermediate pretest probability of CAD who have one of the following baseline electrocardiographic abnormalities:	
	a. Preexcitation (Wolff-Parkinson-White) syndrome	B
	b. >1 mm of ST-segment depression at rest	B
	2. Exercise myocardial perfusion imaging or exercise echocardiography in patients with prior revascularization (either PCI or CABG)	B
	3. Adenosine or dipyridamole myocardial perfusion imaging in patients with intermediate pretest probability of CAD and one of the following baseline ECG abnormalities:	
	a. Electronically paced ventricular rhythm	C
	b. Left bundle branch block	B
IIa (good supportive evidence)		
IIb (weak supportive evidence)	1. Exercise myocardial perfusion imaging or exercise echocardiography in patients with low or high probability of CAD who have one of the following baseline ECG abnormalities:	
	a. Preexcitation (Wolff-Parkinson-White) syndrome	B
	b. >1 mm of ST-segment depression	B
	2. Adenosine or dipyridamole myocardial perfusion imaging in patients with low or high probability of CAD and one of the following baseline electrocardiographic abnormalities:	
	a. Electronically paced ventricular rhythm	C
	b. Left bundle branch block	B
	3. Exercise myocardial perfusion imaging or exercise echocardiography in patients with intermediate probability of CAD who have one of the following:	
	a. Digoxin use with <1 mm ST-segment depression on the baseline ECG	B
	b. LVH with <1 mm ST-segment depression on the baseline ECG	B
	4. Exercise myocardial perfusion imaging, exercise echocardiography, adenosine or dipyridamole myocardial perfusion imaging, or dobutamine echocardiography as the initial stress test in a patient with a normal rest ECG who is not taking digoxin	B
	5. Exercise or dobutamine echocardiography in patients with left bundle branch block	C
III (not indicated)		

*See guidelines text for definitions of level of evidence.

TABLE 57G-5 ACC/AHA Guidelines for Cardiac Stress Imaging as Initial Diagnostic Test for Patients with Chronic Stable Angina Who Are Unable to Exercise

CLASS	INDICATION	LEVEL OF EVIDENCE*
I (indicated)	1. Adenosine or dipyridamole myocardial perfusion imaging or dobutamine echocardiography in patients with intermediate pretest probability of CAD	B
	2. Adenosine or dipyridamole myocardial perfusion imaging or dobutamine echocardiography in patients with prior revascularization (either PCI or CABG)	B
IIa (good supportive evidence)		
IIb (weak supportive evidence)	1. Adenosine or dipyridamole myocardial perfusion imaging or dobutamine echocardiography in patients with low or high probability of CAD in absence of electronically paced ventricular rhythm or left bundle branch block	B
	2. Adenosine or dipyridamole myocardial perfusion imaging in patients with low or high probability of CAD and one of the following baseline ECG abnormalities:	
	a. Electronically paced ventricular rhythm	C
	b. Left bundle branch block	B
	3. Dobutamine echocardiography in patients with left bundle branch block	C
III (not indicated)		

*See guidelines text for definitions of level of evidence.

significance of coronary lesions will guide management (**Tables 57G-8 and 57G-9**). Dipyridamole or adenosine myocardial perfusion imaging is recommended for patients with left bundle branch block or electronically paced ventricular rhythms because of higher rates of false-positive septal perfusion defects with exercise than with dipyridamole or adenosine. Relatively few data exist on the performance of dobutamine echocardiography in this setting, so this approach is not endorsed by the guidelines for patients with left bundle branch block or electronically paced ventricular rhythms. Stress imaging studies are also supported for assessment of the functional significance of coronary lesions in planning PCI.

The guidelines discourage the use of noninvasive testing for risk stratification of patients who have no symptoms of coronary disease. No Class I or IIa indications exist for the use of cardiac stress imaging as an initial test for risk stratification. Supporting evidence is considered weak for the use of cardiac stress imaging for asymptomatic patients with severe coronary calcification on electron beam CT or who had undergone an exercise ECG and had inadequate tests or intermediate- or high-risk Duke treadmill scores.

Coronary Angiography

In the ACC/AHA guidelines, the decision to proceed to coronary angiography should be based on symptomatic status and risk stratification derived from clinical data and noninvasive test results. The guidelines define noninvasive findings that predict a high (>3%), intermediate (1%

TABLE 57G-6 ACC/AHA Guidelines for Coronary Angiography to Establish a Diagnosis in Patients with Suspected Angina*

CLASS	INDICATION	LEVEL OF EVIDENCE†
I (indicated)	Patients with known or possible angina pectoris who have survived sudden cardiac death	B
IIa (good supportive evidence)	1. Patients with an uncertain diagnosis after noninvasive testing for whom the benefit of a more certain diagnosis outweighs the risk and cost of coronary angiography	C
	2. Patients who cannot undergo noninvasive testing because of disability, illness, or morbid obesity	C
	3. Patients with an occupational requirement for a definitive diagnosis	C
	4. Patients who because of young age at onset of symptoms, noninvasive imaging, or other clinical parameters are suspected of having a nonatherosclerotic cause for myocardial ischemia (e.g., coronary artery anomaly, Kawasaki disease, primary coronary artery dissection, radiation-induced vasculopathy)	C
	5. Patients in whom coronary artery spasm is suspected and provocative testing may be necessary	C
	6. Patients with high pretest probability of left main or triple-vessel CAD	C
IIb (weak supportive evidence)	1. Patients with recurrent hospitalization for chest pain in whom a definite diagnosis is judged necessary	C
	2. Patients with an overriding desire for a definitive diagnosis and intermediate or high probability of CAD	C
III (not indicated)	1. Patients with significant comorbidity in whom the risk of coronary arteriography outweighs the benefit of the procedure	C
	2. Patients with an overriding personal desire for a definitive diagnosis and a low probability of CAD	C

*Including those with known CAD who have a significant change in anginal symptoms.
†See guidelines text for definitions of level of evidence.

TABLE 57G-7 ACC/AHA Guidelines for Exercise Testing Risk Assessment and Prognosis in Patients with an Intermediate or High Probability of Coronary Artery Disease

CLASS	INDICATION	LEVEL OF EVIDENCE*
I (indicated)	1. Patients undergoing initial evaluation (exceptions are listed below in Classes IIb and III)	B
	2. Patients after a significant change in cardiac symptoms	C
IIa (good supportive evidence)		
IIb (weak supportive evidence)	1. Patients with the following electrocardiographic abnormalities:	
	a. Preexcitation (Wolff-Parkinson-White) syndrome	B
	b. Electronically paced ventricular rhythm	B
	c. >1 mm of ST-segment depression at rest	B
	d. Complete left bundle branch block	B
	2. Patients who have undergone cardiac catheterization to identify ischemia in the distribution of coronary lesion of borderline severity	C
	3. Postrevascularization patients who have a significant change in anginal pattern suggestive of ischemia	C
III (not indicated)	Patients with severe comorbidity likely to limit life expectancy or prevent revascularization	C

*See guidelines text for definitions of level of evidence.

TABLE 57G-8 ACC/AHA Guidelines for Cardiac Stress Imaging as Initial Test for Risk Stratification of Patients with Chronic Stable Angina Who Are Able to Exercise

CLASS	INDICATION	LEVEL OF EVIDENCE*
I (indicated)	1. Exercise myocardial perfusion imaging or exercise echocardiography to identify the extent, severity, and location of ischemia in patients who do not have left bundle branch block or an electronically paced ventricular rhythm, and who have an abnormal rest ECG or are using digoxin	B
	2. Dipyridamole or adenosine myocardial perfusion imaging in patients with left bundle branch block or electronically paced ventricular rhythm	B
	3. Exercise myocardial perfusion imaging or exercise echocardiography to assess the functional significance of coronary lesions (if not already known) when planning PCI	B
IIa (good supportive evidence)		
IIb (weak supportive evidence)	1. Exercise or dobutamine echocardiography in patients with left bundle branch block	C
	2. Exercise, dipyridamole, or adenosine myocardial perfusion imaging, or exercise or dobutamine echocardiography, as the initial test in patients who have a normal rest ECG and are not taking digoxin	B
III (not indicated)	1. Exercise myocardial perfusion imaging in patients with left bundle branch block	C
	2. Exercise, dipyridamole, or adenosine myocardial perfusion imaging, or exercise or dobutamine echocardiography, in patients with severe comorbidity likely to limit life expectation or prevent revascularization	C

*See guidelines text for definitions of level of evidence.

TABLE 57G-9 ACC/AHA Guidelines for Cardiac Stress Imaging as Initial Test for Risk Stratification of Patients with Chronic Stable Angina Who Are Unable to Exercise

CLASS	INDICATION	LEVEL OF EVIDENCE*
I (indicated)	1. Dipyridamole or adenosine myocardial perfusion imaging or dobutamine echocardiography to identify the extent, severity, and location of ischemia in patients who do not have left bundle branch block or electronically paced ventricular rhythm	B
	2. Dipyridamole or adenosine myocardial perfusion imaging in patients with left bundle branch block or electronically paced ventricular rhythm	B
	3. Dipyridamole or adenosine myocardial perfusion imaging or dobutamine echocardiography to assess the functional significance of coronary lesions (if not already known) when planning PCI	B
IIa (good supportive evidence)		
IIb (weak supportive evidence)	Dobutamine echocardiography in patients with left bundle branch block	C
III (not indicated)	Dipyridamole or adenosine myocardial perfusion imaging or dobutamine echocardiography in patients with severe comorbidity likely to limit life expectation or prevent revascularization	C

*See guidelines text for definitions of level of evidence.

TABLE 57G-10 ACC/AHA Guideline Criteria for Noninvasive Risk Stratification

High Risk (>3% Annual Mortality Rate)

1. Severe resting left ventricular dysfunction (LV ejection fraction [LVEF] < 0.35)
2. High-risk treadmill score (score ≤ −11)
3. Severe exercise left ventricular dysfunction (exercise LVEF < 0.35)
4. Stress-induced large perfusion defect (particularly if anterior)
5. Stress-induced multiple perfusion defects of moderate size
6. Large, fixed perfusion defect with LV dilation or increased lung uptake (thallium-201)
7. Stress-induced moderate perfusion defect with LV dilation or increased lung uptake (thallium-201)
8. Echocardiographic wall motion abnormality (involving more than two segments) developing at low dose of dobutamine (≤10 μg/kg/min) or at low heart rate (<120 beats/min)
9. Stress echocardiographic evidence of extensive ischemia

Intermediate Risk (1%-3% Annual Mortality Rate)

1. Mild or moderate resting LV dysfunction (LVEF = 0.35-0.49)
2. Intermediate-risk treadmill score (−11 < score < 5)
3. Stress-induced moderate perfusion defect without LV dilation or increased lung intake (thallium-201)
4. Limited stress echocardiographic ischemia with a wall motion abnormality only at higher doses of dobutamine involving two segments or less

Low Risk (<1% Annual Mortality Rate)

1. Low-risk treadmill score (score ≥ 5)
2. Normal or small myocardial perfusion defect at rest or with stress*
3. Normal stress echocardiographic wall motion or no change of limited resting wall motion abnormalities during stress*

*Although the published data are limited, patients with these findings will probably not be at low risk in the presence of a high-risk treadmill score or severe resting LV dysfunction (LVEF < 0.35).

From Gibbons RJ, Abrams J, Chatterjee K, et al: ACC/AHA 2002 guideline update for the management of patients with chronic stable angina: A report of the American College of Cardiology/American Heart Association Task Force on Practice Guidelines (Committee to update the 1999 guidelines for the management of patients with chronic stable angina) (http://www.acc.org/clinical/guidelines/stable/stable.pdf).

to 3%), and low (<1%) expected annual mortality rate (**Table 57G-10**). Coronary angiography for risk stratification and as a prelude to intervention is endorsed for patients with high-risk criteria, as well as those with disabling chronic stable angina despite medical therapy or other clinical characteristics suggesting high risk (**Table 57G-11**). The committee considered evidence to be generally supportive (Class IIa) for coronary angiography for patients with milder angina in the setting of left ventricular dysfunction even if they do not have high-risk criteria on noninvasive testing, for asymptomatic patients with high-risk criteria, and for patients whose risk status is uncertain despite noninvasive testing.

Conversely, coronary angiography is discouraged (Class III) for patients who have mild angina and no evidence of ischemia on noninvasive testing or would not undergo revascularization. Only weak support (Class IIb) exists for coronary angiography for patients with mild angina and good left ventricular function in the absence of high-risk criteria on noninvasive testing, for patients with severe angina whose symptoms were controlled with medical therapy, or for patients with mild angina but unacceptable side effects to adequate medical therapy.

TREATMENT

ACC/AHA guidelines for the medical therapy of patients with chronic stable angina are oriented toward preventing myocardial infarction and death and reducing symptoms. When coronary revascularization has been shown to extend life, it is the recommended approach, but in many settings there are a variety of reasonable options including medical therapy, PCI, and CABG. Cost-effectiveness and patient preference are considered important components of the decision making process.

The guidelines assert that the goal of treatment of patients with chronic stable angina should be the complete or almost complete elimination of anginal chest pain and return to normal activities, with minimal side effects. They recommend that the initial treatment of the patient should include all the elements in the following mnemonic:

A = Aspirin and antianginal therapy
B = Beta blocker and blood pressure
C = Cigarette smoking and cholesterol
D = Diet and diabetes
E = Education and exercise

Pharmacologic Therapy

The guidelines emphasize the importance of aspirin and beta blockers for patients with coronary disease in the absence of contraindications (**Table 57G-12**). Absolute contraindications to beta blockers include severe bradycardia, pre-existing high degree of atrioventricular block, sick sinus syndrome, and severe, unstable left ventricular failure. Relative contraindications to beta blockers include asthma and bronchospastic disease, severe depression, and peripheral vascular disease. The guidelines note that most patients with diabetes tolerate beta blockers, although these drugs should be used with caution in patients who require insulin.

Angiotensin-converting enzyme (ACE) inhibitors are recommended (Class I indication) for patients with diabetes, hypertension, chronic kidney disease and/or left ventricular systolic dysfunction, and may be considered for their use in other patients with coronary disease (Class IIa). The guidelines recommend that nitrates and/or calcium antagonists should be used for symptom control but indicate that short-acting dihydropyridine calcium antagonists should be avoided. Low-density lipoprotein cholesterol (LDL-C) should be controlled with a target of less than 100 mg/dL (see later, "Risk Reduction"). Further reduction of LDL-C to less than 70 mg/dL is reasonable (Class IIa).[3]

TABLE 57G-11 ACC/AHA Guidelines for Coronary Angiography for Risk Stratification in Patients with Chronic Stable Angina

CLASS	INDICATION	LEVEL OF EVIDENCE*
I (indicated)	1. Patients with disabling (Canadian Cardiovascular Society [CCS] Classes III and IV) chronic stable angina despite medical therapy	B
	2. Patients with high-risk criteria on noninvasive testing regardless of anginal severity	B
	3. Patients with angina who have survived sudden cardiac death or serious ventricular arrhythmia	B
	4. Patients with angina and symptoms and signs of CHF	C
	5. Patients with clinical characteristics that indicate a high likelihood of severe CAD	C
IIa (good supportive evidence)	1. Patients with significant LV dysfunction (ejection fraction > 0.45), CCS Class I or II angina, and demonstrable ischemia but no high-risk criteria on noninvasive testing	C
	2. Patients with inadequate prognostic information after noninvasive testing	C
	3. Patients with high-risk criteria suggesting ischemia on noninvasive testing	C
IIb (weak supportive evidence)	1. Patients with CCS Class I or II angina, preserved LV function (ejection fraction > 0.45), but no high-risk criteria on noninvasive testing	C
	2. Patients with CCS Class III (not indicated) or IV angina, which improves to Class I or II with medical therapy	C
	3. Patients with CCS Class I or II angina but intolerance (unacceptable side effects) to adequate medical therapy	C
III (not indicated)	1. Patients with CCS Class I or II angina who respond to medical therapy and who have no evidence of ischemia on noninvasive testing	C
	2. Patients who prefer to avoid revascularization	C

*See guidelines text for definitions of level of evidence.
CHF = congestive heart failure.

TABLE 57G-12 ACC/AHA Guidelines for Pharmacotherapy for Chronic Stable Angina

CLASS	INDICATION	LEVEL OF EVIDENCE*
I (indicated)	1. Aspirin in the absence of contraindications	A
	2. Beta blockers as initial therapy in the absence of contraindications in patients with prior myocardial infarction or without prior myocardial infarction	A,B
	3. ACE inhibitor in all patients with CAD who also have diabetes and/or LV systolic dysfunction	A
	4. LDL-lowering therapy in patients with documented or suspected CAD and LDL-C > 130 mg/dL, with a target LDL < 100 mg/dL	A
	5. Sublingual nitroglycerin or nitroglycerin spray for the immediate relief of angina	B
	6. Calcium antagonists† or long-acting nitrates as initial therapy for reduction of symptoms when beta blockers are contraindicated	B
	7. Calcium antagonists† or long-acting nitrates in combination with beta blockers when initial treatment with beta blockers is not successful	B
	8. Calcium antagonists† and long-acting nitrates as a substitute for beta blockers if initial treatment with beta blockers leads to unacceptable side effects	C
IIa (good supportive evidence)	1. Clopidogrel when aspirin is absolutely contraindicated	B
	2. Long-acting nondihydropyridine calcium antagonists† instead of beta blockers as initial therapy	B
	3. In patients with documented or suspected CAD and LDL-C 100-129 mg/dL, several therapeutic options are available:	B
	a. Lifestyle and/or drug therapies to lower LDL to <100 mg/dL; further reduction to <70 mg/dL is reasonable	
	b. Weight reduction and increased physical activity in persons with the metabolic syndrome	
	c. Institution of treatment of other lipid or nonlipid risk factors; consider use of nicotinic acid or fibric acid for elevated triglyceride or low HDL cholesterol levels	
	4. ACE inhibitor in patients with CAD or other vascular disease	B
IIb (weak supportive evidence)	Low-intensity anticoagulation with warfarin in addition to aspirin	B
III (not indicated)	1. Dipyridamole	B
	2. Chelation therapy	B

*See guidelines text for definitions of level of evidence.
†Short-acting dihydropyridine calcium antagonists should be avoided.
LDL = low-density lipoprotein.

Several recommendations about pharmacologic therapy may be altered in future revisions of these guidelines because of further research providing insight into the effects of these agents. Use of dipyridamole or chelation therapy is discouraged.

For asymptomatic patients with known coronary disease (e.g., patients with prior myocardial infarction), the guidelines recommend aspirin and beta blockers in the absence of contraindications and the use of lipid-lowering therapies and ACE inhibitors as described earlier.

Risk Reduction

For patients with chronic stable angina, the ACC/AHA guidelines support intensive management of risk factors, including hypertension (target BP < 130/80 mm Hg),[4] cigarette smoking, diabetes, LDL-C, and obesity (**Table 57G-13**). The guidelines support the use of pharmacologic therapy for patients with LDL levels higher than 130 mg/dL, with a target of 100 mg/dL. Further reduction of LDL-C to less than 70 mg/dL is reasonable (Class IIa).[3] For patients with coronary disease who have an LDL of 100 to

TABLE 57G-13 ACC/AHA Guidelines for Treatment of Risk Factors

CLASS	INDICATION	LEVEL OF EVIDENCE*
I (indicated)	1. Treatment of hypertension according to Joint National Conference VI guidelines	A
	2. Smoking cessation therapy	B
	3. Management of diabetes	C
	4. Comprehensive cardiac rehabilitation program (including exercise)	B
	5. LDL-lowering therapy in patients with documented or suspected CAD and LDL-C ≥ 130 mg/dL, with a target LDL < 100 mg/dL	A
	6. Weight reduction in obese patients in the presence of hypertension, hyperlipidemia, or diabetes mellitus	C
IIa (good supportive evidence)	1. In patients with documented or suspected CAD and LDL-C = 100-129 mg/dL, several therapeutic options are available:	B
	a. Lifestyle and/or drug therapies to lower LDL-C to <100 mg/dL; further reduction to below 70 mg/dL is reasonable	B
	b. Weight reduction and increased physical activity in persons with the metabolic syndrome	B
	c. Institution of treatment of other lipid or nonlipid risk factors; consider use of nicotinic acid or fibric acid for elevated triglyceride or low HDL cholesterol levels	B
	2. Therapy to lower non–HDL-C in patients with documented or suspected CAD and triglyceride > 200 mg/dL, with a target non- HDL-C < 130 mg/dL	B
	3. Weight reduction in obese patients in the absence of hypertension, hyperlipidemia, or diabetes mellitus	C
IIb (weak supportive evidence)	1. Folate therapy in patients with elevated homocysteine levels	C
	2. Identification and appropriate treatment of clinical depression to improve CAD outcomes	C
	3. Interventions directed at psychosocial stress reduction	C
III (not indicated)	1. Initiation of hormone replacement therapy in postmenopausal women to reduce cardiovascular risk	A
	2. Vitamins C and E supplementation	A
	3. Chelation therapy	C
	4. Garlic	C
	5. Acupuncture	C
	6. Coenzyme Q	C

*See guidelines text for definitions of level of evidence.

TABLE 57G-14 Specific Goals for Risk Reduction Strategies in Patients with Chronic Stable Angina

RISK FACTOR OR STRATEGY	GOAL
Smoking	Complete cessation
Blood pressure	130/80 mm Hg*
Lipid management	Primary goal: LDL < 100 mg/dL; further reduction of LDL-C to <70 mg/dL is reasonable (Class IIa) Secondary goal: If triglycerides ≥ 200 mg/dL, then non–HDL-C should be <130 mg/dL
Physical activity	Minimum goal: 30 min, 3 or 4 days/wk Optimal goal: daily
Weight management	BMI: 18.5-24.9 kg/m^2
Diabetes management	HbA1c < 7%
Antiplatelet agents, anticoagulants	All patients—indefinite use of aspirin 75-325 mg/day if not contraindicated. Consider clopidogrel as an alternative if aspirin is contraindicated. Manage warfarin to international normalized ratio = 2.0-3.0 in patients after MI when clinically indicated or for those not able to take aspirin or clopidogrel
ACE inhibitors	Start and continue indefinitely in all patients with LVEF ≤ 40% and in those with hypertension, diabetes, or chronic kidney disease, unless contraindicated. Consider chronic therapy for all other patients with coronary or other vascular disease unless contraindicated. Use as needed to manage blood pressure or symptoms in all other patients
Beta blockers	Start in all postmyocardial infarction and acute patients (arrhythmia, LV dysfunction, inducible ischemia) at 5-28 days. Continue for 6 mo minimum. Observe usual contraindications. Use as needed to manage angina, rhythm, or blood pressure in all patients

BMI = body mass index; CHF = congestive heart failure; HbA1c = hemoglobin A1c.
*Rosendorff C, Black HR, Cannon CP, et al: Treatment of hypertension in the prevention and management of ischemic heart disease: A scientific statement from the American Heart Association Council for High Blood Pressure Research and the Councils on Clinical Cardiology and Epidemiology and Prevention. Circulation 115:2761, 2007.

129 mg/dL, the guidelines consider several options reasonable (Class IIa), including lifestyle modifications and drug therapies.

In changes from prior guidelines, initiation of hormone therapy for the purpose of reducing cardiovascular risk is considered inappropriate (Class III), as is use of vitamins C and E supplementation, chelation therapy, garlic, acupuncture, and coenzyme Q for this purpose. Evidence to support interventions based on lipoprotein (a) and homocysteine levels are considered inconclusive.

Specific goals for key risk reduction interventions are summarized in **Table 57G-14**.

Revascularization

ACC/AHA guidelines for revascularization with PCI or CABG for patients with chronic stable angina focus on improvement of survival for patients with high clinical risk of mortality on medical therapy and on controlling symptoms in patients who have an inadequate quality of life on medical therapy. Recommendations include the use of CABG for patients with significant left main coronary artery disease and in those with triple-vessel disease, particularly those with abnormal left ventricular function (**Table 57G-15**). PCI and CABG are supported for patients with double- and triple-vessel coronary disease who do not have treated diabetes. Revascularization is also supported for patients with single- or double-vessel coronary disease who have a large area of viable myocardium and high-risk criteria on noninvasive testing.

The guidelines discourage the use of PCI or CABG for single- or double-vessel coronary disease without significant proximal left anterior descending (LAD) coronary artery disease if they have mild symptoms or have not received an adequate trial of medical therapy, particularly if noninvasive testing data indicate that they have only a small area of viable myocardium or have no demonstrable ischemia on noninvasive testing. PCI for patients with diabetes is considered a second-choice strategy compared with CABG.

For asymptomatic patients, the guidelines for revascularization with PCI or CABG are identical to those for other patients with chronic stable angina (see Table 57G-15), except that the following indications that were considered Class IIa are regarded as weaker (Class IIb) in asymptomatic patients:

- Use of PCI or CABG for patients with single- or double-vessel CAD without significant proximal LAD disease but with a moderate area of viable myocardium and demonstrable ischemia on noninvasive testing
- Use of PCI or CABG for patients with single-vessel disease with significant proximal LAD disease

Alternative Therapies

The guidelines do not consider alternative therapies to be sufficiently supported by evidence to warrant a Class I indication for patients with chronic stable angina. Surgical laser transmyocardial revascularization is given a Class IIa indication, and enhanced external counterpulsation and spinal cord stimulation are given Class IIb indications.

PATIENT FOLLOW-UP

The ACC/AHA guidelines recommend that patients with chronic stable angina have follow-up evaluations every 4 to 12 months during the first year of therapy; subsequently, annual evaluations are recommended if the patient is stable and reliable enough to call when angina symptoms become worse or other symptoms occur. The guidelines urge restraint in the use of routine testing in follow-up of patients with chronic stable

TABLE 57G-15 ACC/AHA Guidelines for Revascularization with Percutaneous Coronary Intervention and Coronary Artery Bypass Grafting in Patients with Stable Angina

CLASS	INDICATION	LEVEL OF EVIDENCE*
I (indicated)	1. CABG for patients with significant left main coronary disease	A
	2. CABG for patients with triple-vessel disease. The survival benefit is greater in patients with abnormal LV function (LVEF < 0.50).	A
	3. CABG for patients with double-vessel disease with significant proximal LAD CAD and either abnormal LV function (ejection fraction <50%) or demonstrable ischemia on noninvasive testing	A
	4. PCI for patients with double- or triple-vessel disease with significant proximal LAD CAD, who have anatomy suitable for catheter-based therapy and normal LV function and who do not have treated diabetes	B
	5. PCI or CABG for patients with single- or double-vessel CAD without significant proximal LAD CAD but with a large area of viable myocardium and high-risk criteria on noninvasive testing	B
	6. CABG for patients with single- or double-vessel CAD without significant proximal LAD CAD who have survived sudden cardiac death or sustained ventricular tachycardia	C
	7. In patients with prior PCI, CABG, or PCI for recurrent stenosis associated with a large area of viable myocardium or high-risk criteria on noninvasive testing	C
	8. PCI or CABG for patients who have not been successfully treated by medical therapy and can undergo revascularization with acceptable risk	B
IIa (good supportive evidence)	1. Repeat CABG for patients with multiple saphenous vein graft stenoses, especially when there is significant stenosis of a graft supplying the LAD; it may be appropriate to use PCI for focal saphenous vein graft lesions or multiple stenoses in poor candidates for reoperative surgery.	C
	2. Use of PCI or CABG for patients with single- or double-vessel CAD without significant proximal LAD disease but with a moderate area of viable myocardium and demonstrable ischemia on noninvasive testing	B
	3. Use of PCI or CABG for patients with single-vessel disease with significant proximal LAD disease	B
IIb (weak supportive evidence)	1. Compared with CABG, PCI for patients with double- or triple-vessel disease with significant proximal LAD CAD, who have anatomy suitable for catheter-based therapy and who have treated diabetes or abnormal LV function	B
	2. Use of PCI for patients with significant left main coronary disease who are not candidates for CABG	C
	3. PCI for patients with single- or double-vessel CAD without significant proximal LAD CAD who have survived sudden cardiac death or sustained ventricular tachycardia	C
III (not indicated)	1. Use of PCI or CABG for patients with single- or double-vessel CAD without significant proximal LAD CAD, who have mild symptoms that are unlikely to be caused by myocardial ischemia, or who have not received an adequate trial of medical therapy and a. have only a small area of viable myocardium *or* b. have no demonstrable ischemia on noninvasive testing	C
	2. Use of PCI or CABG for patients with borderline coronary stenoses (50%-60% diameter in locations other than the left main coronary artery) and no demonstrable ischemia on noninvasive testing	C
	3. Use of PCI or CABG for patients with insignificant coronary stenosis (<50% diameter)	C
	4. Use of PCI for patients with significant left main coronary artery disease who are candidates for CABG	B

*See guidelines text for definitions of level of evidence.

TABLE 57G-16 ACC/AHA Guidelines for Echocardiography, Treadmill Exercise Testing, Stress Radionuclide Imaging, Stress Echocardiography Studies, and Coronary Angiography During Patient Follow-up

CLASS	INDICATION	LEVEL OF EVIDENCE*
I (indicated)	1. Chest radiograph for patients with evidence of new or worsening CHF	C
	2. Assessment of LVEF and segmental wall motion by echocardiography or radionuclide imaging in patients with new or worsening CHF or evidence of intervening myocardial infarction by history or ECG	C
	3. Echocardiography for evidence of new or worsening valvular heart disease	C
	4. Treadmill exercise test for patients without prior revascularization who have a significant change in clinical status, are able to exercise, and do not have any of the electrocardiographic abnormalities listed in indication 5	C
	5. Stress radionuclide imaging or stress echocardiography procedures for patients without prior revascularization who have a significant change in clinical status and are unable to exercise or have one of the following electrocardiographic abnormalities: a. Preexcitation (Wolff-Parkinson-White) syndrome b. Electronically paced ventricular rhythm c. >1 mm of ST-segment depression at rest d. Complete left bundle branch block	C
	6. Stress radionuclide imaging or stress echocardiography procedures for patients who have a significant change in clinical status and required a stress imaging procedure on their initial evaluation because of equivocal or intermediate-risk treadmill results	C
	7. Stress radionuclide imaging or stress echocardiography procedures for patients with prior revascularization who have a significant change in clinical status	C
	8. Coronary angiography in patients with marked limitation of ordinary activity (CCS Class III) despite maximal medical therapy	C
IIa (good supportive evidence)		
IIb (weak supportive evidence)	Annual treadmill exercise testing in patients who have no change in clinical status, can exercise, have none of the electrocardiographic abnormalities listed in Class I, indication 5, and have an estimated annual mortality rate > 1%	C
III (not indicated)	1. Echocardiography or radionuclide imaging for assessment of LVEF and segmental wall motion in patients with a normal ECG, no history of MI, and no evidence of CHF	C
	2. Repeat treadmill exercise testing in <3 yr in patients who have no change in clinical status and estimated annual mortality rate <1% on their initial evaluation, as demonstrated by one of the following: a. Low-risk Duke treadmill score (without imaging) b. Low-risk Duke treadmill score with negative imaging c. Normal LV function and normal coronary angiogram d. Normal LV function and insignificant CAD	C
	3. Stress imaging or echocardiographic procedures for patients who have no change in clinical status, a normal rest ECG, are not taking digoxin, are able to exercise, and did not require a stress imaging or echocardiographic procedure on their initial evaluation because of equivocal or intermediate-risk treadmill results	C
	4. Repeat coronary angiography in patients with no change in clinical status, no change on repeat exercise testing or stress imaging, and insignificant CAD on initial evaluation	

*See guidelines text for definitions of level of evidence.

angina if they have not had a change in clinical status (**Table 57G-16**). All the Class I indications for testing are for patients who have had a significant change in clinical status, except for the use of coronary angiography for patients with marked limitations of ordinary activity despite maximal medical therapy.

REFERENCES

1. Gibbons RJ, Abrams J, Chatterjee K, et al: ACC/AHA 2002 guideline update for the management of patients with chronic stable angina—summary article: A report of the American College of Cardiology/American Heart Association Task Force on practice guidelines (Committee on the Management of Patients With Chronic Stable Angina). J Am Coll Cardiol 41:159, 2003.
2. Greenland P, Bonow RO, Brundage BH, et al: ACCF/AHA 2007 clinical expert consensus document on coronary artery calcium scoring by computed tomography in global cardiovascular risk assessment and in evaluation of patients with chest pain: A report of the American College of Cardiology Foundation Clinical Expert Consensus Task Force (ACCF/AHA Writing Committee to Update the 2000 Expert Consensus Document on Electron Beam Computed Tomography). Circulation. 115:402, 2007.
3. Smith SC Jr, Allen J, Blair SN, et al: AHA/ACC guidelines for secondary prevention for patients with coronary and other atherosclerotic vascular disease: 2006 update: Endorsed by the National Heart, Lung, and Blood Institute. Circulation 113:2363, 2006.
4. Rosendorff C, Black HR, Cannon CP, et al: Treatment of hypertension in the prevention and management of ischemic heart disease: A scientific statement from the American Heart Association Council for High Blood Pressure Research and the Councils on Clinical Cardiology and Epidemiology and Prevention. Circulation 115:2761, 2007.

CHAPTER 58 Percutaneous Coronary Intervention

Jeffrey J. Popma and Deepak L. Bhatt

The use of percutaneous coronary intervention (PCI) to treat ischemic coronary artery disease (CAD) has expanded dramatically during the past three decades. In the absence of left main or complex multivessel CAD, PCI is the preferred method of revascularization in the United States for most patients with ischemic CAD. The estimated 1,000,000 PCI procedures performed annually in the United States now exceed the number of coronary artery bypass graft (CABG) procedures.[1] During the past several years, however, the growth of PCI slowed because of the effectiveness of risk factor modification, prevention of restenosis with drug-eluting stents (DES), and better understanding of patients who benefit from revascularization.[2,3] The number of PCIs is expected to grow modestly (1% to 5%) during the next decade because of the aging population and increased frequency of obesity and diabetes in the United States. Other key enablers of the expanded use of PCI in patients with complex CAD include improvements in equipment design (e.g., catheters with lower profile and enhanced deliverability), adjunctive pharmacologic strategies (e.g., adenosine diphosphate receptor antagonists, glycoprotein IIb/IIIa inhibitors, and direct thrombin inhibitors) to improve safety, and better hemodynamic support devices in ultrahigh-risk patients.[4] "Hybrid" procedures for the treatment of CAD and valvular heart disease have also been performed with collaboration of interventional cardiologists and cardiac surgeons.[5,6]

Coronary balloon angioplasty, or percutaneous transluminal coronary angioplasty, was first performed by Andreas Gruentzig in 1977 with use of a fixed-wire balloon catheter. The procedure was initially limited to the less than 10% of patients with symptomatic CAD who had a single, focal, noncalcified lesion of a proximal coronary vessel. As equipment design and operator experience evolved during the next decade, the use of PCI expanded to include an increasing spectrum of coronary anatomy, including multivessel CAD, total occlusions, diseased saphenous vein grafts (SVGs), and patients with acute ST-segment elevation myocardial infarction (STEMI; see Chap. 55), among other complexities. Two limitations prevented the widespread use of balloon angioplasty for CAD: abrupt closure of the treated vessel occurred in 5% to 8% of cases, requiring emergency CABG surgery in 3% to 5% of patients; and restenosis resulted in symptom recurrence in 30% of patients within the ensuing year.

New coronary devices were developed in the late 1980s to improve on the limitations associated with balloon angioplasty. Coronary stents scaffold the inner arterial wall to prevent early and late vascular remodeling. Rotational atherectomy ablates calcific atherosclerotic plaque and was developed as stand-alone therapy for undilatable coronary stenoses or used in combination with coronary stents after calcific plaque ablation. By early 2000, a number of other devices were developed to protect the distal circulation from atherothrombotic embolization (i.e., embolic protection devices). Aspiration and thrombectomy catheters were developed to remove medium and large thrombi from within the coronary artery, thereby preventing distal embolization. The term *percutaneous coronary intervention* now encompasses the broad array of the balloons, stents, and adjunct devices required to perform a safe and effective percutaneous revascularization in complex coronary artery lesions.

This chapter reviews the indications and clinical considerations for the selection of patients for PCI; discusses the current array of coronary devices, antithrombotic therapy, and vascular closure devices used for PCI; and details the short- and long-term outcomes of PCI and requirements for operator and institutional proficiency.

Indications for Percutaneous Coronary Intervention

The major value of percutaneous or surgical coronary revascularization is the relief of symptoms and signs of ischemic CAD (see Chap. 57 and PCI Guidelines). PCI reduces risk of mortality and subsequent myocardial infarction (MI) compared with medical therapy in patients with acute coronary syndromes. However, optimal medical therapy is as effective as PCI in reducing death and MI in patients with stable angina, although symptom relief[2] and ischemia improvement[7] are better with PCI. Improvement in ischemia burden >5% was achieved more often with PCI, and the magnitude of the residual ischemia has been correlated with less frequent death and MI.[7] Further studies comparing the use of coronary arteriography and PCI in patients with moderate degrees of myocardial ischemia are planned (e.g., ISCHEMIA Investigators). Irrespective of the indication for revascularization, it is recommended that PCI be coupled with optimal medical therapy after the procedure, such as hypertension and diabetes control, exercise, and smoking cessation (see Chap. 49). Lipid management is also an important component of optimal medical therapy. Compared with medical therapy alone, CABG prolongs life in certain anatomic subsets, such as in patients with left main disease, three-vessel CAD and reduced ventricular function, or left anterior descending artery disease with involvement of one or two additional vessels irrespective of left ventricular function.[8] The risks and benefits of coronary revascularization need careful review with the patient and family members, and the relative options of PCI, CABG, or optimal medical therapy should be discussed before performance of these procedures. A Task Force of the American College of Cardiology (ACC) and the American Heart Association (AHA) has published guidelines for the performance of PCI and CABG,[8-11] and a multispecialty writing committee has developed appropriateness guidelines for revascularization for a number of clinical and lesion-specific subsets[12] (see PCI Guidelines).

ASYMPTOMATIC PATIENTS OR THOSE WITH MILD ANGINA. Asymptomatic patients or those who have only mild symptoms are generally best treated with medical therapy unless one or more high-grade lesions subtend a moderate to large area of viable myocardium, the patient prefers to maintain an aggressive lifestyle or has a high-risk occupation, and the procedure can be performed with a high chance of success and low likelihood of complications (see PCI Guidelines).[10,12] Coronary revascularization should not be performed in patients with absent or mild symptoms if only a small area of myocardium is at risk, if no objective evidence of ischemia can be found, or if the likelihood of success is low or the chance of complications is high.[10,12]

PATIENTS WITH MODERATE TO SEVERE ANGINA (see Chap. 57). Patients with Canadian Cardiovascular Society (CCS) Class III angina, particularly those who are refractory to medical therapy, can benefit from coronary revascularization, provided the lesion subtends a moderate to large area of viable myocardium as determined by noninvasive testing (see PCI Guidelines).[13,14] Patients with recurrent symptoms while receiving medical therapy are candidates for revascularization even if they have a higher risk for an adverse outcome with revascularization. Patients with Class III symptoms should not undergo revascularization without noninvasive evidence of myocardial ischemia or a trial of medical therapy, particularly if only a small region of myocardium is at risk, the likelihood of success is low, or the chance of complications is high.[12]

PATIENTS WITH UNSTABLE ANGINA, NON–ST-SEGMENT ELEVATION MI, AND ST-SEGMENT ELEVATION MI (see Chaps. 55 and 56). Cardiac catheterization and coronary revascularization in moderate- to high-risk patients who present with unstable angina or non–ST-segment MI (NSTEMI) may improve mortality and reduce the rate of reinfarction.[15] In a meta-analysis of seven trials with 8375 patients observed for up to 2 years, the incidence of all-cause mortality was 4.9% in the early invasive group compared with 6.5% in the conservative group (risk ratio [RR] = 0.75; $P = 0.001$)[16] (**Fig. 58-1**). The 2-year incidence of nonfatal MI was 7.6% in the invasive group versus 9.1% in the conservative group (RR = 0.83; $P = 0.012$).[16] At a mean of 13 months of follow-up, there was a reduction in rehospitalization for unstable angina as well (RR = 0.69; $P < 0.0001$).[16] Current guidelines suggest that an early invasive strategy should be pursued in patients with recurrent ischemia despite therapy, elevated troponin levels, new ST depression, new or worsening symptoms of congestive heart failure, depressed left ventricular function, hemodynamic instability, sustained ventricular tachycardia, or recent PCI or CABG[15] (see PCI Guidelines).

A number of clinical scenarios associated with STEMI, including primary PCI, rescue PCI, facilitated PCI, and PCI after successful thrombolysis, have been published[17] (see PCI Guidelines). Timely PCI in patients with STEMI improves survival compared with medical therapy, provided the PCI is performed within 90 minutes of the patient's arrival to the medical facility, the PCI is performed by a physician who performs PCI on a routine basis, and the hospital has a sufficient PCI volume to support its proficiency. Patients with cardiogenic shock or severe congestive heart failure also benefit from primary PCI, irrespective of their age at presentation.

PATIENTS WITHOUT OPTIONS FOR REVASCULARIZATION. Patients who suffer from substantial angina yet are poor candidates for conventional revascularization have limited therapeutic options. These patients generally have a single, proximal vessel occlusion that subtends a large amount of myocardium or have undergone one or more prior CABG operations with stenoses or occlusions of the SVGs poorly suited for conventional repeated revascularization. "Limited options" patients represent approximately 4% to 12% of those undergoing coronary angiography; a larger percentage of patients (20% to 30%) have incomplete revascularization because of unsuitable coronary anatomy for surgical or percutaneous techniques.

Creation of new blood vessels in the ischemic tissue with use of laser injury, also known as therapeutic angiogenesis, may provide symptom relief in these patients. Both surgical and percutaneous approaches have been used to improve regional blood flow to the ischemic myocardium in these patients, although these strategies vary with respect to the depth of myocardial injury, the laser-tissue interactions, the presence or absence of guidance, and the number of channels created. Laser therapy has not yet proved efficacious in blinded clinical trials. Enhanced external counterpulsation support may provide improvement of angina in patients with refractory ischemia[18] (see Chap. 57), although the mechanism of benefit by this technique is not clear.[19]

Patient-Specific Considerations for Percutaneous Coronary Intervention

Assessment of the potential risks and benefits of PCI must address five fundamental patient-specific risk factors: extent of jeopardized myocardium, baseline lesion morphology, underlying cardiac function (including left ventricular function, rhythm stability, and coexisting valvular heart disease), presence of renal dysfunction, and pre-existing medical comorbidities that may render the patient at higher risk for PCI. Each of these factors contributes independently to the risk and benefit attributable to PCI. Proper planning for a PCI procedure requires careful attention to each of these factors.

EXTENT OF JEOPARDIZED MYOCARDIUM. The proportion of viable myocardium subtended by the treated coronary artery is the principal consideration in assessing the acute risk of the PCI procedure. PCI interrupts coronary blood flow for a period of seconds to minutes, and the ability of the patient to hemodynamically tolerate a sustained coronary occlusion depends on both the extent of "downstream" viable myocardium and the presence and grade of collaterals to the ischemic region. Although the risk for abrupt closure has been reduced substantially with the availability of coronary stents, when other procedural complications develop, such as a large side branch occlusion, distal embolization, perforation, or no-reflow, there may be rapid clinical deterioration that is proportionate to the extent of jeopardized myocardium. In the unlikely event that out-of-hospital stent thrombosis develops, the clinical sequelae of the episode relate to the extent of myocardium subtended by the occluded stent. Predictors for the occurrence of cardiovascular collapse with a failed PCI include the percentage of myocardium at risk,

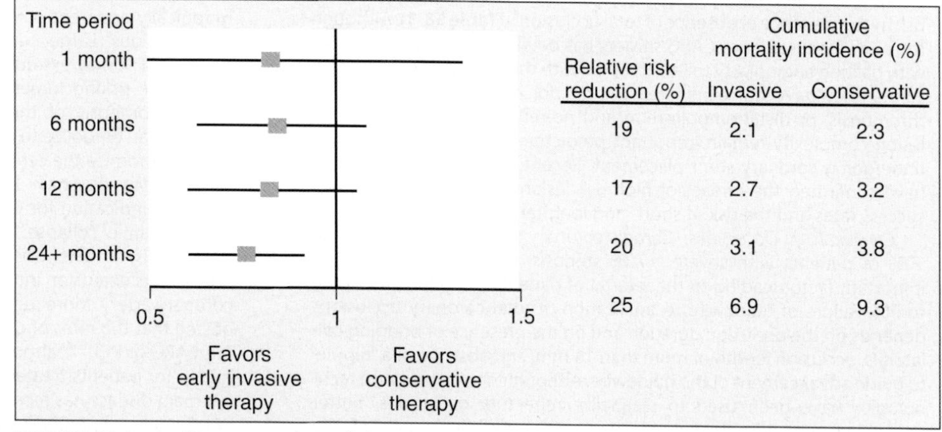

FIGURE 58-1 In this meta-analysis of the contemporary randomized clinical trials of patients with non–ST-segment elevation acute coronary syndromes, a significant reduction in mortality emerges with longer durations of follow-up with an initial invasive versus conservative approach. *(From Bavry AA, Kumbhani DJ, Rassi AN, et al: Benefit of early invasive therapy in acute coronary syndromes: A meta-analysis of contemporary randomized clinical trials. J Am Coll Cardiol 48:1319, 2006.)*

TABLE 58-1 SCAI Lesion Classification System for Risk Assessment

Type I Lesion (Highest Success Expected; Lowest Risk)
1. Does not meet criteria for C lesion
2. Patent
Type II Lesions
1. Meets any of these criteria for ACC/AHA C lesion
Diffuse (>2-cm length)
Excessive tortuosity of proximal segment
Extremely angulated segments greater than 90 degrees
Inability to protect major side branches
Degenerated vein grafts with friable lesions
2. Patent
Type III Lesions
1. Does not meet criteria for C Lesion
2. Occluded
Type IV Lesions (Lowest Success Expected; Highest Risk)
1. Meets any of these criteria for ACC/AHA C lesion
Diffuse (>2-cm length)
Excessive tortuosity of proximal segment
Extremely angulated segments greater than 90 degrees
Inability to protect major side branches
Degenerated vein grafts with friable lesions
2. Occluded

Modified from Krone RJ, Shaw RE, Klein LW, et al: Evaluation of the American College of Cardiology/American Heart Association and the Society for Coronary Angiography and Interventions lesion classification system in the current "stent era" of coronary interventions (from the ACC–National Cardiovascular Data Registry). Am J Cardiol 92:389, 2003.

the severity of the baseline stenosis, multivessel CAD, and the presence of diffuse disease.

Whether complete revascularization in patients with multivessel CAD should be performed in a single or staged setting remains controversial. In patients presenting with STEMI, revascularization of only the culprit infarct-related artery is generally recommended,[12] unless there is ongoing cardiogenic shock because of jeopardized myocardium in other regions. In other nonacute situations, the number of vessels treated in a single setting will depend on whether procedural complications have occurred, the length of time required for additional vessel treatment, the underlying renal function, and the general ability of the patient to tolerate long procedures. Staged procedures can be safely performed up to 4 to 8 weeks after the initial procedure. In the setting of NSTEMI, observational data suggest that multivessel versus culprit-only stenting reduces subsequent need for revascularization but does not affect death or MI rates.[20]

Baseline Lesion Morphology. Several angiographic findings increase the technical complexity of PCI and elevate the risk for acute and long-term complications. The initial ACC/AHA lesion classification system has been recently refined by the Society for Cardiovascular Angiography and Interventions (SCAI) risk system, which further characterizes risk by the presence or absence of total occlusion[21] (**Table 58-1**). Although the need for emergency CABG surgery has been reduced from 3% to 8% with balloon angioplasty to less than 1% with the availability of coronary stents, they have not eliminated the risk for periprocedural MI, stent thrombosis, or distal embolization and no-reflow. Vessel patency and lesion complexity remain important predictors of outcome in patients undergoing coronary stent placement. Recent reviews of registry data have confirmed the impact of high-risk lesion features on procedural success rates and the risk of short- and long-term complications.

Chronic Total Occlusions. Chronic coronary occlusions are present in 50% of patients with severe (>70% stenosis) CAD and are the most important factor leading to the referral of patients to CABG rather than to PCI. Failure of guidewire recanalization of total coronary occlusions depends on the occlusion duration and on the presence of bridging collaterals, occlusion length of more than 15 mm, and absence of a "nipple" to guide advancement of the guidewire. Although newer guidance technologies have been used to recanalize refractory occlusions, better guidewires and wire techniques have accounted for much of the improvement in crossing success during recent years.[22] Once the chronic total occlusion has been crossed, DES may be used to reduce late clinical recurrence.[23]

Saphenous Vein Grafts. SVG interventions represent approximately 8% of PCI procedures and pose an increased risk of postprocedural MI caused by atheroembolization that occurs during PCI. When no-reflow occurs, administration of arterial vasodilators (e.g., nitroprusside, verapamil, or adenosine) into the SVG may improve the flow into the distal native circulation, but there is still a substantially increased risk for death and MI. More extensive SVG degeneration and bulkier lesions (larger estimated plaque volume) are associated with higher complication rates than SVGs that have less extensive disease. In the setting of "high-risk" SVG anatomy, alternative approaches using the native coronary artery should be pursued whenever possible. Lower rates of restenosis in SVG lesions are found after coronary stent placement than after balloon angioplasty. Although DES may provide even lower angiographic restenosis rates, the current DES are poorly suited to SVGs larger than 4.5 mm in diameter, and bare metal stents (BMS) are preferred in this setting. Embolic protection devices are recommended in patients treated for SVG stenoses to lessen the risk of distal embolization of atherothrombotic debris.

Bifurcation Lesions. Optimal management of lesions involving both branches of a coronary bifurcation remains controversial. "Snowplowing" of plaque into the adjacent parent vessel or side branch is a major limitation of conventional balloon angioplasty. Atheroablative devices, such as rotational atherectomy, have only partially reduced this risk. Risk stratification for bifurcation PCI includes assessment of the extent of atherosclerotic disease in both vessels, estimation of the relative vessel size and distribution in the parent vessel and side branch, and determination of the orientation of the vessels to one another. Side branch compromise may also occur in up to 30% of bifurcation lesions without apparent branch vessel disease.

Stent placement in one vessel rather than in both the parent vessel and side branch is generally preferred.[24] In a meta-analysis of six randomized trials including 1642 patients with coronary bifurcation lesions who were randomly selected to undergo PCI by either double or single stenting, there was increased risk of MI with double stenting (RR, 1.78; P = 0.001).[24]

When there is extensive disease in both vessels, a number of strategies have been used, including simultaneous kissing stents and "crush," culotte, T stenting, and TAP (T and small protrusion) techniques (**Fig. 58-2**). Irrespective of the bifurcation stenting strategy used, a final "kissing" balloon inflation in the parent vessel and side branch should generally be performed. DES appear to reduce restenosis compared with BMS, but when recurrence develops in patients treated with a DES, it generally occurs at the origin of the side branch. New dedicated bifurcation stents and side branch access main vessel stents are in development.

Lesion Calcification. The presence of extensive coronary calcification poses unique challenges for PCI because calcium in the vessel wall leads to irregular and inflexible lumens and makes the delivery of guidewires, balloons, and stents much more challenging. Extensive coronary calcification also renders the vessel wall rigid, necessitating higher balloon inflation pressures to obtain complete stent expansion and, on occasion, leading to "undilatable" lesions that resist any achievable balloon expansion pressure. Rotational atherectomy effectively ablates vessel wall calcification and facilitates stent delivery and complete stent expansion (**Fig. 58-3**).

Thrombus. Conventional angiography has poor sensitivity for the detection of coronary thrombus, but the presence of a large, angiographically apparent coronary thrombus heightens risk for procedural complications. Large coronary thrombi may fragment and embolize during PCI or may extrude through gaps between stent struts placed in the vessel, risking lumen compromise or thrombus propagation and acute thrombosis of the treated vessel. In addition, large coronary thrombi can embolize to other coronary branches or vessels or dislodge and compromise the cerebral or other vascular beds (**Fig. 58-4**).

Left Main Coronary Artery Disease. Left main CAD has been an accepted indication for CABG surgery on the basis of the potential for hemodynamic collapse in the setting of acute complications, stent thrombosis, or restenosis involving the body of the left main coronary artery or its extension into the left anterior descending or left circumflex coronary artery. More recent registry and randomized studies have suggested that the rates of death and MI are similar with patients undergoing CABG or PCI,[25,26] although the need for repeated revascularization is higher for patients treated with PCI[3,27-37] (**Table 58-2**). The use of PCI for left main disease has recently been elevated to a Class IIb indication (see PCI Guidelines) pending additional planned randomized study.

Underlying Cardiac Function. Left ventricular function is an important predictor of outcome during PCI. For each 10% decrement in resting left ventricular ejection fraction, the risk of in-hospital mortality after PCI increases by approximately twofold. Associated valvular disease or ventricular arrhythmia further increases the risk for PCI in the

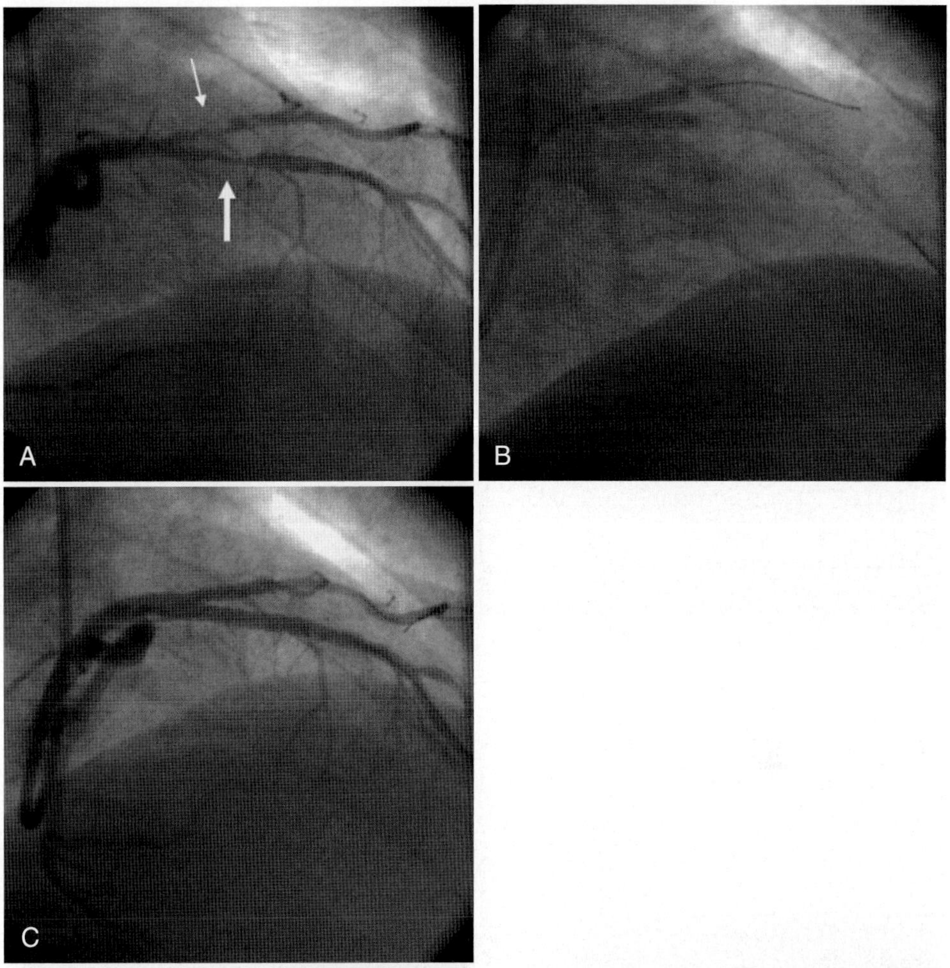

FIGURE 58-2 Bifurcation lesion treated with simultaneous kissing stents. **A,** A complex bifurcation lesion involves both the left anterior descending artery (large arrow) and its diagonal branch (small arrow). **B,** After predilation with balloons in both branches, simultaneous inflation of two 3.0 ×18-mm CYPHER stents (Cordis Corp., Bridgewater, NJ) in the left anterior descending and diagonal branches is performed. **C,** Following postdilation of both branches with simultaneous inflations to expand the stents, an excellent angiographic result is obtained.

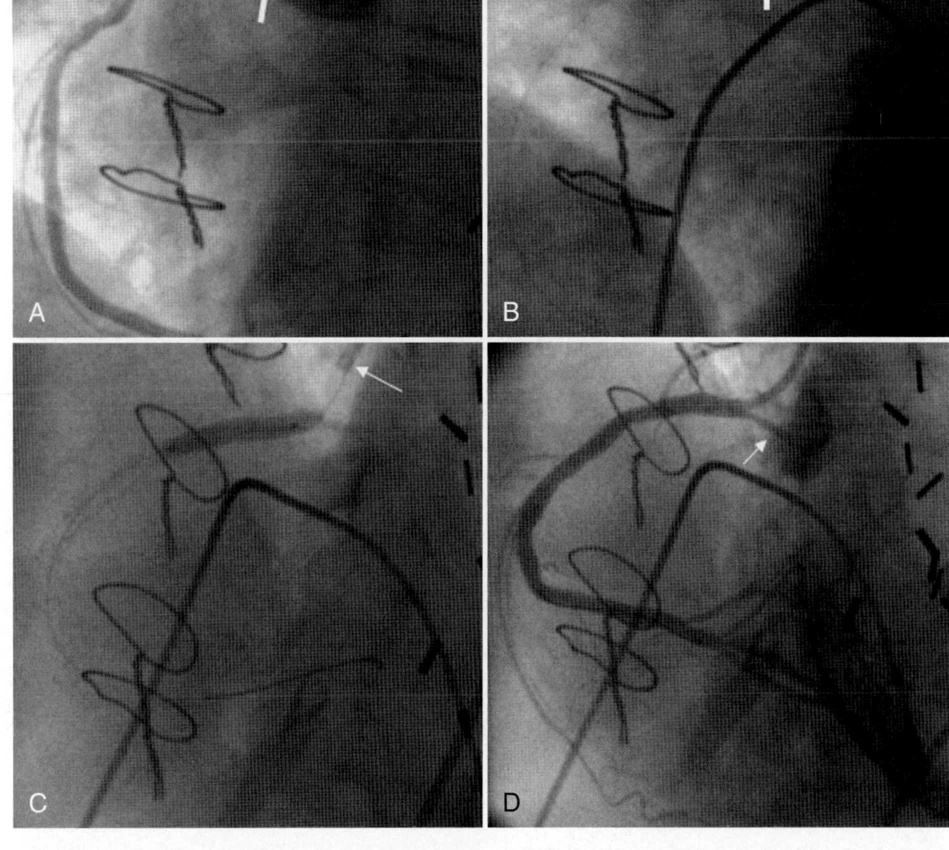

FIGURE 58-3 Rotational atherectomy of an ostial right coronary artery stenosis. **A,** A heavily calcified stenosis of the ostium of the right coronary artery (arrow) precludes conventional balloon angioplasty and stent placement. **B,** A 1.25-mm rotational atherectomy burr (arrow) was advanced to ablate the calcium in the ostium. An additional 1.50-mm rotational atherectomy burr was used to further ablate the calcific plaque. **C,** After predilation with a 2.5-mm balloon, a 3.50 × 23-mm CYPHER stent was advanced and inflated to 16 atm. Note that the guiding catheter is withdrawn (arrow) to allow stent placement just at the origin of the right coronary artery. **D,** An excellent final angiographic result is obtained with no residual stenosis. Note the free reflux of contrast agent from the right coronary artery ostium after stent placement (arrow).

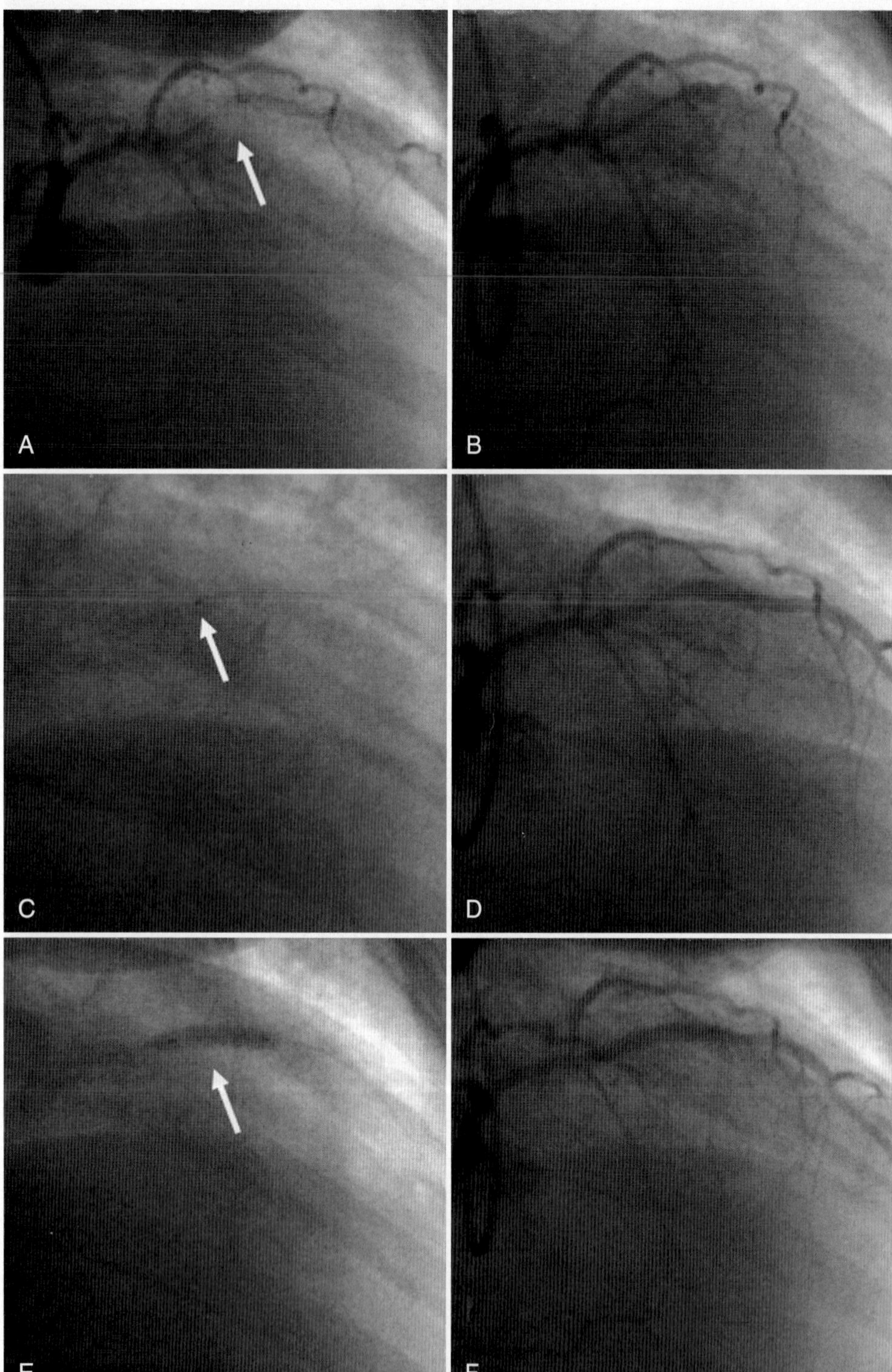

FIGURE 58-4 Aspiration thrombectomy for STEMI. A thrombotic occlusion of the proximal left anterior descending artery is shown (**A,** arrow). There is minimal improvement in flow after a 2.5-mm balloon inflation, with the suspicion of thrombus precluding flow **(B).** An Export catheter is used to remove the thrombus **(C),** and anterograde flow is reestablished and the thrombus is removed **(D).** A 3.0-mm drug-eluting stent was placed **(E),** resulting in no residual stenosis and TIMI 3 flow into the distal vessel **(F).**

setting of left ventricular dysfunction. Intra-aortic balloon pump support may be useful when there is severe compromise of left ventricular function (i.e., ejection fraction less than 35%) or when the PCI target lesion supplies a substantial portion of viable myocardium. Routine use of an intra-aortic balloon pump has limited benefit in patients with STEMI,[38] although it is recommended in patients with cardiogenic shock. Other percutaneous cardiopulmonary support devices that do not effectively reduce left ventricular pressures have been replaced by percutaneous left ventricular assist devices that are positioned in the left atrium (e.g., TandemHeart, CardiacAssist Inc., Pittsburgh, Pa)[39,40] or directly in the left ventricle (Impella LP 2.5, Abiomed Inc., Danvers, Mass)[4,41,42] (**Fig. 58-5**). These devices permit ultrahigh-risk PCI without the risk of hemodynamic collapse during the procedure, although further data are needed to see if they are superior to intra-aortic balloon pumps.

Renal Insufficiency. The morbidity and mortality associated with PCI relate directly to the extent of baseline renal disease (see also Chap. 93). Patients with evidence of mild renal dysfunction have a 20% higher risk of death at 1 year after PCI than do patients with preserved renal function.[43] Renal dysfunction after the administration of contrast material during angiography may relate to contrast-induced nephropathy cholesterol embolization syndrome (see Chaps. 61 and 93), or both. The risk of contrast-induced nephropathy is dependent on the dose of the contrast agents used, hydration status at the time of the procedure, pre-existing renal function of the patient, age, hemodynamic stability, anemia, and diabetes. The risk for cholesterol embolization syndrome relates to catheter manipulation in an ascending or descending atherosclerotic aorta that releases cholesterol crystals. Although the risk of hemodialysis is less than 3% in cases of uncomplicated contrast-induced nephropathy, the in-hospital mortality in the setting of hemodialysis exceeds 30%. Mild renal dysfunction after PCI is associated with an increased risk of death up to fourfold at 1 year after PCI compared with patients with preserved renal function.

Associated Medical Comorbidities. A number of pre-existing medical conditions may increase short- or long-term risks of PCI and should be considered in evaluation of the risks, benefits, and strategic approach for patients undergoing PCI. Patients with diabetes have higher recurrence rates with BMS and with DES, and a long-term survival benefit was shown in diabetic patients undergoing CABG compared with multivessel balloon angioplasty in an older era (see Chap. 64). Contemporary series have shown no early difference in mortality but a substantial increase in the need for early repeated revascularization.[3] Whether there is a long-term surgical survival benefit with CABG compared with multivessel DES placement is the subject of ongoing studies.

A bleeding diathesis or need for chronic warfarin therapy may preclude the patient from tolerating long-term combination aspirin and clopidogrel therapy after DES placement, thereby placing the patient at higher risk for stent thrombosis. The need for discontinuation of dual antiplatelet therapy before impending noncardiac surgery soon after stent implantation may also predispose to stent thrombosis. In each of these circumstances, BMS placement may be the preferred approach, particularly if the surgery can be deferred for approximately 6 weeks after stent placement.

TABLE 58-2 Comparative Trials Between Drug-Eluting Stents and Coronary Bypass Surgery in Unprotected Left Main Coronary Revascularization

TRIAL	N	STUDY DURATION	DEATH	MYOCARDIAL INFARCTION	REPEATED REVASCULARIZATION	STROKE	MACCE	COMMENTS
Chieffo[29]	107 PCI 142 CABG	12 months	PCI 2.8% CABG 6.4%	PCI 0.9% CABG 1.4%	PCI 15.8% CABG 3.6%	PCI 0.9% CABG 0.7%	N/A	Significantly lower adjusted death, myocardial infarction, and stroke with PCI versus CABG Significantly lower repeated revascularization with CABG
Lee[28]	50 PCI 123 CABG	12 months	PCI 4.0% CABG 15.0%	N/A	PCI 13.0% CABG 5.0%	N/A	PCI 17.0% CABG 25.0%	Parsonnet score, diabetes, and CABG independent predictors of MACCE
Palmerini[27]	157 PCI 154 CABG	430 days	PCI 13.4% CABG 12.3%	PCI 8.3% CABG 4.5%	PCI 25.5% CABG 2.6%	N/A	N/A	60% of PCI cohort treated with DES Only 68% determined appropriate for either PCI or CABG
Palmerini[30]	98 PCI 161 CABG	2 years	PCI 18.0% CABG 17.0%	PCI 4.0% CABG 6.0%	PCI 25.0% CABG 3.0%	PCI 28.8% CABG 9.4%	N/A	Study limited to patients ≥75 years
Sanmartin[31]	96 PCI 245 DES	12 months	PCI 5.2% CABG 8.4%	PCI 0% CABG 1.3%	PCI 5.2% CABG 0.8%	PCI 0% CABG 0.8%	PCI 10.4% CABG 11.4%	Significantly higher 30-day MACCE with CABG (2.1% versus 9.0%; $P = 0.03$)
Brener[32]	97 PCI 190 CABG	3 years	PCI 20.0% CABG 15.0%	N/A	N/A	N/A	N/A	57% of PCI cohort treated with DES Higher EuroSCORE and diabetes independent predictors of 3-year mortality
Buszman[33]	Randomized 52 PCI 53 CABG	12 months	PCI 1.9% CABG 7.5%	PCI 1.9% CABG 5.7%	PCI 0% CABG 3.8%	PCI 28.8% CABG 9.4%	PCI 30.8% CABG 24.5%	PCI associated with significant increase in left ventricular ejection fraction at 12 months compared with CABG Trend toward lower mortality with PCI at 28-month follow-up (3 versus 7 events; $P = 0.08$)
Hsu[34]	20 PCI 39 CABG	12 months	PCI 5.0% CABG 20.5%	PCI 0% CABG 0%	PCI 0% CABG 10.3%	PCI 0% CABG 2.6%	PCI 5.0% CABG 33.3%	50% of PCI cohort treated with DES
Rodes-Cabau[35]	104 PCI 145 CABG	23 ± 16 months	PCI 16.3% CABG 12.4%*	PCI 23.1% CABG 19.3%	PCI 9.6% CABG 4.8%	PCI 8.7% CABG 6.2%	PCI 43.3% CABG 35.2%	Study limited to patients ≥80 years; 48% DES in PCI cohort EuroSCORE independent predictor of MACCE regardless of revascularization strategy
Seung[36]	542 PCI 542 CABG	3 years	PCI 7.9% CABG 7.8%	N/A	PCI 12.6% CABG 2.6%	N/A	PCI 9.3% CABG 9.2%†	Propensity matched analysis of 396 PCI and CABG patient pairs demonstrates no significant difference in death, myocardial infarction, or stroke but significantly higher repeated revascularization with DES
Wu[37]	135 PCI 135 CABG	2 years	PCI 18.0% CABG 5.9%	N/A	PCI 27.4% CABG 5.9%	N/A	N/A	Matched analysis of DES and CABG patients (N = 56 pairs) showed no survival difference and higher repeated revascularization with DES
Serruys[3]	357 PCI 348 CABG	12 months	PCI 4.2% CABG 4.4%	PCI 4.3% CABG 4.1%	PCI 11.8% CABG 6.5%	PCI 0.3% CABG 2.7%	PCI 15.8% CABG 13.7%	No significant differences overall in MACCE or death, myocardial infarction, or stroke PCI associated with significantly higher MACCE in highest SYNTAX tercile

*Cardiovascular death.
†Composite endpoint of death, Q-wave myocardial infarction, or stroke.
MACCE = major adverse cardiac and cerebrovascular events.
Modified from Kandzari DE, Colombo A, Park SJ, et al: Revascularization for unprotected left main disease: Evolution of the evidence basis to redefine treatment standards. J Am Coll Cardiol 54:1576, 2009.

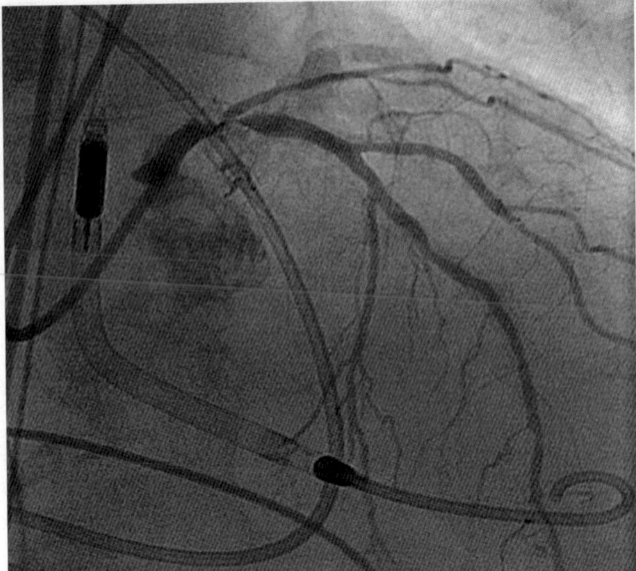

FIGURE 58-5 Impella device position in the left ventricle before left main intervention in a sole remaining artery.

Vascular Access

The most frequently used vascular access sites for PCI include the common femoral artery, the brachial artery, and more recently the radial artery (see Chaps. 20 and 21). The femoral approach (either right or left sided) is the most commonly used vascular access site in the United States and provides the advantages of large vessel size (typically 6 to 8 mm in diameter) and the ability to accommodate larger (>6 French) sheath sizes including intra-aortic balloon pump catheters. In addition, because of the typically straight path from the femoral artery to the ascending aorta, the femoral approach provides excellent guide catheter support and manipulability and access to the venous system through the adjacent femoral vein. Severe peripheral arterial disease, peripheral vascular bypass grafts, and requirement for immobilization after the procedure limit the use of the femoral approach in some patients.

The brachial arterial approach was historically used as the principal alternative to femoral access. However, because the brachial artery provides the only circulation to the forearm and hand (i.e., it is a functional end-artery), any compromise of the brachial artery can lead to severe ischemic complications of the hand.

The radial arterial approach (see Chaps. 20 and 21) has gained in popularity as an alternative to femoral access in patients with significant peripheral vascular disease and particularly in obese patients, in whom direct compression of the radial artery reduces bleeding complications[44,45] (**Table 58-3**). The radial approach provides direct access to the ascending aorta and the unique advantage of allowing immediate mobilization after PCI. An Allen test is useful to assess flow to the hand before radial artery cannulation. Tortuosity of the brachiocephalic trunk may limit the use of the approach in some patients (2% to 3%). The small size of the radial artery limits the size of guiding catheters used during PCI (typically 5F or 6F for women and 7F for men). Transradial access is associated with a generally lower rate (2%) of vascular complications.[46] A meta-analysis has suggested that radial access reduced major bleeding compared with femoral access[47] (**Table 58-4**). A randomized study of 1024 patients undergoing coronary arteriography and PCI found a reduction in major vascular complications (0.58% versus 3.7% in patients accessed by the femoral artery; $P = 0.0008$), albeit at the expense of longer procedure duration and higher radiation exposure.[48] Predictors of failure with the transradial access include age >75 years, prior CABG surgery, and short stature.[49]

TABLE 58-3 Comparison of Radial and Femoral Artery Access

	FEMORAL	RADIAL
Access site bleeding	3%-4%	0%-0.6%
Artery complications	Pseudoaneurysm, retroperitoneal hemorrhage, arteriovenous fistula, painful hematoma	Rare local irritation, pulse loss 3%-9%, forearm hematoma
Patient comfort	Acceptable	Favored
Ambulation	2-4 hours	Immediate
Extra costs	Closure device	Band
Procedure time	Perceived shorter	Perceived longer
Estimated radiation exposure	Perceived shorter	Perceived longer
Access to left internal mammary artery	Easy	Difficult from right radial
Use of artery for CABG	Not applicable	Unknown
Learning curve	Short	Longer
>8F catheter	Acceptable	Maximum 7F (in men)
Peripheral vascular disease, obese	Problematic	Acceptable

Modified from Kern MJ: Cardiac catheterization on the road less traveled. J Am Coll Cardiol Intv 2:1055, 2009.

TABLE 58-4 Outcomes in Radial Versus Femoral Access in Meta-Analysis

	FEMORAL N/TOTAL (%)	RADIAL N/TOTAL (%)	ODDS RATIO (95% CI)	P VALUE
Major bleeding	48/2068 (2.3)	13/2390 (0.05)	0.27 (0.16, 0.45)	<0.001
Death, MI, or stroke	71/1874 (3.8)	56/2209 (2.5)	0.71 (0.49, 1.01)	0.058
Death	28/1874 (1.8)	22/1906 (1.2)	0.74 (0.42, 1.30)	0.29
Myocardial infarction	46/1595 (2.9)	39/1931 (2.0)	0.76 (0.49, 1.17)	0.21
Stroke	5/1107 (0.5)	2/1428 (0.1)	0.39 (0.09, 1.75)	0.22
Access site crossover	34/1107 (1.4)	150/2542 (5.9)	3.82 (2.83, 5.15)	<0.001
Inability to cross the lesion with a wire, balloon, or stent during PCI	40/1186 (3.4)	60/1274 (4.7)	1.31 (0.87, 1.96)	0.20

Modified from Jolly SS, Amlani S, Hamon M, et al: Radial versus femoral access for coronary angiography or intervention and the impact on major bleeding and ischemic events: A systematic review and meta-analysis of randomized trials. Am Heart J 157:132, 2009.

Vascular Access Complications

Vascular access site complications occur after 3% to 7% of PCIs and lead to significantly increased length of hospital stay, total costs, and morbidity and mortality.[50] Complications range from relatively minor access site hematomas to life-threatening retroperitoneal bleeds requiring emergent blood transfusion to damage to the vasculature requiring prompt surgical intervention.[51] Factors predisposing patients to an increased risk of serious vascular complications after PCI include age, female gender, larger vascular sheath size, low body mass index, renal insufficiency, and degree of anticoagulation during the procedure. The location of the entry point for transfemoral access predicts the risk and type of vascular complication (see Chap. 20). If the access site is above the level of the inguinal ligament, the risk of retroperitoneal hemorrhage is substantially increased.[51] If the access site is distal to the femoral bifurcation, pseudoaneurysms (0.4%) and arteriovenous fistulas (0.2%) may occur. Major vascular complications of the femoral approach include limb-threatening ischemia (0.1%) and retroperitoneal hemorrhage (0.4%), which are associated with increased risk of death by 2- to 10-fold in the first 30 days after the PCI procedure.[52]

Vascular Closure Devices

Vascular access closure devices were introduced in the mid-1990s as a new way of managing the access site after femoral access procedures. Vascular closure devices reduce the time to ambulation, increase the patient's comfort after PCI, and provide efficiencies of patient flow in the catheterization laboratory.[53-59]

Currently approved vascular closure devices fall into three categories. Sealant devices include collagen- and thrombin-based systems that leave no mechanical anchor inside or outside the vessel. Mechanical closure devices include suture-mediated and nitinol clip–based systems and provide immediate secure closure to the vessel. Hybrid closure devices, such as the dissolvable AngioSeal device (St. Jude Medical, Minneapolis, Minn), use a combination of collagen sealant with an internal mechanical closure to cause rapid hemostasis.[60] Although each device has proved relatively safe and effective, few comparative data permit evaluation of the relative risks and benefits of each device. Two recent meta-analyses concluded that vascular closure devices do not lower the risk of vascular complications compared with manual hemostasis (**Table 58-5**), but infections may occur more often with suture-based closure devices, and occlusions are found more often with hybrid devices.[61,62]

Coronary Devices

During the past three decades, steady improvements in the equipment used for coronary revascularization (e.g., reductions in device profile and improvements in catheter flexibility) have been supplemented with the introduction of periodic "transformational technology," such as coronary stents and more recently DES, which have extended the scope and breadth of clinical practice. The type of lesions amenable to PCI has become progressively more complex during this period, and the outcomes associated with the use of these devices have progressively improved. A brief overview of the currently available coronary devices follows.

Balloon Angioplasty

Balloon angioplasty expands the coronary lumen by stretching and tearing the atherosclerotic plaque and vessel wall and, to a lesser extent, by redistributing atherosclerotic plaque along its longitudinal axis. Elastic recoil of the stretched vessel wall generally leaves a 30% to 35% residual diameter stenosis, and the vessel expansion can result in propagating coronary dissections, leading to abrupt vessel closure in 5% to 8% of patients. Although stand-alone balloon angioplasty is rarely used other than for very small (<2.25 mm) vessels, balloon angioplasty remains integral to PCI for predilation of lesions before stent placement, deployment of coronary stents, and further expansion of stents after deployment.

Most of the enhancements in balloon technology relate to the development of low-profile (deflated diameter = 0.7 mm) balloons that are more trackable through tortuous anatomy and noncompliant balloons that can inflate to pressures in excess of 20 atm without overexpansion or rupture. A modification of balloon angioplasty includes a focused-force dilation in which a scoring blade or guidewire external to the balloon concentrates dilating force and resists balloon slippage during inflation. The Cutting Balloon (Boston Scientific, Natick, Mass) and the AngioScore catheter (AngioScore, Inc., Fremont, Calif) are focused-force balloon angioplasty systems that are currently used in a small minority (less than 5%) of PCIs.

Coronary Atherectomy

Atherectomy refers to removal (rather than simple displacement) of the obstructing atherosclerotic plaque. By removal of plaque or improving lesion wall compliance in calcified or fibrotic lesions, atherectomy can provide a larger final minimal lumen diameter than that achieved by balloon angioplasty alone. Atherectomy was performed

TABLE 58-5 Complications Associated with Vascular Closure Devices

AUTHOR	STUDY TYPE	N	ENDPOINT	VASCULAR CLOSURE DEVICE	MANUAL COMPRESSION	*P* VALUE
Cura[a]	Registry	2918	Vascular complications	$2.9\%^{AS}$ $3.2\%^{Per}$	3.1%	NS
Dangas[b]	Registry	5093	Surgical repair	2.5%	1.5%	0.03
Resnic[c]	Registry	3027	Vascular complications	3.0%	5.5%	0.002
Dangas[d]	Pooled RCT	2095	Device complications	8.5%	5.9%	0.02
Tavris[53]	ACC Registry	166,680	Vascular complications	1.05-1.48%	1.7%	<0.001
Exaire[54]	TARGET	4736	Transfusions	1.0%	0.8%	NS
Koreny[55]	Meta-analysis	4000	Hematoma	RR = 1.14		NS
Vaitkus[56]	Meta-analysis	5045	Vascular complications	RR = 0.89		<0.05
Nikolsky[57]	Meta-analysis	37,066	Vascular complications	Benefit^{AS}		0.06
Applegate[58]	Registry	4699	Vascular complications	$1.5\%^{AS}$	1.7%	NS
Arora[58a]	Registry	12,937	Vascular complications	↓ 42%-58%		<0.05

[a]Cura FA, Kapadia SR, L'Allier PL, et al: Safety of femoral closure devices after percutaneous coronary interventions in the era of glycoprotein IIb/IIIa platelet blockade. Am J Cardiol 86:780, 2000.
[b]Dangas G, Mehran R, Kokolis S, et al: Vascular complications after percutaneous coronary interventions following hemostasis with manual compression versus arteriotomy closure devices. J Am Coll Cardiol 38:638, 2001.
[c]Resnic FS, Blake GJ, Ohno-Machado L, et al: Vascular closure devices and the risk of vascular complications after percutaneous coronary intervention in patients receiving glycoprotein IIb-IIIa inhibitors. Am J Cardiol 88:493, 2001.
[d]Dangas G, Mehran R, Fahy M, et al: Complications of vascular closure devices—not yet evidence based [reply]. J Am Coll Cardiol 39:1706, 2002.
ACC = American College of Cardiology; AS = Angioseal; NS = not significant; PER = Perclose; RCT = randomized controlled trials; RR = relative risk ratio.
Modified from Dauerman HL, Applegate RJ, Cohen DJ: Vascular closure devices: The second decade. J Am Coll Cardiol 50:1617, 2007.

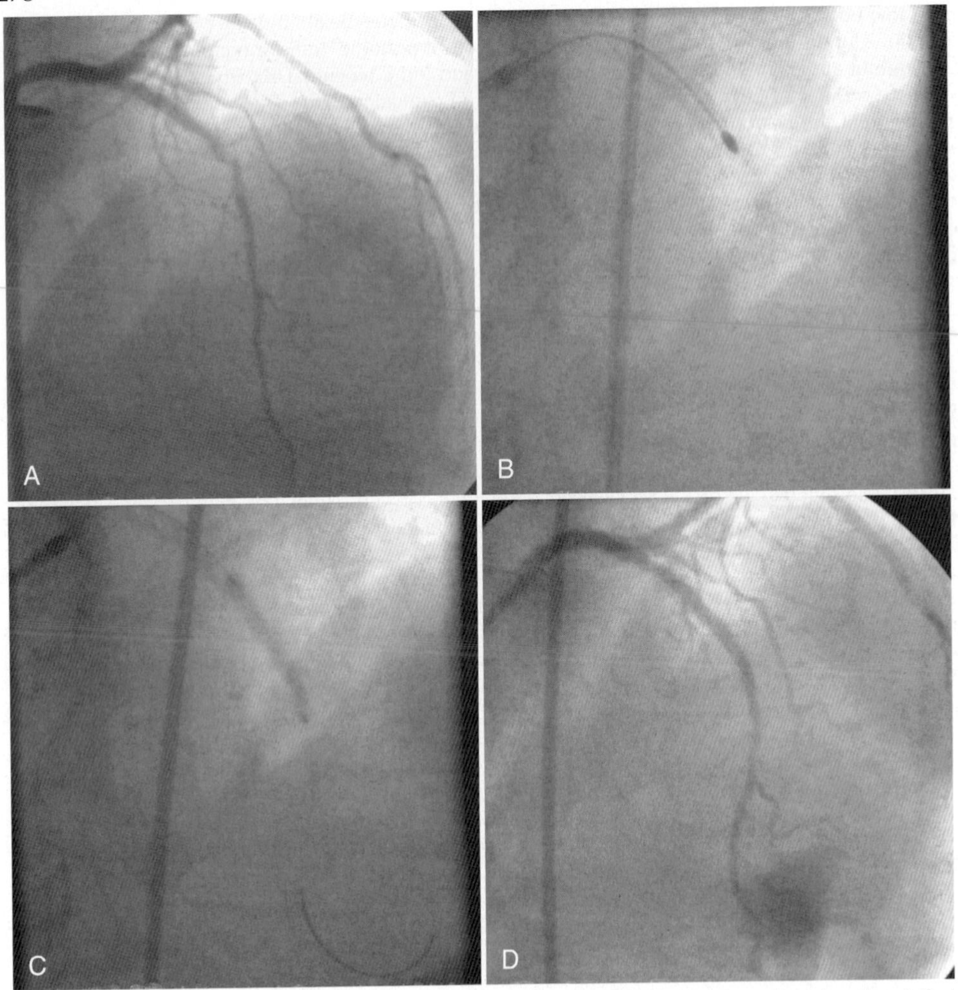

1.5- or 1.75-mm burr to improve lesion compliance (plaque modification) before the lesion is treated definitively by balloon dilation and stent placement. Rotational coronary atherectomy is currently used in less than 5% of PCI procedures (**Fig. 58-6**).

Thrombectomy and Aspiration Devices

The AngioJet rheolytic thrombectomy catheter (Possis Medical, Inc., Minneapolis, Minn) was introduced as a dedicated device for thrombus removal through the dissolution and aspiration of the thrombus. High-speed saline jets within the tip of the catheter create intense local suction by the Venturi effect, pulling surrounding blood, thrombus, and saline into the lumen of the catheter opening, propelling the debris proximally through the catheter lumen. Rheolytic thrombectomy was superior to a prolonged intraluminal urokinase infusion in patients with a large thrombus, but its routine use in patients with STEMI was not associated with improvement in infarct size by single-photon emission computed tomography (SPECT) imaging and may have caused more complications.[63] Rheolytic thrombectomy may still be useful in clinical practice when there is a large angiographic thrombus in a native vessel or SVG.

Newer lower profile aspiration catheters that use 6F and 7F guiding catheters have been developed as alternatives to rheolytic thrombectomy in patients with thrombus-containing lesions. These techniques may be slightly less effective (particularly against partially organized thrombus) than rheolytic thrombectomy, although the risk of distal particulate embolization and device trauma in smaller vessels may be less with these aspiration catheters. In a multicenter study of 1071 patients with STEMI who were randomly assigned to the thrombus-aspiration group or the conventional-PCI group, a myocardial blush grade of 0 or 1 occurred in 17.1% of the patients in the thrombus-aspiration group and in 26.3% of those in the conventional-PCI group ($P < 0.001$).[64] At 30 days, the rate of death in patients with a myocardial blush grade of 0 or 1, 2, and 3 was 5.2%, 2.9%, and 1.0%, respectively ($P = 0.003$), and the rate of adverse events was 14.1%, 8.8%, and 4.2%, respectively ($P < 0.001$).[64] Meta-analysis of the data suggests that simple manual thrombus aspiration before PCI reduces mortality in patients undergoing primary PCI (**Table 58-6** and **Fig. 58-7**)[65] (see PCI Guidelines).

Embolic Protection Devices

The advent of embolic protection systems has reduced the risk of postprocedural adverse events after SVG PCI. Although embolization of atherosclerotic debris was not considered a major complication during the early years of native coronary balloon angioplasty, it is now recognized as one potential cause of distal myocardial necrosis after PCI,[66] particularly in friable SVG lesions. Distal embolization causes postprocedural cardiac enzyme elevation in nearly 20% of cases after SVG PCI, and this enzyme elevation is associated with substantial morbidity and mortality. Numerous additional occlusive and filter-based distal protection systems as well as novel proximal occlusion devices have undergone evaluation and approval for use in SVG interventions. Despite their potential benefit in preventing thromboembolization in patients with STEMI, none of the embolic protection devices has reduced MI size with primary intervention, possibly relating to the high profile of the devices. Embolic protection devices fall into three broad categories: distal occlusion devices, distal embolic filters, and proximal occlusion devices.

A B C D

FIGURE 58-6 Rotational atherectomy of an undilatable left anterior descending artery. **A,** A heavily calcified diffuse lesion in the left anterior descending artery is generally considered undilatable by conventional balloon techniques. **B,** A 1.5-mm rotational atherectomy burr revolving at 160,000 rpm is advanced to ablate the calcified lesion. **C,** A 3.0 × 28-mm stent can then be advanced across the blockage and inflated to 16 atm. It is unlikely that full stent expansion could have occurred without pretreatment with rotational atherectomy. **D,** The final angiographic result shows no residual stenosis and normal flow into the distal vessel.

in 30% of interventional procedures between 1992 and 1994, but its use fell dramatically with the availability of coronary stents. Less than 5% of current procedures involve the use of atherectomy devices, most often rotational atherectomy in combination with coronary stents.

The most commonly used atherectomy device is rotational coronary atherectomy (Boston Scientific), which removes the atheromatous plaque by the abrasion of inelastic calcified plaque using microscopic (20 to 50 μm) diamond chips on the surface of a rapidly rotating (160,000 rpm) olive-shaped atherectomy burr. This abrasion generates 2- to 5-μm microparticles that pass through the coronary microcirculation for removal by the reticuloendothelial system. Burrs travel over a specialized 0.009-inch guidewire and are available in diameters ranging from 1.25 to 2.50 mm. In the setting of severe calcification, smaller (1.25 mm) burrs can be used initially, followed by larger burrs in 0.25- to 0.50-mm increments up to 70% of the reference vessel diameter. Aggressive rotational coronary atherectomy techniques do not provide a restenosis advantage over more conservative methods and tend to increase acute procedural complications, such as distal embolization or coronary perforation. Rotational atherectomy does not appear to reduce restenosis compared with balloon angioplasty in noncalcified vessels. Current use of rotational atherectomy is reserved for ostial and heavily calcified lesions that cannot be dilated with balloon angioplasty or those that prevent delivery of coronary stents. Rotational coronary atherectomy is generally limited to abrasion of superficial calcification with a single

TABLE 58-6 Clinical Benefits from Reperfusion Device from Meta-Analysis

	RISK RATIO	95% CI	P VALUE
Catheter Aspiration Devices			
Mortality	0.63	0.43-0.93	0.018
Myocardial infarction	0.65	0.37-1.12	0.13
Target vessel revascularization	0.83	0.64-1.08	0.16
Stroke	3.43	0.85-14	0.085
MACE	0.76	0.62-0.95	0.013
TIMI blush grade	1.69	1.26-2.28	<0.001
ST-segment resolution	1.41	1.21-1.64	<0.001
Mechanical Thrombectomy Devices			
Mortality	1.93	1.00-3.72	0.05
Myocardial infarction	0.67	0.19-3.01	0.53
Target vessel revascularization	1.14	0.43-3.01	0.79
Stroke	2.67	0.71-10	0.14
MACE	1.64	0.71-1.90	0.55
ST-segment resolution	1.25	0.99-1.58	0.061
Embolic Protection Devices			
Mortality	0.92	0.60-1.40	0.69
Myocardial infarction	0.82	0.44-1.51	0.52
Target vessel revascularization	1.04	0.74-1.47	0.82
Stroke	0.99	0.34-2.92	0.99
MACE	0.95	0.69-1.30	0.73
TIMI blush grade	1.18	1.02-1.38	0.031
ST-segment resolution	1.07	0.98-1.16	0.13

MACE = major adverse cardiac event.
Modified from Bavry AA, Kumbhani DJ, Bhatt DL: Role of adjunctive thrombectomy and embolic protection devices in acute myocardial infarction: A comprehensive meta-analysis of randomized trials. Eur Heart J 29:2989, 2008.

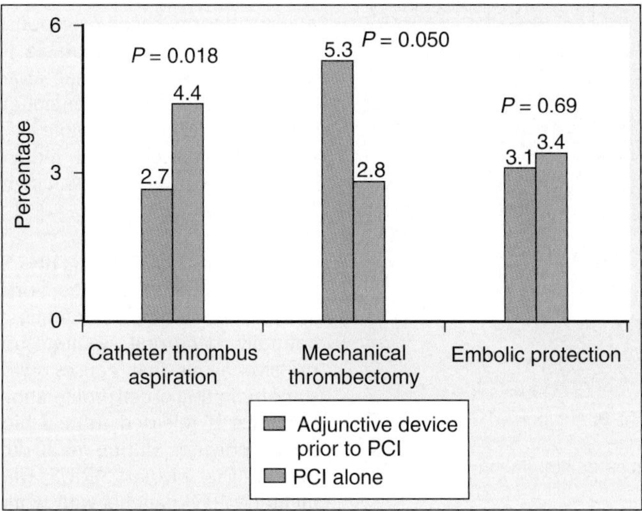

FIGURE 58-7 In this meta-analysis of patients with STEMI undergoing primary PCI, simple manual thrombus aspiration is associated with lower mortality, whereas mechanical aspiration and embolic protection devices are not. *(From Bavry AA, Kumbhani DJ, Bhatt DL: Role of adjunctive thrombectomy and embolic protection devices in acute myocardial infarction: A comprehensive meta-analysis of randomized trials. Eur Heart J 29:2989, 2008.)*

Distal Occlusion Devices. The GuardWire (Medtronic Vascular, Santa Rosa, Calif) is a low-pressure balloon mounted on a hollow guidewire shaft. The device is passed across the target lesion and inflated with a saline contrast admixture to occlude flow; the debris liberated by intervention remains trapped in the stagnant column of blood and is aspirated with a specially designed aspiration catheter before the occlusion balloon is deflated to restore anterograde flow. Compared with SVG intervention without distal occlusion, use of the GuardWire reduced 30-day major adverse clinical events and no-reflow. The major disadvantage of this device is that blood flow is stopped during SVG intervention while the balloon is inflated.

Distal Embolic Filters. Distal filters are advanced across the target lesion in their smaller collapsed state, and a retaining sheath is withdrawn, allowing the filters to open and to expand against the vessel wall. The filters then remain in place to catch any liberated embolic material larger than the filter pore size (usually 120 to 150 μm) during intervention. At the end of the intervention, the filters are collapsed by use of a sheath, and the captured embolic material is removed from the body. This type of device has the advantages of maintaining anterograde flow during the procedure and allowing intermittent injection of contrast material to visualize underlying anatomy, but it has the potential disadvantage of allowing the component of debris with a diameter less than the filter pore size to pass (**Fig. 58-8**). Newer filter devices with reduced crossing profiles and more efficient capture of embolic debris have been developed (**Fig. 58-9**).

Proximal Occlusion Devices. The third type of embolic protection device occludes flow into the vessel with a balloon on the tip of or just beyond the tip of the guiding catheter. Two proximal occlusion devices are currently in use: the Proxis catheter (St. Jude Medical) and Kerberos embolic protection system (Kerberos, Sunnyvale, Calif). With such inflow occlusion, retrograde flow generated by distal collaterals or infusion through a "rinsing" catheter can propel any liberated debris back into the lumen of the guiding catheter. These approaches have the potential advantage of providing embolic protection even before the first wire crosses the target lesion.

Coronary Stents

Coronary stents have emerged as the predominant form of PCI and are currently used in more than 90% of PCI procedures worldwide. Coronary stents scaffold arterial dissection flaps, thereby lowering the incidence of vessel closure and need for emergency CABG surgery, and lessen the frequency of restenosis because of their effect on preventing arterial constriction that is the primary mechanism of restenosis with balloon angioplasty. Despite late clinical improvement compared with balloon angioplasty, restenosis after coronary stent placement occurs in some patients because of excessive intimal hyperplasia within the stent. A number of second-generation balloon-expandable stents were introduced between 1997 and 2003, varying in metallic composition (i.e., cobalt chromium or layered metals versus solid 316 L stainless steel), strut design, stent length, delivery and deployment system, and arterial surface coverage, among other factors. These modifications enhanced flexibility and ease of delivery of the stent while also improving vessel scaffolding and side branch access.

The early use of coronary stents was limited by high (3% to 5%) subacute thrombosis rates, despite aggressive antithrombotic therapy with aspirin (≤325 mg daily), dipyridamole (225 mg daily), and periprocedural low-molecular-weight dextran and an uninterrupted transition from intravenous heparin to oral warfarin. Subacute thrombosis produced profound clinical consequences, resulting in an untoward outcome (e.g., death, MI, or emergency revascularization) in virtually every such patient. Lower frequencies of subacute stent thrombosis (roughly 0.5% to 1.0%) have resulted from use of high-pressure stent deployment and with a drug regimen that includes aspirin and a thienopyridine (e.g., clopidogrel or prasugrel) started just before or after stent placement.

Whereas coronary BMS reduce the incidence of angiographic and clinical restenosis compared with balloon angioplasty, angiographic restenosis (follow-up diameter stenosis >50%) still occurred in 20% to 30% of patients and clinical restenosis (recurrent angina due to restenosis in the treated segment) developed in 10% to 15% of patients in the first year after treatment. Restenosis with BMS occurred more often in patients with small vessels, long lesions, and diabetes mellitus, among other factors. Adjunctive pharmacologic therapy has not prevented restenosis after stent placement.

Several mechanical treatments of in-stent restenosis were attempted, including balloon redilation, removal of in-stent hyperplasia by means of atherectomy, and repeated bare metal stenting. Brachytherapy with use of beta or gamma sources did modestly improve this outcome for in-stent restenosis, but brachytherapy has several limitations, including the requirement for a radiation therapist, a tendency for late "catch-up" restenosis, and the inhibition of endothelialization that markedly

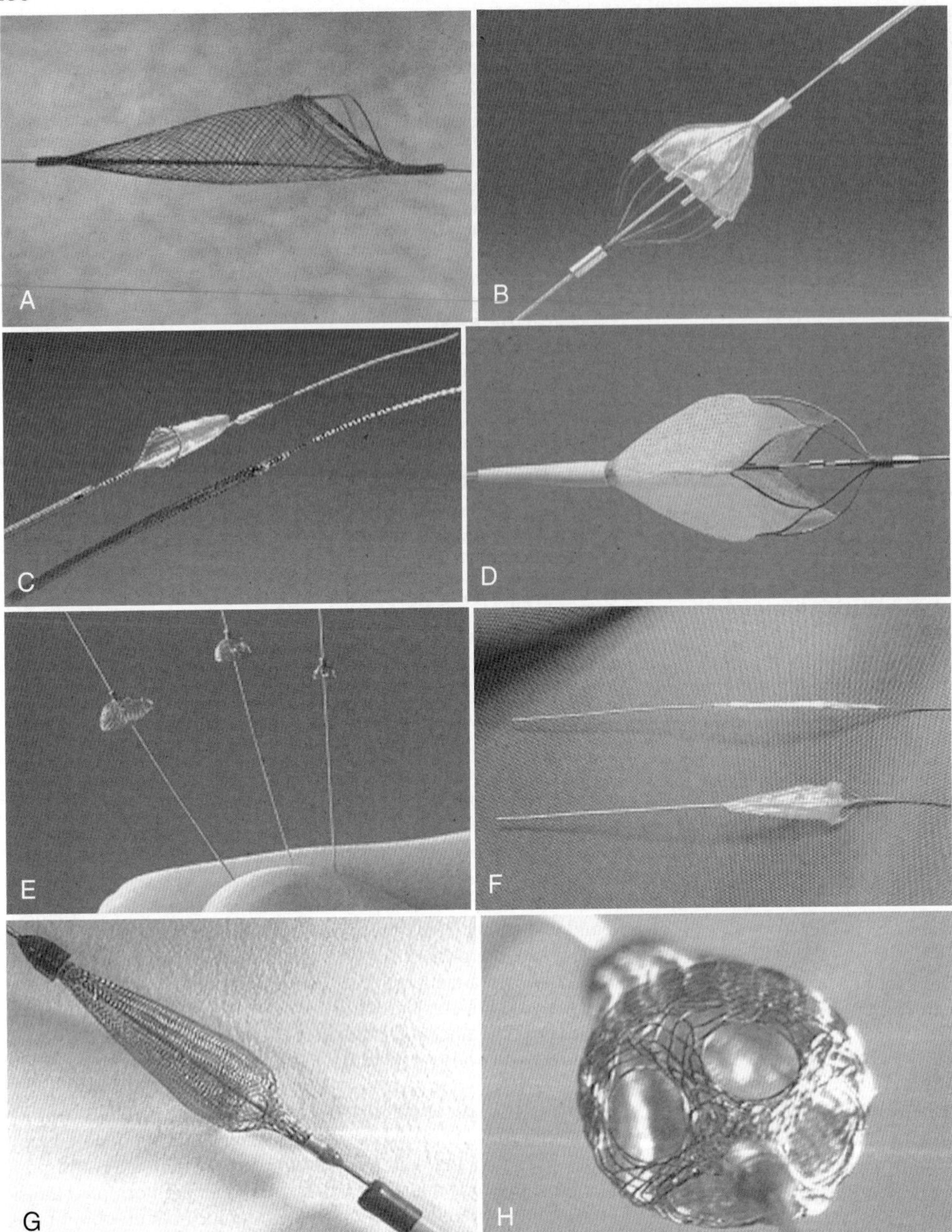

FIGURE 58-8 Filters for distal protection. **A,** The Spider filter (ev3, Minneapolis, Minn). **B,** Angioguard device (Cordis Corp., Warren, NJ). **C,** EPI FilterWire (Boston Scientific, Natick, Mass). **D,** Accunet device (Guidant, Santa Clara, Calif). **E,** MedNova (Abbott, Chicago, Ill). **F,** Rubicon filter (Boston Scientific). **G, H,** The Interceptor filter (Medtronic Vascular, Santa Rosa, Calif) in longitudinal view **(G)** and axial view **(H).**

increases the risk of thrombosis if another stent is implanted in the same vessel segment. Brachytherapy was inferior to DES placement for treatment of restenosis in two randomized studies.[67,68]

BMS are currently used in 10% to 30% of patients undergoing PCI. This is most often due to the inability to take long-term dual antiplatelet therapy; larger (>4.0 mm) vessels, in which the restenosis risk is lower; and acute MI, wherein the issues related to compliance of the patient are more difficult to ascertain.

Drug-Eluting Stents

DES were developed in the early 2000s to provide sustained local delivery of an antiproliferative agent at the site of vessel wall injury. The three components of current DES are the balloon-expandable stent, a durable or resorbable polymer coating that provides sustained drug delivery, and the pharmacologic agent employed to limit intimal hyperplasia (**Fig. 58-10**).

DES have proven efficacy in patients with focal, de novo, and "workhorse" lesions that include reference vessel diameters between 2.5 and 3.5 mm and lesion lengths between 15 and 30 mm. Additional randomized trials and registries have also demonstrated the benefit of DES in patients with long (>30 mm) and small (<2.5 mm) vessels, chronic total occlusions, SVG and internal mammary disease, and in-stent restenosis and in patients with STEMI.[69] With the expanded follow-up of patients receiving DES, it has become apparent that DES placement requires extended (up to 1 year) therapy with the combination of aspirin and clopidogrel to prevent stent thrombosis.[70] Moreover, even after 1 year, there is an infrequent (0.2% to 0.6%) annual rate of very late stent thrombosis, warranting a careful discussion of the risks, benefits, and alternative therapies in candidates for PCI.[71] The risk of late and very late stent thrombosis appears related to endothelial dysfunction and an abnormal healing response to the vessel wall attributable to the durable stent polymer. More biocompatible second-generation polymers may promote a re-endothelialization and reduce the risk of very late stent thrombosis.[72]

SIROLIMUS-ELUTING STENTS. The CYPHER stent (Cordis Corp., Warren, NJ) contains sirolimus, a naturally occurring immunosuppressive agent that causes cytostatic inhibition of cell proliferation. Sirolimus is released from a biostable polymer during a 30-day period. The pivotal SIRIUS trial included 1058 patients with workhorse lesions who were randomized to treatment with a sirolimus-eluting stent or a BMS. The primary clinical endpoint of 8-month target vessel failure, composed of target vessel revascularization, death, or MI, was reduced from 21% in patients treated with BMS to 8.6% in patients with sirolimus-eluting stents ($P < 0.001$). Angiographic restenosis rates were also lower in patients assigned to treatment with the sirolimus-eluting stents within the stent (35.4% with BMS versus 3.2% with sirolimus-eluting stents; $P < 0.001$) and within the treated segment including 5-mm proximal and distal margins (36.3% with BMS versus 8.9% with sirolimus-eluting stents; $P < 0.001$). Target vessel revascularization was reduced from 16.6% in BMS to 4.1% in sirolimus-eluting stents ($P < 0.001$). Reduction in intimal hyperplasia endured for at least 2 years after the procedure. At 5 years, there were significant reductions in target lesion revascularization for sirolimus-eluting stents compared with BMS (cumulative incidence: 12.5% versus 28.8%, respectively; $P < 0.001$).[73,74] There was no difference in the cumulative incidence of MI or revascularization attributed to

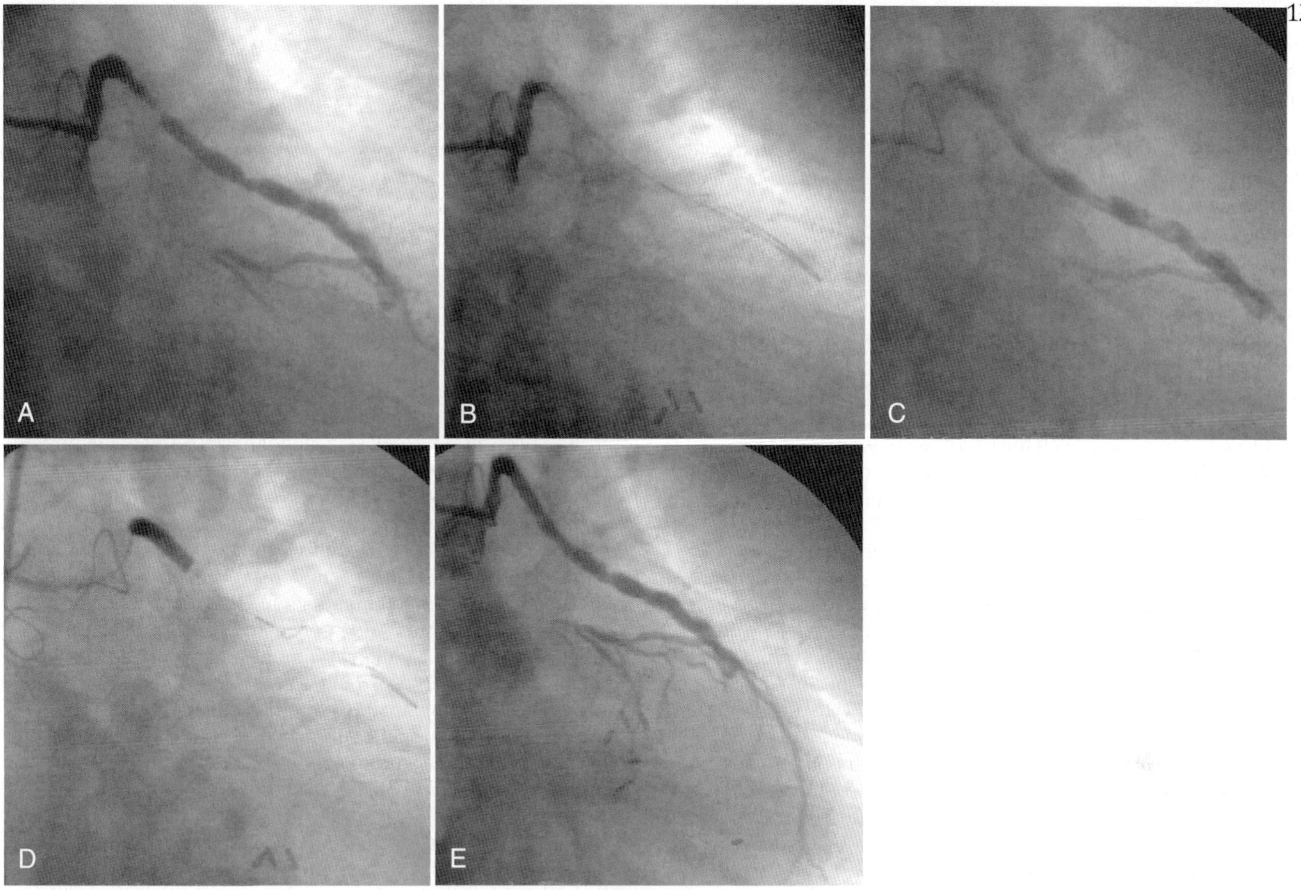

FIGURE 58-9 SVG percutaneous intervention with FilterWire distal protection. **A,** A degenerated SVG to the left anterior descending artery has a stenosis in its proximal segment. **B,** The FilterWire is positioned across the stenosis and deployed against the wall of the SVG. **C,** Flow is shown through the SVG. **D,** A stent is deployed in the proximal segment of the SVG. **E,** The FilterWire is removed, and there is excellent flow into the distal SVG without evidence of distal embolization.

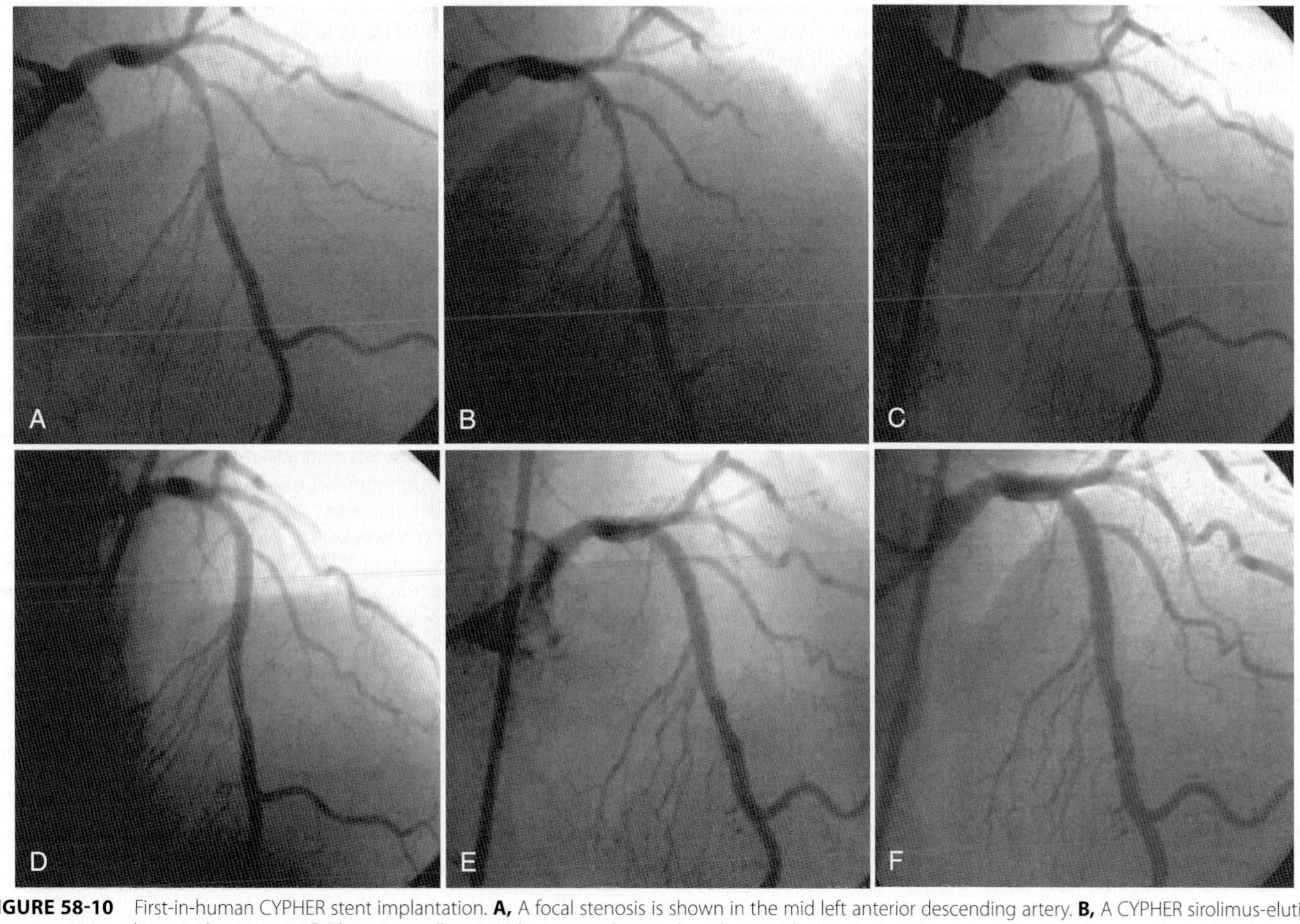

FIGURE 58-10 First-in-human CYPHER stent implantation. **A,** A focal stenosis is shown in the mid left anterior descending artery. **B,** A CYPHER sirolimus-eluting stent is positioned across the stenosis. **C,** There is excellent initial angiographic result and no residual stenosis. Follow-up angiography was performed at 4 months **(D),** 1 year **(E),** and 2 years **(F)** after the procedure without evidence of lumen renarrowing. *(Courtesy of Eduardo Sousa, São Paulo, Brazil.)*

remote segments of the target vessel. Events attributed to the nontarget vessel were frequent and not different for sirolimus-eluting stents versus BMS (25.7% versus 25.8%).[73,74]

PACLITAXEL-ELUTING STENTS. The TAXUS stent (Boston Scientific) is composed of a stainless steel stent platform, a polyolefin polymer derivative, and the microtubular stabilizing agent paclitaxel that has anti-inflammatory effects while also inhibiting both cell migration and division. Paclitaxel release is completed within 30 days of implantation, although a substantial portion (>90%) of the paclitaxel remains within the polymer indefinitely. The pivotal TAXUS IV trial randomly assigned 1314 patients with single de novo coronary lesions to either a TAXUS stent or an identical-appearing BMS. The ischemia-driven target vessel revascularization at 9 months was reduced from 11.3% to 3% and remained significantly reduced at 12 months (from 17.1% to 7.1%) in patients with the paclitaxel-eluting stents ($P < 0.001$). The rate of binary angiographic restenosis was reduced both within the stent (24.4% with BMS versus 5.5% with the paclitaxel-eluting stent; $P < 0.001$) and within the treated segment including 5-mm proximal and distal margins (26.6% and 7.9%, respectively; $P < 0.001$).

ZOTAROLIMUS-ELUTING STENTS. Zotarolimus (previously known as ABT-578) is another rapamycin analogue released from a phosphorylcholine (PC)–coated stent that has been evaluated with use of the Endeavor stent (Medtronic Vascular). In the Endeavor II trial, 1197 patients were assigned to treatment with the Endeavor zotarolimus-eluting PC polymer–coated stent or the same BMS but without the drug or the polymer coating.[75] The 9-month primary endpoint of target vessel failure was reduced from 15.1% with the BMS to 7.9% with the Endeavor ($P < 0.0001$).[75] In-stent late loss was reduced from 1.03 mm to 0.61 mm in patients treated with the Endeavor stent ($P < 0.001$), and the rate of in-segment restenosis was reduced from 35% to 13.2% with the Endeavor stent ($P < 0.0001$). There was a significant reduction associated with the use of the Endeavor stent that persisted to 4 years.[75] The ENDEAVOR III trial compared the Endeavor stent with CYPHER in a 436-patient study (3:1 randomization) and failed to meet the primary endpoint of noninferior in-segment late loss at 8 months (0.34 mm with zotarolimus-eluting stents versus 0.13 mm with sirolimus-eluting stents) with higher late loss (0.60 and 0.15 mm, respectively; $P < 0.001$). There was no significant difference in target lesion revascularization between the two groups (6.3% and 3.5%, respectively; $P = 0.34$). At 3-year follow-up, there was a reduction in the occurrence of death and MI in patients treated with the Endeavor stent but no difference in the occurrence of target vessel revascularization.[76] The Endeavor IV trial, a prospective, randomized, single-blind, controlled trial, compared the safety and efficacy of the zotarolimus-eluting stent with the paclitaxel-eluting stent in 1548 patients with single de novo coronary lesions. The primary endpoint was a composite of cardiac death, MI, or target vessel revascularization, and Endeavor was noninferior to the TAXUS stent. In addition, there were fewer periprocedural MIs with zotarolimus-eluting stents (0.5% versus 2.2%; $P = 0.007$) because of less side branch occlusion in patients with zotarolimus-eluting stents.[77] Although 8-month angiographic restenosis was improved after paclitaxel-eluting stent therapy, at 12 months the frequency of target lesion revascularization was similar comparing zotarolimus- with paclitaxel-eluting stents (4.5% versus 3.8%; $P = 0.228$), especially in those without planned angiographic follow-up (3.6% versus 3.2%; $P = 0.756$), and these results persisted for 2 years.[78]

EVEROLIMUS-ELUTING STENT. The Xience stent (Abbot Vascular, Santa Rosa, Calif) uses the cobalt chromium Vision stent, a durable fluoropolymer, and everolimus, which is a rapamycin analogue that has both immunosuppressive and antiproliferative effects. On the basis of initial studies that evaluated use of an absorbable poly-L-lactic acid polymer, the SPIRIT program has shown reduction in late lumen loss comparable to the CYPHER stent. The SPIRIT III, a prospective, randomized, single-blind, controlled trial, enrolled 1002 patients undergoing PCI in lesions 28 mm or less in length and with reference vessel diameter between 2.5 and 3.75 mm.[79] Angiographic in-segment late loss was significantly less in the everolimus-eluting stent group compared with the paclitaxel group (0.14 mm versus 0.28 mm; $P = 0.004$).[79] The everolimus stent was noninferior to the paclitaxel stent for target vessel failure at 9 months (7.2% versus 9.0%, respectively; $P < 0.001$ for noninferiority).[79] The everolimus stent resulted in significant reductions in composite major adverse cardiac events both at 9 months compared with the paclitaxel stent (4.6% versus 8.1%; $P = 0.03$) and at 1 year (6.0% versus 10.3%; $P = 0.02$) because of fewer MIs and target lesion revascularization procedures.[79]

Antiplatelet Agents (see Chap. 87)

ASPIRIN. Aspirin irreversibly inhibits cyclooxygenase and thus blocks the synthesis of thromboxane A_2, a vasoconstricting agent that promotes platelet aggregation. Aspirin substantially reduces periprocedural MI caused by thrombotic occlusions compared with placebo and has been established as a standard for all patients undergoing PCI. The inhibitory effect of aspirin occurs within 60 minutes, and its effect on platelets lasts for up to 7 days after discontinuation. Although the minimum effective aspirin dosage in the setting of PCI remains uncertain, patients taking daily aspirin should receive 75 to 325 mg aspirin before PCI (see PCI Guidelines). Patients not already taking daily long-term aspirin therapy should be given 300 to 325 mg of aspirin at least 2 hours and preferably 24 hours before PCI is performed. After PCI, in patients without allergy or increased risk of bleeding, aspirin 162 to 325 mg daily should be given for at least 1 month after BMS implantation, 3 months after sirolimus-eluting stent implantation, and 6 months after paclitaxel-eluting stent implantation, after which daily long-term aspirin use should be continued indefinitely at a dose of 75 to 162 mg (see PCI Guidelines).

THIENOPYRIDINE DERIVATIVES. Thienopyridine derivatives cause irreversible platelet inhibition because of their effects on the $P2Y_{12}$ adenosine diphosphate (ADP) receptor that can activate the glycoprotein IIb/IIIa complex. Because aspirin and thienopyridine derivatives have distinct mechanisms of action, their combination inhibits platelet aggregation to a greater extent than either agent alone does. The combination of aspirin and clopidogrel (or previously ticlopidine) was essential for 14 to 28 days to prevent stent thrombosis after BMS placement. The combination of aspirin and clopidogrel also reduces death, MI, and urgent revascularization within 12 months in patients undergoing PCI in the setting of NSTEMI and unstable angina and in those undergoing elective PCI. Recent studies have suggested that a loading dose of 600 mg rather than 300 mg of clopidogrel results in more rapid (<2 hours) platelet inhibition[80,81] and improved clinical outcomes, including lower rates of stent thrombosis. Additional clopidogrel loading with 300 mg or 600 mg may also be used in patients on chronic maintenance clopidogrel therapy.[82] The need for pretreatment with clopidogrel is more controversial, balancing improved clinical outcomes with the potential risk for bleeding should CABG surgery be needed. Current guidelines recommend that a 600-mg loading dose of clopidogrel be administered before or during PCI (see PCI Guidelines). For all post-PCI patients who receive a DES, clopidogrel 75 mg daily should be given for at least 12 months if patients are not at high risk for bleeding. For post-PCI patients receiving a BMS, clopidogrel should be given for a minimum of 1 month and ideally up to 12 months (unless the patient is at increased risk for bleeding; then it should be given for a minimum of 2 weeks) (see PCI Guidelines).

Prasugrel is a more potent $P2Y_{12}$ ADP receptor inhibitor that has a more rapid onset of action and higher levels of platelet inhibition than higher dose clopidogrel.[83] In a study of 13,608 patients with moderate- to high-risk acute coronary syndromes undergoing scheduled PCI and randomly assigned to receive prasugrel (60-mg loading dose and 10-mg daily maintenance dose) or clopidogrel (300-mg loading dose and 75-mg daily maintenance dose) for 6 to 15 months, the primary efficacy endpoint, a composite of death from cardiovascular causes, nonfatal MI, or nonfatal stroke, occurred in 12.1% of patients receiving clopidogrel and 9.9% of patients receiving prasugrel ($P < 0.001$).[84] There were also significant reductions in the prasugrel group in the rates of MI (9.7% for clopidogrel versus 7.4% for prasugrel; $P < 0.001$), urgent target vessel revascularization (3.7% versus 2.5%; $P < 0.001$), and stent thrombosis (2.4% versus 1.1%; $P < 0.001$).[84] On the other hand, major bleeding was observed in 2.4% of patients receiving prasugrel and in 1.8% of patients receiving clopidogrel ($P = 0.03$), with more frequent rates of life-threatening bleeding in the prasugrel group (1.4% versus 0.9% with clopidogrel; $P = 0.01$), including fatal bleeding (0.4% versus 0.1%, respectively; $P = 0.002$).[84,85] Among persons treated with clopidogrel, carriers of reduced-function CYP2C19 alleles had significantly lower levels of active metabolite, diminished platelet inhibition, and higher rates of adverse cardiovascular events.[86] A similar relationship was not found in patients treated with prasugrel. Further research will be necessary to determine if measurement of point-of-care platelet assays of genetic polymorphisms can help in allocating therapy.[87] In patients with an acute coronary syndrome undergoing PCI who are at low bleeding risk, prasugrel 60-mg loading dose should be given as soon as possible after definition of the coronary anatomy and continued for 12 to 15 months after stent placement (see PCI Guidelines).

Ticagrelor, a reversible oral $P2Y_{12}$ receptor antagonist, provides faster, greater, and more consistent ADP-receptor inhibition than clopidogrel.[88] In a multicenter, double-blind trial of 18,624 patients presenting with an acute coronary syndrome, with or without ST-segment elevation, random assignment was made to treatment with ticagrelor (180-mg loading dose, 90 mg twice daily thereafter) or clopidogrel (300- to 600-mg loading dose, 75 mg daily thereafter) for 12 months. The primary endpoint, a composite of death from vascular causes, MI, or stroke at 12 months, occurred in 9.8% of patients receiving ticagrelor and 11.7% of those receiving clopidogrel (hazard ratio, 0.84; $P < 0.001$).[89] There was also a significant reduction in MI alone (5.8% in the ticagrelor group versus 6.9% in the clopidogrel group; $P = 0.005$) and death from vascular causes (4.0% versus 5.1%; $P = 0.001$).[89] No significant difference in the overall rates of major bleeding was found between the ticagrelor and clopidogrel groups (11.6% and 11.2%, respectively; $P = 0.43$), but ticagrelor was associated with a higher rate of major bleeding not related to CABG (4.5% versus 3.8%, $P = 0.03$).[89]

Current evidence suggests that in the absence of risk factors for bleeding, dual antiplatelet therapy should continue for at least 12 months after BMS and DES placement. Prolonged thienopyridine therapy not only reduces late stent thrombosis but also prevents MI by thrombi that complicate plaques remote from the initial intervention. Indefinite aspirin and clopidogrel therapy is recommended in patients receiving brachytherapy, and higher doses (150 mg daily) of chronic clopidogrel are recommended in those patients in whom stent thrombosis may be catastrophic, such as patients with unprotected left main artery stenting or those with stenting of the last remaining vessel if there is less than 50% inhibition of platelet aggregation on platelet assays.[10,11]

Glycoprotein IIb/IIIa Inhibitors. Thrombin and collagen are potent platelet agonists that can cause ADP and serotonin release and activate glycoprotein (GP) IIb/IIIa fibrinogen receptors on the platelet surface. Functionally active GP IIb/IIIa serves in the "final common pathway" of platelet aggregation by binding fibrinogen and other adhesive proteins that bridge adjacent platelets. There are three GP IIb/IIIa inhibitors approved for clinical use. Studies supporting the use of these agents during PCI were performed before the widespread use of dual antiplatelet therapy, and the use of these agents has been reevaluated in this context.

Abciximab is a chimeric human-murine monoclonal antibody that irreversibly binds to the platelet GP IIb/IIIa receptor of human platelets. It also binds to the vitronectin ($\alpha_v\beta_3$) receptor found on platelets and vessel wall endothelial and smooth muscle cells. The recommended dosage of abciximab is an intravenous bolus of 0.25 mg/kg, followed by a continuous intravenous infusion of 0.125 μg/kg/min (to a maximum of 10 μg/min) for 12 hours. Abciximab can be safely administered in patients with renal insufficiency, and platelet infusions can reverse the effect of this agent.

Eptifibatide is a cyclic peptide derivative that reversibly binds GP IIb/IIIa. A double eptifibatide bolus, 180 μg/kg boluses 10 minutes apart, and an infusion dose, 2.0 μg/kg/min for 18 to 24 hours, result in sufficient platelet inhibition to prevent ischemic events in patients undergoing PCI. Addition of eptifibatide to clopidogrel, 600-mg loading dose, also results in incremental platelet inhibition. A reduction of the eptifibatide infusion to 1 μg/kg/min is necessary in patients with a creatinine clearance <50 mL/min. Platelet transfusions do not reverse the platelet inhibition with eptifibatide, although by 4 hours after cessation of the infusion, patients have safely undergone CABG.

Tirofiban, a peptidomimetic small molecule, has also undergone evaluation for its adjunctive benefit during urgent PCI and is inferior to abciximab for the prevention of ischemic events during PCI. The recommended dosage is an initial rate of 0.4 μg/kg/min for 30 minutes and then continued at 0.1 μg/kg/min. Patients with severe renal insufficiency (creatinine clearance <30 mL/min) should receive half the usual rate of infusion. Subsequent studies have suggested that the tirofiban bolus dose given in the initial PCI studies may not have produced optimal antiplatelet effect during PCI, and larger bolus doses can improve the inhibition of platelet aggregation.[90] Tirofiban is generally used for patients with acute coronary syndrome before PCI.

The GP IIb/IIIa inhibitors have demonstrated benefit in improving clinical outcomes within the first 30 days after PCI, primarily by reducing ischemic complications, including periprocedural MI and recurrent ischemia. They are particularly useful in patients with troponin-positive acute coronary syndromes[91] but have no consistent effect on reducing late restenosis. Although GP IIb/IIIa inhibitors differ in their structure, reversibility, and duration, two meta-analyses found no difference between their clinical effects in patients undergoing primary PCI.[92,93] Bleeding is the major risk of GP IIb/IIIa inhibitors, and a downward adjustment of the unfractionated heparin dose has been recommended. GP IIb/IIIa inhibitors are recommended in patients with NSTEMI and unstable angina who are not pretreated with clopidogrel, and it is reasonable to administer them to patients who have a troponin-positive acute coronary syndrome who have also been pretreated with clopidogrel[91] (see PCI Guidelines). Although GP IIb/IIIa inhibitors are recommended in selected patients at the time of PCI, the value of GP IIb/IIIa inhibitors as part of a routine preparatory strategy in patients with STEMI before their transport to the catheterization laboratory has been questioned on the basis of the results of three studies that failed to show benefit of GP IIb/IIIa inhibitors in patients who were pretreated with dual antiplatelet therapy.[90,94,95]

Antithrombin Agents

Unfractionated heparin (see Chap. 87) is the most commonly used thrombin inhibitor during PCI. Point-of-care activated clotting time (ACT) monitoring has facilitated heparin dose titration during PCI, and retrospective studies with balloon angioplasty have related the ACT value to clinical outcome after PCI. An ACT in the range of 350 to 375 seconds provided the lowest composite ischemic event rate, although any level of ACT <250 seconds had no further reductions in ischemic complications with concomitant use of GP IIb/IIIa inhibitors. More recent studies in the thienopyridine era have failed to correlate ischemic outcomes with the level of anticoagulation achieved with unfractionated heparin during coronary stent placement. Weight-adjusted heparin dosing regimens of 50 to 70 IU/kg help avoid "overshooting" the ACT. Sufficient unfractionated heparin should be administered during PCI to achieve an ACT >250 seconds if no GP IIb/IIIa inhibitor is given and >200 seconds if GP IIb/IIIa inhibitors are given. Routine use of intravenous heparin after PCI is no longer indicated. Early sheath removal is encouraged when the ACT falls to less than 150 to 180 seconds (see PCI Guidelines).

LOW-MOLECULAR-WEIGHT HEPARIN (see Chap. 87). Enoxaparin is considered a reasonable alternative to unfractionated heparin in patients with non–ST-segment elevation acute coronary syndromes undergoing PCI (see Chap. 56), but difficulty in monitoring the levels of anticoagulation in the event that PCI is performed has limited its clinical use at many centers.[96] The Superior Yield of the New Strategy of Enoxaparin, Revascularization and Glycoprotein IIb/IIIa Inhibitors (SYNERGY) trial prospectively randomized 10,027 high-risk patients with non–ST-segment elevation acute coronary syndrome with an intended early invasive strategy to treatment with subcutaneous enoxaparin or intravenous unfractionated heparin.[97] The 30-day primary efficacy outcome, a composite clinical endpoint of all-cause death or nonfatal MI, occurred in 14% of patients assigned to enoxaparin and 14.5% of patients assigned to unfractionated heparin. More TIMI (Thrombolysis in Myocardial Infarction) major bleeding was observed in patients treated with enoxaparin (9.1% versus 7.6%; $P = 0.008$). The bleeding risk was highest in those patients who received "crossover" therapy with unfractionated heparin and enoxaparin. When enoxaparin is given before PCI, empiric dose algorithms have been designed to guide additional anticoagulation therapy during PCI. If the last dose of enoxaparin was less than 8 hours before PCI, no additional antithrombin is needed. If the last dose of enoxaparin was given between 8 and 12 hours, a 0.3 mg/kg bolus of intravenous enoxaparin should be given.[97] If the dose was administrated more than 12 hours before PCI, conventional anticoagulation therapy is indicated.

BIVALIRUDIN. Bivalirudin is a direct thrombin inhibitor that has been used as an alternative to unfractionated heparin in patients undergoing PCI. Bivalirudin generally causes fewer bleeding complications than unfractionated heparin because of its shorter half-life (25 minutes) and more predictable bioavailability.[98] Bivalirudin is also accessible to clot-bound thrombin because its anticoagulant effect does not depend on binding with antithrombin. Bivalirudin was not inferior to the combination of unfractionated heparin and a GP IIb/IIIa inhibitor in one trial of 6010 "low-risk" patients in the REPLACE-2 study.[99] In a larger study of 13,819 patients with unstable angina and NSTEMI, bivalirudin alone was compared with bivalirudin with a GP IIb/IIIa inhibitor and heparin with a GP IIb/IIIa inhibitor. With use of a composite ischemia endpoint of death, MI, or unplanned revascularization for ischemia and major bleeding to determine net clinical benefit, bivalirudin alone, compared with heparin plus a GP IIb/IIIa inhibitor, showed noninferiority in the composite ischemia endpoint (7.8% and 7.3%, respectively) and significantly reduced rates of major bleeding (3.0% versus 5.7%; $P < 0.001$), resulting in a better net clinical outcome endpoint (10.1% versus 11.7%; $P = 0.02$).[100] Bivalirudin is considered a reasonable alternative to unfractionated heparin in low-risk patients undergoing PCI and may reduce bleeding complications in higher risk patients with unstable angina and NSTEMI. Bivalirudin may safely be substituted for unfractionated heparin in patients with acute coronary syndromes[101] and is a cost-effective alternative to unfractionated heparin and a GP IIb/IIIa inhibitor.[102] In a randomized study of 3602 patients with STEMI undergoing primary PCI (see Chap. 55), anticoagulation with bivalirudin alone, compared with heparin plus GP IIb/IIIa inhibitors, resulted in significantly reduced 30-day rates of major bleeding and net adverse clinical events, including a lower rate of mortality.[95] Adjunctive clopidogrel should be given as soon as possible (<30 minutes) before PCI in patients with acute coronary syndromes if possible.[103]

FACTOR Xa INHIBITORS. Fondaparinux is a pentasaccharide that has anti-Xa activity without effects on factor IIa and may cause less bleeding when it is used for the treatment of patients with acute coronary syndromes. The OASIS-5 trial randomly assigned 20,078 patients with acute coronary syndromes to receive either fondaparinux (2.5 mg daily) or enoxaparin (1 mg/kg of body weight twice daily) for a mean of 6 days.[104] The occurrence of the 9-day primary study endpoint (death, MI, or refractory ischemia) was similar in the two groups (5.8% with fondaparinux and 5.7% with enoxaparin), although the risk of major bleeding at 9 days was markedly lower with fondaparinux (2.2%) than with enoxaparin (4.1%; $P < 0.001$).[104] This reduction in bleeding was accompanied by an improvement in late mortality in patients treated with fondaparinux. Potential limitations of this approach are the relatively long half-life of fondaparinux and the need for adjunct anticoagulation with heparin during PCI to avoid the occurrence of catheter thrombi. Fondaparinux was not effective in reducing ischemic events in patients undergoing primary PCI for STEMI[105] (see PCI Guidelines).

Outcomes After Percutaneous Coronary Intervention

Procedural success and complication rates are used to measure outcomes after PCI. Early (<30 days) success (e.g., relief of angina; freedom from death, MI, and urgent revascularization) generally relates to the safety and effectiveness of the initial procedure, whereas late (30 days to 1 year) success (e.g., freedom from recurrence of angina, target vessel revascularization, MI, or death) depends on both clinical restenosis and progressive atherosclerosis at remote sites. Substantial improvements in coronary devices (e.g., DES), adjunct antithrombotics used during PCI (e.g., ADP antagonists, GP IIb/IIIa inhibitors, direct thrombin inhibitors), and secondary prevention after PCI (e.g., therapy with lipid-lowering agents, beta-adrenergic blockers, antiplatelet drugs; see Chap. 49) have markedly improved early and late clinical outcomes after PCI over time.[106]

EARLY CLINICAL OUTCOME. Anatomic (or angiographic) success after PCI is defined as the attainment of residual diameter stenosis less than 50%, which is generally associated with at least a 20% improvement in diameter stenosis and relief of ischemia.[10] With the widespread use of coronary stents, the angiographic criterion for success is a 20% stenosis or less when stents are used.[10] Procedural success is defined as angiographic success without the occurrence of major complications (death, MI, or CABG surgery) within 30 days of the procedure. Clinical success is defined as procedural success without the need for urgent repeated PCI or surgical revascularization within the first 30 days of the procedure.[10] A number of clinical, angiographic, and technical variables predict risk of procedural failure in patients undergoing PCI. Major complications include death, MI, or stroke; minor complications include transient ischemic attacks, vascular complications, contrast-induced nephropathy, and a number of angiographic complications (**Table 58-7**).[10]

Mortality

Although mortality after PCI is rare (less than 1%), it is higher in the setting of STEMI, in cardiogenic shock, and in patients who develop an occlusion with prior poor left ventricular function.[10] A number of risk factors for early mortality after PCI have been identified[107-109] (**Table 58-8**).

Myocardial Infarction

Periprocedural MI is one of the most common complications of PCI.[110] Two classification systems were previously used to classify MI after PCI: the World Health Organization (WHO) classification system that defines MI as a total creatine kinase (CK) elevation more than two times normal in association with the elevation of the CK-MB isoform; and a second definition that was more commonly used with evaluations of adjunct pharmacologic agents by the Food and Drug

TABLE 58-7 Variables Associated with Early Failure and Complications After Percutaneous Coronary Intervention

Clinical Variables
Women
Advanced age
Diabetes mellitus
Unstable or Canadian Cardiovascular Society (CCS) Class IV angina
Congestive heart failure
Cardiogenic shock
Renal insufficiency
Preprocedural instability requiring intra-aortic balloon pump support
Preprocedural elevation of C-reactive protein
Multivessel coronary artery disease
Anatomic Variables
Multivessel CAD
Left main disease
Thrombus
SVG intervention
ACC/AHA type B2 and C lesion morphology
Chronic total coronary occlusion
Procedural Factors
A higher final percentage diameter stenosis
Smaller minimal lumen diameter
Presence of a residual dissection or transstenotic pressure gradient

Administration, in which MI was defined as an elevation in CK-MB three times normal or higher after the procedure. A consensus definition for MI has now been reached, in which a cardiac biomarker elevated more than three times normal is used.[111] In clinical practice, asymptomatic CK-MB elevations (<5 times the upper normal limits) occur after 3% to 11% of technically successful PCIs and have little apparent clinical consequence. Larger degrees of myonecrosis (CK-MB ≥5 times the upper normal limits) predict higher 1-year mortality rates and should be considered a periprocedural MI. Many of these clinically silent infarcts may reflect a higher atherosclerotic burden in patients who suffer such events. Troponin T and I elevations occur more commonly than CK-MB elevations, but their prognostic significance over that of the CK-MB elevation is not known. Spontaneous MI after PCI has much more prognostic importance than periprocedural enzyme elevation.[112]

TABLE 58-8 Factors Associated with Early Mortality After Percutaneous Coronary Intervention

Clinical Variables
Advanced age
Female gender
Diabetes mellitus
Chronic lung disease
Prior myocardial infarction
Impairment of left ventricular function
Renal dysfunction
Cardiogenic shock
Salvage, urgent, or emergent PCI
Anatomic Variables
Multivessel CAD
Left main disease
Proximal left anterior descending disease
Large area of myocardium at risk
PCI of artery supplying collaterals to large artery
Higher SCAI lesion classification

Urgent Revascularization

Emergent or urgent CABG surgery after PCI is now uncommon and, in the era of coronary stents, results from catastrophic complications during PCI, such as coronary perforation or severe dissection and abrupt closure. Chest pain after PCI is relatively common, and its evaluation requires an immediate 12-lead electrocardiogram. Recurrent ischemia after PCI manifested by chest pain, electrocardiographic abnormalities, and elevation of cardiac biomarkers may occur as a result of acute or subacute stent thrombosis, residual dissections, plaque prolapse, side branch occlusion, or thrombus at the treatment site or may relate to residual disease not treated with the initial procedure. In the presence of suspected recurrent ischemia, coronary arteriography is the most expeditious way to identify the cause of the residual ischemia.

Angiographic Complications

A number of complications may occur during PCI and, depending on their severity and duration, may result in periprocedural MI. If coronary dissections that extend deeper into the media or adventitia begin to compromise the true lumen of the vessel, clinical ischemia may develop (**Fig. 58-11**). Whereas most intraprocedural dissections can be treated promptly with stenting, significant residual dissections of the treated artery occur in 1.7% of patients. These residual dissections

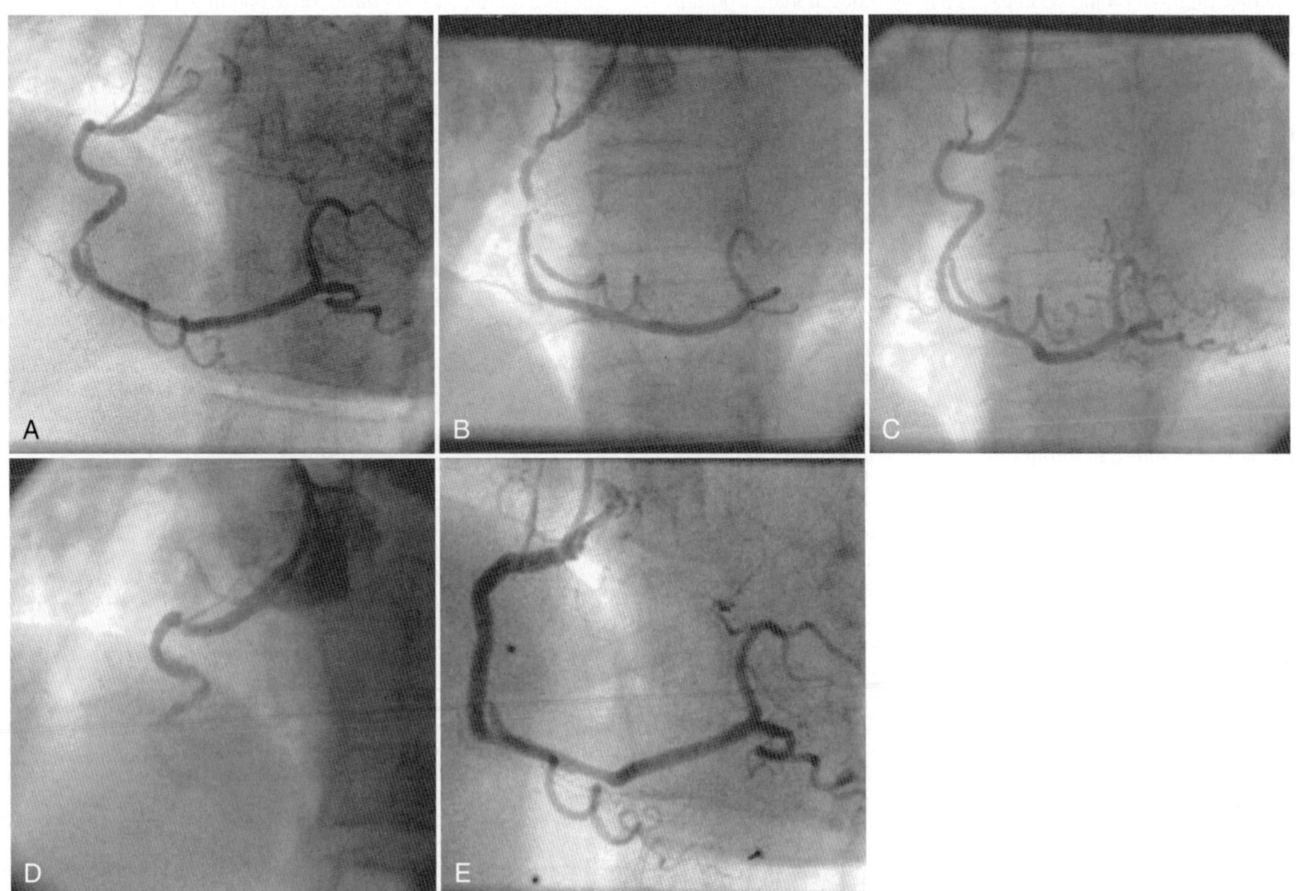

FIGURE 58-11 Abrupt closure after coronary stent placement. **A,** An extremely tortuous right coronary artery has a stenosis in its midportion, **B,** After crossing with a coronary guidewire, there is marked straightening of the vessel. **C,** After a stent is placed and the guidewire is removed, there is an excellent result. **D,** Abrupt closure develops because of a guide catheter dissection, resulting in typical chest pain and ST-segment elevation. **E,** Coronary stents are placed to "bail out" the severe coronary dissection, and normal flow is reestablished to the vessel. Without the availability of coronary stents, it is highly likely that coronary artery bypass graft surgery would have been needed to reverse the abrupt closure event.

raise the risk of postprocedure MI, need for emergent CABG surgery, and stent thrombosis and increase mortality threefold.[113] In addition to barotrauma-induced dissections, guiding catheter dissections represent another mechanism for disruption of the coronary vessel and compromise of distal flow.

Coronary perforation develops in 0.2% to 0.5% of patients undergoing PCI and is more common with atheroablative devices and hydrophilic wires than with balloon angioplasty or with conventional guidewires. Depending on the rate of flow through the vessel perforation, cardiac tamponade and hemodynamic collapse can occur within minutes, requiring immediate recognition and treatment of the perforation. Strategies to control coronary perforations include reversal of intraprocedural anticoagulation and prolonged inflation (at least 10 minutes) of an oversized balloon at low pressure at the site of the perforation to encourage sealing of the tear in the vessel. Management strategies for perforations include the use of perfusion balloons, which provide for a small amount of distal perfusion, and polytetrafluoroethylene (PTFE)–covered stents, which may control free perforations, in addition to decompression of the pericardial pressure with prompt pericardiocentesis. Approximately one third of cases of PCI-associated coronary artery perforation require emergent cardiac surgery.

No-reflow, defined as reduced anterograde perfusion in the absence of a flow-limiting stenosis, occurs in up to 2% to 3% of PCI procedures, typically occurring during interventions on degenerated SVGs, during rotational atherectomy, and during acute MI interventions.[114] No-reflow is likely to be caused by distal embolization of atheromatous and thrombotic debris dislodged by balloon inflation, atherectomy, or stent implantation. Once it occurs, no-reflow can cause severe short- and long-term consequences including a fivefold increased risk of periprocedural MI and threefold increased risk of death. Although numerous pharmacologic strategies such as intracoronary sodium nitroprusside have been used to treat no-reflow, their efficacy in reducing the frequency of subsequent adverse events remains debated.

STENT THROMBOSIS. With the routine use of high-pressure stent postdilation and dual antiplatelet therapy after stent implantation, the rate of stent thrombosis has declined to approximately 1% within the first year after stenting. A number of clinical, angiographic, and procedural factors predispose to its occurrence. Lesion-specific factors that increase the likelihood of stent thrombosis include a residual dissection at the margin of the stent, impaired flow into or out of the stent, small stent diameters (<3 mm), long stent lengths, and treatment of an acute MI, among other factors. Noncompliance of the patient with dual antiplatelet therapy, resistance to the antiplatelet effects of aspirin and clopidogrel, and hypercoagulability may also play important roles in the development of stent thrombosis (**Table 58-9**).

The timing of the stent thrombosis is defined as acute (<24 hours), subacute (24 hours to 30 days), late (30 days to 1 year), and very late (after 1 year). Traditional definitions of stent thrombosis have included only those episodes associated with an acute coronary syndrome and angiographic or pathologic demonstration of thrombosis within the stent or its margins. The Academic Research Consortium has proposed new criteria for documentation of all possible stent thrombosis in clinical studies, including the categories of definite stent thrombosis, probable stent thrombosis, and possible stent thrombosis.[115]

Early reports suggested an incremental risk (0.2% to 0.5% per year) of very late stent thrombosis occurring 1 year or more after DES implantation.[116] Inhibition of endothelialization caused by the potent antiproliferative effect of the drugs delivered by DES may significantly prolong the period of risk for patients to develop stent thrombosis. Although concerning, these events have not yet been shown to cause a significant increase in late morbidity or mortality, probably owing to the benefits of DES in reducing the need for repeated revascularization procedures and the avoidance of the complications associated with the development of in-stent restenosis.[117-120] Ongoing evaluation of the long-term safety of DES has engendered intense investigation, with efforts focused on determining whether patient- and lesion-specific risk factors (such as insensitivity to aspirin or thienopyridine derivatives) may contribute, whether these risks are device- or drug-specific phenomena, and whether prolonged dual antiplatelet therapy may ameliorate these risks. Preliminary data suggest that second-generation DES have lower rates of stent thrombosis than the first-generation DES.

TABLE 58-9 Variables Associated with Stent Thrombosis

Clinical Variables
Acute myocardial infarction
Clopidogrel noncompliance and discontinuation
Clopidogrel bioavailability
Diabetes mellitus
Renal failure
Congestive heart failure
Prior radiation brachytherapy
Anatomic Variables
Long lesions
Smaller vessels
Multivessel disease
Acute myocardial infarction
Bifurcation lesions
Procedural Factors
Stent underexpansion
Incomplete wall apposition
Residual inflow and outflow disease
Margin dissections
Crush technique
Overlapping stent
Polymer materials

The not infrequent scenario of a patient's requiring noncardiac surgery in the weeks after PCI can markedly increase the risk of stent thrombosis. Studies of outcomes in patients undergoing noncardiac surgery soon after PCI with BMS have documented stent thrombosis occurring in up to 8% of patients in the first 2 weeks after PCI, with risks declining to baseline rates by 8 weeks. This increased risk probably results from the frequent cessation of thienopyridine therapy before surgery as well as the hypercoagulable state in the perioperative period.

LATE CLINICAL OUTCOMES. Ischemic events within the first year after PCI result from one of three processes. Lumen renarrowing that requires repeated revascularization (i.e., target lesion revascularization) occurs in 20% to 30% of patients undergoing balloon angioplasty because of reparative arterial constriction, also known as negative remodeling. Clinical restenosis after stent implantation is less common (10% to 20%) and is attributable to intimal hyperplasia within the stent. Clinical recurrence caused by restenosis is least common (3% to 5%) after DES placement because of focal tissue growth within the stent or at its margins. A second cause of clinical events after PCI is the progression of coronary atherosclerosis at a site remote from that treated earlier by PCI. Death and MI can also result from sudden rupture of a plaque that is remote from the site of the initial intervention.

These processes can be partially distinguished by the timing of their occurrence. Clinical restenosis resulting from lumen renarrowing at the site of PCI generally develops within the first 6 to 9 months after PCI, whereas death and MI due to plaque instability may occur at any point after PCI at a low but constant rate (1% to 2% risk per year). Predictors of higher risk of all-cause late mortality include advanced age, reduced left ventricular function, congestive heart failure, diabetes mellitus, number of diseased vessels, inoperable disease, and severe comorbid conditions. A 95% 10-year survival rate can be expected in patients with single-vessel CAD, and an 80% survival rate after PCI can be achieved in those with multivessel CAD. In a 5-year follow-up study of patients treated with the TAXUS stent, target vessel revascularization during the first year was driven by target lesion revascularization, and target vessel revascularization after 1 year involved similar numbers of target lesion and non–target lesion revascularization events, primarily due to the progression of atherosclerotic disease.[121] The annualized hazard ratio for non–target lesion revascularization and other major adverse events (including death, MI, and stent thrombosis) was relatively constant beyond 1 year and not significantly different between paclitaxel-eluting stents and BMS.[121]

Outcomes Benchmarking and Procedural Volumes

Along with CABG surgery, PCI ranks among the most studied of all procedures in the United States. National structured outcomes registries such as the National Heart, Lung and Blood Institute (NHLBI) Dynamic Registry[122-126] and the ACC National Cardiovascular Data Registry (NCDR) have been examined.[9,127-130] The NCDR CathPCI Registry also provides contemporary risk-adjusted outcomes benchmarking to hundreds of participating institutions. Participants in such national, regional, or statewide outcomes reporting initiatives can compare their risk-adjusted clinical outcomes with institutions of similar patient mix and size. The detailed nature of these data sets, in which the data collected span the range of patient clinical characteristics, lesion descriptors, and device level information, provides centers with a comprehensive comparison of their practice patterns and outcomes compared with peer institutions. More than 50% of hospitals in the United States participate in the NCDR CathPCI Registry. It is recommended that centers performing PCI participate in a prospective quality assessment and outcomes registry (see PCI Guidelines).

Current guidelines recommend that physicians undergo a 3-year comprehensive cardiac training program with 12 months of training in diagnostic catheterization, during which the trainee performs 300 diagnostic catheterizations, including 200 as the primary operator.[131] Interventional training requires a fourth year of training, including more than 250 interventional procedures but not more than 600, a level that is also required for physicians to be eligible for the American Board of Internal Medicine certifying examination in interventional cardiology.

The guidelines favor performance of PCI by higher volume operators, defined as those performing more than 75 procedures per year at high-volume centers, defined as those in which more than 400 procedures are performed each year. These recommendations are based on the ongoing observation that higher volume operators have lower adverse event rates than lower volume operators.[132,133] In one analysis of 1338 PCIs performed in the United States and Canada, operators with fewer than 100 cases per year had higher rates of 30-day death, MI, or target vessel revascularization (13.2% versus 8.7%; $P = 0.18$) and large MI (7.7% versus 3.3%; $P = 0.06$) than those with 100 or more cases per year.[133] However, a recent analysis of primary PCI found no relationship between hospital PCI volume and mortality in hospitals participating in a quality improvement initiative.[134]

Although PCI has traditionally been performed at centers that offer on-site surgical back-up, more recent analyses have shown that PCI can be performed for STEMI and elective PCI safely, provided PCI is performed by high-volume operators with minimal institutional volumes requirements.[9,135] Off-site PCI is best suited for underserved areas that are geographically far removed from major centers.[136]

Institutions must have a system for quality measurement and improvement that includes valid peer review. The guidelines recommend that quality assessment reviews take into consideration risk adjustment, statistical power, and national benchmark statistics. They should also include tabulation of adverse event rates for comparison with benchmark values and case review of complicated procedures and some uncomplicated procedures.

Future Directions

After three decades of rapid growth and dissemination of coronary interventional techniques and the associated dramatic refinement in the devices used for revascularization, there are still many challenges remaining for the percutaneous treatment of CAD. Ongoing large-scale multicenter randomized trials will assess the safety and efficacy of PCI with DES for patients with unprotected left main coronary artery stenosis and for patients with diabetes and multivessel CAD. Additional technologies are currently in clinical testing for the treatment of complex bifurcation stenosis with use of dedicated bifurcation stent systems. Better techniques to treat chronic total occlusions are being developed.

Continued evolution of drug-eluting design will attempt to optimize effective early endothelialization of the stented segment without sacrificing the long-term benefits of DES in terms of reducing target lesion revascularization.

Determination of the optimal duration of antiplatelet therapy after DES deployment requires further study. Bioabsorbable stents, produced from bioerodable polymers or magnesium alloys, show promise as a mechanism of providing short-term scaffolding to prevent abrupt closure of the vessel and leaving nothing permanent in the vessel wall after 6 months, thereby potentially reducing the risks of stent thrombosis.

Early investigation into myocardial regeneration after acute MI by percutaneous delivery of autologous stem cell or progenitor cell lines has generated great interest in the potential of such therapies to improve myocardial recovery. Continued refinement of ventricular support devices offers hope for myocardial recovery in the setting of severe myocardial dysfunction.

Acknowledgments

The authors acknowledge Donald Baim, MD, and Fred Resnic, MD, for their prior contribution to this chapter and Thomas Lee, MD, for his prior contribution to the Guidelines section.

REFERENCES

1. Lloyd-Jones D, Adams RJ, Brown TM, et al: Heart disease and stroke statistics—2010 update. A report from the American Heart Association. Circulation 121:948, 2010.
2. Boden WE, O'Rourke RA, Teo KK, et al: Optimal medical therapy with or without PCI for stable coronary disease. N Engl J Med 356:1503, 2007.
3. Serruys PW, Morice MC, Kappetein AP, et al: Percutaneous coronary intervention versus coronary-artery bypass grafting for severe coronary artery disease. N Engl J Med 360:961, 2009.
4. Henriques JP, Remmelink M, Baan J Jr, et al: Safety and feasibility of elective high-risk percutaneous coronary intervention procedures with left ventricular support of the Impella Recover LP 2.5. Am J Cardiol 97:990, 2006.
5. Byrne JG, Leacche M, Unic D, et al: Staged initial percutaneous coronary intervention followed by valve surgery ("hybrid approach") for patients with complex coronary and valve disease. J Am Coll Cardiol 45:14, 2005.
6. Popma JJ, Nathan S, Hagberg RC, Khabbaz KR: Hybrid myocardial revascularization: An integrated approach to coronary revascularization. Catheter Cardiovasc Interv 75(Suppl 1):S28, 2010.

Indications for Percutaneous Coronary Intervention

7. Shaw LJ, Berman DS, Maron DJ, et al: Optimal medical therapy with or without percutaneous coronary intervention to reduce ischemic burden: Results from the Clinical Outcomes Utilizing Revascularization and Aggressive Drug Evaluation (COURAGE) trial nuclear substudy. Circulation 117:1283, 2008.
8. Eagle KA, Guyton RA, Davidoff R, et al: ACC/AHA 2004 guideline update for coronary artery bypass graft surgery: Summary article: A report of the American College of Cardiology/American Heart Association Task Force on Practice Guidelines (Committee to Update the 1999 Guidelines for Coronary Artery Bypass Graft Surgery). Circulation 110:1168, 2004.
9. Kutcher MA, Klein LW, Ou FS, et al: Percutaneous coronary interventions in facilities without cardiac surgery on site: A report from the National Cardiovascular Data Registry (NCDR). J Am Coll Cardiol 54:16, 2009.
10. Smith SC Jr, Feldman TE, Hirshfeld JW Jr, et al: ACC/AHA/SCAI 2005 Guideline Update for Percutaneous Coronary Intervention—summary article: A report of the American College of Cardiology/American Heart Association Task Force on Practice Guidelines (ACC/AHA/SCAI Writing Committee to Update the 2001 Guidelines for Percutaneous Coronary Intervention). Circulation 113:156, 2006.
11. King SB 3rd, Smith SC Jr, Hirshfeld JW Jr, et al: 2007 Focused Update of the ACC/AHA/SCAI 2005 Guideline Update for Percutaneous Coronary Intervention: A report of the American College of Cardiology/American Heart Association Task Force on Practice Guidelines: 2007 Writing Group to Review New Evidence and Update the ACC/AHA/SCAI 2005 Guideline Update for Percutaneous Coronary Intervention, Writing on Behalf of the 2005 Writing Committee. Circulation 117:261, 2008.
12. Patel MR, Dehmer GJ, Hirshfeld JW, et al: ACCF/SCAI/STS/AATS/AHA/ASNC 2009 Appropriateness Criteria for Coronary Revascularization: A report by the American College of Cardiology Foundation Appropriateness Criteria Task Force, Society for Cardiovascular Angiography and Interventions, Society of Thoracic Surgeons, American Association for Thoracic Surgery, American Heart Association, and the American Society of Nuclear Cardiology Endorsed by the American Society of Echocardiography, the Heart Failure Society of America, and the Society of Cardiovascular Computed Tomography. J Am Coll Cardiol 53:530, 2009.
13. Smith SC Jr, Feldman TE, Hirshfeld JW Jr, et al: ACC/AHA/SCAI 2005 guideline update for percutaneous coronary intervention: A report of the American College of Cardiology/American Heart Association Task Force on Practice Guidelines (ACC/AHA/SCAI Writing Committee to Update the 2001 Guidelines for Percutaneous Coronary Intervention). J Am Coll Cardiol 47:e1, 2006.
14. King SB 3rd, Smith SC Jr, Hirshfeld JW Jr, et al: 2007 focused update of the ACC/AHA/SCAI 2005 guideline update for percutaneous coronary intervention: A report of the American College of Cardiology/American Heart Association Task Force on Practice guidelines. J Am Coll Cardiol 51:172, 2008.
15. Antman EM, Hand M, Armstrong PW, et al: 2007 Focused Update of the ACC/AHA 2004 Guidelines for the Management of Patients With ST-Elevation Myocardial Infarction: A report of the American College of Cardiology/American Heart Association Task Force on Practice Guidelines: Developed in collaboration with the Canadian Cardiovascular Society endorsed by the American Academy of Family Physicians: 2007 Writing Group to Review New Evidence and Update the ACC/AHA 2004 Guidelines for the Management of Patients With ST-Elevation Myocardial Infarction, Writing on Behalf of the 2004 Writing Committee. Circulation 117:296, 2008.
16. Bavry AA, Kumbhani DJ, Rassi AN, et al: Benefit of early invasive therapy in acute coronary syndromes: A meta-analysis of contemporary randomized clinical trials. J Am Coll Cardiol 48:1319, 2006.

17. Kushner FG, Hand M, Smith SC Jr, et al: 2009 Focused Updates: ACC/AHA Guidelines for the Management of Patients With ST-Elevation Myocardial Infarction (updating the 2004 Guideline and 2007 Focused Update) and ACC/AHA/SCAI Guidelines on Percutaneous Coronary Intervention (updating the 2005 Guideline and 2007 Focused Update): A report of the American College of Cardiology Foundation/American Heart Association Task Force on Practice Guidelines. Circulation 120:2271, 2009.
18. Cohn PF: Enhanced external counterpulsation for the treatment of angina pectoris. Prog Cardiovasc Dis 49:88, 2006.
19. Nichols WW, Estrada JC, Braith RW, et al: Enhanced external counterpulsation treatment improves arterial wall properties and wave reflection characteristics in patients with refractory angina. J Am Coll Cardiol 48:1208, 2006.
20. Shishehbor MH, Lauer MS, Singh IM, et al: In unstable angina or non–ST-segment acute coronary syndrome, should patients with multivessel coronary artery disease undergo multivessel or culprit-only stenting? J Am Coll Cardiol 49:849, 2007.
21. Krone RJ, Shaw RE, Klein LW, et al: Evaluation of the American College of Cardiology/American Heart Association and the Society for Coronary Angiography and Interventions lesion classification system in the current "stent era" of coronary interventions (from the ACC–National Cardiovascular Data Registry). Am J Cardiol 92:389, 2003.
22. Thompson CA, Jayne JE, Robb JF, et al: Retrograde techniques and the impact of operator volume on percutaneous intervention for coronary chronic total occlusions an early U.S. experience. J Am Coll Cardiol Intv 2:834, 2009.
23. Migliorini A, Moschi G, Vergara R, et al: Drug-eluting stent–supported percutaneous coronary intervention for chronic total coronary occlusion. Catheter Cardiovasc Interv 67:344, 2006.
24. Katritsis D, Siontis G, Ioannidis J: Double versus single stenting for coronary bifurcation lesions: A meta-analysis. Circ Cardiovasc Interv 2:409, 2009.
25. Tamburino C, Angiolillo DJ, Capranzano P, et al: Long-term clinical outcomes after drug-eluting stent implantation in unprotected left main coronary artery disease. Catheter Cardiovasc Interv 73:291, 2009.
26. Kandzari DE, Colombo A, Park SJ, et al: Revascularization for unprotected left main disease: Evolution of the evidence basis to redefine treatment standards. J Am Coll Cardiol 54:1576, 2009.
27. Palmerini T, Marzocchi A, Marrozzini C, et al: Comparison between coronary angioplasty and coronary artery bypass surgery for the treatment of unprotected left main coronary artery stenosis (the Bologna Registry). Am J Cardiol 98:54, 2006.
28. Lee MS, Kapoor N, Jamal F, et al: Comparison of coronary artery bypass surgery with percutaneous coronary intervention with drug-eluting stents for unprotected left main coronary artery disease. J Am Coll Cardiol 47:864, 2006.
29. Chieffo A, Morici N, Maisano F, et al: Percutaneous treatment with drug-eluting stent implantation versus bypass surgery for unprotected left main stenosis: A single-center experience. Circulation 113:2542, 2006.
30. Palmerini T, Barlocco F, Santarelli A, et al: A comparison between coronary artery bypass grafting surgery and drug eluting stent for the treatment of unprotected left main coronary artery disease in elderly patients (aged > or =75 years). Eur Heart J 28:2714, 2007.
31. Sanmartin M, Baz JA, Claro R, et al: Comparison of drug-eluting stents versus surgery for unprotected left main coronary artery disease. Am J Cardiol 100:970, 2007.
32. Brener SJ, Galla JM, Bryant R 3rd, et al: Comparison of percutaneous versus surgical revascularization of severe unprotected left main coronary stenosis in matched patients. Am J Cardiol 101:169, 2008.
33. Buszman PE, Kiesz SR, Bochenek A, et al: Acute and late outcomes of unprotected left main stenting in comparison with surgical revascularization. J Am Coll Cardiol 51:538, 2008.
34. Hsu JT, Chu CM, Chang ST, et al: Percutaneous coronary intervention versus coronary artery bypass graft surgery for the treatment of unprotected left main coronary artery stenosis: In-hospital and one year outcome after emergent and elective treatments. Int Heart J 49:355, 2008.
35. Rodes-Cabau J, Deblois J, Bertrand OF, et al: Nonrandomized comparison of coronary artery bypass surgery and percutaneous coronary intervention for the treatment of unprotected left main coronary artery disease in octogenarians. Circulation 118:2374, 2008.
36. Seung KB, Park DW, Kim YH, et al: Stents versus coronary-artery bypass grafting for left main coronary artery disease. N Engl J Med 358:1781, 2008.
37. Wu C, Hannan EL, Walford G, et al: Utilization and outcomes of unprotected left main coronary artery stenting and coronary artery bypass graft surgery. Ann Thorac Surg 86:1153, 2008.
38. Sjauw KD, Engstrom AE, Vis MM, et al: A systematic review and meta-analysis of intra-aortic balloon pump therapy in ST-elevation myocardial infarction: Should we change the guidelines? Eur Heart J 30:459, 2009.
39. Vranckx P, Otten A, Schultz C, et al: Assisted circulation using the TandemHeart, percutaneous transseptal left ventricular assist device, during percutaneous aortic valve implantation: The Rotterdam experience. EuroIntervention 5:465, 2009.
40. Vranckx P, Schultz CJ, Valgimigli M, et al: Assisted circulation using the TandemHeart during very high-risk PCI of the unprotected left main coronary artery in patients declined for CABG. Catheter Cardiovasc Interv 74:302, 2009.
41. Dixon SR, Henriques JP, Mauri L, et al: A prospective feasibility trial investigating the use of the Impella 2.5 system in patients undergoing high-risk percutaneous coronary intervention (the PROTECT I Trial): Initial U.S. experience. J Am Coll Cardiol Intv 2:91, 2009.
42. Lam K, Sjauw KD, Henriques JP, et al: Improved microcirculation in patients with an acute ST-elevation myocardial infarction treated with the Impella LP2.5 percutaneous left ventricular assist device. Clin Res Cardiol 98:311, 2009.
43. McCullough P: Outcomes of contrast-induced nephropathy: Experience in patients undergoing cardiovascular intervention. Catheter Cardiovasc Interv 67:335, 2006.

Vascular Access

44. Vavalle JP, Rao SV: The association between the transradial approach for percutaneous coronary interventions and bleeding. J Invasive Cardiol 21(Suppl A):21A, 2009.
45. Kern MJ: Cardiac catheterization on the road less traveled. J Am Coll Cardiol Intv 2:1055, 2009.
46. Eichhofer J, Horlick E, Ivanov J, et al: Decreased complication rates using the transradial compared to the transfemoral approach in percutaneous coronary intervention in the era of routine stenting and glycoprotein platelet IIb/IIIa inhibitor use: A large single-center experience. Am Heart J 156:864, 2008.
47. Jolly SS, Amlani S, Hamon M, et al: Radial versus femoral access for coronary angiography or intervention and the impact on major bleeding and ischemic events: A systematic review and meta-analysis of randomized trials. Am Heart J 157:132, 2009.
48. Brueck M, Bandorski D, Kramer W, et al: A randomized comparison of transradial versus transfemoral approach for coronary angiography and angioplasty. J Am Coll Cardiol Intv 2:1047, 2009.
49. Degghani P, Mohammad A, Bajaj R, et al: Mechanism and predictors of failed transradial approach for percutaneous coronary interventions. J Am Coll Cardiol Intv 2:1057, 2009.
50. Kugelmass AD, Cohen DJ, Brown PP, et al: Hospital resources consumed in treating complications associated with percutaneous coronary interventions. Am J Cardiol 97:322, 2006.
51. Ellis SG, Bhatt D, Kapadia S, et al: Correlates and outcomes of retroperitoneal hemorrhage complicating percutaneous coronary intervention. Catheter Cardiovasc Interv 67:541, 2006.
52. Eikelboom JW, Mehta SR, Anand SS, et al: Adverse impact of bleeding on prognosis in patients with acute coronary syndromes. Circulation 114:774, 2006.
53. Tavris DR, Gallauresi BA, Lin B, et al: Risk of local adverse events following cardiac catheterization by hemostasis device use and gender. J Invasive Cardiol 16:459, 2004.
54. Exaire JE, Dauerman HL, Topol EJ, et al: Triple antiplatelet therapy does not increase femoral access bleeding with vascular closure devices. Am Heart J 147:31, 2004.
55. Koreny M, Riedmuller E, Nikfardjam M, et al: Arterial puncture closing devices compared with standard manual compression after cardiac catheterization: Systematic review and meta-analysis. JAMA 291:350, 2004.
56. Vaitkus PT: A meta-analysis of percutaneous vascular closure devices after diagnostic catheterization and percutaneous coronary intervention. J Invasive Cardiol 16:243, 2004.
57. Nikolsky E, Mehran R, Halkin A, et al: Vascular complications associated with arteriotomy closure devices in patients undergoing percutaneous coronary procedures: A meta-analysis. J Am Coll Cardiol 44:1200, 2004.
58. Applegate RJ, Sacrinty M, Kutcher MA, et al: Vascular complications with newer generations of angioseal vascular closure devices. J Interv Cardiol 19:67, 2006.
58a. Arora N, Matheny ME, Sepke C, Resnic FS: A propensity analysis of the risk of vascular complications after cardiac catheterization procedures with the use of vascular closure devices. Am Heart J 153:606, 2007.
59. Dauerman HL, Applegate RJ, Cohen DJ: Vascular closure devices: The second decade. J Am Coll Cardiol 50:1617, 2007.
60. Wong SC, Bachinsky W, Cambier P, et al: A randomized comparison of a novel bioabsorbable vascular closure device versus manual compression in the achievement of hemostasis after percutaneous femoral procedures: The ECLIPSE (Ensure's Vascular Closure Device Speeds Hemostasis Trial). J Am Coll Cardiol Intv 2:785, 2009.
61. Chhatriwalla AK, Bhatt DL: You can't keep a good man (or woman) down. J Invasive Cardiol 18:109, 2006.
62. Chhatriwalla AK, Bhatt DL: Walk this way: Early ambulation after cardiac catheterization—good for the patient and the health care system. Mayo Clin Proc 81:1535, 2006.

Coronary Devices

63. Ali A, Cox D, Dib N, et al: Rheolytic thrombectomy with percutaneous coronary intervention for infarct size reduction in acute myocardial infarction: 30-day results from a multicenter randomized study. J Am Coll Cardiol 48:244, 2006.
64. Svilaas T, Vlaar PJ, van der Horst IC, et al: Thrombus aspiration during primary percutaneous coronary intervention. N Engl J Med 358:557, 2008.
65. Bavry AA, Kumbhani DJ, Bhatt DL: Role of adjunctive thrombectomy and embolic protection devices in acute myocardial infarction: A comprehensive meta-analysis of randomized trials. Eur Heart J 29:2989, 2008.
66. Mauri L, Rogers C, Baim DS: Devices for distal protection during percutaneous coronary revascularization. Circulation 113:2651, 2006.
67. Holmes DR Jr, Teirstein P, Satler L, et al: Sirolimus-eluting stents vs vascular brachytherapy for in-stent restenosis within bare-metal stents: The SISR randomized trial. JAMA 295:1264, 2006.
68. Stone GW, Ellis SG, O'Shaughnessy CD, et al: Paclitaxel-eluting stents vs vascular brachytherapy for in-stent restenosis within bare-metal stents: The TAXUS V ISR randomized trial. JAMA 295:1253, 2006.
69. Stone GW, Lansky AJ, Pocock SJ, et al: Paclitaxel-eluting stents versus bare-metal stents in acute myocardial infarction. N Engl J Med 360:1946, 2009.
70. Chhatriwalla AK, Bhatt DL: Should dual antiplatelet therapy after drug-eluting stents be continued for more than 1 year? Dual antiplatelet therapy after drug-eluting stents should be continued for more than one year and preferably indefinitely. Circ Cardiovasc Interv 1:217, 2008.
71. Bavry AA, Kumbhani DJ, Helton TJ, et al: Late thrombosis of drug-eluting stents: A meta-analysis of randomized clinical trials. Am J Med 119:1056, 2006.
72. Pendyala LK, Yin X, Li J, et al: The first-generation drug-eluting stents and coronary endothelial function. J Am Coll Cardiol Intv 2:1169, 2009.
73. Caixeta A, Leon MB, Lansky AJ, et al: 5-Year clinical outcomes after sirolimus-eluting stent implantation insights from a patient-level pooled analysis of 4 randomized trials comparing sirolimus-eluting stents with bare-metal stents. J Am Coll Cardiol 54:894, 2009.
74. Weisz G, Leon MB, Holmes DR Jr, et al: Five-year follow-up after sirolimus-eluting stent implantation results of the SIRIUS (Sirolimus-Eluting Stent in De-Novo Native Coronary Lesions) trial. J Am Coll Cardiol 53:1488, 2009.
75. Eisenstein E, Wijns W, Fajadet J, et al: Long-term clinical and economic analysis of the Endeavor drug-eluting stent versus the Driver bare metal stent. J Am Coll Cardiol Intv 2:1178, 2009.
76. Eisenstein EL, Leon MB, Kandzari DE, et al: Long-term clinical and economic analysis of the Endeavor zotarolimus-eluting stent versus the Cypher sirolimus-eluting stent. J Am Coll Cardiol Intv 2:1199, 2009.
77. Popma JJ, Mauri L, O'Shaughnessy C, et al: Frequency and clinical consequences associated with sidebranch occlusion during stent implantation using zotarolimus-eluting and paclitaxel-eluting coronary stents. Circ Cardiovasc Interv 2:133, 2009.
78. Leon MB, Kandzari DE, Eisenstein EL, et al: Late safety, efficacy, and cost-effectiveness of a zotarolimus-eluting stent compared with a paclitaxel-eluting stent in patients with de novo coronary lesions. J Am Coll Cardiol Intv 2:1208, 2009.
79. Stone GW, Midei M, Newman W, et al: Comparison of an everolimus-eluting stent and a paclitaxel-eluting stent in patients with coronary artery disease: A randomized trial. JAMA 299:190, 2008.

Antiplatelet Agents

80. Cuisset T, Frere C, Quilici J, et al: Benefit of a 600-mg loading dose of clopidogrel on platelet reactivity and clinical outcomes in patients with non–ST-segment elevation acute coronary syndrome undergoing coronary stenting. J Am Coll Cardiol 48:1339, 2006.
81. Montalescot G, Sideris G, Meuleman C, et al: A randomized comparison of high clopidogrel loading doses in patients with non–ST-segment elevation acute coronary syndromes: The ALBION (Assessment of the Best Loading Dose of Clopidogrel to Blunt Platelet Activation, Inflammation and Ongoing Necrosis) trial. J Am Coll Cardiol 48:931, 2006.
82. Mehta SR, Bassand JP, Chrolavicius S, et al: Design and rationale of CURRENT-OASIS 7: A randomized, 2 × 2 factorial trial evaluating optimal dosing strategies for clopidogrel and aspirin in patients with ST and non–ST-elevation acute coronary syndromes managed with an early invasive strategy. Am Heart J 156:1080, 2008.
83. Wiviott SD, Trenk D, Frelinger AL, et al: Prasugrel compared with high loading- and maintenance-dose clopidogrel in patients with planned percutaneous coronary intervention: The Prasugrel in Comparison to Clopidogrel for Inhibition of Platelet Activation and Aggregation-Thrombolysis in Myocardial Infarction 44 trial. Circulation 116:2923, 2007.
84. Wiviott SD, Braunwald E, McCabe CH, et al: Prasugrel versus clopidogrel in patients with acute coronary syndromes. N Engl J Med 357:2001, 2007.
85. Bhatt DL: Intensifying platelet inhibition—navigating between Scylla and Charybdis. N Engl J Med 357:2078, 2007.
86. Mega JL, Close SL, Wiviott SD, et al: Cytochrome P450 genetic polymorphisms and the response to prasugrel: Relationship to pharmacokinetic, pharmacodynamic, and clinical outcomes. Circulation 119:2553, 2009.
87. Bhatt DL: Prasugrel in clinical practice. N Engl J Med 361:940, 2009.
88. James S, Akerblom A, Cannon CP, et al: Comparison of ticagrelor, the first reversible oral $P2Y_{12}$ receptor antagonist, with clopidogrel in patients with acute coronary syndromes: Rationale, design, and baseline characteristics of the PLATelet inhibition and patient Outcomes (PLATO) trial. Am Heart J 157:599, 2009.
89. Wallentin L, Becker RC, Budaj A, et al: Ticagrelor versus clopidogrel in patients with acute coronary syndromes. N Engl J Med 361:1045, 2009.
90. Van't Hof AW, Ten Berg J, Heestermans T, et al: Prehospital initiation of tirofiban in patients with ST-elevation myocardial infarction undergoing primary angioplasty (On-TIME 2): A multicentre, double-blind, randomised controlled trial. Lancet 372:537, 2008.
91. Kastrati A, Mehilli J, Neumann FJ, et al: Abciximab in patients with acute coronary syndromes undergoing percutaneous coronary intervention after clopidogrel pretreatment: The ISAR-REACT 2 randomized trial. JAMA 295:1531, 2006.
92. Gurm HS, Tamhane U, Meier P, et al: A comparison of abciximab and small-molecule glycoprotein IIb/IIIa inhibitors in patients undergoing primary percutaneous coronary intervention: A meta-analysis of contemporary randomized controlled trials. Circ Cardiovasc Interv 2:230, 2009.
93. De Luca G, Ucci G, Cassetti E, et al: Benefits from small molecule administration as compared with abciximab among patients with ST-segment elevation myocardial infarction treated with primary angioplasty: A meta-analysis. J Am Coll Cardiol 3:166, 2009.
94. Mehilli J, Kastrati A, Schulz S, et al: Abciximab in patients with acute ST-segment-elevation myocardial infarction undergoing primary percutaneous coronary intervention after clopidogrel loading: A randomized double-blind trial. Circulation 119:1933, 2009.
95. Stone GW, Witzenbichler B, Guagliumi G, et al: Bivalirudin during primary PCI in acute myocardial infarction. N Engl J Med 358:2218, 2008.

Antithrombin Agents

96. Gurm HS, Eagle KA: Use of anticoagulants in ST-segment elevation myocardial infarction patients; a focus on low-molecular-weight heparin. Cardiovasc Drugs Ther 22:59, 2008.
97. Ferguson JJ, Califf RM, Antman EM, et al: Enoxaparin vs unfractionated heparin in high-risk patients with non–ST-segment elevation acute coronary syndromes managed with an intended early invasive strategy: Primary results of the SYNERGY randomized trial. JAMA 292:45, 2004.
98. Kastrati A, Neumann FJ, Mehilli J, et al: Bivalirudin versus unfractionated heparin during percutaneous coronary intervention. N Engl J Med 359:688, 2008.
99. Lincoff AM, Bittl JA, Harrington RA, et al: Bivalirudin and provisional glycoprotein IIb/IIIa blockade compared with heparin and planned glycoprotein IIb/IIIa blockade during percutaneous coronary intervention: REPLACE-2 randomized trial. JAMA 289:853, 2003.
100. Stone G, McLaurin B, Cox D, et al: Bivalirudin for patients with acute coronary syndromes. N Engl J Med 355:2203, 2006.
101. White HD, Chew DP, Hoekstra JW, et al: Safety and efficacy of switching from either unfractionated heparin or enoxaparin to bivalirudin in patients with non–ST-segment elevation acute coronary syndromes managed with an invasive strategy: Results from the ACUITY (Acute Catheterization and Urgent Intervention Triage strategY) trial. J Am Coll Cardiol 51:1734, 2008.
102. Pinto DS, Stone GW, Shi C, et al: Economic evaluation of bivalirudin with or without glycoprotein IIb/IIIa inhibition versus heparin with routine glycoprotein IIb/IIIa inhibition for early invasive management of acute coronary syndromes. J Am Coll Cardiol 52:1758, 2008.
103. Lincoff AM, Steinhubl SR, Manoukian SV, et al: Influence of timing of clopidogrel treatment on the efficacy and safety of bivalirudin in patients with non–ST-segment elevation acute coronary syndromes undergoing percutaneous coronary intervention: An analysis of the ACUITY (Acute Catheterization and Urgent Intervention Triage strategY) trial. J Am Coll Cardiol Intv 1:639, 2008.
104. Yusuf S, Mehta SR, Chrolavicius S, et al: Comparison of fondaparinux and enoxaparin in acute coronary syndromes. N Engl J Med 354:1464, 2006.
105. Yusuf S, Mehta SR, Chrolavicius S, et al: Effects of fondaparinux on mortality and reinfarction in patients with acute ST-segment elevation myocardial infarction: The OASIS-6 randomized trial. JAMA 295:1519, 2006.

Outcomes After Percutaneous Coronary Intervention

106. Williams DO, Abbott JD, Kip KE: Outcomes of 6906 patients undergoing percutaneous coronary intervention in the era of drug-eluting stents: Report of the DEScover Registry. Circulation 114:2154, 2006.
107. Hannan EL, Wu C, Bennett EV, et al: Risk index for predicting in-hospital mortality for cardiac valve surgery. Ann Thorac Surg 83:921, 2007.
108. MacKenzie TA, Malenka DJ, Olmstead EM, et al: Prediction of survival after coronary revascularization: Modeling short-term, mid-term, and long-term survival. Ann Thorac Surg 87:463, 2009.
109. Hamburger JN, Walsh SJ, Khurana R, et al: Percutaneous coronary intervention and 30-day mortality: The British Columbia PCI risk score. Catheter Cardiovasc Interv 74:377, 2009.
110. Bhatt DL, Topol EJ: Does creatinine kinase–MB elevation after percutaneous coronary intervention predict outcomes in 2005? Periprocedural cardiac enzyme elevation predicts adverse outcomes. Circulation 112:906, 2005.
111. Thygesen K, Alpert JS, White HD, et al: Universal definition of myocardial infarction. Circulation 116:2634, 2007.
112. Prasad A, Gersh BJ, Bertrand ME, et al: Prognostic significance of periprocedural versus spontaneously occurring myocardial infarction after percutaneous coronary intervention in patients with acute coronary syndromes: An analysis from the ACUITY (Acute Catheterization and Urgent Intervention Triage Strategy) trial. J Am Coll Cardiol 54:477, 2009.
113. Javaid A, Buch AN, Satler LF, et al: Management and outcomes of coronary artery perforation during percutaneous coronary intervention. Am J Cardiol 98:911, 2006.
114. Harding SA: The role of vasodilators in the prevention and treatment of no-reflow following percutaneous coronary intervention. Heart 92:1191, 2006.
115. Cutlip DE, Windecker S, Mehran R, et al: Clinical end points in coronary stent trials: A case for standardized definitions. Circulation 115:2344, 2007.
116. Mauri L, Hsieh WH, Massaro JM, et al: Stent thrombosis in randomized clinical trials of drug-eluting stents. N Engl J Med 356:1020, 2007.
117. Bavry AA, Bhatt DL: Appropriate use of drug-eluting stents: Balancing the reduction in restenosis with the concern of late thrombosis. Lancet 371:2134, 2008.
118. Chen MS, John JM, Chew DP, et al: Bare metal stent restenosis is not a benign clinical entity. Am Heart J 151:1260, 2006.
119. Sarkees ML, Bavry AA, Galla JM, et al: Bare metal stent thrombosis 13 years after implantation. Cardiovasc Revasc Med 10:58, 2009.
120. Roukoz H, Bavry AA, Sarkees ML, et al: Comprehensive meta-analysis on drug-eluting stents versus bare-metal stents during extended follow-up. Am J Med 122:581, 2009.
121. Leon MB, Allocco DJ, Dawkins KD, et al: Late clinical events after drug-eluting stents: The interplay between stent-related and natural history-driven events. J Am Coll Cardiol Intv 2:504, 2009.
122. Mulukutla SR, Vlachos HA, Marroquin OC, et al: Impact of drug-eluting stents among insulin-treated diabetic patients: A report from the National Heart, Lung, and Blood Institute Dynamic Registry. J Am Coll Cardiol Intv 1:139, 2008.
123. Srinivas VS, Selzer F, Wilensky RL, et al: Completeness of revascularization for multivessel coronary artery disease and its effect on one-year outcome: A report from the NHLBI Dynamic Registry. J Interv Cardiol 20:373, 2007.
124. Abbott JD, Voss MR, Nakamura M, et al: Unrestricted use of drug-eluting stents compared with bare-metal stents in routine clinical practice: Findings from the National Heart, Lung, and Blood Institute Dynamic Registry. J Am Coll Cardiol 50:2029, 2007.
125. Abbott JD, Ahmed HN, Vlachos HA, et al: Comparison of outcome in patients with ST-elevation versus non–ST-elevation acute myocardial infarction treated with percutaneous coronary intervention (from the National Heart, Lung, and Blood Institute Dynamic Registry). Am J Cardiol 100:190, 2007.
126. Abbott JD, Vlachos HA, Selzer F, et al: Gender-based outcomes in percutaneous coronary intervention with drug-eluting stents (from the National Heart, Lung, and Blood Institute Dynamic Registry). Am J Cardiol 99:626, 2007.
127. Frutkin AD, Lindsey JB, Mehta SK, et al: Drug-eluting stents and the use of percutaneous coronary intervention among patients with class I indications for coronary artery bypass surgery undergoing index revascularization: Analysis from the NCDR (National Cardiovascular Data Registry). J Am Coll Cardiol Intv 2:614, 2009.
128. Diercks DB, Kontos MC, Chen AY, et al: Utilization and impact of pre-hospital electrocardiograms for patients with acute ST-segment elevation myocardial infarction: Data from the NCDR (National Cardiovascular Data Registry) ACTION (Acute Coronary Treatment and Intervention Outcomes Network) Registry. J Am Coll Cardiol 53:161, 2009.
129. Akhter N, Milford-Beland S, Roe MT, et al: Gender differences among patients with acute coronary syndromes undergoing percutaneous coronary intervention in the American College of Cardiology–National Cardiovascular Data Registry (ACC-NCDR). Am Heart J 157:141, 2009.
130. Wang TY, Peterson ED, Dai D, et al: Patterns of cardiac marker surveillance after elective percutaneous coronary intervention and implications for the use of periprocedural myocardial infarction as a quality metric: A report from the National Cardiovascular Data Registry (NCDR). J Am Coll Cardiol 51:2068, 2008.
131. Beller GA, Bonow RO, Fuster V: ACCF 2008 Recommendations for Training in Adult Cardiovascular Medicine Core Cardiovascular Training (COCATS 3). Revision of the 2002 COCATS training statement. J Am Coll Cardiol 51:335, 2008.
132. Kansagra SM, Curtis LH, Anstrom KJ, et al: Trends in operator and hospital procedure volume and outcomes for percutaneous transluminal coronary angioplasty, 1996 to 2001. Am J Cardiol 99:339, 2007.
133. Madan M, Nikhil J, Hellkamp AS, et al: Effect of operator and institutional volume on clinical outcomes after percutaneous coronary interventions performed in Canada and the United States: A brief report from the Enhanced Suppression of the Platelet glycoprotein IIb/IIIa Receptor with Integrilin Therapy (ESPRIT) study. Can J Cardiol 25:e269, 2009.
134. Pottenger BC, Diercks DB, Bhatt DL: Regionalization of care for ST-segment elevation myocardial infarction: Is it too soon? Ann Emerg Med 52:677, 2008.
135. Singh M, Gersh BJ, Lennon RJ, et al: Outcomes of a system-wide protocol for elective and nonelective coronary angioplasty at sites without on-site surgery: The Mayo Clinic experience. Mayo Clin Proc 84:501, 2009.
136. Kumbhani DJ, Cannon CP, Fonarow GC, et al: Association of hospital primary angioplasty volume in ST-segment elevation myocardial infarction with quality and outcomes. JAMA 302:2207, 2009.

GUIDELINES JEFFREY J. POPMA AND DEEPAK L. BHATT

Percutaneous Coronary Intervention

The American College of Cardiology/American Heart Association (ACC/AHA) published their initial guidelines for the performance of percutaneous coronary intervention (PCI) in 2001[1] and have since provided a series of focused updates that revised selected recommendations on the basis of the ever-expanding clinical evidence base and evolving practice patterns.[2-4] In aggregate, these guidelines have provided clinicians with the tools required to enhance their clinical decision making in patients undergoing percutaneous revascularization.

Like other ACC/AHA guidelines, these use the standard ACC/AHA classification system for indications:

Class I: conditions for which there is evidence and/or general agreement that the test is useful and effective

Class II: conditions for which there is conflicting evidence and/or a divergence of opinion about the usefulness or efficacy of performing the test

Class IIa: weight of evidence or opinion is in favor of usefulness or efficacy

Class IIb: usefulness or efficacy is less well established by evidence/opinion

Class III: conditions for which there is evidence and/or general agreement that the test is not useful or effective and in some cases may be harmful

Three levels are used to rate the evidence on which recommendations have been based.

Level A: recommendations are derived from data from multiple randomized clinical trials.

Level B: recommendations are derived from a single randomized trial or nonrandomized studies.

Level C: recommendations are based on the consensus opinion of experts.

CLINICAL PRESENTATION

Guidelines relevant to the use of PCI for stable ischemic heart disease (**Table 58G-1**), unstable angina with ST elevation myocardial infarction (UA/NSTEMI) (**Table 58G-2**), and ST elevation myocardial infarction (STEMI) (**Table 58G-3**) are provided. Guidelines are also included for patients undergoing PCI with left main stenoses or prior coronary bypass surgery, for patients with acute myocardial infarction complicated by thrombus, and for those undergoing drug-eluting stent placement (**Table 58G-4**).

TABLE 58G-1 ACC/AHA Recommendations for Percutaneous Coronary Intervention in Patients with Stable Coronary Artery Disease[2-4]

INDICATION	CLASS	RECOMMENDATION	LOE
Asymptomatic ischemia or CCS Class I or II angina	Class IIa	Patients with one or more significant lesions in 1 or 2 coronary arteries suitable for PCI with a high likelihood of success and a low risk of morbidity and mortality. The vessels to be dilated must subtend a moderate to large area of viable myocardium or be associated with a moderate to severe degree of ischemia on noninvasive testing.	B
		Recurrent stenosis after PCI with a large area of viable myocardium or high-risk criteria on noninvasive testing	C
		Significant left main CAD (>50% diameter stenosis) in patients who are candidates for revascularization but are not eligible for CABG	B
	Class IIb	Effectiveness of PCI for patients with 2- or 3-vessel CAD with significant proximal LAD disease who are otherwise eligible for CABG with one arterial conduit and who have treated diabetes or abnormal LV function is not well established	B
		Nonproximal LAD stenosis that subtends a moderate area of viable myocardium and ischemia on noninvasive testing	C
	Class III	Not recommended in patients with one or more of the following: • Only a small area of viable myocardium at risk • No objective evidence of ischemia • Lesions that have a low likelihood of successful dilation • Mild symptoms that are unlikely to be due to myocardial ischemia • Factors associated with increased risk of morbidity or mortality • Left main disease and eligibility for CABG • Insignificant disease (<50% coronary stenosis)	C
CCS Class III angina	Class IIa	Patients with single-vessel or multivessel CAD who are undergoing medical therapy and who have one or more significant lesions in one or more coronary arteries suitable for PCI with a high likelihood of success and low risk of morbidity or mortality	B
		Patients with single-vessel or multivessel CAD who are undergoing medical therapy with focal saphenous vein graft lesions or multiple stenoses and are poor candidates for reoperative surgery	C
		Patients with significant left main CAD (>50% diameter stenosis) who are candidates for revascularization but are not eligible for CABG	B
	Class IIb	Patients with single-vessel or multivessel CAD who are undergoing medical therapy and who have one or more lesions to be dilated with a reduced likelihood of success	B
		Patients with no evidence of ischemia on noninvasive testing or who are undergoing medical therapy and have 2- or 3-vessel CAD with significant proximal LAD stenosis and treated diabetes or abnormal LV function	B
	Class III	Not recommended for patients with single-vessel or multivessel CAD, no evidence of myocardial injury or ischemia on objective testing, and no trial of medical therapy or who have one of the following: • Only a small area of myocardium at risk • All lesions or the culprit lesion to be dilated with morphology that conveys a low likelihood of success • A high risk of procedure-related morbidity or mortality • Insignificant disease (<50% coronary stenosis) • Significant left main CAD and candidacy for CABG	C

CABG = coronary artery bypass graft surgery; CAD = coronary artery disease; CCS = Canadian Cardiovascular Society; LAD = left anterior descending coronary artery; LOE = level of evidence; LV = left ventricular; PCI = percutaneous coronary intervention.

TABLE 58G-2 ACC/AHA Recommendations for Percutaneous Coronary Intervention in Patients with Unstable Angina or NSTEMI[2-4]

INDICATION	CLASS	RECOMMENDATION	LOE
Unstable angina or non–ST-segment myocardial infarction	Class I	Early invasive PCI strategy for patients who have no serious comorbidity and who have coronary lesions amenable to PCI and who have characteristics for invasive therapy	A
		Patients with 1- or 2- vessel CAD with or without significant proximal LAD disease but with a large area of viable myocardium and high-risk criteria on noninvasive testing[3]	B
		Patients with multivessel CAD with suitable coronary anatomy, normal LV function, and without diabetes mellitus	A
		An intravenous platelet GP IIb/IIIa inhibitor is useful in UA/NSTEMI patients undergoing PCI.	A
		An early invasive strategy (i.e., diagnostic angiography with intent to perform PCI) is indicated in patients who have refractory angina or hemodynamic or electrical instability (without serious comorbidities or contraindications to such procedures).	B
		Patients selected for an invasive approach should receive dual antiplatelet therapy. • Aspirin should be initiated on presentation. • The recommended second agent is clopidogrel (before or at the time of PCI) or prasugrel (at the time of PCI).	A A A B
	Class IIa	Patients with focal saphenous vein graft lesions or multiple stenoses who are undergoing medical therapy and who are poor candidates for reoperative surgery	C
		Patients with 1- or 2-vessel CAD with or without significant proximal LAD disease but with a moderate area of viable myocardium and ischemia on noninvasive testing	B
		Patients with 1-vessel CAD with significant proximal LAD disease	B
		Patients with significant left main CAD (>50% diameter stenosis) who are candidates for revascularization but are not eligible for CABG or who require emergency intervention at angiography for hemodynamic instability	B
		It is reasonable for initially stabilized high-risk patients with GRACE (Global Registry of Acute Coronary Events) risk score above 140 to undergo an early invasive strategy within 12 to 24 hours of admission. For patients not at high risk, an early invasive approach is also reasonable.	B
	Class IIb	Patients with 1-vessel or multivessel CAD, in the absence of high-risk features associated with UA/NSTEMI, who are undergoing medical therapy and who have one or more lesions to be dilated with a reduced likelihood of success	B
		Patients who are undergoing medical therapy who have 2- or 3-vessel CAD, significant proximal LAD disease, and treated diabetes or abnormal LV function, with anatomy suitable for catheter-based therapy	B
		In initially stabilized patients, an initially conservative (i.e., a selectively invasive) strategy may be considered as a treatment strategy for patients (without serious comorbidities or contraindications to such procedures) who have an elevated risk for clinical events including those who are troponin positive.	B
		The decision to implement an initial conservative (versus initial invasive) strategy may be made by considering physician and patient preference.	C
	Class III	Not recommended for patients with 1- or 2-vessel CAD without significant proximal LAD disease with no current symptoms or symptoms that are unlikely to be due to myocardial ischemia and who have no ischemia on noninvasive testing	C
		In the absence of high-risk features associated with UA/NSTEMI, PCI is not recommended for patients with UA/NSTEMI who have single-vessel or multivessel CAD and no trial of medical therapy or who have 1 or more of the following: • Only a small area of myocardium at risk • All lesions or the culprit lesion to be dilated with morphology that conveys a low likelihood of success • A high risk of procedure-related morbidity or mortality • Insignificant disease (<50% coronary stenosis) • Significant left main CAD and candidacy for CABG	C C C C B B
		A PCI strategy in stable patients with persistently occluded infarct-related coronary arteries after NSTEMI is not indicated.	B

CABG = coronary artery bypass graft surgery; CAD = coronary artery disease; GP = glycoprotein; LAD = left anterior descending coronary artery; LOE = level of evidence; LV = left ventricular; NSTEMI = non–ST-segment elevation myocardial infarction; PCI = percutaneous coronary intervention; UA = unstable angina.

TABLE 58G-3 ACC/AHA Recommendations for Percutaneous Coronary Intervention in Patients with STEMI[2-5]

INDICATION	CLASS	RECOMMENDATION	LOE
ST-segment myocardial infarction	Class I	If immediately available, primary PCI should be performed in patients with STEMI (including true posterior MI) or MI with new or presumably new left bundle branch block who can undergo PCI of the infarct artery within 12 hours of symptom onset, if performed in a timely fashion (balloon inflation goal within 90 minutes of presentation) by persons skilled in the procedure (individuals who perform more than 75 PCI procedures per year, ideally at least 11 PCIs per year for STEMI). The procedure should be supported by experienced personnel in an appropriate laboratory environment (one that performs more than 200 PCI procedures per year, of which at least 36 are primary PCI for STEMI, and that has cardiac surgery capability).	A
		Primary PCI should be performed as quickly as possible, with a goal of a medical contact-to-balloon or door-to-balloon time within 90 minutes.	B
		Primary PCI should be performed in patients with severe congestive heart failure and/or pulmonary edema (Killip Class III) and onset of symptoms within 12 hours. The medical contact-to-balloon or door-to-balloon time should be as short as possible (i.e., goal within 90 minutes).	B
	Class IIa	It is reasonable to perform primary PCI for patients with onset of symptoms within the prior 12 to 24 hours and 1 or more of the following: • Severe congestive heart failure • Hemodynamic or electrical instability • Evidence of persistent ischemia	C
	Class IIb	The benefit of primary PCI for STEMI patients eligible for fibrinolysis when performed by an operator who performs fewer than 75 PCI procedures per year (or fewer than 11 PCIs for STEMI per year) is not well established.	C
	Class III	Elective PCI should not be performed in a non–infarct-related artery at the time of primary PCI of the infarct-related artery in patients without hemodynamic compromise.	C
		Primary PCI should not be performed in asymptomatic patients more than 12 hours after onset of STEMI who are hemodynamically and electrically stable.	C
PCI in fibrinolytic-ineligible patients	Class I	Primary PCI should be performed in fibrinolytic-ineligible patients who present with STEMI within 12 hours of symptom onset.	C
	Class IIa	It is reasonable to perform primary PCI for fibrinolytic-ineligible patients with onset of symptoms within the prior 12 to 24 hours and 1 or more of the following: • Severe congestive heart failure • Hemodynamic or electrical instability • Evidence of persistent ischemia	C
Facilitated PCI	Class IIb	Patients who are not at high risk who receive fibrinolytic therapy as primary reperfusion therapy at a non–PCI-capable facility may be considered for transfer as soon as possible to a PCI-capable facility where PCI can be performed either when needed or as a pharmacoinvasive strategy. Consideration should be given to initiating a preparatory antithrombotic (anticoagulant plus antiplatelet) regimen before and during patient transfer to the catheterization laboratory.	C
	Class III	A planned reperfusion strategy using full-dose fibrinolytic therapy followed by immediate PCI may be harmful.	C
Rescue PCI	Class I	A strategy of coronary angiography with intent to perform PCI (or emergency CABG) is recommended for patients who have received fibrinolytic therapy and have any of the following:	
		• Cardiogenic shock in patients younger than 75 years who are suitable candidates for revascularization	B
		• Severe congestive heart failure and/or pulmonary edema (Killip Class III)	B
		• Hemodynamically compromising ventricular arrhythmias	C
	Class IIa	A strategy of coronary angiography with intent to perform PCI (or emergency CABG) is reasonable in patients 75 years of age or older who have received fibrinolytic therapy and are in cardiogenic shock, provided they are suitable candidates for revascularization.	B
		It is reasonable to perform rescue PCI for patients with 1 or more of the following: • Hemodynamic or electrical instability • Persistent ischemic symptoms	C
		A strategy of coronary angiography with intent to perform rescue PCI is reasonable for patients in whom fibrinolytic therapy has failed (ST-segment elevation <50% resolved after 90 minutes following initiation of fibrinolytic therapy in the lead showing the worst initial elevation) and a moderate or large area of myocardium is at risk (anterior MI, inferior MI with right ventricular involvement or precordial ST-segment depression).	B
	Class III	A strategy of coronary angiography with intent to perform PCI (or emergency CABG) is not recommended in patients who have received fibrinolytic therapy if further invasive management is contraindicated or the patient or designee does not wish further invasive care.	C

TABLE 58G-3 ACC/AHA Recommendations for Percutaneous Coronary Intervention in Patients with STEMI[2-5]—cont'd

INDICATION	CLASS	RECOMMENDATION	LOE
PCI after successful fibrinolysis or for patients not undergoing primary reperfusion	Class I	In patients whose anatomy is suitable, PCI should be performed when there is objective evidence of recurrent MI.	C
		In patients whose anatomy is suitable, PCI should be performed for moderate or severe spontaneous or provokable myocardial ischemia during recovery from STEMI.	C
		In patients whose anatomy is suitable, PCI should be performed for cardiogenic shock or hemodynamic instability.	C
	Class IIa	It is reasonable to perform routine PCI in patients with LV ejection fraction ≤0.40, heart failure, or serious ventricular arrhythmias.	C
		It is reasonable to perform PCI when there is documented clinical heart failure during the acute episode, even though subsequent evaluation shows preserved LV function (LV ejection fraction >0.40).	C
	Class IIb	PCI of a hemodynamically significant stenosis in a patent infarct artery longer than 24 hours after STEMI may be considered as part of an invasive strategy.	B
	Class III	PCI of a totally occluded infarct artery longer than 24 hours after STEMI is not recommended in asymptomatic patients with 1- or 2-vessel disease if they are hemodynamically and electrically stable and do not have evidence of severe ischemia.	C
Cardiogenic shock	Class I	Primary PCI should be performed for patients younger than 75 years with ST elevation or presumably new left bundle branch block who develop shock within 36 hours of MI and are suitable for revascularization that can be performed within 18 hours of shock, unless further support is futile because of the patient's wishes or contraindications/unsuitability for further invasive care.	A
	Class IIa	Primary PCI is reasonable for selected patients 75 years or older with ST elevation or left bundle branch block or who develop shock within 36 hours of MI and are suitable for revascularization that can be performed within 18 hours of shock. Patients with good prior functional status who are suitable for revascularization and agree to invasive care may be selected for such an invasive strategy.	B

CABG = coronary artery bypass graft surgery; LOE = level of evidence; LV = left ventricular; MI = myocardial infarction; PCI = percutaneous coronary intervention; STEMI = ST-segment elevation myocardial infarction.

TABLE 58G-4 ACC/AHA Recommendations for Percutaneous Coronary Intervention in Specific Clinical Circumstances[2-4]

INDICATION	CLASS	RECOMMENDATION	LOE
Prior coronary artery bypass surgery	Class I	When technically feasible, PCI should be performed in patients with early ischemia (usually within 30 days) after CABG.*	B
		It is recommended that distal embolic protection devices be used when technically feasible in patients undergoing PCI to saphenous vein grafts.	B
	Class IIa	Patients with ischemia that occurs 1 to 3 years after CABG and who have preserved LV function with discrete lesions in graft conduits*	B
		Patients with disabling angina secondary to new disease in a native coronary circulation after CABG. (If angina is not typical, objective evidence of ischemia should be obtained.*)	B
		Patients with diseased vein grafts more than 3 years after CABG	B
		When technically feasible in patients with a patent left internal mammary artery graft who have clinically significant obstructions in other vessels*	C
	Class III	Not recommended in patients with prior CABG for chronic total vein graft occlusions	B
		Not recommended in patients who have multiple target lesions with prior CABG and who have multivessel disease, failure of multiple saphenous vein grafts, and impaired LV function unless repeated CABG poses excessive risk due to severe comorbid conditions	B
Left main	Class IIb	PCI of the left main coronary artery with stents as an alternative to CABG may be considered in patients with anatomic conditions that are associated with a low risk of PCI procedural complications and clinical conditions that predict an increased risk of adverse surgical outcomes.	B

TABLE 58G-4 ACC/AHA Recommendations for Percutaneous Coronary Intervention in Specific Clinical Circumstances[2-5]—cont'd

INDICATION	CLASS	RECOMMENDATION	LOE
Aspiration thrombectomy	Class IIa	Aspiration thrombectomy is reasonable for patients undergoing primary PCI.	B
Drug-eluting stent	Class I	A DES should be considered as an alternative to a BMS in those patients for whom clinical trials indicate a favorable effectiveness/safety profile.	A
		Before implanting a DES, the interventional cardiologist should discuss with the patient the need for and duration of dual antiplatelet therapy and confirm the patient's ability to comply with the recommended therapy for DES.	C
		In patients who are undergoing preparation for PCI and are likely to require invasive or surgical procedures for which dual antiplatelet therapy must be interrupted during the next 12 months, consideration should be given to implantation of a BMS or performance of balloon angioplasty with a provisional stent implantation instead of the routine use of a DES.	B
	Class IIa	It is reasonable to use a DES as an alternative to a BMS for primary PCI in STEMI.	B
	Class IIb	A DES may be considered for clinical and anatomic settings in which the efficacy/safety profile appears favorable in STEMI.	B
Contrast medium	Class I	In patients with chronic kidney disease undergoing angiography who are not undergoing chronic dialysis, either an isosmolar contrast medium	A
		or a low-molecular-weight contrast medium other than ioxaglate or iohexol is indicated.	B

*Note: Elective PCI should not be performed at institutions that do not provide on-site cardiac surgery.

BMS = bare metal stent; CABG = coronary artery bypass graft surgery; DES = drug-eluting stent; LOE = level of evidence; LV = left ventricular; MI = myocardial infarction; PCI = percutaneous coronary intervention; STEMI = ST-segment elevation myocardial infarction.

ADJUNCTIVE PHARMACOTHERAPY

The expanding number of antiplatelet and antithrombotic agents available for use during PCI has provided clinicians with a number of competing therapeutic options. Guidelines for antithrombotic therapy during (**Table 58G-5**) and after (**Table 58G-6**) PCI are provided. There is also an increasing awareness that providing optimal medical therapy after PCI is mandatory, including secondary risk factor modifications with lipid-lowering therapy (see Chap. 49).

APPROPRIATENESS CRITERIA FOR PERCUTANEOUS CORONARY INTERVENTION

An ongoing challenge for the application of guidelines to clinical practice is the creation of relevant clinical scenarios that the clinician faces on a daily basis and the construction of expert opinion for the appropriateness of revascularization based on the integration of the clinical presentation, noninvasive testing, coronary anatomy, and intensiveness of medical therapy. Appropriateness criteria for revascularization have been published with a consensus opinion of interventionalists, cardiac surgeons, and noninvasive cardiologists.[6] Risk stratification for cardiac events was established (**Table 58G-7**), and a series of clinical scenarios were graded on a scale of 1 to 9 on the basis of the following appropriateness definitions:

Score 7-9: Appropriate (A) when the expected benefits, in terms of survival or health outcomes (symptoms, functional status, and/or quality of life), exceed the expected negative consequences of the procedure.

Score 4-6: Uncertain (U) for the indication provided, meaning coronary revascularization may be acceptable and may be a reasonable approach for the indication but with uncertainty, implying that more research and/or patient information is needed to further classify the indication.

Score 1-3: Inappropriate (I) for the indication provided, meaning coronary revascularization is not generally acceptable and is not a reasonable approach for the indication and is unlikely to improve the patient's health outcomes or survival.

The appropriateness for revascularization in various manifestations of acute coronary syndromes is listed in **Table 58G-8**. In general, the guidelines support a prominent role for revascularization in patients with acute coronary syndrome. The criteria for stable coronary artery disease are based on extent of coronary artery disease, complexity of coronary anatomy, severity of angina, degree of ischemia, and extent of antianginal medical therapy (**Tables 58G-9 to 58G-11**). These key factors must be weighed before deciding on the appropriateness of revascularization. Patients with prior coronary artery bypass grafting (CABG) who require repeated revascularization merit special consideration, as the risks of repeated bypass surgery are higher than with the initial surgery. In patients with prior CABG, the guidelines recommend revascularization for severe angina (Canadian Class III or IV), especially with large areas or ischemia and when medical therapy has already been maximized. The appropriate mode of revascularization by PCI versus CABG for various anatomic subsets incorporates diabetic status and left ventricular status into the decision making. Importantly, three-vessel disease is categorized as having uncertain appropriateness for PCI, even in the absence of diabetes and depressed left ventricular function (**Table 58G-12**). Similarly, isolated left main stenosis is deemed inappropriate for treatment by PCI. These last two evaluations are controversial, as a substantial amount of data supports PCI in these two scenarios, with a large number of such procedures already performed worldwide.

GUIDELINES FOR TRAINING

The guidelines recommend that physicians undergo a 3-year comprehensive cardiac training program before dedicated interventional training in an accredited program. Interventional training requires a fourth year of training, including more than 250 interventional procedures, a level that is required for physicians to be eligible for the American Board of Internal Medicine certifying examination in interventional cardiology.[7,8] Maintenance of certification requires performance of 150 procedures in the 2 years before the 10-year certification lapses, in addition to retaking of the added qualification examination in interventional cardiology.

TABLE 58G-5 ACC/AHA Recommendations for Medical Therapy During Percutaneous Coronary Intervention[2-4]

INDICATION	CLASS	RECOMMENDATION	LOE
Aspirin	Class I	Patients already taking daily long-term ASA therapy should take 75 to 325 mg of ASA before PCI is performed.	A
		Patients not already taking daily long-term ASA therapy should be given 300 to 325 mg of ASA at least 2 hours and preferably 24 hours before PCI is performed.	C
Clopidogrel/prasugrel	Class I	A loading dose of clopidogrel, generally 600 mg, should be administered before or when PCI is performed.	C
		When a loading dose of clopidogrel is administered, a regimen of more than 300 mg is reasonable to achieve higher levels of antiplatelet activity more rapidly, but the efficacy and safety compared with a 300-mg loading dose are less established.	C
		In patients undergoing PCI within 12 to 24 hours of receiving fibrinolytic therapy, a clopidogrel oral loading dose of 300 mg may be considered.	C
		A loading dose of thienopyridine is recommended for STEMI patients for whom PCI is planned. Regimens should be one of the following:	
		• At least 300 to 600 mg of clopidogrel should be given as early as possible before or at the time of primary or nonprimary PCI.	C
		• Prasugrel 60 mg should be given as soon as possible for primary PCI.	B
		For STEMI patients undergoing nonprimary PCI, the following regimens are recommended:	
		• If the patient has received fibrinolytic therapy and has been given clopidogrel, clopidogrel should be continued as the thienopyridine of choice.	C
		• If the patient has received fibrinolytic therapy without a thienopyridine, a loading dose of 300 to 600 mg of clopidogrel should be given as the thienopyridine of choice.	C
		• If the patient did not receive fibrinolytic therapy, either a loading dose of 300 to 600 mg of clopidogrel should be given or, once the coronary anatomy is known and PCI is planned, a loading dose of 60 mg of prasugrel should be given promptly and no later than 1 hour after the PCI.	B
	Class III	In STEMI patients with a prior history of stroke and transient ischemic attack for whom primary PCI is planned, prasugrel is not recommended as part of a dual antiplatelet therapy regimen.	C
GP IIb/IIIa inhibitors	Class IIa	In patients with UA/NSTEMI undergoing PCI with clopidogrel administration, it is reasonable to administer a GP IIb/IIIa inhibitor (abciximab, eptifibatide, or tirofiban).	B
		In patients undergoing elective PCI with stent placement, it is reasonable to administer a GP IIb/IIIa inhibitor (abciximab, eptifibatide, or tirofiban).	B
		It is reasonable to start treatment with GP IIb/IIIa receptor antagonists at the time of primary PCI (with or without stenting) in selected patients with STEMI. GP IIb/IIIa inhibitors include	
		• Abciximab	A
		• Tirofiban	B
		• Eptifibatide	C
	Class IIb	The usefulness of GP IIb/IIIa receptor antagonists (as part of a preparatory pharmacologic strategy for patients with STEMI before their arrival in the cardiac catheterization laboratory for angiography and PCI) is uncertain.	B
Unfractionated heparin	Class I	UFH should be administered to patients undergoing PCI.	C
		For prior treatment with UFH, administer additional boluses of UFH as needed to support the procedure, taking into account whether GP IIb/IIIa receptor antagonists have been administered.	C
		For patients proceeding to primary PCI who have been treated with aspirin, a thienopyridine, and UFH, additional boluses of UFH should be administered as needed to maintain therapeutic activated clotting time levels, taking into account whether GP IIb/IIIa receptor antagonists have been administered.	C
Bivalirudin	Class I	For patients with heparin-induced thrombocytopenia, it is recommended that bivalirudin or argatroban be used to replace heparin.	B
		For patients proceeding to primary PCI who have been treated with aspirin and a thienopyridine, recommended supportive anticoagulation includes bivalirudin with or without prior treatment with UFH.	B
	Class IIa	It is reasonable to use bivalirudin as an alternative to UFH and GP IIb/IIIa antagonists in low-risk patients undergoing elective PCI.	B
		In STEMI patients undergoing PCI who are at high risk of bleeding, bivalirudin anticoagulation is reasonable.	B
Enoxaparin	Class I	For prior treatment with enoxaparin, if the last subcutaneous dose was administered at least 8 to 12 hours earlier, an IV dose of 0.3 mg/kg of enoxaparin should be given; if the last subcutaneous dose was administered within the prior 8 hours, no additional enoxaparin should be given.	B
	Class IIa	Low-molecular-weight heparin is a reasonable alternative to UFH in patients with UA/NSTEMI undergoing PCI.	B
	Class IIb	Low-molecular-weight heparin may be considered as an alternative to UFH in patients with STEMI undergoing PCI.	B
Fondaparinux	Class I	For prior treatment with fondaparinux, administer additional intravenous treatment with an anticoagulant possessing anti-IIa activity, taking into account whether GP IIb/IIIa receptor antagonists have been administered.	C
		Because of the risk of catheter thrombosis, fondaparinux should not be used as the sole anticoagulant to support PCI. An additional anticoagulant with anti-IIa activity should be administered.	C

ASA = aspirin; GP = glycoprotein; LOE = level of evidence; NSTEMI = non–ST-segment elevation myocardial infarction; PCI = percutaneous coronary intervention; STEMI = ST-segment elevation myocardial infarction; UA = unstable angina; UFH = unfractionated heparin.

TABLE 58G-6 ACC/AHA Recommendations for Medical Therapy After Percutaneous Coronary Intervention[2-4]

INDICATION	CLASS	RECOMMENDATION	LOE
Aspirin	Class I	In patients without allergy or increased risk of bleeding, aspirin 162 to 325 mg daily should be given for at least 1 month after BMS implantation, 3 months after sirolimus-eluting stent implantation, and 6 months after paclitaxel-eluting stent implantation, after which long-term aspirin use should be continued indefinitely at a dose of 75 to 162 mg daily.	B
	Class IIa	In patients for whom the physician is concerned about risk of bleeding, lower dose 75 to 162 mg of aspirin is reasonable during the initial period after stent implantation.	C
Clopidogrel/prasugrel: elective PCI	Class I	For all post-PCI patients who receive a DES, clopidogrel 75 mg daily should be given for at least 12 months if patients are not at high risk of bleeding. For post-PCI patients receiving a BMS, clopidogrel should be given for a minimum of 1 month and ideally up to 12 months (unless the patient is at increased risk of bleeding; then it should be given for a minimum of 2 weeks).	B
Clopidogrel/prasugrel: STEMI and unstable angina/NSTEMI	Class I	The duration of thienopyridine therapy should be as follows:	
		• In patients receiving a stent (BMS or DES) during PCI for ACS, clopidogrel 75 mg daily or prasugrel 10 mg daily should be given for at least 12 months.	B
		• If the risk of morbidity because of bleeding outweighs the anticipated benefit afforded by thienopyridine therapy, earlier discontinuation should be considered.	C
		In patients in whom subacute thrombosis may be catastrophic or lethal (unprotected left main, bifurcating left main, or last patent coronary vessel), platelet aggregation studies may be considered and the dose of clopidogrel increased to 150 mg/day if less than 50% inhibition of platelet aggregation is demonstrated.	C
		In patients taking a thienopyridine in whom CABG is planned and can be delayed, it is recommended that the drug be discontinued to allow dissipation of the antiplatelet effect. The period of withdrawal should be	
		• At least 5 days in patients receiving clopidogrel	B
		• At least 7 days in patients receiving prasugrel	C
		unless the need for revascularization and/or the net benefit of the thienopyridine outweighs the potential risks of excess bleeding	C
	Class IIa	Continuation of clopidogrel or prasugrel beyond 15 months may be considered in patients undergoing DES placement.	B
	Class IIb	For all post-PCI nonstented STEMI patients, treatment with clopidogrel should continue for at least 14 days.	C
		Long-term maintenance therapy (e.g., 1 year) with clopidogrel (75 mg/day orally) is reasonable in STEMI and non-STEMI patients who undergo PCI without reperfusion therapy.	C
		It is reasonable that patients undergoing brachytherapy be given daily clopidogrel 75 mg indefinitely and daily aspirin 75 to 325 mg indefinitely unless there is significant risk for bleeding.	C

ACS = acute coronary syndrome; BMS = bare metal stent; CABG = coronary artery bypass graft surgery; DES = drug-eluting stent; LOE = level of evidence; NSTEMI = non–ST-segment elevation myocardial infarction; PCI = percutaneous coronary intervention; STEMI = ST-segment elevation myocardial infarction.

TABLE 58G-7 Noninvasive Risk Stratification

High Risk (>3% annual mortality rate)

Severe resting left ventricular dysfunction (LVEF <35%)
High-risk treadmill score (score ≤ −11)
Severe exercise left ventricular dysfunction (exercise LVEF <35%)
Stress-induced large perfusion defect (particularly if anterior)
Stress-induced multiple perfusion defects of moderate size
Large, fixed perfusion defect with left ventricular dilation or increased lung uptake (thallium-201)
Stress-induced moderate perfusion defect with left ventricular dilation or increased lung uptake (thallium-201)
Echocardiographic wall motion abnormality (involving more than two segments) developing at low-dose dobutamine (≤10 mg/kg/min) or at a low heart rate (<120 beats/min)
Stress echocardiographic evidence of extensive ischemia

Intermediate Risk (1%-3% annual mortality rate)

Mild to moderate resting left ventricular dysfunction (LVEF = 35%-49%)
Intermediate-risk treadmill score (score > −11 to < 5)
Stress-induced moderate perfusion defect without LV dilation or increased lung uptake (thallium-201)
Limited stress echocardiographic ischemia with a wall motion abnormality only at higher doses of dobutamine involving two segments or less

Low Risk (<1% annual mortality rate)

Low-risk treadmill score (score ≥5)
Normal or small myocardial perfusion defect at rest or with stress
Normal stress echocardiographic wall motion or no change or limited resting wall motion abnormalities during stress

Modified from Patel MR, Dehmer GJ, Hirshfeld JW, et al: ACCF/SCAI/STS/AATS/AHA/ASNC 2009 Appropriateness Criteria for Coronary Revascularization: A Report of the American College of Cardiology Foundation Appropriateness Criteria Task Force, Society for Cardiovascular Angiography and Interventions, Society of Thoracic Surgeons, American Association for Thoracic Surgery, American Heart Association, and the American Society of Nuclear Cardiology: Endorsed by the American Society of Echocardiography, the Heart Failure Society of America, and the Society of Cardiovascular Computed Tomography. J Am Coll Cardiol 53:530, 2009.

TABLE 58G-8 Appropriateness Criteria for Revascularization in Patients with Acute Coronary Syndromes

INDICATION		APPROPRIATENESS SCORE (1-9)
1.	• STEMI • Onset of symptoms within the prior 12 to 24 hours • Severe HF, persistent ischemic symptoms, or hemodynamic or electrical instability present	A (9)
2.	• STEMI • Onset of symptoms within the prior 12 to 24 hours • Severe HF, persistent ischemic symptoms, or hemodynamic or electrical instability present	A (9)
3.	• STEMI • Greater than 12 hours from symptom onset • Asymptomatic; no hemodynamic instability and no electrical instability	I (3)
4.	• STEMI with presumed successful treatment with fibrinolysis • Evidence of HF, recurrent ischemia, or unstable ventricular arrhythmias present • One-vessel CAD, presumed to be the culprit artery	A (9)
5.	• STEMI with presumed successful treatment with fibrinolysis • Asymptomatic; no HF or no recurrent ischemic symptoms, or no unstable ventricular arrhythmias • Normal LVEF • One-vessel CAD presumed to be the culprit artery	U (5)
6.	• STEMI with presumed successful treatment with fibrinolysis • Asymptomatic; no HF, no recurrent ischemic symptoms, or no unstable ventricular arrhythmias at time of presentation • Depressed LVEF • Three-vessel CAD • Elective/semi-elective revascularization	A (8)
7.	• STEMI with successful treatment of the culprit artery by primary PCI or fibrinolysis • Asymptomatic; no HF, no evidence of recurrent or provokable ischemia or no unstable ventricular arrhythmias during index hospitalization • Normal LVEF • Revascularization of a non-infarct related artery during index hospitalization	I (2)
8.	• STEMI or NSTEMI and successful PCI of culprit artery during index hospitalization • Symptoms of recurrent myocardial ischemia and/or high-risk findings on noninvasive stress testing performed after index hospitalization • Revascularization of 1 or more additional coronary arteries	A (8)
9.	• UA/NSTEMI and high-risk features for short-term risk of death or nonfatal MI • Revascularization of the presumed culprit artery	A (9)
10.	• UA/NSTEMI and high-risk features for short-term risk of death or nonfatal MI • Revascularization of multiple coronary arteries when the culprit artery cannot be clearly determined	A (9)
11.	• Patients with acute myocardial infarction (STEMI or NSTEMI) • Evidence of cardiogenic shock • Revascularization of 1 or more coronary arteries	A (8)

CAD = coronary artery disease; HF = heart failure; LVEF = left ventricular ejection fraction; MI = myocardial infarction; NSTEMI = non–ST-segment elevation myocardial infarction; PCI = percutaneous coronary intervention; STEMI = ST-segment elevation myocardial infarction; UA = unstable angina.

From Patel MR, Dehmer GJ, Hirshfeld JW, et al: ACCF/SCAI/STS/AATS/AHA/ASNC 2009 Appropriateness Criteria for Coronary Revascularization: A Report of the American College of Cardiology Foundation Appropriateness Criteria Task Force, Society for Cardiovascular Angiography and Interventions, Society of Thoracic Surgeons, American Association for Thoracic Surgery, American Heart Association, and the American Society of Nuclear Cardiology: Endorsed by the American Society of Echocardiography, the Heart Failure Society of America, and the Society of Cardiovascular Computed Tomography. J Am Coll Cardiol 53:530, 2009.

TABLE 58G-9 Low-Risk Findings on Noninvasive Testing and Asymptomatic Patients

SYMPTOMS MEDICAL THERAPY	CTO OF 1 VESSEL; NO OTHER DISEASE	1 OR 2 VESSELS; NO OTHER DISEASE; NO PROXIMAL LAD	1-VESSEL DISEASE OF PROXIMAL LAD	2-VESSEL DISEASE WITH PROXIMAL LAD	3-VESSEL DISEASE; NO LEFT MAIN DISEASE
Class III or IV Maximum treatment	U	A	A	A	A
Class I or II Maximum treatment	U	U	A	A	A
Asymptomatic Maximum treatment	I	I	U	U	U
Class III or IV No or minimal treatment	I	U	A	A	A
Class I or II No or minimal treatment	I	I	U	U	U
Asymptomatic No or minimal treatment	I	I	U	U	U

TABLE 58G-9 Low-Risk Findings on Noninvasive Testing and Asymptomatic Patients—cont'd

EXERCISE STRESS TEST MEDICAL THERAPY	CTO OF 1 VESSEL; NO OTHER DISEASE	1 OR 2 VESSELS; NO OTHER DISEASE; NO PROXIMAL LAD	1-VESSEL DISEASE OF PROXIMAL LAD	2-VESSEL DISEASE WITH PROXIMAL LAD	3-VESSEL DISEASE; NO LEFT MAIN DISEASE
High risk Maximum treatment	U	A	A	A	A
High risk No or minimal treatment	U	U	A	A	A
Intermediate risk Maximum treatment	U	U	U	U	A
Intermediate risk No or minimal treatment	I	I	U	U	A
Low risk Maximum treatment	I	I	U	U	U
Low risk No or minimal treatment	I	I	U	U	U

CTO = chronic total occlusion; LAD = left anterior descending coronary artery.
Modified from Patel MR, Dehmer GJ, Hirshfeld JW, et al: ACCF/SCAI/STS/AATS/AHA/ASNC 2009 Appropriateness Criteria for Coronary Revascularization: A Report of the American College of Cardiology Foundation Appropriateness Criteria Task Force, Society for Cardiovascular Angiography and Interventions, Society of Thoracic Surgeons, American Association for Thoracic Surgery, American Heart Association, and the American Society of Nuclear Cardiology: Endorsed by the American Society of Echocardiography, the Heart Failure Society of America, and the Society of Cardiovascular Computed Tomography. J Am Coll Cardiol 53:530, 2009.

TABLE 58G-10 Intermediate-Risk Findings on Noninvasive Study and CCS Class I or II Angina

SYMPTOMS MEDICAL THERAPY	CTO OF 1 VESSEL; NO OTHER DISEASE	1 OR 2 VESSELS; NO OTHER DISEASE; NO PROXIMAL LAD	1-VESSEL DISEASE OF PROXIMAL LAD	2-VESSEL DISEASE WITH PROXIMAL LAD	3-VESSEL DISEASE; NO LEFT MAIN DISEASE
Class III or IV Maximum treatment	A	A	A	A	A
Class I or II Maximum treatment	U	A	A	A	A
Asymptomatic Maximum treatment	U	U	U	U	A
Class III or IV No or minimal treatment	U	U	A	A	A
Class I or II No or minimal treatment	U	U	U	A	A
Asymptomatic No or minimal treatment	I	I	U	U	A
EXERCISE STRESS TEST MEDICAL THERAPY	**CTO OF 1 VESSEL; NO OTHER DISEASE**	**1 OR 2 VESSELS; NO OTHER DISEASE; NO PROXIMAL LAD**	**1-VESSEL DISEASE OF PROXIMAL LAD**	**2-VESSEL DISEASE WITH PROXIMAL LAD**	**3-VESSEL DISEASE; NO LEFT MAIN DISEASE**
High risk Maximum treatment	A	A	A	A	A
High risk No or minimal treatment	U	A	A	A	A
Intermediate risk Maximum treatment	U	A	A	A	A
Intermediate risk No or minimal treatment	U	U	U	A	A
Low risk Maximum treatment	U	U	A	A	A
Low risk No or minimal treatment	I	I	U	U	U

CCS = Canadian Cardiovascular Society; CTO = chronic total occlusion; LAD = left anterior descending coronary artery.
Modified from Patel MR, Dehmer GJ, Hirshfeld JW, et al: ACCF/SCAI/STS/AATS/AHA/ASNC 2009 Appropriateness Criteria for Coronary Revascularization: A Report of the American College of Cardiology Foundation Appropriateness Criteria Task Force, Society for Cardiovascular Angiography and Interventions, Society of Thoracic Surgeons, American Association for Thoracic Surgery, American Heart Association, and the American Society of Nuclear Cardiology: Endorsed by the American Society of Echocardiography, the Heart Failure Society of America, and the Society of Cardiovascular Computed Tomography. J Am Coll Cardiol 53:530, 2009.

TABLE 58G-11 High-Risk Findings on Noninvasive Study and CCS Class III or IV Angina

SYMPTOMS MEDICAL THERAPY	CTO OF 1 VESSEL; NO OTHER DISEASE	1 OR 2 VESSELS; NO OTHER DISEASE; NO PROXIMAL LAD	1-VESSEL DISEASE OF PROXIMAL LAD	2-VESSEL DISEASE WITH PROXIMAL LAD	3-VESSEL DISEASE; NO LEFT MAIN DISEASE
Class III or IV Maximum treatment	A	A	A	A	A
Class I or II Maximum treatment	A	A	A	A	A
Asymptomatic Maximum treatment	U	A	A	A	A
Class III or IV No or minimal treatment	A	A	A	A	A
Class I or II No or minimal treatment	U	A	A	A	A
Asymptomatic No or minimal treatment	U	U	A	A	A
EXERCISE STRESS TEST MEDICAL THERAPY	**CTO OF 1 VESSEL; NO OTHER DISEASE**	**1 OR 2 VESSELS; NO OTHER DISEASE; NO PROXIMAL LAD**	**1-VESSEL DISEASE OF PROXIMAL LAD**	**2-VESSEL DISEASE WITH PROXIMAL LAD**	**3-VESSEL DISEASE; NO LEFT MAIN DISEASE**
High risk Maximum treatment	A	A	A	A	A
High risk No or minimal treatment	A	A	A	A	A
Intermediate risk Maximum treatment	A	A	A	A	A
Intermediate risk No or minimal treatment	U	U	A	A	A
Low risk Maximum treatment	U	A	A	A	A
Low risk No or minimal treatment	I	U	A	A	A

CCS = Canadian Cardiovascular Society; CTO = chronic total occlusion; LAD = left anterior descending coronary artery.
Modified from Patel MR, Dehmer GJ, Hirshfeld JW, et al: ACCF/SCAI/STS/AATS/AHA/ASNC 2009 Appropriateness Criteria for Coronary Revascularization: A Report of the American College of Cardiology Foundation Appropriateness Criteria Task Force, Society for Cardiovascular Angiography and Interventions, Society of Thoracic Surgeons, American Association for Thoracic Surgery, American Heart Association, and the American Society of Nuclear Cardiology: Endorsed by the American Society of Echocardiography, the Heart Failure Society of America, and the Society of Cardiovascular Computed Tomography. J Am Coll Cardiol 53:530, 2009.

TABLE 58G-12 Appropriateness of Coronary Artery Bypass Surgery and Percutaneous Coronary Intervention

	CABG			PCI		
	NO DIABETES AND NORMAL LVEF	DIABETES	DEPRESSED LVEF	NO DIABETES AND NORMAL LVEF	DIABETES	DEPRESSED LVEF
Two-vessel coronary artery disease with proximal LAD stenosis	A	A	A	A	A	A
Three-vessel coronary artery disease	A	A	A	U	U	U
Isolated left main stenosis	A	A	A	I	I	I
Left main stenosis and additional coronary artery disease	A	A	A	I	I	I

CABG = coronary artery bypass graft surgery; LAD = left anterior descending coronary artery; LVEF = left ventricular ejection fraction; PCI = percutaneous coronary intervention.
Modified from Patel MR, Dehmer GJ, Hirshfeld JW, et al: ACCF/SCAI/STS/AATS/AHA/ASNC 2009 Appropriateness Criteria for Coronary Revascularization: A Report of the American College of Cardiology Foundation Appropriateness Criteria Task Force, Society for Cardiovascular Angiography and Interventions, Society of Thoracic Surgeons, American Association for Thoracic Surgery, American Heart Association, and the American Society of Nuclear Cardiology: Endorsed by the American Society of Echocardiography, the Heart Failure Society of America, and the Society of Cardiovascular Computed Tomography. J Am Coll Cardiol 53:530, 2009.

REFERENCES

1. Smith SC Jr, Dove JT, Jacobs AK, et al: ACC/AHA guidelines for percutaneous coronary intervention (revision of the 1993 PTCA guidelines)—executive summary: A report of the American College of Cardiology/American Heart Association task force on practice guidelines (Committee to revise the 1993 guidelines for percutaneous transluminal coronary angioplasty) endorsed by the Society for Cardiac Angiography and Interventions. Circulation 103:3019, 2001.
2. Smith SC Jr, Feldman TE, Hirshfeld JW Jr, et al: ACC/AHA/SCAI 2005 guideline update for percutaneous coronary intervention: A report of the American College of Cardiology/American Heart Association Task Force on Practice Guidelines (ACC/AHA/SCAI Writing Committee to Update the 2001 Guidelines for Percutaneous Coronary Intervention). J Am Coll Cardiol 47:e1, 2006.
3. King SB 3rd, Smith SC Jr, Hirshfeld JW Jr, et al: 2007 Focused Update of the ACC/AHA/SCAI 2005 Guideline Update for Percutaneous Coronary Intervention: A report of the American College of Cardiology/American Heart Association Task Force on Practice Guidelines: 2007 Writing Group to Review New Evidence and Update the ACC/AHA/SCAI 2005 Guideline Update for Percutaneous Coronary Intervention, Writing on Behalf of the 2005 Writing Committee. Circulation 117:261, 2008.
4. Kushner FG, Hand M, Smith SC Jr, et al: 2009 Focused Updates: ACC/AHA Guidelines for the Management of Patients With ST-Elevation Myocardial Infarction (updating the 2004 Guideline and 2007 Focused Update) and ACC/AHA/SCAI Guidelines on Percutaneous Coronary Intervention (updating the 2005 Guideline and 2007 Focused Update): A report of the American College of Cardiology Foundation/American Heart Association Task Force on Practice Guidelines. Circulation 120:2271, 2009.
5. Antman EM, Anbe DT, Armstrong PW, et al: ACC/AHA guidelines for the management of patients with ST-elevation myocardial infarction: A report of the American College of Cardiology/American Heart Association Task Force on Practice Guidelines (Committee to Revise the 1999 Guidelines for the Management of Patients with Acute Myocardial Infarction). Circulation 110:e82, 2004.
6. Patel MR, Dehmer GJ, Hirshfeld JW, et al: ACCF/SCAI/STS/AATS/AHA/ASNC 2009 Appropriateness Criteria for Coronary Revascularization: A Report of the American College of Cardiology Foundation Appropriateness Criteria Task Force, Society for Cardiovascular Angiography and Interventions, Society of Thoracic Surgeons, American Association for Thoracic Surgery, American Heart Association, and the American Society of Nuclear Cardiology: Endorsed by the American Society of Echocardiography, the Heart Failure Society of America, and the Society of Cardiovascular Computed Tomography. J Am Coll Cardiol 53:530, 2009.
7. American Board of Internal Medicine: Interventional Cardiology Policies. American Board of Internal Medicine 2010. Available at: http://www.abim.org/certification/policies/imss/icard.aspx#tpr. Accessed January 10, 2010.
8. American Board of Internal Medicine: Interventional Cardiology Policies. American Board of Internal Medicine 2010. Available at: http://www.abim.org/specialty/icard.aspx. Accessed January 10, 2010.

CHAPTER 59 Percutaneous Therapies for Structural Heart Disease in Adults

John G. Webb

This chapter will review transcatheter interventional therapy of structural heart disease in adults. Although the focus is primarily on acquired conditions, some conditions that are not acquired typically become apparent in adulthood and will also be briefly reviewed here.

Non-Valvular Therapies

Patent Foramen Ovale

The foramen ovale, which allows blood flow across the atrial septum in utero, normally closes shortly after birth as pulmonary blood flow increases and the flaplike septum primum is forced against the septum secundum. However, in approximately 25% of adults, closure of the foramen ovale is not complete. The presence of a patent foramen ovale (PFO) has been implicated in paradoxical embolism, cryptogenic stroke, platypnea-orthodeoxia syndrome, arterial gas embolism in decompression illness, high-altitude pulmonary edema, and migraine.[1,2]

Several lines of evidence suggest a role in the pathogenesis of cryptogenic stroke, including documented instances of paradoxical embolism of venous thrombi into the arterial system, a higher than expected incidence of PFO in stroke patients with otherwise unexplained stroke or who are young, and a lower than expected incidence of recurrent stroke after PFO closure. Factors that appear to increase the risk of paradoxical embolism include the presence of a large transatrial shunt at rest, a mobile atrial septal aneurysm, and elevated right atrial pressures. Several lines of evidence also suggest a role in the pathogenesis of migraine, particularly in patients with aura. These include a high incidence of PFO in migraine sufferers, a reduction in migraine frequency and severity following PFO closure for stroke, and anecdotal reports of marked benefit.

Percutaneous PFO closure involves femoral venous access and passage of a long sheath into the right atrium and through the defect into the left atrium. A large number of occlusion devices are available, some of which are shown in **Figure 59-1**. A double-umbrella or double-disk device is most often used. A left atrial disk is first introduced into the left atrium and withdrawn against the septum primum. Withdrawal of the sheath then releases the waist and right atrial disk elements. Most operators use transesophageal or intracardiac echocardiographic guidance in addition to fluoroscopy to confirm positioning, and the device is then released.[3,4]

Serious complications are rare in the hands of experienced operators, but may include cardiac perforation or embolization of thrombus or air, or of the device itself. Episodic atrial fibrillation may occur in up to 5% of patients in the first weeks after implantation, but tends to resolve spontaneously. Late cardiac perforation caused by device erosion is a rare late occurrence.

The indications for PFO closure for the prevention of recurrent thromboembolic stroke remain controversial. However, the low rate of serious complications and multiple nonrandomized studies suggesting a reduction in recurrent thromboembolic events have led to widespread adoption of this therapy, particularly for patients who have failed a trial of anticoagulation. PFO closure is a definitive treatment for systemic deoxygenation syndromes involving right-to-left shunts across a PFO and for documented paradoxical arterial embolism in the setting of venous thrombosis. The randomized Migraine Intervention with StarFlex Technology (MIST) trial has suggested a possible role for PFO closure in patients with refractory migraine, although further evaluation is needed.[5]

Atrial Septal Defect

Although patients with atrial septal defects (ASDs) often remain asymptomatic until early adulthood, they may present at any age with exertional dyspnea, fatigue, right ventricular failure, pulmonary hypertension, atrial arrhythmias, or paradoxical embolism (see Chap. 65). The functional significance of an ASD is primarily determined by the presence of right atrial or ventricular enlargement in the presence of an echocardiographic defect diameter larger than 10 mm or documentation of an elevated left-to-right shunt ratio ($Q_p/Q_s > 1.5{:}1$), determined from oxygen saturation at the time of catheterization.

Ostium secundum ASDs involve the fossa ovalis and account for approximately two thirds of all ASDs. Less common are ostium primum ASDs, typically associated with mitral valve or ventricular septal anomalies, and sinus venosus ASDs, typically involving the junction of the right atrium and superior vena cava. Ostium secundum ASDs are often well suited to percutaneous repair, whereas primum and sinus venosus ASDs generally are not. Surgical repair is generally favored in the presence of additional intracardiac anomalies, deficient rims over a large portion of the circumference of the defect, very large ASDs (diameter > 35 to 40 mm) or proximity to the atrioventricular valves.[3]

The most common device used for percutaneous closure is the Amplatzer ASO atrial septal occluder, consisting of two self-expanding nitinol disks, with each containing embedded synthetic fabric patches and joined by a central waist (**Fig. 59-2**). A device with a waist diameter slightly larger than the defect is selected to be occlusive and to center the device. The procedural approach to percutaneous ASD closure is similar to that for PFO closure. However, the variable size of ASDs requires more accurate sizing, which often involves inflating a calibrated sizing balloon within the defect to aid in measurement. Technical complexities are common, particularly when ASDs are large or multiple, are adjacent to other cardiac structures, or have deficient rims.

Successful defect closure is commonly associated with an improvement in functional class, exercise capacity, and often by a reduction in right heart chamber size and normalization of intracardiac pressures. Complications from ASD closure are rare, but may include device embolization, atrial arrhythmias, stroke, chamber perforation, and exacerbation of headaches. Late and potentially catastrophic device erosion through the atrial or aortic wall may rarely occur, usually as a consequence of device under- or oversizing. Thrombus

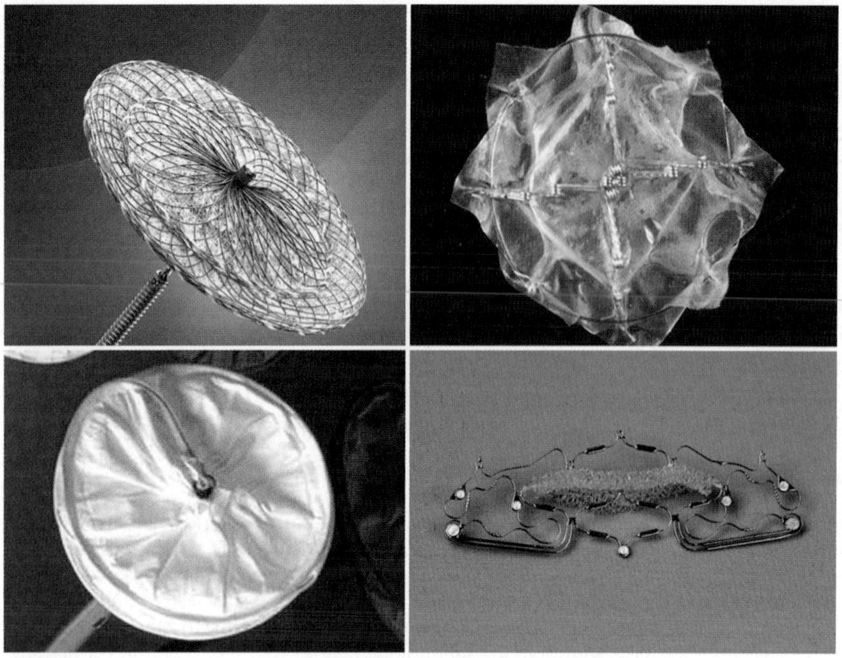

FIGURE 59-1 Patent foramen ovale occluders. **Clockwise from upper left:** (1) Amplatzer PFO occluder (AGA Medical, Plymouth, Minn) fashioned of two nitinol alloy disks, each with embedded fabric and connected by a central waist; (2) BioSTAR device (NMT Medical, Boston), which incorporates biodegradable collagenous disks fashioned similarly to its predecessors, the CardioSEAL and StarFlex devices; (3) Coherex device (Coherex Medical, Salt Lake City), which stretches the defect in one dimension while approximating the edges of the defect; and (4) Helex device (WL Gore & Associates, Newark, Del) with a single spiral coil of nitinol wire covered in fabric.

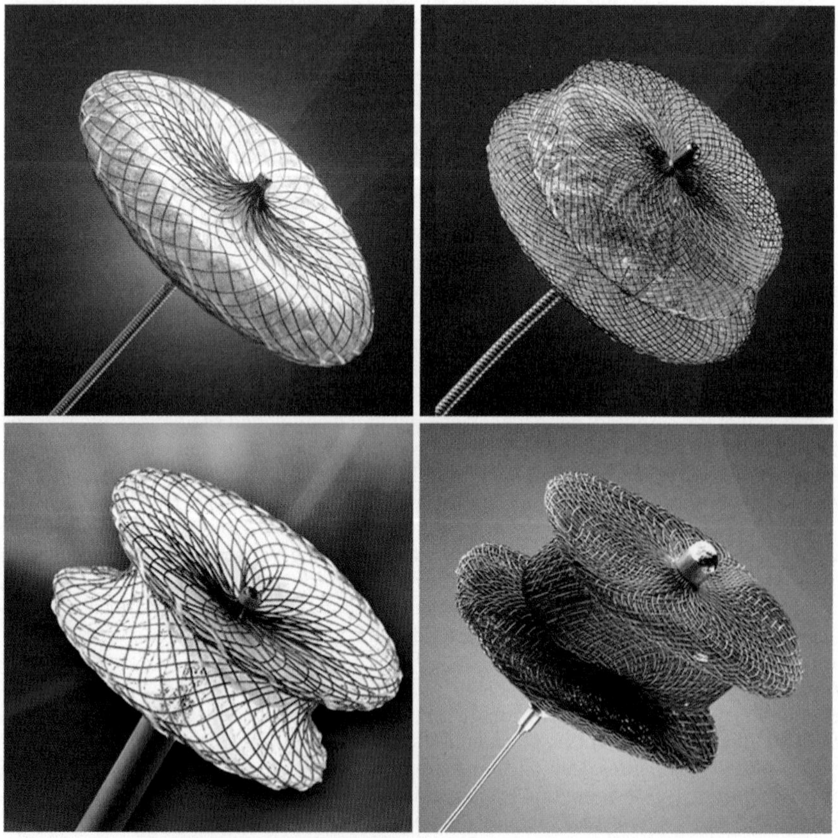

FIGURE 59-2 **Clockwise from upper left:** Amplatzer devices (AGA Medical) designed to occlude an atrial septal defect, left atrial appendage, paravalvular leak, and ventricular septal defect.

formation on the atrial disks may occur, with the potential for thromboembolism.

Ventricular Septal Defects

Acquired ventricular septal defects (VSDs) in adults are relatively rare. They can occur as a consequence of trauma or cardiac surgery, although the most common association is with infarction.[6] Postinfarction rupture of the interventricular septum complicates approximately 0.2% of patients, typically between days 2 to 7, when the large necrotic zone weakens and ruptures (see Chap. 55). Defects that develop in this setting are often irregular, serpiginous, sometimes multiple, and prone to further expansion with time or manipulation. Cardiogenic shock is the norm and mortality exceeds 90% if left untreated. Even in patients undergoing emergent surgical patch exclusion of the VSD, reported mortality ranges from 30 to 60%. Percutaneous closure of postinfarction VSDs has been accomplished with various devices, although usually a specialized Amplatzer occluder is used (see Fig. 59-2).[4] An experienced operator can generally implant an occluder safely, but success is variable, residual leaks are common, and mortality caused by progressive shock remains high.[6,7] The choice between surgical and percutaneous options must take into account the relative risks, likelihood of successful closure, and the need for additional revascularization or valve procedures.[1]

Left Atrial Appendage

Atrial fibrillation is the most common cause of cardioembolic stroke, with an annual stroke rate of approximately 5% (see Chap. 40). Although warfarin may reduce the risk of stroke, its narrow therapeutic range, variable dosing, monitoring requirements, and reported risk of major bleeding rates of 2% to 7%/ year are limitations. Most thromboemboli caused by atrial fibrillation appear to originate in the left atrial appendage (LAA) and surgical exclusion of the appendage at the time of cardiac surgery is believed to reduce the risk of subsequent cardioembolic stroke. The feasibility and efficacy of percutaneous LAA exclusion was demonstrated with a prototypic percutaneous LAA occlusion system (PLAATO).[8] Most experience has been with the subsequent Watchman device (Atritech, Plymouth, Minn), incorporating a self-expanding nitinol frame, barbs for fixation, and a polyester fabric cover (**Fig. 59-3**). In the randomized PROTECT-AF trial, LAA exclusion appeared noninferior to warfarin therapy for stroke prevention.[9] However, short-term complications were increased in this early experience, particularly pericardial effusions caused by transseptal access. LAA occlusion may be a reasonable option in patients intolerant to, or who have failed, warfarin. Long-term safety and efficacy remain to be established.[10]

Paravalvular Leak

Paravalvular regurgitation after valve replacement surgery may occur as a consequence of an incomplete seal between the sewing ring of the prosthetic valve and the annulus (see Chap. 66). Annular calcification, infection, and technical factors may predispose to paravalvular dehiscence. Most small leaks that develop early after surgery seal spontaneously, and most that do not require no treatment. However, when regurgitation is severe, congestive heart failure may result, and hemolysis may occur in the presence of high-velocity left ventricular to left atrial jets associated with mitral leaks, even when relatively small.

The great majority of symptomatic leaks occur in association with mitral valves and, much more rarely, in association with aortic valves. Reoperation for such leaks is associated with significant morbidity and mortality, as well as a high likelihood of recurrent leaks.

Percutaneous closure of paravalvular leaks may be achievable in many patients.[11-13] To date, the role of percutaneous closure has been limited by technical difficulty and modest efficacy. However, recent advances in imaging (particularly three-dimensional transesophageal echocardiography; see Chap. 15), technique (steerable catheters, apical access), and availability of newer closure devices specifically designed for paravalvular leaks offer increasing clinical efficacy.[4] A large number of devices have been used to occlude paravalvular leaks. Most of this experience has been with round plugs designed for closure of a septal defect or patent ductus arteriosus (see Chap. 65). Problems, although rare, include device embolization, interference with mechanical leaflets, and incomplete closure, with worsening of hemolysis. Newer devices specifically designed for the typical crescenteric shape of paravalvular defects (Amplatzer Vascular Plug III) may offer safer and more effective sealing (see Fig. 59-2). Regardless of which device is used, the defect must first be imaged and cannulated using transesophageal echocardiographic and fluoroscopic imaging. Aortic and some mitral leaks can be cannulated retrograde from the aorta. However, most mitral leaks require a transseptal puncture to access the left atrium, after which cannulation of the leak may be a difficult and lengthy process. Direct puncture of the left ventricle with percutaneous or minithoracotomy access has been found to facilitate access to mitral paravalvular leaks (**Fig. 59-4**).

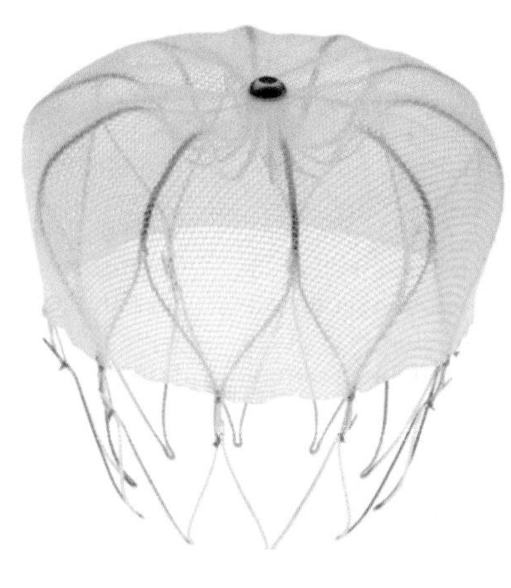

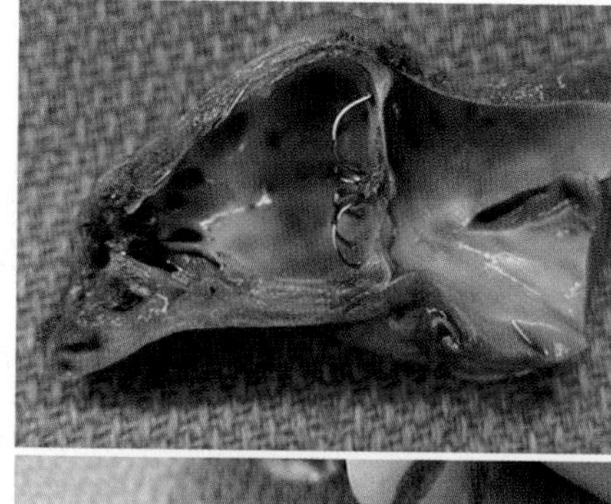

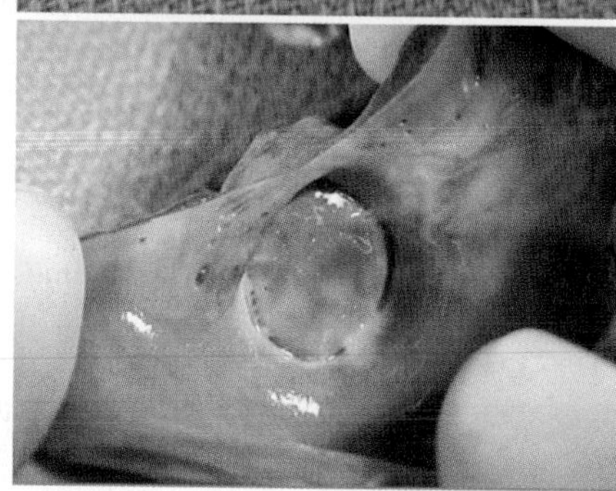

FIGURE 59-3 Left atrial appendage closure with the Watchman device (Atritech, Plymouth, Minn) at 45 days in an animal model.

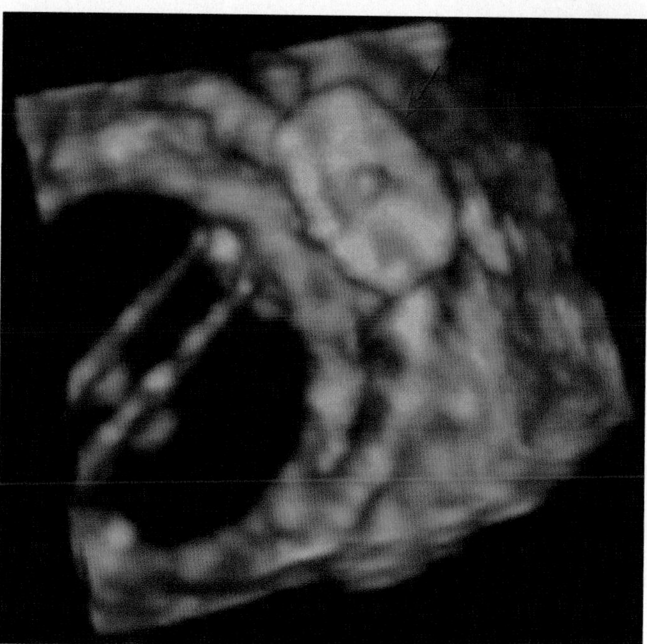

FIGURE 59-4 Transesophageal three-dimensional image of mitral double leaflet mechanical valve. An Amplatzer vascular plug III (AGA Medical) *(arrow)* was implanted to occlude a paravalvular leak using a transapical puncture.

Septal Ablation

Asymmetric hypertrophy of the basal interventricular septum and systolic anterior motion (SAM) of the anterior mitral leaflet (AML) may result in severe obstruction of the left ventricular outflow tract (LVOT) in patients with hypertrophic cardiomyopathy (see Chap. 69). Surgical myectomy has an established role in the palliation of severely symptomatic patients. More recently, percutaneous chemical ablation of the basal septum has been demonstrated to offer similar benefit in selected patients.[14]

Typically, the first septal perforator branch of the left anterior descending artery provides the blood supply to the anterior two thirds of the basal septum (**Fig. 59-5**). This branch is identified angiographically and cannulated. Selective injection of contrast allows demarcation of the area perfused by the chosen artery and echocardiographic confirmation that this is adjacent to the area of mitral valve–septal contact and maximal flow acceleration.[3] A small amount of absolute alcohol (1 to 2 mL) is injected slowly through the central lumen of a balloon catheter, during which the balloon is kept inflated to prevent reflux of alcohol back into the left anterior descending artery. Transient chest discomfort typically accompanies the controlled infarction that occurs.[15,16] Ethanol ablation results in coagulative necrosis of the septal perforator artery and adjacent myocardium. There is typically an immediate reduction in left ventricular systolic function, but diastolic function improves as the LVOT gradient is reduced. A gradual further reduction in gradient commonly occurs over a period of months as the infarcted ventricular septum thins.

Conduction abnormalities may occur as a consequence of temporary or permanent damage to septal conduction tissue. QRS lengthening, first-degree atrioventricular (AV) block, and new bundle branch blocks are common (see Chap. 69). Because complete heart block may occur, a temporary transvenous pacemaker lead is placed prior to the procedure, and permanent pacemaker implantation may be required in approximately 10% of patients. Serious myocardial injury may occur if ethanol refluxes into the left anterior descending artery or passes through septal collaterals to remote areas. Although periprocedural arrhythmias may occur, an increase in late arrhythmias has not been observed. In a pooled analysis of 42 published studies, with a mean follow-up of approximately 1 year, there was a decrease in resting LVOT gradient from 65 to 16 mm Hg, provocable gradient from 125 to 32 mm Hg, and basal septal diameter from 20.9 to 13.9 mm. This was associated with significant improvement in functional class, exercise capacity, and peak oxygen consumption. Mean 30-day mortality was 1.5%.[17]

Valvular Therapies

Mitral Balloon Valvotomy

Percutaneous valvotomy using inflatable balloon catheters was first developed as a therapeutic option for congenital pulmonary and aortic valvular stenosis almost 30 years ago. Percutaneous mitral balloon valvotomy has subsequently become a mainstay of the management of rheumatic mitral stenosis (see Chap. 66). In the past, closed or open commissurotomy (after the advent of cardiopulmonary bypass) was the mainstay of therapy for rheumatic mitral stenosis. However, in the early 1980s, several techniques of mitral balloon valvotomy were developed incorporating single or double cylindrical balloons, and even a mechanical dilator. Currently, this procedure is most often performed using transseptal access to the left atrium and a balloon catheter developed by a Japanese surgeon, Kanji Inoue. The dumbbell-shaped Inoue balloon catheter allows stable and sequential dilation of the stenotic mitral valve (see Fig. 66-24). Although rheumatic valvular disease is increasingly rare in the developed countries, it remains common in less developed countries, where mitral balloon valvotomy remains a common procedure.[18]

A favorable response to mitral dilation is predicated on the presence of fused mitral commissures, as seen in rheumatic disease. Dilation is relatively ineffective in the absence of commissural fusion. Dilation of congenital, prosthetic, or calcific stenosis is generally ineffective and the risk of severe regurgitation generally contraindicates this procedure. Patient selection for mitral valvotomy is largely based on echocardiographic assessment of the mitral valve apparatus.[3] The most widely used tool is the echocardiographic Wilkins score, which attempts to consider the anatomic characteristics of the leaflets, commissures, and chordal apparatus (**Table 59-1**).[19] This system assigns a point value from 1 to 4 for each of the following: (1) leaflet calcification; (2) leaflet mobility; (3) leaflet thickness; and (4) subvalvular apparatus degeneration. A score less than 8 suggests a favorable response to valvotomy (see Fig. 66-26), whereas a score of 9 to 16 suggests that surgical replacement may be needed. Even in the presence of a low score, adverse baseline factors to be considered include increasing severity of regurgitation, advanced age, prior commissurotomy, absence of commissural fusion, and presence of commissural calcification.[4]

A favorable result is evidenced by a reduction in mean transmitral gradient from more than 10 to less than 5 mm Hg, without development of severe mitral regurgitation. Complications, although uncommon, may include pericardial tamponade as a consequence of transseptal puncture, stroke caused by thromboembolism, and severe mitral regurgitation. Consequently, contraindications to valvotomy include anticoagulation, left atrial thrombus, and unfavorable valve anatomy, which might predispose to mitral regurgitation. Multiple lines of evidence, including randomized comparisons with open surgical commissurotomy, have demonstrated that the procedure can be performed with a relatively low rate of complications and a durable benefit (**Table 59-2**). Freedom from restenosis has been reported to be approximately 85% at 5 years, comparable to that for open surgical commissurotomy (see Fig. 66-25). When restenosis does occur, redilation may often be feasible.

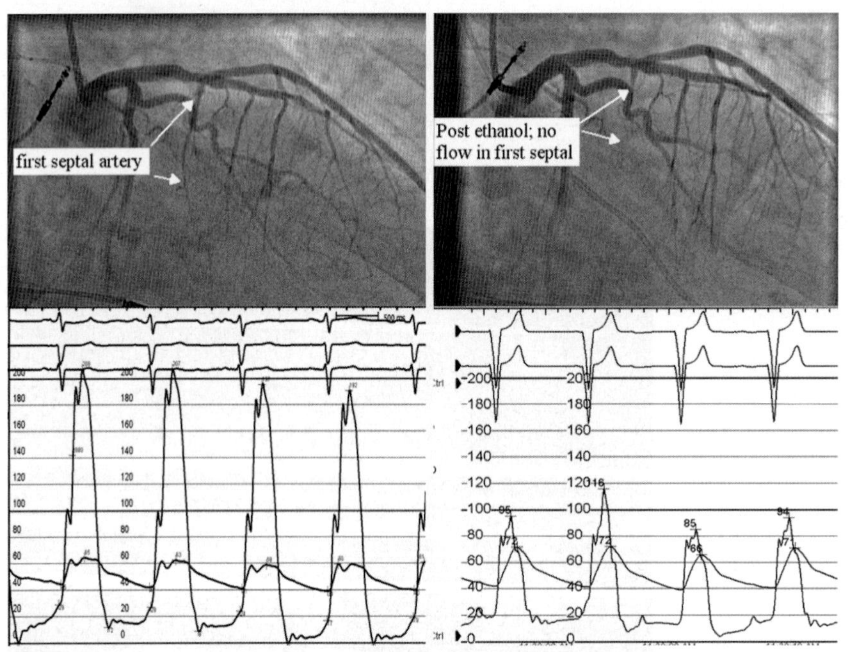

FIGURE 59-5 Septal ablation for obstructive hypertrophic cardiomyopathy. **Left,** Large pressure gradient between the left ventricle and aorta. A large proximal septal perforating artery is identified. **Right,** Following selective injection of ethanol, there is no flow within the septal artery and the gradient is dramatically reduced.

Aortic Balloon Valvotomy

Percutaneous aortic balloon valvotomy for degenerative aortic stenosis was initially described in 1985. Initial enthusiasm was tempered by reports documenting significant risk, limited benefit, and lack of durability.[20] Periprocedural complications included stroke in 1% to 3% of patients, severe aortic regurgitation in 1% to 2%, access site injury in 5% to 20%, and in-hospital mortality of 5% to 10%. More recent

TABLE 59-1 Echocardiographic Determinants of Suitability for Mitral Balloon Valvotomy.

GRADE	MOBILITY	THICKENING	CALCIFICATION	SUBVALVULAR THICKENING
1	Highly mobile valve with only leaflet tips restricted	Minimal thickening just below the mitral leaflets	Leaflets almost normal in thickness (4-5 mm)	Single area of increased echo brightness
2	Leaflet mid and base portions have normal mobility	Thickening of chordal structures, extending up to one third of chordal length	Midleaflets normal, considerable thickening of margins (5-8 mm)	Scattered areas of brightness confined to leaflet margins
3	Valve continues to move forward in diastole, mainly from the base	Thickening, extending to the distal third of the chords	Thickening extending through entire leaflet (5-8 mm)	Brightness extending into midportion of the leaflets
4	No or minimal forward movement of the leaflets in diastole	Extensive thickening and shortening of all chordal structures, extending down to the papillary muscles	Considerable thickening of all leaflet tissue (>8-10 mm)	Extensive brightness throughout much of the leaflet tissue

From Wilkins GT, Weyman AE, Abascal AM, et al: Percutaneous balloon dilation of the mitral valve: An analysis of echocardiographic variables related to outcome and the mechanism of dilatation. Br Heart J 60:299, 1988.

TABLE 59-2 Indications for Percutaneous Mitral Balloon Valvotomy

Class I

1. Percutaneous mitral balloon valvotomy is effective for symptomatic patients (NYHA functional Class II, III, or IV), with moderate or severe mitral stenosis (MS)* and valve morphology favorable for percutaneous mitral balloon valvotomy in the absence of left atrial thrombus or moderate to severe MR (level of evidence: A).
2. Percutaneous mitral balloon valvotomy is effective for asymptomatic patients with moderate or severe MS* and valve morphology that is favorable for percutaneous mitral balloon valvotomy who have pulmonary hypertension (pulmonary artery systolic pressure > 50 mm Hg at rest or > 60 mm Hg with exercise) in the absence of left atrial thrombus or moderate to severe mitral regurgitation (MR) (level of evidence: C).

Class IIa

Percutaneous mitral balloon valvotomy is reasonable for patients with moderate or severe MS* who have a nonpliable calcified valve, are in NYHA functional Class III or IV, and are either not candidates for surgery or are at high risk for surgery (level of evidence: C).

Class IIb

1. Percutaneous mitral balloon valvotomy may be considered for asymptomatic patients with moderate or severe MS* and valve morphology favorable for percutaneous mitral balloon valvotomy who have new onset of atrial fibrillation in the absence of left atrial thrombus or moderate to severe MR (level of evidence: C).
2. Percutaneous mitral balloon valvotomy may be considered for symptomatic patients (NYHA functional Class II, III, or IV) with mitral valve (MV) area greater than 1.5 cm^2 if there is evidence of hemodynamically significant MS based on pulmonary artery systolic pressure higher than 60 mm Hg, pulmonary artery wedge pressure of 25 mm Hg or more, or mean MV gradient higher than 15 mm Hg during exercise (level of evidence: C).
3. Percutaneous mitral balloon valvotomy may be considered as an alternative to surgery for patients with moderate or severe MS who have a nonpliable calcified valve and are in NYHA Class III or IV (level of evidence: C).

Class III

1. Percutaneous mitral balloon valvotomy is not indicated for patients with mild MS (level of evidence: C).
2. Percutaneous mitral balloon valvotomy should not be performed in patients with moderate to severe MR or left atrial thrombus (level of evidence: C).

From Bonow RO, Carabello BA, Chatterjee K, et al: 2008 focused update incorporated into the ACC/AHA 2006 guidelines for the management of patients with valvular heart disease: A report of the American College of Cardiology/American Heart Association Task Force on Practice Guidelines (Writing Committee to Revise the 1998 Guidelines for the Management of Patients With Valvular Heart Disease). J Am Coll Cardiol 52:e1, 2008.

reports have suggested improving outcomes with technical advances and increased experience.[21,22]

Aortic valvotomy may offer modest clinical benefit (see Chap. 66). Most reports have shown that balloon valvotomy in patients with critical aortic stenosis results in significant residual stenosis with valve areas typically between 0.7 and 1 cm^2. In the largest series to date, valve area increased less than 0.4 cm^2 in 77% of patients. Unfortunately, the clinical benefit of aortic balloon valvotomy is not durable. Restenosis, with loss of symptomatic benefit, occurs in approximately 50% of patients by 6 months and in most by 1 year.[21] Pathologic data has shown that balloon valvotomy improves leaflet mobility by fracturing calcified nodules and creating cleavage planes within collagenous stroma. Restenosis appears to occur as a result of granulation tissue, fibrosis, and active osteoblast-mediated calcification. Procedural improvements do not appear to have increased this durability. However, it does appear that external beam radiation early following aortic balloon valvotomy may reduce the rate of restenosis.[23]

Reported survival at 1 year following aortic balloon valvotomy ranges from 38% to 75% and at 2 years is 28% to 60%, comparable to survival in older patients with untreated aortic stenosis. Because balloon valvotomy may offer early benefit but has limited durability, repeat valvotomy has been proposed as a palliative approach.[21] Although repeat aortic balloon valvotomy is reported to provide symptomatic benefit with repeated dilation, the durability and degree of benefit appear to be progressively reduced.

TABLE 59-3 Indications for Aortic Balloon Valvulotomy.

Class IIb

1. Aortic balloon valvotomy might be reasonable as a bridge to surgery in hemodynamically unstable adult patients with aortic stenosis (AS) who are at high risk for aortic valve replacement (AVR) (level of evidence: C).
2. Aortic balloon valvotomy might be reasonable for palliation in adult patients with AS in whom AVR cannot be performed because of serious comorbid conditions (level of evidence: C).

Class III

Aortic balloon valvotomy is not recommended as an alternative to AVR in adult patients with AS; certain younger adults without valve calcification may be an exception (level of evidence: B).

From Bonow RO, Carabello BA, Chatterjee K, et al: 2008 focused update incorporated into the ACC/AHA 2006 guidelines for the management of patients with valvular heart disease: A report of the American College of Cardiology/American Heart Association Task Force on Practice Guidelines (Writing Committee to Revise the 1998 Guidelines for the Management of Patients With Valvular Heart Disease). J Am Coll Cardiol 52:e1, 2008.

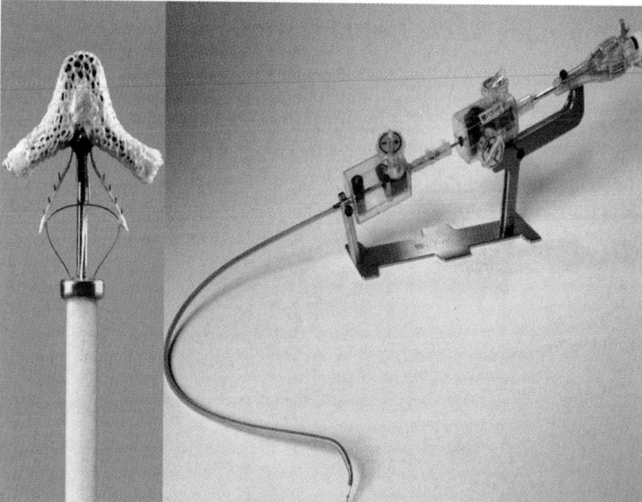

FIGURE 59-6 MitraClip and delivery system (Abbott Laboratories, Abbott Park, Ill).

Current American College of Cardiology/American Heart Association (ACC/AHA) guidelines recognize the possibility that aortic balloon valvotomy may have a limited therapeutic role (**Table 59-3**).[24] Valvotomy remains a Class I therapeutic option in young patients with congenital aortic stenosis. Class IIB recommendations include the following: (1) a bridge to surgery in hemodynamically unstable patients who are at high risk for surgery; and (2) for palliation in adult patients in whom surgery cannot be performed because of serious comorbid conditions. More recently, balloon valvotomy has found an expanded role as part of a transcatheter aortic valve implantation strategy.

Mitral Valve Repair

The potential for less invasive repair of the mitral valve without the need for open heart surgery has generated considerable interest. For the most part, these new approaches are modeled after established surgical strategies (see Chap. 66). The relatively simple but, in selected patients, effective surgical repair originally described by Alfieri can be reproduced percutaneously. Using transesophageal echocardiographic and fluoroscopic guidance, the anterior and posterior mitral leaflets are approximated with a small clip (MitraClip, Abbott Laboratories, Abbott Park, Ill) resulting in a double-orifice or edge to edge repair (**Fig. 59-6**).[4] Although initially intended for structural mitral regurgitation caused by prolapse, the procedure has also proven effective in patients with functional regurgitation and central malcoaptation.[25,26] Success is associated with a sustained, sometimes marked, clinical benefit and a reduction in left ventricular dimensions.[27-30] Potential concerns with respect to a percutaneous edge to edge procedure relate to long-term durability, the potential requirement for adjunctive annuloplasty, and the implications for subsequent surgical repair. The outcome of the now completed pivotal EVEREST II trial, randomized to MitraClip or surgical therapy, will help define the appropriate role for this procedure.

Percutaneous mitral annuloplasty remains investigational at present. Various coronary sinus implants, such as the MONARC (Edwards Lifesciences, Irvine, Calif) and CARILLON (Cardiac Dimensions, Kirkland, Wash) devices, have been evaluated; the objective is to displace the adjacent posterior mitral annulus anteriorly, thus improving leaflet coaptation. Concerns relate to the suboptimal and variable relationship between the coronary sinus and mitral annulus, possibility of left circumflex coronary artery compression, and modest efficacy. Other more direct approaches to modification of the mitral annulus, such as suture plication of the posterior mitral annulus from the left ventricle (Accucinch, Guided Delivery Systems, Santa Clara, Calif) are under active investigation. Although implantation of a valved stent within the native mitral valve is problematic because of the complexities of the mitral apparatus, a number of groups are pursuing transcatheter mitral valve replacement.

Pulmonary Valve Implantation

The use of valved conduits to reconstruct the right ventricular outflow tract in patients with congenital heart disease has allowed most of these patients to survive to adulthood (see Chap. 65). However, calcification leading to valve stenosis and/or regurgitation invariably occurs, often requiring multiple open heart operations over a lifetime. Balloon valvotomy may offer some palliation.[31] Stenting these conduits may relieve stenosis and delay the need for surgery, but the development of free pulmonary regurgitation results in progressive right ventricular dysfunction. Bonhoeffer and colleagues[32] and Zahn and associates[33] have demonstrated the possibility of percutaneous catheter implantation of stented valves in these pulmonary conduits. This initial experience was with a bovine jugular venous valve sutured inside a balloon-expandable stent (Melody, Medtronic, Minneapolis; **Fig. 59-7**).[33a] Late stent fracture with this device has been common, although generally well tolerated. Recently, the bovine pericardial balloon-expandable SAPIEN aortic valve has been used in the pulmonary position.[34]

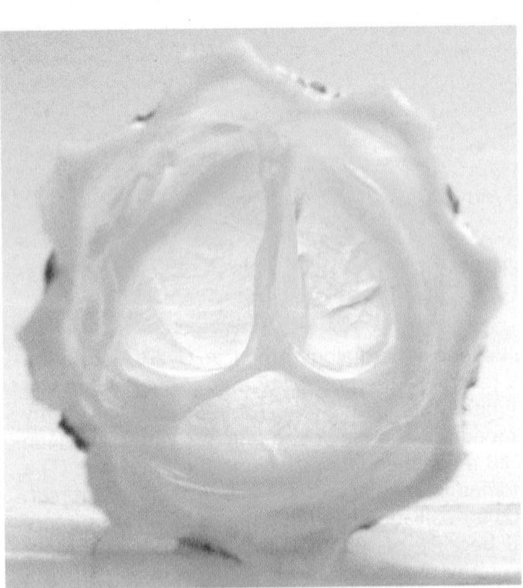

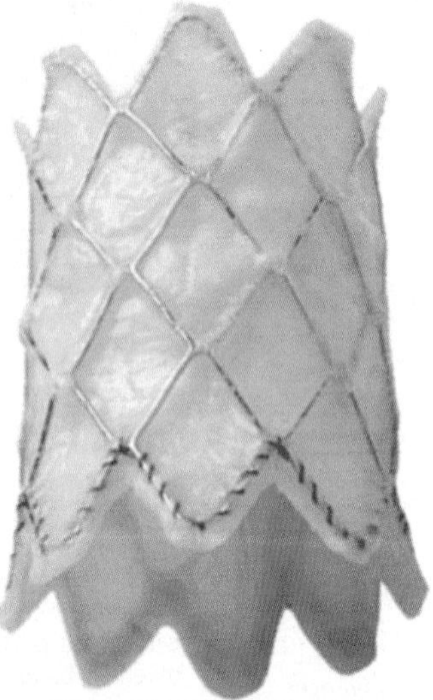

FIGURE 59-7 Transcatheter pulmonary valve implant. The Melody valve (Medtronic, Minneapolis) is constructed of a balloon-expandable metallic frame and a bovine jugular venous valve.

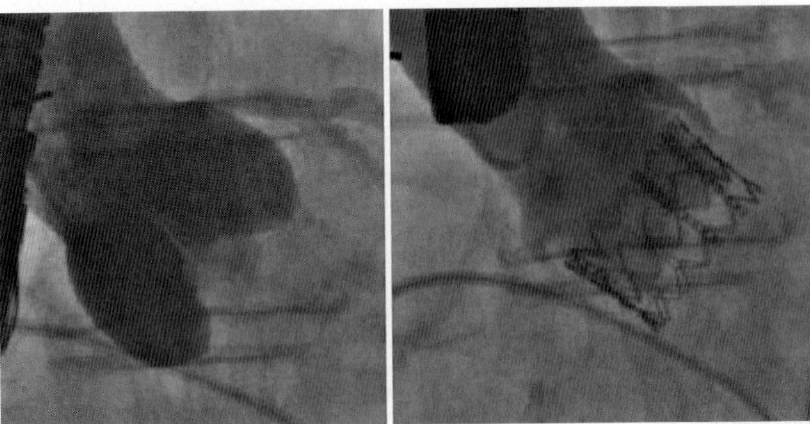

FIGURE 59-8 Aortic root angiogram in a patient with aortic stenosis before **(left)** and after **(right)** implantation of a SAPIEN valve (Edwards Lifesciences, Irvine, Calif).

Aortic Valve Implantation

Early experience with percutaneous valve implantation for aortic stenosis used an antegrade delivery technique with femoral vein access followed by a transseptal puncture to allow passage through the left atrium, mitral valve, and left ventricle.[35] However widespread application required the development of a reproducible transarterial procedure; with which aortic valve implantation has grown rapidly in popularity (**Fig. 59-8**).[36]

Currently, two valve systems are widely available (**Fig. 59-9**)—the balloon-expandable SAPIEN valve (Edwards Lifesciences, Irvine, Calif) and the self-expanding CoreValve device (Medtronic, Minneapolis). The SAPIEN valve consists of a stainless steel balloon-expandable stent frame to which bovine pericardial leaflets and a synthetic fabric sealing cuff to prevent paravalvular leaks are attached. The subsequently developed SAPIEN XT valve uses a cobalt chromium alloy frame with other features to facilitate its use, with a low-profile delivery system.[37] The CoreValve ReValving System (Medtronic) incorporates a self-expanding nitinol alloy frame constrained within a delivery sheath. As the sheath is withdrawn, the frame expands to assume its predetermined shape. The lower portion of the frame, with its sealing cuff, is positioned within the aortic annulus, displacing the native leaflets. The middle portion contains a trileaflet porcine pericardial valve. The upper portion extends above the coronaries to anchor the prosthesis against the ascending aorta.[38,39]

Although initial arterial procedures required a femoral artery cutdown, percutaneous access and closure are becoming the norm using various preclosure suture techniques. In the presence of small or diseased femoral arteries, direct access to the left ventricle through an intercostal incision (transapical approach) or to the subclavian artery through an axillary incision has been widely used.[40]

The hemodynamic characteristics of current transcatheter valves compare favorably with surgical valves (see Chap. 66). Valvular regurgitation is rare. However, paravalvular regurgitation is common, although for the most part relatively mild and well tolerated. Clinical hemolysis has not been reported. Clinically significant paravalvular leaks may sometimes occur because of poor sealing as a consequence of prosthesis undersizing or poor alignment. If severe, this may require redilation, implantation of a second overlapping valve or, rarely, surgical replacement.

Arterial injury has been the major cause of morbidity and mortality complicating transarterial aortic valve implantation. Consequently, detailed iliofemoral angiography and multislice computed tomography have become routine components of the screening process; a major focus of ongoing development has been to reduce the profile of delivery systems. AV block may occur because of compression of the conduction system as it passes through the periaortic septum. Predisposing factors may include preexisting conduction abnormalities, prosthesis oversizing, and extension of the prosthesis into the outflow tract. Permanent pacemakers are required in 5% to 30% of patients, varying with the valve type implanted and local practice. Coronary obstruction may rarely occur when a bulky native leaflet is displaced over the left main coronary ostium (<1%), and stroke may occur because of embolization from the native valve or aortic arch (1% to 4%).[38,39,41,42]

Current transcatheter valves appear sufficiently durable to provide benefit in the mostly elderly patients with comorbid conditions who are currently considered candidates.[41] Accelerated wear testing has demonstrated in vitro durability longer than 10 years and late structural valve failure has not been reported, although clinical follow-up remains limited. Whether durability is sufficient for patients with greater longevity and less comorbidity remains to be determined. However, the feasibility of transcatheter valve implantation in failing aortic, pulmonary, tricuspid, and mitral bioprosthetic surgical valves has recently been demonstrated.[43] Repeat valve in valve implants appear likely to prove to be a commonly used modality for managing late valve failure when this occurs.

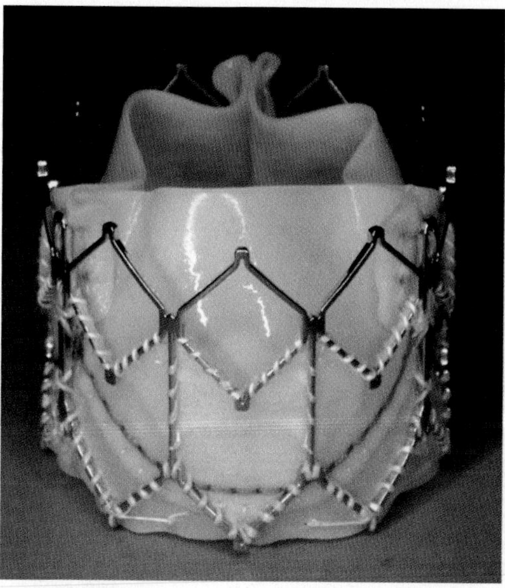

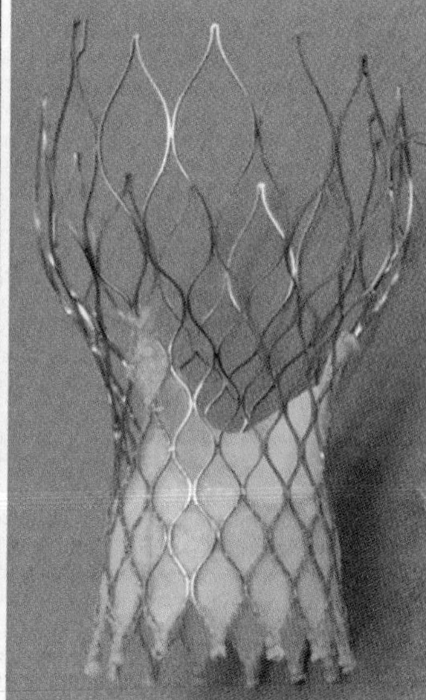

FIGURE 59-9 Transcatheter aortic valves. **Left,** SAPIEN XT valve (Edwards Lifesciences). **Right,** CoreValve (Medtronic).

Multiple single and multicenter high-risk registries have documented survival rates higher than predicted with conventional surgery and associated with a reduction in morbidity.[38,39,41,44] The large randomized North American PARTNER trial compared the Edwards SAPIEN valve to medical management (including balloon valvotomy) in patients considered to be at too high risk for surgical valve replacement and demonstrated substantial reduction in death and hospitalization with transcatheter valve implantation associated with significant improvement in symptoms.[44a] This study will have a major impact on defining the role of transcatheter aortic valve implantation.[45]

Surgical aortic valve replacement remains the current standard of care for symptomatic aortic stenosis because of a large body of favorable experience. In the absence of more studies, transcatheter aortic valve implantation is currently recommended only for patients in whom the risks of surgical morbidity or mortality are high. Logistic EuroSCORE estimates (www.euroscore.org) of a 30-day mortality exceeding 20% or Society of Thoracic Surgeons (STS) estimates (www.sts.org) exceeding 10% have been widely used to determine high surgical risk. However, both risk models commonly overestimate surgical risk in surgical candidates, but underestimate risk in patients with many important comorbidities, such as porcelain aorta, multivalve disease, and frailty, for whom clinical data allowing incorporation into these risk models is lacking. Moreover, the reduced morbidity of a transcatheter procedure may be more important to many older patients than the potential for reduced mortality. Often, the opinion of an experienced surgeon is the best estimate of risk.[46]

Future Perspectives

Percutaneous closure of intracardiac defects is now relatively common. Transcatheter valve implantation is rapidly becoming routine for the management of aortic and pulmonary valve disease, and may play a prominent role in the management of degenerated bioprosthetic valves. It appears likely that edge to edge repair for mitral regurgitation and left atrial appendage exclusion for atrial fibrillation may become widely accepted therapeutic options. New transcatheter procedures for chronic heart failure are on the horizon. Transcatheter approaches to adult structural heart disease have seen dramatic advances over the past decade, and this trend appears likely to continue.

REFERENCES

Closure Devices

1. Kim MS, Klein AJ, Carroll JD: Transcatheter closure of intracardiac defects in adults. J Interv Cardiol 20:524, 2007.
2. Kedia G, Tobis J, Lee MS: Patent foramen ovale: Clinical manifestations and treatment. Rev Cardiovasc Med 9:168, 2008.
3. Kim SS, Hijazi ZM, Lang RM, Knight BP: The use of intracardiac echocardiography and other intracardiac imaging tools to guide noncoronary cardiac interventions. J Am Coll Cardiol 53:2117, 2009.
4. Silvestry FE, Kerber RE, Brook MM, et al: Echocardiography-guided interventions. J Am Soc Echocardiogr 22:213, 2009.
5. Dowson A, Mullen MJ, Peatfield R, et al: Migraine intervention with STARFlex Technology (MIST) trial: A prospective, multicenter, double-blind, sham-controlled trial to evaluate the effectiveness of patent foramen ovale closure with STARFlex septal repair implant to resolve refractory migraine headache. Circulation 117:1397, 2008.
6. Martinez MW, Mookadam F, Sun Y, et al: Transcatheter closure of ischemic and post-traumatic ventricular septal ruptures. Cathet Cardiovasc Interv 69:403, 2007.
7. Butera G, Chessa M, Carminati M: Percutaneous closure of ventricular septal defects. State of the art. J Cardiovasc Med 8:39, 2007.
8. Sievert H, Bayard YL: Percutaneous closure of the left atrial appendage: A major step forward. JACC Cardiovasc Interv 2:601, 2009.
9. Holmes DR, Reddy VY, Turi ZG, et al: Percutaneous closure of the left atrial appendage versus warfarin therapy for prevention of stroke in patients with atrial fibrillation: A randomized non-inferiority trial. Lancet 374:534, 2009.
10. McCabe DJH, Kinsella JA, Tobin WO: Left atrial appendage occlusion in non-valvular atrial fibrillation. Lancet 374:504, 2009.

Paravalvular Leaks

11. Pate GE, Al Zubaidi A, Chandavimol M, et al: Percutaneous closure of prosthetic paravalvular leaks: Case series and review. Catheter Cardiovasc Interv 68:528, 2006.
12. Pate GE, Thompson CR, Munt BI, Webb JG: Techniques for percutaneous closure of prosthetic paravalvular leaks. Cathet Cardiovasc Interv 67:158, 2006.
13. Hein R, Wunderlich N, Wilson N, Sievert H: New concepts in transcatheter closure of paravalvular leaks. Future Cardiology 4:373, 2008.

Septal Ablation

14. Fifer MA: Most fully informed patients choose septal ablation over septal myectomy. Circulation 116:207, 2007.
15. Sorajja P, Valeti U, Nishimura RA, et al: Outcome of alcohol septal ablation for obstructive hypertrophic cardiomyopathy. Circulation 118:131, 2008.
16. van der Lee C, Scholzel B, ten Berg JM, et al: Usefulness of clinical, echocardiographic, and procedural characteristics to predict outcome after percutaneous transluminal septal myocardial ablation. Am J Cardiol 101:1315, 2008.
17. Alam M, Dokainsh H, Lakkis N: Alcohol septal ablation for hypertrophic obstructive cardiomyopathy: A systematic review of published studies. J Interv Cardiol 19:319, 2006.

Mitral Balloon Valvotomy

18. Nobuyoshi M, Arita T, Shirai S, et al: Percutaneous balloon mitral valvuloplasty: A review. Circulation 119:e211, 2009.
19. Wilkins GT, Weyman AE, Abascal AM, et al: Percutaneous balloon dilation of the mitral valve: An analysis of echocardiographic variables related to outcome and the mechanism of dilatation. Br Heart J 60:299,1988.

Aortic Balloon Valvotomy

20. Boone RH, Webb J: Nonsurgical aortic valve therapy: Balloon valvuloplasty and transcatheter aortic valve replacement. In Yusuf S, Cairns, J, Camm J, et al (eds): Evidence-Based Cardiology. 3rd ed. Oxford, Blackwell Publishing, 2010, pp 896-912.
21. Agarwal A, Kini AS, Attanti S, et al: Results of repeat balloon valvuloplasty for treatment of aortic stenosis in patients aged 59 to 104 years. Am J Cardiol 95:43, 2005.
22. Klein A, Lee K, Gera A, et al: Long-term mortality, cause of death, and temporal trends in complications after percutaneous aortic balloon valvuloplasty for calcific aortic stenosis. J Interv Cardiol 19:269, 2006.

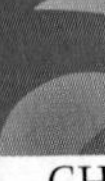

23. Pedersen WR, Block P, Feldman T: The iCoapsys Repair System for the percutaneous treatment of functional mitral insufficiency (http://www.northshore.org/uploadedfiles/cardiology/forphysicians/InterventionalRadiology/5_2006_IntCardioArticle2.pdf).
24. Bonow RO, Carabello BA, Chatterjee K, et al: 2008 focused update incorporated into the ACC/AHA 2006 guidelines for the management of patients with valvular heart disease: A report of the American College of Cardiology/American Heart Association Task Force on Practice Guidelines (Writing Committee to Revise the 1998 Guidelines for the Management of Patients With Valvular Heart Disease). J Am Coll Cardiol 52:e1, 2008.

Mitral Valve Repair

25. Foster E, Wasserman HS, Gray W, et al: Quantitative assessment of severity of mitral regurgitation by serial echocardiography in a multicenter clinical trial of percutaneous mitral valve repair. Am J Cardiol 100:1577, 2007.
26. Feldman T: EVEREST Registry (Endovascular Valve Edge-to-edge REpair Studies). Reduction in mitral regurgitation 12 months following percutaneous mitral valve repair. Clin Cardiol 30:416, 2007.
27. Herrmann HC, Kar S, Fail P, et al: Stability of mitral valve area and gradient following percutaneous repair of mitral regurgitation with the Mitraclip device. J Am Coll Cardiol 51(Suppl B):79, 2008.
28. Feldman T , Kar S, Rinaldi M, et al: Percutanesous mitral repair with the MitraClip system. J Am Coll Cardiol 54:686, 2009.
29. Silvestry FE, Rodriguez LL, Herrmann HC, et al: Echocardiographic guidance and assessment of percutaneous repair for mitral regurgitation with the Evalve MitraClip: Lessons learned from EVEREST I. J Am Soc Echocardiogr 20:1131, 2007.
30. Feldman T, Glower D: Patient selection for percutaneous mitral valve repair: Insight from early clinical trial applications. Nat Clin Pract Cardiovasc Med 5:84, 2008.

Pulmonary Valve Implantation

31. Rao PS: Percutaneous balloon pulmonary valvuloplasty: State of the art. Cathet Cardiovasc Interv 69:747, 2007.
32. Bonhoeffer P, Boudjemline Y, Qureshi SA, et al: Percutaneous insertion of the pulmonary valve. J Am Coll Cardiol 39:1664, 2002.
33. Zahn EM, Hellenbrand WE, Lock JE, McElhinney DB: Implantation of the Melody transcatheter pulmonary valve in patients with a dysfunctional right ventricular outflow tract conduit. J Am Coll Cardiol 54:1722, 2009.
33a. McElhinney DB, Hellenbrand WE, Zahn EM, et al: Short-term outcomes after transcatheter pulmonary valve placement in the expanded multicenter US Melody valve trial. Circulation 122:507, 2010.
34. Boone RH, Webb JG, Horlick E, et al: Transcatheter pulmonary valve implantation using the Edwards SAPIEN transcatheter heart valve (THV). Cathet Cardiovasc Interv 75:286, 2010.

Aortic Valve Implantation

35. Eltchaninoff H, Zajarias A, Tron C, Litzlerb PY, et al: Transcatheter aortic valve implantation: Technical aspects, results and indications. Arch Cardiovasc Dis 101:126, 2008.
36. Webb JG, Chandavimol M, Thompson C, et al: Percutaneous aortic valve implantation retrograde from the femoral artery. Circulation 113:842, 2006.
37. Nietlispach F, Wijesinghe N, Wood D, Carere RG, Webb JG. Current balloon-expandable transcatheter heart valve and delivery systems. Cathet Cardiovasc Intv. 75:295,2010.
38. Grube E, Buellesfeld L, Mueller R, et al: Progress and current status of percutaneous aortic valve replacement: results of three device generations of the CoreValve revalving system. Circ Cardiovasc Intervent 1:167, 2008.
39. Piazza N, Grube E, Gerckens U, et al: Procedural and 30-day outcomes following transcatheter aortic valve implantation using the third generation (18Fr) CoreValve ReValving System: Results from the multicentre, expanded evaluation registry 1-year following CE mark approval. EuroIntery 4:242, 2008.
40. Wong D, Ye J, Cheung A, et al: Technical considerations to avoid pitfalls during transapical aortic valve implantation. J Thorac Cardiovasc Surg 140:196, 2010.
41. Webb JG, Altwegg L, Boone RH, et al: Transcatheter aortic valve implantation: Impact on clinical and valve-related outcomes. Circulation 119:3009, 2009.
42. Masson JB, Kovac J, Schuler G, et al: Transcatheter aortic valve implantation: review of the nature, management and avoidance of procedural complications. JACC Cardiovasc Interv 2:811, 2009.
43. Webb JG, Wood DA, Ye J, et al: Transcatheter valve-in-valve implantation for failed bioprosthetic valves. Circulation 121:1848, 2010.
44. Thomas M, Schymik G, Walter T, et al: 30-day results of the SOURCE Registry: A European registry of transcatheter aortic valve implantation using the Edwards SAPIEN valve. Circulation122:62, 2010.
44a. Leon MB, Smith CR, Mack Met al: Transcatheter aortic-valve implantation for aortic stenosis in patients who cannot undergo surgery. N Engl J Med 2010 [E-pub ahead of print Sep. 22 (10.1056/NEJMoa1008232].
45. Zuckerman BD, Saperstein W, Swain JA: The FDA role in the development of percutaneous valve technology. EuroIntery Suppl A 1:A75, 2006.
46. Dewey TM, Brown D, Ryan WH, et al: Reliability of risk algorithms in predicting early and late operative outcomes in high-risk patients undergoing aortic valve replacement. J Thorac Cardiovasc Surg 135:180, 2008.

CHAPTER 60 Diseases of the Aorta

Alan C. Braverman, Robert W. Thompson, and Luis A. Sanchez

The Normal Aorta

Anatomy and Physiology

The aorta, the body's largest artery, extends from the aortic valve in the chest to the midabdomen, where it bifurcates into the common iliac arteries. Along its course the aorta is divided anatomically into thoracic and abdominal components. The thoracic aorta is further subdivided into the ascending, arch, and descending segments and the abdominal aorta into the suprarenal and infrarenal segments.

The ascending thoracic aorta has two distinct portions. The lower portion is the aortic root, which begins at the level of the aortic valve and extends to the sinotubular junction. The aortic root supports the bases of the three aortic valve leaflets, which bulge outward into the sinuses of Valsalva to allow for full valve cusp excursion during systole. The right and left coronary artery origins arise from within the sinuses of Valsalva. The upper portion of the ascending aorta begins at the sinotubular junction and rises to join the aortic arch. The proximal portion of ascending aorta lies within the pericardial cavity, anterior to the pulmonary artery bifurcation. The aortic arch gives rise to the arch vessels, innominate artery, left common carotid artery, and left subclavian artery.

The descending thoracic aorta begins just past the origin of the left subclavian artery. The point at which the aortic arch joins the descending aorta is called the aortic isthmus and is marked by the location of the ligamentum arteriosum. The aortic isthmus is especially vulnerable to deceleration trauma, because at this site, the relatively mobile portion of the aorta—the ascending aorta and arch—becomes relatively fixed to the thoracic cage. The descending aorta gradually courses downward, where it gives rise to paired intercostal arteries from the posterior aortic wall at each level of the spine. At its distal extent, the thoracic aorta passes through the diaphragm, usually at the level of the 12th thoracic vertebra, and becomes the abdominal aorta.

The abdominal aorta continues downward, giving rise to the celiac axis and the superior mesenteric artery from its anterior wall, followed within several centimeters by the posterolateral origins of the right and left renal arteries. This segment of the aorta is described as the suprarenal or visceral segment. The infrarenal aorta continues along the anterior surface of the lumbar spine, where it gives origin to the paired lumbar artery braches from its posterior wall. The aorta ends by bifurcation into common iliac arteries, usually at the level of the fourth lumbar vertebra.

MICROSCOPIC STRUCTURE. The aortic wall is comprised of three layers—the innermost tunica intima, which contacts the blood through its thin layer of endothelium, the musculoelastic tunica media, which is the thickest layer of the aortic wall, and the fibrous tunica adventitia, which forms its outermost layer (see Chap. 43). The intima consists of endothelial cells and the immediate subendothelial space, and is demarcated from the media by the internal elastic lamina. The media contains concentric layers of elastic fibers alternating with vascular smooth muscle cells (SMCs), with each layer of elastin and SMC constituting a lamellar unit of medial structure. In addition to SMCs, the aortic media normally contains a small number of fibroblasts, mast cells, and other cell types and, although dominated by elastic fibers, the extracellular matrix of the media includes collagen fibers, proteoglycans, and glycosaminoglycans. The microscopic architecture of the media gives the aorta its circumferential resilience (elasticity), necessary to resist hemodynamic stress. The outer portion of the aortic media is delineated from the adventitial layer by the external elastic lamina, which is normally thinner than the internal elastic lamina. The aortic adventitia is composed of a loose network of collagen fibers and fibroblasts, as well as small nerves and capillary-sized blood vessels. The adventitial collagen fibers ultimately govern the tensile strength of the aortic wall.

The human ascending aorta normally contains approximately 55 to 60 elastic lamellae, with a gradual decrease in the number of elastic lamellae down the length of the aorta to approximately 26 at the aortic bifurcation. Despite this regional variation in medial thickness, there appears to be a relatively consistent relationship between the number of elastic lamellae and the estimated amount of hemodynamic stress placed on the vessel wall, except for in the infrarenal aorta, with fewer elastic lamellae than predicted for its hemodynamic load.

Oxygen and nutrients reach the aortic wall by simple diffusion from the lumen, at least in segments of the aorta that contain up to about 29 elastic lamellae. In the proximal aortic segments that contain a greater number of elastic lamellae, additional nutrient supply is provided by an independent network of microvessels, the vasa vasorum, which extends from the adventitia to the outer layers of the elastic media. The outer third of the aortic media in the thoracic aorta contains many vasa vasorum, but the infrarenal aorta normally lacks an independent microvascular supply.

The compliance of the aortic wall under normal conditions results from the reversible extension of the elastic lamellar units in the media. This extensibility derives primarily from the properties of elastic fibers, whereas SMCs make only a minor contribution. At mechanical strain levels that exceed the extensile capacity of medial elastic fibers, the aortic tensile strength becomes dependent on the collagen fiber meshwork of the media and adventitia. Although not functionally significant under normal circumstances or in systemic hypertension, the dependence on adventitial collagen in accommodating greater hemodynamic stress is an important feature of abdominal aortic aneurysms (AAAs), where estimates of wall tension within the dilated segment may exceed that in the normal aorta by several orders of magnitude. In AAAs, collagen fibers are reorganized to accommodate higher degrees of tensile stress. In addition, there is evidence that aneurysmal dilation is accompanied by an active process characterized by a marked increase in collagen production. Surgical experience has shown that much of the inner arterial wall (endothelium and tunica media) can be removed, as is performed during an endarterectomy, without resulting in aneurysmal dilation. This observation illustrates that the structures conferring resistance aneurysmal dilation reside principally within the outer aspect of the media and the adventitia.

PHYSIOLOGY. The aorta is responsible for transmitting pulsatile arterial blood pressure to all points in the arterial tree, a function that depends on its properties as an elastic conduit. The aortic wall therefore requires properties of resilience to cyclic deformation, resistance to structural failure, and durability. The biomechanical properties attributable to elastin and collagen in the media and adventitia serve these demands. The aortic wall pressure-diameter relationship is nonlinear, demonstrating a more distensible component at lower pressures and a stiffer component at higher pressures, with the transition from distensible to stiff behavior occurring at pressures above 80 mm Hg. Thus, the more distensible elastin is the principal load bearer at low pressures and small distentions, whereas at higher pressures and large distentions, both elastin and the stiffer collagen are load bearing.

It is important to point out that the pressure-diameter curve of the aorta becomes less steep with increasing age (i.e., the aorta stiffens and aortic diameter increases). One explanation for this is an increase in the collagen-to-elastin ratio because of an age-related decrease in elastin and a simultaneous increase in collagen. Another factor is a gradual alteration of aortic wall architecture with age, characterized by progressively disordered medial elastic fibers and lamellae displaying thinning, splitting, and fragmentation in older individuals. A third factor is an increase in aortic wall thickness with age because of increased deposition of collagen and proteoglycan, as well as age-related calcification of elastic fibers. Finally, atherosclerotic changes are associated with aging, and may contribute to aortic wall stiffening. In addition to the direct effects of aortic wall plaque, stiffening may occur through compensatory increases in distensibility in areas free of disease (i.e., expansive arterial wall remodeling).

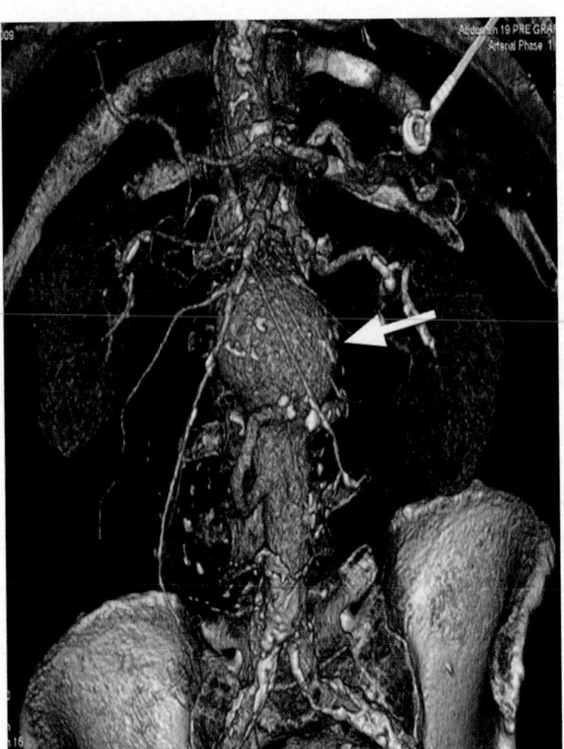

FIGURE 60-1 Three-dimensional reconstruction of a CT scan in a patient with an infrarenal abdominal aortic aneurysm (arrow).

Evaluation of the Aorta

The only location in which the aorta can normally be palpated is in the midabdomen, where in some individuals (depending on body habitus) it may be detected on deep palpation adjacent to the spine. Plain radiography is insensitive for evaluating the thoracic and abdominal aorta. Much more diagnostic detail regarding the aorta is obtained through imaging modalities, such as ultrasound (including echocardiography), computed tomography (CT) and CT angiography, magnetic resonance imaging (MRI), or aortography.

Aortic Aneurysms

The term *aortic aneurysm* refers to a pathologic segment of aortic dilation that has a propensity to expand and rupture. The extent of aortic dilation required to be considered aneurysmal is debated, but one criterion is an increase in diameter at least 50% greater than that expected for the same aortic segment in unaffected individuals of the same age and sex. Aortic aneurysms are usually described in terms of their size, location, morphology, and etiology. Size criteria are usually focused on cross-sectional diameter, as measured in imaging studies. Aortic aneurysms are either fusiform or saccular. Fusiform aneurysms are most common and are characterized by a general symmetric dilation with a fairly uniform shape involving the entire aortic wall circumference. Saccular aneurysms exhibit localized dilation involving only a portion of the aortic wall circumference, appearing as a focal outpouching. These lesions represent true aneurysms in that the aortic wall is intact but dilated, involving all layers of aortic structure. In contrast, pseudoaneurysms (false aneurysms) represent lesions in which there has been bleeding through the aortic wall, resulting in a contained periaortic hematoma in continuity with the aortic lumen. These lesions may result from trauma or from contained rupture of an aortic aneurysm, dissection, or penetrating ulcer.

Abdominal Aortic Aneurysms

AAAs are defined by an increase in size of the abdominal aorta to more than 3.0 cm in diameter. AAAs occur in 3% to 9% of men older than 50 years and are the most common form of aortic aneurysms. Most AAAs arise in the infrarenal aorta (**Fig. 60-1**), but up to 10% may involve the pararenal or visceral aorta, and some extend into the thoracoabdominal segment. The overall incidence of AAAs appears to have increased steadily over the past several decades. AAAs are approximately five times more prevalent in men than in women, and the incidence strongly associates with age, with most occurring in those older than 60 years. AAAs strongly associate with cigarette smoking; current and former smokers have a fivefold increase in risk compared with nonsmokers. Additional risk factors include emphysema, hypertension, and hyperlipidemia. Up to 20% of patients with AAAs describe a family history of aortic aneurysms, suggesting an inherited predisposition in some cohorts. AAAs are a multifactorial disease of aging without a known specific cause.

PATHOGENESIS. Aneurysm formation closely associates with chronic aortic wall inflammation, increased local expression of proteinases, and degradation of connective tissue proteins.[1] Aneurysmal dilation and rupture result from mechanical failure of medial elastin and adventitial collagen, the fibrillar matrix proteins normally responsible for maintaining aortic wall tensile strength, resilience, and structural integrity. Infiltration of the aortic wall by inflammatory cells occurs commonly in AAAs. In contrast to occlusive atherosclerosis, in which inflammation concentrates within the diseased intimal plaque, the distribution of inflammatory cells is transmural in AAAs, with dense focal infiltrates and scattered inflammatory cells centered within the elastic media and adventitia. In some patients with inflammatory AAAs, this process extends to the periaortic retroperitoneal tissues. Because inflammatory cells can elaborate matrix-degrading enzymes thought to be involved in medial degeneration, this process may be responsible for aneurysmal dilation and rupture.

Although the initial events responsible for inflammatory cell recruitment into the aortic media are unknown, they may include signals elaborated by medial SMCs in response to hemodynamic stress and/or ischemia, autoimmune processes, or an extension of intimal atherosclerosis. AAA tissues produce a large number of chemotactic peptides, including chemokines and biologically active products released during matrix degradation that could amplify the mononuclear inflammatory response. The tissue environment of AAAs also includes proinflammatory cytokines capable of stimulating macrophage expression of connective tissue proteinases, such as tumor necrosis factor-α, interleukin-1β, interleukin-6, and interferon-γ. Direct cell-to-cell interactions may be another local mechanism amplifying macrophage proteinase production. Although a response to foreign antigens or microbial infection has been postulated in the development of AAAs, the chronic inflammation in aneurysm tissue also exhibits features of an autoimmune response. AAA tissues thereby contain focal infiltrates of T and B lymphocytes, as well as large amounts of immunoglobulin, which is reactive with a number of matrix protein-related antigens. Whereas the autoimmune response in AAAs suggests a primary mechanism of disease, this response may represent a secondary consequence of extensive matrix degradation, leading to exposure of previously hidden epitopes and amplifying aortic wall inflammation.

Loss of medial elastin both morphologically and biochemically occurs consistently in AAAs. Experimental studies have demonstrated that damage to the elastic lamellae leads to aneurysmal dilation and tortuosity. Because elastin is extremely durable, and its degradation requires the activity of potent substrate-specific enzymes, the elastolytic proteinases produced within aneurysm tissues probably play a critical role in aneurysm development. Experimental studies have shown that maintenance of aortic wall tensile strength is principally attributable to interstitial collagen, and that AAAs are generally associated with an increase in collagen content. This finding manifests clinically as increased wall stiffness, exhibited by aortic aneurysms and elevations in type III procollagen fragments, which can be measured in the plasma as a marker of collagen turnover. Increased collagen production may thereby help preserve the dilated aneurysm wall, whereas enzymes that can initiate cleavage of interstitial collagens are an important factor in rapid aneurysm expansion and rupture.

The most prominent elastin- and collagen-degrading enzymes produced in human AAA tissues are matrix metalloproteinases (MMPs). MMPs degrade a broad range of matrix proteins, with four exhibiting specific activity against elastin (72-kDa gelatinase type IV collagenase [MMP-2], matrilysin [MMP-7], 92-kDa gelatinase type IV collagenase [MMP-9], and macrophage metalloelastase [MMP-12]). At least three MMPs can initiate the degradation of intact fibrillar collagen (MMP-1, MMP-8, and MMP-13), and several others act against denatured collagen (gelatin). Cellular production of MMPs is closely regulated at the level of gene transcription, and most MMPs are secreted into the extracellular space as inactive proenzymes; once secreted, pro-MMPs are regulated by local factors in the pericellular environment, such as proteases that mediate their extracellular activation, oxidative protein modifications, and interaction with secreted tissue inhibitors of metalloproteinases (TIMPs) and other proteinase scavengers.

MMP-9 has an especially important role in human and experimental AAAs. Aneurysm tissue contains abundant MMP-9, and mice lacking expression of MMP-9 show suppression of experimental AAAs. Moreover, treatment of experimental animals with tetracyclines and other MMP inhibitors has consistently suppressed aneurysm development in almost every animal model tested. Other experimental interventions found to suppress AAAs, such as treatment with statins and anti-inflammatory agents, induce a decrease in aortic tissue MMP-9. These observations have suggested the use of doxycycline and other MMP-inhibiting agents as therapeutic approaches to suppress the progression of aneurysmal degeneration in patients with small AAAs.

The development and natural history of AAAs involves a balance between degradative and reparative processes. Because vascular SMCs normally produce elastin and collagen during aortic development, and SMCs are the dominant cell type within the elastic media, SMCs are ideally positioned to mediate connective tissue repair within AAAs. Human AAAs show a pronounced depletion of medial SMCs. Mechanisms underlying the loss of SMCs in AAAs include apoptotic cell death, which may be initiated by medial ischemia, signaling molecules prevalent in AAA tissue, or cellular immune responses. Medial SMC ischemia may also participate in aneurysmal degeneration, because in the absence of vasa vasorum, the nutrient supply to the media depends on diffusion from the aortic lumen, a process jeopardized by intimal thickening and atherosclerotic plaques.

CLINICAL FEATURES. AAAs develop insidiously over a period of several years and rarely cause symptoms in the absence of distal thromboembolism, rapid expansion, or overt rupture. Although large AAAs are at substantial risk of rupture and thereby attract most clinical attention, the vast majority of AAAs are small. Most AAAs are thereby detected by screening, or as an incidental finding on imaging studies performed for other purposes.

Physical examination is notoriously inaccurate in the detection of AAAs, but abdominal palpation may reveal a pulsatile epigastric or periumbilical mass, particularly in relatively thin patients with large aneurysms. Mural thrombus associated with AAAs may lead to thromboembolism, which may be the presenting symptom in 2% to 5% of patients. Because AAAs are frequently associated with peripheral artery aneurysms, physical examination should also include palpation of the femoral and popliteal arteries.

DIAGNOSTIC IMAGING

Ultrasound

Abdominal ultrasound can detect AAAs with a high degree of accuracy, with sensitivities and specificities that approach 100%. Abdominal ultrasound is preferred in screening for AAAs because it is also inexpensive, noninvasive, and avoids radiation exposure. In approximately 2% to 3% of patients, visualization of the infrarenal aorta by ultrasound may be limited by overlying bowel gas or obesity, and alternate imaging studies are necessary. Abdominal ultrasound is also used for serial measurements of AAA size during follow-up surveillance of patients with small AAAs. Because the accuracy of ultrasound-derived aneurysm diameter measurements is not as great as those obtained by CT or MRI, many recommend the use of ultrasound for follow-up of AAAs up to 4.5 cm in diameter, with the use of alternative modalities for larger AAAs. The wide availability of ultrasound has suggested its use in emergency room detection of ruptured AAAs. Despite reports indicating a high degree of accuracy, up to half of ruptured AAAs may be missed in the emergency setting.

Computed Tomography

Abdominal CT is extremely accurate for the detection of AAAs and measurement of aneurysmal diameter (**Fig. 60-2**). Particularly when combined with radiographic contrast enhancement, thin-slice techniques, and three-dimensional reconstructions with measurements

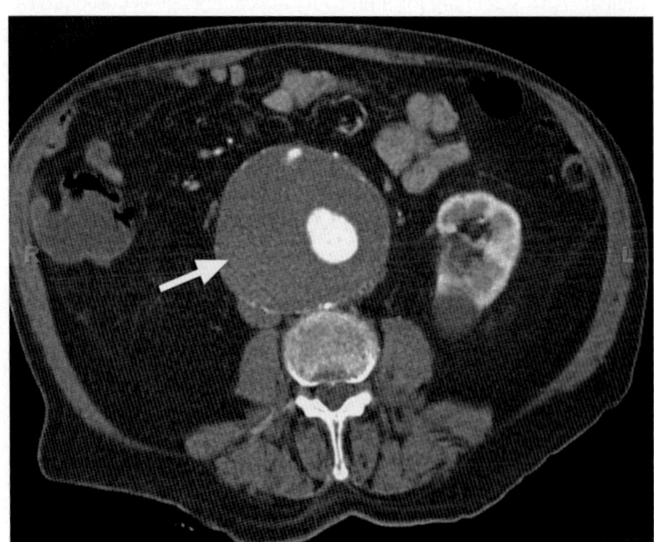

FIGURE 60-2 Contrast CT scan of a large, thrombus-filled abdominal aortic aneurysm (arrow). Contrast fills the lumen of the aneurysm.

obtained perpendicular to the center line of the aorta, CT angiography (CTA) is more accurate than ultrasound and has superseded the need for catheter-based aortography in preoperative planning. CTA is especially useful for demonstrating the extent of aneurysm disease; the relationship of the AAA to the renal, visceral, and iliac arteries; and patterns of mural thrombus, calcification, or coexisting occlusive atherosclerosis that might influence surgical AAA repair. CT imaging is also preferred for the assessment of unusual variants of AAAs, such as inflammatory AAAs and mycotic aneurysms, and AAAs associated with anatomic variations, such as vena cava or renal vein anomalies and pelvic or horseshoe kidneys.

Magnetic Resonance Aortography

Like CT imaging, magnetic resonance aortography (MRA) is extremely accurate for the detection of AAAs, the measurement of aneurysm diameter, and the delineation of aortic anatomy for planning treatment. MRA has the distinct advantage of avoiding exposure to radiation and iodine-based contrast materials. Although MRA is preferred in some centers, where it may be readily available, in most institutions CT imaging remains the preferred imaging modality for the evaluation of AAAs.

As noted, CT angiography now generally supersedes aortography, which is rarely used in this setting. For patients undergoing endovascular AAA repair, aortography is one of the initial steps in the operative procedure. It is also used in subsequent interventions following AAA stent-graft repair, such as embolization of lumbar or iliac artery branches. An unsuspected AAA may occasionally be identified during transfemoral angiography performed for another reason (e.g., cardiac catheterization). The characteristics of an AAA include an enlarged abdominal aortic segment, marked by calcification and occlusion of lumbar branch vessels. The aortic lumen may or may not appear enlarged because of the presence of mural thrombus.

SCREENING. Screening for AAAs with ultrasound, coupled with repair for AAAs above a given size threshold, can reduce AAA-related deaths.[2] The overall incidence of screening-detected AAAs ranges from 1:1000 in adults younger than 60 years of age to 7:1000 in those in their mid-60s, but may be as high as 10% in the presence of risk factors such as older age, male sex, smoking, family history, history of other aneurysms, hypertension, atherosclerotic diseases, and hypercholesterolemia. In asymptomatic U.S. veterans 50 to 79 years of age participating in the Aneurysm Detection and Management Trial, 66% of AAAs identified by screening were smaller than 4.0 cm in diameter. Randomized trials have demonstrated that AAA screening is associated with a 50% reduction in AAA rupture and a 50% decrease in aneurysm-related mortality. Whereas overall there was a 6% reduction in mortality, the presence of a significant reduction in all-cause mortality remains unclear.[3] AAA screening for men 65 to 74 years of age is cost-effective, but the cost-effectiveness of screening for AAAs in women remains debated. Whereas the prevalence of AAAs is lower in women than in men, AAAs occur about 10 years later in women, and the rupture rate and mortality of AAA rupture are both higher. In 2005, the U.S. Preventative Services Task Force reported a recommendation for one-time ultrasound screening for AAA for men 65 to 75 years of age with a history of smoking.[4] The Society for Vascular Surgery also recommends AAA screening in men and women with a family history of AAAs.[5]

GENETICS AND MOLECULAR GENETICS. Several well-defined but relatively uncommon genetic disorders are associated with aortic aneurysms, typically involving the ascending thoracic aorta, but less commonly the abdominal aorta, including Marfan syndrome (MFS), Loeys-Dietz syndrome (LDS), and vascular Ehlers-Danlos syndrome (see later, "Thoracic Aortic Aneurysms"). Up to 20% of patients with an infrarenal AAA describe a family history of AAAs, suggesting an inherited component. A number of genetic variants appear to link with AAAs through analysis of single nucleotide polymorphisms (SNPs) in relatively large populations. One example is a common sequence variant on chromosome 9p21 (rs10757278-G) that is associated with a 31% increased risk of AAAs, as well as increased risks for intracranial aneurysms.[6] Although further work is needed to help validate these findings in additional populations, broader use of genome-wide screening will undoubtedly help identify additional SNPs associated with AAAs.

NATURAL HISTORY. AAAs usually gradually expand over a period of years, and eventually rupture. The risk of AAA rupture is closely correlated with aneurysm size, with the 5-year risk of rupture being approximately 5% for AAAs 3.0 to 4.0 cm in diameter, 10% to 20% for AAAs 4.0 to 5.5 cm in diameter, and 30% to 40% for AAAs 5.5 to 6.0 cm in diameter.[5] The risk of rupture for AAAs larger than 6.0 cm in diameter rises even more rapidly, exceeding 80% for AAAs larger than 7.0 cm. The average rate of aneurysm expansion is approximately 0.3 to 0.5 cm/year, although there is considerable individual variation. Not all AAAs follow a linear or consistent rate of expansion, and many factors may influence AAA growth patterns. Thus, whereas some patients have stable AAAs that grow slowly for many years, others can have a stable AAA size for many years followed by a sudden increase within a short period of time.

Ruptured Abdominal Aortic Aneurysm

Symptoms directly attributable to AAAs usually occur with overt aneurysm rupture or rapid recent expansion presumed to indicate impending rupture. Rupture of an AAA into the peritoneal cavity results in rapid hemorrhage, with severe abdominal pain and cardiovascular collapse because of exsanguination. Rupture into the retroperitoneum may result in a temporarily contained periaortic hematoma, with severe abdominal or back pain that may radiate into the flank or groin. A tender pulsatile abdominal or flank mass is often present, along with hypotension or loss of consciousness. An estimated 30% to 50% of patients with ruptured AAAs die before reaching a hospital, and an additional 30% to 40% die after reaching a hospital but before operative treatment.[5] Whereas immediate surgical treatment is necessary for all ruptured AAAs, the operative mortality rate after rupture is 40% to 50%. Recent evidence has indicated that the mortality rate for repair of ruptured AAAs can be markedly diminished by the use of endovascular repair as compared with open surgical techniques.[7] Hemodynamically stable patients presenting with symptomatic but unruptured AAAs should undergo CT to determine whether rupture has occurred. In the absence of rupture, in some cases it may be prudent to delay surgical repair for 4 to 24 hours until optimal conditions can be achieved, with the patient closely monitored.

MANAGEMENT

Medical Therapy

Patients with small AAAs can be safely observed with imaging surveillance and little risk of rupture and, in general, AAA repair is reserved for aneurysms at least 5.0 to 5.5 cm in diameter.[8] For those with AAAs 3.0 to 4.0 cm in diameter, the rate of growth is less than 10% per year, and annual imaging with abdominal ultrasound is recommended. For those with AAAs larger than 4.0 cm in diameter, variability in growth is greater, so that imaging is recommended at 6-month intervals. For those with AAAs larger than 4.5 cm in diameter, CT may be preferred over ultrasound for more accurate measurement of AAA size.

For patients with small AAAs undergoing imaging surveillance, several steps may help minimize the risk of aneurysm expansion and improve overall health. The most important of these is smoking cessation, because there is strong evidence that ongoing tobacco use is associated with more rapid rates of AAA expansion and rupture. Appropriate management should also be undertaken for hypertension, hyperlipidemia and, diabetes. Almost all patients with small AAAs should take a statin, based on the presence of coexisting atherosclerotic disease, and although randomized data are lacking, these medications may suppress AAA growth.[9] Animal model data have demonstrated a favorable influence of angiotensin-converting enzyme (ACE) inhibitors or angiotensin receptor blockers (ARBs), but interpretable data in humans with AAAs are not yet available. Patients with small AAAs should be encouraged to exercise regularly, because moderate physical activity does not adversely influence the risk of rupture and may even limit the rate of AAA growth.

EXPERIMENTAL THERAPY. Based on laboratory research conducted over the past two decades, interest has accelerated in the potential use of medical (pharmacologic) therapies to suppress the growth rate of small AAAs, thereby reducing the need for surgical repair.[8] One of the earliest approaches suggested was the use of beta-adrenergic receptor blockers (beta blockers) to diminish mechanical stress on the aortic wall. Although several reports have indicated successful use of propranolol in animal models of AAAs, two large clinical trials have demonstrated no benefit to propranolol treatment in patients with small AAAs.[8] A second approach is to suppress proteinases involved in extracellular matrix degradation through the use of doxycycline as a MMP inhibitor. Treatment with doxycycline suppresses or prevents AAAs in a spectrum of animal models in association with MMP inhibition, particularly of MMP-9. Doxycycline is well tolerated by patients with small AAAs, in whom it also appears to decrease MMP activities in aneurysmal aortic tissue and in the circulation. Further clinical investigation is needed to determine whether doxycycline treatment can reduce the rate of AAA expansion. A third experimental approach is the use of angiotensin receptor antagonists, such as losartan, as a means to modify aortic wall connective tissue metabolism. Treatment with losartan suppresses aneurysm formation in mouse models of Marfan syndrome. Because losartan and other ARBs are also effective in other animal models of AAAs, it will be important to determine whether ARBs are useful in suppressing the growth of AAAs in humans.

SURGERY. The decision to repair an asymptomatic AAA electively is based on life expectancy and the estimated risk of rupture, balanced against the estimated risks of AAA repair. Factors significantly influencing operative morbidity and mortality include coronary artery disease (the leading cause of early and late mortality after AAA repair), chronic kidney disease, chronic pulmonary disease, and diabetes mellitus.[5] Thus, evaluation for these conditions is warranted before elective AAA repair, along with optimization of perioperative status wherever possible.

Because many patients with AAAs have underlying coronary artery disease, and postoperative myocardial infarction has a substantial risk of death or later cardiovascular events, special attention is directed toward coronary disease prior to elective AAA repair. Although guidelines to minimize perioperative cardiac risk have been recently updated (see Chap. 85), the first step is to identify those patients with an active cardiac condition that warrants urgent treatment or even precludes repair. In the absence of an active cardiac condition, further noninvasive testing is only indicated if it will change management, in accord with current guidelines. Some patients benefit from preoperative coronary ischemic evaluation and treatment. Perioperative medical management to reduce cardiac risks in patients undergoing AAA repair may include titrated administration of beta blockers, and treatment with statins and/or aspirin, in accord with the individual patient's risk factors and medical findings.[5,9]

Invasive treatment for AAAs can be performed by one of two general approaches—open surgical repair (OSR) or endovascular aneurysm repair (EVAR). The selection of approach depends on the individual anatomy and on secondary factors, such as patient age and estimated risks for anesthesia and surgery.[10]

Techniques and Outcomes. For open surgical repair (OSR) of infrarenal AAAs, the abdominal aorta may be approached through a transperitoneal exposure, using a full midline laparotomy incision, or a left retroperitoneal exposure. A tube or bifurcated prosthetic graft is attached with suture directly to the proximal aorta, followed by sutured anastomosis to the distal aorta (tube graft) or common iliac arteries (bifurcation graft). Following restoration of lower extremity flow through the aortic graft, the aneurysm sac is sewn together to prevent contact between the prosthetic graft and the gastrointestinal tract. The operative mortality rate for conventional OSR ranges from 1% to 4% in reports from single-institution centers of excellence, whereas mortality rates in statewide or national data bases range from 4% to 8%. Operative complication rates range from 10% to 30% and include morbidity related to cardiac, pulmonary, and renal complications, as well as colonic ischemia. Based on recent evidence that outcomes for OSR are related to hospital and surgeon volumes, there has been a trend to recommend that OSR for AAAs be performed at centers with demonstrable operative mortality rates less than 5%.

A number of late complications may develop during long-term follow-up after OSR for AAAs. The most significant of these include problems related to the abdominal incision, para-anastomotic aneurysms (including false aneurysms secondary to suture line disruptions and true aneurysms secondary to proximal aortic degeneration), graft infection, graft-enteric erosions or fistula, and graft limb occlusions with lower extremity ischemia. Annual clinical follow-up and CT at 5-year intervals are generally recommended after open AAA repair.

Endovascular Abdominal Aortic Aneurysm Repair. For patients with suitable anatomy, endovascular aortic aneurysm repair (EVAR) offers a less invasive alternative than open surgical repair (see Chap. 63). EVAR is performed in the operating room or angiographic suite under fluoroscopic guidance, and most patients are discharged within 24 hours. There are currently five U.S. Food and Drug Administration (FDA)-approved endografts commercially available, each with its own design and method of fixation to the aortic wall. The Open Versus Endovascular Repair (OVER) Veterans Affairs Cooperative Study Group randomized 881 veterans 49 years of age or older with a minimum aneurysm diameter of 5.0 cm. The perioperative mortality was lower for endovascular repair compared with open repair (0.5% to 3.0%).[11] High-risk patients can also benefit from endovascular repair. Using high-risk criteria from five multicenter investigational device exemption clinical trials, 565 EVAR patients and 61 open surgical controls were identified. The 30-day operative mortality was 2.9% in EVAR and 5.1% in the open surgical group ($P = 0.32$). The aneurysm-related death rate after EVAR was 3.0% at 1 year and 4.2% at 4 years compared with 5.1% at both time points for the open surgical group ($P = 0.58$). The overall survival at 4 years after EVAR was 56% versus 66% in the open surgical group ($P = 0.23$). After treatment, EVAR successfully prevented rupture in 99.5% at 1 year and 97.2% at 4 years.[12] Patients with ruptured aneurysms also benefit significantly from endovascular repair. In evaluating 27,750 hospital discharges for ruptured AAA, EVAR had a lower overall in-hospital mortality than open surgical repair (32% to 41%; $P < 0.0001$).[13] Data from 13 centers were collected on 1037 patients treated by EVAR and 763 patient treated by open surgical repair. The overall 30-day mortality in all EVAR patients was 21%. In centers performing EVAR whenever possible, almost 50% of patients underwent EVAR. The 30-day mortality rates for these centers were 20% for EVAR compared with 36% for open surgical repair.[14] With appropriate patient selection and accurate graft deployment, low perioperative mortality rates (~1%) and complication rates (10% to 15%) can be achieved irrespective of the endograft used. These results have led to the increased application of EVAR to patients with AAAs that have suitable anatomy. The options of endovascular and open surgical repair with their advantages and disadvantages currently are considered in medically fit patients with suitable anatomy. Most patients select endovascular treatment because of its early perioperative advantages and its less invasive nature.

The development of endoleaks (incomplete exclusion of blood flow from the aneurysm sac) can complicate EVAR. In addition, various other late complications (e.g., endograft migration, limb thrombosis, and implant-related complications such as fractures, component separation, and fabric tears) and graft infection can occur. Long-term radiographic surveillance is essential following EVAR. Imaging with contrast-enhanced CTA is typically performed at 1 month, at 6 months, and annually post–device implantation. A reduced surveillance regimen may be appropriate in cases in which there is early success with newer devices, but this approach has not been validated in a randomized prospective trial setting. In patients for whom contrast use is prohibited (e.g., renal insufficiency, allergy), duplex ultrasound may be combined with noncontrast CT for complete evaluation.

Thoracic Aortic Aneurysms

Thoracic aortic aneurysms (TAAs) occur much less commonly than AAAs, with an estimated incidence of at least 10/100,000 person-years.[15] TAAs may involve the ascending arch and/or the descending aorta. Their cause, natural history, and treatment varies, depending on their location. Ascending aortic aneurysms are most common (~60%), followed by aneurysms of the descending aorta (~35%) and arch (<10%). The term *thoracoabdominal aortic aneurysm* refers to descending thoracic aneurysms that extend distally to involve the abdominal aorta. *Annuloaortic ectasia*, an enlargement of the aorta at the sinuses of Valsalva with normal aortic dimensions above the sinotubular junction, often occurs in genetically triggered aortic diseases.

CAUSES AND PATHOGENESIS. Aneurysms involving the aortic root and ascending aorta can be genetically triggered, degenerative or atherosclerotic, inflammatory, or can result from infectious diseases (see Table 60-e1 on website). Cystic medial degeneration (CMD) describes degeneration and fragmentation of elastic fibers, smooth muscle cell loss, increase in collagen deposition, and replacement with interstitial cysts of mucoid appearing basophilic-staining ground substance (see Fig. 60-e1 on website). CMD of the aorta is present in MFS and many other genetically triggered TAA diseases. In addition, aging associates with some degree of CMD, a process that may be accelerated by hypertension. These changes cause progressive weakening of the aortic wall, leading to dilation and aneurysm formation.

Genetically Triggered Thoracic Aortic Aneurysm Diseases

There are many disorders of the thoracic aorta with an underlying genetic trigger, some of which associate with widespread syndromic features, whereas others associate with thoracic aortic disease alone (see Chap. 8). These include MFS, LDS, vascular Ehlers-Danlos syndrome (vEDS), familial thoracic aortic aneurysm and dissection syndrome (FTAA/D), bicuspid aortic valve (BAV) disease, Turner syndrome (TS), and the aortopathy associated with many congenital heart diseases.

MFS, an autosomal dominant disorder of connective tissue, is caused by abnormal fibrillin-1 resulting from mutations in the *FBN1* gene. In addition to directing elastogenesis and providing structural support to tissues, fibrillin-1 interacts with latent transforming growth factor-β (TGF-β)–binding proteins and controls TGF-β activation and signaling. Mutations in *FBN1* result in abnormal elastin content and function in the aortic wall. Aortic dilation in MFS involves the sinuses of Valsalva (**Fig. 60-3**; see Video 60-1 on website and Fig. 15-81), with the ascending aorta above the sinotubular junction usually being normal in dimension. Angiotensin is important in TGF-β signaling and blocking TGF-β, whether by neutralizing antibody or by the angiotensin II type I receptor blocker (ARB), losartan, attenuating or preventing aortic aneurysm formation in genetically engineered Marfan mice with abnormal fibrillin. In Marfan children with very aggressive aortic disease, ARB therapy resulted in a dramatic stabilization of aortic root size. A trial of beta blockade versus ARB therapy (losartan) in MFS is being conducted to examine the effects of these agents on aortic growth.

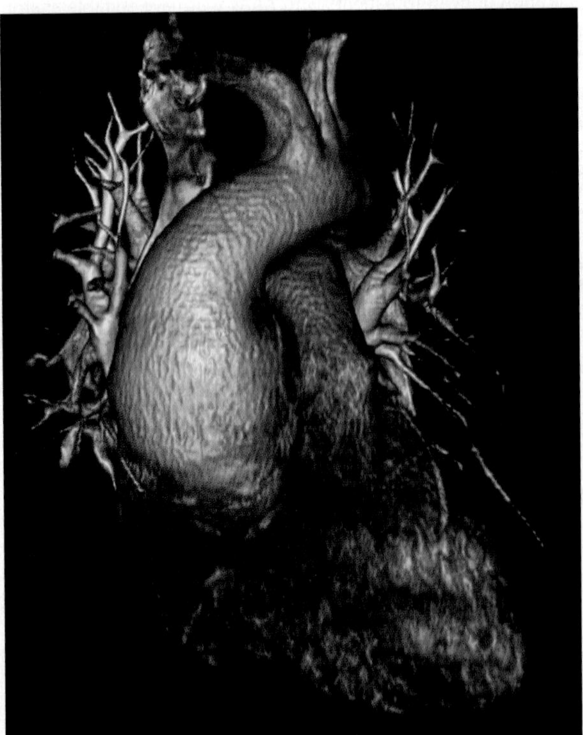

FIGURE 60-3 Three-dimensional CT reconstruction of an aortic root aneurysm in a patient with Marfan syndrome. *(Courtesy of Dr. Kristopher Cummings, Washington University School of Medicine, St. Louis.)*

LDS, an autosomal dominant disorder caused by mutations in *TGFBR1* and *TGFBR2*, is associated with craniofacial features (hypertelorism, bifid-broad uvula, cleft palate, craniosynostosis), arterial tortuosity, and aneurysms and dissections of the aorta and branch vessels.[16] Excess TGF-β signaling is suggested in the diseased tissues of LDS. Importantly, LDS has a much more aggressive vascular phenotype than MFS, and prophylactic aortic surgery at a smaller aortic root dimension is recommended.[17]

Mutations in *COL3A1* leading to abnormal collagen synthesis cause vEDS, an autosomal dominant condition that may be associated with aortic aneurysm and dissection. Individuals with vEDS are at risk for sudden death from spontaneous arterial dissection and rupture, often involving medium-sized arteries. Aortic root involvement is less common, with the descending and abdominal aorta and aortic branch vessels more frequently involved. Unlike MFS and LDS, the abnormal arteries in vEDS are friable, making surgical repair difficult and complicated, with increased risk.

Ascending TAAs, in the absence of other genetic syndromes, may be familial and associated with CMD. When TAA and dissection (TAAD) occur in the absence of other syndromic features, it is often inherited as an autosomal dominant trait with decreased penetrance and variable expression, a disorder known as familial TAAD.[18] Pedigree studies have emphasized the familial nature of TAA disease, highlighting the variable age of onset and variable expression in these families. An inherited pattern for TAA is present in 20% of TAA patients.[19] Among familial TAAD kindreds, 66% had TAAs, 25% had AAAs, and 8% had cerebral aneurysms. Several genes associated with TAAD have been identified to date, including *FBN1*, *TGFBR1*, *TGFBR2*, *MYH11*, and *ACTA2*. Whereas TGF-β signaling abnormalities underlie the pathogenesis in *FBN1*, *TGFBR1*, and *TGFBR2* mutations, defects in SMC contractile function leading to aortic aneurysm and dissection are related to *MYH11* and *ACTA2* mutations. Fibrillin-1 microfibrils may be a component of the mechanotransduction system of vascular SMCs, linking fibrillin-1 in the matrix to intracellular actin filaments. In most families with TAAD, the disorder is autosomal dominant, with decreased penetrance and variable expression with respect to the age of onset of aortic disease, location of the aneurysm, and degree of aortic enlargement prior to dissection. Histopathology of the aortic tissue in TAAD reveals CMD. Imaging of the aorta in family members often reveals asymptomatic aneurysms, and the incidence of aortic disease increases with advancing age. Decreased penetrance complicates the evaluation in this disorder. Some family members with TAAD have associated bicuspid aortic valve (BAV), cerebral aneurysm, and/or patent ductus arteriosus (PDA). *ACTA2* mutations have associated with livedo reticularis, iris flocculi, PDA, and BAV.[20] *MYH11* mutations may be associated with PDA and livedo reticularis. First-degree relatives of the individual with unexplained TAA or dissection should undergo thoracic aortic imaging. If a mutation in a gene associated with TAA or dissection is found, first-degree relatives should undergo testing for the same gene mutation.

BAV affects approximately 1% of the population and may associate with abnormalities of the aorta, including ascending aortic aneurysm, coarctation of the aorta, and aortic dissection (see Chaps. 65 and 66). The aortopathy associated with BAV is one of the most common causes of ascending aortic aneurysm. Ascending aortic dilation is not caused by poststenotic dilation, but instead relates to underlying abnormalities of the aortic media. Ascending aortic aneurysm associated with BAV may occur without associated aortic stenosis or regurgitation, and may occur late after aortic valve replacement. Compared with patients with tricuspid aortic valves, those with BAVs have larger aortic dimensions, even in childhood.[21] The aortic enlargement in BAV often arises in the proximal to mid-ascending aorta, emphasizing the importance of visualizing the entire extent of the ascending aorta in BAV patients to evaluate for aneurysms above the sinotubular junction (**Fig. 60-4**).

CMD underlies the aortic aneurysm and risk of dissection associated with BAV, and has been demonstrated in the aortic wall of patients with BAV, even without significant aneurysm formation.[21] Compared with tricuspid aortic valve aneurysms, patients with BAV aneurysms exhibit a distinct pattern of CMD, increased apoptosis, increased MMP-2 activity, and greater expression of death-promoting mediators by infiltrating lymphocytes.[21] Fibrillin-1 content is reduced in BAV aortas, compared with that seen in tricuspid aortic valve aortas. Polymorphisms in MMP-9 may play a role in thoracic aortic aneurysms and dissections in certain individuals.

BAV and ascending aortic aneurysm may be familial and associate with the risk of aortic dissection, inherited as an autosomal dominant

Medical Management

Because risk factors for TAA formation and rupture include hypertension and cigarette smoking, treating hypertension and smoking cessation are important tenets of management. Long-term surveillance of the aorta with imaging is imperative (see Table 60-e2 on website). Beta blockers are recommended for patients with MFS. Although there have been no randomized trials, beta blockers are often recommended for non-Marfan patients with TAAs and for patients after aneurysm repair. Lifestyle modification is necessary for those with TAAs, including awareness of the condition and risk for aortic dissection and rupture. Avoidance of strenuous physical activity, especially isometric exercise and weightlifting, is important. Pregnancy is associated with an increased risk of aortic dissection in MFS and related disorders, and management strategies must encompass this risk. Because TGF-β signaling is related to the pathogenesis of MFS, and probably LDS, drugs that affect this signaling pathway, such as ARBs, may provide benefit in these conditions. Results of clinical trials of ARBs and matrix metalloproteinase inhibitors, such as doxycycline, are needed to confirm any benefit in humans. Because many diseases that lead to TAAs are familial and have a genetic trigger, it is important to screen for TAAs in first-degree relatives of the patient with a thoracic aneurysm.

Aortic Dissection

Acute aortic dissection is the most common catastrophic event affecting the aorta, with an estimated annual incidence of approximately 5 to 30 per million.[41] In a necropsy series, the prevalence of aortic dissection ranged from 0.2% to 0.8%.[42] The early mortality rate in acute aortic dissection is very high, with a mortality rate up to 1% to 2% per hour reported in the first several hours after dissection occurs.[43] Aortic dissection occurs at least twice as frequently in men than in women.[40] Ascending aortic dissection occurs most commonly between 50 and 60 years of age, whereas descending aortic dissection is more common in older individuals, peaking at 60 to 70 years of age. Because dissection is far less common than other conditions associated with chest or back pain, a high index of suspicion of acute aortic dissection must be maintained when evaluating the patient with unexplained chest or back pain or a syndrome complex compatible with this diagnosis. Improved survival requires immediate recognition of the disorder and timely institution of medical and/or surgical therapy.

There are two main hypotheses for acute aortic dissection (see Fig. 60-e6 on website). The first is that an aortic dissection may be related to a primary tear in the aortic intima, with blood from the aortic lumen penetrating into the diseased media, leading to dissection and creating the true and false lumen. The second main hypothesis is that a primary rupture of the vasa vasorum leads to hemorrhage in the aortic wall, with subsequent intimal disruption, creating the intimal tear and aortic dissection. The pressure of the pulsatile blood within the aortic wall after dissection leads to extension of the dissection. Aortic dissections usually propagate in an antegrade direction related to the pressure pulse from the aortic blood, but occasionally extend in a retrograde direction. The dissection flap may be localized or may spiral the entire length of the aorta. Arterial pressure and shear forces may lead to further tears in the intimal flap (the inner portion of the dissected aortic wall), producing exit sites or additional entry sites for blood flow into the false lumen. Distention of the false lumen with blood causes the intimal flap to compress the true lumen, narrowing its caliber and distorting its shape, which leads to malperfusion. Classic aortic dissection (see earlier) occurs in approximately 80% to 90% of acute aortic syndromes. The variants of aortic dissection, aortic intramural hematoma, and penetrating atherosclerotic ulcers (**Fig. 60-8**), are discussed later.

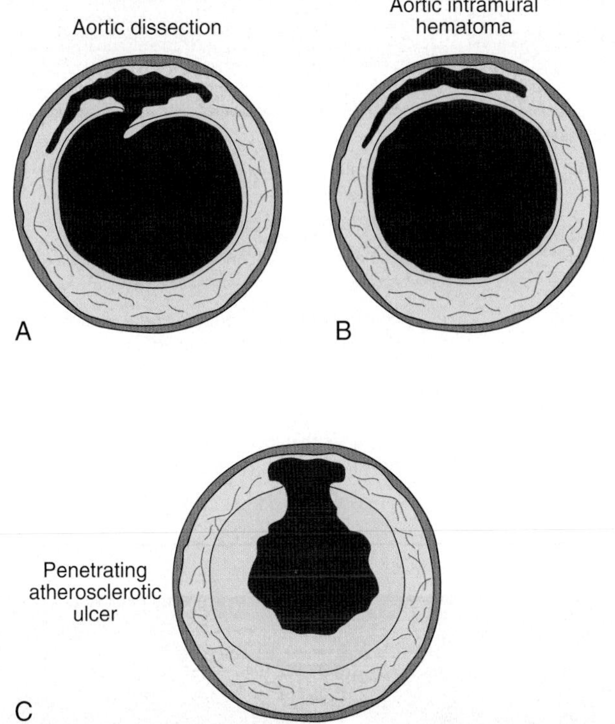

FIGURE 60-8 Acute aortic syndromes. **A,** Classic aortic dissection. **B,** Aortic intramural hematoma. **C,** Penetrating atherosclerotic aortic ulcer.

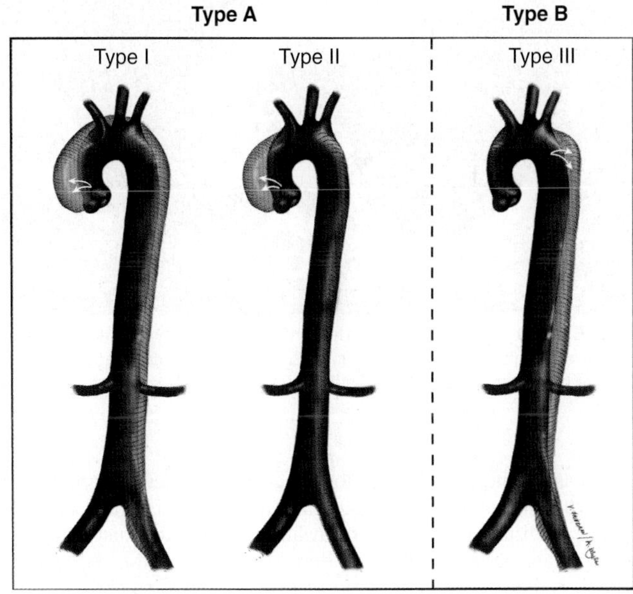

FIGURE 60-9 Classification schemes of acute aortic dissection.

CLASSIFICATION. There are two major classification schemes of aortic dissection, based on the location of the dissection—the DeBakey and Stanford classifications (**Fig. 60-9** and **Table 60-1**). The DeBakey classification system divides dissections into types I, II, and III. DeBakey type I dissections originate in the ascending aorta and extend at least to the aortic arch and often to the descending aorta, frequently all the way to the iliac arteries (**Fig. 60-10**). DeBakey type II dissections involve the ascending aorta alone. DeBakey type III dissections begin in the descending aorta, usually just distal to the left subclavian artery. Type III dissections may be classified further, depending on whether the dissection stops above the diaphragm (IIIa) or extends below the diaphragm (IIIb). Infrequently, a type III dissection may propagate in a retrograde manner into the arch and ascending aorta. The Stanford classification categorizes dissections into types A and B, based on whether the ascending aorta is involved. Stanford type A dissections involve the ascending aorta, with or without extension into the descending aorta, and Stanford type B dissections are those that do not involve the ascending aorta.

TABLE 60-1 Classification Schemes of Acute Aortic Dissection

CLASSIFICATION	SITE OF ORIGIN AND EXTENT OF AORTIC INVOLVEMENT
DeBakey	
Type I	Originates in the ascending aorta and extends at least to the aortic arch and often to the descending aorta (and beyond)
Type II	Originates in the ascending aorta; confined to this segment
Type III	Originates in the descending aorta, usually just distal to the left subclavian artery, and extends distally
Stanford	
Type A	Dissections that involve the ascending aorta (with or without extension into the descending aorta)
Type B	Dissections that do not involve the ascending aorta

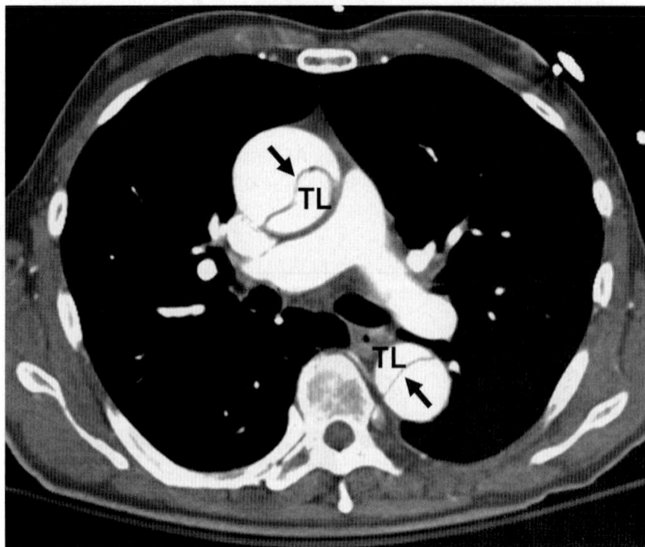

FIGURE 60-10 Contrast CT scan demonstrating acute type A aortic dissection with enlargement of the ascending aorta and intimal flaps (arrows) in the ascending and descending aorta. Both the true lumen (TL) and false lumen are opacified with contrast in this example.

Most ascending aortic dissections begin within a few centimeters of the aortic valve, and most descending aortic dissections have their origin just distal to the left subclavian artery. Approximately 65% of intimal tears occur in the ascending aorta, 30% in the descending aorta, less than 10% in the aortic arch, and approximately 1% in the abdominal aorta. The treatment depends on the site, with emergency surgery recommended for acute type A dissections and initial medical therapy for type B dissections. Aortic dissection is also classified according to its duration, being acute when present for less than 2 weeks and chronic when present for more than 2 weeks. The morbidity and mortality rates of acute dissection are highest in the first 2 weeks, especially within the first 24 hours.

CAUSES AND PATHOGENESIS. Several conditions predispose the aorta to dissection (**Table 60-2**), with most resulting from disruption of the normal architecture and integrity of the aortic wall. Approximately 75% of all patients with aortic dissection have hypertension, which promotes aortic intimal thickening, calcification, and adventitial fibrosis. These structural changes can affect the elastic properties of the arterial wall, increasing stiffness and predisposing to aneurysm or dissection, but hypertension alone usually does not associate with aortic root dilation. Genetically-triggered thoracic aortic syndromes, congenital heart diseases, atherosclerosis, inflammatory vascular diseases, cocaine use, and iatrogenic causes are also risk factors for aortic dissection. CMD is the most common underlying factor in aortic dissection (see Fig. 60-e1 on website). Any disease process that undermines the integrity of the elastic or muscular components of the media predisposes the aorta to dissection (see earlier discussion in TAA section). CMD is an underlying pathophysiologic feature of several genetically triggered disorders of connective tissue, including MFS, LDS, FTAA/D syndrome, and vEDS, and is also common among patients with a congenital BAV (see Table 60-e3 on website). Excessive signaling in the TGF-β pathway and abnormalities in SMC contractile element function may underlie certain aortic dissections.[18] Patients with MFS have a high risk for aortic root aneurysm, especially type A aortic dissection. Although only present in approximately 1 in 5000 individuals, MFS accounts for approximately 5% of all aortic dissections.[31,41]

TABLE 60-2 Risk Factors for Aortic Dissection

Hypertension
Genetically triggered thoracic aortic disease
- Marfan syndrome
- Bicuspid aortic valve
- Loeys-Dietz syndrome
- Hereditary thoracic aortic aneurysm or dissection
- Vascular Ehlers-Danlos syndrome

Congenital diseases or syndromes
- Coarctation of the aorta
- Turner syndrome
- Tetralogy of Fallot

Atherosclerosis
- Penetrating atherosclerotic ulcer

Trauma, blunt or iatrogenic
- Catheter or stent
- Intra-aortic balloon pump
- Aortic or vascular surgery
- Motor vehicle accident
- Coronary artery bypass surgery or aortic valve replacement

Cocaine use
Inflammatory or infectious disease
- Giant cell arteritis
- Takayasu arteritis
- Behçet disease
- Aortitis
- Syphilis

Pregnancy

CMD may accompany many other conditions and factors affecting the aorta, including aging and hypertension. Although hypertension is a very common disorder, the vast majority of hypertensive patients, even severely hypertensive ones, never suffer TAA or dissection. Whether the preponderance of cases of aortic dissection will eventually be related to an underlying genetic trigger is yet unknown, and is the subject of active investigation. Among the 464 patients in the IRAD, hypertension was present in 72%, atherosclerosis in 31%, known aortic aneurysm in 16%, prior aortic dissection in 6%, prior cardiac surgery in 18% (including aortic valve replacement [AVR] in 5% and coronary artery bypass grafting [CABG] in 4%), and iatrogenic dissection in 4%.[41]

When encountering a young patient with aortic dissection, one must consider genetically triggered aortic disease (e.g., MFS, LDS, vEDS, FTAA/D, BAV, TS), pregnancy, cocaine use, congenital heart disease (coarctation of the aorta, tetralogy of Fallot), and prior AVR. The mortality rate for acute dissection is no different for those younger than 40 years of age compared with those older than 40 years of age.[31]

A BAV is an often underrecognized risk factor for ascending aortic aneurysm and dissection and is present in 5% to 7% of aortic dissections, even more commonly among ascending dissections in younger patients. Aortic dissection may occur in the setting of a BAV that functions normally and, importantly, may occur years after BAV replacement.[21] Other congenital disorders associated with dissection include unicuspid aortic valve, supravalvular aortic stenosis, coarctation of the aorta, and TS. Weightlifting, especially in the setting of underlying aortic dilation, may be associated with acute aortic dissection.[26]

Rarely, aortic dissection complicates arteritis involving the aorta, particularly giant cell arteritis. Nonspecific aortitis, Takayasu arteritis, and Behçet disease have all been associated with aortic dissection (see Chap. 89). Syphilitic aortitis is a rare cause of dissection. Cocaine abuse accounts for less than 1% of aortic dissection and is associated with crack cocaine use. Cocaine-related dissection is most typical in young, African American, and hypertensive men who smoke cigarettes.[44] Underlying elastic medial abnormalities and severe sheer forces related to hypertension and tachycardia may play a role.

Aortic dissection can occur during pregnancy or the postpartum period (see Chap. 82). The relationship between pregnancy and aortic dissection is difficult to reconcile based on hemodynamic factors alone. When pregnancy-related dissection occurs, one must diligently search for an underlying genetic trigger, such as mutations in *FBN1*, *TGFBR1*, *TGFBR2*, *ACTA2*, and *MYH11*. Dissections during pregnancy typically occur in the third trimester, but occasionally occur in the early postpartum period. In addition to hemodynamic factors, hormonal changes in aortic wall composition have been described. Women with MFS, LDS, FTAA/D syndrome, vEDS, TS, and BAV with a dilated aorta have increased risk for acute aortic dissection during pregnancy. In MFS, the risk of type A dissection is greatest when the aortic root is enlarged; it has been estimated at 1% when the aortic diameter is smaller than 40 mm and at 10% in high-risk patients (aortic diameter > 40 mm, rapid dilation, or previous dissection of the aorta).[45] Postpartum type B aortic dissection has occurred in MFS, even in the setting of a relatively normal descending aortic dimension, and has occurred late after aortic root repair.

Blunt aortic trauma usually leads to localized tears, periaortic hematomas, or frank aortic transection, and only rarely causes classic aortic dissection. Iatrogenic trauma accounts for approximately 4% of aortic dissections.[41] Intra-arterial catheterization, stent placement, and the insertion of intra-aortic balloon pumps may induce aortic dissection related to intimal disruption. Retrograde ascending aortic dissection occurs in approximately 1% of patients undergoing thoracic endovascular aortic repair (TEVAR) for acute or chronic type B aortic dissection, and associates with a 40% mortality rate.[46] Cardiac surgery also entails a very small risk (0.12% to 0.16%) of acute aortic dissection.[47] But aortic dissection may occur late (months to years) after cardiac surgery. Of cardiac surgical patients, those undergoing AVR and those with prior aortic aneurysm or dissection have the highest risk for aortic dissection as a late complication. Persistent abnormalities of the aortic wall, such as the aortopathy seen with BAV, untreated or recurrent dissection, and injuries to the aortic wall and intima related to cross clamping, suture lines, or cannulation during surgery, account for the increased risk of subsequent aortic dissection.

Individuals with TAA are at risk for aortic dissection, with increased risk of dissection and rupture as aneurysm size increases,[29] but many aortic dissections occur in patients without severely dilated aortic dimensions. Of 591 type A aortic dissections in the IRAD, the maximum aortic diameter averaged 5.3 cm, with 349 patients (59%) having aortic diameters smaller than 5.5 cm and 229 patients (40%) having aortic diameters smaller than 5.0 cm.[48] In a series of 177 non-Marfan patients with tricuspid aortic valves with acute type A aortic dissection, 62% of patients had a maximum aortic diameter smaller than 5.5 cm, 42% had a maximum aortic diameter smaller than 5.0 cm, and more than 20% had a maximum aortic diameter smaller than 4.5 cm, at the time of dissection.[49] Thus, the absolute size of the aorta is not the only factor important in triggering acute dissection. Age, sex, body size, and rate of aortic growth also play a role. Underlying genetic triggers may lead to dissection at differing aortic sizes. The mechanisms responsible for individual susceptibility for acute dissection at a certain aortic size are poorly understood. Mechanical factors and aortic curvature may also affect risk of dissection and location of entry tears.[50] The biomechanical properties (distensibility and wall stress) of the aorta may be assessed noninvasively, and studies are in progress to aid in the prediction of patients at increased risk of aortic complications.[26]

CLINICAL MANIFESTATIONS. (see Chaps. 12 and 53)

Symptoms

The symptoms of aortic dissection can be variable and may mimic those of more common conditions, emphasizing the importance of a high index of suspicion. The most common symptom of acute aortic dissection is pain, which is present in up to 96% of cases.[41] The pain is typically severe and of sudden onset, being at maximum intensity at its inception. This pattern contrasts with the pain of myocardial infarction, which usually has a crescendo-like onset and is not as intense. The pain is often accompanied by a "sense of doom" and may force the patient to writhe in distress or pace restlessly in an attempt to gain relief. The quality of the pain is most commonly described as "sharp" or "severe," and adjectives such as "tearing," "ripping," or "stabbing" are used in about half the cases. Cataclysmic descriptors that are suggestive of aortic dissection, such as being "stabbed in the chest with a knife" or "hit in the back with a baseball bat" are sometimes reported. Some aortic dissections present with chest burning, pressure, or pleuritic discomfort; in others, the symptoms related to a complication from the dissection dominate the clinical scenario, and the pain is not mentioned or is downplayed. In some instances (<5%), no pain is reported at all. Those with painless dissections are often found to have chronic dissections, significant neurologic symptoms, or heart failure dominating their presentation.

The pain of acute aortic dissection is migratory in approximately 17% of patients, tending to follow the path of the dissection through the aorta.[41] The pain of dissection may radiate from chest to back or vise versa. The presence of any pain in the neck, throat, jaw, or head predicts involvement of the ascending aorta (and often the great vessels), whereas pain in the back, abdomen, or lower extremities usually indicates descending aortic involvement.

Other clinical features at initial evaluation, occurring with or without associated chest pain, may include congestive heart failure (7%), syncope (9%), acute stroke (6%), acute myocardial infarction, ischemic peripheral neuropathy, paraplegia, and cardiac arrest or sudden death.[39] Acute congestive heart failure in this setting is usually caused by acute severe aortic regurgitation because of the ascending aortic dissection (see Chap. 66). Syncope is much more common in ascending aortic dissection and is usually associated with hemopericardium, rupture, or stroke. Patients with aortic dissection may have abdominal pain and, on occasion, develop severe nausea and vomiting related to abdominal visceral involvement. These symptoms may delay diagnosis and increase mortality rate.[51] Painless aortic dissection was reported in 6% of patients in one study and was more commonly associated with diabetes, prior aortic aneurysm, and prior cardiac surgery.[52] Painless aortic dissections present with syncope in one third, heart failure in 20%, and stroke in 11%, and are associated with a higher mortality rate (33%).

PHYSICAL FINDINGS. The physical examination findings in acute aortic dissection vary widely, ranging from almost unremarkable to cardiac arrest from hemopericardium or rupture. The findings may demonstrate complications related to the dissection such as aortic regurgitation, abnormal peripheral pulses (see Chap. 12), stroke, or heart failure. Such findings must heighten one's clinical suspicion of aortic dissection. The absence of these findings, however, does not exclude dissection and should not dissuade one from pursuing the diagnosis when suspected. Hypertension is present in approximately 70% of patients with acute aortic dissection. Although most patients with type B dissections are hypertensive, many patients with type A dissections are normotensive or hypotensive on presentation.[41] Hypotension complicating acute dissection is usually the result of cardiac tamponade, acute aortic rupture, or heart failure related to acute severe aortic regurgitation. Hypotension is associated with altered mental status and neurologic deficits; visceral, limb, and myocardial ischemia; and death in 55% of patients.[42] Dissection involving the brachiocephalic vessels may result in pseudohypotension, an inaccurate measurement of blood pressure caused by compromise of the brachial artery circulation.

The physical findings most typically associated with aortic dissection—pulse deficits, aortic regurgitation, and neurologic manifestations—are more characteristic of ascending than descending dissection. Acute chest or back pain associated with these findings strongly suggest the possibility of aortic dissection. In the IRAD, pulse deficit was reported in 19% of type A and only 9% of type B dissections.[41] When acute lower extremity vascular insufficiency occurs and

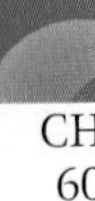

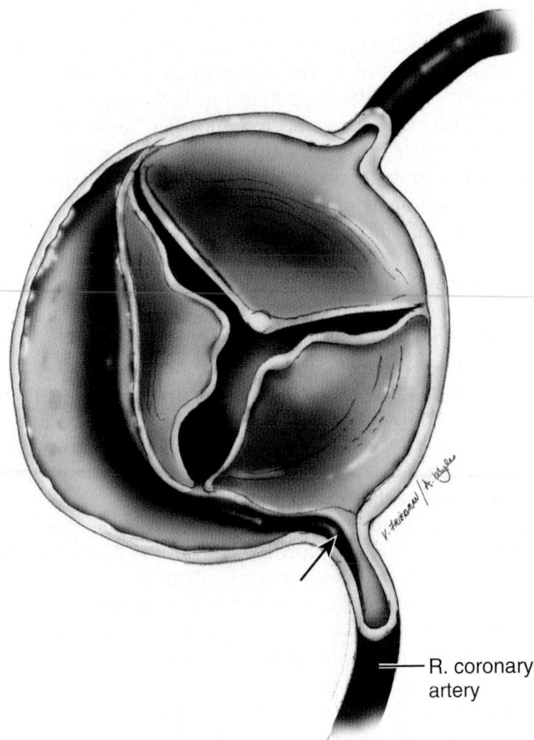

FIGURE 60-11 Aortic regurgitation complicating acute type A aortic dissection. The dissection flap distorts the normal aortic leaflet alignment, leading to malcoaptation of the aortic valve and subsequent aortic regurgitation. In this example, the dissection flap extends into the ostium of the right coronary artery (arrow).

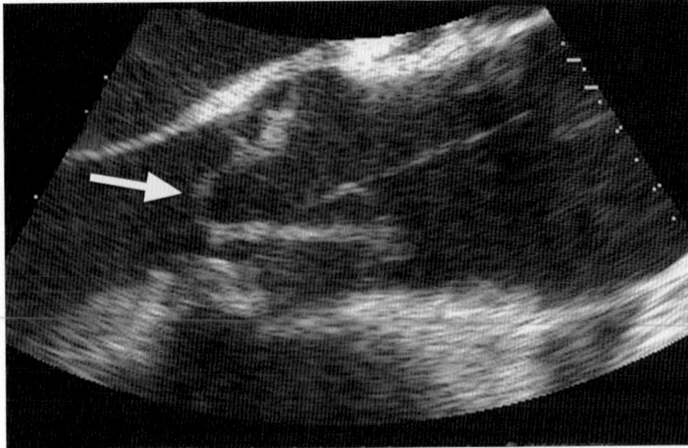

FIGURE 60-12 Transesophageal echocardiogram demonstrating ascending aortic dissection. Prolapse of the dissection flap across the aortic valve into the left ventricular outflow tract (arrow) leads to severe aortic regurgitation.

is not relieved with emergency embolectomy, one should consider the possibility of acute dissection. Vascular insufficiency related to aortic dissection may result from the dissection flap propagating into a branch artery, leading to compression of the true lumen by the distended false lumen and limiting blood flow, or from obstruction of flow into the orifice of the artery by a mobile intimal flap. The pulse deficits may be intermittent because the intimal flap movement sporadically obstructs the arterial orifice or because of distal reentry of blood into the true lumen, which decompresses the false channel. Acute limb ischemia, a marker for more extensive and severe dissection, is associated with a threefold increase in mortality in type B dissection.[53]

Aortic regurgitation is an important diagnostic feature in type A aortic dissection (**Fig. 60-11**). The diastolic murmur of aortic regurgitation accompanying acute chest pain should make one suspect aortic dissection. The murmur of aortic regurgitation is present in 44% of type A dissections and 12% of type B dissections.[41] When aortic regurgitation accompanies type B dissection, this usually indicates coexisting aortic valve disease, aortic root aneurysm, or retrograde dissection. The murmur of aortic regurgitation can vary in intensity, depending on the blood pressure and degree of heart failure and, in some cases, may be inaudible. Aortic regurgitation complicating type A dissection may lead to acute decompensated heart failure (see Chap. 66).

Several mechanisms may explain acute aortic regurgitation in the setting of type A aortic dissection. First, there may be incomplete coaptation of the aortic leaflets because of concurrent dilation of the aortic root and annulus, leading to central aortic regurgitation. Second, and most commonly, the dissection may lead to aortic leaflet prolapse because of the dissection flap into the aortic leaflets or commissures, or from distortion of proper leaflet alignment by an asymmetric dissection flap, leading to eccentric aortic regurgitation (see Fig. 60-11 and Videos 60-2 and 60-3 on website). Third, an extensive or circumferential dehiscing intimal flap may prolapse into the left ventricular outflow tract during diastole, interfere with valve coaptation, and cause severe aortic regurgitation (**Fig. 60-12**; see Videos 60-4 and 60-5 on website).[54] Additionally, there may be preexisting aortic regurgitation related to underlying aortic root aneurysm or BAV.

Neurologic manifestations occur in 17% to 40% of aortic dissections, more commonly in type A dissections. Variability in incidence likely results from a failure to record a detailed neurologic examination in such critically ill patients. The findings may be evanescent, with rapid improvement related to transient arterial occlusion. Syncope, painless aortic dissection, and dissections with predominantly neurologic symptoms may lead to difficulty or delay in diagnosis. Neurologic syndromes include persistent or transient ischemic stroke, spinal cord ischemia, ischemic neuropathy, and hypoxic encephalopathy. These are related to malperfusion to one or more branches supplying the brain, spinal cord, or peripheral nerves (see Table 60-e4 on website).[55] Ischemic stroke occurs in approximately 6% of ascending dissections and more commonly in the left hemisphere, because the left-sided arch vessels are more susceptible to the advancing false lumen.[41,55] Syncope is relatively common in aortic dissection, affecting 9% in one large series (13%, type A; 4%, type B) and may occur without pain or other neurologic findings.[41] Syncope may be related to acute hypotension caused by cardiac tamponade or aortic rupture, cerebral vessel obstruction, or activation of cerebral baroreceptors. It is important to consider aortic dissection in the differential diagnosis in cases of unexplained syncope. Less common neurologic manifestations of dissection include seizures, transient global amnesia, ischemic neuropathy, disturbances of consciousness and coma, and paraparesis or paraplegia related to spinal cord ischemia. Some studies have failed to identify brain malperfusion as an independent risk factor for an adverse outcome after surgical repair,[41,55,56] whereas other reports have associated cerebral malperfusion with poor outcomes.[57]

Acute myocardial infarction, related to involvement of the dissection flap into the ostium of a coronary artery, occurs in 1% to 2% of acute type A aortic dissections, and was more commonly reported in older series.[43] This usually involves the right coronary artery (see Fig. 60-11), leading to acute inferior myocardial infarction. Because coronary ischemia and myocardial infarction are much more common than aortic dissection, when acute infarction complicates acute dissection, the diagnosis of dissection might not be considered. This type of patient may be taken emergently to the catheterization laboratory, and the acute dissection may be recognized only after angiography. Not only does the time delay increase morbidity and mortality, but the use of antiplatelet, anticoagulant, and thrombolytic therapy may have disastrous consequences, including cardiac tamponade and death. Aortic dissection always should be considered in the differential diagnosis of patients presenting with acute infarction, particularly inferior infarction, especially when their risk factors, symptoms, or examination are compatible with this diagnosis.

Types A and B dissections may extend into the abdominal aorta, leading to vascular complications involving one or more branch

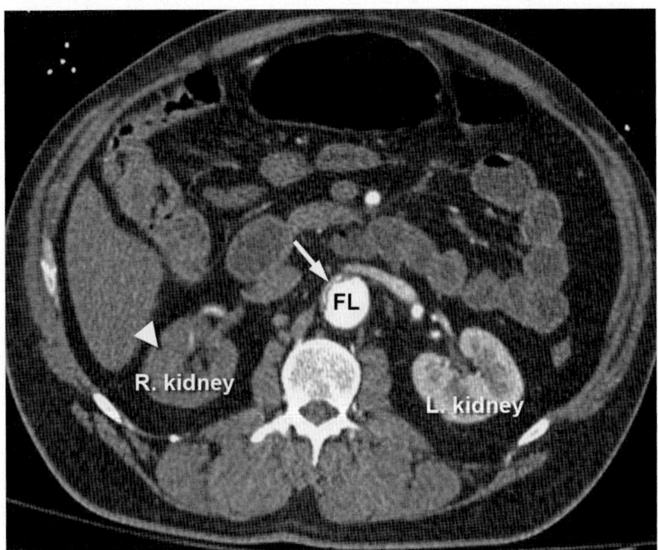

FIGURE 60-13 Contrast CT scan of aortic dissection with malperfusion to the right kidney (arrowhead), which demonstrates less opacification with contrast than the left kidney. The left kidney fills from the collapsed and underfilled true lumen (arrow). The false lumen (FL) is larger than the true lumen.

vessels. Renal artery involvement occurs in at least 5% to 10% of patients and may lead to renal ischemia, infarction, renal insufficiency, or refractory hypertension (**Fig. 60-13**). Mesenteric ischemia or infarction, complications associated with a high level of morbidity and mortality, occurs in approximately 5% of aortic dissections and are associated with acute limb ischemia and renal ischemia.[53] A high index of suspicion is required for this diagnosis, and identifying and correcting visceral malperfusion may improve outcomes. Aortic dissection may extend into the iliac arteries and cause diminished femoral pulses (12%) and acute lower extremity ischemia. Acute limb ischemia and malperfusion syndromes are associated with extensive and severe dissection and a higher mortality rate.[57]

Additional clinical manifestations of aortic dissection include the presence of left-sided pleural effusion, usually related to an inflammatory response. On occasion, acute hemothorax occurs from rupture, contained rupture, or leaking of the descending aortic dissection (**Fig. 60-14**). Type A aortic dissection may present with acute pericarditis, including characteristic electrocardiographic changes (see Chap. 75). Isolated abdominal aortic dissection is rare, accounting for approximately 1% of dissections, and is associated with an existing AAA or has an iatrogenic cause. Acute abdominal pain, mesenteric ischemia, and limb ischemia are more common in this subset of dissections.[58] Rare clinical manifestations of aortic dissection include hoarseness, upper airway obstruction, dysphagia, superior vena cava syndrome, pulsatile neck or abdominal masses, hematemesis (from rupture into the esophagus), hemoptysis (from rupture into the trachea or bronchus), ischemic pancreatitis, and unexplained fever (from the inflammatory reaction).

Aortic dissection may not be considered during the evaluation of a patient with chest, back, or abdominal pain. The signs and symptoms associated with aortic dissection are highly variable and depend on the underlying cause and extent and involvement of the heart and branch vessels from the dissection. Dissection may mimic many other more common disorders, including pleurisy, pericarditis, pulmonary embolism, coronary ischemia, stroke, esophageal disease, gastric gallbladder or pancreatic disease, and acute mesenteric or limb ischemia. In some cases, the diagnosis is immediately suspected on presentation, whereas at other times the diagnosis is made when imaging studies are performed for another reason. Thus, one of the most important factors in making the diagnosis of aortic dissection is a high index of suspicion.

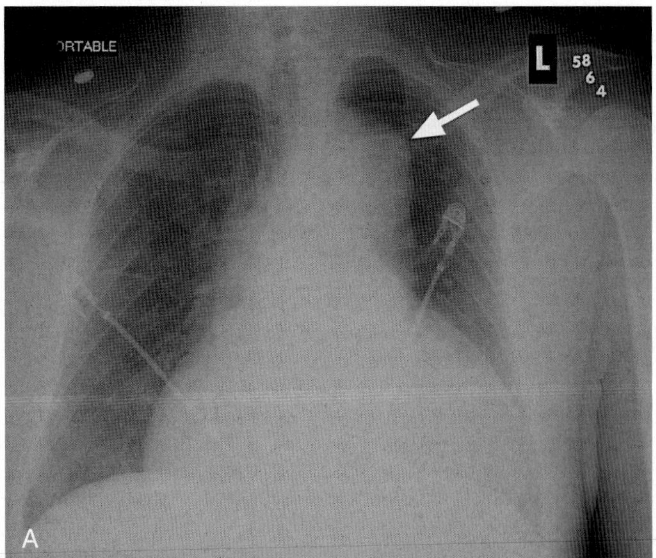

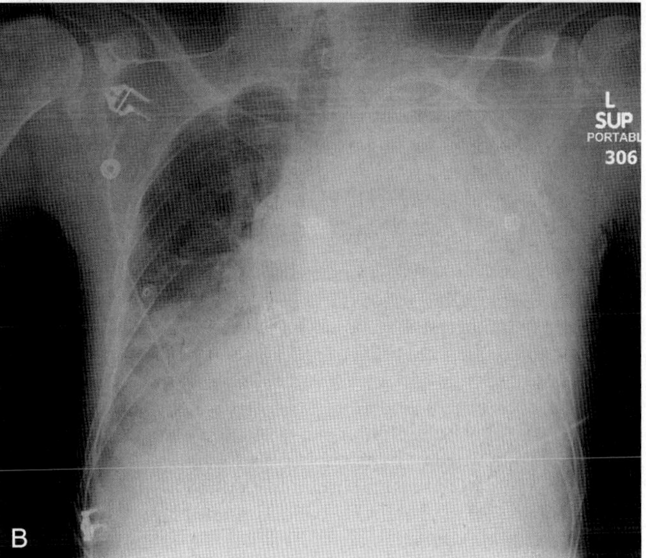

FIGURE 60-14 Chest radiograph in aortic dissection. **A,** Widened mediastinum with abnormal aortic knob and enlarged cardiac silhouette is present. **B,** Acute hemothorax occurred from rupture of the aortic dissection, with rapid opacification of the left hemithorax.

CHRONOBIOLOGY. Like other cardiovascular disorders, aortic dissection demonstrates significant circadian and seasonal or monthly variations. In the IRAD, the onset of aortic dissection was most common in the morning. There was a seasonal variation also, with more dissections being reported in the winter and fewest in the summer. Chronobiologic periodicity may be explained by changes in sympathetic tone and hemorrheologic properties of the blood.[42]

LABORATORY FINDINGS. The chest radiograph may be the first clue to the diagnosis of aortic dissection (see Fig. 60-14 and Fig. 60-e7 on website), but the findings on the chest radiograph are nonspecific, subject to interobserver variability and, in many cases, completely normal. The dissected aorta may not be dilated, and its image between the sternum and vertebrae may not be displaced or widened on the chest radiograph. The most common abnormality seen on a chest radiograph in cases of aortic dissection is an abnormal aortic contour or widening of the aortic silhouette, which appears in 80% to 90% of cases (83%, type A; 72%, type B).[41] Nonspecific widening of the superior mediastinum may be present. If calcification of the aortic knob is present, one may detect a separation of the intimal calcification from the outer aortic soft tissue border by more than 0.5 to 1.0 cm—the calcium sign (see Fig. 60-e8 on website). Comparison of the current chest radiograph with a previous study may reveal acute changes in the aortic or mediastinal silhouettes that would otherwise have gone unrecognized. Pleural effusions are reported in approximately 20% of dissections. Most effusions relate to an inflammatory reaction, but acute hemothorax may occur from aortic rupture (see Fig. 60-14). Most patients with aortic dissection will have an abnormal chest radiograph, but 12% to 15% have normal chest radiographs. Thus, a normal chest radiograph cannot exclude the presence of an aortic dissection.

The electrocardiographic findings in patients with aortic dissection are nonspecific, but may indicate acute complications such as myocardial ischemia or infarction related to coronary artery involvement, or low-voltage QRS complexes (or rarely, acute pericarditis) related to hemopericardium. Three quarters of electrocardiograms (ECGs) on dissection are normal or demonstrate nonspecific ST-segment or T wave changes, and 25% have left ventricular hypertrophy.[41] Acute myocardial infarction is present in 1% to 2% of type A dissections. These are particularly dangerous because the presence of acute coronary ischemia may lead the clinician away from the evaluation of dissection.

Biomarkers

Biomarkers could reliably diagnose or exclude acute aortic dissection. Release of smooth muscle proteins, soluble elastin fragments, and myosin heavy chain and creatine kinase BB isoforms have been reported after aortic dissection.[59] These assays have limited usefulness because of sensitivity, specificity, or time delay, and are not currently available clinically.

D-dimer levels are elevated in pulmonary embolism and can rise in aortic dissection. In a prospective study, D-dimer levels were markedly elevated in patients proven to have aortic dissection (and pulmonary embolism).[59] A D-dimer level higher than 1600 ng/mL within the first 6 hours of presentation showed a positive likelihood ratio of 12.8, suggesting that this test may be useful for identifying patients with a high probability of acute aortic dissection. In patients within the first 24 hours of onset, a D-dimer level less than 500 ng/mL had a negative likelihood ratio of 0.07 and a negative predictive value of 95%. The D-dimer assay may be useful for ruling out acute aortic dissection in this time window, with a diagnostic performance similar to that reported for pulmonary embolism. An elevated D-dimer level may assist clinicians in risk-stratifying patients presenting with chest pain or dyspnea for appropriate imaging. D-dimer levels, however, may not be as useful in various forms of acute aortic syndromes. The patency of the false lumen affects D-dimer levels in acute dissection. In addition, the dissection variants, aortic intramural hematoma and penetrating aortic ulcer, may not have elevated D-dimer levels. Moreover, patients may present more than 24 hours after symptom onset, affecting D-dimer levels. More studies are required to determine the sensitivity and specificity of this assay in acute aortic syndromes, and how best to integrate D-dimer testing into the diagnostic algorithm of aortic dissection.

DIAGNOSTIC IMAGING. When aortic dissection is suspected, it is imperative to confirm the diagnosis quickly and accurately. Diagnostic methods include contrast-enhanced CT, MRI, transthoracic and transesophageal echocardiography (TEE), and aortography. Each modality has advantages and disadvantages with respect to diagnostic accuracy, speed, convenience, and risk. The choice of imaging study often depends on local availability and expertise, with contrast-enhanced CT and TEE being the most commonly performed. Many patients undergo multiple studies in the diagnostic evaluation of suspected aortic dissection. If the probability of dissection is very high, a second diagnostic test should be performed if the first test is negative or nondiagnostic.

When comparing imaging modalities, one must consider the diagnostic information required (see Table 60-e5 on website). Most importantly, the study must confirm the diagnosis of aortic dissection and its variants (intramural hematoma and penetrating atherosclerotic ulcer). Second, it must determine the location of the dissection and whether the dissection involves the ascending aorta (type A) or is confined to the descending aorta or arch. Additional useful information includes anatomic features and complications related to the dissection, including its extent, sites of entry and reentry, presence of thrombus in the false lumen, branch vessel involvement, presence and severity of aortic regurgitation, presence or absence of pericardial effusion and hemopericardium, any coronary artery involvement by the intimal flap, and any signs of rupture or leaking.

Computed Tomography

Contrast-enhanced CT scanning has become the most commonly used modality in evaluating aortic dissection (see Chap. 19). It is best performed as an electrocardiographically gated CT on a multidetector (16 or more) row scanner, which may eliminate aortic pulsation artifacts. On CT, an aortic dissection is diagnosed by the presence of two distinct lumens with a visible intimal flap, which is seen in most cases, or by the detection of two lumens by their differing rates of opacification with contrast (see Fig. 60-10). If the false lumen is completely thrombosed, it demonstrates low attenuation. Acute aortic intramural hematoma, a dissection variant discussed later, demonstrates only a thickened aortic wall with high attenuation on noncontrast CT and no entry tears or visible intimal flap. Spiral (helical) contrast CT allows for three-dimensional reconstruction to evaluate the dissection and branch vessels with enhanced anatomic definition (**Fig. 60-15**) and is critical for decision making, especially when planning endovascular repair (see Fig. 60-e9 on website). Contrast CT is highly accurate for diagnosing aortic dissection, with a sensitivity and specificity of 95% to 98% being reported.

CT scanning does require intravenous contrast; without contrast enhancement, aortic dissection may go undetected (see Fig. 60-e10 on website). CT is also useful for identifying thrombus (partial or complete) in the false lumen, pericardial effusion, hemopericardium, periaortic hematoma, aortic rupture, and branch vessel involvement, and blood supply from the true and false lumens (see Fig. 60-13). Major limitations to CT include the inability to evaluate the coronary arteries and aortic valve reliably, motion artifact related to cardiac movement, streak artifact related to implanted devices, and

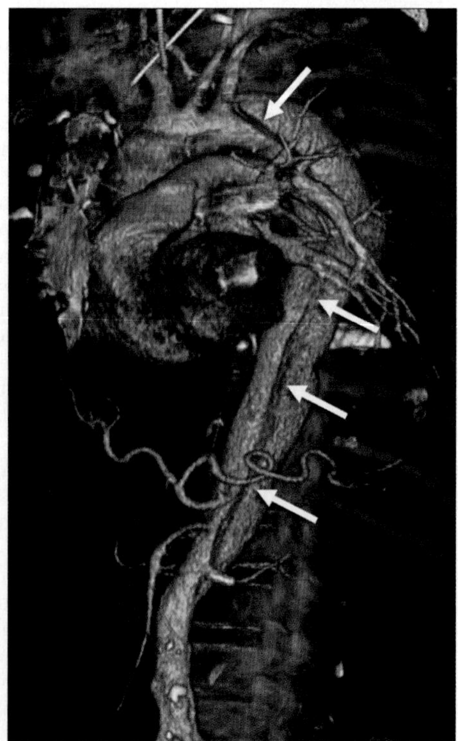

FIGURE 60-15 Three-dimensional CT reconstruction of a type B aortic dissection. The intimal flap is denoted by the arrows.

complications associated with the use of iodinating contrast agents, especially in renal failure.

Magnetic Resonance Imaging

MRI is a highly accurate noninvasive technique for evaluating aortic dissection (see Chap. 18), which does not require intravenous iodinated contrast or ionizing radiation (see Fig. 60-e11 on website). MRI is capable of multiplanar imaging with three-dimensional reconstruction and cine MRI to visualize blood flow, differentiating slow flow and clot and detecting aortic regurgitation. Most MRI protocols involve techniques to assess branch vessel morphology combined with contrast-enhanced MRA. Studies have demonstrated a high sensitivity (95% to 100%) and specificity (94% to 98%) for the detection of aortic dissection. Contrast-enhanced MRI using intravenous gadolinium is highly accurate for the evaluation of dissection and branch vessel involvement. Like CT, MRI may detect pericardial effusion, aortic rupture, entry and exit points, and intramural hematoma with high levels of accuracy. MRA may detect and quantify aortic regurgitation. MRI has important limitations in acute aortic dissection. First, MRI is contraindicated in patients with certain implantable devices (e.g., pacemaker, defibrillator) and other metallic implants. Additionally, MRI has limited availability on an emergency basis in many hospitals and emergency rooms and takes longer for image acquisition than CT. Gadolinium contrast should not be used in those with renal impairment. MRI is rarely used as the initial test for diagnostic evaluation of acute dissection. However, because of the imaging detail and lack of ionizing radiation, MRI is particularly attractive for the long-term follow-up of aortic dissection.

Echocardiography

Echocardiography is well suited for the evaluation of patients with suspected aortic dissection because it is readily available in most hospitals and is noninvasive and quick to perform, and the full examination can be completed at the bedside (see Chap. 15). The echocardiographic finding considered diagnostic of an aortic dissection is the presence of an undulating intimal flap within the aortic lumen that separates the true and false channels (see Fig. 15-84; see Videos 60-6, 60-7, and 60-8 on website). Reverberations and other artifacts can cause linear echodensities within the aortic lumen that mimic aortic dissection. In cases in which the false lumen is thrombosed, displacement of intimal calcification or thickening of the aortic wall may suggest aortic dissection.

TRANSTHORACIC ECHOCARDIOGRAPHY. Transthoracic echocardiography (TTE) is less sensitive (59% to 83%) and less specific (63% to 93%) for the diagnosis of aortic dissection than other modalities (see Fig. 60-e12 and Videos 60-9, 60-10, and 60-11 on website). Thus, it has limited usefulness in the diagnosis of aortic dissection. TTE may demonstrate an intimal flap, thickened aortic wall, aortic regurgitation, and pericardial effusion or tamponade. It has a sensitivity of 78% to 100% for type A aortic dissection, but only 31% to 55% in type B dissection; therefore, a negative TTE does not exclude acute aortic dissection. If dissection is suspected, TTE should not be chosen as a first test for evaluation because a delay in diagnosis may occur. In the emergency setting, however, TTE may be performed rapidly and can help assess features complicating dissection, such as aortic regurgitation, pericardial effusion and tamponade, and associated wall motion abnormalities.

TRANSESOPHAGEAL ECHOCARDIOGRAPHY. TEE is highly accurate for the evaluation and diagnosis of acute aortic dissection (sensitivity of ~98% and specificity of 94% to 97% (**Fig. 60-16**; see Videos 60-2 to 60-8 on website; see Fig. 15-84). The distal ascending aorta and proximal aortic arch may not be well visualized by TEE, but the remaining thoracic aortic segments are well visualized. Adequate sedation is important to avoid a hypertensive response to the procedure, often related to patient discomfort. TEE is less sensitive for detecting the intimal tear (see Fig. 60-e13 and Video 60-12 on website), but it is 100% sensitive in detecting aortic regurgitation complicating dissection and may define its mechanism (see Fig. 60-12 and Videos 60-2 to 60-5 on website).[54] Additionally, TEE provides information about wall motion and left ventricular function and the presence or absence of pericardial effusion. TEE allows visualization of the coronary ostia and determination of whether they arise from the true or false lumen and whether the dissection extends into the coronary artery.

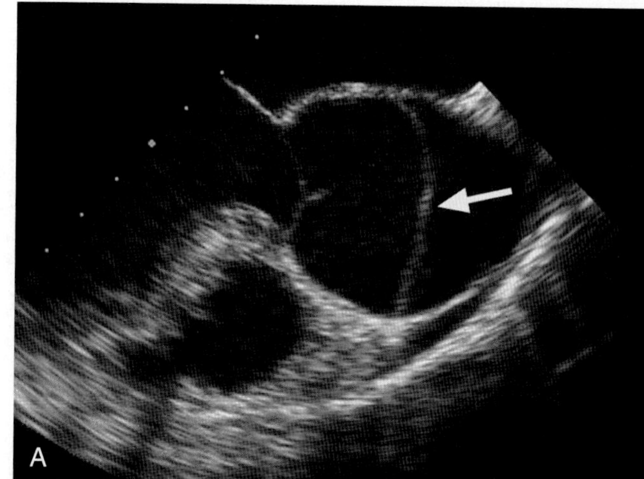

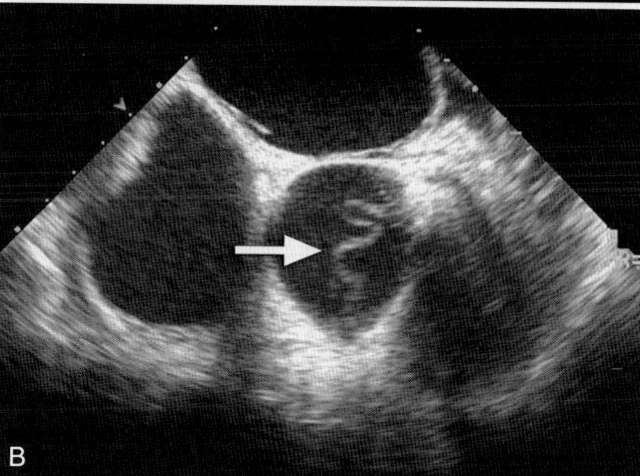

FIGURE 60-16 Transesophageal echocardiogram in acute aortic dissection. **A,** Acute type A dissection in a patient with Marfan syndrome. The dissection flap (arrow) is present in the dilated aortic root. **B,** Serpiginous intimal flap (arrow) immediately distal to the aortic valve in a patient with a type A aortic dissection.

Aortography

Aortography is now rarely used for the diagnosis of acute aortic dissection; it is currently used most often for anatomic imaging and planning before endovascular therapy. Aortography has limited availability in the emergency setting and carries risk because of the procedure itself and the time required to assemble an angiography team. The diagnosis of dissection by aortography is based on imaging the two lumens or an intimal flap (see Fig. 60-e14 on website). Other features may include an undulating deformation of the aortic lumen, aortic wall thickening, branch vessel involvement, and aortic regurgitation. Compared with other imaging modalities, aortography is less accurate in the diagnosis of aortic dissection (sensitivity, 90%; specificity, 94%). A false-negative aortogram may be obtained in the setting of false lumen thrombosis, equal and simultaneous opacification of true and false lumina, and an aortic intramural hematoma.

Selecting an Imaging Modality

Because of its high level of sensitivity and specificity and availability on an emergency basis, contrast CT is usually the test of first choice for the diagnosis of aortic dissection. The risk of contrast nephropathy often complicates the decision about which test to perform, especially in emergency rooms or hospitals in which TEE or MRI is unavailable. It is important to remember than a noncontrast CT scan may fail to diagnose aortic dissection (see Fig. 60-e10 on website). If TEE or MRI is not available on an urgent basis, one must weigh the risks of intravenous contrast versus the potentially fatal consequences of failing to diagnose aortic dissection. A TTE may occasionally diagnose acute ascending aortic dissection, and if there is any concern about time delay for the other imaging modalities to be performed, an emergency bedside TTE may be useful. A negative TTE, however, does not exclude aortic dissection.

In the IRAD, CT was the most commonly used initial imaging study (63%), whereas TEE was used as the initial study in 32% of cases.[41] MRI is less available on an emergent basis, requires a longer time for imaging acquisition and processing, and poses potential risk because of restricted monitoring and accessibility to the patient during imaging. Aortography requires an angiography team and is subject to the risks associated with an invasive procedure, including time delay and intravenous contrast. The diagnostic approach to the patient with suspected aortic dissection must be based on each institution's available resources and expertise, and the rapidity and accuracy with which procedures may be performed.

Role of Coronary Angiography

Routine coronary angiography is not recommended before surgery for acute type A aortic dissection because of concern about delay in emergency surgery.[57,60] Coronary artery involvement in aortic dissection may have various causes. The aortic dissection flap may obstruct the orifice of the coronary artery, leading to coronary ischemia or infarction. Additionally, the dissection flap may propagate down the coronary artery for a variable length, leading to obstruction of flow (see Fig. 60-11), or the patient may have coexisting atherosclerotic coronary artery disease. The presence of occlusive coronary artery disease has been identified in approximately 20% of patients with ascending dissection. At present, preoperative catheterization is only infrequently performed before emergency ascending aortic dissection repair, being carried out in only 10% of patients in one recent report.[60] In IRAD, approximately 10% of patients with acute type A dissection underwent coronary angiography. Preoperative identification of coronary disease by catheterization has not proved to alter survival in patients with acute aortic dissection. In addition to the time delay incurred, coronary angiography may be technically difficult in the setting of dissection. Arterial access may fail to gain entry into the true lumen. Potential complications of catheterization include catheter or guidewire injury to the aorta, leading to an extension of the dissection or perforation of the aorta.

In specific patients, further evaluation for coronary artery disease or coronary artery involvement before aortic dissection surgery may be indicated. Individuals with a history of coronary disease, prior coronary artery bypass surgery, and those with acute ischemic electrocardiographic changes are subgroups in which this decision is usually contemplated. Usually, coronary artery involvement by the dissection may be identified and rectified at surgery, so angiography is not required. One has to make individual decisions based on the specific circumstances. These patients must be hemodynamically stable to be candidates for preoperative cardiac catheterization. The presence of cardiac tamponade and aortic rupture are contraindications to coronary angiography.

Direct inspection of the coronary ostia may be performed once the aorta has been opened at surgery, and any obstruction or involvement of the coronary arteries by the dissection process may then be corrected. TEE may evaluate the ostia of the coronary arteries before surgery or intraoperatively and may assess wall motion, suggesting ischemia. Additionally, coronary atherosclerosis may be identified intraoperatively by inspection, probing, or palpation of the coronary arteries. There is very limited experience in intraoperative coronary angiography in aortic dissection.

MANAGEMENT. The goals of medical management are to stabilize the patient, control pain, lower blood pressure, and reduce the rate of rise or force (dP/dt) of left ventricular ejection. These measures are undertaken immediately while the patient is undergoing diagnostic evaluation. Lowering blood pressure may help prevent further propagation of the dissection and lessen risk of aortic rupture. Aortic dissection is a highly lethal condition. Early literature reported that more than 25% of untreated individuals with acute dissection died in the first 24 hours, 50% died within the first week, and more than 75% died within the first month.[43] Emergency surgery improves survival in acute type A dissections, whereas initial medical therapy is recommended for acute type B dissections. Patients with acute aortic dissection require urgent multidisciplinary evaluation and management. They should be transferred emergently to a tertiary medical center with access to cardiovascular surgery, vascular surgery, interventional radiology, and cardiology. Surgical consultation is recommended, regardless of the anatomic location of the dissection.[32]

Surgical therapy for type A aortic dissection has dramatically improved survival for this lethal condition. The goals of surgical therapy are to treat or prevent the common complications of dissection, such as cardiac tamponade, aortic regurgitation, aortic rupture, stroke, and visceral ischemia. The immediate surgical goals are as follows: (1) excise the intimal tear; (2) obliterate the false channel by oversewing the edges of the aorta; and (3) reconstitute the aorta directly, or more commonly with placement of an interposition graft. In type A dissection, aortic regurgitation is also treated by resuspension of the aortic valve leaflets or by prosthetic aortic valve replacement.

Blood Pressure Reduction

Reduction of systolic blood pressure to levels of approximately100 to 120 mm Hg, or the lowest level appropriate for adequate perfusion to vital organs, is recommended. Beta-blocking agents should be administered, regardless of whether systolic hypertension is present, with a goal of attaining a heart rate of 60 beats/min or lower. For rapid administration of agents to reduce the rate of rise of ventricular force (dP/dt) and stress on the aorta, intravenous beta blockers should be given. The short-acting beta blocker esmolol is often the first choice, and is given as an initial bolus of 500 μg/kg and then a continuous infusion of 50 to 200 μg/kg/min. Labetolol is an alpha- and beta-adrenergic blocker and may be administered intravenously in the acute setting or orally. Labetolol is given at an initial dose of 20 mg IV over 2 minutes, and then at a dose of 40 to 80 mg IV every 15 minutes (maximum dose 300 mg), until an adequate response is achieved. Labetolol is then given by continuous intravenous infusion at a rate of 2 to 8 mg/min. Propranolol and metoprolol may be used intravenously or orally for acute aortic dissection. When acute severe aortic regurgitation complicates aortic dissection, caution should be exercised with beta blocker use.[32]

When beta blockers are contraindicated, one may consider the calcium channel blockers verapamil or diltiazem. These agents have negative inotropic and chronotropic effects and may be administered intravenously, making them advantageous in the acute setting. Intravenous diltiazem is given as 0.25 mg/kg over 2 minutes and then continued as an infusion at a rate of 5 to 15 mg/hr, depending on the effect.

Sodium nitroprusside leads to a rapid reduction of blood pressure, but when used alone may lead to an increase in dP/dt, which could contribute to propagation of the dissection. In the setting of acute aortic dissection, sodium nitroprusside must be used together with beta blockade. Sodium nitroprusside is initiated with a dose of 20 μg/min, with titration to 0.5 to 5 μg/kg/min as required. Caution must be exercised in the setting of renal insufficiency or prolonged use. Because of the risk of cyanide toxicity, nitroprusside is used only for short periods.

Often, multiple agents are required for adequate blood pressure and heart rate control in acute aortic dissection. Intravenous ACE inhibitors (such as IV enalaprilat) and intravenous nitroglycerin may be useful.

When the patient with acute dissection has hypertension that is refractory or difficult to control, there are many considerations. First, the patient may have underlying severe hypertension and may have gone without medications, with medication withdrawal playing a role, especially beta blockers or clonidine. Uncontrolled pain may exacerbate hypertension. Additionally, acute cocaine use may lead to tachycardia and hypertension. Finally, the patient may have renal artery involvement by the dissection flap, leading to hypertension. Renal artery hypertension due to the dissection process may respond favorably to ACE inhibitor therapy, and in some cases requires endovascular therapy. When the patient with suspected aortic dissection has significant hypotension, rapid volume expansion should be considered, given the possible presence of cardiac tamponade or aortic rupture with hemorrhage into the mediastinum, pleural space, or abdomen.

Management of Cardiac Tamponade (See Chap. 75)

Cardiac tamponade, occurring in 19% of acute type A dissections, is one of the most common mechanisms for death in this disorder (**Fig. 60-17**).[61] Patients with tamponade are more likely to present with hypotension, syncope, or altered mental status. The in-hospital mortality rate among patients with cardiac tamponade is twice as high as that among those without tamponade (54% versus 25%). Because hemodynamic instability with hypotension often complicates hemopericardium in acute dissection, pericardiocentesis is commonly considered as initial therapy in this condition, to attempt to stabilize these patients before surgery. But sudden death from pulseless electrical activity has been reported minutes after pericardiocentesis in this setting. The relative increase in intra-aortic pressure that occurs after pericardiocentesis may lead to a reopening or resurgence of blood under pressure from the false channel into the pericardial space, resulting in acute hemorrhage and fatal cardiac tamponade. Therefore, in the relatively stable patient with acute type A dissection and cardiac tamponade, the risks of pericardiocentesis likely outweigh its benefits. The initial strategy should be to proceed emergently to the operating room for open surgical repair of the aorta and drainage of the pericardium under direct visualization, but when managing such a patient, with pulseless electrical activity or refractory hypotension, an attempt at resuscitation with pericardiocentesis may be lifesaving. In this case, one should attempt to aspirate only enough pericardial fluid to stabilize the patient, and then proceed to emergency surgery. Reports of successful pericardiocentesis in acute type A intramural hematoma from the Asian population have suggested that this may be effective in this subset of acute aortic syndrome[32] (see later, "Aortic Intramural Hematoma").

Definitive Therapy

Definitive therapy for acute aortic dissection includes emergency surgery for all patients with acute ascending aortic dissection who are considered surgical candidates. Patients with acute type A aortic dissection are at risk of progression of the disease, including aortic rupture, aortic regurgitation with heart failure, stroke, cardiac tamponade, and visceral ischemia. Compared with medical therapy, immediate surgical treatment improves survival in acute type A aortic dissection. In the IRAD, the mortality rate of patients with type A aortic dissection undergoing surgery was 26%, and was 58% for those treated medically (typically because of advanced age and comorbid conditions) (**Fig. 60-18**).[41] Thus, almost 25% of patients with acute ascending aortic dissection will die, even after presenting to centers with extensive experience with aortic dissection. Other single-center series have reported even lower mortality rates for surgical patients.[60,62] In the IRAD, 526 patients underwent surgical treatment for acute ascending aortic dissection, and the mortality rate was variable, depending on risk factors present preoperatively. In patients considered unstable (e.g., with shock, congestive heart failure, cardiac tamponade, myocardial infarction, renal failure, or mesenteric ischemia), the mortality rate was 31% versus 17% for those considered stable.[42,56] Independent predictors for operative mortality included prior aortic valve replacement, migrating chest pain, hypotension, shock or cardiac tamponade, and limb ischemia. Mortality for patients with a preoperative malperfusion syndrome in type A dissection was fivefold greater (30% versus 6%) than for those without malperfusion.

A bedside preoperative and postoperative risk prediction tool of mortality has been developed to understand better the expected risks of surgery in acute type A aortic dissection (**Table 60-3**).[63] Intraoperative variables, including hypotension, right ventricular dysfunction, and surgical aspects (CABG, partial arch resection), are also used in obtaining a postoperative score (see Table 60-e6 on website). One may use these data to estimate an individual's expected mortality rate with acute type A aortic dissection (**Fig. 60-19**; see Fig. 60-e15 on website).

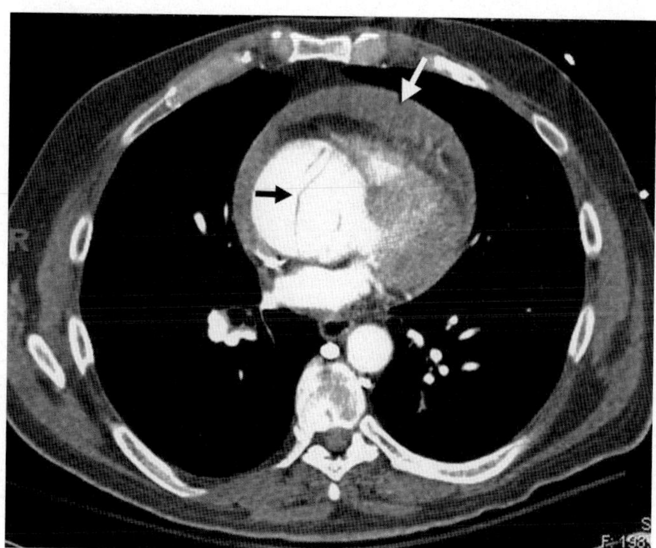

FIGURE 60-17 Contrast CT scan of acute type A aortic dissection (black arrow), with associated hemopericardium (white arrow).

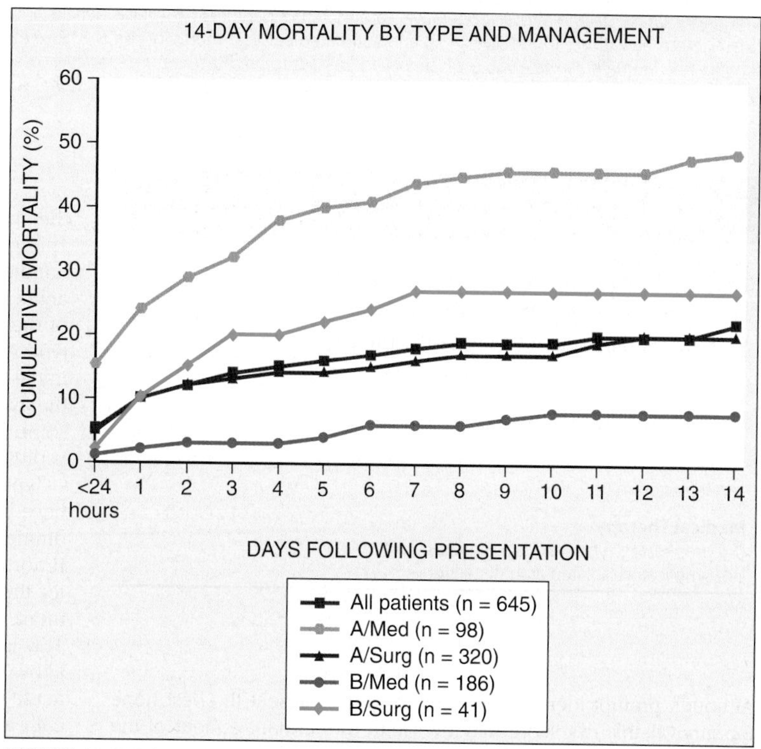

FIGURE 60-18 Two-week mortality rates for acute aortic dissection according to dissection type and medical or surgical treatment. *(From Hagan PG, Nienaber CA, Isselbacher EM, et al: The International Registry of Acute Aortic Dissection [IRAD]: New insights into an old disease. JAMA 283:897, 2000.)*

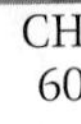

CH 60

TABLE 60-3 Preoperative Prediction Model of Surgical Mortality Risk

VARIABLE	OVERALL TYPE A (%)	AMONG SURVIVORS (%)	AMONG DEATH (%)	COEFFICIENT	SCORE ASSIGNED	P VALUE	ODDS RATIO, DEATH (95% CI)
Age ≥ 70 yr	27.3	24.1	37.4	0.68	0.7	<0.01	1.98 (1.19-3.29)
History of aortic valve replacement	4.5	3.8	6.6	1.44	1.5	<0.01	4.21 (1.56-.34)
Presenting hypotension, shock, or tamponade	28.8	22.4	49.0	1.17	1.2	<0.01	3.23 (1.95-5.37)
Migrating chest pain	13.8	12.1	19.3	0.88	0.9	<0.01	2.42 (1.32-4.45)
Preoperative cardiac tamponade	15.5	11.7	28.2	0.97	1.0	<0.01	2.65 (1.48-4.75)
Any pulse deficit	28.6	25.7	37.8	0.56	0.6	0.03	1.75 (1.06-2.88)

From Rampoldi V, Trimarchi S, Eagle KA, et al: Simple risk models to predict surgical mortality in acute type A aortic dissection: The International Registry of Acute Aortic Dissection score. Ann Thorac Surg 83:55, 2007.

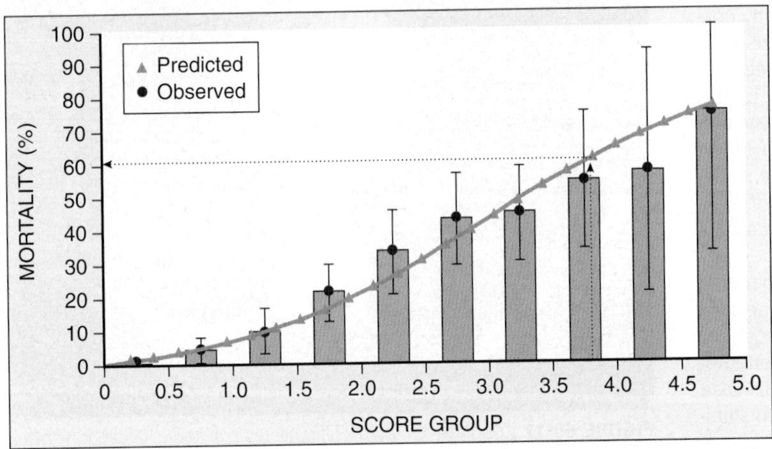

FIGURE 60-19 Observed versus model probabilities of death by preoperative score. This example is of a 77-year-old woman with migrating chest pain, preoperative cardiac tamponade, a pulse deficit, and ST-segment elevation. Her model score is 0.7 (age > 70 years) + 0.9 (migratory chest pain) + 1.0 (preoperative cardiac tamponade) + 0.6 (pulse deficit) + 0.6 (ST-segment elevation). Total score = 3.8 and estimated surgical mortality risk is 61%. *(From Rampoldi V, Trimarchi S, Eagle, KA, et al: Simple risk models to predict surgical mortality in acute type A aortic dissection: The International Registry of Acute Aortic Dissection score. Ann Thorac Surg 83:55, 2007.)*

TABLE 60-4 Indications for Surgical, Endovascular, and Medical Therapy in Acute Aortic Dissection

Surgical Therapy
Acute type A aortic dissection
Retrograde dissection into the ascending aorta

Surgical Therapy and/or Endovascular Therapy
Acute type B aortic dissection complicated by:
- Visceral ischemia
- Limb ischemia
- Rupture or impending rupture
- Aneurysmal dilation
- Refractory pain

Medical Therapy
Uncomplicated type B aortic dissection
Uncomplicated isolated arch dissection

Although prompt identification and surgery represent the best hope for survival, this risk score may be useful in the management of the truly moribund patient who, regardless of surgery, has a very poor chance of survival.

Patients with acute type B aortic dissection have a lower risk of early death than those with acute type A dissection. In the IRAD, the mortality rate of patients with type B dissection treated medically was 10.7% (see Fig. 60-18). However, most series of acute aortic descending dissection have reported a mortality rate of 25% to 50% for those requiring surgery. In patients with uncomplicated type B dissection, the in-hospital mortality rate is very low.[64] However, complicated type B dissection carries a much higher mortality rate, especially when accompanied by shock or malperfusion. In the IRAD, surgery was performed in 20% of type B dissections, with a mortality rate of 31%.[41] Independent predictors for surgical mortality in type B dissection include age older than 70 years and preoperative shock or hypotension. In a series of 129 acute type B aortic dissections treated with the strategy of initial medical therapy, the in-hospital mortality rate was 10%; it was 19% when early vascular intervention was required, and 8% when medical management was maintained.[65] This series and other large retrospective series have demonstrated that in general, initial medical therapy provides an outcome superior to that of initial surgical therapy for uncomplicated type B aortic dissection. Typical indications for surgical or endovascular intervention in type B aortic dissection are complications that develop, such as visceral or limb ischemia, aortic rupture or impending rupture, rapid expansion of the aortic diameter, uncontrollable pain, or retrograde extension of the dissection into the ascending aorta (**Table 60-4**). Often, endovascular therapy for certain complications may be preferred.[66]

Primary arch dissections are uncommon, and management of this condition requires individualization. Mortality for surgical repair of acute arch dissection has been reported as 15% to 29%. If involvement of the ascending aorta is present, then the dissection is classified as type A and emergency surgery is recommended. Many recommend initial medical therapy for primary arch dissections that do not involve the ascending aorta, whereas others advocate emergency surgery for some primary arch dissections, especially if aneurysmal enlargement is present.

Type B dissections that extend retrograde into the transverse arch have been managed variably. For most, initial medical therapy is recommended. In the IRAD population of almost 500 patients with type B aortic dissections, 25% had aortic arch involvement, and mortality for these patients was no different from those without arch involvement.[67] In one series, when extension into the arch is observed, a TEE is performed to characterize the intimal flap and aortic tear, allowing exclusion of ascending aortic involvement.[65] In this series, acute type B dissections with arch involvement were managed medically, and 7% in that subpopulation had cerebral complications.

Surgical Management

Generally accepted indications for definitive surgical therapy are summarized in Table 60-4. Operative therapy for acute aortic dissection is technically very demanding. The aortic wall is thin and friable, and Teflon felt and pledgeted sutures are used to buttress the wall and prevent sutures from tearing through the fragile aortic wall.

TYPE A AORTIC DISSECTION. Open surgery, performed as expediently as possible, is the treatment of choice for ascending aortic dissection to prevent life-threatening complications.[28,41,66] The early mortality rate for surgical treatment in acute type A dissection is typically approximately 25%, whereas single-center experience is often lower.[60] A median sternotomy is routinely performed, and cannulation for cardiopulmonary bypass usually involves the axillary or femoral approach to avoid trauma to the weakened aortic wall. Surgical therapy includes excision of the intimal tear when possible, obliteration of entry into the false lumen proximally and distally, and interposition graft replacement of the ascending aorta. Most patients can be treated by obliteration of the false lumen by placement of Teflon felt as a neomedium and resuspension of the native aortic valve. When aortic regurgitation complicates dissection, repair of the aortic wall and decompression of the false lumen and resuspension of the commissures usually restore valve competence. When aortic leaflet disease precludes repair, aortic valve replacement and associated ascending aortic replacement are indicated. When the sinuses are significantly dilated, composite valve and root replacement is often performed using the modified Bentall procedure. When the aortic root and sinuses are dilated but the aortic leaflets are normal, many have achieved success by performing a valve-sparing root replacement, typically using the reimplantation technique (see Fig. 60-7).[33] At present, no data support the use of endovascular repair for type A dissection. Arch replacement using deep hypothermic circulatory arrest is also performed if the aortic arch is aneurysmal or ruptured or has a primary arch tear at the time of surgical treatment, and is done for some patients with genetically triggered aneurysm syndromes.[68]

TYPE B AORTIC DISSECTION. The treatment of patients with type B aortic dissections is currently evolving with the increased use of endovascular devices. In general, stable patients with uncomplicated type B dissections should be treated medically because of the high mortality rates associated with surgery.[15,41,68] Patients with complicated type B aortic dissections caused by aortic rupture, intractable chest or back pain, and/or visceral ischemia resulting from aortic branch vessel involvement require an intervention, but open surgical repair is associated with high mortality rates. Endovascular techniques have been increasingly used to treat this patient population, with encouraging results (**Fig. 60-20**).

Aortic fenestration techniques with or without additional aortic branch stenting have been used with reasonable success for the treatment of patients with aortic branch vessel involvement and malperfusion syndromes. The first technique is balloon fenestration of the intimal flap, which allows blood to flow from the false lumen into the true lumen, thereby decompressing the distended false lumen. The second technique involves percutaneous stenting of an affected arterial branch whose flow has been compromised by the dissection process. Recently, Patel and colleagues[69] reported the treatment of 69 patients over a period of 10 years, with a 30-day mortality rate of 17%. The freedom from aortic rupture or open surgical repair rates were 80% at 1 year, 68% at 5 years, and 54% at 8 years. These endovascular techniques can address some complications of type B dissections, but are associated with a high rate of conversion to open surgery in the long term.

Endovascular grafts have the potential to treat most, if not all, complications of type B dissections, with relatively low morbidity and mortality rates. The rationale behind this technique is that covering the area of the primary intimal tear with the endovascular graft redirects flow to the true lumen and promotes false lumen thrombosis, allowing aortic remodeling (**Fig. 60-21**).[65] This treatment often corrects branch vessel ischemia and is useful in the treatment of enlarging symptomatic dissections and ruptured aortas. STABLE and other trials are starting to evaluate prospectively the treatment of acute complicated type B dissections with endovascular grafts. The persistence of a perfused false lumen, which can occur in up to two thirds of patients treated, is concerning, as it can lead to reinterventions and surgical conversions. The Petticoat technique, in which the entry point is sealed

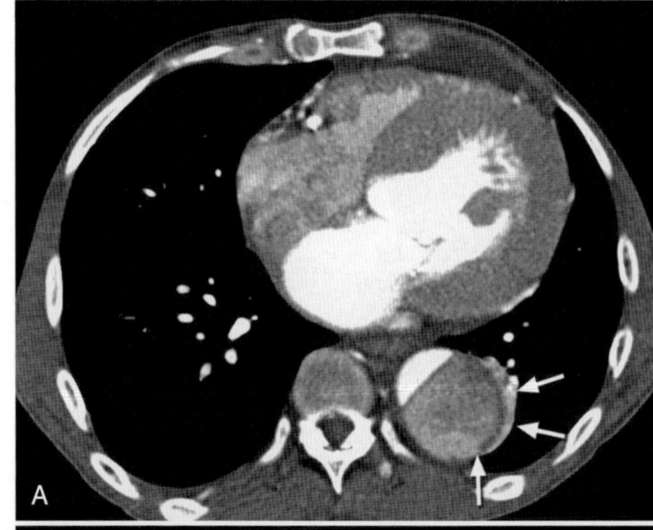

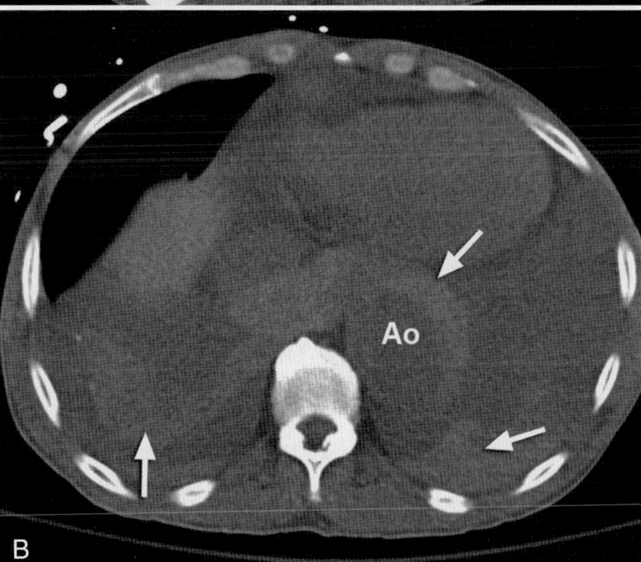

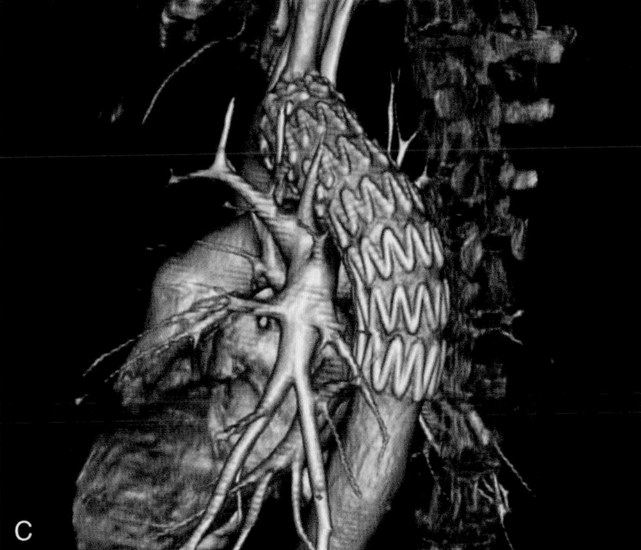

FIGURE 60-20 Rupture of a type B aortic dissection. **A,** Contrast CT scan demonstrating early leaking of blood from the dilated false lumen (arrows). The small true lumen is densely opacified with contrast. **B,** Noncontrast CT scan demonstrating acute hemorrhage from the ruptured type B dissection. **C,** Three-dimensional reconstruction of the descending thoracic aorta after emergency endovascular repair of the ruptured aortic dissection. Ao = aorta.

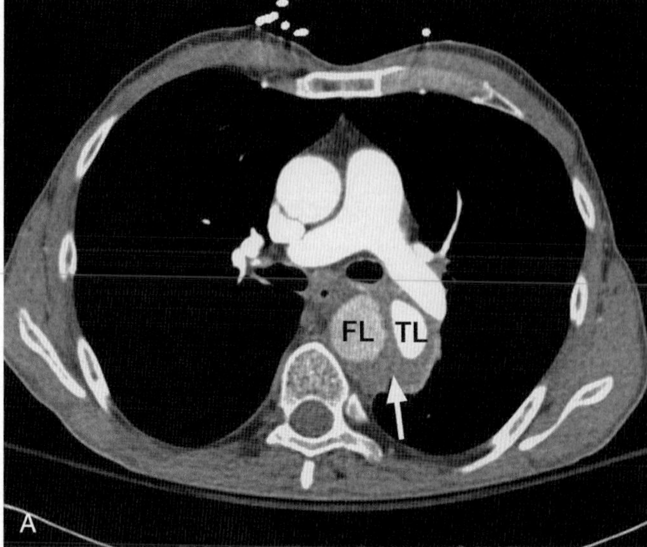

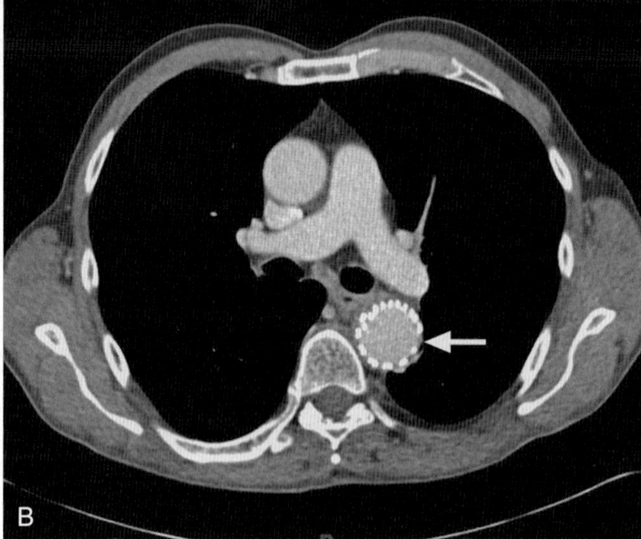

FIGURE 60-21 **A,** Type B aortic dissection with partial thrombosis of the false lumen (arrow). **B,** After endovascular repair of the type B dissection, the false lumen (arrow) has collapsed and remodeled and is no longer visualized. FL = false lumen; TL = true lumen.

with an endograft and the remaining thoracic and potentially the abdominal aorta is stented open, may address this problem.[70] This technique can decrease the chance of true lumen collapse, enhance aortic remodeling, and promote false lumen thrombosis. In addition, various methods of hybrid approaches to the surgical and endovascular repair of dissections involving the arch and descending aorta are being studied, with promising early results but no long-term data as of yet.

Patients with uncomplicated type B aortic dissections are at risk for long-term complications of aneurysm formation, late rupture, and dissection. Whether early endovascular grafting of the uncomplicated type B dissection will change this natural history is under investigation. The first comparison study between endovascular and open surgical repair for patients with subacute or chronic descending thoracic aortic dissections has reported periprocedural mortality rates of 0% and 33% for the endovascular and surgical groups, respectively.[68] This initial experience led to the organization of the INSTEAD trial in Europe, randomizing 140 patients with stable, uncomplicated, chronic type B dissections to endovascular grafting versus medical therapy. At 2 years, there was no significant difference in all-cause mortality,[71] but patients treated with endovascular grafts had a significantly higher rate of aortic remodeling and false lumen thrombosis compared with the medically treated group. The ADSORB trial is enrolling patients with acute uncomplicated type B dissections and will examine various endpoints, including false lumen thrombosis and the prevention of aortic dilation and rupture. The indications for endovascular therapy are evolving and must be balanced against the advances in open therapy, especially when performed by highly skilled surgical teams.

Definitive Medical Management

Hypertension is common in the setting of acute dissection and is related to underlying hypertension, renal artery involvement, pain, or systemic inflammation accompanying the dissection process. Difficult to control or refractory hypertension is not usually considered as an indication for surgical repair of type B dissection. Whereas many patients require multiple antihypertensive agents to control blood pressure acutely, blood pressure often falls over the first several days as the inflammatory response resolves. When severe hypertension persists or there are signs of renal ischemia, one should evaluate the patient for renal artery involvement. It is important to follow the patient closely for malperfusion syndromes involving the viscera or extremities and for evidence of aortic rupture. Mesenteric ischemia may be difficult to recognize, and identification of this serious complication requires vigilance.

LONG-TERM THERAPY AND FOLLOW-UP. Short- and long-term survival in type A aortic dissections has ranged from 52% to 94% at 1 year and 45% to 88% at 5 years.[72] The 10-year actuarial survival rate among patients with acute aortic dissection who survive initial hospitalization has been between 30% and 60% in various studies. In a single-center study of long-term follow-up after type A aortic dissection, 10-year survival was 55% and 20-year survival was 30%.[60]

Among 303 patients who survived acute type A aortic dissection to hospital discharge, 273 were treated surgically and 30 were treated medically. With a mean follow-up of 2.8 years, the survival for patients treated surgically was 96% ± 2% at 1 year and 90% ± 4% at 3 years, versus 89% ± 12% at 1 year and 69% ± 20% at 3 years without surgery.[72] During the 5-year follow-up period, patients managed surgically had a significantly lower mortality rate of 14%, versus 37% for those treated medically. Predictors of increased mortality rate in follow-up include age older than 70 years, renal or cardiac failure, prior cardiac surgery, stroke, and Marfan syndrome.

Medically treated patients with type A aortic dissection have a very high mortality rate, with death rates in excess of 50% reported early after presentation. Little information exists in the literature about the natural history and management of chronic type A aortic dissection. There are some reports of dismal survival with medical therapy alone, even in those who survive initial hospitalization. A few patients are discovered in the subacute stage, and surgery is recommended for them. On occasion, however, patients are discovered incidentally to have a chronic type A dissection in the evaluation of aortic regurgitation or a dilated ascending aorta. Most have advocated surgical treatment for all appropriate candidates with chronic type A dissection, whereas some have reserved surgery for those with aneurysmal dilation of the ascending aorta, aortic regurgitation, or relatively young age. In the IRAD experience, two thirds of patients who survived hospitalization for acute type A aortic dissection with medical therapy alone were still alive at 3 years.[70] In-hospital mortality rate for surgical therapy of chronic type A aortic dissection has ranged from 8% to 17%, depending on the series. Long-term survival after surgical repair of chronic type A aortic dissection has been reported at 42% to 71% at 12 years, depending on whether operative mortality is included and the extent of the dissection.[73]

The long-term survival rates in acute type B dissection have varied, with reports ranging from 56% to 92% at 1 year and from 48% to 82% at 5 years.[74] These studies have included single-center reports with heterogeneous enrollment criteria and lack of endovascular therapy. Nonetheless, the long-term follow-up after type B aortic dissection is worse than that of type A dissection, with about one in four patients dying within 3 years. Studies have demonstrated that many deaths in follow-up are related to subsequent aortic complications, such as rupture, extension of the dissection, and risks of subsequent aortic and vascular surgery. An IRAD study reported the 3-year survival rates for those patients discharged after initial hospitalization for acute type B aortic dissection. The survival for patients treated medically, surgically, or with endovascular therapy were 78% ± 7%, 83% ± 19%, and 76% ± 25%, respectively.[75] Independent predictors of increased mortality in follow-up included in-hospital hypotension or shock, pleural effusion, renal failure, history of atherosclerosis or prior aneurysm, and female sex.

Tenets of long-term management after aortic dissection include the following: (1) medical therapy, including antihypertensive therapy; (2) screening the individual and first-degree relatives for genetically triggered disorders associated with aortic dissection; (3) serial imaging of the aorta over time; (4) lifestyle modifications; and (5) education.

One important goal in long-term management after dissection is treating hypertension, with a blood pressure goal of less than 120/80 mm Hg in most individuals. Studies have demonstrated a dramatic increase in late morbidity and mortality in dissection patients with poorly controlled hypertension. Beta blockers are the drugs of first choice because of their effect on aortic stress and dP/dt, and are recommended even in the absence of hypertension. ARBs, by antagonizing TGF-β, have demonstrated benefit in a mouse model of Marfan syndrome and are the subject of investigation in people with Marfan syndrome. A Japanese trial in patients with hypertension and other types of heart disease has demonstrated a reduction in aortic dissection in patients treated with the ARB valsartan.[32] Whether these or alternative antihypertensive agents have a special role in management after dissection is unknown. Smoking cessation and risk factor modification for atherosclerotic disease are also important in management.

Although most patients who experience acute aortic dissection have underlying hypertension, only a small fraction of hypertensive patients ever suffer a dissection. Many with dissection will eventually be found to have a genetic trigger for the aortic disease. Some have syndromic features recognized as MFS or LDS. Features of these disorders should be sought on examination. The recognition of dural ectasia in the lumbosacral spine on the CT or MRI scan will often provide a clue to such a genetically triggered disorder. Some patients will have an underlying BAV, a condition that is familial in almost 10% of cases. Others will have familial thoracic aortic aneurysm or dissection syndromes. Comprehensive family studies have recognized that almost one in five individuals with a TAA or dissection will have another first-degree relative with thoracic aortic disease.[19] Thus, it is important to evaluate the patient with aortic dissection for a genetically triggered disorder and to evaluate and image first-degree relatives for the presence of familial thoracic aortic disease.[32]

Long-term management after dissection also includes regular imaging of the aorta and its branches for complications (see Fig. 60-e16 on website). Up to one third of patients require additional surgery on the aorta or its branches in the first several years after dissection to address aneurysm formation at the site of dissection, recurrent dissection, rupture, aneurysm formation at a remote site, graft dehiscence or pseudoaneurysm formation, aortic valve regurgitation, or infection. Typical protocols for follow-up after acute dissection include cross-sectional imaging with CT or MRI at 1 to 3, 6, 12, 18, and 24 months, with variability depending on the size of the aorta and changes in aortic dimension over time (see Table 60-e2 on website). One advantage of MRI for long-term follow-up is the avoidance of repeated radiation exposure. Reevaluation at least yearly thereafter is important to survey for aneurysmal dilation or false lumen expansion.

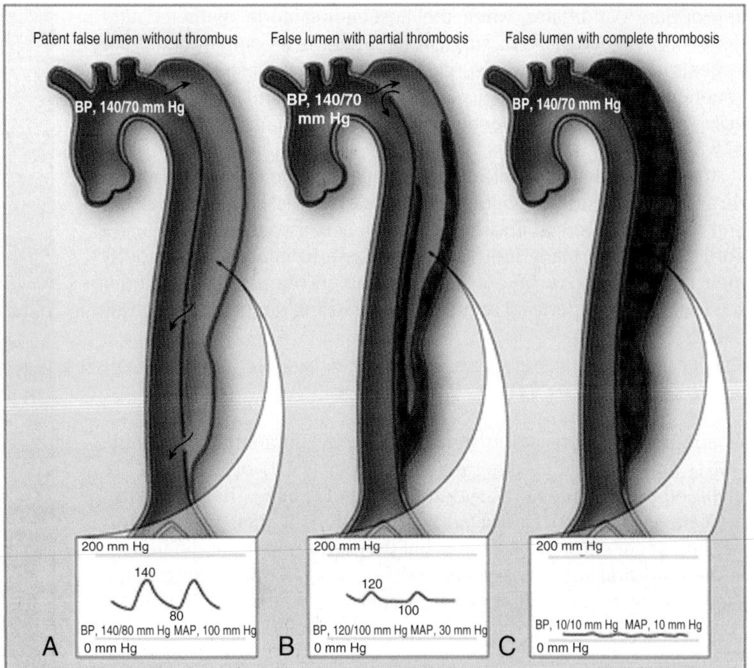

FIGURE 60-22 Conceptual model of risk according to the status of the false lumen. The figure shows a proposed model of the physiologic consequences of false lumen patency or thrombosis, based on hemodynamic studies in ex vivo models and in patients with aortic dissection. **A,** Type B aortic dissection with patent proximal and patent distal reentry tears in the absence of thrombus. The blood pressure tracing shows systolic, diastolic, and mean arterial pressures in the false lumen similar to the pressures in the true lumen. **B,** Type B aortic dissection with a patent entry tear and partial thrombosis that occupies the inner circumference of the false lumen and obstructs the reentry tears, forming a blind sac. The blood pressure tracing shows diastolic and mean arterial pressures in the false lumen that exceed the pressures seen in **A**, with identical pressures in the true lumen. **C,** Type B aortic dissection with a false lumen filled with thrombus and no longer communicating with the true lumen. The pressure within the false lumen is likely to be low and nonpulsatile. BP = blood pressure; MAP = mean arterial pressure. *(From Tsai TT, Evangelista A, Nienaber CA, et al; International Registry of Acute Aortic Dissection: Partial thrombosis of the false lumen in patients with acute type B aortic dissection. N Engl J Med 357:349, 2007.)*

The status of the false lumen is a significant predictor of late outcomes after acute type B aortic dissection.[75] Aortic dilation and patency of the false lumen are associated with subsequent aneurysmal dilation and late complications. Patients with partial false lumen thrombosis (see Fig. 60-21 and Fig. 19-23A) have higher mortality rates at follow-up than patients with completely patent or completely thrombosed false lumen. Increased pressure may occur in the false lumen in the setting of partial thrombosis because of lack of distal reentry tears, leading to subsequent expansion and increased risk of rupture. Additionally, false lumen thrombus may cause arterial wall hypoxemia, resulting in localized wall weakening (**Fig. 60-22**). Whether endovascular intervention used as a primary therapy for certain patients with uncomplicated type B dissection will alter their natural history is unknown. To date, studies of subacute and chronic type B dissections have not found established benefit of prophylactic endovascular stent placement.[71]

Many late deaths following surgery for aortic dissection result from rupture of the aorta at the site of prior dissection or another aneurysm at a remote site (see Fig. 60-20 and Fig. 19-23A). The proximal descending aorta is the most common site of aneurysmal enlargement.[76] Aneurysms related to false lumen expansion have relatively thin walls and have a higher risk of rupture than atheromatous aneurysms. Thus, continued surveillance of the entire aorta and surgical treatment (or endovascular, when appropriate) of aneurysms at appropriate size thresholds is important for long-term survival. The timing of surgical repair for aneurysmal involvement of the residual aorta depends on several factors, including age and general medical condition of the individual, comorbidities, underlying disease process, rate of aneurysmal enlargement, and absolute size of the aorta. In general, for appropriate candidates, when the descending aorta diameter after dissection exceeds 5.5 cm, surgical treatment is recommended.[32] For patients at relatively lower surgical risk and for those with certain genetically triggered thoracic aortic aneurysms and dissection diseases, repair may be appropriate when the aortic diameter exceeds 5.0 to 5.5 cm.

After aortic dissection, lifestyle modifications are necessary. Isometric activities, including weightlifting, leads to increased blood pressure and aortic wall stress, and have rarely been associated with acute aortic dissection. Many individuals will have to change jobs, modify their type of work, or be considered disabled because of aortic dissection and/or underlying aortic disease causing limitations on physical activity.

Aortic Dissection Variants

In addition to acute aortic dissection, aortic intramural hematoma (IMH) and penetrating atherosclerotic ulcer (PAU) of the aorta are included in the acute aortic syndromes (see Fig. 60-8). These disorders may be identical to classic aortic dissection in their presentation, causing acute chest or back pain, but they have important differences in their imaging and management. IMH is associated with many of the same risk factors as classic aortic dissection, whereas PAU is more common in the descending aorta and is associated with heavy calcification and atherosclerosis.

Aortic Intramural Hematoma

In approximately 5% to 25% of cases of acute aortic syndrome, a hematoma develops within the medial layer of the aortic wall with no evidence of an intimal flap or false lumen visualized by imaging study, surgery, or autopsy. These noncommunicating dissections are labeled as aortic IMH. Most consider IMH to be the result of a primary rupture of the vasa vasorum leading to mural hemorrhage. When an aortic atheromatous plaque ruptures into the media—that is, a PAU—a secondary IMH often accompanies the acute ulceration. PAU with IMH formation is a separate entity than a spontaneous IMH (see later).

IMH is an important variant of aortic dissection and must be recognized. In the IRAD experience, approximately 6% of aortic dissections were classified as IMH.[77] In Asian studies, approximately 25% of acute aortic syndromes are IMHs.[78] Compared with classic aortic dissection, patients with IMH are older and more likely to have descending aortic involvement.

IMHs may be localized or may propagate the length of the aorta. They are classified as type A or B, using the same classification scheme as for classic aortic dissection. The presenting symptoms and risk factors associated with IMH resemble those of aortic dissection, with acute chest and/or back pain predominating. The proximity of the intramural hemorrhage to the adventitia may explain the frequent coexistence of pleural and pericardial effusion and underlie the higher risk of subsequent aortic rupture associated with IMH. Ascending IMH may lead to aortic regurgitation, hemopericardium, or rupture, but because there is no intimal flap or false lumen, stroke and visceral ischemia appear less common. There may be a geographic difference in incidence, because IMH is a more common diagnosis among acute aortic syndromes in Asian countries than in Western countries.[79]

Imaging studies that can diagnose IMH include TEE, CT, and MRI. TEE features of IMH include focal crescentic or circumferential aortic wall thickening, eccentric aortic lumen, displaced intimal calcification, and areas of echolucency within the aortic wall (**Fig. 60-23**; see Video 60-13 on website; see Fig. 15-85). There is no evidence of an intimal flap, false lumen, or flow in the aortic wall. The aortic wall thickness in IMH ranges from 5 to 25 mm. On noncontrast CT, IMH appears as an area of high attenuation in the wall of the aorta (see Fig. 60-e17 on website), whereas on contrast CT, the aortic wall demonstrates low attenuation because no contrast enters the wall (**Fig. 60-24**; see Fig. 19-23B). MRI demonstrates focal thickening of the aortic wall with phase contrast cine and gradient echo demonstrating no flow in the aortic wall (see Fig. 60-e18 on website). High signal intensity on

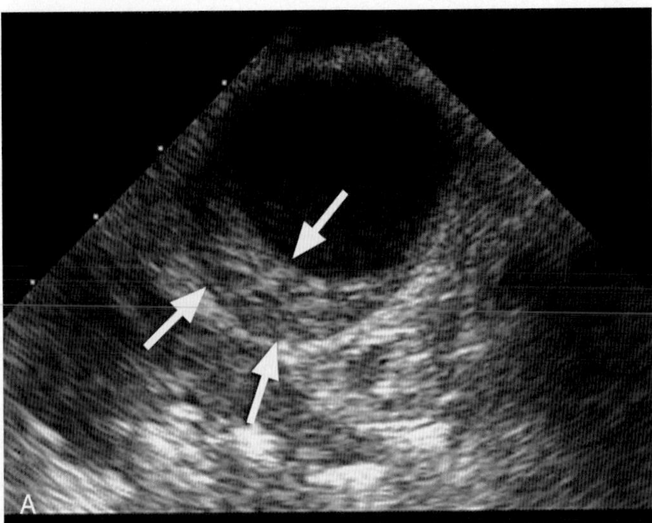

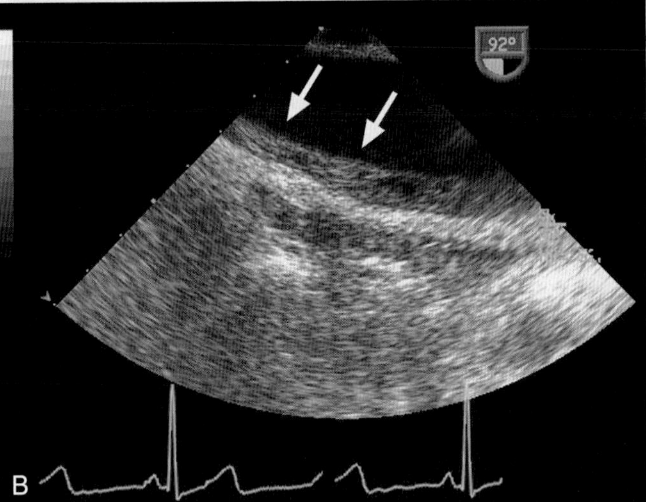

FIGURE 60-23 Transesophageal echocardiographic images of acute type B IMH (arrows). **A,** Short-axis views of the descending aorta demonstrating typical crescentic thickening of the aortic wall in IMH. **B,** Longitudinal views of the aorta demonstrating IMH (arrows).

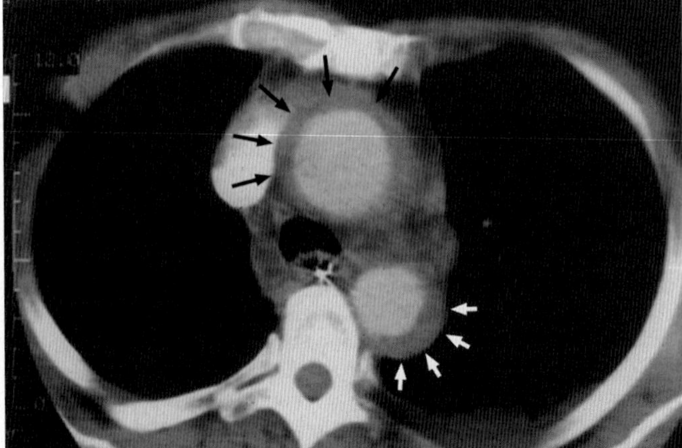

FIGURE 60-24 Contrast CT scan demonstrating type A IMH of the aorta. Note the circumferential hematoma involving the ascending aorta (black arrows) and the crescentic hematoma involving the descending aorta (white arrows).

T2-weighted imaging may be visualized related to blood in the aortic wall in acute IMH, but signal intensity varies, depending on the age of the hemorrhage. Aortography has a poor sensitivity to detect IMH, because this disease involves the aortic wall and not the lumen.

Distinct from an aneurysm with mural thrombus, the IMH has a smooth lumen and curvilinear wall (see Figs. 60-23 and 60-24). In certain cases, it may be difficult to differentiate IMH from aortic dissection with thrombosis of the false lumen, mural thrombus within an aortic aneurysm, or severe aortic atherosclerosis. By TEE, identifying the intima, which is often calcified and echodense, is helpful in this distinction. Thickening beneath the intima is suggestive of IMH, whereas thickening above the intima (on the luminal side) occurs with mural thrombus formation in an aneurysm. In contrast to aortic atherosclerosis, IMH typically is not associated with diffuse irregularities of the aortic intima surface, unless accompanying a penetrating ulcer.

IMH may have several fates: (1) progression to acute, classic aortic dissection or aortic rupture; (2) complete resolution of the hematoma with no evidence of the disorder on follow-up imaging; (3) persistence without progression of the hematoma; or (4) progressive aortic dilation and aneurysm formation.

Early studies from Western Europe and the United States have reported that patients with type A IMH were at high risk for complications, including aortic dissection (25% to 50%), hemopericardium, and rupture, with a mortality in excess of 30% with medical therapy alone.[77,79] In a review of 160 patients from 11 studies, mortality for type A IMH treated medically was almost 50% and was 24% when treated surgically. Type B IMH is associated with a lower mortality rate, 10% to 13% with medical therapy and 15% with surgical repair. These data have led most authorities to recommend emergency cardiac surgery in type A IMH and initial medical therapy in type B IMH. Cardiac surgery in type B IMH is reserved for complications such as progression, impending rupture, or rupture. Descending IMH may progress to frank dissection and late aneurysm formation, or may also reabsorb completely (see Fig. 60-e19 on website).

Reports from Japan and South Korea have suggested much different approaches for the management of type A IMH—medical therapy, serial imaging, and careful observation, with prolonged hospitalization as an initial strategy.[78] In a series of 101 patients with type A IMH from Korea, 16 patients underwent emergency surgery for hemodynamic instability, whereas 85 patients had initial medical therapy.[79] Medically treated patients underwent weekly imaging studies, prolonged hospitalization, and delayed surgery in 29% of patients at a median of 27 days, with a mortality rate of 4%. Predictors of adverse outcomes in these patients included syncope, enlarged aortic diameter (>55 mm), and increased hematoma thickness (>16 mm).

With this approach, however, many patients with type A IMH have progressed to frank dissection, hemopericardium, or rupture requiring emergency surgery (see Fig. 60-e20 on website). In a pooled analysis of 309 type A IMH cases, clinical outcomes were available for 160 patients from North America (NA) and Europe and for 149 patients from Asia.[79] The Asian population was usually treated with initial medical therapy. The overall mortality was lower (9%) for the Asian group compared with the NA-European group (21%). The Asian group also had a lower mortality for patients treated medically compared with the NA-European group. The mortality rates for patients undergoing early surgery for type A IMH were lower in the NA-European group than the Asian group.

Important differences in IMH in these different geographic regions may influence outcomes. IMH causes more frequent acute aortic syndromes in Asia compared with NA-Europe. This variation may be related to more subtle cases being recognized in Asia or because of genetic or environmental issues. In a pooled analysis, those sent for early surgery had lower in-hospital mortality (10%) than those with early medical treatment (18%). In a prior meta-analysis of 143 cases of type A IMH, early surgery associated with a lower mortality than did medical therapy (14% versus 36%, respectively).[79] In the Asian population treated medically, rates of pericardial tamponade were four times more common, and progression to frank aortic dissection was twice as frequent as in NA-European patients. With the strategy of medical therapy for ascending IMH, 30% of those initially treated medically, and more than 50% of IMH overall, eventually underwent surgical repair.[78-80] The IRAD population included 23 patients with ascending IMH. Progression to aortic dissection occurred in 16%, and the mortality rate for type A IMH was 39%.[77] In a series of 36 type A IMHs, 7 patients underwent immediate surgery, 28 underwent initial medical therapy with subsequent conversion to surgical repair (33% of these progressed to acute dissection), and 1 was treated medically, with resolution of the IMH.[81]

Given the potential for unpredictable and catastrophic complications, most authorities continue to recommend immediate surgical therapy for type A IMH in patients at reasonable risk and at experienced surgical centers, and medical management for type B IMH.[77] Management of localized arch IMH must be individualized, with some advocating initial medical therapy for this group.[78] Patients with IMH require continued surveillance after surgery and while on medical therapy for type B IMH. Complete resolution of type B IMH has been described in more than 50% in some series, whereas others have led to frank dissection, rupture, or late aneurysm formation.[82] In one series of type B IMH, almost one third of cases were referred for surgical repair, initially or in follow-up.[83] Although information is limited, predictors of resolution of type B hematoma have included younger age, smaller aortic diameters (<4 to 4.5 cm), hematoma thickness (<1 cm), and postoperative beta blocker use.

Penetrating Atherosclerotic Ulcer

PAU (penetrating aortic ulcer) is a condition in which an atherosclerotic lesion penetrates the internal elastic lamina into the media, often associated with a variable degree of intramural hematoma formation.[83] PAU may lead to pseudoaneurysm formation, aortic rupture, or late aneurysm (**Fig. 60-25**). Aortic ulcers may be single or multiple and range from 5 mm to 25 mm in diameter and 4 mm to 30 mm in depth. PAUs can occur throughout the aorta, but are more common in the thoracic and abdominal aorta than in the arch or ascending aorta.

The incidence of PAU is unknown. Among symptomatic patients with suspected acute aortic syndrome, PAUs are present in 2% to 8%.[83] Patients with PAU are typically older and hypertensive, with multiple coronary risk factors and coexisting vascular disease. Many patients have concomitant aneurysmal dilation of the aorta elsewhere. Whereas up to 25% of PAUs are found incidentally on imaging studies, typical symptoms of PAU include acute chest or back pain, similar in description to those of classic aortic dissection. Because acute PAU may have a higher propensity to rupture, it is imperative to recognize this condition. Although PAU may lead to aortic dissection, most patients do not have aortic regurgitation, pulse deficits, or visceral ischemia.

Imaging techniques for PAU include aortography, CT, MRI, and TEE. Although aortography is no longer the preferred method for diagnosis, the ulcer-like appearance on angiography gave this entity its name. Findings on CT include focal aortic ulceration, associated IMH, and a calcified displaced intima (**Fig. 60-26**). Typically, there is a crater-like outpouching with irregular edges in the setting of heavy atherosclerosis (see Fig. 60-e21 on website). CT findings may also demonstrate pleural effusions, mediastinal hemorrhage, coexisting aneurysms, contained rupture, pseudoaneurysm, and frank rupture (see Fig. 60-24). Approximately 80% of patients have some degree of IMH formation.[83] When PAU occurs with aortic dissection, the dissection often involves a short segment of aorta and has a thick intimal flap. MRI findings in PAU include localized areas of high signal intensity in the aorta wall consistent with IMH, focal intimal thickening, and ulcer-like projections. TEE demonstrates aortic atherosclerosis with focal ulceration of the intima and can demonstrate complications.

The natural history of PAU is uncertain, and descriptions in the literature vary depending on patient selection. A PAU may stabilize or lead to complications, including IMH, distal embolization, aortic rupture, pseudoaneurysm (contained rupture), aortic dissection, and development of a saccular or fusiform aneurysm. In one study, the annual growth rate of PAU was 0.31 cm/year. Some studies have reported gradual aortic enlargement and a low incidence of acute or

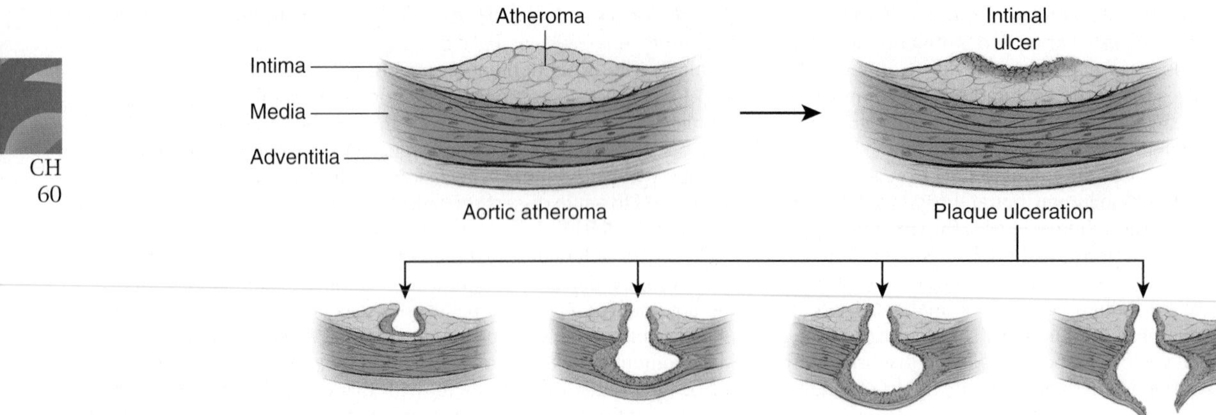

FIGURE 60-25 Evolution of a penetrating atherosclerotic ulcer of the aorta. Once an intimal ulcer has formed, it may then progress to a variable length. Penetration through the intima causes a medial hematoma, whereas penetration through the media leads to the formation of a pseudoaneurysm, and perforation through the adventitial layer results in an aortic rupture. *(From Stanson AW, Kazmier FJ, Hollier LH, et al: Penetrating atherosclerotic ulcers of the thoracic aorta: Natural history and clinicopathologic correlations. Ann Vasc Surg 1:15, 1986.)*

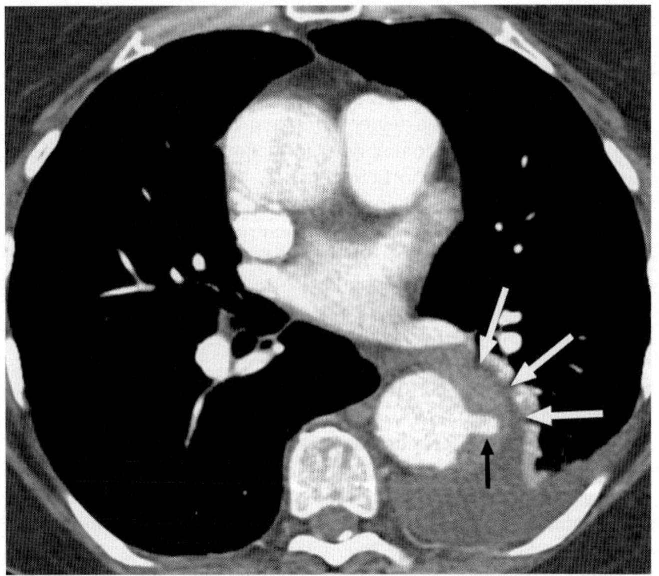

FIGURE 60-26 Contrast CT scan of a penetrating atherosclerotic ulcer of the aorta. Note the ulcer-like projection (black arrow) from the aortic lumen in the proximal descending aorta and the associated intramural hematoma (white arrows). A small pleural effusion is also present. *(Courtesy of Dr. Sanjeev Bhalla, Washington University School of Medicine, St. Louis.)*

life-threatening complications, whereas others have reported a high incidence of acute complications.[82,84] In a report of 26 patients with PAU, more than one third presented with rupture, 46% had ascending involvement, and two thirds underwent surgical repair.[82] In another series of 107 PAU patients, only 2% involved the ascending aorta, 9% presented with rupture, and 72% were treated medically. Only rupture at presentation and maximum aortic diameter predicted failure of medical therapy, defined as death from an aortic cause or caused by aortic surgery.

The management of the patient with PAU must be individualized. In general, patients with ascending PAUs are treated with surgical resection. Stable patients with type B PAUs may be managed medically, with strict follow-up and serial imaging. Patients with refractory or recurrent pain have increased risk of disease progression. Those with a rapid increase in aortic dimension are at risk for rupture and should be treated surgically or with endovascular stent grafts. Indications for surgery or endovascular therapy may include features on imaging that include interval development of hemorrhage, periaortic hematoma, expanding pseudoaneurysm, and rupture. Other predictors of progression of disease include increasing aortic wall thickness, ulcer craters more than 20 mm in diameter or 10 mm in depth, increasing aortic hematoma, and increasing pleural effusion. In a retrospective review, one third of patients with PAU required surgical repair during follow-up for complications.[82] Many have recommended a more aggressive approach to type B PAU than classic type B dissection because of concern of increased risk of rupture.[84]

Because of the relatively focal aortic segment involved in PAU, this acute aortic syndrome may be suitable for endovascular therapy in many cases (see Fig. 60-e22A and 60-e22B on website).[66,82] Patients with PAU are usually older, with multiple comorbidities, which increases their risk for open surgical repair. In a series of 19 patients with complications related to PAU (including aortic rupture in seven patients, aneurysmal enlargement > 55 mm in nine patients, rapid expansion > 10 mm/year, and recurrent pain in three patients), endovascular stent-graft implantation was successful in 95%.[84]

Bacterial Infections of the Aorta

Infected aortic aneurysms are a rare but lethal condition comprising less than 1% of all aneurysms undergoing operation.[85] Although the disease may be insidious in onset, it may also have a fulminant course, with frequent aneurysm rupture (>50%) and a high mortality rate (>25% to 50%). Even in the current era, with medical therapy alone, in-hospital mortality exceeds 50%. The treatment involves aneurysm resection, débridement of infected soft tissues, antibiotics, and arterial reconstruction. Most patients receive in situ aortic grafting, and others undergo extra-anatomic bypass. Endovascular repair has been performed selectively in high-risk patients.[86] The cause of infected aneurysms is most commonly related to direct invasion of circulating microorganisms into an atherosclerotic or disrupted arterial wall. Contiguous spread of microbes from adjacent infection may occur and, occasionally, septic embolization from bacterial endocarditis may seed the aorta, resulting in septic aneurysm formation.

Most patients with an infected aortic aneurysm are symptomatic, with fever, abdominal, back, or chest pain, and a pulsatile tender mass being pathognomonic. But this classic triad is only present in the minority of patients. Patients are febrile, have leukocytosis, and have a high erythrocyte sedimentation rate. Symptoms that arise from involvement of adjacent organs include odynophagia, hematemesis, and hemoptysis. Most patients have positive blood cultures, but in some patients the organism is established only at the time of operative repair with culture and Gram stain of the aortic wall. The average patient in most series is in his or her 70s, and many patients have comorbidities, including diabetes and chronic disease, an underlying immunocompromised state, or chronic steroid therapy. Many have recently undergone gastrointestinal operations or invasive procedures. Infected aneurysms most commonly involve the infrarenal aorta, with the paravisceral and juxtarenal aorta involved less commonly. Infected thoracic aortic aneurysms are rare, most commonly affecting the descending aorta, and usually present with rupture or pseudoaneurysm.[87] Infections of prosthetic aortic grafts occur in 1% to 2% of such reconstructions and present with abdominal or back pain and fever. Aortic graft-enteric erosion or fistula occur in 50%.[85,88]

The most common microorganisms associated with infected aortic aneurysms include *Staphylococcus aureus* and *Salmonella* species, but almost any organism may be responsible. *Escherichia coli*, *Streptococcus* species, *Neisseria* species, and gram-negative bacilli and fungi have been associated. Although *Salmonella* may infect an underlying atherosclerotic aortic aneurysm, this microbe may directly penetrate an intact intima of a normal aortic wall, leading to arteritis and aneurysm formation. Thus, one should always be suspicious of underlying aortic seeding when *Salmonella* bacteremia is present.

CT, MRI, and aortography may be diagnostic in infected aortic aneurysms, with most series describing saccular aneurysms in 70% to 90% and fusiform aneurysms in 10% to 30%.[88] Features on CT scan include disruption of calcification, irregular wall thickening, periaortic mass, rim enhancement, and periaortic stranding. The presence of gas and vertebral body erosion are highly suggestive of infection. Other findings may include periaortic hematoma and associated dissecting aneurysm.[89] Aortocaval or aortoenteric fistulae may complicate infected aneurysms. The aorta is typically enlarged and aneurysmal on diagnosis but, importantly, the aorta is not always significantly dilated on presentation. These aneurysms may be rapidly expanding and have a propensity to rupture—hence, the importance of diagnosis. Because most descending or abdominal aneurysms are atherosclerotic, the lack of calcium in an involved aorta may suggest an infected aneurysm.[89] MRI features of infected aneurysms include soft tissue mass, stranding fluid retention, and rim enhancement. Imaging studies with indium-111–labelled white blood cells have been used in some cases.

The natural history of infected aortic aneurysms is that of expansion and eventual rupture, often with rapid progression. *Salmonella* and other gram-negative infections have a greater tendency for early rupture and death. Overall mortality from infected aortic aneurysms has been reported to be in excess of 50% with medical therapy alone.

The treatment of infected abdominal aortic aneurysms involves excision or exclusion of infected aortic tissue, in situ or extra-anatomic bypass of the aorta and branches, débridement of infected periaortic tissues, and prolonged antibiotic therapy. In the past, most operations included extra-anatomic bypass because of concern about the risk of postoperative aortic graft infection. Many infected aneurysms are in locations not amenable to conventional extra-anatomic reconstruction. In general, when infrarenal aortic aneurysms are associated with extensive aortic and periaortic purulence, extra-anatomic bypass is performed. In situ bypass is more commonly performed in the setting of suprarenal aneurysms or infrarenal aneurysms with minimal purulence. Recent surgical series have reported operative mortality of 12% to 21%.[85,87,88]

In a series of 43 patients with infected aneurysms, 53% had ruptured at the time of surgery, with 60% located at or above the renal arteries. The average aneurysm size was 5.9 cm (range, 3 to 12 cm), and most had periaortic extension of infection. In this series, 85% of patients underwent in situ prosthetic graft placement and 15% had extra-anatomic bypass. The operative mortality was 21%. Antibiotics were continued for 1 to 6 months in 60%, and for life in many.[85] In a series of 32 patients with infected aortic aneurysms, 25 patients underwent open repair with a mortality rate of 12%, compared with 57% on medical therapy alone.[87] Because many patients are considered at high risk of complications of surgery for infected aortic aneurysms, some have advocated endovascular repair as an option for those who are not suitable for open repair, either as a bridge to open repair or as definitive therapy.[86]

Prosthetic stent-graft infections are uncommon, with true incidence unknown. *Staphylococcus*, *Streptococcus*, and *Enterococcus* species are the most common microorganism involved. Risk factors include wound infections, immunosuppression, diabetes, and intestinal ischemia. Pseudoaneurysm and aneurysm expansion and rupture may occur. Treatment includes removal of the infected stent-graft. Axillofemoral bypass with total graft excision and oversewing of the aorta stump has been the traditional repair, but more recently, in situ prosthetic reconstruction has had a more favorable outcome in selected cases. Operative mortality is reported at approximately 10% to 15%, with graft reinfections complicating approximately 10%.[88]

Primary Tumors of the Aorta

Aortic tumors are rare and almost always malignant. They typically present with embolism or arterial obstruction and are often not suspected until histologic analysis reveals malignancy. In one literature review, the average age was 60 years, with a male predominance.[90] Risk factors for aortic tumors are unknown, with prior radiation, prosthetic grafts, and atherosclerosis being hypothesized. Locations of these tumors include the descending thoracic aorta (35%), abdominal aorta (27%), thoracoabdominal aorta (27%), and ascending aorta and arch (11%).[90] Presenting symptoms include pain, embolism, intermittent claudication, renovascular hypertension, and visceral ischemia. Less commonly, these tumors present as stroke, hemorrhagic complications, or invasion of adjacent structures. Aortic tumors fall into three groups—intraluminal (polypoid), intimal, and adventitial (mural). Intraluminal and intimal tumors are the most common. These tumors spread along the aortic inner wall and may appear polypoid on imaging. They may present with acute arterial embolization, with the embolus being a mixture of tumor and thrombus, or lead to arterial obstruction or involvement of visceral arteries. Widely metastatic emboli may occur. Adventitial (mural) tumors are rare and grow to involve periaortic tissue and adjacent organs.

Aortic tumors are of mesenchymal origin and include intimal sarcoma (21%), malignant fibrous histiocytoma (15%), angiosarcoma (26%), leiomyosarcoma (15%), and undifferentiated sarcoma. The diagnosis is usually made by pathologic examination of tumor emboli or at surgery or autopsy, and metastatic spread is present in most patients at diagnosis. Aortography findings are nonspecific and imitate an aneurysm or mural thrombus. Intimal tumors may be detected by CT (**Fig. 60-27**), but the findings may mimic those of protruding atheroma. MRI is considered most reliable for diagnosis and may differentiate between tumor and atheromatous material. TEE has been useful in some cases. If no metastases are present, resection with prosthetic graft replacement is recommended. Because of difficulties in achieving wide margins, local recurrence of tumor may occur. Palliative treatment of obstructive tumors has included endarterectomy, endovascular grafts, and extra-anatomic bypass. Chemotherapy and radiation have been used in some cases, with limited success. The average survival has been about 1 year, with adventitial (mural) tumors having a better prognosis than intimal tumors. In surgically treated patients, 3-year survival has been reported at 16%.[90]

Future Perspectives

Because of dedicated individuals across multiple disciplines, remarkable discovery and progress have occurred in the understanding of aortic disease. Basic and translational research with experimental and animal models of aneurysms and genetically triggered aortic syndromes have led to enhanced understanding of the pathophysiologic events underlying these disorders. This knowledge may lead to direct clinical application with pharmacologic interventions that may well change the course of these diseases. Advances in biomarker development hold promise in identifying disease activity, disease progression, and response to therapy. New biomarkers may allow the rapid identification of patients with a high likelihood of acute aortic dissection.

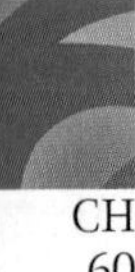

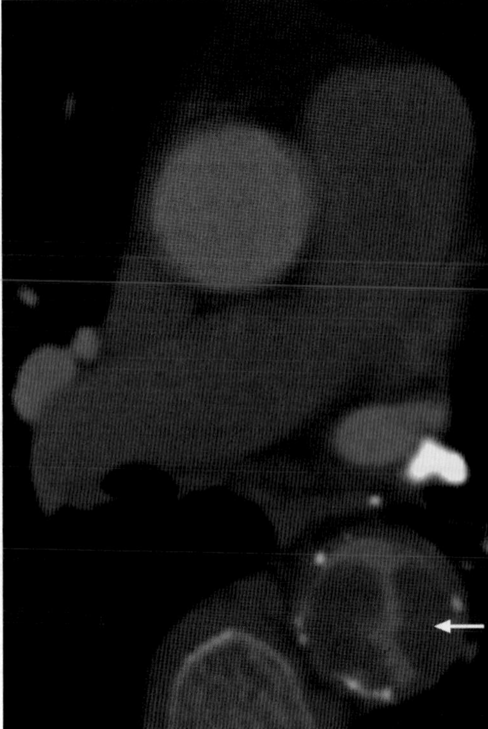

FIGURE 60-27 Contrast CT scan demonstrating an intimal tumor of the descending aorta (arrow). The tumor has the appearance of an intraluminal filling defect with septations.

Advances in imaging the aorta structurally and functionally, using techniques to understand biomechanical forces and biologic activity in the aortic wall, hold promise in following patients with aortic disease. These techniques may allow better individual decision making about the timing of preventive intervention.

Finally, rapid advances in surgical and endovascular therapy have revolutionized the management of complex aortic disease, greatly reducing the morbidity and mortality rates of elective and emergency procedures.

ACKNOWLEDGMENT

The authors gratefully acknowledge the contributions of Dr. Eric Isselbacher to previous versions of this chapter in earlier editions of this text.

REFERENCES

Abdominal Aortic Aneurysms

1. Golledge J, Norman PE: Pathophysiology of abdominal aortic aneurysm relevant to improvements in patients' management. Curr Opin Cardiol 24:532, 2009.
2. Kim LG, P Scott RA, Ashton HA, Thompson SG; Multicentre Aneurysm Screening Study Group: A sustained mortality benefit from screening for abdominal aortic aneurysm. Ann Intern Med 146:699, 2007.
3. Cosford PA, Leng GC: Screening for abdominal aortic aneurysm. Cochrane Database Syst Rev (2):CD002945, 2007.
4. Fleming C, Whitlock EP, Beil TL, Lederle FA: Screening for abdominal aortic aneurysm: A best-evidence systematic review for the U.S. Preventive Services Task Force. Ann Intern Med 142:203, 2005.
5. Chaikof EL, Brewster DC, Dalman RL, et al: The care of patients with an abdominal aortic aneurysm: The Society for Vascular Surgery practice guidelines. J Vasc Surg 50(Suppl):S2, 2009.
6. Helgadottir A, Thorleifsson G, Magnusson KP, et al: The same sequence variant on 9p21 associates with myocardial infarction, abdominal aortic aneurysm and intracranial aneurysm. Nat Genet 40:217, 2008.
7. Rayt HS, Sutton AJ, London NJ, et al: A systematic review and meta-analysis of endovascular repair (EVAR) for ruptured abdominal aortic aneurysm. Eur J Vasc Endovasc Surg 36:536, 2008.
8. Baxter BT, Terrin MC, Dalman RL: Medical management of small abdominal aortic aneurysms. Circulation 117:1883, 2008.
9. Sukhija R, Aronow WS, Sandhu R, et al: Mortality and size of abdominal aortic aneurysm at long-term follow-up of patients not treated surgically and treated with and without statins. Am J Cardiol 97:279, 2006.
10. Schermerhorn ML, O'Malley AJ, Jhaveri A, et al: Endovascular vs. open repair of abdominal aortic aneurysms in the Medicare population. N Engl J Med 358:464, 2008.
11. Lederle FA, Freischlag JA, Kyriakides TC, et al: Open Versus Endovascular Repair (OVER) Veterans Affairs Cooperative Study Group. Outcomes following endovascular vs open repair of abdominal aortic aneurysm: A randomized trial. JAMA 302:1535, 2009.
12. Sicard GA, Zwolak RM, Sidawy AN, et al: Endovascular abdominal aortic aneurysm repair: Long-term outcome measures in patients at high risk for open surgery. J Vasc Surg 44:229, 2006.
13. McPhee J, Eslami MH, Arous EJ, et al: Endovascular treatment of ruptured abdominal aortic aneurysms in the United States (2001-2006): A significant survival benefit over open repair is independently associated with increased institutional volume. J Vasc Surg 49:817, 2009.
14. Veith FJ, Lachat M, Mayer D, et al: Collected world and single center experience with endovascular treatment of ruptured abdominal aortic aneurysms. Ann Surg 250:818, 2009.

Thoracic Aortic Aneurysms

15. Ramanath VS, Oh JK, Sundt TM, Eagle KA: Acute aortic syndromes and thoracic aortic aneurysm. Mayo Clin Proc 84:465, 2009.
16. Loeys BL, Schwarze U, Holm T, et al: Aneurysm syndromes caused by mutations in the TGF-β receptor. N Engl J Med 355:788, 2006.
17. Williams JA, Loeys BL, Nwakanma LU, et al: Early surgical experience with Loeys-Dietz: A new syndrome of aggressive thoracic aortic aneurysm disease. Ann Thorac Surg 83:S757, 2007.
18. Milewicz DM, Guo DG, Tran-Fadulu V, et al: Genetic basis of thoracic aortic aneurysms and dissections: Focus on smooth muscle cell contractile dysfunction. Annu Rev Genomics Hum Genet 9:283, 2008.
19. Albornoz G, Coady MA, Roberts M, et al: Familial thoracic aortic aneurysms and dissections: Incidence, modes of inheritance, and phenotypic patterns. Ann Thorac Surg 82:1400, 2006.
20. Guo DC, Pannu H, Papke CL, et al: Mutations in smooth muscle α-actin (*ACTA2*) lead to thoracic aortic aneurysms and dissections. Nat Genet 39:1488, 2007.
21. Braverman AC, Beardslee MA: The bicuspid aortic valve. *In* Otto C, Bonow R (eds): Valvular Heart Disease: A Companion to Braunwald's Heart Disease. Philadelphia, Saunders Elsevier, 2009, pp 169-186.
22. Loscalzo ML, Goh D, Loeys B, et al: Familial thoracic aortic dilation and bicommissural aortic valve: A prospective analysis of the natural history and inheritance. Am J Med Genet A 143A:1960, 2007.
23. Biner S, Rafique AM, Ray I, et al: Aortopathy is prevalent in relatives of bicuspid aortic valve patients. J Am Coll Cardiol 53:2288, 2009.
24. Bondy CA: Aortic dissection in Turner syndrome. Curr Opin Cardiol 23:519, 2008.
25. Tan JL, Gatzoulis MA, Ho SY: Aortic root disease in tetralogy of Fallot. Curr Opin Cardiol 1:569, 2007.
26. Elefteriades JA, Farkas EA: Thoracic aortic aneurysm. Clinical pertinent controversies and uncertainties. J Am Coll Cardiol 55:841, 2010.
27. Davies RR, Goldstein LJ, Coady MA, et al: Yearly rupture or dissection rates for thoracic aortic aneurysms: Simple prediction based on size. Ann Thorac Surg 2002;73:17-27
28. Patel HJ, Deeb GM: Ascending and arch aorta: Pathology, natural history, and treatment. Circulation 118:188, 2008.
29. Davies RR, Gallo A, Coady MA, et al: Novel measurement of relative aortic size predicts rupture of thoracic aortic aneurysms. Ann Thorac Surg 81:169, 2006.
30. Davies RR, Kaple RK, Mandapati D, et al: Natural history of ascending aortic aneurysms in the setting of an unreplaced bicuspid aortic valve. Ann Thorac Surg 83:1338, 2007.
31. Januzzi JL, Isselbacher EM, Fattori R, et al: Characterizing the young patient with aortic dissection: Results from the International Registry of Acute Aortic Dissection (IRAD). J Am Coll Cardiol 43:665, 2004.
32. Hiratzka LF, Bakris GL, Beckman JA, et al: 2010 ACCF/AHA/AATS/ACR/ASA/SCA/ SCAI/SIR/STS/ SVM guidelines for the diagnosis and management of patients with Thoracic Aortic Disease: A report of the American College of Cardiology Foundation/American Heart Association Task Force on Practice Guidelines, American Association for Thoracic Surgery, American College of Radiology, American Stroke Association, Society of Cardiovascular Anesthesiologists, Society for Cardiovascular Angiography and Interventions, Society of Interventional Radiology, Society of Thoracic Surgeons, and Society for Vascular Medicine. Circulation 121:e266, 2010.
33. Fazel SS, David TE: Aortic valve-sparing operations for aortic root and ascending aortic aneurysms. Curr Opin Cardiol 22: 497, 2007.
34. Luciani GB, Mazzucco A: Aortic root disease after the Ross procedure. Curr Opin Cardiol 21:555, 2006.
35. Elefteriades JA, Botta DM: Indications for the treatment of thoracic aortic aneurysms. Surg Clin North Am 89:845, 2009.
36. Estrera AL, Miller CC 3rd, Chen EP, et al: Descending thoracic aortic aneurysm repair: 12-year experience using distal aortic perfusion and cerebrospinal fluid drainage. Ann Thor Surg 80:1290, 2005.
37. Makaroun MS, Dillavou ED, Kee ST, et al: Endovascular treatment of thoracic aortic aneurysms: Results of the phase II multicenter trial of the Gore TAG thoracic endoprosthesis. J Vasc Surg 41:1, 2005.
38. Fairman RM, Criado F, Farber M, et al: Pivotal results of the Medtronic vascular talent thoracic stent graft system: The Valor Trial. J Vasc Surg 48:546, 2008.
39. Matsumura JS, Cambria RP, Dake MD, et al: International controlled clinical trial of the thoracic endovascular aneurysm repair with the Zenith TX2 endovascular graft: 1 year results. J Vasc Surg 47:247, 2008.
40. Rizvi AZ, Murad MH, Fairman RM, et al: The effect of left subclavian artery coverage on morbidity and mortality in patients undergoing endovascular thoracic aortic interventions: A systematic review and meta-analysis. J Vasc Surg 50:1159, 2009.

Aortic Dissection

41. Hagan PG, Nienaber CA, Isselbacher EM, et al: International Registry of Acute Aortic Dissection (IRAD): New insights from an old disease. JAMA 283:897, 2000.
42. Tsai TT, Trimarchi S, Neinaber CA: Acute aortic dissection: Perspectives from the international registry of acute aortic dissection (IRAD). Eur J Vasc Endovasc Surg 37:149, 2009.
43. Hirst AE Jr, Johns VJ Jr, Kime SW Jr: Dissecting aneurysm of the aorta: A review of 505 cases. Medicine (Baltimore) 37:217, 1958.
44. Hsue PY, Salinas C, Bolger AF, et al: Acute aortic dissection induced by crack cocaine. Circulation 105:1592, 2002.

45. Goland S, Elkayam U: Cardiovascular problems in pregnant women with Marfan syndrome. Circulation 119:619, 2009.
46. Eggebrecht H, Thompson M, Rousseau H, et al: Retrograde ascending aortic dissection during or after thoracic aortic stent-graft placement: Insight from the European registry on endovascular aortic repair complications. Circulation 120(Suppl):S276, 2009.
47. Collins JS, Evangelista A, Nienaber CA, et al: Differences in clinical presentation, management, and outcomes of acute type A aortic dissection in patients with and without previous cardiac surgery. Circulation 110 (Suppl II):II-237, 2004.
48. Pape LA, Tsai TT, Isselbacher EM, et al: Aortic diameter >5.5 cm is not a good predictor of type A aortic dissection. Observations from the international registry of acute aortic dissection. Circulation 116:1120, 2007.
49. Parish LM, Gorman JH III, Kahn S, et al: Aortic size in acute type A dissection: Implications for preventative ascending aortic replacement. Eur J Cardiothorac Surg 35:941, 2009.
50. Poullis M, Warwick R, Oo A, Poole RJ: Ascending aortic curvature as an independent risk factor for type A aortic dissection, and ascending aortic aneurysm formation: A mathematical model. Eur J Cardiovasc Surg 33:995, 2008.
51. Upchurch GR, Nienaber C, Fattori R, et al: Acute aortic dissection presenting with primarily abdominal pain: A rare manifestation of a deadly disease. Ann Vasc Surg 19:367, 2005.
52. Park SW, Hutchinson S, Mehta RH, et al: Association of painless aortic dissection with increased mortality. Mayo Clin Proc 79:1252, 2004.
53. Henke PK, Williams DM, Upchurch GR Jr, et al: Acute limb ischemia associated with type B aortic dissection: Clinical relevance and therapy. Surgery 140:532, 2006.
54. Chow JL, Marian ER, Liang D: Transesophageal echocardiography assessment of severe aortic regurgitation in type A aortic dissection caused by a prolapsed circumferential intimal flap. J Cardiothorac Vasc Anesth 21:85, 2007.
55. Gaul C, Dietrich W, Erbguth FJ: Neurologic symptoms in acute aortic dissection: A challenge for neurologists. Cerebrovasc Dis 26:1, 2008.
56. Trimarchi S, Nienaber CA, Rampoldi V, et al: Contemporary results of surgery in acute type A aortic dissection: The international registry of acute aortic dissection experience. J Thorac Cardiovasc Surg 129:112, 2005.
57. Geirsson A, Szeto Wilson Y, Pochettino A, et al: Significance of malperfusion syndromes prior to contemporary surgical repair for acute type A dissection: Outcomes and need for additional revascularizations. Eur J Cardiothorac Surg 32:255, 2007.
58. Trimarchi S, Tsai T, Eagle KA, et al: Acute abdominal aortic dissection: insight from the international registry of acute aortic dissection (IRAD). J Vasc Surg 46:913, 2007.
59. Suzuki T, Distante A, Zizza A, et al: Diagnosis of acute aortic dissection by D-dimer: The international registry of acute aortic dissection substudy on biomarkers (IRAD-bio) experience. Circulation 119:2702, 2009.
60. Stevens LM, Madsen JC, Isselbacher EM, et al: Surgical management and long-term outcomes of acute ascending aortic dissection. J Thorac Cardiovasc Surg 138:1349, 2009.
61. Gilon D, Mehta RH, Oh JK, et al: Characteristics and in-hospital outcomes of patients with cardiac tamponade complicating type A acute aortic dissection. Am J Cardiol 103:1029, 2009.
62. Geirsson A, Szeto WY, Pochettino A, et al: Significance of malperfusion syndromes prior to contemporary surgical repair for acute type A dissection: Outcomes and need for additional revascularizations. Eur J Cardiothorac Surg 32:255, 2007.
63. Rampoldi V, Trimarchi S, Eagle, KA, et al: Simple risk models to predict surgical mortality in acute type A aortic dissection: The International Registry of Acute Aortic Dissection score. Ann Thorac Surg 83:55, 2007.
64. Trimarchi S, Nienaber CA, Rampoldi V, et al: Role and results of surgery in acute type B aortic dissection. Insights from the international registry of acute aortic dissection (IRAD). Circulation 114(Suppl I):1-357, 2006.
65. Estrera AL, Miller CC, Safi HJ, et al: Outcomes of medical management of acute type B aortic dissection. Circulation 114(Supp I):I-384, 2006.
66. Svensson LG, Kouchoukos NT, Miller DC, et al: Expert consensus document on the treatment of descending thoracic aortic disease using endovascular stent-grafts. Ann Thorac Surg 85:(Suppl):1, 2008.
67. Tsai TT, Isselbacher EM, Trimarchi S, et al: Acute type B aortic dissection: Does aortic arch involvement affect management and outcomes? Insights from the International Registry of Acute Aortic Dissection (IRAD). Circulation 116:I-150, 2007.
68. Lin PH, Huynh TT, Kougias P, et al: Descending thoracic aortic dissection: Evaluation and management in the era of endovascular technology. Vasc Endovasc Surg 43:5, 2009.
69. Patel HJ, Williams DM, Meerkov M, et al: Long-term results of percutaneous management of malperfusion in acute Type B aortic dissection: Implications of thoracic aortic endovascular repair. J Thorac Cardiovasc Surg 38:300, 2009.
70. Nienaber CA, Kische S, Zeller T, et al: Provisional extension to induce complete attachment after stent-graft placement in type B aortic dissection: The PETTICOAT concept. J Endovasc Ther 13:738, 2006.
71. Nienaber CA, Rousseau H, Eggbrecht H, et al: Randomized comparison of strategies for type B aortic dissection. The Investigation of STEnt grafts in Aortic Dissection (INSTEAD) Trial. Circulation 120:2519, 2009.
72. Tsai TT, Evangelista A, Nienaber CA, et al: Long-term survival in patients presenting with type A acute aortic dissection. Insights from the International Registry of Acute Aortic Dissection. Circulation 114(Suppl I):I-350, 2006.
73. Jault F, Rama A, Lievre L, et al: Chronic dissection of the ascending aorta: Surgical results during a 20-year period. Eur J Cardiothorac Surg 29:1041, 2006.
74. Tsai TT, Fattori R, Trimarchi S, et al: Long-term survival in patients presenting with type B acute aortic dissection. Insights from the international registry of acute aortic dissection. Circulation 114:2226, 2006.
75. Tsai TT, Evangelista A, Nienaber CA, et al: Partial thrombosis of the false lumen in patients with acute type B dissection. N Engl J Med 357:349, 2007.
76. Song J, Kim S, Kim J, et al: Long-term predictors of descending aorta aneurysmal change in patients with aortic dissection. J Am Coll Cardiol 50:799, 2007.
77. Evangelista A, Mukherjee D, Mehta RH, et al: Acute intramural hematoma of the aorta. Circulation 111:1063, 2005.
78. Song JK, Yim JH, Ahn JM, Kim DH, et al: Outcomes of patients with acute type A aortic intramural hematoma. Circulation 120:2046, 2009.
79. Pelzel JM, Braverman AC, Hirsch AT, Harris KM: International heterogeneity in diagnostic frequency and clinical outcomes of ascending aortic intramural hematoma. J Am Soc Echo 20:1260, 2007.
80. Moizumi Y, Komatsu T, Motoyoshi N, Tabayashi K: Clinical features and long-term outcome of type A and type B intramural hematoma. J Thorac Cardiovasc Surg 127:421, 2004.
81. Kitai T, Kaji S, Tani T, et al: Clinical outcomes of medical therapy and timely operation in initially diagnosed type A intramural hematoma: a 20 year experience. Circulation 120(Suppl):S292, 2009.
82. Estrera A, Miller C 3rd, Lee TY, et al: Acute type A intramural hematoma: Analysis of current management strategy. Circulation 120(Suppl):S287, 2009.
83. Sundt TM: Intramural hematoma and penetrating atherosclerotic ulcer of the aorta. Ann Thorac Surg 83:S835, 2007.
84. Botta L, Buttazzi K, Russo V, et al: Endovascular repair for penetrating atherosclerotic ulcers of the descending aorta: Early and mid-term results. Ann Thorac Surg 85:987, 2008.
85. Oderich GS, Panneton JM, Bower TC et al: Infected aortic aneurysms: Aggressive presentation, complicated early outcome, but durable results. J Vasc Surg 34:900, 2001.
86. Patel HJ, Williams DM, Upchurch GR Jr, et al: Late outcomes of endovascular aortic repair for the infected thoracic aorta. Ann Thorac Surg 87:1366, 2009.
87. Hsu RB, Lin FY: Infected aneurysm of the thoracic aorta. J Vasc Surg 47:270, 2008.
88. Oderich GS, Bower TC, Cherry KJ Jr, et al: Evolution from axillofemoral to in situ prosthetic reconstruction for the treatment of aortic graft infections at a single center. J Vasc Surg 43:1166, 2006.
89. Lin MP, Chang SC, Wu RH, et al: A comparison of computed tomography, magnetic resonance imaging, and digital subtraction angiography findings in the diagnosis of infected aortic aneurysm. J Comput Assist Tomogr 32:616, 2008.

Primary Tumors of the Aorta

90. Chiche L, Mongredien B, Brocheriou I, Kieffer E: Primary tumors of the thoracoabdominal aorta: Surgical treatment of 5 patients and review of the literature. Ann Vasc Surg 17:354, 2003.

CHAPTER 61 Peripheral Artery Diseases

Mark A. Creager and Peter Libby

Peripheral artery disease (PAD) generally refers to a disorder that obstructs the blood supply to the lower or upper extremities.[1] Most commonly caused by atherosclerosis, it may also result from thrombosis, embolism, vasculitis, fibromuscular dysplasia, or entrapment. The term *peripheral vascular disease* is less specific because it encompasses a group of diseases affecting blood vessels, including other atherosclerotic conditions such as renal artery disease and carotid artery disease, as well as vasculitides, vasospasm, venous thrombosis, venous insufficiency, and lymphatic disorders.

PAD correlates strongly with risk of major cardiovascular events, as it frequently associates with coronary and cerebral atherosclerosis.[2] Moreover, symptoms of PAD, including intermittent claudication, jeopardize quality of life and independence for many patients. PAD is commonly underdiagnosed and undertreated; thus, practitioners of cardiology have increasing interest in its diagnosis and management. This chapter provides a framework for the diagnosis and management of the patient with PAD.

Epidemiology

The prevalence of PAD varies according to the population studied, the diagnostic method used, and whether symptoms are included to derive estimates. Most epidemiologic studies have used a noninvasive measurement, the ankle-brachial index (ABI), to diagnose PAD. The ABI is the ratio of the ankle to brachial systolic blood pressure (described in greater detail later). The prevalence of PAD based on abnormal ABI ranges from approximately 4% among persons 40 years of age and older to 15% to 20% among those 65 years of age and older.[3-6] PAD prevalence is greater in men than in women in some studies, and greater in blacks than in non-Hispanic whites.[7] In the Multi-Ethnic Study of Atherosclerosis (MESA), the odds for development of PAD were 1.47 times higher in blacks than in non-Hispanic whites, whereas it was less than 0.5 times higher in Hispanics and Chinese.[8] These aggregate data indicate that some 8 to 10 million individuals in the United States have PAD.

Questionnaires specifically designed to elicit symptoms of intermittent claudication can assess the prevalence of symptomatic disease in these populations. Estimates vary by age and sex but generally indicate that only 10% to 30% of patients with PAD have claudication. Overall, the estimated prevalence of claudication ranges from 1.0% to 4.5% of a population older than 40 years.[6,9] The prevalence and incidence of claudication increase with age and are greater in men than in women in most studies (**Fig. 61-1**).[3,6,9,10] Less information exists about the incidence of critical limb ischemia, but it is estimated at 400 to 450 per million population per year.[6] The incidence of amputation ranges from 112 to 250 per million population per year.

Risk Factors for Peripheral Artery Disease

(see Chap. 44)

The well-known modifiable risk factors associated with coronary atherosclerosis also contribute to atherosclerosis of the peripheral circulation. Cigarette smoking, diabetes mellitus, dyslipidemia, and hypertension increase the risk of PAD[11] (**Table 61-1**). Data from observational studies indicate a twofold to threefold increase in the risk for development of PAD in smokers.[6] Approximately 84% to 90% of patients with claudication are current or former smokers.[12] Progression of disease to critical limb ischemia and limb loss is more likely to occur in patients who continue to smoke than in those who stop. Smoking can even increase the risk for development of PAD more than it does coronary artery disease (CAD). Current smoking dose-dependently correlates with the presence of PAD in both men and women, and smoking cessation lowers PAD risk.[13] Patients with diabetes mellitus often have extensive and severe PAD and a greater propensity for arterial calcification.[14,15] Involvement of the femoral and popliteal arteries resembles that of nondiabetic persons, but distal disease affecting the tibial and peroneal arteries occurs more frequently. The risk for development of PAD increases twofold to fourfold in patients with diabetes mellitus.[6,16] Among patients with PAD, diabetic patients are more likely to have an amputation than are nondiabetic patients.

Abnormalities in lipid metabolism also associate with an increased prevalence of PAD. Elevations in total or low-density lipoprotein (LDL) cholesterol increase the risk for development of PAD and claudication in most studies. Hypertriglyceridemia independently predicts risk for

PAD.[16] Some epidemiologic studies have found a link between hypertension and PAD.[17] Insulin resistance is associated with a greater prevalence of PAD.[18] Chronic kidney disease also increases the risk for development of PAD.[19] The risk for development of PAD and intermittent claudication increases progressively with the burden of contributing factors. Contemporary views of atherogenesis emphasize inflammation as a link between risk factors and the formation and complication of lesions. Strong evidence supports the concept that the pathobiology of PAD also involves inflammation. Classic studies associated high levels of fibrinogen with risk not only for coronary events but also for the development of PAD. Current analyses suggest that adjustment for the trigger of the acute-phase response, interleukin-6, or for inflammatory markers, such as C-reactive protein, eliminates the risk for PAD associated with fibrinogen.[20] Thus, the elevated fibrinogen levels in PAD may reflect inflammation as much as or more than a procoagulant effect. Considerable evidence links leukocytes, the crucial cellular mediators of the inflammatory response, with the development of PAD. Levels of the soluble forms of leukocyte adhesion molecules correlate with the development and extent of PAD and with the risk of complications.[21-25] Levels of C-reactive protein and of monocytes in peripheral blood independently associate with PAD, consistent with a role for innate immunity and chronic inflammation in its pathogenesis.[23,26] Conversely, serum bilirubin, an endogenous antioxidant with anti-inflammatory properties, associates with reduced PAD prevalence.[27] Inflammation provides the mechanistic link between many of the common risk factors for atherosclerosis and the pathophysiologic processes in the arterial wall that lead to PAD. Ongoing studies will determine whether biomarkers of inflammation add to traditional risk factors in gauging susceptibility to PAD.

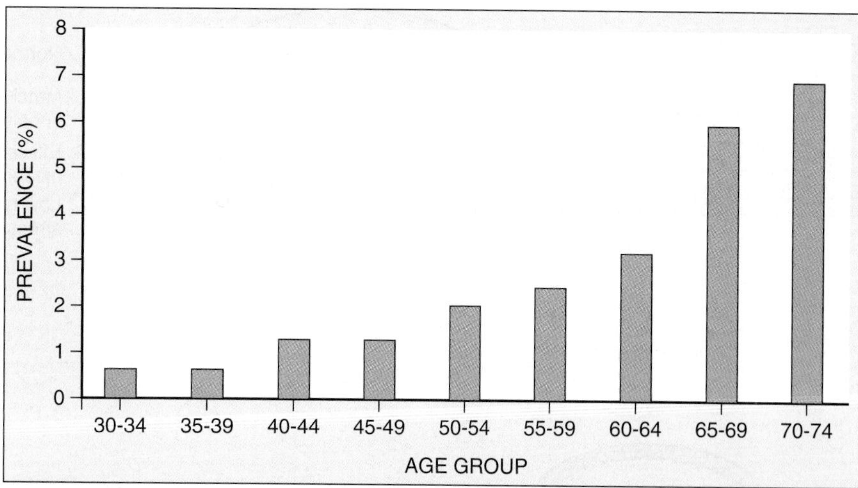

FIGURE 61-1 Age-related prevalence of intermittent claudication, derived from large population-based studies. *(From Norgren L, Hiatt WR, Dormandy JA, et al: Inter-Society Consensus for the Management of Peripheral Arterial Disease [TASC II]. Eur J Vasc Endovasc Surg 33:S1, 2007.)*

TABLE 61-1 Odds Ratio of Peripheral Artery Disease in Persons with Risk Factors

RISK FACTOR	ODDS RATIO (95% CONFIDENCE INTERVAL)
Cigarette smoking	4.46 (2.25-8.84)
Diabetes mellitus	2.71 (1.03-7.12)
Hypertension	1.75 (0.97-3.13)
Hypercholesterolemia	1.68 (1.09-2.57)
Hyperhomocysteinemia	1.92 (0.95-3.88)
Chronic kidney disease	2.00 (1.08-3.70)
Insulin resistance	2.06 (1.10-4.00)
C-reactive protein	2.20 (1.30-3.60)

Data derived from reports of the National Health and Nutrition Examination (Selvin E, Erlinger TP: Prevalence of and risk factors for peripheral arterial disease in the United States: Results from the National Health and Nutrition Examination Survey, 1999-2000. Circulation 110:738, 2004; Pande RL, Perlstein TS, Beckman JA, Creager MA: Association of insulin resistance and inflammation with peripheral arterial disease: The National Health and Nutrition Examination Survey, 1999 to 2004. Circulation 118:33, 2008; O'Hare AM, Glidden DV, Fox CS, Hsu CY: High prevalence of peripheral arterial disease in persons with renal insufficiency: Results from the National Health and Nutrition Examination Survey 1999-2000. Circulation 109:320, 2004; Guallar E, Silbergeld EK, Navas-Acien A, et al: Confounding of the relation between homocysteine and peripheral arterial disease by lead, cadmium, and renal function. Am J Epidemiol 163:700, 2006.)

Pathophysiology of Peripheral Artery Disease

Pathophysiologic considerations in patients with PAD must take into account the balance of circulatory supply of nutrients to the skeletal muscle and the oxygen and nutrient demand of the skeletal muscle (**Table 61-2**). Intermittent claudication occurs when skeletal muscle oxygen demand during effort exceeds blood oxygen supply and results from activation of local sensory receptors by accumulation of lactate or other metabolites. Patients with intermittent claudication may have single or multiple occlusive lesions in the arteries supplying the limb. Blood flow and leg oxygen consumption are normal at rest, but the obstructive lesions limit blood flow and oxygen delivery so that the metabolic needs of the exercising muscle during exercise outstrip the available supply of oxygen and nutrients. Patients with critical limb ischemia typically have multiple occlusive lesions that often affect proximal and distal limb arteries. As a result, even the resting blood supply diminishes and cannot meet the nutritional needs of the limb.

Factors Regulating Blood Supply (see Chap. 52)

The primary determinant of inadequate blood supply to an extremity is a flow-limiting lesion of a conduit artery (**Fig. 61-2**). Flow through an artery is directly proportional to perfusion pressure and inversely proportional to vascular resistance. If atherosclerosis causes a stenosis, flow through the artery is reduced, as described in Poiseuille's equation:

$$Q = \frac{\Delta P \pi r^4}{8 \eta l}$$

where ΔP is the pressure gradient across the stenosis, r is the radius of the residual lumen, η is blood viscosity, and l is the length of the vessel affected by the stenosis. As the severity of a stenotic lesion increases, flow becomes progressively reduced. The pressure gradient across the stenosis increases in a nonlinear manner, emphasizing the importance of a stenosis at high blood flow rates. Usually, a blood pressure gradient

TABLE 61-2 Pathophysiologic Considerations in Peripheral Artery Disease

Factors Regulating Blood Supply to Limb
- Flow-limiting lesion (stenosis severity, inadequate collateral vessels)
- Impaired vasodilation (decreased nitric oxide and reduced responsiveness to vasodilators)
- Accentuated vasoconstriction (thromboxane, serotonin, angiotensin II, endothelin, norepinephrine)
- Abnormal rheology (reduced red blood cell deformability, increased leukocyte adhesivity, platelet aggregation, microthrombosis, increased fibrinogen)

Altered Skeletal Muscle Structure and Function
- Axonal denervation of skeletal muscle
- Loss of type II, glycolytic fast-twitch fibers
- Impaired mitochondrial enzymatic activity

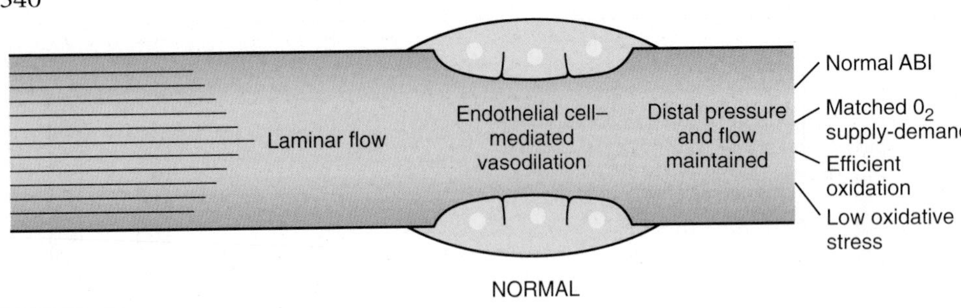

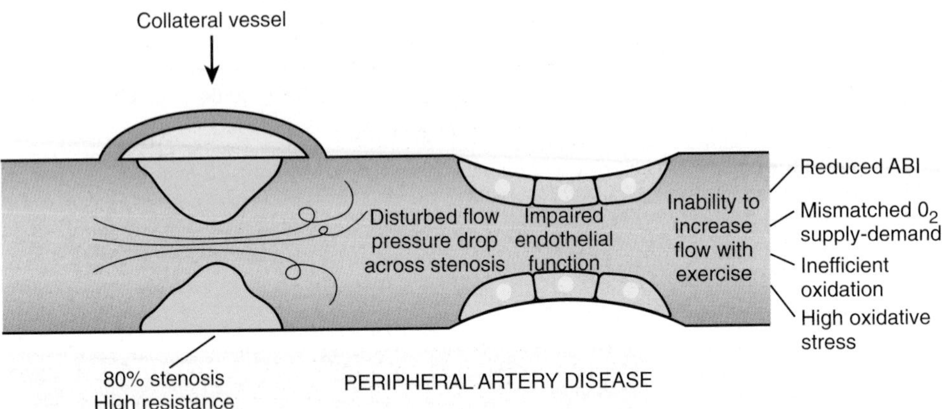

FIGURE 61-2 Pathophysiology of intermittent claudication. In healthy arteries **(top)**, flow is laminar and endothelial function is normal; therefore, blood flow and oxygen delivery match muscle metabolic demand at rest and during exercise. Muscle metabolism is efficient, resulting in low oxidative stress. In contrast, in peripheral artery disease **(bottom)**, the arterial stenosis results in disturbed flow, and the loss of kinetic energy results in a pressure drop across the stenosis. Collateral vessels have high resistance and only partially compensate for the arterial stenosis. In addition, endothelial function is impaired, resulting in further loss of vascular function. These changes limit the blood flow response to exercise, resulting in a mismatch of oxygen delivery to muscle metabolic demand. Changes in skeletal muscle metabolism further compromise the efficient generation of high-energy phosphates. Oxidant stress, the result of inefficient oxidation, further impairs endothelial function and muscle metabolism. *(From Hiatt WR, Brass EP: Pathophysiology of intermittent claudication.* In *Creager MA, Dzau VJ, Loscalzo J [eds]: Vascular Medicine. A Companion to Braunwald's Heart Disease. Philadelphia, Elsevier, 2006.)*

exists at rest if the stenosis reduces the lumen diameter by more than 50% because as distorted flow develops, kinetic energy is lost. A stenosis that does not cause a pressure gradient at rest may cause one during exercise, when blood flow increases from higher cardiac output and vascular resistance decreases. Thus, as flow through a stenosis increases, distal perfusion pressure drops. As the metabolic demand of exercising muscle outstrips its blood supply, local metabolites (including adenosine, nitric oxide, potassium, and hydrogen ion) accumulate, and peripheral resistance vessels dilate. Perfusion pressure then drops further because the stenosis limits flow. In addition, intramuscular pressure rises during exercise and may exceed the arterial pressure distal to an occlusion, causing blood flow to cease. Flow through collateral blood vessels can usually meet the resting metabolic needs of the skeletal muscle tissue at rest but does not suffice during exercise.

Functional abnormalities in vasomotor reactivity also may interfere with blood flow. Vasodilator capability of both conduit and resistance vessels is reduced in patients with peripheral atherosclerosis. Normally, arteries dilate in response to pharmacologic and biochemical stimuli, such as acetylcholine, serotonin, thrombin, and bradykinin, as well as to shear stress induced by increases in blood flow. This vasodilator response results from the release of biologically active substances from the endothelium, particularly nitric oxide (see Chap. 48). The vascular relaxation of a conduit vessel that occurs after a flow stimulus, such as that induced by exercise, may facilitate the delivery of blood to exercising muscles in healthy persons. Endothelium-dependent vasodilation subsequent to flow or pharmacologic stimuli is impaired in the atherosclerotic femoral arteries and calf resistance vessels of patients with PAD. This failure of vasodilation might prevent an increase in nutritive blood supply to exercising muscle because endothelium-derived nitric oxide can contribute to hyperemic blood volume after an ischemic stimulus. It is not known whether vasodilator function with respect to prostacyclin, adenosine, or ion channels is abnormal in atherosclerotic peripheral arteries. Endogenous vasoconstrictor substances, such as prostanoids and other lipid mediators, thrombin, serotonin, angiotensin II, endothelin, and norepinephrine, may interfere with vasodilation.

Abnormalities in the microcirculation contribute to the pathophysiology of critical limb ischemia. Patients with severe limb ischemia have a reduced number of perfused skin capillaries. Other potential causes of decreased capillary perfusion in this condition include reduced red blood cell deformability, increased leukocyte adhesivity, platelet aggregates, fibrinogen, microvascular thrombosis, excessive vasoconstriction, and interstitial edema. Intravascular pressure may also decrease because of precapillary arteriolar dilation due to locally released vasoactive metabolites.[28]

Skeletal Muscle Structure and Metabolic Function

Electrophysiologic and histopathologic examination has found evidence of partial axonal denervation of the skeletal muscle in legs affected by PAD. There is preservation of type I, oxidative slow-twitch fibers but a loss of type II, or glycolytic, fast-twitch fibers in the skeletal muscle of patients with PAD.[10] The loss of type II fibers correlates with decreased muscle strength and reduced exercise capacity. In skeletal muscle distal to PAD, there is a shift to anaerobic metabolism earlier during exercise, and it persists longer after cessation of exercise. Patients with claudication have increased lactate release and accumulation of acylcarnitines during exercise and slowed oxygen desaturation kinetics, indicative of ineffective oxidative metabolism.[29,30] Moreover, mitochondrial respiratory activity and phosphocreatine and adenosine triphosphate recovery time are delayed in the calf muscles of PAD patients, as assessed after submaximal exercise by ^{31}P magnetic resonance spectroscopy.[31]

Clinical Presentation

Symptoms

The cardinal symptoms of PAD include intermittent claudication and rest pain. The term *claudication* is derived from the Latin word *claudicare*, "to limp." Intermittent claudication refers to a pain, ache, sense of fatigue, or other discomfort that occurs in the affected muscle group with exercise, particularly walking, and resolves with rest. The location of the symptom often relates to the site of the most proximal stenosis. Buttock, hip, or thigh claudication typically occurs in patients with obstruction of the aorta and iliac arteries. Calf claudication characterizes femoral or popliteal artery stenoses. The gastrocnemius muscle consumes more oxygen during walking than other muscle groups in the leg and hence causes the most frequent symptom reported by patients. Ankle or foot claudication occurs in patients with tibial and peroneal artery disease. Similarly, stenoses of the subclavian, axillary, or brachial arteries may cause shoulder, biceps, or forearm claudication, respectively. Symptoms should resolve several minutes after cessation of effort. Calf and thigh pain that occurs at rest, such as nocturnal cramps, should not be confused with claudication and is not a symptom of PAD. The history obtained from persons reporting claudication should note the walking distance, speed, and incline that precipitate claudication. This baseline assessment evaluates disability and provides an initial qualitative measure with which to determine stability, improvement, or deterioration during subsequent encounters with the patient. Symptoms other than claudication can limit functional capacity.[32] Patients with PAD walk more slowly and have less walking endurance than patients who do not have PAD.[33]

Several questionnaires have been developed to assess the presence and severity of claudication. The Rose Questionnaire was developed initially to diagnose both angina and intermittent claudication in epidemiologic surveys. It questions whether the patient develops pain in either calf with walking and whether the pain occurs at rest, while walking at an ordinary or hurried pace, or on walking uphill. There have been several modifications to this questionnaire, including the Edinburgh Claudication Questionnaire and the San Diego Claudication Questionnaire,[34] both of which are more sensitive and specific than a physician's diagnosis of intermittent claudication based on walking distance, walking speed, and nature of symptoms. Another validated instrument, the Walking Impairment Questionnaire, asks a series of questions and develops a point score based on walking distance, walking speed, and nature of symptoms.[35]

Symptoms resembling limb claudication occasionally result from nonatherosclerotic causes of arterial occlusive disease (**Table 61-3**). These other causes include arterial embolism; vasculitides such as thromboangiitis obliterans, Takayasu arteritis, and giant cell arteritis; aortic coarctation; fibromuscular dysplasia; irradiation; endofibrosis of the external iliac artery; and extravascular compression due to arterial entrapment or adventitial cyst (see Chap. 89). Several nonvascular causes of exertional leg pain should be considered in patients who present with symptoms suggestive of intermittent claudication (see Table 61-3). Lumbosacral radiculopathy resulting from degenerative joint disease, spinal stenosis, and herniated discs can cause pain in the buttock, hip, thigh, calf, or foot with walking, often after very short distances, or even with standing. This symptom has been called neurogenic pseudoclaudication. Lumbosacral spine disease and PAD both preferentially affect the elderly and hence may coexist in the same individual. Arthritis of the hips and knees also provokes leg pain with walking. Typically, the pain localizes to the affected joint and can be elicited on physical examination through palpation and range-of-motion maneuvers. Exertional compartment syndrome is most often seen in athletes with large calf muscles; increased tissue pressure during exercise limits microvascular flow and results in calf pain or tightness. Symptoms improve after cessation of exercise. Rarely, skeletal muscle disorders such as myositis can cause exertional leg pain. Muscle tenderness, an abnormal neuromuscular examination finding, elevated skeletal muscle enzyme levels, and a normal pulse examination finding should distinguish myositis from PAD. McArdle syndrome, in which there is a deficiency of skeletal muscle phosphorylase, can cause symptoms mimicking the claudication of PAD. Patients with chronic venous insufficiency sometimes report leg discomfort with exertion, which is designated venous claudication. Venous hypertension during exercise increases arterial resistance in the affected limb and limits blood flow. In the case of venous insufficiency, elevated extravascular pressure caused by interstitial edema further diminishes capillary perfusion. A physical examination demonstrating peripheral edema, venous stasis pigmentation, and occasionally venous varicosities will identify this unusual cause of exertional leg pain.

Symptoms may occur at rest in patients with critical limb ischemia. Typically, patients complain of pain or paresthesias in the foot or toes of the affected extremity. This discomfort worsens on leg elevation and improves with leg dependency, as might be anticipated by the effect of gravity on perfusion pressure. The pain can be particularly severe at sites of skin fissuring, ulceration, or necrosis. Often the skin is very sensitive, and even the weight of bedclothes or sheets elicits pain. Patients may sit on the edge of the bed and dangle their legs to alleviate the discomfort. Patients with ischemic or diabetic neuropathy can experience little or no pain despite the presence of severe ischemia.

Critical limb and digital ischemia can result from arterial occlusions other than those caused by atherosclerosis. These include conditions such as thromboangiitis obliterans, vasculitides such as systemic lupus erythematosus or scleroderma, vasospasm, atheromatous embolism, and acute arterial occlusion caused by thrombosis or embolism (see later). Acute gouty arthritis, trauma, and sensory neuropathy such as that caused by diabetes mellitus, lumbosacral radiculopathies, and complex regional pain syndrome (previously known as reflex sympathetic dystrophy) can cause foot pain. Leg ulcers also occur in patients with venous insufficiency and sensory neuropathy, particularly that related to diabetes. These ulcers are easily distinguished from those caused by arterial disease. The ulcer of venous insufficiency usually localizes near the medial malleolus and has an irregular border and a pink base with granulation tissue. Ulcers due to venous disease produce milder pain than those caused by arterial disease. Neurotrophic ulcers occur where there is pressure or trauma, usually on the sole of the foot. These ulcers are deep, frequently infected, and usually not painful because of the loss of sensation (**Fig. 61-3**).

TABLE 61-3 Differential Diagnosis of Exertional Leg Pain

Vascular Causes
Atherosclerosis
Thrombosis
Embolism
Vasculitis
Thromboangiitis obliterans
Takayasu arteritis
Giant cell arteritis
Aortic coarctation
Fibromuscular dysplasia
Irradiation
Endofibrosis of the external iliac artery
Extravascular compression
Arterial entrapment (e.g., popliteal artery entrapment, thoracic outlet syndrome)
Adventitial cysts
Nonvascular Causes
Lumbosacral radiculopathy
Degenerative arthritis
Spinal stenosis
Herniated disc
Arthritis
Hips, knees
Venous insufficiency
Myositis
McArdle syndrome

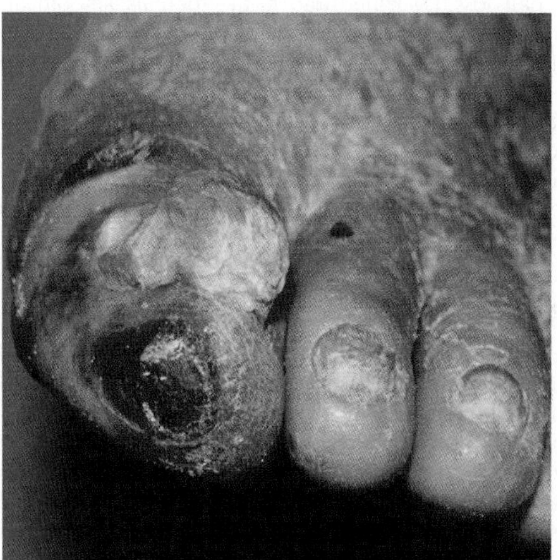

FIGURE 61-3 A typical arterial ulcer. It is a discrete, circumscribed, necrotic ulcer, located on the great toe.

TABLE 61-4 Fontaine Classification of Peripheral Artery Disease

STAGE	SYMPTOMS
I	Asymptomatic
II	Intermittent claudication
IIa	Pain free, claudication walking >200 m
IIb	Pain free, claudication walking <200 m
III	Rest and nocturnal pain
IV	Necrosis, gangrene

TABLE 61-5 Clinical Categories of Chronic Limb Ischemia

GRADE	CATEGORY	CLINICAL DESCRIPTION
	0	Asymptomatic, not hemodynamically correct
I	1	Mild claudication
	2	Moderate claudication
	3	Severe claudication
II	4	Ischemic rest pain
	5	Minor tissue loss: nonhealing ulcer, focal gangrene with diffuse pedal ulcer
III	6	Major tissue loss extending above transmetatarsal level, functional foot no longer salvageable

Modified from Rutherford RB, Baker JD, Ernst C, et al: Recommended standards for reports dealing with lower extremity ischemia: Revised version. J Vasc Surg 26:517, 1997.

Physical Findings

The complete cardiovascular examination includes palpation of pulses and auscultation of accessible arteries for bruits (see also Fig. 12-4). Pulse abnormalities and bruits increase the likelihood of PAD.[36] Readily palpable pulses in healthy individuals include the brachial, radial, and ulnar arteries of the upper extremities and the femoral, popliteal, dorsalis pedis, and posterior tibial arteries of the lower extremities. The aorta also can be palpated in thin people. A decreased or absent pulse provides insight into the location of arterial stenoses. For example, a normal right femoral pulse but absent left femoral pulse suggests the presence of left iliofemoral arterial stenosis. A normal femoral artery pulse but absent popliteal artery pulse would indicate a stenosis in the superficial femoral artery or proximal popliteal artery. Similarly, disease of the anterior and posterior tibial arteries can be inferred when the popliteal artery pulse is present but the dorsalis pedis and posterior tibial pulses, respectively, are not palpable. Bruits often indicate accelerated blood flow velocity and flow disturbance at sites of stenosis. A stethoscope should be used to auscultate the supraclavicular and infraclavicular fossae for evidence of subclavian artery stenosis; the abdomen, flank, and pelvis for evidence of stenoses in the aorta and its branch vessels; and each groin for evidence of femoral artery stenoses. Pallor can be elicited on the soles of the feet of some patients with PAD by performing a maneuver in which the feet are elevated above the level of the heart and the calf muscles are exercised by repeated dorsiflexion and plantar flexion of the ankle. The legs are then placed in the dependent position, and the time to the onset of hyperemia and venous distention is measured. Each of these variables depends on the rate of blood flow, which in turn reflects the severity of stenosis and adequacy of collateral vessels.

The legs of patients with chronic aortoiliac disease may show muscle atrophy. Additional signs of chronic low-grade ischemia include hair loss, thickened and brittle toenails, smooth and shiny skin, and subcutaneous fat atrophy of the digital pads. Patients with severe limb ischemia have cool skin and may also have petechiae, persistent cyanosis or pallor, dependent rubor, pedal edema resulting from prolonged dependency, skin fissures, ulceration, or gangrene. Ulcers due to PAD typically have a pale base with irregular borders and usually involve the tips of the toes or the heel of the foot or develop at sites of pressure (Fig. 61-3). These ulcers vary in size and may be as small as 3 to 5 mm.

Categorization

Classification of patients with PAD depends on the severity of the symptoms and abnormalities detected on physical examination. Categorization of the clinical manifestations of PAD improves communication among professionals caring for these patients and provides a structure for defining guidelines for therapeutic interventions. Fontaine described one widely used scheme that classified patients in one of four stages progressing from asymptomatic to critical limb ischemia (**Table 61-4**). Several professional vascular societies have adopted a contemporary, more descriptive classification that includes asymptomatic patients, three grades of claudication, and three grades of critical limb ischemia ranging from rest pain alone to minor and major tissue loss (**Table 61-5**).[37]

Testing in Peripheral Artery Disease

Segmental Pressure Measurement

The measurement of systolic blood pressure along selected segments of each extremity furnishes one of the simplest and most useful noninvasive tests to evaluate the presence and severity of stenoses in the peripheral arteries. In the lower extremities, pneumatic cuffs are placed on the upper and lower portions of the thigh, on the calf, above the ankle, and often over the metatarsal area of the foot. Likewise, for the upper extremities, pneumatic cuffs are placed on the upper arm over the biceps, on the forearm below the elbow, and at the wrist. Systolic blood pressure at each respective limb segment is measured by first inflating the pneumatic cuff to suprasystolic pressure, then determining the pressure at which blood flow occurs during cuff deflation. The onset of flow is assessed by placing a Doppler ultrasound flow probe over an artery distal to the cuff. In the lower extremities, it is most convenient to place the Doppler probe on the foot over the posterior tibial artery, as it courses inferior and posterior to the medial malleolus, or over the dorsalis pedis artery on the dorsum of the metatarsal arch. In the upper extremities, the Doppler probe can be placed over the brachial artery in the antecubital fossa or over the radial and ulnar arteries at the wrist.

Left ventricular contraction imparts kinetic energy to blood, which is maintained throughout the large and medium-sized vessels. Systolic blood pressure may be higher in the more distal vessels than in the aorta and proximal vessels because of amplification and reflection of blood pressure waves. A stenosis can cause loss of pressure energy, as a result of increased frictional forces and flow disturbance at the site of the stenosis. Approximately 90% of the cross-sectional area of the aorta must be narrowed before a pressure gradient develops. In smaller vessels, such as the iliac and femoral arteries, a 70% to 90% decrease in cross-sectional area will cause a resting pressure gradient sufficient to decrease systolic blood pressure distal to the stenosis. Taking into consideration the precision of this noninvasive method and the variability in blood pressure during even short periods, a blood pressure gradient in excess of 20 mm Hg between successive cuffs is generally used as evidence of arterial stenosis in the lower extremity, whereas a gradient of 10 mm Hg indicates a stenosis between sequential cuffs in the upper extremity. Systolic blood pressure in the toes and fingers approximates 60% of the systolic blood pressure at the ankle and wrist, respectively, as pressure diminishes further in the smaller distal vessels.

Figure 61-4 gives examples of leg segmental pressure measurements in a patient with bilateral calf claudication. In the right leg, there are pressure gradients between the upper and lower thigh and between the calf and ankle. These gradients indicate stenoses in the superficial femoral artery and in the tibioperoneal arteries. In the left leg, pressure gradients between the upper and lower thigh, between

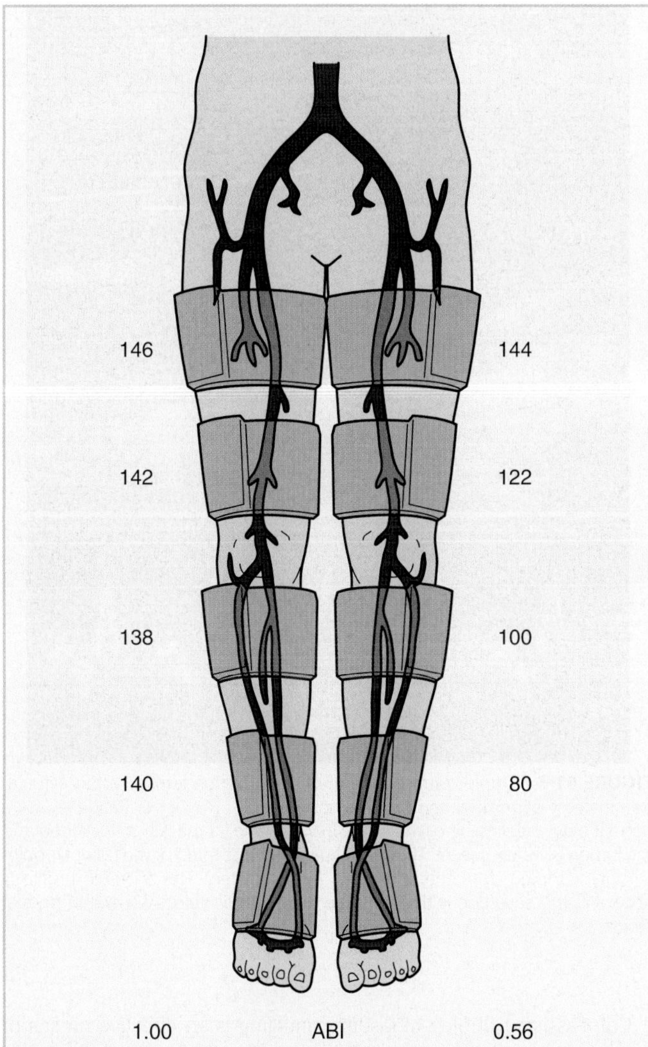

FIGURE 61-4 Segmental pressure measurements in a patient with left calf intermittent claudication. Pressure gradient is present between the left upper and lower thigh cuffs, lower thigh and calf cuffs, and calf and ankle cuffs, consistent with multisegmental disease affecting the femoral-popliteal and tibial arteries. The left ankle-brachial index is 0.56, which is abnormal. The segmental pressure measurements and ankle-brachial index in the right leg are normal.

the lower thigh and calf, and between the calf and ankle indicate stenoses in the superficial femoral and popliteal arteries and in the tibioperoneal arteries.

Ankle-Brachial Index

Determination of the ABI furnishes a simplified application of leg segmental blood pressure measurements readily used at the bedside (see Fig. 61-4 and Fig. 12-4). This index is the ratio of the systolic blood pressure measured at the ankle to the systolic blood pressure measured at the brachial artery. A pneumatic cuff placed around the ankle is inflated to suprasystolic pressure and subsequently deflated while the onset of flow is detected with a Doppler ultrasound probe placed over the dorsalis pedis and posterior tibial arteries, thus denoting ankle systolic blood pressure. Brachial artery systolic pressure can be assessed in a routine manner, with use of either a stethoscope to listen for the first Korotkoff sound or a Doppler probe to listen for the onset of flow during cuff deflation. The normal ABI should be 1.0 or greater; recognizing the variability intrinsic to sequential blood pressure measurements, however, an ABI of less than 0.90 is considered abnormal and is 90% to 95% sensitive and 98% to 100% specific for angiographically verified peripheral arterial stenosis.[6] The ABI is often used to gauge the severity of PAD. Patients with symptoms of leg claudication often have ABIs ranging from 0.5 to 0.8, and patients with critical limb ischemia usually have an ABI of less than 0.5. The ABI correlates inversely with walking distance and speed. Fewer than 40% of patients whose ABI is less than 0.40 can complete a 6-minute walk.[38] In patients with skin ulcerations, an ankle pressure of less than 55 mm Hg would predict poor ulcer healing. One limitation of leg blood pressure recordings is that they cannot be used reliably in patients with calcified vessels, as might occur in persons with diabetes mellitus or renal insufficiency. The calcified vessel cannot be compressed during inflation of the pneumatic cuff, and therefore the Doppler probe indicates continuous blood flow, even when the pressure exceeds 250 mm Hg.

Treadmill Exercise Testing

Treadmill exercise testing can evaluate the clinical significance of peripheral artery stenoses and provide objective evidence of the patient's walking capacity. The claudication onset time is defined as the time at which symptoms of claudication first develop, and the peak walking time is when the patient is no longer able to continue walking because of severe leg discomfort. This standardized and more objective measurement of walking capacity supplements the patient's history and provides a quantitative assessment of his or her disability, as well as a metric for monitoring therapeutic interventions.

Treadmill exercise protocols use a motorized treadmill that incorporates fixed or progressive speeds and angles of incline. A fixed workload test usually maintains a constant grade of 12% and speed of 1.5 to 2.0 miles per hour. A progressive, or graded, treadmill protocol typically maintains a constant speed of 2 miles per hour while the grade is gradually increased by 2% every 2 to 3 minutes. Reproducibility of repeated treadmill test results is reportedly better with progressive than with constant grade protocols.[39]

Treadmill testing can determine whether arterial stenoses contribute to the patient's symptoms of exertional leg pain. During exercise, blood flow through a stenosis increases as vascular resistance falls in the exercising muscle. According to Poiseuille's equation, described previously, the pressure gradient across the stenosis increases in direct proportion to flow. Thus, ankle and brachial systolic blood pressures are measured under resting conditions before treadmill exercise, within 1 minute after exercise, and repeatedly until baseline values are reestablished. Normally, the blood pressure increase that occurs during exercise should be the same in both the upper and lower extremities, maintaining a constant ABI of 1.0 or greater. In the presence of peripheral artery stenoses, the ABI decreases because the increase in blood pressure observed in the arm is not matched by a comparable increase in ankle blood pressure. A 25% or greater decrease in ABI after exercise in a patient whose walking capacity is limited by claudication is considered diagnostic, implicating PAD as a cause of the patient's symptoms.

Many patients with PAD also have coronary atherosclerosis. The addition of cardiac monitoring to the exercise protocol may provide adjunctive information about the presence of myocardial ischemia. A workload sufficient to increase myocardial oxygen demand and to provoke myocardial ischemia may not be achieved in patients whose exercise capacity is limited by claudication. Nonetheless, electrocardiographic changes, particularly during low levels of treadmill exercise, may provide evidence of severe CAD.

Pulse Volume Recording

The pulse volume recording graphically illustrates the volumetric change in a segment of the limb that occurs with each pulse. Plethysmographic instruments, typically using strain gauges or pneumatic cuffs, can transduce volumetric changes in the limb, which can be displayed on a graphic recorder. These transducers are strategically placed along the limb to record the pulse volume in its different segments, such as the thigh, calf, ankle, metatarsal region, and toes or the upper arm, forearm, and fingers. The normal pulse volume contour depends on both local arterial pressure and vascular wall distensibility and resembles a blood pressure waveform. It consists of a sharp systolic upstroke rising rapidly to a peak, a dicrotic notch, and a concave downslope that drops off gradually toward the baseline. The contour of the pulse wave changes distal to a stenosis, with loss of the dicrotic notch, a slower rate of rise, a more rounded peak, and a slower descent. The amplitude becomes lower with increasing severity of disease, and the pulse wave may not be recordable at all in the critically ischemic limb. Segmental analysis of the pulse wave may indicate the location of an arterial stenosis, which is likely to be sited in the artery between a normal and an abnormal pulse volume recording. The pulse volume wave also provides information about the integrity of blood flow when blood pressure measurements cannot be accurately obtained because of noncompressible vessels.

Doppler Ultrasonography

Continuous-wave and pulsed-wave Doppler systems transmit and receive high-frequency ultrasound signals. The Doppler frequency shift caused by moving red blood cells varies directly with the velocity of blood flow. Typically, the perceived frequency shift is between 1 and 20 kHz and is within the audible range of the human ear. Therefore, placement of a Doppler probe along an artery enables the examiner to hear whether blood flow is present and the vessel is patent. Processing and graphic recording of the Doppler signal permit a more detailed analysis of the frequency components.

Doppler instruments can be used without or with gray-scale imaging to evaluate an artery for the presence of stenoses. The Doppler probe is positioned at approximately a 60-degree angle over the common femoral, superficial femoral, popliteal, dorsalis pedis, and posterior tibial arteries. The normal Doppler waveform has three components: a rapid forward flow component during systole, a transient flow reversal during early diastole, and a slow anterograde component during late diastole. The Doppler waveform becomes altered if the probe is placed distal to an arterial stenosis and is characterized by deceleration of systolic flow, loss of the early diastolic reversal, and diminished peak frequencies. Arteries in a limb with critical ischemia may not show any Doppler frequency shift. As with pulse volume recordings, a change from a normal to an abnormal Doppler waveform as the artery is interrogated more distally provides inferential evidence of the location of a stenosis.

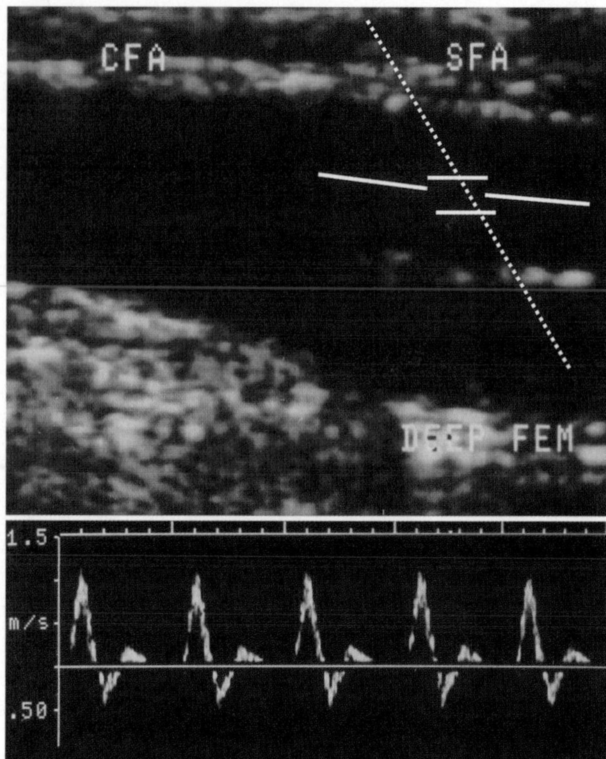

FIGURE 61-5 Duplex ultrasonogram of the common femoral artery bifurcation into the superficial and deep femoral arteries. The upper image shows a normal gray-scale image of the artery in which the intima is not thickened and the lumen is widely patent. The lower image is a recording of the pulse Doppler velocity sampled from the superficial femoral artery. The triphasic profile is apparent, the envelope is thin, and the peak systolic velocity is within normal limits.

Duplex Ultrasound Imaging

Duplex ultrasound imaging provides a direct, noninvasive means of assessing both the anatomic characteristics of peripheral arteries and the functional significance of arterial stenoses. The methodology incorporates gray-scale B-mode ultrasound imaging, pulsed Doppler velocity measurements, and color coding of the Doppler-shift information (**Fig. 61-5**). Real-time ultrasonography scanners emit and receive high-frequency sound waves, typically ranging from 2 to 10 MHz, to construct an image. The acoustic properties of the vascular wall differ from those of the surrounding tissue, enabling them to be imaged easily. Atherosclerotic plaque may be present and visible on gray-scale images. Pulsed-wave Doppler systems emit ultrasound beams at precise times and can therefore sample the reflected ultrasound waves at specific depths, enabling the examiner to determine the blood cell velocity within the lumen of the artery. Positioning the pulsed Doppler beam at a known angle, the examiner can calculate blood flow velocity according to the equation

$$Df = 2VF\cos\theta/C$$

where Df is the frequency shift, V is the velocity, F is the frequency of the transmitted sound, θ is the angle between the transmitted sound and the velocity vector, and C is the velocity of sound and tissue. For optimal measurements, the angle of the pulsed Doppler beam should be less than 60 degrees. With color Doppler, the frequency shift information within the entire field sampled by the ultrasound beam can be superimposed on the gray-scale image. This approach provides a composite real-time display of flow velocity within the vessel.

Color-assisted duplex ultrasound imaging is an effective means of localizing peripheral arterial stenoses (**Fig. 61-6**). Normal arteries have laminar flow, with the highest velocity at the center of the artery. The corresponding color image is usually homogeneous, with relatively constant hue and intensity. In the presence of an arterial stenosis, blood flow velocity increases through the narrowed lumen. As the velocity increases, there is progressive desaturation of the color display, and flow disturbance distal to the stenosis causes changes in hue and color. Pulsed Doppler velocity measurements can be made along the length of the artery and particularly at areas of flow abnormalities suggested by the color images. A twofold or greater increase in peak systolic velocity at the site of an atherosclerotic plaque indicates a 50% or greater stenosis (see Fig. 61-6). A threefold increase in velocity suggests 75% or greater stenosis. An occluded artery generates no Doppler signal. With contrast angiography as a reference standard, duplex ultrasound imaging for identification of sites of arterial stenoses has approximately 89% to 99% specificity and 80% to 98% sensitivity.[40]

Magnetic Resonance Angiography

Magnetic resonance angiography (MRA) can visualize noninvasively the aorta and the peripheral arteries (see Chaps. 18 and 60). The resolution of the vascular anatomy with gadolinium-enhanced MRA approaches that of conventional contrast digital subtraction angiography (**Fig. 61-7**). Comparative studies have reported excellent interobserver agreement, sensitivity of 93% to 100%, and specificity of 96% to 100% for the aorta, iliac, femoropopliteal, and tibioperoneal arteries.[40-42] MRA currently has greatest utility for the evaluation of symptomatic patients to assist decision making before endovascular and surgical intervention or in patients at risk for renal, allergic, or other complications during conventional angiography.

Computed Tomographic Angiography

Computed tomographic angiography (CTA) uses intravenous administration of radiocontrast material to opacify and visualize the aorta and peripheral arteries (see Chap. 19). New computed tomography scanners use multidetector technology to acquire cross-sectional images. This advance permits imaging of peripheral arteries with excellent spatial resolution during a relatively short time, with a reduced amount of radiocontrast material (**Fig. 61-8**).[43] Images can be displayed in three dimensions and rotated to optimize visualization of arterial stenoses. Compared with conventional contrast angiography, the sensitivity and specificity for stenoses greater than 50% or occlusion reported for CTA using multiple detector technology are 95% (95% CI, 92% to 97%) and 96% (95% CI, 93% to 97%), respectively.[44] CTA offers an advantage over MRA in that it can be used in patients with stents, metal clips, and pacemakers, although it has the disadvantage of requiring radiocontrast and ionizing radiation.

Contrast Angiography

Conventional angiography, using a radioiodinated or other contrast agent, can aid in the evaluation of the arterial anatomy before a revascularization procedure. It still has occasional utility when the diagnosis is in doubt. Most contemporary angiography laboratories

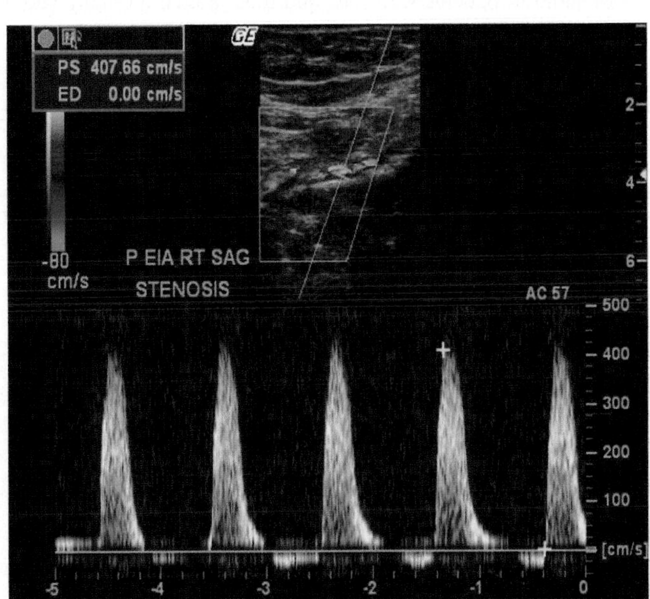

FIGURE 61-6 Duplex ultrasonogram of the external iliac artery. The **upper image** shows a color image of the artery in which there is heterogeneity and desaturation of color, indicative of high-velocity flow through a stenosis. The **lower image** is a recording of the pulse Doppler velocity sampled from the right external iliac artery. The peak velocity of 350 cm/sec is elevated. These features are consistent with a significant stenosis.

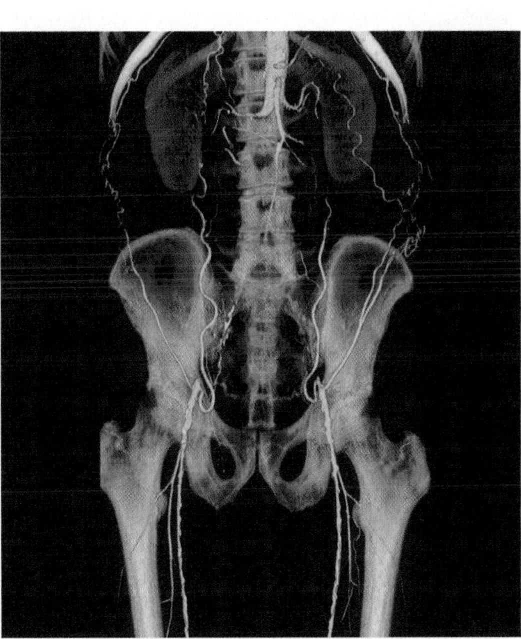

FIGURE 61-8 Computed tomographic angiogram of a patient with complete occlusion of the aorta and both iliac arteries. There is reconstitution of the common femoral arteries. *(Courtesy of the 3D and Image Processing Center of Brigham and Women's Hospital, Boston, Mass.)*

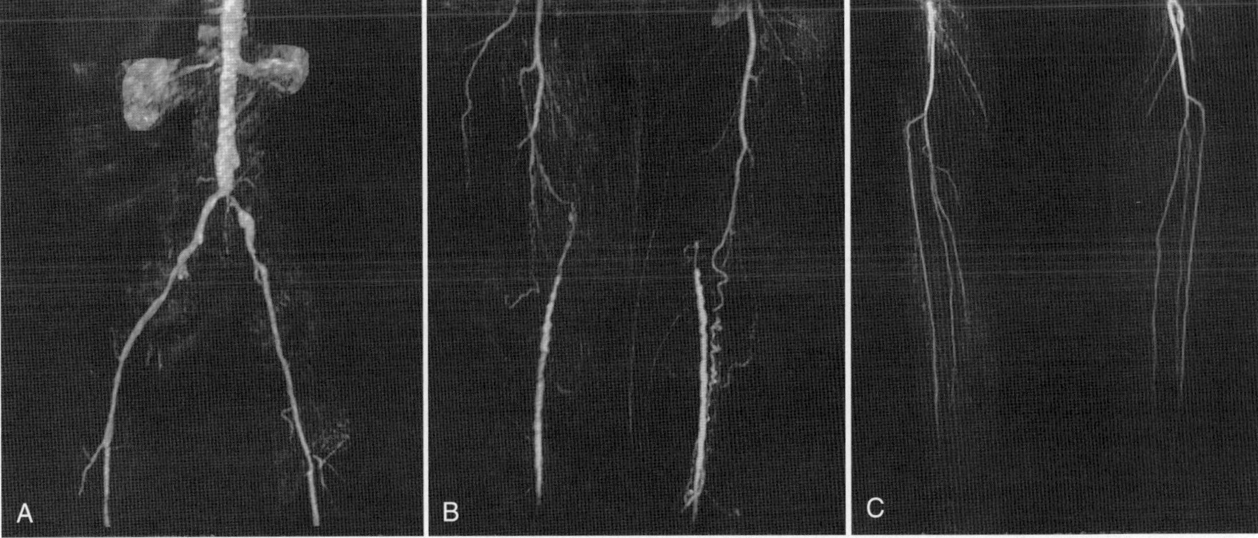

FIGURE 61-7 Gadolinium-enhanced two-dimensional magnetic resonance angiogram of the aorta and both legs, extending from the thighs to above the ankle. **A,** Aortoiliac atherosclerosis with stenosed left common iliac artery. **B,** Bilateral superficial femoral artery occlusion with reconstitution of the distal portion of the right and left superficial femoral arteries. **C,** The anterior tibial, posterior tibial, and peroneal arteries, which are patent in each leg.

use digital subtraction techniques after intra-arterial administration of contrast material to enhance resolution. Injection of the radiocontrast material into the aorta permits visualization of the aorta and iliac arteries, and injection of contrast material into the iliofemoral segment of the involved leg permits optimal visualization of the femoral, popliteal, tibial, and peroneal arteries (**Fig. 61-9**). In patients with aortic occlusion, catheterization of the femoral arteries is not feasible. The aorta can be approached by brachial or axillary artery cannulation or, if necessary, directly by a translumbar approach.

Prognosis

Patients with PAD have an increased risk for adverse cardiovascular events, as well as the risk of limb loss and impaired quality of life.[2,9,11,33] Patients with PAD frequently have concomitant CAD and cerebrovascular disease.[6,9] The relative prevalence of each of these manifestations of atherosclerosis depends in part on the diagnostic criteria used to establish their diagnosis. Patients with abnormal ABIs are twofold to fourfold more likely than those with normal ABIs to have a history of myocardial infarction (MI), angina, congestive heart failure, or cerebrovascular ischemia.[6,9] Coronary calcium scores and carotid artery intima-media thickness are greater in patients with PAD than in those without PAD.[45] Angiographically significant CAD occurs in approximately 60% to 80% of patients with PAD,[9] and 15% to 25% of patients with PAD have significant carotid artery stenoses as detected by duplex ultrasonography. Two international registries have detected a high coprevalence of CAD and cerebrovascular disease in patients with PAD. In the Reduction of Atherothrombosis for Continued Health (REACH) registry, 62% of patients had either or both coronary and cerebrovascular disease.[46] Approximately 25% of the patients with PAD had a history of MI, 30% had angina, 16% had a prior stroke, and 15% had a prior transient ischemic attack. In the AGATHA (A Global Atherothrombosis Assessment) registry, approximately 50% of patients with PAD had established CAD, and 50% had prior stroke, transient ischemic attack, or carotid artery revascularization.[47] The specificity of an abnormal ABI to predict future cardiovascular events is approximately 90%.[48] The risk of death from cardiovascular causes increases 2.5- to 6-fold in patients with PAD, and their annual mortality rate is 4.3% to 4.9%.[6,9,49] The risk of death is greatest in those with the most severe PAD, and mortality correlates with decreasing ABI (**Fig. 61-10**).[50-52] Approximately 25% of patients with critical limb ischemia die within 1 year, and the 1-year mortality rate among patients who have undergone amputation for PAD may be as high as 45%.[6]

Approximately 25% of patients with claudication develop worsening symptoms. Moreover, mobility loss occurs more commonly in patients with PAD than in those without PAD, even among patients who do not

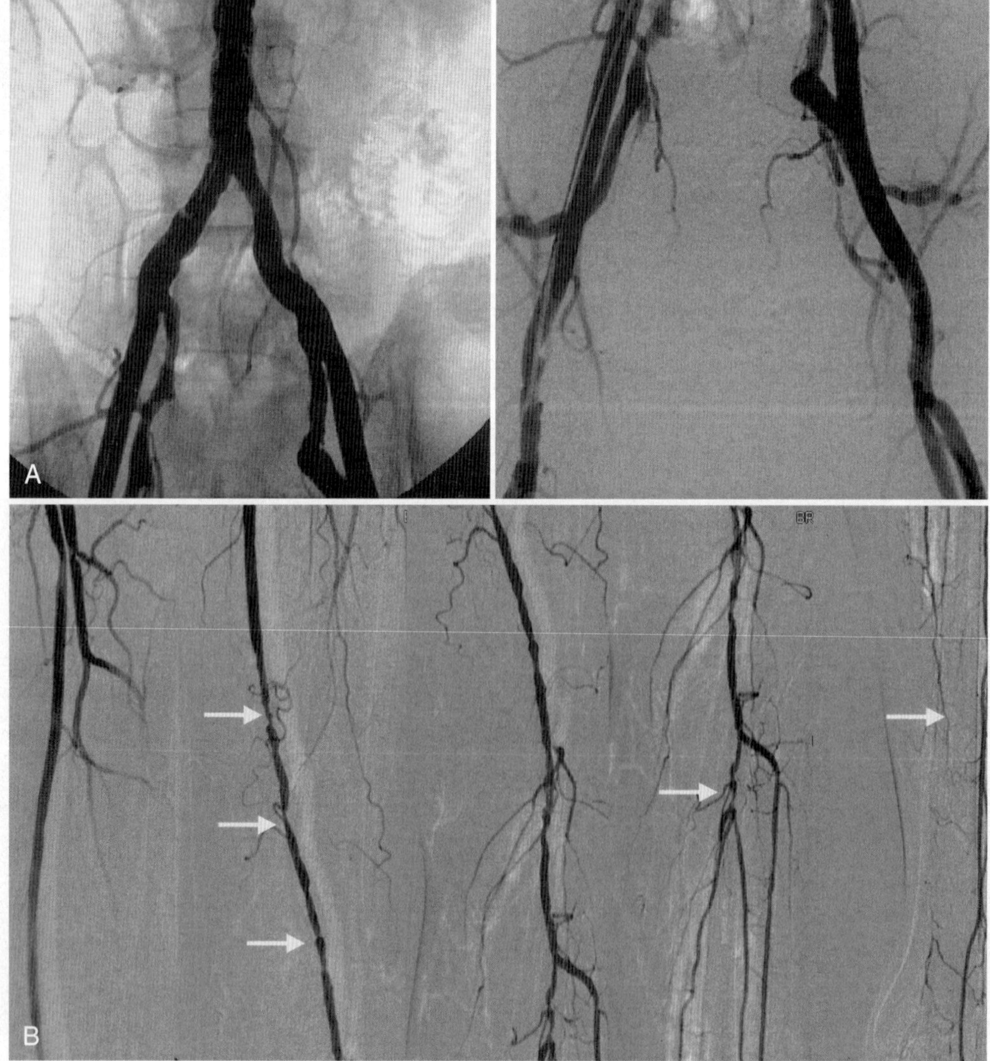

FIGURE 61-9 Angiogram of a patient with disabling left calf claudication. **A,** The aorta and bilateral common iliac arteries are patent. **B,** The left superficial femoral artery has multiple stenotic lesions (arrows). There is a significant stenosis of the left tibioperoneal trunk and left posterior tibial artery (arrows).

have classic symptoms of claudication.[32] Clinical progression to critical limb ischemia occurs in 7% to 9% of patients with claudication in the first year after diagnosis and in approximately 2% to 3% each year thereafter.[6,9,53] Both smoking and diabetes mellitus independently predict progression of disease.[6,9] The risk of amputation in those with diabetes mellitus is at least 12-fold higher than in nondiabetic persons.[54]

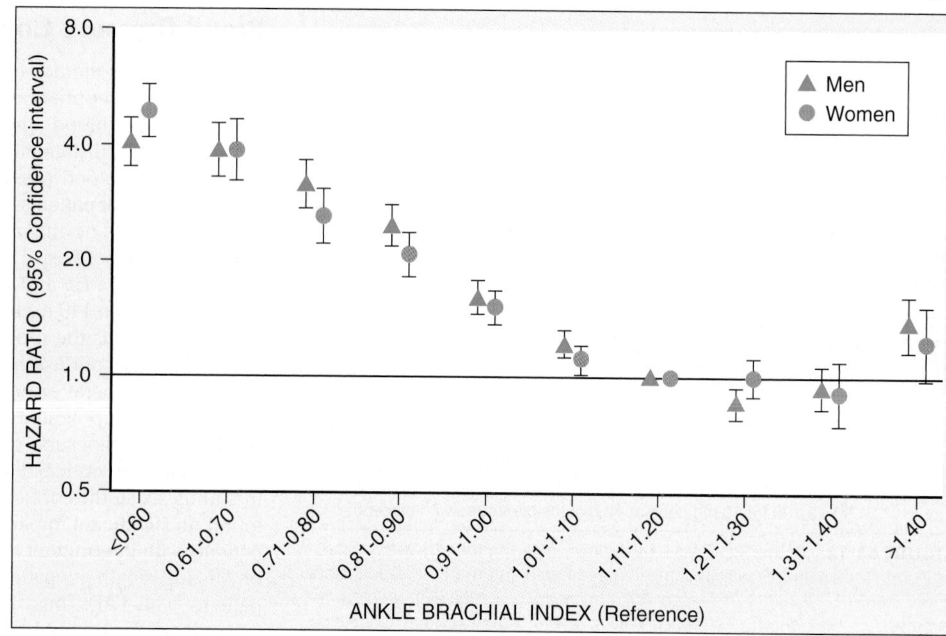

FIGURE 61-10 Association of ABI with all-cause mortality in a meta-analysis of 16 cohort studies. *(From Fowkes FG, Murray GD, Butcher I, et al: Ankle brachial index combined with Framingham Risk Score to predict cardiovascular events and mortality: A meta-analysis. JAMA 300:197, 2008.)*

Treatment

The goal for treatment of PAD is reduction in cardiovascular morbidity and mortality, as well as improvement in quality of life by decreasing symptoms of claudication, eliminating rest pain, and preserving limb viability. Therapeutic considerations therefore include risk factor modification by lifestyle measures and pharmacologic therapy to reduce the risk of adverse cardiovascular events, such as MI, stroke, and death. Symptoms of claudication can improve with pharmacotherapy or exercise rehabilitation. Optimal management of critical limb ischemia often includes endovascular interventions or surgical reconstruction to improve blood supply and to maintain limb viability. Revascularization is also indicated in some patients with disabling symptoms of claudication that persist despite exercise therapy and pharmacotherapy.[6,9]

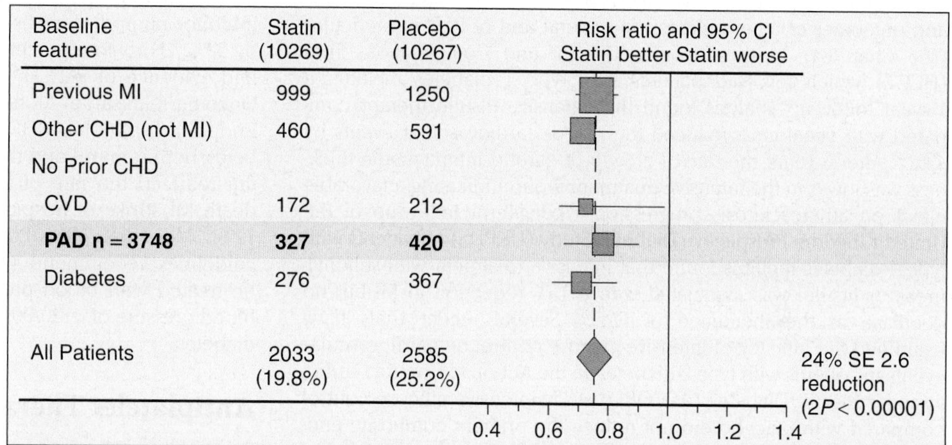

FIGURE 61-11 Relative risk of adverse cardiovascular events in participants of the Heart Protection Study, based on treatment with statin or placebo. Included in this study were 6700 patients with PAD, including 3748 patients who had no prior coronary heart disease (CHD), in whom there was an approximate 24% risk reduction of vascular events. CVD = cardiovascular disease; MI = myocardial infarction. *(From MRC/BHF Heart Protection Study of cholesterol lowering with simvastatin in 20,536 high-risk individuals: A randomized placebo-controlled trial. Lancet 360:7, 2002.)*

Risk Factor Modification

(see Chaps. 47 and 49)

Lipid-lowering therapy can reduce the risk of adverse cardiovascular events (see Chap. 47). The Heart Protection Study found that lipid-lowering therapy with simvastatin reduced the risk of adverse cardiovascular outcomes by 25% in patients with atherosclerosis, including more than 6700 patients with PAD (**Fig. 61-11**).[55] Pooled results from 17 lipid-lowering trials found that lipid-lowering therapy reduced the risk of cardiovascular events in patients with PAD by 26%.[56] Thus, patients with PAD should receive diet and drug therapy to achieve a target LDL-cholesterol level of 100 mg/dL or less.[9] Also, several prospective trials have found that statins improve walking distance in patients with PAD.[57-59] In the Treatment of Peripheral Atherosclerotic Disease with Moderate or Intensive Lipid Lowering (TREADMILL) trial, atorvastatin (80 mg) increased pain-free walking distance by more than 60%, compared with a 38% increase with placebo (**Fig. 61-12**).[58] Additional trials support these findings.[60] Also, patients treated with statins have superior leg functioning, as assessed by walking speed and distance, compared with those not treated.[61] It is not known whether other lipid-lowering therapies (such as niacin, ezetimibe, or fibrates) reduce the risk for cardiovascular events in patients with PAD. In the Fenofibrate and Event Lowering Intervention in Diabetes (FIELD) study, fenofibrate reduced the risk of minor amputation, primarily among patients who did not have known PAD.[62]

Smoking Cessation

Prospective trials examining the benefits of smoking cessation are lacking, but observational evidence unequivocally shows that cigarette smoking increases the risk of atherosclerosis and its clinical sequelae. Nonsmokers with PAD have lower rates of MI and mortality than those who have smoked or continue to smoke, and PAD patients who discontinue smoking have approximately twice the 5-year survival rate of those who continue to smoke.[12] Smoking cessation also lowers the risk for the development of critical limb ischemia. In addition to frequent physician advice, pharmacologic interventions that effectively promote smoking cessation include nicotine replacement therapy, bupropion, and varenicline.[63,64]

Treatment of Diabetes (see Chap. 64)

Aggressive treatment of diabetes decreases the risk for microangiopathic events such as nephropathy and retinopathy, but current data

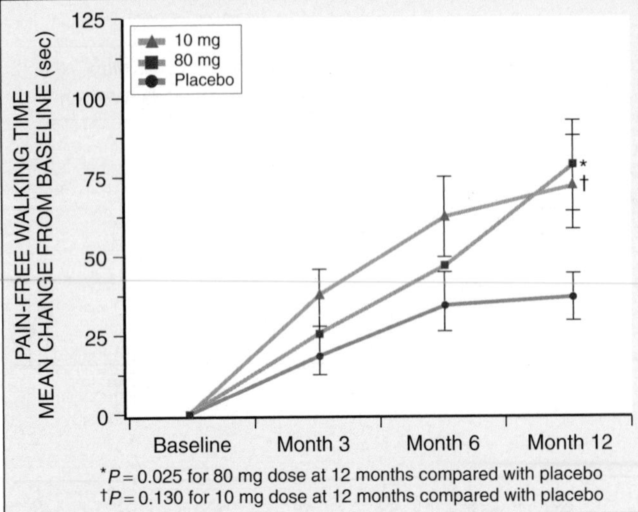

FIGURE 61-12 In the TREADMILL study, lipid-lowering therapy with atorvastatin improved pain-free walking time in patients with intermittent claudication. *(From Mohler ER III, Hiatt WR, Creager MA: Cholesterol reduction with atorvastatin improves walking distance in patients with arterial artery disease. Circulation 108:1481, 2003.)*

fail to support the notion that aggressive treatment of diabetes with glucose-lowering agents favorably affects the clinical manifestations and outcomes of atherosclerosis in general and of PAD in particular (see Chap. 64). In the Diabetes Control and Complications Trial (DCCT), which involved patients with type 1 diabetes mellitus, a 13-year follow-up analysis found that intensive insulin therapy, compared with usual care, reduced the risk of cardiovascular events by 42%.[65] After 6 years, the rate of growth of carotid intima-media thickness was lower in the intensive treatment group, indicating a favorable effect on atherosclerosis progression.[66] Long-term follow-up of the United Kingdom Prospective Diabetes Study (UKPDS) of patients with type 2 diabetes mellitus found that intensive treatment with sulfonylureas or insulin was associated with a 15% reduction in MI but no decrease in the incidence of PAD.[67] Several recent trials have examined the efficacy of intensive glucose control on cardiovascular events in patients with type 2 diabetes. In the Action to Control Cardiovascular Risk in Diabetes (ACCORD) study, intensive glucose control compared with placebo did not reduce the primary composite endpoint of nonfatal MI, nonfatal stroke, or cardiovascular death,[68] but intensive glucose control increased the risk of death and decreased the risk of nonfatal MI, which were secondary outcome measures. In the ADVANCE study, intensive glucose control reduced microvascular events, primarily the incidence of nephropathy, but did not affect macrovascular events, notably cardiovascular death.[69] In the Veterans Affairs Diabetes Trial (VADT), intensive glucose control did not affect the primary composite endpoint of MI, stroke, cardiovascular death, congestive heart failure, revascularization, and amputation for ischemic gangrene.[70] The PROactive (Prospective Pioglitazone Clinical Trial in Macrovascular Events) study assessed the effect of pioglitazone versus placebo on a broad range of cardiovascular endpoints in patients with type 2 diabetes and established atherosclerosis, including CAD, cerebrovascular disease, and PAD, and found no significant benefit of pioglitazone on the primary outcome.[71] Among patients with no PAD at baseline, composite primary and secondary event rates were less with pioglitazone than with placebo treatment. In the PAD patients, however, pioglitazone did not affect these cardiovascular events in patients with PAD.[72] A meta-analysis of five prospective randomized controlled trials found that intensive glycemic control resulted in a 17% reduction in events of nonfatal MI and a 15% reduction in coronary heart disease events, but it had no significant effect on stroke or all-cause mortality.[73] Current guidelines recommend that patients with PAD and diabetes be treated with glucose-lowering agents to achieve a hemoglobin A1c of <7.0%.[9,74]

Blood Pressure Control

Antihypertensive therapy reduces the risk of stroke, CAD, and vascular death. In the Appropriate Blood Pressure Control in Diabetes (ABCD) trial, intensive blood pressure control to levels approximating 128/75 mm Hg substantially reduced cardiovascular events compared with moderate blood pressure control in patients with PAD.[75] In the ACCORD study of patients with diabetes at high risk for cardiovascular events, there was no difference in cardiovascular outcomes between intensive antihypertensive therapy to achieve a systolic blood pressure less than 120 mm Hg and standard therapy to a target systolic blood pressure less than 140 mm Hg.[76] It is not known whether antihypertensive therapy limits the progression of PAD. Treatment of hypertension might decrease perfusion pressure to extremities already compromised by peripheral artery stenoses. In addition, concern has been raised about the potential adverse affects of beta-adrenergic receptor blockers (beta blockers) on peripheral blood flow and symptoms of claudication or critical limb ischemia. A recent systematic review including six studies of beta blocker therapy compared with placebo found no significant impairment on walking capacity in a total of 119 patients with intermittent claudication.[77] Beta blockers reduce the risk of MI and death in patients with CAD, a problem affecting many patients with PAD. Thus, if clinically indicated for other conditions, these drugs should not be withheld in patients with PAD. The balance of evidence supports the treatment of hypertension in patients with PAD according to established clinical guidelines (see Chap. 46).[78]

Angiotensin-converting enzyme inhibitors reduce cardiovascular events in patients with atherosclerosis. In the Heart Outcomes Prevention Evaluation (HOPE) study, the angiotensin-converting enzyme inhibitor ramipril decreased the risk for vascular death, MI, or stroke by 22%.[79] Forty-four percent of the patients enrolled in the HOPE trial had evidence of PAD, as manifested by an ABI less than 0.9. In the Ongoing Telmisartan Alone and in Combination with Ramipril Global Endpoint Trial (ONTARGET) of patients with vascular disease or diabetes, both ramipril and the angiotensin receptor antagonist telmisartan reduced the rate of the composite endpoint of cardiovascular death, MI, stroke, or hospitalization for heart failure by approximately 17%.[80] More than 13% of the patients in ONTARGET had PAD. Current guidelines recommend that patients with PAD and hypertension be treated with blood pressure–lowering agents to achieve a target blood pressure of <140/90 mm Hg, or <130/80 mm Hg in patients with diabetes.[9]

Antiplatelet Therapy (see Chap. 87)

Substantial evidence supports the use of antiplatelet agents to reduce adverse cardiovascular outcomes in patients with atherosclerosis. A meta-analysis that included approximately 135,000 high-risk patients with atherosclerosis, including those with acute and prior MI, stroke, or transient cerebrovascular ischemia, and other high-risk groups including those with PAD, found that antiplatelet therapy yielded a 22% reduction in subsequent vascular death, MI, or stroke.[81] Among the 9214 patients with PAD, included in this analysis, antiplatelet therapy reduced the risk of MI, stroke, or death by 22%. The majority of the PAD trials in this report, however, included antiplatelet therapy other than aspirin. A recent meta-analysis that included 18 prospective, randomized controlled trials, comprising 5269 persons with PAD, found that aspirin therapy compared with placebo was not associated with significant reductions in all-cause or cardiovascular mortality, MI, or major bleeding.[82] Included in this analysis was the Prevention of Progression of Arterial Disease and Diabetes (POPADAD) trial of diabetic patients with asymptomatic PAD, which found that aspirin did not decrease the risk of a composite primary endpoint including death from coronary heart disease or stroke, nonfatal MI or stroke, or amputation above the ankle for critical limb ischemia.[83] Within the Aspirin for Asymptomatic Atherosclerosis trial, in the 3350 participants with ABI ≤0.95, aspirin (100 mg daily) did not significantly reduce vascular events (**Fig. 61-13**).[84] The Clopidogrel versus Aspirin in Patients at Risk of Ischemic Events (CAPRIE) trial compared clopidogrel with aspirin for efficacy in preventing ischemic events in patients with recent MI,

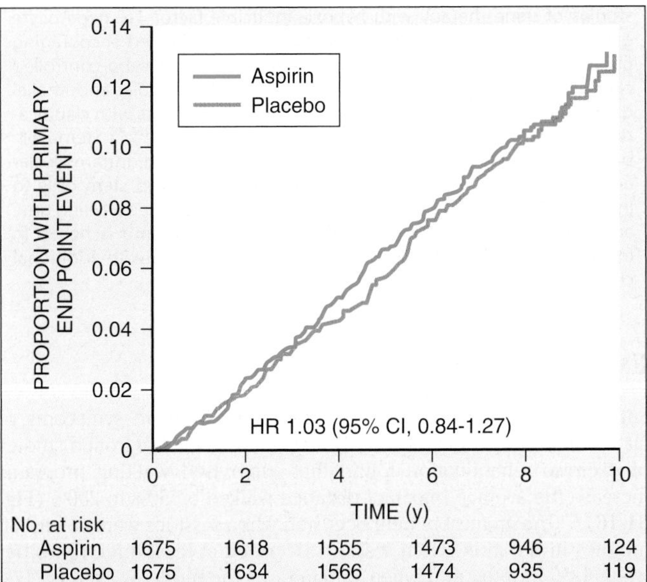

FIGURE 61-13 The primary endpoint event according to treatment group and duration of follow-up in the subset of participants in the Aspirin for Asymptomatic Atherosclerosis Trial with ABI ≤0.95 (fatal or nonfatal coronary event, stroke, or revascularization). CI indicates confidence interval; HR, hazard ratio. *(From Fowkes FG, Price JF, Stewart MC, et al: Aspirin for prevention of cardiovascular events in a general population screened for a low ankle brachial index: A randomized controlled trial. JAMA 303:841, 2010.)*

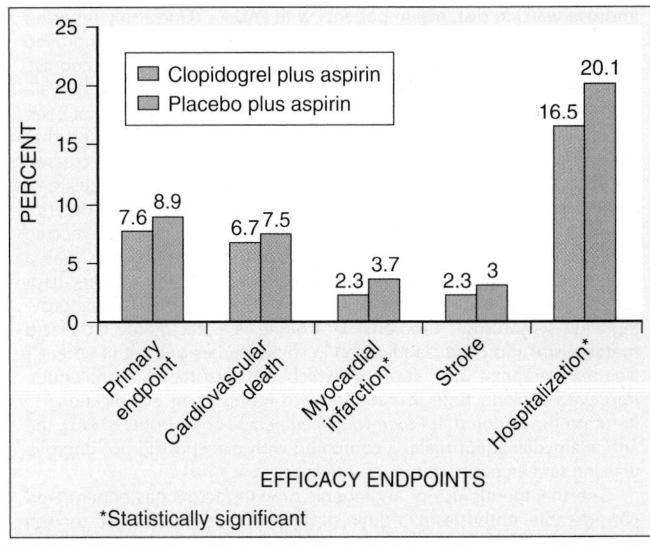

FIGURE 61-14 The effect of clopidogrel plus aspirin versus placebo plus aspirin on the rate of the composite endpoint (cardiovascular death, myocardial infarction, or stroke), cardiovascular death, myocardial infarction, stroke, and hospitalization (for unstable angina, transient ischemic attack, or revascularization procedure). *(From Cacoub PP, Bhatt DL, Steg PG, et al: Patients with peripheral arterial disease in the CHARISMA trial. Eur Heart J 30:192, 2009.)*

recent ischemic stroke, or PAD. Overall, there was an 8.7% relative risk reduction for MI, ischemic stroke, or vascular death in the group treated with clopidogrel.[85] Notably, among the 6452 patients in the PAD subgroup, clopidogrel treatment reduced adverse cardiovascular events by 23.8%. The Clopidogrel for High Atherothrombotic Risk and Ischemic Stabilization, Management, and Avoidance (CHARISMA) trial compared the efficacy of dual antiplatelet therapy with clopidogrel plus aspirin to aspirin alone in patients with established CAD, cerebrovascular disease, or PAD, as well as in patients with multiple atherosclerotic risk factors.[86] Overall, dual antiplatelet therapy produced no significant benefit compared with aspirin alone on the primary efficacy endpoint, a composite of MI, stroke, or cardiovascular death. Among the 3096 patients with PAD in the CHARISMA trial, dual antiplatelet therapy reduced the rates of MI and hospitalization for ischemic events (**Fig. 61-14**).[87] The Warfarin Antiplatelet Vascular Evaluation (WAVE) trial compared combination antiplatelet and oral anticoagulant therapy with antiplatelet therapy alone in patients with PAD.[88] There was no significant difference between the two treatments on the primary composite endpoint of MI, stroke, or cardiovascular death, but life-threatening bleeding occurred more frequently in patients receiving combination antiplatelet and anticoagulant therapy.

Current guidelines recommend that patients with PAD be treated with an antiplatelet drug, such as aspirin or clopidogrel.[9] Oral anticoagulation with warfarin is not recommended to reduce cardiovascular events in patients with PAD because it is no more effective than antiplatelet therapy and confers a higher risk of bleeding. Antiplatelet therapy also prevents occlusion in the peripheral circulation after revascularization procedures. Of approximately 3000 patients with peripheral arterial procedures previously analyzed by the Antiplatelet Trialists Collaboration, the odds reduction for arterial or graft occlusion by antiplatelet therapy (primarily aspirin or aspirin plus dipyridamole) was 43%.

Pharmacotherapy

The development of effective pharmacotherapy for symptoms of PAD has lagged substantially behind drug treatment for CAD. Most studies of vasodilator therapy have failed to demonstrate any efficacy in patients with intermittent claudication. Several pathophysiologic explanations may account for the failure of vasodilator therapy in patients with PAD. During exercise, resistance vessels distal to a stenosis dilate in response to ischemia. Vasodilators would have minimal if any effect on these endogenously dilated vessels but would decrease resistance in other vessels and create a relative steal phenomenon, reducing blood flow and perfusion pressure to the affected leg. Moreover, in contrast to their effects on myocardial oxygen consumption in patients with CAD (due to afterload reduction), vasodilators do not reduce skeletal muscle oxygen demand.

The U.S. Food and Drug Administration (FDA) has approved two drugs, pentoxifylline (Trental) and cilostazol (Pletal), for the treatment of claudication in patients with PAD. Licensing bodies in Europe, Asia, and South America have approved additional drugs. Pentoxifylline is a xanthine derivative used to treat patients with intermittent claudication. Its action may be mediated through its hemorheologic properties, including its ability to decrease blood viscosity and to improve erythrocyte flexibility. It may have anti-inflammatory and antiproliferative effects. Pentoxifylline has marginal efficacy,[6,9] increasing maximum walking distance by only 14% compared with placebo in one study.[89] Cilostazol is a quinolinone derivative that inhibits phosphodiesterase 3, thereby decreasing cyclic adenosine monophosphate degradation and increasing its concentration in platelets and blood vessels. Although cilostazol inhibits platelet aggregation and causes vasodilation in experimental animals, its mechanism of action in patients with PAD is not known. Several trials have reported that cilostazol improves absolute claudication distance by 40% to 50% compared with placebo (**Fig. 61-15**).[90,91] Quality of life measures, assessed by the Medical Outcomes Scale (SF-36) and Walking Impairment Questionnaire, also demonstrated improvement. An FDA advisory stated that cilostazol should not be used in patients with congestive heart failure because other phosphodiesterase 3 inhibitors have been shown to decrease survival in these patients. A long-term safety trial found that cilostazol compared with placebo did not increase the risk of total or cardiovascular mortality, but the study was limited because more than 60% of patients discontinued treatment before study completion.[92]

Other classes of drugs—including statins, angiotensin-converting enzyme inhibitors, serotonin (5-HT_2) antagonists, alpha-adrenergic antagonists, L-arginine, carnitine derivatives, vasodilator prostaglandins, antibiotics, and angiogenic growth factors—have been studied or are currently under investigation for treatment of either claudication or critical limb ischemia. As noted previously, three trials have found that statins improve walking distance in patients with PAD.[57-59] One study reported that the angiotensin-converting enzyme inhibitor ramipril improved maximal claudication time.[93] Naftidrofuryl, a serotonin antagonist, improved symptoms of claudication in some trials and is currently available for use in Europe.[6] Selective serotonin 2A antagonists have not been effective in improving claudication distance.[94,95] One study found that buflomedil, a drug with adrenoceptor antagonist properties, decreased the risk of critical cardiovascular events—defined as the composite of cardiovascular death, nonfatal MI, nonfatal stroke, symptomatic deterioration of PAD, or leg amputation—by 26% compared with placebo in patients with claudication.[96] Notable among these outcomes was a reduction in symptomatic deterioration of PAD. L-Arginine, the precursor for endothelium-derived nitric oxide, has not proved useful for improving PAD symptoms.[97] Propionyl L-carnitine, a cofactor for fatty acid metabolism, improved claudication in some studies but not in others.[98] Neither beraprost nor iloprost, which are prostacyclin analogues, improved walking time in patients with intermittent claudication.[89,99] Refuting the notion that *Chlamydia pneumoniae* contributes to PAD, the antichlamydial agent rifalazil, compared with placebo, did not improve walking time in patients with claudication.[100]

The therapeutic use of angiogenic growth factors has engendered considerable enthusiasm. Administration of basic fibroblast growth factor and vascular endothelial growth factor as protein or gene therapy increases collateral blood vessel development, capillary number, and blood flow in experimental models of hindlimb ischemia. Preliminary studies of gene therapy with hypoxia-inducible factor 1α, hepatocyte growth factor, and fibroblast growth factor 1 have yielded encouraging findings in patients with critical limb ischemia.[101-103] Placebo-controlled clinical trials of angiogenic growth factors, such as vascular endothelial growth factor and hypoxia inducible factor 1α, in patients with claudication have failed to show improvement in walking time.[104,105] Stem cell–based therapies for PAD, including intra-arterial and intramuscular administration of peripheral and bone marrow–derived stem cells to induce angiogenesis, improved ABI, rest pain, and pain-free walking time and prevented amputation in patients with chronic limb ischemia in initial reports.[106-109] These findings require confirmation with additional clinical trials.

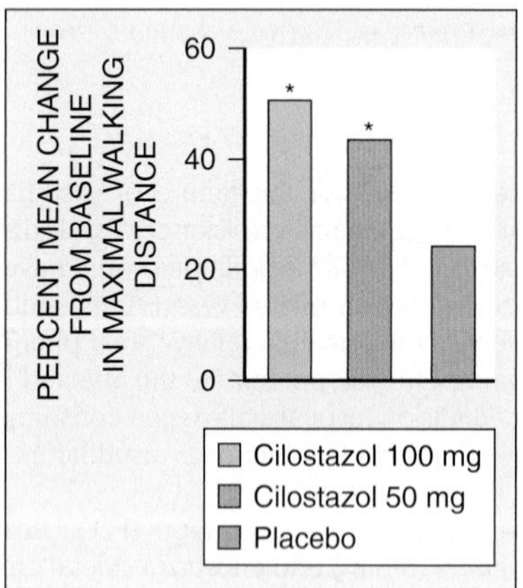

FIGURE 61-15 The effect of cilostazol compared with placebo on maximal walking distance, based on a meta-analysis of nine randomized trials. *(Modified from Pande RL, Hiatt WR, Zhang P, et al: A pooled analysis of the durability and predictors of treatment response of cilostazol in patients with intermittent claudication. Vasc Med 15:181, 2010.)*

Exercise Rehabilitation (see Chaps. 50 and 83)

Supervised exercise rehabilitation programs improve symptoms of claudication in patients with PAD. Meta-analyses of controlled studies of exercise rehabilitation found that supervised walking programs increase the average maximal distance walked by 50% to 200% (**Fig. 61-16**).[110] The greatest benefit occurred when sessions were at least 30 minutes in duration, when sessions occurred at least three times per week for 6 months, and when walking was the mode of exercise. Leg strength training also improves walking time, although not as much as treadmill exercise training.[111] Postulated mechanisms through which exercise training improves claudication include the formation of collateral vessels and improvement in endothelium-dependent vasodilation, hemorheology, muscle structure and metabolism, and walking efficiency.[112,113] Studies in experimental hindlimb ischemia have suggested that regular exercise increases the development of collateral blood vessels.[112] Exercise increases the expression of angiogenic factors, particularly in hypoxic tissue.[114,115] Exercise training may improve endothelium-dependent vasodilation in patients with PAD, as it does in patients with coronary atherosclerosis.[116] Improvement in calf blood flow has not been demonstrated consistently in patients with claudication after exercise training, although one study found that maximal calf blood flow increased commensurate with improvement in walking distance.[112,117] To date, no imaging studies have demonstrated increased collateral blood vessels after exercise training in patients with PAD.

The benefits of exercise training in patients with PAD may result from changes in skeletal muscle structure or function, such as increased muscle mitochondrial enzyme activity, oxidative metabolism, and ATP production rate. In patients with PAD, improvement in exercise performance is associated with a decrease in plasma and skeletal muscle short-chain acylcarnitine concentrations, which

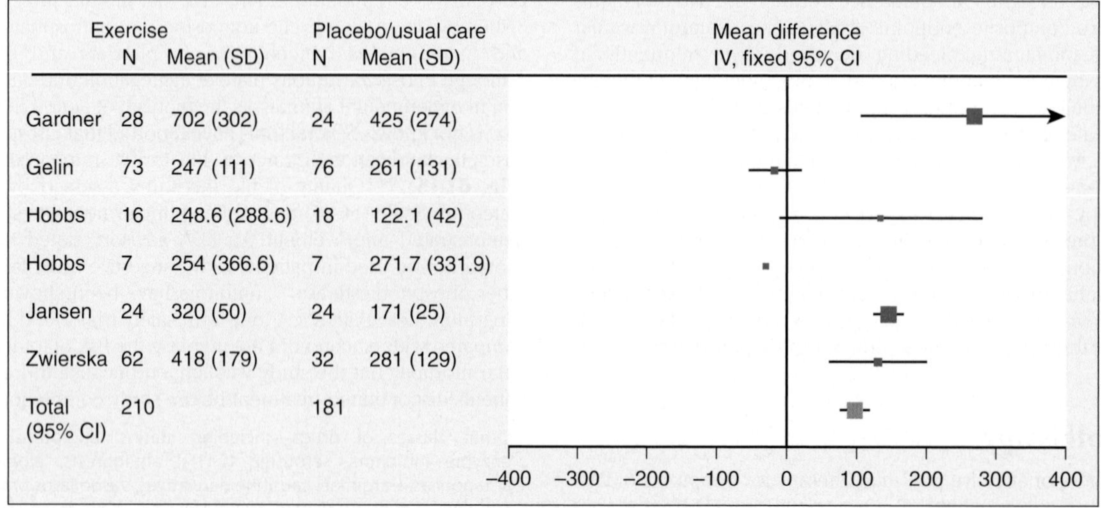

FIGURE 61-16 A meta-analysis of the effect of exercise training versus usual care on maximum walking distance in patients with intermittent claudication. *(From Watson L, Ellis B, Leng GC: Exercise for intermittent claudication. Cochrane Database Syst Rev [4]:CD000990, 2008.)*

indicates improvement in oxidative metabolism and increased peak oxygen consumption. Higher physical activity levels in patients with PAD are associated with greater calf muscle area and density.[38] Training may also enhance biomechanical performance, enabling patients to walk more efficiently with less energy expenditure. Current guidelines recommend that patients with intermittent claudication undergo supervised exercise rehabilitation as initial therapy. Supervised exercise training should consist of 30- to 45-minute sessions, at least three times per week, for a minimum of 12 weeks.[9]

Percutaneous Transluminal Angioplasty and Stents (see Chap. 63)

Peripheral catheter-based interventions are indicated for patients with lifestyle-limiting claudication, despite a trial of exercise rehabilitation or pharmacotherapy.[6,9,118] Endovascular intervention should be considered in symptomatic patients with clinical evidence of inflow disease, manifested by buttock or thigh claudication and diminished femoral pulses. Patients with critical limb ischemia whose anatomy is amenable to catheter-based therapy should also receive endovascular intervention.

Peripheral Artery Surgery

Surgical revascularization generally improves quality of life in patients with disabling claudication on maximal medical therapy and is indicated to relieve rest pain and to preserve limb viability in patients with critical limb ischemia that is not amenable to percutaneous interventions. The specific operation must take into account the anatomic location of the arterial lesions and the presence of comorbid conditions. The surgical procedure is planned after identification of the arterial obstruction by imaging, ensuring that there is sufficient arterial inflow to and outflow from the graft to maintain patency. A preoperative evaluation to assess the risk of vascular surgery should be performed because many of these patients have coexisting CAD. Guidelines for this evaluation exist (see Chap. 85).[119]

Aorto-bifemoral bypass is the most frequent operation for patients with aortoiliac disease. Typically, a knitted or woven prosthesis made of Dacron or polytetrafluoroethylene (PTFE) is anastomosed proximally to the aorta and distally to each common femoral artery. On occasion, the iliac artery is used for the distal anastomosis to maintain anterograde flow into at least one hypogastric artery.

Extra-anatomic surgical reconstructive procedures for aortoiliac disease include axillo-bifemoral bypass, ilio-bifemoral bypass, and femoral-femoral bypass. These bypass grafts, made of Dacron or PTFE, circumvent the aorta and iliac arteries and are generally used in high-risk patients with critical limb ischemia. Long-term patency rates are inferior to those of aorto-bifemoral bypass procedures. Five-year patency rates range from 50% to 70% for axillo-bifemoral bypass operations and from 70% to 80% for femoral-femoral bypass grafts.[9] The operative mortality rate for extra-anatomic bypass procedures is 3% to 5% and reflects, in part, the serious comorbid conditions and advanced atherosclerosis of many of the patients who undergo these procedures.

Reconstructive surgery for infrainguinal arterial disease includes femoral-popliteal and femoral-tibial or femoral-peroneal artery bypass. In situ or reversed autologous saphenous veins or synthetic grafts made of PTFE are used for the infrainguinal bypass. Patency rates for autologous saphenous vein bypass grafts exceed those with PTFE grafts,[6,9] and patency rates are better for grafts in which the distal anastomosis is placed in the popliteal artery above the knee, compared with below the knee.[6] Five-year primary patency rates for femoral-popliteal reconstruction in patients with claudication are approximately 80% and 75% for autogenous vein grafts or PTFE grafts, respectively, and approximately 65% and 45%, respectively, in patients with critical limb ischemia. For femoral below-knee bypass, including tibioperoneal artery reconstruction, the 5-year patency rates for saphenous vein grafts in patients with claudication or critical limb ischemia are comparable to those for femoral-popliteal above-knee grafts (60% to 80%). The 5-year patency rate for PTFE grafts in the infrapopliteal position is considerably lower, approximating 65% in patients with claudication and 33% in patients with critical limb ischemia. The operative mortality rate for infrainguinal bypass operations is 1% to 2%.

Graft stenoses can result from technical errors at the time of surgery, such as retained valve cuffs or intimal flap or valvotome injury; from fibrous intimal hyperplasia, usually within 6 months of surgery; or from atherosclerosis, usually occurring within the vein graft at least 1 to 2 years after surgery. Institution of graft surveillance protocols with the use of color-assisted duplex ultrasonography has enabled the identification of graft stenoses, prompting graft revision and avoiding complete graft failure.[9] Graft outcome is improved as a result of routine ultrasonographic surveillance. Antithrombotic agents, including antiplatelet drugs and coumarin derivatives, also improve graft patency. Several studies have suggested that antiplatelet drugs may be more effective in preserving synthetic grafts, whereas coumarin derivatives may be more effective for vein bypass grafts.[120-122]

Algorithm for Treatment of the Symptomatic Leg

Figure 61-17 provides a management algorithm for the treatment of intermittent claudication.

Vasculitis (see Chap. 89)

Thromboangiitis Obliterans

Thromboangiitis obliterans (TAO) is a segmental vasculitis that affects the distal arteries, veins, and nerves of the upper and lower extremities. It typically occurs in young persons who smoke.[123]

Pathology and Pathogenesis

TAO primarily affects the medium and small vessels of the arms, including the radial, ulnar, palmar, and digital arteries, and their counterparts in the legs, including the tibial, peroneal, plantar, and digital arteries. Involvement can extend to the cerebral, coronary, renal, mesenteric, aortoiliac, and pulmonary arteries.[123] The pathologic findings include an occlusive, highly cellular thrombus incorporating polymorphonuclear leukocytes, microabscesses, and occasionally multinucleated giant cells. The inflammatory infiltrate can also affect the vascular wall, but the internal elastic membrane remains intact. In the chronic phase of the disease, the thrombus becomes organized and the vascular wall becomes fibrotic.

The precise cause of TAO is not known. Tobacco use or exposure is present in virtually every patient. Potential immunologic mechanisms include increased cellular sensitivity to types I and III collagen and the presence of antiendothelial cell antibodies. CD4 T cells have been identified in cellular infiltrates of vessels of patients with TAO.[123,124] Decreased endothelium-dependent vasodilation to acetylcholine can occur in both affected and unaffected limbs of patients with TAO, raising the possibility that reduced bioavailability of nitric oxide contributes to the disorder.[124]

Clinical Presentation

The prevalence of TAO is greater in Asia than in North America or western Europe. In the United States, TAO occurs in approximately 13 per 100,000 population.[123,124] Most patients develop symptoms before 45 years of age, and 75% to 90% are men. Patients can have claudication of the hands, forearms, feet, or calves. The majority of patients with TAO present with rest pain and digital ulcerations; often, more than one extremity is affected. Raynaud phenomenon occurs in approximately 45% of patients, and superficial thrombophlebitis,

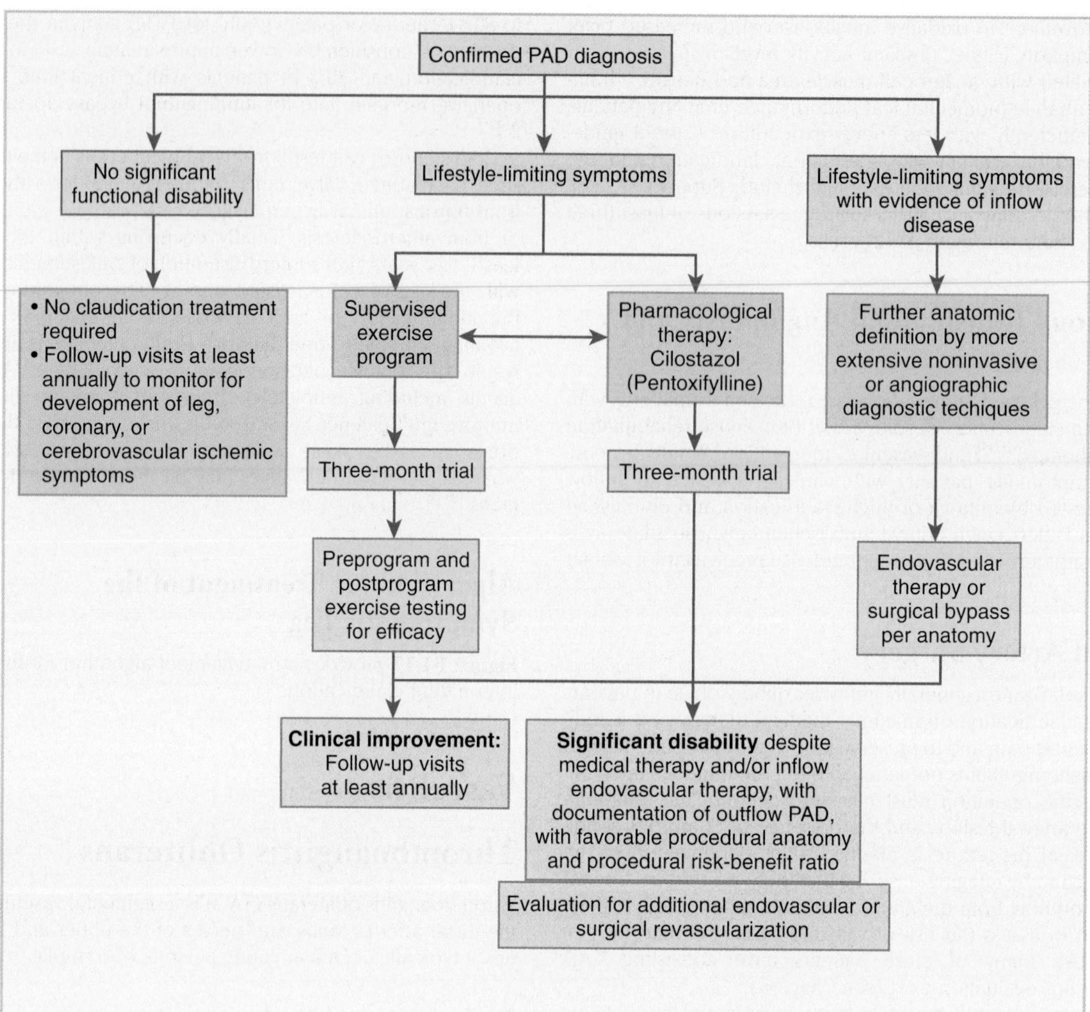

FIGURE 61-17 Management algorithm for the treatment of symptomatic PAD. *(From Hirsch AT, Haskal ZJ, Hertzer NR, et al: ACC/AHA 2005 guidelines for the management of patients with peripheral arterial disease [lower extremity, renal, mesenteric, and abdominal aortic]: Executive summary a collaborative report from the American Association for Vascular Surgery/Society for Vascular Surgery, Society for Cardiovascular Angiography and Interventions, Society for Vascular Medicine and Biology, Society of Interventional Radiology, and the ACC/AHA Task Force on Practice Guidelines [Writing Committee to Develop Guidelines for the Management of Patients With Peripheral Arterial Disease] endorsed by the American Association of Cardiovascular and Pulmonary Rehabilitation; National Heart, Lung, and Blood Institute; Society for Vascular Nursing; TransAtlantic Inter-Society Consensus; and Vascular Disease Foundation. J Am Coll Cardiol 47:1239, 2006.)*

which may be migratory, occurs in approximately 40%. The risk of amputation within 5 years is approximately 25%.[125]

The radial, ulnar, dorsalis pedis, and posterior tibial pulses may be absent if the corresponding vessel is involved. The clinical characteristics of critical limb ischemia and ischemic digital ulcerations are described earlier in this chapter. The Allen test result is abnormal in two thirds of patients. To perform the Allen test, both radial and ulnar arteries are compressed while the hand is clenched and then opened. This maneuver causes palmar blanching. Release of compression from either pulse should normally produce palmar erythema if the palmar arches are patent. If these are occluded, pallor persists on the side where compression is maintained. The distal aspects of the extremities may have discrete, tender, erythematous subcutaneous cords, indicating a superficial thrombophlebitis.

Diagnosis

No specific laboratory tests, other than biopsy, can diagnose TAO. Most tests, therefore, aim to exclude other diseases that might have similar clinical presentations, including autoimmune diseases such as scleroderma or systemic lupus erythematosus, hypercoagulable states, diabetes, and acute arterial occlusion due to embolism. Acute-phase indicators, such as the erythrocyte sedimentation rate or C-reactive protein, are usually normal. Serum immunologic markers, including antinuclear antibodies and rheumatoid factor, should not be present, and serum complement levels should be normal. If it is clinically indicated, a proximal source of embolism should be excluded by cardiac and vascular ultrasonography or by computed tomography, magnetic resonance angiography, or conventional arteriography. Arteriography of an affected limb supports the diagnosis of TAO if there is segmental occlusion of small and medium arteries, absence of atherosclerosis, and corkscrew collateral vessels circumventing the occlusion (**Fig. 61-18**). These same findings, however, can occur in patients with scleroderma, systemic lupus erythematosus, mixed connective tissue disease, and antiphospholipid antibody syndrome. The conclusive test is a biopsy showing the classic pathologic findings. This procedure is rarely indicated, and biopsy sites may fail to heal because of severe ischemia. The diagnosis, therefore, usually depends on an age at onset of younger than 45 years, a history of tobacco use, physical examination demonstrating distal limb ischemia, exclusion of other diseases, and if necessary, angiographic demonstration of typical lesions.

Treatment

The cornerstone of treatment is cessation of tobacco use. Patients without gangrene who stop smoking rarely require amputation.[123,125] In contrast, one or more amputations may ultimately be required in 40% to 45% of patients with TAO who continue to smoke.

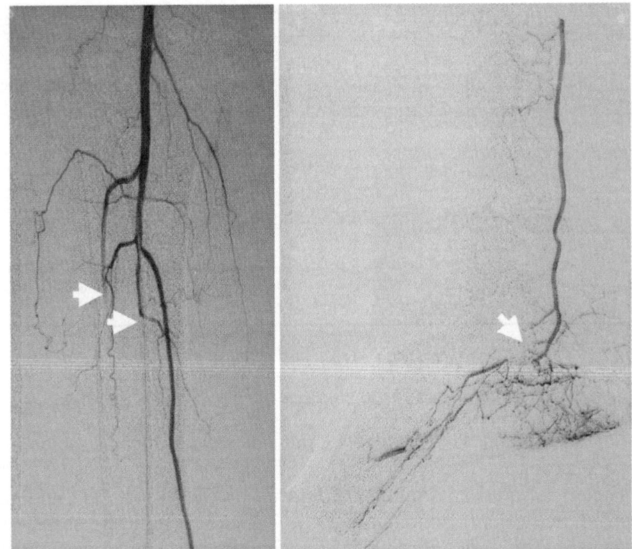

FIGURE 61-18 Angiogram of a young woman with thromboangiitis obliterans. The **left panel** demonstrates occlusion of the anterior tibial and peroneal arteries (arrows). The **right panel** demonstrates an occlusion of the distal portion of the posterior tibial artery (arrow) with bridging collateral vessels.

There is no definitive drug therapy for limb ischemia in patients with TAO. Vascular reconstructive surgery is usually not a viable option because of the segmental nature of this disease and the involvement of distal vessels. An autogenous saphenous vein bypass graft can be considered if a target vessel for the distal anastomosis is available. Long-term patency rates are better in ex-smokers than in smokers.[126]

Takayasu Arteritis and Giant Cell Arteritis (see Chap. 89)

Fibromuscular Dysplasia

Fibromuscular dysplasia is a disease of medium and large arteries. It typically affects the renal and carotid arteries. It may affect the arteries supplying the leg, particularly the iliac arteries and less so the femoral, popliteal, tibial, and peroneal arteries.[127] Fibromuscular dysplasia is a rare cause of either intermittent claudication or critical limb ischemia. It most often occurs in young white women but can occur at any age in both sexes. The histopathologic examination shows fibroplasia that most often affects the media but can involve the intima or adventitia. The histologic classification of fibromuscular dysplasia includes the medial subtypes (medial fibroplasia, perimedial fibroplasia, and medial hyperplasia) as well as intimal fibroplasia and adventitial hyperplasia.[10,127] Depending on the histopathologic type, stenosis results from hyperplasia of fibrous or muscular components of the vessel wall. Angiography demonstrates a beaded appearance of arteries affected by medial and perimedial fibroplasia and focal or tubular stenosis in arteries affected by intimal fibroplasia. Symptomatic patients should be treated with percutaneous transluminal angioplasty.

Popliteal Artery Entrapment Syndrome

Popliteal artery entrapment syndrome is an uncommon cause of intermittent claudication. It occurs when an anatomic variation in the configuration or insertion of the medial head of the gastrocnemius muscle compresses the popliteal artery.[128,129] The popliteus muscle can also compress the popliteal artery and cause this syndrome. Popliteal artery entrapment is bilateral in approximately one third of affected patients. It should be suspected when a young, typically athletic, usually male person presents with claudication. Potential consequences include popliteal artery thrombosis, embolism, and aneurysm formation.

The peripheral pulse examination findings may be normal unless provocative maneuvers are performed. Walking or repeated ankle dorsiflexion and plantar flexion maneuvers may cause attenuation or disappearance of pedal pulses and a decrease in the ABI in patients with popliteal artery entrapment. Imaging studies, such as duplex ultrasonography, computed tomography, and magnetic resonance angiography or conventional angiography, performed at rest and during ankle flexion maneuvers, can confirm the diagnosis. Magnetic resonance and computed tomography imaging will also provide information about the relationship of the gastrocnemius muscle to the popliteal artery.

Treatment of popliteal artery entrapment syndrome involves release of the popliteal artery. This may require division and reattachment of the medial head of the gastrocnemius muscle. On occasion, if the popliteal artery is occluded, surgical bypass is required.

Acute Limb Ischemia

Acute limb ischemia occurs when an arterial occlusion suddenly reduces blood flow to the arm or leg. The metabolic needs of the tissue outstrip perfusion, placing limb viability in jeopardy. The clinical presentation of patients with acute limb ischemia relates to the location of the arterial occlusion and the resulting decrease in blood flow. Depending on the severity of ischemia, patients may note disabling claudication or pain at rest. Pain may develop during a short period and is manifested in the affected extremity distal to the site of obstruction. It is not necessarily confined to the foot or toes, or hand or fingers, as is usually the case in chronic limb ischemia. Concurrent ischemia of peripheral nerves causes sensory loss and motor dysfunction. The physical findings can include absence of pulses distal to the occlusion, cool skin, pallor, delayed capillary return and venous filling, diminished or absent sensory perception, and muscle weakness or paralysis. This constellation of symptoms and signs is often recalled as the five *p*'s: pain, pulselessness, pallor, paresthesias, and paralysis.

Prognosis

Patients presenting with acute limb ischemia usually have comorbid cardiovascular disorders, which may even be responsible for the ischemia. This population therefore has a poor long-term outcome. The 5-year survival rate after acute limb ischemia caused by thrombosis approximates 45%, and after embolism, it is less than 20%.[6] The 1-month survival rate in persons older than 75 years with acute limb ischemia is approximately 40%.[130] The risk of limb loss depends on the severity of the ischemia and the elapsed time before a revascularization procedure is performed.

A classification scheme that takes into consideration the severity of ischemia and the viability of the limb, along with related neurologic findings and Doppler signals, has been developed by the Society for Vascular Surgery and the International Society for Cardiovascular Surgery (**Table 61-6**).[37] A viable limb, category I, is not immediately threatened, has neither sensory nor motor abnormalities, and has blood flow detectable by Doppler interrogation. Threatened viability, category II, indicates that the severity of ischemia will cause limb loss unless the blood supply is restored promptly. The category is subdivided into marginally and immediately threatened limbs, the latter characterized by pain, sensory deficits, and muscle weakness. Doppler interrogation cannot detect arterial blood flow. Irreversible limb ischemia leading to tissue loss and requiring amputation, category III, is characterized by loss of sensation, paralysis, and the absence of Doppler-detected blood flow in both arteries and veins distal to the occlusion.

Pathogenesis

The causes of acute limb ischemia include arterial embolism, thrombosis in situ, dissection, and trauma. Most arterial emboli arise from thrombotic sources in the heart. Atrial fibrillation complicating valvular heart disease, congestive heart failure, CAD, and hypertension accounts

TABLE 61-6 Clinical Categories of Acute Limb Ischemia

		FINDINGS		DOPPLER SIGNALS	
CATEGORY	DESCRIPTION/PROGNOSIS	SENSORY LOSS	MUSCLE WEAKNESS	ARTERIAL	VENOUS
I. Viable	Not immediately threatened	None	None	Audible	Audible
II. Threatened					
a. Marginally	Salvageable if promptly treated	Minimal (toes) or none	None	(Often) inaudible	Audible
b. Immediately	Salvageable with immediate revascularization	More than toes, rest pain	Mild, moderate	(Usually) inaudible	Audible
III. Irreversible	Major tissue loss or permanent nerve damage inevitable	Profound, anesthetic	Profound, paralysis (rigor)	Inaudible	Inaudible

Modified from Rutherford RB, Baker JD, Ernst C, et al: Recommended standards for reports dealing with lower extremity ischemia: Revised version. J Vasc Surg 26:517, 1997.

for approximately 50% of cardiac emboli to the limbs. Other sources include rheumatic or prosthetic cardiac valves, ventricular thrombus resulting from MI or left ventricular aneurysm, paradoxical embolism of venous thrombi through the intra-atrial or intraventricular communications, and cardiac tumors such as left atrial myxomas. Aneurysms of the aorta or peripheral arteries may harbor thrombi, which subsequently embolize to more distal arterial sites, usually lodging at branch points where the artery decreases in size.

Thrombosis in situ occurs in atherosclerotic peripheral arteries, infrainguinal bypass grafts, peripheral artery aneurysms, and normal arteries of patients with hypercoagulable states. In patients with peripheral atherosclerosis, thrombosis in situ may complicate plaque rupture, causing acute arterial occlusion and limb ischemia, in a manner analogous to that which occurs in coronary arteries in patients with acute MI. Thrombosis complicating popliteal artery aneurysms is a much more common complication than rupture and may account for 10% of cases of acute limb ischemia in elderly men.[6] One of the most common causes of acute limb ischemia is thrombotic occlusion of an infrainguinal bypass graft, as discussed previously. Acute thrombotic occlusion of a normal artery is unusual but may occur in patients with acquired thrombophilic disorders, such as antiphospholipid antibody syndrome, heparin-induced thrombocytopenia, disseminated intravascular coagulation, and myeloproliferative diseases. There is limited evidence that inherited thrombophilic disorders such as activated protein C resistance (factor V Leiden), prothrombin G20210 gene mutation, or deficiencies of antithrombin III and protein C and S increase the risk of acute peripheral arterial thrombosis.

Diagnostic Tests

The history and physical examination usually establish the diagnosis of acute limb ischemia. Time available for diagnostic tests is often limited, and tests should not delay urgent revascularization procedures if limb viability is immediately threatened. The pressure in the affected limb and corresponding ABI can be measured if flow is detectable by Doppler ultrasonography. A Doppler probe can interrogate the presence of blood flow in peripheral arteries, particularly when pulses are not palpable. Color-assisted duplex ultrasonography can determine the site of occlusion. It is particularly applicable to evaluate the patency of infrainguinal bypass grafts. Magnetic resonance, computed tomography, and conventional contrast arteriography can demonstrate the site of occlusion and provide an anatomic guide for revascularization.

Treatment

Analgesic medications should be administered to reduce pain. For patients with acute leg ischemia, the bed should be positioned such that the feet are lower than chest level, thereby increasing limb perfusion pressure by gravitational effects. This goal can be accomplished by putting blocks under the posts at the head of the bed. Efforts should be made to reduce pressure on the heels, on bone prominences, and between the toes by appropriate placement of soft material on the bed (such as sheepskin) and between the toes (such as lamb's wool). The room should be kept warm to prevent cold-induced cutaneous vasoconstriction.

Heparin should be administered intravenously as soon as the diagnosis of acute limb ischemia is made. The dose should be sufficient to increase the partial thromboplastin time by 1.5 to 2.5 times control values to prevent thrombus propagation or recurrent embolism. It is not known whether low-molecular-weight heparin is as effective as unfractionated heparin in patients with acute limb ischemia.

Revascularization is indicated when the viability of the limb is threatened or when symptoms of ischemia persist. Options for revascularization include intra-arterial thrombolytic therapy, percutaneous mechanical thrombectomy, and surgical revascularization. Catheter-directed intra-arterial thrombolysis is an initial treatment option for patients presenting with either category I or II acute limb ischemia, if there is no contraindication to thrombolysis.[131] Catheter-based thrombolysis can also be considered for patients who are considered at high risk for surgical intervention. Long-term patency after thrombolysis is greater in patients with category I and II critical limb ischemia than in those with category III ischemia, greater in native arteries than in grafts, and greater in vein grafts than in prosthetic grafts.[132] Identification and repair of a graft stenosis after successful thrombolysis improve long-term graft patency. Thrombolytic regimens have employed streptokinase, urokinase, recombinant tissue plasminogen activator, reteplase, and tenecteplase. The duration of catheter-based thrombolytic therapy should generally not exceed 48 hours to achieve optimal benefit and to limit the risk of bleeding. It is not known whether adjuvant use of platelet glycoprotein IIb/IIIa inhibitors shortens thrombolysis time or improves outcome.[133] Percutaneous, catheter-based mechanical thrombectomy, with devices that apply hydrodynamic forces or rotating baskets, can be used alone or in addition to pharmacologic thrombolysis to treat patients with acute limb ischemia. Surgical thromboembolectomy is no longer common.[134] Surgical reconstruction, bypassing the occluded area, is an option for restoration of blood flow to an ischemic limb. These techniques were discussed previously in this chapter.

Five prospective randomized trials, comprising 1283 patients, have compared the benefits and risks of thrombolysis and surgical reconstruction in patients presenting with acute limb ischemia.[135] Overall, there was no difference in the rate of death or amputation during 1 year between the two interventions, although the risk of major bleeding within 30 days was greater in patients receiving thrombolysis. The findings from the individual trials suggest that catheter-based thrombolysis is an appropriate initial option in patients with category I and IIa acute limb ischemia of less than 14 days' duration, especially those with thrombosed bypass grafts, whereas surgical revascularization is more appropriate for those with category IIb and III acute limb ischemia and in those whose symptoms have lasted for more than 14 days (**Fig. 61-19**).[136]

Atheroembolism

Atheroembolism refers to the occlusion of arteries resulting from detachment and embolization of atheromatous debris, including fibrin, platelets, cholesterol crystals, and calcium fragments. Other terms include atherogenic embolism and cholesterol embolism. Atheroemboli originate most frequently from shaggy protruding atheromas of the aorta and less frequently from atherosclerotic branch arteries. The atheroemboli typically occlude small downstream arteries and arterioles of the extremities, brain, eye, kidneys, or mesentery.[137,138] The prevalence of atheroembolism in the general population is not known. Most affected individuals are men older than 60 years with clinical evidence of atherosclerosis.

Pathogenesis

The risk of atheroembolism is greatest in patients with aortic atherosclerosis characterized by large protruding atheromas (**Fig. 61-20**). Large aortic plaques identified by ultrasonography strongly associate with previous embolic disease.[137] Similarly, identification of large protruding atheromas by transesophageal ultrasound predicts future embolic events.[137,139] Atheroemboli typically occlude arterioles and small arteries. Approximately 50% of atheroemboli involve vessels in the lower extremities. Catheter manipulation causes a large proportion of atheroemboli, affecting approximately 1% to 2% of patients undergoing endovascular procedures.[138,140] Similarly, surgical manipulation of the aorta during cardiac or vascular operations may precipitate atheroembolism. Controversy remains as to whether anticoagulants or thrombolytic drugs contribute to atheroembolism.[139] Recent clinical trials of anticoagulant drugs have found a relatively low incidence of atheroembolism in patients with large aortic plaques.[137]

Clinical Presentation

The most notable clinical features of atheroembolism to the extremities include painful cyanotic toes, called blue toe syndrome (**Fig. 61-21**). Livedo reticularis occurs in approximately 50% of patients. Local areas of erythematous or violaceous discoloration may be present on the lateral aspects of the feet and the soles, and also on the calves. Other findings include digital and foot ulcerations, nodules, purpura, and petechiae. Pedal pulses are typically present because the emboli tend to lodge in the more distal digital arteries and arterioles. Symptoms and signs indicating additional organ involvement with atheroemboli should be sought. Funduscopy can visualize Hollenhorst plaques in patients with visual loss secondary to retinal ischemia or infarction. Renal involvement, manifested by increased blood pressure and azotemia, commonly occurs in patients with peripheral atheroemboli. Patients also sometimes show evidence of mesenteric or bladder ischemia and splenic infarction.

The clinical setting and findings are usually sufficient for diagnosis of atheroembolism, but some of the manifestations of

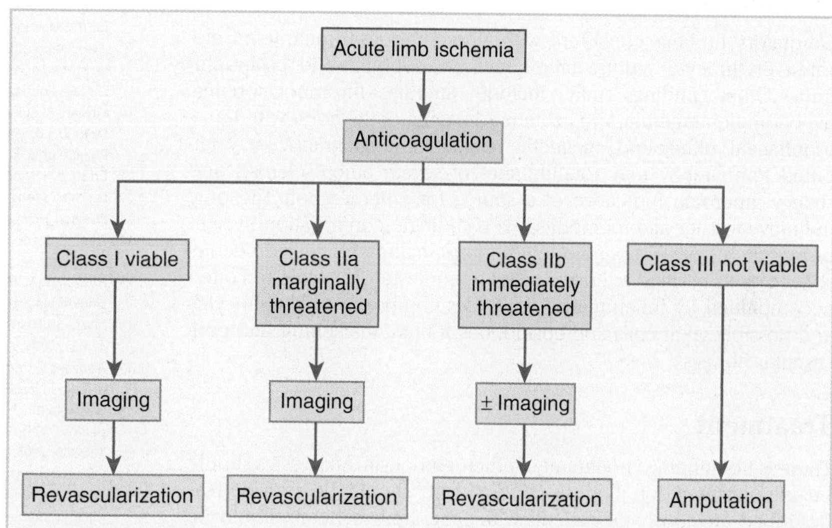

FIGURE 61-19 Management algorithm for the treatment of acute limb ischemia. *(Modified from Norgren L, Hiatt WR, Dormandy JA, et al: Inter-Society Consensus for the Management of Peripheral Arterial Disease [TASC II]. J Vasc Surg 45[Suppl S]:S5, 2007.)*

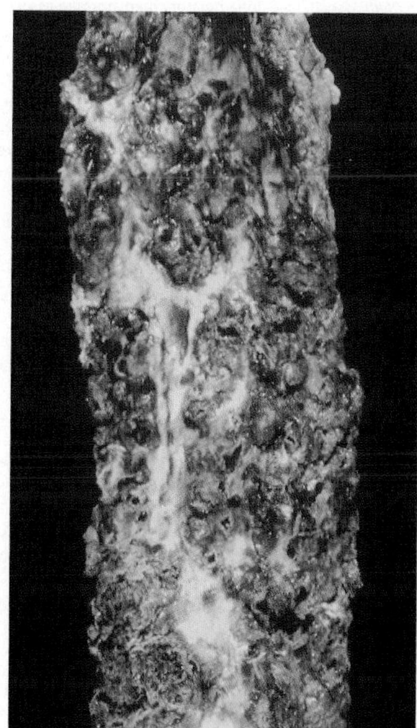

FIGURE 61-20 Atherosclerotic aorta of a patient with atheroemboli. There are multiple, protruding, shaggy atheromas with superimposed mural thrombi. *(Courtesy of R.N. Mitchell, MD, PhD, Department of Pathology, Brigham and Women's Hospital, Boston, Mass.)*

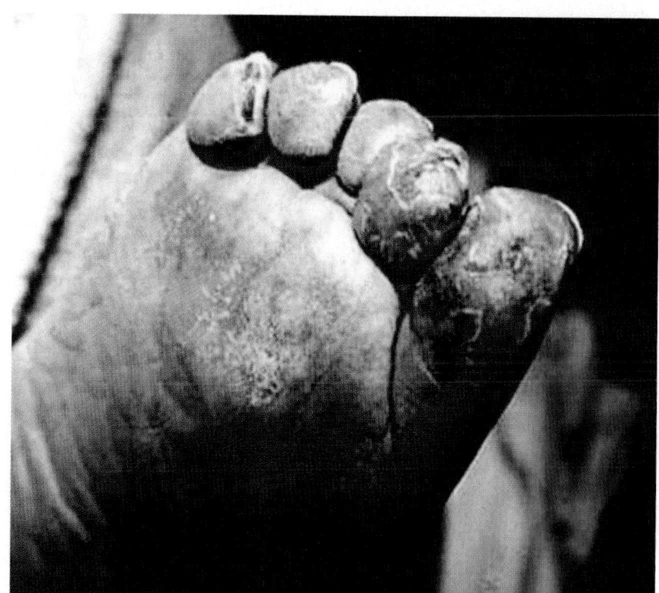

FIGURE 61-21 Atheroemboli to the foot or "blue toe syndrome." There is cyanotic discoloration of toes, with localized areas of violaceous discoloration. *(Modified from Beckman JA, Creager MA: Peripheral arterial disease: Clinical evaluation. In Creager MA, Dzau VJ, Loscalzo J [eds]: Vascular Medicine: A Companion to Braunwald's Heart Disease. Philadelphia, Elsevier, 2006, p 259.)*

atheroemboli may be present with other diseases. As discussed previously, critical limb ischemia occurs in patients with severe peripheral atherosclerosis, and acute limb ischemia is a consequence of thromboembolism, each of which would be characterized by an abnormal pulse examination. Hypersensitivity vasculitides secondary to connective tissue diseases, infections, drugs, polyarteritis nodosa, or cryoglobulinemia, for example, may be manifested with multisystem organ damage and cutaneous findings of purpura, ulcers, and digital ischemia similar to those resulting from atheroemboli (see Chap. 89). Procoagulant disorders such as antiphospholipid antibody syndrome, heparin-induced thrombocytopenia, and myeloproliferative disorders such as essential thrombocythemia can cause digital artery thrombosis with resultant digital ischemia, cyanosis, and ulceration.

Diagnostic Tests

Laboratory findings consistent with atheroembolism include an elevated erythrocyte sedimentation rate, eosinophilia, and eosinophiluria. Other findings may include anemia, thrombocytopenia, hypocomplementemia, and azotemia. Imaging of the aorta with transesophageal ultrasound, magnetic resonance angiography, or computed tomography may identify sites of severe atherosclerosis and shaggy atheroma indicative of a source for atheroemboli. The only definitive test for atheroembolism is pathologic confirmation by skin or muscle biopsy. Pathognomonic findings include elongated needle-shaped clefts in small arteries, caused by cholesterol crystals and often accompanied by inflammatory infiltrates composed of lymphocytes and possibly giant cells and eosinophils, intimal thickening, and perivascular fibrosis.

Treatment

There is no definitive treatment of atheroembolism. Analgesics should be administered for pain. Local foot care should be provided as described previously for patients with acute limb ischemia. It may be necessary to excise or to amputate necrotic areas.

Patients with this condition are subject to recurrent atheroembolic events. Risk factor modification, such as lipid-lowering therapy with statins and smoking cessation, can favorably affect overall outcome from atherosclerosis, but whether such intervention will prevent recurrent atheroembolism is unknown. The use of antiplatelet drugs to prevent recurrent atheroembolism remains controversial. It is reasonable, however, to administer antiplatelet agents even in the absence of strong clinical evidence of efficacy, because the agents will prevent other adverse cardiovascular events in patients with atherosclerosis. The use of warfarin also engenders controversy, and some investigators have even suggested that anticoagulants precipitate atheroemboli, whereas others have found that warfarin reduces atheroembolic events, particularly in patients with mobile aortic atheroma.[139] The use of corticosteroids to treat atheroembolism also is controversial.

Surgical removal of the source should be considered in patients with atheroembolism, particularly in those in whom it recurs. Surgical procedures include excision and replacement of affected portions of the aorta, endarterectomy, and bypass operations. Operative intervention is targeted to the site of the aorta and iliac or femoral arteries where there is aneurysm formation or obvious shaggy friable atherosclerotic plaque. Often, the aorta is diffusely affected by severe atherosclerosis, and it is not possible to identify the precise segment that is responsible for atheroembolism. In addition, many of these patients are elderly and have coexisting CAD, which increases the risk of major vascular operations. Endovascular placement of stents and stent grafts to prevent recurrent atheroembolism has been reported in several small case series.[138]

REFERENCES

Epidemiology

1. Hiatt WR, Goldstone J, Smith SC Jr, et al: Atherosclerotic Peripheral Vascular Disease Symposium II: Nomenclature for vascular diseases. Circulation 118:2826, 2008.
2. Steg PG, Bhatt DL, Wilson PW, et al: One-year cardiovascular event rates in outpatients with atherothrombosis. JAMA 297:1197, 2007.
3. Criqui MH: Peripheral arterial disease—epidemiological aspects. Vasc Med 6(Suppl):3, 2001.
4. Diehm C, Schuster A, Allenberg JR, et al: High prevalence of peripheral arterial disease and co-morbidity in 6880 primary care patients: Cross-sectional study. Atherosclerosis 172:95, 2004.
5. Selvin E, Erlinger TP: Prevalence of and risk factors for peripheral arterial disease in the United States: Results from the National Health and Nutrition Examination Survey, 1999-2000. Circulation 110:738, 2004.
6. Norgren L, Hiatt WR, Dormandy JA, et al: Inter-Society Consensus for the Management of Peripheral Arterial Disease (TASC II). J Vasc Surg 45(Suppl S):S5, 2007.
7. Criqui MH, Vargas V, Denenberg JO, et al: Ethnicity and peripheral arterial disease: The San Diego Population Study. Circulation 112:2703, 2005.
8. Allison MA, Criqui MH, McClelland RL, et al: The effect of novel cardiovascular risk factors on the ethnic-specific odds for peripheral arterial disease in the Multi-Ethnic Study of Atherosclerosis (MESA). J Am Coll Cardiol 48:1190, 2006.
9. Hirsch AT, Haskal ZJ, Hertzer NR, et al: ACC/AHA 2005 guidelines for the management of patients with peripheral arterial disease (lower extremity, renal, mesenteric, and abdominal aortic): Executive summary a collaborative report from the American Association for Vascular Surgery/Society for Vascular Surgery, Society for Cardiovascular Angiography and Interventions, Society for Vascular Medicine and Biology, Society of Interventional Radiology, and the ACC/AHA Task Force on Practice Guidelines (Writing Committee to Develop Guidelines for the Management of Patients With Peripheral Arterial Disease) endorsed by the American Association of Cardiovascular and Pulmonary Rehabilitation; National Heart, Lung, and Blood Institute; Society for Vascular Nursing; TransAtlantic Inter-Society Consensus; and Vascular Disease Foundation. J Am Coll Cardiol 47:1239, 2006.
10. Virmani R, Burke AP, Taylor AJ: Congenital malformations of the vasculature. *In* Creager MA, Dzau VJ, Loscalzo J (eds): Vascular Medicine: A Companion to Braunwald's Heart Disease. Philadelphia, Elsevier, 2006, pp 934-960.
11. Criqui MH, Ninomiya J: The epidemiology of peripheral arterial disease. *In* Creager MA, Dzau VJ, Loscalzo J (eds): Vascular Medicine: A Companion to Braunwald's Heart Disease. Philadelphia, Elsevier, 2006, pp 223-238.
12. Lu JT, Creager MA: The relationship of cigarette smoking to peripheral arterial disease. Rev Cardiovasc Med 5:189, 2004.
13. He Y, Jiang Y, Wang J, et al: Prevalence of peripheral arterial disease and its association with smoking in a population-based study in Beijing, China. J Vasc Surg 44:333, 2006.
14. Marso SP, Hiatt WR: Peripheral arterial disease in patients with diabetes. J Am Coll Cardiol 47:921, 2006.
15. Aboyans V, Criqui MH, Denenberg JO, et al: Risk factors for progression of peripheral arterial disease in large and small vessels. Circulation 113:2623, 2006.
16. Wattanakit K, Folsom AR, Selvin E, et al: Risk factors for peripheral arterial disease incidence in persons with diabetes: The Atherosclerosis Risk in Communities (ARIC) Study. Atherosclerosis 180:389, 2005.
17. Olin JW: Hypertension and peripheral arterial disease. Vasc Med 10:241, 2005.
18. Pande RL, Perlstein TS, Beckman JA, Creager MA: Association of insulin resistance and inflammation with peripheral arterial disease: The National Health and Nutrition Examination Survey, 1999 to 2004. Circulation 118:33, 2008.
19. Wattanakit K, Folsom AR, Selvin E, et al: Kidney function and risk of peripheral arterial disease: Results from the Atherosclerosis Risk in Communities (ARIC) Study. J Am Soc Nephrol 18:629, 2007.
20. Tzoulaki I, Murray GD, Lee AJ, et al: C-reactive protein, interleukin-6, and soluble adhesion molecules as predictors of progressive peripheral atherosclerosis in the general population: Edinburgh Artery Study. Circulation 112:976, 2005.
21. Barani J, Nilsson JA, Mattiasson I, et al: Inflammatory mediators are associated with 1-year mortality in critical limb ischemia. J Vasc Surg 42:75, 2005.
22. Brevetti G, Schiano V, Chiariello M: Cellular adhesion molecules and peripheral arterial disease. Vasc Med 11:39, 2006.
23. Wildman RP, Muntner P, Chen J, et al: Relation of inflammation to peripheral arterial disease in the national health and nutrition examination survey, 1999-2002. Am J Cardiol 96:1579, 2005.
24. Owens CD, Ridker PM, Belkin M, et al: Elevated C-reactive protein levels are associated with postoperative events in patients undergoing lower extremity vein bypass surgery. J Vasc Surg 45:2, 2007.
25. Pradhan AD, Shrivastava S, Cook NR, et al: Symptomatic peripheral arterial disease in women: Nontraditional biomarkers of elevated risk. Circulation 117:823, 2008.
26. Nasir K, Guallar E, Navas-Acien A, et al: Relationship of monocyte count and peripheral arterial disease: Results from the National Health and Nutrition Examination Survey 1999-2002. Arterioscler Thromb Vasc Biol 25:1966, 2005.
27. Perlstein TS, Pande RL, Beckman JA, Creager MA: Serum total bilirubin level and prevalent lower-extremity peripheral arterial disease: National Health and Nutrition Examination Survey (NHANES) 1999 to 2004. Arterioscler Thromb Vasc Biol 28:166, 2008.
28. Hiatt WR, Brass EP: Pathophysiology of claudication. *In* Creager MA (ed): Peripheral Arterial Disease. 2nd ed. London, Remedica, 2008, pp 49-70.
29. Hiatt WR, Brass EP: Pathophysiology of intermittent claudication. *In* Creager MA, Dzau VJ, Loscalzo J (eds): Vascular Medicine: A Companion to Braunwald's Heart Disease. Philadelphia, Elsevier, 2006, pp 239-247.
30. Bauer TA, Brass EP, Barstow TJ, Hiatt WR: Skeletal muscle StO_2 kinetics are slowed during low work rate calf exercise in peripheral arterial disease. Eur J Appl Physiol 100:143, 2007.
31. Isbell DC, Berr SS, Toledano AY, et al: Delayed calf muscle phosphocreatine recovery after exercise identifies peripheral arterial disease. J Am Coll Cardiol 47:2289, 2006.

Clinical Presentation

32. McDermott MM, Liu K, Greenland P, et al: Functional decline in peripheral arterial disease: Associations with the ankle brachial index and leg symptoms. JAMA 292:453, 2004 .
33. McDermott MM, Hoff F, Ferrucci L, et al: Lower extremity ischemia, calf skeletal muscle characteristics, and functional impairment in peripheral arterial disease. J Am Geriatr Soc 55:400, 2007.
34. Golomb BA, Criqui MH: Epidemiology. *In* Creager MA (ed): Peripheral Arterial Disease. 2nd ed. London, Remedica, 2008, pp 1-21.

35. Coyne KS, Margolis MK, Gilchrist KA, et al: Evaluating effects of method of administration on Walking Impairment Questionnaire. J Vasc Surg 38:296, 2003.
36. Khan NA, Rahim SA, Anand SS, et al: Does the clinical examination predict lower extremity peripheral arterial disease? JAMA 295:536, 2006.
37. Rutherford RB, Baker JD, Ernst C, et al: Recommended standards for reports dealing with lower extremity ischemia: Revised version. J Vasc Surg 26:517, 1997.

Testing in Peripheral Arterial Drsease

38. McDermott MM, Guralnik JM, Ferrucci L, et al: Physical activity, walking exercise, and calf skeletal muscle characteristics in patients with peripheral arterial disease. J Vasc Surg 46:87, 2007.
39. Chaudhry H, Holland A, Dormandy J: Comparison of graded versus constant treadmill test protocols for quantifying intermittent claudication. Vasc Med 2:93, 1997.
40. Collins R, Cranny G, Burch J, et al: A systematic review of duplex ultrasound, magnetic resonance angiography and computed tomography angiography for the diagnosis and assessment of symptomatic, lower limb peripheral arterial disease. Health Technol Assess 11:iii, xi, 1, 2007.
41. Ouwendijk R, Kock MC, Visser K, et al: Interobserver agreement for the interpretation of contrast-enhanced 3D MR angiography and MDCT angiography in peripheral arterial disease. AJR Am J Roentgenol 185:1261, 2005.
42. Ouwendijk R, de Vries M, Pattynama PM, et al: Imaging peripheral arterial disease: A randomized controlled trial comparing contrast-enhanced MR angiography and multi-detector row CT angiography. Radiology 236:1094, 2005.
43. Flohr TG, Schaller S, Stierstorfer K, et al: Multi-detector row CT systems and image-reconstruction techniques. Radiology 235:756, 2005.
44. Met R, Bipat S, Legemate DA, et al: Diagnostic performance of computed tomography angiography in peripheral arterial disease: A systematic review and meta-analysis. JAMA 301:415, 2009.

Prognosis

45. McDermott MM, Liu K, Criqui MH, et al: Ankle-brachial index and subclinical cardiac and carotid disease: The multi-ethnic study of atherosclerosis. Am J Epidemiol 162:33, 2005.
46. Cacoub PP, Abola MT, Baumgartner I, et al: Cardiovascular risk factor control and outcomes in peripheral artery disease patients in the Reduction of Atherothrombosis for Continued Health (REACH) Registry. Atherosclerosis 204:e86, 2009.
47. Fowkes FG, Low LP, Tuta S, Kozak J: Ankle-brachial index and extent of atherothrombosis in 8891 patients with or at risk of vascular disease: Results of the international AGATHA study. Eur Heart J 27:1861, 2006.
48. Doobay AV, Anand SS: Sensitivity and specificity of the ankle-brachial index to predict future cardiovascular outcomes: A systematic review. Arterioscler Thromb Vasc Biol 25:1463, 2005.
49. Fowkes FG, Murray GD, Butcher I, et al: Ankle brachial index combined with Framingham Risk Score to predict cardiovascular events and mortality: A meta-analysis. JAMA 300:197, 2008.
50. O'Hare AM, Katz R, Shlipak MG, et al: Mortality and cardiovascular risk across the ankle-arm index spectrum: Results from the Cardiovascular Health Study. Circulation 113:388, 2006.
51. Resnick HE, Lindsay RS, McDermott MM, et al: Relationship of high and low ankle brachial index to all-cause and cardiovascular disease mortality: The Strong Heart Study. Circulation 109:733, 2004.
52. Criqui MH, Ninomiya JK, Wingard DL, et al: Progression of peripheral arterial disease predicts cardiovascular disease morbidity and mortality. J Am Coll Cardiol 52:1736, 2008.
53. Aquino R, Johnnides C, Makaroun M, et al: Natural history of claudication: Long-term serial follow-up study of 1244 claudicants. J Vasc Surg 34:962, 2001.
54. Fosse S, Hartemann-Heurtier A, Jacqueminet S, et al: Incidence and characteristics of lower limb amputations in people with diabetes. Diabet Med 26:391, 2009.

Treatment

55. Randomized trial of the effects of cholesterol-lowering with simvastatin on peripheral vascular and other major vascular outcomes in 20,536 people with peripheral arterial disease and other high-risk conditions. J Vasc Surg 45:645; discussion 653, 2007.
56. Aung PP, Maxwell HG, Jepson RG, et al: Lipid-lowering for peripheral arterial disease of the lower limb. Cochrane Database Syst Rev (4):CD000123, 2007.
57. Aronow WS, Nayak D, Woodworth S, Ahn C: Effect of simvastatin versus placebo on treadmill exercise time until the onset of intermittent claudication in older patients with peripheral arterial disease at six months and at one year after treatment. Am J Cardiol 92:711, 2003.
58. Mohler ER 3rd, Hiatt WR, Creager MA: Cholesterol reduction with atorvastatin improves walking distance in patients with peripheral arterial disease. Circulation 108:1481, 2003.
59. Mondillo S, Ballo P, Barbati R, et al: Effects of simvastatin on walking performance and symptoms of intermittent claudication in hypercholesterolemic patients with peripheral vascular disease. Am J Med 114:359, 2003.
60. Momsen AH, Jensen MB, Norager CB, et al: Drug therapy for improving walking distance in intermittent claudication: A systematic review and meta-analysis of robust randomised controlled studies. Eur J Vasc Endovasc Surg 38:463, 2009 .
61. McDermott MM, Guralnik JM, Greenland P, et al: Statin use and leg functioning in patients with and without lower-extremity peripheral arterial disease. Circulation 107:757, 2003.
62. Rajamani K, Colman PG, Li LP, et al: Effect of fenofibrate on amputation events in people with type 2 diabetes mellitus (FIELD study): A prespecified analysis of a randomised controlled trial. Lancet 373:1780, 2009.
63. Gonzales D, Rennard SI, Nides M, et al: Varenicline, an $\alpha 4\beta 2$ nicotinic acetylcholine receptor partial agonist, vs sustained-release bupropion and placebo for smoking cessation: A randomized controlled trial. JAMA 296:47, 2006.
64. Jorenby DE, Hays JT, Rigotti NA, et al: Efficacy of varenicline, an $\alpha 4\beta 2$ nicotinic acetylcholine receptor partial agonist, vs placebo or sustained-release bupropion for smoking cessation: A randomized controlled trial. JAMA 296:56, 2006.
65. Nathan DM, Cleary PA, Backlund JY, et al: Intensive diabetes treatment and cardiovascular disease in patients with type 1 diabetes. N Engl J Med 353:2643, 2005.
66. Nathan DM, Lachin J, Cleary P, et al: Intensive diabetes therapy and carotid intima-media thickness in type 1 diabetes mellitus. N Engl J Med 348:2294, 2003.
67. Holman RR, Paul SK, Bethel MA, et al: 10-year follow-up of intensive glucose control in type 2 diabetes. N Engl J Med 359:1577, 2008.
68. Gerstein HC, Miller ME, Byington RP, et al: Effects of intensive glucose lowering in type 2 diabetes. N Engl J Med 358:2545, 2008.
69. Patel A, MacMahon S, Chalmers J, et al: Intensive blood glucose control and vascular outcomes in patients with type 2 diabetes. N Engl J Med 358:2560, 2008.
70. Duckworth W, Abraira C, Moritz T, et al: Glucose control and vascular complications in veterans with type 2 diabetes. N Engl J Med 360:129, 2009.
71. Dormandy JA, Charbonnel B, Eckland DJ, et al: Secondary prevention of macrovascular events in patients with type 2 diabetes in the PROactive Study (PROspective pioglitAzone Clinical Trial In macroVascular Events): A randomised controlled trial. Lancet 366:1279, 2005.
72. Dormandy JA, Betteridge DJ, Schernthaner G, et al: Impact of peripheral arterial disease in patients with diabetes—results from PROactive (PROactive 11). Atherosclerosis 202:272, 2009.
73. Ray KK, Seshasai SR, Wijesuriya S, et al: Effect of intensive control of glucose on cardiovascular outcomes and death in patients with diabetes mellitus: A meta-analysis of randomised controlled trials. Lancet 373:1765, 2009.
74. Skyler JS, Bergenstal R, Bonow RO, et al: Intensive glycemic control and the prevention of cardiovascular events: Implications of the ACCORD, ADVANCE, and VA diabetes trials: A position statement of the American Diabetes Association and a scientific statement of the American College of Cardiology Foundation and the American Heart Association. Circulation 119:351, 2009.
75. Mehler PS, Coll JR, Estacio R, et al: Intensive blood pressure control reduces the risk of cardiovascular events in patients with peripheral arterial disease and type 2 diabetes. Circulation 107:753, 2003.
76. The ACCORD Study Group: Effects of intensive blood-pressure control in type 2 diabetes mellitus. N Engl J Med 362:1575, 2010.
77. Paravastu SC, Mendonca D, Da Silva A: Beta blockers for peripheral arterial disease. Cochrane Database Syst Rev (4):CD005508, 2008.
78. Chobanian AV, Bakris GL, Black HR, et al: The Seventh Report of the Joint National Committee on Prevention, Detection, Evaluation, and Treatment of High Blood Pressure: The JNC 7 report. JAMA 289:2560, 2003.
79. Bosch J, Lonn E, Pogue J, et al: Long-term effects of ramipril on cardiovascular events and on diabetes: Results of the HOPE study extension. Circulation 112:1339, 2005.
80. Yusuf S, Teo KK, Pogue J, et al: Telmisartan, ramipril, or both in patients at high risk for vascular events. N Engl J Med 358:1547, 2008.
81. Collaborative meta-analysis of randomised trials of antiplatelet therapy for prevention of death, myocardial infarction, and stroke in high risk patients. BMJ 324:71, 2002.
82. Berger JS, Krantz MJ, Kittelson JM, Hiatt WR: Aspirin for the prevention of cardiovascular events in patients with peripheral artery disease: A meta-analysis of randomized trials. JAMA 301:1909, 2009.
83. Belch J, MacCuish A, Campbell I, et al: The prevention of progression of arterial disease and diabetes (POPADAD) trial: Factorial randomised placebo controlled trial of aspirin and antioxidants in patients with diabetes and asymptomatic peripheral arterial disease. BMJ 337:a1840, 2008.
84. Fowkes FG, Price JF, Stewart MC, et al: Aspirin for prevention of cardiovascular events in a general population screened for a low ankle brachial index: A randomized controlled trial. JAMA 303:841, 2010.
85. A randomised, blinded, trial of clopidogrel versus aspirin in patients at risk of ischaemic events (CAPRIE). CAPRIE Steering Committee. Lancet 348:1329, 1996.
86. Bhatt DL, Fox KA, Hacke W, et al: Clopidogrel and aspirin versus aspirin alone for the prevention of atherothrombotic events. N Engl J Med 354:1706, 2006.
87. Cacoub PP, Bhatt DL, Steg PG, et al: Patients with peripheral arterial disease in the CHARISMA trial. Eur Heart J 30:192, 2009.
88. Anand S, Yusuf S, Xie C, et al: Oral anticoagulant and antiplatelet therapy and peripheral arterial disease. N Engl J Med 357:217, 2007.
89. Creager MA, Pande RL, Hiatt WR: A randomized trial of iloprost in patients with intermittent claudication. Vasc Med 13:5, 2008.
90. Robless P, Mikhailidis DP, Stansby GP: Cilostazol for peripheral arterial disease. Cochrane Database Syst Rev (1):CD003748, 2007.
91. Pande RL, Hiatt WR, Zhang P, et al: A pooled analysis of the durability and predictors of treatment response of cilostazol in patients with intermittent claudication. Vasc Med 15:181, 2010.
92. Hiatt WR, Money SR, Brass EP: Long-term safety of cilostazol in patients with peripheral artery disease: The CASTLE study (Cilostazol: A Study in Long-term Effects). J Vasc Surg 47:330, 2008.
93. Ahimastos AA, Lawler A, Reid CM, et al: Brief communication: Ramipril markedly improves walking ability in patients with peripheral arterial disease: A randomized trial. Ann Intern Med 144:660, 2006.
94. Hiatt WR, Hirsch AT, Cooke JP, et al: Randomized trial of AT-1015 for treatment of intermittent claudication. A novel 5-hydroxytryptamine antagonist with no evidence of efficacy. Vasc Med 9:18, 2004.
95. Norgren L, Jawien A, Matyas L, et al: Sarpogrelate, a 5-hT2A receptor antagonist in intermittent claudication. A phase II European study. Vasc Med 11:75, 2006.
96. Leizorovicz A, Becker F: Oral buflomedil in the prevention of cardiovascular events in patients with peripheral arterial obstructive disease: A randomized, placebo-controlled, 4-year study. Circulation 117:816, 2008.
97. Wilson AM, Harada R, Nair N, et al: L-Arginine supplementation in peripheral arterial disease: No benefit and possible harm. Circulation 116:188, 2007.
98. Hiatt WR: Carnitine and peripheral arterial disease. Ann N Y Acad Sci 1033:92, 2004.
99. Mohler ER 3rd, Hiatt WR, Olin JW, et al: Treatment of intermittent claudication with beraprost sodium, an orally active prostaglandin I_2 analogue: A double-blinded, randomized, controlled trial. J Am Coll Cardiol 41:1679, 2003.
100. Jaff MR, Dale RA, Creager MA, et al: Anti-chlamydial antibiotic therapy for symptom improvement in peripheral artery disease: Prospective evaluation of rifalazil effect on vascular symptoms of intermittent claudication and other endpoints in *Chlamydia pneumoniae* seropositive patients (PROVIDENCE-1). Circulation 119:452, 2009.

101. Rajagopalan S, Olin J, Deitcher S, et al: Use of a constitutively active hypoxia-inducible factor-1α transgene as a therapeutic strategy in no-option critical limb ischemia patients: Phase I dose-escalation experience. Circulation 115:1234, 2007.
102. Nikol S, Baumgartner I, Van Belle E, et al: Therapeutic angiogenesis with intramuscular NV1FGF improves amputation-free survival in patients with critical limb ischemia. Mol Ther 16:972, 2008.
103. Powell RJ, Simons M, Mendelsohn FO, et al: Results of a double-blind, placebo-controlled study to assess the safety of intramuscular injection of hepatocyte growth factor plasmid to improve limb perfusion in patients with critical limb ischemia. Circulation 118:58, 2008.
104. Rajagopalan S, Mohler ER 3rd, Lederman RJ, et al: Regional angiogenesis with vascular endothelial growth factor in peripheral arterial disease: A phase II randomized, double-blind, controlled study of adenoviral delivery of vascular endothelial growth factor 121 in patients with disabling intermittent claudication. Circulation 108:1933, 2003.
105. Creager MA: Treatment of intermittent claudication with hypoxia-inducible factor-1α. Paper presented at Late Breaking Clinical Trials Session of the American College of Cardiology 58th Annual Scientific Sessions; March 2009; Orlando, Florida.
106. Bartsch T, Brehm M, Zeus T, et al: Transplantation of autologous mononuclear bone marrow stem cells in patients with peripheral arterial disease (the TAM-PAD study). Clin Res Cardiol 96:891, 2007.
107. Burt RK, Loh Y, Pearce W, et al: Clinical applications of blood-derived and marrow-derived stem cells for nonmalignant diseases. JAMA 299:925, 2008.
108. Burt RK, Testori A, Oyama Y, et al: Autologous peripheral blood $CD133^+$ cell implantation for limb salvage in patients with critical limb ischemia. Bone Marrow Transplant 45:111, 2010.
109. Matoba S, Tatsumi T, Murohara T, et al: Long-term clinical outcome after intramuscular implantation of bone marrow mononuclear cells (Therapeutic Angiogenesis by Cell Transplantation [TACT] trial) in patients with chronic limb ischemia. Am Heart J 156:1010, 2008.
110. Watson L, Ellis B, Leng GC: Exercise for intermittent claudication. Cochrane Database Syst Rev (4):CD000990, 2008.
111. McDermott MM, Ades P, Guralnik JM, et al: Treadmill exercise and resistance training in patients with peripheral arterial disease with and without intermittent claudication: A randomized controlled trial. JAMA 301:165, 2009.
112. Stewart KJ, Hiatt WR, Regensteiner JG, Hirsch AT: Exercise training for claudication. N Engl J Med 347:1941, 2002.
113. Brass EP, Hiatt WR, Green S: Skeletal muscle metabolic changes in peripheral arterial disease contribute to exercise intolerance: A point-counterpoint discussion. Vasc Med 9:293, 2004.
114. Sandri M, Adams V, Gielen S, et al: Effects of exercise and ischemia on mobilization and functional activation of blood-derived progenitor cells in patients with ischemic syndromes: Results of 3 randomized studies. Circulation 111:3391, 2005.
115. Arany Z, Foo SY, Ma Y, et al: HIF-independent regulation of VEGF and angiogenesis by the transcriptional coactivator PGC-1α. Nature 451:1008, 2008.
116. Hambrecht R, Adams V, Erbs S, et al: Regular physical activity improves endothelial function in patients with coronary artery disease by increasing phosphorylation of endothelial nitric oxide synthase. Circulation 107:3152, 2003.
117. Gardner AW, Katzel LI, Sorkin JD, et al: Exercise rehabilitation improves functional outcomes and peripheral circulation in patients with intermittent claudication: A randomized controlled trial. J Am Geriatr Soc 49:755, 2001.
118. White CJ, Gray WA: Endovascular therapies for peripheral arterial disease: An evidence-based review. Circulation 116:2203, 2007.
119. Fleisher LA, Beckman JA, Brown KA, et al: ACC/AHA 2007 Guidelines on Perioperative Cardiovascular Evaluation and Care for Noncardiac Surgery: Executive Summary: A Report of the American College of Cardiology/American Heart Association Task Force on Practice Guidelines (Writing Committee to Revise the 2002 Guidelines on Perioperative Cardiovascular Evaluation for Noncardiac Surgery): Developed in Collaboration With the American Society of Echocardiography, American Society of Nuclear Cardiology, Heart Rhythm Society, Society of Cardiovascular Anesthesiologists, Society for Cardiovascular Angiography and Interventions, Society for Vascular Medicine and Biology, and Society for Vascular Surgery. Circulation 116:1971, 2007.
120. Dorffler-Melly J, Buller HR, Koopman MM, Prins MH: Antithrombotic agents for preventing thrombosis after infrainguinal arterial bypass surgery. Cochrane Database Syst Rev (4):CD000536, 2003.

Thromboangitis, Obliterans, Fibromuscular Dysplasia, and Popliteal Artery Entrapment Syndrome

121. Dorffler-Melly J, Koopman MM, Adam DJ, et al: Antiplatelet agents for preventing thrombosis after peripheral arterial bypass surgery. Cochrane Database Syst Rev (3):CD000535, 2003.
122. Brown J, Lethaby A, Maxwell H, et al: Antiplatelet agents for preventing thrombosis after peripheral arterial bypass surgery. Cochrane Database Syst Rev (4):CD000535, 2008.
123. Olin JW: Thromboangiitis obliterans (Buerger's disease). *In* Creager MA, Dzau VJ, Loscalzo J (eds): Vascular Medicine: A Companion to Braunwald's Heart Disease. Philadelphia, Elsevier, 2006, pp 641-656.
124. Olin JW, Shih A: Thromboangiitis obliterans (Buerger's disease). Curr Opin Rheumatol 18:18, 2006.
125. Cooper LT, Tse TS, Mikhail MA, et al: Long-term survival and amputation risk in thromboangiitis obliterans (Buerger's disease). J Am Coll Cardiol 44:2410, 2004.
126. Sasajima T, Kubo Y, Inaba M, et al: Role of infrainguinal bypass in Buerger's disease: An eighteen-year experience. Eur J Vasc Endovasc Surg 13:186, 1997.
127. Slovut DP, Olin JW: Fibromuscular dysplasia. N Engl J Med 350:1862, 2004.
128. Rigberg DA, Freischlag JA, Machleder HE: Vascular compression syndromes. *In* Creager MA, Dzau VJ, Loscalzo J (eds): Vascular Medicine: A Companion to Braunwald's Heart Disease. Philadelphia, Elsevier, 2006, pp 920-933.
129. Korngold EC, Jaff MR: Unusual causes of intermittent claudication: Popliteal artery entrapment syndrome, cystic adventitial disease, fibromuscular dysplasia, and endofibrosis. Curr Treat Options Cardiovasc Med 11:156, 2009.

Acute Limb Ischemia

130. Braithwaite BD, Davies B, Birch PA, et al: Management of acute leg ischaemia in the elderly. Br J Surg 85:217, 1998.
131. Ouriel K: Acute arterial occlusion. *In* Creager MA, Dzau VJ, Loscalzo J (eds): Vascular Medicine: A Companion to Braunwald's Heart Disease. Philadelphia, Elsevier, 2006, pp 669-676.
132. Thrombolysis in the management of lower limb peripheral arterial occlusion—a consensus document. J Vasc Interv Radiol 14(pt 2):S337, 2003.
133. Kessel DO, Berridge DC, Robertson I: Infusion techniques for peripheral arterial thrombolysis. Cochrane Database Syst Rev (1):CD000985, 2004.
134. Dormandy J, Heeck L, Vig S: Acute limb ischemia. Semin Vasc Surg 12:148, 1999.
135. Berridge DC, Kessel D, Robertson I: Surgery versus thrombolysis for acute limb ischaemia: Initial management. Cochrane Database Syst Rev (3):CD002784, 2002.
136. Sobel M, Verhaeghe R: Antithrombotic therapy for peripheral artery occlusive disease: American College of Chest Physicians Evidence-Based Clinical Practice Guidelines (8th Edition). Chest 133(Suppl):815S, 2008.

Artheroembolism

137. Tunick PA, Kronzon I: Atheroembolism. *In* Creager MA, Dzau VJ, Loscalzo J (eds): Vascular Medicine: A Companion to Braunwald's Heart Disease. Philadelphia, Elsevier, 2006, pp 677-687.
138. Liew YP, Bartholomew JR: Atheromatous embolization. Vasc Med 10:309, 2005.
139. Molisse TA, Tunick PA, Kronzon I: Complications of aortic atherosclerosis: Atheroemboli and thromboemboli. Curr Treat Options Cardiovasc Med 9:137, 2007.
140. Fukumoto Y, Tsutsui H, Tsuchihashi M, et al: The incidence and risk factors of cholesterol embolization syndrome, a complication of cardiac catheterization: A prospective study. J Am Coll Cardiol 42:211, 2003.

CHAPTER 62 Prevention and Management of Stroke

Larry B. Goldstein

Each year, more than 795,000 Americans have strokes and more than 150,000 die, making stroke the country's third leading cause of death.[1] More than 25% of stroke survivors older than 65 years of age are institutionalized 6 months later. Stroke disproportionately affects minority populations (see Chap. 2). Over 60% of stroke-related deaths occur in women, and women have greater poststroke disability than men (see Chap. 81). Advancing age is a major risk factor for stroke, but more than one third of strokes occur in persons younger than 65 years of age, and even children can be affected. Many of the risk factors for stroke overlap with those of cardiac and peripheral vascular disease (consistent with the concept of global risk), yet stroke represents a variety of conditions and can reflect a diverse set of pathophysiologic processes, and specific therapeutic interventions can confer levels of benefit and risk that differ from those for other forms of vascular disease. This discussion focuses on therapeutic interventions for stroke prevention and treatment of particular relevance to cardiologists. The American Stroke Association and American Heart Association have provided detailed, current, evidence-based guidelines for the primary prevention of ischemic stroke,[2] prevention of ischemic stroke in patients with prior stroke or transient ischemic attack,[3,4] and early management of patients with ischemic stroke, including the use of thrombolytic therapy.[5-7]

Medical Therapy for Stroke Prevention

Approximately 77% of strokes are first events, making primary prevention of paramount importance.[1] Prevention of recurrent events is also critical. Depending on age and race or ethnicity, approximately 10% to 30% of survivors will have a second stroke within 5 years. The period soon after the stroke entails the highest rate of recurrence. The risk of ischemic stroke after a transient ischemic attack (TIA, a condition frequently misdiagnosed, that has been defined as a brief episode of neurologic dysfunction that results from focal brain or retinal ischemia, with clinical symptoms that typically last less than 1 hour and with no radiologic evidence of infarction) is as high as 10.5% over 90 days, with the highest risk over the first week.[3] The ABCD^2 score is helpful in assessing the short-term risk of stroke in patients with TIA (**Table 62-1**).[8] The risk of stroke within 2 days is low (1%) in those with a score of 0 to 3, moderate (4%) in those with a score of 4 or 5, and high (8%) in those with a score of 6 or 7. The risks and benefits of therapeutic interventions differ for primary and secondary stroke prevention.

Platelet Antiaggregants

PRIMARY PREVENTION. The use of antiplatelet agents for primary stroke prevention requires consideration in the context of the patient's global risk for cardiovascular events and stroke. No evidence has shown that antiplatelet therapy reduces stroke in persons at low risk.[2]

The benefit of aspirin for primary cardiovascular prophylaxis outweighs its associated risk of bleeding complications in persons with a 10-year risk of coronary heart events of 6% to 10%, but does not reduce stroke risk even in men, and aspirin is not recommended for this purpose.[2] Although the Women's Health Study found no reduction in its prespecified primary endpoint (nonfatal myocardial infarction [MI], nonfatal stroke, or cardiovascular death) with aspirin (100 mg on alternate days), stroke fell 17%, although the risk of bleeding increased.[9] This benefit accrued primarily in women at elevated stroke risk because of other factors (e.g., hypertension, diabetes). Thus, aspirin may be considered for women whose risk of stroke outweighs its associated bleeding risk. Evidence does not support the benefit of any other antiplatelet agent in reducing the risk of a first stroke.

Anticoagulation is generally recommended for stroke prevention in patients with atrial fibrillation who are at high risk of systemic embolization (see later and Chap. 40).[2] Aspirin plus clopidogrel may decrease the risk of major vascular events (MVEs, predominately stroke) and stroke (**Fig. 62-1**) as compared with aspirin alone in patients with atrial fibrillation judged not to be candidates for anticoagulation, but the combination increases the risk of major bleeding complications—so there was no overall net benefit (MVEs decreased 0.8%/year, major hemorrhages increased 0.7%/year; relative risk [RR], 0.97; 95% confidence interval [CI], 0.89 to 1.06; $P = 0.54$).[10]

SECONDARY PREVENTION. Aspirin (lowest effective dose compared with placebo is 50 mg/day) lowers the risk of recurrent stroke in persons with a noncardioembolic ischemic stroke by approximately 18%.[3] Sustained-release dipyridamole (200 mg twice daily) is as effective as aspirin in reducing the risk of recurrent stroke, with a further reduction (approximately 37%) when the two drugs are combined.[11] Aspirin–sustained-release dipyridamole is available in the United States in a fixed-dose combination (25 mg aspirin plus 200 mg dipyridamole) given twice daily. Cardiologists often worry that dipyridamole might increase the risk of cardiac ischemia, but clinical trials have not substantiated this reservation. There is also concern that the total dose of aspirin (50 mg/day), although effective for secondary stroke prophylaxis, is below the dose shown to be effective for cardiac prophylaxis. To address this potential limitation, a small additional dose of aspirin can be added (e.g., 81 mg/day) to the fixed combination of aspirin-dipyridamole.

Clopidogrel monotherapy given to patients with a history of MI, stroke, or symptomatic peripheral arterial disease reduces the combined risk of MI, stroke, or vascular death as compared with aspirin by 8.7%.[3] Although based on a potentially underpowered subgroup analysis, there is no evidence of a significant reduction in stroke among those with prior stroke. There was no reduction in a composite endpoint of MI, stroke, or cardiovascular death in patients with cardiovascular disease (including stroke) or multiple risk factors with aspirin plus clopidogrel as compared with aspirin alone.[12] When tested directly in patients with stroke, the combination of aspirin and clopidogrel increased bleeding complications without reducing ischemic stroke.[13] Aspirin and clopidogrel should not be used in combination for stroke prophylaxis in patients at high risk or in patients with recent stroke.

CH 62

TABLE 62-1 Short-Term Risk of Stroke After Transient Ischemic Attack: ABCD² Score

FACTOR	POINTS
Age ≧ 60 years	1
BP ≧ 140/90 mm Hg	1
Clinical features	
• Speech deficit, no weakness	1
• Unilateral weakness	2
Diabetes	1
Duration (minutes)	
• 0-59	1
• ≧60	2

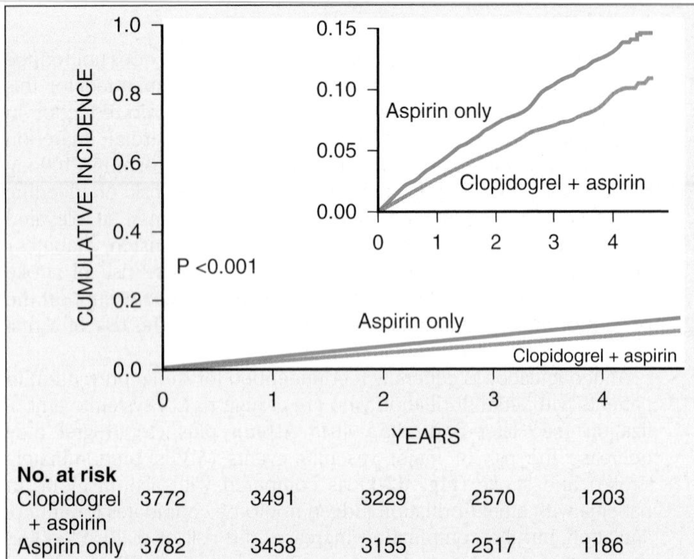

FIGURE 62-1 Clopidogrel plus aspirin versus aspirin alone in patients with atrial fibrillation judged not to be candidates for anticoagulation and risk of stroke. *(From ACTIVE Investigators: Effect of clopidogrel added to aspirin in patients with atrial fibrillation. N Engl J Med 360:2066, 2009.)*

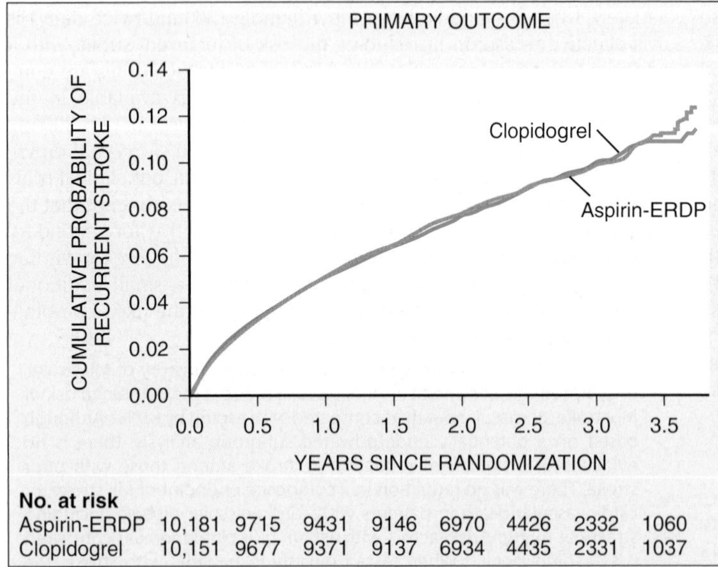

FIGURE 62-2 Clopidogrel versus aspirin plus extended-release dipyridamole (ERDP) for secondary stroke prevention. The primary outcome is time to first recurrent stroke. *(From Sacco RL, Diener HC, Yusuf S, et al: Aspirin and extended-release dipyridamole versus clopidogrel for recurrent stroke. N Engl J Med 359:1238, 2008.)*

A direct comparison found that aspirin plus dipyridamole was comparable to clopidogrel monotherapy for secondary stroke prevention in patients with noncardioembolic stroke (**Fig. 62-2**).[14] Aspirin, aspirin plus sustained-release dipyridamole, and clopidogrel are reasonable options for secondary prevention in these types of patients.[4]

Anticoagulation

PRIMARY PREVENTION. The use of long-term anticoagulation to reduce the risk of a first cardiogenic embolism in patients at increased risk caused by conditions such as mechanical heart valves, atrial fibrillation, and cardiomyopathy is addressed in Chaps. 28, 40, and 66. The combination of aspirin and clopidogrel is inferior to warfarin for stroke prevention in patients with atrial fibrillation (**Fig. 62-3**).[15]

SECONDARY PREVENTION. The evidence supporting the use of anticoagulation for prevention of recurrent stroke in patients without atrial fibrillation or other high-risk cardiogenic sources is uncertain, or the evidence suggests that the benefit does not outweigh the risk of warfarin-associated bleeding complications.

For patients with noncardioembolic stroke, the Warfarin-Aspirin Recurrent Stroke Study (WARSS) directly compared warfarin (international normalized ratio [INR], 2 to 3) and aspirin (325 mg/day).[16] There was a nonsignificant advantage associated with aspirin treatment (17.8% rate of recurrent stroke or death for warfarin, versus 16.0% for aspirin, $P = 0.25$; **Fig. 62-4**). Given the increased costs and monitoring associated with warfarin, there is no reason to use this drug for this purpose.

Although based on a post hoc analysis, data from WARSS also evaluated the problem of what has been termed *aspirin failures*. This term is used variably to refer to patients taking aspirin who have no measurable platelet antiaggregant effect, or to patients who have a recurrent ischemic event such as stroke despite treatment. The latter definition was used in the WARSS analysis. Of the patients who had a history of stroke before the study index stroke, those taking aspirin before randomization (i.e., aspirin failures) and randomized to receive aspirin had a 31.8% rate of recurrent stroke as compared with a 16.9% rate in those who were randomized to aspirin but had not been taking aspirin before randomization (i.e., the rate of recurrent stroke was higher in those who had failed aspirin). The rate of recurrent stroke, however, was 29% in those who had failed aspirin and were randomized to warfarin. Therefore, based on the data from WARSS, despite a high rate of recurrent stroke in patients failing aspirin who subsequently received aspirin, treatment with warfarin showed no advantage. No data show that patients who fail aspirin benefit from an alternative antiplatelet regimen.

A retrospective data analysis has suggested that patients with symptomatic, intracranial, large-vessel stenotic disease benefited from warfarin as compared with aspirin.[17] This hypothesis was subsequently tested in the Warfarin-Aspirin Symptomatic Intracranial Disease (WASID) trial comparing warfarin (INR, 2 to 3) with aspirin (1300 mg/day).[18] The rate of recurrent ischemic stroke, intracerebral hemorrhage, or nonstroke vascular death did not differ between the two treatment regimens (22% with warfarin versus 21% with aspirin; $P = 0.83$), but there was a higher rate of major hemorrhages with warfarin (8.3% versus 3.2%; $P = 0.01$). Because of a lack of efficacy and higher rate of bleeding complications, warfarin should generally not be used for patients with symptomatic large-vessel intracranial stenotic disease. Angioplasty and stenting may also be considered for patients with this condition who fail medical therapy, but no prospective randomized trial has compared this approach with medical therapy.

Although a patent foramen ovale (PFO, with or without an atrial septal aneurysm) is found more commonly in young patients with cryptogenic stroke, optimal medical therapy for secondary stroke prophylaxis is uncertain, and randomized trials assessing the potential benefits of endovascular closure as compared with medical therapy are underway (see Chap. 59). Uncertainty about appropriate management exists in part because of the unclear relationship between the presence of PFO (whether large or small, and with or without an atrial septal aneurysm) and the risk of recurrent stroke and death. A systematic literature review of 129 articles identified four meeting minimal quality criteria and found, as compared with those without a PFO, that there was no significant increase in recurrent stroke or death for those with PFO (odds ratio [OR], 0.95; 95% CI, 0.62 to 1.44), small PFO (OR, 1.23; 95% CI, 0.76 to 2.00), large PFO (OR, 0.59; 95% CI, 0.28 to 1.24), or combined PFO and atrial septal aneurysm (OR, 2.10; 95% CI, 0.86 to 5.06).[19] This finding agrees with the results of the subsequently reported PFO in Cryptogenic Stroke Study (PICSS) that found almost identical rates of recurrent stroke or death, regardless of the presence of a PFO.[20] Essentially, no prospective randomized trials have compared antiplatelet and anticoagulant therapy in this setting, and PICSS found almost identical rates of recurrent stroke or death with aspirin or warfarin in those with and without a PFO.

Patients with low ejection fraction (EF) congestive heart failure are also at risk for systemic embolization, but data from large prospective randomized trials were previously unavailable to determine optimal antithrombotic therapy. The Warfarin and Antiplatelet Therapy in Chronic Heart Failure (WATCH) trial compared open-label warfarin (target INR, 2.5 to 3.0) with double-blind treatment with clopidogrel or aspirin in patients in sinus rhythm with chronic congestive heart failure (EF < 35%).[21] There were no differences between warfarin and aspirin (hazard ratio [HR], 0.98; 95% CI, 0.86 to 1.12; $P = 0.77$), between warfarin and clopidogrel (HR, 0.89; 95% CI, 0.68 to 1.16; $P = 0.39$), or between clopidogrel and aspirin (HR, 1.08; 95% CI, 0.83 to 1.40; $P = 0.57$) for the primary outcome (time to nonfatal stroke, nonfatal MI, or death). There was also no evidence that warfarin is superior to aspirin or that clopidogrel is superior to aspirin for stroke prevention in patients with low ejection fraction congestive heart failure.

The various inherited (e.g., protein C, protein S, antithrombin III deficiency, factor V Leiden, prothrombin G20210A mutation) and acquired (e.g., lupus anticoagulant, anticardiolipin, or antiphospholipid antibodies) coagulopathies are more commonly associated with venous as compared with arterial thromboses (see Chap. 87).[3] Although occasionally these disorders associate with ischemic stroke, particularly in children or young adults, causal relationships remain controversial. For example, in another substudy of the WARSS trial, the Antiphospholipid Antibody Stroke Study (APASS), 41% of 1770 subjects were positive for one or more antiphospholipid antibodies.[22] Rates of recurrent thromboembolic events were somewhat higher for those who were antiphospholipid antibody–positive, but there was no difference for those antibody-positive patients who were treated with warfarin as compared with aspirin. Patients with venous thromboembolic events who have an underlying coagulopathy, or those with stroke or TIA otherwise fulfilling the criteria for the antiphospholipid antibody syndrome (venous and arterial occlusive disease in multiple organs, miscarriages, and livedo reticularis) are appropriately treated with warfarin. Because coagulopathies, especially the genetic forms listed, are more commonly associated with venous thromboses, cryptogenic stroke in this setting should prompt an evaluation for sources of paradoxical embolism. The yield of magnetic resonance imaging (MRI) of the pelvic and lower extremities is higher than with ultrasound, and should be considered in patients with a presumed paradoxical embolus.[23] Those with arterial stroke who are found to have only elevated antiphospholipid antibody levels may reasonably be treated with aspirin.

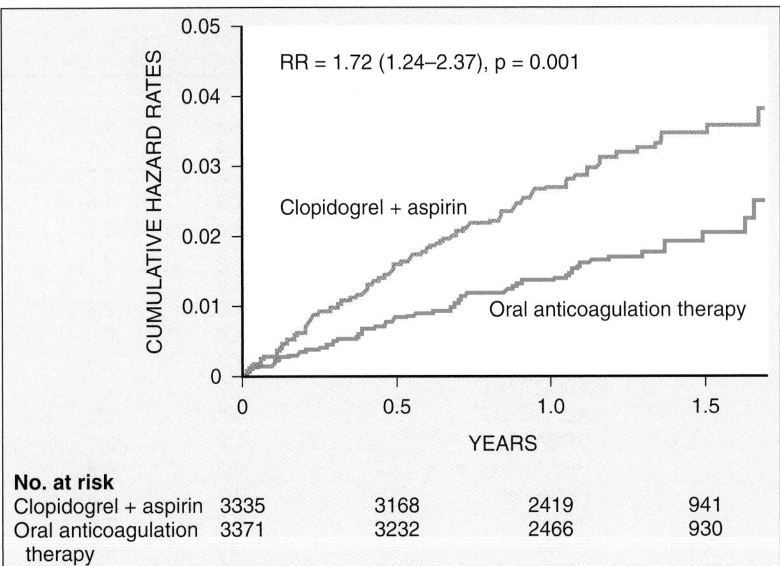

FIGURE 62-3 Clopidogrel plus aspirin versus anticoagulation in patients with atrial fibrillation and risk of stroke. *(From the Active Writing Group of the ACTIVE Investigators; Connolly S, Pogue J, Hart R, et al: Clopidogrel plus aspirin versus oral anticoagulation for atrial fibrillation in the Atrial Fibrillation Clopidogrel Trial with Irbesartan for prevention of Vascular Events (ACTIVE W): A randomised controlled trial. Lancet 367:1903, 2006.)*

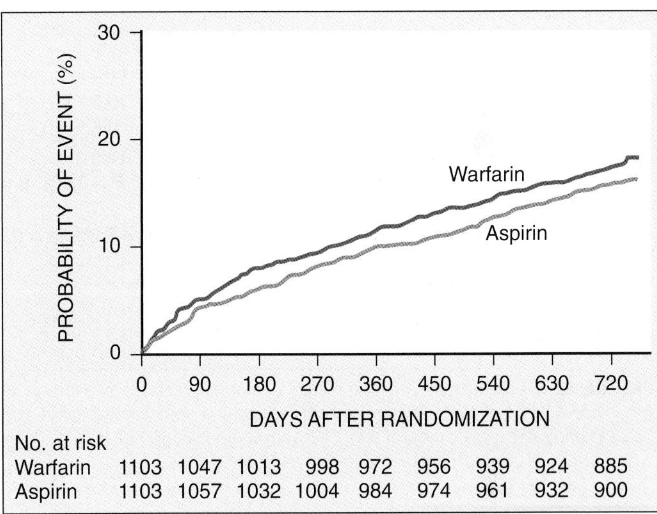

FIGURE 62-4 Kaplan-Meier analyses of the time to recurrent ischemic stroke or death according to treatment assignment. *(From Mohr JP, Thompson JL, Lazar RM, et al: A comparison of warfarin and aspirin for the prevention of recurrent ischemic stroke. N Engl J Med 345:1444, 2001.)*

HMG-CoA Reductase Inhibitors (Statins)

(See Chaps. 47 and 49.)

PRIMARY PREVENTION. Statins not only reduce cardiac events, but also the risk of a first stroke in patients at risk (**Fig. 62-5**). A meta-analysis of randomized trials of statins including 165,792 subjects found that each 40-mg/dL decrease in low-density lipoprotein (LDL) cholesterol was associated with a 21.1% (95% CI, 6.3 to 33.5%; $P = 0.009$) reduction in the risk of a first stroke (**Fig. 62-6**).[24]

Some studies have shown a reduction in the risk of first stroke with statin treatment among diabetics,[25,26] hypertensives,[27] and older adults.[28] The Justification for the Use of Statins in Prevention: An Intervention Trial Evaluating Rosuvastatin (JUPITER) evaluated the effect of a statin in persons with an elevated (more than 2 mg/dL) high sensitivity C-reactive protein level, but with LDL cholesterol below 130 mg/dL (see Chap. 47).[29] Statin treatment resulted in a 44% reduction in the time to the primary endpoint (combined risk of MI, stroke, arterial revascularization, hospitalization for unstable angina, or death from cardiovascular causes [HR, 0.56; 95% CI, 0.46 to 0.69; $P < 0.00001$) including an approximate 50% reduction in stroke (**Fig. 62-7**). The implications of the results of the trial for patient management have engendered debate.[30]

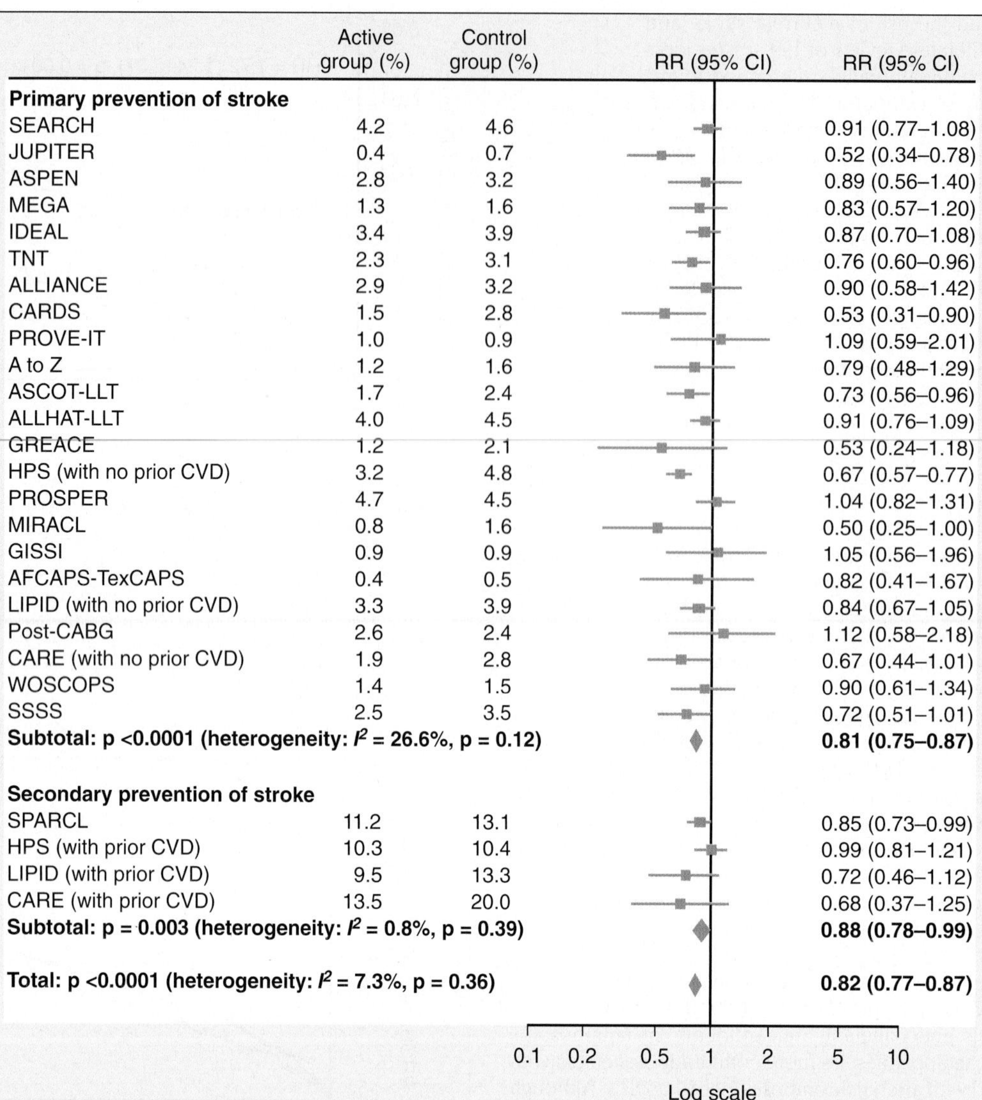

FIGURE 62-5 Meta-analysis of the effects of statins on stroke prevention. Results are from 24 trials with 165,792 patients with fatal and nonfatal stroke. *(From Amarenco P, Labreuche J: Lipid management in the prevention of stroke: Review and updated meta-analysis of statins for stroke prevention. Lancet Neurol 8:453, 2009; data on LIPID and CARE with or without prior CVD from Vergouwen MD, de Haan RJ, Vermeulen M, Roos YB: Statin treatment and the occurrence of hemorrhagic stroke in patients with a history of cerebrovascular disease. Stroke 39:497, 2008.)*

SECONDARY PREVENTION. In contrast to the large amount of data showing a reduction in the risk of a first stroke in patients with coronary heart disease (CHD) or at high CHD risk who are treated with a statin, until recently there has been no evidence that treatment with a statin reduces the risk of a second stroke. The Heart Protection Study (HPS) included 3280 subjects with a history of stroke (including 1820 with stroke and no history of CHD) who were treated with a statin or placebo.[31] Among those with a prior history of stroke, statin treatment reduced the frequency of MVEs (e.g., MI, stroke, revascularization procedure, or vascular death) by 20%, but did not lower the risk of recurrent stroke (occurring in 10.5% in those treated with placebo versus 10.4% in those treated with the statin). Among several plausible reasons for the lack of effect on recurrent stroke, the most important might be that patients were randomized an average of approximately 4 years after the index event. Most recurrent strokes occur within the first few years, so those randomized in the HPS were at relatively low risk of recurrent stroke.

The Stroke Prevention with Aggressive Reduction in Cholesterol Levels (SPARCL) trial randomized over 4700 subjects who were within 6 months of a noncardioembolic stroke or TIA and with no known CHD to high-dose statin or placebo, for a primary endpoint of the first occurrence of a nonfatal or fatal stroke.[32] Those randomized to high-dose statin treatment had a 16% relative reduction in nonfatal or fatal stroke, as well as a 35% relative reduction in major coronary events. Added to the previous data on prevention of a first stroke, SPARCL showed that treatment with a high-dose statin can reduce the risk of recurrent stroke after a stroke or TIA (**Fig. 62-8**). On the basis of this trial, statin therapy with intensive lipid-lowering effects is recommended for patients with atherosclerotic ischemic stroke or TIA and without known CHD to reduce the risk of stroke and cardiovascular events.[4] The results suggest that noncardioembolic stroke might be considered as a CHD equivalent because of the dramatic reduction in CHD events, despite the subjects having no known CHD at the time of randomization.

Antihypertensives (see Chap. 46)

PRIMARY PREVENTION. Hypertension is one of the most important treatable risk factors for both ischemic stroke and parenchymal intracerebral hemorrhage. The Seventh Report of the Joint National Committee on Prevention, Detection, Evaluation, and Treatment of High Blood Pressure (JNC 7) has provided comprehensive,

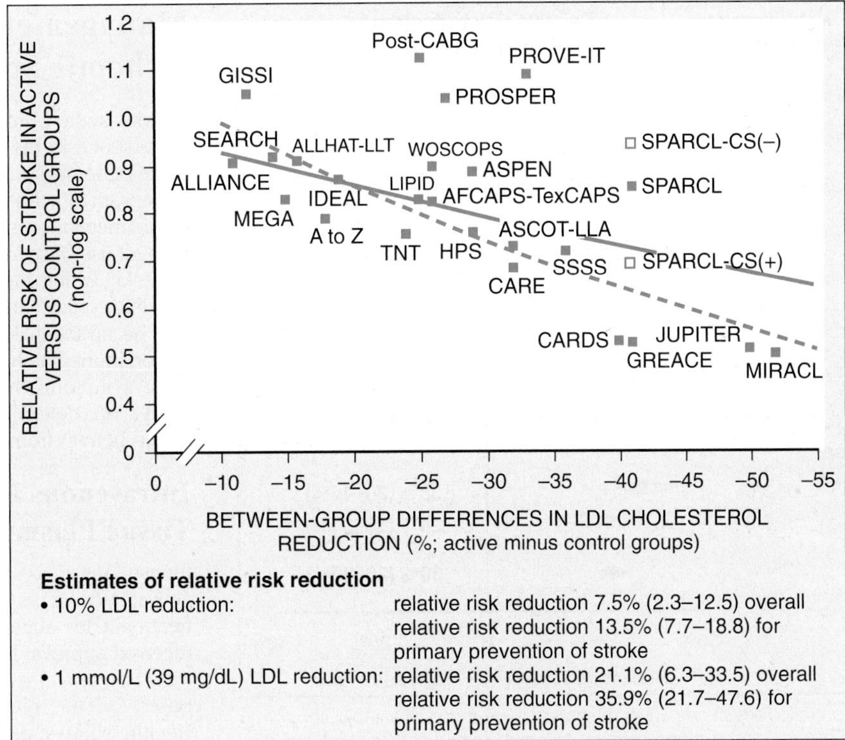

FIGURE 62-6 Cholesterol lowering with statins and stroke risk. Inverse variance-weighted regression lines have been plotted after including all 24 trials (165,792 patients; solid line) and after excluding trials with clearly identified groups of patients in secondary stroke prevention (SPARCL; HPS, LIPID, and CARE subgroups with previous cerebrovascular disease; dashed line). The underlying causes of stroke are important when considering the association between lipid and stroke risk, so the SPARCL results are also shown in accordance with the presence or absence of documented CS. The data for the SEARCH trial were presented at the 2008 American Heart Association meeting. CS = carotid stenosis. *(From Amarenco P, Labreuche J: Lipid management in the prevention of stroke: Review and updated meta-analysis of statins for stroke prevention. Lancet Neurol 8:453, 2009.)*

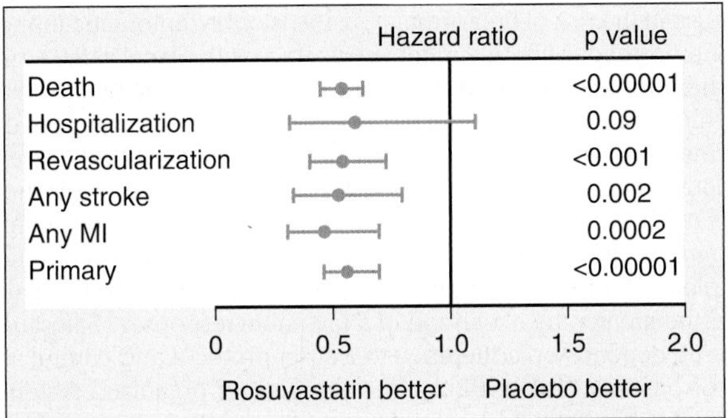

FIGURE 62-7 Results of the JUPITER trial evaluating the effects of statin treatment in patients with high-sensitivity C-reactive protein (hs-CRP) > 2 mg/dL and no other indication for statin therapy. Numbers indicate point estimate; horizontal lines indicate 95% CI. *(From Goldstein LB: JUPITER and the world of stroke medicine. Lancet Neurol 8:130, 2009; data from Ridker PM: Rosuvastatin in the primary prevention of cardiovascular disease among patients with low levels of low-density lipoprotein cholesterol and elevated high-sensitivity C-reactive protein: Rationale and design of the JUPITER trial. Circulation 108:2292, 2003.)*

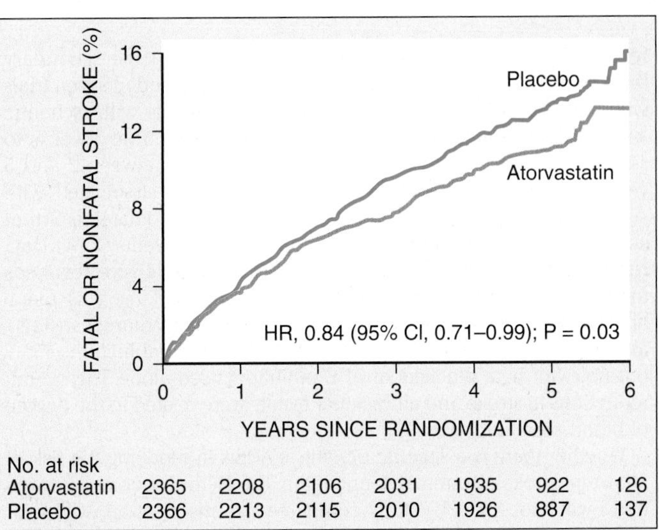

FIGURE 62-8 Kaplan-Meier curve for stroke or TIA in SPARCL. The data report an intention-to-treat analysis with prespecified adjustments for geographic region, entry event, time since entry event, sex, and baseline age for the first occurrence of a fatal or nonfatal stroke or TIA. *(From Amarenco P, Bogousslavsky J, Callahan A III, et al: High-dose atorvastatin after stroke or transient ischemic attack. N Engl J Med 355:549, 2006.)*

evidence-based guidelines for the classification and treatment of hypertension, reiterated in the current American Stroke Association Primary Stroke Prevention Guidelines.[2,33] Both guidelines support individualization of the choice of a specific antihypertensive regimen, and suggest that the reduction in blood pressure is generally more important than the specific agent(s) used to achieve this goal. A meta-analysis of randomized controlled trials comparing antihypertensive drugs with placebo or no treatment on stroke, including more than 73,500 participants and almost 2900 stroke events, found similar risk reductions for angiotensin-converting enzyme (ACE) inhibitors (28%), beta-adrenergic receptor blockers (beta blockers) or diuretics (35%), and calcium channel antagonists (39%), corresponding to blood pressure reductions of 5/2, 13/6 and 10/5 mm Hg, respectively (**Fig. 62-9**).[34]

SECONDARY PREVENTION. Only limited data directly address the role of blood pressure treatment in secondary prevention for those with a history of stroke or TIA. A systematic review focused on the

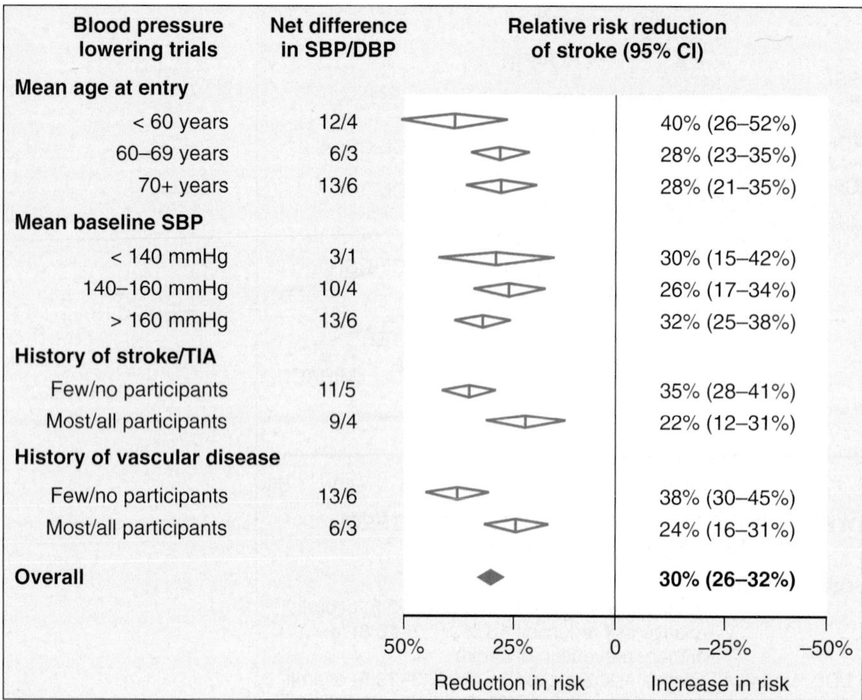

FIGURE 62-9 Randomized controlled trials comparing antihypertensive drugs with a placebo (or no treatment) by subgroup. The meta-analyses of blood pressure–lowering trials were stratified into subgroups on the basis of mean age of trial participants at entry, baseline systolic blood pressure level, and whether trial participants predominantly had a history of stroke-TIA or vascular disease. The diamonds are centered on the pooled estimate of effect and represent a 95% CI. The solid diamond represents the pooled relative risk and 95% CI for all contributing trials. BP = blood pressure; DBP = diastolic blood pressure; SBP = systolic blood pressure. *(From Lawes CM, Bennett DA, Feigin FL, Rodgers A: Blood pressure and stroke: An overview of published reviews. Stroke 35:1024, 2004.)*

relationship between blood pressure reduction and the secondary prevention of stroke and other vascular events; it included seven trials with a combined sample size of 15,527 participants with ischemic stroke, TIA, or intracerebral hemorrhage randomized from 3 weeks to 14 months after the index event and followed for between 2 and 5 years.[35] Treatment with antihypertensive drugs was associated with significant reductions in all recurrent strokes (24%), nonfatal recurrent stroke (21%), MI (21%; **Fig. 62-10**), and all vascular events (21%). Data regarding the relative benefits of specific antihypertensive regimens for secondary stroke prevention are generally lacking. This meta-analysis found a reduction in recurrent stroke with diuretics (32%), and with diuretics and ACE inhibitors (ACEIs) in combination (45%), but not with beta blockers or ACE inhibitors used alone. The overall reductions in stroke and all vascular events were related to the degree of blood pressure lowering.

Whether there is a specific benefit of ACEIs in reducing the risk of recurrent stroke also remains uncertain. The Heart Outcomes Prevention Evaluation (HOPE) study compared the effects of an ACEI with placebo in high-risk persons and found a 24% risk reduction in the risk of stroke, MI, or vascular death among the 1013 patients with a history of stroke or TIA.[3] The Perindopril Protection Against Recurrent Stroke Study (PROGRESS) tested the effects of a blood pressure–lowering regimen, including an ACEI, in 6105 patients with stroke or TIA within the prior 5 years.[3] Randomization was stratified by intention to use single (ACEI) or combination (ACEI plus the diuretic indapamide) therapy in hypertensive (>160 mm Hg systolic or >90 mm Hg diastolic) and nonhypertensive patients. The combination (lowering blood pressure by an average of 12/5 mm Hg) reduced the risk of recurrent stroke by 43% and of major vascular events by 40% in both the hypertensive and normotensive groups. However, there was no significant benefit of either antihypertensive given alone. The choice of a specific antihypertensive regimen should be guided by specific patient characteristics and comorbid conditions.

Management of Acute Ischemic Stroke

As with acute coronary syndromes, time is of the essence in the treatment of patients with acute ischemic stroke. Stroke has a large variety of causative factors and potential pathophysiologic mechanisms that critically influence the rational use of secondary preventive therapies, some of which were reviewed earlier. Some conditions may cause symptoms and signs that can be mistaken for those of a stroke. In the period immediately following the onset of ischemic symptoms, however, evaluation should center on determining whether the patient would benefit from reperfusion therapy.

Intravenous Recombinant Tissue Plasminogen Activator

Intravenous recombinant tissue plasminogen activator (rt-PA) is currently the only specific treatment for acute ischemic stroke that has received approval from the FDA. The treatment aims to lyse a clot occluding a cerebral artery. Based on the pivotal National Institutes of Health (NIH)–sponsored randomized clinical trial, treatment of appropriate patients is associated with an approximate 13% absolute (32% relative) increase in the proportion of patients free of disability 3 months later.[6] Benefits are similar for patients with small penetrating artery distribution ischemic stroke and for those with occlusion of larger intracranial arteries. Although treatment is also associated with an increase in the risk of hemorrhage (6.4% risk of symptomatic intracerebral hemorrhage with treatment versus 0.6% with placebo; 2.9% risk of fatal hemorrhage versus 0.3% with placebo), the overall benefit includes these adverse events. The drug must be given within 3 hours of the onset of symptoms, which means that the patient must generally arrive at a properly equipped and organized hospital within 2 hours of symptom onset to have the necessary evaluations (including a brain computed tomography [CT] scan to exclude hemorrhage or other conditions) completed. Within the 3-hour window, the sooner treatment can be given, the greater the likelihood of a favorable response.[36] Safest use of the drug depends on adherence to a strict protocol and careful selection of patients (**Table 62-2**). Development of organized systems of stroke care has been advocated to perform rapidly the necessary clinical evaluations, to minimize delays in treatment, to institute other interventions associated with improved outcomes, and ensure that patients receive appropriate secondary prevention.[37]

Secondary analyses of prior thrombolytic trials have suggested a benefit, albeit reduced, with treatment up to 4 to 5 hours after symptom onset.[36] This hypothesis was tested in a separate clinical trial that included restrictions in addition to those of the NIH-sponsored three-hour trial (see Table 62-2).[38] Treatment resulted in an increase in the proportion of patients with excellent outcomes (Rankin index, 0 to 1) after 3 months (52.4% versus 45.2% with placebo; OR, for global favorable outcome, 1.28; 95% CI, 1.00 to 1.65). Although not FDA-approved, guidelines have been modified to extend treatment to this restricted group of patients who can be treated between 3 to 4.5 hours of symptom onset, but stress that treatment must be given as soon as possible after symptom onset to derive the greatest benefit.[7]

Up to one third of patients may have early arterial reocclusion after intravenous thrombolysis.[6] One study has suggested that clot lysis might be facilitated by concomitant exposure to ultrasound provided by transcranial Doppler, which can also be used to monitor clot dissolution.[39] A prospective trial is evaluating the usefulness of this approach.

Endovascular Therapy

Endovascular approaches that are catheter-based for acute reperfusion have the theoretical advantages of allowing for direct clot visualization and localized rather than systemic administration of thrombolytics, as well as the opportunity for mechanical clot disruption. No prospective randomized trials have directly compared endovascular therapy with intravenous rt-PA. In addition, endovascular therapy can only be accomplished in centers with immediate access to neurovascular interventionalists, is not generally feasible in patients with distal arterial occlusions, and might entail longer times to reperfusion (e.g., related to the need for access to an interventional suite, catheter placement time).

Prospective randomized data comparing intra-arterial thrombolysis with nonthrombolytic medical therapy have come primarily from a single clinical trial.[6] This study evaluated intra-arterial thrombolysis with prourokinase in patients within 6 hours of angiographically proven proximal middle cerebral artery occlusion, and found a significant improvement in 3-month outcome (40% of treated versus 25% of control patients had little or no disability), despite a trend toward an increase in symptomatic intracerebral hemorrhages (10% versus 2%, respectively). Prourokinase has not been approved by the FDA and is not currently available in the United States. Intra-arterial rt-PA is commonly used for this purpose in patients who do not qualify for treatment with intravenous rt-PA (usually because of arriving at the hospital too late) and otherwise fulfills the inclusion criteria for the prourokinase trial cited. In addition to patients with middle cerebral artery occlusions up to 6 hours earlier, based on case series data, selected patients with basilar artery occlusion up to 12 hours or longer may also be treated with this approach. Several ongoing studies are evaluating intra-arterial thrombolysis with rt-PA, but the FDA has not yet approved this approach.

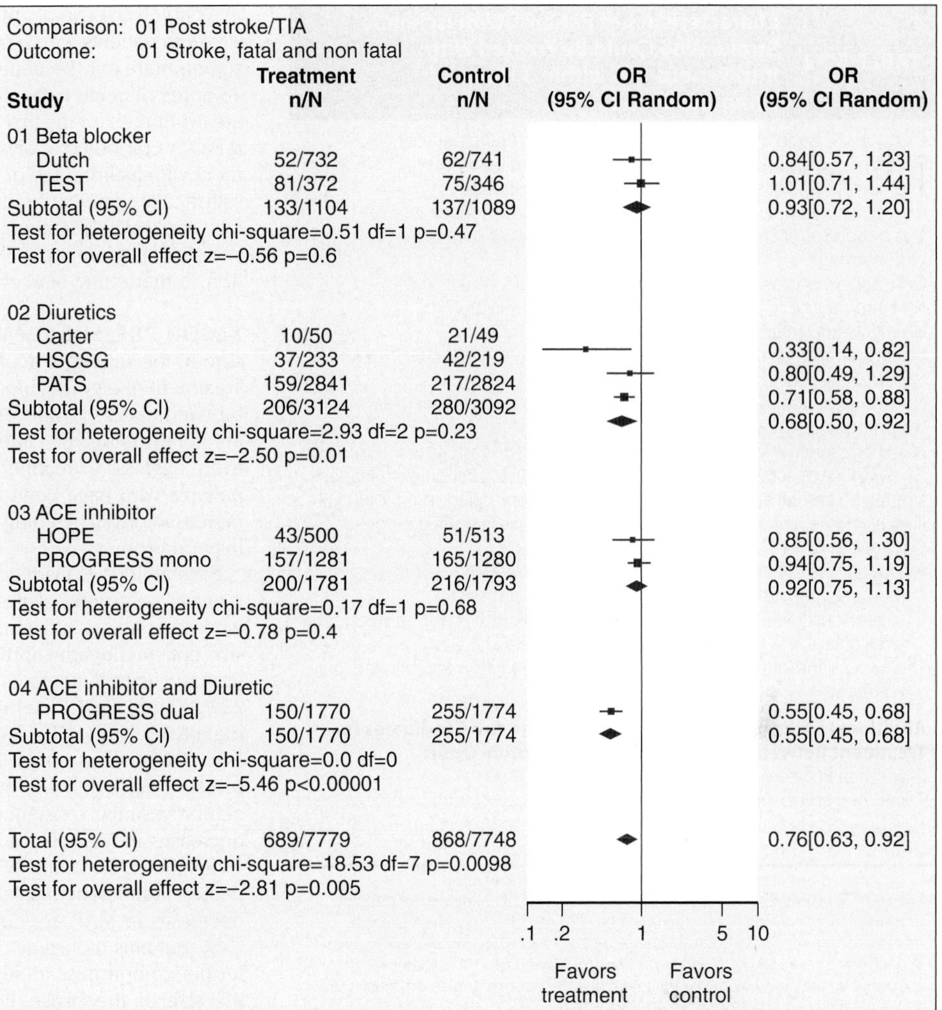

FIGURE 62-10 Forrest plot of the effect of antihypertensive therapy in patients with prior stroke or TIA on subsequent fatal and nonfatal stroke. *(From Rashid P, Leonardi-Bee J, Bath P: Blood pressure reduction and secondary prevention of stroke and other vascular events: A systematic review. Stroke 34:2741, 2003.)*

Mechanical clot retrieval has the theoretical advantage of avoiding the bleeding risk associated with thrombolytic drugs. The MERCI clot retriever was the first approved by the FDA for the removal of blood clots from brain blood vessels, but not as a specific treatment for acute stroke. This approval was based on the results of a noncontrolled case series involving 151 enrolled patients (141 of whom could be treated) with proximal (internal carotid, middle cerebral, or vertebrobasilar) arterial occlusions within 6 hours (mean, 4.3 hours to catheterization).[40] Recanalization was achieved in 48%, of whom 30% died or had a second stroke or MI within 30 days. Approximately 30% died within 90 days, but 46% of those surviving at 90 days had little or no disability. Procedural complications occurred in 13% (six arterial perforations, four arterial dissections, three cases of embolization to another artery, three subarachnoid hemorrhages, and three groin hematomas), with 28% having asymptomatic intracerebral hemorrhages and 8% symptomatic hemorrhages. The frequency of parenchymal hemorrhages might at first seem surprising; however, the arterial endothelium can be subject to ischemia-related damage, and reperfusion of a damaged artery (with or without a thrombolytic) can lead to bleeding. This study had no concurrent controls, leaving open whether outcomes would be similar, better, or worse than with other reperfusion treatments. Other devices have since been approved, also based on case series lacking concurrent controls. The approach has the same logistic limitations as endovascular thrombolytic therapy, but does offer the possibility of treatment for selected patients who cannot be treated with a thrombolytic drug (e.g., patients already anticoagulated, having a recent operation or invasive procedure, or having an embolus complicating cardiac or other catheterization after the catheter sheath has been removed).

Other Measures for Stroke Treatment

Several other important questions often arise concerning the management of patients with acute ischemic stroke and other interventions that are generally used, even without definitive supporting data.

ANTICOAGULATION AND ANTIPLATELET THERAPY. The indications for acute anticoagulation of patients with ischemic stroke are extremely limited. The most recent American Heart Association/American Academy of Neurology guidelines specifically discourage emergent anticoagulation with the goal of improving neurologic outcomes or preventing early recurrent stroke in patients with acute ischemic stroke because of a high risk of intracranial bleeding complications, and do not recommend the initiation of anticoagulant therapy within 24 hours of treatment with intravenously administered rt-PA.[41] Patients with atrial fibrillation–associated stroke benefit from long-term anticoagulation, unless contraindicated because of high bleeding risk (e.g., prior intracerebral hemorrhage, falls). The risk of early recurrence in patients with stroke related to atrial fibrillation is generally low (approximately 0.3 to 0.5%/day for the first 2 weeks), so the timing of the initiation of anticoagulation needs to be balanced

CH 62

TABLE 62-2 Characteristics of Patients With Ischemic Stroke Who Could Be Treated With Intravenous-tPA within 3 Hours of Symptom Onset

Diagnosis of ischemic stroke causing measurable neurologic deficit
The neurologic signs should not be clearing spontaneously.
The neurologic signs should not be minor and isolated.
Caution should be exercised in treating a patient with major deficits.
The symptoms of stroke should not be suggestive of subarachnoid hemorrhage.
Onset of symptoms < 3 hours before beginning treatment
No head trauma or prior stroke in the previous 3 months
No myocardial infarction in the previous 3 months
No gastrointestinal or urinary tract hemorrhage in the previous 21 days
No major surgery in the previous 14 days
No arterial puncture at a noncompressible site in the previous 7 days
No history of previous intracranial hemorrhage
Blood pressure not elevated (systolic > 185 mm Hg; diastolic > 110 mm Hg)
No evidence of active bleeding or acute trauma (fracture) on examination
Not taking an oral anticoagulant, or if anticoagulant being taken, INR< 1.7
If receiving heparin in previous 48 hr, aPTT must be in normal range
Platelet count > 100,000 mm^3
Blood glucose concentration > 50 mg/dL (2.7 mmol/liter)
No seizure with postictal residual neurologic impairments
CT does not show a multilobar infarction (hypodensity one third of cerebral hemisphere).
The patient and/or family understands the potential risks and benefits of treatment.

Additional Exclusion Criteria for Patients Who Are Candidates for Treatment Between 3 and 4.5 Hours of Symptom Onset

Older than 80 years
Taking oral anticoagulants regardless of INR
NIHSS score > 25
History of both prior stroke and diabetes

aPTT = activated partial thromboplastin time; NIHSS = NIH stroke scale.
Modified from Adams HP, Adams R, Del Zoppo G, Goldstein LB: Guidelines for the early management of patients with ischemic stroke: 2005 guidelines update. A scientific statement from the Stroke Council of the American Heart Association/American Stroke Association. Stroke 36:916, 2005; and Del Zoppo G, Saver J, Jauch EC, Adams HP: Expansion of the time window for treatment of acute ischemic stroke with intravenous tissue plasminogen activator. Stroke 40:2945, 2009.

against the risk of bleeding. Those with large strokes and those with uncontrolled hypertension generally have the highest risk of spontaneous hemorrhagic transformation of an ischemic stroke.

The use of anticoagulants in patients with stroke related to infective endocarditis is problematic (see Chap. 67). Systemic embolization occurs in 22% to 50% of patients with infective endocarditis, with up to 65% of emboli affecting the central nervous system; most of these (90%) involve the middle cerebral artery.[42] There is no demonstrated benefit for anticoagulation in patients with native valve endocarditis, and it is generally not recommended for at least the first 2 weeks of antibiotic therapy in patients with stroke related to *Staphylococcus aureus* prosthetic valve endocarditis. Of particular concern is the possible development of mycotic intracranial aneurysms. These are often multiple and can be asymptomatic, associated with focal neurologic signs, or can affect distal branches of the middle cerebral artery, associated with signs and symptoms of subarachnoid hemorrhage or a sterile meningitis. Although CT angiography in patients without renal insufficiency or MR angiography can be useful screening tests in patients with symptoms suggesting the presence of a mycotic aneurysm, because distal portions of the artery are most commonly affected, catheter angiography is the gold standard for the detection of these lesions; distal portions of the middle cerebral artery can be difficult to visualize by CT or MR angiography. The management of patients with intracranial mycotic aneurysms is complex; many regress with antibiotic treatment. Depending on a variety of factors, surgical clipping or endovascular obliteration can also be considered. Anticoagulation is generally avoided in patients with known mycotic aneurysms because of their propensity to rupture.

As noted, the use of antiplatelet agents reduces the risk of recurrent stroke in patients with a history of ischemic stroke or TIA. In the acute setting, there may be benefit from treatment with aspirin begun within 48 hours of acute ischemic stroke (these platelet antiaggregant drugs are prohibited for the first 24 hours in patients treated with intravenous rt-PA). A combined analysis of two relevant trials has found that treatment with aspirin (160 or 325 mg daily) is associated with a small but statistically significant reduction of nine (±three) fewer deaths or nonfatal strokes/1000 treated patients.[41] There remain no data showing the benefit of any other platelet antiaggregant, given alone or in combination, in the setting of acute ischemic stroke.

BLOOD PRESSURE MANAGEMENT. Management of blood pressure in the setting of acute ischemic stroke remains largely empiric.[6] Treatment of elevated blood pressure in patients who might otherwise be candidates for intravenous rt-PA differs from that of patients who are not thrombolytic candidates, and follows a specific protocol. Relatively aggressive treatment for elevated blood pressure is used for patients who have been treated with a thrombolytic because of an increased risk of bleeding complications associated with uncontrolled hypertension.

Several lines of evidence suggest cautious blood pressure management in nonthrombolytic-treated patients with acute ischemic stroke who do not have malignant hypertension (i.e., patients with hypertensive encephalopathy, aortic dissection, acute renal failure, acute pulmonary edema, acute myocardial infarction, or blood pressures > 220/120 mm Hg).[6] Cerebral autoregulation maintains constant cerebral blood flow (CBF) despite fluctuations in systemic blood pressure (see Chaps. 45 and 46). CBF is determined by the cerebral perfusion pressure (generally the mean arterial pressure, MAP) divided by the cerebrovascular resistance (CVR).[43] As reflected by this relationship, decreases in MAP lead to dilation of cerebral arterioles (decreased CVR), thereby keeping CBF constant. The local acidosis that accompanies brain ischemia leads to maximal vasodilatation. As a result, decreases in MAP are directly reflected in changes in local CBF (if CVR remains constant). Therefore, lowering blood pressure may further compromise an already ischemic brain, potentially increasing the size of the stroke. If treatment is necessary, precipitous drops should be avoided.

Stroke after Percutaneous Coronary Intervention and Thrombolytic Treatment for Myocardial Infarction

Although occurring infrequently, stroke can be a major complication of percutaneous coronary intervention (PCI) (see Chap. 58). The same principles outlined for the management of acute stroke in other settings apply. If neurologic symptoms are recognized while the catheter sheath is still in place, the patient might be treated with intravenous rt-PA, provided that all the other inclusion criteria are met and there are no other contraindications to the therapy. If symptoms are first noted after the catheter sheath has been removed, then the patient could be evaluated for catheter-based endovascular treatment. It is important to have a system in place to ensure the rapid evaluation and treatment of patients with stroke after PCI.

Intracerebral hemorrhage following thrombolytic administration for acute myocardial MI is another serious treatment-related complication (see Chap. 55). The infusion should be stopped and heparin discontinued for any patient developing acute neurologic symptoms. Because these symptoms might result from hemorrhage or ischemia, a brain imaging study is mandatory before proceeding with further treatment. Treatments to reduce the amount of thrombolytic-associated intracerebral hemorrhage once it has occurred are not well established. The administration of cryoprecipitate and/or fresh-frozen plasma has been advocated. Those with brainstem compression related to cerebellar hemorrhage may benefit from surgical evacuation of the hematoma. Patients should be transferred to a setting with expertise in neurologic intensive care as soon as feasible.

REFERENCES

1. Lloyd-Jones D, Adams R, Carnethon M, et al: Heart disease and stroke statistics—2009 update: A report from the American Heart Association Statistics Committee and Stroke Statistics Subcommittee. Circulation 119:480, 2009.

Guidelines

2. Goldstein LB, Adams R, Alberts MJ, et al: Primary prevention of ischemic stroke: A guideline from the American Heart Association/American Stroke Association Stroke Council. Stroke 37:1583, 2006.
3. Sacco RL, Adams R, Albers G, et al: Guidelines for prevention of stroke in patients with ischemic stroke or transient ischemic attack. A statement for healthcare professionals from the American Heart Association/ American Stroke Association Council on Stroke. Stroke 37:577, 2006.
4. Adams RJ, Albers G, Alberts MJ, et al: Update to the AHA/ASA recommendations for the prevention of stroke in patients with stroke and transient ischemic attack. Stroke 39:1647, 2008.
5. Adams HP, Adams RJ, Brott T, et al: Guidelines for the early management of patients with ischemic stroke: A scientific statement from the Stroke Council of the American Stroke Association. Stroke 34:1056, 2003.
6. Adams HP, Adams R, Del Zoppo G, Goldstein LB: Guidelines for the early management of patients with ischemic stroke: 2005 guidelines update. A scientific statement from the Stroke Council of the American Heart Association/American Stroke Association. Stroke 36:916, 2005.
7. Del Zoppo G, Saver J, Jauch EC, Adams HP: Expansion of the time window for treatment of acute ischemic stroke with intravenous tissue plasminogen activator. Stroke 40:2945, 2009.

Medical Therapy for Stroke Prevention

8. Johnston SC, Rothwell PM, Nguyen-Huynh MN, et al: Validation and refinement of scores to predict very early stroke risk after transient ischaemic attack. Lancet 369:283, 2007.
9. Ridker PM, Cook NR, Lee I-M, et al: A randomized trial of low-dose aspirin in the primary prevention of cardiovascular disease in women. N Engl J Med 352:1293, 2005.
10. ACTIVE Investigators: Effect of clopidogrel added to aspirin in patients with atrial fibrillation. N Engl J Med 360:2066, 2009.
11. ESPRIT Study Group: Aspirin plus dipyridamole versus aspirin alone after cerebral ischaemia of arterial origin (ESPRIT): Randomised controlled trial. Lancet 367:1665, 2006.
12. Bhatt DL, Fox KA, Hacke W, et al: Clopidogrel and aspirin versus aspirin alone for the prevention of atherothrombotic events. N Engl J Med 354:1706, 2006.
13. Diener H-C, Bogousslavsky J, Brass LM, et al: Aspirin and clopidogrel compared with clopidogrel alone after recent ischaemic stroke or transient ischaemic attack in high-risk patients (MATCH): Randomised, double-blind, placebo-controlled trial. Lancet 364:331, 2004.
14. Sacco RL, Diener HC, Yusuf S, et al: Aspirin and extended-release dipyridamole versus clopidogrel for recurrent stroke. N Engl J Med 359:1238, 2008.
15. Active Writing Group of the ACTIVE Investigators: Clopidogrel plus aspirin versus oral anticoagulation for atrial fibrillation in the Atrial fibrillation Clopidogrel Trial with Irbesartan for prevention of Vascular Events (ACTIVE W): A randomised controlled trial. Lancet 367:1903, 2006.
16. Mohr JP, Thompson JLP, Lazar RM, et al: Comparison of warfarin and aspirin for the prevention of recurrent ischemic stroke. N Engl J Med 345:1444, 2001.
17. Chimowitz MI, Kokkinos J, Strong J, et al: The Warfarin-Aspirin Symptomatic Intracranial Disease study. Neurology 45:1488, 1995.
18. Chimowitz MI, Lynn MJ, Howlett-Smith H, et al: Comparison of warfarin and aspirin for symptomatic intracranial arterial stenosis. N Engl J Med 352:1305, 2005.
19. Messé SR, Silverman IE, Kizer JR, et al: Practice parameter: Recurrent stroke with patent foramen ovale and atrial septal aneurysm: Report of the Quality Standards Subcommittee of the American Academy of Neurology. Neurology 62:1042, 2004.
20. Homma S, Sacco RL, Di Tullio MR, et al: Effect of medical treatment in stroke patients with patent foramen ovale: Patent Foramen Ovale in Cryptogenic Stroke Study. Circulation 105:2625, 2002.
21. Massie BM, Collins JF, Ammon SE, et al: Randomized trial of warfarin, aspirin, and clopidogrel in patients with chronic heart failure: The Warfarin and Antiplatelet Therapy in Chronic Heart Failure (WATCH) Trial. Circulation 119:1616, 2009.
22. Levine SR, Brey RL, Tilley BC, et al: Antiphospholipid antibodies and subsequent thrombo-occlusive events in patients with ischemic stroke. JAMA 291:576, 2004.
23. Cramer SC, Rordorf G, Maki JH, et al: Increased pelvic vein thrombi in cryptogenic stroke. Results of the Paradoxical Emboli from Large Veins in Ischemic Stroke (PELVIS) study. Stroke 35:46, 2004.
24. Amarenco P, Labreuche J: Lipid management in the prevention of stroke: Review and updated meta-analysis of statins for stroke prevention. Lancet Neurol 8:453, 2009.
25. Collins R, Armitage J, Parish S, et al; Heart Protection Study Collaborative Group: MRC/BHF Heart Protection Study of cholesterol-lowering with simvastatin in 5963 people with diabetes: A randomized placebo-controlled trial. Lancet 361:2005, 2003.
26. Colhoun HM, Betteridge DJ, Durrington PN, et al: Primary prevention of cardiovascular disease with atorvastatin in type 2 diabetes in the Collaborative Atorvastatin Diabetes Study (CARDS): Multicentre randomised placebo-controlled trial. Lancet 364:685, 2004.
27. Sever PS, Dahlof B, Poulter NR, et al: Prevention of coronary and stroke events with atorvastatin in hypertensive patients who have average or lower-than-average cholesterol concentrations, in the Anglo-Scandinavian Cardiac Outcomes Trial—Lipid Lowering Arm (ASCOT-LLA): A multicentre randomised controlled trial. Lancet 361:1149, 2003.
28. Shepherd J, Blauw GJ, Murphy MB, et al: Pravastatin in elderly individuals at risk of vascular disease (PROSPER): A randomised controlled trial. Lancet 360:1623, 2002.
29. Ridker PM, Danielson E, Fonseca FAH, et al: Rosuvastatin to prevent vascular events in men and women with elevated C-reactive protein. N Engl J Med 359:2195, 2009.
30. Goldstein LB: JUPITER and the world of stroke medicine. Lancet Neurol 8:130, 2009.
31. Collins R, Armitage J, Parish S, et al: Effects of cholesterol-lowering with simvastatin on stroke and other major vascular events in 20536 people with cerebrovascular disease or other high-risk conditions. Lancet 363:757, 2004.
32. Amarenco P, Bogousslavsky J, Callahan AS, et al: Design and baseline characteristics of the stroke prevention by aggressive reduction in cholesterol levels (SPARCL) study. Cerebrovasc Dis 16:389, 2003.
33. Chobanian AV, Bakris GL, Black HR, et al: The Seventh Report of the Joint National Committee on Prevention, Detection, Evaluation, and Treatment of High Blood Pressure: The JNC 7 report. JAMA 289:2560, 2003.
34. Lawes CMM, Bennett DA, Feigin VL, Rodgers A: Blood pressure and stroke. An overview of published reviews. Stroke 35:776, 2004.
35. Rashid P, Leonardi-Bee J, Bath P: Blood pressure reduction and secondary prevention of stroke and other vascular events: a systematic review. Stroke 34:2741, 2003.

Management of Acute Ischemic Stroke

36. Hacke W, Donnan G, Fieschi C, et al: Association of outcome with early stroke treatment: Pooled analysis of ATLANTIS, ECASS, and NINDS rt-PA stroke trials. Lancet 363:768, 2004.
37. Schwamm LH, Pancioli A, Acker JE 3rd, et al: Recommendations for the establishment of stroke systems of care: Recommendations from the American Stroke Association's Task Force on the Development of Stroke Systems. Circulation 111:1078, 2005.
38. Hacke W, Kaste M, Bluhmki E, et al: Thrombolysis with alteplase 3 to 4.5 hours after acute ischemic stroke. N Engl J Med 359:1317, 2008.
39. Alexandrov AV, Molina CA, Grotta JC, et al: Ultrasound-enhanced systemic thrombolysis for acute ischemic stroke. N Engl J Med 351:2170, 2004.
40. Smith WS, Sung G, Starkman S, et al: Safety and efficacy of mechanical embolectomy in acute ischemic stroke: Results of the MERCI trial. Stroke 36:1432, 2005.
41. Coull BM, Williams LS, Goldstein LB, et al: Anticoagulants and antiplatelet agents in acute ischemic stroke. Report of the Joint Stroke Guideline Development Committee of the American Academy of Neurology and the American Stroke Association. Neurology 59:13, 2002.
42. Baddour LM, Wilson WR, Bayer AS, et al: Infective endocarditis: diagnosis, antimicrobial therapy, and management of complications. Circulation 111:e394, 2005.
43. Goldstein LB: Blood pressure management in patients with acute ischemic stroke. Hypertension 43:137, 2004.

CHAPTER 63 Endovascular Treatment of Noncoronary Obstructive Vascular Disease

Andrew C. Eisenhauer, Christopher J. White, and Deepak L. Bhatt

Noncoronary, peripheral vascular disease encompasses a very broad range of arterial, venous, and lymphatic diseases. This chapter focuses on percutaneous, catheter-based, endovascular treatment of atherosclerotic peripheral arterial disease (upper and lower extremity, renal, mesenteric, aortic arch vessels, carotid and vertebral arteries) and venous disease. Recognition is increasing that atherosclerotic peripheral arterial disease (PAD) has a high prevalence and clinical importance (see Chap. 61). As the population ages, the number of people with both symptomatic and asymptomatic PAD increases. Physicians and patients are becoming more aware of the ramifications of PAD, including its associated morbidity and mortality. Revascularization strategies are shifting from open surgery to percutaneous or endovascular procedures. Percutaneous transluminal angioplasty (PTA) was initially developed as a treatment for PAD. Recent improvements in technology have generally led to better and much more reliable clinical results. These advances in technology have combined with patient demand for less invasive therapies and revolutionized revascularization therapies for PAD. The widespread availability of high-resolution noninvasive diagnostic imaging, capable of accurately identifying pathology and arterial obstructions that are amenable to less invasive treatment, has further enabled percutaneous therapies for symptomatic PAD.

Although historically, the primary method of revascularization therapy for PAD has involved surgery, percutaneous catheter-based or endovascular therapies now provide patients with a less invasive and equally effective modality for the treatment of atheromatous disease in almost all vascular territories. Effective therapies for arterial aneurysmal disease and venous conditions are currently available and offer advantages over surgical treatments. The American College of Cardiology (ACC) and American Heart Association (AHA) guidelines and recommendations for the diagnosis and treatment of atherosclerotic peripheral arterial disease have recently been published.[1] To provide optimal therapy, clinicians must understand the specific disease state being managed and consider the full range of treatment options. In complicated cases, the patient will benefit from the input of those in vascular-related specialties.

Endovascular Therapy for Atherosclerotic Peripheral Artery Disease

Atherosclerotic Lower Extremity Disease

Lower extremity intermittent claudication is caused by stenosis or occlusion of the iliac, femoral-popliteal, or tibioperoneal vessels (see Chap. 61). Claudication is an exertion-related discomfort affecting specific muscle groups and is relieved with rest. Symptoms affect the muscle groups below the level of the arterial narrowing. For example, vascular blockages (occlusions or stenoses) of the iliac vessels typically cause hip, thigh, and calf pain, whereas femoral and popliteal artery obstructions cause symptoms in the calf and foot muscles. Patients with typical symptoms of intermittent claudication represent fewer than 20% of patients with objective evidence of PAD. The clinician must distinguish pseudoclaudication (discomfort from spinal stenosis, compartment syndromes, venous congestion, or arthritis) from claudication (**Table 63-1**).

The initial therapy for patients with claudication should be atherosclerosis risk factor modification, antiplatelet therapy, and supervised exercise training (see Chap. 61). Because patients with claudication progress to limb-threatening ischemia uncommonly, revascularization is reserved for those patients who have failed a trial of medical therapy, or those with lifestyle-limiting symptoms and favorable anatomy for revascularization. Patients with more advanced disease—that is, vocation-limiting claudication or limb-threatening ischemia (rest pain, nonhealing ulcers, or gangrene)—require a more aggressive approach and are considered candidates for revascularization.

Therapy in patients with claudication aims to relieve symptoms, resulting in an increased walking distance and improvement in quality of life. A durable revascularization solution is important, because symptoms will likely return if restenosis occurs. In contrast, in patients with limb-threatening ischemia, the goal of therapy is limb salvage. The best treatment option will offer a high success rate for restoration of pulsatile flow to the distal limb, with a low procedural morbidity. Less blood flow is required to maintain tissue integrity than to heal a wound; restenosis will generally not result in recurrent limb-threatening ischemia without a subsequent reinjury to the limb. For the clinician caring for patients with lower extremity vascular disease, it is important to weigh improvement in functional capacity and quality of life, as well as long-term results, when considering revascularization.

Basic noninvasive testing includes determining the ankle-brachial index (ABI) at rest and potentially after exercise. Pulse volume recordings with segmental Doppler pressures are helpful in confirming the presence of obstructive disease and estimating its level and severity (see Chaps. 12 and 61). Normal ABIs at rest may miss significant aortoiliac disease, so if clinical suspicion is high, exercise ABIs should be determined. In general, lower extremity angiography is reserved for patients who meet criteria for revascularization, if suitable anatomy is found. Magnetic resonance angiography (MRA) and computed tomography angiography (CTA) enable remarkable noninvasive definition of the vascular anatomy; invasive angiography confirms the diagnosis and helps formulate a strategy and approach to revascularization. For

TABLE 63-1 Intermittent Claudication Versus Pseudoclaudication

FEATURE	INTERMITTENT CLAUDICATION	PSEUDOCLAUDICATION
Character of discomfort	Cramping, tightness, or tiredness	Same or tingling, weakness, clumsiness
Location of discomfort	Buttock, hip, thigh, calf, foot	Same
Exercise induced	Yes	Yes or no
Distance to claudication	Same each time	Variable
Occurs with standing	No	Yes
Relief	Stop walking	Often must sit or change body position

critical limb ischemia, anatomic definition is required in almost all cases to plan therapy. For claudication, imaging should be performed as outlined in **Figure 63-1**.

The probability of clinical success and the technical approach to percutaneous revascularization will vary according to anatomic site. These aspects are best considered separately for aortoiliac, femoropopliteal, and tibioperoneal segments.

AORTOILIAC OBSTRUCTIVE DISEASE. Ischemia producing lesions (stenosis or occlusion) of the aorta and iliac vessels is most commonly atherosclerotic in origin and treatment for both sites, typically referred to as inflow vessels to the leg, is similar. Lower extremity vascular disease frequently involves multiple levels. Patients with aortoiliac occlusive disease will often also have femoral and/or tibial disease. In patients with claudication and multilevel disease, correction of any hemodynamically significant inflow lesions may be undertaken as the first stage in revascularization. Aorto-iliac revascularization will often result in symptomatic improvement, by increasing inflow to the limb, and thus collateral blood flow to the distal extremity.

The preferred mode of revascularization of the aortoiliac vessels has shifted from predominantly surgical to almost completely catheter-based percutaneous therapies. This change is based on the less invasive nature of PTA and the excellent rate of clinical success, which now rivals surgical bypass for many patients. The primary use of stents, as opposed to balloon angioplasty alone, has become the clinical standard of care in the aortoiliac vessels.

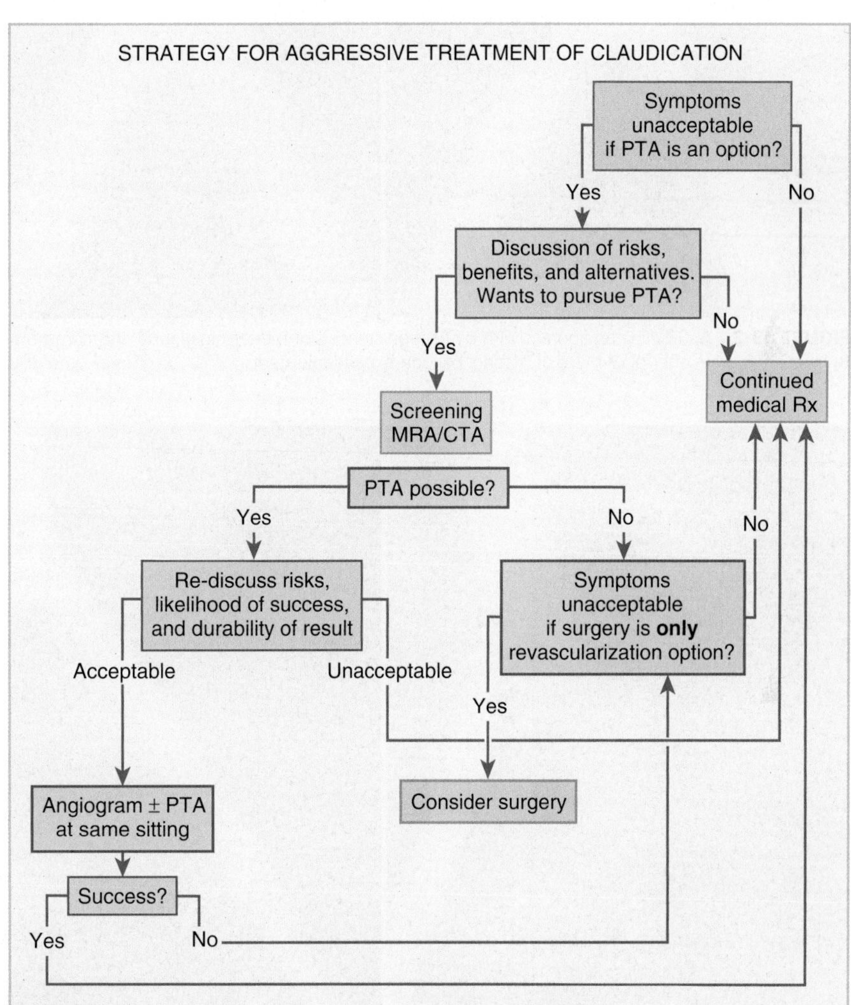

FIGURE 63-1 Strategy for aggressive treatment of claudication. The strategy is based on assessment of symptoms and frank discussion with patients about the risks and benefits of available therapies. Currently, noninvasive diagnostic imaging is used not to make a diagnosis but to ascertain the anatomic suitability for intervention and to assess the patient's procedural risk profile. Rx = treatment. See Figure 61-17 for a management scheme for less lifestyle-limiting claudication.

Treatment

Because experience has suggested that when excellent angiographic and hemodynamic results are obtained from PTA alone, patency rates and clinical success rates at 2 years are similar to stent placement. Some interventionalists favor a strategy of provisional stenting, wherein stents are reserved for cases of failed balloon angioplasty, but many patients ultimately receive stents. The immediate success rate and 4-year patency are superior for stents versus PTA alone. Longer lesions, diffuse disease, and occlusions, in particular, will likely benefit from primary stenting. The current guidelines recommend primary stent placement in the iliac arteries.[1] As is the case with all revascularization techniques, limited or compromised runoff seems to predict higher failure rates. For the subset of patients with stenotic or occlusive disease that involves the terminal aorta and compromises the origins of the common iliac arteries, the preferred therapy is placement of "kissing" balloon-expandable stents (**Fig. 63-2**).

Finally, with regard to the composition of stent selected, there is no advantage of self-expanding nitinol over balloon-expandable stainless steel.[2] Balloon expandable stents offer stronger radial force and more precise placement, whereas self-expanding stents offer flexible diameters that accommodate a tapering and sometimes tortuous vessel.

The most serious complications of endovascular aortoiliac repair remain distal embolizations, with rates reportedly as high as 7%, although most operators' experience suggests lower rates of significant

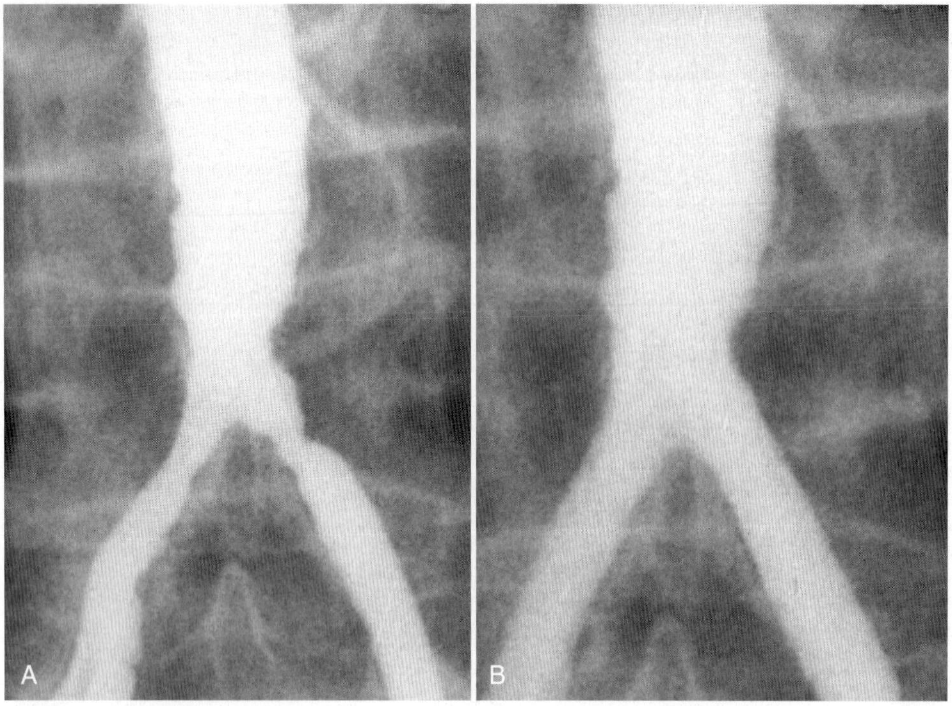

FIGURE 63-2 **A,** Baseline angiogram with bifurcation stenosis of the terminal aorta and common iliac arteries. **B,** Final angiogram after placement of "kissing" balloon-expandable stents.

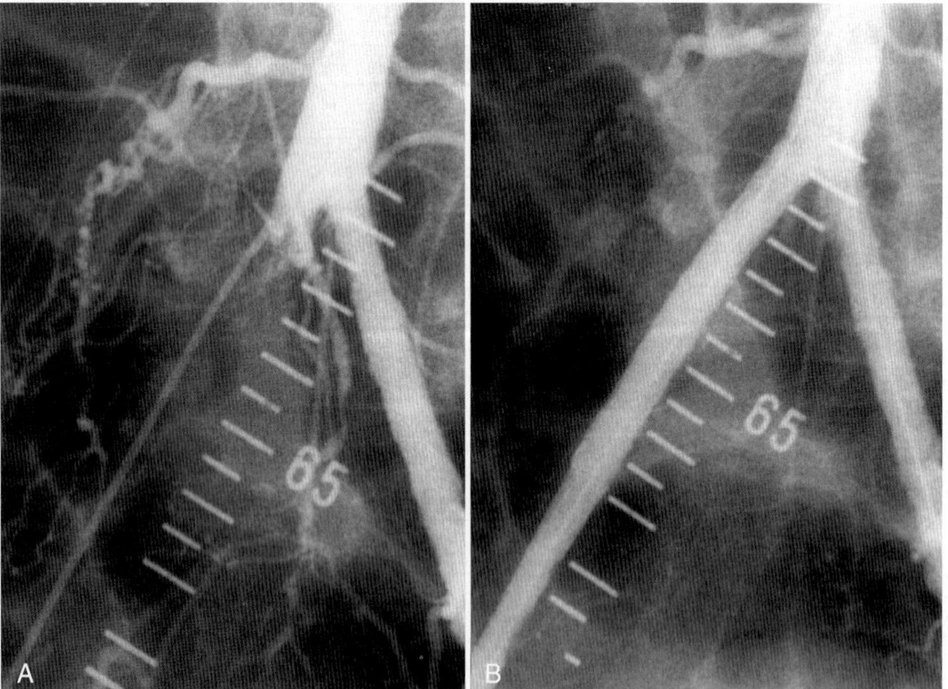

FIGURE 63-3 **A,** Occlusion of right common iliac artery. **B,** Recanalization and stent placement of right common iliac artery.

embolization. Arterial perforation or rupture is rare. Covered stents, or stent grafts, are available for treating vessel rupture. Based on these improved outcomes, percutaneous treatment is generally attempted for short occlusions and for longer iliac stenosis or occlusions that are technically suitable (**Fig. 63-3**). Total occlusions of the abdominal aorta are more often treated surgically, although thrombolysis followed by PTA remains an option.

In summary, primary stent placement represents appropriate first-line therapy for aortoiliac obstructive disease. Stent placement offers high procedural success and durability similar to that of surgical reconstruction, with less risk and at reduced cost. In the small percentage of patients in whom patency cannot be maintained, surgery remains a feasible option. The availability of these effective, less invasive techniques has lowered the threshold for performing intervention in patients with aortoiliac disease who are disabled by claudication or limb ischemia. Technical success and durability of results remain high (**Table 63-2**).[3-18]

FEMOROPOPLITEAL OBSTRUCTIVE DISEASE. Because the results of endovascular therapy for the superficial femoral artery (SFA) or popliteal artery differ little, this chapter will consider their indications and results together. The SFA, particularly within the adductor canal of the thigh, has a propensity to accumulate atherosclerotic plaque. Procedural success for femoropopliteal recanalization now exceeds 90%. The advent of hydrophilic guidewires and reentry catheters, including those with ultrasound guidance, has greatly enhanced the ability to traverse femoropopliteal occlusions.

Despite such technologic advances, the rate of restenosis remains more than twofold that for iliac disease and far exceeds what would be expected, considering the size (mean lumen diameter, 5 to 6 mm) of the SFA. A variety of adjunct technologies have been attempted to improve long-term patency. Cryotherapy, cutting balloons, and debulking devices such as directional atherectomy, excimer laser, and rotational atherectomy, although sometimes providing a better immediate angiographic result, have not demonstrated a reduction in restenosis in any controlled comparative trials.[19]

Treatment

Multiple small trials failed to demonstrate an advantage for first-generation stent placement over PTA in the femoropopliteal vessels, until more collective experience demonstrated that stents have superior long-term patency compared with PTA. Good clinical evidence from a randomized trial by Schillinger and colleagues[20] has indicated that a strategy of primary stent placement in the femoropopliteal vessels yields superior patency rates and functional outcomes compared with provisional stent placement (i.e., placement of stents for failed PTA). Restenosis at 1 year was 63% in the PTA group, but 37% in the stent arm. Functionally, both walking distance and ABI were increased significantly in the stent arm compared with the PTA group. These benefits accrued, even though 32% of the PTA group crossed over and received a stent after a suboptimal balloon angioplasty result.

A second trial by Krankenberg and associates[21] randomized 244 patients with relatively discrete SFA lesions (mean length, 45 mm) to

TABLE 63-2 Evolution of Results of Iliac Artery Stent Placement*

STUDY (YEAR)	NO. OF PATIENTS TREATED	NO. OF LESIONS STENTED	TOTAL OCCLUSIONS (%)	TECHNICAL SUCCESS (%)	*ABI* BEFORE	AFTER	MEAN LESION LENGTH (cm)	STENT(S) USED	PRIMARY PATENCY AT 2 yr (%)	CUMULATIVE PATENCY AT 2 yr (%)
Reyes et al (1997)[3]	59	61	100	92	0.51	0.9	10	SES	73	88
Dyet (1997)[4]	72	72	100	93	NA	NA	6.7	BES, SES	85	85
Murphy et al (1998)[5]	65	90	31	97	0.62	0.9	5.6	BES, SES	69	80
Tetteroo et al (1998)[6]	143	187	9	NA	0.78	NA	NA	BES	NA	71.3
Powell et al (2000)[7]	87	210	NA	97	0.56	0.75	NA	Various	43	72
Saha et al (2001)[8]	50	61	4	97	NA	NA	NA	BES, SES	97	100
Timaran et al (2001)[9]	189	247	NA	97	NA	NA	NA	BES, SES	NA	—
Haulon et al (2002)[10]	106	212	NA	100	NA	NA	NA	BES, SES	79.4	97.7
Siskin et al (2002)[11]	42	59	8.5	95	0.68	0.99	NA	BES, SES	72	88
Mohamed et al (2002)[12]	24	48	42	100	NA	NA	5.2	BES, SES	58	84
Reekers et al (2002)[13]	126	143	10	100	0.67	0.92	3.3	BES	84[†]	89[†]
Funovics et al (2002)[14]	78	94	100	96	NA	NA	6.2	Various	74.5	88.8
Hans et al (2008)[15]	40	68	48	95	0.55/0.52[‡]	0.82/0.77[‡]	NA	Various	69	89
Kashyap et al (2008)[16]	83	127	59	96	0.36	0.82	NA	Various	74	97
Sixt et al (2008)[17]	375	354	26	97	0.36	NA	4.9	Various	86[†]	98[†]
Uberol et al (2009)[18]	2233	—	—	98	—	—	—	—	—	—

BES = balloon-expandable stainless steel; SES = self-expanding stainless steel; SEN = self-expanding nitinol; SESG = self-expanding stent graft; — = not assessed or reported.

*Historical and contemporary results of iliac artery stent placement. The difficulty in interpreting the literature is that these reports of experience include patients with widely varying degrees of disease and incorporate a variety of stent types and techniques. Nevertheless, cumulative 2-year patency is approximately 90% in most series.

†At 12 months.

‡Separate report for right and left legs.

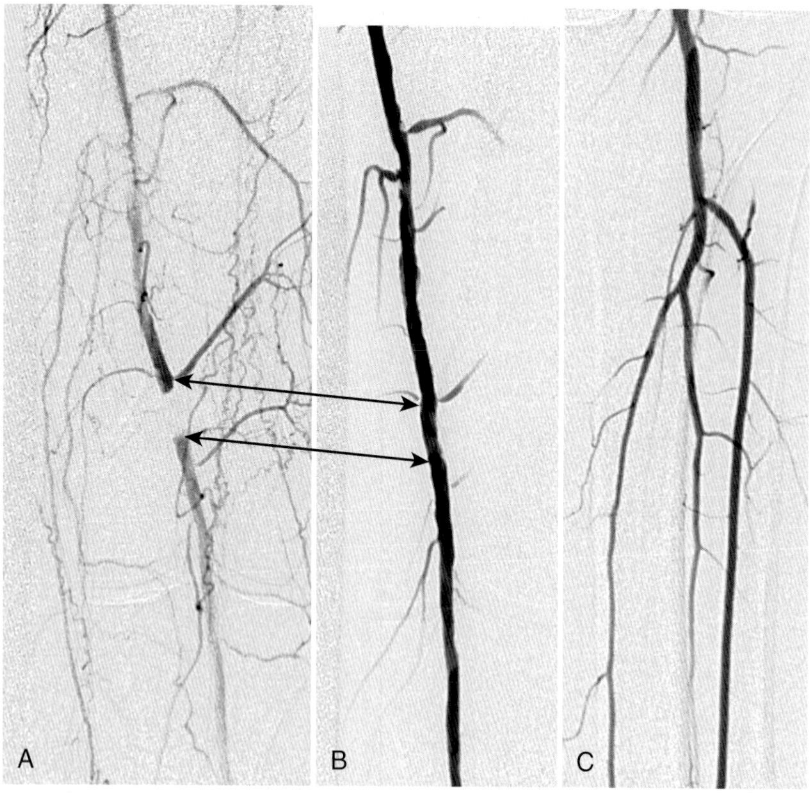

FIGURE 63-4 Result of recanalization and balloon dilation of a short-segment femoropopliteal occlusion. **A,** Digital subtraction angiogram illustrating the area of total occlusion and comparing it with that in **B,** which shows the results of balloon dilation only. Both areas are indicated by the double-ended black arrows. **C,** Intact three-vessel runoff without evidence of distal embolization.

balloon angioplasty or primary stent placement. Only 11% of the PTA patients crossed over to receive a stent, which improves the validity of the intention-to-treat analysis that showed no restenosis benefit for stent over PTA. The major difference between the Schillinger and Krankenburg trials was lesion length. The stent group in both trials had restenosis rates ranging from 30% to 39%, whereas the PTA restenosis rate in the long lesions was 67%, compared with only 38% for the shorter SFA lesions. A current meta-analysis of 10 randomized controlled trials included data on 1442 limbs, with an average length lesion similar to the Krankenberg trial (stent, 45.8 mm; PTA, 43.3 mm). No benefit was found for primary stent placement over provisional stent placement for SFA lesions. Thus, longer SFA lesions and total occlusions are more likely to benefit from primary stenting, whereas more discrete stenoses do just as well with PTA.

Two recently published multicenter randomized controlled trials in 87 and 154 patients have demonstrated significant benefit for paclitaxel-coated balloons compared with controls out to 18 and 24 months.[22,23] The next step will be a study of drug-coated balloons with provisional stenting, compared with drug-coated balloons with primary stenting.

The use of endovascular approaches to recanalize and stent diffuse femoropopliteal disease is reemerging (**Figs. 63-4 to 63-7**). With the success of drug-eluting coronary stents, strong interest has been rekindled in the development of stent coatings such as rapamycin for lower extremity use. In a randomized series of long-segment SFA disease patients, the results for those receiving rapamycin-coated nitinol self-expanding stents were no different than those in the bare-metal stent control group.[24] One concern raised in this trial was a high incidence of stent fractures, which appear to be related to restenosis.[25] After a period of study, fracture-resistant stent designs and modified coatings are emerging. Recent reports of paclitaxel-coated self-expanding stents are more favorable, with few fractures and preserved results at 12 and 24 months.[26] So far, the results of drug-eluting stents in the lower limbs have been mixed, but this work remains in its preliminary stages. In general, multiple modalities have been used successfully to treat a wide variety of femoropopliteal lesions in multiple series (**Table 63-3**).[20,26-42]

When weighing the risks and benefits of invasive therapy, each patient and lesion requires individual consideration. When comparing medical therapy with revascularization, quality-of-life measures for treatment of claudication have suggested that PTA is more effective than exercise alone, with a cost-effectiveness ratio generally within the acceptable range. If one compares surgery to PTA in patients with claudication, remembering that late patency is the key to long-term symptom relief, PTA emerges as the preferred strategy if the 5-year patency rate for PTA is more than 30%. An initial endovascular approach may also benefit patients with critical limb ischemia and femoropopliteal vascular disease.[43] In a large (*N* = 452) randomized trial, a surgery-first strategy, was compared with a PTA-first strategy, with follow-up over 5 years. PTA and surgery resulted in similar outcomes for amputation-free survival, and PTA was less expensive, leading to a recommendation for a PTA-first strategy when feasible.

To summarize, in many cases, surgery or interventional techniques can ameliorate symptoms. The decision about which is the most appropriate therapy can be made by the patient and physician, taking into account the risks and discomforts of the proposed procedure, its probable durability and reproducibility, the degree to which a procedure closes the door to other therapies, the degree of lifestyle limitation, and the individual patient's tolerance for risk.

The treatment of symptomatic femoropopliteal disease should favor a percutaneous approach over an open surgical procedure, and provisional stent placement appears to be the preferred strategy. Controversy exists about the correct approach for longer lesions (>10 cm) and chronic total occlusions. The advent of fracture-resistant stent designs, better recanalization techniques for occlusions, and perhaps the future development of effective drug-eluting stents, holds promise for further enhancements in the future.

TIBIOPERONEAL OBSTRUCTIVE DISEASE. PAD often involves multiple levels, from proximal to distal, in the extremity. When disease affects the proximal vessels, the infrapopliteal arteries often also have significant occlusive disease (anterior tibial, peroneal, and posterior tibial). Similarly, when tibioperoneal narrowing is present, proximal disease probably coexists. A symptomatic lesion is rarely isolated to a single vessel below the knee. Revascularization strategies for below-knee lesions must take into account the extent, severity, and distribution of disease in more proximal vessels.

For patients with claudication and multilevel disease, correction of inflow obstructive disease in a proximal vessel may be sufficient for symptom relief. This differs from critical limb ischemia, which usually requires restoration of uninterrupted (pulsatile flow) patency to at least one vessel to the foot to heal the lesion. In the absence of severe and flow-limiting proximal disease, significant disease of all three crural vessels is usually required to provoke symptomatic calf claudication or higher grades of ischemia (rest pain or tissue loss).

Treatment

Historically, revascularization of tibioperoneal vessels has been reserved for patients with critical limb ischemia. Endovascular approaches are rapidly replacing traditional surgical bypass. Technologic advances and the use of coronary equipment allow for routine and uncomplicated access to the infrapopliteal vessels. Numerous reports have confirmed the feasibility, safety, and efficacy of tibioperoneal PTA. Primary success rates are generally 80% to 95%, and cumulative 2-year patency rates can approximate 75% (**Table 63-4**).[44-53] Limb salvage rates for percutaneous intervention can rival those of surgical

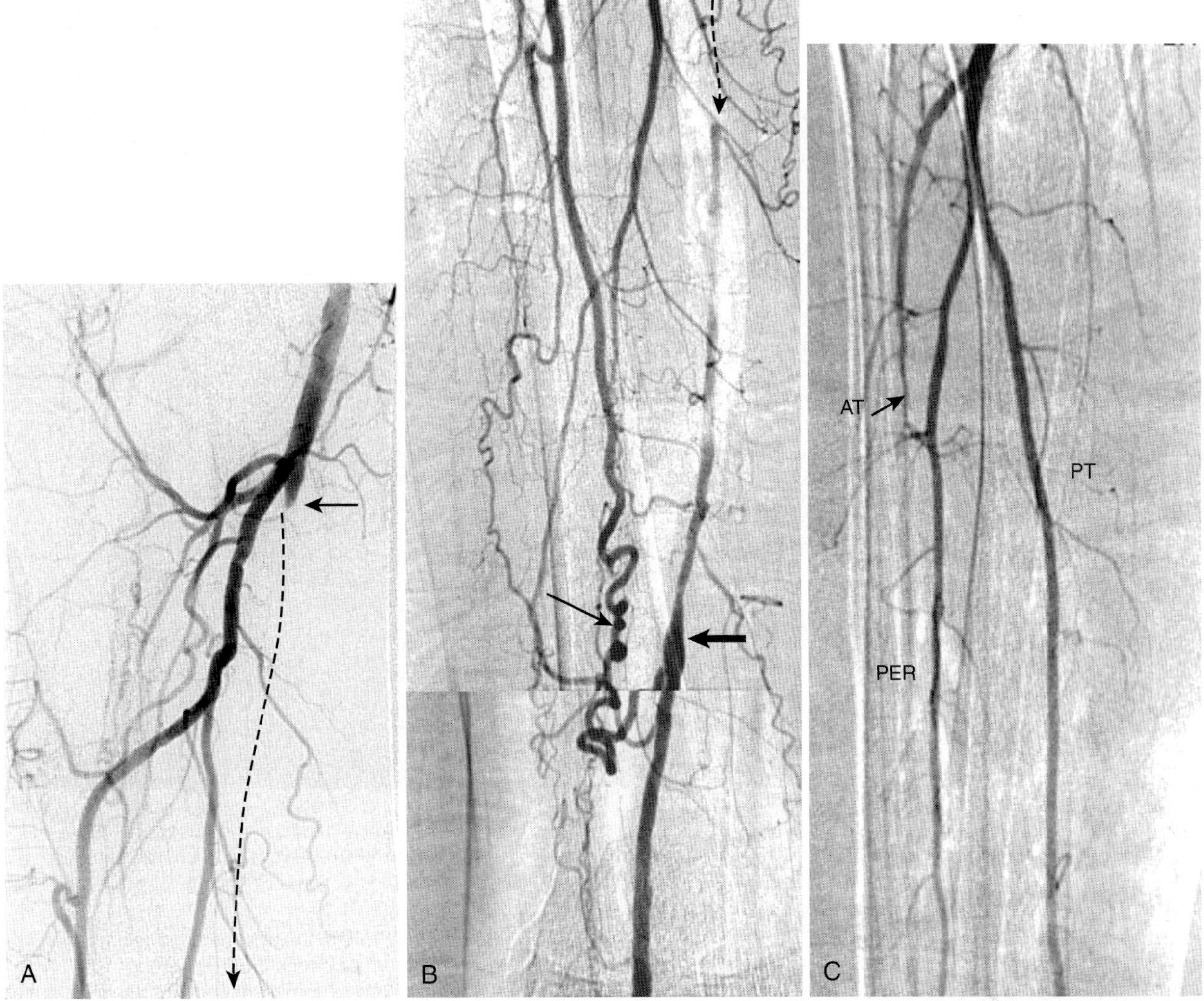

FIGURE 63-5 Long-segment chronic total occlusion. In contrast to the short-segment disease in Figure 63-4, this lesion requires recanalization from the origin of the SFA (**A,** solid arrow) along the path of the SFA (dashed arrow), continuing to the level of the most significant collateral inflow (**B,** thin arrow) and reconstitution of the vessel (**B,** thick arrow). **C,** Crural vessels and occlusion of the anterior tibial (AT) with patent peroneal (PER) and posterior tibial (PT) runoff.

reconstruction. PTA can also effectively salvage ischemic limbs in diabetic patients with small-vessel disease.[54,55]

For tibioperoneal PTA, focal stenoses have the best outcomes, and patients with fewer than five separate lesions have a higher success rate. The success of endovascular therapy is measured by relief of rest pain, healing of ulcers, and avoiding amputation, and not necessarily by long-term vessel patency. It requires more oxygenated blood to heal a wound than to maintain tissue integrity.

The safe and effective revascularization of tibioperoneal vessels with the percutaneous approach in this higher risk cohort has changed the management of patients with critical limb ischemia. When anatomically feasible, a strategy of PTA first is a reasonable and appropriate strategy for revascularization in all patients, even those with low surgical risk for infrapopliteal bypass (**Figs. 63-8 and 63-9**).[43]

The changing approach to revascularization also relates to the indications for intervention in patients with symptomatic but less critical tibioperoneal disease. The threshold for revascularization had traditionally been very high, largely because of the risk of the surgical approach. The availability of effective, less-invasive options permits a lower threshold for intervention. Specifically, in the subset of patients who claudicate solely because of infrapopliteal disease, PTA offers favorable acute and intermediate-term patency and clinical results. Such a strategy should be limited to patients who have severe symptoms (Rutherford category 3) and straightforward anatomy. Infrapopliteal PTA may also help claudicants undergoing proximal revascularization, either with surgery or PTA, with severely impaired runoff. When tibial outflow is a major determinant of long-term patency, recanalizing the runoff vessels may provide benefit.

In summary, optimal management of patients with lower extremity arterial occlusive disease and associated symptoms requires the input of practitioners knowledgeable about the capabilities of percutaneous and surgical revascularization. A strategy of PTA first should be considered if the anatomy is favorable and is certainly preferable to primary amputation.[56] The physician must explain the risks, potential symptomatic benefit, and durability of the proposed intervention. For patients with claudication, there is little evidence that early and aggressive revascularization alters the natural history of lower extremity occlusive disease. Thus, treatment should be guided by the patient's degree of functional impairment.

Limb-threatening ischemia, in contrast, requires prompt treatment, using the modality that will provide the most complete revascularization with the lowest procedural risk. The principal of restoring straight line pulsatile flow to the extremity affected by diffuse disease or long-segment femoropopliteal obstruction may be accomplished with traditional bypass surgery or an endovascular approach. Current evidence supports a PTA-first approach, in selected patients with limb-threatening ischemia and obstructive infrainguinal PAD.[43] As the short and long-term outcomes of catheter-based interventions continue to improve, these endovascular techniques will assume an even more

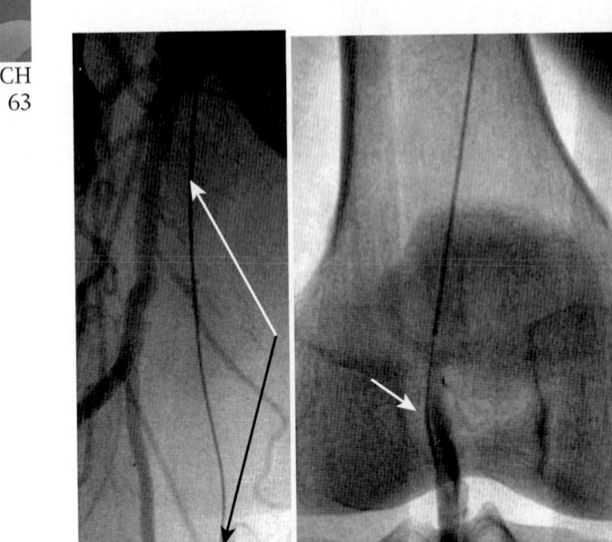

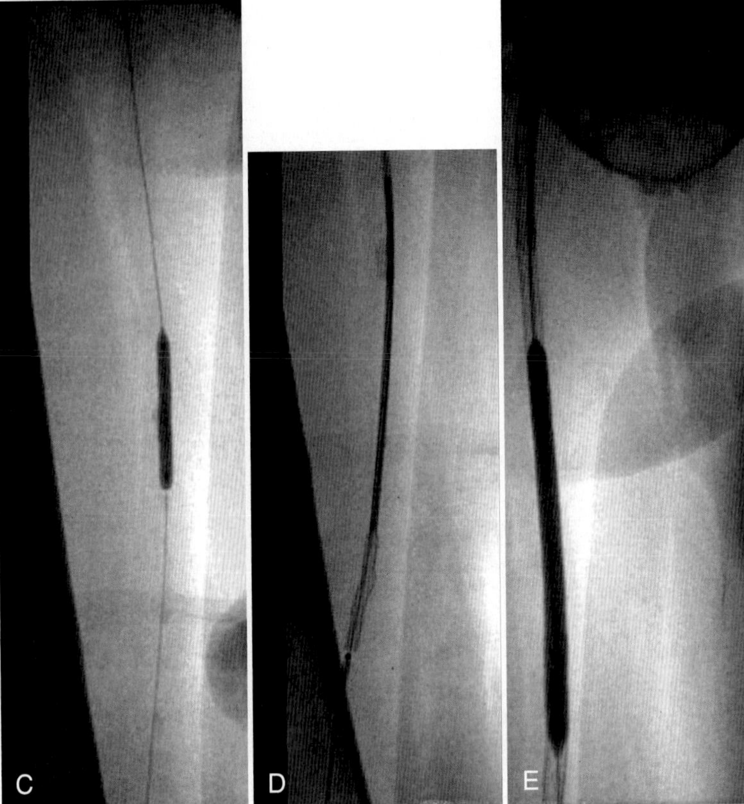

FIGURE 63-6 **A,** Recanalization of this lesion was accomplished from the contralateral approach, using a hydrophilic guidewire advanced into the occluded segment (arrows). **B,** Once the guidewire is free in the distal vessel, a small catheter is passed over the wire and a contrast agent is injected to confirm the intravascular position (arrow). This is followed by predilation **(C),** self-expanding stent placement from distal to proximal **(D),** and finally postdilation to the appropriate size **(E).**

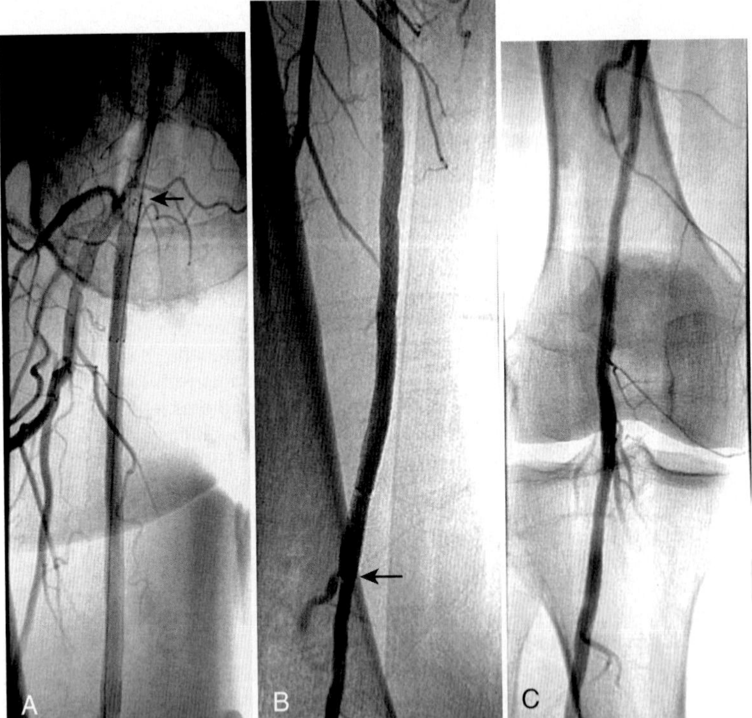

FIGURE 63-7 Recanalization of this long-segment occlusion and stenting from the origin of the SFA in **A** (arrow) to the level of collateral reconstitution in **B** (arrow) resulted in reconstitution of the normal anatomy, **(C),** return of pedal pulses, and healing of digital ulcers. Care was taken to preserve the collateral vessel ostia so that in the event of restenosis, collateral pathways could be reestablished. This anatomy should be contrasted with total occlusion of the SFA but short-segment disease, shown in Figure 63-4. These cases illustrate the anatomic variations that commonly occur and emphasize the difficulty in characterizing the true extent of disease in patients with total occlusions of this vessel.

prominent role in the treatment of patients presenting with claudication or critical limb ischemia.

Regardless of initial treatment strategy, optimum long-term outcome requires diligent follow-up and intrinsic risk factor management. Although surveillance strategies for surgical bypass grafts exist, formal guidelines for monitoring patients following percutaneous therapy are lacking. Pending such guidelines, these individuals should undergo regular evaluation, including clinical examination of the affected limb and performance of duplex sonographic studies.

Atherosclerotic Renal Artery Disease

RENAL ARTERY STENOSIS. Atherosclerosis of the renal artery resulting in renal artery stenosis (RAS) associates with increased cardiovascular events and mortality (see Chap. 93). Assessment of a general population by renal duplex ultrasound in individuals older than 65 years of age has revealed an approximately 7% prevalence of RAS, which increases to 20% to 30% in high-risk populations (e.g., patients with known atherosclerotic vascular disease). Atherosclerotic RAS is a progressive disease associated with a loss of renal mass over time, despite control of hypertension. Progression of RAS to occlusion is more likely with more severe (>60%) lesions and may occur at a rate of up to 20%/year.

Atherosclerotic RAS is an important cause of renal insufficiency, refractory hypertension, and cardiac destabilization syndromes (unstable angina and flash pulmonary edema). Unilateral RAS manifests clinically as a vasoconstrictor-mediated hypertension, whereas bilateral RAS causes hypertension caused by volume overload. Up to 20% of patients older than 50 years of age entering renal dialysis

TABLE 63-3 Evolution of Results of Femoropopliteal Artery Stenting*

STUDY (YEAR)	NO. OF LESIONS	TOTAL OCCLUSIONS (%)	TECHNICAL SUCCESS (%)	*ABI* BEFORE	*ABI* AFTER	MEAN LESION LENGTH (cm)	DEVICES USED	PRIMARY SUCCESS (%)†	CUMULATIVE DURATION (MO)	SUCCESS (%)†	DURATION (mo)
Gray et al (1997)[27]	58	NA	NA	0.48	0.71	16.5	SES, BES	22	24	46	24
Martin (1999)[28]	NA	6	100	NA	NA	NA	PTA	NA	–	57	24
Kessel et al (1999)[29]	NA	—	95	0.6	1	17	SG	29	12	64	12
Conroy et al (2000)[30]	61	100	100	NA	NA¶	13.5	SES, BES	47	12	79	12
Cheng et al (2001)[31]	69	NA	92	NA	NA	13.8	SEN, SES	52.8	24	72.1	24
Gordon et al (2001)[32]	71	100	NA	0.59	0.86	14.4	SES	38.2	24	76.2	24
Scheinert et al (2001)[33]	411	100	83	0.62	NA	19.4	LPTA, SEN	33.6†	12	75.9	12
Lofberg et al (2001)[34]	121	47	88	NA	NA	NA	PTA	27	60	34	60
Bauermeister (2001)[35]	NA	100	100	0.25	0.87	22	SG§	73.2	12	82.6	12
Duda et al (2002)[36]	36	57	100	NA	NA	8.5	DEN/SEN	100/77	6	NA	–
Steinkamp et al (2002)[37]	312	100	91.7	0.56	0.88	7.5	LPTA, SEN	61.5	24	90.2	24
Gray et al (2002)[38]	NA	84	88	0.54	0.84	6.2	LPTA	33	24	75	24
Jamsen et al (2002)[39]	218	NA	83.5	NA	NA	NA	PTA	25	60	4.1	60
Cho et al (2003)[40]	40	100	100	0.61	0.93	NA	SEN	NA	–	NA	–
Becquemin et al (2003)[41]	277	NA	90	0.52	NA	2.5	BES vs. PTA	65/67‡	12	NA	–
Jahnke et al (2003)[42]	63	83	100	0.54	0.89	10.9	SG	74.1	24	83.2	24
Duda et al (2005)[24]	57	65	—	0.61	0.87	81.5	DEN vs. SEN	20.7/17.9	18	NA	–
Schillinger et al (2006)[20]	104	35	100	0.58	0.84	13.2	SEN vs. PTA	37/63	12	NA	–
Dake (2009)[26]	843	—	—	—	—	—	DEN	82	24	78 (EFS)	24

*Summary of reports of femoropopliteal interventions from the literature. A wide variety of anatomic situations are represented here, including many with chronic long-segment total occlusions. Of note is that primary patency of 2 years, when reported, is considerably lower than that for iliac interventions, yet cumulative patency ranges from approximately 75% to 90%. This emphasizes the need for both postprocedure surveillance and consideration of the performance of a femoral intervention when embarking on a course of therapy.

†Clinical or objective patency.

‡Angiographic patency (<50% stenosis) in mandatory stent group versus PTA with selective stenting group.

§Devices placed surgically.

¶Average increase of 0.26.

BES = balloon-expandable stainless steel; DEN = drug-eluting nitinol; EFS = event-free survival; LPTA = excimer laser-assisted PTA; NA = not assessed or reported; PTA = percutaneous transluminal (balloon) angioplasty; SEN = self-expanding nitinol; SES = self-expanding stainless steel; SG = stent graft.

TABLE 63-4 Evolution of Results of Tibioperoneal Artery Interventions

STUDY (YEAR)*	NO. OF PATIENTS TREATED	NO. OF LESIONS TREATED	TOTAL OCCLUSION (%)	TECHNICAL SUCCESS (%)	*ABI* BEFORE	*ABI* AFTER	MEAN LESION LENGTH (cm)	PRIMARY DEVICE	PRIMARY PATENCY (%)	DURATION (MO)	CUMULATIVE PATENCY (%)	DURATION (mo)	EVENT-FREE SURVIVAL (%)	DURATION (mo)	LIMB SALVAGE (%)	DURATION (mo)
Sivananthan et al (1994)[44]	38	73	24	96	—	—	—	PTA	—	—	—	—	—	—	—	—
Varty et al (1995)[45]	38	40	17	98	0.55	0.84	1	PTA	59	24	68	24	—	—	77	12
Dorros et al (1998)[46]	312	657	27	98	—	—	—	PTA	—	—	—	—	—	—	—	—
Desgranges et al (2000)[47]	33	—	—	82	—	—	—	PTA	66	12	77	12	94	12	91	12
Soder et al (2000)[48]	60	72	35	84/61[†]	—	—	—	PTA	68/48[†]	10	56	18	—	—	80	18
Dorros et al (2001)[49]	235	529	28.9	92	—	—	—	PTA	—	—	—	—	31	60	91	60
Tsetis et al (2002)[50]	12	13	100	92.3	0.35	0.68	7	VPTA	—	—	—	—	—	—	—	—
Feiring et al (2004)[51]	82	92	—	94	0.32	0.9	—	SE	—	—	—	—	92	12	96	12
Giles et al (2008)[52]	163	176	29	93	—	—	—	PTA	24	24	61	24	35	24		
Sioablis et al (2009)[53]	75	153	24.2	98.7	—	—	5.5	DES	36	36	—	—	78	36	84	36

*Selected recent literature on tibial artery interventions. Most reports are of single-center experience and procedural results.

[†]Stenosis or occlusion.

DES = drug-eluting stent; PTA = percutaneous transluminal (balloon) angioplasty; VPTA = vibrational PTA; — = not assessed or reported.

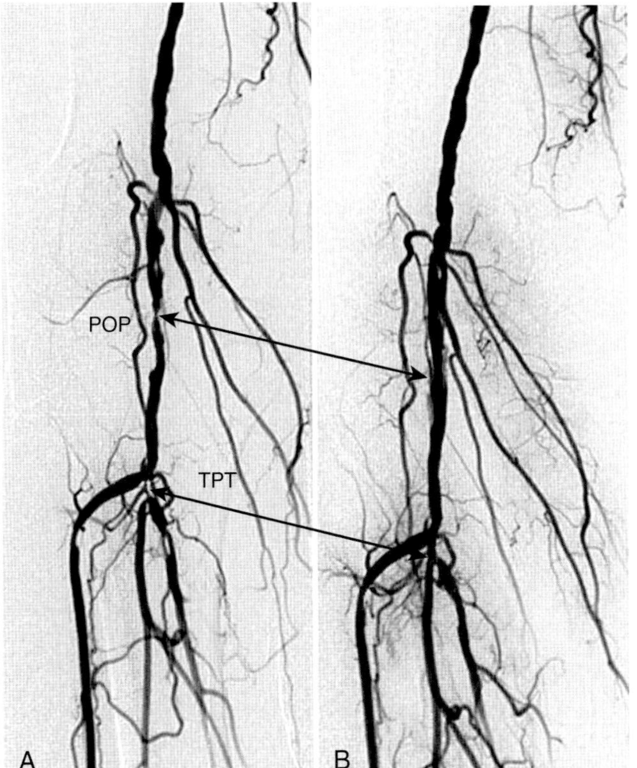

FIGURE 63-8 Intervention in tibial disease. Lesions in the below-knee popliteal artery (POP; **A**) and in the very short tibioperoneal trunk (TPT; **B**) were identified and successfully treated with PTA.

programs in the United States have atherosclerotic RAS (ischemic nephropathy) as the cause of their renal failure. The 2-, 5-, and 10-year survival rates are about 60%, 20%, and 5%, respectively, for dialysis-dependent patients with RAS. The mortality risk depends on the severity of RAS (**Table 63-5**). The median survival for dialysis patients with atherosclerotic RAS was 25 months, compared with 133 months for patients with polycystic kidney disease. Clearly, the early diagnosis of RAS and the prevention of end-stage renal disease (ESRD) is an important goal.

Diagnosis

Clinical clues to the diagnosis of RAS (**Table 63-6**) include the onset of diastolic hypertension after 55 years of age refractory or malignant hypertension, resistant hypertension in a previously well-controlled patient, and/or an increasing serum creatinine level. These should alert the clinician and prompt further diagnostic testing (**Figs. 63-10 and 63-11**). Imaging best diagnoses RAS. Duplex renal artery ultrasound, CTA, and MRA are all recommended as noninvasive screening tests for patients suspected of having RAS.[1] Invasive renal angiography is recommended when the clinical suspicion is high and noninvasive testing is inconclusive or inconsistent with the clinical evidence. Some advocate renal angiography at the time of cardiac catheterization or peripheral vascular angiography for patients who are at increased risk for RAS. Screening modalities that are no longer recommended include captopril renal scintigraphy, measurement of plasma renin activity (with or without captopril stimulation), and selective renal vein renin measurements.

Treatment

After establishing the anatomic diagnosis of RAS, one must consider the most appropriate management. The goals of treatment include blood pressure control, preserving or improving renal function, and reducing the risk of flash pulmonary edema, refractory heart failure, and difficult to control angina pectoris. The indications for revascularization require the presence of clinical findings related to RAS with a hemodynamically significant stenosis, defined as the following: (1) 50% diameter or larger stenosis, with a systolic translesional gradient (measured with a 5Fr or smaller catheter or pressure wire) of 20 mm Hg or more or a mean pressure gradient of 10 mm Hg or more; (2) 70% diameter or larger stenosis by quantitative angiographic methods; or (3) 70% diameter or larger stenosis by intravascular ultrasound measurement.[57]

Although PTA alone remains the treatment of choice for fibromuscular dysplasia (FMD) lesions, primary stent placement for atherosclerotic RAS is the current standard of care (**Fig. 63-12**).[1] Stents have been proven to yield more predictable and hemodynamically favorable results in renal revascularization, and studies have suggested that restenosis rates for renal stenting are generally very low (**Table 63-7**).[58-65]

The strongest predictor of late renal stent patency is acute gain, or maximizing the stent lumen. Larger diameter (≥6 mm) renal arteries have lower restenosis rates than smaller (<4.5 mm) vessels. Long-term follow-up has suggested primary patency rates of approximately 80% to 85% and secondary patency rates of more than 90%. Almost all in-stent restenosis occurs during the first year after stent implantation, with restenosis later than 2 years an unusual occurrence.

Despite technical success rates in excess of 95% using stents, angiographic stenosis does not predict clinical benefit (**Table 63-8**).[58-61,63-66] This implies that either the renal artery stenosis is not causally related to the hypertension, or the successful revascularization procedure did not relieve the renal hypoperfusion. A major difficulty in predicting a treatment response in patients with renovascular disease is that they commonly have other nephrotoxic conditions that could confound their response to revascularization, such as diabetes, essential hypertension, atheroemboli, and medication-related insults.

Patient Selection

Analogous to the coronary technique of fractional flow reserve (FFR), the renal fractional flow reserve serves as a lesion-specific functional assessment of a renal artery stenosis (see Chap. 52). Consistent with the unpredictable clinical results, quantitative angiography correlates poorly with hemodynamic gradients (peak, mean, and hyperemic), whereas an excellent correlation has been shown for the renal FFR and the baseline pressure gradient.[67] Renal FFR, determined in 17 patients with poorly controlled hypertension, correlated with clinical improvement. An abnormal renal FFR (<0.8) predicted blood pressure improvement (86%), compared with a 30% improvement if the FFR was normal ($P = 0.04$).[68]

Brain natriuretic peptide (BNP) promotes diuresis, natriuresis, and arterial vasodilation; antagonizes the renin-angiotensin system and angiotensin II; and may serve as a biomarker of response to renal revascularization. In 27 patients with uncontrolled hypertension and RAS (≥70% diameter stenosis), hypertension improved in 77% of those with elevated BNP levels, compared with 0 of 5 patients with a baseline BNP of 80 pg/mL or less ($P = 0.001$). If BNP levels decreased to more than 30% after successful stent placement, 94% (16 of 17) had improvement in their blood pressure control.[69]

The renal artery resistive index (RI), measured noninvasively by Doppler ultrasound, may also stratify patients likely to respond to renal intervention. Data conflict, however, regarding the ability of RI to predict treatment response in patients with RAS. A retrospective study in which most patients were treated with balloon angioplasty, not stents, has suggested that an elevated RI is associated with a low probability of improved blood pressure or renal function after revascularization.[70] In a prospective study of renal stent placement in 241 patients, however, patients with an abnormal RI experienced blood pressure response and renal functional improvement at 1 year after renal arterial intervention (**Figs. 63-13 and 63-14**).[71] The preponderance of evidence and scientific quality of the latter studies favors the conclusion that an elevated RI should not preclude the performance of renal artery intervention for obstructive RAS.

Several clinical trials have demonstrated that successful renal artery stent placement improves or stabilizes renal function in patients with atherosclerotic renovascular renal insufficiency. Patients with renal insufficiency and hemodynamically significant RAS improve after

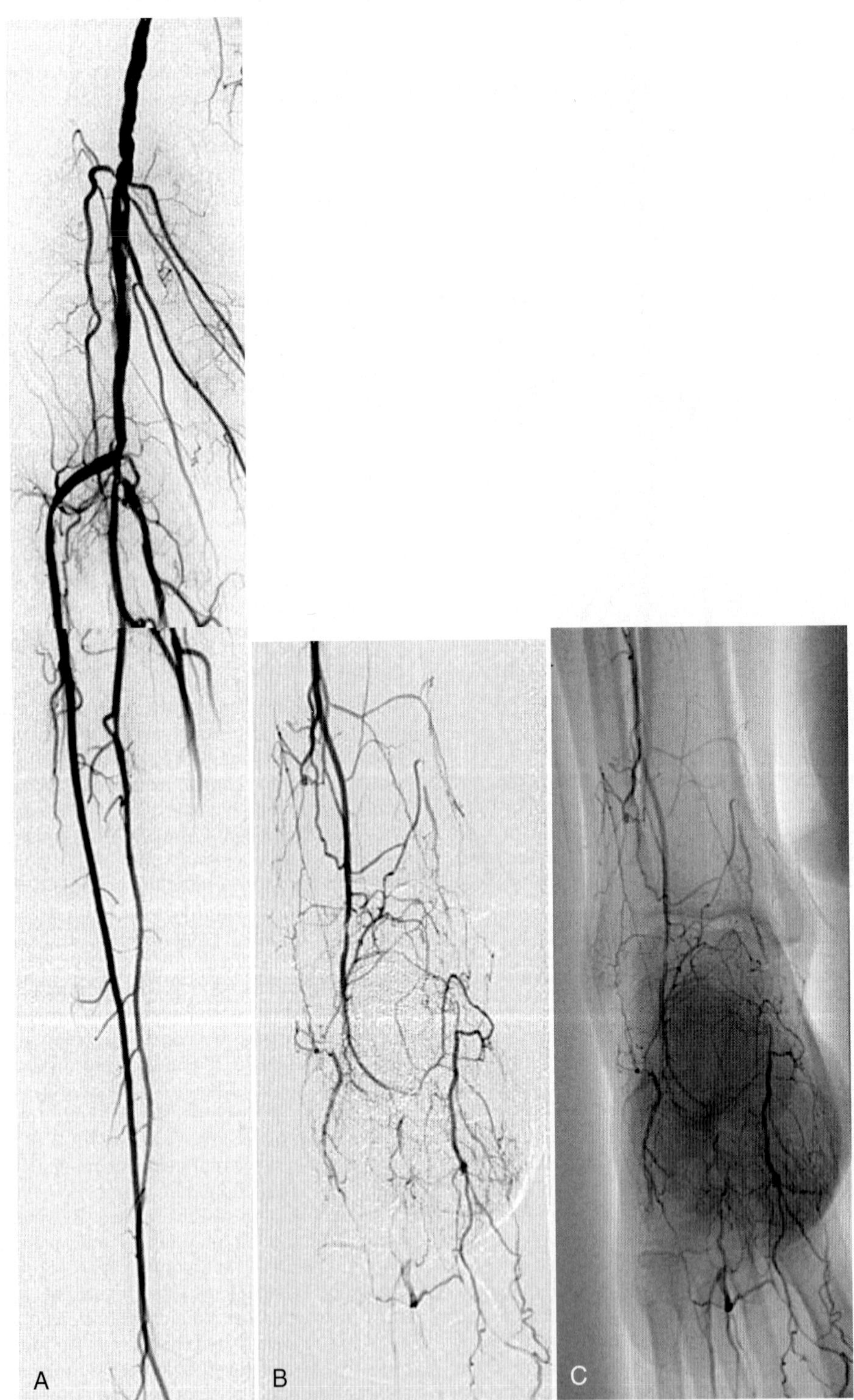

FIGURE 63-9 **A,** Composite angiogram from the patient depicted in Figure 63-8 demonstrating the intact anterior tibial runoff in the calf. The peroneal normally attenuates by the level of the malleoli and, in this case, the posterior tibial is also occluded. **B, C,** Pedal circulation in digital subtraction angiography and native views. Although straight line flow to the foot was reconstituted and the patient's ulcers healed, the evident diffuse small-vessel disease in the pedal vessels still places the foot in long-term jeopardy. Careful surveillance and compulsive continuing medical management are critical for this group of patients, even in the context of technical procedural success.

stent placement. Successful renal artery stent placement can significantly slow the progression of renal failure. Calculation of the mean slope of the reciprocal of serum creatinine levels before and after stent placement shows a fourfold slowing in the progression of renal insufficiency after renal artery stent placement. One of the best predictors of improvement in renal function following percutaneous revascularization is a rapid rate of decline in renal function immediately prior to intervention, suggesting that the rapid decline in renal function reflects a more acute injury, which is more likely to be reversible.[72] Alternatively, approximately 20% of patients who undergo renal intervention will have a decline or worsening in their renal function. One contributing factor may be atheroembolism, resulting from the trauma to the bulky aortic plaque (**Fig. 63-15**). Work is ongoing to adapt embolic protection for renal interventions.[73]

TABLE 63-5 Severity of Renal Artery Stenosis and Survival

SEVERITY OF RAS	4-YEAR SURVIVAL
No RAS	90%
50% to 75%	70%
76% to 95%	68%
> 95%	48%

Modified from Conlon PJ, Little MA, Pieper K, Mark DB: Severity of renal vascular disease predicts mortality in patients undergoing coronary angiography. Kidney Int 60:1490, 2001.

TABLE 63-6 Clinical Predictors of Renal Artery Stenosis

1. Onset of hypertension in patients ≤30 yr or >55 yr
2. Malignant, accelerated, or resistant hypertension
3. Unexplained renal dysfunction
4. Development of azotemia or worsening renal function after ACE inhibitor or ARB
5. "Flash" pulmonary edema
6. Atrophic kidney or size discrepancy between kidneys of >1.5 cm
7. Multivessel coronary disease or peripheral arterial disease

Modified from Hirsch AT, Haskal ZJ, Hertzer NR, et al: ACC/AHA 2005 guidelines for the management of patients with peripheral arterial disease (lower extremity, renal, mesenteric, and abdominal aortic): Executive summary: A collaborative report from the American Association for Vascular Surgery/Society for Vascular Surgery, Society for Cardiovascular Angiography and Interventions, Society for Vascular Medicine and Biology, Society of Interventional Radiology, and the ACC/AHA Task Force on Practice Guidelines (Writing Committee to Develop Guidelines for the Management of Patients with Peripheral Arterial Disease) endorsed by the American Association of Cardiovascular and Pulmonary Rehabilitation; National Heart, Lung and Blood Institute; Society for Vascular Nursing; TransAtlantic Inter-Society Consensus; and Vascular Disease Foundation. J Am Coll Cardiol 47:1239, 2006.

Unilateral Renal Artery Stenosis and Nephropathy

Traditional teaching holds that unilateral RAS does not cause ischemic nephropathy when the contralateral renal artery is patent. However, revascularization of unilateral RAS can improve or stabilize renal function. Revascularization of unilateral RAS can result in measurable improvement in the split renal function of the stenotic kidney. Restoring flow to the stenotic kidney can reverse the hyperfiltration of the nonstenotic kidney, resulting in decreased proteinuria. Thus, in patients with abnormal renal function, treatment of unilateral RAS may improve and/or stabilize renal function.

Percutaneous treatment of renovascular disease, in summary, offers a safe and effective therapy that is preferable to open surgical revascularization. Renal artery stenting can ameliorate hypertension and improve or stabilize renal function, and may delay the need for hemodialysis in appropriately selected patients. Finally, the advent of distal protection devices to limit atheroembolic complications may further improve safety and renal parenchymal preservation. The current recommended systematic approach to the investigation and treatment of this condition is outlined in Figures 63-10 and 63-11. Despite many reports of clinical success in selected and carefully chosen patient groups, the enthusiasm for widespread treatment of mild or moderate renovascular disease has waned. Recent published data from the ASTRAL trial, in which patients were randomized to revascularization versus continued medical therapy alone, did not show a clear benefit of renal revascularization,[65] although its design and conclusions have been criticized.[74] The ongoing CORAL trial is randomizing patients with RAS to renal stenting versus medical therapy alone to determine whether an even broader population might benefit from revascularization.[75]

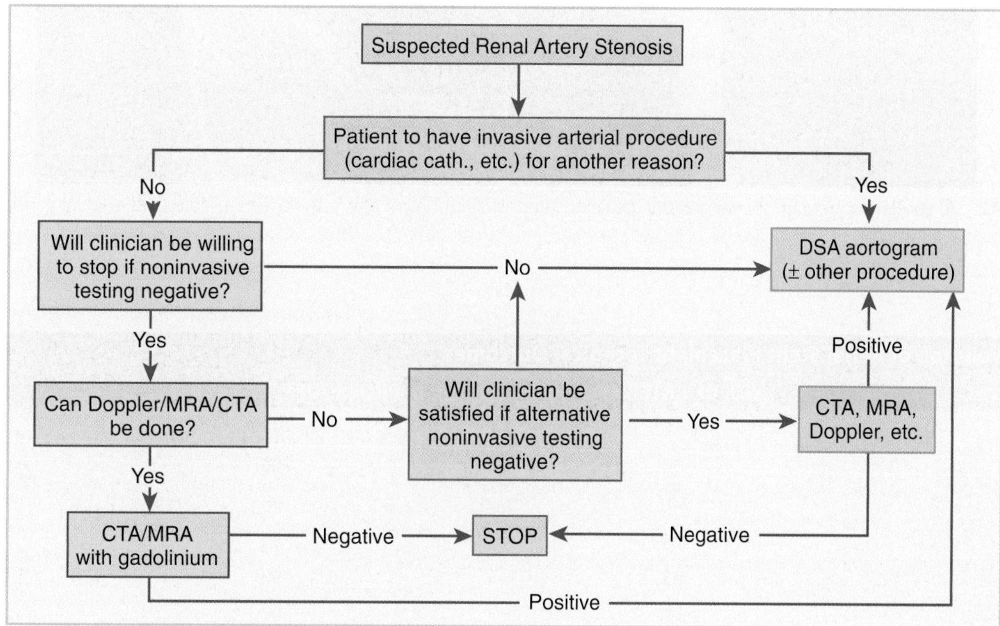

FIGURE 63-10 Approach to the anatomic evaluation of RAS. Once stenosis is suspected, if the patient is to have another invasive arterial procedure, noninvasive imaging is deferred and low-volume DSA is performed at the time of that procedure. In other cases, the clinician should assess whether a negative noninvasive test would be sufficient evidence to acquit the renal arteries. If so, noninvasive testing should be performed. If not, consideration should be given to DSA and selective angiography. Cath = catheterization.

CH 63

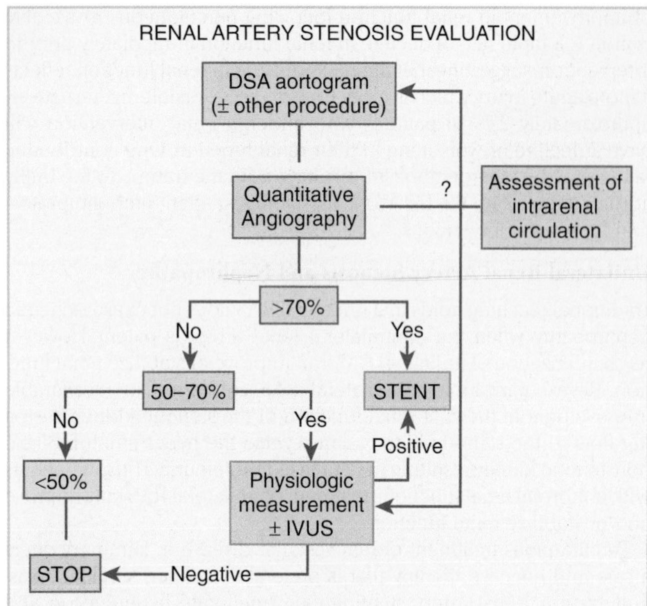

FIGURE 63-11 Approach to the angiographic evaluation and treatment of renal artery stenosis. Once DSA is performed, confirming the presence of renovascular disease, quantitative angiography and objective evaluation of the severity of stenosis should be performed. Very severe (>70% diameter stenosis) lesions are subjected to revascularization, and mild lesions (<50% diameter stenosis) are not. We believe that the intermediate lesion should be assessed with physiologic evaluation and/or additional anatomic documentation of severity, such as intravascular ultrasound (IVUS) or fractional flow reserve. The absence of translesional flow acceleration or a pressure gradient should mitigate the desire to intervene (see Fig. 45-14).

Chronic Mesenteric Ischemia

The clinical syndrome of chronic mesenteric ischemia (CMI) is surprisingly uncommon, given the high frequency of atherosclerotic disease of the aorta and the common finding of aorto-ostial stenosis of the visceral vessels.[76] The mesenteric circulation consists of the celiac trunk, the superior mesenteric artery (SMA), and the inferior mesenteric artery (IMA). The rarity of this clinical syndrome probably reflects the redundancy of the visceral circulation with multiple pathways from the SMA and IMA. Females are disproportionately affected (70%), and the classic presentation is postprandial abdominal discomfort; patients with CMI typically avoid food and usually have significant weight loss. Even in advanced cases, multiple other causes of the weight loss and abdominal pain are often entertained before intestinal angina comes into focus as the diagnosis of exclusion. Significant obstruction of two or more of these vessels usually underlies classic symptoms. Endoscopic findings suggest bowel ischemia, although single-vessel disease, usually of the SMA, can sometimes cause CMI, particularly if collateral connections have been disrupted by prior abdominal surgery.

Diagnosis

The relatively common application of CTA and MRA for these abdominal symptoms now enables the anatomic diagnosis without invasive angiography. Invasive angiography is useful for diagnosis, but requires a lateral aortogram to visualize the ostia of the mesenteric vessels (**Figs. 63-16 and 63-17**). When the symptoms are typical, the anatomic findings severe, and the alternative pathologic explanations few, the diagnosis is confirmed and revascularization is in order. As might be expected, however, this patient group has a high incidence of coronary artery disease and the surgical mortality and morbidity ranges from 5% to 8%, with the highest incidence of complications occurring in older patients.

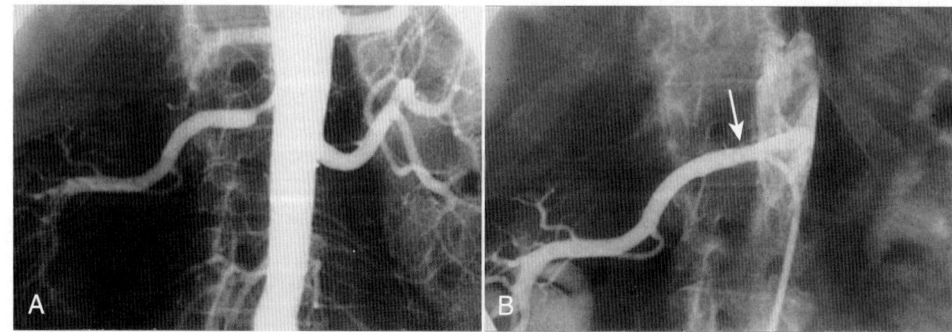

FIGURE 63-12 **A,** Baseline aortogram showing ≥70% diameter stenosis of right renal artery. **B,** Poststent. Note mild residual narrowing (arrow).

TABLE 63-7 Evolution of Renal Stent Placement Technical Outcomes

STUDY (YEAR)	NO. OF ARTERIES	PROCEDURE SUCCESS (%)	RESTENOSIS
White et al (1997)[58]	133	99	18.8
Blum et al (1997)[59]	74	100	11.0
Tuttle et al (1998)[60]	148	98	14.0
Henry et al (1999)[61]	209	99	11.4
van de Ven et al (1999)[62]	43	90	14.0
Rocha-Singh et al (1999)[63]	180	97	12.0
Lederman et al (2001)[64]	358	100	21.0
Wheatley et al (2009)[65]	335	95	NR

NR = not reported.

TABLE 63-8 Blood Pressure Response to Renal Artery Stenting

STUDY (YEAR)	NO. OF PATIENTS	ARTERIES	CURED (%)	IMPROVED (%)	BENEFIT (%)
Blum et al 1997)[59]	68	74	16	62	78
Tuttle et al (1998)[60]	129	148	2	55	57
Henry et al (1999)[61]	210	244	19	61	78
Rocha-Singh et al (1999)[63]	150	180	6	50	56
Dorros et al (1993)[66]	76	92	7	52	59
White et al (1997)[58]	100	133	NR	76	76
Lederman et al (2001)[64]	261	NR	<1	70	70

NR = not reported.

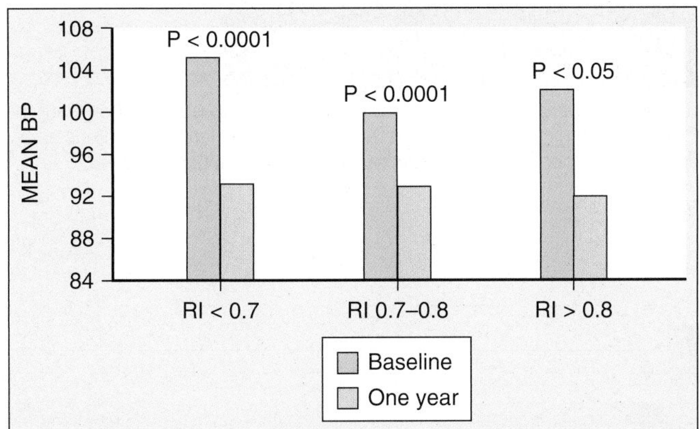

FIGURE 63-13 Blood pressure (BP) response in patients with normal RI (<0.7), moderate elevation (RI = 0.7-0.8), and severe nephrosclerosis (>0.8) at 1 year after stent placement. *(Data from Zeller T, Frank U, Müller C, et al: Predictors of improved renal function after percutaneous stent-supported angioplasty of severe atherosclerotic ostial renal artery stenosis. Circulation 108:2244, 2003.)*

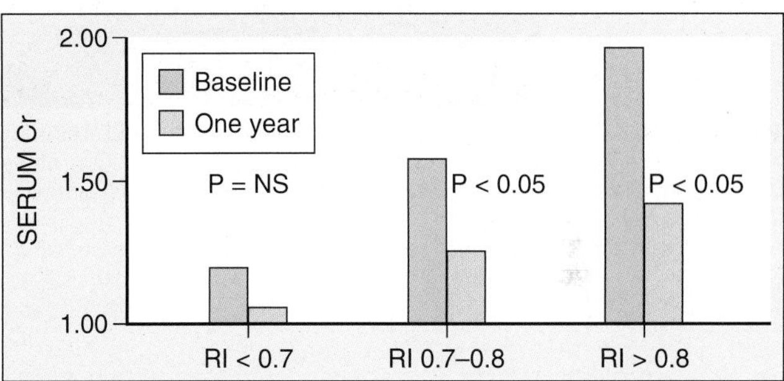

FIGURE 63-14 Renal function change in patients with normal RI (<0.7), moderate elevation (RI = 0.7-0.8), and severe nephrosclerosis (>0.8) at 1 year after stent placement. Cr = creatinine. *(Data from Zeller T, Frank U, Müller C, et al: Predictors of improved renal function after percutaneous stent-supported angioplasty of severe atherosclerotic ostial renal artery stenosis. Circulation 108:2244, 2003.)*

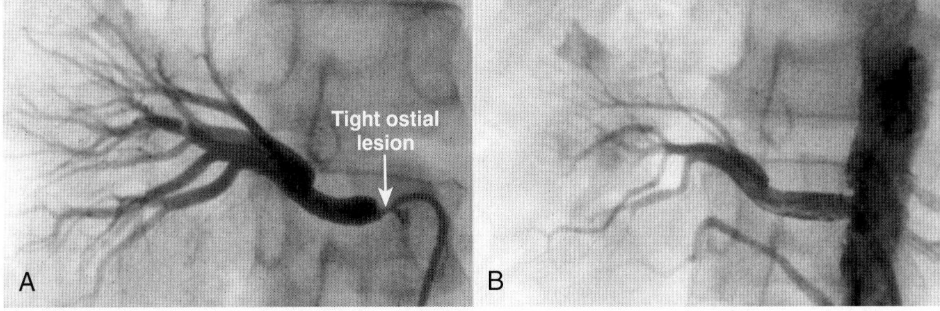

FIGURE 63-15 Distal embolization post intervention: **A,** Baseline selective right renal angiogram. Note normal cortical vessels. **B,** Poststent. Note the absence of distal filling because of atheroembolization.

Treatment

Obstructions of the visceral vessels resemble those of the renal arteries. The technical considerations for PTA and stent placement are similar to those for renal artery intervention. The endovascular approach circumvents the need for general anesthesia and the operative trauma associated with open surgery, and may result in a lower acute mortality and morbidity.[77,78]

Because of the relative infrequency of this disease, there are no comparative trials of surgery versus endovascular treatment for CMI. Interpretation of the literature, which reports successful case series of surgical and interventional treatment, is confounded by the obvious case selection and other inherent biases. Interventional treatment offers an alternative for the management of chronic visceral ischemia that may have advantages over surgery, especially for those patients of advanced age or with additional increased risk of morbidity and mortality (see Fig. 63-17).

The single largest series of endovascular therapy for CMI was recently reported, with a technical success rate of 96% and symptom relief in 88% of 63 patients (79 vessels).[79] At a mean follow-up of 38 ± 15 months, 17% had recurrence of symptoms but none developed acute mesenteric ischemia, and all underwent successful revascularization without complication. Follow-up was carried out in 90% of patients and 90% of the vessels with angiographic CT, conventional angiography, or Duplex ultrasound, showing an in-stent restenosis rate of 29%.

In summary, although no prospective controlled data compare outcomes of balloon angioplasty versus stent placement for the treatment of mesenteric arterial stenoses, recent studies have suggested that endovascular stent placement confers immediate and long-term results superior to balloon angioplasty alone. Therefore,

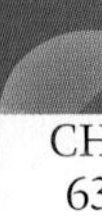

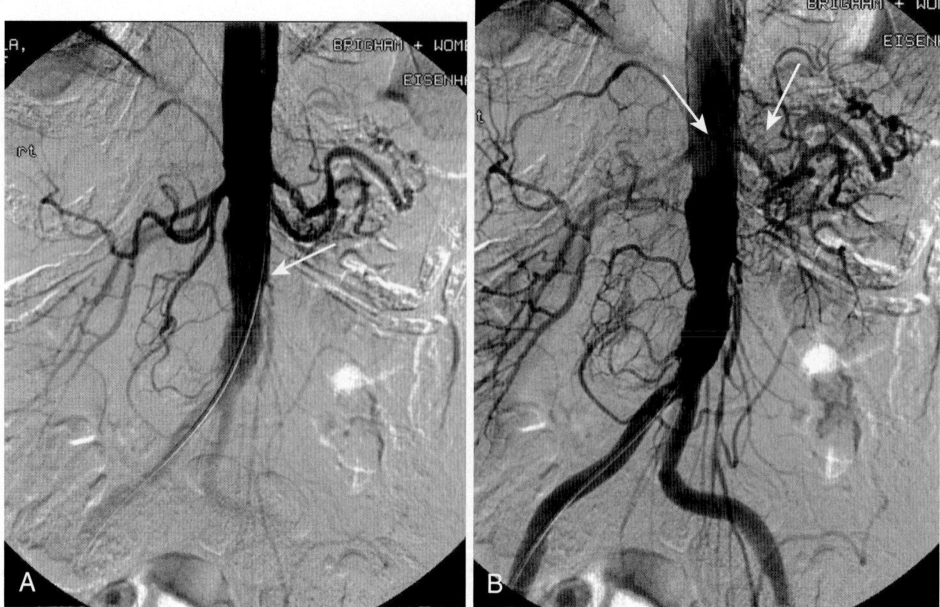

FIGURE 63-16 Visceral angiogram from a patient with postprandial abdominal pain, weight loss, and abdominal bruits. This projection does not demonstrate the origins of the celiac or superior mesenteric arteries. **A,** Early in the run, however, the thin arrow indicates a stenosis at the origin of the inferior mesenteric artery. **B,** Then, from a later frame, the origins of the renal arteries are seen (arrows); although potentially not seen in absolute profile, they appear unobstructed.

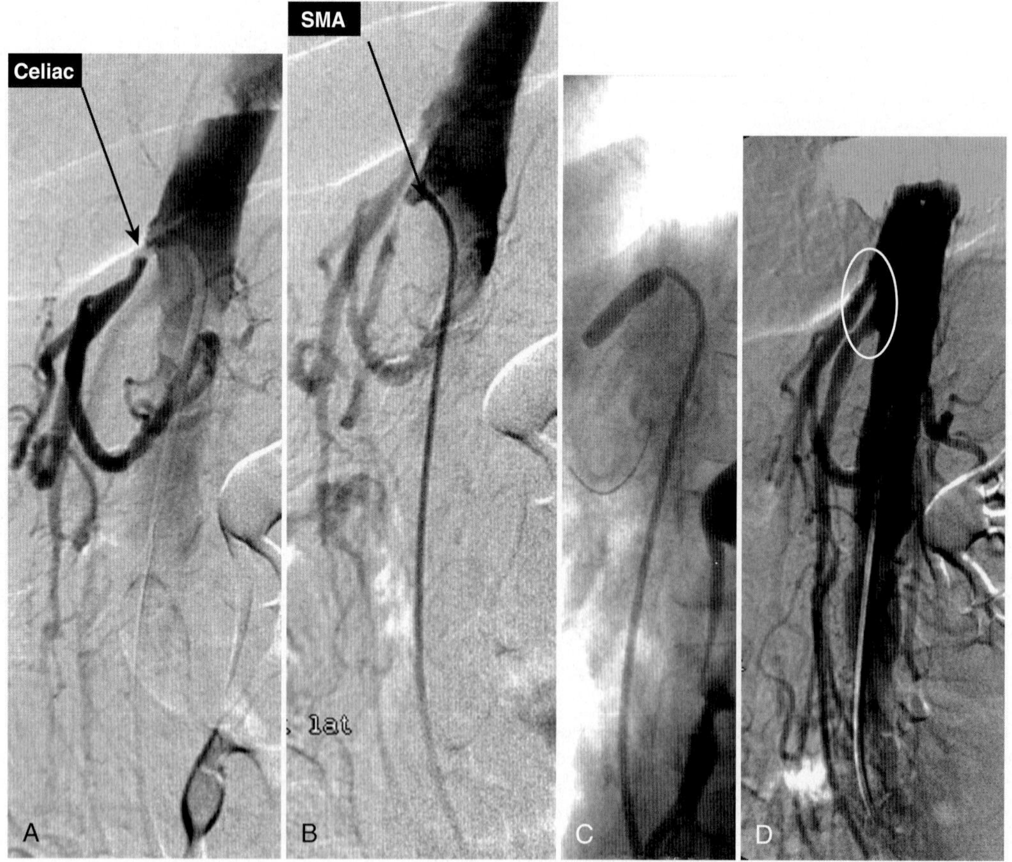

FIGURE 63-17 Selective evaluation of the celiac arteries and SMA in the lateral projection of the patient in Figure 63-16. **A, B,** Both these vessels proved to be critically stenosed. **C,** They were treated interventionally, restoring wide patency to both, as outlined in **D.** The patient's symptoms abated and she began to gain weight.

stent revascularization should be the percutaneous treatment of choice.

Brachiocephalic and Subclavian Obstructive Disease

Once considered relatively rare, brachiocephalic and subclavian artery obstructions have received increased attention recently because of the use of internal mammary conduits for coronary bypass surgery. Asymptomatic differences in systolic arm pressures (≥10 mm Hg) are the most common presentation of brachiocephalic or subclavian stenosis. Subclavian steal syndrome arises because of reversal of flow in the vertebral artery as blood is shunted to the upper extremity circulation. Vertebrobasilar symptoms of dizziness, syncope, and vertigo are most common, along with upper extremity claudication of the ipsilateral limb. In coronary subclavian steal, there is reversal of flow within the left internal mammary artery because of proximal subclavian stenosis. These patients often come to clinical attention with myocardial ischemia. Although conservative therapy offers some clinical improvement, the problem usually requires relief of the anatomic obstruction.

Treatment

Balloon angioplasty for subclavian artery stenosis was described in the early 1980s, with subsequent reports showing acute success and patency rates at follow-up comparable to those of surgery. Furthermore, there was a low rate of complications and infrequent mortality. There was initial concern about the potential for distal embolization and stroke, uncertain long-term patency, and difficulty in treating total occlusions. With continued improvements in anesthetic and operative technique, short hospital stays, and early discharge, many practitioners continue to regard surgery as the standard against which endovascular methods must be compared.

Clinical data regarding long-term patency of the subclavian or brachiocephalic vessels are limited (**Fig. 63-18**). An evaluation of the reports of surgery versus angioplasty or stenting of this condition has described technical success (with the planned procedure yielding target lesion revascularization and survival to discharge), patient death, stroke, and patency of the treated segment.[80] There was no uniformity or standardization for evaluating or reporting complications in the studies in which stenting was performed; however, adverse events were reported in approximately 6% of patients.

Similarly, the overall incidence of postprocedure complications, such as vascular access bleeding, hemorrhage, pseudoaneurysm, transfusion, or contrast-mediated transient renal insufficiency, is not known. Technical success has been reported in 97% of cases. No strokes or deaths occurred. Follow-up data were available in about two thirds of cases at a mean of 16.8 months. Occlusion or restenosis was found in less than 10%.[80] Additional reports of subclavian stent placement continue to suggest that perioperative strokes are uncommon and the results are favorable.[81] There have been some concerns not only about long-term patency, but also about durability of the stent because of strut fracture at the site of flexion and compression.

A European series reviewed 115 patients with subclavian disease who were treated percutaneously.[82] Successful revascularization was achieved in 98% of patients. There were no periprocedural deaths, but 1 patient had a transient ischemic attack from the left vertebral artery and 2 patients had emboli—1 to the renal artery and 1 to the mesenteric artery. All 3 patients recovered completely from these events. Whereas patency rates were significantly higher at 1 year in the stent group, compared with those treated only with angioplasty (95% versus 76%), by 4 years of follow-up there was more restenosis in the stent patients.[82] Another recent report[83] on 170 symptomatic patients with 177 subclavian and innominate arteries treated with catheter-based stent therapy had a procedure success rate of 98.3%, no mortalities occurred within 30 days, and the periprocedural stroke rate was less than 1%. At 3 years of follow-up, 82% of patients remained asymptomatic, with a primary patency rate of 83% and a secondary patency rate of 96%.

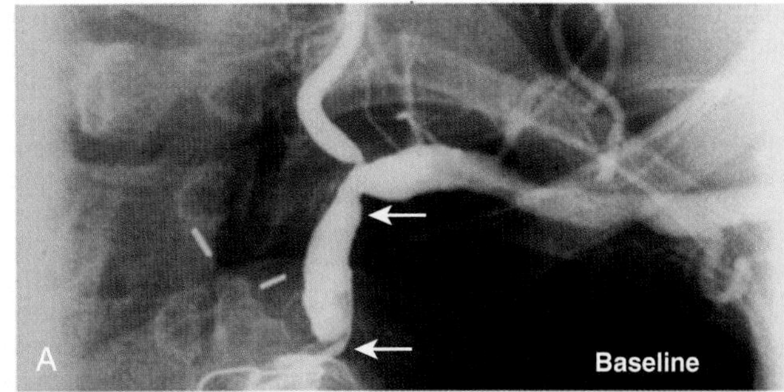

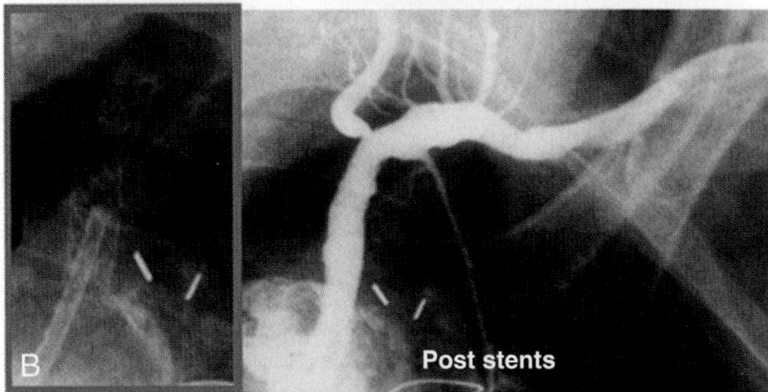

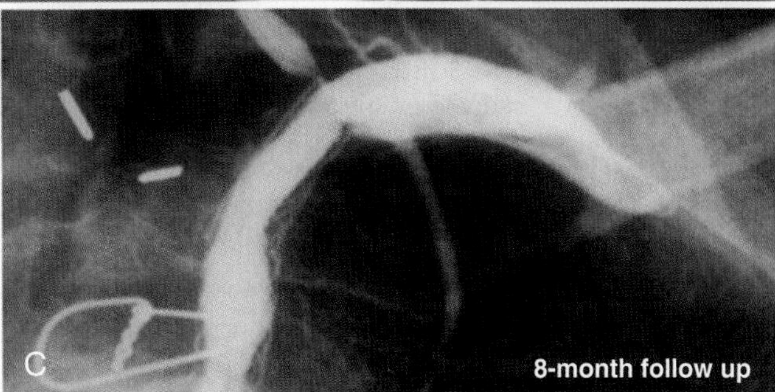

FIGURE 63-18 **A,** Baseline angiogram of a left subclavian artery with a tight proximal stenosis and a moderate stenosis just proximal to the vertebral artery. **B,** After placement of two balloon expandable stents. Note the position of the stents in the inset. **C,** Follow-up angiogram at 8 months with patent stents.

In summary, it is unlikely that a large well-designed trial comparing surgical and interventional treatment of patients with brachiocephalic and subclavian disease will be carried out because of the relative infrequency of this disease. At present, experience and examination of the literature support the consideration of a primary percutaneous approach in most patients with symptomatic obstructive disease.

Carotid and Vertebral Disease

CAROTID ARTERY DISEASE. Slightly more than 50% of the 731,000 strokes/year in the United States result from extracranial atherosclerotic carotid artery disease. Stroke is the leading cause of disability and the third leading cause of death after coronary artery disease and cancer in the United States (see Chap. 62). Atherosclerotic extracranial carotid artery disease usually causes symptoms as a result of embolic events. In contrast to acute coronary syndromes, a minority of ischemic strokes are caused by thrombotic occlusion.

The two internal carotid arteries and two vertebral arteries come together at the base of the skull to form the circle of Willis, which is an ideal anastomotic network. In theory, a single vessel could supply the circulatory needs of the entire brain. However, although a circle of Willis is present in every brain, there is a huge amount of individual variability, and fewer than half are complete.

Cerebrovascular events are classified as transient ischemic attacks (TIAs) if they are transient and do not result in an infarction, or as strokes if they cause an acute infarction[84] (see Chap. 62). Patients with a TIA have a 1 in 20 (5%) chance of stroke within 30 days, and almost 25% will have a recurrent cerebrovascular event within 1 year. Hemispheric symptoms refer to a single carotid distribution, typically causing contralateral hemiparesis or hemiparesthesia, aphasia, and/or ipsilateral monocular blindness (amaurosis fugax). Nonhemispheric symptoms include dysarthria, diplopia, vertigo, syncope, and/or transient confusion.

Noninvasive Imaging

Doppler ultrasound of the carotid arteries is cost-effective, accurate, and reproducible. Blood flow velocity measurements translate into estimates of lesion severity that have clinical relevance. There is controversy regarding the ability of ultrasound imaging to serve as the sole imaging criteria to select patients for carotid revascularization and, although ultrasound is an excellent screening tool, its accuracy in a community setting has been debated. However, many patients are revascularized based solely on their carotid ultrasound findings. MRA and CTA are being used to image the extracranial carotid arteries and intracerebral vessels (**Fig. 63-19**). The images can be reconstructed into noninvasive angiograms that have the advantage of imaging the circle of Willis with excellent resolution and clarity. If the ultrasound, MRA, and CTA results agree, many proceed directly to revascularization without angiography if the clinical indications are also appropriate.

Invasive Angiography

All the revascularization trials that have informed carotid artery treatment decisions have used angiographic criteria for patient selection. Digital subtraction angiography (DSA) is the gold standard for the diagnosis of vascular pathology of the aortic arch, cervical, and cerebral vessels (**Fig. 63-20**). Invasive angiography can cause adverse events, including a 0.5% stroke rate.

Surgical Treatment

Treatment of carotid artery disease aims to prevent disabling stroke and death. All therapeutic modalities should be judged ultimately on their ability to achieve these endpoints rather than surrogates. For revascularization to benefit patients, the strokes prevented by the procedure must exceed the strokes caused by the procedure. Similarly, procedure-related mortality cannot obliterate the late benefit of surgery. This concept is important, because the longer patients live after a revascularization procedure, the greater the benefit they will enjoy. Very old or very ill patients may not live long enough to justify placing them at risk of a procedure-related death.[85]

Carotid endarterectomy (CEA) is an established surgical procedure for stroke prevention in patients with extracranial carotid artery disease (**Table 63-9**). Randomized controlled trials in selected populations have demonstrated benefit in both symptomatic (>50%) and asymptomatic (≥60%) patients for stroke prevention with CEA compared with medical therapy.[86]

The applicability of these surgical trial results to daily patient outcomes has generated controversy. Results in the Medicare population have not been as good as those reported in the trials. The AHA expert consensus panel suggested that indications for CEA include good surgical risk candidates with symptoms related to a 50% or greater stenosis, and asymptomatic patients with an 80% or greater stenosis; however, the perioperative risk of stroke and death should not exceed 3% for asymptomatic patients, 6% for symptomatic patients, or 10% for repeat CEA.[87]

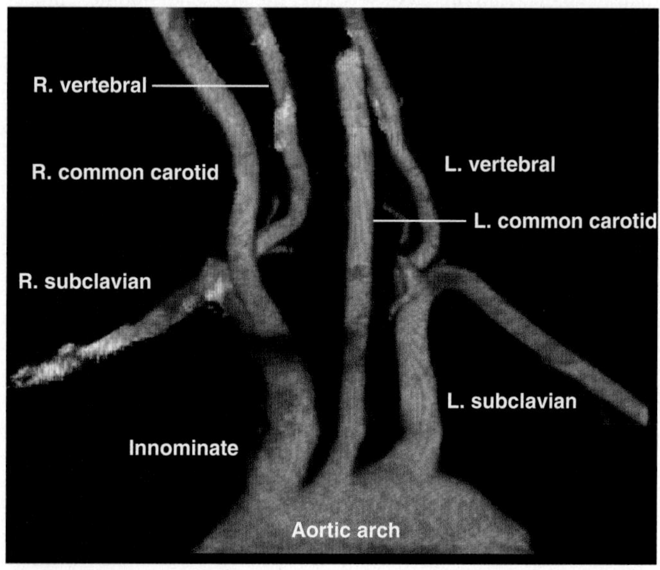

FIGURE 63-19 CTA depiction of aortic arch and arch vessels.

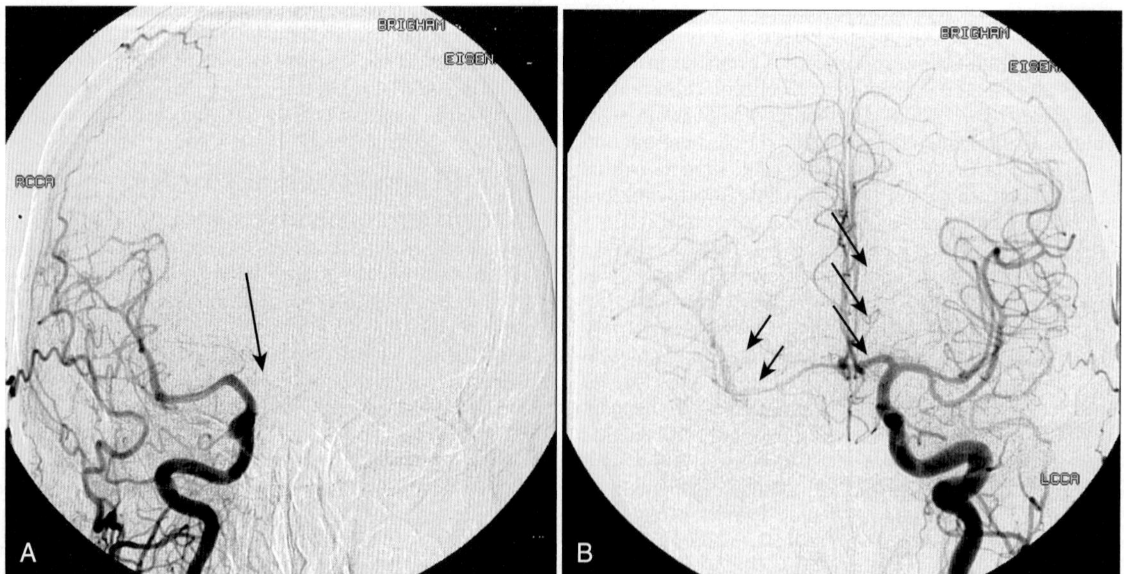

FIGURE 63-20 Corresponding anteroposterior (Townes) view of the right **(A)** and left **(B)** intracranial carotid angiograms. **A,** Perfusion of the right middle cerebral territory only. No flow is seen into the anterior cerebral vessel, the expected location of which is delineated by the arrow. **B,** Injection of the left carotid artery, demonstrating filling of both hemispheres, including the right anterior cerebral (three long arrows) and middle cerebral (two short arrows) territories.

TABLE 63-9 Carotid Surgery Versus Medical Therapy Trials

TRIAL	MEDICAL RISK OF STROKE (%)	CEA RISK OF STROKE (%)	PERIOPERATIVE 30-DAY INCIDENCE OF STROKE AND DEATH (%)
NASCET, 70%-99%	25.1	8.9	5.8
NASCET, 50%-69%	16.2	11.3	7.1
ECST, 70%-99%	16.8	10.3	7.5
ACAS, ≥60%	11.0	5.1	2.3
ACST, ≥60%	11.0	3.8	3.1

ACAS = Asymptomatic Carotid Atherosclerosis Study; ACST = Asymptomatic Carotid Surgery Trial; ECST = European Carotid Surgery Trial; NASCET = North American Symptomatic Carotid Endarterectomy Trial.

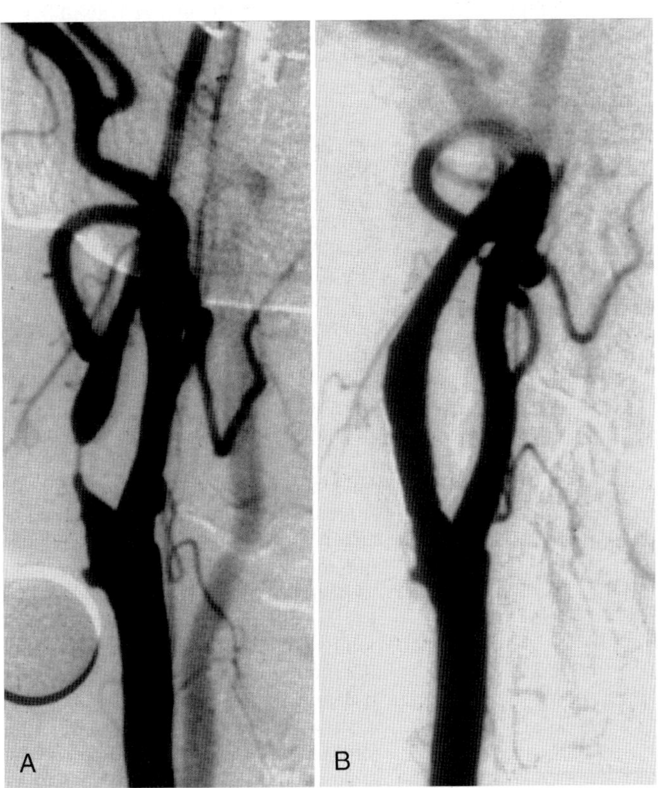

FIGURE 63-21 **A,** Baseline selective carotid angiogram showing critical stenosis of the internal carotid artery. The external carotid is identified as the vessel that gives off branches. **B,** Following stent deployment.

Catheter-Based Treatment

Carotid artery stent (CAS) placement has evolved over the past 20 years to become an accepted method for treating selected patients (**Fig. 63-21**).[88] Self-expanding stents are used to avoid stent deformation and compression. Concern over the potential release of atheroemboli has led to the development of several emboli protection systems, including the following: (1) distal balloon occlusion with aspiration[89]; (2) proximal occlusion with aspiration[90]; and (3) distal filter systems.[91]

Several large contemporary, nonrandomized, prospective registry studies (e.g., BEACH, ARCHeR 2, SECuRITY) have investigated the safety and efficacy of CAS, with embolic protection in symptomatic and asymptomatic patients at increased risk for surgical treatment.[92-96] All these trials have met their targets for safety and efficacy (**Fig. 63-22**).

The Stenting and Angioplasty with Protection in Patients at High Risk for Endarterectomy (SAPPHIRE) trial was a randomized controlled trial that compared CAS with distal emboli protection to CEA in patients at increased risk for CEA.[97] A total of 747 patients were entered into the trial, with 159 randomized to CAS with distal protection and 151 randomized to CEA. An additional 406 patients were refused surgery and were treated in a stent registry, but only 7 patients were refused CAS and were treated in a surgery registry.

In the randomized patients, the 30-day incidence of stroke, death, or myocardial infarction was lower for CAS (4.8%) than for CEA (9.6%; $P = 0.14$). The CEA group also had cranial nerve injuries (5.3%), which were not seen in the CAS group. The 1-year combined endpoint for the CAS group was 12%, compared with 20.1% ($P = 0.048$) in the CEA group (**Fig. 63-23**). This trial met the criteria for noninferiority, and led to the first U.S. Food and Drug Administration (FDA) approval of a carotid stent. This randomized trial provides compelling evidence that CAS with distal protection is the procedure of choice for patients at increased risk for carotid surgery.

Recently, three large peer-reviewed reports considered CAS in high-surgical-risk postmarket surveillance trials reporting on more than 8000 patients treated outside the clinical investigational setting. The Stenting and Angioplasty with Protection of Patients with High Risk for Endarterectomy World-Wide (SAPPHIRE WW) postmarket approval registry trial evaluated 30-day outcomes after CAS in high-surgical-risk patients.[98] Independent neurologic assessment was used for outcomes assessment. The investigators reported 30-day safety and efficacy outcomes in 2001 symptomatic and asymptomatic high-surgical-risk patients (anatomic = 716; comorbid = 918; both = 327) treated by carotid stent operators with varying clinical experience. Approximately 72% were asymptomatic and 28% were symptomatic. The criteria for anatomic or comorbid surgical risk features were based on the FDA labeling for the devices. The primary endpoint of composite adverse outcomes included combined stroke (based on independent neurologic assessment using the National Institutes of Health Stroke Scale [NIHSS] and Rankin scale), death, and myocardial infarction. The overall independently adjudicated 30-day stroke and death rate for CAS in the high-surgical-risk patients was 4.0%. In the asymptomatic SAPPHIRE WW patients, the adverse outcome rate was 1.8% in the anatomic subgroup and 3.0% in the comorbid subgroup, within the 3% limit required by the AHA Expert Consensus group. For symptomatic patients, the overall adverse event rate was again lower than the 6% rate described by the AHA consensus document—4.5% for the anatomic subgroup, which rose to 8.3% in the comorbid high-risk group. This study involved almost 350 sites and operators with a wide variety of experience, suggesting that the outcomes from prior premarket approval (PMA) trials are generalizable.

Two other large postmarket registry trials, EXACT and CAPTURE-2, reported on more than 6000 high-surgical-risk patients treated by CAS operators with varying levels of experience in large prospective, multicenter registries (EXACT, $N = 2145$; CAPTURE-2, $N = 4175$).[99] Both trials included independent neurologic assessment of outcomes to reinforce the rigor for ascertaining adverse events. The overall incidence of 30-day stroke and death for the EXACT patients was 4.1%, and for the CAPTURE-2 patients it was only 3.4%. Importantly, for patients who would have been comparable to patients included in the 2006 AHA published guidelines (<80 years), the CAS results met the threshold recommendations for 30-day stroke and death rates for symptomatic patients (≥50% stenosis) at 5.3% (benchmark for CEA, ≤6%), and for

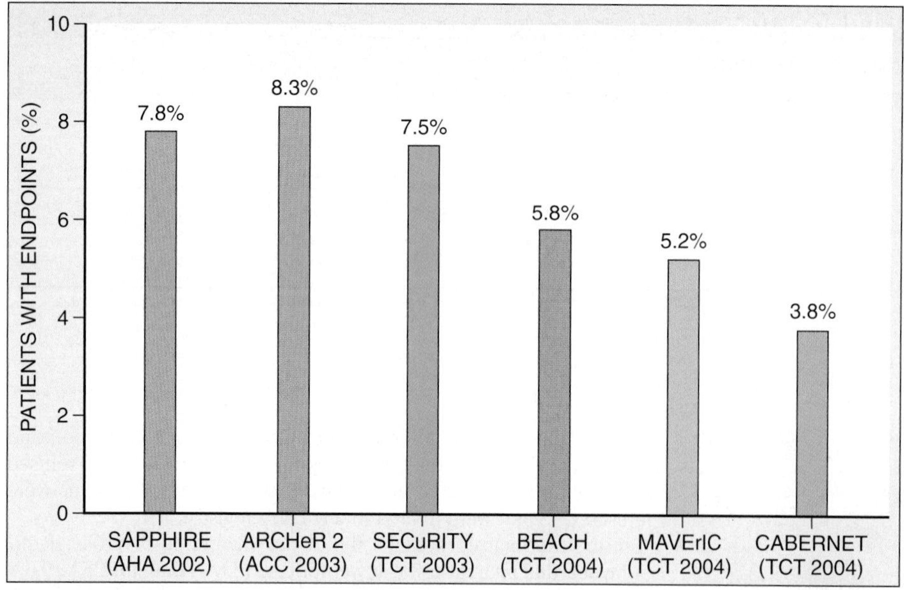

FIGURE 63-22 Bar graph showing 30-day composite endpoint (stroke, death, myocardial infarction) for U.S. carotid stent trials.

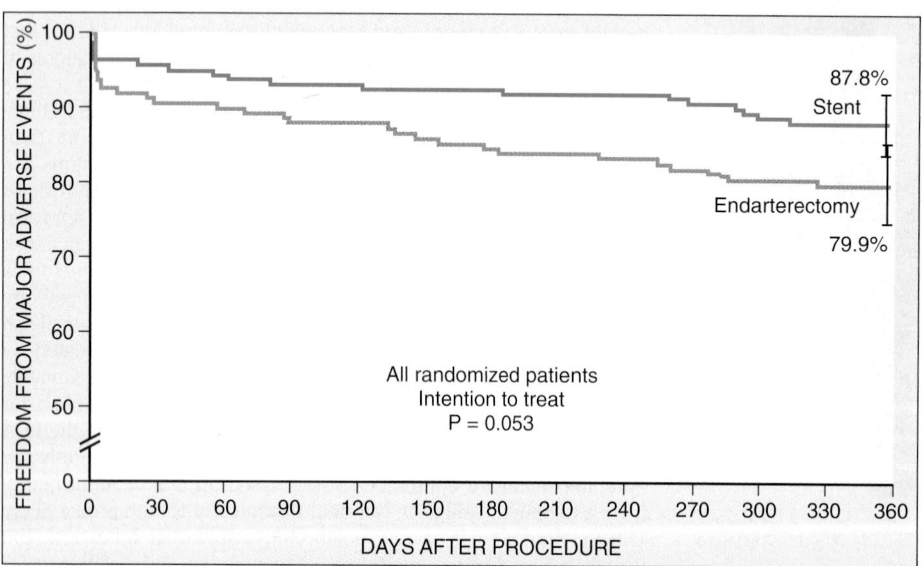

FIGURE 63-23 Outcome at 1 year for freedom from major adverse events, showing superiority for carotid stent over carotid surgery in randomized patients by intention to treat in the SAPPHIRE trial. *(From Yadav JS, Wholey MH, Kuntz RE, et al: Protected carotid-artery stenting versus endarterectomy in high-risk patients. N Engl J Med 351:1493, 2004.)*

asymptomatic patients (≥80% stenosis) at 2.9% (benchmark for CEA, ≤ 3%).

Four randomized trials of CEA versus CAS in usual-surgical-risk patients have been reported. The Endarterectomy versus Stenting in Patients with Symptomatic Severe Carotid Stenosis (EVA-3S) trial compared CAS with a variety of techniques and variable cerebral embolic protection with CEA. The results showed statistically lower rates of stroke and death at 6 months in the endarterectomy group.[100,101] This trial was carried out by experienced vascular surgeons and inexperienced interventionalists, and it used a much wider variety of techniques for CAS than other trials.

The 30-day results of the Stent-Supported Percutaneous Angioplasty versus Endarterectomy of the Carotid Artery versus Endarterectomy (SPACE) trial showed no difference in stroke or death, but it enrolled too few patients to demonstrate noninferiority of carotid stenting compared with endarterectomy. The rate of ipsilateral stroke or death was 6.84% among patients who underwent carotid stenting, compared with 6.38% among those who had endarterectomy.[102] The SPACE study actually demonstrated superior (log rank, $P = 0.001$) outcomes in average- or low-surgical-risk patients for CAS compared with CEA for patients 68 years of age or younger.[103] These two trials reflect the current controversies in carotid revascularization, the interpretation of which depends on the bias of the reader.

The International Carotid Stent Study (ICSS) randomized 1713 usual-risk patients to CAS ($N = 855$) versus CEA ($N = 858$).[104] The primary endpoint for the trial, disabling stroke or death, was no different between the two groups, but there was an excess of nondisabling strokes and fatal strokes in the CAS arm. These three European trials (EVA-3S, SPACE, and ICSS) all contain a significant bias against CAS by allowing very inexperienced operators to be tutored in the technique while enrolling patients and requiring emboli protection devices. These two issues, which did not occur in the Carotid Revascularization Endarterectomy versus Stenting Trial (CREST), contributed to the excess in strokes seen in the CAS arm.

Currently, CREST is widely viewed as the definitive comparison of these two techniques of carotid revascularization.[105] This study randomized over 2500 patients with significant carotid stenosis to stenting with embolic protection or surgery. More than one third were female, and more than 50% of the population consisted of symptomatic patients. There was no difference in the primary endpoint of periprocedural stroke, myocardial infarction, death, or postprocedural ipsilateral stroke up to 4 years (7.2% versus 6.8%; $P = 0.51$). There were significantly more myocardial infarctions with surgery and significantly more strokes with carotid stenting, although no significant difference in periprocedural major strokes. Of note, the periprocedural event rates were remarkably low in both arms of the study. As expected, periprocedural cranial nerve palsies were significantly lower with carotid stenting (0.3% versus 4.8%; $P < 0.0001$). There was no evidence of differential efficacy based on sex or symptomatic status. There was, however, an interaction by age that appeared significant, such that carotid stenting provided superior results in patients younger than 70 years of age, whereas those older than 70 years of age appeared to have better results with surgery. Further research is needed to define the optimal treatment of older patients,[85] but the results of CREST have shown that when performed by well-trained operators, carotid stenting with embolic protection and carotid surgery both provide excellent periprocedural outcomes and freedom from ipsilateral stroke. The choice of which form of revascularization is best likely depends on patient characteristics and individual preferences, which for many patients will be carotid stenting. At present, the moderate viewpoint is that the techniques are not very different, and that much still remains to be learned about their safe and effective applications.

Current indications for carotid artery stent placement are both in symptomatic (diameter > 50%) and asymptomatic (diameter ≥ 60% to

TABLE 63-10	Factors Associated with Increased Risk of Complications from Carotid Artery Stent Placement
• Tortuous aortic arch	
• Platelet or clotting disorder	
• Difficult vascular access	
• Lesion or vessel calcification	
• Visible thrombus	
• Advanced age (>75-80 yr)*	

*Risk of cerebrovascular accident (CVA) with CAS increased and risk of myocardial infarction (MI) with CEA increased.

TABLE 63-11	Factors Associated with Increased Risk from Carotid Artery Surgery
Anatomic Criteria	
• High cervical or intrathoracic lesion	
• Prior neck surgery or radiation therapy	
• Contralateral carotid artery occlusion	
• Prior ipsilateral CEA	
• Contralateral laryngeal nerve palsy	
• Tracheostomy	
Medical Comorbidities	
• Age > 80 yr*	
• Class III or IV congestive heart failure	
• Class III or IV angina pectoris	
• Left main coronary disease	
• Two- or three-vessel coronary artery disease	
• Need for open heart surgery	
• Ejection fraction ≤30%	
• Recent myocardial infarction	
• Severe chronic obstructive lung disease	

*Risk of CVA with CAS increased and risk of MI with CEA increased.

80%) stenoses in patients at increased risk for carotid surgery who are anatomically good candidates for CAS (**Table 63-10**). Currently, patients who do not meet high-surgical-risk criteria (**Table 63-11**) should have their treatment individualized and may be offered surgery[106] or stenting. Trials and registries are continuing to enroll low-surgical-risk patients and are hoping to readdress the issue of whether prophylactic medical therapy, which itself is improving, may be equivalent or superior to stenting and/or endarterectomy for asymptomatic patients. The best patient care will continue to require knowledge, skill, and the best application of the physician's judgment.

VERTEBRAL ARTERY DISEASE. People can tolerate ligature of one of the two vertebral arteries well, making the clinical presentation of vertebrobasilar insufficiency infrequent. Atherosclerotic occlusive disease of the origin of both vertebral arteries is the most common clinical lesion culprit; however, other combinations of carotid, subclavian, and innominate stenoses can compromise the posterior circulation and precipitate symptoms of vertebrobasilar insufficiency. In patients presenting with symptoms of cerebrovascular disease, 40% will have evidence of at least vertebral stenosis and 10% will have a vertebral occlusion. Of those with posterior circulation symptoms (e.g., dizziness, ataxia, drop attacks, or diplopia), up to 35% will have a stroke within 5 years.

Treatment

Although initial treatment with platelet inhibitors and anticoagulants is warranted, arch and four-vessel study (CTA, MRA, or DSA) is indicated if posterior circulation symptoms continue despite medical management. Surgical therapy is difficult and associated with significant perioperative morbidity. Transection of the vertebral artery above the stenosis and reimplantation into the ipsilateral subclavian or carotid artery, vertebral artery endarterectomy, or vein patch angioplasty are the surgical techniques for treatment of this disease.

In one series, 174 patients undergoing proximal vertebral artery reconstruction had no in-hospital deaths, and reported complications were as follows: recurrent laryngeal nerve palsy, 2%; Horner's syndrome, 15%; lymphocele, 4%; chylothorax, 0.5%; and immediate thrombosis, 1%. Secondary patency rates were 95% and 91% at 5 and 10 years, respectively. Seventy-five patients undergoing reconstruction of the distal vertebral artery had a mortality rate of 4% and an immediate graft thrombosis rate of 8%. Secondary patency rates for distal vertebral artery reconstruction were 87% and 82% at 5 and 10 years, respectively. Mortality rates for surgical treatment of this disease are acceptable, but excessive morbidity restricts this technique from widespread use for the treatment of vertebral artery disease. Percutaneous treatment of this disease is not associated with the excessive morbidity that accompanies surgical correction.

The safety and efficacy of stent placement in treating atherosclerotic vertebral artery disease has been demonstrated by Jenkins and coworkers,[107] who reported 105 consecutive symptomatic patients treated with stents (112 arteries, 71% male) for extracranial (91%) and intracranial (9%) vertebral artery stenosis (VAS). Of these, 57 patients (54%) had bilateral VAS, 71 patients (68%) had concomitant carotid disease, and 43 patients (41%) had a prior stroke. Procedural and clinical success was achieved in 105 patients (100%) and 95 patients (90.5%), respectively (**Fig 63-24**). At 1-year follow-up in 87 patients (82.9%), 69 patients (79.3%) remained symptom-free. At 1 year, 6 patients (5.7%) had died and 5 patients (5%) had a posterior circulation stroke. Target vessel revascularization occurred in 7.4% at 1 year. At a median follow-up of 29.1 months, 13.1% had target vessel revascularization, 71.4% were alive, and 70.5% remained symptom-free.

Concern about the risk of distal embolization of debris renders debulking devices inappropriate for use in the cerebral circulation. Because the most common location for vertebral artery stenoses is at or near its origin from the subclavian artery, considerable recoil often accompanies PTA alone. Embolic protection devices have been used, although whether they improve outcomes remains uncertain.

Endoluminal stenting of vertebral artery lesions is safe and effective with a durable result, as evidenced by the low recurrence rate. Primary stent placement is an attractive treatment option for atherosclerotic vertebral artery disease.

Obstructive Venous Disease

Extremity Deep Venous Thrombosis

Unlike atherosclerotic arterial obstructive disease, the major presenting obstructive element in venous obstruction is thrombus (see Chaps. 77 and 87). Thus, dissolution or removal of the offending thrombus is the most evident goal of interventions for extremity venous thrombosis. However, underlying the thrombus is almost always a predisposing factor, such as a hypercoagulable state, external obstruction, venous stricture, scarring, or an indwelling foreign body. As a result, the treatment of venous thrombosis is comprised not only of the removal of the thrombus but also an attempt to correct the underlying cause.

Treatment

For most patients, anticoagulation and/or thrombolytic therapy are the mainstays of therapy (see Chaps. 77 and 87). Both systemic and catheter-directed thrombolysis have achieved some success (**Fig. 63-25**). Mechanical thrombectomy, balloon venoplasty, and stenting have all been reported, but evidence supporting the use of catheter-directed therapy is limited.

Because of the possibility of a reduction in the incidence of post-thrombotic syndrome with lysis compared with anticoagulation alone, and because of the possibility of reduced major bleeding, catheter-directed therapy seems reasonable in patients at higher risk for the complications of systemic lysis and in those who have a large thrombus burden and/or a high risk of developing a post-thrombotic syndrome. In addition, more interventional concepts are emerging. There are reports of experience with rheolytic thrombectomy[108] or mechanical clot disruption. The ATTRACT trial will randomize patients with DVT to medical therapy with anticoagulation or catheter-directed therapy.[109] Additional experience with stents suggests that in patients

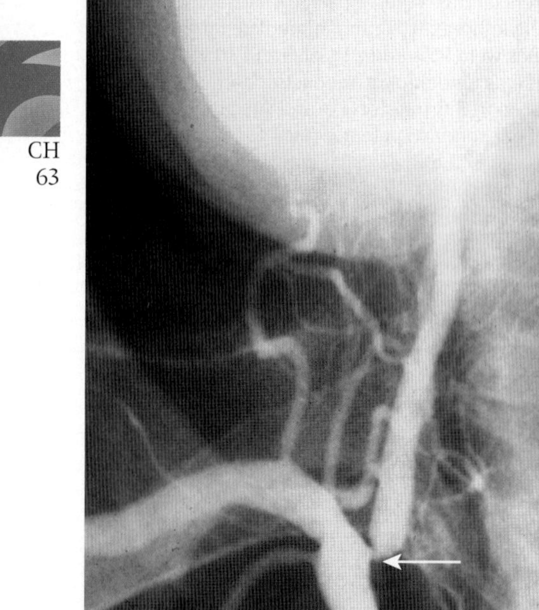

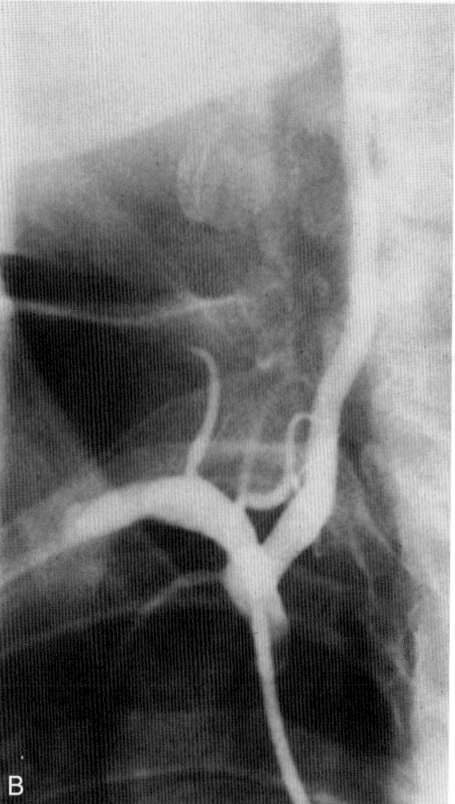

FIGURE 63-24 **A,** Angiogram of a tight stenosis at the ostium of the right vertebral artery (arrow). **B,** After balloon-expandable stent placement.

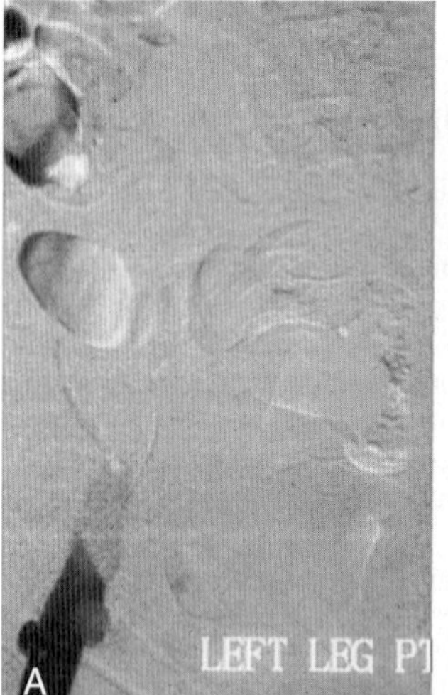

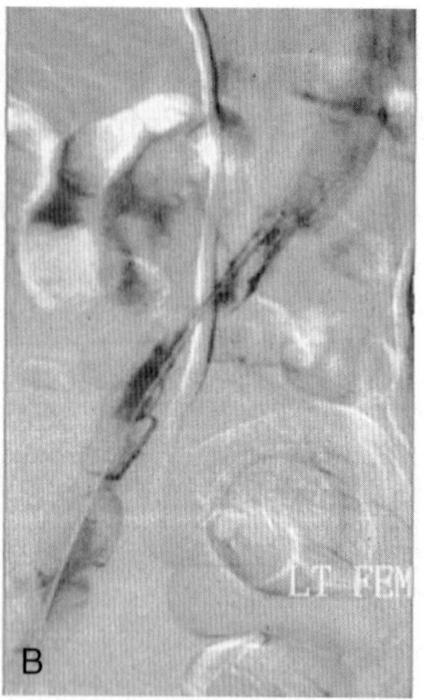

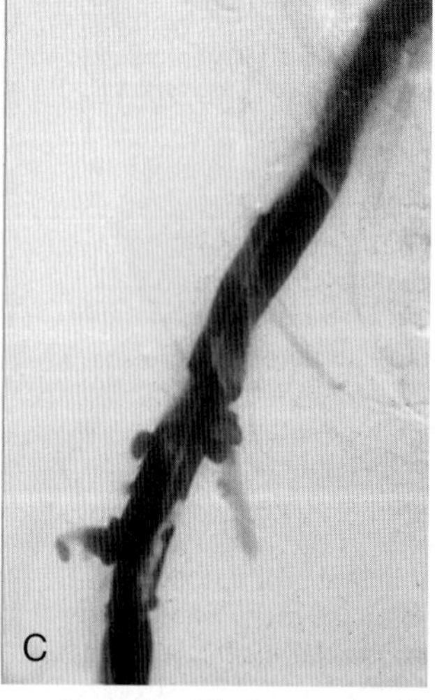

FIGURE 63-25 Venogram of the left femoral vein after gaining access at the popliteal vein with ultrasound guidance. The patient is lying face down on the table to allow access to the popliteal vein. **A,** Baseline shows occlusion of the left femoral vein. **B,** Multiholed catheter across the venous occlusion; the administration of lytic agents is started. **C,** 4 hours after lysis following PTA and placement of a self-expanding stent to restore patency.

in whom there is residual venous obstruction from scarring or external compression, relief of that obstruction with self-expanding stents may be important to maintain venous patency and prevent recurrent thrombosis. This is particularly true after relief of the initial insult, such as an indwelling port infusion catheter. Balloon venoplasty is also increasingly used to provide temporary relief of venous obstruction to facilitate the placement of transvenous pacing and/or defibrillator leads.

The mainstay of venous thrombosis of the extremities is anticoagulation. However, the selective application of catheter-based thrombolysis, thrombectomy, and venous stenting to relieve symptoms and help prevent postphlebitic syndromes is appropriate based on individual circumstances.

Central Venous Obstruction

SUPERIOR VENA CAVA SYNDROME. Superior vena cava (SVC) syndrome results from the obstruction of the blood flow in the superior vena cava. Pathologic processes from contiguous structures can compress or directly invade the SVC. Superimposed venous thrombosis may contribute to the development of SVC syndrome in up to 50% of patients. Historically, SVC syndrome was most frequently caused by direct tumor compression (see Chap. 90). The use of indwelling venous access catheters, coupled with the improved survival of chemotherapy patients, has increased the occurrence of nonmalignant SVC syndrome in patients following cure of their cancer. The explosion in the use of the automatic implantable cardioverter-defibrillator (AICD) and sophisticated multilead pacing systems has increased the incidence and recognition of this condition.

Percutaneous Treatment

Medical and surgical options for the treatment of superior vena cava obstruction are well established (see Chap. 90). Since the initial description of successful percutaneous treatment of SVC syndrome in the adult, the use of angioplasty alone was limited by a high rate of initial failure and early restenosis because of recoil of the highly elastic SVC wall. Stenting therefore quickly gained acceptance in this area of vascular intervention after its introduction in the 1980s. Stenting in malignant SVC syndrome results in rapid improvement of symptoms. Patients report almost immediate resolution of headache, visual disturbances, and other central nervous system symptoms. Dyspnea, cough, and edema usually resolve within 1 to 3 days, but occasionally may take up to 1 week. Stenting results in complete resolution of symptoms in most patients with malignant SVC syndrome. In the largest series,[110] 76 consecutive patients with SVC syndrome were treated with stents and compared with historical controls of patients treated with radiation. Procedural success was 100%, and all patients had improvement of symptoms within 48 hours. Of patients treated with a stent, 90% had no symptoms of SVC obstruction at the time of death, compared with 12% of patients treated with radiation. The recurrence rate of SVC syndrome after percutaneous intervention has been reported to vary widely, occurring in up to 45% of patients. This variability likely results from diverse mechanisms. Acute stent thrombosis can develop shortly after stent placement in patients on insufficient anticoagulation or antiplatelet therapy; tumor ingrowth through stent struts or intimal

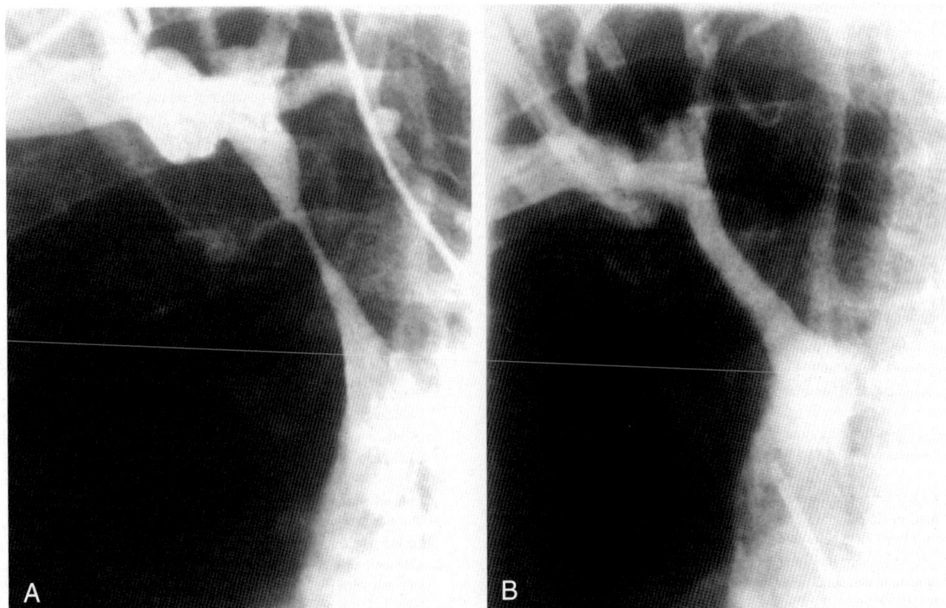

FIGURE 63-26 SVC syndrome and its treatment. **A,** Baseline venogram showing a tight stenosis of the SVC, which was crossed with a 0.035-in. guidewire from the femoral vein. The stenosis was predilated with a balloon and a large self-expanding stent was then placed to overcome recoil. **B,** Final venogram.

hyperplasia or fibrous scarring can occur. Stent length oversizing may prevent recurrence of SVC syndrome because of stent edge overgrowth, but may increase the risk of SVC stent thrombosis or restenosis. Patients with total SVC occlusion have the highest recurrence rate of SVC syndrome, but repeat procedures in these patients are uniformly successful; additional stent placement, angioplasty, and/or thrombolysis can be used alone or in combination.[111]

In the developed world, SVC syndrome of nonmalignant cause (benign SVC syndrome) is usually iatrogenic in origin, most frequently as a result of indwelling intravenous catheters and pacing leads. Complications of pacemaker lead placement, such as venous thrombosis or stenosis, occur in up to 30% of patients. Only a few patients become symptomatic, but the presence of multiple leads, retention of severed lead(s), and previous lead infection may increase the risk of SVC syndrome. The largest series of percutaneous therapy in benign SVC syndrome included 16 patients.[112] In this series, 10 patients had SVC syndrome because of the indwelling catheter, 2 because of the pacemaker wire, and 1 each because of goiter, fibrous mediastinitis, heart-lung transplantation, and spontaneous thrombosis. The patency rate in 13 patients who were followed for a mean of 17 months was 85%. Similar results can be expected in patients with SVC syndrome associated with central venous infusion catheters. Ideally, interventional treatment should also include removal of the inciting lead or catheter. Combination laser sheath extraction of pacemaker and defibrillator leads followed by venous angioplasty and stenting with subsequent lead reimplantation can be performed successfully.

Superior vena cava stenting is a low-risk procedure that provides fast and durable symptomatic relief in malignant caval obstruction, often in combination with chemotherapy or radiation. It provides patients with the benefit of life prolongation together with effective symptom control. In patients with SVC syndrome of nonmalignant cause, based on mid-term follow-up results, stenting is the treatment of choice (**Fig. 63-26**). Surgical therapy should be reserved for patients with benign SVC syndrome refractory to percutaneous therapy. Only a few patients become truly refractory; most patients with recurrent SVC syndrome can undergo repeated percutaneous intervention.

Conclusion

Although the specific tools and techniques vary, the theme of endovascular intervention is similar across many vascular territories. In general, vascular stenting has become the mainstay of percutaneous revascularization for relief of symptoms. The challenge for the future will be to continue to improve the long-term durability of endovascular therapy and to explore its potential for preventing the complications of progressive vascular disease.

REFERENCES

1. Hirsch AT, Haskal ZJ, Hertzer NR, et al: ACC/AHA 2005 guidelines for the management of patients with peripheral arterial disease (lower extremity, renal, mesenteric, and abdominal aortic): Executive summary: A collaborative report from the American Association for Vascular Surgery/Society for Vascular Surgery, Society for Cardiovascular Angiography and Interventions, Society for Vascular Medicine and Biology, Society of Interventional Radiology, and the ACC/AHA Task Force on Practice Guidelines (Writing Committee to Develop Guidelines for the Management of Patients With Peripheral Arterial Disease) endorsed by the American Association of Cardiovascular and Pulmonary Rehabilitation; National Heart, Lung and Blood Institute; Society for Vascular Nursing; TransAtlantic Inter-Society Consensus; and Vascular Disease Foundation. J Am Coll Cardiol 47:1239, 2006.

Atherosclerotic Lower Extremity Disease

2. Ponec D, Jaff MR, Swischuk J, et al: The nitinol SMART stent vs wallstent for suboptimal iliac artery angioplasty: CRISP US trial results. J Vasc Interv Radiol 9:911, 2004.
3. Reyes R, Maynar M, Lopera J, et al: Treatment of chronic iliac artery occlusions with guide wire recanalization and primary stent placement. J Vasc Interv Radiol 8:1049, 1997.
4. Dyet JF: Endovascular stents in the arterial system—current status. Clin Radiol 52:83, 1997.
5. Murphy TP, Khwaja AA, Webb MS: Aortoiliac stent placement in patients treated for intermittent claudication. J Vasc Interv Radiol 9:421, 1998.
6. Tetteroo E, van der Graaf Y, Bosch JL, et al: Randomised comparison of primary stent placement versus primary angioplasty followed by selective stent placement in patients with iliac artery occlusive disease. Lancet 351:1153, 1998.
7. Powell RJ, Fillinger M, Bettmann M, et al: The durability of endovascular treatment of multisegment iliac occlusive disease. J Vasc Surg 31:1178, 2000.
8. Saha S, Gibson M, Magee TR, et al: Early results of retrograde transpopliteal angioplasty of iliofemoral lesions. Cardiovasc Intervent Radiol 24:378, 2001.
9. Timaran CH, Stevens SL, Freeman MB, Goldman MH: External iliac and common iliac artery angioplasty and stenting in men and women. J Vasc Surg 34:440, 2001.
10. Haulon S, Mounier-Véhier C, Gaxotte V, et al: Percutaneous reconstruction of the aortoiliac bifurcation with the "kissing stents" technique: Long-term follow-up in 106 patients. J Endovasc Ther 9:363, 2002.
11. Siskin GP, Englander M, Roddy S, et al: Results of iliac artery stent placement in patients younger than 50 years of age. J Vasc Interv Radiol 13:785, 2002.
12. Mohamed F, Sarkar B, Timmons G, et al: Outcome of "kissing stents" for aortoiliac atherosclerotic disease, including the effect on the non-diseased contralateral iliac limb. Cardiovasc Intervent Radiol 25:472, 2002.
13. Reekers JA, Vorwerk D, Rousseau H, et al: Results of a European multicentre iliac stent trial with a flexible balloon expandable stent. Eur J Vasc Endovasc Surg 24:511, 2002.
14. Funovics MA, Lackner B, Cejna M, et al: Predictors of long-term results after treatment of iliac artery obliteration by transluminal angioplasty and stent deployment. Cardiovasc Intervent Radiol 25:397, 2002.
15. Hans SS, DeSantis D, Siddiqui R, Khoury M: Results of endovascular therapy and aortobifemoral grafting for Transatlantic Inter-Society type C and D aortoiliac occlusive disease. Surgery 144:583, 2008.

16. Kashyap VS, Pavkov ML, Bena JF, et al: The management of severe aortoiliac occlusive disease: Endovascular therapy rivals open reconstruction. J Vasc Surg 48:1451, 2008.
17. Sixt S, Alawied AK, Rastan A, et al: Acute and long-term outcome of endovascular therapy for aortoiliac occlusive lesions stratified according to the TASC classification: A single-center experience. J Endovasc Ther 15:408, 2008.
18. Uberoi R, Milburn S, Moss J, et al: British Society of Interventional Radiology Iliac Artery Angioplasty-Stent Registry III. Cardiovasc Intervent Radiol 32:887, 2009.
19. Amighi J, Schillinger M, Dick P, et al: De novo superficial femoropopliteal artery lesions: peripheral cutting balloon angioplasty and restenosis rates—randomized controlled trial. Radiology 247:267, 2008.
20. Schillinger M, Sabeti S, Loewe C, et al: Balloon angioplasty versus implantation of nitinol stents in the superficial femoral artery. N Engl J Med 354:1879, 2006.
21. Krankenberg H, Schlüter M, Steinkamp HJ, et al: Nitinol stent implantation versus percutaneous transluminal angioplasty in superficial femoral artery lesions up to 10 cm in length: The femoral artery stenting trial (FAST). Circulation 116:285, 2007.
22. Tepe G, Zeller T, Albrecht T, et al: Local delivery of paclitaxel to inhibit restenosis during angioplasty of the leg. N Engl J Med 358:689, 2008.
23. Werk M, Langner S, Reinkensmeier B, et al: Inhibition of restenosis in femoropopliteal arteries: paclitaxel-coated versus uncoated balloon: Femoral paclitaxel randomized pilot trial. Circulation 118:1358, 2008.
24. Duda SH, Bosiers M, Lammer J, et al: Sirolimus-eluting versus bare nitinol stent for obstructive superficial femoral artery disease: The SIROCCO II trial. J Vasc Interv Radiol 16:331, 2005.
25. Scheinert D, Scheinert S, Sax J, et al: Prevalence and clinical impact of stent fractures after femoropopliteal stenting. J Am Coll Cardiol 45:312, 2005.
26. Dake M: Interim report on the Zilver PTX clinical study. J Vasc Surg 50:447, 2009.
27. Gray BH, Sullivan TM, Childs MB, et al: High incidence of restenosis/reocclusion of stents in the percutaneous treatment of long-segment superficial femoral artery disease after suboptimal angioplasty. J Vasc Surg 25:74, 1997.
28. Martin DR, Katz SG, Kohl RD, Qian D: Percutaneous transluminal angioplasty of infrainguinal vessels. Ann Vasc Surg 13:184, 1999.
29. Kessel DO, Wijesinghe LD, Robertson I, et al: Endovascular stent-grafts for superficial femoral artery disease: Results of 1-year follow-up. J Vasc Interv Radiol 10:289, 1999.
30. Conroy RM, Gordon IL, Tobis JM, et al: Angioplasty and stent placement in chronic occlusion of the superficial femoral artery: Technique and results. J Vasc Interv Radiol 11:1009, 2000.
31. Cheng SW, Ting AC, Wong J: Endovascular stenting of superficial femoral artery stenosis and occlusions: Results and risk factor analysis. Cardiovasc Surg 9:133, 2001.
32. Gordon IL, Conroy RM, Arefi M, et al: Three-year outcome of endovascular treatment of superficial femoral artery occlusion. Arch Surg 136:221, 2001.
33. Scheinert D, Laird JR Jr, Schröder M, et al: Excimer laser-assisted recanalization of long, chronic superficial femoral artery occlusions. J Endovasc Ther 8:156, 2001.
34. Löfberg AM, Karacagil S, Ljungman C, et al: Percutaneous transluminal angioplasty of the femoropopliteal arteries in limbs with chronic critical lower limb ischemia. J Vasc Surg 34:114, 2001.
35. Bauermeister G: Endovascular stent-grafting in the treatment of superficial femoral artery occlusive disease. J Endovasc Ther 8:315, 2001.
36. Duda SH, Pusich B, Richter G, et al: Sirolimus-eluting stents for the treatment of obstructive superficial femoral artery disease: Six-month results. Circulation 106:1505, 2002.
37. Steinkamp HJ, Wissgott C, Rademaker J, et al: Short (1-10 cm) superficial femoral artery occlusions: Results of treatment with excimer laser angioplasty. Cardiovasc Intervent Radiol 25:388, 2002.
38. Gray BH, Laird JR, Ansel GM, Shuck JW: Complex endovascular treatment for critical limb ischemia in poor surgical candidates: A pilot study. J Endovasc Ther 9:599, 2002.
39. Jämsén TS, Manninen HI, Jaakkola PA, Matsi PJ: Long-term outcome of patients with claudication after balloon angioplasty of the femoropopliteal arteries. Radiology 225:345, 2002.
40. Cho L, Roffi M, Mukherjee D, et al: Superficial femoral artery occlusion: Nitinol stents achieve better flow and reduce the need for medications than balloon angioplasty alone. J Inv Cardiol 15:198, 2003.
41. Becquemin JP, Favre JP, Marzelle J, et al: Systematic versus selective stent placement after superficial femoral artery balloon angioplasty: A multicenter prospective randomized study. J Vasc Surg 37:487, 2003.
42. Jahnke T, Andresen R, Müller-Hülsbeck S, et al: Hemobahn stent-grafts for treatment of femoropopliteal arterial obstructions: Midterm results of a prospective trial. J Vasc Interv Radiol 14:41, 2003.
43. Adam DJ, Beard JD, Cleveland T, et al: Bypass versus angioplasty in severe ischaemia of the leg (BASIL): Multicentre, randomised controlled trial. Lancet 366:1925, 2005.
44. Sivananthan UM, Browne TF, Thorley PJ, Rees MR: Percutaneous transluminal angioplasty of the tibial arteries. Br J Surg 81:1282, 1994.
45. Varty K, Bolia A, Naylor AR, et al: Infrapopliteal percutaneous transluminal angioplasty: A safe and successful procedure. Eur J Vasc Endovasc Surg 9:341, 1995.
46. Dorros G, Jaff MR, Murphy KJ, Mathiak L: The acute outcome of tibioperoneal vessel angioplasty in 417 cases with claudication and critical limb ischemia. Cathet Cardiovasc Diagn 45:251, 1998.
47. Desgranges P, Kobeiter K, d'Audiffret A, et al: Acute occlusion of popliteal and/or tibial arteries: The value of percutaneous treatment. Eur J Vasc Endovasc Surg 20:138, 2000.
48. Söder HK, Manninen HI, Jaakkola P, et al: Prospective trial of infrapopliteal artery balloon angioplasty for critical limb ischemia: Angiographic and clinical results. J Vasc Interv Radiol 11:1021, 2000.
49. Dorros G, Jaff MR, Dorros AM, et al: Tibioperoneal (outflow lesion) angioplasty can be used as primary treatment in 235 patients with critical limb ischemia: Five-year follow-up. Circulation 104:2057, 2001.
50. Tsetis DK, Michalis LK, Rees MR, et al: Vibrational angioplasty in the treatment of chronic infrapopliteal arterial occlusions: Preliminary experience. J Endovasc Ther 9:889, 2002.
51. Feiring AJ, Wesolowski AA, Lade S: Primary stent-supported angioplasty for treatment of below-knee critical limb ischemia and severe claudication: Early and one-year outcomes. J Am Coll Cardiol 44:2307, 2004.
52. Giles KA, Pomposelli FB, Spence TL, et al: Infrapopliteal angioplasty for critical limb ischemia: Relation of TransAtlantic InterSociety Consensus class to outcome in 176 limbs. J Vasc Surg 48:128, 2008.
53. Siablis D, Karnabatidis D, Katsanos K, et al: Infrapopliteal application of sirolimus-eluting versus bare metal stents for critical limb ischemia: Analysis of long-term angiographic and clinical outcome. J Vasc Interv Radiol 20:1141, 2009.
54. Faglia E, Mantero M, Caminiti M, et al: Extensive use of peripheral angioplasty, particularly infrapopliteal, in the treatment of ischaemic diabetic foot ulcers: Clinical results of a multicentric study of 221 consecutive diabetic subjects. J Intern Med 252:225, 2002.
55. Faglia E, Dalla Paola L, Clerici G, et al: Peripheral angioplasty as the first-choice revascularization procedure in diabetic patients with critical limb ischemia: Prospective study of 993 consecutive patients hospitalized and followed between 1999 and 2003. Eur J Vasc Endovasc Surg 29:620, 2005.
56. Tefera G, Hoch J, Turnipseed WD: Limb-salvage angioplasty in vascular surgery practice. J Vasc Surg 41:988-993.

Atherosclerotic Renal Artery Disease

57. Rundback JH, Sacks D, Kent KC, et al: AHA Councils on Cardiovascular Radiology, High Blood Pressure Research, Kidney in Cardiovascular Disease, Cardio-Thoracic and Vascular Surgery, and Clinical Cardiology, and the Society of Interventional Radiology FDA Device Forum Committee: Guidelines for the reporting of renal artery revascularization in clinical trials. American Heart Association. Circulation 106:1572, 2002.
58. White CJ, Ramee SR, Collins TJ, et al: Renal artery stent placement: Utility in lesions difficult to treat with balloon angioplasty. J Am Coll Cardiol 30:1445, 1997.
59. Blum U, Krumme B, Flügel P, et al: Treatment of ostial renal-artery stenoses with vascular endoprostheses after unsuccessful balloon angioplasty. N Engl J Med 336:459, 1997.
60. Tuttle KR, Chouinard RF, Webber JT, et al: Treatment of atherosclerotic ostial renal artery stenosis with the intravascular stent. Am J Kidney Dis 32:611, 1998.
61. Henry M, Amor M, Henry I, et al: Stents in the treatment of renal artery stenosis: Long-term follow-up. J Endovasc Surg 6:42, 1999.
62. van de Ven PJ, Kaatee R, Beutler JJ, et al: Arterial stenting and balloon angioplasty in ostial atherosclerotic renovascular disease: a randomised trial. Lancet 353:282, 1999.
63. Rocha-Singh KJ, Mishkel GJ, Katholi RE, et al: Clinical predictors of improved long-term blood pressure control after successful stenting of hypertensive patients with obstructive renal artery atherosclerosis. Catheter Cardiovasc Interv 47:167, 1999.
64. Lederman RJ, Mendelsohn FO, Santos R, et al: Primary renal artery stenting: Characteristics and outcomes after 363 procedures. Am Heart J 142:314, 2001.
65. ASTRAL Investigators: Revascularization versus medical therapy for renal-artery stenosis. N Engl J Med 361:1953, 2009.
66. Dorros G, Prince C, Mathiak L: Stenting of a renal artery stenosis achieves better relief of the obstructive lesion than balloon angioplasty. Cathet Cardiovasc Diagn 29:191, 1993.
67. Subramanian R, White CJ, Rosenfield K, et al: Renal fractional flow reserve: A hemodynamic evaluation of moderate renal artery stenoses. Catheter Cardiovasc Interv 64:480, 2005.
68. Mitchell JA, Subramanian R, Stewart R, White CJ: Pressure-derived renal fractional flow reserve with clinical outcomes following intervention. Catheter Cardiovasc Interv 65:135, 2005.
69. Silva JA, Chan AW, White CJ, et al: Elevated brain natriuretic peptide predicts blood pressure response after stent revascularization in patients with renal artery stenosis. Circulation 111:328, 2005.
70. Radermacher J, Chavan A, Bleck J, et al: Use of Doppler ultrasonography to predict the outcome of therapy for renal-artery stenosis. N Eng J Med 344:410, 2001.
71. Zeller T, Frank U, Müller C, et al: Predictors of improved renal function after percutaneous stent-supported angioplasty of severe atherosclerotic ostial renal artery stenosis. Circulation 108:2244, 2003.
72. Muray S, Martín M, Amoedo ML, et al: Rapid decline in renal function reflects reversibility and predicts the outcome after angioplasty in renal artery stenosis. Am J Kidney Dis 39:60, 2002.
73. White CJ: Catheter-based therapy for atherosclerotic renal artery stenosis. Circulation 113:1464, 2006.
74. Dworkin LD, Cooper CJ: Clinical practice. Renal-artery stenosis. N Engl J Med 361:1972, 2009.
75. National Heart, Lung and Blood Institute: Benefits of Medical Therapy Plus Stenting for Renal Atherosclerotic Lesions (CORAL), 2010 (http://clinicaltrials.gov/ct2/show/NCT00081731).

Chronic Mesenteric Disease

76. Hansen KJ, Wilson DB, Craven TE, et al: Mesenteric artery disease in the elderly. J Vasc Surg 40:45, 2004.
77. Cercueil JP, Weiller M, Tatou E, et al: Chronic mesenteric ischemia: Imaging and percutaneous treatment. Radiographics 22:863, 2002.
78. Matsumoto AH, Angle JF, Spinosa DJ, et al: Percutaneous transluminal angioplasty and stenting in the treatment of chronic mesenteric ischemia: Results and long-term followup. J Am Coll Surg 194(1 Suppl):S22, 2002.
79. Silva JA, White CJ, Collins TJ, et al: Endovascular therapy for chronic mesenteric ischemia. J Am Coll Cardiol 47:944, 2006.

Brachiocephalic and Subclavian Obstructive Disease

80. Eisenhauer AC, Shaw JA: Atherosclerotic subclavian artery disease and revascularization. *In* Abella G (ed): Peripheral Vascular Disease: Basic Diagnostic and Therapeutic Approaches. Philadelphia, Lippincott Williams & Wilkins, 2004, pp 283:294.
81. Amor M, Eid-Lidt G, Chati Z, Wilentz JR: Endovascular treatment of the subclavian artery: Stent implantation with or without predilatation. Catheter Cardiovasc Interv 63:364, 2004.
82. Schillinger M, Haumer M, Schillinger S, et al: Risk stratification for subclavian artery angioplasty: Is there an increased rate of restenosis after stent implantation? J Endovasc Ther 8:550, 2001.
83. Patel SN, White CJ, Collins TJ, et al: Catheter-based treatment of the subclavian and innominate arteries. Catheter Cardiovasc Interv 71:963, 2008.

Carotid and Vertebral Disease

84. Easton JD, Saver JL, Albers GW, et al: Definition and evaluation of transient ischemic attack: A scientific statement for healthcare professionals from the American Heart Association/

American Stroke Association Stroke Council; Council on Cardiovascular Surgery and Anesthesia; Council on Cardiovascular Radiology and Intervention; Council on Cardiovascular Nursing; and the Interdisciplinary Council on Peripheral Vascular Disease. The American Academy of Neurology affirms the value of this statement as an educational tool for neurologists. Stroke 40:2276, 2009.
85. Belkin M, Bhatt DL: Carotid stenting in the elderly: Is 80 the new 60? Circulation 119:2302, 2009.
86. MRC Asymptomatic Carotid Surgery Trial (ACST) Collaborative Group: Prevention of disabling and fatal strokes by successful carotid endarterectomy in patients without recent neurological symptoms: Randomised controlled trial. Lancet 363:1491, 2004.
87. Biller J, Feinberg WM, Castaldo JE, et al: Guidelines for carotid endarterectomy: A statement for healthcare professionals from a Special Writing Group of the Stroke Council, American Heart Association. Circulation 97:501, 1998.
88. Helton TJ, Bavry AA, Rajagopal V, et al: The optimal treatment of carotid atherosclerosis: A 2008 update and literature review. Postgrad Med 120:103, 2008.
89. Henry M, Amor M, Henry I, et al: Carotid stenting with cerebral protection: First clinical experience using the PercuSurge GuardWire system. J Endovasc Surg 6:321, 1999.
90. Grunwald IQ, Dorenbeck U, Axmann C, et al: Proximal protection systems using carotid artery stent. Radiologe 44:998, 2004.
91. Müller-Hülsbeck S, Jahnke T, Liess C, et al: Comparison of various cerebral protection devices used for carotid artery stent placement: An in vitro experiment. J Vasc Interv Radiol 14:613, 2003.
92. Gray W: Two-year composite endpoint results for the Archer Trials: Acculink for revascularization of carotids in high risk patients. Am J Cardiol 94(Suppl 6A):62E, 2004.
93. Gray WA: A cardiologist in the carotids. J Am Coll Cardiol 43:1602, 2004.
94. White CJ, for the Beach Investigators: 30 day outcomes of carotid wallstent and filterwire EX/EZ distal protection system placement for treatment of high surgical risk patients. J Am Coll Cardiol 45(Suppl A):28A, 2005.
95. Whitlow P: Security: More good data for protected carotid stenting in high-risk surgical patients, 2003 (http://www.medscape.com/viewarticle/461721_print).
96. Ramee S, Higashida R: Evaluation of the Medtronic self-expanding carotid stent system with distal protection in the treatment of carotid artery stenosis. Am J Cardiol 94(Suppl 6A):61E, 2004.
97. Yadav JS, Wholey MH, Kuntz RE, et al: Protected carotid-artery stenting versus endarterectomy in high-risk patients. N Engl J Med 351:1493, 2004.
98. Massop D, Dave R, Metzger C, et al: Stenting and angioplasty with protection in patients at high-risk for endarterectomy: SAPPHIRE Worldwide Registry first 2,001 patients. Catheter Cardiovasc Interv 73:129, 2009.
99. Gray WA, Chaturvedi S, Verta P: Thirty-day outcomes for carotid artery stenting in 6320 patients from 2 prospective, multicenter, high-surgical-risk registries. Circ Cardiovasc Interv 2:159, 2009.
100. Mas JL, Chatellier G, Beyssen B, et al: Endarterectomy versus stenting in patients with symptomatic severe carotid stenosis. N Engl J Med 355:1660, 2006.
101. Furlan AJ: Carotid-artery stenting—case open or closed? N Engl J Med 355:1726, 2006.
102. SPACE Collaborative Group; Ringleb PA, Allenberg J, Brückmann H, et al: 30 day results from the SPACE trial of stent-protected angioplasty versus carotid endarterectomy in symptomatic patients: A randomised non-inferiority trial. Lancet 368:1239, 2006.
103. Stingele R, Berger J, Alfke K, et al: Clinical and angiographic risk factors for stroke and death within 30 days after carotid endarterectomy and stent-protected angioplasty: A subanalysis of the SPACE study. Lancet Neurol 7:216, 2008.
104. International Carotid Stenting Study investigators: Carotid artery stenting compared with endarterectomy in patients with symptomatic carotid stenosis (International Carotid Stenting Study): An interim analysis of a randomised controlled trial. Lancet 375:985, 2010.
105. Brott T, Roubin GS, Howard G: The randomized carotid revascularization endarterectomy versus stenting trial (CREST): Primary results. Presented at the American Stroke Association's International Stroke Conference, A29: Plenary Session II: Late-Breaking Science. San Diego, Calif, February 2009.
106. Coward LJ, Featherstone RL, Brown MM: Safety and efficacy of endovascular treatment of carotid artery stenosis compared with carotid endarterectomy: A Cochrane systematic review of the randomized evidence. Stroke 36:905, 2005.
107. Jenkins JS, Patel SN, White CJ, et al: Endovascular stenting for vertebral artery stenosis. J Am Coll Cardiol 55:538, 2010.

Obstructive Venous Disease

108. Kasirajan K, Gray B, Beavers FP, et al: Rheolytic thrombectomy in the management of acute and subacute limb-threatening ischemia. J Vasc Interv Radiol 12:413, 2001.
109. Washington University School of Medicine: Acute Venous Thrombosis: Thrombus Removal With Adjunctive Catheter-Directed Thrombolysis (ATTRACT), 2010 (http://clinicaltrials.gov/ct2/show/NCT00790335).
110. Nicholson AA, Ettles DF, Arnold A, et al: Treatment of malignant superior vena cava obstruction: Metal stents or radiation therapy. J Vasc Interv Radiol 8:781, 1997.
111. Schifferdecker B, Shaw JA, Piemonte TC, Eisenhauer AC: Nonmalignant superior vena cava syndrome: pathophysiology and management. Catheter Cardiovasc Interv 65:416, 2005.
112. Kee ST, Kinoshita L, Razavi MK, et al: Superior vena cava syndrome: Treatment with catheter-directed thrombolysis and endovascular stent placement. Radiology 206:187, 1998.

CHAPTER 64 Diabetes and the Cardiovascular System

Darren K. McGuire

Scope of the Problem

Diabetes Mellitus

Diabetes mellitus is a group of diseases characterized by insufficient production of insulin or by the failure to respond appropriately to insulin, resulting in hyperglycemia. The diagnostic criteria are summarized in **Table 64-1**.[1] Importantly, new to the diagnostic criteria in 2010, a glycosylated hemoglobin (A1c) level ≥6.5% has been added. Diabetes is typically classified as type 2 diabetes, characterized by relative insulin deficiency with a backdrop of insulin resistance and representing >90% of all diabetes cases, or type 1 diabetes, characterized by absolute insulin deficiency.

Diabetes is among the most common chronic diseases in the world, affecting an estimated 180 million people in 2008.[2] Confounding this high global burden is the increasing incidence and prevalence of type 2 diabetes, driven by increasing population age, obesity, and physical inactivity (see Chaps. 1 and 44), as well as by the increasing longevity of patients with diabetes; estimates project that more than 360 million persons will be affected by diabetes by 2030 (**Fig. 64-1**).

Whereas much attention historically has focused on the prevention and treatment of microvascular disease complications of diabetes (i.e., retinopathy, nephropathy, and neuropathy), cardiovascular disease (CVD) remains the principal morbidity and driver of mortality in the setting of diabetes—most commonly in the form of coronary heart disease (CHD), but also in the incremental risk associated with diabetes for cerebrovascular disease, peripheral vascular disease, and heart failure. For these reasons, continual efforts toward mitigating the risk of CVD in diabetes remain a global public health imperative.

Atherosclerosis

Compared with nondiabetic individuals, patients with diabetes have a twofold to fourfold increased risk for development and dying of CHD (**Fig. 64-2**).[3] Whereas older studies have suggested a diabetes-associated CVD risk similar to that observed among nondiabetic patients with a prior myocardial infarction (MI)—that is, a "coronary disease equivalent"—more recent observations from clinical trials including patients with diabetes suggest a substantially lower CHD risk, most likely reflecting the effectiveness of contemporary therapeutic interventions.[4-6]

Diabetes is associated with an increased risk for MI; and across the spectrum of acute coronary syndrome (ACS) events, in which diabetes may affect more than one in three patients,[7] patients with diabetes have worse CVD outcomes after ACS events (**Fig. 64-3**; see Chaps. 54 to 56).[8] Despite overall improvements in outcomes during the past several decades for patients with and without diabetes, the gradient of risk associated with diabetes persists (**Fig. 64-4**).[8] Furthermore, the graded association of increased risk observed with diabetes in the setting of ACS events extends to glucose values in the range well below the diabetes threshold, whether it is analyzed by glucose values at the time of presentation or those observed throughout hospitalization (**Fig. 64-5**).[9]

In addition to CHD, diabetes increases the risks of stroke and peripheral arterial disease. The diagnosis of diabetes portends a twofold increased stroke risk compared with nondiabetic individuals (see Chap. 62), with hyperglycemia affecting approximately one in three patients with acute stroke, associated with a twofold to sixfold increased risk for adverse clinical outcomes after stroke.[10] Among patients with symptomatic peripheral arterial disease, diabetes prevalence ranges from 20% to 30% and accounts for approximately 50% of all lower extremity amputations (see Chap. 61).[11]

Heart Failure

In the ambulatory setting, diabetes associates independently with a twofold to fivefold increased risk of heart failure (HF) compared with those without diabetes, comprising both systolic and diastolic HF, and diabetes patients have worse outcomes once HF has developed.[12] In addition, diabetes is associated with an increased HF risk in the setting of ACS events.[13] The increased risk of HF observed in diabetes is multifactorial, caused by ischemic, metabolic, and functional myocardial perturbations.[14]

Coronary Heart Disease in the Patient with Diabetes

Mechanistic Considerations Linking Diabetes and Atherosclerosis

Traditional CHD risk factors such as hypertension, dyslipidemia, and adiposity cluster in patients with impaired glucose tolerance or diabetes, and each condition directly influences atherosclerotic disease risk (see Chaps. 44 to 47). However, this clustering does not completely account for the increased risk observed among patients with diabetes, with numerous other implicated mechanisms (**Table 64-2**).[15]

The pathobiologic attribution of hyperglycemia to CVD risk per se remains poorly understood; but given the clear associations between severity of hyperglycemia and CVD risk in both type 1 and type 2 diabetes (sharing hyperglycemia as the common pathophysiologic

TABLE 64-1 American Diabetes Association Diagnostic Criteria for Diabetes Mellitus[1]

Fasting plasma glucose ≥ 7.0 mmol/liter (126 mg/dL)
or
2-hour plasma glucose ≥ 11.1 mmol/liter (200 mg/dL) during standardized 75-g oral glucose tolerance test
or
Symptoms of hyperglycemia plus nonfasting plasma glucose ≥ 11.1 mmol/liter
or
A1c ≥ 6.5% (200 mg/dL)

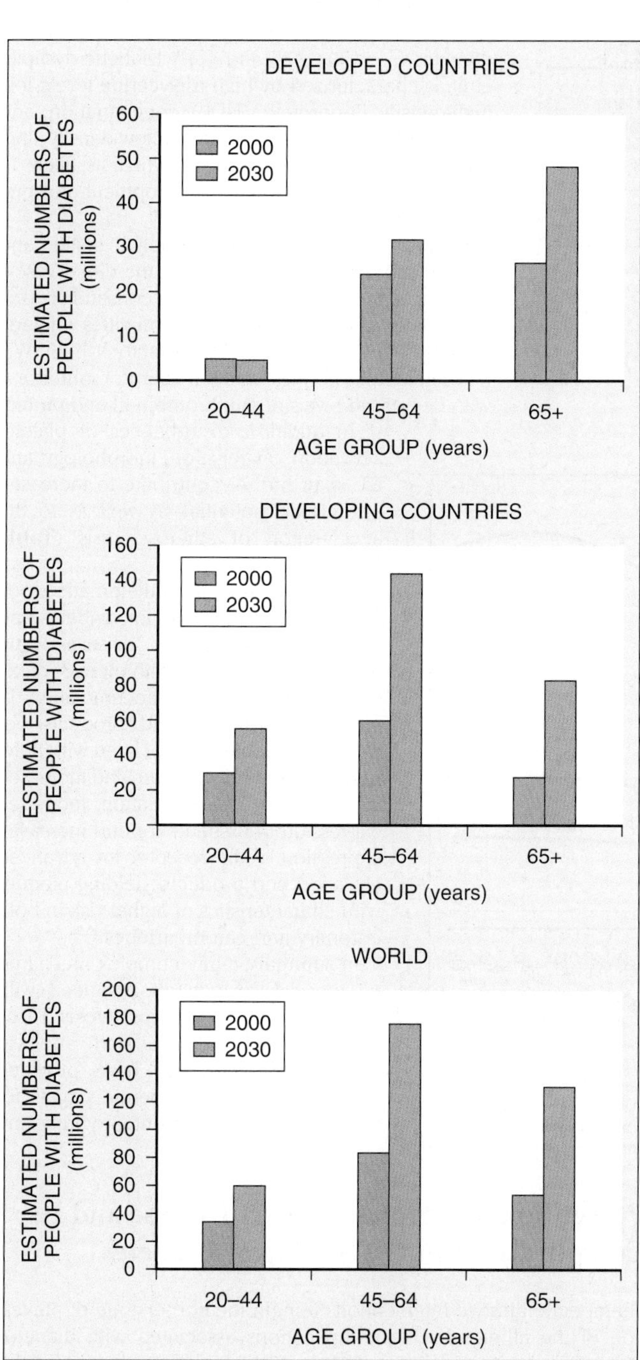

FIGURE 64-1 Estimated number of adults with diabetes in 2000 and projected for 2030 stratified by age group, with projections for the overall global population and by developed and developing country categories. *(From Wild S, Roglic G, Green A, et al: Global prevalence of diabetes: Estimates for the year 2000 and projections for 2030. Diabetes Care 27:1047, 2004.)*

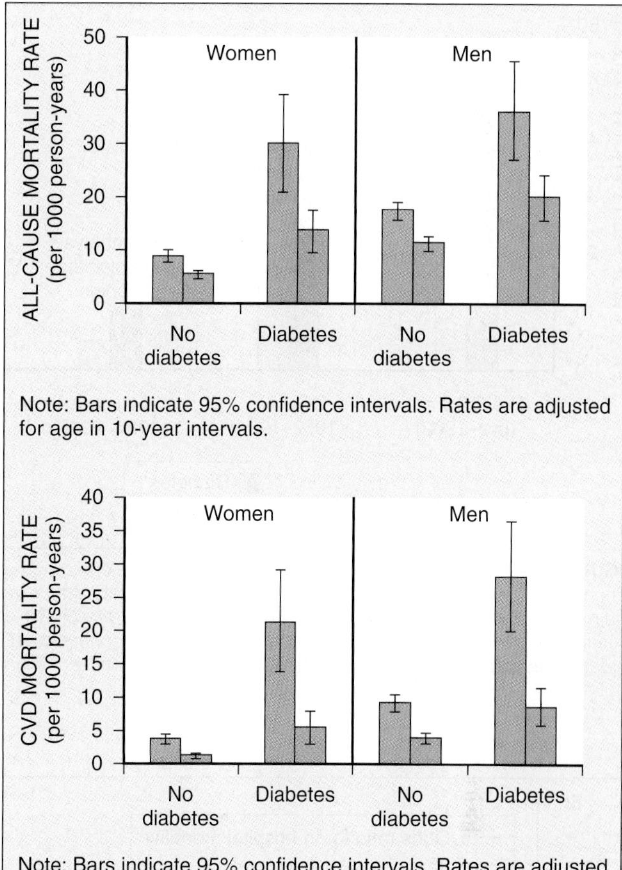

FIGURE 64-2 Age-adjusted all-cause **(top)** and CVD **(bottom)** mortality rates among participants with and without diabetes mellitus by sex and time period. Pink bars represent earlier time period (1950 to 1975); blue bars represent later time period (1976 to 2001). *(From Preis SR, Hwang SJ, Coady S, et al: Trends in all-cause and cardiovascular disease mortality among women and men with and without diabetes mellitus in the Framingham Heart Study, 1950 to 2005. Circulation 119:1728, 2009.)*

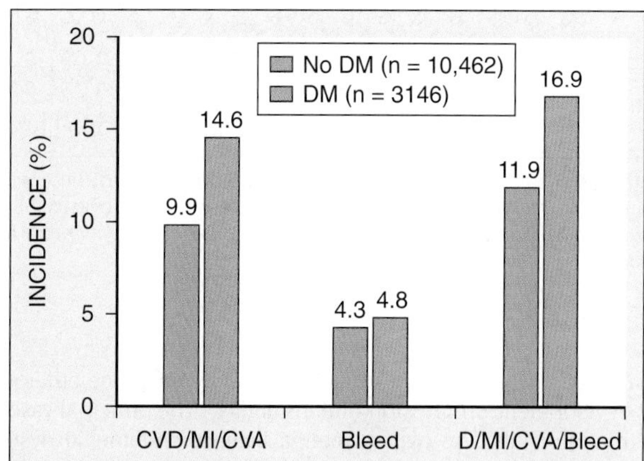

FIGURE 64-3 Adverse clinical outcomes after acute coronary syndromes during more than 1 year of follow-up, according to diabetes status, among patients participating in the TRITON–TIMI 38 randomized trial.[8] CVA = cerebrovascular accident; CVD = cardiovascular death; D = death; DM = diabetes mellitus; MI = myocardial infarction.

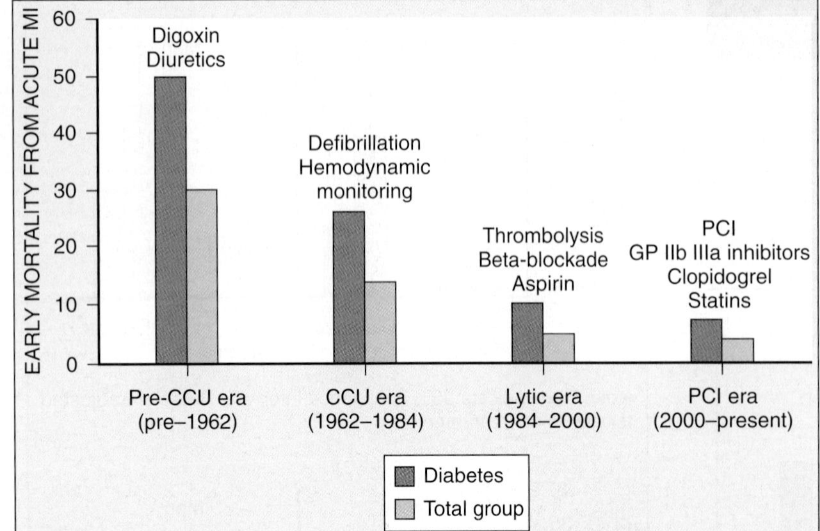

FIGURE 64-4 People with diabetes have an increased prevalence of atherosclerosis and coronary heart disease and experience higher morbidity and mortality after acute coronary syndrome and myocardial infarction than do people without diabetes. CCU = coronary care unit; GP = glycoprotein; PCI = percutaneous coronary intervention. *(Modified from Braunwald E: Cardiovascular medicine at the turn of the millennium: Triumphs, concerns, and opportunities. N Engl J Med 337:1360, 1997.)*

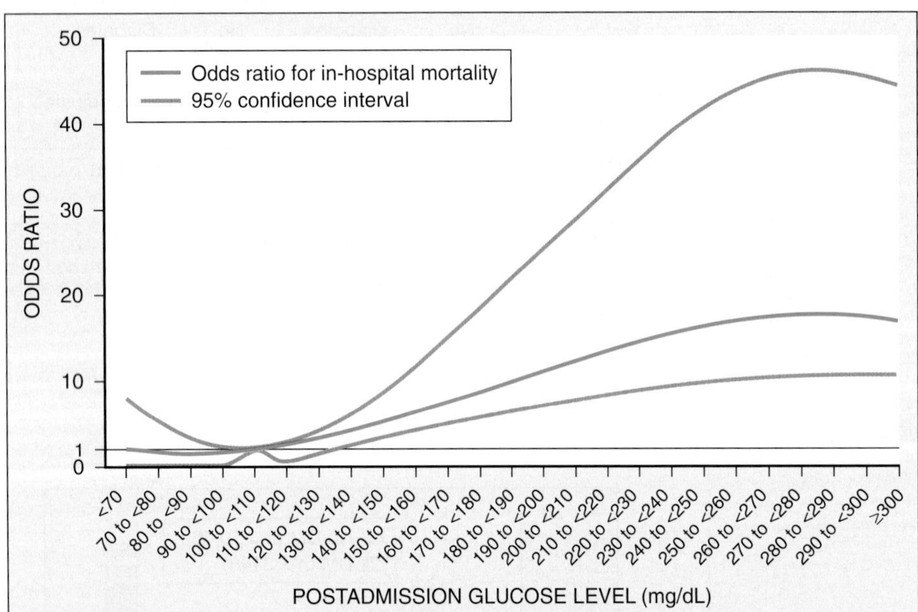

FIGURE 64-5 Postadmission glucose levels and mortality in the entire patient cohort after multivariable adjustment (to convert glucose to millimoles per liter, multiply by 0.0555). *(From Kosiborod M, Inzucchi SE, Krumholz HM, et al: Glucose normalization and outcomes in patients with acute myocardial infarction. Arch Intern Med 169:438, 2009.)*

disturbance), hyperglycemia is likely to directly influence atherosclerosis development, progression, and instability.[15] The principal vascular perturbations linked to hyperglycemia include endothelial dysfunction, vascular effects of advanced glycation end products, adverse effects of circulating free fatty acids, and increased systemic inflammation. In addition, the pernicious effects of hypoglycemia complicating diabetes therapy, the sympathovagal imbalance due to diabetic autonomic neuropathy, and the vascular effects of constitutive exposure to excess insulin may further contribute to atherosclerotic risk.

Endothelial dysfunction, a hallmark of diabetic vascular disease,[16] is associated with increased hypertension and adverse CVD outcomes. The myriad mechanisms contributing to endothelial dysfunction include abnormal nitric oxide biology, increased endothelin and angiotensin II, and reduced prostacyclin activity, all of which contribute to abnormal control of blood flow. In the setting of ACS events, no-reflow after percutaneous intervention reflecting acute endothelial dysfunction occurs more commonly in the presence of diabetes or hyperglycemia and may contribute to increased myocardial jeopardy, resulting in larger infarcts, increased arrhythmia, and worse systolic function.

Abnormalities in lipid metabolism also contribute to the increased atherosclerotic risk associated with diabetes (see Chaps. 44 and 47).[17] Diabetic dyslipidemia is characterized by high triglyceride levels, low high-density lipoprotein (HDL) concentration, and increased atherogenic small dense low-density lipoprotein (LDL) particles, each of which is likely to contribute to the accelerated development and progression of atherosclerosis.

Perturbations in the proteo-fibrinolytic system and platelet biology further compound the direct vascular effects of diabetes, yielding a constitutive prothrombotic milieu.[18] These abnormalities include increased circulating tissue factor, factor VII, von Willebrand factor, and plasminogen activator inhibitor 1, with decreased levels of antithrombin III and protein C. In addition, disturbances of platelet activation, aggregation, morphology, and life span further contribute to increased thrombotic potential, as well as to the acceleration of atherosclerosis (**Table 64-3**).

Increased systemic inflammation portends an increased risk for diabetes and diabetic atherosclerotic disease,[19] and diabetes is associated with increased oxidative stress and the accumulation of advanced glycation end products. For example, diabetes is associated with lipid-rich atherosclerotic plaque and increased inflammatory cell infiltration, increased expression of tissue factor, and increased expression of the receptor for advanced glycation end products, yielding plaques with characteristics of higher risk in both coronary and carotid arteries.[15,20]

In summary, many complex mechanistic theories have been advanced with regard to diabetic atherosclerosis. These considerations have yielded an avid investigative field and have provided myriad potential therapeutic targets for which drug development programs are currently under way.

Prevention of Coronary Heart Disease and Its Complications in the Setting of Diabetes

Therapeutic lifestyle interventions remain the cornerstone of prevention of the atherosclerotic complications associated with diabetes; therapeutic targets similar to those reviewed in Chap. 49 are effective both for the prevention of type 2 diabetes and for the mitigation of atherosclerotic risk in the setting of diabetes. As recommended by the American Diabetes Association (ADA) and the American Heart Association (AHA), overarching therapeutic lifestyle targets include smoking abstinence, at least 150 minutes of moderate-intensity aerobic activity weekly, and medical nutrition therapy recommendations for weight control and dietary composition.[21,22]

TABLE 64-2 Examples of Mechanisms Implicated in Diabetic Vascular Disease

Endothelium	↑ NF-κβ activation ↓ Nitric oxide production ↓ Prostacyclin bioavailability ↑ Endothelin 1 activity ↑ Angiotensin II activity ↑ Cyclooxygenase 2 activity ↑ Thromboxane A_2 activity ↑ Reactive oxygen species ↑ Lipid peroxidation products ↓ Endothelium-dependent relaxation ↑ RAGE expression
Vascular smooth muscle cells and vascular matrix	↑ Proliferation and migration into intima ↑ Increased matrix degradation Altered matrix components
Inflammation	↑ IL-1β, IL-6, CD36, MCP-1 ↑ ICAMs, VCAMs, and selectins ↑ Activity of protein kinase C ↑ AGEs and AGE/RAGE interactions

AGEs = advanced glycation end products; ICAMs = intracellular adhesion molecules; IL = interleukin; MCP = monocyte chemoattractant protein; NF = nuclear factor; RAGE = receptor for advanced glycation end products; VCAMs = vascular cell adhesion molecules.
Modified from Orasanu G, Plutzky J: The pathologic continuum of diabetic vascular disease. J Am Coll Cardiol 53:S35, 2009.

Beyond lifestyle, a number of pharmacologic strategies have proven effective for CVD risk reduction in diabetes and are recommended for routine prescription for patients with diabetes.[21,22] Such interventions include intensive blood pressure and lipid management, consideration for angiotensin-converting enzyme (ACE) inhibitors independent of blood pressure, and daily antiplatelet therapy for patients with prevalent CVD or increased primary risk. In the context of these evidence-based CVD interventions, the accumulated data regarding the effects of glucose control on CVD risk mitigation remain less robust.[23,24]

LIPID THERAPY. Insulin resistance and type 2 diabetes are associated with a characteristic pattern of dyslipidemia, reviewed in detail in Chap. 47. Each component of diabetic lipid abnormality independently associates with adverse cardiovascular outcomes, including increased small dense LDL particles, increased apolipoprotein B concentration, increased triglycerides, and decreased HDL cholesterol.[17] Despite extensive research in modifying triglyceride and HDL cholesterol levels with a variety of pharmacologic agents, however, the net influence on CVD risk of these strategies remains uncertain, and the modification of LDL cholesterol remains the cornerstone of therapeutic lipid intervention in patients with diabetes.[22]

STATIN THERAPY. Contemporary guidelines for the management of diabetic dyslipidemia focus on the use of statin medications,[21,22] based on results from randomized clinical trials enrolling large numbers of patients with diabetes and supported by a recent meta-analysis yielding estimates of numbers needed to treat to prevent major adverse CVD complications in the setting of diabetes: 39 for primary prevention and 19 among patients with prevalent CVD.[25] Recommendations from many contemporary professional societies do not require elevation of LDL cholesterol as a requisite for the initiation of a statin; instead they use the aggregate risk assessment recommending statins for all patients with diabetes older than 40 years of age with one or more other CVD factors, or younger in the setting of prevalent CVD or clustering of CVD risk, endorsing the lower target of LDL <100 mg/dL or 35% to 40% reduction from baseline.[21] In addition, considering diabetes as a coronary disease risk equivalent, an optional target for LDL cholesterol of <70 mg/dL should be considered for patients with diabetes.[22]

Once LDL cholesterol targets have been achieved through lifestyle modification and statin therapy, the principal secondary therapeutic lipid target for patients with diabetes who have persistent fasting triglyceride elevation >200 mg/dL is non–HDL cholesterol (i.e., total cholesterol – HDL cholesterol = non–HDL cholesterol). Therapeutic targets for this parameter are 30 mg/dL higher than the corresponding LDL cholesterol target for the individual patient.[22] The preferred method to achieve the secondary non-HDL target is by intensification of statin monotherapy as tolerated, with the secondary option to add another lipid-modifying agent such as niacin, fish oil, ezetimibe, bile acid binders, or fibric acid derivatives. The net CVD efficacy and overall safety associated with add-on therapy, however, remain poorly defined. Large-scale randomized clinical trials are currently under way, assessing the addition of fibrates, niacin, and omega-3 fatty acids.

TABLE 64-3 Perturbations of Platelet Structure and Function Associated with Diabetes

Reduced membrane fluidity
Altered Ca^{2+} and Mg^{2+} homeostasis
Increased arachidonic acid metabolism
Increased thromboxane A_2 synthesis
Decreased nitric oxide and prostacyclin production
Decreased antioxidant levels
Increased expression of activation-dependent adhesion molecules (e.g., glycoprotein IIb/IIIa, P-selectin)
Increased platelet microparticle formation
Increased platelet turnover

Modified from Colwell JA, Nesto RW: The platelet in diabetes: Focus on prevention of ischemic events. Diabetes Care 26:2181, 2003.

OMEGA-3 FATTY ACIDS. (see Chap. 48) Given the principal lipid effect of long-chain omega-3 fatty acids (predominantly fish oil preparations in clinical use) of lowering circulating triglycerides by up to 40%, such therapy holds particular promise in the treatment of diabetic dyslipidemia. In addition, in the absence of reported interactions with statins, fish oil is particularly attractive as an add-on therapy to statins if incremental triglyceride reduction is desired once LDL targets have been achieved with statin medication. Fish oil has minimal effects on HDL and total cholesterol and modestly raises LDL with no adverse glycemic effects in patients with diabetes, despite early concerns to the contrary.[17] In addition, a series of randomized clinical trials have demonstrated beneficial effects on CVD outcomes with fish oil, such as data from a subanalysis of 4565 patients with impaired fasting glucose or diabetes participating in the Japan EPA Lipid Intervention Study (JELIS), a randomized trial comparing treatment with 1800 mg of eicosapentaenoic acid (EPA) plus simvastatin daily versus simvastatin alone.[26] In this subset, EPA treatment conferred a 22% risk reduction ($P = 0.048$) for major adverse CVD events compared with simvastatin alone. On the basis of the accumulated data, fish oil has emerged as the primary consideration for add-on therapy in patients with diabetes who do not achieve non-HDL targets with maximally tolerated statin monotherapy.

FIBRIC ACID DERIVATIVES (FIBRATES). Fibrates are agonists of the nuclear transcriptional regulator peroxisome proliferator–activated receptor (PPAR) α that lower triglycerides and modestly increase HDL cholesterol. Although they favorably affect two of the fundamental abnormalities of diabetic dyslipidemia, the net CVD effects of this class of drugs remain uncertain. Randomized trials of gemfibrozil versus placebo have demonstrated efficacy among subjects with diabetes, but these trials were executed before the use of statins became prevalent in the populations studied, and the use of gemfibrozil with statins is limited by an increased risk of myopathy.[17,27] More recently, the Fenofibrate Intervention and Event Lowering in Diabetes (FIELD) trial evaluated the CVD effect of fenofibrate versus placebo in a population of 9795 patients with type 2 diabetes and failed to demonstrate a statistically significant reduction in the primary endpoint of coronary death or nonfatal MI, despite accumulating 544 primary outcome events for evaluation (5.2% versus 5.9%; HR = 0.89; 95% CI, 0.75-1.05).[28] The interpretation of this trial is confounded by the prevalent drop-in of statin use in the placebo arm, which may have contributed to the negative results; but in the present era, when statins are indicated for all patients eligible for the FIELD trial, the trial results have limited generalizability and challenge the utility of fenofibrate add-on therapy for CVD risk mitigation. In the more recently completed ACCORD-Lipid trial that included 5518 patients with type 2 diabetes at high cardiovascular risk, fenofibrate, compared with placebo each added to simvastatin background therapy, likewise failed to yield significant improvements on major adverse cardiovascular outcomes, despite the accumulation of 601 primary endpoint events of CV death, MI, and stroke.[29]

In summary, fibrates remain an option for patients with intolerance to statin medications, for isolated hypertriglyceridemia in diabetic patients at otherwise low CVD risk, and as add-on therapy to maximally tolerated statin monotherapy when patients do not achieve therapeutic targets (noting some increased myopathy risk).

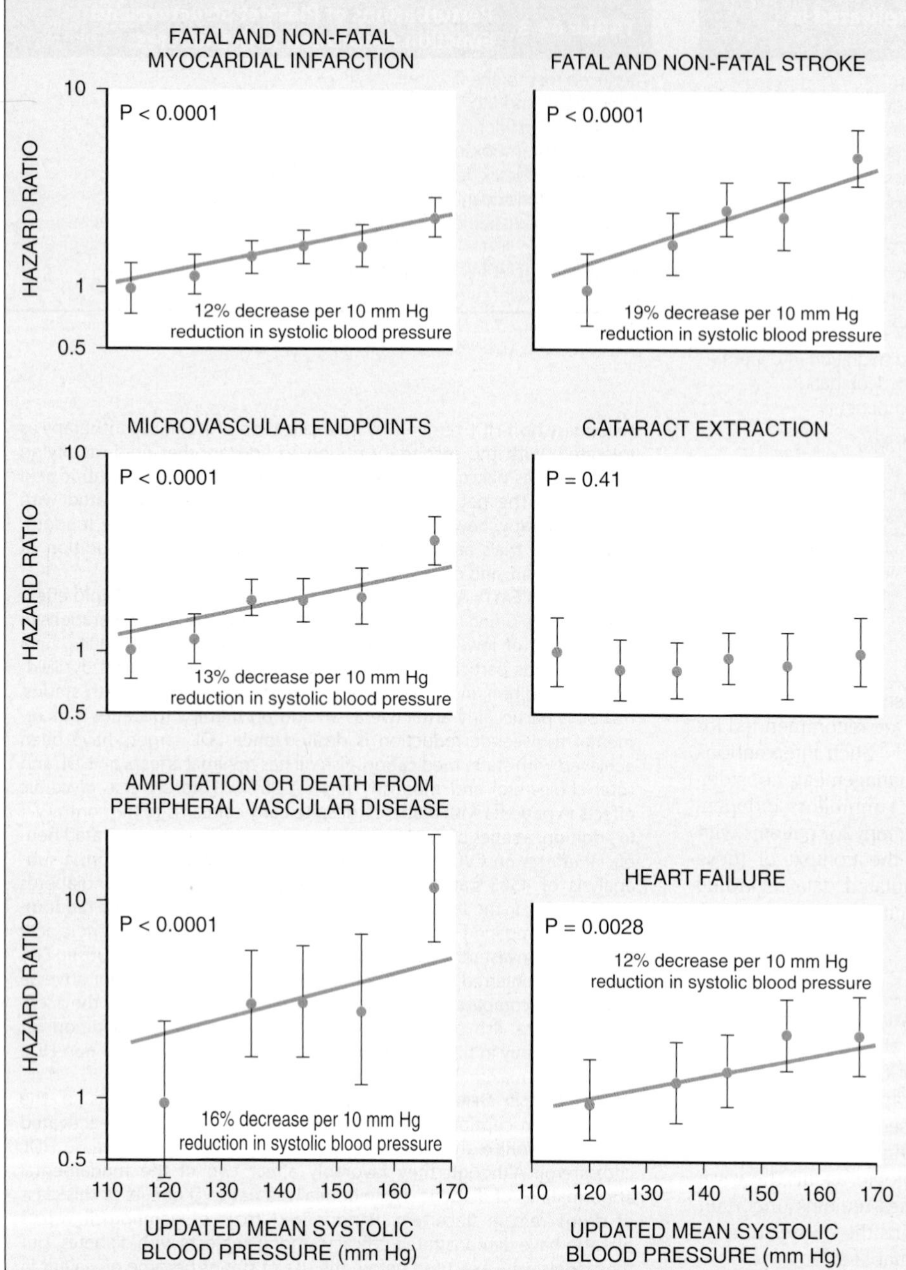

FIGURE 64-6 Hazard rates (95% confidence intervals as floating absolute risks) as estimate of association between category of updated mean systolic blood pressure and myocardial infarction, stroke, and heart failure, with log linear scales. Reference category (hazard ratio 1.0) is systolic blood pressure <120 mm Hg for myocardial infarction and <130 mm Hg for stroke and heart failure; *P* value reflects contribution of systolic blood pressure to multivariate model. Data adjusted for age at diagnosis of diabetes, ethnic group, smoking status, presence of albuminuria, hemoglobin A1c, high- and low-density lipoprotein cholesterol, and triglyceride. *(Modified from Adler AI, Stratton IM, Neil HA, et al: Association of systolic blood pressure with macrovascular and microvascular complications of type 2 diabetes [UKPDS 36]: Prospective observational study. BMJ 321:412, 2000.)*

NIACIN. Niacin is a potent modulator of lipid metabolism (although the mechanism of action remains poorly understood) and has the greatest effect among currently available drugs on increasing HDL-cholesterol while also lowering triglycerides. However, the net CVD effects and safety of niacin, especially in the context of background statin therapy, remain to be determined.[17,27] As with fibrates, the accumulated data set regarding the net CVD effects of niacin remains limited by small studies with substantial dropout rates; a recent meta-analysis estimated a 27% relative risk reduction associated with niacin in the absence of statin background therapy.[27] The incremental CVD efficacy and safety of niacin added to simvastatin therapy, compared with simvastatin alone, are presently being evaluated in two large, ongoing randomized trials: the National Heart, Lung, and Blood Institute (NHLBI)–sponsored Atherothrombosis Intervention in Metabolic Syndrome with Low HDL/High Triglycerides and Impact on Global Health Outcomes (AIM HIGH) trial, comprising 3300 patients with vascular disease and atherogenic dyslipidemia; and the Heart Protection Study 2-Treatment of HDL to Reduce the Incidence of Vascular Events (HPS2-THRIVE) trial, coordinated by the Oxford University Clinical Trial Service Unit, that has completed enrollment of over 25,000 patients with CVD.

Like fibrates, niacin remains an option for patients with intolerance to statin medications, for isolated hypertriglyceridemia in diabetic patients with an otherwise low CVD risk, and as add-on therapy to maximally tolerated statin monotherapy when patients do not achieve therapeutic targets.

HYPERTENSION. (see Chap. 46) Hypertension affects approximately 70% of diabetic patients (twice the rate observed in nondiabetic subjects), with a steep graded association between blood pressure and adverse cardiovascular outcomes (**Fig. 64-6**). In this context, numerous classes of antihypertensive medications reduce diabetic CVD risk,[29a] and given the potent benefits for both macrovascular and microvascular disease complications, blood pressure management is of principal importance in this high-risk population. Furthermore, blood pressure targets for patients with diabetes are more aggressive than for the overall population, with a goal of <130/80 mm Hg.[21,22]

ANTAGONISTS OF THE RENIN-ANGIOTENSIN-ALDOSTERONE SYSTEM (RAAS). ACE inhibitors and angiotensin II receptor blockers (ARBs) have become keystones of therapy for hypertension in diabetes because of their broadly demonstrated favorable effects on diabetic nephropathy and CVD outcomes, as well as their modest favorable effects on measures of glucose metabolism.[21,22,29a,30]

ACE INHIBITORS. The recommendation for ACE inhibitors as first-line hypertension therapy in the setting of diabetes is supported by data from randomized trials of patients with and without hypertension. For example, in the Heart Outcomes Prevention Evaluation (HOPE) study, which compared ramipril versus placebo among patients at increased risk for CVD, ramipril was superior to placebo in the diabetes subset of 3577 HOPE patients for the primary outcome of cardiovascular death, MI, and stroke (25% RRR; $P = 0.004$) and for overt nephropathy (24% RRR; $P = 0.027$). Similar observations derive from the diabetes subanalysis of the EUROPA trial, which tested perindopril versus placebo; the point estimate of treatment effect with perindopril, compared with placebo, of 19% relative risk reduction among the 1502 participants with diabetes was similar to the 20% risk reduction observed in the overall trial. On the basis of these results and support from a meta-analysis of reported trials, ACE inhibitors are the first-line treatment for hypertension in the setting of diabetes and should be considered for all diabetic patients with prevalent CVD or a clustering of CVD risk factors.[21,22]

ANGIOTENSIN II RECEPTOR BLOCKERS. Cardiovascular outcomes data for ARBs are much less robust than for ACE inhibitors and are particularly lacking for patients with diabetes. The Telmisartan Randomized AssessmeNt Study in ACE iNtolerant subjects with cardiovascular Disease (TRANSCEND) trial enrolled 5926 patients with intolerance to ACE inhibitors, randomized to telmisartan 80 mg daily versus placebo, including 2118 patients with diabetes.[31] In the overall trial, telmisartan failed to achieve statistical superiority over placebo in reducing the primary composite of CVD death, MI, stroke, or HF hospitalization (HR = 0.92; 95% CI, 0.81-1.05), but it significantly reduced the secondary composite of CV death, MI, or stroke (HR = 0.87; 95% CI, 0.76-1.00). Although the results in the subgroup with diabetes lacked statistical power, the point estimates of effect for both the primary and key secondary outcomes were markedly attenuated in the subset with diabetes. Although guidelines from the ADA and AHA have endorsed ARBs and ACE inhibitors with similar levels of recommendation,[21,22] such recommendations for ARB use are based almost entirely on trials assessing ARB effects on intermediate outcomes, especially intermediate measures of nephropathy, with little evidence available with regard to CVD outcomes—excepting demonstrated superiority in the randomized trial meta-analysis of ARBs compared with non–RAAS-blocking drugs in the prevention of HF among patients with diabetes.[29a] Therefore, ARBs should be considered second-line therapy, and their use reserved for those patients who cannot tolerate ACE inhibitors because of cough, angioedema, or rash.

Calcium Channel Blockers. Dihydropyridine calcium channel blockers, such as nifedipine, nitrendipine, nisoldipine, and amlodipine, are well tolerated and effective at lowering blood pressure. Analyses of diabetes subsets of randomized clinical trials have suggested CVD clinical benefits of a magnitude similar to or greater than those observed in the nondiabetic cohorts, including evaluations of nitrendipine, nisoldipine, and amlodipine.[29a] In active controlled comparisons, amlodipine has been proven superior to hydrochlorothiazide when it is added to a background of benazepril therapy,[32] but in randomized trials directly comparing the efficacy of calcium channel blockers versus ACE inhibitors, superior outcomes were observed with ACE inhibitors.

Beta Blockers. Antagonists of the beta-adrenergic receptors (beta blockers) are another key component of effective CVD risk reduction in diabetes. Early in the course of clinical use, beta blockers were considered relatively contraindicated in the setting of diabetes because of concerns about masking hypoglycemia symptoms and adverse effects on glucose and lipid metabolism. These concerns have been mitigated by the results of CVD outcomes trials supporting the benefit of beta blockers for patients with diabetes in the chronic ambulatory setting[33] and in the post-ACS population.[34] In addition, the metabolic effects of various beta blockers differ, which suggests improved metabolic parameters with noncardioselective beta blockers that also have alpha receptor–blocking properties; the clinical relevance of these differential effects remains to be determined. The utility of beta blockers in the treatment of patients with diabetes has most recently been supported by a meta-analysis of randomized clinical trials.[29a]

Thiazide Diuretics. Concern about the adverse glycometabolic effects of the thiazide diuretic class of medications—including hydrochlorothiazide, chlorthalidone, indapamide, and bendroflumethiazide—has resulted in some degree of hesitancy to use these medications in the setting of diabetes or in patients at increased risk for development of diabetes. However, randomized trials of thiazide diuretics that included substantial numbers of patients with diabetes have consistently demonstrated CVD benefits despite their adverse metabolic effects. In a subanalysis of the Antihypertensive and Lipid-Lowering Treatment to Prevent Heart Attack Trial (ALLHAT), the CVD effects of chlorthalidone compared with both lisinopril and amlodipine were similar in patients with diabetes or impaired fasting glucose, despite modest but statistically significant increases in incident diabetes associated with chlorthalidone.[35] A meta-analysis of randomized trials further supported the benefits of thiazide diuretics in the treatment of patients with diabetes.[29a]

Combination Therapy for Hypertension. In addition to demonstrated efficacy with individual drugs, a number of studies have also demonstrated the benefits of combination therapy in patients with diabetes. In the Action in Diabetes and Vascular disease: preterAx and diamicroN-MR Controlled Evaluation (ADVANCE) trial, which compared combination therapy with perindopril and indapamide versus placebo in 11,140 patients with type 2 diabetes,[36] the combination therapy was associated with a 9% relative reduction in a composite primary outcome combining microvascular and macrovascular disease endpoints, compared with placebo. In the Anglo-Scandinavian Cardiac Outcomes Trial–Blood Pressure Lowering Arm (ASCOT-BPLA),[37] which randomized treatment to amlodipine with perindopril added as needed versus atenolol with bendroflumethiazide added as needed, the amlodipine-perindopril combination yielded a significant 13% relative risk reduction (P = 0.028) in major CVD outcomes in the 923 patients with diabetes, compared with atenolol-bendroflumethiazide. Finally, in the Avoiding Cardiovascular Events through Combination Therapy in Patients Living with Systolic Hypertension (ACCOMPLISH) trial,[32] in which all patients were treated with benazepril, with randomization to add-on amlodipine versus add-on hydrochlorothiazide, treatment with benazepril-amlodipine versus benazepril-hydrochlorothiazide was associated with a 21% reduction in CVD outcomes among the 6946 patients with diabetes (60.4% of the study cohort; P = 0.003). Therefore, in combination with thiazide diuretics and with amlodipine, ACE inhibitors are associated with improved CVD outcomes, with the combination with amlodipine proving superior in head-to-head comparison.

Blood Pressure Targets for Patients with Diabetes. Given the incremental CVD risk associated with hypertension in DM, and the clearly demonstrated graded association between magnitude of blood pressure reduction and CVD clinical risk reduction, patients with DM have been identified as a special population warranting more aggressive than usual blood pressure control, with targets for patients with DM of <130/80 mm Hg being endorsed by a number of professional guidelines.[21,37a,37b] These recommendations, based largely on epidemiologic data, have been supported by observations of more recent randomized clinical trials. In the Hypertension Optimal Treatment (HOT) trial, participants with elevated diastolic blood pressure were randomized to treatment to three different targets: 90, 85, and 80 mm Hg.[37c] While the overall trial failed to demonstrate significant differences by intensity of blood pressure treatment, a post hoc analysis of the subset of patients with DM exhibited a significant intensity-dependent reduction in CVD, including a 50% relative risk reduction for major adverse CVD events in the group with the lowest compared with the highest blood pressure target. Likewise, the average systolic blood pressure achieved in the diabetic subset of HOPE (139/77 mm Hg) and in the ADVANCE trial (136/73 mm Hg) provide further support for the safety and efficacy of such intensified blood pressure targets in the high-risk population of patients with DM. More recently, results were reported from the NHLBI-sponsored Action to Control Cardiovascular Risk in Diabetes (ACCORD) trial, in which 4733 patients with type 2 diabetes at high cardiovascular risk were randomized to treatment to systolic blood pressure goals of <120 mm Hg versus <140 mm Hg.[37d] In a comparison of the more intensive versus less intensive arm, the point estimate of a 12% relative risk reduction in the primary composite endpoint of CV death, MI, and stroke failed to achieve statistical significance (HR = 0.88; 95% CI, 0.73-1.06); more intensive control was associated with a significant 41% reduction in stroke (HR = 0.59; 95% CI, 0.39-0.89). Of note, at the time of randomization, when clinical guidelines endorsed systolic blood pressure targets of <130/80 mm Hg, the average blood pressure at study entry was 139/76 mm Hg in this high-risk cohort. During the trial, the average blood pressure achieved in the <120 mm Hg arm was 119.3 mm Hg, contrasted with an average of 133.5 mm Hg in the patients randomized to a target of <140 mm Hg requiring an average of 3.4 and 2.3 medications, respectively. Therefore, though the trial failed to prove the benefit of more intensive blood pressure control than contemporary targets, the blood pressure achieved in the less intensive group fell quite close to such targets, and in the context of favorable secondary outcomes with no prohibitive safety signals observed, the present target of <130/80 mm Hg seems prudent, with no clear imperative to target more aggressive control.

Antihypertensive Therapy Summary

In summary, five classes of medications have substantial evidence basis for CVD efficacy in the setting of diabetes, including ACE inhibitors, calcium channel blockers, beta blockers, thiazide diuretics, and ARBs. In addition, evidence supports an aggressive blood pressure target of <130/80 mm Hg for patients with diabetes to achieve optimal CVD risk mitigation, with most patients requiring a combination of multiple blood pressure medications to achieve such targets.

ANTIPLATELET THERAPY. As discussed earlier, patients with diabetes have a number of aberrations of platelet structure, function, and activity, yielding in aggregate a prothrombotic milieu. On the basis of these observations, much interest and investigation have been focused on optimizing antiplatelet therapy for this high-risk cohort of patients.

Aspirin Therapy

The ADA and AHA presently recommend daily aspirin (75 to 162 mg/day) for all patients with diabetes who have prevalent CVD or for primary prevention in all patients older than 40 years with additional CVD risk factors (or younger in the presence of prevalent CVD risk).[21,22] Whereas these recommendations are supported by a substantial evidence base in the setting of secondary CVD risk modification,[38] they have been challenged to some degree by the absence of statistically significant benefits observed in two recent meta-analyses of primary prevention with aspirin in patients with diabetes,[38,39] and uncertainties remain about the optimal population of patients to treat and the optimal dose of aspirin to use for patients with diabetes.[18] In addition to the spectrum of platelet abnormalities associated with diabetes, absolute or relative aspirin resistance may occur in up to 40% of patients with diabetes, with increasing prevalence associated with poor metabolic control.[40]

On the basis of this ongoing uncertainty with regard to the role of aspirin in the setting of primary CVD risk prevention in type 2 diabetes, two large-scale randomized clinical trials are currently under way. A Study of Cardiovascular Events In Diabetes (ASCEND) plans to enroll 10,000 patients with type 1 or type 2 diabetes without CVD, randomized factorially to treatment with 100 mg acetylsalicylic acid (ASA) daily versus placebo or with omega-3 fatty acid 1 g daily versus placebo, with a primary endpoint of major adverse cardiovascular events *(http://www.ctsu.ox.ac.uk/ascend/)*. The Aspirin and Simvastatin Combination for Cardiovascular Events Prevention Trial in Diabetes (ACCEPT-D) plans to enroll 4700 patients with type 1 or type 2 diabetes to receive 100 mg ASA plus simvastatin versus simvastatin alone in a prospective, open-label, blinded endpoint evaluation (PROBE) design trial to assess the cardiovascular efficacy of ASA in primary prevention for patients with diabetes that has been treated with statins.[41]

In summary, until further evidence becomes available, the present recommendations—as outlined by guidelines from diabetes and cardiovascular professional societies—remain the most evidence-based approach. Daily aspirin (75 to 162 mg) is recommended for all patients with diabetes who have prevalent CVD, or increased CVD risk assessed by >50 years of age for men and >60 years of age for women with additional CVD risk factors present.[21,22]

Thienopyridines

In aggregate, the epidemiologic, mechanistic, and primary or secondary prevention clinical trial data support the hypothesis that patients with type 2 diabetes may require more aggressive antiplatelet treatment to yield commensurate antiplatelet effects to affect CVD risk reduction, and that more aggressive antiplatelet dosing in this setting may not increment bleeding risk. The thienopyridines irreversibly bind to $P2Y_{12}$ ADP receptors and inhibit ADP-induced activation of glycoprotein (GP) IIb/IIIa, preventing the binding of fibrinogen and platelet thrombus formation, thus yielding more potent antiplatelet effects than achieved with aspirin alone.

Observations from trials of the thienopyridines clopidogrel and prasugrel provide support for the concept of incremental efficacy in diabetes with more potent platelet inhibition in the chronic ambulatory setting and, as reviewed later in this chapter, in the setting of ACS.[18] In the CAPRIE trial, which compared outcomes in patients with non–ST-segment elevation MI, ischemic stroke, or established peripheral artery disease randomized to treatment with aspirin versus clopidogrel, 3866 patients with diabetes were enrolled. In the subset of patients with diabetes, the 12.5% reduction in major adverse CVD events with clopidogrel versus aspirin was comparable to the effect observed in the overall study cohort. Given the incremental expense of clopidogrel and its associated increment in bleeding risk, however, this strategy is not routinely recommended over the use of aspirin alone for most patients.

Diabetes is associated with an increased prevalence of resistance to clopidogrel, a prodrug requiring metabolic conversion that appears to be impaired in diabetes, resulting in decreased circulating active metabolite.[42,43] These observations have led some investigators to explore the effects of increased dosing of clopidogrel in patients with diabetes, with preliminary data suggesting increased antiplatelet effects with such a strategy.[43] However, the net clinical safety and efficacy of increased dosing of clopidogrel requires further evaluation before application in clinical practice.

GLUCOSE MANAGEMENT. For the treatment of hyperglycemia associated with diabetes, there are numerous drug classes comprising oral and injectable glucose-lowering medications approved for clinical use (**Table 64-4**). These drugs work by stimulating endogenous insulin release, impairing hepatic glucose production, improving the body's response to insulin, or delaying intestinal carbohydrate absorption.

Cardiovascular Effects of Selected Drugs for Diabetes

To date, the approval of drugs for diabetes has been based almost exclusively on the demonstration of proof of concept for efficacy of glucose lowering without requirement of demonstration of efficacy on clinical outcomes. The regulatory landscape for diabetes drugs has recently undergone major changes, such that all future diabetes drugs (and probably those currently on the market) will be required to demonstrate designated margins of CVD safety to achieve or to maintain regulatory approval, leading to a rapid proliferation of clinical trials under way or in planning to assess CVD outcomes associated with these therapies.[44] In this context, few data are available with regard to the net CVD safety and efficacy of such medications, and current management strategies and guidelines remain grounded on the proven microvascular disease benefits demonstrated with glucose control.[21,45]

METFORMIN. Metformin, in the biguanide class, lowers blood glucose primarily by decreasing hepatic glucose output and with some improvement in insulin sensitivity.[46] In addition to improved glucose control, metformin is also associated with weight reduction, favorable effects on lipid parameters, improved coagulation profiles, and low risk for hypoglycemia. In the United Kingdom Prospective Diabetes Study (UKPDS) of various glucose-lowering strategies in a population of patients with newly diagnosed type 2 diabetes, patients who were overweight at study entry were eligible to randomization to metformin therapy in addition to the other treatments, which included sulfonylureas, insulin, and usual care. Those treated with metformin had statistically superior outcomes for all diabetes endpoints, MI, and all-cause mortality compared with either of the other two drug treatment strategies or with usual care.[4]

Delaying the regulatory approval of metformin in the United States and hindering its clinical uptake were concerns about its potential to cause lactic acidosis, based primarily on observations with the earlier use of another biguanide, phenformin, that clearly caused lactic acidemia and was removed from the market on that basis. In response to this concern, metformin has been contraindicated for use in the setting of renal compromise including chronic kidney disease (CKD), for 48 to 72 hours after the administration of iodinated contrast material, and in symptomatic HF. However, in the context of widespread global use of metformin for more than five decades and a substantial aggregated data base of comparative clinical trials, no convincing signal for increased lactic acidemia has been observed.[47] Whereas the CKD and contrast agent exposure contraindications remain in the product label, with their relevance remaining uncertain, the contraindication for use in HF was recently removed on the basis of demonstrated clinical safety.[46]

On the basis of safety, tolerability, low hypoglycemia risk, outcomes data, and relatively low cost of the generic medication, metformin should be the first-line drug for type 2 diabetes in the absence of CKD contraindications.[21,46] It is the only oral therapy routinely recommended to be continued once insulin therapy has been initiated.

SULFONYLUREAS. Sulfonylurea medications, in clinical use since 1950, are the oldest oral glucose-lowering drugs. They lower glucose by augmenting insulin release through inhibition of ATP-dependent potassium (K_{ATP}) channels in pancreatic beta cells. Although these drugs are typically well tolerated and are relatively potent, their use results in the highest rate of hypoglycemia of any available oral drug and is associated with weight gain. Whereas tolbutamide, a first-generation sulfonylurea, was shown to increase cardiovascular risk and mortality in an early randomized trial,[48] no such adverse cardiovascular safety signals have emerged from subsequent trials with randomized assignment to second- and third-generation sulfonylureas. On the basis of the extensive clinical experience, the availability of low-cost generics, and the efficacy of glucose control demonstrated in a number of clinical trials, sulfonylureas have been endorsed as a second-line drug (after metformin) for the treatment of type 2 diabetes.[45]

Some concerns persist about the use of sulfonylureas in CVD cohorts, driven by the weight gain associated with the drugs, the increased risk for hypoglycemia and commensurate stimulation of the

TABLE 64-4 Glucose-Lowering Medications for Type 2 Diabetes Mellitus

AGENT	MECHANISM OF ACTION	EXPECTED A1C REDUCTION	ADVERSE EFFECTS	CARDIOVASCULAR ISSUES
Sulfonylureas Glyburide Glipizide Glimepiride Gliclazide Chlorpropamide Tolbutamide	Bind to sulfonylurea receptors on pancreatic islet beta cells, closing K_{ATP} channels, stimulating insulin release Relatively long duration of action	~1%-2%	Hypoglycemia Weight gain	Hypoglycemia may precipitate ischemia, arrhythmia Cardiac K_{ATP} channel closure may impair ischemic preconditioning
Meglitinides Repaglinide Nateglinide	Bind to sulfonylurea receptors on pancreatic islet beta cells, closing K_{ATP} channels, stimulating insulin release Relatively short duration of action	~1%-2%	Hypoglycemia Weight gain	Hypoglycemia may precipitate ischemia, arrhythmia Cardiac K_{ATP} channel closure may impair ischemic preconditioning
Biguanides Metformin	Decrease hepatic glucose production	~1%-2%	Diarrhea, nausea Lactic acidosis Decreases B_{12} levels	May improve CVD outcomes[105] Should not be used in acute or unstable HF because of lactic acidosis risk
α-Glucosidase inhibitors Acarbose Miglitol	Slow gut carbohydrate absorption	~0.5%-1.0%	Gas, bloating	Improves postprandial glucose excursions, which are more tightly associated with CVD than fasting glucose May reduce MI risk[106]
Thiazolidinediones Rosiglitazone Pioglitazone	Activate the nuclear receptor PPAR-γ, increasing peripheral insulin sensitivity Also reduces hepatic glucose production	~1%-1.5%	Weight gain Edema ? Bone loss in women	May precipitate clinical HF in predisposed individuals Contraindicated in NYHA Class III-IV HF (because of fluid retention); not recommended in Class II HF[107] Pioglitazone may reduce MI, stroke risk[51] Rosiglitazone may increase MI risk[108]
Incretin modulators GLP-1 mimetics Exenatide	Increase glucose-dependent insulin secretion, decrease glucagon secretion, and delay gastric emptying	~1%	Nausea, vomiting	Very preliminary data suggest possible benefit in patients with cardiomyopathy[109]
Dipeptidyl peptidase 4 inhibitors Sitagliptin Saxagliptin	Inhibit degradation of endogenous GLP-1 (and GIP-1), thereby enhancing the effects of these incretins	~0.6%-0.8%	—	—
Amylin analogues Pramlintide	Decrease glucagon secretion and delay gastric emptying	~0.4%-0.6%	Nausea, vomiting	—
Insulins Glargine, Detemir NPH, Lente Regular Lispro, Aspart, Glulisine Premixed Inhaled	Increase insulin supply	No limit (theoretically)	Hypoglycemia Weight gain Edema (at high doses)	Retrospective data in HF suggest worse clinical outcomes in HF patients who require and are treated with insulin

CVD = cardiovascular disease; GLP-1 = glucagon-like peptide 1; GIP-1 = glucose-dependent insulinotropic peptide; HF = heart failure; MI = myocardial infarction; NPH = neutral protamine Hagedorn.

Reprinted from Inzucchi SE, McGuire DK: New drugs for the treatment of diabetes: Part II: Incretin-based therapy and beyond. Circulation 117:574, 2008.

adrenergic stress-response system with potential adverse CVD effects,[46] and their potential to inhibit ischemic preconditioning via blockade of myocardial K_{ATP} channels.[49] In experimental MI, activation of myocardial K_{ATP} channels reduces infarct size, an effect termed ischemic preconditioning, that is blocked by sulfonylureas. The relevance of these observations to humans remains poorly understood[49] but is one potential explanation of the increased MI case-fatality rate observed in the more intensively treated patients of the ACCORD trial (summarized later), a conjecture that remains speculative, with limited ability to analyze outcomes according to drugs used in that trial.[5] Observations from the UKPDS trial counter the likelihood of such an effect, as an intensive glucose control policy with two different sulfonylureas—chlorpropamide and glyburide—yielded similar MI and cardiovascular death outcomes, as did insulin in a trial that accumulated 595 MI events.[48] On the basis of these concerns, sulfonylureas that are relatively specific for pancreatic K_{ATP} channels have been developed,[49] although no cardiovascular clinical outcomes trials have yet been executed to evaluate the cardiovascular safety and efficacy resulting from such evolution of the class.

THIAZOLIDINEDIONES. Thiazolidinediones (i.e., rosiglitazone and pioglitazone) decrease glucose levels in type 2 diabetes by increasing the insulin sensitivity of target tissues and induce a wide variety of nonglycemic effects mediated through activation of the nuclear receptor PPAR-γ, including a number of favorable effects on intermediate markers of CVD risk and disease, leading to much interest in their effects on CVD morbidity and mortality.[50] In the Prospective Pioglitazone Clinical Trial in Macrovascular Events (PROactive study), the first randomized trial designed to assess the effect of any glucose-lowering medication on cardiovascular clinical outcomes, treatment with pioglitazone significantly reduced the composite endpoint of all-cause mortality, nonfatal MI, and stroke compared with placebo in patients with type 2 diabetes and prevalent CVD at study entry, treated during a 34.5-month follow-up, although the effect on the primary endpoint was not significant.[51] In contrast, rosiglitazone may increase CVD risk—and, specifically, increase MI risk (**Fig. 64-7**).[50,52] Though the data are not definitive, the signal for increased MI risk with rosiglitazone has led to severe product-label restrictions for use in the United States and withdrawal of the drug from the European market.

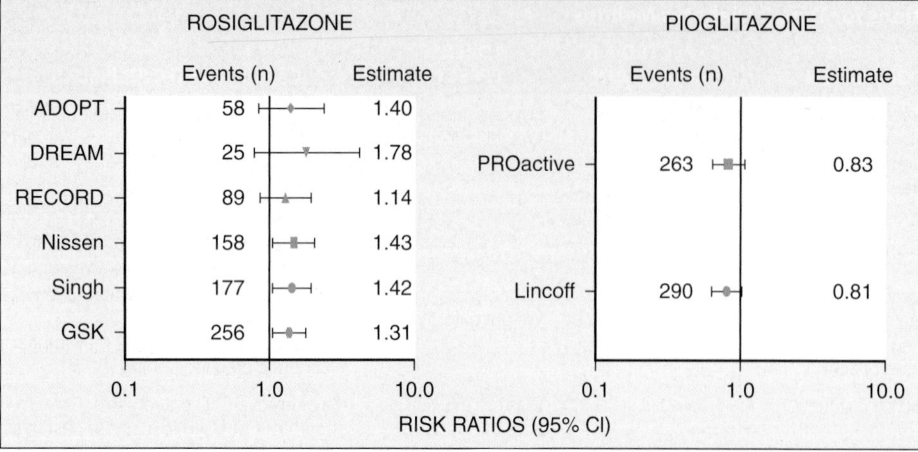

FIGURE 64-7 Relative risk of myocardial infarction associated with rosiglitazone **(left)** and pioglitazone **(right)** versus comparator in randomized clinical trials and meta-analyses. *(Modified from Rohatgi A, McGuire DK. Effects of the thiazolidinedione medications on micro- and macrovascular complications in patients with diabetes—update 2008. Cardiovasc Drugs Ther 22:233, 2008.)*

Both available thiazolidinediones increase the risk for peripheral edema, with a small but consistent increase in risk for new or worsening HF.[50] On that basis, the product labels for both agents caution against their use in patients with HF, with a contraindication for initiation in patients with New York Heart Association (NYHA) Class III or IV HF.[53] Although the mechanism of the observed increase in edema and HF remains unclear, it appears to be primarily due to increased renal sodium reclamation and plasma volume expansion, with no evidence to date of pernicious cardiac effects of these drugs.[50,53a]

OTHER GLUCOSE-LOWERING MEDICATIONS. Few data are available with regard to the CVD effects of other glucose-lowering medications.[46] Suggested CVD benefits with insulin derive from selected trials including both type 2 and type 1 diabetes, but these studies all had limited statistical power to assess such effects.[4,54] On this backdrop, and in the wake of increased regulatory scrutiny with regard to safety and efficacy assessment of drugs being developed for diabetes,[44] numerous randomized CVD clinical outcomes trials are currently under way or in advanced planning.

Cardiovascular Effects of Intensive Glucose Control Strategies

UKPDS[4,48] randomized 5102 patients with newly diagnosed type 2 diabetes to intensive glucose control with sulfonylurea or insulin compared with diet alone; those overweight at study entry (n = 795) could also be randomized in the intensive arm to receive metformin. In the insulin and sulfonylurea analyses, achieving A1c levels of 7.0% versus 7.9% during an average of 10 years, intensive control decreased risk for a composite endpoint of all diabetes-related complications (RRR = 12%; $P = 0.029$) and significantly improved microvascular disease risk (RRR = 25%; $P = 0.01$). Whereas a trend toward decreased risk of MI was observed with intensive control (14.8% versus 16.8%; $P = 0.052$), stroke was numerically increased, although the difference was not statistically significant (5.6% versus 5.2%; $P = 0.52$). In overweight subjects, metformin had better glucose control (A1c 7.4% versus 8.0%) as well as significantly improved risk for MI (RRR = 39%; $P = 0.01$) and for all-cause mortality (RRR = 36%; $P = 0.011$). These observations have recently been extended by the publication of results derived from long-term post-trial follow-up of the UKPDS trial cohort, with an average duration of 10 years after completion of the trial,[4] during which glucose control converged rapidly after the study treatment discontinuation. These analyses reveal a significantly reduced risk for MI in those originally randomized to intensive control, both in the insulin and sulfonylurea group (RRR = 15%; $P = 0.01$) and in the metformin group (RRR = 33%; $P = 0.005$).

More recently, the results from three trials assessing the CVD effects of more intensive glucose control among patients with type 2 diabetes at high CVD risk have become available (**Table 64-5**).[5,6,55] Comprising

TABLE 64-5 Baseline Characteristics and Main Results from Three Large Randomized Cardiovascular Trials in Patients with Type 2 Diabetes Mellitus

	ACCORD		ADVANCE		VADT	
N	10,251		11,140		1791	
Age (mean, years)	62		66		60	
BMI (mean, kg/m²)	32		28		31	
Follow-up (mean, years)	3.5		5		5.6	
A1c target	<6.0% versus 7.0%-7.9%		≤6.5% versus "standard"		<6% versus 8%-9%	
Baseline A1c (mean)	8.3%		7.5%		9.4%	
Endpoint A1c (mean)	Intensive 6.4%	Standard 7.5%	Intensive 6.43%	Standard 7.0%	Intensive 6.9%	Standard 8.4%
Severe hypoglycemic events	Intensive 10.5%	Standard 3.5%	Intensive 2.7%	Standard 1.5%	Intensive 8.5%	Standard 2.1%
Weight change	Intensive +3.5 kg	Standard +0.4 kg	Intensive −0.1 kg	Standard −1.0 kg	Intensive +8.1%	Standard +4.1%
Major macrovascular or microvascular event	Not reported		0.9 (0.82-0.98), $P = 0.01$		0.88 (0.74-1.05), $P = 0.14$	
Nonfatal MI/stroke, CV death	HR 0.9 (0.78-1.04), $P = 0.16$		0.94 (0.84-1.06), $P = 0.32$		Not reported	
All-cause mortality	HR 1.22 (1.01-1.46), $P = 0.04$		0.93 (0.83-1.06), $P = 0.28$		1.07 (0.81-1.42), $P = 0.62$	
Nonfatal MI	HR 0.76 (0.62-0.92), $P = 0.004$		0.98 (0.77-1.22), P = NS		0.82 (059-1.14), $P = 0.24$	

ACCORD = Action to Control Cardiovascular Risk in Diabetes trial[5]; ADVANCE = Action in Diabetes and Vascular disease: preterAx and diamicroN-MR Controlled Evaluation trial[6]; A1c = glycosylated hemoglobin; BMI = body mass index; CV = cardiovascular; MI = myocardial infarction; VADT = Veterans Affairs Diabetes Trial[55].
From Gore MO, Inzucchi SE, McGuire DK. *In* Prevention of Cardiovascular Disease: Companion to Braunwald's Heart Disease. Philadelphia, Elsevier, 2010.

more than 23,000 patients treated on study protocol from 3 to 5 years, all three trials showed no significant CVD benefit of intensified glucose control.

The ACCORD trial compared intensive versus standard glucose control in 10,251 patients with type 2 diabetes who were at high CVD risk, achieving A1c contrast of 6.4% versus 7.5%.[5] This trial was stopped early at the recommendation of the Data Safety Monitoring Committee because of an excess of all-cause mortality (257 versus 203 events; $P = 0.04$) in the intensively treated group, with no significant difference observed in the primary composite CVD endpoint of cardiovascular death, MI, and stroke (HR = 0.90; 95% CI, 0.78-1.04). The explanation for the incremental mortality remains unresolved; possible explanations currently being explored include increased hypoglycemia precipitating cardiovascular death, pernicious effects of specific drugs or drug combinations, and a chance finding in the context of the other recently reported trials. More than 75% of the intensively treated patients were treated with insulin during the trial, and most patients were prescribed three or more oral agents simultaneously; in the absence of randomization to specific therapies, post hoc analysis of cause is especially difficult.

The ADVANCE trial enrolled 11,140 patients with type 2 diabetes who had CVD, microvascular disease, or another vascular risk factor at study entry. The patients were randomized to intensive versus standard glucose control with gliclazide plus other drugs in the intensive arm, compared with other drugs in the standard control group.[6] Similar to the ACCORD trial, the ADVANCE trial failed to achieve statistically significant improvement in the composite CVD outcome of cardiovascular death, MI, and stroke with intensive control (achieved A1c 6.4% versus 7.0%), despite the ascertainment of 1147 events (10.0% versus 10.6%; RRR = 6%; 95% CI, –6% to 16%).

In the Veterans Affairs Diabetes Trial (VADT), 1791 U.S. veterans with type 2 diabetes and inadequate glucose control were randomized to intensive versus standard glucose control. Despite a wide separation in glucose control values (A1c 6.9% versus 8.4%) and ascertainment of 499 primary major adverse cardiovascular events, this trial also failed to demonstrate significant improvement in cardiovascular outcomes with intensive control (29.5% versus 33.5%; $P = 0.14$).

From post hoc analyses of each of these recent trials, and supported by the long-term observations reported from UKPDS of patients with newly diagnosed diabetes at study entry, the concept has emerged that more intensive glycemic control may both be safer and have more favorable cardiovascular effects when it is used in patients earlier in the course of diabetes, particularly among those without prevalent CVD. This hypothesis requires confirmation in additional clinical trials.

In summary, whereas these recent randomized trials failed to demonstrate significant incremental cardiovascular benefits with more intensive glucose control, the analyses of the primary composite endpoints for each trial revealed point estimates of relative risk reductions ranging from 6% to 12%, each with upper 95% confidence limits ranging from 1.04 to 1.06. Such results provide significant assurance of a margin of cardiovascular safety with more intensive glucose control, supported by a recently published meta-analysis of the available data, demonstrating statistically significant reductions in MI (HR = 0.83; 95% CI, 0.75-0.93), with no significant effects on stroke (HR = 0.93; 95% CI, 0.81-1.06) or all-cause mortality (HR = 1.02; 95% CI, 0.87-1.19).[24] These observed upper confidence limits are well within the noninferiority margins recently adopted as acceptable by U.S. and European regulatory agencies for diabetes drug registration[44] to exclude the upper noninferiority confidence limit of 1.3 (or no greater than 30% worse than comparator) for cardiovascular safety.

Comparative Effectiveness of Insulin Provision Versus Insulin Sensitization

In a randomized trial comparing two strategies for glucose control (as opposed to different intensities), the Bypass Angioplasty Revascularization Investigation 2 Diabetes (BARI 2D) trial enrolled patients with type 2 diabetes and prevalent obstructive coronary disease, randomized to insulin provision therapy (IP; insulin or sulfonylurea) versus insulin sensitization (IS; metformin or thiazolidinedione), with a factorial randomization to prompt revascularization with intensive medical therapy versus intensive medical therapy alone.[56] Comprising a sample of 2368 patients with the co-primary endpoints of all-cause mortality and the composite of cardiovascular death, MI, and stroke (major adverse cardiovascular events [MACE]), and with an average study treatment duration of 5.3 years, there was no statistical difference between the two glucose treatment strategies in either of the primary endpoints, in the context of a difference in achieved A1c of 0.5% favoring IS (7.0% versus 7.5%; $P < 0.001$). All-cause mortality occurred in 115 patients in the IP group versus 117 in the IS group (11.8% versus 12.1%; $P = 0.89$), and the primary MACE composite occurred in 218 versus 238 patients (22.3% versus 24.6%; $P = 0.13$). Peripheral edema was more common in the IS group (56.6% versus 51.9%; $P = 0.02$), and hypoglycemia was much more common in the IP group (53.3% versus 73.8%; $P < 0.001$). Confounding interpretation of this trial, however, was the nearly exclusive use of rosiglitazone as the thiazolidinedione treatment, given its uncertain cardiovascular effects (as outlined earlier) and a relatively high rate of crossover treatment between the randomized groups—especially in the IS group, requiring the addition of sulfonylurea or insulin to maintain targeted glucose control.

Summary of Glucose Management

In the context of these recently accumulated data, the ADA, the AHA, and the American College of Cardiology (ACC) continue to endorse a treatment target for glucose control in diabetes of A1c <7%,[23] based predominantly on microvascular disease mitigation with acknowledged uncertainty regarding the effects of intensive glucose control on CVD risk and with little evidence from a CVD standpoint to support a lower target. Similar targets have been endorsed in a consensus statement from the ADA and the European Association for the Study of Diabetes, with recommendations for drug therapies summarized in their published algorithm (**Fig. 64-8**).[45] Key among these recommendations is the use of metformin as foundation therapy in all patients without contraindications, and combination therapy including the early use of insulin to achieve A1c targets expeditiously. From a CVD standpoint, the early use of metformin is justifiable, but recommendations beyond that are less certain. Among other considerations are the demonstrated CVD benefits of pioglitazone and continued uncertainty with rosiglitazone; the risk of weight gain, peripheral edema, and HF observed with thiazolidinediones; the risk of hypoglycemia and weight gain with both insulin and insulin secretagogues; and the limited data regarding cardiovascular safety and efficacy of other diabetes medications currently available.

Acute Coronary Syndromes

Given the high risk associated with diabetes in the setting of ACS, much investigation has focused on this population. In general, as endorsed by the most recent ACS guidelines,[34] the treatment of patients with diabetes should mimic that of the overall population (see Chaps. 54 to 56). Some specific therapies also are recommended in patients with diabetes.

INSULIN AND GLUCOSE CONTROL. The myocardium preferentially metabolizes free fatty acids under physiologic conditions,[14] but it can also metabolize a variety of substrates during periods of stress (such as ischemia), and glucose is principal among these. Countering the metabolic switch to glucose metabolism during ischemia, the myocardium develops a relative insulin resistance, underpinning extensive research into metabolic modulation of the ischemic myocardium, with insulin as the primary focus of investigation.[57] However, it is critical to differentiate study results deriving from protocols designed to deliver high-dose insulin supported by exogenous glucose administration (i.e., glucose-insulin-potassium or GIK therapy), comprising virtually the entirety of data in this area, contrasted with the evaluation of insulin administration to achieve targeted glucose control, for which no large-scale clinical outcomes trials exist to date (**Table 64-6**).

Glucose-Insulin-Potassium Therapy

The use of insulin for ACS was first described in 1963 by Sodi-Pallares, with the intention of facilitating potassium flux in the ischemic myocardium, the so-called polarizing therapy. After decades of investigation, this combination of glucose, insulin, and potassium has become

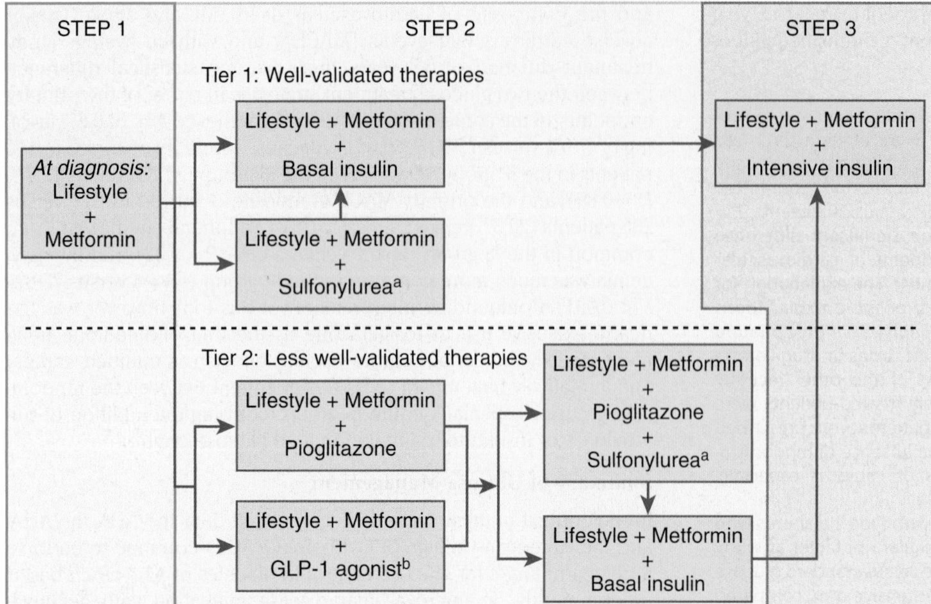

FIGURE 64-8 Algorithm for the metabolic management of type 2 diabetes. Reinforce lifestyle interventions at every visit. Check A1c every 3 months until A1c is <7%, and then at least every 6 months. Interventions should be changed if A1c is ≥7%. *(From Nathan DM, Buse JB, Davidson MB, et al: Medical management of hyperglycaemia in type 2 diabetes mellitus: A consensus algorithm for the initiation and adjustment of therapy: A consensus statement from the American Diabetes Association and the European Association for the Study of Diabetes. Diabetologia 52:17, 2009.)*

known as GIK therapy, and the focus of attention has shifted from the polarizing effects to the direct effects of insulin, including promotion of myocardial glucose oxidation, reduction of circulating nonesterified free fatty acids that may contribute to myocardial injury through an increased oxygen demand associated with free fatty acid metabolism and resultant accumulation of toxic free fatty acid metabolites, improved coagulation parameters, and anti-inflammatory effects (**Fig. 64-9**).[58] Despite these proposed mechanistic benefits of GIK therapy and the suggestion of clinical benefit derived from numerous small trials,[57] the strategy recently has been proven futile in a trial comprising 20,201 patients with MI, randomized to GIK therapy versus usual care and accumulating 1980 mortality events—demonstrating no benefit of GIK therapy compared with usual care (10.0% versus 9.7%; HR = 1.03; 95% CI, 0.95-1.13).[59] The GIK therapy protocol specifies high-dose insulin supported by glucose administration to maintain modest levels of hyperglycemia (to avoid hypoglycemia), notably contrasted with targeting tight glucose control with insulin (see Table 64-6).

Targeted Glucose Control

To date, no large-scale clinical trial has assessed the effect of intensive glucose control in the setting of ACS events. The Diabetes Mellitus Insulin-Glucose Infusion in Acute Myocardial Infarction (DIGAMI) trial enrolled 620 patients with hyperglycemia at presentation with MI, randomized to insulin infusion acutely followed by multidose subcutaneous insulin injection compared with usual care, demonstrating significant mortality reduction in the insulin-treated group during long-term follow-up.[60] DIGAMI, however, used an acute infusion of high-dose insulin (5 units/hour), coupled with intravenous glucose administration with protocol targeted hyperglycemia ranging from 126 to 198 mg/dL, a GIK insulin dosing protocol that has been used in each subsequent GIK trial (see Table 64-6). Often misinterpreted as a trial of intensive glucose control, this study has been cited as the basis of guideline recommendations for intensive glucose control in the management of ACS events since 2004, advocating normalization or near-normalization of blood glucose concentration.[34,61] However, in the wake of numerous randomized trials in noncardiac intensive care unit (ICU) populations demonstrating, at best, no benefit and, at worst, increased mortality associated with insulin infusions to normalize blood glucose concentration (**Table 64-7**),[62-66] professional guidelines have evolved substantially toward much more conservative targets in the care of patients with ACS events, recommending insulin infusion to achieve targets of <180 mg/dL.[67,68]

The risk of hypoglycemia associated with intensive glucose control in acutely ill patients remains an important concern, with an incidence of severe hypoglycemia as high as 19% observed in the recently reported trials. This concern may be especially important in the treatment of ACS events, in which the counter–hormone response associated with hypoglycemia may be particularly deleterious to ischemic and infarcting myocardium. Data from observational studies have shown increased risk associated with hypoglycemia among ACS cohorts,[69,70] but it remains unclear whether hypoglycemia is simply a marker of disease severity or contributes to adverse outcomes.[71] In the Normoglycemia in Intensive Care Evaluation–Survival Using Glucose Algorithm Regulation (NICE-SUGAR) trial,[66] the incidence of hypoglycemia associated with the insulin infusion was the lowest (6.8%) of all the trials reported, yet it is the only trial to demonstrate statistically significant increased mortality with intensive glycemic control in the ICU setting, raising the possibility that alternative mechanisms may mediate the adverse effects of the insulin infusion. The importance of

TABLE 64-6 Summary of Selected Randomized Trials Assessing the Effect of Insulin Infusion on Major Adverse Cardiovascular Outcomes Among Patients with Acute Coronary Syndrome Events

	DIGAMI	ECLA	GIPS	CREATE	HI-5	POL-GIK
N	620	407	940	20,000+	240	954
Dose (units/hr)	5	1.4/5.2	5	5	2.0	1.3→0.8
Infusion	24-72 hr	24 hr	8-12 hr	24 hr	24 hr	24 hr
Glucose target	126-198	126-198	126-198	126-198	72-180	(<300)
Results	↓ Mortality	↓ Mortality	↓ Mortality*	Neutral	↑ Mortality*	↑ Mortality

*Not significant.

DIGAMI = Diabetes Mellitus Insulin-Glucose Infusion in Acute Myocardial Infarction trial[60]; ECLA = Estudios Cardiológicos Latinoamérica glucose-insulin-potassium pilot trial[110]; GIPS = glucose-insulin-potassium study[111]; CREATE = Clinical Trial of REviparin and Metabolic Modulation in Acute Myocardial Infarction Treatment Evaluation[59]; Hi-5 = The Hyperglycemia: Intensive Insulin Infusion in Infarction study[112]; Pol-GIK = The Poland glucose-insulin-potassium trial[113]; units/hr = units per hour of intravenous insulin.

this observation is that the ability to avoid excess hypoglycemia should no longer be justification for the continued use of insulin infusions targeting tight glycemic control.

Few of the reported trials assessing targeted glucose control in ICU settings included patients with ACS events, and therefore the generalizability of the observations remains uncertain. In this context, and with the paucity of data in the ACS setting, a more conservative approach to glucose management should be used for patients with ACS events than has previously been recommended. The most recently recommended glucose targets of <180 mg/dL are reasonable, based on existing data.[67,68]

ANTIPLATELET DRUGS. Aspirin therapy is effective in an ACS setting, including in patients with diabetes. However, because of the aberrations of platelet function associated with diabetes, significant interest and investigation have centered on the unique potential for more intensive antiplatelet therapies to be especially beneficial in patients with diabetes who are experiencing ACS events. Support for this concept derives from clinical trial data of thienopyridine medications and GP IIb/IIIa antagonists.

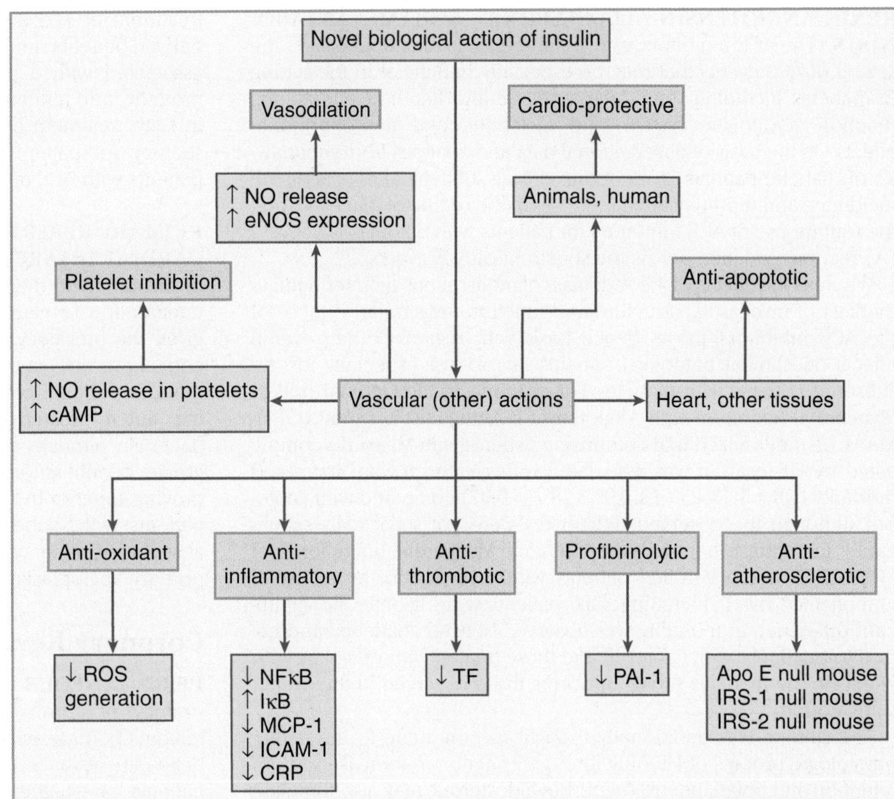

FIGURE 64-9 Novel biologic effects of insulin. CRP = C-reactive protein; cAMP = cyclic adenosine monophosphate; eNOS = endothelial nitric oxide synthase; IκB = inhibitor of nuclear factor κB; ICAM = intercellular adhesion molecule; MCP = monocyte chemotactic protein; NFκB = nuclear factor κB; NO = nitric oxide; PAI-1 = plasmin activator inhibitor type 1; ROS = reactive oxygen species; TF = tissue factor. *(Modified from Dandona P, Aljada A, Chaudhuri A, et al: Metabolic syndrome: A comprehensive perspective based on interactions between obesity, diabetes, and inflammation. Circulation 111:1448, 2005.)*

Thienopyridines

The incremental efficacy of adding thienopyridines (clopidogrel or prasugrel) to aspirin therapy in the treatment of ACS has been demonstrated in randomized clinical trials that included significant enrollment of patients with diabetes.[18,72] In the Clopidogrel in Unstable Angina to Prevent Recurrent Events (CURE) trial, which included 2840 patients with diabetes, the estimate of treatment benefit of clopidogrel in this subpopulation of 15% relative risk reduction was numerically similar to the overall trial results (14.2% versus 16.7%; $P > 0.05$). More recently, prasugrel (a third-generation thienopyridine) added to aspirin therapy, compared with aspirin alone, demonstrated significantly reduced CVD risk in the diabetes subset of the Trial to Assess Improvement in Therapeutic Outcomes by Optimizing Platelet Inhibition With Prasugrel–Thrombolysis In Myocardial Infarction 38 (TRITON–TIMI 38) trial, including patients with ACS undergoing a primary invasive management strategy (12.2% versus 17.0%; $P < 0.001$).[8] Most notably, the incremental CVD risk-benefit with prasugrel within the diabetes subset did not entail a significant increase in major bleeding complications (2.6% versus 2.5%). In aggregate, these observations support the incremental benefits of thienopyridine treatment added to aspirin therapy in diabetes patients with ACS events, and they should be part of routine clinical management.

Glycoprotein IIb/IIIa Blockers

The GP IIb/IIIa inhibitors potently inhibit platelet aggregation (see Chap. 87). In current clinical practice, eptifibatide and tirofiban are approved for use in the setting of ACS; abciximab is approved for percutaneous coronary intervention (PCI) but not specifically for ACS. On the basis of results from a meta-analysis of the GP IIb/IIIa antagonists trials for the treatment of ACS events, demonstrating a significant mortality benefit with GP IIb/IIIa blockers in the subset with diabetes but not in the nondiabetic subjects,[18] the use of GP IIb/IIIa antagonists for patients with diabetes suffering an ACS event is a level I (A) recommendation in the ACC/AHA guidelines.[34]

TABLE 64-7 Summary of Randomized Trials Comparing Normalization of Blood Glucose Concentration with Insulin Infusion, Compared with Standard of Care in a Variety of Intensive Care Unit Settings

STUDY	POPULATION	GLUCOSE TARGET	PRIMARY ENDPOINT	RESULT	HYPOGLYCEMIA
Van den Berghe—1	SICU (n = 1548)	80-110 versus 180-200	ICU death	42% RRR	7.2% (<40 mg/dL)
Van den Berghe—2	MICU (n = 1200)	80-110 versus 180-215	Hospital death	No difference	18.7% (mean 32 mg/dL)
VISEP*	MICU, sepsis (n = 488)	80-110 versus 180-200	28-day death	↑ Mortality trend	17.0% (<40 mg/dL)
GIST-UK*	Stroke ICU (n = 933)	72-126 versus usual care	90-day death	No difference	15.7% (<70 mg/dL)
European Glucontrol*	MICU (n = 1101)	80-110 versus 140-180	Hospital death	↑ Mortality trend	8.6% (<40 mg/dL)
NICE-SUGAR	MICU	81-108 versus <180	90-day death	14% ↑ Mortality	6.8% (<40 mg/dL)

*Stopped early/futility.

Van den Berghe—1 = trial of intensive insulin in the SICU[114]; Van den Berghe—2 = trial of intensive insulin in the MICU[62]; VISEP = Efficacy of Volume Substitution and Insulin Therapy in Severe Sepsis trial[63]; GIST-UK = UK Glucose Insulin in Stroke Trial[64]; European Glucontrol = Glucontrol study[65]; NICE-SUGAR = Normoglycemia in Intensive Care Evaluation–Survival Using Glucose Algorithm Regulation[66]; SICU = surgical intensive care unit; MICU = medical intensive care unit; RRR = relative risk reduction.

RENIN-ANGIOTENSIN-ALDOSTERONE SYSTEM ANTAGONISTS. The ACE inhibitors have a number of favorable effects in the setting of ACS events that may be especially beneficial in the setting of diabetes, including ventricular structure and function, endothelial function, fibrinolytic system, and metabolic and neurohormonal effects. On the basis of observational data and analyses from subanalysis of diabetic patients in randomized trials, beneficial effects on HF incidence and mortality appear greater in the setting of diabetes. Thus, the routine use of ACE inhibitors for patients with diabetes is a level I (A) recommendation across the spectrum of ACS events.[34,61]

Whereas the effects of the ARB class of medications on intermediate markers of myocardial structure and function are similar to those of the ACE inhibitors, the evidence basis with regard to their overall effects on clinical outcomes remains less robust, especially for the subset of patients with diabetes. For example, in the Optimal Trial in Myocardial Infarction with Angiotensin II Antagonist Losartan (OPTIMAAL), a randomized trial comprising patients with MI events complicated by HF, losartan was associated with a trend toward increased mortality (RR = 1.13; 95% CI, 0.99-1.28; $P = 0.07$) compared with captopril, although the observed differences were not statistically significant.[73] In contrast, in the Valsartan in Acute Myocardial Infarction Trial (VALIANT), which enrolled patients within 10 days of an acute MI complicated by HF, including 3400 patients with diabetes, no significant difference in mortality was observed between patients randomized to treatment with captopril and those treated with valsartan, with effects in the diabetes subset mirroring those observed in the overall study cohort.[74]

Aldosterone was traditionally thought to contribute to the pathophysiologic process of HF only through its action to increase sodium retention and potassium excretion. But aldosterone may also stimulate directly the production of inflammatory mediators, cause myocardial fibrosis, and promote endothelial dysfunction and vascular stiffening, and the role of aldosterone blockade in the setting of ACS has been a subject of recent investigation.[75] In the Eplerenone Post–Acute Myocardial Infarction Heart Failure Efficacy and Survival Study (EPHESUS) trial, the mineralocorticoid-selective aldosterone antagonist eplerenone was compared with placebo, added to optimal therapy, in a population of 6632 MI patients with decreased ejection fraction who had either clinical HF or, in the absence of manifest HF, diabetes.[76] In the overall study cohort, treatment with eplerenone compared with placebo reduced the risk of cardiovascular death by 17% (RR = 0.83; 95% CI, 0.72, 0.94), with numerically similar observations in the subset of 2232 patients with diabetes. On the basis of this trial, the use of an aldosterone antagonist for patients with diabetes and reduced ejection fraction after MI is recommended across the spectrum of ACS events,[34,61] with the important caveat that such therapy should not be used in patients with impaired renal function (creatinine >2.0 mg/dL) or hyperkalemia (>5.0 mEq/liter). In addition, serial monitoring of potassium concentration is recommended for patients with diabetes, given the high prevalence of type 4 renal tubular acidosis in the diabetes population.

BETA-ADRENERGIC BLOCKING AGENTS. As discussed earlier, despite evidence of their incremental effectiveness in the treatment of patients with diabetes after ACS events, beta blockers continue to be underprescribed in this group.[77] As discussed in the previous section on hypertension, such observations are likely to have resulted in part from the ongoing perception of relative contraindications in the setting of diabetes because of metabolic effects. To the contrary, beta blockers have magnified benefits in post-ACS care of the diabetic patient,[78] probably owing to several factors. Beta blockers can help restore sympathovagal balance in diabetic patients with autonomic neuropathy and may decrease fatty acid use within the myocardium, thus reducing oxygen demand. Therefore, they should be prescribed for all patients after ACS events, independent of diabetes status, unless other contraindications exist.[34,61]

PRIMARY INVASIVE STRATEGY FOR NON–ST ELEVATION ACUTE CORONARY SYNDROMES. (See Chap. 56.) In randomized trials comparing primary invasive versus noninvasive strategies for treatment of ACS events, the subsets of patients with diabetes have derived benefits similar to or greater than those of nondiabetic patients associated with a primary invasive management strategy, although mortality and reinfarction were still higher in the groups with diabetes in both treatment arms.[34] Despite these benefits, a primary invasive strategy for patients with diabetes continues to be underused in patients with ACS events.[77]

PRIMARY REPERFUSION THERAPY FOR ST ELEVATION MYOCARDIAL INFARCTION. (See Chap. 55.) Early in the development of thrombolytic therapy, concern arose about the potential for such intervention to cause retinal hemorrhage in patients with diabetes, given the prevalence of background diabetic retinopathy. Such concerns have not been borne out in analyses of diabetic subsets in the randomized trials of thrombolytics, with the group with diabetes deriving much greater absolute benefit compared with nondiabetic patients.[79] Similarly, analyses from trials of primary angioplasty suggest greater benefit among patients with diabetes, with primary angioplasty proving superior to thrombolysis in patients with diabetes.[80] Therefore, patients with diabetes should undergo reperfusion therapy in the absence of other contraindications, preferentially with a strategy of primary angioplasty when it is available.

Coronary Revascularization Considerations

PERCUTANEOUS CORONARY INTERVENTION. The optimal strategy of coronary revascularization for patients with diabetes remains controversial (see Chap. 57). Although diabetic and nondiabetic patients have similar rates of initial angioplasty success, diabetic patients have higher restenosis rates after percutaneous transluminal coronary angioplasty (PTCA) and worse long-term outcomes.[81] The mechanism underlying the increased restenosis rate in diabetes after coronary intervention is unclear. A variety of metabolic and anatomic abnormalities associated with diabetes and a greater degree of plaque burden may contribute to restenosis in diabetic patients.

Although drug-eluting stents have reduced the need for target lesion revascularization in diabetic patients,[82] diabetic patients still have more restenosis (see Chap. 58).[81] Most trials have included relatively few patients with diabetes and have excluded patients with multivessel disease. Despite these limitations, the favorable outcomes with drug-eluting stents compared with bare metal stents in the high-risk subset of patients with diabetes supports their preferential use.

The GP IIb/IIIa antagonists have demonstrated similar or increased efficacy in the setting of PCI in patients with diabetes compared with nondiabetic patients, including a suggestion of improved long-term mortality in diabetic patients treated with abciximab.[83] Given the relatively small sample sizes of diabetic patients participating in the reported studies, however, the power to evaluate fully this treatment interaction with diabetes status is limited, and these drugs should be considered adjunctive therapy for PCI in the presence or absence of diabetes.

CORONARY ARTERY BYPASS GRAFT SURGERY. Most studies comparing outcomes in diabetic and nondiabetic patients undergoing coronary artery bypass graft (CABG) surgery show an increased risk of postoperative death and 30-day and long-term mortality, and an increased need for subsequent reoperation in the diabetic population.[81] Although diabetic patients have a worse risk profile, tend to be older, and have more extensive coronary artery disease and poorer left ventricular function than do nondiabetic patients, their higher long-term mortality does not depend entirely on these factors and continues to diverge from that of nondiabetic patients during long-term follow-up, a difference that probably reflects accelerated disease progression in both bypassed and untreated coronary vessels.

Perioperative Glucose Control

The utility of intensive glucose control for the improvement of outcomes among patients undergoing cardiac surgery has been extensively studied, including assessment of longitudinal cohort studies[84] and randomized trial comparisons.[85] The Society of Thoracic Surgeons recently has published guideline recommendations for the perioperative glucose management of patients undergoing cardiac surgery,[86] advocating insulin infusions for patients with or without diabetes to maintain glucose ≤180 mg/dL, with a more stringent target of ≤150 mg/dL advocated for those patients with anticipated ICU stays exceeding 3 days.

CORONARY ARTERY BYPASS GRAFT VERSUS PERCUTANEOUS CORONARY INTERVENTION. In general, randomized trials comparing PTCA with CABG have reported similar outcomes. However, in patients with diabetes, CABG yields superior mortality outcomes compared with PCI, with incremental benefit associated with increasing severity of underlying coronary artery disease.[81,87] This interaction of the mode of revascularization with diabetes status was first observed in the Bypass Angioplasty Revascularization Investigation (BARI) trial, which compared balloon angioplasty with bypass surgery in patients with multivessel coronary disease (see Chap. 57). Whereas the outcomes were comparable in the overall trial and in the subset of patients without diabetes, patients with diabetes had a significantly lower mortality in the bypass arm compared with angioplasty (19% versus 34%; $P < 0.003$), prompting an NHLBI clinical alert advocating CABG over angioplasty for all such diabetic patients.[81] Subsequently, despite the widespread availability of drug-eluting stents and other advances in devices, techniques, and adjunctive pharmacotherapy, the mortality benefit of CABG over PCI remains, and it continues to be recommended as the preferred mode of revascularization for patients with diabetes and multivessel coronary disease.[87]

REVASCULARIZATION VERSUS OPTIMAL MEDICAL THERAPY. In the BARI 2D trial, 2368 patients with type 2 diabetes and obstructive coronary artery disease were randomized to receive prompt revascularization plus intensive medical therapy for CVD risk reduction compared with intensive medical therapy alone.[56] The mode of revascularization was left to the discretion of the treating physician and was determined before randomization, with randomization stratified by the planned mode of revascularization. During 5 years of study follow-up, the overall mortality rates between the two groups did not differ significantly—11.7% in those undergoing revascularization and 12.2% in those treated with intensive medical therapy alone ($P = 0.97$). In secondary analyses stratified according to the mode of revascularization, all cardiovascular outcomes were statistically similar between the PCI and medical therapy groups, but CABG compared with medical therapy was associated with a significant reduction in major adverse cardiovascular events (22.4% versus 30.5%; $P = 0.01$). These data provide support for a primary strategy of intensive medical therapy, as well as additional suggestion of the benefit of bypass surgery, although direct comparisons between PCI and CABG are not possible from this study design.

Applying Coronary Heart Disease Risk Reduction to Practice

Whereas myriad lifestyle and pharmacologic interventions can improve CVD risk of diabetes in the chronic and the acute setting, clinical use of such therapies remains suboptimal,[77,88,89] probably contributing to a portion of the excess CVD risk associated with diabetes. Systematic application of global CVD risk modification to patients with diabetes measurably improves CVD outcomes. For example, in a large registry study in Germany, total hospital mortality of diabetic patients hospitalized for MI declined from 29% in 1999 to 17% in 2001, and mortality within 24 hours of admission fell from 16% to 4% during the same period.[90] This reduction was associated with the increased use of therapeutic approaches (e.g., coronary angiography, stenting, antiplatelet therapy) in diabetic patients during this period. Similarly, in the chronic stable population, in a randomized trial comprising a cohort of patients with diabetes and increased CVD risk defined by the presence of albuminuria, an intensive strategy of global CVD risk modification (including intensive lifestyle, glucose, lipid, and blood pressure interventions) reduced major CVD events by 50% compared with usual care.[91]

Although much of the gap between the outcomes evidence and its clinical application remains poorly understood, some contributing factors may pertain. For example, patients with diabetes have been commonly denied beta blockers because of concerns about their adverse effects on glucose measures and lipid metabolism and the potential masking of symptoms of hypoglycemia. As discussed previously, however, numerous studies have demonstrated clinical benefits of beta blockers among diabetes cohorts similar to or exceeding those observed in the nondiabetic population.[33] Underuse of antiplatelet and anticoagulant therapies has been attributed to concerns for increased risk for retinal hemorrhage, yet these concerns have not been borne out in clinical trials.[48] Therefore, continued diligence to the application of evidence-based therapies with proven benefit in the diabetes population remains a key public health imperative.

Heart Failure in the Patient with Diabetes (see Chaps. 25 to 28)

Scope of the Problem

HF is the pathophysiologic state in which the heart cannot maintain cardiac output sufficient to meet the metabolic needs of the body. Although MI and hypertension are the most common risk factors associated with HF, diabetes mellitus and measures of insulin resistance before the development of diabetes are also strong and independent risk factors for HF, with associated twofold to fivefold increased risk.[12,14] In addition, once HF is present, diabetes portends especially adverse prognosis for subsequent morbidity and mortality, with estimates of relative increases in mortality hazard ranging from 30% to 60% based on subanalyses of data from a series of randomized clinical trials.[13,92] Given these observations, improved understanding of the pathobiologic underpinnings linking diabetes with HF and optimization of strategies for the prevention and treatment of HF in this population remain key public health considerations.

Mechanistic Considerations

Diabetic and nondiabetic subjects share common causes of HF, such as ischemic heart disease, hypertension, left ventricular hypertrophy, atrial fibrillation, and valvular disease. The incremental HF risk with diabetes is not completely attributable to these common risk factors, however, suggesting increased myocardial vulnerability in the setting of diabetes and probable synergistic effects between such factors and diabetes that increase HF risk, yielding the concept of "diabetic cardiomyopathy." The pathologic underpinnings of abnormal cardiac structure and function in diabetes remain poorly understood (**Table 64-8**).

ISCHEMIC HEART DISEASE AND HYPERTENSION. Given the high prevalence in patients with diabetes, ischemic heart disease remains the principal risk factor for HF in patients with diabetes both in the chronic ambulatory setting and after ACS events. In addition to the burden of coronary atherosclerosis, other contributors to this

TABLE 64-8 Pathophysiologic Abnormalities Associated with Cardiac Dysfunction, Congestive Heart Failure, and Adverse Outcomes in Diabetes

Sympathetic nervous system activation
Renin-angiotensin system activation
Increased sodium and free water retention
Decreased vascular compliance
Elevated endothelin levels (in diabetes)
Loss of "dipping" nocturnal blood pressure pattern
Increased free fatty acid levels
Dysregulated myocardial glucose and fatty acid metabolism
Increased left ventricular hypertrophy or mass via myocyte hypertrophy
Deposition of advanced glycation end products in extracellular matrix
Increased cardiac fibrosis
Increased cardiac steatosis

increased risk may include increased prevalence of silent or atypical symptoms of ischemia delaying diagnosis and intervention, suboptimal use of therapeutic interventions, disturbed sympathovagal balance, prothrombotic milieu that may attenuate benefit of antithrombotic therapies, impaired coronary endothelial function, and disordered ischemic myocardial metabolism.[14,93] In aggregate, these effects and others probably increase ischemic burden, increase infarct size, and adversely affect remodeling in the setting of ischemic heart disease and ACS events. Affecting both ischemic heart disease and HF risk, hypertension prevalence exceeds 70% in populations with diabetes. Among patients with type 2 diabetes, HF risk increases 12% for every increment of 10 mm Hg in systolic blood pressure (see Fig. 64-6).[94]

MYOCARDIAL METABOLISM AND STRUCTURE. (see Chap. 24) The direct effects of hyperglycemia and insulin resistance on myocardial cellular metabolism may contribute to cardiac dysfunction in diabetes,[14] with altered energy substrate supply and impairment of metabolic substrate switching under conditions of stress. The myocardium uses predominantly free fatty acids under aerobic conditions but increasingly shifts to glycolysis and pyruvate oxidation during ischemia (**Fig. 64-10**). In the diabetic heart, insulin resistance impairs such substrate switching and glucose transport into cells, resulting in anaerobic fatty acid oxidation and compromising the efficiency of myocardial energetics, as well as generating pernicious oxidative byproducts. Systemic free fatty acid excess, combined with cellular dysregulation of lipid metabolism in type 2 diabetes, contributes to accumulation of myocellular triglyceride (myocardial steatosis), resulting in further perturbations of myocyte metabolism and inducing apoptosis due to lipotoxicity, in addition to the adverse influence of cardiac mechanical function attributable to the increased myocardial mass.[95,96]

Diabetes causes a variety of morphologic changes in the myocardium, with abnormalities in myocytes, extracellular matrix, and microvasculature.[14] Whereas such abnormalities are commonly present across causes of cardiomyopathy, they tend to be more common and more severe in the setting of diabetes. In addition, more specific to diabetes, the myocardial accumulation of advanced glycation end products (AGEs)—which are products of macromolecules, the formation and accumulation of which depend on the severity of hyperglycemia—may contribute to HF risk. Deposition of AGEs within the myocardial extracellular matrix adversely affects both systolic and diastolic cardiac function, largely attributable to AGE cross-linking of matrix collagen.[97]

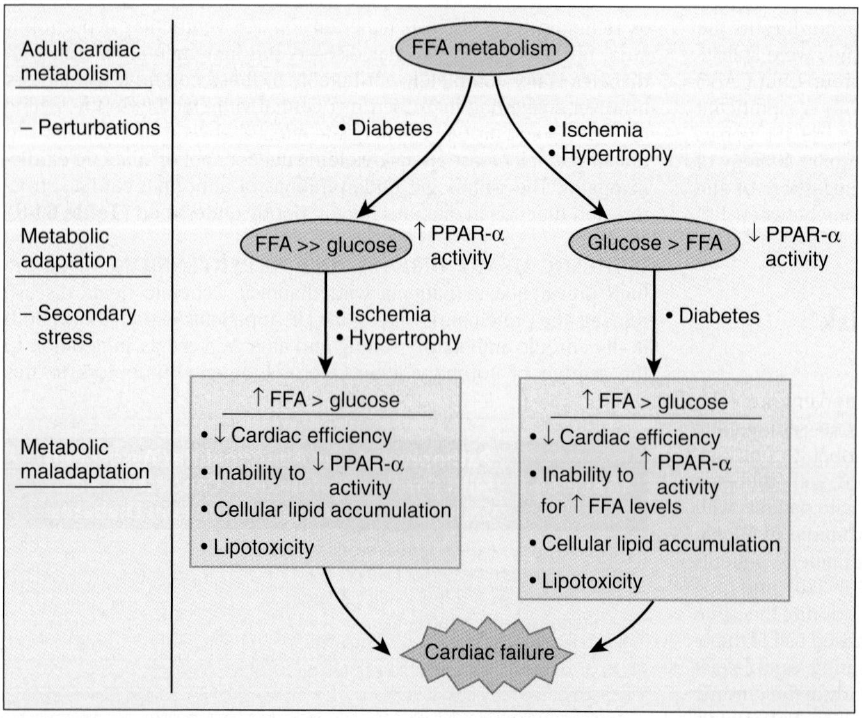

FIGURE 64-10 Schematic summary of cardiac adaptive and maladaptive metabolic modifications occurring in response to diabetes with or without superimposed ischemia or hypertrophy, culminating in overt cardiomyopathy. FFA = free fatty acid; PPAR-α = peroxisome proliferator–activated receptor α. *(From Saunders J, Mathewkutty S, Drazner MH, McGuire DK: Cardiomyopathy in type 2 diabetes: Update on pathophysiological mechanisms. Herz 33:184, 2008.)*

Prevention and Management of Heart Failure in Diabetes

The goals of prevention and treatment of HF in diabetic patients resemble those in nondiabetic patients: preservation of myocardial function, relief of pulmonary congestion, slowing of the progression of the disease, and prolongation of survival. In general, drug therapies for HF evaluated in the overall population of patients with risk and disease generally have similar if not better efficacy in patients with diabetes compared with those without diabetes (see Chap. 28).[98]

MODULATION OF THE RENIN-ANGIOTENSIN-ALDOSTERONE SYSTEM. Whereas diabetes patients were underrepresented in early studies of ACE inhibitors in HF cohorts, yielding little insight into specific effects in diabetes, more recent studies have enrolled increasingly higher numbers of patients with diabetes, demonstrating marked benefit of ACE inhibitors in patients with diabetes for the prevention and treatment of HF.[29a] Meta-analysis of the effect of ACE inhibitors for primary prevention of HF in high-risk cohorts of patients with diabetes demonstrates an 18% relative risk reduction (HR = 0.82; 95% CI, 0.69-0.98).[29a] Likewise, in a meta-analysis of trials comprising patients with moderate to severe systolic dysfunction, ACE inhibitors compared with placebo were associated with a significant mortality benefit among patients with diabetes (RR = 0.84; 95% CI, 0.7-1.0),[99] numerically similar to that observed among the nondiabetic group. Therefore, ACE inhibitors should be first-line therapy for the prevention and treatment of HF in patients with diabetes.[100]

Fewer data are available regarding the effect of ARBs for the prevention and treatment of HF among patients with diabetes. In the context of primary prevention of HF in patients with diabetes, in a meta-analysis of placebo-controlled trials, ARBs were associated with significant reduction for incident HF commensurate with the treatment effect observed with ACE inhibitors (HR = 0.70; 95% CI, 0.59-0.83).[29a] In the treatment of patients with prevalent HF, the data for the ARB class of medications are less consistent.[29a] On the basis of accumulated data, ARBs may be considered alternatives to ACE inhibitors for the prevention and treatment of HF,[100] with losartan having the most rigorous data for HF prevention, and both candesartan and valsartan having been proven effective in the setting of prevalent HF with decreased ejection fraction.

The effect of aldosterone antagonists (e.g., spironolactone and eplerenone) among patients with diabetes and systolic HF has not been extensively studied. In the EPHESUS randomized trial of 6632 patients with acute MI and decreased ejection fraction complicating acute MI who had either clinical HF or prevalent diabetes, eplerenone was associated with a significant 15% reduction in all-cause mortality in the overall study (HR = 0.85; 95% CI, 0.75-0.96), with similar observations in the diabetes subset of 2122 patients. On the basis of these results, eplerenone is recommended for all patients with diabetes and acute MI with decreased ejection fraction, except in the presence of contraindications such as renal insufficiency or hyperkalemia, as described before.[34]

BETA-ADRENERGIC BLOCKING AGENTS. Beta blockers and diuretic medications have been demonstrated to significantly reduce incident HF among patients with diabetes.[29a] In addition, a number of beta blockers, including metoprolol succinate, carvedilol, and bisoprolol, have demonstrated benefit in the setting of HF with systolic dysfunction (see Chap. 28), and these effects appear to be similar independent of diabetes status.[98,99] Carvedilol may offer advantages in diabetic patients because of its favorable effects on insulin sensitivity and plasma lipid profiles,[101] but the clinical relevance of these observations remains uncertain. In summary, all beta blockers proven effective in the treatment of HF appear to yield similar effects in patients with diabetes.[100]

GLUCOSE MANAGEMENT. Poor glycemic control is associated with the risk for development of HF in diabetes, with the association stronger in women than in men. Whether dysglycemia is causal or is simply associated as a marker of underlying CVD risk remains poorly understood.[12] No trials to date have rigorously assessed the effect of targeting glucose control to any specific therapeutic targets, or the comparative effect of existing therapies alone or in combination with regard to their influence on major adverse HF events. Therefore, the role of glucose control in the prevention and treatment of HF remains poorly understood, and pending further data, patients with HF should be treated to the same A1c goals as the overall population of patients with diabetes, with a target of A1c <7%.[23]

Some specific considerations warrant attention with regard to drugs and strategies used to treat hyperglycemia in the setting of HF.[46] Drugs with a propensity to precipitate hypoglycemia, especially sulfonylureas and exogenous insulin administration, should be used with some caution, as the stress response to hypoglycemia stimulates the neurohormonal axis that has been linked to clinical adversity in the setting of HF. Thiazolidinedione medications have a propensity to increase plasma volume and to precipitate incident or worsening HF, and their use is cautioned for patients with any degree of HF and contraindicated for initiation in patients with NYHA Class III or IV HF.[50] Whereas the modulators of the incretin axis that have most recently come to clinical use, including incretin mimetics and dipeptidyl peptidase 4 inhibitors, appear to have some favorable effects on a variety of intermediate markers associated with myocardial dysfunction and HF, research and clinical experience remain limited with regard to their overall safety and efficacy in cardiovascular cohorts, including those at risk for HF or with HF.[46]

Metformin has been contraindicated in the setting of HF on the basis of concern about the development of lactic acidosis resulting from observations of its predecessor phenformin, which was withdrawn from clinical use because of this risk. Extensive surveillance of metformin in widespread global use for decades and approved for use in the United States in 1995, as well as meta-analysis of existing comparative clinical trials, has yielded no signal for lactic acidosis with metformin, with estimates suggesting an incidence of no more than 1 in 300,000 patient-years of exposure.[47] Given this information, as well as a number of observational studies in populations with HF yielding no signal of lactic acidosis risk and suggesting net clinical benefit,[102,103] the boxed product label contraindicating metformin use in the setting of HF has been removed, retaining a caution for use specifically in the setting of acute or decompensated HF.[46] The best available evidence supports consideration of the use of metformin in patients with stable and compensated HF, especially in the context of the available CVD outcomes data, low risk of hypoglycemia, low cost, and tolerability profile.

Insulin therapy remains an option in patients failing conventional oral glucose-lowering therapies; some concern persists with regard to effects in patients with HF on the basis of observational analyses, in which the effect of insulin cannot be resolved from the confounding and incremental risk based on underlying disease severity of those patients treated with insulin.[104] Plausibility exists, however, whereby insulin may exacerbate signs and symptoms of HF by its effects of increasing renal sodium reclamation, contributing to increased intravascular volume.[46] Nonetheless, in HF patients failing to achieve acceptable A1c targets with oral agents, insulin remains an acceptable option.

In summary, HF is common among patients with diabetes, and in addition to usual pathologic contributors to HF in common with the overall population, numerous metabolic and pathologic abnormalities associated with diabetes may explain the increased HF risk and inform drug development efforts toward new therapeutic targets. Whereas the safety and efficacy of drugs and strategies of glucose control in patients with HF remain uncertain, the bulk of the evidence accumulated for the broader therapeutic arsenal for HF treatment in the overall population suggests that patients with diabetes derive at least as much and often more benefit from such evidence-based therapies. Therefore, in addition to ongoing research in this area, clinical efforts should focus on the optimal application of existing risk-mitigating therapies in patients with diabetes and HF.

Summary and Future Directions

Overall, diabetes increases risk for virtually all CVD complications and, most notably, atherosclerotic vascular disease and HF. Virtually all the advances in the care of patients at risk for CVD complications during the past few decades apply to patients with diabetes, with similar or even greater benefit in this high-risk population. Nonetheless, the gradient of risk associated with diabetes persists. Further progress requires continued efforts in two domains. First, increased and optimal application of the existing evidence for CVD risk reduction has paramount importance, with studies consistently demonstrating a substantial gap between the accumulated evidence and its application in patients with diabetes. Second, continued investigation into specific therapies and strategies targeting the unique risks for CVD associated with diabetes remains a critical global public health imperative. In that light, driven largely by the regulatory evolution toward requiring CVD safety and efficacy evaluations for all drugs developed for diabetes management, a proliferation of randomized CVD clinical outcomes trials is currently under way or under development, providing great promise for the future management of diabetic CVD.

Acknowledgment

The author gratefully acknowledges the contributions of Dr. Richard W. Nesto to previous versions of this chapter in earlier editions of this text.

REFERENCES

General

1. American Diabetes Association: Diagnosis and classification of diabetes mellitus. Diabetes Care 33(Suppl 1):S62, 2010.
2. Wild S, Roglic G, Green A, et al: Global prevalence of diabetes: Estimates for the year 2000 and projections for 2030. Diabetes Care 27:1047, 2004.
3. Preis SR, Hwang SJ, Coady S, et al: Trends in all-cause and cardiovascular disease mortality among women and men with and without diabetes mellitus in the Framingham Heart Study, 1950 to 2005. Circulation 119:1728, 2009.
4. Holman RR, Paul SK, Bethel MA, et al: 10-year follow-up of intensive glucose control in type 2 diabetes. N Engl J Med 359:1577, 2008.
5. Gerstein HC, Miller ME, Byington RP, et al: Effects of intensive glucose lowering in type 2 diabetes. N Engl J Med 358:2545, 2008.
6. Patel A, MacMahon S, Chalmers J, et al: Intensive blood glucose control and vascular outcomes in patients with type 2 diabetes. N Engl J Med 358:2560, 2008.
7. Fang J, Alderman MH: Impact of the increasing burden of diabetes on acute myocardial infarction in New York City: 1990-2000. Diabetes 55:768, 2006.
8. Wiviott SD, Braunwald E, Angiolillo DJ, et al: Greater clinical benefit of more intensive oral antiplatelet therapy with prasugrel in patients with diabetes mellitus in the trial to assess improvement in therapeutic outcomes by optimizing platelet inhibition with prasugrel–Thrombolysis in Myocardial Infarction 38. Circulation 118:1626, 2008.
9. Kosiborod M, Inzucchi SE, Krumholz HM, et al: Glucose normalization and outcomes in patients with acute myocardial infarction. Arch Intern Med 169:438, 2009.
10. Martini SR, Kent TA: Hyperglycemia in acute ischemic stroke: A vascular perspective. J Cereb Blood Flow Metab 27:435, 2007.
11. Canavan RJ, Unwin NC, Kelly WF, Connolly VM: Diabetes- and nondiabetes-related lower extremity amputation incidence before and after the introduction of better organized diabetes foot care: Continuous longitudinal monitoring using a standard method. Diabetes Care 31:459, 2008.
12. Aguilar D: Management of type 2 diabetes in patients with heart failure. Curr Treat Options Cardiovasc Med 10:465, 2008.
13. Aguilar D, Solomon SD, Kober L, et al: Newly diagnosed and previously known diabetes mellitus and 1-year outcomes of acute myocardial infarction: The VALsartan In Acute myocardial iNfarcTion (VALIANT) trial. Circulation 110:1572, 2004.
14. Saunders J, Mathewkutty S, Drazner MH, McGuire DK: Cardiomyopathy in type 2 diabetes: Update on pathophysiological mechanisms. Herz 33:184, 2008.

15. Orasanu G, Plutzky J: The pathologic continuum of diabetic vascular disease. J Am Coll Cardiol 53:S35, 2009.
16. Rask-Madsen C, King GL: Mechanisms of disease: Endothelial dysfunction in insulin resistance and diabetes. Nat Clin Pract Endocrinol Metab 3:46, 2007.
17. Khera A, McGuire DK: Management of diabetic dyslipidemia: Need for reappraisal of the goals. Am J Cardiovasc Drugs 5:83, 2005.
18. Mathewkutty S, McGuire DK: Platelet perturbations in diabetes: Implications for cardiovascular disease risk and treatment. Expert Rev Cardiovasc Ther 7:541, 2009.
19. Libby P, Plutzky J: Inflammation in diabetes mellitus: Role of peroxisome proliferator–activated receptor-alpha and peroxisome proliferator–activated receptor-gamma agonists. Am J Cardiol 99:27B, 2007.
20. Lindsey JB, Cipollone F, Abdullah SM, McGuire DK: Receptor for advanced glycation end-products (RAGE) and soluble RAGE (sRAGE): Cardiovascular implications. Diab Vasc Dis Res 6:7, 2009.
21. American Diabetes Association: Standards of medical care in diabetes—2010. Diabetes Care 33(Suppl 1):S11, 2010.
22. Pignone M, Alberts MJ, Colwell JA, et al: Aspirin for primary prevention of cardiovascular events in people with diabetes: A position statement of the American Diabetes Association, a scientific statement of the American Heart Association, and an expert consensus document of the American College of Cardiology Foundation. Circulation 121:2694, 2010.
23. Skyler JS, Bergenstal R, Bonow RO, et al: Intensive glycemic control and the prevention of cardiovascular events: Implications of the ACCORD, ADVANCE, and VA Diabetes Trials: A position statement of the American Diabetes Association and a Scientific Statement of the American College of Cardiology Foundation and the American Heart Association. J Am Coll Cardiol 53:298, 2009.

Risk Factor Control

24. Ray KK, Seshasai SR, Wijesuriya S, et al: Effect of intensive control of glucose on cardiovascular outcomes and death in patients with diabetes mellitus: A meta-analysis of randomised controlled trials. Lancet 373:1765, 2009.
25. Kearney PM, Blackwell L, Collins R, et al: Efficacy of cholesterol-lowering therapy in 18,686 people with diabetes in 14 randomised trials of statins: A meta-analysis. Lancet 371: 117, 2008.
26. Oikawa S, Yokoyama M, Origasa H, et al: Suppressive effect of EPA on the incidence of coronary events in hypercholesterolemia with impaired glucose metabolism: Sub-analysis of the Japan EPA Lipid Intervention Study (JELIS). Atherosclerosis 206:535, 2009.
27. Birjmohun RS, Hutten BA, Kastelein JJ, Stroes ES: Efficacy and safety of high-density lipoprotein cholesterol–increasing compounds: A meta-analysis of randomized controlled trials. J Am Coll Cardiol 45:185, 2005.
28. Keech A, Simes RJ, Barter P, et al: Effects of long-term fenofibrate therapy on cardiovascular events in 9795 people with type 2 diabetes mellitus (the FIELD study): Randomised controlled trial. Lancet 366:1849, 2005.
29. Ginsberg HN, Elam MB, Lovato LC, et al: Effects of combination lipid therapy in type 2 diabetes mellitus. N Engl J Med 362:1563, 2010.
29a. Turnbull F, Neal B, Algert C, et al: Effects of different blood pressure–lowering regimens on major cardiovascular events in individuals with and without diabetes mellitus: Results of prospectively designed overviews of randomized trials. Arch Intern Med 165: 1410, 2005.
30. McGuire DK, Winterfield JR, Rytlewski JA, Ferrannini E: Blocking the renin-angiotensin-aldosterone system to prevent diabetes mellitus. Diab Vasc Dis Res 5:59, 2008.
31. Yusuf S, Teo K, Anderson C, et al: Effects of the angiotensin-receptor blocker telmisartan on cardiovascular events in high-risk patients intolerant to angiotensin-converting enzyme inhibitors: A randomised controlled trial. Lancet 372:1174, 2008.
32. Jamerson K, Weber MA, Bakris GL, et al: Benazepril plus amlodipine or hydrochlorothiazide for hypertension in high-risk patients. N Engl J Med 359:2417, 2008.
33. Holman RR, Paul SK, Bethel MA, et al: Long-term follow-up after tight control of blood pressure in type 2 diabetes. N Engl J Med 359:1565, 2008.
34. Anderson JL, Adams CD, Antman EM, et al: ACC/AHA 2007 guidelines for the management of patients with unstable angina/non ST-elevation myocardial infarction: A report of the American College of Cardiology/American Heart Association Task Force on Practice Guidelines (Writing Committee to Revise the 2002 Guidelines for the Management of Patients With Unstable Angina/Non ST-Elevation Myocardial Infarction): developed in collaboration with the American College of Emergency Physicians, the Society for Cardiovascular Angiography and Interventions, and the Society of Thoracic Surgeons: endorsed by the American Association of Cardiovascular and Pulmonary Rehabilitation and the Society for Academic Emergency Medicine. Circulation 116:e148, 2007.
35. Barzilay JI, Davis BR, Cutler JA, et al: Fasting glucose levels and incident diabetes mellitus in older nondiabetic adults randomized to receive 3 different classes of antihypertensive treatment: A report from the Antihypertensive and Lipid-Lowering Treatment to Prevent Heart Attack Trial (ALLHAT). Arch Intern Med 166:2191, 2006.
36. Patel A, MacMahon S, Chalmers J, et al: Effects of a fixed combination of perindopril and indapamide on macrovascular and microvascular outcomes in patients with type 2 diabetes mellitus (the ADVANCE trial): A randomised controlled trial. Lancet 370:829, 2007.
37. Dahlof B, Sever PS, Poulter NR, et al: Prevention of cardiovascular events with an antihypertensive regimen of amlodipine adding perindopril as required versus atenolol adding bendroflumethiazide as required, in the Anglo-Scandinavian Cardiac Outcomes Trial–Blood Pressure Lowering Arm (ASCOT-BPLA): A multicentre randomised controlled trial. Lancet 366:895, 2005.
37a. Buse JB, Ginsberg HN, Bakris GL, et al: Primary prevention of cardiovascular diseases in people with diabetes mellitus: a scientific statement from the American Heart Association and the American Diabetes Association. Circulation 115:114, 2007.
37b. Chobanian AV, Bakris GL, Black HR, et al: The Seventh Report of the Joint National Committee on Prevention, Detection, Evaluation, and Treatment of High Blood Pressure: The JNC 7 report. JAMA 289:2560, 2003.
37c. Hansson L, Zanchetti A, Carruthers SG, et al: Effects of intensive blood-pressure lowering and low-dose aspirin in patients with hypertension: Principal results of th Hypertension Optimal Treatment (HOT) randomised trial. HOT Study Group. Lancet 351:1755, 1998.
37d. Cushman WC, Evans GW, Byington RP, et al: Effects of intensive blood-pressure control in type 2 diabetes mellitus. N Engl J Med 362:1575, 2010.
38. Baigent C, Blackwell L, Collins R, et al: Aspirin in the primary and secondary prevention of vascular disease: Collaborative meta-analysis of individual participant data from randomised trials. Lancet 373:1849, 2009.
39. De Berardis G, Sacco M, Strippoli GF, et al: Aspirin for primary prevention of cardiovascular events in people with diabetes: Meta-analysis of randomised controlled trials. BMJ 339:b4531, 2009.
40. Fateh-Moghadam S, Plockinger U, Cabeza N, et al: Prevalence of aspirin resistance in patients with type 2 diabetes. Acta Diabetol 42:99, 2005.
41. De Berardis G, Sacco M, Evangelista V, et al: Aspirin and Simvastatin Combination for Cardiovascular Events Prevention Trial in Diabetes (ACCEPT-D): Design of a randomized study of the efficacy of low-dose aspirin in the prevention of cardiovascular events in subjects with diabetes mellitus treated with statins. Trials 8:21, 2007.
42. Erlinge D, Varenhorst C, Braun OO, et al: Patients with poor responsiveness to thienopyridine treatment or with diabetes have lower levels of circulating active metabolite, but their platelets respond normally to active metabolite added ex vivo. J Am Coll Cardiol 52:1968, 2008.
43. Angiolillo DJ, Capranzano P, Desai B, et al: Impact of $P2Y_{12}$ inhibitory effects induced by clopidogrel on platelet procoagulant activity in type 2 diabetes mellitus patients. Thromb Res 124:318, 2009.

Glycemic Control

44. Gore MO, McGuire DK: Cardiovascular disease and type 2 diabetes mellitus: Regulating glucose and regulating drugs. Curr Cardiol Rep 11:258, 2009.
45. Nathan DM, Buse JB, Davidson MB, et al: Medical management of hyperglycaemia in type 2 diabetes mellitus: A consensus algorithm for the initiation and adjustment of therapy: A consensus statement from the American Diabetes Association and the European Association for the Study of Diabetes. Diabetologia 52:17, 2009.
46. Inzucchi SE, McGuire DK: New drugs for the treatment of diabetes: Part II: Incretin-based therapy and beyond. Circulation 117:574, 2008.
47. Salpeter S, Greyber E, Pasternak G, Salpeter E: Risk of fatal and nonfatal lactic acidosis with metformin use in type 2 diabetes mellitus. Cochrane Database Syst Rev (1):CD002967, 2006.
48. Stancoven A, McGuire DK: Preventing macrovascular complications in type 2 diabetes mellitus: Glucose control and beyond. Am J Cardiol 99:5H, 2007.
49. Quast U, Stephan D, Bieger S, Russ U: The impact of ATP-sensitive K^+ channel subtype selectivity of insulin secretagogues for the coronary vasculature and the myocardium. Diabetes 53(Suppl 3):S156, 2004.
50. McGuire DK, Inzucchi SE: New drugs for the treatment of diabetes mellitus: Part I: Thiazolidinediones and their evolving cardiovascular implications. Circulation 117:440, 2008.
51. Dormandy JA, Charbonnel B, Eckland DJ, et al: Secondary prevention of macrovascular events in patients with type 2 diabetes in the PROactive Study (PROspective pioglitAzone Clinical Trial In macroVascular Events): A randomised controlled trial. Lancet 366:1279, 2005.
52. Rohatgi A, McGuire DK: Effects of the thiazolidinedione medications on micro- and macrovascular complications in patients with diabetes—update 2008. Cardiovasc Drugs Ther 22:233, 2008.
53. Nathan DM, Buse JB, Davidson MB, et al: Management of hyperglycemia in type 2 diabetes: A consensus algorithm for the initiation and adjustment of therapy: Update regarding thiazolidinediones: A consensus statement from the American Diabetes Association and the European Association for the Study of Diabetes. Diabetes Care 31:173, 2008.
53a. McGuire DK, Abdullah SM, See R, et al: Randomized comparison of the effects of rosiglitazone vs. placebo on peak integrated cardiovascular performance, cardiac structure, and function. Eur Heart J 31:2262, 2010.
54. Nathan DM, Cleary PA, Backlund JY, et al: Intensive diabetes treatment and cardiovascular disease in patients with type 1 diabetes. N Engl J Med 353:2643, 2005.
55. Duckworth W, Abraira C, Moritz T, et al: Glucose control and vascular complications in veterans with type 2 diabetes. N Engl J Med 360:129, 2009.
56. Frye RL, August P, Brooks MM, et al: A randomized trial of therapies for type 2 diabetes and coronary artery disease. N Engl J Med 360:2503, 2009.

Acute Coronary Syndromes and Cardiac Surgery

57. Gnaim CI, McGuire DK: Glucose-insulin-potassium therapy for acute myocardial infarction: What goes around comes around. Am Heart J 148:924, 2004.
58. Dandona P, Aljada A, Chaudhuri A, et al: Metabolic syndrome: A comprehensive perspective based on interactions between obesity, diabetes, and inflammation. Circulation 111:1448, 2005.
59. Mehta SR, Yusuf S, Diaz R, et al: Effect of glucose-insulin-potassium infusion on mortality in patients with acute ST-segment elevation myocardial infarction: The CREATE-ECLA randomized controlled trial. JAMA 293:437, 2005.
60. Malmberg K: Prospective randomised study of intensive insulin treatment on long term survival after acute myocardial infarction in patients with diabetes mellitus. DIGAMI (Diabetes Mellitus, Insulin Glucose Infusion in Acute Myocardial Infarction) Study Group. BMJ 314:1512, 1997.
61. Antman EM, Anbe DT, Armstrong PW, et al: ACC/AHA guidelines for the management of patients with ST-elevation myocardial infarction: A report of the American College of Cardiology/American Heart Association Task Force on Practice Guidelines (Committee to Revise the 1999 Guidelines for the Management of Patients with Acute Myocardial Infarction). Circulation 110:e82, 2004.
62. Van den Berghe G, Wilmer A, Hermans G, et al: Intensive insulin therapy in the medical ICU. N Engl J Med 354:449, 2006.
63. Brunkhorst FM, Engel C, Bloos F, et al: Intensive insulin therapy and pentastarch resuscitation in severe sepsis. N Engl J Med 358:125, 2008.
64. Gray CS, Hildreth AJ, Sandercock PA, et al: Glucose-potassium-insulin infusions in the management of post-stroke hyperglycaemia: The UK Glucose Insulin in Stroke Trial (GIST-UK). Lancet Neurol 6:397, 2007.

65. Preiser JC, Devos P, Ruiz-Santana S, et al: A prospective randomised multi-centre controlled trial on tight glucose control by intensive insulin therapy in adult intensive care units: The Glucontrol study. Intensive Care Med 35:1738, 2009.
66. Finfer S, Chittock DR, Su SY, et al: Intensive versus conventional glucose control in critically ill patients. N Engl J Med 360:1283, 2009.
67. Deedwania P, Kosiborod M, Barrett E, et al: Hyperglycemia and acute coronary syndrome: A scientific statement from the American Heart Association Diabetes Committee of the Council on Nutrition, Physical Activity, and Metabolism. Circulation 117:1610, 2008.
68. Kushner FG, Hand M, Smith SC Jr, et al: 2009 Focused Updates: ACC/AHA Guidelines for the Management of Patients With ST-Elevation Myocardial Infarction (Updating the 2004 Guideline and 2007 Focused Update) and ACC/AHA/SCAI Guidelines on Percutaneous Coronary Intervention (Updating the 2005 Guideline and 2007 Focused Update). A Report of the American College of Cardiology Foundation/American Heart Association Task Force on Practice Guidelines. Circulation 120:2271, 2009.
69. Svensson AM, McGuire DK, Abrahamsson P, Dellborg M: Association between hyper- and hypoglycaemia and 2 year all-cause mortality risk in diabetic patients with acute coronary events. Eur Heart J 26:1255, 2005.
70. Pinto DS, Skolnick AH, Kirtane AJ, et al: U-shaped relationship of blood glucose with adverse outcomes among patients with ST-segment elevation myocardial infarction. J Am Coll Cardiol 46:178, 2005.
71. Kosiborod M, Inzucchi SE, Goyal A, et al: Relationship between spontaneous and iatrogenic hypoglycemia and mortality in patients hospitalized with acute myocardial infarction. JAMA 301:1556, 2009.
72. Wiviott SD, Braunwald E, McCabe CH, et al: Prasugrel versus clopidogrel in patients with acute coronary syndromes. N Engl J Med 357:2001, 2007.
73. Dickstein K, Kjekshus J: Effects of losartan and captopril on mortality and morbidity in high-risk patients after acute myocardial infarction: The OPTIMAAL randomised trial. Optimal Trial in Myocardial Infarction with Angiotensin II Antagonist Losartan. Lancet 360:752, 2002.
74. Pfeffer MA, McMurray JJ, Velazquez EJ, et al: Valsartan, captopril, or both in myocardial infarction complicated by heart failure, left ventricular dysfunction, or both. N Engl J Med 349:1893, 2003.
75. Brandimarte F, Blair JE, Manuchehry A, et al: Aldosterone receptor blockade in patients with left ventricular systolic dysfunction following acute myocardial infarction. Cardiol Clin 26:91, vii, 2008.
76. Pitt B, Remme W, Zannad F, et al: Eplerenone, a selective aldosterone blocker, in patients with left ventricular dysfunction after myocardial infarction. N Engl J Med 348:1309, 2003.
77. Brogan GX Jr, Peterson ED, Mulgund J, et al: Treatment disparities in the care of patients with and without diabetes presenting with non–ST-segment elevation acute coronary syndromes. Diabetes Care 29:9, 2006.
78. McDonald CG, Majumdar SR, Mahon JL, Johnson JA: The effectiveness of beta-blockers after myocardial infarction in patients with type 2 diabetes. Diabetes Care 28:2113, 2005.
79. Collet JP, Montalescot G: The acute reperfusion management of STEMI in patients with impaired glucose tolerance and type 2 diabetes. Diab Vasc Dis Res 2:136, 2005.
80. Timmer JR, Ottervanger JP, de Boer MJ, et al: Primary percutaneous coronary intervention compared with fibrinolysis for myocardial infarction in diabetes mellitus: Results from the Primary Coronary Angioplasty vs Thrombolysis-2 trial. Arch Intern Med 167:1353, 2007.
81. Flaherty JD, Davidson CJ: Diabetes and coronary revascularization. JAMA 293:1501, 2005.
82. Garg P, Normand SL, Silbaugh TS, et al: Drug-eluting or bare-metal stenting in patients with diabetes mellitus: Results from the Massachusetts Data Analysis Center Registry. Circulation 118:2277, 2008.
83. Smith SC Jr, Feldman TE, Hirshfeld JW Jr, et al: ACC/AHA/SCAI 2005 guideline update for percutaneous coronary intervention: A report of the American College of Cardiology/American Heart Association Task Force on Practice Guidelines (ACC/AHA/SCAI Writing Committee to Update 2001 Guidelines for Percutaneous Coronary Intervention). Circulation 113:e166, 2006.
84. Furnary AP, Wu Y: Clinical effects of hyperglycemia in the cardiac surgery population: The Portland Diabetic Project. Endocr Pract 12(Suppl 3):22, 2006.
85. Van den Berghe G: Does intensive insulin therapy during cardiac surgery improve postoperative outcome? Nat Clin Pract Endocrinol Metab 3:630, 2007.
86. Lazar HL, McDonnell M, Chipkin SR, et al: The Society of Thoracic Surgeons practice guideline series: Blood glucose management during adult cardiac surgery. Ann Thorac Surg 87:663, 2009.
87. Hlatky MA, Boothroyd DB, Bravata DM, et al: Coronary artery bypass surgery compared with percutaneous coronary interventions for multivessel disease: A collaborative analysis of individual patient data from ten randomised trials. Lancet 373:1190, 2009.

Heart Failure

88. Das SR, Vaeth PA, Stanek HG, et al: Increased cardiovascular risk associated with diabetes in Dallas County. Am Heart J 151:1087, 2006.
89. Saydah SH, Fradkin J, Cowie CC: Poor control of risk factors for vascular disease among adults with previously diagnosed diabetes. JAMA 291:335, 2004.
90. Schnell O, Schafer O, Kleybrink S, et al: Intensification of therapeutic approaches reduces mortality in diabetic patients with acute myocardial infarction: The Munich registry. Diabetes Care 27:455, 2004.
91. Gaede P, Lund-Andersen H, Parving HH, Pedersen O: Effect of a multifactorial intervention on mortality in type 2 diabetes. N Engl J Med 358:580, 2008.
92. Pocock SJ, Wang D, Pfeffer MA, et al: Predictors of mortality and morbidity in patients with chronic heart failure. Eur Heart J 27:65, 2006.
93. Prior JO, Quinones MJ, Hernandez-Pampaloni M, et al: Coronary circulatory dysfunction in insulin resistance, impaired glucose tolerance, and type 2 diabetes mellitus. Circulation 111:2291, 2005.
94. Adler AI, Stratton IM, Neil HA, et al: Association of systolic blood pressure with macrovascular and microvascular complications of type 2 diabetes (UKPDS 36): Prospective observational study. BMJ 321:412, 2000.
95. Saunders SA, Wallymhamed M, Macfarlane IA: Improvements in glycaemic control and cardiovascular risk factors in a cohort of patients with type 1 diabetes over a 5-year period. QJM 102:29, 2009.
96. McGavock JM, Victor RG, Unger RH, Szczepaniak LS: Adiposity of the heart, revisited. Ann Intern Med 144:517, 2006.
97. Zieman S, Kass D: Advanced glycation end product cross-linking: Pathophysiologic role and therapeutic target in cardiovascular disease. Congest Heart Fail 10:144, 2004.
98. Masoudi FA, Inzucchi SE: Diabetes mellitus and heart failure: Epidemiology, mechanisms, and pharmacotherapy. Am J Cardiol 99:113B, 2007.
99. Shekelle PG, Rich MW, Morton SC, et al: Efficacy of angiotensin-converting enzyme inhibitors and beta-blockers in the management of left ventricular systolic dysfunction according to race, gender, and diabetic status: A meta-analysis of major clinical trials. J Am Coll Cardiol 41:1529, 2003.
100. Hunt SA, Abraham WT, Chin MH, et al: 2009 focused update incorporated into the ACC/AHA 2005 Guidelines for the Diagnosis and Management of Heart Failure in Adults: A report of the American College of Cardiology Foundation/American Heart Association Task Force on Practice Guidelines: Developed in collaboration with the International Society for Heart and Lung Transplantation. Circulation 119:e391, 2009.
101. Bakris GL, Fonseca V, Katholi RE, et al: Metabolic effects of carvedilol vs metoprolol in patients with type 2 diabetes mellitus and hypertension: A randomized controlled trial. JAMA 292:2227, 2004.
102. Masoudi FA, Inzucchi SE, Wang Y, et al: Thiazolidinediones, metformin, and outcomes in older patients with diabetes and heart failure: An observational study. Circulation 111:583, 2005.
103. Eurich DT, Majumdar SR, McAlister FA, et al: Improved clinical outcomes associated with metformin in patients with diabetes and heart failure. Diabetes Care 28:2345, 2005.
104. Smooke S, Horwich TB, Fonarow GC: Insulin-treated diabetes is associated with a marked increase in mortality in patients with advanced heart failure. Am Heart J 149:168, 2005.
105. UK Prospective Diabetes Study (UKPDS) Group: Effect of intensive blood-glucose control with metformin on complications in overweight patients with type 2 diabetes (UKPDS 34). Lancet 352:854, 1998.
106. Chiasson JL, Josse RG, Gomis R, et al: Acarbose treatment and the risk of cardiovascular disease and hypertension in patients with impaired glucose tolerance: The STOP-NIDDM trial. JAMA 290:486, 2003.
107. Nesto RW, Bell D, Bonow RO, et al: Thiazolidinedione use, fluid retention, and congestive heart failure: A consensus statement from the American Heart Association and American Diabetes Association. Circulation 108:2941, 2003.
108. Nissen SE, Wolski K: Effect of rosiglitazone on the risk of myocardial infarction and death from cardiovascular causes. N Engl J Med 356:2457, 2007.
109. Nikolaidis LA, Mankad S, Sokos GG, et al: Effects of glucagon-like peptide-1 in patients with acute myocardial infarction and left ventricular dysfunction after successful reperfusion. Circulation 109:962, 2004.
110. Diaz R, Paolasso EA, Piegas LS, et al: Metabolic modulation of acute myocardial infarction. The ECLA (Cardiológicos Latinoamérica) Collaborative Group. Circulation 98:2227, 1998.
111. van der Horst IC, Zijlstra F, van't Hof AW, et al: Glucose-insulin-potassium infusion in patients treated with primary angioplasty for acute myocardial infarction: The glucose-insulin-potassium study: A randomized trial. J Am Coll Cardiol 42:784, 2003.
112. Cheung NW, Wong VW, McLean M: The Hyperglycemia: Intensive Insulin Infusion in Infarction (HI-5) study: A randomized controlled trial of insulin infusion therapy for myocardial infarction. Diabetes Care 29:765, 2006.
113. Ceremuzynski L, Budaj A, Czepiel A, et al: Low-dose glucose-insulin-potassium is ineffective in acute myocardial infarction: Results of a randomized multicenter Pol-GIK trial. Cardiovasc Drugs Ther 13:191, 1999.
114. van den Berghe G, Wouters P, Weekers F, et al: Intensive insulin therapy in the critically ill patients. N Engl J Med 345:1359, 2001.

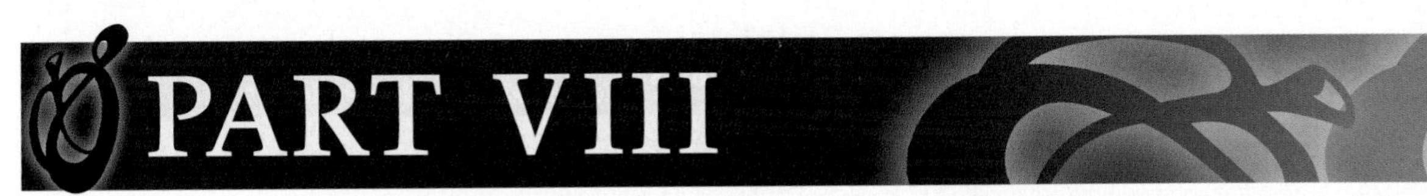

DISEASES OF THE HEART, PERICARDIUM, AND PULMONARY VASCULATURE BED

CHAPTER 65 Congenital Heart Disease

Gary D. Webb, Jeffrey F. Smallhorn, Judith Therrien, and Andrew N. Redington

This chapter has been written for the practicing cardiologist and is compatible with the existing expert management recommendations[1] for the care of adult patients with congenital cardiac defects. Additional information can be found in other sources.[2] *Congenital cardiovascular disease* is defined as an abnormality in cardiocirculatory structure or function that is present at birth, even if it is discovered much later. Congenital cardiovascular malformations usually result from altered embryonic development of a normal structure or failure of such a structure to progress beyond an early stage of embryonic or fetal development. The aberrant patterns of flow created by an anatomic defect can, in turn, significantly influence the structural and functional development of the remainder of the circulation. For instance, the presence in utero of mitral atresia can prohibit normal development of the left ventricle, aortic valve, and ascending aorta. Similarly, constriction of the fetal ductus arteriosus can result in right ventricular dilation and tricuspid regurgitation in the fetus and newborn, contribute importantly to the development of pulmonary arterial aneurysms in the presence of a ventricular septal defect (VSD) and absent pulmonary valve, or result in an alteration in the number and caliber of fetal and newborn pulmonary vascular resistance vessels.

Postnatal events can markedly influence the clinical presentation of a specific "isolated" malformation. Infants with Ebstein malformation of the tricuspid valve may improve dramatically as the magnitude of tricuspid regurgitation diminishes with the normal fall in pulmonary vascular resistance after birth; and infants with pulmonary atresia or severe stenosis may not become cyanotic until normal spontaneous closure of a patent ductus arteriosus (PDA) occurs. Ductal constriction many days after birth also may be a central factor in some infants in the development of coarctation of the aorta. Still later in life, patients with a VSD may experience spontaneous closure of the abnormal communication or can develop right ventricular outflow tract obstruction, aortic regurgitation, or pulmonary vascular obstructive disease. These selected examples serve to emphasize that anatomic and physiologic changes in the heart and circulation can continue indefinitely from prenatal life in association with any specific congenital cardiocirculatory lesion.

Incidence. The true incidence of congenital cardiovascular malformations is difficult to determine accurately, partly because of difficulties in definition. About 0.8% of live births are complicated by a cardiovascular malformation. This figure does not take into account what may be the two most common cardiac anomalies: the congenital, functionally normal bicuspid aortic valve and prolapse of the mitral valve.

Specific defects can show a definite gender preponderance. PDA, Ebstein anomaly of the tricuspid valve, and atrial septal defect (ASD) are more common in females, whereas aortic valve stenosis, coarctation of the aorta, hypoplastic left heart syndrome, pulmonary and tricuspid atresia, and transposition of the great arteries (TGA) are more common in males.

Extracardiac anomalies occur in about 25% of infants with significant cardiac disease, and their presence may significantly increase mortality. The extracardiac anomalies are often multiple. One third of infants with both cardiac and extracardiac anomalies have some established syndrome.

Adult Patient. Thanks to the great successes of pediatric cardiac care, the overall number of adult patients with congenital heart disease (CHD) is now greater than the number of pediatric cases. In 2000, there were about 485,000 American adults with moderately complex to very complex CHD. There were another 300,000 patients with simple forms of CHD, for a total population of 785,000 adult CHD patients in the United States. The 485,000 patients with moderately to very complex CHD are at significant risk of premature mortality, reoperation, or future complications of their conditions and their treatments. Many patients, especially those with moderately to very complex conditions, should see a specialist. At present, there are not enough such practitioners or facilities to always make this possible. Adult patients should have been taught in adolescence about their condition, their future outlook, and the

CH 65

TABLE 65-1 Types of Simple Congenital Heart Disease in Adult Patients*

Native Disease
Isolated congenital aortic valve disease
Isolated congenital mitral valve disease (except parachute valve, cleft leaflet)
Isolated patent foramen ovale or small atrial septal defect
Isolated small ventricular septal defect (no associated lesions)
Mild pulmonic stenosis

Repaired Conditions
Previously ligated or occluded ductus arteriosus
Repaired secundum or sinus venosus atrial septal defect without residua
Repaired ventricular septal defect without residua

*These patients can usually be cared for in the general medical community.
From Webb G, Williams R, Alpert J, et al: 32nd Bethesda Conference: Care of the Adult with Congenital Heart Disease, October 2-3, 2000. J Am Coll Cardiol 37:1161, 2001.

TABLE 65-2 Types of Congenital Heart Disease of Moderate Severity in Adult Patients*

Aorto–left ventricular fistulas
Anomalous pulmonary venous drainage, partial or total
Atrioventricular septal defects (partial or complete)
Coarctation of the aorta
Ebstein anomaly
Infundibular right ventricular outflow obstruction of significance
Ostium primum atrial septal defect
Patent ductus arteriosus (not closed)
Pulmonary valve regurgitation (moderate to severe)
Pulmonic valve stenosis (moderate to severe)
Sinus of Valsalva fistula or aneurysm
Sinus venosus atrial septal defect
Subvalvular or supravalvular aortic stenosis (except HOCM)
Tetralogy of Fallot
Ventricular septal defect with the following:
- Absent valve or valves
- Aortic regurgitation
- Coarctation of the aorta
- Mitral disease
- Right ventricular outflow tract obstruction
- Straddling tricuspid or mitral valve
- Subaortic stenosis

*These patients should be seen periodically at regional adult congenital heart disease centers.
HOCM = hypertrophic obstructive cardiomyopathy.
From Webb G, Williams R, Alpert J, et al: 32nd Bethesda Conference: Care of the Adult with Congenital Heart Disease, October 2-3, 2000. J Am Coll Cardiol 37:1161, 2001.

possibility of further surgery and complications if appropriate, and they also should have been advised about their responsibilities in ensuring self-care and professional surveillance. Copies of operative reports should accompany patients being transferred for adult care, along with other key documents from the pediatric file.

Table 65-1 lists the types of simple CHD in adult patients which are suitable for community care. **Tables 65-2 and 65-3** show the diagnoses for adults with moderately complex and very complex CHD. Patients with moderately complex and very complex CHD should be monitored throughout their lives.

CHD in the adult is not simply a continuation of the childhood experience. The patterns of many lesions change in adult life. Arrhythmias are more frequent and of a different character (see Chap. 39). Cardiac chambers often enlarge, and ventricles tend to develop systolic dysfunction. Bioprosthetic valves, prone to early failure in childhood, last longer when they are implanted at an older age. The comorbidities that tend to develop in adult life often become important factors needing attention. As a result, the needs of these adult CHD patients are often best met by a physician or a team familiar with both pediatric and adult cardiology issues. Congenital heart surgery and interventional catheterization procedures should be performed at centers with adequate surgical and institutional volumes of congenital heart cases at any age.

Echocardiographic studies, diagnostic heart catheterizations, electrophysiologic studies, and cardiac magnetic resonance (CMR) and other imaging of complex cases (see Chaps. 15 to 20) are best done where

TABLE 65-3 Types of Congenital Heart Disease of Great Complexity in Adult Patients*

Conduits, valved or nonvalved
Cyanotic congenital heart (all forms)
Double-outlet ventricle
Eisenmenger syndrome
Fontan procedure
Mitral atresia
Single ventricle (also called double inlet or outlet, common or primitive)
Pulmonary atresia (all forms)
Pulmonary vascular obstructive diseases
Transposition of the great arteries
Tricuspid atresia
Truncus arteriosus or hemitruncus
Other abnormalities of atrioventricular or ventriculoarterial connection not included above (i.e., crisscross heart, isomerism, heterotaxy syndromes, ventricular inversion)

*These patients should be seen regularly at adult congenital heart disease centers.
From Webb G, Williams R, Alpert J, et al: 32nd Bethesda Conference: Care of the Adult with Congenital Heart Disease, October 2-3, 2000. J Am Coll Cardiol 37:1161, 2001.

qualified staff has relevant training, experience, and equipment. Ideally, patient care should be multidisciplinary. Special cardiology and echocardiography skills are essential, but individuals with other special training, experience, and interest should also be accessible. These include congenital heart surgeons and their teams, nurses, reproductive health staff, mental health professionals, medical imaging specialists, respiratory consultants, and others.

ETIOLOGY

Congenital cardiac malformations can occur with mendelian inheritance directly as a result of a genetic abnormality, be strongly associated with an underlying genetic disorder (e.g., trisomy), be related directly to the effect of an environmental toxin (e.g., alcohol), or result from an interaction between multifactorial genetic and environmental influences too complex to allow a single definition of cause (e.g., CHARGE syndrome; see Syndromes in Congenital Heart Disease later). The last group is shrinking as genetic research identifies new genetic abnormalities underlying many conditions.

Genetic. A single gene mutation can be causative in the familial forms of ASD with prolonged atrioventricular (AV) conduction; mitral valve prolapse; VSD; congenital heart block; situs inversus; pulmonary hypertension; and the syndromes of Noonan, LEOPARD, Ellis–van Creveld, and Kartagener (see Syndromes in Congenital Heart Disease later). The genes responsible for several defects have now been identified (e.g., long-QT syndrome, Holt-Oram syndrome, Marfan syndrome, hypertrophic cardiomyopathy, supravalvular aortic stenosis), and contiguous gene defects on the long arm of chromosome 22 underlie the conotruncal malformations of DiGeorge and velocardiofacial syndromes. However, at present, less than 15% of all cardiac malformations can be accounted for by chromosomal aberrations or genetic mutations or transmission (see Chaps. 7 to 9).

It is interesting, but unexplained, that several different gene defects may lead to the same cardiac malformation (e.g., atrioventricular septal defect). Furthermore, the finding that, with some exceptions, only one of a pair of monozygotic twins is affected by CHD indicates that most cardiovascular malformations are not inherited in a simple manner. However, this observation may have led, in the past, to an underestimation of the genetic contribution because most recent twin studies reveal more than double the incidence of heart defects in monozygotic twins but usually in only one of the pair. Family studies indicate a 2-fold to 10-fold increase in the incidence of CHD in siblings of affected patients or in the offspring of an affected parent. Malformations are often concordant or partially concordant within families. Routine fetal cardiac screening of subsequent pregnancies should be performed in such circumstances.

Environmental. Maternal rubella, ingestion of thalidomide and isotretinoin early during gestation, and chronic maternal alcohol abuse are environmental insults known to interfere with normal cardiogenesis in humans. Rubella syndrome consists of cataracts; deafness; microcephaly; and, either singly or in combination, PDA, pulmonary valve or arterial stenosis, and ASD. Thalidomide exposure is associated with major limb deformities and, occasionally, with cardiac malformations without a predilection for a specific lesion. Tricuspid valve anomalies are associated with ingestion of lithium during pregnancy. The fetal alcohol syndrome consists of microcephaly, micrognathia, microphthalmia, prenatal growth retardation, developmental delay, and cardiac defects (often defects of the ventricular septum) in about 45% of affected infants.

PREVENTION

Physicians who treat pregnant women (see Chap. 82) should be aware of the effects of known teratogens as well as drugs (e.g., angiotensin-converting enzyme [ACE] inhibition and fetal renal development) that may have a functional rather than a structural damaging influence on the fetal and newborn heart and circulation. They should also recognize that for many drugs, information about their teratogenic potential is inadequate. Similarly, appropriate radiologic equipment and techniques for reducing gonadal and fetal radiation exposure should always be used to reduce the hazards of this potential cause of birth defects.

Detection of genetic abnormalities during fetal life is becoming an increasing reality. Fetal cells are obtained from amniotic fluid or chorionic villus biopsy. Many fetuses in whom CHD is detected will undergo genetic testing, and fetal echocardiography is frequently indicated when a chromosomal abnormality is diagnosed for other reasons. Many social, religious, and legal considerations influence whether termination of pregnancy is performed under these circumstances, but the improved outcomes for even the most complex CHDs frequently argue against the cardiac condition being used as the sole reason. Immunization of children with rubella vaccine has been one of the most effective preventive strategies against fetal rubella syndrome and its associated congenital cardiac abnormalities.

ANATOMY AND EMBRYOLOGY

Embryology

Normal Cardiac Development. During the first month of gestation, the primitive, straight cardiac tube is formed, comprising the sinuatrium (most cephalad), the primitive ventricle, the bulbus cordis, and the truncus arteriosus (most caudad) in series. In the second month of gestation, there is rightward looping of the heart tube. By the end of the fifth week, parts of the ventricles are visible and the left ventricle supports most of the circumference of the AV canal. The superior and inferior cushions fuse by the sixth week into the left and right AV junctions. Migration of the AV canal to the right and of the ventricular septum to the left serves to align each ventricle with its appropriate AV valve. At the distal end of the cardiac tube, the bulbus cordis divides into a subaortic muscular conus and a subpulmonary muscular conus; the subpulmonary conus elongates and the subaortic conus resorbs, allowing the aorta to move posteriorly and to connect with the left ventricle.

Abnormal Development. A host of anomalies can result from defects in this basic developmental pattern. Double-inlet left ventricle is observed if the tricuspid orifice does not align over the right ventricle. The various types of persistent truncus arteriosus result from failure of the truncus to divide into main pulmonary artery and aorta. Double-outlet anomalies of the right ventricle are produced by failure of either the subpulmonary or subaortic conus to resorb, whereas resorption of the subpulmonary instead of the subaortic conus may lead to TGA.

Atria. The primitive sinuatrium is separated into right and left atria by the downgrowth from its roof of the septum primum toward the AV canal, fusing with the cushions. Numerous perforations form in the anterosuperior portion of the septum primum. After this, there is a superior infolding of the roof of the atria, which has traditionally been called the septum secundum. The remnant of the septum primum forms the fossa ovalis.

Fusion of the endocardial cushions anteriorly and posteriorly divides the AV canal into tricuspid and mitral inlets. The inferior portion of the atrial septum, the superior portion of the ventricular septum, and portions of the septal leaflet of the tricuspid and aortic leaflet of the mitral valve are formed from the endocardial cushions. The posterior or mural leaflet of the mitral valve is mainly formed from a sheet of AV myocardium that protrudes into the lumen of the ventricle, rather than by delamination, as was previously thought. The integrity of the atrial septum depends on growth of the septum primum and the superior infolding and proper fusion of the endocardial cushions. ASDs and various degrees of AV defect are the result of developmental deficiencies of this process.

Ventricles. Partitioning of the ventricles occurs as cephalic growth of the main ventricular septum results in its fusion with the endocardial cushions and the infundibular or conus septum. Defects in the ventricular septum may occur because of a deficiency of septal substance; malalignment of septal components in different planes, preventing their fusion; or an overly long conus, keeping the septal components apart. Isolated defects probably result from the first mechanism, whereas the last two appear to generate the VSDs in tetralogy of Fallot and transposition complexes.

Pulmonary Veins. These structures arise from the primitive foregut and are drained early in embryogenesis by channels from the splanchnic plexus to the cardinal and umbilicovitteline veins. When the pulmonary vein is first recognized as a channel entering the heart, it is a solitary structure, entering the atrial component close to the AV junction. After closure of the interventricular communication, the pulmonary veins migrate to the roof of the left atrium. This communicates with the splanchnic plexus, establishing pulmonary venous drainage to the left atrium. The umbilicovitteline and anterior cardinal vein communications atrophy as the common pulmonary vein is incorporated into the left atrium. Anomalous pulmonary venous connections to the umbilicovitteline (portal) venous system or to the cardinal system (superior vena cava) result from failure of the common pulmonary vein to develop or to establish communications to the splanchnic plexus.

Great Arteries. The truncus arteriosus is connected to the dorsal aorta in the embryo by six pairs of aortic arches. Partition of the truncus arteriosus into two great arteries is a result of the fusion of tissue arising from the back wall of the vessel and the truncus septum. Rotation of the truncus coils the aortopulmonary septum and creates the normal spiral relation between aorta and pulmonary artery. Semilunar valves and their related sinuses are created by absorption and hollowing out of tissue at the distal side of the truncus ridges. Aortopulmonary septal defect and persistent truncus arteriosus represent various degrees of partitioning failure.

Although the six aortic arches appear sequentially, portions of the arch system and dorsal aorta disappear at different times during embryogenesis. The first, second, and fifth sets of paired arches regress completely. The proximal portions of the sixth arches become the right and left pulmonary arteries, and the distal left sixth arch becomes the ductus arteriosus. The third aortic arch forms the connection between internal and external carotid arteries, and the left fourth arch becomes the arterial segment between left carotid and subclavian arteries. The proximal portion of the right subclavian artery forms from the right fourth arch. An abnormality in regression of the arch system in a number of sites can produce a wide variety of arch anomalies, whereas a failure of regression usually results in a double aortic arch malformation.

Normal Cardiac Anatomy

The key to understanding CHD is an appreciation of the segmental approach to the diagnosis of both simple and complex lesions.

CARDIAC SITUS. This refers to the status of the atrial appendages. The normal left atrial appendage is a finger-like structure with a narrow base and no guarding crista. On the other hand, the right atrial appendage is broad based and has a guarding crista and pectinate muscles. *Situs solitus* or *inversus* refers to hearts with both a morphologic left and right atrium. *Situs ambiguus* refers to hearts with two morphologic left or right atrial appendages. These are dealt with in the section on isomerism and have implications with regard to associated intracardiac and extracardiac abnormalities.

ATRIOVENTRICULAR CONNECTIONS. This refers to the connections between the atria and ventricles. The AV connections are said to be concordant if the morphologic left atrium is connected to a morphologic left ventricle via the mitral valve, with the morphologic right atrium connecting to the morphologic right ventricle via a tricuspid valve. They are said to be discordant in other circumstances, such as in congenitally corrected TGA (cc-TGA).

VENTRICULOARTERIAL CONNECTIONS. This refers to the connections between the semilunar valve and the ventricles. Ventriculoarterial concordance occurs when the morphologic left ventricle is connected to the aorta and the morphologic right ventricle is connected to the pulmonary artery. Ventriculoarterial discordance occurs when the morphologic left ventricle is connected to the pulmonary artery, with the aorta being connected to the morphologic right ventricle. Double-outlet right ventricle occurs when more than 50% of both great arteries is connected to the morphologic right ventricle. A single-outlet heart has only one great artery connected to the heart.

ATRIA. The assignment of either a morphologic left or right atrium is determined by the morphology of the atrial appendages and not by the status of the systemic or pulmonary venous drainage. The right atrial appendage is broad and triangular; the left is smaller and fingerlike. The internal architecture is the key feature to an accurate diagnosis, with the right having extensive pectinate muscles, unlike its left counterpart. Although the pulmonary veins usually drain to a morphologic left atrium and the systemic veins drain into a morphologic right atrium, this is not always the case.

ATRIOVENTRICULAR VALVES. The morphologic mitral valve is a bileaflet valve with the anterior or aortic leaflet in fibrous continuity with the noncoronary cusp of the aortic valve. The mitral valve leaflets are supported by two papillary muscle groups located in the anterolateral and posteromedial positions. Each papillary muscle supports the adjacent part of both valve leaflets, with considerable variation in the morphology of the papillary muscles.

The tricuspid valve is a trileaflet valve, although it can frequently be difficult to identify all three leaflets because of variability in the anteroposterior commissure. With close inspection, the commissural chordae that arise from the papillary muscles may permit the identification of the three leaflets. The three leaflets occupy a septal anterior, superior, and inferior position. The commissures between the leaflets are the anterior septal, anterior inferior, and inferior. The papillary muscles supporting the valve leaflets arise mostly from the trabecula septomarginalis and its apical ramifications.

MORPHOLOGIC RIGHT VENTRICLE. The morphologic right ventricle is a triangular structure with an inlet, trabecular, and outlet component. The inlet component of the right ventricle has attachments from the septal leaflet of the tricuspid valve. Inferior to this is the moderator band, which arises at the base of the trabecula septomarginalis, with extensive trabeculations toward the apex of the right ventricle. The outlet component of the right ventricle consists of a fusion of three structures (i.e., the infundibular septum separating the aortic from the pulmonary valve, the ventriculoinfundibular fold separating the tricuspid valve from the pulmonary valve, and finally the anterior and posterior limbs of the trabecula septomarginalis).

MORPHOLOGIC LEFT VENTRICLE. The morphologic left ventricle is an elliptical structure with a fine trabecular pattern, with absent septal attachments of the mitral valve in the normal heart. It consists of an inlet portion containing the mitral valve and a tension apparatus, with an apical trabecular zone that is characterized by fine trabeculations and an outlet zone that supports the aortic valve.

SEMILUNAR VALVES. The aortic valve is a trileaflet valve with the left and right cusps giving rise to the left and right coronary arteries, respectively; the noncoronary cusp lacks a coronary artery connection. Of note, the noncoronary cusp is in fibrous continuity with the anterior leaflet of the mitral valve. The aortic valve has a semilunar attachment to the junction of the ventricular outlet and its great arteries. The aortic cusps have a main core of fibrous tissue with endocardial linings on each surface. The cusps are thickened at the midpoint to form a nodule. The characteristics of the pulmonary valve are similar to those of its aortic counterpart, noting the absence of the coronary ostia arising at the superior portion of the sinuses.

AORTIC ARCH AND PULMONARY ARTERIES. In the normal heart, the aortic arch usually points to the left, with the first branch, the innominate artery, giving rise to the right carotid and subclavian arteries. In general, the left carotid and left subclavian arteries arise separately from the aortic arch. By definition, the ascending aorta is proximal to the origin of the innominate artery, with the transverse aortic arch being from the innominate artery to the origin of the left subclavian artery. The aortic isthmus is the area between the left subclavian artery and a PDA or ligamentum arteriosum.

SYSTEMIC VENOUS CONNECTIONS. In the normal heart, the left and right innominate veins form the superior caval vein, which connects to the roof of the right atrium. The inferior caval vein connects to the inferior portion of the morphologic right atrium, with hepatic veins joining the inferior caval vein before its insertion into the atrium. The coronary veins drain into the flow of the coronary sinus, with the latter running in the posterior AV groove and terminating in the right atrium. The inferior caval vein is guarded by the eustachian valve, which may vary in size among hearts.

PULMONARY VENOUS DRAINAGE IN THE NORMAL HEART. The pulmonary veins drain to the left-sided atrium. Usually three pulmonary veins arise from the trilobed right lung and two pulmonary veins from the bilobed left lung. The pulmonary veins drain into the left atrium in superior and inferior locations. There is a short segment of extraparenchymal pulmonary vein before it disappears into the adjacent hila of the lungs.

Fetal and Transitional Circulations (Fig. 65-1)

CHD is being diagnosed with increasing frequency during fetal life. Our ability to modify the evolution of structural (by fetal intervention) and physiologic (by drug therapy) heart disease is increasing. Knowledge of the changes in cardiovascular structure, function, and metabolism that occur during fetal development is perhaps more important today than at any time in the past.

FETAL CIRCULATORY PATHWAYS. Dynamic alterations occur in the circulation during the transition from fetal to neonatal life when the lungs take over the function of gas exchange from the placenta. The fetal circulation consists of parallel pulmonary and systemic pathways in contrast to the "in-series" circuit of the normal postnatal circulation. Oxygenated blood returns from the placenta through the umbilical vein and enters the portal venous system. A variable amount of this stream bypasses the hepatic microcirculation and enters the inferior vena cava by way of the ductus venosus. Inferior vena caval blood is from the

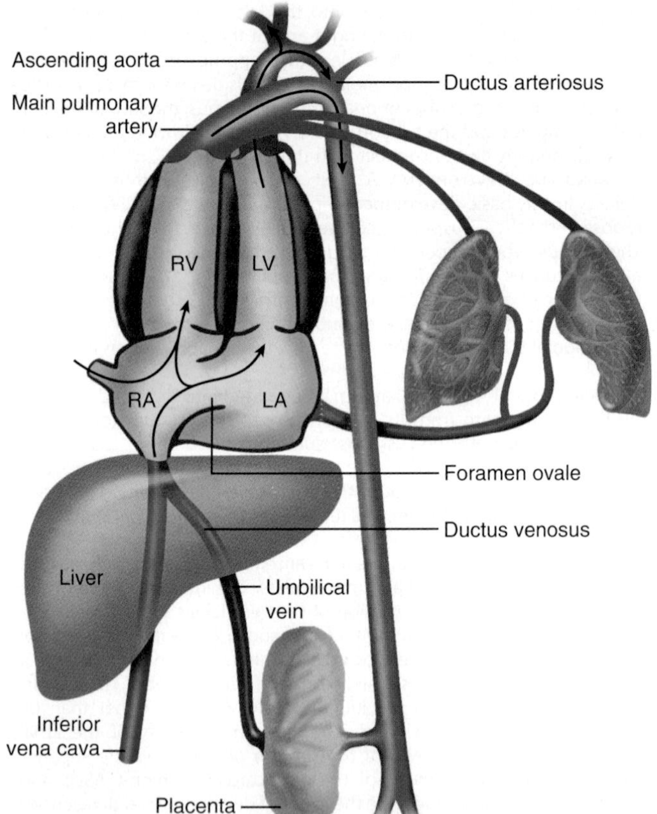

FIGURE 65-1 The fetal circulation, with arrows indicating the directions of flow. A fraction of umbilical venous blood enters the ductus venosus and bypasses the liver. This relatively highly oxygenated blood flows across the foramen ovale to the left side of the heart, preferentially perfusing the coronary arteries, head, and upper trunk. The output of the right ventricle flows preferentially across the ductus arteriosus and circulates to the placenta as well as to the abdominal viscera and lower trunk. *(Courtesy of Dr. David Teitel.)*

ductus venosus, hepatic veins, and lower body venous drainage and is partly deflected across the foramen ovale into the left atrium. Because of a streaming effect, almost all superior vena caval blood passes directly through the tricuspid valve, entering the right ventricle. Most of the blood that reaches the right ventricle bypasses the high-resistance, unexpanded lungs and passes through the ductus arteriosus into the descending aorta. The right ventricle contributes about 55% and the left ventricle 45% to the total fetal cardiac output. The major portion of blood ejected from the left ventricle supplies the brain and upper body, with lesser flow to the coronary arteries; the balance passes across the aortic isthmus to the descending aorta, where it joins with the large stream from the ductus arteriosus before flowing to the lower body and back to the placenta.

Fetal Pulmonary Circulation. In fetal life, the alveoli are fluid filled, and the pulmonary arteries and arterioles have relatively thick walls and a small lumen, similar to arteries in the systemic circulation. The low pulmonary blood flow in the fetus (7% to 10% of the total cardiac output) is the result of high pulmonary vascular resistance. Fetal pulmonary vessels are highly reactive to changes in oxygen tension or in the pH of blood perfusing them as well as to a number of other physiologic and pharmacologic influences.

Effects of Cardiac Malformations on the Fetus. Although fetal somatic growth may be unimpaired, the hemodynamic effects of many cardiac malformations can alter the development and structure of the fetal heart and circulation. For example, although lesions associated with left-to-right shunts in postnatal life rarely influence fetal cardiac size and function, regurgitant AV valves can lead to chamber dilation, hydrops, and fetal death. Ventricular obstructive lesions (e.g., aortic valve stenosis) may variably lead to hypertrophy, dilation, and failure. The secondary effects of congenital lesions are also important. Reduced flow through the left side of the heart can result in aortic hypoplasia and coarctation. Reduced anterograde pulmonary blood flow is associated with pulmonary artery hypoplasia. These effects rarely affect the fetal circulation overtly, however, and often only become exposed as problems after birth as the ductus arteriosus closes.

Function of the Fetal Heart. Compared with the adult heart, the fetal and newborn heart is unique with respect to its ultrastructural appearance, its mechanical and biochemical properties, and its autonomic innervation. During late fetal and early neonatal development, there is maturation of the excitation-contraction coupling process and changes in the biochemical composition of the heart's energy-using myofibrillar proteins and of adenosine triphosphate and creatine phosphate energy-producing proteins. Moreover, fetal and neonatal myocardial cells are small in diameter and reduced in density so that the immature heart contains relatively more noncontractile mass (primarily mitochondria, nuclei, and surface membranes) than later in postnatal life. As a result, force generation and the extent and velocity of shortening are decreased, and stiffness and water content of ventricular myocardium are increased in the fetal and early newborn periods. The fetal heart is surrounded by fluid-filled rather than air-filled lungs. As a result, the fetal and neonatal heart has limited ability to increase cardiac output in the presence of either a volume load or a lesion that increases resistance to emptying. Ultimately, cardiac output is much more dependent on changes in heart rate, explaining why bradycardia is so poorly tolerated by the fetal circulation. Tachycardia can also rapidly lead to heart failure in the fetus, whether it is due to the hemodynamic issues discussed earlier or a manifestation of energy substrate use.

Changes at Birth. Inflation of the lungs at the first inspiration produces a marked reduction in pulmonary vascular resistance. The reduced extravascular pressure and increased alveolar oxygen content, as fluid is removed from the lungs and replaced by air, lead to pulmonary vasodilation and recruitment. As a result, pulmonary artery pressure falls, and pulmonary blood flow increases greatly, raising left atrial pressure and closing the flap valve of the foramen ovale. Conversely, systemic vascular resistance rises. This is related to loss of the low-resistance placental circulation and gradual closure of the ductus arteriosus. It is also related to a sudden increase in arterial blood oxygen tension, subsequent to the lack of mixing of oxygenated and deoxygenated blood that characterizes the fetal milieu. In healthy, mature infants, the ductus arteriosus is profoundly constricted at 10 to 15 hours and is closed functionally by 72 hours, with total anatomic closure following within a few weeks by a process of thrombosis, intimal proliferation, and fibrosis. Preterm infants have a high incidence of persistent patency of the ductus arteriosus because of an immaturity of those mechanisms responsible for constriction.

The ductus venosus, ductus arteriosus, and foramen ovale remain potential channels for blood flow after birth. Thus, persistent patency of the ductus venosus is capitalized on during balloon atrial septostomy performed through the umbilical vein. Lesions producing right or left atrial volume or pressure overload can stretch the foramen ovale and render incompetent the flap valve mechanism for its closure. Anomalies that depend on patency of the ductus arteriosus for preservation of pulmonary or systemic blood flow may remain latent until the ductus arteriosus constricts. A common example is the rapid intensification of cyanosis observed in infants with tetralogy of Fallot when the magnitude of pulmonary hypoperfusion is unmasked by spontaneous closure of the ductus arteriosus. Moreover, increasing evidence shows that ductal constriction is a key factor in the postnatal development of coarctation of the aorta and is clearly the most important factor governing the presentation in babies with a duct-dependent systemic circulation. The management of these conditions is discussed in the appropriate sections later.

Neonate and Infant. Most management decisions in patients with significant CHD occur during the first few months of life. An increase in the prenatal diagnosis of major congenital heart defects has resulted in earlier admission and intervention in the neonate with CHD. These neonates are, in general, healthier than in the past because of the administration of prostaglandins at the time of delivery, thus maintaining hemodynamic stability. With improved surgery and interventional catheterization techniques, many of these neonates undergo intervention within the first days or weeks of life. Indeed, there has been a trend toward complete repair in the neonate and young infant because of an improvement in myocardial preservation and surgical techniques. In most major cardiac centers, the surgical mortality for this age group is in the range of 2% to 4%, which is an improvement on the results of the past, when a palliative procedure often preceded a complete repair.

With increasing experience in this age group, the focus has now shifted from mortality to morbidity. Because the expectation is that most of these neonates and young infants will survive into their adult years, their neurodevelopmental outcome has become as important as the results of the cardiac intervention.[3] It is also being recognized that systemic venous obstruction is a major cause of ongoing morbidity, being directly related to the use of central and peripheral lines in the immediate postoperative period.

Child and Adolescent. The rapid somatic growth rates of infancy and adolescence are periods of rapid hemodynamic change. Stenotic lesions that may be relatively slowly progressive throughout early childhood need more frequent surveillance during adolescence. Childhood and adolescence is a time to begin educating patients, not just their parents, about their heart disease and the responsibilities that go with it. Issues such as the need for compliance with medications, avoidance of smoking and illicit drug use, and pregnancy and contraception counseling are by no means exclusively issues of the adult with CHD and increasingly require discussion in the pediatric cardiac clinic.

Indeed, the early teenage years should be regarded as part of the transition process before transfer to adult follow-up. The management of the older adolescent and follow-up of adults with newly discovered or previously treated CHD is a burgeoning new subspecialty that will require careful planning to ensure adequate resources for the increasing number of adult "graduates" of pediatric programs. A coordinated approach with specialists in an affiliated adult congenital clinic is clearly desirable.

Adult. Patients, and often family members, should understand their cardiac condition in terms of both what has been done so far and what could happen in the future. This is important for a young patient graduating into the adult world. Patients need information and should become partners in their own care.

Potential long-term complications in adults with CHD (such as arrhythmias, ventricular failure, conduit obstruction, and endocarditis) should be explained to patients who are at relatively high risk. The possible need for future therapy—medical (antiarrhythmics, anticoagulation, heart failure therapy), catheter based (valve dilation, stents, arrhythmia ablation), or surgical (redo surgery, transplantation)—should be discussed if the patient may require treatment in the short or intermediate future. Day-to-day issues of concern for these young adults need to be addressed, such as exercise prescriptions, driving restrictions, and traveling limitations. Many young people with CHD need advice about career choices, entering the work force, insurability, and life expectancy.

Many will want to start a family, and reproductive issues will need to be addressed. Discussion of appropriate contraception methods for any given patient should be offered.[4] Counseling before conception as to the risk to the mother and the fetus for any given pregnancy should be done by specialized physicians. They will take into account the maternal cardiac anatomy, maternal functional status, maternal life expectancy, risk of CHD transmission to the offspring, and risk of premature birth. High-risk patients (e.g., Marfan with aortic root dilation, severe pulmonary hypertension, New York Heart Association [NYHA] Class III or IV, and severe aortic stenosis) should be advised against pregnancy. Intermediate-risk patients (e.g., cyanotic, mechanical valve and other warfarin-requiring patients, moderate left ventricular outflow tract obstruction, moderate to severe left ventricular dysfunction) need to know that pregnancy, although possible, may be complicated and that they will require careful follow-up.

Last but not least, comorbidities such as obesity, smoking, high blood pressure, diabetes, and high cholesterol add new levels of complexity to these adults as they age and must be part of the mandate of the patient's cardiologist.

Pathologic Consequences of Congenital Cardiac Lesions

Congestive Heart Failure (see Chaps. 25 to 30)

Although the basic mechanisms of cardiac failure are similar for all ages, the common causes, the time of onset, and often the approach to treatment vary with age (see Chaps. 31 to 34 and Chap. 80). Fetal echocardiography now allows the diagnosis of intrauterine cardiac failure. The cardinal findings of fetal heart failure are scalp edema, ascites, pericardial effusion, and decreased fetal movements. In preterm infants, especially of less than 1500 g birth weight, persistent patency of the ductus arteriosus is the most common cause of cardiac decompensation, and other forms of structural heart disease are rare. In full-term newborns, the earliest important causes of heart failure are the hypoplastic left heart and aortic coarctation syndromes, sustained tachyarrhythmia, cerebral or hepatic arteriovenous fistula, and myocarditis. Among the lesions commonly producing heart failure beyond age 1 to 2 weeks, when diminished pulmonary vascular resistance allows substantial left-to-right shunting, are VSDs and AV septal defects, TGA, truncus arteriosus, and total anomalous pulmonary venous connection. Infants younger than 1 year who have cardiac malformations account for 80% to 90% of pediatric patients who develop congestive failure. In older children, heart failure is often due to acquired disease or is a complication of open heart surgical procedures. In the acquired category are rheumatic and endomyocardial diseases, infective endocarditis, hematologic and nutritional disorders, and severe cardiac arrhythmias.

The distinction between left-sided and right-sided heart failure is less obvious in infants than in older children or adults. Conversely, augmented filling or elevated pressure of the right ventricle in infants reduces left ventricular compliance disproportionately compared with older children or adults and gives rise to signs of both systemic and pulmonary venous congestion.

Care of infants with heart failure must include careful consideration of the underlying structural or functional disturbance. The general aims of treatment are to achieve an increase in cardiac performance, to augment peripheral perfusion, and to decrease pulmonary and systemic venous congestion. In many conditions, medical management cannot control the effects of the abnormal loads imposed by a host of congenital cardiac lesions. Under these circumstances, cardiac diagnosis and interventional catheter or operative intervention may be urgently required.

Congestive heart failure is not common in adult congenital heart practice, although prevention of myocardial dysfunction is a common concern. The adult patient with CHD may develop heart failure in the presence of a substrate (e.g., myocardial dysfunction, valvular regurgitation) and a precipitant (e.g., sustained arrhythmia, pregnancy, hyperthyroidism). Patients prone to congestive failure include those with longstanding volume loads (e.g., valvular regurgitation and left-to-right shunts) and those with a primary depression of myocardial function (e.g., systemic right ventricles, ventricles damaged during surgery or because of late treatment of ventricular overload). Treatment depends on a clear understanding of the elements contributing to decompensation and addressing each of the treatable components. The greatest success is achieved when the main elements can be eliminated. When this is not possible, standard palliative adult heart failure regimens are applied and may include ACE inhibitors, angiotensin receptor blockers, beta blockers, diuretics, resynchronization pacing, transplantation, or other novel therapies.

CHD accounts for 40% of pediatric heart transplants but only 2% of adult heart transplants.[5] Adult CHD heart transplant recipients have a mean survival of 11 years, similar to that of patients with other forms of heart disease. Patients who have had Fontan surgery tend to have worse outcomes, presumably because they have multiorgan disease.[6] About one third of heart-lung transplants are done for CHD. Three-year survival is about 50% and better in patients with Eisenmenger syndrome.

Cyanosis

DEFINITION. Central cyanosis refers to arterial oxygen desaturation resulting from the shunting or mixing of systemic venous blood into the arterial circulation. The magnitude of shunting or mixing and the amount of pulmonary blood flow determine the severity of desaturation.

MORPHOLOGY. Cardiac defects that result in central cyanosis can be divided into two categories: (1) those with increased pulmonary blood flow and (2) those with decreased pulmonary blood flow (**Table 65-4**).

PATHOPHYSIOLOGY. Hypoxemia increases renal production of erythropoietin, which in turn stimulates bone marrow production of circulating red blood cells, enhancing oxygen-carrying capacity. Secondary erythrocytosis should be present in all cyanotic patients because it is a physiologic response to tissue hypoxia. The improved tissue oxygenation that results from this adaptation may be sufficient to reach a new equilibrium at a higher hematocrit. However, adaptive failure can occur if the increased whole blood viscosity rises so much that it impairs oxygen delivery.

CLINICAL FEATURES

Hyperviscosity Syndrome

Erythrocytosis, by virtue of increasing whole blood viscosity, can cause hyperviscosity symptoms including headaches, faintness, dizziness, fatigue, altered mentation, visual disturbances, paresthesias, tinnitus, and myalgias. Iron deficiency, a common finding in cyanotic adult patients if repeated phlebotomies or excessive bleeding occurs, may cause hyperviscosity symptoms at hematocrit levels well below 65%.

Hematologic

Hemostatic abnormalities have been documented in cyanotic patients with erythrocytosis and can occur in up to 20% of patients. A bleeding tendency can be mild and superficial, leading to easy bruising, skin petechiae, and mucosal bleeding, or it can be moderate or life-threatening with hemoptysis or intracranial, gastrointestinal, or postoperative bleeding. Elevated prothrombin and partial thromboplastin times, decreased factor levels (factors V, VII, VIII, and IX), qualitative and quantitative platelet disorders, increased fibrinolysis, and systemic endothelial dysfunction from increased shear stress have all been implicated.[7]

TABLE 65-4 Cardiac Defects Causing Central Cyanosis

Transposition of the great arteries	**E**bstein anomaly
Tetralogy of Fallot	**E**isenmenger physiology
Tricuspid atresia	Critical pulmonary stenosis or atresia
Truncus arteriosus	Functionally single ventricle
Total anomalous pulmonary venous return	

Note five T's and two E's.

Central Nervous System

Neurologic complications including cerebral hemorrhage can occur secondary to hemostatic defects and can be seen in patients taking anticoagulants. Patients with right-to-left shunts may be at risk for paradoxical cerebral emboli, especially if they are iron deficient. A brain abscess should be suspected in a cyanotic patient with a new or different headache or new neurologic symptoms. Air filters should be used in peripheral and central venous lines in cyanotic patients to avoid paradoxical emboli through a right-to-left shunt.

Renal

Renal dysfunction can be manifested as proteinuria, hyperuricemia, or renal failure. Pathologic studies at the level of the glomeruli show evidence of vascular abnormalities as well as increased cellularity and fibrosis. Hyperuricemia is common and is thought to be due mainly to the decreased reabsorption of uric acid rather than to overproduction with erythrocytosis. Urate nephropathy, uric acid nephrolithiasis, and gouty arthritis may occur.

Arthritic

Rheumatologic complications include gout and, especially, hypertrophic osteoarthropathy, which is thought to be responsible for the arthralgias and bone pain affecting up to one third of patients. In patients with right-to-left shunting, megakaryocytes released from the bone marrow can bypass the lung. The entrapment of megakaryocytes in the systemic arterioles and capillaries induces the release of platelet-derived growth factor, promoting local cell proliferation. New osseous formation with periostitis ensues and gives rise to arthralgia and bone pain.

Coronary Arteries

Patients with central cyanosis display dilated coronaries with no obstruction. Their level of total cholesterol is also lower than that of the general population.[8]

INTERVENTIONAL OPTIONS AND OUTCOMES

Physiologic Repair

Physiologic repair results in total or near-total anatomic and physiologic separation of the pulmonary and systemic circulations in complex cyanotic lesions that leads to relief of cyanosis. Such procedures should be performed whenever feasible.

Palliative Surgical Intervention

Palliative surgical interventions can be performed in patients with cyanotic lesions to increase pulmonary blood flow while allowing cyanosis to persist. Palliative surgical shunts are summarized in **Table 65-5**. Blalock-Taussig, central, and Glenn (also called cavopulmonary) shunts are still in use today. Blalock-Taussig shunts seldom have caused pulmonary hypertension compared with central shunts and are less likely to cause pulmonary artery distortion. Glenn shunts have the advantage of increasing pulmonary flow without imposing a volume load on the systemic ventricle. Glenn shunts require low pulmonary artery pressures to work, and they may be associated with the development over time of pulmonary arteriovenous fistulas, which can worsen cyanosis.

TABLE 65-5 Palliative Systemic to Pulmonary Shunts

Arterial

Blalock-Taussig shunt (subclavian artery to pulmonary artery)
- Classic: end-to-side, no or reduced ipsilateral arm pulses
- Current: side-to-side tubular grafts, preserved arm pulses

Central shunt (side-to-side tubular graft, aorta to pulmonary artery)
Potts shunt (descending aorta to left pulmonary artery)
Waterston shunt (ascending aorta to right pulmonary artery)

Venous

Glenn shunt (superior vena cava to ipsilateral pulmonary artery without cardiac or other pulmonary artery connection)
Bidirectional cavopulmonary (Glenn) shunt (end-to-side superior vena cava to left pulmonary artery and right pulmonary artery shunt)

Transplantation (see Chap. 31)

Transplantation of heart, one or both lungs with surgical cardiac repair, and heart-lung transplantation have been performed in cyanotic patients with or without palliation who were no longer candidates for other forms of intervention. Pulmonary vascular obstructive disease precludes isolated heart transplantation. An increasing number of CHD patients with previous palliation and ventricular failure are successfully undergoing cardiac transplantation.[5] Timing of transplantation in these patients remains difficult.

OTHER MANAGEMENT

Phlebotomy

The goal of phlebotomy is symptom control. When patients have troubling symptoms of hyperviscosity, are iron replete (normal mean corpuscular volume, hematocrit >65%), and are not dehydrated, removal of 250 to 500 mL of blood during 30 to 45 minutes should be performed with concomitant quantitative volume replacement. The procedure may be repeated every 24 hours until symptomatic improvement occurs or the hemoglobin level has fallen below 18 to 19 g/dL. Phlebotomy is not indicated for asymptomatic patients.

Iron Replacement

If iron deficiency anemia is found, iron supplements should be prescribed. Cyanotic patients should avoid iron deficiency, which can cause functional deterioration and is associated with an increased risk of stroke.

Bleeding Diathesis

Platelet transfusions, fresh frozen plasma, vitamin K, cryoprecipitate, and desmopressin can be used to treat severe bleeding. Given the inherent tendency to bleed, aspirin, heparin, and warfarin should be avoided in the cyanotic patient unless the risks of treatment are outweighed by the risks of nontreatment. Likewise, nonsteroidal anti-inflammatory drugs should be avoided to prevent bleeding.

Gouty Arthritis

Symptomatic hyperuricemia and gouty arthritis can be treated as needed with colchicine, probenecid, or allopurinol.

REPRODUCTIVE ISSUES. Pregnancy in cyanotic CHD (excluding Eisenmenger syndrome) results in a 32% incidence of maternal cardiovascular complications and a 37% incidence of fetal prematurity. Pregnant women with a resting oxygen saturation greater than 85% fare better than do women with an oxygen saturation less than 85%.

FOLLOW-UP. All cyanotic patients should be observed by a CHD cardiologist, and particular attention should be paid to the following: underlying heart condition; symptoms of hyperviscosity; systemic complications of cyanosis; change in exercise tolerance; change in saturation levels; and prophylaxis against endocarditis, influenza, and pneumococcal infections. The clinician should remember to measure oxygen saturation only after the patient has been resting for at least 5 minutes. In stable cyanotic patients, yearly follow-up is recommended and should include annual influenza vaccination, periodic pneumococcal vaccination, yearly blood work (complete blood count, ferritin, clotting profile, renal function, uric acid), and regular echocardiographic Doppler studies. Home oxygen therapy may have a role in increasing oxygen saturation through its pulmonary vasodilatory effect, but clinical indications and outcomes are not clear.[9]

Pulmonary Hypertension

Pulmonary hypertension is a common accompaniment of many congenital cardiac lesions,[10] and the status of the pulmonary vascular bed is often the principal determinant of the clinical manifestations, the course, and whether corrective treatment is feasible (see Chap. 78). Recent consensus statements provide important information on this general topic.[11,12] Increases in pulmonary arterial pressure result from elevations of pulmonary blood flow or resistance, the latter sometimes caused by an increase in vascular tone but usually the result of underdevelopment or obstructive or obliterative structural changes within the pulmonary vascular bed. Although pulmonary hypertension usually affects the entire pulmonary vascular bed, it may occur focally. For example, unilateral pulmonary hypertension may occur in an overshunted lung (the other lung perhaps protected and fed by a cavopulmonary Glenn shunt) or in lung segments supplied by aortopulmonary collateral flow.

Pulmonary vascular resistance normally falls rapidly immediately after birth because of the onset of ventilation and subsequent pulmonary vasodilation. Subsequently, the medial smooth muscle of pulmonary arterial resistance vessels thins gradually. In infants with large aortopulmonary or ventricular communications, this process is often delayed by several months, at which time levels of pulmonary vascular resistance are still somewhat elevated. In patients with high pulmonary arterial pressures from birth, failure of normal growth of the pulmonary circulation may occur, and anatomic changes in the pulmonary vessels in the form of proliferation of intimal cells and intimal and medial thickening often progress, so in an older child or adult, vascular resistance ultimately may become relatively fixed by obliterative changes in the pulmonary vascular bed. The causes of pulmonary vascular obstructive disease remain unknown, although increased pulmonary arterial blood pressure, elevated pulmonary venous pressure, erythrocytosis, systemic hypoxia, acidemia, and the nature of the bronchial circulation have been implicated. Quite likely, injury to pulmonary vascular endothelial cells initiates a cascade of events that involves the release or activation of factors that alter the extracellular matrix, induces hypertrophy, causes proliferation of vascular smooth muscle cells, and promotes connective tissue protein synthesis. Considered together, these may permanently alter vessel structure and function.

Mechanisms of Development. Intimal damage appears to be related to shear stresses because endothelial cell damage occurs at high shear rates. A reduction in pulmonary arteriolar lumen size due to either thickened medial muscle or vasoconstriction increases the velocity of flow. Shear stress also increases as blood viscosity rises; therefore, infants with hypoxemia and high hematocrit levels as well as increased pulmonary blood flow are at increased risk for development of pulmonary vascular disease. In patients with left-to-right shunts, pulmonary arterial hypertension, if it is not present in infancy or childhood, may never occur or may not develop until the third or fourth decade or later. Once developed, intimal proliferative changes with hyalinization and fibrosis are not reversible by repair of the underlying cardiac defect. In severe pulmonary vascular obstructive disease, arteriovenous malformations may develop and predispose to massive hemoptysis.

Most vexing is the variability among patients with the same or similar cardiac lesions in both the time of appearance and the rate of progression of the pulmonary vascular obstructive process. Although genetic influences may be operative (an example is the apparent acceleration of pulmonary vascular disease in patients with CHD and trisomy 21), evidence is now accumulating for important prenatal and postnatal modifiers of the pulmonary vascular bed that appear, at least in part, to be lesion dependent. Thus, a quantitative variability exists in the pulmonary vascular bed related to the number, not just the size and wall structure, of arterial vessels within the pulmonary circulation.

Modeling of the blood vessels occurs proximal to and within terminal bronchioles (preacinar and intra-acinar vessels, respectively) continuously from before birth. The intra-acinar vessels, in particular, increase in size and number from late fetal life throughout childhood, with minimal muscularization of their walls. The ensuing increase in the cross-sectional area of the pulmonary arterial circulation allows the cardiac output to rise substantially without an increase in pulmonary arterial pressure. If, however, the presence of a cardiac lesion interferes with the normal growth and multiplication of these peripheral arteries, the resulting elevation of pulmonary vascular resistance may first be related to failure of the intra-acinar pulmonary circulation to develop fully and then secondarily to the morphologic changes of obliterative vascular disease: medial thickening, intimal proliferation, hyalinization and fibrosis, angiomatoid and plexiform lesions, and, ultimately, arterial necrosis.

Eisenmenger Syndrome

DEFINITION. Eisenmenger syndrome, a term coined by Paul Wood, is defined as pulmonary vascular obstructive disease that develops as a consequence of a large preexisting left-to-right shunt such that pulmonary artery pressures approach systemic levels and the direction of the flow becomes bidirectional or right-to-left. Congenital heart defects that can result in Eisenmenger syndrome include simple defects, such as ASD, VSD, and PDA, as well as more complex defects, such as AV septal defect, truncus arteriosus, aortopulmonary window, and univentricular heart. The high pulmonary vascular resistance is usually established in infancy (by the age of 2 years, except in ASD) and is sometimes present from birth.

NATURAL HISTORY OF THE UNREPAIRED PATIENT. Patients with defects that allow free communication between the pulmonary and systemic circuits at the aortic or ventricular levels usually have a fairly healthy childhood and gradually become overtly cyanotic during their second or third decade. Exercise intolerance (dyspnea and fatigue) is proportional to the degree of hypoxemia or cyanosis. In the absence of complications, these patients generally have an excellent to good functional capacity up to their third decade and thereafter usually experience a slowly progressive decline in their physical abilities. Most patients survive to adulthood, with a reported 77% and 42% survival rate at 15 and 25 years of age, respectively.

Congestive heart failure in patients with Eisenmenger syndrome usually occurs after 40 years of age. The most common modes of death are sudden death (≈30%; see Chap. 41), congestive heart failure (≈25%), and pulmonary hemorrhage (≈15%). Pregnancy, perioperative mortality after noncardiac surgery, and infectious causes (brain abscesses and endocarditis) account for most of the remainder.

CLINICAL MANIFESTATIONS. Patients can present with the following complications: those related to the cyanotic state; palpitations in nearly half the patients (atrial fibrillation or flutter in 35%, ventricular tachycardia in up to 10%); hemoptysis in about 20%; pulmonary thromboembolism, angina, syncope, and endocarditis in about 10% each; and congestive heart failure. Hemoptysis is usually due to bleeding bronchial vessels or pulmonary infarction. Physical examination reveals central cyanosis and clubbing of the nailbeds. Patients with Eisenmenger PDA can have pink nailbeds on the right (>left) hand and cyanosis and clubbing of both feet, so-called differential cyanosis. This occurs because venous blood shunts through the ductus and enters the aorta distal to the subclavian arteries. The jugular venous pressure in patients with Eisenmenger syndrome can be normal or elevated, especially with prominent v waves when tricuspid regurgitation is present. Signs of pulmonary hypertension—right ventricular heave, palpable and loud P_2, and right-sided S_4—are typically present. In many patients, a pulmonary ejection click and a soft and scratchy systolic ejection murmur, attributable to dilation of the pulmonary trunk, and a high-pitched decrescendo diastolic murmur of pulmonary regurgitation (Graham Steell) are audible. Peripheral edema is absent until right-sided heart failure ensues.

Laboratory Investigations

Electrocardiography. Peaked P waves consistent with right atrial overload and evidence of right ventricular hypertrophy with right-axis deviation are the rule. Atrial arrhythmias can be present.

Chest Radiography. Dilated central pulmonary arteries with rapid tapering of the peripheral pulmonary vasculature are the radiographic hallmarks of Eisenmenger syndrome. Pulmonary artery calcification may be seen and is diagnostic of longstanding pulmonary hypertension. Eisenmenger syndrome due to VSD or PDA usually has a normal or slightly increased cardiothoracic ratio. Eisenmenger syndrome due to an ASD typically has a large cardiothoracic ratio because of right atrial and ventricular dilation, along with an inconspicuous aorta. Calcification of the duct may be seen in Eisenmenger PDA.

Echocardiography. The intracardiac defect should be seen readily along with bidirectional shunting. A pulmonary hypertensive PDA is not easily seen. Evidence of pulmonary hypertension is found. Assessment of pulmonary right ventricular function adds prognostic value.

Cardiac Catheterization. Cardiac catheterization not only provides direct measurement of the pulmonary artery pressure, documenting the existence of severe pulmonary hypertension, but also can allow assessment of reactivity of the pulmonary vasculature. Administration of pulmonary arterial vasodilators (oxygen, nitric oxide, prostaglandin I_2 [epoprostenol]) can discriminate patients in whom surgical repair is contraindicated and those with reversible pulmonary hypertension who may benefit from surgical repair. Radiographic contrast material may cause hypotension and worsening cyanosis and should be used cautiously.

Open Lung Biopsy. Open lung biopsy should be considered only when reversibility of the pulmonary hypertension is uncertain from the hemodynamic data. An expert opinion will be necessary to determine the severity of the changes, often by use of the Heath-Edwards classification.

INDICATIONS FOR INTERVENTION. The underlying principle of clinical management in patients with Eisenmenger syndrome is to avoid any factors that may destabilize the delicately balanced physiology. In general, an approach of nonintervention has been traditionally recommended, although research in the treatment of pulmonary hypertension may alter this approach in the future.[13] The main interventions, therefore, are directed toward prevention of complications (e.g., influenza vaccine and pneumococcal vaccine to reduce the morbidity of respiratory infections) or restoration of the physiologic balance (e.g., iron replacement for iron deficiency, antiarrhythmic management of atrial arrhythmias, diuretics for right-sided heart failure). As a general rule, the first episode of hemoptysis should be considered an indication for investigation. Bed rest is usually recommended; and although it is usually self-limited, each such episode should be regarded as potentially life-threatening, and a treatable cause should be sought. When patients are seriously incapacitated from severe hypoxemia or congestive heart failure, the main intervention available is lung transplantation (plus repair of the cardiac defect) or, with somewhat better results, heart-lung transplantation. This is generally reserved for individuals without contraindications who are thought to have a 1-year survival of less than 50%. Such assessment is fraught with difficulty because of the unpredictability of the time course of the disease and the risk of sudden death.

Noncardiac surgery should be performed only when it is absolutely necessary because of its high associated mortality. Eisenmenger syndrome patients are particularly vulnerable to alterations in hemodynamics induced by anesthesia or surgery, such as a minor decrease in systemic vascular resistance that can increase right-to-left shunting and possibly potentiate cardiovascular collapse. Local anesthesia should be used whenever possible. Avoidance of prolonged fasting and especially dehydration, use of antibiotic prophylaxis when appropriate, and careful intraoperative monitoring are recommended. The choice of general versus epidural-spinal anesthesia is controversial. An experienced cardiac anesthetist with an understanding of Eisenmenger syndrome physiology should administer anesthesia. Additional risks of surgery include excessive bleeding, postoperative arrhythmias, and deep venous thrombosis with paradoxical emboli. An air filter or "bubble trap" should be used for most intravenous lines in cyanotic patients. Early ambulation is recommended. Postoperative care in an intensive care unit setting is optimal.

INTERVENTIONAL OPTIONS AND OUTCOMES

Oxygen

Supplemental nocturnal oxygen has recently been shown to have no impact on exercise capacity or on survival in adult patients with Eisenmenger syndrome. Supplemental oxygen during commercial air travel is often recommended, but the scientific basis for this recommendation is lacking.

Transplantation

Lung transplantation may be undertaken in association with repair of existing cardiovascular defects. Alternatively, heart-lung transplantation may be required if the intracardiac anatomy is not correctable. The 3-year survival rate after heart-lung transplantation for CHD is 50%.[14] The subgroup of patients with Eisenmenger syndrome may do better, with a 50% 5-year survival. These procedures offer the best hope to individuals with end-stage CHD who are confronting death and have an intolerable quality of life.

Medical Therapy

ENDOTHELIN RECEPTOR ANTAGONISTS. A randomized trial of a nonselective endothelin receptor antagonist (bosentan) in patients with Eisenmenger syndrome[15] showed that pulse oximetry was not reduced. Compared with placebo, bosentan reduced the pulmonary vascular resistance index and pulmonary artery pressure and improved 6-minute walk and functional class. A smaller observational study of bosentan 125 mg twice a day in nine Eisenmenger patients showed an improvement in functional class and increased resting oxygen saturation levels.[16] In another study, bosentan was less effective in patients with Down syndrome.[17]

PHOSPHODIESTERASE INHIBITORS. Sildenafil (Viagra), in a large double-blind, placebo-controlled study administered in varying doses to 278 patients with symptomatic pulmonary arterial hypertension of different causes, improved the 6-minute walk distance (maintained for the 1 year of the trial), increased functional class, and modestly improved pulmonary arterial pressures and cardiac output.[18] A second randomized, placebo-controlled, double-blind crossover study of a smaller group of patients produced similar improvements.[19] Additional experience has recently been reported,[20,21] and the importance of considering safety issues in treating these patients has been highlighted.[22]

FOLLOW-UP. Education of the patient is critical. Avoidance of over-the-counter medications, dehydration, smoking, high-altitude exposure, and excessive physical activity should be stressed. Avoidance of pregnancy is of paramount importance. Annual influenza vaccination, a single dose of pneumococcal vaccine, and use of endocarditis prophylaxis together with proper skin hygiene (avoidance of nail biting) are recommended. A yearly assessment of complete blood cell count and uric acid, creatinine, and ferritin levels should be done to monitor treatable causes of deterioration.

Cardiac Arrhythmias (see Chaps. 35 to 39)

In teenagers and young adults, most arrhythmias (see Chap. 39) are in association with previously repaired CHD. Arrhythmias can be a major clinical challenge in adolescent and adult congenital heart patients. They are the most frequent reason for emergency department visits and hospital admissions, and they are usually recurrent and may worsen or become less responsive to treatment with time. Treatment may be challenging.

ATRIAL ARRHYTHMIAS. Atrial flutter and, to a lesser degree, atrial fibrillation are most common. Atrial flutter tends to reflect right atrial abnormalities, and atrial fibrillation, left atrial abnormalities. Atrial flutter in such patients is often atypical in appearance and behavior and is better called intra-atrial reentrant tachycardia. Recognition of atrial flutter can be difficult, and the observer must be vigilant in recognizing 2:1 conduction masquerading as sinus rhythm. Recurrence is likely and should not necessarily be assumed to represent failure of the management strategy. The conditions in which atrial flutter is most likely are Mustard or Senning repairs of TGA, repaired or unrepaired ASDs, repaired tetralogy of Fallot, Ebstein anomaly of the tricuspid valve, and after a Fontan operation. Atrial flutter may reflect hemodynamic deterioration in patients who have had Mustard, Senning, tetralogy of Fallot, or Fontan repairs. Its arrival is usually associated with more symptoms and functional limitation.

The pharmaceutical agents most commonly used in therapy are warfarin, beta blockers, amiodarone, sotalol, propafenone, and digoxin. As a rule, patients with good ventricular function can receive sotalol or propafenone, whereas those with depressed ventricular function should receive amiodarone. Other therapies including pacemakers, ablative procedures, and innovative surgery are being both applied and refined. Sustained ventricular tachycardia or ventricular fibrillation occurs less often, usually in the setting of ventricular dilation, dysfunction, and scarring. Although sudden death is common in several conditions, the mechanism is poorly understood.

VENTRICULAR TACHYCARDIA. This arrhythmia can be seen as a manifestation of proarrhythmic effects of various agents in patients with acute myocardial injury or infarction, and in CHD patients with severe ventricular dysfunction. In particular, sustained ventricular tachycardia has been seen in patients with repaired tetralogy of Fallot as a manifestation of hemodynamic problems requiring repair, as a reflection of right ventricular dilation and dysfunction, and in relation to ventricular scarring.

SUDDEN DEATH. In contrast to adults, children seldom die suddenly and unexpectedly of cardiovascular disease. Nonetheless, sudden death has been reported with arrhythmias, aortic stenosis, hypertrophic obstructive cardiomyopathy, primary pulmonary hypertension, Eisenmenger syndrome, myocarditis, congenital complete heart block, and primary endocardial fibroelastosis and when there are certain anomalies of the coronary arteries. Sudden death is more frequent in older patients with postoperative heart disease, particularly after atrial switch procedures and repair of tetralogy of Fallot.

ATRIOVENTRICULAR BLOCK. First-degree AV block is commonly seen in patients with AV septal defects, Ebstein anomaly, complete TGA (D-TGA), and in the older ASD patient. Complete heart block may develop spontaneously in patients with cc-TGA and may develop postoperatively in these and other patients. When pacing is required, epicardial leads are usually placed in cyanotic patients. Many adult patients with CHD are prone to problems of vascular access because of prior surgeries and pacing leads.

Infective Endocarditis (see Chap. 67)

Infective endocarditis complicating CHD is uncommon before 2 years of age, except in the immediate postoperative period. Recent guidelines for endocarditis prophylaxis have substantially altered clinical practice.[23,24] Maintenance of excellent oral hygiene is encouraged most strongly. Antibiotic prophylaxis before dental procedures is recommended for patients with prosthetic heart valves or prosthetic material used for cardiac valve repair; for patients with a prior history of infective endocarditis, persistently cyanotic CHD, or residual defects that are adjacent to a prosthetic patch or prosthetic device; for the first 6 months after placement of prosthetic material or device for CHD; and for cardiac transplant recipients who develop cardiac valvulopathy.

Chest Pain (see Chap. 53)

Angina pectoris is an uncommon symptom of cardiac disease in young infants and children, although it probably explains the irritability and crying during or after feeding in babies with coronary ischemia resulting from anomalous origin of the coronary artery from the pulmonary artery. In older children and young adults with severe left or right ventricular outflow tract obstruction and pulmonary hypertension, chest pain commonly occurs with or follows effort and may be identical to effort angina of coronary artery disease in older adults. A sensation of chest discomfort or cardiac awareness is frequently interpreted as pain by the parents of children with cardiac arrhythmias. Careful questioning serves to identify palpitations rather than pain as the symptom and often elicits an additional history of anxiety, pallor, and sweating. Pain caused by pericarditis is commonly of acute onset and associated with fever, and it can be identified by specific physical, radiographic, and echocardiographic findings. Most commonly, late postoperative chest pain is musculoskeletal in origin and may be reproduced on upper extremity movement or by palpation. Finally, children and adults may suffer chest pain of nonspecific form as a result of anxiety, with or without hyperventilation.

Syndromes in Congenital Heart Disease

ALCAPA SYNDROME. The acronym stands for *a*nomalous *l*eft *co*ronary *a*rtery *a*rising from the *p*ulmonary *a*rtery. It is also called Bland-White-Garland syndrome.

ALAGILLE SYNDROME. This is a hereditary syndrome consisting of intrahepatic cholestasis, characteristic facies, butterfly-like vertebral anomalies, and varying degrees of peripheral pulmonary artery stenoses or diffuse hypoplasia of the pulmonary artery and its branches. It is associated with a deletion in chromosome 20p.

DIGEORGE SYNDROME. This syndrome is caused by a microdeletion at chromosome 22q11, resulting in a wide clinical spectrum. It was previously referred to as CATCH 22 syndrome, with CATCH standing for cardiac defect, *a*bnormal facies, *t*hymic hypoplasia, cleft palate, and *h*ypocalcemia. Cardiac defects include conotruncal defects such as interrupted aortic arch, tetralogy of Fallot, truncus arteriosus, and double-outlet right ventricle. This umbrella grouping also encompasses patients with velocardiofacial syndrome.

CHARGE ASSOCIATION. This anomaly is characterized by the presence of coloboma or choanal atresia and three of the following defects: CHD, nervous system anomaly or mental retardation, genital abnormalities, ear abnormality, or deafness. Congenital heart defects seen in the CHARGE association are tetralogy of Fallot with or without other cardiac defects, AV septal defect, double-outlet right ventricle, double-inlet left ventricle, TGA, interrupted aortic arch, and others.

DOWN SYNDROME. This is the most common genetic malformation and is caused by trisomy 21. Most of the patients (95%) have complete trisomy of chromosome 21; some have translocation or mosaic forms. The phenotype is diagnostic (short stature, characteristic facial appearance, mental retardation, brachydactyly, atlantoaxial instability, and thyroid and white blood cell disorders). Congenital heart defects are frequent (40%), with AV septal defect, VSD, and PDA being the most common. Patients with Down syndrome are prone to earlier and more severe pulmonary vascular disease than otherwise expected as a result of the lesions identified. Hypothyroidism is common in later life, and patients should be screened intermittently.

ELLIS-VAN CREVELD SYNDROME. This is an autosomal recessive syndrome in which common atrium, primum ASD, and partial AV septal defects are the most common cardiac lesions.

HOLT-ORAM SYNDROME. This is an autosomal dominant syndrome consisting of radial abnormalities of the forearm and hand associated with secundum ASD (most common), VSD, or, rarely, other cardiac malformations.

LEOPARD SYNDROME. This autosomal dominant condition is a close cousin of Noonan syndrome and shares a similar genetic substrate (deletion of the *PTPN11* gene). It includes *l*entigines, *e*lectrocardiographic abnormalities, *o*cular hypertelorism, *p*ulmonary stenosis, *a*bnormal genitalia, *r*etardation of growth, and *d*eafness. Rarely, cardiomyopathy or complex CHD may be present.

NOONAN SYNDROME. This is an autosomal dominant syndrome, phenotypically somewhat similar to Turner syndrome but with a normal chromosomal complement. Noonan syndrome is associated with congenital cardiac anomalies, especially dysplastic pulmonary valve stenosis, pulmonary artery stenosis, and ASD. Hypertrophic cardiomyopathy is less common. Congenital lymphedema is a commonly associated anomaly that may be unrecognized.

RUBELLA SYNDROME. This is a wide spectrum of malformations caused by rubella infection early in pregnancy, including cataracts, retinopathy, deafness, CHD, bone lesions, and mental retardation. The spectrum of congenital heart lesions is wide and includes pulmonary artery stenosis, PDA, tetralogy of Fallot, and VSD.

SCIMITAR SYNDROME. This is a constellation of anomalies including total or partial anomalous pulmonary venous connection (PAPVC) of the right lung to the inferior vena cava, often associated with hypoplasia of the right lung and right pulmonary artery. The lower portion of the right lung (sequestered lobe) tends to receive its arterial supply from the abdominal aorta. The name of the syndrome derives from the appearance on the posteroanterior chest radiograph of the shadow formed by the anomalous pulmonary venous connection that resembles a Turkish sword or scimitar (see Fig. 18-19).

SHONE COMPLEX (SYNDROME). This is an association of multiple levels of left ventricular inflow and outflow obstruction (subvalvular and valvular left ventricular outflow tract obstruction, coarctation of the aorta, and mitral stenosis [parachute mitral valve and supramitral ring]).

TURNER SYNDROME. This is a clinical syndrome due to the 45 XO karyotype in about 50% of cases, with various other X chromosome abnormalities in the remainder. There is a characteristic but variable phenotype and an association with congenital cardiac anomalies, especially postductal coarctation of the aorta and other left-sided obstructive lesions, as well as PAPVC without ASD. The female phenotype varies with the age at presentation and is somewhat similar to that of Noonan syndrome.

WILLIAMS SYNDROME. This is a congenital syndrome frequently associated with inherited or sporadic mutations of 7q11.23. It is associated with intellectual deficit, infantile hypercalcemia, characteristic phenotype, and CHD, especially supravalvular aortic stenosis and multiple peripheral pulmonary stenoses. An identical vascular phenotype is sometimes seen in otherwise phenotypically and intellectually normal families.

Evaluation of the Patient with Congenital Heart Disease

Physical Examination

Although the advances in technology have profoundly improved our diagnostic abilities, there is still a role for detailed clinical examination in the assessment and follow-up of patients with unrepaired, palliated, and repaired CHD. The relevant findings pertaining to specific abnormalities are outlined in the appropriate sections that follow, but some general principles bear consideration (see Chap. 12).

PHYSICAL ASSESSMENT. The presence of characteristic facial or somatic features of an underlying syndrome may be a strong clue to the type of heart disease (e.g., Williams, Noonan, Down) at any age. Central cyanosis can be difficult to diagnose clinically when it is mild but should be actively excluded by oximetry in any patient with suspected CHD. One should assess both cardiac and visceral situs and not assume that the heart will be left sided. Careful surveillance of the chest wall for scars is also important in older patients and adults, who do not always know or report the type and sequence of their surgical interventions. The thin chest wall of children and many young adults with CHD assists the detection of chamber enlargement by palpation as well as the detection of systolic or diastolic thrills.

The infant or child with hemodynamically significant heart disease may show signs of failure to thrive (underweight, small, or both). The weight and height should therefore be plotted sequentially against normal growth curves appropriate to race, sex, and underlying syndrome (e.g., Down syndrome growth chart). The manifestations of "heart failure" vary with age and the underlying problem. In children, peripheral edema is rare, but intercostal recession, nasal flaring, and grunting with respiration are signs of congestive heart failure. In small children, an excellent barometer of cardiac function is liver size and pulsatility, reflecting right atrial pressure, right ventricular filling time, and diastolic dysfunction or tricuspid regurgitation. The jugular venous pressure is difficult to assess in young children but is a fundamental part of the examination of the older child, teenager, and adult.

Examination of the upper and lower limb peripheral pulses is important at any age. Delay, absence, or reduction of a pulse is an important clue to the presence of arterial obstruction and its site. The left brachial pulse is often compromised by surgery for coarctation, and blood pressure measurements should not be taken in only the left arm. Similarly, other palliative procedures (Blalock-Taussig shunt, interposition grafts) may affect either or both upper limb pulses. Assessment of the femoral and carotid pulses in addition to the upper limb pulses is important in such patients. Just as in acquired disease, the pulse volume and character also provide important information about the severity of obstructive or regurgitant left-sided heart disease. A low-volume pulse (usually with a narrow pulse pressure) reflects a low cardiac output. Pulsus alternans signifies severe systemic ventricular dysfunction. Pulsus paradoxus points to cardiac tamponade. In adolescents and adults, the jugular venous pressure examination is often important. It may indicate cardiac decompensation, cardiac chamber hypertrophy or restriction, valvular regurgitation or stenosis, arrhythmia or conduction disturbance, cardiac tamponade, pericardial constriction, and other phenomena.

AUSCULTATION. The rules of auscultation also follow those developed for acquired heart disease. However, cardiac and vascular malposition may significantly affect the appreciation of heart sounds and murmurs. For example, in TGA treated by an atrial switch procedure, the aorta remains anterior to the pulmonary artery. Consequently, the aortic component of the second sound can be exceptionally loud, and the pulmonary component may be virtually inaudible, making it difficult to estimate the pulmonary artery pressure clinically under such circumstances. Conversely, when there is a valved conduit between the right ventricle and pulmonary artery, the pulmonary closure sound may be extremely loud, even though the pulmonary artery diastolic pressure is low. This is because the conduit is frequently adherent to the chest wall, assisting sound transmission to the stethoscope placed close to it. Calcification of semilunar valves is relatively unusual in childhood and early adult life, making the differentiation of valve stenosis from subvalve or supravalve narrowing, by the presence of an ejection click, more precise in these patients. The differentiation of multiple murmurs is sometimes a challenge. Systolic or diastolic murmurs in an individual may have several causes, and supplementary clinical information may be required to establish their significance in some cases. Auscultation over the entire anterior and posterior chest wall is important. The continuous murmurs of aorto-aortic collateral arteries in coarctation may be audible only between the shoulder blades posteriorly, for example; similarly, a localized distal pulmonary artery stenosis or an aortopulmonary collateral artery may be detected only in a localized area of the chest wall, particularly in adults.

Electrocardiography

The electrocardiogram (ECG; see Chap. 13) remains an important tool in the assessment of CHD. Heart rhythm and rate as well as AV conduction can be evaluated. The dominant theme that runs through ECGs in CHD is the prevalence of right-sided heart disease. This often takes the form of right-axis deviation along with right atrial and right ventricular hypertrophy. Right ventricular hypertrophy may reflect pulmonary hypertension, right ventricular outflow tract obstruction, or a subaortic right ventricle. Incomplete right bundle branch block often indicates right ventricular hypertrophy due to pressure (e.g., pulmonary hypertension or pulmonary stenosis) or volume (e.g., ASD) overload. Right ventricular volume overload is likely when the r′ in V_1 is less than 7 mm. Very wide QRS complexes should be seen as possible manifestations of dilated and dysfunctional ventricles, most specifically in patients with repaired tetralogy, complete right bundle branch block, and severe pulmonary regurgitation. The ECG may be uninterpretable in patients with abnormal cardiac or visceral situs unless it is clear where the leads were placed.

Atrial flutter (often in an atypical form, so-called intra-atrial reentrant tachycardia) is much more common in young patients than is atrial fibrillation. First-degree block is often seen in AV septal defects, cc-TGA, and Ebstein anomaly. Complete heart block is most often seen in patients with cc-TGA as well as in those with older VSD repairs.

Left atrial overload may reflect increased pulmonary blood flow as well as AV valve dysfunction and myocardial failure. Left-axis deviation should make one think of AV septal defect, a univentricular heart, and a hypoplastic right ventricle. Deep Q waves in the left chest leads can be caused by left ventricular volume overload in a young person with aortic or mitral regurgitation. Pathologic Q waves can be evidence of the anomalous origin of the left coronary from the pulmonary artery.

Chest Radiography

The chest radiograph (see Chap. 16) is another valuable tool for the discerning physician caring for patients with congenital heart defects. Although more recent technologies have rightly attracted much attention, there is value in learning how to interpret the chest radiograph. Some teaching points can be made that may anchor the interpretation of chest radiographs of some CHD patients. The following sections provide a number of clinical and radiographic differential diagnoses.

CRITERIA FOR SHUNT VASCULARITY (see Fig. 16-14). These include (1) uniformly distributed vascular markings with absence of the normal lower lobe vascular predominance, (2) right descending pulmonary artery diameter that exceeds 17 mm, and (3) pulmonary artery branch that is larger than its accompanying bronchus (best noted in the right parahilar area). Prominent vascularity is apparent only if the pulmonary-to-systemic flow ratio is greater than 1.5 : 1. As a rule, cardiac enlargement usually implies a shunt greater than 2.5 : 1. Anemia, pregnancy, thyrotoxicosis, and a pulmonary AV fistula may mimic shunt vascularity.

Cyanotic Patients with Shunt Vascularity. This group includes single ventricle with transposition, persistent truncus arteriosus, tricuspid atresia without significant pulmonary outflow obstruction, total anomalous pulmonary venous connection, double-outlet right ventricle, and a common atrium.

Cyanotic Patients with a VSD and Normal or Decreased Pulmonary Vascularity. This group includes tetralogy of Fallot, tricuspid atresia with pulmonary stenosis, single ventricle and pulmonary stenosis, D-TGA with pulmonary stenosis, cc-TGA with pulmonary stenosis, double-outlet right ventricle with pulmonary stenosis, pulmonary atresia, and asplenia syndrome.

Causes of Retrosternal Filling on Lateral Chest Radiograph. These include right ventricular dilation, TGA, ascending aortic aneurysm, and noncardiovascular masses (e.g., lymphoma, thymoma, teratoma, thyroid).

Causes of a Straight Left-Sided Heart Border. These include right ventricular dilation, left atrial dilation, cc-TGA, pericardial effusion, Ebstein anomaly, and congenital absence of the left pericardium.

Cardiovascular Diseases Associated with Scoliosis. These include cyanotic CHD, Eisenmenger syndrome, Marfan syndrome, and occasionally mitral prolapse.

Causes of Large Central Pulmonary Arteries. These include increased pulmonary flow (main pulmonary artery and branches), increased pulmonary pressure (main pulmonary artery and branches), pulmonary stenosis (main and left pulmonary artery), and idiopathic dilation of the pulmonary artery (main pulmonary artery).

Situs Solitus with Cardiac Dextroversion. Situs solitus with cardiac dextroversion is associated with CHD in more than 90% of cases. Up to 80% have a congenitally corrected transposition with a high incidence of associated VSD, pulmonary stenosis, and tricuspid atresia. Situs inversus with dextrocardia carries a low incidence of CHD, whereas situs inversus with levocardia is virtually always associated with severe CHD.

Cardiovascular Magnetic Resonance Imaging

CMR (see Chap. 18) in adolescents and adults with CHD has become of ever-increasing importance in the past decade. CMR can circumvent the echocardiographic problem of suboptimal visualization of the heart in adult patients, especially those who have had surgery. This technique can now generate information never previously available and do so more easily and more accurately than by other means. New magnetic resonance image acquisition methods are faster and provide improved temporal and spatial resolution. Major advances in hardware design, new pulse sequences, and faster image reconstruction techniques now permit rapid high-resolution imaging of complex cardiovascular anatomy. CMR can produce quantitative measures of ventricular volumes, mass, and ejection fraction. CMR can quantify blood flow in any vessel.

CMR is of particular value when transthoracic echocardiography cannot provide the needed diagnostic information; as an alternative to diagnostic cardiac catheterization; and for its unique capabilities, such as tissue imaging, myocardial tagging, and vessel-specific flow quantification. The value of CMR over echocardiography in the evaluation of the right ventricle is becoming increasingly appreciated. The capability of CMR to assess the right ventricle is of great importance because the right ventricle is a key component of many of the more complex CHD lesions. In addition, CMR can evaluate valve regurgitation, postoperative systemic and pulmonary venous pathways, Fontan pathways, and the great vessels. CMR should be considered the main imaging modality in adolescents and adults with repaired tetralogy of Fallot, TGA, Fontan procedure, and diseases of the aorta. In the near future, we will see real-time CMR to allow magnetic resonance–guided interventional procedures and molecular imaging that will further expand the capabilities of CMR.

Transthoracic Echocardiography (see Chap. 15)

FETAL ECHOCARDIOGRAPHY

General Considerations

Fetal echocardiography has graduated from being a special area of interest to some pediatric cardiologists to one of standard care. As early as 16 weeks' gestation, excellent images of the fetal cardiac structures can be obtained by the transabdominal route, along with an appreciation of cardiac and placental physiology through the use of Doppler technology. Transvaginal ultrasound is a newer approach that permits the echocardiographer to obtain images at approximately 13 to 14 weeks' gestation. Data are beginning to emerge as to the benefit of this approach, although current opinion would support a follow-up cardiac screen at 18 weeks' gestation. Although it has some application for cases with a higher risk of recurrent CHD (e.g., obstructive left-sided lesions), its accuracy has yet to be determined. This is in part due to the limited number of views that are possible because of a relatively fixed position of the transducer. Although there are specific indications for fetal echocardiographic scanning, the highest number of cases arise from anatomic or functional abnormalities detected at routine obstetric screening. A routine anatomic screen has become a standard of care in many obstetric practices throughout the world. As a result, there has been a tremendous push by pediatric fetal echocardiographers to improve the standard of routine screening of the prenatal heart. A rapid rise has occurred in the number of abnormalities that are detected by general obstetric ultrasonographers and subsequently referred in a timely manner to the pediatric cardiologist and echocardiographer. Nevertheless, the routine detection rate in unselected populations is still less than 50%.

Impact of Fetal Echocardiography

Most major structural congenital heart defects are now accurately categorized through fetal echocardiography. Once the abnormalities are identified, families and obstetric caregivers can be counseled as to the impact of the abnormality on both the fetus and the family. Decisions appropriate to the individual family and fetus can then be made. Although termination of pregnancy is one of the consequences of prenatal diagnosis, it is not the main objective. In fact, data are starting to appear in the literature indicating that prenatal diagnosis of some major cardiac malformations has a direct impact on outcome, from a survival, morbidity, and cost standpoint. This is in part due to the fact that when a prenatal diagnosis is made, subsequent caregivers are prepared for the immediate postnatal effects of the defect. For example, in hypoplastic left heart syndrome and other duct-dependent lesions, prostaglandin E_1 can be started immediately after birth, in a hospital within or attached to a pediatric cardiology facility.

Fetal echocardiography has also permitted an improved understanding of the evolution of certain congenital cardiac malformations. For example, although the fetal heart is fully formed by the time a prenatal scan is performed, tremendous growth of the cardiac structures still must occur. Therefore, in some circumstances, a cardiac chamber that may appear only mildly hypoplastic at 16 weeks' gestation may be profoundly affected at the time of birth. This has a major impact on the management of the newborn as well as on the counseling process at 16 weeks' gestation.

Direct Fetal Intervention

The next step is direct intervention for specific cardiac lesions. This has initially involved obstructive lesions, thus far mainly being limited to the left ventricle.[25] The rationale behind this therapy is based on the notion that the relief of obstructive outflow tract lesions will permit growth of the affected ventricle, potentially changing a neonatal pathway from univentricular to biventricular. Cardiac surgery to the fetus is also a future option, and indeed there is already a considerable amount of research on the impact of this in fetal animal models.

SEGMENTAL APPROACH TO ECHOCARDIOGRAPHY IN CONGENITAL HEART DISEASE. The following four echocardiographic steps of segmental analysis are crucial in any patient with CHD. Starting from a standard subcostal view, one should determine the position of the apex, the situs of the atria, and the atrioventricular and ventriculoarterial relationships.

1. *Apex position.* From a standard subcostal view, determine if the apex of the heart is pointing to the right (dextrocardia), to the left (levocardia), or to the middle (mesocardia).

2. *Situs of the atria* (**Fig. 65-2**). The right and left atria differ morphologically with regard to their appendages. A morphologic right atrium has a broad right atrial appendage, whereas a morphologic left atrium has a narrow left atrial appendage. Right and left atrial appendages, however, are difficult to visualize by transthoracic echocardiography, and one often has to rely on abdominal situs to determine the atrial situs. Atrial situs follows abdominal situs in about 70% to 80% of the cases. From a standard subcostal view with the probe pointing at a right angle to the spine, one can visualize the abdominal aorta as well as the inferior vena cava and the spine at the back. When the aorta is to the left of the spine and the inferior vena cava to the right of the spine, there is abdominal situs solitus and, in all probability, corresponding atrial situs solitus (meaning the morphologic right atrium is on the right side and the morphologic left atrium is on the left side). When the aorta is to the right of the spine and the inferior vena cava is to the left of the spine, there is abdominal situs inversus and, in all probability, corresponding atrial situs inversus (morphologic right atrium on the left side and morphologic left atrium on the right side). When both the aorta and inferior vena cava are to the left of the spine, there is abdominal and atrial left isomerism (two morphologic left atria). When both the aorta and inferior vena cava are to the right of the spine, there is abdominal and atrial right isomerism (two morphologic right atria).

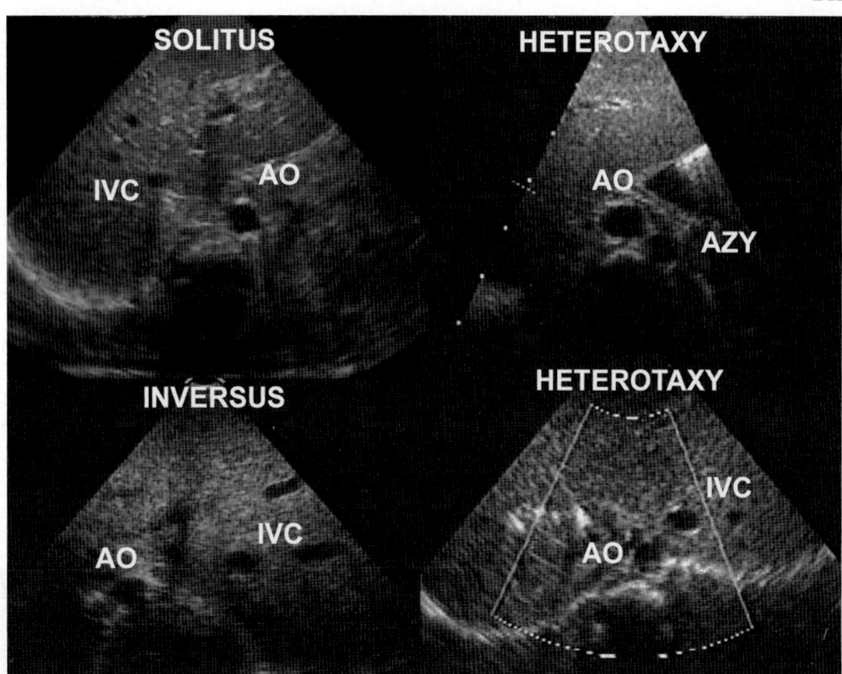

FIGURE 65-2 Montage of the different types of situs as seen by a subcostal echocardiographic scan. Note that situs solitus and inversus are just the mirror image of each other. The upper right picture is in the setting of heterotaxy with an interrupted intrahepatic inferior vena cava, with azygos continuation on the left. This is seen more frequently in left atrial isomerism. The lower right picture is also in the setting of heterotaxy with an intrahepatic inferior vena cava that is positioned closer to the aorta than in solitus or inversus. Note also the midline liver. This pattern is seen more commonly in right atrial isomerism. AO = aorta; AZY = azygos; IVC = inferior vena cava.

3. *Atrioventricular relationship.* Once the situs of the atria is determined, one must assess the position of the ventricles in relation to the atria. The morphologic right ventricle has four characteristic features that distinguish it from the morphologic left ventricle: a trabeculated apex, a moderator band, a septal attachment of the tricuspid valve, and a lower (apical) insertion of the tricuspid valve. The tricuspid valve is always attached to the morphologic right ventricle. The morphologic left ventricle has the following characteristics: a smooth apex, no moderator band, no septal attachment of the mitral valve, and a higher (basal) insertion of the mitral valve. The mitral valve is always attached to the morphologic left ventricle. Once the position of the ventricles is determined, one can then establish the AV relationship. When the morphologic right atrium empties into the morphologic right ventricle and the morphologic left atrium empties into the morphologic left ventricle, there is AV concordance. When the morphologic right atrium empties into the morphologic left ventricle and the morphologic left atrium empties into the morphologic right ventricle, there is AV discordance. When both atria predominantly empty into one ventricle (right or left), the AV connection is called a double-inlet.
4. *Ventriculoarterial relationship.* Once the AV relationship has been determined, one should assess the position of the great arteries in relation to the ventricles. The pulmonary artery can be distinguished by its early branching pattern into the left and right pulmonary arteries; the pulmonary valve is always attached to the pulmonary artery. Similarly, the aorta can be distinguished by its "candy cane" shape and the takeoff of its three head and neck vessels (innominate, carotid, and subclavian arteries). The aortic valve is always attached to the aorta. Once the position of the great arteries is determined, one can then establish the ventriculoarterial relationship. When the morphologic right ventricle ejects into the pulmonary artery and the morphologic left ventricle ejects into the aorta, there is ventriculoarterial concordance. When the morphologic right ventricle ejects into the aorta and the morphologic left ventricle ejects into the pulmonary artery, there is ventriculoarterial discordance. When more than 50% of both great arteries exit from one ventricle (right or left), this is called a double-outlet (right or left) ventricle.

Once segmental analysis has been completed, one can then proceed to the usual echocardiographic windows to determine the nature of the specific lesions as well as their hemodynamic relevance.

ECHOCARDIOGRAPHY IN THE NEONATE AND INFANT. Echocardiography is of immense value in differentiating between heart disease and lung disease in newborns. Indeed, it has become the standard for the diagnosis of virtually all cardiovascular malformations. Most neonates and infants needing intervention are now referred directly after ultrasound study for repair, without intervening cardiac catheterization. It is simpler to list those lesions for which it cannot be used as the sole mode of investigation before a management decision is made. For example, in pulmonary atresia and VSD with multiple aortopulmonary collaterals, echocardiography is used as an adjunct to angiocardiography. Echocardiography provides details about the intracardiac disease, whereas angiocardiography is necessary to delineate the sources of pulmonary blood supply. In pulmonary atresia with intact ventricular septum, the presence or absence of a right ventricle–dependent coronary circulation is best assessed by angiocardiography. Apart from these two lesions, there are few other preoperative decisions that cannot be made by echocardiography alone in the newborn and infant. Postoperative management is different, particularly for those defects that are on a Fontan track, when precise hemodynamic measurements are of key importance in the decision process.

Transesophageal echocardiography (TEE) is usually unnecessary for the preoperative evaluation of the neonate or infant with heart disease. This technique has now become a standard in the immediate postoperative period for the evaluation of residual anatomic or functional abnormalities. Newer techniques, such as tissue Doppler and three-dimensional echocardiography, are being applied to this age group and will be used more widely in the future.

ECHOCARDIOGRAPHY IN THE OLDER CHILD AND ADOLESCENT. This technique still plays a key role in the diagnosis and follow-up of the older child and adolescent with congenital or acquired heart disease. Because many of the patients underwent surgery in the neonatal or infant period, they often have suboptimal ultrasound windows that necessitate other modes of investigation, especially magnetic resonance angiography. The application of newer technologies, such as tissue Doppler and three-dimensional echocardiography, is already possible in this population and provides additional information that has thus far not been obtainable from standard techniques. For example, force-frequency relationships have been obtained in postoperative patients to try to predict optimal heart rates for maintaining maximum cardiac efficiency. On the other hand, three-dimensional echocardiography can provide new insights into congenital and acquired heart disease[26] that have not been possible from standard two-dimensional techniques. Despite the new information from this technique, it is still limited by the quality of the transthoracic window, which is more of a problem in the older and previously repaired patient. This limitation has been partially overcome by the recent introduction of a real-time three-dimensional TEE matrix array probe, which can be used in children with a weight of >16 to 18 kg (**Fig. 65-3**).

ECHOCARDIOGRAPHY IN THE ADULT. Advances in cardiac ultrasonography now allow comprehensive noninvasive assessment of cardiovascular structure and function in adults with CHD. Because of its widespread availability, easy use, and quick interpretation, transthoracic echocardiography remains the technique of choice for the initial diagnosis and for follow-up in adults with CHD. The general initial approach to the diagnosis of CHD by transthoracic echocardiography starts with a segmental approach to ascertain the relative position of the various cardiac chambers. Once the segmental approach has been completed, a more lesion-specific approach can then be carried out, as discussed in the individual lesion sections.

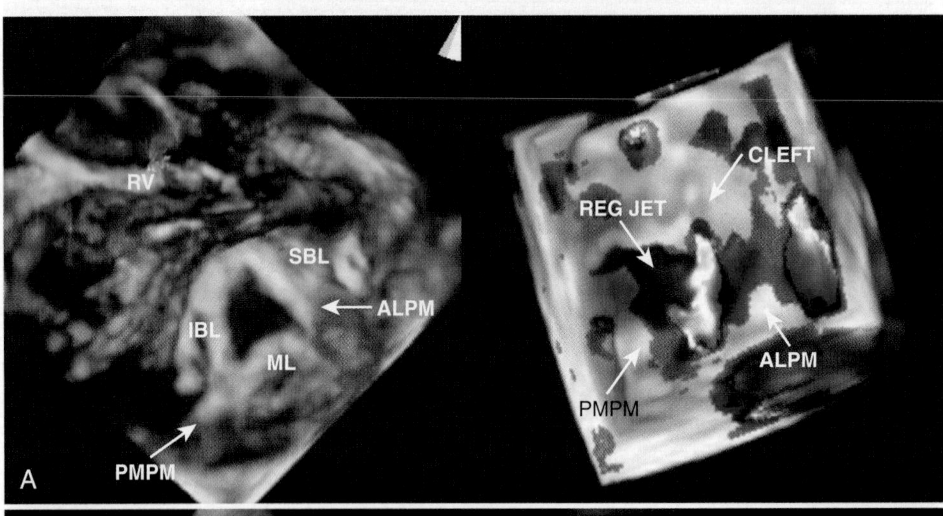

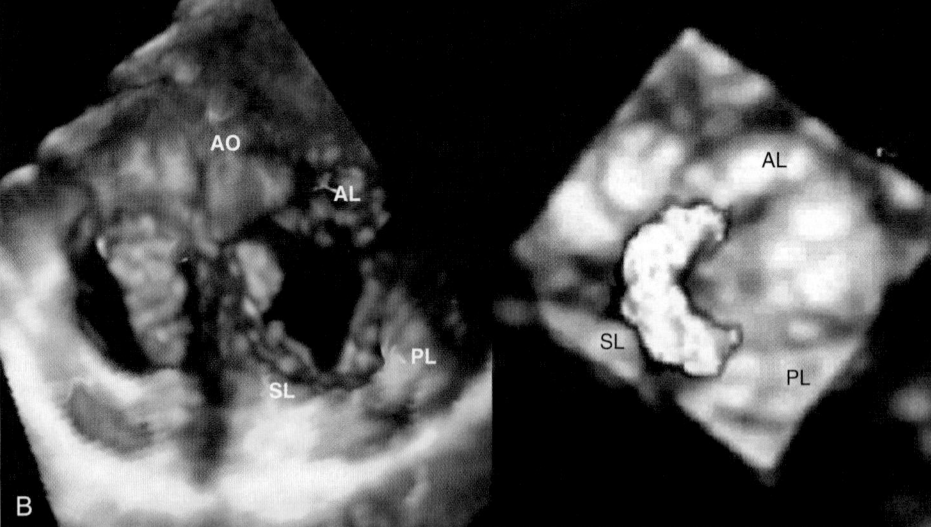

FIGURE 65-3 **A,** This montage is from a child with an atrioventricular septal defect with left atrioventricular valve regurgitation. This was acquired by real-time three-dimensional echocardiography from the transthoracic approach. The valve is viewed from beneath and the three leaflets that constitute the left atrioventricular valve can be clearly identified. The image on the right, also viewed from below, demonstrates the left atrioventricular valve regurgitation that originates at the cleft, directed toward the inferior bridging leaflet and mural leaflet commissure. ALPM = anterolateral papillary muscle; IBL = inferior bridging leaflet; ML = mural leaflet; PMPM = posteromedial papillary muscle; RV = right ventricle; SBL = superior bridging leaflet. **B,** These images were obtained with the real-time transesophageal three-dimensional probe in an adolescent. They demonstrate the tricuspid valve, as seen from above in a surgical view, with evidence of a cleft in the septal leaflet, which is the site of regurgitation seen in the right-hand image. Note the detail with the regurgitation involving the coaptation of the whole septal leaflet. AO = aorta; AL = anterior leaflet; PL = posterior leaflet; SL = septal leaflet.

Transesophageal Echocardiography

DIAGNOSTIC ASSESSMENT. TEE offers a better two-dimensional resolution than transthoracic echocardiography. This is especially important in adult patients with multiple previous cardiac operations, when adequate transthoracic windows are often difficult to obtain.

TEE should be used whenever transthoracic echocardiography does not provide adequate two-dimensional, color, or Doppler information. The addition of real-time three-dimensional TEE has opened up a new window in this age group.[13] TEE should be considered in the setting of the conditions discussed in the following sections.

Secundum Atrial Septal Defect. Use TEE for assessment of device closure feasibility, measurement of ASD size, assessment of adequacy of margins for device anchoring, and ruling out of anomalous pulmonary venous connection. This information can be enhanced by real-time three-dimensional imaging, which provides precise anatomic detail of the ASD.

Mitral Regurgitation. Use TEE for preoperative evaluation of mitral valve leaflet morphology and suitability for mitral valve repair versus replacement. Real-time three-dimensional TEE is rapidly becoming the reference standard for evaluation of mitral valve form and function before surgical or catheter intervention.[13]

Ebstein Anomaly. Use TEE for preoperative assessment of tricuspid valve morphology and the potential for tricuspid valve repair.

Fontan. Use TEE when a right atrial clot is suspected on clinical grounds or by transthoracic echocardiography or when circuit obstruction is suspected.

Before Cardioversion. For any patient who is not anticoagulated, presenting with atrial flutter or fibrillation longer than 24 hours, TEE should be performed before chemical or electrical cardioversion. Patients with a Fontan circuit should undergo TEE irrespective of the duration of atrial tachyarrhythmia to rule out a right or left atrial thrombus.

Guidance of Therapeutic Intervention. Both standard two-dimensional TEE and, more recently, real-time three-dimensional TEE can be instrumental in helping guide therapy at the time of transcatheter or surgical procedures. TEE is particularly helpful in the following situations.

Percutaneous Device Closure. TEE is performed at the time of transcatheter ASD closure to assist ASD stretched balloon sizing and device deployment, unless intracardiac echocardiography (see later) is available.

Intraoperative and Postoperative Assessment. TEE is often required for the intraoperative and postoperative assessment of the adult patient undergoing congenital cardiac surgery. It has a particular role in the intraoperative assessment of adequacy of valve repair. A TEE service by an experienced echocardiographer is an essential requirement for centers performing adult congenital cardiac surgery.

Three-Dimensional Echocardiography

Diagnostic Assessment. Three-dimensional echocardiography has advanced from the research arena to a clinical tool with the advent of transthoracic and transesophageal real-time systems.[13] Although much of it still depends on an adequate transthoracic window, this is readily overcome in the adult population through the application of real-time three-dimensional TEE techniques. Indeed, for mitral valve assessment, this technique has already established itself as the standard before intervention (**Fig. 65-4**).[14] In addition, this technique can be used to improve the accuracy of left ventricular volume calculation by echocardiography.[27,28]

Intracardiac Echocardiography

Intracardiac echocardiography (ICE) uses lower frequency transducers that have been miniaturized and mounted into catheters capable of percutaneous insertion into the heart.[29] ICE not only provides high-resolution two-dimensional and hemodynamic data with full Doppler capabilities but also eliminates the need for general anesthesia, which is often required for TEE.

Current Applications

Percutaneous ASD Device Closure. ICE supports percutaneous ASD device closure by adequately sizing the defect and assisting device positioning while avoiding the need for general anesthesia. More recently, real-time three-dimensional TEE is being used not only to assess the size and suitability for ASD device closure but to monitor the procedure, either in an interventional setting or surgically by use of robotic procedures.[30]

Electrophysiologic Studies. ICE assists electrophysiologic procedures by guiding transseptal puncture, enabling endocardial visualization, and ensuring electrode-tissue contact at the time of ablative procedures. More recently, a forward-looking imaging and ablation probe has been developed, which would enable precise localization of energy delivery to an arrhythmogenic focus[31] (see Chap. 36).

Cardiac Catheterization

With the development of cross-sectional echocardiography and the subsequent introduction of CMR and fast computed tomography (CT) methods, truly diagnostic cardiac catheterization (see Chap. 20) is becoming a thing of the past for both children and adults. "Diagnostic" catheterization is reserved for resolving unanswered questions from the less-invasive techniques and measuring hemodynamics. A good example of this is the assessment of major aortopulmonary collateral arteries in tetralogy of Fallot with pulmonary atresia; their presence and distribution may be shown beautifully by magnetic resonance angiography, but cardiac catheterization may be required to demonstrate the presence of communications with the central pulmonary arteries and to measure the pressure within them. There is no adequate substitute for cardiac catheterization to measure ventricular end-diastolic pressures or pulmonary artery pressures and resistance with the precision required to plan for or to assess the Fontan circulation. Furthermore, diagnostic testing may also be needed to evaluate possible coronary artery disease, especially before heart surgery in the adult.

THERAPEUTIC CATHETERIZATION. Balloon atrial septostomy was the first catheter intervention that proved useful in treating heart disease, and it remains the standard initial palliation in many infants with D-TGA. Many transcatheter techniques are now used successfully to treat CHD: blade atrial septostomy; device or coil closure of PDA; closure of ASD and patent foramen ovale; transluminal balloon dilation of pulmonary and aortic valve stenosis; radiofrequency perforation of pulmonary valve atresia; balloon-expandable intravascular stents for right ventricular outflow tract, pulmonary artery, aortic coarctation, and other vascular stenoses; and device occlusion of unwanted collateral vessels and AV fistulas. These have all become treatments of choice in centers with these capabilities. Some are universally accepted as the standard of care (e.g., balloon pulmonary valvuloplasty), whereas debate continues for other interventions (e.g., unrepaired coarctation). One of the most exciting recent developments has been that of transcatheter valved stents for the treatment of right ventricular outflow stenosis and regurgitation in patients with congenital defects, which has led to an explosion of transcatheter valve techniques for acquired disease.

Going along with the extraordinary expansion of interventional techniques for the treatment of structural abnormalities, ablative techniques for the treatment of tachycardias are now performed routinely in centers with congenital heart electrophysiology programs and are crucial to the management of the adult with repaired and unrepaired CHD, in whom arrhythmias are such a burden in terms of their morbidity as well as a significant cause of late mortality.

The indications, outcomes, and current status of each of these techniques are discussed in detail in the sections concerning specific lesions.

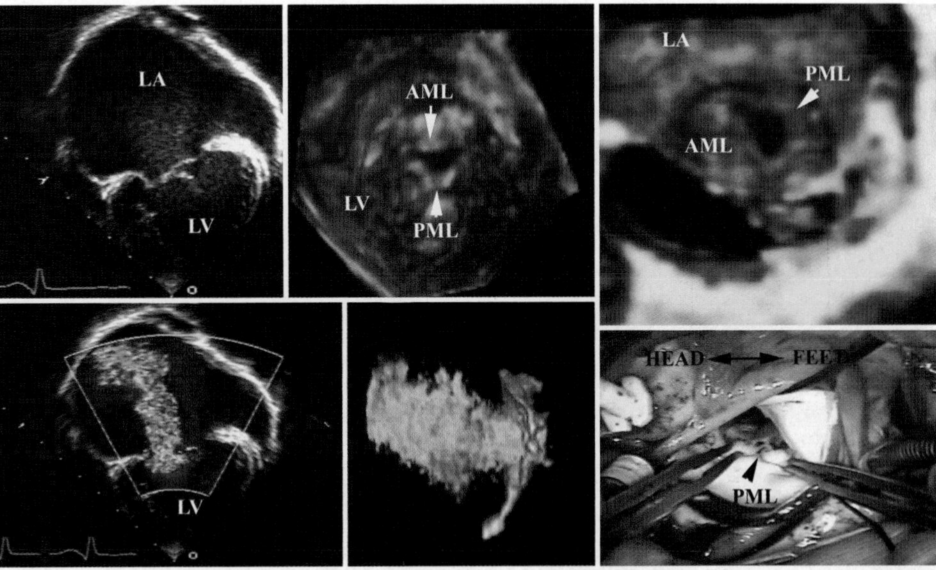

FIGURE 65-4 This montage is from a patient with a congenitally dysplastic mitral valve and significant mitral valve regurgitation. The two left-hand images show the transthoracic four-chamber view during systole. Note the large central jet of regurgitation. The upper middle panel is a real-time three-dimensional image of the mitral valve as seen from below. Note the tethered posterior leaflet. The lower middle panel shows the three-dimensional regurgitant jet. The upper right-hand panel views the mitral valve from above. Note the poor coaptation of the two leaflets. The lower right-hand panel is the surgical view of the valve that demonstrates the tethering of the posterior leaflet. AML = anterior mitral leaflet; LA = left atrium; LV = left ventricle; PML = posterior mitral leaflet.

Specific Cardiac Defects

Left-to-Right Shunts

Atrial Septal Defect

MORPHOLOGY. Four types of ASDs or interatrial communications exist: ostium primum, ostium secundum, sinus venosus, and coronary sinus defects (**Fig. 65-5**). (Ostium primum is discussed in the section on AV septal defect.) Ostium secundum defects occur from either excessive resorption of the septum primum or deficient growth of the septum secundum and are occasionally associated with anomalous pulmonary venous connection (<10%). Sinus venosus defects of the superior vena cava type occur at the cardiac junction of the superior vena cava, giving rise to a superior vena cava connected to both atria, and are almost always associated with anomalous pulmonary venous connection (right » left). Sinus venosus–inferior vena cava defects are very uncommon and abut the junction of the inferior vena cava, inferior to the fossa ovalis. Coronary sinus septal defects are rare and arise from an opening of its wall with the left atrium, allowing left-to-right atrial shunting.

PATHOPHYSIOLOGY. In any type of ASD, the degree of left-to-right atrial shunting depends on the size of the defect and the relative diastolic filling properties of the two ventricles. Any condition causing reduced left ventricular compliance (e.g., systemic hypertension, cardiomyopathy, myocardial infarction) or increased left atrial pressure (mitral stenosis or regurgitation) tends to increase the left-to-right shunt. If similar forces are present in the right side of the heart, this will diminish the left-to-right shunt and promote right-to-left shunting.

NATURAL HISTORY. A large ASD (pulmonary artery blood flow relative to systemic blood flow $[Q_p/Q_s] > 2.0:1.0$) may cause congestive heart failure and failure to thrive in an infant or child. An undetected ASD with a significant shunt ($Q_p/Q_s > 1.5:1.0$) probably causes symptoms over time in adolescence or adulthood, and symptomatic patients usually become progressively more physically limited as they age. Effort dyspnea is seen in about 30% of patients by the third decade and in more than 75% of patients by the fifth decade. Supraventricular arrhythmias (atrial fibrillation or flutter) and right-sided heart failure develop by 40 years of age in about 10% of patients and become more prevalent with aging. Paradoxical embolism resulting in a transient ischemic attack or stroke can call attention to the diagnosis. The development of pulmonary hypertension, although probably not as common as originally thought, can occur at an early age.[32] If pulmonary hypertension is severe, a second causative diagnosis should be sought. Life expectancy is clearly reduced in ASD patients, although not as severely as was quoted in earlier papers because only patients with large ASDs were described.

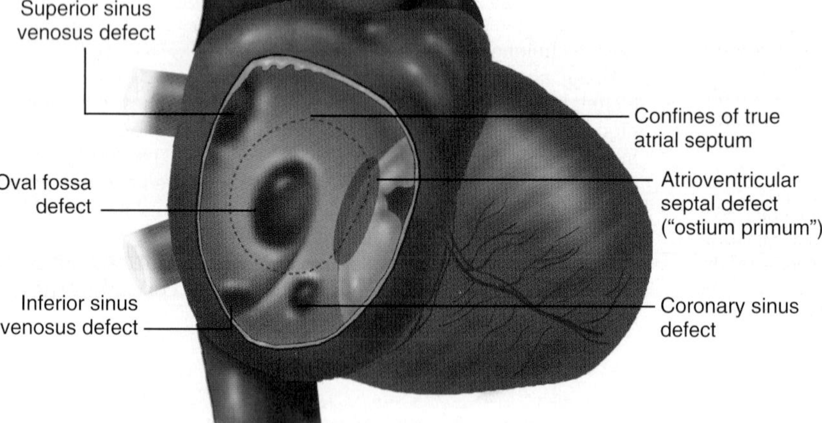

FIGURE 65-5 **A,** Schematic diagram outlining the different types of interatrial shunting that can be encountered. Note that only the central defect is suitable for device closure. **B,** Subcostal right anterior oblique view of a secundum atrial septal defect (asterisk) that is suitable for device closure. The right panel is a specimen as seen in a similar view, outlining the landmarks of the defect.

CLINICAL FEATURES

Pediatrics

Most children are asymptomatic, and the diagnosis is made after the discovery of a murmur. On occasion, increased pulmonary blood flow may be so great that congestive heart failure, recurrent chest infections, chronic wheezing, or even pulmonary hypertension may necessitate closure in infancy. Spontaneous closure of an ASD may occur within the first year of life. Even quite substantial defects diagnosed in the neonatal period (>7 mm) may reduce in size and not require later intervention. Thus, in asymptomatic children with an isolated secundum ASD, intervention is usually deferred so that elective device closure becomes an option if indicated.

Adults

The most common presenting symptoms in adults are exercise intolerance (exertional dyspnea and fatigue) and palpitations (typically from atrial flutter, atrial fibrillation, or sick sinus syndrome). Right ventricular failure can be the presenting symptom in older patients. The presence of cyanosis should alert one to the possibility of shunt reversal and Eisenmenger syndrome or, alternatively, to a prominent eustachian valve directing inferior vena cava flow to the left atrium via a secundum ASD or sinus venosus ASD of the inferior vena cava type.

On examination, there is "left atrialization" of the jugular venous pressure (A wave = V wave). A hyperdynamic right ventricular impulse may be felt at the left sternal border at the end of expiration or in the subxiphoid area on deep inspiration. A dilated pulmonary artery trunk may be palpated in the second left intercostal space. A wide and fixed split of S_2 is the auscultatory hallmark of ASD, although it is not always present. A systolic ejection murmur, usually grade 2 and often scratchy, is best heard at the second left intercostal space, and a mid-diastolic rumble, from increased flow through the tricuspid valve, may be present at the left lower sternal border. When right ventricular failure occurs, a pansystolic murmur of tricuspid regurgitation is usual.

Laboratory Investigations

Electrocardiography. Sinus rhythm or atrial fibrillation or flutter may be present. The QRS axis is typically rightward in secundum ASD. Negative P waves in the inferior leads indicate a low atrial pacemaker often seen in sinus venosus–superior vena cava defects, which are located in the area of the sinoatrial node and render it deficient. Complete right bundle branch block appears as a function of age. Tall R or R′ waves in V_1 often indicate pulmonary hypertension.

Chest Radiography. The classic radiographic features are of cardiomegaly (from right atrial and ventricular enlargement), dilated central pulmonary arteries with pulmonary plethora indicating increased pulmonary flow, and a small aortic knuckle (reflecting a chronic low cardiac output state).

Echocardiography. Transthoracic echocardiography documents the type and size (defect diameter) of the ASD (see Figs. 15-95, 15-96, and 15-97), the direction of the shunt (Fig. 65-5B), and sometimes the presence of anomalous pulmonary venous return. The functional importance of the defect can be estimated by the size of the right ventricle (see Fig. 15-94), the presence or absence of right ventricular volume overload (paradoxical septal motion), and the estimation of Q_p/Q_s. Indirect measurement of the pulmonary artery pressure can be obtained from the Doppler velocity of the tricuspid regurgitation jet. TEE permits better visualization of the interatrial septum and is usually required when device closure is contemplated, partly to ensure that pulmonary venous drainage is normal. ICE can be used instead of TEE during device closure to help guide device insertion, reducing the fluoroscopy and procedural time and forgoing the need for general anesthesia.[33]

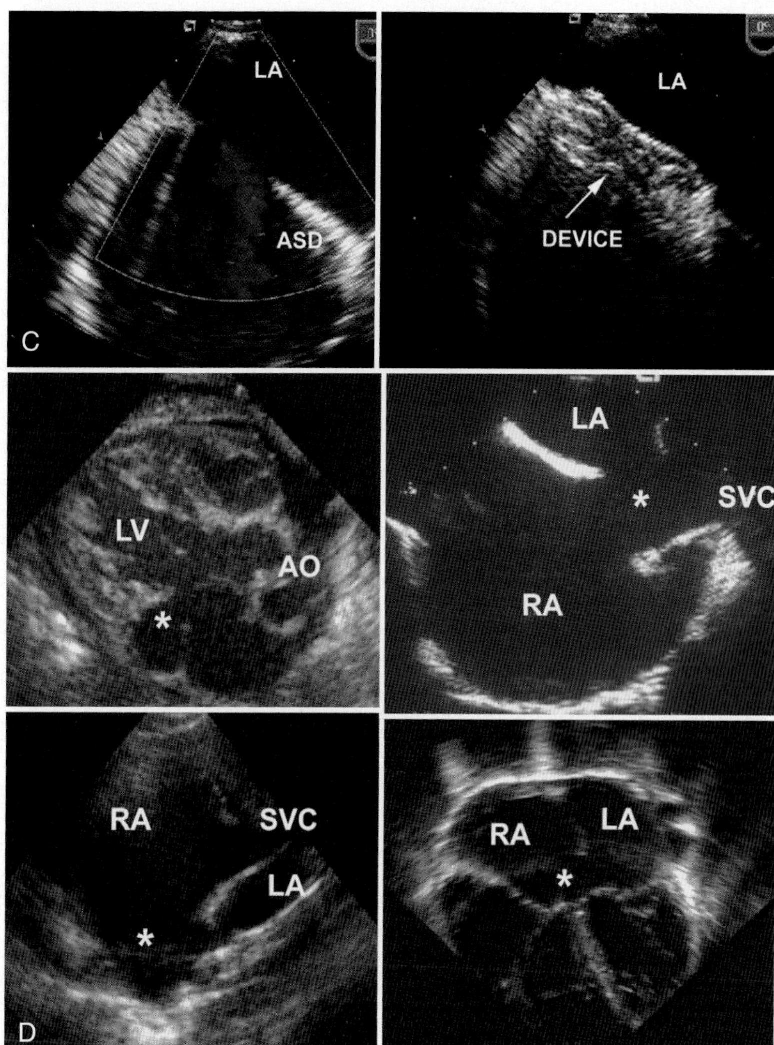

FIGURE 65-5, cont'd C, Transesophageal echocardiogram with color flow before device closure (left) and after release of an Amplatzer device (right). **D,** Montage of interatrial communications that are not atrial septal defects (asterisks) and therefore not suitable for device closure. The upper left is a coronary sinus defect due to unroofing; the top right is a superior sinus venosus defect; the bottom left is an inferior sinus venosus defect; and the bottom right is an atrial septal defect in the setting of an atrioventricular septal defect. AO = aorta; ASD = atrial septal defect; CS = coronary sinus; Eust = eustachian; IVC = inferior vena cava; LA = left atrium; LV = left ventricle; RA = right atrium; SVC = superior vena cava; Tric = tricuspid.

INDICATIONS FOR INTERVENTION. In asymptomatic children, the decision to intervene is based on the presence of right-sided heart dilation and a significant ASD (>5 mm) that shows no sign of spontaneous closure. Shunt fractions are now rarely measured and are reserved for "borderline" cases. Hemodynamically insignificant ASDs ($Q_p/Q_s < 1.5$) do not require closure, with the possible exception of trying to prevent paradoxical emboli in older patients after a stroke. "Significant" ASDs ($Q_p/Q_s > 1.5$, or ASDs associated with right ventricular volume overload) should be closed, especially if device closure is available and appropriate. For patients with pulmonary hypertension (pulmonary artery pressure > ⅔ systemic arterial blood pressure or pulmonary arteriolar resistance > ⅔ systemic arteriolar resistance), closure can be recommended if there is a net left-to-right shunt of at least 1.5:1 or evidence of pulmonary artery reactivity on challenge with a pulmonary vasodilator (e.g., oxygen or nitric oxide).

Device Closure

Device closure of secundum ASDs percutaneously under fluoroscopy and TEE or with intracardiac echocardiographic guidance is the therapy of choice when appropriate (Fig. 65-5C). Indications for device closure are the same as for surgical closure, but the selection criteria are stricter. Depending on the device, this technique is available only for patients with a secundum ASD with a stretched diameter of less than 41 mm and with adequate rims to enable secure deployment of the device. Anomalous pulmonary venous connection or proximity of the defect to the AV valves or coronary sinus or systemic venous drainage usually precludes the use of this technique. It is a safe and effective procedure in experienced hands, with major complications (e.g., device embolization, atrial perforation, thrombus formation[34]) occurring in less than 1% of patients and clinical closure achieved in more than 90% of patients. Device closure of an ASD improves functional status in symptomatic patients and exercise capacity in asymptomatic and symptomatic patients. Intermediate follow-up data have proved ASD device closure to be safe and effective,[35] with better preservation of right ventricular function[36] and lower complication rates than with surgery.[37]

Surgery

Device closure is not an option for those with sinus venosus or ostium primum defects or with secundum defects with unsuitable anatomy. Surgical closure of ASDs can be performed by primary suture closure or by use of a pericardial or synthetic patch. The procedure is usually performed through a midline sternotomy, but the availability of an inframammary or minithoracotomy approach to a typical secundum ASD should be made known to cosmetically sensitive patients. Surgical mortality in the adult without pulmonary hypertension should be less than 1%. Surgical closure of an ASD improves functional status and exercise capacity in symptomatic patients and improves (but usually does not normalize) survival and improves or eliminates congestive heart failure, especially when patients are operated on at an earlier age. However, surgical closure of ASD in adult life does not prevent atrial fibrillation or flutter or stroke, especially when patients are operated on after the age of 40 years. The role of a concomitant Cox maze procedure in patients with a prior history of atrial flutter or fibrillation should be considered[38] (see Chaps. 37 and 39).

REPRODUCTIVE ISSUES. Pregnancy is well tolerated in patients after ASD closure (see Chap. 82). Pregnancy is also well tolerated in women with unrepaired ASDs, but the risk of paradoxical embolism is increased (still only to a very low risk) during pregnancy and in the postpartum period. Pregnancy is contraindicated in Eisenmenger syndrome because of the high maternal (≈50%) and fetal (≈60%) mortality.

FOLLOW-UP. Most children with isolated secundum defect can be discharged to the care of their family physician 6 months after complete closure is confirmed, no matter whether it is surgical or by device. After device closure, patients require 6 months of aspirin and endocarditis prophylaxis until the device endothelializes, after which, assuming there is no residual shunt, they do not require any special precautions or endocarditis prophylaxis. Patients with sinus venosus defect are at risk for development of caval or pulmonary vein stenosis and should be kept under intermittent review. Patients who have had surgical or device repair as adults, patients with atrial arrhythmias preoperatively or postoperatively, and patients with ventricular dysfunction should remain under long-term cardiology surveillance.

Patent Foramen Ovale

ANATOMY. The foramen ovale is a tunnel-like space between the overlying septum secundum and septum primum and typically closes in 75% of people at birth by fusion of the septum primum and secundum. In utero, the foramen ovale is necessary for blood flow across the fetal atrial septum. Oxygenated blood from the placenta returns to the inferior vena cava, crosses the foramen ovale, and enters the systemic circulation. In about 25% of people, a patent foramen ovale (PFO) persists into adulthood. PFOs may be associated with atrial septal aneurysms (a redundancy of the interatrial septum), eustachian valves (a remnant of the sinus venosus valve), and Chiari networks (filamentous strands in the right atrium).

PATHOPHYSIOLOGY. PFOs have recently been scrutinized for their implication in the mechanism of cryptogenic stroke. Many of the basic tenets linking PFO and stroke seem plausible but have not been demonstrated. The current views may be summarized as follows. PFOs may serve either as a conduit for paradoxical embolization from the venous side to the systemic circulation or, because of their tunnel-like structure and propensity to stagnant flow, as a nidus for in situ thrombus formation. Variation in PFO size, right atrial anatomy, varying hemodynamic conditions, and occurrence of venous thrombi may all contribute to the chances of paradoxical embolization. The risk of a cryptogenic stroke seems increased for larger PFOs. The presence of an interatrial septal aneurysm in combination with a PFO also increases the risk of an adverse event, perhaps because of increased in situ thrombus formation in the aneurysmal tissue or simply because PFOs associated with an interatrial septal aneurysm tend to be larger. Eustachian valves and a Chiari network may direct blood flow from the inferior vena cava toward the atrial septum, encouraging right-to-left shunting in the presence of an interatrial communication. Physiologic (Valsalva maneuvers) and pathologic conditions increasing right ventricular pressure will raise the right atrial pressure, favoring right-to-left shunting. Finally, pelvic vein thrombi are found more frequently in young patients with cryptogenic stroke than in patients with a known cause of stroke[39] and may provide the source of venous thrombi.

PFOs have also been implicated in the pathophysiologic mechanism of decompression sickness (arterial gas embolism from the venous side) as well as more recently in the pathogenesis of migraine headaches.[40] Platypnea-orthodeoxia syndrome (dyspnea and arterial desaturation in the upright position, which improves on lying down) has also been attributed to the presence of a PFO.

CLINICAL IMPACT. The cause-and-effect relationship between PFO and cryptogenic stroke is still tentative and needs clarification. The recent body of literature would suggest a strong association, if not a causative link, especially in younger patients. Indeed, young patients with cryptogenic stroke have a significantly higher incidence of PFO (36% to 54%) than normal controls (15% to 25%). The association is more controversial in the population of older patients. Older patients often have more risk factors for stroke, and the causative role of a PFO in these patients is more difficult to establish.

When a patient presents with a stroke and a PFO is discovered, the usual causes of stroke must first be eliminated. Potential causes of stroke include carotid artery disease, ascending aortic atherosclerosis, atrial fibrillation, neurovascular abnormalities, and prothrombotic tendencies. If, after an exhaustive investigation (see later), no other cause of the stroke can be found, the PFO may be seen to have possibly had a causative role. The diagnosis of a PFO as a cause of cryptogenic stroke is, at best, a diagnosis of exclusion.

INVESTIGATIONS. A PFO is usually detected by transthoracic echocardiography, transesophageal echocardiography, or transcranial Doppler study. Transesophageal echocardiography is the most sensitive test, especially when it is performed with contrast media injected during a cough or Valsalva maneuver (see Fig. 15-17). A PFO is judged to be present if microbubbles are seen in the left-sided cardiac chambers within three cardiac cycles from the maximum right atrial opacification.

Screening for prothrombotic states (e.g., protein C or S deficiency, antithrombin III, or lupus anticoagulant), atrial fibrillation, significant carotid atherosclerosis by carotid Doppler imaging, and neurovascular abnormalities by brain magnetic resonance angiography must be undertaken in each patient before a PFO can be considered a possible culprit.

THERAPEUTIC OPTIONS. Once the presumptive diagnosis of a cryptogenic stroke caused by a PFO is determined, treatment modalities to prevent recurrent events include antiplatelet or anticoagulant agents, percutaneous device closure (see Fig. 59-1),[41,42] and surgical PFO closure. Medical therapy for secondary prevention of stroke with warfarin or antiplatelet agents is often used as "first-line" therapy with similar efficacy, a yearly recurrence rate of about 2%. Patients with PFO and atrial septal aneurysm who have had strokes seem to be at higher risk of recurrent stroke (as high as 15% per year), and a preventive strategy other than aspirin or warfarin should perhaps be considered. Device closure is safe and seems effective, with a recurrence rate of stroke between 0% and 3.8% per year (see Chap. 59). Surgical closure of PFO is usually performed when cardiac surgery is required for other reasons.

Recent nonrandomized trials comparing anticoagulation and antiplatelet treatment showed a lower risk of recurrent events with anticoagulation.[41,42] Regarding medical management after a cryptogenic stroke, the available nonrandomized trials support anticoagulation for patients with PFO and atrial septal aneurysm and at least antiplatelet treatment for patients with PFO without atrial septal aneurysm. The recurrence rate of stroke after transcatheter closure of PFO is lower compared with trials that used medical treatment. For patients with atrial septal aneurysm or those with recurrent cryptogenic ischemic events, closure of the PFO should be considered to provide a lower recurrence rate of ischemic events and to avoid the bleeding risk associated with long-term anticoagulation.[43]

Randomized clinical trials comparing various treatment options are necessary before definitive recommendations for the optimal treatment of cryptogenic stroke can be made.

Atrioventricular Septal Defect

TERMINOLOGY. The terms *atrioventricular septal defect, atrioventricular canal defect,* and *endocardial cushion defect* can be used interchangeably to describe this group of defects. The variable components of these lesions are explained in the following sections.

MORPHOLOGY. The basic morphology of AV septal defect is common to all types and is independent of the presence or absence of an ASD or VSD. These common features (**Figs. 65-6** and **65-7**) are absence of the muscular AV septum (resulting in the AV valves being at the same level on echocardiographic examination), inlet/outlet disproportion (resulting in an elongated left ventricular outflow tract, the so-called goose-neck deformity), abnormal lateral rotation of the posteromedial papillary muscle, and abnormal configuration of the AV valves. The left AV valve is a trileaflet valve made of superior and inferior bridging leaflets separated by a mural leaflet. The space between the superior and inferior leaflets as they bridge the interventricular septum is called the cleft in the left AV valve. The bridging leaflets may be completely adherent to the crest of the interventricular septum, free floating, or attached by chordal apparatus.

Partitioned Versus Complete Atrioventricular Septal Defects. A partitioned orifice is one in which the superior and inferior leaflets are joined by a connecting tongue of tissue as they bridge the interventricular septum. This partitions the valve into separate left and right orifices. A common AV valve orifice is one in which there is no such connecting tongue, resulting in one large orifice that encompasses the left- and right-sided components. Interatrial (ostium primum) and interventricular defects are common in AV septal defect.

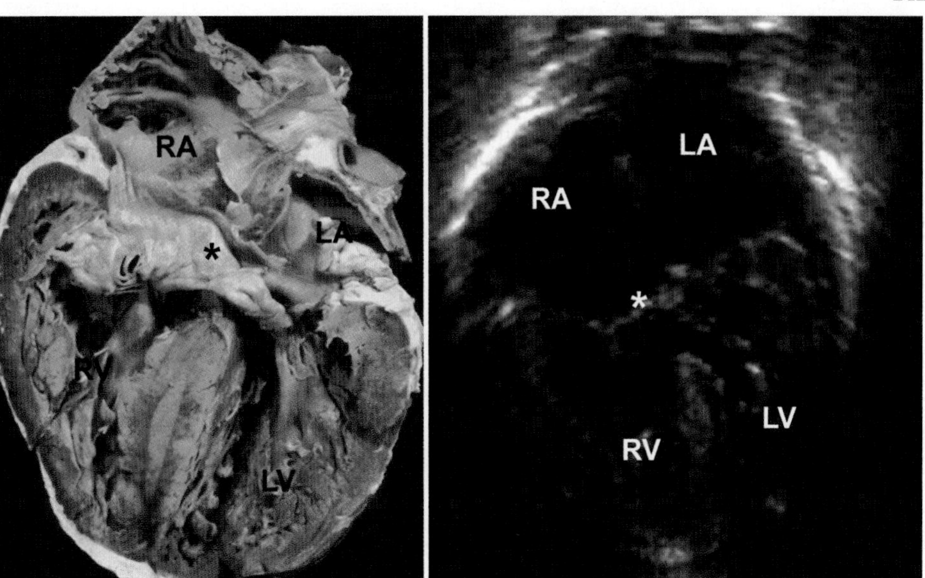

FIGURE 65-6 Apical four-chamber view in a complete atrioventricular septal defect with a common atrioventricular valve orifice (asterisk). Note the large interatrial and interventricular communications and the large free-floating superior bridging leaflet. LA = left atrium; LV = left ventricle; RA = right atrium; RV = right ventricle.

The left ventricular outflow tract is elongated and predisposes to subaortic stenosis. The papillary muscles are closer together than normal. The term *unbalanced AV septal defect* refers to cases in which one ventricle is hypoplastic. This is seen more commonly in patients with heterotaxy and those with left-sided obstructive defects.

Pathophysiology

Native. The pathophysiology of an isolated shunt at atrial level (commonly referred to as a primum ASD) is similar to that of a large secundum ASD, with unrestricted left-to-right shunting through the primum ASD, leading to right-sided atrial and ventricular volume overload. Chronic left AV valve regurgitation may produce left-sided ventricular and atrial volume overload. Complete AV septal defect has a greater degree of left-to-right shunting from the primum ASD as well as the nonrestrictive VSD, which triggers earlier left ventricular dilation and a greater degree of pulmonary hypertension.

After Correction. Residual significant left AV valve regurgitation may occur and cause significant left atrial as well as left ventricular dilation. Left AV valve stenosis from overzealous repair of the valve may also occur. The long, narrow left ventricular outflow tract of AV septal defect promotes left ventricular outflow tract obstruction and leads to subaortic stenosis in about 5% of patients.

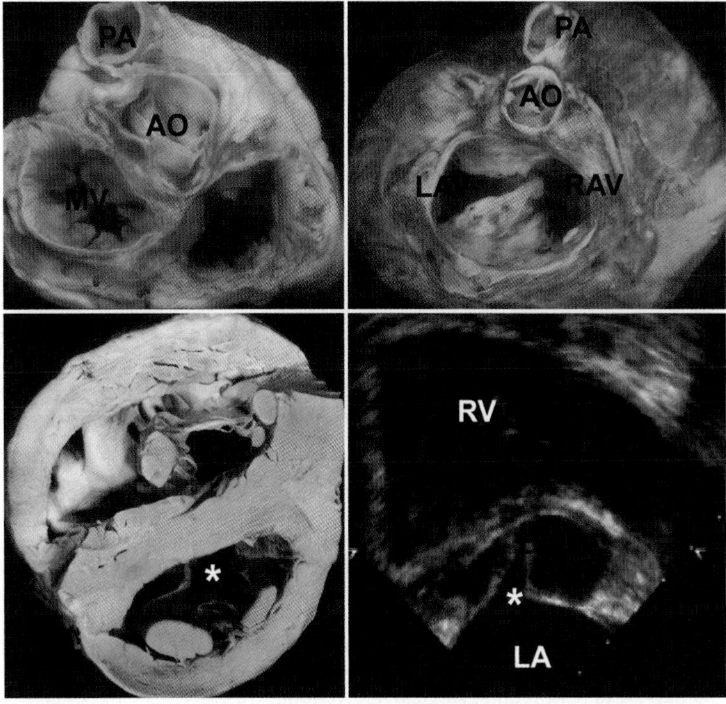

FIGURE 65-7 Montage comparing the normal atrioventricular junction with that seen in an atrioventricular septal defect. The upper left picture is the normal atrioventricular junction as seen from above. Note the normal morphology of the mitral and tricuspid valves, with the aorta wedged between them. The upper right picture is a similar view in an atrioventricular septal defect. Note the unwedged aorta, the trileaflet left atrioventricular valve, and the cleft between the superior and inferior bridging leaflets. The lower left picture is a specimen of an atrioventricular septal defect demonstrating the cleft. The lower right picture is an echocardiogram showing the cleft. AO = aorta; LA = left atrium; LAV = left atrioventricular valve; MV = mitral valve; PA = pulmonary artery; RAV = right atrioventricular valve; RV = right ventricle; TV = tricuspid valve.

NATURAL HISTORY. Patients with an isolated primum ASD have a course similar to that of those with large secundum ASDs, although symptoms may appear sooner when significant left AV valve regurgitation is present. Patients may be asymptomatic until their third or fourth decade, but progressive symptoms related to congestive heart failure, atrial arrhythmias, complete heart block, and variable degrees of pulmonary hypertension develop in virtually all of them by the fifth decade.

Most patients with complete AV septal defect have had surgical repair in infancy. Infants present with dyspnea, congestive heart failure, and failure to thrive. When presenting unrepaired, most adults have established pulmonary vascular disease. Patients with Down syndrome have a propensity for development of pulmonary hypertension at an even earlier age than do other patients with AV septal defect.

CLINICAL ISSUES

Down Syndrome

Down syndrome occurs in 35% of patients with AV septal defect. These patients more commonly have a complete AV septal defect with a common AV valve orifice and a large associated VSD. They often present in infancy with pulmonary hypertension. Clinical features are cardiomegaly, right ventricular heave, and pulmonary outflow tract murmur. If associated AV valve regurgitation exists, there is a pansystolic murmur.

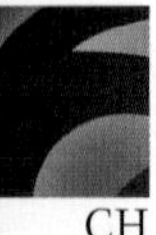

Non–Down Syndrome

Clinical presentation depends on the presence and size of the ASD and the VSD and on the competence of the left AV valve. A large left-to-right shunt gives rise to symptoms of heart failure (exertional dyspnea or fatigue) or pulmonary vascular disease (exertional syncope, cyanosis). In adulthood, palpitations from atrial arrhythmias are common. Cardiac findings on physical examination for patients with an isolated shunt at atrial level are similar to those of patients with secundum ASD, with the important addition of a prominent left ventricular apex and pansystolic murmur when significant left AV valve regurgitation is present. Cases with a primum ASD and a restrictive VSD have similar findings but with the addition of a pansystolic VSD murmur heard best at the left sternal border. Complete AV septal defects have a single S_1 (common AV valve), a mid-diastolic murmur from augmented AV valve inflow, and findings of pulmonary hypertension or a right-to-left shunt.

LABORATORY INVESTIGATIONS

ELECTROCARDIOGRAPHY. Most patients have left-axis deviation. Complete AV block and atrial fibrillation or flutter can be present in older patients. Partial or complete right bundle branch block is usually associated with right ventricular dilation or prior surgery.

CHEST RADIOGRAPHY. If the defect is unrepaired, this demonstrates cardiomegaly with right atrial and right ventricular prominence with increased pulmonary vascular markings. In those cases with a small interatrial communication and important left AV valve regurgitation, there is cardiomegaly due to left ventricular enlargement and normal pulmonary vascular markings. Findings of Eisenmenger syndrome are also possible. When the defect has been repaired, the study may be normal with sternal wires.

ECHOCARDIOGRAPHY. This has replaced angiography in assessing virtually all cases with AV septal defect. The cardinal and common features discussed in the morphology section are readily recognized by echocardiography. In the four-chamber view, the AV valves appear at the same level, irrespective of the presence or absence of a VSD. The typical inferior ASD and the posteriorly positioned VSD will be sought. The degree of associated AV valve regurgitation, the left-to-right shunt, and the estimated right ventricular systolic pressure should be determined. When the right AV valve is used to assess right ventricular pressure, care must be taken to ensure that the jet is not contaminated by an obligatory left ventricle to right atrial shunt.

CARDIAC CATHETERIZATION. In general, this technique has been replaced by echocardiography for the evaluation of patients with an AV septal defect. The one role it still has is in the evaluation of the patient who presents late and may have associated pulmonary vascular or coronary disease.

INDICATIONS FOR INTERVENTION. The patient with an unrepaired or newly diagnosed AV septal defect and significant hemodynamic defects requires surgical repair. Equally, patients with persistent left AV valve regurgitation (or stenosis from previous repair) causing symptoms, atrial arrhythmia, or deterioration in ventricular function, and patients with significant subaortic obstruction (a mean gradient >50 mm Hg at rest) require surgical intervention.

In the presence of severe pulmonary hypertension (pulmonary artery pressure > ⅔ systemic blood pressure or pulmonary arteriolar resistance > ⅔ systemic arteriolar resistance), there must be a net left-to-right shunt of at least 1.5:1 or evidence of pulmonary artery reactivity on challenge with a pulmonary vasodilator (e.g., oxygen, nitric oxide, prostaglandins).

INTERVENTIONAL OPTIONS AND OUTCOMES

Isolated Shunt at Atrial Level (Primum Atrial Septal Defect)

Pericardial patch closure of the primum ASD with concomitant suture (with or without annuloplasty) of the "cleft" left AV valve is usually performed. When left AV valve repair is not possible, replacement may be necessary. In the short term, the results of repair of partial AV septal defect are similar to those after closure of secundum ASD, but sequelae of left AV ("mitral") valve regurgitation,[44,45] subaortic stenosis, and AV block may develop or progress.

Complete Atrioventricular Septal Defect

The "staged approach" (pulmonary artery banding followed by intracardiac repair) has been supplanted by primary intracardiac repair in infancy. The goals of intracardiac repair are ventricular and atrial septation with adequate mitral and tricuspid reconstruction. Both single- and double-patch techniques to close ASDs and VSDs have been described with comparable results. On occasion, left AV valve replacement is necessary when valve repair is not possible. The intermediate results of repair of complete AV septal defect are good for Down syndrome patients as well as for non–Down syndrome patients,[46,47] with problems similar to those of partial AV septal defect.

REPRODUCTIVE ISSUES. Pregnancy is well tolerated in patients with complete repair and no significant residual lesions. Women in NYHA Classes I and II with unrepaired, isolated primum ASD usually tolerate pregnancy well. Pregnancy is contraindicated in Eisenmenger syndrome because of the high maternal (≈50%) and fetal (≈60%) mortality.

FOLLOW-UP ISSUES. All patients require periodic follow-up by an expert cardiologist because of the possibility of postoperative complications, which include patch dehiscence or residual septal defects (1%), development of complete heart block (3%), late atrial fibrillation or flutter, significant left AV valve dysfunction (10%), and subaortic stenosis (5% to 10%). Left AV valve regurgitation requires reoperation in at least 10% of patients. Subaortic stenosis develops or progresses in 5% to 10% of patients after repair, particularly in patients with primum ASD, especially if the left AV ("mitral") valve has been replaced. Particular attention should be paid to those patients with pulmonary hypertension preoperatively. Antibiotic prophylaxis is necessary only in the first 6 months after surgery unless there is residual patch leak or a prosthetic valve.

Isolated Ventricular Septal Defect

MORPHOLOGY. The ventricular septum can be divided into three major components—inlet, trabecular, and outlet—all abutting on a small membranous septum lying just underneath the aortic valve. VSDs (**Fig. 65-8**) are classified into three main categories according to their location and margins (**Fig. 65-9**). Muscular VSDs are bordered entirely by myocardium and can be trabecular, inlet, or outlet in location. Membranous VSDs often have inlet, outlet, or trabecular extension and are bordered in part by fibrous continuity between the leaflets of an AV valve and an arterial valve. Doubly committed subarterial VSDs are more common in Asian patients, are situated in the outlet septum, and are bordered by fibrous continuity of the aortic and pulmonary valves. This section deals with VSDs occurring in isolation from major associated cardiac anomalies.

PATHOPHYSIOLOGY. A restrictive VSD is a defect that produces a significant pressure gradient between the left ventricle and the right ventricle (pulmonary-to-aortic systolic pressure ratio < 0.3) and is accompanied by a small (≤1.4:1) shunt. A moderately restrictive VSD is accompanied by a moderate shunt (Q_p/Q_s of 1.4 to 2.2:1) with a pulmonary-to-aortic systolic pressure ratio less than 0.66. A large or nonrestrictive VSD is accompanied by a large shunt ($Q_p/Q_s > 2.2$) and a pulmonary-to-aortic systolic pressure ratio greater than 0.66. An Eisenmenger VSD has a systolic pressure ratio of 1 and Q_p/Q_s less than 1:1 or a net right-to-left shunt.

NATURAL HISTORY. A restrictive VSD does not cause significant hemodynamic derangement and may close spontaneously during childhood and sometimes in adult life. A perimembranous defect in an immediately subaortic position, or any doubly committed VSD, may be associated with progressive aortic regurgitation. Late development of subaortic and subpulmonary stenosis (see section on double-chambered right ventricle) and the formation of a left ventricular to right atrial shunt are well described and should be excluded at follow-up. A moderately restrictive VSD imposes a hemodynamic burden on the left ventricle, which leads to left atrial and ventricular dilation and dysfunction as well as a variable increase in pulmonary vascular resistance. A large or nonrestrictive VSD features left ventricular volume overload early in life with a progressive rise in pulmonary artery pressure and a fall in left-to-right shunting. In turn, this leads to higher pulmonary vascular resistance and eventually to Eisenmenger syndrome.

CLINICAL FEATURES

Pediatrics

Neonatal presentation with a murmur is increasingly frequent. Most of these patients have a restrictive defect, and the murmur becomes apparent only as the pulmonary vascular resistance falls. Paradoxically, those infants with large nonrestrictive defects tend to present later. This is because equalization of pressures across the defect obviates the generation of a pansystolic murmur. Instead, pulmonary blood flow increases progressively as the pulmonary vascular resistance falls. Presentation with breathlessness, congestive heart failure, and failure to thrive in the second and third months of life are usual. At that time, a pulmonary ejection murmur and a mitral rumble may be heard, reflecting increased pulmonary flow and pulmonary venous return. Cyanosis is rare in early childhood, and if it is present, other causes of a raised pulmonary vascular resistance should be excluded (e.g., mitral stenosis or coexisting lung disease).

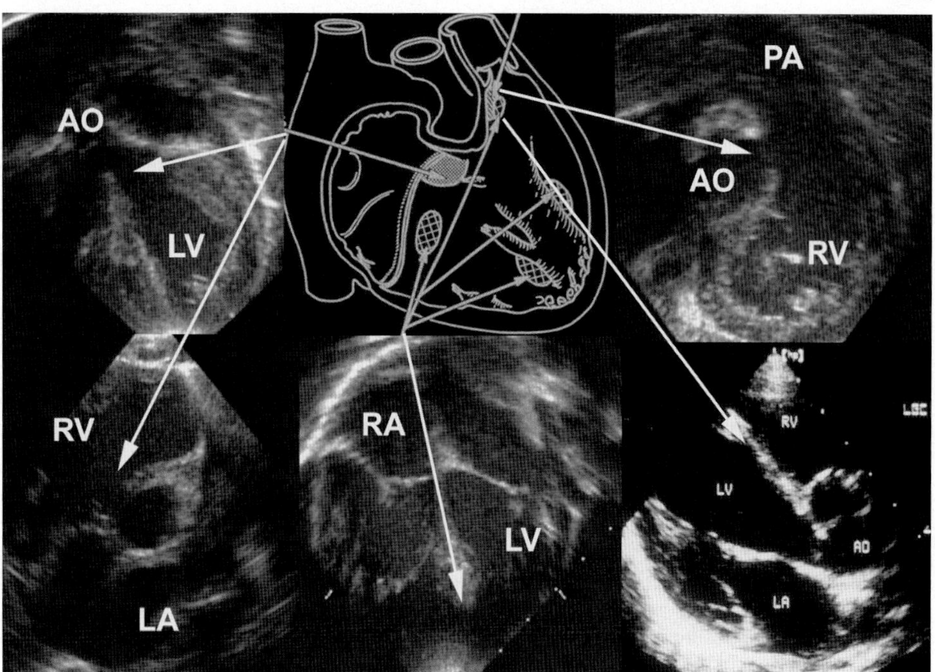

FIGURE 65-8 Montage of the different types of ventricular septal defects. The central diagram outlines the location of the various types of defects as seen from the right ventricle. The two left images show a perimembranous ventricular septal defect as seen in the five-chamber and short-axis views. Note that the defect is roofed by the aorta and is next to the tricuspid valve. The bottom middle echocardiogram is a muscular apical defect. The upper right image is a right anterior oblique view in a doubly committed ventricular septal defect. The lower right image is a short-axis view showing an outlet ventricular septal defect with prolapse of the right coronary cusp. AO = aorta; LA = left atrium; LV = left ventricle; PA = pulmonary artery; RA = right atrium; RV = right ventricle.

Medical management of the symptomatic infant is directed at improving symptoms before surgery or "buying time" while spontaneous closure or diminution in size occurs. Treatment with diuretics is universally accepted, and increasingly, the successful use of ACE inhibition is being reported.

Adults

Most adult patients with a small restrictive VSD are asymptomatic. Physical examination reveals a harsh or high-frequency pansystolic murmur, usually grade 3 to 4/6, heard with maximal intensity at the left sternal border in the third or fourth intercostal space. Patients with a moderately restrictive VSD often present with dyspnea in adult life, perhaps triggered by atrial fibrillation. Physical examination typically reveals a displaced cardiac apex with a similar pansystolic murmur as well as an apical diastolic rumble and third heart sound at the apex from the increased flow through the mitral valve. Patients with large nonrestrictive Eisenmenger VSDs present as adults with central cyanosis and clubbing of the nailbeds. Signs of pulmonary hypertension–a right ventricular heave, a palpable and loud P_2, and a right-sided S_4—are typically present. A pulmonary ejection click, a soft and scratchy systolic ejection murmur, and a high-pitched decrescendo diastolic murmur of pulmonary regurgitation (Graham Steell) may be audible. Peripheral edema usually reflects right-sided heart failure.

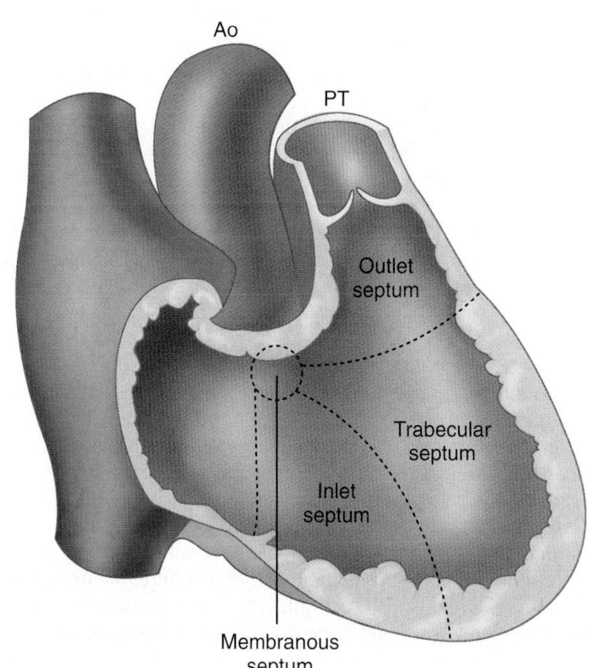

FIGURE 65-9 Four components of the ventricular septum shown here from the right ventricular aspect are now described by Anderson and associates as inlet and outlet components of the right ventricle because these areas do not correspond to septal structures as initially suggested. Ao = aorta; PT = pulmonary trunk. *(Modified from Anderson RH, Becker AE, Lucchese E, et al: Morphology of Congenital Heart Disease. Baltimore, University Park Press, 1983.)*

LABORATORY INVESTIGATIONS

ELECTROCARDIOGRAPHY. The ECG mirrors the size of the shunt and the degree of pulmonary hypertension. Small, restrictive VSDs usually produce a normal tracing. Moderate-sized VSDs produce a broad, notched P wave characteristic of left atrial overload as well as evidence of left ventricular volume overload, namely, deep Q and tall R waves with tall T waves in leads V_5 and V_6 and perhaps eventually atrial fibrillation. After repair, the ECG is usually normal with right bundle branch block.

CHEST RADIOGRAPHY. The chest radiograph reflects the magnitude of the shunt as well as the degree of pulmonary hypertension. A moderate-sized shunt causes signs of left ventricular dilation with some pulmonary plethora.

ECHOCARDIOGRAPHY. (See Figs. 15-97 and 15-98.) Transthoracic echocardiography can identify the location, size, and hemodynamic consequences of the VSD as well as any associated lesions (aortic regurgitation, right ventricular outflow tract obstruction, or left ventricular outflow tract obstruction).

CARDIAC CATHETERIZATION. Cardiac catheterization may be required when the hemodynamic significance of a VSD is questioned or when assessment of pulmonary artery pressures and resistances is necessary. In some centers, therapeutic catheterization is performed for percutaneous closure (see later).

INDICATIONS FOR INTERVENTION. The presence of a significant VSD (the symptomatic patient shows a $Q_p/Q_s > 1.5:1$, pulmonary artery systolic pressure > 50 mm Hg, increased left ventricular and left atrial size, or deteriorating left ventricular function) in the absence of irreversible pulmonary hypertension warrants surgical closure. If severe pulmonary hypertension (see ASD section) is present, closure is seldom feasible. Other relative indications for VSD closure are the presence of a perimembranous or outlet VSD with more than mild aortic regurgitation and a history of recurrent endocarditis.

In children, a nonrestrictive VSD and a smaller VSD with significant symptoms failing to respond to medication are indications for surgical or device closure. Elective surgery is usually performed between 3 and 9 months of age. Some patients have pulmonary hypertension. If pulmonary arteriolar resistance is less than 7 Wood units, closure can be safely undertaken if there is a net left-to-right shunt of at least 1.5:1 or strong evidence of pulmonary reactivity on challenge with a pulmonary vasodilator (oxygen, nitric oxide).

INTERVENTIONAL OPTIONS AND OUTCOMES

Surgery

Surgical closure by direct suture or with a patch has been used for more than 50 years with a low perioperative mortality—even in adults—and a high closure rate. Patch leaks are not uncommon but seldom need reoperation. Late sinus node disease may occur.[48]

Device Closure

Successful transcatheter device closure of trabecular (muscular) and perimembranous VSDs has been reported. Trabecular VSDs have proven more amenable to this technique because of their relatively straightforward anatomy and muscular rim to which the device attaches well and, as such, result in excellent closure rates with a low procedural mortality.[49,50] Immediate as well as short-term results are good. The closure of a perimembranous VSD is technically more challenging because of its proximity to valve structures, and careful selection of patients is required. It should be performed only in centers with appropriate expertise. Short-term follow-up data show complete closure in 96% of patients, with the development of aortic or tricuspid regurgitation or the development of complete heart block in less than 5% of patients.[50] No long-term follow-up data are available yet.

REPRODUCTIVE ISSUES. Pregnancy is well tolerated in women with small or moderate VSDs and in women with repaired VSDs. Pregnancy is contraindicated in Eisenmenger syndrome because of high maternal (≈50%) and fetal (≈60%) mortality.

FOLLOW-UP. For patients with good to excellent functional class and good left ventricular function before surgical closure, life expectancy after surgical correction is close to normal.[48] The risk of progressive aortic regurgitation is reduced after surgery, as is the risk of endocarditis, unless a residual VSD persists. Yearly cardiac evaluation is suggested for patients with right ventricular outflow tract obstruction, left ventricular outflow tract obstruction, and aortic regurgitation not undergoing surgical repair; for patients with Eisenmenger syndrome; and for adults with significant atrial or ventricular arrhythmias. Cardiac surveillance is also recommended for patients who had late repair of moderate or large defects, which are often associated with left ventricular impairment and elevated pulmonary artery pressure at the time of surgery.

Patent Ductus Arteriosus

MORPHOLOGY. The ductus arteriosus derives from the left sixth primitive aortic arch and connects the proximal left pulmonary artery to the descending aorta, just distal to the left subclavian artery.

PATHOPHYSIOLOGY. The ductus is widely patent in the normal fetus, carrying unoxygenated blood from the right ventricle through the descending aorta to the placenta, where the blood is oxygenated. Functional closure of the ductus from vasoconstriction occurs shortly after a term birth, whereas anatomic closure from intimal proliferation and fibrosis takes several weeks to be completed. Some patients have "ductus-dependent" physiology as neonates. This means their circulation depends on the ductus for pulmonary blood flow, such as in severe aortic coarctation, hypoplastic left heart syndrome, and sometimes D-TGA. If spontaneous closure of the ductus occurs in such neonates, clinical deterioration and death usually follow.

Isolated PDAs, the subject of this section, are often categorized according to the degree of left-to-right shunting, which is determined by both the size and length of the duct and the difference between systemic and pulmonary vascular resistances, as follows:

- Silent: tiny PDA detected only by nonclinical means (usually echocardiography)
- Small: continuous murmur common; $Q_p/Q_s < 1.5:1$
- Moderate: continuous murmur common; Q_p/Q_s of 1.5 to 2.2:1
- Large: continuous murmur present; $Q_p/Q_s > 2.2:1$
- Eisenmenger: continuous murmur absent; substantial pulmonary hypertension, differential hypoxemia, and differential cyanosis (pink fingers, blue toes)

NATURAL HISTORY

Premature Infants

Patency of a ductus arteriosus is common in a preterm infant who lacks the normal mechanisms for postnatal ductal closure because of immaturity. A PDA is thus an expected finding in a premature infant, and delayed spontaneous closure of the ductus may be anticipated if the infant does not succumb to other problems.

Full-Term Infants

In a full-term newborn, patency of a ductus is a true congenital malformation. On occasion, some full-term newborns have persistent patency of the ductus arteriosus because their relative hypoxemia contributes to vasodilation of the channel. This includes infants born at high altitude; those with congenital malformations causing hypoxemia; or malformations in which ductal flow supplies the systemic circulation, such as hypoplastic left heart syndrome, interrupted aortic arch, or aortic coarctation.

Children and Adults

Children and adults with silent PDAs are detected by nonclinical means, usually echocardiography, and face virtually no long-term complications. An exception occurs if the patient's murmur is inaudible because of obesity or other somatic factors. A small ductus accompanied by a small shunt does not cause a significant hemodynamic derangement but may predispose to endarteritis,[51] especially when a murmur is present. A moderate-sized duct and shunt pose a volume load on the left atrium and ventricle with resultant left ventricular dilation and dysfunction and perhaps eventual atrial fibrillation. A large duct results initially in left ventricular volume overload but develops a progressive rise in pulmonary artery pressures and eventually irreversible pulmonary vascular changes by 2 years of age.

CLINICAL FEATURES

Premature Infants

Most preterm infants with a birth weight less than 1500 g have a PDA, and about one third have a large enough shunt to cause significant cardiopulmonary deterioration. Clinical findings in these patients include bounding peripheral pulses, infraclavicular and interscapular systolic murmur (occasionally a continuous murmur), precordial hyperactivity, hepatomegaly, and either multiple episodes of apnea and bradycardia or ventilator dependence.

Full-Term Infants, Children, and Adults

A small audible duct usually causes no symptoms but may rarely be manifested as an endovascular infection. Physical examination may reveal a grade 1 or 2 continuous murmur peaking in late systole and best heard in the first or second left intercostal space. Patients with a moderate-sized duct may present with dyspnea or palpitations from atrial arrhythmias. A louder continuous or "machinery" murmur in the first or second left intercostal space is typically accompanied by a wide systemic pulse pressure from aortic diastolic runoff into the pulmonary trunk and signs of left ventricular volume overload, such as a displaced left ventricular apex and sometimes a left-sided S_3 (meaningful in adults only). With a moderate degree of pulmonary hypertension, the diastolic component of the murmur disappears, leaving a systolic murmur. Adults with a large uncorrected PDA eventually present with a short systolic ejection murmur, hypoxemia in the feet more than in the hands (differential cyanosis), and Eisenmenger physiology.

Laboratory Investigations in Premature Infants

Electrocardiography. This may be normal or demonstrate right or left ventricular hypertrophy or both, depending on the amount of left-to-right shunting and the degree of associated pulmonary hypertension.

Chest Radiography. This may demonstrate cardiomegaly and increased pulmonary vascular markings that may be difficult to interpret in the setting of hyaline membrane disease.

Echocardiography. This is the key to diagnosis. The ductus arteriosus can be imaged in its entirety and its size estimated. Doppler study demonstrates the shunt and permits an accurate assessment of mean pulmonary artery pressure. This is achieved by calculating the mean left-to-right spectral trace and subtracting it from the mean blood pressure. Measurements of the left atrial and left ventricular size provide indirect evidence of the magnitude of left-to-right shunting.

Laboratory Investigations in Full-Term Infants, Children, and Adults

Electrocardiography. The ECG reflects the size and degree of shunting occurring through the duct. A small duct produces a normal ECG. A moderate duct may show left ventricular volume overload with broad, notched P waves together with deep Q waves, tall R waves, and peaked T waves in V_5 and V_6. A large duct with Eisenmenger physiology produces findings of right ventricular hypertrophy.

Chest Radiography. A small duct produces a normal chest radiograph. A moderate-sized duct causes moderate cardiomegaly with left-sided heart enlargement, a prominent aortic knuckle, and increased pulmonary perfusion. Ring calcification of the ductus may be seen through the soft tissue density of the aortic arch or pulmonary trunk in older adults. The large PDA produces an Eisenmenger appearance with a prominent aortic knuckle.

Echocardiography. (See Fig. 15-99.) This determines the presence, size, and degree of shunting and the physiologic consequences of the shunt. The PDA is seen with difficulty in an Eisenmenger context. A bubble study shows the communication.

INDICATIONS FOR INTERVENTION

Premature Infants

Treatment of preterm infants with a PDA varies with the magnitude of shunting and the severity of hyaline membrane disease because the ductus may contribute importantly to mortality in infants with respiratory distress syndrome. Intervention in an asymptomatic infant with a small left-to-right shunt is unnecessary because the PDA almost invariably undergoes spontaneous closure. Those infants who demonstrate unmistakable signs of a significant ductal left-to-right shunt during the course of the respiratory distress syndrome are often unresponsive to medical measures to control congestive heart failure and require closure of the PDA to survive. These infants are best treated by pharmacologic inhibition of prostaglandin synthesis with indomethacin or ibuprofen to constrict and to close the ductus. Surgical ligation is required in the estimated 10% of infants who are unresponsive to indomethacin.

Full-Term Infants

In the clinical settings in which the ductus preserves pulmonary blood flow, the inevitable spontaneous closure of the vessel is associated with profound clinical deterioration and often death. Undesirable ductal closure may be reversed medically within the first 4 or 5 days of life by an infusion of prostaglandin E_1. By dilation of the constricted ductus arteriosus, a temporary increase should occur in arterial blood oxygen tension and saturation and correct acidemia.

Children and Adults

There is no debate about the desirability of closing a hemodynamically important PDA. There is debate about the merits of closing an inaudible or small PDA strictly to reduce the risk of endarteritis. In the presence of severe pulmonary hypertension (see ASD earlier), closure is seldom indicated. Contraindications to ductal closure include irreversible pulmonary hypertension and active endarteritis.

INTERVENTIONAL OPTIONS AND OUTCOMES

Transcatheter Treatment (Fig. 65-10)

During the past 20 years, the efficacy and safety of transcatheter device closure for ducts smaller than 8 mm have been established, with complete ductal closure achieved in more than 85% of patients by 1 year after device placement at a mortality rate of less than 1%. In centers with appropriate resources and experience, transcatheter device occlusion should be the method of choice for ductal closure.[52]

Surgical Treatment

Surgical closure, by ductal ligation or division, has been performed for more than 50 years with a marginally greater closure rate than by device closure but with somewhat greater morbidity and mortality. Immediate clinical closure (no shunt audible on physical examination) is achieved in more than 95% of patients. Surgical closure is a low-risk procedure in children. Surgical mortality in adults is 1% to 3.5% and relates to the presence of pulmonary arterial hypertension and difficult ductal morphology (calcified or aneurysmal) often seen in adults. Surgical closure should be reserved for those in whom the PDA is too large for device closure or at centers without access to device closure.

REPRODUCTIVE ISSUES. Pregnancy is well tolerated in women with silent and small PDAs and in patients who were asymptomatic before pregnancy. In the woman with a hemodynamically important PDA, pregnancy may precipitate or worsen heart failure. Pregnancy is contraindicated in Eisenmenger syndrome because of the high maternal (≈50%) and fetal (≈60%) mortality.

FOLLOW-UP. Patients with device occlusion or after surgical closure should be examined periodically for possible recanalization. Silent residual shunts may be found by transthoracic echocardiography. Endocarditis prophylaxis is recommended for 6 months after PDA device closure or for life if any residual defect persists. Patients with a silent or small PDA probably do not require endocarditis prophylaxis or follow-up.

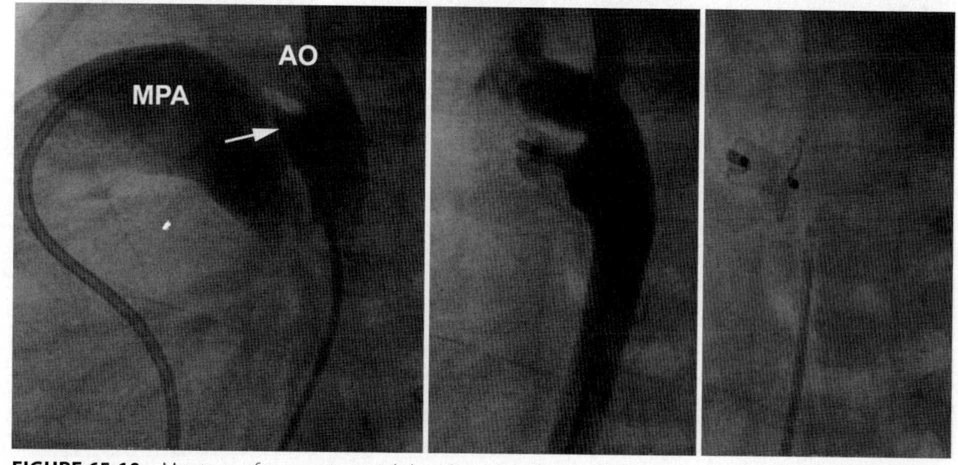

FIGURE 65-10 Montage of a patent arterial duct (arrow), before and after device occlusion. AO = aorta; MPA = main pulmonary artery.

Persistent Truncus Arteriosus

Morphology. Persistent truncus arteriosus is an anomaly in which a single vessel forms the outlet of both ventricles and gives rise to the systemic, pulmonary, and coronary arteries. It is always accompanied by a VSD and frequently with a right-sided aortic arch. The truncal valve is usually tricuspid but is quadricuspid in about one third of patients. Truncal valve regurgitation and truncal valve stenosis are each seen in 10% to 15% of patients. There can be a single coronary artery.

Truncus malformations can be classified either anatomically according to the mode of origin of pulmonary vessels from the common trunk or from a functional point of view on the basis of the magnitude of blood flow to the lungs. In the common type (type I) of truncus arteriosus, a partially separate pulmonary trunk of variable length exists and gives rise to left and right pulmonary arteries. In type II, each pulmonary artery arises separately but close to the other from the posterior aspect of the truncus. In type III, each pulmonary artery arises from the lateral aspect of the truncus. Less commonly, one pulmonary artery branch may be absent, with aortopulmonary collateral arteries supplying the lung that does not receive a pulmonary artery branch from the truncus.

Pathophysiology. Pulmonary blood flow is governed by the size of the pulmonary arteries and the pulmonary vascular resistance. In infancy, pulmonary blood flow is usually excessive because pulmonary vascular resistance is not greatly increased. Thus, in the neonate, only minimal cyanosis is present. With time, pulmonary vascular resistance increases, relieving the left ventricular volume load but at the price of increasing cyanosis. When pulmonary vascular resistance reaches systemic levels, Eisenmenger physiology and bidirectional shunting occur. Significant truncal valve regurgitation produces a volume load on both right and left ventricles because of the biventricular origin of the truncal artery.

NATURAL HISTORY. Most deaths from congestive heart failure occur before 1 year of age. Unrepaired patients who survive past 1 year most likely present with established pulmonary hypertension. The prevalence of truncal valve regurgitation increases with age, causing biventricular heart failure and increasing susceptibility to endocarditis.

CLINICAL FEATURES

Pediatrics

Infants with truncus arteriosus usually present with mild cyanosis coexisting with the cardiac findings of a large left-to-right shunt. This is the result of excessive pulmonary blood flow due to a low pulmonary vascular resistance. Symptoms of heart failure and poor physical development usually appear in the first weeks or months of life. The most frequent physical findings include cardiomegaly, collapsing peripheral pulses, loud single second heart sound, harsh systolic murmur preceded by an ejection click, and low-pitched mid-diastolic rumbling murmur and bounding pulses. A decrescendo diastolic murmur suggests associated truncal valve regurgitation.

DiGeorge syndrome may be seen with truncus arteriosus. Facial dysmorphism, high incidence of extracardiac malformations (particularly of the limbs, kidneys, and intestine), atrophy or absence of the thymus gland, T-lymphocyte deficiency, and predilection to infection also may be features of the clinical presentation.

The physical findings are different if pulmonary blood flow is restricted by a high pulmonary vascular resistance. Cyanosis is prominent, and only a short systolic murmur may be heard in association with an ejection click. Pulmonary vascular obstruction usually does not restrict pulmonary blood flow before 1 year of age.

Adults

Adults presenting with an unrepaired truncus arteriosus have Eisenmenger syndrome and its typical findings.

Laboratory Investigations (Unrepaired)

Electrocardiography. This demonstrates biventricular hypertrophy with strain as the pulmonary resistance rises.

Chest Radiography. This demonstrates cardiomegaly with prominent pulmonary arterial markings and unusually high hilar areas. A right aortic arch occurs in 50% of cases.

Echocardiography (**Fig. 65-11**). In most cases, two-dimensional echocardiography provides a complete diagnosis. The study should demonstrate the overriding truncal root, the origin of the pulmonary arteries, the number of truncal cusps, the origin of the coronary arteries, the functional status of the truncal valve, and the size of the VSD.

Cardiac Catheterization and Angiography. This is rarely necessary and in fact carries a risk of both morbidity and mortality. In general, significant arterial desaturation in the absence of branch pulmonary artery stenosis indicates that the lesion cannot be repaired.

INDICATIONS FOR INTERVENTION. Early surgical intervention is indicated in all cases within the first 2 months of life. In the presence of severe pulmonary hypertension (see ASD section), surgical intervention is usually not performed.

INTERVENTIONAL OPTIONS AND OUTCOMES. Operation consists of closure of the VSD, leaving the aorta arising from the left ventricle; excision of the pulmonary arteries from their truncus origin; and placement of a valve-containing prosthetic conduit or aortic homograft valve conduit between the right ventricle and the pulmonary arteries to establish circulatory continuity. Truncal valve insufficiency is a challenging problem and may require valve replacement or repair.

Important risk factors for perioperative death are severe truncal valve regurgitation, interrupted aortic arch, coronary artery anomalies, and age at initial operation older than 100 days. Patients with only one pulmonary artery are especially prone to early development of severe pulmonary vascular disease.

REPRODUCTIVE ISSUES. Patients with a repaired truncus arteriosus and no hemodynamically important residual lesions should tolerate pregnancy well. Patients with significant conduit obstruction or important truncal valve regurgitation need pre-pregnancy counseling, with consideration of correction of the lesions before pregnancy and careful follow-up throughout pregnancy. Pregnancy is contraindicated in patients with Eisenmenger syndrome, given its 50% maternal mortality.

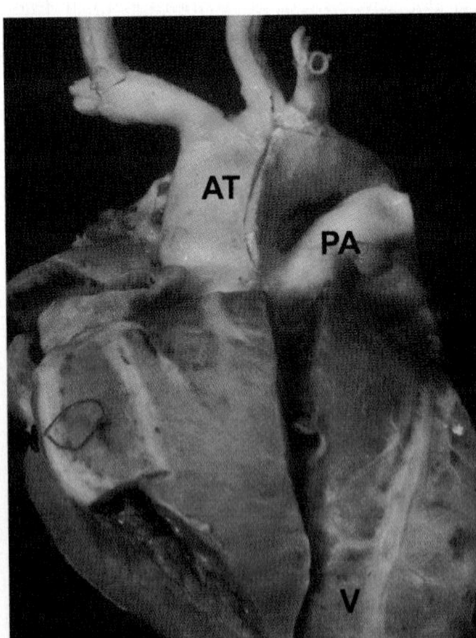

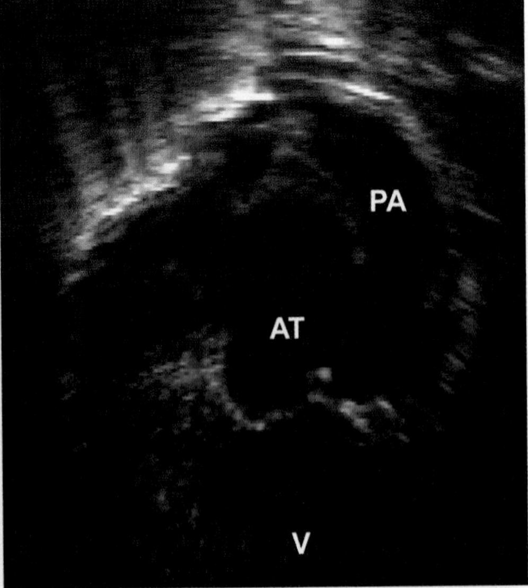

FIGURE 65-11 View of the origin of the pulmonary artery in truncus arteriosus. Note the lateral origin of the pulmonary artery. AT = ascending trunk; PA = pulmonary artery; V = ventricle.

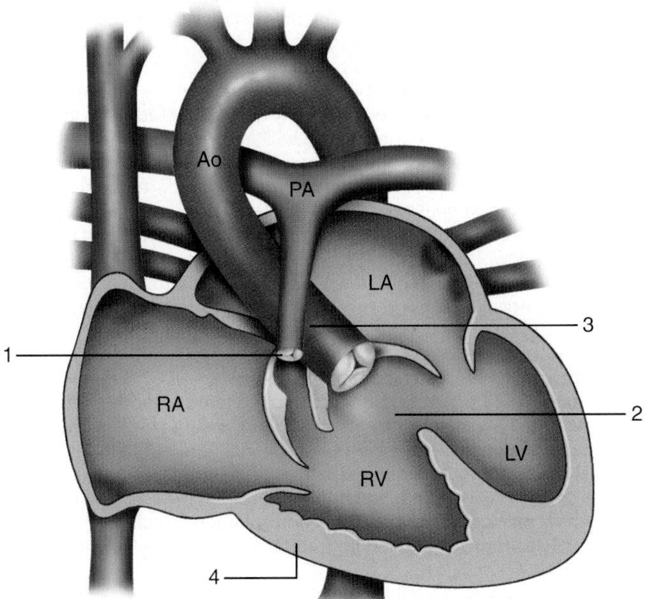

FIGURE 65-12 Diagrammatic representation of tetralogy of Fallot: 1, pulmonary stenosis; 2, ventricular septal defect; 3, overriding aorta; 4, right ventricle hypertrophy. Ao = aorta; LA = left atrium; LV = left ventricle; PA = pulmonary artery; RA = right atrium; RV = right ventricle. *(From Mullins CE, Mayer DC: Congenital Heart Disease: A Diagrammatic Atlas. New York, Wiley-Liss, 1988.)*

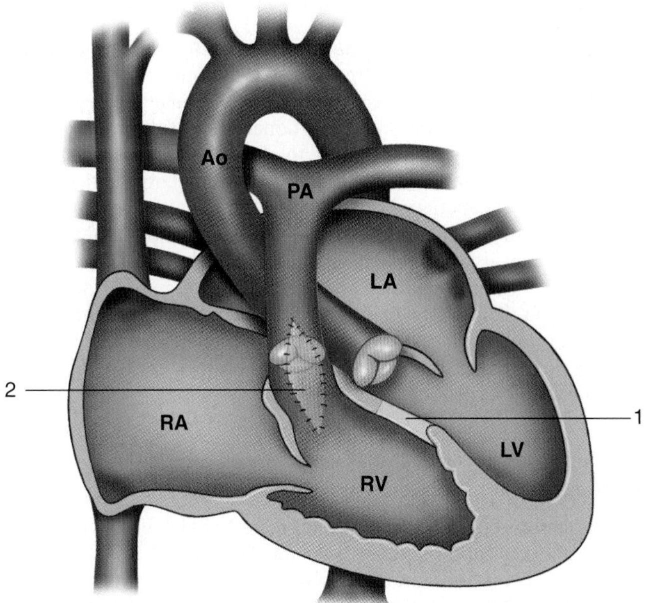

FIGURE 65-13 Diagrammatic representation of the surgical repair of tetralogy of Fallot: 1, patch closure of ventricular septal defect; 2, right ventricular outflow–main pulmonary artery outflow patch (transannular patch). Ao = aorta; LA = left atrium; LV = left ventricle; PA = pulmonary artery; RA = right atrium; RV = right ventricle. *(From Mullins CE, Mayer DC: Congenital Heart Disease: A Diagrammatic Atlas. New York, Wiley-Liss, 1988.)*

FOLLOW-UP. Patients operated on early (<1 year of age) generally do well. However, conduit change is often indicated within the first few years after repair as the patient outgrows its size. Those cases with significant truncal valve stenosis or regurgitation may eventually require truncal valve replacement. Patients operated on late (>1 year of age) require careful follow-up for any signs of pulmonary hypertension progression. Endocarditis prophylaxis is required in all patients.

Cyanotic Heart Disease

Tetralogy of Fallot (Including Tetralogy with Pulmonary Atresia)

MORPHOLOGY (Figs. 65-12 and 65-13). The four components of tetralogy of Fallot are an outlet VSD, obstruction to right ventricular outflow, overriding of the aorta (>50%), and right ventricular hypertrophy. The fundamental abnormality contributing to each of these features is anterior and cephalad deviation of the outlet septum, which is malaligned with respect to the trabecular septum. Thus, tetralogy may occur in the setting of double-outlet right ventricle (aortic override >50%) and may coexist with an AV septal defect, for example. Right ventricular outflow tract obstruction is variable. Often, a stenotic, bicuspid pulmonary valve with supravalvular hypoplasia exists. The dominant site of obstruction is usually at the subvalve level. In some cases, the outflow tract is atretic, and the heart can be diagnosed as having tetralogy of Fallot with pulmonary atresia (also known as complex pulmonary atresia when major aortopulmonary collateral arteries are present). The management and outcome of patients with major aortopulmonary collateral arteries are significantly different from those of patients with less extreme forms of tetralogy and are discussed separately.

ASSOCIATED ANOMALIES. A right aortic arch occurs in about 25% of patients, and abnormalities of the course of the coronary arteries occur in approximately 5%. In the most common anomaly, the anterior descending artery originates from the right coronary artery and courses anteriorly to cross the infundibulum of the right ventricle. Absent pulmonary valve syndrome is a rare form of tetralogy in which stenosis and regurgitation of the right ventricular outflow tract are due to a markedly stenotic pulmonary valve ring with poorly formed or absent valve leaflets. The pulmonary arteries are usually markedly dilated or aneurysmal and may produce airway compression at birth, a poor prognostic feature.

PATHOPHYSIOLOGY. In the absence of alternative sources of pulmonary blood flow, the degree of cyanosis reflects the severity of right ventricular outflow tract obstruction and the level of systemic vascular resistance. There is right-to-left shunting across the VSD. A tetralogy "spell" is an acute fall in arterial saturation, and it may be life-threatening. Its treatment is aimed at relieving obstruction and increasing systemic resistance. Relief of hypoxia with oxygen and morphine, intravenous propranolol, and systemic vasoconstriction (e.g., squatting, knee-chest position, vasoconstrictor drugs) usually reverses the cyanosis.

NATURAL HISTORY. Progressive hypoxemia in the first years of life is expected. Survival to adult life is rare without palliation or correction. The presence of additional sources of blood supply (see later) modifies the rate of progression of cyanosis and its complications.

CLINICAL FEATURES

Unrepaired Patients

Variable cyanosis exists. A right ventricular impulse and systolic thrill are often palpable along the left sternal border. An early systolic ejection sound that is aortic in origin may be heard at the lower left sternal border and apex; the second heart sound is usually single. The intensity and duration of the systolic ejection murmur vary inversely with the severity of subvalve obstruction, the opposite of the relation that exists in patients with pulmonary valve stenosis. With extreme outflow tract stenosis or pulmonary atresia and during an attack of paroxysmal hypoxemia, no murmur or only a short, faint murmur may be detected. A continuous murmur faintly audible over the anterior or posterior chest reflects flow through aortopulmonary collateral vessels or a duct.

After Surgery, Palliated

Progressive cyanosis with its complications can result from worsening right ventricular outflow tract obstruction, gradual stenosis and occlusion of palliative aortopulmonary shunts, or the development of pulmonary hypertension (sometimes seen after Waterston or Potts shunts). Progressive aortic dilation and aortic regurgitation are becoming increasingly recognized. Central cyanosis and clubbing are invariably present.

After Surgery, Repaired

After intracardiac repair, more than 85% of patients are asymptomatic on follow-up, although objective testing will usually demonstrate a reduction in maximal exercise performance. Palpitations from atrial and ventricular arrhythmias and exertional dyspnea from progressive right ventricular dilation secondary to chronic pulmonary regurgitation or severe residual right ventricular outflow tract obstruction occur in 10% to 15% of patients within 20 years after initial repair. An ascending aortic aneurysm and progressive aortic regurgitation from a dilated aortic root may also be present. A parasternal right ventricular lift and a soft and delayed P_2 with a low-pitched diastolic murmur from pulmonary regurgitation may exist. A systolic ejection murmur from right ventricular outflow tract obstruction, a high-pitched diastolic murmur from aortic regurgitation, and a pansystolic murmur from a VSD patch leak may also be heard.

Tetralogy of Fallot with Pulmonary Atresia and Major Aortopulmonary Collateral Arteries

This subgroup represents one of the greatest challenges in CHD. The aim of unifocalization surgery is to amalgamate all the sources of pulmonary blood flow and to establish unobstructed right ventricular to pulmonary artery continuity while achieving a normal pulmonary artery pressure and a closed ventricular septum. When this is not possible, a combined interventional catheterization and surgical approach may be indicated. Balloon dilation and stenting of stenosed arteries and anastomoses can "rehabilitate" segmental supply and allow subsequent VSD closure or, if it is already closed, reduce right ventricular pressure.

Laboratory Investigations

Electrocardiography. Right-axis deviation with right ventricular and right atrial hypertrophy is common. In adults with repaired tetralogy of Fallot, a complete right bundle branch block after repair has been the rule. QRS width may reflect the degree of right ventricular dilation and, when extreme (>180 milliseconds) or rapidly progressive, may be a risk factor for sustained ventricular tachycardia and sudden death.

Chest Radiography. Characteristically, there is a normal-sized, boot-shaped heart *(coeur en sabot)* with prominence of the right ventricle and a concavity in the region of the underdeveloped right ventricular outflow tract and main pulmonary artery. The pulmonary vascular markings are typically diminished, and the aortic arch may be on the right side (25%). The ascending aorta is often prominent.

Echocardiography (**Fig. 65-14**). A complete diagnosis can usually be established by Doppler echocardiography alone. The study should identify the malaligned and nonrestrictive VSD and overriding aorta (>50% override) and the presence and degree of right ventricular outflow tract obstruction (infundibular, valvular, or pulmonary arterial stenosis). Cardiac catheterization is now rarely required before corrective surgery. The exception to this rule is when there are additional sources of pulmonary blood flow. In patients with repaired tetralogy of Fallot, residual pulmonary stenosis and regurgitation (see Fig. 66-42), residual VSD, right and left ventricular size and function, aortic root size, and degree of aortic regurgitation should be assessed.

Cardiac Catheterization and Angiocardiography. Although echocardiography, magnetic resonance angiography, and fast CT may delineate the presence and proximal course of the pulmonary blood vessels, the preoperative assessment of tetralogy with pulmonary atresia with major aortopulmonary collateral arteries usually includes delineation of the arterial supply to both lungs by selective catheterization and angiography to show the course and segmental supply from the collateral arteries and central pulmonary arteries. Major aortopulmonary collateral arteries usually arise from the descending aorta at the level of the tracheal bifurcation.

CMR. The goals of CMR examination after tetralogy of Fallot repair include the quantitative assessment of left and particularly right ventricular volumes, stroke volumes, and ejection fraction; imaging of the anatomy of the right ventricular outflow tract, pulmonary arteries, aorta, and aortopulmonary collaterals; and quantification of pulmonary, aortic, and tricuspid regurgitation (see Fig. 66-42).

INDICATIONS FOR INTERVENTION

Children

Symptomatic infants are now repaired at any age, and elective repair in asymptomatic infants during the first 6 months is advocated by many. This is often at the expense of a transannular patch enlargement of the right ventricular outflow tract, which is a risk factor for later reintervention. Marked hypoplasia of the pulmonary arteries, small body size, and prematurity are relative contraindications for early corrective operation, and these patients may be successfully palliated by balloon dilation of the right ventricular outflow tract (with or without stenting) and pulmonary arteries.

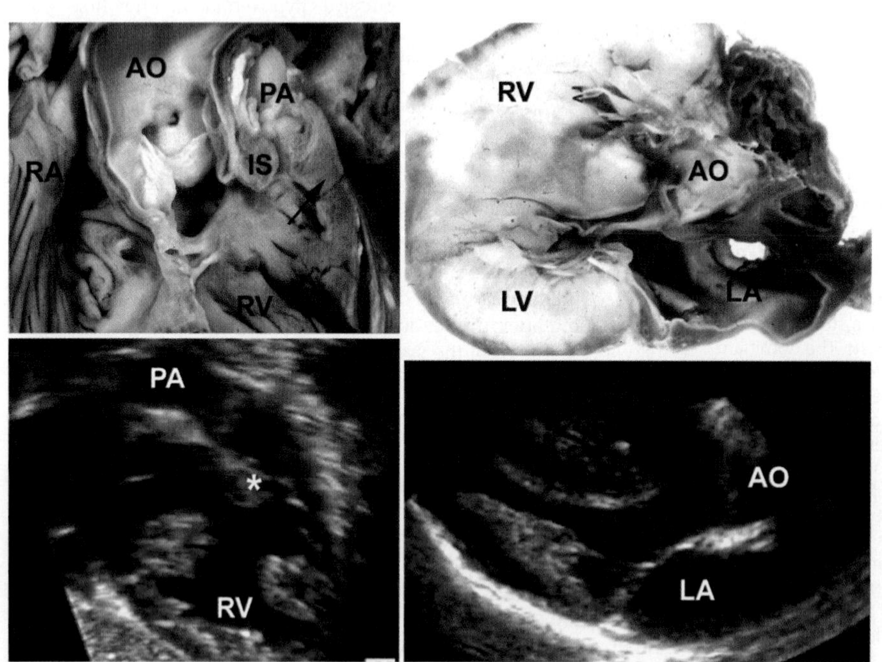

FIGURE 65-14 Montage of tetralogy of Fallot. The two left images are in the right anterior oblique view that demonstrates the anteriorly deviated infundibular septum (asterisk) and the ventricular septal defect. The arrow on the specimen points to the hypertrophied septoparietal trabeculations. The right images demonstrate the overriding aorta and the ventricular septal defect. AO = aorta; IS = infundibular septum; LA = left atrium; PA = pulmonary artery; RA = right atrium; RV = right ventricle.

Adults, Unrepaired

For unrepaired adults, surgical repair is still recommended because the results are gratifying and the operative risk is comparable to that of pediatric series, provided there is no serious coexisting morbidity.

Palliated

Palliation was seldom intended as a permanent treatment strategy, and most of these patients should undergo surgical repair. In particular, palliated patients with increasing cyanosis and erythrocytosis (from gradual shunt stenosis or development of pulmonary hypertension), left ventricular dilation, or aneurysm formation in the shunt should undergo intracardiac repair with takedown of the shunt unless irreversible pulmonary hypertension has developed.

Repaired

The following situations *may* warrant intervention after repair: a residual VSD with a shunt greater than 1.5:1; residual pulmonary stenosis (either the native right ventricular outflow or valved conduit if one is present) with right ventricular systolic pressure two thirds or more of systemic pressure; or severe pulmonary regurgitation associated with substantial right ventricular dilation or dysfunction (i.e., right ventricular diastolic volume index >150 to 170 mL/m^2 or a right ventricular ejection fraction <45%),[53,54] exercise intolerance, or sustained arrhythmias. The coexistence of substantial left ventricular dysfunction or a QRS duration >180 milliseconds offers additional support when other indications are present. The development of major cardiac arrhythmias, most commonly atrial flutter or fibrillation or sustained ventricular tachycardia, usually reflects hemodynamic deterioration and should be treated accordingly. Surgery is occasionally necessary for significant aortic regurgitation associated with symptoms or progressive left ventricular dilation and for aortic root enlargement of 55 mm or more.[55] Rapid enlargement of a right ventricular outflow tract aneurysm needs surgical attention.

INTERVENTIONAL OPTIONS

Surgery

Reparative surgery involves closure of the VSD with a Dacron patch and relief of the right ventricular outflow tract obstruction. The latter may involve resection of infundibular muscle and insertion of a right ventricular outflow tract or transannular patch—a patch across the pulmonary valve annulus that disrupts the integrity of the pulmonary valve and causes important pulmonary regurgitation. When an anomalous coronary artery crosses the right ventricular outflow tract and precludes a patch, an extracardiac conduit is placed between the right ventricle and pulmonary artery, bypassing the right ventricular outflow tract obstruction. A PFO or secundum ASD may be closed. Additional treatable lesions, such as muscular VSDs, PDAs, and aortopulmonary collaterals, should also be addressed at the time of surgery.

Reoperation is necessary in 10% to 15% of patients after reparative surgery during a 20-year follow-up. For persistent right ventricular outflow tract obstruction, resection of residual infundibular stenosis or placement of a right ventricular outflow or transannular patch, with or without pulmonary arterioplasty, can be performed. On occasion, an extracardiac valved conduit may be necessary. Pulmonary valve replacement (either homograft or xenograft) is used to treat severe pulmonary regurgitation. Concomitant tricuspid valve annuloplasty may be performed for moderate or severe tricuspid regurgitation. Concomitant cryoablation may be performed at the time of surgery for patients with preexisting atrial or ventricular arrhythmias.

Transcatheter

Percutaneous pulmonary valve replacement can be performed with mortality similar to that of surgical pulmonary valve replacement and favorable hemodynamic short- and intermediate-term results with less morbidity to the patient,[56,57] but it should be done only in adult CHD centers with expertise in the procedure.[57] At present, these therapies are reserved primarily for those patients with circumferential right ventricle–pulmonary artery conduits (i.e., homografts, valved conduits) measuring ≤22 mm.[58] Significant branch pulmonary artery stenosis can be managed with balloon dilation and usually stent insertion.

Implantable Cardioverter-Defibrillator (see Chap. 38)

The selection of appropriate candidates for primary prevention implantable-cardioverter defibrillators (ICDs) remains controversial. ICDs are probably most beneficial in "high-risk patients" (e.g., prior palliative shunt, QRS >180 milliseconds, inducible ventricular tachycardia, and left ventricular dysfunction) and are probably best reserved for those with a high annual risk (≥3.5% per year) of sudden cardiac death. When a patient presents with ventricular tachycardia and no underlying significant hemodynamic lesion, ICD implantation should be considered a secondary prevention measure.

INTERVENTIONAL OUTCOMES. The overall survival of patients who have had initial operative repair is excellent, provided the VSD has been closed and the right ventricular outflow tract obstruction has been relieved. A 25-year survival of 94% has been reported. Pulmonary valve replacement for chronic pulmonary regurgitation or right ventricular outflow tract obstruction after initial intracardiac repair can be done safely with a mortality rate of 1%. Pulmonary valve replacement, when it is performed for significant pulmonary regurgitation, leads to an improvement in exercise tolerance as well as favorable right ventricular remodeling. Sudden death can occur. Ventricular tachycardia can arise at the site of the right ventriculotomy, from VSD patch sutures, or from the right ventricular outflow tract. Patients at high risk for sudden death include those with right ventricular dilation and a QRS duration of 180 milliseconds or more on the ECG. Moderate to severe left ventricular dysfunction is another risk factor for sudden death. The reported incidence of sudden death is approximately 5%, which accounts for approximately one third of late deaths during the first 20 years of follow-up.

FOLLOW-UP. All patients should have expert cardiology follow-up every 1 to 2 years.

Fontan Procedure–Requiring Lesions

The next four sections describe lesions usually or often treated with a Fontan procedure. These include tricuspid atresia, hypoplastic left heart syndrome, double-inlet ventricle, and isomerism. *Fontan procedure* has become a generic term to describe a palliative surgical procedure that redirects the systemic venous return directly to the pulmonary arteries without passing through a subpulmonary ventricle. It is performed in patients having a "functionally single" ventricle or when a biventricular intracardiac repair is not possible, even though there are two good-sized ventricles. Although it is undoubtedly imperfect, the Fontan circuit restores an in-series pulmonary-to-systemic circulation, removing the chronic volume load of the systemic ventricle previously supporting a parallel circuit of pulmonary and systemic circulations. The earliest iteration of the Fontan procedure was a simple "atriopulmonary" connection, whereby the right atrium or its appendage was anastomosed to the pulmonary arteries. Because of the long-term problems of atrial dilation, arrhythmia, and thrombosis, this procedure has been abandoned in favor of hemodynamically superior versions. In the early 1990s, the total cavopulmonary anastomosis or lateral tunnel Fontan was introduced. This consisted of a direct, end-to-side superior cavopulmonary anastomosis (bidirectional Glenn operation) in combination with an intra-atrial baffle or tube connection of the inferior vena cava to the underside of the confluent pulmonary arteries. More recently, the inferior vena cava has been directed to the pulmonary arteries via an extracardiac conduit, completely excluding the atrium from the circuit. It remains to be seen whether these modifications will have the desired effect of reducing late morbidity, and all patients will require regular and careful review in special centers.

Tricuspid Atresia (Absent Right Atrioventricular Connection)

MORPHOLOGY. Classic tricuspid atresia is best described as absence of the right AV connection (**Figs. 65-15** and **65-16**). Consequently, there must be an ASD. There is usually hypoplasia of the morphologic right ventricle, which communicates to the dominant ventricle via a VSD. Patients may be subdivided into those with concordant ventriculoarterial connections and normally related great arteries (70% to 80% of cases) and those with discordant connections, in which the aorta arises from the small right ventricle and is fed via the VSD. Associated lesions in the latter group include subaortic stenosis and aortic arch anomalies.

PATHOPHYSIOLOGY. The clinical picture and management are dominated by issues related to the ventriculoarterial connections. All patients have "mixing" of atrial blood, and thus their degree of cyanosis is governed by the amount of pulmonary blood flow and systemic venous saturations. Patients with concordant ventriculoarterial connections tend to be more cyanosed (depending on the size of the VSD), whereas those with discordant connections are pinker and tend to develop heart failure (because the unobstructed pulmonary circulation arises directly from the left ventricle). Some present with a critical reduction of systemic blood flow because of obstruction at the VSD or associated aortic arch anomalies and behave much like hypoplastic left heart syndrome.

LABORATORY INVESTIGATIONS

ELECTROCARDIOGRAPHY. Left-axis deviation, right atrial enlargement, and left ventricular hypertrophy often occur. Left atrial enlargement may be present if pulmonary flow is high.

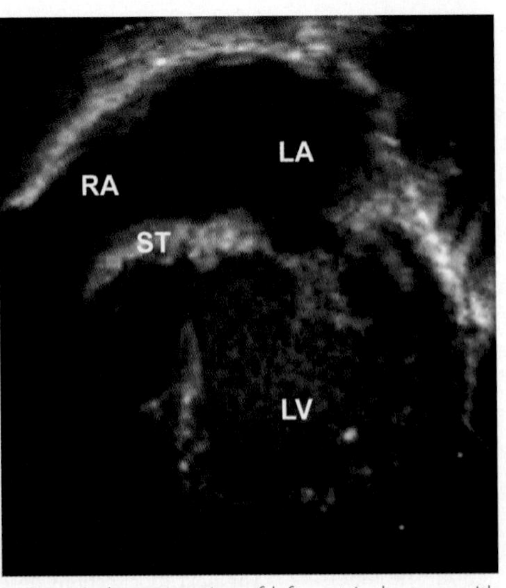

FIGURE 65-15 Apical four-chamber view in univentricular connection of left ventricular type with absent right connection (tricuspid atresia). Note the wedge of sulcus tissue in the floor of the right atrium. LA = left atrium; LV = left ventricle; RA = right atrium; ST = sulcus tissue.

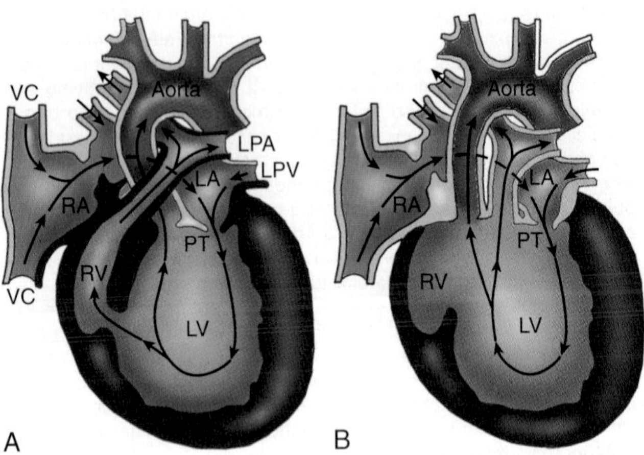

FIGURE 65-16 **A,** Tricuspid atresia with normally related great arteries, a small ventricular septal defect, diminutive right ventricular chamber, and narrowed outflow tract. **B,** An example of tricuspid atresia and complete transposition of the great arteries in which the left ventricular chamber is essentially a common ventricle, with the aorta arising from an infundibular component (RV) of the common ventricle. LA = left atrium; LPA = left pulmonary artery; LPV = left pulmonary vein; LV = left ventricle; PT = pulmonary trunk; RA = right atrium; RV = right ventricle; VC = vena cava. *(**A** and **B** modified from Edwards JE, Burchell HB: Congenital tricuspid atresia: Classification. Med Clin North Am 33:1177, 1949.)*

Chest Radiography. Situs solitus, levocardia, and a left-sided aortic arch usually occur. The heart size and pulmonary vascular markings vary with the amount of pulmonary blood flow. The main pulmonary trunk is inapparent. A right aortic arch exists in 25% of patients.

Echocardiography. This establishes the full segmental diagnosis. The size of the ASD, VSD, and aortic arch must be carefully assessed.

Cardiac Catheterization. This is rarely required for initial diagnosis or management. It can be useful to assess the degree of subaortic stenosis (by assessing the change in left ventricle to aortic pressure gradient while performing an isoprenaline or dobutamine challenge) and is usually performed to measure the pulmonary artery pressure and resistance before venopulmonary connections.

MANAGEMENT OPTIONS. In those with concordant ventriculoarterial connections and severe cyanosis, a systemic to pulmonary shunt is performed in the first 6 to 8 weeks of life, and in older children, a primary bidirectional Glenn procedure can be considered. In infants with discordant arterial connections, early palliation ranges from pulmonary artery banding to reduce pulmonary blood flow when there is no subaortic narrowing to a full Norwood stage 1 procedure in those presenting with severe stenosis and a hypoplastic ascending aorta and arch.

The aim of early palliation is to prepare for a Fontan procedure. This should be performed only when there is good ventricular function, unobstructed systemic blood flow, and minimal AV valve regurgitation. Candidates for these corrective procedures must also have a low pulmonary resistance, a mean pulmonary artery pressure less than 15 mm Hg, and pulmonary arteries of adequate size.

Hypoplastic Left Heart Syndrome

DEFINITION. Hypoplastic left heart syndrome is a generic term used to describe a group of closely related cardiac anomalies characterized by underdevelopment of the left cardiac chambers, in association with atresia or stenosis of the aortic or the mitral orifice and hypoplasia of the aorta. The term should be restricted to those with normally connected hearts with concordant atrioventricular and ventriculoarterial connections. Hypoplastic left heart syndrome (**Fig. 65-17**) is characterized by duct-dependent systemic blood flow and so tends to present with severe symptoms within the first week of life, as ductal constriction occurs. Untreated, the disease is almost uniformly fatal in infancy. In the past, many infants would present with severe acidemic circulatory collapse, but this is becoming less frequent as fetal ultrasound screening for cardiac

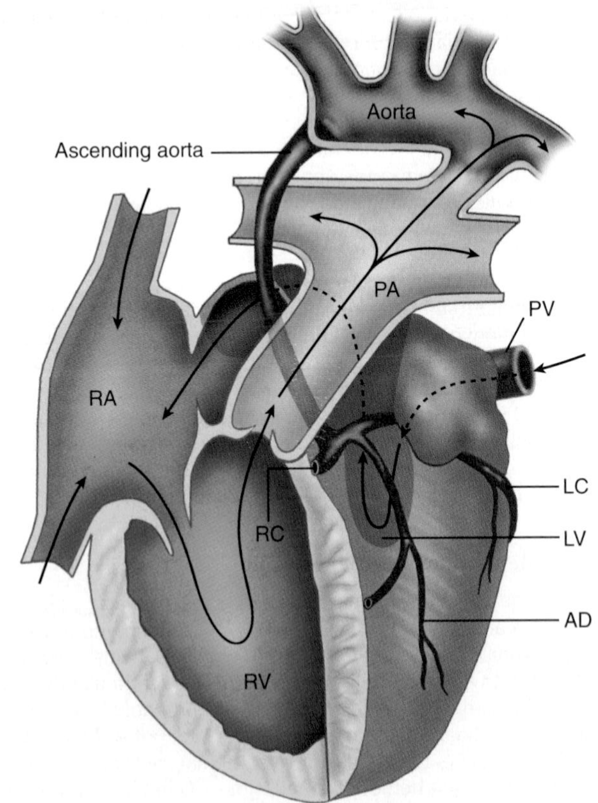

FIGURE 65-17 Hypoplastic left heart with aortic hypoplasia, aortic valve atresia, and a hypoplastic mitral valve and left ventricle. AD = anterior descending; LC = left circumflex; LV = left ventricle; PA = pulmonary artery; PV = pulmonary vein; RA = right atrium; RC = right coronary artery; RV = right ventricle. *(From Neufeld HN, Adams P Jr, Edwards JE, et al: Diagnosis of aortic atresia by retrograde aortography. Circulation 25:278, 1962.)*

anomalies becomes more generally available and successful. Fetal diagnosis allows a planned delivery and institution of prostaglandin therapy from birth and has now been proven to reduce subsequent preoperative morbidity and perioperative mortality during the first stage of surgical repair.

PATHOPHYSIOLOGY. It remains uncertain whether hypoplastic left heart syndrome reflects a primary myocardial disease or is a consequence of a structural or hemodynamic abnormality. There is no doubt that in some patients, an apparently isolated dilated cardiomyopathy in early fetal life may evolve (as a result of a subsequent lack of left ventricular growth) into hypoplastic left heart syndrome later in gestation. Congenital structural abnormalities clearly play a significant role as well. This is exemplified by the effect of isolated valvular stenosis to produce a continuum of hypoplastic left heart syndrome to critical aortic stenosis with a normal-sized left ventricle. Therefore, hypoplastic left heart syndrome is likely to be multifactorial in origin.

CLINICAL FEATURES. The diagnosis should be considered in any infant with the sudden onset of circulatory collapse and severe lactic acidosis. As such, it must be distinguished from neonatal sepsis and metabolic disorders. Until it is excluded, any child presenting in this way should be treated with prostaglandin, which may have a dramatically positive effect if there is an underlying cardiac abnormality and little effect if there is not.

LABORATORY INVESTIGATIONS

ELECTROCARDIOGRAPHY. This frequently shows right-axis deviation, right atrial and ventricular enlargement, and ST and T wave abnormalities in the left precordial leads.

CHEST RADIOGRAPHY. This usually shows some cardiac enlargement shortly after birth; but with clinical deterioration, there may be marked cardiomegaly and increased pulmonary venous and arterial vascular markings.

ECHOCARDIOGRAPHY (**Fig. 65-18**). Cross-sectional echocardiography provides a full segmental diagnosis. In its classic form, the left ventricular cavity is small, with a diminutive mitral valve. The myocardium may be thinned or be of normal thickness, but the endocardium is usually thickened, consistent with endocardial fibroelastosis. There may be fistulous communications between the left ventricular cavity and the coronary arteries, a feature much more likely when the mitral valve is patent rather than atretic. The aortic root is usually diminutive, less than 4 to 5 mm in diameter at the level of the sinuses of Valsalva and narrowed in its ascending portion. The aortic arch is usually larger, but there is often a juxtaductal coarctation. The duct varies in size according to treatment, and assessment of this and the size of the interatrial communication is crucial to management. There may be profound desaturation and rapid demise (because of a combination of reduced pulmonary blood flow and pulmonary edema) in children with an intact atrial septum or restrictive PFO.

MANAGEMENT OPTIONS. Early treatment with prostaglandin is mandatory. Those presenting in shock require paralysis, mechanical ventilation, and inotropic support. Crucial to management of these patients is maintenance of a balanced pulmonary and systemic blood flow. The cardiac output is fixed and is distributed according to the relative magnitude of the systemic and pulmonary vascular resistance. Thus, measures to elevate the pulmonary resistance (by imposing hypercapnia or by alveolar hypoxia) and to reduce the systemic resistance (using vasodilators) are frequently required.

Surgical Treatment

Staged surgical management now provides long-term palliation to most patients with hypoplastic left heart syndrome. The first stage, often referred to as the Norwood procedure, now has many versions, but its essence is the creation of an unobstructed communication between the right ventricle and an unobstructed aorta. The right ventricular to aortic connection is accomplished by direct connection between the transected proximal pulmonary trunk and ascending aorta, usually with a patch extending around the augmented aortic arch. Pulmonary blood flow is established via a systemic to pulmonary shunt or the more recently introduced right ventricle to pulmonary artery conduit. The PDA is ligated, and a large interatrial communication is created. Early results of this procedure were poor, but survival rates higher than 85% have recently been published. Institutional variations, the interval mortality, and those unsuitable to progress to stage 2 must also be taken into account, however, and in some centers, the preferred operation is cardiac transplantation.

Stage 2 consists of an end-to-side superior vena cava to pulmonary artery connection (bidirectional Glenn procedure) or a hemi-Fontan (incorporating the roof of the atrium into the pulmonary artery anastomosis). This is performed at approximately 6 months of age as an intermediate step before stage 3, a Fontan operation. A newer innovation is the so-called hybrid procedure, whereby at the first stage each pulmonary artery is banded separately and a stent is placed, by the interventional cardiologist, to maintain ductal patency either directly via the main pulmonary artery in concert with the surgeon or percutaneously. The second stage combines the surgical aortopulmonary anastomosis with the bidirectional Glenn procedure. It remains to be seen whether this approach confers a survival or physiologic advantage.

ADULT ISSUES. The survivors of the earliest attempts at staged Norwood palliation are just now entering adult life. Their issues are likely to be common to all late survivors of Fontan palliation with a systemic right ventricle.

Double-Inlet Ventricle

DEFINITION. Double-inlet connection falls under the umbrella of univentricular AV connections. These hearts are defined by having more than 50% of each AV connection connected to a dominant ventricle. In practice, this usually means that the whole of one and more than 50% of the alternative junction is connected to either a left or right ventricle. When there is a common junction, more than 75% of the junction must be connected to the dominant ventricle.

MORPHOLOGY. In about 75% of patients, the dominant ventricle is a left ventricle that is separated from the right ventricle by a VSD. In 20%, the dominant ventricle is a right ventricle, and the small, incomplete ventricle is of left ventricular apical morphology. In only 5% of cases is there truly only one ventricle in the ventricular mass. In double-inlet left ventricle, the most common ventriculoarterial connection is discordant. Thus, the aorta arises from the small right ventricle and is fed via the VSD, and the generally unobstructed pulmonary artery arises from the left ventricle. Aortic and aortic arch anomalies are frequent in these patients.

PATHOPHYSIOLOGY. The basic circulatory physiology of double-inlet left ventricle is identical to that of tricuspid atresia. Common mixing of systemic and pulmonary venous blood occurs, and the blood is then ejected from the left ventricle into the pulmonary artery (with discordant connections) or aorta (with concordant connections). In the former, the

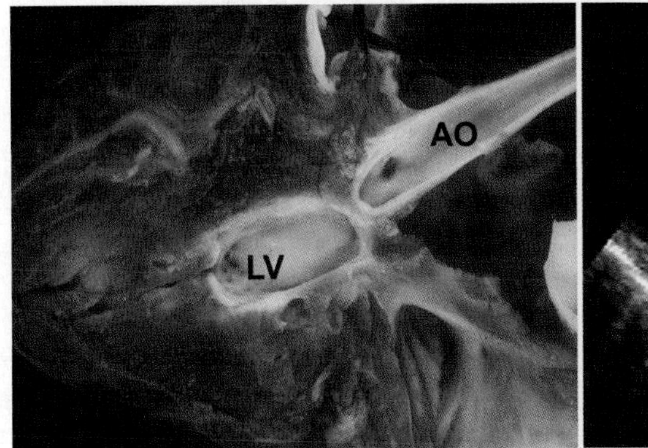

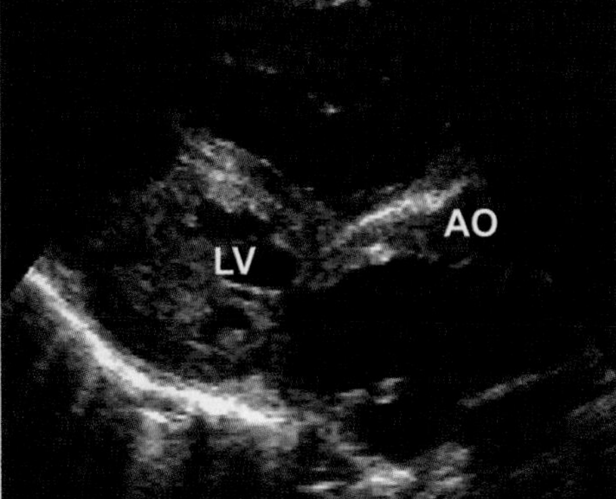

FIGURE 65-18 Long-axis view of the left ventricle and aorta in hypoplastic left heart syndrome. Note the associated endocardial fibroelastosis in the specimen. AO = aorta, LV = left ventricle.

blood must pass through the VSD to gain egress to the aorta. Subaortic stenosis, aortic hypoplasia, and arch anomalies are therefore common. In double-inlet right ventricle, it is those patients with concordant ventriculoarterial connections who are at particular risk of systemic outflow obstruction. One or the other or both of the two AV valves (when present) may be stenotic, atretic, or regurgitant. Under these circumstances, the integrity of the atrial septum becomes important. If there is left or right atrial outflow obstruction, a septectomy or septostomy will be required.

CLINICAL FEATURES. When there is critical reduction of systemic outflow, infants may be duct dependent and present with acidemic shock. Conversely, when pulmonary blood flow is reduced, presentation may be with severe cyanosis or with duct-dependent pulmonary blood flow. Other patients may not present in the neonatal period and will develop heart failure because of increased pulmonary blood flow. Patients undergo the same surgical algorithms as those with tricuspid atresia and so ultimately will undergo a Fontan operation. Their clinical issues are typical of any patient after this procedure.

LABORATORY INVESTIGATIONS

ELECTROCARDIOGRAPHY. This is highly variable. Ventricular hypertrophy appropriate to the dominant ventricle is expected.

CHEST RADIOGRAPHY. This is similarly variable and rarely diagnostic.

ECHOCARDIOGRAPHY (**Fig. 65-19**). A full segmental diagnosis should be possible in all patients. Particular attention should be paid to defining AV valve anomalies and the presence and anatomy of any subaortic obstruction. This may develop, even if it is not present at birth, and should be part of the routine surveillance of these patients.

INDICATIONS AND OPTIONS FOR INTERVENTION. Survival without intervention may be prolonged, but at the expense of increasing cyanosis (when there is restriction to pulmonary blood flow) or pulmonary vascular disease (when there is unrestricted pulmonary blood flow). Those born with restricted systemic blood flow require urgent surgical intervention, usually undergoing a Norwood-type repair to establish the pulmonary valve as the unobstructed systemic outflow tract. Pulmonary artery banding is offered only to those infants with pulmonary overcirculation, heart failure, and unobstructed systemic outflow. Subsequently, and sometimes as the primary procedure, a bidirectional Glenn anastomosis is performed as a prelude to a Fontan procedure.

FOLLOW-UP. These patients should be reviewed frequently and in a center conversant with the issues of the Fontan operation.

Isomerism

DEFINITION. For the purposes of illustrating the cardiac manifestations, isomerism describes the situation in which both atrial appendages have either left or right anatomic features (i.e., bilateral right or bilateral left atrial appendages).

MORPHOLOGY. Experts have made many attempts to describe hearts with complex abnormalities of visceral and atrial situs, whereby normal lateralization is lost. Terms such as *heterotaxy, asplenia,* and *polysplenia* fail to adequately describe either the visceral or cardiac manifestations with enough precision. The left atrial appendage is characterized by its tubular shape and pectinate muscles confined to the appendage. The pectinate muscles of the triangular right atrial appendage extend from its broad junction with the atrium to extend around the vestibule or AV junction. Thus, the arrangement of the atria (usual, mirror image, right or left isomerism) can be defined independently of the venous anatomy.

In left isomerism, it is not unusual to have a biventricular AV connection, with separate AV junctions. A common junction (with an AV septal defect) is seen in approximately 30% of cases of left isomerism and more than 90% of hearts with right isomerism. Concordant ventriculoarterial connections predominate in left isomerism, and a double-outlet right ventricle with an anterior aorta is most frequently seen when there is right isomerism. The venous connections are variable. These variations significantly affect the clinical and interventional management of these patients.

Isomerism of the Right Atrial Appendages

CLINICAL FEATURES. Bilateral "right-sidedness" results in a pattern of visceral abnormalities sometimes described as asplenia syndrome. The liver is midline, and both lungs are trilobed with symmetrically short bronchi on the chest radiograph; the spleen is hypoplastic or absent, which mandates immunization against pneumococcal infection and continuous penicillin prophylaxis against gram-positive sepsis. The diagnosis can be inferred from the bronchial pattern on the chest radiograph but most often is established by cross-sectional echocardiography because of early presentation with severe CHD. Abdominal scanning shows ipsilateral arrangement of the aorta and an anterior inferior vena cava. The intracardiac anatomy is most often that of an AV septal defect with varying degrees of right ventricular dominance, and there is frequently an associated double-outlet right ventricle with an anterior aorta and subpulmonary stenosis or atresia. Thus, cyanosis is the most common presentation. The inferior vena cava may connect to either right atrium, and superior venae cavae are often lateralized and separate. It is the pulmonary venous drainage that is crucial to the presentation and outcome of these children. By definition, the pulmonary veins are draining anomalously to one or other right atrium, but this is frequently indirect or obstructed. Adequate repair of this is fundamental to the outcome of these children, who almost uniformly ultimately require a Fontan procedure.

MANAGEMENT OPTIONS AND OUTCOMES. Initial palliation is usually directed toward regulating pulmonary blood flow and dealing with anomalies of pulmonary venous connection. Subsequently, these patients (even when there are equal-sized ventricles) are treated along a Fontan algorithm. This is because repair of complete AV septal defect in the setting of abnormal ventriculoarterial connections is technically difficult or impossible. Thus, a unilateral or bilateral superior cavopulmonary anastomosis is performed at approximately 6 months of age, followed when possible by a Fontan procedure at 2 to 4 years of age.

The long-term outcome of surgery for right isomerism, however, has been poor. Improved early palliation and a staged approach toward the Fontan procedure have led to improved results. The prognosis for these infants, particularly when there is obstruction to pulmonary venous return, must remain guarded.

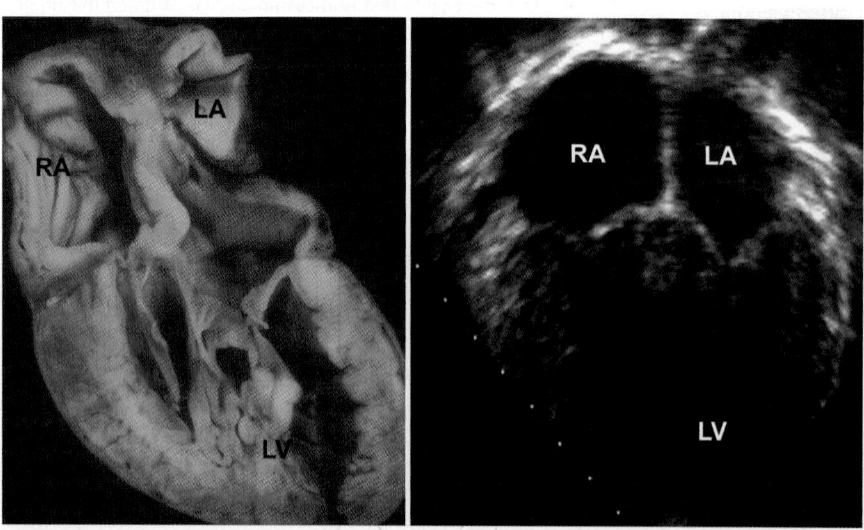

FIGURE 65-19 Apical four-chamber view in a double-inlet univentricular connection of left ventricular type with two atrioventricular valves. LA = left atrium; LV = left ventricle; RA = right atrium.

Isomerism of the Left Atrial Appendages

CLINICAL FEATURES. These patients have bilateral "left-sidedness." Hence, they have two left lungs and bronchi, tend to have polysplenia, and frequently have malrotation of the gut. The cardiac abnormalities tend to be less severe than those of right isomerism. These patients are particularly prone to development of atrial arrhythmias because the normal sinoatrial node is a right atrial structure and is usually absent in these patients. The ECG often shows an abnormal P wave axis, or wandering pacemaker. Complete heart block may also occur. The anatomic diagnosis is usually established by echocardiography. The abdominal great vessels are both to the right or left of the spine, as with right isomerism; but in left isomerism, the vein is a posterior azygos vein that continues to connect to a left- or right-sided superior vena cava. The intrahepatic inferior vena cava is absent in 90%, and under these circumstances, the hepatic veins drain directly to the atria. The pulmonary venous connection needs to be defined precisely before any surgical intervention. Pulmonary arteriovenous malformations are not infrequently seen in patients with left isomerism. These can lead to cyanosis in unrepaired or repaired patients. The intracardiac anatomy varies from essentially normal to complex. Again, AV septal defect (partial and complete) is overrepresented but with less frequent ventricular imbalance and abnormalities of ventriculoarterial connection.

MANAGEMENT OPTIONS. A biventricular repair is achieved in many more of these patients, albeit with the need for complex atrial baffle surgery to separate the systemic and pulmonary venous returns. The long-term outcome for patients with left isomerism is therefore much better than that for patients with right isomerism. The issues are much like those related to the type of surgery, but monitoring for arrhythmia needs to be even more intense than usual.

The Fontan Patient (Fig. 65-20)

BACKGROUND. As stated in the introduction to this section, the uncertain nature of the Fontan circulation and the frequency of its failure require that all patients be followed up regularly in a specialized center for CHD, and new symptoms should prompt early reevaluation in such a center.

Since its description for the surgical management of tricuspid atresia in 1971, the Fontan procedure has become the definitive palliative surgical treatment when a biventricular repair is not possible. The principle is diversion of the systemic venous return directly to the pulmonary arteries without passing through a subpulmonary ventricle. Over the years, many modifications of the original procedure have been described and performed, namely, direct atriopulmonary connection, total cavopulmonary connection, and extracardiac conduit. Fenestration (4- to 5-mm diameter) of the Fontan circuit into the left atrium is sometimes performed at the time of surgery in high-risk patients, permitting right-to-left shunting and decompression of the Fontan circuit.

PATHOPHYSIOLOGY. Elevation of the central venous pressure and a reduced cardiac output (sometimes at rest but always on exercise) are inevitable consequences of the Fontan procedure. Small adverse changes in ventricular function (particularly diastolic) or circuit efficiency (elevated pulmonary resistance, obstruction, thrombosis) and the onset of arrhythmia all potentially lead to major symptomatic deterioration.

Although it is reasonable to describe patients after the Fontan procedure as existing in a form of chronic heart failure (since their right atrial pressure must be high), this is seldom due to marked systolic dysfunction. Indeed, a small elevation in ventricular diastolic pressure may be much more harmful. Thus, it may be incorrect to treat these patients with traditional heart failure medications. In a randomized, blinded placebo-controlled study, ACE inhibition failed to improve functional performance, and some indices worsened.

The more "streamlined" Fontan circulations (total cavopulmonary anastomosis, extracardiac conduit) that exclude the right atrium from the circulation have demonstrably better fluid dynamic properties and improved functional performance. Physical obstruction at surgical anastomoses, distal pulmonary arteries, or pulmonary veins (often due to compression by a dilated right atrium) reduces circulatory efficiency, however. Similarly, elevated pulmonary arteriolar resistances have adverse effects. This is because the pulmonary vascular resistance is the single biggest contributor to impairment of venous return and elevation of venous pressure. Relatively little is known about pulmonary vascular resistance late after the procedure, but it has been shown to be elevated in a significant number of patients and to be reactive to inhaled nitric oxide, suggesting pulmonary endothelial dysfunction. Recently, beneficial effects on exercise performance were shown with sildenafil treatment, but this remains to be confirmed in larger studies.

CLINICAL FEATURES. The majority of patients (≈90%) present in functional Class I or II at 5 years' follow-up after a Fontan procedure. Progressive deterioration of functional status with time is the rule. Supraventricular arrhythmias such as atrial tachycardia, flutter, and fibrillation are common. Physical examination in an otherwise uncomplicated patient reveals an elevated, usually nonpulsatile jugular venous pulse, a quiet apex, a normal S_1, and a single S_2 (the pulmonary artery having been tied off). A heart murmur should not be present, and its identification may suggest the presence of systemic AV valve regurgitation or subaortic obstruction. Generalized edema and ascites may be a sign of protein-losing enteropathy (see later).

COMPLICATIONS AND SEQUELAE

Arrhythmia (see Chap. 39)

Although often associated with marked symptomatic decline, atrial arrhythmias tend to reflect the consequences of the abnormalities of ventricular function and circulatory efficiency described earlier. The

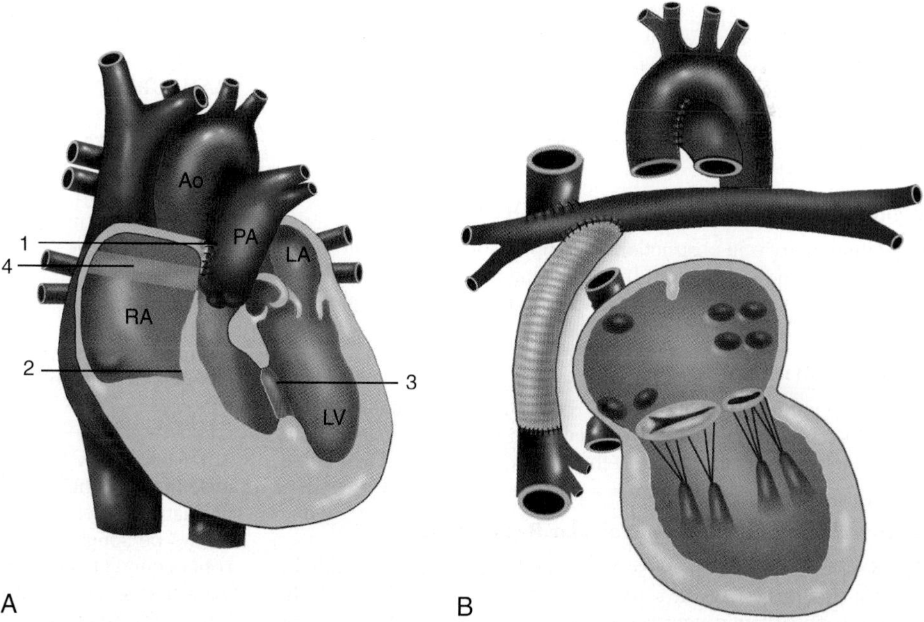

FIGURE 65-20 Modification of the Fontan operation. **A,** Direct atriopulmonary connection (1) for tricuspid valve atresia (2); ventricular septal defect, oversewn (3); patch closure of atrial septal defect (4). **B,** Extracardiac conduit made of a Dacron graft bypassing the right atrium, connecting the inferior vena cava to the inferior aspect of the right pulmonary artery. Superior vena cava is anastomosed to the superior aspect of the right pulmonary artery. Ao = aorta; LA = left atrium; LV = left ventricle; PA = pulmonary artery; RA = right atrium. *(**A** from Mullins CE, Mayer DC: Congenital Heart Disease: A Diagrammatic Atlas. New York, Wiley-Liss, 1988. **B** from Marcelletti C: Inferior vena cava–pulmonary artery extracardiac conduit: A new form of right heart bypass. J Thorac Cardiovasc Surg 100:228, 1990.)*

massively dilated right atrium after an atriopulmonary connection is commonly associated with atrial flutter and fibrillation (15% to 20% at 5 years' follow-up).[59] Atrial flutter or fibrillation carries significant morbidity, can be associated with profound hemodynamic deterioration, and needs prompt medical attention. The combination of atrial incisions and multiple suture lines at the time of Fontan surgery along with increased right atrial pressure and size probably explains the high incidence of atrial arrhythmias in such patients. Patients at greater risk for atrial tachyarrhythmias are those who were operated on at an older age, with poor ventricular function, systemic AV valve regurgitation, or increased pulmonary artery pressure. It has been suggested that the exclusion of the right atrium from elevated systemic venous pressure (as in total cavopulmonary connections or extracardiac conduits) leads to a decrease in the incidence of atrial arrhythmias. This apparent benefit may, however, be due exclusively to the shorter length of follow-up in this group of patients. Sinus node dysfunction and complete heart block can occur and require pacemaker insertion.

Thrombosis and Stroke

The reported incidence of thromboembolic complications in the Fontan circuit varies from 6% to 25%, depending on the diagnostic method used and the length of follow-up. Thrombus formation may relate to the presence of supraventricular arrhythmias, right atrial dilation, right atrial "smoke," and the artificial material used to construct the Fontan circuit. Systemic arterial embolism in patients with and without a fenestrated Fontan has also been reported. Protein C deficiency has been reported in these patients and may explain in part their propensity to thromboembolism. There is continuing debate as to the role of anticoagulation, antiplatelet therapy, or both in the long-term management of these patients, but most receive some form of therapy.

Protein-Losing Enteropathy

Protein-losing enteropathy, defined as severe loss of serum protein into the intestine, occurs in 4% to 13% of patients after a Fontan procedure.[60] Patients present with generalized edema, ascites, pleural effusion, or chronic diarrhea. Protein-losing enteropathy is thought to result principally from chronically elevated systemic venous pressure causing intestinal lymphangiectasia with consequent loss of albumin, protein, lymphocytes, and immunoglobulin into the gastrointestinal tract. The diagnosis is confirmed by the findings of low serum albumin and protein concentrations, low plasma alpha$_1$-antitrypsin level and lymphocyte counts, and, most important, high alpha$_1$-antitrypsin stool clearance. It carries a dismal prognosis, with a 5-year survival of 46% to 59%.

Right Pulmonary Vein Compression or Obstruction

Right pulmonary vein obstruction or compression can occur from the enlarged right atrium or atrial baffle bulging into the left atrium and can lead to a vicious spiral of increased pulmonary artery pressure with further dilation of the right atrium.

Fontan Obstruction

Stenosis or partial obstruction of the Fontan connection leads to exercise intolerance, atrial tachyarrhythmias, and right-sided heart failure. Sudden total obstruction (usually thrombotic) can present as sudden death.

Ventricular Dysfunction and Valvular Regurgitation

Progressive deterioration of systemic ventricular function, with or without progressive AV valve regurgitation, is common. Patients with morphologic systemic right ventricles may fare less well than those with morphologic left ventricles.

Hepatic Dysfunction

Mildly raised hepatic transaminase levels from hepatic congestion are frequent but seldom clinically important. Cirrhosis due to chronic venous hypertension is increasingly recognized, and monitoring for complications of cirrhosis should be initiated.[61]

Cyanosis

Worsening cyanosis may relate to worsening of ventricular function, the development of venous collateral channels draining to the left atrium, or the development of pulmonary arteriovenous malformations (especially if a classic Glenn procedure remains as part of the Fontan circulation). In Fontan patients with cirrhosis, the hepatopulmonary syndrome may occur.[62]

Laboratory Investigations

Electrocardiography. Sinus rhythm, atrial flutter, junctional rhythm, or complete heart block may be present. The QRS complex reflects the basic underlying cardiac anomaly. In patients with tricuspid atresia, left-axis deviation is the norm. In patients with univentricular hearts, the conduction pattern varies widely and depends on the morphology and relative position of the rudimentary chamber.

Chest Radiography. Mild bulging of the right lower heart border from a dilated right atrium is often seen in patients with an atriopulmonary connection.

Echocardiography. The presence or absence of right atrial stasis, thrombus, patency of a fenestration, and Fontan circuit obstruction should be sought. Superior and inferior venae cavae biphasic and pulmonary artery triphasic flow patterns suggest unobstructed flow in the Fontan circuit, whereas a mean gradient between the Fontan circuit and the pulmonary artery of 2 mm Hg or more may represent significant obstruction. Assessment of the pulmonary venous flow pattern is important in detecting pulmonary vein obstruction (right pulmonary vein > left pulmonary vein) sometimes caused by an enlarged right atrium. Concomitant assessment of systemic ventricular function and AV valve regurgitation can be readily accomplished. TEE may be required if there is inadequate visualization of the Fontan anastomosis or to exclude thrombus in the right atrium.

CMR. The objectives of CMR in Fontan patients include assessment of the pathways from the systemic veins to the pulmonary arteries for obstruction and thrombus; detection of Fontan baffle fenestration or leaks; evaluation of the pulmonary veins for compression; assessment of systemic ventricular volume, mass, and ejection fraction; imaging of the systemic ventricular outflow tract for obstruction; and quantitative assessment of the AV and semilunar valves for regurgitation, of the aorta for obstruction or an aneurysm, and for aortopulmonary, systemic venous, or systemic to pulmonary venous collateral vessels.

Diagnostic Catheterization. Complete heart catheterization is advised if surgical reintervention is planned or if adequate assessment of the hemodynamics is not obtained by noninvasive means.

MANAGEMENT OPTIONS AND OUTCOMES. Selection of patients is of utmost importance and has a major impact on clinical outcome. Long-term survival in "ideal" candidates is 81% at 10 years, compared with 60% to 71% in "all comers." Death occurs mostly from congestive heart failure and atrial arrhythmias. The Fontan procedure remains a palliative, not curative, procedure. A more radical approach to the failing atriopulmonary Fontan circulation, including surgical revision of the circuit to an extracardiac conduit, in combination with a Cox maze procedure and, frequently, simultaneous epicardial pacemaker insertion, has recently been shown to provide good early palliation. Ultimately, cardiac transplantation may be required by some of these patients, although outcomes are less favorable in such patients.[5,6]

Arrhythmias

Atrial tachyarrhythmias are difficult to manage and should quickly raise the thought of long-term warfarin therapy. When atrial flutter or fibrillation is present, an underlying hemodynamic cause should always be sought, and, in particular, evidence for obstruction of the Fontan circuit needs to be excluded. Prompt attempts should be made to restore sinus rhythm. Antiarrhythmic medications, alone or combined with an epicardial antitachycardia pacing device, and radiofrequency catheter ablation techniques have had limited success (see Chap. 39). Surgical conversion from an atriopulmonary Fontan to a total cavopulmonary connection with concomitant atrial cryoablation therapy at the time of surgery has been reported with good short-term success.[63] Epicardial pacemaker insertion for sinus node dysfunction or complete heart block may be necessary. Epicardial AV sequential pacing should be employed whenever possible (see Chap. 38).

Anticoagulant Therapy

The use of prophylactic long-term anticoagulation is contentious. Experts recommend that patients with a history of documented arrhythmias, fenestration in the Fontan connection, or spontaneous contrast (smoke) in the right atrium on echocardiography be anticoagulated. For established thrombus, thrombolytic therapy versus surgical removal of the clot and conversion of the Fontan circuit have been described, both with high mortality rates.

Protein-Losing Enteropathy

Treatment modalities include a low-fat, high-protein, medium-chain triglyceride diet to reduce intestinal lymphatic production; albumin infusions to increase intravascular osmotic pressure; and the introduction of diuretics, afterload-reducing agents, and positive inotropic agents to lower central venous pressure. Most often, these therapies are ineffective and should not be continued if indeed they are tried at all. Catheter-based interventions such as balloon dilation of pathway obstruction or creation of an atrial fenestration and surgical interventions from conversion or takedown of the Fontan circuit to cardiac transplantation have also been advocated. Other reportedly effective treatment modalities include subcutaneous heparin, octreotide treatment, and steroid therapy. All therapies have a similar failure rate of about 50%.

Right Pulmonary Vein Compression or Obstruction

When this is hemodynamically significant, Fontan conversion to a total cavopulmonary connection or extracardiac conduit may be recommended.

Fontan Obstruction

Surgical revision of an obstructed right atrium to pulmonary artery or superior and inferior venae cavae to pulmonary artery connections is recommended, usually to an extracardiac Fontan. Alternatively, balloon angioplasty with or without stenting may be used when it is appropriate and feasible.

Ventricular Failure and Valvular Regurgitation

ACE inhibitors are of unproven benefit, do not appear to enhance exercise capacity, and may cause clinical deterioration in Fontan patients. Patients with systemic AV valve regurgitation may require AV valve repair or replacement. Cardiac transplantation should also be considered.

Cyanosis

In the setting of a fenestrated Fontan, surgical or preferably transcatheter closure of the fenestration can be attempted. Pulmonary arteriovenous fistulas from a classic Glenn shunt may be improved by surgical conversion to a bidirectional Glenn connection.

FOLLOW-UP. Close and expert follow-up is recommended, with particular attention to ventricular function and systemic AV valve regurgitation. The development of atrial tachyarrhythmia should instigate a search for possible obstruction at the Fontan anastomosis, right pulmonary vein obstruction, or thrombus within the right atrium.

Total Anomalous Pulmonary Venous Connection

DEFINITION. This describes the situation in which all pulmonary veins fail to connect directly to the morphologic left atrium. As a result, all of the systemic and pulmonary venous return usually drains to the right atrium, albeit by varied routes.

Morphology (Fig. 65-21). The anatomic varieties of total anomalous pulmonary venous connection may be subdivided according to the path of the abnormal drainage. The anomalous connection is most often supradiaphragmatic, connecting via a vertical vein to the left brachiocephalic vein, directly to the right atrium, to the coronary sinus, or directly to the superior vena cava. In about 10% to 15%, the pathway is below the diaphragm. The anomalous trunk then connects into the portal vein or one of its tributaries, the ductus venosus, or, rarely, the hepatic or other abdominal veins.

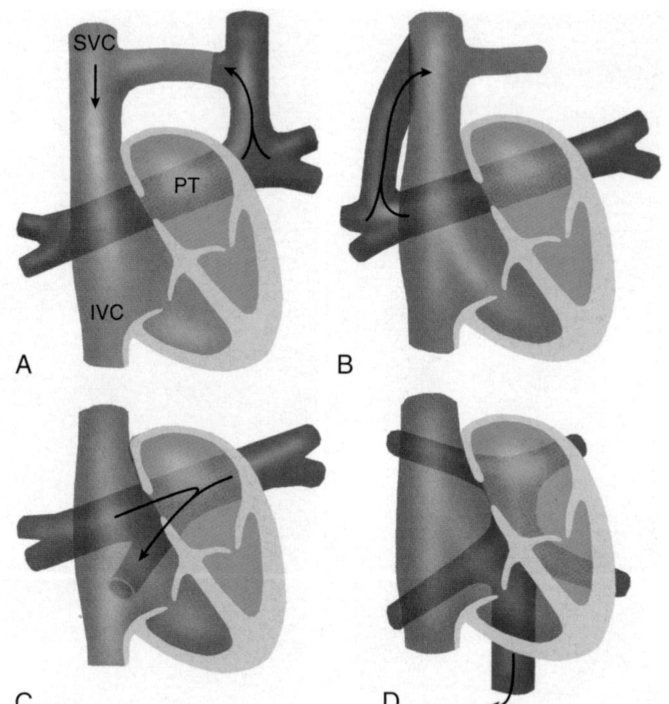

FIGURE 65-21 Anatomic types of total anomalous pulmonary venous return: supracardiac, in which the pulmonary veins drain either via the vertical vein to the anomalous vein **(A)** or directly to the superior vena cava (SVC) with the orifice close to the orifice of the azygos vein **(B)**; drainage into the right atrium via the coronary sinus **(C)**; infracardiac drainage **(D)** via a vertical vein into the portal vein or the inferior vena cava (IVC). PT = pulmonary trunk. *(**A** to **D** from Stark J, deLeval M: Surgery for Congenital Heart Defects. 2nd ed. Philadelphia, WB Saunders, 1994, p 330.)*

Pathophysiology. The physiologic consequences and, accordingly, the clinical picture depend on the size of the interatrial communication and the degree of obstruction elsewhere within the pathway. When the interatrial communication is small, systemic blood flow is severely limited with right-sided heart failure. Obstruction to pulmonary venous return and pulmonary venous hypertension are invariably present in patients with infradiaphragmatic anomalous pulmonary venous connection.

NATURAL HISTORY. Most patients with total anomalous pulmonary venous connection have symptoms during the first year of life, and 80% die before 1 year of age if they are not treated. The presence of obstruction in the pulmonary venous pathway or at the atrial septum leads to earlier presentation. When the obstruction is severe, neonatal presentation with severe cyanosis and cardiovascular collapse may occur. This is incompatible with survival without urgent surgical intervention.

CLINICAL FEATURES. Symptomatic infants with total anomalous pulmonary venous connection present with signs of heart failure or cyanosis. Infants with pulmonary venous obstruction present with the early onset of severe dyspnea, pulmonary edema, cyanosis, and right-sided heart failure. Without obstruction, cyanosis may be minimal and go undetected. On auscultation, there is usually a fixed, widely split second heart sound with an accentuated pulmonic component.

Laboratory Investigations

Electrocardiography. This usually shows right-axis deviation and right atrial and right ventricular hypertrophy.

Chest Radiography. In the unrepaired patient, this usually shows cardiomegaly with increased pulmonary blood flow. The right atrium and ventricle are dilated and hypertrophied, and the pulmonary artery segment is enlarged. The so-called figure-of-8 or "snowman" heart is due to enlargement of the heart and the presence of a dilated right superior vena cava, innominate vein, and left vertical vein.

Echocardiography (**Fig. 65-22**). This usually shows marked enlargement of the right ventricle and a small left atrium. Demonstration of the entire pathway of pulmonary venous drainage is usually possible, and cardiac catheterization (which may be hazardous) is almost never performed now. An echo-free space representing the pulmonary venous confluence can usually be seen behind the left atrium. The drainage of all four pulmonary veins and their connections must be identified.

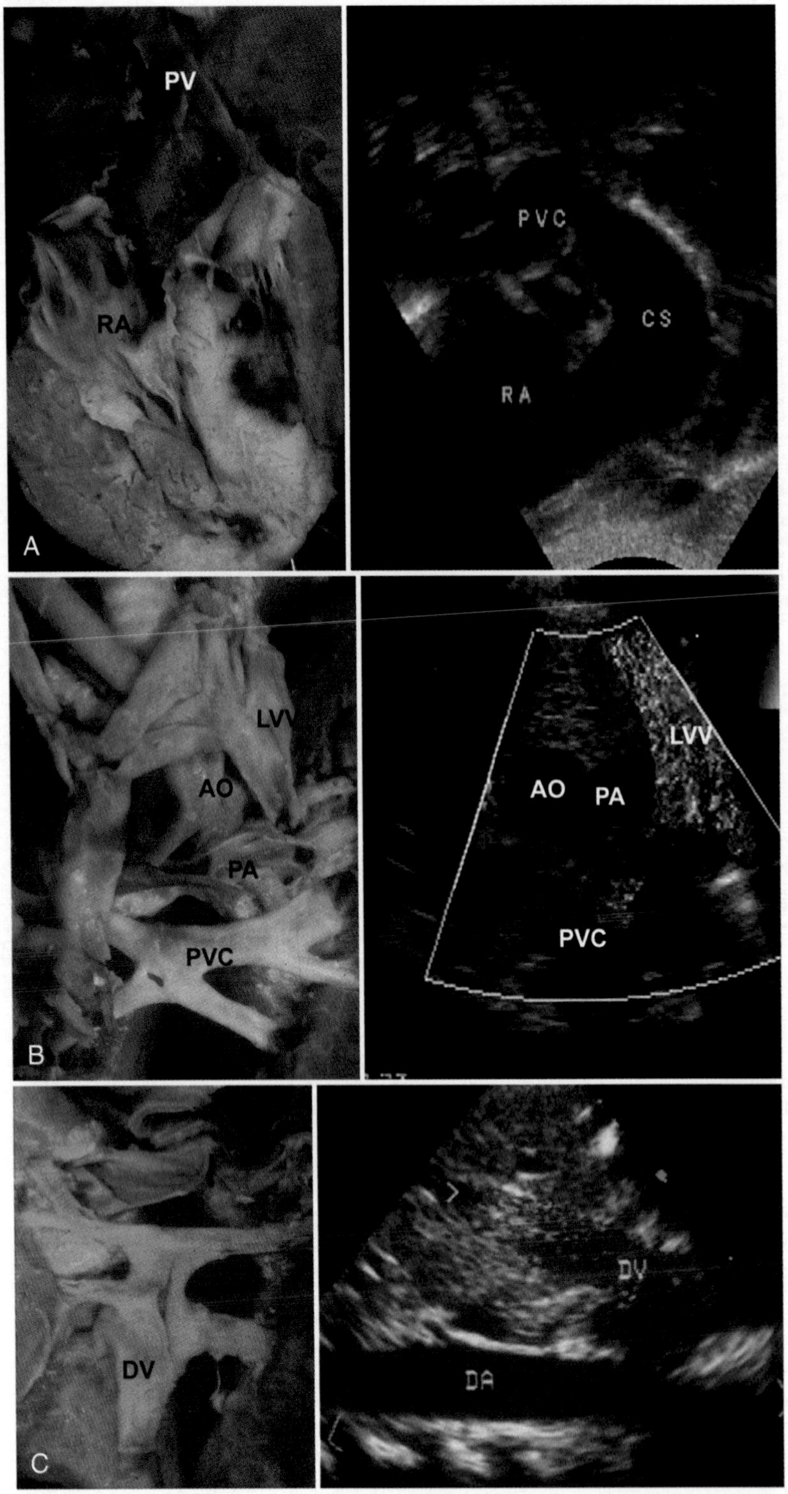

CMR. Although it is not often used, especially in infants, CMR may be helpful in delineation of the site of connections of total anomalous pulmonary venous return, when there are multiple mixed sites, in older children, and for detection of stenosis in postoperative patients.

INDICATIONS FOR INTERVENTION. Medical therapy, other than mechanical ventilation, has a limited role in the symptomatic infant, and corrective surgery should be performed as soon as possible. In asymptomatic children without pulmonary hypertension, surgery can be deferred to 3 to 6 months of age.

INTERVENTIONAL OPTIONS AND OUTCOMES. An urgent balloon atrial septostomy is occasionally required to increase systemic blood flow before surgery. Otherwise, interventional catheterization is restricted to attempts at relief of postoperative pulmonary venous stenosis, although this is often unrewarding. Historically, surgical repair of restenosis was also disappointing. However, the sutureless technique, whereby the pulmonary veins are opened widely into the retroatrial space, has markedly improved the results of such surgery. Adult patients have almost always had surgical repair in childhood. As a rule, they function normally and are not too prone to arrhythmias or other problems. They are seen as low- to moderate-risk adults.

FOLLOW-UP. Early follow-up should be frequent and aimed at early detection of stenosis of the pulmonary veins or the surgical anastomosis. If it is not present within the first year, stenosis is rare, but annual follow-up during childhood is required.

FIGURE 65-22 **A,** Subcostal view demonstrating total anomalous pulmonary drainage to the coronary sinus. Note the dilated coronary sinus in both images. The echocardiogram also demonstrates an associated confluence that connects to the coronary sinus. **B,** Suprasternal view demonstrating total anomalous pulmonary venous drainage to a left vertical vein. Note the direction of flow in the vertical vein that differentiates it from a left superior vena cava. **C,** Total anomalous pulmonary venous drainage below the diaphragm. The specimen shows the pulmonary veins as they enter the confluence, whereas the echocardiogram demonstrates the descending veins as they enter the liver. Note that the direction of flow is away from the heart. AO = aorta; CS = coronary sinus; DA = descending aorta; DV = descending vein; LVV = left vertical vein; PA = pulmonary artery; PV = pulmonary vein; PVC = pulmonary venous confluence; RA = right atrium.

Transposition Complexes

The key anatomic feature that characterizes this group of diagnoses is ventriculoarterial discordance. This is most commonly seen in the context of AV concordance, also known as complete transposition or D-TGA. The second condition that is discussed in this section is the combination of ventriculoarterial discordance with AV discordance, commonly referred to as congenitally corrected TGA or L-TGA. More complicated arrangements are not considered here.

Complete Transposition of the Great Arteries

DEFINITION AND NATURAL HISTORY. This is a common and potentially lethal form of heart disease in newborns and infants. The malformation consists of the origin of the aorta from the morphologic right ventricle and that of the pulmonary artery from the morphologic left ventricle. Consequently, the pulmonary and systemic circulations are connected in parallel rather than the normal in-series connection. In one circuit, systemic venous blood passes to the right atrium, to the right ventricle, and then to the aorta. In the other, pulmonary venous blood passes through the left atrium and ventricle to the pulmonary artery. This situation is incompatible with life unless mixing of the two circuits occurs.

Approximately two thirds of patients have no major associated abnormalities (simple transposition), and one third have associated abnormalities (complex transposition). The most common associated abnormalities are VSD and pulmonary or subpulmonary stenosis. It is increasingly being diagnosed in utero. Without treatment, about 30% of these infants die within the first week of life, and 90% die within the first year.

Morphology. Some communication between the two circulations must exist after birth to sustain life. Almost all patients have an interatrial communication, blood flow across which governs the amount of desaturation. Two thirds have a PDA, and about one third have an associated VSD.

Pathophysiology. The degree of tissue hypoxia, the nature of the associated cardiovascular anomalies, and the anatomic and functional status of the pulmonary vascular bed determine the clinical course. The anatomic arrangement results in two separate and parallel circulations. The systemic arterial oxygen saturation is governed by the amount of blood exchanged between the two circulations. Infants with D-TGA are particularly susceptible to the early development of pulmonary vascular obstructive disease even in the absence of a PDA and even with an intact ventricular septum.

CLINICAL FEATURES

Pediatric

The average birth weight and size of infants born with complete TGA are greater than normal. The usual clinical manifestations are dyspnea and cyanosis from birth, progressive hypoxemia, and congestive heart failure. The most severe cyanosis and hypoxemia are observed in infants who have only a small PFO or ductus arteriosus and an intact ventricular septum or in those infants with relatively reduced pulmonary blood flow because of left ventricular outflow tract obstruction. With a large ASD or PDA or large VSD, cyanosis can be minimal, and heart failure is usually the dominant problem after the first few weeks of life. Cardiac murmurs are of little diagnostic significance.

The two-dimensional echocardiogram should establish the complete diagnosis, including the coronary artery pattern. Prenatal detection is possible and favorably modifies neonatal morbidity and mortality. Ultrasound imaging has become a standard procedure to guide catheter placement and manipulation during balloon atrial septostomy and to assess the anatomic adequacy of the septostomy.

MANAGEMENT OPTIONS. Maintenance of ductal patency by prostaglandin E_1 in the early neonatal period improves the arterial saturation by enhancing mixing at atrial level. This is usually as a prelude to the creation or enlargement of an interatrial communication by a balloon or blade atrial septostomy. Surgical atrial septectomy is seldom required now.

Surgery

Although balloon atrial septostomy is often lifesaving, it is palliative and anticipates "corrective" surgery. Atrial redirection procedures were developed in the 1950s and 1960s but were replaced by the arterial switch operation, which became widely adopted in the 1980s.

Atrial Switch (Fig. 65-23)

The most common surgical procedure in patients who are currently adults is the atrial switch operation. Patients will have had either a Mustard or a Senning procedure. Blood is redirected at the atrial level by a baffle made of Dacron or pericardium (Mustard operation) or atrial flaps (Senning operation), achieving physiologic correction. Systemic venous return is diverted through the mitral valve into the subpulmonary left ventricle, and the pulmonary venous return is rerouted through the tricuspid valve into the subaortic right ventricle. By virtue of this repair, the morphologic right ventricle supports the systemic circulation.

Palliative Atrial Switch

Uncommonly, in patients with a large VSD and established pulmonary vascular disease, a palliative atrial switch operation is done to improve oxygenation. The VSD is left open or enlarged at the time of atrial baffle surgery. These patients resemble patients with Eisenmenger VSDs and should be managed as such.

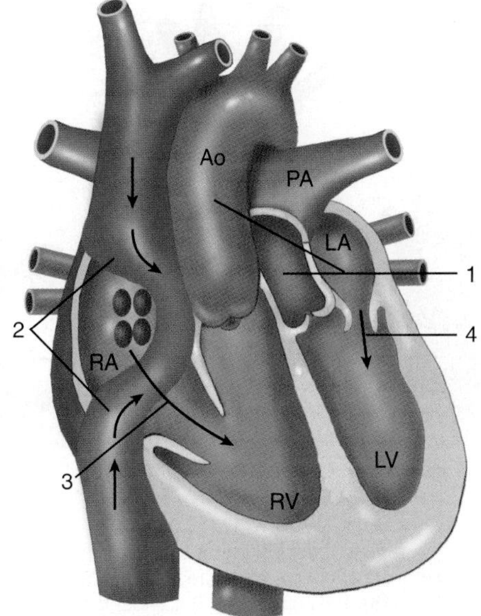

FIGURE 65-23 Diagrammatic representation of atrial switch surgery (Mustard or Senning procedure). Superior vena cava and inferior vena cava blood is redirected into the morphologic left ventricle (LV), which pumps blood into the pulmonary artery (PA), whereas the pulmonary venous blood flow is rerouted to the morphologic right ventricle (RV), which empties into the aorta (Ao). RA = right atrium; LA = left atrium; 1, transposition of the great arteries; 2, atrial baffles; 3, pulmonary vein blood flow through tricuspid valve to right ventricle; 4, inferior vena cava and superior vena cava blood flow through mitral valve to left ventricle. *(From Mullins CE, Mayer DC: Congenital Heart Disease: A Diagrammatic Atlas. New York, Wiley-Liss, 1988.)*

Arterial Switch Operation (Fig. 65-24)

In this operation, the arterial trunks are transected and reanastomosed to the contralateral root. If a VSD is present, it is closed. The coronary arteries must be transposed to the neoaorta. This is the most challenging part of the procedure and accounts for most of the mortality. Nonetheless, this rate has fallen to less than 2% in most large centers. The major advantages of the arterial switch procedure, compared with the atrial switch procedure, are restoration of the left ventricle as the systemic pump and the potential for long-term maintenance of sinus rhythm.

Follow-up studies after the arterial switch operation have demonstrated good left ventricular function and normal exercise capacity. Potential sequelae of the operation include coronary occlusion, supravalvular pulmonary stenosis (which may be treated by either reoperation or balloon angioplasty), supravalvular aortic stenosis, ascending aortic aneurysms, and neoaortic regurgitation (usually mild).[64-66] Long-term patency and growth of the coronary arteries appear satisfactory.

Rastelli Procedure

Infants with TGA plus a VSD and left ventricular outflow tract obstruction may require an early systemic–pulmonary artery shunt when a pronounced diminution in pulmonary blood flow exists. A later corrective procedure for these patients bypasses the left ventricular outflow obstruction with an extracardiac prosthetic conduit between the right ventricle and the distal end of a divided pulmonary artery and uses an intracardiac ventricular baffle to tunnel the left ventricle to the aorta (Rastelli procedure).

MANAGEMENT OUTCOMES

Atrial Switch

After atrial baffle surgery, most patients who reach adulthood are in NYHA Classes I and II, but abnormalities of ventricular filling, due to the abnormal atrial pathways, may be of more direct importance to functional capacity than right ventricular performance issues in many.

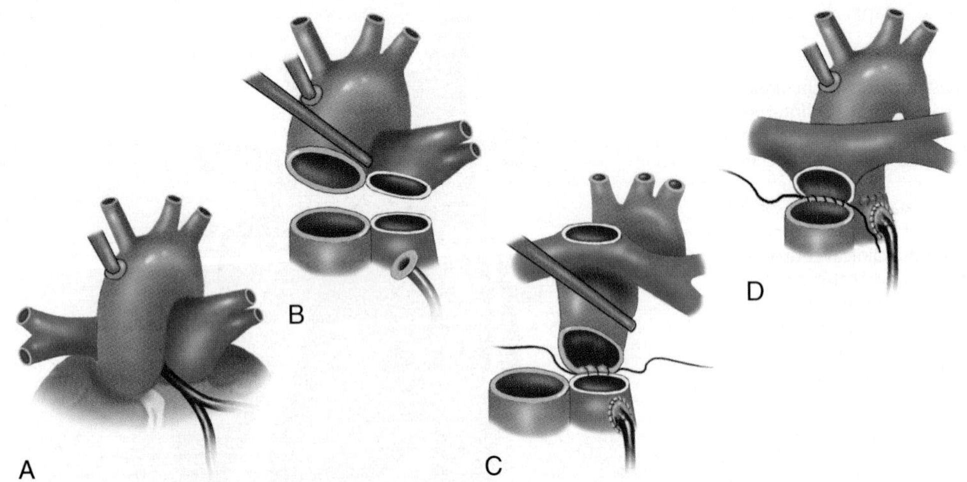

FIGURE 65-24 Complete transposition of the great arteries, corrected by a modified arterial switch operation. The aorta and pulmonary artery are transected **(A),** and the orifices of the coronary arteries are excised with a rim of adjacent aortic wall **(B).** The aorta is brought under the bifurcation of the pulmonary artery, and the pulmonary artery and the aorta are anastomosed without necessitating graft interposition. The coronary arteries are transferred to the pulmonary artery **(C).** The mobilized pulmonary artery is directly anastomosed to the proximal aortic stump **(D).** *(**A** to **D** from Stark J, deLeval M: Surgery for Congenital Heart Defects. New York, Grune & Stratton, 1983, p 379.)*

Some present with symptoms of congestive heart failure (2% to 15%). Echocardiographic evidence of moderate or severe systemic right ventricular dysfunction is present in up to 40% of patients. Relative right ventricular ischemia (supply-demand mismatch) is thought to perhaps play a role in systemic right ventricular dysfunction. More than mild systemic tricuspid regurgitation is present in 10% to 40%, both reflecting and exacerbating right ventricular dysfunction. Palpitations and near-syncope or syncope from rhythm disturbances are fairly common. Atrial flutter occurs in 20% of patients by 20 years of age, and sinus node dysfunction is seen in half of the patients by that time. These rhythm disturbances are a consequence of direct and indirect atrial and sinus node damage at the time of atrial baffle surgery.

A shortened life expectancy is the rule, with 70% to 80% survival at 20 to 30 years' follow-up. Patients with complex TGA in general fare much worse than those with simple TGA. Sudden cardiac death can occur in these patients and may relate to systemic right ventricular dysfunction, the presence of atrial flutter, and pulmonary hypertension. Significant pulmonary vascular disease can develop over time and relates to older age at the time of atrial switch operation, particularly in patients with a substantial VSD as well as in those with long-standing left-to-right shunts through a baffle leak. Superior vena cava or inferior vena cava baffle obstruction often goes undetected because collateral drainage through the azygos vein prevents systemic venous congestion. Pulmonary venous baffle obstruction causes elevated pulmonary artery pressure, and patients can present with dyspnea and pulmonary venous congestive features.

Physical examination of a patient whose condition is otherwise uncomplicated reveals a right ventricular parasternal lift, a normal S_1, a single S_2 (P_2 is not heard because of its posterior location), a pansystolic murmur from tricuspid regurgitation if it is present (best heard at the left lower sternal border, but not increasing with inspiration), and a right-sided S_4 when severe systemic ventricular dysfunction is present.

Arterial Switch

Data on long-term complications in adults who have undergone the arterial switch procedure are emerging. The development of progressive neoaortic valve regurgitation from neoaortic root dilation is the most common long-term sequela. It is time dependent and as such requires periodic follow-up.[65,66] Supra–neopulmonary artery stenosis is a frequent finding but rarely has clinical consequences. The development of ostial coronary artery disease has also been described in some patients.[64] Arrhythmia promises to be less of a problem in this group of patients. Cardiac examination in uncomplicated patients is normal.

Rastelli Procedure

Progressive right ventricular to pulmonary artery conduit obstruction can cause exercise intolerance or right ventricular angina. Left ventricular tunnel obstruction can present as exertional dyspnea or syncope. Conduit replacement or transcatheter stent or stent-valve implantation is inevitably required in surviving patients.[67] Physical examination in uncomplicated patients reveals, in contrast to those after atrial switch, no right ventricular lift, an ejection systolic murmur from the conduit, and two components to the S_2.

Laboratory Investigations

Electrocardiography. Sinus bradycardia or junctional rhythm (without a right atrial overload pattern) with evidence of marked right ventricular hypertrophy is characteristically present in patients after the atrial switch procedure. The ECG is typically normal in patients after the arterial switch procedure. The ECG typically shows right bundle branch block after a Rastelli procedure.

Chest Radiography. On the posteroanterior film, a narrow vascular pedicle with an oblong cardiac silhouette ("egg on side") is typically seen in patients after the atrial switch procedure. On the lateral view, the anterior aorta may be seen to fill the retrosternal space. For the arterial switch, normal mediastinal borders are present despite the Lecompte maneuver. After the Rastelli procedure, the chest radiograph may be normal unless the conduit becomes calcified.

Echocardiography. After the atrial switch procedure, parallel great arteries are the hallmark of TGA (**Fig. 65-25**). They are best visualized from a parasternal long-axis view (running side by side) or from a parasternal short-axis view (seen en face, with the aorta anterior and rightward). Qualitative assessment of systemic right ventricular function, the degree of tricuspid regurgitation, and the presence or absence of subpulmonary left ventricular obstruction (dynamic or fixed) is important. Assessment of baffle leak or obstruction (**Fig. 65-26**) is best done with color and Doppler flow imaging. Normal baffle flow should be phasic in nature and vary with respiration, with a peak velocity less than 1 m/sec. After arterial switch, neoaortic valve regurgitation, supra–neopulmonary valve stenosis, and segmental wall motion abnormality from ischemia due to coronary ostial stenosis should be sought. In patients who have undergone the Rastelli operation, left ventricular to aorta tunnel obstruction as well as right ventricular to pulmonary artery conduit degeneration (stenosis or regurgitation) must be assessed.

CMR. The major role of CMR in patients with atrial switch is to evaluate the baffles and systemic right ventricular volume and ejection fraction. As a rule, CMR reports better right ventricular size and function than does echocardiography. For patients who are claustrophobic or have a pacemaker, CT angiography may serve as a substitute.

Cardiac Catheterization. Diagnostic cardiac catheterization may be required to assess the presence or severity of systemic or pulmonary baffle obstruction, baffle leak, and pulmonary hypertension; coronary ostial stenosis; or tunnel or conduit obstruction when it is not diagnosed by noninvasive means.

INDICATIONS FOR REINTERVENTION. After the atrial switch procedure, severe symptomatic right ventricular dysfunction may warrant surgical treatment in the form of a two-stage arterial switch procedure[68] or cardiac transplantation. Tricuspid valve repair or replacement is rarely performed for severe systemic (tricuspid) AV valve regurgitation, particularly if it is due to a flail leaflet or cusp perforation and provided right ventricular function is adequate. A baffle leak resulting in a significant left-to-right shunt (>1.5:1), any right-to-left shunt, or attributable symptoms require surgical or transcatheter closure. Superior vena cava or inferior vena cava pathway obstruction may require intervention. Superior vena cava stenosis is usually benign, whereas inferior vena cava stenosis may have greater hemodynamic consequences, depending on the adequacy of alternative routes of venous return, usually via the azygos vein to the superior vena cava. Balloon dilation of superior vena cava or inferior vena cava stenosis is an option in expert hands. Stenting usually relieves the stenosis completely.

Pathway obstruction after the Senning operation is usually more amenable to balloon dilation and stenting. Pulmonary venous obstruction, although usually seen early and reoperated on in childhood, may present in adulthood. Symptomatic bradycardia warrants permanent pacemaker implantation, whereas tachyarrhythmias may require catheter ablation, an antitachycardia pacemaker device, or medical therapy. After an atrial switch, transvenous pacing leads must traverse the upper limb of the baffle to enter the morphologic left ventricle. Active fixation is required because coarse trabeculation is absent in the morphologic left ventricle. Transvenous pacing should be avoided in patients with residual intracardiac communications because paradoxical emboli can occur.[69]

After an arterial switch procedure, significant right ventricular outflow tract obstruction at any level (gradient > 50 mm Hg or right-to-left ventricular pressure ratio > 0.6) may require surgical or catheter augmentation of the right ventricular outflow tract. Myocardial ischemia from coronary artery obstruction may require coronary artery bypass grafting, preferably with arterial conduits. Significant neoaortic valve regurgitation may warrant aortic valve replacement.

In patients who have had the Rastelli procedure, significant right ventricle to pulmonary artery conduit stenosis (>50 mm Hg withdrawal gradient or mean echo gradient) or significant regurgitation necessitates intervention. Subaortic obstruction across the left ventricle to aorta tunnel necessitates left ventricle to aorta baffle reconstruction. A significant residual VSD (shunt >1.5:1) may require surgical closure.

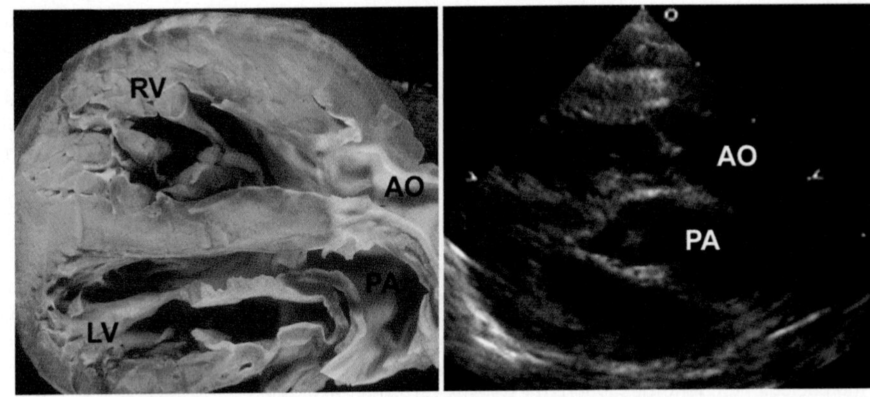

FIGURE 65-25 Parasternal long-axis view in transposition of the great arteries. Note the parallel nature of the aorta and pulmonary artery. AO = aorta; LV = left ventricle; PA = pulmonary artery; RV = right ventricle.

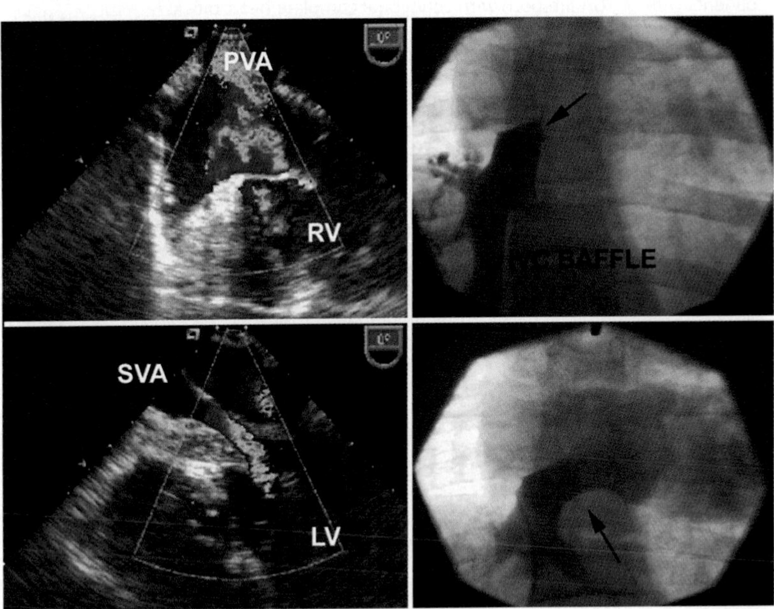

FIGURE 65-26 Montage of post-Mustard cases. The angiogram in the right upper panel shows complete obstruction of the inferior limb of the systemic venous baffle, whereas the lower right panel is the same case after stenting. The upper left image is a transesophageal echocardiogram showing the pulmonary venous baffle with some mild flow acceleration in its midpoint. The lower left panel shows the systemic venous baffle at its left ventricular end. IVC = inferior vena cava; LV = left ventricle; PVA = pulmonary venous atrium; RV = right ventricle; SVA = systemic venous atrium.

REINTERVENTION OPTIONS

Medical Therapy

In patients with an atrial switch, the role of afterload reduction with ACE inhibitors, angiotensin receptor blockers,[70,71] or beta blockade[72,73] to preserve systemic right ventricular function is unknown.

Two-Stage Arterial Switch and Cardiac Transplantation

Patients with symptomatic, severe systemic (right) ventricular dysfunction with or without severe systemic (tricuspid) AV valve regurgitation, following an atrial switch procedure, may require consideration of a conversion procedure to an arterial switch (two-stage arterial switch) or heart transplantation. The two-stage arterial switch, or switch-conversion procedure, consists of banding the pulmonary artery in the first stage to induce subpulmonary left ventricular hypertrophy and to "train" the left ventricle to support systemic pressure. Once left ventricular systolic pressure is more than 75% of systemic pressure and the left ventricular mass is considered adequate, in the second stage the atrial baffles and the pulmonary band are taken down, the atrial septum is reconstructed, and the great arteries are switched, leaving the morphologic left ventricle as the systemic ventricle. This procedure is still experimental in adults, with few data available to assess its short- and long-term efficacy.

REPRODUCTIVE ISSUES. Severe systemic ventricular dysfunction or intractable arrhythmias may be a contraindication to pregnancy, and baffle obstruction should, ideally, be relieved before pregnancy. Women who have had an atrial switch usually tolerate pregnancy well, but about 15% will develop worsening right ventricular function or tricuspid regurgitation during the pregnancy. In half of these cases, the problem does not improve after delivery.[74]

FOLLOW-UP. Regular follow-up by physicians with special expertise in CHD is recommended.

Atrial Switch

Serial follow-up of systemic right ventricular function is warranted. Asymptomatic baffle obstruction should be sought with echocardiography or CMR. Regular Holter monitoring is recommended to diagnose unacceptable bradyarrhythmias or tachyarrhythmias.

Arterial Switch and Rastelli Procedure

Regular follow-up with echocardiography is recommended.

Congenitally Corrected Transposition of the Great Arteries

DEFINITION. The term *congenitally corrected transposition of the great arteries* describes hearts in which there are discordant AV connections in combination with discordant ventriculoarterial connections.

MORPHOLOGY (Fig. 65-27). cc-TGA is a rare condition, accounting for less than 1% of all CHD. When there is the usual atrial arrangement, systemic venous blood passes from the right atrium through a mitral valve to a left ventricle and then to the posteriorly located pulmonary artery. Pulmonary venous blood passes from the left atrium through a tricuspid valve to a left-sided right ventricle and then to an anterior, left-sided aorta. The circulation is thus "physiologically" corrected, but the morphologic right ventricle supports the systemic circulation. Associated anomalies occur in up to 95% of patients and consist of VSD (75%), pulmonary or subpulmonary stenosis (75%), and left-sided (tricuspid and often Ebstein-like) valve anomalies (>75%).

Because of the inherently abnormal conduction system, 5% of patients with cc-TGA are born with congenital complete heart block.

PATHOPHYSIOLOGY. Patients with no associated abnormalities (isolated cc-TGA) can exceptionally survive until the seventh or eighth decade. Progressive systemic (tricuspid) AV valve regurgitation and systemic (right) ventricular dysfunction tend to occur from the fourth decade onward, whereas atrial tachyarrhythmias are more common from the fifth decade onward. In addition to those born with congenital complete heart block, acquired complete AV block continues to develop at a rate of 2% per year, concentrated mainly at the time of cardiac surgery. Patients with associated anomalies (VSD, pulmonary stenosis, left-sided [tricuspid] valve anomaly) often have undergone surgical palliation (systemic to pulmonary artery shunt for cyanosis) or repair of the associated anomalies (see section on surgical procedures), but a significant number of patients are naturally balanced by a combination of their VSD and subpulmonary left ventricular outflow tract obstruction. Although cyanosed, they often remain well, with no intervention for many years.

CLINICAL FEATURES

Unrepaired

Patients with no associated defects can be asymptomatic until late adulthood. Dyspnea, exercise intolerance from developing congestive heart failure, and palpitations from supraventricular arrhythmias most often arise in the fifth decade. Patients with well-balanced VSD and pulmonary stenosis can present with paradoxical emboli or cyanosis, especially if pulmonary stenosis is severe. Physical examination of a patient whose condition is otherwise uncomplicated reveals a somewhat more medial apex due to the side-by-side orientation of the two ventricles. The A_2 is often palpable in the second left intercostal space because of the anterior location of the aorta. A single S_2 (A_2) is heard, with P_2 often being silent because of its posterior location. The murmur of an associated VSD or of left AV valve regurgitation may be heard. The murmur of pulmonary stenosis radiates upward and to the right, given the rightward direction of the main pulmonary artery. If there is complete heart block, cannon *a* waves with an S_1 of variable intensity are present.

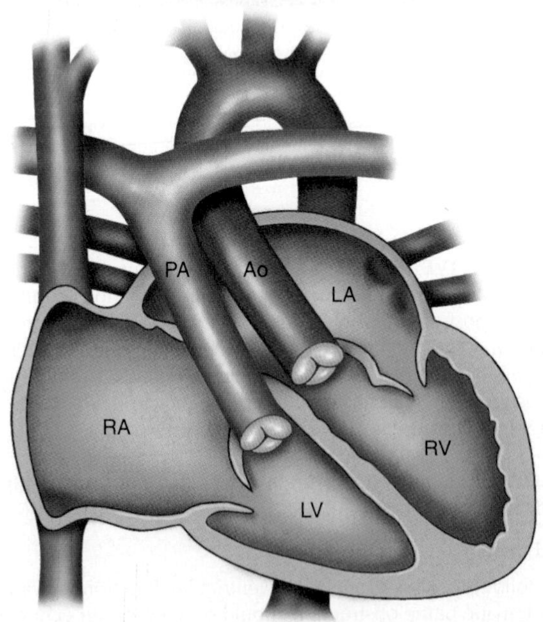

FIGURE 65-27 Diagrammatic representation of congenitally corrected transposition of the great arteries. Ao = aorta; LA = left atrium; LV = left ventricle; PA = pulmonary artery; RA = right atrium; RV = right ventricle. *(From Mullins CE, Mayer DC: Congenital Heart Disease: A Diagrammatic Atlas. New York, Wiley-Liss, 1988.)*

VSD Patch and Left Ventricular to Pulmonary Artery Conduit Repair

Most patients are in functional Class I at 5 to 10 years after surgery despite the common development of systemic tricuspid regurgitation and systemic right ventricular dysfunction after surgical repair. Dyspnea, exercise intolerance, and palpitations from supraventricular arrhythmia often occur in the fourth decade. Complete heart block may complicate surgery in an additional 25%. Physical examination reflects the basic cardiac malformation with or without residual coexisting anomalies.

LABORATORY INVESTIGATIONS

ELECTROCARDIOGRAPHY. An abnormal direction of initial (septal) depolarization from right to left causes reversal of the precordial Q wave pattern (Q waves are often present in the right precordial leads and absent in the left). First-degree AV block occurs in about 50%, and complete AV block occurs in up to 25% of patients. Atrial arrhythmias may be seen.

CHEST RADIOGRAPHY. Chest radiography characteristically reveals absence of the normal pulmonary artery segment in favor of a smooth convexity of the left supracardiac border produced by the left-sided ascending aorta. The main pulmonary trunk is medially displaced and absent from the cardiac silhouette; the right pulmonary hilum is often prominent and elevated compared with the left, producing a right-sided "waterfall" appearance.

ECHOCARDIOGRAPHY (**Fig. 65-28;** see Fig. 15-93B). Echocardiography permits the identification of the basic malformation as well as of any associated anomalies. The right-sided morphologic left ventricle is characterized by its smooth endocardial surface and is guarded by a bileaflet AV (mitral) valve with no direct septal attachment. The morphologic right ventricle is recognized by its apical trabeculation and moderator band and is guarded by a trileaflet apically displaced AV valve (tricuspid valve) with direct attachment to the septum. The AV valves therefore show reversed offsetting, a strong clue to the diagnosis. Ebstein-like malformation of the left (tricuspid) AV valve is defined by excessive (>8 mm/m^2 body surface area) apical displacement of the left (tricuspid) AV valve, with or without dysplasia.

CMR. The major role of CMR in cc-TGA patients is to evaluate the systemic right ventricular volume and ejection fraction. It does so better than echocardiography can at present. For claustrophobic or pacemaker patients, high-quality radionuclide angiography or CT angiography with volume estimates may serve as a substitute. CMR can evaluate other issues as well, including conduit function and AV valve regurgitation.

CARDIAC CATHETERIZATION. This is rarely required for diagnosis but may be indicated before surgical repair to demonstrate the coronary artery anatomy as well as ventricular end-diastolic and pulmonary artery pressures.

INDICATIONS FOR INTERVENTION AND REINTERVENTION. If moderate or severe systemic (tricuspid, left) AV valve regurgitation develops, valve replacement should be considered. Left AV valve replacement should be performed before systemic right ventricular function deteriorates, namely, at an ejection fraction of 45% or more. When tricuspid regurgitation is associated with poor systemic (right) ventricular function, the double-switch procedure should perhaps be considered, although its role remains controversial.[75] Patients with end-stage symptomatic heart failure should be referred for cardiac transplantation. The presence of a hemodynamically significant VSD (Q_p/Q_s > 1.5:1) or residual VSD with significant native or postsurgical (conduit) pulmonary outflow tract stenosis (echo mean or catheter gradient > 50 mm Hg) may require surgical correction, although the latter is sometimes best left alone as it can maintain a neutral septal position and minimize tricuspid regurgitation. Left AV valve replacement at the time of VSD and pulmonary stenosis surgery should be considered if concomitant left AV valve regurgitation is present. Pacemaker implantation is usual when complete AV block is present. The optimal pacing modality is DDD. Active fixation electrodes are required because of the lack of apical trabeculation in the morphologic left ventricle. Transvenous pacing should be avoided if there are intracardiac shunts because paradoxical emboli may occur.[69] Epicardial leads are preferred under these circumstances.

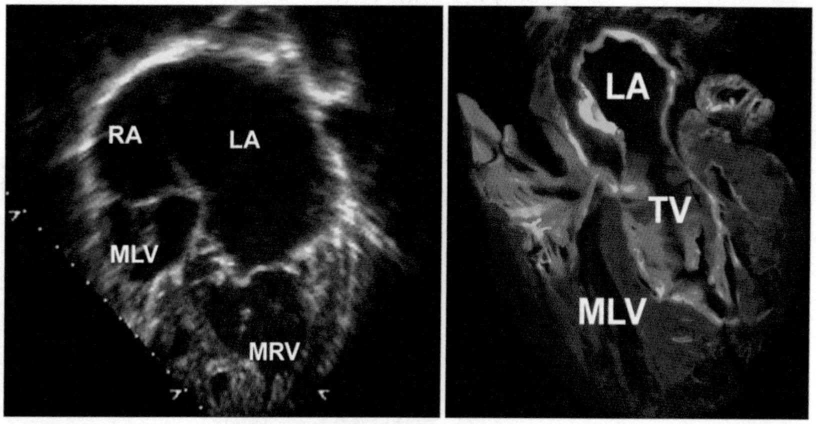

FIGURE 65-28 Four-chamber view in congenitally corrected transposition with dysplasia and displacement of the morphologic left-sided tricuspid valve. LA = left atrium; MLV = morphologic left ventricle; MRV = morphologic right ventricle; RA = right atrium; TV = tricuspid valve.

INTERVENTIONAL OPTIONS

Medical Therapy

ACE inhibitor or beta blocker therapy for patients with systemic ventricular dysfunction may be intuitive, but the role of such agents has not yet been demonstrated conclusively.[70,71,73]

Conduit Replacement or Repair

This is inevitably required in survivors of this type of initial surgery. Fortunately, it is now possible in some patients and in many countries to repair a failing conduit with a percutaneously delivered stented valve.[58]

Tricuspid Valve Replacement

For significant regurgitation, this is preferable to tricuspid valve repair. Valve repair is usually unsuccessful because of the abnormal, often Ebstein-like anatomy of the valve.

Double-Switch Procedure

This procedure has been successfully performed in children and carefully selected adults. It should be considered for patients with severe tricuspid regurgitation and systemic ventricular dysfunction.[75] Its purpose is to relocate the left ventricle into the systemic circulation and the right ventricle into the pulmonary circulation, achieving physiologic correction. An atrial switch procedure (Mustard or Senning), together with either an arterial switch procedure (when pulmonary stenosis is not present) or a Rastelli-type repair, the so-called Ilbawi procedure (left ventricle tunneled to aorta and right ventricle to pulmonary artery valved conduit when VSD and pulmonary stenosis are present), can be performed after adequate left ventricular retraining, leaving the regurgitant tricuspid valve and failing right ventricle on the pulmonary side.

Cardiac Transplantation

Patients with deteriorating systemic (right) ventricular function should be treated aggressively with medical therapy but may need to be considered for transplantation.

INTERVENTIONAL OUTCOMES. After conduit repair and VSD patching, the median survival of patients reaching adulthood is 40 years. The usual causes of death are sudden (presumed arrhythmic) and, more commonly, progressive systemic right ventricular dysfunction with systemic (tricuspid) AV valve regurgitation. The major predictor of poor outcome is the presence of left AV (tricuspid) valve regurgitation. Reoperation is common (15% to 25%), with left AV valve replacement usually being the primary reason. Data in adults who have had the double-switch procedure are lacking, and this procedure should be considered experimental in this population of patients.

FOLLOW-UP. All patients should have at least annual cardiology follow-up with an expert in the care of patients with congenital cardiac defects. Regular assessment of systemic (tricuspid) AV valve regurgitation by serial echocardiographic studies and systemic ventricular function by CMR or radionuclide angiography should be done. Holter recording can be useful if paroxysmal atrial arrhythmias or transient complete AV block is suspected.

Double-Outlet Right Ventricle

DEFINITION. The term *double-outlet right ventricle* describes hearts in which more than 50% of each semilunar valve arises from the morphologic right ventricle. It may coexist with any form of atrial arrangement or AV connection and is independent of infundibular (conal) anatomy.

Morphology (Fig. 65-29). Few morphologic descriptors have invoked more discussion and controversy than double-outlet right ventricle. The definition given earlier is flawed but pragmatic. To some extent, this anatomic definition is less important than the understanding of the relationship between the great vessels and the VSD and the anatomy of the outlets to the great vessels, both of which are crucial determinants of clinical presentation and management.

CLINICAL FEATURES. Three main categories of double-outlet right ventricle exist: (1) double-outlet right ventricle with a subaortic VSD, (2) double-outlet right ventricle with a subpulmonary VSD, and (3) double-outlet right ventricle with a noncommitted VSD.

The position of the infundibular septum further modifies the hemodynamics. Taking double-outlet right ventricle with a subaortic VSD as an example, in which the aorta and its semilunar valve are closest to or overriding the trabecular septum, anterior deviation of the outlet septum causes subpulmonary stenosis, and the clinical scenario and management algorithm are similar or identical to those of tetralogy of Fallot. Conversely, if the outlet septum is deviated posteriorly, there will be subaortic stenosis, often with a coexisting abnormality of the aortic arch. The presentation and management of this variation are therefore entirely different. If there is no deviation of the outlet septum and no outlet obstruction, the clinical scenario will be that of a simple VSD. Double-outlet right ventricle with a subpulmonary VSD (Taussig-Bing anomaly) can be considered along with TGA. This is because the usual position of the pulmonary artery (posterior and leftward to the aorta) means that the streaming of deoxygenated and oxygenated blood is similar to that of transposition, even though most of the pulmonary valve is connected to the right ventricle. Anterior deviation of the outlet septum causes subaortic stenosis and aortic anomalies, and posterior deviation causes subpulmonary stenosis and limits pulmonary blood flow. It is also important to recognize double-outlet right ventricle with a noncommitted VSD. This defines hearts in which the VSD is remote from the outlets, making surgical management particularly difficult.

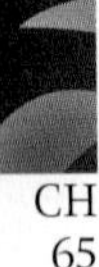

CH 65

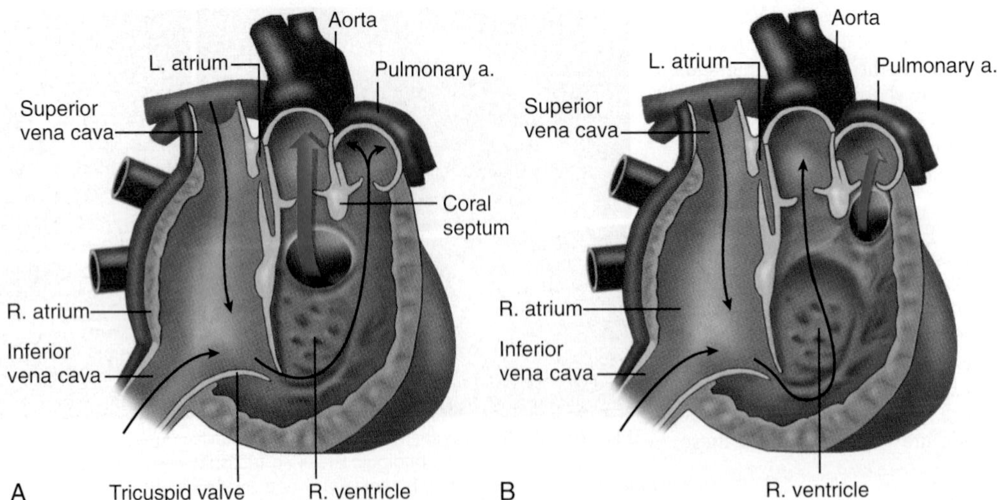

FIGURE 65-29 Double-outlet right ventricle with side-by-side relation of great arteries is illustrated in both panels. **A,** A subaortic ventricular septal defect below the crista supraventricularis favors delivery of left ventricular blood to the aorta. **B,** Subpulmonary location of the ventricular septal defect above the crista favors streaming to the pulmonary trunk. *(**A** and **B** from Castañeda A, Jonas RA, Mayer JE, et al: Cardiac Surgery of the Neonate and Infant. Philadelphia, WB Saunders, 1994, p 446.)*

ASSOCIATED LESIONS. More than half of patients with double-outlet right ventricles have associated anomalies of the AV valves. Mitral valve stenosis or atresia associated with a hypoplastic left ventricle is common. Ebstein anomaly of the tricuspid valve, complete AV septal defect, and overriding or straddling of either AV valve may occur.

LABORATORY INVESTIGATIONS. Because of the diversity of underlying anatomies, discussion of the electrocardiographic and radiographic features is not included here.

ECHOCARDIOGRAPHY. This is the mainstay of diagnosis. The commitment of the semilunar valves to the ventricles is ascertained. When it is present, deviation of the outlet septum beneath a semilunar valve probably has implications for downstream development of the great vessels. For example, when there is subaortic stenosis, the echocardiographic examination is incomplete until abnormalities of the aortic arch have been excluded. Preoperative evaluation must also take into account potential AV valve anomalies and straddling, in particular.

INDICATIONS FOR INTERVENTION. The goals of operative treatment are to establish continuity between the left ventricle and aorta, to create adequate right ventricle to pulmonary continuity, and to repair associated lesions. Palliative surgery is reserved for those in whom biventricular repair is not possible and in those with markedly reduced pulmonary blood flow. In the latter, an aortopulmonary shunt may be placed to temporize before complete correction. For the remainder, complete repair is now performed as a primary procedure in the majority. In double-outlet right ventricle with a subaortic VSD, repair is accomplished by creation of an intraventricular baffle that conducts left ventricular blood to the aorta. If there is coexisting subpulmonary stenosis, the repair is similar to that of tetralogy of Fallot. When the VSD is subpulmonary, but without subpulmonary stenosis, repair is accomplished by closure of the VSD and arterial switch. Subpulmonary stenosis is frequently present in a double-outlet right ventricle with a subpulmonary VSD. In these cases, the aorta is connected to the left ventricle by an intraventricular baffle, and a right ventricle to pulmonary artery conduit is placed to complete the repair (Rastelli procedure). Classic surgical approaches cannot be used when the VSD is remote and uncommitted to either semilunar orifice. On occasion, the VSD can be baffled toward the aorta, but when this is not possible, the right ventricle may be used as the systemic ventricle. This requires a Mustard or Senning atrial redirection procedure, closure of the VSD, and placement of a conduit between the left ventricle and the pulmonary trunk.

INTERVENTIONAL OPTIONS AND OUTCOMES. The late follow-up of the surgical procedures described earlier (e.g., tetralogy of Fallot repair, arterial switch, Rastelli procedure) tends to be less satisfactory when there is a double-outlet right ventricle than when surgery is performed for more classic indications. The development of subaortic stenosis is more likely because of the abnormal geometry of the left ventricular outflow tract that often results after correction. Similarly, right ventricle to pulmonary artery conduit obstruction is more likely because of the spatial difficulties imposed on placement of the conduit with respect to the position on the right ventricle and the sternum. Because of these considerations, the options for catheter interventions are often fairly limited. However, recurrent arch obstruction and distal pulmonary artery obstruction are amenable to balloon dilation with or without stenting.

FOLLOW-UP. All of these patients require at least annual review by a CHD cardiologist.

Ebstein Anomaly

MORPHOLOGY (Fig. 65-30). The common feature in all cases of Ebstein anomaly is apical displacement of the septal tricuspid leaflet in conjunction with leaflet dysplasia. Many but not all have associated displacement of the posterior mural leaflet, with the anterior leaflet never being displaced. Although the anterior leaflet is never displaced apically, it may be adherent to the free wall of the right ventricle, causing right ventricular outflow tract obstruction. The displacement of the tricuspid valve results in "atrialization" (functioning as an atrial chamber) of the inflow tract of the right ventricle and consequently produces a variably small functional right ventricle. Associated anomalies include PFO or ASD in approximately 50% of patients; accessory conduction pathways in 25% (usually right sided); and, occasionally, varying degrees of right ventricular outflow tract obstruction, VSD, aortic coarctation, PDA, or mitral valve disease. Left ventricular abnormalities resembling noncompaction syndrome have also been described.

PATHOPHYSIOLOGY. Varying degrees of tricuspid regurgitation (or exceptionally tricuspid stenosis) result from the abnormal tricuspid leaflet morphology with consequent further right atrial enlargement. Right ventricular volume overload from significant tricuspid regurgitation and infundibular dilation can also be present. Right-to-left shunting through a PFO or ASD occurs if the right atrial pressure exceeds the left atrial pressure (which is often the case when severe tricuspid regurgitation is present).

NATURAL HISTORY. The natural history of patients with Ebstein anomaly depends on its severity. When the tricuspid valve deformity and dysfunction are extreme, death in utero from hydrops fetalis is the norm. When the tricuspid valve deformity is severe, symptoms usually develop in newborn infants. Patients with moderate tricuspid valve deformity and dysfunction usually develop symptoms during late

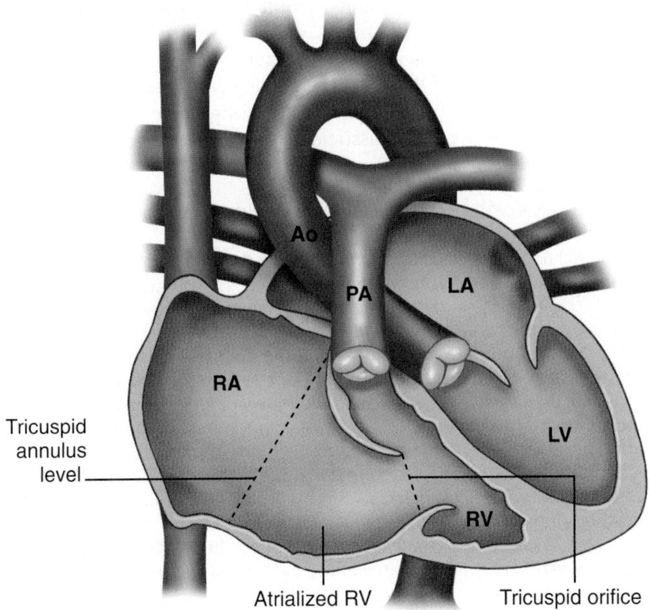

FIGURE 65-30 Diagrammatic representation of Ebstein anomaly. Ao = aorta; LA = left atrium; LV = left ventricle; PA = pulmonary artery; RA = right atrium; RV = right ventricle. *(From Mullins CE, Mayer DC: Congenital Heart Disease: A Diagrammatic Atlas. New York, Wiley-Liss, 1988.)*

adolescence or young adult life. Adults with Ebstein anomaly can occasionally remain asymptomatic throughout their lives if the anomaly is mild; exceptional survival to the ninth decade has been reported.

CLINICAL ISSUES

Pediatrics

With severe tricuspid valve deformity, newborns and infants present with failure to thrive and right-sided congestive heart failure. Most other pediatric patients who present after the neonatal period remain asymptomatic until late adolescence or early adult life.

Adults

Most adult patients present with exercise intolerance (exertional dyspnea and fatigue), palpitations of supraventricular origin, or cyanosis from a right-to-left shunt at atrial level. On occasion, a paradoxical embolus resulting in a transient ischemic attack or stroke can call attention to the diagnosis. Right-sided cardiac failure from severe tricuspid regurgitation and right ventricular dysfunction is possible. Sudden death (presumed to be arrhythmic in nature) is described. Physical examination typically reveals an unimpressive jugular venous pressure because of the large and compliant right atrium and atrialized right ventricle, a widely split S_1 with a loud tricuspid component (the "sail sound"), a widely split S_2 from a right bundle branch block, and a right-sided third heart sound. A pansystolic murmur increasing on inspiration from tricuspid regurgitation is best heard at the lower left sternal border. Cyanosis from a right-to-left shunt at the atrial level may or may not be present.

LABORATORY INVESTIGATIONS

ELECTROCARDIOGRAPHY. The electrocardiographic presentation of Ebstein anomaly varies widely (see Chap. 13). Low voltage is typical. Peaked P waves in leads II and V_1 reflect right atrial enlargement. The PR interval is usually prolonged, but a short PR interval and a delta wave from early activation through an accessory pathway can be present. An rsr′ pattern consistent with right ventricular conduction delay is typically seen in lead V_1, and right bundle branch block is common in adults. Atrial flutter and fibrillation are common. The ECG may be normal.

CHEST RADIOGRAPHY. A rightward convexity from an enlarged right atrium and atrialized right ventricle coupled with a leftward convexity from a dilated infundibulum gives the heart a "water bottle" appearance on the chest radiograph. Cardiomegaly, highly variable in degree, is the rule. The aorta and the pulmonary trunk are inconspicuous. The pulmonary vasculature is usually normal to reduced.

ECHOCARDIOGRAPHY (**Fig. 65-31;** see Fig. 15-93A). The diagnosis of Ebstein anomaly is usually made by echocardiography. Apical displacement of the septal leaflet of the tricuspid valve by 8 mm/m^2 or more, combined with an elongated sail-like appearance of the anterior leaflet, confirms the diagnosis. The size of the atrialized portion of the right ventricle (identified between the tricuspid annulus and the ventricular attachment of the tricuspid valve leaflets) and the systolic performance of the functional right ventricle can be estimated. The degree of tricuspid regurgitation (and more rarely stenosis) can be assessed. Associated defects such as ASDs as well as the presence and direction of shunting can also be identified.

ANGIOGRAPHY. Cardiac catheterization is required mainly when concomitant coronary artery disease is suspected and to determine if pulmonary artery pressures are elevated. When it is performed, selective right ventricular angiography shows the extent of tricuspid valve displacement, the size of the functional right ventricle, and configuration of its outflow tract.

CMR. This investigation can offer insights into functional right ventricular volume and function.

INDICATIONS FOR INTERVENTION. Indications for intervention include substantial cyanosis, right-sided heart failure, poor functional capacity, and perhaps the occurrence of paradoxical emboli. Recurrent supraventricular arrhythmias not controlled by medical or ablation therapy and asymptomatic substantial cardiomegaly (cardiothoracic ratio > 65%) are relative indications.

INTERVENTIONAL OPTIONS. Tricuspid valve repair, when feasible, is preferable to tricuspid valve replacement. The feasibility of tricuspid valve repair depends primarily on the experience and skill of the surgeon as well as on the adequacy of the anterior leaflet of the tricuspid valve to form a monocusp valve. Tricuspid valve repair is possible when the edges of the anterior leaflet of the tricuspid valve are not severely tethered down to the myocardium and when the functional right ventricle is of adequate size (>35% of the total right ventricle). If the tricuspid valve is irreparable, valve replacement will be necessary, usually with a bioprosthetic tricuspid valve.[76]

For high-risk patients (those with severe tricuspid regurgitation, an inadequate functional right ventricle [because of size or function], or chronic supraventricular arrhythmias), a bidirectional

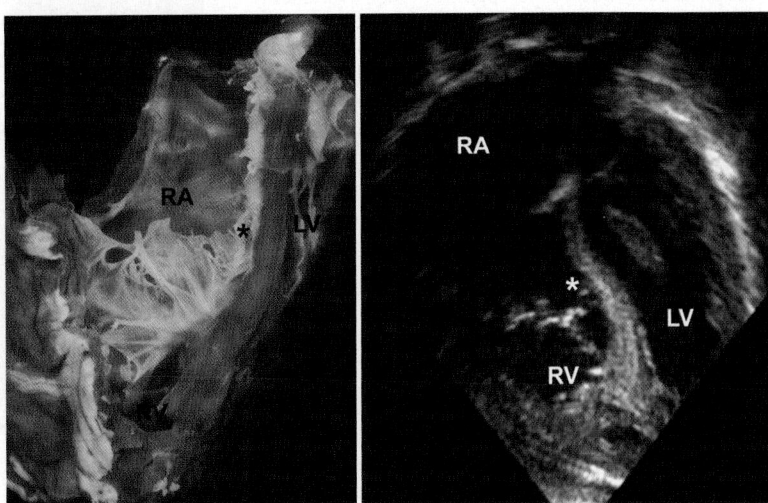

FIGURE 65-31 Apical four-chamber view in Ebstein malformation of the tricuspid valve. Note the significant displacement of the septal tricuspid valve leaflet (asterisk), with associated valve dysplasia. LV = left ventricle; RA = right atrium; RV = right ventricle.

cavopulmonary connection can be added to reduce right ventricular preload if pulmonary artery pressures are low.[77] On occasion, a Fontan operation may be the best option in patients with tricuspid stenosis or a hypoplastic right ventricle.[78] A concomitant right atrial or biatrial maze procedure at the time of surgery should be considered in patients with chronic atrial flutter or fibrillation.[79] If an accessory pathway is present, this should be mapped and obliterated either at the time of surgical repair or preoperatively in the catheterization laboratory. An atrial communication, if present, should be closed. In occasional patients with a resting oxygen saturation >90% and exercise intolerance due to worsening hypoxemia, closure of the PFO or ASD may be indicated without addressing the tricuspid valve itself.

With satisfactory valve repair, with or without plication of the atrialized right ventricle or bidirectional cavopulmonary connection, the medium-term prognosis is excellent. Late arrhythmias can occur.[80] With valve replacement, results are less satisfactory. Valve re-replacement may be necessary because of a failing bioprosthesis or a thrombosed mechanical valve.[76]

REPRODUCTIVE ISSUES. In the absence of maternal cyanosis, right-sided heart failure, or arrhythmias, pregnancy is usually well tolerated.

FOLLOW-UP. All patients with Ebstein anomaly should have regular follow-up, the frequency being dictated by the severity of their disease. Particular attention should be paid to patients with cyanosis, substantial cardiomegaly, poor right ventricular function, and recurrent atrial arrhythmias. Patients with substantial tricuspid regurgitation after tricuspid valve repair need close follow-up, as do patients with recurrent atrial arrhythmias, degenerating bioprostheses, or dysfunctional mechanical valves.

Valvular and Vascular Conditions

(see Chaps. 60, 61, and 66)

LEFT VENTRICULAR OUTFLOW TRACT LESIONS (Fig. 65-32)

Coarctation of the Aorta

Aortic arch obstruction can be divided into (1) localized coarctation close to a PDA or ligamentum, (2) tubular hypoplasia of some part of the aortic arch system, and (3) aortic arch interruption.

Localized Aortic Coarctation

MORPHOLOGY. This lesion consists of a localized shelf in the posterolateral aortic wall opposite the ductus arteriosus. A neonatal presentation is more often associated with a shelf plus transverse aortic arch and isthmic hypoplasia, whereas with a later presentation, these areas are larger.

CLINICAL FEATURES. Coarctation occurs two to five times more commonly in males, and there is a high degree of association with gonadal dysgenesis (Turner syndrome) and bicuspid aortic valve. Other common associated anomalies include VSD and mitral stenosis or regurgitation. Additional lesions have an impact on outcome.

Neonates

Rapid, severe obstruction in infancy is a prominent cause of left ventricular failure and systemic hypoperfusion. Heart failure in this setting is due to a sudden increase in left ventricular wall stress after closure of the arterial duct. Substantial left-to-right shunting across a PFO and pulmonary venous hypertension secondary to heart failure cause pulmonary arterial hypertension. Because little or no aortic obstruction existed during fetal life, the collateral circulation in the newborn period is often poorly developed. In these infants, peripheral pulses are characteristically weak throughout the body until left ventricular function is improved with medical management; a significant pressure difference then develops between the arms and the legs, allowing detection of a pulse discrepancy. Cardiac murmurs are nonspecific in infancy and are commonly derived from associated lesions.

LABORATORY INVESTIGATIONS

ELECTROCARDIOGRAPHY. The ECG shows right-axis deviation and right ventricular hypertrophy.

CHEST RADIOGRAPHY. This shows generalized cardiomegaly and pulmonary arterial and venous engorgement.

ECHOCARDIOGRAPHY (**Fig. 65-33A**). This demonstrates the posterior shelf and the degree of associated isthmic or transverse arch hypoplasia. Doppler echocardiography is helpful if the ductus is closed or partially restrictive and demonstrates a high-velocity jet during systole and diastole. On the other hand, if the ductus is widely patent, the usual right-to-left shunting makes the Doppler assessment invalid because the distal pressure then reflects the high pulmonary artery pressure. With associated tubular hypoplasia, Doppler-derived gradients provide higher and less reliable values compared with those obtained by blood pressure or catheterization measurements.

MAGNETIC RESONANCE ANGIOGRAPHY. Although this is the gold standard for evaluation of the aortic arch in the older child and adult, it is usually unnecessary in the neonate and infant.

MANAGEMENT. Management usually involves prostaglandin therapy in an attempt to reopen or to maintain patency of a ductus arteriosus. After prostaglandin E_1 infusion to dilate the ductus arteriosus, the pressure difference may be obliterated across the site of coarctation because the fetal flow pattern is reestablished. This has the additional benefit of improving renal perfusion, which in turn helps reverse the frequently associated metabolic acidosis.

INTERVENTION. Intervention in this age group usually involves surgical relief of the obstruction with excision of the area of coarctation and extended end-to-end repair or end-to-side anastomosis with absorbable sutures to allow remodeling of the aorta with time. Subclavian flap aortoplasty, which was employed extensively in the past, is now less popular than the earlier-mentioned procedures. Experts generally believe that balloon dilation does not play a role in management in this age group because there is a lower rate of medium-term success.[81] Early surgery is associated with a lower incidence of

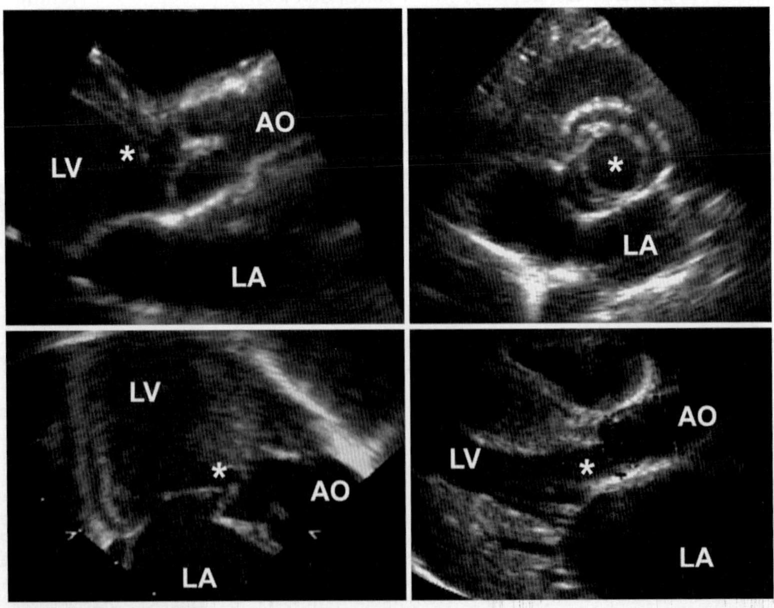

FIGURE 65-32 Montage demonstrating the different types of left ventricular outflow tract obstruction (asterisks). The upper left image shows isolated fibromuscular obstruction; the upper right, stenosis due to a bicuspid aortic valve; the lower left, obstruction because of chordal apparatus from the anterior mitral leaflet; and the lower right, obstruction due to tunnel narrowing at the valve, annular, and subvalve level. AO = aorta; LA = left atrium; LV = left ventricle.

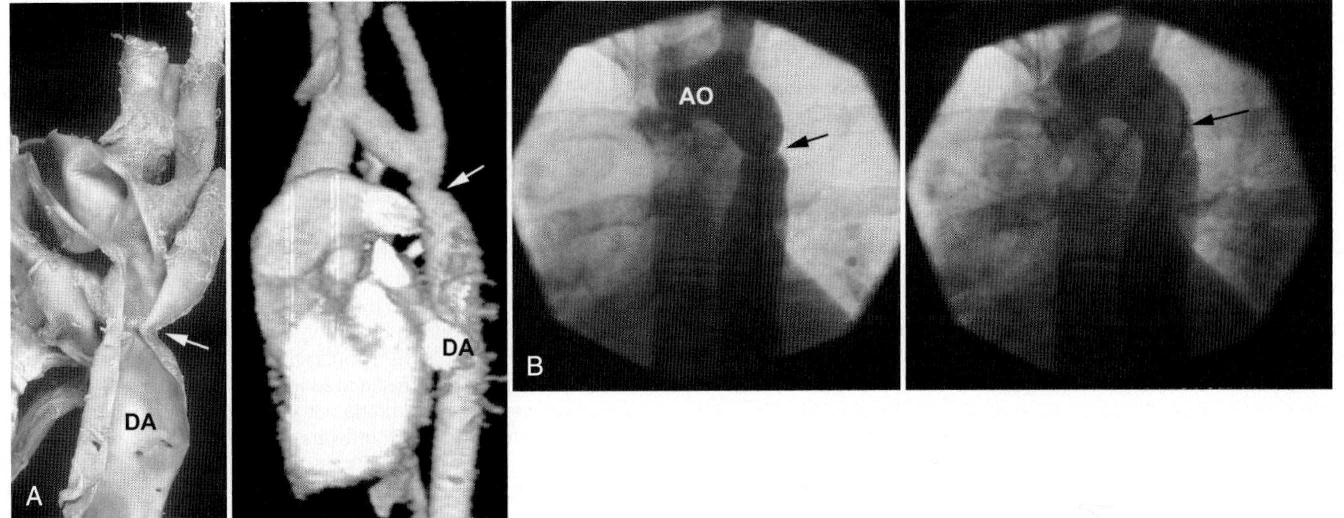

FIGURE 65-33 **A,** Montage of a coarctation of the aorta. The left image is a specimen that shows the site of the posterior shelf, as outlined by the arrow. The right image is from a CMR examination and shows the posterior shelf and some associated transverse arch hypoplasia. **B,** Angiogram of a coarctation of the aorta, before and after stenting. AO, aorta; DA, descending aorta.

long-term hypertension. At time of presentation, transverse arch and isthmal hypoplasia are frequent associations; however, subsequent growth appears to occur, even in neonates weighing less than 2.5 kg.[82]

Infants and Children

PRESENTATION. Most infants and children with isolated coarctation are asymptomatic, with the findings of reduced femoral pulses and hypertension being detected during routine medical care of the pediatric patient. Heart failure is uncommon because the left ventricle has a chance to become hypertrophied, thus maintaining a normal wall stress. Complaints of headache, cold extremities, and claudication with exercise may be noted in the older child and adolescent.

A midsystolic murmur over the anterior chest, back, and spinous processes is most frequent, becoming continuous if the lumen is sufficiently narrowed to result in a high-velocity jet across the lesion throughout the cardiac cycle. Additional systolic and continuous murmurs over the lateral thoracic wall may reflect increased flow through dilated and tortuous collateral vessels, which are commonly not heard until later childhood.

Laboratory Investigations

Electrocardiography. This reveals left ventricular hypertrophy of various degrees, depending on the height of arterial pressure above the obstruction and the patient's age. Coexisting right ventricular hypertrophy usually implies a complicated lesion.

Chest Radiography. The characteristic posteroanterior film feature is the so-called figure-3 configuration of the proximal descending thoracic aorta due to both prestenotic and poststenotic dilation. Rib notching (unilateral or bilateral, second to ninth ribs) is present in 50% of cases. Rib notching is unilateral if the right or left subclavian arteries arise from the aorta distal to the coarctation. Rib notching is noted as an erosion of the undersurface of a posterior rib, usually at its outer third, with a sclerotic margin.

Echocardiography. This demonstrates a posterior shelf, a well-expanded isthmus and transverse aortic arch (in most cases), and a high-velocity continuous jet through the coarctation site. Interestingly, a slow upstroke is observed on the abdominal aortic velocity profile compared with that seen in the ascending aorta.

CMR. This provides detailed information in this age group and may be performed before intervention, particularly if balloon dilation is the treatment of choice. This is the best tool for postintervention imaging and has become routine in many centers.

Angiocardiography. This is reserved for delineating the coarctation at the time of balloon dilation. Primary management in those cases with a well-expanded isthmus and transverse aortic arch invariably involves balloon dilation.

INTERVENTION. Balloon dilation is the current technique in many centers,[83] with surgery being reserved for cases with associated arch hypoplasia. Extended end-to-end anastomosis is the currently favored surgical approach, with patch augmentation being reserved for cases with significant arch hypoplasia.

Paradoxical hypertension of short duration is often noted in the immediate postoperative period, a phenomenon much less common after balloon angioplasty. A resetting of carotid baroreceptors and increased catecholamine secretion appear to be responsible for the initial phase of postoperative systemic hypertension, with a later, second phase of prolonged elevation of systolic and particularly diastolic blood pressure related to activation of the renin-angiotensin system. A necrotizing panarteritis of the small vessels of the gastrointestinal tract of uncertain cause occasionally complicates the course of recovery.

Recoarctation

The risk of recurrent narrowing after repair of coarctation in infancy is 5% to 10%. Such narrowing is best screened for with Doppler ultrasonography, with CMR being the gold standard for imaging. Clinical decisions to intervene are usually based on a cuff blood pressure difference between the right arm and leg (for a left aortic arch and normal innominate artery). Although there are no hard and fast rules for absolute blood pressure difference, it has been common practice to reintervene when the blood pressure difference is more than 25 to 30 mm Hg in the presence of systemic hypertension. Although Doppler measurements can detect a recurrent obstruction, this technique provides an overestimation of the blood pressure–measured gradients because of the phenomenon of pressure recovery. Recoarctation is usually addressed with balloon dilation if the obstruction is relatively localized. In the presence of long-segment narrowings, surgical intervention may be necessary, with the use of patch augmentation of the hypoplastic segment. In the adolescent or adult, balloon-expandable stents are routinely employed with good success (see Fig. 65-33B). This has the advantage of avoiding the risk of potential spinal cord damage perisurgery in patients with poorly developed collaterals.

Long-term Complications

In patients who survive the first 2 years of life without an intervention, complications of juxtaductal coarctation are uncommon before the second or third decade. The chief hazards to patients with coarctation result from severe hypertension and include the development of cerebral aneurysms and hemorrhage, hypertensive encephalopathy, rupture of the aorta, left ventricular failure, and infective endocarditis. In patients with coarctation repaired, systemic hypertension in the absence of residual coarctation has been observed in resting or exercise-stressed patients postoperatively and appears to be related to the duration of preoperative hypertension as well as the architecture of the aortic arch segments.[84] These patients also have abnormalities of vascular reactivity, as demonstrated by flow-mediated studies. Increased left ventricular mass is observed, even in the absence of a residual arm-leg gradient. Life-long observation is desirable because of the late onset of hypertension in some postoperative patients.

In those who have undergone balloon dilation of a native coarctation, the incidence of aneurysm formation at the coarctation site is on the order of 7%.[85]

Adults

Although much of the previous material is also relevant to the adult, there are some differences in the issues faced by adult patients. *Complex coarctation* is used to describe coarctation in the presence of other important intracardiac anomalies (e.g., VSD, left ventricular outflow tract obstruction, and mitral stenosis) and is usually detected in infancy. *Simple coarctation* refers to coarctation in the absence of such lesions. It is the most common form detected de novo in adults. Associated abnormalities include bicuspid aortic valve in most cases (80%), intracranial aneurysms (most commonly of the circle of Willis) in 2% to 10%, and acquired intercostal artery aneurysms. One definition of *significant coarctation* requires a gradient greater than 20 mm Hg across the coarctation site at angiography with or without proximal systemic hypertension. A second definition of significant coarctation requires the presence of proximal hypertension in the company of echocardiographic or angiographic evidence of aortic coarctation. If there is an extensive collateral circulation (see Fig. 82-4), there may be minimal or no pressure gradient and acquired aortic atresia.

Death in patients who do not undergo repair is usually due to heart failure (usually older than 30 years), coronary artery disease, aortic rupture or dissection, concomitant aortic valve disease, infective endarteritis or endocarditis, or cerebral hemorrhage.[86] Of Turner syndrome patients, 35% have aortic coarctation.

CLINICAL FEATURES. Patients can be asymptomatic, or they can present with minimal symptoms of epistaxis, headache, and leg weakness on exertion or more serious symptoms of congestive heart failure, angina, aortic stenosis, aortic dissection, or unexplained intracerebral hemorrhage. Leg claudication (pain) is rare unless there is concomitant abdominal aortic coarctation. A thorough clinical examination reveals upper limb systemic hypertension as well as a differential systolic blood pressure of at least 10 mm Hg (brachial > popliteal artery pressure). Radial-femoral pulse delay is evident unless significant aortic regurgitation coexists. Auscultation may reveal an interscapular systolic murmur emanating from the coarctation site and a widespread crescendo-decrescendo continuous murmur throughout the chest wall from intercostal collateral arteries. Funduscopic examination can reveal "corkscrew" tortuosity of retinal arterioles.

INTERVENTIONAL OUTCOMES

Surgical

After surgical repair of simple coarctation, the obstruction is usually relieved, with minimal mortality (1%). Paraplegia due to spinal cord ischemia is uncommon (0.4%) and may occur in patients who do not have well-developed collateral circulation. The prevalence of recoarctation reported in the literature varies widely from 7% to 60% but is probably about 10%,[87] depending on the definition used, the length of follow-up, and the age at surgery. The appropriateness of the surgical repair for a given anatomy is probably the main factor dictating the chance of recoarctation rather than the type of surgical repair itself. True aneurysm formation at the site of coarctation repair is also a well-recognized entity, with a reported incidence between 2% and 27%. Aneurysms are particularly common after Dacron patch aortoplasty and usually occur in the native aorta opposite the patch.[88] Late dissection at the repair site is rare, but false aneurysms, usually at the suture line, can occur. Long-term follow-up after surgical correction of coarctation of the aorta still reveals an increased incidence of premature cardiovascular disease and death.

Transcatheter

After balloon dilation (see Fig. 65-33B), aortic dissection, restenosis, and aneurysm formation at the site of coarctation have been documented. These complications have been reduced with the now increasing if not exclusive use of primary stenting in the adults with native coarctation as well as recoarctation.[89] The significance of aneurysm formation is often unknown, and longer term data are necessary.

Prior hypertension resolves in up to 50% of patients but may recur later in life, especially if the intervention is performed at an older age. In some of these patients, this may be essential hypertension, but a hemodynamic basis should be sought and blood pressure control should be attained. Systolic hypertension is also common with exercise and is not a surrogate marker for recoarctation of the aorta. It may be related to residual arch hypoplasia or to increased renin and catecholamine activity from residual functional abnormalities of the precoarctation vessels. The criteria for and significance of exertional systolic hypertension are controversial. Late cerebrovascular events occur, notably in those patients undergoing repair as adults and in those with residual hypertension. Endocarditis or endarteritis can occur at the coarctation site or on intracardiac lesions; and if this occurs at the coarctation site, embolic manifestations are restricted to the legs.

FOLLOW-UP. All patients should have a follow-up examination every 1 to 3 years. Particular attention should be directed toward residual hypertension, heart failure, intracardiac disease (such as an associated bicuspid aortic valve (see Chap. 66), which can become stenotic or regurgitant later in life), or an ascending aortopathy sometimes seen in the presence of bicuspid aortic valve. Complications at the site of repair, such as restenosis and aneurysm formation, should also be sought by clinical examination, chest radiography, echocardiography, and periodic CMR or CT scanning. Patients with Dacron patch repair should probably undergo CMR or spiral CT examination every 3 to 5 years or so to detect subclinical aneurysm formation. Hemoptysis from a leaking or ruptured aneurysm is a serious complication requiring immediate investigation and surgery. New or unusual headaches raise the possibility of berry aneurysms.

Aortic Arch Hypoplasia

MORPHOLOGY. The aortic isthmus, the portion of the aorta between the left subclavian artery and the ductus arteriosus, should be narrowed in the fetus and newborn. The lumen of the aortic isthmus is about two thirds that of the ascending and descending portions of the aorta until age 6 to 9 months, when the physiologic narrowing disappears. Pathologic tubular hypoplasia of the aortic arch usually is noted in the aortic isthmus and is most commonly associated with presentation of aortic coarctation in the newborn period. Despite this, in a small group of cases, the arch obstruction is due primarily to tubular hypoplasia, usually involving both the aortic isthmus and transverse aortic arch (between the innominate and subclavian arteries). These cases usually present early in life with findings similar to those with a severe coarctation of the aorta. As with the latter, they are duct dependent and may also be associated with other left-sided obstructive lesions.

MANAGEMENT OPTIONS. Provided the other left-sided structures are formed well enough to sustain life, the management involves arch reconstruction with a patch, in a fashion similar to those cases undergoing a Norwood procedure for hypoplastic left heart syndrome. If the left-sided structures are hypoplastic, palliative surgery with a Norwood procedure and cardiac transplantation are the two treatments of choice.

Complex Coarctation

In some instances, the coarctation of the aorta is part of a more complex spectrum of lesions. This can be seen in cases with double-outlet right ventricle, cc-TGA, D-TGA, functionally single ventricle, truncus arteriosus, and AV septal defect. In these cases, the decision process involves not only the coarctation repair but the management of the associated lesions. The current trend is to complete repair of the intracardiac lesion at the same time as the arch repair.

Aortic Arch Interruption

Aortic arch interruption is a rare and usually lethal anomaly. Unless it is treated surgically, almost all infants die within the first month of life. Interruptions distal to the left subclavian artery (type A) occur with almost equal frequency to interruptions distal to the left common carotid artery (type B). The right subclavian artery is of variable origin, frequently arising from the descending aortic segment distal to the interruption. The clinical presentation resembles that in tubular hypoplasia or severe coarctation of the aorta with a PDA.

Virtually all patients have associated intracardiac anomalies. A PDA almost always connects the main pulmonary artery with the descending aorta. Patients with interrupted aortic arch typically have either a VSD (80% to 90% of cases) or an aortopulmonary window (10% to 20%). Because the ductus arteriosus provides lower body blood flow, its spontaneous constriction results in profound clinical deterioration. The latter may be temporarily managed by prostaglandin E_1 infusion. Other complex intracardiac malformations, such as TGA, aortopulmonary window, and truncus arteriosus, are common.

CLINICAL FEATURES. An association with the genetic 22q11 deletion DiGeorge syndrome is frequent. The major clinical problem is severe congestive heart failure as a consequence of volume overload of the left ventricle from an associated intracardiac left-to-right shunt and of pressure overload imposed by systemic hypertension. Absent upper and lower limb pulses, with a palpable superficial temporal pulse, is a helpful clue to the diagnosis.

LABORATORY INVESTIGATIONS

ELECTROCARDIOGRAPHY. This demonstrates right ventricular hypertrophy with right-axis deviation and ST-T wave changes.

CHEST RADIOGRAPHY. Cardiomegaly is noted with increased pulmonary markings and pulmonary edema.

ECHOCARDIOGRAPHY. This is the gold standard for the diagnosis of aortic arch interruption and associated lesions. The VSD can be characterized, as can the degree of left ventricular outflow tract obstruction.

MANAGEMENT. The perioperative clinical condition of most patients can be improved by intensive medical management with mechanical ventilation, inotropic support, and prostaglandin infusion. There has been increasing success with complete primary repair in infancy as the procedure of choice. In some cases in which the left ventricular outflow tract obstruction is thought to be too severe for standard primary repair, a Norwood procedure is initially performed. This is followed by a complete repair by tunneling the left ventricle through the VSD to the new aorta and placement of a right ventricle to pulmonary artery conduit.

OUTCOME. The medium- and long-term outcomes are reasonable, but there may be a need for reintervention for left ventricular outflow tract obstruction and recurrent arch obstruction.[90]

Sinus of Valsalva Aneurysm and Fistula

MORPHOLOGY. The malformation consists of a separation, or lack of fusion, between the media of the aorta and the annulus fibrosus of the aortic valve. The receiving chamber of a right aortic sinus aortocardiac fistula is usually the right ventricle, but occasionally, when the noncoronary cusp is involved, the fistula drains into the right atrium. From 5% to 15% of aneurysms originate in the posterior or noncoronary sinus. The left aortic sinus is seldom involved. Associated anomalies are common and include a VSD, bicuspid aortic valve, and aortic coarctation.

CLINICAL FEATURES. The deficiency in the aortic media appears to be congenital. Reports in infants are exceedingly rare and are infrequent in children because progressive aneurysmal dilation of the weakened area develops but may not be recognized until the third or fourth decade of life, when rupture into a cardiac chamber occurs. A congenital aneurysm of an aortic sinus of Valsalva, particularly the right coronary sinus, is an uncommon anomaly that occurs three times more often in males. An unruptured aneurysm usually does not produce a hemodynamic abnormality. Rarely, myocardial ischemia may be caused by coronary arterial compression. Rupture is often of abrupt onset, causes chest pain, and creates continuous arteriovenous shunting and acute volume loading of both right and left heart chambers, which promptly results in heart failure. An additional complication is infective endocarditis, which may originate either on the edges of the aneurysm or on those areas in the right side of the heart that are traumatized by the jetlike stream of blood flowing through the fistula.

This anomaly should be suspected in a patient with a combination of chest pain of sudden onset, resting or exertional dyspnea, bounding pulses, and a loud, superficial, continuous murmur accentuated in diastole when the fistula opens into the right ventricle as well as a thrill along the right or left lower sternal border. The physical findings can be difficult to distinguish from those produced by a coronary arteriovenous fistula.

LABORATORY INVESTIGATIONS

ELECTROCARDIOGRAPHY. This may show biventricular hypertrophy, or it may be normal.

CHEST RADIOGRAPHY. This may demonstrate generalized cardiomegaly and usually heart failure.

ECHOCARDIOGRAPHY. Studies based on two-dimensional and pulsed Doppler echocardiography may detect the walls of the aneurysm and disturbed flow within the aneurysm or at the site of perforation. TEE may provide more precise information than the transthoracic approach.

CARDIAC CATHETERIZATION. This reveals a left-to-right shunt at the ventricular or, less commonly, the atrial level. The diagnosis may be established definitively by retrograde thoracic aortography.

MANAGEMENT OPTIONS AND OUTCOMES. Preoperative medical management consists of measures to relieve cardiac failure and to treat coexistent arrhythmias or endocarditis, if present. At operation, the aneurysm is closed and amputated, and the aortic wall is reunited with the heart, either by direct suture or with a prosthesis. All efforts should be made to preserve the aortic valve in children because patch closure of the defect combined with prosthetic valve replacement greatly increases the risk of operation in small patients. Device closure of the ruptured aneurysm has also been attempted.

Vascular Rings

MORPHOLOGY. The term *vascular ring* is used for those aortic arch or pulmonary artery malformations that exhibit an abnormal relation with the esophagus and trachea, often causing dysphagia or respiratory symptoms.

DOUBLE AORTIC ARCH (**Fig. 65-34**). The most common vascular ring is produced by a double aortic arch in which both the right and left fourth embryonic aortic arches persist. In the most common type of double aortic arch, there is a left ligamentum arteriosum or occasionally a ductus arteriosus. Although both arches may be patent at the time of diagnosis, invariably the left arch distal to the left subclavian artery is atretic and is connected to the descending aorta by a fibrous remnant that completes the ring. When both arches are patent, the right arch is usually larger than the left. This usually occurs as an isolated lesion, with the respiratory symptoms being caused by tracheal compression and frequently associated laryngomalacia, usually in the neonate and young infant.

RIGHT AORTIC ARCH. A right aortic arch with a left ductus or ligamentum arteriosum connecting the left pulmonary artery and the upper part of the descending aorta is the next most important vascular ring seen. Although all cases with this lesion have a vascular ring, not all cases are symptomatic. Indeed, those patients who are symptomatic usually have an associated diverticulum of Kommerell. This is a large outpouching at the distal takeoff of the left subclavian artery from the descending aorta. It is the combination of the diverticulum and the ring that causes the airway compression.

ANOMALOUS ORIGIN OF A RIGHT SUBCLAVIAN ARTERY. Anomalous origin of a right subclavian artery is one of the most common abnormalities of the aortic arch. Although the aberrant right subclavian artery runs posterior to the esophagus, it does not form a vascular ring unless there is an associated right-sided ductus or ligamentum to complete the ring. During adulthood, about 5% of patients with an aberrant right subclavian artery (and a left ductus) develop symptoms due to rigidity of the aberrant vessel.

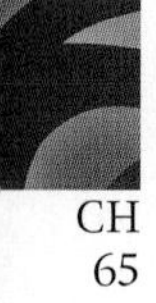

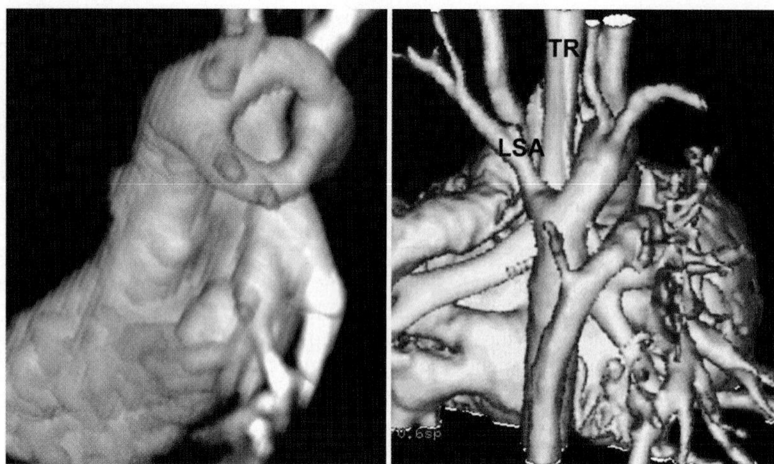

FIGURE 65-34 The left image is a three-dimensional reconstruction of a double aortic arch from a CMR examination. The right image is from an aberrant left subclavian artery as seen by spiral CT. LSA = left subclavian artery; TR = trachea.

Retroesophageal Descending Aorta. This is a rarer but more problematic type of vascular ring. In this setting, there may be either an ascending left and descending right aorta or an ascending right and descending left aorta. The retroesophageal component of the descending aorta causes the tracheal compression, in conjunction with the left- or right-sided ligamentum.

Pulmonary Artery Sling. This is usually made up of the left pulmonary artery arising from the right pulmonary artery and runs posterior to the trachea but anterior to the esophagus. This is usually seen in isolation and is associated with significant hypoplasia of the bronchial tree, which is the predominant cause of the airway symptoms.

CLINICAL FEATURES. The symptoms produced by vascular rings depend on the tightness of anatomic constriction of the trachea and esophagus and consist principally of respiratory difficulties including stridor, cyanosis (especially with feeding), and dysphagia. Not all patients with a vascular ring are symptomatic, and cases with an aberrant left subclavian artery are frequently detected at the time of evaluation for associated CHD. Although most patients with a true ring and some airway compression present early in life, others present later with dysphagia; others escape diagnosis forever.

Laboratory Investigations

Electrocardiography. This appears normal unless associated cardiovascular anomalies are present.

Chest Radiography. If there is evidence of a right aortic arch in a symptomatic patient, a vascular ring should be suspected. In some instances, there is evidence of some airway narrowing. The barium esophagogram is a useful screening procedure. Prominent posterior indentation of the esophagus is observed in many of the common vascular ring arrangements, although the pulmonary artery vascular sling produces an anterior indentation.

Echocardiography. Echocardiography is a sensitive tool for evaluation of the laterality of the aortic arch, including a detailed assessment of the associated brachiocephalic vessels. In general, if there is normal branching of the innominate artery, to the right for a left aortic arch and to the left for a right, along with the correct "sidedness" of the descending aorta, a vascular ring can be excluded. *Most cases with a double aortic arch* have a dominant right arch, with the descending aorta appearing to dip posteriorly as it runs behind the esophagus. A patent ductus or ligamentum can usually be identified by echocardiography. When both arches are patent, a frontal plane sweep from inferior to superior demonstrates both patent arches as well as their brachiocephalic vessels. *A right aortic arch with an aberrant left subclavian artery* is suspected when it is not possible to identify normal branching of the left-sided innominate artery. *A retroesophageal descending aorta* should be suspected when the ascending aorta and its brachiocephalic arteries are readily identified but there is difficulty in identifying the descending aorta as it traverses behind the esophagus. *A left pulmonary artery sling* is suspected when the normal branching pattern of pulmonary arteries cannot be identified. In this setting, color Doppler study permits the identification of the left pulmonary artery as it arises from the right pulmonary artery and runs in a posterior and leftward direction.

CMR and CT. CMR and CT play a major role in the evaluation of patients with a vascular ring. In fact, CMR has become the gold standard for the evaluation of the aorta and its branches. The only disadvantage for infants is that general anesthesia is often required for a successful examination to be achieved. On the other hand, spiral CT is a technique that is fast and provides better definition of the affected airways; this technique is particularly valuable for patients with a pulmonary artery sling, in which the vascular ring plays a secondary role to the airway abnormalities. The advantages of these techniques are that, unlike echocardiography, they permit a precise assessment of the more posterior vascular structures and their relationships to the esophagus and airways. These techniques are particularly valuable in the more complex forms, such as a retroesophageal descending aorta.

MANAGEMENT OPTIONS AND OUTCOMES. The severity of symptoms and the anatomy of the malformation are the most important factors in determining treatment. Patients, particularly infants, with respiratory obstruction require prompt surgical intervention. A left thoracotomy is the surgical approach in most patients with a vascular ring. For the most common vascular rings, such as double aortic arch and aberrant left subclavian artery, the combination of chest radiography, barium swallow study, and echocardiography is all that is necessary before surgical intervention.

Operative repair of the double aortic arch requires division of the minor arch (usually the left) and the ligamentum. Patients with a right aortic arch and a left ductus or ligamentum arteriosum require division of the ductus or ligamentum or ligation and division of the left subclavian artery, which is the posterior component of the ring. Video-assisted thoracoscopy holds promise as an alternative to open thoracotomy for management. In patients with a pulmonary artery vascular sling, operation consists of detachment of the left pulmonary artery at its origin and anastomosis to the main pulmonary artery directly or by way of a conduit with its proximal end brought anterior to the trachea. The addition of tracheal narrowing that requires surgical intervention adds to the mortality in this group of patients, as does the association with intracardiac malformations.[91]

Congenital Aortic Valve Stenosis

GENERAL CONSIDERATIONS. We deal here only with this condition in newborns and children because the adult presentation is described in Chap. 66. Congenital aortic valve stenosis is a relatively common anomaly. Congenital aortic valve stenosis occurs much more frequently in males, with a gender ratio of 4:1. Associated cardiovascular anomalies have been noted in up to 20% of patients. PDA and coarctation of the aorta occur most frequently with aortic valve stenosis; all three of these lesions may coexist.

Morphology. The basic malformation consists of thickening of valve tissue with various degrees of commissural fusion. The valve is most commonly bicuspid. In some patients, the stenotic aortic valve is unicuspid and dome shaped, with no or one lateral attachment to the aorta at the level of the orifice. In infants and young children with severe aortic stenosis, the aortic valve annulus may be relatively underdeveloped. This lesion forms a continuum with the hypoplastic left heart syndrome and the aortic atresia and hypoplasia complexes. Secondary calcification of the valve is rare in childhood. When the obstruction is hemodynamically significant, concentric hypertrophy of the left ventricular wall and dilation of the ascending aorta occur.

NEONATAL PRESENTATION. The newborn presentation is often similar to that seen with other obstructive left-sided lesions, such as coarctation of the aorta and interrupted aortic arch. The infant presents with heart failure and depends on ductal patency for survival. An association with varying degrees of left ventricular hypoplasia, mitral valve abnormalities, and endocardial fibroelastosis occurs frequently. With the advent of good prenatal screening, many are detected before birth, with deliveries being performed in a high-risk obstetric unit attached to a congenital heart facility. The decision process around single versus biventricular repair is a complex one and beyond the scope of this chapter. Suffice it to say that this still poses a challenge in the newborn period.[92]

Clinical Findings

Newborns generally have weak pulses throughout, signs of heart failure, and often little in the way of murmurs, despite the severe left ventricular outflow tract obstruction.

Laboratory Investigations

Electrocardiography. An ECG usually shows right ventricular dominance with evidence of diffuse ST wave changes due to left ventricular strain.

Chest Radiography. Chest radiography usually shows cardiomegaly due to a large right ventricle and varying degrees of pulmonary edema.

Echocardiography. Echocardiography is currently the diagnostic test of choice. It usually shows a poorly contracting left ventricle with varying degrees of endocardial fibroelastosis and frequently hypoplasia of the left ventricle and aortic root. Doppler assessment of gradients is often unreliable because of poor left ventricular function. Right ventricular hypertension and tricuspid valve regurgitation are common associated findings.

Management

Prostaglandin therapy is instituted in this population of patients to maintain the fetal circulation with retrograde ductal flow that permits coronary and cerebral perfusion. The nature of further treatment depends on whether the left ventricle and aortic root are believed to be of a sufficient size to support a biventricular repair. If so, balloon dilation is rapidly becoming the treatment of choice, although surgical intervention is still preferred by some. If the left-sided heart structures are believed to be too small to sustain life, either cardiac transplantation or a Norwood procedure can be undertaken.

PRESENTATION BEYOND THE NEWBORN PERIOD. The diagnosis is invariably made after the detection of a murmur. On occasion, heart failure ensues, usually in the first 1 to 2 months of life, when there is a rapid progression of the obstruction and lack of left ventricular mass to maintain a normal wall stress. Natural history studies performed several years ago demonstrated that more rapid progression of aortic valve stenosis is more likely to happen within the first 2 years of life, after which the rate of progressive obstruction is more uniform.

Clinical Findings

In general, the children are asymptomatic, having normal peripheral pulses if the stenosis is less severe and low-volume, slow-rising pulses when it progresses. Exercise fatigue and chest pain are rare complaints and occur only when the stenosis is severe. With severe stenosis, there is a systolic thrill in the same area that can also be felt in the suprasternal notch and carotid arteries. Beyond the newborn period, there is usually an ejection click at the apex that precedes the murmur. The second heart sound is usually normal in children. An ejection systolic murmur is heard along the left sternal border, with radiation into the right infraclavicular area. Associated aortic regurgitation may be heard.

Laboratory Investigations

Electrocardiography. Left ventricular hypertrophy with or without strain is the hallmark feature.

Chest Radiography. Overall heart size is normal or the degree of enlargement is slight in most children with congenital aortic valve stenosis.

Echocardiography. Two-dimensional echocardiography provides detailed information about the morphology of the valve, the left ventricular function, and the presence of associated left-sided lesions. Doppler echocardiography can be used to determine the severity of stenosis and the presence or absence of associated aortic regurgitation. Doppler study provides peak instantaneous gradients that are higher than the peak-to-peak gradients determined from cardiac catheterization. The importance of this lies in the fact that the natural history studies and clinical decision making have thus far been based on peak-to-peak catheterization gradients in the infant, child, and adolescent. Valve areas are usually not calculated in this age group because there are no good data to support their use in pediatric patients. Mean gradients as derived from Doppler study and catheterization correlate closely, but again, no data support their use in clinical decision making. Some data convert the Doppler-derived mean gradients to peak to peak, with the addition of the pulse pressure as obtained from blood pressure measurements. Whatever absolute number is chosen to work with, the additional finding of left ventricular hypertrophy on electrocardiography and echocardiography provides supportive data about timing for intervention. The pediatric community generally agrees that a peak-to-peak gradient of 60 mm Hg or more probably warrants intervention.

Cardiac Catheterization. Cardiac catheterization is now rarely used to establish the site and severity of obstruction to left ventricular outflow. Instead, catheterization is undertaken when therapeutic interventional balloon aortic valvuloplasty is indicated.

Management Options

In this era, balloon dilation has almost completely replaced primary surgical valvotomy in children.

FOLLOW-UP. Follow-up studies indicate that aortic valvotomy is a safe and effective means of palliative treatment with excellent relief of symptoms. Aortic insufficiency can occasionally be progressive and require valve replacement. Moreover, after commissurotomy, the valve leaflets remain somewhat deformed, and further degenerative changes including calcification will likely lead to significant stenosis in later years. Thus, prosthetic aortic valve replacement is required in approximately 35% of patients within 15 to 20 years of the original operation. For those children and adolescents requiring aortic valve replacement, the surgical options include replacement with a mechanical aortic valve, an aortic homograft, and a pulmonary autograft in the aortic position. Accumulating evidence shows that the pulmonary autograft may ultimately be preferable to the aortic homograft. In the pulmonary autograft, called the Ross procedure, the patient's pulmonary valve is removed and used to replace the diseased aortic valve, and the right ventricular outflow tract is reconstructed with a pulmonary valve homograft. This approach appears to confer a survival advantage in the younger age group, in whom repeated mechanical valve replacement is associated with an increased mortality.[63] Despite this advantage, caution is necessary when it is applied to patients with bicuspid aortic valve and aortic regurgitation. This is due to associated aortic root dilation, which is inherent to this lesion and may complicate the long-term reliability of the Ross procedure. This surgical approach can be applied from neonatal through adult life. Neither homografts nor autografts require anticoagulation.

Subaortic Stenosis

Morphology

Discrete Fibromuscular. This lesion consists of a ridge or fibrous ring encircling the left ventricular outflow tract at varying distances from the aortic valve. The subvalvular fibrous process usually extends onto the aortic valve cusps and almost always makes contact with the ventricular aspect of the anterior mitral leaflet at its base. In other cases with fibrous discontinuity between the mitral and aortic valves, it forms more of a tunnel obstruction.

Focal Muscular. Rarely there is no fibrous element but rather a focal muscular obstruction on the crest of the interventricular septum, which differs from typical cases with hypertrophic cardiomyopathy.

Hypoplasia of the Left Ventricular Outflow Tract. In some cases, valvular and subvalvular aortic stenoses coexist with hypoplasia of the aortic valve annulus and thickened valve leaflets, producing a tunnel-like narrowing of the left ventricular outflow tract. Additional findings often include a small ascending aorta.

Discrete Subaortic Stenosis and VSD. This combination is frequently encountered in the pediatric age group, with the fibromuscular component often being absent at the initial echocardiographic evaluation. The association should be suspected in VSDs with some associated anterior malalignment of the aorta and a more acute aortoseptal angle. These hearts frequently develop subpulmonary stenosis. In a different subset of patients with aortic arch interruption and a VSD, there is muscular subaortic stenosis due to posterior deviation of the infundibular septum.

Complex Subaortic Stenosis. Various anatomic lesions other than a discrete ridge may produce subaortic stenosis. Among these are abnormal adherence of the anterior leaflet of the mitral valve to the septum and the presence in the left ventricular outflow tract of accessory endocardial cushion tissue. These are frequently associated with a "cleft in the anterior mitral valve leaflet," which is to be differentiated from that seen in an AV septal defect. These types of obstruction are seen more commonly in those cases with abnormalities of the ventriculoarterial connection in association with a VSD (e.g., double-outlet right ventricle, transposition, VSD).

CLINICAL FEATURES. These types of obstruction are usually identified as secondary lesions in those cases with associated VSDs, with or without abnormalities of the ventriculoarterial connections or aortic arch obstruction. In general, the substrate for left ventricular outflow tract obstruction is present, although actual physiologic obstruction is absent in some cases. In other cases, the patients are referred for evaluation because of a systolic murmur. In cases with a gradient across the left ventricular outflow tract, there is an ejection systolic murmur heard along the lower left sternal border with the absence of an ejection click.

Laboratory Investigations

Electrocardiography. In those with associated defects, the ECG reflects the major abnormality rather than the associated left ventricular outflow tract obstruction. With isolated forms of left ventricular outflow tract obstruction, there may be left ventricular hypertrophy when the obstruction is significant.

Chest Radiography. This is usually unhelpful in these cases.

Echocardiography. Echocardiography is the standard diagnostic tool in this lesion. Not only can it permit an accurate delineation of the mechanisms of obstruction, but it provides detailed data about associated lesions. In all forms, the parasternal long-axis view is key to providing an accurate diagnosis. The presence of mitral aortic discontinuity, the relationship of a fibromuscular ridge to the aortic valve, the presence of accessory obstructive tissue, and the dimensions of the aortic annulus and root are well imaged in this view. In addition, color flow mapping permits the identification of associated aortic valve regurgitation and provides hemodynamic evidence of the site of onset of obstruction. The extension of a fibromuscular ridge onto the anterior mitral leaflet is best appreciated in the apical five-chamber view. This also provides the best site for pulsed or continuous-wave Doppler assessment of the maximum gradient across the left ventricular outflow tract. In the older patient, TEE plays an important role in delineating the pathologic process. Real-time three-dimensional echocardiography provides additional information, particularly in cases with complex mechanisms of left ventricular outflow tract obstruction (**Fig. 65-35**).

Cardiac Catheterization. This technique is no longer of importance in evaluating this lesion. Although balloon dilation has been attempted, it is generally believed that this is a surgical lesion.

CMR. In general, CMR is unnecessary unless there are problems obtaining the needed information by echocardiography.

INTERVENTIONAL OPTIONS. Surgical intervention is indicated either at the time of the repair of the underlying primary lesion or in those cases with discrete obstruction when the obstruction is severe enough to raise concerns.

Discrete Subaortic Stenosis (Fibrous and Muscular)

The rate of progression is varied and may be slow. In general, the approach to the latter group has been to intervene when there is a mean echo gradient across the left ventricular outflow tract of greater than 30 mm Hg to avoid future aortic leaflet damage. Surgery involves a fibromyectomy, with care to avoid damage to the aortic valve or creation of a traumatic VSD. There is a recurrence rate of subaortic stenosis requiring reoperation in up to 20% of cases.[93] In some cases, the recurrence is in the form of a fibrous ridge; in others, there is acquired disease of the aortic valve in the form of stenosis or regurgitation. Reoperation may involve just repeated resection of a recurrent fibrous ridge, or it may involve surgery for the aortic valve in those cases with significant aortic regurgitation.

Complex Forms of Left Ventricular Outflow Tract Obstruction and an Intact Ventricular Septum

In cases with an intact ventricular septum, the indications for intervention are similar to those in cases with discrete obstruction. The difference lies in the fact that the surgical approach must be modified

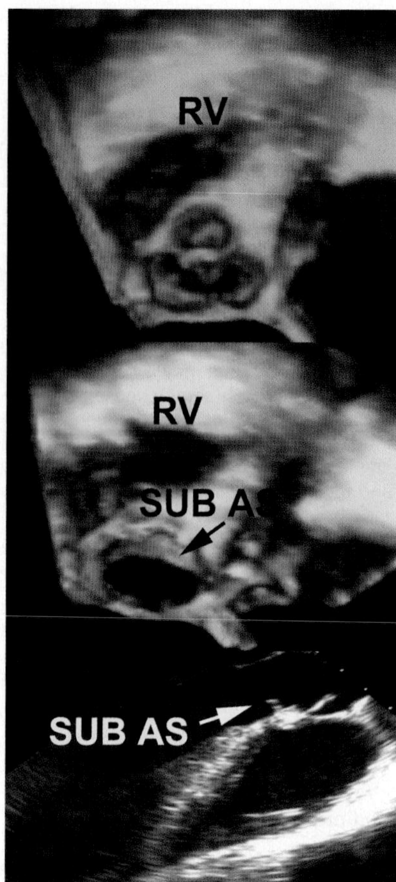

FIGURE 65-35 This montage is from a case with left ventricular outflow tract obstruction, as seen by transesophageal echocardiography in both the two- and three-dimensional modes. **Upper panel,** surgical view of the aortic valve demonstrating the three aortic leaflets. **Middle panel,** is the same case with the aortic valve open. Note the subaortic membrane that is crescentic in shape *(black arrow).* **Bottom panel,** the image seen by two-dimensional echocardiography shows only part of the shelf. RV = right ventricle, SUB AS = subaortic stenosis.

according to the underlying pathologic process. Resection of any fibromuscular component or accessory tissue (provided it is not a primary support mechanism for the mitral valve), a valve-sparing Konno operation, and, in those cases with a hypoplastic aortic annulus, a classic Konno procedure with aortic valve replacement are the potential surgical options.

Left Ventricular Outflow Tract Obstruction and Complex Forms of CHD

In general, surgery to the left ventricular outflow tract is part of the general repair of the lesion and is not dependent on the precise degree of obstruction across this site.

OUTCOMES. Immediate complications related to surgery include complete AV block, creation of a VSD, and mitral regurgitation from intraoperative damage to the mitral valve apparatus. Long-term complications include recurrence of fibromuscular subvalvular left ventricular outflow tract obstruction (up to 20%).[93] Clinically important aortic regurgitation is not uncommon (up to 25% of patients). In some cases with predominant acquired aortic valve stenosis, balloon dilation has been the treatment of choice.

FOLLOW-UP. Particular attention should be paid to patients with residual or recurrent subaortic stenosis and those with an associated bicuspid aortic valve or important aortic regurgitation because they are most likely to require surgery eventually. Reoperation is more likely in cases with complex forms of obstruction, younger age at operation, and incomplete relief of obstruction at the initial procedure.[65] Patients with bioprosthetic aortic valves in the aortic position (after the Konno procedure) or the pulmonary position (after the Ross-Konno procedure) need close follow-up. Endocarditis prophylaxis should be used for prosthetic valves or in the presence of any residual lesions.

Supravalvular Aortic Stenosis

MORPHOLOGY. Three anatomic types of supravalvular aortic stenosis are recognized, although some patients may have findings of more than one type. Most common is the hourglass type, in which marked thickening and disorganization of the aortic media produce a constricting annular ridge at the superior margin of the sinuses of Valsalva. The membranous type is the result of a fibrous or fibromuscular semicircular diaphragm with a small central opening stretched across the lumen of the aorta. Diffuse hypoplasia of the ascending aorta characterizes the third type.

Because the coronary arteries arise proximal to the site of outflow obstruction in supravalvular aortic stenosis, they are subjected to the elevated pressure that exists within the left ventricle. These vessels are often dilated and tortuous, and premature coronary arteriosclerosis has been described. Moreover, if the free edges of some or all of the aortic cusps adhere to the site of supravalvular stenosis, coronary artery inflow may be compromised. The left ventricle may have a "ballerina foot" configuration, which can result in muscular left ventricular outflow tract obstruction, particularly in association with significant supravalvular obstruction.

CLINICAL FEATURES. The clinical picture of supravalvular obstruction differs in major respects from that observed in the other forms of aortic stenosis. Chief among these differences is the association of supravalvular aortic stenosis with idiopathic infantile hypercalcemia, a disease that occurs in the first years of life and can be associated with deranged vitamin D metabolism.

Williams Syndrome

The designation *supravalvular aortic stenosis syndrome, Williams syndrome,* or *Williams-Beuren syndrome* has been applied to the distinctive picture produced by the coexistence of the cardiac features in the setting of a multisystem disorder. Beyond infancy in these patients, a challenge with vitamin D or calcium-loading tests unmasks abnormalities in the regulation of circulating 25-hydroxyvitamin D. Infants with Williams syndrome often exhibit feeding difficulties, failure to thrive, and gastrointestinal problems in the form of vomiting, constipation, and colic. The entire spectrum of clinical manifestations includes auditory hyperacusis, inguinal hernia, hoarse voice, and a typical personality that is outgoing and engaging. Other manifestations of this syndrome include intellectual impairment, "elfin facies," narrowing of peripheral systemic and pulmonary arteries, strabismus, and abnormalities of dental development consisting of microdontia, enamel hypoplasia, and malocclusion.

Many medical conditions can complicate the course of Williams syndrome, including systemic hypertension, gastrointestinal problems, and urinary tract abnormalities. In an older child or adult, progressive joint limitation and hypertonia may become a problem. Adult patients are usually handicapped by their developmental disabilities.

Williams syndrome was previously considered to be nonfamilial; however, a number of families in which parent-to-child transmission of Williams syndrome has occurred have now been identified. All of these families show a parent and child to be affected with Williams syndrome, including one instance of male-to-male transmission. This supports autosomal dominant inheritance as the likely pattern, with most cases of Williams syndrome probably occurring as the result of a new mutation. New information indicates that a genetic defect for supravalvular aortic stenosis is located in the same chromosomal subunit as elastin on chromosome 7q11.23. Elastin is an important component of the arterial wall, but precisely how mutations in elastin genes cause the phenotypes of supravalvular aortic stenosis is not known.

FAMILIAL AUTOSOMAL DOMINANT PRESENTATION. On occasion, the aortic anomaly and peripheral pulmonary arterial stenosis are also found in familial and sporadic forms not associated with the other features of the syndrome. Affected patients have normal intelligence and are normal in facial appearance. Genetic studies suggest that when the anomaly is familial, it is transmitted as autosomal dominant with variable expression. Some family members may have peripheral pulmonary stenosis either as an isolated lesion or in combination with the supravalvular aortic anomaly.

CLINICAL FEATURES. Patients with Williams syndrome are intellectually challenged (**Fig. 65-36**). The typical appearance is similar to that of the elfin facies observed in the severe form of idiopathic infantile hypercalcemia and is characterized by a high prominent forehead, stellate or lacy iris patterns, epicanthal folds, underdeveloped bridge of the nose and mandible, overhanging upper lip, strabismus, and anomalies of dentition. Recognition of this distinctive appearance, even in infancy, should alert the physician to the possibility of underlying multisystem disease. In addition, a positive family history in a patient with a normal appearance and clinical signs suggesting left ventricular outflow obstruction should lead to the suspicion of either supravalvular aortic stenosis or hypertrophic obstructive cardiomyopathy.

Prior studies of the natural history of the principal vascular lesions in these patients—supravalvular aortic stenosis and peripheral pulmonary artery stenosis—indicate that the aortic lesion is usually progressive, with an increase in the intensity of obstruction related often to poor growth of the ascending aorta. This has recently been questioned in a longitudinal single-center study, in which those with smaller gradients at presentation appeared to have evidence of regression of their

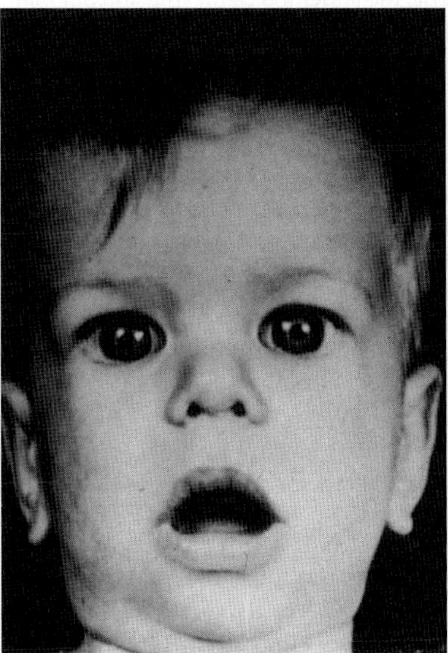
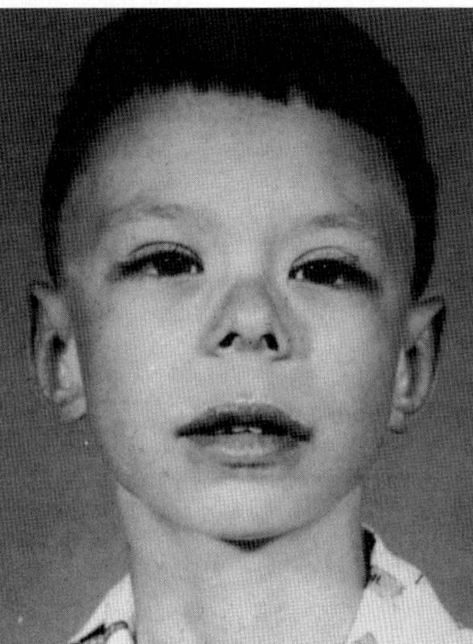
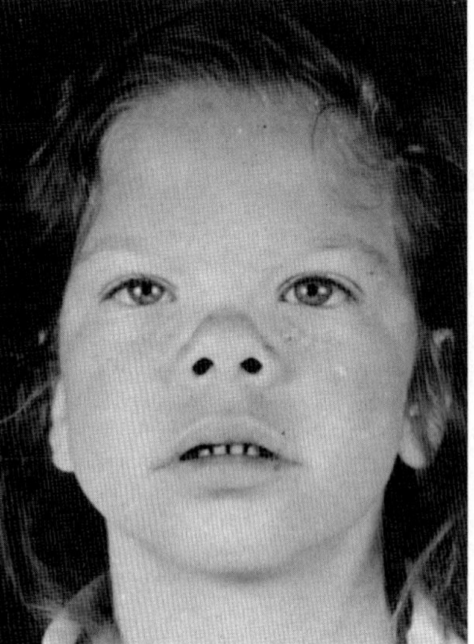

FIGURE 65-36 Typical elfin facies in three patients with supravalvular aortic stenosis. *(From Friedman WF, Kirkpatrick SE: Congenital aortic stenosis. In Adams FH, Emmanouilides GC, Riemenschneider TA, et al [eds]: Moss' Heart Disease in Infants, Children, and Adolescents. 4th ed. Baltimore, Williams & Wilkins, 1989.)*

stenosis.[94] Those with pulmonary branch stenosis, whether associated with the aortic lesion or not, tend to show no change or a reduction in right ventricular pressure with time.

With few exceptions, the major physical findings resemble those observed in patients with aortic valve stenosis. Among these exceptions are an accentuation of aortic valve closure due to elevated pressure in the aorta proximal to the stenosis, an absent ejection click, and the especially prominent transmission of a thrill and murmur into the jugular notch and along the carotid vessels. The narrowing of the peripheral pulmonary arteries may produce a late systolic or continuous murmur heard best in the lung fields and is usually accentuated by inspiration. Another hallmark of supravalvular aortic stenosis is that the systolic pressure in the right arm is usually higher than in the left arm. This pulse disparity may relate to the tendency of a jet stream to adhere to a vessel wall (Coanda effect) and selective streaming of blood into the innominate artery.

Laboratory Investigations

Electrocardiography. This usually reveals left ventricular hypertrophy when the obstruction is severe. Biventricular or even right ventricular hypertrophy may be found if there is significant narrowing of peripheral pulmonary arteries.

Chest Radiography. In contrast to valvular and discrete subvalvular aortic stenosis, dilation of the ascending aorta is absent.

Echocardiography. This is a valuable technique to localize the site of obstruction to the supravalvular area. Most often, the sinuses of Valsalva are dilated, and the ascending aorta and arch appear small or of normal size. The diameter of the aortic annulus is always greater than that of the sinotubular junction. Doppler examination determines the location of obstruction but usually overestimates the gradient compared with that obtained at cardiac catheterization. This results from the obstruction being lengthy, and the Doppler gradient is overestimated because of the phenomenon of pressure recovery.

Angiocardiography. In most cases, this is necessary to define an accurate hemodynamic gradient across the left ventricular outflow tract as well as to determine the status of the coronary arteries. It also usually involves an assessment of the branch pulmonary arteries as well as the brachiocephalic, renal, and mesenteric arteries, all of which can be stenotic. Because of the nature of the anatomic defect, transcatheter balloon angioplasty, with or without stenting, is not an effective treatment option.

INTERVENTIONAL OPTIONS AND OUTCOMES. Surgical intervention for supravalvular aortic stenosis has been successful in most cases with good medium- and long-term results.[95] A variety of surgical procedures may be performed, all of which are tailored to the type of pathologic change. The use of a Y patch, resection with end-to-end anastomosis, and a Ross procedure are the main techniques employed. Additional procedures including coronary bypass of ostial stenosis, aortic valvuloplasty, and subaortic resection may be necessary in some cases.

The cardiac prognosis is good, with some patients requiring further surgery for recurrent supravalvular stenosis. As peripheral pulmonary artery stenosis tends to improve with time, there is a reluctance to attempt intervention, either surgical or by balloon angioplasty. Long-term behavioral and intellectual problems persist.

CONGENITAL MITRAL VALVE ANOMALIES

Congenital Mitral Stenosis

Morphology. Anatomic types of mitral stenosis include the parachute deformity of the valve, in which shortened chordae tendineae converge and insert into a single large papillary muscle; thickened leaflets with shortening and fusion of the chordae tendineae; anomalous arcade of obstructing papillary muscles; accessory mitral valve tissue; and supravalvular circumferential ridge or "ring" of connective tissue arising at the base of the atrial aspect of the mitral leaflets. Associated cardiac defects are common and include endocardial fibroelastosis, coarctation of the aorta, PDA, and left ventricular outflow tract obstruction. An association between persistence of the left superior vena cava and obstructive left-sided lesions also exists.

CLINICAL FEATURES. In most cases, the findings are incidental at the time of evaluation of another left-sided obstructive lesion, such as coarctation of the aorta or aortic valve stenosis. The classic auscultatory findings seen with rheumatic mitral valve stenosis are often absent in the congenital form. Typical findings include a normal S_1, a mid-diastolic murmur with or without some presystolic accentuation, and no opening snap.

Laboratory Investigations

Electrocardiography. In milder forms, this is usually normal, or there may be left atrial overload, with or without right ventricular hypertrophy due to associated pulmonary hypertension.

Chest Radiography. This is normal in milder forms, with evidence of pulmonary edema in those cases with more severe obstruction.

Echocardiography. Two-dimensional and more recently three-dimensional echocardiography, combined with Doppler studies, usually provides a complete analysis of the anatomy and function of congenital mitral stenosis. The status of the papillary muscles is best appreciated in the precordial short-axis view. If two papillary muscles are present, they are usually closer together than is seen in the normal heart. The precordial long-axis view permits identification of a supravalvular mitral ring as well as the degree of mobility of the valve leaflets. Color flow Doppler allows identification of the level of the obstruction as well as the presence of mitral valve regurgitation. Pulsed or continuous-wave Doppler provides an accurate assessment of the mean gradient across the mitral valve. The advantage of the pressure half-time lies in the fact that it is independent of cardiac output, unlike the mean gradient across the mitral valve. Because of the more rapid heart rates in children, the pressure half-time is of less value.

INTERVENTIONAL OPTIONS AND OUTCOMES. In asymptomatic cases, clinical and echocardiographic follow-up is all that is necessary. The presence of a single papillary muscle in itself does not predict progressive stenosis.[96] If the patient starts to develop pulmonary hypertension or symptoms, surgical intervention is usually indicated. Mitral valve balloon dilation is not as successful as it is in rheumatic mitral valve stenosis.[97] Surgery usually involves removal of a supramitral ring if it is present, splitting papillary muscles and fused chordal apparatus in those cases with more common forms of congenital mitral stenosis. In general, surgical intervention provides temporary relief, with many surgical cases requiring valve replacement later in life.

Congenital Mitral Regurgitation

Morphology

Isolated Congenital Mitral Valve Regurgitation. This is usually either due to an isolated cleft of the anterior mitral valve leaflet or the result of leaflet dysplasia. In these cases, there is evidence of shortened chordae in conjunction with dysplastic valve leaflets. In those with an isolated mitral valve *cleft,* the deficiency in the anterior mitral leaflet points toward the left ventricular outflow tract, unlike those cases with an AV septal defect. In general, the larger the cleft in the anterior mitral leaflet, the greater the degree of regurgitation.

In cases with a *dysplastic* mitral valve, the chordal apparatus is shortened with varying degrees of dysplasia of the leaflets. Other anatomic lesions, such as mitral valve arcade resulting in regurgitation, are usually part of a more generalized abnormality of the left side of the heart.

Complex Congenital Mitral Valve Regurgitation

This is seen more frequently in association with abnormalities of the ventriculoarterial connection, such as double-outlet right ventricle, transposition and VSD, and corrected transposition. In the first two, it is frequent to have a cleft in the anterior mitral valve leaflet with some chordal support apparatus that renders the valve less regurgitant than in those cases with an isolated cleft. In cc-TGA, the morphologic mitral valve may have an associated cleft, be dysplastic, or have multiple papillary muscles, all of which increase the tendency for it to be regurgitant.

CLINICAL FEATURES. The presence of symptoms relates to the severity of the regurgitation in cases in which the pathologic change is isolated to the valve. Exercise intolerance, combined with a pansystolic murmur at the apex, with or without a mid-diastolic murmur, is the cardinal clinical feature.

Laboratory Investigations

Electrocardiography. This is either normal or demonstrates left atrial and left ventricular hypertrophy.

Chest Radiography. This demonstrates cardiomegaly predominantly involving the left ventricle and atrium.

Echocardiography. Doppler and two-dimensional echocardiography provide an accurate evaluation of the mechanisms and degree of valvular regurgitation. The cleft in the anterior mitral valve leaflet is best seen in the precordial short-axis view, pointing toward the left ventricular outflow tract. Patients with a dysplastic mitral valve lack mobility of the valve leaflets and have shortened chordae. Color Doppler interrogation helps in locating the site of regurgitation. The severity of regurgitation is assessed in the standard fashion. Three-dimensional echocardiography permits a comprehensive evaluation of the mechanisms of regurgitation, with additional information being obtained about commissural length, leaflet area, and sites of regurgitation from color flow Doppler.[98]

Angiocardiography and MRI. These procedures are seldom helpful in management planning.

INTERVENTIONAL OPTIONS AND OUTCOMES. This depends on the severity of regurgitation and its impact on left ventricular function. Surgery should not be delayed until the patients become symptomatic. Surgery involves suture of an isolated cleft, with or without associated commissuroplasties. In those cases with a dysplastic mitral valve, leaflet extension in conjunction with an annuloplasty and commissuroplasty usually results in effective control of the regurgitation in the short and medium term.[99,100] Despite this, many of these patients require a mitral valve replacement at some stage in the future. Attempted surgical repair, rather than replacement, is important in the pediatric age group because it permits temporary relief that allows the child to grow, such that future surgery can be done into a larger mitral annulus. When it is required, mitral valve replacement has had a good short- and medium-term outcome in cases in which repair is not possible.

RIGHT VENTRICULAR OUTFLOW TRACT LESIONS

Peripheral Pulmonary Artery Stenosis (Fig. 65-37)

Right ventricular outflow tract is a term that applies to patients with both peripheral pulmonary artery stenosis and an intact ventricular septum. It excludes those with an associated VSD, which is dealt with in the sections on tetralogy of Fallot and pulmonary atresia with a VSD. Also excluded is Noonan syndrome, which is dealt with in the subsequent section on pulmonary valve stenosis.

Etiology

Rubella Syndrome. The most important cause of significant pulmonary artery stenoses producing symptoms in newborns used to be intrauterine rubella infection. Other cardiovascular malformations commonly found in association with congenital rubella include PDA, pulmonary valve stenosis, and ASD. Generalized systemic arterial stenotic lesions also may be a feature of the rubella embryopathy, which may involve large and medium-sized vessels such as the aorta and coronary, cerebral, mesenteric, and renal arteries. Cardiovascular lesions are but one manifestation of intrauterine rubella infection because cataracts, microphthalmia, deafness, thrombocytopenia, hepatitis, and blood dyscrasias are also common. The clinical picture in infants with rubella syndrome depends on the severity of the cardiovascular lesions and the associated abnormalities.

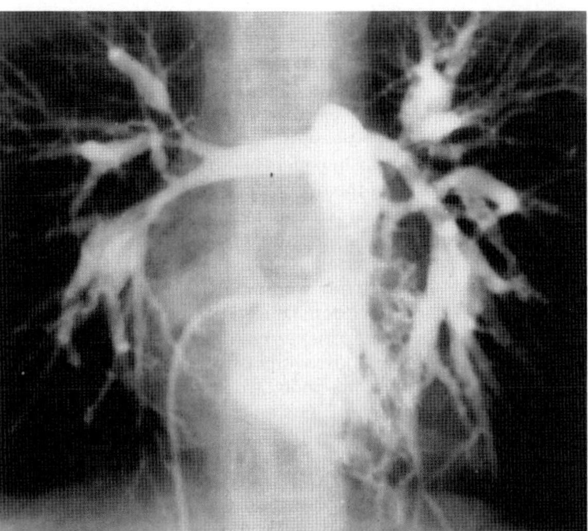

FIGURE 65-37 Right ventricular angiocardiogram showing numerous sites of peripheral pulmonic stenosis and poststenotic dilation of the peripheral pulmonic arteries.

Williams Syndrome. Peripheral pulmonary artery stenosis is also associated with supravalvular aortic stenosis in patients with Williams syndrome, which is discussed in the section on supravalvular aortic stenosis.

Alagille Syndrome. Peripheral pulmonary artery stenosis is a component of this syndrome, with some cases having a *JAG1* mutation.

Isolated Branch Pulmonary Artery Stenosis. This is encountered mainly in the proximal left pulmonary artery and is invariably related to a sling of ductal tissue that causes stenosis when the ductus arteriosus closes after birth. In most cases, this is fairly mild, but a significant obstruction resulting in failure of distal growth of the left pulmonary artery may also be seen.

Morphology. Apart from the isolated form mentioned earlier, the stenoses are usually diffuse and bilateral and extend into the mediastinal, hilar, and intraparenchymal pulmonary arteries.

Clinical Features. The degree of obstruction is the principal determinant of clinical severity. The type of obstruction determines the feasibility of intervention. Most patients are asymptomatic. An ejection systolic murmur heard at the upper left sternal border and well transmitted to the axilla and back is most common. No pulmonary ejection click is heard. The pulmonic component of the second heart sound may be accentuated and is loud only if there is proximal pulmonary hypertension. A continuous murmur is often audible in patients with significant branch stenosis. The murmurs in the lung fields are typically increased by inspiration.

Laboratory Investigations

Electrocardiography. Right ventricular hypertrophy is seen when obstruction is severe. Left-axis deviation with counterclockwise orientation of the frontal QRS vector is common in rubella syndrome and when there is also supravalvular aortic stenosis.

Chest Radiography. Mild or moderate stenosis usually produces normal findings. Detectable differences in vascularity between regions of the lungs or dilated pulmonary artery segments are uncommon. When obstruction is bilateral and severe, right atrial and ventricular enlargement may be seen.

Echocardiography. Echocardiography is helpful in making the diagnosis and excluding associated lesions; however, it is limited in its ability to image the distal pulmonary arteries beyond the hilum of the lung. Right ventricular pressure assessment may be predicted if there is associated tricuspid valve regurgitation.

CMR and Spiral CT. These are valuable diagnostic tests because they permit a more distal evaluation of the branch pulmonary arteries. The advantage of spiral CT in young children is that it can be performed without the need for heavy sedation or even general anesthesia. Although most patients require cardiac catheterization and angiography, these other techniques are excellent for the initial evaluation and for following the progress of the lesions.

Radionuclide Quantitative Lung Perfusion Scan. This is valuable in cases with unilateral stenosis to determine whether intervention is necessary. Similar flow estimates can now be obtained by CMR.

Cardiac Catheterization and Angiocardiography. This permits the assessment of right ventricular pressure and the pressures in the pulmonary arterial tree. Angiocardiography is the key to precise assessment of the extent and severity of the stenoses.

Interventional Options and Outcomes. For those cases with isolated left pulmonary artery stenosis in which there is less than 30% of flow to the lung, balloon dilation with or without stent insertion is effective in relieving the obstruction. In those cases with more diffuse bilateral stenoses, the indications for intervention depend on the right ventricular pressure. As the natural history of diffuse peripheral pulmonary artery stenosis in Williams syndrome is one of potential regression over time, intervention is in general reserved for those cases with systemic or suprasystemic right ventricular pressure. Intervention also depends in part on the extent of the stenosis and the dilation capability of the lesions, with or without stenting. In some cases, several attempts at dilation are required to achieve any improvement in vessel caliber. High-pressure balloons are usually necessary, but some lesions cannot be dilated even with such balloons. Recently, improved results have been reported with use of "cutting" balloons, which may assist dilation in an otherwise

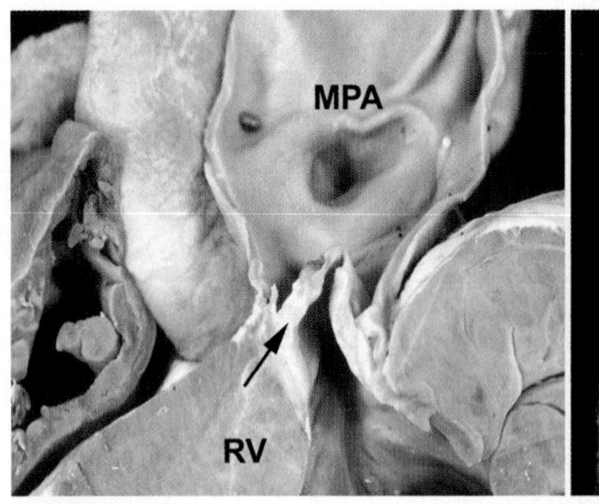

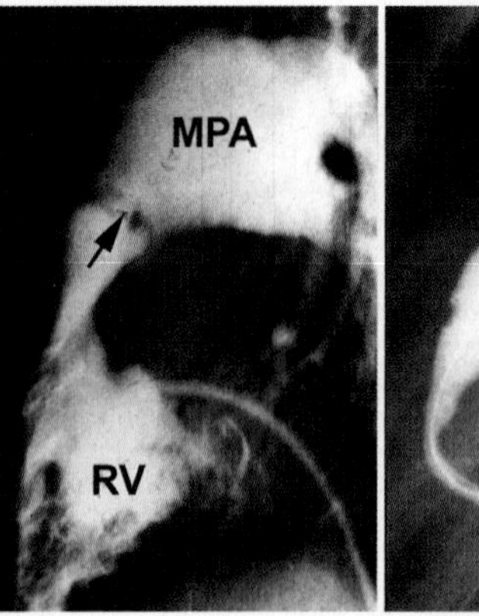

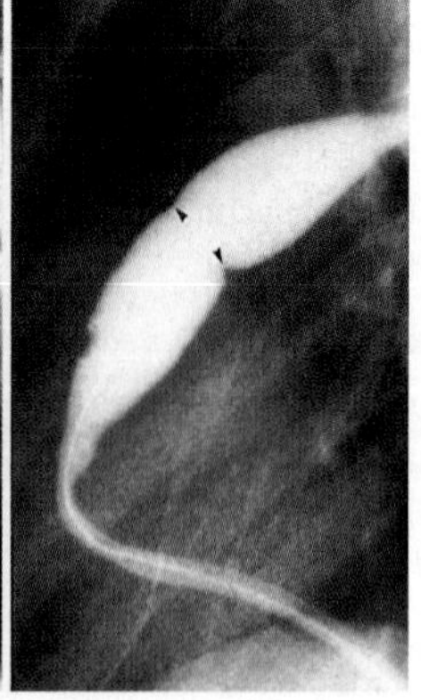

FIGURE 65-38 Montage of pulmonary valve stenosis demonstrating typical pathology (**left,** arrow) with a thickened pulmonary valve and obstruction due to commissural fusion. Note the poststenotic dilation. The angiogram demonstrates a case before (**middle,** arrow) and during (**right**) balloon dilation. MPA = main pulmonary artery; RV = right ventricle.

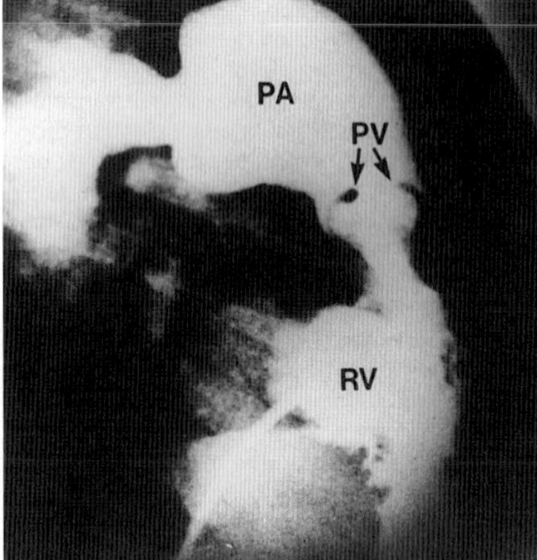

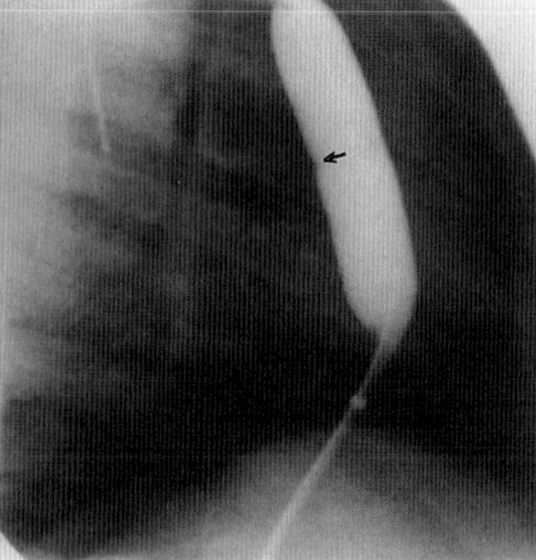

FIGURE 65-39 **Left,** Right ventriculogram (RV) in the lateral projection from a patient with valvular pulmonic stenosis. The pulmonary valve (PV) is thickened and domes in systole (arrows). Poststenotic dilation of the pulmonary artery (PA) is seen. **Right,** Successful balloon valvuloplasty shows almost complete disappearance of the stenotic waist (arrow). *(Courtesy of Dr. Thomas G. DiSessa.)*

undilatable stenosis. As a rule, surgery has little to offer those patients with diffuse peripheral pulmonary artery stenoses and can indeed make the situation worse.

Supravalvular Right Ventricular Outflow Tract Obstruction

Supravalvular right ventricular outflow tract obstruction seldom occurs in isolation. It can occur in tetralogy of Fallot, Williams syndrome, Noonan syndrome, VSD, or arteriohepatic dysplasia (Alagille syndrome). Supravalvular right ventricular outflow tract obstruction can progress in severity and should be monitored. Dilation of the pulmonary trunk is not a feature of subvalvular and supravalvular right ventricular outflow tract obstruction. Intervention is recommended when the peak gradient across the right ventricular outflow tract is more than 50 mm Hg at rest or when the patient is symptomatic.

Pulmonary Stenosis with Intact Ventricular Septum (Figs. 65-38 and 65-39)

This lesion exists as a continuum, ranging from isolated valvular stenosis to complete atresia of the pulmonary outflow tract. Two modes of presentation exist. The first is manifested in the neonatal period, usually with associated disease of the tricuspid valve, right ventricle, or coronary arteries. The second mode of presentation is beyond the neonatal period, when the valvular stenosis is usually isolated. Some cases with severe stenosis diagnosed in utero can present with valvular atresia at the time of birth.

Morphology. The pulmonary valve may vary from a well-formed trileaflet valve with varying degrees of commissural fusion to an imperforate membrane. If stenosis is present, the right ventricle is usually of normal size or only mildly hypoplastic. Patients with an imperforate valve and a patent infundibulum invariably have a larger right ventricular volume than do patients with both infundibular and valve atresia.

Clinical Features

Neonate with Critical Pulmonary Valve Stenosis. The neonate presents with central cyanosis due to right-to-left shunting at the atrial level and depends on a prostaglandin infusion to maintain the patency of the ductus arteriosus. Auscultatory findings include a single second heart sound, no ejection click, and a murmur that, when present, is due to tricuspid valve regurgitation.

Infant and Child. In cases beyond the newborn period, the referral is usually for the assessment of a cardiac murmur. This may be detected within the first few weeks of life, more commonly at the routine 6-week postnatal visit or later. These patients usually have an ejection click and a second heart sound that moves with respiration but with a soft pulmonary component. An ejection murmur of varying intensity and duration is heard best in the pulmonary area.

Adult. Adults with isolated mild to moderate right ventricular outflow tract obstruction of any type usually have no symptoms. Patients with severe right ventricular outflow tract obstruction may present with exertional fatigue, dyspnea, lightheadedness, and chest discomfort (right ventricular angina). Physical examination may reveal a prominent jugular *a* wave, a right ventricular lift, and possibly a thrill in the second left intercostal space. Auscultation reveals a normal S_1, a single or split S_2 with a diminished P_2 (unless the obstruction is supravalvular, in which case the intensity of the P_2 is normal or increased), and a systolic ejection murmur best heard in the second left intercostal space. When the pulmonary valve is thin and pliable, a systolic ejection click will be heard, which decreases on inspiration. As the severity of the pulmonary stenosis progresses, the interval between S_1 and the systolic ejection click becomes shorter, S_2 becomes widely split, P_2 diminishes or disappears, and the systolic ejection murmur lengthens and peaks later in systole, often extending beyond A_2. An ejection click seldom occurs with dysplastic pulmonary stenosis. Cyanosis may be present when a PFO or ASD permits right-to-left shunting.

Adult patients with trivial and mild valvular right ventricular outflow tract obstruction do not become worse with time. Moderate valvular right ventricular outflow tract obstruction can progress in 20% of unrepaired patients, especially in adults because of calcification of the valve, and may require intervention. Some of these patients can also become symptomatic, particularly in later life, because of atrial arrhythmias resulting from right ventricular pressure overload and tricuspid regurgitation. Patients with severe valvular right ventricular outflow tract obstruction will have had balloon or surgical valvotomy to survive to adult life. Long-term survival in patients with repaired pulmonary valve stenosis is similar to that of the general population, with good to excellent functional class at long-term follow-up in most patients. A few patients have severe pulmonary regurgitation.

Laboratory Investigations

Electrocardiography. In the newborn period, this may show left-axis deviation and left ventricular dominance in cases with significant right ventricular hypoplasia. Other patients may have a normal QRS axis. Right atrial overload is present in those with increased right atrial pressure. In the infant, child, and adult, the findings depend on the severity of the stenosis. In milder cases, the ECG should be normal. As the stenosis progresses, evidence of right ventricular hypertrophy appears. Severe stenosis is seen in the form of a tall R wave in lead V_4R or V_1 with a deep S wave in V_6. A tall QR wave in the right precordial leads with T wave inversion and ST-segment depression (right ventricular "strain") reflects severe stenosis. When an rSR′ pattern is observed in lead V_1 (20% of patients), lower right ventricular pressures are found than in patients with a pure R wave of equal amplitude. Right atrial overload is associated with moderate to severe pulmonary stenosis.

Chest Radiography. In the neonate, this demonstrates pulmonary oligemia with a prominent right-sided heart border in those with associated tricuspid valve regurgitation. In the infant, child, and adult with mild or moderate pulmonary stenosis, chest radiography often shows a heart of normal size and normal pulmonary vascularity. Poststenotic dilation of the main and left pulmonary arteries is often seen. Right atrial and right ventricular enlargement is observed in patients with severe obstruction and right ventricular failure. The pulmonary vascularity is usually normal in the absence of a right-to-left atrial shunt but may be reduced in patients with severe stenosis and right ventricular failure.

Echocardiography. Combined two-dimensional echocardiographic and continuous-wave Doppler examination characterizes the anatomic valve abnormality and its severity and has essentially eliminated the requirement for diagnostic cardiac catheterization. Although maximum instantaneous gradients have traditionally been used to select patients for balloon valvuloplasty, recent data would suggest the contrary. Mean Doppler gradients appear to correlate better with catheter-derived peak-peak gradients, with a value of 50 mm Hg being the cut point for intervention.[101] Invasive studies are currently used for balloon valvuloplasty.

Right ventricular size is currently best assessed indirectly from the tricuspid annular dimension. In the absence of a VSD, there is an excellent correlation between the two. Right ventricular pressure can be assessed indirectly from the tricuspid regurgitation gradient. Tricuspid valve morphology and function and the status of the interatrial septum need to be addressed.

Interventional Options and Outcomes

Neonate. In the neonate, prostaglandin E_1 is instituted in cases with ductal dependency. After this, balloon dilation is performed in those with stenosis, whereas radiofrequency perforation in conjunction with dilation may be undertaken in those with pulmonary valve atresia. If relief of the obstruction is successful, the prostaglandins are slowly discontinued to determine if the right ventricle is large enough to support the circulation. If not, a systemic to pulmonary artery shunt is necessary early in the management. In cases with a normal-sized right ventricle, no further therapy is usually necessary in the future because there is a low recurrence rate of stenosis. Newborns with isolated pulmonary stenosis do well after relief of the stenosis.[102]

Infant and Older Child. Balloon dilation of the pulmonary valve is the therapeutic procedure of choice with excellent short- and medium-term results.

Adults. Balloon valvuloplasty is recommended when the gradient across the right ventricular outflow tract is greater than 50 mm Hg at rest[2] or when the patient is symptomatic.

Despite the excellent survival results from the second natural history study (survival after surgical valvotomy of 95.7% compared with sex-matched controls of 96.6%), recent long-term data suggest that this population of patients faces ongoing challenges. After a mean follow-up period of 33 years, 53% of patients had required further intervention and 38% had either atrial or ventricular arrhythmias.[103]

Dysplastic Pulmonary Valve Stenosis

Morphology. In pulmonary valve stenosis due to valvular dysplasia, the obstruction is caused not by commissural fusion but by a combination of thickened and dysplastic pulmonary valve leaflets in combination with varying degrees of supravalvular pulmonary stenosis. The supravalvular stenosis is classically at the distal part of pulmonary valve sinuses, and there is usually no poststenotic pulmonary artery dilation. This entity is associated with Noonan syndrome, which in turn may be associated with hypertrophic cardiomyopathy.

Clinical Features. In most cases, the diagnosis is made either during an evaluation of a systolic murmur or in a child with dysmorphic features who is undergoing clinical evaluation. Children with Noonan syndrome have short stature, webbed necks, and broad-shaped chests in a fashion similar to Turner syndrome. Although this syndrome does not have an associated chromosomal abnormality, it may be familial and affects both sexes equally. A unique association in the newborn is pulmonary lymphangiectasia. The auscultatory finding that differentiates dysplastic valves from simple pulmonary valve stenosis is the lack of an ejection click. The other features of the murmur are similar to those described in pulmonary valve stenosis.

Laboratory Investigations

Electrocardiography. The ECG is helpful in that patients with dysplastic pulmonary stenosis frequently have a leftward QRS axis, particularly in association with hypertrophic cardiomyopathy. The remainder of the ECG is similar to that seen in pulmonary valve stenosis.

Chest Radiography. The findings are similar to typical pulmonary valve stenosis, apart from the lack of poststenotic pulmonary trunk dilation, even in the presence of severe obstruction. In those with pulmonary lymphangiectasia, the chest radiograph has a ground-glass appearance, which can be difficult to differentiate from pulmonary venous obstruction.

Echocardiography. This demonstrates a thickened fleshy pulmonary valve, lack of poststenotic dilation, and varying degrees of supravalvular pulmonary stenosis. The associated diagnosis of hypertrophic cardiomyopathy can be confirmed or excluded. If the initial echocardiogram does not demonstrate hypertrophic cardiomyopathy, further studies should be performed throughout childhood and adolescence, particularly in cases with left-axis deviation.

Interventional Options and Outcomes

Cardiac Catheterization and Angiography. Although the results of balloon valvuloplasty are less rewarding than in those with stenosis due to commissural fusion, it is worth attempting this before considering surgical intervention. Success has been varied, with many cases having some reduction in gradient that can delay surgery.

Surgical Intervention. If balloon valvuloplasty fails, surgical intervention is indicated. This usually involves a partial valvectomy in conjunction with patch repair of the supravalvular stenosis.

Outcomes. Adequate relief of the right ventricular outflow tract obstruction results in an excellent outlook. The greatest long-term risk factor is the presence of hypertrophic cardiomyopathy.

Subpulmonary Right Ventricular Outflow Tract Obstruction (Anomalous Muscle Bundles or a Double-Chambered Right Ventricle)

Morphology. A double-chambered right ventricle is formed by right ventricular obstruction due to anomalous muscle bundles. Although this can occur in isolation, it is more frequently part of a combination of lesions that includes right ventricular muscle bundles, a perimembranous-outlet VSD, and subaortic stenosis with or without aortic valve prolapse.

Clinical Features. Most cases are discovered incidentally during the evaluation of a VSD. In some cases, there may be only an ejection systolic murmur. If the obstruction is isolated, there is an ejection systolic murmur that is heard best in the upper left sternal border. If the VSD is the predominant lesion, the right ventricular outflow tract murmur may not be appreciated. Before the routine use of echocardiography, the diagnosis was often made during follow-up for a VSD when the pansystolic murmur decreased in intensity and a systolic ejection murmur emerged. The patients are usually pink unless there is progression of the subpulmonary stenosis in the setting of a VSD. The diagnosis may be more problematic in adults.

Laboratory Investigations

Electrocardiography. The ECG is similar to that of those with isolated pulmonary valve stenosis beyond the newborn period. In cases with a nonrestrictive VSD and mild subpulmonary stenosis, the ECG typically shows biventricular hypertrophy due to a left-to-right shunt and associated pulmonary hypertension. If the stenosis is more severe, right ventricular hypertrophy will be seen. Those with a restrictive VSD may have a normal ECG or left ventricular hypertrophy, which is replaced with right ventricular hypertrophy if the subpulmonary stenosis increases in severity.

Chest Radiography. This is usually normal in those with isolated subpulmonary stenosis, whereas those with a VSD may have either increased or reduced pulmonary blood flow, depending on the severity of the obstruction.

Echocardiography. Doppler and two-dimensional echocardiography usually provide a complete diagnosis. The level of subpulmonary obstruction is appreciated best in a combination of subcostal right anterior oblique and precordial short-axis views. These views permit the identification of the relationship of the VSD to the muscle bundles as well as the degree of anterior malalignment of the infundibular septum in those with a VSD. The precordial short-axis view is the best position to evaluate the presence of possible subaortic stenosis and aortic cusp prolapse. Color and pulsed or continuous-wave Doppler evaluation usually allows differentiation of the VSD flow jet from that originating from the muscle bundles. This permits an accurate assessment of the hemodynamic effect of the subpulmonary obstruction.

Cardiac Catheterization and Angiocardiography. This technique is rarely necessary. In older patients in whom the echocardiographic images of the subpulmonary region may be suboptimal, a combination of magnetic resonance angiography and echocardiography is all that is generally necessary.

Management Options and Outcomes. Management is dictated by the severity of the subpulmonary stenosis and the presence of associated defects. In patients with isolated subpulmonary stenosis, surgery is indicated when the right ventricular pressure is more than 60% of systemic. This involves resection of the muscle bundles through the right atrium. For those cases with an associated VSD, the decision is based on the size of the VSD, the degree of associated subaortic stenosis, the presence of aortic valve prolapse, and the severity of the subpulmonary stenosis. These patients tend to have a progressive disease, so many cases that are followed up conservatively for several years will eventually require surgery. In general, the outcome is excellent with a low rate of recurrence after surgical resection of obstructive muscle bundles. Infrequently, recurrence of the subaortic obstruction may occur.

Miscellaneous Lesions

Cor Triatriatum

Morphology. In this malformation, failure of resorption of the common pulmonary vein results in a left atrium divided by an abnormal fibromuscular diaphragm into a posterosuperior chamber receiving the pulmonary veins and an anteroinferior chamber giving rise to the left atrial appendage and leading to the mitral orifice. The communication between the divided atrial chambers may be large, small, or absent, depending on the size of the opening in the diaphragm, which determines the degree of obstruction to pulmonary venous return. Elevations of both pulmonary venous pressure and pulmonary vascular resistance may result in severe pulmonary artery hypertension.

Clinical Features. Cor triatriatum may be detected as an incidental finding in a patient who has echocardiography for another reason. In general, this represents the unobstructed form that requires no early intervention. Cases with more severe obstruction present in a fashion similar to patients with congenital pulmonary vein stenosis.

Laboratory Investigations

Electrocardiography. In unobstructed cases, this is normal. In those with significant obstruction, there is right ventricular hypertrophy due to the associated pulmonary hypertension.

Chest Radiography. This may be normal in those with mild obstruction or who demonstrate pulmonary edema in those with significant obstruction.

Echocardiography. The diagnosis is established by two-dimensional echocardiography or TEE, with further insight from three-dimensional reconstruction. The obstructive diaphragm is visualized in the parasternal long- and short-axis and four-chamber views and can be distinguished from a supravalvular mitral ring by its position superior to the left atrial appendage, which forms part of the distal chamber. Also present is diastolic fluttering of the mitral leaflets and high-velocity flow detected by Doppler examination in the distal atrial chamber and at the mitral orifice.

Cardiac Catheterization and Angiocardiography. This technique is usually unnecessary since the advent of echocardiography and CMR.

Management Options and Outcomes. Surgical resection of the membrane is the treatment of choice for patients with significant obstruction. This results in symptom relief and a reduction of pulmonary artery pressure. In general, the outcome after surgery is good. With the advent of more routine echocardiography, a subset of cases with typical but nonobstructive forms has been recognized. Thus far, these cases appear to remain asymptomatic, with an infrequent need for surgical intervention.

Pulmonary Vein Stenosis

Congenital pulmonary vein stenosis may occur as a focal stenosis at the atrial junction or generalized hypoplasia of one or more pulmonary veins. The incidence of associated cardiac malformations, including VSD, ASD, tetralogy of Fallot, tricuspid and mitral atresia, and AV septal defect, is extremely high. In other cases, the pulmonary vein stenosis is acquired after surgical intervention for total anomalous pulmonary venous connection. Children frequently present with recurrent respiratory infections, whereas adults exhibit exercise intolerance. Pulmonary hypertension is one of the consequences of pulmonary vein stenosis, whether it is congenital or acquired. In cases with unilateral pulmonary vein stenosis, clinical symptoms are frequently absent because there is pulmonary blood flow redistribution away from the affected lung.

Laboratory Investigations

Electrocardiography. The ECG is usually normal unless there is evidence of pulmonary hypertension, in which case right ventricular hypertrophy may be seen.

Chest Radiography. With unilateral pulmonary vein stenosis, there is oligemia of the affected lung and increased flow to the contralateral side. If the obstruction is bilateral, pulmonary edema is seen.

Echocardiography. This can usually exclude or confirm the diagnosis of pulmonary vein stenosis. Assessment of pulmonary artery pressure from tricuspid or pulmonary valve regurgitation is possible. Doppler color flow assessment of the right- and left-sided pulmonary veins is the best screening tool. If there is evidence of turbulence or aliasing in the color flow pattern, spectral analysis with pulsed Doppler will help confirm the diagnosis. Usually, pulmonary venous flow is low velocity and phasic. If the pattern is high velocity and turbulent, there is disturbed pulmonary venous flow. Absolute Doppler gradients may or may not be helpful for two reasons. First, the absolute velocity depends on the amount of pulmonary blood flow to that segment of lung. Second, it is often difficult to obtain a parallel line of interrogation of the pulmonary veins that will affect gradient assessment. The absolute velocity is less important than the diagnosis of pulmonary vein stenosis and its effect on pulmonary artery pressure.

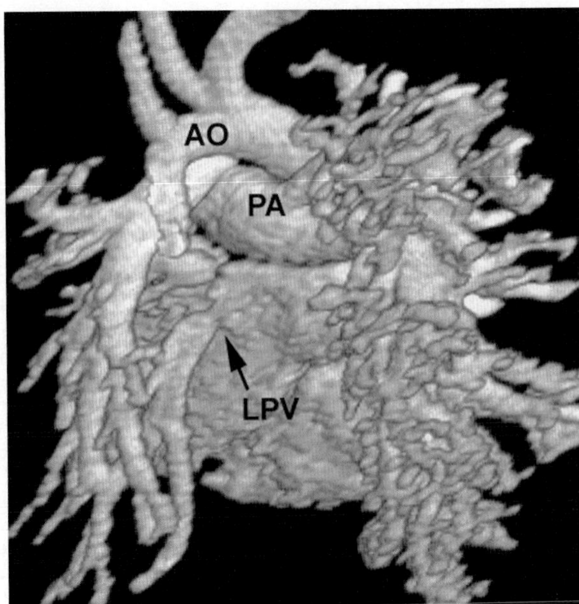

FIGURE 65-40 Three-dimensional CMR demonstrating stenosis of the left lower lobe pulmonary vein. AO = aorta; LPV = left pulmonary vein; PA = pulmonary artery.

CMR (**Fig. 65-40**). This technique has now become the gold standard for the diagnosis of pulmonary vein stenosis. This permits a detailed assessment of the pulmonary veins. Velocity assessment is now possible, although this is in the actual veins themselves rather than at the venoatrial junction, which is the site assessed by Doppler echocardiography.

Cardiac Catheterization and Angiography. In general, a combination of echocardiography and CMR makes invasive procedures unnecessary.

Management Options and Outcomes. If the patient has unilateral pulmonary vein stenosis and normal pulmonary artery pressure, no treatment may be necessary. Continued follow-up is important because this is often a progressive disease that can subsequently affect both sides. In cases with bilateral stenoses, the outlook in the past was believed to be hopeless, with virtually 100% mortality. Stents usually provided only temporary relief. More recently, a pericardial reflection procedure using native tissue has resulted in some early success in this lesion. This involves use of native atrial tissue to form a pocket around the surgically resected stenotic region.

Partial Anomalous Pulmonary Venous Connection

Morphology. This refers to conditions in which part or all of one lung drains to a site other than the left atrium. Sinus venosus defects are associated with PAPVC typically from the right upper and middle lobe pulmonary veins to the superior vena cava. PAPVC may be directed to a left vertical vein, to the superior vena cava at the level of or above the right pulmonary artery, to the azygos vein, or to the coronary sinus. PAPVC to the inferior vena cava (scimitar syndrome) may have associated hypoplasia of the right lung, pulmonary sequestration, and abnormal collateral supply to the sequestered segment. It can be seen in some patients (<10%) with a secundum ASD as well as in association with many other forms of CHD. PAPVC to the right atrium has the pulmonary veins lying in the normal position; however, there is deviation of the septum primum to the left with absence of the septum secundum. This type of lesion is seen more frequently in hearts with visceral heterotaxy.

Clinical Features. In the absence of associated anomalies, the physiologic disturbance is determined by the number of anomalous veins and their site of connection, the presence and size of an ASD, and the state of the pulmonary vascular bed. In the usual patient with isolated partial pulmonary venous connection, the hemodynamic state and physical findings are similar to those in ASD.

Laboratory Investigations

Electrocardiography. In isolated cases, findings similar to a secundum ASD may be seen.

Chest Radiography. Isolated cases show cardiomegaly involving the right ventricle with increased pulmonary vascular markings. In scimitar syndrome, there is typically right lung hypoplasia, with a secondary shift of the heart into the right thorax and a right-sided scimitar sign that represents the anomalous pulmonary vein.

Echocardiography. If there is a significant left-to-right shunt, there is right ventricular volume overload with paradoxical interventricular septal motion. A dilated coronary sinus is seen in PAPVC to the coronary sinus. In scimitar syndrome, the abnormal pulmonary vein can be seen from the subcostal position during evaluation of the inferior vena cava. Associated stenosis of the pulmonary vein may exist. The suprasternal position permits identification of a left vertical vein, and in general it is possible in children to identify the number of connecting veins on that side. Abnormal venous drainage to the right superior vena cava may be more difficult to identify unless a systematic approach is undertaken. The suprasternal frontal plane view allows the identification of veins that connect just above the right pulmonary artery. Those that connect just behind the right pulmonary artery, into either the superior vena cava or the azygos, can be identified with a right anterior oblique view of the superior vena cava, whether from the subcostal position or a high right parasternal location. In adults, TEE may also be useful in detecting PAPVC.

CMR. Although TEE can be used with a considerable degree of accuracy in older patients with a poorer ultrasound window, it is less invasive to obtain the data by CMR. This provides superb images of the connecting veins that can be seen more distally to their connections with the hilum of the lung. The pulmonary-to-systemic flow ratio can be calculated, obviating the need for hemodynamic evaluation. The pulmonary-to-systemic flow ratio can also be calculated by radionuclide techniques.

Management Options. In cases with a volume-loaded right ventricle, surgical intervention should be considered. Surgery is not necessary when a single anomalously draining vein has not produced right ventricular volume loading. Surgery is typically performed at a time similar to an ASD repair, at approximately 3 to 5 years of age. The type of surgery depends on the location of the drainage but in general consists of reconnection of the abnormal veins to the left atrium, either directly in the case of a left vertical vein or by a baffle in most other instances. In scimitar syndrome, occlusion of the collateral arteries as well as redirection of the pulmonary veins may be necessary.

Outcomes. In general, patients with repaired PAPVC have a good outcome similar to that of patients with an isolated ASD. What is unclear is the exact patency rate of the veins that are reconnected or baffled back to the left atrium. Patients with scimitar syndrome fare well if the lesion is relatively isolated but do poorly if there is significant associated intracardiac disease.

Pulmonary Arteriovenous Fistula

Abnormal development of the pulmonary arteries and veins in a common vascular complex is responsible for this congenital anomaly. A variable number of pulmonary arteries communicate directly with branches of the pulmonary veins. Most patients have an associated Weber-Osler-Rendu syndrome; associated problems include bronchiectasis and other malformations of the bronchial tree as well as absence of the right lower lobe. Pulmonary arteriovenous fistulas may also complicate classic Glenn shunts used in the palliation of cyanotic CHD and are believed to be due to the absence of "hepatic factor" in the venous blood feeding the superior vena cava–pulmonary artery connection. Hepatopulmonary syndrome may also be associated with substantial right-to-left intrapulmonary shunting.[62] The amount of right-to-left shunting depends on the extent of the fistulous communications and may result in cyanosis. Paradoxical emboli or a brain abscess may result and cause major neurologic deficits. Patients with hereditary hemorrhagic telangiectasia are often anemic because of repeated blood loss and may have less obvious cyanosis because of anemia. Systolic and continuous murmurs may be audible over areas of the fistula. Rounded opacities of various sizes in one or both lungs on chest radiography may suggest the presence of the lesion.

Laboratory Investigations. Echocardiography is helpful in the initial diagnostic process with the use of a saline contrast injection into a systemic vein. With pulmonary arteriovenous malformations, there is early pulmonary venous return to the left atrium, but not as quickly as for patients with a PFO or ASD and right-to-left atrial shunting. More recently, CT and CMR techniques have provided valuable diagnostic information. Pulmonary angiography reveals the site and extent of the abnormal communication.

Management Options. Unless the lesions are widespread throughout both lungs, surgical treatment aimed at removal of the lesions with preservation of healthy lung tissue is commonly indicated to avoid the complications of massive hemorrhage, bacterial endocarditis, and rupture of arteriovenous aneurysms. Transcatheter balloon or plug or coil occlusion embolotherapy may prove to be the therapeutic procedure of choice in some patients.

Coronary Arteriovenous Fistula

Morphology. A coronary arteriovenous fistula is a communication between one of the coronary arteries and a cardiac chamber or vein. The right coronary artery (or its branches) is the site of the fistula in about 55% of patients; the left coronary artery is involved in about 35%; and both coronary arteries are involved in a few. Connections between the coronary system and a cardiac chamber appear to represent persistence of embryonic intertrabecular spaces and sinusoids. Most of these fistulas drain into the right ventricle, the right atrium, or the coronary sinus. Coronary to pulmonary artery fistulas are an occasional and usually incidental finding in the adult coronary angiography suite.

Clinical Features. The shunt through the fistula is usually small, and myocardial blood flow is not compromised. Potential complications include pulmonary hypertension and congestive heart failure if a large left-to-right shunt exists, bacterial endocarditis, rupture or thrombosis of the fistula or of an associated arterial aneurysm, and myocardial ischemia distal to the fistula due to a "myocardial steal."

Most pediatric patients are asymptomatic and are referred because of a cardiac murmur that is loud, superficial, and continuous at the lower or midsternal border. The site of maximal intensity of the murmur is related to the site of drainage and is usually away from the second left intercostal space, the classic site of the continuous murmur of persistent ductus arteriosus.

Laboratory Investigations

Electrocardiography. This is usually normal unless there is a large left-to-right shunt.

Chest Radiography. Radiographic findings are often normal and seldom show selective chamber enlargement.

Echocardiography. Coronary artery fistulas are now recognized with a high degree of accuracy with the advent of routine coronary artery evaluation during most pediatric echocardiography examinations. A significantly enlarged feeding coronary artery can be detected, and the entire course and site of entry of the arteriovenous fistula can be traced by Doppler color flow mapping. The shunt entry site is characterized by a continuous turbulent systolic and diastolic flow pattern. Multiplane TEE also accurately defines the origin, course, and drainage site of the fistula.

Cardiac Catheterization and Angiocardiography. If echocardiography demonstrates a significant coronary artery fistula, hemodynamic evaluation is warranted. Standard retrograde thoracic aortography, balloon occlusion angiography of the aortic root with a 45-degree caudal tilt of the frontal camera ("laid-back" aortogram), or coronary arteriography can be used reliably to identify the size and anatomic features of the fistulous track.

Management Options and Outcomes. Small fistulas have an excellent long-term prognosis. Untreated larger fistulas may predispose the individual to premature coronary artery disease in the affected vessel. Coil embolization at the time of cardiac catheterization is rapidly becoming the treatment of choice. Surgical treatment is still required in some instances.

REFERENCES

1. Warnes CA, Williams RG, Bashore TM, et al: ACC/AHA 2008 guidelines for the management of adults with congenital heart disease: A report of the American College of Cardiology/American Heart Association Task Force on Practice Guidelines (Writing Committee to Develop Guidelines on the Management of Adults With Congenital Heart Disease). Developed in Collaboration With the American Society of Echocardiography, Heart Rhythm Society, International Society for Adult Congenital Heart Disease, Society for Cardiovascular Angiography and Interventions, and Society of Thoracic Surgeons. J Am Coll Cardiol 52:e1, 2008.
2. Gatzoulis MA, Webb GD, Daubeney PEF: Diagnosis and Management of Adult Congenital Heart Disease. Edinburgh, Churchill Livingstone, 2003.

Anatomy and Embryology

3. Bird GL, Jeffries HE, Licht DJ, et al: Neurological complications associated with the treatment of patients with congenital cardiac disease: Consensus definitions from the Multi-Societal Database Committee for Pediatric and Congenital Heart Disease. Cardiol Young 18(Suppl 2):234, 2008.

4. Thorne S, MacGregor A, Nelson-Piercy C: Risks of contraception and pregnancy in heart disease. Heart 92:1520, 2006.

Pathologic Consequences of Congenital Cardiac Lesions

5. Hosseinpour AR, Cullen S, Tsang VT: Transplantation for adults with congenital heart disease. Eur J Cardiothorac Surg 30:508, 2006.
6. Lamour JM, Kanter KR, Naftel DC, et al: The effect of age, diagnosis, and previous surgery in children and adults undergoing heart transplantation for congenital heart disease. J Am Coll Cardiol 54:160, 2009.

Cyanosis

7. Oechslin E, Kiowski W, Schindler R, et al: Systemic endothelial dysfunction in adults with cyanotic congenital heart disease. Circulation 112:1106, 2005.
8. Fyfe A, Perloff JK, Niwa K, et al: Cyanotic congenital heart disease and coronary artery atherogenesis. Am J Cardiol 96:283, 2005.
9. Walker F, Mullen MJ, Woods SJ, Webb GD: Acute effects of 40% oxygen supplementation in adults with cyanotic congenital heart disease. Heart 90:1073, 2004.

Pulmonary Hypertension

10. Duffels MG, Engelfriet PM, Berger RM, et al: Pulmonary arterial hypertension in congenital heart disease: An epidemiologic perspective from a Dutch registry. Int J Cardiol 120:198, 2007.
11. McLaughlin VV, Archer SL, Badesch DB, et al: ACCF/AHA 2009 expert consensus document on pulmonary hypertension a report of the American College of Cardiology Foundation Task Force on Expert Consensus Documents and the American Heart Association developed in collaboration with the American College of Chest Physicians; American Thoracic Society, Inc.; and the Pulmonary Hypertension Association. J Am Coll Cardiol 53:1573, 2009.
12. Consensus statement on the management of pulmonary hypertension in clinical practice in the UK and Ireland. Thorax 63(Suppl 2):ii1, 2008.
13. Beghetti M, Galie N: Eisenmenger syndrome a clinical perspective in a new therapeutic era of pulmonary arterial hypertension. J Am Coll Cardiol 53:733, 2009.
14. Trulock EP, Christie JD, Edwards LB, et al: Registry of the International Society for Heart and Lung Transplantation: Twenty-fourth official adult lung and heart-lung transplantation report—2007. J Heart Lung Transplant 26:782, 2007.
15. Galie N, Beghetti M, Gatzoulis MA, et al: Bosentan therapy in patients with Eisenmenger syndrome: A multicenter, double-blind, randomized, placebo-controlled study. Circulation 114:48, 2006.
16. Christensen DD, McConnell ME, Book WM, Mahle WT: Initial experience with bosentan therapy in patients with the Eisenmenger syndrome. Am J Cardiol 94:261, 2004.
17. Duffels MG, Vis JC, van Loon RL, et al: Effect of bosentan on exercise capacity and quality of life in adults with pulmonary arterial hypertension associated with congenital heart disease with and without Down's syndrome. Am J Cardiol 103:1309, 2009.
18. Galie N, Ghofrani HA, Torbicki A, et al: Sildenafil citrate therapy for pulmonary arterial hypertension. N Engl J Med 353:2148, 2005.
19. Singh TP, Rohit M, Grover A, et al: A randomized, placebo-controlled, double-blind, crossover study to evaluate the efficacy of oral sildenafil therapy in severe pulmonary artery hypertension. Am Heart J 151:851.e1, 2006.
20. Garg N, Sharma MK, Sinha N: Role of oral sildenafil in severe pulmonary arterial hypertension: Clinical efficacy and dose response relationship. Int J Cardiol 120:306, 2007.
21. Chau EM, Fan KY, Chow WH: Effects of chronic sildenafil in patients with Eisenmenger syndrome versus idiopathic pulmonary arterial hypertension. Int J Cardiol 120:301, 2007.
22. Wort SJ: Sildenafil in Eisenmenger syndrome: Safety first. Int J Cardiol 120:314, 2007.

Infective Endocarditis

23. Wilson W, Taubert KA, Gewitz M, et al: Prevention of infective endocarditis: Guidelines from the American Heart Association: A guideline from the American Heart Association Rheumatic Fever, Endocarditis and Kawasaki Disease Committee, Council on Cardiovascular Disease in the Young, and the Council on Clinical Cardiology, Council on Cardiovascular Surgery and Anesthesia, and the Quality of Care and Outcomes Research Interdisciplinary Working Group. J Am Dent Assoc 139(Suppl):3S, 2008.
24. Gould FK, Elliott TS, Foweraker J, et al: Guidelines for the prevention of endocarditis: Report of the Working Party of the British Society for Antimicrobial Chemotherapy. J Antimicrob Chemother 57:1035, 2006.

Evaluation of the Patient with Congenital Heart Disease

25. Makikallio K, McElhinney DB, Levine JC, et al: Fetal aortic valve stenosis and the evolution of hypoplastic left heart syndrome: Patient selection for fetal intervention. Circulation 113:1401, 2006.
26. Barrea C, Levasseur S, Roman K, et al: Three-dimensional echocardiography improves the understanding of left atrioventricular valve morphology and function in atrioventricular septal defects undergoing patch augmentation. J Thorac Cardiovasc Surg 129:746, 2005.
27. Sawada SG, Thomaides A: Three-dimensional stress echocardiography: The promise and limitations of volumetric imaging. Curr Opin Cardiol 24:426, 2009.
28. van den Bosch AE, Robbers-Visser D, Krenning BJ, et al: Real-time transthoracic three-dimensional echocardiographic assessment of left ventricular volume and ejection fraction in congenital heart disease. J Am Soc Echocardiogr 19:1, 2006.
29. Awad SM, Cao QL, Hijazi ZM: Intracardiac echocardiography for the guidance of percutaneous procedures. Curr Cardiol Rep 11:210, 2009.
30. Suematsu Y, Kiaii B, Bainbridge DT, et al: Robotic-assisted closure of atrial septal defect under real-time three-dimensional echo guide: In vitro study. Eur J Cardiothorac Surg 32:573, 2007.
31. Stephens DN, O'Donnell M, Thomenius K, et al: Experimental studies with a 9F forward-looking intracardiac imaging and ablation catheter. J Ultrasound Med 28:207, 2009.
32. Roberts KE, McElroy JJ, Wong WP, et al: BMPR2 mutations in pulmonary arterial hypertension with congenital heart disease. Eur Respir J 24:371, 2004.
33. Boccalandro F, Baptista E, Muench A, et al: Comparison of intracardiac echocardiography versus transesophageal echocardiography guidance for percutaneous transcatheter closure of atrial septal defect. Am J Cardiol 93:437, 2004.
34. Krumsdorf U, Ostermayer S, Billinger K, et al: Incidence and clinical course of thrombus formation on atrial septal defect and patient foramen ovale closure devices in 1,000 consecutive patients. J Am Coll Cardiol 43:302, 2004.
35. Masura J, Gavora P, Podnar T: Long-term outcome of transcatheter secundum-type atrial septal defect closure using Amplatzer septal occluders. J Am Coll Cardiol 45:505, 2005.
36. Cheung YF, Lun KS, Chau AK: Doppler tissue imaging analysis of ventricular function after surgical and transcatheter closure of atrial septal defect. Am J Cardiol 93:375, 2004.
37. Butera G, Carminati M, Chessa M, et al: Percutaneous versus surgical closure of secundum atrial septal defect: Comparison of early results and complications. Am Heart J 151:228, 2006.
38. Silversides CK, Siu SC, McLaughlin PR, et al: Symptomatic atrial arrhythmias and transcatheter closure of atrial septal defects in adult patients. Heart 90:1194, 2004.
39. Cramer SC, Rordorf G, Maki JH, et al: Increased pelvic vein thrombi in cryptogenic stroke: Results of the Paradoxical Emboli from Large Veins in Ischemic Stroke (PELVIS) study. Stroke 35:46, 2004.
40. Beda RD, Gill EA Jr: Patent foramen ovale: Does it play a role in the pathophysiology of migraine headache? Cardiol Clin 23:91, 2005.
41. Windecker S, Wahl A, Nedeltchev K, et al: Comparison of medical treatment with percutaneous closure of patent foramen ovale in patients with cryptogenic stroke. J Am Coll Cardiol 44:750, 2004.
42. Schuchlenz HW, Weihs W, Berghold A, et al: Secondary prevention after cryptogenic cerebrovascular events in patients with patent foramen ovale. Int J Cardiol 101:77, 2005.
43. Wohrle J: Closure of patent foramen ovale after cryptogenic stroke. Lancet 368:350, 2006.
44. Ten Harkel AD, Cromme-Dijkhuis AH, Heinerman BC, et al: Development of left atrioventricular valve regurgitation after correction of atrioventricular septal defect. Ann Thorac Surg 79:607, 2005.
45. Murashita T, Kubota T, Oba J, et al: Left atrioventricular valve regurgitation after repair of incomplete atrioventricular septal defect. Ann Thorac Surg 77:2157, 2004.
46. Masuda M, Kado H, Tanoue Y, et al: Does Down syndrome affect the long-term results of complete atrioventricular septal defect when the defect is repaired during the first year of life? Eur J Cardiothorac Surg 27:405, 2005.
47. Frid C, Bjorkhem G, Jonzon A, et al: Long-term survival in children with atrioventricular septal defect and common atrioventricular valvar orifice in Sweden. Cardiol Young 14:24, 2004.
48. Roos-Hesselink JW, Meijboom FJ, Spitaels SE, et al: Outcome of patients after surgical closure of ventricular septal defect at young age: Longitudinal follow-up of 22-34 years. Eur Heart J 25:1057, 2004.
49. Thanopoulos BD, Rigby ML: Outcome of transcatheter closure of muscular ventricular septal defects with the Amplatzer ventricular septal defect occluder. Heart 91:513, 2005.
50. Carminati M, Butera G, Chessa M, et al: Transcatheter closure of congenital ventricular septal defect with Amplatzer septal occluders. Am J Cardiol 96:52L, 2005.
51. Sadiq M, Latif F, Ur-Rehman A: Analysis of infective endarteritis in patent ductus arteriosus. Am J Cardiol 93:513, 2004.
52. Moore JW, Levi DS, Moore SD, et al: Interventional treatment of patent ductus arteriosus in 2004. Catheter Cardiovasc Interv 64:91, 2005.

Cyanotic Heart Disease

53. Oosterhof T, van Straten A, Vliegen HW, et al: Preoperative thresholds for pulmonary valve replacement in patients with corrected tetralogy of Fallot using cardiovascular magnetic resonance. Circulation 116:545, 2007.
54. Knauth AL, Gauvreau K, Powell AJ, et al: Ventricular size and function assessed by cardiac MRI predict major adverse clinical outcomes late after tetralogy of Fallot repair. Heart 94:211, 2008.
55. Yetman AT, Graham T: The dilated aorta in patients with congenital cardiac defects. J Am Coll Cardiol 53:461, 2009.
56. Lurz P, Coats L, Khambadkone S, et al: Percutaneous pulmonary valve implantation: Impact of evolving technology and learning curve on clinical outcome. Circulation 117:1964, 2008.
57. Lurz P, Bonhoeffer P, Taylor AM: Percutaneous pulmonary valve implantation: An update. Expert Rev Cardiovasc Ther 7:823, 2009.
58. Khambadkone S, Bonhoeffer P: Percutaneous pulmonary valve implantation. Semin Thorac Cardiovasc Surg Pediatr Card Surg Annu 23, 2006.
59. Wong T, Davlouros PA, Li W, et al: Mechano-electrical interaction late after Fontan operation: Relation between P-wave duration and dispersion, right atrial size, and atrial arrhythmias. Circulation 109:2319, 2004.
60. Rychik J: Protein-losing enteropathy after Fontan operation. Congenit Heart Dis 2:288, 2007.
61. Kiesewetter CH, Sheron N, Vettukattill JJ, et al: Hepatic changes in the failing Fontan circulation. Heart 93:579, 2007.
62. Rodriguez-Roisin R, Krowka MJ: Hepatopulmonary syndrome—a liver-induced lung vascular disorder. N Engl J Med 358:2378, 2008.
63. Mavroudis C, Backer CL, Deal BJ: Late reoperations for Fontan patients: State of the art invited review. Eur J Cardiothorac Surg 34:1034, 2008.
64. Prandstetter C, Hofer A, Lechner E, et al: Early and mid-term outcome of the arterial switch operation in 114 consecutive patients: A single centre experience. Clin Res Cardiol 96:723, 2007.
65. Bove T, De Meulder F, Vandenplas G, et al: Midterm assessment of the reconstructed arteries after the arterial switch operation. Ann Thorac Surg 85:823, 2008.
66. Lange R, Cleuziou J, Horer J, et al: Risk factors for aortic insufficiency and aortic valve replacement after the arterial switch operation. Eur J Cardiothorac Surg 34:711, 2008.
67. Horer J, Schreiber C, Dworak E, et al: Long-term results after the Rastelli repair for transposition of the great arteries. Ann Thorac Surg 83:2169, 2007.
68. Benzaquen BS, Webb GD, Colman JM, Therrien J: Arterial switch operation after Mustard procedures in adult patients with transposition of the great arteries: Is it time to revise our strategy? Am Heart J 147:E8, 2004.
69. Khairy P, Landzberg MJ, Gatzoulis MA, et al: Transvenous pacing leads and systemic thromboemboli in patients with intracardiac shunts: A multicenter study. Circulation 113:2391, 2006.
70. Dore A, Houde C, Chan KL, et al: Angiotensin receptor blockade and exercise capacity in adults with systemic right ventricles: A multicenter, randomized, placebo-controlled clinical trial. Circulation 112:2411, 2005.

71. Therrien J, Provost Y, Harrison J, et al: Effect of angiotensin receptor blockade on systemic right ventricular function and size: A small, randomized, placebo-controlled study. Int J Cardiol 129:187, 2008.
72. Doughan AR, McConnell ME, Book WM: Effect of beta blockers (carvedilol or metoprolol XL) in patients with transposition of great arteries and dysfunction of the systemic right ventricle. Am J Cardiol 99:704, 2007.
73. Josephson CB, Howlett JG, Jackson SD, et al: A case series of systemic right ventricular dysfunction post atrial switch for simple D-transposition of the great arteries: The impact of beta-blockade. Can J Cardiol 22:769, 2006.
74. Guedes A, Mercier LA, Leduc L, et al: Impact of pregnancy on the systemic right ventricle after a Mustard operation for transposition of the great arteries. J Am Coll Cardiol 44:433, 2004.
75. Quinn DW, McGuirk SP, Metha C, et al: The morphologic left ventricle that requires training by means of pulmonary artery banding before the double-switch procedure for congenitally corrected transposition of the great arteries is at risk of late dysfunction. J Thorac Cardiovasc Surg 135:1137, 2008.
76. Brown ML, Dearani JA, Danielson GK, et al: Comparison of the outcome of porcine bioprosthetic versus mechanical prosthetic replacement of the tricuspid valve in the Ebstein anomaly. Am J Cardiol 103:555, 2009.
77. Quinonez LG, Dearani JA, Puga FJ, et al: Results of the 1.5-ventricle repair for Ebstein anomaly and the failing right ventricle. J Thorac Cardiovasc Surg 133:1303, 2007.
78. Dearani JA, Danielson GK: Surgical management of Ebstein's anomaly in the adult. Semin Thorac Cardiovasc Surg 17:148, 2005.
79. Khositseth A, Danielson GK, Dearani JA, et al: Supraventricular tachyarrhythmias in Ebstein anomaly: Management and outcome. J Thorac Cardiovasc Surg 128:826, 2004.
80. Brown ML, Dearani JA, Danielson GK, et al: Functional status after operation for Ebstein anomaly: The Mayo Clinic experience. J Am Coll Cardiol 52:460, 2008.

Valvular and Vascular Conditions

81. Fiore AC, Fischer LK, Schwartz T, et al: Comparison of angioplasty and surgery for neonatal aortic coarctation. Ann Thorac Surg 80:1659, 2005.
82. Karamlou T, Bernasconi A, Jaeggi E, et al: Factors associated with arch reintervention and growth of the aortic arch after coarctation repair in neonates weighing less than 2.5 kg. J Thorac Cardiovasc Surg 137:1163, 2009.
83. Wong D, Benson LN, Van Arsdell GS, et al: Balloon angioplasty is preferred to surgery for aortic coarctation. Cardiol Young 18:79, 2008.
84. Ou P, Celermajer DS, Raisky O, et al: Angular (Gothic) aortic arch leads to enhanced systolic wave reflection, central aortic stiffness, and increased left ventricular mass late after aortic coarctation repair: Evaluation with magnetic resonance flow mapping. J Thorac Cardiovasc Surg 135:62, 2008.
85. Fawzy ME, Fathala A, Osman A, et al: Twenty-two years of follow-up results of balloon angioplasty for discreet native coarctation of the aorta in adolescents and adults. Am Heart J 156:910, 2008.
86. Oliver JM, Gallego P, Gonzalez A, et al: Risk factors for aortic complications in adults with coarctation of the aorta. J Am Coll Cardiol 44:1641, 2004.
87. Hager A, Kanz S, Kaemmerer H, et al: Coarctation Long-term Assessment (COALA): Significance of arterial hypertension in a cohort of 404 patients up to 27 years after surgical repair of isolated coarctation of the aorta, even in the absence of restenosis and prosthetic material. J Thorac Cardiovasc Surg 134:738, 2007.
88. Pacini D, Bergonzini M, Loforte A, et al: Aneurysms after coarctation repair associated with hypoplastic aortic arch: Surgical management through median sternotomy. Ann Thorac Surg 81:758, 2006.
89. Tzifa A, Ewert P, Brzezinska-Rajszys G, et al: Covered Cheatham-platinum stents for aortic coarctation: Early and intermediate-term results. J Am Coll Cardiol 47:1457, 2006.
90. Suzuki T, Ohye RG, Devaney EJ, et al: Selective management of the left ventricular outflow tract for repair of interrupted aortic arch with ventricular septal defect: Management of left ventricular outflow tract obstruction. J Thorac Cardiovasc Surg 131:779, 2006.
91. Chiu PP, Rusan M, Williams WG, et al: Long-term outcomes of clinically significant vascular rings associated with congenital tracheal stenosis. J Pediatr Surg 41:335, 2006.
92. Hickey EJ, Caldarone CA, Blackstone EH, et al: Critical left ventricular outflow tract obstruction: The disproportionate impact of biventricular repair in borderline cases. J Thorac Cardiovasc Surg 134:1429, 2007.
93. Dodge-Khatami A, Schmid M, Rousson V, et al: Risk factors for reoperation after relief of congenital subaortic stenosis. Eur J Cardiothorac Surg 33:885, 2008.
94. Hickey EJ, Jung G, Williams WG, et al: Congenital supravalvular aortic stenosis: Defining surgical and nonsurgical outcomes. Ann Thorac Surg 86:1919, 2008.
95. Scott DJ, Campbell DN, Clarke DR, et al: Twenty-year surgical experience with congenital supravalvar aortic stenosis. Ann Thorac Surg 87:1501, 2009.
96. Schaverien MV, Freedom RM, McCrindle BW: Independent factors associated with outcomes of parachute mitral valve in 84 patients. Circulation 109:2309, 2004.
97. McElhinney DB, Sherwood MC, Keane JF, et al: Current management of severe congenital mitral stenosis: Outcomes of transcatheter and surgical therapy in 108 infants and children. Circulation 112:707, 2005.
98. Macnab A, Jenkins NP, Ewington I, et al: A method for the morphological analysis of the regurgitant mitral valve using three dimensional echocardiography. Heart 90:771, 2004.
99. Oppido G, Davies B, McMullan DM, et al: Surgical treatment of congenital mitral valve disease: Midterm results of a repair-oriented policy. J Thorac Cardiovasc Surg 135:1313, 2008.
100. Chauvaud S: Congenital mitral valve surgery: Techniques and results. Curr Opin Cardiol 21:95, 2006.
101. Silvilairat S, Cabalka AK, Cetta F, et al: Echocardiographic assessment of isolated pulmonary valve stenosis: Which outpatient Doppler gradient has the most clinical validity? J Am Soc Echocardiogr 18:1137, 2005.
102. Karagoz T, Asoh K, Hickey E, et al: Balloon dilation of pulmonary valve stenosis in infants less than 3 kg: A 20-year experience. Catheter Cardiovasc Interv 74:753, 2009.
103. Earing MG, Connolly HM, Dearani JA, et al: Long-term follow-up of patients after surgical treatment for isolated pulmonary valve stenosis. Mayo Clin Proc 80:871, 2005.

CHAPTER 66 Valvular Heart Disease

Catherine M. Otto and Robert O. Bonow

Valvular heart disease accounts for 10% to 20% of all cardiac surgical procedures in the United States. The primary causes of valve disease are age-associated calcific valve changes and inherited or congenital conditions (e.g., a bicuspid aortic valve or myxomatous mitral valve disease). The prevalence of rheumatic valve disease now is very low in the United States and Europe because of primary prevention of rheumatic fever, although rheumatic valve disease remains prevalent in the developing world (see Chap. 88). About two thirds of all heart valve operations are for aortic valve replacement (AVR), most often for aortic stenosis (AS). Mitral valve surgery is most often performed for mitral regurgitation (MR) because most patients with mitral stenosis (MS) are treated by a percutaneous approach.[1,2] In addition to patients with severe valve disease that eventually requires mechanical intervention, there is a larger group of patients with mild to moderate disease who need accurate diagnosis and appropriate medical management.

Aortic Valve Disease

Aortic Stenosis

CAUSES AND PATHOLOGY. Obstruction to left ventricular (LV) outflow is localized most commonly at the aortic valve and is discussed in this section. However, obstruction may also occur above the valve (supravalvular stenosis) or below the valve (discrete subvalvular stenosis; see Chap. 65), or it may be caused by hypertrophic cardiomyopathy (HCM; see Chap. 69). Valvular AS has three principal causes—a congenital bicuspid valve with superimposed calcification, calcification of a normal trileaflet valve, and rheumatic disease (**Fig. 66-1**). In a U.S. series of 933 patients undergoing AVR for AS, a bicuspid valve was present in more than 50% including two thirds of those younger than 70 years and 40% of those older than 70 years.[3]

In addition, AS may be caused by a congenital valve stenosis presenting in infancy or childhood. Rarely, AS is caused by severe atherosclerosis of the aorta and aortic valve; this form of AS occurs most frequently in patients with severe hypercholesterolemia and is observed in children with homozygous type II hyperlipoproteinemia. Rheumatoid involvement of the valve is a rare cause of AS and results in nodular thickening of the valve leaflets and involvement of the proximal portion of the aorta. Ochronosis with alkaptonuria is another rare cause of AS.

Congenital Aortic Valve Disease

Congenital malformations of the aortic valve may be unicuspid, bicuspid, or tricuspid, or there may be a dome-shaped diaphragm (see Chap. 65). Unicuspid valves produce severe obstruction in infancy and are the most frequent malformations found in fatal valvular AS in children younger than 1 year. Congenitally bicuspid valves may be stenotic with commissural fusion at birth, but more often they are not responsible for serious narrowing of the aortic orifice during childhood.[4-6] A subset of patients with a bicuspid aortic valve develops significant aortic regurgitation (AR) requiring valve surgery in young adulthood. However, most patients have normal valve function until late in life, when superimposed calcific changes result in valve obstruction (see later, "Bicuspid Aortic Valve Disease").

Calcific Aortic Valve Disease

Age-related calcific (formerly termed *senile* or *degenerative*) AS of a congenital bicuspid or normal trileaflet valve is now the most common cause of AS in adults. In a population-based echocardiographic study, 2% of persons 65 years of age or older had frank calcific AS (see Chap. 80), whereas 29% exhibited age-related aortic valve sclerosis without stenosis, defined by Otto and colleagues[7,7a] as irregular thickening of the aortic valve leaflets detected by echocardiography without significant obstruction. Aortic sclerosis is the initial stage of calcific valve disease and, even in the absence of valve obstruction, is associated with a 50% increased risk of cardiovascular death and myocardial infarction.[8-10]

Although once considered to represent the result of years of normal mechanical stress on an otherwise normal valve, the evolving concept is that the disease process represents proliferative and inflammatory changes, with lipid accumulation, upregulation of angiotensin-converting enzyme (ACE) activity, increased oxidative stress, and infiltration of macrophages and T lymphocytes (**Fig. 66-2**),[11-15] ultimately leading to bone formation[16] in a manner similar, but not identical, to vascular calcification. Progressive calcification, initially along the flexion lines at their bases, leads to immobilization of the cusps. A high prevalence of calcific AS also exists in patients with Paget disease of bone and end-stage renal disease.

Age-related calcific AS shares common risk factors with mitral annular calcification, and the two conditions often coexist. Genetic polymorphisms have been linked to the presence of calcific AS, including the vitamin D receptor, interleukin-10 alleles, and the apolipoprotein E4 allele. Familial clustering of calcific AS also has been described, suggesting a possible genetic predisposition to valve calcification.[17-19] The risk factors for the development of calcific AS are similar to those for vascular atherosclerosis—elevated serum levels of low-density lipoprotein (LDL) cholesterol and lipoprotein(a) [Lp(a)], diabetes, smoking, and hypertension.[7,7a,10,20] Calcific AS has also been linked to inflammatory markers and components of the metabolic syndrome.[21,22] Retrospective studies have linked treatment with 3-hydroxy-3-methylglutaryl-coenzyme A (HMG-CoA) reductase (statin) medications with a lower rate of progression of calcific AS, and this effect has been demonstrated in animal models of hypercholesterolemia.[14,23] Hence there is growing consensus that "degenerative" calcific AS

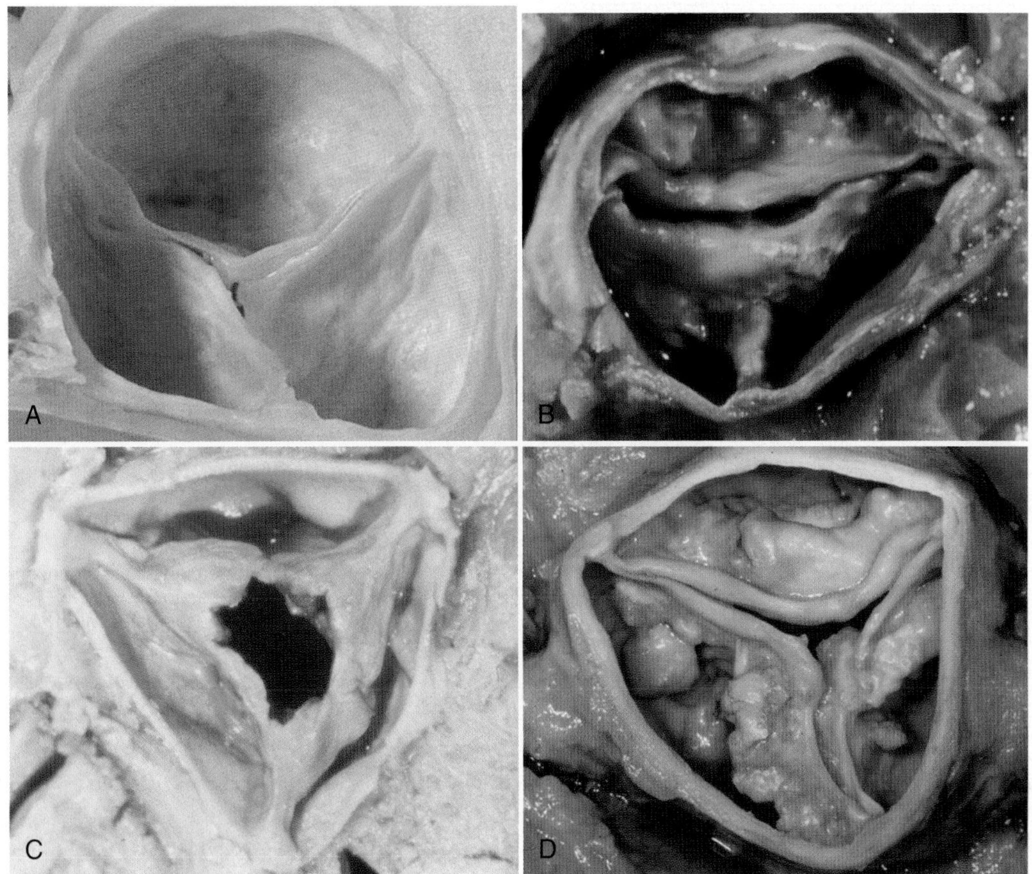

FIGURE 66-1 Major types of aortic valve stenosis. **A,** Normal aortic valve. **B,** Congenital bicuspid aortic stenosis. A false raphe is present at 6 o'clock. **C,** Rheumatic aortic stenosis. The commissures are fused with a fixed central orifice. **D,** Calcific degenerative aortic stenosis. *(**A,** From Manabe H, Yutani C [eds]: Atlas of Valvular Heart Disease. Singapore, Churchill Livingstone, 1998, pp 6, 131;* ***B, C, D,*** *Courtesy of Dr. William C. Roberts, Baylor University Medical Center, Dallas, Tex.)*

shares many pathophysiologic features with atherosclerosis and that specific pathways might be targeted to prevent or retard disease progression.[11,16,24]

However, no benefit was seen in a small prospective randomized trial of atorvastatin versus placebo, despite a significant lowering of serum LDL levels, in patients with relatively advanced calcific AS,[25] and a subsequent prospective study in patients with less severe AS demonstrated only a slight reduction in the rate of progression of AS with rosuvastatin.[26] The Simvastatin and Ezetimibe for Aortic Stenosis (SEAS) Trial[27] and the Aortic Stenosis Progression Observation: Measuring Effects of Rosuvastatin (ASTRONOMER) Trial[28] randomized 1800 and 269 adults, respectively, with mild to moderate AS to intensive lipid-lowering therapy versus placebo. These studies convincingly showed no improvement in mortality, time to valve replacement, or rate of AS progression in the treatment versus placebo groups. Current interest is focused on other disease pathways in calcific valve disease that may be amenable to medical therapy.[16,29]

Rheumatic Aortic Stenosis

Rheumatic AS results from adhesions and fusions of the commissures and cusps and vascularization of the leaflets of the valve ring, leading to retraction and stiffening of the free borders of the cusps. Calcific nodules develop on both surfaces, and the orifice is reduced to a small round or triangular opening (see Fig. 66-1C). As a consequence, the rheumatic valve is often regurgitant, as well as stenotic. Patients with rheumatic AS invariability have rheumatic involvement of the mitral valve (see Chap. 88). With the decline in rheumatic fever in developed nations, rheumatic AS is decreasing in frequency, although it continues to be a major problem on a worldwide basis.

PATHOPHYSIOLOGY. In adults with AS, outflow obstruction usually develops and increases gradually over a prolonged period (**Fig. 66-3**). In infants and children with congenital AS, the valve orifice shows little change as the child grows, thereby intensifying the relative obstruction gradually. LV function can be well maintained in experimentally produced, gradually developing subcoronary AS in animals. In the experimental model, as well as in children and adults with chronic severe AS, LV output is maintained by the presence of LV hypertrophy, which may sustain a large pressure gradient across the aortic valve for many years without a reduction in cardiac output, LV dilation, or development of symptoms.

Severe obstruction to LV outflow is usually characterized by the following: (1) an aortic jet velocity greater than 4 m/sec; (2) a mean systolic pressure gradient exceeding 40 mm Hg in the presence of a normal cardiac output; or (3) an effective aortic orifice (calculated by the continuity equation; see Chap. 15) less than approximately 1.0 cm^2 in an average-sized adult (i.e., $<0.6\ cm^2/m^2$ of body surface area, approximately 25% of the normal aortic orifice of 3.0 to 4.0 cm^2). An aortic valve orifice of 1.0 to 1.5 cm^2 is considered moderate stenosis, and an orifice of 1.5 to 2.0 cm^2 is referred to as mild stenosis[1,30,30a] (**Table 66-1**). However, the degree of stenosis associated with symptom onset varies among patients, and there is no single number that defines severe or critical AS in an individual patient. Clinical decisions are based on consideration of symptom status and the LV response to chronic pressure overload, in conjunction with hemodynamic severity. In some cases, additional measures of hemodynamic severity, such as stroke work loss or valvular impedance, or evaluation with changing loading conditions (e.g., dobutamine stress) or with exercise, are necessary to evaluate disease severity fully.[31-33a]

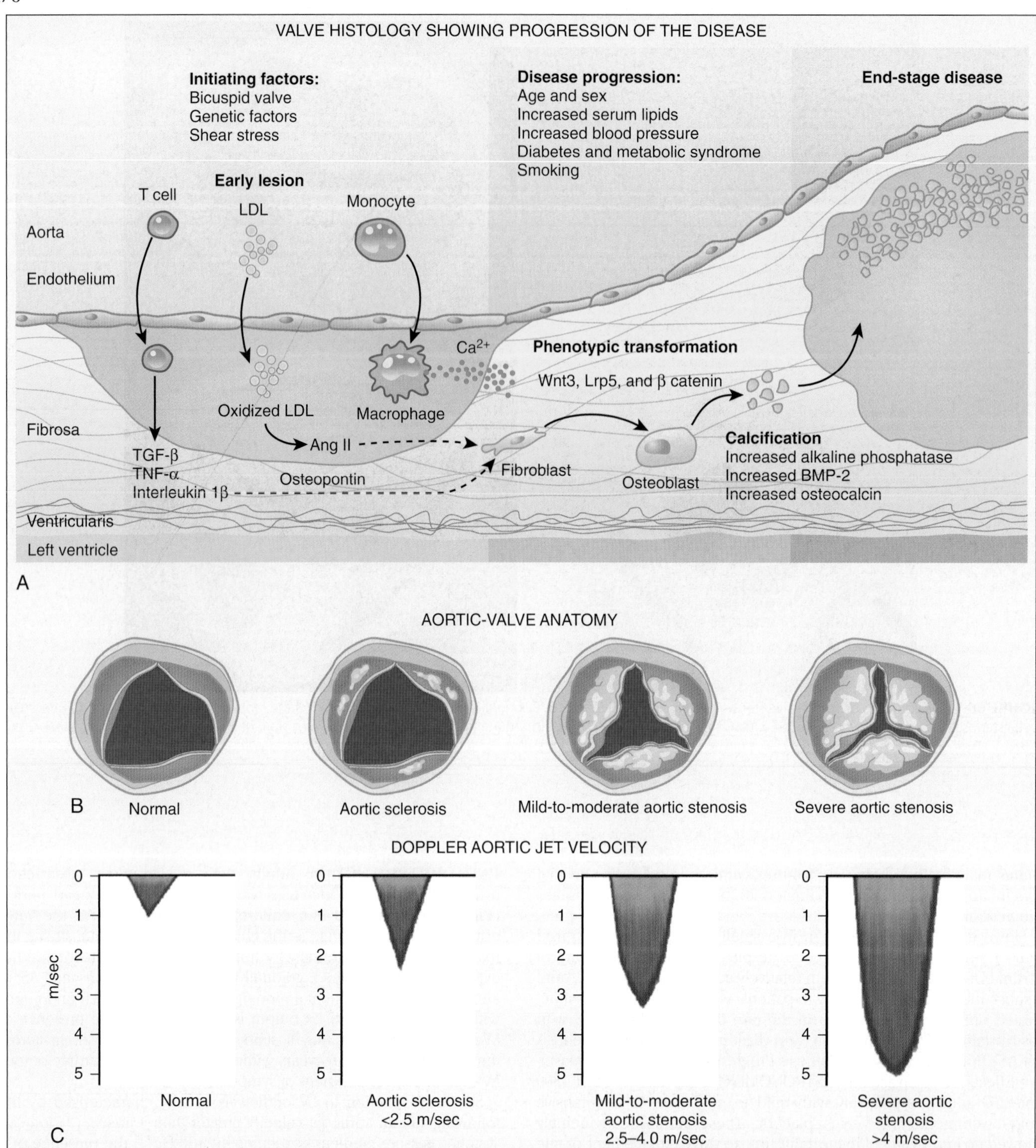

FIGURE 66-2 Disease progression in calcific aortic stenosis, showing changes in aortic valve histologic features, leaflet opening in systole, and Doppler velocities. **A,** The histology of the early lesion is characterized by a subendothelial accumulation of oxidized LDL, production of angiotensin (Ang) II, and inflammation with T lymphocytes and macrophages. Disease progression occurs by several mechanisms, including local production of proteins, such as osteopontin, osteocalcin, and bone morphogenic protein 2 (BMP-2), which mediate tissue calcification; activation of inflammatory signaling pathways, including tumor necrosis factor (TNF), tumor growth factor-β (TGF-β), the complement system, C-reactive protein, and interleukin-1β; and changes in tissue matrix, including the accumulation of tenascin C, and upregulation of matrix metalloproteinase 2 and alkaline phosphatase activity. In addition, leaflet fibroblasts undergo phenotypic transformation into osteoblasts, regulated by the Wnt3-Lrp5-β catenin signaling pathway. Microscopic accumulations of extracellular calcification (Ca^{2+}) are present early in the disease process, with progressive calcification as the disease progresses and areas of frank bone formation in end-stage disease. **B,** The corresponding changes in aortic valve anatomy are viewed from the aortic side with the valve open in systole. **C,** Corresponding changes in Doppler aortic jet velocity. *(From Otto CM: Calcific aortic stenosis—time to look more closely at the valve. N Engl J Med 359:1395, 2008.)*

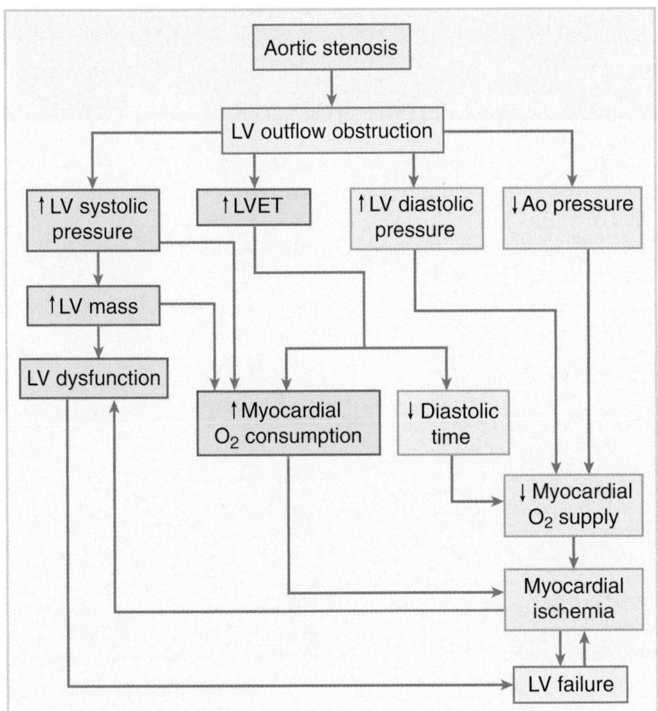

FIGURE 66-3 Pathophysiology of aortic stenosis. LV outflow obstruction results in an increased LV systolic pressure, increased LV ejection time (LVET), increased LV diastolic pressure, and decreased aortic (Ao) pressure. Increased LV systolic pressure with LV volume overload increases LV mass, which may lead to LV dysfunction and failure. Increased LV systolic pressure, LV mass, and LVET increase myocardial oxygen (O_2) consumption. Increased LVET results in a decrease of diastolic time (myocardial perfusion time). Increased LV diastolic pressure and decreased Ao diastolic pressure decrease coronary perfusion pressure. Decreased diastolic time and coronary perfusion pressure decrease myocardial O_2 supply. Increased myocardial O_2 consumption and decreased myocardial O_2 supply produce myocardial ischemia, which further deteriorates LV function. *(From Boudoulas H, Gravanis MB: Valvular heart disease.* In *Gravanis MB [ed]: Cardiovascular Disorders: Pathogenesis and Pathophysiology. St. Louis, CV Mosby, 1993, p 64.)*

Chronic pressure overload typically results in concentric LV hypertrophy, with increased wall thickness and a normal chamber size. The increased wall thickness allows normalization of wall stress (afterload) so that LV contractile function is maintained. However, the increased myocardial cell mass and increased interstitial fibrosis result in diastolic dysfunction, which may persist even after relief of AS. Gender differences in the LV response to AS have been reported, with women more frequently exhibiting normal LV performance and a smaller, thicker walled, concentrically hypertrophied left ventricle with diastolic dysfunction (see later) and normal or even subnormal systolic wall stress. Men more frequently have eccentric LV hypertrophy, excessive systolic wall stress, systolic dysfunction, and chamber dilation.

The LV changes caused by chronic pressure overload are reflected in the LV and left atrial pressure waveforms and Doppler velocity curves. As contraction of the left ventricle becomes progressively more isometric, the LV pressure pulse exhibits a rounded, rather than flattened, summit and the Doppler velocity curve exhibits a progressively later systolic peak. The elevated LV end-diastolic pressure and the corresponding Doppler changes in LV filling, which are characteristic of severe AS, reflect delayed relaxation and eventually decreased compliance of the hypertrophied LV wall. In patients with severe AS, large *a* waves usually appear in the left atrial pressure pulse and Doppler LV filling curve because of the combination of enhanced contraction of a hypertrophied left atrium and diminished LV compliance. Atrial contraction plays a particularly important role in filling of the left ventricle in AS. It raises LV end-diastolic pressure without causing a concomitant elevation of mean left atrial pressure. This "booster pump" function of the left atrium prevents the pulmonary venous and capillary pressures from rising to levels that would produce pulmonary congestion, whereas at the same time maintaining LV end-diastolic pressure at the elevated level necessary for effective contraction of the hypertrophied left ventricle. These changes in diastolic function are reflected in the Doppler parameter of LV filling and noninvasive measures of diastolic function, such as strain and strain rate (see Chap. 15). Loss of appropriately timed, vigorous atrial contraction, as occurs in atrial fibrillation (AF) or atrioventricular dissociation, may result in rapid clinical deterioration in patients with severe AS.

Systemic vascular resistance also contributes to total LV afterload in adults with AS. Concurrent hypertension increases total LV load and may affect the evaluation of AS severity.[34] Mild pulmonary hypertension is present is about one third of adults with AS because of the chronic elevation of LV end-diastolic pressure; more severe pulmonary hypertension is seen in about 15% of AS patients.

Exercise physiology is abnormal in adults with moderate to severe AS, and even asymptomatic patients have a reduced exercise tolerance. Although cardiac output at rest is within normal limits, the normal increase in cardiac output with exercise is blunted and is mediated primarily by increased heart rate, with little change in stroke volume. Even though stroke volume is unchanged, transvalvular flow rate increases because of the shortened systolic ejection period so that aortic jet velocity and transvalvular gradient increase proportionally. Prior to symptom onset, valve area increases slightly with exercise (by 0.2 cm^2 on average) but as AS becomes more severe and symptoms are imminent, valve area becomes fixed, resulting in an even greater rise in jet velocity and pressure gradient with exercise. At this point, there is an abnormal blood pressure response to exercise (rise in systolic blood pressure < 10 mm Hg), signifying severe valve obstruction.

Myocardial Function in Aortic Stenosis. When the aorta is suddenly constricted in experimental animals, LV pressure rises, wall stress increases significantly, and both the extent and velocity of shortening decline. As noted in Chap. 24, the development of LV hypertrophy is one of the principal mechanisms whereby the heart adapts to such an increased hemodynamic burden. The increased systolic wall stress induced by AS leads to parallel replication of sarcomeres and concentric hypertrophy. The increase in LV wall thickness is often sufficient to counterbalance the increased pressure so that peak systolic wall tension returns to normal, or remains normal, if the obstruction develops slowly. An inverse correlation between wall stress and ejection fraction has been described in patients with AS. This suggests that the depressed ejection fraction and velocity of fiber shortening that occur in some patients are a consequence of inadequate wall thickening, resulting in afterload mismatch. In others, the lower ejection fraction is secondary to a true depression of contractility; in this group, surgical treatment is less effective. Thus, both increased afterload and altered contractility are operative to varying extents in depressing LV performance. To evaluate myocardial function in patients with AS, ejection phase indices, such as ejection fraction and myocardial fiber shortening, should be related to the existing wall tension.

Diastolic Properties. Although LV hypertrophy is a key adaptive mechanism to the pressure load imposed by AS, it has an adverse pathophysiologic consequence (i.e., it increases diastolic stiffness; see Chaps. 24 and 30). As a result, greater intracavitary pressure is required for LV filling. Some patients with AS manifest an increase in stiffness of the left ventricle (increased chamber stiffness) simply because of increased muscle mass with no alteration in the diastolic properties of each unit of myocardium (normal muscle stiffness); others exhibit increases in chamber and muscle stiffness. This increased stiffness, however produced, contributes to the elevation of LV diastolic filling pressure at any level of ventricular diastolic volume. Diastolic dysfunction may revert toward normal with regression of hypertrophy following surgical relief of AS, but some degree of long-term diastolic dysfunction typically persists.

Ischemia. In patients with AS, coronary blood flow at rest is elevated in absolute terms but is normal when corrections are made for myocardial mass. Reduced coronary blood flow reserve may produce inadequate myocardial oxygenation in patients with severe AS, even in the absence of coronary artery disease. The hypertrophied LV muscle mass, increased systolic pressure, and prolongation of ejection all elevate myocardial oxygen consumption. The abnormally heightened pressure

TABLE 66-1 Classification of the Severity of Valve Disease in Adults

		Severity	
VALVE DISEASE	**MILD**	**MODERATE**	**SEVERE**
Aortic Stenosis			
Jet velocity (m/sec)	<3.0	3.0-4.0	>4.0
Mean gradient (mm Hg)*	<25	25-40	>40
Valve area (cm^2)	>1.5	1.0-1.5	<1.0
Valve area index (cm^2/m^2)			<0.6
Mitral Stenosis			
Mean gradient (mm Hg)*	<5	5-10	>10
Pulmonary artery systolic pressure (mm Hg)	<30	30-50	>50
Valve area (cm^2)	>1.5	1.0-1.5	<1.0
Aortic Regurgitation			
Qualitative			
Angiographic grade	1+	2+	3-4+
Color Doppler jet width	Central jet, width < 25% of LVOT	> Mild but no signs of severe AR	Central jet, width >65% LVOT
Doppler vena contracta width (cm)	<0.3	0.3-0.6	>0.6
Quantitative (cath or echo)			
Regurgitant volume (mL/beat)	<30	30-59	≥60
Regurgitant fraction (%)	<30	30-49	≥50
Regurgitant orifice area (cm^2)	<0.10	0.10-0.29	≥0.30
Additional Essential Criteria			
Left ventricular size			Increased
Mitral Regurgitation			
Qualitative			
Angiographic grade	1+	2+	3-4+
Color Doppler jet area	Small, central jet (<4 cm^2 or <20% LA area)	Signs of MR > mild present, but no criteria for severe MR	Vena contracta width >0.7 cm with large central MR jet (area >40% of LA area) or with a wall-impinging jet of any size, swirling in LA
Doppler vena contracta width (cm)	<0.3	0.3–0.69	≥0.70
Quantitative (cath or echo)			
Regurgitant volume (mL/beat)	<30	30-59	≥60
Regurgitant fraction (%)	<30	30-49	≥50
Regurgitant orifice area (cm^2)	<0.20	0.2-0.39	≥0.40
Additional Essential Criteria			
Left atrial size			Enlarged
Left ventricular size			Enlarged
Right-Sided Valve Disease			
Severe tricuspid stenosis		Valve area <1.0 cm^2	
Severe tricuspid regurgitation		Vena contracta width >0.7 cm and systolic flow reversal in hepatic veins	
Severe pulmonic stenosis		Jet velocity >4 m/sec or maximum gradient >60 mm Hg	
Severe pulmonic regurgitation		Color jet fills outflow tract Dense continuous wave Doppler signal with a steep deceleration slope	

*Valve gradients are flow-dependent and, when used as estimates of severity of valve stenosis, should be assessed with knowledge of cardiac output or forward flow across the valve.

LA = left atrial, left atrium; LVOT = left ventricular outflow tract.

From Zoghbi WA, Enriquez-Sarano M, Foster E, et al: Recommendations for evaluation of the severity of native valvular regurgitation with two-dimensional and Doppler echocardiography. J Am Soc Echocardiogr 16:777, 2003; and from Bonow RO, Carabello BA, Chatterjee K, et al: ACC/AHA 2006 guidelines for the management of patients with valvular heart disease: A report of the American College of Cardiology/American Heart Association Task Force on Practice Guidelines (writing Committee to Revise the 1998 guidelines for the management of patients with valvular heart disease) developed in collaboration with the Society of Cardiovascular Anesthesiologists endorsed by the Society for Cardiovascular Angiography and Interventions and the Society of Thoracic Surgeons. J Am Coll Cardiol 48:e1, 2006.

compressing the coronary arteries may exceed the coronary perfusion pressure and the shortening of diastole interferes with coronary blood flow, thus leading to an imbalance between myocardial oxygen supply and demand (see Fig. 66-3). Myocardial perfusion is also impaired by the relative decrease in myocardial capillary density as myocardial mass increases and by the elevation of LV end-diastolic pressure, which lowers the aortic-LV pressure gradient in diastole (i.e., the coronary perfusion pressure gradient). This underperfusion may be responsible for the development of subendocardial ischemia, especially when oxygen demand is increased or the diastolic filling period is reduced (e.g., tachycardia, anemia, infection, pregnancy).

CLINICAL PRESENTATION

Symptoms

The cardinal manifestations of acquired AS are exertional dyspnea, angina, syncope, and ultimately heart failure.[31,35] Many patients now are diagnosed before symptom onset on the basis of the finding of a systolic murmur on physical examination, with confirmation of the diagnosis by echocardiography. Symptoms typically occur at age 50 to 70 years with bicuspid aortic valve stenosis and in those older than 70 years with calcific stenosis of a trileaflet valve, although even in this age group about 40% of AS patients have a congenital bicuspid valve.[3]

The most common clinical presentation in patients with a known diagnosis of AS who are followed prospectively is a gradual decrease in exercise tolerance, fatigue, or dyspnea on exertion. The mechanism of exertional dyspnea may be LV diastolic dysfunction, with an excessive rise in end-diastolic pressure leading to pulmonary congestion. Alternatively, exertional symptoms may be a result of the limited ability to increase cardiac output with exercise. More severe exertional dyspnea, with orthopnea, paroxysmal nocturnal dyspnea, and pulmonary edema reflects varying degrees of pulmonary venous hypertension. These are relatively late symptoms in patients with AS, and intervention now is typically undertaken before this disease stage.

Angina occurs in approximately two thirds of patients with severe AS, about 50% of whom have associated significant coronary artery obstruction. It usually resembles the angina observed in patients with coronary artery disease (see Chap. 53) in that it is commonly precipitated by exertion and relieved by rest. In patients without coronary artery disease, angina results from the combination of the increased oxygen needs of hypertrophied myocardium and reduction of oxygen delivery secondary to the excessive compression of coronary vessels. In patients with coronary artery disease, angina is caused by a combination of epicardial coronary artery obstruction and the oxygen imbalance characteristic of AS. Very rarely, angina results from calcium emboli to the coronary vascular bed.

Syncope is most commonly caused by the reduced cerebral perfusion that occurs during exertion when arterial pressure declines consequent to systemic vasodilation in the presence of a fixed cardiac output. Syncope has also been attributed to malfunction of the baroreceptor mechanism in severe AS (see Chap. 94), as well as to a vasodepressor response to a greatly elevated LV systolic pressure during exercise. Premonitory symptoms of syncope are common. Exertional hypotension may also be manifested as graying out spells or dizziness on effort. Syncope at rest may be caused by transient AF with loss of the atrial contribution to LV filling, which causes a precipitous decline in cardiac output, or to transient atrioventricular block caused by extension of the calcification of the valve into the conduction system.

Other late findings in patients with isolated AS include AF, pulmonary hypertension, and systemic venous hypertension. Although AS may be responsible for sudden death (see Chap. 41), this usually occurs in patients who had previously been symptomatic.

Gastrointestinal bleeding may develop in patients with severe AS, often associated with angiodysplasia (most commonly of the right colon) or other vascular malformations. This complication arises from shear stress–induced platelet aggregation with a reduction in high-molecular-weight multimers of von Willebrand factor and increases in proteolytic subunit fragments. These abnormalities correlate with the severity of AS and are correctable by AVR.

Infective endocarditis is a greater risk in younger patients with milder valvular deformity than in older patients with rocklike calcific aortic deformities. Cerebral emboli resulting in stroke or transient ischemic attacks may be caused by microthrombi on thickened bicuspid valves. Calcific AS may cause embolization of calcium to various organs, including the heart, kidneys, and brain.

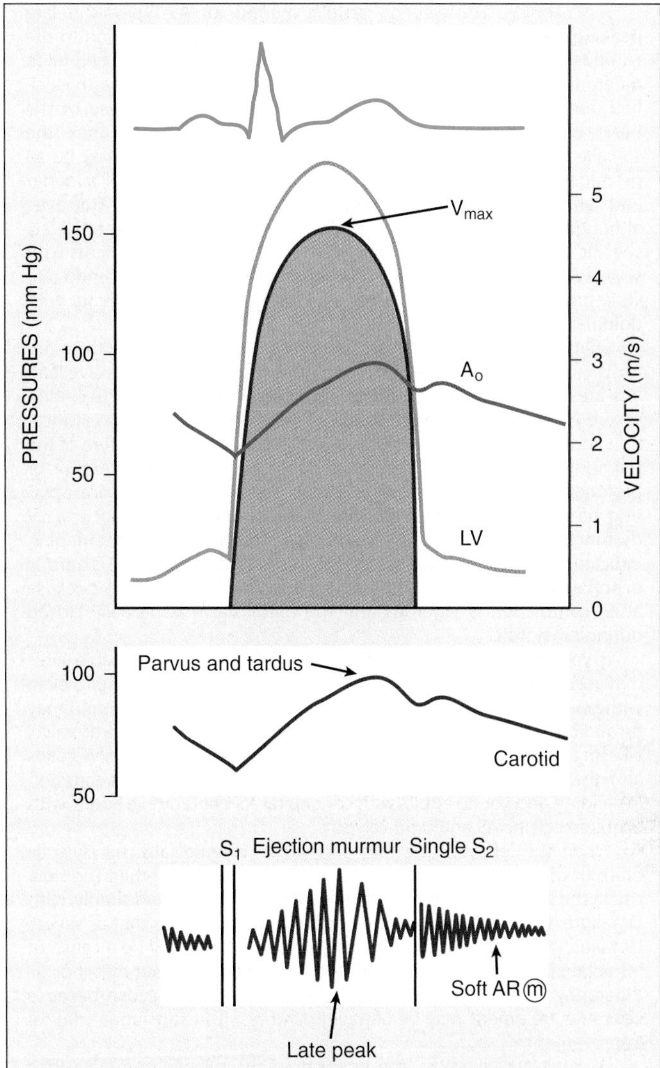

FIGURE 66-4 Relationship between LV and aortic (Ao) pressures and the Doppler aortic stenosis velocity curve (in red). The pressure difference between the left ventricle and aorta in systole is four times the velocity squared (the Bernoulli equation). Thus, a maximum velocity (V_{max}) of 4.3 m/sec corresponds to a maximum LV to Ao pressure difference of 74 mm Hg and a mean systolic gradient of 44 mm Hg. On physical examination, the slow rate of rise and delayed peak in the carotid pulse (or parvus and tardus) matches the contour of the aortic pressure waveform. The murmur corresponds to the Doppler velocity curve with a harsh crescendo-decrescendo late-peaking systolic murmur, best heard at the aortic region (upper right sternal border). Often, a soft, high-pitched diastolic decrescendo murmur of aortic regurgitation also is appreciated.

PHYSICAL EXAMINATION. The key features of the physical examination in patients with AS are palpation of the carotid upstroke, evaluation of the systolic murmur, assessment of splitting of the second heart sound, and examination for signs of heart failure (see Chap. 12).

The carotid upstroke directly reflects the arterial pressure waveform. The expected finding with severe AS is a slow-rising, late-peaking, low-amplitude carotid pulse, the parvus and tardus carotid impulse (**Fig. 66-4**). When present, this finding is specific for severe AS. However, many adults with AS have concurrent conditions, such as AR or systemic hypertension, that affect the arterial pressure curve and the carotid impulse. Thus, an apparently normal carotid impulse is not reliable for excluding the diagnosis of severe AS. Similarly, blood pressure is not a helpful method for evaluation of AS severity. When severe AS is present, systolic blood pressure and pulse pressures may be reduced. However, in patients with associated AR or in older patients with an inelastic arterial bed, systolic and pulse pressures may be normal or even increased. With severe AS, radiation of the murmur to the carotids may result in a palpable thrill or carotid shudder.

The cardiac impulse is sustained and becomes displaced inferiorly and laterally with LV failure. Presystolic distention of the left ventricle (i.e., a prominent precordial *a* wave) is often visible and palpable. A hyperdynamic left ventricle suggests concomitant AR and/or MR. A systolic thrill is usually best appreciated when the patient leans forward during full expiration. It is palpated most readily in the second right intercostal space or suprasternal notch and is frequently transmitted along the carotid arteries. A systolic thrill is specific, but not sensitive, for severe AS.

Auscultation. The ejection systolic murmur of AS typically is late peaking and heard best at the base of the heart, with radiation to the carotids (see Fig. 66-4). Cessation of the murmur before A_2 is helpful in differentiation from a pansystolic mitral murmur. In patients with calcified aortic valves, the systolic murmur is loudest at the base of the heart, but high-frequency components may radiate to the apex (the so-called Gallavardin phenomenon), in which the murmur may be so prominent that it is mistaken for the murmur of MR. In general, a louder and later peaking murmur indicates more severe stenosis. However, although a systolic murmur of grade 3 intensity or greater is relatively specific for severe AS, this finding is insensitive and many patients with severe AS have only a grade 2 murmur. High-pitched decrescendo diastolic murmurs secondary to AR are common in many patients with dominant AS.

Splitting of the second heart sound is helpful in excluding the diagnosis of severe AS because normal splitting implies the aortic valve leaflets are flexible enough to create an audible closing sound (A_2). With severe AS, the second heart sound (S_2) may be single because calcification and immobility of the aortic valve make A_2 inaudible, closure of the pulmonic valve (P_2) is buried in the prolonged aortic ejection murmur, or prolongation of LV systole makes A_2 coincide with P_2. Paradoxical splitting of S_2, which suggests associated left bundle branch block or LV dysfunction, may also occur. Thus, in older adults, normal splitting of S_2 indicates a low likelihood of severe AS. The first heart sound (S_1) is normal or soft and a fourth heart sound (S_4) is prominent, presumably because atrial contraction is vigorous and the mitral valve is partially closed during presystole.

In young patients with congenital AS (see Chap. 65), the flexible valve may result in an accentuated A_2 so that S_2 may be normally split, even with severe valve obstruction. In addition, an aortic ejection sound may be audible because of the halting upward movement of the aortic valve. Like an audible A_2, this sound is dependent on mobility of the valve cusps and disappears when they become severely calcified. Thus, it is common in children and young adults with congenital AS but is rare in adults with acquired calcific AS and rigid valves.

When the left ventricle fails and stroke volume falls, the systolic murmur of AS becomes softer; rarely, it disappears altogether. The slow rise in the arterial pulse is more difficult to recognize. Stated simply, with LV failure, the clinical picture changes from typical AS to that of severe LV failure with a low cardiac output. Thus, occult AS may be a cause of intractable heart failure, and severe AS should be ruled out by echocardiography in patients with heart failure of unknown cause because operative treatment may be lifesaving and result in substantial clinical improvement.

Dynamic Auscultation. The intensity of the systolic murmur varies from beat to beat when the duration of diastolic filling varies, as in AF or following a premature contraction. This characteristic is helpful in differentiating AS from MR, in which the murmur is usually unaffected. The murmur of valvular AS is augmented by squatting, which increases stroke volume. It is reduced in intensity during the strain of the Valsalva maneuver and when standing, which reduce transvalvular flow.

Echocardiography

Echocardiography is the standard approach for evaluating and following patients with AS and selecting them for operation (see Chap. 15 and Figs. 15-36 to 15-38, and 15-43 to 15-45).

Echocardiographic imaging allows accurate definition of valve anatomy, including the cause of AS and the severity of valve calcification, and sometimes allows direct imaging of the orifice area.[30,36] Echocardiographic imaging also is invaluable for the evaluation of LV hypertrophy and systolic function, with calculation of the ejection fraction, and for measurement of aortic root dimensions and detection of associated mitral valve disease.[37]

Doppler echocardiography allows measurement of the transaortic jet velocity, which is the most useful measure for following disease severity and predicting clinical outcome. The effective orifice area is calculated using the continuity equation, and mean transaortic pressure gradient is calculated using the modified Bernoulli equation (see Fig. 15-38).[37,38] Both valve area and pressure gradient calculations from Doppler data have been well validated compared with invasive hemodynamics and in terms of their ability to predict clinical outcome. However, the accuracy of these measures requires an experienced laboratory with meticulous attention to technical details.

The combination of pulsed, continuous wave and color flow Doppler echocardiography is helpful in detecting and determining the severity of AR (which coexists in about 75% of patients with predominant AS) and in estimating pulmonary artery pressure. In some patients, additional measures of AS severity may be necessary, such as correction for poststenotic pressure recovery or transesophageal imaging of valve anatomy.[31,39] Evaluation of AS severity is affected by the presence of systemic hypertension so that reevaluation after blood pressure control may be necessary.[34] In patients with LV dysfunction and low cardiac output, assessing the severity of AS can be enhanced by assessing hemodynamic changes during dobutamine infusion (see later).

Other Diagnostic Evaluation Modalities

Electrocardiography. The principal electrocardiographic change is LV hypertrophy (see Chap. 13), which is found in approximately 85% of patients with severe AS. The absence of LV hypertrophy does not exclude the presence of critical AS, and the correlation between the absolute electrocardiographic voltages in precordial leads and the severity of obstruction is poor in adults but good in children with congenital AS. T wave inversion and ST-segment depression in leads with upright QRS complexes are common. There is evidence of left atrial enlargement in more than 80% of patients with severe isolated AS. AF occurs in only 10% to 15% of AS patients. The extension of calcific infiltrates from the aortic valve into the conduction system may cause various forms and degrees of atrioventricular and intraventricular block in 5% of patients with calcific AS. Such conduction defects are more common in patients who have associated mitral annular calcification.

Radiography. On chest radiography (see Figs. 16-10 and 16-23), the heart is usually of normal size or slightly enlarged, with a rounding of the LV border and apex, unless regurgitation or LV failure is present and causes substantial cardiomegaly. Dilation of the ascending aorta is a common finding, particularly in patients with a bicuspid aortic valve. Calcification of the aortic valve is found in almost all adults with hemodynamically significant AS but is rarely visible on the chest radiograph, although readily detected by fluoroscopy or cardiac computed tomography (CT; see Fig. 19-21). The left atrium may be slightly enlarged in patients with severe AS, and there may be radiologic signs of pulmonary venous hypertension. However, when left atrial enlargement is marked, the presence of associated mitral valvular disease should be suspected.

Cardiac Catheterization and Angiography. In almost all patients, the echocardiographic examination provides the important hemodynamic information required for patient management, and cardiac catheterization is now recommended only when noninvasive tests are inconclusive, when clinical and echocardiographic findings are discrepant, and for coronary angiography prior to surgical intervention.[1,2,40] Hemodynamic or echocardiographic assessment of AS severity at rest and with dobutamine is reasonable when AS is associated with low cardiac output and impaired LV function (see later).

Chest Computed Tomography. In addition to assessing aortic valve calcification, CT (see Chap. 19) is useful for evaluating aortic dilation in patients with evidence of aortic root disease by echocardiography or chest radiography. Measurement of aortic dimensions at several levels, including the sinuses of Valsalva, sinotubular junction, and ascending aorta, is necessary for clinical decision making and surgical planning.

Cardiac Magnetic Resonance. Cardiac magnetic resonance (CMR) is useful for assessing LV volume, function, and mass, especially in settings in which this information cannot be obtained readily from echocardiography (see Chap. 18). AS severity also can be quantitated by CMR, although this approach is not widely used.[41]

DISEASE COURSE

Clinical Outcome

ASYMPTOMATIC PATIENTS. The severity of outflow tract obstruction gradually increases over 10 to 15 years, so there is a long latent period during which stenosis severity is only mild to moderate and clinical outcomes are similar to those of age-matched normal patients.[42] In patients with mild valve thickening but no obstruction to outflow (e.g., aortic sclerosis), 16% will develop valve obstruction at 1 year of follow-up, but only 2.5% will develop severe valve obstruction at an average of 8 years after the diagnosis of aortic sclerosis.

Once moderate to severe AS is present, prognosis remains excellent as long as the patient remains asymptomatic.[43] However, retrospective studies of survival in adults with severe AS diagnosed by echocardiography emphasize the progressive nature of the disease and the need

TABLE 66-2 Clinical Outcomes in Prospective Studies of Asymptomatic Aortic Stenosis in Adults

STUDY (YEAR)	NO. OF PATIENTS	SEVERITY OF AORTIC STENOSIS	AGE (YR)	MEAN FOLLOW-UP	EVENT-FREE SURVIVAL WITHOUT SYMPTOMS
Kelly et al (1988)	51	V_{max} > 3.6 m/sec	63 ± 8	5-25 mo	Overall: 59% at 15 mo
Pellikka et al (1990)	113	V_{max} ≥ 4.0 m/sec	40-94	20 mo	Overall: 86% at 1 yr; 62% at 2 yr
Kennedy et al (1991)	66	AVA = 0.7-1.2 cm^2	67 ± 10	35 mo	Overall: 59% at 4 yr
Otto et al (1997)	123	V_{max} > 2.6 m/sec	63 ± 16	2.5 ± 1.4 yr	Overall: 93 ± 5% at 1 yr; 62 ± 8% at 3 yr; 26 ± 10% at 5 yr *Subgroups:* V_{max} < 3 m/sec, 84% ± 16% at 2 yr V_{max} 3-4 m/sec, 66% ± 13% at 2 yr V_{max} > 4 m/sec, 21% ± 18% at 2 yr
Rosenhek et al (2000)	128	V_{max} > 4.0 m/sec	60 ± 18	22 ± 18 mo	Overall: 67 ± 5% at 1 yr; 56 ± 55% at 2 yr; 33 ± 5% at 4 yr *Subgroups:* No or mild Ca^{++}, 75% ± 9% at 4 yr Mod-severe Ca^{++}, 20% ± 5% at 4 yr
Amato et al (2001)	66	AVA ≥ 1.0 cm^2	18-80 (50 ± 15)	15 ± 12 mo	Overall: 57% at 1 yr; 38% at 2 yr *Subgroups:* AVA ≥ 0.7 cm^2, 72% at 2 yr AVA < 0.7 cm^2, 21% at 2 yr Negative exercise test 85% at 2 yr Positive exercise test* 19% at 2 yr
Das et al (2005)	125	AVA < 1.4 cm^2	56-74 (mean, 65)	12 mo	Overall: 71% at 1 yr *Subgroups:* AVA ≥ 1.2 cm^2, 100% at 1 yr AVA ≤ 0.8 cm^2, 46% at 1 yr No symptoms on exercise test,* 89% at 1 yr Symptoms on exercise test, 49% at 1 yr
Pellikka et al (2005)	622	V_{max} 4.0 ≥ m/sec	72 ± 11	5.4 ± 4.0 yr	Overall: 82% at 1 yr; 67% at 2 yr; 33% at 5 yr
Monin et al (2009)	211	V_{max} = 3.5-4.4 (mean, 4.1) m/sec	63-77 (mean, 72)	21 mo	Risk score = $2V_{max} + 1.5\ ln_{BNP} + 1.5$ (if female)† 24 mo event rate < 10% in lowest risk quartile compared with >75% in highest risk quartile (score > 15)

*Positive exercise test = symptoms, abnormal ST-segment response, or abnormal blood pressure response (less than 20 mmHg increase) with exercise.

†V_{max} measured in m/sec.

AVA = aortic valve area; BNP = blood natriuretic peptide level (pg/mL); Ca^{++} = aortic valve calcification; ln = logarithm; Mod = moderate; V_{max} = maximum aortic velocity.

From Bonow RO, Carabello BA, Chatterjee K, et al: ACC/AHA 2006 guidelines for the management of patients with valvular heart disease: A report of the American College of Cardiology/American Heart Association Task Force on Practice Guidelines (writing Committee to Revise the 1998 guidelines for the management of patients with valvular heart disease) developed in collaboration with the Society of Cardiovascular Anesthesiologists endorsed by the Society for Cardiovascular Angiography and Interventions and the Society of Thoracic Surgeons. J Am Coll Cardiol 48:e1, 2006.

Data from Kelly TA, Rothbart RM, Cooper CM, et al: Comparison of outcome of symptomatic to symptomatic patients older that 20 years of age with valvular aortic stenosis. Am J Cardiol 61:123,1988; Pellikka PA, Nishimura RA, Bailey KR, Tajik AJ: The natural history of adults with asymptomatic, hemodynamically significant aortic stenosis. J Am Coll Cardiol 15:1012, 1990; Kennedy KD, Nishimura RA, Holmes DRJ, Bailey KR: Natural history of moderate aortic stenosis. J Am Coll Cardiol 17:313, 1991; Otto CM, Burwash IG, Legget ME, et al: A prospective study of asymptomatic valvular aortic stenosis: Clinical, echocardiographic, and exercise predictors of outcome. Circulation 95:2262, 1997; Rosenhek R, Binder T, Porenta G, et al: Predictors of outcome in severe asymptomatic aortic valve stenosis. N Engl J Med 343:611, 2000; Amato MC, Moffa PJ, Werner KE, Ramires JA: Treatment decision in asymptomatic aortic valve stenosis: Role of exercise testing. Heart 86:381, 2001; Das P, Rimington H, Chambers J: Exercise testing to stratify risk in aortic stenosis. Eur Heart J 26:1309, 2005; Pellikka PA, Sarano ME, Nishimura RA, et al: Outcome of 622 adults with asymptomatic, hemodynamically significant aortic stenosis during prolonged follow-up. Circulation 111:3290, 2005; and Monin JL, Lancellotti P, Monchi M, et al: Risk score for predicting outcome in patients with asymptomatic aortic stenosis. Circulation 120:69, 2009.)

for close follow-up.[44] Although stenosis severity on average is more severe in symptomatic versus asymptomatic patients, there is marked overlap in all measures of severity between these two groups. Prospective studies evaluating the rate of progression to symptomatic AS in initially asymptomatic patients are summarized in **Table 66-2**. The strongest predictor of progression to symptoms is the Doppler aortic jet velocity.[45,46,46a] Survival free of symptoms is 84% at 2 years when jet velocity is less than 3 m/sec compared with only 21% when jet velocity is greater than 4 m/sec (**Fig. 66-5**).[31] In adults with severe AS (Doppler velocity > 4 m/sec), outcome can be further predicted by the magnitude of the Doppler velocity and also by the severity of aortic valve calcification.[47,47a] Event-free survival at 5 years is 75% ± 9% in those with little valve calcification compared with 20% ± 5% in those with moderate to severe valve calcification. Retrospective studies have reported some cases of sudden death in apparently asymptomatic adults with severe AS. However, more recent prospective studies have suggested that sudden death in asymptomatic patients is very unlikely, with an estimated risk of less than 1%/year.[46]

SYMPTOMATIC PATIENTS. Once even mild symptoms are present, survival is poor unless outflow obstruction is relieved. Survival curves derived from older retrospective studies show that the interval from the onset of symptoms to the time of death is approximately 2 years in patients with heart failure, 3 years in those with syncope, and 5 years in those with angina. More recent series have confirmed this poor prognosis, with an average survival of only 1 to 3 years after symptom onset.[48] Among symptomatic patients with severe AS, the outlook is poorest when the left ventricle has failed and the cardiac output and transvalvular gradient are both low. The risk of sudden death is high with symptomatic severe AS, so these patients should be promptly referred for surgical intervention. In patients who do not undergo surgical intervention, recurrent hospitalizations for angina and decompensated heart failure are common.

Hemodynamic Progression

The average rate of hemodynamic progression is an annual decrease in aortic valve area of 0.12 cm^2/year,[31] an increase in aortic jet velocity of 0.32 m/sec/year, and an increase in mean gradient of 7 mm Hg/year. However, the rate of progression is highly variable and difficult to predict in individual patients. In clinical studies, the factors associated with more rapid hemodynamic progression included older age, more severe leaflet calcification, renal insufficiency, hypertension, smoking, and hyperlipidemia. The role of genetic factors remains unclear.

Because of the variability in hemodynamic severity at symptom onset and because many patients fail to recognize symptom onset resulting from the insidious rate of disease progression, both exercise testing (see Table 66-2)[32,49,50] and serum brain natriuretic peptide

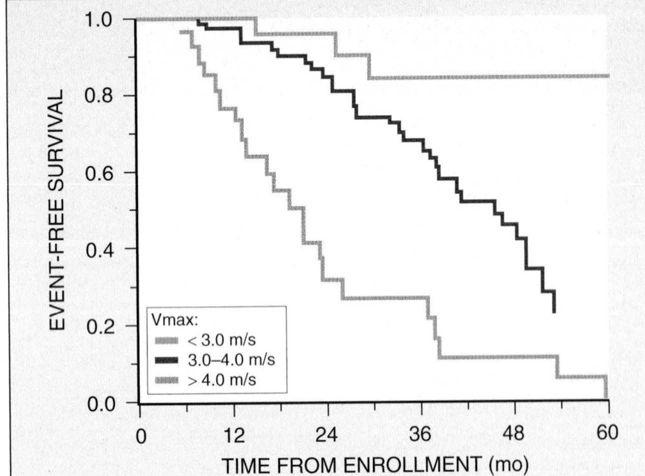

FIGURE 66-5 Natural history of asymptomatic patients with aortic stenosis. Initial aortic jet velocity (Vmax) stratifies patients according to the likelihood that symptoms requiring valve replacement will develop over time. Most events in this series were the onset of symptoms warranting aortic valve replacement. *(From Otto CM, Burwarsh IG, Legget ME, et al: A prospective study of asymptomatic valvular aortic stenosis: Clinical, echocardiographic, and exercise predictors of outcome. Circulation 95:2262, 1997.)*

(BNP) levels[51-53a] have been evaluated as measures of disease progression and predictors of symptom onset. Clearly, patients who develop symptoms on treadmill exercise or who have a decrease in blood pressure with exertion show evidence of severe symptomatic disease. An elevated BNP level may be helpful when symptoms are equivocal or when stenosis severity is only moderate, but the role of BNP in evaluation of disease progression has not been fully defined.

MANAGEMENT

Medical Treatment

The most important principle in the management of adults with AS is patient education regarding the disease course and typical symptoms.[31,39] Patients should be advised to promptly report the development of any symptoms possibly related to AS. Patients with severe AS should be cautioned to avoid vigorous athletic sports and physical activity.[54] However, such restrictions do not apply to patients with mild obstruction. Although medical therapy has not been shown to affect disease progression, adults with AS (as with any other adult) should be evaluated and treated for conventional coronary disease risk factors, as per established guidelines.

Echocardiography is recommended for the initial diagnosis and assessment of AS severity, assessment of LV hypertrophy and systolic function, reevaluation in patients with changing signs or symptoms, and reevaluation annually for severe AS, every 1 to 2 years for moderate AS, and every 3 to 5 years for mild AS.[1,2] Because patients may tailor their lifestyle to minimize symptoms or may ascribe fatigue and dyspnea to deconditioning or aging, they may not recognize early symptoms as important warning signals, although these symptoms often can be elicited by a careful history. Exercise testing may be helpful in apparently asymptomatic patients to detect covert symptoms, limited exercise capacity, or an abnormal blood pressure response.[31] Exercise stress testing should be absolutely avoided in symptomatic patients.

Symptomatic patients with severe AS are usually operative candidates because medical therapy has little to offer. However, medical therapy may be necessary for patients considered to be inoperable, usually because of comorbid conditions that preclude surgery. Some of these patients may be candidates for transcatheter valve implantation, but others will not be candidates for or will decline this procedure. Although diuretics are beneficial when there is abnormal accumulation of fluid, they must be used with caution because hypovolemia may reduce the elevated LV end-diastolic pressure, lower cardiac output, and produce orthostatic hypotension. ACE inhibitors should be used with caution but are beneficial in treating patients with symptomatic LV systolic dysfunction who are not candidates for surgery. They should be initiated at low doses and increased slowly to target doses, avoiding hypotension. Beta-adrenergic blockers can depress myocardial function and induce LV failure, and should be avoided in patients with AS.

AF or atrial flutter occurs in less than 10% of patients with severe AS, perhaps because of the late occurrence of left atrial enlargement in this condition. When such an arrhythmia is observed in a patient with AS, the possibility of associated mitral valvular disease should be considered. When AF occurs, the rapid ventricular rate may cause angina pectoris. The loss of the atrial contribution to ventricular filling and a sudden fall in cardiac output may cause serious hypotension. Therefore, AF should be treated promptly, usually with cardioversion. New-onset AF in a previously asymptomatic patient with severe AS may be a marker of impending symptom onset.

Management of concurrent cardiac conditions, such as hypertension and coronary disease, is complicated in patients with asymptomatic AS by the concern that the vasodilatory effects of medications may not be offset by a compensatory increase in cardiac output. Despite this concern, AS patients should receive appropriate treatment for concurrent disease, although medications should be started at low doses and slowly titrated upward, with close monitoring of blood pressure and symptoms. Adults with asymptomatic severe AS can undergo noncardiac surgery and pregnancy, with careful hemodynamic monitoring and optimization of loading conditions. However, when stenosis is very severe, elective AVR prior to noncardiac surgery or a planned pregnancy may be considered.[55]

Surgical Treatment

CHILDREN. In the adolescent or young adult with severe congenital AS, balloon aortic valvotomy is recommended for all symptomatic patients and asymptomatic patients with a transvalvular gradient higher than 60 mm Hg or electrocardiographic ST-segment changes at rest or with exercise.[56] The same indications are appropriate for surgical intervention, although balloon valvotomy is probably preferable at experienced centers. At surgery, simple commissural incision under direct vision usually leads to substantial hemodynamic improvement with low risk (i.e., mortality rate < 1%; see Chap. 65). Despite the salutary hemodynamic results following percutaneous or surgical valvotomy, the valve is not rendered entirely normal anatomically. The turbulent blood flow through the valve may subsequently lead to further deformation, calcification, development of regurgitation, and restenosis after 10 to 20 years, often requiring reoperation and valve replacement later.

ADULTS. AVR is recommended for adults with symptomatic severe AS, even if symptoms are mild. Despite this clear guideline recommendation,[1,2] many patients with symptomatic AS are not referred appropriately for surgery, even when the operative risk is low.[48,57] AVR also is recommended for severe AS with an ejection fraction less than 50% and for patients with severe asymptomatic AS who are undergoing coronary bypass grafting (CABG) or other forms of heart surgery (**Fig. 66-6**).[1,2,58,59] In addition, AVR may be considered for apparently asymptomatic patients with severe AS when exercise testing provokes symptoms or a fall in blood pressure. In asymptomatic patients with severe AS and a low operative risk, AVR may be considered when markers of rapid disease progression are present (e.g., severe valve calcification) or when AS is very severe, depending on patient preferences regarding the risk of earlier intervention versus careful monitoring with intervention promptly at symptom onset. Coronary angiography should be performed before valve replacement in most adults with AS.

Surgical AVR is the procedure of choice for relief of outflow obstruction in adults with valvular AS. Surgical repair is not feasible because attempts at débridement of valve calcification have not been successful. Balloon aortic valvotomy has only a modest hemodynamic effect in patients with calcific AS and does not favorably affect long-term outcome. Thus, balloon aortic valvotomy is not recommended as an alternate to AVR for calcific AS. In selected cases, balloon valvotomy might be reasonable as a bridge to surgery in unstable patients or as a palliative procedure when surgery is very high risk. Transcatheter aortic

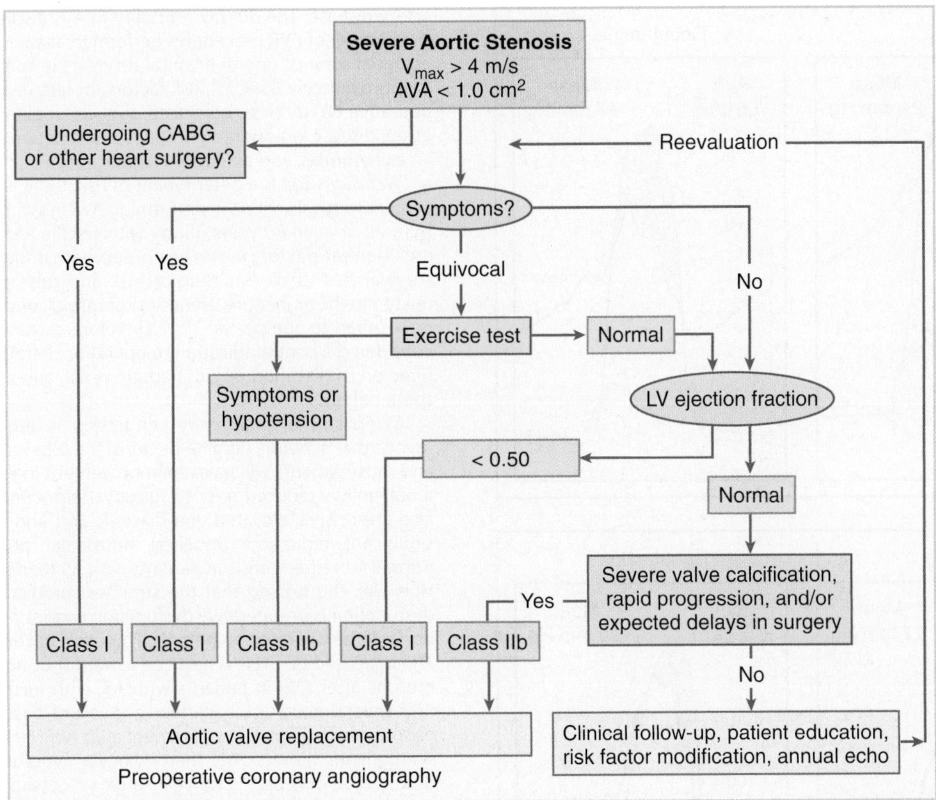

FIGURE 66-6 Management strategy for patients with severe aortic stenosis. Preoperative coronary angiography should be performed routinely as determined by age, symptoms, and coronary risk factors. Cardiac catheterization and angiography may also be helpful when there is discordance between clinical findings and echocardiography. AVA = aortic valve area; BP = blood pressure; V_{max} = maximal velocity across aortic valve by Doppler echocardiography. *(From Bonow RO, Carabello BA, Chatterjee K, et al: ACC/AHA 2006 guidelines for the management of patients with valvular heart disease: A report of the American College of Cardiology/American Heart Association Task Force on Practice Guidelines [writing committee to revise the 1998 Guidelines for the Management of Patients With Valvular Heart Disease]: Developed in collaboration with the Society of Cardiovascular Anesthesiologists: Endorsed by the Society for Cardiovascular Angiography and Interventions and the Society of Thoracic Surgeons. Circulation 114:e84, 2006.)*

valve implantation (TAVI) by a percutaneous or transapical approach is a rapidly evolving technology that is available in Europe and under investigation in the US for seriously ill patients who are not candidates for conventional surgery.[60-64a] In the Canadian multicenter registry of TAVI in 339 patients, the procedure was successful in 93% with a 30 day mortality of 10%. At a median followup of 8 months, overall mortality was 22%, and the procedure was effective in both frail elderly adults and in those with a porcelain aorta.[60,63] The US randomized prospective PARTNER trial, comparing TAVI with medical therapy (including balloon valvotomy) in patients considered to be at too high risk for conventional AVR, demonstrated substantial reduction in death and hospitalization with TAVI, associated with significant improvement in symptoms.[64a]

AORTIC STENOSIS WITH LEFT VENTRICULAR DYSFUNCTION. Surgical risk is higher in patients with impaired LV function (ejection fraction < 35%).[32,65-68] However, their prognosis is extremely poor without operation, overall survival is improved with AVR, and many patients in this group have significant clinical and functional recovery following AVR. Hence, AVR should generally be offered to these patients. Even octogenarians with LV dysfunction can have improved survival after AVR, although their operative risks are higher. Exceptions are patients with advanced congestive heart failure or LV dysfunction that can be related to previous myocardial infarction rather than to AS. In acutely ill patients with decompensated heart failure, nitroprusside has been reported to be safe and effective for improving hemodynamics rapidly and may be used in bridging critically ill patients to AVR. The role of TAVI for severe AS with significant LV systolic dysfunction has not been studied.

AORTIC STENOSIS WITH LOW GRADIENT AND LOW CARDIAC OUTPUT. Patients with critical AS, severe LV dysfunction, and low cardiac output (and hence a low transvalvular pressure gradient) often create diagnostic dilemmas for the clinician because their clinical presentation and hemodynamic data may be indistinguishable from those of patients with a dilated cardiomyopathy and a calcified valve that is not stenotic.[38,65] Low-flow, low-gradient AS is defined as a valve area smaller than 1.0 cm², LV ejection fraction less than 40% and mean gradient less than 30 to 40 mm Hg. Because aortic valve velocities and estimates of aortic valve area are dependent on flow, an important method for distinguishing between those with severe AS versus those with primary LV dysfunction is to reassess hemodynamics during transient increases in flow, usually by increasing cardiac output with dobutamine while measuring hemodynamics with Doppler or invasive approaches. (**Fig. 66-7**; see Fig. 15-45).[69,70] Severe AS is present if there is an increase in aortic velocity to at least 4 m/sec at any flow rate, with a valve area less than 1.0 cm²; AS is not severe if the valve area is increased to more than 1.0 cm².[30] Dobutamine echocardiography also provides evidence of myocardial contractile reserve (an increase in stroke volume or ejection fraction > 20% from baseline), which is an important predictor of operative risk, improvement in LV function, and survival after AVR in these patients. However, even in patients with a lack of contractile reserve, AVR should be considered if the mean gradient is over 20 mm Hg because survival after AVR is better (≈50% at 5 years) than with medical therapy.[66,67]

RESULTS. Successful replacement of the aortic valve results in substantial clinical and hemodynamic improvement in patients with AS, AR, or combined lesions. In patients without frank LV failure, the operative risk ranges from 2% to 5% in most centers[71] and, in patients younger than 70 years, the operative risk has been reported to be as low as 1%. The STS National Database Committee has reported an overall operative mortality rate of 3.2% in 67,292 patients undergoing isolated AVR and 5.6% in 66,074 patients undergoing AVR and coronary artery bypass grafting (**Table 66-3**).[72,73] Risk factors associated with a higher mortality rate include a high New York Heart Association (NYHA) class, impairment of LV function, advanced age, and the presence of associated coronary

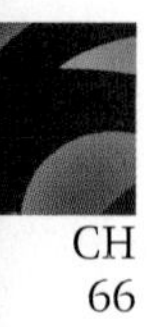

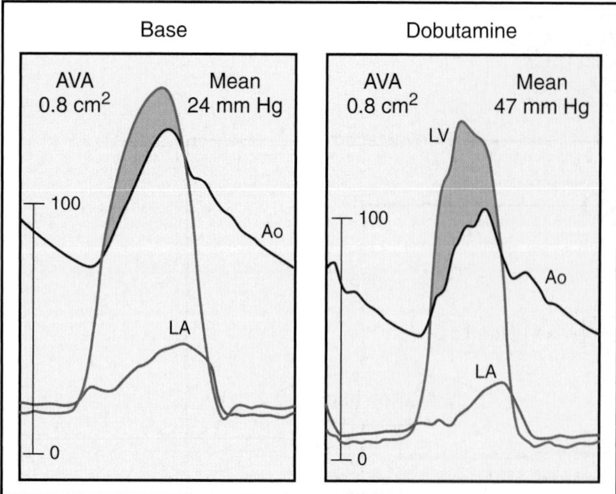

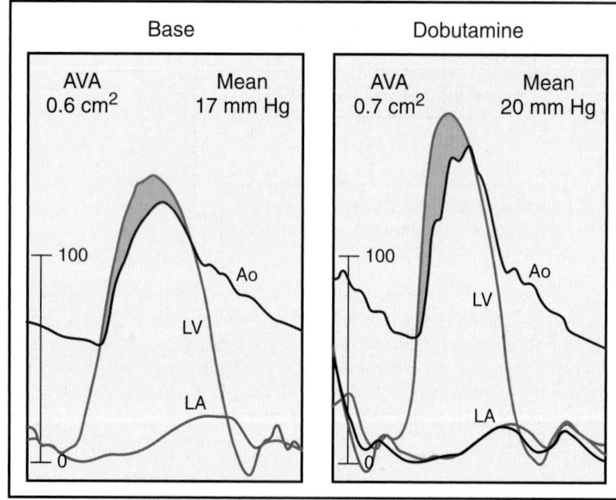

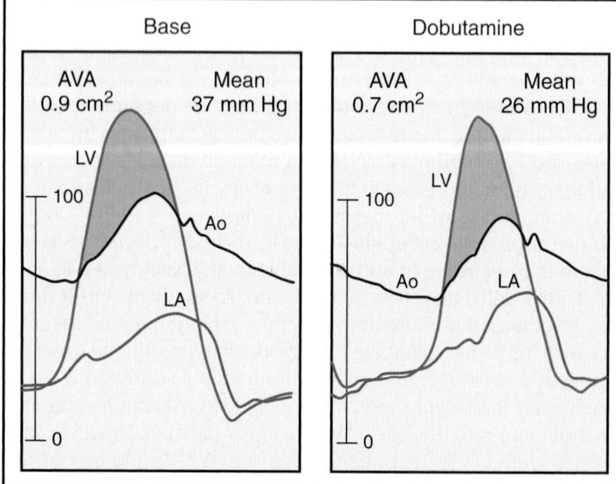

FIGURE 66-7 Hemodynamic tracings from three patients with left ventricular dysfunction, low cardiac output, and low aortic valve gradient, demonstrating three different responses to dobutamine. **A,** Increase in cardiac output and in mean aortic valve gradient from 24 to 47 mm Hg. Aortic valve area (AVA) remained 0.8 cm^2. This patient underwent successful valve replacement. **B,** Increase in cardiac output and minimal increase in mean pressure gradient from 17 to 20 mm Hg. The final calculated aortic valve area was 0.7 cm^2. The patient was found to have only minimal AS at the time of surgery. **C,** No change in cardiac output, with decrease in mean pressure gradient from 37 to 26 mm Hg in response to dobutamine. The test was terminated because of hypotension. The patient was found to have severe AS at the time of surgery. Ao = aortic; LA = left atrial; LV = left ventricular. *(From Nishimura RA, Grantham A, Connolly HM, et al: Low-output, low-gradient aortic stenosis in patients with depressed left ventricular systolic function: The clinical utility of the dobutamine challenge in the catheterization laboratory. Circulation 106:809, 2002.)*

artery disease. The 30-day mortality rate is also significantly related to the number of AVR procedures performed at each hospital.[74] The 10-year actuarial survival rate of hospital survivors in surgically treated patients is approximately 85%.[75,76] Risk factors for late death include higher preoperative NYHA class, advanced age, concomitant untreated coronary artery disease, preoperative impaired LV function, preoperative ventricular arrhythmias, and associated significant AR.[77-80]

Although age is a determinant of risk, there is increasing experience at most surgical centers in performing AVR in symptomatic patients older than 70 or even 80 years of age with calcific AS.[81,81a] The results of AVR are often satisfactory in this age group, with improved quality of life and survival (see Chap. 80). Surgical risk and postoperative morbidity are related to the higher prevalence of comorbid conditions in older patients, rather than to age per se.[75,82,82a] Therefore, advanced age should not be considered a contraindication to operation. Particular attention must be directed to the adequacy of hepatic, renal, and pulmonary functions in these patients.

Symptoms of pulmonary congestion (exertional dyspnea) and of myocardial ischemia (angina pectoris) are relieved in almost all patients, and most patients will have an improvement in exercise tolerance, even if only mildly reduced prior to surgery. Hemodynamic results of AVR are also impressive; elevated end-diastolic and end-systolic volumes show significant reduction. Impaired ventricular performance returns to normal more frequently in patients with AS than in those with AR or MR. However, the finding that the strongest predictor of postoperative LV dysfunction is preoperative dysfunction suggests that patients should, if possible, be operated on before LV function becomes seriously impaired. The increased LV mass is reduced toward (but not to) normal within 18 months after AVR in patients with AS, with further reduction over the next several years. Coronary flow reserve and diastolic function also demonstrate considerable improvement after AVR. However, interstitial fibrosis regresses more slowly than myocyte hypertrophy, so that diastolic dysfunction may persist for years after successful valve replacement.

When operation is carried out in patients with critical AS, frank LV failure, depressed ejection fraction, or low cardiac output (and hence a reduced transaortic pressure gradient), the operative risk is higher, and the mortality rate ranges from 8% to 20% , depending on the skill of the surgical team and the severity of heart failure. Obviously, performing surgery before heart failure develops is desirable, but emergency operation, even in patients with severe heart failure, is sometimes lifesaving. In view of the extremely poor prognosis of such patients who are treated medically, unless serious comorbid conditions exist that preclude surgery, there is usually little choice but to advise immediate mechanical relief of obstruction.

In patients with AS and obstructive coronary artery disease—a relatively common combination—AVR and myocardial revascularization should be performed together. Although the risk of AVR is increased when accompanied by CABG (see Table 66-3), the surgical risk increases even more when severe coronary artery disease is left untreated. The ability to avoid serious myocardial ischemia in the perioperative period is a major factor that has served to reduce operative mortality in these patients. Characteristics of patients that have been shown to increase the risk of AVR, as reported in different series, are shown in **Table 66-4**.

Aortic Regurgitation

CAUSES AND PATHOLOGY. AR may be caused by primary disease of the aortic valve leaflets and/or the wall of the aortic root (**Fig. 66-8**).[83-85] Among patients with isolated AR who undergo valve replacement, the percentage with aortic root disease has been increasing steadily during the past few decades; it now represents the most common cause and accounts for more than 50% of all such patients in some series.

Valvular Disease

Primary valvular causes of AR include the following: calcific AS in older patients, in whom some degree (usually mild) of AR is present (in 75% of patients); infective endocarditis (see Chap. 67), in which the infection may destroy or cause perforation of a leaflet, or the vegetations may interfere with proper coaptation of the cusps; and trauma that results in a tear of the ascending aorta, in which loss of commissural support can cause prolapse of an aortic cusp. Although the most common complication of a congenitally bicuspid valve in adults is stenosis, incomplete closure and/or prolapse of a bicuspid valve may also cause isolated regurgitation or a combination of stenosis and regurgitation.[6] Rheumatic fever remains a common cause of primary

TABLE 66-3 Operative Mortality Rates Following Valve Replacement and Repair (2002-2006 STS Data Base)*

OPERATIVE CATEGORY	NUMBER	OPERATIVE MORTALITY (%)	CVA (%)	RENAL FAILURE (%)	PROLONGED VENTILATION (%)	REOPERATION (%)	ANY ADVERSE EVENT (%)	PROLONGED LENGTH OF STAY (%)
AVR	67,292	3.2	1.5	4.1	10.9	8.0	17.4	7.9
AVR + CABG	66,074	5.6	2.7	7.6	17.6	10.7	26.3	12.7
MVR	21,229	5.7	2.1	6.4	18.9	11.5	26.7	15.3
MVR + CABG	13.663	11.6	3.7	13.6	32.7	16.6	43.2	24.0
MV repair	21,238	1.6	1.4	2.6	7.3	6.3	12.7	5.5
MV repair + CABG	21,924	7.4	3.1	10.3	25.0	12.6	33.5	17.8

*Operative mortality = death during hospitalization or within 30 days of valve surgery. Other endpoints are during initial hospitalization for valve surgery: CVA = permanent stroke (neurologic deficit persisting > 72 hr); Renal Failure = new need for dialysis, increase in serum creatinine level to > 2.0 mg/dL or increase to twice preoperative baseline; Prolonged Ventilation = need for ventilatory support > 24 hours postoperatively; Reoperation = reoperation during initial hospitalization; Any Adverse Event = any of the above endpoints plus deep sternal wound infection (occurred in <1%); Prolonged length of stay = postoperative hospitalization > 14 days.

Data from Shahian DM, O'Brien SM, Filardo G, et al: The Society of Thoracic Surgeons 2008 cardiac surgery risk models: Part 3—valve plus coronary artery bypass grafting surgery. Ann Thorac Surg 88:S43, 2009; and O'Brien SM, Shahian DM, Filardo G, et al: The Society of Thoracic Surgeons 2008 cardiac surgery risk models: Part 2—isolated valve surgery. Ann Thorac Surg 88:S23, 2009.

TABLE 66-4 Predictors of Poor Outcome After Aortic Valve Replacement for Aortic Stenosis

- Advanced age (>70 yr)
- Female gender
- Emergent surgery
- Coronary artery disease
- Previous CABG
- Hypertension
- Left ventricular dysfunction (ejection fraction <45% or 50%)
- Heart failure
- Atrial fibrillation
- Concurrent mitral valve replacement or repair
- Renal failure

disease of the aortic valve that leads to regurgitation. The cusps become infiltrated with fibrous tissues and retract a process that prevents cusp apposition during diastole; this usually leads to regurgitation into the left ventricle through a defect in the center of the valve (see Fig. 66-1C). The associated fusion of the commissures may restrict the opening of the valve, resulting in combined AS and AR; some associated mitral valve involvement is also common. Progressive AR may occur in patients with a large ventricular septal defect, as well as in patients with membranous subaortic stenosis (see Chap. 65) and as a complication of percutaneous aortic balloon valvotomy. Progressive regurgitation may also occur in patients with myxomatous proliferation of the aortic valve. An increasingly common cause of valvular AR is structural deterioration of a bioprosthetic valve.

Less common causes of AR include various forms of congenital AR, such as unicommissural and quadricuspid valves, or rupture of a congenitally fenestrated valve, particularly in the presence of hypertension. Other less common causes of AR occur in association with systemic lupus erythematosus, rheumatoid arthritis, ankylosing spondylitis, Jaccoud arthropathy, Takayasu disease, Whipple disease, Crohn disease, and, in the past, the use of certain anorectic drugs. Isolated congenital AR is an uncommon lesion on necropsy studies but, when present, is usually associated with a bicuspid valve.

Aortic Root Disease

AR secondary to marked dilation of the ascending aorta is now more common than primary valve disease in patients undergoing AVR for isolated AR (see Chap. 60).[86] The conditions responsible for aortic root disease include age-related (degenerative) aortic dilation, cystic medial necrosis of the aorta (either isolated or associated with classic Marfan syndrome; see Fig. 15-81), aortic dilation related to bicuspid valves,[87] aortic dissection, osteogenesis imperfecta, syphilitic aortitis, ankylosing spondylitis, the Behçet syndrome, psoriatic arthritis, arthritis associated with ulcerative colitis, relapsing polychondritis, reactive arthritis, giant cell arteritis, and systemic hypertension, and exposure to some appetite suppressant drugs.[88]

When the aortic annulus becomes greatly dilated, the aortic leaflets separate and AR may ensue. Dissection of the diseased aortic wall may occur and aggravate the AR. Dilation of the aortic root may also have secondary effects on the aortic valve because dilation causes tension and bowing of the individual cusps, which may thicken, retract, and become too short to close the aortic orifice. This leads to intensification of the AR, further dilating the ascending aorta and thus leading to a vicious circle in which, as is the case for MR, regurgitation leads to regurgitation. AR, regardless of its cause, produces dilation and hypertrophy of the left ventricle, dilation of the mitral valve ring, and sometimes hypertrophy and dilation of the left atrium. Endocardial pockets frequently develop in the LV cavity at sites of impact of the regurgitant jet.

CHRONIC AORTIC REGURGITATION

Pathophysiology

In contrast to MR, in which a fraction of the LV stroke volume is ejected into the low-pressure left atrium, in AR the entire LV stroke volume is ejected into a high-pressure chamber (i.e., the aorta), although the low aortic diastolic pressure does facilitate ventricular emptying during early systole (**Fig. 66-9**). In MR, especially acute MR, the reduction of wall tension (i.e., reduced afterload) allows more complete systolic emptying; in AR the increase in LV end-diastolic volume (i.e., increased preload) provides hemodynamic compensation.[89,90]

Severe AR may occur with a normal effective forward stroke volume and a normal ejection fraction ([forward plus regurgitant stroke volume]/[end-diastolic volume]), together with an elevated LV end-diastolic volume, pressure, and stress (**Fig. 66-10**).[91] In accord with Laplace's law, which indicates that wall tension is related to the product of the intraventricular pressure and radius divided by wall thickness, LV dilation also increases the LV systolic tension required to develop any level of systolic pressure. Thus, in AR, there is an increase in preload and afterload. LV systolic function is maintained through the combination of chamber dilation and hypertrophy. This leads to eccentric hypertrophy, with replication of sarcomeres in series and elongation of myocytes and myocardial fibers. In compensated AR, there is sufficient wall thickening so that the ratio of ventricular wall thickness to cavity radius remains normal. This maintains or returns end-diastolic wall stress to normal levels. AR contrasts with AS, in which there is pressure overload (concentric) hypertrophy with replication of sarcomeres, largely in parallel, and an increased ratio of wall thickness to radius but, like AS, there is an increase in interstitial connective tissue. In AR, LV mass is usually greatly increased, often to levels even higher than in isolated AS. As AR persists and increases in severity over time, wall thickening fails to keep pace with the hemodynamic load and end-systolic wall stress rises. At this point, the afterload mismatch results in a decline in systolic function, and the ejection fraction falls.[90]

Patients with severe chronic AR have the largest end-diastolic volumes of those with any form of heart disease, resulting in so-called cor bovinum. However, end-diastolic pressure is not uniformly elevated

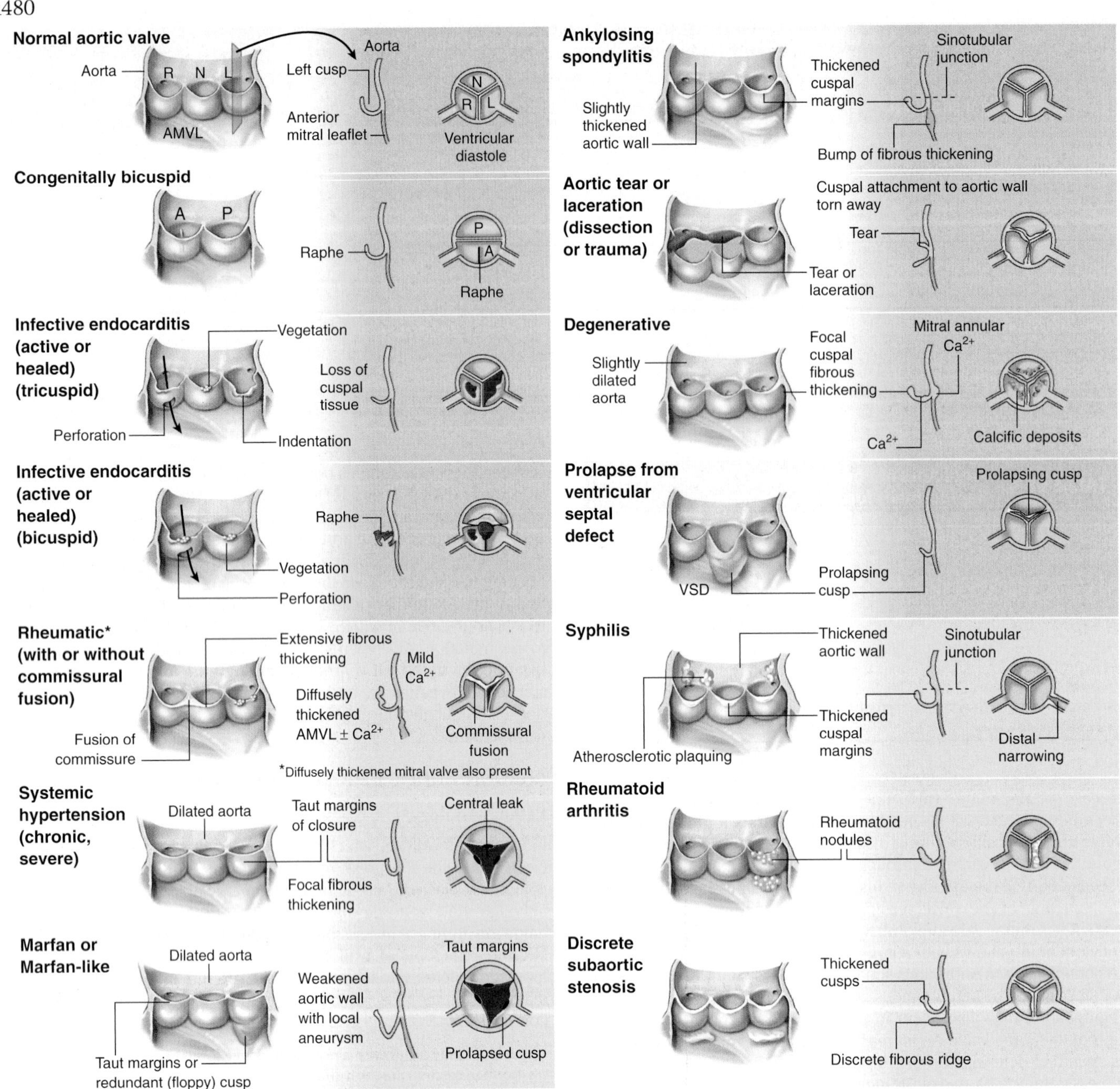

FIGURE 66-8 Diagram of various causes of pure aortic regurgitation. A = anterior; AMVL = anterior mitral valve leaflet; P = posterior; VSD = ventricular septal defect. *(From Waller BF: Rheumatic and nonrheumatic conditions producing valvular heart disease. Cardiovasc Clin 16:30, 1986.)*

(i.e., LV compliance is often increased; see Fig. 66-10). In more severe cases of AR, the regurgitant flow may exceed 20 liters/min, so the total LV output at rest approaches 25 liters/min, a level that can be achieved acutely only by a trained endurance runner during maximal exercise. Thus, the adaptive response to gradually increasing, chronic AR permits the ventricle to function as an effective high-compliance pump, handling a large stroke volume, often with little increase in filling pressure. During exercise, peripheral vascular resistance declines and, with an increase in heart rate, diastole shortens and the regurgitation per beat decreases, facilitating an increment in effective (forward) cardiac output without substantial increases in end-diastolic volume and pressure. The ejection fraction and related ejection phase indices are often within normal limits, both at rest and during exercise, even though myocardial function, as reflected in the slope of the end-systolic pressure-volume relationship, is depressed.

Left Ventricular Function. As the left ventricle decompensates, interstitial fibrosis increases, compliance declines, and LV end-diastolic pressure and volume rise (see Fig. 66-10). In advanced stages of decompensation, left atrial, pulmonary artery wedge, pulmonary arterial, right ventricular (RV), and right atrial pressures rise and the effective (forward) cardiac output falls, at first during exercise and then at rest. The normal decline in end-systolic volume or the rise in ejection fraction fails to occur during exercise. Symptoms of heart failure develop, particularly those secondary to pulmonary congestion.

Myocardial Ischemia. When acute AR is induced experimentally, myocardial oxygen requirements rise substantially, secondary to an increase in wall tension. In patients with chronic severe AR, total myocardial oxygen requirements are also augmented by the increase in LV mass. Because the major portion of coronary blood flow occurs during diastole, when arterial pressure is lower than normal in AR, coronary perfusion pressure is reduced. Studies in experimentally induced AR have shown a reduction in coronary flow reserve, with a change in forward coronary flow from diastole to systole. The result—a combination of increased oxygen demands and reduced supply—sets the stage for the development of myocardial ischemia, especially during exercise. Thus, patients with severe AR exhibit a reduction of coronary reserve, which may be responsible for myocardial ischemia and which may in turn play a role in the deterioration of LV function.

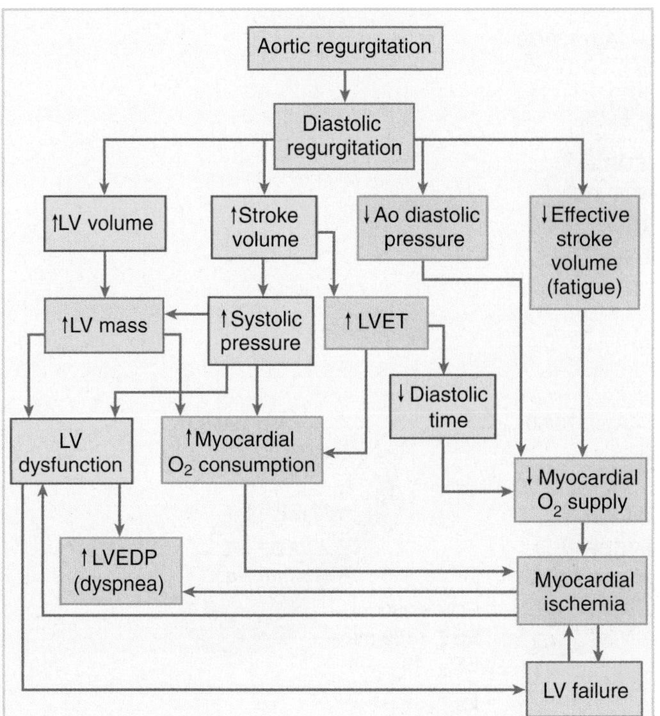

FIGURE 66-9 Pathophysiology of aortic regurgitation. Aortic regurgitation results in an increased LV volume, increased stroke volume, increased aortic (Ao) systolic pressure, and decreased effective stroke volume. Increased LV volume results in an increased LV mass, which may lead to LV dysfunction and failure. Increased LV stroke volume increases systolic pressure and prolongation of LV ejection time (LVET). Increased LV systolic pressure results in a decrease in diastolic time. Decreased diastolic time (myocardial perfusion time), diastolic aortic pressure, and effective stroke volume reduce myocardial O_2 supply. Increased myocardial O_2 consumption and decreased myocardial O_2 supply produce myocardial ischemia, which further deteriorates LV function. LVEDP = LV end-diastolic pressure. *(From Boudoulas H, Gravanis MB: Valvular heart disease.* In *Gravanis MB [ed]: Cardiovascular Disorders: Pathogenesis and Pathophysiology. St. Louis, CV Mosby, 1993, p 64.)*

Clinical Presentation

SYMPTOMS. In patients with chronic severe AR, the left ventricle gradually enlarges while the patient remains asymptomatic.[83,91] Symptoms of reduced cardiac reserve or myocardial ischemia develop, most often in the fourth or fifth decade and usually only after considerable cardiomegaly and myocardial dysfunction have occurred. The principal complaints of exertional dyspnea, orthopnea, and paroxysmal nocturnal dyspnea usually develop gradually. Angina pectoris is prominent late in the course; nocturnal angina may be troublesome and is often accompanied by diaphoresis, which occurs when the heart rate slows and arterial diastolic pressure falls to extremely low levels. Patients with severe AR often complain of an uncomfortable awareness of the heartbeat, especially on lying down, and disagreeable thoracic pain caused by pounding of the heart against the chest wall. Tachycardia, occurring with emotional stress or exertion, may cause troubling palpitations and head pounding. Premature ventricular contractions are particularly distressing because of the great heave of the volume-loaded left ventricle during the postextrasystolic beat. These complaints may be present for many years before symptoms of overt LV dysfunction develop.

Physical Examination

In patients with chronic, severe AR, the head may bob with each heartbeat (de Musset sign), and there are water hammer pulses, with abrupt distention and quick collapse (Corrigan pulse). The arterial pulse is often prominent and can be best appreciated by palpation of the radial artery with the patient's arm elevated (see Chap. 12). A bisferiens pulse may be present and is more readily recognized in the brachial and femoral arteries than in the carotid arteries. A variety of auscultatory findings provide confirmation of a wide pulse pressure. The Traube sign (also known as pistol shot sounds) refers to booming systolic and diastolic sounds heard over the femoral artery, the Müller sign consists of systolic pulsations of the uvula, and the Duroziez sign consists of a systolic murmur heard over the femoral artery when it is compressed proximally and a diastolic murmur when it is compressed distally. Capillary pulsations (the Quincke sign) can be detected by transmitting a light through the patient's fingertips or exerting gentle pressure on the tip of a fingernail.

Systolic arterial pressure is elevated, and diastolic pressure is abnormally low. Korotkoff sounds often persist to zero even though the intra-arterial pressure rarely falls below 30 mm Hg. The point of change in Korotkoff sounds (i.e., the muffling of these sounds in phase IV) correlates with the diastolic pressure. As heart failure develops, peripheral vasoconstriction may occur and arterial diastolic pressure may rise, even though severe AR is present. The Hill sign (an exaggerated difference in systolic blood pressure between the upper and lower extremities) is an artifact of sphygmomanometric measurements and is no longer considered a sign of severe AR.

The apical impulse is diffuse and hyperdynamic and is displaced laterally and inferiorly; there may be systolic retraction over the parasternal region. A rapid ventricular filling wave is often palpable at the apex. The augmented stroke volume may create a systolic thrill at the base of the heart or suprasternal notch, and over the carotid arteries. In many patients, a carotid shudder is palpable.

AUSCULTATION. The aortic regurgitant murmur, the principal physical finding of AR, is high frequency and begins immediately after A_2. It may be distinguished from the murmur of pulmonic regurgitation by its earlier onset (i.e., immediately after A_2 rather than after P_2) and usually by the presence of a widened pulse pressure. The murmur is heard best with the diaphragm of the stethoscope while the patient is sitting up and leaning forward, with the breath held in deep exhalation. In severe AR, the murmur reaches an early peak and then has a dominant decrescendo pattern throughout diastole.

The severity of AR correlates better with the duration than with the intensity of the murmur. In mild AR, the murmur may be limited to early diastole and is typically high-pitched and blowing. In severe AR, the murmur is holodiastolic and may have a rough quality. When the murmur is musical (cooing dove murmur), it usually signifies eversion or perforation of an aortic cusp. In patients with severe AR and LV decompensation, equilibration of aortic and LV pressures in late diastole abolishes the late diastolic component of the regurgitant murmur. When regurgitation is caused by primary valvular disease, the diastolic murmur is heard best along the left sternal border in the third and fourth intercostal spaces. However, when it is caused mainly by dilation of the ascending aorta, the murmur is often more readily audible along the right sternal border.

Many patients with chronic AR have a harsh systolic outflow murmur caused by the increased total LV stroke volume and ejection rate, which often radiates to the carotid vessels. The systolic murmur is often more readily audible than the diastolic murmur. It may be higher pitched and less rasping than the murmur of AS but is often accompanied by a systolic thrill. Palpation of the carotid pulses will elucidate the cause of the systolic murmur and differentiate it from the murmur of AS.

A_2 may be normal or accentuated when AR is caused by disease of the aortic root but is soft or absent when the valve is causing AR. P_2 may be obscured by the early diastolic murmur. Thus, S_2 may be absent or single or exhibit narrow or paradoxical splitting. A systolic ejection sound, presumably related to abrupt distention of the aorta by the augmented stroke volume, is frequently audible. A third heart sound (S_3) correlates with an increased LV end-diastolic volume. Its development may be a sign of impaired LV function, which is useful in identifying patients with severe AR who are candidates for surgical treatment.

A mid-diastolic and late diastolic apical rumble, the Austin Flint murmur, is common in severe AR and may occur in the presence of a normal mitral valve. This murmur appears to be created by severe aortic reflux impinging on the anterior leaflet of the mitral valve or the free LV wall; there is no convincing evidence for obstruction to mitral inflow in these patients.

ECHOCARDIOGRAPHY. Echocardiography (see Chap. 15) is helpful in identifying the cause of AR (see Figs. 15-48 and 15-49) and may demonstrate a bicuspid valve, thickening of the valve cusps, other

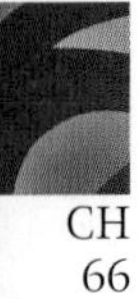

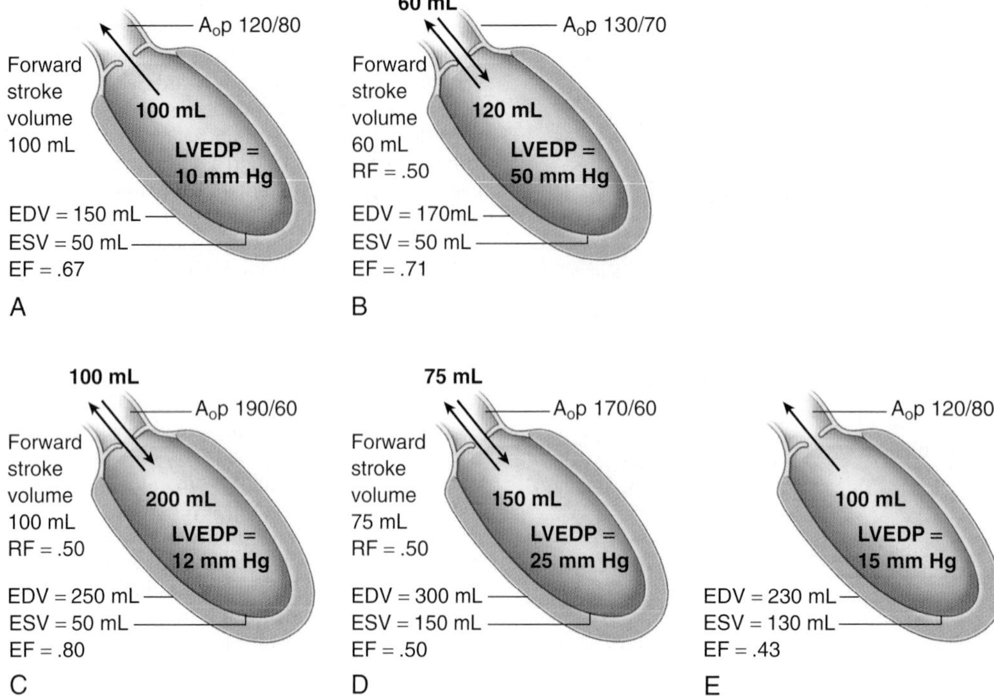

FIGURE 66-10 Hemodynamics of aortic regurgitation. **A,** Normal conditions. **B,** The hemodynamic changes that occur in severe acute aortic regurgitation. Although total stroke volume is increased, forward stroke volume is reduced. Left ventricular end-diastolic pressure (LVEDP) rises dramatically. **C,** Hemodynamic changes occurring in chronic compensated aortic regurgitation are shown. Eccentric hypertrophy produces increased end-diastolic volume (EDV), which permits an increase in total, as well as forward, stroke volume. The volume overload is accommodated, and left ventricular filling pressure is normalized. Ventricular emptying and end-systolic volume (ESV) remain normal. **D,** In chronic decompensated aortic regurgitation, impaired left ventricular emptying produces an increase in end-systolic volume and a fall in ejection fraction (EF), total stroke volume, and forward stroke volume. There is further cardiac dilation and reelevation of left ventricular filling pressure. **E,** Immediately following valve replacement, preload estimated by EDV decreases, as does filling pressure. ESV also is decreased, but to a lesser extent. The result is an initial fall in EF. Despite these changes, elimination of regurgitation leads to an increase in forward stroke volume, and with time ejection fraction increases. Aop = aortic pressure; RF = regurgitant fraction. *(From Carabello BA: Aortic regurgitation: Hemodynamic determinants of prognosis.* In *Cohn LH, DiSesa VJ [eds]: Aortic Regurgitation: Medical and Surgical Management. New York, Marcel Dekker, 1986, p 99-101.)*

congenital abnormalities, prolapse of the valve, a flail leaflet, or vegetation. In addition to leaflet anatomy and motion, the size and shape of the aortic root can be evaluated, although visualization of the ascending aorta is not always adequate and may require additional imaging procedures. Transthoracic imaging is usually satisfactory, but transesophageal echocardiography (TEE) often provides more detail, particularly of the aortic root.

Transthoracic echocardiography is useful for the measurement of LV end-diastolic and end-systolic dimensions and volumes, ejection fraction, and mass.[36] Two-dimensional guided M-mode measurements of LV dimensions are recommended when possible, because the high temporal resolution of this modality allows more accurate identification of endocardial borders. Care is needed to ensure that measurements are not oblique and are at the same site on subsequent studies. When the M-line is oblique, two-dimensional measurements are made in conjunction with the calculation of biplane ventricular end-diastolic and end-systolic volumes. Recent studies have suggested that end-systolic volume is a strong predictor of adverse clinical outcomes.[92,93] These measurements, when made serially, are of great value in selecting the optimal time for surgical intervention.

High-frequency fluttering of the anterior leaflet of the mitral valve during diastole may be seen in acute and chronic AR. However, it does not develop when the mitral valve is rigid, as occurs with rheumatic involvement. This sign, unlike the Austin Flint murmur, occurs even in mild AR and results from the movement imparted to the anterior leaflet of the mitral valve by the jet of blood regurgitating from the aorta.

Doppler echocardiography and color flow Doppler imaging are the most sensitive and accurate noninvasive techniques for the diagnosis and evaluation of AR. They readily detect mild degrees of AR that may be inaudible on physical examination. Both the aortic regurgitant orifice size and aortic regurgitant flow can be estimated quantitatively (**Fig. 66-11**; see Figs. 15-48 and 15-49)[36,94] and are strongly recommended.[1] These quantitative data provide the basis for the definitions of mild, moderate, and severe AR (see Table 66-1). Serial studies permit determination of the progression of AR and its effect on the left ventricle.

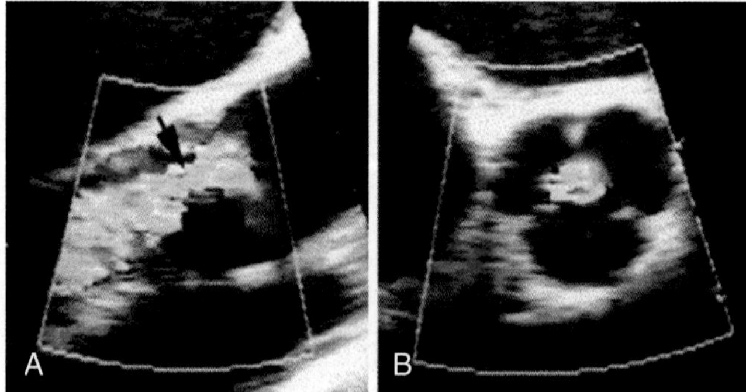

FIGURE 66-11 Transesophageal color Doppler imaging of the aortic regurgitant jet. **A,** Long-axis view. The black arrow indicates the vena contracta, the narrowest portion of the jet located at or just distal to its orifice. The width (in millimeters) of the vena contracta correlates well with volumetric measurement of regurgitant fraction and regurgitant volume. **B,** Short-axis view in the same patient. *(From Willett DL, Hall SA, Jessen ME, et al: Assessment of aortic regurgitation by transesophageal color Doppler imaging of the vena contracta: Validation against an intraoperative aortic flow probe. J Am Coll Cardiol 37:1450, 2001.)*

OTHER DIAGNOSTIC EVALUATION MODALITIES

Electrocardiography. Chronic severe AR results in left axis deviation and a pattern of LV diastolic volume overload, characterized by an increase in initial forces (prominent Q waves in leads I, aVL, and V_3 through V_6) and a relatively small wave in lead V_1. With the passage of time, these initial forces diminish, but the total QRS amplitude increases. The T waves may be tall and upright in the left precordial leads early in the course, but more commonly they are inverted, with ST-segment depressions. An LV strain pattern correlates with the presence of dilation and hypertrophy (see Chap. 13). Intraventricular conduction defects occur late in the course and are usually associated with LV dysfunction. The electrocardiogram (ECG) is not an accurate predictor of the severity of AR or cardiac weight. When AR is caused by an inflammatory process, prolongation of the PR interval may be present.

Radiography. Cardiac size is a function of the duration and severity of regurgitation and the state of LV function (see Fig. 16-22). In acute AR, there may be minimal cardiac enlargement, but marked enlargement is a common finding in chronic AR. Typically, the left ventricle enlarges in an inferior and leftward direction, causing a significant increase in the long axis but sometimes causing little or no increase in the transverse diameter of the heart. Calcification of the aortic valve is uncommon in patients with isolated AR but is often present in patients with combined AS and AR. Distinct left atrial enlargement in the absence of heart failure suggests associated mitral valve disease. Aneurysmal dilation of the aorta suggests that aortic root disease (e.g., the Marfan syndrome, cystic medial necrosis, annuloaortic ectasia) is responsible for the AR. Linear calcifications in the wall of the ascending aorta are seen in syphilitic aortitis but are nonspecific and are also observed in degenerative disease.

Angiography. For angiographic assessment of AR, contrast material should be injected rapidly (i.e., 25 to 35 mL/sec) into the aortic root, and filming should be carried out in the right and left anterior oblique projections (see Chap. 20). Opacification may be improved by filming during a Valsalva maneuver. In acute AR, there is only a slight increase in LV end-diastolic volume but, with the passage of time, both the end-diastolic volume and thickness of the LV wall increase, usually in parallel.[87]

Cardiac Magnetic Resonance Imaging. CMR provides accurate measurements of regurgitant volumes and the regurgitant orifice in AR (see Fig. 18-20). It is the most accurate noninvasive technique for assessing LV end-systolic volume, diastolic volume, and mass (see Chap. 18). CMR accurately quantifies the severity of AR on the basis of the antegrade and retrograde flow volumes in the ascending aorta and is recommended when echocardiographic evaluation of regurgitation is suboptimal.[41,95]

Disease Course

NATURAL HISTORY OF CHRONIC AORTIC REGURGITATION. Moderately severe or even severe chronic AR often is associated with a generally favorable prognosis for many years. Quantitative measures of AR severity predict clinical outcome, and LV size and systolic function also are strong predictors of clinical outcome. In a study of 251 asymptomatic patients (mean age, 61 years), the 10-year survival was 94% ± 4% in those with mild AR, compared with 69% ± 9% in those with severe AR (**Fig. 66-12**).[94] In contrast, in series involving younger asymptomatic patients (mean age, 39 years) with severe AR and normal LV ejection fractions, the mortality rate was less than 1%/year[1,91] and more than 45% remained asymptomatic with normal LV function at 10 years. The average rate of developing symptoms or LV systolic dysfunction in these latter series was less than 6%/year (**Fig. 66-13** and **Table 66-5**).

However, as is the case for AS, once the patient becomes symptomatic, the downhill course becomes rapidly progressive. Congestive heart failure, punctuated by episodes of acute pulmonary edema, and sudden death may occur, usually in previously symptomatic patients who have considerable LV dilation. Data compiled in the presurgical

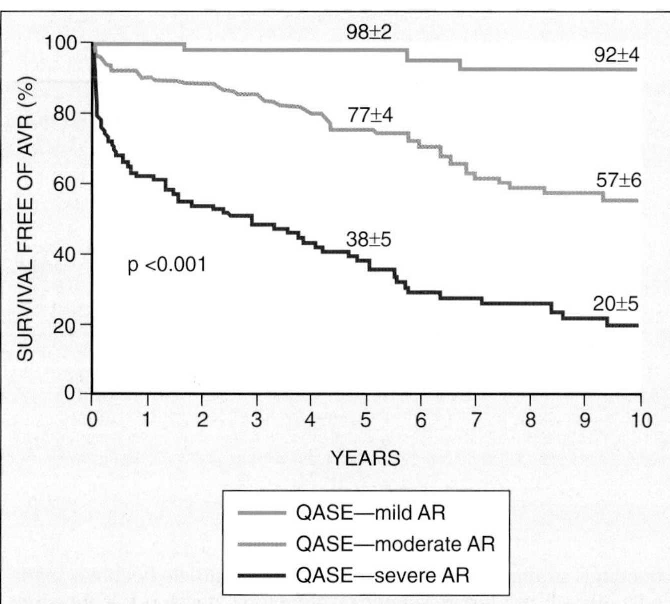

FIGURE 66-12 Composite end point of survival free of surgery for AR after diagnosis in asymptomatic patients. Patients are stratified according to quantitative criteria of the American Society of Echocardiography (QASE AR grading). The QASE-severe AR is defined as RV > 60 mL/beat or effective regurgitant orifice (ERO) > 30 mm² (red line). The QASE-mild AR is defined as RV < 30 mL/beat and ERO < 10 mm² (blue line) and QASE-moderate AR (yellow line) as larger than mild (RV, 30 mL/beat, or ERO, 10 mm²), but not reaching QASE-severe criteria. The 5- and 10-year rates of the endpoint ± standard error are indicated. Note the wide difference in outcome according to QASE grading at baseline. *(From Detaint D, Messika-Zeitoun D, Maalouf J, et al: Quantitative echocardiographic determinants of clinical outcome in asymptomatic patients with aortic regurgitation: A prospective study. J Am Coll Cardiol Img 1:1, 2008.)*

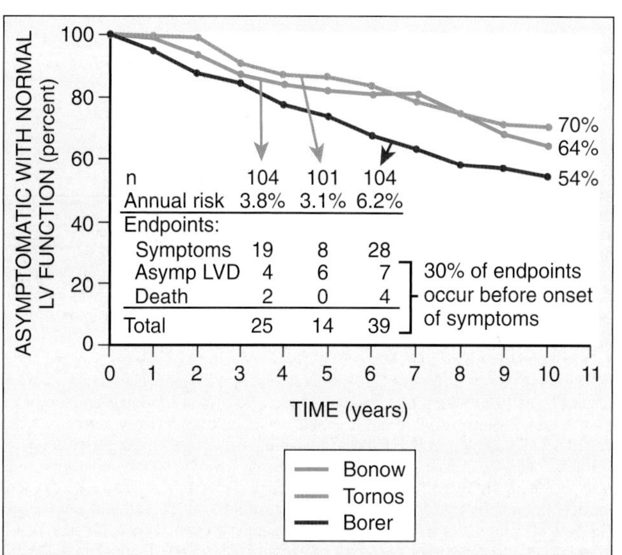

FIGURE 66-13 Natural history of chronic asymptomatic aortic regurgitation in patients with normal LV ejection fraction at rest in three series reported by Bonow and associates (blue line), Tornos and associates (yellow line), and Borer and colleagues (red line), each enrolling more than 100 patients. At 10 years, 54% to 70% of patients remained asymptomatic with normal LV function, such that the risk of developing symptoms, LV dysfunction (LVD), or death is approximately 3% to 6%/year. The endpoints encountered in these series are indicated. Most patients who deteriorated developed symptoms leading to aortic valve replacement. However, 25% to 30% of the endpoints, either asymptomatic LVD (Asymp LVD) or death, occurred without warning symptoms. *(Modified from Bonow RO, Lakatos E, Maron BJ, et al: Serial long-term assessment of the natural history of asymptomatic patients with chronic aortic regurgitation and normal left ventricular systolic function. Circulation 84:1625, 1991; Tornos MP, Olona M, Permanyer-Miralda G, et al: Clinical outcome of severe asymptomatic chronic aortic regurgitation: A long term prospective follow up study. Am Heart J 130:333, 1995; and Borer JS, Hochreiter C, Herrold EM, et al: Prediction of indications for valve replacement among asymptomatic and minimally symptomatic patients with chronic aortic regurgitation and normal left ventricular performance. Circulation 97:525, 1998.)*

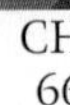

TABLE 66-5 Studies of the Natural History of Asymptomatic Aortic Regurgitation

	Progression to Symptoms, Death, or LV Dysfunction			*Progression to Asymptomatic LV Dysfunction*			
STUDY (YEAR)	NO. OF PATIENTS	MEAN FOLLOW-UP (yr)	RATE/ yr (%)	NO. OF PATIENTS	RATE/ yr (%)	MORTALITY (NO. OF PATIENTS)	COMMENTS
Bonow et al (1983, 1991)	104	8.0	3.8	4	0.5	2	Outcome predicted by LV ESD, EDD, change in EF with exercise, rate of change in ESD and EF at rest with time
Scognamiglio et al (1986)*	30	4.7	2.1	3	2.1	0	Three patients developing asymptomatic LV dysfunction initially had lower PAP/ESV ratios and trend toward higher LV ESD and EDD and lower FS.
Siemienczuk et al (1989)	50	3.7	4.0	1	0.5	0	Patients included those receiving placebo and medical dropouts in a randomized drug trial; included some patients with NYHA FC II symptoms; outcome predicted by LV ESV, EDV, change in EF with exercise, and end-systolic wall stress
Scognamiglio et al (1994)*	74	6.0	5.7	15	3.4	0	All patients received digoxin as part of a randomized trial.
Tornos et al (1995)	101	4.6	3.0	6	1.3	0	Outcome predicted by pulse pressure, LV ESD, EDD, and EF at rest
Ishii et al (1996)	27	14.2	3.6	—	—	0	Development of symptoms predicted by systolic BP, LV ESD, EDD, mass index, and wall thickness; LV function not reported in all patients
Borer et al (1998)	104	7.3	6.2	7	0.9	4	20% of patients in NYHA FC II; outcome predicted by initial FC II symptoms, change in LV EF with exercise, LV ESD, and LV FS
Tarasoutchi et al (2003)	72	10	4.7	1	0.1	0	Development of symptoms predicted by LV ESD and EDD; LV function not reported in all patients
Evangelista et al (2005)	31	7	3.6	—	—	1	Placebo control group in 7-year vasodilator clinical trial
Detaint et al (2008)	251	8.0	5.0	17	2.1	33	10-year actuarial survival free of AVR: 92 ± 4% with mild AR (RV <30 mL and ERO < 0.1cm^2) 57 ± 5% with moderate AR 20 ± 5% with severe AR (RV ≥ 60 mL and ERO ≥ 0.3 cm^2)

*Two studies by same authors involved separate patient groups.

BP = blood pressure, EDD = end-diastolic dimension; EDV = end-diastolic volume; EF = ejection fraction; ESD = end-systolic dimension; ESV = end-systolic volume; FC = functional class; FS = fractional shortening; PAP = pulmonary artery pressure.

Modified from Bonow RO, Carabello BA, Chatterjee K, et al: ACC/AHA 2006 guidelines for the management of patients with valvular heart disease: A report of the American College of Cardiology/American Heart Association Task Force on Practice Guidelines (writing Committee to Revise the 1998 guidelines for the management of patients with valvular heart disease) developed in collaboration with the Society of Cardiovascular Anesthesiologists endorsed by the Society for Cardiovascular Angiography and Interventions and the Society of Thoracic Surgeons. J Am Coll Cardiol 48:e1, 2006

Data from Bonow RO, Rosing DR, McIntosh CL, et al: The natural history of asymptomatic patients with aortic regurgitation and normal left ventricular function. Circulation 68:509,1983; Bonow RO, Lakatos E, Maron BJ, Epstein SE: Serial long-term assessment of the natural history of asymptomatic patients with chronic aortic regurgitation and normal left ventricular systolic function. Circulation 84:1625, 1991; Scognamiglio R, Fasoli G, Dalla Volta S: Progression of myocardial dysfunction in asymptomatic patients with severe aortic insufficiency. Clin Cardiol 9:151, 1986; Siemienczuk D, Greenberg B, Morris C, et al: Chronic aortic insufficiency: Factors associated with progression to aortic valve replacement. Ann Intern Med 110:587, 1989; Scognamiglio R, Rahimtoola SH, Fasoli G, et al: Nifedipine in asymptomatic patients with severe aortic regurgitation and normal left ventricular function. N Engl J Med 331:689, 1994; Tornos MP, Olona M, Permanyer Miralda G, et al: Clinical outcome of severe asymptomatic chronic aortic regurgitation: A long-term prospective follow-up study. Am Heart J 130:333; 1995; Ishii K, Hirota Y, Suwa M, et al: Natural history and left ventricular response in chronic aortic regurgitation. Am J Cardiol 78:357, 1996; Borer JS, Hochreiter C, Herrold EM, et al: Prediction of indications for valve replacement among asymptomatic or minimally symptomatic patients with chronic aortic regurgitation and normal left ventricular performance. Circulation 97:525, 1998; Tarasoutchi F, Grinberg M, Spina GS, et al: Ten-year clinical laboratory follow-up after application of a symptom-based therapeutic strategy to patients with severe chronic aortic regurgitation of predominant rheumatic etiology. J Am Coll Cardiol 41:1316, 2003; Evangelista A, Tornos P, Sambola A, et al: Long-term vasodilator therapy in patients with severe aortic regurgitation. N Engl J Med 353:1342, 2005; Detaint D, Messika-Zeitoun D, Maalouf J, et al: Quantitative echocardiographic determinants of clinical outcome in asymptomatic patients with aortic regurgitation: a prospective study. J Am Coll Cardiol Img 1:1, 2008.

era indicated that without surgical treatment, death usually occurred within 4 years after the development of angina pectoris and within 2 years after the onset of heart failure. Even in the current era, 4-year survival without surgery in patients with NYHA Class III or IV symptoms is only approximately 30% (**Fig. 66-14**).

Gradual deterioration of LV function may occur even during the asymptomatic period, and some patients may develop significant impairment of systolic function before the onset of symptoms. Numerous surgical series over the past two decades have indicated that depressed LV ejection fraction is among the most important determinants of mortality after AVR, particularly when LV dysfunction is irreversible and does not improve after operation.[1,2] LV dysfunction is more likely to be reversible if detected early, before ejection fraction becomes severely depressed, before the left ventricle becomes markedly dilated, and before significant symptoms develop. It is therefore important to intervene surgically before these changes have become irreversible.[30a,85,91]

Management

MEDICAL TREATMENT. There is no specific therapy to prevent disease progression in chronic AR. Patients with mild or moderate AR who are asymptomatic with normal or only minimally increased cardiac size require no therapy but should be followed clinically and by echocardiography every 12 or 24 months. Asymptomatic patients with chronic severe AR and normal LV function should be examined at intervals of approximately 6 months. In addition to clinical

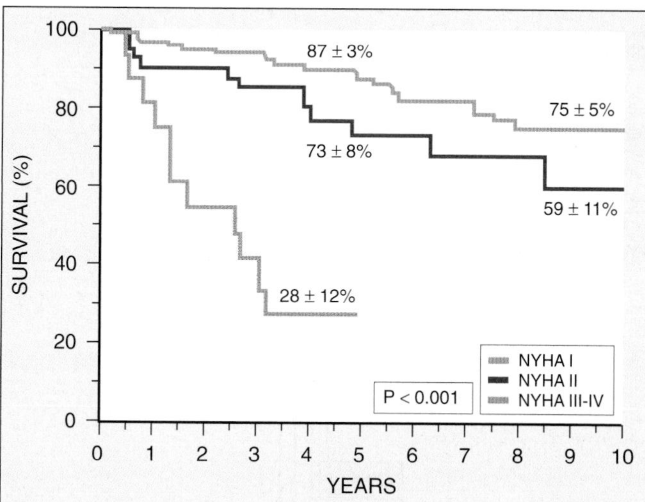

FIGURE 66-14 Survival without surgery in 242 patients with chronic aortic regurgitation, demonstrating the importance of symptoms in determining outcome. Patients with NYHA Class III or IV symptoms had a survival of only 28% at 4 years. In contrast, the 10-year survival in patients in Class I was 75%, which was identical to that of an age-matched normal population (75% at 10 years). *(From Dujardin KS, Enriquez-Sarano M, Schaff HV, et al: Mortality and morbidity of aortic regurgitation in clinical practice: A long-term follow-up study. Circulation 99:1851, 1999.)*

examination, serial echocardiographic assessments of LV size and ejection fraction should be made. CMR imaging is usually not necessary but may be useful for patients whose noninvasive test results are inconclusive or discordant with clinical findings or when further evaluation of aortic size is needed (see Fig 18-20). Patients with mild to moderate AR and those with severe AR with a normal ejection fraction and only mild ventricular dilation may engage in aerobic forms of exercise. However, patients with AR who have limitations of cardiac reserve and/or evidence of declining LV function should not engage in vigorous sports or heavy exertion.[54] Systemic arterial diastolic hypertension, if present, should be treated because it increases the regurgitant flow; vasodilating agents such as nifedipine or ACE inhibitors are preferred, and beta-blocking agents should be used with great caution. AF and bradyarrhythmias are poorly tolerated and should be prevented, if possible. If these arrhythmias occur, they must be treated promptly and vigorously. Recommendations for antibiotic prophylaxis for infective endocarditis have changed recently, and most patients with AR do not need prophylaxis (see Chap. 67).

Vasodilator Therapy. There is considerable uncertainty about whether patients with chronic AR and evidence of significant volume overload (increased end-diastolic dimension or volume) should be considered for vasodilator therapy.[96] Short-term studies spanning 6 months to 2 years have demonstrated beneficial hemodynamic effects of oral hydralazine, nifedipine, felodipine, and ACE inhibitors. One randomized study followed asymptomatic patients with severe AR for 6 years, comparing the effects of long-acting nifedipine (69 patients) and digoxin (74 patients) on LV function and symptoms. Nifedipine delayed the need for operation: at 6 years, 85% of patients receiving nifedipine remained asymptomatic, with a normal LV ejection fraction, compared with only 65% of patients receiving digoxin. However, a second randomized trial compared placebo, long-acting nifedipine, and enalapril in 95 consecutive patients who were followed for 7 years.[97] Neither nifedipine nor enalapril reduced the development of symptoms or LV dysfunction warranting AVR compared with placebo. Moreover, neither drug significantly altered LV dimension, ejection fraction, or mass over the course of time compared with placebo. In view of this equipoise, definitive recommendations regarding the indications for long-active nifedipine or ACE inhibitors are not possible.[1]

Symptomatic Patients

AVR is the treatment of choice for symptomatic patients. Chronic medical therapy may be necessary for some patients who refuse surgery or are considered to be inoperable because of comorbid conditions. These patients should receive an aggressive heart failure regimen (see Chap. 28) with ACE inhibitors (and perhaps other vasodilators), digoxin, diuretics, and salt restriction; beta blockers may also be beneficial.[98] Even though nitroglycerin and other nitrates are not as helpful in relieving anginal pain in patients with AR as they are in patients with coronary artery disease or AS, they are worth a try.

In patients who are candidates for surgery but who have severely decompensated LV dysfunction, vasodilator therapy may be particularly helpful in stabilizing patients while preparing for operation.

SURGICAL TREATMENT

Indications for Operation

Because of their excellent prognosis in the short and medium term, operative correction should be deferred in patients with chronic severe AR who are asymptomatic, have good exercise tolerance, and have an ejection fraction greater than 50% without severe LV dilation (i.e., end-diastolic diameter ≤75 mm; end-systolic diameter ≤55 mm) or progressive LV dilation on serial echocardiograms. In the absence of obvious contraindications or serious comorbidity, surgical treatment is advisable for symptomatic patients with severe AR and for asymptomatic patients with an ejection fraction of 50% or less, severe LV dilation (end-diastolic diameter > 75 mm or end-systolic diameter > 55 mm) or less severe dilation (end-diastolic diameter > 70 mm or end-systolic diameter > 50 mm), with evidence of progressive LV enlargement on serial echocardiograms.[1] Between these two ends of the clinical-hemodynamic spectrum are many patients in whom it may be difficult to balance the immediate risks of operation and the continuing risks of an implanted prosthetic valve, on the one hand, against the hazards of allowing a severe volume overload to damage the left ventricle, on the other.[85,90,91]

A proposed management strategy for patients with chronic severe AR is shown in **Figure 66-15**. Because severe symptoms (NYHA Class III or IV) and LV dysfunction with an ejection fraction less than 50% are independent risk factors for poor postoperative survival (**Fig. 66-16**), surgery should be carried out in NYHA Class II patients before severe LV dysfunction has developed.[1,2,83,92] Even after successful correction of AR, patients with severe LV dysfunction may have persistent cardiomegaly and depressed LV function. Such patients often exhibit persistent histologic changes in the left ventricle, including massive fiber hypertrophy and increased interstitial fibrous tissue. Therefore, it is highly desirable to operate on patients before irreversible LV changes have occurred.

Because AR has complex effects on preload and afterload, the selection of appropriate indices of ventricular contractility to identify patients for operation is challenging. The relationship between end-systolic wall stress and ejection fraction or percentage fractional shortening is a useful measurement,[35] as are more load-independent measures of LV contractility. However, in the absence of such complex measurements, serial changes in ventricular end-diastolic and end-systolic volumes or dimensions can be used to detect the relative deterioration of ventricular function.[90] Although LV end-diastolic volume and ejection phase indices (e.g., ejection fraction, ventricular fraction shortening) are strongly influenced by loading conditions, they are nonetheless useful empirical predictors of postoperative function.

Serial echocardiograms should be obtained to detect changes in LV size and function in asymptomatic patients with severe AR (see Fig. 66-15). Impaired LV function at rest is the basis for selecting patients for operation; normal LV function at rest with failure of the ejection fraction to rise normally with exercise is not considered an indication for surgery per se, but is an early warning sign that portends impaired function at rest. Echocardiographic measurements of LV size also are important, with M-mode LV end-diastolic and end-systolic dimensions, when possible, and with biplane apical calculations of the end-systolic volume index. Echocardiographic measurements should be made with side-by-side comparison of previous serial studies. A consistent change in dimensions or volumes, greater than measurement variability, must be ensured before recommending AVR for asymptomatic patients on the basis of these numbers alone.

CH 66

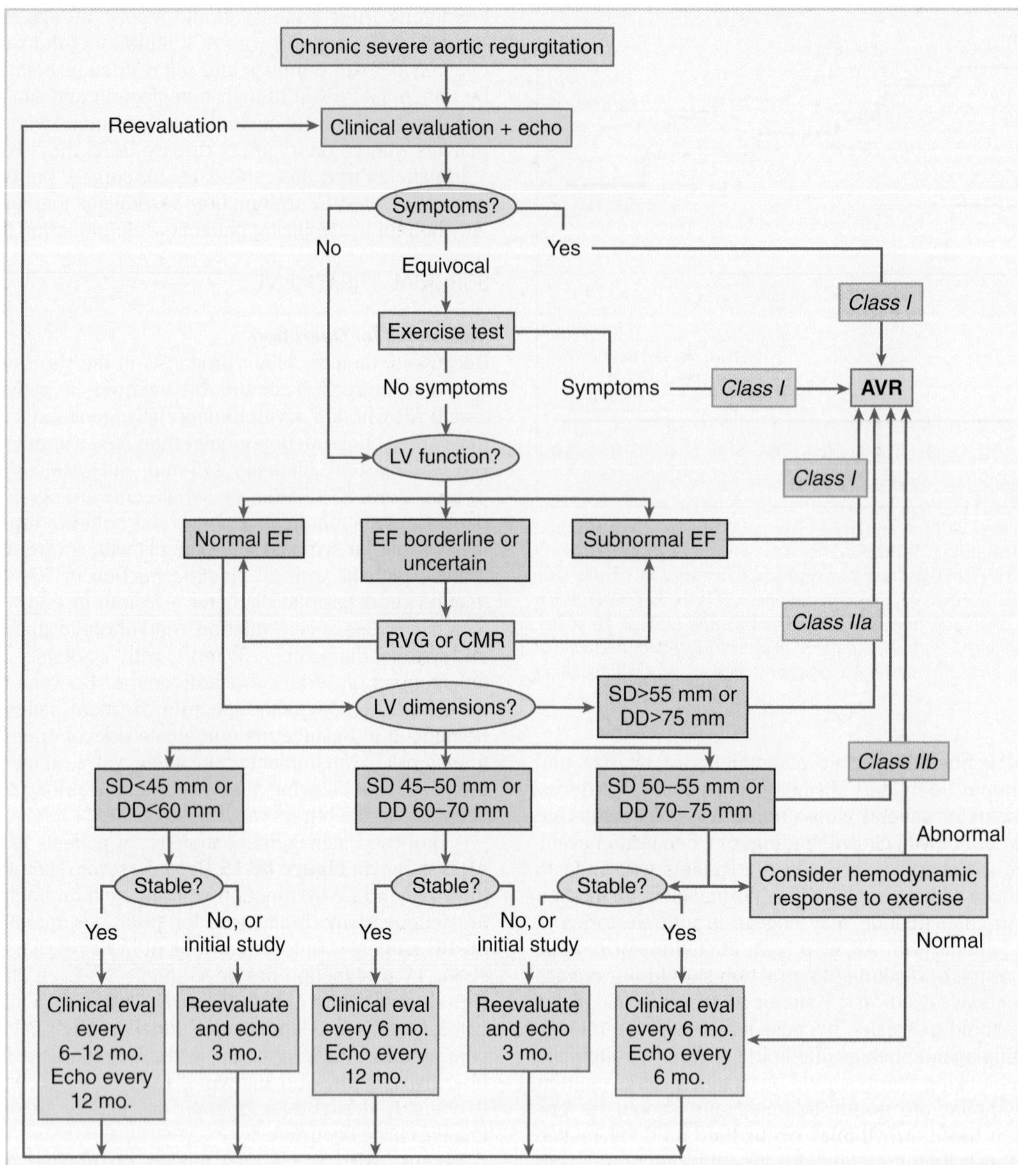

FIGURE 66-15 Management strategy for patients with chronic severe aortic regurgitation. Preoperative coronary angiography should be performed routinely as determined by age, symptoms, and coronary risk factors. Cardiac catheterization and angiography may also be helpful when there is discordance between clinical findings and echocardiography. "Stable" refers to stable echocardiographic measurements. In some centers, serial follow-up may be performed with radionuclide ventriculography (RVG) or CMR rather than echocardiography to assess LV volume and systolic function. DD = end-diastolic dimension; EF = ejection fraction; SD = end-systolic dimension. *(From Bonow RO, Carabello BA, Chatterjee K, et al: ACC/AHA 2006 guidelines for the management of patients with valvular heart disease: A report of the American College of Cardiology/American Heart Association Task Force on Practice Guidelines [writing committee to revise the 1998 Guidelines for the Management of Patients With Valvular Heart Disease]. Circulation 114:e84, 2006.)*

Asymptomatic patients with severe AR but normal LV function have an excellent prognosis and do not warrant prophylactic operation (see Table 66-5). On average, less than 6% of patients/year require operation because of the development of symptoms or of LV dysfunction (see Fig. 66-13), although the rate of symptom development is higher in patients older than 60 years.[94] The LV end-systolic dimension determined by echocardiography is valuable in predicting outcome in asymptomatic patients. Patients with severe AR and an end-systolic diameter less than 40 mm almost invariably remain stable and can be followed without immediate surgery. However, patients with an end-systolic diameter more than 50 mm have a 19% likelihood/year of developing symptoms of LV dysfunction, and those with an end-systolic diameter more than 55 mm have an increased risk of irreversible LV dysfunction if they are not operated on. Postoperative function and survival in this latter group is determined by the severity of symptoms, severity of LV dysfunction, and duration of LV dysfunction.[83,91] Indexed end-systolic dimension or volume (ESVI) may be a more robust indicator for timing of surgical intervention.[93,94] Patients with an ESVI ≥45 mL/m^2 are at higher risk of adverse outcomes.[94] Further data on the use of ESVI is needed before this approach becomes standard.

In summary, the following considerations apply to the selection of patients with chronic AR for surgical treatment.[1] Operation should be deferred in asymptomatic patients with normal and stable LV function and should be recommended for symptomatic patients (see Fig 66-15). In asymptomatic patients with LV dysfunction, a decision should be based not on a single abnormal measurement but rather on several observations of depressed performance and impaired exercise tolerance, carried out at intervals of 2 to 4 months. If evidence of LV dysfunction is borderline or inconsistent, continued close follow-up is indicated. If abnormalities are progressive and consistent (i.e., LV ejection fraction ≤ 50%, LV end-systolic diameter rises to >55 mm, or LV end-diastolic dimension rises to >75 mm), operation should be strongly considered, even in asymptomatic patients. It is also

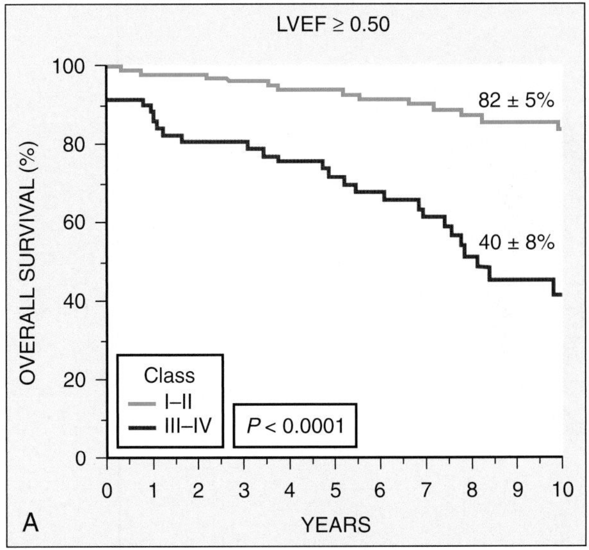

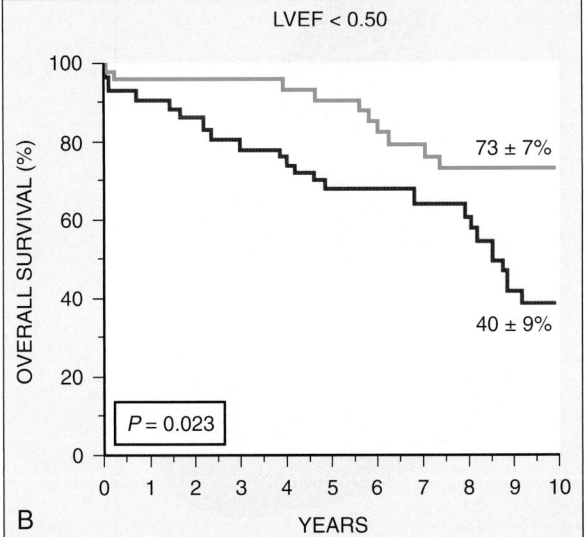

FIGURE 66-16 Long-term postoperative survival in patients with aortic regurgitation, stratified according to the severity of preoperative symptoms and preoperative left ventricular ejection fraction (LVEF). Patients with NYHA Class III or IV symptoms experienced significantly worse survival than those with Class I or II symptoms whether the echocardiographic LVEF was higher than 0.50 **(A)** or less than 0.50 **(B)** without associated coronary artery disease. *(From Klodas E, Enriquez-Sarano M, Tajik AJ, et al: Optimizing timing of surgical correction in patients with severe aortic regurgitation: Role of symptoms. J Am Coll Cardiol 30:746, 1997.)*

reasonable to consider AVR at lower levels of LV dilation (end-systolic dimension >50 mm; end-diastolic dimension >70 mm) in patients with progressive LV dilation on serial imaging studies. Symptomatic patients with severe AR who have normal, mildly depressed, or moderately depressed LV function should be operated on. Patients with severely impaired LV function (ejection fraction < 25%) are at high surgical risk and have a guarded prognosis, even after successful AVR. However, their outlook is also extremely poor when they receive medical therapy alone, and their management should be considered on an individual basis.

The indications for surgery for patients with severe AR secondary to aortic root disease are similar to those for patients with primary valvular disease. However, progressive expansion of the aortic root and/or a diameter more than 50 mm by echocardiography with any degree of regurgitation in patients with a bicuspid valve (or other connective tissue disorder) or with a diameter more than 55 mm in other patients is also an indication for aortic root replacement surgery.[1,98a]

As is the case for patients with other valvular lesions, adult surgical candidates who may have underlying coronary artery disease, based on symptoms, age, gender, and risk factors, should undergo preoperative coronary arteriography. Those with coronary artery stenoses should undergo revascularization at the time of AVR.

Operative Procedures

The standard surgical approach for chronic AR is valve replacement. Concurrent aortic root replacement is performed when aortic dilation is the cause or accompanies valve dysfunction. However, there is growing experience with surgical aortic valve repair, which is a viable option for selected patients in experienced centers.[99,100] Occasionally, when a leaflet has been torn from its attachments to the aortic annulus by trauma, surgical repair may be possible and, in patients with AR secondary to prolapse of an aortic leaflet, aortic cusp resuspension or cusp resection may be used. When AR is caused by leaflet perforation resulting from healed infective endocarditis, a pericardial patch can be used for repair. However, unlike patients with chronic MR, the large majority of patients with pure AR will require AVR rather than repair.

Because an increasing proportion of patients with severe isolated AR coming to operation now have primary aortic root rather than primary valvular disease, an increasing number can be treated surgically by correcting the dilated aortic root.[100,101] Aneurysmal dilation of the ascending aorta requires excision, replacement with a graft that includes a prosthetic valve, and reimplantation of the coronary arteries. In some patients with aortic root disease, the native valve can be spared when the aortic root is replaced or repaired (**Fig. 66-17**).

When AVR is performed in patients with severe AR, the aortic annulus often is larger than in patients with AS. Hence, a larger prosthetic valve can be inserted, and mild postoperative obstruction to LV outflow is less of a problem than it is in some patients with AS. In general, the risks and results of AVR in patients with AR are similar to those in patients with AS, with a large percentage of patients exhibiting striking improvement in symptoms. Reductions in heart size and in LV diastolic volume and mass occur in most patients.[90] Exceptions are patients who are in NYHA Class III or IV heart failure and/or patients who have severe LV dysfunction preoperatively. As is true for patients with AS, the operative risk of AVR for patients with AR depends on the general condition of the patient, state of LV function, and skill and experience of the surgical team. The mortality rate ranges from 3% to 8% in most medical centers (see Table 66-3). A late mortality of approximately 5% to 10%/year is observed in survivors who had marked cardiac enlargement and/or prolonged LV dysfunction preoperatively. Follow-up studies have shown both early rapid and then slower long-term reductions of LV mass, ejection fraction, myocyte hypertrophy, and ventricular fibrous content following relief of AR. By extending the indications for operation to symptomatic patients with normal LV function, as well as to asymptomatic patients with LV dysfunction, early and late results are improving. With the continued improvement of surgical techniques and results, it will likely become possible to extend the recommendation for operative treatment to asymptomatic patients with severe AR, normal LV systolic function, and only mild LV dilation. However, given the risks of operation and the long-term complications of presently available prosthetic valves, we do not believe that the time for such a policy has yet arrived.

ACUTE AORTIC REGURGITATION. Acute AR is caused most commonly by infective endocarditis, aortic dissection, or trauma (see Chaps. 60, 67, and 76).[102] The characteristic features of acute AR are tachycardia and an increase in LV diastolic pressures. In contrast to the pathophysiologic events in chronic AR just described, in which the left ventricle can adapt to the increased hemodynamic load, in acute AR the regurgitant volume fills a ventricle of normal size that cannot accommodate the combined large regurgitant volume and inflow from the left atrium. Because the ability of total stroke volume to rise acutely is limited, forward stroke volume declines. The sudden increase in LV filling causes the LV diastolic pressure to rise rapidly above left atrial pressure during early diastole (see Fig. 66-10), causing the mitral valve to close prematurely in diastole. Premature closure of the mitral valve, together with tachycardia that also shortens diastole, reduces the time interval during which the mitral valve is open. The tachycardia may compensate for the reduced forward stroke volume, and the LV and aortic systolic pressures may exhibit little change.

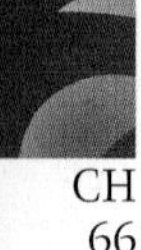

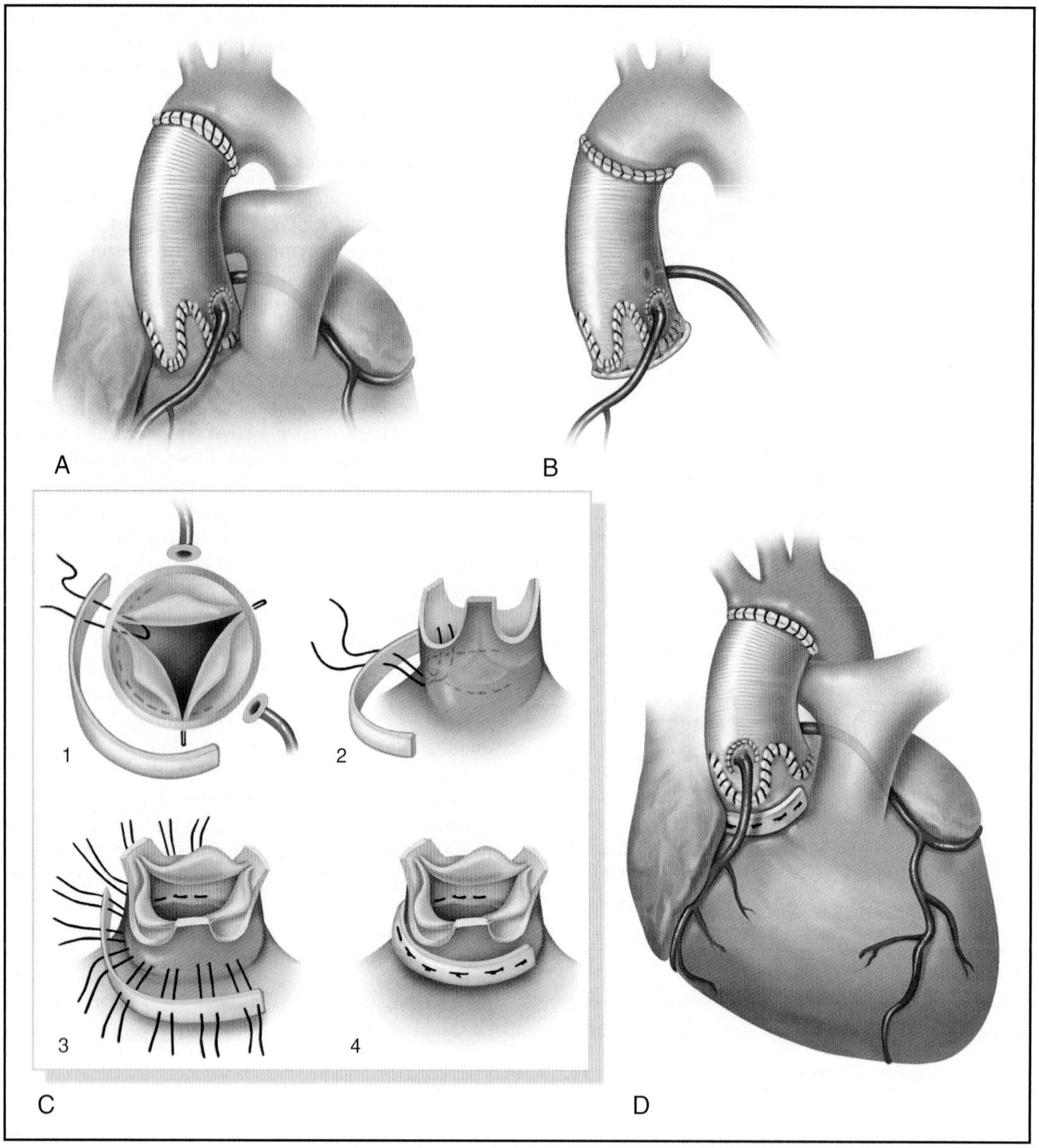

FIGURE 66-17 Repair of aortic regurgitation caused by aortic root dilation. **A,** Remodeling of the aortic root with replacement of all three aortic sinuses. **B,** Reimplantation of the aortic valve in patients with annuloaortic ectasia and aortic root aneurysm. **C, D,** Aortic annuloplasty in patients with annuloaortic ectasia. *(From David TE: Aortic root aneurysms: Remodeling or composite replacement? Ann Thorac Surg 64:1564, 1997.)*

However, acute severe AR may cause profound hypotension and cardiogenic shock. In light of the limited ability of the left ventricle to tolerate acute severe AR, patients with this valvular lesion often develop clinical manifestations of sudden cardiovascular collapse, including weakness, severe dyspnea, and profound hypotension secondary to the reduced stroke volume and elevated left atrial pressure. In some patients, the aortic diastolic pressure equilibrates with the elevated LV diastolic pressure.

Physical Examination. Patients with acute severe AR characteristically appear gravely ill, with tachycardia, severe peripheral vasoconstriction, and cyanosis, and sometimes pulmonary congestion and edema. The peripheral signs of AR are often not impressive and certainly not as dramatic as in patients with chronic AR. The normal or only slightly widened pulse pressure may lead to serious underestimation of the severity of the valvular lesion. The LV impulse is normal or almost normal, and the rocking motion of the chest characteristic of chronic AR is not apparent. S_1 may be soft or absent because of premature closure of the mitral valve, and the sound of mitral valve closure in mid or late diastole is occasionally audible. However, closure of the mitral valve may be incomplete, and diastolic MR may occur. Evidence of pulmonary hypertension, with an accentuated P_2, S_3, and S_4, is frequently present.

The early diastolic murmur of acute AR is lower pitched and shorter than that of chronic AR because as LV diastolic pressure rises, the (reverse) pressure gradient between the aorta and left ventricle is rapidly reduced. A systolic murmur is common, resulting in to and fro sounds. The Austin Flint murmur is often present, but is brief and ceases when LV pressure exceeds left atrial pressure in diastole. With premature diastolic closure of the mitral valve, the presystolic portion of the Austin Flint murmur is eliminated.

Echocardiography. In acute AR the echocardiogram reveals a dense, diastolic Doppler signal with an end-diastolic velocity approaching zero and premature closure and delayed opening of the mitral valve. LV size and ejection fraction are normal. This contrasts with the findings in chronic AR, in which end-diastolic dimensions and wall motion are increased. Occasionally, with equilibration of aortic and LV pressures in diastole, premature opening of the aortic valve may be detected.

Other Diagnostic Evaluation Modalities

Electrocardiography. In acute AR, the ECG may or may not show LV hypertrophy, depending on the severity and duration of the regurgitation. However, nonspecific ST-segment and T wave changes are common.

Radiography. In acute AR, there is often evidence of marked pulmonary venous hypertension and pulmonary edema. The cardiac silhouette is usually remarkably normal, although left atrial enlargement may be present and, depending on the cause of the AR, there may be enlargement of the ascending aorta.

Management of Acute Aortic Regurgitation. Because early death caused by LV failure is frequent in patients with acute severe AR despite intensive medical management, prompt surgical intervention is indicated. Even a normal ventricle cannot sustain the burden of acute, severe volume overload. Therefore, the risk of acute AR is much greater than that of chronic AR.[1] While the patient is being prepared for surgery, treatment with an intravenous positive inotropic agent (dopamine or dobutamine) and/or a vasodilator (nitroprusside) is often necessary. The agent and dosage should be selected on the basis of arterial pressure (see Chap. 27). Beta-blocking agents and intra-aortic balloon counterpulsation are contraindicated, because either lowering the heart rate or augmenting peripheral resistance during diastole can lead to rapid hemodynamic decompensation. In hemodynamically stable patients with acute AR secondary to active infective endocarditis, operation may be deferred to allow 5 to 7 days of intensive antibiotic therapy (see Chap. 67). However, AVR should be undertaken at the earliest sign of hemodynamic instability or if echocardiographic evidence of diastolic closure of the mitral valve develops.

Bicuspid Aortic Valve Disease

EPIDEMIOLOGY. A congenital bicuspid aortic valve is present in about 1% to 2% of the population and is more prevalent in men, accounting for 70% to 80 % of cases. A subset of bicuspid aortic valve patients have familial clustering consistent with an autosomal dominant inheritance with incomplete penetrance.[4,6] In some families with bicuspid aortic valve and associated congenital anomalies, a mutation in the *NOTCH1* gene has been described.[103]

PATHOPHYSIOLOGY. The most prevalent anatomy for a bicuspid valve is two cusps with a right-left systolic opening, consistent with congenital fusion of the right and left coronary cusps, seen in 70% to 80% of patients. An anterior-posterior orientation, with fusion of the right and noncoronary cusps, is less common, seen in about 20% to 30% of cases.[104,105] Fusion of the left and noncoronary cusps is rarely seen. A prominent ridge of tissue or raphe may be present in the larger of the two cusps so that the closed valve in diastole may mimic a trileaflet valve. Echocardiographic diagnosis relies on imaging the systolic leaflet opening with only two aortic commissures. Unicuspid valves are distinguished from a bicuspid valve by having only one aortic commissure.

Bicuspid aortic valve disease is associated with an aortopathy, with dilation of the ascending aorta related to accelerated degeneration of the aortic media (see Chap. 60).[4-6,86,104] The presence, location, and severity of aortic dilation is related to valve morphology but does not appear to be related to the severity of valve dysfunction per se. The risk of aortic dissection in patients with a bicuspid aortic valve is five to nine times higher than the general population.[101,105a] Some studies have also suggested an association between bicuspid aortic valve disease (anterior-posterior leaflet opening) and mitral valve prolapse.[106]

CLINICAL PRESENTATION. Patients with a bicuspid valve may be diagnosed at any age based on the presence of an aortic ejection sound or a systolic or diastolic murmur. However, some patients are initially diagnosed on echocardiography requested for other reasons. Often, the diagnosis is unknown until the patient develops valve dysfunction with physical examination findings and/or clinical symptoms.

Disease Course. Most bicuspid valves function normally until late in life, although a subset of patients present in childhood or adolescence with valve dysfunction. Overall, survival is not different than population estimates.[107,108] Risk factors for cardiac events are age older than 30 years, moderate or severe AR, and moderate or severe AS. Over a mean follow-up of 9 years, primary cardiac events occurred in 25% of 642 ambulatory adults with a bicuspid valve. Events included aortic valve or root replacement (22%), hospitalization for heart failure (2%), and cardiac death (3%; **Fig. 66-18**). Over their lifetime, approximately 20% of patients with bicuspid valves develop severe AR requiring AVR between 10 and 40 years of age. Patients with a bicuspid aortic valve also are at increased risk for endocarditis (0.4/100,000), accounting for about 1200 deaths/year in the United States. However, most patients with a bicuspid valve develop calcific valve stenosis later in life, typically presenting with severe AS after 50 years of age. Although the histopathology of calcific stenosis of a bicuspid aortic valve is no different than that of a trileaflet

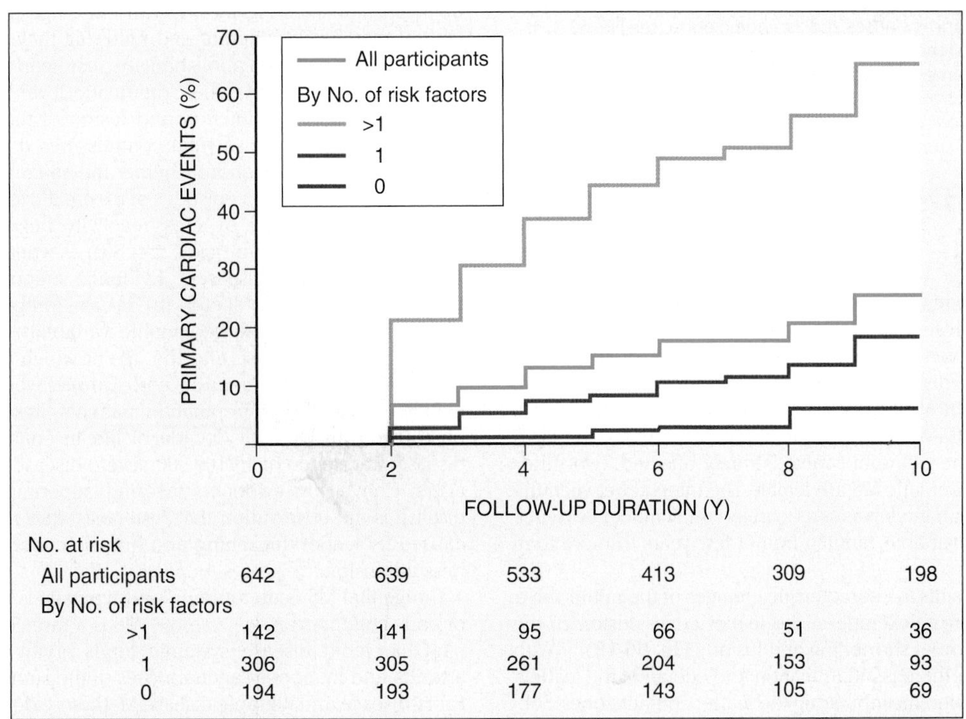

FIGURE 66-18 Outcome of patients with bicuspid aortic valves. The frequency of primary cardiac events in patients with more than one risk factor at baseline (*n* = 142) was 65% (standard deviation [SD] = 5%); in all participants (*N* = 642), 25% (SD = 2%); in patients with one risk factor at baseline (*n* = 306), 18% (SD = 3%); and in patients with no risk factors at baseline (*n* = 194), 6% (SD = 2%). The risk factors for primary cardiac events were age older than 30 years, moderate or severe aortic regurgitation, and moderate or severe aortic stenosis. *(From Tzemos N, Therrien J, Yip J, et al: Outcomes in adults with bicuspid aortic valves. JAMA 300:1317, 2008.)*

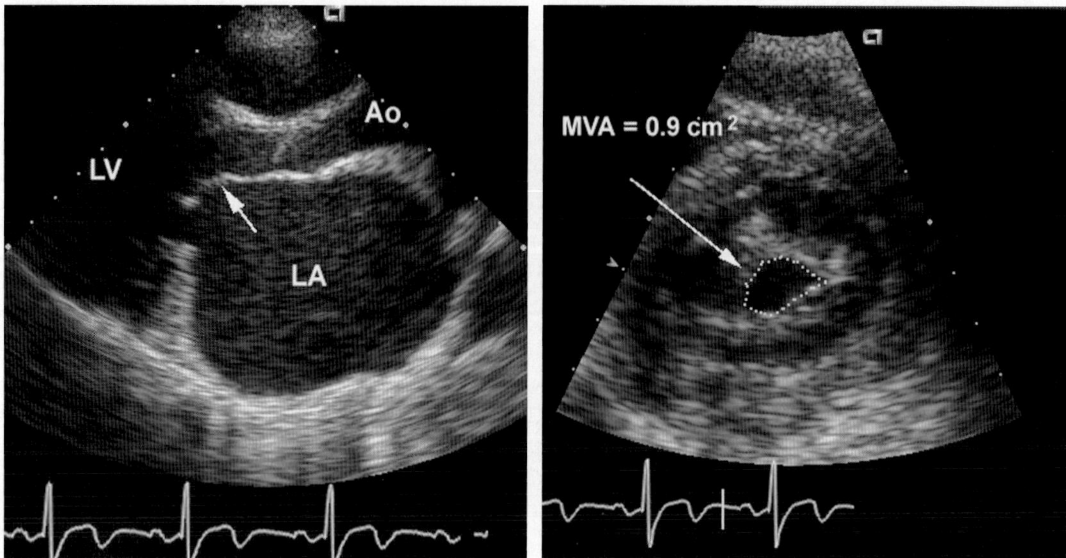

FIGURE 66-19 Parasternal long-axis **(left)** and short-axis **(right)** two-dimensional echocardiographic views showing the characteristic findings in rheumatic mitral stenosis. Note the commissural fusion that results in doming of the leaflets in the long-axis view and in a decrease in the width of the mitral orifice in the short-axis view. This patient has relatively thin, flexible leaflets with little subvalvular involvement. Ao = aorta; LA = left atrium; LV = left ventricle. *(From Otto CM: Valvular Heart Disease. Elsevier, Philadelphia, 2004.)*

valve, the turbulent flow and increased leaflet stress caused by the abnormal architecture is postulated to result in accelerated valve changes, providing an explanation for the earlier average age at presentation of patients with a bicuspid, compared with trileaflet, stenotic valve. Bicuspid valve disease accounts for over 50% of AVRs in the United States[3] and is a common cause of calcific AS, even in older individuals.

MANAGEMENT. The management of bicuspid aortic valve disease is directed toward the hemodynamic consequences of valve dysfunction—AS or AR—as discussed in these sections earlier. Currently, there are no effective medical therapies to prevent progressive valve deterioration when a bicuspid valve is diagnosed. In addition to appropriate follow-up for valve dysfunction, evaluation of the ascending aorta is needed, often with CT or CMR imaging to ensure adequate visualization and accurate measurement of the aortic sinuses and ascending aorta (see Fig. 60-4). If AVR is needed for stenosis or regurgitation, concurrent aortic root replacement is recommended if the maximum aortic dimension (measured at end-diastole) exceeds 45 mm. Even in the absence of aortic valve disease, aortic root replacement is recommended when the aortic dimension exceeds 50 mm in adults with a bicuspid aortic valve.[1,98a]

Mitral Valve Disease

Mitral Stenosis

CAUSE. The predominant cause of MS is rheumatic fever,[109] with rheumatic changes present in 99% of stenotic mitral valves excised at the time of mitral valve (MV) replacement. About 25% of all patients with rheumatic heart disease have isolated MS, and about 40% have combined MS and MR. Multivalve involvement is seen in 38% of MS patients, with the aortic valve affected in about 35% and the tricuspid valve in about 6%. The pulmonic valve is rarely affected. Two thirds of all patients with rheumatic MS are female. The interval between the initial episode of rheumatic fever (see Chap. 88) and clinical evidence of MV obstruction is variable, ranging from a few years to more than 20 years.[110]

Rheumatic fever results in characteristic changes of the mitral valve; diagnostic features are thickening at the leaflet edges, fusion of the commissures, and chordal shortening and fusion (**Fig. 66-19**).[111] With acute rheumatic fever, there is inflammation and edema of the leaflets, with small fibrin-platelet thrombi along the leaflet contact zones. Subsequent scarring leads to the characteristic valve deformity, with obliteration of the normal leaflet architecture by fibrosis, neovascularization and increased collagen and tissue cellularity. Aschoff bodies, the pathologic hallmark of rheumatic disease, are most frequently seen in the myocardium, not the valve tissue, with Aschoff bodies identified in only 2% of autopsied patients with chronic valve disease.

These anatomic changes lead to a typical functional appearance of the rheumatic mitral valve. In earlier stages of the disease, the relatively flexible leaflets snap open in diastole into a curved shape because of restriction of motion at the leaflet tips. This diastolic doming is most evident in the motion of the anterior leaflet and becomes less prominent as the leaflets become more fibrotic and calcified. The symmetrical fusion of the commissures results in a small central oval orifice in diastole that on pathologic specimens is shaped like a fish mouth or buttonhole because the anterior leaflet is not in the physiological open position (see Fig. 66-19). With end-stage disease, the thickened leaflets may be so adherent and rigid that they cannot open or shut, reducing or, rarely, even abolishing the first heart sound and leading to combined MS and MR. When rheumatic fever results exclusively or predominantly in contraction and fusion of the chordae tendineae, with little fusion of the valvular commissures, dominant MR results.

A debate continues about whether the anatomic changes in severe MS result from recurrent episodes of rheumatic fever, a chronic autoimmune process caused by cross-reactivity between a streptococcal protein and valve tissue (see Chap. 88), or whether there is superimposed calcific valve disease.[112] Evidence supporting recurrent infection as an important factor in disease progression includes the correlation between the geographic variability in the prevalence of rheumatic heart disease and the age at which patients present with severe MS. In North America and Europe, where there is approximately 1 case/100,000 population, patients present with severe valve obstruction in the sixth decade of life. In contrast, in Africa, with a disease prevalence of 35/100,000, severe disease often is seen in teenagers. Conversely, evidence favoring superimposed calcific valve disease is the observation that restenosis after mitral valvuloplasty is caused by leaflet thickening and fibrosis rather than recurrent commissural fusion.[113]

Congenital MS is uncommon and typically is diagnosed in infancy or early childhood (see Chap. 65). MS is a rare complication of malignant carcinoid disease, systemic lupus erythematosus, rheumatoid arthritis, and mucopolysaccharidoses of the Hunter-Hurler phenotype, Fabry disease, and Whipple disease. Methysergide therapy is an unusual but documented cause of MS. The association of atrial septal defect with rheumatic MS is called Lutembacher syndrome.

Other conditions may result in obstruction to LV inflow, including a left atrial tumor, particularly myxoma (see Chap. 74), ball valve thrombus in the left atrium (usually associated with MS), infective endocarditis with large vegetations (see Chap. 67), or a congenital membrane in the left atrium (i.e., cor triatriatum; see Chap. 65). In older patients, extensive mitral annular calcification may result in restriction of the size and motion of the annulus and may extend onto the base of the mitral leaflets, resulting in functional MS, although obstruction rarely is severe.

PATHOPHYSIOLOGY. The most useful descriptor of the severity of mitral valve obstruction is the degree of valve opening in diastole, or the mitral valve orifice area. In normal adults, the cross-sectional area of the mitral valve orifice is 4 to 6 cm^2 (see Table 66-1). When the orifice is reduced to approximately 2 cm^2, which is considered to represent mild MS, blood can flow from the left atrium to the left ventricle only if propelled by a small, although abnormal, pressure gradient. When the mitral valve opening is reduced to 1 cm^2, which is considered to represent severe MS,[114] a left atrioventricular pressure gradient of approximately 20 mm Hg (and therefore, in the presence of a normal LV diastolic pressure, a mean left atrial pressure >25 mm Hg) is required to maintain normal cardiac output at rest (**Fig. 66-20**; see Fig. 20-14).

The transvalvular pressure gradient for any given valve area is a function of the square of the transvalvular flow rate.[114] Thus, a doubling of flow rate quadruples the pressure gradient. The elevated left atrial pressure, in turn, raises pulmonary venous and capillary pressures, resulting in exertional dyspnea. The first bouts of dyspnea in patients with MS are usually precipitated by tachycardia resulting from exercise, pregnancy, hyperthyroidism, anemia, infection, or AF. All these (1) increase the rate of blood flow across the mitral orifice, resulting in further elevation of the left atrial pressure, and (2) decrease the diastolic filling time, resulting in a reduction in forward cardiac output. Because diastole shortens proportionately more than systole as heart rate increases, the time available for flow across the mitral valve is reduced at higher heart rates. Therefore, at any given stroke volume, tachycardia results in a higher instantaneous volume flow rate and higher transmitral pressure gradient, which elevates left atrial pressures further. This higher transmitral gradient, often in combination with inadequate ventricular filling (because of the shortened diastolic filling time), explains the sudden occurrence of dyspnea and pulmonary edema in previously asymptomatic patients with MS who develop AF with a rapid ventricular rate. It also accounts for the equally rapid improvement in these patients when the ventricular rate is slowed.

Atrial contraction augments the presystolic transmitral valvular gradient by approximately 30% in patients with MS. AF is common in patients with MS, with an increasing prevalence with age. In patients with severe MS younger than 30 years, only about 10% are in AF compared with approximately 50% of those older than 50 years. Withdrawal of atrial transport when AF develops reduces cardiac output by approximately 20%, often resulting in symptom onset.

Obstruction at the mitral valve level has other hemodynamic consequences, which account for many of the adverse clinical outcomes associated with this disease. Elevated left atrial pressure results in pulmonary artery hypertension, with secondary effects on the pulmonary vasculature and right heart. In addition, left atrial enlargement and stasis of blood flow is associated with an increased risk of thrombus formation and systemic embolism. Typically, the left ventricle is relatively normal, unless there is coexisting MR, with the primary abnormalities of the left ventricle being a small underfilled chamber and paradoxical septal motion caused by RV enlargement and dysfunction.

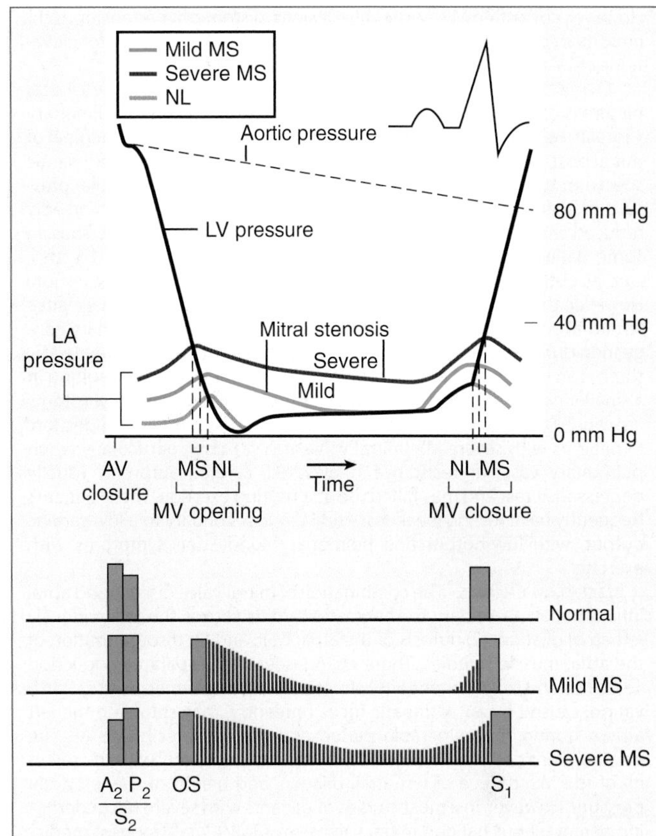

FIGURE 66-20 Schematic representation of LV, aortic, and left atrial (LA) pressures, showing normal relationships and alterations with mild and severe MS. Corresponding classic auscultatory signs of MS are shown at the bottom. The higher left atrial v wave of severe MS causes earlier pressure crossover and earlier MV opening, leading to a shorter time interval between aortic valve (AV) closure and the opening snap (OS). The higher left atrial end-diastolic pressure with severe MS also results in later closure of the mitral valve. With severe MS, the diastolic rumble becomes longer and there is accentuation of the pulmonic component (P_2) of the second heart sound (S_2) in relation to the aortic component (A_2).

Hemodynamic Consequences of Mitral Stenosis

Pulmonary Hypertension. In patients with MS and sinus rhythm, mean left atrial pressure is elevated (see Fig. 66-20), and the left atrial pressure curve shows a prominent atrial contraction (*a* wave), with a gradual pressure decline after mitral valve opening (*y* descent). In patients with mild to moderate MS without elevated pulmonary vascular resistance, pulmonary arterial pressure may be normal or only minimally elevated at rest but rises during exercise. However, in patients with severe MS and those in whom the pulmonary vascular resistance is significantly increased, pulmonary arterial pressure is elevated when the patient is at rest. Rarely, in patients with extremely elevated pulmonary vascular resistance, pulmonary arterial pressure may exceed systemic arterial pressure. Further elevations of left atrial and pulmonary vascular pressures occur during exercise and/or tachycardia.

Pulmonary hypertension in patients with MS results from the following: (1) passive backward transmission of the elevated left atrial pressure; (2) pulmonary arteriolar constriction, which presumably is triggered by left atrial and pulmonary venous hypertension (reactive pulmonary hypertension); and (3) organic obliterative changes in the pulmonary vascular bed, which may be considered to be a complication of long-standing and severe MS (see Chap. 78). With moderately elevated pulmonary arterial pressure (systolic pressure 30 to 60 mm Hg), RV performance is usually maintained. In time, severe pulmonary hypertension results in right-sided heart failure, with dilation of the right ventricle and its annulus, secondary tricuspid regurgitation (TR), and sometimes pulmonic regurgitation. These changes in the pulmonary vascular bed may also exert a protective effect; the elevated precapillary resistance makes the development of symptoms of pulmonary congestion less likely to occur by tending to prevent blood from surging into the pulmonary capillary bed and damming up behind the stenotic mitral valve. However, this protection occurs at the expense of a reduced cardiac output. In patients with severe MS, pulmonary vein–bronchial vein shunts occur. Their rupture may cause hemoptysis. Patients with severe MS manifest a reduction in pulmonary compliance, increase in the work of breathing, and redistribution of pulmonary blood flow from the base to the apex.

Left Ventricular Function. The LV chamber typically is normal or small, with normal systolic function and normal LV end-diastolic pressure.

However, coexisting MR, aortic valve lesions, systemic hypertension, ischemic heart disease, and cardiomyopathy may all be responsible for elevations of LV diastolic pressure

Exercise Hemodynamics. At any given severity of stenosis, the clinical picture is dictated largely by the levels of cardiac output and pulmonary vascular resistance with exertion. The response to a given degree of mitral obstruction may be characterized at one end of the hemodynamic spectrum by a normal cardiac output and high left atrioventricular pressure gradient or, at the opposite end of the spectrum, by a markedly reduced cardiac output and low transvalvular pressure gradient. Thus, in some patients with moderate MS (mitral valve area = 1.0 to 1.5 cm^2), cardiac output at rest may be normal and rises normally during exertion. However, the high transvalvular pressure gradient with exertion elevates left atrial and pulmonary capillary pressures, leading to pulmonary congestion during exertion. In contrast, in other patients with moderate MS, there is an inadequate rise in cardiac output during exertion, resulting in a smaller rise in pulmonary venous pressure. In these patients, symptoms are caused by a low cardiac output rather than by pulmonary congestion. In patients with severe MS (mitral valve area < 1 cm^2), particularly when pulmonary vascular resistance is elevated, cardiac output is usually depressed at rest and may fail to rise at all during exertion. These patients frequently have resting weakness and fatigue secondary to a low cardiac output, with low-output and pulmonary congestion symptoms with exercise.

Left Atrial Changes. The combination of mitral valve disease and atrial inflammation secondary to rheumatic carditis causes the following: (1) left atrial dilation; (2) fibrosis of the atrial wall; and (3) disorganization of the atrial muscle bundles. These changes lead to disparate conduction velocities and inhomogeneous refractory periods. Premature atrial activation, caused by an automatic focus or reentry, may stimulate the left atrium during the vulnerable period and thereby precipitate AF. The development of this arrhythmia correlates independently with the severity of the MS, degree of left atrial dilation, and height of the left atrial pressure. However, in a most studies of patients with severe MS undergoing percutaneous balloon mitral valvotomy (BMV), the strongest predictor of AF is older age. AF is often episodic at first but then becomes more persistent. AF per se causes diffuse atrophy of atrial muscle, further atrial enlargement, and further inhomogeneity of refractoriness and conduction. These changes, in turn, lead to irreversible AF.

CLINICAL PRESENTATION

Symptoms

DYSPNEA. The most common presenting symptoms of MS are dyspnea, fatigue, and decreased exercise tolerance.[115] Symptoms may be caused by a reduced ability to increase cardiac output normally with exercise or elevated pulmonary venous pressures and reduced pulmonary compliance. Dyspnea may be accompanied by cough and wheezing. Vital capacity is reduced, presumably because of the presence of engorged pulmonary vessels and interstitial edema. Patients who have critical obstruction to left atrial emptying and dyspnea with ordinary activity (NYHA functional Class III) generally have orthopnea as well and are at risk of experiencing attacks of frank pulmonary edema. The latter may be precipitated by effort, emotional stress, respiratory infection, fever pregnancy, or AF with a rapid ventricular rate or other tachyarrhythmia. Pulmonary edema may be caused by any condition that increases the flow rate across the stenotic mitral valve, either because of an increase in total cardiac output or a reduction in the time available for blood flow across the mitral orifice to occur. In patients with a markedly elevated pulmonary vascular resistance, RV function is often impaired and the presentation may also include symptoms and signs of right heart failure.

MS is a slowly progressive disease, and many patients remain seemingly asymptomatic merely by readjusting their lifestyles to a more sedentary level. Usually, symptom status can be accurately assessed by a directed history, asking the patient to compare current levels of maximum exertion to specific time points in the past. Exercise testing may be useful for selected patients to determine functional status in an objective manner and may be combined with Doppler echocardiography (see later) to assess exercise hemodynamics.

HEMOPTYSIS. Hemoptysis is rare in patients with a known diagnosis of MS because intervention is performed before severe obstruction becomes chronic. When hemoptysis does occur, it can be sudden and severe, caused by rupture of thin-walled, dilated bronchial veins, usually as a consequence of a sudden rise in left atrial pressure, or it may be milder, with only blood-stained sputum associated with attacks of paroxysmal nocturnal dyspnea. MS patients also may have pink frothy sputum characteristic of acute pulmonary edema with rupture of alveolar capillaries. Hemoptysis also may be caused by pulmonary infarction, a late complication of MS associated with heart failure.

CHEST PAIN. Chest pain is not a typical symptom of MS, but a small percentage, perhaps 15%, of patients with MS experience chest discomfort that is indistinguishable from that of angina pectoris. This symptom may be caused by severe RV hypertension secondary to the pulmonary vascular disease or by concomitant coronary atherosclerosis. Rarely, chest pain may be secondary to coronary obstruction caused by coronary embolization. In many patients, however, a satisfactory explanation for the chest pain cannot be uncovered, even after complete hemodynamic and angiographic studies.

PALPITATIONS AND EMBOLIC EVENTS. Patients with AF often are initially diagnosed when they present with AF or an embolic event.

OTHER SYMPTOMS. Compression of the left recurrent laryngeal nerve by a greatly dilated left atrium, enlarged tracheobronchial lymph nodes, and dilated pulmonary artery may cause hoarseness (Ortner syndrome). A history of repeated hemoptysis is common in patients with pulmonary hemosiderosis. Systemic venous hypertension, hepatomegaly, edema, ascites, and hydrothorax are all signs of severe MS with elevated pulmonary vascular resistance and right-sided heart failure.

PHYSICAL EXAMINATION. The most common findings on physical examination in patients with MS are an irregular pulse caused by AF and signs of left and right heart failure (see Chap. 12). The classic diastolic murmur and loud first heart sound are often difficult to appreciate. Patients with severe chronic MS, a low cardiac output, and systemic vasoconstriction may exhibit the so-called mitral facies, characterized by pinkish-purple patches on the cheeks. The arterial pulse is usually normal, but in patients with a reduced stroke volume, the pulse may be low in volume. The jugular venous pulse usually exhibits a prominent *a* wave in patients with sinus rhythm and elevated pulmonary vascular resistance. In patients with AF, the *x* descent of the jugular venous pulse disappears, and there is only one crest, a prominent *v* or *c-v* wave, per cardiac cycle. Palpation of the cardiac apex usually reveals an inconspicuous left ventricle; the presence of a palpable presystolic expansion wave or an early diastolic rapid filling wave speaks strongly against serious MS. A readily palpable, tapping S_1 suggests that the anterior mitral valve leaflet is pliable. When the patient is in the left lateral recumbent position, a diastolic thrill of MS may be palpable at the apex. Often, a RV lift is felt in the left parasternal region in patients with pulmonary hypertension. A markedly enlarged right ventricle may displace the left ventricle posteriorly and produce a prominent RV apex beat that can be confused with a LV lift. A loud P_2 may be palpable in the second left intercostal space in patients with MS and pulmonary hypertension.

Auscultation. The auscultatory features of MS (see Fig. 66-20) include an accentuated S_1 with prolongation of the Q-S_1 interval, correlating with the level of the left atrial pressure. Accentuation of S_1 occurs when the mitral valve leaflets are flexible. It is caused, in part, by the rapidity with which LV pressure rises at the time of mitral valve closure, as well as by the wide closing excursion of the leaflets. Marked calcification and/or thickening of the mitral valve leaflets reduce the amplitude of S_1, probably because of diminished motion of the leaflets. As pulmonary arterial pressure rises, P_2 at first becomes accentuated and widely transmitted and can often be readily heard at both the mitral and the aortic areas. With further elevation of pulmonary arterial pressure, splitting of S_2 narrows because of reduced compliance of the pulmonary vascular bed, with earlier pulmonic valve closure. Finally, S_2 becomes single and accentuated. Other signs of severe pulmonary hypertension include a nonvalvular pulmonic ejection sound that diminishes during inspiration, because of dilation of the pulmonary artery, a systolic murmur of TR, a Graham Steell murmur of pulmonic regurgitation, and an S_4 originating from the right ventricle. An S_3 gallop originating from the left ventricle is absent in patients with MS unless significant MR or AR coexists.

The opening snap (OS) of the mitral valve is caused by a sudden tensing of the valve leaflets after the valve cusps have completed their opening excursion. The OS occurs when the movement of the mitral dome into the left ventricle suddenly stops. It is most readily audible at the apex, using the diaphragm of the stethoscope. The OS can usually be differentiated from P_2 because the OS occurs later, unless right bundle branch block is present. In addition, the OS usually is loudest at the apex, whereas S_2 is best heard at the cardiac base. The mitral valve cannot be totally rigid if it produces an OS, so an OS is usually accompanied by an accentuated S_1. Calcification confined to the tip of the mitral valve leaflets does not preclude an OS, although calcification of the body and tip does. The mitral OS follows A_2 by 0.04 to 0.12 second; this interval varies inversely with the left atrial pressure. A short A_2-OS interval is a reliable indicator of severe MS but accurate estimation of this time interval requires considerable experience.

The diastolic, low-pitched, rumbling murmur of MS is best heard at the apex, with the bell of the stethoscope (low-frequency mode on electronic stethoscopes) and with the patient in the left lateral recumbent position. When this murmur is soft, it is limited to the apex but, when louder, it may radiate to the left axilla or the lower left sternal area. Although the intensity of the diastolic murmur is not closely related to the severity of stenosis, the duration of the murmur is a guide to the severity of mitral valve narrowing. The murmur persists for as long as the left atrioventricular pressure gradient exceeds approximately 3 mm Hg. The murmur usually commences immediately after the OS. In mild MS, the early diastolic murmur is brief but, in the presence of sinus rhythm, it resumes in presystole. In severe MS, the murmur persists until end-diastole, with presystolic accentuation while sinus rhythm is maintained (see Figs. 66-20 and 12-8F).

Other Auscultatory Findings. A pansystolic murmur of TR and an S_3 originating from the right ventricle may be audible in the fourth intercostal space in the left parasternal region in patients with severe MS. These signs, which are secondary to pulmonary hypertension, may be confused with the findings of MR. However, the inspiratory augmentation of the murmur and of the S_3 and the prominent *v* wave in the jugular venous pulse aid in establishing that the murmur originates from the tricuspid valve. A high-pitched decrescendo diastolic murmur along the left sternal border in patients with MS and pulmonary hypertension may be audible pulmonic regurgitation (Graham Steell murmur), but more often is caused by concomitant AR.

DIAGNOSIS AND EVALUATION

Differential Diagnosis. MS is a rare diagnosis in developed countries and most apical diastolic murmurs have other causes. In older patients, an apical diastolic rumble most likely is caused by mitral annular calcification, and 90% of patients with a diastolic apical murmur have no evidence of MS on echocardiography. In severe MR—indeed, in any condition in which flow across a nonstenotic mitral valve is increased (e.g., a ventricular septal defect)—there may also be a short diastolic murmur following an S_3. Left atrial myxoma (see Chap. 74) may produce auscultatory findings similar to those in rheumatic valvular MS. A diastolic rumble may also be present in some patients with HCM, caused by early diastolic flow into the hypertrophied, nondistensible left ventricle (see Chap. 69).

Echocardiography

Echocardiography is the most accurate approach to the diagnosis and evaluation of MS (see Chap. 15).[36] It is recommended for all patients with MS at initial presentation, for reevaluation of changing symptoms or signs, and at regular intervals (depending on disease severity) for monitoring disease progression (see Table 66-1). Imaging shows the characteristic anatomy with leaflet thickening and restriction of opening caused by symmetric fusion of the commissures, resulting in "doming" of the leaflets in diastole (see Fig. 66-19 and Fig 15-46). As disease becomes more severe, thickening extends from the leaflet tips toward the base with further restriction of motion and less curvature of the leaflet in diastole. The mitral chords are variably thickening, fused, and shortened and there may be superimposed calcification of the valve apparatus (see Figs. 15-4C and 15-5C).

Mitral valve area is measured by direct planimetry from two-dimensional short-axis images and calculated by the Doppler pressure half-time method (see Figs. 15-39 and 15-47). The transmitral gradient is also calculated (see Fig. 15-36B) and any coexisting MR is quantitated on the basis of the accepted guidelines.[30] Evaluation of the morphology of the valve is helpful for predicting the hemodynamic results and outcome of percutaneous BMV. A score of 0 to 4+ is given for leaflet thickness, mobility, calcification, and chordal involvement to provide an overall score that is favorable (low) or unfavorable (high) for valvuloplasty (see Table 15-11). Other important anatomic features of the valve are the degree of anterior leaflet doming, symmetry of commissural fusion, and distribution of leaflet calcification.[114]

Other key features on echocardiography are left atrial size, pulmonary artery pressures, LV size and systolic function, and RV size and systolic function. When pulmonary hypertension is present, the right ventricle is frequently dilated, with reduced systolic function. TR may be secondary to RV dysfunction and annular dilation or may be caused by rheumatic involvement of the tricuspid valve. Complete evaluation of aortic valve anatomy and function is also important because the aortic valve is affected in approximately one third of patients with MS. When transthoracic images are suboptimal, TEE is appropriate. TEE is also necessary to exclude left atrial thrombus and evaluate MR severity when percutaneous BMV is considered.

Exercise Testing with Doppler Echocardiography

Exercise testing is useful for many patients with MS to ascertain the level of physical conditioning and elicit covert cardiac symptoms. The exercise test can be combined with Doppler echocardiography to assess exercise pulmonary pressure,[70,114] usually with the Doppler examination performed at rest after termination of exercise. Exercise Doppler testing is recommended when there is a discrepancy between resting echocardiographic findings and the severity of clinical symptoms.[1] Useful parameters on exercise testing include the following: (1) exercise duration; (2) blood pressure and heart rate response; and (3) increase in pulmonary pressures with exercise, compared with the expected normal changes. An exercise pulmonary systolic pressure greater than 60 mm Hg is a key decision point in the management of these patients.

Other Diagnostic Evaluation Modalities.

Electrocardiography. The ECG is relatively insensitive for detecting mild MS, but it does show characteristic changes in moderate or severe obstruction (see Chap. 13). Left atrial enlargement (P wave duration in lead II >0.12 second and/or a P wave axis between +45 and −30 degrees) is a principal electrocardiographic feature of MS and is found in 90% of patients with significant MS and sinus rhythm. The electrocardiographic signs of left atrial enlargement correlate more closely with left atrial volume than with left atrial pressure and often regress following successful valvotomy. AF is common with long-standing MS, as noted.

Electrocardiographic evidence of RV hypertrophy correlates with RV systolic pressure. When RV systolic pressure is 70 to 100 mm Hg, approximately 50% of patients manifest ECG criteria for RV hypertrophy, including a mean QRS axis greater than 80 degrees in the frontal plane and an R:S ratio greater than 1 in lead V_1. Other patients with this degree of pulmonary hypertension have no frank evidence of RV hypertrophy, but the R:S ratio fails to increase from the right to the midprecordial leads. When RV systolic pressure is greater than 100 mm Hg in patients with isolated or predominant MS, electrocardiographic evidence of RV hypertrophy is consistently found.

Radiography. Patients with hemodynamically significant MS almost invariably have evidence of left atrial enlargement on the lateral and left anterior oblique views (see Chap. 16 and Figs. 16-10, 16-17, and 16-18), although the cardiac silhouette may be normal in the frontal projection. Extreme left atrial enlargement rarely occurs in isolated MS; when present, MR is usually severe (see Fig. 16-15). Enlargement of the pulmonary artery, right ventricle, and right atrium (as well as the left atrium) is commonly seen in patients with severe MS. Occasionally, calcification of the mitral valve is evident on the chest roentgenogram but, more commonly, fluoroscopy is required to detect valvular calcification.

Radiologic changes in the lung fields indirectly reflect the severity of MS. Interstitial edema, an indication of severe obstruction, is manifested as Kerley B lines (dense, short, horizontal lines most commonly seen in the costophrenic angles). This finding is present in 30% of patients with resting pulmonary arterial wedge pressures less than 20 mm Hg and in 70% of patients with pressures greater than 20 mm Hg. Severe long-standing mitral obstruction often results in Kerley A lines (straight, dense lines up to 4 cm in length, running toward the hilum), as well as the findings of pulmonary hemosiderosis and rarely of parenchymal ossification.

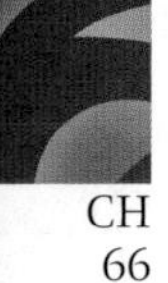

CARDIAC CATHETERIZATION. Catheter-based measurement of left atrial and LV pressures shows the expected hemodynamics (see Fig. 20-14) and allows measurement of the mean transmitral pressure gradient and, in conjunction with measurement of transmitral volume flow rate, calculation of the valve area using the Gorlin formula (see Chap. 20). Occasionally, diagnostic cardiac catheterization is necessary when echocardiography is nondiagnostic or results are discrepant with clinical findings.[116] More often, these measurements now are recorded for monitoring before, during, and after percutaneous BMV. Routine diagnostic cardiac catheterization is not recommended for the evaluation of MS.

DISEASE COURSE

Interval Between Acute Rheumatic Fever and Mitral Valve Obstruction

In temperate zones, such as the United States and Western Europe, patients who develop acute rheumatic fever have an asymptomatic period of approximately 15 to 20 years before symptoms of MS develop. It then takes approximately 5 to 10 years for most patients to progress from mild disability (i.e., early NYHA Class II) to severe disability (i.e., NYHA functional Class III or IV; **Fig. 66-21**). The progression is much more rapid in patients in tropical and subtropical areas, in Polynesians, and in Native Alaskans. In India, critical MS may be present in children as young as 6 to 12 years old. In North America and Western Europe, however, symptoms develop more slowly and occur most commonly between the ages of 45 and 65 years. The most likely causes for these differences are the relative prevalence of rheumatic fever and lack of primary and secondary prevention in developing countries, resulting in recurrent episodes of valve scarring (see Chap. 88).

Hemodynamic Progression

Serial echocardiographic data have described the rate of hemodynamic progression in patients with mild MS.[113-115] The two largest series followed a combined total of 153 adults, with a mean age of approximately 60 years, for an average of slightly more than 3 years. As in most series of MS patients, 75% to 80% were women. The initial valve area was 1.7 ± 0.6 cm^2 and the overall rate of progression was a decrease in valve area of 0.09 cm^2/yr. Approximately one third of patients showed rapid progression, defined as a decrease in valve area greater than 0.1 cm^2/yr. These data apply to the older MS patients seen in developed countries. There are little data on the rate of hemodynamic progression of rheumatic MS in underdeveloped countries in which the age of symptom onset is much younger.

Clinical Outcomes

Natural history data obtained in the presurgical era indicate that symptomatic patients with MS have a poor outlook, with 5-year survival rates of 62% among patients with MS in NYHA Class III but only 15% among those in Class IV. Data from unoperated patients in the surgical era still reported a 5-year survival rate of only 44% in patients with symptomatic MS who refused valvotomy (**Fig. 66-22**).

Overall clinical outcomes are greatly improved in patients who undergo surgical or percutaneous relief of valve obstruction on the basis of current guidelines. However, longevity is still shortened compared with that expected for age, largely because of complications of the disease process (AF, systemic embolism, pulmonary hypertension) and side effects of therapy (e.g., prosthetic valves, anticoagulation).

COMPLICATIONS

ATRIAL FIBRILLATION. The most common complication of MS is AF (see Chap. 40).[113,115] The prevalence of AF in patients with MS is related to the severity of valve obstruction and patient age. In historical series, AF was present in 17% of those 21 to 30 years, 45% of those 31 to 40 years, 60% of those 41 to 50 years, and 80% of those older than 51 years. Even when MS is severe, the prevalence of AF is related to age. In more recent BMV studies, the prevalence of AF ranged from 4% in a series of 600 patients from India, with a mean age of 27 years, and 27% in a series of 4832 patients from China, with a mean age of 37 years, to 40% in a series of 1024 patients from France, with a mean age of 49 years.

AF may precipitate or worsen symptoms caused by loss of the atrial contribution to filling and to a short diastolic filling period when the ventricular rate is not well controlled. In addition, AF predisposes to left atrial thrombus formation and systemic embolic events. AF conveys a worse overall prognosis in MS patients than in the general population. In patients with AF and MS, 5-year survival is only 64% compared with 85% in AF patients without MS.

SYSTEMIC EMBOLISM. Systemic embolism in patients with MS is caused by left atrial thrombus formation. Although systemic embolization most often occurs in patients with AF, 20% of patients with MS and a systemic embolic event are in sinus rhythm. When embolization occurs in patients in sinus rhythm, the possibility of transient AF or underlying infective endocarditis should be considered. However, up to 45% of patients with MS who are in normal sinus rhythm have prominent spontaneous left atrial contrast (a marker of embolic risk) seen by TEE (see Chap. 15). Atrial thrombi have been documented in a few MS patients in sinus rhythm, and many patients with new-onset AF have left atrial thrombi. It is postulated that the loss of atrial appendage contractile function,

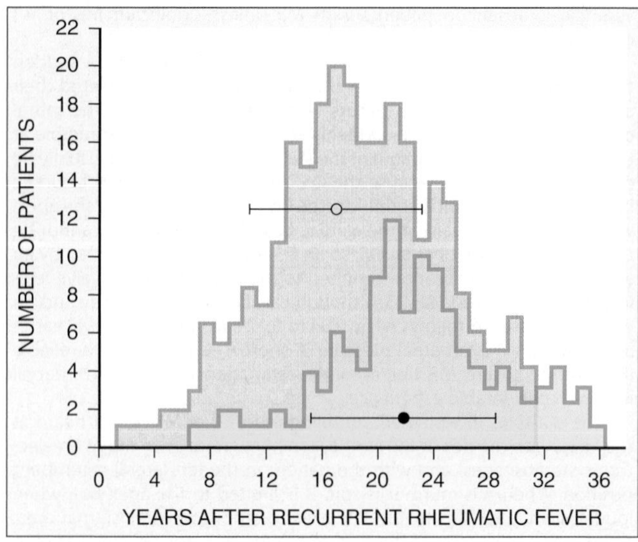

FIGURE 66-21 Interval between active rheumatic fever and clinical symptoms of valve disease in 177 patients with mitral stenosis (yellow bars) and 121 with aortic stenosis (blue bars). *(From Horstkotte D, Niehues R, Strauer BE: Pathomorphological aspects, aetiology, and natural history of acquired mitral valve stenosis. Eur Heart J 12[Suppl B]:55, 1991.)*

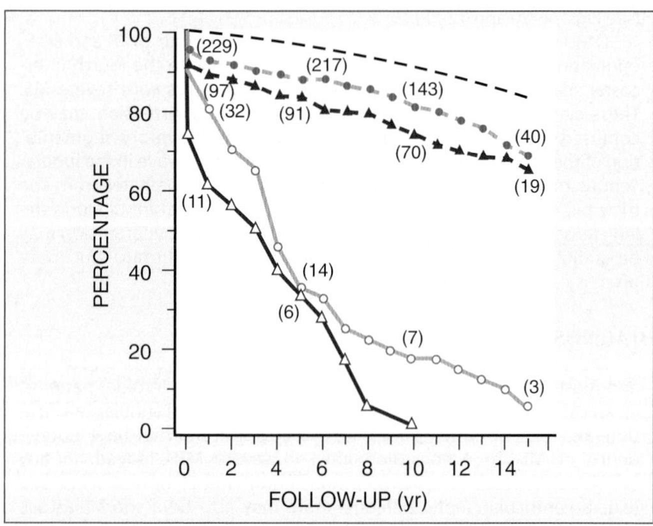

FIGURE 66-22 Natural history of 159 patients with isolated mitral stenosis (solid blue line) or mitral regurgitation (solid purple line) who were not operated on, even though the operation was indicated, compared with patients treated with valve replacement for mitral stenosis (dashed blue line) or mitral regurgitation (dashed purple line). The expected survival rate in the absence of mitral valve disease is indicated by the upper curve (dashed black line). *(From Horstkotte D, Niehues R, Strauer BE: Pathomorphological aspects, aetiology, and natural history of acquired mitral valve stenosis. Eur Heart J 12[Suppl B]:55, 1991.)*

despite electrical evidence of sinus rhythm, leads to blood flow stasis and thrombus formation.

The risk of embolism correlates directly with patient age and left atrial size and inversely with the cardiac output. Before the advent of surgical treatment, this serious complication of MS developed in at least 20% of patients at some time during the course of their disease. Before the era of anticoagulant therapy and surgical treatment, approximately 25% of all fatalities in patients with mitral valve disease were secondary to systemic embolism.

Approximately half of all clinically apparent emboli are found in the cerebral vessels. Coronary embolism may lead to myocardial infarction and/or angina pectoris, and renal emboli may be responsible for the development of systemic hypertension. Emboli are recurrent and multiple in approximately 25% of patients who develop this complication. Rarely, massive thrombosis develops in the left atrium, resulting in a pedunculated ball valve thrombus, which may suddenly aggravate obstruction to left atrial outflow when a specific body position is assumed or may cause sudden death. Similar consequences occur in patients with free-floating thrombi in the left atrium. These two conditions are usually characterized by variability in the physical findings, often on a positional basis. They are very hazardous and require surgical treatment, often as an emergency.

INFECTIVE ENDOCARDITIS. MS is a predisposing factor for endocarditis (see Chap. 67) in less than 1% of cases in clinical series of bacterial endocarditis. The estimated risk of endocarditis in patients with MS is 0.17/1000 patient-years, which is much lower than the risk in patients with MR or aortic valve disease.

MANAGEMENT

Medical Treatment

The medical management of MS is primarily directed toward the following: (1) prevention of recurrent rheumatic fever; (2) prevention and treatment of complications of MS; and (3) monitoring disease progression to allow intervention at the optimal time point.[113,115] Patients with MS caused by rheumatic heart disease should receive penicillin prophylaxis for beta-hemolytic streptococcal infections to prevent recurrent rheumatic fever, per established guidelines (see Chap. 88). Prophylaxis for infective endocarditis is no longer recommended (see Chap. 67). Anemia and infections should be treated promptly and aggressively in patients with valvular heart disease. However, blood cultures should always be considered before beginning antibiotic therapy in patients with valve disease because the presentation of endocarditis often is mistaken for a noncardiac infection.

Anticoagulant therapy is indicated for prevention of systemic embolism in MS patients with AF (persistent or paroxysmal), any prior embolic events (even if in sinus rhythm), and documented left atrial thrombus. Anticoagulation also may be considered for patients with severe MS and sinus rhythm when there is severe left atrial enlargement (diameter >55 mm) or spontaneous contrast on echocardiography. Treatment with warfarin is used to maintain the international normalized ratio (INR) between 2 and 3.[117]

Asymptomatic patients with mild to moderate rheumatic mitral valve disease should have a history and physical examination annually, with echocardiography every 3 to 5 years for mild stenosis, every 1 to 2 years for moderate stenosis, and annually for severe stenosis. More frequent evaluation is appropriate for any change in signs or symptoms. All patients with significant MS should be advised to avoid occupations requiring strenuous exertion.

In patients with severe MS, with persistent symptoms after intervention or when intervention is not possible, medical therapy with oral diuretics and the restriction of sodium intake may improve symptoms. Digitalis glycosides do not alter the hemodynamics and usually do not benefit patients with MS and sinus rhythm, but these drugs are of value in slowing the ventricular rate in patients with AF and in treating patients with right-sided heart failure. Hemoptysis is managed by measures designed to reduce pulmonary venous pressure, including sedation, assumption of the upright position, and aggressive diuresis. Beta-blocking agents and rate-slowing calcium antagonists may increase exercise capacity by reducing heart rate in patients with sinus rhythm, especially in patients with AF.

TREATMENT OF ARRHYTHMIAS. AF is a frequent complication of severe MS. Management of AF for patients with MS is similar to management for AF of any cause (see Chap. 40). However, it typically is more difficult to restore and maintain sinus rhythm because of pressure overload of the left atrium in conjunction with effects of the rheumatic process on atrial tissue and the conducting system.

Immediate treatment of AF includes administration of intravenous heparin followed by oral warfarin. The ventricular rate should be slowed, as stated in the American College of Cardiology/American Heart Association (ACC/AHA) guidelines for the management of AF,[117] initially with an intravenous beta blocker or nondihydropyridine calcium channel antagonist, followed by long-term rate control with oral doses of these agents. When these medications are ineffective or when additional rate control is necessary, digoxin or amiodarone may be considered. Digoxin alone for long-term management of AF may be considered in patients with concurrent LV dysfunction or a sedentary lifestyle. An effort should be made to reestablish sinus rhythm by a combination of pharmacologic treatment and cardioversion. If cardioversion is planned in a patient who has had AF for more than 24 hours before the procedure, anticoagulation with warfarin for more than 3 weeks is indicated. Alternatively, if TEE results show no atrial thrombus, immediate cardioversion can be carried out provided the patient is effectively anticoagulated with intravenous heparin before and during the procedure, and with warfarin chronically thereafter. Paroxysmal AF and repeated conversions, spontaneous or induced, carry the risk of embolization. In patients who cannot be converted or maintained in sinus rhythm, digitalis should be used to maintain the ventricular rate at rest at approximately 60 beats/min. If this is not possible, small doses of a beta-blocking agent, such as atenolol (25 mg daily) or metoprolol (50 to 100 mg daily), may be added. Beta blockers are particularly helpful in preventing rapid ventricular responses that develop during exertion. Multiple repeat cardioversions are not indicated if the patient fails to sustain sinus rhythm while on adequate doses of an antiarrhythmic.

Patients with chronic AF who undergo surgical MV repair or MV replacement may undergo the maze procedure (atrial compartment operation).[118,119] More than 80% of patients undergoing this procedure can be maintained in sinus rhythm postoperatively and can regain normal atrial function, including a satisfactory success rate in those with significant left atrial enlargement. Early intervention with percutaneous valvotomy may prevent the development of AF.[120]

Mitral Valvotomy

PERCUTANEOUS BALLOON MITRAL VALVOTOMY. Patients with mild to moderate MS who are asymptomatic frequently remain so for years, and clinical outcomes are similar to age-matched normal patients. However, severe or symptomatic MS is associated with poor long-term outcomes if the stenosis is not relieved mechanically (see Fig. 66-22). Percutaneous BMV (see Chap. 59) is the procedure of choice for the treatment of MS so that surgical intervention is now reserved for patients who require intervention and are not candidates for a percutaneous procedure.[113]

BMV is recommended for symptomatic patients with moderate to severe MS (i.e., a mitral valve area < 1 cm^2/m^2 body surface area [BSA] or <1.5 cm^2 in normal-sized adults) and with favorable valve morphology, no or mild MR, and no evidence of left atrial thrombus (**Fig. 66-23**). Even mild symptoms, such as a subtle decrease in exercise tolerance, are an indication for intervention because the procedure relieves symptoms and improves long-term outcome with a low procedural risk. In addition, BMV is recommended for asymptomatic patients with moderate to severe MS when mitral valve obstruction has resulted in pulmonary hypertension with a pulmonary systolic pressure greater than 50 mm Hg at rest or 60 mm Hg with exercise.

BMV also is reasonable for symptomatic patients who are at high risk for surgery, even when valve morphology is not ideal, including patients with restenosis after a previous BMV or previous commissurotomy who are unsuitable for surgery because of very high risk. These include very old frail patients, patients with associated severe ischemic heart disease, patients in whom MS is complicated by pulmonary, renal, or neoplastic disease, women of childbearing age

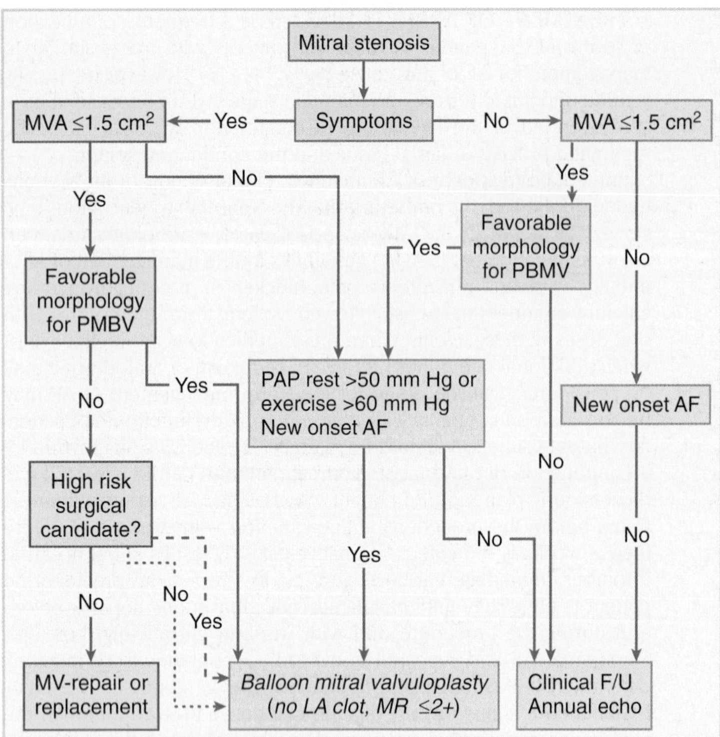

FIGURE 66-23 Management strategy for patients with mitral stenosis. F/U = follow-up; LA = left atrial; MVA = mitral valve area; PAP = pulmonary artery systolic pressure; PBMV = percutaneous balloon mitral valvotomy. *(Modified from Bonow RO, Carabello BA, Chatterjee K, et al: ACC/AHA 2006 guidelines for the management of patients with valvular heart disease: A report of the American College of Cardiology/American Heart Association Task Force on Practice Guidelines [writing committee to revise the 1998 Guidelines for the Management of Patients With Valvular Heart Disease]. Circulation 114:e84, 2006.)*

in whom MV replacement is undesirable, and pregnant women with MS.

BMV may be considered for patients with moderate to severe MS and new-onset AF and those with mild MS when significant pulmonary hypertension is present (see Fig. 66-23). In this last group, it is likely that valve obstruction is the cause of pulmonary hypertension, even when stenosis severity does not meet the valve area criteria for severe obstruction.

This percutaneous technique consists of advancing a small balloon flotation catheter across the interatrial septum (after transseptal puncture), enlarging the opening, advancing a large (23- to 25-mm) hourglass-shaped balloon (the Inoue balloon), and inflating it within the orifice (**Fig. 66-24**).[121] Alternatively, two smaller (15- to 20-mm) side by side balloons across the mitral orifice may be used. A third technique involves retrograde, nontransseptal dilation of the mitral valve, in which the balloon is positioned across the mitral valve using a steerable guidewire.

Commissural separation and fracture of nodular calcium appear to be the mechanisms responsible for improvement in valvular function. In several series, the hemodynamic results of BMV have been favorable (**Fig. 66-25**), with reduction of the transmitral pressure gradient from an average of approximately 18 to 6 mm Hg (see Chap. 59), a small (average, 20%) increase in cardiac output, and an average doubling of the calculated mitral valve area, from 1 to 2 cm^2.[113-115] Results are especially impressive in younger patients without severe valvular thickening or calcification (see Fig. 66-19). Elevated pulmonary vascular resistance declines rapidly, although usually not completely. The reported mortality rate has ranged from 1% to 2%. Complications include cerebral emboli and cardiac perforation, each in approximately 1% of patients, and the development of MR severe enough to require operation in another 2% (approximately 15% develop lesser, but still undesirable, degrees of MR). Approximately 5% of patients are left with a small residual atrial septal defect, but this closes or decreases in size in most. Rarely, the defect is large enough to cause right-sided heart failure; this complication most often is seen in conjunction with an unsuccessful mitral valvotomy.

The likelihood of hemodynamic benefit and the risk of complication with BMV are predicted by anatomic features of the stenosed valve. Rigid thickened valves with extensive subvalvular fibrosis and calcification lead to suboptimal results. One echocardiographic scoring system divides patients into three groups—those with a pliable, noncalcified anterior leaflet and little chordal disease (group 1); those with a pliable, noncalcified anterior leaflet but with chordal thickening and shortening (<10 mm long; group 2); and those with fluoroscopic evidence of calcification of any extent of the valve apparatus (group 3).[113] Event-free survival at 3 years is highest for group 1 (89%) compared with group 2 (78%) or group 3 (65%).[113,114] With an alternate echocardiographic scoring system, leaflet rigidity, leaflet thickening, valvular calcification, and subvalvular disease are each scored from 0 to 4 (see Table 15-11).[1,113] A score of 8 or lower is usually associated with an excellent immediate and long-term result, whereas scores exceeding 8 are associated with less impressive results (**Fig. 66-26**) including the risk of development of MR. Commissural calcification also is a predictor of poor outcomes.

TEE should be performed just prior to BMV to exclude left atrial thrombus and confirm that MR is not moderate or severe. TEE also is appropriate for the evaluation of MS severity and mitral valve morphology when transthoracic images are suboptimal, but the chordal apparatus is less well visualized compared with transthoracic imaging. During the procedure, transthoracic, transesophageal, or intracardiac echocardiography is used to monitor placement of the catheters and balloon, assess hemodynamic results after each inflation, and detect complications such as MR.

In patients with suitable anatomic findings, long-term results are favorable, with excellent survival rates without functional disability or need for surgery or repeat BMV.[113,115,121] A prospective randomized trial in which patients with severe MS were randomized to undergo BMV, closed surgical valvotomy, or open surgical valvotomy had similar clinical outcomes with BMV and the open surgical technique that were superior to the results of the closed surgical valvotomy. After 7 years, mitral valve area was equivalent in the BMV and open surgical groups, both significantly greater than in the closed valvotomy group (see Fig. 66-25). In another randomized study that included older patients with less favorable valve morphology, compared with open surgical commissurotomy, patients randomized to BMV had a smaller increase in valve area and higher likelihood of restenosis (28% versus 18% at 4 years). Excellent results have also been reported in children and adolescents in developing nations, where patients tend to be younger. These young patients usually have pliable valves, which are ideal for BMV.

Surgical Valvotomy. Three operative approaches are available for the treatment of rheumatic MS: (1) closed mitral valvotomy using a transatrial or transventricular approach; (2) open valvotomy (i.e., valvotomy carried out under direct vision with the aid of cardiopulmonary bypass, which may be combined with other repair techniques, such as leaflet resection, chordal procedures, and annuloplasty when MR is present; and (3) MV replacement (**Table 66-6**). Surgical intervention for MS is recommended for patients with severe MS and significant symptoms (NYHA Class III or IV) when BMV is not available, BMV is contraindicated because of persistent left atrial thrombus or moderate to severe MR, or when the valve is calcified and surgical risk is acceptable.[122] The preferred surgical approach is valve repair (open valvotomy, with or without additional procedures) whenever possible. Surgery also is reasonable for patients with severe MS and severe pulmonary hypertension when BMV is not possible and may be considered for patients with moderate to severe MS with recurrent embolic events despite anticoagulation.

Closed Mitral Valvotomy. Closed mitral valvotomy is rarely used in the United States today, having been replaced by BMV, which is more effective in patients who are candidates for closed mitral valvotomy. Closed mitral valvotomy is more popular in developing nations, where

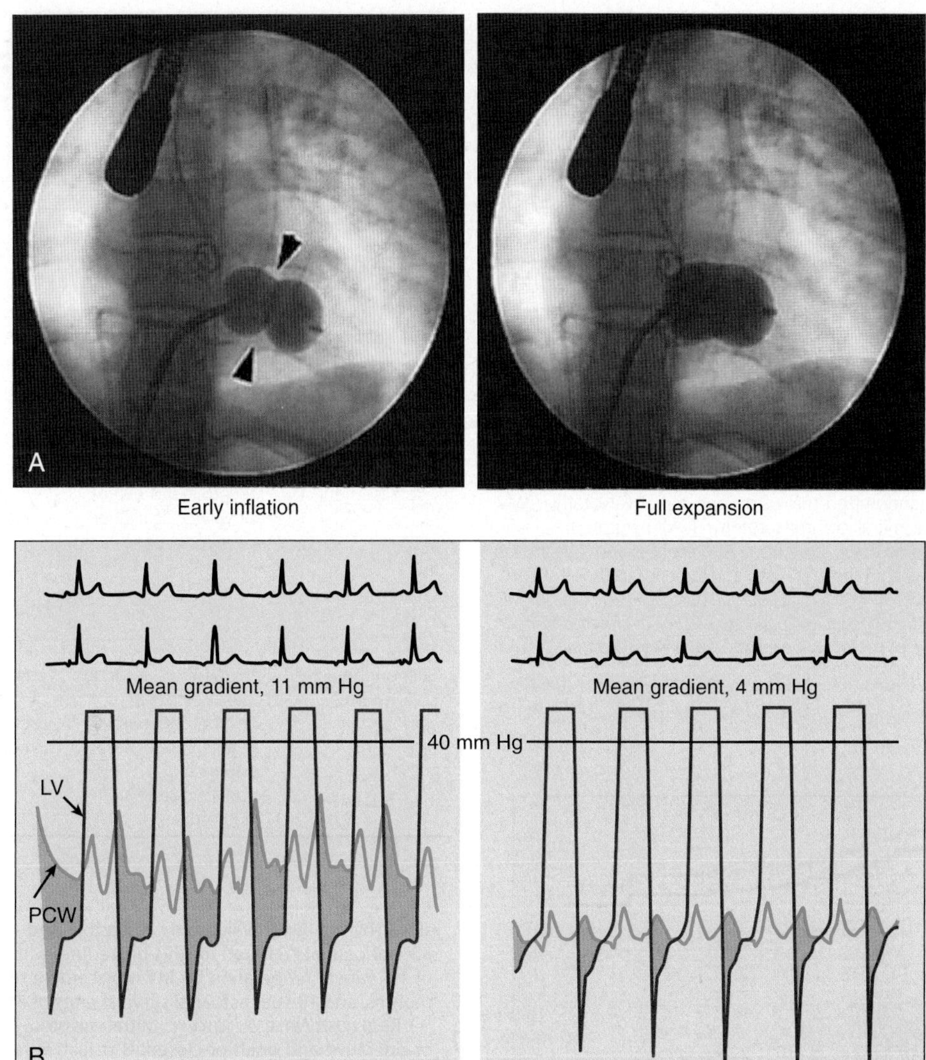

FIGURE 66-24 Percutaneous balloon mitral valvotomy (BMV) for mitral stenosis using the Inoue technique (see Chap. 59). **A,** The catheter is advanced into the left atrium via the transseptal technique and guided antegrade across the mitral orifice. As the balloon is inflated, its distal portion expands first and is pulled back so that it fits snugly against the orifice. With further inflation, the proximal portion of the balloon expands to center the balloon within the stenotic orifice **(left).** Further inflation expands the central "waist" portion of the balloon **(right),** resulting in commissural splitting and enlargement of the orifice. **B,** Successful BMV results in significant increase in mitral valve area, as reflected by a reduction in the diastolic pressure gradient between left ventricle (magenta) and pulmonary capillary wedge (blue) pressure, as indicated by the shaded area. *(From Delabays A, Goy JJ: Images in clinical medicine: Percutaneous mitral valvuloplasty. N Engl J Med 345:e4, 2001.)*

the expense of open heart surgery and even of balloon catheters for BMV is an important factor and where patients with MS are younger and therefore have more pliable valves. However, even in these nations, closed mitral valvotomy is being replaced by BMV.

This procedure is performed without cardiopulmonary bypass but with the aid of a transventricular dilator. It is an effective operation, provided that MR, atrial thrombosis, or valvular calcification is not serious and that chordal fusion and shortening are not severe. Echocardiography is useful for selecting suitable candidates for this procedure by identifying patients without valvular calcification or dense fibrosis. If possible, closed mitral valvotomy should be carried out with pump standby; if the surgeon is unable to achieve a satisfactory result, the patient can be placed on cardiopulmonary bypass and the valvotomy carried out under direct vision or the valve replaced.

On average, the mitral valve area is increased by 1 cm^2, with only 20% to 30% of patients requiring MV replacement within 15 years. The hospital mortality rate is 1% to 2% in experienced centers. Marked symptomatic improvement occurs in most patients, and there is excellent long-term survival in patients selected with low echo scores.[122] Long-term follow-up has shown that the results are best if the operation is carried out before chronic AF and/or heart failure has occurred, and complication rates are higher when valves are calcified and/or severely thickened.

Open Valvotomy. Most surgeons now prefer to carry out direct vision or open valvotomy. This operation is most frequently performed in patients with MS whose mitral valves are too distorted or calcified for BMV. Cardiopulmonary bypass is established and, to obtain a dry, quiet heart, body temperature is usually lowered, the heart is arrested, and the aorta is occluded intermittently. Thrombi are removed from the left atrium and its appendage, and the latter is often amputated to remove a potential source of postoperative emboli. The commissures are incised and, when necessary, fused chordae tendineae are separated, the underlying papillary muscle is split, and the valve leaflets are débrided of calcium. Mild or even moderate MR may be corrected using similar repair approaches as for primary MR. Left atrial and LV pressures are measured after bypass has been discontinued to confirm that the valvotomy has been effective. When it has not been effective, another attempt can be made. When repair is not possible—usually because of severe distortion and calcification of the valve and subvalvular apparatus, with accompanying MR that cannot be corrected—MV replacement should be carried out. In patients with AF, a left atrial maze or AF ablation procedure typically is done at the time of surgery to increase the likelihood of long-term

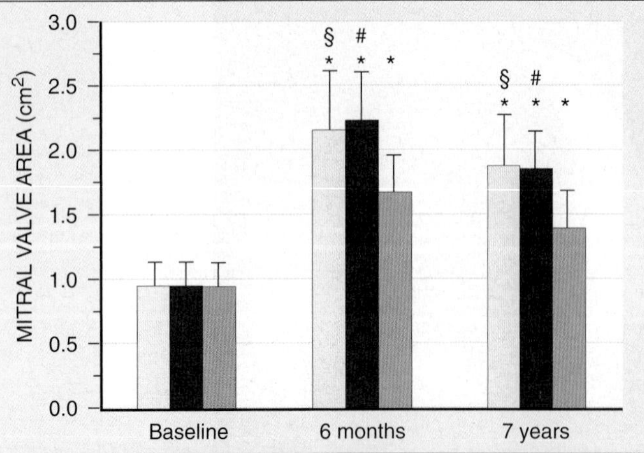

FIGURE 66-25 Mitral valve area before and 6 months and 7 years after valvotomy in a prospective, randomized trial of balloon mitral valvotomy (BMV, yellow bars), open surgical mitral commissurotomy (OMC, purple bars) and closed mitral commissurotomy (CMC, blue bars). At 6 months and 7 years, the results of BMV were equivalent to those of OMC and superior to those of CMC. §P<.001 for BMC versus CMC; #P<.001 for OMC versus CMC. *(From Farhat MB, Ayari M, Maatouk F, et al: Percutaneous balloon versus surgical closed and open mitral commissurotomy: Seven-year follow-up results of a randomized trial. Circulation 97:245, 1998.)*

TABLE 66-6 Approaches to Mechanical Relief of Mitral Stenosis

APPROACH	ADVANTAGES	DISADVANTAGES
Closed surgical valvotomy	Inexpensive Relatively simple Good hemodynamic results in selected patients Good long-term outcome	No direct visualization of valve Only feasible with flexible, noncalcified valves Contraindicated if MR > 2+ Surgical procedure with general anesthesia
Open surgical valvotomy	Visualization of valve allows directed valvotomy Concurrent annuloplasty for MR is feasible	Best results with flexible, noncalcified valves Surgical procedure with general anesthesia
Valve replacement	Feasible in all patients regardless of extent of valve calcification or severity of MR	Surgical procedure with general anesthesia Effect of loss of annular-papillary muscle continuity on LV function Prosthetic valve Chronic anticoagulation
Balloon mitral valvotomy	Percutaneous approach Local anesthesia Good hemodynamic results in selected patients Good long-term outcome	No direct visualization of valve Only feasible with flexible noncalcified valves Contraindicated if MR > 2+

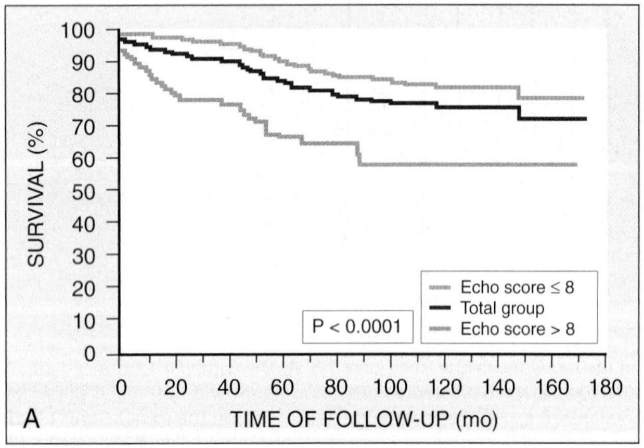

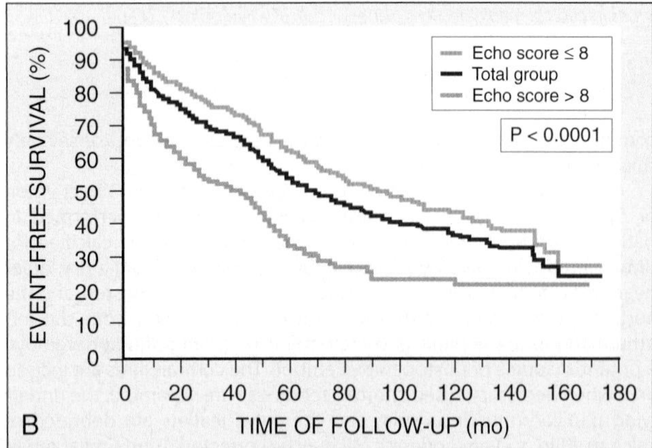

FIGURE 66-26 Long-term survival **(A)** and event-free survival **(B)** after balloon mitral valvotomy for 879 patients who were stratified by baseline echocardiographic morphology score, 8 or less (blue line) or more than 8 (gold line). Patients with the lower echo score had a significantly better outcome initially and over the next 12 to 13 years. *(From Palacios IF, Sanchez PL, Harrell LC, et al: Which patients benefit from percutaneous mitral balloon valvuloplasty? Prevalvuloplasty and postvalvuloplasty variables that predict long-term outcome. Circulation 105:1465, 2002.)*

sinus rhythm. Open valvotomy is feasible and successful in more than 80% of patients referred for this procedure, with an operative mortality of 1%, rate of reoperation for MV replacement of 0% to 16% at 36 to 53 months, and 10-year actuarial survival rates of 81% to 100%.

Restenosis After Valvotomy. Mitral valvotomy, whether percutaneous or operative and open or closed, is palliative rather than curative and, even when successful, there is some degree of residual mitral valve dysfunction. Because the valve is not normal postoperatively, turbulent flow usually persists in the paravalvular region, and the resultant trauma may play a role in restenosis. These changes are analogous to the gradual development of obstruction in a congenitally bicuspid aortic valve and are not usually the result of recurrent rheumatic fever. It is likely that the process of superimposed leaflet calcification and increased stiffness superimposed on the rheumatic valve is similar to the calcific changes seen in aortic valve stenosis.

On clinical grounds alone, based on the reappearance of symptoms, the incidence of restenosis has been estimated to range widely, from 2% to 60%. Recurrence of symptoms is usually not caused by restenosis but may be caused by one or more of the following conditions: (1) an inadequate first operation with residual stenosis; (2) increased severity of MR, either at operation or as a consequence of infective endocarditis; (3) progression of aortic valve disease; or (4) development of coronary artery disease. True restenosis occurs in less than 20% of patients who are followed for 10 years.[113]

Thus, in properly selected patients, mitral valvotomy, however performed—percutaneous BMV, closed or open surgical valvotomy—is a low-risk procedure that results in a significant increase in the size of the mitral orifice and favorably alters the clinical course of an otherwise progressive disease. Pulmonary arterial pressure falls promptly and decisively when mitral obstruction is effectively relieved. Most patients maintain clinical improvement for 10 to 15 years of follow-up. When a second procedure is required because of symptomatic deterioration, the valve is usually calcified and more seriously deformed than at the time of the first operation, and adequate reconstruction may not be possible. Accordingly, MV replacement is often necessary at that time.

Mitral Valve Replacement

MV replacement is recommended for symptomatic patients with severe MR when BMV or surgical MV repair is not possible. Usually, MV replacement is required for patients with combined MS and moderate or severe MR, those with extensive commissural calcification, severe fibrosis, and subvalvular fusion, and those who have undergone previous valvotomy. The operative mortality rate for isolated MV replacement ranges from 3% to 8% in most centers and averaged 6.04% in the large data base of 16,105 such operations for patients with MS and/or MR reported in the Society of Thoracic Surgeons (STS) National Database (see Table 66-3). Prosthetic valves are associated with increased risk because of valve deterioration and chronic anticoagulation, so the threshold for operation should be higher in patients in whom preoperative evaluation suggests that MV replacement may be required than in patients in whom valvotomy alone appears to be indicated.

Generally, a mechanical valve is preferred when MV replacement for MS is necessary when AF is present because of the need for chronic anticoagulation. In patients younger than 65 years who are in sinus rhythm, a mechanical valve is reasonable because of the risk of tissue valve deterioration and likely need for a second operation in the future. However, some younger patients may choose a bioprosthetic valve for lifestyle considerations, despite the risk of valve deterioration. A bioprosthetic valve is appropriate in patients who cannot take warfarin and is reasonable in all patients older than 65 years.

MV replacement is indicated in two groups of patients with MS whose valves are not suitable for valvotomy: (1) those with a mitral valve area smaller than 1.5 cm^2 in NYHA Class III or IV; and (2) those with severe MS (mitral valve area ≤1 cm^2), NYHA Class II, and severe pulmonary hypertension (pulmonary artery systolic pressure >60 mm Hg). Because the operative mortality risk may be high (10% to 20%) in patients in NYHA Class IV, surgery should be carried out before patients reach this stage if possible. On the other hand, even such high-risk patients should not be denied this option unless they have comorbid conditions that preclude surgery or a satisfactory outcome.

Mitral Regurgitation

CAUSES AND PATHOLOGY. The mitral valve apparatus involves the mitral leaflets, chordae tendineae, papillary muscles, and mitral annulus (**Fig. 66-27**). Abnormalities of any of these structures may cause MR.[123] The major causes of MR include mitral valve prolapse (MVP), rheumatic heart disease, infective endocarditis, annular calcification, cardiomyopathy, and ischemic heart disease (**Table 66-7**). Specific aspects of the MVP syndrome, the most important cause of significant MR in the United States, are discussed later. Less common causes of MR include collagen vascular diseases, trauma, the hypereosinophilic syndrome, carcinoid, and exposure to certain drugs.

Abnormalities of Valve Leaflets

MR caused by involvement of the valve leaflets occurs in many situations.[124] MR in patients with chronic rheumatic heart disease, in contrast to MS, is more frequent in men than in women. It is a consequence of shortening, rigidity, deformity, and retraction of one or both mitral valve cusps and is associated with shortening and fusion of the chordae tendineae and papillary muscles. MVP involves both leaflets and chordae and is usually associated with annular dilation. Infective endocarditis can cause MR by perforating valve leaflets (see Chap. 67); vegetations can prevent leaflet coaptation, and valvular retraction during the healing phase of endocarditis can cause MR. Destruction of the mitral valve leaflets can also occur in patients with penetrating and nonpenetrating trauma (see Chap. 76). MR associated with drug exposure also results from anatomic changes in the valve leaflets.[125-127]

Abnormalities of the Mitral Annulus

DILATION. In a normal adult, the mitral annulus measures approximately 10 cm in circumference. It is soft and flexible, and contraction of the surrounding LV muscle during systole causes the annular constriction that contributes importantly to valve closure. MR secondary to dilation of the mitral annulus can occur in any form of heart disease characterized by dilation of the left ventricle, especially dilated cardiomyopathy. LV submitral aneurysm has been reported as a cause of annular MR in sub-Saharan Africa and appears to be caused by a congenital defect in the posterior portion of the annulus. Diagnosis by TEE and surgical repair have been reported.

CALCIFICATION. Idiopathic (degenerative) calcification of the mitral annulus is one of the most common cardiac abnormalities found at autopsy; in most hearts, it is of little functional consequence. However, when severe (see Fig. 16-21), it may be an important cause of MR and, in contrast to MR secondary to rheumatic fever, is more common in women than in men. The development of degenerative calcification of the mitral annulus shares common risk factors with atherosclerosis, including systemic hypertension, hypercholesterolemia, and diabetes. Hence, mitral annular calcification is associated with coronary and carotid atherosclerosis and identifies patients at higher risk for cardiovascular morbidity and mortality.[128-130] Annular calcification may also be accelerated by an intrinsic defect in the fibrous skeleton of the heart, as in the Marfan and Hurler syndromes. In these two syndromes, the mitral annulus is not only calcified but dilated, further contributing to MR. The incidence of mitral annular calcification is also increased in patients who have chronic renal failure with secondary hyperparathyroidism. The annulus may also become thick, rigid, and calcified secondary to rheumatic involvement; when this process is severe, it also can interfere with valve closure.

With severe annular calcification, a rigid curved bar or ring of calcium encircles the mitral orifice, and calcific spurs may project into the adjacent LV myocardium. The calcification may immobilize the basal portion of the mitral leaflets, preventing their normal excursion in diastole and coaptation in systole, and aggravating the MR that results from loss of the normal sphincteric action of the mitral ring. Rarely, obstruction to LV filling may occur when severe calcification encroaches on or protrudes into the mitral orifice. In patients with severe calcification, the conduction system may be invaded by calcium, leading to atrioventricular and/or intraventricular conduction defects. Calcification of the aortic valve cusps is an associated finding in approximately 50% of patients with severe mitral annular calcification, but this rarely causes AS. Occasionally, calcific deposits extend into the coronary arteries.

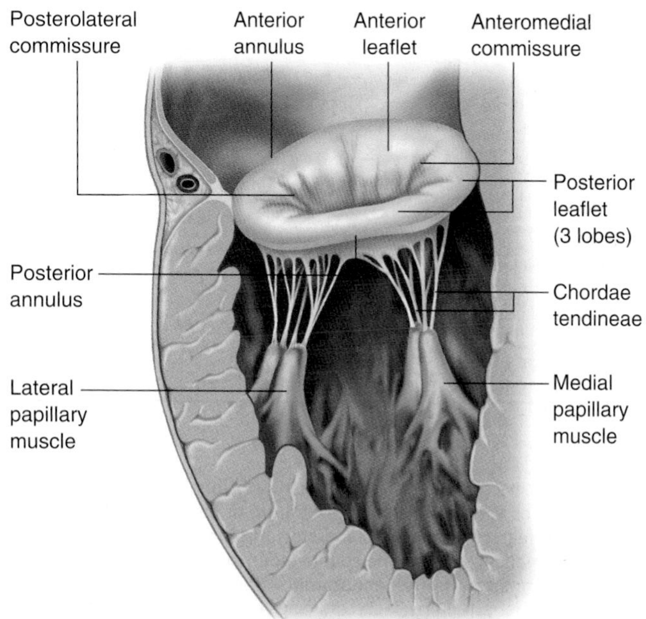

FIGURE 66-27 Continuity of the mitral apparatus and the left ventricular myocardium. MR may be caused by any condition that affects the leaflets or the structure and function of the left ventricle. Similarly, a surgical procedure that disrupts the mitral apparatus in an attempt to correct MR has adverse effects on left ventricular geometry, volume, and function. *(From Otto CM: Evaluation and management of chronic mitral regurgitation. N Engl J Med 345:740, 2001.)*

TABLE 66-7 Causes of Acute and Chronic Mitral Regurgitation

Acute

Mitral Annulus Disorders

- Infective endocarditis (abscess formation)
- Trauma (valvular heart surgery)
- Paravalvular leak caused by suture interruption (surgical technical problems or infective endocarditis)

Mitral Leaflet Disorders

- Infective endocarditis (perforation or interfering with valve closure by vegetation)
- Trauma (tear during percutaneous balloon mitral valvotomy or penetrating chest injury)
- Tumors (atrial myxoma)
- Myxomatous degeneration
- Systemic lupus erythematosus (Libman-Sacks lesion)

Rupture of Chordae Tendineae

- Idiopathic (e.g., spontaneous)
- Myxomatous degeneration (mitral valve prolapse, Marfan syndrome, Ehlers-Danlos syndrome)
- Infective endocarditis
- Acute rheumatic fever
- Trauma (percutaneous balloon valvotomy, blunt chest trauma)

Papillary Muscle Disorders

- Coronary artery disease (causing dysfunction and rarely rupture)
- Acute global left ventricular dysfunction
- Infiltrative diseases (amyloidosis, sarcoidosis)
- Trauma

Primary Mitral Valve Prosthetic Disorders

- Porcine cusp perforation (endocarditis)
- Porcine cusp degeneration
- Mechanical failure (strut fracture)
- Immobilized disc or ball of the mechanical prosthesis

Chronic

Inflammatory

- Rheumatic heart disease
- Systemic lupus erythematosus
- Scleroderma

Degenerative

- Myxomatous degeneration of mitral valve leaflets (Barlow click-murmur syndrome, prolapsing leaflet, mitral valve prolapse)
- Marfan syndrome
- Ehlers-Danlos syndrome
- Pseudoxanthoma elasticum
- Calcification of mitral valve annulus

Infective

- Infective endocarditis affecting normal, abnormal, or prosthetic mitral valves

Structural

- Ruptured chordae tendineae (spontaneous or secondary to myocardial infarction, trauma, mitral valve prolapse, endocarditis)
- Rupture or dysfunction of papillary muscle (ischemia or myocardial infarction)
- Dilation of mitral valve annulus and left ventricular cavity (congestive cardiomyopathies, aneurysmal dilation of the left ventricle)
- Hypertrophic cardiomyopathy
- Paravalvular prosthetic leak

Congenital

- Mitral valve clefts or fenestrations
- Parachute mitral valve abnormality in association with:
  Endocardial cushion defects
  Endocardial fibroelastosis
  Transposition of the great arteries
  Anomalous origin of the left coronary artery

Data from Jutzy KR, Al-Zaibag M: Acute mitral and aortic valve regurgitation. *In* Al-Zaibag M, Duran CMG (eds): Valvular Heart Disease. New York, Marcel Dekker, 1994, pp 345-362; and Haffajee CI: Chronic mitral regurgitation. In Dalen JE, Alpert JS (eds): Valvular Heart Disease. 2nd ed. Boston, Little, Brown, 1987, p 112.

Abnormalities of the Chordae Tendineae. Such abnormalities are important causes of MR. Lengthening and rupture of the chordae tendineae are cardinal features of the MVP syndrome. The chordae may be congenitally abnormal; rupture may be spontaneous (primary) or may occur as a consequence of infective endocarditis, trauma, rheumatic fever or, rarely, osteogenesis imperfecta or relapsing polychondritis. In most patients, no cause for chordal rupture is apparent other than increased mechanical strain. Chordae to the posterior leaflet rupture more frequently than those to the anterior leaflet. Patients with idiopathic rupture of mitral chordae tendineae frequently exhibit pathologic fibrosis of the papillary muscles. It is possible that the dysfunction of the papillary muscles may cause stretching and ultimately rupture of the chordae tendineae. Chordal rupture may also result from acute LV dilation, regardless of the cause. Depending on the number of chordae involved in rupture and the rate at which rupture occurs, the resultant MR may be mild, moderate, or severe and acute, subacute, or chronic.

Involvement of the Papillary Muscles. Diseases of the LV papillary muscles are a frequent cause of MR. Because these muscles are perfused by the terminal portion of the coronary vascular bed, they are particularly vulnerable to ischemia, and any disturbance in coronary perfusion may result in papillary muscle dysfunction. When ischemia is transient, it results in temporary papillary muscle dysfunction and may cause transient episodes of MR that are sometimes associated with attacks of angina pectoris or pulmonary edema.[131] When ischemia of papillary muscles is severe and prolonged, it causes papillary muscle dysfunction and scarring, as well as chronic MR. The posterior papillary muscle, which is supplied by the posterior descending branch of the right coronary artery, becomes ischemic and infarcted more frequently than the anterolateral papillary muscle; the latter is supplied by diagonal branches of the left anterior descending coronary artery and often by marginal branches from the left circumflex artery as well. Ischemia of the papillary muscles is usually caused by coronary atherosclerosis, but may also occur in patients with severe anemia, shock, coronary arteritis of any cause, or an anomalous left coronary artery. MR occurs frequently in patients with healed myocardial infarcts[132,133] and is most frequently caused by regional dysfunction of the LV myocardium at the base of a papillary muscle, resulting in tethering of the mitral leaflets and incomplete leaflet coaptation. Although necrosis of a papillary muscle is a frequent complication of myocardial infarction, frank rupture is far less common; the latter is usually fatal because of the extremely severe MR that it produces (see Chap. 55). However, rupture of one or two of the apical heads of a papillary muscle results in a lesser degree of MR and thus makes survival possible, usually following surgical therapy.

Various other disorders of the papillary muscles may also be responsible for the development of MR (see Chaps. 25, 57, and 68). These include congenital malposition of the muscles, absence of one papillary muscle, resulting in the so-called parachute mitral valve syndrome, and involvement or infiltration of the papillary muscles by a variety of processes, including abscesses, granulomas, neoplasms, amyloidosis, and sarcoidosis.

Left Ventricular Dysfunction

Ischemic LV dysfunction and dilated cardiomyopathy are important causative factors in the development of MR (see Fig. 66-27) and represent the second leading cause of MR after MVP in the United States. LV dilation of any cause including ischemia can alter the spatial relationships between the papillary muscles and chordae tendineae and thereby result in functional MR (see Fig. 66-27; see Fig 15-53).[133,134]

Some degree of MR is found in approximately 30% of patients with coronary artery disease who are being considered for coronary artery bypass surgery. In most of these patients, MR develops from tethering of the posterior leaflet because of regional LV dysfunction. The outlook for the patient with ischemic MR is substantially worse than that for MR from other causes because of the associated LV remodeling and systolic dysfunction. There may be additional ischemic damage to the papillary muscles, dilation of the mitral valve ring, and/or loss of systolic annular contraction contributing further to MR. In most of these patients, MR is mild; however, in the small percentage with severe MR (3% in one large series of patients with coronary artery disease proved by coronary arteriography), it is associated with a poor prognosis. The incidence and severity of regurgitation vary inversely with the LV ejection fraction and directly with the LV end-diastolic pressure. MR occurs in approximately 20% of patients following acute myocardial infarction and, even when mild, is associated with a higher risk of adverse outcomes.[135]

Other causes of MR, discussed in greater detail elsewhere, include obstructive HCM (see Chap. 69), the hypereosinophilic syndrome, endomyocardial fibrosis, trauma affecting the leaflets and/or papillary muscles, Kawasaki disease, left atrial myxoma, and various congenital anomalies, including cleft anterior leaflet and ostium secundum atrial septal defect (see Chaps. 65, 74, 76, and 89).

PATHOPHYSIOLOGY. Because the regurgitant mitral orifice is functionally in parallel with the aortic valve, the impedance to ventricular emptying is reduced in patients with MR. Consequently, MR enhances LV emptying. Almost 50% of the regurgitant volume is ejected into the left atrium before the aortic valve opens. The volume of MR flow depends on a combination of the instantaneous size of the regurgitant orifice and the (reverse) pressure gradient between the left ventricle and left atrium.[136] Both the orifice size and pressure gradient are labile. LV systolic pressure, and therefore the LV–left atrial gradient, depends on systemic vascular resistance and, in patients in whom the mitral annulus has normal flexibility, the cross-sectional area of the mitral annulus may be altered by many interventions. Thus, increase of preload and afterload and depression of contractility increase LV size and enlarge the mitral annulus, and thereby the regurgitant orifice. When LV size is reduced by treatment with positive inotropic agents, diuretics, and particularly vasodilators, the regurgitant orifice size decreases, and the volume of regurgitant flow declines, as reflected in the height of the v wave in the left atrial pressure pulse and in the intensity and duration of the systolic murmur. Conversely, LV dilation, regardless of cause, may increase MR.[137]

Left Ventricular Compensation

The left ventricle initially compensates for the development of acute MR by emptying more completely and by increasing preload (i.e., by use of the Frank-Starling principle).[137] Because acute MR reduces late systolic LV pressure and radius, LV wall tension declines markedly (and proportionately to a greater extent than LV pressure), permitting a reciprocal increase in the extent and velocity of myocardial fiber shortening, leading to a reduced end-systolic volume (**Fig. 66-28**). Because regurgitation, particularly severe regurgitation, becomes chronic, the LV end-diastolic volume increases and the end-systolic volume returns to normal. By means of the Laplace principle, which states that myocardial wall tension is related to the product of intraventricular pressure and radius, the increased LV end-diastolic volume increases wall tension to normal or supranormal levels in the so-called chronic compensated stage of severe MR.[90] The resultant increase in LV end-diastolic volume and mitral annular diameter may create a vicious circle, in which MR leads to more MR. In patients with chronic MR, LV end-diastolic volume and mass are increased; that is, typical

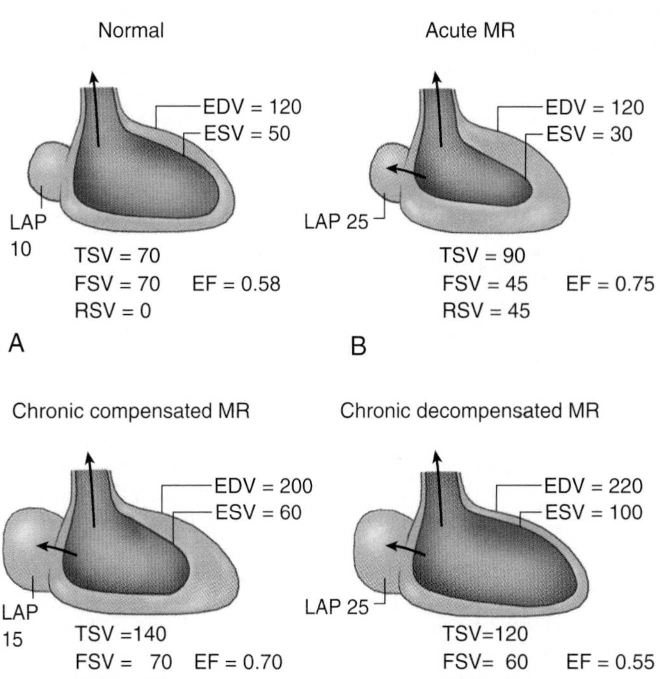

FIGURE 66-28 Three phases of MR are depicted and compared with normal physiology **(A). B,** In acute MR, an increase in preload and a decrease in afterload cause an increase in end-diastolic volume (EDV) and a decrease in end-systolic volume (ESV), producing an increase in total stroke volume (TSV). However, forward stroke volume (FSV) is diminished because 50% of the TSV regurgitates as the regurgitant stroke volume (RSV), resulting in an increase in left atrial pressure (LAP). **C,** In the chronic compensated phase, eccentric hypertrophy has developed and EDV is now increased substantially. Afterload has returned toward normal as the radius term of the Laplace relationship increases with the increase in EDV. Normal muscle function and a large increase in EDV permit a substantial increase in TSV from the acute phase. This, in turn, permits a normal FSV. Left atrial enlargement now accommodates the regurgitant volume at lower LAP. Ejection fraction (EF) remains greater than normal. **D,** In the chronic decompensated phase, muscle dysfunction has developed, impairing ejection fraction, diminishing both TSV and FSV. The EF, although still normal, has decreased to 0.55, and LAP is reelevated because less volume is ejected during systole, causing a higher ESV. *(From Carabello BA: Progress in mitral and aortic regurgitation. Curr Probl Cardiol 28:553, 2003.)*

volume overload (eccentric) hypertrophy develops. However, the degree of hypertrophy is often not proportional to the degree of LV dilation, so the ratio of LV mass to end-diastolic volume may be less than normal. Nonetheless, the reduced afterload permits maintenance of ejection fraction in the normal to supranormal range. The reduced LV afterload allows a greater proportion of the contractile energy of the myocardium to be expended in shortening than in tension development, and explains how the left ventricle can adapt to the load imposed by MR.

The eccentric ventricular hypertrophy that accompanies the elevated end-diastolic volume of chronic MR is secondary to new sarcomeres laid down in series. A shift to the right (greater volume at any pressure) occurs in the LV diastolic pressure-volume curve in patients with chronic MR. With decompensation, chamber stiffness increases, raising the diastolic pressure at any volume.

In most patients with severe primary MR, compensation is maintained for years, but in some patients the prolonged hemodynamic overload ultimately leads to myocardial decompensation.[137] End-systolic volume, preload, and afterload all increase, whereas ejection fraction and stroke volume decline. In such patients, there is evidence of neurohormonal activation and elevation of circulating proinflammatory cytokines. Plasma natriuretic peptide levels also increase in response to the volume load—more in patients with symptomatic decompensation.

Coronary flow rates may be increased in patients with severe MR, but the increases in myocardial oxygen consumption ($M\dot{V}O_2$) are relatively modest compared with patients with AS and AR, because myocardial fiber shortening, which is elevated in patients with MR, is not one of the principal determinants of $M\dot{V}O_2$ (see Chap. 24). One of these determinants, mean LV wall tension, may actually be reduced in patients with MR, whereas the other two, contractility and heart rate, may be little affected. Thus, patients with MR have a low incidence of clinical manifestations of myocardial ischemia compared with the much higher incidence in those with AS and AR, conditions in which $M\dot{V}O_2$ is greatly augmented.

Assessment of Myocardial Contractility in Mitral Regurgitation

Because the ejection phase indices of myocardial contractility are inversely correlated with afterload, patients with early MR (with reduced LV afterload) often exhibit elevations in ejection phase indices of myocardial contractility, such as ejection fraction, fractional fiber shortening, and velocity of circumferential fiber shortening (VCF).[35,137] Many patients ultimately develop symptoms because of elevated left atrial and pulmonary venous pressures related to the regurgitant volume and with no change in these ejection phase indices, which remain elevated. However, in other patients, major symptoms reflect serious contractile dysfunction, at which time ejection fraction, fractional shortening, and mean VCF have declined to low-normal or below-normal levels (see Fig. 66-28). As MR persists, the reduction in afterload, which increases myocardial fiber shortening and the aforementioned ejection phase indices, is opposed by the impairment of myocardial function characteristic of severe chronic diastolic overload. However, even in patients with overt heart failure secondary to MR, the ejection fraction and fractional shortening may be only modestly reduced. Therefore, values in the low-normal range for the ejection phase indices of myocardial performance in patients with chronic MR may actually reflect impaired myocardial function, whereas moderately reduced values (e.g., ejection fraction 40% to 50%) generally signify severe, often irreversible, impairment of contractility, identifying patients who may do poorly after surgical correction of the MR (**Fig. 66-29**). An ejection fraction of less than 35% in patients with severe MR usually represents advanced myocardial dysfunction; such patients are high operative risks and may not experience satisfactory improvement following MV replacement.

End-Systolic Volume

Preoperative myocardial contractility is an important determinant of the risk of operative death, cardiac failure perioperatively, and postoperative level of LV function. Therefore, it is not surprising that the end-systolic pressure-volume (or stress-dimension) relationship

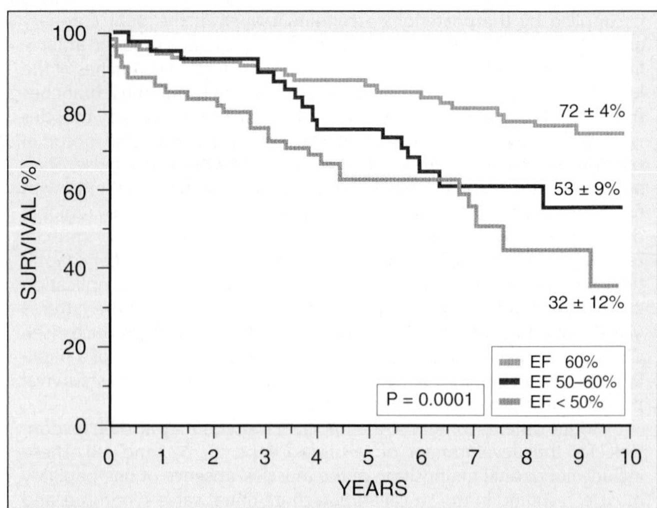

FIGURE 66-29 Late survival of patients after surgical correction of mitral regurgitation subdivided on the basis of the preoperative echocardiographic ejection fraction (EF). *(From Enriquez-Sarano M, Tajik AJ, Schaff HV, et al: Echocardiographic prediction of survival after surgical correction of organic mitral regurgitation. Circulation 90:833, 1994.)*

has emerged as a useful index for evaluating LV function in patients with MR. The simple measurement of end-systolic volume or diameter has been found to be a useful predictor of function and survival following mitral valve surgery.[136-138] A preoperative LV end-systolic diameter that exceeds 40 mm identifies a patient with a high likelihood of impaired LV systolic function following surgery.[1,139]

Hemodynamics

Effective (forward) cardiac output is usually depressed in severely symptomatic patients with MR, whereas total LV output (the sum of forward and regurgitant flow) is usually elevated until late in the patient's course. The cardiac output achieved during exercise, not the regurgitant volume, is the principal determinant of functional capacity. The atrial contraction *a* wave in the left atrial pressure pulse is usually not as prominent in MR as in MS, but the *v* wave is characteristically much taller (see Chap. 20) because it is inscribed during ventricular systole, when the left atrium is being filled with blood from the pulmonary veins and from the left ventricle. Occasionally, backward transmission of the tall *v* wave into the pulmonary arterial bed may result in an early diastolic pulmonary arterial *v* wave (**Fig. 66-30**). In patients with isolated MR, the *y* descent in the pulmonary capillary pressure pulse is particularly rapid because the distended left atrium empties rapidly during early diastole. However, in patients with combined MS and MR, the *y* descent is gradual. Although a left atrioventricular pressure gradient persisting throughout diastole signifies the presence of significant associated MS, a brief early diastolic gradient may occur in patients with isolated severe MR as a result of the rapid flow of blood across a normal-sized mitral orifice early in diastole, often accompanied by an early diastolic murmur at the apex.

Left Atrial Compliance. The compliance of the left atrium (and pulmonary venous bed) is an important determinant of the hemodynamic and clinical picture in patients with severe MR. Three major subgroups of patients with severe MR based on left atrial compliance have been identified and are characterized as follows.

Normal or Reduced Compliance. In this subgroup, there is little enlargement of the left atrium but marked elevation of the mean left atrial pressure, particularly of the *v* wave, and pulmonary congestion is a prominent symptom. Severe MR usually develops acutely, as occurs with rupture of the chordae tendineae, infarction of one of the heads of a papillary muscle, or perforation of a mitral leaflet as a consequence of trauma or endocarditis. In patients with acute MR, the left atrium initially operates on the steep portion of its pressure-volume curve, with a marked rise in pressure for a small increase in volume. Sinus rhythm is usually present; after the passage of weeks or a few months, the left atrial wall becomes hypertrophied, is capable of contracting vigorously, and

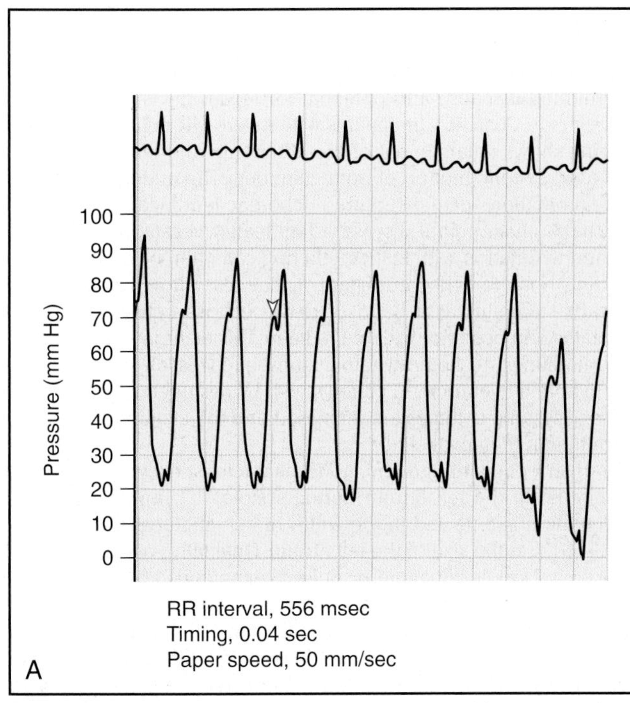

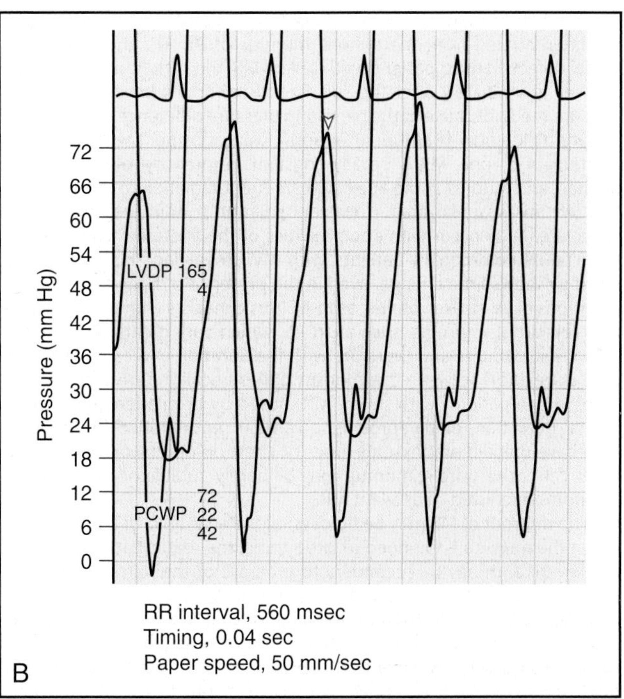

FIGURE 66-30 Hemodynamic tracings in a 45-year-old woman with acute mitral regurgitation from bacterial endocarditis. **A,** Pulmonary artery pressure. **B,** Simultaneous left ventricular diastolic pressure (LVDP) and pulmonary capillary wedge pressure (PCWP). The PCWP demonstrates a markedly elevated v wave (arrowhead, **B**) that transmits to the pulmonary artery pressure (arrowhead, **A**). *(Modified from Wisse B, Sniderman AD: Severe mitral regurgitation. N Engl J Med 343:1386, 2000.)*

facilitates LV filling. The thicker atrium is less compliant than normal, which further increases the height of the *v* wave. Thickening of the walls of the pulmonary veins and proliferative changes in the pulmonary arteries, as well as marked elevations of pulmonary vascular resistance and pulmonary artery pressure, usually develop over the course of 6 to 12 months after the onset of acute severe MR.

Markedly Increased Compliance. At the opposite end of the spectrum from patients in the first group are those with severe long-standing MR with massive enlargement of the left atrium and normal or only slightly elevated left atrial pressure. The atrial wall contains only a small remnant of muscle surrounded by fibrous tissue. Long-standing MR in these patients has altered the physical properties of the left atrial wall and thereby displaced the atrial pressure-volume curve to the right, allowing a normal or almost normal pressure to exist in a greatly enlarged left atrium. Pulmonary arterial pressure and pulmonary vascular resistance may be normal or only slightly elevated at rest. AF and a low cardiac output are almost invariably present.

Moderately Increased Compliance. This most common subgroup consists of patients between the ends of the spectrum represented by the first and second groups. These patients have severe chronic MR and exhibit variable degrees of enlargement of the left atrium, associated with significant elevation of the left atrial pressure, and these two factors (in association with age) determine the likelihood that AF will ensue.

CLINICAL PRESENTATION

Symptoms

The nature and severity of symptoms in patients with chronic MR are functions of a combination of interrelated factors, including the severity of MR, rate of its progression, level of left atrial, pulmonary venous, and pulmonary arterial pressure, presence of episodic or chronic atrial tachyarrhythmias, and presence of associated valvular, myocardial, or coronary artery disease. Symptoms may occur with preserved LV contractile function in patients with chronic MR who have severely elevated pulmonary venous pressures or AF. In other patients, symptoms herald LV decompensation. In patients with rheumatic MR, the time interval between the initial attack of rheumatic fever and development of symptoms tends to be longer than in those with MS, and often exceeds two decades. Hemoptysis and systemic embolization are less common in patients with isolated or predominant MR than in those with MS. The development of AF affects the course adversely but perhaps not as dramatically as in MS. Conversely, chronic weakness and fatigue secondary to a low cardiac output are more prominent features in MR.

Most patients with MR of rheumatic origin have only mild disability, unless regurgitation progresses as a result of chronic rheumatic activity, infective endocarditis, or rupture of the chordae tendineae. However, the indolent course of MR may be deceptive. By the time that symptoms secondary to a reduced cardiac output and/or pulmonary congestion become apparent, serious and sometimes even irreversible LV dysfunction may have developed.

In patients with severe chronic MR who have a greatly enlarged left atrium and relatively mild left atrial hypertension (patients with increased left atrial compliance), pulmonary vascular resistance does not usually rise markedly. Instead, the major symptoms, fatigue and exhaustion, are related to the depressed cardiac output. Right-sided heart failure, characterized by congestive hepatomegaly, edema, and ascites, may be prominent in patients with acute MR, elevated pulmonary vascular resistance, and pulmonary hypertension. Angina pectoris is rare unless coronary artery disease coexists.

PHYSICAL EXAMINATION. Palpation of the arterial pulse is helpful in differentiating AS from MR, both of which may produce a prominent systolic murmur at the base of the heart and apex (see Chap. 12). The carotid arterial upstroke is sharp in severe MR and delayed in AS; the volume of the pulse may be normal or reduced in the presence of heart failure. The cardiac impulse, like the arterial pulse, is brisk and hyperdynamic. It is displaced to the left, and a prominent LV filling wave is frequently palpable. Systolic expansion of the enlarged left atrium may result in a late systolic thrust in the parasternal region, which may be confused with RV enlargement.

Auscultation. When chronic severe MR is caused by defective valve leaflets, S_1, produced by mitral valve closure, is usually diminished. Wide splitting of S_2 is common and results from the shortening of LV ejection and an earlier A_2 as a consequence of reduced resistance to LV ejection. In patients with MR who have severe pulmonary hypertension, P_2 is louder than A_2. The abnormal increase in the flow rate across the mitral orifice during the rapid filling phase is often associated with an S_3, which should not be interpreted as a feature of heart failure in these patients, and this may be accompanied by a brief diastolic rumble.

The systolic murmur is the most prominent physical finding; it must be differentiated from the systolic murmur of AS, TR, and ventricular septal defect. In most patients with severe MR, the systolic murmur commences immediately after the soft S_1 and continues beyond and may obscure the A_2 because of the persisting pressure difference between the left ventricle and left atrium after aortic valve closure. The holosystolic murmur of chronic MR is usually constant in intensity, blowing, high-pitched, and loudest at the apex, with frequent radiation to the left axilla and left infrascapular area. However, radiation toward the sternum or aortic area may occur with abnormalities of the posterior leaflet and is particularly common in patients with MVP involving this leaflet. The murmur shows little change, even in the presence of large beat to beat variations of LV stroke volume, as in AF. This contrasts with most midsystolic (ejection) murmurs, such as in AS, which vary greatly in intensity with stroke volume and therefore with the duration of diastole. There is little correlation between the intensity of the systolic murmur and severity of MR. In patients with severe MR caused by LV dilation, acute myocardial infarction, or paraprosthetic valvular regurgitation, or in those who have marked emphysema, obesity, chest deformity, or a prosthetic heart valve, the systolic murmur may be barely audible or even absent, a condition referred to as silent MR.

The murmur of MR may be holosystolic, late systolic, or early systolic. When the murmur is confined to late systole, the regurgitation is usually not severe and may be secondary to prolapse of the mitral valve or to papillary muscle dysfunction. These causes of MR are frequently associated with a normal S_1 because initial closure of the mitral valve cusps may be unimpaired. The late systolic murmur of papillary muscle dysfunction is particularly variable; it may become accentuated or holosystolic during acute myocardial ischemia and often disappears when ischemia is relieved. A midsystolic click preceding a mid to late systolic murmur, and the response of that murmur to a number of maneuvers, helps establish the diagnosis of MVP. Early systolic murmurs are typical of acute MR. When the left atrial *v* wave is markedly elevated in acute MR, the murmur may diminish or disappear in late systole as the reverse pressure gradient declines. As noted, a short, low-pitched diastolic murmur following S_3 may be audible in patients with severe MR, even without accompanying MS.

Dynamic Auscultation. The holosystolic murmur of MR varies little during respiration. However, sudden standing usually diminishes the murmur, whereas squatting augments it. The late systolic murmur of MVP behaves in the opposite direction, decreasing in duration with squatting and increasing in duration with standing. The holosystolic MR murmur is reduced during the strain of the Valsalva maneuver and shows a left-sided response (i.e., a transient overshoot that occurs six to eight beats following release of the strain). The murmur of MR is usually intensified by isometric exercise, differentiating it from the systolic murmurs of valvular AS and obstructive HCM, both of which are reduced by this intervention. The murmur of MR caused by LV dilation decreases in intensity and duration following effective therapy with cardiac glycosides, diuretics, rest, and particularly vasodilators.

DIAGNOSIS AND EVALUATION

Differential Diagnosis. The holosystolic murmur of MR resembles that produced by a ventricular septal defect. However, the latter is usually loudest at the sternal border rather than the apex and is often accompanied by a parasternal, rather than an apical, thrill. The murmur of MR may also be confused with that of TR, but the latter is usually heard best along the left sternal border, is augmented during inspiration, and is accompanied by a prominent *v* wave and *y* descent in the jugular venous pulse.

When the chordae tendineae to the posterior leaflet of the mitral valve rupture, the regurgitant jet is often directed anteriorly, so that it impinges on the atrial septum adjacent to the aortic root and causes a systolic murmur that is most prominent at the base of the heart. This murmur can be confused with that of AS. On the other hand, when the chordae tendineae to the anterior leaflet rupture, the jet is usually directed to the posterior wall of the left atrium and the murmur may be transmitted to the spine or even the top of the head.

Patients with rheumatic disease of the mitral valve exhibit a spectrum of abnormalities, ranging from pure MS to pure MR. The presence of an S_3, a rapid LV filling wave and LV impulse on palpation, and a soft S_1 all favor predominant MR. In contrast, an accentuated S_1, a prominent OS with a short A_2-OS interval, and a soft, short systolic murmur all indicate predominant MS. Elucidation of the predominant valvular lesion may be complicated by the presence of a holosystolic murmur of TR in patients with pure MS and pulmonary hypertension; this murmur may sometimes be heard at the apex when the right ventricle is greatly enlarged and may therefore be mistaken for the murmur of MR.

Echocardiography

Echocardiography plays a central role in the diagnosis of MR, in determining its cause and potential for repair, and in quantifying its severity (see Chap. 15). In patients with severe MR, echocardiographic imaging shows enlargement of the left atrium and left ventricle, with increased systolic motion of both chambers. The underlying cause of the regurgitation, such as rupture of chordae tendineae, MVP (see Fig. 15-52), rheumatic mitral disease, a flail leaflet, vegetations (see Chap. 67), and LV dilation with leaflet tethering can often be determined on the transthoracic echocardiogram. It may also show calcification of the mitral annulus as a band of dense echoes between the mitral apparatus and posterior wall of the heart. This technique is also useful for estimating the hemodynamic consequences of MR on the left atrium and left ventricle; in patients with LV dysfunction, end-diastolic and end-systolic volumes are increased and the ejection fraction and shortening rate may decline.[138]

Doppler echocardiography in MR characteristically reveals a high-velocity jet in the left atrium during systole.[36,140] The severity of the regurgitation is reflected in the width of the jet across the valve (see Fig. 15-50) and the size of the left atrium. Qualitative assessment using color flow Doppler imaging or pulsed techniques correlates reasonably well with angiographic methods in estimating the severity of MR. However, color flow jet areas are significantly influenced by the cause of the regurgitation and jet eccentricity, thus limiting the accuracy of this approach. Quantitative methods to measure regurgitant fraction, regurgitant volume, and regurgitant orifice area have greater accuracy in comparison with angiography[141,142] (see Figs. 15-40, 15-41, 15-50, and 15-51), and these methods are strongly recommended (see Table 66-1).[1] The vena contracta, defined as the narrowest cross-sectional areas of the regurgitant jet as mapped by color flow Doppler echocardiography, also predicts the severity of MR (**Fig. 66-31**). The proximal isovelocity surface area (PISA) method estimates MR severity with isovelocity hemispheric shells as regurgitant flow accelerates toward the mitral orifice. Reversal of flow in the pulmonary veins during systole and a high peak mitral inflow velocity are also useful signs of severe MR.

Doppler echocardiography is also an important tool to estimate the pulmonary artery systolic pressure and to determine the presence and severity of associated AR or TR.

TEE (see Chap. 15) may be needed in addition to transthoracic echocardiography for assessment of the detailed anatomy of the regurgitant mitral valve (see Fig. 15-54) and the severity of MR in some patients. TEE is useful when the transthoracic images are suboptimal and also when determining whether MV repair is feasible or whether MV replacement is necessary. Three-dimensional transthoracic echocardiography and three-dimensional color Doppler[142] have also been reported to help elucidate the mechanism of MR.

Exercise echocardiography is helpful in determining severity of MR and hemodynamic abnormalities (e.g., pulmonary hypertension) during exercise.[70] This is a useful objective means to evaluate symptoms in patients who appear to have only mild MR at rest and, alternatively, to determine functional status and dynamic changes in hemodynamics in patients who otherwise appear stable and asymptomatic.

Other Diagnostic Evaluation Modalities

Electrocardiography. The principal electrocardiographic findings are left atrial enlargement and AF. Electrocardiographic evidence of LV enlargement occurs in about one third of patients with severe MR. Approximately 15% of patients exhibit electrocardiographic evidence of RV hypertrophy, a change that reflects the presence of pulmonary hypertension of sufficient severity to counterbalance the hypertrophied left ventricle of MR.

Radiography. Cardiomegaly with LV enlargement, and particularly with left atrial enlargement, is a common finding in patients with chronic severe MR (see Fig. 16-20). Although the left atrium may be severely enlarged, there is little correlation between left atrial size and pressure. Interstitial edema with Kerley B lines is frequently seen in patients with acute MR or with progressive LV failure.

In patients with combined MS and MR, overall cardiac enlargement and particularly left atrial dilation are prominent findings (see Fig. 16-15).

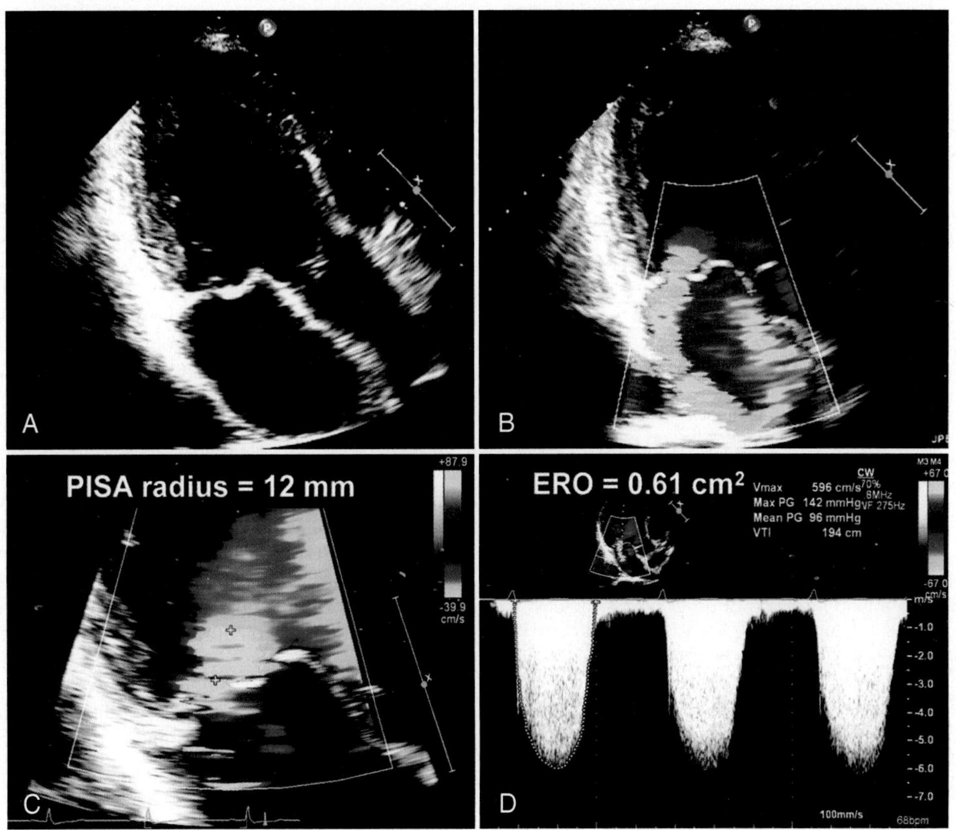

FIGURE 66-31 Severe MR caused by mitral valve prolapse with quantitative determination of effective regurgitant orifice area (ERO) on echocardiography. **A, B,** Severe prolapse of the mitral valve with severe MR was observed. **C, D,** ERO was calculated with the PISA radius and peak velocity of the MR jet. *(From Kang DH, Kim JH, Rim JH, et al: Comparison of early surgery versus conventional treatment in asymptomatic severe mitral regurgitation. Circulation 119:797, 2009.)*

Predominant MS is suggested by relatively mild cardiomegaly (principally straightening of the left cardiac border) and significant changes in the lung fields, whereas predominant MR is more likely when the heart is greatly enlarged and the changes in the lungs are relatively inconspicuous. Calcification of the mitral annulus, an important cause of MR in the elderly, is most prominent in the posterior third of the cardiac silhouette. The lesion is best visualized on chest films exposed in the lateral or right anterior oblique projections, in which it appears as a dense, coarse, C-shaped opacity (see Fig. 16-21).

Cardiac Magnetic Resonance. CMR (see Chap. 18) provides accurate measurements of regurgitant flow that correlate well with quantitative Doppler imaging.[41,95] It is also the most accurate noninvasive technique for measuring LV end-diastolic volume, end-systolic volume, and mass. Although detailed visualization of mitral valve structure and function is obtained more reliably with echocardiography, CMR offers a promising approach for more accurate assessment of regurgitant severity.

Left Ventricular Angiography. The prompt appearance of contrast material in the left atrium following its injection into the left ventricle indicates the presence of MR. The injection should be rapid enough to permit LV opacification but slow enough to avoid the development of premature ventricular contractions, which can induce spurious regurgitation (see Chap. 20). The regurgitant volume can be determined from the difference between the total LV stroke volume, estimated by angiocardiography, and the simultaneous measurement of the effective forward stroke volume by the Fick method. In patients with severe MR, the regurgitant volume may approach, and even exceed, the effective forward stroke volume. Qualitative but clinically useful estimates of the severity of MR may be made by cineangiographic observation of the degree of opacification of the left atrium and pulmonary veins following the injection of contrast material into the left ventricle.

DISEASE COURSE

The natural history of MR is highly variable and depends on a combination of the volume of regurgitation, state of the myocardium, and cause of the underlying disorder. Asymptomatic patients with mild primary MR usually remain in a stable state for many years. Severe MR develops in only a small percentage of these patients, usually because of intervening infective endocarditis or rupture of the chordae tendineae. In patients with mild MR related to MVP, the rate of progression in severity of MR is highly variable; in most patients, progression is gradual unless a ruptured chordae or flail leaflet supervenes. Regurgitation tends to progress more rapidly in patients with connective tissue diseases, such as the Marfan syndrome, than in those with chronic MR of rheumatic origin. Acute rheumatic fever is a frequent cause of isolated severe MR in adolescents in developing nations, and these patients often have a rapidly progressive course.

AF is a common arrhythmia in patients with chronic MR, associated with age and left atrial dilation, and its onset is a marker for disease progression. Patients with AF have an adverse outcome compared with patients who remain in sinus rhythm,[143,144] and development of AF is considered an indication for operative intervention, especially in patients who are candidates for MV repair.[1]

Because the natural history of severe MR has been altered greatly by surgical intervention, it is difficult now to predict the course of patients who receive medical therapy alone. However, a 5-year survival of only 30% was reported in patients who were candidates for operation, presumably because of symptoms, but who declined (see Fig. 66-22). Among patients with severe MR resulting from flail leaflets, the annual mortality rate is as high as 6.3%,[145] and at 10 years 90% have died or undergone surgical correction (**Fig. 66-32**). This latter series included many patients who were initially symptomatic or had LV dysfunction or AF, and thus might be considered to be a higher risk.

Whether patients with severe MR who are asymptomatic, with normal LV function, are at risk of death is a subject of debate. One long-term retrospective study has demonstrated that patients with severe MR, defined quantitatively as an effective orifice area lager than 40 mm^2 (see Table 66-1), had a 4%/year risk of cardiac death.[141] In contrast, a second study reported the outcomes of 132 patients with

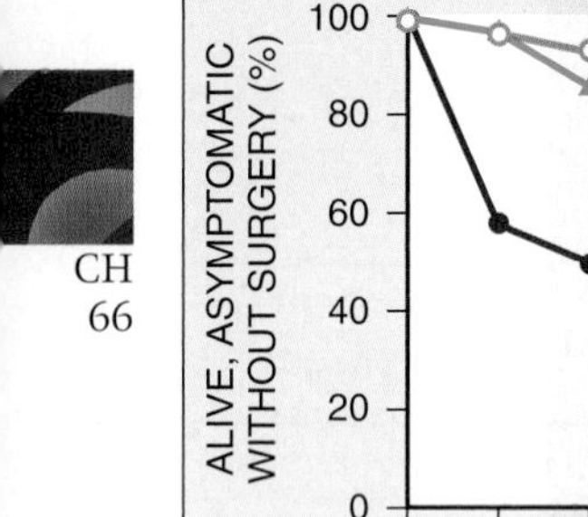

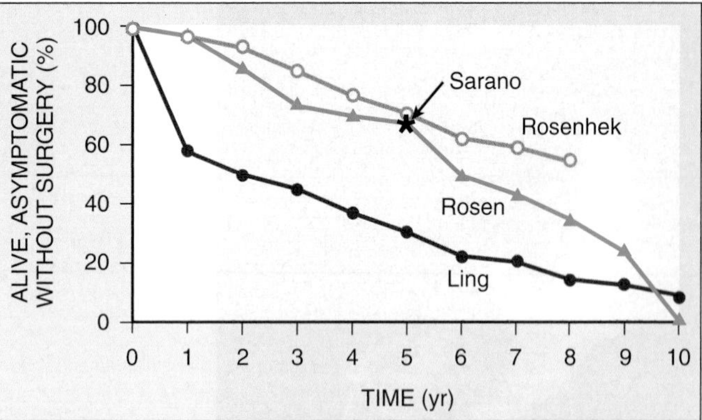

FIGURE 66-32 Four series examining the natural history of patients with severe MR, including a series of patients with flail mitral leaflets reported by Ling and associates (magenta), many of whom were symptomatic, had atrial fibrillation, or had evidence of left ventricular (LV) dysfunction, and three series reported by Rosen and colleagues (blue triangles), Sarano and coworkers (black asterisk), and Rosenhek and associates (gold open circles) in patients who initially were asymptomatic with normal LV function. Although the patients with flail leaflets had a steeper initial attrition rate, all series demonstrated that patients with severe MR have a high likelihood of developing symptoms or other indications for surgery over the course of 6 to 10 years. *(Modified from Ling LH, Enriquez-Sarano M, Seward JB, et al: Clinical outcome of mitral regurgitation due to flail leaflet. N Engl J Med 335:1417, 1996; Rosen SF, Borer JS, Hochreiter C, et al: Natural history of the asymptomatic patient with severe mitral regurgitation secondary to mitral valve prolapse and normal right and left ventricular performance. Am J Cardiol 74:374, 1994; Enriquez-Sarano M, Avierinos JF, Messika-Zeitoun D, et al: Quantitative determinants of the outcome of asymptomatic mitral regurgitation. N Engl J Med 352:875, 2005; and Rosenhek R, Rader F, Klaar U, et al: Outcome of watchful waiting in asymptomatic severe mitral regurgitation. Circulation 113:2238, 2006.)*

severe MR followed prospectively for 5 years,[146] during which the indications for surgery were symptoms or the development of LV dysfunction (ejection fraction < 0.60), LV end-systolic dimension larger than 45 mm, AF, or pulmonary hypertension. Only 2 patients in this latter study had cardiac death, both of whom met criteria for surgery but refused this intervention. A third study followed 286 asymptomatic patients with severe MR and normal LV function without surgery and reported an annual mortality less than 1% (5% mortality at 7 years); in 127 propensity score-matched patients in that study, the estimated actuarial 7 year survival was 99% ± 1% in those treated with early surgery compared with only 85% ± 4% for those treated according to current guidelines for watchful waiting.[147,148] However, mortality arguments aside, all studies uniformly indicated that among asymptomatic patients with initially normal LV ejection fractions, severe MR is associated with a high likelihood of requiring surgery over the next 6 to 10 years because of heart failure symptoms, LV dysfunction, or AF (see Fig. 66-32).

MANAGEMENT OF CHRONIC MITRAL REGURGITATION

Medical Treatment

DEGENERATIVE MITRAL REGURGITATION. The role of pharmacologic therapy for MR remains another subject of uncertainty and some debate.[137,145] Although there is no doubt that afterload reduction therapy is indicated, and may be lifesaving, in patients with acute MR, the indications for such therapy in patients with chronic MR are much less clear. Because afterload is not excessive in most patients with chronic MR, in whom systolic shortening is facilitated by the reduced systolic wall stress, systemic vasodilator therapy to reduce afterload further may not provide additional benefit. Acute administration of nitroprusside, nifedipine, and ACE inhibitors to severely symptomatic patients has been demonstrated to alter hemodynamics favorably in some studies, but these effects may not pertain to asymptomatic patients with preserved systolic function. Several small studies of chronic therapy with ACE inhibitors, ranging from 4 weeks to 6 months, have failed to provide evidence of hemodynamic benefit, and there are no long-term studies and no randomized trials with which to make definitive recommendations. At present, there is a lack of convincing data that vasodilator therapy affects LV volumes or systolic function favorably in the absence of symptoms or hypertension, and current guidelines do not recommend the use of these agents for chronic therapy of primary degenerative MR. An exception would be those patients with severe chronic MR, with symptoms or LV dysfunction (or both) who are not candidates for surgery because of age or other comorbidities. These patients should receive standard, aggressive management for heart failure with ACE inhibitors and beta adrenergic blocking agents (see Chap. 28). Antibiotic prophylaxis to prevent infective endocarditis is no longer recommended routinely for patients with MR (see Chap. 67). All patients with AF, paroxysmal or chronic, should receive chronic anticoagulation.

FUNCTIONAL MITRAL REGURGITATION. Patients with secondary, functional MR stemming from LV dilation and dysfunction should undergo evidence-based aggressive medical management for LV systolic dysfunction (see Chap. 28). There is evidence that beneficial reverse remodeling with medical therapy will reduce the severity of MR in many patients.

RESYNCHRONIZATION THERAPY. In patients with a dilated or ischemic cardiomyopathy and secondary MR, resynchronization therapy with dual ventricular chamber pacing has been observed to decrease mitral regurgitant severity. The mechanism of this effect likely is similar to that achieved in some patients with medical management—LV remodeling with a reduction in ventricular size and associated improvement in alignment of the papillary muscles (see Chap. 29). This leads to improved leaflet coaptation and decreased backflow across the mitral valve.[145]

Surgical Treatment

Surgical treatment should be considered for patients with functional disability and/or for patients with no symptoms or only mild symptoms but with progressively deteriorating LV function or progressively increasing LV dimensions, as documented by noninvasive studies.[30a,136] In patients considered for surgery, two-dimensional transthoracic or TEE with Doppler evaluation and color flow Doppler imaging provide detailed assessment of mitral valve structure and function.[36,138] However, left heart catheterization, LV angiocardiography, and coronary arteriography are indicated for the following: (1) evaluating a discrepancy between echocardiographic findings and the clinical picture; (2) detecting and assessing the severity of any associated valvular lesions; and (3) determining the presence and assessing the extent of coronary artery disease.

Without surgical treatment, the prognosis for patients with MR and heart failure is poor (see Fig. 66-22), and hence MV repair or replacement is indicated for symptomatic patients. When operative treatment is being considered, the chronic and often slowly but relentlessly progressive nature of MR must be weighed against the immediate risks and long-term uncertainties attendant on surgery, especially if MV replacement is required. Surgical mortality depends on the following: patient's clinical and hemodynamic status (particularly the function of the left ventricle); patient's age (see Chap. 80)[149,150]; presence of comorbid conditions such as renal, hepatic, or pulmonary disease[82]; and the skill and experience of the surgical team.[151-153] The decision to replace or to repair the valve (**Fig. 66-33**) is of critical importance, and MV repair is strongly recommended whenever possible.[152-154] Replacement involves the operative risk, as well as the risks of thromboembolism and anticoagulation in patients receiving mechanical prostheses, of late structural valve deterioration in patients receiving bioprostheses, and of late mortality, especially in patients with associated coronary artery disease who require coronary artery bypass grafting (see Table 66-3). Surgical mortality in patients requiring MV replacement does not depend significantly on which of the currently used tissue or mechanical valve prostheses is selected.

Repair of the mitral valve is most often successful in the following: (1) children and adolescents with pliable valves; (2) adults with degenerative MR secondary to MVP; (3) annular dilation; (4) papillary muscle dysfunction secondary to ischemia or rupture; (5) chordal rupture; or (6) perforation of a mitral leaflet caused by infective endocarditis. This represents the vast majority of patients with MR in the United States and other developed countries. These procedures are less likely to be successful in older patients with the rigid, calcified, deformed valves of rheumatic heart disease or those with severe subvalvular chordal thickening and major loss of leaflet substance; many of these latter patients require MV replacement. Younger patients in developing countries who have severe rheumatic MR in the absence of active carditis may undergo successful repair.[152]

MV repair for degenerative MR consists of reconstruction of the valve, which is usually accompanied by a mitral annuloplasty using a rigid or flexible prosthetic ring (see Fig. 66-33). Prolapsed valves causing severe MR are usually treated with resection of the prolapsing segment(s) with plication and reinforcement of the annulus. Replacing, reimplanting, elongating, or shortening of the chordae tendineae, splitting the papillary muscles, and repairing the subvalvular apparatus have been successful in selected patients with pure or predominant MR in whom subvalvular pathology contributes to the MR.[152,155] Repair of anterior and posterior prolapsing leaflets has been successful in experienced centers.[153,156]

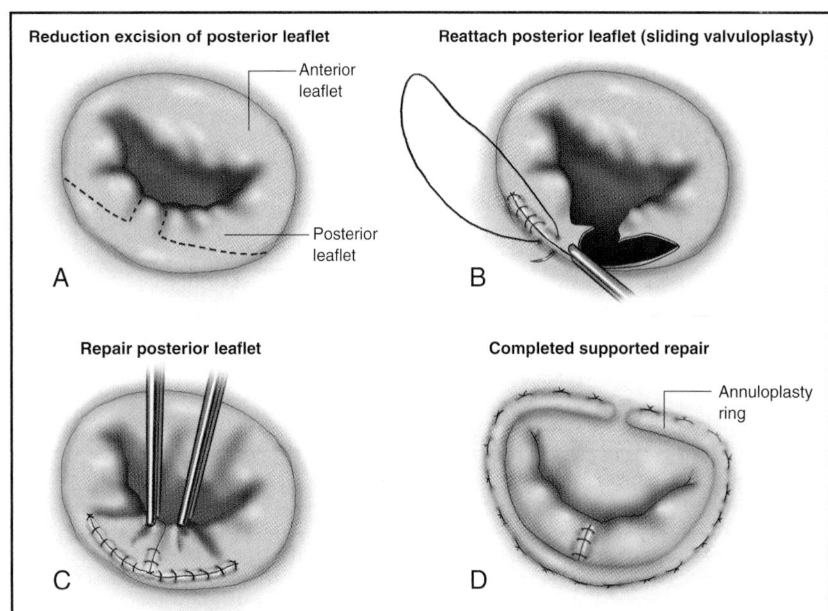

FIGURE 66-33 A-D, Mitral valve repair using reduction excision and reattachment of the posterior leaflet with implantation of an annuloplasty ring. *(From Doty DB [ed]: Cardiac Surgery: Operative Technique. St. Louis, Mosby Year Book, 1997, p 259.)*

Ischemic MR secondary to regional LV dysfunction with annular dilation may be treated by annuloplasty (see Chap. 31). Annuloplasty is also successful in many patients with significant functional MR resulting from dilated cardiomyopathy. Episodic MR caused by transient ischemia is often eliminated by coronary revascularization, whereas moderate to severe chronic MR secondary to ischemic heart disease usually requires MV repair or replacement.[157,158] In patients undergoing coronary artery bypass surgery, some investigators recommend that concomitant MV repair be considered for even mild MR.[159]

Intraoperative TEE and Doppler is extremely useful for assessing the adequacy of MV repair.[160] In the minority of patients with persistent severe MR in whom the operative results are unsatisfactory, the problem can usually be corrected immediately or, if necessary, the valve can be replaced. LV outflow tract obstruction caused by systolic anterior motion of the mitral valve occurs in 5% to 10% of patients following MV repair for degenerative MR. The causes are not clear but may include excess valvular tissue with severe leaflet redundancy and/or an interventricular septum bulging into a small left ventricle. These complications may also be recognized intraoperatively by TEE. Treatment with volume loading and beta-blocking agents is often helpful. The obstruction usually disappears with time; if it does not, reoperation and rerepair or MV replacement may be necessary.

Preoperative AF is an independent predictor of reduced long-term survival after MV surgery for chronic MR.[144] The persistence of AF postoperatively requires long-term anticoagulation, thereby partially nullifying the advantages of MV repair. In patients who have developed AF, whether chronic or paroxysmal, outcomes are improved if a maze procedure is performed at the time of MV repair or replacement,[119,155] with reduced risk of postoperative stroke. The decision to perform a maze procedure should be based on surgical expertise as well as patient age and comorbidities, because this procedure may add to the length and complexity of the operation.

Mitral Valve Repair Versus Replacement. Although MV replacement has been used successfully in treating MR for almost four decades, there has been some dissatisfaction with the results of this operation. First, LV function often deteriorates following MV replacement, contributing to early and late mortality and late disability. The increase in afterload consequent to abolishing the low impedance leak was first believed to be responsible, but now it is clear that the loss of annular-chordal-papillary muscle continuity (see Fig. 66-27) interferes with LV geometry, volume, and function in patients who have undergone MV replacement. This does not occur after MV repair. Animal experiments have shown convincingly that the normal function of the MV apparatus primes the left ventricle for normal contraction that is prevented when surgery causes discontinuity of this apparatus. There is evidence from animal experiments and from human patients that preservation of the papillary muscle and its chordal attachments to the mitral annulus is beneficial to postoperative LV function after MV reconstruction and replacement. Thus, preservation of these tissues, whenever possible, is now considered a critical feature of MV replacement.[145]

A second disadvantage of MV replacement is the prosthesis itself, including the risks of thromboembolism or hemorrhage associated with mechanical prostheses, late structural deterioration of bioprostheses, and infective endocarditis with all prostheses.

For these reasons, increasing efforts are being made to repair the mitral valve whenever possible in patients with isolated or predominant MR.[152-155] The STS National Database Committee reported an operative mortality rate of less than only 1.6% of 21,229 patients undergoing mitral valve repair from 2002 to 2006.[73] This compares favorably with the 5.7% operative mortality for the 12,238 patients undergoing isolated MV replacement. However, risk is high when concurrent CABG is necessary. Operative mortality for combining CABG and mitral valve replacement is 11.6% compared with 7.4% for mitral valve repair and CABG.[72] Long-term postoperative outcomes are also more favorable with MV repair versus MV replacement, whether or not concomitant CABG is required (**Fig. 66-34**).

With growing experience in MV repair for degenerative causes of MR, including MVP and rupture of chordae tendineae, as well as for ischemic MR, the number of patients in whom valve reconstruction is carried out is increasing on a yearly basis. In many centers in the United States, over two thirds of all patients requiring operation for pure or predominant MR now undergo MV repair. However, in 2003, only 42% of patients undergoing surgery for pure MR in the STS National Cardiac Surgery Database underwent repair and 58% underwent MV replacement. This percentage has steadily increased, and currently 69% of patients in the STS Database undergoing surgery for isolated MR undergo MV repair.[161] However, many patients who are candidates for repair continue to undergo MV replacement. MV repair is technically a more demanding procedure than MV replacement, with a distinct learning curve for the surgeon. In addition, MR recurs after MV repair in a subset of patient with degenerative valve disease that is predicted, in part, by the presence of residual MR immediately following repair. Hence, there is growing emphasis of referral of patients requiring surgery for pure MR to centers of excellence in performing MV repair.[1,152,162]

Minimally invasive surgical techniques using a small, low, asymmetrical sternotomy or anterior thoracotomy and percutaneous cardiopulmonary bypass[162,163] have been found to be less traumatic and can be used for MV repair and replacement. This approach has been reported to reduce cost, improve cosmetic results, and shorten the recovery time. However, it also is demanding technically and is successfully performed

CH 66

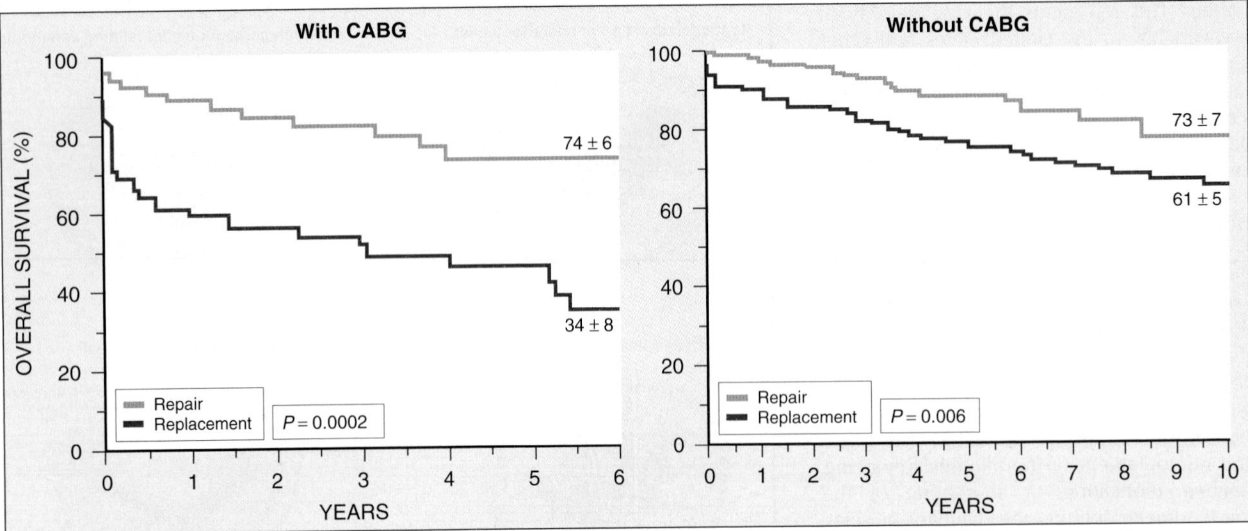

FIGURE 66-34 Plots of overall survival compared for mitral repair and replacement groups in patients who had **(left)** or did not have **(right)** associated CABG. Note that the outcome is better with repair than with replacement in both groups and that the outcome is worse in patients who underwent CABG and mitral valve replacement. *(From Enriquez-Sarano M, Schaff HV, Orszulak TA, et al: Valve repair improves the outcome of surgery for mitral regurgitation: A multivariate analysis. Circulation 91:1022, 1995.)*

by only a minority of cardiac surgeons. There is now growing interest in the development of percutaneous approaches to MV repair[164] using either the edge to edge technique[165] or the coronary sinus approach for percutaneous mitral annuloplasty.[166,167]

Surgical Results. Operative mortality rates of 3% to 9% are now common in many centers for patients with pure or predominant MR (NYHA Class II or III) who undergo elective isolated MV replacement. The overall mortality rate was 5.7% in the STS National Database of more than 20,000 patients undergoing isolated MV replacement between 2002 and 2006 and 1.6% for the 21,000 patients undergoing MV repair.[72,73] In comparison, the operative mortality rate for isolated AVR during the same period was 3.2%. The combination of MV replacement with CABG, however, is associated with a mortality rate of 7% to 12% , and the mortality rate is higher (up to 25%) in patients with severe LV dysfunction, especially when MR is secondary to myocardial ischemia, when pulmonary or renal function is impaired, or when the operation must be carried out as an emergency.[82] Age per se is no barrier to successful surgery; MV repair or replacement can be performed in patients older than 75 years if their general health status is adequate[149-150a]; however, surgery in these patients has a higher risk than in younger patients (see Chap. 80). A review of Medicare data involving 684 U.S. hospitals and more than 61,000 patients has indicated that the average in-hospital mortality for isolated MV replacement in patients older than 65 years is 14.1% (20.5% in low-volume centers and 10.1% in high-volume centers).

Surgical treatment substantially improves survival in patients with symptomatic MR. Preoperative factors, such as age younger than 60 years, NYHA Class I or II, cardiac index exceeding 2.0 liters/min/m^2, LV end-diastolic pressure less than 12 mm Hg, and a normal ejection fraction and end-systolic volume, all correlate with excellent immediate and long-term survival rates. Both preoperative LV ejection fraction (see Fig. 66-29) and end-systolic diameter are important predictors of short- and long-term outcomes.[136,139] Excellent outcome is anticipated in patients with end-systolic diameters less than 40 mm and ejection fractions of 60% or more. Intermediate outcomes are observed in patients with end-systolic diameters between 40 and 50 mm and ejection fractions between 50% and 60%. Poor outcomes are associated with values beyond these limits.

A large proportion of operative survivors have improved clinical status, quality of life, and exercise tolerance following MV repair or replacement. Severe pulmonary hypertension is reduced, LV end-diastolic volume and mass decrease, and coronary flow reserve increases. Depressed contractile function improves, especially if the papillary muscles and chordal attachment to the annulus remain intact. However, patients with MR who have marked LV dysfunction preoperatively sometimes remain symptomatic, with depressed LV function, despite a technically satisfactory surgical procedure. Progressive LV dysfunction and death from heart failure may occur, presumably because LV dysfunction may be advanced and largely irreversible by the time patients with pure MR develop serious symptoms. Thus, every effort should be made to operate on patients before they develop serious symptoms, and even asymptomatic patients with severe MR may be considered for surgery in an experienced center if there is a high likelihood (>90%) that the valve can be repaired successfully without residual MR.[1,2]

Even though surgical results are suboptimal in patients with MR who have developed severe symptoms or marked LV dysfunction,[145] operation is still indicated for most of these patients because conservative therapy has little to offer. Postoperative survival rates are lower in patients in AF than in those in sinus rhythm.[143,144] As with patients with MS, the arrhythmia by itself does not unfavorably influence outcome, but is a marker for older age and other clinical and hemodynamic features associated with less optimal results.

The cause of MR clearly plays an important role in determining outcome following surgical treatment.[152,156,158,168] In patients with primary degenerative disease of the mitral valve, MV repair or replacement has the potential to improve LV performance. However, in those with functional MR, the primary problem is disease of the LV myocardium, and prognosis is strongly influenced by the degree of LV dysfunction. MV repair or replacement in these latter patients has less beneficial effects on long-term outcome, particularly in those with ischemic MR, compared with patients with degenerative MR. Occlusive coronary artery disease coexisting with MR, but not the primary cause of MR, requires simultaneous coronary CABG and MV repair or replacement.[169] Coronary artery disease is associated with decreased perioperative and long-term postoperative survival (see Fig. 66-34).

INDICATIONS FOR OPERATION. A proposed management strategy for patients with chronic severe MR is shown in **Figure 66-35**.[1] The threshold for surgical treatment of MR is declining for several reasons. These include the reductions in operative mortality, the improvements in MV repair procedures, long-term results indicating stability of repair in experienced centers, and the recognition of the poor long-term results in many patients when MR is corrected only after a long history of symptoms, impaired LV function, AF, or pulmonary hypertension. A detailed echocardiographic examination should be carried out to assess the likelihood that MV repair, rather than MV replacement, is possible, and the difference in outcomes between these procedures should be weighed when deciding whether or not to proceed.

Asymptomatic Patients

Asymptomatic patients (NYHA Class I) should be considered for MV repair if they have LV systolic dysfunction (ejection fraction ≤60% and/or LV end-systolic diameter ≥40 mm).[1,2] It is also reasonable to

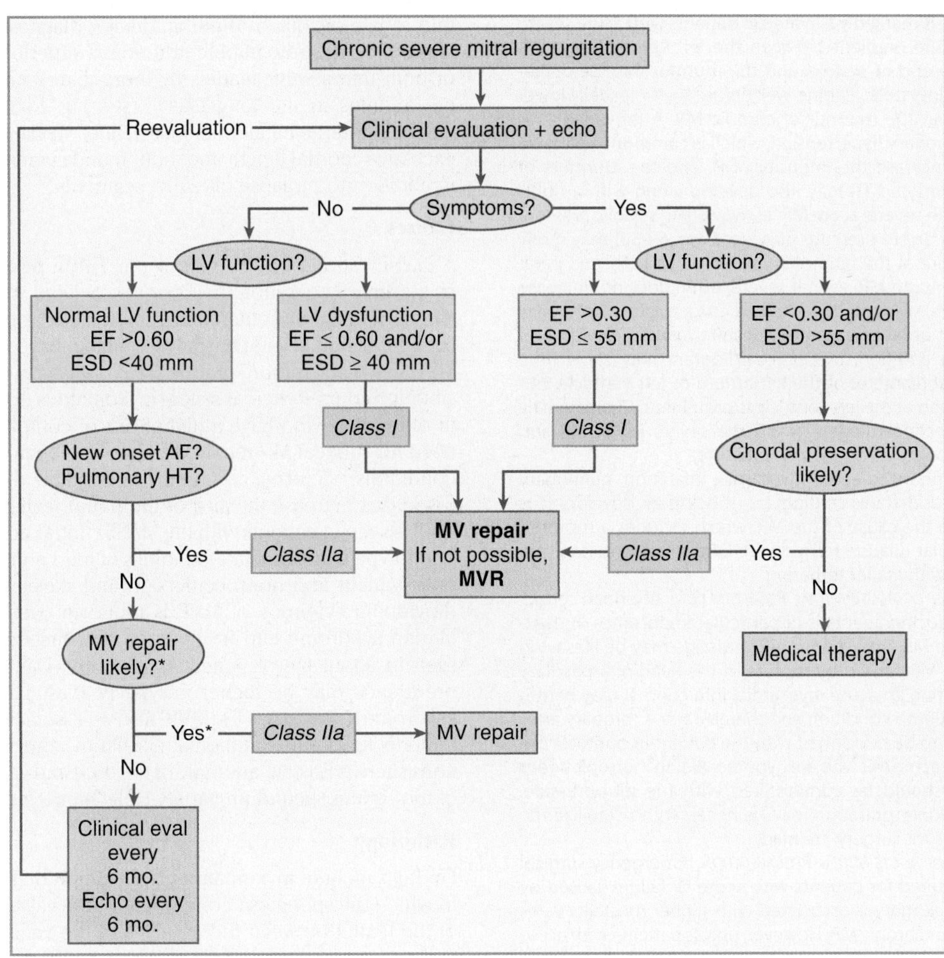

FIGURE 66-35 Management strategy for patients with chronic severe mitral regurgitation. EF = ejection fraction, ESD = end-systolic dimension, HT = hypertension; MVR = mitral valve replacement. *Mitral valve repair may be performed in asymptomatic patients with normal LV function if performed by an experienced surgical team and the likelihood of successful MV repair is greater than 90%. *(From Bonow RO, Carabello BA, Chatterjee K, et al: ACC/AHA 2006 guidelines for the management of patients with valvular heart disease: A report of the American College of Cardiology/American Heart Association Task Force on Practice Guidelines [writing committee to revise the 1998 Guidelines for the Management of Patients With Valvular Heart Disease]: Developed in collaboration with the Society of Cardiovascular Anesthesiologists: Endorsed by the Society for Cardiovascular Angiography and Interventions and the Society of Thoracic Surgeons. Circulation 114:e84, 2006.)*

consider MV repair in asymptomatic patients when AF or pulmonary hypertension is present.

A number of centers are moving toward a more aggressive surgical approach in which MV repair is recommended to all patients with severe MR, independent of symptoms or LV function. However, such a recommendation should be considered only for patients with severe MR (see Table 66-1) who are referred to centers in which the surgical experience indicates that the patient will undergo successful MV repair with a very high degree of certainty. Unfortunately, successful MV repair cannot be guaranteed and, even in the best of circumstances, some young asymptomatic patients may be subjected to the risks of prosthetic valves prematurely and unnecessarily with this approach.

When MV repair is not recommended, asymptomatic patients with normal LV function should be followed clinically and by echocardiography every 6 to 12 months. At times, a careful history and performance of an exercise test often reveal that these patients are not truly asymptomatic.

If MV replacement is likely to be necessary, a higher threshold for clinical and hemodynamic impairment should be used than if MV repair is contemplated, and there are few indications for MV replacement in asymptomatic patients other than LV systolic dysfunction (see Fig 66-35). Because of the higher operative mortality, older patients (>75 years) should, in general, undergo surgery only if they are symptomatic.

Symptomatic Patients

Patients with severe MR and moderate or severe symptoms (NYHA Classes II, III, and IV) should generally be considered for surgery. One exception is a patient in whom the LV ejection fraction is less than 30% and echocardiography suggests that MV replacement will be required and that the subvalvular apparatus cannot be preserved. Because of the high risk of operation and the poor long-term results in these patients, medical therapy is usually advised, but the outcome is poor in any event. However, when MV repair appears possible, even patients with serious LV dysfunction may be considered for operation (see Fig 66-35).

ACUTE MITRAL REGURGITATION. The causes of acute MR (see Table 66-7) are diverse and represent acute manifestations of disease processes that may, under other circumstances, cause chronic MR. Especially important causes of acute MR are spontaneous rupture of chordae tendineae, infective endocarditis with disruption of valve leaflets or chordal rupture, ischemic dysfunction or rupture of a papillary muscle, and malfunction of a prosthetic valve.[102]

Acute severe MR causes a marked reduction of forward stroke volume, slight reduction of end-systolic volume, and increase in end-diastolic volume. One major hemodynamic difference between acute and chronic MR derives from the differences in left atrial compliance. Patients who develop acute severe MR usually have a normal-sized left atrium, with normal or reduced left atrial compliance. The left atrial pressure rises abruptly, which often leads to pulmonary edema, marked elevation of pulmonary vascular resistance, and right-sided heart failure.

Because the *v* wave is markedly elevated in patients with acute severe MR, the reverse pressure gradient between the left ventricle and left atrium declines at the end of systole, and the murmur may be decrescendo rather than holosystolic, ending well before A_2. It is usually lower pitched and softer than the murmur of chronic MR. A left-sided S_4 is frequently found. Pulmonary hypertension, which is common in patients with acute MR, may increase the intensity of P_2 and the murmurs of pulmonary regurgitation and TR may also develop along with a right-sided S_4. In patients with severe, acute MR, a *v* wave (late systolic pressure rise) in the pulmonary artery pressure pulse (see Fig. 66-30) may rarely cause premature closure of the pulmonary valve, an early P_2, and paradoxical splitting of S_2. Acute MR, even if severe, often does not increase overall cardiac size, as seen on the chest roentgenogram, and may produce only mild left atrial enlargement despite marked elevation of left atrial pressure. In addition, the echocardiogram may show little increase in the internal diameter of the left atrium or left ventricle, but increased systolic motion of the left ventricle is prominent. Characteristic features on Doppler echocardiography are the severe jet of MR and elevation of the pulmonary artery systolic pressure.

In severe MR secondary to acute myocardial infarction, pulmonary edema, hypotension, and frank cardiogenic shock may develop. It is essential to determine the cause of the MR, which includes a ruptured papillary muscle, annular dilation from severe LV dilation, and papillary muscle displacement with leaflet tethering.

Medical Management of Acute Mitral Regurgitation. Afterload reduction with afterload-reducing agents is of particular importance in treating patients with acute MR. Intravenous nitroprusside may be lifesaving in patients with acute MR caused by rupture of the head of a papillary muscle that occurs during an acute myocardial infarction. It may permit stabilization of the patient's condition and thereby allow coronary arteriography and surgery to be performed with the patient in optimal condition. In patients with acute MR who are hypotensive, an inotropic agent such as dobutamine should be administered with the nitroprusside. Intra-aortic balloon counterpulsation may be necessary to stabilize the patient as preparations for surgery are made.

Surgical Treatment of Acute Mitral Regurgitation. Emergency surgical treatment may be required for patients with acute LV failure caused by acute MR. Emergency surgery is associated with higher mortality rates than elective surgery for chronic MR. However, unless patients with acute severe MR and heart failure are treated aggressively, a fatal outcome is almost certain.

Acute papillary muscle rupture requires emergency surgery with MV repair or replacement. In patients with papillary muscle dysfunction, initial treatment should consist of hemodynamic stabilization, usually with the aid of an intra-aortic balloon pump, and surgery should be considered for those patients who do not improve with aggressive medical therapy. If patients with MR can be stabilized by medical treatment, it is preferable to defer operation until 4 to 6 weeks after the infarction. Vasodilator treatment may be useful during this period. However, medical management should not be prolonged if multisystem (renal and/or pulmonary) failure develops.[102]

Surgical mortality rates are also higher in patients with acute MR and refractory heart failure (NYHA Class IV), those with prosthetic valve dysfunction, and those with active infective endocarditis (of a native or prosthetic valve). Despite the higher surgical risks, the efficacy of early operation has been established in patients with infective endocarditis complicated by medically uncontrollable congestive heart failure and/or recurrent emboli (see Chap. 67).[170]

Mitral Valve Prolapse

CAUSES AND PATHOLOGY. MVP has been given many names, including the systolic click-murmur syndrome, Barlow syndrome, billowing mitral cusp syndrome, myxomatous mitral valve syndrome, floppy valve syndrome, and redundant cusp syndrome.[171,172] It is a variable clinical syndrome that results from diverse pathogenic mechanisms of one or more portions of the mitral valve apparatus, valve leaflets, chordae tendineae, papillary muscle, and valve annulus. MVP is one of the most prevalent cardiac valvular abnormalities. Using standardized echocardiographic diagnostic criteria, community-based studies have shown that MVP syndrome occurs in 2.4% of the population. MVP is twice as frequent in women as in men. However, serious MR occurs more frequently in older men (>50 years) with MVP than in young women with this disorder.

The clinical and echocardiographic criteria for the diagnosis of MVP have been well established. The characteristic systolic click and mid to late systolic murmur is a major diagnostic criterion. The most specific echocardiographic criterion is superior displacement of one or both mitral valve leaflets by more than 2 mm above the plane of the annulus in the long axis[171] (see Fig. 15-52). Other echocardiographic criteria include diffuse leaflet thickening and redundancy, excessive chordal length and motion, and evidence of ruptured chords, in addition to prolapse of leaflet segments.

Causes

A classification of MVP is shown in **Table 66-8**. Usually, MVP occurs as a primary condition that is not associated with other diseases and can be familial or nonfamilial. Familial MVP is transmitted as an autosomal trait and several chromosomal loci have been identified.[173] The MVP syndrome is more prevalent in young women, who generally have a benign course, whereas severe myxomatous disease is more common in older men, who have a higher risk of complications, including the need for surgical MV repair. MVP has also been associated with many conditions, occurring commonly in heritable disorders of connective tissue that increase the size of the mitral leaflets and apparatus.[171,172] MVP is seen in patients with the MASS (mitral, aortic, skin, and skeletal) phenotype, with associated findings of mild nonprogressive aortic root enlargement and nonspecific skin and skeletal changes.[174] Echocardiographic evidence of MVP is found in over 90% of patients with Marfan syndrome and in many of their first-degree relatives. MVP is seen in about 6% of patients with Ehlers-Danlos syndrome, but the prevalence may be higher in type IV (vascular type) Ehlers-Danlos syndrome (see Chap. 8). MVP also is associated with osteogenesis imperfecta, pseudoxanthoma elasticum, and congenital malformations such as Ebstein anomaly of the tricuspid valve, atrial septal defect of the ostium secundum variety, Holt-Oram syndrome, and HCM.

Pathology

Findings include myxomatous proliferation of the mitral valve leaflets, in which the spongiosa component of the valve (i.e., the middle layer of the leaflet between the atrialis and the ventricularis composed of loose, myxomatous material) is unusually prominent[111,171] and the quantity of acid mucopolysaccharide is increased. Electron microscopy shows a haphazard arrangement of cells with disruption and fragmentation of collagen fibrils. Secondary effects include fibrosis of the surface of the MV leaflets, thinning and/or elongation of the chordae tendineae, and ventricular friction lesions.

In mild cases, the valvular myxoid stroma is enlarged on histologic examination, but the leaflets are grossly normal. However, with increasing quantities of myxoid stroma, the leaflets become grossly abnormal, redundant, and prolapsed. There is interchordal hooding caused by leaflet redundancy that includes the rough and clear zones of the

TABLE 66-8 Classification of Mitral Valve Prolapse

Mitral Valve Prolapse Syndrome
- Younger age (20-50 yr)
- Predominantly female
- Click or click-murmur on physical examination
- Thin leaflets with systolic displacement on echocardiography
- Associated with low blood pressure, orthostatic hypotension, palpitations
- Benign long-term course

Myxomatous Mitral Valve Disease
- Older age (40-70 yr)
- Predominantly male
- Thickened, redundant valve leaflets
- Mitral regurgitation on physical exam and echocardiography
- High likelihood of progressive disease requiring mitral valve surgery

Secondary Mitral Valve Prolapse
- Marfan syndrome
- Hypertrophic cardiomyopathy
- Ehlers-Danlos syndrome
- Other connective tissue diseases

Modified from Otto CM: Valvular Heart Disease. 2nd ed. Philadelphia, WB Saunders, 2004, p 369.

involved leaflets. Regions of endothelial disruption are common and are possible sites of endocarditis or thrombus formation. The severity of MR depends on the extent of the prolapse. The cusps of the mitral valve, chordae tendineae, and annulus may all be affected by myxomatous proliferation. Degeneration of collagen and myxomatous changes within the central core of the chordae tendineae, with associated decreases in tensile strength,[124] are primarily responsible for chordal rupture, which often occurs and may intensify the severity of MR. Increased chordal tension resulting from the enlarged area of the valve cusps may play a contributory role. Myxomatous changes in the annulus may result in annular dilation and calcification, further contributing to the severity of MR.

Myxomatous proliferation, although most commonly affecting the mitral valve, has also been described in the tricuspid, aortic, and pulmonic valves, particularly in patients with the Marfan syndrome, and may lead to regurgitation of these valves and the mitral valve.

CLINICAL PRESENTATION. The clinical presentations of the MVP syndrome are diverse. The condition has been observed in patients of all ages and both genders. Despite the overestimation of prevalence in the population referred to earlier, MVP is the most common cause of isolated MR requiring surgical treatment in the United States and the most common cardiac condition predisposing patients to infective endocarditis (see Chap. 67).

Symptoms

The vast majority of patients with MVP are asymptomatic and remain so throughout their lives. Although early studies called attention to an MVP syndrome, with a characteristic systolic nonejection click and various nonspecific symptoms, such as fatigability, palpitations, postural orthostasis, and anxiety and other neuropsychiatric symptoms, as well as symptoms of autonomic dysfunction, these associations have not been confirmed in carefully controlled studies.[171] How and even whether these symptoms relate to the presence of MVP is not clear.

Patients may complain of syncope, presyncope, palpitations, chest discomfort and, when MR is severe, symptoms of diminished cardiac reserve. Chest discomfort may be typical of angina pectoris but is more often atypical in that it is prolonged, not clearly related to exertion, and punctuated by brief attacks or severe stabbing pain at the apex. The discomfort may be secondary to abnormal tension on papillary muscles. In patients with MVP and severe MR, the symptoms of the latter (fatigue, dyspnea, and exercise limitation) may be present. Patients with MVP may also develop symptomatic arrhythmias (see later).

PHYSICAL EXAMINATION. The body weight is often low and the habitus may be asthenic (see Chap. 12). Blood pressure is usually normal or low; orthostatic hypotension may be present. As noted below, patients with MVP have a higher than expected prevalence of straight back syndrome, scoliosis, and pectus excavatum. MR ranges from absent to severe.

Auscultation. The auscultatory findings unique to the MVP syndrome are best elicited with the diaphragm of the stethoscope. The patient should be examined in the supine, left decubitus, and sitting positions. The most important finding is a nonejection systolic click at least 0.14 second after S_1.[172] This can be differentiated from an aortic ejection click because it occurs after the beginning of the carotid pulse upstroke. Occasionally, multiple mid and late systolic clicks are audible, most readily along the lower left sternal border. The clicks are believed to be produced by sudden tensing of the elongated chordae tendineae and of the prolapsing leaflets. They are often, although not invariably, followed by a mid to late crescendo systolic murmur that continues to A_2. This murmur is similar to that produced by papillary muscle dysfunction, which is readily understandable because both result from mid to late systolic MR. In general, the duration of the murmur is a function of the severity of the MR. When the murmur is confined to the latter portion of systole, MR usually is not severe. However, as MR becomes more severe, the murmur commences earlier and ultimately becomes holosystolic.

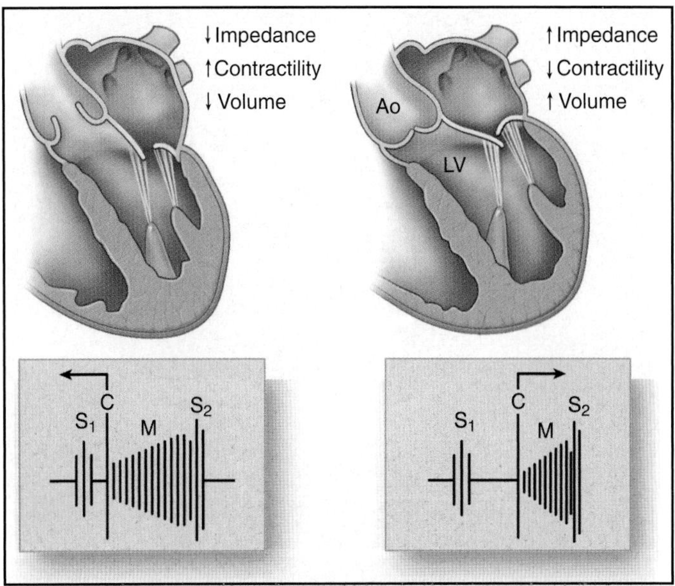

FIGURE 66-36 Dynamic auscultation in mitral valve prolapse. Any maneuver that decreases LV volume (e.g., decreased venous return, tachycardia, decreased outflow impedance, increased contractility) worsens the mismatch in size between the enlarged mitral valve and LV chamber, resulting in prolapse earlier in systole and movement of the click (C) and murmur (M) toward the first heart sound (S_1). Conversely, maneuvers that increase LV volume (e.g., increased venous return, bradycardia, increased outflow impedance, decreased contractility) delay the occurrence of prolapse, resulting in movement of the click and murmur toward the second heart sound (S_2). Ao = aorta. *(Modified from O'Rourke RA, Crawford MH: The systolic click-murmur syndrome: Clinical recognition and management. Curr Probl Cardiol 1:9, 1976.)*

There is considerable variability of the physical findings in the MVP syndrome. Some patients exhibit both a midsystolic click and a mid to late systolic murmur, others present with only one of these two findings, and still others have only a click on one occasion and only a murmur on another, both on a third examination, and no abnormality at all on a fourth. Conditions other than MVP that may cause midsystolic clicks include tricuspid valve prolapse, atrial septal aneurysms, and extracardiac factors.

Dynamic Auscultation. The auscultatory findings are exquisitely sensitive to physiologic and pharmacologic interventions, and recognition of the changes induced by these interventions is of great value in the diagnosis of the MVP syndrome (**Fig. 66-36**). The mitral valve begins to prolapse when the reduction of LV volume during systole reaches a critical point at which the valve leaflets no longer coapt; at that instant, the click occurs and the murmur commences. Any maneuver that decreases LV volume, such as a reduction of impedance to LV outflow, reduction in venous return, tachycardia, or augmentation of myocardial contractility, results in an earlier occurrence of prolapse during systole. As a consequence, the click and onset of the murmur move closer to S_1. When prolapse is severe and/or LV size is markedly reduced, prolapse may begin with the onset of systole. As a consequence, the click may not be audible, and the murmur may be holosystolic. On the other hand, when LV volume is augmented by an increase in the impedance to LV emptying, an increase in venous return, reduction of myocardial contractility, or bradycardia, both the click and onset of the murmur will be delayed.

During the straining phase of the Valsalva maneuver and on sudden standing, cardiac size decreases, and the click and onset of the murmur occur earlier in systole. In contrast, a sudden change from the standing to the supine position, leg raising, squatting, maximal isometric exercise and, to a lesser extent, expiration will delay the click and the onset of the murmur. During the overshoot phase of the Valsalva maneuver (i.e., six to eight cycles following release), and with prolongation of the R-R interval, either following a premature contraction or in AF, the click and onset of the murmur are usually delayed, and the intensity of the murmur is reduced. Maneuvers that elevate arterial pressure, such as isometric exercise, increase the intensity of the click and murmur. In general, when the onset of the murmur is delayed, both its duration and intensity are diminished, reflecting a reduction in the severity of MR.

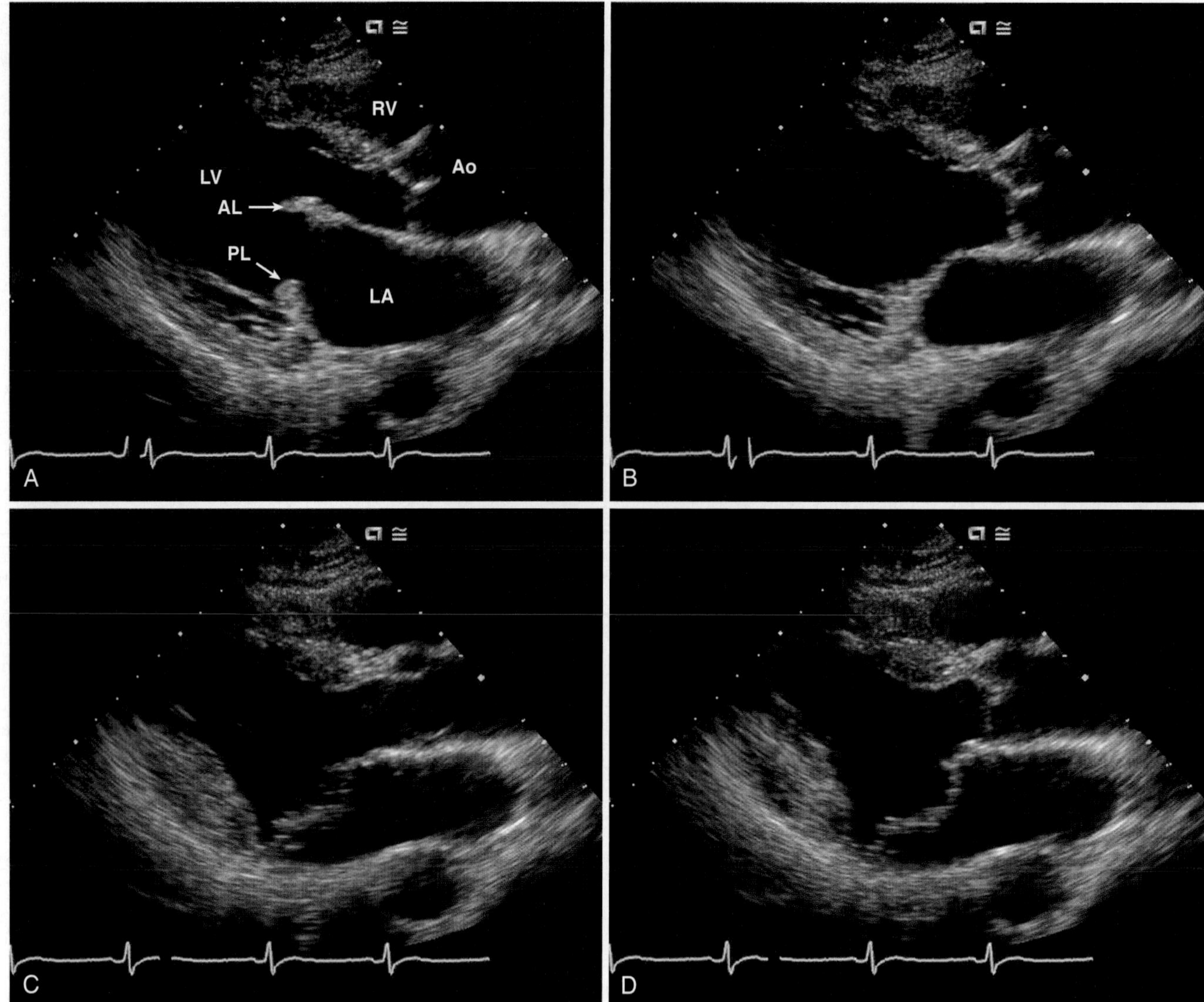

FIGURE 66-37 Parasternal long-axis two-dimensional echocardiographic images in a 41-year-old man with MVP and auscultatory findings of a midsystolic click and MR. **A,** End-diastolic image. The mitral valve leaflets are severely thickened, and the anterior leaflet (AL) is elongated. **B-D,** Serial images from early systole to midsystole demonstrating bileaflet prolapse. Color flow imaging in this patient demonstrated severe MR. Patients with these findings are at increased risk of complications, such as infective endocarditis, systemic emboli, and heart failure. Ao = aorta; LA = left atrium; LV = left ventricle; PL = posterior leaflet; RV = right ventricle.

The response to several interventions may be helpful in differentiating obstructive HCM from MVP (see Chap. 69). During the strain of the Valsalva maneuver, the murmur of HCM increases in intensity, whereas the murmur of MVP becomes longer but usually not louder. Following a premature beat, the murmur of HCM increases in intensity and duration, whereas that caused by MVP usually remains unchanged or decreases.

Echocardiography

Echocardiography (see Chap. 15) plays an essential role in the diagnosis of MVP and has been instrumental in the delineation of this syndrome (**Fig. 66-37**; see Fig. 15-52).[175] To establish the diagnosis, the two-dimensional echocardiogram must show that one or both mitral valve leaflets billow by at least 2 mm into the left atrium during systole in the long-axis view. Thickening of the involved leaflet to more than 5 mm supports the diagnosis. Findings of more severe myxomatous disease include increased leaflet area, leaflet redundancy, chordal elongation, and annular dilation. These findings are also helpful in identifying patients at significant risk for developing severe MR or infective endocarditis (**Table 66-9**). The mitral annular diameter is often abnormally increased. TEE provides additional details regarding integrity of the mitral valve apparatus, such as rupture of the chordae tendineae. In MR secondary to MVP, the echocardiogram also provides valuable information regarding LV size and function.

The echocardiographic findings of MVP may be observed in patients without a click or murmur. Others have typical echocardiographic and auscultatory features. The echocardiographic findings of MVP have been reported to occur in a large number of first-degree relatives of patients with established MVP. Two-dimensional echocardiography has also revealed prolapse of the tricuspid and aortic valves in approximately 20% of patients with MVP. Conversely, however, prolapse of the tricuspid and aortic valves occurs uncommonly in patients without prolapse of the mitral valve.

Doppler echocardiography frequently reveals mild MR that is not always associated with an audible murmur. Moderate to severe MR is present in about two thirds of patients with posterior leaflet prolapse and in about 25% of patients with anterior leaflet prolapse. The severity of MR should be assessed quantitatively, as noted earlier (see Table 66-1).

Other Diagnostic Evaluation Modalities

Electrocardiography. The ECG is usually normal in asymptomatic patients with MVP. In a minority of asymptomatic patients and in many symptomatic patients, the ECG shows inverted or biphasic T waves and

TABLE 66–9 Predictors of Clinical Outcome in Mitral Valve Prolapse

PREDICTOR	SURVIVAL	VALVE SURGERY	ARRHYTHMIAS OR SUDDEN DEATH	ENDOCARDITIS
Age	+++	+++	–	–
Gender	++	++	–	–
Leaflet thickness or redundancy	+++	+++	++++	++++
Severity of mitral regurgitation	++++	++++	++++	++++
Systolic click	+	–	–	–
Left ventricular dilation	+	++++	++	–
Left atrial dilation	–	++	+	–

Symbols indicate the relative predictive value of each variable for the listed clinical outcomes on a scale of no predictive value (–) to strongly predictive (++++).

nonspecific ST-segment changes in leads II, III, and aVf and occasionally in the anterolateral leads as well.

ARRHYTHMIAS. A spectrum of arrhythmias has been observed in patients with MVP. These include atrial and ventricular premature contractions and supraventricular and ventricular tachyarrhythmias,[172] as well as bradyarrhythmias caused by sinus node dysfunction or varying degrees of atrioventricular block. The mechanism of the arrhythmias is not clear. Diastolic depolarization of muscle fibers in the anterior mitral leaflet in response to stretch has been demonstrated experimentally, and the abnormal stretch of the prolapsed leaflet may be of pathogenetic significance.

Paroxysmal supraventricular tachycardia is the most common sustained tachyarrhythmia in patients with MVP and may be related to an increased incidence of left atrioventricular bypass tracts. The incidence of MVP in patients with the Wolff-Parkinson-White syndrome is increased. There is also an increased association between MVP and prolongation of the QT interval, which may play a role in the pathogenesis of serious ventricular arrhythmias. Patients with MVP have an increased incidence of abnormal late potentials on signal-averaged ECGs, as well as reduced heart rate variability.

ANGIOGRAPHY. Angiography is not recommended for the diagnostic evaluation of MVP. However, if angiography is performed for other indications, there are features of the left ventriculogram that are characteristic of MVP. The right anterior oblique projection is most useful for defining the posterior leaflet of the mitral valve and the left anterior oblique projection is most useful for studying the anterior leaflet. The most helpful sign is extension of the mitral leaflet tissue inferiorly and posteriorly to the point of attachment of the mitral leaflets to the mitral annulus. Angiography may also reveal scalloped edges of the leaflets, reflecting redundancy of tissue. Other angiographic abnormalities in some patients with MVP include LV dilation, decreased systolic contraction (especially of the basal portion of the ventricle), and calcification of the mitral annulus.

MAGNETIC RESONANCE IMAGING AND CARDIAC COMPUTED TOMOGRAPHY. These advanced imaging techniques can help in determining the extent of MVP and LV function in patients with suboptimal echocardiographic examinations. CMR is also useful for evaluating the presence and severity of MR.

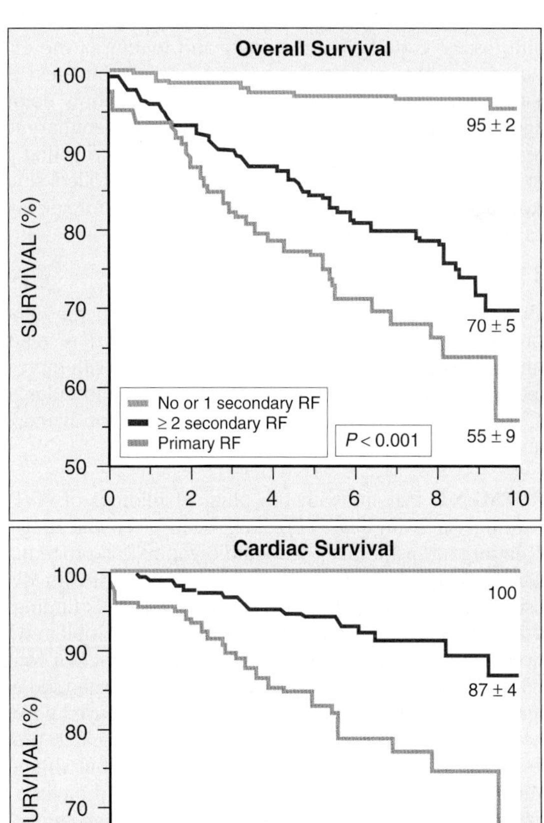

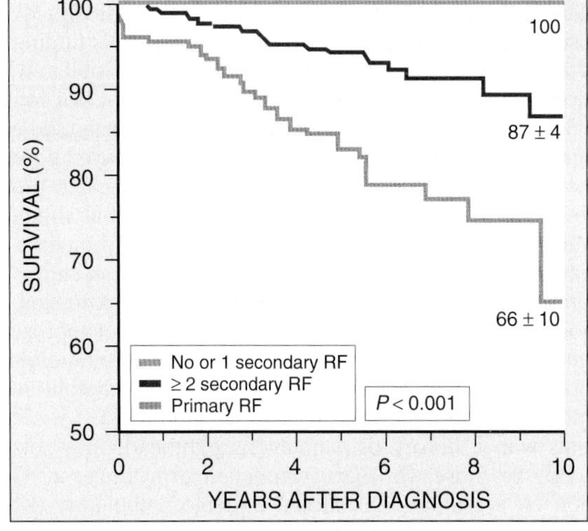

FIGURE 66-38 Survival in patients with mitral valve prolapse according to categories of baseline risk factors (RFs). Primary RFs were moderate to severe MR and ejection fraction <50%. Secondary RFs were mild MR, left atrium larger than 40 mm, flail leaflet, atrial fibrillation, and age older than 50 years. *(Modified from Avierinos JF, Gersh BJ, Melton LJ, et al: Natural history of asymptomatic mitral valve prolapse in the community. Circulation 106:1355, 2002.)*

DISEASE COURSE. The outlook for patients with MVP in general is excellent; a large majority remain asymptomatic for many years without any change in clinical or laboratory findings.[171,172] Serious complications (need for cardiac surgery, acute infective endocarditis, or cerebral embolic events) occur at a rate of only 1/100 patient-years. In one study, 4% of patients died over an 8-year period. In contrast, another study reported a much more aggressive course in 833 patients with MVP, with a 19% mortality rate at 10 years and a 20% rate of MVP-related events, including heart failure, AF, cerebrovascular events, arterial thromboembolism, and endocarditis. The apparent explanation for these latter observations is that patients with MVP could be risk-stratified on the basis of several factors (**Fig. 66-38**). The primary risk factors were moderate to severe MR and/or LV ejection fraction less than 50% , and secondary risk factors included mild MR, left atrial dimension 40 mm or greater, flail leaflet, and age 50 years or older. Patients with a primary risk factor had excessive mortality and morbidity, as did those with two or more secondary risk factors. Other series have supported these observations, demonstrating greater risk of cardiac death or MVP-related complications in men, those older than 45 years, those with holosystolic murmurs, those with severe MR, and those with left atrial dimension more than 40 mm. Those studies that reported a lower prevalence of adverse sequelae of MVP included relatively fewer patients with these risk factors. Variables associated with an adverse outcome are summarized in Table 66-9.

Progressive MR, with a gradual increase in left atrial and LV size, AF, pulmonary hypertension, and the development of congestive heart failure, is the most frequent serious complication, occurring in about

15% of patients over a 10- to 15-year period, with age and initial MR severity being the primary predictors of progression.[176] Patients with the MVP syndrome are also at risk of developing infective endocarditis. Both severe MR and endocarditis develop more frequently in patients with murmurs and clicks compared with those with an isolated click, patients with thickened (greater than 5 mm) and redundant mitral valve leaflets, and men older than 50 years (see Table 66-9). In many patients, rupture of the chordae tendineae is responsible for the precipitation and/or intensification of the MR. Infective endocarditis often aggravates the severity of MR and therefore precipitates the need for surgical treatment.

Acute hemiplegia, transient ischemic attacks, cerebellar infarcts, amaurosis fugax, and retinal arteriolar occlusions have been reported to occur more frequently in patients with the MVP syndrome, suggesting that cerebral emboli are unusually common in this condition. It has been proposed that these neurologic complications are associated with loss of endothelial continuity and tearing of the endocardium overlying the myxomatous valve, which initiates platelet aggregation and the formation of mural platelet-fibrin complexes. Although it has been proposed that embolization secondary to MVP may be a significant cause for unexplained strokes in young people without cerebrovascular disease, a large case-controlled study has show no association between MVP and ischemic neurologic events in persons younger than 45 years.[171]

Mitral Valve Prolapse and Sudden Death

The risk of sudden death is about twice normal in patients with mitral valve prolapse, most likely because of an increased risk of ventricular arrhythmias.[171] The risk of sudden death is increased with more severe MR or severe valvular deformity and with complex ventricular arrhythmias, QT interval prolongation, AF, and a history of syncope and palpitations.[158]

MANAGEMENT. Patients with the physical findings of MVP—and those without such findings who have been given the diagnosis—should undergo transthoracic echocardiography. This procedure also should be performed in first-degree relatives of patients with MVP.[1] The diagnosis of MVP requires definitive echocardiographic findings; overdiagnosis and incorrect labeling have been a major problem with this condition. Asymptomatic patients, or those whose principal complaint is anxiety, with no arrhythmias evident on a routine extended electrocardiographic tracing and without evidence of MR, have an excellent prognosis. They should be reassured about the favorable prognosis and be encouraged to engage in normal lifestyles, but should have follow-up examinations every 3 to 5 years. This should include a two-dimensional echocardiogram and a color flow Doppler study.

Patients with a long systolic murmur may show progression of MR and should be evaluated more frequently, at intervals of approximately 12 months. Endocarditis prophylaxis is no longer recommended routinely for patients with MVP, including those with a systolic murmur and typical echocardiographic findings (see Chap. 67).

Patients with a history of palpitations, lightheadedness, dizziness, or syncope, or those who have ventricular arrhythmias or QT prolongation on a routine ECG, should undergo ambulatory (24-hour) electrocardiographic monitoring and/or exercise electrocardiography to detect arrhythmias. Because of the risk, albeit very low, of sudden death, further electrophysiologic studies may be carried out to characterize arrhythmias, if they exist. Beta-adrenergic blockers are useful in the treatment of palpitations secondary to frequent premature ventricular contractions and for self-terminating episodes of supraventricular tachycardia. These drugs may also be useful in the treatment of chest discomfort, both for patients with associated coronary artery disease and those with normal coronary vessels in whom the symptoms may be caused by regional ischemia secondary to MVP. Radiofrequency ablation of atrioventricular bypass tracts is useful for frequent or prolonged episodes of supraventricular tachycardia.

Aspirin should be given to patients with MVP who have had a documented focal neurologic event and in whom no other cause, such as a left atrial thrombus or AF, is apparent.

Patients with MVP and severe MR should be treated similarly to other patients with severe MR and may require MV surgery. MV repair without replacement is possible in over 90% of patients (see Fig. 66-33). Therefore, the threshold for surgical treatment in these patients is lower than in patients with MR in whom MV replacement may be necessary, providing that patients are referred to a surgical team with established success in MV repair, as noted. Most of all MV repairs for MR are now carried out in patients with MVP. Resection of the most deformed leaflet segment, usually the middle scallop of the posterior leaflet, and insertion of an annuloplasty ring to reduce the dilated annulus is the most commonly used procedure. Repair of anterior leaflet prolapse is more challenging. Rupture of the chordae tendineae to the anterior leaflet can sometimes be treated by chordal transfer from the posterior leaflet. In other patients, shortening of the chordae tendineae and/or papillary muscle is necessary. The average operative mortality is 1.6%, and long-term studies demonstrate excellent durability of MV repair in most patients.[152-155] However, MR recurs in a subset of patients, at which point it may be necessary to perform repeat MV repair or replacement.

Although this discussion has focused attention on complications of MVP, it should not be forgotten that, on the whole, this is a benign condition. The vast majority of patients with this syndrome remain asymptomatic for their entire lives and require, at most, observation every few years and reassurance.

Tricuspid, Pulmonic, and Multivalvular Disease

Tricuspid Stenosis

CAUSES AND PATHOLOGY

Tricuspid stenosis (TS) is almost always rheumatic in origin.[177] Other causes of obstruction to right atrial emptying are unusual and include congenital tricuspid atresia (see Chap. 65), right atrial tumors, which may produce a clinical picture suggesting rapidly progressive TS (see Chap. 74), and the carcinoid syndrome (see Chap. 68), which more frequently produces TR. Rarely, obstruction to RV inflow can be caused by endomyocardial fibrosis, tricuspid valve vegetations, a pacemaker lead, or extracardiac tumors.

Most patients with rheumatic tricuspid valve disease present with TR or a combination of TS and TR. Isolated rheumatic TS is uncommon and almost never occurs as an isolated lesion but generally accompanies mitral valve disease. In many patients with TS, the aortic valve is also involved (i.e., trivalvular stenosis is present). TS is found at autopsy in about 15% of patients with rheumatic heart disease but is of clinical significance in only about 5%. Organic tricuspid valve disease is more common in India, Pakistan, and other developing nations near the equator than in North America or Western Europe. The anatomic changes of rheumatic TS resemble those of MS, with fusion and shortening of the chordae tendineae and fusion of the leaflets at their edges, producing a diaphragm with a fixed central aperture. However, valvular calcification is rare. As is the case with MS, TS is more common in women. The right atrium is often greatly dilated in TS, and its walls are thickened. There may be evidence of severe passive congestion, with enlargement of the liver and spleen.

PATHOPHYSIOLOGY. A diastolic pressure gradient between the right atrium and ventricle—the hemodynamic expression of TS—is augmented when the transvalvular blood flow increases during inspiration or exercise and is reduced when the blood flow declines during expiration. A relatively modest diastolic pressure gradient (i.e., a mean gradient of only 5 mm Hg) is usually sufficient to elevate the mean right atrial pressure to levels that result in systemic venous congestion and, unless sodium intake has been restricted or diuretics have been given, is associated with jugular venous distention, ascites, and edema.

In patients with sinus rhythm, the right atrial *a* wave may be very tall and may even approach the level of the RV systolic pressure. Resting

TABLE 66-10 Clinical and Laboratory Features of Rheumatic Tricuspid Stenosis

History
- Progressive fatigue, edema, anorexia
- Minimal orthopnea, paroxysmal nocturnal dyspnea
- Rheumatic fever in two thirds of patients
- Female preponderance
- Pulmonary edema and hemoptysis rare

Physical Findings
- Signs of multivalvular involvement
- Diastolic rumble at lower left sternal border, increasing in intensity with inspiration
- Often confused with mitral stenosis
- Peripheral cyanosis
- Neck vein distention, with prominent *a* waves and slow *y* descent
- Absent right ventricular lift
- Associated murmurs of mitral and aortic valve disease
- Hepatic pulsation
- Ascites, peripheral edema

Imaging Findings
- ECG—tall right atrial P waves and no right ventricular hypertrophy
- Chest roentgenogram—dilated right atrium without enlarged pulmonary artery segment
- Echocardiogram—diastolic doming of tricuspid valve leaflet

Modified from Ockene IS: Tricuspid valve disease. In Dalon JE, Alpert JS (eds): Valvular Heart Disease. 2nd ed. Boston, Little Brown, 1987, pp 356, 390.

cardiac output is usually markedly reduced and fails to rise during exercise. This accounts for the normal or only slightly elevated left atrial, pulmonary arterial, and RV systolic pressures, despite the presence of accompanying mitral valvular disease.

A mean diastolic pressure gradient across the tricuspid valve as low as 2 mm Hg is sufficient to establish the diagnosis of TS. However, exercise, deep inspiration, and the rapid infusion of fluids or the administration of atropine may greatly enhance a borderline pressure gradient in a patient with TS. Therefore, when this diagnosis is suspected, right atrial and ventricular pressures should be recorded simultaneously, using two catheters or a single catheter with a double lumen, with one lumen opening on either side of the tricuspid valve. The effects of respiration on any pressure difference should be examined.

CLINICAL PRESENTATION

Symptoms

The low cardiac output characteristic of TS causes fatigue, and patients often experience discomfort caused by hepatomegaly, ascites, and anasarca (**Table 66-10**). The severity of these symptoms, which are secondary to an elevated systemic venous pressure, is out of proportion to the degree of dyspnea. Some patients complain of a fluttering discomfort in the neck, caused by giant *a* waves in the jugular venous pulse. Despite the coexistence of MS, the symptoms characteristic of this valvular lesion (severe dyspnea, orthopnea, and paroxysmal nocturnal dyspnea) are usually mild or absent in the presence of severe TS because the latter prevents surges of blood into the pulmonary circulation behind the stenotic mitral valve. The absence of symptoms of pulmonary congestion in a patient with obvious MS should suggest the possibility of TS.

PHYSICAL EXAMINATION. Because of the high frequency with which MS occurs in patients with TS and the similarity in the physical findings between the two valvular lesions, the diagnosis of TS is commonly missed. The physical findings are mistakenly attributed to MS, which is more common and may be more obvious. Therefore, a high index of suspicion is required to detect the tricuspid valvular lesion. In the presence of sinus rhythm, the *a* wave in the jugular venous pulse is tall, and a presystolic hepatic pulsation is often palpable. The *y* descent is slow and barely appreciable. The lung fields are clear and, despite engorged neck veins and the presence of ascites and anasarca, the patient may be comfortable while lying flat. Thus, the diagnosis of TS may be suspected from inspection of the jugular venous pulse in a patient with MS but without clinical evidence of pulmonary hypertension. This suspicion is strengthened when a diastolic thrill is palpable at the lower left sternal border, particularly if the thrill appears or becomes more prominent during inspiration.

The auscultatory findings of the accompanying MS are usually prominent and often overshadow the more subtle signs of TS. A tricuspid OS may be audible but is often difficult to distinguish from a mitral OS. However, the tricuspid OS usually follows the mitral OS and is localized to the lower left sternal border, whereas the mitral OS is usually most prominent at the apex and radiates more widely. The diastolic murmur of TS is also commonly heard best along the lower left parasternal border in the fourth intercostal space and is usually softer, higher pitched, and shorter in duration than the murmur of MS. The presystolic component of the TS murmur has a scratchy quality and a crescendo-decrescendo configuration that diminishes before S_1. The diastolic murmur and OS of TS are both augmented by maneuvers that increase transtricuspid valve flow, including inspiration, the Mueller maneuver (forced inspiration against a closed glottis), assumption of the right lateral decubitus position, leg raising, inhalation of amyl nitrite, squatting, and isotonic exercise. They are reduced during expiration or the strain of the Valsalva maneuver and return to control levels immediately (i.e., within two to three beats) after Valsalva release.

Echocardiography

The echocardiographic changes (see Chap. 15)of the tricuspid valve in TS resemble those observed in the mitral valve in MS.[177] Two-dimensional echocardiography characteristically shows diastolic doming of the leaflets (especially the anterior tricuspid valve leaflet), thickening and restricted motion of the other leaflets, reduced separation of the tips of the leaflets, and a reduction in diameter of the tricuspid orifice. TEE allows added delineation of the details of valve structure. Doppler echocardiography shows a prolonged slope of antegrade flow and compares well with cardiac catheterization in the quantification of TS and assessment of associated TR. Doppler evaluation of TS has largely replaced the need for catheterization to assess severity.

Other Diagnostic Evaluation Modalities

ELECTROCARDIOGRAPHY. In the absence of AF in a patient with valvular heart disease, TS is suggested by the presence of electrocardiographic evidence of right atrial enlargement (see Chap. 13). The P wave amplitude in leads II and V_1 exceeds 0.25 mV. Because most patients with TS have mitral valvular disease, the electrocardiographic signs of biatrial enlargement are commonly found. The amplitude of the QRS complex in lead V_1 may be reduced by the dilated right atrium.

RADIOGRAPHY. The key radiologic finding is marked cardiomegaly with conspicuous enlargement of the right atrium (i.e., prominence of the right heart border), which extends into a dilated superior vena cava and azygos vein, but without conspicuous dilation of the pulmonary artery. The vascular changes in the lungs characteristic of mitral valvular disease may be masked, with little or no interstitial edema or vascular redistribution, but left atrial enlargement may be present.

Angiography following injection of contrast material into the right atrium and filming in the 30-degree right anterior oblique projection characteristically shows thickening and decreased mobility of the leaflets, a diastolic jet through the constricted orifice, and thickening of the normal atrial wall.

MANAGEMENT. Although the fundamental approach to the management of severe TS is surgical treatment, intensive sodium restriction and diuretic therapy may diminish the symptoms secondary to the accumulation of excess salt and water. A preparatory period of diuresis may diminish hepatic congestion and thereby improve hepatic function sufficiently to diminish the risks of subsequent operation.

Most patients with TS have coexisting valvular disease that requires surgery. In patients with combined TS and MS, the former must not be corrected alone because pulmonary congestion or edema may ensue. Surgical treatment of TS should be carried out at the time of MV repair or replacement in patients with TS in whom the mean diastolic pressure gradient exceeds 5 mm Hg and the tricuspid orifice is less than approximately 2.0 cm^2. The final decision concerning surgical treatment is often made at the operating table.

Because TS is almost always accompanied by some TR, simple finger fracture valvotomy may not result in significant hemodynamic

TABLE 66-11 Causes and Mechanisms of Pure Tricuspid Regurgitation

Causes

- Anatomically abnormal valve
  - Rheumatic
  - Nonrheumatic
    - Infective endocarditis
    - Ebstein anomaly
    - Floppy (prolapse)
    - Congenital (non-Ebstein)
    - Carcinoid
    - Papillary muscle dysfunction
    - Trauma
    - Connective tissue disorders (Marfan)
    - Rheumatoid arthritis
    - Radiation injury
- Anatomically normal valve (functional)
  - Elevated right ventricular systolic pressure (dilated annulus)

Mechanisms

CONDITION	LEAFLET AREA	ANNULAR CIRCUMFERENCE	LEAFLET INSERTION
Floppy	↑	↑	Normal
Ebstein anomaly	↑	↑	Abnormal
Pulmonary/right ventricular systolic hypertension	Normal	↑	Normal
Papillary muscle dysfunction	Normal	Normal	Normal
Carcinoid	↓/Normal	Normal	Normal
Rheumatic	↓/Normal	Normal	Normal
Infective endocarditis	↓/Normal	Normal	Normal

Modified from Waller BF: Rheumatic and nonrheumatic conditions producing valvular heart disease. *In* Frankl WS, Brest AN (eds): Cardiovascular Clinics: Valvular Heart Disease: Comprehensive Evaluation and Management. Philadelphia, FA Davis, 1989, pp 35, 95.

improvement but may merely substitute severe TR for TS. However, open valvotomy in which the stenotic tricuspid valve is converted into a functionally bicuspid valve may result in substantial improvement. The commissures between the anterior and septal leaflets and between the posterior and septal leaflets are opened. It is not advisable to open the commissure between the anterior and posterior leaflets for fear of producing severe TR. If open valvotomy does not restore reasonably normal valve function, the tricuspid valve may have to be replaced. A large bioprosthesis is preferred to a mechanical prosthesis in the tricuspid position because of the high risk of thrombosis of the latter and the longer durability of bioprostheses in the tricuspid than in the mitral or aortic positions. The feasibility of tricuspid balloon valvuloplasty has been demonstrated, and this procedure may be combined with mitral balloon valvuloplasty.

Tricuspid Regurgitation

CAUSES AND PATHOLOGY. The most common cause of TR is not intrinsic involvement of the valve itself (i.e., primary TR) but rather dilation of the right ventricle and of the tricuspid annulus causing secondary (functional) TR (**Table 66-11**).[177,178] This may be a complication of RV failure of any cause. It is observed in patients with RV hypertension secondary to any form of cardiac or pulmonary vascular disease, most commonly mitral valve disease.[179] In general, a RV systolic pressure greater than 55 mm Hg will cause functional TR. TR can also occur secondary to RV infarction, congenital heart disease (e.g., pulmonic stenosis and pulmonary hypertension secondary to Eisenmenger syndrome; see Chap. 65), primary pulmonary hypertension (see Chap. 78) and, rarely, cor pulmonale. In infants, TR may complicate RV failure secondary to neonatal pulmonary diseases and pulmonary hypertension with persistence of the fetal pulmonary circulation. In all these cases, TR reflects the presence of, and in turn aggravates, severe RV failure. Functional TR may diminish or disappear as the right ventricle decreases in size with the treatment of heart failure. TR can also occur as a consequence of dilation of the annulus in the Marfan syndrome, in which RV dilation secondary to pulmonary hypertension is not present.

A variety of disease processes can affect the tricuspid valve apparatus directly and lead to regurgitation (primary TR).[177] Thus, organic TR may occur on a congenital basis (see Chap. 65), as part of Ebstein anomaly, defects involving the atrioventricular canal, when the tricuspid valve is involved in the formation of an aneurysm of the ventricular septum, or in corrected transposition of the great arteries, or it may occur as an isolated congenital lesion. Rheumatic fever may involve the tricuspid valve directly. When this occurs, it usually causes scarring of the valve leaflets and/or chordae tendineae, leading to limited leaflet mobility and either isolated TR or a combination of TR and TS. Rheumatic involvement of the mitral, and often aortic, valves coexist.

TR or the combination of TR and TS is an important feature of the carcinoid syndrome (**Fig. 66-39**), which leads to focal or diffuse deposits of fibrous tissue on the endocardium of the valvular cusps and cardiac chambers and on the intima of the great veins and coronary sinus (see Chap. 68). The white, fibrous carcinoid plaques are most extensive on the right side of the heart, where they are usually deposited on the ventricular surfaces of the tricuspid valve and cause the cusps to adhere to the underlying RV wall, thereby producing TR. Endomyocardial fibrosis with shortening of the tricuspid leaflets and chordae tendineae is an important cause of TR in tropical Africa. TR may result from prolapse of the tricuspid valve caused by myxomatous changes in the valve and chordae tendineae (**Fig. 66-40**); prolapse of the mitral valve is usually present in these patients as well. Prolapse of the tricuspid valve occurs in about 20% of all patients with MVP. Tricuspid valve prolapse may also be associated with atrial septal defect. Other causes of TR include penetrating and nonpenetrating trauma, dilated cardiomyopathy, infective endocarditis (particularly staphylococcal endocarditis in IV drug users), and following surgical excision of the tricuspid valve in patients with infective endocarditis that is unresponsive to medical management. Less common causes of TR include cardiac tumors (particularly right atrial myxoma), transvenous pacemaker leads, repeated endomyocardial biopsy in a transplanted heart, endomyocardial fibrosis, methysergide-induced valvular disease, exposure to fenfluramine-phentermine, and systemic lupus erythematosus involving the tricuspid valve.

CLINICAL PRESENTATION

Symptoms

In the absence of pulmonary hypertension, TR is generally well tolerated. However, when pulmonary hypertension and TR coexist, cardiac output declines and the manifestations of right-sided heart failure become intensified. Thus, the symptoms of TR result from a reduced cardiac output and from ascites, painful congestive hepatomegaly, and massive edema. Occasionally, patients have throbbing pulsations in the neck, which intensify on effort and are caused by jugular venous distention, and systolic pulsations of the eyeballs have also been described. In the many patients with TR who have mitral valve disease, the symptoms of the latter usually predominate. Symptoms of pulmonary congestion may abate as TR develops but are replaced by weakness, fatigue, and other manifestations of a depressed cardiac output.

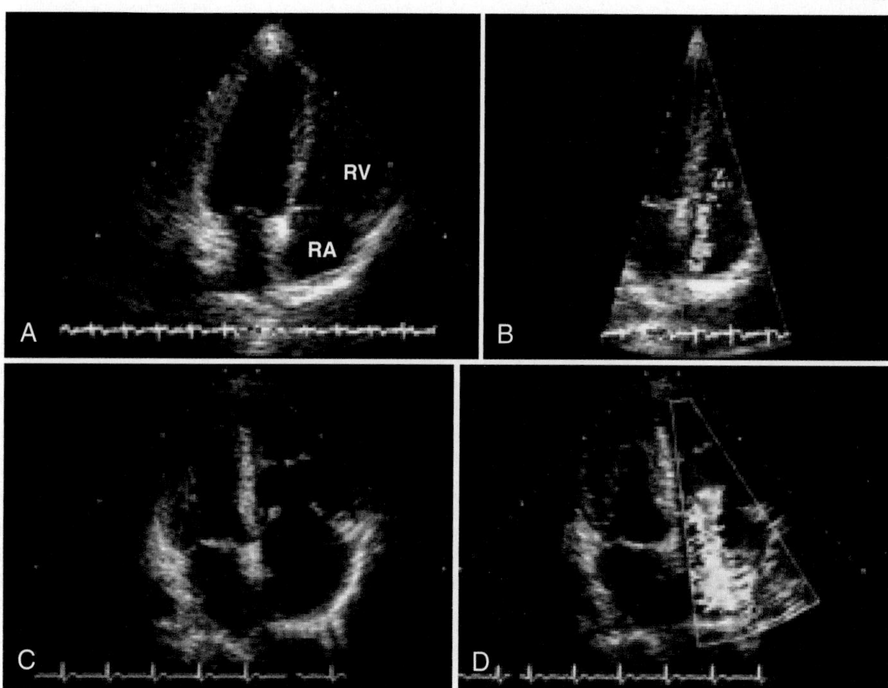

FIGURE 66-39 TR caused by carcinoid involvement of the tricuspid valve. Serial two-dimensional echocardiograms (**A** and **C**) and color Doppler studies (**B** and **D**), separated by 3 years are shown. **C,** After 3 years, there is severe thickening and fixation of the tricuspid leaflets, leading to severe TR and associated right ventricular (RV) and right atrial (RA) enlargement. *(From Møller JE, Connolly HM, Rubin J, et al: Factors associated with progression of carcinoid heart disease. N Engl J Med 348:1005, 2003.)*

PHYSICAL EXAMINATION. Evidence of weight loss and cachexia, cyanosis, and jaundice are often present on inspection in patients with severe TR. AF is common. There is jugular venous distention, the normal *x* and *x′* descents disappear, and a prominent systolic wave—a *c-v* wave (or *s* wave)—is apparent. The descent of this wave, the *y* descent, is sharp and becomes the most prominent feature of the venous pulse unless there is coexisting TS, in which case it is slowed. A venous systolic thrill and murmur in the neck may be present in patients with severe TR. The RV impulse is hyperdynamic and thrusting in quality. Systolic pulsations of an enlarged tender liver are commonly present initially. However, in patients with chronic TR and congestive cirrhosis, the liver may become firm and nontender. Ascites and edema are frequent.

Auscultation usually reveals an S_3 originating from the right ventricle, which is accentuated by inspiration. When TR is associated with and secondary to pulmonary hypertension, P_2 is accentuated as well. When TR occurs in the presence of pulmonary hypertension, the systolic murmur is usually high-pitched, pansystolic, and loudest in the fourth intercostal space in the parasternal region but occasionally is loudest in the subxiphoid area. When TR is mild, the murmur may be short. When TR occurs in the absence of pulmonary hypertension (e.g., in infective endocarditis or following trauma), the murmur is usually of low intensity and limited to the first half of systole. When the right ventricle is greatly dilated and occupies the anterior surface of the heart, the murmur may be prominent at the apex and difficult to distinguish from that produced by MR.

The response of the systolic murmur to respiration and other maneuvers is of considerable aid in establishing the diagnosis of TR. The murmur is characteristically augmented during inspiration (Carvallo sign). However, when the failing ventricle can no longer increase its stroke volume in the recumbent or sitting positions, the inspiratory augmentation may be elicited by standing. The murmur also increases during the Mueller maneuver (see earlier), exercise, leg raising, and hepatic compression. It demonstrates an immediate overshoot after release of the Valsalva strain but is reduced in intensity and duration in the standing position and during the strain of the Valsalva maneuver. Increased atrioventricular flow across the tricuspid orifice in diastole may cause a short early diastolic flow rumble in the left parasternal region following S_3. Tricuspid valve prolapse, like MVP, causes nonejection systolic clicks and late systolic murmurs. However, in tricuspid valve prolapse, these findings are more prominent at the lower left sternal border. With inspiration, the clicks occur later and the murmurs intensify and become shorter in duration

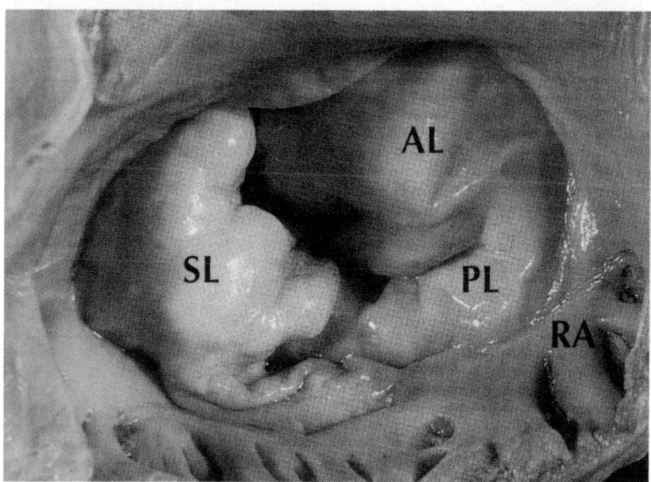

FIGURE 66-40 Tricuspid valve prolapse, viewed from the right atrium (RA). AL = anterior leaflet; PL = posterior leaflet; SL = septal leaflet. *(From Virmani R, Burke AP, Farb A: Pathology of valvular heart disease. In Rahimtoola SH [ed]: Valvular Heart Disease. In Braunwald E [series ed]: Atlas of Heart Diseases. Vol 11. Philadelphia, Current Medicine, 1997, p 1.17.)*

Echocardiography

The goal of echocardiography (see Figs. 15-55 and 15-56) is to detect TR, estimate its severity, and assess pulmonary arterial pressure and RV function. In patients with TR secondary to dilation of the tricuspid annulus, the right atrium, right ventricle, and tricuspid annulus are all usually greatly dilated on echocardiography. There is evidence of RV diastolic overload with paradoxical motion of the ventricular septum similar to that observed in atrial septal defect. Exaggerated motion and delayed closure of the tricuspid valve are evident in patients with Ebstein anomaly (see Fig. 15-93). Prolapse of the tricuspid valve caused by myxomatous degeneration may be evident on echocardiography. Echocardiographic indications of tricuspid valve abnormalities, especially TR by Doppler examination, can be detected in most patients with carcinoid heart disease (see Fig. 66-39). In patients with TR caused by endocarditis, echocardiography may reveal vegetations on the valve or a flail valve. TEE enhances detection of TR. Doppler

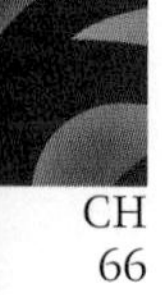

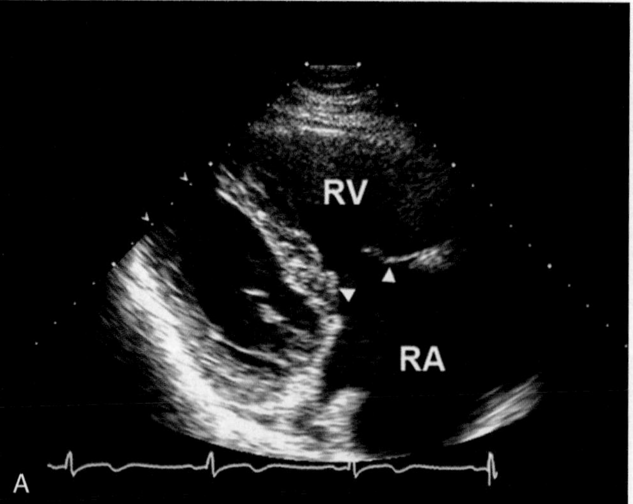

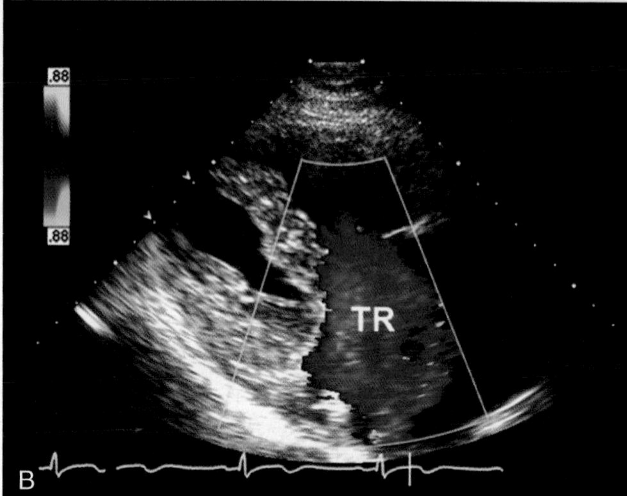

FIGURE 66-41 **A,** Two-dimensional echocardiographic systolic image (right ventricular inflow view) demonstrates thickened septal and anterior tricuspid valve leaflets (arrowheads) and enlargement of the right ventricle (RV) and right atrium (RA) in a patient with carcinoid heart disease. **B,** Color flow Doppler image demonstrates severe TR in the same patient. Note laminar color flow (blue) filling an enlarged right atrium. *(From Bruce CJ, Connolly HM: Right sided valve disease.* In *Otto CM, Bonow RO [eds]: Valvular Heart Disease: A Companion to Braunwald's Heart Disease. Philadelphia, Elsevier, 2009, pp 334-335.)*

echocardiography is a sensitive technique for visualizing the TR jet. The magnitude of TR can be quantified using techniques similar to those used to evaluation MR (**Fig. 66-41**).

Other Diagnostic Evaluation Modalities

Electrocardiography. The ECG is usually nonspecific and characteristic of the lesion causing TR. Incomplete right bundle branch block, Q waves in lead V_1, and AF are commonly found.

Radiography. In patients with functional TR, marked cardiomegaly is usually evident, and the right atrium is prominent. Evidence of elevated right atrial pressure may include distention of the azygos vein and the presence of a pleural effusion. Ascites with upward displacement of the diaphragm may be present. Systolic pulsations of the right atrium may be present on fluoroscopy.

Hemodynamic Findings. The right atrial and RV end-diastolic pressures are often elevated in TR whether the condition is caused by organic disease of the tricuspid valve or is secondary to RV systolic overload. The right atrial pressure tracing usually reveals absence of the *x* descent and a prominent *v* or *c-v* wave (ventricularization of the atrial pressure). Absence of these findings essentially excludes moderate or severe TR. As the severity of TR increases, the contour of the right atrial pressure pulse increasingly resembles that of the RV pressure pulse. A rise or no change in right atrial pressure on deep inspiration, rather than the usual fall, is a characteristic finding. Determination of the pulmonary arterial (or RV) systolic pressure may be helpful in deciding whether the TR is primary (caused by disease of the valve or its supporting structures) or functional (secondary to RV dilation). A pulmonary arterial or RV systolic pressure less than 40 mm Hg favors a primary cause, whereas a pressure greater than 55 mm Hg suggests that TR is secondary.

MANAGEMENT. TR in the absence of pulmonary hypertension usually is well tolerated and may not require surgical treatment. Both human patients and experimental animals with normal pulmonary arterial pressure may tolerate total excision of the tricuspid valve as long as the RV systolic pressure is normal. Dilation of the right side of the heart usually occurs months or years after tricuspid valvectomy (usually carried out for acute infective endocarditis).

Surgical treatment of acquired TR secondary to annular dilation was greatly improved with the development of annuloplasty techniques, with or without an annuloplasty ring. At the time of mitral valve surgery in patients with TR secondary to pulmonary hypertension, the severity of the regurgitation should be assessed by palpation of the tricuspid valve. In addition, it should be determined whether the TR is secondary to pulmonary hypertension, in which case the valve is normal, or whether it is secondary to other disease processes. Patients with mild TR without annular dilation usually do not require surgical treatment; pulmonary vascular pressures decline following successful mitral valve surgery, and the mild TR tends to disappear. However, even mild TR should be repaired if there is dilation of the tricuspid annulus, because the TR is likely to progress in severity if left untreated.[180,181] Excellent results have been reported in patients with mild to moderate TR with the use of suture annuloplasty of the posterior (unsupported) portion of the annulus. Patients with severe TR, with or without annular dilation, require valvotomy and ring annuloplasty. A surgical mortality rate of 13.9% has been reported (see Table 66-3). Residual TR after tricuspid annuloplasty is determined principally by the degree of preoperative tricuspid leaflet tethering.[182] If these procedures do not provide a good functional result at the operating table, as assessed by TEE, valve replacement using a large bioprosthesis may be required.

When organic disease of the tricuspid valve (Ebstein anomaly or carcinoid heart disease) causes TR severe enough to require surgery, valve replacement is usually needed. The risk of thrombosis of mechanical prostheses is greater in the tricuspid than in the mitral or aortic positions, presumably because pressure and flow rates are lower in the right side of the heart. For this reason, the artificial valve of choice for the tricuspid position in adults is a bioprosthesis. Anticoagulants are not required, and a graft durability of more than 10 years has been established.

In treating the difficult problem of tricuspid endocarditis in IV drug users (see Chap. 67), total excision of the tricuspid valve without immediate replacement can generally be tolerated by these patients, who usually do not have associated pulmonary hypertension. When antibiotic therapy is unsuccessful, valve replacement frequently results in reinfection or continued infection. Therefore, diseased valvular tissue should be excised to eradicate the endocarditis, and antibiotic treatment can then be continued. Initially, most patients tolerate loss of the tricuspid valve without great difficulty. However, RV dysfunction usually occurs subsequently. A bioprosthetic valve may therefore be inserted 6 to 9 months after valve excision and control of the infection.

Pulmonic Valve Disease

CAUSES AND PATHOLOGY

Pulmonic Stenosis

The congenital form is the most common cause of pulmonic stenosis (PS). Manifestations in children and adults are discussed in Chap. 65. Rheumatic inflammation of the pulmonic valve is very uncommon, is usually associated with involvement of other valves, and rarely leads to serious deformity. Carcinoid plaques, similar to those involving the tricuspid valve, are often present in the outflow tract of the right ventricle of patients with malignant carcinoid. The plaques result in constriction of the pulmonic valve ring, retraction and fusion of the valve cusps, and either PS or the combination of PS and pulmonic regurgitation. Obstruction in the region of the pulmonic valve may be extrinsic to the valve apparatus and may be produced by cardiac tumors or by aneurysm of the sinus of Valsalva (see Fig. 15-82). Management of congenital PS focuses on balloon dilation (see Chap. 59).

Pulmonic Regurgitation

Pulmonic regurgitation (PR) can result from dilation of the valve ring secondary to pulmonary hypertension (of any cause) or from dilation of the pulmonary artery. Infective endocarditis can involve the pulmonic valve, resulting in valve regurgitation. As more patients with congenital heart disease survive to adulthood, there is an increasing population of young adults with residual pulmonic regurgitation after surgical treatment of congenital PS or tetralogy of Fallot (**Fig. 66-42**). PR may also result from various lesions that directly affect the pulmonic valve. These include congenital malformations, such as absent, malformed, fenestrated, or supernumerary leaflets. These anomalies may occur as isolated lesions but more often are associated with other congenital anomalies, particularly tetralogy of Fallot, ventricular septal defect, and pulmonic valvular stenosis. Less common causes include trauma, carcinoid syndrome, rheumatic involvement, injury produced by a pulmonary artery flow-directed catheter, syphilis, and chest trauma.

CLINICAL PRESENTATION. Like TR, isolated PR causes RV volume overload and may be tolerated for many years without difficulty unless it complicates, or is complicated by, pulmonary hypertension. In this case, PR is usually accompanied by and aggravates RV failure. Patients with PR caused by infective endocarditis who develop septic pulmonary emboli and pulmonary hypertension often exhibit severe RV

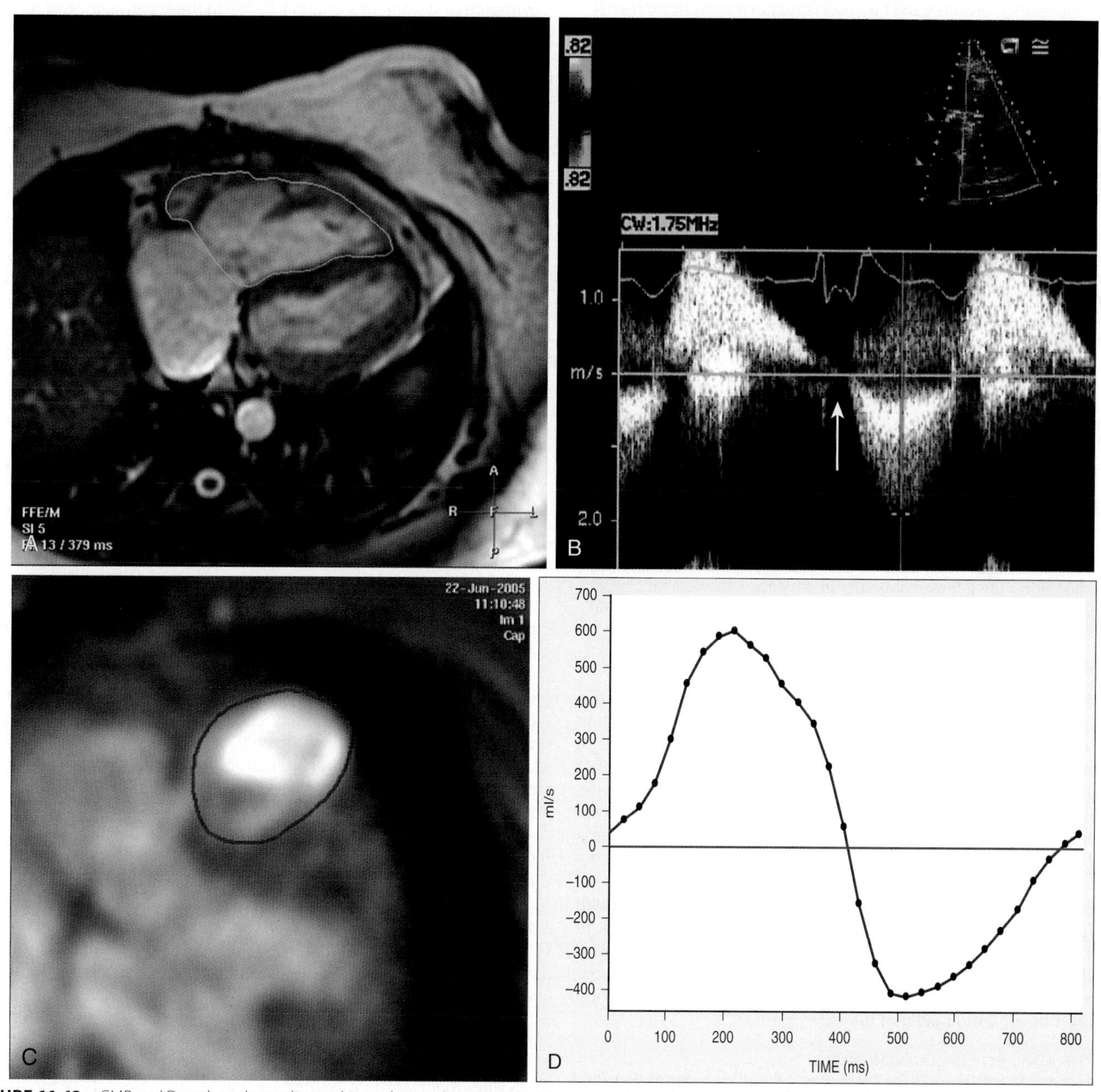

FIGURE 66-42 CMR and Doppler echocardiographic evaluation in a 40-year-old woman who underwent repair of tetralogy of Fallot as a child. She is asymptomatic but has significant right ventricular (RV) enlargement on echocardiography. **A,** RV dilation is confirmed in the CMR images, with a calculated RV end-diastolic volume of 444 mL. **B,** The Doppler tracing shows a dense signal in diastole with a steep deceleration slope that reaches the baseline before the end of diastole (arrow). **C,** Interrogation of pulmonary artery flow in the CMR phase-velocity images is performed by drawing a region of interest (red) around the pulmonary artery. **D,** Graph of the pulmonary artery flow within the region of interest indicated in **C** demonstrates both antegrade and retrograde flow. The total RV stroke volume was 245 mL, with antegrade flow of 98 mL, yielding a regurgitant fraction of 67%.

failure. In most patients, the clinical manifestations of the primary disease are severe and usually overshadow the PR, which often results only in incidental auscultatory findings.

PHYSICAL EXAMINATION. The right ventricle is hyperdynamic and produces palpable systolic pulsations in the left parasternal area, and an enlarged pulmonary artery often produces systolic pulsations in the second left intercostal space. Sometimes systolic and diastolic thrills are felt in the same area. A tap reflecting pulmonic valve closure is usually easily palpable in the second intercostal space in patients with pulmonary hypertension and secondary PR.

AUSCULTATION. P_2 is not audible in patients with congenital absence of the pulmonic valve; however, this sound is accentuated in patients with PR secondary to pulmonary hypertension. There may be wide splitting of S_2 caused by prolongation of RV ejection accompanying the augmented RV stroke volume. A nonvalvular systolic ejection click due to the sudden expansion of the pulmonary artery by the augmented RV stroke volume frequently initiates a midsystolic ejection murmur, most prominent in the second left intercostal space. An S_3 and S_4 originating from the right ventricle are often audible, most readily in the fourth intercostal space at the left parasternal area, and are augmented by inspiration.

In the absence of pulmonary hypertension, the diastolic murmur of PR is low-pitched and usually heard best at the third and fourth left intercostal spaces adjacent to the sternum. The murmur commences when pressures in the pulmonary artery and right ventricle diverge, approximately 0.04 second after P_2. It is diamond-shaped in configuration and brief, reaching a peak intensity when the gradient between these pressures is maximal, and ending with equilibration of the pressures. The murmur becomes louder during inspiration.

When systolic pulmonary arterial pressure exceeds approximately 55 mm Hg, dilation of the pulmonic annulus results in a high-velocity regurgitant jet resulting in the audible murmur of PR, or Graham Steell murmur. (Doppler ultrasonography reveals pulmonary regurgitation at much lower pulmonary arterial pressures.) This murmur is high-pitched, blowing, and decrescendo, beginning immediately after P_2 and is most prominent in the left parasternal region in the second to fourth intercostal spaces. Thus, although it resembles the murmur of AR, it is usually accompanied by severe pulmonary hypertension—that is, an accentuated P_2 or fused S_2, an ejection sound, and a systolic murmur of TR, and not by a widened arterial pulse pressure. Sometimes, a low-frequency presystolic murmur is present, originating from increased diastolic flow across the tricuspid valve.

The murmur of PR secondary to pulmonary hypertension usually increases in intensity with inspiration, is diminished during the Valsalva strain, and returns to baseline intensity almost immediately after release of the Valsalva strain. This PR murmur resembles and may be confused with the diastolic blowing murmur of AR. However, a diastolic blowing murmur along the left sternal border in patients with rheumatic heart disease and pulmonary hypertension (even in the absence of peripheral signs of AR) is usually caused by AR rather than PR.

Echocardiography

Two-dimensional echocardiography shows RV dilation and, in patients with pulmonary hypertension, RV hypertrophy as well. RV function can be evaluated. Abnormal motion of the septum characteristic of volume overload of the right ventricle in diastole and/or septal flutter may be evident. The motion of the pulmonic valve may point to the cause of the PR. Absence of *a* waves and systolic notching of the posterior leaflet suggest pulmonary hypertension; large *a* waves indicate pulmonic stenosis. Doppler echocardiography is extremely accurate in detecting PR and in helping estimate its severity (see Fig. 66-42 and Fig. 15-57). Abnormal Doppler signals in the RV outflow tract with velocity sustained throughout diastole are generally observed in patients in whom PR is caused by dilation of the valve ring secondary to pulmonary hypertension. When the velocity falls during diastole, the pulmonary artery pressure is usually normal, and the regurgitation is caused by an abnormality of the valve itself.

OTHER DIAGNOSTIC EVALUATION MODALITIES

ELECTROCARDIOGRAPHY. In the absence of pulmonary hypertension, PR often results in an ECG that reflects RV diastolic overload—an rSr (or rsR) configuration in the right precordial leads. PR secondary to pulmonary hypertension is usually associated with ECG evidence of RV hypertrophy.

RADIOGRAPHY. Both the pulmonary artery and right ventricle are usually enlarged, but these signs are nonspecific. Fluoroscopy may demonstrate pronounced pulsation of the main pulmonary artery. PR can be diagnosed by observing opacification of the right ventricle following injection of contrast material into the main pulmonary artery, but this diagnosis is made in almost all patients with echocardiography or cardiac magnetic resonance.

CARDIAC MAGNETIC RESONANCE. CMR plays an important role in assessing pulmonary artery dilation, imaging the regurgitant jet and quantifying PR severity (see Fig. 66-42). CMR also is useful in evaluating RV dilation and systolic function.[41,184]

MANAGEMENT. Except in patients with previous surgery for tetralogy of Fallot, PR alone is seldom severe enough to require specific treatment. Treatment of the primary condition, such as infective endocarditis, or the lesion responsible for the pulmonary hypertension, such as surgery for mitral valvular disease, often ameliorates the PR. The timing of surgery for severe PR after tetralogy of Fallot is controversial with current recommendations based on the degree of RV dilation and evidence of systolic dysfunction.[56,183,185] In these patients, valve replacement may be carried out, preferably with a pulmonary allograft. There is growing experience with catheter-based approaches to pulmonic valve replacement in native pulmonic valve disease and in PR following surgical correction of congenital heart defects (see Chap. 59).[186]

Multivalvular Disease

Multivalvular involvement is caused frequently by rheumatic fever and various clinical and hemodynamic syndromes can be produced by different combinations of valvular abnormalities. Myxomatous MR and associated pulmonary hypertension is a leading cause of concomitant TR, often with dilation of the tricuspid annulus. The Marfan syndrome and other connective tissue disorders may cause multivalve prolapse and dilation, resulting in multivalvular regurgitation. Degenerative calcification of the aortic valve may be associated with degenerative mitral annular calcification and cause AS and MR. Different pathologic conditions may affect two valves in the same patient (e.g., infective endocarditis on the aortic valve causing AR and ischemia causing MR).

In patients with multivalvular disease, the clinical manifestations depend on the relative severity of each of the lesions. When the valvular abnormalities are of approximately equal severity, clinical manifestations produced by the more proximal (upstream) of the two valvular lesions (i.e., the mitral valve in patients with combined mitral and aortic valvular disease and the tricuspid valve in patients with combined tricuspid and mitral valvular disease) are generally more prominent than those produced by the distal lesion. Thus, the proximal lesion tends to mask the distal lesion.

It is important to recognize multivalvular involvement preoperatively because failure to correct all significant valvular disease at the time of operation increases mortality considerably. In patients with multivalvular disease, the relative severity of each lesion may be difficult to estimate by clinical examination and noninvasive techniques because one lesion may mask the manifestations of the other. Therefore, patients suspected of having multivalvular involvement and who are being considered for surgical treatment should undergo careful clinical evaluation and full Doppler echocardiographic evaluation and right and left cardiac catheterization and angiography. If there is any question concerning the presence of significant AS in patients undergoing mitral valve surgery, the aortic valve should be inspected because overlooking this condition can lead to a high perioperative mortality. Similarly, it is useful to palpate the tricuspid valve at the time of mitral valve surgery.

MITRAL STENOSIS AND AORTIC VALVE DISEASE. Aortic valve involvement is present in about one third of patients with rheumatic MS. Rheumatic aortic valve disease may result in primary regurgitation, stenosis, or mixed stenosis and regurgitation. AR is evident on physical examination in about two thirds of patients with severe MS but only about 10% of patients with MS have severe rheumatic AR. On physical examination, a proximal lesion may mask signs of a distal lesion. For example, significant AR may be missed in patients with severe MS because the widened pulse pressure may be absent. On the other hand, MS may be missed or, conversely, may be falsely diagnosed on clinical examination of patients with obvious AR. An accentuated S_1 and an OS in a patient with AR should suggest the possibility of mitral valvular disease. AS is evident on physical examination based on the typical murmur, even when MS is present; however, cardiac output tends to be reduced more than in patients with isolated AS. On physical examination, an S_4 (which is common in patients with pure AS) is usually not present. The midsystolic murmur characteristic of AS may be reduced in intensity and duration because the stroke volume is reduced by the MS.

Echocardiography is of decisive value in the evaluation of patients with rheumatic disease and allows accurate diagnosis of the presence and severity of multivalve involvement, taking into consideration the altered flow conditions with serial lesions. For example, the gradient across the stenotic aortic valve may be relatively low when MS is present because of a low cardiac output; valve area calculations are especially helpful in this setting.

Because double-valve replacement is associated with increased short- and long-term risks, balloon mitral valvotomy can be the first procedure if MS is the predominant lesion, with subsequent AVR when needed. If percutaneous balloon valvotomy is not an option or concurrent AVR is needed, surgical valvotomy may be considered as an option.

It is vital to recognize the presence of hemodynamically significant aortic valvular disease (i.e., AS and/or AR) preoperatively in patients who are to undergo mitral valvotomy. This procedure may be hazardous because it can impose a sudden hemodynamic load on the left ventricle that had previously been protected by the MS and may lead to acute pulmonary edema.

AORTIC STENOSIS AND MITRAL REGURGITATION. AS is often accompanied by MR caused by mitral valve prolapse, annular calcification, rheumatic disease, or functional MR. The increased LV pressure secondary to LV outflow obstruction may augment the volume of MR flow, whereas the presence of MR may diminish the ventricular preload necessary for maintenance of the LV stroke volume in patients with AS. The result is a reduced forward cardiac output and marked left atrial and pulmonary venous hypertension. The development of AF (caused by left atrial enlargement) has an adverse hemodynamic effect in the presence of AS. Physical findings may be confusing because it may be difficult to recognize two distinct systolic murmurs. However, on echocardiography, the cause and severity of AS and MR can be accurately diagnosed. In most cases, MR is mild to moderate and it is appropriate to treat AS alone. When MR is severe or there is significant structural mitral valve disease, concurrent mitral repair (whenever possible) or valve replacement at the time of AVR should be considered.

AORTIC AND MITRAL REGURGITATION. This relatively infrequent combination of lesions may be caused by rheumatic heart disease, prolapse of both the aortic and the mitral valves because of myxomatous degeneration, or dilation of both annuli in patients with connective tissue disorders. The left ventricle is usually greatly dilated. The clinical features of AR usually predominate, and it is sometimes difficult to determine whether the MR is caused by organic involvement of this valve or dilation of the mitral valve ring secondary to LV enlargement. When both valvular leaks are severe, this combination of lesions is poorly tolerated. The normal mitral valve ordinarily serves as a backup to the aortic valve, and premature (diastolic) closure of the mitral valve limits the volume of reflux that occurs in patients with acute AR. With severe combined regurgitant lesions, regardless of the cause of the mitral lesion, blood may reflux from the aorta through both chambers of the left side of the heart into the pulmonary veins. Physical and laboratory examinations usually show evidence of both lesions. An S_3 and a brisk arterial pulse are frequently present. The relative severity of each lesion can be assessed best by Doppler echocardiography and contrast angiography. This combination of lesions leads to severe LV dilation. MR that occurs in patients with AR secondary to LV dilation often regresses following AVR alone. If severe, the MR may be corrected by annuloplasty at the time of AVR. An intrinsically normal mitral valve that is regurgitant because of a dilated annulus should not be replaced.

SURGICAL TREATMENT OF MULTIVALVULAR DISEASE. Combined AVR and MV replacement is usually associated with a higher risk and poorer survival than replacement of either of the valves alone. The operative risk of double-valve replacement is about 70% higher than for single-valve replacement. The STS National Database Committee has reported an overall operative mortality rate of 9.6% for multiple (usually double) valve replacement in 3840 patients, compared with 3.2% and 5.7% for isolated AVR and MV replacement, respectively[72,73] (see Table 66-3). The long-term survival depends strongly on the preoperative functional status. Patients operated on for combined AR and MR have poorer outcomes than patients undergoing double-valve replacement for any of the other combinations of lesions, presumably because both AR and MR may produce irreversible LV damage. MV repair or balloon valvotomy in combination with AVR is preferable to double-valve replacement and should be carried out whenever possible. Risk factors that reduce long-term survival after double-valve replacement include advanced age, higher NYHA class, lower LV ejection fraction, greater LV enlargement, and accompanying ischemic heart disease requiring coronary artery bypass grafting.[73,82]

Given the higher risks, a higher threshold is required for multivalvular versus single-valve surgery. Thus, patients are generally advised not to undergo multivalvular surgery until they reach late NYHA Class II or Class III, unless there is evidence of declining LV function. Despite a detailed noninvasive and invasive workup, the decision to treat more than one valve is often made by palpation or by direct inspection at the operating table.

TRIPLE-VALVE DISEASE. Hemodynamically significant disease involving the mitral, aortic, and tricuspid valves is uncommon and typically is caused by rheumatic heart disease. Patients with trivalvular disease may present in advanced heart failure with marked cardiomegaly, and surgical correction of all three valvular lesions is imperative. However, triple-valve replacement is a long and complex operation. Early in the experience with this procedure, the mortality rate was 20% for patients in NYHA Class III and 40% for patients in Class IV. More recently, the mortality rate has declined, but nevertheless triple-valve replacement should be avoided if possible. In many patients with trivalvular disease, it is possible to replace the aortic valve, repair the mitral valve, and perform a tricuspid annuloplasty or valvuloplasty.

Patients who survive triple-valve replacement surgery usually show substantial clinical improvement during the early postoperative period, and postoperative catheterization studies show marked reductions in pulmonary arterial and capillary pressures. However, some patients die of arrhythmias or congestive heart failure in the late postoperative period despite three normally functioning prostheses. The cause of cardiac failure in this situation is unknown, but may be related to intraoperative myocardial ischemia, microemboli from the multiple prostheses, or continued subclinical episodes of rheumatic myocarditis.

When multiple prosthetic valves must be inserted, it is logical to select two bioprostheses or two mechanical prostheses for the left side of the heart. If the patient is to be exposed to the hazards of anticoagulants for one mechanical prosthesis, it seems unreasonable to add the potential risks of early failure of a bioprosthesis. However, if two mechanical prostheses are selected for the left side of the heart, the use of a bioprosthesis in the tricuspid position is suggested.

Prosthetic Cardiac Valves

The first successful human replacements of cardiac valves were accomplished in 1960 by Nina Braunwald and colleagues, Dwight Harken and coworkers, and Albert Starr and Lowell Edwards. Two major groups of prosthetic valves are currently available in models designed for the atrioventricular (mitral and tricuspid) and aortic positions, mechanical prostheses and bioprostheses (tissue valves; **Fig. 66-43**). The major differences are related to the risk of thromboembolism (higher with mechanical valves) and the risk of structural deterioration of the prosthesis (higher with bioprostheses).[187,188]

Mechanical Prostheses

Mechanical prosthetic valves are classified into three major groups—bileaflet, tilting disc, and ball cage. The bileaflet valves are the most

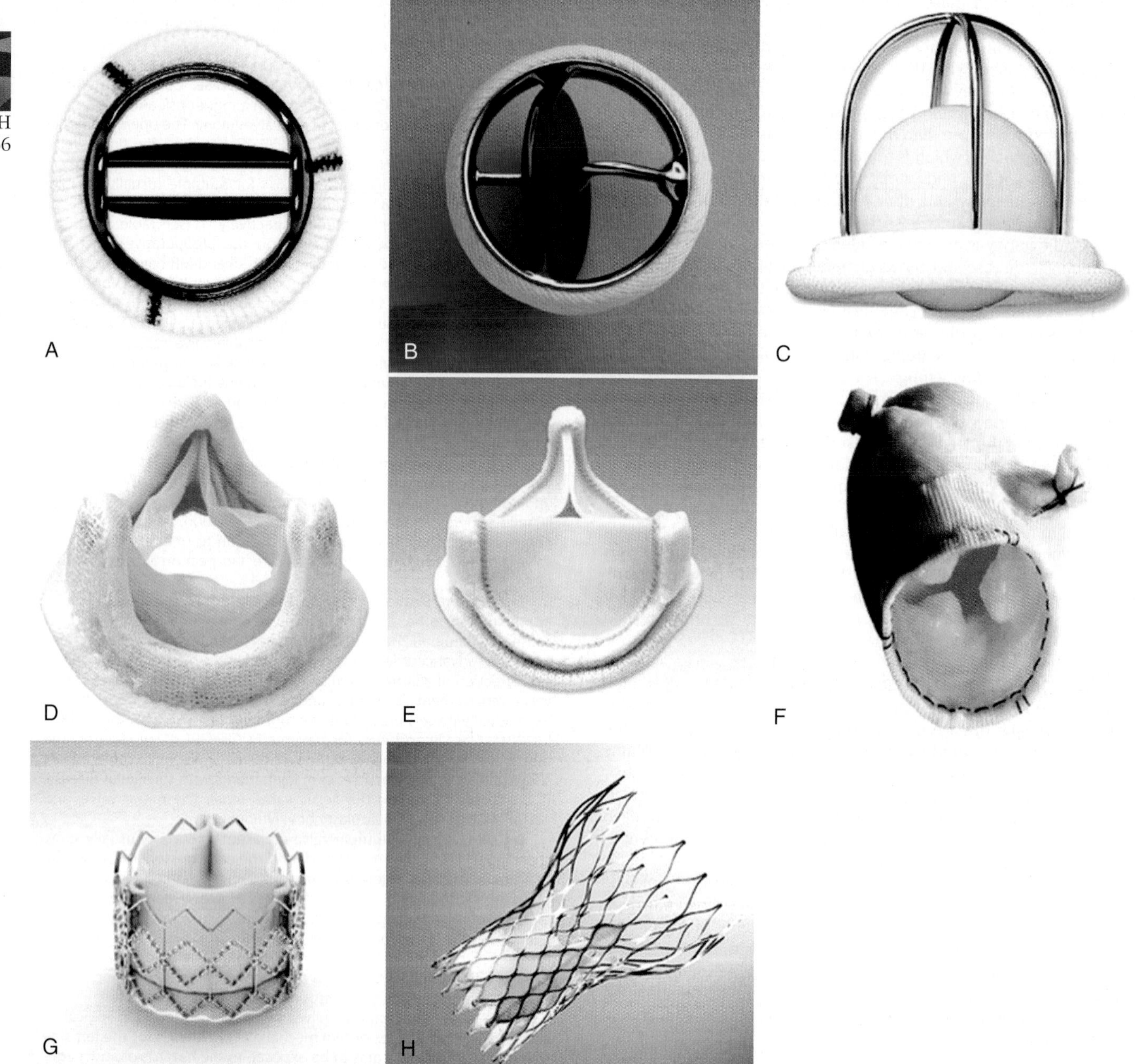

FIGURE 66-43 Different types of prosthetic valves. **A,** Bileaflet mechanical valve (St. Jude Medical, West Berlin, NJ). **B,** Monoleaflet mechanical valve (Medtronic-Hall, Medtronic, Minneapolis). **C,** Caged ball valve (Starr-Edwards,). **D,** Stented porcine bioprosthesis (Medtronic Mosaic). **E,** Stented pericardial bioprosthesis (Carpentier-Edwards Magna, Edwards Lifesciences, Irvine, Calif). **F,** Stentless porcine bioprosthesis (Medtronic Freestyle). **G,** Transcatheter bioprosthesis expanded over a balloon (Edwards SAPIEN). **H,** Self-expandable percutaneous bioprosthesis (CoreValve, Medtronic). *(From Pibarot P, Dumesnil JG: Prosthetic heart valves: Selection of the optimal prosthesis and long-term management. Circulation 119:1034, 2009.)*

commonly implanted mechanical valves because of their low bulk and flat profile and superior hemodynamics. Bileaflet valves are currently the most widely used mechanical prosthesis. The St. Jude bileaflet mechanical valve (St. Jude Medical, West Berlin, NJ) is coated with pyrolytic carbon and has two semicircular discs that pivot between open and closed positions without the need for supporting struts.[187-189] It has favorable flow characteristics and causes a lower transvalvular pressure gradient at any outer diameter and cardiac output than caged ball or tilting disc valves. Bileaflet valves appear to have particularly favorable hemodynamic characteristics in the smaller sizes. Thrombogenicity in the mitral position may be less than that associated with other prosthetic valves, although, as with other mechanical prostheses, lifelong anticoagulation is needed. A variation of the St. Jude valve, the CarboMedics prosthesis (Sorin group, Milan, Italy), is also a bileaflet valve composed of pyrolytic carbon with a titanium housing that can be rotated to avoid interference with disc excursion by subvalvular tissue.

An example of a tilting disc valve in current use is the Medtronic-Hall valve (Medtronic, Minneapolis, Minn), which has a Teflon sewing ring and titanium housing; its thin, carbon-coated pivoting disc has a central perforation that allows improved hemodynamics. Thrombogenicity appears to be low (less than one episode/100 patient-years in the mitral position), and mechanical performance is excellent over the long term. Mechanical valves, both bileaflet and tilting disc, are associated with small (5 to 10 mL/beat) obligatory (normal) regurgitation. All have distinctive auscultatory features (**Fig. 66-44**).

Production of the Starr-Edwards caged-ball valve was discontinued in 2007, but patients in whom this valve was implanted are still encountered frequently in clinical practice. The poppet is made of silicone rubber, the cage of Stellite alloy, and the sewing ring

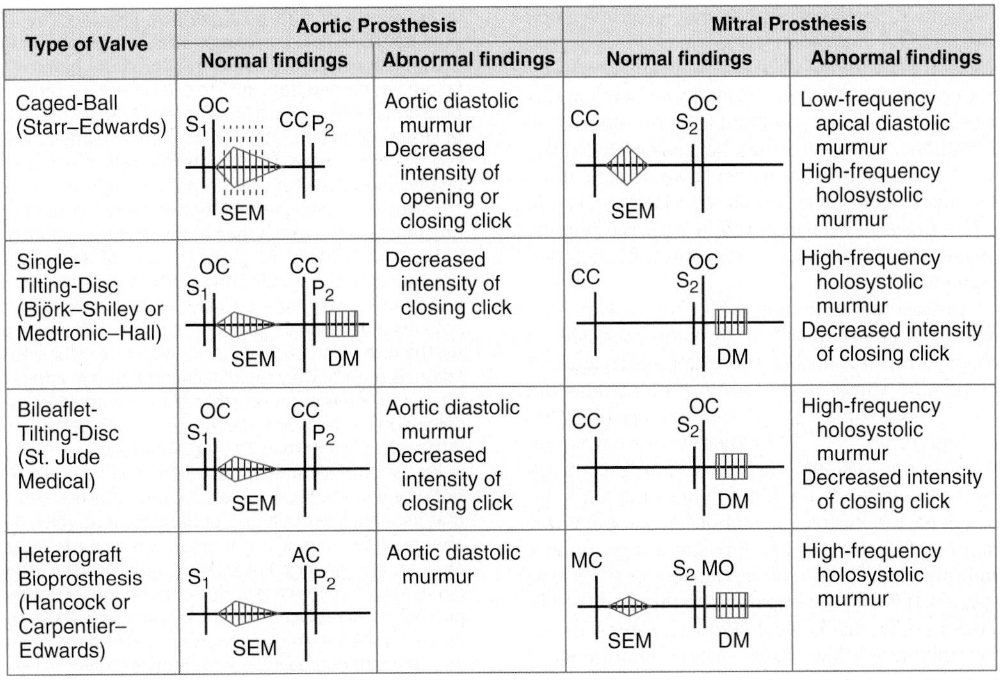

Type of Valve	Aortic Prosthesis		Mitral Prosthesis	
	Normal findings	Abnormal findings	Normal findings	Abnormal findings
Caged-Ball (Starr–Edwards)	OC, S_1, CC, P_2, SEM	Aortic diastolic murmur Decreased intensity of opening or closing click	CC, OC, S_2, SEM	Low-frequency apical diastolic murmur High-frequency holosystolic murmur
Single-Tilting-Disc (Björk–Shiley or Medtronic–Hall)	OC, CC, S_1, P_2, SEM, DM	Decreased intensity of closing click	CC, OC, S_2, DM	High-frequency holosystolic murmur Decreased intensity of closing click
Bileaflet-Tilting-Disc (St. Jude Medical)	OC, CC, S_1, P_2, SEM	Aortic diastolic murmur Decreased intensity of closing click	CC, OC, S_2, DM	High-frequency holosystolic murmur Decreased intensity of closing click
Heterograft Bioprosthesis (Hancock or Carpentier–Edwards)	AC, S_1, P_2, SEM	Aortic diastolic murmur	MC, S_2 MO, SEM, DM	High-frequency holosystolic murmur

FIGURE 66-44 Auscultatory characteristics of various prosthetic valves in the aortic and mitral positions, with schematic diagrams of normal findings and descriptions of abnormal findings. AC = aortic closure; CC = closing click; DM = diastolic murmur; MC = mitral valve closure; MO = mitral opening; OC = opening click; SEM = systolic ejection murmur. *(From Vongpatanasin W, Hillis LD, Lange RA: Prosthetic heart valves. N Engl J Med 335:407, 1996.)*

of Teflon and polypropylene cloth. Because of the bulky cage design, the Starr-Edwards valve is not suitable for the mitral position in patients with a small LV cavity, for the aortic position in those with a small aortic annulus, or for those requiring a valve–aortic arch composite graft. In a small number of patients, this valve induces hemolysis, which may be greatly exaggerated and become clinically important if a perivalvular leak develops. When they are of small size, Starr-Edwards valves may cause mild obstruction, and the incidence of thromboembolism is slightly higher than with the tilting disc or bileaflet valve.

Durability and Thrombogenicity. All mechanical prosthetic valves have an excellent record of durability, up to 40 years for the Starr-Edwards valve and over 25 years for the St. Jude valve.[187,188] In the mitral position, perivalvular regurgitation appears to occur more frequently with mechanical than with tissue valves. Thrombosis and thromboembolism risks are greater with any mechanical valve in the mitral than in the aortic position, and higher doses of warfarin are generally recommended for mitral prostheses.[1] However, patients with any mechanical prosthesis, regardless of design or site of placement, require long-term anticoagulation and aspirin administration because of the hazard of thromboembolism, which is greatest in the first postoperative year. Without anticoagulants and aspirin, the incidence of thromboembolism is three- to sixfold higher than when proper doses of these medications are administered. Very rarely, thrombosis of the mechanical valve occurs. This may be a fatal event, but when nonfatal, it interferes with prosthetic valve function.

Warfarin should begin about 2 days after operation, and the INR should be in the range of 2.0 to 3.0 for patients with the bileaflet disc and the Medtronic-Hall valve in the aortic position. The INR should be between 2.5 and 3.5 for patients at higher risk for thrombosis (e.g., AF, previous thromboembolism) as well as for patients with other mechanical valves in the aortic position and for all valves in the mitral position (see Chap. 87).[1] This relatively conservative approach reduces the risk of anticoagulant hemorrhage but does not appear to be associated with a greater frequency of thromboembolism than an INR of 3.0 to 4.0. Antiplatelet agents without anticoagulants do not provide adequate protection. However, the addition of aspirin, 75 to 100 mg daily, together with warfarin may reduce the risk of thromboembolism and should be given to all patients with prosthetic valves.[1] Although this approach does increase the risk of bleeding slightly, there is a favorable risk-benefit profile.

Prosthetic valve thrombosis should be suspected by the sudden appearance of dyspnea and muffled sounds or new murmurs on auscultation. This serious complication is diagnosed by two-dimensional TEE and Doppler echocardiography (see Fig. 15-59). Unless surgical risk is high, the preferred treatment for left-sided valve thrombosis is emergency surgery when NYHA Class III-IV symptoms are present or there is a large clot burden. Fibrinolytic therapy is reasonable for right-sided valve thrombosis, left-sided valve thrombosis with a small clot burden, and only mild symptoms. Fibrinolytic therapy is followed by intravenous heparin and aspirin until the INR is therapeutic.[1,102,190]

The following must be recognized: (1) the administration of warfarin has an estimated mortality risk of 0.2/100 patient-years and serious hemorrhage of 2.2 episodes/100 patient-years; and (2) despite treatment with anticoagulants, the incidence of thromboembolic complications with the best mechanical prosthesis is still about 0.2 fatal complications and 1.0 to 2.0 nonfatal complications/100 patient-years for aortic valves and 2.0 to 3.0 nonfatal complications for mitral valves. Valve thrombosis, a particularly hazardous complication, occurs at an incidence of about 0.1%/year in the aortic position and 0.35%/year in the mitral position. Thrombosis of mechanical prostheses in the tricuspid position is high, and therefore bioprostheses are preferred at this site. The incidence of embolization in patients who have experienced repeated emboli from a prosthetic valve despite anticoagulants may be reduced by replacement with a tissue valve. Mechanical prostheses regularly cause mild hemolysis, but this is not severe enough to be of clinical importance unless the patient develops paraprosthetic regurgitation.

Bioprosthetic Valves

Tissue valves (bioprostheses) were developed primarily to overcome the risk of thromboembolism that is inherent in all mechanical prosthetic valves and the attendant hazards and inconvenience of permanent anticoagulant therapy.

STENTED BIOPROSTHETIC VALVES. A stented tissue valve consists of three tissue leaflets mounted on a ring with semirigid stents that facilitate implantation and maintain the three-dimensional relationship between the leaflets. Stented porcine aortic heterografts were developed for the mitral and aortic positions and have been in wide clinical use since 1965. Over the past 45 years, stented bioprosthetic valve design has improved to maximize orifice area by reconfiguration of the sewing ring and stents and improve durability by the use of other biologic tissues, improved fixation techniques, and anticalcification treatments. Bioprosthetic valves may be constructed from porcine valve tissue fixed and preserved in glutaraldehyde and mounted on a Dacron cloth–covered flexible polypropylene strut—for example the Hancock porcine bioprosthesis (Medtronic, Minneapolis, Minn), which was approved by the U.S. Food and Drug Administration (FDA) in 1989. Bioprosthetic valves also may be constructed using bovine pericardium—for example, the Carpentier-Edwards pericardial valve (Edwards Lifesciences, Irvine, Calif), which was FDA-approved in 1991. The Medtronic Mosaic valve, FDA-approved in 2000, is a porcine valve fixed at zero pressure to preserve leaflet function with an added anticalcification treatment.

During the first 3 postoperative months, while the sewing ring becomes endothelialized, there is a risk of thromboembolism so that warfarin anticoagulation is reasonable. Thereafter, anticoagulants are not required for porcine valves in the aortic position, and the thromboembolic rate is approximately one or two episodes/100 patient-years without these drugs.[1,187,188] When these valves have been placed in the mitral position in patients who are in sinus rhythm, do not have heart failure or thrombus in the left atrium or the left atrial appendage, and do not have a history of embolism preoperatively, anticoagulants are not needed after the first 3 postoperative months, and the thromboembolic rate is also approximately one or two episodes/100 patient-years. This rate is comparable to that observed in patients with the St. Jude or other mechanical valves who are receiving anticoagulants and are therefore subject to the risks of hemorrhage. It is unlikely that any MV replacement can be associated with a thromboembolic rate much below 0.5 episodes/100 patient-years because some of the emboli in patients with long-standing mitral disease are derived from the left atrium rather than from the valve itself. In patients undergoing MV replacement with a bioprosthesis who have experienced a previous embolism, in whom thrombus is found in the left atrium at operation, or who remain in AF postoperatively (approximately one third of all patients receiving MV replacement), the hazard of thromboembolism and the need for anticoagulants persist. This negates the principal advantage of the tissue valves and mechanical prostheses would appear to be preferable to bioprostheses in these patients.

The major problem with porcine bioprostheses is their limited durability (**Fig. 66-45**). Cuspal tears, degeneration, fibrin deposition, disruption of the fibrocollagenous structure, perforation, fibrosis, and calcification sufficiently severe to require reoperation begin to appear in some patients in the fourth or fifth postoperative year, and by 10 years the rate of primary tissue failure averages 30%. It then accelerates and, by 15 years postoperatively, the actuarial freedom from bioprosthetic primary tissue failure has ranged from 30% to 60% in several series. In contrast, stented pericardial valves have a lower rate of primary tissue failure with 86% free of structural deterioration at 12 years. Prosthetic valve endocarditis is a serious, often grave, illness with the risk of endocarditis highest in the first few months after valve implantation (see Chap. 67).

Structural valve deterioration is more frequent in patients with bioprostheses in the mitral than in the aortic position, presumably because of the higher closing pressure. The rate of structural valve failure is age-dependent and is significantly lower in patients older than 65 years than in younger patients, especially in the aortic position (**Fig. 66-46**). In patients older than 65 years undergoing AVR with a porcine bioprosthesis, the rate of structural deterioration is less than 10% at 10 years. Valve failure is prohibitively rapid in children and in adults younger than 35 to 40 years. Therefore, bioprostheses are not advisable for these age groups. On the other hand, degeneration is rare when these valves are implanted into patients older than 70 years. Bioprostheses also have been reported to have extremely limited durability in patients with chronic renal failure, but recent studies have called this into question (see later). Other factors that increase the likelihood of bioprosthetic valve deterioration include abnormalities of calcium metabolism and, possibly, hypercholesterolemia and pregnancy. Fortunately, tissue valves usually do not fail suddenly, as is often the case for structural failure or thrombosis of mechanical prostheses. Rereplacement of a bioprosthetic valve should be carried out when significant and/or progressive structural deterioration is evident and standard criteria for intervention for native valve disease are present. The second operation, when carried out on an elective basis, may be associated with a surgical mortality rate that is two to three times higher than the initial valve replacement.

Echocardiographic evaluation is extremely helpful in the early detection of bioprosthetic valve malfunction. TEE is more sensitive than transthoracic imaging in detecting bioprosthetic mitral valve deterioration. A baseline echocardiographic study is recommended 2 to 4 weeks after hospital discharge for valve replacement. Annual cardiology follow-up is recommended with echocardiography during the first 5 years only if there are changes in symptoms or examination findings. After 5 years, annual echocardiography is reasonable, even in the absence of clinical findings, to evaluate for bioprosthetic valve deterioration.

STENTLESS BIOPROSTHETIC VALVES. Because the stent adds to the obstruction and thereby increases stress on the leaflets, stentless valves have been developed for the aortic position and are especially

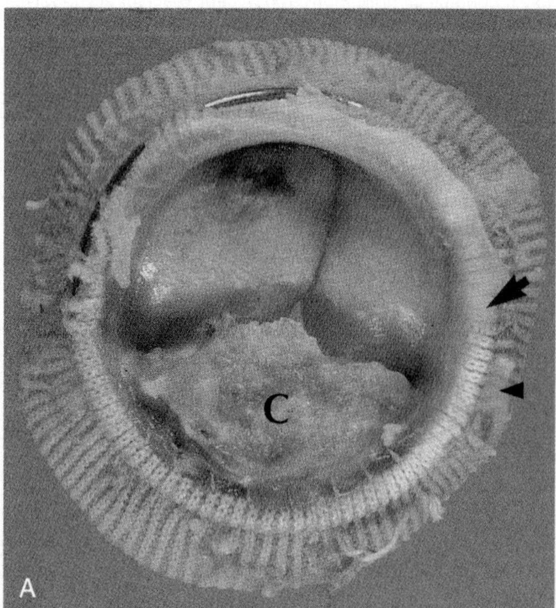

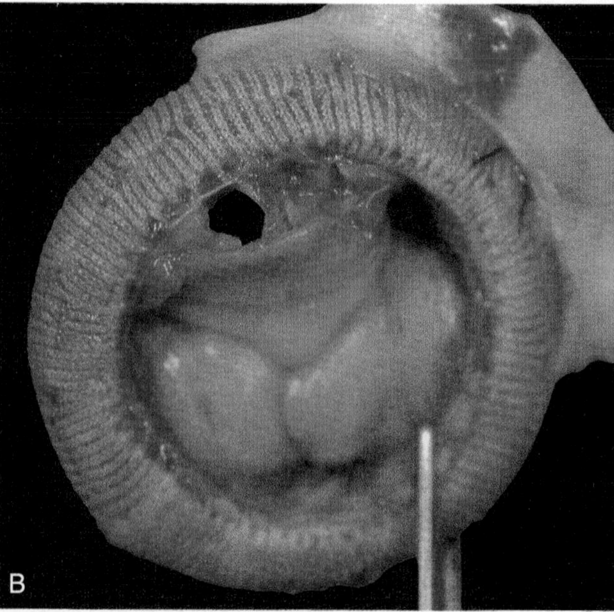

FIGURE 66-45 Structural deterioration of bioprosthetic valves. **A,** Valve failure related to mineralization and collagen degeneration. **B,** Cuspal tears and perforations. These processes may occur independently, or they may be synergistic. (**A,** *From Virmani R, Burke AP, Farb A: Pathology of valvular heart disease. In Rahimtoola SH [ed]: Valvular Heart Disease. In Braunwald E [series ed]: Atlas of Heart Diseases. Vol 11. Philadelphia, Current Medicine, 1997, p 1.26;* **B,** *from Manabe H, Yutani C [eds]: Atlas of Valvular Heart Disease. Singapore, Churchill Livingstone, 1998, p 158.)*

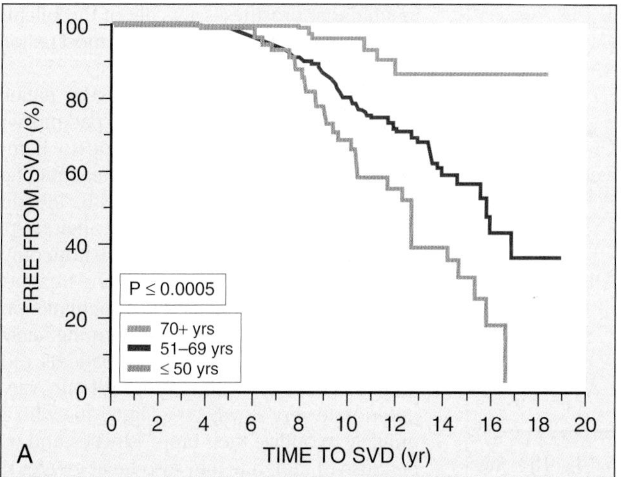

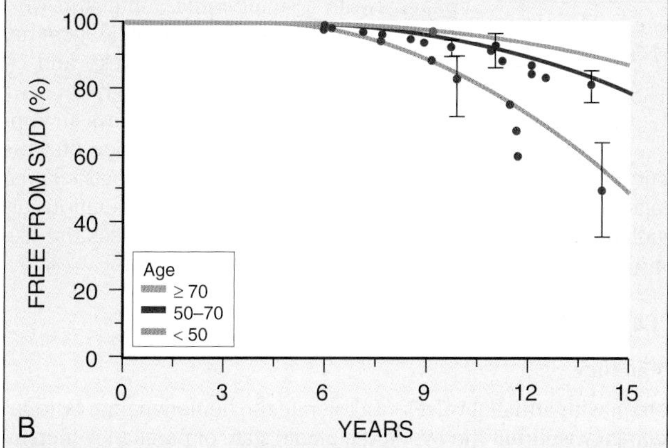

FIGURE 66-46 Estimates of freedom from structural valve deterioration (SVD) for patients undergoing porcine **(A)** and bovine pericardial **(B)** aortic valve replacement who are stratified according to age. *(**A,** From Cohn LH, Collins JJ Jr, Rizzo RJ, et al: Twenty-year follow-up of the Hancock modified orifice porcine aortic valve. Ann Thorac Surg 66:S30, 1998; **B,** from Banbury MK, Cosgrove DM, White JA, et al: Age and valve size effect on the long-term durability of the Carpentier-Edwards aortic pericardial bioprosthesis. Ann Thorac Surg 72:753, 2001.)*

useful for patients with small aortic roots. These include the Toronto SPV stentless valve (St. Jude Medical valve), Edwards stentless valve, and Medtronic Freestyle valve. These valves have been reported to have more physiologic flow and lower transvalvular gradients than stented porcine valves, with the potential for enhanced regression of LV hypertrophy and improved LV function. However, long-term outcome appears to be similar to that for other currently implanted tissue valves, in part because current generation stented bioprosthetic valves have better durability than older generation valves.[187,191,192]

TRANSCATHETER BIOPROSTHESES (see Chap. 59). Bioprosthetic valves that can be placed via a catheter in the aortic valve position are currently undergoing clinical trials in the United States and have been approved for use in Europe. These trileaflet bioprosthetic valves are mounted in a wire mesh stent that can be crimped to allow delivery of the valve over a catheter. Transcatheter aortic valve implantation (TAVI) may be performed using a catheter advanced from the femoral artery retrograde across the aortic valve, or from a small thoracotomy with the catheter positioned in the LV apex and passed antegrade across the aortic valve. This procedure is used for calcific AS with the native valve remaining in place, which helps anchor the valve stent. TAVI clinical trials have focused on adults with a high risk of cardiac surgery. In this subset of high-risk patients, procedural results and short-term outcomes are promising. The U.S. prospective randomized PARTNER trial, comparing TAVI with medical therapy (including balloon valvotomy) in patients considered to be at too high risk for conventional AVR, demonstrated substantial reduction in death and hospitalization with TAVI, associated with significant improvement in symptoms.[64a] Long-term durability of these valves has not yet been evaluated in clinical trials.[61-64] Transcatheter valve implantation also holds promise for treating patients with failing bioprosthetic valves in the aortic and mitral positions, using a valve in valve approach.[193]

HOMOGRAFT (ALLOGRAFT) AORTIC VALVES. These are harvested from cadavers, usually within 24 hours of donor death. They are sterilized with antibiotics and cryopreserved for long periods at −196°C. They are inserted directly, usually in the aortic position, without being placed into a prosthetic stent. In the aortic position, the isolated valve is implanted in the subcoronary position or the valve and a portion of attached aorta are implanted as a root replacement, with reimplantation of the coronary arteries into the graft. Homograft hemodynamics are superior to those of stented porcine valves and similar to those of stentless porcine valves. Like porcine xenografts, their thrombogenicity is low, but cryopreserved valves appear to have similar issues with structural deterioration, with evidence that this rate is reduced with the use of freshly harvested valves, approximate matching of donor's and patient's ages, and use of the root replacement technique. The subcoronary technique is associated with a higher incidence of prosthetic AR and reoperation. In addition, the homograft valve and root are prone to severe calcification, making reoperation difficult. One possible advantage of homografts is in the avoidance of early endocarditis, and homografts are commonly used in the treatment of aortic valve endocarditis, particularly complex aortic root endocarditis, However, in randomized studies, there was no benefit of homografts compared with other tissue valves in outcome after endocarditis.[194]

PULMONARY AUTOGRAFTS. In this operation, the Ross procedure, the patient's own pulmonary valve and adjacent main pulmonary artery are removed and used to replace the diseased aortic valve and often the neighboring aorta, with reimplantation of the coronary arteries into the graft.[195] A human pulmonary or aortic homograft is then inserted into the pulmonary position. The autograft is nonthrombogenic. In children and adolescents, there is evidence that the autograft grows along with the patient.[196] The risk of endocarditis is very low, anticoagulants are not required and, perhaps most importantly, the long-term durability appears to be excellent. A high incidence of pulmonary homograft stenosis has been reported in some series, which may represent a postoperative inflammatory reaction. The pulmonary artery tissue adapts to the aortic pressure and usually does not dilate. However, this procedure should not be performed in patients with bicuspid valves and dilated aortic roots, because the implanted pulmonary artery tissue exposed to the higher aortic pressures may also undergo degenerative changes, leading to significant dilation of the autograft. A subcoronary technique, in which the pulmonary autograft is inserted without a root replacement, may circumvent this problem, but late dilation of the autograft remains a concern.[197] The pulmonary autograft is the replacement valve of choice in children, adolescents, and younger adults who have a long (>20-year) life expectancy, particularly young women who wish to become pregnant. A prospective randomized clinical trial has demonstrated improved long-term survival in patients undergoing AVR who received a pulmonary autograft compared to those receiving a homograft.[197a] However, its use has been limited because the operation is technically much more demanding than a simple AVR. The procedure should be carried out only by highly experienced surgeons.

Hemodynamics of Valve Replacements. The most commonly used prosthetic valves—mechanical prostheses and stented porcine or pericardial xenografts—have an effective in vitro orifice size that is smaller than the normal valve at the same site.[187,189] Current generation tissue and mechanical valves have larger effective valve areas than older valves, particularly stented, valves, but still do not restore valve area or hemodynamics to normal. Although all prosthetic valves are inherently mildly stenotic, postoperative hemodynamic measurements show reasonably good function, with effective mitral valve orifice areas averaging 1.7 to 2.0 cm^2 and mitral valve gradients of 4 to 8 mm Hg at rest (see Tables 15-12 to 15-15). Aortic valve effective orifice areas and transvalvular gra-

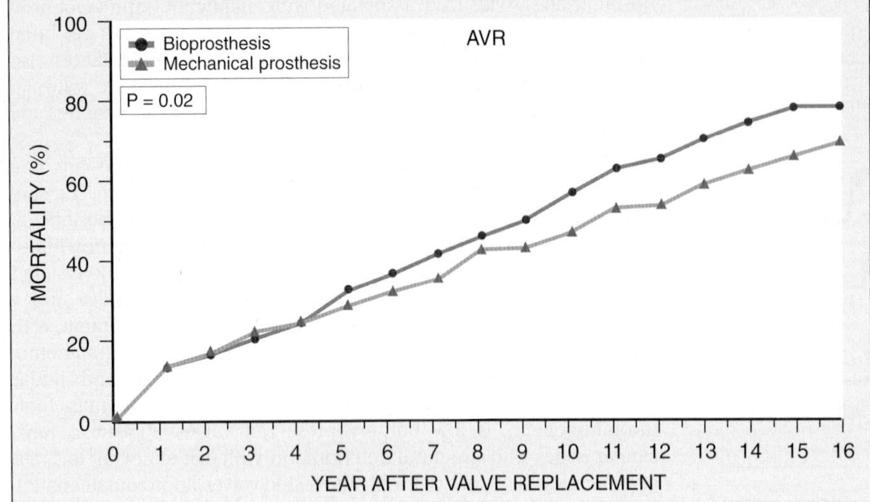

FIGURE 66-47 Mortality after AVR with the Björk-Shiley (Pfizer, New York) and porcine valves from the Department of Veterans Affairs trial. *(From Hammermeister KE, Sethi GK, Henderson WG, et al: Outcomes 15 years after valve replacement with a mechanical versus a bioprosthetic valve: Final report of the Veterans Affairs randomized trial. J Am Coll Cardiol 36:1152, 2000.)*

dients depend on valve size and type and have been detailed in published tables of normal values and guidelines.[187,188,198]

The degree of physiologic stenosis of a normally functioning prosthetic valve is considered significant (often called patient-prosthesis mismatch) when the effective valve orifice is 0.85 cm^2/m^2 or less and is severe when the effective orifice area is less than 0.65 cm^2/m^2. Patient prosthetic mismatch adversely affects short- and long-term survival after valve surgery.[199] Mismatch can be avoided by choosing a valve with an adequate orifice area for the patient's body size. In some cases, an annular enlarging procedure may be necessary. Rarely, reoperation to correct a malfunctioning prosthesis may be necessary.

Selection of an Artificial Valve

Most comparisons of mechanical and bioprosthetic valves indicate similar overall results in terms of early and late mortality, prosthetic valve endocarditis and other complications, and the need for reoperation, at least for the first 5 years postoperatively.[200] As indicated, there appear to be no significant differences when a valve size appropriate for the patient's body size is implanted.[187] Patients with a small aortic annulus may be better candidates for unstented homografts, heterografts, or pulmonary autografts. In general, patient outcome after valve surgery is related more to preoperative factors, such as age, LV function, associated coronary artery disease, and comorbid conditions, than to the prosthesis itself.

The major task when selecting an artificial valve is to weigh the advantage of durability and the disadvantages of the risks of thromboembolism and anticoagulant treatment inherent in mechanical prostheses on the one hand with the advantage of low thrombogenicity and the disadvantage of abbreviated durability of bioprostheses on the other.[200a] Overall survival after AVR is better with a mechanical compared with a bioprosthetic aortic valve (**Fig. 66-47**), principally because of the higher rate of structural deterioration of the bioprosthesis (especially in patients younger than 65 years). Much of the increased mortality in patients receiving a tissue valve is because of reoperation, which is associated with about twice the mortality of the initial procedure. With MV replacement, the prosthetic valve type does not influence survival nor the probability of developing other valve-related complications, including endocarditis, valve thrombosis, and systemic embolism, although anticoagulant-related bleeding is higher in patients receiving mechanical valves. Patients with mechanical valves also have a higher incidence of perivalvular regurgitation in the mitral position and a trend for this complication in the aortic position. The higher survival rates with mechanical compared with bioprosthetic valves have been confirmed in other studies as well. Therefore, mechanical prostheses, usually of the bileaflet variety, are the valves of choice for most patients younger than 65 years.

However, the following groups of patients should receive bioprostheses: (1) patients with coexisting disease who are prone to hemorrhage and who therefore tolerate anticoagulants poorly, such as those with bleeding disorders, intestinal polyposis, and angiodysplasia; (2) patients who are likely to be noncompliant with permanent anticoagulant treatment, who are unwilling to take anticoagulants on a regular basis, or who live in developing nations and cannot be monitored; (3) patients older than 65 years in whom bioprosthetic valves deteriorate very slowly (see Fig. 66-46), who are unlikely to outlive their bioprostheses, and who because of their age may also be at greater risk of hemorrhage while taking anticoagulants; (4) patients with a small aortic annulus in whom an unstented (free) bioprosthetic graft may provide superior hemodynamics; and (5) younger women wishing to bear children, who require AVR. Patient preference plays an important role in determining the choice of a prosthetic valve. A bioprosthesis is reasonable for AVR in patients <65 years of age who elect to receive this valve for lifestyle considerations after detailed discussions of the risks of anticoagulation versus the likelihood that a second AVR may be necessary in the future.

SPECIAL CONSIDERATIONS

Pregnancy

Women with artificial valves can tolerate the hemodynamic burden of pregnancy well, but the hypercoagulable state of pregnancy increases the risk of thromboembolism in pregnant patients with mechanical prostheses (see Chap. 82).[201,202] Anticoagulation must not be interrupted, although an increased risk of fatal fetal hemorrhage occurs in women in whom anticoagulants are continued. There is also a risk of fetal malformation caused by the probable teratogenic effect of warfarin. Although these problems represent rationales for the use of tissue valves in all women of childbearing age, their limited durability in young adults makes their use unacceptable. Therefore, every effort should be made to defer valve replacement until after childbirth. In pregnant women with critical MS or AS, balloon valvuloplasty should be considered and, if at all possible, MV repair instead of replacement should be undertaken for patients with MR. Women of childbearing potential who have a mechanical prosthesis should be counseled against pregnancy.

When a woman who already has a mechanical prosthetic valve becomes pregnant, the risk of fetal defects with oral anticoagulants must be balanced against the risk of inadequate anticoagulation if oral therapy is interrupted. The management of anticoagulation in pregnant women with mechanical valves is controversial. All agree that the goal is continuous, effective, monitored anticoagulation and avoidance of fetal defects. In pregnant patients who receive warfarin, oral therapy is discontinued at week 36 of gestation and replaced with continuous intravenous unfractionated heparin. Heparin should be discontinued at the onset of labor but may be restarted, along with warfarin, several hours after delivery. Between weeks 1 to 36, the options include the following: (1) continued oral therapy with warfarin to maintain a therapeutic INR; (2) replacement of warfarin with dose-adjusted subcutaneous heparin or dose-adjusted subcutaneous low-molecular-weight heparin between weeks 6 and 12 (when the risk of fetal defects is highest); and (3) continuous intravenous or dose-adjusted subcutaneous heparin or dose-adjusted subcutaneous low-molecular-weight heparin for the duration of pregnancy.[1] The most important management principle is to ensure that anticoagulation is not interrupted and that the dose of anticoagulation is adequate based on frequent monitoring of the partial thromboplastin time (PTT; for intravenous or subcutaneous heparin), INR (for warfarin), or anti-Xa levels (for low-molecular-weight heparin).

Noncardiac Surgery

When noncardiac surgery is required for patients with prosthetic valves who are receiving anticoagulants, the risk depends on the valve type, location, and associated risk factors. In patients with an isolated AVR and no associated risk factors, the anticoagulant is stopped 1 to 3 days preoperatively and resumed as soon as possible postoperatively without the need for heparin therapy. However, when the risk of thromboembolism is higher, intravenous heparin is started when the INR falls below 2.0 and resumed postoperatively until the INR is again therapeutic. High-risk patients include those with a mechanical mitral valve prosthesis, AF, previous thromboembolism, LV dysfunction, hypercoagulable condition, older generation thrombotic valve, mechanical tricuspid valve, or more than one mechanical valve. The use of subcutaneous low-molecular-weight heparin in this situation has been advocated by some experts, but this topic represents another area of controversy.[1,203-205]

Children and Patients Receiving Chronic Hemodialysis

The high incidence of bioprosthetic valve failure in children and adolescents almost prohibits their use in these groups. In young adults between the ages of 25 and 35 years, the failure of bioprosthetic valves is somewhat higher than in older adults; this serves as a relative, but not an absolute, contraindication to their use in this age group.

In children, a mechanical prosthesis (generally the St. Jude valve), with its favorable hemodynamics and established durability, is preferred despite the disadvantages inherent in the need for anticoagulants in this age group. Alternatively, if an experienced surgical team is available and the patient requires an AVR, a pulmonary autograft is an excellent alternative.

Previous studies indicated a high rate of bioprosthetic structural deterioration in patients receiving chronic renal dialysis. However, several studies have reported no difference in survival of patients with a bioprosthesis or a mechanical valve, coupled with an unacceptably high rate of stroke and major bleeding in patients with the mechanical valves. Current guidelines no longer recommend mechanical valves for these patients, but this clearly is an area in which physician judgment is important for individual patients.

Tricuspid Position

The risk of thrombosis for all valves is highest in the tricuspid position because of the lower pressures and velocity of blood flow. This complication appears to be highest for tilting disc valves, intermediate for caged ball valves, and lowest for bioprostheses, which are the valves of choice as tricuspid replacements. Fortunately, bioprostheses exhibit a much slower rate of mechanical deterioration in the tricuspid position than in the mitral or aortic positions.

REFERENCES

1. Bonow RO, Carabello BA, Chatterjee K, et al: ACC/AHA 2006 guidelines for the management of patients with valvular heart disease: A report of the American College of Cardiology/American Heart Association Task Force on Practice Guidelines (Writing Committee to Revise the 1998 guidelines for the management of patients with valvular heart disease) developed in collaboration with the Society of Cardiovascular Anesthesiologists: Endorsed by the Society for Cardiovascular Angiography and Interventions and the Society of Thoracic Surgeons. J Am Coll Cardiol 48:e1, 2006.
2. Vahanian A, Baumgartner H, Bax J, et al: Guidelines on the management of valvular heart disease: The Task Force on the Management of Valvular Heart Disease of the European Society of Cardiology. Eur Heart J 28:230, 2007.

Aortic Stenosis

3. Roberts WC, Ko JM: Frequency by decades of unicuspid, bicuspid, and tricuspid aortic valves in adults having isolated aortic valve replacement for aortic stenosis, with or without associated aortic regurgitation. Circulation 111:920, 2005.
4. Braverman AC, Guven H, Beardslee MA, et al: The bicuspid aortic valve. Curr Probl Cardiol 30:470, 2005.
5. Lewin MB, Otto CM: The bicuspid aortic valve: Adverse outcomes from infancy to old age. Circulation 111:832, 2005.
6. Braverman AC: The bicuspid aortic valve. *In* Otto CM, Bonow RO (eds): Valvular Heart Disease: A Companion to Braunwald's Heart Disease. Philadelphia, Saunders/Elsevier, 2009, pp 169-186.
7. Stewart BF, Siscovick D, Lind BK, et al: Clinical factors associated with calcific aortic valve disease. J Am Coll Cardiol 29:630, 1997.

7a. Freeman RV, Otto CM: Spectrum of calcific aortic valve disease: Pathogenesis, disease progression, and treatment strategies. Circulation 111:3316, 2005.

8. Olsen MH, Wachtell K, Bella JN, et al: Aortic valve sclerosis relates to cardiovascular events in patients with hypertension (a LIFE substudy). Am J Cardiol 95:132, 2005.
9. Taylor HA Jr, Clark BL, Garrison RJ, et al: Relation of aortic valve sclerosis to risk of coronary heart disease in African-Americans. Am J Cardiol 95:401, 2005.
10. Owens DS, Otto CM: Is it time for a new paradigm in calcific aortic valve disease? J Am Coll Cardiol Img 2:928, 2009.
11. Rajamannan NM, Otto CM: Targeted therapy to prevent progression of calcific aortic stenosis. Circulation 110:1180, 2004.
12. Helske S, Otto CM: Lipid lowering in aortic stenosis: Still some light at the end of the tunnel? Circulation 119:2653, 2009.
13. O'Brien KD: Pathogenesis of calcific aortic valve disease: A disease process comes of age (and a good deal more). Arterioscler Thromb Vasc Biol 26:1721, 2006.
14. Miller JD, Chu Y, Brooks RM, et al: Dysregulation of antioxidant mechanisms contributes to increased oxidative stress in calcific aortic valvular stenosis in humans. J Am Coll Cardiol 52:843, 2008.
15. Rajamannan NM: Calcific aortic stenosis: Lessons learned from experimental and clinical studies. Arterioscler Thromb Vasc Biol 29:162, 2009.
16. Otto CM: Calcific aortic stenosis—time to look more closely at the valve. N Engl J Med 359:1395, 2008.
17. Bella JN, Tang W, Kraja A, et al: Genome-wide linkage mapping for valve calcification susceptibility loci in hypertensive sibships: The Hypertension Genetic Epidemiology Network Study. Hypertension 49:453, 2007.
18. Bosse Y, Mathieu P, Pibarot P: Genomics: The next step to elucidate the etiology of calcific aortic valve stenosis. J Am Coll Cardiol 51:1327, 2008.
19. Probst V, Le Scouarnec S, Legendre A, et al: Familial aggregation of calcific aortic valve stenosis in the western part of France. Circulation 113:856, 2006.
20. Ngo DTM, Sverdlov AL, Willoughby SR, et al: Determinants of occurrence of aortic sclerosis in an aging population. J Am Coll Cardiol Img 2:919, 2009.
21. Katz R, Wong ND, Kronmal R, et al: Features of the metabolic syndrome and diabetes mellitus as predictors of aortic valve calcification in the Multi-Ethnic Study of Atherosclerosis. Circulation 113:2113-2119, 2006.
22. Briand M, Dumesnil JG, Kadem L, et al: Reduced systemic arterial compliance impacts significantly on left ventricular afterload and function in aortic stenosis: Implications for diagnosis and treatment. J Am Coll Cardiol 46:291, 2005.
23. Rajamannan NM: Cellular, molecular and genetic mechanisms of valvular heart disease. *In* Otto CM, Bonow RO (eds): Valvular Heart Disease: A Companion to Braunwald's Heart Disease. Philadelphia, Saunders/Elsevier. 2009, pp 39-54.
24. Miller JD, Weiss RM, Serrano KM, et al: Lowering plasma cholesterol levels halts progression of aortic valve disease in mice. Circulation 119:2693, 2009.
25. Cowell SJ, Newby DE, Prescott RJ, et al: A randomized trial of intensive lipid-lowering therapy in calcific aortic stenosis. N Engl J Med 352:2389, 2005.
26. Moura LM, Ramos SF, Zamorano JL, et al: Rosuvastatin affecting aortic valve endothelium to slow the progression of aortic stenosis. J Am Coll Cardiol 49:554, 2007.
27. Rossebo AB, Pedersen TR, Boman K, et al: Intensive lipid lowering with simvastatin and ezetimibe in aortic stenosis. N Engl J Med 359:1343, 2008.
28. Chan KL, Teo K, Dumesnil JG, et al: Effect of lipid lowering with rosuvastatin on progression of aortic stenosis: Results of the Aortic Stenosis Progression Observation: Measuring Effects of Rosuvastatin (ASTRONOMER) Trial. Circulation 121:306, 2010.
29. Busseuil D, Shi Y, Mecteau M, et al: Regression of aortic valve stenosis by apo A-I mimetic peptide infusions in rabbits. Br J Pharmacol 154:765, 2008.
30. Baumgartner H, Hung J, Bermejo J, et al: Echocardiographic assessment of valve stenosis: EAE/ASE recommendations for clinical practice. Eur J Echocardiogr 10:1, 2009.

30a. Maganti K, Rigolin VH, Enriquez-Sarano M, Bonow RO. Heart valve disease: Diagnosis and management. Mayo Clin Proc 85:453, 2010.

31. Otto CM: Valvular aortic stenosis: Disease severity and timing of intervention. J Am Coll Cardiol 47:2141, 2006.
32. Monin JL, Lancellotti P, Monchi M, et al: Risk score for predicting outcome in patients with asymptomatic aortic stenosis. Circulation 120:69, 2009.
33. Coglianese EE, Davidoff R: Predicting outcome in patients with asymptomatic aortic stenosis. Circulation 120:9, 2009.

33a. Maréchaux S, Hachicha Z, Bellouin A, et al: Usefulness of exercise-stress echocardiography for risk stratification of true asymptomatic patients with aortic valve stenosis. Eur Heart J 31:1390, 2010.

34. Kadem L, Dumesnil JG, Rieu R, et al: Impact of systemic hypertension on the assessment of aortic stenosis. Heart 91:354, 2005.
35. Carabello BA, Paulus WJ: Aortic stenosis. Lancet 373:956, 2009.
36. Otto CM (ed): Textbook of Clinical Echocardiography. 4th ed. Philadelphia, Saunders/Elsevier, 2009.
37. Rosenhek R, Baumgartner H: Aortic stenosis. *In* Otto CM, Bonow RO (eds): Valvular Heart Disease: A Companion to Braunwald's Heart Disease. Philadelphia, Saunders/Elsevier, 2009, pp 127-154.
38. Rosenhek R: Aortic stenosis: Evaluation of disease severity, disease progression, and the role of echocardiography in clinical decision making. *In* Otto CM (ed): The Clinical Practice of Echocardiography. Philadelphia, Saunders/Elsevier, 2007, pp 516-551.
39. Baumgartner H: What influences the outcome of valve replacement in critical aortic stenosis? Heart 91:1254, 2005.
40. Chambers J, Bach D, Dumesnil J, et al: Crossing the aortic valve in severe aortic stenosis: No longer acceptable? J Heart Valve Dis 13:344, 2004.
41. Cawley PJ, Maki JH, Otto CM: Cardiovascular magnetic resonance imaging for valvular heart disease: Technique and validation. Circulation 119:468, 2009.
42. Otto CM: Calcific aortic valve disease: Outflow obstruction is the end stage of a systemic disease process. Eur Heart J 2009.
43. Dal-Bianco JP, Khandheria BK, Mookadam F, et al: Management of asymptomatic severe aortic stenosis. J Am Coll Cardiol 52:1279, 2008.
44. Varadarajan P, Kapoor N, Bansal RC, Pai RG: Clinical profile and natural history of 453 nonsurgically managed patients with severe aortic stenosis. Ann Thorac Surg 82:2111, 2006.

45. Rosenhek R, Klaar U, Schemper M, et al: Mild and moderate aortic stenosis. Natural history and risk stratification by echocardiography. Eur Heart J 25:199, 2004.
46. Pellikka PA, Sarano ME, Nishimura RA, et al: Outcome of 622 adults with asymptomatic, hemodynamically significant aortic stenosis during prolonged follow-up. Circulation 111:3290, 2005.
46a. Stewart RA, Kerr AJ, Walley GA, et al: Left ventricular systolic and diastolic function assessed by tissue Doppler imaging and outcome in asymptomatic aortic stenosis. Eur Heart J 31:2191, 2010.
47. Rosenhek R, Zilberszac R, Schemper M, et al: Natural history of very severe aortic stenosis. Circulation 121:151, 2010.
47a. Lancellotti P, Donal E, Magne J, et al: Risk stratification in asymptomatic moderate to severe aortic stenosis: The importance of the valvular, arterial and ventricular interplay. Heart 96:1364, 2010.
48. Bach DS, Siao D, Girard SE, et al: Evaluation of patients with severe symptomatic aortic stenosis who do not undergo aortic valve replacement: The potential role of subjectively overestimated operative risk. Circ Cardiovasc Qual Outcomes 2:533, 2009.
49 Das P, Rimington H, Chambers J: Exercise testing to stratify risk in aortic stenosis. Eur Heart J 26:1309, 2005.
50. Lancellotti P, Lebois F, Simon M, et al: Prognostic importance of quantitative exercise Doppler echocardiography in asymptomatic valvular aortic stenosis. Circulation 112:I377, 2005.
51. Bergler-Klein J, Klaar U, Heger M, et al: Natriuretic peptides predict symptom-free survival and postoperative outcome in severe aortic stenosis. Circulation 109:2302, 2004.
52. Lim P, Monin JL, Monchi M, et al: Predictors of outcome in patients with severe aortic stenosis and normal left ventricular function: Role of B-type natriuretic peptide. Eur Heart J 25:2048, 2004.
53. Gerber IL, Legget ME, West TM, et al: Usefulness of serial measurement of N-terminal pro-brain natriuretic peptide plasma levels in asymptomatic patients with aortic stenosis to predict symptomatic deterioration. Am J Cardiol 95:898, 2005.
53a. Monin JL, Lancellotti P, MD, Monchi M, et al: Risk score for predicting outcome in patients with asymptomatic aortic stenosis. Circulation 120:69, 2009.
54. Bonow RO, Cheitlin MD, Crawford MH, Douglas PS: Task Force 3: Valvular heart disease. J Am Coll Cardiol 45:1334, 2005.
55. Christ M, Sharkova Y, Geldner G, Maisch B: Preoperative and perioperative care for patients with suspected or established aortic stenosis facing noncardiac surgery. Chest 128:2944, 2005.
56. Warnes CA, Williams RG, Bashore TM, et al: ACC/AHA 2008 guidelines for the management of adults with congenital heart disease: A report of the American College of Cardiology/American Heart Association Task Force on Practice Guidelines (writing committee to develop guidelines on the management of adults with congenital heart disease). Circulation 118:e714, 2008.
57. Iung B, Cachier A, Baron G, et al: Decision-making in elderly patients with severe aortic stenosis: Why are so many denied surgery? Eur Heart J 26:2714, 2005.
58. Pereira JJ, Balaban K, Lauer MS, et al: Aortic valve replacement in patients with mild or moderate aortic stenosis and corbnary bypass surgery. Am J Med 118:735, 2005.
59. Gillinov AM, Garcia MJ: When is concomitant aortic valve replacement indicated in patients with mild to moderate stenosis undergoing coronary revascularization? Curr Cardiol Rep 7:101, 2005.
60. Munt B: Percutaneous aortic valve implantation. *In* Otto CM, Bonow RO (eds): Valvular Heart Disease: A Companion to Braunwald's Heart Disease. Philadelphia, Saunders/Elsevier, 2009, pp 209-220.
61. Rosengart TK, Feldman T, Borger MA, et al: Percutaneous and minimally invasive valve procedures: A scientific statement from the American Heart Association Council on Cardiovascular Surgery and Anesthesia, Council on Clinical Cardiology, Functional Genomics and Translational Biology Interdisciplinary Working Group, and Quality of Care and Outcomes Research Interdisciplinary Working Group. Circulation 117:1750, 2008.
62. Vahanian A, Alfieri O, Al-Attar N, et al: Transcatheter valve implantation for patients with aortic stenosis: A position statement from the European association of cardio-thoracic surgery (EACTS) and the European Society of Cardiology (ESC), in collaboration with the European Association of Percutaneous Cardiovascular Interventions (EAPCI). EuroIntervention 4:193, 2008.
63. Rodés-Cabau J, Webb JG, Cheung A, et al: Transcatheter aortic valve implantation for the treatment of severe symptomatic aortic stenosis in patients at very high or prohibitive surgical risk: Acute and late outcomes of the multicenter Canadian experience. J Am Coll Cardiol 55:1080, 2010.
64. Webb JG, Altwegg L, Boone RH, et al: Transcatheter aortic valve implantation: Impact on clinical and valve-related outcomes. Circulation 119:3009, 2009.
64a. Leon MB, Smith CR, Mack M, et al: Transcatheter aortic-valve implantation for aortic stenosis in patients who cannot undergo surgery. N Engl J Med 363:1667, 2010.
65. Chambers J: Low "gradient," low flow aortic stenosis. Heart 92:554, 2006.
66. Tribouilloy C, Levy F, Rusinaru D, et al: Outcome after aortic valve replacement for low-flow/low-gradient aortic stenosis without contractile reserve on dobutamine stress echocardiography. J Am Coll Cardiol 53:1865, 2009.
67. Levy F, Laurent M, Monin JL, et al: Aortic valve replacement for low-flow/low-gradient aortic stenosis operative risk stratification and long-term outcome: A European multicenter study. J Am Coll Cardiol 51:1466, 2008.
68. Quere JP, Monin JL, Levy F, et al: Influence of preoperative left ventricular contractile reserve on postoperative ejection fraction in low-gradient aortic stenosis. Circulation 113:1738, 2006.
69. Clavel MA, Fuchs C, Burwash IG, et al: Predictors of outcomes in low-flow, low-gradient aortic stenosis: Results of the multicenter TOPAS Study. Circulation 118:S234, 2008..
70. Picano E, Pibarot P, Lancellotti P, et al: The emerging role of exercise testing and stress echocardiography in valvular heart disease. J Am Coll Cardiol 54:2251, 2009.
71. Brown JM, O'Brien SM, Wu C, et al: Isolated aortic valve replacement in North America comprising 108,687 patients in 10 years: Changes in risks, valve types, and outcomes in the Society of Thoracic Surgeons National Database. J Thorac Cardiovasc Surg 137:82, 2009.
72. Shahian DM, O'Brien SM, Filardo G, et al: The Society of Thoracic Surgeons 2008 cardiac surgery risk models: Part 3—valve plus coronary artery bypass grafting surgery. Ann Thorac Surg 88:S43, 2009.
73. O'Brien SM, Shahian DM, Filardo G, et al: The Society of Thoracic Surgeons 2008 cardiac surgery risk models: Part 2—isolated valve surgery. Ann Thorac Surg 88:S23, 2009.
74. Goodney PP, O'Connor GT, Wennberg DE, Birkmeyer JE: Do hospitals with low mortality rates in coronary artery bypass also perform well in valve replacement? Ann Thorac Surg 76:1131, 2003.
75. Vahanian A, Otto CM: Risk stratification in aortic stenosis. Eur Heart J 31:416, 2010.
76. Dewey TM, Brown D, Ryan WH: Reliability of risk algorithms in predicting early and late operative outcomes in high-risk patients undergoing aortic valve replacement. J Thorac Cardiovasc Surg 135:180, 2008.
77. Wendt D, Osswald BR, Kayser K, et al: Society of Thoracic Surgeons score is superior to the EuroSCORE determining mortality in high risk patients undergoing isolated aortic valve replacement. Ann Thorac Surg 88:468, 2009.
78. Hannan EL, Wu C, Bennett EV, et al: Risk index for predicting in-hospital mortality for cardiac valve surgery. Ann Thorac Surg 83:921, 2008.
79. Pedrazzini GB, Masson S, Latini R, et al: Comparison of brain natriuretic peptide plasma levels versus logistic EuroSCORE in predicting in-hospital and late postoperative mortality in patients undergoing aortic valve replacement for symptomatic aortic stenosis. Am J Cardiol 102:749, 2008.
80. Kolh P, Kerzmann A, Honore C,et al: Aortic valve surgery in octogenarians: Predictive factors for operative and long-term results. Eur J Cardiothorac Surg 31:600, 2007.
81. Lung B: Management of the elderly patient with aortic stenosis. Heart 94:519, 2008.
81a. Malaisrie SC, McCarthy PM, McGee EC, et al: Contemporary perioperative results of isolated aortic valve replacement for aortic stenosis: Implications for referral of patients for valve replacement. Ann Thorac Surg 89:751, 2010.
82. Ambler G, Omar RZ, Royston P, et al: Generic, simple risk stratification model for heart valve surgery. Circulation 112:224, 2005.
82a. Maillet JM, Sommeb D, Hennel E, et al: Frailty after aortic valve replacement (AVR) in octogenarians. Arch Gerontol Geriatrics 48:391, 2009.

Aortic Regurgitation

83. Maurer G: Aortic regurgitation. Heart 92:994, 2006.
84. Bekeredjian R, Grayburn PA: Valvular heart disease: Aortic regurgitation. Circulation 112:125, 2005.
85. Enriquez-Sarano M, Tajik AJ: Clinical practice. Aortic regurgitation. N Engl J Med 351:1539, 2004.
86. Roberts WC, Ko JM, Moore TR, Jones WH III: Causes of pure aortic regurgitation in patients having isolated aortic valve replacement at a single U.S. tertiary hospital (1993 to 2005). Circulation 114:422, 2006.
87. Tadros TM, Klein MD, Shapira OM: Ascending aortic dilation associated with bicuspid aortic valve: Pathophysiology, molecular biology, and clinical implications. Circulation 119:880, 2009.
88. Palazzi C, D' AS, Lubrano E, Olivieri I: Aortic involvement in ankylosing spondylitis. Clin Exp Rheumatol 26:S13, 2008.
89. Bermudez EA, Gaasch WH: Regurgitant lesions of the aortic and mitral valves: Considerations in determining the ideal timing of surgical intervention. Heart Fail Clin 2:473, 2006.
90. Rigolin VH, Bonow RO: Hemodynamic characteristics and progression to heart failure in regurgitant lesions. Heart Fail Clin 2:453, 2006.
91. Tornos P, Bonow RO: Aortic regurgitation. *In* Otto CM, Bonow RO (eds): Valvular Heart Disease: A Companion to Braunwald's Heart Disease. Philadelphia, Saunders/Elsevier, 2009, pp 155-168.
92. Tornos P, Sambola A, Permanyer-Miralda G, et al: Long-term outcome of surgically treated aortic regurgitation: Influence of guideline adherence toward early surgery. J Am Coll Cardiol 47:1012, 2006.
93. Sambola A, Tornos P, Ferreira-Gonzalez I, Evangelista A: Prognostic value of preoperative indexed end-systolic left ventricle diameter in the outcome after surgery in patients with chronic aortic regurgitation. Am Heart J 155:1114, 2008.
94. Detaint D, Messika-Zeitoun D, Maalouf J, et al: Quantitative echocardiographic determinants of clinical outcome in asymptomatic patients with aortic regurgitation: A prospective study. J Am Coll Cardiol Img 1:1, 2008.
95. Gelfand EV, Hughes S, Hauser TH, et al: Severity of mitral and aortic regurgitation as assessed by cardiovascular magnetic resonance: optimizing correlation with Doppler echocardiography. J Cardiovasc Magn Reson 8:503, 2006.
96. Mahajerin A, Gurm HS, Tsai TT, et al: Vasodilator therapy in patients with aortic insufficiency: A systematic review. Am Heart J 153:454, 2007.
97. Evangelista A, Tornos P, Sambola A,et al: Long-term vasodilator therapy in patients with severe aortic regurgitation. N Engl J Med 353:1342, 2005.
98. Sampat U, Varadarajan P, Turk R, et al: Effect of beta-blocker therapy on survival in patients with severe aortic regurgitation: Results from a cohort of 756 patients. J Am Coll Cardiol 54;452, 2009.
98a. Hiratzka FD, Bakris GL, Beckman JA, et al: 2010 ACCF/AHA/AATS/ACR/ASA/SCA/SCAI/SIR/STS/SVM Guidelines for the diagnosis and management of patients with thoracic aortic disease: Executive summary. A Report of the American College of Cardiology Foundation/American Heart Association Task Force on Practice Guidelines, American Association for Thoracic Surgery, American College of Radiology, American Stroke Association, Society of Cardiovascular Anesthesiologists, Society for Cardiovascular Angiography and Interventions, Society of Interventional Radiology, Society of Thoracic Surgeons, and Society for Vascular Medicine. Circulation 121:1544, 2010.
99. Minakata K, Schaff HV, Zehr KJ, et al: Is repair of aortic valve regurgitation a safe alternative to valve replacement? J Thorac Cardiovasc Surg 127:645, 2004.
100. Stelzer P, Adams DH: The surgical approach to aortic valve disease. *In* Otto CM, Bonow RO (eds): Valvular Heart Disease: A Companion to Braunwald's Heart Disease. Philadelphia, Saunders/Elsevier, 2009, pp 187-208.
101. Borger MA, Preston M, Ivanov J, et al: Should the ascending aorta be replaced more frequently in patients with bicuspid aortic valve disease? J Thorac Cardiovasc Surg 128:677, 2004.
102. Stout KK, Verrier ED: Acute valvular regurgitation. Circulation 119:3232, 2009.

Bicuspid Aortic Valve

103. Garg V, Muth AN, Ransom JF, et al: Mutations in NOTCH1 cause aortic valve disease. Nature 437:270, 2005.
104. Schaefer BM, Lewin MB, Stout KK, et al: Usefulness of bicuspid aortic valve phenotype to predict elastic properties of the ascending aorta. Am J Cardiol 99:686, 2007.
105. Fernandez B, Duran AC, Fernandez-Gallego T, et al: Bicuspid aortic valves with different special orientations of the leaflets are distinct etiological entities. J Am Coll Cardiol 54:2312, 2009.
105a. Bonow RO: Bicuspid aortic valves and dilated aortas: A critical review of the critical review of the ACC/AHA guidelines recommendations. Am J Cardiol 102:111, 2008.

106. Schaefer BM, Lewin MB, Stout KK, et al: The bicuspid aortic valve: an integrated phenotypic classification of leaflet morphology and aortic root shape. Heart 94:1634, 2008.
107. Tzemos N, Therrien J, Yip J, et al: Outcomes in adults with bicuspid aortic valves. JAMA 300:1317, 2008.
108. Michelena HI, Desjardins VA, Avierinos JF, et al: Natural history of asymptomatic patients with normally functioning or minimally dysfunctional bicuspid aortic valve in the community. Circulation 117:2776, 2008.

Mitral Stenosis

109. Mensah GA: The burden of valvular heart disease. *In* Otto CM, Bonow RO (eds): Valvular Heart Disease: A Companion to Braunwald's Heart Disease. Philadelphia, Saunders/Elsevier, 2009, pp 1-18.
110. Essop MR, Nkomo VT: Rheumatic and nonrheumatic valvular heart disease: Epidemiology, management, and prevention in Africa. Circulation 112:3584, 2005.
111. Roberts WC, Ko JM: Clinical pathology of valvular heart disease. *In* Otto CM, Bonow RO (eds): Valvular Heart Disease: A Companion to Braunwald's Heart Disease. Philadelphia, Saunders/Elsevier, 2009, pp 19-38.
112. Rajamannan NM, Subramaniam M, Caira F, et al: Atorvastatin inhibits hypercholesterolemia-induced calcification in the aortic valves via the Lrp5 receptor pathway. Circulation 112 (suppl I):I-229, 2005.
113. Iung B, Vahanian A: Rheumatic mitral valve disease. *In* Otto CM, Bonow RO (eds): Valvular Heart Disease: A Companion to Braunwald's Heart Disease. Philadelphia, Saunders/Elsevier, 2009, pp 221-242.
114. Iung B, Vahanian A: Echocardiography in the patient undergoing catheter balloon mitral valvuloplasty: Patient selection, hemodynamic results, complications and long term outcome. *In* Otto CM (ed): The Clinical Practice of Echocardiography. Philadelphia, Saunders/Elsevier, 2007, pp 481-501.
115. Carabello BA: Modern management of mitral stenosis. Circulation 112:432, 2005.
116. Shavelle DM: Evaluation of valvular heart disease by cardiac catheterization and angiography. *In* Otto CM, Bonow RO (eds): Valvular Heart Disease: A Companion to Braunwald's Heart Disease. Philadelphia, Saunders/Elsevier, 2009, pp. 85-100
117. Fuster V, Ryden LE, Cannom DS, et al: ACC/AHA/ESC 2006 guidelines for the management of patients with atrial fibrillation: A report of the American College of Cardiology/American Heart Association Task Force on Practice Guidelines and the European Society of Cardiology Committee for Practice Guidelines (Writing Committee to Revise the 2001 Guidelines for the Management of Patients With Atrial Fibrillation): Developed in collaboration with the European Heart Rhythm Association and the Heart Rhythm Society. Circulation 114:e257, 2006.
118. Abreu Filho CA, Lisboa LA, Dallan LA, et al: Effectiveness of the maze procedure using cooled-tip radiofrequency ablation in patients with permanent atrial fibrillation and rheumatic mitral valve disease. Circulation 112(Suppl I):I-20, 2005.
119. Doukas G, Samani NJ, Alexiou C, et al: Left atrial radiofrequency ablation during mitral valve surgery for continuous atrial fibrillation: A randomized controlled trial. JAMA 294:2357, 2005.
120. Krasuski RA, Assar MD, Wang A, et al: Usefulness of percutaneous balloon mitral commissurotomy in preventing the development of atrial fibrillation in patients with mitral stenosis. Am J Cardiol 93:936, 2004.
121. Song JK, Song JM, Kang DH, et al: Restenosis and adverse clinical events after successful percutaneous mitral valvuloplasty: Immediate post-procedural mitral valve area as an important prognosticator. Eur Heart J 30:1254, 2009.
122. Zakkar M, Amirak E, Chan KM, Punjabi PP: Rheumatic mitral valve disease: Current surgical status. Prog Cardiovasc Dis 51:478, 2009.

Mitral Regurgitation

123. Enriquez-Sarano M, Akins CW, Vahanian A: Mitral regurgitation. Lancet 373:1382, 2009.
124. Schoen FJ: Evolving concepts of cardiac valve dynamics: The continuum of development, functional structure, pathobiology, and tissue engineering. Circulation 118:1864, 2008.
125. Van CG, Flamez A, Cosyns B, et al: Treatment of Parkinson's disease with pergolide and relation to restrictive valvular heart disease. Lancet 363:1179, 2004.
126. Schade R, Andersohn F, Suissa S, et al: Dopamine agonists and the risk of cardiac-valve regurgitation. N Engl J Med 356:29-••, 2007.
127. Zanettini R, Antonini A, Gatto G, et al: Valvular heart disease and the use of dopamine agonists for Parkinson's disease. N Engl J Med 356:39, 2007.
128. Barasch E, Gottdiener JS, Larsen EK, et al: Clinical significance of calcification of the fibrous skeleton of the heart and aortosclerosis in community dwelling elderly: The Cardiovascular Health Study (CHS). Am Heart J 151:39, 2006.
129. Kizer JR, Wiebers DO, Whisnant JP, et al: Mitral annular calcification, aortic valve sclerosis, and incident stroke in adults free of clinical cardiovascular disease: The Strong Heart Study. Stroke 36:2533, 2005.
130. Allison MA, Cheung P, Criqui MH, et al: Mitral and aortic annular calcification are highly associated with systemic calcified atherosclerosis. Circulation 113:861, 2006.
131. Pierard LA, Lancellotti P: The role of ischemic mitral regurgitation in the pathogenesis of acute pulmonary edema. N Engl J Med 351:1627, 2004.
132. Levine RA: Dynamic mitral regurgitation—more than meets the eye. N Engl J Med 351:1681, 2004.
133. Levine RA, Schwammenthal E: Ischemic mitral regurgitation on the threshold of a solution: from paradoxes to unifying concepts. Circulation 112:745, 2005.
134. Agricola E, Galderisi M, Mele D, et al: Mechanical dyssynchrony and functional mitral regurgitation: Pathophysiology and clinical implications. J Cardiovasc Med (Hagerstown) 9:461, 2008.
135. Bursi F, Enriquez-Sarano M, Nkomo VT, et al: Heart failure and death after myocardial infarction in the community: The emerging role of mitral regurgitation. Circulation 111:295, 2005.
136. Nishimura RA, Schaff HV: Mitral regurgitation: timing of surgery. *In* Otto CM, Bonow RO (eds): Valvular Heart Disease: A Companion to Braunwald's Heart Disease. Philadelphia, Saunders/Elsevier, 2009, pp 274-290.
137. Gaasch WH, Meyer TE: Left ventricular response to mitral regurgitation: Implications for management. Circulation 118:2298, 2008.
138. Otto CM: Timing of intervention for chronic valve regurgitation: the role of echocardiography. *In* Otto CM (ed): The Clinical Practice of Echocardiography. Philadelphia, Saunders/Elsevier, 2007, pp 430-458.
139. Tribouilloy C, Grigioni F, Avierinos JF, et al: Survival implication of left ventricular end-systolic diameter in mitral regurgitation due to flail leaflets: A long-term follow-up multicenter study. J Am Coll Cardiol 54:1961, 2009.
140. Otto CM: Evaluation of valvular heart disease by echocardiography. *In* Otto CM, Bonow RO (eds): Valvular Heart Disease: A Companion to Braunwald's Heart Disease. Philadelphia, Saunders/Elsevier, 2009, pp 62-84.
141. Enriquez-Sarano M, Avierinos JF, Messika-Zeitoun D, et al: Quantitative determinants of the outcome of asymptomatic mitral regurgitation. N Engl J Med 352:875, 2005.
142. Hung J, Lang R, Flachskampf F, et al: 3D echocardiography: A review of the current status and future directions. J Am Soc Echocardiogr 20:213, 2007.
143. Bando K, Kasegawa H, Okada Y, et al: Impact of preoperative and postoperative atrial fibrillation on outcome after mitral valvuloplasty for nonischemic mitral regurgitation. J Thorac Cardiovasc Surg 129:1032, 2005.
144. Eguchi K, Ohtaki E, Matsumura T, et al: Pre-operative atrial fibrillation as the key determinant of outcome of mitral valve repair for degenerative mitral regurgitation. Eur Heart J 26:1866, 2005.
145. Carabello BA: The current therapy for mitral regurgitation. J Am Coll Cardiol 52:319, 2008.
146. Rosenhek R, Rader F, Klaar U, et al: Outcome of watchful waiting in asymptomatic severe mitral regurgitation. Circulation 113:2238, 2006.
147. Kang DH, Kim JH, Rim JH, et al: Comparison of early surgery versus conventional treatment in asymptomatic severe mitral regurgitation. Circulation 119:797, 2009.
148. Schaff HV: Asymptomatic severe mitral valve regurgitation: Observation or operation? Circulation 119:768, 2009.
149. DiGregorio V, Zehr KJ, Orszulak TA, et al: Results of mitral surgery in octogenarians with isolated nonrheumatic mitral regurgitation. Ann Thorac Surg 78:807, 2004.
150. Nagendran J, Norris C, Maitland A, et al: Is mitral valve surgery safe in octogenarians? Eur J Cardiothorac Surg 28:83, 2005.
150a. Chikwe J, Goldstone AB, Passage J, et al: A propensity score-adjusted retrospective comparison of early and mid-term results of mitral valve repair versus replacement in octogenarians. Eur Heart J. Published ahead of print doi:10.1093/eurheartj/ehq331.
151. Nowicki ER, Birkmeyer NJ, Weintraub RW, et al: Multivariable prediction of in-hospital mortality associated with aortic and mitral valve surgery in Northern New England. Ann Thorac Surg 77:1966, 2004.
152. Fedak PW, McCarthy PM, Bonow RO: Evolving concepts and technologies in mitral valve repair. Circulation 117:963, 2008.
153. Adams DH, Anyanwu AC: Seeking a higher standard for degenerative mitral valve repair: Begin with etiology. J Thorac Cardiovasc Surg 136:551, 2008.
154. Verma S, Mesana TG: Mitral-valve repair for mitral-valve prolapse. N Engl J Med 361:2261, 2009.
155. McCarthy PM, Malaisrie SC: Mitral valve repair and replacement, including associated atrial fibrillation and tricuspid regurgitation. *In* Otto CM, Bonow RO (eds): Valvular Heart Disease: A Companion to Braunwald's Heart Disease. Philadelphia, Saunders/Elsevier, 2009, pp. 291-306.
156. DeBonis M, Lorusso R, Lapenna E, et al: Similar long-term results of mitral valve repair for anterior compared with posterior leaflet prolapse. J Thorac Cardiovasc Surg 131:364, 2006.
157. Lam BK, Gillinov AM, Blackstone EH, et al: Importance of moderate ischemic mitral regurgitation. Ann Thorac Surg 79:462, 2005.
158. Bax JJ, Braun J, Somer ST, et al: Restrictive annuloplasty and coronary revascularization in ischemic mitral regurgitation results in reverse left ventricular remodeling. Circulation 110(Suppl II):II-103, 2004.
159. Schroder JN, Williams ML, Hata JA, et al: Impact of mitral valve regurgitation evaluated by intraoperative transesophageal echocardiography on long-term outcomes after coronary artery bypass grafting. Circulation 112:I293, 2005.
160. Shah PM: Intraoperative echocardiography for mitral valve disease. *In* Otto CM, Bonow RO (eds): Valvular Heart Disease: A Companion to Braunwald's Heart Disease. Philadelphia, Saunders/Elsevier, 2009, pp 322-333.
161. Gammie JS, Sheng S, Griffith BP, et al: Trends in mitral valve surgery in the United States: Results from the Society of Thoracic Surgeons Adult Cardiac Database. Ann Thorac Surg 87:1431, 2009.
162. Bridgewater B, Hooper T, Munsch C, et al: Mitral repair best practice: proposed standards. Heart 92:939, 2006.
163. Dogan S, Aybek T, Risteski PS, et al: Minimally invasive port access versus conventional mitral valve surgery: prospective randomized study. Ann Thorac Surg 79:492, 2005.
164. Vassiliades TA Jr, Block PC, Cohn LH, et al: The clinical development of percutaneous heart valve technology: A position statement of the Society of Thoracic Surgeons (STS), the American Association for Thoracic Surgery (AATS), and the Society for Cardiovascular Angiography and Interventions (SCAI) Endorsed by the American College of Cardiology Foundation (ACCF) and the American Heart Association (AHA). J Am Coll Cardiol 45: 1554, 2005.
165. Feldman T, Wasserman HS, Herrmann HC, et al: Percutaneous mitral valve repair using the edge-to-edge technique: Six-month results of the EVEREST Phase I Clinical Trial. J Am Coll Cardiol 46:2134, 2005.
166. Webb JG, Harnek J, Munt BI, et al: Percutaneous transvenous mitral annuloplasty: initial human experience with device implantation in the coronary sinus. Circulation 113:851, 2006.
167. Block PC: Percutaneous transcatheter intervention for mitral regurgitation. *In* Otto CM, Bonow RO (eds): Valvular Heart Disease: A Companion to Braunwald's Heart Disease. Philadelphia, Saunders/Elsevier, 2009, pp 307-321.
168. Iung B, Rousseau-Paziaud J, Cormier B, et al: Contemporary results of mitral valve repair for infective endocarditis. J Am Coll Cardiol 43:386, 2004.
169. Beeri R, Otsuji Y, Schwammenthal E, Levine RA: Ischemic mitral regurgitation. *In* Otto CM, Bonow RO (eds): Valvular Heart Disease: A Companion to Braunwald's Heart Disease. Philadelphia, Saunders/Elsevier, 2009, pp 260-273.
170. Zegdi R, Debieche M, Latremouille C, et al: Long-term results of mitral valve repair in active endocarditis. Circulation 111:2532, 2005.

Mitral Valve Prolapse

171. Griffin BP: Myxomatous mitral valve disease. *In* Otto CM, Bonow RO (eds): Valvular Heart Disease: A Companion to Braunwald's Heart Disease. Philadelphia, Saunders/Elsevier, 2009, pp 243-259.

172. Hayek E, Gring CN, Griffin BP: Mitral valve prolapse. Lancet 365:507, 2005.
173. Nesta F, Leyne M, Yosefy C, et al: New locus for autosomal dominant mitral valve prolapse on chromosome 13: clinical insights from genetic studies. Circulation 112:2022, 2005.
174. Judge DP, Dietz HC: Marfan's syndrome. Lancet 366:1965, 2005.
175. Stewart WJ, Griffin BP: Intraoperative echocardiography in mitral valve repair. *In* Otto CM (ed): The Clinical Practice of Echocardiography. Philadelphia, Saunders/Elsevier, 2007, pp 459-480.
176. Avierinos JF, Detaint D, Messika-Zeitoun D, et al: Risk, determinants, and outcome implications of progression of mitral regurgitation after diagnosis of mitral valve prolapse in a single community. Am J Cardiol 101:662, 2008.

Tricuspid, Pulmonic, and Multivalve Disease

177. Bruce CJ, Connolly HM: Right-sided valve disease deserves a little more respect. Circulation 119:2726, 2009.
178. Rogers JH, Bolling SF: The tricuspid valve: Current perspective and evolving management of tricuspid regurgitation. Circulation 119:2718, 2009.
179. Forfia PR, Weigers SE: Echocardiographic findings in acute and chronic respiratory disease. *In* Otto CM (ed): The Clinical Practice of Echocardiography. Philadelphia, Saunders/Elsevier, 2007, pp 848-876.
180. McCarthy PM, Bhudia SK, Rajeswaran J, et al: Tricuspid valve repair: Durability and risk factors for failure. J Thorac Cardiovasc Surg 127:674, 2004.
181. Dreyfus GD, Corbi PJ, Chan KM, Bahrami T: Secondary tricuspid regurgitation or dilation: Which should be the criteria for surgical repair? Ann Thorac Surg 79:127, 2005.
182. Fukuda S, Song JM, Gillinov AM, et al: Tricuspid valve tethering predicts residual tricuspid regurgitation after tricuspid annuloplasty. Circulation 111:975, 2005.
183. Huehnergarth KV, Gurvitz M, Stout KK, Otto CM: Repaired tetralogy of Fallot in the adult: Monitoring and management. Heart 94:1663, 2008.
184. Therrien J, Siu SC, McLaughlin PR, et al: Pulmonary valve replacement in adults late after repair of tetralogy of fallot: Are we operating too late? J Am Coll Cardiol 36:1670, 2000.
185. Sommer RJ, Hijazi ZM, Rhodes JF: Pathophysiology of congenital heart disease in the adult: Part III: Complex congenital heart disease. Circulation 117:1340, 2008.
186. McElhinney DB, Hellenbrand WE, Zahn EM, et al: Short- and medium-term outcomes after transcatheter pulmonary valve placement in the expanded multicenter US melody valve trial. Circulation 122:507, 2010.

Prosthetic Cardiac Valves

187. Pibarot P, Dumesnil JG: Prosthetic heart valves: Selection of the optimal prosthesis and long-term management. Circulation 119:1034, 2009.
188. O'Gara PT, Bonow RO, Otto CM: Prosthetic heart valves. *In* Otto CM, Bonow RO (eds): Valvular Heart Disease: A Companion to Braunwald's Heart Disease. Philadelphia, Saunders/Elsevier, 2009, pp 383-398.
189. Yoganathan AP, Travis BR: Fluid dynamics of prosthetic valves. *In* Otto CM (ed): The Clinical Practice of Echocardiography. Philadelphia, Saunders/Elsevier, 2007, pp 552-576.
190. Tong AT, Roudaut R, Ozkan M, et al: Transesophageal echocardiography improves risk assessment of thrombolysis of prosthetic valve thrombosis: Results of the international PRO-TEE registry. J Am Coll Cardiol 43:77, 2004.
191. Schoen FJ, Levy RJ: Calcification of tissue heart valve substitutes: Progress toward understanding and prevention. Ann Thorac Surg 79:1072, 2005.
192. Ruel M, Kulik A, Rubens FD, et al: Late incidence and determinants of reoperation in patients with prosthetic heart valves. Eur J Cardiothorac Surg 25:364, 2004.
193. Webb JG, Wood DA, Ye J, et al: Transcatheter valve-in-valve implantation for failed bioprosthetic heart valves. Circulation 121:1848, 2010.
194. Leyh RG, Knobloch K, Hagl C, et al: Replacement of the aortic root for acute prosthetic valve endocarditis: Prosthetic composite versus aortic allograft root replacement. J Thorac Cardiovasc Surg 127:1416, 2004.
195. Takkenberg JJM, Klieverik LMA, Schoof PH, et al: The Ross procedure: A systematic review and meta-analysis. Circulation 119:222, 2009.
196. Raja SG, Pozzi M: Ross operation in children and young adults: The Alder Hey case series. BMC Cardiovasc Disord 4:3, 2004.
197. de Kerchove L, Rubay J, Pasquet A, et al: Ross operation in the adult: long-term outcomes after root replacement and inclusion techniques. Ann Thorac Surg 87:95, 2009.
197a. El-Hamamsy J, Eryigit A, Stevens LM, et al. Long-term outcomes after autograft versus homograft aortic root replacement in adults with aortic valve disease: A randomized controlled trial. Lancet 376:524, 2010.
198. Zabalgiotia M: Echocardiographic recognition and quantitation of prosthetic valve dysfunction. *In* Otto CM (ed): The Clinical Practice of Echocardiography. Philadelphia, Saunders/Elsevier, 2007, pp 577-604.
199. Pibarot P, Dumesnil JG: Prosthesis-patient mismatch: Definition, clinical impact, and prevention. Heart 92:1022, 2006.
200. Seiler C: Management and follow up of prosthetic heart valves. Heart 90:818, 2004.
200a. Rahimtoola SH: Choice of prosthetic heart valve in adults: An update. J Am Coll Cardiol 55:2413, 2010.
201. Elkayam U, Bitar F: Valvular heart disease and pregnancy part I: Native valves. J Am Coll Cardiol 46:223, 2005.
202. Stout KK: Valvular heart disease in pregnancy. *In* Otto CM, Bonow RO (eds): Valvular Heart Disease: A Companion to Braunwald's Heart Disease. Philadelphia, Saunders/Elsevier, 2009, pp 424-436.
203. Spyropoulos AC, Frost FJ, Hurley JS, Roberts M: Costs and clinical outcomes associated with low-molecular-weight heparin vs unfractionated heparin for perioperative bridging in patients receiving long-term oral anticoagulant therapy. Chest 125:1642, 2004.
204. Kovacs MJ, Kearon C, Rodger M, et al: Single-arm study of bridging therapy with low-molecular-weight heparin for patients at risk of arterial embolism who require temporary interruption of warfarin. Circulation 110:1658, 2004.
205. Salem DN, O'Gara PT, Madias C, Pauker SG, American College of Chest Physicians: Valvular and structural heart disease: American College of Chest Physicians Evidence-Based Clinical Practice Guidelines (8th Edition). Chest 133:593S, 2008.

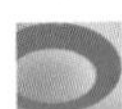

GUIDELINES Robert O. Bonow and Catherine M. Otto*

Management of Valvular Heart Disease

The American College of Cardiology and the American Heart Association (ACC/AHA) first published guidelines for the management of patients with valvular heart disease in 1998.[1] These were revised in 2006[2] and updated in 2008.[3] Some material from the 2008 guidelines is presented elsewhere in other chapters. In addition to the guidelines tables and figures in Chap. 66, guidelines for the prevention and treatment of infective endocarditis are summarized in the appendix to Chap. 67 and guidelines for the management of anticoagulation in pregnancy are included in the appendix to Chap. 82. Other recommendations for valvular heart diseases are included in the ACC/AHA guidelines for the use of echocardiography,[4] appropriate use criteria for echocardiography from the ACC and other organizations,[5] ACC recommendations for assessment of athletes with cardiovascular abnormalities,[6] and AHA recommendations for cardiovascular assessment of athletes.[7]

The ACC/AHA guidelines emphasize that the clinical assessment should be based on the patient's symptomatic status and findings from the physical examination. Cardiac auscultation remains the most widely used method of screening for valvular heart disease. The chest radiograph and electrocardiogram (ECG), if normal, can often provide reassurance that a murmur is clinically insignificant. Echocardiography should be considered after assessment of these more routine data, and echocardiography is determined to be inappropriate for the evaluation of murmurs that experienced observers consider innocent or functional. In contrast, echocardiography is considered appropriate even in asymptomatic patients with murmurs suggesting significant valvular disease or with other signs or symptoms of cardiovascular disease (**Table 66G-1**), and there is emphasis on the use of Doppler echocardiography to quantify the severity of valvular stenosis and regurgitation (see Table 66-1). In some cases, cardiac catheterization and angiography are appropriate, as is exercise stress testing.

As with other ACC/AHA guidelines, these use the standard ACC/AHA classification system for indications:

Class I: Conditions for which there is evidence and/or general agreement that the test is useful and effective
Class II: Conditions for which there is conflicting evidence and/or a divergence of opinion about the usefulness or efficacy of performing the test
Class IIa: Weight of evidence or opinion in favor of usefulness or efficacy
Class IIb: Usefulness or efficacy less well established by evidence or opinion
Class III: Conditions for which there is evidence and/or general agreement that the test is not useful or effective and in some cases may be harmful

Three levels are used to rate the evidence on which recommendations have been based. Level A recommendations are derived from data from multiple randomized clinical trials, level B recommendations are derived from a single randomized trial or nonrandomized studies, and level C recommendations are based on the consensus opinion of experts.

AORTIC STENOSIS

The guidelines indicate that Doppler echocardiography is a highly appropriate test for diagnosis and assessment of aortic stenosis (AS) and for evaluation of left ventricular (LV) function in patients with this condition. Yearly echocardiograms are helpful for the management of asymptomatic patients with severe AS, but intervals of 1 to 2 years are recommended for asymptomatic patients with moderate AS and 3 to 5 years for those with

*Dr. Thomas H. Lee contributed to this section in previous editions of this book.

TABLE 66G-1 ACC/AHA Guidelines for Echocardiography in Patients with a Cardiac Murmur

CLASS	INDICATION	LOE
I	Asymptomatic patients with diastolic, continuous, holosystolic, and late systolic murmurs, murmurs associated with ejection clicks, or those that radiate to the neck or back	C
	Patients with heart murmurs and symptoms or signs of heart failure, myocardial ischemia or infarction, syncope, thromboembolism, infective endocarditis, or other clinical evidence of structural heart disease	C
	Asymptomatic patients who have grade 3 or louder midpeaking systolic murmurs	C
IIa	Asymptomatic patients with murmurs associated with other abnormal cardiac physical findings or murmurs associated with an abnormal ECG or chest radiograph	C
	Patients whose symptoms and/or signs are likely noncardiac in origin but in whom a cardiac basis cannot be excluded by standard evaluation	C
III	Not recommended for patients with grade 2 or softer midsystolic murmurs identified as innocent or functional by an experienced observer	C

LOE = level of evidence.

TABLE 66G-2 ACC/AHA Guidelines for Management of Patients with Aortic Valve Stenosis

INDICATION	CLASS	RECOMMENDATION	LOE
Echocardiography	I	Diagnosis and assessment of AS severity	B
		Assessment of LV wall thickness, size, and function	B
		Diagnosis and assessment of AS severity	B
		Reevaluating patients with known AS and changing symptoms or signs	B
		Assessment changes in AS severity and LV function in patients with known AS during pregnancy	B
		Serial testing in asymptomatic patients—severe AS, every yr; moderate AS, every 1-2 yr; mild AS: every 3-5 yr	B
Exercise stress testing	IIb	Consider for asymptomatic patients to elicit exercise-induced symptoms and abnormal blood pressure responses	B
	III	Should not be performed in symptomatic patients with AS	B
Cardiac catheterization for hemodynamic assessment	I	Hemodynamic measurements for assessment of AS severity in symptomatic patients when noninvasive tests are inconclusive, or when there is a discrepancy between noninvasive tests and clinical findings regarding severity of AS	C
	III	Not recommended for assessment of AS severity when noninvasive tests are adequate and concordant with clinical findings	C
Coronary angiography	I	Indicated before AVR in patients at risk for CAD	B
		Indicated before AVR when pulmonary autograft (Ross procedure) is contemplated and origin of the coronary arteries is not identified by noninvasive techniques	C
Low-flow, low-gradient aortic stenosis	IIa	Dobutamine infusion during echocardiography or cardiac catheterization for evaluation of low-flow, low-gradient AS and LV dysfunction	B
Aortic valve replacement	I	Symptomatic patients with severe AS	B
		Patients with severe AS undergoing CABG or surgery on the aorta or other heart valves	C
		Patients with severe AS and LV systolic dysfunction (ejection fraction < 0.50)	B
	IIa	Patients with moderate AS undergoing CABG or surgery on the aorta or other heart valves	B
	IIb	Asymptomatic patients with severe AS and abnormal response to exercise	C
		Patients undergoing CABG who have mild AS and evidence that progression may be rapid	C
		Patients with severe asymptomatic AS if there is a high likelihood of rapid progression (age, calcification, and CAD) or if surgery might be delayed at the time of symptom onset	C
		Asymptomatic patients with extremely severe AS (aortic valve area < 0.6 cm^2, mean gradient > 60 mm Hg, and jet velocity > 5 m/sec) if expected operative mortality is ≤1%	C
	III	Not useful for the prevention of sudden death in asymptomatic patients with AS who have none of the findings listed under the Class IIa or IIb recommendations	B
Aortic balloon valvotomy	IIb	Bridge to surgery in hemodynamically unstable patients with AS who are at high risk for AVR	C
		Palliation in patients with AS in whom AVR cannot be performed because of serious comorbid conditions	C
	III	Not recommended as an alternative to AVR in adult patients with AS; certain younger adults without valve calcification may be exception	B

LOE = level of evidence.

mild AS (**Table 66G-2**). For patients with severe AS and low cardiac output (low-flow, low-gradient AS), dobutamine stress echocardiography may be a reasonable tool for evaluation.

Exercise testing of asymptomatic patients can be performed safely and may be a reasonable approach for eliciting symptoms, but it should not be performed in symptomatic patients. An experienced physician should supervise exercise tests for patients with AS and closely monitor blood pressure and the ECG. Physical activity should not be restricted in asymptomatic patients with mild AS. However, the 36th Bethesda Conference on Eligibility Recommendations for Competitive Athletes With Cardiovascular Abnormalities has recommended that patients with mild to moderate AS avoid competitive sports with high dynamic and static muscular demands.[6]

Cardiac Catheterization

The ACC/AHA guidelines indicate that coronary angiography is appropriate in patients with possible coronary artery disease (CAD), and catheterization may be necessary to assess the hemodynamic severity of AS in symptomatic patients when other data are not conclusive (see Table 66G-2). Catheterization is discouraged solely for the purposes of confirming information available from noninvasive tests or assessing LV function and severity of AS in asymptomatic patients. Cardiac catheterization with infusion of dobutamine may be useful for hemodynamic evaluation in patients with low-flow, low-gradient AS and LV dysfunction.

Aortic Valve Replacement

Surgery is recommended for almost all symptomatic patients with severe AS, and the ACC/AHA guidelines are generally supportive (Class IIa) of aortic valve replacement (AVR) for patients with moderate disease who are undergoing coronary artery bypass grafting (CABG) or surgery on the aorta or other heart valves. The guidelines are less supportive of AVR in patients who are asymptomatic despite severe AS (see Table 66G-2), although subgroups with a high likelihood of progressive disease are identified in whom this might be considered. Aortic balloon valvotomy was given qualified support as a bridge to surgery for hemodynamically unstable patients who cannot undergo immediate aortic valve replacement or as palliation for those who cannot undergo valve replacement. It is not recommended as an alternative to AVR except in the case of some younger patients with congenital AS without valve calcification.

AORTIC REGURGITATION

Doppler echocardiography is a highly appropriate test for the diagnosis and serial assessment of patients with aortic regurgitation (AR; **Table 66G-3**). Serial echocardiography is indicated to evaluate LV size and function periodically in asymptomatic patients with severe AR and to reevaluate AR in patients with new or changing symptoms to ensure that rapid progression is not underway. Asymptomatic patients with mild AR, normal LV function, and little or no LV dilation can be seen on an annual basis, and echocardiography can be performed every 2 to 3 years in the absence of changes in symptoms. However, the guidelines support echocardiography every 6 to 12 months for patients with severe AR and significant LV dilation, such as end-diastolic dimension more than 60 mm. For patients with even more advanced LV dilation, echocardiography as often as every 3 months is endorsed.

TABLE 66G-3 ACC/AHA Guidelines for Management of Patients with Aortic Regurgitation

INDICATION	CLASS	RECOMMENDATION	LOE
Echocardiography	I	Confirm presence and severity of acute or chronic AR.	B
		Assess cause of chronic AR (including valve morphology and aortic root size and morphology) and LV hypertrophy, LV dimension (or volume), and LV systolic function.	B
		Assess AR severity and severity of aortic dilation in patients with enlarged aortic root.	B
		Periodically reevaluate LV size and function in asymptomatic patients with severe AR.	B
		Reevaluate mild, moderate, or severe AR in patients with new or changing symptoms.	B
Exercise stress testing	IIa	Assess functional capacity and symptomatic response in patients with a history of equivocal symptoms.	B
		Evaluate symptoms and functional capacity before participation in athletic activities.	C
	IIb	Perform exercise testing with radionuclide angiography for assessment of LV function in asymptomatic or symptomatic patients with chronic AR.	B
Radionuclide imaging or CMR	I	Radionuclide angiography or CMR is indicated for the initial and serial assessment of LV volume and function at rest in patients with AR and suboptimal echocardiograms.	B
	IIa	Perform CMR for estimation of AR severity in patients with unsatisfactory echocardiograms	B
Vasodilator therapy	I	Chronic therapy in patients with severe AR who have symptoms or LV dysfunction when AVR is not recommended because of additional cardiac or noncardiac factors	B
	IIa	Short-term therapy to improve the hemodynamic profile of patients with severe heart failure symptoms and severe LV dysfunction before proceeding with AVR	C
	IIb	Long-term therapy for asymptomatic patients with severe AR and LV dilation but normal systolic function	B
	III	Not indicated for long-term therapy in asymptomatic, mild to moderate AR and normal LV systolic function	B
		Not indicated for long-term therapy in asymptomatic patients with LV systolic dysfunction who are otherwise candidates for AVR	C
		Not indicated for long-term therapy in symptomatic patients with either normal LV function or mild to moderate LV systolic dysfunction who are otherwise candidates for AVR	C
Cardiac catheterization for hemodynamic assessment and aortic root angiography	I	Assessment of AR severity, LV function, or aortic root size when noninvasive tests are inconclusive or discordant with clinical findings	B
	III	Not indicated for assessment of LV function, aortic root size, or AR severity before AVR when noninvasive tests are adequate and concordant with clinical findings	C
		Not indicated for assessment of LV function and severity of regurgitation in asymptomatic patients when noninvasive tests are adequate	C
Coronary angiography	I	Indicated before AVR in patients at risk for CAD	C
AVR or aortic valve repair	I	Symptomatic patients with severe AR irrespective of LV systolic function	B
		Asymptomatic patients with severe AR and LV systolic dysfunction (EF ≤ 0.50) at rest	B
		Patients with chronic severe AR undergoing CABG or surgery on the aorta or other heart valves	C
	IIa	Asymptomatic patients with severe AR and normal LV systolic function (EF > 0.50) but with severe LV dilation (EDD > 75 mm or ESD > 55 mm)*	B
	IIb	Patients with moderate AR while undergoing CABG or surgery on the ascending aorta	C
		Asymptomatic patients with severe AR and normal LV systolic function at rest (EF > 0.50) with LVEDD > 70 mm or LVESD >50 mm,* when there is evidence of progressive LV dilation, declining exercise tolerance, or abnormal hemodynamic response to exercise	C
	III	Not indicated for asymptomatic patients with mild, moderate, or severe AR and normal LV systolic function at rest (EF > 0.50) when LV dilation is not moderate or severe (EDD < 70 mm; ESD < 50 mm)*	B

*Consider lower thresholds for patients of small stature, regardless of gender.
EDD = end-diastolic dimension; EF = ejection fraction; ESD = end-systolic dimension; LOE = level of evidence.

Exercise testing is considered appropriate for the assessment of functional capacity in patients in whom the history is not definitive, but the impact of this test on management is not otherwise strongly supported. Cardiac magnetic resonance (CMR) is reasonable for estimating the severity of AR and LV volume and function in patients with equivocal echocardiograms. Radionuclide angiography is less positively endorsed as an alternative to echocardiography for the assessment of LV volume and function.

Medical Therapy

The ACC/AHA guidelines consider vasodilator therapy appropriate for patients with hypertension, with weak endorsement for those with severe AR, normal LV function, and evidence of LV dilation. However, there is no endorsement for long-term vasodilator therapy in normotensive patients with normal LV function and mild AR. Vasodilator therapy is not an alternative to surgery for patients who are appropriate candidates for valve replacement, including those with asymptomatic LV dysfunction.

Cardiac Catheterization

Cardiac catheterization is not routinely needed to confirm the diagnosis or assess the severity of AR when echocardiographic studies are adequate. The most common appropriate indication for cardiac catheterization is coronary angiography as a prelude to surgery.

Aortic Valve Replacement

The ACC/AHA guidelines deem AVR to be clearly appropriate for patients with symptoms (New York Heart Association [NYHA] Class II, III or IV), progressive LV dilation, mild to moderate LV systolic dysfunction, or declining exercise tolerance (see Table 66G-3). The guidelines were not supportive of surgery solely because of a decline in ejection fraction during exercise. Following AVR, close follow-up is necessary to evaluate both the function of the new valve and LV function. This usually includes an echocardiogram soon after surgery to be used as a baseline. Patients should be followed clinically at 6 months, 12, months, and then annually if the clinical course is uncomplicated. Serial postoperative echocardiograms after the initial early postoperative study are usually not indicated if the clinical course is uncomplicated. Patients with persistent LV dilation on the initial postoperative echocardiogram should be treated as any other patient with symptomatic or asymptomatic LV dysfunction, including treatment with angiotensin-converting enzyme (ACE) inhibitors and beta-adrenergic blocking agents.

BICUSPID AORTIC VALVE WITH DILATED ASCENDING AORTA

Transthoracic echocardiography should be used initially to evaluate patients with known bicuspid aortic valves (**Table 66G-4**). CMR or computed tomography (CT) should be used when echocardiography cannot adequately assess the aortic root or ascending aorta or to quantify the severity of dilation and involvement of the ascending aorta further. Surgical repair or replacement is indicated if the diameter of the aortic root or ascending aorta is more than 5 cm (or smaller in patients of small stature) or if the rate of increase in diameter is 0.5 cm/year or more.

MITRAL STENOSIS

Transthoracic echocardiography is endorsed in the ACC/AHA guidelines as the first-line test for the diagnosis and follow-up of patients with mitral stenosis (MS). Transesophageal echocardiography has a role for the detection of left atrial thrombus in patients being considered for percutaneous mitral balloon valvotomy or cardioversion (**Table 66G-5**) but not for routine evaluation of mitral valve morphology or hemodynamics, unless transthoracic echocardiography has been unsuccessful.

Medical Management

Patients with more than mild MS should be counseled to avoid unusual physical stresses. Anticoagulation is recommended for patients with MS if they have a history of atrial fibrillation, prior embolic event, or left atrial thrombus. The guidelines are not strongly supportive of anticoagulation on the basis of left atrial size alone.

Cardiac Catheterization

The guidelines support the use of cardiac catheterization for hemodynamic evaluation when noninvasive tests are not conclusive or yield discrepant results.

Percutaneous Mitral Balloon Valvotomy

In centers with skilled operators, the guidelines indicate that percutaneous mitral balloon valvotomy is the initial procedure of choice for symptomatic patients (NYHA functional Classes II to IV) with moderate or severe MS and favorable valve morphology, and for asymptomatic patients with pulmonary hypertension (see Table 66G-5). It is not indicated for patients with mild MS, left atrial thrombus, or moderate to severe mitral regurgitation (MR).

Surgical Options

When possible, mitral valve repair is indicated for patients with symptomatic (NYHA functional Classes II to IV) moderate or severe mitral valve stenosis when percutaneous mitral valve balloon valvotomy is not possible. Mitral valve repair may be considered for asymptomatic patients who experience recurrent embolic events despite adequate anticoagulation. Mitral valve replacement is an option when repair is not feasible.

MITRAL VALVE PROLAPSE

The diagnosis of mitral valve prolapse (MVP) should be made by physical examination; two-dimensional and Doppler echocardiography should be used primarily for evaluation of MR and ventricular compensation, as well as for excluding the diagnosis of MVP in patients who have been given the diagnosis inappropriately (**Table 66G-6**). Serial use of echocardiography in stable patients with mild or no regurgitation is discouraged.

Management

Reassurance is an important element of the management of patients with MVP. A normal lifestyle and regular exercise are encouraged, especially in patients with mild or no symptoms and mild MVP.

TABLE 66G-4 ACC/AHA Guidelines for Management of Patients with Bicuspid Aortic Valves and Dilated Ascending Aortas

INDICATION	CLASS	RECOMMENDATION	LOE
Echocardiography, CMR and cardiac CT	I	Initial transthoracic echo to assess the diameters of the aortic root and ascending aorta	B
		CMR or CT when morphology of the aortic root or ascending aorta cannot be assessed accurately by echo	C
		Serial evaluation of aortic root, ascending aorta size and morphology by echo, CMR, or cardiac CT annually when dilation of the aortic root or ascending aorta > 4 cm*	C
	IIa	CMR or cardiac CT in patients with bicuspid aortic valves when aortic root dilation is detected by echo to quantify severity of dilation and involvement of the ascending aorta further	B
Medical therapy	IIa	Beta-adrenergic blocking agents for patients with bicuspid valves and dilated aortic roots (diameter > 4 cm*) who are not candidates for surgical correction and who do not have moderate to severe AR	C
Surgery	I	Surgery to repair the aortic root or replace the ascending aorta indicated for patients with bicuspid aortic valves if the diameter of the aortic root or ascending aorta >5 cm* or rate of increase in diameter ≥ 0.5 cm/yr	C
		Repair of aortic root or replacement of ascending aorta if the diameter of the aortic root or ascending aorta > 4.5 cm* in patients with bicuspid valves undergoing AVR or repair because of severe AS or AR	C

*Consider lower thresholds for patients of small stature, regardless of gender .
Echo = echocardiography.

TABLE 66G-5 ACC/AHA Guidelines for Management of Patients with Mitral Stenosis

INDICATION	CLASS	RECOMMENDATION	LOE
Echocardiography	I	Diagnosis of MS, assessment of hemodynamic severity, assessment of concomitant valvular lesions, assessment of valve morphology (to determine suitability for PMBV)	B
		Reevaluation in patients with known MS and changing symptoms or signs	B
		Assess hemodynamic response of the mean gradient and PA pressure by exercise Doppler echo when there is a discrepancy among resting Doppler echo findings, clinical findings, symptoms, and signs.	C
		Transesophageal echo to assess presence or absence of left atrial thrombus and evaluate the severity of MR further in patients considered for PMBV	C
		Transesophageal echo to evaluate MV morphology and hemodynamics when transthoracic echo provides suboptimal data	C
	IIa	Reevaluation of asymptomatic patients with MS and stable clinical findings to assess PA pressure—severe MS, every yr; moderate MS, every 1-2 yr; mild MS, every 3-5 yr	C
	III	Transesophageal echo not indicated for routine evaluation of MV morphology and hemodynamics when complete transthoracic echo data are satisfactory	C
Anticoagulation therapy	I	Patients with MS and atrial fibrillation (paroxysmal, persistent, or permanent)	B
		Patients with MS and prior embolic event, even in sinus rhythm	B
		Patients with MS with left atrial thrombus	B
	IIb	Asymptomatic patients with severe MS and left atrial dimension ≥ 55 mm by echo	B
		Patients with severe MS, enlarged left atrium, and spontaneous contrast on echo	C
Cardiac catheterization for hemodynamic assessment	I	Assess severity of MS when noninvasive tests are inconclusive or when there is discrepancy between noninvasive tests and clinical findings.	C
		Hemodynamic evaluation (including left ventriculography to evaluate severity of MR) when there is a discrepancy between Doppler-derived mean gradient and valve area	C
	IIa	Assess PA and left atrial pressures during exercise when clinical symptoms and resting hemodynamics are discordant.	C
		Assess the cause of severe PA hypertension when out of proportion to severity of MS as determined by noninvasive testing.	C
	III	Not recommended when two-dimensional and Doppler echo data are concordant with clinical findings	C
PMBV	I	Indicated for symptomatic patients with moderate or severe MS and valve morphology favorable for PMBV in the absence of left atrial thrombus or moderate to severe MR	A
	IIa	Patients with moderate or severe MS who have a nonpliable calcified valve, are in NYHA functional Class III or IV, and are not candidates for surgery or are at high risk for surgery	C
	IIb	Asymptomatic patients with moderate or severe MS and valve morphology favorable for PMBV who have new-onset of atrial fibrillation in the absence of left atrial thrombus or moderate to severe MR	C
		Symptomatic patients with MV area >1.5 cm^2 if there is evidence of significant MS based on exercise PA systolic pressure > 60 mm Hg, exercise PA wedge pressure ≥ 25 mm Hg, or exercise mean MV gradient >15 mm Hg	C
		Alternative to surgery for patients with moderate or severe MS who have a nonpliable calcified valve and are in NYHA functional Class III or IV	C
	III	Not indicated for patients with mild MS	C
		Not indicated for patients with moderate to severe MR or left atrial thrombus	C
Surgery (repair if possible)	I	Indicated for symptomatic (NYHA functional Class III or IV) moderate or severe MS when PMBV is unavailable or contraindicated because of left atrial thrombus, despite anticoagulation or because concomitant moderate to severe MR is present	B
		Indicated for symptomatic (NYHA functional Class III or IV) moderate or severe MS when valve morphology is not favorable for PMBV in patients with acceptable operative risk	B
		Indicated for moderate to severe MS when there is moderate to severe MR	C
	IIa	MV replacement for severe MS and severe PA hypertension (PA systolic pressure > 60 mm Hg) with NYHA functional Class I or II symptoms in patients who are not candidates for PMBV or surgical MV repair	C
	IIb	MV replacement for symptomatic patients with moderate or severe MS who have had recurrent embolic events while receiving adequate anticoagulation and who have valve morphology favorable for repair	C
	III	Not indicated for patients with mild MS	C
		Closed commissurotomy should not be performed in patients undergoing MV repair; open commissurotomy is preferred approach	C

Echo = echocardiography; LOE = level of evidence; MV = mitral valve; PA = pulmonary artery; PMBV = percutaneous mitral balloon valvotomy.

In general, asymptomatic athletes with MVP need not have any restrictions, but recommendations from the ACC[6] and AHA[7] include restriction of patients to low-intensity competitive sports (e.g., golf and bowling) if any of the following are present: (1) history of syncope, judged probably arrhythmogenic in origin; (2) family history of sudden death caused by MVP; (3) repetitive supraventricular or complex ventricular tachyarrhythmias, particularly if exacerbated by exercise; (4) moderate to severe MR; and (5) prior embolic event.

Daily low-dose aspirin therapy is recommended for patients with MVP who have experienced transient ischemic attacks, as well as younger patients with atrial fibrillation but without MR, hypertension, or heart failure. Anticoagulation with warfarin is recommended for poststroke patients with MVP who have MR, atrial fibrillation, or left atrial thrombus. Warfarin is also recommended for poststroke patients with echocardiographic evidence of thickening or redundancy of the valve leaflets and those who experience recurrent transient ischemic attacks while taking aspirin.

Antibiotic prophylaxis is not considered appropriate for patients with the characteristic click-murmur complex or with echocardiographic evidence of MVP with MR (see summary of revised recommendations in Chap. 67 Guidelines).

TABLE 62G-6 ACC/AHA Guidelines for Management of Patients with Mitral Valve Prolapse

INDICATION	CLASS	RECOMMENDATION	LOE
Echocardiography	I	Diagnosis of MVP and assessment of MR, leaflet morphology, and LV compensation in asymptomatic patients with physical signs of MVP	B
	IIa	Exclude MVP in asymptomatic patients who have been diagnosed without clinical evidence to support the diagnosis.	C
		Risk stratification in asymptomatic patients with physical signs of MVP or known MVP	C
	III	Not indicated to exclude MVP in asymptomatic patients with ill-defined symptoms in the absence of a constellation of clinical symptoms or physical findings suggestive of MVP or a positive family history	B
		Not indicated for asymptomatic patients with MVP and no MR or with MVP and mild MR with no changes in clinical signs or symptoms	C
Antithrombotic therapy	I	Aspirin (75-325 mg/day) for patients with MVP who experience cerebral transient ischemic attacks	C
		Warfarin for patients with MVP and AF who are >65 yr or who have hypertension, MR murmur, or history of heart failure	C
		Aspirin (75-325 mg/day) for patients with MVP and AF < 65 yr and with no history of MR, hypertension, or heart failure	C
		Warfarin for patients with MVP and history of stroke who have MR, AF, or left atrial thrombus	C
	IIa	Warfarin for patients with MVP and history of stroke who do not have MR, AF, or left atrial thrombus when there is echo evidence of thickening (≥5 mm) and/or redundancy of the valve leaflets	C
		Aspirin (75-325 mg/day) for patients with MVP and history of stroke who do not have MR, AF, left atrial thrombus, or echo evidence of thickening (≥5 mm) or redundancy of the valve leaflets	C
	IIb	Aspirin (75-325 mg/day) for patients in sinus rhythm with echo evidence of high-risk MVP	C

AF = atrial fibrillation; echo = echocardiography; LOE= level of evidence.

MITRAL REGURGITATION

The ACC/AHA guidelines consider transthoracic echocardiography to be appropriate for the diagnosis of acute or chronic MR, as well as for annual or semiannual surveillance of LV function in patients with severe MR, even if asymptomatic (**Table 66G-7**). Serial use of chest radiographs and ECGs are considered to be of less value. In asymptomatic patients with mild MR and no evidence of LV dysfunction, the guidelines recommend annual evaluations to detect worsening symptomatic status but do not support annual echocardiography. Transesophageal echocardiography is considered most appropriate for intraoperative guidance and when transthoracic studies are inadequate.

Cardiac Catheterization

Catheterization is usually performed as a prelude to surgery in patients with MR, or when noninvasive tests yield discordant results or do not provide adequate information to guide management. The ACC/AHA guidelines do not consider catheterization routinely necessary in patients with MR when valve surgery is not planned.

Surgery

The guidelines consider mitral valve repair to be the operation of choice for patients with suitable valves when performed by an experienced operator. Surgery is deemed appropriate for acute symptomatic MR and for patients with chronic severe MR and symptoms of congestive heart failure, even if they have normal LV function (see Table 66G-7). Among asymptomatic patients, surgery is appropriate when there is evidence of mild or greater LV dysfunction (ejection fraction = 0.30 to 0.60 and/or end-systolic dimension >40 mm).

The 2006 and 2008 guidelines contained two important new recommendations regarding mitral valve repair. The first applies to asymptomatic patients with severe MR and normal LV function. The guidelines indicate that it is reasonable to consider mitral valve repair in such patients if they undergo surgery in experienced surgical centers in which the likelihood of successful repair without residual regurgitation is greater than 90% (Class IIa). A stronger recommendation (class I) indicates that mitral valve repair is recommended over mitral valve replacement for most patients who undergo surgery, and patients should be referred to surgical centers experienced in mitral valve repair.

OTHER VALVULAR DISEASE

Multiple Valve Disease

Given the large number of possible combinations and the slim evidence base for diagnosis and management, the ACC/AHA guidelines offer no specific recommendations for the management of mixed valve disease.

Tricuspid Valve Disease

Tricuspid valve repair is appropriate for correcting severe tricuspid regurgitation (TR) in patients with mitral valve disease requiring valve repair or replacement (**Table 66G-8**). Tricuspid valve replacement or annuloplasty is considered reasonable for patients with symptomatic severe primary TR. Annuloplasty may be considered for patients with mild to moderate TR who are undergoing surgery for mitral valve disease if they have pulmonary hypertension or dilation of the tricuspid annulus.

SURGICAL CONSIDERATIONS

Numerous options are available for the surgical management of valvular heart disease. The ACC/AHA guidelines generally favor mitral valve repair over replacement. The standard surgical approach usually entails a median sternotomy with cardiopulmonary bypass. However, numerous alternatives are gaining acceptance. These include minimally invasive approaches to valve repair such as ministernotomy, small right thoracotomy, or robotic surgery. Percutaneous approaches to mitral valve repair, pulmonary valve implantation, and aortic valve replacement have been conducted, with generally successful results,[8-10] and percutaneous devices are now approved for clinical use in Europe. Whether such catheter-based approaches gain widespread acceptance will depend on larger and longer-term clinical trial results and advances in device technology.

When replacement is necessary, several variables influence the selection of a bioprosthetic versus a mechanical valve (**Table 66G-9**). Patient preference plays an important role in determining the choice of a prosthetic valve. In the 1998 guidelines, bioprosthetic valves were considered appropriate only for patients older than 65 years for AVR and older than 70 years for mitral valve replacement. The 2006 and 2008 guidelines emphasize that a bioprosthesis is reasonable for patients younger than 65 years who elect to receive this valve for lifestyle considerations after detailed discussion of the risks of anticoagulation versus the likelihood that a second valve replacement may be necessary in the future.

The 1998 guidelines also considered bioprosthetic valves inappropriate for patients with end-stage renal failure, especially those undergoing chronic dialysis, because of concerns of accelerated calcification of bioprosthetic valves. Subsequent clinical studies have not demonstrated a difference in outcomes between mechanical and bioprosthetic valves in these patients, and this recommendation was removed in 2006.

Intraoperative Assessment

The ACC/AHA guidelines emphasize the importance of intraoperative transesophageal echocardiography by recommending its use during valve repair; valve replacement with a stentless xenograft, homograft, or autograft valve; or valve surgery for infective endocarditis. It may

TABLE 66G-7 ACC/AHA Guidelines for Management of Patients with Mitral Regurgitation

INDICATION	CLASS	RECOMMENDATION	LOE
Transthoracic echocardiography	I	Baseline evaluation of LV size and function, RV and LA size, PA pressure, and severity of MR in any patient suspected of having MR	C
		Delineation of the mechanism of MR	B
		Annual or semiannual surveillance of LV function (estimated by EF and ESD) in asymptomatic patients with moderate to severe MR	C
		Evaluate the MV apparatus and LV function after a change in signs or symptoms	C
		Initial evaluation of LV size and function and MV hemodynamics after MV replacement or repair	C
	IIa	Exercise Doppler echo in asymptomatic severe MR to assess exercise tolerance and effects of exercise on PA pressure and MR severity	C
	III	Not indicated for routine follow-up of asymptomatic mild MR with normal LV size and systolic function	C
Transesophageal echocardiography	I	Indicated when transthoracic echo provides nondiagnostic information regarding severity of MR, mechanism of MR, and/or status of LV function	B
		Preoperative or intraoperative assessment of the anatomic basis for severe MR to assess feasibility of repair and guide repair when surgery is recommended	B
	IIa	Preoperative assessment in asymptomatic patients with severe MR who are considered for surgery to assess feasibility of repair	C
	III	Not indicated for routine follow-up or surveillance of asymptomatic native valve MR	C
Cardiac catheterization for hemodynamic assessment and left ventriculography	I	Indicated when noninvasive tests are inconclusive regarding severity of MR, LV function, or need for surgery	C
		Indicated when PA pressure is out of proportion to the severity of MR as assessed by noninvasive testing	C
		Indicated when there is a discrepancy between clinical and noninvasive findings regarding severity of MR	C
	III	Not indicated in patients with MR in whom valve surgery is not contemplated	C
Coronary angiography	I	Indicated before MV repair or MV replacement in patients at risk for CAD	C
Surgery	I	Symptomatic patients with acute severe MR	B
		Patients with chronic severe MR and NYHA functional Class II, III, or IV symptoms in the absence of severe LV dysfunction (defined as EF < 0.30 and/or ESD > 55 mm)	B
		Asymptomatic patients with chronic severe MR and mild to moderate LV dysfunction, EF = 0.30 to 0.60, and/or ESD ≥ 40 mm	B
		MV repair recommended over MV replacement for most patients with severe chronic MR who require surgery; patients should be referred to surgical centers experienced in MV repair	C
	IIa	MV repair in experienced surgical centers for asymptomatic patients with chronic severe MR with preserved LV function (EF > 0.60 and ESD < 40 mm) in whom the likelihood of successful repair without residual MR is >90%	B
		Asymptomatic patients with chronic severe MR, preserved LV function, and new onset of atrial fibrillation or pulmonary hypertension (PA systolic pressure > 50 mm Hg at rest or > 60 mm Hg with exercise)	C
		Patients with chronic severe MR caused by primary abnormality of the mitral apparatus, NYHA functional Class III or IV symptoms, and severe LV dysfunction (EF < 0.30 and/or ESD > 55 mm) in whom MV repair is highly likely	C
	IIb	Patients with chronic severe secondary MR caused by severe LV dysfunction (EF < 0.30) who have persistent NYHA functional Class III or IV symptoms despite optimal therapy for heart failure, including biventricular pacing	C
	III	Not indicated for asymptomatic patients with MR and preserved LV function (EF > 0.60 and ESD < 40 mm) if there is significant doubt about the feasibility of repair	C
		Not indicated for patients with mild or moderate MR	C

Echo = echocardiography; EF = ejection fraction; ESD = end-systolic dimension; LA = left atrial; LOE = level of evidence; PA = pulmonary artery; RV = right ventricular.

TABLE 66G-8 ACC/AHA Guidelines for Management of Patients with Tricuspid Valve Disease

INDICATION	CLASS	RECOMMENDATION	LOE
Surgery	I	Severe TR in patients with MV disease requiring MV surgery	B
	IIa	Severe primary TR when symptomatic	C
		Tricuspid valve replacement for severe TR secondary to diseased or abnormal tricuspid valve leaflets not amenable to annuloplasty or repair	C
	IIb	Patients undergoing MV surgery when TR is not severe but there is pulmonary hypertension or tricuspid annular dilatation	C
	III	Not indicated in asymptomatic TR when PA systolic pressure < 60 mm Hg and MV is normal	C
		Not indicated in patients with mild primary TR	C

LOE= level of evidence.

also be reasonable for all patients undergoing cardiac valve surgery. The guidelines committee recommends that centers performing valve surgery establish consistent and credible intraoperative echocardiography programs capable of providing accurate anatomic and functional information relevant to valve operations. Given that even a generally safe procedure such as transesophageal echocardiography has risks, preoperative screening for risk factors and obtaining informed consent should be a routine part of each intraoperative transesophageal study.

Patients with Prosthetic Heart Valves

The ACC/AHA guidelines recommend warfarin therapy for patients with mechanical valves. For patients with aortic valve prostheses, those with bileaflet mechanical valves and Medtronic-Hall valves should maintain an international normalized ratio (INR) between 2 and 3, whereas those with Starr-Edwards valves or mechanical disc valves should maintain an INR between 2.5 and 3.5 (**Table 66G-10**). The same target is indicated following mitral valve replacement with a mechanical valve. Aspirin (75 to

TABLE 66G-9 ACC/AHA Major Criteria for the Selection of Replacement Valves for Individuals with Valvular Heart Disease

INDICATION	CLASS	RECOMMENDATION	LOE
Aortic valve replacement	I	Mechanical prosthesis in patients with a mechanical valve in the mitral or tricuspid position	C
		Bioprosthesis in patients of any age who will not take warfarin or who have major medical contraindications to warfarin therapy.	C
	IIa	Patient preference is a reasonable consideration in the selection of valve prosthesis. Mechanical prosthesis is reasonable for AVR in patients < 65 yr who do not have a contraindication to anticoagulation. A bioprosthesis is reasonable for AVR in patients < 65 yr who elect to receive this valve for lifestyle considerations after detailed discussions of the risks of anticoagulation versus the likelihood that a second AVR may be necessary in the future.	C
		Bioprosthesis is reasonable for patients ≥ 65 yr without risk factors for thromboembolism.	C
		Homograft is reasonable for patients undergoing repeat AVR with active prosthetic valve endocarditis.	
	IIb	Bioprosthesis might be considered for a woman of childbearing age.	C
Mitral valve replacement	I	Bioprosthesis in patients who will not take warfarin, is incapable of taking warfarin, or has a clear contraindication to warfarin therapy.	C
	IIa	Mechanical prosthesis reasonable for patients younger than 65 years of age with longstanding AF	C
		Bioprosthesis is reasonable in patients ≥ 65 yr	C
		Bioprosthesis is reasonable in patients < 65 yr in sinus rhythm who elect to receive this valve for life-style considerations after detailed discussions of the risks of anticoagulation versus the likelihood that a second MV replacement may be necessary in the future.	C

ACC/AHA = American College of Cardiology/American Heart Association; AF = atrial fibrillation; AVR = aortic valve replacement; LOE = level of evidence; MV = mitral valve.

TABLE 66G-10 Recommendations for Antithrombotic Therapy in Patients with Prosthetic Heart Valves*

PROSTHESIS	LOCATION	RISK*		ASPIRIN (75-100 mg)	WARFARIN (INR, 2-3)	WARFARIN (INR, 2.5-3.5)	NO WARFARIN
Mechanical prosthetic valves	AVR	Low	<3 mo	Class I	Class I	Class IIa	
			>3 mo	Class I	Class I		
		High		Class I		Class I	
	MVR			Class I		Class I	
Bioprosthetic valves	AVR	Low	<3 mo	Class I	Class IIa		Class IIb
			>3 mo	Class I			Class IIa
		High		Class I	Class I		
	MVR	Low	<3 mo	Class I	Class IIa		
			>3 mo	Class I			Class IIa
		High		Class I	Class I		

*Antithrombotic therapy must be individualized depending on a patient's clinical status. For patients receiving warfarin, aspirin is recommended in almost all situations. Risk factors include atrial fibrillation, left ventricular dysfunction, previous thromboembolism, and hypercoagulable condition. INR should be maintained between 2.5 and 3.5 for aortic disc valves and Starr-Edwards valves.

AVR = aortic valve replacement; INR = international normalized ratio; MVR = mitral valve replacement.

325 mg/day) is indicated for patients who are unable to take warfarin. Low-dose aspirin (75 to 100 mg/day) is recommended in addition to warfarin for all patients with mechanical heart valves and those with biologic valves who have risk factors such as atrial fibrillation, prior thromboembolism, LV dysfunction, or a hypercoagulable condition. Clopidogrel may be considered for those who cannot take aspirin.

Bridging Therapy

Antithrombotic medications must sometimes be interrupted in patients with mechanical valve prostheses for noncardiac surgery, invasive procedures, or dental care. In patients at low risk of thrombosis, warfarin should be stopped 48 to 72 hours before the procedure and started no more than 24 hours after the procedure (**Table 66G-11**). The ACC/AHA guidelines indicate that the use of heparin is usually unnecessary for patients at low risk of thrombosis, defined as those with a bileaflet mechanical aortic valve prosthesis with no risk factors. They recommend bridging anticoagulant therapy for higher risk individuals, including those with a mechanical mitral or tricuspid prosthesis or a mechanical aortic prosthesis who have risk factors such as atrial fibrillation, a recent thrombosis or embolus, LV dysfunction, or an older generation thrombogenic valve, and those with demonstrated thrombotic problems when previously off therapy. The recommended bridging therapy is intravenous unfractionated heparin (Class I), but subcutaneous doses of unfractionated heparin or low-molecular weight heparin may also be considered (Class IIb). The use of low-molecular-weight heparin remains controversial for this indication.

Prosthetic Valve Thrombosis

Emergency surgery is reasonable for patients with a thrombosed left-sided prosthetic valve and moderate to severe symptoms (NYHA Class III or IV) or a large clot burden. Fibrinolytic therapy may be considered for patients with less severe symptoms, smaller clot burdens, or when surgery is high risk or unavailable (**Table 66G-12**).

Follow-up

After prosthetic valve implantation, asymptomatic patients should be seen 2 to 4 weeks after hospital discharge and then at 6-month or 1-year intervals (**Table 66G-13**). Routine annual echocardiography is not indicated in the absence of changes in clinical status. All patients should also receive primary and secondary prevention measures to reduce the risk of future cardiovascular events.

Patients who do not improve after receiving a prosthetic heart valve or who later show deterioration of functional capacity should undergo appropriate testing to determine the cause. Patients with postoperative LV systolic dysfunction, even if it is asymptomatic, should receive standard medical therapy for systolic heart failure indefinitely, even if systolic function or symptoms improve.

EVALUATION AND MANAGEMENT OF CORONARY ARTERY DISEASE IN PATIENTS WITH VALVULAR HEART DISEASE

Concomitant CAD is common in patients with valvular disease. Because of the impact of untreated CAD on perioperative and long-term

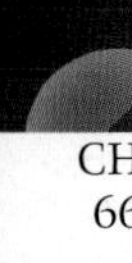

TABLE 66G-11 ACC/AHA Recommendations for Bridging Therapy in Patients with Mechanical Valves*

INDICATION	CLASS	RECOMMENDATION	LOE
Planned noncardiac invasive procedure	I	In patients at low risk of thrombosis,† warfarin should be stopped 48 to 72 hr before the procedure (so that the INR falls to <.5) and restarted within 24 hr after the procedure. Heparin is usually unnecessary.	B
	I	In patients at high risk of thrombosis,‡ start therapeutic doses of IV UFH when INR falls below 2 (typically 48 hr before surgery), stop 4 to 6 hr before the procedure, restart as early after surgery as bleeding stability allows, and continue until INR is again therapeutic with warfarin therapy.	B
	IIb	In patients at high risk of thrombosis,‡ therapeutic doses of subcutaneous UFH (15,000 U/12 hr) or LMWH (100 U/kg/12 hr) may be considered during the period of a subtherapeutic INR.	B
	III	High-dose vitamin K_1 should not be given routinely because this could create a hypercoagulable condition.	B
Emergency noncardiac surgery	IIa	Reasonable to give fresh-frozen plasma to patients with mechanical valves who require emergency interruption of warfarin therapy. Fresh frozen plasma is preferable to high-dose vitamin K_1.	B

*Who require interruption of warfarin therapy for noncardiac surgery, invasive procedures, or dental care.
†Low risk of thrombosis—bileaflet mechanical AVR with no risk factors (see below).
‡High risk of thrombosis—any mechanical MV replacement or mechanical AVR with any risk factor. Risk factors include atrial fibrillation, previous thromboembolism, LV dysfunction, hypercoagulable conditions, older generation thrombogenic valves, mechanical tricuspid valves, or more than one mechanical valve.
INR = international normalized ratio; IV = intravenous; LMWH = low-molecular-weight heparin; LOE = level of evidence; MV = mitral valve; UFH = unfractionated heparin.

TABLE 66G-12 ACC/AHA Guidelines for Management of Prosthetic Heart Valve Thrombosis

INDICATION	CLASS	RECOMMENDATION	LOE
Echocardiography	I	Indicated in patients with suspected prosthetic valve thrombosis to assess hemodynamic severity	B
	I	Transesophageal echo and/or fluoroscopy in patients with suspected valve thrombosis to assess valve motion and clot burden	B
Emergency operation	IIa	Reasonable for patients with thrombosed left-sided prosthetic valves and NYHA Class III or IV symptoms	C
	IIa	Reasonable for patients with thrombosed left-sided prosthetic valves and a large clot burden	C
Fibrinolytic therapy	IIa	Reasonable for patients with thrombosed right-sided prosthetic valves with NYHA Class III or IV symptoms or large clot burden	C
	IIb	May be considered as first-line therapy for patients with thrombosed left-sided prosthetic valves, NYHA Class I or II symptoms, and small clot burden	B
	IIb	May be considered as first-line therapy for patients with thrombosed left-sided prosthetic valves, NYHA Class III or IV symptoms, and a small clot burden if surgery is high risk or not available	B
	IIb	May be considered for patients with obstructed, thrombosed left-sided prosthetic valves, NYHA Class II or IV symptoms, and large clot burden if emergency surgery is high risk or not available	C
	IIb	May consider intravenous UFH as an alternative to fibrinolytic therapy for patients with thrombosed prosthetic valves, NYHA functional Class I or II, and small clot burden	C

Echo = echocardiography; LOE = level of evidence; UFH = unfractionated heparin.

TABLE 66G-13 ACC/AHA Guidelines for Patient Follow-up after Prosthetic Valve Implantation

INDICATION	CLASS	RECOMMENDATION	LOE
General patient follow-up	I	History, physical examination, and appropriate tests should be performed at the first postoperative outpatient evaluation, 2 to 4 wk after hospital discharge. This includes a transthoracic Doppler echo if a baseline echo was not obtained before hospital discharge.	C
		Routine annual follow-up visits, with earlier reevaluations (with echo) if there is a change in clinical status	C
	IIb	Consider annual echos after the first 5 yr in patients with bioprostheses in the absence of a change in clinical status.	C
	III	Routine annual echos not indicated in the absence of a change in clinical status in patients with mechanical valves or during the first 5 yr after valve replacement with a bioprosthesis	C
Follow-up of patients with complications	I	Patients with LV systolic dysfunction after valve surgery should receive standard medical therapy for systolic heart failure. This therapy should be continued even if there is improvement of LV dysfunction.	B

Echo = echocardiogram; LOE = level of evidence.

postoperative survival, preoperative identification of CAD is of great importance in patients with aortic or mitral valve disease. Thus, in symptomatic patients and/or those with LV dysfunction, the guidelines recommend preoperative coronary angiography in men 35 years and older, premenopausal women older than 35 years with coronary risk factors, and postmenopausal women.

The guidelines support the practice of bypassing all significant coronary artery stenoses when possible in patients undergoing AVR.

REFERENCES

1. Bonow RO, Carabello B, De Leon AC Jr, et al: ACC/AHA guidelines for the management of patients with valvular heart disease: A report of the American College of Cardiology/American Heart Association Task Force on Practice Guidelines (Committee on Management of Patients with Valvular Heart Disease). J Am Coll Cardiol 32:1486, 1998.
2. Bonow RO, Carabello BA, Chatterjee K, et al: ACC/AHA 2006 guidelines for the management of patients with valvular heart disease: A report

of the American College of Cardiology/American Heart Association Task Force on Practice Guidelines (writing committee to revise the 1998 guidelines for the management of patients with valvular heart disease) developed in collaboration with the Society of Cardiovascular Anesthesiologists and endorsed by the Society for Cardiovascular Angiography and Interventions and the Society of Thoracic Surgeons. J Am Coll Cardiol 48:e1, 2006.

3. Bonow RO, Carabello B, Chatterjee K, et al: 2008 focused update incorporated into the ACC/AHA 2006 Guidelines for the Management of Patients with Valvular Heart Disease. J Am Coll Cardiol 52:e1, 2008.
4. Cheitlin MD, Armstrong WF, Aurigemma GP, et al: ACC/AHA/ASE 2003 guideline update for the clinical application of echocardiography: A report of the American College of Cardiology/American Heart Association Task Force on Practice Guidelines (ACC/AHA/ASE Committee to Update the 1997 Guidelines for the Clinical Application of Echocardiography). J Am Coll Cardiol 42:954, 2003.
5. Douglas PS, Khandheria B, Stainback RF, et al: ACCF/ASE/ACEP/ASNC/SCAI/SCCT/SCMR 2007 Appropriateness criteria for transthoracic and transesophageal echocardiography: A report of the American College of Cardiology Foundation Quality Strategic Directions Committee Appropriateness Criteria Working Group, American Society of Echocardiography, American College of Emergency Physicians, American Society of Nuclear Cardiology, Society for Cardiovascular Angiography and Interventions, Society of Cardiovascular Computed Tomography, and the Society for Cardiovascular Magnetic Resonance Endorsed by the American College of Chest Physicians and the Society of Critical Care Medicine. J Am Coll Cardiol 50;187, 2007.
6. Bonow RO, Cheitlin MD, Crawford MH, Douglas PS: Task Force 3: Valvular heart disease. J Am Coll Cardiol 45:1334, 2005.
7. Maron BJ, Araujo CG, Thompson PD, et al: Recommendations for preparticipation screening and the assessment of cardiovascular disease in masters athletes: An advisory for healthcare professionals from the working groups of the World Heart Federation, the International Federation of Sports Medicine, and the American Heart Association Committee on Exercise, Cardiac Rehabilitation, and Prevention. Circulation 103:327, 2001.
8. Feldman T, Wasserman HS, Herrmann HC, et al: Percutaneous mitral valve repair using the edge-to-edge technique: Six-month results of the EVEREST Phase I Clinical Trial. J Am Coll Cardiol 46:2134, 2005.
9. Rosengart TK, Feldman T, Borger MA, et al: Percutaneous and minimally invasive valve procedures: A scientific statement from the American Heart Association Council on Cardiovascular Surgery and Anesthesia, Council on Clinical Cardiology, Functional Genomics and Translational Biology Interdisciplinary Working Group, and Quality of Care and Outcomes Research Interdisciplinary Working Group. Circulation 117:1750, 2008.
10. Webb JG, Altwegg L, Boone RH, et al: Transcatheter aortic valve implantation: Impact on clinical and valve-related outcomes. Circulation 119:3009, 2009.

CHAPTER 67 Infective Endocarditis

Adolf W. Karchmer

The characteristic lesion of infective endocarditis (IE), the vegetation, is a variably sized amorphous mass of platelets and fibrin with abundant enmeshed microorganisms and moderate inflammatory cells. Infections involve heart valves most commonly but may occur at the site of a septal defect, on chordae tendineae, or on mural endocardium. Infections of arteriovenous shunts, arterioarterial shunts (patent ductus arteriosus), or coarctation of the aorta are clinically and pathologically similar to IE. Many species of bacteria cause IE; nevertheless, streptococci, staphylococci, enterococci, and fastidious gram-negative coccobacilli cause the majority of cases of IE.

IE is often called acute or subacute. Acute IE is caused typically by *Staphylococcus aureus*. It presents with marked toxicity and progresses during days to several weeks to valvular destruction and metastatic infection. Subacute IE, usually caused by viridans streptococci, enterococci, coagulase-negative staphylococci, or gram-negative coccobacilli, evolves during weeks to months with only modest toxicity and rarely causes metastatic infection.

Epidemiology

The incidence of IE remained relatively stable from 1950 through 2000 at about 3.6 to 7.0 cases per 100,000 patient-years.[1,2] In selected areas, the incidence may be increased because of the concentration of populations at uniquely high risk of infection, specifically intravenous (IV) drug users. For example, from 1988 to 1990, 11.6 episodes per 100,000 population were reported from metropolitan Philadelphia (Delaware Valley), with injection drug abuse accounting for approximately half of the cases. The stable incidence is illustrated in Olmsted County, Minnesota, where from 1970 to 2000 the 5-year interval IE incidence ranged from 5.0 to 7.0 per 100,000 person-years; and in France, the IE incidence in 1991 and 1999 was 3.1 and 2.6 per 100,000 population, respectively.[2] Risk factors in industrialized countries have shifted, however, from rheumatic and congenital heart disease to IV drug use, degenerative valve disease in the elderly, intracardiac devices, health care–associated infection, and hemodialysis. Endocarditis continues to occur more frequently in men than in women, with a 2:1 ratio, but the median age of patients has gradually increased and now is 57.9 years (interquartile range, 43.2 to 71.8 years).[3] The age-specific incidence of endocarditis increases from 5 cases per 100,000 person-years among persons younger than 50 years to 15 to 30 cases per 100,000 person-years in the sixth through eighth decades of life.[1] From 50% to 75% of patients with native valve endocarditis (NVE) have predisposing valve conditions. The nature of the predisposing conditions and, in part, the microbiology of IE correlate with the age of patients (**Table 67-1**). Recent case series from large tertiary care referral centers have illustrated not only the previously noted shift in risk factors but also concomitant changes in microbiology, in particular that *S. aureus* exceeds streptococci as a causative agent (**Fig. 67-1**).[3-5] In contrast, population-based series, particularly if they are not dominated by cases among drug abusers, illustrate the continued importance of rheumatic and congenital valvular disease as predispositions and the predominance of streptococci as causal agents.[2,6] Where NVE among adults is not skewed dramatically by IV drug abuse and nosocomial infection, the microbiology is as shown in Table 67-1.

Groups of Patients

CHILDREN. In the Netherlands, IE was noted in 1.7 and 1.2 per 100,000 male and female children younger than 10 years, respectively. IE among neonates often involves the tricuspid valve of structurally normal hearts and arises as a consequence of infected intravascular catheters or cardiac surgery. Most children with IE occurring after the neonatal period have identifiable structural cardiac abnormalities; congenital heart abnormalities are present in 75% to 90% of cases. In many cases, IE occurs at the site of surgical repair and reflects the persistent risk for infection after complex reconstructive surgery. Neither secundum atrial septal defect nor patent ductus arteriosus or pulmonic stenosis after repair is associated with IE. Mitral valve prolapse in association with a regurgitant murmur predisposes to IE in children. The clinical features and echocardiographic findings of IE in children are similar to those noted among adults with native or prosthetic valve endocarditis.

ADULTS. Mitral valve prolapse, a prominent predisposing structural cardiac abnormality in adults, accounts for 7% to 30% of NVE not related to drug abuse or nosocomial infection. The frequency of mitral valve prolapse in IE is not entirely a direct reflection of relative risk but rather a function of the frequency of the lesion in the general population. This increased risk of endocarditis is largely confined to patients with prolapse, thickened valve leaflets (>5 mm), and mitral regurgitation murmur, especially among men and patients older than 45 years (see Chap. 66). Among patients with mitral valve prolapse and a systolic murmur, the incidence of IE is 52 per 100,000 person-years, compared with a rate of 4.6 per 100,000 person-years among those with prolapse and no murmur or among the general population. The microbiology and morbidity of IE engrafted on mitral valve prolapse are similar to those of NVE that is not associated with drug abuse.

TABLE 67-1 Conditions Predisposing to and Microbiology of Native Valve Endocarditis

	Children (%)		*Adults (%)*	
CONDITIONS AND MICROBIOLOGY	**NEONATES**	**2 MONTHS-15 YEARS**	**15-60 YEARS**	**>60 YEARS**
Predisposing Conditions				
Rheumatic heart disease		2-10	25-30	8
Congenital heart disease	28	75-90*	10-20	2
Mitral valve prolapse		5-15	10-30	10
Degenerative heart disease			Rare	30
Parenteral drug abuse			15-35	10
Other			10-15	10
None	72†	2-5	25-45	25-40
Microbiology				
Streptococci	15-20	40-50	33-65‡	30-45‡
Enterococci		4	5-8	15
Staphylococcus aureus	40-50	25	30-40‡	25-30‡
Coagulase-negative staphylococci	10	5	3-10	5-10
Gram-negative bacteria§	10	5	4-8	5
Fungi	10	1	1	Rare
Polymicrobial	4		1	Rare
Other			1	2
Culture negative	4	0-15	3-10	5

*50% of cases follow surgery and may involve implanted devices and foreign material.
†Often tricuspid valve IE.
‡In recent large series from tertiary centers, the referral bias combined with health care–associated IE and prevalent IV drug abuse result in a reversal in the relative frequency of IE caused by *S. aureus* and streptococci (see text).
§Frequently *Haemophilus* species, *Aggregatibacter* species, *Cardiobacterium hominis* in cases after the neonatal period.

Rheumatic heart disease as a predisposing cardiac lesion for IE has become less prevalent in industrialized nations.[3] In patients with rheumatic heart disease, endocarditis occurs most frequently on the mitral valve, followed by the aortic valve.

Congenital heart disease is the substrate for IE in 10% to 20% of younger adults and 8% of older adults. Among adults, the common predisposing lesions are patent ductus arteriosus, ventricular septal defect, and bicuspid aortic valve, the last particularly found among older men (>60 years).

Infection with human immunodeficiency virus (HIV) is not a significant risk factor for IE (see Chap. 72). Among HIV-infected persons who are not IV drug abusers, organisms typical of NVE and those that are uniquely associated with AIDS, such as *Bartonella* species, *Salmonella* species, and *Streptococcus pneumoniae*, cause IE. In an urban cohort of HIV-infected patients, the incidence of first episodes of IE was 4.4 per 1000 patient-years. IE was associated with injection drug use, was caused commonly by *S. aureus*, recurred frequently, and resulted in high mortality rates.[7]

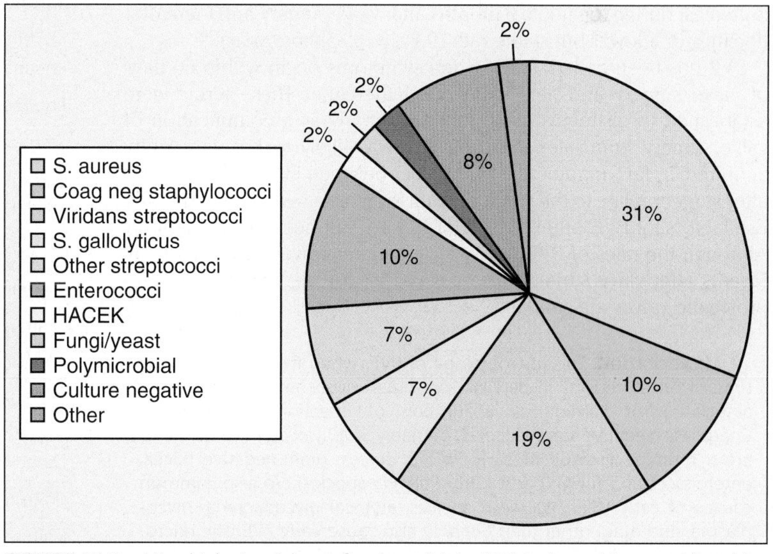

FIGURE 67-1 Microbiologic etiology of endocarditis in 1558 patients, 18 years old or older, admitted directly to 58 hospitals in 25 countries between June 2000 and September 2005. *(Data from Murdoch DR, Corey CR, Hoen B, et al: Clinical presentation, etiology, and outcome of infective endocarditis in the 21st century. Arch Intern Med 169:463, 2009.)*

INTRAVENOUS DRUG ABUSERS. The risk for IE among IV drug abusers is several-fold greater than that for patients with rheumatic heart disease or prosthetic valves. From 65% to 80% of such cases of IE occur in men, aged 27 to 37 years. IE is located on the tricuspid valve in 46% to 78%, mitral valve in 24% to 32%, and aortic valve in 8% to 19%; as many as 16% of patients have infection at multiple sites. The valves were normal before infection in 75% to 93% of patients. IV drug abuse is a risk factor for recurrent NVE.

MICROBIOLOGY. *S. aureus* causes more than 50% of IE occurring in IV drug abusers overall and 60% to 70% of infections involving the tricuspid valve (**Table 67-2**).[3] The well-established predilection for *S. aureus* to infect normal heart valves is noted in addicts with frequent infection of normal tricuspid valves. Streptococci and enterococci infect previously abnormal mitral or aortic valves in addicts. Infection of right- and left-sided heart valves by *Pseudomonas aeruginosa* and other gram-negative bacilli and left-sided heart valves by fungi occurs with increased frequency among drug abusers. Unusual organisms related to injection of contaminated materials cause endocarditis in these patients (e.g., *Corynebacterium* species, *Lactobacillus, Bacillus cereus,* and nonpathogenic *Neisseria* species). Polymicrobial endocarditis accounts for 3% to 5% of cases of IE.[3]

The clinical manifestations of IE in IV drug abusers depend on the valves involved and, to a lesser degree, on the infecting organism. Pleuritic chest pain, shortness of breath, cough, and hemoptysis occur with tricuspid valve endocarditis, particularly when it is caused by *S. aureus*. In 65% to 75% of patients, chest radiographs reveal abnormalities related to septic pulmonary emboli. Murmurs of tricuspid regurgitation are noted in less than half of these patients. Infection of the aortic or mitral valve in addicts clinically resembles IE seen in patients who are not drug abusers. HIV infection has been noted in 27% to 73% of IV drug abusers with IE (see Chap. 72).

TABLE 67-2 Microbiology of Endocarditis Associated with Intravenous Drug Abuse

	Number of Cases (%) of Endocarditis in Drug Addicts*			
ORGANISMS	RIGHT SIDED (N = 346)	LEFT SIDED (N = 204)	TOTAL (N = 675)	SPAIN, 1977-1993† (N = 1529)
Streptococci‡	17 (5)	31 (15)	80 (12)	131 (8.5)
Enterococci	7 (2)	49 (24)	59 (9)	21 (1)
Staphylococcus aureus	267 (77)	47 (23)	396 (57)	1138 (74)
Coagulase-negative staphylococci	—	—		44 (3)
Gram-negative bacilli§	7 (5)	26 (13)	45 (7)	23 (1.5)
Fungi (predominantly *Candida* species)	—	25 (12)	26 (4)	18 (1)
Polymicrobial/miscellaneous	28 (8)	20 (10)	49 (7)	48 (3)
Culture negative	10 (3)	6 (3)	20 (3)	106 (7)

*Ten patients with right- and left-sided infective endocarditis are counted twice.
†Data from Miro JM, del Rio A, Mestres CA: Infective endocarditis in intravenous drug abusers and HIV-1 infected patients. Infect Dis Clin North Am 16:273, 2002.
‡Includes viridans streptococci, *Streptococcus gallolyticus*, other non–group A groupable streptococci, *Abiotrophia* and *Granulicatella* species (nutritionally variant streptococci).
§*Pseudomonas aeruginosa, Serratia marcescens,* and Enterobacteriaceae.

Prosthetic Valve Endocarditis

Epidemiologic studies suggest that prosthetic valve endocarditis (PVE) constitutes 10% to 30% of all cases of IE in developed countries.[4,6,8,9] In patients undergoing valve surgery between 1965 and 1995, the cumulative incidence of PVE estimated actuarially ranged from 1.4% to 3.1% at 12 months and 3.0% to 5.7% at 5 years.[10] The frequency is greatest during the initial 6 months after valve surgery and thereafter declines to a lower but stable rate (0.2% to 0.35% per year).[10]

PVE has been called "early" when symptoms begin within 60 days of valve surgery and "late" with onset thereafter. These terms were established to distinguish PVE that arose early as a complication of valve surgery from later infection that was likely to be community acquired. In fact, many cases with onset between 60 days and 1 year after surgery relate to the surgical admission or to health care. Specific risk factors for PVE, other than prior IE, have not been clearly defined. Although the rates of PVE vary with time after valve implantation, by 5 years after valve surgery the rates of PVE for mechanical and bioprosthetic valves are similar.[10]

Microbiology. The microbiology of PVE, when it is considered by time of onset, reflects in part the presumed nosocomial, health care–associated, or community acquisition of infection (**Table 67-3**). Coagulase-negative staphylococci, primarily *Staphylococcus epidermidis,* are a prominent cause of early PVE. *S. aureus,* gram-negative bacilli, enterococci, and fungi (particularly *Candida* species) are also common causes of early PVE. *Legionella* species, atypical mycobacteria, mycoplasma, and fungi other than *Candida* also cause early PVE. The microbiology of late PVE resembles that of community-acquired NVE; streptococci, *S. aureus*, enterococci, and coagulase-negative staphylococci are the major causes. Nosocomial and health care–associated late PVE has increased recently with attendant increases in infection caused by *S. aureus,* coagulase-negative staphylococci, and enterococci.[8,11]

Pathology. In contrast to the largely leaflet-confined pathology of NVE, infection on bioprostheses during the year after implantation or on mechanical prostheses commonly extends into the annulus and periannular tissue, causing dehiscence of the prosthesis with hemodynamically significant paravalvular regurgitation and conduction disturbances. Bulky vegetations can interfere with valve function at the mitral site and cause valve stenosis (**Fig. 67-2**).

Among 85 patients with mechanical valve PVE in whom the site of infection was examined at surgery or autopsy, annulus invasion was noted in 42%, myocardial abscess in 14%, valve obstruction in 4%, and pericarditis in 2%.[10] Among 49 patients with bioprosthetic PVE, 29 (59%) had later onset infection. Aortic site and clinical onset within a year of valve surgery correlate with an increased risk of invasive infection. Infected prosthetic valves can be distinguished from uninfected valves on histologic examination.

Signs and symptoms in patients developing PVE within 60 days of cardiac surgery may be obscured by surgery or postoperative complications. Peripheral signs of endocarditis (5% to 14%) and central nervous system emboli (10%) occur less frequently in these patients than in those with PVE occurring later. Among patients with later onset PVE, congestive heart failure (CHF) occurs in 40%, cerebrovascular complications in 26% to 28%, and peripheral signs in 15% to 28%.[10] Among patients with PVE treated since 1980, in-hospital mortality overall ranges from 14% to 41% and that for early and late infection from 30% to 46% and 19% to 34%, respectively.[9,11] Mortality for *S. aureus* PVE regardless of time of onset remains high, 36% to 47%.[8,12,13] Mortality is associated with age and complications of PVE, including CHF, stroke, intracardiac abscess, and persistent bacteremia.

TABLE 67-3 Microbiology of Prosthetic Valve Endocarditis, 1970-2006

	Number of Cases (%)* with Time of Onset After Valve Surgery	
ORGANISMS	EARLY (N = 290) <12 MONTHS	LATE (N = 331) > 12 MONTHS
Streptococci†	7 (2)	93 (28)
Pneumococci	—	—
Enterococci	29 (10)	46 (14)
Staphylococcus aureus	72 (25)	57 (17)
Coagulase-negative staphylococci	85 (29)	41 (12)
Fastidious gram-negative coccobacilli (HACEK group)‡	—	13 (4)
Gram-negative bacilli	38 (13)	18 (5)
Fungi, *Candida* species	21 (7)	5 (2)
Polymicrobial/ miscellaneous	6 (2)	15 (5)
Diphtheroids	10 (3)	7 (2)
Coxiella burnetii	—	5 (2)
Culture negative	22 (8)	31 (9)

*Data from Karchner AW, Longworth DL: Infections of intracardiac devices. Infect Dis Clin North Am 16:477, 2002; Rivas P, Alonso J, Moya J, et al: The impact of hospital-acquired infections on the microbial etiology and prognosis of late-onset prosthetic valve endocarditis. Chest 128:764, 2005; Hill EE, Herregods MC, Vanderschueren S, et al: Management of prosthetic valve endocarditis. Am J Cardiol 101:1174, 2008; Wang A, Athan E, Pappas P, et al: Contemporary clinical profile and outcome of prosthetic valve endocarditis. JAMA 297:1354, 2007.
†Includes viridans streptococci, *Streptococcus gallolyticus*, other non–group A groupable streptococci, *Abiotrophia* and *Granulicatella* species (nutritionally variant streptococci).
‡Includes *Haemophilus* species, *Aggregatibacter* species, *Cardiobacterium hominis, Eikenella* species, and *Kingella* species.

Health Care–Associated Endocarditis

Health care–associated endocarditis includes nosocomial IE as well as IE arising in the community after a recent hospitalization or as a direct consequence of long-term indwelling devices, such as central venous lines and hemodialysis catheters. Health care–associated IE, unrelated to concurrent cardiac surgery, makes up 24% to 34% of cases in recent series and accounts for an even larger proportion of cases in the United States.[3,4,14] Infection may involve normal valves, including the tricuspid, as well as implanted intracardiac devices and valves.[3,5,6,10,11,14] Onset of health care–associated NVE is nosocomial or community based in 54% and 46%, respectively.[14]

The onset of health care–associated IE is usually acute, and although a changing murmur may be heard, other classic signs of endocarditis are infrequent. Mortality rates among these patients, many of whom are elderly and have serious underlying diseases, are high (27% to 38%).[6,14]

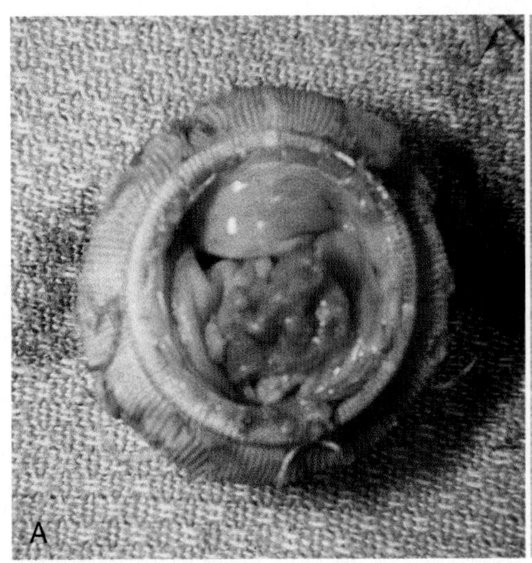

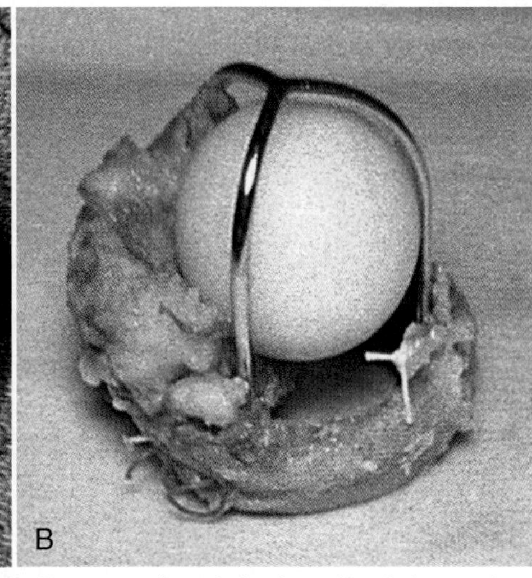

FIGURE 67-2 **A,** A large vegetation caused by *Candida albicans* partially occludes the orifice of a bioprosthetic valve removed from the mitral position. **B,** A Starr-Edwards prosthesis removed from the aortic position, where this large vegetation related to *Aspergillus* infection partially obstructed the outflow tract but also allowed regurgitation by preventing valve closure. (***A*** *reproduced from Karchmer AW: Infections of prosthetic heart valves. In Korzeniowski OM [ed]: Cardiovascular Infection, vol X, Atlas of Infectious Diseases. Philadelphia, Churchill Livingstone, 1998, p 5.7.)*

Microbiology. Among 660 episodes of health care–associated IE from five series, *S. aureus* caused 305 (46%) infections (47% of *S. aureus* were methicillin resistant); coagulase-negative staphylococci, 94 (14%); enterococci, 105 (16%); streptococci, 72 (11%); *Candida* species, 18 (3%); gram-negative bacilli, 24 (4%); and other organisms, 6 (1%). Culture was negative in 36 cases (5%).

Catheter-associated and hemodialysis-associated *S. aureus* bacteremia occurs with sufficient frequency to be the predominant predisposing factor for health care–associated IE. Transesophageal echocardiography is recommended to exclude IE in patients with catheter-related *S. aureus* bacteremia (see Chap. 15). Patients with *S. aureus* catheter-related bacteremia who have abnormal heart valves, prosthetic valves, or persisting fever or bacteremia for 3 or 4 days after catheter removal and initiation of therapy should be treated for presumed IE.

Etiologic Microorganisms

Viridans Streptococci

These streptococci, which in developed countries cause 18% to 30% of NVE cases unrelated to drug abuse and health care, are normal inhabitants of the oropharynx, characteristically produce alpha-hemolysis when grown on sheep blood agar, and are usually nontypable by the Lancefield system.[2,6] By earlier taxonomy, the non–beta-hemolytic streptococci causing NVE were distributed as follows: *Streptococcus mitior,* 31% of cases; *Streptococcus sanguis,* 24%; *Streptococcus bovis,* 27%; *Streptococcus mutans,* 7%; *Streptococcus milleri* (now called *Streptococcus anginosus* group and includes *Streptococcus intermedius, anginosus,* and *constellatus*), 4%; *Streptococcus faecalis* (now *Enterococcus faecalis*), 7%; and *Streptococcus salivarius* and other species, 2%. Nutritional variant organisms that require media supplemented with either pyridoxal hydrochloride or L-cysteine for growth, previously speciated as *Streptococcus adjacens* or *Streptococcus defectivus,* cause 5% of cases of streptococcal NVE. These organisms have been reclassified as *Granulicatella* species and *Abiotrophia defectiva* species, respectively. *Gemella morbillorum,* previously called *Streptococcus morbillorum,* shares some characteristics with nutritionally variant organisms and should be treated with similar antibiotic therapy.[15]

The viridans streptococci causing IE have been, in general, highly susceptible to penicillin; 5% to 8% of these have penicillin minimum inhibitory concentrations (MICs) >0.1 µg/mL. These streptococci are killed in a synergistic manner by penicillin plus gentamicin.

Streptococcus bovis and Other Streptococci

Streptococcus gallolyticus (formerly *S. bovis*), part of the gastrointestinal tract normal flora, causes 20% to 40% of the episodes of streptococcal NVE. Although it superficially resembles the enterococci, the distinction is important because *S. gallolyticus* is highly penicillin susceptible, in contrast to the relative penicillin resistance of enterococci. *S. gallolyticus* type I endocarditis is frequently associated with coexistent polyps or malignant disease in the colon; accordingly, colonoscopy is warranted in these patients.

Group A streptococci cause rare episodes of endocarditis. Among IV drug abusers, group A streptococci have caused tricuspid valve IE similar to that noted with *S. aureus.* Group B organisms (*Streptococcus agalactiae,* part of the normal flora of the mouth, genital tract, and gastrointestinal tract) infect normal and abnormal valves and cause a morbid NVE syndrome with a high incidence of systemic emboli and septic musculoskeletal complications (arthritis, discitis, osteomyelitis). The *S. anginosus* group cause destructive extracardiac infections and IE with intracardiac complications. Beta-hemolytic (groups A, B, C, and G) streptococcal IE often occurs in the absence of valvular disease and causes frequent intracardiac or extracardiac complications. Surgical intervention is often necessary in treatment of beta-hemolytic streptococcal and *S. anginosus* IE.

Streptococcus pneumoniae

S. pneumoniae accounts for only 1% to 3% of NVE cases. Pneumococcal IE frequently involves a normal aortic valve and progresses rapidly with valve destruction, myocardial abscess formation, and acute CHF. The diagnosis of IE is often delayed until intracardiac complications or systemic emboli are evident. The clinical presentation, complications, and outcome of endocarditis caused by penicillin-susceptible and penicillin-resistant *S. pneumoniae* are similar. Patients commonly require cardiac surgery because of valve dysfunction, CHF, or persisting fever. Mortality (35%) is related to left-sided heart failure and not to the penicillin susceptibility of the infecting strain.

Enterococci

E. faecalis and *Enterococcus faecium* cause 85% and 10% of cases of enterococcal IE, respectively. Enterococci, which are part of the normal gastrointestinal flora and cause genitourinary tract infection, account for 5% to 15% of cases of both NVE and PVE (see Tables 67-2 and 67-3).[2,4,6,14,16] Disease typically occurs with equal frequency in older men (often from a urinary tract portal of entry) and women, and 15% to 25% of cases are nosocomial.[16] Enterococci infect abnormal valves and prosthetic valves. IE may be acute or subacute. Mortality rates are comparable to those noted with viridans streptococcal IE.

Enterococci are resistant to cephalosporins, semisynthetic penicillinase-resistant penicillins (oxacillin and nafcillin), and therapeutic concentrations of aminoglycosides. Most enterococci are inhibited by modest concentrations of the cell wall–active antibiotics: penicillin, ampicillin, vancomycin, teicoplanin (not licensed in the United States), daptomycin, and linezolid. Bactericidal antienterococcal activity can be achieved by combining an inhibitory cell wall–active agent and streptomycin or gentamicin. This bactericidal activity, called synergy, is essential for optimal treatment of enterococcal IE. Strains of enterococci that are resistant to penicillin and ampicillin, resistant to vancomycin, or highly resistant to streptomycin or gentamicin have been identified as causes of IE. These resistant strains of enterococci may be unresponsive to standard antienterococcal regimens and defy development of synergistic bactericidal therapy.[17] The antibiotic susceptibility of any enterococcus causing IE must be thoroughly evaluated if optimal therapy is to be ensured.

Staphylococci

The coagulase-positive staphylococci are a single species: *S. aureus*. Of the 13 species of coagulase-negative staphylococci that colonize humans, *S. epidermidis* has emerged as an important pathogen in the setting of implanted devices and health care–associated infection.

S. aureus

This organism is a major cause of IE in all population groups (see Fig. 67-1 and Tables 67-1 to 67-3). *S. aureus* is the most common cause of IE noted in large international series from tertiary care centers.[3,4,18] In general, 25% to 30% of isolates are methicillin resistant; however, among nosocomial and health care–associated cases, rates of methicillin resistance are 57% and 40%, respectively.[14] *S. aureus* IE is characterized by a highly toxic febrile illness, frequent focal metastatic infection, 30% to 50% rate of CHF, and central nervous system complications.[4] A cerebrospinal fluid polymorphonuclear pleocytosis, with or without *S. aureus* cultured from the cerebrospinal fluid, is common. Heart murmurs as a consequence of intracardiac damage are ultimately heard in 75% to 85%. The mortality rate in nonaddicts with left-sided *S. aureus* endocarditis ranges from 16% to 65% overall and is increased with age, with significant underlying diseases, or when IE is complicated by a major neurologic event, perivalvular abscess and valve dysfunction, or CHF.[4,18] Among addicts, left-sided *S. aureus* IE resembles that in nonaddicts. With *S. aureus* IE limited to the tricuspid valve (see Fig. 15-e21 on website), systemic complications are rare and mortality rates are only 2% to 4%, although occasional patients suffer overwhelming septic pulmonary emboli, pyopneumothorax, and severe respiratory insufficiency.

Coagulase-Negative Staphylococci

These organisms, particularly *S. epidermidis*, are a major cause of PVE, an important cause of nosocomial IE, and the cause of 8% to 10% of NVE, usually in the setting of prior valve abnormalities (see Fig. 67-1).[3,14,19] Non-*epidermidis* species cause NVE that is not associated with health care. Coagulase-negative staphylococcal NVE is often complicated and fatal.[19] *Staphylococcus lugdunensis*, a community-acquired, antibiotic-susceptible coagulase-negative species, causes valve damage and frequently requires surgical intervention.

Gram-Negative Bacteria

The HACEK organisms (*Haemophilus parainfluenzae, Aggregatibacter* [previously *Haemophilus*] *aphrophilus, Aggregatibacter* [previously *Actinobacillus*] *actinomycetemcomitans, Cardiobacterium hominis, Eikenella corrodens,* and *Kingella kingae*), which are part of the upper respiratory tract and oropharyngeal flora, infect abnormal cardiac valves, causing subacute NVE and PVE that occurs a year or more after valve surgery. Although fastidious and slow growing, HACEK organisms are usually detected in blood cultures within 5 days of incubation; more prolonged incubation is occasionally required. HACEK NVE has been associated with large vegetations and a high incidence of systemic emboli.

Gram-negative bacilli, despite causing frequent episodes of bacteremia, are implicated in only sporadic cases of IE. *Escherichia coli* and *P. aeruginosa* are the most commonly implicated species.[20] Mortality rates are high (25% to 50%).

Neisseria gonorrhoeae, a rare cause of endocarditis today, causes acute IE with valve destruction and intracardiac abscesses. Antibiotic resistance is widespread among *N. gonorrhoeae;* accordingly, treatment must be based on the susceptibility of the implicated isolate. Other *Neisseria* species (nongonococcal, nonmeningococcal) cause rare episodes of subacute IE, usually in the setting of preexisting valvulopathy.

Other Organisms

Corynebacterium species, called diphtheroids, although often contaminants in blood cultures, cannot be ignored when they are isolated from multiple blood cultures. They are an important cause of PVE and cause endocarditis involving abnormal valves. *Listeria monocytogenes* occasionally infects abnormal left-sided heart valves and prosthetic devices. *Tropheryma whipplei,* the cause of Whipple disease, causes a cryptic afebrile form of IE with associated arthralgias but without diarrhea as well as valvular disease as part of typical Whipple disease. The diagnosis has been established by identification of the organism on excised valves by periodic acid–Schiff stain or by polymerase chain reaction (PCR). IE caused by *T. whipplei* often does not fulfill the Duke criteria for diagnosis (**Table 67-4**); thus, detection requires a high index of suspicion.

The rickettsia *Coxiella burnetii,* an uncommon cause of IE in the United States, is a prominent cause of IE in other parts of the world. IE follows acute infection by *C. burnetii* (Q fever) in persons with abnormal mitral or aortic valves and particularly those with prosthetic valves. Patients with acute Q fever and echocardiographically confirmed valvulopathy should receive prolonged antibiotic treatment with doxycycline plus hydroxychloroquine to prevent IE.[21] IE commonly is manifested with low-grade fever, fatigue, weight loss, hepatosplenomegaly, digital clubbing, and an immune complex vasculitis-induced purpuric rash. Vegetations are small, have smooth surfaces, and are not uniformly visible on the echocardiogram. The diagnosis is typically based on high immunoglobulin G antibody titers to phase I *C. burnetii* antigens plus immunoglobulin A antibody or demonstration of the organism in excised cardiac valves by immunohistologic or Gimenez staining or by PCR testing.

Bartonella quintana and *Bartonella henselae* together may cause 3% of NVE. In the absence of special blood culturing efforts, PCR detection of genetic material in excised vegetations, or serologic testing, many cases would have been "culture negative." *B. henselae,* the etiologic agent of cat-scratch disease, causes IE in patients with prior valve injury and cat exposure. *B. quintana,* the agent of trench fever, causes IE on normal valves largely in homeless people who are exposed to infected body lice. *Bartonella* IE arises insidiously; diagnosis is often delayed, and CHF and systemic emboli frequently complicate infection. Treatment commonly requires valve surgery.

Fungi

Candida species, *Histoplasma,* and *Aspergillus* species are the most common of the many fungal organisms identified as causing IE. Unusual so-called emerging fungi and molds account for 25% of cases. Risk factors include previous valve surgery, antibiotic use, injection drug abuse, intravascular catheters, surgery other than cardiac, and immunocompromised state. Fever, murmurs, embolization including major limb artery occlusion, neurologic abnormalities, and CHF are common. Blood cultures are positive commonly when IE is caused by *Candida* species but rarely when it is caused by molds. Culture and histologic examination of vegetations and peripheral emboli yield a microbiologic diagnosis in 75% to 95% of cases.

Pathogenesis

The interactions between the human host and selected microorganisms that culminate in IE involve the vascular endothelium, hemostatic mechanisms, host immune system, gross anatomic abnormalities in the heart, surface properties of microorganisms, enzyme and toxin production by microorganisms, and peripheral events that initiate bacteremia. Each component is in itself complex, influenced by many factors. On occasion, these interactions result in a pathogenetic sequence wherein microorganisms gain access to the bloodstream, rapidly adhere to valve surfaces, become persistent at the site of adherence, proliferate

TABLE 67-4 Diagnosis of Infective Endocarditis (Modified Duke Criteria)

Definite Infective Endocarditis

Pathologic criteria
Microorganisms: demonstrated by culture or histology in a vegetation, *or* in a vegetation that has embolized, *or* in an intracardiac abscess, *or*
Pathologic lesions: vegetation or intracardiac abscess present, confirmed by histology showing active endocarditis
Clinical criteria, using specific definitions listed below
Two major criteria, *or*
One major criterion and three minor criteria, *or*
Five minor criteria

Possible Infective Endocarditis

One major criterion and one minor criterion or three minor criteria

Rejected

Firm alternative diagnosis for manifestations of endocarditis, *or*
Sustained resolution of manifestations of endocarditis, with antibiotic therapy for 4 days or less, *or*
No pathologic evidence of infective endocarditis at surgery or autopsy, after antibiotic therapy for 4 days or less

Criteria for Diagnosis of Infective Endocarditis
Major Criteria

Positive blood culture
Typical microorganism for infective endocarditis from two separate blood cultures
Viridans streptococci, *Streptococcus bovis*, HACEK group *or* *Staphylococcus aureus* or community-acquired enterococci in the absence of a primary focus, *or*
Persistently positive blood culture, defined as recovery of a microorganism consistent with infective endocarditis from:
Blood cultures (≥2) drawn more than 12 hr apart, *or*
All of three or a majority of four or more separate blood cultures, with first and last drawn at least 1 hr apart
Single positive blood culture for *Coxiella burnetii* or anti–phase I IgG antibody titer >1 : 800
Evidence of endocardial involvement
Positive echocardiogram (TEE advised for PVE or complicated infective endocarditis)
Oscillating intracardiac mass, on valve or supporting structures, *or* in the path of regurgitant jets, *or* on implanted material, in the absence of an alternative anatomic explanation, *or*
Abscess, *or*
New partial dehiscence of prosthetic valve, *or*
New valvular regurgitation (increase or change in preexisting murmur not sufficient)

Minor Criteria

Predisposition: predisposing heart condition *or* intravenous drug use
Fever ≥38.0°C (100.4°F)
Vascular phenomena: major arterial emboli, septic pulmonary infarcts, mycotic aneurysm, intracranial hemorrhage, conjunctival hemorrhages, Janeway lesions
Immunologic phenomena: glomerulonephritis, Osler nodes, Roth spots, rheumatoid factor
Microbiologic evidence: positive blood culture but not meeting major criterion as noted previously* *or* serologic evidence of active infection with organism consistent with infective endocarditis

*Excluding single positive cultures for coagulase-negative staphylococci and organisms that do not cause endocarditis commonly.
IgG = immunoglobulin G; PVE = prosthetic valve endocarditis; TEE = transesophageal echocardiography.
Modified from Durack DT, Lukes AS, Bright DK: New criteria for diagnosis of infective endocarditis: Utilization of specific echocardiographic findings. Am J Med 96:200, 1994; modified per Li JS, Sexton DJ, Mick N, et al: Proposed modifications to the Duke criteria for the diagnosis of infective endocarditis. Clin Infect Dis 30:633, 2000.

to cause local damage and vegetation growth, and ultimately disseminate hematogenously with or without emboli. Studies have begun to elucidate the pathogenesis of IE caused by viridans streptococci and *S. aureus*.[1] The rarity of endocarditis in spite of frequent bacteremia indicates that the intact endothelium is relatively resistant to infection. It is hypothesized that platelet-fibrin deposition occurs spontaneously on abnormal valves and at sites of cardiac endothelium injury or inflammation and that these deposits, called nonbacterial thrombotic endocarditis (NBTE), are the sites at which microorganisms adhere during bacteremia to initiate IE.[1]

Development of Nonbacterial Thrombotic Endocarditis

Two major mechanisms appear pivotal in the formation of NBTE: endothelial injury and a hypercoagulable state. Marantic NBTE, thought to be a result of hypercoagulability, has been found in 1.3% of patients at autopsy and is more common with increasing age and in patients with malignant disease, disseminated intravascular coagulation, uremia, burns, systemic lupus erythematosus (see Fig. 15-62), valvular heart disease, and intracardiac catheters. NBTE occurs at the valve closure contact line on the atrial surfaces of the mitral and tricuspid valves and on the ventricular surfaces of the aortic and pulmonic valves. Three hemodynamic circumstances may injure the endothelium, initiating NBTE: (1) a high-velocity jet striking endothelium; (2) flow from a high-pressure to a low-pressure chamber; and (3) flow across a narrow orifice at high velocity.

During bacteremia, blood flow through a narrowed orifice deposits bacteria maximally at the low-pressure sink immediately beyond an orifice as a consequence of the Venturi effect or at the site where a jet stream strikes a surface. These are the same sites where NBTE forms as a result of endothelial injury or hypercoagulability. The superimposition of NBTE formation and preferential deposition of bacteria helps explain the distribution of infected vegetations.

Conversion of Nonbacterial Thrombotic Endocarditis to Infective Endocarditis

Bacteremia is the event that converts NBTE to IE. The frequency and magnitude of bacteremia associated with daily activities and health care procedures appear related to the specific mucosal surfaces and skin, the density of colonizing bacteria, the disease state of the surface, and the extent of the local trauma. Bacteremia rates are highest for events that traumatize the oral mucosa, particularly the gingiva, and progressively decrease with procedures involving the genitourinary tract and the gastrointestinal tract. For viable circulating microorganisms to reach NBTE, they must be resistant to the complement-mediated bactericidal activity of serum.

The adherence of microorganisms to the NBTE or to apparently intact valve endothelium, a pivotal early event in the development of IE, is mediated by bacterial surface molecules (adhesins). Collectively, these adhesins are known as microbial surface components recognizing adhesive matrix molecules (MSCRAMMs). Streptococci that produce surface polysaccharides called glucans or dextran cause endocarditis more frequently than strains that do not. Surface dextran mediates the adherence of streptococci to platelet-fibrin lattices and injured valves and facilitates the development of endocarditis in experimental models.[1] Dextran production, however, is not universal among the major microbial causes of IE; thus, other mechanisms of adherence are likely. FimA protein of *Streptococcus parasanguis* facilitates adherence to fibrin and development of experimental endocarditis. Collagen adhesins and biofilm-associated pili on the surface of *E. faecalis* and *E. faecium* similarly facilitate development of endocarditis in experimental models.[22,23]

Fibronectin, an important factor in the pathogenesis of IE, has been identified in lesions on heart valves and is produced by endothelial cells, platelets, and fibroblasts in response to vascular injury; a soluble form binds with fibrinogen and fibrin to exposed subendothelial collagen. Receptors for fibronectin, MSCRAMMs, are present on the surface of *S. aureus;* viridans streptococci; groups A, C, and G streptococci; enterococci; *S. pneumoniae;* and *C. albicans.* Fibronectin has numerous binding domains and thus can bind simultaneously to fibrin, collagen, cells, and microorganisms and facilitate adherence of bacteria to the valve at the site of injury or NBTE. Fibronectin-binding proteins A and B in *S. aureus* are critical in the induction of experimental endocarditis. Clumping factor (or fibrinogen-binding surface protein) of *S. aureus* also mediates the binding of these organisms to platelet-fibrin thrombi and to aortic valves in models of endocarditis.[1] The glycocalyx or slime on the surface of *S. epidermidis* does not appear to function as an adhesin but may render organisms more virulent by enhancing their ability to avoid eradication by host defenses.

The mechanism by which virulent organisms colonize and infect intact valvular endothelium is less clearly understood. Degenerative valve sclerosis may be associated with local inflammation that in turn may promote endothelial cell expression of integrins that bind fibronectin and other extracellular matrix molecules. Particulate material injected during IV drug abuse might stimulate similar endothelial events. These endothelial changes could allow *S. aureus* adherence through MSCRAMMs to apparently normal valves.[1] Adherent *S. aureus* triggers its own internalization by intact endothelial cells. Multiplication of the organism intracellularly results in cell death, which in turn disrupts the endothelial surface and initiates formation of platelet-fibrin deposits and additional sites for bacterial adherence and subsequently IE.

After adherence to NBTE or the endothelium, bacteria must persist and multiply if IE is to develop. Resistance of viridans streptococci and *S. aureus* to platelet antimicrobial proteins is associated with increased ability to cause experimental endocarditis.[1] Persistence and multiplication result in a complex dynamic process during which the infected vegetation increases in size by platelet-fibrin aggregation, microorganisms multiply and are shed into the blood, and vegetation fragments embolize. Staphylococcal and streptococcal surface proteins bind to platelets and promote aggregation and growth of the vegetation. Organisms that bind and aggregate platelets are more virulent in experimental models. Streptococci and staphylococci increase local procoagulant activity by inducing fibrin-adherent monocytes to elaborate tissue factor (a tissue thromboplastin that binds to activated factor VII to initiate clotting). Also, *S. aureus* can induce tissue factor production by endothelial cells, which would facilitate endocarditis development on normal valves. Multiple replications of this cycle from adherence to multiplication and platelet-fibrin deposition result in clinical IE.

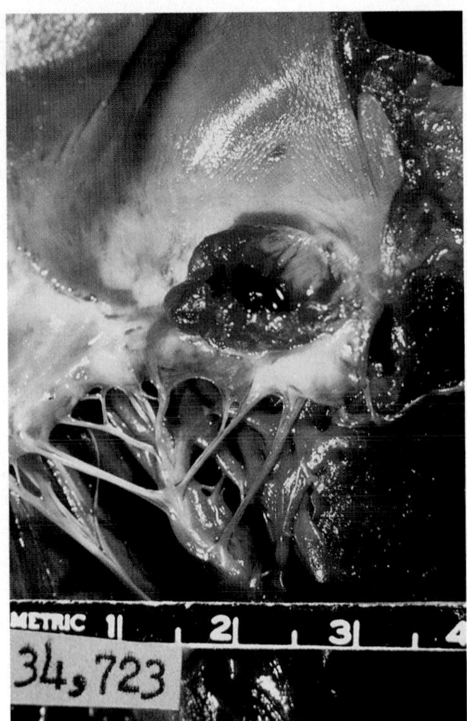

FIGURE 67-3 A normal valve with a large, bulky vegetation caused by *S. aureus* infection. Clot is present centrally in the vegetation, obscuring a valve fenestration.

Pathophysiology

Aside from the constitutional symptoms of infection, which are probably mediated by cytokines, the clinical manifestations of IE result from (1) the local destructive effects of intracardiac infection; (2) the embolization of bland or septic fragments of vegetations to distant sites, resulting in infarction or infection; (3) the hematogenous seeding of remote sites during continuous bacteremia; and (4) an antibody response to the infecting organism with subsequent tissue injury caused by deposition of preformed immune complexes or antibody-complement interaction with antigens deposited in tissues.

The intracardiac consequences of IE range from an infected vegetation with no attendant tissue damage to destruction of valves and adjacent structures. Distortion or perforation of valve leaflets, rupture of chordae tendineae, and fistulas between major vessels and cardiac chambers or between chambers themselves may result in CHF that is progressive (**Fig. 67-3**). Infection may extend into paravalvular tissue and result in abscesses and consequent persistent fever, disruption of the conduction system with electrocardiographic conduction abnormalities and arrhythmias, or purulent pericarditis. Large vegetations, particularly at the mitral valve, can result in functional valvular stenosis. In general, intracardiac complications involving the aortic valve evolve more rapidly than those associated with the mitral valve; nevertheless, the progression is highly variable and unpredictable in individual patients.

Clinically apparent emboli, half of which cause strokes, occur in 11% to 43% of patients.[24,25] Pathologic evidence of emboli at autopsy is more frequent (45% to 65%). Pulmonary emboli, which are often septic, occur in 66% to 75% of IV drug abusers with tricuspid valve IE. IE caused by virulent organisms, particularly *S. aureus,* beta-hemolytic streptococci, or other pyogenic organisms, is complicated more frequently by metastatic infection, often with local signs and symptoms or persistent fever during therapy, than IE due to avirulent bacteria (e.g., viridans streptococci). Metastatic infection assumes particular importance when the required therapy is more than the antibiotics indicated for IE (e.g., when abscesses require drainage or meningitis requires antibiotics penetrating into the cerebrospinal fluid).

Clinical Features

The interval between the presumed initiating bacteremia and the onset of symptoms of IE is estimated to be less than 2 weeks in more than 80% of patients with NVE. Interestingly, in some patients with candidemia causing IE or with intraoperative or perioperative infection of prosthetic valves, the incubation period may be prolonged (5 months or more).

Fever is almost universal (**Table 67-5**). However, it may be absent or minimal in those with CHF, severe debility, or chronic renal failure. Heart murmurs are usually emblematic of the lesion predisposing to IE. Murmurs are commonly not audible in patients with tricuspid valve IE. The new or changing regurgitant murmurs indicative of valve damage are relatively infrequent in subacute NVE and are more prevalent in acute IE and PVE (e.g., that due to *S. aureus*). They are frequently harbingers of CHF. Enlargement of the spleen is more common in subacute IE of long duration.

The classic peripheral manifestations of IE are encountered infrequently today and are virtually absent in IE restricted to the tricuspid valve. Petechiae, the most common of these manifestations, are found on the palpebral conjunctiva, the buccal and palatal mucosa, and the extremities. Splinter or subungual hemorrhages are dark red, linear, or occasionally flame-shaped streaks in the proximal nailbed. Distal lesions at the nail tip are probably caused by trauma. Osler nodes are small, tender subcutaneous nodules in the pulp of the digits, or occasionally more proximal, that persist for hours to several days. Janeway lesions are small erythematous or hemorrhagic macular nontender lesions on the palms and soles and are the consequence of septic embolic events. Embolic infarcts in the digits (**Fig. 67-4**) are common in left-sided *S. aureus* IE. Roth spots, oval retinal hemorrhages with pale

TABLE 67-5 Clinical Features of Infective Endocarditis

SYMPTOMS	PERCENTAGE OF PATIENTS	SIGNS	PERCENTAGE OF PATIENTS
Fever	80-85	Fever	80-96
Chills	42-75	Murmur	80-85
Sweats	25	Changing or new murmur	10-40
Anorexia	25-55	Neurologic abnormalities†	30-40
Weight loss	25-35	Embolic event	20-40
Malaise	25-40	Splenomegaly	15-50
Dyspnea	20-40	Clubbing	10-20
Cough	25	Peripheral manifestations	
Stroke	13-20	Osler nodes	7-10
Headache	15-40	Splinter hemorrhage	5-15
Nausea or vomiting	15-20	Petechiae	10-40
Myalgia arthralgia	15-30	Janeway lesion	6-10
Chest pain*	8-35	Retinal lesion or Roth spots	4-10
Abdominal pain	5-15		
Back pain	7-10		
Confusion	10-20		

*More common in intravenous drug abusers with right-sided infective endocarditis.
†Central nervous system.

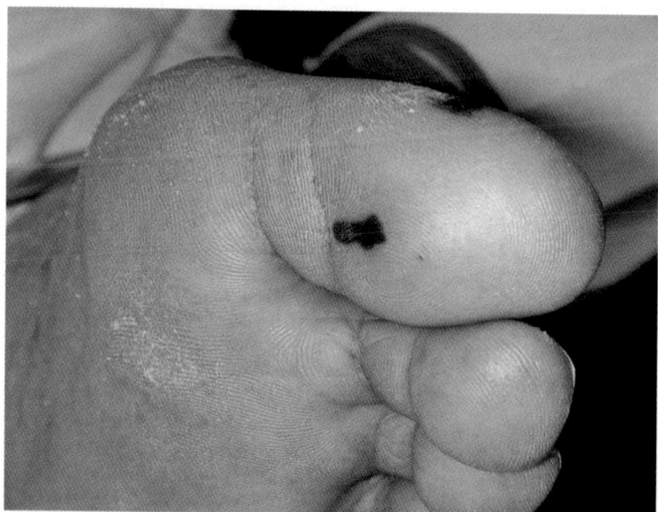

FIGURE 67-4 Digit infarcts in a patient with infective endocarditis due to *S. aureus*. *(Courtesy of Alan J. Lesse, MD.)*

centers, are infrequent findings in IE. Neither these nor Osler nodes nor conjunctival petechiae are pathognomonic for IE.

Musculoskeletal symptoms, unrelated to focal infection, are relatively common in patients with IE. These include arthralgias and myalgias, occasional true arthritis with nondiagnostic but inflammatory synovial fluid findings, and prominent back pain without demonstrable infection of vertebrae, disc space, epidural space, or sacroiliac joint. In patients with arthritis or back pain, focal infection must be excluded because additional therapy may be required.

Symptomatic systemic emboli frequently antedate or coincide with the diagnosis of IE; the incidence decreases promptly during administration of effective antibiotic therapy. Embolic events are infrequent after 2 weeks of therapy.[25] The risks of emboli generally increase with large vegetations (>10 mm), mitral vegetations, *S. aureus* IE, and increasing vegetation size during therapy.[4,24,25] Embolic stroke syndromes (clinically evident), predominantly involving the middle cerebral artery territory, occur in 15% to 35% of patients with NVE and PVE. A similar additional frequency of asymptomatic embolic infarcts may be detected with careful routine imaging. Coronary artery emboli, common findings at autopsy, rarely cause transmural infarction. Emboli to the extremities may produce pain and overt ischemia, and emboli to mesenteric arteries may cause abdominal pain, ileus, and guaiac-positive stools.

Neurologic symptoms and signs are caused most commonly by embolic strokes, are more frequent when IE is caused by *S. aureus*, and are associated with increased mortality rates.[24-26] Intracranial hemorrhage, which occurs in 5% of patients, results from rupture of a mycotic aneurysm, rupture of an artery related to septic arteritis at the site of embolic occlusion, or hemorrhage into an infarct. Cerebritis with microabscesses complicates IE caused by invasive pathogens such as *S. aureus*, but large brain abscesses are rare. Purulent meningitis complicates some episodes of IE caused by *S. aureus* or *S. pneumoniae*, but more typically the cerebrospinal fluid, if abnormal, has an aseptic profile. Other neurologic manifestations include severe headache (a potential clue to a mycotic aneurysm), seizures, and encephalopathy.

CHF primarily results from valve destruction or distortion or rupture of chordae tendineae. Intracardiac fistulas, myocarditis, or coronary artery embolization may occasionally contribute to the genesis of CHF, as obviously can underlying cardiac disease.

Renal insufficiency as a result of immune complex–mediated glomerulonephritis occurs in less than 15% of patients with IE. Azotemia as a result of this process may develop or progress during initial therapy but usually improves with continued administration of effective antibiotic therapy. Focal glomerulonephritis and embolic renal infarcts cause hematuria but rarely result in azotemia. The most common cause of renal dysfunction in patients with IE is impaired hemodynamics or antimicrobial toxicities (interstitial nephritis or aminoglycoside toxicity).

Diagnosis

The symptoms and signs of endocarditis are often constitutional and, when localized, may result from a remote complication rather than reflect the intracardiac infection itself (see Table 67-5). Consequently, to avoid overlooking the diagnosis of IE, a high index of suspicion must be maintained. The diagnosis must be investigated when patients with fever present with one or more of the cardinal elements of IE: predisposing cardiac lesion or behavior pattern, bacteremia, embolic phenomenon, and evidence of an active endocardial process or new prosthetic valve dysfunction. Among patients with a predisposition to IE, unexplained weight loss, malaise, azotemia, and anemia should prompt consideration of IE even in the absence of fever. Even when the illness seems typical of endocarditis, the definitive diagnosis requires positive blood cultures or positive cultures (or histology or PCR recovery of the DNA of a microorganism) from the vegetation or an embolus. There are many mimics of IE: atrial myxoma (see Chap. 74), acute rheumatic fever (see Chap. 88), systemic lupus erythematosus or other collagen-vascular disease (see Chap. 89), marantic endocarditis, antiphospholipid syndrome, carcinoid syndrome, renal cell carcinoma with increased cardiac output, and thrombotic thrombocytopenic purpura.

The modified Duke criteria provide a schema that facilitates evaluation of patients for endocarditis (see Table 67-4).[27] Clinical and laboratory data, including echocardiography, should be collected to assess the presence or absence of the listed major and minor criteria. Finding evidence of two major criteria or one major criterion plus three minor criteria or five minor criteria establishes a clinical diagnosis of "definite endocarditis," whereas finding one major criterion plus one minor criterion or three minor criteria indicates "possible endocarditis." When used judiciously over the entire evaluation (i.e., not limited to initial findings), these criteria are sensitive and specific for the diagnosis of IE.[27] Erroneous rejection of the diagnosis of endocarditis is unlikely. When the criteria are used to guide therapy, patients who are categorized with possible endocarditis should be treated as if they have IE. Requiring at least one major criterion plus one minor criterion or three minor criteria to designate possible endocarditis reduces the potential for overdiagnosis (failure to reject the diagnosis).[27] Nevertheless, because the echocardiogram cannot fully distinguish healed vegetations and other valvular masses from actively infected vegetations, these guidelines are vulnerable to misidentification of patients as having culture-negative IE when vegetations that complicate marasmus, malignant disease, cryptic collagen-vascular disease, antiphospholipid antibody syndrome, or previously treated IE are detected. To use bacteremia caused by coagulase-negative staphylococci or diphtheroids (organisms that may cause IE but more often contaminate blood cultures) to support the diagnosis of endocarditis, blood cultures must be persistently positive or the organisms recovered in several sporadically positive cultures must be proved to represent a single clone.[27]

Echocardiography

Inclusion of echocardiographic evidence of endocardial infection in these criteria recognizes the high sensitivity of two-dimensional echocardiography with color Doppler study, especially if biplane or multiplanar transesophageal echocardiography (TEE) and transthoracic echocardiography (TTE) are combined (see Chap. 15), and the relative infrequency of false-positive studies when experienced operators use specific definitions for vegetations.[28] TEE provides improved resolution and allows visualization of smaller vegetations compared with TTE (see Fig. 15-60). The sensitivity of TTE for the detection of vegetations, even with the use of harmonic imaging and other modern techniques, in patients with NVE is approximately 45% to 65%, whereas that of TEE in these patients is 85% to 95%. The likelihood of a false-negative study can be reduced to 5% to 10% if TEE is repeated.[15] TEE is the preferred approach in patients in whom TTE is technically suboptimal and is the procedure of choice for imaging of the pulmonic valve and patients with suspected PVE.[28,29] Among patients with PVE, the diagnostic sensitivity of TTE is 15% to 45%. In contrast, the sensitivity of TEE for detection of signs of PVE ranges from 82% to 96% with mechanical or bioprosthetic devices in the aortic or mitral position. Thus, the highly sensitive TEE helps preclude the diagnosis of IE when the clinical suspicion is low; when the clinical suspicion is high, even these studies cannot exclude the diagnosis or need for treatment.[28] When initial TEE is normal and the clinical suspicion of IE remains, repeating TEE in 7 to 10 days is advocated.[15,30]

The American Heart Association (AHA) and the American College of Cardiology (ACC) guidelines recommend echocardiographic evaluation in all patients with suspected IE (see Table 67G-2).[15,30a] Echocardiography should not be used as a screening test for IE in unselected patients with positive blood cultures or in evaluating patients with fevers of unknown origin when the clinical probability of IE is low.[28,29] A decision analysis evaluation assessed the use of echocardiography to make the diagnosis and to initiate treatment of NVE in patients with bacteremia; the study suggests that, assuming the diagnostic enhancement of TEE over TTE is 15%, the most cost-effective strategies are as follows: (1) if prior probability of IE is less than 2%, treat for bacteremia without echocardiography; (2) if prior probability is 2% to 4%, use TTE; and (3) if prior probability is 5% to 45%, use TEE initially in lieu of TTE. If the prior probability of IE is greater than 45%, therapy for IE without echocardiography is cost-effective, although imaging is preferred to evaluate for complications and other risks. The approach for use of echocardiography advocated by the AHA is outlined in **Figure 67-5**. The ACC 2007 appropriateness criteria for transthoracic and transesophageal echocardiography also endorse TEE as a highly appropriate initial study to aid in the management of patients with a moderate or high pretest probability of IE.[31]

Studies suggest that among patients with a high prior probability of NVE, data derived from TEE rarely alter the decisions to treat for endocarditis based on the clinical presentation and TTE. Exceptions to this, when TEE provides pivotal information, include when TTE is technically inadequate, when PVE is suspected, and when there is *S. aureus* or enterococcal bacteremia. In patients with clinically uncomplicated catheter-associated *S. aureus* bacteremia, in whom the risk of IE ranges from 6% to 23%, use of TEE to seek vegetations and to determine the duration of antibiotic therapy (4 to 6 weeks versus 2 weeks, i.e., treatment for IE or not) is more cost-effective and less morbid than empiric selection of either treatment duration.

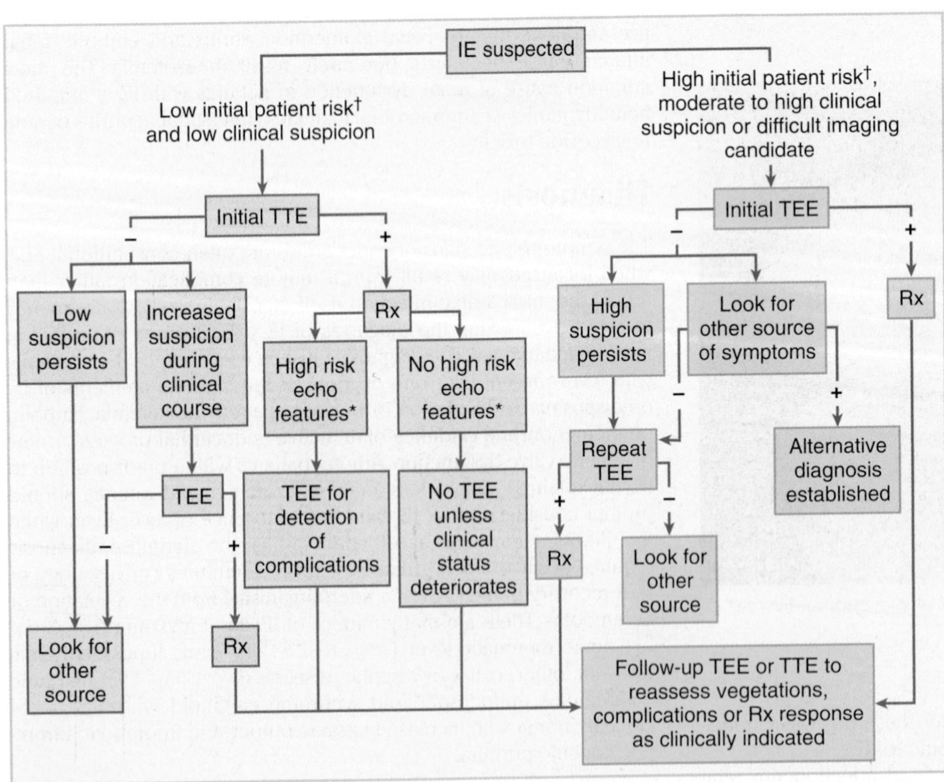

FIGURE 67-5 Schematic approach to the diagnostic use of echocardiography for infective endocarditis (IE). *High-risk echocardiographic features include large vegetations, valve insufficiency, suggestion of perivalvular extension, and ventricular dysfunction. †Patients with high initial risk include those with prosthetic heart valves, complex congenital heart disease, prior IE, new murmur, and heart failure. Rx indicates initiation of antibiotic therapy for IE. TEE = transesophageal echocardiography; TTE = transthoracic echocardiography. *(Reproduced from Bayer AS, Bolger AF, Taubert KA, et al: Diagnosis and management of infective endocarditis and its complications. Circulation 98:2936, 1998.)*

Despite the sensitivity of TEE in detecting vegetations in patients with proven IE, echocardiography does not itself provide a definite diagnosis. Vegetations and valve dysfunction may be demonstrated, but determination of causality requires clinical or direct anatomic and microbiologic confirmation. In addition to noninfected vegetations, thickened valves, ruptured chordae or valves, valve calcification, and nodules may be mistaken for infected vegetations.

Establishing the Microbial Cause

A microbial cause of IE is established by recovering the infecting agent from the blood or by identifying it in vegetations or embolic material. In detecting the continuous bacteremia of IE, there is no advantage to obtaining blood cultures in relation to fever or from arterial blood. In patients who have not received prior antibiotics and who will ultimately have blood culture–positive IE, it is likely that 95% to 100% of all cultures obtained will be positive and that one of the first two cultures will be positive in at least 95% of patients. Prior antibiotic therapy is a major cause of blood culture–negative IE, particularly when the causative microorganism is highly antibiotic susceptible. After subtherapeutic antibiotic exposure, the time required for reversion to positive cultures is directly related to the duration of antimicrobial therapy and the susceptibility of the causative agent; days to a week or more may be required.

Obtaining Blood Culture Specimens

Three separate sets of blood cultures, each from a separate venipuncture, obtained during 24 hours, are recommended to evaluate patients with suspected endocarditis.[28] Each set should include a bottle containing an aerobic medium and one containing thioglycollate broth (anaerobic medium); at least 10 mL of blood should be placed into each bottle. If a clinically stable patient has received an antimicrobial agent during the past several weeks, it is prudent to delay therapy so that repeated cultures can be performed on successive days without further confounding by antibiotics. If endocarditis caused by fungi or unusual bacteria (*Legionella* species or *Bartonella* species) is suspected, the laboratory should be consulted for guidance regarding optimal culture techniques. Serologic tests can be used to make the presumptive diagnosis of endocarditis caused by *Brucella* species, *Legionella* species, *Bartonella* species, *C. burnetii*, *Aspergillus* species, or *Chlamydia* species. By use of special techniques, including PCR and antigen detection, these agents and others that are difficult to recover in blood culture can be identified in blood or vegetations.[28,32]

In evaluation of positive blood cultures, sustained bacteremia, which is typical of IE, should be distinguished from transient bacteremia. When several blood culture samples obtained during 24 hours or more are positive, the diagnosis of IE must be considered. The identity of the organism is also helpful in determining the intensity with which the diagnosis is entertained. Organisms can be divided into those that commonly or rarely cause IE and the intermediate-behaving organisms, such as enterococci and *S. aureus*, which, when in the blood, may or may not indicate IE. Finally, the presence or absence of alternative sources for the bacteremia aids in the assessment of bacteremia.

Laboratory Tests

Anemia, with normochromic normocytic red blood cell indices, low serum iron level, and low serum iron-binding capacity, is found in 70% to 90% of patients. Anemia worsens with increased duration of illness and thus in acute IE may be absent. In subacute IE, the white blood cell count is usually normal; in contrast, a leukocytosis with increased segmented granulocytes is common in acute IE. Thrombocytopenia occurs only rarely. The erythrocyte sedimentation rate is elevated (average approximately 55 mm/hr) in almost all patients with IE; the exceptions are those with CHF, renal failure, or disseminated intravascular coagulation. The C-reactive protein is elevated with mean concentrations ranging from 67 to 179 mg/liter, depending on the causative organism. The rheumatoid factor is increased in 50% of patients. Proteinuria and microscopic hematuria are noted in 50% of patients even when renal function remains normal. In patients with diffuse immune complex glomerulonephritis, circulating immune complexes are detectable and complement is depressed.

Imaging

ECHOCARDIOGRAPHY. In addition to its role in diagnosis, echocardiography (see Chap. 15) may identify complications or a need for surgery and provide information central to the management of IE. Valve dysfunction, obstructing vegetations, or evidence of decompensated CHF can be visualized and quantitated by echocardiography with Doppler study. Some degree of regurgitation by Doppler evaluation is almost universal early in the course of NVE and PVE and does not necessarily predict progressive hemodynamic deterioration. Extension of infection beyond the valve leaflet results in abscesses in the annulus or adjacent structures, mycotic aneurysms of the sinus of Valsalva or mitral valve, intracardiac fistulas, and purulent pericarditis. Myocardial abscesses are more readily detected by TEE than by TTE in patients with NVE or PVE (see Fig. 15-61). The sensitivity and specificity for abscess detection are 28% and 98% for TTE, compared with 87% and 95% for TEE. TEE is also more sensitive and accurate than TTE for recognizing subaortic invasive disease and valve perforations. Progressive CHF, new electrocardiographic conduction changes, changes in heart murmurs, and evidence of pericarditis warrant prompt evaluation by TEE to plan care. To facilitate long-term care, valve morphology and function, vegetation size, and ventricular function should be determined by TTE at the conclusion of treatment.

OTHER IMAGING. Scintigraphy is insufficiently sensitive to be clinically useful. Magnetic resonance imaging and multislice computed tomography (CT) can define cardiac anatomy and supplement TEE evaluation (see Chaps. 18 and 19). Multislice CT with contrast media may be comparable to TEE in the diagnosis of IE and provide better paravalvular anatomic detail (see Fig. 19-22), as well as visualization of the coronary arteries.[33]

Treatment

Two major objectives must be achieved to treat IE effectively. The infecting microorganism in the vegetation must be eradicated. Failure to accomplish this results in relapse of infection. Also, invasive, destructive intracardiac and focal extracardiac complications of infection must be resolved if morbidity and mortality are to be minimized. The second objective often exceeds the capacity of effective antimicrobial therapy and requires cardiac or other surgical intervention.

Bacteria in vegetations multiply to population densities approaching 10^9 to 10^{10} organisms per gram of tissue, become metabolically dormant, and are difficult to eradicate. Clinical experience and animal model experiments suggest that optimal therapy requires bactericidal antibiotics or antibiotic combinations rather than bacteriostatic agents. To reach effective antibiotic concentrations in avascular vegetations by passive diffusion, high serum concentrations must be achieved. Parenteral antimicrobial therapy is used whenever feasible to achieve suitable serum antibiotic concentrations and to avoid the potentially erratic absorption of orally administered therapy. Treatment is continued for prolonged periods to ensure eradication of dormant microorganisms.

In selecting antimicrobial therapy for patients with IE, one must consider the MIC and the ability of potential agents to kill the causative organism. The MIC is the lowest concentration that inhibits growth, and the minimum bactericidal concentration (MBC) is the lowest concentration that decreases a standard inoculum of organisms 99.9% during 24 hours. For most streptococci and staphylococci, the MIC and MBC of penicillins, cephalosporins, or vancomycin are the same or differ by only a factor of 2 to 4. Organisms for which the MBC for these antibiotics is 10-fold or greater than the MIC are occasionally encountered. This phenomenon has been termed tolerance. Most of the tolerant strains are simply killed more slowly than nontolerant strains, and with prolonged incubation (48 hours) their MICs and MBCs are similar. Enterococci exhibit what superficially appears to be tolerance when tested against penicillins and vancomycin; however, these organisms are, in fact, not killed by these agents but are merely inhibited even after longer incubation times. Enterococci can be killed by the synergistic activity of selected penicillins or vancomycin and an aminoglycoside. A similar effect can be seen with these combinations against streptococci and staphylococci.

A synergistic bactericidal effect is required for optimal therapy for enterococcal endocarditis and has been used to achieve more effective therapy or effective short-course therapy for IE caused by other organisms. Tolerance in streptococci or staphylococci has not been correlated with decreased cure rates or delayed responses to treatment with penicillins, cephalosporins, or vancomycin and is not an indication for combination therapy. In fact, regimens are designed using the MICs of these organisms.[15]

The regimens recommended for the treatment of IE caused by specific organisms are designed to provide concentrations of antibiotics in serum and deep in vegetations that exceed the organism's MIC throughout most of the interval between doses. Although antibiotic concentrations in vegetations of patients with IE have been measured infrequently, the success of the recommended regimens suggests that this goal is achieved. Accordingly, for optimal therapy, it is important that the recommended regimens be followed carefully.

Antimicrobial Therapy for Specific Organisms

Optimal antimicrobial therapy, which is based on the susceptibility of the causative organism, should sterilize the vegetation while causing little or no toxicity. Antibiotic modifications may be needed to accommodate end-organ dysfunction, allergies, or anticipated toxicities. In anticipation of the possible need to modify therapy, the organism causing endocarditis should be saved until successful therapy has been completed. With the exception of staphylococcal endocarditis, the antimicrobial regimens recommended for the treatment of NVE and PVE are similar, although more prolonged treatment is often advised for PVE.[10,15]

Penicillin-Susceptible Viridans Streptococci or *Streptococcus gallolyticus (bovis)*

Multiple regimens provide highly effective, comparable therapy for patients with uncomplicated NVE caused by penicillin-susceptible streptococci and *S. gallolyticus* (**Table 67-6**). The 4-week regimens yield bacteriologic cure rates of 98%. The synergistic combination of penicillin or ceftriaxone plus gentamicin for 2 weeks is as effective in selected cases as treatment with the 4-week regimens.[15] The short-course combination regimens are recommended for patients who have uncomplicated NVE and who are not at increased risk for aminoglycoside toxicity. Patients with endocarditis caused by nutritionally variant organisms (*Granulicatella* species, *Abiotrophia defectiva*, *G. morbillorum*) and patients with PVE or endocarditis complicated by a mycotic aneurysm, myocardial abscess, perivalvular infection, or an extracardiac focus of infection should not be treated with a short-course regimen.

From 2% to 8% of viridans streptococci and *S. gallolyticus* causing endocarditis are highly resistant to streptomycin (MIC >2000 µg/mL) and are not killed synergistically by penicillin plus streptomycin but are killed synergistically by penicillin plus gentamicin. Consequently, gentamicin is recommended for use in the short-course combination regimen. Ceftriaxone 2 g once daily plus either gentamicin (3 mg/kg) or netilmicin (4 mg/kg) given as a single daily dose for 14 days has effectively treated endocarditis caused by penicillin-susceptible streptococci. The nutritionally variant organisms are generally more resistant to penicillin than viridans streptococci are; thus, IE caused by these organisms is treated with regimens recommended for enterococcal endocarditis (see later); however, outcome remains unsatisfactory.

For the treatment of streptococcal endocarditis in patients with a history of urticarial or anaphylactic reactions to a penicillin or cephalosporin, vancomycin is recommended (see Table 67-6). Patients with other forms of penicillin allergy (delayed maculopapular rash) may be treated cautiously with the ceftriaxone regimens (see Table 67-6). For patients with PVE caused by penicillin-susceptible streptococci, treatment with 6 weeks of penicillin is recommended, with or without gentamicin 3 mg/kg/day in three divided doses given during the initial 2 weeks.[10,15]

Relatively Penicillin Resistant Streptococci. Treatment with 4 weeks of high-dose parenteral penicillin or ceftriaxone plus an aminoglycoside (primarily gentamicin for the reasons noted previously) during the initial 2 weeks is recommended for endocarditis caused by streptococci with MICs for penicillin between >0.1 and 0.5 µg/mL (**Table 67-7**). Patients who cannot tolerate penicillin because of immediate hypersensitivity reactions can be treated with vancomycin alone. For those with non-immediate penicillin hypersensitivity, effective treatment can be accomplished either with vancomycin alone or with the ceftriaxone-gentamicin regimen (see Table 67-7). NVE caused by streptococci that are "fully" resistant to penicillin (MIC >0.5 µg/mL; *Granulicatella* species, *Abiotrophia defectiva*, and *G. morbillorum*) or PVE caused by relatively or fully penicillin-resistant organisms should be treated for 6 weeks with penicillin or ceftriaxone plus gentamicin (doses per Table 67-7 or Table 67-8) or vancomycin alone.[15,34]

Streptococcus Pyogenes, Streptococcus Pneumoniae, and Group B, C, and G Streptococci. Endocarditis caused by these streptococci has been either refractory to antibiotic therapy or associated with extensive valvular damage. Penicillin G in a dose of 3 million units intravenously every 4 hours for 4 weeks is recommended for the treatment of group A streptococcal endocarditis. Ceftriaxone and vancomycin, depending on the degree of penicillin allergy, are treatment alternatives (see Table 67-7).

IE caused by group G, C, or B streptococci is more difficult to treat than that caused by penicillin-susceptible viridans streptococci. Consequently, the addition of gentamicin to the first 2 weeks of a 4-week regimen using high doses of penicillin is often advocated (see Table 67-7). Early cardiac surgery to correct intracardiac complications is needed in almost half of these cases and may improve outcome.

In selecting treatment for pneumococcal IE, both antibiotic resistance in the infecting strain and coexisting meningitis are important considerations.[15] The treatment of IE caused by penicillin-susceptible pneumococci (MIC ≤0.1 µg/mL) with or without concomitant meningitis is penicillin G 4 million units intravenously every 4 hours, ceftriaxone 2 g

TABLE 67-6 Treatment of Native Valve Endocarditis Caused by Penicillin-Susceptible Viridans Streptococci and *Streptococcus gallolyticus (bovis)* (MIC <0.1 µg/mL)*

ANTIBIOTIC	DOSAGE AND ROUTE†	DURATION
Aqueous penicillin G	12-18 million units/24 hr IV either continuously or every 4 hr in six equally divided doses	4 weeks
or		
Ceftriaxone	2 g once daily IV or IM	4 weeks
Aqueous penicillin G	12-18 million units/24 hr IV either continuously or every 4 hr in six equally divided doses	2 weeks
or		
Ceftriaxone	2 g once daily IV or IM	2 weeks
plus		
Gentamicin	3 mg/kg/day IM or IV as a single daily dose or divided in equal doses every 8 hr	2 weeks
Vancomycin	30 mg/kg/24 hr IV in two equally divided doses, not to exceed 2 g/24 hr unless serum levels are monitored	4 weeks

Three treatment options are recommended.

*For nutritionally variant organisms (*Granulicatella* species, *Gemella morbillorum*, *Abiotrophia defectiva*), see text and Table 67-8.

†Dosages given are for patients with normal renal function. Vancomycin and gentamicin doses must be reduced for treatment of patients with renal dysfunction. Gentamicin doses are calculated by ideal body weight (men = 50 kg + 2.3 kg per inch over 5 feet; women = 45.5 kg + 2.3 kg per inch over 5 feet). Vancomycin doses are based on actual body weight. Vancomycin doses are adjusted to yield 1-hour postinfusion serum concentration of 30 to 45 µg/mL and trough of 15 µg/mL. Gentamicin administered every 8 hours should be adjusted to achieve a 1-hour peak concentration of 3 to 3.5 µg/mL and a trough of <1.0 µg/mL. Lengthening of the dose-to-dose interval may be required to achieve these parameters in patients with renal dysfunction.

Modified from Baddour LM, Wilson WR, Bayer AS, et al: Infective endocarditis: Diagnosis, antimicrobial therapy, and management of complications. Circulation 111:3167, 2005.

TABLE 67-7 Treatment of Native Valve Endocarditis Caused by Strains of Viridans Streptococci and *Streptococcus gallolyticus (bovis)* Relatively Resistant to Penicillin G (MIC >0.1 µg/mL and <0.5 µg/mL)*

ANTIBIOTIC	DOSAGE AND ROUTE†	DURATION
Aqueous penicillin G	24 million units/24 hr IV either continuously or every 4 hr in six equally divided doses	4 weeks
or		
Ceftriaxone	2 g once daily IV or IM	
plus		
Gentamicin	3 mg/kg/day IM or IV as a single daily dose or divided in equal doses every 8 hr	2 weeks
Vancomycin	30 mg/kg/24 hr IV in two equally divided doses, not to exceed 2 g/24 hr unless serum levels are monitored	4 weeks

Two treatment options are recommended.

*For streptococci with penicillin MIC > 0.5 µg/mL, see text and Table 67-8.

†Dosages are for patients with normal renal function; see Table 67-6 footnote.

Modified from Baddour LM, Wilson WR, Bayer AS, et al: Infective endocarditis: Diagnosis, antimicrobial therapy, and management of complications. Circulation 111:3167, 2005.

intravenously every 12 hours, or cefotaxime 4 g intravenously every 6 hours. In the absence of meningitis, these regimens are effective for IE caused by pneumococci that are relatively penicillin resistant (MIC 0.1 to 1.0 μg/mL). If IE, including that caused by relatively penicillin resistant isolates when complicated by meningitis, is caused by a penicillin-resistant (MIC = 2.0 μg/mL) or cefotaxime-resistant (MIC = 2.0 μg/mL) pneumococcus, therapy with ceftriaxone 2 g intravenously every 12 hours or cefotaxime 4 g intravenously every 6 hours plus vancomycin 15 mg/kg intravenously every 12 hours and rifampin is preferred. CHF rather than penicillin resistance is associated with mortality; thus, intervention early with cardiac surgery may be essential for an optimal outcome.

Enterococci

Optimal therapy for enterococcal endocarditis requires synergistic bactericidal interaction of an antimicrobial targeted against the bacterial cell wall (penicillin, ampicillin, or vancomycin) and an aminoglycoside that is able to exert a lethal effect (streptomycin or gentamicin). High-level resistance, defined as the inability of high concentrations of streptomycin (1000 or 2000 μg/mL) or gentamicin (500 to 2000 μg/mL) to inhibit the growth of an enterococcus, predicts the agent's inability to exert this lethal effect and to participate in the bactericidal synergistic interaction. Similarly, resistance to the cell wall–targeted agents indicates their inability to contribute to synergistic killing. The standard regimens recommended for the treatment of enterococcal endocarditis (**Table 67-8**) are designed to achieve bactericidal synergy and to result in cure rates of approximately 85%, compared with 40% with single-agent, nonbactericidal treatment. Isolates with high-level gentamicin resistance are not routinely high-level streptomycin resistant. In the absence of high-level resistance to streptomycin in a causative strain, streptomycin, 7.5 mg/kg intramuscularly or intravenously every 12 hours to achieve a 1-hour peak serum concentration of approximately 20 to 35 μg/mL and a trough of <10 μg/mL, can be substituted for gentamicin in the standard regimens. The streptomycin dose must be reduced if renal function is decreased. The vancomycin-aminoglycoside regimen (see Table 67-8) is recommended only for patients allergic to penicillin. Desensitization to penicillin may be desirable when preexisting renal dysfunction favors avoidance of the potentially more nephrotoxic vancomycin-aminoglycoside combination. Therapy is administered for 4 to 6 weeks, with the longer course used to treat patients with PVE or IE that was symptomatic for more than 3 months or is complicated. Careful monitoring of patients clinically and of serum creatinine and aminoglycoside levels is required to prevent nephrotoxicity and ototoxicity.

Favorable outcomes with regimens using shortened courses of aminoglycosides suggest that the aminoglycoside component of combination therapy can be abbreviated if toxicity becomes significant. Of 93 patients treated for enterococcal IE (66 with NVE, 27 with PVE), 75 (81%) were cured, 15 (16%) died, and 3 (3%) relapsed. Cure was achieved with a median duration of cell wall–active antimicrobial therapy and aminoglycoside therapy of 42 and 15 days, respectively. In 39 of the patients who were cured, aminoglycosides were administered for 21 days or less. Experimental data and limited clinical data suggest that double beta-lactam antibiotic therapy (ceftriaxone or cefotaxime plus ampicillin) may be bactericidal and provide a non-nephrotoxic alternative for treatment of *E. faecalis* infection.[15,35]

Enterococci causing endocarditis must be tested for high-level resistance to both streptomycin and gentamicin and susceptibility to penicillin, ampicillin, and vancomycin (**Table 67-9**). High-level resistance to gentamicin predicts resistance to all other aminoglycosides except streptomycin. With use of these data, an attempt should be made to design a regimen containing a cell wall–active agent to which the isolate is susceptible plus gentamicin or streptomycin, depending on the absence of high-level resistance. If a bactericidal synergistic regimen is not feasible, an alternative treatment plus possible surgery should be considered (see Table 67-9).[15,17]

TABLE 67-8 Standard Therapy for Endocarditis Caused by Enterococci*

ANTIBIOTIC	DOSAGE AND ROUTE†	DURATION
Aqueous penicillin G	18-30 million units/24 hr IV given continuously or every 4 hr in six equally divided doses	4-6 weeks
plus		
Gentamicin	1 mg/kg IM or IV every 8 hr	4-6 weeks
Ampicillin	12 g/24 hr IV given continuously or every 4 hr in six equally divided doses	4-6 weeks
plus		
Gentamicin	1 mg/kg IM or IV every 8 hr	4-6 weeks
Vancomycin‡	30 mg/kg/24 hr IV in two equally divided doses not to exceed 2 g/24 hr unless serum levels are monitored	4-6 weeks
plus		
Gentamicin	1 mg/kg IM or IV every 8 hr	4-6 weeks

Three treatment options are recommended.

*All enterococci causing endocarditis must be tested for antimicrobial susceptibility for selection of optimal therapy. These regimens are for treatment of endocarditis caused by enterococci that are susceptible to penicillin, ampicillin, or vancomycin and not highly resistant to gentamicin. These may also be used for treatment of endocarditis caused by penicillin-resistant (MIC > 0.5 μg/mL) viridans streptococci and nutritionally variant organisms or enterococcal prosthetic valve endocarditis.

†Dosages are for patients with normal renal function; see Table 67-6 footnote.

‡For patients allergic to penicillin or ampicillin. Alternatively, desensitize to penicillin. For enterococcal IE, cephalosporins are not alternatives to penicillin or ampicillin in penicillin-allergic patients.

Modified from Baddour LM, Wilson WR, Bayer AS, et al: Infective endocarditis: Diagnosis, antimicrobial therapy, and management of complications. Circulation 111:3167, 2005.

TABLE 67-9 Strategy to Select Therapy for Enterococcal Endocarditis Caused by Strains Resistant to Components of the Standard Regimen

I. Ideal therapy includes a cell wall–active agent plus an effective aminoglycoside to achieve bactericidal synergy (see text)

II. Cell wall–active antimicrobial
   A. Determine MIC for ampicillin and vancomycin; test for beta-lactamase production (nitrocefin test)
   B. If ampicillin and vancomycin susceptible, use ampicillin
   C. If ampicillin resistant (MIC ≥16 μg/mL) and vancomycin susceptible, use vancomycin
   D. If beta-lactamase produced, use vancomycin or consider ampicillin-sulbactam
   E. If ampicillin resistant and resistant to vancomycin (MIC > 8 μg/mL) and teicoplanin* (MIC ≥ 8 μg/mL), see IV C, D†

III. Aminoglycoside to be used with cell wall–active antimicrobial
   A. If no high-level resistance to streptomycin (MIC < 1000 or 2000 μg/mL) or gentamicin (MIC < 500-2000 μg/mL), use gentamicin or streptomycin
   B. If high-level resistance to gentamicin (MIC > 500-2000 μg/mL), test streptomycin; if no high-level resistance to streptomycin, use streptomycin (see IV B)
   C. If high-level resistance to gentamicin and streptomycin, omit aminoglycoside therapy; use prolonged therapy (8-12 wk) with cell wall–active antimicrobial if the organism is susceptible (see II A-E) or alternative therapy (see IV C, D, E)†

IV. Alternative regimens and approaches (use with consultative assistance of infectious disease specialist)
   A. Single-drug therapy (see III C) and possible surgical intervention
   B. Consider ampicillin, vancomycin (or teicoplanin), streptomycin based on absence of high-level resistance
   C. Consider quinupristin-dalfopristin therapy for infective endocarditis caused by susceptible *Enterococcus faecium* and surgical intervention
   D. Consider linezolid therapy for *E. faecalis* or *E. faecium* with or without surgical intervention
   E. Daptomycin active in vitro against vancomycin-resistant enterococci but few clinical data for this treatment

*Not approved by the Food and Drug Administration for use in the United States.

†See Stevens MP, Edmond MB: Endocarditis due to vancomycin-resistant enterococci: Case report and review of the literature. Clin Infect Dis 41:1134, 2005.

MIC = minimum inhibitory concentration.

Staphylococci

ANTIBIOTIC RESISTANCE. In excess of 90% of *S. aureus* and coagulase-negative staphylococci, whether acquired in the hospital or community, produce beta-lactamase and thus are resistant to penicillin, ampicillin, and the ureidopenicillins. Penicillin-resistant *S. aureus* can be further subdivided into isolates that are either methicillin susceptible, that is, susceptible to penicillinase-resistant beta-lactam antibiotics (nafcillin, oxacillin, cloxacillin, and cefazolin), or methicillin-resistant, that is, resistant to all beta-lactam antibiotics but susceptible, with rare exceptions, to vancomycin, teicoplanin (not approved for use in the United States), and daptomycin. Previously, the majority of *S. aureus* infections were caused by methicillin-susceptible isolates. Currently, methicillin-resistant *S. aureus* (MRSA) have become a common cause of staphylococcal infections that are nosocomial or community acquired (both health care associated and not health care associated). Accordingly, empiric therapy for suspected *S. aureus* IE should be effective against MRSA. Coagulase-negative staphylococci causing community-acquired infections are frequently methicillin susceptible, whereas those causing nosocomial IE are commonly methicillin resistant. Methicillin-resistant coagulase-negative staphylococci may not always phenotypically express this resistance (a property called heteroresistance) and require special testing. Most methicillin-resistant strains of *S. aureus* and coagulase-negative staphylococci remain susceptible to vancomycin, teicoplanin, and daptomycin. *S. aureus* and coagulase-negative staphylococci with reduced susceptibility (and occasionally overt resistance) to vancomycin, teicoplanin, and daptomycin have emerged as pathogens.[36] Reduced susceptibility to vancomycin among MRSA is manifested as vancomycin intermediate *S. aureus* (VISA, MIC 4 to 16 μg/mL) or heteroresistant vancomycin intermediate *S. aureus* (hVISA). In hVISA, although the MIC suggests that the isolate is vancomycin susceptible (MIC ≤2.0 μg/mL), there are subpopulations that require higher concentrations for inhibition and killing.[37] VISA and hVISA may emerge during vancomycin treatment and result in failure.[38] MRSA that develop reduced susceptibility to vancomycin may be nonsusceptible to daptomycin. Thus, the antibiotic susceptibility of MRSA recovered from patients who have failed vancomycin therapy must be carefully reassessed.

Among staphylococci killed by beta-lactam antibiotics or vancomycin, the bactericidal effects of these agents can be enhanced by aminoglycosides. Combinations of semisynthetic penicillinase-resistant penicillins or vancomycin with rifampin do not result in predictable bactericidal synergism; nevertheless, rifampin has unique activity against staphylococcal infections that involve foreign material and is included in regimens for staphylococcal PVE.[39]

STAPHYLOCOCCAL NATIVE VALVE ENDOCARDITIS. The semisynthetic penicillinase-resistant penicillins are the preferred treatment of endocarditis caused by methicillin-susceptible staphylococci. When patients have a non-immediate penicillin allergy, a first-generation cephalosporin can be used. Treatment with beta-lactam antibiotics plus gentamicin has not increased the cure rates for staphylococcal endocarditis, although this combination has modestly accelerated the eradication of staphylococci in vegetations and in the blood.[39] The potential benefit from adding gentamicin to beta-lactam therapy for *S. aureus* IE, even when it is limited to the initial 3 to 5 days of therapy, however, is offset by nephrotoxicity. Thus, routine use of this combination is not advised.[36,40] The role for combination therapy is less well defined in NVE caused by coagulase-negative staphylococci.

In IV drug addicts, methicillin-susceptible *S. aureus* endocarditis that is uncomplicated and limited to the right-sided heart valves has been effectively treated with 2 weeks of semisynthetic penicillinase-resistant penicillin (but not vancomycin) given alone or in combination with gentamicin 1 mg/kg intravenously or intramuscularly every 8 hours (normal renal function). Patients with right-sided *S. aureus* who develop peripheral signs suggesting left-sided infection or with other localized infection are not candidates for abbreviated therapy. Vancomycin or daptomycin (6 mg/kg once daily) for 4 weeks is recommended when right-sided IE is caused by MRSA.[15,36]

Left-sided NVE caused by MRSA requires treatment with vancomycin (**Table 67-10**) or daptomycin. Vancomycin doses to achieve trough serum concentrations of 15 to 20 μg/mL are recommended even though this may be associated with nephrotoxicity.[41] Vancomycin killing of MRSA with a vancomycin MIC of 1.5 to 2.0 μg/mL may be suboptimal even with aggressive dosing. Accordingly, in this setting, some experts prefer treatment with daptomycin (doses from 6 to 10 mg/kg daily, normal renal function) even though this indication is not approved by the Food and Drug Administration. Bacteremia in MRSA IE often persists for 5 to 7 days in spite of treatment.[36,38] With vancomycin therapy, persistent bacteremia or later relapse may be accompanied by emergence of reduced susceptibility (see earlier) and requires infectious disease consultation. Experience in treating MRSA IE with linezolid, although the isolates are usually susceptible, is limited. Teicoplanin (not available in the United States) is a possible alternative, but its efficacy is potentially less than that of vancomycin. Combining gentamicin with vancomycin to enhance activity against MRSA is associated with nephrotoxicity and is not recommended routinely.[15] The addition of rifampin to vancomycin for treatment of methicillin-resistant *S. aureus* NVE has not been beneficial.

STAPHYLOCOCCAL PROSTHETIC VALVE ENDOCARDITIS. *S. aureus* and coagulase-negative staphylococcal PVE should be treated with three antibiotics in combination (**Table 67-11**).[15,39] Rifampin provides unique antistaphylococcal activity when infection involves foreign bodies. However, rifampin-resistant staphylococci rapidly emerge when rifampin is used alone or in combination with only vancomycin or a beta-lactam antibiotic. Consequently, staphylococcal PVE is treated with two antimicrobials plus rifampin.[10,15,39]

For PVE caused by methicillin-resistant staphylococci, start treatment with vancomycin plus gentamicin and add rifampin after 2 or 3 days if the organism is susceptible to gentamicin. If the organism is resistant to gentamicin, an effective alternative antibiotic, such as another aminoglycoside or a quinolone, should be used in lieu of gentamicin.[10,15] Trimethoprim-sulfamethoxazole or linezolid could be considered also. For treatment of PVE caused by methicillin-susceptible staphylococci, a semisynthetic penicillinase-resistant penicillin should be substituted for vancomycin in the combination regimen (see Table 67-11). Because heteroresistance may confound detection of methicillin resistance in coagulase-negative staphylococci, these organisms should be considered methicillin resistant, particularly when PVE occurs during the initial postoperative year, until susceptibility is conclusively established.

Coagulase-negative staphylococcal PVE that occurs within the initial year after valve placement and *S. aureus* PVE are often complicated by perivalvular extension of infection. Their outcome is improved if early surgical intervention is combined with appropriate combination antimicrobial therapy.[12,13,15]

TABLE 67-10 Treatment of Staphylococcal Endocarditis in the Absence of Prosthetic Material

ANTIBIOTIC	DOSAGE AND ROUTE*	DURATION
Methicillin-susceptible staphylococci†		
Nafcillin or oxacillin	2 g IV every 4 hr	4-6 weeks
or		
Cefazolin	2 g IV every 8 hr	4-6 weeks
or		
Vancomycin	15 to 20 mg/kg actual body weight, IV every 8 to 12 hr	4-6 weeks
Methicillin-resistant staphylococci‡		
Vancomycin§	15 to 20 mg/kg actual body weight, IV every 8 to 12 hr	4-6 weeks

*Dosages are for patients with normal renal function; see Table 67-6 footnote.

†For treatment of endocarditis caused by penicillin-susceptible staphylococci (MIC ≤ 0.1 μg/mL), aqueous penicillin G 18-24 million units/24 hr) can be used for 4 to 6 weeks instead of nafcillin or oxacillin. Cefazolin or vancomycin may be used in selected penicillin-allergic patients contingent on degree of allergic response.

‡For staphylococcal infection, vancomycin target trough serum concentration is 15 to 20 μg/mL.

§If vancomycin MIC > 1.5 μg/mL, see text for daptomycin use.

Modified from Baddour LM, Wilson WR, Bayer AS, et al: Infective endocarditis: Diagnosis, antimicrobial therapy, and management of complications. Circulation 111:3167, 2005.

TABLE 67-11 Treatment of Staphylococcal Endocarditis in the Presence of a Prosthetic Valve or Other Prosthetic Material

ANTIBIOTIC	DOSAGE AND ROUTE*	DURATION
Regimen for methicillin-resistant staphylococci†		
Vancomycin‡	15 to 20 mg/kg actual body weight, IV every 8 to 12 hr	≥6 weeks
plus		
Rifampin	300 mg PO every 8 hr	≥6 weeks
and		
Gentamicin§	1.0 mg/kg IM or IV every 8 hr	2 weeks
Regimen for methicillin-susceptible staphylococci		
Nafcillin or oxacillin¶	2 g IV every 4 hr	≥6 weeks
plus		
Rifampin	300 mg PO every 8 hr	≥6 6weeks
and		
Gentamicin§	1.0 mg/kg IM or IV every 8 hr	2 weeks

*Dosages are for patients with normal renal function. See Table 67-6 footnote for gentamicin dosing.
†If vancomycin MIC >1.5 μg/mL, see text for daptomycin use.
‡For staphylococcal infection, vancomycin trough serum concentration is 15 to 20 μg/mL.
§Use during initial 2 weeks of treatment. If strain is gentamicin resistant, see text for alternatives.
¶Cefazolin 2 g IV every 8 hours can be used in lieu of these agents in patients with non–immediate-type penicillin allergy. Vancomycin is used with immediate-type allergy.
Modified from Baddour LM, Wilson WR, Bayer AS, et al: Infective endocarditis: Diagnosis, antimicrobial therapy, and management of complications. Circulation 111:3167, 2005.

TABLE 67-12 Treatment of Endocarditis Caused by HACEK Microorganisms*

ANTIBIOTIC	DOSAGE AND ROUTE†	DURATION
Ceftriaxone‡	2 g once daily IV or IM	4 weeks
or		
Ampicillin-sulbactam	12 g/24 hr IV given every 4 hr in six equally divided doses	4 weeks

*HACEK microorganisms are *Haemophilus* species, *Aggregatibacter aphrophilus* or *actinomycetemcomitans, Cardiobacterium hominis, Eikenella corrodens,* and *Kingella* species.
†Dosages are for those with normal renal function; see Table 67-6 footnote.
‡Cefotaxime or another third- or fourth-generation cephalosporin in comparable doses may be substituted for ceftriaxone. See text for treatment of patients unable to take beta-lactam antibiotics.
Modified from Baddour LM, Wilson WR, Bayer AS, et al: Infective endocarditis: Diagnosis, antimicrobial therapy, and management of complications. Circulation 111:3167, 2005.

Haemophilus species, *Aggregatibacter* (previously *Actinobacillus*) *actinomycetemcomitans, Cardiobacterium hominis, Eikenella corrodens,* and *Kingella* species (HACEK organisms)

HACEK organisms may produce beta-lactamase, resulting in ampicillin resistance. HACEK organisms are highly susceptible to third-generation cephalosporins; accordingly, these agents are recommended for treatment of NVE or PVE (**Table 67-12**).[15] Treatment with a fluoroquinolone has been recommended for patients who cannot tolerate a beta-lactam antibiotic.[15]

Other Pathogens

Recommendations for therapy of IE caused by unusual organisms are contained in the AHA Scientific Statement and the guidelines of the European Society of Cardiology.[15,42] Amphotericin desoxycholate or a less toxic liposomal amphotericin formulation, at full doses, often combined with 5-fluorocytosine, is recommended for treatment of *Candida* endocarditis. Although it is not of proven benefit, surgical intervention shortly after beginning of medical treatment is advised. Sporadic cases of *Candida* NVE and PVE have been successfully treated with caspofungin, a fungicidal echinocandin agent. Prolonged or indefinite oral azole therapy has been advocated for patients treated either medically or surgically.[15]

Many corynebacteria (diphtheroids) causing IE remain susceptible to penicillin, vancomycin, and aminoglycosides. Strains susceptible to aminoglycosides are killed synergistically by penicillin in combination with an aminoglycoside. *Corynebacterium jeikeium*, although often resistant to penicillin and aminoglycosides, is killed by vancomycin. NVE or PVE caused by *Corynebacterium* species can be treated with the combination of penicillin plus an aminoglycoside or vancomycin, contingent on the susceptibilities of the causative strain.

The antibiotic susceptibility of Enterobacteriaceae (*Escherichia coli, Klebsiella, Enterobacter, Serratia, Salmonella,* and *Proteus* species) and *P. aeruginosa* is unpredictable. IE caused by these organisms is treated with high doses of a highly active beta-lactam plus full doses of an aminoglycoside (i.e., gentamicin 1.7 mg/kg every 8 hours).[15] If *P. aeruginosa* is susceptible, the preferred treatment of IE is tobramycin (8 mg/kg/day intravenously once daily with peak and trough serum concentrations of 15 to 20 μg/mL and <2 μg/mL, respectively) plus piperacillin, ceftazidime, or cefipime.[15]

C. burnetii IE is difficult to eradicate. Treatment for at least 4 years using doxycycline (100 mg twice daily) combined with a quinolone has been advocated. Treatment with doxycycline combined with hydroxychloroquine for 18 to 48 months (mean, 31 months; median, 26 months) may be more effective than longer courses of doxycycline plus a quinolone. Surgery is important in effective treatment.

Culture-Negative Endocarditis. Special studies must be performed to diagnose IE caused by fastidious bacteria and other organisms (see Obtaining Blood Culture Specimens) and to distinguish these from noninfectious mimics of IE (marantic endocarditis, atrial myxoma, antiphospholipid antibody syndrome, acute rheumatic fever, hypernephroma, carcinoid syndrome, and so on). Clinical and epidemiologic clues, such as acute versus subacute presentation, partial response to prior antibiotics, or presence and duration of prosthetic valve, are important in designing therapy. Recommended therapy for patients with suspected NVE who received confounding antibiotic therapy is either ampicillin-sulbactam plus gentamicin (3 mg/kg/day) or vancomycin plus gentamicin and ciprofloxacin; for those with suspected PVE, it is vancomycin plus gentamicin, cefepime, and rifampin.[15] For patients with suspected IE in whom negative cultures are not confounded by prior antibiotics, fastidious organisms must be considered. *Bartonella* species and *C. burnetii* may be the most common of these causes. Suspected *Bartonella* IE is treated with 6 weeks of ceftriaxone plus gentamicin (1 mg/kg every 8 hours for at least 2 weeks) with an additional 6 weeks of doxycycline (100 mg intravenously or orally every 12 hours) if diagnostic studies are confirmatory (see Diagnosis).[43] For those who do not fully respond to empiric antimicrobial therapy, surgical intervention both as therapy and to obtain vegetations for a detailed microbiologic, PCR, and pathologic examination is recommended (see Diagnosis).

Timing the Initiation of Antimicrobial Therapy

Cost-containment pressures frequently result in initiation of antimicrobial therapy for suspected endocarditis immediately after blood culture specimens have been obtained. This practice is appropriate for patients with acute IE that is highly destructive and rapidly progressive and for those presenting with hemodynamic decompensation requiring urgent surgical intervention. Precipitous initiation of therapy in hemodynamically stable patients with suspected subacute endocarditis does not prevent early complications and may, by compromising subsequent blood cultures, obscure the etiologic diagnosis. In the latter patients, particularly in those who have received antibiotics recently, delay of antibiotic therapy briefly pending the results of the initial blood cultures is prudent. If these cultures are not immediately positive, this delay provides an important opportunity to perform additional blood cultures without the confounding effect of empiric treatment.

Monitoring Therapy for Endocarditis. Patients must be carefully monitored during therapy and for several months thereafter. Failure of antimicrobial therapy, myocardial or metastatic abscess, emboli, hypersensitivity to antimicrobial agents, and other complications of therapy (catheter-related infection, thrombophlebitis) or intercurrent illness may be manifested by persistent or recurrent fever. Adverse reactions (fever, rash, neutropenia, and hepatic or renal toxicity) occur in 33% of patients treated for IE with beta-lactam antimicrobials. The serum concentration of vancomycin or aminoglycosides should be measured periodically and doses adjusted to ensure optimal therapy and to avoid adverse events.

Renal function should be monitored in patients receiving these two antimicrobials, and the complete blood count should be monitored in patients receiving high-dose beta-lactam antibiotics or vancomycin. Repeated blood cultures should be performed during the initial days of therapy or if fever persists or recurs to determine whether the bacteremia has been controlled and to detect relapse or new infections.

Outpatient Antimicrobial Therapy. Technical advances allowing safe administration of complex antimicrobial regimens combined with well-developed home care systems that provide supplies and monitor treatment make outpatient treatment feasible. However, only patients who have responded to initial therapy and are free of fever, who are not experiencing threatening complications, who will be compliant with therapy, and who have a home situation that is physically suitable should be considered for outpatient treatment. Because most threatening complications of IE occur during the initial 2 weeks of therapy, some clinicians have suggested that treatment during this period be administered in the inpatient setting or an outpatient setting that provides daily physician oversight. Patients must be instructed to seek advice promptly on encountering unexpected or untoward clinical events and to have regular physician supervision and laboratory monitoring. Outpatient therapy must not result in compromises leading to suboptimal treatment.

Surgical Treatment of Intracardiac Complications

INDICATIONS FOR SURGICAL INTERVENTION. Cardiac surgical intervention has an important role in the treatment of infection that is unresponsive to antibiotics as well as the intracardiac complications of endocarditis (see Table 67G-3). Retrospective data suggest that mortality is unacceptably high when these aspects of IE are treated medically, whereas mortality is reduced when treatment combines antibiotics and surgical intervention.[44,45] The indications for cardiac surgery evolve from these experiences (see Table 67G-3). Surgical intervention for these indications has not been evaluated in randomized prospective trials. However, most retrospective studies of patients with left-sided IE, particularly NVE, wherein the analysis of outcome of surgical versus medical treatment is adjusted for predictors of mortality and the presence of surgical indications, demonstrate improved survival rates with surgery. Benefit of surgery measured at hospital discharge is apparent in those with the most urgent need for intervention and among all patients if the cohort is observed for at least 6 months.[45-49]

Congestive Heart Failure

Medical therapy for NVE that is complicated by moderate to severe (New York Heart Association [NYHA] Class III and IV) CHF related to new or worsening valvular dysfunction results in mortality rates of 50% to 90% versus 20% to 40% for a similar group of patients treated with antibiotics and cardiac surgery.[44] In an analysis controlled for bias against operating on severely ill patients with NVE, surgery on those with moderate to severe CHF was associated with a significantly improved 6-month survival compared with medical treatment.[45] Survival rates among surgically treated patients with PVE complicated by valvular dysfunction and CHF are 45% to 85%; in contrast, few patients with these complications are alive at 6 months when they are treated with antibiotics alone.[10] Patients with aortic valve dysfunction require surgery on a more urgent basis when CHF supervenes. Severe mitral valve insufficiency, nevertheless, results in inexorable CHF and ultimately requires surgical intervention. Echocardiography indicating significant valvular regurgitation during the initial week of endocarditis treatment does not reliably predict the patients who require valve replacement during active endocarditis. Alternatively, despite the absence of significant valvular regurgitation on early echocardiography, marked CHF may still develop. Thus, decisions about surgical intervention should be based on careful serial monitoring.

Unstable Prostheses

Dehiscence of an infected prosthetic valve is a manifestation of paravalvular infection and often results in hemodynamically significant valvular dysfunction. Surgical intervention is recommended for PVE patients with these complications. The risk of invasive infection is increased among patients with onset of PVE within the year after valve implantation and in those with infection of aortic valve prostheses, endocarditis, and PVE caused by invasive antimicrobial-resistant organisms. Clinically stable patients who have overtly unstable and hypermobile prostheses, a finding indicative of dehiscence in excess of 40% of the circumference, are likely to experience progressive valve instability and warrant urgent surgery. Occasional patients with PVE caused by noninvasive, highly antibiotic-susceptible organisms (e.g., streptococci), despite a favorable clinical course, experience minor valve dehiscence without prosthesis instability or hemodynamic deterioration. Surgical treatment of these patients can be deferred unless clear indications arise.

Uncontrolled Infection or Unavailable Effective Antimicrobial Therapy

Surgical intervention has improved the outcome of IE when maximal antibiotic therapy fails to eradicate infection. Surgical intervention is recommended for fungal PVE or NVE, particularly with intracardiac complications; endocarditis caused by some gram-negative bacilli (e.g., *P. aeruginosa, Burkholderia cepacia, Brucella* species); and enterococcal endocarditis caused by a strain resistant to synergistic bactericidal therapy when antibiotic therapy is failing. Perivalvular invasive infection is in some instances a form of ineradicable infection. Relapse of PVE after optimal antimicrobial therapy reflects invasive disease or the difficulty in eradicating infection involving foreign devices and merits surgical intervention. In contrast, patients with uncomplicated NVE who relapse, unless infected with a highly resistant microorganism, are often treated again with intensified, prolonged antimicrobial therapy.

S. aureus Prosthetic Valve Endocarditis. Crude mortality rates for *S. aureus* PVE treated medically range from 48% to 73% as contrasted to 28% to 48% for treatment with antibiotics plus surgery.[9,12,13] Assessment of management strategy is undoubtedly distorted by selection bias, the most ill patients often being denied surgery. Among 33 cases of *S. aureus* PVE analyzed in a multivariate model to adjust for confounding variables, the presence of intracardiac complications was associated with a 13.7-fold increased risk of death, and surgical intervention during active disease was accompanied by a 20-fold reduction in mortality. Data suggest that early surgical treatment can improve outcome of patients with *S. aureus* PVE and intracardiac complications.[9,12] Some patients younger than 50 years, with an American Society of Anesthesiologists score of 3 and neither intracardiac nor central nervous system complications, may do well with medical therapy.[13]

Perivalvular Invasive Infection. Perivalvular abscess or intracardiac fistula formation occurs in 10% to 14% of patients with NVE and 45% to 60% of those with PVE. Persistent, otherwise unexplained fever despite appropriate antimicrobial therapy or pericarditis in patients with aortic valve endocarditis suggests infection extending beyond the valve leaflet. New-onset and persistent electrocardiographic conduction abnormalities, although not a sensitive indicator of perivalvular infection (28% to 53%), are relatively specific (85% to 90%). TEE is superior to TTE for detection of invasive infection in patients with NVE and PVE. Abscesses suspected but not detected by initial and repeated TEE may be detected by cardiac magnetic resonance imaging or multislice CT scans. Cardiac catheterization adds little to these imaging studies and is not recommended unless coronary angiography is needed.

Cardiac surgery should be considered to débride abscesses, allowing eradication of uncontrolled infection, and to reconstruct cardiac structures, restoring hemodynamics and alleviating CHF. Sporadic patients with small, structurally insignificant abscesses in which the cavity is open to the circulatory stream have been treated medically.[15]

Left-Sided S. aureus Endocarditis. Because this infection is difficult to control, highly destructive, and associated with high mortality (25% to 47%), some investigators have suggested that these patients should be considered for surgical treatment when the response to antimicrobial therapy is not prompt and complete. Patients with *S. aureus* left-sided NVE and vegetations that are visible by TTE (versus requiring TEE) are at increased risk for arterial emboli and death and thus should be considered for surgery. IV drug abusers with *S. aureus* endocarditis limited to the tricuspid or pulmonary valves often experience prolonged fever during antimicrobial therapy; nevertheless, most respond to antimicrobial therapy and do not require surgery.

UNRESPONSIVE CULTURE-NEGATIVE ENDOCARDITIS. Patients who have culture-negative endocarditis and do not respond to empiric antimicrobial therapy, particularly those with PVE, should be considered for surgical intervention. If endocarditis is not marantic, persistent fever likely represents either unrecognized perivalvular infection or ineffective antimicrobial therapy. Surgery may help clarify the cause as well as facilitate treatment.

LARGE VEGETATIONS (>10 MM) AND THE PREVENTION OF SYSTEMIC EMBOLI. Systemic embolization is increased in patients with vegetations larger than 10 mm versus those with smaller or undetectable vegetations (33% to 37% versus 19%). In addition, mitral valve location and *S. aureus* infection increase the risk of an embolic event.[25] Although a relation may exist between vegetation characteristics—including size, mobility, and extent (number of leaflets involved)—and embolic complications, the implications for surgical intervention are not clear. The recommendation for valve surgery to prevent arterial emboli based on vegetation characteristics or after two major arterial emboli can be questioned.[15,17,42]

In deciding to intervene with cardiac surgery to prevent arterial emboli, many factors must be considered carefully. The rate of systemic or cerebral emboli in patients with NVE and PVE decreases rapidly during the course of effective antibiotic therapy. Thus, maximum benefit requires early surgery.[25,42] Also, it is not clear that valve replacement reduces the frequency of systemic emboli. The morbidity and mortality caused by cerebral and coronary emboli, the major events to be prevented, must be compared with the immediate and long-term risks of valve replacement or, if feasible, vegetectomy and valve repair. The sum of the clinical findings, risk of embolization, and other surgically correctable intracardiac complications may be sufficient to justify surgery in spite of these immediate and remote hazards. However, only on rare occasions is vegetation size alone or a prior systemic embolus a sufficient independent indication for surgical intervention.[15,28,42]

REPAIR OF INTRACARDIAC DEFECTS

Timing of Surgical Intervention

When endocarditis is complicated by valvular regurgitation and significant CHF, surgical intervention before the development of severe intractable hemodynamic dysfunction is recommended, regardless of the duration of antimicrobial therapy.[15,44,45,50] Postoperative mortality correlates with the severity of preoperative hemodynamic dysfunction; consequently, this approach is justified.[15] In patients who have valvular dysfunction and in whom infection is controlled and cardiac function is compensated, surgery may be delayed until antimicrobial therapy has been completed.

More specific recommendations for timing of surgery have been presented.[44] Strong clinical evidence suggests emergent (same day) surgery for acute aortic regurgitation with mitral valve preclosure, acute severe mitral or aortic valve regurgitation with pulmonary edema or cardiogenic shock, sinus of Valsalva rupture into the right side of the heart, and fistula to the pericardial sac; urgent (1 to 2 days) surgery for valve obstruction, unstable prosthesis, acute aortic or mitral regurgitation with CHF (NYHA Class III to IV), septal perforation, perivalvular extension of infection, and no effective antimicrobial therapy; and early elective surgery for progressive paravalvular regurgitation, valve dysfunction and persistent fever, and fungal IE.[42,44]

It may be desirable to delay surgical intervention to avoid worsening of neurologic status or death in patients who have sustained recent neurologic injury. Among patients who have had a nonhemorrhagic embolic stroke, exacerbation of cerebral dysfunction occurs during cardiac surgery in 44% of cases when the interval between the stroke and surgery is 7 days or less but decreases progressively with time to 10% or less when more than 2 weeks has elapsed. After hemorrhagic intracerebral events, the risk for neurologic worsening or death with cardiac surgery persists at 20% even after 1 month.[51] Thus, when the response of IE to antimicrobial therapy and hemodynamic status permit, delay of cardiac surgery for 2 to 3 weeks after a significant embolic infarct and at least a month after intracerebral hemorrhage (with prior repair of a mycotic aneurysm) has been recommended.[42,51] Alternatively, in patients at immediate risk of death in the absence of cardiac surgery, operation during the early days after cerebral infarction has been advocated as lifesaving in spite of potential neurologic risk.[42] Urgent surgery should not be delayed by the fortuitous discovery of an asymptomatic cerebral infarct, nor is routine screening for asymptomatic infarcts recommended as a guide for timing surgery.

Duration of Antimicrobial Therapy After Surgical Intervention

Inflammatory changes and bacteria visible with Gram stain have been found in vegetations removed from patients who had successfully completed standard recommended antibiotic therapy for IE: 29 of 53 (55%) still taking antibiotics; 7 of 15 (47%) without antibiotics for less than a month; and 4 of 18 (22%) without antibiotics for 1 to 6 months. Cultures of these vegetations yielded bacteria in 5, 0, and 1 instances, respectively. If vegetation cultures are negative, neither visible bacteria nor PCR detection of bacterial DNA indicates that antimicrobial therapy has failed or that a full course of antibiotic therapy is needed postoperatively. The duration of antimicrobial therapy after surgery depends on the length of preoperative therapy, the antibiotic susceptibility of the causative organism, the presence of paravalvular invasive infection, and the culture status of the vegetation. In general, for uncomplicated NVE caused by relatively antibiotic-responsive organisms with negative cultures of operative specimens, the duration of preoperative plus postoperative therapy should at least equal a full course of recommended therapy with perhaps 2 weeks or less of therapy postoperatively.[52] For patients with prostheses sewn into a débrided abscess cavity or with positive intraoperative cultures, a full course of therapy should be given postoperatively.[15] Patients with PVE should receive a full course of antimicrobial therapy postoperatively when the causative organism is seen or cultured in resected material.

Treatment of Extracardiac Complications

SPLENIC ABSCESS. Three percent to 5% of patients with IE develop a splenic abscess.[15] Although splenic defects can be identified by ultrasonography and computed tomography, these tests in isolation usually cannot reliably discriminate between abscess and the far more common infarct. Persistent fever and progressive enlargement of the lesion during antimicrobial therapy suggest that it is an abscess. Successful therapy for splenic abscesses requires drainage percutaneously or a splenectomy.[15,28,42] If possible, abscesses in the spleen should be treated effectively before valve replacement surgery; alternatively, splenectomy should be performed as soon thereafter as surgical risks permit.[28,42]

MYCOTIC ANEURYSMS AND SEPTIC ARTERITIS. Two percent to 10% of patients with IE have mycotic aneurysms, and half of these involve cerebral vessels. Cerebral mycotic aneurysms occur at the branch points in cerebral vessels and are generally located distally over the cerebral cortex, particularly in branches of the middle cerebral artery. Aneurysms arise either from occlusion of vessels by septic emboli with secondary arteritis and vessel wall destruction or from injury caused by bacteremia seeding the vessel wall through the vasa vasorum. *S. aureus* is commonly implicated in the former mechanism and viridans streptococci in the latter. Devastating intracranial hemorrhage is the initial clinical event in many patients with mycotic aneurysms. Focal deficits from embolic events, persistent focal headache, unexplained neurologic deterioration, or cerebrospinal fluid with erythrocytes and xanthochromia may be premonitory. Magnetic resonance or spiral computed tomographic angiography, each of which has a 90% to 95% sensitivity for aneurysms >5 mm, has been recommended for patients experiencing premonitory symptoms, especially if cardiac surgery or anticoagulant therapy is planned.[28] Cerebral angiography is required to evaluate patients with suspected small (≤2 mm) aneurysms or intracerebral hemorrhage. Rupture or leakage may occur at any point before or during early antibiotic therapy or rarely later. Mortality is 80% with aneurysm rupture.

Unruptured mycotic aneurysms should be observed during antimicrobial therapy. Half of these may resolve.[28] If it is feasible anatomically, aneurysms that have ruptured should be repaired.[53] Surgery should be considered for a single aneurysm that enlarges during or after antimicrobial therapy. Anticoagulant therapy should be avoided in patients with a persisting mycotic aneurysm. There is no accurate estimation of risk for late rupture of persisting aneurysms. Prevailing opinion favors the resection of single aneurysms, particularly those larger than 7 mm, that persist after therapy whenever possible without serious neurologic injury.[53] The potential existence of occult aneurysms in patients without neurologic symptoms or in those who have had a nondiagnostic angiographic evaluation is not considered a contraindication to anticoagulant therapy after completion of antimicrobial therapy.

Extracranial mycotic aneurysms should be managed as outlined for cerebral aneurysms. Those that leak, that are expanding during therapy, or that persist after therapy should be repaired. Particular attention should be given to aneurysms that involve intra-abdominal arteries, rupture of which could result in life-threatening hemorrhage.[28]

ANTICOAGULANT THERAPY. Patients with PVE involving devices that would usually warrant maintenance anticoagulation are continued on careful anticoagulant therapy with either warfarin or heparin. Some investigators advise that anticoagulant therapy be withdrawn from patients with *S. aureus* PVE during the initial 2 weeks of treatment.[15] In the absence of an accepted indication, anticoagulation is not initiated as prophylaxis against IE-related thromboembolism in patients with PVE involving devices that do not usually require this therapy. Anticoagulant therapy in patients with NVE is limited to patients for whom there is a clear indication and no increased risk for intracranial hemorrhage. If central nervous system complications occur in patients who are receiving anticoagulant therapy, anticoagulation should be reversed immediately. In a randomized blinded trial, initiation of aspirin, 325 mg daily, did not reduce the risk of emboli and was likely associated with increased bleeding.[54] Data are inconclusive about the benefits or risks of continued aspirin in patients who were using this medication before having IE diagnosed.

Response to Therapy

Within a week after initiation of effective antimicrobial therapy, almost 70% of patients with NVE or PVE are afebrile, and 90% have defervesced by the end of the second week of treatment. Fever persists longer in patients with *S. aureus, P. aeruginosa,* or culture-negative IE as well as IE characterized by microvascular phenomena and major embolic complications. Persistence (or recurrence) of fever or a low percentage decline in C-reactive protein more than 10 days after initiation of antibiotic therapy identifies patients with increased mortality rates and with complications of infection or therapy.[55] These patients should be evaluated for intracardiac complications, focal extracardiac septic complications, intercurrent nosocomial infections, recurrent pulmonary emboli (patients with right-sided IE), drug-associated fever, additional underlying illnesses, and, if appropriate, in-hospital substance abuse. Blood cultures should be repeated and the antimicrobial susceptibility of the causative organism should be reevaluated. Fever attributed to the antimicrobial therapy may warrant revision of treatment if a suitable alternative is available. In the absence of effective alternative therapy, treatment can be continued despite drug fever if there is no significant end-organ toxicity. The increased erythrocyte sedimentation rate and anemia may not correct until after therapy has been completed.

Mortality rates for large series of patients with NVE treated since 1980 ranged from 13% to 20%.[3,6,18] Death from IE has been associated with increased age (>65 to 70 years), underlying diseases, infection involving the aortic valve, development of CHF, nosocomial origin, *S. aureus* infection, renal failure, and central nervous system complications.[6,26] Early surgical treatment of CHF due to valve dysfunction has decreased the mortality associated with CHF. As a result, neurologic events, uncontrolled infection, and myocardial abscess have accounted for a larger proportion of deaths in recent series.

Mortality rates among patients with IE caused by viridans streptococci, enterococci, and *S. gallolyticus* have ranged from 4% to 16%. Mortality rates are higher with left-sided NVE caused by other organisms: *S. aureus,* 25% to 47%; non-viridans streptococci (groups B, C, and G), 13% to 50%; *C. burnetii,* 5% to 37%; *P. aeruginosa,* Enterobacteriaceae, and fungi, >50%.

Outcome for patients with PVE, as contrasted with NVE, has been less favorable. Before 1980, mortality rates for PVE with onset less than 60 days after surgery and PVE with later onset averaged 70% and 45%, respectively. With the recognition that PVE outcome would benefit from surgical intervention, mortality rates have decreased to 14% to 36%.[9,11] Among patients with PVE treated surgically, survival rates at 4 to 6 years ranged from 50% to 82%. Long-term survival was adversely affected by the presence of moderate or severe CHF at discharge. Survival rates are not related to time of onset after cardiac surgery.

Among patients with NVE (nonaddicts) discharged after medical or medical-surgical therapy, survival was 71% to 88% at 5 years and 61% to 81% at 10 years. Among patients treated surgically for NVE, survival at 5 years ranged from 70% to 80%.

RELAPSE AND RECURRENCE. Relapse of IE usually occurs within 2 months of discontinuation of antibiotic treatment. Patients who have NVE caused by penicillin-susceptible viridans streptococci and who receive a recommended course of therapy experience less than 2% relapse. From 8% to 20% of patients with enterococcal IE relapse after standard therapy. Patients with IE caused by *S. aureus*, Enterobacteriaceae, or fungi are more likely to experience overt failure of therapy rather than relapse; nevertheless, 4% of patients with *S. aureus* IE suffer relapse. Relapse of fungal endocarditis, which occurs in at least 17% to 30% of cases, may be seen at long intervals after treatment. Relapse occurs in 10% of patients with PVE overall and in 6% to 15% of those treated surgically.

Among nonaddicts with an initial episode of NVE or PVE, 4.5% to 7% experience one or more additional episodes. Recurrent IE episodes share the clinical and microbiologic features and response to therapy noted in primary episodes. IV drug abuse is now the most common predisposing factor for recurrent IE.

Prevention

The AHA has dramatically restricted its recommendations for the chemoprophylaxis for IE.[56] These recommendations reflect an evaluation of data documenting procedure-related bacteremia, the antibiotic susceptibility of procedure-related bacteremic organisms that cause endocarditis most commonly, the results of prophylaxis studies in animal models of endocarditis, population-based studies of endocarditis and the prevalence of valvulopathy at risk for endocarditis, the association of excess morbidity with specific forms of endocarditis, and retrospective and prospective studies of endocarditis prophylaxis. The committee recommends that prophylactic antibiotics be used in conjunction with dental and oral procedures only in those patients with underlying cardiac conditions at the highest risk for a severe morbid outcome as a consequence of endocarditis. The recommendations are acknowledged to be "less well established by evidence" and to represent the consensus opinion of experts. The committee's reasoning is summarized here.

GENERAL METHODS. The incidence of IE can be significantly reduced by total surgical correction of some congenital lesions, such as patent ductus arteriosus, ventricular septal defect, and pulmonary stenosis. Maintaining good oral hygiene, which decreases the frequency of bacteremia that accompanies daily activities, is an important preventive measure. Oral hygiene and dental health should be addressed before prosthetic valves are placed electively. Some activities or procedures likely to induce bacteremia should be avoided. Oral irrigating devices are not recommended. The use of central intravascular catheters and urinary catheters should be minimized. Infections associated with bacteremia must be treated promptly and, if possible, eradicated before the involved tissues are incised or manipulated.

CHEMOPROPHYLAXIS. Transient bacteremia occurs commonly after manipulation of the teeth and periodontal tissues and various dental procedures. In addition, transient bacteremia frequently develops during routine daily activities involving the oral cavity: brushing and flossing teeth, using water irrigation devices, and chewing. Considering the relative infrequency of dental visits or oral surgery, the cumulative exposure of cardiac structures to bacteremia is dramatically greater from routine daily activities than from dental procedures. It has been estimated that brushing teeth twice daily for a year results in 154,000 times greater bacteremia exposure than extraction of a single tooth, the dental procedure that induces the greatest risk of bacteremia. Thus, the risk of seeding cardiac structures is far greater from routine daily activities than from dental manipulations. Furthermore, the ability of antibiotics or topical antiseptics to prevent or to reduce bacteremia precipitated by dental procedures is not established and is impaired even further by the gradual increase in the frequency of resistance of viridans streptococci to antibiotics advocated for prophylaxis.

The causal association of dental manipulations with endocarditis is not established, and in fact, the often implied association may result from biased observations. Population-based studies in the Netherlands concluded that dental procedures caused at best only a small fraction of IE cases and that prophylaxis, even if totally effective, would prevent only a small number of cases. Strom and associates did not find that premorbid dental procedures increased in patients with endocarditis compared with uninfected controls.[57] In France, the estimate of IE related to unprotected procedures was 1 per 10,700 and 1 per 54,300, with prosthetic and native valve predispositions, respectively.[58] Thus, a huge prophylaxis effort may be required to prevent one case of IE.

The committee recognized the absence of data documenting that antibiotic prophylaxis prevents endocarditis as a result of procedure-induced bacteremia; however, it could not exclude that a small number of IE cases could be prevented by antibiotic prophylaxis. Nevertheless, in weighing the benefits, potential adverse events, and cost associated with antibiotic prophylaxis, the committee considered that prophylaxis is not warranted on the basis of a lifetime increased risk of IE related to cardiac disease but rather that prophylaxis should be restricted to those patients whose cardiac abnormality places them at the highest risk for a morbid outcome from IE (see Table 67G-1). Notably, prophylaxis is no longer recommended for patients with mitral valve prolapse or for cardiac conditions other than those noted (see Table 67G-1).

The new guidelines advise that prophylaxis be used in the high-risk group before any dental procedures that involve gingival tissue or the periapical region of a tooth or that perforate oral mucosa. Procedures and events not warranting prophylaxis include routine intraoral anesthetic injection through uninfected tissue, taking of dental radiographs, placement or adjustment of removable prosthodontic or orthodontic brackets or appliances, shedding of deciduous teeth, or bleeding due to lip or oral mucosa trauma.[56] The regimens recommended are single-dose modifications of those previously advocated (**Table 67-13**). These same regimens are considered appropriate for at-risk patients (see Table 67G-1) who will undergo incision or biopsy of the respiratory mucosa, such as tonsillectomy, adenoidectomy, or bronchoscopy.

The causal relationship between gastrointestinal and genitourinary tract procedures and IE is less well defined than that for dental procedures. Consequently, antibiotics are not recommended to prevent endocarditis when at-risk patients undergo these procedures.[56] When at-risk patients with gastrointestinal or genitourinary tract infection are to receive antibiotic therapy to prevent wound infections or procedure-induced sepsis, it is reasonable to include an agent active against enterococci. Eradication of genitourinary tract infection, especially that caused by enterococci, before manipulation is advised. Similarly, in at-risk patients undergoing surgery on infected skin or musculoskeletal tissue, antibiotic therapy should include an agent active against anticipated or documented *S. aureus* (including methicillin-resistant strains) and beta-hemolytic streptococci.

TABLE 67-13 Regimens for Prophylaxis Against Endocarditis: Use with Dental, Oral, and Upper Respiratory Tract Procedures

SETTING PROCEDURE	REGIMEN ADMINISTERED 30-60 MINUTES BEFORE*
Standard regimen†	Amoxicillin 2.0 g PO
Amoxicillin- or penicillin-allergic patients	Cephalexin 2 g PO† *or* Azithromycin or clarithromycin 500 mg PO *or* Clindamycin 600 mg PO
Patients unable to take oral medications	Ampicillin 2.0 g IM or IV *or* Cefazolin or ceftriaxone 1 g IV†
Ampicillin-, amoxicillin-, or penicillin-allergic patients unable to take oral medications	Clindamycin 300 mg IV 30 min before procedure, then 150 mg 6 hr after initial dose

*Dosages for adults. Initial pediatric dosages are as follows: ampicillin or amoxicillin, 50 mg/kg; clindamycin, 20 mg/kg; azithromycin or clarithromycin, 15 mg/kg.
†Cephalosporins are not used in patients with history of anaphylaxis, angioedema, or urticaria associated with penicillin, ampicillin, or cephalosporins.
Modified from Wilson W, Taubert KA, Gewitz M, et al: Prevention of infective endocarditis: Guidelines from the American Heart Association. Circulation 116:1736, 2007.

Patients with at-risk cardiac lesions should be given written material about their predisposing lesion and the recommended antibiotic prophylaxis.

Future Perspectives

The continued significant mortality and morbidity associated with IE stimulate ongoing efforts to improve diagnostic, preventive, and therapeutic strategies. Molecular detection of nonviable, nonculturable, and even routine causative organisms is likely and will provide more rapid, efficient, and sensitive diagnostic tests. The increasing prominence of *S. aureus* as a cause of IE and its increasing resistance to antibiotics have stimulated efforts to develop staphylococcal vaccines. If it is proven to be efficacious, a vaccine could protect patients at continuous high risk for *S. aureus* IE (e.g., patients with chronic health care exposure [hemodialysis] and implanted cardiac devices). New antibiotics are under development for treatment of resistant gram-positive bacteria, including MRSA. Groups of investigators are collaborating to develop large prospectively collected endocarditis data bases. Using sophisticated analytic techniques, these investigators will address therapeutic questions that are not amenable to randomized clinical trials and thus provide data for evidenced-based decision making in difficult areas of treatment, such as surgical indications for and treatment of unusual causes of IE.

REFERENCES

Epidemiology

1. Moreillon P, Que YA: Infective endocarditis. Lancet 363:139, 2004.
2. Tleyjeh IM, Steckelberg JM, Murad HS, et al: Temporal trends in infective endocarditis: A population-based study in Olmsted County, Minnesota. JAMA 293:3022, 2005.
3. Murdoch DR, Corey GR, Hoen B, et al: Clinical presentation, etiology, and outcome of infective endocarditis in the 21st century. Arch Intern Med 169:463, 2009.
4. Fowler VG Jr, Miro JM, Hoen B, et al: *Staphylococcus aureus* endocarditis: A consequence of medical progress. JAMA 293:3012, 2005.
5. Hill EE, Herijgers P, Claus P, et al: Infective endocarditis: Changing epidemiology and predictors of 6-month mortality: A prospective cohort study. Eur Heart J 28:196, 2007.
6. Martin-Davila P, Fortun J, Navas E, et al: Nosocomial endocarditis in a tertiary hospital: An increasing trend in native valve cases. Chest 128:772, 2005.
7. Gebo KA, Burkey MD, Lucas GM, et al: Incidence of, risk factors for, clinical presentation, and 1-year outcomes of infective endocarditis in an urban HIV cohort. J AIDS 43:426, 2006.

Etiologic Microorganisms

8. Wang A, Athan E, Pappas PA, et al: Contemporary clinical profile and outcome of prospective valve endocarditis. JAMA 297:1354, 2007.
9. Habib G, Tribouilloy C, Thuny F, et al: Prosthetic valve endocarditis: Who needs surgery? A multicentre study of 104 cases. Heart 91:954, 2005.
10. Karchmer AW, Longworth DL: Infections of intracardiac devices. Cardiol Clin 21:253, 2003.
11. Rivas P, Alonso J, Moya J, et al: The impact of hospital-acquired infections on the microbial etiology and prognosis of late-onset prosthetic valve endocarditis. Chest 128:764, 2005.
12. Chirouze C, Cabell CH, Fowler VG Jr, et al: Prognostic factors in 61 cases of *Staphylococcus aureus* prosthetic valve infective endocarditis from the International Collaboration on Endocarditis merged database. Clin Infect Dis 38:1323, 2004.
13. Sohail MR, Martin KR, Wilson WR, et al: Medical versus surgical management of *Staphylococcus aureus* prosthetic valve endocarditis. Am J Med 119:147, 2006.
14. Benito N, Miro JM, de Lazzari E, et al: Health care–associated native valve endocarditis: Importance of non-nosocomial acquisition. Ann Intern Med 150:586, 2009.
15. Baddour LM, Wilson WR, Bayer AS, et al: Diagnosis, antimicrobial therapy, and management of complications. A statement for healthcare professionals from the Committee on Rheumatic Fever, Endocarditis, and Kawasaki Disease, Council on Cardiovascular Disease in the Young, and the Councils on Clinical Cardiology, Stroke, and Cardiovascular Surgery and Anesthesia, American Heart Association. Circulation 111:e394, 2005.
16. McDonald JR, Olaison L, Anderson DJ, et al: Enterococcal endocarditis: 107 cases from the international collaboration on endocarditis merged database. Am J Med 118:759, 2005.
17. Stevens MP, Edmond MB: Endocarditis due to vancomycin-resistant enterococci: Case report and review of the literature. Clin Infect Dis 41:1134, 2005.
18. Miro JM, Anguera I, Cabell CH, et al: *Staphylococcus aureus* native valve infective endocarditis: Report of 566 episodes from the International Collaboration on Endocarditis merged database. Clin Infect Dis 41:507, 2005.
19. Chu VH, Woods CW, Miro JM, et al: Emergence of coagulase-negative staphylococci as a cause of native valve endocarditis. Clin Infect Dis 46:232, 2008.
20. Morpeth S, Murdoch D, Cabell CH, et al: Non-HACEK gram-negative bacillus endocarditis. Ann Intern Med 147:829, 2007.
21. Fenollar F, Thuny F, Xeridat B, et al: Endocarditis after acute Q fever in patients with previously undiagnosed valvulopathies. Clin Infect Dis 42:818, 2006.

Pathogenesis, Clinical Features, Diagnosis

22. Nallapareddy SR, Singh KV, Sillanpaa J, et al: Endocarditis and biofilm-associated pili of *Enterococcus faecalis*. J Clin Invest 116:2799, 2006.
23. Nallapareddy SR, Singh KV, Murray BE: Contribution of the collagen adhesin Acm to pathogenesis of *Enterococcus faecium* in experimental endocarditis. Infect Immun 76:4120, 2010.

24. Thuny F, DiSalvo G, Belliard O, et al: Risk of embolism and death in infective endocarditis: Prognostic value of echocardiography. A prospective multicenter study. Circulation 112:69, 2005.
25. Dickerman SA, Abrutyn E, Barsic B, et al: The relationship between the initiation of antimicrobial therapy and the incidence of stroke in infective endocarditis: An analysis from the ICE prospective cohort study (ICE-PCS). Am Heart J 154:1086, 2007.
26. Hasbun R, Vikram HR, Barakat LA, et al: Complicated left-sided native valve endocarditis in adults: Risk classification for mortality. JAMA 289:1933, 2003.
27. Li JS, Sexton DJ, Mick N, et al: Proposed modifications to the Duke criteria for the diagnosis of infective endocarditis. Clin Infect Dis 30:633, 2000.
28. Bayer AS, Bolger AF, Taubert KA, et al: Diagnosis and management of infective endocarditis and its complications. Circulation 98:2936, 1998.
29. Kini V, Logani S, Ky B, et al: Transthoracic and transesophageal echocardiography for the indication of suspected infective endocarditis: Vegetations, blood cultures and imaging. J Am Soc Echocardiograph 23:396, 2010.
30. Vieira MLC, Grinberg M, Pomerantzeff PM, et al: Repeated echocardiographic examinations of patients with suspected infective endocarditis. Heart 90:1020, 2004.
30a. Bonow RO, Carabello B, Chatterjee K, et al: 2008 focused update incorporated into the ACC/AHA 2006 guidelines for the management of patients with valvular heart disease. Circulation 118:e523, 2008.
31. Douglas PS, Khandheria B, Stainback RF, et al: ACCF/ASE,ACEP/ASNC/SCAI/ SCCT/SCMR 2007 appropriateness criteria for transthoracic and transesophageal echocardiography. J Am Coll Cardiol 50:187, 2007.
32. Grijalva M, Horvath R, Dendis M, et al: Molecular diagnosis of culture negative infective endocarditis: Clinical validation in a group of surgically treated patients. Heart 89:263, 2003.
33. Feuchtner GM, Stolzmann P, Dichtl W, et al: Multislice computed tomography in infective endocarditis. J Am Coll Cardiol 53:436, 2009.

Treatment

34. Knoll B, Tleyjeh IM, Steckelberg JM, et al: Infective endocarditis due to penicillin-resistant viridans group streptococci. Clin Infect Dis 44:1585, 2007.
35. Gavalda J, Len O, Miro JM, et al: Treatment of *Enterococcus faecalis* endocarditis with ampicillin plus ceftriaxone. Ann Intern Med 146:574, 2007.
36. Fowler VG Jr, Boucher HW, Corey GR, et al: Daptomycin versus standard therapy for bacteremia and endocarditis caused by *Staphylococcus aureus*. N Engl J Med 355:653, 2006.
37. Tenover FC, Moellering RC Jr: The rationale for revising the Clinical and Laboratory Standards Institute vancomycin minimal inhibitory concentration interpretive criteria for *Staphylococcus aureus*. Clin Infect Dis 44:1208, 2007.
38. Hawkins C, Huang J, Jin N, et al: Persistent *Staphylococcus aureus* bacteremia. Arch Intern Med 167:1861, 2007.
39. Drinkovic D, Morris AJ, Pottumarthy S, et al: Bacteriological outcome of combination versus single-agent treatment for staphylococcal endocarditis. J Antimicrob Chemother 52:820, 2003.
40. Cosgrove SE, Vigliani GA, Campion M, et al: Initial low-dose gentamicin for *Staphylococcus aureus* bacteremia and endocarditis is nephrotoxic. Clin Infect Dis 48:713, 2009.
41. Rybak MJ, Lomaestro BM, Rotschafer JC, et al: Vancomycin therapeutic guidelines. A summary of consensus recommendations from the Infectious Diseases Society of America, the American Society of Health-System Pharmacists and the Society of Infectious Disease Pharmacists. Clin Infect Dis 49:325, 2009.
42. Habib G, Hoen B, Tornos P, et al: Guidelines on the prevention, diagnosis, and treatment of infective endocarditis (new version 2009). Eur Heart J 30:2369, 2009.
43. Rolain JM, Brouqui P, Koehler JE, et al: Recommendations for treatment of human infections caused by *Bartonella* species. Antimicrob Agents Chemother 48:1921, 2004.
44. Olaison L, Pettersson G: Current best practices and guidelines indications for surgical intervention in infective endocarditis. Cardiol Clin 21:235, 2003.
45. Vikram HR, Buenconsejo J, Hasbun R, et al: Impact of valve surgery on 6-month mortality in adults with complicated, left-sided native valve endocarditis: A propensity analysis. JAMA 290:3207, 2003.
46. Bannay A, Hoen B, Duval X, et al: The impact of valve surgery on short- and long-term mortality in left-sided infective endocarditis: Do differences in methodological approaches explain previous conflicting results? Eur Heart J doi:10.1093/eurheartj/ehp008:2009.
47. Aksoy O, Sexton DJ, Wang A, et al: Early surgery in patients with infective endocarditis: A propensity score analysis. Clin Infect Dis 44:364, 2007.
48. Nadji G, Goissen T, Brahim A, et al: Impact of early surgery on 6-month outcome in acute infective endocarditis. Int J Cardiol 129:227, 2009.
49. Cabell CH, Abrutyn E, Fowler VG Jr, et al: Use of surgery in patients with native valve infective endocarditis: Results from the International Collaboration on Endocarditis merged database. Am Heart J 150:1092, 2005.
50. Thuny F, Beurtheret S, Mancini J, et al: The timing of surgery influences mortality and morbidity in adults with severe complicated infective endocarditis: A propensity analysis. Eur Heart J doi:10.1093/eurheartj/ehp089:2009.
51. Eishi K, Kawazoe K, Kuriyama Y, et al: Surgical management of infective endocarditis associated with cerebral complications: Multicenter retrospective study in Japan. J Thorac Cardiovasc Surg 110:1745, 1995.
52. Morris AJ, Drinkovic D, Pottumarthy S, et al: Bacteriological outcome after valve surgery for active infective endocarditis: Implications for duration of treatment after surgery [abstract]. Clin Infect Dis 41:187, 2005.
53. Phuong LK, Link M, Wijdicks E: Management of intracranial infectious aneurysms: A series of 16 cases. Neurosurgery 51:1145, 2002.
54. Chan KL, Dumesnil JG, Cujec B, et al: A randomized trial of aspirin on the risk of embolic events in patients with infective endocarditis. J Am Coll Cardiol 42:775, 2003.
55. Verhagen DWM, Hermanides J, Korevaar JC, et al: Prognostic value of serial C-reactive protein measurements in left-sided native valve endocarditis. Arch Intern Med 168:302, 2008.

Prevention

56. Wilson W, Taubert KA, Gewitz M, et al: Prevention of infective endocarditis. Guidelines from the American Heart Association. Circulation 116:1736, 2007.
57. Strom BL, Abrutyn E, Berlin JA, et al: Dental and cardiac risk factors for infective endocarditis: A population-based, case-control study. Ann Intern Med 129:761, 1998.
58. Duval X, Alla F, Hoen B, et al: Estimated risk of endocarditis in adults with predisposing cardiac conditions undergoing dental procedures with or without antibiotic prophylaxis. Clin Infect Dis 42:e102, 2006.

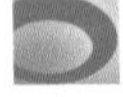

GUIDELINES ROBERT O. BONOW

Infective Endocarditis

The American Heart Association (AHA) guidelines for prevention of infective endocarditis have been evolving for the last 50 years, with the most recent key updates providing recommendations for antibiotic prophylaxis published in 2007.[1] The AHA scientific statement regarding the recommendations for diagnosis and management of this condition were published in 1997.[2] Other guidelines with recommendations relevant to this condition include the American College of Cardiology/American Heart Association (ACC/AHA) guidelines for management of patients with valvular heart disease, updated most recently in 2008.[3]

PREVENTION

The 2007 AHA guidelines represent a marked departure from prior recommendations, previously published in 1997,[4] and greatly reduce the patient population for which prophylactic antibiotics are recommended. These new guidelines note that prior recommendations were based on research showing that antimicrobial prophylaxis is effective for prevention of experimental infective endocarditis in animal models but also acknowledge the lack of evidence that antimicrobial prophylaxis is effective in humans for prevention of endocarditis after dental, gastrointestinal, or genitourinary procedures. The expert committee also considered the complexity of prior guidelines, which required stratification of patients and procedures on their risk for infective endocarditis.

The 2007 AHA guidelines committee concluded that only an extremely small number of cases of infective endocarditis might be prevented by antibiotic prophylaxis for dental procedures even if such prophylaxis was 100% effective. Accordingly, the revised guidelines recommend infective endocarditis prophylaxis for dental procedures only for patients with underlying cardiac conditions associated with the highest risk of adverse outcomes from infective endocarditis (**Table 67G-1**). These new recommendations were incorporated in the 2008 ACC/AHA guidelines update for management of patients with valvular heart disease.[3] That guidelines update, however, also included the following statement regarding individualization of preventive strategies based on physician and patient preference:

> The committee recognizes that decades of previous recommendations for patients with most forms of valvular heart disease and other conditions have been abruptly changed by the new AHA guidelines. Because this may cause consternation among patients, clinicians should be available to discuss the rationale for these new changes with their patients, including the lack of scientific evidence to demonstrate a proven benefit for infective endocarditis prophylaxis. In select circumstances, the committee also understands that some clinicians and some patients may still feel more comfortable continuing with prophylaxis for infective endocarditis, particularly for those with bicuspid aortic valve or coarctation of the aorta, severe mitral valve prolapse, or hypertrophic obstructive cardiomyopathy. In those settings, the clinician should determine that the risks associated with antibiotics are low before continuing a prophylaxis regimen. Over time, and with continuing education, the committee anticipates increasing acceptance of the new guidelines among both provider and patient communities.

For patients with the conditions in which antibiotic prophylaxis is recommended, the antibiotics are intended for dental procedures that involve manipulation of gingival tissue or the periapical region of teeth or

TABLE 67G-1 Cardiac Conditions and Dental Procedures for Which Antibiotic Prophylaxis Is Recommended

Cardiac Conditions Associated with the Highest Risk of Adverse Outcome from Endocarditis for which Prophylaxis with Dental Procedures is Recommended

Prosthetic cardiac valve
Previous infective endocarditis
Congenital heart disease (CHD)
- Unrepaired cyanotic CHD, including those with palliative shunts and conduits
- Completely repaired CHD with prosthetic material or device either by surgery or by catheter intervention during the first 6 months after the procedure
- Repaired CHD with residual defects at the site or adjacent to the site of a prosthetic patch or prosthetic device (which inhibit endothelialization)
- Except for the conditions listed above, antibiotic prophylaxis is no longer recommended for any other form of CHD

Cardiac transplantation recipients who develop cardiac valvulopathy

Dental Procedures for which Endocarditis Prophylaxis is Recommended for High-Risk Patients (see above)

All dental procedures and events that involve manipulation of gingival tissue or the periapical region of teeth or perforation of the oral mucosa **except** the following:
- Routine anesthetic injections through noninfected tissue
- Taking dental radiographs
- Placement of removable prosthodontic or orthodontic appliances
- Adjustment of orthodontic appliances
- Placement of orthodontic brackets
- Shedding of deciduous teeth and bleeding from trauma to the lips or oral mucosa

From Wilson W, Taubert KA, Gewitz M, et al: Prevention of infective endocarditis. Recommendations by the American Heart Association. Circulation 116:1736, 2007.

perforation of the oral mucosa. The guidelines recommend a single dose of amoxicillin or ampicillin as the preferred prophylactic agent for individuals who do not have a history of type I hypersensitive reactions to a penicillin. For individuals who are allergic to penicillins or amoxicillin, alternative recommendations include first-generation oral cephalosporins, clindamycin, azithromycin, or clarithromycin.

Antibiotic administration is not recommended for patients undergoing genitourinary or gastrointestinal tract procedures solely for the purpose of preventing endocarditis. This recommendation is in contrast with previous guidelines that recommended endocarditis antibiotic prophylaxis before some procedures and not others. Antibiotic prophylaxis for bronchoscopy is not recommended unless the procedure involves incision of the respiratory tract mucosa.

INDICATIONS FOR ECHOCARDIOGRAPHY

Echocardiography is strongly supported in virtually all patients with suspected or known infective endocarditis (**Table 67G-2**).[3] The guidelines urge use of transesophageal echocardiography (TEE) when specific questions are not adequately addressed by an initial transthoracic echocardiographic evaluation, such as when the transthoracic study is of poor quality, if the transthoracic echocardiogram is negative despite a high clinical suspicion of endocarditis, if a prosthetic valve is involved, and if there is a high suspicion such as in a patient with staphylococcal bacteremia or in an elderly patient with valvular abnormalities that make diagnosis by transthoracic imaging difficult.

Diagnosis of prosthetic valve endocarditis with transthoracic echocardiography is more difficult than diagnosis of endocarditis of native valves. Thus, the ACC/AHA guidelines suggest a lower threshold for performance of TEE in patients with prosthetic valves and suspected endocarditis (see Table 67G-2).[3]

SURGERY FOR ACTIVE ENDOCARDITIS

The ACC/AHA guidelines for valvular heart disease support performance of surgery for patients with life-threatening congestive heart failure or cardiogenic shock related to active endocarditis.[3] Indications for surgery for patients with stable endocarditis are considered less clear (**Table 67G-3**).

ACKNOWLEDGMENT

Thomas H. Lee, MD, contributed to this section in previous editions of this book.

TABLE 67G-2 ACC/AHA Guidelines for Echocardiography in Endocarditis

INDICATION	CLASS	RECOMMENDATION	LOE
Transthoracic echocardiography	Class I	Detection and characterization of valvular lesions, their hemodynamic severity, and/or ventricular compensation	B
		Detection of vegetations and characterization of lesions in patients in whom IE is suspected	B
		Detection of associated complications (e.g., abscesses, shunts)	B
		Reevaluation in complex IE (e.g., virulent organism, severe hemodynamic lesion, aortic valve involvement, new murmur, persistent or recurrent fever or bacteremia, clinical change, or symptomatic deterioration)	C
	Class IIa	Persistent fever without bacteremia or a new murmur in patients with prosthetic heart valves	C
	Class IIb	Reevaluation of prosthetic valve IE during antibiotic therapy in the absence of clinical deterioration	C
	Class III	Not indicated to reevaluate uncomplicated (including no regurgitation on baseline echocardiogram) native valve IE during antibiotic treatment in the absence of clinical deterioration, new physical findings, or persistent fever	C
Transesophageal echocardiography	Class I	Assess severity of valvular lesions in symptomatic patients with IE, if transthoracic echocardiography is nondiagnostic	C
		Diagnose IE in patients with valvular heart disease and positive blood cultures, if transthoracic echocardiography is nondiagnostic	C
		Assess complications of IE with potential impact on prognosis and management (e.g., abscesses, perforation, and shunts)	C
		First-line diagnostic study to diagnose prosthetic valve IE and assess for complications	C
		Preoperative evaluation in patients with known IE, unless the need for surgery is evident on transthoracic imaging and unless preoperative imaging will delay surgery in urgent cases	C
		Intraoperative monitoring of patients undergoing valve surgery for IE	C
	Class IIa	Diagnose possible IE in patients with persistent staphylococcal bacteremia without a known source	C
	Class IIb	Detection of IE in patients with nosocomial staphylococcal bacteremia	C

IE = infective endocarditis; LOE = level of evidence.

From Bonow RO, Carabello B, Chatterjee K, et al: 2008 focused update incorporated into the ACC/AHA 2006 guidelines for the management of patients with valvular heart disease. Circulation 118:e1, 2008.

CH 67

TABLE 67G-3 ACC/AHA Guidelines for Surgery in Endocarditis

INDICATION	CLASS	RECOMMENDATION	LOE
Surgery for native valve endocarditis	Class I	Acute valve stenosis or regurgitation with heart failure	B
		Acute AR or MR with evidence of elevated filling pressures (such as early closure of the mitral valve in acute AR or moderate or severe pulmonary hypertension)	B
		Fungal endocarditis or IE caused by other highly resistant organisms	B
		IE complicated by heart block, annular or aortic abscess, or destructive penetrating lesions	B
	Class IIa	Recurrent emboli and persistent vegetations despite appropriate antibiotic therapy	C
	Class IIb	Mobile vegetations >10 mm	C
Surgery for prosthetic valve endocarditis	Class I	IE of a prosthetic valve resulting in heart failure	B
		IE of a prosthetic valve with evidence of dehiscence by cine fluoroscopy or echocardiography	B
		IE of a prosthetic valve with evidence of increasing obstruction or worsening regurgitation	C
		IE of a prosthetic valve with complications, such as abscess formation	C
		Consultation with a cardiac surgeon is indicated for patients with IE of a prosthetic valve.	C
	Class IIa	IE of a prosthetic valve with evidence of persistent bacteremia or recurrent emboli despite appropriate antibiotic treatment	C
		IE of a prosthetic valve with relapsing infection	C
	Class III	Routine surgery is not indicated for patients with uncomplicated IE of a prosthetic valve caused by first infection with a sensitive organism	C

AR = aortic regurgitation; IE = infective endocarditis; LOE = level of evidence; MR = mitral regurgitation.

From Bonow RO, Carabello B, Chatterjee K, et al: 2008 focused update incorporated into the ACC/AHA 2006 guidelines for the management of patients with valvular heart disease. Circulation 118:e1, 2008.

REFERENCES

1. Wilson W, Taubert KA, Gewitz M, et al: Prevention of infective endocarditis. Recommendations by the American Heart Association. Circulation 116:1736, 2007.
2. Bayer AS, Bolger AF, Taubert KA, et al: Diagnosis and management of infective endocarditis and its complications. Circulation 98:2936, 1998.
3. Bonow RO, Carabello B, Chatterjee K, et al: 2008 focused update incorporated into the ACC/AHA 2006 guidelines for the management of patients with valvular heart disease. Circulation 118:e1, 2008.
4. Dajani AS, Taubert KA, Wilson W, et al: Prevention of bacterial endocarditis: Recommendations by the American Heart Association. Circulation 96:363, 1997.

CHAPTER 68 The Dilated, Restrictive, and Infiltrative Cardiomyopathies

Joshua M. Hare

Cardiomyopathies are diseases of heart muscle that result from myriad insults, such as genetic defects, cardiac myocyte injury, and infiltration of myocardial tissues. Thus, cardiomyopathies result from both insults to cellular elements of the heart, notably the cardiac myocyte, and processes that are external to cells, such as deposition of abnormal substances into the extracellular matrix. Cardiomyopathies are traditionally defined on the basis of structural and functional phenotypes (**Tables 68-1 and 68-2**), notably dilated (characterized primarily by an enlarged ventricular chamber and reduced cardiac performance),[1] hypertrophic (characterized primarily by thickened, hypertrophic ventricular walls and enhanced cardiac performance), and restrictive (characterized primarily by thickened, stiff ventricular walls that impede diastolic filling of the ventricle; cardiac systolic performance is typically close to normal).[2] A fourth and increasingly appreciated structural and functional phenotype is a cardiomyopathy that primarily involves the right ventricle—arrhythmogenic right ventricular dysplasia/cardiomyopathy. The dilated cardiomyopathy phenotype is often viewed as a "final common pathway" of numerous types of cardiac injuries and is the most common cardiomyopathic phenotype.[3]

The use of the term *cardiomyopathy* was previously reserved for primary diseases of the heart, not including processes affecting valvular structures, coronary vasculature, or pericardium. Because of the recognition of the final common pathway phenomenon, the term *cardiomyopathy* has entered into common use to denote specific cardiomyopathies, such as ischemic cardiomyopathy[4] or valvular cardiomyopathy (see Table 68-1). There is biologic support for this because there is substantial (but clearly not complete[5]) overlap in the altered signaling pathways and compensatory mechanisms in the failing heart, regardless of underlying cause.[3]

Specific Causes. Classification of the causes of cardiomyopathy continues to be a challenge, and a satisfactory and uniformly agreed on classification system remains in evolution.[6] Classification schemes are plagued by the fact that as the causal basis of heart muscle disease becomes increasingly understood, it is also appreciated that for a given etiology, there may be a spectrum of phenotypes that can overlap or evolve. For example, both myocarditis and amyloidosis can have a spectrum of phenotypes ranging from restrictive to dilated. Recently, a new classification of cardiomyopathies that incorporates molecular insights was proposed by an American Heart Association Scientific Statement panel.[6] This classification divides cardiomyopathy into primary and secondary causes, in a manner similar to traditional classification schemes, but adds important subcharacterization of the primary cardiomyopathies into genetic, mixed, and acquired groups (**Fig. 68-1**). From the clinical perspective, where the objective is diagnosis and delivery of effective therapy that may be cause-specific, there is major overlap with the concept of an acquired primary cardiomyopathy and a secondary cardiomyopathy. An important new addition to the genetic subgroup is that of ion channel disorders, which often are not accompanied by structural heart disease but clearly can be considered a primary disorder of the heart (see Chap. 9 for further discussion). Ischemic heart disease can also lead to a cardiomyopathy and is discussed in Chaps. 25, 52, and 54. The hypertrophic cardiomyopathies are discussed in Chaps. 8 and 69.

Operationally, disagreement about classification of cardiomyopathies does not necessarily impede patient management. Rather, the disagreement reinforces the key principle in patient evaluation—there are many primary, secondary, and systemic disorders that manifest with cardiac dysfunction or congestive heart failure. Accordingly, the patient with an abnormality in cardiac structure or function requires comprehensive evaluation for a broad array of disorders. The main goal of this approach is to identify disorders that cause reversible cardiac dysfunction, capable of significant improvement with treatment of the underlying cause of the heart failure.[7,8] Thus, a key principle for management of the cardiomyopathy patient is an exhaustive evaluation to determine the underlying etiologic diagnosis. Throughout this chapter, the issue of reversibility will be addressed (see Chap. 25). In contrast to the principle that the underlying etiologic basis of cardiomyopathy is broad is the therapeutic concept that therapies for heart failure are somewhat similar. A common approach of addressing the patient's volume status and use of neurohormonal blockade is appropriate management regardless of etiology (see Chap. 28). Only now are specific etiology-based therapies entering into clinical testing.

CH 68

TABLE 68-1 Classification of the Cardiomyopathies

DISORDER	DESCRIPTION
Dilated cardiomyopathy	Dilation and impaired contraction of the left ventricle or both ventricles Caused by familial-genetic, viral, immune, alcoholic-toxic, or unknown factors or is associated with recognized cardiovascular disease
Hypertrophic cardiomyopathy	Left and/or right ventricular hypertrophy, often asymmetric, which usually involves the interventricular septum Mutations in sarcoplasmic proteins cause the disease in many patients
Restrictive cardiomyopathy	Restricted filling and reduced diastolic size of either ventricle or both ventricles with normal or near-normal systolic function Idiopathic or associated with other disease (e.g., amyloidosis, endomyocardial disease)
Arrhythmogenic right ventricular cardiomyopathy	Progressive fibrofatty replacement of the right, and to some degree the left, ventricular myocardium Familial disease is common
Unclassified cardiomyopathy	Diseases that do not fit readily into any category; examples include systolic dysfunction with minimal dilation, mitochondrial disease, and fibroelastosis
Specific Cardiomyopathies	
Ischemic cardiomyopathy	Arises as dilated cardiomyopathy with depressed ventricular function not explained by the extent of coronary artery obstructions or ischemic damage
Valvular cardiomyopathy	Arises as ventricular dysfunction that is out of proportion to the abnormal loading conditions produced by the valvular stenosis and/or regurgitation
Hypertensive cardiomyopathy	Arises with left ventricular hypertrophy with features of cardiac failure related to systolic or diastolic dysfunction
Inflammatory cardiomyopathy	Cardiac dysfunction as a consequence of myocarditis
Metabolic cardiomyopathy	Includes a wide variety of causes, including endocrine abnormalities, glycogen storage disease, deficiencies (such as hypokalemia), and nutritional disorders
General systemic disease	Includes connective tissue disorders and infiltrative diseases such as sarcoidosis and leukemia
Muscular dystrophies	Includes Duchenne, Becker-type, and myotonic dystrophies
Neuromuscular disorders	Includes Friedreich ataxia, Noonan syndrome, and lentiginosis
Sensitivity and toxic reactions	Includes reactions to alcohol, catecholamines, anthracyclines, irradiation, and others
Peripartum cardiomyopathy	First becomes manifested in the peripartum period, but it is probably a heterogeneous group

Derived from Richardson P, McKenna W, Bristow M, et al: Report of the 1995 World Health Organization/International Society and Federation of Cardiology Task Force on the Definition and Classification of Cardiomyopathies. Circulation 93:841, 1996. Copyright 1996, American Heart Association.

TABLE 68-2 Functional Classification of the Cardiomyopathies

DILATED	RESTRICTIVE	HYPERTROPHIC
Symptoms		
Congestive heart failure, particularly left sided Fatigue and weakness Systemic or pulmonary emboli	Dyspnea, fatigue Right-sided congestive heart failure Signs and symptoms of systemic disease, e.g., amyloidosis, iron storage disease	Dyspnea, angina pectoris Fatigue, syncope, palpitations
Physical Examination		
Moderate to severe cardiomegaly; S_3, S_4 Atrioventricular valve regurgitation, especially mitral	Mild to moderate cardiomegaly; S_3 or S_4 Atrioventricular valve regurgitation; inspiratory increase in venous pressure (Kussmaul sign)	Mild cardiomegaly Apical systolic thrill and heave; brisk carotid upstroke S_4 common Systolic murmur that increases with Valsalva maneuver
Chest Radiography		
Moderate to marked cardiac enlargement, especially left ventricular Pulmonary venous hypertension	Mild cardiac enlargement Pulmonary venous hypertension	Mild to moderate cardiac enlargement Left atrial enlargement
Electrocardiography		
Sinus tachycardia Atrial and ventricular arrhythmias ST-segment and T wave abnormalities Intraventricular conduction defects	Low voltage Intraventricular conduction defects Atrioventricular conduction defects	Left ventricular hypertrophy ST-segment and T wave abnormalities Abnormal Q waves Atrial and ventricular arrhythmias
Echocardiography		
Left ventricular dilation and dysfunction Abnormal diastolic mitral valve motion secondary to abnormal compliance and filling pressures	Increased left ventricular wall thickness and mass Small or normal-size left ventricular cavity Normal systolic function Pericardial effusion	Asymmetric septal hypertrophy Narrow left ventricular outflow tract Systolic anterior motion of the mitral valve Small or normal-sized left ventricle
Radionuclide Studies		
Left ventricular dilation and dysfunction (RVG)	Infiltration of myocardium (^{201}Tl) Small or normal-sized left ventricle (RVG) Normal systolic function (RVG)	Small or normal-sized left ventricle (RVG) Vigorous systolic function (RVG) Asymmetric septal hypertrophy (RVG or ^{201}Tl)
Cardiac Catheterization		
Left ventricular enlargement and dysfunction Mitral and/or tricuspid regurgitation Elevated left- and often right-sided filling pressures Diminished cardiac output	Diminished left ventricular compliance "Square root" sign in ventricular pressure recordings Preserved systolic function Elevated left- and right-sided filling pressures	Diminished left ventricular compliance Mitral regurgitation Vigorous systolic function Dynamic left ventricular outflow gradient

RVG = radionuclide ventriculogram; ^{201}Tl = thallium-201.

Dilated Cardiomyopathy

The hallmarks of dilated cardiomyopathy (DCM), the most common cardiomyopathy, are enlargement of one or both of the ventricles and systolic dysfunction (**Fig. 68-2**; see Fig. 68-e1 on website). It is not uncommon for chamber enlargement to precede signs and symptoms of congestive heart failure. Recent classification revision attempts recognize that chamber dilation is part of the spectrum of genetic and environmental disorders affecting the heart; thus, a patient presenting with DCM may have a broad array of cardiac or systemic conditions. Nevertheless, DCM is an important and frequent clinical presentation. In 50% or more of patients with a DCM, an etiologic basis will not be identified, in which case the patient is referred to as having an idiopathic DCM.[1,7]

Natural History

The natural history of DCM remains incompletely understood. This is because this diagnosis clearly contains a variety of causes and patients have highly variable presentations. The presentations of patients can range from asymptomatic left ventricular dysfunction to mild, moderate, or severe congestive heart failure. Different studies report wide-ranging estimates of annual mortality that are between 10% and 50%.[9] Traditionally, it is held that symptomatic heart failure is invariably progressive. However, several factors suggest that this concept should be reexamined and that biologic factors may determine favorable or unfavorable long-term outcomes.[10] First, there has been an impact of therapy on the natural history of patients. Whereas the 1-year mortality in the placebo arm was approximately 50% in the Cooperative North Scandinavian Enalapril Survival Study (CONSENSUS) conducted in the 1980s, similar patients experienced ~20% annual mortality in the Carvedilol Prospective Randomized Cumulative Survival (COPERNICUS) trial conducted in the 1990s, and this dropped further in the 2000s to ~10% (see Chap. 28). There is also growing awareness that treatment with pharmacologic therapies that antagonize the neurohormonal system can lead to myocardial recovery or "reverse left ventricular remodeling" in some patients with DCM (see Chap. 25). Finally, it is reported that between

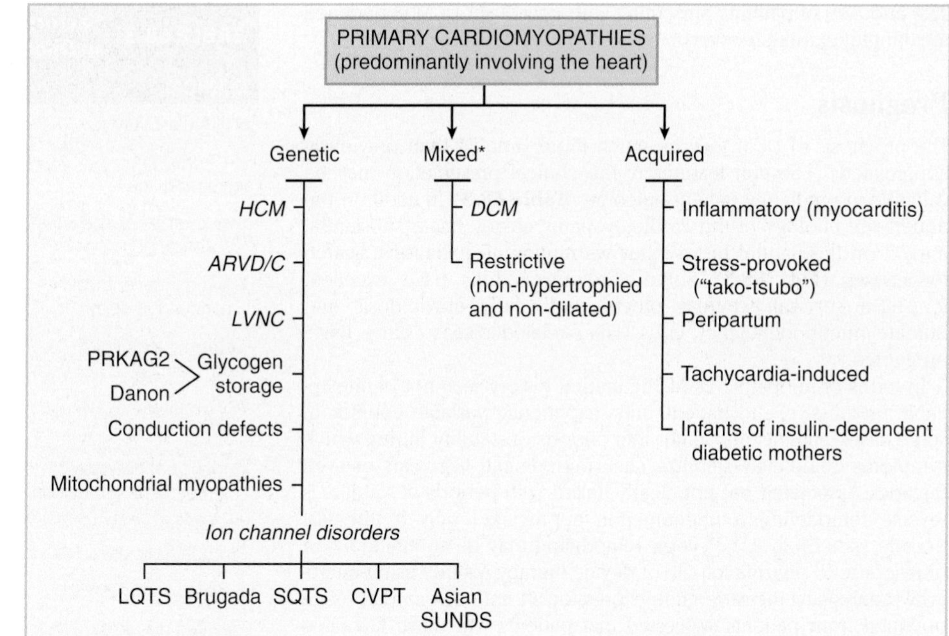

FIGURE 68-1 Primary and specific cardiomyopathies that are primarily manifested with cardiac involvement. *The mixed group comprises predominantly nongenetic causes; however, within this group, familial disease with a genetic origin has been reported in a minority of cases. ARVD/C = arrhythmogenic right ventricular dysplasia/cardiomyopathy; CVPT = catecholaminergic polymorphic ventricular tachycardia; DCM = dilated cardiomyopathy; HCM = hypertrophic cardiomyopathy; LQTS = long-QT syndrome; LVNC = left ventricular noncompaction; PRKAG2 = gene encoding the γ_2 regulatory subunit of the AMP-activated protein kinase; SQTS = short-QT syndrome; SUNDS = sudden unexplained nocturnal death syndrome. *(From Maron BJ, Towbin JA, Thiene G, et al: Contemporary definitions and classification of the cardiomyopathies: An American Heart Association Scientific Statement from the Council on Clinical Cardiology, Heart Failure and Transplantation Committee; Quality of Care and Outcomes Research and Functional Genomics and Translational Biology Interdisciplinary Working Groups; and Council on Epidemiology and Prevention. Circulation 113:1807, 2006.)*

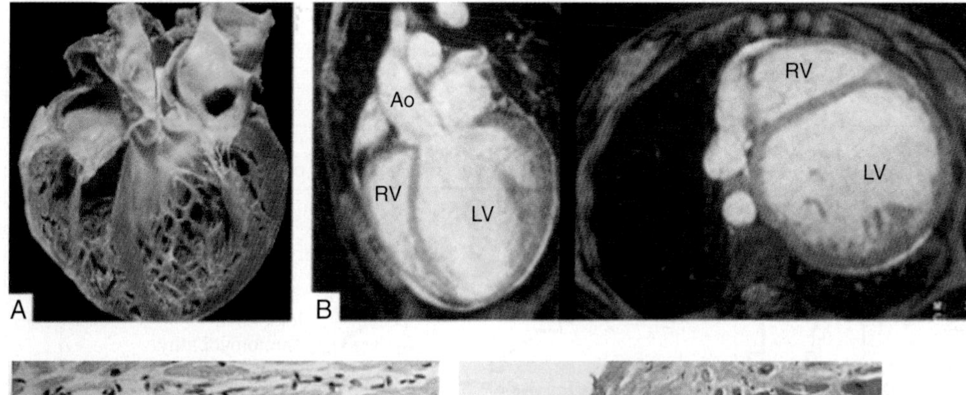

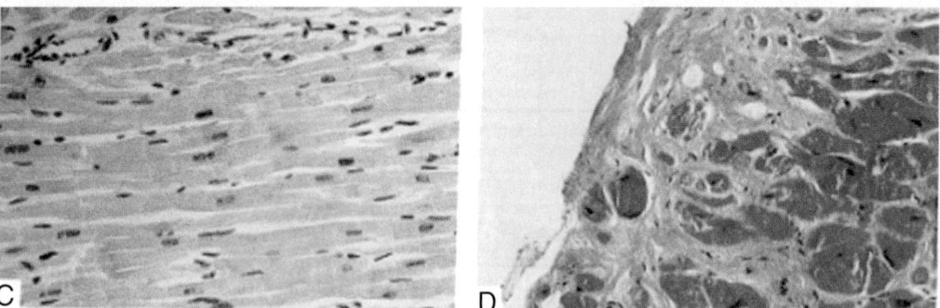

FIGURE 68-2 Dilated cardiomyopathy, gross and microscopic appearance. Affected hearts exhibit four-chamber enlargement as shown by gross cardiac specimen **(A)** and with cardiac magnetic resonance imaging **(B)**. Cardiac myocytes are hypertrophied **(D)** with variable size and enlarged nuclei compared with normally aligned myocytes **(C)**. In addition, there is significant interstitial deposition of fibrotic tissue **(D)**. Ao = aorta; LV = left ventricle; RV = right ventricle. *(From Hare JM: Etiologic basis of congestive heart failure. In Colucci WS [ed]: Atlas of Heart Failure. 5th ed. Philadelphia, Springer, Current Medicine Group, 2008, pp 29-56. Copyright 2008, Current Medicine LLC.)*

25% and 33% of patients presenting with new-onset DCM experience meaningful cardiac recovery.[11]

Prognosis

The prognosis of DCM may be much more variable than previously appreciated.[9,10] Several features of the clinical presentation may be valuable in predicting patient outcome (**Table 68-3**). In addition, the underlying etiology of the cardiomyopathy clearly has a substantial impact on the natural history, thus warranting an exhaustive search for causes (**Fig. 68-3**). Some cardiomyopathies have excellent long-term survival, whereas others, particularly amyloidosis and human immunodeficiency virus (HIV)–related disease, carry grave prognoses.[7]

In terms of idiopathic DCM, the natural history may not be inextricably progressive, and patients may experience variable courses. In some cases, patients may enter into periods of stability during which symptoms completely stabilize; such periods can last years or even decades. Associated but not clearly linked with periods of stability is reverse remodeling, a phenomenon appreciated only in the last decade (see Chap. 25). Reverse remodeling may be spontaneous or in response to pharmacologic or device therapy. A study using microarray analysis to measure gene expression in endomyocardial tissue obtained from patients suggested that patients who have favorable long-term outcomes accompanied by reverse remodeling can be detected at the time of clinical presentation[10] (**Fig. 68-4**). Alternatively, it is clear that some patients may experience sudden deterioration after a period of stability or never experience a quiescent time.[12] It is also critical to appreciate that certain patients may have severe and life-threatening hemodynamic embarrassment at initial presentation. For these patients, a diagnostic evaluation including endomyocardial biopsy should be rapidly performed[13]; these patients are critically ill and frequently require inotropic or mechanical support as a lifesaving therapy.

The determinants of the natural history are not entirely clear, but several studies suggest that biomarkers or panels of laboratory values may have prognostic value.[9,10] As discussed subsequently, there is growing appreciation for the genetic component of DCM, and it is likely that inherited predisposition plays a major role in the natural history of this disorder.

TABLE 68-3 Factors Associated with an Adverse Outcome in Dilated Cardiomyopathy

CLINICAL	NONINVASIVE	INVASIVE
NYHA Class III/IV	Low LV ejection fraction	High LV filling pressures
Increasing age	Marked LV dilation	
Low exercise peak oxygen consumption	Low LV mass	
Marked intraventricular conduction delay	≥Moderate mitral regurgitation	
Complex ventricular arrhythmias	Abnormal diastolic function	
Abnormal signal-averaged ECG	Abnormal contractile reserve	
Evidence of excessive sympathetic stimulation	Right ventricular dilation or dysfunction	
Protodiastolic gallop (S_3)		
Elevated serum BNP		
Elevated uric acid		
Decreased serum sodium		

BNP = brain natriuretic peptide; ECG = electrocardiogram; LV = left ventricular; NYHA = New York Heart Association.

Pathology

MACROSCOPIC EXAMINATION. Gross inspection of the heart demonstrates four-chamber enlargement (see Fig. 68-2). Most often, the ventricular walls are increased in thickness consistent with the myocyte hypertrophy that accompanies this disorder. Increasing chamber thickness is attributed to a compensatory mechanism aimed at reducing wall stress and is thus thought to play a beneficial role, averting further chamber remodeling.[3] The valvular structures themselves are normal, although chamber enlargement frequently leads to a dilation of the valvular orifice. Intracavitary thrombi are often noted and are preferentially located in the ventricular apices. The coronary circulation is most commonly normal, although the presence of nonocclusive epicardial disease can raise a diagnostic conundrum wherein the degree of cardiomyopathy is "out of proportion to the underlying coronary artery disease." A definition for ischemic cardiomyopathy has been arbitrarily set at a requirement for a greater than 70% stenosis in a major epicardial coronary artery, although pathologic studies have reported greater degrees of disease.[4] Preferential involvement of the right ventricle should suggest the diagnoses of arrhythmogenic right ventricular dysplasia/cardiomyopathy (ARVD/C)[14] or cor pulmonale (secondary to pulmonary hypertension).

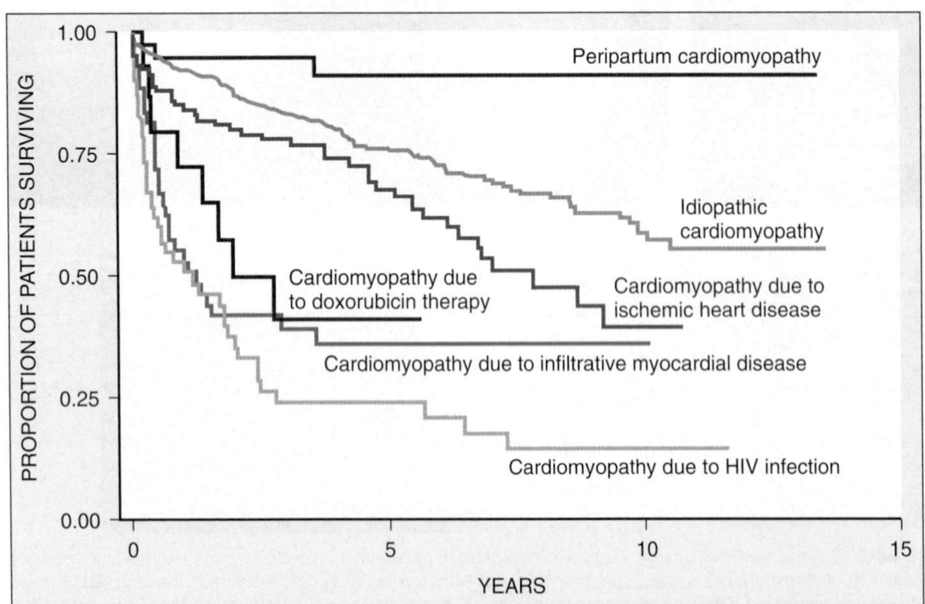

FIGURE 68-3 Variable survival in patients with dilated cardiomyopathy depending on underlying etiologic basis. HIV = human immunodeficiency virus. *(From Felker GM, Thompson RE, Hare JM, et al: Underlying causes and long-term survival in patients with initially unexplained cardiomyopathy. N Engl J Med 342:1077, 2000.)*

HISTOLOGIC EXAMINATION. Histologic evaluation of the myocardium reveals varying degrees of myocyte hypertrophy and interstitial fibrosis (see Fig. 68-2).[4] Fibrosis most often affects the left ventricular subendocardium or throughout the myocardium in interstitial or perivascular patterns. A finding of replacement fibrosis, an island of fibrotic tissue, often signifies a small area of tissue necrosis and suggests an ischemic etiology. It has been difficult to identify characteristic immunologic or infectious findings; however, progress is being made, particularly with regard to viral persistence within the heart (see later). Scattered cells considered to be lymphocytes are a frequent observation and may lead to a diagnosis of borderline myocarditis. This does not appear to affect prognosis.[15]

Etiology

DCM accounts for approximately 25% of the cases of congestive heart failure in the United States.[16] The majority of the additional cases are due to specific cardiomyopathies, most notably ischemic or hypertensive cardiomyopathies,[16] or nonsystolic heart failure.[17] The DCM phenotype can be manifested from specific systemic diseases or primary acquired processes, and intensive diagnostic evaluations in referral centers can reveal a specific associated cause of cardiomyopathy in ~50% of patients; the remaining 50% are assigned the diagnosis of exclusion, idiopathic DCM.[7,8] It is increasingly being appreciated that many of the so-called cases of idiopathic DCM result from underlying genetic abnormalities or previous environmental insults that are difficult to detect at the time of clinical presentation. With the advent of sophisticated molecular and imaging technologies in clinical medicine, it is likely in the future that an increasing number of the idiopathic cases will have a specific diagnosis assigned.

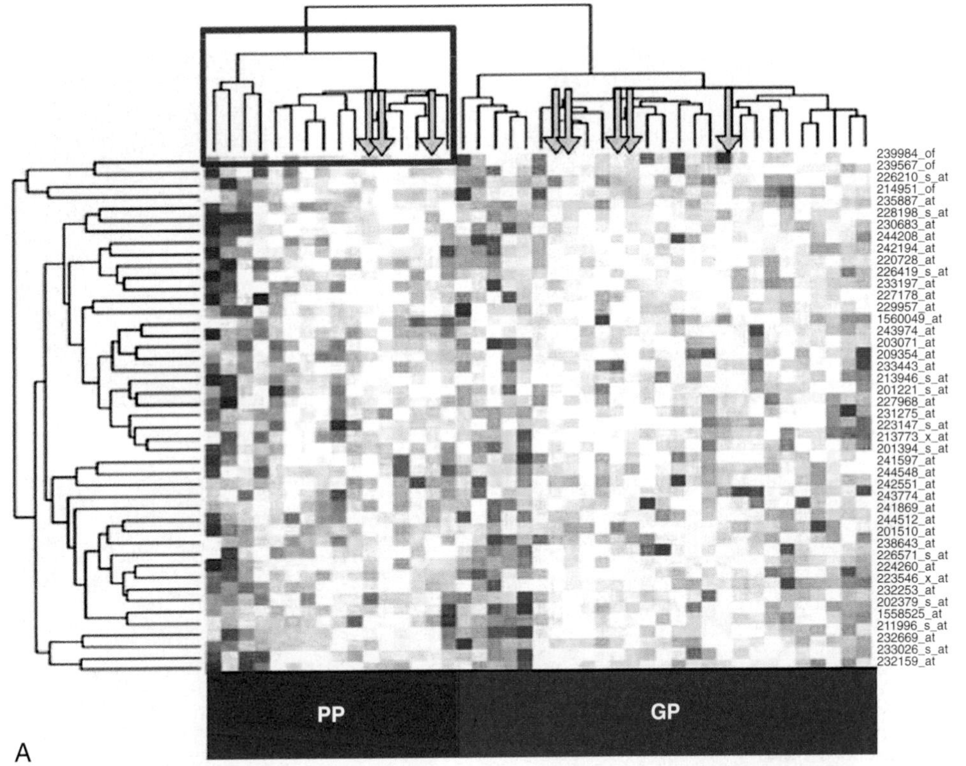

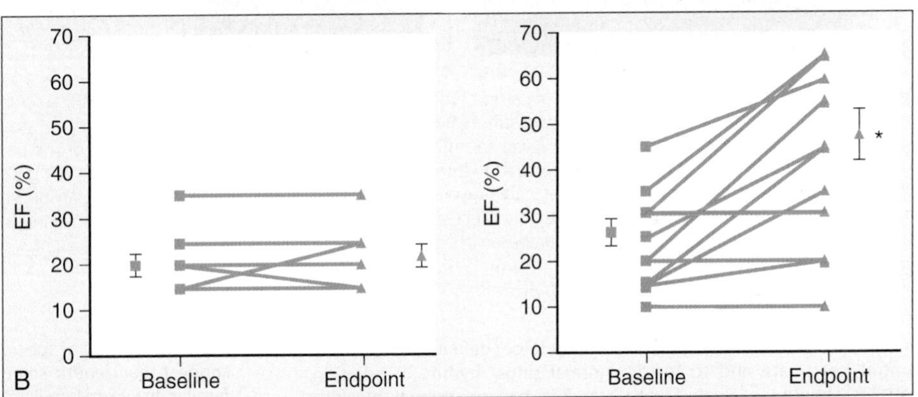

FIGURE 68-4 Inherent biologic processes affect long-term survival in patients with idiopathic dilated cardiomyopathy. **A,** Microarray transcriptomic analysis revealed a gene signature that predicted long-term event-free survival compared with poor prognosis manifesting as death or need for heart transplantation within 2 years. The dendograms depict individual signatures in specific columns and specific genes in rows. **B,** Patients with gene signature predicting favorable outcome undergo reverse remodeling and improvement in ejection fraction (EF). Yellow arrows in **A** and green line in **B** (at right) denote misclassified samples. GP = good prognosis; PP = poor prognosis. *(From Heidecker B, Kasper EK, Wittstein IS, et al: Transcriptomic biomarkers for individual risk assessment in new-onset heart failure. Circulation 118:238, 2008.)*

Specific Cardiomyopathies with a Dilated Phenotype

Clinically, there are a host of important causes of secondary DCM (see Table 68-1) that include alcohol and cocaine abuse (see Chap. 73), HIV infection (see Chap. 72), and metabolic abnormalities as well as the cardiotoxicity of anticancer drugs (see Chap. 90), most notably doxorubicin and newly introduced drugs that inhibit tyrosine kinases (e.g., herceptin and imitinab). The following four specific disorders are particularly important to recognize in that correct diagnosis has a major impact on patient management and chance for recovery.

Stress (Tako-tsubo or Broken Heart Syndrome).[18] An acute cardiomyopathy can be provoked by a stressful or emotional situation or exposure to high doses of catecholamines (sympathomimetic drugs)[18,19] (see Chap. 28). This cardiomyopathy is most common among middle-aged women, appears to be related to catecholamine release, and in most cases is fully reversible with supportive care (**Fig. 68-5**; see Fig. 15-32). Electrocardiographic findings of myocardial infarction in the presence of left ventricular dysfunction and absence of epicardial coronary stenoses should prompt the diagnosis. Endomyocardial biopsy is of value to exclude myocarditis, which can also mimic acute myocardial infarction, and demonstrates contraction band necrosis.

Peripartum Cardiomyopathy. Peripartum cardiomyopathy[20,21] is defined as a cardiomyopathy manifesting between the last month of pregnancy and 6 months post partum. The etiology is unclear, but inflammatory factors are highly implicated, and some studies reveal a high incidence of lymphocytic inflammation. Peripartum cardiomyopathy is common in Africa but also is manifested in the developed world; it has an excellent long-term natural history if patients survive the initial period (see Fig. 68-4), during which time hemodynamic compromise may be severe.[22] Prognosis is worse in the developing world and among indigent patients in the United States.[23] It is important to differentiate peripartum cardiomyopathy from a chronic cardiomyopathy exacerbated by the volume load occurring during pregnancy.[20] Women who recover are at increased risk of recurrences with subsequent pregnancies; women with full recovery are more likely to tolerate a subsequent pregnancy than are those with residual left ventricular dysfunction.[21]

Tachycardia-Induced Cardiomyopathy. Patients may develop a DCM with congestive heart failure in the face of recurrent or persistent tachycardias. The most common association is with atrial fibrillation or supraventricular tachycardia. There is a high rate of full recovery with control of the arrhythmia.[24] This cardiomyopathy is notable for the degree to which it resembles idiopathic DCM phenotypically, yet it is characterized by a remarkable degree of recovery in left ventricular function once the arrhythmia is controlled. Patients presenting with an atrial

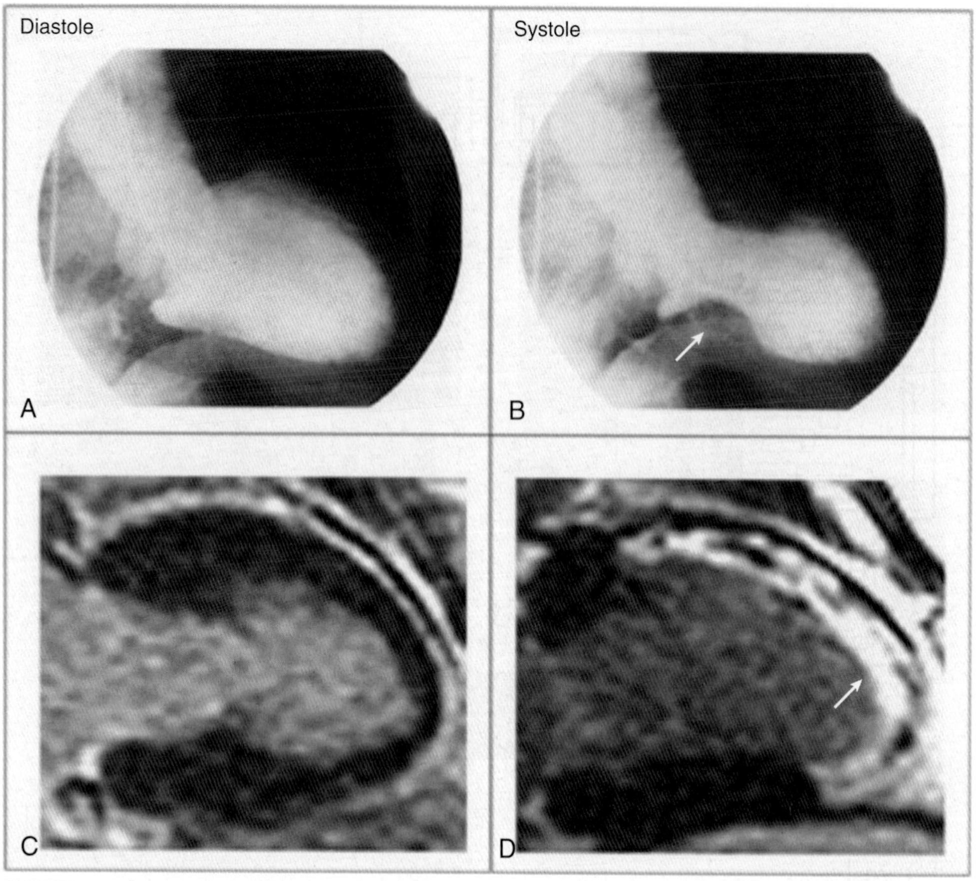

FIGURE 68-5 Ventriculographic assessment of cardiac function and cardiac magnetic resonance (CMR) assessment of myocardial viability at admission in a patient with stress cardiomyopathy. Contrast-enhanced ventriculography during diastole, in **A,** and systole, in **B,** demonstrates apical and midventricular akinesis, with relative sparing of the base of the heart (arrow). **C,** CMR in the long-axis view reveals that the akinetic regions seen on ventriculography are dark and hypoenhanced, consistent with the presence of viable myocardium. **D,** presented for purposes of comparison, shows hyperenhancement (arrow), indicative of necrosis and decreased viability, after an acute anterior myocardial infarction. *(From Wittstein IS, Thiemann DR, Lima JA, et al: Neurohumoral features of myocardial stunning due to sudden emotional stress. N Engl J Med 352:539, 2005.)*

or supraventricular arrhythmia should undergo definitive therapy to control heart rate and to restore normal sinus rhythm. In addition, patients should be treated with standard neurohormonal blocking agents and carefully monitored with echocardiography in the weeks to months after presentation for signs of recovery.

Alcoholic Cardiomyopathy. Alcoholic cardiomyopathy is a common cause of DCM and the most common secondary cardiomyopathy. Phenotypically and clinically, it closely resembles idiopathic DCM (see also Chap. 73). The disorder is linked to ongoing excessive alcohol consumption and appears to be both dose related and responsive to cessation of alcohol exposure. Alcohol exposure also increases risk for comorbidities that can contribute to cardiovascular disease, such as hypertension, stroke, arrhythmias, and sudden death. Alcoholic cardiomyopathy is discussed in Chap. 73.

Etiologic Basis for Idiopathic Dilated Cardiomyopathy

Rapidly advancing knowledge in four areas is shedding light on pathophysiologic mechanisms that may contribute to DCM and may in turn lead to new therapeutic approaches. These areas include (1) familial and genetic factors,[25] (2) inflammatory and infectious factors, particularly viral infection,[26] (3) cytotoxicity, and (4) cell loss and abnormalities in endogenous repair mechanisms.[27,28]

Genetic and Familial Factors. Studies of the genetics of DCM offer major insights into the etiology of the disease. Two general lines of evidence initially suggested a genetic component to DCM.[25] Familial studies indicated that in excess of 20% of patients with DCM had other family members with the condition, and conversely, certain inherited conditions, particularly muscular dystrophies, had cardiomyopathy as a component.[25,29] There are now abundant gene linkage studies with multiple genes identified; autosomal dominant and recessive as well as X-linked modes of inheritance exist (see Chap. 8).[25]

Most of the genes encode structural elements of the cell, notably members of the dystrophin-associated glycoprotein complex, or components of the sarcomeric contractile machinery. A mutation in the gene encoding phospholamban[30] implicates abnormalities in the excitation-contraction cascade as a cause of cardiomyopathy and supports attempts to treat cardiomyopathy with other elements of the calcium cycling machinery (i.e., delivery of the gene encoding the sarcoplasmic reticulum calcium pump [SERCA]).[31]

The fact that genetic abnormalities play a role offers insights into the phenotype in general. Clearly, genetic predisposition may be a central factor in the development of primary and secondary DCMs. Genetic defects may be primary causes of DCM, or they may act as predisposing factors in the setting of an environmental stressor-host-environment interaction. Primary examples of the latter are viral infections and hypertension, wherein exposure may lead to DCM only in subpopulations of exposed individuals. Genetic predisposition may be of fundamental importance in the variable natural history of DCM and may contribute to responsiveness to therapy.[32]

Knowledge of the genetics of DCM has led to the entry of genetic screening into the clinical arena and the development of specialty clinics at referral centers. Recent guidelines suggest that genetic screening and counseling should be considered in families in whom familial DCM is suspected, as a means of early detection of cardiomyopathy in family members.[25]

Inflammatory and Infectious Myocarditis. The diagnosis and management of infectious myocarditis are discussed in Chap. 70 and reviewed here only briefly. Myocarditis may result from viral (or other pathogen) infection, autoimmune disease, or a combination (autoimmune reaction stimulated by a viral infection).[33] It is also increasingly possible that genetic factors increase the risk for development of cardiac disease after viral infection.

It has long been postulated that viral infection in susceptible hosts may be a proximate cause of cardiomyopathy and may serve as a precursor to the development of DCM. This hypothesis has been difficult to prove because of challenges in confirming viral infection in affected individuals coupled with the fact that common viruses are implicated in viral cardiomyopathy, leading to concerns of a high false-positive rate when viruses are detected in patients with heart failure. Lymphocytic myocarditis with or without myocyte necrosis has been considered the hallmark diagnostic finding necessary for a diagnosis, and criteria established for the histologic evaluation are termed the Dallas criteria.[33] The link between myocarditis and viral heart disease is problematic because true inflammatory myocarditis can occur in the absence of an infectious agent (see later). As discussed in Chap. 70, the application of the polymerase chain reaction (PCR) to detect viral particles in myocardial samples taken from patients with DCM has provided important insights into the role played by viruses in heart muscle disease.

Two general mechanisms for postviral cardiac injury have been invoked: autoimmune reactions and direct tissue injury resulting from viral infection of the heart (see Chap. 70). Both of these mechanisms are incompletely proved and remain controversial. The presence or absence of inflammation on endomyocardial biopsy, which varies greatly from study to study, is used to substantiate immunologic injury. However, other studies have suggested different criteria (e.g., complement or immunoglobulin deposition). The postviral hypothesis has increasing support, and viral material has been detected on the basis of elevated viral titers, presence of viral genomic material by PCR, and detection of viral particles.

Autoimmunity. Studies support abnormalities of humoral and cellular immunity in DCM. Two general theories are proposed for an autoimmune cause of DCM: (1) viral components incorporate into the cardiac myocyte membrane, stimulating an antigenic response; and (2) anti–heart antibodies are generated as a result of myocardial damage as opposed to being the proximate cause. Certain specific human leukocyte antigen (HLA) class II antigens (particularly DR4) are associated with DCM. In addition, numerous circulating antimyocardial antibodies have been measured in DCM patients that react with a variety of antigens, including the myosin heavy chain, the beta adrenoceptor, the muscarinic receptor, sarcolemmal sodium-potassium adenosine triphosphatase, laminin, and mitochondrial proteins. Whether anti-inflammatory therapies have efficacy in treating DCM has been difficult to prove; corticosteroid trials performed in the 1980s have been neutral, but there are ongoing attempts to test the value of immunoabsorption strategies. A regimen of prednisone and azathioprine has recently been shown to improve ejection fraction in patients with virus-negative myocarditis.[34]

Cytotoxicity and Deranged Intracellular Signaling. The direct action of various circulating factors is implicated in the pathophysiology of myocyte dysfunction. For example, tumor necrosis factor and endothelin levels are elevated in DCM. The exact role of these factors remains incompletely understood, and therapies to antagonize their effects have not been definitively established.

An additional molecular mechanism gaining increased experimental and clinical support is that of nitroso-redox imbalance, an intracellular phenomenon characterized by dysregulation of nitric oxide production coupled with increased production of reactive oxygen species.[35] This imbalance is described in experimental animal models and in humans with DCM and causes cellular dysfunction and possibly cytotoxicity. Although not definitively proved, one mechanism postulated to explain the response of DCM patients to hydralazine–isosorbide dinitrate is a restoration of nitroso-redox balance (see Chap. 25).

Injury, Cell Loss, and Endogenous Repair. A variety of other causes related to damage to cellular constituents of the heart are proposed as etiologic factors. Although none is accepted as the absolute cause, the variety of mechanisms highlights the notion of a final common pathway, with various insults converging on a set of mechanisms that all result in a common phenotypic response to injury. Many of the mechanisms, such as endocrine disturbances and toxic exposures, derive from the existence of specific examples of secondary cardiomyopathies. The appearance of DCM in only a small fraction of subjects with a common disorder is supportive of the idea that specific host (gene)–environment interactions lead to the cardiac manifestations of the exposure.

Ischemia due to hyperreactivity or spasm of the microvasculature may contribute to diffuse myocyte necrosis and replacement fibrosis. The classic disorder in which this is manifested is scleroderma heart disease. Increased myocyte apoptosis is described in DCM and ARVD/C, leading to the suggestion that augmented cell loss may contribute to the development of left ventricular remodeling in DCM processes. Although there are an increasing number of experimental studies supporting cardiac recovery when antiapoptotic agents are administered in animal models,[36] the exact role of apoptosis in these conditions is not known. Further, the role of cell loss in DCM has become more interesting in light of recent accumulating data supporting the idea that endogenous cardiac stem cells repopulate cardiac myocytes throughout life,[28] thereby serving a homeostatic balancing mechanism for ongoing cell loss and cell replacement after tissue injury (see Chap. 11). Indeed, studies already support the idea of cardiac stem cell senescence contributing to the development of human cardiomyopathy.[27] Thus, depletion or dysfunction of endogenous cells with capacity to divide and to differentiate in cardiac cellular constituents may be a central pathophysiologic contributor to cardiomyopathic processes.[27]

Clinical Evaluation of the Dilated Cardiomyopathies

HISTORY. DCM affects individuals of all ages, including neonates and children.[37,38] In adults, the incidence of DCM is estimated to be between 5 and 8 per 100,000 persons per year. DCM is most frequent in middle age and affects men to a greater degree than women. Although the incidence of ischemic cardiomyopathy is higher than that of DCM, these two diagnoses account for an equal number of heart transplantations performed.

The clinical presentation of patients with heart failure is discussed in Chap. 26. In the case of DCM, the clinical presentation of patients can vary substantially. In some patients, symptoms develop very gradually and diagnosis can result from the detection of cardiomegaly on routine chest radiography. Patients presenting with clear-cut symptoms of congestive heart failure report the development of progressive symptoms for periods varying from weeks to months. Intercurrent illnesses frequently precipitate congestive heart failure in individuals with DCM. A significant minority of patients with DCM present with aggressive, life-threatening congestive heart failure (fulminant heart failure) that can require the most intensive forms of mechanical intervention.[15] The causes of the fulminant presentation vary from idiopathic cardiomyopathy to fulminant lymphocytic myocarditis to giant cell myocarditis (see Chap. 70).[13,16] The determinants of these various forms of clinical presentation are poorly understood.

EVALUATION FOR SECONDARY CARDIOMYOPATHIES. An initial history must focus on identifying etiologic factors[7] (see Table 68-1). A past or associated history of rheumatologic, endocrine, or infectious diseases or of previous neoplasia should be sought.[7] In patients with a history of cancer, treatment with anthracyclines, tyrosine kinase inhibitors, or irradiation is particularly relevant. The family history can often reveal heritable forms of cardiomyopathy. Patients should be questioned about the consumption of alcohol, tobacco, and illicit drugs. Travel history can reveal exposure to geographically related infectious pathogens.

The most typical symptoms are those of congestive heart failure and include dyspnea, fatigue, and volume gain. A minority of patients report chest pain, which can signify epicardial coronary disease, subendocardial disease, or pulmonary embolism. A report of abdominal discomfort or anorexia is frequent in late stages of the disease and suggests hepatomegaly or bowel edema, respectively.

Common late complications include thromboembolic events, which may be systemic, originating from dislodgment of left atrial and ventricular intracardiac or pulmonary thrombi from the lower extremity venous system.

PHYSICAL EXAMINATION. The physical examination for patients with heart failure is discussed in Chaps. 12 and 26. Particular attention should be paid in the physical examination to excluding findings of valvular heart disease. S_3 and S_4 gallops are invariably present in DCM. The S_3 must be differentiated from a pericardial knock or an opening snap of mitral stenosis, both of which are higher pitched sounds than the S_3. Patients with fulminant heart failure of new onset will frequently be tachycardic and will develop a gallop rhythm in which S_3 and S_4 fuse. Attention should be paid to differentiation of right-sided gallops and murmurs to consider the possibility of right-sided involvement.

NONINVASIVE EVALUATION. The diagnostic evaluation of patients with heart failure is discussed in Chap. 26. For patients presenting with DCM, the initial evaluation should focus on identification of reversible and secondary causes. Even though the presentation of the patient with a dilated ventricle and heart failure may be fairly uniform, a wide array of specific and secondary cardiomyopathies may cause a clinical presentation of a DCM. The first step in the diagnostic evaluation involves screening biochemical testing, including serum electrolytes, phosphorus, calcium, and markers of renal function (serum creatinine and urea).[7] Endocrine function should be screened, notably thyroid function (hyperthyroidism and hypothyroidism) and possibly urinary evaluation of catecholamine levels to exclude pheochromocytoma. To screen for rheumatologic conditions, an antinuclear antibody and erythrocyte sedimentation rate should be obtained. When suspected, rarer causes of cardiomyopathy can be excluded with blood testing. For example, Lyme titers can be a useful screen for

Lyme carditis. Iron studies may assist in evaluating hemochromatosis, and HIV testing is valuable.

The use of biomarkers (such as troponin) to assess myocardial necrosis and the use of circulating brain natriuretic peptide (BNP or pro-BNP) levels may serve as useful adjunctive strategies to help determine diagnosis or prognosis (see Chap. 26). Further, there is increasing support for the use of serum uric acid levels as a prognostic marker.[9,39] A chest radiograph offers supporting evidence for the diagnosis and in some cases is the initial mode of detection. Cardiomegaly may be appreciated, as may evidence of pulmonary vascular redistribution. Rarely, interstitial and alveolar edema are present on initial presentation. With advancing heart failure, pleural effusions are present, and dilated azygos veins and superior vena cava indicate right-sided volume overload.

ELECTROCARDIOGRAPHY. There are no specific electrocardiographic findings signifying DCM. Sinus tachycardia is often present in proportion to the degree of heart failure. Typical changes in the QRS complex include poor R wave progression, intraventricular conduction delays, and left bundle branch block. A wide QRS complex portends a worse prognosis and has now emerged as a clinical indicator of responsiveness to cardiac resynchronization therapy (see Chaps. 28 and 29). Patients with substantial left ventricular fibrosis may exhibit anterior Q waves even in the absence of a discrete scar or epicardial coronary artery obstructions. A broad array of abnormalities may be manifested, such as nonspecific ST-segment and T wave abnormalities as well as P wave alterations, notably left atrial abnormality. Nonsustained ventricular tachycardia is extremely common on 24-hour ambulatory monitoring and represents a predictor of all-cause mortality. Persistent supraventricular or ventricular tachyarrhythmias represent an important etiologic factor for ventricular dysfunction,[24] and restoration of sinus rhythm or heart rate control may lead to recovery of ventricular function. Control of atrial fibrillation is also important because of atrial transport issues contributing to cardiac output. In addition, atrial fibrillation should prompt consideration of tachycardia-induced cardiomyopathy.

ECHOCARDIOGRAPHY. Echocardiography is a cornerstone in the evaluation and management of patients with DCM (see Chaps. 15 and 26). Two-dimensional echocardiography is a highly useful and readily available technique to assess ventricular size and performance and to exclude associated valvular or pericardial abnormalities. Doppler echocardiography permits the evaluation of valvular regurgitation or stenosis and the quantification of cardiac output (see Figs. 15-53 and 15-63). Doppler detection of restrictive filling patterns may indicate disease of greater severity (see Fig. 15-64). Pericardial effusion may be present. Performing echocardiography during dobutamine stimulation may identify occult coronary artery disease by provoking regional wall motion abnormalities, differentiating these patients from those with idiopathic DCM. Moreover, significant contractile reserve during dobutamine infusion represents a positive prognostic finding. Three-dimensional echocardiography may be of additional value in assessing mitral valve orifice remodeling and determining ventricular dyssynchrony.

RADIONUCLIDE IMAGING. Nuclear imaging protocols for myocardial perfusion stress imaging may be useful to exclude an ischemic cause of dilated heart failure. Radionuclide ventriculography also provides evidence of cardiac structure and function, showing increased chamber volumes at end diastole and end systole; it provides quantification of reduced ejection fraction in either or both ventricles, and it can elucidate the regional nature of wall motion abnormalities (see Chap. 17). Not always necessary, this technique can be of particular value if echocardiography is technically suboptimal.

CARDIAC MAGNETIC RESONANCE IMAGING AND MULTIDETECTOR COMPUTED TOMOGRAPHY (see Fig. 68-2). Cardiac magnetic resonance imaging (CMR) and multidetector computed tomography are relatively new imaging modalities that are likely to become increasingly useful to evaluate patients with cardiomyopathies (see Chap. 18).[40] Specific cardiomyopathic disorders in which CMR has proved particularly valuable include ARVD/C,[41] endocardial fibroelastosis, myocarditis,[42] amyloidosis,[43] and sarcoidosis. CMR evaluation is also emerging as a critical tool to understand DCM pathophysiology and may contribute to identification of patients at particular risk for complications, such as sudden cardiac death (e.g., within DCM subsets, those with or without areas of replacement fibrosis that may predispose to electrical instability and sudden cardiac death).[44] CMR is also emerging as an important tool in the delineation of infiltrative and inflammatory cardiomyopathies.

INVASIVE EVALUATION INCLUDING ENDOMYOCARDIAL BIOPSY. Catheterization for the exclusion of epicardial coronary disease is essential in the management of the patient presenting with DCM. Because DCM and heart failure increase the false-positive and false-negative rates of noninvasive nuclear assessment for myocardial ischemia, performance of coronary angiography is often necessary to exclude epicardial coronary obstructive disease.[4] It is increasingly relevant to obtain hemodynamic assessments in individuals presenting with acute or worsening heart failure. Use of these diagnostic tests is currently nonuniform.[45] Catheterization usually reveals elevated left ventricular end-diastolic and pulmonary artery wedge pressures. Pulmonary arterial hypertension may be of variable degrees, ranging from mild to severe. The right ventricle is frequently involved and enlarged, hemodynamically manifesting with increased right ventricular end-diastolic, right atrial, and central venous pressures.

Left ventriculography demonstrates varying degrees of ventricular dilation and diffuse chamber hypokinesis. There may be a degree of regionality to the decreased function resembling ischemic heart disease, although a diffuse pattern is frequently present. Filling defects may be present because of left ventricular thrombi, and mild mitral regurgitation is not unusual. It is not always possible to distinguish between left ventricular dilation due to severe mitral regurgitation associated with primary mitral valve disease and DCM with secondary mitral regurgitation.

Coronary arteriography is particularly important to exclude coronary obstructive disease. In patients with DCM, the arterial circulation is typically normal although vasodilator function may be abnormal.

BIOPSY. The role of endomyocardial biopsy to evaluate the myocardium histologically has been historically controversial in the evaluation of the patient presenting with structural heart disease or symptoms of heart failure.[8,46] Recently, however, expert guidelines have been published that offer significant guidance as to the indications for endomyocardial biopsy (see Table 70-4).[13] This procedure, which is routine in the management of heart transplant recipients, allows the acquisition of small pieces of myocardium by use of a flexible bioptome. Currently available bioptomes are advanced transvenously, most commonly by a right internal jugular venous approach, to the right ventricular septum. If it is required, the left ventricular septum may be sampled by a transarterial approach. This procedure is currently performed with either fluoroscopic or echocardiographic guidance. Although not reported in the literature, the widespread use of disposable bioptomes, which have replaced reusable Stanford-Caves devices, has led to a reduction of complications, particularly right ventricle perforation.

Perhaps the most compelling reason in favor of routine biopsy is the detection of a few relatively rare diseases in which accurate diagnosis yields a life-threatening disease with specific management.[15,47] For example, lymphocytic and giant cell myocarditis must be detected early in the course of the presentation for patients to survive and can be separated from each other only by histologic evaluation.[34,48] Biopsy is also an established method for grading the severity of anthracycline cardiomyopathy and has potential similar value for cardiac amyloidosis. A biopsy finding that is negative for inflammation is also valuable in patients with rapidly progressive severe decompensated heart failure, insofar as it may prompt advancement to aggressive mechanical support earlier in the patient's clinical course. Whereas widespread use of the myocardial biopsy is no longer routinely recommended, recent guidelines and treatment trials continue to add clarity around appropriate selection of patients. As reflected in the guidelines, the determination of whether to perform the procedure remains a balance between exposing a patient to a low-yield procedure in the entire population versus the lifesaving potential in a relatively fewer number of patients. In patients with fulminant heart failure, particularly those with new-onset cardiomyopathy, the risk-benefit assessment is more clearly in favor of performing a biopsy to more rationally allocate patients for emergent heart transplantation listing or for insertion of a mechanical assist device. Patients who have fulminant lymphocytic myocarditis have excellent long-term prognosis after short-term hemodynamic support[15]; those with giant cell myocarditis should be aggressively immunosuppressed or listed for heart transplantation[48]; and those with idiopathic cardiomyopathy (suggested by the absence of myocardial inflammation on biopsy) should be aggressively supported and converted to conventional therapy once stabilized. Not infrequently, the endomyocardial biopsy reveals an unsuspected cause of cardiomyopathy.

Management

PHARMACOLOGIC AND DEVICE THERAPY. Whereas the concept of specific etiology-based therapies represents an ongoing quest for patients with DCM, the general treatment of these patients should follow the practice guidelines for all patients with heart failure (see Guidelines: Management of Heart Failure[49] and Chaps. 27, 28, and 30). Indeed, treatment with neurohormonal antagonists to prevent disease progression and the use of diuretics to maintain the volume balance are the therapeutic cornerstones for the management of patients with DCM.[49] Similarly, the use of prophylactic implantable cardiac defibrillators and biventricular pacemakers is indicated in appropriate patients with nonischemic and ischemic DCM (see Chaps. 28, 29, and 38).[49,50]

SURGERY. The surgical management for patients with heart failure is discussed in Chap. 31. Patients with valvular heart disease, coronary artery disease, pericardial disease, or congenital heart defects should have these conditions corrected surgically, when appropriate. Other specific operations geared toward the cardiomyopathic heart include approaches motivated by the concept of restoring chamber geometry or interventions to provide mechanical support. Approaches to achievement of reverse remodeling surgically include left ventricular reconstruction and implantation of external restraint devices (see Chap. 31). Left ventricular assist devices provide aggressive mechanical support to patients with advanced decompensated heart failure (see Chap. 32).

EMERGING SPECIFIC THERAPIES. Only recently are specific etiology-based therapies being evaluated. These include agents to eradicate persistent viral infections and immunomodulatory agents (see Chap. 70). Stem cells for cardiac regeneration and gene therapy approaches are in clinical trials (see Chaps. 11 and 33).

Restrictive and Infiltrative Cardiomyopathy

Relative to the dilated and hypertrophic cardiomyopathies, restrictive cardiomyopathy occurs with lower frequency in the developed world. Specific forms of restrictive cardiomyopathy, such as endomyocardial disease (**Table 68-4**), are important causes of morbidity and mortality common in specific geographic locales, especially in underdeveloped countries.[51-53] The pathophysiologic feature that defines restrictive cardiomyopathy is the increase in stiffness of the ventricular walls, which causes heart failure because of impaired diastolic filling of the ventricle (see also Chaps. 24 and 26).[16] In early stages of the syndrome, systolic function may be normal, although deterioration in systolic function is usually observed as the disease progresses.[2]

Restrictive cardiomyopathy must be distinguished from constrictive pericarditis, which is also characterized by normal or nearly normal systolic function but abnormal ventricular filling (see Chap. 75).[2] Differentiation of these two conditions represents a classic diagnostic challenge and is one of significant clinical importance because pericardial constriction may be treated successfully with pericardiectomy.

TABLE 68-4 Classification of Types of Restrictive Cardiomyopathy According to Cause

Myocardial
Noninfiltrative
Idiopathic cardiomyopathy*
Familial cardiomyopathy
Hypertrophic cardiomyopathy
Scleroderma
Pseudoxanthoma elasticum
Diabetic cardiomyopathy
Infiltrative
Amyloidosis*
Sarcoidosis*
Gaucher disease
Hurler disease
Fatty infiltration
Storage Disease
Hemochromatosis
Fabry disease
Glycogen storage disease
Endomyocardial
Endomyocardial fibrosis*
Hypereosinophilic syndrome
Carcinoid heart disease
Metastatic cancers
Radiation*
Toxic effects of anthracycline*
Drugs causing fibrous endocarditis (serotonin, methysergide, ergotamine, mercurial agents, busulfan)

*These conditions are more likely than the others to be encountered in clinical practice.
From Kushwaha S, Fallon JT, Fuster V: Restrictive cardiomyopathy. N Engl J Med 336:267, 1997. Copyright 1997, Massachusetts Medical Society.

Approximately 50% of cases of restrictive cardiomyopathy result from specific clinical disorders, whereas the remainder represents an idiopathic process. The most common specific cause of restrictive cardiomyopathy is infiltration caused by amyloidosis; there are both acquired and genetic causes of amyloid.[54] Although there are other specific pathologic presentations associated with restrictive cardiomyopathy, their precise etiology often remains obscure. Like DCM, there are inflammatory and genetic factors important in the etiology of restrictive cardiomyopathy. The identification of specific infiltrative processes may have prognostic and therapeutic implications (**Fig. 68-6**).[7] The abnormal diastolic properties of the ventricle are attributable to myocardial fibrosis, infiltration, or scarring of the endomyocardial surface. Myocyte hypertrophy is common, particularly in idiopathic restrictive cardiomyopathy (**Fig. 68-7**).

Clinical Evaluation

CARDIAC CATHETERIZATION AND ENDOMYOCARDIAL BIOPSY. A classic diagnostic challenge is to differentiate restrictive cardiomyopathy from constrictive pericarditis, which is manifested with similar clinical and hemodynamic features. Cardiac catheterization is a key step in this evaluation (see Chaps. 20 and 75). Whereas there is equalization of diastolic pressures in constrictive pericarditis (pressures differ by no more than 5 mm Hg), they may vary to a greater extent in restrictive cardiomyopathy (see Fig. 20-15). Pulmonary hypertension is worse in restrictive cardiomyopathy, with systolic pulmonary pressures often exceeding 50 mm Hg. In constrictive pericarditis, the plateau of right ventricular diastolic pressure is usually at least one third of peak systolic pressure; in restrictive cardiomyopathy, this is most often lower. Hemodynamically, both conditions have a rapid early diastolic pressure decline followed by a rapid rise and plateau

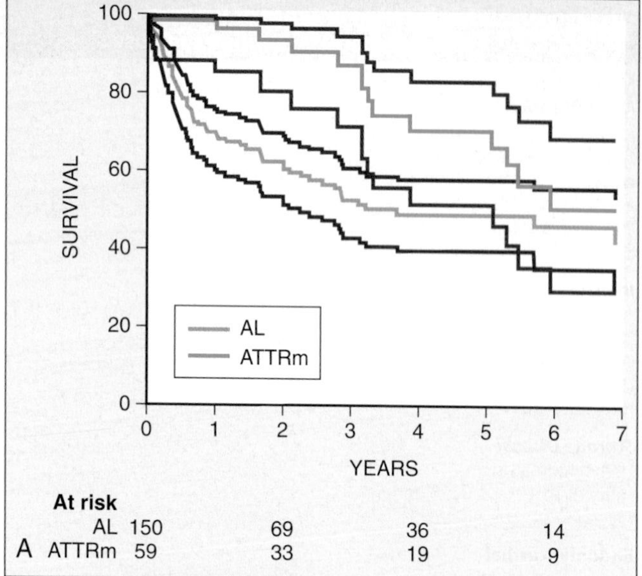

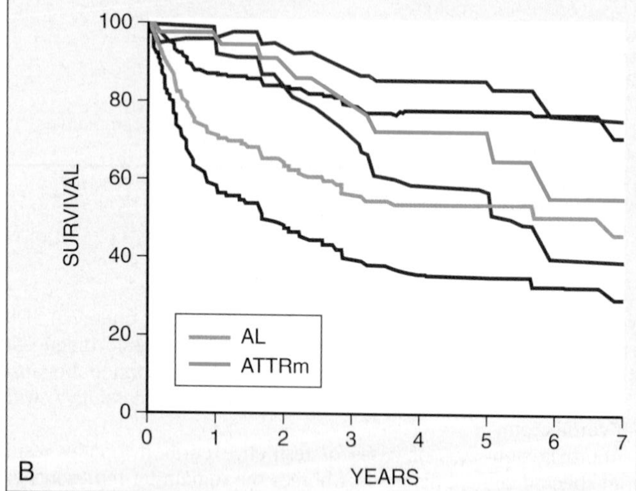

FIGURE 68-6 Variable prognosis in patients with cardiac amyloidosis based on the specific etiology. Overall survival (with 95% confidence intervals) of patients with transthyretin-related (ATTRm) and light chain (AL) amyloidosis before **(A)** and after **(B)** adjustment for renal involvement or insufficiency. *(From Rapezzi C, Merlini G, Quarta CC, et al: Systemic cardiac amyloidoses. Disease profiles and clinical courses of the 3 main types. Circulation 120:1203, 2009.)*

in early diastole, the so-called square root sign. The atrial pressure tracing is manifested as either a classic square root pattern or an M or W waveform when the *x* descent is also rapid. Both *a* and *v* waves are prominent and frequently have the same amplitude. Right- and left-sided atrial filling pressures are elevated, although in the case of restrictive cardiomyopathy, the left ventricular filling pressure typically is 5 mm Hg, or more, greater than the right ventricular diastolic pressure. This difference may be accentuated by Valsalva maneuver, exercise, or a fluid challenge.

Endomyocardial biopsy can also be valuable in the evaluation of these patients to exclude an infiltrative process or cardiomyopathic-appearing myocytes and received a Class IIa recommendation in the guidelines.[13] A normal-appearing biopsy specimen supports the diagnosis of a pericardial process. Surgical exploration is needed far less often, given the availability of biopsy and imaging technology (see later).

Prognosis

Restrictive cardiomyopathy carries a variable prognosis dependent on etiology (see Fig. 68-e2 on website). Most often, especially in the case

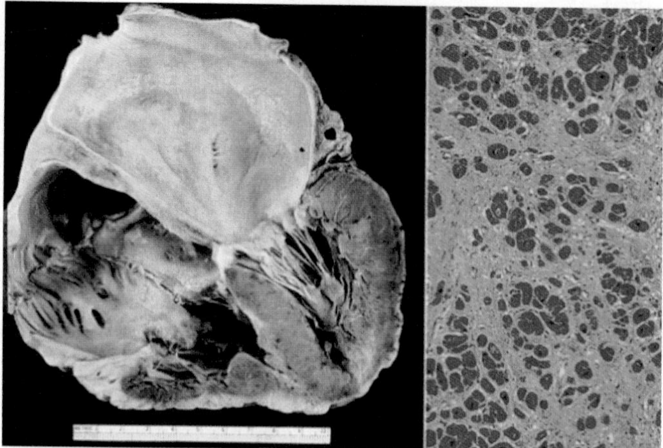

FIGURE 68-7 Pathology of idiopathic restrictive cardiomyopathy in a 63-year-old woman. **Left,** Gross cardiac specimen, shown in four-chamber format, demonstrating prominent biatrial enlargement, with normal-sized ventricles. **Right,** Light microscopy showing marked interstitial fibrosis (light pink areas). Hematoxylin and eosin; magnification ×120. *(From Ammash NM, Seward JB, Bailey KR, et al: Clinical profile and outcome of idiopathic restrictive cardiomyopathy. Circulation 101:2490, 2000.)*

of amyloidosis, it is invariably progressive with an accelerated mortality.[55] A longitudinal study of 233 patients revealed the importance of the underlying type of amyloidosis in outcome; patients fared better with the transthyretin-related form of amyloid than with immunoglobulin associated (see Fig. 68-6).[54] There is no specific therapy for the idiopathic form of restrictive cardiomyopathy, but intensive fluid and supportive management are required to maintain a patient with a reasonable quality of life. There are ongoing aggressive attempts to devise therapies for secondary forms of restrictive cardiomyopathy tailored to the etiology (e.g., iron removal in hemochromatosis or enzyme replacement therapy in Fabry disease).

Clinical Manifestations

Patients with restrictive cardiomyopathy frequently present with exercise intolerance that results from an impaired ability to augment cardiac output during increasing heart rate because of the restriction of diastolic filling. Other notable symptoms are weakness, dyspnea, and edema, and exertional chest pain is reported by some but not all patients. With advancing disease, profound edema occurs that includes peripheral edema, hepatomegaly, ascites, and anasarca. These patients represent the most difficult volume management because of the balance between volume status and hypotension that can result during diuresis by reduced preload filling of the ventricles. Physical examination is notable for an elevated jugular venous pulse, often with the Kussmaul sign, a rising jugular pressure during inspiration (because of the restriction to filling). Both S_3 and S_4 gallops are common, and the apical pulse is palpable (in contrast to constrictive pericarditis). Patients with restrictive cardiomyopathy are highly prone to development of atrial fibrillation.[2]

Laboratory Studies

Computed tomography and CMR are valuable for differentiation of constrictive and restrictive disease. (see Chaps. 18 and 19). A thickened pericardium supports the diagnosis of pericardial constriction. Other ancillary tests also may be helpful. For example, chest radiography may detect pericardial calcification. The electrocardiogram may disclose atrial fibrillation. Echocardiography (see Fig. 15-68) should be routinely performed in patients suspected of restrictive cardiomyopathy or constriction and may reveal biatrial dilation and increasing wall thickness associated with myocardial infiltration as well as alterations in the appearance of the myocardium (e.g., speckling). Doppler echocardiography supplemented with tissue Doppler reveals evidence of impaired myocardial relaxation with increased early left ventricular filling velocity, decreased atrial filling velocity, and decreased isovolumetric relaxation time (see Figs. 15-69 and 15-70); these findings are additionally useful for the discrimination from constrictive disease.[2,56] BNP levels may be used to discriminate between restrictive cardiomyopathy and constrictive disease, with concentrations approximately five times greater in the former compared with the latter.[57]

Amyloidosis

Etiology and Types

Amyloidosis is a unique disease process that results from tissue deposition of proteins that have a unique secondary structure (twisted beta-pleated sheet fibrils; **Fig. 68-8**). Amyloid may be found in almost any organ but does not produce clinically evident disease unless tissue infiltration is extensive. Several classification systems have been used to characterize the different clinical presentations of amyloidosis. Primary (acquired) amyloidosis results from the deposition of portions of immunoglobulin light chains (designated AL amyloid) within tissues. In most cases, the excess production of this protein results from a monoclonal expansion of plasma cells in the setting of multiple myeloma. Rarely, a patient with a plasma cell dyscrasia may develop restrictive cardiomyopathy due to deposition of light chains in a nonamyloid manner. Importantly, the latter form of disease may be reversible. Historically, primary amyloidosis occurred from other chronic untreated inflammatory conditions. Secondary amyloidosis (also known as reactive systemic amyloidosis) results from the excess production of a nonimmunoglobulin protein known as AA.

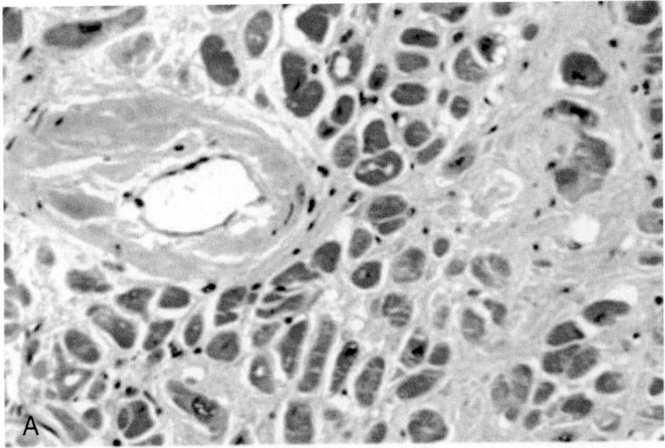

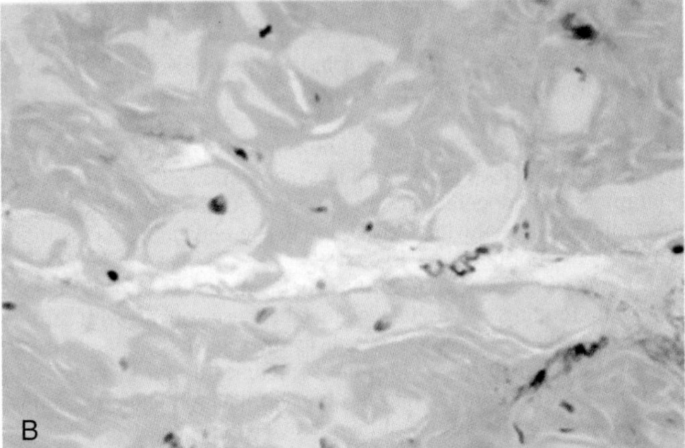

FIGURE 68-8 Histologic phenotype of cardiac amyloidosis. **A,** Endomyocardial biopsy specimen, stained with hematoxylin and eosin, from a patient with cardiac amyloidosis. The amyloid stains light pinkish red and is seen as an amorphous material that separates the darker-staining myocytes. **B,** Staining of the tissue from the same patient with sulfated Alcian blue. The amyloid stains turquoise green and the myocytes stain yellow, characteristic of amyloid. *(From Falk RH: Diagnosis and management of the cardiac amyloidoses. Circulation 112:2047, 2005.)*

FAMILIAL (HEREDITARY) AMYLOIDOSIS. In the past decade, there has been growing recognition that various familial diseases can lead to amyloid deposition in the heart. An autosomal dominant form results from the deposition of a variant form of prealbumin serum carrier termed transthyretin in tissues. Multiple (>100) point mutations in the transthyretin gene are associated with amyloidosis.[54] Transthyretin amyloidosis usually produces one of three different clinical scenarios—nephropathy, neuropathy, or cardiomyopathy. Isolated cardiomyopathy occurring with older age, associated with the Ile 122 variant, is more common in individuals of African American descent.[58] Given that transthyretin is produced within the liver, liver transplantation may be contemplated in affected individuals who are detected early.

SENILE SYSTEMIC AMYLOIDOSIS. This form of amyloidosis results from amyloid deposition of proteins that are like either atrial natriuretic peptide or transthyretin.[59] This form of amyloidosis is increasing in incidence as the population ages, with a predilection for elderly men. Although it affects individuals of older age, the prognosis is better than that of AL disease.[59] Deposition of amyloid in the atria and pulmonary vessels is often found at autopsy in octogenarians and may be a risk factor for atrial fibrillation.

CARDIAC AMYLOIDOSIS. Cardiac amyloidosis is an invariably progressive infiltrative cardiomyopathy that carries a grave prognosis.[55] Cardiac involvement may be present in up to one third of patients with primary amyloidosis resulting from plasma cell dyscrasias. When the heart is studied pathologically, AL protein deposits are present invariably at necropsy even if clinically silent in life. Myocardial infiltration tends to be less with secondary amyloidosis, in which the AA protein deposits tend to be smaller and more perivascular in location, where they are less likely to produce myocardial dysfunction.

Approximately one quarter of patients with transthyretin-induced (familial) amyloidosis experience clinically significant cardiac involvement that is often marked by involvement of the conduction system. Neurologic or renal involvement may also predominate in this form of amyloidosis. Patients will typically present with clinical symptoms after the age of 35 years. In half of the cases involving deposition of transthyretin, the mode of death is cardiac, from either heart failure or sudden cardiac death. In senile amyloidosis, deposits vary from isolated atrial involvement to extensive ventricular infiltration causing severe restrictive cardiomyopathy. Cardiac amyloidosis is observed more frequently in men than in women and is rare before the age of 40 years.

Pathology

The term *amyloidosis* was coined by Virchow and means "starch-like." The heart infiltrated with amyloid appears tan and waxy and is rubbery in consistency. The atria are also significantly enlarged (see Fig. 68-8). On histologic examination, amyloid deposits can be detected with Congo red or Sirius red staining and are present between cardiac myocytes.[16,55] Amyloidosis may cause focal thickening of the cardiac valves but infrequently leads to valvular dysfunction. In addition, amyloid may deposit within the media and adventitia of intramural coronary arteries and may cause impairment in coronary perfusion.

Clinical Manifestations

There are four overlapping cardiovascular syndromes that may occur with cardiovascular involvement of amyloidosis, including restrictive cardiomyopathy, systolic heart failure, orthostatic hypotension, and presentation with conduction system disease.

RESTRICTIVE CARDIOMYOPATHY. Amyloid infiltration and circulating immunoglobulins produce classic restrictive physiology leading to increased diastolic chamber stiffness with a resultant impairment of left ventricular filling. The impairment of chamber filling leads to fluid retention and peripheral edema, hepatomegaly, and elevated jugular venous pressure. Hemodynamic measurements reveal the classic dip and plateau square root sign. One feature differentiating amyloidosis from constrictive pericarditis is the rate of early diastolic filling, which is accelerated in pericardial disease but is diminished in amyloidosis.

Systolic Heart Failure. Although systolic function may be normal early in the disease, it frequently deteriorates late in the disease as the degree of amyloid deposition increases. Deposition of amyloid in the atrium can also lead to atrial arrest, even though the sinus node is fully functional. The loss of atrial transport function may contribute to worsening heart failure, particularly in the face of restrictive cardiac physiology. Patients may also exhibit angina pectoris, although epicardial coronary arteries are normal angiographically. This form of the disease is usually relentlessly progressive.

Orthostatic Hypotension. Approximately 10% of affected individuals will exhibit orthostasis caused by amyloid infiltration of the autonomic nervous system, blood vessels, or both.[60] Infiltration of the heart and adrenal glands may contribute to the pathogenesis of this variant. Renal failure resulting in the nephrotic syndrome and volume retention can worsen the postural hypotension. Patients with amyloidosis frequently experience frank syncope often associated with emotional or physical stress, a phenomenon that may be associated with left ventricular outflow obstruction. Syncope during exertion represents an extremely poor prognosis, with demise likely within 3 months.

Conduction System Disease. Abnormal propagation of cardiac electrical signals is the least common form of amyloidosis and may result in arrhythmias and conduction disturbances. Sudden cardiac death, caused by malignant arrhythmias or conduction block, is an important mode of death. Episodes of syncope may herald more severe events, such as sudden cardiac death.

Physical Examination

Most commonly, patients with cardiac amyloidosis present with signs of congestive heart failure. The jugular venous pulse is elevated, often massively, and there are signs of systemic edema with hepatomegaly, ascites, and edema. On auscultation, apical systolic murmurs due to mitral regurgitation and S_3 gallops are frequently present, although the S_4 is typically absent when there is atrial infiltration with amyloid that leads to impaired atrial contraction. The blood pressure is normal to reduced, and the pulse pressure may be quite narrow, consistent with low cardiac output.

Noninvasive Testing

Cardiomegaly is present on chest radiography in patients with systolic dysfunction but not in those with restrictive presentations. Pulmonary congestion will be detected if heart failure is present. The electrocardiogram most often reveals low QRS voltage, and bundle branch block and abnormal axis are also common. A pattern of old anterior myocardial infarction may be simulated by diminutive or absent R waves in the right precordial leads or by inferior Q waves. Amyloid infiltration of the atrium predisposes to atrial fibrillation, and ventricular arrhythmias are also common. Signal-averaged electrocardiography has proved valuable in predicting increased risk for sudden cardiac death. Atrioventricular conduction defects are common, are particularly prominent in familial amyloidosis with polyneuropathy, and may portend a poor prognosis. Electrophysiologic testing is usually necessary to detect significant intrahisian block. Sinus node dysfunction is also common, and the electrocardiogram may show sick sinus syndrome.

ECHOCARDIOGRAPHY. Echocardiography is valuable and reveals increased ventricular wall thickness with small intracavitary chambers, enlarged atria, and a thickened interatrial septum (see Fig. 15-78). As noted, systolic function is normal early in the course of the disease, but progressive left ventricular dysfunction ensues with advancing amyloid deposition. The walls of the ventricles often reveal a distinctive appearance with a sparkling and granular texture, most likely resulting from the amyloid deposition itself. The cardiac valves may have a thickened appearance but typically have normal excursion. Pericardial effusions may be present but do not advance to tamponade. Patterns of chamber hypertrophy are, on occasion, regional, leading to a pattern reminiscent of hypertrophic cardiomyopathy. The echocardiographic appearance of thickened left ventricular walls associated with low voltage on electrocardiography is valuable for differentiation from pericardial disease. Both Doppler echocardiography and radionuclide ventriculography are valuable to evaluate diastolic dysfunction (see Fig. 15-79), the degree of which offers prognostic information.

RADIONUCLIDE AND MAGNETIC RESONANCE CARDIAC IMAGING. Technetium-99m pyrophosphate scintigraphy and other agents that bind to calcium may be valuable for amyloid detection. This tool is frequently strongly positive when amyloidosis is extensive and correlates with the degree of cardiac infiltration; however, false-negative results may occur. Both CMR and indium-labeled antimyosin antibody imaging are useful for the detection of cardiac amyloid involvement. CMR has a very high sensitivity for the detection of cardiac amyloid (see Fig. 18-14) and may also be valuable in measuring the extent of amyloid deposition in the heart, which may be of significant prognostic importance.[43] There are specialized agents that may detect sympathetic denervation in patients with cardiac amyloidosis.

Diagnosis

In the past, systemic amyloidosis was frequently diagnosed at autopsy. However, the increasing awareness and the availability of endomyocardial biopsy now allow antemortem diagnosis in the majority of patients. Biopsy of alternative tissue locations, such as the abdominal fat pad, rectum, gingiva, bone marrow, liver, and kidney, is also useful for the detection of systemic amyloidosis. For the diagnosis of cardiac amyloidosis, endomyocardial biopsy performed by an experienced operator is safe and definitive and allows evaluation of the extent of tissue infiltration, which may offer prognostic information.[61] Tissue may be examined by immunohistochemistry to identify specific amyloid proteins, which is increasingly important for targeted therapy. Measurement of circulating serum proteins may also be diagnostically valuable. The importance of seeking the identity of the specific amyloidogenic protein is underscored by a study showing that unsuspected hereditary amyloidosis was detected in nearly 10% of patients initially thought to have primary (AL) amyloidosis. In addition, the specific type of transthyretin amyloidosis has prognostic implications.[54]

Management

Patients with cardiac amyloidosis have few treatment options, although there are ongoing attempts to modify the severe natural history of this disorder (**Fig. 68-9**).[62] Approaches for patients with AL amyloidosis involve chemotherapy with alkylating agents alone or in combination with autologous bone marrow stem cell transplantation. Heart transplantation with concomitant autologous bone marrow transplants has been reported with variable degrees of success with a 39% 4-year survival in one study and 30% 5-year survival in another, although amyloid is likely to recur in the transplanted heart.[63] Nevertheless, survival rates may exceed those if the patient is left untreated. Moreover, combination bone marrow and cardiac transplantation may offer better survival rates in the future. For patients with transthyretin amyloid, liver transplantation may remove the source of the abnormal amyloidogenic protein.[64] No form of therapy is effective in the senile form of amyloidosis, although the clinical course is more benign than in primary amyloidosis.

In terms of conventional cardiac medications, the use of digitalis glycosides requires additional vigilance because patients with cardiac amyloidosis have increased sensitivity to digitalis preparations. In spite of this, digitalis glycosides are sometimes useful for successful control of the ventricular rate in atrial fibrillation. Calcium channel antagonists also require caution because their negative inotropic effect has the potential to exacerbate heart failure. Pacemakers are frequently indicated for conduction system disturbances, and implantable cardioverter-defibrillators (ICDs) should be considered for appropriate patients. Perhaps the mainstay of symptom relief in volume overloaded patients is the judicious use of diuretics, which requires very careful titration, in combination with rigorous fluid restriction. Vasodilator agents may also afford symptom relief and enhance diuresis but must be used cautiously to avoid systemic hypotension.

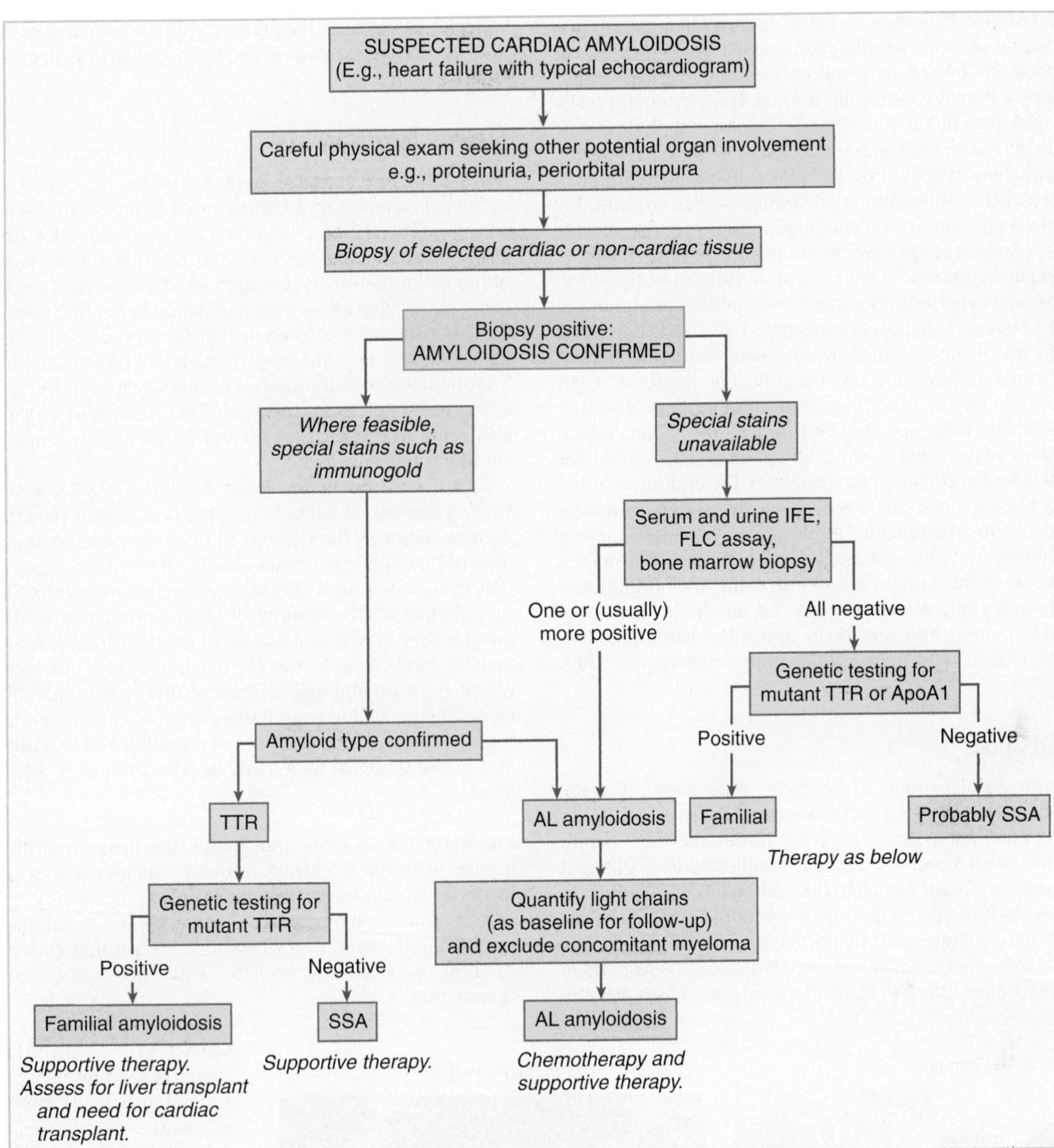

FIGURE 68-9 Flow diagram outlining the evaluation of a patient with suspected cardiac amyloidosis. Clinical evaluation may reveal clues that strengthen the likelihood of amyloidosis, but a tissue diagnosis is mandatory. Although special staining of the biopsy specimen may confirm the type of amyloid, further workup of amyloid (AL) is required to exclude myeloma and to quantify free light chains. If the biopsy specimen stains positive for transthyretin, further testing is needed to determine whether this is a wild-type or mutant transthyretin. ApoA1 = apoprotein type A1; FLC = free light chain; IFE = immunofixation electrophoresis; SSA = senile systemic amyloidosis; TTR = transthyretin. *(From Falk RH: Diagnosis and management of the cardiac amyloidoses. Circulation 112:2047, 2005.)*

Anticoagulation should be considered in the case of atrial standstill or atrial fibrillation.

Inherited and Acquired Infiltrative Disorders Causing Restrictive Cardiomyopathy

The heritable metabolic disorders resulting from the myocardial accumulation or infiltration of abnormal metabolic products represent an important cause of restrictive cardiomyopathy. These disorders produce classic restrictive cardiomyopathy with diastolic impairment and variable degrees of systolic dysfunction. The heritable metabolic disorders include Fabry disease, Gaucher disease, the glycogenoses, and the mucopolysaccharidoses. Early diagnosis is increasingly important because of the availability, in some cases, of effective enzyme replacement therapy.

Fabry Disease

Fabry disease, also referred to as angiokeratoma corporis diffusum universale, is an X-linked recessive disorder that results in deficiency of alpha-galactosidase A, a lysosomal enzyme, and the resultant accumulation of glycosphingolipids (most notably globotriaosylceramide) in lysosomes.[65,66] The major clinical features result from the accumulation of glycolipid substrate in the endothelium. More than 160 different mutations are described that have varying impact, ranging from absence of alpha-galactosidase activity to an attenuated level of activity of this enzyme. Patients with absent alpha-galactosidase activity exhibit widespread systemic manifestations with prominent kidney and cutaneous manifestations, whereas those with an attenuated level of enzyme activity have atypical variants of Fabry disease that may cause isolated myocardial disease. Histologic evaluation of the heart demonstrates diffuse involvement of the myocardium, vascular endothelium, conduction system, and valves, most notably the mitral valve (see Fig. 68-e3 on website).

CARDIAC FINDINGS. Patients with Fabry disease often experience angina pectoris and myocardial infarction caused by the accumulation of lipid species in the coronary endothelium, although epicardial coronary arteries are angiographically normal. The ventricular walls are thickened and have mildly diminished diastolic compliance with normal systolic function. Mild mitral regurgitation may be present. Diastolic abnormalities detected by Doppler echocardiography may be one of the earlier manifestations preceding cardiac hypertrophy. Males almost always present with symptomatic cardiovascular involvement, whereas female carriers may be completely asymptomatic or have only minimal symptoms.[67] Other common features of the disorder include systemic hypertension, congestive heart failure, and mitral valve prolapse. Echocardiography demonstrates increased ventricular wall thickness, which may mimic hypertrophic cardiomyopathy.[65] Whereas echocardiography may not be sufficient to do so, CMR may be able to differentiate Fabry disease from other infiltrative processes such as amyloidosis (see Fig. 68-e4 on website).[68] The surface electrocardiogram may reveal a short PR interval, atrioventricular block, and ST-segment and T wave abnormalities. The endomyocardial biopsy and low plasma alpha-galactosidase A activity offer a definitive diagnosis, which has therapeutic implications because enzyme replacement therapy for Fabry disease is safe and effective; moreover, heart biopsy may be used to monitor response to therapy.[69] Administration of recombinant alpha-galactosidase A can ameliorate the stores of globotriaosylceramide from the heart and other tissues, leading to symptomatic, clinical, and echocardiographic improvement (**Fig. 68-10**).[69]

Gaucher Disease

Gaucher disease results from a heritable deficiency of beta-glucosidase, which leads to an accumulation of cerebrosides in diffuse organs including spleen, liver, bone marrow, lymph nodes, brain, and heart. Cardiac disease is manifested as a stiffened ventricle caused by reduced chamber compliance, leading to impaired cardiac performance. Other manifestations include left ventricular failure and enlargement, hemorrhagic pericardial effusion, and sclerotic, calcified left-sided valves. Gaucher disease is responsive to enzyme replacement therapy or, in more extreme cases, hepatic transplantation; both therapies contribute to reducing tissue infiltration by cerebrosides and can lead to varying degrees of clinical improvement.[70]

Hemochromatosis

Hemochromatosis results from excessive deposition of iron in a variety of parenchymal tissues, notably the heart, liver, gonads, and pancreas. The classic pentad is a symptom complex of heart failure, cirrhosis, impotence, diabetes, and arthritis. The most frequent form of hemochromatosis is inherited as an autosomal recessive disorder (see Chap. 8) that arises from a mutation in the *HFE* gene, which codes for a transmembrane protein that is responsible for regulating iron uptake in the intestine and liver. Hemochromatosis may also arise from ineffective erythropoiesis secondary to a defect in hemoglobin synthesis as well as from chronic liver disease, or it may be acquired as a result of chronic and excessive oral or parenteral intake of iron (or blood transfusions).[71]

Iron deposition in the heart is almost always accompanied by varying degrees of infiltration of the liver, spleen, pancreas, and bone marrow, although the degrees of different organ system involvement may not parallel each other. Cardiac involvement produces a mixed pattern of systolic and diastolic dysfunction that is often accompanied by arrhythmias. The severity of hemochromatosis is less and age at onset is later in women because of the menstrual loss of iron. Cardiac toxicity results directly from the free iron moiety in addition to adverse effects of tissue infiltration. Death results most frequently from cirrhosis and hepatocellular carcinoma, whereas cardiac mortality accounts for an additional one third of the mortality and is particularly important in the group of male patients who present at relatively younger ages.

PATHOLOGY. In gross appearance, the hearts are dilated and ventricular walls are thickened. Iron deposits locate preferentially in the myocyte sarcoplasmic reticulum, more frequently in ventricular versus atrial cardiomyocytes. Frequently, the conduction system is involved, and loss of myocytes with fibrosis is often present. The degree of iron deposition correlates with the extent of myocardial dysfunction.

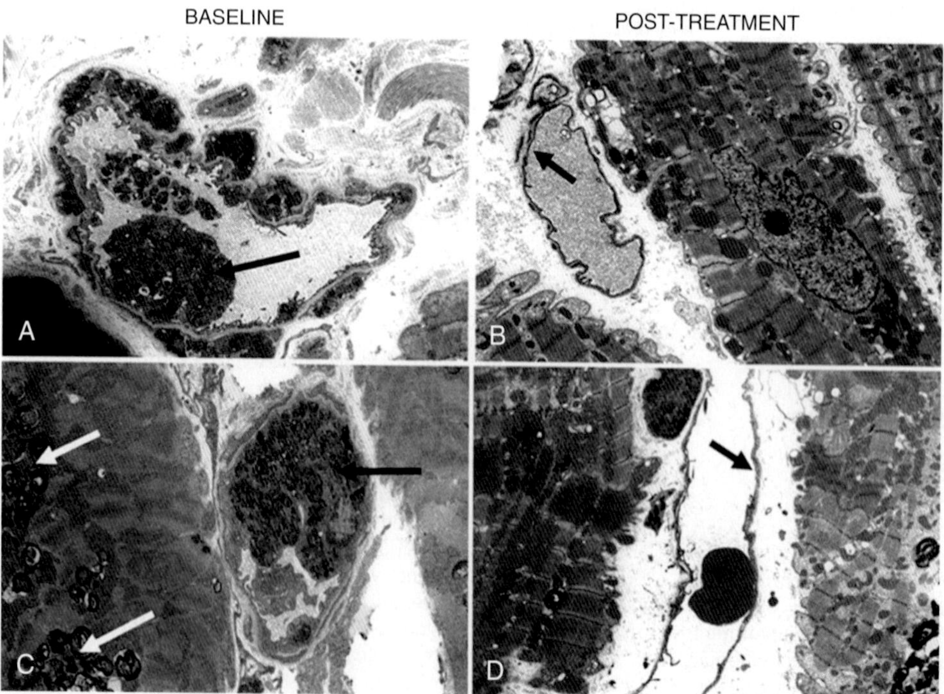

FIGURE 68-10 Electron microscopy demonstrates clearance of GL-3 from cardiac capillaries. *(From Thurberg BL, Fallon JT, Mitchell R, et al: Cardiac microvascular pathology in Fabry disease: Evaluation of endomyocardial biopsies before and after enzyme replacement therapy. Circulation 119:2561, 2009.)*

CLINICAL MANIFESTATIONS. Symptoms at presentation vary widely, and some patients are asymptomatic although evidence exists for myocardial involvement. Echocardiography reveals increased left ventricular wall thickness, ventricular dilation, and ventricular dysfunction. Both computed tomography and CMR are useful to detect early subclinical myocardial involvement at a time when therapy is most effective.[72] Electrocardiographic manifestations occur with advancing cardiac involvement and include ST-segment and T wave abnormalities and supraventricular arrhythmias.

Clinical and echocardiographic features usually are diagnostic, and endomyocardial biopsy is confirmatory but because of false negativity cannot definitively rule out the diagnosis. Evaluation of iron metabolism may aid in the diagnosis. Plasma iron levels are elevated, total iron-binding capacity is low or normal, and serum ferritin, urinary iron, liver iron, and especially saturation of transferrin are markedly elevated. Management should include repeated phlebotomies or treatment with chelating agents such as deferoamine. For advanced disease, cardiac transplantation carries acceptable 5- and 10-year survival rates.[73]

Glycogen Storage Disease

Patients with type II, III, IV, and V glycogen storage diseases may have cardiac involvement. However, survival to adulthood is rare with the exception of patients with type III disease (glycogen debranching enzyme deficiency). The most typical cardiac involvement is left ventricular hypertrophy, with electrocardiographic and echocardiographic findings, often with the absence of symptoms. A subset of patients may present with overt cardiac dysfunction, arrhythmias, and presentation of a DCM.

Inflammatory Causes of Infiltrative Cardiomyopathy

SARCOIDOSIS

Sarcoidosis is a systemic inflammatory condition characterized by the formation of noncaseating granulomas, most commonly involving the lungs, reticuloendothelial system, and skin. Sarcoid has been reported to involve essentially all tissues including the heart, which is recognized in 20% to 30% of autopsies of affected patients. Cardiac impairment may also arise secondary to pulmonary sarcoidosis, in which case extensive pulmonary fibrosis leads to advancing right-sided heart failure. The main clinical manifestations of sarcoid heart disease result from infiltration of the conduction system and myocardium, producing heart block, malignant arrhythmias, heart failure, and sudden cardiac death. Patients with cardiac sarcoidosis may also present with a restrictive cardiomyopathy caused by increased ventricular chamber stiffness.[47]

PATHOLOGY. Noncaseating granulomas surrounded by multinucleated giant cells are the diagnostic feature of the disorder and are found in multiple organs. In the heart, they infiltrate the myocardium and lead to the formation of fibrotic scars. The condition must be separated from two other inflammatory conditions of the heart—chronic active myocarditis and giant cell myocarditis (see Chap. 70). Giant cell myocarditis, which is characterized by diffuse giant cell inflammation in the absence of discrete granulomas, has a much more fulminant course than cardiac sarcoid (**Fig. 68-11**).[13,48] In sarcoidosis, the granulomas may involve discrete areas of the ventricular walls in a patchy fashion, increasing the likelihood of a false-negative endomyocardial biopsy result. Granulomas are most commonly observed in the interventricular septum and left ventricular free wall, and patients with conduction system disease typically have involvement of the basal portion of the interventricular septum. Left ventricular aneurysm formation may occur with extensive transmural free wall involvement. In terms of the coronary anatomy, the large conductance vessels are usually spared, but small coronary artery branches may be involved.

CLINICAL MANIFESTATIONS. The clinical manifestations result from infiltration of the conduction system and myocardium. The most devastating presentation is that of sudden death due to malignant ventricular arrhythmia. Patients may also present with heart block, congestive heart failure, and syncope. Both atrial and ventricular arrhythmias are common.[74] Patients may be asymptomatic despite significant cardiac involvement. Heart failure may result from direct myocardial involvement or cor pulmonale due to extensive pulmonary fibrosis. Survival may range from months to years, with a positive endomyocardial biopsy finding heralding a grave outcome.[75] Excellent long-term outcome may be achieved with aggressive immunosuppression. Isolated cardiac sarcoid has been reported.

The initial detection of cardiac sarcoidosis often results from the presence of bilateral hilar lymphadenopathy on chest radiographs in individuals with clinical or electrocardiographic findings suggesting myocardial disease. Endomyocardial biopsy should be performed if it is available because of the importance of positive findings, but it has a high false-negative rate.[13,75] Multiple imaging modalities assist in assessing diagnosis and prognosis. Echocardiography may demonstrate either global or regional left ventricular dysfunction and rarely may reveal aneurysm formation. Echocardiography is also valuable to evaluate right ventricular hypertrophy and to estimate pulmonary artery systolic pressures. CMR is emerging as a highly sensitive and specific test (see Fig. 18-13).[76] Other modalities include myocardial nuclear imaging with thallium-201 or technetium-99m, which can reveal segmental perfusion defects due to granulomatous inflammation, and [^{18}F]-fluorodeoxyglucose positron emission tomography, which can reveal focal uptake consistent with sarcoid. Uptake of technetium pyrophosphate, gallium, or labeled antimyosin antibody may also contribute to making the diagnosis.

The physical examination may show evidence of extracardiac sarcoid or may be totally normal. An apical systolic murmur due to mitral regurgitation is frequently present, often arising from cardiac chamber dilation as opposed to direct papillary muscle infiltration. Murmurs of tricuspid regurgitation, pulmonic regurgitation, and right-sided third heart sounds suggest pulmonary hypertension and cor pulmonale. Both S_3 and S_4 are frequently appreciated.

Electrocardiography typically demonstrates nonspecific findings suggestive of myocardial involvement, with T wave abnormalities commonly present. The electrocardiogram is highly valuable to assess the degree of conduction system involvement in terms of intraventricular delays and atrioventricular block (see Fig. 68-e5 on website). Q waves may be present, indicating severe and extensive myocardial replacement and fibrosis. Typical findings on echocardiography include left ventricular dilation with global or regional hypokinesis, right-sided enlargement and hypertrophy, possible left ventricular aneurysm formation, and, not infrequently, pericardial effusion. On occasion, increased echogenicity suggests an infiltrative process.

MANAGEMENT. Sarcoidosis is generally treated with immunosuppression.[13,47] Conduction disturbance, arrhythmias, and myocardial dysfunction may all respond to corticosteroids. Steroids effectively halt the progression of inflammation, and some studies suggest that therapy may offer improved survival. Other drugs that may be of benefit in sarcoidosis include hydroxychloroquine, methotrexate, and cyclophosphamide. It is important to distinguish cardiac sarcoidosis from giant cell myocarditis, a much more aggressive disorder that requires intensive immunosuppression and frequently mechanical support or heart transplantation (see Chap. 70). Whereas antiarrhythmic therapy is often ineffective for control of malignant arrhythmias,

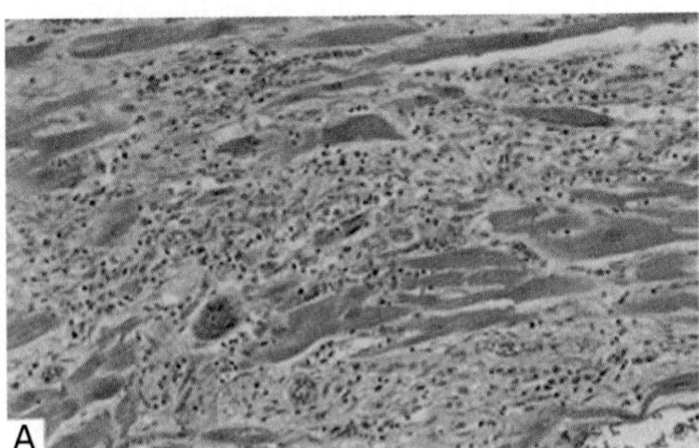

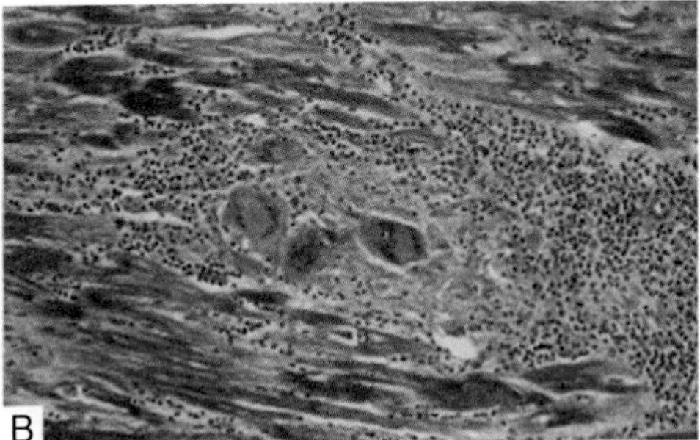

FIGURE 68-11 Sarcoid versus giant cell myocarditis. Giant cell myocarditis **(A)** is characterized by lymphocytic infiltration, myocyte necrosis, and giant cells. Sarcoidosis **(B)** is characterized by the presence of true noncaseating granulomas. *(From Hare JM: Etiologic basis of congestive heart failure. In Colucci WS [ed]: Atlas of Heart Failure. 5th ed. Philadelphia, Springer, Current Medicine Group, 2008, pp 29-56. Copyright 2008, Current Medicine LLC.)*

ICD therapy is appropriate for patients at risk for sudden cardiac death. Implantation of a permanent pacemaker is often required in the case of conduction system disease. Heart or heart-lung transplantation should be considered in the case of intractable heart failure, although sarcoid may recur in the grafted organ.

Endomyocardial Disease

DEFINITION AND PATHOGENESIS. A common form of restrictive cardiomyopathy found in a geographic location close to the equator is known as endomyocardial disease. Endomyocardial disease is common in equatorial Africa and is manifested less frequently in South America, Asia, and nontropical countries, including the United States. Two variants are described that, despite similar phenotypes, are likely unique processes, both manifesting as aggressive endocardial scarring obliterating the ventricular apices and subvalvular regions. Endomyocardial fibrosis or Davies disease is the first variant and occurs primarily in tropical regions; the second, Löffler endocarditis parietalis fibroplastica, or the hypereosinophilic syndrome, is encountered in more temperate zones. Although the pathologic appearance of these two disorders is similar, there are sufficient differences between the two disorders to suggest that they indeed are two distinct entities. Löffler endocarditis is more aggressive and rapidly progresses, affects mainly males, and is associated with hypereosinophilia, thromboemboli, and systemic arteritis; endomyocardial fibrosis occurs in a younger distribution, affects young children, and is only variably associated with eosinophilia.

Differences Between Löffler Endocarditis and Endomyocardial Fibrosis. Overlap between Löffler endocarditis and endomyocardial fibrosis is suggested by the observation that both diseases are attributable to the direct toxic effects of eosinophils in the myocardium. It is suggested that hypereosinophilia (regardless of cause) produces the first phase of endomyocardial disease, which is characterized by necrosis, intense myocarditis, and arteritis (i.e., Löffler endocarditis). This phase lasts for a period of months and is then followed by a thrombotic stage a year after the initial presentation, in which nonspecific thickening of the myocardium with a layer of thrombus replaces the inflammatory portion of myocardium. In the late phase, final healing is achieved by the formation of fibrosis, at which point the clinical features of endomyocardial fibrosis are present. Most of the support for this three-stage pathophysiologic process, namely, necrotic, thrombotic, and fibrotic, comes from autopsy studies. Nonetheless, definitive evidence that each patient passes sequentially through these stages is lacking.

Role of Eosinophils. The mechanism by which eosinophils participate in the development of cardiac disease remains incompletely understood. These cells have the capacity to directly infiltrate tissues or to release factors that may exert toxicity. The observation that patients with Löffler endocarditis have degranulated eosinophils in their peripheral blood supports the idea that these granules contain cardiotoxic substances, capable of causing the necrotic phase of endomyocardial disease, which leads to the thrombotic and fibrotic phases once the eosinophilia resolves. It is conceivable that this effect may occur only in temperate zones of the world, as the link between eosinophilia and endomyocardial fibrosis is less clear (although parasitic diseases have increased incidence), suggesting that endomyocardial fibrosis may result from a different mechanism in tropical countries. Factors implicated include elevated cerium levels and hypomagnesemia.

Löffler Endocarditis: The Hypereosinophilic Syndrome

In temperate climates, endomyocardial disease is closely associated with significant hypereosinophilia, which can have several different causes. Hypereosinophilia associated with Löffler endocarditis usually is characterized by eosinophil counts exceeding 1500/mm^3 for at least 6 months. Most patients with this degree of hypereosinophilia will have cardiac involvement. The eosinophilia may be secondary to leukemia, reactive disorders such as parasite infection, allergies, granulomatous syndromes, hypersensitivity, or neoplastic disorders. In addition, patients with Churg-Strauss syndrome, characterized by asthma or allergic rhinitis and a necrotizing vasculitis, often have cardiac involvement.[77]

PATHOLOGY. The hypereosinophilic syndrome involves several organ systems beyond the heart, including the lungs, brain, and bone marrow. Both chambers of the heart are involved and show endocardial thickening of the inflow regions and ventricular apices. On histologic examination, there are variable degrees of eosinophilic myocarditis of the myocardium and subendocardium, thrombosis and inflammation of small intramural coronary vessels, mural thrombosis containing eosinophils, and endocardial fibrotic thickening of several millimeters.

CLINICAL MANIFESTATIONS. Patients with hypereosinophilic syndrome exhibit weight loss, fever, cough, rash, and congestive heart failure. Early in the course of cardiac involvement, patients may be asymptomatic; but with progression, in excess of 50% of patients will have overt congestive heart failure or cardiomegaly. Murmurs of mitral regurgitation are common. Systemic emboli occur frequently, resulting in neurologic and renal sequelae. Death results from heart failure associated with renal, hepatic, or pulmonary involvement. Sudden cardiac death and syndromes mimicking acute myocardial infarction are described.

LABORATORY EXAMINATION. Chest radiography may demonstrate an enlarged cardiac silhouette accompanied by evidence of pulmonary congestion or, less frequently, pulmonary infiltrates. Changes on the electrocardiogram are nonspecific and include ST-segment and T wave abnormalities. Atrial fibrillation and conduction defects, most notably right bundle branch block, are often noted. The echocardiogram often shows regional thickening of the posterobasal portion of the left ventricular wall, with substantial impairment in the motion of the posterior leaflet of the mitral valve. The apex may be obliterated by thrombus (see Fig. 15-80). The atria are often dilated, and there is Doppler ultrasound evidence of atrioventricular regurgitation. As is typical for restrictive cardiomyopathy, systolic function is often normal. Hemodynamic measurements support a restrictive cardiomyopathic appearance with abnormal diastolic filling, secondary to the dense endocardial scarring and reduced size of the ventricular cavity from the organized thrombus. Regurgitation through atrioventricular valves results from involvement of their respective supporting structures. Cardiac catheterization reveals markedly elevated ventricular filling pressures, and there may be evidence of tricuspid or mitral regurgitation. A characteristic feature on angiocardiography is largely preserved systolic function with obliteration of the apex of the ventricles. Endomyocardial biopsy can provide diagnostic confirmation but is not always positive.

MANAGEMENT. There is a role for both medical and surgical therapy in improving quality and quantity of life in patients with Löffler endocarditis. There is evidence that both corticosteroids and cytotoxic drugs such as hydroxyurea may have an important favorable effect on survival. In refractory patients, treatment with interferon may offer a valuable adjunctive therapy. Routine supportive cardiac therapy with diuretics, neurohormonal blockade, and anticoagulation as indicated is appropriate for management of these patients. Surgical therapy consisting of endocardiectomy and valve replacement or repair appears to provide significant symptomatic palliation once the fibrotic stage of the disease is manifested.

Endomyocardial Fibrosis

Endomyocardial fibrosis is a disorder found typically in tropical and subtropical Africa, notably in Uganda, Nigeria, and Mozambique, and is a major cause of morbidity and mortality, accounting for 25% of cases of congestive heart failure and death in equatorial Africa.[53,78,79] A population-based study in rural Mozambique revealed a prevalence of the disorder affecting 19.8% of the population.[53] In this study, only 48 of 211 patients were symptomatic at time of detection, and familial occurrence was high.

The disease is increasingly recognized in other tropical and subtropical regions within 15 degrees of the equator, including India, Brazil, Colombia, and Sri Lanka.[52] Importantly, it is also recognized in the Middle East, particularly Saudi Arabia.[79] Cardiac dysfunction occurs because of fibrous lesions that affect the inflow of the right and left ventricles and that may also involve the atrioventricular valves, thereby producing regurgitant lesions. Endomyocardial fibrosis has increased incidence among the Rwanda tribe of Uganda and in individuals of low socioeconomic status.[51] It has a slight male preponderance, is most common in children[78] and young adults,[53] but has been described in individuals into the sixth decade of life (see Fig. 68-e6 on website). Although most cases occur in black individuals, there are occasional presentations in white subjects residing in temperate climates. There are rare reports of endomyocardial fibrosis in individuals who have not resided in tropical areas.

PATHOLOGY. Endomyocardial fibrosis affects both the right and left ventricles in approximately 50% of patients, purely the left in 40%, and the right ventricle alone in the remaining 10%.[52,79] The typical gross appearance is that of a normal to slightly enlarged heart. The right atrium may be dilated in proportion to the severity of right ventricular involvement. There is often a pericardial effusion, which may be large. The right-sided heart border may be indented because of apical scarring. The hallmark feature of the disorder is fibrotic obliteration of the apex of the affected ventricles (**Fig. 68-12**). The fibrosis involves the papillary muscles and chordae tendineae, leading to atrioventricular valve distortion and regurgitation. In the left ventricle, the fibrosis extends from the apex to the posterior mitral valve leaflet, usually sparing the anterior mitral leaflet and the ventricular outflow tract. Endocardial calcific deposits can be present involving diffuse areas of the ventricle. The fibrotic tissue often creates a nidus for thrombus formation, which can be extensive. Atrial thrombi also occur. The process usually does not involve the epicardium, and the coronary artery obstruction is distinctly uncommon.

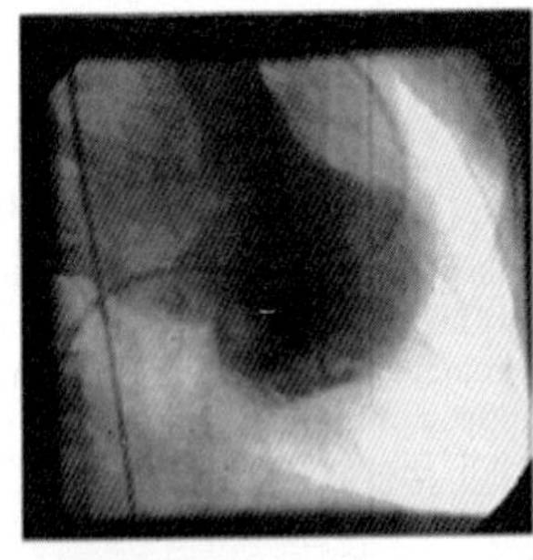

A

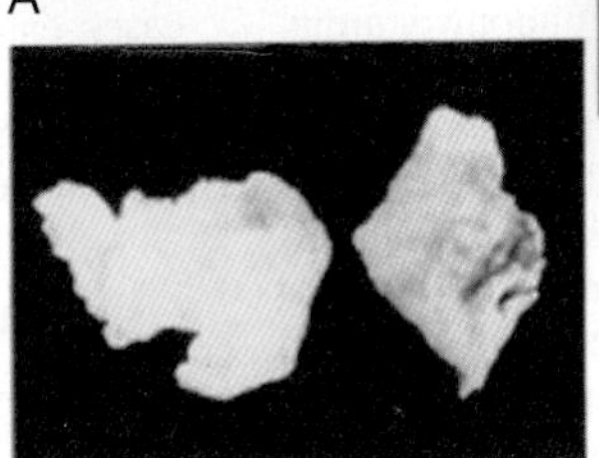

B

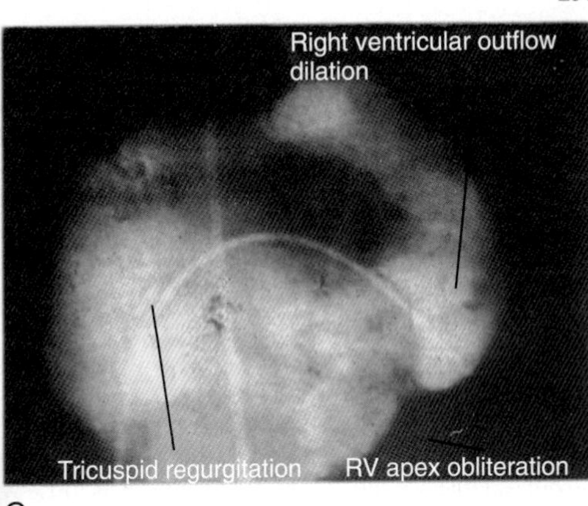

C

FIGURE 68-12 Right- and left-sided endomyocardial fibrosis. **A,** Left-sided endomyocardial fibrosis is characterized by apical obliteration, patchy filling defects, and severe mitral regurgitation. **B,** The management of endomyocardial fibrosis often requires surgical excision of the endocardial fibrosis. Depicted are pieces of excised endocardial fibrosis. **C,** Right ventricular (RV) angiogram of a patient with RV endomyocardial fibrosis showing RV outflow tract dilation, RV apex obliteration, and tricuspid regurgitation. *(**A** and **B** from Joshi R, Abraham S, Kumar AS: New approach for complete endocardiectomy in left ventricular endomyocardial fibrosis. J Thorac Cardiovasc Surg 125:40, 2003. **C** from Seth S, Thatai D, Sharma S, et al: Clinico-pathological evaluation of restrictive cardiomyopathy [endomyocardial fibrosis and idiopathic restrictive cardiomyopathy] in India. Eur J Heart Fail 6:723, 2004.)*

HISTOLOGIC FINDINGS. Endomyocardial fibrosis is clearly apparent histologically, presenting as a thick layer of collagen overlying loosely arranged connective tissue.[79] In addition, there are fibrous and granular septations extending into the underlying myocardial tissue. Myocyte hypertrophy is common.[52] Whereas cellular infiltration is uncommon, interstitial edema is frequently present. Fibroelastosis that is found in the ventricular outflow tracts beneath the semilunar valves often represents a secondary process caused by local trauma. Examination of intramural coronary arteries may show involvement with medial degeneration, the deposition of fibrin, and fibrosis.

CLINICAL MANIFESTATIONS. The symptomatic status of patients at presentation relates to which ventricles are involved. Pulmonary congestion signals left-sided involvement, whereas predominantly right-sided disease may mimic restrictive cardiomyopathy or constrictive pericarditis. Atrioventricular valve regurgitation is common. The disease may be heralded by an acute febrile illness or may be simply insidious. Endomyocardial fibrosis is a relentless and progressive process, although the time course of decline may vary considerably, with some patients appearing to have periods of stability. Modes of death include progressive heart failure, infection, infarction, sudden cardiac death, and complications of surgery. Atrial fibrillation and ascites are reported to be poor prognostic indicators.[80,81]

Right Ventricular Endomyocardial Fibrosis. In pure or predominant right ventricular involvement, the right ventricular apex is characterized by fibrous obliteration, which may extend to involve the supporting structures of the tricuspid valve, with ensuing tricuspid regurgitation. Patients exhibit an elevated jugular venous pressure, a prominent *v* wave with rapid *y* descent, and a right-sided S_3 gallop. There is prominent hepatomegaly with a pulsatile liver, ascites, splenomegaly, and peripheral edema, but pulmonary congestion is typically absent because of the lack of left-sided involvement. In this regard, pulmonary artery and pulmonary capillary wedge pressures are normal. A large pericardial effusion is often present. The right atrium may be enormously dilated. The electrocardiogram often has findings consistent with right-sided enlargement, especially a qR pattern in lead V_1, and supraventricular arrhythmias are common. The chest radiograph often demonstrates obvious right atrial prominence, a pericardial effusion, and calcification in the walls of the right and, less frequently, the left ventricle. Echocardiography demonstrates thickening of the right ventricle with obliteration of the apex, a dilated atrium, hyperechoic endocardial surfaces, and abnormal septal motion in patients with tricuspid regurgitation. On angiography, the right ventricular apex is typically not visualized because of fibrous obliteration; tricuspid regurgitation, right atrial enlargement, and filling defects in the right atrium caused by thrombi may be present.

Left Ventricular Endomyocardial Fibrosis. In cases of predominant left-sided disease, fibrosis involves the ventricular apex and often the chordae tendineae or the posterior mitral valve leaflet, producing mitral regurgitation. The associated murmur may be late systolic, characteristic of a papillary muscle dysfunction murmur, or pansystolic. Findings of pulmonary hypertension may be prominent, and an S_3 protodiastolic gallop is frequently present. The electrocardiogram usually shows ST-segment and T wave abnormalities, low-voltage QRS complexes if a pericardial effusion is present, or left ventricular hypertrophy. Left atrial abnormality is often noted. As with right-sided involvement, atrial fibrillation is often present and portends a poor prognosis. Echocardiography reveals increased endocardial echoreflectivity, preserved systolic function, apical obliteration, enlarged atrium, pericardial effusion of varying size, and Doppler ultrasound evidence of mitral regurgitation. Pulmonary hypertension is typically observed during cardiac catheterization, as well as left atrial hypertension and a reduced cardiac index. Left ventriculography shows mitral regurgitation, and ventricular filling defects caused by intracavitary thrombi may be present. Coronary arteriography usually excludes obstructive epicardial vessel stenoses.

Biventricular Endomyocardial Fibrosis. Biventricular endomyocardial fibrosis is more common then either isolated right- or left-sided disease. The typical clinical presentation of endomyocardial fibrosis resembles right ventricular endomyocardial fibrosis; however, a murmur of mitral regurgitation is indicative of left-sided involvement. Unless left ventricular involvement is extensive, severe pulmonary hypertension is absent and the right-sided findings are the predominant mode of presentation. Approximately 15% of patients will experience systemic embolization, and only 2% will have infective endocarditis.

DIAGNOSIS. Detection of endomyocardial fibrosis in individuals from the appropriate geographic area requires typical clinical and laboratory findings as well as angiography. Eosinophilia is variably present and may result from parasitic infection.[51] Endomyocardial biopsy is diagnostic, but false negatives can occur because of the patchy nature of the disease. Insofar as myocardial biopsy may be complicated by systemic emboli, left-sided myocardial biopsy is contraindicated.

MANAGEMENT. The medical management of endomyocardial fibrosis remains challenging. One third to one half of patients with advanced disease die within 2 years, whereas those who are less symptomatic fare better. The development of atrial fibrillation is a poor prognostic indicator, although symptomatic relief can be achieved with rate control.[80] Heart failure is difficult to control, and diuretics are effective only in early stages of disease, losing efficacy with advanced ascites. Once endomyocardial fibrosis progresses to severe endocardial fibrosis, surgical resection with atrioventricular valve replacement on affected sides is the treatment of choice.[82] Surgical therapy consisting of endocardiectomy and valve replacement or repair usually results in hemodynamic improvement with reductions in ventricular filling pressures, increased cardiac output, and normalized angiographic appearance (see Fig. 68-12). Operative mortality is high, between 15% and 25%, and may be lower if valve replacement is not necessary.[83] Fibrosis may recur, although there are case reports of excellent long-term survival.[84]

Endocardial Fibroelastosis

Endocardial fibroelastosis is a disorder of fetuses and infants of unclear etiology that is characterized by deposition of collagen and elastin, leading to ventricular hypertrophy and diffuse endocardial thickening (see Fig. 68-e7 on website). Causes are incompletely understood, and there are reports of associations with viral infections (especially mumps), metabolic disorders, autoimmune disease, and congenital left-sided obstructive lesions. Two recent reports implicate mitochondrial disorders and placental insufficiency.[85,86] Like DCM, endocardial fibroelastosis usually progresses to severe congestive heart failure and subsequent death. The echocardiographic finding of a highly reflective endocardial surface of the ventricular myocardium suggests endocardial fibroelastosis.

Neoplastic Infiltrative Cardiomyopathy—Carcinoid Heart Disease

The carcinoid syndrome results from the metastasis of carcinoid tumors from the gut to the heart.[87] The symptoms include marked cutaneous flushing, diarrhea, bronchoconstriction, and endocardial plaques composed of a unique type of fibrous tissue. The symptom complex is caused in large part by the release of serotonin and other circulating substances secreted by the tumor. Essentially all patients experience diarrhea and flushing, 50% have cardiac lesions detected echocardiographically, and about 25% of the patients have severe right-sided involvement.

Carcinoid tumors originate largely from the gut, with 60% to 90% being found in the small bowel and appendix and the remainder arising from other regions of the gastrointestinal tract or the bronchi. Carcinoid tumors arising in the ileum pose the greatest risk of metastasis, most likely affecting regional lymph nodes and the liver. The carcinoid tumors arising in the liver affect the heart. The severity of the cardiac lesions is related to the circulating concentrations of serotonin and 5-hydroxyindoleacetic acid (its primary metabolite), which are produced primarily by the carcinoid tumors in the liver. The observation that the right side of the heart is preferentially affected in the carcinoid syndrome reflects inactivation of the circulating toxic substances in the lung; the 5% to 10% of individuals presenting with left-sided lesions are likely to have right-to-left shunts or tumor involvement of the lungs.

Pathology

The characteristic lesions are fibrous plaques involving locations "downstream" of the tricuspid and pulmonic valves, the endocardium, and the intima of the venae cavae, pulmonary artery, and coronary sinus. Both stenotic and regurgitant valvular lesions result from fibrotic distortion originating in the plaques.[87] The plaque material appears as a layer of fibrous tissue composed of smooth muscle cells, collagen, and mucopolysaccharides overlying the endocardium and in some cases extending into the underlying regions. Interestingly, identical pathology results from exposure to the anorectic drugs fenfluramine and dexfenfluramine. On occasion, there is actual metastasis of the tumor to one or both of the ventricles.

Clinical Manifestations

Cardiac murmurs indicating right-sided valve involvement are widely appreciated. A systolic murmur of tricuspid regurgitation along the left sternal border is almost always present, and pulmonic valve murmurs of either stenosis or regurgitation may also be present (see Chap. 66). The chest radiograph may be normal or may show cardiac enlargement and pleural effusions or nodules. The pulmonary artery trunk is most often not enlarged, and poststenotic dilation is also absent, differentiating pulmonic involvement from congenital pulmonic stenosis. Although there are no specific changes on the electrocardiogram diagnostic of carcinoid heart disease, it is not uncommon to encounter right atrial enlargement without other findings of right ventricular hypertrophy, nonspecific ST-segment and T wave abnormalities, and sinus tachycardia. Patients with advanced disease are likely to have low QRS voltage. Echocardiography often reveals tricuspid or pulmonary valve thickening and enlargement of the right atrium and ventricle (see Figs. 66-39 and 66-41); a minority of patients may have a small pericardial effusion. CMR may offer additional value in evaluating the right side of the heart that may be difficult to image with echocardiography.[88]

Management

For mild congestive heart failure, standard therapy with diuretics and neurohormonal antagonists is appropriate. Both somatostatin analogues and chemotherapy can lead to improved symptoms and possibly enhanced survival, but neither is effective at amelioration of progressive cardiac disease in patients with carcinoid syndrome. A key element of management is relief of stenotic lesions of the tricuspid and pulmonary valves. This may be achieved with either balloon valvuloplasty or surgery, both of which can achieve symptomatic relief. Operative mortality is traditionally high, but it has improved significantly in experienced centers.[87]

Arrhythmogenic Right Ventricular Dysplasia/Cardiomyopathy

Arrhythmogenic right ventricular dysplasia/cardiomyopathy (ARVD/C), first described in 1977 by Fontaine and coworkers, is a genetic form of cardiomyopathy characterized prototypically by fibrofatty infiltration of the right ventricle (**Figs. 68-13** and **68-14**). ARVD/C accounts for 20% of cases of sudden cardiac death, and importantly, among young athletes dying suddenly, the prevalence of this condition is higher.[89,90]

Presenting Symptoms and Natural History

Patients typically present between the teenage years and the forties, with only 10% falling outside of this age range. The natural history of the disorder is characterized by four phases: a concealed phase in which patients are asymptomatic, a phase characterized by an overt clinical manifestation of an electrical system disturbance, progression

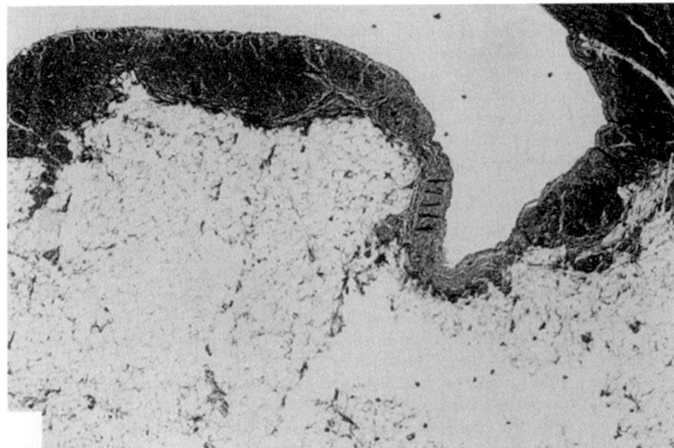

FIGURE 68-13 Arrhythmogenic right ventricular dysplasia/cardiomyopathy (ARVD/C). Histologic appearance of ARVD/C showing fibrosis, adipose infiltration, and myocardial thinning. *(From Hare JM: Etiologic basis of congestive heart failure.* In *Colucci WS [ed]: Atlas of Heart Failure. 5th ed. Philadelphia, Springer, Current Medicine Group, 2008, pp 29-56. Copyright 2008, Current Medicine LLC.)*

to signs and symptoms of right ventricular failure, and finally frank biventricular congestive heart failure. Accordingly, presenting symptoms range from palpitations to syncope and sudden cardiac death. A majority of patients who subsequently experience sudden cardiac death have a history of syncope, which thus represents an important prognostic event.[90] Progression to heart failure occurs in the minority of patients but is the predominant mode of death in individuals who are protected from sudden cardiac death by ICD implantation.

Pathology

Characteristically, a heart affected with ARVD/C exhibits fatty or fibrofatty replacement of the myocardium predominantly affecting the right ventricle. Rarely, the process extends to the left ventricle (see Fig. 18-11).

Genetics

Several genes and gene loci are associated with ARVD/C, and both autosomal dominant and recessive modes of inheritance are described. Most but not all genes encode desmosomal proteins.[91] Implicated genes include desmoplakin, junctional plakoglobin (*JUP*), the cardiac ryanodine receptor plakophilin 2 (*PKP2*), and transforming growth factor-β3. *JUP* mutations are causally implicated in Naxos disease, a syndrome characterized by ARVD/C, wooly hair, and palmoplantar keratoderma. Individuals with mutations in *PKP2* present at younger ages and are more likely to have malignant arrhythmias.[89] This finding suggests the prognostic importance of genetic testing for ARVD/C. In addition, immunohistochemical detection of plakoglobin is proposed to be of value in diagnosis.[91]

Diagnosis

A task force has set diagnostic criteria to aid in the study and characterization of ARVD/C. The diagnostic criteria involve features obtained from imaging, electrocardiography, signal-averaged electrocardiography, and histologic evaluation as well as a positive family history and a history of arrhythmias.[14] Early diagnosis of ARVD/C remains challenging. Whereas endomyocardial biopsy may offer valuable diagnostic information, CMR is emerging as a more definitive diagnostic tool.[41] The main limitation of endomyocardial biopsy is a high false-negative rate because of sampling error and the fact that the right ventricle septum may lack the characteristic histologic changes; however, immunohistochemical detection of plakoglobin may enhance the value of tissue diagnosis.[91] Tandri and colleagues[41] have reported that characterization of the ventricular wall morphology with delayed enhancement gadolinium CMR correlated well with

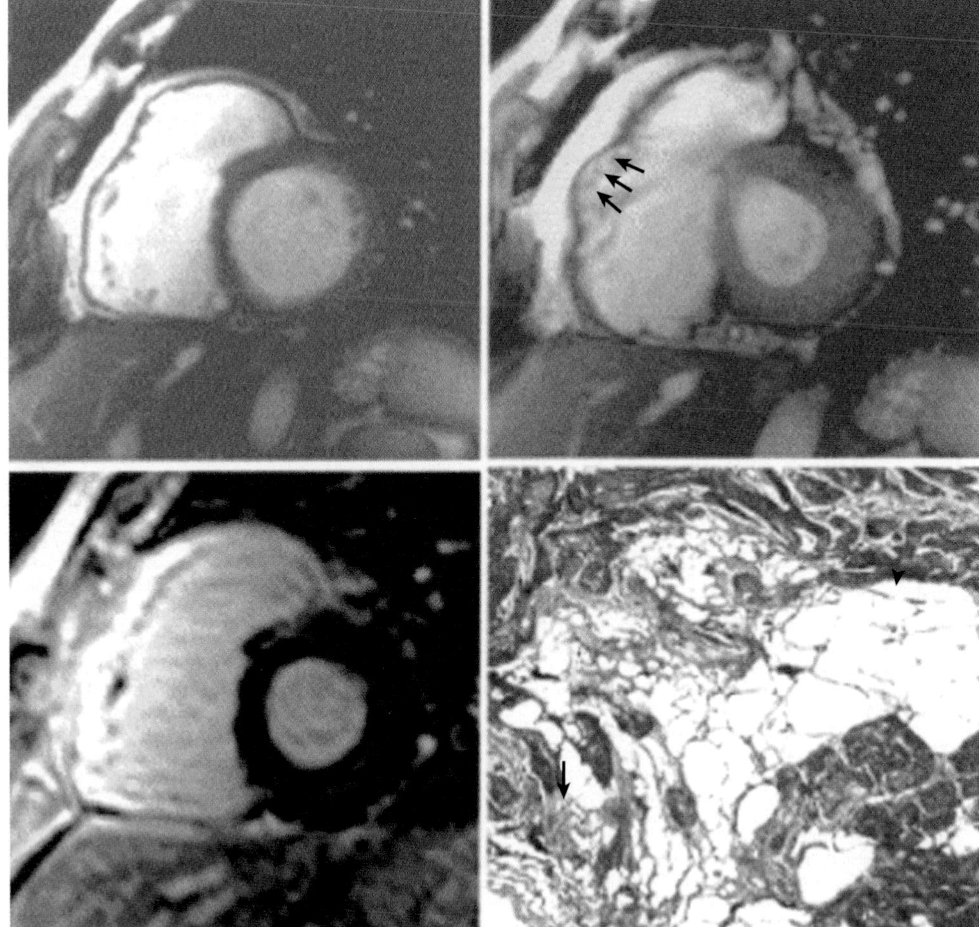

FIGURE 68-14 Arrhythmogenic right ventricular dysplasia/cardiomyopathy (ARVD/C). The **top left and right panels** represent the end-diastolic and end-systolic frames of a short-axis cine magnetic resonance image showing an area of dyskinesia on right ventricular free wall characterizing a focal ventricular aneurysm (arrows). The **bottom left panel** displays the delayed-enhanced magnetic resonance image with increased signal intensity within the right ventricular myocardium (arrows), at the location of right ventricular aneurysms. The **bottom right panel** shows the corresponding endomyocardial biopsy. Trichrome stain of the right ventricle at high magnification shows marked replacement of the ventricular muscle by adipose tissue. The adipose tissue cells (arrowhead) are irregular in size and infiltrate the ventricular muscle. There is also abundant replacement fibrosis (arrow). There is no evidence of inflammation. *(From Tandri H, Saranathan M, Rodriguez ER, et al: Noninvasive detection of myocardial fibrosis in arrhythmogenic right ventricular cardiomyopathy using delayed-enhancement magnetic resonance imaging. J Am Coll Cardiol 45:98, 2005.)*

histologic findings as well as with inducibility of ventricular tachycardia during electrophysiologic testing.

Management

Patients diagnosed with ARVD/C should receive an ICD. Antiarrhythmic therapy is appropriate before ICD insertion and in some cases after, in patients who have recurrent ICD firings. Use of an ICD can have an enormous clinical impact on reducing the major cause of mortality in affected individuals. It is also recommended that patients receive neurohormonal blockade with angiotensin-converting enzyme inhibitors and beta adrenoreceptor antagonists. In individuals progressing to overt heart failure, management involves the same principles for the treatment of other forms of cardiomyopathy. Consideration of heart transplantation is indicated for patients with overt biventricular failure.

Summary and Future Perspectives

Our current understanding of cardiomyopathic processes is still fairly rudimentary as evidenced by the large percentage of patients who are assigned as having idiopathic disease. Continual advances are being made with respect to genetics and cellular biology (stem cells) that are revealing important insights into the etiology, natural history, and potentially the management of dilated, restrictive, and right ventricular cardiomyopathy. The strong genetic basis of several cardiomyopathic disorders coupled with new high-throughput technologies will allow the possibility of widespread genetic testing of affected individuals and their family members. Genetic testing will also facilitate understanding of which patients have a genetic cause of their disease as opposed to a genetic predisposition to an environmental insult. In addition to genetics, measurement of expressed genes (transcriptomics), microRNA abnormalities,[92] and proteins (proteomics) has the potential to aid in understanding etiology, prognosis, and individualized responses to therapy (personalized medicine). A key example of the last is the attempt to identify patients with a viral cause of cardiomyopathy and to treat those patients with appropriate antiviral therapy, on the one hand, and those without viral infection with immunosuppressive therapy, on the other hand. The most recent advance with significant future implications is the observation that the body, including the bone marrow and the heart, possesses reservoirs of endogenous stem cells regulated in stem cell niches; the discovery of these cells and their niches offers new insights into the causes of cardiomyopathy and may, in the future, provide a new therapeutic avenue.

REFERENCES

Dilated Cardiomyopathy

1. Dec GW, Fuster V: Idiopathic dilated cardiomyopathy. N Engl J Med 331:1564, 1994.
2. Ammash NM, Seward JB, Bailey KR, et al: Clinical profile and outcome of idiopathic restrictive cardiomyopathy. Circulation 101:2490, 2000.
3. Mann DL, Bristow MR: Mechanisms and models in heart failure: The biomechanical model and beyond. Circulation 111:2837, 2005.
4. Hare JM, Walford GD, Hruban RH, et al: Ischemic cardiomyopathy: Endomyocardial biopsy and ventriculographic evaluation of patients with congestive heart failure, dilated cardiomyopathy and coronary artery disease. J Am Coll Cardiol 20:1318, 1992.
5. Kittleson MM, Minhas KM, Irizarry RA, et al: Gene expression analysis of ischemic and nonischemic cardiomyopathy: Shared and distinct genes in the development of heart failure. Physiol Genomics 21:299, 2005.
6. Maron BJ, Towbin JA, Thiene G, et al: Contemporary definitions and classification of the cardiomyopathies: An American Heart Association Scientific Statement from the Council on Clinical Cardiology, Heart Failure and Transplantation Committee; Quality of Care and Outcomes Research and Functional Genomics and Translational Biology Interdisciplinary Working Groups; and Council on Epidemiology and Prevention. Circulation 113:1807, 2006.
7. Felker GM, Thompson RE, Hare JM, et al: Underlying causes and long-term survival in patients with initially unexplained cardiomyopathy. N Engl J Med 342:1077, 2000.
8. Ardehali H, Qasim A, Cappola T, et al: Endomyocardial biopsy plays a role in diagnosing patients with unexplained cardiomyopathy. Am Heart J 147:919, 2004.
9. Levy WC, Mozaffarian D, Linker DT, et al: The Seattle Heart Failure Model: Prediction of survival in heart failure. Circulation 113:1424, 2006.
10. Heidecker B, Kasper EK, Wittstein IS, et al: Transcriptomic biomarkers for individual risk assessment in new-onset heart failure. Circulation 118:238, 2008.
11. McNamara DM, Holubkov R, Starling RC, et al: Controlled trial of intravenous immune globulin in recent-onset dilated cardiomyopathy. Circulation 103:2254, 2001.
12. Teuteberg JJ, Lewis EF, Nohria A, et al: Characteristics of patients who die with heart failure and a low ejection fraction in the new millennium. J Card Fail 12:47, 2006.
13. Cooper LT, Baughman KL, Feldman AM, et al: The role of endomyocardial biopsy in the management of cardiovascular disease: A scientific statement from the American Heart Association, the American College of Cardiology, and the European Society of Cardiology. Circulation 116:2216, 2007.
14. Marcus FI, Zareba W, Calkins H, et al: Arrhythmogenic right ventricular cardiomyopathy/dysplasia clinical presentation and diagnostic evaluation: Results from the North American Multidisciplinary Study. Heart Rhythm 6:984, 2009.
15. McCarthy RE, Boehmer JP, Hruban RH, et al: Long-term outcome of fulminant myocarditis as compared with acute (nonfulminant) myocarditis. N Engl J Med 342:690, 2000.
16. Hare JM: The etiologic basis of congestive heart failure. *In* Colucci WS (ed): Atlas of Heart Failure. 5th ed. Philadelphia, Springer, Current Medicine Group, 2008, pp 29-56.
17. Owan TE, Hodge DO, Herges RM, et al: Trends in prevalence and outcome of heart failure with preserved ejection fraction. N Engl J Med 355:251, 2006.
18. Wittstein IS, Thiemann DR, Lima JA: et al: Neurohumoral features of myocardial stunning due to sudden emotional stress. N Engl J Med 352:539, 2005.
19. Abraham J, Mudd JO, Kapur NK, et al: Stress cardiomyopathy after intravenous administration of catecholamines and beta-receptor agonists. J Am Coll Cardiol 53:1320, 2009.
20. Elkayam U, Akhter MW, Singh H, et al: Pregnancy-associated cardiomyopathy: Clinical characteristics and a comparison between early and late presentation. Circulation 111:2050, 2005.
21. Elkayam U, Tummala PP, Rao K, et al: Maternal and fetal outcomes of subsequent pregnancies in women with peripartum cardiomyopathy. N Engl J Med 344:1567, 2001.
22. Felker GM, Jaeger CJ, Klodas E, et al: Myocarditis and long-term survival in peripartum cardiomyopathy. Am Heart J 140:785, 2000.
23. Modi KA, Illum S, Jariatul K, et al: Poor outcome of indigent patients with peripartum cardiomyopathy in the United States. Am J Obstet Gynecol 201:171, 2009.
24. Redfield MM, Kay GN, Jenkins LS, et al: Tachycardia-related cardiomyopathy: A common cause of ventricular dysfunction in patients with atrial fibrillation referred for atrioventricular ablation. Mayo Clinic Proc 75:790, 2000.
25. Hershberger RE, Lindenfeld J, Mestroni L, et al: Genetic evaluation of cardiomyopathy—a Heart Failure Society of America practice guideline. J Card Fail 15:83, 2009.
26. Poller W, Kuhl U, Tschoepe C, et al: Genome-environment interactions in the molecular pathogenesis of dilated cardiomyopathy. J Mol Med 83:579, 2005.
27. Chimenti C, Kajstura J, Torella D, et al: Senescence and death of primitive cells and myocytes lead to premature cardiac aging and heart failure. Circ Res 93:604, 2003.
28. Kajstura J, Urbanek K, Perl S, et al: Cardiomyogenesis in the adult human heart. Circ Res 107:305, 2010.
29. Lee DS, Pencina MJ, Benjamin EJ, et al: Association of parental heart failure with risk of heart failure in offspring. N Engl J Med 355:138, 2006.
30. Schmitt JP, Kamisago M, Asahi M, et al: Dilated cardiomyopathy and heart failure caused by a mutation in phospholamban. Science 299:1410, 2003.
31. Lyon AR, Sato M, Hajjar RJ, et al: Gene therapy: Targeting the myocardium. Heart 94:89, 2008.
32. McNamara DM, Tam SW, Sabolinski ML, et al: Aldosterone synthase promoter polymorphism modulates outcome in black patients with heart failure: Results from the A-HeFT trial. J Am Coll Cardiol 48:1277, 2006.
33. Cooper LT Jr: Myocarditis. N Engl J Med 360:1526, 2009.
34. Frustaci A, Russo MA, Chimenti C: Randomized study on the efficacy of immunosuppressive therapy in patients with virus-negative inflammatory cardiomyopathy: The TIMIC study. Eur Heart J 30:1995, 2009.
35. Zimmet JM, Hare JM: Nitroso-redox interactions in the cardiovascular system. Circulation 114:1531, 2006.
36. Dorn GW: Apoptotic and non-apoptotic programmed cardiomyocyte death in ventricular remodelling. Cardiovasc Res 81:465, 2009.
37. Towbin JA, Lowe AM, Colan SD, et al: Incidence, causes, and outcomes of dilated cardiomyopathy in children. JAMA 296:1867, 2006.
38. Cox GF, Sleeper LA, Lowe AM, et al: Factors associated with establishing a causal diagnosis for children with cardiomyopathy. Pediatrics 118:1519, 2006.
39. Hare JM, Mangal B, Brown J, et al: Impact of oxypurinol in patients with symptomatic heart failure. Results of the OPT-CHF study. J Am Coll Cardiol 51:2301, 2008.
40. Williams TJ, Manghat NE, Kay-Ferguson A, et al: Cardiomyopathy: Appearances on ECG-gated 64-detector row computed tomography. Clin Radiol 63:464, 2008.
41. Tandri H, Saranathan M, Rodriguez ER, et al: Noninvasive detection of myocardial fibrosis in arrhythmogenic right ventricular cardiomyopathy using delayed-enhancement magnetic resonance imaging. J Am Coll Cardiol 45:98, 2005.
42. Friedrich MG, Sechtem U, Schulz-Menger J, et al: Cardiovascular magnetic resonance in myocarditis: A JACC White Paper. J Am Coll Cardiol 53:1475, 2009.
43. Maceira AM, Joshi J, Prasad SK, et al: Cardiovascular magnetic resonance in cardiac amyloidosis. Circulation 111:186, 2005.
44. Nazarian S, Bluemke DA, Lardo AC, et al: Magnetic resonance assessment of the substrate for inducible ventricular tachycardia in nonischemic cardiomyopathy. Circulation 112:2821, 2005.
45. Kurtz CE, Gerber Y, Weston SA, et al: Use of ejection fraction tests and coronary angiography in patients with heart failure. Mayo Clinic Proc 81:906, 2006.
46. Ardehali H, Kasper EK, Baughman KL: Diagnostic approach to the patient with cardiomyopathy: Whom to biopsy. Am Heart J 149:7, 2005.
47. Okura Y, Dec GW, Hare JM, et al: A clinical and histopathologic comparison of cardiac sarcoidosis and idiopathic giant cell myocarditis. J Am Coll Cardiol 41:322, 2003.
48. Cooper LT Jr, Hare JM, Tazelaar HD, et al: Usefulness of immunosuppression for giant cell myocarditis. Am J Cardiol 102:1535, 2008.
49. Jessup M, Abraham WT, Casey DE, et al: 2009 focused update: ACCF/AHA Guidelines for the Diagnosis and Management of Heart Failure in Adults: A report of the American College of Cardiology Foundation/American Heart Association Task Force on Practice Guidelines: Developed in collaboration with the International Society for Heart and Lung Transplantation. Circulation 119:1977, 2009.
50. Cleland JG, Daubert JC, Erdmann E, et al: The effect of cardiac resynchronization on morbidity and mortality in heart failure. N Engl J Med 352:1539, 2005.

Restrictive and Infiltrative Cardiomyopathy

51. Rutakingirwa M, Ziegler JL, Newton R, et al: Poverty and eosinophilia are risk factors for endomyocardial fibrosis (EMF) in Uganda. Trop Med Int Health 4:229, 1999.
52. Seth S, Thatai D, Sharma S, et al: Clinico-pathological evaluation of restrictive cardiomyopathy (endomyocardial fibrosis and idiopathic restrictive cardiomyopathy) in India. Eur J Heart Fail 6:723, 2004.
53. Mocumbi AO, Ferreira MB, Sidi D, et al: A population study of endomyocardial fibrosis in a rural area of Mozambique. N Engl J Med 359:43, 2008.

Amyloidosis

54. Rapezzi C, Merlini G, Quarta CC, et al: Systemic cardiac amyloidoses. Disease profiles and clinical courses of the 3 main types. Circulation 120:1203, 2009.
55. Falk RH: Diagnosis and management of the cardiac amyloidoses. Circulation 112:2047, 2005.
56. Ha JW, Ommen SR, Tajik AJ, et al: Differentiation of constrictive pericarditis from restrictive cardiomyopathy using mitral annular velocity by tissue Doppler echocardiography. Am J Cardiol 94:316, 2004.
57. Leya FS, Arab D, Joyal D, et al: The efficacy of brain natriuretic peptide levels in differentiating constrictive pericarditis from restrictive cardiomyopathy. J Am Coll Cardiol 45:1900, 2005.
58. Jacobson DR, Pastore RD, Yaghoubian R, et al: Variant-sequence transthyretin (isoleucine 122) in late-onset cardiac amyloidosis in black Americans. N Engl J Med 336:466, 1997.
59. Ng B, Connors LH, Davidoff R, et al: Senile systemic amyloidosis presenting with heart failure: A comparison with light chain–associated amyloidosis. Arch Int Med 165:1425, 2005.
60. Wang AK, Fealey RD, Gehrking TL, et al: Patterns of neuropathy and autonomic failure in patients with amyloidosis. Mayo Clin Proc 83:1226, 2008.
61. Rahman JE, Helou EF, Gelzer-Bell R, et al: Noninvasive diagnosis of biopsy-proven cardiac amyloidosis. J Am Coll Cardiol 43:410, 2004.
62. Palladini G, Merlini G: Current treatment of AL amyloidosis. Haematologica 94:1044, 2009.
63. Sack FU, Kristen A, Goldschmidt H, et al: Treatment options for severe cardiac amyloidosis: Heart transplantation combined with chemotherapy and stem cell transplantation for patients with AL-amyloidosis and heart and liver transplantation for patients with ATTR-amyloidosis. Eur J Cardiothorac Surg 33:257, 2008.
64. Delahaye N, Rouzet F, Sarda L, et al: Impact of liver transplantation on cardiac autonomic denervation in familial amyloid polyneuropathy. Medicine (Baltimore) 85:229, 2006.

Inherited and Acquired Infiltrative Disorders Causing Restrictive Cardiomyopathy

65. Pieroni M, Chimenti C, de Cobelli F, et al: Fabry's disease cardiomyopathy: Echocardiographic detection of endomyocardial glycosphingolipid compartmentalization. J Am Coll Cardiol 47:1663, 2006.
66. Sheppard MN, Cane P, Florio R, et al: A detailed pathologic examination of heart tissue from three older patients with Anderson-Fabry disease on enzyme replacement therapy. Cardiovasc Pathol 19:293, 2010.
67. Glass RBJ, Astrin KH, Norton KI, et al: Fabry disease: Renal sonographic and magnetic resonance imaging findings in affected males and carrier females with the classic and cardiac variant phenotypes. J Comput Assist Tomogr 28:158, 2004.
68. Imbriaco M, Pisani A, Spinelli L, et al: Effects of enzyme-replacement therapy in patients with Anderson-Fabry disease: A prospective long-term cardiac magnetic resonance imaging study. Heart 95:1103, 2009.
69. Thurberg BL, Fallon JT, Mitchell R, et al: Cardiac microvascular pathology in Fabry disease: Evaluation of endomyocardial biopsies before and after enzyme replacement therapy. Circulation 119:2561, 2009.
70. Elstein D, Zimran A: Review of the safety and efficacy of imiglucerase treatment of Gaucher disease. Biologics 3:407, 2009.
71. Hoffbrand AV: Diagnosing myocardial iron overload. Eur Heart J 22:2140, 2001.
72. Ptaszek LM, Price ET, Hu MY, et al: Early diagnosis of hemochromatosis-related cardiomyopathy with magnetic resonance imaging. J Cardiovasc Magn Reson 7:689, 2005.
73. Caines AE, Kpodonu J, Massad MG, et al: Cardiac transplantation in patients with iron overload cardiomyopathy. J Heart Lung Transplant 24:486, 2005.
74. Koplan BA, Soejima K, Baughman K, et al: Refractory ventricular tachycardia secondary to cardiac sarcoid: Electrophysiologic characteristics, mapping, and ablation. Heart Rhythm 3:924, 2006.
75. Ardehali H, Howard DL, Hariri A, et al: A positive endomyocardial biopsy result for sarcoid is associated with poor prognosis in patients with initially unexplained cardiomyopathy. Am Heart J 150:459, 2005.
76. Smedema JP, Snoep G, van Kroonenburgh MP, et al: Evaluation of the accuracy of gadolinium-enhanced cardiovascular magnetic resonance in the diagnosis of cardiac sarcoidosis. J Am Coll Cardiol 45:1683, 2005.
77. Pela G, Tirabassi G, Pattoneri P, et al: Cardiac involvement in the Churg-Strauss syndrome. Am J Cardiol 97:1519, 2006.
78. Marijon E, Ou P: What do we know about endomyocardial fibrosis in children of Africa? Pediatr Cardiol 27:523, 2006.
79. Hassan WM, Fawzy ME, Al Helaly S, et al: Pitfalls in diagnosis and clinical, echocardiographic, and hemodynamic findings in endomyocardial fibrosis: A 25-year experience. Chest 128:3985, 2005.
80. Barretto ACP, Mady C, Nussbacher A, et al: Atrial fibrillation in endomyocardial fibrosis is a marker of worse prognosis. Int J Cardiol 67:19, 1998.
81. Barretto AC, Mady C, Oliveira SA, et al: Clinical meaning of ascites in patients with endomyocardial fibrosis. Arq Bras Cardiol 78:196, 2002.
82. Joshi R, Abraham S, Kumar AS: New approach for complete endocardiectomy in left ventricular endomyocardial fibrosis. J Thorac Cardiovasc Surg 125:40, 2003.
83. Moraes F, Lapa C, Hazin S, et al: Surgery for endomyocardial fibrosis revisited. Eur J Cardiothorac Surg 15:309, 1999.
84. Cherian SM, Jagannath BR, Nayar S, et al: Successful reoperation after 17 years in a case of endomyocardial fibrosis. Ann Thorac Surg 82:1115, 2006.
85. Corradi D, Tchana B, Miller D, et al: Dilated form of endocardial fibroelastosis as a result of deficiency in respiratory-chain complexes I and IV. Circulation 120:e38, 2009.
86. Perez MH, Boulos T, Stucki P, et al: Placental immaturity, endocardial fibroelastosis and fetal hypoxia. Fetal Diagn Ther 26:107, 2009.

Carcinoid Heart Disease and Arrhythmogenic Right Ventricular Dysplasia/Cardiomyopathy

87. Moller JE, Pellikka PA, Bernheim AM, et al: Prognosis of carcinoid heart disease: Analysis of 200 cases over two decades. Circulation 112:3320, 2005.
88. Bastarrika G, Cao MG, Cano D, et al: Magnetic resonance imaging diagnosis of carcinoid heart disease. J Comput Assist Tomogr 29:756, 2005.
89. Dalal D, Molin LH, Piccini J, et al: Clinical features of arrhythmogenic right ventricular dysplasia/cardiomyopathy associated with mutations in plakophilin-2. Circulation 113:1641, 2006.
90. Dalal D, Nasir K, Bomma C, et al: Arrhythmogenic right ventricular dysplasia: A United States experience. Circulation 112:3823, 2005.
91. Asimaki A, Tandri H, Huang H, et al: A new diagnostic test for arrhythmogenic right ventricular cardiomyopathy. N Engl J Med 360:1075, 2009.
92. Matkovich SJ, Van Booven DJ, Youker KA, et al: Reciprocal regulation of myocardial microRNAs and messenger RNA in human cardiomyopathy and reversal of the microRNA signature by biomechanical support. Circulation 119:1263, 2009.

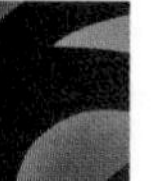

CHAPTER 69 Hypertrophic Cardiomyopathy

Barry J. Maron

Hypertrophic cardiomyopathy (HCM), the most common of the genetic cardiovascular diseases, is caused by a multitude of mutations in genes encoding proteins of the cardiac sarcomere.[1-5] HCM is characterized by heterogeneous clinical expression, unique pathophysiology, and diverse natural history.[6-13] This condition is the most common cause of sudden death in the young, including competitive athletes,[14] and it is responsible for heart failure–related disability at virtually any age.[1,7] Since the modern description of HCM more than 50 years ago, our understanding of the clinical complexity and spectrum of this disease has evolved dramatically. This chapter represents a contemporary summary of HCM with respect to diagnosis, natural history, and management.

Definition, Prevalence, and Nomenclature

HCM is characterized by a thickened but nondilated left ventricle in the absence of other cardiac or systemic conditions (e.g., aortic valve stenosis, systemic hypertension, and some expressions of physiologic athlete's heart) capable of producing the magnitude of left ventricular (LV) hypertrophy evident (**Figs. 69-1 and 69-2**).[1,3,5,7] Several epidemiologic studies have reported a similar prevalence of the HCM phenotype in the general population (e.g., about 0.2%; 1:500), equivalent to 600,000 people in the United States with this disease.[15] This estimated frequency in the general population far exceeds the relatively uncommon occurrence of HCM in cardiology practice, inferring that most affected individuals may remain unidentified and in most cases probably without symptoms or shortened life expectancy.[1,7] HCM is a global disease[16] reported in more than 50 countries from all continents, although most cases have come from the United States and Canada, western Europe, Israel, and Asia (Japan and China).

The first contemporary reports of HCM in 1958 are from Brock in the cardiac catheterization laboratory and from Teare, who described at autopsy "asymmetrical hypertrophy of the heart" as responsible for sudden cardiac death in a small group of young people. The disease rapidly acquired a confusing array of names,[5] with most emphasizing the highly visible feature of LV outflow obstruction.[13,17] However, since obstruction to LV outflow is not invariable and about 30% of patients have the nonobstructive form,[13] names once in common use, such as idiopathic hypertrophic subaortic stenosis, hypertrophic obstructive cardiomyopathy, and muscular subaortic stenosis (as well as their acronyms, IHSS, HOCM, and MSS) have been largely abandoned.[1,5-7] Hence, the preferred and generally accepted name for this condition is now hypertrophic cardiomyopathy (HCM).[1,5,7]

Genetic Basis (see Chap. 8)

HCM is transmitted as a mendelian trait with an autosomal dominant pattern of inheritance.[1-5,7] Molecular studies, conducted intensively during almost two decades, have provided access to definitive laboratory-based diagnosis by identification of pathologic disease-causing mutations (even in patients without obvious clinical evidence of the disease), in the process affording important insights into the broad clinical expression of HCM and genetic counseling, as well as promoting recognition of greater numbers of affected individuals.

Eleven mutated genes encoding proteins of the cardiac sarcomere are presently associated with HCM, accounting for about 50% of patients, most commonly beta-myosin heavy chain (the first identified) and myosin-binding protein C (see Fig. 8-1).[2,4,5] Each of the other nine genes appears to account for far fewer cases; these include troponin T and I, alpha-tropomyosin, regulatory and essential myosin light chains, titin, alpha-actin, alpha-myosin heavy chain, and muscle LIM protein (MLP). This diversity is compounded by considerable intragenetic heterogeneity, with myriad individual mutations identified (total >1000). The characteristic diversity of the HCM phenotype (even among closely related family members) is likely to be attributable to the disease-causing mutations as well as the influence of modifier genes and environmental factors. Neither the complete number of genes nor the number of HCM-causing mutations is known, and many others remain to be identified. Genetic testing is now commercially available, translating genomics into the clinical arena.[4]

Non-sarcomeric protein mutations cause storage diseases that are phenocopies of sarcomeric HCM and require molecular diagnosis, namely, Fabry disease, γ_2 regulatory subunit of adenosine monophosphate–activated protein kinase (*PRKAG2*), and lysosome-associated membrane protein 2 (*LAMP2;* Danon disease; **Fig. 69-3**).[18,19] Clinical presentation is often indistinguishable from sarcomeric HCM, although *PRKAG2* and *LAMP2* are frequently associated with ventricular preexcitation. *LAMP2* cardiomyopathy, which is characterized by massive LV hypertrophy (see Fig. 69-3) and profound clinical course refractory to defibrillator therapy (with survival beyond 25 years unusual), necessitates consideration for early heart transplantation.[19]

Morphology

Left Ventricular Hypertrophy (see Chaps. 15 and 18)

Clinical diagnosis of HCM is usually made with two-dimensional echocardiography (see Fig. 69-1; see Figs. 15-65, 15-66, and 15-67),[1] although more recently cardiovascular magnetic resonance imaging (CMR) has emerged with an expanding role in noninvasive diagnosis by virtue of its high-resolution tomographic imaging capability (see Fig. 69-2; see

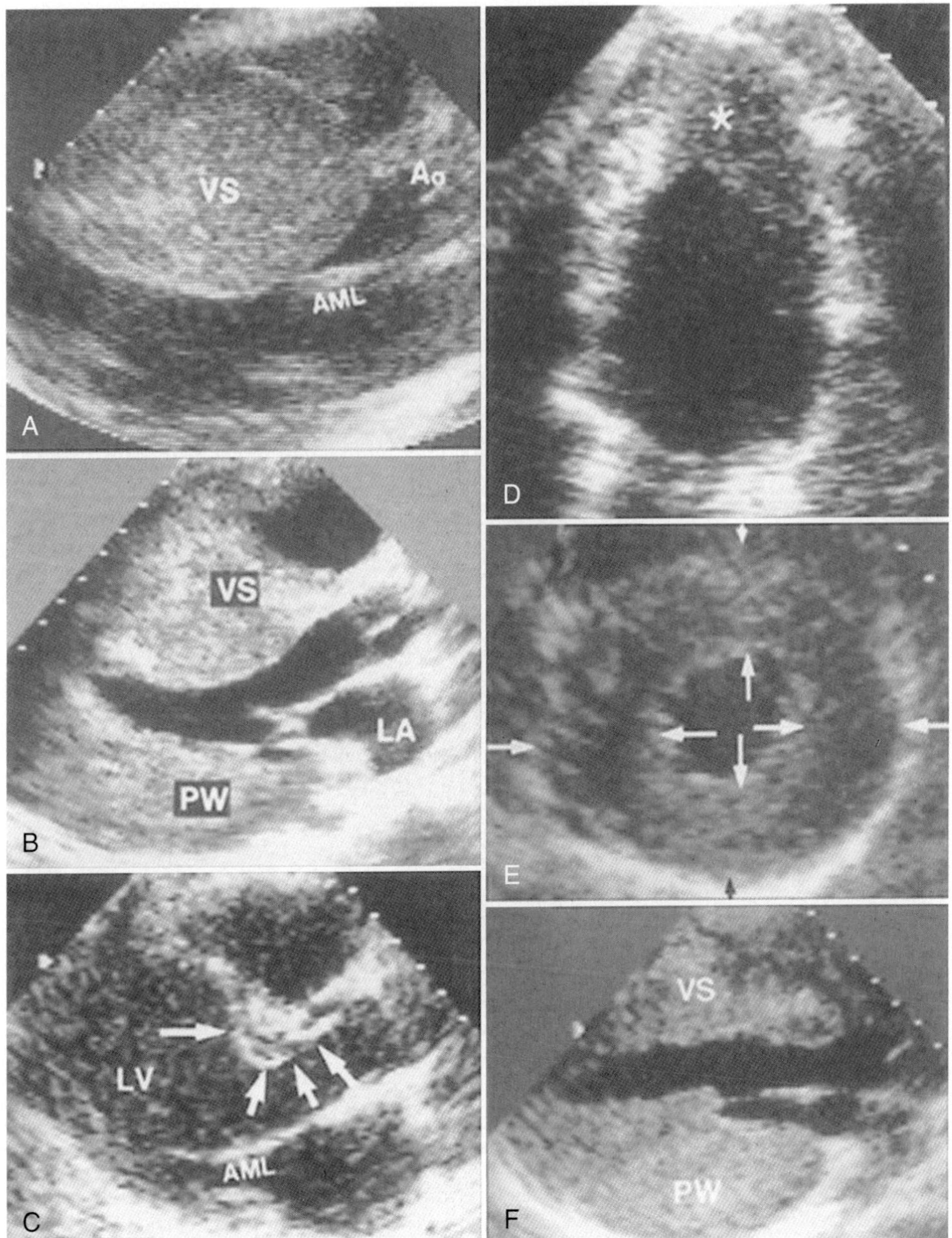

FIGURE 69-1 Patterns of LV hypertrophy in HCM. Heterogeneous distribution and extent of LV wall thickening by echocardiography. **A,** Massive asymmetric hypertrophy of ventricular septum (VS) with thickness >50 mm. **B,** Septal hypertrophy with distal portion considerably thicker than proximal region. **C,** Hypertrophy confined to proximal septum just below aortic valve (arrows). **D,** Hypertrophy localized to LV apex (asterisk), that is, apical HCM. **E,** Relatively mild hypertrophy in symmetric pattern showing similar or identical thicknesses within each segment (paired arrows). **F,** Inverted pattern with posterior free wall (PW) thicker (40 mm) than anterior VS. Calibration marks = 1 cm. Ao = aorta; AML = anterior mitral leaflet; LA = left atrium. *(From Maron BJ: Hypertrophic cardiomyopathy: A systematic review. JAMA 287:1308, 2002. Reproduced with permission of the American Medical Association.)*

Fig. 18-10).[8,9] CMR is complementary to echocardiography by clarifying technically ambiguous LV wall thicknesses, by visualizing abnormalities often not identifiable with echocardiography (e.g., areas of segmental hypertrophy in the anterolateral free wall[8,9]; see Fig. 69-2), or by depicting pathologic changes in the apical region including hypertrophy[9] and aneurysm formation[12] (**Fig. 69-4**) that may clarify diagnosis or in some patients alter management strategies (see Fig. 69-2).

Diverse patterns of asymmetric LV hypertrophy are characteristic of HCM, including dissimilar phenotypes in relatives (with the exception of identical twins; see Fig. 69-1). Typically, one or more regions of the LV wall are of greater thickness than other areas, frequently with sharp transitions in thickness between adjacent areas or noncontiguous patterns of segmental hypertrophy, as well as extension into the right ventricle.[20] However, there is not a single "classic" morphologic form, and virtually all possible patterns of LV hypertrophy have been reported in HCM, including genetically affected children and adults with normal LV wall thicknesses (see Fig. 69-1).[1,7,9] There is no evidence that specific patterns of LV hypertrophy are consistently related to outcome.[1,7]

Hypertrophy is frequently diffuse, involving portions of both ventricular septum and LV free wall, including some patients with the greatest magnitude of LV hypertrophy observed in any cardiac disease with wall thicknesses ranging to 50 to 60 mm (see Fig. 69-1).[9] However, in about 50% of patients, LV hypertrophy is nondiffuse, including a sizeable minority with wall thickening confined to segmental areas of the LV chamber. Wall thickening limited to the most distal portion of the LV chamber (apical HCM) represents a morphologic form characterized by a "spade" deformity of the distal left ventricle and marked T

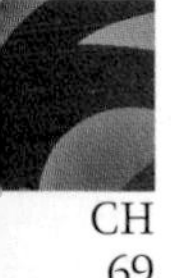

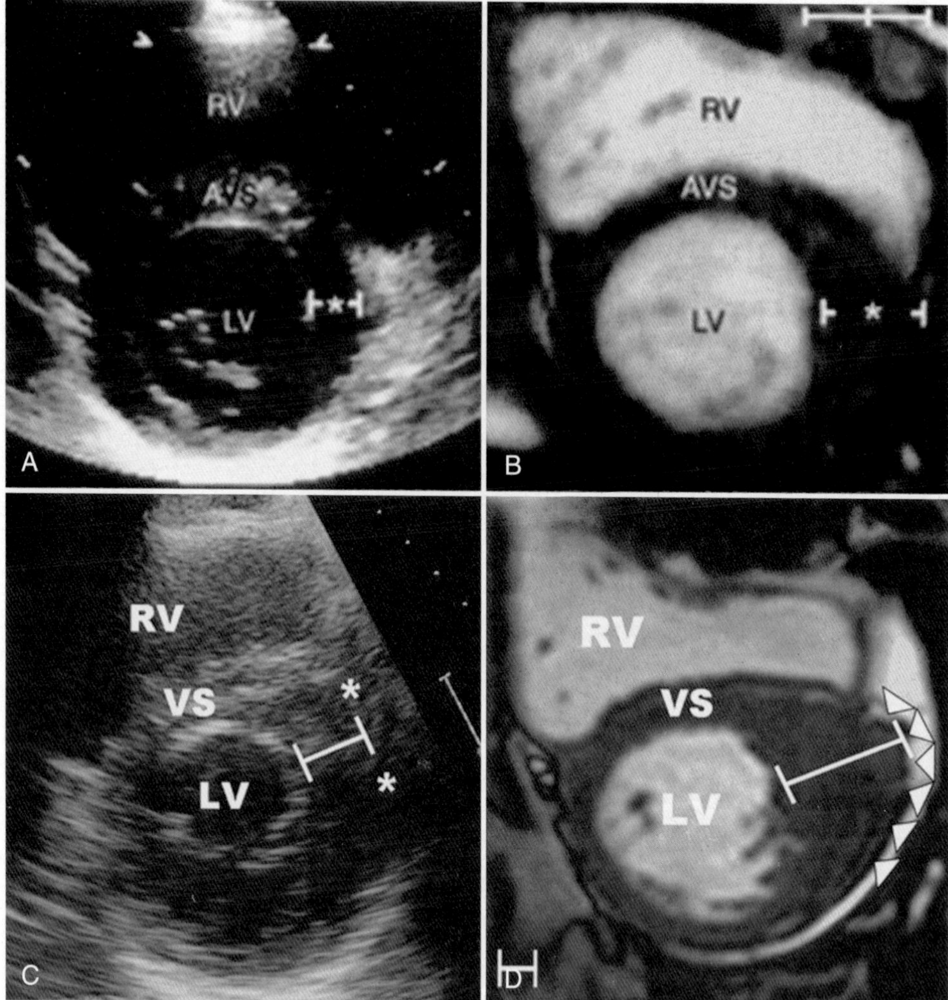

FIGURE 69-2 Cardiovascular magnetic resonance (CMR) identification of segmental LV wall thickening in HCM. Diagnosis: two-dimensional echocardiogram **(A)** and comparative CMR image **(B)** acquired in short-axis plane at end diastole at same level from 13-year-old asymptomatic identical twin. **A,** Echocardiogram shows normal anterolateral free wall thickness (asterisk). **B,** CMR shows segmental area of hypertrophy confined to anterolateral LV free wall (20 mm) and small portion of contiguous anterior septum (asterisk). Calibration marks are 1 cm apart. *(From Rickers C, Wilke NM, Jerosch-Herold M, et al: Utility of cardiac magnetic resonance imaging in the diagnosis of hypertrophic cardiomyopathy. Circulation 112:855, 2005. Reproduced with permission of the American Heart Association.)* Management implications: echocardiogram **(C)** and comparative CMR image **(D)** from 46-year-old man with HCM. **C,** Echocardiographic short-axis image shows anterolateral free wall thickness of 18 mm. **D,** CMR shows focal area of massive LV hypertrophy (wall thickness, 35 mm) in the same region of LV, significantly underestimated by two-dimensional echocardiography. This finding defined high-risk status, prompting altered management strategy with an ICD recommendation for primary prevention of sudden death. Calibration markers are 1 cm apart. AVS = anterior ventricular septum. LV = left ventricle; RV = right ventricle; VS = ventricular septum. *(From Maron MS, Lesser JR, Maron BJ: Management implications of massive left ventricular hypertrophy in hypertrophic cardiomyopathy significantly underestimated by echocardiography but identified by cardiovascular magnetic resonance. Am J Cardiol 105:1842, 2010.)*

wave negativity on electrocardiography that may be due to mutations in proteins of the cardiac sarcomere (see Fig. 69-1; see Fig. 15-67). Increased LV mass (calculated by CMR) is not invariable in HCM and is normal or nearly normal in 20% of patients when hypertrophy is localized and segmental.[10]

LV hypertrophy commonly develops dynamically after a variable period of latency (**Fig. 69-5**). Typically, the HCM phenotype is incomplete until adolescence, when accelerated growth and maturation are often accompanied by spontaneous and striking increases in LV wall thickness (i.e., average 100% change) and more extensive distribution of hypertrophy.[1,7] These structural changes, which occasionally may be delayed until later in midlife, are part of a genetically predetermined remodeling process not usually associated with development of symptoms or arrhythmia-related events. In genetically affected individuals, 12-lead electrocardiographic abnormalities or subtle preclinical evidence of diastolic dysfunction (usually diminished E′ velocity) detectable by tissue Doppler imaging may precede the appearance of LV hypertrophy,[21] including the possibility that some athletes with marked repolarization abnormalities on electrocardiogram may later manifest clinical and phenotypic evidence of HCM.[22]

Mitral Valve Apparatus

Structural abnormalities of the mitral valve apparatus that are responsible for LV outflow obstruction include diverse alterations in valvular size and shape and represent a primary morphologic abnormality in HCM, most frequently evident in younger patients.[1,7] The mitral valve may be as much as twice normal size from elongation of both leaflets or segmental enlargement of only the anterior leaflet or the midportion of the posterior leaflet. In a small subset of patients, congenital and anomalous anterolateral papillary muscle insertion into the anterior mitral leaflet (without the interposition of chordae tendineae) produces muscular midcavity outflow obstruction.[7]

Histopathology

In HCM, cardiac muscle cells (myocytes) in both ventricular septum and LV free wall show increased transverse diameter and bizarre shapes, often maintaining intercellular connections with several adjacent cells.[7] Many myocytes (and myofilaments) are arranged in chaotic, disorganized patterns at oblique and perpendicular angles

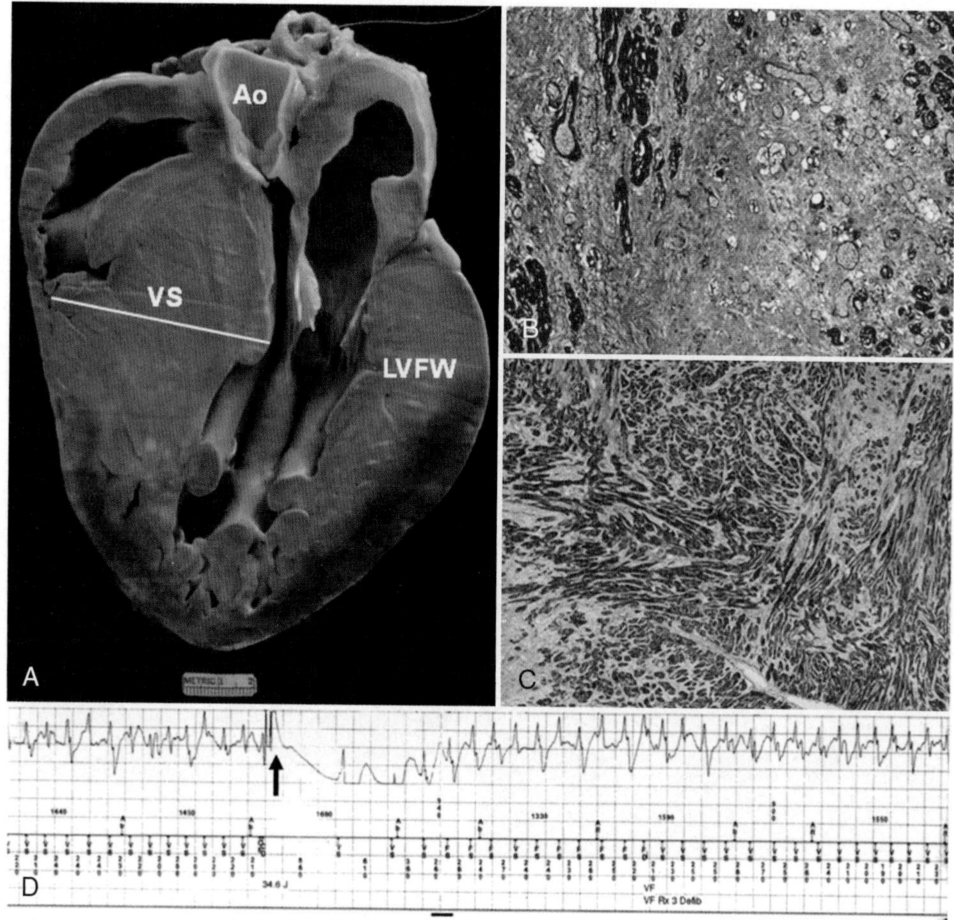

FIGURE 69-3 *LAMP2* cardiomyopathy. **A,** From 14-year-old boy with sudden death and septal thickness of 65 mm (heart weight, 1425 g). Ao = aorta; LVFW = left ventricular free wall; VS = ventricular septum. **B,** Clusters of myocytes with vacuolated sarcoplasm (stained red) embedded in area of scar (stained blue; Masson trichrome). **C,** Disorganized arrangement of myocytes most typical of sarcomeric HCM. **D,** Intracardiac electrogram. ICD elicited five defibrillation shocks that failed to interrupt ventricular fibrillation (280 beats/min). *(From Maron BJ, Roberts WC, Arad M, et al: Clinical outcome and phenotypic expression in LAMP2 cardiomyopathy. JAMA 301:1253, 2009. Reproduced with permission of the American Medical Association.)*

(**Fig. 69-6**). Areas of disorganized architecture are evident in 95% of HCM patients at autopsy, usually occupying substantial portions of hypertrophied (as well as nonhypertrophied) LV myocardium (33% of septum and 25% of free wall).[7]

Abnormal intramural coronary arteries with thickened walls (composed of increased intimal and medial components) and narrowed lumen are present in 80% of patients at necropsy, most frequently within or close to areas of replacement fibrosis[1,7,23] (see Fig. 69-6). This microvascular small-vessel disease[23] is responsible for clinically silent myocardial ischemia[23] and myocyte death, leading to a repair process in the form of replacement (often transmural) with fibrosis[7,11,23,24] (see Fig. 69-6). Also, the volume of the interstitial (matrix) collagen compartment, constituting the structural LV framework, is greatly expanded.

It is likely that the disorganized cellular architecture and replacement fibrosis evident in HCM impair transmission of electrophysiologic impulses and predispose to disordered patterns and increased dispersion of electrical depolarization and repolarization, in turn serving as an electrically unstable substrate and nidus for reentry ventricular tachyarrhythmias and sudden death.

Pathophysiology

Left Ventricular Outflow Obstruction

Longstanding LV outflow tract obstruction (basal gradient,≥30 mm Hg) is a strong determinant of HCM-related progressive heart failure symptoms and cardiovascular death[17,25] (**Fig. 69-7**). However, only a weak relationship is evident between outflow obstruction and specifically the risk for sudden cardiac death (usually in patients without significant heart failure symptoms).[17,25]

Subaortic obstruction in HCM represents true mechanical impedance to LV outflow, producing markedly increased intraventricular pressures that may be detrimental to LV function, probably by increasing myocardial wall stress and oxygen demand.[17,25] In most patients, obstruction is produced in the proximal left ventricle by systolic anterior motion (SAM) of mitral valve and midsystolic ventricular septal contact. Characteristic of SAM, particularly in young patients, is abrupt anterior motion of the mitral valve in which elongated leaflets move toward the septum with a sharp-angled 90-degree bend. SAM appears to be generated largely by a drag effect, that is, hydrodynamic pushing force of flow directly on the leaflets. Magnitude of the outflow gradient, reliably estimated with continuous-wave Doppler, is directly related to duration of mitral valve–septal contact. Mitral regurgitation is a secondary consequence of SAM, with the jet (usually mild to moderate in degree) directed posteriorly.[1] Severe mitral regurgitation suggests an intrinsic valve abnormality, such as myxomatous degeneration.

Subaortic gradients (and systolic ejection murmurs) in HCM are often dynamic, with spontaneous variability,[1] or reduced or abolished by interventions that decrease myocardial contractility (e.g., beta-adrenergic blocking drugs) or increase ventricular volume or arterial pressure (e.g., squatting, isometric handgrip, phenylephrine).[6] Alternatively, gradients can be augmented by circumstances in which arterial pressure or ventricular volume is reduced (e.g., Valsalva maneuver, nitroglycerin or amyl nitrite administration, blood loss, dehydration) or

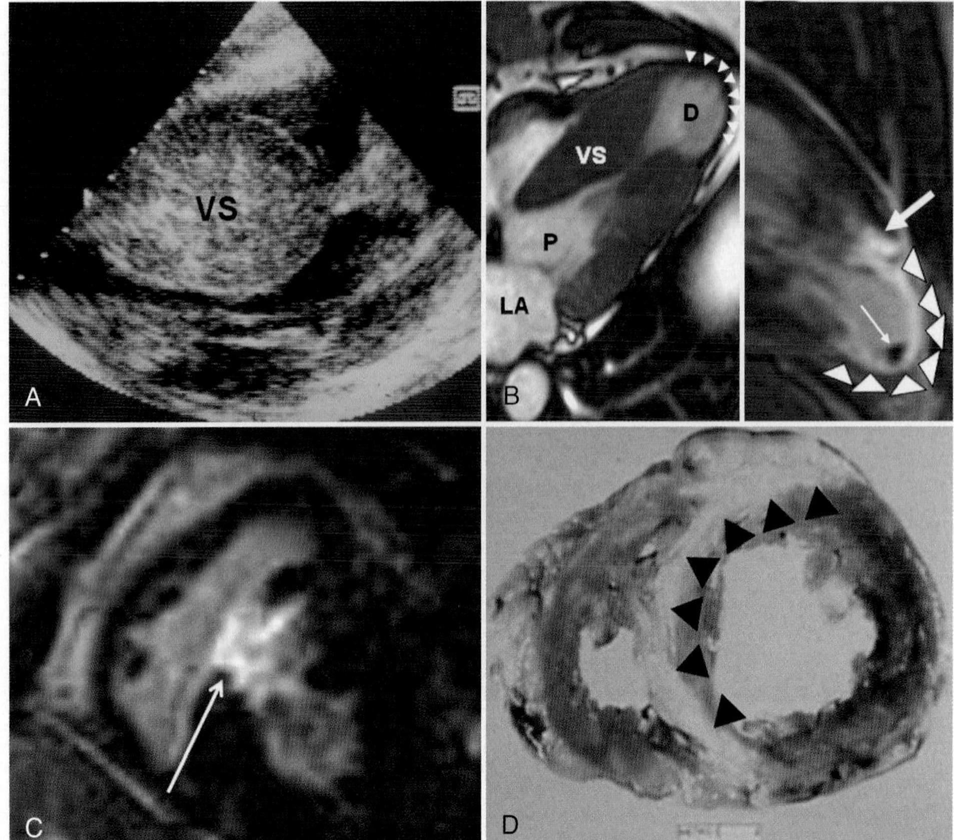

FIGURE 69-4 LV morphology associated with risk for sustained ventricular tachyarrhythmias and sudden death. **A,** Massive hypertrophy with ventricular septal (VS) thickness of 55 mm. **B, left,** Akinetic thin-walled LV apical aneurysm, associated with midcavity muscular apposition; contrast-enhanced CMR images demonstrated substantial, transmural delayed enhancement contiguous with the aneurysm. D = distal (cavity); LA = left atrium; P = proximal (cavity). **B, right,** Contrast-enhanced CMR image showing delayed enhancement (i.e., scar) involving thin aneurysm rim (arrowheads) and contiguous myocardium (large arrow); small apical thrombus is evident (small arrow). **C,** Large transmural ventricular septal scar (arrow), resulting from alcohol septal ablation procedure. *(From Valeti US, Nishimura RA, Holmes DR, et al: Comparison of surgical septal myectomy and alcohol septal ablation by cardiac magnetic resonance imaging in patients with hypertrophic obstructive cardiomyopathy. J Am Coll Cardiol 49:350, 2007. Reproduced with permission of the American College of Cardiology.)* **D,** End-stage heart showing extensive, transmural scarring involving the septum and extending into anterior free wall (arrowheads).

contractility is increased, such as with premature ventricular contractions, infusion of isoproterenol or dobutamine, or exercise.[6]

Consumption of a heavy meal or small amounts of alcohol can also transiently increase subaortic gradient and produce dyspnea. Furthermore, a large proportion of HCM patients without outflow obstruction (or SAM) at rest may generate outflow gradients with physiologic exercise, sometimes associated with severe heart failure symptoms.[13] Fully 70% of a hospital-based HCM cohort have the propensity to develop an outflow gradient ≥30 mm Hg, either at rest or during exercise.[13]

Microvascular

Myocardial ischemia due to microvascular dysfunction occurs in HCM and is an important pathophysiologic component of the disease process, promoting LV myocardial scarring and remodeling and affecting clinical course.[23] Active ischemia, demonstrable with positron emission tomography, is a determinant of progressive heart failure and cardiovascular mortality.[23] However, the relationship between chest pain commonly encountered in HCM and active myocardial ischemia is unresolved.

Diastolic Dysfunction

Evidence of impaired LV relaxation and filling, by mitral inflow pulsed Doppler and tissue Doppler imaging (see Chap. 15), is present in as many as 80% of HCM patients, probably contributing to heart failure symptoms of exertional dyspnea, although not directly related to severity of LV hypertrophy.[1] The rapid filling phase is usually prolonged, associated with decreased rate and volume of LV filling and (in sinus rhythm) a compensatory increase in the contribution of atrial systole to overall filling.[1,21] Parameters of diastolic function have limited applicability to patient management and do not accurately predict prognosis, symptoms, or filling pressures, although restrictive LV filling patterns may be linked to adverse outcome in some HCM patients.

Reduced ventricular compliance in HCM probably results largely from those factors determining passive elastic properties of the LV chamber, such as hypertrophy, replacement scarring and interstitial fibrosis, and disorganized cellular architecture. Diastolic dysfunction is likely to be the fundamental mechanism by which heart failure occurs in nonobstructive HCM with preserved LV systolic function (see Chap. 30).

FAMILY SCREENING STRATEGIES

Clinical screening of relatives in HCM families (in the absence of genetic testing) is performed with two-dimensional echocardiography and 12-lead electrocardiography (also CMR) as well as by history taking and physical examination. Screening evaluations are usually performed on a 12- to 18-month basis, beginning at the age of 12 years.[26] If these studies do not show LV hypertrophy by the time full growth is achieved (18 to 21 years), it is usually reasonable to conclude that an HCM-causing mutation is likely absent. However, morphologic conversions to HCM phenotypes (i.e., LV hypertrophy) can be delayed into adulthood, and it is not possible to provide unequivocal reassurance that a normal echocardiogram at maturity defines a genetically unaffected relative.[1,2,7,26] In such circumstances, it may be prudent to pursue genetic testing[4] or to extend echocardiographic surveillance into adulthood at 5-year intervals.[26]

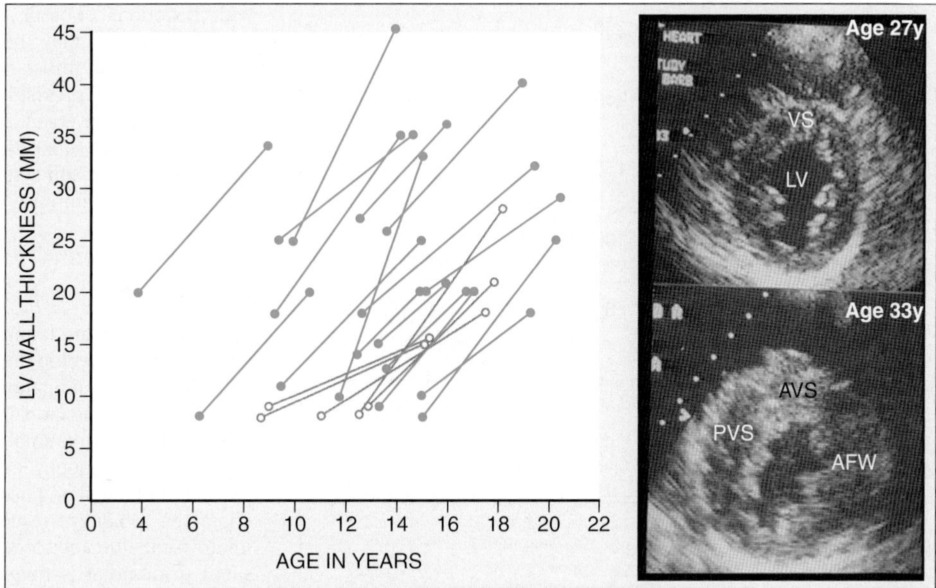

FIGURE 69-5 LV remodeling with development or progression of HCM phenotype. **Left,** Childhood/adolescence. Increased echocardiographic LV wall thickness in patients with familial HCM, unassociated with changes in clinical course. Open symbols denote those without initial evidence of hypertrophy in any LV segment. *(From Maron BJ, Spirito P, Wesley Y, Arce J: Development and progression of left ventricular hypertrophy in children with hypertrophic cardiomyopathy. N Engl J Med 315:610, 1986. Reproduced with permission of the Massachusetts Medical Society.)* **Right,** Adulthood. Woman with myosin-binding protein C mutation at age 27 years, with normal LV thickness (≤12 mm) in all segments of the wall **(top)**; 6 years later, at age 33 years, wall thickness has increased to 20 mm in both anterior ventricular septum and posterior septum as well as anterolateral free wall **(bottom)**. LV wall thickness eventually increased to >30 mm, and the patient was prophylactically implanted with a defibrillator for primary prevention of sudden death. Calibration marks are 10 mm apart. *(From Maron BJ, Niimura H, Casey SA, et al: Development of left ventricular hypertrophy in adults in hypertrophic cardiomyopathy caused by cardiac myosin-binding protein C gene mutations. J Am Coll Cardiol 38:315, 2001. Reproduced with permission of the American College of Cardiology.)*

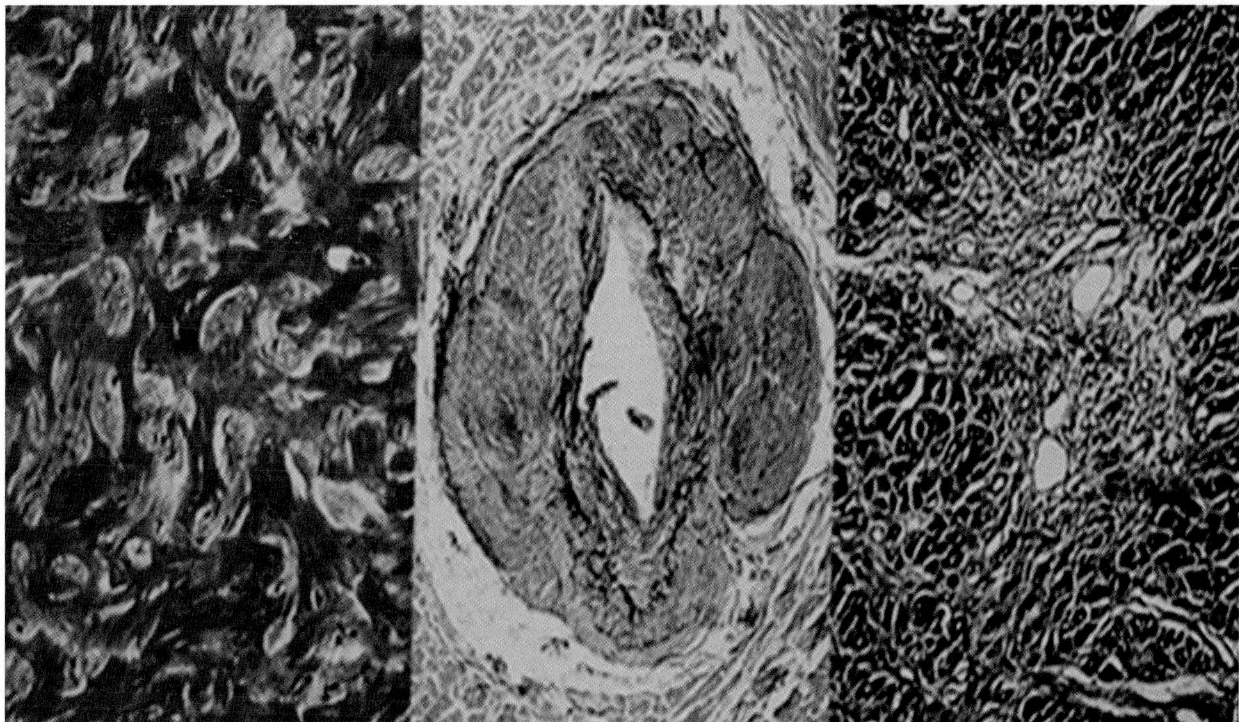

FIGURE 69-6 Arrhythmogenic myocardial substrate. **Left,** Disorganized LV architecture with myocyte disarray. **Center,** Small-vessel disease; remodeled intramural coronary arteriole with thickened media and narrowed lumen. **Right,** Repair process with replacement fibrosis, the consequence of silent myocardial ischemia and myocyte death.

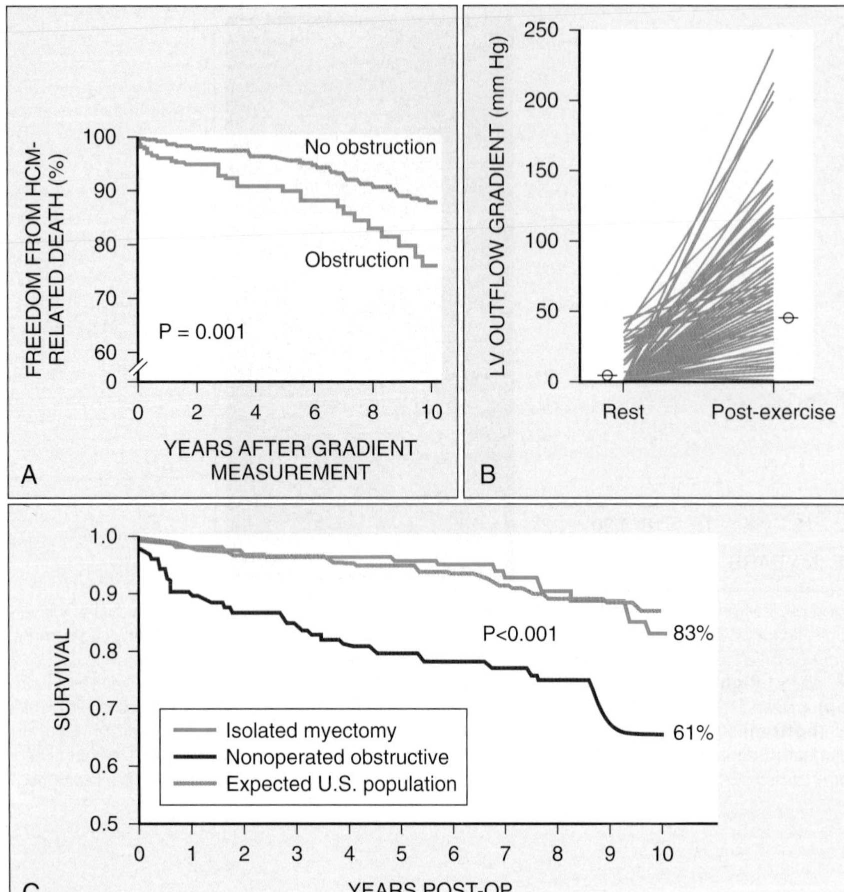

FIGURE 69-7 Left ventricular outflow tract obstruction. **A,** Probability of severe progressive heart failure (NYHA Class III or IV), heart failure death, or stroke in patients with LV outflow obstruction significantly exceeds that in patients without obstruction (relative risk, 4.4; $P < 0.001$). *(From Maron MS, Olivotto I, Betocchi S, et al: Effect of left ventricular outflow tract obstruction on clinical outcome in hypertrophic cardiomyopathy. N Engl J Med 348:295, 2003. Reproduced with permission of the Massachusetts Medical Society.)* **B,** Changes in LV outflow tract gradient from resting (basal) conditions to immediately after termination of treadmill exercise. Each patient is depicted by a line connecting the two gradient measurements. θ indicates the mean. *(From Maron MS, Olivotto I, Zenovich AG, et al: Hypertrophic cardiomyopathy is predominantly a disease of left ventricular outflow tract obstruction. Circulation 114:216, 2006. Reproduced with permission of the American Heart Association.)* **C,** After myectomy with relief of LV outflow obstruction, survival free from all-cause mortality compared with age- and gender-matched U.S. population and also patients with nonoperated obstruction ($P < 0.001$). *(From Ommen SR, Maron BJ, Olivotto I, et al: Long-term effects of surgical septal myectomy on survival in patients with obstructive hypertrophic cardiomyopathy. J Am Coll Cardiol 46:470, 2005. Reproduced with permission of the American College of Cardiology.)*

Clinical Features

Physical Examination

Physical examination findings in patients with HCM are variable and related in large measure to hemodynamic state (see Chap. 12). Initial clinical suspicion of HCM may be triggered by recognition of a heart murmur on routine examination or before sports participation, although the majority of patients are still identified by virtue of clinically overt symptom onset or cardiac events.[27] Patients with outflow obstruction characteristically have a medium-pitch systolic ejection murmur at the lower left sternal border and apex that varies in intensity with the magnitude of the subaortic gradient, increasing with the Valsalva maneuver, during or immediately after exercise, or on standing. Most patients with loud murmurs of at least grade 3/6 are likely to have LV outflow gradients >30 mm Hg; arterial pulses usually rise rapidly with bisferiens contour, and double or triple apical impulses may be palpable, reflecting outward systolic thrust caused by ventricular contraction and presystolic accentuated atrial contraction. Conversely, physical findings in patients without subaortic gradients are more subtle, with no or soft systolic murmur, although a forceful apical impulse may arouse suspicion of HCM.

Symptoms

Symptoms of heart failure (with preserved LV function) may develop unpredictably at any age, with functional limitation due to exertional dyspnea or fatigue, and in advanced stages by orthopnea or paroxysmal nocturnal dyspnea.[1,7] Disability is frequently accompanied by chest pain, either typical angina pectoris or atypical in character, possibly resulting from structural microvasculature abnormalities responsible for silent myocardial ischemia. HCM patients may also experience impaired consciousness with syncope (or near-syncope) and lightheadedness potentially explained by several mechanisms, including arrhythmias and outflow obstruction. Severity of symptoms in HCM may be similar, independent of whether obstruction to LV outflow is present.[1]

Electrocardiographic Findings

The 12-lead electrocardiogram (ECG) is abnormal in more than 90% of probands with HCM and in about 75% of asymptomatic relatives.[1,3] ECGs show a wide variety of abnormal patterns, some of which are distinctly altered or even bizarre, although none is typical or characteristic of the disease. Most common abnormalities include increased voltages consistent with LV hypertrophy, ST-T changes including marked T wave inversion in the lateral precordial leads, left atrial enlargement, deep and narrow Q waves, and diminished R waves in the lateral precordial leads.[28] Normal electrocardiographic patterns (present in about 5% of patients) are associated with less severe phenotype and favorable cardiovascular course[29] but are not predictive of future sudden death events or appropriate defibrillator interventions.[28] Increased voltages (tall R waves or deep S waves) are only weakly correlated with the magnitude of LV hypertrophy evident on echocardiography and do not reliably distinguish the obstructive and nonobstructive forms.[28]

Gender and Race

HCM occurs with equal frequency in men and women.[2] The predominance of men in the literature reflects underdiagnosis in women, who achieve clinical recognition less frequently, at older ages, and with more pronounced symptoms than in men.[30] Furthermore, women have greater risk than men do for progression to advanced heart failure (usually associated with outflow obstruction), although there is no relation between gender and sudden death or overall mortality.[30] HCM has been reported in many races[1] but is underrecognized in African Americans, with most competitive athletes who die suddenly of HCM previously undiagnosed black men.[31] Phenotypic expression of HCM is similar throughout the world, with the possible exception of the morphologic form characterized by hypertrophy confined to the LV apex, most common in Japan.[7,16]

Athletes

Athlete's Heart and Hypertrophic Cardiomyopathy

Long-term athletic training can increase LV diastolic cavity dimension, wall thickness, and calculated mass, known as the athlete's heart.[31] Physiologically induced increases in absolute LV wall thickness are usually modest, are more substantial in some elite and highly trained individuals participating in rowing and cycling, but are not associated with purely isometric sports such as weightlifting.[31] A diagnostic dilemma may arise in distinguishing clinically benign and physiologic LV hypertrophy (as a consequence of athletic training) from pathologic conditions such as HCM. Clinical parameters that favor the diagnosis of HCM in trained athletes in the ambiguous "gray zone" of overlap between the two conditions (maximum LV wall thicknesses, 13 to 15 mm) include identification of a disease-causing sarcomeric protein mutation or recognition of HCM in a relative, transmitral Doppler waveform consistent with altered LV relaxation and filling, and LV end-diastolic cavity dimension <45 mm (**Fig. 69-8**). Parameters favoring physiologic athlete's heart include regression of wall thickness after a short (4- to 6-week) period of deconditioning assessed with CMR and enlarged LV cavity size exceeding 55 mm.

Preparticipation Screening

Detection of cardiovascular abnormalities having the potential for sudden death associated with intense physical training and competition is a major objective of preparticipation screening for high-school and college-aged sports participants.[31,32] In the United States, customary screening practice dictates a personal and family history and physical examination. Although HCM can be suspected and identified by this process, in other instances the disease remains undetected, given that many affected individuals do not have a heart murmur or historical clues (e.g., syncope or family history of HCM). Mandatory incorporation of noninvasive testing (such as with ECGs) into a national screening program for competitive athletes is not practical or feasible within the current U.S. health care system for several reasons, including limited physician resources.[32] The frequency of borderline and false-positive test results (and the uncertainty that accompanies these circumstances), the variations in ECG patterns with respect to race,[33] and the possibility that HCM phenotypes are not always detectable in early adolescence represent other limitations to mass ECG screening. Broad-based screening of athletes with echocardiography would not appear to be cost-effective.[34]

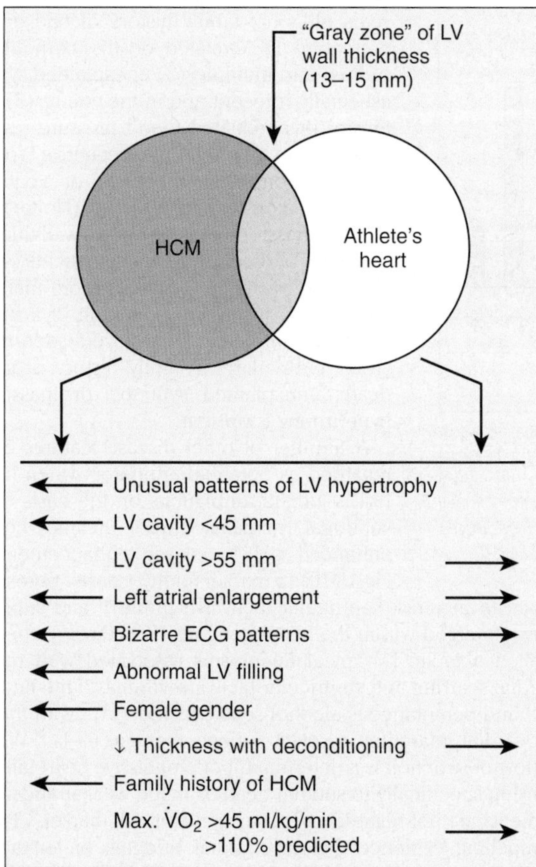

FIGURE 69-8 Differential diagnosis of HCM versus physiologic athlete's heart. Clinical criteria used to distinguish nonobstructive HCM from athlete's heart when maximal LV wall thickness is within the shaded gray area of overlap, consistent with both diagnoses. ↓ = decreased. *(Modified from Maron BJ, Pelliccia A: The heart of trained athletes: Cardiac remodeling and the risks of sports including sudden death. Circulation 114;1633, 2006. Reproduced with permission of the American Heart Association.)*

Clinical Course

Natural History

HCM is perhaps unique among cardiovascular diseases with the potential for clinical presentation during all phases of life, from infancy to old age (birth to >90 years).[1,7,35] Affected patients at either extreme of this age range appear to have the same basic disease process, although not necessarily with the same clinical course. During the last decade, greater clarity and general understanding have emerged regarding the natural history of HCM. Community-based patient populations, uncontaminated by tertiary center referral bias (and most representative of the true disease state), have reported overall HCM-related mortality rates of about 1%/year (**Fig. 69-9**), although somewhat higher in children (i.e., 2%/year).[1,7,14] This characterization of HCM contrasts with the older literature. Previously reported annual mortality rates of 4% to 6% were derived from highly selected cohorts at major referral centers incorporating substantial patient referral bias and skewed toward high-risk patients. This extreme perception of the natural history of HCM patients has been rendered obsolete with respect to the contemporary population.

Although clinical course is typically variable, patients with HCM may remain stable during long periods.[1,7,35] Notably, HCM is compatible with normal life expectancy with little or no disability and without the necessity for major therapeutic interventions to achieve this outcome (see Fig. 69-9).[1,7,29,35] Indeed, adults with HCM have the same overall life expectancy as that of an age- and sex-matched general population, underscoring the important principle that many patients with this disease deserve a large measure of reassurance regarding prognosis.

Nevertheless, subgroups at higher risk for important disease complications and premature death reside within an HCM population. Such patients proceed along specific adverse pathways, punctuated by clinical events that ultimately dictate targeted treatment strategies[1,7,11,14,17,35-40]: (1) sudden and unexpected death; (2) progressive heart failure with exertional dyspnea and functional limitation (often accompanied by chest pain) in the presence of preserved LV systolic function; and (3) atrial fibrillation (AF), with the risk for embolic stroke and heart failure. However, prediction of clinical course and outcome for individual patients with HCM remains encumbered by the markedly diverse disease expression and the long period of potential risk for young patients.[1,7,38,39]

Heart Failure

Whereas some degree of heart failure with exertional dyspnea is common in HCM, progression to severe functional limitation with preserved LV systolic function (i.e., New York Heart Association [NYHA] Class III or IV) is infrequent, occurring in probably 10% to 15% of the overall patient population.[1,7] The principal determinants of progressive heart failure and heart failure–related death appear to be LV outflow obstruction, AF, and diastolic dysfunction.[13,17,20,21,23,25,35] Also, microvascular dysfunction[23] has been advanced as a predictor of long-term outcome and heart failure death. In contrast to the risk specifically for sudden death (which bears a linear relationship to magnitude of LV hypertrophy) greater degrees of LV wall thickness are

CH 69

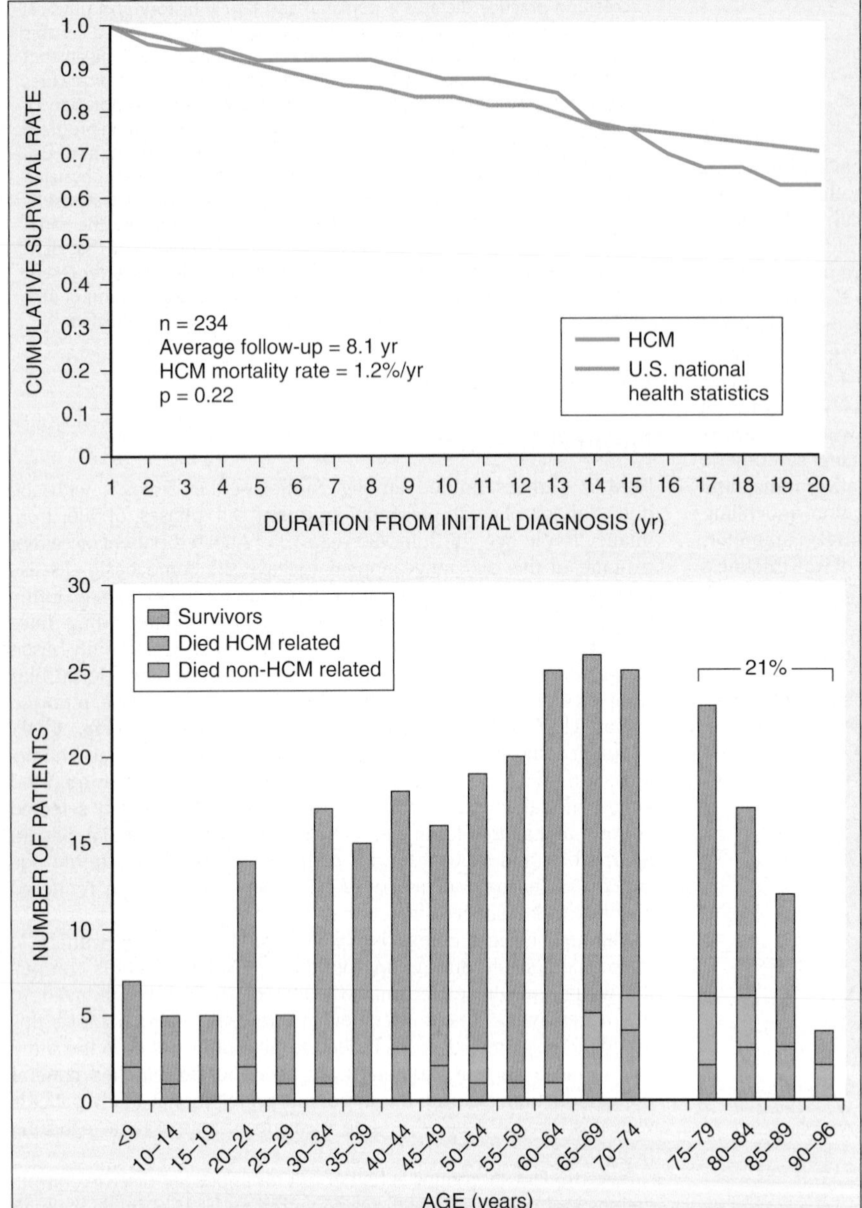

FIGURE 69-9 Clinical course of HCM patients. **Top,** Cumulative survival in a community-based adult HCM population. Total mortality of 1%/year does not differ significantly from that expected in the general U.S. population after adjustment for age, gender, and race. **Bottom,** Age at initial presentation with >20% of patients achieving normal life expectancy (≥75 years). *(From Maron BJ, Casey SA, Poliac LC, et al: Clinical course of hypertrophic cardiomyopathy in a regional United States cohort. JAMA 281:650, 1999. Reproduced with permission of the American Medical Association.)*

not associated with higher likelihood for development of progressive heart failure symptoms.[40] HCM is a rare cause of heart failure in infants and young children, and this presentation is regarded as an unfavorable prognostic sign.[1,3]

About 3% of HCM patients manifest the end stage characterized by systolic dysfunction (ejection fraction <50%; see Fig. 69-4).[11] This profound form of progressive heart failure (often associated with AF) may be expressed by various patterns of LV remodeling, including wall thinning and cavity dilation, associated with diffuse transmural scarring that can be identified in vivo by CMR[11,23,24] (the consequence of small-vessel mediated myocardial ischemia). Clinical course is unpredictable, but progression to refractory heart failure or sudden death is frequent (10%/year). The most reliable risk marker for evolution to the end stage is a family history of the end stage.[11]

Risk Stratification and Sudden Death

Sudden death in HCM may occur at a wide range of ages but most commonly in adolescents and young adults <30 to 35 years of age (**Fig. 69-10**).[1,7,14,31,36,38] These events are arrhythmia based, caused by primary ventricular tachycardia and ventricular fibrillation.[38,39] Sudden death is often the initial clinical manifestation of HCM, occurring commonly in asymptomatic individuals, many of whom are undiagnosed during life. Whereas most sudden deaths occur while sedentary or during modest physical activity, such events are also frequently associated with vigorous exertion, consistent with the observation that HCM is the most common cardiovascular cause of athletic field deaths (see Fig. 69-10).[14] Association of HCM with vigorous exercise and sudden death constitutes the basis for prudent recommendations by the 36th Bethesda Conference to disqualify young athletes with HCM from intense competitive sports to reduce sudden death risk.[41]

The greatest risk for sudden death is associated with specific clinical markers (**Fig. 69-11**). For secondary prevention, these are prior cardiac arrest and sustained ventricular tachycardia. For primary prevention, risk markers include one or more of the following, which assume greater weight in younger patients (<50 years old): (1) family history of one or more premature HCM-related deaths, particularly if sudden and multiple; (2) unexplained syncope, especially if recent and in the young; (3) hypotensive or attenuated blood pressure response to exercise; (4) multiple, repetitive (or prolonged) nonsustained bursts of ventricular tachycardia on serial ambulatory (Holter) ECGs; and (5) massive LV hypertrophy (wall thickness, ≥30 mm), particularly in young patients (see Fig. 69-4). The presence of one or more major risk factors may justify consideration of a primary prevention implantable cardioverter-defibrillator (ICD), particularly if family history of sudden death, unexplained syncope, or massive LV hypertrophy is present.

A number of other disease features can be regarded as potential arbitrators when level of risk is judged ambiguous on the basis of conventional markers. These include contrast-enhanced CMR[24] delayed enhancement (see Fig. 18-10) (a marker for myocardial fibrosis with a relation to high-risk ventricular tachyarrhythmia)[42] and subgroups that have emerged within the heterogeneous HCM disease spectrum: thin-walled akinetic LV apical aneurysms associated with regional myocardial scarring and ventricular tachyarrhythmias,[12] the end-stage phase,[11] and percutaneous alcohol septal ablation[38,43-45] with transmural myocardial infarction in select patients (see Fig. 69-4).[46] Whereas LV outflow obstruction is a determinant of progressive heart failure, its relationship specifically to sudden death is much weaker, and subaortic gradients are not regarded per se as a major risk marker.[17] There is no compelling evidence that myocardial bridging of left anterior descending coronary artery is a sudden death risk factor in HCM.[47]

At present, there is very limited prognostic significance that can be attributed to specific HCM-causing mutations for stratification of risk and clinical decision-making in individual patients.[1] Moreover, prognosis appears to be benign in gene carriers without LV hypertrophy, with little evidence[48] to justify disqualification from most competitive sports or employment opportunities.[41]

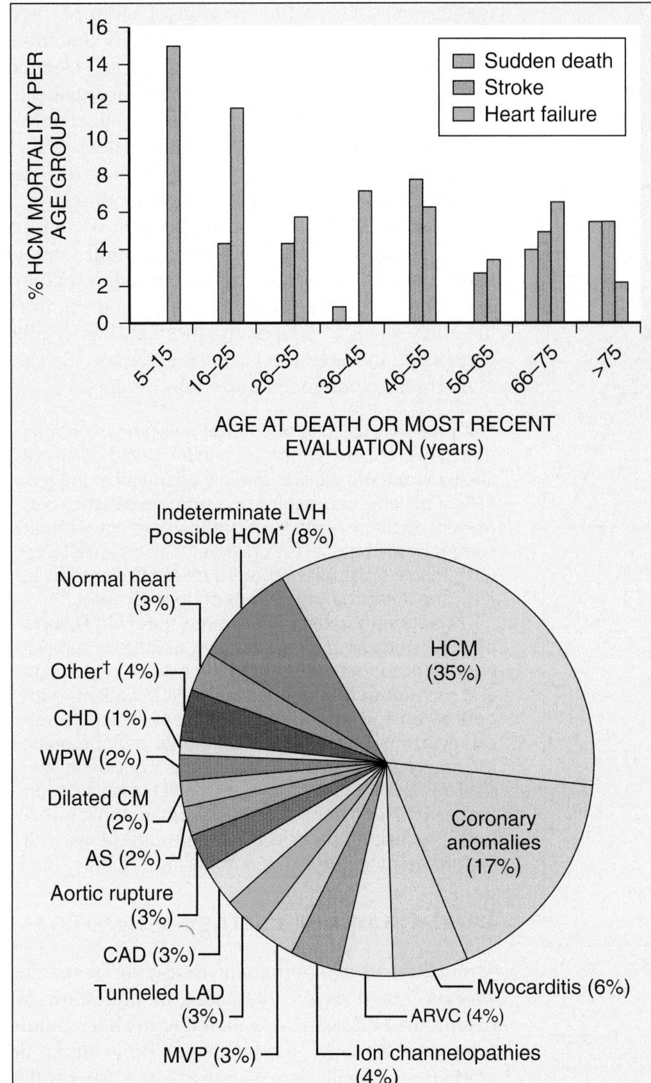

FIGURE 69-10 Clinical profile of sudden death. **Top,** Sudden death is most common in children and young adults before about 25 years of age, whereas heart failure and stroke generally occur later in life. *(From Maron BJ, Olivotto I, Spirito P, et al: Epidemiology of hypertrophic cardiomyopathy–related death: Revisited in a large non-referral-based patient population. Circulation 102:858, 2000. Reproduced with permission of the American Heart Association.)* **Bottom,** HCM is the single most common cause of sudden death in young competitive athletes in the United States. ARVC = arrhythmogenic right ventricular cardiomyopathy; AS = aortic valve stenosis; CAD = coronary artery disease; CHD = congenital heart disease; CM = cardiomyopathy; LAD = left anterior descending; LVH = left ventricular hypertrophy; MVP = mitral valve prolapse; WPW = Wolff-Parkinson-White. *Regarded as possible (but not definitive) evidence for HCM at autopsy with mildly increased LV wall thicknesses (18 ± 4 mm) and heart weight (447 ± 76 g). †Includes most commonly Kawasaki disease, sickle cell trait, and sarcoidosis. *(From Maron BJ, Doerer JJ, Haas TS, et al: Sudden deaths in young competitive athletes: Analysis of 1866 deaths in the U.S., 1980-2006. Circulation 119:1085, 2009. Reproduced with permission of the American Heart Association.)*

Management

Prevention of Sudden Death

The ICD has altered the natural history of HCM for many patients by virtue of effectively and reliably aborting potentially lethal ventricular tachyarrhythmias (see Chap. 38),[38,39,49-52] for both secondary prevention after cardiac arrest (11%/year) and primary prevention for risk factors (4%/year) (see Fig. 69-e1 on website).[38,49] Noteworthy is the extended time (i.e., 5 to 10 years) that may elapse between the clinical decision to implant an ICD and the time at which the device is required to terminate ventricular tachyarrhythmias (**Fig. 69-12**). The unpredictability of arrhythmic events in HCM is underscored by the absence of a distinct circadian pattern, the occurrence of a substantial proportion during sleep,[39] and the long periods that may elapse after cardiac arrest without a recurrent event.[38,49,51] Notably, development of heart failure symptoms appears to be uncommon in the years after an appropriate ICD intervention.[51]

Age may alter the threshold for prophylactic ICD implants; elderly patients are less often targeted for devices, given that HCM-related sudden death is uncommon in this age group and survival to advanced age itself generally declares lower risk status. Whereas it appears that current risk stratification strategy for HCM reliably identifies most high-risk patients, nevertheless this algorithm is probably incomplete, and a small minority of patients without any of the traditional primary prevention risk factors may be susceptible to sudden death.[52] Prophylactic, empiric pharmacologic treatment with amiodarone for asymptomatic high-risk patients to reduce sudden death risk is an obsolete strategy that has been abandoned, given the lack of proven efficacy and the likelihood for important side effects during the long risk period of young HCM patients.[1,7]

Medical Treatment of Heart Failure (see Fig. 69-12)

Symptoms of heart failure, that is, exertional dyspnea (sometimes fatigue) and chest pain, are attributable to diastolic dysfunction, outflow tract obstruction, or microvascular myocardial ischemia or combinations of these pathophysiologic variables. Symptom relief due to medical treatment can be highly variable, and drug administration is often empirically tailored to requirements of individual patients. Since the mid-1960s, beta-adrenergic receptor blocking drugs have been used extensively to relieve symptoms of heart failure in obstructive or nonobstructive HCM by slowing heart rate and reducing force of LV contraction, thus augmenting ventricular filling and relaxation and decreasing myocardial oxygen consumption. Long-acting preparations of propranolol, atenolol, metoprolol, or nadolol are now commonly used. By inhibiting sympathetic stimulation of the heart, beta blockers also have the potential to blunt LV outflow gradient triggered by physiologic exercise.[6]

Verapamil improves symptoms and exercise capacity, largely in patients without marked obstruction to LV outflow, probably because of its beneficial effect on ventricular relaxation and filling. Some investigators favor disopyramide as a third option (in combination with a beta blocker) to ameliorate symptoms when other drugs fail to achieve symptom control.[53] Diuretic agents may be judiciously administered, in conjunction with beta blockers or verapamil, to reduce pulmonary congestion and LV filling pressures. Either beta blockers or verapamil can be administered initially, although there is no evidence that combining these drugs is advantageous, and together they may excessively lower heart rate or blood pressure.

Therapeutic strategies for patients with systolic dysfunction in the end stage are similar to those employed for congestive heart failure in other cardiac diseases, including the administration of beta blockers, angiotensin-converting enzyme inhibitors or angiotensin receptor blockers, and diuretics or possibly spironolactone as well as warfarin.[11] End stage with widespread LV scarring also represents a sudden death risk factor with consideration for ICD as a bridge to heart transplantation.[1,7,11]

Atrial Fibrillation (see Fig. 69-12)

AF is the most common sustained arrhythmia in HCM, frequently accounting for unexpected hospital admissions and lost productivity and on occasion requiring aggressive therapeutic intervention (see Chap. 40).[1,7] AF, either paroxysmal or chronic, occurs in about 20% of HCM patients, increasing in incidence with age and linked to enlargement of the left atrium (a finding that has also been associated with overall adverse outcome in HCM, even independent of AF).[54] AF is well tolerated by about one third of patients but not uncommonly associated with adverse consequences, including embolic stroke (incidence, 1%/year; prevalence, 6%), and progressive heart failure, particularly

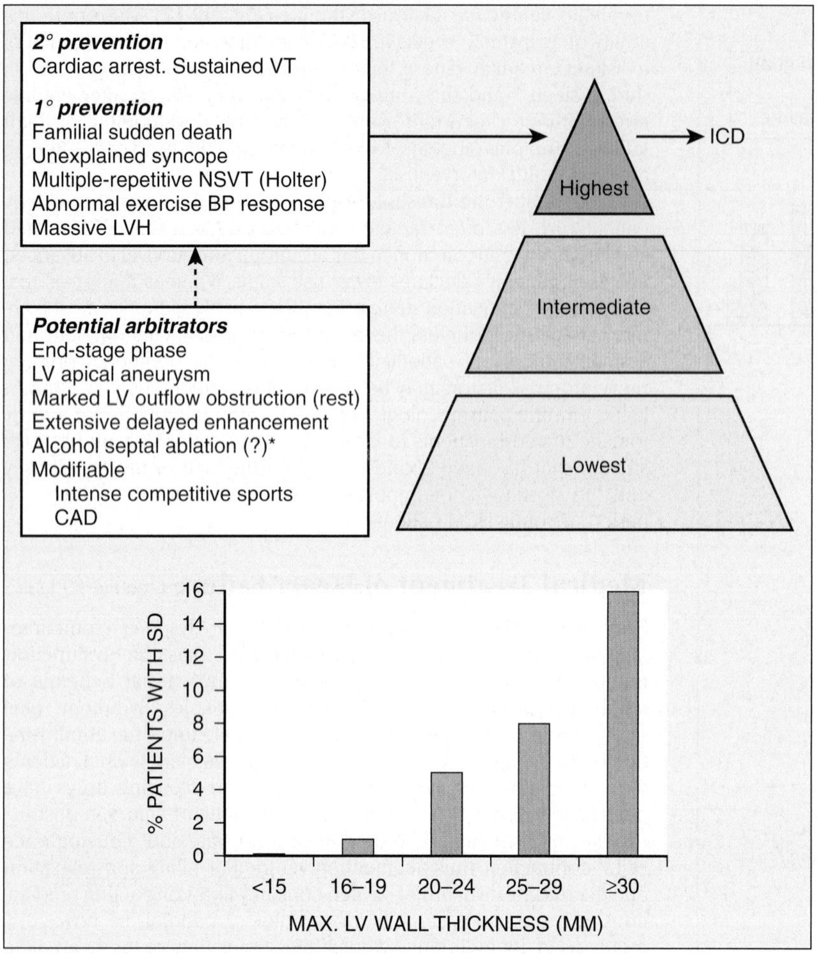

FIGURE 69-11 Sudden death risk stratification. **Top,** Risk pyramid currently used to identify the most likely candidates for prevention of sudden death with ICDs. BP = blood pressure; CAD = coronary artery disease; ICD = implantable cardiac defibrillator; LV = left ventricle. LVH = left ventricular hypertrophy; NSVT = nonsustained ventricular tachycardia; VT = ventricular tachycardia. **Bottom,** Relation between magnitude of LV hypertrophy (maximum [max] wall thickness by echocardiography) and sudden death risk in an unselected HCM cohort. Mild hypertrophy conveys generally lower risk and extreme hypertrophy (wall thickness ≥30 mm) the highest risk. *(From Spirito P, Bellone P, Harris KM, et al: Magnitude of left ventricular hypertrophy and risk of sudden death in hypertrophic cardiomyopathy. N Engl J Med 342:1778-85, 2000. Reproduced with permission of the Massachusetts Medical Society.)* *Sustained ventricular tachyarrhythmias have been reported in a significant minority of patients (10%) short term after the alcohol septal ablation procedure.[43-46,59,60]

when it is associated with outflow obstruction or onset before the age of 50 years.

Because of potential for clot formation and embolization, a low threshold for initiation of anticoagulant therapy with warfarin is prudent, although such decisions should be tailored to individual patients after consideration of lifestyle modifications, hemorrhagic risk, and expectations for compliance. Although data specifically in HCM are limited, amiodarone is considered the most effective drug in reducing AF recurrences. Beta blockers and verapamil are usually administered to control heart rate in chronic AF. Some success in treatment of refractory AF complicating HCM with radiofrequency catheter ablation has been reported in relatively small numbers of patients, but long-term outcome is largely unresolved.[56,58,59]

Surgery (see Fig. 69-12)

On the basis of the extensive worldwide experience during more than 45 years, surgical septal myectomy remains the preferred treatment option for patients with severe drug-refractory heart failure symptoms and marked functional disability (i.e., NYHA Classes III and IV in adults, but less limitation in children) associated with obstruction to LV outflow under basal conditions or with physiologic exercise (i.e., gradient ≥50 mm Hg).[1,7,56-59] Inducing gradients with nonphysiologic maneuvers, such as the infusion of inotropic and catecholamine inducing drugs (e.g., dobutamine and isoproterenol), is not advisable in selecting patients for septal myectomy (or alcohol ablation).

Patients with obstructive HCM have mechanical impedance to LV outflow and a form of heart failure that is reversible by surgery.[1,7,17,25,56-59] Transaortic ventricular septal myectomy (Morrow procedure) involves resection of a small portion of muscle (usually 3 to 10 g) from the basal septum.[57] Some surgeons now perform a more aggressive myectomy, extended in the septum for about 7 cm distal from the aortic valve.[56,58,59] Operative mortality has steadily decreased and is now <1% during the last 15 years at the most experienced myectomy centers.[58,59]

The primary objective of surgical myectomy is reduction in heart failure symptoms and improved quality of life, by virtue of relieving outflow obstruction. Indeed, 95% of patients undergoing myectomy experience permanent abolition of the basal outflow gradient, without compromise of global LV function.[56-59] As a result, long-term follow-up studies reported relief of symptoms in 85% of patients during periods of up to 25 years.[56-59]

Myectomy also beneficially alters the clinical course of HCM; surgical patients achieve long-term survival equivalent to that expected in the general population and superior to that of nonsurgical HCM patients with outflow obstruction[56] (see Fig. 69-6). At present, surgical myectomy is not recommended for asymptomatic (or mildly symptomatic) patients, as conclusive evidence is lacking that prophylactic relief of obstruction is of benefit long term. There is no evidence that myectomy predisposes patients to the end-stage phase with systolic dysfunction and LV remodeling.[11,58,59]

Dual-Chamber Pacing (see Fig. 69-12)

About 20 years ago, permanent dual-chamber pacing was promoted as an alternative to myectomy for obstructive HCM patients with refractory heart failure symptoms. Although modest reduction in subaortic gradient may result from pacing in some patients, this benefit is inconsistent, particularly compared with that achieved by myectomy or alcohol ablation.[1] Several randomized studies demonstrated that the subjectively perceived symptomatic benefit from pacing was not accompanied by objective evidence of improved exercise capacity and appeared to be largely a placebo effect.[1,7] The overall role for pacing in HCM has become particularly limited during the last decade.

Alcohol Septal Ablation (see Chap. 59)

Percutaneous alcohol septal ablation, an alternative to myectomy only in selected patients (see Fig. 69-12; see Fig. 59-5),[1] involves introduction of 1 to 3 mL of 95% alcohol into a major septal perforator coronary artery to create necrosis and a permanent transmural myocardial infarction in the proximal ventricular septum (see Fig. 69-4).[43-46] This scar leads to progressive thinning and restricted septal excursion, outflow tract enlargement, and reduction in LV outflow tract gradient and mitral regurgitation in most patients.

Alcohol ablation resolves heart failure symptoms in many patients, although follow-up is short compared with myectomy, and even in expert centers, it may be associated with procedural mortality and complication rates exceeding those of myectomy.[44,45,59] Nonrandomized, comparative data show that gradient reduction after alcohol ablation is similar to myectomy, although less consistent or complete, and patients ≤65 years experience better symptom resolution with myectomy than with ablation.[45] About 20% of patients require repeated ablations because of unsatisfactory hemodynamic and symptomatic results or permanent pacing for complete heart block.[44]

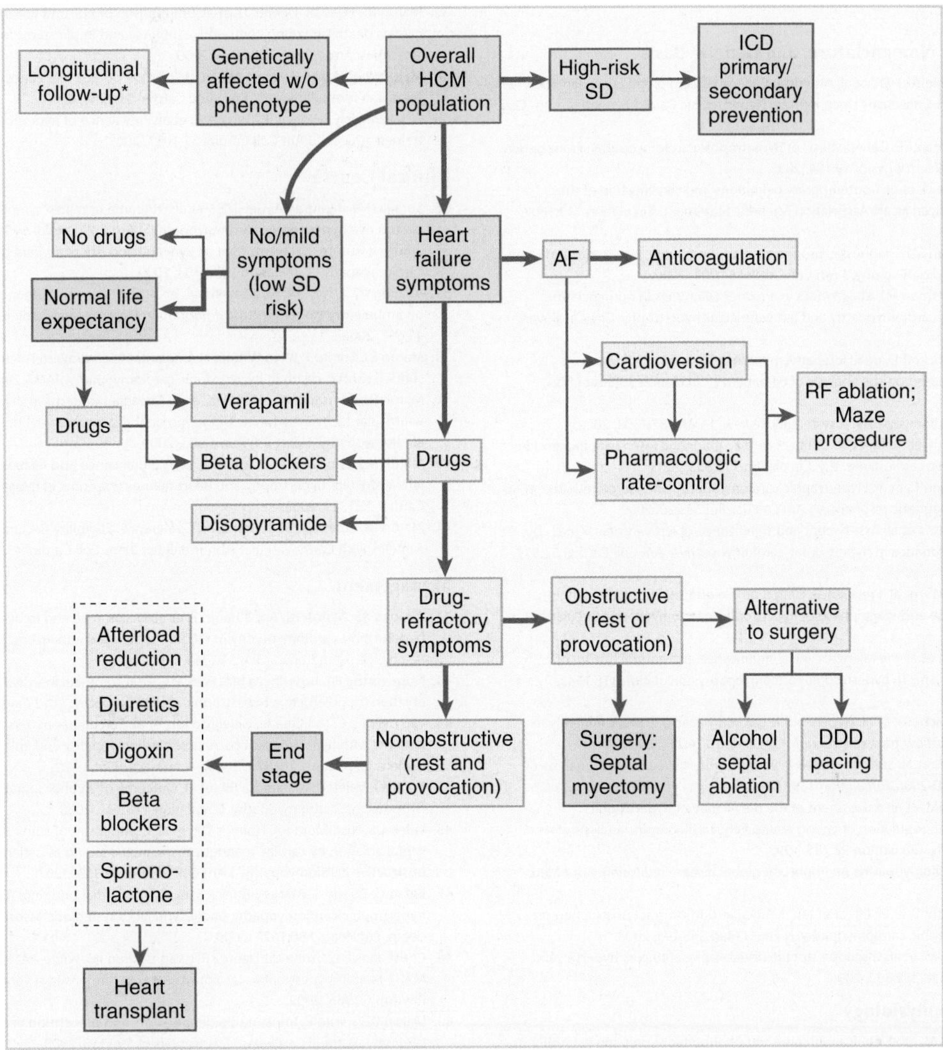

FIGURE 69-12 Management strategies for subgroups of patients within the broad HCM clinical spectrum. *Generally no specific treatment or intervention indicated. AF = atrial fibrillation; DDD = dual-chamber; ICD = implanted cardioverter-defibrillator; RF= radiofrequency; SD = sudden death.

An American College of Cardiology/European Society of Cardiology expert consensus panel[1] recommended surgical myectomy as the preferred and primary management option for patients with severe refractory symptoms and marked outflow obstruction. Alcohol ablation is regarded as an alternative treatment strategy for patients not considered optimal operative candidates (e.g., advanced age, significant comorbidity and increased operative risk, or strongly adverse to surgery personally).

Long-term issues remain unresolved, most importantly the clinical significance of the alcohol-induced transmural scar (occupying about 10% of the LV wall; see Fig. 69-4),[46] which represents a potentially unstable arrhythmogenic substrate that in some patients has triggered potentially lethal ventricular tachyarrhythmias and could raise sudden death risk in some susceptible patients.[43-46,59,60] Indeed, there is a recognized risk for life-threatening sustained ventricular tachyarrhythmias largely during the short term[43-46,59,60] (with postprocedural annual event rates of 3% to 5% involving approximately 10% of reported patients).[43,60] On the basis of this consideration, some practitioners have prudently implanted ICDs prophylactically in selected patients with alcohol septal ablation.[60] It is, however, unlikely that a randomized myectomy versus ablation trial will be carried out to resolve the level of risk conveyed long term by alcohol ablation.[61]

Other Management Issues

There is no evidence that HCM patients are generally at increased risk during pregnancy and delivery. Maternal mortality appears confined to the very small subset of symptomatic women with high-risk clinical profiles, such as severe heart failure, ventricular tachyarrhythmias, or possibly marked LV outflow obstruction, who should be afforded specialized and preventive obstetric care. Otherwise, most women with HCM can undergo normal vaginal delivery, without the necessity for cesarean section.

Bacterial endocarditis is an uncommon complication of HCM (prevalence <1%), virtually confined to patients with LV outflow obstruction. Vegetations most commonly involve anterior mitral leaflet or septal endocardium at the site of mitral valve contact. Prevention of bacterial endocarditis by antimicrobial prophylaxis remains a prudent strategy before dental or surgical procedures for this patient group.[62]

Future Directions

The last decade has witnessed a substantially increased understanding of the diagnosis, clinical profile, and natural history of HCM as well as substantial advances in management. Future clinical directions will include the development of more precise risk stratification strategies to more reliably identify those patients at unacceptably high risk for sudden death and deserving of consideration for ICD therapy. Also, there will be a continuing effort to define the proper role of alcohol septal ablation relative to surgical septal myectomy in the management of severely symptomatic drug-refractory patients with outflow obstruction, as well as the role of commercial genetic testing.

REFERENCES

Definition, Prevalence, Nomenclature, and Genetic Basis

1. Maron BJ, McKenna WJ, Danielson GK, et al: American College of Cardiology/European Society of Cardiology Clinical Expert Consensus Document on Hypertrophic Cardiomyopathy. J Am Coll Cardiol 42:1687, 2003.
2. Alcalai R, Seidman JG, Seidman CE: Genetic basis of hypertrophic cardiomyopathy: From bench to the clinics. J Cardiovasc Electrophysiol 19:104, 2008.
3. Maron BJ, Towbin JA, Thiene G, et al: Contemporary definitions and classification of the cardiomyopathies. An American Heart Association Scientific Statement. Circulation 113:1807, 2006.
4. Bos JM, Towbin JA, Ackerman MJ: Diagnostic, prognostic, and therapeutic implications of gene testing for hypertrophic cardiomyopathy. J Am Coll Cardiol 54:201, 2009.
5. Maron BJ, Seidman CE, Ackerman MJ, et al: What's in a name? Dilemmas in nomenclature characterizing hypertrophic cardiomyopathy and left ventricular hypertrophy. Circ Cardiovasc Genet 2:8, 2009.
6. Braunwald E, Lambrew C, Rockoff D, et al: Idiopathic hypertrophic subaortic stenosis. I. Description of the disease based on the analysis of 64 patients. Circulation 30(Suppl IV):1, 1964.
7. Maron BJ: Hypertrophic cardiomyopathy: A systematic review. JAMA 287:1308, 2002.
8. Rickers C, Wilke NM, Jerosch-Herold M, et al: Utility of cardiac magnetic resonance imaging in the diagnosis of hypertrophic cardiomyopathy. Circulation 112:855, 2005.
9. Maron MS, Maron BJ, Harrigan C, et al: Hypertrophic cardiomyopathy phenotype revisited at 50 years with cardiovascular magnetic resonance. J Am Coll Cardiol 54:220, 2009.
10. Olivotto I, Maron MS, Autore C, et al: Assessment and significance of left ventricular mass by cardiovascular magnetic resonance in hypertrophic cardiomyopathy. J Am Coll Cardiol 52:559, 2008.
11. Harris KM, Spirito P, Maron MS, et al: Prevalence, clinical profile and significance of left ventricular remodeling in the end-stage phase of hypertrophic cardiomyopathy. Circulation 114;216, 2006.
12. Maron MS, Finley JJ, Bos JM, et al: Prevalence, clinical significance and natural history of left ventricular apical aneurysms in hypertrophic cardiomyopathy. Circulation 118:1541, 2008.
13. Maron MS, Olivotto I, Zenovich AG, et al: Hypertrophic cardiomyopathy is predominantly a disease of left ventricular outflow tract obstruction. Circulation 114:216, 2006.
14. Maron BJ, Doerer JJ, Haas TS, et al: Sudden deaths in young competitive athletes: Analysis of 1866 deaths in the U.S., 1980-2006. Circulation 119:1085, 2009.
15. Maron BJ, Gardin JM, Flack JM, et al: Assessment of the prevalence of hypertrophic cardiomyopathy in a general population of young adults: Echocardiographic analysis of 4111 subjects in the CARDIA Study. Circulation 92:785, 1995.
16. Maron BJ: Hypertrophic cardiomyopathy: An important global disease [editorial]. Am J Med 116:63, 2004.
17. Maron MS, Olivotto I, Betocchi S, et al: Effect of left ventricular outflow tract obstruction on clinical outcome in hypertrophic cardiomyopathy. N Engl J Med 348:295, 2003.
18. Arad M, Maron BJ, Gorham JM, et al: Glycogen storage diseases presenting as hypertrophic cardiomyopathy. N Engl J Med 352:362, 2005.

Morphology and Pathophysiology

19. Maron BJ, Roberts WC, Arad M, et al: Clinical outcome and phenotypic expression in LAMP2 cardiomyopathy. JAMA 301:1253, 2009.
20. Maron MS, Hauser TH, Dubrow E, et al: Right ventricular involvement in hypertrophic cardiomyopathy. Am J Cardiol 100:1293, 2007.
21. Ho CY, Carlsen C, Thune JJ, et al: Echocardiographic strain imaging to assess early and late consequences of sarcomere mutations in hypertrophic cardiomyopathy. Circ Cardiovasc Genet 2:14, 2009.
22. Pelliccia A, DiPaolo FM, Quattrini FM, et al: Outcomes in athletes with marked ECG repolarization abnormalities. N Engl J Med 358:152, 2008.
23. Maron MS, Olivotto I, Maron BJ, et al: The case for myocardial ischemia in hypertrophic cardiomyopathy: An emerging but under-recognized pathophysiologic mechanism. J Am Coll Cardiol 54:866, 2009.
24. Maron MS, Appelbaum E, Harrigan C, et al: Clinical profile and significance of delayed enhancement in hypertrophic cardiomyopathy. Circ Heart Fail 1:184, 2008.
25. Maron BJ, Maron MS, Wigle ED, Braunwald E: 50 year history of left ventricular outflow tract obstruction in hypertrophic cardiomyopathy: From idiopathic hypertrophic subaortic stenosis to hypertrophic cardiomyopathy. J Am Coll Cardiol 54:191, 2009.

Family Screening, Clinical Features, and Athletes

26. Maron BJ, Seidman JG, Seidman CE: Proposal for contemporary screening strategies in families with hypertrophic cardiomyopathy. J Am Coll Cardiol 44:2125, 2004.
27. Adabag AS, Kuskowski MA, Maron BJ: Determinants for clinical diagnosis of hypertrophic cardiomyopathy. Am J Cardiol 98:1507, 2006.
28. Montgomery JV, Harris KM, Casey SA, et al: Relation of electrocardiographic patterns to phenotypic expression and clinical outcome in hypertrophic cardiomyopathy. Am J Cardiol 96:270, 2005.
29. McLeod CJ, Ackerman MJ, Nishimura RA, et al: Outcome of patients with hypertrophic cardiomyopathy and a normal electrocardiogram. J Am Coll Cardiol 54:229, 2009.
30. Olivotto I, Maron MS, Adabag AS, et al: Gender-related differences in the clinical presentation and outcome of hypertrophic cardiomyopathy. J Am Coll Cardiol 46:480, 2005.
31. Maron BJ, Pelliccia A: The heart of trained athletes: Cardiac remodeling and the risks of sports including sudden death. Circulation 114:1633, 2006.
32. Maron BJ, Haas TS, Doerer JJ, et al: Comparison of U.S. and Italian experiences with sudden cardiac deaths in young competitive athletes and implications for preparticipation screening strategies. Am J Cardiol 104:276, 2009.
33. Magalski A, Maron BJ, Main ML, et al: Relation of race to electrocardiographic patterns in elite American football players. J Am Coll Cardiol 51:2250, 2008.
34. Basavarajaiah S, Wilson M, Whyte G, et al: Prevalence of hypertrophic cardiomyopathy in highly trained athletes. J Am Coll Cardiol 51:1033, 2008.

Clinical Course

35. Sorajja P, Nishimura RA, Gersh BJ, et al: Outcome of mildly symptomatic or asymptomatic obstructive hypertrophic cardiomyopathy. J Am Coll Cardiol 54:234, 2009.
36. Spirito P, Autore C, Rapezzi C, et al: Syncope and risk of sudden death in hypertrophic cardiomyopathy. Circulation 119:1703, 2009.
37. Adabag AS, Casey SA, Kuskowski MA, et al: Spectrum and prognostic significance of arrhythmias on ambulatory Holter electrocardiogram in hypertrophic cardiomyopathy. J Am Coll Cardiol 45:697, 2005.
38. Maron BJ, Spirito P, Shen W-K, et al: Implantable cardioverter-defibrillators and prevention of sudden cardiac death in hypertrophic cardiomyopathy. JAMA 298:405, 2007.
39. Maron BJ, Semsarian C, Shen W-K, et al: Circadian patterns in the occurrence of malignant ventricular tachyarrhythmias triggering defibrillator interventions in patients with hypertrophic cardiomyopathy. Heart Rhythm 6:603, 2009.
40. Maron MS, Zenovich AG, Casey SA, et al: Significance and relationship between magnitude of left ventricular hypertrophy and heart failure symptoms in hypertrophic cardiomyopathy. Am J Cardiol 95:1329, 2005.
41. Maron BJ, Zipes DP: 36th Bethesda Conference: Eligibility Recommendations for Competitive Athletes with Cardiovascular Abnormalities. J Am Coll Cardiol 45:1312, 2005.

Management

42. Adabag AS, Maron BJ, Appelbaum E, et al: Occurrence and frequency of arrhythmias in hypertrophic cardiomyopathy in relation to delayed enhancement on cardiovascular magnetic resonance. J Am Coll Cardiol 51:1369, 2008.
43. Noseworthy PA, Rosenberg MA, Fifer MA, et al: Ventricular arrhythmia following alcohol septal ablation for obstructive hypertrophic cardiomyopathy. Am J Cardiol 104:128, 2009.
44. van der Lee C, ten Cate FJ, Geleijnse ML, et al: Percutaneous versus surgical treatment for patients with hypertrophic obstructive cardiomyopathy and enlarged anterior mitral valve leaflets. Circulation 112:482, 2005.
45. Sorajja P, Valeti U, Nishimura RA, et al: Outcome of alcohol septal ablation for obstructive hypertrophic cardiomyopathy. Circulation 118:131, 2008.
46. Valeti US, Nishimura RA, Holmes DR, et al: Comparison of surgical septal myectomy and alcohol septal ablation by cardiac magnetic resonance imaging in patients with hypertrophic obstructive cardiomyopathy. J Am Coll Cardiol 49:350, 2007.
47. Basso C, Thiene G, Mackey-Bojack S, et al: Myocardial bridging: A frequent component of the hypertrophic cardiomyopathy phenotype lacks systematic association with sudden cardiac death. Eur Heart J 30:1627, 2009.
48. Christiaans I, Lekanne dit Deprez RH, van Langen IM, Wilde AAM: Ventricular fibrillation in MYH7-related hypertrophic cardiomyopathy before onset of ventricular hypertrophy. Heart Rhythm 6:1366, 2009.
49. Maron BJ, Spirito P: Implantable defibrillators and prevention of sudden death in hypertrophic cardiomyopathy. J Cardiovasc Electrophysiol 19:1118, 2008.
50. Woo A, Monakier D, Harris L, et al: Determinants of implantable defibrillator discharges in high-risk patients with hypertrophic cardiomyopathy. Heart 93:1044, 2007.
51. Maron BJ, Haas TS, Shannon KM, et al: Long-term survival after cardiac arrest in hypertrophic cardiomyopathy. Heart Rhythm 6:993, 2009.
52. Maron BJ, Maron MS, Lesser JR, et al: Sudden cardiac arrest in hypertrophic cardiomyopathy in the absence of conventional criteria for high risk status. Am J Cardiol 101:544, 2008.
53. Sherrid MV, Barac I, McKenna WJ, et al: Multicenter study of the efficacy and safety of disopyramide in obstructive hypertrophic cardiomyopathy. J Am Coll Cardiol 45:1251, 2005.
54. Nistri S, Olivotto I, Betocchi S, et al: Prognostic significance of left atrial size in patients with hypertrophic cardiomyopathy (from the Italian Registry for Hypertrophic Cardiomyopathy). Am J Cardiol 98:960, 2006.
55. Kilicaslan F, Verma A, Saad E, et al: Efficacy of catheter ablation of atrial fibrillation in patients with hypertrophic obstructive cardiomyopathy. Heart Rhythm 3:275, 2006.
56. Ommen SR, Maron BJ, Olivotto I, et al: Long-term effects of surgical septal myectomy on survival in patients with obstructive hypertrophic cardiomyopathy. J Am Coll Cardiol 46:470, 2005.
57. Woo A, Williams WG, Choi R, et al: Clinical and echocardiographic determinants of long-term survival following surgical myectomy in obstructive hypertrophic cardiomyopathy. Circulation 111:2033, 2005.
58. Maron BJ, Dearani JA, Ommen SR, et al: The case for surgery in obstructive hypertrophic cardiomyopathy. J Am Coll Cardiol 44:2044, 2004.
59. Maron BJ: Controversies in cardiovascular medicine. Surgical myectomy remains the primary treatment option for severely symptomatic patients with obstructive hypertrophic cardiomyopathy. Circulation 116:196, 2007.
60. Cuoco FA, Spencer WH III, Fernandes VL, et al: Implantable cardioverter-defibrillator therapy for primary prevention of sudden death after alcohol septal ablation of hypertrophic cardiomyopathy. J Am Coll Cardiol 52:1718, 2008.
61. Olivotto I, Ommen SR, Maron MS, et al: Surgical myectomy versus percutaneous alcohol septal ablation for obstructive hypertrophic cardiomyopathy: Will there ever be a randomized trial? J Am Coll Cardiol 50:831, 2007.
62. Maron BJ, Lever H: In defense of antimicrobial prophylaxis for prevention of infective endocarditis in patients with hypertrophic cardiomyopathy. J Am Coll Cardiol 54:2339, 2009.

CHAPTER 70 Myocarditis

Peter Liu and Kenneth L. Baughman

Myocarditis is defined as inflammation of the heart muscle. The most common causes today are infectious agents such as viruses or parasites and autoimmune conditions. True viral myocarditis is probably more common than currently diagnosed, largely because of its protean manifestations and the reliance on myocardial biopsies for pathologic confirmation. The availability of new diagnostic modalities, such as cardiac magnetic resonance imaging, helps increase the appropriate identification of suspected cases. New molecular tools to identify the viral genome from cardiac tissues also help in defining the appropriate etiology.

The pathogenesis of myocarditis is a classic paradigm of cardiac injury followed by immunologic response from the host as cardiac inflammation. The relative incidence of viral causes is continually evolving as new diagnostic tools based on molecular epidemiology become available. Just as important, if the host immune response is overwhelming or inappropriate, the inflammation may destroy the heart tissue acutely or lingers on and produces cardiac remodeling, leading to dilated cardiomyopathy, heart failure, or death. For the appropriate diagnosis of myocarditis, a heightened clinical suspicion is required. A composite diagnostic criterion is also evolving. Fortunately for the majority of patients, clinical myocarditis is often self-limited if proper support and follow-up are available. The role of endomyocardial biopsy has been evaluated in a recently published consensus report. Ventricular function after myocarditis may recover without residual damage, result in some degree of dysfunction, or progress rapidly to life-threatening cardiac compromise. Because of the high incidence of ultimate recovery, aggressive therapy including ventricular assist is indicated for patients with severe hemodynamic compromise. With the evolution of new understanding of pathophysiology and new therapies for this condition, the outlook for myocarditis is continuing to improve.

Definition and Incidence

Myocarditis

Myocarditis broadly refers to inflammation of the heart muscle. Inflammation can be found after any form of injury to the heart, including ischemic damage, mechanical trauma, and genetic cardiomyopathies. However, classic myocarditis refers to inflammation of the heart muscle as a result of exposure to either discrete external antigens (such as viruses, bacteria, parasites, toxins, or drugs) or internal triggers, such as autoimmune activation against self antigens.[1] The classic Dallas criteria for the pathologic diagnosis of myocarditis require the presence of inflammatory cells simultaneous with evidence of myocyte necrosis on the same microscopic section on examination of a myocardial biopsy specimen. Borderline myocarditis is characterized by inflammatory cell infiltrate without myocardial necrosis (**Fig. 70-1**).[2] However, the Dallas criteria have been criticized as too restrictive. These concerns include sampling error, intraobserver variability of interpretation, and failure of the criteria to be associated with demonstrated viral infection by molecular techniques and clinical outcomes. A broader definition including the presence of viral genome or molecular markers of immune activation has since evolved, but consensus has not yet been achieved on these additional measures.[3]

It is not surprising, then, that the precise incidence of myocarditis is difficult to ascertain, depending on inclusion and diagnostic criteria applied. One estimate has been about 8 to 10 per 100,000 population. However, because of failure to make the appropriate diagnosis or failure to detect subclinical cases, many deaths due to myocarditis may go unrecognized. Therefore, the prevalence of myocarditis among unselected autopsy series is as high as 1 to 5 per 100. Recent pathologic series examining young adults who had suffered sudden deaths suggested an even higher incidence of myocarditis around 8.6%.[4] When patients with idiopathic dilated cardiomyopathy only are considered, myocarditis accounts for 10% to 40% of the cases overall.[5] This suggests that myocarditis is not clinically suspected in a large number of cases, leading to death or severe heart failure.

Dilated Cardiomyopathy (see Chap. 68)

Cardiomyopathy with systolic dysfunction refers to disorders of the heart muscle with decreased contractility and usually increased internal diastolic dimensions of the left ventricular chamber. This generally includes cardiac dysfunction *not* associated with overt ischemic heart disease. About one third of dilated cardiomyopathy cases can be attributed to single-gene mutations involving defects of cytoskeletal proteins, such as actin, dystrophin complex, plakoglobin, or laminin. Myocarditis may also be an antecedent event leading to dilated

Supported in part by grants from the Heart and Stroke Foundation, the Canadian Institutes of Health Research; and National Heart, Lung and Blood Institute, National Institutes of Health.

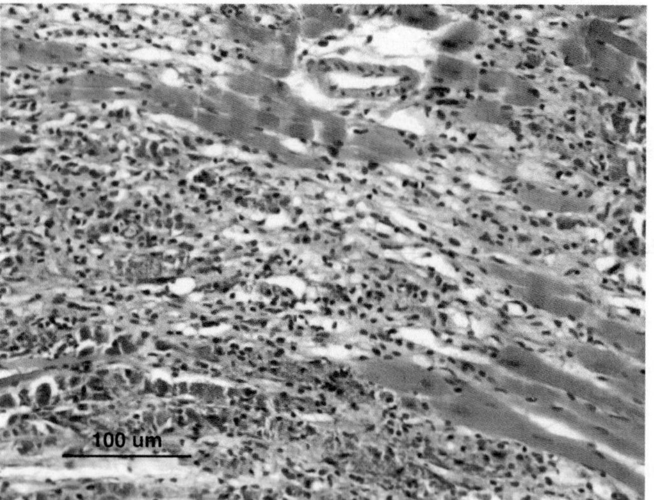

FIGURE 70-1 Myocardial biopsy section under high power (hematoxylin and eosin stain). This section is diagnostic of myocarditis by the Dallas criteria. The Dallas criteria require the presence of a lymphocyte-rich inflammatory infiltrate associated with myocyte degeneration or necrosis in the same view. However, the Dallas criteria are viewed as overly conservative, in view of the patchy nature of the inflammatory foci and less than ideal reproducibility.

cardiomyopathy, with ventricular dilation a consequence of inflammation-induced myocyte loss and interstitial fibrosis. In one pediatric series of patients with dilated cardiomyopathy, 46% of the cases could be attributed to antecedent myocarditis.[6]

In that 50% of patients with new-onset cardiomyopathy or heart failure submitted to endomyocardial biopsy who have no cause of their dysfunction identified, it is conceivable that viral myocarditis or postviral autoimmune activation may cause a large proportion of these cases. Therefore, understanding of myocarditis may allow improved diagnosis of and therapy for patients otherwise destined to the natural history of cardiomyopathy with systolic dysfunction.

Viruses such as coxsackievirus can also elaborate proteases that directly modify the cytoskeleton components, such as the dystrophin complex in the heart, leading to ventricular dilation.[7] Dilated cardiomyopathy is associated with relatively poor prognosis and is one of the most common indications for cardiac transplantation worldwide.

Acute Pericarditis (see Chap. 75)

Acute pericarditis is characterized by typical pericardial chest pain, pericardial friction rub, diffuse ST elevation by standard electrocardiography, and usually an associated pericardial effusion on transthoracic echocardiography. In approximately 15% of patients with pericarditis, myocardial involvement (myopericarditis) is diagnosed when, in addition, there is elevation of cardiac enzymes and diffuse or focal wall motion abnormalities by echocardiography. Patients may have associated supraventricular or ventricular arrhythmias and, less frequently, atrial ventricular block. Most patients respond to treatment with aspirin or nonsteroidal anti-inflammatory agents; however, approximately 15% report recurrence of pain, with or without evidence of myopericarditis. By 12 months after the acute event, virtually all patients will have resolved their symptoms and electrocardiographic and echocardiographic abnormalities. Those who fail to respond to aspirin or nonsteroidal anti-inflammatory drugs and require corticosteroids for relief of pain may have a higher rate of complications.[8]

Epidemiology

Myocarditis has been more often a diagnosis of exclusion rather than a specific diagnosis. However, the incidence of myocarditis is increasing with the advent of newer molecular diagnostic techniques in place of the absolute requirement of inflammatory cell infiltrates on myocardial biopsy. Multiple investigators evaluating heart biopsy samples in patients with clinical myocarditis or new-onset cardiomyopathy have demonstrated cardiotropic viral agents with no evidence of myocardial inflammation or myocyte destruction compatible with myocarditis as required by the Dallas criteria. Other investigators have demonstrated upregulation of immune markers in these populations, suggesting that a postviral autoimmune response is responsible.[9,10]

Meanwhile, the increasing prevalence of human immunodeficiency virus (HIV) infection with the improved survival of patients with acquired immunodeficiency syndromes (AIDS) introduced the new condition of HIV-associated myocarditis (see Chap. 72). This condition is associated with very poor prognosis and is probably related to both the HIV infection and multiple comorbidities in these patients.

Changing Etiology and Divergent Geographic Distribution. The etiologic agents accounting for myocarditis have changed not only temporally but also geographically around the globe. Previously, the most common etiologic agents globally have been enteroviruses, with coxsackieviruses predominating. However, more recent series have indicated that the traditional dominance of coxsackieviruses has been replaced by a broader spectrum of viral causes, including adenoviruses, parvoviruses, and cytomegaloviruses. There is also an evolving distinct viral profile in different regions of the globe.

In Europe, Kuhl and colleagues' recent series of biopsies from 245 patients with dilated cardiomyopathy found that 51.4% of the biopsy samples tested positively for parvovirus B19, 21.6% for human herpesvirus 6, but only 9.4% for enterovirus and 1.6% for adenovirus.[11] Interestingly, 27.3% had evidence of multiple infections.

In contrast, Bowles and coworkers analyzed biopsy specimens from 624 patients with polymerase chain reaction (PCR) and found that overall viral positivity was 38% (or 239/624).[12] On analysis, 22.8% tested positive for adenovirus, 13.6% for enterovirus, but only 1.0% for parvovirus. This group of patients was younger, resided mainly in North America, and certainly showed a distinct viral etiologic profile (see Fig. 70-e1 on website). Meanwhile, in Japan, hepatitis C virus infection of the heart, particularly related to a hypertrophic cardiomyopathy, dominated the etiologic profile. Both hepatitis C virus antibodies and genome have been detected in the serum and myocardial biopsy specimens of patients with myocarditis.[13]

Whereas PCR has expanded our ability to identify viral pathogens, there are limitations to this technology. PCR is performed to identify specific viral pathogens predetermined by the investigator. At this time, there is no proven methodology to screen heart tissue for all viral agents. Doing so may further enhance our ability to associate cardiomyopathy with viral causes.

Globally, a common cause of dilated cardiomyopathy in the Third World is still Chagas' disease, an inflammatory myocarditis caused by the parasite *Trypanosoma cruzi*. Therefore, there are major regional differences in etiologic profile of myocarditis, showing the footprints of genetic and environmental interaction. Some of these differences may be due to the differences in the prevalence of these viruses in the local population, but others may be due to differences of definition and inclusion criteria.

Specific Etiologic Agents

Myocarditis most commonly results from an external inflammatory trigger, such as a virus, inducing host immune response, which may range from a minimally transient response to fulminant overwhelming inflammation. Characterization of the etiologic triggers has benefited significantly from molecular tools such as PCR amplification and in situ hybridization to detect external agents such as viral genome. These techniques have shown that the viral genome may persist in the myocardium for variable periods, with or without the accompaniment of an inflammatory cell infiltrate.

Recent series of molecular analysis in patients with suspected myocarditis have confirmed that indeed viruses are the most common etiologic agents associated with the condition (**Table 70-1**). Meta-analysis of PCR studies in patients who had heart biopsies with clinically suspected myocarditis or cardiomyopathy demonstrated an odds ratio of 3.8 for viral presence compared with control patients. The persistence of viral genome in the myocardium is also associated

TABLE 70-1 Etiologic Agents of Myocarditis

Viral (Most Common)
Adenovirus
Coxsackievirus, enterovirus
Cytomegalovirus
Parvovirus B19
Hepatitis C virus
Influenza virus
Human immunodeficiency virus
Herpesvirus
Epstein-Barr virus
Mixed infections
Bacterial
Mycobacterial species
Chlamydia pneumoniae
Streptococcal species
Mycoplasma pneumoniae
Treponema pallidum
Fungal
Aspergillus
Candida
Coccidioides
Cryptococcus
Histoplasma
Protozoal
Trypanosoma cruzi
Parasitic
Schistosomiasis
Larva migrans
Toxins
Anthracyclines
Cocaine
Hypersensitivity
Clozapine
Sulfonamides
Cephalosporins
Penicillins
Tricyclic antidepressants
Autoimmune Activation
Smallpox vaccination
Giant cell myocarditis
Churg-Strauss syndrome
Sjögren syndrome
Inflammatory bowel disease
Celiac disease
Sarcoidosis
Systemic lupus erythematosus
Takayasu arteritis
Wegener granulomatosis

with progressive ventricular dysfunction and worse outcome during follow-up.[11]

Viruses

ENTEROVIRUSES INCLUDING COXSACKIEVIRUSES. The most common etiologic agent of viral myocarditis has traditionally been the enteroviruses, single-stranded RNA viruses that include the coxsackieviruses and echoviruses. Because coxsackieviruses can also infect susceptible strains of mice, they are the model system on which the current understanding of the pathophysiology of viral myocarditis in humans is based.

Current evidence suggests that coxsackieviruses enter the host gastrointestinal or respiratory system by the coxsackie-adenoviral receptor (CAR), a junctional protein important for cell-cell communication and critical for internalization of the virus.[14,15] CAR localization is particularly concentrated in the cardiovascular, immune, and neurologic systems. Use of the CAR for viral entry also triggers host immune activation through its associated receptor tyrosine kinases, leading to the subsequent inflammatory response. The virus is usually cleared from the host by the immune system in 1 to 2 weeks; however, in some instances, the virus genome can persist in the host myocardium for 6 months or longer, constituting a nidus for chronic inflammatory response and a known risk factor for worse prognosis. There is also evidence to suggest that coxsackieviral infection may contribute to sudden cardiac death in those with acute coronary thrombosis.[16]

More recent series of myocarditic patients have demonstrated a decrease in the prevalence of enteroviruses as an etiologic agent, particularly in western Europe. This could be related to the development of herd immunity after a period of prolonged exposure, leading to temporary decrease in the prevalence of infections in the community.

ADENOVIRUS. Adenovirus is a DNA virus that commonly infects the human mucosal surface, particularly in the pediatric population. Adenoviruses also use the CAR (shared with coxsackievirus) as well as the integrin receptor to gain entry into cells. Adenoviral infections can be much more virulent than coxsackievirus infections and can cause extensive cell death without comparable inflammatory response. The immunologic profile associated with adenovirus is very different from that found with enterovirus, with markedly decreased CD2, CD3, and CD45RO T-lymphocyte counts in those with adenoviral genome present in the myocardium.

PARVOVIRUS. A new entry in the epidemiology of myocarditis is the parvovirus B19 family of viruses. Parvoviruses are single-stranded DNA viruses that cause common childhood infections, such as the fever and exanthem seen in pediatric populations known as fifth disease. However, in recent biopsy series from Europe, parvovirus B19 genome has been found in more than 51% of the patients with dilated cardiomyopathy.[10] Questions have been raised as to whether this is mere association, contamination, or truly causal. By autopsy myocardial analysis, even in those without cardiac dysfunction, parvovirus B19 may persist in most patients who are seropositive for this pathogen. Demonstration of immunoglobulin M parvovirus B19 antibody response may help determine those with an acute as opposed to a chronic inflammation.[17] There have been cases of myocarditis or heart failure reported after clinical fifth disease, and this can be accompanied by persistent detection of parvovirus B19 in the circulation. Patients with parvovirus myocarditis are frequently symptomatic with nonspecific chest pain, and, interestingly, parvovirus is mainly resident and trophic in the endothelial cells of the vasculature. Persistent viral infection, particularly with parvovirus B19, in patients with myocarditis has been associated with decreased flow-mediated vasodilation.[18] There is recent evidence that endothelial dysfunction from the parvovirus infection may contribute to local inflammation and vasospasm, producing the symptoms of chest pain and ventricular dysfunction.[19] This may also be consistent with the high prevalence of parvovirus infection in patients with diastolic dysfunction and myocarditis.[9]

HEPATITIS C VIRUS. In contrast to the high prevalence of parvovirus in Europe, hepatitis C virus appears to be a new etiologic agent mainly seen in Asian countries such as Japan.[13] Myocardial biopsy samples have demonstrated the hepatitis C viral genome; serum samples show confirmatory antibody rise in those patients affected. Hepatitis C infection is also overall much more prevalent in Asia than in other parts of the world and may account for the higher detection rates. The phenotype of myocarditis also appears to be different; many of the patients exhibit a hypertrophic cardiomyopathy phenotype rather than a dilated heart. This may suggest that hepatitis C directly alters the growth and hypertrophy program within the myocardium. Symptomatic myocarditis is generally observed in the first to third week of illness. Patients may have dyspnea, palpitations, and anginal chest pain; fatalities have been reported. Once the virus clears, the heart has been reported to return to normal function and morphology.

HUMAN IMMUNODEFICIENCY VIRUS. With improved survival in patients with HIV infection, the prevalence of ventricular dysfunction and associated myocarditis is also increasing (see Chap. 72). From histologic analysis of postmortem cases infected with HIV, 14 of 21 patients (67%) had criteria for myocarditis, and this increases to 83% in another study when one concentrates only on high-risk patients. In asymptomatic patients with HIV infection, the annual incidence of progression to dilated cardiomyopathy has been estimated to be around 15.9 cases per 1000 individuals. It is often impossible to determine the precise cause of the ventricular dysfunction in a given patient as it may be attributable to the HIV infection itself, immunologic dysregulation, side effects of antiretroviral treatment, opportunistic coinfection or comorbid conditions, or a combination of any of these factors.

INFLUENZA. During epidemics, 5% to 10% of infected patients may experience cardiac symptoms. The presence of pre-existing cardiovascular disease greatly increases the risk of morbidity and mortality. Cardiac involvement typically occurs within 4 days to 2 weeks of the onset of the illness. Death may be associated with massive hemorrhagic pulmonary edema due to viral or bacterial involvement of the lungs.

Mixed Viral Infections. Another interesting new finding is the detection of mixed or multiple etiologic agents from a single myocardial biopsy specimen by multiplexed molecular detection tools. It appears that multiple viruses can enhance each other's virulence in a given host by cooperating as coinfections. This may occur for both coxsackieviruses and adenoviruses as they share the same receptor CAR, which can be upregulated in the presence of cardiomyopathy.[20] Conversely, this may also be an indication that the host's immune system is incapable of clearing multiple types of viruses as a result of a likely genetic defect, which then leads to worse ventricular function and outcome.[11]

Bacteria

Virtually any bacterial agent can cause myocardial dysfunction. This occurs because of activation of inflammatory mediators (see Chap. 25) through specific interactions with toll-like receptors 2 and 4, bacterial invasion, microabscess formation, and toxins elaborated by the pathogen. Other clinical manifestations of the infection mask or delay the appreciation of myocardial involvement. Accordingly, the clinician must always be alert for cardiac involvement during systemic bacterial infections.

Clostridial Infection. Cardiac involvement is common in patients with clostridial infections with multiple organ involvement. The myocardial damage results from the toxin elaborated by the bacteria, with gas bubbles present in the myocardium. An inflammatory infiltrate is usually absent. *Clostridium perfringens* may cause myocardial abscess formation with myocardial perforation and resultant purulent pericarditis.

Diphtheria. Myocardial involvement is a serious complication of diphtheria and occurs in up to half of cases. Indeed, myocardial involvement is the most common cause of death in this infection, and half of the fatal cases demonstrate cardiac involvement. Cardiac damage is due to the liberation of a toxin that inhibits protein synthesis by interfering with the transfer of amino acids from soluble RNA to polypeptide chains under construction. The toxin appears to have a particular affinity for the cardiac conducting system. Antitoxin should be administered as rapidly as possible. Antibiotic therapy is of less urgency. The development of complete atrioventricular block is an ominous complication, and mortality is high despite insertion of a transvenous pacemaker.

Streptococcal Infection. The most commonly detected cardiac finding after beta-hemolytic streptococcal infection is acute rheumatic fever. Involvement of the heart by the streptococcus may produce a myocarditis that is distinct from acute rheumatic carditis. It is characterized by an interstitial infiltrate composed of mononuclear cells with occasional polymorphonuclear leukocytes, and the infiltrate may be focal or diffuse. Electrocardiographic abnormalities, including prolongation of the PR and QT intervals, occur frequently. Rarely, this may result in sudden death, conduction disturbances, and arrhythmias.

Tuberculosis. Involvement of the myocardium by *Mycobacterium tuberculosis* (not tuberculous pericarditis) is rare. Tuberculous involvement of the myocardium occurs by means of hematogenous or lymphatic spread or directly from contiguous structures and may cause nodular, miliary, or diffuse infiltrative disease. On occasion, it may lead to arrhythmias, including atrial fibrillation and ventricular tachycardia, complete atrioventricular block, heart failure, left ventricular aneurysms, and sudden death.

Whipple Disease. Although overt involvement is rare, intestinal lipodystrophy, or Whipple disease, is not uncommonly associated with cardiac involvement, and periodic acid–Schiff–positive macrophages can be found in the myocardium, pericardium, coronary arteries, and heart valves of patients with this disorder. Electron microscopy has demonstrated rod-shaped structures in the myocardium similar to those found in the small intestine, representing the causative agent of the disease, *Tropheryma whipplei*, a gram-negative bacillus related to the actinomycetes. There may be an associated inflammatory infiltrate and foci of fibrosis. The valvular fibrosis may be severe enough to result in aortic regurgitation and mitral stenosis. Although it is usually asymptomatic, nonspecific electrocardiographic changes are most common; systolic murmurs, pericarditis, complete heart block, and even overt congestive heart failure may occur. Antibiotic therapy appears to be effective in treatment of the basic disease, but relapses can occur, often more than 2 years after initial diagnosis.

Spirochetal Infections: Lyme Carditis. Lyme disease is caused by a tick-borne spirochete *(Borrelia burgdorferi)*. It usually begins during the summer months with a characteristic rash (erythema chronicum migrans), followed by acute neurologic, joint, or cardiac involvement and usually few long-term sequelae.[21] About 10% of patients with Lyme disease develop evidence of transient cardiac involvement, the most common manifestation being variable degrees of atrioventricular block. Syncope due to complete heart block is frequent with cardiac involvement because often there is an associated depression of ventricular escape rhythms. Diffuse ST-segment and T wave abnormalities are transient and usually asymptomatic. An abnormal gallium scan is compatible with cardiac involvement, and the demonstration of spirochetes in myocardial biopsy specimens of patients with Lyme carditis suggests a direct cardiac effect. Patients with second-degree or complete heart block should be hospitalized and undergo continuous electrocardiographic monitoring. Temporary transvenous pacing may be required for a week or longer in patients with high-grade block. Although the efficacy of antibiotics is not established, they are used routinely in patients with Lyme carditis. Intravenous antibiotics are suggested, although oral antibiotics can be used when there is only mild cardiac involvement. Corticosteroids may reduce myocardial inflammation and edema, which in turn can shorten the duration of heart block. It is thought that treatment of the early manifestations of the disease will prevent development of late complications.

Protozoal Infections

CHAGAS' DISEASE (see Chap. 71). Chagas' disease is still one of the most common causes of dilated cardiomyopathy worldwide. The World Health Organization estimates that currently there are 18 million infected cases worldwide, and 5 million will develop symptomatic disease.[22] The causative organism is the protozoan *Trypanosoma cruzi*, spread by arthropods as the vector in endemic regions in the world, most notably in South America. Organs other than the heart may also be involved. The parasite incites an intense acquired T lymphocyte–mediated inflammatory response in the host, akin to viral myocarditis, leading to extensive scarring and remodeling of the myocardium, resulting in chagasic cardiomyopathy. Treatment is most effective during the acute phase of the disease. Ultimately, prevention through public health measures will be most cost-effective.

Metazoal Myocardial Diseases

Echinococcosis (Hydatid Cyst). Echinococcosis is endemic in many sheep-raising areas of the world, particularly Argentina, New Zealand, Greece, North Africa, and Iceland; however, cardiac involvement in patients with hydatid disease is uncommon (<2%). The usual host of *Echinococcus granulosus* is the dog, but humans may serve as intermediate hosts if they accidentally ingest ova from contaminated dog feces. When cardiac involvement is present, the cysts usually are intramyocardial in the interventricular septum or left ventricular free wall. A myocardial cyst can degenerate and calcify, develop daughter cysts, or rupture. Rupture of the cyst is the most dreaded complication; rupture into the pericardium can result in acute pericarditis, which may progress to chronic constrictive pericarditis. Rupture into the cardiac chambers can result in systemic or pulmonary emboli. Rapidly progressive pulmonary hypertension can occur with rupture of right-sided cysts, with subsequent embolization of hundreds of scolices into the pulmonary circulation. The liberation of hydatid fluid into the circulation can produce profound, fatal circulatory collapse due to an anaphylactic reaction to the protein constituents of the fluid. It is estimated that only about 10% of patients with cardiac hydatid cysts have clinical symptoms. The electrocardiogram may reflect the location of the cyst. Chest pain is usually due to rupture of the cyst into the pericardial space with resultant pericarditis. Large cystic masses sometimes produce right-sided obstruction. The chest radiograph may show an abnormal cardiac silhouette or a calcified lobular mass adjacent to the left ventricle. Two-dimensional echocardiography, computed tomography, or magnetic resonance imaging may aid in the detection and localization of heart cysts. Eosinophilia, when present, is a useful adjunctive finding. The Casoni skin test, or serologic evaluations for echinococcus, have a limited role in cardiac diagnosis. In terms of therapy, despite the availability of effective drugs such as mebendazole and albendazole, surgical excision is generally recommended, even for asymptomatic patients. This is because of the significant risk of rupture of the cyst and its attendant serious and sometimes fatal consequences.

Trichinosis. Infestation with *Trichinella spiralis* is common, but clinically detectable cardiac involvement occurs in only a minority of patients. Symptomatic involvement is uncommon and may be responsible for the fatalities. Less frequently, death is due to pulmonary embolism secondary to venous thrombosis or neurologic complications. Although the parasite can invade the heart, it does not usually encyst there, and it is rare to find larvae or larval fragments in the myocardium. The heart may be dilated and flabby, and a pericardial effusion may be present. A prominent focal infiltrate composed of lymphocytes and eosinophils can be found, with occasional microthrombi in the intramural arterioles. Areas of muscle degeneration and necrosis are present. The clinical myocarditis in trichinosis is usually mild and goes unnoticed, but in occasional cases it is manifested by heart failure and chest pain, usually appearing around the third week of the disease. Electrocardiographic abnormalities are detected in about 10% of patients with trichinosis and parallel the time course of clinical cardiac involvement, initially appearing in the second or third week and usually resolving by the seventh week of the illness. The most common electrocardiographic abnormalities are repolarization abnormalities and ventricular premature complexes. The diagnosis is usually based on the demonstration of indirect immunofluorescent antibody in a patient with the clinical features of trichinosis. Eosinophilia, when present, is a supportive finding. The skin test result is usually but not invariably positive. Treatment is with anthelmintics and corticosteroids; dramatic improvement in cardiac function has been reported after their use.

Hypersensitivity Reactions: Vaccines and Drugs

Drug-induced hypersensitivity syndrome may involve the heart and be associated with myocarditis. The syndrome usually occurs within 8 weeks of the initiation of a new drug but can occur at any time after drug consumption. Common agents include antiepileptics, antimicrobials, allopurinol, and sulfa-based drugs. Dobutamine, often used as hemodynamic support in patients with failing hearts, may be associated with eosinophilic myocarditis, and the drug should be stopped when eosinophilia appears or there is an unexpected decline in left ventricular function. Presenting characteristics usually include a rash (unless the patient is immunologically compromised), fever, and multiorgan dysfunction (including hepatitis, nephritis, and myocarditis). Diffuse myocardial involvement may result in systemic hypotension and thromboembolic events. Magnetic resonance imaging and cardiac biomarkers may help identify patients with cardiac involvement. Endomyocardial biopsy may demonstrate eosinophils, histiocytes, lymphocytes, myocardial necrosis, and occasionally granuloma and vasculitis. Myocardial involvement is patchy and therefore definitively diagnosed only when the biopsy finding is positive. Corticosteroids and drug withdrawal usually resolve this syndrome; however, some patients may display a prolonged and relapsing course (see Chap. 70 Online Supplement for further details about physical agents).[23]

Physical Agents

A wide variety of substances other than infectious agents can act on the heart and damage the myocardium. In some cases, the damage is acute, transient, and associated with evidence of an inflammatory myocardial infiltrate with myocyte necrosis (e.g., with the arsenicals and lithium). Other agents that damage the myocardium can lead to chronic changes with resulting histologic evidence of fibrosis and a clinical picture of a dilated or restrictive cardiomyopathy. Numerous chemicals and drugs (both industrial and therapeutic) can lead to cardiac damage and dysfunction. Several physical agents (e.g., radiation and excessive heat) can also contribute directly to myocardial damage (see Chap. 70 Online Supplement for further details about physical agents).

Pathophysiology

Our current understanding of the pathogenesis of viral myocarditis is derived mostly from enteroviral models of myocarditis in the mouse, and the principles have been generalized to other types of myocarditis.[1,24] The disease represents a delicate interaction between the virus and the host. Myocarditis can be considered to have three phases in its pathophysiology (**Fig. 70-2**). The first is the viral phase, followed by the immunologic response phase (including innate and acquired immunity components), followed by the cardiac remodeling phase (**Fig. 70-3**).

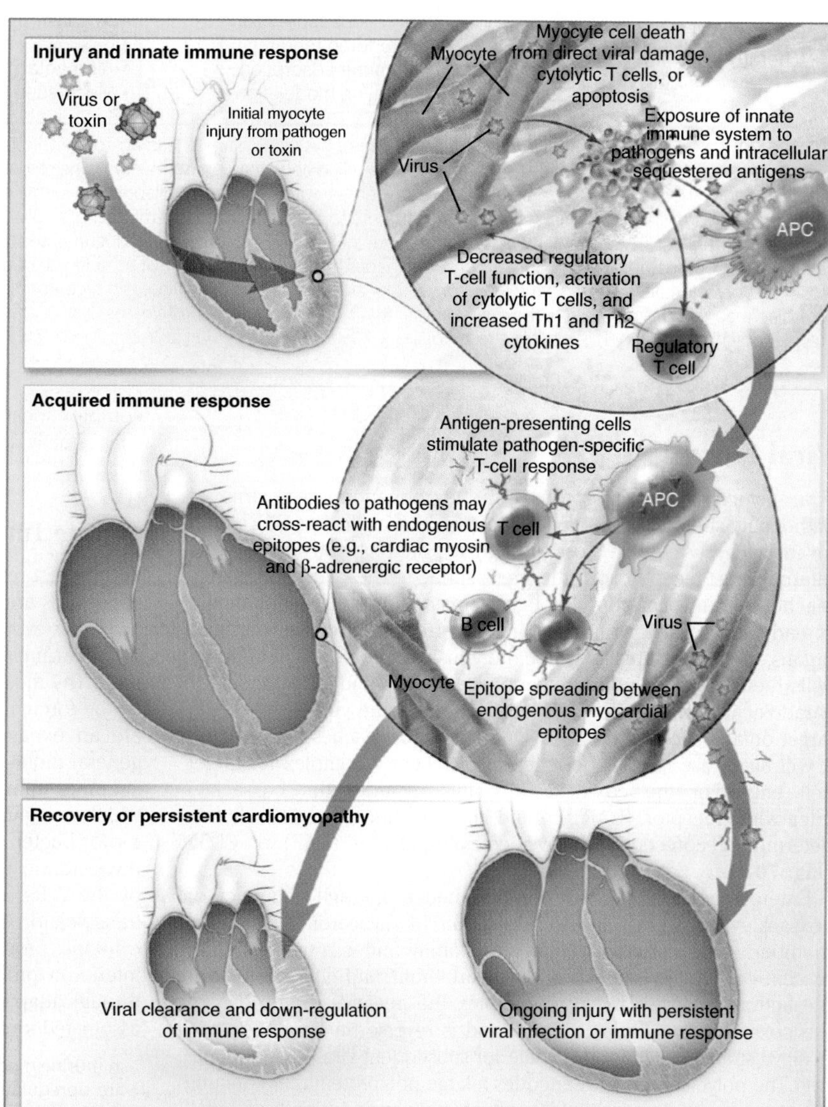

FIGURE 70-2 Pathogenesis of myocarditis. The current understanding of the cellular and molecular pathogenesis of postviral and autoimmune myocarditis is based solely on animal models. In these models, the progression from acute injury to chronic dilated cardiomyopathy may be simplified into a three-stage process. Acute injury leads to cardiac damage, exposure of intracellular antigens such as cardiac myosin, and activation of the innate immune system. During weeks, specific immunity that is mediated by T lymphocytes and antibodies directed against pathogens and similar endogenous heart epitopes causes robust inflammation. In most patients, the pathogen is cleared and the immune reaction is downregulated with few sequelae. However, in other patients, the virus is not cleared and causes persistent myocyte damage, and heart-specific inflammation may persist because of mistaken recognition of endogenous heart antigens as pathogenic entities. APC = antigen-presenting cell. *(From Cooper LT Jr: Myocarditis. N Engl J Med 360:1526, 2009. Copyright © 2009 Massachusetts Medical Society. All rights reserved.)*

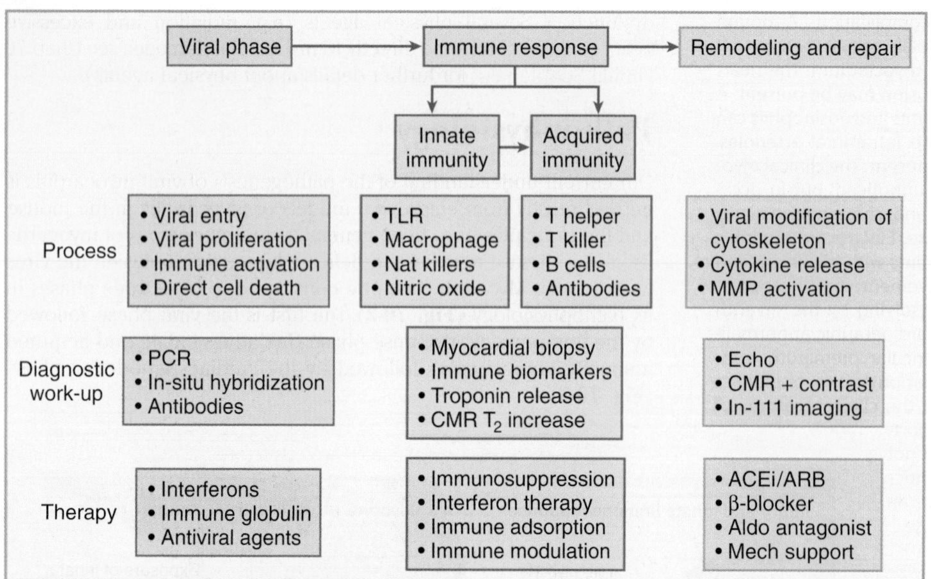

FIGURE 70-3 Conceptual framework of the three pathophysiologic stages leading to chronic myocarditis, including viral phase, immune response phase, and remodeling and repair phase. The immune response can be subdivided into the innate and acquired immune responses, with significant collaboration between the two processes. Both the viral and immune processes contribute to cell death, cardiac remodeling, and inflammatory response by the host. The therapeutic efficacy unfortunately has not been as well documented because of heterogeneity of the population, high rates of spontaneous improvement, and small sample size of the studies. ACEi = angiotensin-converting enzyme inhibitors; Aldo = aldosterone; ARB = angiotensin receptor blocker; CMR = cardiac magnetic resonance; Mech = mechanical; MMP = matrix metalloproteinases; Nat = natural; PCR = polymerase chain reaction; TLR = toll-like receptors.

Viral Entry

Viral myocarditis is initiated by the introduction of a virus of pathogenic strain (e.g., enterovirus such as coxsackievirus B3), which invades the susceptible host through a portal of entry by a virus internalizing receptor on the cell surface. The virus ultimately reaches the myocardium through hematogenous or lymphangitic spread. Many of the viruses are initially processed in the lymphoid organs, such as the spleen, where the virus will proliferate in immune cells themselves, including macrophages and T and B lymphocytes. Paradoxically, through host immune activation, the viruses reach the target organs, such as the heart. Once the virus reaches the myocyte, it will again use its specific receptor or receptor complex for target cell entry. For the coxsackievirus, this includes the coxsackie-adenoviral receptor (CAR)[14,20] and the attachment and virulence-determining coreceptor decay-accelerating factor (DAF) or CD55 (**Fig. 70-4**).

Enteroviruses use the CAR complex, hence the high frequency of coxsackievirus and adenovirus infection in myocarditis. CAR is a member of the immunoglobulin superfamily and is a tight junction protein particularly present in the heart, brain, and gut.[14,24] Through the activation of this receptor complex, the negative strand RNA of the coxsackievirus enters the cell and is reverse transcribed into a positive strand to act as a template for subsequent viral RNA duplication. The polycistronic RNA encodes a large polyprotein that contains its own cleavage enzyme and important viral capsid subunits VP1-VP4. Exuberant viral replication in a susceptible host lacking suitable immunity defenses can cause acute myocardial damage and early death of the host.

Entry of the virus through the receptor also activates its signaling system, including tyrosine kinase p56lck, Fyn, and Abl.[14,15] Activation of these signals modifies the host cell cytoskeleton to permit more viral entry. At the same time, these signals also mediate the activation of T cells, which are critically dependent on p56lck and Fyn. Interestingly, heart tissue damage and inflammation upregulate the CAR receptor and increase the susceptibility of the host to coxsackieviral infection.[20]

Immune Activation and Viral Persistence (see Fig. 70-2)

Whereas viral entry triggers the immune activation, the immune system has a dual role. On one hand, it is activated to eliminate as many virus-infected cells as possible to control the infection. On the other hand, the response needs to be modulated by negative controls; otherwise, there will be excessive tissue damage from the inflammatory response with organ dysfunction. The virus has an elaborate system in place to escape host immunologic surveillance, including molecular mimicry, proliferation in immunocytes, and upregulation of its own receptors, and it can persist in the myocyte for months to years.

Viral persistence can expose the host to persistent antigenic trigger and chronic immune activation and the potential of chronic myocarditis. Persistence of the viral genome, such as coxsackievirus in the myocyte, has been directly linked to the development of dilated cardiomyopathy through cytoskeleton remodeling. Knowlton and colleagues have identified that the enteroviral protease 2A can directly cleave the dystrophin-sarcoglycan complex located at the myocyte–extracellular matrix junction.[7] This can directly lead to myocyte remodeling and subsequent cardiac dilation.[24]

Innate Immunity (see Fig. 70-2)

The earliest responses of the host to the presence of foreign genome sequences are members of the innate immune system. Innate immunity is an evolutionarily ancient host protective system that provides early warnings for the cells to deal with an adverse external environment. The most common pathway for innate immunity to be triggered by the foreign virus is the ubiquitous toll-like receptors (TLRs), which are an expanding family of cell surface receptors that recognize general molecular patterns without the high specificity conferred by acquired immune players, such as T and B cells. For example, TLR3, which recognizes double-stranded RNA, and TLR4, which is the receptor for bacterial lipopolysaccharide, are present in abundance in the myocardium. The presence of foreign genetic material can be detected by the TLRs, leading to signaling activation that ultimately leads to translocation of transcription factors such as NF-κB, with amplified cytokine production, and interferon regulatory factors, leading to interferon production (see Fig. 70-4). The activation of TLRs signals through adaptors and kinases such as MyD88 and interleukin receptor–associated kinases (IRAKs).

In murine models of myocarditis, many components of innate immunity are upregulated immediately on viral exposure, including MyD88 and IRAK-4,[25] leading to NF-κB activation. In turn, the activation of NF-κB appears to be modulated by the interferon production pathways, including interferon regulatory factors such as IRF3.[24,25] Downregulation of MyD88 and in turn of NF-κB and activation of acquired immunity are accompanied by the upregulation of type I interferons (IFN-α and IFN-β). Interferon is critical for host protection and survival, and its absence leads to excessive viral proliferation and direct cardiac damage.[26] Type I interferon thus may have an ideal dual role of control of viral proliferation and downregulation of acquired immune pathways of T-cell activation and clonal expansion. Besides these positive regulators of host defense responses, there are also systems of negative modulators that will counteract the excessive cytokine activation. One system, the intracellular suppressors of cytokine signaling (SOCS), negatively regulates innate immune response.[27] The SOCS system particularly downregulates cytokine signals going through the gp130 receptor on the myocytes. Normal signals through the gp130 receptor serve to stabilize the dystrophin complex and confer protection for the host. This appears to be a SOCS3-dependent phenomenon, as cardiac-restricted overexpression of SOCS3 in a transgenic model led to gp130 instability and worse outcome.

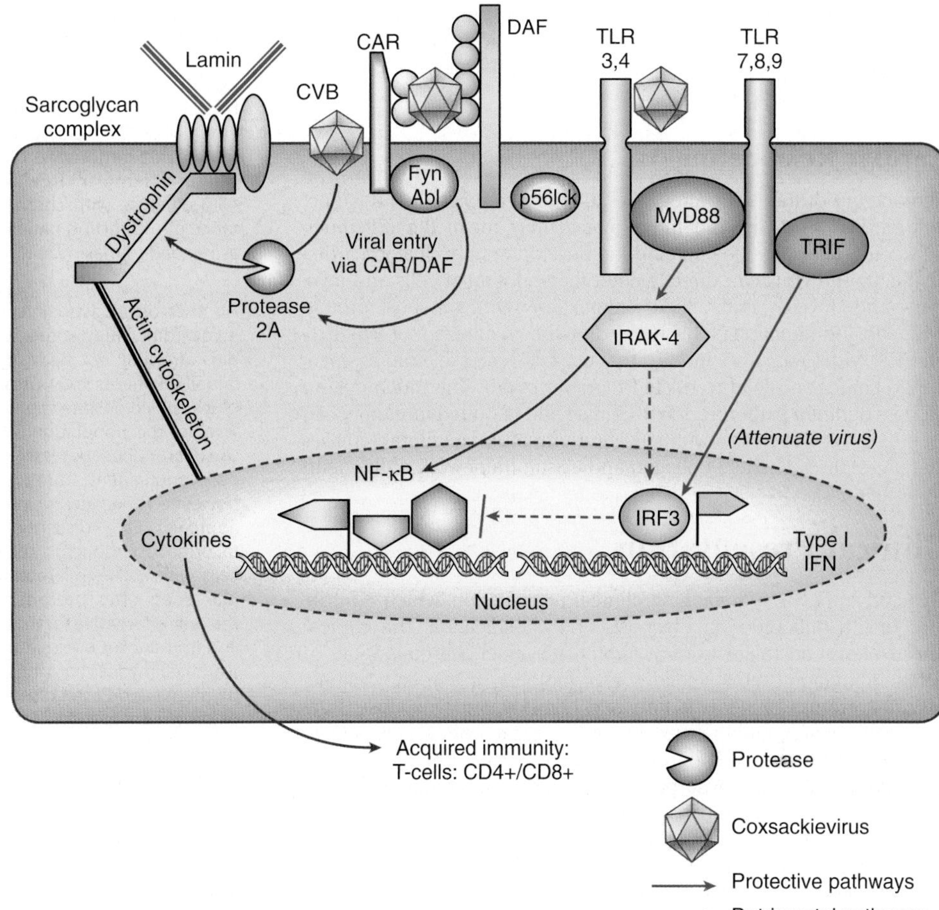

FIGURE 70-4 The pathogenesis of viral myocarditis, such as that caused by coxsackievirus. The virus enters the cell membrane through internalization receptors of coxsackie-adenoviral receptor (CAR), which in turn can trigger receptor-associated kinases such as p56lck, Fyn, and Abl to alter host myocyte cytoskeleton to facilitate viral entry. Viruses such as the coxsackievirus (CVB) can directly produce enzymes such as protease 2A that can disassemble the important cytoskeletal components such as dystrophin-sarcoglycan complex, leading to myocyte remodeling and destruction. Engagement of the receptor also activates tyrosine kinases, which are important for T-cell clonal expansion and linking between the innate and the acquired immune systems. The virus also activates innate immunity by engaging toll-like receptors (TLR) through adaptors such as MyD88 and TRIF. Activation and translocation of NF-κB, on the one hand, will produce cytokines and trigger acquired immunity such as CD4/CD8 T-cell mobilization. On the other hand, this can be attenuated by the activation of IRF3 and type I interferon (IFN) production. The latter may be protective through multiple mechanisms, including attenuation of the virus. DAF = decay-accelerating factor, CVB coreceptor; IRAK = interleukin receptor–associated kinase, a signaling protein in innate immune pathway; IRF = interferon regulatory factor.

Acquired Immunity

Acquired immunity refers to the ability of the immune system to recognize and to respond specifically to a single viral or tissue antigen through T and B cells that recognize very specific peptide sequences. This system is triggered by the recognition of a precise "foreign" molecular pattern by the variable region of the T-cell receptor. The T cell is then stimulated to clonally expand to attack the source of "antigen," which could be from the viral coat protein or sometimes from parts of the myocardium (such as myosin), which may resemble the pattern of the virus (molecular mimicry), triggering autoimmunity. However, this process is very much dependent on costimulation from inflammatory signals, often linked to innate immunity signaling activated earlier in the injury process.

The result of acquired immune activation is the production of T killer cells that can directly attack the virus and virally infected cells. The activation of T cells also leads to B-cell activation and the production of specific antibodies to neutralize the antigen. This results in subacute and chronic inflammation observed in myocarditis and contributes to the subsequent myocyte necrosis, fibrosis, and remodeling. The critical contributory role of the signals through the acquired immune pathways has been examined in mouse models of myocarditis. A common downstream signaling pathway from the T-cell receptor is the tyrosine kinase p56lck. Interestingly, p56lck is the same tyrosine kinase signal attached to the CAR-DAF receptor complex for viral entry. When p56lck is genetically removed from the mouse by transgenic knockout techniques, the mouse is no longer susceptible to the inflammation seen in typical myocarditis, and the mortality is almost completely eliminated.[15] T cells, when present, will attempt to seek out the infected cells and destroy them by mechanisms such as cytokine-mediated signaling[28] or perforin-mediated cell death. This confirms that the T-cell receptor activation sequence ultimately does lead to the detrimental phenotype of the disease and supports the concept that decreasing inflammation from acquired immunity, while finding ways to control the virus through innate immunity, will lead to the most beneficial outcomes of the disease.

A more recently recognized counterregulatory system in acquired immunity is the small population of T-regulatory cells (or Tregs). These cells also derive from part of the T-cell activation process but are present in small numbers to act as a counterbalancing population to T killer cells. This population of cells were known earlier as T helper $CD4^+$ cells. Currently, Tregs are more precisely defined as $CD4^+CD25^+Foxp3^+$ T cells. Enhanced levels of Tregs in models of myocarditis appear to be protective by reducing inflammatory cytokine response and inducing tolerance to self antigens. Therefore, Tregs may one day have a therapeutic potential in viral myocarditis.

To understand why certain individuals develop overwhelming myocarditis after exposure to the virus and rapidly die of the disease and others do not even show inflammation, we have been methodically mapping the major determinants of the host immune system by molecular targeting strategies in knockout mice. Earlier work identified that components of innate immunity, such as interferon and IRF3, are critical for host survival, yet T-cell signaling and activation are injurious to the host. Through $CD4^-/CD8^-$ knockout mice, we have established that both CD4 and CD8 T cells contribute to the host autoimmune inflammatory disease, accompanied by a shift of cytokine profile from Th1 to Th2 response. More recently, we have identified that p56lck triggers downstream ERK activation in the host target cell and appears to be critical for the determinant of host susceptibility.[28] To validate these observations, we have also investigated the function of the associated tyrosine phosphatase CD45 linked in function to the p56lck kinase and confirmed that $CD45^{-/-}$ animals are also resistant to viral myocarditis. After careful dissection, it was apparent that CD45 is an important Src as well as JAK/STAT phosphatase, and virally triggered CD45 activation shuts down interferon production. Interferon levels are markedly increased once CD45 is removed, and the host is indeed rescued through this dual protective process.

Cardiac Remodeling (see Chap. 25)

Remodeling of the heart after cardiac injury can significantly affect that cardiac structure and function and may mean the difference between appropriate healing and the development of dilated cardiomyopathy. The virus can directly enter the endothelial cells and myocytes and through intracellular interactions with the host protein synthetic and signaling pathways lead to direct cell death or hypertrophy. The virus can also modify the myocyte cytoskeleton, as mentioned earlier, and lead to dilated cardiomyopathy. The inflammatory process outlined earlier from both innate and acquired immunity can lead to cytokine release and activation of matrix metalloproteinases that digest the interstitial collagen and elastin framework of the heart (see Chap. 25).

Clinical Presentation

Myocarditis has a wide-ranging clinical presentation, which contributes to the difficulties in diagnosis and classification. The clinical presentation can range from asymptomatic electrocardiographic or echocardiographic abnormalities to symptoms of cardiac dysfunction, arrhythmias or heart failure, and hemodynamic collapse. Transient electrocardiographic or echocardiographic abnormalities have been observed frequently during community viral outbreaks or influenza epidemics, but most patients remain asymptomatic from a cardiac point of view and have few long-term sequelae. Myocarditis typically has a bimodal distribution in terms of age in the population, with the acute presentation more commonly seen in young children and teenagers. In contrast, the presenting symptoms are more subtle and insidious, often with dilated cardiomyopathy and heart failure, in the older adult population. Felker and colleagues have observed earlier in consecutive cases of new-onset dilated cardiomyopathy in adults that 9% to 16% have classic myocarditis on biopsy by the Dallas criteria.[29] The difference in presentation is probably related to the maturity of the immune system, whereby the young tend to have an exuberant response to the initial exposure of a provocative antigen. On the other hand, the older individual would have developed a greater degree of tolerance and show a chronic inflammatory response only to the chronic presence of a foreign antigen or a dysregulated immune system that predisposes to autoimmunity.

Acute Myocarditis

Classically, patients with myocarditis present with nonspecific symptoms related to the heart. In a recent series of 245 patients with clinically suspected myocarditis, the most common symptoms included fatigue (82%), dyspnea on exertion (81%), arrhythmias (55%, both supraventricular and ventricular), palpitations (49%), and chest pain at rest (26%).[10] These can be difficult to distinguish from acute ischemic syndromes because they result in release of troponin, ST-segment elevation on electrocardiography, and segmental wall motion abnormalities on echocardiography. Therefore, the symptoms can be quite nonspecific, although some symptoms indicate cardiac involvement. The viral prodrome of fever, chills, myalgias, and constitutional symptoms occurs in between 20% and 80% of the cases, can be readily missed by the patient, and thus cannot be relied on for diagnosis.

Many cases of myocarditis present with de novo onset of heart failure, particularly when the patient is middle aged or older. When the health care team fails to identify other causes of heart failure, viral myocarditis along with idiopathic dilated cardiomyopathy becomes the diagnosis of exclusion. To distinguish myocarditis from idiopathic dilated cardiomyopathy, almost one third of the cases of viral myocarditis will recover to normal cardiac function with appropriate supportive therapy, which is less frequent in genetic dilated cardiomyopathy.

Fulminant Myocarditis

Approximately 10% of patients with biopsy-proven myocarditis display fulminant myocarditis. This entity is characterized by an abrupt onset, usually within 2 weeks of a viral illness. Patients have hemodynamic compromise and hypotension, often requiring pressors or mechanical support. The echocardiogram reveals diffuse global hypofunction, rarely cardiac dilation, and typically thickening of the ventricular wall probably due to myocardial edema from myocardial inflammation and cytokine release. Endomyocardial biopsy reveals typical and diffuse myocarditis in virtually each histologic section, making endomyocardial biopsy confirmation straightforward. On follow-up, 93% of the original cohort were alive and transplant free 11 years after initial biopsy, compared with only 45% of those with chronic myocarditis.[30] This underscores the importance of supporting patients with fulminant myocarditis as aggressively as needed to maximize time for recovery.

Giant Cell Myocarditis

Another distinctive clinicopathologic form of myocarditis is giant cell myocarditis. This disorder is more subtle in onset than fulminant myocarditis and may not be distinguishable from other forms of myocarditis initially. Patients may present with heart failure, arrhythmia, or heart block, which despite standard medical therapy fails to improve. The survival for this population is less than 6 months and is improved with the use of immunosuppressive therapy.[31] Preliminary data suggest that high-dose multiagent immunosuppression may improve the prognosis; however, there are no prospective randomized trials to confirm this approach. Early discontinuation of immunosuppression may lead to recurrence. Endomyocardial biopsy reveals a distinctive pattern of giant cells with active inflammation and scar tissue. Currently, cardiac transplantation, often preceded by mechanical circulatory support, remains the only alternative for most patients with this disorder. Early recognition and immunosuppressive therapy may alter this approach. Patients with giant cell myocarditis often have other autoimmune disorders including thymoma and Crohn disease. The pathophysiologic mechanism remains unknown but is suspected to be autoimmune in nature.

Chronic Active Myocarditis

This group represents most older adult patients with myocarditis, and the onset is often insidious and difficult to pinpoint. The patient presents with symptoms compatible with moderate ventricular dysfunction, such as fatigue and dyspnea. Pathologic examination of a myocardial biopsy specimen may show active myocarditis, but more frequently it is only borderline or generalized chronic myopathic changes with fibrosis and myocyte dropout. Some may progress to diastolic dysfunction with predominantly fibrosis, resembling ultimately a restrictive cardiomyopathy.

This category encompasses 60% to 70% of patients with active or borderline myocarditis who present with dilated cardiomyopathy of unknown etiology. Use of newer imaging approaches such as magnetic resonance imaging with gadolinium enhancement and positron emission tomography–computed tomography (PET-CT), molecular diagnosis by immunohistopathologic analysis, assessment of upregulation of immune markers, and molecular testing, including PCR and in situ hybridization, may expand this population significantly.

Eosinophilic Myocarditis

The eosinophil may be associated with myocardial inflammation in three distinct forms of myocardial inflammation. Allergic eosinophilic myocarditis is caused by a hypersensitivity reaction to a foreign antigen, almost always a drug. This form of myocarditis requires a high degree of suspicion (related to the initiation of new agents) and subtle declines in left ventricular function. Withdrawal of the offending agent and administration of corticosteroids usually result in resolution. The heart may be inflamed in association with systemic eosinophilic disorders, resulting in myocardial, endocardial, and valvular involvement (Löffler endocarditis). The outcome is dependent on control of the underlying condition. Finally, fulminant necrotic myocarditis presents in a fashion similar to fulminant myocarditis, has no clear etiology, and requires aggressive medical immunosuppression and occasional mechanical support.

Peripartum Cardiomyopathy

Peripartum cardiomyopathy is characterized by the onset of left ventricular dysfunction in the last month of pregnancy or within 5 months of delivery, with no pre-existing cardiac dysfunction and no recognized cause of the cardiomyopathy. There is evidence that patients submitted to endomyocardial biopsy early after presentation have a high frequency of myocarditis.[29] As most patients with this disorder recover with standard therapy, biopsy is recommended only for those with persistent left ventricular dysfunction and symptoms despite heart failure management.

Diagnostic Approaches

The diagnosis of myocarditis has traditionally required a histologic diagnosis according to the classic Dallas criteria.[2] However, because

TABLE 70-2 Expanded Criteria for Diagnosis of Myocarditis

Suggestive of myocarditis:	2 positive categories
Compatible with myocarditis:	3 positive categories
High probability of being myocarditis:	all 4 categories positive

(Any matching feature in category = positive for category)

Category I: Clinical Symptoms
Clinical heart failure
Fever
Viral prodrome
Fatigue
Dyspnea on exertion
Chest pain
Palpitations
Presyncope or syncope

Category II: Evidence of Cardiac Structural or Functional Perturbation *in the absence* of Regional Coronary Ischemia
Echocardiography evidence
Regional wall motion abnormalities
Cardiac dilation
Regional cardiac hypertrophy
Troponin release
High sensitivity (>0.1 ng/mL)
Positive indium In 111 antimyosin scintigraphy
and
Normal coronary angiography *or*
Absence of reversible ischemia by coronary distribution on perfusion scan

Category III: Cardiac Magnetic Resonance Imaging
Increased myocardial T2 signal on inversion recovery sequence
Delayed contrast enhancement after gadolinium-DTPA infusion

Category IV: Myocardial biopsy—Pathologic or Molecular Analysis
Pathology findings compatible with Dallas criteria
Presence of viral genome by polymerase chain reaction or in situ hybridization

DTPA = diethylenetriamine penta-acetic acid.

of low sensitivity due to the patchy nature of the inflammatory infiltrates in the myocardium and the reluctance of clinicians to perform an invasive diagnostic procedure, myocarditis is severely underdiagnosed. Because the incidence of the disease is likely to be much higher than is appreciated, a high level of clinical suspicion, together with hybrid clinical and laboratory criteria and new imaging modalities, may help secure the diagnosis without necessarily resorting to biopsy in all cases.

With the advent of a number of new diagnostic strategies for myocarditis, one may now *strongly suspect myocarditis* if two of the following criteria are present, and the diagnosis is *highly probable as myocarditis* if three or more criteria are present: (1) compatible clinical symptoms; (2) evidence of cardiac structural or functional defect or myocardial damage in the absence of active regional coronary ischemia; (3) regional delayed contrast enhancement or increased T2 signal on cardiac magnetic resonance imaging; and (4) presence of inflammatory cell infiltrate or positive viral genome signals on myocardial biopsy or pathologic examination (**Table 70-2**). Of course, myocardial biopsy still provides the most specific diagnosis for myocarditis.

For example, myocarditis as a diagnosis should be suspected when a young patient presents with unexplained symptoms of heart failure or chest pain but the coronary arteries are found to be normal on angiography. When young patients such as this present with minimal risk factors for coronary disease with acute chest pain or ischemic electrocardiographic abnormalities, 32% will have biopsy evidence of acute myocarditis according to the Dallas criteria. An even higher proportion will also be viral genome positive on molecular analysis. A major limitation to the accurate diagnosis of myocarditis is the lack of a highly sensitive and specific tool that is noninvasive and widely applicable. The common diagnostic modalities and their reported sensitivities and specificities are outlined in **Table 70-3**.

TABLE 70-3 Comparison of Efficacy of Various Diagnostic Modalities for Myocarditis

DIAGNOSTIC MODALITY	SENSITIVITY RANGE (%)	SPECIFICITY RANGE (%)
Electrocardiographic changes (AV block; Q wave, ST changes)	47	?
Troponin (lower threshold of >0.1 ng/mL)	34-53	89-94
Creatine kinase MB isoform	6	?
Antibodies to virus or myosin	25-32	40
Indium 111 antimyosin scintigraphy	85-91	34-53
Echocardiography (ventricular dysfunction)	69	?
Cardiac magnetic resonance	86	95
Myocardial biopsy (Dallas criteria of pathology)	35-50	78-89
Myocardial biopsy (viral genome by PCR)	38-65	80-100

? = indeterminate or poor; AV = atrioventricular; PCR = polymerase chain reaction.

Clinical Symptoms

The clinical symptoms of myocarditis are not specific and very much depend on the mode of presentation as outlined before. Younger patients most often complain of chest pain and fatigue. Patient with cardiac dysfunction may present with new-onset heart failure, dyspnea, or fatigue. Some patients are also symptomatic of the supraventricular or ventricular arrhythmias, including palpitations, presyncope, and syncope. In most severe cases, such as those with fulminant myocarditis, patients may present with cardiogenic shock and intractable arrhythmias. Some patients may present with constitutional symptoms, such as fever and viral prodrome. However, these are infrequent and unreliable for diagnosis.

Laboratory Testing

Severe myocarditis will lead to myocardial damage secondary to the presence of inflammatory cell infiltrates and cytokine activation as well as some contribution directly from virus-mediated cell death. These processes can severely depress cardiac function and produce evidence of cardiac damage. This can be detected as leakage of cardiac enzymes such as creatine kinase and troponin when the damage is severe or chronic (see Table 70-2). However, in most cases, the leakage of enzymes is relatively minor, and standard laboratory testing for creatine kinase or its isoform MB is too insensitive (overall sensitivity for myocarditis is only 8%). Enzyme biomarkers such as troponin are more useful when high sensitivity thresholds are used. For example, when a serum troponin T threshold of >0.1 ng/mL is used as a cutoff, the sensitivity can be increased from 34% to 53% without compromising specificity. Similar findings have been noted for troponin I. Other biomarkers, such as cytokines, complement, and antiviral or anti–heart antibodies, are either too insensitive or inadequately standardized to make them generally useful clinically.

The cardiac damage can also be manifested as electrocardiographic abnormalities (see Chap. 13) that range from T wave inversions to frank ST-segment elevation and bundle branch block, depending on the region and extent of inflammatory damage. Kuhl and associates have noted that arrhythmias may be present in 55% of the patients, including both supraventricular and ventricular arrhythmias.

Imaging techniques such as two-dimensional echocardiography (see Chap. 15) are useful for initial diagnostic evaluation of the patient to detect the regional ventricular dysfunction that often accompanies the condition. Parameters of ventricular remodeling, including chamber dilation, regional hypertrophy, and regional wall motion abnormalities, are often seen with myocarditis, but these changes may be indistinguishable from those of myocardial ischemia or infarction at the outset. The absence of matching regional coronary disease and evidence of rapid recovery of ventricular dysfunction during follow-up are general clues to the diagnosis of myocarditis. Retrospective analysis of echocardiograms from 42 patients with biopsy-proven myocarditis identified ventricular dysfunction in 69% of the patients, but the presence of cardiac dilation is much more variable. Newer techniques such as tissue characterization and tissue Doppler imaging may permit better diagnostic accuracy in the future. Additional validation studies will be needed to determine their ultimate clinical role. However, echocardiography is certainly useful as a follow-up imaging modality to monitor the natural history of the patient's ventricular function or response to treatment. Two-dimensional echocardiography may also help distinguish fulminant from more classic forms of myocarditis; fulminant myocarditis shows less diastolic dimensional increase but increased septal thickness, whereas the more classic forms of myocarditis show a much greater degree of ventricular dilation.

Newer imaging techniques, such as PET-CT, may reveal inflammation of the myocardium and associated mediastinal and thoracic structures. This technique is particularly beneficial in conditions such as sarcoidosis.

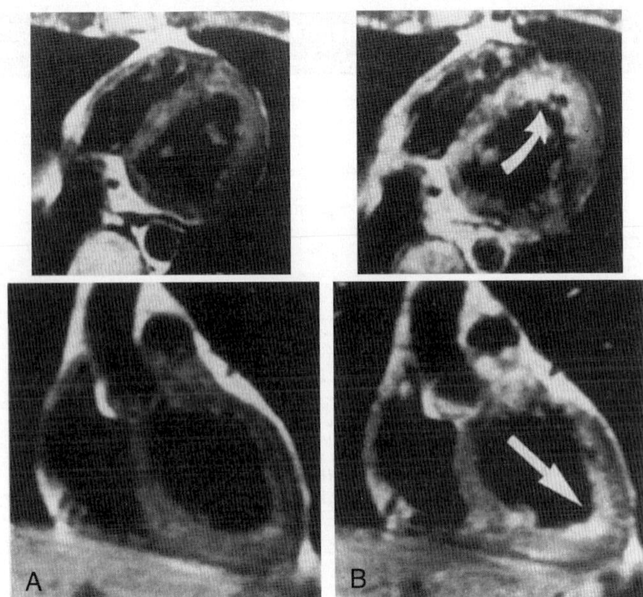

FIGURE 70-5 **A,** Precontrast T1-weighted transaxial **(upper)** and coronal **(lower)** magnetic resonance images through the left ventricle in a patient with myocarditis. **B,** Postcontrast magnetic resonance images at the same levels after injection of contrast material. Note enhancement of the myocardial signal in the septum and apical region (arrows). *(From Matsouka H, Hamada M, Honda T, et al: Evaluation of acute myocarditis and pericarditis by Gd-DTPA enhanced magnetic resonance imaging. Eur Heart J 15:283, 1994.)*

Cardiac Magnetic Resonance Imaging

(see Chap. 18)

A new approach to the diagnosis of myocarditis is cardiac magnetic resonance (CMR). CMR imaging is attractive for the detection of myocarditis because of its ability to characterize tissue according to water content and changes in contrast kinetics. CMR also allows visualization of the entire myocardium and is thus well suited to detect the local patchy nature of the myocarditic lesions.[32] The local inflammatory process in myocarditis leads to cytokine release and mobilization of inflammatory cells to the infected foci. This in turn produces local changes in membrane permeability, tissue edema, and ultimately tissue fibrosis. These changes directly affect the T2 relaxation parameters of the tissues, which are dependent on water content. Furthermore, extracellular contrast agents such as gadolinium-DTPA will also distribute and clear very differently in inflamed or scarred tissue compared with normal tissue, leading to changes in T1 relaxation and thus contrast changes or delayed enhancement on T1 weighted images (**Fig. 70-5**; see Fig. 18-12).

Evaluation of the relative accuracy of the CMR technique in the detection of myocarditis has demonstrated the relative merit of using a T2-weighted imaging strategy, such as the inversion recovery sequence. This approach to detection of myocarditic lesions showed a sensitivity of 84% and specificity of 74% based on biopsy or natural history evidence of myocarditis.[33] The addition of the T2-weighted imaging to the more commonly used gadolinium-DTPA–based extracellular T1-altering contrast agent and the inclusion of local delayed enhancement further increased the diagnostic accuracy to more than 90% by collation of all of the current studies.[32] The delayed contrast enhancement phenomenon is often associated with recent cardiac necrosis or healing of the myocardium after myocardial infarction; but in the setting of myocarditis, it also further increases the sensitivity and specificity of diagnosis. The mechanism is not clear but may be related to the deposition of local collagen bundles during the healing process that can also temporarily bind the gadolinium-DTPA to delay its clearance.

The ability to localize areas of tissue signature abnormality together with regional wall motion abnormality visualized by CMR has permitted contrast-enhanced CMR to also guide subsequent myocardial biopsy. Mahrholdt and coworkers used this CMR-guided cardiac biopsy in 32 patients with suspected myocarditis. Biopsy in these abnormal regions showed remarkable positive and negative predictive values of 71% and 100%, respectively.[34] Interestingly, CMR suggested that the lateral wall may actually be the most common location for lesion development, not the septum, from which most of the biopsy samples have been taken previously.

A consensus document on the role of CMR in myocarditis was published in 2009.[35] The recommended indications for CMR in suspected myocarditis include a combination of (1) new-onset or persisting symptoms suggestive of myocarditis, (2) evidence of recent or ongoing myocardial injury or dysfunction, and (3) suspected viral or nonischemic etiology. The generally agreed on CMR criteria of myocarditis include at least two of the following indicators of inflammation: (1) regional or global myocardial signaling intensity increase in T2-weighted images; (2) increased global myocardial early gadolinium enhancement ratio between myocardium and skeletal muscle in gadolinium-enhanced T1-weighted images; and (3) at least one focal lesion with nonischemic regional distribution in inversion recovery prepared gadolinium-enhanced T1-weighted images (late gadolinium enhancement).

Myocardial Biopsy

HISTOLOGIC EVALUATION. The Dallas criteria for the diagnosis of myocarditis represented the first attempt to standardize the pathologic definition of myocarditis. The Dallas criteria require an inflammatory infiltrate and associated myocyte necrosis or damage not characteristic of an ischemic event. Borderline myocarditis requires a less intense inflammatory infiltrate and no light microscopic evidence of myocyte destruction. Despite insensitivity for detection of myocarditis, the Dallas criteria remain the gold standard for unequivocal diagnosis.

The reasons for the insensitivity of the Dallas criteria are many, and some of them are outlined here. Because of the patchy nature of the myocarditic lesions in the myocardium, standard biopsy sampling of myocardial tissue of about 30 mg in mass is very much a "hit or miss" phenomenon. Chow and McManus first demonstrated this insensitivity by biopsy of postmortem hearts from patients with myocarditis. They demonstrated that with a single endomyocardial biopsy sample, histologic myocarditis could be demonstrated in only 25% of cases. Even with five random biopsy samples, correct diagnosis of myocarditis by the classic Dallas criteria could be reached in only about two thirds of subjects. This is further compounded by a recent magnetic resonance imaging study showing that the earliest myocardial inflammatory abnormalities in myocarditis are located commonly in the lateral wall of the left ventricle, a site difficult to reach with a standard bioptome.[34] Therefore, there is considerable built-in sampling error and insensitivity with the standard diagnosis of myocarditis with endomyocardial biopsies. To compound the situation further, there are also variations in the interpretation of histologic samples by expert pathologists experienced in reading cardiac biopsies. For example, of the 111 patients recruited in the original National Institutes of Health (NIH) Myocarditis Treatment Trial diagnosed with myocarditis by heart biopsy, only 64% had that diagnosis confirmed by the expert pathology panel during consensus reading of the same biopsy samples later.[36]

Indications for Endomyocardial Biopsy. The AHA/ACC/ESC/HFSA guidelines for endomyocardial biopsy in the analysis of patients with new-onset cardiomyopathy or heart failure provide guidance to the clinician in the determination of the appropriateness of endomyocardial biopsy based on the patient's clinicopathologic presentation (**Table 70-4**). Whereas these guidelines are evidence based, there are very few prospective randomized trials to guide management, and most recommendations are the result of expert opinions. Nonetheless, patients presenting with a clinicopathologic picture compatible with fulminant, giant cell, or eosinophilic myocarditis or who are thought to have cardiac sarcoidosis should undergo endomyocardial biopsy. As the diagnosis of cardiomyopathy from a viral pathogen is enhanced by additional molecular techniques, these categories in which biopsy must or should be performed may be expanded in the future.[37]

Risks of Endomyocardial Biopsy. Studies suggest that the complication rate of myocardial biopsy in patients with dilated cardiomyopathy is approximately 2% to 5%. Approximately half of these complications are related to venous access and the remainder to the biopsy procedure itself. Complications related to venous access include inadvertent arterial puncture, pneumothorax, vasovagal reaction, and bleeding after sheath removal. The use of ultrasonographically guided techniques to identify the internal jugular vein or to guide vein cannulation improves the success rate and decreases the complication rate and access time. Complications associated with the procedure include arrhythmias, cardiac conduction abnormalities, and cardiac perforation, which can lead to pericardial tamponade and rarely death. Patients with perforation report pain, which otherwise should not be experienced during the procedure. These patients may deteriorate rapidly because of the rapid accumulation of blood in the pericardial space and underlying left ventricular dysfunction. The rapid accumulation of blood in the pericardial space can form a clot acutely, which may interfere with percutaneous pericardial evacuation of blood. Patients who cannot be immediately resuscitated by percutaneous pericardiocentesis should have open chest evacuation of the hematoma. This requires coordination with cardiovascular surgery and preparation in the laboratory for the occurrence of these rare but expected complications. The complication rate with biopsies through the femoral vein is at least equivalent to that experienced with a jugular venous procedure. Performance of left ventricular biopsies shares similar perforation complication rates, despite the greater wall thickness of the left ventricle. In addition, left ventricular endomyocardial biopsy may be complicated by arterial embolization. Some operators use antiplatelet agents to diminish this complication. If noninvasive techniques continue to reveal evidence of left rather than right ventricular septal involvement, it is likely that more left ventricular biopsy procedures will be done in the future.

Image-Guided Biopsies. Patients with arrhythmogenic right ventricular dysplasia may at times represent underlying chronic active myocarditis, with positive viral signals on molecular analysis of biopsy specimens[38] or contrast enhancement on magnetic resonance imaging. To clarify the diagnosis, patients with suspected arrhythmogenic right ventricular cardiomyopathy are sometimes submitted to endomyocardial biopsy.[39] Image-guided biopsy, usually in the triangle of dysplasia, provides the most useful histology. Whereas fat and fibrosis are

TABLE 70-4 The Role of Endomyocardial Biopsy in 14 Clinical Scenarios

SCENARIO NUMBER	CLINICAL SCENARIO	CLASS OF RECOMMENDATION (I, IIa, IIb, III)	LEVEL OF EVIDENCE (A, B, C)
1	New-onset heart failure of <2 weeks' duration associated with a normal-sized or dilated left ventricle and hemodynamic compromise	I	B
2	New-onset heart failure of 2 weeks' to 3 months' duration associated with a dilated left ventricle and new ventricular arrhythmias, second- or third-degree heart block, or failure to respond to usual care within 1 to 2 weeks	I	B
3	Heart failure of >3 months' duration associated with a dilated left ventricle and new ventricular arrhythmias, second- or third-degree heart block, or failure to respond to usual care within 1 to 2 weeks	IIa	C
4	Heart failure associated with a DCM of any duration associated with suspected allergic reaction and/or eosinophilia	IIa	C
5	Heart failure associated with suspected anthracycline cardiomyopathy	IIa	C
6	Heart failure associated with unexplained restrictive cardiomyopathy	IIa	C
7	Suspected cardiac tumors	IIa	C
8	Unexplained cardiomyopathy in children	IIa	C
9	New-onset heart failure of 2 weeks' to 3 months' duration associated with a dilated left ventricle, without new ventricular arrhythmias or second- or third-degree heart block, that responds to usual care within 1 to 2 weeks	IIb	B
10	Heart failure of >3 months' duration associated with a dilated left ventricle, without new ventricular arrhythmias or second- or third-degree heart block, that responds to usual care within 1 to 2 weeks	IIb	C
11	Heart failure associated with unexplained HCM	IIb	C
12	Suspected ARVD/C	IIb	C
13	Unexplained ventricular arrhythmias	IIb	C
14	Unexplained atrial fibrillation	III	C

ARVD/C = arrhythmogenic right ventricular dysplasia/cardiomyopathy; DCM = dilated cardiomyopathy; HCM = hypertrophic cardiomyopathy.

From Cooper LT, Baughman KL, Feldman AM, et al: The role of endomyocardial biopsy in the management of cardiovascular disease: A scientific statement from the American Heart Association, the American College of Cardiology, and the European Society of Cardiology. Circulation 116:2216, 2007.

considered "diagnostic," PET-CT imaging may reveal inflammation of the myocardium and associated mediastinal and thoracic structures. This technique is particularly beneficial in conditions such as sarcoidosis.

Molecular Evaluation. Whereas the traditional Dallas criteria based on standard pathologic analysis of myocardial biopsy specimens have limitations, advances in molecular techniques in detecting the viral genome and inflammatory activation within the same biopsy sample have expanded our ability to detect viral myocarditis significantly, to delineate the potential viral etiology, and to improve the sensitivity of the biopsy as a diagnostic technique.

Molecular detection techniques for viral genome, such as in situ hybridization seeking the presence of viral genetic signatures in a pathologic sample and multiplexed PCR amplification of the RNA from the biopsy specimen itself, have increased the sensitivity of detecting virus signatures in the heart. These techniques have demonstrated that viral RNA can be significantly associated with symptoms and prognosis. However, the surprise was that the presence of viral genome is entirely independent of the presence or absence of inflammatory cells on the same biopsy specimen. Thus, a tissue sample can be Dallas positive only, molecularly positive only, both, or neither. This underscores that myocarditis is truly a disease of both the molecular trigger by the virus and the immunologic response by the host; either alone will be able to produce the disease syndrome.

PCR is limited by the requirement that the viral pathogen to be searched for must be declared in advance of the analysis, which is usually based on historical demonstration of pathogens in other series of patients. Techniques capable of demonstrating any viral pathogen would greatly enhance the recognition of viral causes of cardiomyopathy and may allow correlation of specific pathogens with clinical pathologic entities.

Analysis of immunologic activation on the biopsy tissues may also provide additional information. The tissues can be analyzed for inflammatory cell infiltration subtypes or signal activation, such as cytokine and complement signals. The tissues can also be analyzed for the upregulation of major histocompatibility complex (MHC) antigens. Whereas the sensitivity and specificity of MHC antigen upregulation have been shown to be 80% and 85%, respectively, from studies of very small sample size, this has not been replicated in larger series. Nevertheless, MHC expression has been used to guide therapy for patients with myocarditis and inflammatory cardiomyopathy in one study evaluating immunosuppressive therapy.

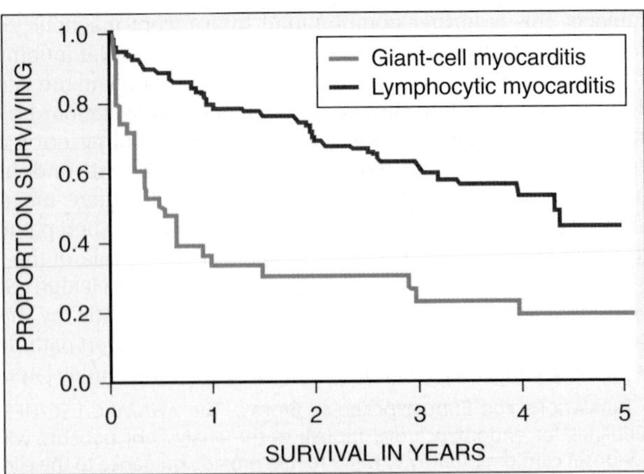

FIGURE 70-6 Prognosis in patients with giant cell myocarditis. Patients with giant cell myocarditis have much worse survival compared with patients with lymphocytic myocarditis, particularly in the acute phase soon after presentation.

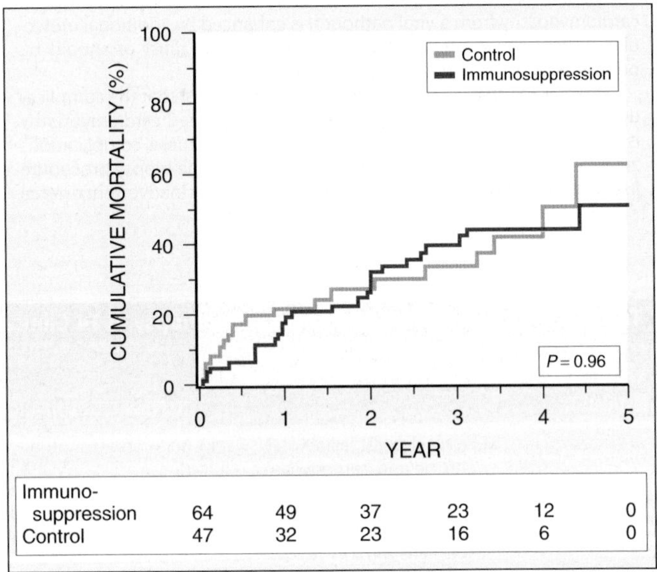

	0	1	2	3	4	5
Immuno-suppression	64	49	37	23	12	0
Control	47	32	23	16	6	0

FIGURE 70-7 The cumulative mortality data from the NIH-sponsored Myocarditis Treatment Trial. The mortality curve confirms the general poor prognosis of patients with myocarditis, who unfortunately did not demonstrate that the immunosuppressive treatment conferred any mortality benefit over standard medical therapy (control). Overall, 20% of the patients were dead in 1 year, and 54% died during 4.3 years of follow-up. There was a temporary improvement in the immunosuppressive arm that was not sustained. *(Modified from Mason JW, O'Connell JB, Herskowitz A, et al: A clinical trial of immunosuppressive therapy for myocarditis. N Engl J Med 333:269, 1995.)*

Prognosis

Patients with acute myocarditis and mild cardiac involvement generally will recover in the majority of cases without long-term sequelae. However, patients with more advanced cardiac dysfunction accompanying myocarditis may have a more varied outlook. Paradoxically, patients with severe hemodynamic collapse at presentation (fulminant myocarditis) have a surprisingly good prognosis, with one series documenting transplant-free survival of 93% in 11 years.[30] Those with chronic myocarditis may recover (30%), maintain some degree of left ventricular compromise, or progress to dilated cardiomyopathy and require intensive medical therapy, mechanical support, or cardiac transplantation.[40] Patients with giant cell myocarditis have extremely poor prognosis, with median survival of less than 6 months, and most will require transplantation to avoid succumbing to the disease (**Fig. 70-6**). On the other hand, patients with chronic active myocarditis with dilated cardiomyopathy, like those recruited into the NIH Myocarditis Treatment Trial, still have a relatively poor prognosis. These patients all had the diagnosis of myocarditis based on the Dallas biopsy criteria and showed a mortality of 20% at 1 year and 56% at 4.3 years, with many cases of chronic heart failure despite optimal medical management (**Fig. 70-7**).[36]

Several studies have attempted to identify clinical variables that can predict adverse outcomes in viral myocarditis. Although many of these variables cannot be replicated from study to study, several factors do appear to predict death or transplantation, including presentation with syncope, bundle branch block on electrocardiography, and ejection fraction of less than 40%. Additional predictors of poor outcome included New York Heart Association Class III or IV, pulmonary capillary wedge pressure greater than 15 mm Hg, immunopathologic evidence of myocardial inflammation, failure to use beta-blocking therapy,[41] biventricular failure, and giant cell or viral genome on biopsy.[42] On the other hand, two-dimensional echocardiographic evidence of a small left atrial and left ventricular size was predictive of myocardial recovery from a small study of 15 patients. Whereas general pathologic features of the biopsy specimen did not predict prognosis in more recent series, the resolution of myocarditis on follow-up biopsy and the absence of azan-Mallory staining of cardiac myocytes (a marker of cellular edema or myocytolysis) do appear to herald functional ventricular recovery.[41,43]

Why and associates reported that of 120 patients with dilated cardiomyopathy, the group (34%) who were positive for enteroviral minus strand RNA had a significantly worse outcome during 2 years (68% versus 92%; $P = 0.02$) compared with those who were enteroviral genome negative.[44] More recent studies have also demonstrated that viral genome persistence on myocardial biopsy predicted more rapid deterioration of ventricular function during follow-up.[11,42] Interestingly, molecular markers of cell apoptosis may turn out to be good prognosticators. Fuse and colleagues from Japan found that serum levels of soluble Fas and Fas ligand were significantly higher in patients with fatal myocarditis than in survivors. Sheppard more recently examined the patients who participated in the Intervention in Myocarditis and Acute Cardiomyopathy (IMAC II) trial. Patients with myocardial expression of Fas ligand or tumor necrosis factor receptor 1 (TNFR1) showed minimal recovery, suggesting again that excessive apoptosis is a poor prognosticator in patients with acute myocarditis. Because of the diversity of outcomes in patients with myocarditis and the general lack of dramatic response to treatment, meticulous follow-up of patients to determine their natural history is very important. This will also help determine the need for continuation or additional therapy and ongoing risk.

Therapeutic Approaches

Supportive Therapy

The first-line therapy for all patients with myocarditis and heart failure is supportive care (see Chap. 28). A very small proportion of patients will require hemodynamic support (**Fig. 70-8**) that ranges from vasopressors (see Chap. 27) to intra-aortic balloon pump and ventricular assist devices (see Chap. 32). These patients should be treated like any patient with clinical heart failure, including initial diuretics to remove excessive volume overload if present. Patients may also benefit from intravenous vasodilators such as nitroglycerin and nesiritide in appropriate doses with appropriate monitoring to improve cardiac output and to lower filling pressures (see Chap. 27). The recommended therapy for heart failure, such as angiotensin modulators (angiotensin-converting enzyme [ACE] inhibitors or angiotensin receptor blockers) and beta blockers, should then be initiated as soon as the patient is clinically stable and able to tolerate these medications (see Chap. 28). The current ACC/AHA/ESC/CCS guidelines for heart failure care should be followed.[45]

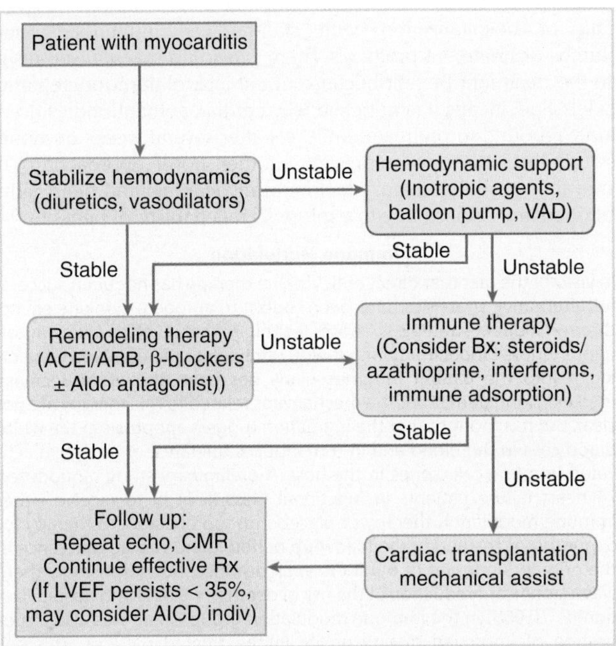

FIGURE 70-8 Treatment algorithms for patients with myocarditis, depending on hemodynamic stability and response to general supportive and remodeling treatment regimen at each step. All patients should have aggressive support and appropriate follow-up. Immune therapy at present is still mainly to support those who have failed to improve spontaneously. ACEi = angiotensin-converting enzyme inhibitors; AICD = automatic implantable cardioverter-defibrillator; Aldo = aldosterone; ARB = angiotensin receptor blockers; Bx = biopsy; CMR = cardiac magnetic resonance; indiv = based on individual assessment of risk versus benefit; LVEF = left ventricular ejection fraction; VAD = ventricular assist device.

There is usually an urgent discussion of whether immunosuppressive therapies should be used for patients with myocarditis, but what is not well recognized is that the traditional heart failure therapies may already have significant anti-inflammatory effect. ACE inhibitors together with beta blockers represent the cornerstones of modern heart failure therapy. It has been previously well documented that angiotensin is a potent proinflammatory and pro-oxidative agent. ACE inhibitors have been shown to decrease the expression of adhesion molecules on the surface of the endothelium. ACE inhibitors also have general anti-inflammatory properties in terms of attenuating inflammatory cell mobilization and cytokine release. The effect of ACE inhibition observed to date in heart failure and atherosclerosis is consistent with its effect on inflammation. Even though beta blockers have traditionally been associated mainly with blockade of the adrenergic system, more recently there is appreciation that they may also have an impact on inflammatory cytokine signaling. In a canine model of heart failure, the effective use of beta blockade in this setting can significantly reduce cytokine gene expression in the myocardium. This is accompanied by improvements in ventricular function and reverses remodeling of the left ventricle.

Immunosuppression

Because inflammatory cell infiltrates have consistently been found on myocardial biopsy or autopsy of patients who have myocarditis, the general belief has been that immunosuppression should be beneficial for myocarditis. However, this is very much an unproven hypothesis, as our current understanding of inflammation suggests that the immune response can be as much protective as harmful and that broad immunosuppressive regimens may produce as much harm as benefit. To date, there is no shortage of small trials evaluating a variety of immunosuppressive regimens. However, all of them are fraught with significant limitations, including (1) the high degree of spontaneous improvement in the control and treatment arms, (2) the small sample size with a heterogeneous collection of recruited patients, (3) the patchy nature of myocardial biopsy detection of myocarditis, and (4) the lack of relationship between pathologic abnormalities and clinical prognosis.

The first systematic approach to evaluate immune modulatory therapy in heart disease is the NIH-sponsored Myocarditis Treatment Trial (see Fig. 70-8). In this trial, patients with biopsy-proven myocarditis according to the Dallas criteria were randomized to receive either conventional therapy, including ACE inhibitors and standard anti–heart failure regimen, or the addition of immunosuppressive therapy. The immunosuppressive therapy regimen consisted of steroids, azathioprine, or cyclosporine. The results showed that there was a significant improvement in ejection fraction in both arms of the randomized trial, such that at the end of the follow-up period at 4.3 years, there was no significant difference between the two arms.[36] The overall outcome of patients with myocarditis and dilated cardiomyopathy is still poor in the trial. Predictors of improvement included high initial left ventricular ejection fraction (LVEF), less intensive conventional therapy, and short duration of symptoms. When the survival was examined in more detail, there was a trend for improvement in the immunosuppressed arm while the treatment was actively being administered. However, because the immunosuppression was given for only 6 months and was discontinued thereafter, the effect was not sustained. In retrospect, during the time in which the Myocarditis Treatment Trial was conducted, the clinical approach was focused on the overly simplified notion of immune activation in myocarditis and heart failure. The immunosuppressive regimen used was nonspecific for the innate or acquired arms of immunity. In addition, there was no delineation of the viral etiology in the trial itself. Finally, the patients entered in the trial were at various stages of development of cardiomyopathy, and the sample size was not adequate in retrospect to detect a transient albeit potentially important benefit during the short term.[1] A series from Italy examined 112 patients with active biopsy-proven

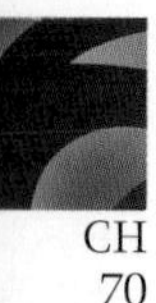

myocarditis, of whom 41 were treated with prednisone and azathioprine because of failure of conventional therapy. The responders to the immunosuppressive regimen were 90% positive for cardiac autoantibodies, and there was no evidence of persisting viral genome. Polish investigators demonstrated improved ejection fraction and subjective symptoms in patients with myocarditis defined by alternative endomyocardial biopsy markers of immunologic activation, as opposed to standard Dallas criteria. This suggested that there may evolve to be predictors of response to immunosuppression.

On the basis of the results of the foregoing studies, immunosuppression should not be routinely considered for patients with myocarditis. However, patients with giant cell myocarditis, myocarditis due to autoimmune or hypersensitivity reactions, or severe hemodynamic compromise and deteriorating conditions may benefit from a trial of immunosuppressive therapy in the hope of stabilizing the hemodynamic condition of the patient. The best responders may be those with active autoimmune response without persisting viral genome. We need to be aware that this is unlikely to influence the ultimate mortality of the patient, but it may improve the short-term natural history.

Interferon

Type I interferons (IFN-α and IFN-β) exert antiviral activity by virtue of their ability to phosphorylate interferon-stimulated genes (ISGs) in the host innate immune system. These ISGs together can lead to degradation of foreign viral RNA, and the small GTPase Mx (a component of the ISG) can interfere with the accumulation of viral RNA and coat protein. IFN-β has been shown to be most effective in animal models of viral myocarditis, and we have demonstrated recently that IFN-β knockout animals ($IFN\text{-}\beta^{-/-}$) have a higher viral titer, increased inflammatory cell infiltrate, increased mortality, and worse cardiac function.[26]

To determine if this strategy can be applied to patients, Kuhl and associates have evaluated 22 patients with dilated cardiomyopathy and biopsy evidence of viral persistence.[46] The patients were treated with subcutaneous IFN-β for a period of 24 weeks. The interferon treatment was able to eliminate the viral genome from all of the patients, and ventricular function improved in 15 of 22 patients. The mean LVEF improved from 44.6% to 53.1% ($P < 0.001$). Overall, the patients also improved in clinical status. These encouraging phase II results have paved the way for a phase IIb trial of IFN-β in patients with dilated cardiomyopathy. Preliminary data in this trial suggested that there was a reduction in viral load from myocardial biopsy samples in the interferon-treated group.[47] There was also improvement in New York Heart Association functional class and quality of life indices in the IFN-β–treated group. However, this is an encouraging and intriguing result. This will need to be replicated to represent a true advancement for the treatment of myocarditis.

Intravenous Immune Globulin

Many causes of acute-onset dilated cardiomyopathy, including peripartum cardiomyopathy, are likely to represent an autoimmune inflammatory process in the myocardium that is triggered by a transient viral infection. Instead of anticytokine therapy or active immune suppression, a possible strategy is passive immunization through the infusion of immune globulins. In cases of pediatric heart failure, particularly myocarditis, uncontrolled studies suggested a potential benefit with intravenous immune globulins.

Retrospective analysis suggested that in patients with peripartum cardiomyopathy, many of whom also had concurrent myocarditis, those who received intravenous immune globulin appear to have better ventricular function during follow-up.[48] To test this hypothesis more thoroughly and prospectively in adults, McNamara and associates conducted a randomized double-blinded trial involving 62 patients with acute heart failure and randomized the patients with 2 g/kg intravenous immune globulin or placebo, followed up for changes in LVEF from the baseline to 6 months and 12 months (IMAC II trial).[40] Overall, there was impressive improvement of LVEF from 25% to 41% at 6 months and to 42% at 12 months; however, the improvement was identical in both the intravenous immune globulin treatment arm and in the placebo arm. The transplant-free survival was 92% at 1 year. In IMAC, the patients spontaneously improved left ventricular ejection significantly with or without immune globulin treatment. The rapid improvement in LVEF in the control precluded any possibility of demonstrating a treatment effect. In retrospect, the evaluation of this agent in a more advanced chronic cardiomyopathy population with evidence of inflammation in the heart may have produced a more definitive result. Accordingly, at present, there is no primary indication for immune globulins in myocarditis, except perhaps in pediatric populations and those refractory to immunosuppressive therapy.

Immune Adsorption Therapy

A physical approach to removal of potential cardiac depressant factors is immune adsorption therapy through plasmapheresis of peripheral blood. There have been previous suggestions that in addition to cytokines, circulating antibodies may target against specific components of the myocyte under stress, such as the beta-adrenergic receptor, the adenosine triphospate (ATP) carrier, or even the myosin molecule, leading to eventual cell dysfunction and cell death. Various strategies have been developed to capture these cardiodepressant factors or antibodies by use of immune adsorption columns.

In one earlier randomized trial using immune adsorption therapy, 34 patients were randomized to standard therapy or immune adsorption therapy aimed at removal of antibodies against the beta-adrenergic receptor. After 1 year of treatment, the treated group demonstrated a change of LVEF from a mean of 22% to 38%, whereas the placebo or standard treatment arm did not show any significant improvement. There was also accompanying improvement in patients' symptomatic status. More recently, other groups have demonstrated further specificity by identifying the IgG3 subclass of antibodies to be particularly responsible for cardiac depression.[49,50] Patients who had effective removal of the IgG3 class of antibodies are particularly the patients who demonstrated improvement in ejection fraction.

However, these innovative approaches have not been subjected to a large randomized trial examining objective endpoints, such as death or hospitalization, with standardized immunoadsorption columns or treatment protocols. There is also no mechanistic insight into the treatment benefit because of the lack of appropriate animal models. Specifically, it is not clear why cardiac autoantibodies do not simply rebound to pretreatment levels after several weeks or months. Nevertheless, this does represent another novel approach to the removal of proinflammatory factors in myocarditis and heart failure and offers the opportunity to explore its mechanism of benefit.

Immune Modulation

In view of the fact that direct anticytokine therapy has not been successful, alternative strategies have been sought to abrogate cytokine effects through indirect strategies. A novel technique that involves taking autologous whole blood, irradiating it with ultraviolet radiation, and reinjecting it into the patient intramuscularly has been shown to decrease markers of inflammation. The mechanisms related to this therapy are not clear, but it is thought that the irradiation triggers apoptosis in the white blood cells in the blood and in turn induces tolerance or anergy in activated immune cell clones in the host. A preliminary study randomized 75 heart failure patients in functional Class III or IV to receive either immune modulation therapy or placebo on top of standard therapy for 6 months. At the end of the follow-up period, there was no difference in the primary endpoint of 6-minute walk distance, but surprisingly there was a significant reduction in the risk of death ($P = 0.022$) and hospitalization ($P = 0.008$) in the immune modulation group. There was also a suggestion of improved quality of life in the treated patients. This has resulted in a large follow-up mortality and morbidity trial involving more than 2400 patients (the ACCLAIM trial).[51] During 10.2 months of follow-up, there was no overall difference in the composite endpoints of time to death or transplantation for cardiovascular reasons. Nonetheless, two prespecified subgroups, those with no history of myocardial infarction and those with Class II New York Heart Association heart failure, displayed significant reductions in the primary endpoint. The failure of immunomodulation therapy to improve left ventricular compromise relates to redundancy of the immune system and alternative effects of TNFR1 and TNFR2 on NF-κB, inflammation, apoptosis, and hypertrophy.

Hemodynamic Support (see Chap. 32)

Whereas there has been no universally applicable specific therapy for patients with myocarditis, general supportive measures, even for those patients with hemodynamic compromise, have been effective because a significant portion of patients recover spontaneously. Patients with myocarditis presenting with profound hemodynamic compromise secondary to fulminant myocarditis or cardiogenic shock can be supported effectively with devices ranging from intra-aortic balloon pumps to full ventricular assist devices (VAD). Indeed, many of the cases of spontaneous recovery after VAD support without the need for transplantation, or so-called bridge to recovery, are in patients with the primary diagnosis of myocarditis. For example, Simon and colleagues reported a single-center series of 154 patients receiving VAD therapy, of whom 10 had successful recovery without transplantation.[52] The majority of cases were nonischemic cardiomyopathy, including myocarditis in three patients and peripartum cardiomyopathy in four patients.

Vaccination

If viruses continue as the most common cause of myocarditis and dilated cardiomyopathy, one may consider in the future the possibility of targeted vaccination. Patients who may be genetically susceptible to myocarditis may receive vaccination against the most common causative agents, thus obviating the risk for development of the disease. One example is the disappearance of endocardial fibroelastosis causing dilated cardiomyopathy in children associated with the mumps vaccination program. If vaccination is effective, this could lead to an effective prevention program of myocarditis and dilated cardiomyopathy, with attendant reduction in cost and improvement in morbidity and mortality.

Future Perspectives

Myocarditis serves as an excellent model for the study of host injury and repair. The outcome is critically dependent on the virulence of the causative agent, the ability of the host immune system to mount an appropriate response, and the ability of the host to repair the injury effectively and efficiently. Future determination of the genetic risk factors leading to the phenotype of myocarditis and its potential interactions with the environment and the ability to predict who will or will not recover will be beneficial in identifying those at particular high risk for development of long-term sequelae of the condition.

Meanwhile, the diagnostic techniques are evolving to identify novel blood-based biomarkers reflecting cardiac inflammation through microarray and proteomic analysis of tissues of both laboratory models and patient samples. The goal in the near future is to develop a blood-based diagnostic tool or panel with sufficient sensitivity and specificity to obviate the need for myocardial biopsies. The combination of blood samples of biomarkers together with imaging techniques such as cardiac magnetic resonance imaging may help properly diagnose and stage the disease and avoid the current problem of severe underdiagnosis due to dependence on the Dallas criteria by biopsy.

With the understanding of new pathophysiologic mechanisms, new therapies are also being developed and evaluated in clinical trials. Ongoing interferon and immune-modifying strategies may become more refined as data determining their relative efficacies compared with traditional therapies become available. This may help develop more evidence-based guidelines for treatment of these very ill patients. In addition, the increased refinement of ventricular assist strategies to support patients and ultimately to wean them from support without necessary transplantation represents another unique opportunity to improve outcomes for the patients presenting with dramatic hemodynamic collapse. One long-term goal would be to identify individuals at risk for myocarditis and to evaluate the opportunity and cost-effectiveness of developing a combination vaccine to prevent the development of disease in these individuals despite exposure to the causative agents.

In Memoriam

Kenneth L. Baughman's scientific contributions to the study of myocarditis, the subject of this chapter, were legion. He was also a consummate clinician, a caring and dedicated physician, a generous mentor, a valued colleague, and a trusted and loyal friend. He was an avid athlete who regularly competed in triathlons. He was also a loving and devoted husband, father, and grandfather. His untimely death while attending the American Heart Association meeting in Orlando, Florida, in November 2009 has had a lasting impact on the editors and his colleagues at the Brigham and Women's Hospital. He is sorely missed, and the editors dedicate this chapter to his memory.

REFERENCES

Definition, Incidence, and Epidemiology

1. Cooper LT Jr: Myocarditis. N Engl J Med 360:1526, 2009.
2. Aretz HT, Billingham ME, Edwards WD, et al: Myocarditis, a histopathologic definition and classification. Am J Cardiovasc Pathol 1:3, 1987.
3. Baughman KL: Diagnosis of myocarditis: Death of Dallas criteria. Circulation 113:593, 2006.
4. Fabre A, Sheppard MN: Sudden adult death syndrome and other non-ischaemic causes of sudden cardiac death. Heart 92:316, 2006.
5. Nugent AW, Daubeney PE, Chondros P, et al: The epidemiology of childhood cardiomyopathy in Australia. N Engl J Med 348:1639, 2003.
6. Towbin JA, Lowe AM, Colan SD, et al: Incidence, causes, and outcomes of dilated cardiomyopathy in children. JAMA 296:1867, 2006.
7. Xiong D, Yajima T, Lim BK, et al: Inducible cardiac-restricted expression of enteroviral protease 2A is sufficient to induce dilated cardiomyopathy. Circulation 115:94, 2007.
8. Imazio M, Cecchi E, Demichelis B, et al: Myopericarditis versus viral or idiopathic acute pericarditis. Heart 94:498, 2008.
9. Tschope C, Bock CT, Kasner M, et al: High prevalence of cardiac parvovirus B19 infection in patients with isolated left ventricular diastolic dysfunction. Circulation 111:879, 2005.
10. Kuhl U, Pauschinger M, Noutsias M, et al: High prevalence of viral genomes and multiple viral infections in the myocardium of adults with "idiopathic" left ventricular dysfunction. Circulation 111:887, 2005.
11. Kuhl U, Pauschinger M, Seeberg B, et al: Viral persistence in the myocardium is associated with progressive cardiac dysfunction. Circulation 112:1965, 2005.
12. Bowles NE, Ni J, Kearney DL, et al: Detection of viruses in myocardial tissues by polymerase chain reaction: Evidence of adenovirus as a common cause of myocarditis in children and adults. J Am Coll Cardiol 42:466, 2003.

Etiologic Agents

13. Matsumori A: Hepatitis C virus infection and cardiomyopathies. Circ Res 96:144, 2005.
14. Coyne CB, Bergelson JM: Virus-induced Abl and Fyn kinase signals permit coxsackievirus entry through epithelial tight junctions. Cell 124:119, 2006.
15. Liu P, Aitken K, Kong YY, et al: Essential role for the tyrosine kinase $p56^{lck}$ in coxsackievirus B3 mediated heart disease. Nat Med 6:429, 2000.
16. Andreoletti L, Venteo L, Douche-Aourik F, et al: Active coxsackieviral B infection is associated with disruption of dystrophin in endomyocardial tissue of patients who died suddenly of acute myocardial infarction. J Am Coll Cardiol 50:2207, 2007.
17. Schenk T, Enders M, Pollak S, et al: High prevalence of human parvovirus B19 DNA in myocardial autopsy samples from subjects without myocarditis or dilative cardiomyopathy. J Clin Microbiol 47:106, 2009.
18. Vallbracht KB, Schwimmbeck PL, Kuhl U, et al: Endothelium-dependent flow-mediated vasodilation of systemic arteries is impaired in patients with myocardial virus persistence. Circulation 110:2938, 2004.
19. Yilmaz A, Mahrholdt H, Athanasiadis A, et al: Coronary vasospasm as the underlying cause for chest pain in patients with PVB19 myocarditis. Heart 94:1456, 2008.
20. Noutsias M, Fechner H, de Jonge H, et al: Human coxsackie-adenovirus receptor is colocalized with integrins $\alpha_v\beta_3$ and $\alpha_v\beta_5$ on the cardiomyocyte sarcolemma and upregulated in dilated cardiomyopathy: Implications for cardiotropic viral infections. Circulation 104:275, 2001.
21. Nowakowski J, Nadelman RB, Sell R, et al: Long-term follow-up of patients with culture-confirmed Lyme disease. Am J Med 115:91, 2003.
22. Barrett MP, Burchmore RJ, Stich A, et al: The trypanosomiases. Lancet 362:1469, 2003.
23. Ben m'rad M, Leclerc-Mercier S, Blanche P, et al: Drug-induced hypersensitivity syndrome: Clinical and biologic disease patterns in 24 patients. Medicine (Baltimore) 88:131, 2009.

Pathophysiology

24. Maekawa Y, Ouzounian M, Opavsky MA, Liu PP: Connecting the missing link between dilated cardiomyopathy and viral myocarditis: Virus, cytoskeleton, and innate immunity. Circulation 115:5, 2007.
25. Fuse K, Chan G, Liu Y, et al: Myeloid differentiation factor-88 plays a crucial role in the pathogenesis of coxsackievirus B3 induced myocarditis and influences type I interferon production. Circulation 112:2276, 2005.
26. Deonarain R, Cerullo D, Fuse K, et al: Protective role for interferon-β in coxsackievirus B3 infection. Circulation 110:3540, 2004.

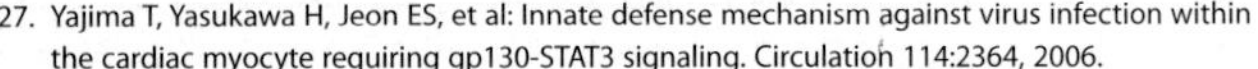

27. Yajima T, Yasukawa H, Jeon ES, et al: Innate defense mechanism against virus infection within the cardiac myocyte requiring gp130-STAT3 signaling. Circulation 114:2364, 2006.
28. Opavsky MA, Martino T, Rabinovitch M, et al: Enhanced ERK-1/2 activation in mice susceptible to coxsackievirus-induced myocarditis. J Clin Invest 109:1561, 2002.

Clinical Presentation and Diagnosis

29. Felker GM, Thompson RE, Hare JM, et al: Underlying causes and long-term survival in patients with initially unexplained cardiomyopathy. N Engl J Med 342:1077, 2000.
30. McCarthy RE 3rd, Boehmer JP, Hruban RH, et al: Long-term outcome of fulminant myocarditis as compared with acute (nonfulminant) myocarditis. N Engl J Med 342:690, 2000.
31. Cooper LT Jr, Hare JM, Tazelaar HD, et al: Usefulness of immunosuppression for giant cell myocarditis. Am J Cardiol 102:1535, 2008.
32. Liu PP, Yan AT: Cardiovascular magnetic resonance for the diagnosis of acute myocarditis: Prospects for detecting myocardial inflammation. J Am Coll Cardiol 45:1823, 2005.
33. Abdel-Aty H, Boye P, Zagrosek A, et al: Diagnostic performance of cardiovascular magnetic resonance in patients with suspected acute myocarditis: Comparison of different approaches. J Am Coll Cardiol 45:1815, 2005.
34. Mahrholdt H, Goedecke C, Wagner A, et al: Cardiovascular magnetic resonance assessment of human myocarditis: A comparison to histology and molecular pathology. Circulation 109:1250, 2004.
35. Friedrich MG, Sechtem U, Schulz-Menger J, et al: Cardiovascular magnetic resonance in myocarditis: A JACC White Paper. J Am Coll Cardiol 53:1475, 2009.
36. Mason JW, O'Connell JB, Herskowitz A, et al: A clinical trial of immunosuppressive therapy for myocarditis. N Engl J Med 333:269, 1995.
37. Cooper LT, Baughman KL, Feldman AM, et al: The role of endomyocardial biopsy in the management of cardiovascular disease: A scientific statement from the American Heart Association, the American College of Cardiology, and the European Society of Cardiology. Circulation 116:2216, 2007.
38. Bowles NE, Ni J, Marcus F, Towbin JA: The detection of cardiotropic viruses in the myocardium of patients with arrhythmogenic right ventricular dysplasia/cardiomyopathy. J Am Coll Cardiol 39:892, 2002.
39. Pieroni M, Dello Russo A, Marzo F, et al: High prevalence of myocarditis mimicking arrhythmogenic right ventricular cardiomyopathy: Differential diagnosis by electroanatomic mapping–guided endomyocardial biopsy. J Am Coll Cardiol 53:681, 2009.
40. McNamara DM, Holubkov R, Starling RC, et al: Controlled trial of intravenous immune globulin in recent-onset dilated cardiomyopathy. Circulation 103:2254, 2001.
41. Kindermann I, Kindermann M, Kandolf R, et al: Predictors of outcome in patients with suspected myocarditis. Circulation 118:639, 2008.
42. Caforio AL, Calabrese F, Angelini A, et al: A prospective study of biopsy-proven myocarditis: Prognostic relevance of clinical and aetiopathogenetic features at diagnosis. Eur Heart J 28:1326, 2007.
43. Mann DL: Determinants of myocardial recovery in myocarditis has the time come for molecular fingerprinting? J Am Coll Cardiol 46:1043, 2005.
44. Why HJ, Meany BT, Richardson PJ, et al: Clinical and prognostic significance of detection of enteroviral RNA in the myocardium of patients with myocarditis or dilated cardiomyopathy. Circulation 89:2582, 1994.
45. Hunt SA, Abraham WT, Chin MH, et al: ACC/AHA 2005 Guideline Update for the Diagnosis and Management of Chronic Heart Failure in the Adult: A report of the American College of Cardiology/American Heart Association Task Force on Practice Guidelines (Writing Committee to Update the 2001 Guidelines for the Evaluation and Management of Heart Failure). Circulation 112:1825, 2005.
46. Kuhl U, Pauschinger M, Schwimmbeck PL, et al: Interferon-β treatment eliminates cardiotropic viruses and improves left ventricular function in patients with myocardial persistence of viral genomes and left ventricular dysfunction. Circulation 107:2793, 2003.
47. Schultheiss HP, Poller W, Kuhl U, et al: Interferon β-1b in patients with chronic viral cardiomyopathy. American Heart Association meeting; New Orleans, La; November 2008.
48. Bozkurt B, Villaneuva FS, Holubkov R, et al: Intravenous immune globulin in the therapy of peripartum cardiomyopathy. J Am Coll Cardiol 34:177, 1999.
49. Staudt A, Schaper F, Stangl V, et al: Immunohistological changes in dilated cardiomyopathy induced by immunoadsorption therapy and subsequent immunoglobulin substitution. Circulation 103:2681, 2001.
50. Staudt A, Bohm M, Knebel F, et al: Potential role of autoantibodies belonging to the immunoglobulin G-3 subclass in cardiac dysfunction among patients with dilated cardiomyopathy. Circulation 106:2448, 2002.
51. Torre-Amione G, Anker SD, Bourge RC, et al: Results of a non-specific immunomodulation therapy in chronic heart failure (ACCLAIM trial): A placebo-controlled randomised trial. Lancet 371:228, 2008.
52. Simon MA, Kormos RL, Murali S, et al: Myocardial recovery using ventricular assist devices: Prevalence, clinical characteristics, and outcomes. Circulation 112:I32, 2005.

CHAPTER 71 Chagas' Disease

José A.F. Ramires, Andrei C. Sposito, Edécio Cunha-Neto, and Maria de Lourdes Higuchi

Chagas' disease, or American trypanosomiasis, is an infection caused by the protozoan *Trypanosoma cruzi* (*T. cruzi*), originally transmitted by hematophagous triatomine insects.[1,2] Triatominae infected by *T. cruzi* inhabit 18 countries in North and South America, ranging from the southern United States to southern Argentina, and the prevalence of the disease relates to the proximity between infected triatomines and humans. The infection can also result from maternal-fetal transmission, from food contaminated with feces or urine from infected Triatominae, from laboratory accidents, and from blood transfusion or organs transplanted from infected donors. Some 20,000 people die annually from Chagas' disease, 16 to 18 million people are infected, and 100 million people are at risk of contracting the infection. During its life cycle, *T. cruzi* can assume three forms (**Fig. 71-1**).

Pathologic Findings

Manifestations of Chagas' disease vary during the course of infection. In the acute phase, at the site of inoculation, local swelling occurs (called a chagoma). The histology typically shows amastigote forms of *T. cruzi* in macrophages, adipose cells, and muscle fibers in the subcutaneous tissue, associated with lymphohystiocytic inflammatory infiltrate, vascular proliferation, edema, and congestion.[3] Some metastatic chagomas (cutaneous nodes showing inflammation without parasites) may occur. The parasites entering the bloodstream (**Fig. 71-2A**) reach almost all organs and infect different types of cells, including macrophages, endothelial cells, smooth and skeletal muscle cells, cardiac myocytes, and fibroblasts.

The most common cause of death in this phase is an acute myocarditis characterized macroscopically by a flabby congested dilated heart, with normal or moderately increased volume, and microscopically by moderate to severe mononuclear inflammatory infiltration with some neutrophils, edema, myocytolysis, and many intramyocyte nests of amastigotes, with no inflammation when cells remain intact (see Fig. 71-2B). An inflammatory infiltrate injures nerves and parasympathetic ganglia. Parasites and mononuclear inflammatory infiltrate can also affect skeletal muscles (see Fig. 71-2C) and smooth muscle of the esophagus and large intestine, destroying myenteric plexus. Meningoencephalitis can also cause death in this phase.[3]

Reactivation of the disease during the chronic phase may occur because of immunosuppression, as in AIDS or neoplasia or after heart transplantation.[4,5] *T. cruzi* may be detected in peripheral blood or bone marrow or in subcutaneous nodes, resembling primary chagomas (see Fig. 71-2D and E). An asymptomatic period called the indeterminate phase follows the acute phase of infection with *T. cruzi*. Endomyocardial biopsies of 15% of patients in this phase show mild lymphocytic myocarditis without substantial structural alterations such as fibrosis, hypertrophy, or myocytolysis.[6]

Several years after initial infection, an estimated 30% of infected people will develop clinical Chagas' cardiomyopathy. In necropsy studies,[3,7] patients who died because of Chagas' cardiomyopathy presented with rounded globe-shaped hearts; severe chamber dilation, mainly on the right side; myocardial hypertrophy; congested epicardial veins; and intracavitary thrombosis, usually in the left ventricular apex and right atrial appendage (**Fig. 71-3A**). Microscopy shows a variable degree of lymphocytic inflammatory infiltrate surrounding nonparasitized myocytes, severe myofiber hypertrophy (see Fig. 71-3B), and fibrosis (see Fig. 71-3C). In this phase, nests of *T. cruzi* are rare. Immunohistochemistry and polymerase chain reaction (PCR) techniques have demonstrated antigens and DNA of the parasite at sites of inflammation (see Fig. 71-3D), but their quantity does not relate to the intensity of myocarditis, suggesting involvement of other factors.[8,9]

Segmental fibrotic lesions often occur in the myocardium of patients with chronic Chagas' disease.[3,8,10] One is the so-called apex lesion, characterized by a thinning of the left ventricular apex, with total or partial disappearance of the myocardium (replaced by fibrosis), a pathognomonic sign of Chagas' disease. In necropsy studies, other segmental thinning of the myocardial wall is usually found at the inferolateral wall of the left ventricle. These lesions are accompanied by mural thrombosis and aneurysm dilatation (**Fig. 71-4**). In patients, myocardial delayed enhancement by contrast cardiac magnetic resonance (CMR)[11] has also demonstrated fibrosis in the inferolateral wall associated with clinical manifestation of sustained ventricular tachycardia. Segmental fibrotic lesions often occur in the watershed zone of coronary circulation (**Fig. 71-5**), and may correspond to healed ischemic injury, explaining also the segmental fibrosis in the conduction system (see Fig. 71-4D).

The apex lesion might result from conduction system fibrosis, which would delay the electric stimulus to the apex,[12] parasympathetic denervation. Altered myocardial perfusion occurs in patients with Chagas' disease who manifest myocardial ischemia in the absence of epicardial coronary stenosis; the imbalance between the sympathetic and parasympathetic nervous systems may account for this coronary flow disturbance.[13-15]

Pathophysiology

Chagas' cardiomyopathy is essentially a myocarditis.[3,8,16,17] The inflammatory process, although more intense in the acute phase, is clinically silent but incessant in patients in the indeterminate and chronic phases of the disease. The T-cell rich mononuclear cell inflammatory infiltrate seems to play a major pathogenic role in the disease.[18,19] Various observations support this view: (1) the worse prognosis of Chagas' disease compared with cardiomyopathies of noninflammatory cause; (2) the relationship between the frequency of myocarditis and the severity of cardiomyopathy; and (3) the correlation between ventricular dilation and the intensity of myocarditis in Syrian hamsters chronically infected by *T. cruzi*.[20] The scarcity of *T. cruzi* parasites in the

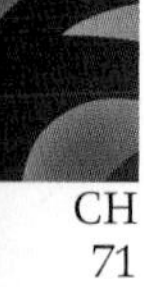

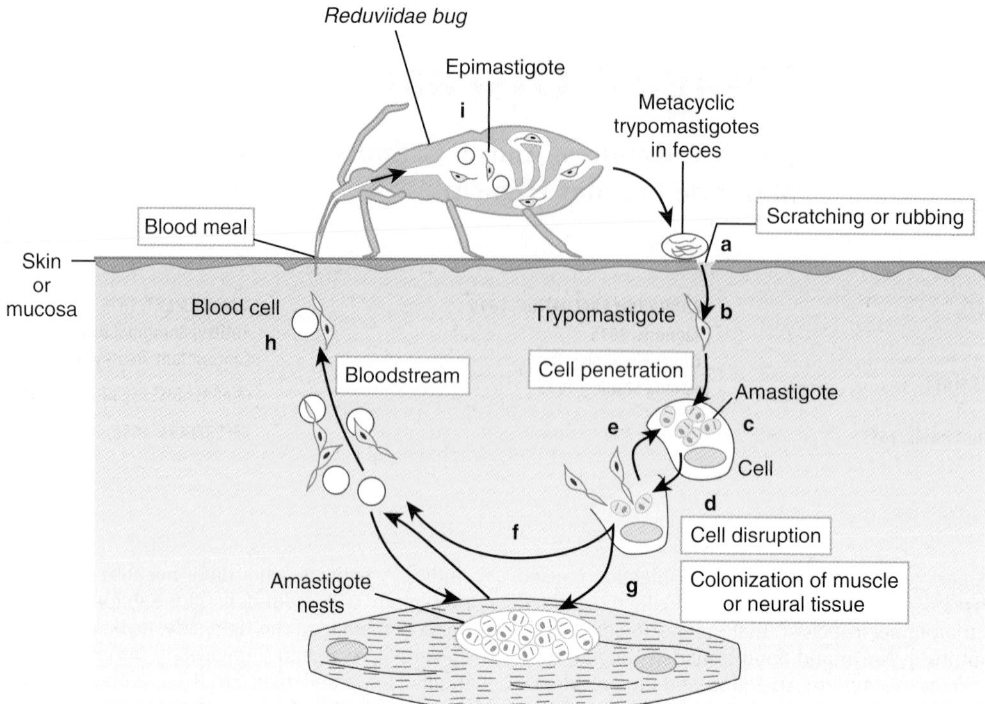

FIGURE 71-1 The life cycle of *Trypanosoma cruzi*. Reduvid bugs transmit *T. cruzi*. While partaking of a blood meal (a), the insect defecates on the host's skin, releasing the infective trypomastigote form of the parasite. The trypomastigotes penetrate the host's skin or mucous membrane through abrasion caused by scratching or rubbing the bitten area (b). Trypomastigotes can infect host cardiac, skeletal, smooth muscle, or neural cells, and give rise to the round amastigote form that can replicate intracellularly (c). Amastigotes can give rise to trypomastigotes that can lyse cells (d). Amastigotes and trypomastigotes released from dying cells can propagate the infection or reenter the circulation (e-g). Insects can pick up the parasite when consuming a blood meal (h), and develop the epimastigote form that replicates in the insect gut (i). *(From Macedo AM, Oliveira RP, Pena SD: Chagas' disease: Role of parasite genetic variation in pathogenesis. Expert Rev Mil Med 4:1, 2002.)*

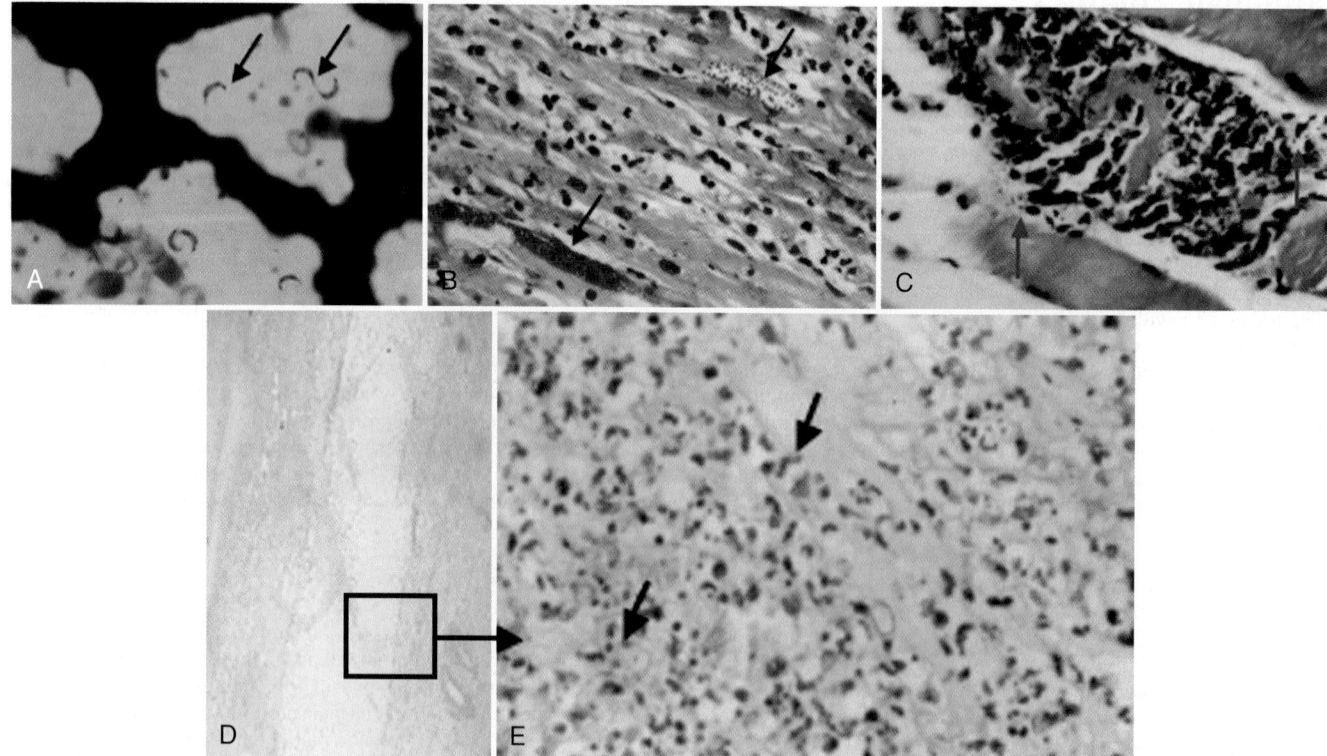

FIGURE 71-2 Microscopic features of acute or reactivation of Chagas' disease. **A,** Diagnosis of the disease is made during the second or third week by microscopic detection of *T. cruzi* organisms in the blood or tissues, appearing in peripheral blood stains as long, slender, C- or S-shaped flagellates, 15 to 20 μm in length (arrows). **B,** Myocardium presenting intracellular nests of amastigotes, which are ovoid, aflagellate forms 2 to 5 μm in length (arrows), and inflammatory mononuclear infiltrate with occasional neutrophils. **C,** Infected ruptured skeletal muscle fiber infiltrated by lymphocytic inflammatory cells, exhibiting many free amastigotes (arrows). **D,** Chagoma-like subcutaneous inflammatory lesion in a reactivation episode of Chagas' disease after heart transplantation. **E,** Close-up view of the lesion in **D**, showing many *T. cruzi* amastigotes in macrophages and endothelial cells stained brown by immunostaining (arrows).

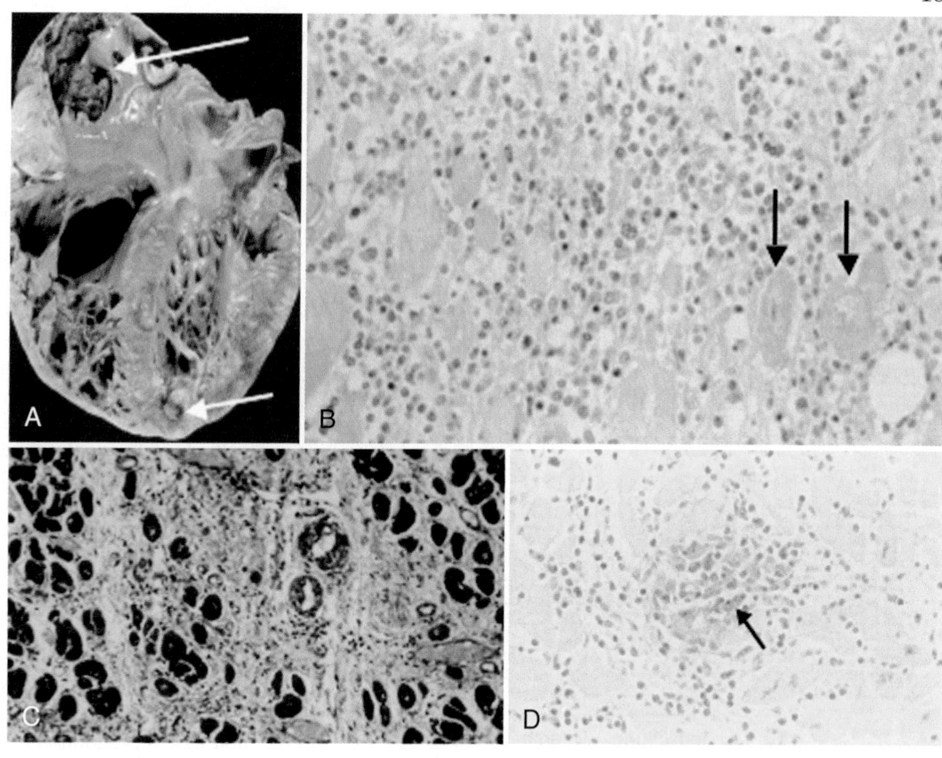

FIGURE 71-3 Macroscopic and microscopic aspects of chronic cardiac Chagas' disease with heart failure. **A,** A dilated globular heart with the most frequent sites of intracavitary thrombosis at the left ventricle apex and right atrial appendage (arrows). **B,** Lymphocytic myocarditis destroying nonparasitized myocardial fibers, suggesting an autoimmune myocarditis. The myofibers exhibit severe hypertrophy with aberrant nuclei (arrows) (H&E stain, ×40). **C,** Ischemic-like fibrotic areas and thin diffuse fibrosis surrounding small groups or individual myocytes (Masson trichrome stain, ×20). **D,** Scarce *T. cruzi* antigens (arrow; immunoperoxidase stain, ×40) surrounded by intense lymphomononuclear inflammatory infiltrate.

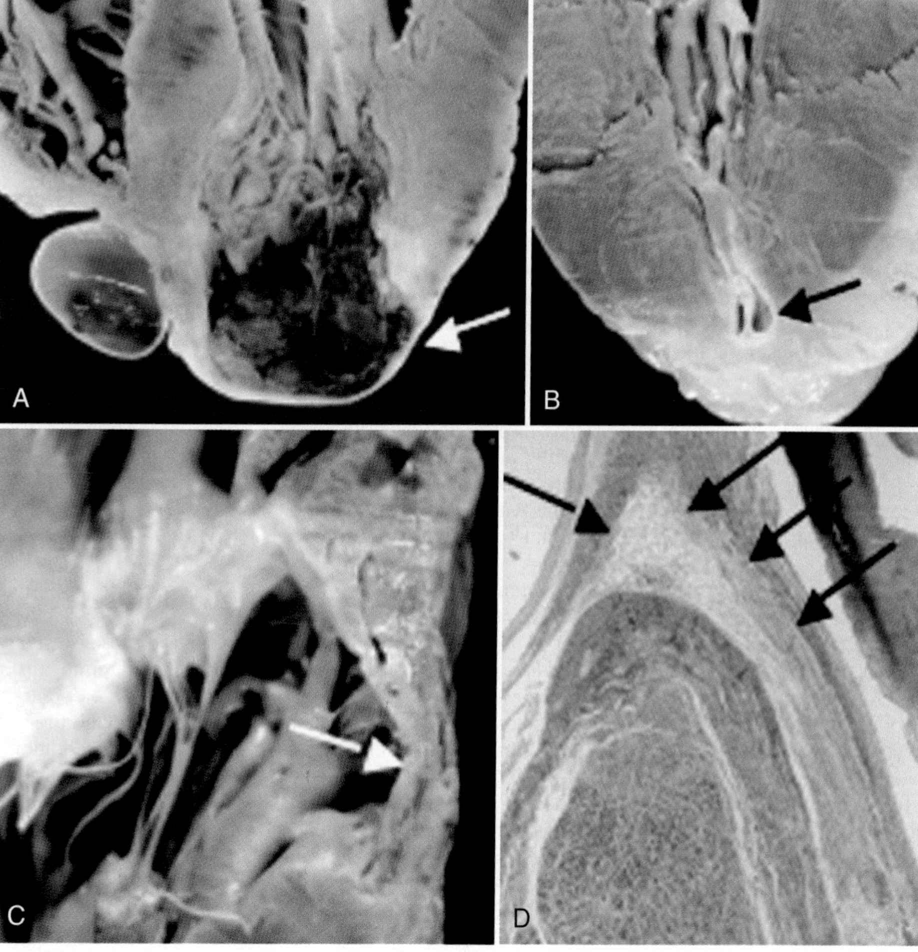

FIGURE 71-4 Necropsy findings of segmental fibrotic chagasic lesions (arrows). **A,** The left ventricle apex lesion shows aneurysm dilation and thrombosis in a patient who died from heart failure. **B,** Focal small apex left ventricular lesion in a sudden death patient. **C,** Lateroposterior basal subvalvar lesion characterized by myocardial wall thinning. **D,** Histology of the conduction system at the His bundle bifurcation, almost completely replaced by fibrosis and adipose tissue (Masson trichrome stain, ×2.5).

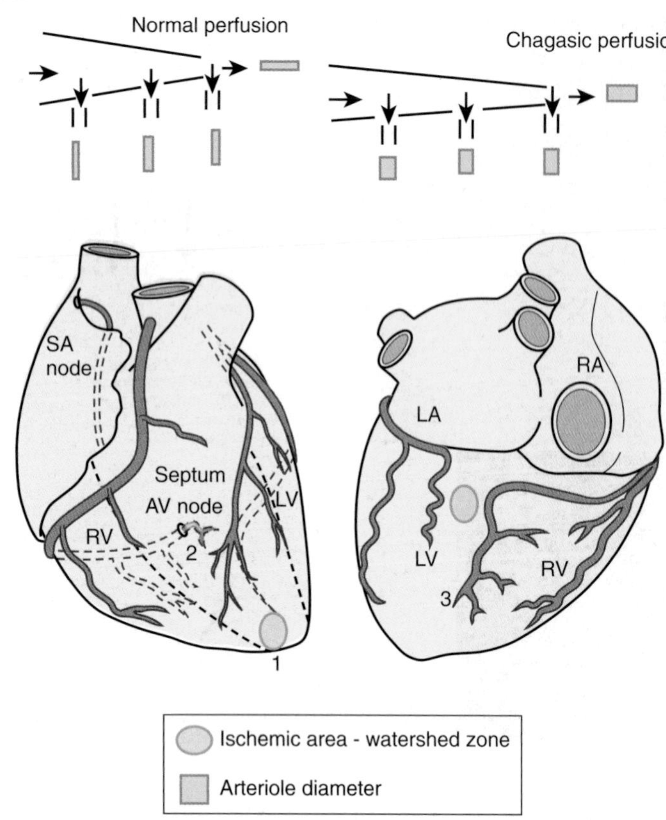

FIGURE 71-5 Schematic representation of three regions that frequently have segmental replacement by fibrosis or adipose tissue in dilated chagasic hearts, and that correspond to watershed regions in the coronary circulation. These lesions may have been caused by ischemia resulting from imbalanced blood flow distribution in the presence of arteriolar vessel dilation. Watershed regions: apex of the left ventricle, irrigated by the anterior and posterior descending interventricular arteries (1); His bundle, irrigated by the crux cordis branch originated from the right coronary artery and septal branch originated from the anterior descending interventricular branch of the left coronary artery (2); lateroposterior basal wall of left ventricle (LV), irrigated by posterior descending right and circumflex coronary arteries. AV = atrioventricular; LA = left atrium; RA = right atrium; RV = right ventricle; SA = sinoatrial.

intensely inflamed heart tissue of patients with Chagas' cardiomyopathy has cast doubt on whether *T. cruzi* antigens trigger myocardial inflammation. The autoimmune hypothesis of pathogenesis has predicted that T cells infiltrating the myocardium should recognize heart proteins as a result of chronic *T. cruzi* infection.[21] Numerous reports have documented autoimmune recognition of neuroantigens, cardiovascular receptors, highly conserved proteins, and cardiac myosin by sera or T cells from patients with Chagas' disease and experimentally infected animals.[22,23] Both *T. cruzi*–specific and autoimmune CD4$^+$ T cells that cross-reactively recognize cardiac myosin and *T. cruzi* proteins populate the myocardium of patients with Chagas' cardiomyopathy, indicating that both antigenic stimuli contribute to sustained inflammation-induced myocardial damage.

Animal studies have shown that inflammatory cytokines play a central part in acute *T. cruzi* infection. Shortly after the acute infection starts, *T. cruzi* components, including DNA and membrane glycoconjugates, trigger innate immunity via Toll-like receptors 2, 4, and 9 in macrophages and dendritic cells.[24] On activation, these cells secrete proinflammatory cytokines and chemokines, express costimulatory receptors, and increase endocytosis and intracellular killing of parasites through the release of reactive oxygen and nitrogen species. The release of proinflammatory cytokines, such as interleukin-1 (IL-1), IL-6, IL-12, IL-18, IL-27, and tumor necrosis factor-α (TNF-α), amplifies and propagates the local inflammatory response. Macrophages and dendritic cells that have endocytosed the parasite subsequently elicit a strong T-cell and antibody response against *T. cruzi*. The resultant *T. cruzi*–specific T cells produce the signature T-helper 1 (Th1) cytokine interferon-γ (IFN-γ)[25] which, together with other inflammatory cells, migrate to sites of *T. cruzi*-induced inflammation in response to chemokines such as CCL2, CCL3, CCL4, CCL5, CXCL9, and CXCL10.[26] This inflammatory T-cell and antibody response leads to control of, but not complete elimination of, tissue and blood parasitism. Immunologic changes found in the indeterminate and chronic phases of Chagas' disease are consistent with low-grade persistent infection by *T. cruzi*. These changes include moderate to high-titer anti–*T. cruzi* immunoglobulin G (IgG) serum antibodies, increased plasma TNF-α levels, IFN-γ–producing *T. cruzi*–specific CD4$^+$ and CD8$^+$ T cells, and suppressed production of the Th2 cytokine IL-4.

The subset of patients that develops Chagas' cardiomyopathy manifest an array of immunologic alterations consistent with an exacerbated Th1 immune response. They display an increased number of peripheral blood IFN-γ–producing T cells,[25] with reduced numbers of IL-10–producing and FoxP3$^+$ regulatory T cells[19] as compared with patients with indeterminant-phase Chagas' disease. Among patients showing ventricular dysfunction, circulating levels of both TNF-α and CCL2 exceed those in indeterminant-phase patients, or those displaying electrocardiographic alterations but no ventricular dysfunction.[25] The exacerbated Th1 response observed in the peripheral blood reflects the nature of the inflammatory infiltrate found in the myocardium of patients with Chagas' cardiomyopathy.[16] The mononuclear cell inflammatory infiltrate contains macrophages, CCR5$^+$, CXCR3$^+$, and IFN-γ–producing T cells, granzyme-expressing cytotoxic CD8$^+$ T cells, and CD4$^+$ T cells. The chemokines CCL2, CXCL9 and CXCL10, also expressed in Chagas' disease myocardium, attract the cell types found in the infiltrate. Local production of cytokines such as IFN-γ, TNF-α, IL-4, IL-6, IL-7, and IL-15 indicates ongoing T-cell or macrophage activation. Enhanced transforming growth factor-β (TGF-β) signaling may contribute to the pronounced fibrosis found in heart lesions.[19] Increased myocardial expression of adhesion molecules and human leukocyte antigen (HLA) classes I and II result from exposure to cytokines such as IFN-γ and facilitate inflammatory-cell influx and antigen presentation. In vitro experiments have shown that IFN-γ can change the cardiomyocyte gene expression program, inducing the hypertrophic gene expression program and modulating energy metabolism pathways.[22] Together, these observations suggest that IFN-γ–producing T cells migrate to the heart, where IFN-γ–mediated chronic myocardial inflammation could sustain inflammation and act directly on cardiomyocyte function.

The reasons why only one third of infected patients develop Chagas' cardiomyopathy are poorly understood. Familial aggregation of cases suggests a genetic component to risk. Single nucleotide polymorphisms (SNPs) in DNA in immune or inflammatory genes (e.g., *MAL/TIRAP*) involved in signal transduction of Toll-like receptors, the proinflammatory cytokines IL-1β, TNF-α, lymphotoxin-α (LTα), and IL-12β, chemokine CCL2, and chemokine receptor CCR5 are all associated with the development of Chagas' cardiomyopathy. Among patients with Chagas' cardiomyopathy who also have overt heart failure, particular TNF-α genotypes are associated with a significantly shortened survival.[25] Given the important role played by such inflammatory molecules in the various stages of pathogenesis, functional genotypic variants likely influence the course of Chagas' disease.

Clinical Manifestations

Acute Phase

Chagas disease is usually acquired after contact between humans and infected triatomines (the vectors). However, the disease can also be acquired by blood transfusion, contaminated food, across the placenta or through the birth canal, laboratory accidents, or organ transplantation.[1] In addition, in patients in the indeterminate or chronic phases of Chagas' disease, HIV infection may induce the elevation of the parasitemia or the manifestation of symptoms of the acute phase.[27,28]

The acute phase of Chagas' disease is frequently asymptomatic and lasts for the first few weeks or months of the infection.[29] Symptoms may include fever, fatigue, body pain, headache, cutaneous rash, diarrhea, and vomiting. Physical examination shows slight hepatosplenomegaly, lymphadenopathy, and the chagoma. The classic chagoma, or swelling of the eyelid on the side of the face nearest the bite wound, is called the Romaña sign. Even in individuals who manifest symptoms in the acute phase, 90% of these symptoms abate spontaneously within 2 to 12 weeks, but the infection persists, leading to the indeterminate phase of the disease.

Indeterminate and Chronic Phases

The indeterminate phase is asymptomatic and may last indefinitely. The appearance of clinical manifestations[20] defines the onset of the chronic phase and may become apparent through the gradual onset of dementia (3%), cardiomyopathy (30%), or dilation of the digestive tract (6%).

Chagas' cardiomyopathy can cause arrhythmias, heart failure, and sudden death.[11,30] Arrythmias occur in about 50% of patients, and constitute the most frequent clinical manifestation in the chronic phase. Extensive myocardial fibrosis creates a substrate for reentry and for delays in cardiac conduction, including the sinus-atrial node, atrioventricular node, His bundle, His bundle branches, and Purkinje fibers.[20] Polymorphic ventricular extrasystoles are a common finding, followed by complete right bundle branch block, left anterior hemiblock, various degrees of atrioventricular block, and changes in ventricular repolarization. These arrhythmias are generally well tolerated or even unapparent. However, depending on its severity, the atrioventricular block can cause fainting, syncope, and seizures caused by reduced cardiac output and cerebral blood flow.

Myocardial fibrosis can also cause malignant ventricular tachyarrhythmias, a major cause of sudden death in patients with chronic Chagas' disease. Structural abnormalities of the myocardium, such as foci of inflammation and fibrosis, can lead to areas of unidirectional block or slow conduction in circumscribed ventricular regions, and to the formation of reentrant circuits. Such reentrant circuits can occur in various regions in both ventricles, but are more often found in regions of fibrotic thinning of the inferolateral wall of the left ventricle. Accordingly, ventricular arrhythmias typically affect individuals with systolic dysfunction, and rarely those with a normal electrocardiogram (ECG) and cardiac anatomy.

The progressive nature of chronic Chagas' myocarditis promotes a slow replacement of myocardial fibers by fibrosis, leading to systolic dysfunction. The onset of heart failure usually follows the development of ventricular arrhythmias late in the course of chagasic myocardial injury. Once present, heart failure generally leads to death in 5 years or less.

In general, systolic dysfunction in Chagas' disease is biventricular, but the initial clinical manifestation with predominantly right ventricular failure characterizes Chagas' cardiomyopathy. These patients often present with elevated jugular venous pressure, painful hepatomegaly, and pedal edema, without signs of pulmonary congestion or orthopnea. Patients at this stage usually have cardiomegaly, electrocardiographic changes, and diffuse and segmental hypokinesis of both ventricles. Several schemes classify the stages of Chagasic cardiomyopathy.[31]

Carlos Chagas recognized the high prevalence of sudden death in the chronic phase in his original description of the disease in 1912. Sustained ventricular tachycardia progressing to ventricular fibrillation most commonly causes sudden death.[32,33] Less commonly, sudden death can result from ventricular asystole, ventricular failure, or systemic embolism. Near-syncope or syncope, systolic dysfunction, ventricular arrhythmias (sustained or unsustained), sinus node dysfunction, and advanced atrioventricular block may predict sudden death.

Laboratory Evaluation

Diagnosis

For decades, the diagnosis of Chagas' disease has been based on the presence of parasites in the blood or tissues. These techniques are especially useful for monitoring drug therapy for *T. cruzi*. In the acute phase, parasites can be easily found through microscopic examination of fresh blood. When parasitemia is low, procedures for parasite concentration (e.g., microhematocrit, Strout) or amplification by indirect methods (e.g., xenodiagnosis, blood culture) can aid in the diagnosis.

In the microhematocrit, blood is centrifuged and the parasite sought in the buffy coat. In the Strout preparation, blood cells are removed by precipitation and centrifugation and the parasites are sought microscopically. The xenodiagnostic method consists of feeding uninfected Triatominae with blood from the patient under examination and searching for *T. cruzi* in the intestinal contents of the insects 30, 60, and 90 days later.[34] In addition to these methods, amplification of *T. cruzi* DNA by PCR assay recently has become feasible and is the method of choice for the detection of parasites in blood and tissues. Although it is more sensitive than xenodiagnosis and blood culture, the sensitivity of PCR also depends on the parasite burden.

Antibodies against *T. cruzi* can also support the diagnosis of Chagas' disease—IgM in the early phase, and IgG after the acute phase. Three methods can be used for the indirect diagnosis—hemagglutination, immunofluorescence, and enzyme-linked immunosorbent assay (ELISA). Despite the possibility of false-positive test results for cross reactions with other pathogens or autoimmune diseases, these tests have high sensitivity, and a positive result in two of these tests is sufficient to diagnose the disease. In conjunction with PCR to estimate parasitemia, serologic tests can be used to monitor patients undergoing causative treatment.

Echocardiography (see Chap. 15)

In the early stages of the disease, diastolic dysfunction commonly occurs, resulting from the presence of myocarditis foci on the ventricular wall that reduces its compliance. With the progression of the disease, these foci eventually become hypokinetic, akinetic, or dyskinetic areas. As noted, the involvement of the right ventricle often precedes, and can occur even in the absence of, any anomaly detectable in the left ventricle. Because echocardiography has a low accuracy for detecting right ventricular dysfunction, CMR or radionuclide angiography is preferred for this evaluation. Initially, global systolic dysfunction may be apparent only during stress induced by dobutamine or phenylephrine, indicating reduced systolic reserve. In advanced stages, the region of myocarditis at the apex becomes an aneurysm, and the global systolic function of the left and right ventricles deteriorates.[11,17]

Imaging Studies

RADIONUCLIDE IMAGING (see Chap. 17). Myocardial ischemia in the absence of coronary obstruction often occurs in patients with Chagas' disease and probably relates to autonomic denervation and inflammatory damage in the coronary endothelium. Transient or permanent perfusion defects are often observed, particularly in the apex and inferolateral segments of the left ventricle. Similar changes in coronary endothelium-dependent or -independent vasodilation may also accompany idiopathic dilated cardiomyopathy, suggesting that microvascular dysfunction is unlikely to be pathogen-dependent, but rather is an early sign of ventricular disease.[13,15]

CARDIAC MAGNETIC RESONANCE (see Chap. 18). CMR with delayed hyperenhancement can demonstrate areas of myocardial fibrosis, even in individuals in the indeterminate phase. Early detection of areas of fibrosis may be useful for the characterization and treatment of arrhythmogenic foci and estimation of the severity of myocardial damage.[11,30]

Management

Antitrypanosomal Drug Treatment

Nitrofuran and nitroimidazole derivatives (nifurtimox and benznidazole, respectively) remain the treatment of choice for Chagas' disease.

These compounds exert their trypanosomicidal action by the generation of superoxide anions, causing oxidative stress and cell death in the parasites.[35] In the acute phase or congenital infection, both compounds significantly reduce the parasite load and improve serologic test results. In the indeterminate phase, however, the results are less promising. Although treatment with nitroimidazole derivatives, especially benznidazole, can reduce the blood parasite load and titers of specific antibodies, their effectiveness in delaying or preventing the onset of chronic symptomatic disease is unknown.

In individuals in the chronic phase of Chagas' disease, the benefit of this type of treatment is even less clear. In these subjects, the disappearance of specific antibodies is not common and can take as long as 10 to 20 years. The DNA of the parasite is present in various tissues, and parasite antigens can induce an immune response during treatment and perhaps even disease progression. Current evidence does not demonstrate substantial clinical benefit in the antiparasitic treatment of patients in the chronic phase of Chagas' disease. Recommendations for antitrypanosomal drug treatment vary among different patient categories.[31]

Concomitant Treatment

In the acute phase of the disease, symptoms disappear spontaneously within 2 months. In rare cases of severe acute myocarditis, concomitant treatment with corticosteroids or immunosuppressants has been attempted empirically, with inconsistent results. Studies are too scarce in this small group of patients to validate this treatment strategy. In the chronic phase, mortality from Chagas' disease is caused primarily by heart failure and life-threatening arrhythmias. The treatment of heart failure should resemble that for other cardiomyopathies (see Chap. 28).[36]

In patients with severe heart failure, cardiac transplantation is feasible. Although immunosuppression may cause some complications in patients with Chagas' disease, including reactivation of the disease[37] or the development of cancer,[38] the clinical complications are well known and preventive strategies are well established. Current strategies for changing the degree of immunosuppression, especially the substitution of mycophenolate mofetil for azathioprine or low doses of mycophenolate mofetil, have proven effective in reducing Chagas' disease reactivation.[39] Monitoring for parasitemia is required and reactivation warrants causative treatment.

Prevention of sudden death is of high priority in patients with heart failure secondary to Chagas' disease. As in other patients with heart failure, treatment with amiodarone reduces the incidence of complex ventricular arrhythmias and sudden death. Its effectiveness, however, is further attenuated in patients with severe systolic dysfunction. Thus, ablation by catheter or surgical procedures and implantation of an implantable cardioverter-defibrillator (ICD) is frequently required (see Chaps. 38 and 41). Reentry is the primary arrhythmogenic substrate for ventricular tachyarrhythmias in Chagas' disease, and the circuits typically localize in the perianeurysmal zone or in focal areas of fibrosis in the inferolateral segment of the left ventricle. Surgical aneurysmectomy associated with myocardial or endocardial resection and/or isolation of reentry sites by endocardectomy or cryoablation guided by electrophysiologic mapping has been a treatment of choice.[32,33] Nevertheless, because the mortality of the procedure is high, surgical ablation should be considered in the absence of severe systolic dysfunction and when other surgical procedures, such as aneurysmectomy, are indicated.

Simultaneous percutaneous ablation of endocardial and epicardial sites is an alternative approach for the treatment of patients with Chagas' disease and recurrent ventricular tachycardia who are unfit for surgery. The sites of reentry could be endocardial, intramural, or epicardial, so this combined approach is essential for the treatment of recurrent ventricular tachycardia in these patients. In addition, in patients with severe systolic dysfunction, especially those with left ventricular ejection fraction below 30%, the implantation of an ICD is recommended.

Symptomatic or high-risk bradycardia is often manifested in these patients and limits antiarrhythmic treatment. Thus, concomitant pacemaker and ICD implantation is often indicated. ICDs can prevent death caused by ventricular tachyarrhythmias, but frequent shocks triggered by tachycardia, whether life-threatening or not, may reduce quality of life. Therefore, a combination of ICD, antiarrhythmic therapy, and catheter ablation is the ideal approach for these patients.[32,33]

Chagas' Disease in the United States

An estimated 100,000 individuals infected with *T. cruzi* are in the United States, placing this nation in the top 10 countries with regard to the prevalence of Chagas' disease. Most infected individuals acquired the infection in endemic areas and then migrated to North America, resulting in many unrecognized chronic infections in the United States. There is a small risk of vector-borne infection; approximately six species of insect vectors inhabit the United States. Many common animal species can provide reservoirs for infections, including rodents, dogs, ungulates, squirrels, and skunks. The major cause of new *T. cruzi* infections in North America is transfusion or aquisition from transplanted organs. Screening of donated blood in the United States using a U.S. Food and Drug Administration (FDA)–approved ELISA for *T. cruzi* was instituted in 2007. This program has identified those with unrecognized infection.

The antitrypanosomal drugs benznidazole and nifurtimox are available from the Centers for Disease Control and Prevention (CDC), through the CDC drug service (http://www.cdc.gov/). An excellent recent review provides details regarding the evaluation and treatment of Chagas' disease in the United States, including an algorithm for evaluation of the patient with newly diagnosed *T. cruzi* infection.[31]

REFERENCES

Background

1. Coura JR: Chagas disease: What is known and what is needed—a background article. Mem Inst Oswaldo Cruz 102(Suppl 1):113, 2007.
2. Moncayo A, Silveira AC: Current epidemiological trends for Chagas disease in Latin America and future challenges in epidemiology, surveillance and health policy. Mem Inst Oswaldo Cruz 104 Suppl 1:17, 2007.
3. Andrade Z, Andrade S: Patologia. *In* Brener Z, Andrade Z (eds): Trypanosoma cruzi e doença de Chagas. Guanabara, Brazil, Koogan, 1979, pp 199-248.
4. Bocchi EA, Bellotti G, Mocelin AO, et al: Heart transplantation for chronic Chagas' heart disease. Ann Thorac Surg 61:1727, 1996.

Pathophysiology

5. Cunningham DS, Grogl M, Kuhn RE: Suppression of antibody responses in humans infected with Trypanosoma cruzi. Infect Immun 30:496, 1980.
6. Pereira Barretto AC, Mady C, Arteaga-Fernandez E, et al: Right ventricular endomyocardial biopsy in chronic Chagas' disease. Am Heart J 111:307, 1986.
7. Rossi MA: Fibrosis and inflammatory cells in human chronic chagasic myocarditis: Scanning electron microscopy and immunohistochemical observations. Int J Cardiol 66:183, 1998.
8. Higuchi Mde L, Benvenuti LA, Martins Reis M, Metzger M: Pathophysiology of the heart in Chagas' disease: Current status and new developments. Cardiovasc Res 60:96, 2003.
9. Jones EM, Colley DG, Tostes S, et al: Amplification of a Trypanosoma cruzi DNA sequence from inflammatory lesions in human chagasic cardiomyopathy. Am J Trop Med Hyg 48:348, 1993.
10. Lopes E, Chapadeiro E, Almeida H, Rocha A: Contribuição ao estudo da anatomia patológica dos corações de chagásicos falecidos subitamente. Rev Soc Bras Med Trop 9:269, 1975.
11. Rochitte CE, Oliveira PF, Andrade JM, et al: Myocardial delayed enhancement by magnetic resonance imaging in patients with Chagas' disease: A marker of disease severity. J Am Coll Cardiol 246:1553, 2005.
12. Andrade ZA, Andrade SG, Oliveira GB, Alonso DR: Histopathology of the conducting tissue of the heart in Chagas' myocarditis. Am Heart J 95:316, 1978.
13. Marin-Neto JA, Marzullo P, Marcassa C, et al: Myocardial perfusion abnormalities in chronic Chagas' disease as detected by thallium-201 scintigraphy. Am J Cardiol 69:780, 1992.
14. Higuchi ML, Fukasawa S, De Brito T, et al: Different microcirculatory and interstitial matrix patterns in idiopathic dilated cardiomyopathy and Chagas' disease: A three-dimensional confocal microscopy study. Heart 82:279, 1999.
15. Torres FW, Acquatella H, Condado JA, et al: Coronary vascular reactivity is abnormal in patients with Chagas' heart disease. Am Heart J 129:995, 1995.
16. Higuchi M de L, Gutierrez PS, Aiello VD, et al: Immunohistochemical characterization of infiltrating cells in human chronic chagasic myocarditis: comparison with myocardial rejection process. Virchows Arch A Pathol Anat Histopathol 423:157, 1993.
17. Higuchi M de L, de Morais CF, Pereira Barreto AC, et al: The role of active myocarditis in the development of heart failure in chronic Chagas' disease: A study based on endomyocardial biopsies. Clin Cardiol 10:665, 1987.
18. Araujo FF, Gomes JA, Rocha MO, et al: Potential role of CD4+CD25HIGH regulatory T cells in morbidity in Chagas' disease. Front Biosci 12:2797, 2007.
19. Araujo-Jorge TC, Waghabi MC, Soeiro M de N, et al: Pivotal role for TGF-beta in infectious heart disease: The case of Trypanosoma cruzi infection and consequent Chagasic myocardiopathy. Cytokine Growth Factor Rev 19:405, 2008.

20. Marin-Neto JA, Cunha-Neto E, Maciel BC, Simoes MV: Pathogenesis of chronic Chagas' heart disease. Circulation 115:1109, 2007.
21. Cunha-Neto E, Coelho V, Guilherme L, et al: Autoimmunity in Chagas' disease. Identification of cardiac myosin-B13 Trypanosoma cruzi protein crossreactive T cell clones in heart lesions of a chronic Chagas' cardiomyopathy patient. J Clin Invest 98:1709, 1996.
22. Cunha-Neto E, Dzau VJ, Allen PD, et al: Cardiac gene expression profiling provides evidence for cytokinopathy as a molecular mechanism in Chagas' disease cardiomyopathy. Am J Pathol 167:305, 2005.
23. Fonseca SG, Moins-Teisserenc H, Clave E, et al: Identification of multiple HLA-A*0201-restricted cruzipain and FL-160 CD8+ epitopes recognized by T cells from chronically Trypanosoma cruzi-infected patients. Microbes Infect 7:688, 2005.
24. Bafica A, Santiago HC, Goldszmid R, et al: Cutting edge: TLR9 and TLR2 signaling together account for MyD88-dependent control of parasitemia in Trypanosoma cruzi infection. J Immunol 177:3515, 2006.
25. Bilate AM, Cunha-Neto E: Chagas disease cardiomyopathy: Current concepts of an old disease. Rev Inst Med Trop Sao Paulo 50:67, 2008.
26. Teixeira MM, Gazzinelli RT, Silva JS: Chemokines, inflammation and Trypanosoma cruzi infection. Trends Parasitol 18:262, 2002.

Clinical Manifestations and Management

27. Rosemberg S, Chaves CJ, Higuchi ML, et al: Fatal meningoencephalitis caused by reactivation of Trypanosoma cruzi infection in a patient with AIDS. Neurology 42(Pt 1):640, 1992.
28. Sartori AM, Ibrahim KY, Nunes Westphalen EV, et al: Manifestations of Chagas' disease (American trypanosomiasis) in patients with HIV/AIDS. Ann Trop Med Parasitol 101:31, 2007.
29. Acquatella H, Perez JE, Condado JA, Sanchez I: Limited myocardial contractile reserve and chronotropic incompetence in patients with chronic Chagas' disease: Assessment by dobutamine stress echocardiography. J Am Coll Cardiol 33:522, 1999.
30. Bocchi EA, Kalil R, Bacal F, et al: Magnetic resonance imaging in chronic Chagas' disease: Correlation with endomyocardial biopsy findings and gallium-67 cardiac uptake. Echocardiography 15:279, 1998.
31. Bern C, Montgomery SP, Herwaldt BL, et al: Evaluation and treatment of Chagas' disease in the United States: A systematic review. JAMA 298:2171, 2007.
32. d'Avila A, Splinter R, Svenson RH, et al: New perspectives on catheter-based ablation of ventricular tachycardia complicating Chagas' disease: Experimental evidence of the efficacy of near infrared lasers for catheter ablation of Chagas' VT. J Interv Card Electrophysiol 7:23, 2002.
33. Sosa E, Scanavacca M, D'Avila A, et al: Radiofrequency catheter ablation of ventricular tachycardia guided by nonsurgical epicardial mapping in chronic Chagasic heart disease. Pacing Clin Electrophysiol 22(Pt 1):128, 1999.
34. Schenone H: Xenodiagnosis. Mem Inst Oswaldo Cruz 94(Suppl 1):289, 1999.
35. Villar JC, Marin-Neto JA, Ebrahim S, Yusuf S: Trypanocidal drugs for chronic asymptomatic Trypanosoma cruzi infection. Cochrane Database Syst Rev (1):CD003463, 2002.
36. Ramires FJ, Salemi VM, Ianni BM, et al: Aldosterone antagonism in an inflammatory state: Evidence for myocardial protection. J Renin Angiotensin Aldosterone Syst 7:162, 2006.
37. Bacal F, Silva CP, Bocchi EA, et al: Mycophenylate mofetil increased Chagas' disease reactivation in heart transplanted patients: Comparison between two different protocols. Am J Transplant 5:2017, 2005.
38. Bocchi EA, Higuchi ML, Vieira ML, et al: Higher incidence of malignant neoplasms after heart transplantation for treatment of chronic Chagas' heart disease. J Heart Lung Transplant 17:399, 1998.
39. Bacal F, Silva CP, Pires PV, et al: Transplantation for Chagas' disease: an overview of immunosuppression and reactivation in the last two decades. Clin Transplant 24:E29, 2010.

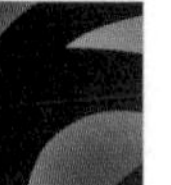

CHAPTER 72 Cardiovascular Abnormalities in HIV-Infected Individuals

Stacy D. Fisher and Steven E. Lipshultz

Background

Infection with the human immunodeficiency virus (HIV) is one of the leading causes of acquired heart disease and specifically of symptomatic heart failure and pulmonary arterial hypertension (**Table 72-1**). Cardiac complications of HIV infection tend to occur late in the disease or are associated with related therapies and are therefore becoming more prevalent as therapy and longevity improve.[1-6] Complicated drug therapies for HIV infection have sustained life but may increase cardiovascular risk and accelerate atherosclerotic disease and events.[7]

Approximately 33 million adults and children were living with HIV infection at the end of 2007. Two million deaths and 2.7 million new infections were reported that year. In the United States, approximately 10% of those infected are older than 50 years and more than 85% of HIV-infected individuals survive more than 10 years.[8,9] The 2- to-5-year incidence of symptomatic heart failure ranges from 4% to 28%,[1,10] suggesting a prevalence of symptomatic HIV-related heart failure of between 4 and 5 million cases worldwide. Among HIV-infected children, up to 10 years of age, 25% die with chronic cardiac disease, and 28% experience serious cardiac events after an AIDS-defining illness.[11] Antiretroviral therapy clearly increases survival, and goals now involve balancing survival and toxicities with therapy. As survival improves, atherosclerotic cardiovascular disease has become an increasingly important cause of morbidity and mortality among patients with HIV infection (**Fig. 72-1**).

A range of cardiac abnormalities (see Table 72-1) associated with HIV infection has been suggested by autopsy studies; the conditions, in order of frequency, are pericardial effusion, lymphocytic interstitial myocarditis, dilated cardiomyopathy (frequently with myocarditis), infective endocarditis, and malignancy (myocardial Kaposi sarcoma and B-cell immunoblastic lymphoma).[3,4] Even more prevalent are drug effects and interactions, which directly challenge the cardiovascular system.

Left Ventricular Dysfunction

Left Ventricular Systolic Dysfunction

CLINICAL PRESENTATION. In HIV-infected patients, concurrent pulmonary infections, pulmonary hypertension, anemia, portal hypertension, malnutrition, or malignancy can alter or confuse the characteristic signs that define heart failure in other populations. Thus, patients with left ventricular systolic dysfunction can be asymptomatic or can present with New York Heart Association Class III or IV heart failure.

Echocardiography (see Chap. 15) is useful for assessing left ventricular systolic function in this population and, in addition to diagnosing left ventricular dysfunction, often reveals low to normal wall thickness or left ventricular hypertrophy and a dilated left ventricle.[5,12] Echocardiography should be performed in any patient at elevated cardiovascular risk, with any clinical manifestations of cardiovascular disease, or with unexplained or persistent pulmonary symptoms or viral coinfections at baseline and every 1 to 2 years thereafter, or as clinically indicated.[11]

Electrocardiography (see Chap. 13) can reveal nonspecific conduction defects or repolarization changes. The chest radiograph has low sensitivity and specificity for congestive heart failure in patients with HIV infection.[13] In small studies of HIV-infected patients and large populations of patients without HIV infection, brain natriuretic peptide levels have been inversely correlated with left ventricular ejection fraction and can be useful in the differential diagnosis of congestive cardiomyopathy in HIV-infected patients.[14]

Patients with encephalopathy are more likely to die of congestive heart failure than those without encephalopathy (hazard ratio, 3.4).[15] HIV persists in reservoir cells in the myocardium and the cerebral cortex, even after antiretroviral therapy. These cells seem to be important in the development and progression of cardiomyopathy and encephalopathy. Reservoir cells may hold HIV on their surfaces for extended periods of time and cause progressive tissue damage by chronic release of cytotoxic cytokines.

INCIDENCE. A 4-year observational study of 296 patients with a spectrum of HIV-related disease before highly active antiretroviral therapy (HAART) found 44 (15%) with dilated cardiomyopathy (fractional shortening < 28%, with global left ventricular hypokinesis), 13 (4%) with isolated right ventricular dysfunction (right ventricle larger than left ventricle on standard two-dimensional views), and 12 (4%) with borderline left ventricular dysfunction (left ventricular end-systolic diameter > 58 mm but fractional shortening > 28%, or global dysfunction reported by one or two but not all three observers).[1] Dilated cardiomyopathy was strongly associated with a CD4 count lower than 100 cells/mL.[5]

Left ventricular (LV) dysfunction is a common consequence of HIV infection in children. In a study of 205 children infected with HIV by maternal-fetal transmission (enrolled at a median age of 22 months and observed with echocardiography every 4 to 6 months and with electrocardiography, Holter monitoring, and chest radiography every year), the prevalence of decreased left ventricular function (fractional shortening < 28%) was 5.7%. The 2-year cumulative incidence was 15.3%.[4] The cumulative incidence of symptomatic congestive heart failure, the use of cardiac medications, or both was 10% over 2 years.[16] Progressive LV dilation is common in HIV-infected children, may be a harbinger of congestive heart failure (CHF; 5-year cumulative incidence, 12.3%), and is associated with inadequate LV hypertrophy, elevated afterload, and reduced LV function.

PATHOGENESIS. A wide variety of possible causative agents has been postulated for HIV-related cardiomyopathy (see Table 72-1), including myocardial infection with HIV itself, opportunistic infections,

TABLE 72-1 Summary of HIV-Associated Cardiovascular Diseases

TYPE OF DISEASE	POSSIBLE CAUSES	INCIDENCE, PREVALENCE	DIAGNOSIS	TREATMENT
Dilated cardiomyopathy	Drug-related: Cocaine, AZT, IL-2, doxorubicin, interferon Infectious: HIV, toxo-plasma, coxsackievirus group B, EBV, CMV, adenovirus Metabolic or endocrine: selenium or carnitine deficiency, anemia, hypocalcemia, hypophosphatemia, hyponatremia, hypokalemia, hypoalbuminemia, hypothyroidism, growth hormone deficiency, adrenal insufficiency, hyperinsulinemia, hemochromatosis, pheochromocytoma, sarcoidosis, amyloidosis Cytokines: TNF-α, nitric oxide, TGF-β, endothelin-I, interleukins Immunodeficiency: CD4 < 100 cells/mm^3 Autoimmune factors	≤8% of asymptomatic patients; ≤25% of autopsy cases; systolic > diastolic	Chest radiograph findings: Nonspecific conduction abnormalities, PVCs, PACs Echocardiographic findings: Low-normal LV wall thickness, increased LV mass, dilated LV, systolic LV dysfunction. Possible laboratory studies: Troponin T, brain natriuretic peptide, CD4 count, viral load, viral PCR, *Toxoplasma* serology, thyroid-stimulating hormone, cortisol, carnitine, selenium, serum ACE, vanillylmandelic acid, amyloid, urinanalysis, stress testing, myocardial biopsy, cardiac catheterization	Diuretics, digoxin, ACE inhibitors, beta blockers Adjunctive treatment in HIV patients: Treatment of infection, nutritional replacement, IVIg Intensify antiretroviral therapy Follow-up: Serial echocardiograms
Pericardial	Bacteria: *Staphylococcus, Streptococcus, Proteus, Klebsiella Enterococcus, Listeria, Nocardia, Mycobacterium* Viral pathogens: HIV, HSV, CMV, adenovirus, echovirus Other pathogens: *Cryptococcus, Toxoplasma, Histoplasma* Malignancy: Kaposi sarcoma, lymphoma, capillary leak, wasting, malnutrition Hypothyroidism Immunodeficiency Uremia	11%/yr; spontaneous resolution in 42% of affected patients; ≈30% increase in 6-mo mortality	Pericardial rub on examination Echocardiogram Fluid analysis for gram stain, and culture, cytology ECG: Low voltage, PR depression Associated pleural and peritoneal fluid analysis Pericardial biopsy	Treat the cause Follow-up: Serial echocardiograms Intensify antiretroviral therapy Pericardiocentesis or window
Infective endocarditis	Autoimmune factors Bacteria: *Staphylococcus aureus* or *Staphylococcus epidermidis, Salmonella, Streptococcus, Haemophilus parainfluenzae, Pseudallescheria boydii*, HACEK (see Chap. 67) Fungal: *Aspergillus fumigatus, Candida, Cryptococcus neoformans*	6% increased incidence in IVDA, regardless of HIV status	Blood cultures; echocardiogram	IV antibiotics, valve replacements
Nonbacterial thrombotic endocarditis	Valvular damage, vitamin C deficiency, malnutrition, wasting, DIC, hypercoagulable state, prolonged acquired immunodeficiency	Rare but clinically relevant emboli in 42% of cases	Echocardiogram	Anticoagulation, treat vasculitis or underlying illness
Malignancy	Kaposi sarcoma, non-Hodgkin lymphoma, leiomyosarcoma, low CD4 count, prolonged immunodeficiency, HHV-8, EBV	Approximately 1% incidence; usually metastatic in HIV-positive patients	Echocardiogram, biopsy	Chemotherapy possible
Right ventricular and pulmonary disease	Recurrent pulmonary infections, pulmonary arteritis, microvascular pulmonary emboli		ECG, echocardiogram, right heart catheterization	Diuretics, treat underlying lung infection or disease, anticoagulation
Primary pulmonary hypertension	Plexogenic pulmonary arteriopathy	0.5%	ECG, echocardiogram, right heart catheterization	Anticoagulation, vasodilators, prostacyclin analogues
Vasculitis	Drug therapy with antibiotics and antivirals	Increasing incidence	Clinical diagnosis	Systemic corticosteroids, withdrawal of drug
Accelerated atherosclerosis	Protease inhibitors, atherogenesis with virus-infected macrophages, chronic inflammation, glucose intolerance, dyslipidemia	≤8% prevalence	Stress testing, echocardiogram, lipid profile, CT angiogram, calcium scoring	Minimize risk factors, exercise, controversial statin use
Autonomic dysfunction	CNS disease, drug therapy, prolonged immunodeficiency, malnutrition	Increased in patients with CNS disease	Tilt-table test, Holter monitoring	Procedural precautions
Arrhythmias	Drug therapy, pentamidine, autonomic dysfunction, acidosis electrolyte abnormalities		ECG: Long-QT, Holter monitoring, exercise stress testing	Discontinue drug, procedural precautions
Lipodystrophy	Drug therapy: Protease inhibitors		Echocardiogram, lipid profile, cardiac catheterization, coronary calcium score	Lipid therapy (beware of drug interactions), aerobic exercise, altered antiretroviral, therapy, cosmetic surgery, fat implantation

CMV = cytomegalovirus; DIC = disseminated intravascular coagulation; EBV = Epstein-Barr virus; ECG = electrocardiogram; HSV = herpes simplex virus; HTN = hypertension; IVDA = intravenous drug abuse; IVIg = intravenous immunoglobulin; PAC = premature atrial complex; PCR = polymerase chain reaction; PVC = premature ventricular complex.

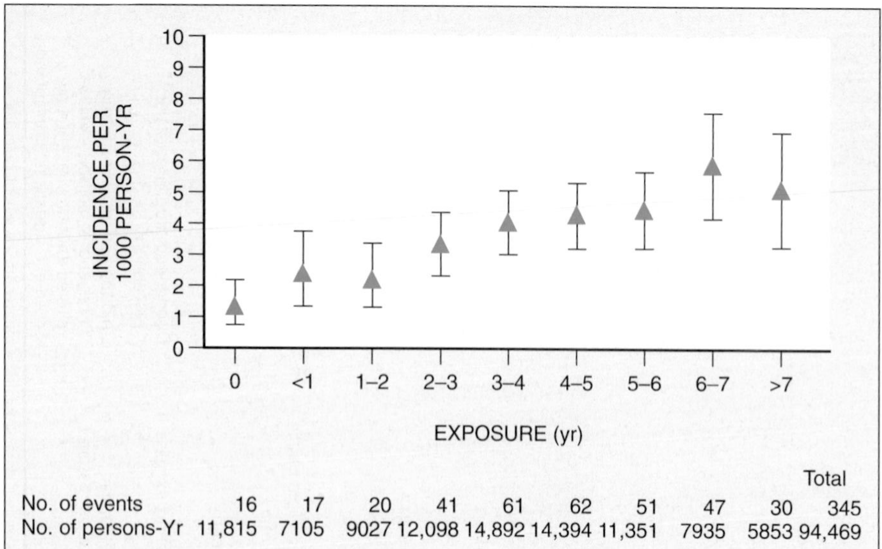

FIGURE 72-1 Risk of myocardial infarction according to exposure to combination antiretroviral therapy. The crude incidence of primary events was assessed beginning at baseline according to the cumulative duration of combination antiretroviral therapy since the initiation of therapy, stratified in 1-year intervals from the initiation of therapy to more than 7 years of exposure. The adjusted relative rate of myocardial infarction according to cumulative exposure to combination antiretroviral therapy was 1.16/year of exposure (95% confidence interval [CI], 1.09 to 1.23). The I bars denote the 95% CIs. *(From DAD Study Group: Class of antiretroviral drugs and the risk of myocardial infarction. N Engl J Med 356:1723, 2007.)*

viral infections, autoimmune response to viral infection, cardiotoxicity or direct mitochondrial injury from therapeutic or illicit drugs, nutritional deficiencies, and cytokine overexpression.

Myocarditis is perhaps the best studied of the possible causes (see Chap. 70). Dilated cardiomyopathy can be related to a direct action of HIV on the myocardial tissue or to proteolytic enzymes or cytokine mediators induced by HIV alone or in conjunction with coinfecting viruses.[16-18] *Toxoplasma gondii*, coxsackievirus group B, Epstein-Barr virus, cytomegalovirus, adenovirus, and HIV in myocytes have been found in biopsy specimens.

Autopsy and biopsy results have revealed only scant and patchy inflammatory cell infiltrates in the myocardium.[11,17] HIV can clearly infect myocardial interstitial cells but not the cardiac myocyte. Increased numbers of infected interstitial cells have been found in patients with confirmed myocarditis in which proteolytic enzymes or increased levels of tumor necrosis factor-α (TNF-α) or interleukin may injure the myocytes. Increased levels of TNF-α, inducible nitric oxide synthase, and interleukin-6 in affected patients and experimental models have been reported.

Notably, HIV-related cardiomyopathy is often not associated with any specific opportunistic infection, and approximately 40% of patients have not experienced any opportunistic infection before the onset of cardiac symptoms.[11]

Pathogenesis in Children

In children with vertically transmitted HIV infection, two mechanisms of pathogenesis have been described. One is dilation of the left ventricle with a reduction in the ratio of thickness to end-systolic dimension of the ventricle. The other is concentric hypertrophy of the muscle; with dilation, the ratio of thickness to end-systolic dimension remains normal or is increased.[5]

CYTOKINE ALTERATIONS. HIV infection increases the production of TNF-α, which alters intracellular calcium homeostasis and increases nitric oxide production, transforming growth factor-β, and endothelin-1 upregulation.[15] High levels of nitric oxide induced experimentally had a negative inotropic effect and were cytotoxic to myocytes.

In one study, HIV-infected individuals with dilated cardiomyopathy were much more likely to have myocarditis and had a broader spectrum of viral infections than HIV-negative patients with idiopathic dilated cardiomyopathy. Also, levels of TNF-α and induced nitric oxide synthase were higher in myocytes from the HIV-infected patients with dilated cardiomyopathy, particularly those with viral coinfections, and levels varied inversely with the CD4 count. Immunodeficiency may favor the selection of those viral variants with increased pathogenicity or enhance the cardiovirulence of viral strains.[15,17]

NUTRITIONAL DEFICIENCIES. Nutritional deficiencies are common in HIV infection, particularly in those with late-stage disease. Poor absorption and diarrhea both lead to electrolyte imbalances and deficiencies in elemental nutrients. Deficiencies of trace elements have been associated with cardiomyopathy. For example, selenium deficiency increases the virulence of coxsackie virus to cardiac tissue.[11] Selenium replacement reverses cardiomyopathy and restores LV function in nutritionally depleted patients. Levels of vitamin B_{12}, carnitine, and growth and thyroid hormone can also be altered in HIV disease; all have been associated with LV dysfunction.

COURSE OF DISEASE. Patients with asymptomatic LV dysfunction (fractional shortening < 28%, with global left ventricular hypokinesis) may have transient disease by echocardiographic criteria. In one serial echocardiographic study, three of six patients with abnormal fractional shortening had normal readings after a mean of 9 months. The three with persistently depressed LV function died within 1 year of baseline.[11]

PROGNOSIS. Mortality in HIV-infected patients with cardiomyopathy is increased, independently of CD4 count, age, gender, and HIV risk group. The median survival to AIDS-related death was 101 days in patients with LV dysfunction and 472 days in patients with a normal heart at a similar stage of infection before HAART (see Fig. 72-1).[1,11] Isolated right ventricular dysfunction or borderline LV dysfunction did not place patients at risk.

In the Pediatric Pulmonary and Cardiovascular Complications of Vertically Transmitted HIV Infection (P2C2 HIV) study of children with vertically transmitted HIV infection (median age, 2.1 years), 5-year cumulative survival was 64%.[10] Mortality was higher in children with baseline measurements showing depressed left ventricular fractional shortening or increased LV dimension, thickness, mass, wall stress, heart rate, or blood pressure. Decreased LV fractional shortening and increased wall thickness also predicted survival after adjustment for age, height, CD4 count, HIV RNA copy number, clinical center, and encephalopathy[3,4] (**Fig. 72-2**).

Fractional shortening was abnormal for up to 3 years before death, whereas wall thickness identified a population at risk only 18 to 24 months before death. Thus, in children, fractional shortening may be a useful long-term predictor, and wall thickness may be a useful short-term predictor of mortality.[19]

Postmortem cardiomegaly was associated with echocardiographic evidence of increased LV mass and documented chronically increased heart rate before death but not with anemia, encephalopathy, or HIV viral load.[12] In HIV-infected children, mild persistent depression of LV function and elevated LV mass were associated with higher all-cause mortality.[19] A 2-SD decrease in LV fractional shortening from 34% to 30% in a 10-year old, levels that most cardiologists would not consider to be action values, is associated with an increase in 5-year mortality from 15% to 55%.

Rapid-onset congestive heart failure has a grim prognosis in HIV-infected adults and children, with more than half of patients dying

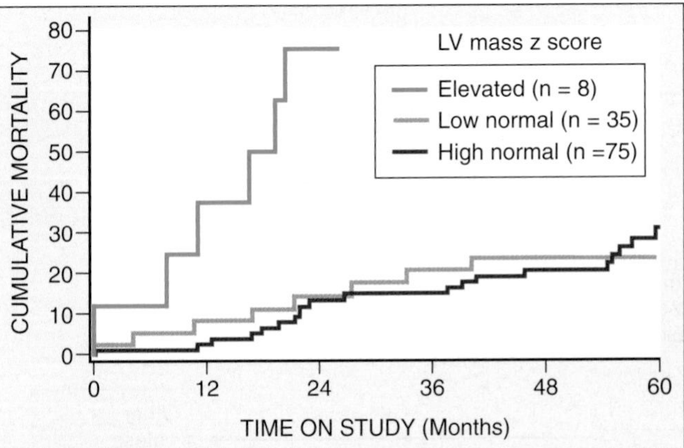

FIGURE 72-2 Mildly increased LV mass is a risk marker for early HIV mortality, even though it is still inadequate for LV dimension. This National Heart, Lung and Blood Institute study shows cumulative mortality in 113 HIV-infected children by degree of LV mass abnormality. *(From Fisher SD, Easley KA, Orav EJ, et al: Mild dilated cardiomyopathy and increased LV mass predict mortality: The prospective P2C2 HIV Multicenter Study. Am Heart J 150:439, 2005.)*

from primary cardiac failure within 12 months of presentation.[10,11] Chronic-onset heart failure may respond better to medical therapy in these patients.

THERAPY. Therapy for dilated cardiomyopathy associated with HIV infection is generally similar to therapy for nonischemic cardiomyopathy. It includes diuretics, digoxin, beta blockers, aldosterone antagonists, and angiotensin-converting enzyme (ACE) inhibitors, as tolerated (see Chap. 28). No studies have investigated the efficacy of specific cardiac therapeutic regimens other than intravenous immunoglobulin.[2] A suggested evaluation of cardiac dysfunction is presented in **Figure 72-3**.

Opportunistic or other infections should be sought aggressively and treated to improve or resolve the cardiomyopathy. Right ventricular biopsy may be useful for identifying infectious causes of failure and to suggest targeted therapy.[11,13] However, right ventricular biopsy is probably underused.

After medical therapy is begun, serial echocardiographic studies should be performed at 4-month intervals (see Fig. 72-3).[13] Monitoring recommendations for testing and timing of follow-up are based on studies relating impairment of fractional shortening to a worse prognosis. If function continues to worsen or the clinical course deteriorates, a biopsy should be considered. Patients with congestive heart failure who have not responded to 2 weeks of medical therapy may benefit from cardiac catheterization and endomyocardial biopsy, which may reveal lymphocytic infiltrates suggesting myocarditis or treatable opportunistic infections (by special stains), permitting aggressive therapy of an underlying pathogen. Tissue should be evaluated for the presence of abnormal mitochondria that could benefit from an antiretroviral drug holiday. Angiography should be performed selectively if there are risk factors for atherosclerotic disease or suggestive clinical symptoms.

Intravenous immunoglobulins have had some success in treating acute congestive cardiomyopathy and nonspecific myocarditis in patients who are not infected with HIV. Monthly immunoglobulin infusions in HIV-infected children have minimized LV dysfunction, increased LV wall thickness, and reduced peak LV wall stress, suggesting that both impaired myocardial growth and LV dysfunction can be immunologically mediated.[2]

Patients should be evaluated for nutritional status, and any patients with deficiencies should receive supplements. Supplementation with selenium, carnitine, multivitamins, or all three can be helpful, especially for anorexic patients or those with wasting or diarrhea syndromes.

Heart transplantation has been reported, including one HIV-infected man believed to have anthracycline-related cardiomyopathy. At 24 months of follow-up, his course was complicated by more frequent and higher grade episodes of rejection than average, but otherwise was relatively uneventful and productive.[20] Transplantation therapy is not currently widely available but is an area of active consideration and discussion.

ANIMAL MODELS. Chronic pathogenic simian immunodeficiency virus (SIV) infection in rhesus macaques has resulted in marked depression of LV ejection fraction and extensive coronary arteriopathy suggestive of a cell-mediated immune response.[21] Notably, 9 of 15 chronically infected macaques who died of SIV had myocardial pathology with lymphocytic myocarditis, and 9 had coronary arteriopathy (6 alone and 3 in combination with myocarditis). Coronary arteriopathy was associated with evidence of vessel occlusion and recanalization, with associated areas of myocardial necrosis in four animals. Two animals had marantic endocarditis, and one had a LV mural thrombus. Animals with cardiac pathology were emaciated to a greater extent than those with SIV and similar periods of infection who did not experience cardiac pathology.

Transgenic mouse models with cardiac pathologic changes have been studied and may help evaluate the impact of environmental factors, therapeutic or illicit drugs, or drug combinations in both the cause and treatment of HIV-associated myocarditis.[22]

Left Ventricular Diastolic Dysfunction

Clinical and echocardiographic findings suggest that diastolic dysfunction (see Chaps. 25 and 27) is relatively common in long-term survivors of HIV infection. LV diastolic dysfunction may precede systolic dysfunction.[7,16,18]

Pericardial Effusion (see Chap. 75)

CLINICAL PRESENTATION. HIV-infected patients with pericardial effusions generally have a lower CD4 count than those without effusions, indicating more advanced disease.[7,18] Effusions are generally small and asymptomatic.

INCIDENCE. Asymptomatic pericardial effusions are common in HIV-infected patients. The 5-year Prospective Evaluation of Cardiac Involvement in AIDS (PRECIA) study found that 16 of 231 patients (59 patients with asymptomatic HIV, 62 with AIDS-related complex, and 74 with AIDS) had pericardial effusions.[18] Three had an effusion on enrollment and 13 experienced effusions during follow-up (12 had AIDS). Pericardial effusions were small (maximum pericardial space < 10 mm at end-diastole) in 13 and asymptomatic in 14 patients. The incidence of pericardial effusion in those with AIDS was 11%/year. The prevalence of effusion in AIDS patients increases over time, reaching a mean in asymptomatic patients of about 22% after 25 months of follow-up.

HIV infection should be suspected whenever young patients have pericardial effusion or tamponade. In a retrospective series of cardiac tamponade cases in a city hospital, 13 of 37 patients (35%) had HIV infection.[11]

PATHOGENESIS. Pericardial effusion may be related to an opportunistic infection, metabolic abnormality, or malignancy (see Table 72-1), but usually the cause is not clear. The effusion is often part of a generalized serous effusive process also involving pleural and peritoneal surfaces. This capillary leak syndrome may be related to enhanced cytokine production in the later stages of HIV disease. Other causes can include uremia from HIV-associated nephropathy or drug nephrotoxicity. Fibrinous pericarditis with or without effusion is also well described, constituting 9% of cardiac lesions found in AIDS patients in one autopsy series.[18]

COURSE OF DISEASE AND PROGNOSIS. Effusion markedly increases mortality. For example, in the PRECIA study, it almost tripled the risk of death among AIDS patients.[17] Also, 2 of 16 patients with effusions experienced pericardial tamponade. Pericardial effusion may, however, resolve spontaneously in up to 42% of patients.[11]

MONITORING AND THERAPY. Screening echocardiography is recommended for HIV-infected individuals, regardless of the stage of disease.[13] All HIV-infected patients with evidence of heart failure, Kaposi sarcoma, tuberculosis, or other pulmonary infections should undergo baseline echocardiography and electrocardiographic testing.

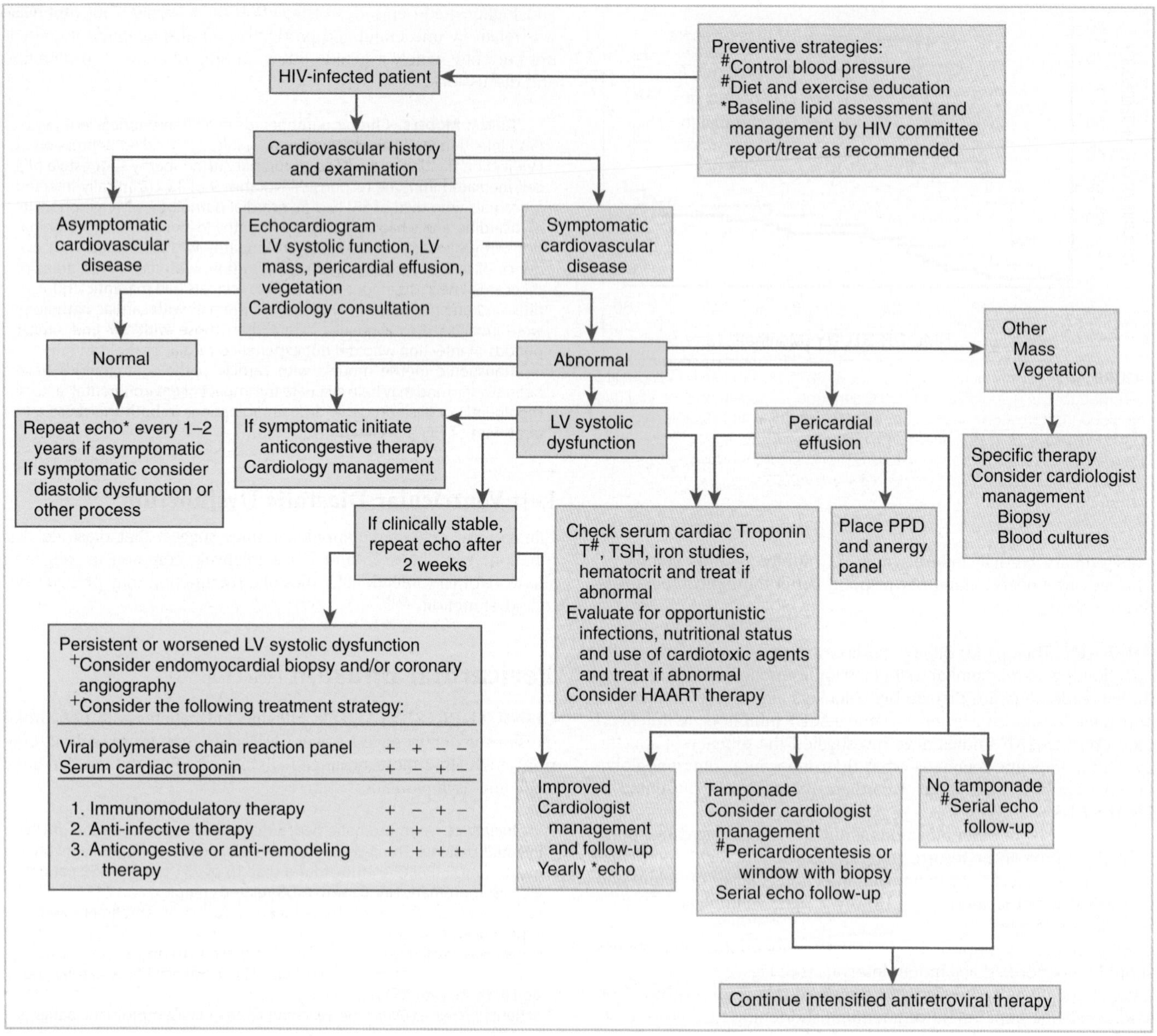

HIV-infected patient

Preventive strategies:
#Control blood pressure
#Diet and exercise education
*Baseline lipid assessment and management by HIV committee report/treat as recommended

Cardiovascular history and examination

Asymptomatic cardiovascular disease

Echocardiogram
LV systolic function, LV mass, pericardial effusion, vegetation
Cardiology consultation

Symptomatic cardiovascular disease

Normal

Abnormal

Other
Mass
Vegetation

Repeat echo* every 1–2 years if asymptomatic
If symptomatic consider diastolic dysfunction or other process

If symptomatic initiate anticongestive therapy
Cardiology management

LV systolic dysfunction

Pericardial effusion

Specific therapy
Consider cardiologist management
Biopsy
Blood cultures

If clinically stable, repeat echo after 2 weeks

Check serum cardiac Troponin T#, TSH, iron studies, hematocrit and treat if abnormal
Evaluate for opportunistic infections, nutritional status and use of cardiotoxic agents and treat if abnormal
Consider HAART therapy

Place PPD and anergy panel

Persistent or worsened LV systolic dysfunction
+Consider endomyocardial biopsy and/or coronary angiography
+Consider the following treatment strategy:

Viral polymerase chain reaction panel	+	+	–	–
Serum cardiac troponin	+	–	+	–
1. Immunomodulatory therapy	+	–	+	–
2. Anti-infective therapy	+	+	–	–
3. Anticongestive or anti-remodeling therapy	+	+	+	+

Improved
Cardiologist management and follow-up
Yearly *echo

Tamponade
Consider cardiologist management
#Pericardiocentesis or window with biopsy
Serial echo follow-up

No tamponade
#Serial echo follow-up

Continue intensified antiretroviral therapy

FIGURE 72-3 Cardiac dysfunction in HIV-infected patients. *Evidence-based; #non-HIV standard of care data; +considered for future research. PPD = purified protein derivative; TSH = thyroid-stimulating hormone. *(From Dolin R, Masur H, Saag MS [eds]: AIDS Therapy. 2nd ed. New York, Churchill Livingstone, 2003, p 817.)*

Patients should undergo pericardiocentesis if they have pericardial effusion and clinical signs of tamponade (e.g., elevated jugular venous pressure, dyspnea, hypotension, persistent tachycardia, pulsus paradoxus) or echocardiographic signs of tamponade (e.g., continuous-wave Doppler evidence of respiratory variation in valvular inflow, septal bounce, right ventricular diastolic collapse, a large effusion).

Patients with pericardial effusion without tamponade should be evaluated for treatable opportunistic infections, such as tuberculosis, and for malignancy. Highly active antiretroviral therapy (HAART) should be considered if therapy has not already been instituted. Repeated echocardiography is recommended after 1 month, or sooner if clinical symptoms direct (see Fig. 72-3).

Other Disorders

Infective Endocarditis

Injection drug users are at greater risk than the general population for infective endocarditis, chiefly of right-sided heart valves (see Chap. 67). Surprisingly, HIV-infected patients may not have a higher incidence of endocarditis than people with similar risk behaviors.[7]

Because the autoimmune response to bacterial endocarditis is often largely responsible for the valvular destruction associated with endocarditis, the course of the disease in HIV-infected patients may vary. For example, HIV-infected patients have a higher risk of salmonella endocarditis than immunocompetent patients because they are more likely to experience salmonella bacteremia during salmonella infection. However, they respond better to antibiotic therapy and may be less likely to sustain valvular damage because of their impaired immune response.[11,18,23]

Common organisms associated with endocarditis in HIV-infected patients include *Staphylococcus aureus* and *Salmonella* species. Fungal endocarditis with organisms such as *Aspergillus fumigatus*, *Candida* species, and *Cryptococcus neoformans* are more common in intravenous drug users with HIV than in those without it, and again may be responsive to therapy (see Table 72-1).[11]

Fulminant courses of infective endocarditis with high mortality can occur in late-stage AIDS patients with poor nutritional status and severely compromised immune systems, but several patients have been successfully treated with antibiotic therapy. Operative indications in HIV-infected patients with endocarditis include hemodynamic instability, failure to sterilize blood cultures after appropriate intravenous antibiotics, and severe valvular destruction in patients with a reasonable life expectancy after recovery from surgery.

Nonbacterial Thrombotic Endocarditis

Nonbacterial thrombotic endocarditis (or marantic endocarditis) involves large, friable, sterile vegetations that form on the cardiac valves. These lesions have been associated with disseminated intravascular coagulation and systemic embolization. Lesions are rarely diagnosed ante mortem; among patients who do receive the diagnosis, clinically relevant emboli occur in a high percentage of cases.[11] In the early HIV epidemic, several case series suggested a high incidence of this uncommon disorder; however, few cases have since been reported, and almost none have been found in prospective series. Marantic endocarditis should be suspected in any patient with systemic embolization, but should be considered rare in AIDS patients.

Treatment of nonbacterial thrombotic endocarditis should focus on reducing the underlying disease causing coagulation abnormalities, valvular endothelial damage, or both. An anticoagulation risk-benefit assessment must be made on an individual basis.

Cardiovascular Malignancy

Malignancy affects many AIDS patients, generally in the later stages of disease (see Chap. 74). Cardiac malignancy is usually metastatic disease.

Kaposi sarcoma (angiosarcoma) is associated with human herpesvirus 8 and affects up to 35% of AIDS patients, particularly homosexuals, with an incidence inversely related to the CD4 count. Autopsy studies have found that 28% of HIV-infected patients with widespread Kaposi sarcoma had cardiac involvement and rarely described it as a primary cardiac tumor.[3] Kaposi sarcoma has not been found invading the coronary arteries but is often an endothelial cell neoplasm, with a predilection in the heart for subpericardial fat around the coronary arteries.

Kaposi sarcoma involving the heart is generally an incidental finding at autopsy and rarely causes cardiac symptoms. Specific symptoms can be related to pericardial effusion associated with the epicardial location of the tumor. Pericardial fluid in patients with cardiac Kaposi sarcoma is typically serosanguineous, without malignant cells or infection.[3]

Kaposi sarcoma is difficult to treat, although most affected patients die from opportunistic infections related to the advanced stage of immunodeficiency rather than from the malignancy. Protease inhibitors have significantly decreased the incidence of Kaposi sarcoma from the reported incidence in the pre-HAART era.[24]

Primary cardiac malignancy associated with HIV infection is generally caused by cardiac lymphoma. Non-Hodgkin lymphomas are 25 to 60 times more common in HIV-infected individuals. They are the first manifestation of AIDS in up to 4% of new cases.[3] Patients with primary cardiac lymphoma can present with dyspnea, right-sided heart failure, biventricular failure, chest pain, or arrhythmias. Cardiac lymphoma is associated with rapid progression to cardiac tamponade, symptoms of congestive heart failure, myocardial infarction (MI), tachyarrhythmias, conduction abnormalities, or superior vena cava syndrome. Pericardial fluid typically reveals malignant cells but can be histologically normal. Systemic multiagent chemotherapy with and without concomitant radiation or surgery has been beneficial for some patients, but overall the prognosis is poor (**Fig. 72-4**). HAART has not substantially affected the incidence of HIV-related non-Hodgkin lymphomas, but cumulative viremia has been associated, even during HAART therapy.[25] An intracardiac mass in late-stage HIV infection is associated with a uniformly poor prognosis.

Isolated Right Ventricular Disease

Isolated right ventricular hypertrophy, with or without right ventricular dilation, is relatively uncommon in HIV-infected individuals and is generally related to pulmonary disease that increases pulmonary vascular resistance. Possible causes include multiple bronchopulmonary infections, pulmonary arteritis from the immunologic effects of HIV disease, or microvascular pulmonary emboli caused by thrombus or contaminants in injected drugs.

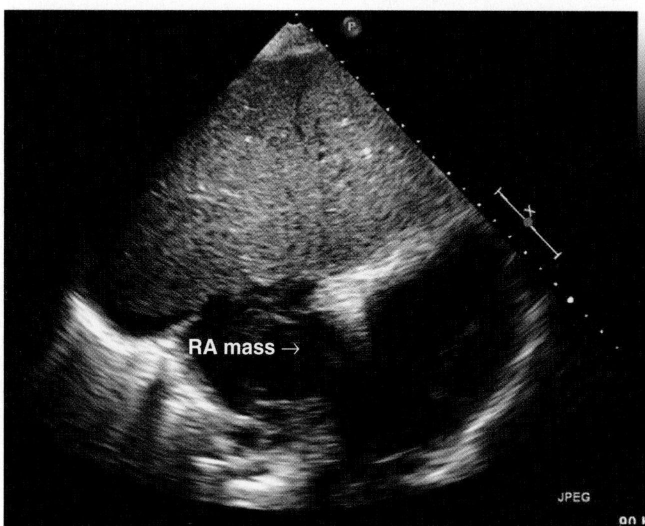

FIGURE 72-4 Burkitt's lymphoma in an AIDS patient. This four-chamber apical echocardiogram view shows near obliteration of the right atrial (RA) cavity, with tumor invading through hepatic veins directly into the right atrium.

Pulmonary Hypertension

Primary pulmonary arterial hypertension (see Chap. 78) has been described in a disproportionate number of HIV-infected individuals, estimated to occur in about 0.5% of hospitalized AIDS patients,[4,7] Histologic analysis often reveals plexogenic pulmonary arteriopathy characterized by remodeling of the pulmonary vasculature, with intimal fibrosis and replacement of normal endothelial structure. All these patients had clear lung fields on examination and chest radiography and normal perfusion scans.

Primary pulmonary arterial hypertension (PAH) has been reported in HIV-infected patients without a history of thromboembolic disease, intravenous drug use, or pulmonary infections associated with HIV.[4] One autopsy and one biopsy specimen revealed precapillary muscular pulmonary artery and arteriole medial hypertrophy, fibroelastosis, and eccentric intimal fibrosis, without direct viral infection of pulmonary artery cells. This finding suggests mediator release from infected cells elsewhere. Primary PAH has also been found in hemophiliacs receiving lyophilized factor VIII, intravenous drug users, and patients with LV dysfunction, obscuring any relationship with HIV. A controversial association is present between human herpesvirus 8 (HHV-8) and PAH. It may be that HIV or a coinfection causes endothelial damage and mediator-related vasoconstriction of the pulmonary arteries.

The CD4 count has been independently associated with survival in HIV PAH patients, and pulmonary hypertension was the direct cause of death in 72% of those affected. Survival rates at 1, 2, and 3 years were 73%, 60%, and 47%, respectively. Survival rates in New York Heart Association functional Class III and IV patients at the time of diagnosis were 60%, 45%, and 28%.[26,27]

A high rate or response has been reported to vasodilator testing (37%) in HIV PAH patients.[27,28] Standard treatments for PAH including prostaglandin E5 (PGE5) inhibitors, endothelin antagonists, and prostacyclin analogues have all been shown effective in the HIV infected population. Therapy also includes anticoagulation (on the basis of individual risk-benefit analysis). HAART has been continued in affected patients. Notably, in HIV PAH patients, the PAH is the immediate threat to life and should be aggressively approached. Best current practice is to follow guidelines set for PAH patients because the morbidity and mortality reflect the PAH more than the HIV infection and respond to current strategies.

Vasculitis

Clinically, suspicion occurs in the setting of fever of unknown origin, unexplained multisystem disease, unexplained arthritis or myositis, glomerulonephritis, peripheral neuropathy, especially mononeuritis multiplex, or unexplained gastrointestinal, cardiac, or central nervous system (CNS) ischemia. Many types of vasculitis (see Chap. 89) have been described in HIV-infected patients, including systemic necrotizing vasculitis, hypersensitivity vasculitis, Henoch-Schönlein purpura, lymphomatoid granulomatosis, and primary angiitis of the CNS. Successful immunomodulatory therapy, chiefly with systemic corticosteroid therapy, has been described.

HIV protein transactivator of transcription (tat) has been implicated in the pathogenesis of vasculitis, where transduction of this gene into a monocyte cell line led to TNF-α and TNF-β production.

Accelerated Atherosclerosis

Accelerated atherosclerosis (see Chap. 43) has been observed in young HIV-infected adults and children without traditional coronary risk factors.[29,30] Pronounced coronary lesions were discovered at autopsy in several HIV-positive patients 23 to 32 years of age who died unexpectedly. Endothelial dysfunction is possibly the most plausible link between HIV infection and atherosclerosis. Increased expression of adhesion molecules such as intercellular adhesion molecule-1 (ICAM)-1 and endothelial adhesion molecule (E-selectin) and inflammatory cytokines such as TNF)-α and interleukin-6 (IL-6) have been reported in HIV-positive patients. Higher plasma TNF-α, IL-6, and von Willebrand factor levels also correlate with viral load, supporting the presence of endothelial response to injury.[31,32] Clinically, this also may manifest after percutaneous coronary interventions; restenosis may be higher in these patients than in other populations.

Premature cerebrovascular disease is common in AIDS patients. The prevalence of stroke in AIDS patients was estimated to be 8% on review of autopsy records between 1983 and 1987. Of the patients with stroke, 4 of 13 had evidence of cerebral emboli, and in 3 of those 4, the embolus had a clear cardiac source.[31]

Protease inhibitor therapy markedly alters lipid metabolism and can be associated with premature atherosclerotic disease. Chronic inflammatory states have also been associated with premature atherosclerotic vascular disease. Atherosclerotic disease in the HIV-infected individual is believed to be multifactorial in cause and prone to plaque rupture, possibly related to the host environment.[32] In a large, prospective observational study, the adjusted risk of MI was 16%/year of protease inhibitor exposure, an approximate doubling over 5 years. The adjusted risk with non-nucleotide reverse transcriptase inhibitors (NNRTIs) increased by 5%/year, but this was not statistically significant. The risk of MI associated with the use of protease inhibitors was attenuated when traditional risk factors were added to the model, suggesting that some but not all of the protease inhibitor–associated MI risk can be attributed to metabolic changes.[32]

Overall, however, protease inhibitor therapy, specifically HAART, have clearly improved morbidity and mortality, with no short-term evidence of increased cardiovascular mortality.[32] Lipodystrophy, including fat redistribution with increased truncal obesity, temporal wasting, increased triglyceride levels, elevated levels of small, dense low-density lipoproteins, and glucose intolerance, should be recognized and treated because of an elevated 10-year cardiovascular risk.[7,31] Risk stratification based on traditional risk factors, plus diet, alcohol intake, physical exercise, hypertriglyceridemia, cocaine use, heroin use, thyroid disease, renal disease, and hypogonadism, should be considered for long-term cardiac preventive care.[13,30]

Fat redistribution is seen in 42% of children after more than 5 years of antiretroviral therapy.[29] Routine physical and laboratory assessment should be part of routine follow-up to balance cardiovascular risk and necessary HIV therapies. Diet and exercise modification are recommended to reduce cardiovascular risk.

Autonomic Dysfunction

Early clinical signs of autonomic dysfunction (see Chap. 94) in HIV-infected patients include syncope and presyncope, diminished sweating, diarrhea, bladder dysfunction, and impotence. In one study, heart rate variability; Valsalva ratio; cold pressor testing; and hemodynamic responses to isometric exercise, tilt-table testing, and standing showed that autonomic dysfunction occurred in patients with HIV and was pronounced in AIDS patients. AIDS patients receiving HAART were relatively protected. Patients with HIV-associated nervous system disease had the most abnormalities in autonomic function (**Fig. 72-5**).[33] Screening and augmented procedural precautions in patients with clinical symptoms need to be applied.

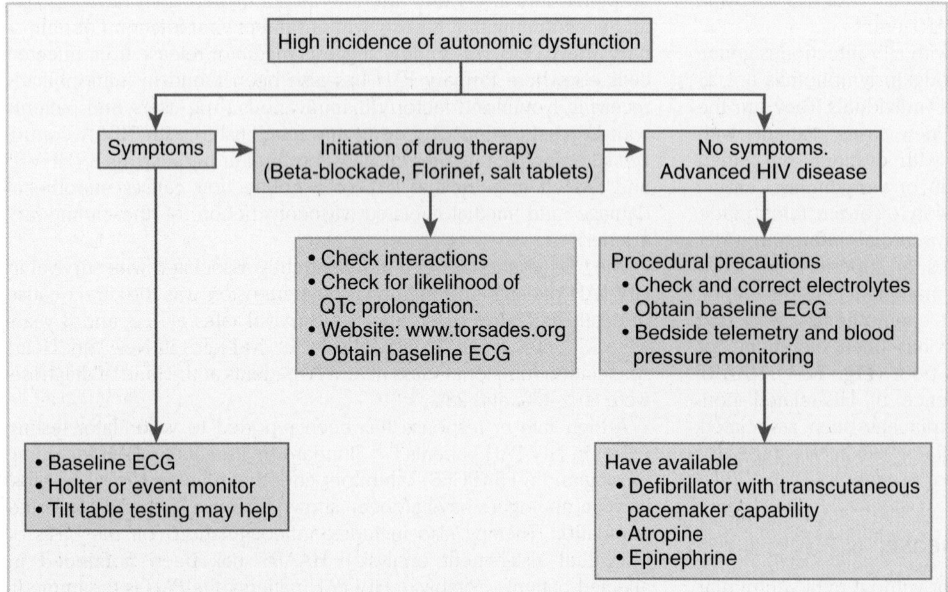

FIGURE 72-5 Evaluation and management of dysautonomia. ECG = electrocardiogram. *(From Dolin R, Masur H, Saag MS [eds]: AIDS Therapy. 2nd ed. New York, Churchill Livingstone, 2003, p 817.)*

Long-QT Interval

HIV infection is associated with QT prolongation and torsades de pointes ventricular tachycardia; the incidence increases with progression to AIDS (see Chaps. 36 and 39).[34] Hepatitis C is independently associated with increased QT duration, and coinfection with HIV almost doubles the risk of clinically important QT prolongation (i.e., QT_c values of 470 milliseconds or longer). The risk of QT prolongation was 16% with HIV alone and 30% with both HIV and hepatitis C infections.[35]

Complications of Therapy for HIV

Complications in Adults

Potent antiretroviral medications and HAART, which generally combines three or more agents and usually includes a protease inhibitor, have clearly increased the life span and quality of life of HIV-infected patients.[9] However, protease inhibitors, particularly when used in combination therapy or in HAART, are associated with lipodystrophy, fat wasting and redistribution, metabolic abnormalities, hyperlipidemia, insulin resistance, and increased atherosclerotic risk (**Fig. 72-6**). HIV-infected patients treated with protease inhibitors have reported substantial decreases in total body fat with peripheral lipodystrophy (fat wasting of the face, limbs, and buttocks) and relative conservation or enhancement of central adiposity (truncal obesity, breast enlargement, and buffalo hump) compared with patients who have not received protease inhibitors. Lipid alterations associated with protease inhibitors include higher triglyceride, total cholesterol, insulin, lipoprotein (a), and C-reactive protein levels and lower high-density lipoprotein levels, all promoting an atherogenic profile.[29]

Lipid abnormalities vary with different protease inhibitors. Ritonavir has the most adverse effects on lipids, with a mean increase in total cholesterol of 2.0 mmol/L and a mean increase in triglyceride level of 1.83 mmol/L. More modest increases of total cholesterol without marked triglyceride increases were found in patients taking indinavir and nelfinavir. Combination with saquinavir did not further elevate total cholesterol. Protease inhibitor therapy increased lipoprotein(a) by 48% in patients with elevated pretreatment values (>20 mg/dL).[36] In some cases, switching protease inhibitors may reverse elevations in triglyceride levels and abnormal fat deposition. Low-level aerobic exercise may also help reverse lipid abnormalities.[7,37]

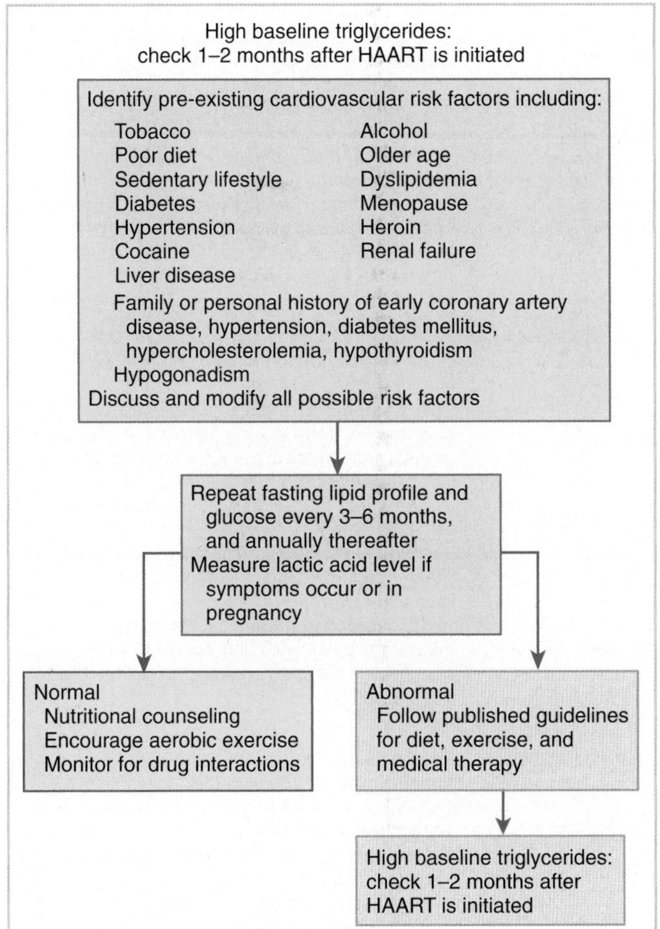

FIGURE 72-6 Cardiovascular considerations when initiating HAART.

Zidovudine (azidothymidine, AZT) has been implicated in skeletal muscle myopathies. In culture, AZT causes a dose-dependent destruction of human myotubes. Human cultured cardiac muscle cells treated with AZT have developed mitochondrial abnormalities, and NNRTIs in general have been associated with altered mitochondrial DNA replication.[38] However, cardiac myopathies have not been evident in clinical data. Rarely, patients with LV dysfunction have improved with cessation of AZT therapy.

Intravenous pentamidine, used to treat *Pneumocystis jiroveci* pneumonia in patients intolerant of trimethoprim-sulfamethoxazole, has been associated with cases of torsades de pointes and refractory ventricular tachycardia.[11,38] Pentamidine should be reserved for patients whose QTc interval is 48 milliseconds or less. Multiple medication reactions and interactions have occurred during the treatment of HIV infection and are a major cause of cardiac emergencies in HIV-infected patients. Common cardiac drug interactions are outlined in **Table 72-2**.

Perinatal Transmission and Vertically Transmitted HIV Infection

Most children with HIV are infected in the perinatal period, but HIV transmission can be minimized if mothers are given antiretroviral therapy in the second and third trimesters or short courses before parturition.[39] The incidence of vertical transmission can be limited to less than 2% with current therapies, some including up to 6 months of neonatal AZT.

Rates of congenital cardiovascular malformations in cohorts of HIV-uninfected and HIV-infected children born to HIV-infected mothers have ranged from 5.6% to 8.9%. These rates were 5 to 10 times higher than those reported in population-based epidemiologic studies but are not higher than in normal populations similarly screened.[11]

In the same cohorts, serial echocardiograms obtained at 4- to 6-month intervals have shown subclinical cardiac abnormalities to be common, persistent, and often progressive.[5] Some dilated cardiomyopathy (LV contractility ≥ 2 SDs below the normal mean; LV end-diastolic dimension ≥2 SDs above the mean) and some had mildly increased cardiac mass for height and weight. Depressed LV function correlated with immune dysfunction at baseline but not longitudinally, suggesting that the CD4 cell count may not be a useful surrogate marker of HIV-associated LV dysfunction. The development of encephalopathy was highly correlated with a decline in fractional shortening.

In children with vertically transmitted HIV-1 infection, disease can progress rapidly or slowly.[10] Rapid progressors have higher heart rates, higher respiratory rates, and lower fractional shortening on serial examinations than nonrapid progressors and HIV-uninfected children who are similarly screened. Rapid progressors have higher 5-year cumulative mortality, higher HIV-1 viral loads, and lower $CD8^+$ (cytotoxic) T-cell counts than nonrapid progressors. Knowing the patterns of disease allows more aggressive therapy to be initiated earlier in rapid progressors.

Evaluating non-HIV infected infants born to HIV infected mothers has shown that fetal exposure to HAART is associated with reduced LV mass, LV dimension, and septal wall thickness and higher LV fractional shortening and contractility during the first 2 years of life. In utero exposure to HAART may impair myocardial growth while initially improving LV function, although LV function was less than normal. These effects are more pronounced in girls. Long-term monitoring of these infants is still needed to define the mechanism of these effects better and to evaluate their long-term clinical importance.[5,40]

Monitoring Recommendations

Routine, systematic cardiac evaluation, including a comprehensive history and thorough cardiac examination, is essential for the care of HIV-infected adults and children. The history should include traditional risk factors, environmental exposures, and therapeutic and illicit drug use. Routine blood pressure monitoring is important because HIV-infected individuals have been reported to experience

TABLE 72-2 Cardiovascular Actions and Interactions of Drugs Commonly Used in HIV Therapy*

CLASS	CARDIAC DRUG INTERACTIONS	CARDIAC SIDE EFFECTS
Antiretroviral		
Nucleotide reverse transcriptase inhibitors	Zidovudine, dipyridamole	Rare—lactic acidosis, hypotension Accelerated risk with cardiopulmonary bypass Zidovudine—skeletal muscle myopathy, myocarditis
Non-nucleotide reverse transcriptase inhibitors	Calcium channel blockers, warfarin, beta blockers, nifedipine, quinidine, steroids, theophylline Delavirdine—can cause serious toxic effects if given with antiarrhythmic drugs and calcium channel blockers	
Protease inhibitors	Metabolized by cytochrome P-450 and interact with other drugs metabolized through this pathway, such as selected antimicrobials, antidepressant, and antihistamine agents; cisapride, HMG-CoA reductase inhibitors (lovastatin, simvastatin), sildenafil Potentially dangerous interactions that require close monitoring or dose adjustment; can occur with amiodarone, disopyramide, flecainide, lidocaine, mexiletine, propafenone, quinidine Ritonavir—most potent cytochrome activator (CYP3A) and P-glycoprotein inhibitor; most likely to interact Indinavir, amprenavir, and nelfinavir—moderate Saquinavir—lowest probability to interact Calcium channel blockers, prednisone, quinine, beta blockers (1.5- to 3-fold increase) Decrease theophylline concentrations	Implicated in premature atherosclerosis, dyslipidemia, insulin resistance, diabetes mellitus, fat wasting and redistribution
Anti-infective		
Antibiotics	Rifampin—reduces therapeutic effect of digoxin by inducing intestinal P-glycoprotein, reduces protease inhibitor concentration and effect Erythromycin—cytochrome P-450 metabolism and drug interactions Trimethoprim-sulfamethoxazole (Bactrim)—increases warfarin effects	Erythromycin—orthostatic hypotension, ventricular tachycardia, bradycardia, torsades (with drug interactions) Clarithromycin—QT prolongation and torsades de pointes Trimethoprim-sulfamethoxazole—orthostatic hypotension, anaphylaxis, QT prolongation, torsades de pointes, hypokalemia Sparfloxacin (fluoroquinolones)— QT prolongation
Antifungal agents	Amphotericin B—digoxin toxicity Ketoconazole or itraconazole—cytochrome P-450 metabolism and drug interactions; increases levels of sildenafil, warfarin, HMG-CoA reductase inhibitors, nifedipine, digoxin	Amphotericin B—hypertension, arrhythmia, renal failure, hypokalemia, thrombophlebitis, bradycardia, angioedema, dilated cardiomyopathy; liposomal formulations still have potential for electrolyte imbalance and QT prolongation Ketoconazole, fluconazole, itraconazole—QT prolongation, torsades de pointes
Antiviral	Ganciclovir—zidovudine	Foscarnet—reversible cardiac failure, electrolyte abnormalities Ganciclovir—ventricular tachycardia, hypotension
Antiparasitic		Pentamidine—hypotension, QT prolongation, arrhythmias (torsades de pointes), ventricular tachycardia, hyperglycemia, hypoglycemia, sudden death; these effects enhanced by hypomagnesemia and hypokalemia
Chemotherapeutic	Vincristine, doxorubicin—decrease digoxin level	Vincristine—arrhythmia, MI, cardiomyopathy, autonomic neuropathy Recombinant human interferon-alfa—hypertension, hypotension, tachycardia, acute coronary events, dilated cardiomyopathy, arrhythmias, sudden death, atrioventricular block, peripheral vasodilation Contraindicated in patients with unstable angina or recent MI IL-2—hypotension, arrhythmia, sudden death, MI, dilated cardiomyopathy, capillary leak, thyroid alterations Anthracyclines (doxorubicin, daunorubicin, mitoxantrone)—myocarditis, cardiomyopathy Liposomal anthracyclines—as above for doxorubicin and vasculitis
Other		
Systemic corticosteroids	Corticosteroids—decrease salicylate levels, increase gastric ulceration in combination with salicylates	Corticosteroids—ventricular hypertrophy, cardiomyopathy, hyperglycemia
Pentoxifylline		Pentoxifylline—decreased triglyceride levels, arrhythmias, chest pain Megestrol acetate—edema, thrombophlebitis, hyperglycemia
Megestrol acetate (Megace)		Epoetin alfa (erythropoietin)—hypertension, ventricular dysfunction
Methadone		Prolonged QT interval
Amphetamines		Increased heart rate and blood pressure

*See Piscitelli SC, Gallicano KD: Interactions among drugs for HIV and opportunistic infections. N Engl J Med 344:984, 2001, for cytochrome P-450 isoforms and selected drugs used in the care of HIV-infected patients.
HMG-CoA = 3-hydroxy-3-methylglutaryl coenzyme A.

hypertension at a younger age and more frequently than in the general population.[11,13,18]

Routine electrocardiographic and Holter monitoring are not warranted unless patients have symptoms such as palpitations, syncope, stroke, or dysautonomia. These tests can also be useful for baseline and monitoring before, during, and after therapies, such as pentamidine, methadone, or antibiotics, that may prolong the QT interval.[13,18]

Asymptomatic cardiac disease related to HIV can be fatal, and cardiac symptoms are often disguised by secondary effects of HIV infection, so systematic echocardiographic monitoring is warranted. We recommend an echocardiogram at the time of HIV diagnosis and every 1 to 2 years thereafter (see Fig. 72-3). Symptomatic patients with HIV infection without cardiovascular abnormalities should have annual echocardiographic follow-up. Echocardiography should also be considered for patients with unexplained or persistent pulmonary symptoms and those with viral coinfection at risk for myocarditis.[13]

An international consensus panel has recommended slightly less aggressive echocardiographic monitoring, with a baseline, for any patient at high risk or with any clinical manifestation of cardiovascular disease, and serial studies repeated every 1 to 2 years or as clinically indicated. Patients with cardiac symptoms should have a formal cardiac assessment, including baseline echocardiography, electrocardiography, and Holter monitoring, and should begin directed therapy.[13] Brain natriuretic peptide levels may be helpful for diagnosing ventricular dysfunction.

In patients with LV dysfunction, serum troponin assays are indicated. Serum troponin level elevations warrant consideration of cardiac catheterization and endomyocardial biopsy. Myocarditis proven by biopsy warrants considering therapy with intravenous immunoglobulin.[2] Cytomegalovirus inclusions on the biopsy specimen support the use of antiviral therapy, and abnormal mitochondria should encourage consideration of a drug holiday from zidovudine. Echocardiography should be repeated after 2 weeks of therapy to allow a more aggressive approach if LV dysfunction persists or worsens and to encourage continued therapy if improvement has occurred.[13]

Because HIV has become a chronic disease, cardiovascular disease will predominate as a cause of mortality and will surface as a vital area of research. Research may translate to other populations if HIV can be used as a model of chronic immunosuppression in a large population. Understanding genetic predispositions to QT prolongation may guide therapy, and determining the causes of cardiomyopathy may benefit diverse research efforts, such as the effects of cytokines, mitochondria, and neurohormonal pathways. Observations such as increased mortality related to LV mass and very mild LV dysfunction may enhance diagnostic testing in at-risk populations affected by other poorly understood cardiomyopathies.

REFERENCES

History

1. Currie PF, Jacob AJ, Foreman AR, et al: Heart muscle disease related to HIV infection: Prognostic implications. BMJ 309:1605, 1994.
2. Lipshultz SE, Orav EJ, Sanders SP, Colan SD: Immunoglobulins and LV structure and function in pediatric HIV infection. Circulation 92:2220, 1995.
3. Jenson HB, Pollock BH: Cardiac cancers in HIV-infected patients. *In* Lipshultz SE (ed): Cardiology in AIDS. New York, Chapman & Hall, 1998, pp 255-263.
4. Saidi A, Bricker JT: Pulmonary hypertension in patients infected with HIV. *In* Lipshultz SE (ed): Cardiology in AIDS. New York, Chapman & Hall, 1998, pp 187-194.
5. Lipshultz SE, Easley KA, Orav EJ, et al: Cardiac dysfunction and mortality in HIV-infected children: The Prospective P2C2 HIV Multicenter Study: Circulation 102:1542, 2000.
6. Felker GM, Thompson RE, Hare JM, et al: Underlying causes and long-term survival in patients with initially unexplained cardiomyopathy. N Engl J Med 342:1077-1084, 2000.

Background

7. Morse CG, Kovacs JA: Metabolic and skeletal complications of HIV infection: The price of success. JAMA 296:844, 2006.
8. UNAIDS (Joint United Nations Programme on HIV/AIDS): 2008 Report on the Global AIDS Epidemic (http://www.unaids.org/en/KnowledgeCentre/HIVData/GlobalReport/2008).
9. Stein JH: Managing cardiovascular risk in patients with HIV infection. J Acquir Immune Defic Syndr 38:115, 2005.
10. Ho JE, Hsue PY: Cardiovascular manifestations of HIV infection. Heart 95:1193, 2009.
11. Al-Attar I, Orav EJ, Exil V, et al: Predictors of cardiac morbidity and related mortality in children with acquired immunodeficiency syndrome. J Am Coll Cardiol 41:1598, 2003.

LV Systolic and Diastolic Dysfunction

12. Kearney DL, Perez-Atayde AR, Easley KA, et al: Postmortem cardiomegaly and echocardiographic measurements of LV size and function in children infected with the human immunodeficiency virus. The Prospective P2C2 HIV Multicenter Study. Cardiovasc Pathol 12:140, 2003.
13. Lipshultz SE, Fisher SD, Lai WW, Miller TL: Cardiovascular risk factors, monitoring, and therapy for HIV-infected patients. AIDS 17:S96, 2003.
14. Mansoor A, Althoff K, Gange S, et al: Elevated NT-pro-BNP levels are associated with comorbidities among HIV-infected women. AIDS Res Hum Retroviruses 25:997, 2009.
15. Fisher SD, Bowles NE, Towbin JA, Lipshultz SE: Mediators in HIV-associated cardiovascular disease: A focus on cytokines and genes. AIDS 17:S29, 2003.
16. Starc TJ, Lipshultz SE, Easley KA, et al: Incidence of cardiac abnormalities in children with human immunodeficiency virus infection: The prospective P2C2 HIV study. J Pediatr 141:327, 2002.
17. Currie PF, Boon NA: Immunopathogenesis of HIV-related heart muscle disease: Current perspectives. AIDS 17:S21, 2003.
18. Sudano I, Spieker LE, Noll G, et al: Cardiovascular disease in HIV infection. Am Heart J 151:1147, 2006.
19. Fisher SD, Easley KA, Orav EJ, et al: Mild dilated cardiomyopathy and increased LV mass predict mortality: The prospective P2C2 HIV Multicenter Study. Am Heart J 150:439, 2005.
20. Calabrese LH, Albrecht M, Young J, et al: Successful cardiac transplantation in an HIV-1–infected patient with advanced disease. N Engl J Med 348:2323, 2003.

Animal Models

21. Yearley JH, Mansfield KG, Carville AA, et al: Antigenic stimulation in the simian model of HIV infection yields dilated cardiomyopathy through effects of TNFalpha. AIDS 22:585, 2008.
22. Kohler JJ, Cucoranu I, Fields E, et al: Transgenic mitochondrial superoxide dismutase and mitochondrially targeted catalase prevent antiretroviral-induced oxidative stress and cardiomyopathy. Lab Invest 89:782, 2009.

Infective Endocarditis

23. Martin-Davila P, Navas E, Fortun J, et al: Analysis of mortality and risk factors associated with native valve endocarditis in drug users: The importance of vegetation size. Am Heart J 150:1099, 2005.

Cardiovascular Malignancy

24. Bruno R, Sacchi P, Filice G: Overview on the incidence and the characteristics of HIV-related opportunistic infections and neoplasms of the heart: Impact of highly active antiretroviral therapy. AIDS 17:S83, 2003.
25. Zoufaly A, Stellbrink HJ, Heiden MA: Cumulative HIV viremia during highly active antiretroviral therapy is a strong predictor of AIDS-related lymphoma. J Infect Dis 200:8, 2009.

Right Ventricular Dysfunction and Pulmonary Hypertension

26. Degano B, Guillaume M, Savale L, et al: HIV-associated pulmonary arterial hypertension: survival and prognostic factors in the modern therapeutic era. AIDS 24:67, 2010.
27. Opravil M, Sereni D: Natural history of HIV-associated pulmonary arterial hypertension: trends in the HAART era. AIDS 22 Suppl 3:S35-S40, 2008.
28. McLaughlin VV, Archer SL, Badesch DB, et al: ACCF/AHA 2009 expert consensus document on pulmonary hypertension: A report of the American College of Cardiology Foundation Task Force on Expert Consensus Documents and the American Heart Association: Developed in collaboration with the American College of Chest Physicians, American Thoracic Society, Inc., and the Pulmonary Hypertension Association. Circulation 119:2250, 2009.

Accelerated Atherosclerosis

29. Grinspoon S, Carr A: Cardiovascular risk and body-fat abnormalities in HIV-infected adults. N Engl J Med 352:48, 2005.
30. Boccara F, Teiger E, Cohen A, et al: Percutaneous coronary intervention in HIV infected patients: Immediate results and long term prognosis. Heart 92:543, 2006.
31. Kotler DP: HIV and antiretroviral therapy: lipid abnormalities and associated cardiovascular risk in HIV-infected patients. J Acquir Immune Defic Syndr 49(Suppl 2):S79, 2008.
32. DAD Study Group, Friis-Møller N, Reiss P, Sabin CA, et al: Class of antiretroviral drugs and the risk of myocardial infarction. N Engl J Med 356:1723, 2007.

Autonomic Dysfunction

33. Correia D, Rodrigues De Resende LA, Molina RJ, et al: Power spectral analysis of heart rate variability in HIV-infected and AIDS patients. Pacing Clin Electrophysiol 29:53, 2006.

Long-QT Interval

34. Sani MU, Okeahialam BN: QTc interval prolongation in patients with HIV and AIDS. J Natl Med Assoc 97:1657, 2005.
35. Nordin C, Kohli A, Beca S, et al: Importance of hepatitis C coinfection in the development of QT prolongation in HIV-infected patients. J Electrocardiol 39:199, 2006.

Complications of Therapy for HIV

36. Fisher SD, Miller TL, Lipshultz SE: Impact of HIV and highly active antiretroviral therapy on leukocyte adhesion molecules, arterial inflammation, dyslipidemia, and atherosclerosis. Atherosclerosis 185:1, 2006.
37. Nanavati KA, Fisher SD, Miller TL, Lipshultz SE: HIV-related cardiovascular disease and drug interactions. Am J Cardiovasc Drugs 4:315, 2004.
38. Zareba KM, Miller TL, Lipshultz SE: Cardiovascular disease and toxicities related to HIV infection and its therapies. Expert Opin Drug Saf 4:1017. 2005.

Perinatal Transmission and Vertically Transmitted HIV Infection

39. Mofenson LM, Brady MT, Danner SP, et al: Guidelines for the Prevention and Treatment of Opportunistic Infections among HIV-exposed and HIV-infected children: Recommendations from CDC, the National Institutes of Health, the HIV Medicine Association of the Infectious Diseases Society of America, the Pediatric Infectious Diseases Society, and the American Academy of Pediatrics. MMWR Recomm Rep 58(RR-11):1, 2009.
40. Lavigne JE, Shearer WT, Thompson B: Cardiovascular outcomes of pediatric seroreverters perinatally exposed to HAART: Design of a longitudinal clinical study. Cardiovasc Toxicol 4:187, 2004.

CHAPTER 73 Toxins and the Heart

Richard A. Lange and L. David Hillis

Because many toxins, some used by a substantial portion of the population, may affect the heart adversely, it is important to understand the myriad of ways in which these substances may influence the cardiovascular system. This chapter focuses on environmental exposures and commonly prescribed pharmacologic agents, as well as frequently used illicit drugs, including cocaine and amphetamines. Chap. 90 discusses the toxicities of various chemotherapeutic agents in greater detail.

Ethanol

An estimated two thirds of Americans occasionally consume ethanol, and approximately 10% are considered to be heavy consumers. Although the ingestion of a moderate amount of ethanol (usually defined as three to nine drinks/week) is associated with a reduced risk of cardiovascular disease, the consumption of excessive amounts has the opposite effect. When ingested in substantial amounts, ethanol may cause ventricular systolic and/or diastolic dysfunction, systemic arterial hypertension, angina pectoris, arrhythmias, and even sudden cardiac death.

Effects of Ethanol on Cardiac Myocyte Structure and Function

Ethanol may cause myocardial damage via several mechanisms (**Table 73-1**).[1] First, ethanol and its metabolites, acetaldehyde and acetate, may exert a direct toxic effect on the myocardium. Second, deficiencies of certain vitamins (e.g., thiamine), minerals (e.g., selenium), or electrolytes (e.g., magnesium, phosphorus, potassium) that sometimes occur in heavy ethanol consumers may adversely affect myocardial function. Third, certain substances that sometimes contaminate alcoholic beverages, such as lead (often found in moonshine) or cobalt, may damage the myocardium.

Ethanol impairs excitation-contraction, mitochondrial oxidative phosphorylation, and cardiac contractility by adversely affecting the function of the sarcolemmal membrane, the sarcoplasmic reticulum, mitochondria, and contractile proteins. Electron microscopic studies of the hearts of experimental animals in close temporal proximity to heavy ethanol ingestion have demonstrated dilated sarcoplasmic reticula and swollen mitochondria, with fragmented cristae and glycogen-filled vacuoles. With sustained exposure to ethanol, myofibrillar degeneration and replacement fibrosis appear. In addition to the effects of ethanol on the myocardial contractile apparatus, acute or chronic consumption may adversely influence myofibrillar protein synthesis. Microscopically, the hearts of chronic heavy consumers of ethanol manifest an increased accumulation of collagen in the extracellular matrix, as well as increased intermolecular cross links.

Effects of Ethanol on Organ Function

Chronic heavy ethanol ingestion may induce left ventricular diastolic and/or systolic dysfunction. Diastolic dysfunction, which is caused at least in part by interstitial fibrosis of the myocardium, is often demonstrable in heavy consumers of ethanol, even in the absence of symptoms or obvious signs. About 50% of asymptomatic chronic alcoholics have echocardiographic evidence of left ventricular hypertrophy with preserved systolic performance. By Doppler echocardiography, the left ventricular relaxation time is often prolonged, the peak early diastolic velocity is reduced, and the acceleration of early diastolic flow is slowed—all manifestations of left ventricular diastolic dysfunction. Abnormal increases in left ventricular filling pressure during volume or pressure loading may be observed.

Ethanol may induce asymptomatic left ventricular systolic dysfunction, even when it is ingested by healthy individuals in relatively small quantities, as occurs in subjects who are considered social drinkers. As many as 30% of asymptomatic chronic alcoholics have echocardiographic evidence of left ventricular systolic dysfunction. With continued heavy ethanol ingestion, these subjects often develop symptoms and signs of congestive heart failure, which is caused by a dilated cardiomyopathy (see Chap. 68). In fact, ethanol abuse is the leading cause of nonischemic dilated cardiomyopathy in industrialized countries, accounting for approximately half of those who carry this diagnosis. The likelihood of developing an ethanol-induced dilated cardiomyopathy correlates with the amount of ethanol that is consumed in a lifetime. Most men who develop an ethanol-induced dilated cardiomyopathy have consumed more than 80 g of ethanol/day (i.e., 1 liter of wine, 8 standard-sized beers, or 0.5 pint of hard liquor) for at least 5 years. Women appear to be even more susceptible to ethanol's cardiotoxic effects, in that they may develop a dilated cardiomyopathy following the consumption of a smaller amount of ethanol daily and over their lifetime when compared with their male counterparts.

Although the heavy intake of ethanol is associated with nonischemic dilated cardiomyopathy, individuals with light to moderate ethanol consumption actually have a lower incidence of congestive

TABLE 73-1 Mechanisms of Ethanol-Induced Myocardial Injury

Direct Toxic Effects
Uncoupling of the excitation-contraction system
Reduced calcium sequestration in sarcoplasmic reticulum
Inhibition of sarcolemmal ATP-dependent Na+/K+ pump
Reduction in mitochondrial respiratory ratio
Altered substrate uptake
Increased interstitial-extracellular protein synthesis
Toxic Effect of Metabolites
Acetaldehyde
Ethyl esters
Nutritional or Trace Metal Deficiencies
Thiamine
Selenium
Electrolyte Disturbances
Hypomagnesemia
Hypokalemia
Hypophosphatemia
Toxic Additives
Cobalt
Lead

heart failure when compared with those who do not drink at all.[2] In patients with left ventricular dysfunction, light to moderate ethanol ingestion does not exacerbate heart failure. In subjects with an ischemic cardiomyopathy, light to moderate ethanol consumption may reduce mortality.[3]

Subjects with markedly symptomatic ethanol-induced dilated cardiomyopathy may manifest a substantial improvement in left ventricular systolic function and symptoms of heart failure with complete abstinence or a dramatic reduction in ethanol consumption (i.e., to less than 60 g of ethanol/day or the equivalent of four standard drinks). Although most of this improvement occurs in the first 6 months of abstinence, it often continues for as long as 2 years of observation.

Ethanol and Systemic Arterial Hypertension

Experts estimate that ethanol is a causative factor in up to 11% of men with hypertension (see Chap. 45). Individuals who consume more than two drinks daily are 1.5 to 2 times more likely to have hypertension when compared with age- and sex-matched nondrinkers. This effect is dose-related and is most prominent when the daily ethanol intake exceeds five drinks (i.e., 30 g of ethanol).[3,4] Social ethanol consumption is associated with a modest rise in systolic arterial pressure, whereas heavy consumption and binge drinking may lead to a substantial increase. Although the mechanism whereby ethanol induces a rise in systemic arterial pressure is poorly understood, studies have demonstrated that ethanol consumption increases plasma levels of catecholamines, renin, and aldosterone, each of which may cause systemic arterial vasoconstriction. In individuals with ethanol-induced hypertension, abstinence often normalizes systemic arterial pressure.

Ethanol and Lipid Metabolism

Ethanol consumption inhibits the oxidation of free fatty acids by the liver, which stimulates hepatic triglyceride synthesis and the secretion of very low-density lipoprotein (LDL) cholesterol. Most commonly, therefore, ethanol consumption causes hypertriglyceridemia. In addition, heavy ingestion may cause an increase in the serum concentrations of total and LDL cholesterol. Regular ethanol consumption increases the serum concentration of high-density lipoprotein (HDL) cholesterol. Subjects with hyperlipidemia should be encouraged to limit their ethanol intake.

TABLE 73-2 Qualitative Effects of Light to Moderate and Heavier Alcohol Intake on Cardiovascular (CV) Risk Factors and Outcomes

CV RISK FACTORS AND OUTCOMES	LIGHT TO MODERATE ALCOHOL INTAKE*	HEAVIER ALCOHOL INTAKE†
Blood pressure	↔	↑↑
HDL-C	↑↑	↑↑↑
Triglycerides	↑	↑↑
LDL-C	↔ or ↓	↑
Platelet aggregability or coagulability	↓	↓↓
Systemic inflammation	↓	↑
CHF	↓	↑↑
CAD (angina, non-fatal MI)	↓↓	↓
Atrial fibrillation	↔	↑↑
Stroke	↓	↑↑
SCD	↓↓	↑

*Less than two drinks/day.
†More than two drinks/day.
↔ = Indicates no or equivocal effect; ↑ = indicates mild effect; ↑↑ = indicates modest effect; ↑↑↑ = indicates substantial effect.

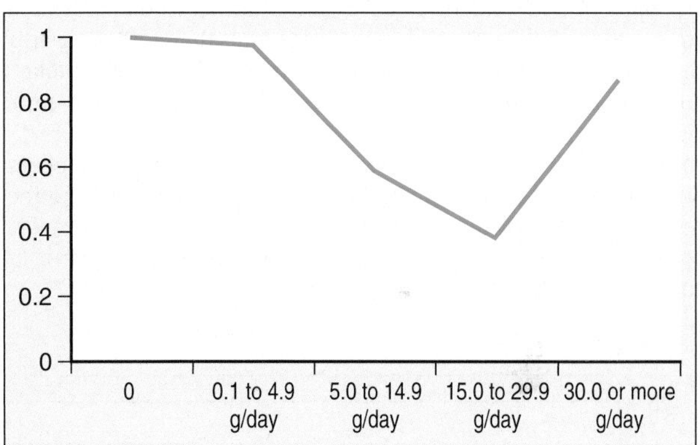

FIGURE 73-1 Relative risk of MI according to daily alcohol intake in men already at low risk for cardiovascular disease on the basis of body mass index, physical activity, smoking, and diet. Moderate alcohol intake is associated with a lower risk of MI.

Coronary Artery Disease

Heavy ethanol use is associated with an increased incidence of atherosclerotic coronary artery disease and resultant cardiovascular morbidity and mortality (see Chaps. 44 and 49). This rise may result at least in part, from the increased likelihood that heavy ethanol consumers (compared with nondrinkers) have systemic arterial hypertension, an increased left ventricular muscle mass (with concomitant diastolic and/or systolic dysfunction), and hypertriglyceridemia (**Table 73-2**). Conversely, light to moderate ethanol intake (two to seven drinks/week) is associated with a decreased risk of cardiovascular morbidity and mortality in men and women.[3-5] Even in men already at low risk for cardiovascular disease on the basis of body mass index, physical activity, smoking, and diet, moderate alcohol intake is associated with a reduced risk of myocardial infarction (MI) (**Fig 73-1**).[6] This lower risk of cardiovascular morbidity and mortality among consumers of moderate amounts of ethanol—when compared with nondrinkers or heavy consumers—is supported by numerous retrospectively and prospectively conducted studies. The French were noted to have a reduced incidence of coronary artery disease when compared with inhabitants of other countries, despite high smoking rates and a diet that is high in fat (the so-called French paradox). Although this diminished incidence initially was attributed to the antioxidant and hemostatic properties of red wine, similar findings subsequently were reported in mild to moderate consumers of other alcoholic beverages and in other study populations.[7] Several prospectively performed cohort studies have demonstrated that drinkers of moderate amounts of ethanol are 40% to 70% less likely to manifest coronary artery disease or ischemic stroke when compared with nondrinkers or heavy consumers.[7] Some studies have suggested that the consumption of all alcoholic beverages exerts such an effect, whereas others have reported that this so-called cardioprotection is strongest with the consumption of wine.[8] The mechanism(s) whereby the consumption of moderate amounts of ethanol reduces cardiovascular risk appear to be multifactorial, in that moderate consumption exerts several beneficial effects, including the following: (1) an increase in the serum concentrations of HDL cholesterol and apolipoprotein A-I; (2) inhibition of platelet aggregation; (3) a decreased serum fibrinogen concentration; (4) increased antioxidant activity (from the phenolic compounds and flavonoids contained in red wine); (5) anti-inflammatory effects (with lower concentrations of white blood cells and C-reactive protein); and (6) improved fibrinolysis resulting from increased concentrations of endogenous tissue plasminogen activator and a concomitant decrease in endogenous plasminogen activator inhibitor activity (**Fig. 73-2**).[5,8]

Men and women manifest a difference in the cardioprotective effect of alcohol (**Fig. 73-3**). The maximal beneficial effect of ethanol occurs at lower doses for women than for men, and the range of alcohol consumption with which it is protective is wider for men than for women. In addition, the relative cardioprotective effect of ethanol is greater for middle-aged and older individuals than for young adults.[8] Light to moderate ethanol consumption is associated with similar risk reductions in coronary artery disease among diabetic and nondiabetic men and women.[9]

In survivors of MI, moderate ethanol consumption appears to reduce subsequent mortality. In the setting of an acute MI, the recent ingestion of ethanol does not appear to reduce infarct size or the propensity for the subsequent appearance of an arrhythmia or heart failure.

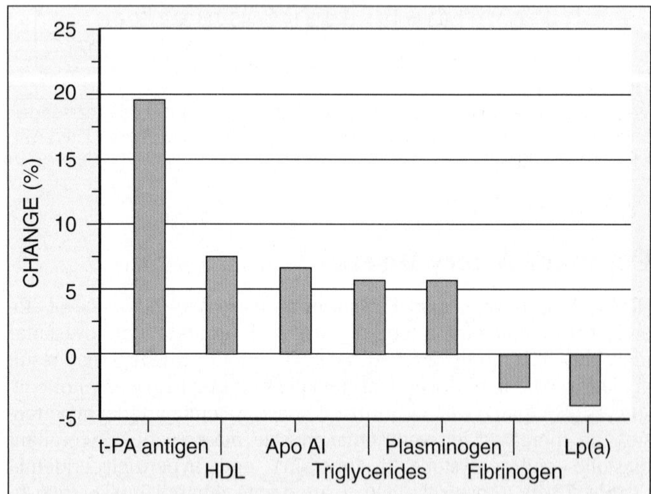

FIGURE 73-2 Percentage change in various serologic variables caused by ethanol ingestion. The ingestion of ethanol, 30 g daily for 1 to 9 weeks, was associated with increased serum concentrations of tissue type plasminogen activator (t-PA) antigen, HDL cholesterol, apolipoprotein A-I (Apo AI), serum triglycerides, and serum plasminogen, as well as decreased concentrations of serum fibrinogen and lipoprotein(a) [Lp(a)]. The reduced risk of cardiovascular events seen in subjects who consume moderate amounts of ethanol may be caused, at least in part, by these beneficial changes in serologic variables. *(From Rimm EB, Williams P, Fosher K, et al: Moderate alcohol intake and lower risk of coronary heart disease: meta-analysis of effects on lipids and haemostatic factors. BMJ 319:1523, 1999.)*

Arrhythmias

Ethanol consumption is associated with a variety of atrial and ventricular arrhythmias, most commonly the following: (1) atrial or ventricular premature beats; (2) supraventricular tachycardia; (3) atrial flutter; (4) atrial fibrillation; (5) ventricular tachycardia; or (6) ventricular fibrillation. The most common ethanol-induced arrhythmia is atrial fibrillation (see Chap. 40). Ethanol is a causative factor in about one third of subjects with new-onset atrial fibrillation; in those younger than 65 years of age, it may be responsible in as many as two thirds. Most episodes occur after binge drinking, usually on weekends or holidays—hence, the term *holiday heart*. Electrophysiologic testing in humans without cardiac disease has shown that ethanol enhances vulnerability to the induction of atrial flutter and fibrillation. The treatment of these ethanol-induced arrhythmias is abstinence.

Ethanol may be arrhythmogenic via several mechanisms. In many ethanol consumers, concomitant factors may predispose to arrhythmias, including cigarette smoking, electrolyte disturbances, metabolic abnormalities, hypertension, or sleep apnea. Acute ethanol ingestion

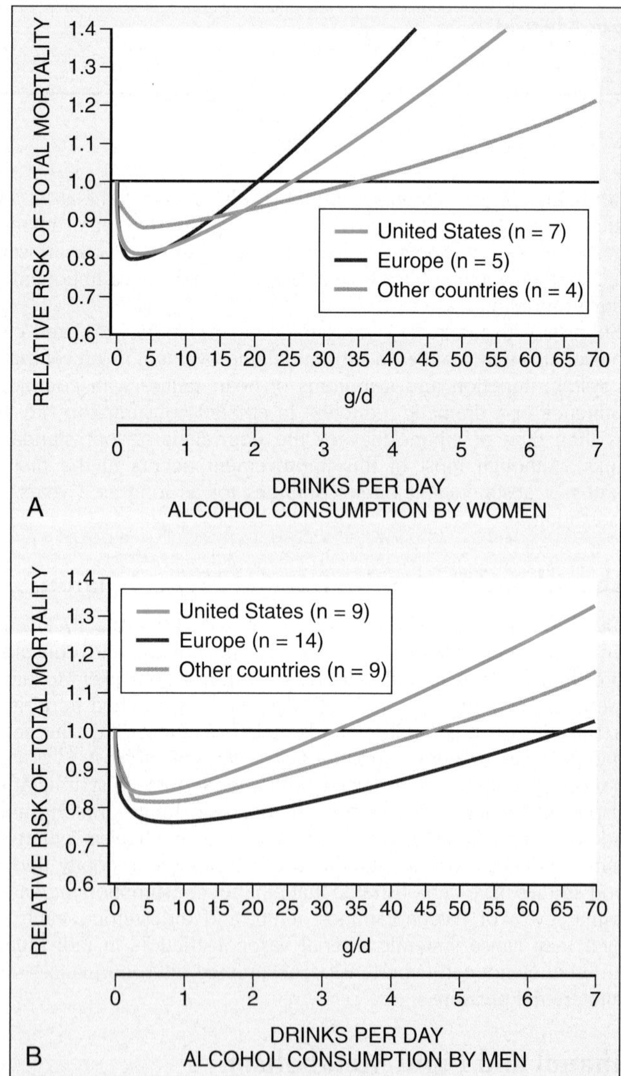

FIGURE 73-3 Relative risk of total mortality and alcohol intake in women **(A)** and men **(B)** in the United States, Europe, and other countries (Australia, Japan, and China). A J-shaped relationship between alcohol consumption and total mortality is observed in men and women. Consumption of alcohol, up to four drinks/day in men and two drinks/day in women, is inversely associated with total mortality. Higher doses of alcohol were associated with increased mortality. The inverse association in women disappears at lower doses than in men. *(From Di Castelnuovo A, Constanzo S, Bagnardi V, et al: Alcohol dosing and total mortality in men and women. An updated meta-analysis of 34 prospective studies. Arch Intern Med 166:2437, 2006.)*

induces a diuresis, which is accompanied by the concomitant urinary loss of sodium, potassium, and magnesium. The presence of myocardial interstitial fibrosis, ventricular hypertrophy, cardiomyopathy, and autonomic dysfunction also may enhance the likelihood of dysrhythmias.

Sudden Death

In subjects without known cardiac disease, the decrease in cardiovascular mortality associated with moderate ethanol intake results largely from a reduction in the incidence of sudden death (**Fig. 73-4**). Of the more than 21,000 men in the Physicians Health Study, those who consumed two to four drinks/week or five to six drinks/week had a significantly reduced risk of sudden death (relative risks, 0.40 and 0.21, respectively) when compared with those who rarely or never drank.[10] In contrast, heavy ethanol consumption (i.e., six or more drinks/day) or binge drinking was associated with an increased risk of sudden death. Heavy ethanol consumption is associated with an increased incidence of sudden death independent of the presence of coronary artery disease (see Chap. 41). The incidence of ethanol-induced sudden death increases with age and the amount of ethanol that is ingested. For example, the daily ingestion of more than 80 g of ethanol is associated with a threefold increased incidence of mortality when compared with a daily consumption of a lesser amount.

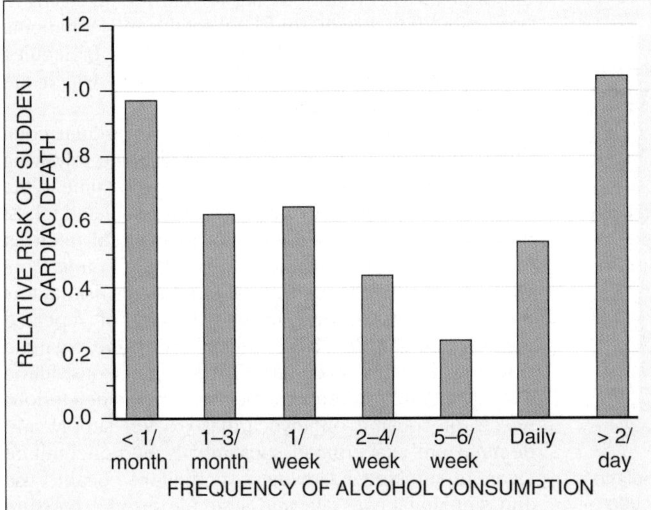

FIGURE 73-4 Ethanol consumption and the risk of sudden cardiac death in U.S. male physicians. In comparison to those who had less than one drink/month (far left bar), those who consumed small or moderate amounts of ethanol (middle bars) had a reduced risk of sudden cardiac death. In contrast, those who consumed at least two drinks/day (far right bar) had an increased risk.

TABLE 73-3 Cardiovascular Complications of Cocaine Use

- Myocardial ischemia
- Angina pectoris
- Myocardial infarction
- Sudden death
- Arrhythmias
- Pulmonary edema
- Myocarditis
- Endocarditis
- Aortic dissection

Cocaine

Cocaine is currently the most commonly used illicit drug among subjects seeking care in hospital emergency departments, and is the most frequent cause of drug-related deaths reported by medical examiners in the United States.[11] Its widespread use is attributable to the following: (1) its ease of administration; (2) the ready availability of relatively pure drug; (3) its relatively low cost; and (4) the misperception that its recreational use is safe. As cocaine abuse has increased in frequency, the number of cocaine-related cardiovascular complications, including angina pectoris, MI, cardiomyopathy, and sudden death, has increased (**Table 73-3**).

Pharmacology and Mechanisms of Action

Cocaine (benzoylmethylecgonine) is an alkaloid extracted from the leaf of the *Erythroxylon coca* bush, which grows primarily in South America. It is available in two forms, the hydrochloride salt and the freebase. Cocaine hydrochloride is prepared by dissolving the alkaloid in hydrochloric acid to form a water-soluble powder or granule, which can be taken orally, intravenously, or intranasally (so-called chewing, mainlining, or snorting, respectively). The freebase form is manufactured by processing the cocaine with ammonia or sodium bicarbonate (baking soda). Unlike the hydrochloride form, freebase cocaine is heat-stable so that it can be smoked. It is known as crack because of the popping sound that it makes when heated.

Cocaine hydrochloride is well absorbed through all mucous membranes; therefore, users may achieve a high blood concentration with intranasal, sublingual, vaginal, or rectal administration. The route of administration determines the rapidity of onset and duration of action (**Table 73-4**). The euphoria associated with smoking crack cocaine occurs within seconds and is short-lived. Crack cocaine is considered the most potent and addictive form of the drug. Cocaine is metabolized by serum and liver cholinesterases to water-soluble metabolites, primarily benzoylecgonine and ecgonine methyl ester, which are excreted in the urine. Because cocaine's serum half-life is only 45 to 90 minutes, it is detectable in blood or urine only for several hours after its use. However, its metabolites persist in blood or urine for 24 to 36 hours after its administration.

When applied locally, cocaine acts as an anesthetic by virtue of its inhibition of membrane permeability to sodium during depolarization, thereby blocking the initiation and transmission of electrical signals. When given systemically, it blocks the presynaptic reuptake of norepinephrine and dopamine, thereby producing an excess of these neurotransmitters at the site of the postsynaptic receptor (**Fig. 73-5**). In short, cocaine acts as a powerful sympathomimetic agent.

Cocaine-Related Myocardial Ischemia and Infarction

Since 1982, numerous reports have associated cocaine use with myocardial ischemia and infarction. In one survey of 10,085 adults 18 to 45 years of age, 25% of nonfatal MIs were attributed to cocaine use.[12] Cocaine-related myocardial ischemia or infarction may result from the following: (1) increased myocardial oxygen demand in the setting of a limited or fixed oxygen supply; (2) marked coronary arterial vasoconstriction; and (3) enhanced platelet aggregation and thrombus formation (**Fig. 73-6**).

TABLE 73-4 Pharmacokinetics of Cocaine According to Route of Administration

ROUTE OF ADMINISTRATION	ONSET OF ACTION	PEAK EFFECT	DURATION OF ACTION
Inhalation (smoking)	3-5 sec	1-3 min	5-15 min
Intravenous	10-60 sec	3-5 min	20-60 min
Intranasal or other mucosal	1-5 min	15-20 min	60-90 min

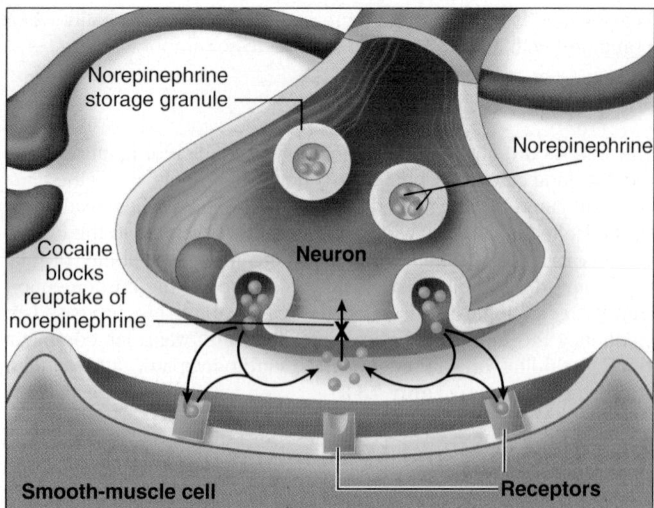

FIGURE 73-5 Mechanism whereby cocaine alters sympathetic tone. Cocaine blocks the reuptake of norepinephrine by the preganglionic neuron, resulting in excess amounts of this neurotransmitter at postganglionic receptor sites.

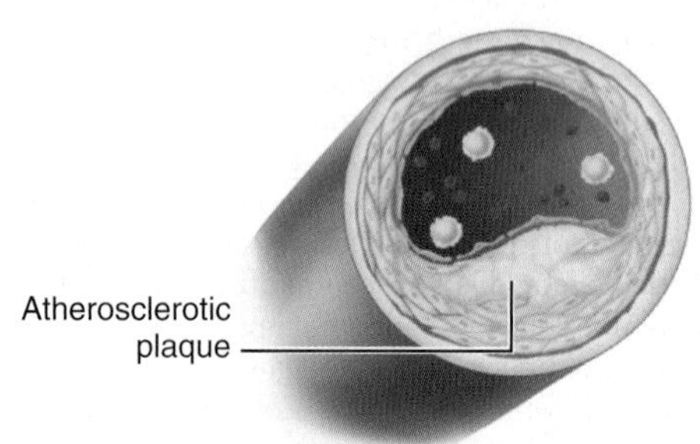

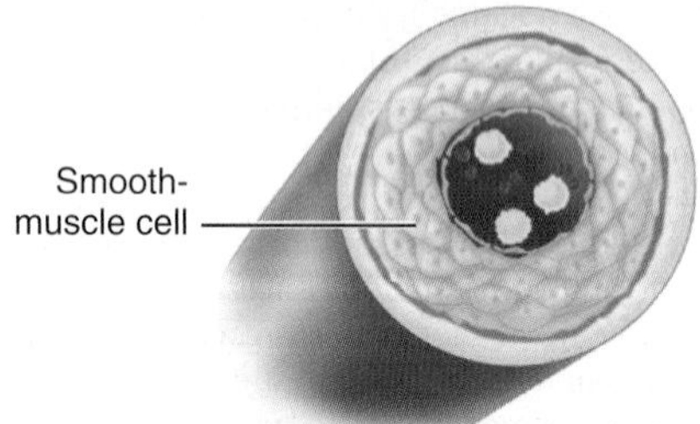

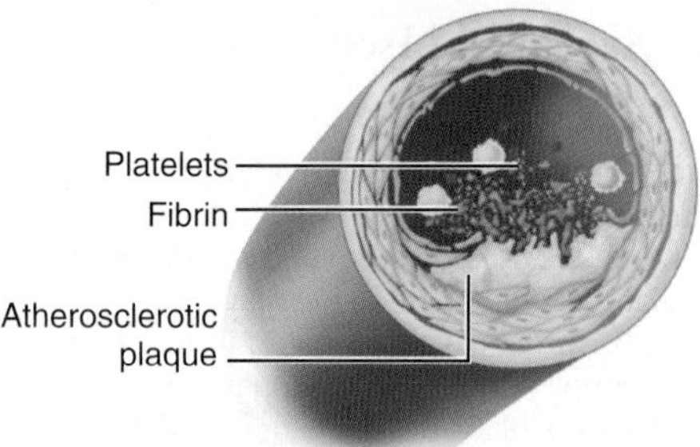

FIGURE 73-6 Mechanisms whereby cocaine may induce myocardial ischemia or infarction. Cocaine may increase the determinants of myocardial oxygen demand in the setting of limited oxygen supply **(top),** cause intense coronary arterial vasoconstriction **(middle),** or induce accelerated atherosclerosis and thrombosis **(bottom).** *(From Lange RA, Hills LD: Cardiovascular complications of cocaine use. N Engl J Med 345:351, 2001.)*

By virtue of its sympathomimetic effects, cocaine increases the three major determinants of myocardial oxygen demand—heart rate, left ventricular wall tension, and left ventricular contractility. At the same time, the ingestion of even small amounts of the drug causes vasoconstriction of the epicardial coronary arteries (so-called inappropriate vasoconstriction), in that myocardial oxygen supply decreases as demand increases. Cocaine induces vasoconstriction in normal coronary arteries but exerts a particularly marked vasoconstrictive effect in diseased segments. As a result, cocaine users with atherosclerotic coronary artery disease probably have an especially high risk for an ischemic event after cocaine use. Cocaine-induced coronary arterial vasoconstriction results primarily from the stimulation of coronary arterial alpha-adrenergic receptors, because it is reversed by phentolamine (an alpha-adrenergic antagonist) and exacerbated by propranolol (a beta-adrenergic antagonist). In addition, cocaine causes increased endothelial production of endothelin (a potent vasoconstrictor) and decreased production of nitric oxide (a potent vasodilator), which also may promote vasoconstriction.

Cocaine use may enhance platelet activation and aggregability, as well as increase concentrations of plasminogen activator inhibitor, which may promote thrombus accumulation. The presence of premature atherosclerotic coronary artery disease, as observed in postmortem studies of long-term cocaine users, may provide a nidus for thrombosis. In vitro studies have shown that cocaine causes structural abnormalities in the endothelial cell barrier, increasing its permeability to low-density lipoprotein and enhancing the expression of endothelial adhesion molecules, thereby favoring leukocyte migration, all of which are associated with atherogenesis.

Chest pain is the most common cardiovascular complaint of patients seeking medical assistance following cocaine use. Approximately 6% of those who come to the emergency department with cocaine-associated chest pain have enzymatic evidence of myocardial necrosis. Most subjects with cocaine-related MI are young, nonwhite, male cigarette smokers, without other risk factors for atherosclerosis, who have a history of repeated cocaine use (**Table 73-5**). Similar to cocaine, cigarette smoking induces coronary arterial vasoconstriction through an alpha-adrenergic mechanism. The deleterious effects of cocaine on myocardial oxygen supply and demand are exacerbated substantially by concomitant cigarette smoking. Following concomitant cocaine use and smoking, heart rate and systemic arterial pressure increase markedly, and coronary arterial vasoconstriction is more intense than with either alone.

In subjects who are considered otherwise to be at low risk for MI, the risk of infarction increases 24-fold during the first 60 minutes after cocaine use. The occurrence of MI after cocaine use appears to be unrelated to the amount ingested, its route of administration, and the frequency of its use; cocaine-related infarction has been reported with doses ranging from 200 to 2000 mg, after ingestion by all routes, and in habitual and first-time users. About 50% of patients with cocaine-related MI have no angiographic evidence of atherosclerotic coronary artery disease. Therefore, when subjects with no or few risk factors for atherosclerosis, particularly those who are young or have a history of substance abuse, present with acute MI, urine and blood samples should be analyzed for cocaine and its metabolites.

Cardiovascular complications resulting from cocaine-related MI are relatively uncommon, with ventricular arrhythmias occurring in 4% to 17%, congestive heart failure in 5% to 7%, and death in less than 2%. This low incidence of complications is caused, at least in part, by the young age and absence of extensive multivessel coronary artery disease of most patients with cocaine-related infarction. If complications develop, most occur within 12 hours of presentation to the hospital.[13]

TABLE 73-5 Characteristics of Patients with Cocaine-Induced Myocardial Infarction

Dose of Cocaine
Five or six lines (150 mg), up to 2 g
Serum concentration, 0.01-1.02 mg/liter
Frequency of Use
Reported in chronic, recreational, and first-time users
Route of Administration
Occurs with all routes of administration
75% of reported MIs occurred after intranasal use
Age
Mean, 34 yr (range, 17-71 yr)
20% younger than 25 yr
Sex
80%-90% male
Timing
Often within minutes of cocaine use
Reported as late as 5-15 hr after use

TABLE 73-6 Cardiac Dysrhythmias and Conduction Disturbances Reported with Cocaine Use

Sinus tachycardia
Sinus bradycardia
Supraventricular tachycardia
Bundle branch block
Complete heart block
Accelerated idioventricular rhythm
Ventricular tachycardia
Ventricular fibrillation
Asystole
Torsades de pointes
Brugada pattern (right bundle branch block with ST-segment elevation in leads V_1, V_2, and V_3)

Following hospital discharge, continued cocaine use and recurrent chest pain are common. Occasionally, a patient has recurrent nonfatal or fatal MI.

Most subjects with cocaine-related myocardial ischemia or infarction have chest pain within an hour of cocaine use, when the blood cocaine concentration is highest. Occasionally some individuals note the onset of symptoms several hours after the administration of the drug, when the blood cocaine concentration is low or even undetectable. With cocaine ingestion, the diameter of the coronary arteries decreases as the drug concentration increases. Then, as the drug concentration declines, the vasoconstriction resolves. Thereafter, as the concentrations of cocaine's major metabolites (benzoylecgonine and ecgonine methyl ester) rise, delayed (i.e., recurrent) coronary arterial vasoconstriction occurs, thereby explaining why myocardial ischemia or infarction has been reported to occur several hours after drug use.

Cocaethylene

In individuals who use cocaine in temporal proximity to the ingestion of ethanol, hepatic transesterification leads to the production of a unique metabolite, cocaethylene. Cocaethylene is often detected postmortem in subjects who are presumed to have died of cocaine and ethanol toxicity. Similar to cocaine, cocaethylene blocks the reuptake of dopamine at the synaptic cleft, thereby possibly potentiating the systemic toxic effects of cocaine. In experimental animals, in fact, cocaethylene is more lethal than cocaine. In humans, the combination of cocaine and ethanol causes a substantial increase in myocardial oxygen demand. The concomitant use of cocaine and ethanol is associated with a higher incidence of disability and death than either agent alone. Individuals presumably dying of a combined cocaine-ethanol overdose have much lower blood cocaine concentrations than those presumably dying of a cocaine overdose alone, thereby suggesting an additive or synergistic effect of ethanol on the catastrophic cardiovascular events that are induced by cocaine.

Cocaine-Induced Myocardial Dysfunction

Long-term cocaine abuse has been associated with left ventricular hypertrophy, as well as with left ventricular diastolic and/or systolic dysfunction. Several reports have described dilated cardiomyopathy in long-term cocaine abusers, and others have described profound but reversible myocardial depression after binge cocaine use. Approximately 7% of long-term chronic users without cardiac symptoms have radionuclide ventriculographic evidence of left ventricular systolic dysfunction.

Cocaine may adversely affect left ventricular systolic function by several mechanisms. First, as noted, cocaine may induce myocardial ischemia or infarction. Second, the profound repetitive sympathetic stimulation induced by cocaine is similar to that observed in patients with pheochromocytoma; either may induce a cardiomyopathy and characteristic microscopic changes of subendocardial contraction band necrosis. Third, the concomitant administration of adulterants or infectious agents may cause myocarditis, which has been seen on occasion in intravenous cocaine users studied post mortem. Fourth, studies in experimental animals have shown that cocaine increases the production of reactive oxygen species, alters cytokine production in the endothelium and in circulating leukocytes, induces the transcription of genes responsible for changes in the composition of myocardial collagen and myosin, and induces myocyte apoptosis.

Aside from the effects of long-term cocaine use on myocardial performance, it may cause an acute deterioration of left ventricular systolic and/or diastolic function or transient apical ballooning (also called takotsubo cardiomyopathy, or broken heart syndrome). In some subjects, this deterioration results from neurohormonal, metabolic, and/or acid-base disturbances that accompany cocaine intoxication, whereas in others it may be caused by a direct toxic effect of the drug. The intracoronary infusion of cocaine, in an amount sufficient to produce a concentration in coronary sinus blood similar in magnitude to the peripheral blood concentration found in abusers presumably dying of cocaine intoxication, exerts a deleterious effect on left ventricular systolic and diastolic function.

Arrhythmias

Cardiac dysrhythmias may occur with cocaine (**Table 73-6**), but the precise arrhythmogenic potential of the drug is poorly defined. In many cases, the dysrhythmias ascribed to cocaine occur in the setting of profound hemodynamic or metabolic derangements, such as hypotension, hypoxemia, seizures, or MI. Nonetheless, because of cocaine's sodium and potassium channel–blocking properties and its ability to enhance sympathetic activation, it is considered a likely cause of cardiac arrhythmias.[14] The development of lethal arrhythmias with cocaine use may require an underlying substrate of abnormal myocardium. Studies in experimental animals have shown that cocaine precipitates ventricular arrhythmias only in the presence of myocardial ischemia or infarction. In humans, life-threatening arrhythmias and sudden death associated with cocaine use occur most often in those with myocardial ischemia or infarction, or in those with nonischemic myocellular damage. Long-term cocaine use is associated with increased left ventricular mass and wall thickness, which are known risk factors for ventricular dysrhythmias. In some cocaine users, such an increased mass may provide the substrate for arrhythmias.

Cocaine may affect the generation and conduction of cardiac impulses by several mechanisms. First, its sympathomimetic properties may increase ventricular irritability and lower the threshold for fibrillation. Second, it inhibits action potential generation and conduction (i.e., it prolongs the QRS and QT intervals) as a result of its sodium channel–blocking effects. In so doing, it acts in a manner similar to that of a Class I antiarrhythmic agent. Accordingly, Brugada-type electrocardiographic features and torsades de pointes have been observed following cocaine use. Third, cocaine increases the intracellular calcium concentration, which may result in afterdepolarizations and triggered ventricular arrhythmias. Fourth, it reduces vagal activity, thereby potentiating its sympathomimetic effects.

Endocarditis

Although the intravenous administration of any illicit drug associates with an increased risk of bacterial endocarditis, the intravenous use of cocaine appears to be accompanied by a greater risk of endocarditis than the intravenous administration of other drugs. The reason for this enhanced risk of endocarditis in intravenous cocaine users is unknown, but several hypotheses have been proposed. The increases in heart rate and systemic arterial pressure that accompany cocaine use may induce valvular injury that predisposes to bacterial invasion. Cocaine's immunosuppressive effects may increase the risk of infection. The manner in which cocaine is manufactured, as well as the adulterants that are often present in it, may increase the risk of endocarditis. In contradistinction to the endocarditis associated with other drugs, the endocarditis of cocaine users more often involves the left-sided cardiac valves.

Aortic Dissection

Because aortic dissection or rupture has been temporally related to cocaine use, it should be considered as a possible cause of chest pain in cocaine users. In one study of 38 patients with acute aortic dissection, 14 (37%) were related to cocaine use, with an average interval from cocaine use to the onset of symptoms of 12 hours (range, 0 to 24 hours).[15] Dissection probably results from a cocaine-induced increase in systemic arterial pressure. In addition to aortic rupture, the cocaine-related rupture of mycotic and intracerebral aneurysms has been reported.

Amphetamines

Amphetamines were previously prescribed for the treatment of obesity, attention deficit disorder, and narcolepsy; at present, their use is strictly limited. The most frequently abused amphetamines are dextroamphetamine, methcathinone, methamphetamine, methylphenidate, ephedrine, propylhexedrine, phenmetrazine, and 3,4-methylenedioxymethamphetamine (MDMA, also known as ecstasy). Ice is a freebase form of methamphetamine that can be inhaled, smoked, or injected. Because amphetamines are sympathomimetic agents, their use has been associated with systemic arterial hypertension, premature coronary artery disease, acute coronary syndromes, MI, myocardial damage consistent with catecholamine excess, aortic dissection, and lethal arrhythmias.[16,17] Similar to cocaine, amphetamines may induce intense coronary arterial vasoconstriction, with or without thrombus formation.[18] Finally, dilated cardiomyopathy following repetitive amphetamine can occur, with recovery of cardiovascular function after drug discontinuation.[17]

Catecholamines and Beta-Adrenergic Receptor Agonists

Catecholamines, administered exogenously or secreted by a neuroendocrine tumor (e.g., pheochromocytoma or neuroblastoma), may produce acute myocarditis (with focal myocardial necrosis and inflammation), cardiomyopathy, tachycardia, and arrhythmias. Similar abnormalities have been described with the excessive use of beta-adrenergic receptor agonist inhalants and methylxanthines in patients with severe pulmonary disease. The administration of beta receptor agonists or catecholamines (i.e., dobutamine or epinephrine, respectively) has been associated with the appearance of transient left ventricular apical dyskinesis and anterior electrocardiographic T wave inversions. This entity, known as takotsubo or stress cardiomyopathy, is more likely to occur in women than in men. It resolves spontaneously when catecholamine secretion abates.[19,20]

Several mechanisms may be responsible for the acute and chronic myocardial damage associated with catecholamines. They may exert a direct toxic effect on the myocardium through changes in autonomic tone, enhanced lipid mobility, calcium overload, free radical production, or increased sarcolemmal permeability. Alternatively, myocardial damage may be secondary to a sustained increase in myocardial oxygen demands and/or decrease in myocardial oxygen supply—the latter caused by catecholamine-induced coronary arterial vasoconstriction or platelet aggregation.

Inhalants

Inhalants may be classified as organic solvents, organic nitrites (e.g., amyl nitrite or amyl butyl), and nitrous oxide. The organic solvents include toluene (airplane glue, rubber cement, paint thinner), Freon, kerosene, gasoline, carbon tetrachloride, acrylic paint sprays, shoe polish, degreasers, nail polish remover, typewriter correction fluid, adhesives, permanent markers, room freshener, deodorants, dry-cleaning agents, and lighter fluid. These solvents are most often inhaled by children or young adolescents. Acute or chronic inhalant use occasionally has been reported to induce cardiac abnormalities, most commonly dysrhythmias; rarely, inhalant use has been associated with myocarditis, MI, and sudden death. The inhalation of Freon, for example, can sensitize the myocardium to catecholamines; in these individuals, fatal arrhythmias have been reported to occur when the user is startled during inhalation.

Pharmaceuticals

Antiretroviral Agents

Subjects treated with highly active antiretroviral therapy (HAART; see Chap. 72) have been observed to have severe hypertriglyceridemia (serum triglyceride levels >1000 mg/dL), marked elevations in lipoprotein(a), hypercholesterolemia, increased LDL and decreased HDL cholesterol levels, and insulin resistance.[21] Not surprisingly, therefore, patients who are maintained on these agents have an increased risk of atherosclerosis.[22] Dilated cardiomyopathy in association with HIV antiretroviral therapy has been reported.[23-25] In mice, zidovudine produces a cardiomyopathy, with pathologic changes demonstrable in the mitochondria, and similar ultrastructural mitochondrial changes have been observed in myocardial biopsy specimens from HIV-infected patients treated with this agent.[25] In one individual, discontinuation of zidovudine resulted in a reversal of cardiac dysfunction.

Serotonin Agonists

The medicinal use of serotonin agonists, such as ergotamine and methysergide (migraine therapy); bromocriptine, cabergoline, and pergolide (Parkinson's disease therapy); and fenfluramine and dexfenfluramine (appetite suppressants) has been associated with left- and right-sided valvular disease.[26-29] Echocardiographic and histopathologic findings resemble those described in patients with carcinoid syndrome. Grossly, the valve leaflets and chordae tendineae are thickened and have a glistening white appearance. Histologically, leaflet architecture is intact, but a plaque-like encasement of the leaflets and chordal structures occurs, and proliferative myofibroblasts surround an abundant extracellular matrix.

Two medications used to treat subjects with migraine headaches, ergotamine and sumatriptan, have been associated with acute MI. Ergotamine causes vasoconstriction of intracerebral and extracranial arteries; rarely, its use has been associated with coronary arterial vasospasm and acute MI. Its vasoconstrictor effects are exaggerated by concomitant caffeine ingestion or beta-adrenergic blocker use. Sumatriptan, a selective 5-hydroxytryptamine agonist, also exerts its therapeutic effects by inducing cerebral arterial vasoconstriction. There have been several reports of patients in whom coronary vasospasm and acute MI occurred following the administration of therapeutic doses of sumatriptan, some of which were complicated by ventricular tachycardia or fibrillation and sudden cardiac death.

Chemotherapeutic Agents

Several chemotherapeutic agents may adversely affect cardiac function (see Chap. 90). Some of these substances have been reported to induce hypertension, acute cardiomyopathy, myocardial ischemia or infarction, dysrhythmias, QT prolongation, and/or sudden death (**Table 73-7**; see Table 90-2).[30,31] Among the agents that cause cardiotoxicity, the anthracyclines are known to induce acute myocarditis and longstanding cardiomyopathy. Tyrosine kinase inhibitors may cause a decrease in left ventricular ejection fraction, which is especially likely to occur if administered in conjunction with paclitaxel or anthracyclines. In contrast to anthracycline cardiotoxicity, however, the cardiotoxicity associated with a tyrosine kinase inhibitor is not cumulative or dose-dependent, and cardiac function often returns to normal after the agent is discontinued. As a result, its repeat administration is acceptable once cardiac function has normalized.

Up to 31% of patients who receive paclitaxel as a chemotherapeutic agent develop transient asymptomatic bradycardia. More substantial cardiac disturbances, including atrioventricular block, left bundle branch block, ventricular tachycardia, and myocardial ischemia, occur in up to 5% of subjects. Finally, 5-fluorouracil and capecitabine may cause myocardial ischemia or infarction by inducing coronary vasospasm.

TABLE 73-7 Cardiotoxic Effects of Chemotherapeutic Agents

AGENT	INCIDENCE (%)
Chemotherapy Associated with Left Ventricular Dysfunction	
Anthracyclines	
Doxorubicin (Adriamycin)*	3-26*
Epirubicin (Ellence)	0.9-3.3
Idarubicin (Idamycin)	5-18
Alkylating Agents	
Cyclophosphamide (Cytoxan)	7-28
Ifosfamide (Ifex)	17
Antimetabolites	
Clofarabine (Clolar)	27
Antimicrotubule Agents	
Docetaxel (Taxotere)	2.3-8
Monoclonal Antibody–Based Tyrosine Kinase Inhibitors	
Bevacizumab (Avastin)	1.7-3
Trastuzumab (Herceptin)	2-28
Proteasome Inhibitors	
Bortezomib (Velcade)	2-5
Small-Molecule Tyrosine Kinase Inhibitors	
Dasatinib (Sprycel)	2-4
Imatinib mesylate (Gleevec)	0.5-1.7
Lapatinib (Tykerb)	1.5-2.2
Sunitinib (Sutent)	2.7-11
Chemotherapy Associated with Ischemia	
Antimetabolites	
Capecitabine (Xeloda)	3-9
Fluorouracil (Adrucil)	1-68
Antimicrotubule Agents	
Paclitaxel (Taxol)	<1-5
Docetaxel (Taxotere)	1.7
Monoclonal Antibody–Based Tyrosine Kinase Inhibitors	
Bevacizumab (Avastin)	0.6-1.5
Small-Molecule Tyrosine Kinase Inhibitors	
Erlotinib (Tarceva)	2.3
Sorafenib (Nexavar)	2.7-3
Chemotherapy Associated with Bradycardia	
Angiogenesis Inhibitors	
Thalidomide (Thalomid)	0.12-55
Antimicrotubule Agents	
Paclitaxel (Taxol)	<0.1-31
Chemotherapy Associated with QT Prolongation	
Histone Deacetylase Inhibitors	
Vorinostat (Zolinza)	3.5-6
Miscellaneous	
Arsenic trioxide (Trisenox)	26-93
Small-Molecule Tyrosine Kinase Inhibitors	
Dasatinib (Sprycel)	<1-3
Lapatinib (Tykerb)	16
Nilotinib (Tasigna)	1-10

*At a cumulative dose of 550 mg/m^2.

Environmental Exposures

Cobalt

In the mid-1960s, an acute and fulminant form of dilated cardiomyopathy was described in heavy beer drinkers. It was suggested that the cobalt chloride that was added to the beer as a foam stabilizer was the causative agent; therefore, its addition was discontinued. Subsequently, this acute and severe form of cardiomyopathy disappeared. More recently, several reports of dilated cardiomyopathy after occupational exposure to cobalt have appeared; in these individuals, high concentrations of cobalt were demonstrated in endomyocardial biopsy specimens.

Lead

Patients with lead poisoning typically have complaints that are referable to the gastrointestinal and central nervous systems. On occasion, subjects with lead poisoning have electrocardiographic abnormalities, atrioventricular conduction defects, and overt congestive heart failure. Rarely, myocardial involvement may contribute to or be the principal cause of death.

Mercury

Occupational exposure to metallic mercuric vapors may cause systemic arterial hypertension and myocardial failure. Although some studies have suggested that a high mercury content of fish may counteract the beneficial effects of its omega-3 fatty acids, thereby increasing the risk of atherosclerotic cardiovascular disease, more recent assessments have not supported an association between total mercury exposure and the risk of coronary artery disease.

Antimony

Various antimony compounds have been used in the treatment of patients with schistosomiasis. Their use is often associated with electrocardiographic abnormalities, including prolongation of the QT interval and T wave flattening or inversion. Rarely, chest pain, bradycardia, hypotension, ventricular arrhythmias, and sudden death have been reported.

Arsenic

Arsenic exposure typically occurs from pesticide poisoning. Its cardiac manifestations include pericardial effusion, myocarditis, and various electrocardiographic abnormalities, including QT interval prolongation with T wave inversion.

Carbon Monoxide

Carbon monoxide has a higher affinity for hemoglobin than oxygen; as a result, elevated blood concentrations of carbon monoxide lead to reduced tissue oxygen delivery. Although central nervous system symptoms are the predominant manifestations of carbon monoxide poisoning, cardiac toxicity may occur because of myocardial hypoxia or a direct toxic effect of the gas on myocardial mitochondria. Such cardiac involvement may appear promptly after carbon monoxide exposure or may be delayed for several days. Sinus tachycardia and various arrhythmias, including ventricular extrasystoles and atrial fibrillation, are common; bradycardia and atrioventricular block may occur in more severe cases. Angina pectoris or MI may be precipitated by carbon monoxide exposure in patients with or without underlying coronary artery disease. Electrocardiographic ST-segment and T wave abnormalities occur commonly, and transient ventricular dysfunction may occur. The administration of 100% oxygen or treatment in a hyperbaric oxygen chamber usually results in rapid resolution of the cardiac abnormalities.

Thallium

Thallium salts are toxic when inhaled, ingested, or absorbed through the skin. Gastrointestinal and neurologic symptoms of poisoning occur within 12 to 24 hours of a single toxic dose (>1 g in adults). Several weeks after acute exposure, individuals are predisposed to cardiac arrhythmias and sudden death.

Cardenolides

Cardenolides are naturally occurring plant toxins that act primarily on the heart, causing serious dysrhythmias—including second- or third-degree heart block—and cardiac arrest. Poisoning with the digitalis cardenolides (digoxin and digitoxin) is reported worldwide. Cardiotoxicity from other cardenolides, such as the yellow, pink, or white oleander and sea mango tree, is a major problem in South Asia. In India and Sri Lanka, yellow oleander has become a popular means of self-injury, with tens of thousands of ingestions annually and a case fatality ratio of 5% to 10%.[32] Prolonged hospitalization and observation is recommended, because the occurrence of dangerous dysrhythmias may be delayed up to 72 hours after ingestion.

"Mad Honey"

Honey produced from the nectar of rhododendrons growing on the mountains of the eastern Black Sea region of Turkey may contain grayanotoxins, which bind to voltage-dependent sodium channels in the heart and lead to bradycardia and atrioventricular block.[33] Symptoms of "mad honey" poisoning (e.g., nausea, vomiting, hypotension, syncope) occur a few minutes to several hours after honey ingestion, with the severity of the poisoning dependent on the amount ingested. Grayanotoxins are metabolized and excreted rapidly, so the toxic effects of honey poisoning are rarely fatal and typically resolve in 2 to 9 hours.

Scombroid

Acute severe myocardial dysfunction caused by histamine poisoning has been reported within 1 hour of the ingestion of spoiled scombroid fish, such as tuna or bonito.[34] The flesh of these fish is rich in histidine, which is metabolized by gastrointestinal flora to histamine. The diagnosis is mainly based on clinical findings, but can be documented by the determination of histamine concentrations in the ingested fish or increased plasma histamine levels in the patient within 4 hours of fish ingestion.

Envenomations

Black widow spider, bee, wasp, jellyfish, cobra, and scorpion envenomation have been associated with cardiac complications, including MI, acute cardiac failure, myocarditis, bradyarrhythmias, heart block, ventricular tachyarrhythmias, and sudden death.[35,36] The mechanisms whereby these adverse outcomes occur include the systemic release of catecholamines, cardiac ion channel modulation, coronary arterial vasoconstriction, and direct myotoxic effects.

REFERENCES

Ethanol

1. Lucas DL, Brown RA, Wassef M, Giles TD: Alcohol and the cardiovascular system: Research challenges and opportunities. J Am Coll Cardiol 45:1916, 2005.
2. Djousse L, Gaziano JM: Alcohol consumption and heart failure: A systematic review. Curr Atheroscler Rep 10:117, 2008.
3. Kloner RA, Rezkalla SH: To drink or not to drink? That is the question. Circulation 116:1306, 2007.
4. di Castelnuovo A, Constanza S, Bagnardi V, et al: Alcohol dosing and total mortality in men and women. An updated meta-analysis of 34 prospective studies. Arch Intern Med 166:2437, 2006.
5. Mukanal KJ, Rimm EB: Alcohol consumption: risks and benefits. Curr Atheroscler Rep 10:536, 2008.
6. Mukamal KJ, Chiuve SE, Rimm EB: Alcohol consumption and risk for coronary heart disease in men with healthy lifestyles. Arch Intern Med 166:2145, 2006.
7. Mukamal KJ, Conigrave KM, Mittleman MA, et al: Roles of drinking pattern and type of alcohol consumed in coronary heart disease in men. N Engl J Med 348:109, 2003.
8. Tolstrup J, Gronbaek M: Alcohol and atherosclerosis: Recent insights. Curr Atheroscler Rep 9:116, 2007.
9. Koppes LL, Dekker JM, Hendriks HF, et al: Meta-analysis of the relationship between alcohol consumption and coronary heart disease and mortality in type 2 diabetic patients. Diabetologia 49:648, 2006.
10. Albert CM, Manson JE, Cook NR, et al: Moderate alcohol consumption and the risk of sudden cardiac death among US male physicians. Circulation 31:944, 1999.

Cocaine

11. Drug Abuse Warning Network (DAWN): National Estimates of Drug-Related Emergency Department Visits, 2006. DHHS Publication No. 08-4339. Substance Abuse and Mental Health Services Administration, Office of Applied Studies. Rockville, MD, 2008.
12. Qureshi AI, Suri MF, Guterman LR, et al: Cocaine use and the likelihood of nonfatal myocardial infarction and stroke: Data from the Third National Health and Nutrition Examination Survey. Circulation 103:502, 2001.
13. Weber JE, Shofer FS, Larkin GL, et al: Validation of a brief observation period for patients with cocaine-associated chest pain. N Engl J Med 348:510, 2003.
14. Bauman JL, DiDomenico RJ: Cocaine-induced channelopathies: Emerging evidence on the multiple mechanisms of sudden death. J Cardiovasc Pharmacol Ther 7:195, 2002.
15. Hsue PY, Salinas CL, Bolger AF, et al: Acute aortic dissection related to crack cocaine. Circulation 105:1592, 2002.

Amphetamines and Methamphetamines

16. Jacobs W: Fatal amphetamine-associated cardiotoxicity and its medicolegal implications. Am J Forens Med Pathol 27:156, 2006.
17. Kaye S, McKEtin R, Duflou J, Darke S: Methamphetamine and cardiovascular pathology. Addiction 102:1204, 2007.
18. Costa G, Pizzi C, Bresciani B, et al: Acute myocardial infarction caused by amphetamines: A case report and review of the literature. Ital Heart J 2:478, 2001.

Catecholamines and Beta-Adrenergic Receptor Agonists

19. Abraham J, Mudd JO, Kapur N, et al: Stress cardiomyopathy after intravenous administration of catecholamines and beta-receptor agonists. J Am Coll Cardiol 53:1320, 2009.
20. Akashi YJ, Nakazawa K, Sakakibara M, et al: Reversible left ventricular dysfunction "takotsubo" cardiomyopathy related to catecholamine cardiotoxicity. J Electrocardiol 35: 351, 2002.

Antiretroviral Agents (Protease Inhibitors)

21. Calza L, Manfredi R, Pocaterra D, Chiodo R: Risk of premature atherosclerosis and ischemic heart disease associated with HIV infection and antiretroviral therapy. J Infect 57:16, 2008.
22. Kulasekaram R, Peters BS, Wiersbicki AS: Dyslipidemia and cardiovascular risk in HIV infection. Curr Med Res Opin 21:1717, 2005.
23. Sudano I, Spieker LE, Noll G, et al: Cardiovascular disease in HIV infection. Am Heart J 151: 1147, 2006.
24. Zareba KM, Lavigne JE, Lipshultz SE: Cardiovascular effects of HAART in infants and children of HIV-infected mothers. Cardiovasc Toxicol 4:271, 2004.
25. Lewis W: Mitochondrial DNA replication, nucleoside reverse-transcriptase inhibitors, and AIDS cardiomyopathy. Prog Cardiovasc Dis 45:305, 2003.

Serotonin Agonists

26. Connolly Antonini A, Poewe W: Fibrotic heart-valve reactions to dopamine-agonist treatment in Parkinson's disease. Lancet Neurol 6:826, 2007.
27. Zanettini R, Antonini A, Gatto G, et al: Valvular heart disease and the use of dopamine agonists for Parkinson's disease. N Engl J Med 356:39, 2007.
28. Schade R, Andersohn F, Suissa S, et al: Dopamine agonists and the risk of cardiac-valve regurgitation. N Engl J Med 356:29, 2007.
29. Weissman NJ, Panza JA, Tighe JF, et al: Natural history of valvular regurgitation 1 year after discontinuation of dexfenfluramine therapy. A randomized, double-blind, placebo-controlled trial. Ann Intern Med 134:267, 2001.

Chemotherapeutic Agents

30. Force T, Kerkela R: Cardiotoxicity of the new cancer therapeutics— mechanisms of, and approaches to, the problem. Drug Disc Today 13:778, 2008.
31. Yeh ET: Cardiotoxicity induced by chemotherapy and antibody therapy. Ann Rev Med 57:485, 2006.

Environmental Exposures

32. Roberts DM, Buckley N: Antidotes for acute cardenolide (cardiac glycoside) poisoning. Cochrane Database Syst Rev (4):CD005490, 2006.
33. Gunduz A, Turedi S, Uzun H, Topbas M: Mad honey poisoning. Am J Emerg Med 24:595, 2006.
34. Grinda J-m, Bellenfant F, Bribet FG, et al: Biventricular assist device for scombroid poisoning with refractory myocardial dysfunction: A bridge to recovery. Crit Care Med 32:1957, 2004.
35. Valkanas MA, Bowman S, Dailey M: Electrocardiographic myocardial infarction without structural lesion in the setting of acute hymenoptera envenomation. Am J Emerg Med 25:1082, 2007.
36. Tibbals J: Australian venomous jellyfish, envenomation syndromes, toxins, and therapy. Toxicon 48:830, 2006.

CHAPTER 74 Primary Tumors of the Heart

Bruce McManus

Primary tumors of the heart are rare across all age groups, with a reported prevalence of 0.001% to 0.03% in autopsy series.[1] Secondary involvement of the heart by extracardiac tumors is 20 to 40 times more common than by primary cardiac tumors.[1-3] Despite rarity, multiple histologic types of primary cardiac tumors are recognized. Excluding tumors that are primarily based in the pericardium, like mesotheliomas and teratomas (see Chap. 75), the overwhelming majority of primary cardiac tumors are mesenchymal tumors that display the full spectrum of differentiation as those in the soft tissue do. Non-neoplastic hamartomatous lesions represent the majority of pediatric tumors; in the fetus, there is a higher proportion of germ cell tumors.[4] About 75% of all primary cardiac tumors are regarded as benign neoplasms; cardiac myxoma accounts for at least half of them. However, the oncologic designation of benignity understates the potentially devastating effect any benign primary cardiac tumor may impose on the patient. By virtue of their anatomic locations, primary cardiac tumors are capable of producing myriad cardiac, embolic, and systemic symptoms, sometimes with fatal consequences. Of the remaining 25% of primary cardiac tumors that are considered to be malignant neoplasms, the majority are sarcomas; lymphomas are the next most common. Because many symptoms of malignant primary cardiac tumors occur relatively late in the disease course, findings of locally infiltrative or systemically widespread disease at initial presentation are not uncommon.

The diagnosis of primary cardiac tumors is frequently challenging. The symptoms associated with most primary cardiac tumors are nonspecific, and they often mimic far more commonly encountered disease entities. Furthermore, many tumors are manifested with mild and vague symptoms such that most routine workups will fail to identify the underlying abnormality. This elusiveness often results in a delay in the diagnosis of disease. Fortunately, the more widespread use of noninvasive and relatively sensitive imaging modalities such as echocardiography, computed tomography (CT), cardiac magnetic resonance (CMR), and positron emission tomography (PET) (see Chaps. 15, 17, 18, and 19) should facilitate the identification of cardiac lesions. However, the consideration of primary cardiac tumor in the differential diagnosis combined with a high index of suspicion is also paramount in arriving at the correct diagnosis. In addition to the diagnostic challenges, the management of some primary cardiac tumors is also not straightforward even when the histologic diagnosis has been made. Many benign primary cardiac tumors are now found incidentally in asymptomatic individuals. Therefore, the treatment decision requires a thorough analysis of the potential benefits and harms of surgery versus conservative management. Because of our limited experience with the natural clinical course of many primary cardiac tumors, this treatment decision may be difficult to reach.

Clinical Presentations

Primary cardiac tumors are great masqueraders of many commonly encountered cardiac and systemic diseases. Depending on the location, size, mobility, friability, and histologic type of the lesions, cardiac tumors can produce a variety of symptoms and clinical findings. The clinical manifestations that are produced by primary cardiac tumors overall can be divided into four general mechanistic categories: systemic manifestations, embolic manifestations, cardiac manifestations, and phenomena secondary to metastatic diseases.

Systemic Manifestations

Primary cardiac tumors, whether benign or malignant, are capable of producing a multitude of systemic symptoms that can add to the challenge of reaching the proper diagnosis. Patients with primary cardiac tumors may experience constitutional symptoms of fever, chills, fatigue, malaise, and weight loss. In addition, these symptoms mimic those of several connective tissue diseases and vasculitides such as myalgia, arthralgia, muscle weakness, and Raynaud phenomenon.[5,6] Routine laboratory tests may reveal evidence of leukocytosis, polycythemia, anemia, thrombocytosis, thrombocytopenia, hypergammaglobulinemia, and increased erythrocyte sedimentation rate. These systemic manifestations are believed to be produced by secretory products released by the tumor or by tumor necrosis. Among the benign primary cardiac tumors, cardiac myxomas are the most notorious for causing systemic symptoms, and an elevated serum interleukin-6 (IL-6) frequently found in these patients is believed to mediate such symptoms.[7,8] Malignant primary cardiac tumors, similar to their counterparts from extracardiac sites, are also frequently associated with constitutional findings.

Embolic Phenomena

Primary cardiac tumors can cause systemic or pulmonary embolism by way of tumor emboli or thromboemboli that are released from or formed on the surface of the tumor, respectively. The propensity for cardiac tumors to cause embolic phenomena depends largely on the predominant origin of the tumor (intramural or intracavitary), the type of the tumor, and the friability of the intraluminal tumor surface.[9] Among the benign primary cardiac neoplasms, cardiac myxomas are most frequently associated with embolic findings, especially when the tumor possesses a villous surface.[9] Other benign primary cardiac neoplasms that are known to produce emboli include papillary fibroelastomas, hemangiomas, and lymphangiomas.[10-12] Embolism related to malignant primary cardiac tumors is not uncommon because many malignant tumors have a friable and sometimes necrotic luminal surface. However, systemic and pulmonary metastases from the malignant tumor must be excluded because they can produce similar manifestations. Primary cardiac tumors can embolize to almost any organ, resulting in ischemia, infarction, and even delayed aneurysm formation in the organs or the body sites involved.[1,6,13,14] The brain is the most common site of involvement for systemic emboli produced by primary cardiac tumors, and the involvement of both hemispheres and multiple regions is seen more than 40% of the time.[13] The multifocal nature of cerebral involvement should therefore prompt a search for embolic origin with echocardiography and carotid Doppler ultrasound in these instances. Cerebral embolism most commonly results in a transient ischemic attack or an ischemic stroke, but intracranial hemorrhage may occur as well. Depending on the region of the brain involved, patients may experience a variety of psychiatric and neurologic disturbances that range in severity from mild vertigo to seizure and even coma. Delayed aneurysm formation presumably at the site of previous cerebral tumor emboli represents another dreadful complication of the disease.[14] In addition to the brain, the tumor emboli or tumor-associated thromboemboli can occur in almost any organ or tissue. This includes tumor emboli to a coronary artery that result in clinical findings of myocardial infarction, which can further conceal the underlying abnormality. Careful examination of embolectomy specimens is therefore important because it may reveal evidence of tumor emboli. Pulmonary embolization is typically caused by a right-sided tumor, although emboli from a left-sided tumor located proximal to the site of a left-to-right intracardiac shunt can also result in pulmonary embolism in rare instances. Consideration should be given to the possibility of a primary cardiac tumor in patients presenting with findings of pulmonary embolism when no identifiable source of emboli surfaces after conventional assessment.

Cardiac Manifestations

The cardiac manifestations of primary cardiac tumors can result from direct mechanical interference with myocardial or valvular function, interruption of coronary blood flow, interference with electrophysiologic conduction, and accumulation of pericardial fluid. The propensity for various cardiac manifestations depends primarily on the location of the tumor (pericardial, intramural, or intracavitary), the chamber involved, the size, and the infiltrative nature. Pericardial tumors are not addressed in this chapter because they are dealt with elsewhere (see Chap. 75).

Primary cardiac tumors that are completely or predominantly intramural or myocardial are typically asymptomatic, especially if the sizes are small. Large intramural tumors that are within or pressing on major cardiac conduction pathways may, however, cause a wide variety of arrhythmias, including complete heart block and asystole in more severe cases.[5] In addition, large intramural tumors may also compress the cardiac cavities, obstruct the ventricular outflow tract, or contribute to insufficiency of the mitral valve.

In contrast to intramural tumors, primary cardiac tumors with a significant intracavitary component tend to cause more symptoms for patients. Furthermore, intracavitary tumors that are pedunculated and mobile can be especially problematic because of their tendency to interfere with valvular and myocardial function. The precise cardiac manifestations depend also on the locale of a tumor in the heart. For left atrial tumors, intracavitary lesions that are pedunculated and mobile can interfere with the mitral valve and produce clinical findings typical of mitral regurgitation that include fatigue, dyspnea, orthopnea, paroxysmal nocturnal dyspnea, cough, hemoptysis, chest pain, pulmonary edema, and peripheral edema. However, findings atypical for mitral regurgitation, such as the aforementioned systemic and constitutional symptoms, should prompt further investigation. These symptoms can be sudden in onset, intermittent, and positional. Physical examination may reveal signs of pulmonary congestion with an S_3 and loud and widely split S_1, a holosystolic murmur most prominent at the apex with radiation to the axilla, a diastolic murmur from turbulent blood flow through the mitral orifice, and a tumor "plop." Such tumor plop is thought to result from the tumor's striking the endocardial wall or the abrupt halt of tumor excursions. It occurs later than an opening snap but earlier than an S_3. For intracavitary tumors located in the right atrium, findings of right-sided heart failure that include fatigue, peripheral edema, ascites, hepatosplenomegaly, and elevated jugular venous pressure with a prominent *a* wave are the most common cardiac presentations.

Because of the right atrial location, the diagnosis is often delayed, with an average time interval from presentation to the correct diagnosis of 3 years. Patients frequently present with rapidly progressive right-sided heart failure and also new-onset heart murmurs because of mechanical interference with the tricuspid valve. In patients with a patent foramen ovale, the buildup of right atrial pressure can produce right-to-left intracardiac shunting with resulting systemic hypoxia, cyanosis, clubbing, and polycythemia. On occasion, patients may also present with superior vena cava syndrome caused by a large right atrial tumor. Physical examination may reveal findings of peripheral edema, hepatosplenomegaly, ascites, elevated jugular venous pressure with prominent *a* wave and steep *y* descent, and an early diastolic murmur or holosystolic murmur that exhibits significant respiratory or positional variation.

Right ventricular tumors with a significant intracavitary component may obstruct the filling or the outflow of the right ventricle and as such can produce right-sided heart failure that includes dyspnea, peripheral edema, ascites, and hepatosplenomegaly. Precordial auscultation may reveal a systolic ejection murmur at the left sternal border, an S_3, and a delayed P_2. An elevated jugular venous pressure and Kussmaul sign may also be present. These findings may vary significantly, depending on the position of the patient. In addition, left ventricular tumors with a significant intracavitary component can obstruct the left ventricular outflow tract and produce findings of left-sided heart failure and syncope as well as atypical chest pain from obstruction of a coronary artery by either direct tumor involvement or tumor emboli. Physical examination may reveal evidence of pulmonary edema, low blood pressure, and systolic murmurs that mimic the findings of aortic or subaortic stenosis. The murmurs and blood pressure may display considerable positional variation. In the case of malignant primary cardiac tumors, such as angiosarcomas and primary cardiac lymphomas, malignant hemorrhagic pericardial effusion may be present. Life-threatening cardiac tamponade and cardiac rupture leading to sudden death may also occur.[15-17]

Metastatic Diseases

Truly metastatic diseases are by definition features of malignant primary cardiac tumors. Most malignant primary cardiac tumors are detected at a late stage with systemic dissemination present. In some cases, symptoms secondary to the metastatic disease may represent the initial clinical manifestation of the malignant primary cardiac tumor.[18] Common sites of metastases for most primary cardiac sarcomas like angiosarcomas and rhabdomyosarcomas include lung, brain, and bone,[15,19,20] although metastases to the liver, lymph node, adrenal gland, spleen, and skin have also been reported.

DIAGNOSTIC APPROACH

Primary cardiac tumors are among the most challenging disease entities to diagnose because of their rarity and their highly variable and usually nonspecific clinical presentations. Therefore, it is understandable that clinicians who first encounter a patient with a primary cardiac tumor generally attribute the findings to other, more commonly encountered disease entities and proceed with the investigation accordingly. Thus, the key to proper and timely diagnosis of a primary cardiac tumor lies not necessarily in its immediate diagnostic recognition but rather in the consideration of primary cardiac tumor in the differential diagnosis. In addition, clinicians need to maintain a high index of suspicion for rare entities like primary cardiac tumors, especially when atypical features are present. A thorough clinical evaluation including a complete history and physical examination coupled with appropriate laboratory tests is necessary because pertinent information may be present to help support a possible diagnosis of primary cardiac tumor (see Table 74-e1 on website) or secondary cardiac tumor. When cardiac tumor is considered in the differential diagnosis, the most ideal initial method of evaluation is echocardiography (see Chap. 15), either transthoracic or transesophageal, depending on the clinical circumstances. The sensitivities of transthoracic and transesophageal echocardiography for detection of a cardiac mass are 93% and 97%, respectively.[21] Thus, transesophageal echocardiography is more comprehensive and accurate in assessment compared with transthoracic echocardiography, and transesophageal echocardiography is especially advantageous in evaluating right atrial tumors. Three-dimensional echocardiography can assess the size of cardiac masses and describe complex anatomy of the heart.[22] If a cardiac lesion is identified, chest CT with contrast enhancement and CMR with contrast are superior modalities for characterization of the lesions and delineation of the extent of tumor involvement (see Chaps. 18 and 19). They can also help exclude the possibility of direct cardiac extension of a tumor that originates from adjacent mediastinal structures. CT and CMR are particularly good at depicting the pericardium and great vessels and evaluating the extent of disease, and CT can also detect calcification, which is important in the differential diagnosis.[23] Features suggestive of malignant cardiac tumors include a large broad-based lesion occupying most of the affected cardiac chamber, hilar lymphadenopathy, extensive pericardial involvement, and hemorrhagic pericardial effusions. However, the diagnosis of a cardiac tumor, whether benign or malignant, cannot be made with imaging studies alone, and histologic evaluation is necessary for definitive diagnosis. Depending on the clinical settings, tissue diagnosis may be made with less invasive methods such as cytologic evaluation of pericardial or pleural fluids, echocardiographically guided percutaneous cardiac biopsy, or echocardiographically guided transvenous cardiac biopsy.[15,24,25] However, a negative finding on biopsy performed through these less invasive methods does not rule out a diagnosis of malignancy because the false-negative rate of these methods can be significant. Therefore, more invasive methods of tumor biopsy through mediastinoscopy or even thoracotomy may be necessary to obtain a definitive diagnosis. In the scenarios in which the presence of a malignant cardiac tumor is confirmed through tissue diagnosis or strongly suspected on the basis of clinical and imaging findings, a full metastatic workup should be performed if it is clinically feasible. Of note, the great majority of malignant cardiac tumors represent local or distant metastases by an extracardiac tumor, and most malignant primary cardiac tumors are diagnosed at an advanced stage with distant metastases already present. Therefore, a thorough physical examination and a complete series of imaging may help locate probable extracardiac origin of the primary tumor or identify potential metastatic lesions from the primary cardiac tumor. This information will help in the disease staging and prognostication as well as in the planning of a treatment course.

Benign Tumors

Myxomas

Myxoma, the most common type of primary cardiac tumor, accounts for 30% to 50% of all primary tumors of the heart.[1] It has an annual incidence of 0.5 per million population and most commonly presents in adults 30 to 50 years of age, although it can occur in nearly all age groups ranging from 1 to 83 years.[8] Sixty-five percent of cardiac myxomas occur in women, and 4.5% to 10% of cardiac myxomas are familial[8]; thus, routine screening of first-degree relatives of myxoma patients is recommended.[22] Although there was debate in the past about whether cardiac myxoma was, indeed, a neoplastic entity or an organized thrombus, recent gene expression and immunohistochemical studies have shown that cardiac myxoma is a neoplasm with tumor cells arising most likely from multipotent mesenchymal cells.[26-32] Other features suggestive of its being a neoplastic process include its ability to recur, occurrence in multiple sites, and occurrence in families. Despite several documented reports of metastases to various anatomic sites, the typical cardiac myxoma is regarded as a benign neoplasm in a conventional sense, and the reported metastases most likely represent tumor growth from embolic tumor fragments that are deposited along the arterial circulation in different remote sites. Thus, although histopathologically benign, cardiac myxomas can cause chronic systemic inflammation, embolism, or intracardiac obstructions, leading to increased morbidity.[33]

The pathogenesis of cardiac myxoma is poorly understood, especially for those tumors that occur sporadically. Studies have, however, shed more light on the pathogenesis of familial cases of cardiac myxomas. Carney syndrome accounts for the majority of familial cases of cardiac myxoma and for 7% of all cardiac myxomas.[27] Carney syndrome or complex is an autosomal dominant syndrome characterized by myxoma formation in cardiac and several extracardiac locations, spotty skin pigmentation, endocrine hyperactivity, and other tumors (such as testicular Sertoli cell tumor, psammomatous melanotic schwannoma, pituitary adenoma, and thyroid tumors).[27] The cardiac myxomas occurring in the setting of Carney syndrome and sporadic cases are histologically indistinguishable. However, cardiac myxomas associated with Carney syndrome show no age or gender predilection, can be single or multiple, can occur in any intracardiac location, and tend to recur with a rate of 20% despite adequate surgical excision. In contrast, sporadic cases of cardiac myxoma tend to occur in women of middle age and as isolated lesions in the left atrial aspect of interatrial septum. Sporadic cases have a lower recurrence rate (roughly 3%) than those mentioned previously. Mutations in *PRKAR1A*, a regulatory subunit 1A of cAMP-dependent protein kinase A (PKA), and in *MYH8*, a non-PKA phosphorylated perinatal myosin isoform, are believed to be responsible for cardiac myxoma formation in most individuals with Carney syndrome. The precise mechanism of tumorigenesis involving these mutations is unknown. However, there may be a role for genetic testing for these mutations in asymptomatic kindreds of individuals with myxomas to guide further investigation and management.[34]

Clinically, patients with symptomatic cardiac myxoma can have a variety of nonspecific findings, depending on its size, location, and mobility. However, the majority of the patients will present with at least one of the classic triad of obstructive cardiac, embolic, and constitutional or systemic signs.[1,5] The obstructive cardiac findings including dizziness, dyspnea, cough, pulmonary edema, and heart failure are the result of mechanical interference with the mitral valve by the tumor and account for the most common presenting findings in the triad. Tumor embolism is another common basis for clinical presentation and can affect the systemic or pulmonary circulation, depending on the location of the tumor and the patency of the foramen ovale. Cardiac myxoma is the most common primary cardiac tumor to produce tumor emboli, and it has been reported to embolize to virtually any organ or tissue. Constitutional and nonembolic systemic findings secondary to cardiac myxoma include several nonspecific symptoms, such as fever, weight loss, fatigue, myalgia, arthralgia, muscle weakness, and Raynaud syndrome. These nonspecific symptoms often create the most confusion and difficulty in the diagnosis because they may mimic immunologic diseases.[6,7,35] They are believed to be related to IL-6 release by the myxoma tumor cells. A significant subset (approximately two thirds) of patients with cardiac myxoma have abnormal electrocardiograms (ECGs), commonly showing evidence of left atrial enlargement, although a variety of abnormalities can be seen.[6,9,36] However, atrial arrhythmias or conduction disturbances are rare. On chest radiography, about one third of patients have normal findings. Evidence of elevated left atrial pressure, such as left atrial enlargement, vascular redistribution, prominent pulmonary trunk, and pulmonary edema, is found in 53% of patients with left atrial myxoma.[5] Cardiomegaly is seen in 37% and 50% of left and right atrial myxomas, respectively. Intracardiac tumor calcification is a rare finding in left atrial myxomas but is found in 56% of patients with right atrial myxoma. The typical imaging modalities used for diagnostic and preoperative assessment purposes include CT, CMR, and echocardiography. Most cardiac myxomas appear as spherical or ovoid masses with lobular contour on CT and CMR scans.[5] Two thirds of myxomas are heterogeneous, whereas one third appear homogeneous on CT.

Contrast-enhanced CT reveals that most myxomas have an overall attenuation lower than that of myocardium; few such tumors have equivalent attenuation, but in no instance have the tumors shown higher attenuation. CMR shows heterogeneous signal intensity in 90% of cardiac myxomas; the T1-weighted images show isointense signal in 79% and hyperintense signal in 14% of the cases (see Chap. 18). Cine gradient-echo CMR appears to be superior to other imaging modalities in the assessment of cardiac tumors because it allows better visualization of the size, location, and point of attachment of the tumor.[5] Echocardiography is the most commonly used modality for diagnostic purposes, and transesophageal echocardiography is the recommended method for initial assessment of suspected cardiac lesions.[3]

Cardiac myxoma most commonly occurs in the left atrium (**Fig. 74-1**). A recent meta-analysis showed that 83% of cardiac myxomas occur in the left atrium (see Fig. 15-86), 12.7% occur in the right atrium, and 1.3% are biatrial.[8] Occurrence in the ventricles is uncommon; only 1.7% and 0.6% of myxomas occur in the left ventricle and the right ventricle, respectively.[1] The majority (>90%) of myxomas are solitary, although multiple synchronous cardiac myxomas can occur, especially in the setting of Carney syndrome. Cardiac myxomas are generally pedunculated tumors with a fibrovascular stalk attaching to the subendothelial base. The usual site of attachment is the interatrial septum in the region of the fossa ovalis.[6,37] Rarely, cardiac myxoma can involve heart valves directly. Most have sizes ranging from 4 to 8 cm in diameter, although they can reach a size of 16 cm.[4,5,8] The mean weight is 37 g, with a range of 15 to 180 g. Approximately half of the cardiac myxomas have a smooth compact surface, whereas the remaining half have a villous surface. Evidence suggests that myxomas with a villous surface are more likely to embolize.[9] On cross section, cardiac myxomas have a gelatinous appearance, although foci of hemorrhage, calcification (see Fig. 74-e1 on website), ossification, and cystic change can also be present.[5] On histologic examination, the myxoma contains sparsely distributed uniform spindle- and stellate-shaped cells within an extensive myxoid stroma. Although generally hypocellular, the degree of cellularity can vary from tumor to tumor. Tumor spindle- and stellate-shaped cells typically possess round or oval nuclei, with indistinct nucleoli and indistinct cell borders. Binucleate or multinucleate cells may be seen. Mitotic figures are rarely present. The myxoid stroma is composed of acid mucopolysaccharides that are hyaluronidase sensitive. The stroma typically contains prominent thin-walled vessels. Necrosis, calcification, and Gamna bodies (calcified elastic fibers) can be seen in a small subset of cardiac myxomas.[4,5] Smooth muscle cells and fibroblasts are occasionally present in the stroma.[32] A mixed inflammatory infiltrate is also commonly seen. Although infrequent, cardiac myxomas may contain epithelial or glandular, hematopoietic, chondroid, and thymic elements.[32,38,39] Experts suspect that these heterotopic elements represent a form of choristoma. Even more rarely, malignant transformation of these heterotopic elements can occur, giving rise to various malignant neoplasms.[38] On histochemical evaluation, both the stroma and the tumor cells stain positive with periodic acid–Schiff, whereas only the stroma shows positive staining with alcian blue. On immunohistochemical evaluation, the stromal tumor cells show vimentin positivity and variable S100 and NSE positivity, but never keratin positivity.[32] When embolic myxoma is suspected in embolectomy specimens, calretinin and IL-6 may be useful in differentiating between embolic myxoma and myxoid thrombus.[9,40]

The treatment of symptomatic cardiac myxoma is prompt surgical resection of the tumor with the patient placed on cardiopulmonary bypass.[41] Complete excision is the goal, although this may not be possible in all instances.[42] Immediate postoperative mortality in most series ranges from 0% to 7.5%.[6,37,43] Other common postoperative complications include arrhythmias, which may require long-term medication.[37] Recurrence develops in about 3% of tumors, although the rate is higher with familial cardiac myxomas and can occur anywhere from 3 months up to 14 years postoperatively.[5,23-25] Recurrences can be local or in extracardiac locations, such as the brain, lung, skeletal muscle, bone, kidney, gastrointestinal tract, skin, and other soft tissue sites. Recurrence of myxoma in the brain, which probably represents growth of the embolized tumor fragments, can be difficult to manage, but chemotherapy is not recommended because embolic myxomas do not truly represent metastatic diseases.[44] A particularly rare but potentially life-threatening complication is the development of cerebral aneurysm secondary to embolic tumor fragments.[14]

Lipomas and Lipomatous Hypertrophy of the Atrial Septum

Benign lipomatous tumor is the second most common primary neoplasm of the heart and can be divided into two major groups primarily on the basis of the degree of encapsulation—lipoma and lipomatous hypertrophy of the atrial septum (LHAS). Cardiac lipomas (**Fig. 74-2**) can occur sporadically at all ages with equal frequency in both sexes.[45] Although lipomas from other body sites, such as skin, frequently show cytogenetic abnormalities involving chromosome 12 in q15,[46] the molecular and genetic basis of cardiac lipomas is not elucidated. Clinically, most cardiac lipomas are asymptomatic and typically are incidental findings. However, the tumor can produce a variety of symptoms, depending on its size and location. Cardiac lipomas can occur at any atrial or ventricular surface.[1] They originate most commonly in the subepicardial and subendocardial locations, although intramyocardial lesions have also been reported. Subendocardial lipomas with a prominent intracavitary component can interfere with mechanical function of the heart, resulting in symptoms of heart failure.[47] Subepicardial tumors are usually asymptomatic, but large lesions may cause compression of the heart and produce pericardial effusion.[1] Intramyocardial lipoma may interfere with electrical conduction in the heart and cause arrhythmias. Diagnostically, even though transesophageal echocardiography can be used to assess the location, size, and mobility of these cardiac lesions, it may not be possible to accurately determine the tissue type because typical cardiac lipomas have a nonspecific appearance on ultrasound examination.[45,48] CT can provide better tissue characterization because cardiac lipomas display a low attenuation signal similar to subcutaneous or mediastinal fat.[45] In gross appearance, cardiac lipomas usually are single well-encapsulated masses, although multiple lesions can occur, especially in patients with tuberous sclerosis.[45] Size typically ranges from 1 to 8 cm in diameter. Similar to lipomas found in other sites, cardiac lipoma is histopathologically composed of mature fat cells with occasional fibrous connective tissue (fibrolipoma) and vacuolated brown fat (hibernoma-like). Areas of degeneration and extensive radiographically apparent calcification may be present.[49] The treatment of symptomatic cardiac lipomas is surgical resection, and the postoperative prognosis is excellent.[1,47]

In contrast to lipoma, LHAS (**Fig. 74-3**), also known as massive fatty deposits of the atrial septum, is a nonencapsulated excessive accumulation of fat in the atrial septum at the level of the fossa ovalis that is more than 2 cm in thickness and typically occurs in elderly, obese patients; the mean age at diagnosis in most series is about 70 years.[48] A study revealed that this disease as diagnosed by CT scan may have an incidence as high as 2.2%, which is considerably higher than previously estimated.[48] The cause of LHAS is unknown, and there is controversy about whether the condition truly represents a neoplasm in most instances.[1,48,50] Its apparent association with advanced age and obesity has led to the suggestion that it may represent a metabolic process. However, the observed occurrence in nonobese patients suggests otherwise.[1] Clinically, the great majority of LHAS does not cause any symptoms. On occasion, it can result in a variety of rhythm disturbances and even sudden death.[45] These rhythm disturbances are speculated to involve fatty tissue infiltration into atrial myocyte tissue, which alters the architecture and function of the myocytes.[51] In rare instances in which the tumor protrudes into the right atrium and the superior vena cava, patients can present with symptoms related to blood flow obstruction.[52] CT and CMR are the most desirable modalities for the diagnosis of LHAS because they are superior to echocardiography in differentiating between fat and connective tissue. Multislice CT is the most advantageous method of diagnosis because it has greater coverage, has a decreased number of motion artifacts, and provides sharper images (see Fig. 15-90).[51] On imaging, the atrial septum is thickened to up to 7 cm, whereas normally it is less than 1 cm,[48,53] but this thickening always avoids the fossa ovalis, giving the atrial septum a dumbbell or hourglass shape.[51] The lipomatous hypertrophy appears macroscopically as circumscribed, nonencapsulated, slightly firm adipose tissue and cannot be differentiated from epicardial fat.[51] Accumulation of the fat beneath the atrial septal endocardium may bulge into the right atrium. On histologic examination, LHAS contains an infiltrating mixture of mature fat and vacuolated adipose cells resembling brown fat with enlarged cardiac myocytes. There is a focal excess of fibrous tissue. No mitotic activity is observed in the fat cells in contrast to liposarcoma.[1] Occasional mononuclear cells are present, and mast cells are also not uncommon in association with the adipose cells. LHAS with symptomatic arrhythmias can be managed medically; surgical excision should be restricted to the rare cases in which the disease causes symptomatic hemodynamic obstruction.[48,54]

Papillary Tumors of the Heart Valves

Papillary fibroelastoma is the third most common primary cardiac tumor with an incidence of up to 0.33% in autopsy series.[55] It is believed to be an acquired lesion of fibroblastic origin with a slow growth rate that is distinct from Lambl excrescences.[12,56] It does not spontaneously regress. It also may have focal calcification and occasionally cystic degeneration.[33] Clinically, most patients with papillary fibroelastoma are asymptomatic. However, a review of the literature shows that nearly half of

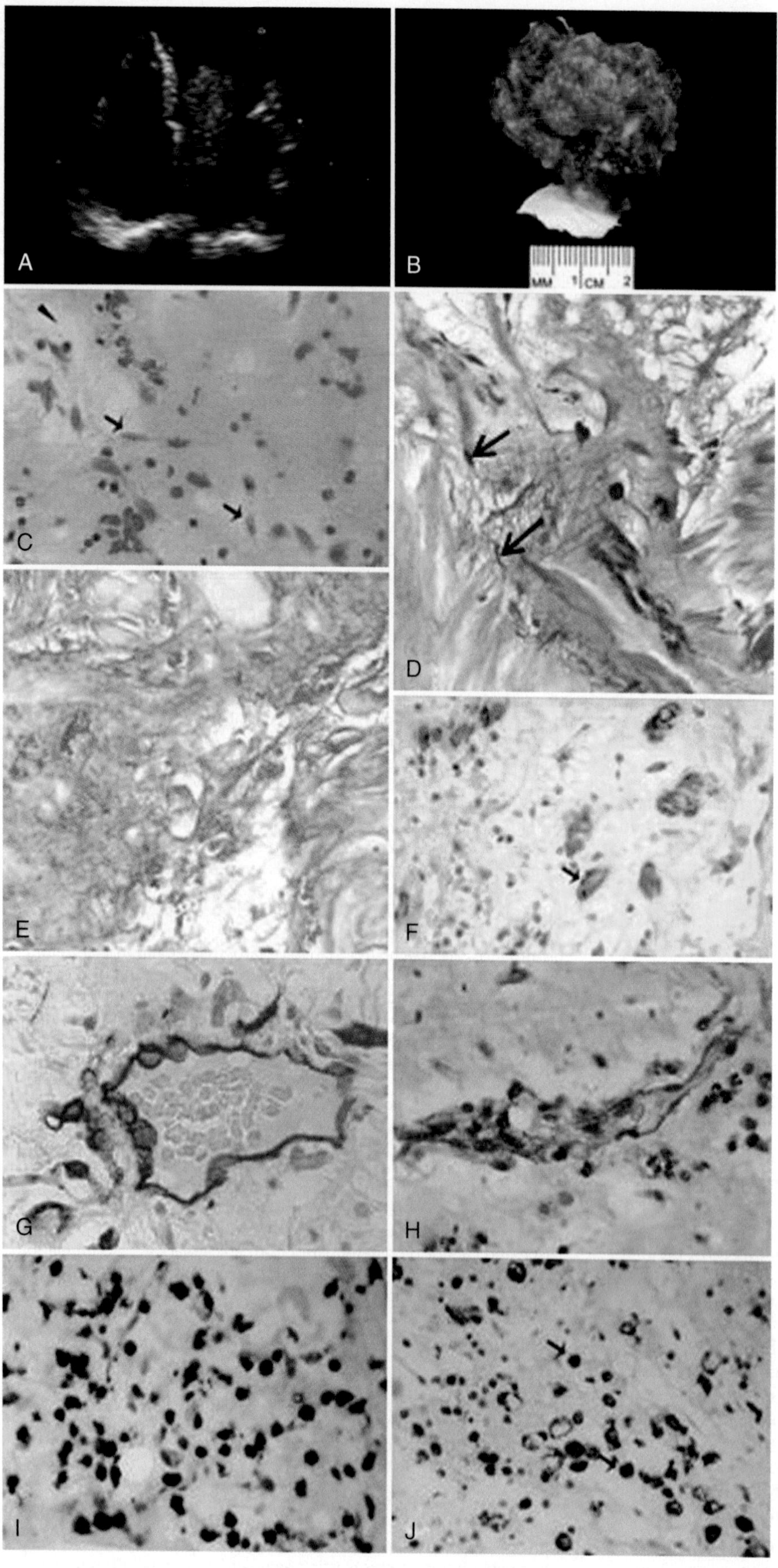

FIGURE 74-1 **A,** Four-chamber echocardiogram of a left atrial myxoma in a 71-year-old woman showing a mass on the left side of the heart projecting from the atrial septum through the mitral valve into the left ventricle. **B,** Gross photograph of the left atrial myxoma that was surgically excised from the same woman. The tumor is a pedunculated, variegated mass with a friable, gelatinous texture. **C,** Hematoxylin and eosin staining of the loose, proteoglycan-rich tumor (×200). The tumor is highly vascular, with vessels containing red blood cells admixed with lipidic cells present in a network throughout the tumor matrix (arrows). **D,** Movat pentachrome staining aids in defining the composition of a myxoma (×400). A variably loose (bubbly turquoise appearance) glycosaminoglycan-rich connective tissue is interspersed with collagen (yellow), rare mononuclear cells, and lipidic mesenchymal cells (arrows, magenta). **E,** Immunohistochemical staining indicates prominent expression of versican (golden brown), a major proteoglycan in myxomas (×400). **F**, **G**, and **H**, Immunohistochemical staining for vessels was positive for alpha smooth muscle actin (arrow), CD34, and CD31, respectively (×400). **I**, Staining for leukocyte common antigen is positive for mononuclear cells (×400). **J**, Staining for CD68 shows several macrophages (arrows), some of which are hemosiderin laden, reflecting previous hemorrhage, a common occurrence in myxomas (×400).

patients can be symptomatic[55] with transient ischemic attacks, stroke, angina, myocardial infarction, and dyspnea. Cerebral embolic symptoms are present in more than half of the symptomatic patients.[55] Rarely, patients present with subacute bacterial endocarditis–like findings, and pulmonary embolism and sudden death have also been reported. Cardiac papillary fibroelastomas are usually firmly attached to the valvular or mural endocardium. In contrast to other cardiac neoplasms like cardiac myxoma, the embolic material from papillary fibroelastoma is believed to be fibrin or a thrombus originating from the fragile papillary fronds of the tumor surface because fragments of tumor have only rarely been found in the vessels involved.[57] Transesophageal echocardiography is the recommended imaging modality for the diagnosis and characterization of papillary fibroelastoma (see Fig. 15-88), with a sensitivity and specificity of 89% and 88%, respectively, for lesions measuring 2 cm or more.[58] A papillary fibroelastoma generally appears as a round, oval, or irregular lesion that is well demarcated and homogeneous on echocardiography. A diagnosis is supported by the echodensity of the tumor's central collagen core. CMR can differentiate between a tumor and a thrombus by the delayed enhancement after the administration of extracellular contrast media. With multislice scanners, CT is just as effective as echocardiography in depicting small moving structures. Cine CMR can also assess myocardial and valvular function, but the spatial resolution is reduced.[33] Even though papillary fibroelastoma can be found anywhere in the heart, 80% to 90% are found on the valvular endocardium.[58] The aortic valve is the most common site (37% to 45%), although fibroelastomas can also originate on the mitral, tricuspid, or pulmonary valves and less commonly on the left atrial and left ventricular endocardium.[55,58-60] The lesions are single in 91% of the cases,[58] although multiple papillary fibroelastomas from different sites can be found in a small subset of patients.[61,62] The average size of a reported papillary fibroelastoma is about 1 cm in diameter, and it can range from 0.2 to 4.6 cm. In gross appearance, the papillary fibroelastoma has often been compared with the sea anemone because of the numerous and delicate papillary fronds. The tumor is soft, white to tan, and often friable with adherent thrombus, which likely represents the source of the emboli. Forty-four percent of papillary fibroelastomas have a 1- to 3-mm stalk, and this mobile type of papillary fibroelastoma appears more likely to give rise to embolism.[55,58,63] Papillary fibroelastoma has a distinct histologic appearance with multiple narrow, elongated, avascular papillary villous fronds radiating from a central stalk. Each frond has a surface that is covered by a single hyperplastic layer of endothelial cells frequently with attached fibrin thrombi, and the matrix of the papillary fronds consists of variable amounts of mucopolysaccharides, collagen, elastic fibers, and rare spindle cells resembling smooth muscle cells or fibroblasts. The treatment of papillary fibroelastoma is surgical excision or tumor shaving from the valvular leaflets with either reconstitution or, less commonly, replacement of the valve.[33,50,58] In prospective studies involving 45 patients with suspected papillary fibroelastomas based on transesophageal echocardiography, 6.6% of the patients went on to develop embolic-type symptoms in a 1-year follow-up period.[58] However, the risk of papillary fibroelastoma–related complication must be weighed against the risk of surgery from patient to patient. Asymptomatic patients with small, left-sided, nonmobile-type papillary fibroelastomas can be cautiously observed, whereas excision

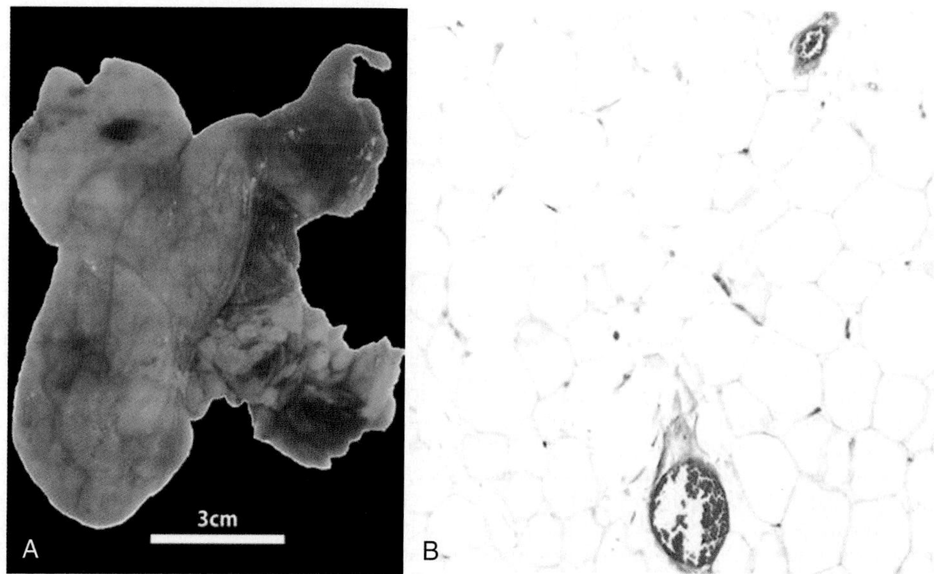

FIGURE 74-2 A, Gross photograph of a pericardial lipoma from a 71-year-old man. **B,** Hematoxylin and eosin staining depicts mature adipocytes in the tumor with associated vascular supply (×200).

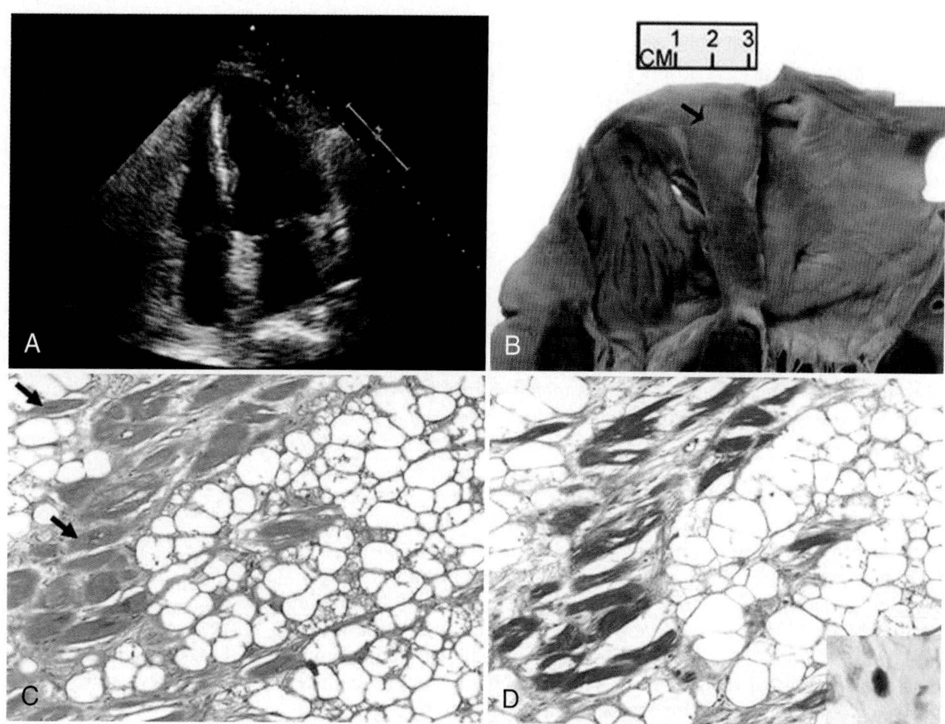

FIGURE 74-3 A, Four-chamber echocardiogram demonstrating lipomatous hypertrophy of the atrial septum in a 72-year-old woman. **B,** Lipomatous hypertrophy of the atrial septum in a heart from a 62-year-old man. The atrial septum superior to the fossa ovale was measured to have a thickness greater than 3 cm (arrow). **C,** Hematoxylin and eosin staining depicts variably hypertrophied and atrophied cardiac myocytes (arrows), with associated fibrous tissue and an admix of mature (larger) and immature (smaller and granular) adipocytes (×200). **D,** Movat pentachrome staining highlights the myocytes (red) and associated excess collagen (yellow) as well as the unusual adipose tissue (×200). **D, inset,** Chloracetate esterase staining shows the presence of mast cells (×400). *(**A** and **B** courtesy of Dr. Kenneth Gin, University of British Columbia, Division of Cardiology.)*

should be considered for patients with larger (≥1 cm) or mobile-type papillary fibroelastomas.[50,53,58] Aortic valve location and tumor mobility are good predictors for cardiac papillary fibroelastoma–related deaths.[33] No data are currently available to support the use of systemic anticoagulation to prevent the embolic complications of papillary fibroelastoma. The prognosis for patients with surgically resectable papillary fibroelastoma is excellent, and there is no reported case of recurrence to date.[58]

Rhabdomyomas

Cardiac rhabdomyomas are the most frequently encountered primary cardiac tumor in infants and children. Nearly 80% of the reported cases of cardiac rhabdomyomas occur in patients younger than 1 year,[29] but rare cases of cardiac rhabdomyomas occurring in adults have been encountered.[64] Arrhythmias represent the most common presentation for adult-type rhabdomyomas.[64,65] However, for both fetal-type and adult-type rhabdomyomas, patients may be asymptomatic if the lesions are small. Rhabdomyomas appear as well-circumscribed masses with hyperintense T1- and T2-weighted spin-echo images and hypointense images after the administration of gadolinium. Cardiac rhabdomyoma arises more commonly in the ventricles, although up to 30% of cases can involve either atrium.[1,66] On histologic examination, cardiac rhabdomyoma is a well-demarcated lesion composed of enlarged cells with clear cytoplasm and occasional "spider cells."[1] Adult-type cardiac rhabdomyoma histologically resembles the extracardiac rhabdomyoma found in the head and neck region of adults, with a high degree of cellularity, foci of tightly packed small cells, and inconspicuous vacuolated spider cells.[59,61] Mitotic activity is absent in adult-type rhabdomyoma.

In symptomatic patients with arrhythmias, antiarrhythmic drugs may be used, and surgical excision with removal of the culprit portion of the lesion is indicated if the drugs fail to control symptoms.[4] No recurrence has been documented to date for cardiac rhabdomyomas, and the prognosis of this disease is excellent.

Fibromas and Hamartomas

Cardiac fibroma is the second most common primary cardiac neoplasm in infants and children after rhabdomyomas.[1] About 90% of the reported cases occur in children before the age of 1 year, although fibromas can occur in any age group ranging from a few days to 83 years. Some cases of cardiac fibroma have also been diagnosed prenatally by ultrasound.[67] There is no sex predilection, and the majority of cases appear to be nonfamilial.[1] The exact nature of cardiac fibroma is unknown, and it is unclear whether it represents a hamartoma or a true neoplasm. The majority of cardiac fibromas behave like hamartomas with no tendency to recur or to grow aggressively.[1] Of note, hamartomas usually cause arrhythmogenic disorders such as ventricular tachycardia, atrial fibrillation, and right or left bundle branch block.[4] They typically appear as subendocardial yellow-tan nodules or plaques. Histologic findings show multifocal hamartomatous proliferation of cardiac cells with oncocytic features, such as nests of foamy-appearing myocytes resembling macrophages.[4] The first line of treatment is antiarrhythmic drugs, allowing the regression of lesions. Other treatments include surgical excision, electrophysiologic mapping and cryoablation, or direct-vision cryoablation of nodular tumors. The survival rate is approximately 80%.[4] Some cardiac fibromas behave like benign neoplasms with the ability to recur but never metastasize. Although most cardiac fibromas appear to occur sporadically, some appear to develop as part of the Gorlin syndrome (nevoid basal cell carcinoma syndrome), which is a result of germline mutations in the *PTC* gene that maps to chromosome 9q22.3 and is homologous to the Drosophila *patched* gene.[4,68]

Clinically, heart failure, heart murmurs, arrhythmias, and syncope are the more common presenting findings in patients with cardiac fibroma.[1] Less common presenting findings include sudden death and atypical chest pain. However, up to one third of patients with cardiac fibroma can remain asymptomatic. The ECG can show a number of abnormalities, including evidence of left ventricular hypertrophy, right ventricular hypertrophy, bundle branch block, and atrioventricular (AV) block as well as ventricular tachycardia.[69] Chest radiography may reveal cardiomegaly with or without a focal bulge, and calcification is visible in 15% of cases. Because of its tendency to occur in children, cardiac fibroma must be considered in the differential diagnosis for children with unexplained heart failure, arrhythmias, cardiomegaly, murmur, and pericardial effusion. On echocardiography, cardiac fibroma usually appears as a solitary homogeneous echogenic lesion (see Fig. 15-87).[67] For preoperative assessment, CT and CMR are more desirable for evaluating the "resectability" of the lesion. CT can delineate the heterogeneity of the mural mass, the degree of calcification, and its three-dimensional characteristics.[23] In gadolinium-enhanced CMR and first-pass perfusion imaging, fibromas demonstrate a hypoperfused tumor core that is readily distinguishable from the surrounding myocardium.[4] Cardiac fibromas typically appear grossly as solitary, rounded, intramural masses with a fibrous, whorled cut surface.[1] The mass can be grossly circumscribed or infiltrative with a pushing margin. The average size of the tumor is 5 cm, although lesions up to 10 cm have been reported.[1] Cardiac fibromas are generally single lesions, and they are commonly found in the ventricular septum or the left ventricular free wall, with occurrence in the right ventricle or the atria in less than 10% of cases. On histologic examination, cardiac fibroma shows a proliferation of monomorphic fibroblasts with little or no cellular atypia and resembles fibromatoses with infiltrating margins. The degree of cellularity decreases with age, whereas the amount of collagen deposition increases with age.[1]

Mitotic activity is usually absent but can be present in infants who are only a few months old.[1] A variable amount of elastic fibers and lymphocytic and histiocytic infiltrates may exist. Immunohistochemical examination may demonstrate some degree of smooth muscle actin positivity, but staining for desmin, CD34, and S100 should be negative.[70] The differential diagnosis, especially in the more cellular cases, includes low-grade fibrosarcoma and inflammatory myofibroblastic tumors. The differential feature favoring fibroma over rhabdomyoma is calcification, which occurs in fibromas but not in rhabdomyomas.[4] Because of the potential for cardiac fibroma to cause arrhythmias and occasionally to recur, complete surgical resection in symptomatic cases is recommended. The postoperative prognosis is typically good, although some surgical attempts in infants younger than 4 months have resulted in death.[1] If complete resection is not feasible, palliative partial resection may be considered. Periodic echocardiography may be necessary to monitor for recurrence of the tumor. For large, unresectable tumors, cardiac transplantation may be considered if symptoms such as arrhythmias persist.

Hemangiomas and Lymphangiomas

Primary benign vascular tumors of the heart include hemangiomas, lymphangiomas, and hemangioendotheliomas. Lymphangiomas and hemangioendotheliomas are extremely rare, with only a few reported cases in the literature.[1] In comparison, cardiac hemangioma is more frequent but accounts for less than 2% of primary cardiac neoplasms.[10] Hemangioma can occur in any age group ranging from a few months to the seventh decade of life.[1] Cardiac hemangiomas are considered to be benign neoplasms with potential for recurrence, but the etiology is not defined. Patients with cardiac hemangioma may remain asymptomatic. In symptomatic patients, the clinical presentation of cardiac hemangioma is variable. Depending on the nature and location of the tumor, patients can present with palpitations,[71] arrhythmias,[1,10] heart failure,[1,10] pericardial effusion, ventricular outflow tract obstruction, pseudoangina,[11] cerebral embolism,[9,10] and, in more extreme cases, sudden death. In some instances, giant cardiac hemangioma can result in Kasabach-Merritt syndrome, characterized by thrombosis, consumptive thrombocytopenia, and coagulopathy. Cardiac hemangioma can occasionally be associated with hemangioma in extracardiac sites, such as the gastrointestinal tract and on the skin or face. Echocardiography is a sensitive, noninvasive method for detection of the tumor, with cardiac hemangioma appearing typically as a hyperechoic lesion.[3] Coronary angiography can sometimes demonstrate blood supply to the tumor, with the presence of "tumor blush."[3,10] On chest CT, cardiac hemangioma is characterized by heterogeneous signal with intense enhancement in most cases after contrast material administration.[3,68] On CMR, cardiac hemangiomas appear as masses with intermediate signal intensity on T1-weighted images and hypointense signal on T2-weighted images, and there may be rapid enhancement during infusion of the contrast agent.[72] In gross appearance, cardiac hemangiomas can range from less than 1 cm to 8 cm in size and can occur as intracavitary, intramural, epicardial, or pericardial lesions. They can occur in any chamber, although occurrences in the ventricles are more frequent than in the atria. Multiple tumors are seen in about 30% of cases.[73] Although usually well demarcated, some cardiac hemangiomas can have an infiltrative border, which makes complete surgical resection difficult.[1] The histologic appearance of cardiac hemangiomas is similar to that of hemangiomas arising in other sites. Three main histologic subtypes exist: (1) the cavernous hemangioma, which is composed of multiple thin- or thick-walled dilated vessels; (2) the capillary hemangioma, which is composed of lobules of endothelial cells forming small, capillary-like vessels; and (3) the arteriovenous hemangioma, which is composed of dysplastic thick-walled arterioles, venous-like vessels, and capillaries. The cavernous type of cardiac hemangioma tends not to show a rapid signal enhancement with administration of contrast material on imaging because of the slow blood flow.[3] In contrast to angiosarcoma, necrosis, marked nuclear atypia, and mitotic activity are not seen in hemangioma. In symptomatic patients, radical resection of the tumor is recommended because of the potential for recurrence, especially if the resection is incomplete.[11] The postoperative prognosis is excellent in patients with resectable tumors.[74] Because cardiac hemangiomas may regress spontaneously, conservative management may be considered in asymptomatic patients, particularly if complex and potentially hazardous excision is required.[3] In instances in which surgical resection is high risk, treatment of a congenital pericardial hemangioma next to the coronary artery with high-dose corticosteroid therapy may lead to regression of the tumor.[75] Notably, a single case of cardiac angiosarcoma developing 7 years after surgical excision of a cardiac hemangioma has been reported.[76] As such, in all cases of cardiac hemangioma, periodic echocardiography is recommended to examine for recurrence of tumor growth.

Malignant Tumors

Approximately one fourth of all cardiac tumors are considered malignant, and about one half to three quarters of all malignant primary cardiac tumors are sarcomas; primary cardiac lymphomas are the next most common group.[1,77] Of note is that metastatic tumors to the heart are 20 to 40 times more common (see Chap. 90). Most common malignant neoplasms that involve the heart or pericardium include lung and breast cancer. However, Hodgkin disease, non-Hodgkin lymphomas, malignant melanoma (see Fig. 18-18), numerous primary gastrointestinal malignant neoplasms, and various types of sarcomas arising from extracardiac locations can also secondarily involve the heart. Therefore, it is important as well as logical to consider the possibility that a cardiac lesion confirmed histologically to be a sarcoma may actually be a metastasis from a sarcoma in another anatomic location. A thorough clinical examination combined with a series of imaging studies should help rule out this possibility. The more common malignant primary tumors of the heart (excluding malignant mesothelioma that arises from the pericardium) include angiosarcomas, leiomyosarcomas, rhabdomyosarcomas, malignant fibrous histiocytomas, undifferentiated sarcomas, fibrosarcomas, and malignant lymphomas. Other rarely encountered primary cardiac sarcomas include liposarcomas, synovial sarcomas, and malignant peripheral nerve sheath tumors. In general, the individual histologic subtypes of primary cardiac sarcomas do not appear to influence the outcome as significantly as the histologic grade of the sarcomas, which is evaluated on the basis of a combination of mitotic activity, amount of necrosis, and degree of cellular differentiation. Sarcomas showing high mitotic activity (>5 mitotic figures/10 high-power fields), extensive tumor necrosis, and poor cellular differentiation have a worse prognosis than sarcomas without these features.[1] The presence of metastases also confers a poorer prognosis. In terms of imaging studies, nearly all sarcomas occurring in the heart are aggressive tumors that show a highly infiltrative pattern of growth. They often appear on CT or CMR as large, heterogeneous, broad-based masses that frequently occupy most of the affected cardiac chambers.[3] CMR is usually the method of choice for imaging of sarcomas because it provides excellent tissue characterization and local extent of the tumor.[23] The tumors may also show evidence of extension into other cardiac chambers and the pericardium, and there may also be associated pericardial effusions and hilar lymphadenopathy.

Angiosarcomas

Primary cardiac angiosarcoma is the most common primary cardiac sarcoma in adults, accounting for 30% to 37% of the cases.[1,2,78] Other malignant vascular tumors, such as Kaposi sarcoma and malignant epithelioid hemangioendothelioma, are even rarer by comparison. Cardiac angiosarcomas typically occur in adults 30 to 50 years old but can occur in almost any age group from 2 to 80 years. A slight male predilection exists.[2,18] With the exception of a single report of familial occurrence of cardiac angiosarcomas, all others appear to occur sporadically.[79] Little is known about the oncogenesis of angiosarcoma. Complex cytogenetic changes and mutations in *p53* have been identified in some angiosarcomas.[79,80] Clinically, patients with primary cardiac angiosarcomas typically present with advanced disease, with 66% to 89% of patients already demonstrating evidence of metastatic disease at initial presentation.[2] Initial findings may include dyspnea, chest pain, heart murmur, constitutional symptoms, arrhythmias, superior vena cava syndrome, and evidence of heart failure.[1,2,15,81,82] Because of the propensity for cardiac angiosarcoma to involve pericardium, pericardial effusion and cardiac tamponade may also be the presentation.[14,15,72] Hemorrhagic pericardial tamponade usually indicates tumor infiltration through the myocardium.[23] Less commonly, symptoms related to the metastatic disease, such as stroke-like neurologic symptoms secondary to cerebral metastases, are the initial presentation in patients with cardiac angiosarcoma.[2,83] The ECG may reveal nonspecific ST changes, arrhythmias, and AV block. The chest radiograph may show nonspecific changes like cardiomegaly, widened mediastinum, hilar lymphadenopathy, and pleural effusion.[78] Transesophageal echocardiography is the initial imaging modality of choice[14,73] for detection of the lesion, but echocardiography has limited ability to demonstrate tumor infiltration and cannot depict mediastinal and extracardiac involvement. CT and CMR are therefore required[78] for a better characterization of the tumor growth and involvement (**Fig. 74-4**). Angiosarcomas typically appear as low-attenuation, invasive, irregular nodular masses showing heterogeneous enhancement with the administration of contrast media on CT and heterogeneous mass on CMR. They frequently show extensive pericardial involvement and hemorrhagic pericardial effusions.[3] For histologic diagnosis, invasive methods like echocardiographically guided transvenous cardiac biopsy may provide diagnostic material, but a negative biopsy finding does not rule out the possibility of angiosarcoma.[14,21] Alternatively, biopsy of the metastatic lesion in a more accessible location or cytology examination on pericardiocentesis fluid may also assist in the diagnosis.[15] In gross appearance, angiosarcomas are typically large, multilobular, dark brown intramural masses that may protrude into or replace most of the atrial cavity.[1] About 90% of angiosarcomas arise in the right atrium, and this is thought to contribute to the late onset of symptoms. Involvement of adjacent structures such as the tricuspid valve, pulmonary valve, and vena cava as well as extension into the pericardium may occur. On histologic examination, cardiac angiosarcomas usually exhibit evidence of endothelial differentiation with formation of vascular channels or papillary structures.[1] In contrast to benign vascular lesions, the lining cells are atypical and form irregular anastomosing sinusoid structures. Moderate nuclear and mitotic pleomorphisms are also observed. In some cases, the tumor is composed primarily of anaplastic or spindle cells with little evidence of endothelial derivation, and the identification of poorly formed vascular channels or intracytoplasmic vacuoles containing red blood cells can aid in the diagnosis. Immunohistochemical study can be used to further support evidence of endothelial differentiation by demonstrating CD31, CD34, and von Willebrand factor positive immunophenotype in the tumor cells.[84] Novel lymphatic endothelial markers including D2-40 and LYVE-1 can further identify tumors showing more lymphatic endothelial differentiation than vascular endothelial differentiation.[85-87]

Cardiac angiosarcomas are aggressive-behaving neoplasms that are associated with a poor prognosis and mean survival of 9 to 10 months.[82]

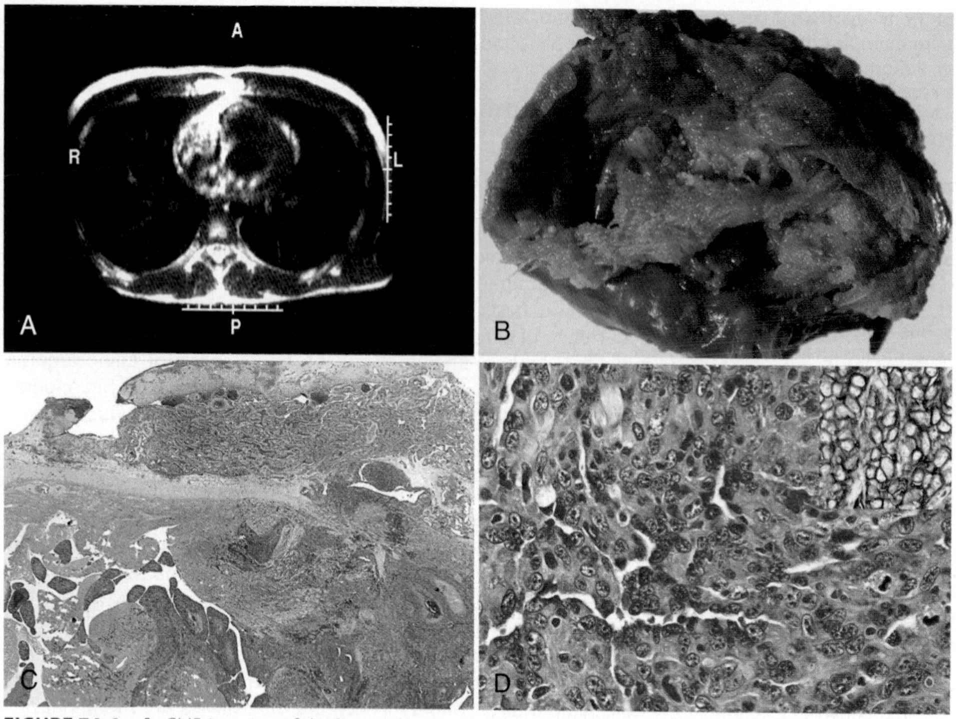

FIGURE 74-4 **A,** CMR imaging of the heart of a 20-year-old man with an angiosarcoma in the right atrium. CMR confirmed findings from a transesophageal echocardiogram that showed a 3 × 3 × 3.5-cm intra-arterial mass with extension toward the inferior vena cava. **B,** Angiosarcoma tumor resected from the right atrium of a 20-year-old man. This tumor was surgically resected from the superior vena cava down to the annulus of the tricuspid valve. The surgical resected specimen shows a tan-red, multilobulated tumor mass. **C** and **D,** Section of angiosarcoma (hematoxylin and eosin; **D** ×400). **D, inset,** Brightly positive staining for CD31 in tumor cells. *(**A** and **C** courtesy of Drs. Gerald Berry and Kizhake Kurian, Department of Pathology, Stanford University, Calif., and Department of Cardiovascular Medicine, UFSHC at Jacksonville, Fla., respectively. **B** and **D** from Kurian KC, Weisshaar D, Parekh H, et al: Primary cardiac angiosarcoma: Case report and review of the literature. Cardiovasc Pathol 15:110, 2006.)*

This is partially because of the late detection of the disease; most patients present with advanced-stage disease. Common sites of metastases include lung, liver, brain, and bone, although metastases to lymph nodes, adrenal glands, spleen, and skin have also been reported.[14,18] Even though no consistent, effective treatment has been identified for cardiac angiosarcoma to date,[82] a multidisciplinary approach to the treatment of cardiac angiosarcoma is advocated.[15,18] Such an integrated approach includes a combination of surgery, irradiation, adjuvant or neoadjuvant chemotherapy, and immunotherapy with interleukin-12 (IL-12). Chemotherapy with doxorubicin, an anthracycline antibiotic with antineoplastic activity, has been shown to improve the survival of patients.[88] The aim of the surgery is still complete tumor resection.[89] Neoadjuvant chemotherapy may be administered to reduce the tumor mass and to facilitate surgical excision.[90] However, the prognosis for patients with angiosarcomas is still poor. The use of heart transplantation remains controversial in this setting.[2] For patients with advanced-stage unresectable disease, palliative treatment including the use of metallic stents for superior vena cava syndrome and for severe right ventricular outflow tract obstruction may help improve the patient's short-term quality of life.[2,90] It has been shown that the MDM2 protein binds to and inhibits p53 activity. The *MDM2* gene is often overexpressed in angiosarcomas even when the p53 expression is normal. MDM2 directly induces cellular transformation and is associated with vascular endothelial growth factor overproduction and angiogenesis. Thus, inhibition of angiogenesis through MDM2 may potentially be a therapeutic target used to treat angiosarcomas.[91]

Rhabdomyosarcomas

Cardiac rhabdomyosarcomas are the most common primary sarcoma of the heart in children. The average age at disease presentation is in the second decade of life, but it can also occur in young adults. A slight male predominance, especially in the pediatric population, exists.[1] Because of its rarity, the etiology of primary cardiac rhabdomyosarcomas remains elusive. Heart failure, arrhythmias, cardiac murmurs, and constitutional symptoms are common manifestations of the disease.[1] Occasional cases are also associated with hypereosinophilia, hypertrophic osteoarthropathy, and polyarthritis.[92,93] Nonspecific electrocardiography and chest radiography findings are often present. As with other cardiac sarcomas, transthoracic echocardiography and transesophageal echocardiography are reasonable imaging modalities in the initial workup of the patient thought to have a cardiac lesion.[20,93] Chest CT or CMR is necessary for better delineation of the nature, origin, and extent of the lesion, especially if a malignant lesion is suspected.[20,93] Although echocardiographically guided transvenous cardiac biopsy may be attempted for tissue diagnosis, a negative result cannot be relied on because there is a high rate of false negatives. In contrast to angiosarcomas, cardiac rhabdomyosarcomas show no predilection for a specific cavity, and multiple lesions are frequently present (60%).[20,93] The histologic features of cardiac rhabdomyosarcomas are similar to those of their extracardiac counterparts. The embryonal type and pleomorphic type of rhabdomyosarcomas are more commonly seen as primary tumors in the heart, whereas the alveolar type of rhabdomyosarcomas is typically found as a metastatic disease to the heart.[1] Cardiac rhabdomyosarcomas are aggressive neoplasms with a tendency to produce local and distant metastases, most commonly to the lung and lymph nodes, although spread to various other organs has also been documented previously.[20] Cardiac rhabdomyosarcomas have a dismal prognosis, and survival is usually less than 1 year. Tumors demonstrating a high mitotic activity, extensive tumor necrosis, lack of cellular differentiation, and extensive myocardial and pericardial extension are associated with the worst prognosis.[1,93] The primary aim of treatment is complete surgical resection, but the highly infiltrative nature of tumor often precludes this. Furthermore, the tumor has a poor response to radiation therapy and chemotherapy.[94] In selected cases, heart transplantation may be considered if no obvious distant metastases are present.[93]

Leiomyosarcomas

Leiomyosarcomas are malignant mesenchymal tumors that demonstrate histologic and immunophenotypic evidence of smooth muscle differentiation. The mean age at presentation is in the fourth decade, and there is no apparent sex predilection.[1] The exact oncogenesis of leiomyosarcomas is not known. The common clinical presentations include dyspnea, pericardial effusions, chest pain, atrial arrhythmias, and heart failure.[1,95,96] Approximately 70% to 80% of leiomyosarcomas arise from the left atrium, and they tend to extend into the pulmonary trunk.[95] The tumor is typically solitary but can be multiple in 30% of patients.[1,96] Echocardiography can help identify the cardiac lesion, and contrast-enhanced CT or CMR can help to further characterize the nature and extent of tumor growth.[96,97] On histologic examination, typical leiomyosarcomas show intersecting fascicles of spindle cells with blunt-ended nuclei and well-defined eosinophilic cytoplasm with longitudinal striations. Some leiomyosarcomas contain a large number

Diagnostic Approach

21. Meng Q, Lai H, Lima J, et al: Echocardiographic and pathologic characteristics of primary cardiac tumors: A study of 149 cases. Int J Cardiol 84:69, 2002.
22. Ekmektzoglou KA, Samelis GF, Xanthos T: Heart and tumors: Location, metastasis, clinical manifestations, diagnostic approaches and therapeutic considerations. J Cardiovasc Med (Hagerstown) 9:769, 2008.
23. van Beek EJ, Stolpen AH, Khanna G, et al: CT and MRI of pericardial and cardiac neoplastic disease. Cancer Imaging 7:19, 2007.
24. Nitta R, Sakomura Y, Tanimoto K, et al: Primary cardiac angiosarcoma of the right atrium undiagnosed by transvenous endocardial tumor biopsy. Intern Med 37:1023, 1998.
25. Anghel G, Zoli V, Petti N, et al: Primary cardiac lymphoma: Report of two cases occurring in immunocompetent subjects. Leuk Lymphoma 45:781, 2004.

Benign Tumors

26. Terracciano LM, Mhawech P, Suess K, et al: Calretinin as a marker for cardiac myxoma. Diagnostic and histogenetic considerations. Am J Clin Pathol 114:754, 2000.
27. Wilkes D, Charitakis K, Basson CT: Inherited disposition to cardiac myxoma development. Nat Rev Cancer 6:157, 2006.
28. Orlandi A, Ciucci A, Ferlosio A, et al: Cardiac myxoma cells exhibit embryonic endocardial stem cell features. J Pathol 209:231, 2006.
29. Amano J, Kono T, Wada Y, et al: Cardiac myxoma: Its origin and tumor characteristics. Ann Thorac Cardiovasc Surg 9:215, 2003.
30. Kodama H, Hirotani T, Suzuki Y, et al: Cardiomyogenic differentiation in cardiac myxoma expressing lineage-specific transcription factors. Am J Pathol 161:381, 2002.
31. Kono T, Koide N, Hama Y, et al: Expression of vascular endothelial growth factor and angiogenesis in cardiac myxoma: A study of fifteen patients. J Thorac Cardiovasc Surg 119:101, 2000.
32. Pucci A, Gagliardotto P, Zanini C, et al: Histopathologic and clinical characterization of cardiac myxoma: Review of 53 cases from a single institution. Am Heart J 140:134, 2000.
33. Sydow K, Willems S, Reichenspurner H, et al: Papillary fibroelastomas of the heart. Thorac Cardiovasc Surg 56:9, 2008.
34. Aspres N, Bleasel NR, Stapleton KM: Genetic testing of the family with a Carney-complex member leads to successful early removal of an asymptomatic atrial myxoma in the mother of the patient. Australas J Dermatol 44:121, 2003.
35. Mochizuki Y, Okamura Y, Iida H, et al: Interleukin-6 and "complex" cardiac myxoma. Ann Thorac Surg 66:931, 1998.
36. Komiya N, Isomoto S, Hayano M, et al: The influence of tumor size on the electrocardiographic changes in patients with left atrial myxoma. J Electrocardiol 35:53, 2002.
37. Ipek G, Erentug V, Bozbuga N, et al: Surgical management of cardiac myxoma. J Card Surg 20:300, 2005.
38. Miller DV, Tazelaar HD, Handy JR, et al: Thymoma arising within cardiac myxoma. Am J Surg Pathol 29:1208, 2005.
39. Pucci A, Bartoloni G, Tessitore E, et al: Cytokeratin profile and neuroendocrine cells in the glandular component of cardiac myxoma. Virchows Arch 443:618, 2003.
40. Val-Bernal JF, Acebo E, Gomez-Roman JJ, et al: Anticipated diagnosis of left atrial myxoma following histological investigation of limb embolectomy specimens: A report of two cases. Pathol Int 53:489, 2003.
41. Rosenberg FM, Chan A, Lichtenstein SV, et al: Cardiac neoplasms. Curr Treat Options Cardiovasc Med 1:243, 1999.
42. Bjessmo S, Ivert T: Cardiac myxoma: 40 years' experience in 63 patients. Ann Thorac Surg 63:697, 1997.
43. Selkane C, Amahzoune B, Chavanis N, et al: Changing management of cardiac myxoma based on a series of 40 cases with long-term follow-up. Ann Thorac Surg 76:1935, 2003.
44. Altundag MB, Ertas G, Ucer AR, et al: Brain metastasis of cardiac myxoma: Case report and review of the literature. J Neurooncol 75:181, 2005.
45. Salanitri JC, Pereles FS: Cardiac lipoma and lipomatous hypertrophy of the interatrial septum: Cardiac magnetic resonance imaging findings. J Comput Assist Tomogr 28:852, 2004.
46. Mitelman F: Catalog of Chromosome Aberrations in Cancer. New York, Wiley-Liss, 1998.
47. Akram K, Hill C, Neelagaru N, Parker M: A left ventricular lipoma presenting as heart failure in a septuagenarian: A first case report. Int J Cardiol 114:386, 2007 .
48. Heyer CM, Kagel T, Lemburg SP, et al: Lipomatous hypertrophy of the interatrial septum: A prospective study of incidence, imaging findings, and clinical symptoms. Chest 124:2068, 2003.
49. Nova M, Steiner I: A rationale for a stone on the heart—subepicardial lipoma. Cardiovasc Pathol 15:176, 2006.
50. Meaney JF, Kazerooni EA, Jamadar DA, et al: CT appearance of lipomatous hypertrophy of the interatrial septum. AJR Am J Roentgenol 168:1081, 1997.
51. Xanthos T, Giannakopoulos N, Papadimitriou L: Lipomatous hypertrophy of the interatrial septum: A pathological and clinical approach. Int J Cardiol 121:4, 2007.
52. Christiansen S, Stypmann J, Baba HA, et al: Surgical management of extensive lipomatous hypertrophy of the right atrium. Cardiovasc Surg 8:88, 2000.
53. Roberts WC: Primary and secondary neoplasms of the heart. Am J Cardiol 80:671, 1997.
54. Nadra I, Dawson D, Schmitz SA, et al: Lipomatous hypertrophy of the interatrial septum: A commonly misdiagnosed mass often leading to unnecessary cardiac surgery. Heart 90:e66, 2004.
55. Howard RA, Aldea GS, Shapira OM, et al: Papillary fibroelastoma: Increasing recognition of a surgical disease. Ann Thorac Surg 68:1881, 1999.
56. Sumino S, Paterson HS: No regrowth after incomplete papillary fibroelastoma excision. Ann Thorac Surg 79:e3, 2005.
57. Roberts WC: Papillary fibroelastomas of the heart. Am J Cardiol 80:973, 1997.
58. Sun JP, Asher CR, Yang XS, et al: Clinical and echocardiographic characteristics of papillary fibroelastomas: A retrospective and prospective study in 162 patients. Circulation 103:2687, 2001.
59. Saad RS, Galvis CO, Bshara W, et al: Pulmonary valve papillary fibroelastoma. A case report and review of the literature. Arch Pathol Lab Med 125:933, 2001.
60. Georghiou GP, Erez E, Vidne BA, et al: Tricuspid valve papillary fibroelastoma: An unusual cause of intermittent dyspnea. Eur J Cardiothorac Surg 23:429, 2003.
61. Davoli G, Bizzarri F, Enrico T, et al: Double papillary fibroelastoma of the aortic valve. Tex Heart Inst J 31:448, 2004.
62. Eslami-Varzaneh F, Brun EA, Sears-Rogan P: An unusual case of multiple papillary fibroelastoma, review of literature. Cardiovasc Pathol 12:170, 2003.
63. Nawaz MZ, Lander AR, Schussler JM, et al: Tumor excision versus valve replacement for papillary fibroelastoma involving the mitral valve. Am J Cardiol 97:759, 2006.
64. Burke AP, Gatto-Weis C, Griego JE, et al: Adult cellular rhabdomyoma of the heart: A report of 3 cases. Hum Pathol 33:1092, 2002.
65. Krasuski RA, Hesselson AB, Landolfo KP, et al: Cardiac rhabdomyoma in an adult patient presenting with ventricular arrhythmia. Chest 118:1217, 2000.
66. Chen X, Hoda SA, Edgar MA: Cardiac rhabdomyoma. Arch Pathol Lab Med 126:1559, 2002.
67. Kim TH, Kim YM, Han MY, et al: Perinatal sonographic diagnosis of cardiac fibroma with MR imaging correlation. AJR Am J Roentgenol 178:727, 2002.
68. Bossert T, Walther T, Vondrys D, et al: Cardiac fibroma as an inherited manifestation of nevoid basal-cell carcinoma syndrome. Tex Heart Inst J 33:88, 2006.
69. Wong JA, Fishbein MC: Cardiac fibroma resulting in fatal ventricular arrhythmia. Circulation 101:E168, 2000.
70. de Montpreville VT, Serraf A, Aznag H, et al: Fibroma and inflammatory myofibroblastic tumor of the heart. Ann Diagn Pathol 5:335, 2001.
71. Eftychiou C, Antoniades L: Cardiac hemangioma in the left ventricle and brief review of the literature. J Cardiovasc Med (Hagerstown) 10:565, 2009.
72. Oshima H, Hara M, Kono T, et al: Cardiac hemangioma of the left atrial appendage: CT and MR findings. J Thorac Imaging 18:204, 2003.
73. Moniotte S, Geva T, Perez-Atayde A, et al: Images in cardiovascular medicine. Cardiac hemangioma. Circulation 112:e103, 2005.
74. Kojima S, Sumiyoshi M, Suwa S, et al: Cardiac hemangioma: A report of two cases and review of the literature. Heart Vessels 18:153, 2003.
75. Wu G, Jones J, Sequeira IB, et al: Congenital pericardial hemangioma responding to high-dose corticosteroid therapy. Can J Cardiol 25:e139, 2009.
76. Chalet Y, Mace L, Franc B, et al: Angiosarcoma 7 years after surgical excision of histiocytoid haemangioma in left atrium. Lancet 341:1217, 1993.

Malignant Tumors

77. Farah HH, Jacob M, Aragam J: Images in cardiology: A case of cardiac angiosarcoma presenting as pericardial tamponade. Heart 86:665, 2001.
78. Deetjen AG, Conradi G, Mollmann S, et al: Cardiac angiosarcoma diagnosed and characterized by cardiac magnetic resonance imaging. Cardiol Rev 14:101, 2006.
79. Casha AR, Davidson LA, Roberts P, et al: Familial angiosarcoma of the heart. J Thorac Cardiovasc Surg 124:392, 2002.
80. Zu Y, Perle MA, Yan Z, et al: Chromosomal abnormalities and p53 gene mutation in a cardiac angiosarcoma. Appl Immunohistochem Mol Morphol 9:24, 2001.
81. Amonkar GP, Deshpande JR: Cardiac angiosarcoma. Cardiovasc Pathol 15:57, 2006.
82. Kurian KC, Weisshaar D, Parekh H, et al: Primary cardiac angiosarcoma: Case report and review of the literature. Cardiovasc Pathol 15:110, 2006.
83. Liassides C, Katsamaga M, Deretzi G, et al: Cerebral metastasis from heart angiosarcoma presenting as multiple hematomas. J Neuroimaging 14:71, 2004.
84. Weiss SW, Goldblum J: Enzinger and Weiss's Soft Tissue Tumors. 4th ed. St. Louis, Mosby, 2001.
85. Arai E, Kuramochi A, Tsuchida T, et al: Usefulness of D2-40 immunohistochemistry for differentiation between kaposiform hemangioendothelioma and tufted angioma. J Cutan Pathol 33:492, 2006.
86. Khan MA, Mujahed MA: Atrial myxoma producing a saddle embolus in a child. Thorax 25:634, 1970.
87. Xu H, Edwards JR, Espinosa O, et al: Expression of a lymphatic endothelial cell marker in benign and malignant vascular tumors. Hum Pathol 35:857, 2004.
88. Pigott C, Welker M, Khosla P, et al: Improved outcome with multimodality therapy in primary cardiac angiosarcoma. Nat Clin Pract Oncol 5:112, 2008.
89. Hoffmeier A, Scheld HH, Tjan TD, et al: Ex situ resection of primary cardiac tumors. Thorac Cardiovasc Surg 51:99, 2003.
90. Totaro M, Miraldi F, Ghiribelli C, et al: Cardiac angiosarcoma arising from pulmonary artery: Endovascular treatment. Ann Thorac Surg 78:1468, 2004.
91. Neragi-Miandoab S, Kim J, Vlahakes GJ: Malignant tumours of the heart: A review of tumour type, diagnosis and therapy. Clin Oncol (R Coll Radiol) 19:748, 2007.
92. Lo Re V 3rd, Fox KR, Ferrari VA, et al: Hypereosinophilia associated with cardiac rhabdomyosarcoma. Am J Hematol 74:64, 2003.
93. Grandmougin D, Fayad G, Decoene C, et al: Total orthotopic heart transplantation for primary cardiac rhabdomyosarcoma: Factors influencing long-term survival. Ann Thorac Surg 71:1438, 2001.
94. Aksoylar S, Kansoy S, Bakiler AR, et al: Primary cardiac rhabdomyosarcoma. Med Pediatr Oncol 38:146, 2002.
95. Ishikawa K, Takanashi S, Mihara W, et al: Surgical treatment for primary cardiac leiomyosarcoma causing right ventricular outflow obstruction. Circ J 69:121, 2005.
96. Clarke NR, Mohiaddin RH, Westaby S, et al: Multifocal cardiac leiomyosarcoma. Diagnosis and surveillance by transoesophageal echocardiography and contrast enhanced cardiovascular magnetic resonance. Postgrad Med J 78:492, 2002.
97. Ogimoto A, Hamada M, Ohtsuka T, et al: Rapid progression of primary cardiac leiomyosarcoma with obstruction of the left ventricular outflow tract and mitral stenosis. Intern Med 42:827, 2003.
98. Rockwell L, Hetzel P, Freeman JK, et al: Cardiac involvement in malignancies. Case 3. Primary cardiac lymphoma. J Clin Oncol 22:2744, 2004.
99. Nart D, Nalbantgil S, Yagdi T, et al: Primary cardiac lymphoma in a heart transplant recipient. Transplant Proc 37:1362, 2005.
100. Binder J, Pfleger S, Schwarz S: Images in cardiovascular medicine. Right atrial primary cardiac lymphoma presenting with stroke. Circulation 110:e451, 2004.
101. Quigley MM, Schwartzman E, Boswell PD, et al: A unique atrial primary cardiac lymphoma mimicking myxoma presenting with embolic stroke: A case report. Blood 101:4708, 2003.

102. Engelen MA, Juergens KU, Breithardt G, et al: Interatrial conduction delay and atrioventricular block due to primary cardiac lymphoma. J Cardiovasc Electrophysiol 16:926, 2005.
103. Fujisaki J, Tanaka T, Kato J, et al: Primary cardiac lymphoma presenting clinically as restrictive cardiomyopathy. Circ J 69:249, 2005.
104. Giunta R, Cravero RG, Granata G, et al: Primary cardiac T-cell lymphoma. Ann Hematol 83:450, 2004.
105. Rolla G, Bertero MT, Pastena G, et al: Primary lymphoma of the heart. A case report and review of the literature. Leuk Res 26:117, 2002.
106. Dawson MA, Mariani J, Taylor A, et al: The successful treatment of primary cardiac lymphoma with a dose-dense schedule of rituximab plus CHOP. Ann Oncol 17:176, 2006.
107. Nakagawa Y, Ikeda U, Hirose M, et al: Successful treatment of primary cardiac lymphoma with monoclonal CD20 antibody (rituximab). Circ J 68:172, 2004.

Management of Primary Cardiac Tumors

108. Messa C, Di Muzio N, Picchio M, et al: PET/CT and radiotherapy. Q J Nucl Med Mol Imaging 50:4, 2006.
109. von Schulthess GK, Steinert HC, Hany TF: Integrated PET/CT: Current applications and future directions. Radiology 238:405, 2006.
110. Nielsen TO, West RB, Linn SC, et al: Molecular characterisation of soft tissue tumours: A gene expression study. Lancet 359:1301, 2002.
111. Fletcher CD: The evolving classification of soft tissue tumours: An update based on the new WHO classification. Histopathology 48:3, 2006.
112. Fletcher CD, Gustafson P, Rydholm A, et al: Clinicopathologic re-evaluation of 100 malignant fibrous histiocytomas: Prognostic relevance of subclassification. J Clin Oncol 19:3045, 2001.

CHAPTER 75 Pericardial Diseases

Martin M. LeWinter and Marc D. Tischler

Anatomy and Physiology of the Pericardium

The pericardium is composed of two layers,[1,2] the visceral pericardium, a monolayer membrane of mesothelial cells and associated collagen and elastin fibers that is adherent to the epicardial surface of the heart, and the fibrous parietal layer, which is about 2 mm thick in normal humans and surrounds most of the heart. The parietal pericardium is largely acellular and also contains both collagen and elastin fibers. Collagen is the major structural component and appears as wavy bundles at low levels of stretch. With further stretch, the bundles straighten, resulting in increased stiffness. The visceral pericardium reflects back near the origins of the great vessels, becoming continuous with and forming the inner layer of the parietal pericardium. The pericardial space or sac is contained within these two layers and normally contains up to 50 mL of serous fluid. The reflection of the visceral pericardium is a few centimeters proximal to the junctions of the caval vessels with the right atrium; portions of these vessels lie within the pericardial sac (**Fig. 75-1**). Posterior to the left atrium, the reflection occurs at the oblique sinus of the pericardium. The left atrium is largely extrapericardial. The parietal pericardium has ligamentous attachments to the diaphragm, sternum, and other structures. These ensure that the heart occupies a fixed position within the thoracic cavity regardless of respiration and body position. The only noncardiovascular macrostructures associated with the pericardium are the phrenic nerves enveloped by the parietal pericardium.

Although pericardiectomy does not result in obvious negative consequences, the normal pericardium does have functions. As noted before, it maintains the position of the heart relatively constant. It may also be a barrier to infection and provides lubrication between visceral and parietal layers. The pericardium is well innervated with mechanoreceptors and chemoreceptors and phrenic afferents. The roles of these receptors are incompletely understood, but they probably participate in reflexes arising from the pericardium and epicardium (e.g., the Bezold-Jarisch reflex) as well as in transmission of pericardial pain. The pericardium also secretes prostaglandins and related substances that may modulate neural traffic and coronary tone by effects on coronary receptors.

The best-characterized mechanical function of the pericardium is its restraining effect on cardiac volume. This reflects the mechanical properties of the pericardial tissue. The parietal pericardium has a tensile strength similar to that of rubber. At low applied stresses similar to those at physiologic or subphysiologic cardiac volumes, it is very elastic (see Fig. 75-e1, top, on website). As stretch increases, the tissue fairly abruptly becomes stiff and resistant to further stretch. The point on the pericardial stress-strain relation (see Fig. 75-e1, top, on website) where this transition occurs probably corresponds to stresses present around the upper range of physiologic cardiac volumes and is likely related to straightening of collagen bundles.

The pressure-volume relation of the parietal pericardial sac parallels the properties of the isolated tissue (see Fig. 75-e1, bottom, left curve, on website), that is, a relatively flat, compliant segment transitioning relatively abruptly to a noncompliant segment, with the transition in the range of the upper limit of normal total cardiac volume. Thus, the pericardial sac has a relatively small reserve volume. When it is exceeded, the pressure within the sac operating on the surface of the heart increases rapidly and is transmitted to the inside of the cardiac chambers. The shape of the pericardial pressure-volume relation accounts for the fact that once a critical level of effusion is reached, relatively small amounts of additional fluid cause large increases in intrapericardial pressure and have marked effects on cardiac function. Conversely, removal of small amounts of fluid can result in striking benefit.

The shape of the pericardial pressure-volume relation suggests that it can normally restrain cardiac volume, that is, the force it exerts on the surface of the heart can limit filling, with a component of intracavitary filling pressure representing transmission of the pericardial pressure. This has been examined with flattened balloons designed to measure surface contact pressures. These studies demonstrate a substantial pericardial contact pressure, especially when the upper limit of normal cardiac volume is exceeded. This pressure is proportionally more important for the right side of the heart, whose filling pressures are normally lower than the left.

Pericardial contact pressure has also been estimated by quantifying the change in the right- and left-sided heart diastolic pressure-volume relation before and after pericardiectomy. A decrease in pressure at a given volume is the effective pericardial pressure at that volume. Studies in canine hearts using this approach indicate negligible pericardial restraint at low normal filling volumes, with contact pressures in the range of 2 to 4 mm Hg at the upper end of the normal range. With additional filling, contact pressure rapidly increases. At left-sided filling pressure of ~25 mm Hg, estimated contact pressure is ~10 mm Hg, accounting for most of the right-sided heart pressure at this level of filling. Thus, the normal pericardium can acutely restrain cardiac volume and influences intracavitary filling pressure. Moreover, patients with normal preoperative cardiac volumes undergoing pericardiotomy in conjunction with heart surgery develop mild postoperative increases in cardiac mass and volume (similar to chronic volume overload), consistent

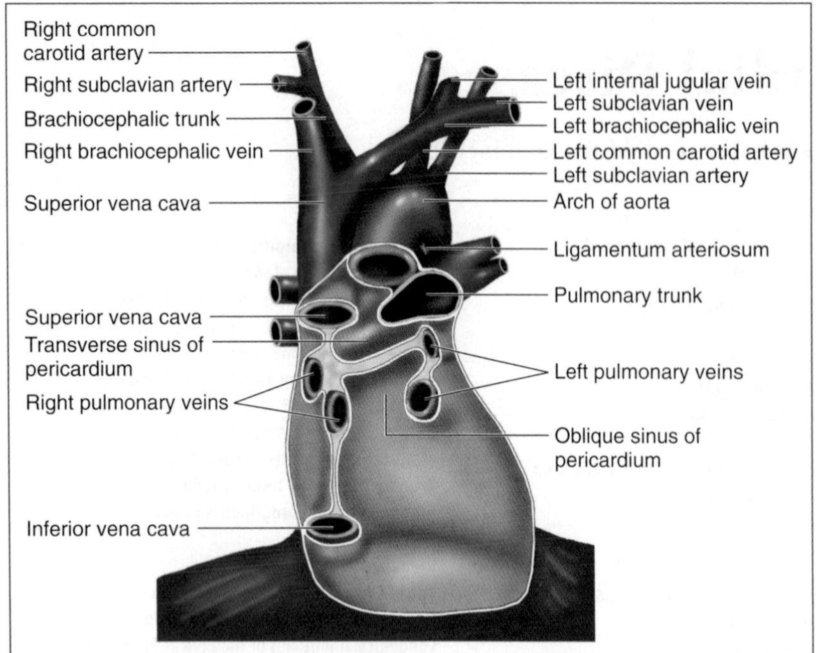

FIGURE 75-1 The pericardial reflections near the origins of the great vessels shown after removal of the heart. Note that portions of the caval vessels are within the pericardial space. *(From Johnson D: The pericardium. In Standring S, et al [eds]: Gray's Anatomy. New York, Elsevier Churchill Livingstone, 2005, pp 995-996.)*

with relief of underlying, normally occurring restraint to filling by the pericardium. It has recently been shown that the visceral pericardium also restrains cardiac volume.[2]

The normal pericardium also contributes to diastolic interaction, the transmission of intracavitary filling pressure to adjoining chambers. Thus, for example, a portion of right ventricular diastolic pressure is transmitted to the left ventricle across the interventricular septum and contributes to left ventricular diastolic pressure. Because its presence increases right ventricular intracavitary pressure, the normal pericardium amplifies diastolic interaction. Thus, as cardiac volume increases above the physiologic range, the pericardium contributes increasingly to intracavitary filling pressures, directly because of the external contact pressure and indirectly because of increased diastolic interaction.

The Passive Role of the Normal Pericardium in Heart Disease

When the cardiac chambers dilate rapidly, the restraining effect of the pericardium and its contribution to diastolic interaction become markedly augmented, resulting in a hemodynamic picture with features of both cardiac tamponade and constrictive pericarditis. The most common example is right ventricular myocardial infarction (MI),[3] usually in conjunction with inferior left ventricular MI. Here, the right side of the heart dilates markedly and rapidly such that total heart volume exceeds the pericardial reserve volume. As a result of increased pericardial constraint and augmented interaction, left- and right-sided filling pressures equilibrate at elevated levels, and a paradoxical pulse and inspiratory increase in systemic venous pressure (Kussmaul sign) may be observed (see Chap. 12). Other conditions with similar effects include acute pulmonary embolus and subacute mitral regurgitation.

Chronic cardiac dilation due to dilated cardiomyopathy or regurgitant valvular disease can result in cardiac volumes well in excess of the normal pericardial reserve volume. Despite this, exaggerated restraining effects are not ordinarily encountered. This implies that the pericardium undergoes chronic adaptation to accommodate marked increases in cardiac volume. In experimental chronic volume overload, the pericardial pressure-volume relation shifts to the right and its slope decreases (see Fig. 75-e1, bottom, right curve, on website), that is, it becomes more compliant in association with increased pericardial area and mass and a decreased effect on the left ventricular diastolic pressure-volume relation. Thus, apparent growth of pericardial tissue occurs in response to chronic stretch. A similar effect presumably occurs with very large, slowly accumulating effusions.

Acute Pericarditis

Etiology, Epidemiology, and Pathophysiology

Table 75-1 is a partial list of diseases that can involve the pericardium. Acute pericarditis, defined as symptoms or signs resulting from pericardial inflammation of no more than 1 to 2 weeks in duration, can occur in a variety of these diseases (denoted by asterisks in Table 75-1), but the majority of cases are idiopathic.[4,5] The term *idiopathic* is used to denote acute pericarditis for which no specific cause can be found with routine diagnostic testing as outlined later. Most cases of acute idiopathic pericarditis are presumed to be viral in etiology, but testing for specific viruses is not routine because of cost and the fact that this knowledge rarely alters management.

The incidence of acute pericarditis is difficult to quantify because there are undoubtedly many undiagnosed cases. At autopsy, the frequency is ~1%.[6] Pericarditis is common in patients presenting to the emergency department, accounting for up to 5% of those with nonischemic chest pain. The fraction of all acute cases accounted for by idiopathic pericarditis is also uncertain and is influenced by population demographics and regional and seasonal variation in viral infections. However, 80% to 90% seems a reasonable estimate.[4-6] This percentage is lower in patients with pericarditis who require hospitalization and higher in young, previously healthy patients. Tuberculous pericarditis is included in Table 75-1 as a cause of acute pericarditis, but it usually presents with more chronic symptoms. Bacterial pericarditis is also included because it can present with signs and symptoms of acute pericardial inflammation, but these patients are usually critically ill, and other components of their illness, including pericardial effusions, sepsis, and pneumonias, typically dominate the picture. Pericarditis occurring 24 to 72 hours after transmural MI caused by local inflammation and the delayed pericarditis of Dressler syndrome used to be common (see Chap. 54). Their incidence has markedly declined during the era of early reperfusion. Other than this, the etiologic distribution of acute pericarditis has changed little over time. In contrast, the epidemiology of pericardial effusion and constriction has changed considerably.

The pathophysiology of uncomplicated acute pericarditis is straightforward, that is, symptoms and signs result from inflammation of pericardial tissue. A minority of cases are complicated, as discussed later, and some are associated with myocarditis.[4-6] Coexistent myocarditis is usually manifested solely by modest release of biomarkers such as troponin I (see Chap. 70). Rarely, however, myocardial dysfunction occurs in conjunction with clinically manifested pericarditis.

History and Differential Diagnosis

Acute pericarditis almost always presents with chest pain.[4] A few cases are diagnosed during evaluation of symptoms, such as dyspnea and fever, or incidentally in conjunction with noncardiac manifestations of systemic diseases, such as systemic lupus erythematosus (SLE). The pain of pericarditis can be quite severe. It is variable in quality but almost always pleuritic. It usually does not have the viselike, constricting or oppressive features of myocardial ischemia. Pericardial pain typically has a relatively rapid onset and sometimes begins remarkably abruptly. It is most commonly substernal but can be

TABLE 75-1 Categories of Pericardial Disease and Selected Specific Causes

Idiopathic*
Infectious
Viral* (echovirus, coxsackievirus, adenovirus, cytomegalovirus, hepatitis B, infectious mononucleosis, HIV/AIDS)
Bacterial* (pneumococcus, staphylococcus, streptococcus, mycoplasma, Lyme disease, *Haemophilus influenzae, Neisseria meningitidis,* and others)
Mycobacterial* *(Mycobacterium tuberculosis, Mycobacterium avium-intracellulare)*
Fungal (histoplasmosis, coccidioidomycosis)
Protozoal
Immune-inflammatory
Connective tissue disease* (systemic lupus erythematosus, rheumatoid arthritis, scleroderma, mixed)
Arteritis (polyarteritis nodosa, temporal arteritis)
Inflammatory bowel disease
Early post–myocardial infarction
Late post–myocardial infarction (Dressler syndrome),* late post-cardiotomy/thoracotomy*
Late post-trauma*
Drug induced* (procainamide, hydralazine, isoniazid, cyclosporine, others)
Neoplastic disease
Primary: mesothelioma, fibrosarcoma, lipoma, others
Secondary*: breast and lung carcinoma, lymphomas, Kaposi sarcoma
Radiation induced*
Early post–cardiac surgery and post–orthotopic heart transplantation
Hemopericardium
Trauma
Post–myocardial infarction free wall rupture
Device and procedure related: percutaneous coronary procedures, implantable defibrillators, pacemakers, post–arrhythmia ablation, post–atrial septal defect closure, post–valve repair or replacement
Dissecting aortic aneurysm
Trauma
Blunt and penetrating,* post–cardiopulmonary resuscitation*
Congenital
Cysts, congenital absence
Miscellaneous
Cholesterol ("gold paint" pericarditis)
Chronic renal failure, dialysis related
Chylopericardium
Hypothyroidism and hyperthyroidism
Amyloidosis
Aortic dissection

*Causes that can present as acute pericarditis.

centered in the left anterior chest or epigastrium. Left arm radiation is not unusual. The most characteristic radiation is to the trapezius ridge, which is highly specific for pericarditis. Pericardial pain is almost always relieved by sitting forward and worsened by lying down. Associated symptoms can include dyspnea, cough, and occasionally hiccoughs. An antecedent history of symptoms suggesting a viral syndrome is common. It is important to review the past medical history for clues to specific etiologic diagnoses. A history of cancer or an autoimmune disorder, high fevers with shaking chills, rash, or weight loss should alert the physician to specific diseases that can cause pericarditis.

The differential diagnosis of chest pain is extensive (see Chaps. 12 and 53). Diagnoses most easily confused with pericarditis include pneumonia or pneumonitis with pleurisy (which may coexist with pericarditis), pulmonary embolus or infarction, costochondritis, and gastroesophageal reflux disease. Acute pericarditis is usually relatively easily distinguished from myocardial ischemia or infarction, but coronary angiography is occasionally required to resolve this issue. Other considerations include aortic dissection, intra-abdominal processes, pneumothorax, and herpes zoster pain before skin lesions appear. Finally, acute pericarditis is occasionally the presenting manifestation of a preceding, silent MI.

Physical Examination

Patients with uncomplicated acute pericarditis often appear uncomfortable and anxious and may have low-grade fever and sinus tachycardia. Otherwise, the only abnormal physical finding is the friction rub caused by contact between visceral and parietal pericardium. The classic rub is easily recognized and pathognomonic of pericarditis. It consists of three components corresponding to ventricular systole, early diastolic filling, and atrial contraction and is similar to the sound made when walking on crunchy snow. The rub is usually loudest at the lower left sternal border and is best heard with the patient leaning forward. It is often dynamic, disappearing and returning during short periods. Thus, it is often rewarding to listen frequently to a patient with suspected pericarditis who does not have an audible rub initially. Sometimes what is considered a pericardial rub has only two components or even one component. Such findings should be labeled rubs with caution because the sound may actually represent a murmur. It is important to perform a careful, complete physical examination in a patient with acute pericarditis and to look for clues to specific etiologic diagnoses. The examiner must also be alert to findings indicating significant pericardial effusion, as discussed subsequently.

Laboratory Testing

ELECTROCARDIOGRAPHY. The electrocardiogram (ECG) is the most important laboratory test for diagnosis of acute pericarditis (see Chap. 13). The classic finding is diffuse ST-segment elevation (**Fig. 75-2**; see Fig. 13-45).[4-6] The ST-segment vector typically points leftward, anterior, and inferior, with ST-segment elevation in all leads except aVR and often V_1. The ST segment is usually coved upward and resembles the current of injury of acute, transmural ischemia. However, the distinction between acute pericarditis and transmural ischemia is usually not difficult because of more extensive lead involvement in pericarditis and the presence of much more prominent reciprocal ST-segment depression in ischemia. However, ST elevation in pericarditis sometimes involves a smaller number of leads, in which case the distinction is more difficult. In other cases, the ST segment more closely resembles early repolarization. Here again, pericarditis usually involves more leads than typical early repolarization. As with the rub, electrocardiographic changes can be dynamic. Frequent recordings can yield a diagnosis in patients with suspected pericarditis who present initially with neither rub nor ST elevation. PR-segment depression is also common (see Fig. 75-2). PR depression can occur without ST elevation and be the initial or sole electrocardiographic manifestation of acute pericarditis. Electrocardiographic abnormalities other than ST elevation and PR depression are unusual in patients presenting soon after the onset of symptoms of acute pericarditis. Subsequent electrocardiographic changes are variable.[4-6] In some, the ECG reverts to normal during days or weeks. In others, the elevated ST segment passes through the isoelectric point and progresses to ST-segment depression and T wave inversions in leads with upright QRS complexes. These changes can persist for weeks or even months but have no known significance in patients who have otherwise recovered. In patients presenting late after the onset of symptoms, these electrocardiographic changes can be difficult to distinguish from ischemia.

Electrocardiographic abnormalities other than these should be considered carefully because they suggest diagnoses other than idiopathic pericarditis or the presence of complications. As examples, atrioventricular block may indicate Lyme disease, pathologic Q waves can signify a previous silent MI with pericardial pain as its first manifestation, and low voltage or electrical alternans points toward significant effusion.

HEMOGRAM. Modest elevations of the white blood cell count with mild lymphocytosis are common in acute idiopathic pericarditis. Higher counts are an alert for the presence of other causes, as is anemia.

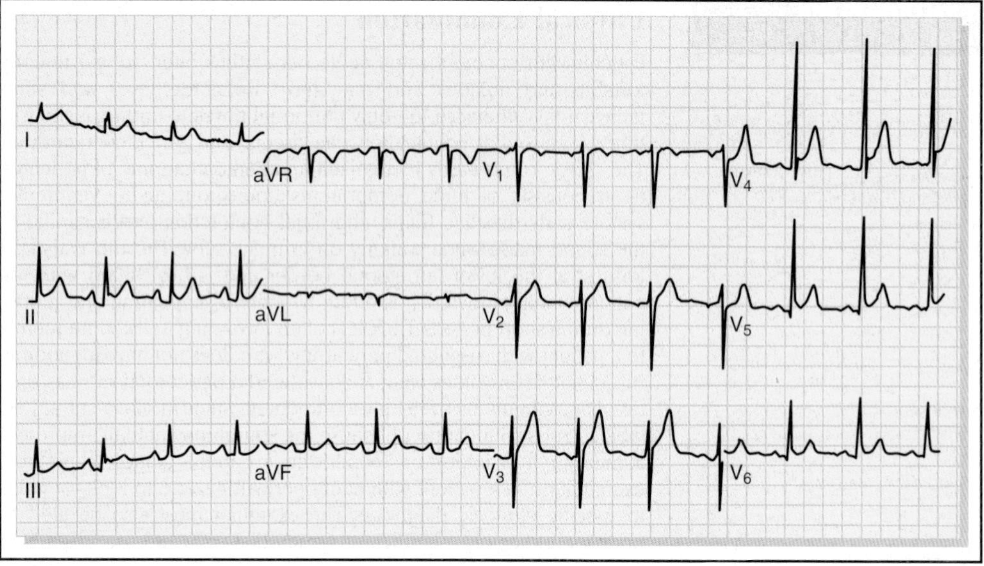

FIGURE 75-2 The electrocardiogram in acute pericarditis. Note both diffuse ST-segment elevation and PR-segment depression.

CARDIAC ENZYMES AND TROPONIN MEASUREMENTS. A significant fraction of patients with a diagnosis of acute pericarditis without other evidence of myocarditis (see Chap. 70) or MI (see Chap. 54) have elevated creatine kinase MB fraction or troponin I values. This suggests a significant incidence of concomitant, otherwise silent myocarditis. Pericarditis patients with elevated biomarkers of myocardial injury almost always have ST-segment elevation. Another concern in patients with elevated biomarkers is silent MI presenting with subsequent pericarditis. Post-MI pericarditis usually (but not always) occurs after MIs with transmural electrocardiographic changes.

CHEST RADIOGRAPHY (see Chap. 16). The chest radiograph is usually normal in uncomplicated acute idiopathic pericarditis. On occasion, small pulmonary infiltrates or pleural effusions are present, presumably due to viral or possibly mycoplasmal infections. Other than this, pulmonary parenchymal or other abnormalities suggest diagnoses other than idiopathic pericarditis. Thus, bacterial pericarditis often occurs in conjunction with severe pneumonia. Tuberculous pericarditis can occur with or without associated pulmonary disease. Mass lesions and enlarged lymph nodes suggestive of neoplastic disease also have great significance. Small to even moderate effusions may not cause an abnormal cardiac silhouette; thus, even modest enlargement is a cause for concern.

ECHOCARDIOGRAPHY (see Chap. 15). The echocardiogram is normal in most patients with acute idiopathic pericarditis. The main reason for its performance is to exclude an otherwise silent effusion. There are no modern data delineating the incidence of effusions. Most patients do not have effusions, but small ones are fairly common and not a cause for concern. Moderate or larger effusions are unusual and may signal a diagnosis other than idiopathic pericarditis. Echocardiography is also useful in delineating whether associated myocarditis is severe enough to alter ventricular function as well as in detection of MI.

Natural History and Management

The European Society of Cardiology has published guidelines for the diagnosis and management of pericardial diseases.[5] Although these are useful, there have been few randomized clinical trials devoted to the diagnosis or management of pericardial disease. It is therefore important to keep in mind that objective data to support the following recommendations for management of acute pericarditis as well as other pericardial diseases are limited.

Initial management should be focused on screening for specific causes that would alter management, detection of effusion and other echocardiographic abnormalities, alleviation of symptoms, and appropriate treatment if a specific cause is discovered. Initially, we recommend obtaining the laboratory data discussed before, that is, ECG, hemogram, chest radiograph, serum creatine kinase and troponin I, and echocardiogram. In young women, it is not unreasonable to test for SLE. However, low antinuclear antibody (ANA) titers appear to be common in patients with recurrent idiopathic pericarditis who do not meet other criteria for SLE.[7] Thus, the significance of low ANA titers in the setting of an initial presentation is somewhat uncertain. **Table 75-2** summarizes our recommendations for initial assessment and treatment of patients with definite or suspected acute pericarditis.

Acute idiopathic pericarditis is a self-limited disease without significant complications or recurrence in 70% to 90% of patients.[4-6,8,9] If laboratory data support the clinical diagnosis, symptomatic treatment with nonsteroidal anti-inflammatory drugs (NSAIDs) should be initiated.[4-6] Because of its excellent safety profile, we prefer ibuprofen (600 to 800 mg orally three times daily) with discontinuation if pain is no longer present after 2 weeks. Many patients have very gratifying responses to the first dose or two of the NSAID, and most respond fully and need no additional treatment. Reliable patients with no more than small effusions who respond well to NSAIDs need not be admitted to the hospital.[10] Patients who do not respond well initially, have larger effusions, or have a suspected cause other than idiopathic pericarditis should be hospitalized for additional observation, diagnostic testing, and treatment as necessary.

Patients who respond slowly or inadequately to NSAIDs may require supplementary narcotic analgesics to allow time for a full response or a course of colchicine. Colchicine is administered as a 2- to 3-mg oral loading dose followed by 1 mg daily for 10 to 14 days.[5,11,12] It is unusual not to achieve a satisfactory response to a regimen of an NSAID, with colchicine added if necessary. On the basis of two randomized trials,[11,12] colchicine has been proposed as a standard adjuvant to NSAIDs for initial treatment. However, these trials have uncertain applicability as they were open label, and the treatment arms consisted of aspirin versus aspirin plus colchicine for either 3 or 6 months, much longer than the usual recommendation for acute pericarditis. Poorly

TABLE 75-2 Initial Approach to the Patient with Definite or Suspected Acute Pericarditis

If the diagnosis is suspected but not certain, listen frequently for pericardial rub and obtain frequent ECGs to look for diagnostic findings.

If the diagnosis is suspected or certain, obtain the following tests to determine if a specific etiologic diagnosis is likely or significant associated conditions or complications are present:

- Chest radiograph
- Hemogram
- Echocardiogram
- Creatine kinase with MB fraction, troponin I
- Echocardiogram
- Consider serum antinuclear antibody if patient is young woman

If diagnosis is certain, initiate therapy with a nonsteroidal anti-inflammatory drug.

responding patients have typically been treated with short courses of corticosteroids. However, corticosteroids should be avoided as they appear to encourage recurrences.[5,6,13] If they simply cannot be avoided to manage an initial episode, we recommend prednisone 60 mg orally daily for 2 days with tapering to zero during a week.

Complications of acute pericarditis include effusion, tamponade, and constriction (myocarditis is best considered an associated condition rather than a complication). As noted earlier, small effusions are common. Relatively little is known about the incidence of more significant complications. In the largest modern report on this topic,[9] a specific cause was identified in 17% of patients with acute pericarditis. During an average 31-month follow-up period, 3.1% developed tamponade and 1.5% developed constriction. Most complications occurred in patients with identified causes. Thus, in patients without an identified cause, the incidence of complications (including larger effusions) is extremely low during the acute episode and for the longer term.

Relapsing and Recurrent Pericarditis

Perhaps 15% to 30% of patients with acute, apparently idiopathic pericarditis who respond satisfactorily to treatment as outlined before suffer a relapse.[4-6,9] Women and patients in whom initial therapy with NSAIDs fails are at increased risk.[9] A minority develop recurrent bouts of pericardial pain, which can be chronic and debilitating. Recurrent pain is often not associated with objective signs of pericardial inflammation. Evidence of a specific cause is manifested in some patients with what is initially thought to be idiopathic pericarditis as they develop recurrences. Accordingly, repeated evaluation for specific causes, especially autoimmune disorders, is appropriate. A pericardial biopsy to look for a specific cause in patients with recurrent pain *without effusion* is rarely indicated because it is unlikely that a diagnosis will actually result or that the information obtained will alter management. The complication rate, including constrictive pericarditis, is very low in patients with recurrent pericarditis, and the long-term prognosis is good; most patients eventually have a full remission.[14,15]

Treatment of recurrent pain is empiric. For an initial relapse, a second 2-week course of an NSAID is often effective. A course of colchicine may be at least as effective.[11] For bouts of recurrent pain beyond an initial relapse, we recommend colchicine prophylaxis.[11,16] There is now a substantial experience with colchicine as prophylaxis for recurrent pericardial pain due to idiopathic pericarditis and other causes (e.g., after thoracotomy, SLE). This experience indicates that colchicine is at least as effective as corticosteroid therapy and has a much more favorable side effect profile. The usual dose is a 2- to 3-mg oral load followed by 1 mg orally daily. Initiation of prophylactic therapy does not preclude simultaneous use of NSAIDs. The most common difficulty in using colchicine is nausea or diarrhea, which results in dose reduction or termination in 10% to 15% of patients.

Patients with recurrent pericardial pain despite NSAIDs and colchicine (or who cannot tolerate colchicine) are a challenging problem. One option is a brief course of prednisone as outlined before whenever symptoms first appear. Maintenance corticosteroid therapy should be avoided if at all possible. If prednisone therapy must be continued for longer periods, lower doses appear to be preferable. In a retrospective study,[17] 0.2 to 0.5 mg/kg of oral prednisone daily was associated with a lower recurrence and hospitalization rate than an average of 1.0 mg/kg daily; only the higher dose range was associated with severe side effects. Nonsteroidal immunosuppressive therapy with drugs such as azathioprine and cyclophosphamide is another alternative, but there has been no systematic, published experience. Pericardiectomy has occasionally been employed for recurrent pericarditis but appears to be effective in only a minority of patients.[4-6]

Pericardial Effusion and Tamponade

Etiology

Idiopathic pericarditis and any infection, neoplasm, and autoimmune or inflammatory process that can cause pericarditis can cause an effusion (see Table 75-1).[5,6,18] Effusions are common early after both routine cardiac surgery and orthotopic heart transplantation,[19] but tamponade is unusual, and they almost always resolve within several weeks to a few months. A lengthy list of miscellaneous, noninflammatory diseases can cause effusion (see Table 75-1). Patients with severe circulatory congestion can have small to moderate transudative effusions. Bleeding into the pericardial sac occurs after blunt and penetrating trauma (see Chap. 76), following post-MI rupture of the free wall of the left ventricle, and as a complication of percutaneous cardiac procedures and device implantation. Retrograde bleeding is an important cause of death due to aortic dissection (see Chap. 60). Last, occasional patients are encountered with large, silent pericardial effusion.[20] These are generally stable, but instances of tamponade do occur over time.

Those causes of effusion with a high incidence of progression to tamponade include bacterial (including mycobacterial) infections, fungal infections, human immunodeficiency virus (HIV)–associated infections (see Chap. 72), bleeding, and neoplastic involvement. Whereas large effusions due to acute idiopathic pericarditis are unusual, this form of pericarditis accounts for a significant percentage of tamponade cases because of its high frequency. About 20% of large, symptomatic effusions without an obvious cause after routine evaluation constitute the initial presentation of a previously unrecognized cancer.[21] Details of pericardial effusion pertinent to specific disease entities are discussed later.

Pathophysiology and Hemodynamics

Formation of an effusion is a component of the inflammatory response when there is an inflammatory or infectious process affecting the pericardium. This is also the likely mechanism with pericardial tumor implants (see Chap. 74). Lymphomas occasionally cause effusion in association with enlarged mediastinal lymph nodes by obstructing pericardial lymph drainage. The pathophysiologic mechanism of effusions in situations in which there is no obvious inflammation (e.g., uremia) is very poorly understood.

Cardiac tamponade represents a continuum from an effusion causing minimal effects to full-blown circulatory collapse. Clinically, the most critical point occurs when an effusion reduces the volume of the cardiac chambers such that cardiac output begins to decline. Determinants of the hemodynamic consequences of an effusion are the pressure in the pericardial sac and the ability of the heart to compensate for elevated pressure. The pressure in turn depends on the amount of fluid and the pericardial pressure-volume relation. As discussed earlier, the pericardium normally has little reserve volume. As a result, relatively modest amounts of rapidly accumulating fluid can have major effects on cardiac function. Large, slowly accumulating effusions are often well tolerated, presumably because of chronic changes in the pericardial pressure-volume relation described earlier. The compensatory response to a significant pericardial effusion includes increased adrenergic stimulation and parasympathetic withdrawal, which cause tachycardia and increased contractility[22] and can maintain cardiac output and blood pressure for a time. Eventually, however, cardiac output and blood pressure progressively decline. Patients who cannot mount a normal adrenergic response (e.g., those receiving beta-adrenergic blocking drugs) are more susceptible to the effects of an effusion. In terminal tamponade, a depressor reflex with paradoxical bradycardia can supervene.

The hemodynamic consequences of pericardial effusion have fascinated physiologists and physicians for years.[18,22] Non–steady-state responses to an abrupt increase in pericardial pressure provide insights into the mechanisms of these derangements. **Figure 75-3** shows an experiment in a dog in which aortic and pulmonary arterial flow (stroke volume) were measured beat to beat before and after a large amount of fluid was abruptly introduced into the pericardial sac, indicated by the arrow. This causes an immediate decrease in pulmonary arterial stroke volume but no change in aortic stroke volume. Two beats later, aortic stroke volume decreases, and eventually a new steady state is achieved with equivalent decreases in aortic and pulmonary arterial stroke volume. During the time required to achieve a new steady state, pulmonary stroke volume is less than aortic stroke volume. The transient inequality in left- and

CH 75

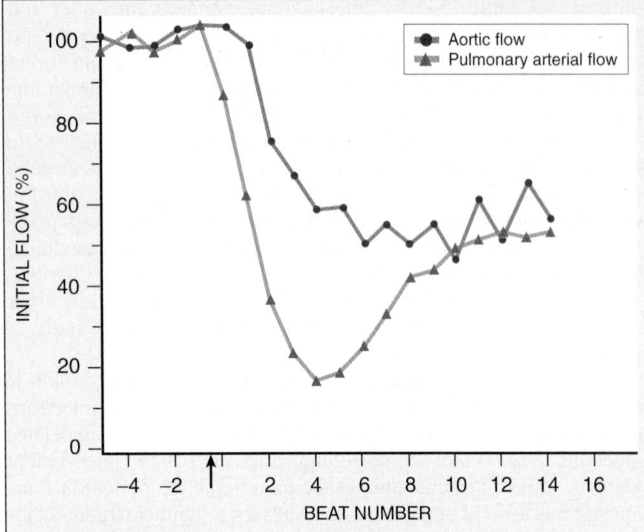

FIGURE 75-3 Beat-to-beat changes in pulmonary arterial and aortic stroke volume (as percentage of control) after abrupt production of cardiac tamponade (at arrow). Note that pulmonary arterial stroke volume decreases immediately, but there is a brief lag before aortic stroke volume decreases. Pulmonary arterial stroke volume is lower than aortic stroke volume until new steady state is reached. *(From Ditchey R, Engler R, LeWinter M, et al: The role of the right heart in acute cardiac tamponade in dogs. Circ Res 48:701, 1981.)*

right-sided heart output results in transfer of blood out of the pulmonary and into the systemic circulation and may explain the decrease in pulmonary vascularity on the chest radiograph in tamponade. In parallel studies, right-sided heart volume was shown to decrease more than left-sided heart volume in response to a given increase in pericardial pressure. These results indicate that high pericardial pressure exerts its effect mainly by impeding right-sided heart filling, with much of the effect on the left side of the heart due to secondary underfilling.

As fluid accumulates, left- and right-sided atrial and ventricular diastolic pressures rise and in severe tamponade equalize at a pressure similar to that in the pericardial sac, typically 15 to 20 mm Hg (**Fig. 75-4**). Equalization is closest during inspiration. Thus, the pericardial pressure dictates the intracavitary pressure, and the transmural filling pressures of the cardiac chambers are very low. Correspondingly, cardiac volumes progressively decline. The small end-diastolic ventricular volume (decreased preload) mainly accounts for the small stroke volume. Because of compensatory increases in contractility, end-systolic volume also decreases, but not enough to normalize stroke volume (hence, the importance of tachycardia in maintaining cardiac output). Because transmural right-sided heart filling pressure is normally lower than left-sided heart filling pressure (upper limit of right atrial pressure ~7 mm Hg, left atrial pressure ~12 mm Hg), as fluid accumulates, filling pressure increases more rapidly in the right side than in the left side of the heart.

In addition to elevated and equal intracavitary filling pressures, low transmural filling pressures, and small cardiac volumes, two other hemodynamic abnormalities are characteristic of tamponade. One is loss of the *y* descent of the right atrial or systemic venous pressure (see Fig. 75-4). The *x* and *y* descents of the venous pressure waveform correspond to periods when flow is increasing. Loss of the *y* descent has been explained on the basis of the concept that total heart volume is fixed in severe tamponade.[18,22] Thus, blood can enter the heart only when blood is simultaneously leaving. The right atrial *y* descent begins when the tricuspid valve opens, that is, when blood is not leaving the heart. Thus, no blood can enter, and the *y* descent is lost. In contrast, the *x* descent occurs during ventricular ejection. Because blood is leaving the heart, venous inflow can increase and the *x* descent is retained. Loss of the *y* descent can be difficult to discern at the bedside but is easily appreciated in recordings of systemic venous or right atrial pressure and provides a useful clue to the presence of very significant tamponade.

The second characteristic hemodynamic finding is the paradoxical pulse (**Fig. 75-5**), an abnormally large decline in systemic arterial pressure during inspiration (usually defined as a drop of >10 mm Hg in systolic pressure). Other causes of pulsus paradoxus include constrictive pericarditis, pulmonary embolus, and pulmonary disease with large variations in intrathoracic pressure. In severe tamponade, the arterial pulse is impalpable during inspiration. The mechanism of the paradoxical pulse is multifactorial, but respiratory changes in systemic venous return are certainly important.[18,22] In tamponade, in contrast to constriction, the normal inspiratory increase in systemic venous return is retained. Therefore, the normal decline in systemic venous pressure on inspiration is present (and Kussmaul sign is absent). The increase in right-sided heart filling occurs, once again, under conditions in which total heart volume is fixed and left-sided heart volume is markedly reduced to start. The interventricular septum shifts to the left in exaggerated fashion on inspiration, encroaching on the left ventricle such that its stroke volume and pressure generation are further reduced (see Fig. 75-5). Although the inspiratory increase in right-sided heart volume (preload) causes an increase in right ventricular stroke volume, this requires several cardiac cycles to increase left ventricular filling and stroke volume and to counteract the septal shift. Other factors that may contribute to the paradoxical pulse include increased afterload caused by transmission of negative intrathoracic pressure to the aorta and traction on the pericardium caused by descent of the diaphragm, which increases pericardial pressure. Associated with these mechanisms are the striking findings that left- and right-sided heart pressure and stroke volume variations are exaggerated and 180 degrees out of phase (see Fig. 75-5). **Table 75-3** lists the major hemodynamic findings of tamponade in comparison with constrictive pericarditis.

When there are pre-existing elevations in diastolic pressures or volume, tamponade can occur without a paradoxical pulse.[18,22] Examples are patients with left ventricular dysfunction, aortic regurgitation, and atrial septal defect. In patients with retrograde bleeding into the pericardial sac due to aortic dissection, tamponade can occur without a paradoxical pulse because of aortic valve disruption and regurgitation.

Although left- and right-sided filling pressures are usually 15 to 20 mm Hg in severe tamponade, tamponade can occur at lower levels of filling pressure, which is termed low-pressure tamponade.[18,22,23] Low-pressure tamponade occurs when there is a decrease in blood volume in the setting of a pre-existing effusion that would not otherwise cause significant hemodynamic consequences. A relatively modestly elevated pericardial pressure can then lower transmural filling pressure to levels at which stroke volume is compromised. Because the venous pressure is only modestly elevated or even normal, the diagnosis may not be suspected. Low-pressure tamponade is typically observed during hemodialysis, when it may be signaled by hypotension; in patients with blood loss and dehydration; and when diuretics are administered to patients with effusions (see Chap. 93). In the only large published experience with this entity,[23] about 20% of patients undergoing combined cardiac catheterization and closed pericardiocentesis met criteria for low-pressure tamponade. Compared with high-pressure tamponade, low-pressure tamponade patients were less often critically ill and signs of tamponade were less prominent. Echocardiographic findings were similar to those of high-pressure tamponade, and substantial hemodynamic benefit was derived from pericardiocentesis.

Pericardial effusions can be loculated or localized, resulting in regional tamponade, which is most commonly encountered after cardiac surgery.[22] Regional tamponade can cause atypical hemodynamic findings, that is, reduced cardiac output with unilateral filling pressure elevation. However, reports of hemodynamics are scarce, and it is difficult to generalize about this entity. Regional tamponade should be considered whenever there is hypotension in a setting in which a loculated effusion is present or suspected. Large pleural effusions can also compress the heart and even cause clinical cardiac tamponade.[24]

Clinical Presentation

Obviously, in patients with pericardial effusions, a history pertinent to a specific cause can often be elicited. On occasion, large, asymptomatic chronic effusions are discovered when a chest imaging study is performed for an unrelated reason.[20] As discussed earlier, specific causes are usually not found in these cases. Effusions do not cause symptoms unless tamponade is present, although many patients with effusions have pericardial pain because of associated pericarditis. Patients with tamponade may complain of true dyspnea, whose mechanism is uncertain because there is no pulmonary congestion. They almost always are more comfortable sitting forward. Other symptoms reflect the severity of cardiac output and blood pressure reduction. Pericardial pain or a nonspecific sense of discomfort may dominate the clinical picture.

A complete physical examination of patients with pericardial effusion can provide clues to a specific cause (see Chap. 12). In pericardial effusion without tamponade, the cardiovascular examination findings are normal except that if the effusion is large, the cardiac impulse can be difficult to palpate and the heart sounds muffled. A friction rub can of course also be present. Tubular breath sounds may be heard in the left axilla or left base due to bronchial compression. The Beck triad of hypotension, muffled heart sounds, and elevated jugular venous pressure remains a useful clue to the presence of severe tamponade. Patients with tamponade almost always appear uncomfortable, with signs reflecting varying degrees of reduced cardiac output and shock, including tachypnea, diaphoresis, cool extremities, peripheral cyanosis, depressed sensorium, and, rarely, yawning.[25] Hypotension with reduced pulse pressure is usually present, although compensatory mechanisms maintain the blood pressure in early stages. A paradoxical pulse is the rule, but it is important to be alert to those situations in which it may not be present. It is quantified by cuff sphygmomanometry by noting the difference between the pressure at which Korotkoff sounds first appear and that at which they are present with each heart beat. In severe tamponade, the inspiratory decrease in arterial pressure is palpable and most obvious in arteries distant from the heart. Tachycardia is also the rule unless heart rate–lowering drugs have been administered, conduction system disease coexists, or a preterminal bradycardic reflex has supervened. The jugular venous pressure is markedly elevated except in low-pressure tamponade, and the *y* descent is absent (see Fig. 75-4). The normal decrease in venous pressure on inspiration is retained. Examination of the heart itself is simply consistent with an effusion, as outlined before. Tamponade can be confused with anything that causes hypotension, shock, and elevated jugular venous pressure, including myocardial failure, right-sided heart failure due to pulmonary embolus or other causes of pulmonary hypertension, and right ventricular MI.

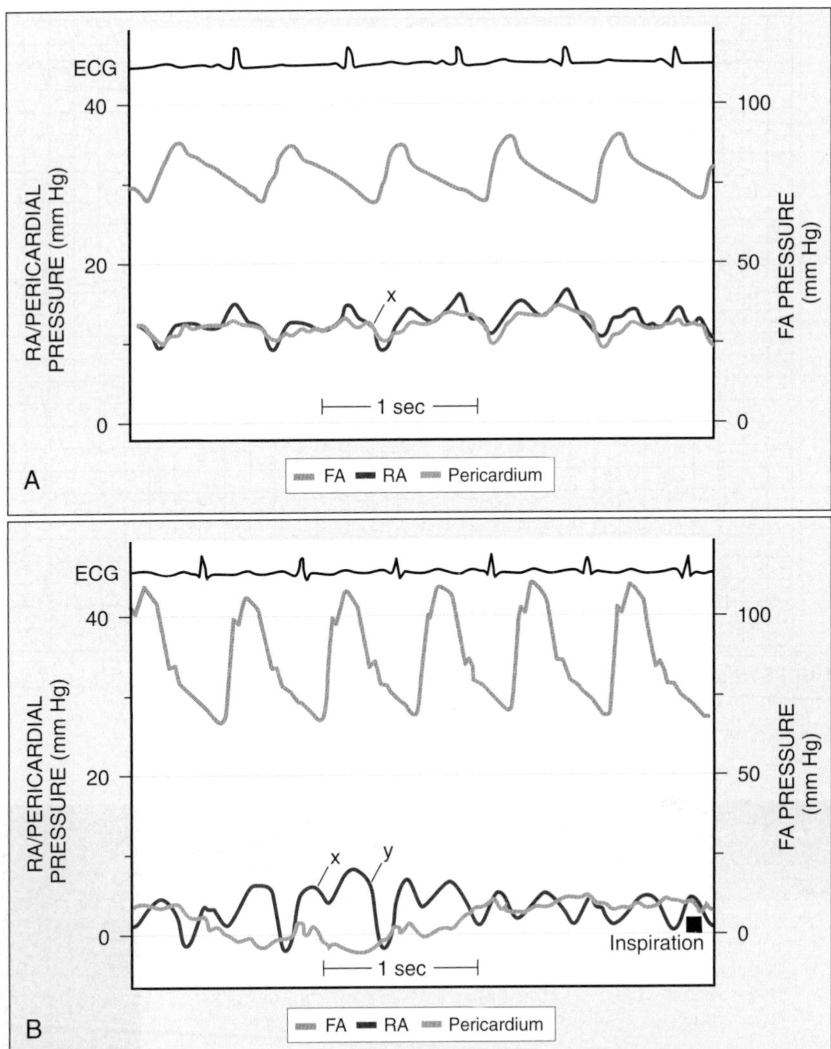

FIGURE 75-4 Femoral arterial (FA), right atrial (RA), and pericardial pressure before **(A)** and after **(B)** pericardiocentesis in a patient with cardiac tamponade. Both right atrial and pericardial pressures are about 15 mm Hg before pericardiocentesis. In this case, there was a negligible paradoxical pulse. Note presence of *x* descent but absence of *y* descent before pericardiocentesis. Pericardiocentesis results in marked increase in femoral arterial pressure and marked decrease in right atrial pressure. During inspiration, pericardial pressure becomes negative, there is clear separation between right atrial and pericardial pressures, and *y* descent is now prominent, suggesting the possibility of an effusive-constrictive picture. *(Modified from Lorell BH, Grossman W: Profiles in constrictive pericarditis, restrictive cardiomyopathy and cardiac tamponade.* In *Baim DS, Grossman W [eds]: Grossman's Cardiac Catheterization, Angiography, and Intervention. Philadelphia, Lippincott Williams & Wilkins, 2000, p 840.)*

Laboratory Testing

ELECTROCARDIOGRAPHY. Electrocardiographic abnormalities characteristic of pericardial effusion and tamponade are reduced voltage and electrical alternans[22] (**Fig. 75-6**; see Fig. 13-51). Reduced voltage is nonspecific and can be caused by several other conditions (e.g., emphysema, infiltrative myocardial disease, pneumothorax). Electrical alternans is specific but relatively insensitive for large effusions. It is caused by anterior-posterior swinging of the heart with each heart beat. When pericarditis coexists, the usual electrocardiographic findings may be present (see Chap. 13).

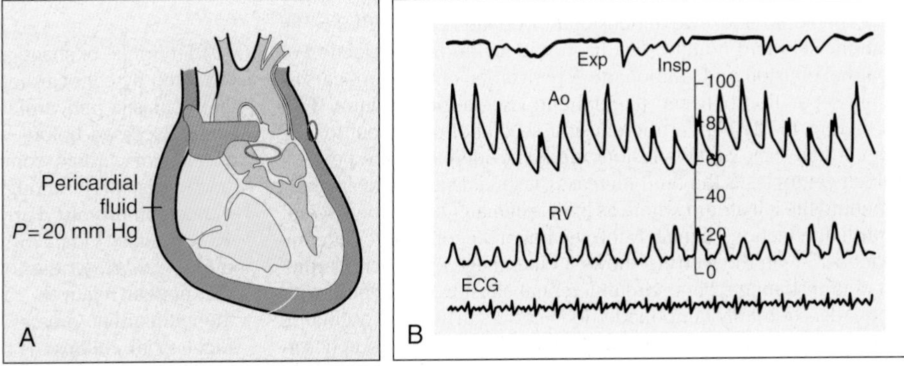

FIGURE 75-5 **A,** Schematic illustration of leftward septal shift with encroachment of left ventricular volume during inspiration in cardiac tamponade. **B,** Respiration marker and aortic and right ventricular pressure tracings in cardiac tamponade. Note paradoxical pulse and marked, 180-degree out-of-phase respiratory variation in right- and left-sided pressures. *(From Shabetai R: The Pericardium. New York, Grune & Stratton, 1981, p 266.)*

CHEST RADIOGRAPHY (see Chap. 16). The cardiac silhouette is normal until effusions are at least moderate in size. With moderate and larger effusions, the anteroposterior cardiac silhouette assumes a rounded, flasklike

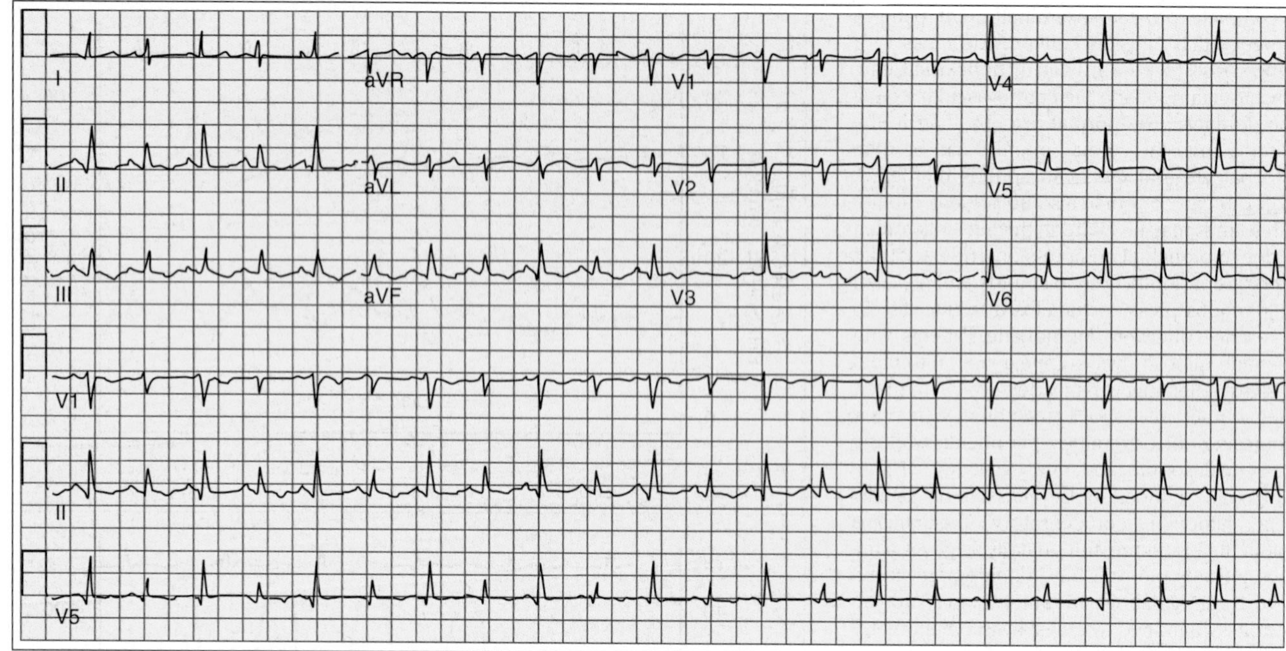

FIGURE 75-6 ECG in cardiac tamponade showing electrical alternans. *(From Lau TK, Civitello AB, Hernandez A, Coulter SA: Cardiac tamponade and electrical alternans. Tex Heart Inst J 48:67, 2002.* Copyright 2002 Texas Heart Institute.)

TABLE 75-3 Hemodynamics in Cardiac Tamponade and Constrictive Pericarditis

	TAMPONADE	CONSTRICTION
Paradoxical pulse	Usually present	Present in ~⅓
Equal left- and right-sided filling pressures	Present	Present
Systemic venous wave morphology	Absent *y* descent	Prominent *y* descent (M or W shape)
Inspiratory change in systemic venous pressure	Decrease (normal)	Increase or no change (Kussmaul sign)
"Square root" sign in ventricular pressure	Absent	Present

appearance (see Fig. 75-e2 on website). Lateral views may reveal the pericardial fat pad sign, a linear lucency between the chest wall and the anterior surface of the heart representing separation of parietal pericardial fat from epicardium. The lungs appear oligemic.

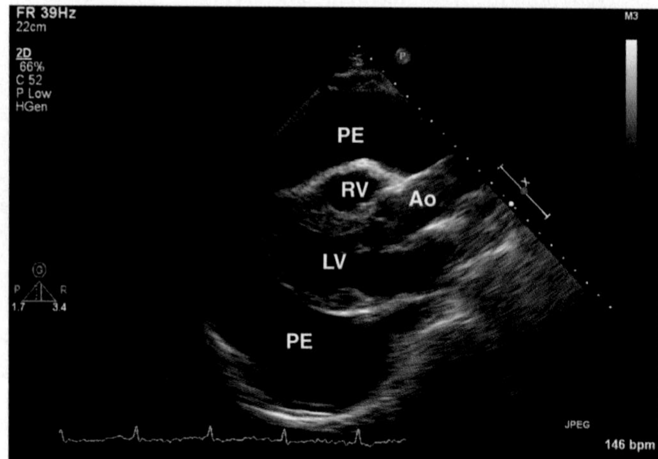

FIGURE 75-7 Two-dimensional echocardiogram of a large, circumferential pericardial effusion (PE). Ao = aorta; LV = left ventricle; RV = right ventricle. *(From Kabbani SS, LeWinter M: Cardiac constriction and restriction. In Crawford MH, DiMarco JP [eds]: Cardiology. St. Louis, Mosby, 2001, p 5, 15.5.)*

ECHOCARDIOGRAPHY (see Chap. 15). Because of their convenience, M-mode and two-dimensional Doppler echocardiography remain the standard noninvasive diagnostic methods for detection of pericardial effusion and tamponade. A pericardial effusion appears as a lucent separation between parietal and visceral pericardium (**Fig. 75-7**; see Fig. 15-72). With a true effusion, separation is present for the entire cardiac cycle. Small effusions are first evident over the posterobasal left ventricle. As the fluid increases, it spreads anteriorly, laterally, and behind the left atrium, where its limit is demarcated by the visceral pericardial reflection. Ultimately, the separation becomes circumferential. Video 75-1 on the website shows a cine image of an echocardiogram demonstrating a large, circumferential effusion in a patient with tamponade. Ordinarily, tamponade does not occur without a circumferential effusion, and the diagnosis should be viewed with skepticism if this is not the case. However, as discussed earlier, loculated effusions can cause regional tamponade. Computed tomography (CT) scanning and cardiac magnetic resonance (CMR) are more precise than echocardiography for imaging of the pericardium itself (see Chaps. 18 and 19). Frondlike or shaggy-appearing structures in the pericardial space detected by echocardiography suggest clots or chronic inflammatory or neoplastic pericardial processes.

As discussed before, tamponade is best considered a spectrum of severity of cardiac compression. Several findings indicate that tamponade is severe enough to cause at least some degree of hemodynamic compromise. Early diastolic collapse of the right ventricle (**Fig. 75-8**; see also Video 75-1 on website) and right atrium (which occurs during *ventricular* diastole; **Fig. 75-9**) are sensitive and specific signs that appear relatively early during tamponade.[18,22] Both occur when the pericardial pressure transiently exceeds intracavitary pressure. Right atrial collapse is more sensitive and right ventricular collapse more specific for tamponade.[18] As noted earlier, a large pleural effusion can also cause right-sided chamber collapse. Rarely, left ventricular collapse and left atrial collapse occur with loculated effusions after cardiac surgery.[18] The cardiac chambers are small in tamponade, and as discussed before, the heart may swing anteroposteriorly within the effusion. Distention of the caval vessels that does not diminish with inspiration is also a useful sign.

Reflecting the hemodynamic abnormalities discussed earlier, Doppler velocity recordings demonstrate exaggerated respiratory variation in right- and left-sided venous and valvular flow, with inspiratory increases on the right and decreases on the left (see Fig. 15-73).[18,22] As a result of reduced systemic venous inflow during early diastole with loss of the *y* descent, most caval and pulmonary venous inflow occurs during ventricular systole. These flow patterns were found to have good sensitivity and high specificity for diagnosis of tamponade. The absence of chamber collapse is especially useful in excluding tamponade in patients with effusions, but its presence is less well correlated with tamponade than abnormal venous flow patterns are. Newer techniques such as tissue Doppler do not as yet have a well-defined, additive role in cardiac tamponade. In most cases of pericardial effusion, transthoracic echocardiography provides sufficient diagnostic information for informed management decisions to be made. Transesophageal studies provide better quality images but are often impractical in sick patients unless they are intubated.

OTHER IMAGING MODALITIES. Fluoroscopy is useful in the cardiac catheterization laboratory for detection of procedure-related effusions because they may cause damping or abolition of cardiac pulsation.

CT (see Chap. 19) and CMR (see Chap. 18) are useful adjuncts to echocardiography in the characterization of effusion and tamponade.[26,27] Neither is ordinarily required or advisable in sick patients who require prompt management and treatment decisions. They have an important ancillary role in situations in which hemodynamics are atypical, other conditions complicate interpretation, and the presence and severity of tamponade are less certain. They are of course invaluable when echocardiography is technically inadequate. Video 75-2 on the website shows a CMR cine image revealing a large, circumferential pericardial effusion and a small, underfilled left ventricle. In this case, the right ventricle is not compressed because of longstanding pulmonary hypertension as evidenced by significant right ventricular hypertrophy.

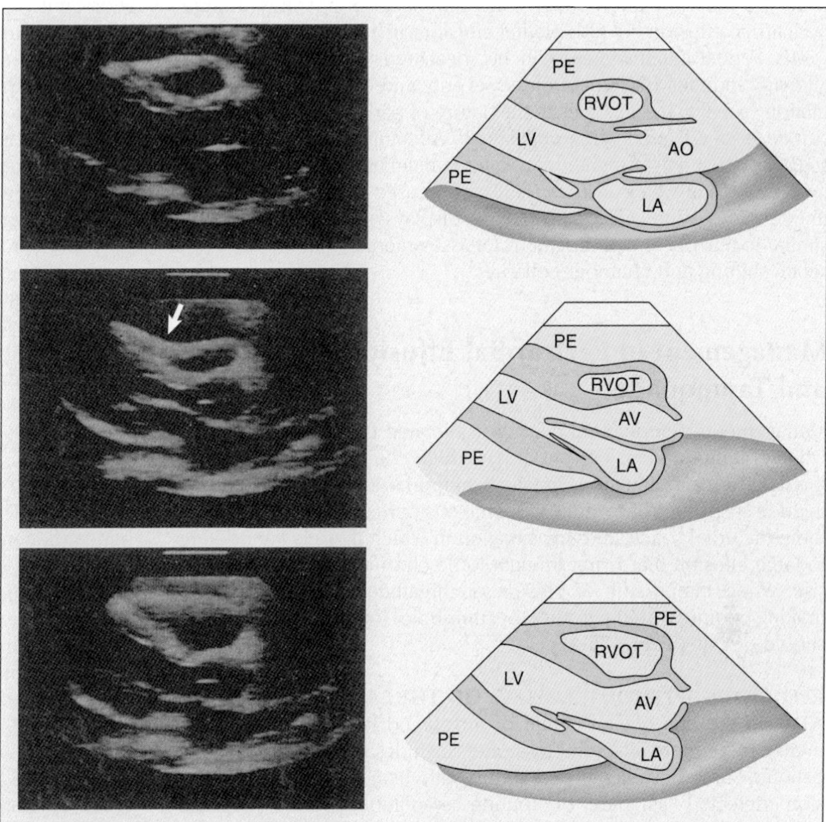

FIGURE 75-8 Two-dimensional echocardiogram illustrating diastolic collapse or indentation of the right ventricle in cardiac tamponade. **Top,** Systole. **Middle,** Early diastole with indentation indicated by arrow. **Bottom,** Late diastole with return of normal configuration. AO = aorta; AV = aortic valve; LA = left atrium; LV = left ventricle; PE = pericardial effusion; RVOT = right ventricular outflow tract. *(From Weyman AE: Principles and Practice of Echocardiography. Philadelphia, Lea & Febiger, 1994, p 1119.)*

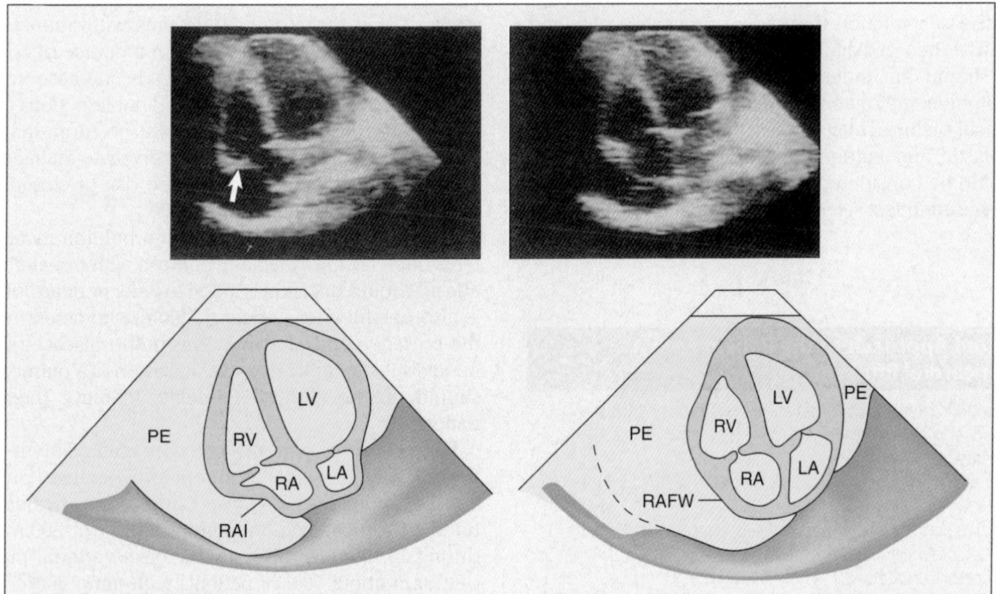

FIGURE 75-9 Two-dimensional echocardiogram illustrating right atrial collapse or indentation in cardiac tamponade. LA = left atrium; LV = left ventricle; PE = pericardial effusion; RA = right atrium; RAFW = right atrial free wall; RAI = right atrial inversion; RV = right ventricle. *(From Gillam LD, Guyer DE, Gibson TC, et al: Hemodynamic compression of the right atrium: A new echocardiographic sign of cardiac tamponade. Circulation 68:294, 1983.)*

It is important to recognize this constellation of findings because coexistent pulmonary hypertension reduces the accuracy of echocardiographic signs of cardiac tamponade. CT and CMR provide more detailed quantitation and regional localization than echocardiography does and are especially useful for loculated effusions and in the presence of coexistent pleural effusions. In Video 75-3 on the website, the wide field of view afforded by CMR demonstrates not only a large pericardial effusion but also pleural effusions in a patient with polyserositis. Pericardial thickness can be measured with both methods, allowing indirect assessment of the severity and chronicity of inflammation (see Fig. 18-17). Clues to the nature of pericardial fluid can be gained from CT attenuation coefficients. Attenuation similar to water suggests transudative; higher than water, malignant, bloody, or purulent; and lower than water, chylous. CMR can be used to make similar distinctions. Real-time CT or CMR cine displays provide information similar to that of echocardiography for assessment of tamponade (e.g., septal shifting and chamber collapse).

Management of Pericardial Effusion and Tamponade

Management of pericardial effusion is dictated first and foremost by whether tamponade is present or has a high chance of developing in the near term.[18,22] Situations in which tamponade is a near-term threat include suspected bacterial or tuberculous pericarditis, bleeding into the pericardial space, and any situation in which there is a moderate to large effusion that is not thought to be chronic or is increasing in size. When tamponade is present or threatened, clinical decision making requires urgency, and the threshold for pericardiocentesis should be low (**Table 75-4**).

EFFUSIONS WITHOUT ACTUAL OR THREATENED TAMPONADE. In the absence of actual or threatened tamponade, management can be more leisurely. This cohort includes several categories of patients. Some have acute pericarditis with a small to moderate effusion detected as part of routine evaluation. Others undergo echocardiography because of diseases known to involve the pericardium. The rest are asymptomatic and have effusions detected when diagnostic tests are performed for reasons other than suspected pericardial disease, such as when echocardiography is performed to evaluate an enlarged cardiac silhouette on the chest radiograph or CT or CMR is used to investigate thoracic disease.

In many cases of effusion when tamponade is neither present nor threatened, a cause will be evident or suggested by the history (e.g., known neoplastic disease, radiation therapy) or previously obtained diagnostic test results. When a diagnosis is not clear, an assessment of specific causes should be undertaken. This should include the diagnostic tests recommended for acute pericarditis and anything else dictated by the clinical picture. Thus, skin testing for tuberculosis and screening for neoplastic and autoimmune diseases, infections, and hypothyroidism should be considered. At the same time, careful judgment should be exercised in test selection. Thus, a patient with severe heart failure and circulatory congestion with a small, asymptomatic effusion does not need testing. In contrast, patients with evidence of a systemic disease deserve very careful attention. Titers of serum antibodies to viruses usually are not helpful in these cases because results may be nonspecific or negative despite a viral etiology. However, situations occasionally arise in which evidence of a viral etiology, if present, is helpful in clarifying diagnostic dilemmas, providing reassurance, and avoiding unnecessary diagnostic testing or treatments. Thus, it may be useful to save serum obtained at presentation should there be a need to measure viral titers at a later date.

In most of these patients, pericardiocentesis (closed or open with biopsy) needs to be undertaken only for diagnostic purposes and is usually not required. As discussed before, in many cases, a diagnosis will either be obvious when the effusion is first noted or become evident as part of initial investigations. Moreover, in this setting, analysis of pericardial fluid alone in general has a low yield for providing a specific diagnosis.[18] In occasional situations in which pericardiocentesis is thought to be necessary for diagnostic purposes, consideration should be given to open drainage with biopsy.

Occasional patients with large, asymptomatic effusions and no evidence of tamponade or a specific cause are a special category.[20] The effusions are by definition chronic because tamponade would be present if this were not the case. They are in general stable, and specific causes usually are not evident. However, a minority develop tamponade unpredictably. After closed pericardiocentesis, the effusions typically do not reaccumulate.[20] Thus, there is a rationale for pericardiocentesis after routine evaluation for specific causes as outlined before. This decision can be individualized, however, as little is lost by conservative management in reliable patients. Before pericardiocentesis is undertaken, a course of NSAID or colchicine should be considered because this will shrink some of these effusions. A course of corticosteroids may have the same effect, but this is controversial because of the possibility of an increased likelihood of recurrence.

EFFUSIONS WITH ACTUAL OR THREATENED TAMPONADE. These patients should be considered a true or potential medical emergency. With the exception of those who do not wish prolongation of life (mainly those with metastatic cancer), hospital admission and hemodynamic and echocardiographic monitoring are mandatory. Most patients require pericardiocentesis to treat or to prevent tamponade. Treatment should be individualized, and thoughtful clinical judgment is critical. Thus, for example, patients with acute, apparently idiopathic pericarditis who have no more than mild tamponade can be treated with a course of NSAID or colchicine in the hope that their effusions will shrink rapidly. Patients with autoimmune diseases can be treated in the same way or with a course of corticosteroids (there is no evidence that corticosteroids increase recurrence in these patients). Those with possible bacterial infections or bleeding into the pericardial sac whose effusions are no more than moderate in size may be suitable for initial conservative management and careful monitoring, especially because the risk of closed pericardiocentesis is increased with smaller effusions.

Hemodynamic monitoring with a pulmonary artery balloon catheter is often useful, especially in those with threatened or mild tamponade in whom a decision is made to defer pericardiocentesis. Monitoring is also helpful after pericardiocentesis to assess reaccumulation and the presence of underlying constrictive disease (see Fig. 75-4), as discussed subsequently. However, insertion of a pulmonary artery catheter should not be allowed to delay definitive therapy in critically ill patients.

For most patients in this category, management should be oriented toward urgent or emergent pericardiocentesis. Once actual or threatened tamponade is diagnosed, intravenous hydration should be instituted. In a recent report, administration of 500 mL of normal saline during 10 minutes modestly increased arterial pressure and cardiac output in about 50% of patients with tamponade.[28] Positive inotropes can also be employed but are of limited efficacy. Hydration and positive inotropes are temporizing measures and should not be allowed to substitute for or to delay pericardiocentesis.

TABLE 75-4 Initial Approach to the Patient with a Pericardial Effusion

Determine if tamponade is present or threatened on the basis of history, physical examination, and echocardiogram.

If tamponade is not present or threatened:
- If the cause is not apparent, consider diagnostic tests as for acute pericarditis.
- If the effusion is large, consider course of NSAID or corticosteroid; if no response, consider closed pericardiocentesis.

If tamponade is present or threatened:
- Urgent or emergent closed pericardiocentesis or careful monitoring is indicated if a trial of medical treatment to reduce effusion is considered appropriate.

In most circumstances, closed pericardiocentesis is the treatment of choice. Before proceeding, it is important to be confident that there is an effusion large enough to cause tamponade, especially if hemodynamics are atypical. Loculated effusions or effusions containing clots or fibrinous material are also of concern because the risk and difficulty of closed pericardiocentesis are increased. In these situations, if removal of fluid is thought to be necessary, an open approach should be considered for safety and to obtain pericardial tissue and to create a window. One of the more difficult management decisions is whether to perform closed versus open pericardiocentesis in patients with known or suspected bleeding into the pericardial space. The danger of a closed approach is that lowering the intrapericardial pressure will simply encourage more bleeding without affording an opportunity to correct its source. In cases of trauma or rupture of the wall of the left ventricle after MI, closed pericardiocentesis should in general be avoided. However, if bleeding is slower (e.g., due to a procedural coronary perforation or puncture of a cardiac chamber), closed pericardiocentesis is often appropriate because bleeding may stop spontaneously or the procedure can provide temporary relief before definitive repair.

The most commonly employed approach to closed pericardiocentesis is subxiphoid needle insertion with echocardiographic guidance to minimize the risk of myocardial puncture and to assess completeness of fluid removal. Once the needle has entered the pericardial space, a modest amount of fluid should be immediately removed (perhaps 50 to 150 mL) in an effort to produce immediate hemodynamic improvement. A guidewire is then inserted, and the needle is replaced with a pigtail catheter. The catheter is manipulated with continuing echocardiographic guidance to maximize fluid removal. In a large series from the Mayo Clinic,[29] procedural success rate was 97% and complication rate 4.7% (major, 1.2%; minor, 3.5%). Whenever possible, the procedure should be performed in the cardiac catheterization laboratory with experienced personnel in attendance. If echocardiographic guidance is unavailable, the needle should be directed toward the left shoulder and then replaced with a catheter for subsequent fluid removal. Fluoroscopy-guided drainage is an alternative when echocardiography cannot be used.

If a pulmonary artery catheter has been inserted, pulmonary capillary wedge and systemic arterial pressures and cardiac output should be monitored before, during, and after the procedure. Ideally, pericardial fluid pressure should also be measured. As discussed before, removal of relatively small amounts of fluid can result in substantial hemodynamic improvement. Hemodynamic monitoring before and after pericardiocentesis is useful for several reasons. Initial measurements confirm and document the severity of tamponade. Assessment after completion establishes a baseline to assess reaccumulation. As discussed later, some patients presenting with tamponade have a coexisting component of constriction (i.e., effusive-constrictive pericarditis),[30] which is difficult to detect when an effusion dominates the picture. Filling pressures that remain elevated after pericardiocentesis and the appearance of venous waveforms typical of constriction (rapid *x* and *y* descents) indicate coexistent constriction.

After pericardiocentesis, repeated echocardiography and in many cases continued hemodynamic monitoring are useful to assess reaccumulation. The duration of monitoring is a matter of judgment, but 24 hours is typically sufficient. A follow-up echocardiogram should be obtained immediately before hemodynamic monitoring is discontinued. We recommend consideration of leaving intrapericardial catheters in place for several days to allow continued fluid removal. This has been shown to minimize recurrences[5,18] and facilitates delivery of intrapericardial drugs if indicated.

Open pericardiocentesis is occasionally preferred for initial removal of pericardial fluid. Bleeding due to trauma and rupture of the left ventricular free wall has been mentioned previously in this regard. Loculated effusions or effusions that are borderline in size are drained more safely in the operating room. Recurring effusions, especially those causing tamponade, may initially be drained by a closed approach because of logistical considerations. However, open pericardiocentesis with biopsy and establishment of a pericardial window are preferred for most recurrences that are severe enough to cause tamponade. Creation of a window reliably eliminates future tamponade and provides pericardial tissue to assist in diagnosis. The surgeon should inspect the pericardium carefully and obtain multiple biopsy specimens.

More recently, percutaneous balloon techniques have been used for drainage. These methods are safe and effective for producing pericardial windows but are available at relatively few centers. Balloon pericardiotomy appears to be particularly useful in patients with malignant effusions,[31] in whom the incidence of recurrence is high and a definitive approach without a surgical procedure is desirable.

ANALYSIS OF PERICARDIAL FLUID. Normal pericardial fluid in general has the features of a plasma ultrafiltrate.[32] However, the lactate dehydrogenase level is 2.4 times and the mean protein level is 0.6 times that of plasma. Lymphocytes are the predominant cell type.

Although analysis of pericardial fluid does not have a high yield in identifying the cause of pericardial disease, careful analysis can be rewarding. Assuming that a diagnosis is not known before fluid removal, routine pericardial fluid measurements should include specific gravity, white blood cell count and differential, hematocrit, and protein content.[5,18,32] Although most effusions are exudates, detection of a transudate reduces the diagnostic possibilities considerably. Sanguinous fluid is nonspecific and does not necessarily indicate bleeding. Chylous effusions can occur after traumatic or surgical injury to the thoracic duct or obstruction by a neoplastic process. On occasion, they are idiopathic. Cholesterol-rich ("gold paint") effusions occur in severe hypothyroidism.

Pericardial fluid should routinely be stained and cultured for detection of bacteria, including tuberculosis, and fungi. As much fluid as possible should be submitted for detection of malignant cells as there is a reasonably high diagnostic yield. In tuberculous pericardial disease, several tests other than culture of fluid and examination of biopsy specimens are useful.[5,18,32-35] These include adenosine deaminase (ADA), interferon-γ, and the polymerase chain reaction (PCR), discussed in more detail later. Unless some other cause is evident, we believe that some relatively rapid test for tuberculosis (ADA, PCR) should be routine because of the difficulty in diagnosis of tuberculous pericarditis and the delays involved in making a diagnosis by culture. There may also be a role for routine measurement of selected tumor markers as a general screen for malignant effusion and an adjunct to direct detection of malignant cells.[5]

PERICARDIOSCOPY AND PERCUTANEOUS BIOPSY. Some experts advocate the routine use of pericardioscopy-guided biopsy in patients with pericardial effusion without an etiologic diagnosis. Seferovic and colleagues[35] compared the diagnostic yield of percutaneous, fluoroscopy-guided parietal biopsy (3 to 6 samples) with that of targeted, pericardioscopy-guided biopsy with either limited (3 to 6 samples) or extended (18 to 20 samples) sampling. Tissue was examined by routine histology. Pericardioscopic biopsy was found to have a higher sampling efficiency than fluoroscopic guidance and a much higher diagnostic yield. Extended sampling performed best, leading to a new diagnosis in 41% and a specific etiology in 53% of cases. The technique was especially useful in detecting malignant involvement, and few complications occurred. However, pericardioscopy is technically challenging, and few individuals have significant experience. Moreover, in earlier reports, major complications were occasionally encountered, and it is as yet uncertain whether its use will significantly improve long-term outcomes. Thus, this procedure should be undertaken only by individuals with appropriate training and experience.

Constrictive Pericarditis

Etiology

Constrictive pericarditis is the end stage of an inflammatory process involving the pericardium. Virtually any process listed in Table 75-1 can cause constriction. In the developed world, the etiology is most commonly idiopathic, postsurgical, or radiation injury[6,18] (**Table 75-5**). Tuberculosis was the most common cause in the developed world before the advent of effective drug therapy and remains important in developing countries. Although constriction can follow an initial insult by as little as several months, it usually takes years to develop. The end result is dense fibrosis, often calcification, and adhesions of the parietal and visceral pericardium. Scarring is usually more or less symmetric and impedes filling of all heart chambers. In a subset of patients, the process develops relatively rapidly and is reversible. This variant is seen most commonly after cardiac surgery.[36]

Pathophysiology

The pathophysiologic consequence of pericardial scarring is markedly restricted filling of the heart.[18] This results in elevation and equilibration of filling pressures in all chambers and the systemic and pulmonary veins. In early diastole, the ventricles fill abnormally rapidly because of markedly elevated atrial pressures and accentuated early diastolic ventricular suction, the latter related to small end-systolic volumes. During early to mid diastole, ventricular filling abruptly ceases when intracardiac volume reaches the limit set by the stiff pericardium. As a result, almost all ventricular filling occurs early in diastole. Systemic venous congestion results in hepatic congestion, peripheral edema, ascites and sometimes anasarca, and cardiac cirrhosis. Reduced cardiac output is a consequence of impaired ventricular filling and causes fatigue, muscle wasting, and weight loss. In "pure" constriction, contractile function is preserved, although ejection fraction can be reduced because of reduced preload. The myocardium is occasionally involved in the chronic inflammation and fibrosis, leading to true contractile dysfunction that can at times be quite severe and predicts a poor response to pericardiectomy.

Failure of transmission of intrathoracic respiratory pressure changes to the cardiac chambers is an important contributor to the pathophysiologic process of constrictive pericarditis (**Fig. 75-10**). These pressure changes continue to be transmitted to the pulmonary circulation. Thus, on inspiration, the drop in intrathoracic pressure (and therefore pulmonary venous pressure) is not transmitted to the left side of the heart.[18] Consequently, the small pulmonary venous to left atrial pressure gradient that normally drives left-sided heart filling is reduced, resulting in decreased transmitral inflow. The inspiratory decrease in left ventricular filling allows an increase in right ventricular filling and an interventricular septal shift to the left. The opposite sequence occurs with expiration.

High systemic venous pressure and reduced cardiac output result in compensatory retention of sodium and water by the kidneys. Inhibition of natriuretic peptides also may contribute to renal sodium retention, further exacerbating increased filling pressures.[37]

TABLE 75-5 Causes of Constrictive Pericarditis

Idiopathic
Irradiation
Postsurgical
Infectious
Neoplastic
Autoimmune (connective tissue) disorders
Uremia
Post-trauma
Sarcoid
Methysergide therapy
Implantable defibrillator patches

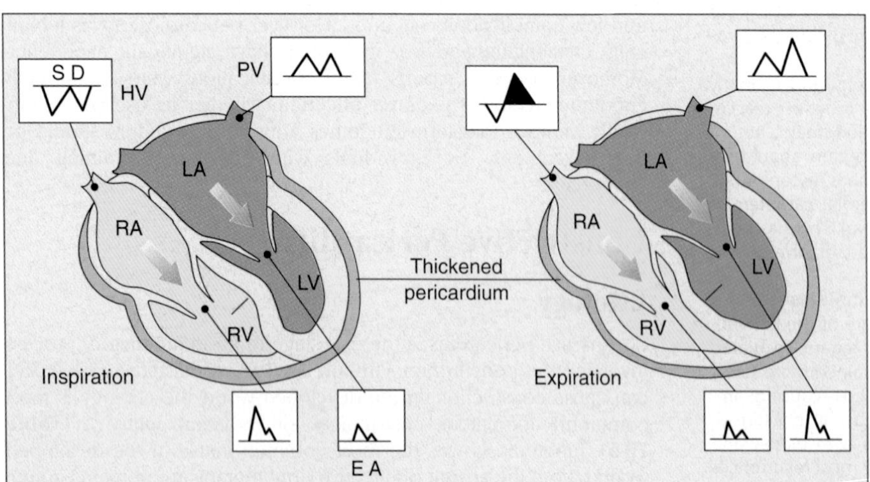

FIGURE 75-10 Schematic representation of transvalvular and central venous flow velocities in constrictive pericarditis. During inspiration, the decrease in left ventricular filling results in a leftward septal shift, allowing augmented flow into the right ventricle. The opposite occurs during expiration. D = diastole; EA = mitral inflow; HV = hepatic vein; LA = left atrium; LV = left ventricle; PV = pulmonary venous flow; RA = right atrium; RV = right ventricle; S = systole.

Clinical Presentation

The usual presentation consists of signs and symptoms of right-sided heart failure. At a relatively early stage, these include lower extremity edema, vague abdominal complaints, and passive hepatic congestion. As the disease progresses, hepatic congestion worsens and can progress to ascites, anasarca, and jaundice due to cardiac cirrhosis. Signs and symptoms ascribable to elevated pulmonary venous pressures, such as exertional dyspnea, cough, and orthopnea, may also appear with progressive disease. Atrial fibrillation and tricuspid regurgitation, which further exacerbate venous pressure elevation, may also appear at this stage. In end-stage constrictive pericarditis, the effects of a chronically low cardiac output are prominent, including severe fatigue, muscle wasting, and cachexia. Other findings include recurrent pleural effusions and syncope. Constrictive pericarditis can be mistaken for any cause of right-sided heart failure as well as end-stage primary hepatic disease. Of course, venous pressure is not elevated in the latter circumstance.

Physical Examination

Physical findings include markedly elevated jugular venous pressure with a prominent, rapidly collapsing *y* descent. This, combined with a normal *x* descent, results in an M- or W-shaped venous pressure contour. At the bedside, this is best appreciated as two prominent descents with each cardiac cycle. In patients in atrial fibrillation, the *x* descent is lost, leaving only the prominent *y* descent (see Fig. 12-3). The latter is very difficult to distinguish from tricuspid regurgitation, which, as noted before, may itself be due to constrictive pericarditis. Kussmaul sign, an inspiratory increase in systemic venous pressure, is usually present,[18] or the venous pressure may simply fail to decrease on inspiration. Kussmaul sign reflects loss of the normal increase in right-sided heart venous return on inspiration, even though tricuspid flow increases. These characteristic abnormalities of the venous waveform contrast with tamponade. A paradoxical pulse occurs in perhaps one third of patients with constriction, especially when there is an effusive-constrictive picture (see later). It is best explained by the aforementioned lack of transmission of decreased intrathoracic pressure to the left-sided heart chambers. Table 75-3 is a comparison of hemodynamic findings in tamponade and constrictive pericarditis.

In cases with extensive calcification and adhesion of the heart to adjacent structures, the position of the cardiac point of maximal impulse may fail to change with changes in body position. However, the most notable cardiac finding is the pericardial knock, an early diastolic sound best heard at the left sternal border or the cardiac apex (see Fig. 12-3). It occurs slightly earlier and has a higher frequency content than a typical third heart sound. The knock corresponds to the early, abrupt cessation of ventricular filling. Widening of second heart sound splitting may also be present. As noted, patients may have secondary tricuspid regurgitation with its characteristic murmur.

Abdominal examination reveals hepatomegaly, often with palpable venous pulsations, with or without ascites. Other signs of hepatic congestion or cardiac cirrhosis include jaundice, spider angiomas, and palmar erythema. Lower extremity edema is the rule. As noted before, with end-stage constriction, muscle wasting, cachexia, and massive ascites and anasarca may appear.

Laboratory Testing

ELECTROCARDIOGRAPHY. There are no specific electrocardiographic findings. Nonspecific T wave abnormalities, reduced voltage, and left atrial abnormality may be present. Atrial fibrillation is also common.

CHEST RADIOGRAPHY (see Chap. 16). The cardiac silhouette can be enlarged secondary to a coexisting pericardial effusion. Pericardial calcification is seen in a minority of patients and suggests tuberculosis (**Fig. 75-11**; see Fig. 16-11), but calcification per se is not diagnostic of constrictive physiology. The lateral view may reveal pericardial calcification along the right-sided heart border and in the atrioventricular groove. Isolated calcification of the left ventricular apex or posterior wall suggests ventricular aneurysm rather than pericardial calcification. Pleural effusions are occasionally noted and can be a presenting sign of constrictive pericarditis. When left-sided heart filling pressures are markedly elevated, pulmonary vascular congestion and redistribution can be present.

ECHOCARDIOGRAPHY (see Chap. 15). M-mode and two-dimensional transthoracic echocardiographic findings include pericardial thickening, abrupt displacement of the interventricular septum during early diastole (septal "bounce"),[5,18] and signs of systemic venous congestion such as dilation of hepatic veins and distention of the inferior vena cava with blunted respiratory fluctuation. Premature pulmonic valve opening as a result of elevated right ventricular early diastolic pressure may also be observed. Exaggerated septal shifting during respiration is often present.

Lack of transmission of intrathoracic pressure to the cardiac chambers and resulting mitral and tricuspid inflow patterns have been discussed earlier. In accordance with these patterns, Doppler measurements often reveal exaggerated respiratory variation in both mitral inflow velocity and tricuspid-mitral inflow velocity, with the latter 180 degrees out of phase (see Fig. 15-73). Although there is some overlap with tamponade, these inflow patterns have good sensitivity and specificity for diagnosis of constrictive pericarditis and also help distinguish restrictive cardiomyopathy from constriction.[5,18] Typically, patients with constriction demonstrate a ≥25% increase in mitral E velocity during expiration compared with inspiration and increased diastolic flow reversal with expiration in the hepatic veins. Mitral E wave deceleration time is usually but not always <160 milliseconds. However, up to 20% of patients with constriction do not exhibit typical respiratory changes, most likely because of markedly increased left atrial pressure or possibly a mixed constrictive-restrictive pattern due to myocardial involvement by the constrictive process. In patients without typical respiratory mitral-tricuspid flow findings, examination after maneuvers that decrease preload (head-up tilt, sitting) can unmask characteristic respiratory variation in mitral E velocity.[18] Tissue Doppler examination reveals increased E′ velocity of the mitral annulus as well as septal abnormalities corresponding to the bounce.[38,39] Tissue Doppler appears to be at least as sensitive as mitral-tricuspid inflow Doppler for diagnosis of constriction.

Similar patterns of respiratory variation in mitral inflow velocity can be observed in chronic obstructive lung disease, right ventricular infarction, pulmonary embolism, and pleural effusion. These conditions have other clinical and echocardiographic features that differentiate them from constrictive pericarditis. Superior vena caval flow velocities are helpful in distinguishing constrictive pericarditis from chronic obstructive pulmonary disease. Patients with pulmonary disease display a marked increase in inspiratory superior vena caval systolic forward flow velocity, which is not seen in constriction.

Transesophageal echocardiography is superior to transthoracic echocardiography for measuring pericardial thickness and has an excellent correlation with CT. When mitral inflow velocities by transthoracic echocardiography are technically inadequate or equivocal, measurement of transesophageal pulmonary venous Doppler velocity demonstrates pronounced respiratory variation, larger than that observed across the mitral valve.

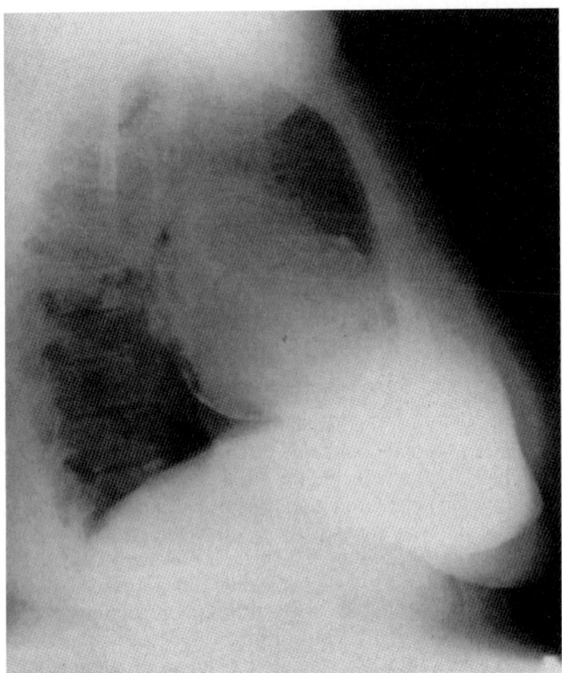

FIGURE 75-11 Chest radiograph showing marked pericardial calcification in a patient with constrictive pericarditis.

CARDIAC CATHETERIZATION AND ANGIOGRAPHY (see Chap. 20). Cardiac catheterization in patients with suspected constriction provides documentation of the hemodynamics of constrictive physiology and assists in discriminating between constrictive pericarditis and restrictive cardiomyopathy.[5,18] Whereas there is limited need for contrast ventriculography, coronary angiography should ordinarily be performed in patients being considered for pericardiectomy. On rare occasions, external pinching or compression of the coronary arteries by the constricting pericardium is detected.

Right atrial, right ventricular diastolic, pulmonary capillary wedge, and pre-*a* wave left ventricular diastolic pressures are elevated and equal, or nearly so, at around 20 mm Hg. Differences of more than 3 to 5 mm Hg between left- and right-sided heart filling pressures are rarely encountered. The right atrial pressure tracing shows a preserved *x* descent, a prominent *y* descent, and roughly equal *a* and *v* wave height, with the resultant M or W configuration. Both right and left ventricular pressures reveal an early, marked diastolic dip followed by a plateau ("dip and plateau" or "square root" sign; **Fig. 75-12**). Pulmonary artery and right ventricular systolic pressures are often modestly elevated, in the range of 35 to 45 mm Hg. Greater elevation of the pulmonary artery systolic pressure is not a feature of constrictive pericarditis and casts doubt on the diagnosis. Hypovolemia (e.g., secondary to diuretic therapy) can mask typical hemodynamic findings. Rapid volume challenge of 1000 mL of normal saline during 6 to 8 minutes may reveal typical hemodynamic features. Stroke volume is almost always reduced, but resting cardiac output can be preserved because of tachycardia. Depression of stroke volume is primarily caused by reduced diastolic filling. In the absence of extensive coexisting myocardial involvement, left ventricular ejection fraction is normal or slightly reduced.

COMPUTED TOMOGRAPHY AND CARDIAC MAGNETIC RESONANCE. CT (see Chap. 19) provides detailed pericardial images and is helpful in detecting even minute amounts of pericardial calcification[26,27] (see Fig. 75-e3 on website). Its major disadvantage is the frequent need for iodinated contrast medium to best display pericardial disease. The thickness of the normal pericardium measured by CT is <2 mm. CMR[26,27] (see Chap. 18) provides a detailed and comprehensive examination of the pericardium without the need for contrast material

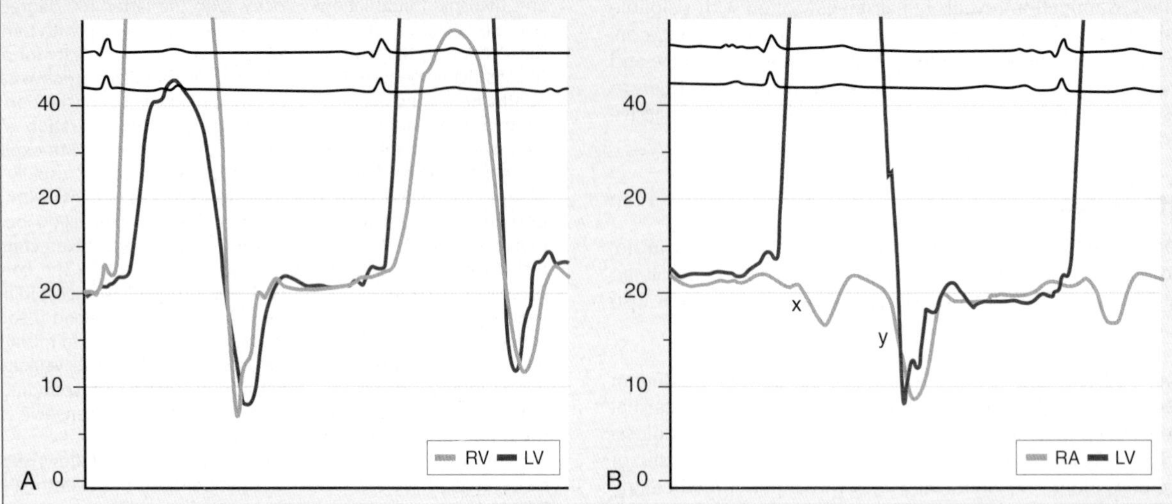

FIGURE 75-12 Pressure recordings in a patient with constrictive pericarditis. **A,** Simultaneous right ventricular (RV) and left ventricular (LV) pressure tracings with equalization of diastolic pressure as well as "dip and plateau" morphology. **B,** Simultaneous right atrial (RA) and LV pressure tracings with equalization of RA and LV diastolic pressure. Note the prominent *y* descent. *(From Vaitkus PT, Cooper KA, Shuman WP, Hardin NJ: Images in cardiovascular medicine: Constrictive pericarditis. Circulation 93:834, 1996.)*

or ionizing radiation. It is somewhat less sensitive than CT for detection of calcification. The "normal" pericardium visualized by CMR is up to 3 to 4 mm in thickness. This measurement most likely reflects the entire pericardial "complex," with physiologic fluid representing a component of the measured thickness.

Demonstration of a thickened pericardium indicates acute or chronic pericarditis. If there is clinical evidence of impaired diastolic filling, pericardial thickening, especially with calcification, is virtually diagnostic of constriction. Absence of pericardial thickening argues against the diagnosis of constriction but does not completely rule it out. The pericardium can be globally or focally thickened. Localized compression of the heart caused by focal thickening is reported and is much more common on the right than on the left side. In patients being considered for pericardiectomy, delineation of the location and severity of thickening and calcification aids the surgeon with respect to both risk stratification and planning of surgery. Additional findings include distorted ventricular contours, hepatic venous congestion, ascites, pleural effusions, and occasionally pericardial effusion. Cine acquisition (CMR or CT) shows abnormal motion of the interventricular septum (septal bounce) in early diastole (see Video 75-4 on website). Finally, enhanced uptake of gadolinium appears useful for detection of pericardial inflammation.[40]

There is a cohort of patients with well-documented constriction who have no pericardial thickening on the basis of measurements in pathologic specimens despite histologic evidence of inflammation and calcification. These patients constituted 18% of those with constrictive pericarditis in a Mayo Clinic series.[41] Almost all had normal pericardial thickness by CT. Calcification and distorted ventricular contours occurred in a majority, providing clues to the diagnosis despite normal thickness.

TABLE 75-6 Hemodynamic and Echocardiographic Features of Constrictive Pericarditis Compared with Restrictive Cardiomyopathy

	CONSTRICTION	RESTRICTION
Prominent *y* descent in venous pressure	Present	Variable
Paradoxical pulse	~⅓ of cases	Absent
Pericardial knock	Present	Absent
Equal right- and left-sided filling pressures	Present	Left at least 3-5 mm Hg > right
Filling pressures >25 mm Hg	Rare	Common
Pulmonary artery systolic pressure >60 mm Hg	No	Common
"Square root" sign	Present	Variable
Respiratory variation in left- and right-sided pressures or flows	Exaggerated	Normal
Ventricular wall thickness	Normal	Usually increased
Atrial size	Possible left atrial enlargement	Biatrial enlargement
Septal bounce	Present	Absent
Tissue Doppler E′ velocity	Increased	Reduced
Pericardial thickness	Increased	Normal

Differentiation of Constrictive Pericarditis from Restrictive Cardiomyopathy

Because their treatment is radically different, distinguishing constrictive pericarditis from restrictive cardiomyopathy is extremely important (**Table 75-6**). Their presentation and course overlap in many respects. A pericardial knock points to constriction, but prominent third heart sounds in restrictive disease can be confusing. Electrocardiographic and chest radiographic findings are mostly nonspecific. However, a calcified pericardium indicates constriction, whereas low QRS voltage suggests amyloidosis. There are some useful echocardiographic distinctions. Patients with restrictive cardiomyopathy usually have thick-walled ventricles due to infiltrative processes such as amyloidosis (see Fig. 15-77). Marked biatrial enlargement is also common in restriction (see Fig. 68-7). In constriction, the most distinctive finding is the septal bounce. As discussed before, the pericardium is usually thickened in constriction, but this may be difficult to assess with transthoracic echocardiography. As noted, transesophageal echocardiographic measurements of pericardial thickness correlate well with CT, although they are limited by their narrow field of view. With use of two-dimensional speckle tracking, differences in contraction mechanics that are useful in distinguishing constriction from restriction have been described.[42] In constriction, deformation of the left ventricle and early diastolic recoil velocity were attenuated in the circumferential direction, whereas in restriction, they were attenuated in the longitudinal direction.

Doppler measurements are also useful in differentiating constrictive from restrictive physiology.[18,38,39] Enhanced respiratory variation in mitral inflow velocity (>25%) is seen in constriction; in restriction, velocity varies by <10% (see Fig. 75-10; see Fig. 15-75). In restriction, pulmonary venous systolic flow is markedly blunted and diastolic flow is increased. This is not observed in constriction. Hepatic veins demonstrate enhanced expiratory flow reversal with constriction, in contrast to increased inspiratory flow reversal in restriction (see Figs. 15-70 and 15-76). Tissue Doppler echocardiography and color M-mode flow propagation are complementary to mitral Doppler respiratory variation in distinguishing constriction from restrictive cardiomyopathy. Higher tissue Doppler mitral annulus E′ values in constriction versus restrictive cardiomyopathy (see Figs. 15-69 and 15-77) are reported to have a higher sensitivity than mitral inflow parameters for making the distinction.[38,39]

Hemodynamic differentiation between constrictive pericarditis and restrictive cardiomyopathy in the cardiac catheterization laboratory can be difficult. However, careful attention to the hemodynamic profile usually allows successful distinction (see Table 75-6). In both conditions, right and left ventricular diastolic pressures are markedly elevated. In restrictive cardiomyopathy, diastolic pressure in the left ventricle is usually higher than in the right ventricle by at least 3 to 5 mm Hg; in constrictive pericarditis, left- and right-sided diastolic pressures typically track closely and rarely differ by more than 3 to 5 mm Hg. Pulmonary hypertension is common with restrictive cardiomyopathy but rare in constriction. The absolute level of atrial or ventricular diastolic pressure elevation is also sometimes useful in distinguishing the two conditions, with extremely high pressures (>25 mm Hg) much more common in restrictive cardiomyopathy.[5,18] Finally, the ratio of right ventricular to left ventricular systolic pressure-time area during inspiration versus expiration[43] is greater in constriction versus restriction (reflecting exaggerated ventricular interaction) and is reported to have a high sensitivity and specificity for distinguishing between them (see Fig. 20-15).

CT and CMR, because of their ability to provide detailed assessment of pericardial thickness and calcification, are useful in differentiating constriction from restriction.[26,27] Occasional patients with constriction and normal pericardial thickness have been discussed before. Pericardial calcification or distorted ventricular contour is helpful in making the correct diagnosis in these patients. Endomyocardial or abdominal fat pad biopsy establishes the diagnosis of restrictive cardiomyopathy due to amyloidosis. Brain natriuretic peptide (BNP) levels may be useful in distinguishing constriction from restriction. BNP is reported to be elevated in restrictive cardiomyopathy and normal in constriction.[37] More recent data[43] indicate that this difference is more useful in secondary constriction (e.g., postoperative, irradiation) than in idiopathic cases.

Availability of the multiple diagnostic modalities discussed before has made it very rare to have to resort to exploratory thoracotomy to distinguish constriction from restriction.

Management

Constrictive pericarditis is a progressive disease but has a variable course. With the exception of patients with transient constriction, surgical pericardiectomy is the definitive treatment. Transient constriction should be suspected in patients presenting relatively earlier after cardiac surgery or with relatively rapid development of symptoms. Such patients can be monitored for several months to look for spontaneous improvement. They may respond to a course of corticosteroids, and there is little to lose by managing them in this way. Patients with major comorbidities or severe debilitation are often at too high risk to undergo pericardiectomy. Radiation-induced disease is also considered a relative contraindication to pericardiectomy. Healthy older patients with very mild constriction may also be managed nonsurgically, with pericardiectomy held in reserve until there is disease progression. Otherwise, surgery should not be delayed once the diagnosis is made. Medical management with diuretics and salt restriction is useful for relief of fluid overload and edema, but patients ultimately become refractory. Because sinus tachycardia is a compensatory mechanism, beta-adrenergic blockers and calcium antagonists that slow the heart rate should be avoided. In patients with atrial fibrillation and a rapid ventricular response, digoxin is recommended as initial treatment to slow the ventricular rate before resorting to beta blockers or calcium antagonists. In general, the rate should not be allowed to drop below 80 to 90 beats/min.

Pericardiectomy can be performed through either a median sternotomy or a left fifth interspace thoracotomy and involves radical excision of as much of the parietal pericardium as possible.[5] The visceral pericardium is then inspected and resection considered if it is involved in the disease process. Most surgeons initially attempt to perform pericardiectomy without cardiopulmonary bypass. Cardiopulmonary bypass is available as backup and is frequently required to facilitate access to the lateral and diaphragmatic surfaces of the left ventricle and to allow safe removal of a maximal amount of pericardial tissue. Ultrasonic or laser débridement[5,44] is useful as an adjunct to conventional surgical débridement or as the sole technique in high-risk patients with extensive, calcified adhesions between pericardium and epicardium. Occasional patients may be candidates for video-assisted thoracoscopic pericardiectomy in centers with appropriate expertise.

Hemodynamic and symptomatic improvement is achieved in some patients immediately after operation. In others, improvement may be delayed for weeks to months. Videos 75-5 and 75-6 on the website show cine CMR images before and after successful pericardial stripping, demonstrating relief of exaggerated variations in right- and left-sided heart volume. After pericardiectomy, 70% to 80% of patients remain free from adverse cardiovascular outcomes at 5 years and 40% to 50% at 10 years.[45] Long-term results are worse in patients with radiation-induced disease, impaired renal function, relatively high pulmonary artery systolic pressure, reduced left ventricular ejection fraction, moderate or severe tricuspid regurgitation, low serum sodium, and advanced age.[45,46] Left ventricular diastolic function based on echocardiography returns to normal in about 40% of patients early and in nearly 60% late after pericardiectomy. Persistence of abnormal filling was correlated with postoperative symptoms. Delayed or inadequate responses to pericardiectomy have been attributed to longstanding disease with myocardial atrophy or fibrosis, incomplete pericardial resection, and development of recurrent cardiac compression by mediastinal inflammation and fibrosis. Lack of improvement after pericardiectomy may also be due to inadequate resection of visceral pericardium. Tricuspid regurgitation usually does not improve after surgery[47] and can cause postoperative hemodynamic deterioration.

Pericardiectomy has a 5% to 15% perioperative mortality in patients with constriction. In a Cleveland Clinic series,[45] 63% of patients were alive after a median follow-up of 6.9 years, but long-term results were variable. Early mortality results primarily from low cardiac output, often in debilitated patients with prolonged cardiopulmonary bypass and difficult dissections. Sepsis, uncontrolled hemorrhage, and renal and respiratory insufficiency also contribute to early mortality.[45,46] The highest mortality occurs in patients with Class III or IV symptoms, supporting the recommendation of early pericardiectomy.

Effusive-Constrictive Pericarditis

A number of patients with pericardial disease present with a syndrome combining elements of effusion or tamponade and constriction. They often have a subacute course initially. An inflammatory effusion may dominate early, with constriction more prominent later. As noted previously, these patients are often identified when hemodynamics fail to normalize after pericardiocentesis. Sagrista-Sauleda and coworkers[30] defined effusive-constrictive pericarditis as a failure of the right atrial pressure to decline by at least 50% to a level below 10 mm Hg when the pericardial pressure is reduced to near 0 mm Hg by pericardiocentesis. In their series at a referral center, 8% of those undergoing pericardiocentesis met these criteria. Causes are diverse. The most common are idiopathic, malignant disease, radiation, and tuberculosis. Physical, hemodynamic, and echocardiographic findings are often mixtures of those associated with effusion and constriction and may vary with time as the syndrome progresses. Diagnosis may require acquisition of pericardial fluid and biopsy specimens if the cause is not obvious and tamponade does not mandate pericardiocentesis. It is important to be cautious in performing closed pericardiocentesis in patients without large effusions. Management is tailored to the specific cause, if it is known. Pericardiectomy is often ultimately required.

Specific Causes of Pericardial Disease

The pericardium is involved in a wide variety of diseases. Some are relatively common, but pericardial involvement is rare (e.g., inflammatory bowel disease). Conversely, there are a number of very rare diseases in which pericardial involvement is often common. Following is a discussion of the most significant categories of diseases affecting the pericardium.

Viral Pericarditis

ETIOLOGY AND PATHOPHYSIOLOGY. Viral pericarditis is the most common form of pericardial infection.[5,6,48] It is caused by either direct damage resulting from viral replication or immune responses. Numerous viruses have been implicated (HIV is discussed separately later). Echoviruses and coxsackieviruses are the most common. Cytomegalovirus has a predilection for immunocompromised patients. Other than identification of specific viral particles, the most definitive way to diagnose viral pericarditis is by detection of DNA by PCR or in situ hybridization in pericardial fluid or tissue. As discussed earlier, this is rarely necessary.

CLINICAL FEATURES AND MANAGEMENT. These have been discussed earlier in conjunction with the syndrome of acute pericarditis.

Bacterial Pericarditis

ETIOLOGY AND PATHOPHYSIOLOGY. Bacterial pericarditis is usually characterized by a purulent effusion. A wide variety of organisms can be causative.[5,6,48,49] Direct extension from pneumonia or empyema accounts for a majority of cases. The most common agents are staphylococci, pneumococci, and streptococci. Hematogenous spread during bacteremia and contiguous spread after thoracic surgery or trauma are also important. Hospital-acquired, post–thoracic surgery methicillin-resistant staphylococcal pericarditis has been increasing. Anaerobic organisms have also been increasing in frequency,[49] usually in association with concomitant infection in the mediastinum, head, or neck.

Bacterial pericarditis can also result from rupture of perivalvular abscesses into the pericardial space (see Chap. 67). Rarely, pericardial invasion spreads along fascial planes from the oral cavity (e.g., periodontal and peritonsillar abscesses). The pericardium can become infected in the course of meningococcal sepsis with or without concurrent meningitis. In contrast to the usual purulent fluid, *Neisseria* can evoke a sterile effusion accompanied by systemic reactions such as arthritis, pleuritis, and ophthalmitis. This responds to anti-inflammatory drugs.

CLINICAL FEATURES. The clinical presentation of bacterial pericarditis is usually high-grade fever with shaking chills, but these may be absent in debilitated patients. Patients may complain of dyspnea and chest pain. A pericardial friction rub is present in the majority. Bacterial pericarditis can take a fulminant course with rapid development of tamponade and may be unsuspected because associated illnesses dominate the clinical picture. Laboratory findings include leukocytosis with marked left shift. Pericardial fluid shows polymorphonuclear leukocytosis and low glucose, high protein, and elevated lactate dehydrogenase levels. Frank pus is occasionally drained. The chest radiograph shows widening of the cardiac silhouette if the effusion is large. With gas-producing organisms, an air-fluid interface may be observed. The ECG shows typical ST-T wave changes of acute pericarditis along with low voltage if there is a large effusion. Echocardiography almost always demonstrates a significant pericardial effusion with or without adhesions.

MANAGEMENT. Suspected or proven bacterial pericarditis should be considered a medical emergency and prompt closed pericardiocentesis or surgical drainage performed.[5,6,48] We recommend at least 3 to 4 days of subsequent catheter drainage. Fluid should be Gram stained and cultured for aerobic and anaerobic bacteria with appropriate antibiotic sensitivity testing. Fungal and tuberculosis staining and cultures should also be performed. Blood, sputum, urine, and surgical wounds should all be cultured. Broad-spectrum antibiotics should be started promptly and modified according to culture results. Anaerobic coverage is critical when pericarditis associated with head and neck infections is suspected.

Purulent pericardial effusions are likely to recur. Thus, surgical drainage with construction of a window is often needed. In patients with thick, purulent effusions and dense adhesions, extensive pericardiectomy may be required to achieve adequate drainage and to prevent the development of constriction. Early surgical drainage may also help prevent late constriction. Intrapericardial streptokinase has been administered to selected patients with purulent or loculated effusions and may obviate the need for a window.[50] The prognosis of bacterial pericarditis is poor,[6] with survival in the range of 30% even in modern series.

Pericardial Disease and Human Immunodeficiency Virus (see Chap. 72)

ETIOLOGY AND PATHOPHYSIOLOGY. A wide variety of pericardial diseases have been reported in patients infected with HIV. About 20% of HIV-infected patients have pericardial involvement at some time. Pericardial disease is the most common cardiac manifestation, and the most common abnormality is an effusion.[51,52] Most are small, asymptomatic, and, in the developed world, idiopathic. Effusions may also be part of a generalized seroeffusive process. This "capillary leak" syndrome is likely related to enhanced cytokine expression in the later stages of HIV disease. Moderate to large effusions are more frequent with more advanced stages of infection. Congestive heart failure, Kaposi sarcoma, tuberculosis, and other pulmonary infections are independently associated with moderate to large effusions, but most remain idiopathic. In some cases, the virus itself appears to be the cause. Tuberculosis is the most common etiology of pericardial effusion in African HIV-infected patients.[34,53] Other, less frequent forms of pericardial disease include involvement by various neoplasms, classic acute pericarditis, and myopericarditis. Constrictive pericarditis is rare; when present, it is usually due to *Mycobacterium tuberculosis*.

CLINICAL FEATURES. Symptomatic patients with pericardial disease usually present with dyspnea or chest pain secondary to pericardial inflammation or a large effusion. Large effusions are often caused by infection or neoplasm. The most common agents identified in symptomatic effusions are *M. tuberculosis* and *M. avium-intracellulare*. However, a wide variety of organisms, often unusual, have been implicated. Lymphomas and Kaposi sarcoma are the most common neoplasms associated with effusion (see Chap. 74).

MANAGEMENT. Asymptomatic patients with small to moderate pericardial effusions do not require treatment. Most are idiopathic and usually remain asymptomatic or resolve spontaneously. Symptomatic, large effusions should be drained and an identifiable cause sought. Even though it is often small and asymptomatic, effusion in HIV disease often occurs in the context of or heralds the onset of full-blown acquired immunodeficiency syndrome and is strongly associated with a shortened survival.[51] Importantly, highly active antiretroviral therapy has substantially reduced the incidence and severity of the myopericardial complications of HIV disease.[52,53]

Tuberculous Pericarditis

ETIOLOGY AND PATHOPHYSIOLOGY. The incidence of pericardial tuberculosis has decreased markedly in the developed world. Of patients with pulmonary tuberculosis, 1% to 8% develop pericardial involvement.[5,34,54] In a modern series of acute to subacute pericardial disease, tuberculosis was diagnosed in only 4% overall and 7% of patients who developed cardiac tamponade. Similarly, tuberculosis is now a rare cause of constrictive pericarditis. However, pericardial tuberculosis remains a major problem in immunocompromised hosts and the Third World. It is estimated to account for 70% of large pericardial effusions and most cases of constrictive pericarditis in developing countries.[34,54] Mortality is estimated to be 17% to 40%, with a similar proportion going on to constriction after development of an effusion.[34] Tuberculous pericarditis is by far the most common cause of pericardial disease in African HIV-infected patients. Evidence of pericardial involvement in patients with HIV infection in African countries where tuberculosis and HIV infection are endemic is sufficient to prompt antituberculous therapy.[54] Pericardial involvement is usually secondary to retrograde spread from peribronchial, peritracheal, or mediastinal lymph nodes or hematogenous spread from the primary focus. Less commonly, the pericardium is involved by breakdown and contiguous spread of a necrotic lesion in the lung.

CLINICAL FEATURES. The clinical presentation of tuberculous pericarditis is usually subacute to chronic, with fever, malaise, and dyspnea in association with an effusion. Cough, night sweats, orthopnea, weight loss, and ankle edema are also common. The most frequent findings are radiographic cardiomegaly, pericardial rub, fever, and tachycardia. Evidence of cardiac tamponade with severe hemodynamic compromise, paradoxical pulse, increased venous pressure, pleural effusion, and distant heart sounds is common. Many patients have a subacute, effusive-constrictive syndrome.[30] Late constrictive pericarditis may develop despite antituberculous treatment.[30,34,54] Clinical evidence of pulmonary tuberculosis may be absent or subtle, a chief reason that the diagnosis is sometimes unsuspected.

Diagnosis of tuberculous pericardial disease has been notoriously difficult.[5,34,48] A definitive diagnosis is made by isolating the organism from pericardial fluid or a biopsy specimen or identifying it histologically. However, the yield for isolation from pericardial fluid is low.[54] The probability of making a diagnosis is increased if both pericardial fluid and biopsy specimens are examined early in the effusive stage of the disease. Thus, there is a definite role for pericardial biopsy. Pericardial tissue reveals either granulomas or organisms in 80% to 90% of cases. The optimal diagnostic workup (as well as management) of suspected tuberculous pericarditis includes a pericardial window with fluid and tissue sent for culture and histopathologic examination. The presence of granulomas without bacilli in biopsy tissue is helpful but not diagnostic of tuberculous pericarditis because granulomas can be found in rheumatoid and sarcoid disease. A positive skin test response increases suspicion, but a negative test response does not exclude the diagnosis, especially in immunocompromised hosts. A positive skin test response is also less helpful in populations with a high endemic incidence of tuberculosis. Unexplained pericarditis in a patient with proven tuberculosis elsewhere makes the diagnosis highly likely.

Measurement of ADA, an enzyme produced by white blood cells in pericardial fluid, was the first modern test to markedly improve the accuracy and speed of diagnosis of tuberculous pericarditis.[5,34,55] A recent systematic review[55] indicates that ADA >40 units/liter in pericardial fluid has a sensitivity of 88% and a specificity of 83%. Increased interferon-γ in pericardial fluid is an additional marker. Combined with ADA, it provides even greater diagnostic accuracy. Most recently, PCR to detect *M. tuberculosis* DNA has been used and can be performed in minute amounts of fluid or tissue, even in patients with constriction.[56] Use of one or more of these modern tests should be routine whenever tuberculous pericarditis is suspected.

MANAGEMENT. The goals of therapy are to treat symptoms as well as tamponade and to prevent progression to constriction. Multidrug antimycobacterial treatment is mandatory and has greatly decreased mortality.[55] The role of corticosteroids and the issue of open surgical drainage versus closed pericardiocentesis have been debated for some time. In studies performed in the 1980s in South Africa,[34,54] patients were randomly allocated to open biopsy and complete surgical drainage of fluid or percutaneous pericardiocentesis and further randomized to receive or not to receive prednisolone. All patients were treated with isoniazid, streptomycin, rifampin, and pyrazinamide. The outcomes suggested that patients who undergo open drainage are less likely to require repeated pericardiocentesis, and there was a trend in the open drainage group toward reduced constriction. Corticosteroids did not influence the risk of death or progression to constriction but did speed the resolution of symptoms and decrease fluid reaccumulation. Subsequent meta-analyses[5] tend to support these conclusions, but individual studies have been inconclusive, and there are no modern, appropriately powered, controlled trials of corticosteroids. In contrast, a recent prospectively performed trial[57] in patients with large effusions concluded that there is no benefit from the use of systemic or intrapericardial triamcinolone, but the total number of patients was only 57. No studies have specifically addressed the use of corticosteroids in HIV-positive patients with tuberculous pericarditis, in whom outcomes could be different. If corticosteroids are administered, high doses (1 to 2 mg/kg/day with tapering during 6 to 8 weeks) are recommended[5,54] because rifampin induces their hepatic metabolism. Because data are inconclusive, selection of closed versus open drainage and corticosteroid use are necessarily based on clinical judgment. There is no rationale for corticosteroids once established constriction is present.

Fungal Pericarditis

ETIOLOGY AND PATHOPHYSIOLOGY. Fungal infections can rarely cause pericarditis. They are mainly due to locally endemic organisms such as *Histoplasma* and *Coccidioides* or opportunistic fungi such as *Candida* and *Aspergillus*,[5,48] although a number of other organisms have been reported. Histoplasmosis is the most common. It is endemic in Ohio, the Mississippi River valley, and the western Appalachians; it is acquired by inhalation and can infect otherwise healthy patients living in endemic areas. Coccidioidomycosis is endemic in the Southwest. The organism is acquired by inhalation.[58] Immunocompromised patients, those taking corticosteroids or broad-spectrum antibiotics, and drug addicts are at increased risk.

CLINICAL FEATURES AND MANAGEMENT. Pericardial histoplasmosis usually occurs in a previously healthy patient and is thought to represent an inflammatory process in response to infection of adjacent mediastinal lymph nodes.[5,48] Accordingly, isolation of organisms from pericardial fluid is unusual. The fluid is serous, xanthochromic, or hemorrhagic. The disease usually begins with respiratory symptoms followed by pericardial pain. Effusion leading to tamponade occurs in almost half the cases. The diagnosis must be considered in endemic zones and is aided by rising complement fixation titers. Provided effusions are drained as needed, pericardial involvement eventually resolves with or without anti-inflammatory drugs. Antifungal agents are indicated only for disseminated histoplasmosis.

Coccidioidomycosis pericarditis occurs as a complication of progressive, disseminated infection[5,48,58] in chronically ill, debilitated patients. Pericardial involvement does not occur in the self-limited influenza-like form of the infection. Physical findings suggestive of cardiac compression may be the first clues to the diagnosis. Treatment is directed at the disseminated infection with intravenous amphotericin B. Pericardiocentesis is of course indicated when tamponade occurs.

Pericarditis due to opportunistic fungi such as *Candida* and *Aspergillus* usually occurs in patients who are immune suppressed or receiving broad-spectrum antibiotics as well as in patients recovering from open heart surgery,[5,48] typically in the setting of disseminated infection. The prognosis is poor, and the diagnosis is often made at autopsy.

Pericarditis in Patients with Renal Disease

(see Chap. 93)

ETIOLOGY AND PATHOPHYSIOLOGY. The incidence of classic uremic pericarditis has decreased markedly since the advent of widespread dialysis. Its pathophysiology was never fully elucidated, but it is correlated with levels of blood urea nitrogen and creatinine. Toxic metabolites, hypercalcemia, hyperuricemia, and hemorrhagic, viral, and autoimmune mechanisms have all been proposed as etiologic factors.[5,59] The acute or subacute phase is characterized by shaggy, hemorrhagic, fibrinous exudates on both parietal and visceral surfaces with minimal inflammatory reaction. Subacute or chronic constriction may develop with organization of the effusion and formation of thick adhesions within the pericardial space. Large, gradually accumulating effusions are typical.

What we term *dialysis-associated pericardial disease* is now much more common than classic uremic pericarditis.[5,59] It is characterized by de novo appearance of pericardial disease in patients undergoing chronic dialysis, despite normal or mildly elevated blood urea nitrogen and creatinine. Its mechanisms and relation to classic uremic pericarditis are unclear. Small pericardial effusions are often caused by volume overload.

An increased incidence of asymptomatic pericardial effusion has been found in patients with autosomal dominant polycystic kidney disease.[60] About half are moderate to large. They do not appear to cause tamponade and are not correlated with renal function.

CLINICAL FEATURES. In modern populations of dialysis patients, the clinical presentation is sometimes that of acute pericarditis with chest pain, fever, leukocytosis, and pericardial friction rub. Small, asymptomatic effusions are common. Alternatively, patients can present with a pericardial effusion causing hypotension during or after ultrafiltration (low-pressure tamponade). Although conventional cardiac tamponade with acute or subacute hemodynamic compromise can occur, the extremely large, asymptomatic effusions typical of classic uremic pericarditis are unusual today.

The ECG most often is not markedly affected and reflects a high incidence of associated abnormalities (left ventricular hypertrophy, previous MI, electrolyte abnormalities). The chest radiograph may demonstrate cardiac enlargement related to myocardial dysfunction, volume overload, or pericardial effusion.

MANAGEMENT. The management of classic uremic pericarditis is intensive hemodialysis and drainage in patients with effusions causing hemodynamic compromise[5,48,59] Patients with symptomatic pericarditis almost always respond. Heparin should be used cautiously during hemodialysis because of the possibility of causing hemorrhagic pericarditis. Pericardial effusions without hemodynamic compromise usually resolve after several weeks of intensive hemodialysis.

Treatment of pericardial disease appearing de novo in patients on chronic dialysis is empiric.[5,48,59] Tamponade of course requires drainage. In our experience, intensification of dialysis is variably beneficial, presumably because these patients are already receiving most of its benefits. Use of NSAIDs for pericardial pain is appropriate. Corticosteroids are probably ineffective. There is little experience with colchicine, but its use is not unreasonable. A pericardial window may be required and is usually the most effective approach in patients with recurring effusions. For patients requiring drainage, instillation of a nonabsorbable corticosteroid in the pericardial space was found beneficial in small series of patients.

Early Post–Myocardial Infarction Pericarditis and Dressler Syndrome (see Chap. 54)

ETIOLOGY AND PATHOPHYSIOLOGY. Early post-MI pericarditis occurs during the first 1 to 3 days and no more than a week after the index event.[5] It is due to transmural necrosis with inflammation affecting the adjacent visceral and parietal pericardium. Pericardial involvement is correlated with infarct size. At autopsy, around 40% of patients with large, Q-wave MIs have pericarditis. Thrombolysis and mechanical revascularization have markedly reduced the incidence of this form of pericarditis. Thus, in a recent report,[61] only 4% of patients undergoing primary percutaneous intervention for acute MI had clinical evidence of early post-MI pericarditis.

Late pericarditis is characterized by polyserositis with pericardial or pleural effusions.[5,48] The syndrome was initially described by Dressler and had an estimated incidence of 3% to 4%. Its incidence has also markedly diminished since the onset of early revascularization and was only 0.1% in the same recent report.[61] Dressler syndrome is believed to have an autoimmune etiology due to sensitization to myocardial cells at the time of MI. Antimyocardial antibodies have been demonstrated. In contrast to early post-MI pericarditis, inflammation is diffuse and not localized to the myocardial injury site.

CLINICAL FEATURES. Most commonly, early post-MI pericarditis is asymptomatic and identified by auscultation of a rub, usually within 1 to 3 days after presentation. Many are monophasic (usually systolic) and can be confused with murmurs of mitral regurgitation or ventricular septal defect. Early post-MI pericarditis virtually never causes tamponade by itself. However, tamponade does occur with left ventricular free wall rupture. Because of its association with large MIs, early post-MI pericarditis should alert the clinician to this possibility, especially if an effusion is present. Symptomatic patients develop pleuritic chest pain within the above time frame. It is important to distinguish pericardial pain from recurrent ischemic discomfort. Ordinarily, this is not difficult on clinical grounds. However, typical electrocardiographic changes of acute pericarditis are uncommon after MI. Pericardial inflammation is localized to the infarcted area; hence, electrocardiographic changes usually involve subtle re-elevation of the ST segment in originally involved leads. An atypical T wave evolution consisting of persistent upright T waves or early normalization of inverted T waves may occur and appears to be highly sensitive for early post-MI pericarditis.

Dressler syndrome occurs as early as 1 week to a few months after acute MI. Symptoms include fever and pleuritic chest pain. The physical examination may reveal pleural or pericardial friction rubs. The chest radiograph may show a pleural effusion or enlargement of the cardiac silhouette, and the ECG often demonstrates ST elevation and T wave changes typical of acute pericarditis. Although pericardial effusions are common, tamponade is unusual.

MANAGEMENT. Although it is associated with large, transmural MIs, early post-MI pericarditis per se is almost invariably a benign process that does not *independently* affect in-hospital mortality. Treatment is therefore based on symptoms. Augmentation of usual post-MI aspirin doses (650 mg orally three or four times per day for 2 to 5 days) or acetaminophen is usually effective.[5,48] Corticosteroids and perhaps some nonaspirin NSAIDs interfere with conversion of MI into a scar, resulting in greater wall thinning and a higher incidence of post-MI rupture.[5,18] Thus, these drugs should be avoided. Because significant hemopericardium is extremely rare with early post-MI pericarditis and there is no evidence that heparin or other antithrombotic drugs increase its risk, their administration need not be modified.

Although Dressler syndrome is a self-limited disorder, admission to the hospital for observation and monitoring should be considered if there is a substantial pericardial effusion or other conditions (e.g., pulmonary infarction) are also being considered. Aspirin or other NSAIDs are effective for symptomatic relief.[5,48] Colchicine is also likely effective. A short course of prednisone, 40 to 60 mg orally per day with a 7- to 10-day taper, can be used in patients not responding to treatment or for recurrent symptoms.

Post-Pericardiotomy and Post–Cardiac Injury Pericarditis

(see Chap. 76)

Blunt or penetrating injury of the chest and heart with myocardial contusion can cause acute pericarditis. The pericarditis is rarely of clinical significance compared with other effects of the trauma. However, pericarditis can develop days to months after cardiac surgery, thoracotomy, or chest trauma. The pathogenesis of this syndrome is thought to involve production of anti-heart antibodies in response to myocardial injury.[5] A systemic inflammatory response occurs and is characterized by low-grade fever, mild leukocytosis, and pleuropericardial inflammation with associated chest discomfort. The chest radiograph typically shows pleural effusions. A few patients demonstrate pulmonary infiltrates. The ECG reveals changes consistent with acute pericarditis in about 50% of cases. The echocardiogram usually shows a small to moderate pericardial effusion, but tamponade is rare. NSAIDs are first-line treatment, with an excellent response usually occurring within 48 hours. Colchicine is also likely effective. Treatment should be maintained for 2 to 3 weeks. Corticosteroid therapy is reserved for patients with unresponsive, severe, or recurrent symptoms.

Radiation-Induced Pericarditis

Mediastinal and thoracic radiation therapy remains standard treatment of a variety of thoracic neoplasms. Hodgkin disease, non-Hodgkin lymphoma, and breast carcinoma are most commonly associated with radiation pericarditis (see Chap. 90). Factors that influence pericardial injury include the total dose, the amount of cardiac silhouette exposed, the nature of the radiation source, and the duration and fractionation of therapy. There is about a 2% incidence of clinically evident pericarditis in conjunction with modern radiation delivery.[5,48] However, the incidence can be as high as 20% when the entire pericardium is exposed.

Radiation pericarditis takes one of two forms, an acute illness with chest pain and fever and a delayed form that can occur years after treatment. Self-limited, asymptomatic effusions are common soon after radiation therapy, but tamponade is unusual. Late manifestations of radiation injury occur from about a year to up to 20 years after exposure. Patients can present with symptomatic pericarditis and effusion with or without cardiac compression or circulatory congestion due to constrictive pericarditis. Effusions can evolve into constriction (i.e., an effusive-constrictive syndrome).[30]

Radiation-induced pericarditis and effusion can be confused with malignant effusions. The malignant effusions are usually associated with other evidence of disease recurrence. Hypothyroidism induced by mediastinal irradiation can also contribute to pericardial effusion. Pericardiocentesis with fluid analysis for malignant cells and thyroid function tests differentiate radiation-induced effusion from other causes. Large, symptomatic pericardial effusions may be drained either percutaneously or surgically. Recurrent pericardial effusions are usually best treated surgically with either a window or pericardiectomy. Pericardiectomy is the treatment of choice for patients with constriction. However, perioperative mortality is higher than with idiopathic constrictive pericarditis.

Metastatic Pericardial Disease (see Chaps. 74 and 90)

Pericardial tumor implants are the usual cause of effusion in patients with known malignant neoplasms, although as noted earlier, obstruction of lymphatic drainage by enlarged mediastinal nodes is occasionally observed.[5,21,48,62] Malignant disease is a leading cause of cardiac tamponade in developed countries. Lung carcinoma is the most common, accounting for about 40% of malignant effusions; breast carcinoma and lymphomas are responsible for about another 40%. Gastrointestinal carcinoma, melanoma, sarcomas, and other cancers are less common. With the advent of HIV disease, the incidence of Kaposi sarcoma and lymphomatous involvement of the pericardium increased, but highly active antiretroviral therapy has reduced their incidence (see Chap. 72).

Pericardial tumor implants can cause pericardial pain. However, the dominant feature is usually an effusion. Effusive-constrictive patterns are common. An asymptomatic, incidentally discovered pericardial effusion can be the presenting sign of a malignant neoplasm. However, most patients present with symptomatic effusions or tamponade. In a recent series,[63] 18% of large, symptomatic effusions represented the first presentation of a malignant neoplasm after exclusion of those with an easily identifiable cause. The ECG in malignant effusions is variable but usually shows nonspecific T wave abnormalities with low-voltage QRS. ST-segment elevation is somewhat unusual but can occur. In addition to echocardiography, CT and CMR are useful in evaluating the extent of metastatic disease to the pericardium and adjacent structures.

In most cancer patients with effusions, it is important that metastatic involvement of the pericardium be confirmed by identification of malignant cells or tumor markers in pericardial fluid. This is because of occasional patients with obstructed lymphatic drainage, the possibility of confusion with radiation-induced disease, and the fact that other forms of pericardial disease can occur in patients who have cancer. However, there are many exceptions when clinical judgment dictates that pericardial fluid need not be obtained, especially when effusions are not large and specific treatment (e.g., instillation of drugs in the pericardial space) is not being contemplated.

It is essential to evaluate the life expectancy of patients before performing pericardiocentesis and choosing treatment modalities. In terminally ill patients, drainage should be performed only to aid in relief of symptoms. However, patients with better prognoses deserve a more aggressive approach, which can be gratifying in a surprisingly large number. In many cases, a single drainage will provide prolonged relief as well as fluid for analysis, although it is likely that the only factor to ultimately influence survival is successful treatment of the underlying cancer. For this reason, pericardiocentesis should be the initial step in most patients, with several days of drainage and careful attention to detection of reaccumulation. For recurrences and perhaps in some cases of a first effusion, intrapericardial instillation of tetracycline or chemotherapeutic agents has a reasonable record.[5] Cisplatin appears effective in treating pericardial involvement by lung adenocarcinoma[64]; bleomycin is useful for non–small cell lung cancer.[65] Thiotepa[66] has a good record with a variety of malignant neoplasms. External beam radiation therapy is an option in patients with radiation-sensitive tumors. A pericardial window or even complete surgical pericardiectomy should be considered in unusual patients with unresponsive, recurrent effusions who continue to have a good prognosis otherwise.

Primary Pericardial Tumors

A number of primary pericardial neoplasms, all exceedingly rare, have been reported. They include malignant mesotheliomas, fibrosarcomas, lymphangiomas, hemangiomas, teratomas, neurofibromas, and lipomas.[5,67] Because of their rarity, it is difficult to generalize about their clinical presentation and course. They are usually either locally invasive or compress cardiac structures or are detected because of an abnormal cardiac silhouette on the chest radiograph. Mesotheliomas and fibrosarcomas are lethal. Others, such as lipomas, are benign. CT and CMR are helpful in delineating the anatomy of these tumors, but surgery is usually required for diagnosis and treatment.

Autoimmune and Drug-Induced Pericardial Disease

Pericardial involvement can occur in virtually any autoimmune disease, but the bulk of cases occur in rheumatoid arthritis, SLE, and progressive systemic sclerosis (scleroderma).[5,48] In addition, many drugs have been reported to cause pericarditis as part of an autoimmune process. Maisch and colleagues[68] coined the general term *autoreactive pericarditis* when an autoimmune mechanism is thought to be involved as the cause of pericarditis. Assignment to this group is not dependent on establishment of a specific diagnosis (e.g., SLE); rather, evaluation includes analysis of pericardial fluid that is designed to systematically exclude nonautoimmune causes. In a selected cohort, 32% of patients with pericardial effusion were found to have autoreactive pericarditis. Maisch and colleagues[68] advocate treatment of these patients with intrapericardial instillation of triamcinolone. However, theirs was not a controlled study, follow-up was relatively short, and a significant number of patients suffered transient Cushing syndrome. Thus, the overall effectiveness of this approach is uncertain.

Rheumatoid Arthritis. Pericardial involvement is common in rheumatoid arthritis[5,48] (see Chap. 89). Older autopsy studies revealed pericardial inflammation in about 50% of patients. There are no contemporary pathologic or clinical studies addressing the incidence of pericardial involvement. Clinically evident pericardial involvement is reported in up to 25% of patients. Patients can present with chest pain, fever, and dyspnea due to acute pericarditis, which usually occurs in conjunction with exacerbation of underlying disease. Asymptomatic pericardial effusion and cardiac tamponade can also be presenting manifestations. Pericardial fluid is characterized by low glucose concentration, neutrophilic leukocytosis, elevated titers of rheumatoid factor, low complement levels, and, rarely, high cholesterol levels. Constrictive pericarditis also can occur as the result of longstanding pericardial inflammation. In patients with joint exacerbations, management of acute pericarditis or asymptomatic effusion is first and foremost effective treatment of the exacerbation. Pericardial manifestations seem to respond well to high-dose aspirin or NSAIDs. Effusions causing tamponade should be drained both to treat tamponade and to establish with confidence that there is no other cause (e.g., infection) in patients who may be receiving immunosuppressive drugs. In general, the response to treatment of underlying disease exacerbations is too slow and uncertain to advocate a period of watchful waiting in the hope that large effusions will shrink. Recurrent tamponade and large effusions are good indications for a pericardial window. Therapy with colchicine has also been shown to be effective for recurrences.[5] In some patients receiving anti–tumor necrosis factor therapy, pericardial effusion may be drug rather than disease related.[69]

Systemic Lupus Erythematosus. Pericarditis is the most common cardiovascular manifestation of SLE (see Chap. 89).[5,48] Acute pericarditis can be the first manifestation of the disease. About 40% of patients with SLE develop pericarditis at some time, usually in conjunction with a flare and involvement of other serosal surfaces. Typical patients present with pleuritic chest pain and low-grade fever. Large effusions can occur but are unusual. The ECG often shows typical findings of acute pericarditis. The chest radiograph may show enlargement of the cardiac silhouette if effusion is present, along with pleural effusions and often parenchymal infiltrates. Pericardial effusions have high protein and low glucose contents and a white blood cell count below 10,000/mL^3. As with rheumatoid arthritis, it is important to exclude purulent, fungal, or tuberculous pericarditis because many patients are immunosuppressed. Most patients respond to corticosteroids or immunosuppressive therapy used to treat disease flares. Hemodynamic compromise secondary to cardiac tamponade may occur in as many as 10% to 20% of patients with SLE.[70] Accordingly, we recommend hospitalization to monitor for hemodynamic complications until stability is ensured. Closed drainage combined with corticosteroids is reported to have a good outcome in these patients.[6,70] However, a significant proportion of patients with tamponade may require a window despite high-dose corticosteroids.

Progressive Systemic Sclerosis (Scleroderma) (see Chap. 89). There is about a 10% incidence of acute pericarditis with chest pain and pericardial rub in progressive systemic sclerosis.[5,48] Pericardial involvement is found at autopsy in about 50% of patients. Pericardial effusion is detected by echocardiography in up to 40%. Most are small and asymptomatic, but there are occasional instances of large effusions. Late constrictive pericarditis has been described. Treatment of acute pericarditis in scleroderma patients is often unrewarding, with an unpredictable response to aspirin and NSAIDs. Although there is no published experience, colchicine should be considered. Right-heart catheterization is useful in patients presenting with dyspnea or right-sided heart failure to evaluate pulmonary vascular disease, which is relatively common and can be confused with pericardial involvement. Moreover, various pericardial CT scan abnormalities are associated with pulmonary hypertension due to systemic sclerosis.[71]

Drug-Induced Pericarditis. The great majority of cases of drug-induced pericardial disease occur as a component of drug-induced SLE syndromes.[5] There are no recent studies of the epidemiology or etiology of drug-induced SLE, and the list of offending agents is long. Isoniazid and hydralazine are probably the most common current offenders. Large effusions, tamponade, and even constriction have been reported but are rare in drug-induced SLE pericarditis. In addition to drug cessation, management is dictated by the specific elements of the SLE syndrome present as well as usual efforts aimed at detection and treatment of effusions. Rarely, drug-induced pericarditis due to agents such as penicillin and cromolyn involves eosinophilic hypersensitivity reactions without an SLE picture.

Hemopericardium

Any form of chest trauma can cause hemopericardium[5,48] (see Chap. 76). Post-MI free wall rupture with hemopericardium occurs within several days of transmural MI and is discussed in Chap. 54. Hemopericardium due to retrograde bleeding into the pericardial sac is an important complication and frequent cause of death in type I dissecting aortic aneurysm (see Chap. 60). These patients may also have the combination of acute volume overload due to disruption of the aortic valve and tamponade without a paradoxical pulse.

Puncture of atrial or ventricular walls can occur during mitral valvuloplasty and is signaled by abrupt chest pain.[5,48] Tamponade commonly ensues and can occur rapidly or with a delayed course. It is usually managed with percutaneous drainage. Small pericardial effusions are occasionally observed after device closure of atrial septal defects, but tamponade appears to be rare.[72]

Pericardial effusion with tamponade is a rare but important complication of percutaneous coronary intervention[73] (see Chap. 58). The incidence is 0.1% to 0.6% and may have increased in the 1990s in relation to aggressive treatment of complex lesions with atherectomy and debulking devices and stiff or hydrophilic guidewires. With more modern equipment and experience, the incidence may be decreasing or at least stabilizing. Cardiac tamponade during percutaneous coronary intervention is almost always a result of coronary perforation. The clinical presentation is usually rapidly progressive cardiac decompensation and severe hypotension, although it can occasionally be delayed and more insidious. The diagnosis of perforation is usually made by detection of extravasation of dye from the coronary circulation into the pericardial space. Loss of cardiac pulsation on fluoroscopy indicates that a significant pericardial effusion is present. Management of tamponade requires sealing of the perforation, pericardiocentesis, and reversal of anticoagulation.[5,73] If perforation cannot be managed percutaneously, emergency surgery is indicated.

Pericardial effusion and tamponade can also occur as a complication of catheter-based arrhythmia procedures, especially atrial fibrillation ablations. In a large, prospective series,[74] 0.8% of patients had pericardial effusions that did not require pericardiocentesis and 0.6% had cardiac tamponade, which was successfully drained in all. Reduction of energy appears to reduce the incidence. Management is similar to that for coronary perforations. Right ventricular perforation is an occasional immediate complication of pacemaker and implantable defibrillator lead insertion but rarely causes tamponade. The risk of delayed right ventricular perforation (>5 days after implantation) by small-diameter active fixation pacing and implantable defibrillator leads has recently been emphasized.[75] The clinical presentation is variable, but cardiac tamponade occurs in a significant number of cases.

Last, right ventricular perforation remains an occasional complication of right ventricular endomyocardial biopsy but very rarely causes tamponade.[76]

Thyroid-Associated Pericardial Disease (see Chap. 86)

Of patients with severe hypothyroidism, 25% to 35% develop pericardial effusions.[5] These can be large but rarely if ever cause tamponade. Effusions occasionally occur in subclinical hypothyroidism. Hypothyroid effusions often have high concentrations of cholesterol. The effusions gradually resolve with thyroid replacement. Rarely, effusion can occur in hyperthyroidism.

Pericardial Disease in Pregnancy (see Chap. 82)

Small, clinically insignificant pericardial effusions are observed in about 40% of healthy pregnant women.[5] There is no evidence that pregnancy per se influences the incidence, etiology, or course of pericardial disease, and it is in general managed no differently than in nonpregnant patients. However, colchicine is contraindicated, and pericardiocentesis should be performed only for effusions causing tamponade or if a treatable infectious cause is suspected. Early during pregnancy, fluoroscopically guided pericardiocentesis should be avoided.

Congenital Anomalies of the Pericardium

Pericardial Cysts. Pericardial cysts are rare, benign congenital malformations.[5,67] They are usually fluid filled, located at the right costophrenic angle, and identified as an incidental finding on a chest radiograph. The diagnosis is usually confirmed by echocardiography. Management is conservative.

Congenital Absence of the Pericardium. Congenital absence of the pericardium is rare (see Chap. 65). Usually part or all of the left parietal pericardium is absent, but partial absence of the right side has also been reported.[5] Partial absence of the left pericardium is associated with other anomalies, including atrial septal defect, bicuspid aortic valve, and pulmonary malformations. It is often symptomatic and may allow herniation of portions of the heart through the defect or torsion of the great vessels, with potentially life-threatening consequences. Recurrent pulmonary infections are occasionally seen. Patients can present with chest pain, syncope, or even sudden death. The ECG typically reveals incomplete right bundle branch block. Absence of all or most of the left pericardium results in a characteristic chest radiograph with a leftward shift of the cardiac silhouette, elongated left-sided heart border, and radiolucent bands between the aortic knob and the main pulmonary artery and the left diaphragm and the base of the heart. Echocardiography reveals paradoxical septal motion and right ventricular enlargement. CT or CMR can be employed to establish a definitive diagnosis. Pericardiectomy should be advised to ameliorate symptoms and to prevent herniation.

REFERENCES

Classic Reading List

Ditchey R, Engler R, LeWinter M, et al: The role of the right heart in acute cardiac tamponade in dogs. Circ Res 48:701, 1981.

Hatle LK, Appleton CP, Popp RL: Differentiation of constrictive pericarditis and restrictive cardiomyopathy by Doppler echocardiography. Circulation 79:357,1989.

LeWinter MM, Myhre EESP, Slinker BK: Influence of the pericardium and ventricular interaction on diastolic function. *In* Gaasch WH, LeWinter MM (eds): Heart Failure and Left Ventricular Diastolic Function. Philadelphia, Lea & Febiger, 1993, pp 103-117.

Shabetai R: The Pericardium. New York, Grune & Stratton, 1981.

Singh S, Wann LS, Schuchard GH, et al: Right ventricular and right atrial collapse in patients with cardiac tamponade—a combined echocardiographic and hemodynamic study. Circulation 70:966, 1984.

Anatomy and Physiology of the Pericardium

1. Johnson D: The pericardium. *In* Standring S, et al (eds): Gray's Anatomy. New York, Elsevier Churchill Livingstone, 2005, pp 995-996.
2. Jöbsis PD, Ashikaga H, Wen H, et al: The visceral pericardium: Macromolecular structure and contribution to passive mechanical properties of the left ventricle. Am J Physiol 293:H3379, 2007.

The Passive Role of the Normal Pericardium in Heart Disease

3. O'Rourke RA, Dell'Italia LJ: Diagnosis and management of right ventricular myocardial infarction. Curr Probl Cardiol 29:6, 2004.

Acute Pericarditis

4. Lange RA, Hillis LD: Clinical practice. Acute pericarditis. N Engl J Med 351:2195, 2004.
5. Maisch B, Seferovic PM, Ristic AD, et al: Guidelines on the diagnosis and management of pericardial diseases executive summary; the Task force on the diagnosis and management of pericardial diseases of the European Society of Cardiology. Eur Heart J 25:587, 2004.
6. Troughton RW, Asher CR, Klein AL: Pericarditis. Lancet 363:717, 2004.
7. Imazio M, Brucato A, Doria A, et al: Antinuclear antibodies in recurrent idiopathic pericarditis: Prevalence and clinical significance. Int J Cardiol 136:289, 2009. Epub 2008 Jul 31.
8. Imazio M, Demichelis B, Parrini I, et al: Management, risk factors, and outcomes in recurrent pericarditis. Am J Cardiol 96:736, 2005.
9. Imazio M, Cecchi E, Demichelis B, et al: Indicators of poor prognosis of acute pericarditis. Circulation 115:2739, 2007.
10. Imazio M, Demichelis B, Parrini I, et al: Day-hospital treatment of acute pericarditis: A management program for outpatient therapy. J Am Coll Cardiol 43:1042, 2004.

11. Imazio M, Bobbio M, Cecchi E, et al: Colchicine as first-choice therapy for recurrent pericarditis: Results of the CORE (COlchicine for REcurrent pericarditis) trial. Arch Intern Med 165:1987, 2005.
12. Imazio M, Bobbio M, Cecchi E, et al: Colchicine in addition to conventional therapy for acute pericarditis: Results of the COlchicine for acute PEricarditis (COPE) trial. Circulation 112:2012, 2005.
13. Artom G, Koren-Morag N, Spodick DH, et al: Pretreatment with corticosteroids attenuates the efficacy of colchicine in preventing recurrent pericarditis: A multi-centre all-case analysis. Eur Heart J 26:723, 2005.
14. Brucato A, Brambilla G, Moreo A, et al: Long-term outcomes in difficult-to-treat patients with recurrent pericarditis. Am J Cardiol 98:267, 2006.
15. Imazio M, Brucato A, Adler Y, et al: Prognosis of idiopathic recurrent pericarditis as determined from previously published reports. Am J Cardiol 100:1026, 2007.
16. Imazio M, Brucato A, Trinchero R, et al: Colchicine for pericarditis: Hype or hope? Eur Heart J 30:532, 2009.
17. Imazio M, Brucato A, Cumetti D, et al: Corticosteroids for recurrent pericarditis: High versus low doses: A nonrandomized observation. Circulation 118:667, 2008.

Pericardial Effusion and Tamponade

18. Little WC, Freeman GL: Pericardial disease. Circulation 113:1622, 2006.
19. Al-Dadah AS, Guthrie TJ, Pasque MK, et al: Clinical course and predictors of pericardial effusion following cardiac transplantation. Transplant Proc 39:1589, 2007.
20. Goland S, Caspi A, Malnick S, et al: Idiopathic chronic pericardial effusion. N Engl J Med 342:1449, 2000.
21. Ben-Horin S, Bank I, Guetta V, Livneh A: Large symptomatic pericardial effusion as the presentation of unrecognized cancer: A study in 173 consecutive patients undergoing pericardiocentesis. Medicine (Baltimore) 85:49, 2006.
22. Spodick DM: Acute cardiac tamponade. N Engl J Med 349:684, 2003.
23. Sagristà-Sauleda J, Angel J, Sambola A, et al: Low-pressure cardiac tamponade: Clinical and hemodynamic profile. Circulation 114:945, 2006.
24. Kopterides P, Lignos M, Papanikolaou S, et al: Pleural effusion causing cardiac tamponade: Report of two cases and review of the literature. Heart Lung 35:66, 2006.
25. Krantz MJ, Lee JK, Spodick DH: Repetitive yawning associated with cardiac tamponade. Am J Cardiol 94:701, 2004.
26. Wang ZJ, Reddy GP, Gotway MB, et al: CT and MR imaging of pericardial disease. Radiographics 23:S167, 2003.
27. Oyama N, Oyama N, Komuro K, et al: Computed tomography and magnetic resonance imaging of the pericardium: Anatomy and pathology. Magn Res Med Sci 3:145, 2004.
28. Sagristà-Sauleda J, Angel J, Sambola A, Permanyer-Miralda G: Hemodynamic effects of volume expansion in patients with cardiac tamponade. Circulation 117:1545, 2008.
29. Tsang TS, Enriquez-Sarano M, Freeman WK, et al: 1127 consecutive therapeutic echocardiographically guided pericardiocenteses: Clinical profile, practice patterns, and outcomes spanning 21 years. Mayo Clin Proc 77:429, 2002.
30. Sagrista-Sauleda J, Angel J, Sanchez A, et al: Effusive-constrictive pericarditis. N Engl J Med 350:469, 2004.
31. Swanson N, Mirza I, Wijesinghe N, Devlin G: Primary percutaneous balloon pericardiotomy for malignant pericardial effusion. Catheter Cardiovasc Interv 71:504, 2008.
32. Ben-Horin S, Shinfeld A, Kachel E, et al: The composition of normal pericardial fluid and its implications for diagnosing pericardial effusions. Am J Med 118:636, 2005.
33. Permanyer-Miralda G: Acute pericardial disease: Approach to the aetiologic diagnosis. Heart 90:252, 2004.
34. Mayosi BM, Burgess LJ, Doubell AF: Tuberculous pericarditis. Circulation 112:3608, 2005.
35. Seferovic PM, Ristic AD, Maksimovic R, et al: Diagnostic value of pericardial biopsy: Improvement with extensive sampling enabled by pericardioscopy. Circulation 107:978, 2003.

Constrictive Pericarditis

36. Haley JH, Tajik AJ, Danielson GK, et al: Transient constrictive pericarditis: Causes and natural history. J Am Coll Cardiol 43:271, 2004.
37. Leya FS, Arab D, Joyal D, et al: The efficacy of brain natriuretic peptide levels in differentiating constrictive pericarditis from restrictive cardiomyopathy. J Am Coll Cardiol 45:1900, 2005.
38. Ha JW, Ommen SR, Tajik AJ, et al: Differentiation of constrictive pericarditis from restrictive cardiomyopathy using mitral annular velocity by tissue Doppler echocardiography. Am J Cardiol 94:316, 2004.
39. Sengupta PP, Mohan JC, Mehta V, et al: Doppler tissue imaging improves assessment of abnormal interventricular septal and posterior wall motion in constrictive pericarditis. J Am Soc Echocardiogr 18:226, 2005.
40. Taylor AM, Dymarkowski S, Verbeken EK, Bogaert J: Detection of pericardial inflammation with late-enhancement cardiac magnetic resonance imaging: Initial results. Eur Radiol 16:569, 2006.
41. Talreja DR, Edwards WD, Danielson GK, et al: Constrictive pericarditis in 26 patients with histologically normal pericardial thickness. Circulation 108:1852, 2003.
42. Sengupta PP, Krishnamoorthy VK, Abhayaratna WP, et al: Disparate patterns of left ventricular mechanics differentiate constrictive pericarditis from restrictive cardiomyopathy. JACC Cardiovasc Imaging 1:29, 2008.
43. Talreja DR, Nishimura RA, Oh JK, Holmes DR: Constrictive pericarditis in the modern era: Novel criteria for diagnosis in the cardiac catheterization laboratory. J Am Coll Cardiol 22:315, 2008.
44. Hirai S, Hamanaka Y, Mitsui N, et al: Surgical treatment of chronic constrictive pericarditis using an ultrasonic scalpel. Ann Thorac Cardiovasc Surg 11:204, 2005.
45. Ling LH, Oh JK, Schaff HV, et al: Constrictive pericarditis in the modern era: Evolving clinical spectrum and impact on outcome after pericardiectomy. Circulation 100:1380, 1999.
46. Bertog SC, Thambidorai SK, Parakh K, et al: Constrictive pericarditis: Etiology and cause-specific survival after pericardiectomy. J Am Coll Cardiol 43:1445, 2004.
47. Góngora E, Dearani JA, Orszulak TA: Tricuspid regurgitation in patients undergoing pericardiectomy for constrictive pericarditis. Ann Thorac Surg 85:163, 2008.

Specific Causes of Pericardial Disease

48. Maisch B, Ristic AD: Practical aspects of the management of pericardial disease. Heart 89:1096, 2003.
49. Brook I: Pericarditis caused by anaerobic bacteria. Int J Antimicrob Agents 33:297, 2009.
50. Tomkowski WZ, Gralec R, Kuca P, et al: Effectiveness of intrapericardial administration of streptokinase in purulent pericarditis. Herz 29:802, 2004.
51. Barbaro G: Pathogenesis of HIV-associated cardiovascular disease. Adv Cardiol 40:49, 2003.
52. Ntsekhe M, Hakim J: Impact of human immunodeficiency virus infection on cardiovascular disease in Africa. Circulation 112:3602, 2005.
53. Sudano I, Spieker LE, Noll G, et al: Cardiovascular disease in HIV infection. Am Heart J 151:1147, 2006.
54. Syed FF, Mayosi BM: A modern approach to tuberculous pericarditis. Prog Cardiovasc Dis 50:218, 2007.
55. Tuon FF, Litvoc MN, Lopes MI: Adenosine deaminase and tuberculous pericarditis—a systematic review with meta-analysis. Acta Trop 99:67,2006.
56. Zamirian M, Mokhtarian M, Motazedian MH, et al: Constrictive pericarditis: Detection of *Mycobacterium tuberculosis* in paraffin-embedded pericardial tissues by polymerase chain reaction. Clin Biochem 40:355,2007.
57. Reuter H, Burgess LJ, Louw VJ, Doubell AF: Experience with adjunctive corticosteroids in managing tuberculous pericarditis. Cardiovasc J S Afr 17:233, 2006.
58. Arsura EL, Bobba RK, Reddy CM: Coccidioidal pericarditis. Int J Infect Dis 10:86, 2006.
59. Alpert MA, Ravenscraft MD: Pericardial involvement in end-stage renal disease. Am J Med Sci 325:228, 2003.
60. Qian Q, Hartman RP, King BF, Torres VE: Increased occurrence of pericardial effusion in patients with autosomal dominant polycystic kidney disease. Clin J Am Soc Nephrol 2:1223, 2007.
61. Imazio M, Negro A, Belli R, et al: Frequency and prognostic significance of pericarditis following acute myocardial infarction treated by primary percutaneous coronary intervention. Am J Cardiol 103:1525, 2009.
62. Imazio M, Demichelis B, Parrini I, et al: Relation of acute pericardial disease to malignancy. Am J Cardiol 95:1393, 2005.
63. Ben-Horin S, Bank I, Guetta V, Livneh A: Large symptomatic pericardial effusion as the presentation of unrecognized cancer: A study in 173 consecutive patients undergoing pericardiocentesis. Medicine (Baltimore) 85:49, 2006.
64. Bischiniotis TS, Lafaras CT, Platogiannis DN, et al: Intrapericardial cisplatin administration after pericardiocentesis in patients with lung adenocarcinoma and malignant cardiac tamponade. Hellenic J Cardiol 46:324, 2005.
65. Maruyama R, Yokoyama H, Seto T, et al: Catheter drainage followed by the instillation of bleomycin to manage malignant pericardial effusion in non–small cell lung cancer: A multi-institutional phase II trial. J Thorac Oncol 2:65, 2007.
66. Martinoni A, Cipolla CM, Cardinale D, et al: Long-term results of intrapericardial chemotherapeutic treatment of malignant pericardial effusions with thiotepa. Chest 126:1412, 2004.
67. Duwe BV, Sterman DH, Musani AI: Tumors of the mediastinum. Chest 128:2893, 2005.
68. Maisch B, Ristic AD, Pankuweit S: Intrapericardial treatment of autoreactive pericardial effusion with triamcinolone; the way to avoid side effects of systemic corticosteroid therapy. Eur Heart J 23:1503, 2002.
69. Edwards MH, Leak AM: Pericardial effusions on anti-TNF therapy for rheumatoid arthritis—a drug side effect or uncontrolled systemic disease? Rheumatology (Oxford) 48:316, 2009.
70. Rosenbaum E, Krebs E, Cohen M, et al: The spectrum of clinical manifestations, outcome and treatment of pericardial tamponade in patients with systemic lupus erythematosus: A retrospective study and literature review. Lupus 18:608, 2009.
71. Fischer A, Misumi S, Curran-Everett D, et al: Pericardial abnormalities predict the presence of echocardiographically defined pulmonary arterial hypertension in systemic sclerosis–related interstitial lung disease. Chest 131:988, 2007.
72. Elshershari H, Cao QL, Hijazi ZM: Transcatheter device closure of atrial septal defects in patients older than 60 years of age: Immediate and follow-up results. J Invasive Cardiol 20:177, 2008.
73. Fasseas P, Orford JL, Panetta CJ, et al: Incidence, correlates, management, and clinical outcome of coronary perforation: Analysis of 16,298 procedures. Am Heart J 147:140, 2004.
74. Bertaglia E, Zoppo F, Tondo C, et al: Early complications of pulmonary vein catheter ablation for atrial fibrillation: A multicenter prospective registry on procedural safety. Heart Rhythm 4:1265, 2007.
75. Laborderie J, Barandon L, Ploux S, et al: Management of subacute and delayed right ventricular perforation with a pacing or an implantable cardioverter-defibrillator lead. Am J Cardiol 102:1352, 2008.
76. Holzmann M, Nicko A, Kühl U, et al: Complication rate of right ventricular endomyocardial biopsy via the femoral approach: A retrospective and prospective study analyzing 3048 diagnostic procedures over an 11-year period. Circulation 118:1722, 2008.

CHAPTER 76 Traumatic Heart Disease

Matthew J. Wall, Jr., Peter I. Tsai, and Kenneth L. Mattox

Incidence

Thoracic trauma is responsible for 25% of the deaths from vehicular accidents. These can be comprised of six lethal injuries—airway obstruction, tension pneumothorax, cardiac tamponade, open pneumothorax, massive hemothorax, and flail chest. There are six hidden injuries, which can be potentially lethal; these should be detected during secondary survey and include thoracic aortic disruption, tracheobronchial disruption, blunt cardiac injury, traumatic diaphragmatic tear, esophageal disruption, and pulmonary contusion.[1] Of motor vehicle fatalities, 10% to 70% may have been the result of blunt cardiac rupture. Penetrating cardiac trauma is a highly lethal injury, with relatively few victims surviving long enough to reach the hospital. In a series of 1198 patients with penetrating cardiac injuries in South Africa, only 6% of patients reached the hospital with any signs of life.[2] With improvements in organized emergency medical transport systems, up to 45% of those who sustain significant heart injury may reach the emergency department with signs of life. Transport times shorter than 5 minutes and successful endotracheal intubation are positive factors for survival when the patient suffers a pulseless cardiac injury.[3] However, the overall mortality for penetrating cardiac trauma has not changed significantly, even in the major trauma centers.[4]

Traumatic heart disease can be categorized on the basis of the mechanism of injury (**Table 76-1**). Knowledge of the various types of cardiac injuries, methods available to facilitate rapid diagnosis, and familiarity of the techniques for surgical repair are no longer an academic exercise but a lifesaving necessity.[5] This chapter deals primarily with the presentation, evaluation, and treatment of penetrating, nonpenetrating, and miscellaneous cardiac injuries.

Penetrating Cardiac Injury

Causes

Penetrating trauma is the most common cause of significant cardiac injury seen in the hospital setting, with the predominant cause being firearms and knives.[6,7] Other mechanisms, such as shotguns, ice picks, and fence post impalement, have also been reported.

The location of injury to the heart often correlates with the location of injury on the chest wall. Because of their anterior location, the anatomic chambers at greatest risk for injury are the right and left ventricles. A review of 711 patients with penetrating cardiac trauma has reported 54% sustained stab wounds and 42% gunshot wounds. The right ventricle was injured in 40% of cases, the left ventricle in 40%, the right atrium in 24%, and the left atrium in 3%.[6]

In one study, one third of cardiac injuries involved multiple cardiac structures.[6] Significant complex cardiac injuries involved the coronary arteries ($n = 39$), valvular apparatus (mitral; $n = 2$), intracardiac fistulas (i.e., ventricular septal defects [VSDs]; $n = 14$), and unusual injuries ($n = 10$). Only 2% of patients surviving the initial injury and undergoing an operation required reoperation for a residual defect, and most of these repairs were performed on a semielective basis.

Thus, most injuries are to the myocardium. These are readily managed by the general, trauma, or acute care surgeon.

Clinical Presentation and Pathophysiology

Wounds involving the epigastrium and precordium should raise suspicion for cardiac injury. Stab wounds present a more predictable path of injury than gunshot wounds. Patients with cardiac injury can present with a clinical spectrum from full cardiac arrest with no vital signs to asymptomatic with normal vital signs. Up to 80% of stab wounds that injure the heart eventually manifest tamponade. The weapon injures the pericardium and heart but as the weapon is removed, the pericardium may not allow the blood to escape. Rapid bleeding into the pericardium favors clotting rather than defibrination.[8] As pericardial fluid accumulates, a decrease in ventricular filling occurs, leading to a decrease in stroke volume. A compensatory rise in catecholamine levels leads to tachycardia and increased right heart filling pressures. The limits of distensibility are reached as the pericardium is filled with blood and the septum shifts toward the left side, further compromising left ventricular function. If this cycle persists, ventricular output can continue to deteriorate, leading to irreversible shock. As little as 60 to 100 mL of blood in the pericardial sac can produce the clinical picture of tamponade.

The rate of accumulation depends on the location of the wound. Because it has a thicker wall, wounds to the right ventricle seal themselves more readily than wounds to the right atrium. Patients with penetrating injuries to the coronary arteries present with rapid onset of tamponade combined with cardiac ischemia.

The classic findings of Beck's triad (muffled heart sounds, hypotension, and distended neck veins) are seen in only 10% of trauma patients. Pulsus paradoxus (a substantial fall in systolic blood pressure during inspiration) and Kussmaul's sign (increase in jugular venous distention on inspiration) may be present but are not reliable signs.[9] A valuable and reproducible sign of pericardial tamponade is a narrowing of the pulse pressure. An elevation of the central venous pressure often accompanies rapid and cyclic hyperresuscitation with crystalloid solutions, but in such cases a widening of the pulse pressure occurs.

In contrast to stab wounds, gunshot wounds to the heart are more frequently associated with hemorrhage than with tamponade. Of gunshot wounds to the heart, 20% manifest as tamponade. With firearms, the kinetic energy is greater and the wounds to the heart and pericardium are frequently larger. Thus, these patients present with exsanguination into a pleural cavity and arrest more often.[9]

TABLE 76-1 Causes of Traumatic Heart Diseases

I. Penetrating
  A. Stab wounds—knives, swords, ice picks, fence posts, wire, sports
  B. Gunshot wounds—handguns, rifles, nail guns, lawnmower projectiles
  C. Shotgun wounds—pellets, close versus distant range
II. Nonpenetrating (blunt)
  A. Motor vehicle accident
    1. Seat belt
    2. Air bag
    3. Dashboard, steering wheel
  B. Vehicle-pedestrian accident
  C. Falls from height
  D. Crushing—industrial accident
  E. Blasts—improvised explosive devices, grenades, fragments (combined blunt and penetrating)
  F. Assault
  G. Sternal or rib fractures
  H. Recreational—sporting events, rodeo, baseball
III. Iatrogenic
  A. Catheter-induced
  B. Pericardiocentesis-induced
  C. Percutaneous
IV. Metabolic
  A. Traumatic response to injury
  B. "Stunning"
  C. Systemic inflammatory response syndrome
V. Other
  A. Burn
  B. Electrical
  C. Factitious—needles, foreign bodies
  D. Embolic—missiles

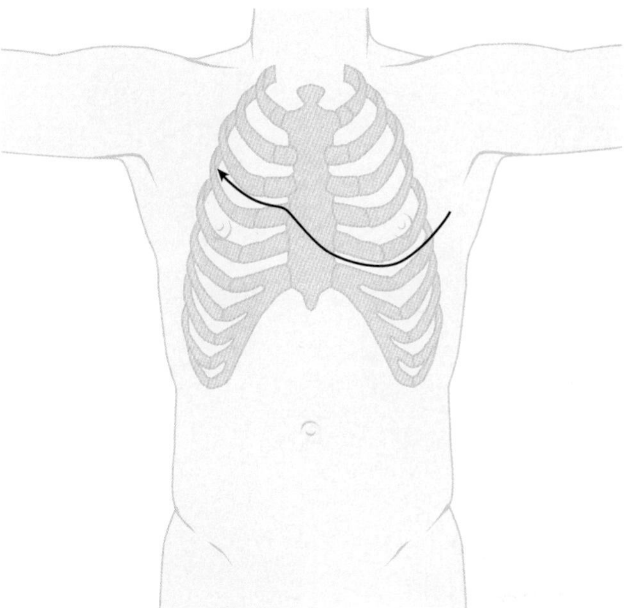

FIGURE 76-1 Left anterior thoracotomy (extension across the sternum if required). See text for details. *(Redrawn from Baylor College of Medicine, 2005.)*

Evaluation

The evaluation of suspected heart injury differs, depending on whether the presenting patient is clinically stable or in extremis. The diagnosis of heart injury requires a high index of suspicion. On initial presentation to the emergency center, airway, breathing, and circulation (ABCs) under the Advanced Trauma Life Support protocol are evaluated and established.[10] Intravenous access is obtained and blood is typed and cross-matched. The patient undergoes chest radiography[11] followed by focused abdominal sonography for trauma (FAST)[12] and can be examined for Beck's triad of muffled heart sounds, hypotension, and distended neck veins, as well as for pulsus paradoxus and Kussmaul's sign. These findings suggest cardiac injury but are present in only 10% of patients with cardiac tamponade. If the FAST results demonstrates pericardial fluid in an unstable patient (systemic blood pressure < 90 mm Hg), transfer of the patient to the operating room to address the injury is recommended.

Patients in extremis often require emergency thoracotomy for resuscitation. The clear indications for emergency department thoracotomy by surgical personnel include the following[13,14]:

1. Salvageable postinjury cardiac arrest (e.g., patients who have experienced cardiac arrest with a high likelihood of intrathoracic injury, particularly penetrating cardiac wounds)
2. Severe postinjury hypotension (i.e., systolic blood pressure < 60 mm Hg) caused by cardiac tamponade, air embolism, or thoracic hemorrhage

If vital signs are regained after resuscitative thoracotomy, the patient can be transferred to the operating room for definitive repair. The patient with confirmed pericardial fluid by FAST, with normal vital signs (systemic blood pressure > 90 mm Hg), may undergo a thorough evaluation to identify associated injuries. If other injuries are excluded, open exploration may then proceed to exclude cardiac injury. In the absence of known causes of the presence of pericardial fluid (e.g., malignant pericardial effusion), a missed cardiac injury can lead to delayed bleeding, deterioration, or death.

Surgeons are increasingly performing ultrasonography for thoracic trauma, paralleling the use of ultrasonography for blunt abdominal trauma. The FAST examination evaluates four anatomic windows for the presence of intra-abdominal or pericardial fluid.[12] Ultrasonography in this setting is not intended to reach the precision of studies performed in the radiology or cardiology suite but is merely intended to determine the presence of abnormal fluid collections, which aids in surgical decision making. Ultrasonography is safe, portable, and expeditious and can be repeated as indicated. If performed by a trained surgeon, the FAST examination has a sensitivity of almost 100% and a specificity of 97.3%. As the use of FAST evolves, the most universally agreed indication is evaluation for pericardial blood.

Chest radiography is nonspecific, but can identify hemothorax or pneumothorax. Other possibly indicated examinations include ultrasonography, central venous pressure measurements, computed tomography (CT) scan for trajectory, thoracoscopy, and laparoscopy.

Treatment

Definitive treatment involves surgical exposure through an anterior thoracotomy or median sternotomy. The goals of treatment are relief of tamponade and hemorrhagic control. Concomitantly, correction of acidosis and hypothermia and reestablishment of effective coronary perfusion are addressed by appropriate resuscitation.

Exposure of the heart is accomplished via a left anterolateral thoracotomy (**Fig. 76-1**), which allows access to the pericardium and heart and exposure for aortic cross-clamping if necessary. This incision can be extended across the sternum to gain access to the right side of the chest and for better exposure of the right atrium or right ventricle. Once the left pleural space is entered, the lung is retracted to expose the descending thoracic aorta for cross-clamping. The amount of blood present in the left chest indicates whether one is dealing with hemorrhage or tamponade. The pericardium anterior to the phrenic nerve is opened, injuries are rapidly identified, and repair is performed. In selected cases, particularly stab wounds to the precordium, median sternotomy can be used. This incision allows excellent exposure to the anterior structures of the heart, but difficulty with access to the posterior mediastinal structures and descending thoracic aorta for cross-clamping may be encountered.

Cardiorrhaphy should be carefully performed. Poor technique can result in enlargement of the lacerations or injury to the coronary arteries. If the initial treating physician is uncomfortable with the suturing technique, digital pressure can be applied until a more experienced surgeon arrives. Other techniques that have been described include

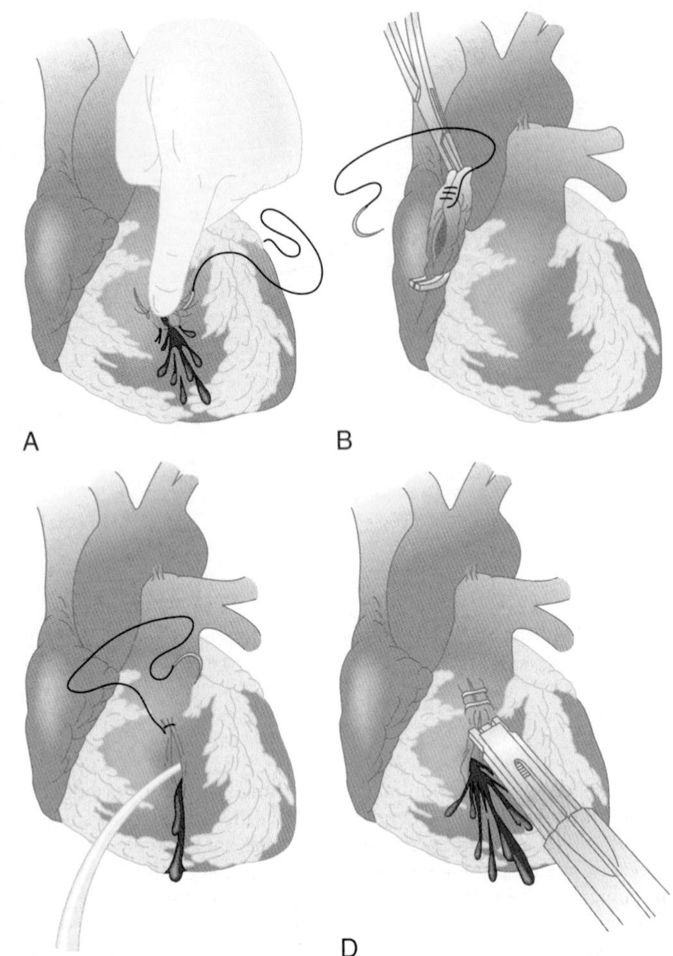

FIGURE 76-2 Temporary techniques to control bleeding. **A,** Finger occlusion. **B,** Partial occluding clamp. **C,** Foley balloon catheter. **D,** Skin staples. *(Redrawn from Baylor College of Medicine, 2005.)*

the use of a Foley balloon catheter and a skin stapler (**Fig. 76-2**). Injuries adjacent to coronary arteries can be managed by placing the sutures deep to the artery (**Fig. 76-3**).

Complex cardiac injuries include coronary artery injury, valvular apparatus injury (annulus, papillary muscles, and chordae tendineae), intracardiac fistulas, arrhythmias, and delayed tamponade. These delayed sequelae have been reported to have a broad incidence (4% to 56%), depending on the definition.

Coronary artery injury is a rare injury, occurring in 5% to 9% of patients with cardiac injuries, with a 69% mortality rate.[6] A coronary artery injury is most often controlled by simple ligation, but bypass grafting using a saphenous vein may be required for proximal left anterior descending injuries (with cardiopulmonary bypass). With a resurrection of the old concept of coronary artery bypass grafting without cardiopulmonary bypass (off-pump bypass), this technique can theoretically be used for these injuries in the highly unlikely event that the patient is hemodynamically stable.

Valvular apparatus dysfunction is rare (0.2% to 9%) and can occur with blunt and penetrating trauma. The aortic valve is most frequently injured, followed by the mitral and tricuspid valves, although many victims of aortic valve injuries die at the scene. Often, these injuries are identified after the initial cardiorrhaphy and resuscitation have been performed. Timing of repair depends on the patient's condition. If severe cardiac dysfunction exists at the time of the initial operation, immediate valve repair or replacement may be required; otherwise, delayed repair is usually advised.[6]

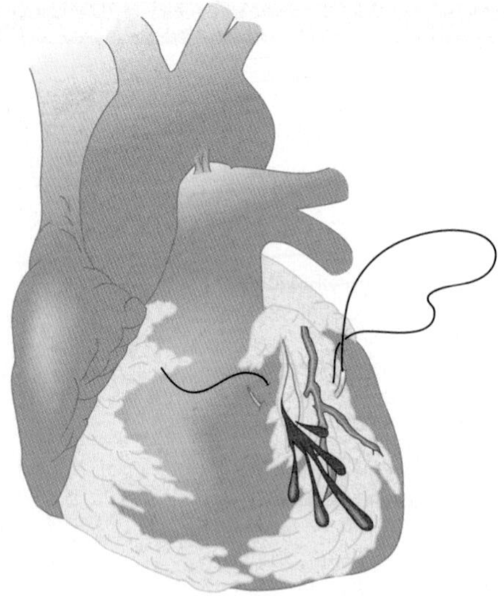

FIGURE 76-3 Injuries adjacent to coronary arteries can be addressed by placing sutures deep, avoiding injury to the artery. *(Redrawn from Baylor College of Medicine, 2005.)*

Intracardiac fistulas include VSDs, atrial septal defects, and atrioventricular fistulas, with an incidence of 1.9% among cardiac injuries. Management depends on symptoms and degree of cardiac dysfunction, with only a minority of these patients requiring repair. These injuries are often identified after primary repair is carried out, and they can be repaired after the patient has recovered from the original and associated injuries. Cardiac catheterization and detailed echocardiography should be performed before repair so that specific anatomic sites of injury and incision planning can be addressed.

The overall hospital survival rate for patients with penetrating heart injuries ranges from 30% to 90%. The survival rate for patients with stab wounds is 70% to 80%, whereas survival after gunshot wounds is 30% to 40%.[4]

Blunt Cardiac Injury

Causes

The term *nonpenetrating* or *blunt cardiac trauma* has replaced the term *cardiac contusion* and describes injury ranging from minor bruises of the myocardium to cardiac rupture. It can be caused by direct energy transfer to the heart or compression of the heart between the sternum and vertebral column at the time of the accident. It can even include cardiac contusion and cardiac rupture during external cardiac massage as part of cardiopulmonary resuscitation (CPR).[15,16] Within this spectrum, blunt cardiac injuries can manifest as septal rupture, free wall rupture, coronary artery thrombosis, cardiac failure, complex and simple dysrhythmias, and/or rupture of chordae tendineae or papillary muscles.[17-19] The incidence can be as high as 75% of patients with severe bodily trauma. Mechanisms include motor vehicle accidents, vehicle-pedestrian accidents, falls, crush injuries, blasts, assaults, CPR, and recreational events. Such injuries can be associated with sternal or rib fractures. A fatal cardiac dysrhythmia can occur when the sternum is struck by a ball,[20] which may be a form of commotio cordis.[21,22]

Cardiac rupture carries a significant risk of mortality. The biomechanics of cardiac rupture include the following: (1) direct transmission of increased intrathoracic pressure to the chambers of the heart; (2) hydraulic effect from a large force applied to the abdominal or extremity veins, causing force to be transmitted to the right atrium; (3) decelerating force between fixed and mobile areas, explaining atriocaval tears; (4) direct force causing myocardial contusion, necrosis, and delayed rupture; and (5) penetration from a broken rib or fractured sternum.[8,23]

Blunt rupture of the cardiac septum occurs most frequently near the apex of the heart when the injury occurs in late diastole or early systole. Multiple ruptures as well as disruption of the conduction system have been reported.[19] From autopsy data, blunt cardiac trauma with ventricular rupture most often involves the left ventricle, followed by the right ventricle. In contrast, in patients who arrive alive to the hospital, right atrial disruption is more common.[24] This is seen at the superior vena cava–atrial junction, inferior vena cava–atrial junction, or the appendage. VSDs can occur, with the most common tear involving the membranous and muscular portions of the septum. Injury to only the membranous portion of the septum is the least common type of blunt VSD. Traumatic rupture of the thoracic aorta is associated with lethal cardiac rupture in almost 25% of cases.[25] Blunt pericardial rupture results from pericardial tears secondary to increased intra-abdominal pressure or lateral decelerative forces. Tears can occur on the left side, most often parallel to the phrenic nerve, to the right of the pleuropericardium, to the diaphragmatic surface of the pericardium, and finally to the mediastinum. Cardiac herniation with cardiac dysfunction can occur in conjunction with these tears.[26] The heart can be displaced into either pleural cavity or even into the abdomen. In the case of right pericardial rupture, the heart can become twisted, leading to the surprising discovery of an empty pericardial cavity at resuscitative left anterolateral thoracotomy. With a left-sided cardiac herniation through a pericardial tear, a trapped distending heart prevents the heart from returning to the pericardium, and the term *strangulated heart* has been applied. Venous filling is impaired and, unless the cardiac herniation is reduced, hypotension and cardiac arrest can occur.[27] One clue to the presence of cardiac herniation is sudden loss of pulse when the patient is repositioned, such as when moved to a stretcher.

Clinical Presentation and Pathophysiology

As in penetrating cardiac trauma, clinically severe blunt cardiac trauma (e.g., cardiac rupture) manifests as tamponade or hemorrhage into the pleural cavity, depending on the status of the pericardium. If the pericardium is intact, tamponade develops; if it is not intact, extrapericardial bleeding occurs and hypovolemic shock ensues. Tamponade is sometimes combined with hypovolemia, thus complicating the clinical presentation.

Blunt cardiac injury can be divided into clinically significant and insignificant injuries. Clinically significant injuries include cardiac rupture (ventricular or atrial), septal rupture, valvular dysfunction, coronary thrombosis, and caval avulsion. These injuries manifest as tamponade, hemorrhage, or severe cardiac dysfunction. Septal rupture and valvular dysfunction (e.g., leaflet tear, papillary muscle, chordal rupture) can initially appear without symptoms but later demonstrate the delayed sequelae of heart failure.[8,17] Blunt cardiac injury can also appear as a dysrhythmia, most commonly premature ventricular contractions, the precise mechanism of which is unknown. Ventricular tachycardia can occur and degenerate into ventricular fibrillation. Supraventricular tachyarrhythmias can also occur. These symptoms commonly occur within the first 24 to 48 hours after injury.

A major difficulty in managing blunt cardiac injury relates to definitions. *Cardiac contusion* is a nonspecific term that should likely be abandoned. It is best to describe these injuries as "blunt cardiac trauma with ..." followed by the clinical manifestation, such as dysrhythmia or heart failure.[28]

Evaluation

Blunt cardiac injury can often present like a penetrating injury, especially if there is tear and laceration to the heart resulting in pericardial tamponade. The routine ABCs and FAST used for penetrating cardiac injury apply here as well. A high suspicion of the mechanism of injury leads to monitoring for blunt cardiac injury.[29-31]

ELECTROCARDIOGRAPHY. In cases of blunt cardiac injury, conduction disturbances are common.[29,30] Thus, a screening 12-lead electrocardiogram (ECG) can be helpful for evaluation. Sinus tachycardia is the most common rhythm disturbance seen.

Other common disturbances include T wave and ST-segment changes, sinus bradycardia, first- and second-degree atrioventricular block, right bundle branch block, right bundle branch block with hemiblock, third-degree block, atrial fibrillation, premature ventricular contractions, ventricular tachycardia, and ventricular fibrillation.[29,30]

CARDIAC ENZYMES. Much has been written previously about the use of cardiac enzyme level determinations in evaluating blunt cardiac injury. However, no correlation among serum assays (e.g., creatine phosphokinase–myocardial band, cardiac troponin T, cardiac troponin I) and identification and prognosis of injury have been demonstrated with blunt cardiac injury. Therefore, cardiac enzyme level assays are not helpful unless one is evaluating concomitant coronary artery disease, or are considered with other diagnostic modalities (e.g., 12-lead ECG, echocardiography) to improve the diagnosis.[29-32]

ECHOCARDIOGRAPHY. Transthoracic echocardiography (TTE) has limited use in evaluating blunt cardiac trauma because most patients also have significant chest wall injury, thus rendering the test suboptimal. Its major use is in diagnosing intrapericardial blood, suggesting an injury or chamber rupture. To evaluate more subtle findings of blunt cardiac injury, such as wall motion, valvular, or septal abnormalities in the stable patient, transesophageal echocardiography (TEE) is a more sensitive test for evaluating blunt cardiac injury.[29,30] Cardiac septal defects and valvular insufficiency are readily diagnosed with TEE. Because echocardiography is operator-dependent, the approach is often based on the local expertise available.

Ventricular dysfunction can often mimic cardiac tamponade in its clinical presentation. Echocardiography is particularly useful for older patients with preexisting ventricular dysfunction. However, most blunt cardiac injuries identified by echocardiography in stable patients rarely require acute treatment.[33]

Treatment

Much debate and discussion has occurred about the clinical relevance of cardiac contusion. Most trauma surgeons conclude that this diagnosis should be eliminated because it does not affect how these injuries are treated. Thus, a normotensive patient with a normal initial ECG and suspected blunt cardiac injury is managed in observation units, with no expected clinical significance. Patients with an abnormal ECG are admitted for monitoring and treated accordingly. Patients who present in cardiogenic shock are evaluated for a structural injury, which is then repaired.[28]

Dysrhythmias can occur as a result of blunt injury, ischemia, or electrolyte abnormalities and are addressed according to the injury (**Table 76-2**). Complex cardiac injuries from blunt trauma remain rare, and treatment is similar to that for penetrating cardiac injuries of the valvular, septal, and atrial-ventricular apparatus. Cardiac rupture has a worse prognosis than penetrating injuries to the heart, with a survival rate of approximately 20%.

Miscellaneous Cardiac Trauma

Iatrogenic Cardiac Injury

Iatrogenic cardiac injury can occur with central venous line insertion, cardiac catheterization procedures, endovascular interventions, percutaneous pericardiocentesis, or while creating an open pericardial window.[34] Cardiac injuries caused by central venous lines usually occur with placement from the left subclavian or left internal jugular vein.

Perforation causing tamponade has also been reported with a right internal jugular introducer sheath for transjugular intrahepatic portocaval shunts. Vigorous insertion of left-sided central lines, especially during dilation of the line tract, can lead to cardiac perforations.

Even appropriate technique carries a discrete rate of iatrogenic injury secondary to central venous catheterization. Common sites of

TABLE 76-2 Dysrhythmias Associated with Cardiac Injury

Penetrating Cardiac Injury
Sinus tachycardia
ST-segment changes associated with ischemia
Supraventricular tachycardia
Ventricular tachycardia, fibrillation
Blunt Cardiac Injury
Sinus tachycardia
ST-segment, T wave abnormalities
Atrioventricular conduction alterations, bradycardia
Ventricular tachycardia, fibrillation
Electrical Injury
Sinus tachycardia
ST-segment, T wave abnormalities
Bundle branch blocks
Axis deviation
Prolonged QT
Paroxysmal supraventricular tachycardia
Atrial fibrillation
Ventricular tachycardia, fibrillation (alternating current)
Asystole (lightning strike)

cardiac injury include the superior vena cava–atrium junction and superior vena cava–innominate junction. These small perforations often lead to a compensated cardiac tamponade. Drainage by pericardiocentesis is often unsuccessful, and evacuation via a subxiphoid pericardial window or full median sternotomy is sometimes required. Once access to the pericardial space is gained, the site of injury has sometimes sealed and may be difficult to find.

Complications from cardiac catheterization are fortunately relatively rare, but include perforation of the coronary arteries, cardiac perforation, and aortic dissection. These can be catastrophic and require emergency surgical intervention. Other potential iatrogenic causes of cardiac injury include external and internal cardiac massage, endovascular interventions, transthoracic percutaneous interventions, right ventricular injury during pericardiocentesis, and intracardiac injections.[35]

Intracardiac Foreign Bodies and Missiles

Intrapericardial and intracardiac foreign bodies can cause complications of acute suppurative pericarditis, chronic constrictive pericarditis, foreign body reaction, and hemopericardium.[36] Intrapericardial foreign bodies that have been reported to result in complications include bullets,[37] explosive device and missile fragments, knitting needles, and hypodermic needles. Needles and similar foreign bodies have been noted after deliberate insertion by patients, usually those with psychiatric diagnoses. A report by LeMaire and colleagues[36] has advocated removal of those intrapericardial foreign bodies that are larger than 1 cm, contaminated, or produce symptoms.

Intracardiac missiles are foreign bodies that are embedded in the myocardium, retained in the trabeculations of the endocardial surface, or free in a cardiac chamber. These are the result of direct penetrating thoracic injury or injury to a peripheral venous structure, with embolization to the heart. Location and other conditions determine the type of complications that can occur and the treatment required. Observation might be considered when the missile is small, right-sided, embedded completely in the wall, contained within a fibrous covering, not contaminated, and/or producing no symptoms. Right-sided missiles can embolize to the lung, at which point they can be removed if large. In rare cases they can embolize paradoxically through a patent foramen ovale or atrial septal defect. Left-sided missiles can manifest as systemic embolization shortly after the initial injury. Diagnosis is pursued with radiography in two projections, fluoroscopy, echocardiography, or angiography. More recently, rapid CT scanning can be used to diagnose and locate these fragments.

The full body topogram can help identify all missiles and then the cross-sectional images can locate them precisely. Treatment of retained missiles is individualized. Removal is recommended for missiles that are left-sided, larger than 1 to 2 cm, rough in shape, or produce symptoms. Although a direct approach, with or without cardiopulmonary bypass, has been advocated in the past, a large percentage of right-sided foreign bodies can now be removed by endovascular techniques.

Metabolic Cardiac Injury and Burns

Metabolic cardiac injury refers to cardiac dysfunction in response to injury and may be associated with injuries caused by burns, electrical injury, sepsis, the systemic inflammatory response syndrome, and multisystem trauma.[38,39] Intraoperatively, myocardial depression can occur shortly after restoring blood flow to an ischemic extremity. The exact mechanism responsible for this dysfunction is unclear, but responses to trauma can induce a release of cytokines that may have a direct effect on the myocardium, with gender differences in response.[40] Endotoxin, tumor necrosis factor-α, tumor necrosis factor-β, interleukin-1, interleukin-6, interleukin-10, catecholamines (epinephrine, norepinephrine), cell adhesion molecules, and nitric oxide are all possible mediators.[41-43]

Metabolic cardiac injury can manifest clinically as conduction disturbances or decreased contractility leading to decreased output. Myocardial depression can occur in response to the mediator storm and can alter calcium uptake and depression of the myocyte responsiveness to beta-adrenergic stimulation.[44]

Myocytes have altered calcium uptake in patients with injuries from burns. The activation of constitutive nitric oxide synthase can modulate cardiac responsiveness to cholinergic and adrenergic stimulation, and production of inducible nitric oxide synthase can depress myocyte contractile responsiveness to beta-adrenergic agonists. The myocardial depressive effects appear to be reversible.[39]

Treatment of metabolic cardiac injury has been supportive, with correction of the initiating insults, but some practitioners have attempted to address the involved mediators using intravenous phosphodiesterase inhibitors, corticosteroids, arginine, granulocyte-macrophage colony-stimulating factor, and glutamate.[44,45] Use of an intra-aortic counterpulsation balloon pump can be considered to treat such myocardial depression, but no controlled series have tested this hypothesis.

Cardiac complications in the early postburn period are a major cause of death. The initial cardiovascular effect of burn injury is attributable to the profound reduction in cardiac output that can occur within minutes of injury. The overall cardiac response has been described as an ebb and flow pattern, with the initial ebb phase lasting between 1 and 3 days, marked by hypovolemia and myocardial depression, and the flow phase characterized by a prolonged period of increased metabolic demand, with increased cardiac output and peripheral blood flow. The reduction in cardiac output observed in the initial period of burn injury is the result of a dramatic and rapid decrease in intravascular volume and of direct myocardial depression.

Hypovolemia results from the capillary leak caused by endothelial injury and may be mediated by platelet-activating factor, complement, cytokines, arachidonic acid, or oxygen free radicals. Myocardial depression manifested by a decrease in myocardial contractility and abnormalities in ventricular compliance becomes apparent with a total body surface area burn of 20% to 25%. Myocardial depressant factor, tumor necrosis factor-α, vasopressin, oxygen free radicals, and interleukins may be responsible for the depression.[46-48]

Electrical Injury

Cardiac complications are a common cause of death after electrical injury. An estimated 1100 to 1300 deaths occur annually in the United States from electrical injury, including lightning strikes.

The cardiac complications after electrical injury include immediate cardiac arrest, acute myocardial necrosis with or without ventricular failure, myocardial ischemia, dysrhythmias, conduction abnormalities, acute hypertension with peripheral vasospasm, and asymptomatic nonspecific abnormalities evident on the ECG. Damage from electrical injury is caused by direct effects on the excitable tissues, heat generated from the electrical current, and accompanying associated injuries (e.g., falls, explosions, fires).[49] Thus, electrical injuries can result in later complications and algorithms have been developed for monitoring after the event.[50,51]

Pericardial Injury

Small isolated tears in the pericardium can lead to cardiac herniation. This is a rare complication of pericardial rupture and depends on the size of the pericardial tear. If large enough, cardiac herniation can occur, leading to acute cardiac dysfunction.[8,27,52] Traumatic pericardial rupture is rare. Most patients with pericardial rupture do not survive transport to the hospital because of other significant associated injuries. The overall mortality of those who are treated at trauma centers with such injury remains as high as 64%.[53] Motor vehicle accidents are is the most common causes of pericardial rupture. Sixty percent of pericardial ruptures occur along the left pleuropericardial surface.[53] Most of these cases are diagnosed intraoperatively or on autopsy.[27] The clinical presentation of pericardial rupture can mimic that of pericardial tamponade with associated cardiac electrical-mechanical dissociation caused by impaired venous return. When the heart returns to its normal position in the pericardium, venous return resumes.

Positional hypotension is a manifestation of cardiac herniation caused by pericardial rupture,[27] whereas pericardial tamponade is associated with persistent hypotension until the pericardium is decompressed. Therefore, a high index of suspicion should be maintained when evaluating polytrauma patients with unexplained positional hypotension.

Late Sequelae

Secondary sequelae in survivors of cardiac trauma include valvular abnormalities and intracardiac fistulas.[6,54,55] These abnormalities can be identified intraoperatively by gross palpation of a thrill[5] or with the use of TEE. TEE may not be feasible, however, in the acutely injured patient. Early postoperative clinical examination and electrocardiographic findings are unreliable. Thus, echocardiography is recommended during the initial hospitalization to identify occult injury and establish a baseline study. Because the incidence of late sequelae can be as high as 56%, follow-up echocardiography 3 to 4 weeks after injury has been recommended by some.

Summary

The approach to the injured patient follows a well-defined plan. Patients with penetrating trauma who arrive alive at a trauma center can have hemopericardium diagnosed by FAST. Urgent operation performed in the trauma resuscitation area or the operating room can result in survival. Blunt cardiac trauma can produce a range of presentation, from minor electrocardiographic changes to frank rupture of the septum, free wall, or cardiac valves. Associated injuries are common. Stable patients can undergo more extensive evaluation, but unstable patients require rapid imaging and urgent operation. Late sequelae of fistula, valve dysfunction, coronary occlusion, and heart failure are rare and are most often detected by echocardiography or catheterization within the first year after injury.

REFERENCES

Incidence

1. Yamamoto L, Schroeder C, Morley D, Beliveau C: Thoracic trauma: The deadly dozen. Crit Care Nurs Q 28:22, 2005.
2. Campbell NC, Thomsen SR, Murkart DJ, et al: Review of 1198 cases of penetrating cardiac trauma. Br J Surg 84:1737, 1997.
3. Durham LA, Richardson R, Wall MJ, et al: Emergency center thoracotomy: Impact of prehospital resuscitation. J Trauma 32:779, 1992.
4. Thourani VH, Feliciano DV, Cooper WA, et al: Penetrating cardiac trauma at an urban trauma center: A 22-year perspective. Am Surg 65: 811, 1999.
5. Embrey R: Cardiac trauma. Thorac Surg Clin 17:87, 2007.

Penetrating Cardiac Injury

6. Wall MJ Jr, Mattox KL, Chen CD, Baldwin JC: Acute management of complex cardiac injuries. J Trauma 42:905, 1997.
7. Degiannis E, Loogna P, Doll D, et al: Penetrating cardiac injuries: Recent experience in South Africa. World J Surg 30:1258, 2006.
8. Ivatury RR: The injured heart. *In* Moore ES, Feliciano DV, Mattox KL (eds): Trauma. 5th Ed. New York, McGraw Hill, 2004, pp 555-568.
9. Brown J, Grover FL: Trauma to the heart. Chest Surg Clin North Am 7:325, 1997.
10. American College of Surgeons, Committee on Trauma: Advanced Trauma Life Support. Chicago, American College of Surgeons, 2008.
11. Ho ML, Gutierrez FR: Chest radiography in thoracic polytrauma. AJR Am J Roentgenol 192:599, 2009.
12. Rozycki GS, Schmidt JA, Oschner MG, et al: The role of surgeon-performed ultrasound in patients with possible penetrating wounds: A prospective multicenter study. J Trauma 45:190, 1998.
13. Biffl WD, Moore EE, Johnson JL: Emergency department thoracotomy. *In* Moore EE, Feliciano DV, Mattox KL (eds): Trauma. 5th ed. New York, McGraw-Hill, 2004, pp 239-252.
14. Working Group, Ad Hoc Subcommittee on Outcomes, American College of Surgeons-Committee on Trauma: Practice management guidelines for emergency department thoracotomy. J Am Coll Surg 193:303, 2001.

Blunt Cardiac Injury

15. Hashimoto Y, Moriya F, Furumiya J: Forensic aspects of complications resulting from cardiopulmonary resuscitation. Leg Med (Tokyo) 9:94, 2007.
16. Bansal MK, Maraj S, Chewaproug D, Amanullah A: Myocardial contusion injury: Redefining the diagnostic algorithm. Emerg Med J 22:465, 2005.
17. Choi JS, Kim EJ: Simultaneous rupture of the mitral and tricuspid valves with left ventricular rupture caused by blunt trauma. Ann Thorac Surg 86:1371, 2008.
18. Varahan SL, Farah GM, Caldeira CC, et al: The double jeopardy of blunt chest trauma: A case report and review. Echocardiography 23:235, 2006.
19. Schaffer RB, Berdat PA, Seiler C, Carrel TP: Isolated rupture of the ventricular septum after blunt chest trauma. Ann Thorac Surg 67:853, 1999.
20. Wahl P, Schreyer N, Yersin B: Injury pattern of the Flash-Ball, a less-lethal weapon used for law enforcement: Report of two cases and review of the literature. J Emerg Med 31:325, 2006.
21. Maron BJ, Link MS, Wang PJ, et al: Clinical profile of commotio cordis: An underappreciated cause of sudden death in young during sports and other activities. J Cardiovasc Electrophysiol 10:114, 1999.
22. Hsing DD, Madikians A: True-true, unrelated: A case report. Pediatr Emerg Care 21:755, 2005.
23. Bakaeen FG, Wall MJ Jr, Mattox KL: Successful repair of an avulsion of the superior vena cava from the right atrium inflicted by blunt trauma. J Trauma 59:1486, 2005.
24. Vougiouklakis T, Peschos D, Doulis A, et al: Sudden death from contusion of the right atrium after blunt chest trauma: Case report and review of the literature. Injury 36:213, 2005.
25. Howanitz EP, Buckley D, Galbraith TA, et al: Combined blunt traumatic rupture of the heart and aorta: Two case reports and review of the literature. J Trauma 30:506, 1990.
26. Nassiri N, Yu A, Statkus N, Gosselin M: Imaging of cardiac herniation in traumatic pericardial rupture. J Thorac Imaging 24:69, 2009.
27. Wall MJ Jr, Mattox KL, Wolf DA: The cardiac pendulum—blunt rupture of the pericardium with strangulation of the heart. J Trauma 59:136, 2005.
28. Mattox KL, Flint LM, Carrico CJ, et al: Blunt cardiac injury (formerly termed "myocardial contusion") [editorial]. J Trauma 31:653, 1992
29. Holanda MS, Domínguez MJ, López-Espadas F, et al: Cardiac contusion following blunt chest trauma. Eur J Emerg Med 13:373, 2006.
30. Elie MC: Blunt cardiac injury. Mt Sinai J Med 73:542, 2006.
31. Jackson L, Stewart A: Best evidence topic report. Use of troponin for the diagnosis of myocardial contusion after blunt chest trauma. Emerg Med J 22:193, 2005.
32. Bertinchant JP, Polge A, Mohty D, et al: Evaluation of incidence, clinical significance and prognostic value of circulating cardiac troponin I and T elevation in hemodynamically stable patients with suspected myocardial contusion after blunt chest trauma. J Trauma 48:924, 2000.
33. Karalis DG, Victor MF, Davis GA, et al: The role of echocardiography in blunt chest trauma: A transthoracic and transesophageal echocardiographic study. J Trauma 36:53, 1994.

Iatrogenic Cardiac Injury

34. Barleben A, Huerta S, Mendoza R, et al: Left ventricle injury with a normal pericardial window: Case report and review of the literature. J Trauma. 63:414, 2007.
35. Ivatury RR, Simon RJ, Rohman M: Cardiac complications. *In* Mattox KL (ed): Complications of Trauma. New York, Churchill Livingstone, 1994, pp 409-428.

Intracardiac Foreign Bodies and Missiles

36. LeMaire SA, Wall MJ Jr, Mattox KL: Needle embolus causing cardiac puncture and chronic constrictive pericarditis. Ann Thorac Surg 65:1786, 1998.
37. Davis RE, Bruno AD 2nd, Larsen WB, et al: Mobile intrapericardial bullet: Case report and review of the literature. J Trauma 58:378, 2005.

Metabolic Cardiac Injury and Burns

38. Huang YS, Yang ZC, Tan BG, et al: Pathogenesis of early cardiac myocyte damage after sear burns. J Trauma 46:428, 1999.
39. Sharkey SW, Shear W, Hodges M, Herzog CA: Reversible myocardial contraction abnormalities in patients with an acute non-cardiac illness. Chest 114:98, 1998.
40. Kher A, Wang M, Tsai BM, et al: Sex differences in the myocardial inflammatory response to acute injury. Shock 23:1, 2005.
41. Kumar A, Thota V, Dee L, et al: TNF-alpha and IL-1 are regulators for depression of in vitro myocardial cell contractility induced by serum from humans with septic shock. J Exp Med 183:949, 1996.
42. Meldrum DR, Shenkar R, Sheridan BC, et al: Hemorrhage activates myocardial NF-kappa and increases TNF-alpha in the heart. J Mol Cell Cardiol 29:2849, 1997.

43. Horton JW, Lin C, Maass D: Burn trauma and tumor necrosis factor alpha alter calcium handling by cardiomyocytes. Shock 10:270, 1998.
44. Heinz G, Geppert A, Delle Karth G, et al: IV milrinone for cardiac output increase and maintenance: Comparison in nonhyperdynamic SIRS/sepsis and congestive heart failure. Intensive Care Med 25:620, 1999.
45. Flohe S, Borgermann J, Dominquez FE, et al: Influence of granulocyte-macrophage colony-stimulating factor (GM-CSF) on whole blood endotoxin responsiveness following trauma, cardiopulmonary bypass, and severe sepsis. Shock 12:17, 1999.
46. Maass DL, White J, Horton JW: IL-1beta and IL-6 act synergistically with TNF-alpha to alter cardiac contractile function after burn trauma. Shock 18:360, 2002.
47. Horton JW: Oxygen free radicals contribute to post-burn cardiac cell membrane dysfunction. J Surg Res 61:97, 1996.
48. Horton JW: Cellular basis for burn-mediated cardiac dysfunction in adult rabbits. Am J Physiol 271:H2615, 1996.
49. Lee RC: Injury by electrical forces: Pathophysiology, manifestations, and therapy. Curr Probl Surg 34:677, 1997.
50. Chen EH: Do children require ECG evaluation and inpatient telemetry after household electrical exposures? Ann Emerg Med 49:64, 2007.
51. Arnoldo B, Klein M, Gibran NS: Practice guidelines for the management of electrical injuries. J Burn Care Res 27:439, 2006.

Pericardial Injury

52. Nassiri N, Yu A, Statkus N, Gosselin M: Imaging of cardiac herniation in traumatic pericardial rupture. J Thorac Imaging 24:69, 2009.
53. Galindo Gallego M, Lopez-Cambra MJ, Fernandez-Acenero MJ, et al: Traumatic rupture of the pericardium. Case report and literature review. J Cardiovasc Surg (Torino) 37:187, 1996.

Late Sequelae

54. Meyer DM, Jessen ME, Grayburn PA: Use of echocardiography to detect occult cardiac injury after penetrating thoracic trauma: A prospective study. J Trauma 39:902, 1995.
55. Mattox KL, Limacher MC, Feliciano DV, et al: Cardiac evaluation following heart injury. J Trauma 25:758, 1985.

CHAPTER 77 Pulmonary Embolism

Samuel Z. Goldhaber

Pulmonary embolism (PE) and deep venous thrombosis (DVT) constitute one of the "big three" cardiovascular killers, along with myocardial infarction and stroke. Known collectively as venous thromboembolism (VTE), PE and DVT account for several hundred thousand deaths annually in the United States and afflict millions of individuals worldwide. The case fatality rate for PE, approximately 15%, exceeds the mortality rate for acute myocardial infarction. PE survivors may have to deal with an impaired quality of life because of chronic thromboembolic pulmonary hypertension or chronic venous insufficiency (also called post-thrombotic syndrome) of the legs. During the past decade, VTE has become integrated into the curriculum for cardiovascular medicine training. The American Heart Association, the American College of Cardiology, and the European Society of Cardiology have targeted PE as an area requiring special guidelines[1] and professional education. The U.S. government has created VTE policies both with a "big stick" (exacting penalties on hospitals that do not optimize prophylaxis) and simultaneously with a "carrot" (increasing federal funding for basic and clinical VTE research projects as well as educational outreach programs for health care professionals and the public). The U.S. Surgeon General has issued a call to action to prevent DVT and PE in which he describes VTE as the most preventable cause of death among hospitalized patients.[2] New nonprofit organizations have formed and include patient advocacy as part of their core mission to improve public education and awareness of VTE and to support innovative research on VTE prevention and treatment.[3] Momentum from these activities is beginning to reap rewards because the case fatality rate for PE is decreasing in the United States.[4]

VTE is a common problem, yet it is often difficult to diagnose. It strikes a wide range of individuals, from teenagers to nonagenarians. Its onset is usually unpredictable. The likelihood of recurrence after completion of a time-limited course of anticoagulation is high, especially when surgery, trauma, or estrogens do not precipitate the initial event. VTE exacts a psychological toll on patients, who wonder whether they will suffer a recurrent event, whether it will affect their family members, and whether it will diminish their quality of life and shorten their life span.

No diagnostic test for PE has utility unless PE is considered in the differential diagnosis. Therefore, clinicians must remain vigilant to detect PE, which has been known for generations as the great masquerader because it mimics other illnesses such as pneumonia and congestive heart failure. For imaging of PE, chest computed tomography (CT) scanning has virtually replaced ventilation-perfusion lung scanning. When the clinical likelihood of PE is low and the result of a screening blood test, the plasma D-dimer assay, is negative, the exclusion of PE is usually straightforward and accurate. The principal challenge now is to confront runaway technology that has led to overuse of CT scanning, with too little attention paid to history, physical examination, and clinical likelihood scoring systems. This trend toward relying on advanced imaging technology, typical of many aspects of contemporary medicine, has led to excessive exposure to radiation and to intravenous contrast material, with its attendant complications of renal dysfunction, anaphylaxis, and exponential increases in cost.

As soon as the diagnosis of acute PE is established, rapid and precise risk stratification is of paramount importance. Effective anticoagulation serves as the foundation of therapy. High-risk patients may also benefit from thrombolysis, catheter embolectomy, surgical embolectomy, or placement of an inferior vena caval filter. Accurate prognostication relies on classic clinical assessment of general appearance, heart rate, blood pressure, and respiratory rate, as well as a new array of poor prognosis indicators that include elevation of cardiac biomarkers, right ventricular hypokinesis assessed by echocardiography, and right ventricular enlargement detected by chest CT. These risk stratification variables can predict the development of clinical deterioration and adverse outcomes that occur several days after admission to the hospital, despite an initial presentation of hemodynamic stability.

The selection of immediately active parenteral anticoagulant drugs has expanded beyond unfractionated heparin (UFH). Low-molecular-weight heparins (LMWH) and fondaparinux provide convenient fixed-dose, weight-based therapy as an alternative to an adjusted-dose continuous intravenous infusion of UFH monitored by the activated partial thromboplastin time (aPTT). Three direct thrombin inhibitors—argatroban, lepirudin, and bivalirudin—are available for use in patients with suspected or proven heparin-induced thrombocytopenia. Although warfarin is the only oral anticoagulant approved for the treatment of acute PE, its effectiveness and safety are improving with a combination of centralized anticoagulation management services (often run by pharmacists or nurses), more widespread use of self-testing fingerstick machines for rapid turnaround of coagulation results, development of computer-driven dosing nomograms that factor clinical variables and response to prior warfarin doses into the algorithm, and use of rapid turnaround genetic testing during warfarin dose initiation.[5] Meanwhile, novel oral anticoagulants have immediate action and fixed-dose administration and do not require routine coagulation monitoring.[6] Two are approved in Canada and Europe for VTE prevention after orthopedic surgery—the anti-Xa agent rivaroxaban[7,8] and the direct thrombin inhibitor dabigatran[9] (see Chap. 87). In a primary prevention trial of cardiovascular disease, rosuvastatin 20 mg daily reduced the symptomatic VTE rate by 43% within 2 years compared with placebo.[10] This finding points to emerging pharmacologic approaches to VTE prevention other than standard anticoagulation.

A key to reducing VTE incidence will be the implementation of prophylaxis measures that have proven safe and effective in rigorously executed trials.[11] Currently, a wide gap exists between extensive evidence-based knowledge of VTE prevention and meager prescription of anticoagulants or mechanical measures. At-risk

TABLE 77-1 Modifiable Risk Factors for Venous Thromboembolism

Obesity
Metabolic syndrome
Cigarette smoking
Hypertension
Abnormal lipid profile
High consumption of red meat and low consumption of fish, fruits, and vegetables

TABLE 77-2 Major Risk Factors for Venous Thromboembolism That Are Not Readily Modifiable

Advancing age
Arterial disease, including carotid and coronary disease
Personal or family history of venous thromboembolism
Recent surgery, trauma, or immobility, including stroke
Congestive heart failure
Chronic obstructive pulmonary disease
Acute infection
Air pollution
Long-haul air travel
Pregnancy, oral contraceptive pills, or postmenopausal hormone replacement therapy
Pacemaker, implantable cardiac defibrillator leads, or indwelling central venous catheter
Hypercoagulable states
Factor V Leiden resulting in activated protein C resistance
Prothrombin gene mutation 20210
Antithrombin deficiency
Protein C deficiency
Protein S deficiency
Antiphospholipid antibody syndrome

patients hospitalized[12] on medical services[13] and medical subspecialty services, including cardiology and heart failure patients,[14] less often receive guideline-approved prophylaxis[15] than surgical service patients do.[16] Yet, prevention is much easier than diagnosis and treatment of PE or DVT and is far more cost-effective.[17] Failure to prevent VTE has important ramifications after hospital discharge because hospitalized patients receiving inadequate prophylaxis contribute to the burden of out-of-hospital PE and DVT, where three of every four VTE events occur.[18] Universal VTE prophylaxis among at-risk hospitalized patients will bring us toward the goal of near eradication of PE, both in the hospital setting and in the community after hospital discharge of high-risk patients. Strategies to improve implementation of prophylaxis include enhanced education, performance-based incentives, financial penalties if VTE occurs, electronic computerized alerts,[19] and "human alerts" from a hospital staff member to the responsible physicians[20] whose high-risk patients are not receiving prophylaxis.

Epidemiology

The incidence of VTE is about 1.5 per 1000 person-years. There are approximately twice as many DVT as PE cases. Although children and adolescents are susceptible,[21] incidence rises with age[22] and is similar in men and women. About half the cases are idiopathic and occur without antecedent trauma, surgery, immobilization, or the diagnosis of cancer.[23] Several gene polymorphisms associate independently with an increased risk of VTE apart from those with widely known prothrombotic effects, such as factor V Leiden. These include polymorphisms in the beta$_2$-adrenergic receptor and lipoprotein lipase genes.[24] Clinical predictors for fatal PE include anatomically massive PE, neurologic disease, age older than 75 years, and cancer.[25]

A major breakthrough in epidemiology is the discovery that VTE and arterial thrombosis share many identical risk factors, including increasing age, obesity, cigarette smoking, diabetes mellitus, and unfavorable lipid profile.[26] In a cohort of 5451 patients with ultrasound-confirmed DVT from 183 U.S. hospitals, the five most frequent comorbidities were hypertension (50%), surgery within 3 months (38%), immobility within 30 days (34%), cancer (32%), and obesity (27%).[27] Patients with newly diagnosed VTE have an increased long-term risk for development of myocardial infarction or stroke.[28] A meta-analysis of 63,552 patients with VTE and control subjects found that the relative risk for VTE was 2.3 for obesity, 1.5 for hypertension, 1.4 for diabetes mellitus, 1.2 for cigarette smoking, and 1.2 for hypercholesterolemia. High-density lipoprotein (HDL) cholesterol levels were lower in VTE patients.[29] The metabolic syndrome is a risk factor for VTE.[30] Persistent stress also predisposes to VTE.[31] Eating less red meat and more fish, fruit, and vegetables is associated with a lower incidence of VTE.[32] An especially problematic VTE risk factor is obesity, which has become pandemic in the United States. Obesity doubles or triples the likelihood of VTE.[33] The overlap between venous and arterial thrombosis means that the cardiovascular medicine practitioner can counsel patients on steps to reduce VTE and coronary heart disease risk simultaneously. **Table 77-1** lists modifiable VTE risk factors.

Many risk factors for VTE are not readily modifiable (**Table 77-2**). Acute urinary tract infection or respiratory infection may precipitate VTE.[34] Heart failure is a common problem in patients with VTE. The combination of higher medical acuity, increased frequency of VTE risk factors, and low rate of VTE prophylaxis constitutes a "triple threat" to patients with heart failure.[14] As patients survive longer with cancer, the frequency of VTE is increasing because cancer patients have twice the incidence of VTE (see Chap. 90).[35] This increased risk of VTE not only accompanies adenocarcinomas of the pancreas, stomach, lung, esophagus, prostate, and colon, but also threatens patients with "liquid tumors" such as myeloproliferative disease, lymphoma, and leukemia. In patients with a first VTE and without the diagnosis of cancer, the risk for detection of a subsequent new cancer is 1% to 2% per year and is higher in patients with unprovoked VTE and in those with advanced age.[36]

Pregnancy,[37] hormonal contraception,[38] and postmenopausal hormonal therapy[39] each contribute to increased risk. Less well known risk factors include chronic obstructive pulmonary disease,[40] nephrotic syndrome,[41] and air pollution.[42]

Perhaps the most frequently discussed acquired risk factor is long-haul air travel. The risk of fatal PE in this setting is less than 1 in 1 million. However, when death occurs, it is dramatic and especially tragic because the victim is often an otherwise healthy young person. It appears that among some individuals, there is activation of the coagulation system during air travel.[43] For each 2-hour increase in travel duration, there appears to be an 18% higher risk of VTE.[44]

Hospitalized patients with medical illnesses[13] such as pneumonia and congestive heart failure have a high risk for development of VTE. The stasis and immobilization associated with postoperative venous thrombosis may paradoxically increase after hospital discharge because with short hospital lengths of stay, patients may be too weak and debilitated at home to ambulate after surgery. Vigilance is required to ensure that appropriate patients receive extended VTE prophylaxis at the time of hospital discharge.

Upper extremity DVT is an increasingly important clinical entity because of more frequent placement of pacemakers and internal cardiac defibrillators, as well as more frequent use of chronic indwelling catheters for chemotherapy and nutrition. Patients with upper extremity DVT are at risk for PE, superior vena caval syndrome, and loss of vascular access.[45]

Risk factors for VTE in the community include advancing age, cancer, prior VTE, venous insufficiency, pregnancy, trauma, frailty, and immobility. Of those suffering VTE in the community in the Worcester Venous Thromboembolism Study, 23% had undergone surgery and 36% had been hospitalized within the preceding 3 months. Among those patients, fewer than half had received anticoagulant prophylaxis.[18] More than half of VTE events occurred in subjects 65 years of age or older.[46]

Pathophysiology

Hypercoagulable States (see Chap. 90)

In 1856, Rudolf Virchow postulated a triad of factors that predispose to intravascular coagulation: local trauma to the vessel wall, hypercoagulability, and stasis. Classically, the pathogenesis of PE has been dichotomized as caused by either inherited (primary) or acquired (secondary) risk factors. It appears likely, however, that a combination of thrombophilia and acquired risk factors (see Table 77-2) often precipitates overt thrombosis.

The two most common genetic causes of thrombophilia are factor V Leiden and the prothrombin gene mutation. Normally, a specified amount of activated protein C (aPC) can be added to plasma to prolong the aPTT. Patients with "aPC resistance" have a blunted aPTT prolongation and a predisposition to development of PE and DVT. The phenotype of aPC resistance is associated with a single point mutation, designated factor V Leiden, in the factor V gene. Factor V Leiden triples the risk for development of VTE. This genetic mutation is also a risk factor for recurrent pregnancy loss, possibly caused by placental vein thrombosis. Use of oral contraceptives by patients with factor V Leiden increases the risk of VTE by at least 10-fold. A single point mutation in the 3′ untranslated region of the prothrombin gene (G-to-A transition at nucleotide position 20210) is associated with increased levels of prothrombin. In the Physicians' Health Study, the prevalence of the prothrombin gene mutation was 3.9%, and this mutation doubled the risk of venous thrombosis. The Agency for Healthcare Research and Quality concluded that there is no direct evidence that testing for these mutations leads to improved clinical outcomes in adults with a history of VTE or their adult family members. The test results have variable clinical validity for predicting VTE in these populations and have only weak clinical utility.[47]

The most common acquired thrombophilia is the antiphospholipid syndrome.[48] It can cause venous or arterial thrombosis, thrombocytopenia, recurrent fetal loss, or acute ischemic encephalopathy.[49] A careful family history remains the most rapid and cost-effective method of identifying a predisposition to venous thrombosis. Investigation with blood tests can be misleading. For example, consumption coagulopathy caused by venous thrombosis may be misdiagnosed as deficiency of antithrombin, protein C, or protein S. Heparin administration can depress antithrombin levels. Use of warfarin ordinarily causes a mild deficiency of protein C or protein S. Both oral contraceptives and pregnancy depress protein S levels.

Relationship Between Deep Venous Thrombosis and Pulmonary Embolism

When venous thrombi detach from their sites of formation, they flow through the venous system toward the vena cava. They pass through the right atrium and right ventricle and then enter the pulmonary arterial circulation. An extremely large embolus may lodge at the bifurcation of the pulmonary artery, forming a saddle embolus (**Fig. 77-1**). More commonly, a major pulmonary vessel is occluded. Many patients with large PEs do not have ultrasonographic evidence of DVT, probably because the clot has already embolized to the lungs.

RIGHT VENTRICULAR DYSFUNCTION. The extent of pulmonary vascular obstruction and the presence of underlying cardiopulmonary disease are probably the most important factors determining whether right ventricular dysfunction ensues.[50] As obstruction increases, pulmonary artery pressure rises. Further increases in pulmonary vascular resistance and pulmonary hypertension are caused by secretion of vasoconstricting compounds such as serotonin, reflex pulmonary artery vasoconstriction, and hypoxemia.[51] The overloaded right ventricle[51] releases cardiac biomarkers such as pro–brain natriuretic peptide (pro-BNP), brain natriuretic peptide (BNP), and troponin, all of which predict an increased likelihood of an adverse clinical outcome.

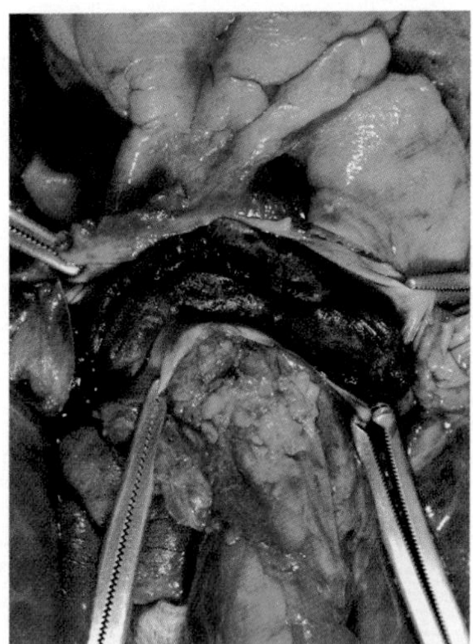

FIGURE 77-1 A 41-year-old woman with poorly controlled hypertension suffered an intracerebral hemorrhage, complicated 6 days later by acute pulmonary embolism. Emergency catheter embolectomy was unsuccessful, and she suffered cardiac arrest. At autopsy, a large saddle embolus extended from the root of the pulmonary artery into the left and right lungs.

VENTRICULAR INTERDEPENDENCY. The sudden rise in pulmonary artery pressure abruptly increases right ventricular afterload, with consequent elevation of right ventricular wall tension followed by right ventricular dilation and dysfunction (**Fig. 77-2**). As the right ventricle dilates, the interventricular septum shifts toward the left, with resultant underfilling and decreased left ventricular diastolic distensibility. With underfilling of the left ventricle, systemic cardiac output and systolic arterial pressure both decline, potentially impairing coronary perfusion and producing myocardial ischemia. Elevated right ventricular wall tension after massive PE[52] reduces right coronary artery flow, increases right ventricular myocardial oxygen demand, and causes ischemia. Perpetuation of this cycle can lead to right ventricular infarction, circulatory collapse, and death.[53]

Summary of Pathophysiology

PE can have the following pathophysiologic effects: increased pulmonary vascular resistance caused by vascular obstruction, neurohumoral agents, or pulmonary artery baroreceptors; impaired gas exchange caused by increased alveolar dead space from vascular obstruction and hypoxemia from alveolar hypoventilation, low ventilation-perfusion units, and right-to-left shunting as well as impaired carbon monoxide transfer caused by loss of gas exchange surface; alveolar hyperventilation caused by reflex stimulation of irritant receptors; increased airway resistance due to bronchoconstriction; and decreased pulmonary compliance due to lung edema, lung hemorrhage, and loss of surfactant.

Diagnosis

Diagnosis of PE is more difficult than treatment or prevention. Fortunately, noninvasive diagnostic approaches have become increasingly reliable and streamlined. The greatest challenge is to remember to consider the possible diagnosis of PE and to realize that it can masquerade as many other illnesses, such as asthma, pneumonia, and congestive heart failure. PE can occur concomitantly with other illnesses, thereby confounding the diagnostic workup. The most useful approach is the clinical assessment of likelihood, based on presenting symptoms and signs, in conjunction with judicious diagnostic testing. When PE is not highly suspected, a normal plasma D-dimer enzyme-linked immunosorbent assay (ELISA) usually suffices to rule out this condition. When PE is highly suspected, especially with an elevated D-dimer ELISA, chest CT scanning is the best imaging test. Another problem is that patients often delay seeking medical attention.[54] Among 1152 patients with confirmed DVT or PE at 70 North American

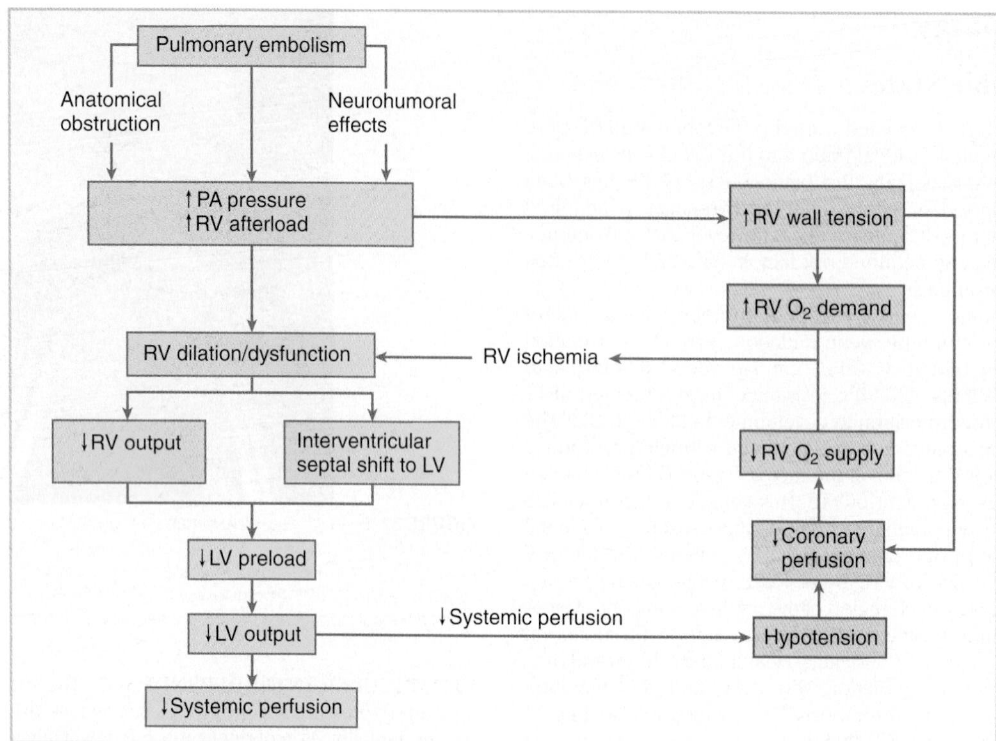

FIGURE 77-2 Pathophysiology of right ventricular dysfunction. LV = left ventricular; PA = pulmonary artery; RV = right ventricular.

TABLE 77-3 Most Common Symptoms and Signs of Pulmonary Embolism

Symptoms
Otherwise unexplained dyspnea
Chest pain, either pleuritic or "atypical"
Anxiety
Cough
Signs
Tachypnea
Tachycardia
Low-grade fever
Left parasternal lift
Tricuspid regurgitant murmur
Accentuated P_2
Hemoptysis
Leg edema, erythema, tenderness

medical centers, 21% of DVT patients and 17% of PE patients received diagnoses more than 1 week after symptom onset.

CLINICAL PRESENTATION. Symptoms and signs of PE are nonspecific. Hence, clinical suspicion of PE is of paramount importance in guiding diagnostic testing. Clinical gestalt and clinical experience are helpful, but the incremental gain in diagnostic accuracy is small when comparing attending physicians with interns.[55] Dyspnea is the most frequent symptom and tachypnea is the most frequent sign of PE (**Table 77-3**). In general, severe dyspnea, syncope, or cyanosis portends a major life-threatening PE, which is often devoid of chest pain. Paradoxically, severe pleuritic pain often signifies that the embolism is small and located in the distal pulmonary arterial system, near the pleural lining.

PE should be suspected in hypotensive patients when (1) there is evidence of venous thrombosis or predisposing factors for it and (2) there is clinical evidence of acute cor pulmonale (acute right ventricular failure), such as distended neck veins, right-sided S_3 gallop, right ventricular heave, tachycardia, or tachypnea, especially if (3) there are echocardiographic findings of right ventricular dilation and hypokinesis or electrocardiographic evidence of acute cor pulmonale manifested by a new $S_1Q_3T_3$ pattern, new right bundle branch block, or right ventricular ischemia (**Fig. 77-3** and see Fig. 13-21).

A reliable set of clinical decision rules can stratify patients into high clinical likelihood or non–high clinical likelihood of PE with a set of seven bedside assessment questions (**Table 77-4**). This approach was validated in a large Dutch study in which almost half of the patients could be categorized as "PE unlikely." In this low-risk group, only about 5% of patients were subsequently diagnosed with PE.[56] But the problem with this scoring system, known as the Wells criteria, is that it appears at first glance to be time-consuming and, therefore, has not been adopted into everyday use. Simplified Wells criteria have been developed and validated[57] (**Table 77-5**).

DIFFERENTIAL DIAGNOSIS. The differential diagnosis of PE is broad and covers a wide spectrum from life-threatening disease such as acute myocardial infarction to innocuous anxiety states (**Table 77-6**). Some patients have concomitant PE and other illnesses. For example, if pneumonia or heart failure does not respond to appropriate therapy, the possibility of coexisting PE should be considered. Idiopathic pulmonary hypertension may present with sudden exacerbations that mimic acute PE.

Clinical Syndromes of Pulmonary Embolism

Classification of acute PE (**Table 77-7**) can assist with prognostication and clinical management. Massive PE occurs rarely in most hospitals. Submassive PE is more common, and small to moderate PE is most common.

MASSIVE PULMONARY EMBOLISM. Patients with massive PE are susceptible to cardiogenic shock and multisystem organ failure. Renal insufficiency, hepatic dysfunction, and altered mentation are common findings. Thrombosis is widespread, affecting at least half of the pulmonary arterial vasculature. Clot is typically present bilaterally. Dyspnea is usually the most noticeable symptom; chest pain is unusual, transient cyanosis is common, and systemic arterial hypotension requiring pressor support is frequent. Excessive fluid boluses may worsen right-sided heart failure and render therapy more difficult.

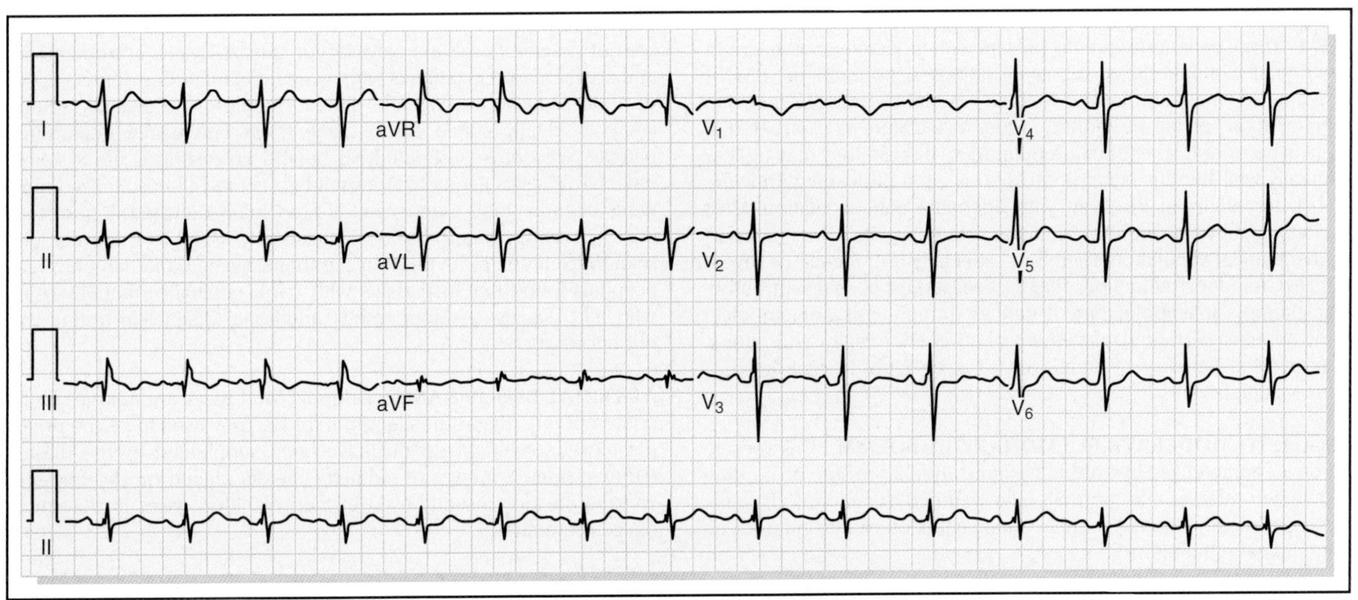

FIGURE 77-3 Electrocardiogram from a 33-year-old man who presented with a left main pulmonary artery embolism on chest CT scan. He was hemodynamically stable and had normal right ventricular function on echocardiography. His troponin and brain natriuretic peptide levels were normal. He was managed with anticoagulation alone. On the initial electrocardiogram, he has a heart rate of 90/min, $S_1Q_3T_3$, and incomplete right bundle branch block, with inverted or flattened T waves in leads V_1 through V_4.

TABLE 77-4 Classic Wells Criteria to Assess Clinical Likelihood of Pulmonary Embolism

>4 score points = high probability

≤4 score points = non–high probability

	SCORE POINTS
DVT symptoms or signs	3
An alternative diagnosis is less likely than PE	3
Heart rate >100/min	1.5
Immobilization or surgery within 4 weeks	1.5
Prior DVT or PE	1.5
Hemoptysis	1
Cancer treated within 6 months or metastatic	1

TABLE 77-5 Simplified Wells Criteria to Assess Clinical Likelihood of Pulmonary Embolism

>1 score point = high probability

≤1 score point = non–high probability

	SCORE POINTS
DVT symptoms or signs	1
An alternative diagnosis is less likely than PE	1
Heart rate >100/min	1
Immobilization or surgery within 4 weeks	1
Prior DVT or PE	1
Hemoptysis	1
Cancer treated within 6 months or metastatic	1

TABLE 77-6 Differential Diagnosis of Pulmonary Embolism

Anxiety, pleurisy, costochondritis
Pneumonia, bronchitis
Myocardial infarction
Pericarditis
Congestive heart failure
Idiopathic pulmonary hypertension

TABLE 77-7 Classification of Acute Pulmonary Embolism

CLASSIFICATION	PRESENTATION	THERAPY
Massive PE	Systolic blood pressure <90 mm Hg or poor tissue perfusion or multisystem organ failure plus right or left main pulmonary artery thrombus or "high clot burden"	Thrombolysis or embolectomy or inferior vena caval filter plus anticoagulation
Submassive PE	Hemodynamically stable but moderate or severe right ventricular dysfunction or enlargement	Addition of thrombolysis, embolectomy, or filter remains controversial
Small to moderate PE	Normal hemodynamics and normal right ventricular size and function	Anticoagulation

MODERATE TO LARGE (SUBMASSIVE) PULMONARY EMBOLISM. These patients frequently present with moderate or severe right ventricular hypokinesis as well as elevations in troponin, pro-BNP, or BNP, but they maintain normal systemic arterial pressure. Usually, one third or more of the pulmonary artery vasculature is obstructed. If there is no prior history of cardiopulmonary disease, they may appear clinically well, but this initial impression is often misleading. They are at risk for recurrent PE, even with adequate anticoagulation. Most survive, but they may require escalation of therapy with pressor support or mechanical ventilation. Therefore, especially if moderate or severe right ventricular dysfunction persists, one should consider thrombolytic therapy or embolectomy. If neither thrombolysis nor embolectomy appears warranted, placement of an inferior vena caval filter is controversial but may be employed as a "back-up" in case heparin anticoagulation fails.

SMALL TO MODERATE PULMONARY EMBOLISM. This presentation is characterized by normal systemic arterial pressure, no cardiac biomarker release, and normal right ventricular function. Patients appear clinically stable. Adequate anticoagulation results in an excellent clinical outcome.

PULMONARY INFARCTION. This syndrome (**Table 77-8**) is characterized by pleuritic chest pain that may be unremitting or may wax and wane. The pleurisy is occasionally accompanied by hemoptysis. The embolus usually lodges in the peripheral pulmonary arterial tree, near the pleura. Tissue infarction usually occurs 3 to 7 days after embolism. The syndrome often includes fever, leukocytosis, elevated erythrocyte sedimentation rate, and radiologic evidence of infarction.

PARADOXICAL EMBOLISM. This syndrome may present with a sudden stroke. The cause is a small DVT that embolizes to the arterial system, usually through a patent foramen ovale. VTE is rarely detected in patients who suffer paradoxical embolism; the DVT is small and breaks away from a tiny leg vein completely, leaving no residual evidence of thrombosis that can be imaged on venous ultrasound examination. After a "cryptogenic stroke," echocardiography with bubble study may diagnose a patent foramen ovale. Contemporary management requires choosing between indefinite duration of anticoagulation and closure of the patent foramen ovale, usually percutaneously.

NONTHROMBOTIC PULMONARY EMBOLISM. Sources of embolism other than thrombus are uncommon. They include fat, tumor, air, and amniotic fluid. Fat embolism syndrome is most often observed after blunt trauma complicated by long bone fractures. Air embolus can occur during placement or removal of a central venous catheter. Amniotic fluid embolism may be catastrophic and is characterized by respiratory failure, cardiogenic shock, and disseminated intravascular coagulation. Intravenous drug abusers sometimes self-inject hair, talc, and cotton that contaminate the drug they have acquired. These patients also have susceptibility to septic PE, which can cause endocarditis of the tricuspid or pulmonic valves.

Nonimaging Diagnostic Methods

PLASMA D-DIMER ASSAY. This blood screening test relies on the principle that most patients with PE have ongoing endogenous fibrinolysis that is not effective enough to prevent PE but that does break down some of the fibrin clot to D-dimers. Although elevated plasma concentrations of D-dimers are sensitive for the presence of PE, they are not specific. Levels are elevated for at least 1 week postoperatively and are increased in patients with myocardial infarction, sepsis, cancer, or almost any other systemic illness. Therefore, the plasma D-dimer assay is ideally suited for outpatients or emergency department patients who have suspected PE but no coexisting acute systemic illness. This test is generally not useful for acutely ill hospitalized inpatients because their D-dimer levels are usually elevated. A normal D-dimer assay appears to be as diagnostically useful as a normal lung scan to exclude PE.[58] A randomized trial at seven Canadian university hospitals found that in patients with a low clinical probability of PE who had negative D-dimer results, additional diagnostic testing was not necessary.[59]

ARTERIAL BLOOD GASES. Arterial blood gases are not part of the contemporary diagnostic algorithm for PE. They used to be the principal blood screening test but have been supplanted by the plasma D-dimer assay. Noninvasive oximetry meters placed on the finger or earlobe are now usually used instead of blood gases to determine oxygen saturation.

ELECTROCARDIOGRAM. The electrocardiogram (ECG) helps exclude acute myocardial infarction and may raise suspicion or help confirm the diagnosis of PE among patients with electrocardiographic manifestations of right-sided heart strain (**Table 77-9**), which is an ominous prognostic finding.[60] Right-sided heart strain is not specific, however, and may be observed in patients with asthma or idiopathic pulmonary hypertension. Patients with massive PE may have sinus tachycardia, slight ST and T wave abnormalities, or even entirely normal ECGs. Other abnormalities include incomplete or complete right bundle branch block or an $S_1Q_3T_3$ complex (see Fig. 77-3). T wave inversion in leads V_1 to V_4 has the greatest accuracy for identification of right ventricular dysfunction in patients with acute PE.

Imaging Methods

CHEST RADIOGRAPHY. The chest radiograph is usually the first imaging study obtained in patients with suspected PE. A near-normal radiograph in the setting of severe respiratory compromise is highly suggestive of massive PE. Major chest radiographic abnormalities are uncommon. Focal oligemia (Westermark sign) indicates massive central embolic occlusion. A peripheral wedge-shaped density above the diaphragm (Hampton hump) usually indicates pulmonary infarction. Subtle abnormalities suggestive of PE include enlargement of the descending right pulmonary artery. The vessel often tapers rapidly after the enlarged portion. The chest radiograph can also help identify patients with diseases that can mimic PE, such as lobar pneumonia and pneumothorax, but patients with these illnesses can also have concomitant PE.

CHEST COMPUTED TOMOGRAPHY. Chest CT has supplanted pulmonary radionuclide perfusion scintigraphy as the initial imaging test in most patients with suspected PE (**Fig. 77-4**, Fig. 19-23C).[61] Lung scans have caused consternation because most are nondiagnostic. An unequivocal normal or high probability scan is the exception, not the rule. Lung scans depend on expert interpretation, and there is a great deal of interobserver variability even among experts. Therefore, the medical community has welcomed the advent of chest CT to provide definitive diagnosis or exclusion of PE. Only three indications to obtain

TABLE 77-8 Pulmonary Infarction Syndrome
Caused by a tiny peripheral pulmonary embolism
Pleuritic chest pain, often not responsive to narcotics
Low-grade fever
Pleural rub
Occasional scant hemoptysis
Leukocytosis

TABLE 77-9 Electrocardiographic Signs of Pulmonary Embolism
Sinus tachycardia
Incomplete or complete right bundle branch block
Right-axis deviation
T wave inversions in leads III and aVF or in leads V_1-V_4
S wave in lead I and a Q wave and T wave inversion in lead III ($S_1Q_3T_3$)
QRS axis greater than 90 degrees or an indeterminate axis
Atrial fibrillation or atrial flutter

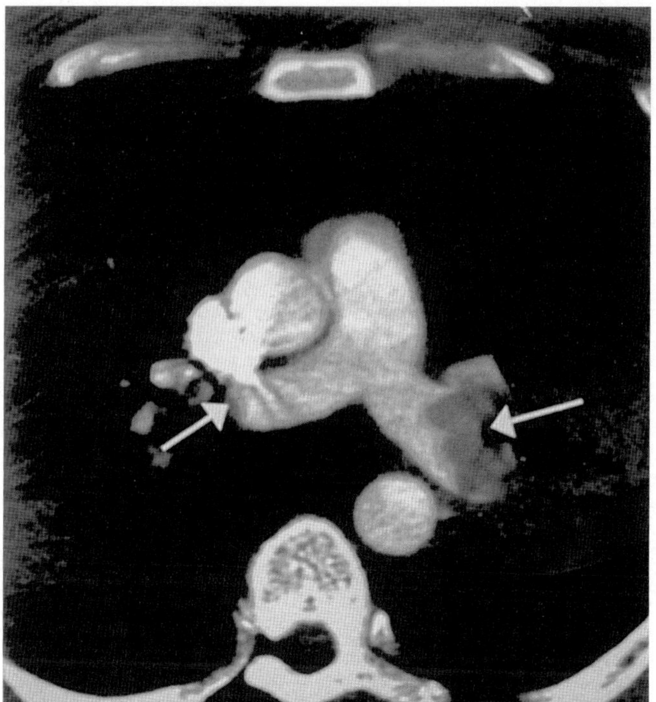

FIGURE 77-4 A 62-year-old physician suffered a massive pulmonary embolism 2 weeks after prostatectomy. Spiral chest CT with contrast enhancement provided a definitive diagnosis, with a large thrombus burden apparent in the right and left main pulmonary arteries (arrows).

a lung scan exist: (1) renal insufficiency, (2) anaphylaxis to intravenous contrast agent that cannot be suppressed with high-dose corticosteroids, and (3) pregnancy (lower radiation exposure to the fetus).

CT scanners are technologic marvels for patients with suspected PE.[62] Multiple generations of CT scanners exist. Even first-generation "single-slice" machines provide images that are clear, rapidly acquired, and accurate in delineating the proximal pulmonary arterial tree. Massive PE can easily be visualized and can confirm surgical or catheter accessibility to the centrally located thrombus. Multidetector-row CT scanners can rapidly image the entire chest with submillimeter resolution. The latest generation of scanners can image thrombus in sixth-order vessels. These thrombi are so tiny that their clinical significance is uncertain.

A meta-analysis of chest CT for suspected PE comprised 3500 patients. All patients were followed for at least 3 months. The overall negative predictive value of a chest CT scan was 99.4%.[63] A validated outcome strategy is D-dimer testing followed by multidetector-row chest CT for patients with abnormally elevated D-dimer levels. With use of this strategy, only 1.5% of patients in whom PE was ruled out developed DVT or PE during 3-month follow-up.[64] For patients with PE, the CT scan serves as a prognostic and diagnostic test. Right ventricular enlargement on CT portends a complicated hospital course. Thus, the CT scan can serve as a "one-stop shop" for diagnosis, detection of source of thrombus, and prognosis. The chest CT scan can also detect other pulmonary diseases that are present in conjunction with PE or that explain a clinical presentation that mimics PE. These include pneumonia, atelectasis, pneumothorax, and pleural effusion that might not be well visualized on the chest radiograph. At times, the chest CT scan detects an incidental but critical finding, such as a small lung carcinoma.

When ordering a CT scan, it is of paramount importance to know what generation of scanners is available (**Table 77-10**). Routine use of CT leg venography increases radiation exposure and rarely changes clinical management.[65] The CT scan reports should always comment on the size of the right ventricle compared with the left ventricle. Three-dimensional images can be reconstructed, and color can be added electronically to enhance details of thrombus localization.[66] Clinical outcome studies differ from studies testing the accuracy of a particular diagnostic modality. The Prospective Investigation of Pulmonary Embolism Diagnosis II (PIOPED II) trial found that the accuracy of CT plummeted on the rare occasions when the imaging results and clinical probability assessment were discordant.[67]

TABLE 77-10 Chest Computed Tomography

When reviewing results, the clinician should *learn* the following:
The type of scanner used (single-slice versus multislice) and the resolution for visualizing thrombus
Whether the bolus of injected contrast material was technically adequate
Whether a CT protocol specific for PE was used, versus an aortic dissection protocol or a cancer staging protocol
Whether the images extend to the pelvic and deep leg veins
When reviewing results, the clinician should *look for* the following:
Size, location, and extent of thrombus
Other diagnoses that may coexist with PE or explain PE symptoms:
Pneumonia
Atelectasis
Pericardial effusion
Pneumothorax
Left ventricular enlargement
Pulmonary artery enlargement, suggestive of pulmonary hypertension
Age of thrombus: acute, subacute, chronic
Location of thrombus: pulmonary arteries, pelvic veins, deep leg veins, upper extremity veins
Right ventricular enlargement
Contour of the interventricular septum: whether it bulges toward the left ventricle, thus indicating right ventricular pressure overload
Incidental masses or nodules in lung

TABLE 77-11 Echocardiographic Signs of Pulmonary Embolism

Right ventricular enlargement or hypokinesis, especially free wall hypokinesis, with sparing of the apex (the McConnell sign)
Interventricular septal flattening and paradoxical motion toward the left ventricle, resulting in a D-shaped left ventricle in cross section
Tricuspid regurgitation
Pulmonary hypertension with a tricuspid regurgitant jet velocity >2.6 m/sec
Loss of respiratory-phasic collapse of the inferior vena cava with inspiration
Dilated inferior vena cava without physiologic inspiratory collapse
Direct visualization of thrombus (more likely with transesophageal echocardiography)

ECHOCARDIOGRAPHY. Echocardiography (**Table 77-11**) is normal in about half of unselected patients with acute PE. Therefore, echocardiography is not recommended as a routine diagnostic test for PE. However, it is a rapid, practical, and sensitive technique for detection of right ventricular overload among patients with established and large PE. Moderate or severe right ventricular hypokinesis, persistent pulmonary hypertension, patent foramen ovale, and free-floating thrombus in the right atrium or right ventricle help identify patients at high risk of death or recurrent thromboembolism. Echocardiography can also help identify illnesses that may mimic PE, such as myocardial infarction and pericardial disease. For those patients in whom transthoracic imaging is unsatisfactory, transesophageal echocardiography can be carried out.

VENOUS ULTRASONOGRAPHY. The primary diagnostic criterion for DVT is loss of vein compressibility. Normally, the vein collapses completely when gentle pressure is applied to the skin overlying it. Upper extremity DVT can be more difficult to diagnose than leg DVT because the clavicle can hinder attempts to compress the subclavian vein. When PE is suspected, venous ultrasonography is useful if it demonstrates DVT, because DVT can be considered a surrogate for PE. But at least half of patients with PE have no imaging evidence of DVT. *Therefore, if clinical suspicion of PE is moderate or high, patients without evidence of DVT should undergo further investigation for PE.*

LUNG SCANNING. Pulmonary radionuclide perfusion scintigraphy (lung scanning) uses radiolabeled aggregates of albumin or microspheres that lodge in the pulmonary microvasculature. Patients with large PE often have multiple perfusion defects. If ventilation scanning is performed on a patient with PE but no intrinsic lung disease, a normal ventilation study is expected, yielding a ventilation-perfusion mismatch and a lung scan interpreted as high probability for PE. However, many patients with low-probability scans but high clinical suspicion for PE do, in fact, have PE proven by invasive pulmonary angiography. Therefore, the term *low-probability scan* is a potentially lethal misnomer.

Magnetic Resonance Imaging. Gadolinium-enhanced magnetic resonance angiography (MRA) is far less sensitive than CT for the detection of PE. However, unlike chest CT or catheter-based pulmonary angiography, MRA does not require ionizing radiation or injection of iodinated contrast agent. In addition, magnetic resonance pulmonary angiography can assess right ventricular size and function. Three-dimensional MRA can be carried out during a single breath-hold and may provide high resolution from the main pulmonary artery through the segmental pulmonary artery branches.[68]

Pulmonary Angiography. Invasive pulmonary angiography was formerly the reference standard for diagnosis of PE, but it is now rarely performed. It is an uncomfortable and potentially risky procedure. However, pulmonary angiography is required when interventions are planned, such as suction catheter embolectomy, mechanical clot fragmentation, or catheter-directed thrombolysis. In cases of chronic thromboembolic PE, pulmonary arteries appear pouched. The thrombus usually organizes with a concave edge. Bandlike defects called webs may be present, in addition to intimal irregularities and abrupt narrowing or occlusion of lobar vessels.

Contrast Venography. Although contrast phlebography was once the reference standard for DVT diagnosis, venograms are now rarely obtained. Venography is costly, invasive, and potentially harmful. It can cause contrast-induced renal failure, anaphylaxis, or chemical phlebitis. Furthermore, difficulty in interpretation of contrast venograms causes considerable disagreement among experienced readers. Invasive contrast phlebography is required, of course, for interventional procedures such as catheter-directed thrombolysis, suction embolectomy, angioplasty, stenting, and placement of an inferior vena caval filter. In patients undergoing total hip or knee replacement, contrast venography is more sensitive than venous ultrasonography for the diagnosis of acute DVT. In one large study of orthopedic surgery patients, sensitivity of venous ultrasound compared with contrast venography was about 30%.[69]

TABLE 77-12 Diagnostic Tests for Suspected Pulmonary Embolism

TEST	COMMENTS
Oxygen saturation	Nonspecific, but suspect PE if there is a sudden, otherwise unexplained decrement
D-dimer	An excellent "rule-out" test if normal, especially if accompanied by non–high clinical probability
Electrocardiography	May suggest an alternative diagnosis, such as myocardial infarction or pericarditis
Lung scanning	Usually provides ambiguous result; used in lieu of chest CT for patients with anaphylaxis to contrast agent, renal insufficiency, or pregnancy
Chest CT	The most accurate diagnostic imaging test for PE (see Table 77-10); beware if CT result and clinical likelihood probability are discordant
Pulmonary angiography	Invasive, costly, uncomfortable; used primarily when local catheter intervention is planned
Echocardiography	Best used as a prognostic test in patients with established PE rather than as a diagnostic test (see Table 77-11); many patients with large PE will have normal echocardiograms
Venous ultrasonography	Excellent for diagnosis of acute symptomatic proximal DVT; a normal study does not rule out PE because a recent leg DVT may have embolized completely; calf vein imaging is operator dependent
Magnetic resonance	Reliable only for imaging of proximal segmental pulmonary arteries; requires gadolinium but does not require iodinated contrast agent

Overall Strategy: An Integrated Diagnostic Approach

A wide array of diagnostic tests is available for the investigation of suspected PE (**Table 77-12**). Familiarity with each test's strengths and weaknesses will enable a concise and streamlined workup. The key to success is to consider PE a possible diagnosis in assessing symptoms, signs, and associated clinical circumstances and comorbidities (**Fig. 77-5**). The first step in an integrated diagnostic strategy is a directed history and physical examination to assess the clinical likelihood of acute PE. An assessment of non–high clinical probability is followed by D-dimer testing. A normal D-dimer assay usually concludes the workup for PE. If the D-dimer is elevated, chest CT usually provides the definitive diagnosis or exclusion of PE. If the CT scan is normal, there is no need to obtain venous ultrasonography of the leg to exclude the diagnosis of PE.[70] For patients in whom the clinical likelihood of PE is high, skip the D-dimer testing and proceed directly to chest CT scanning. For the rare equivocal CT result, venous ultrasonography of the legs may help. Diagnostic pulmonary angiography may be useful if PE is strongly suspected and both the chest CT and the venous ultrasound study of the legs are normal.

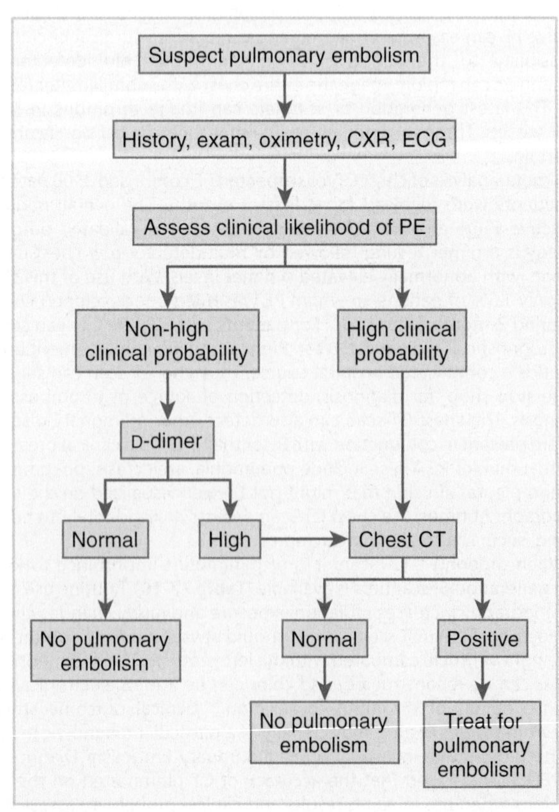

FIGURE 77-5 Integrated diagnostic approach. CXR = Chest x-ray.

Management

Risk Stratification

PE presents with a wide spectrum of illness ranging from mild to severe. Therefore, rapid and accurate risk stratification is of paramount importance. Appropriate care can range from prevention of recurrent PE with anticoagulation alone in low-risk patients to thrombolysis or embolectomy in high-risk patients. High-risk patients may require intensive hemodynamic and respiratory support with pressors or mechanical ventilation while the PE itself is managed with aggressive medical, percutaneous interventional, or surgical therapy (**Fig. 77-6**). The three key components for risk stratification are (1) clinical

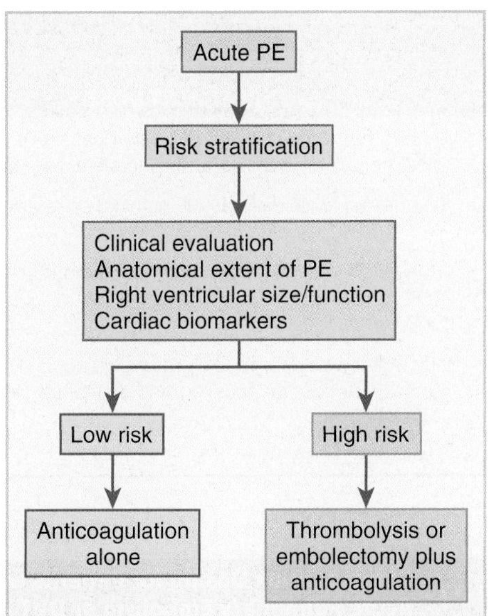

FIGURE 77-6 Management strategy for acute PE, based on risk stratification.

TABLE 77-13 The Pulmonary Embolism Severity Index: Predictors of Low Prognostic Risk

PREDICTOR	SCORE POINTS
Age, per year	Age, in years
Male sex	10
History of cancer	30
History of heart failure	10
History of chronic lung disease	10
Pulse ≥110/min	20
Systolic blood pressure <100 mm Hg	30
Respiratory rate ≥30/min	20
Temperature <36°C	20
Altered mental status	60
Arterial oxygen saturation <90%	20

Low prognostic risk is defined as ≤85 points.

evaluation, (2) assessment of right ventricular size and function, and (3) analysis of cardiac biomarkers such as troponin, pro-BNP, and BNP (even though troponin-based risk stratification has been challenged).[71]

Clinical evaluation is straightforward if the patient looks and feels well and has no evidence of right ventricular dysfunction. The Pulmonary Embolism Severity Index has identified 11 features from demographics, history, and clinical findings that can be weighted and scored to predict good prognosis and to identify low-risk patients[72] (**Table 77-13**). The practitioner can detect right ventricular dysfunction on physical examination by seeking distended jugular veins, a systolic murmur of tricuspid regurgitation, or an accentuated P_2. Obese necks may make jugular vein assessment difficult. Noisy emergency departments can obscure the subtle auscultatory findings of right ventricular dysfunction. Clinical assessment should be supplemented by electrocardiography to look for a right ventricular strain pattern (right bundle branch block, $S_1Q_3T_3$, negative T waves in V_1 through V_4),[60] echocardiography,[73] or chest CT[74] for evidence of right ventricular enlargement, which predicts increased 30-day mortality, and elevated cardiac biomarkers, which indicate right ventricular microinfarction or right ventricular pressure overload and a potentially

TABLE 77-14 Predictors of Increased Mortality

Hemodynamic instability
Right ventricular hypokinesis on echocardiogram
Right ventricular enlargement on echocardiogram or chest CT scan
Right ventricular strain on electrocardiogram
Elevated cardiac biomarkers

TABLE 77-15 Intravenous Unfractionated Heparin "Raschke Nomogram"

VARIABLE	ACTION
Initial heparin bolus	80 units/kg bolus, then 18 units/kg/hr
aPTT <35 seconds (<1.2 times control)	80 units/kg bolus, then increase by 4 units/kg/hr
aPTT 35 to 45 seconds (1.2 to 1.5 times control)	40 units/kg bolus, then increase by 2 units/kg/hr
aPTT 46 to 70 seconds (1.5 to 2.3 times control)	No change
aPTT 71 to 90 seconds (2.3 to 3 times control)	Decrease infusion rate by 2 units/kg/hr
aPTT >90 seconds (>3 times control)	Hold infusion 1 hr, then decrease infusion rate by 3 units/kg/hr

From Raschke RA, Reilly BM, Guidry JR, et al: The weight-based heparin dosing nomogram compared with a "standard care" nomogram: A randomized controlled trial. Ann Intern Med 119:874, 1993.

ominous prognosis[75] (**Table 77-14**). The combination of right ventricular hypokinesis and elevated cardiac biomarkers identifies the highest-risk group of PE patients.[76]

Certain hospital, patient, and socioeconomic factors portend high risk and poor outcome. Patients with PE admitted on weekends have a higher short-term mortality than those admitted on weekdays.[77] Those with a very short length of stay had a greater postdischarge mortality compared with those with a typical length of stay.[78] In a study of 14,426 PE patients discharged from 186 hospitals in Pennsylvania, early readmission after PE occurred in 14% and was associated with black race, Medicaid insurance, and high baseline PE Severity Index (see Table 77-13).[79]

Anticoagulation (see Chap. 87)

UNFRACTIONATED HEPARIN. Heparin is the cornerstone for treatment of acute PE. For patients with average bleeding risk, begin with an intravenous UFH bolus of 80 units/kg, followed by a continuous infusion at 18 units/kg per hour. Target the aPTT between 1.5 and 2.5 times the control value.[80] Commonly, the therapeutic range is 60 to 80 seconds. A nomogram may be helpful for heparin dose adjustment (**Table 77-15**). Although there is a trend toward the use of LMWH for patients who present with acute PE, the shorter half-life of UFH is advantageous for patients who might require insertion of an inferior vena caval filter, thrombolysis, or embolectomy. In patients with active major bleeding, withhold heparin and consider nonpharmacologic treatment with insertion of an inferior vena caval filter. Alternative UFH dosing regimens, used rarely, employ fixed-dose weight-adjusted subcutaneous UFH[81] or adjusted-dose subcutaneous UFH.[82]

UFH is a highly sulfated glycosaminoglycan that is partially purified, most often from porcine intestinal mucosa. Heparin acts primarily by binding to antithrombin, a protein that inhibits the coagulation factors thrombin (factor IIa), Xa, IXa, XIa, and XIIa. Heparin subsequently promotes a conformational change in antithrombin that accelerates its activity approximately 100- to 1000-fold. This prevents additional thrombus formation and permits endogenous fibrinolytic mechanisms

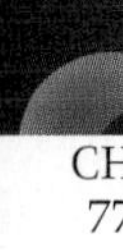

CH 77

TABLE 77-16 Low-Molecular-Weight Heparins

NAME	STATUS	MOLECULAR WEIGHT	ANTI-Xa/ANTI-IIa RATIO	TREATMENT DOSE
Enoxaparin	FDA approved for DVT treatment	4800	3.9	1 mg/kg twice daily (approved as an inpatient or outpatient dose), or 1.5 mg/kg once daily (inpatient dose only)
Dalteparin	FDA approved for cancer-associated DVT	5000	2.2	100 units/kg twice daily, or 200 units/kg once daily
Nadroparin	Not available in the United States	4500	3.5	4100 units twice daily for patients weighing <50 kg, 6150 units twice daily for 50-70 kg, and 9200 units twice daily for >70 kg
Reviparin	Not available in the United States	3900	3.3	3500 units twice daily for patients weighing 35-45 kg, 4200 units twice daily for 46-60 kg, and 6300 units twice daily for >60 kg
Tinzaparin	FDA approved for DVT treatment	4500	1.5	175 units/kg once daily

to lyse clot that has already formed. Heparin does *not* directly dissolve thrombus that already exists. The world's heparin supplies were temporarily contaminated by oversulfated chondroitin sulfate, which caused severe anaphylactoid reactions in some patients.[83,84] Contamination ended after closer factory inspection and additional analytic testing were instituted.

LOW-MOLECULAR-WEIGHT HEPARIN. LMWH consists of fragments of UFH that exhibit less binding than UFH to plasma proteins and endothelial cells. Therefore, LMWH has greater bioavailability, a more predictable dose response, and a longer half-life than UFH. These features permit weight-based LMWH dosing without laboratory tests for dose adjustment in most instances. Consequently, LMWHs have revolutionized the management of DVT and converted the treatment from a mandatory minimum 5-day hospitalization to either an overnight stay or outpatient therapy for most patients (**Table 77-16**). Whereas this approach has been shown to be feasible, safe, and cost-effective in DVT treatment, further data are needed before the strategy of shortened hospital stay can be endorsed for the management of PE.[85]

In 2007, the Food and Drug Administration (FDA) approved the LMWH dalteparin as monotherapy without warfarin in cancer patients with acute VTE. In a trial of 672 patients with VTE and cancer, those randomized to dalteparin monotherapy had a much lower VTE recurrence rate than did patients receiving dalteparin as a "bridge" to warfarin: 8.8% versus 17.4%.[86] At times, LMWH is used off label as monotherapy without warfarin to treat VTE patients without cancer who cannot tolerate warfarin or who suffer recurrent VTE despite warfarin.[87]

LMWH is usually dosed according to weight. However, if a quantitative assay is desired, an anti-Xa level can be obtained. Whether use of anti-Xa levels improves efficacy and safety remains controversial. The plasma anti-Xa level may be useful in five situations: (1) UFH anticoagulation with baseline elevated aPTT caused by a lupus anticoagulant or anticardiolipin antibodies, (2) LMWH dosing in obese patients, (3) LMWH dosing in patients with renal dysfunction, (4) pregnancy, and (5) determination of the origin of an unexpected bleeding or clotting problem in patients receiving what appeared to be appropriate anticoagulant dosing.

FONDAPARINUX. Fondaparinux is an anticoagulant pentasaccharide that specifically inhibits activated factor X. By selectively binding to antithrombin, fondaparinux potentiates (about 300 times) the neutralization of factor Xa by antithrombin. Its predictable and sustained pharmacokinetic properties allow a fixed-dose, once-daily subcutaneous injection, without the need for coagulation laboratory monitoring or dose adjustment. Fondaparinux does not cross-react with heparin-induced antibodies. The FDA has approved fondaparinux for initial treatment of acute PE and acute DVT as a bridge to oral anticoagulation with warfarin.[88] The subcutaneous dosing regimen to treat VTE is straightforward (**Table 77-17**). Fondaparinux is often used off label for the management of suspected or proven heparin-induced thrombocytopenia[89] (see later). At times, fondaparinux is used off label as monotherapy without warfarin to treat VTE patients without cancer who cannot tolerate warfarin or who suffer recurrent VTE despite warfarin.[90] The dose for VTE prophylaxis is a fixed low dose of 2.5 mg once daily, regardless of body weight. However, fondaparinux elimination is prolonged in patients with renal impairment.

TABLE 77-17 Fondaparinux Dosing for Patients with Acute Pulmonary Embolism or DVT

Patient weight	<50 kg	50-100 kg	>100 kg
Daily dose of fondaparinux*	5 mg	7.5 mg	10 mg

*Assumes normal renal function.

HEPARIN-INDUCED THROMBOCYTOPENIA. Heparin-induced thrombocytopenia is a serious,[91] costly,[92] and perhaps increasingly frequent immune-mediated complication.[93] It occurs about 10 times more often with UFH than with LMWH. Immunoglobulin G antibodies bind to a heparin–platelet factor 4 complex and activate platelets, causing release of prothrombotic microparticles, platelet consumption, and thrombocytopenia. The microparticles promote excessive thrombin generation, which can result in paradoxical thrombosis. The thrombosis is usually extensive DVT or PE but can be manifested as myocardial infarction, stroke, or unusual arterial thrombosis such as mesenteric arterial thrombosis. Suspect heparin-induced thrombocytopenia when the platelet count decreases to less than 100,000 or to less than 50% of baseline. Typically, heparin-induced thrombocytopenia occurs after 5 to 10 days of heparin exposure. UFH or LMWH should be immediately discontinued, and platelets should not be transfused. A direct thrombin inhibitor[94] such as argatroban, bivalirudin, or lepirudin should be used.

WARFARIN. Warfarin is a vitamin K antagonist that prevents gamma-carboxylation activation of coagulation factors II, VII, IX, and X. The full anticoagulant effect of warfarin may not be apparent for 5 to 7 days, even if the prothrombin time, used to monitor warfarin's effect, becomes elevated more rapidly. Elevation in the prothrombin time, used to adjust the dose of warfarin, may initially reflect depletion of coagulation factor VII, which has a short half-life of about 6 hours, whereas factor II has a long half-life of about 5 days. The prothrombin time should be standardized and reported according to the international normalized ratio (INR), not the prothrombin time ratio or the prothrombin time expressed in seconds. For VTE patients, the usual target INR range is between 2.0 and 3.0.

WARFARIN OVERLAP WITH HEPARIN. Initiation of warfarin as monotherapy to treat acute VTE without UFH, LMWH, or fondaparinux may paradoxically exacerbate hypercoagulability, increasing the likelihood of recurrent thrombosis. Warfarin monotherapy decreases the levels of two endogenous anticoagulants, proteins C and S, thus increasing thrombogenic potential. Overlapping warfarin for at least 5 days with an immediately effective parenteral anticoagulant counteracts the procoagulant effect of unopposed warfarin.

DOSING AND MONITORING OF WARFARIN. Dosing of warfarin is both an art and a science. Warfarin is traditionally dosed by an "educated guess" coupled with trial and error. Controversy exists over the optimal initial warfarin dose, and whether it should be 5 mg or 10 mg. One open-label, randomized trial compared two warfarin initiation nomograms (5 mg versus 10 mg) in 50 patients with acute VTE.[95] The median time to two consecutive target INRs was 5 days in both groups ($P = 0.69$), whether the initial dose was 5 mg or 10 mg. Nevertheless, most practitioners begin with warfarin 5 mg daily. A new and promising approach is to use computer-assisted warfarin dosing,[96] which appears to be at least as accurate and cost-effective as conventional dosing.[97]

Some patients have unexplained variability in their INR response to warfarin. Large body stores of phylloquinone allow steady clotting factor activation and stable control of anticoagulation. Therefore, although it seems paradoxical and counterintuitive, administration of vitamin K supplementation can improve anticoagulation control in patients with unexplained instability of response to warfarin.[98]

Monitoring of warfarin requires walking a tightrope. High INRs predispose to bleeding complications,[99] but subtherapeutic dosing makes patients vulnerable to recurrent VTE. An overview of more than 22,000 warfarin-treated patients found that their time within the therapeutic INR range was only about 50%.[100] All patients taking warfarin should wear a medical alert bracelet or necklace. This allows emergency medical personnel to reverse warfarin quickly if major trauma causes catastrophic bleeding.

Warfarin is plagued by multiple drug-drug and drug-food interactions. Most antibiotics increase the INR, but some, like rifampin, lower the INR. Even benign-sounding drugs such as acetaminophen increase the INR in a dose-dependent manner. The warfarin dose should be reduced in the management of debilitated or elderly patients. On the other hand, green leafy vegetables have vitamin K and lower the INR. Concomitant medications with antiplatelet effects may increase the bleeding risk without increasing the INR. These include fish oil supplements, vitamin E, and alcohol.

Centralized anticoagulation clinics, staffed by nurses or pharmacists, have eased the administrative burden of prescribing warfarin and have facilitated safer and more effective anticoagulation. In a report encompassing 50,208 patients from 67 studies, patients managed by anticoagulation clinics or clinical trials remained in the therapeutic INR range 66% of the time. However, patients managed by community practices were therapeutic for only 57% of the study period.[101] "Point-of-care" devices provide the INR result within 2 minutes by use of a drop of whole blood obtained from a fingertip puncture. Appropriately selected patients can be taught to obtain their own INRs and to self-manage their warfarin dosing at home. In a meta-analysis of self-monitoring and self-adjustment of oral anticoagulation among 3049 patients in 14 trials, self-monitoring of INR was associated with a 55% reduction in thromboembolic events and a 39% reduction in all-cause mortality compared with conventional management. Those patients capable of both self-monitoring and self-adjustment of therapy had fewer thromboembolic events (73% less) and 63% lower mortality compared with those who undertook self-monitoring alone compared with, conventional management.[102]

WARFARIN PHARMACOGENOMICS. (See Chap. 10.) Genetic determinants of warfarin dose response include CYP2C9 variant alleles, which impair the hydroxylation of *S*-warfarin, resulting in extremely low warfarin dose requirements, and variants in the gene encoding vitamin K epoxide reductase complex 1 (VKORC1). Variability in the INR response to warfarin appears more strongly associated with VKORC1 than with CYP2C9.[103] A multiple regression model using the predictors of CYP2C9, VKORC1, age, sex, and drug interactions explains about half of the variance in warfarin dose.[104] Use of a pharmacogenetic algorithm for initiation of warfarin dosing appears to be of greatest benefit among those patients requiring very high or very low doses of warfarin.[5] This approach may be cost-effective when warfarin is initiated in patients at high risk for hemorrhage.[105] The largest randomized trial to date studied 206 patients who received either pharmacogenetic-guided or standard warfarin dosing. The primary endpoint, reduction in out-of-range INRs, was not achieved in the group undergoing rapid turnaround genetic testing.[106] The National Heart, Lung and Blood Institute (NHLBI) is sponsoring a larger trial (NCT00839657) with more than 1200 patients who will be randomized to a genotype-guided versus clinical-guided warfarin dosing algorithm. The primary endpoint is the percentage of time that participants spend within the therapeutic INR range. Results should be available in 2012.

COMPLICATIONS OF ANTICOAGULATION. The most important adverse effect of anticoagulation is hemorrhage. Major bleeding during anticoagulation may unmask a previously silent lesion, such as bladder or colon cancer. Resumption of anticoagulation at a lower dose or implementation of alternative therapy depends on the severity of the bleeding, the risk of recurrent thromboembolism, and the extent to which bleeding may have resulted from excessive anticoagulation. For management of bleeding caused by heparin, cessation of UFH or LMWH will usually suffice. However, the anticoagulation effect will persist longer with LMWH than with UFH. With life-threatening or intracranial hemorrhage, protamine sulfate can be administered at the time heparin is discontinued. With warfarin, the risk of bleeding increases as the INR increases. The dose of warfarin should be adjusted downward when an "intranormal rise" in the INR occurs, such as an increase from 2.2 to 2.8 in patients whose target INR range is 2 to 3. Ironically, for patients who develop warfarin-associated intracerebral hemorrhage, the INR is often less than 3 at the time of diagnosis.[107] Be aware that an INR specimen that is not assayed promptly after blood collection can be spuriously high. In addition, point-of-care machines generally have higher INRs than central laboratories when the INR value exceeds 4. These abnormally high INR results should be verified with standard central laboratory instrumentation.[108] Life-threatening bleeding caused by warfarin can be managed with enough cryoprecipitate or fresh frozen plasma to normalize the INR and to achieve immediate hemostasis. Recombinant human factor VIIa concentrate can also be used to achieve rapid warfarin reversal.

NOVEL ANTICOAGULANTS. Novel oral anticoagulants[6] promise immediate onset of action and administration in fixed doses without routine laboratory coagulation monitoring. They will compete against warfarin, the only oral anticoagulant licensed in the United States since 1954. These drugs have few drug-drug or drug-food interactions, making them more "user friendly" than warfarin for patients and for health care providers. The onset of action of these new drugs is rapid, and the half-life is short. Therefore, when they must be stopped for a diagnostic or surgical procedure, no "bridging" is needed with a parenteral anticoagulant. Dabigatran is a direct thrombin inhibitor. It has proven noninferior to enoxaparin in three major orthopedic surgery trials of total knee or hip arthroplasty.[9,109] In a large-scale trial of acute VTE, dabigatran was noninferior to warfarin. Rivaroxaban is a factor Xa inhibitor with 80% bioavailability and a 5- to 9-hour half-life. Its efficacy has proven superior to enoxaparin to prevent VTE after total knee[8] and hip[7] arthroplasty. Both dabigatran and rivaroxaban are approved in Canada and Europe for VTE prevention after knee or hip arthroplasty.

OPTIMAL DURATION OF ANTICOAGULATION.

Provoked VTE (Including Cancer)

Management is more straightforward and less controversial for provoked rather than unprovoked VTE (**Table 77-18**). For patients with first-time PE or proximal leg DVT provoked by surgery, trauma, oral contraceptives, pregnancy, or hormone replacement, the optimal

TABLE 77-18 Optimal Duration of Anticoagulation

CLINICAL SETTING	RECOMMENDATION
First provoked PE/proximal leg DVT	3 to 6 months
First provoked upper extremity DVT or isolated calf DVT	3 months
Second provoked VTE	Uncertain
Third VTE	Indefinite duration
Cancer and VTE	Consider indefinite duration or until cancer is resolved
Unprovoked PE/proximal leg DVT	Consider indefinite duration
First unprovoked calf DVT	3 months
Second unprovoked calf DVT	Uncertain

duration of anticoagulation is 3 to 6 months, with a target INR between 2.0 and 3.0. For patients with a first-time isolated calf or upper extremity DVT, with any of the same provoking factors, the optimal duration of anticoagulation is 3 months, with a target INR between 2.0 and 3.0. For a second VTE with the same provoking factors, many clinicians double the duration of anticoagulation, and a few favor indefinite-duration anticoagulation. For a third VTE, a broad and strong consensus supports lifelong anticoagulation.

For patients with cancer and a first episode of DVT, there is now a consensus from the American College of Chest Physicians,[110] the National Comprehensive Cancer Network,[111] and the American Society of Clinical Oncology[112] to manage the first 3 to 6 months of treatment with LMWH as monotherapy without warfarin. Consider continuation of anticoagulation indefinitely or until the cancer has resolved. There is uncertainty as to whether subsequent anticoagulation should be continued with LMWH as monotherapy or whether cancer patients should be switched to warfarin.

Unprovoked VTE

No area of VTE management is more hotly debated than the optimal duration of anticoagulation for idiopathic and unprovoked VTE, which accounts for about half of all PE and DVT cases. Unprovoked VTE includes patients who develop VTE during long-haul air travel or "out of the blue." Recurrent VTE develops more often after discontinuation of anticoagulant therapy among patients with unprovoked events than among those who had provoked VTE. The emerging concept is that VTE is a chronic illness, with latent periods between flares of acute PE or DVT. Those who favor a population-based approach anticoagulate unprovoked VTE patients indefinitely, whereas those who favor a personalized approach consider each patient's clinical profile—including age, sex, comorbid conditions, and thrombophilia workup—to devise an individualized plan for the duration of anticoagulation.[113] Debate also surrounds the intensity of anticoagulation after the first 6 months of therapy. Whereas many continue to use standard-intensity warfarin, with a target INR range between 2.0 and 3.0, a low-intensity anticoagulant regimen with a target INR range between 1.5 and 2.0 is effective and safe.[114]

Recurrent VTE has a high fatality rate, especially when it occurs despite ongoing anticoagulation within the first week of diagnosis.[115] Even after completion of a 6-month course of anticoagulation, the case fatality rate for recurrent PE remains high.[116] Risk factors for recurrent VTE can be subdivided into variables that increase the likelihood of recurrence either while anticoagulants are being taken or after anticoagulants are discontinued (**Table 77-19**). Persistent right ventricular dysfunction on echocardiography after acute PE is an independent risk factor for recurrent VTE.[117] However, it is surprising and counterintuitive that most thrombophilias do not appear to increase the risk of recurrent VTE.[118] Risk factors for recurrent VTE after anticoagulants are discontinued include male sex,[119,120] overweight,[121] initial presentation with symptomatic PE rather than symptomatic DVT,[122] low levels of HDL-cholesterol,[123] and residual DVT with failure to recanalize the deep veins on subsequent venous ultrasonography.[124] Persistent thrombus imaged on chest CT does not predict recurrent PE.

TABLE 77-19 Risk Factors for Recurrent Venous Thromboembolism

While anticoagulants are being taken
Increasing age
Immobilization
Cancer
Chronic obstructive pulmonary disease
Right ventricular enlargement or right ventricular dyskinesis
After anticoagulants are discontinued
Male sex
Overweight
Presenting symptoms of PE rather than DVT
Low levels of HDL-cholesterol
Lack of leg vein recanalization on venous ultrasound examination

About half of PE patients have persistent imaging defects on chest CT 6 months after the initial event.[125]

Persistent abnormally elevated D-dimer levels after withdrawal of anticoagulation may reflect an ongoing hypercoagulable state. In the placebo group of the PREVENT trial, patients with unprovoked VTE received only 6 months of anticoagulation. D-dimer was measured 7 weeks after discontinuation of warfarin.[126] The subsequent recurrence rate was twice as high in those with elevated D-dimer levels. Thus, D-dimer might be useful to identify patients at particularly high risk of recurrence if warfarin is withdrawn after an initial 6 months of anticoagulation. However, an overview of 1888 patients who had unprovoked VTE showed that they had a high 3.5% annual risk of recurrence despite normal D-dimer levels after stopping of anticoagulation.[127] In a separate meta-analysis of patients with idiopathic VTE, those with normal D-dimer levels measured 1 month after discontinuation of oral anticoagulation had a clinically important 7.2% recurrence rate.[128] No guideline committee has endorsed the use of D-dimer levels to direct the optimal duration of anticoagulation.

INFERIOR VENA CAVAL FILTERS. The two major indications for placement of an inferior vena caval filter are major hemorrhage that precludes anticoagulation, and recurrent PE despite well-documented anticoagulation. Eight-year follow-up of a randomized controlled trial of filters shows that filters reduce the risk of PE, increase the risk of DVT, and have no long-term impact on survival.[129] Nevertheless, insertion of filters has markedly increased, with a 25-fold increase in use in the United States during the past two decades.[130] In a prospective DVT registry of 5451 patients at 183 U.S. sites, 14% underwent insertion of filters.[131] Some patients have a temporary contraindication to anticoagulation. Under these circumstances, placement of a nonpermanent, retrievable filter may be appropriate. Retrievable filters can be left in place for weeks to months or can remain permanently, if necessary, because of a trapped large clot or a persistent contraindication to anticoagulation.[132]

FIBRINOLYSIS. When it is successfully used, thrombolysis will reverse right-sided heart failure by physical dissolution of anatomically obstructing pulmonary arterial thrombus, thereby reducing right ventricular pressure overload; prevent the continued release of serotonin and other neurohumoral factors that can worsen pulmonary hypertension; and dissolve thrombus in the pelvic or deep leg veins, thereby at least theoretically decreasing the likelihood of recurrent PE. Thrombolysis may also improve pulmonary capillary blood flow and reduce the likelihood for development of chronic thromboembolic pulmonary hypertension. The American College of Chest Physicians advises: "For patients with evidence of hemodynamic compromise, we recommend use of thrombolytic therapy unless there are major contraindications owing to bleeding risk (Grade 1B).... In selected high-risk patients without hypotension who are judged to have a low risk of bleeding, we suggest administration of thrombolytic therapy (Grade 2B)."[110]

The FDA has approved alteplase for massive PE, in a dose of 100 mg as a continuous infusion during 2 hours, without concomitant heparin. Unlike patients receiving myocardial infarction thrombolysis, patients with PE have a wide "window" for effective use of thrombolysis. Those who receive thrombolysis up to 14 days after new symptoms or signs maintain an effective response, probably because of the bronchial collateral circulation. Guidelines for heparin before and after alteplase are provided in **Table 77-20**.

Thrombolysis in normotensive high-risk PE patients remains controversial.[133] The fear is that the risk of bleeding complications, especially intracranial hemorrhage, outweighs any potential benefit. Women may not gain as much benefit from PE thrombolysis as men do. In a German multicenter PE registry, thrombolysis was associated with a 79% reduction in 30-day mortality in men but no statistically significant reduction in women. Women had a 27% rate of major bleeding compared with 15% in men.[134] The rationale in favor of thrombolysis is that improved survival will ensue. However, a study of patients who received thrombolysis within a cohort of 15,116 PE patients from Pennsylvania does not support this concept.[135] In the International

TABLE 77-20 Use of Heparin Before and After Thrombolysis

1. Discontinue the continuous infusion of intravenous UFH as soon as the decision has been made to administer thrombolysis.
2. Proceed to order thrombolysis. Use the U.S. Food and Drug Administration–approved regimen of alteplase 100 mg as a continuous infusion during 2 hours.
3. Do not delay the thrombolysis infusion by obtaining an activated partial thromboplastin time (aPTT).
4. Infuse thrombolysis as soon as it becomes available.
5. At the conclusion of the 2-hour infusion, obtain a stat aPTT.
6. If the aPTT is 80 seconds or less (which is almost always the case), resume UFH as a continuous infusion without a bolus.
7. If the aPTT exceeds 80 seconds, hold off from resuming heparin for 4 hours and repeat the aPTT. At this time, the aPTT has virtually always declined to <80 seconds. If this is the case, resume continuous infusion of intravenous UFH without a bolus.

Cooperative Pulmonary Embolism Registry, 108 patients presented with massive PE and hypotension. Counterintuitively, among those with massive PE who received thrombolysis, mortality was not reduced.[136]

Thrombolysis is being tested in high-risk normotensive PE patients in an ambitious multicentered European randomized trial that plans to enroll about 1000 patients (NCT00639743). The primary clinical composite endpoint is all-cause mortality or hemodynamic collapse. At Brigham and Women's Hospital, we tend to prescribe thrombolysis when patients have elevation in cardiac biomarkers as well as moderate or severe right ventricular hypokinesis. Despite more than two decades of experience with thrombolysis for acute PE, review of our alteplase-treated patients revealed a major bleeding rate of 19%.[137]

Deep Venous Thrombosis Interventions. Indications for catheter-directed DVT thrombolysis remain controversial because no convincing reduction in post-thrombotic syndrome has yet been demonstrated. Common indications for thrombolysis include extensive iliofemoral or upper extremity venous thrombosis. Totally occlusive venous thrombosis usually does not improve if the agent is infused through a peripheral vein. Therefore, DVT thrombolysis is almost always administered locally through a catheter. This intervention frequently accompanies catheter-directed suction embolectomy, venous angioplasty, or venous stenting. The American College of Chest Physicians guidelines endorse catheter-directed thrombolysis in selected patients with extensive acute proximal DVT (e.g., iliofemoral DVT, symptoms for <14 days, good functional status, life expectancy ≥1 year) who have a low risk of bleeding.[110] The NHLBI is funding a randomized trial of pharmacomechanical catheter-directed thrombolysis versus conventional anticoagulation in approximately 700 patients with iliac or femoral vein DVT (NCT00790335). The primary endpoint is the incidence of post-thrombotic syndrome in each group. Results are expected in 2014.

Catheter Embolectomy. Interventional catheterization techniques[138] for massive PE include mechanical fragmentation of thrombus with a standard pulmonary artery catheter, clot pulverization with a rotating basket catheter, percutaneous rheolytic thrombectomy,[139] and pigtail rotational catheter embolectomy. Another approach is mechanical clot fragmentation and aspiration,[140] which can be combined if necessary with pharmacologic thrombolysis[141] (**Fig. 77-7**). Pulmonary artery balloon dilation and stenting can also be considered. Successful catheter embolectomy rapidly restores normal blood pressure and decreases hypoxemia. Catheter techniques have been limited by poor maneuverability, mechanical hemolysis, macroembolization, and microembolization.

Surgical Embolectomy. Emergency surgical embolectomy with cardiopulmonary bypass has reemerged as an effective strategy for management of patients with massive PE and systemic arterial hypotension or submassive PE with right ventricular dysfunction[142] in whom contraindications preclude thrombolysis (**Fig. 77-8**). This operation is also suited for acute PE patients who require surgical excision of a right atrial thrombus or closure of a patent foramen ovale. Surgical embolectomy can also rescue patients refractory to thrombolysis.[143] The results of embolectomy will be optimized if patients are referred before the onset of cardiogenic shock. In one study, 47 patients underwent surgical embolectomy in a 4-year period, with a 96% survival rate.[144] We perform the procedure off bypass, with normothermia, without aortic cross-clamping or cardioplegic or fibrillatory arrest. Avoidance of blind instrumentation of the fragile pulmonary arteries is imperative. Extraction is limited to directly visible clot, which can be accomplished through the segmental pulmonary arteries.

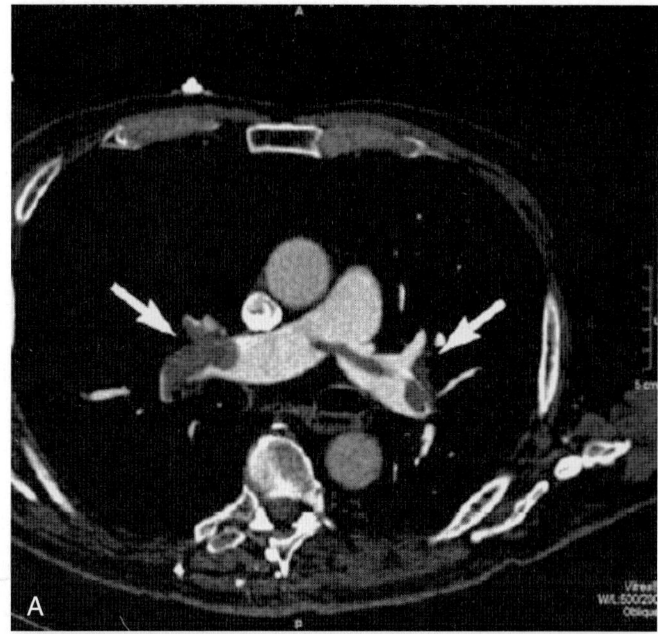

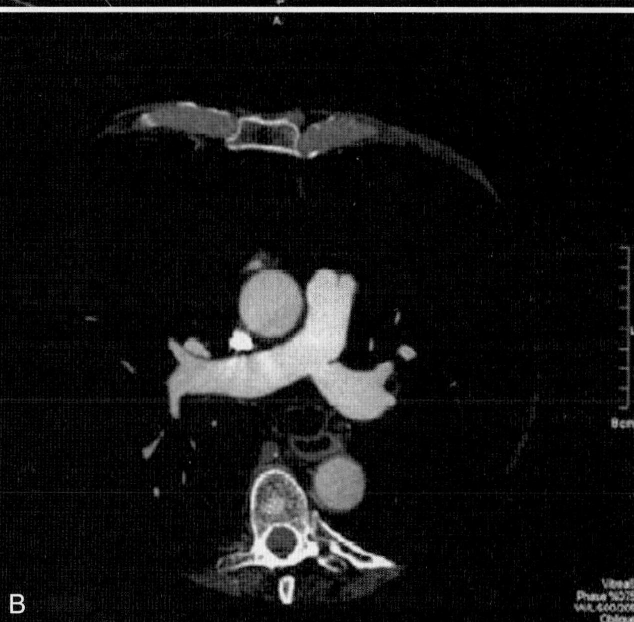

FIGURE 77-7 **A,** Chest CT demonstrates thrombus in the right and left main stem pulmonary arteries, with clot extending into lobar and segmental branches (arrows). **B,** One month after catheter-directed intrapulmonary administration of tissue plasminogen activator and rheolytic thrombectomy, the thrombus has resolved.

Emotional Support. Patients find PE to be emotionally draining. They and their families seek constant reassurance that most patients have good outcomes once the diagnosis has been established. They must confront PE-related issues such as genetic predisposition, potential long-term disability, changes in lifestyle related to anticoagulation, and the possibility of suffering a recurrent event. By discussing the implications of PE with patients and their families, we can help allay the emotional burden. A Pulmonary Embolism Support Group for patients can fill this need. Our group meets at the hospital once monthly in the evening. We discuss the anxieties and day-to-day difficulties that occur in the aftermath of PE.

Massive Pulmonary Embolism. Hospitals should establish written protocols and rehearse interdisciplinary management for patients with

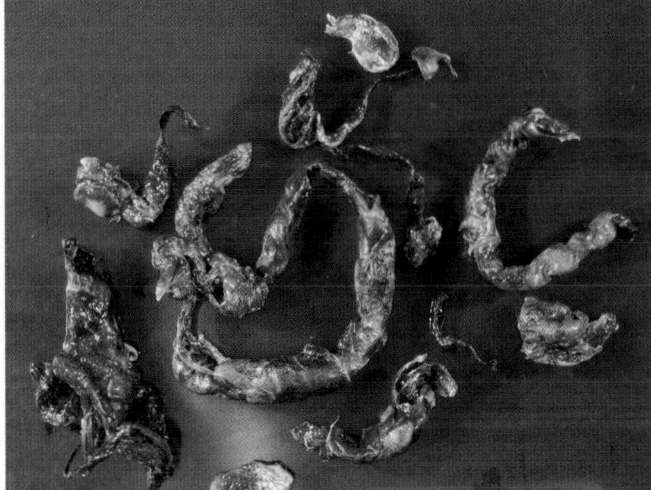

FIGURE 77-8 This 72-year-old woman presented with presyncope, hypotension, and hypoxia. She was diagnosed with massive pulmonary embolism by chest CT scan and underwent emergency pulmonary embolectomy.

TABLE 77-21 Massive Pulmonary Embolism

- Begin bolus high-dose intravenous unfractionated heparin as soon as massive pulmonary embolism is suspected.
- Begin continuous infusion of unfractionated heparin to achieve a target aPTT of at least 80 seconds.
- Try volume resuscitation with no more than 500 to 1000 mL of fluid.
- Excessive volume resuscitation will worsen right ventricular failure.
- Have a low threshold for administration of vasopressors and inotropes.
- Decide whether thrombolysis can be safely administered, without a high risk of major hemorrhage.
- If thrombolysis is too risky, consider placement of an inferior vena caval filter, catheter embolectomy, or surgical embolectomy.
- Do not use a combination of thrombolysis and vena caval filter insertion. The prongs of the filter insert into the caval wall. Concomitant thrombolysis predisposes to caval wall hemorrhage.
- Consider immediate referral to a tertiary care hospital specializing in massive pulmonary embolism.

TABLE 77-22 Regimens for Venous Thromboembolism Prevention

CONDITION	PROPHYLAXIS
Hospitalization with medical illness	Unfractionated heparin 5000 units SC bid or tid *or* Enoxaparin 40 mg SC qd *or* Dalteparin 5000 units SC qd *or* Fondaparinux 2.5 mg SC qd (in patients with a heparin allergy such as heparin-induced thrombocytopenia) *or* Graduated compression stockings or intermittent pneumatic compression for patients with contraindications to anticoagulation Consider combination pharmacologic and mechanical prophylaxis for high-risk patients Consider surveillance lower extremity ultrasonography for intensive care unit patients
General surgery	Unfractionated heparin 5000 units SC bid or tid *or* Enoxaparin 40 mg SC qd *or* Dalteparin 2500 or 5000 units SC qd
Major orthopedic surgery	Warfarin (target INR 2 to 3) *or* Enoxaparin 30 mg SC bid *or* Enoxaparin 40 mg SC qd *or* Dalteparin 2500 or 5000 units SC qd *or* Fondaparinux 2.5 mg SC qd Rivaroxaban 10 mg qd (in Canada and Europe) Dabigatran 220 mg bid (in Canada and Europe)
Neurosurgery	Unfractionated heparin 5000 units SC bid *or* Enoxaparin 40 mg SC qd *and* Graduated compression stockings or intermittent pneumatic compression Consider surveillance lower extremity ultrasonography
Oncologic surgery	Enoxaparin 40 mg SC qd
Thoracic surgery	Unfractionated heparin 5000 units SC tid *and* Graduated compression stockings or intermittent pneumatic compression

INR = international normalized ratio; qd = daily; SC = subcutaneous; bid = twice daily; tid = three times daily.

massive PE.[52] The policies and procedures to treat massive PE should become as firmly established and enforced as those for acute ST-segment elevation myocardial infarction. **Table 77-21** presents some management tips. Rapid integration of historical information, physical findings, and laboratory data and coordination with a team composed of cardiologists, cardiac surgeons, emergency department physicians, radiologists, and other specialists are crucial to maximize success. Immediate patient referral to hospitals specializing in massive PE should be considered.

Post-Thrombotic Syndrome and Chronic Venous Insufficiency. Dysfunction of the valves of the deep venous system often results from damage due to prior DVT.[145] Obstruction of the deep veins may limit the outflow of blood, causing increased venous pressure with muscle contraction. Abnormal hemodynamics in the large veins of the leg are transmitted into the microcirculation. The eventual result is venous microangiopathy. Physical findings may include varicose veins, abnormal pigmentation of the medial malleolus, and skin ulceration. The economic impact is high because of time lost from work and the expense of medical diagnosis and treatment. Chronic venous disease is associated with a reduced quality of life due to pain, decreased physical function, and decreased mobility. A mainstay of therapy is vascular compression stockings, below knee, 30 to 40 mm Hg. Compression stockings improve venous hemodynamics, reduce edema, and minimize skin discoloration. By alleviation of calf discomfort, stockings improve the quality of life. Risk factors for development of post-thrombotic syndrome include proximal (rather than calf) DVT, male sex, and high D-dimer levels after completion of a course of anticoagulation.[146]

Chronic Thromboembolic Pulmonary Hypertension. Chronic thromboembolic pulmonary hypertension occurs much more frequently after acute PE than previously believed.[147] The old teaching was that chronic thromboembolic pulmonary hypertension had a prevalence of 1 in 500 or 1 in 1000 cases of acute PE. New data indicate that the frequency is between 1% and 4%. Although acute PE is the initiating event, pulmonary vascular remodeling may cause severe pulmonary hypertension out of proportion to the pulmonary vascular obliteration observed on pulmonary angiography.[148] Primary therapy is pulmonary thromboendarterectomy, which, if successful, can reduce and at times even cure pulmonary hypertension.[149] The operation involves a median sternotomy, institution of cardiopulmonary bypass, and deep hypothermia with circulatory arrest periods. Incisions are made in both pulmonary arteries into the lower lobe branches. Sildenafil[150] and bosentan,[151] which are established therapies for idiopathic pulmonary hypertension, also appear promising for the treatment of chronic thromboembolic pulmonary hypertension.

Prevention

PE is the most preventable cause of in-hospital death. However, once it occurs, PE is difficult to diagnose, expensive to treat, and potentially lethal despite therapy. Therefore, VTE prevention is of paramount importance. Low fixed-dose anticoagulant prophylaxis is effective.[152] Fortunately, numerous prophylaxis options are available (**Table 77-22**). North American[15] and European[153] consensus conferences have recommended detailed guidelines using various mechanical measures and pharmacologic agents. Often, multiple options are available for each category of risk. Computer-generated alerts to physicians whose hospitalized patients are not receiving prophylaxis can reduce the frequency of symptomatic PE and DVT[19] and maintain effectiveness over time.[154]

There appears to be a failure-to-use-prophylaxis phenomenon. The problem is more widespread among medical service patients than among surgical service patients. For example, 227 American hospitals were surveyed for medical patients 40 years of age or older and requiring at least 6 days of hospitalization without contraindications to anticoagulation.[155] Almost 200,000 patients were identified, all of whom should have received VTE prophylaxis. However, only 62% received any preventive measures, and only 38% received prophylaxis administered in accordance with the American College of Chest Physicians 8th Edition guidelines (2008).

Failure to use prophylaxis during hospitalization has adverse effects that continue after hospital discharge.[18] In a survey of 1897 patients with VTE in the Worcester, Massachusetts, area, 74% developed DVT or PE in the outpatient setting. Of the 516 who had been hospitalized within the prior 3 months and subsequently developed VTE, 67% developed VTE within 1 month after the hospitalization. These findings indicate the need to consider extension of VTE prophylaxis after hospital discharge.

Medicare will not pay the incremental cost to manage a "never event," defined as a medical complication that should never happen. Rather, the hospital bears the additional financial burden. In 2008, Medicare selected the occurrence of VTE after total knee or hip replacement to be listed as a never event.[156] It is now clear that the fiercely independent practitioner, who used to be free to accept or to reject VTE prophylaxis without oversight, is a fading memory destined to become a footnote in the history of medicine.

Mechanical Measures

Mechanical measures consist of intermittent pneumatic compression devices, which enhance endogenous fibrinolysis and increase venous blood flow, and graduated compression stockings. Mechanical measures are prescribed for patients who have an absolute contraindication to anticoagulation. A meta-analysis of intermittent pneumatic compression devices was undertaken in 2270 postoperative patients from 15 studies. In comparison to no prophylaxis, intermittent pneumatic compression devices reduced the risk of DVT by 60%.[157] They also appear to be cost-effective.[158] However, in a large study of stroke patients, thigh-high graduated compression did not confer protection.[159] Pharmacologic prophylaxis appears to be more effective.[160]

Pharmacologic Agents

Pharmacologic prophylaxis options include low fixed-dose UFH, LMWH, fondaparinux, and full-dose warfarin. The American College of Chest Physicians does not consider aspirin to confer meaningful prophylaxis against VTE.

Unconventional Approaches

VITAMIN E. The Women's Health Study randomized 39,876 women to receive 600 units of vitamin E or placebo.[161] After a median follow-up of 10 years, there was a 21% reduction in VTE among women assigned to vitamin E. The reduction was most striking among women with VTE before randomization (44% reduction) and in women with either the factor V Leiden mutation or the prothrombin gene mutation (49% reduction). These data suggest that supplementation with vitamin E may reduce VTE risk in women, especially those with a prior history of VTE or with a genetic predisposition.

STATINS. Observational studies suggest that statins as a class reduce VTE. In the JUPITER study, 17,802 apparently healthy men and women with both low-density lipoprotein cholesterol levels of less than 130 mg/dL and high-sensitivity C-reactive protein levels of 2.0 mg/dL or higher were randomized to receive rosuvastatin, 20 mg/day, or placebo.[10] During a median follow-up period of 1.9 years, the prespecified endpoint of symptomatic VTE was reduced by 43% in the rosuvastatin group ($P = 0.007$). Thus, rosuvastatin appears to prevent VTE. Notably, statins do not increase bleeding risk, in contrast to most other pharmacologic approaches to VTE prevention.

Future Perspectives

PE and DVT are major cardiovascular illnesses that cause suffering and death. VTE has much in common with coronary heart disease—risk factors are similar, prevention has not received adequate emphasis, and drug therapy has not been adequately integrated with lifestyle modification. During the next several years, we will witness widespread institution of electronic decision support to prevent in-hospital VTE. Hospitalized patients will subsequently be observed closely after discharge to ensure that preventive efforts are maintained in the community. Public and professional education and awareness of PE and DVT will increase. These trends should reduce the delay in seeking medical assistance and will lead to more rapid diagnosis, risk stratification, and effective therapy. For the minority of patients requiring advanced therapy for massive PE, specialized hospitals modeled after trauma centers will offer catheter-directed thrombolysis, pharmacomechanical thrombectomy, and surgical embolectomy. Novel anticoagulants will be introduced into clinical medicine and will provide increased convenience for the patient and practitioner, and perhaps superior efficacy. Translational and clinical research in VTE will intensify and flourish.

REFERENCES

1. Torbicki A, Perrier A, Konstantinides S, et al: Guidelines on the diagnosis and management of acute pulmonary embolism: The Task Force for the Diagnosis and Management of Acute Pulmonary Embolism of the European Society of Cardiology (ESC). Eur Heart J 29:2276, 2008.
2. Galson S: The Surgeon General's Call to Action to Prevent Deep Vein Thrombosis and Pulmonary Embolism. Available at: http://www.surgeongeneral.gov/topics/deepvein/.
3. North American Thrombosis Forum (www.natfonline.org).
4. Park B, Messina L, Dargon P, et al: Recent trends in clinical outcomes and resource utilization for pulmonary embolism in the United States: Findings from the nationwide inpatient sample. Chest 136:983, 2009.
5. Klein TE, Altman RB, Eriksson N, et al: Estimation of the warfarin dose with clinical and pharmacogenetic data. N Engl J Med 360:753, 2009.
6. Gross PL, Weitz JI: New anticoagulants for treatment of venous thromboembolism. Arterioscler Thromb Vasc Biol 28:380, 2008.
7. Eriksson BI, Borris LC, Friedman RJ, et al: Rivaroxaban versus enoxaparin for thromboprophylaxis after hip arthroplasty. N Engl J Med 358:2765, 2008.
8. Lassen MR, Ageno W, Borris LC, et al: Rivaroxaban versus enoxaparin for thromboprophylaxis after total knee arthroplasty. N Engl J Med 358:2776, 2008.
9. Wolowacz SE, Roskell NS, Plumb JM, et al: Efficacy and safety of dabigatran etexilate for the prevention of venous thromboembolism following total hip or knee arthroplasty. A meta-analysis. Thromb Haemost 101:77, 2009.
10. Glynn RJ, Danielson E, Fonseca FA, et al: A randomized trial of rosuvastatin in the prevention of venous thromboembolism. N Engl J Med 360:1851, 2009.
11. Dentali F, Douketis JD, Gianni M, et al: Meta-analysis: Anticoagulant prophylaxis to prevent symptomatic venous thromboembolism in hospitalized medical patients. Ann Intern Med 146:278, 2007.
12. Anderson FA Jr, Zayaruzny M, Heit JA, et al: Estimated annual numbers of US acute-care hospital patients at risk for venous thromboembolism. Am J Hematol 82:777, 2007.
13. Piazza G, Seddighzadeh A, Goldhaber SZ: Double trouble for 2,609 hospitalized medical patients who developed deep vein thrombosis: Prophylaxis omitted more often and pulmonary embolism more frequent. Chest 132:554, 2007.
14. Piazza G, Seddighzadeh A, Goldhaber SZ: Heart failure in patients with deep vein thrombosis. Am J Cardiol 101:1056, 2008.
15. Geerts WH, Bergqvist D, Pineo GF, et al: Prevention of venous thromboembolism: American College of Chest Physicians Evidence-Based Clinical Practice Guidelines (8th Edition). Chest 133:381S, 2008.
16. Cohen AT, Tapson VF, Bergmann JF, et al: Venous thromboembolism risk and prophylaxis in the acute hospital care setting (ENDORSE study): A multinational cross-sectional study. Lancet 371:387, 2008.
17. Deitelzweig SB, Becker R, Lin J, et al: Comparison of the two-year outcomes and costs of prophylaxis in medical patients at risk of venous thromboembolism. Thromb Haemost 100:810, 2008.
18. Spencer FA, Lessard D, Emery C, et al: Venous thromboembolism in the outpatient setting. Arch Intern Med 167:1471, 2007.
19. Kucher N, Koo S, Quiroz R, et al: Electronic alerts to prevent venous thromboembolism among hospitalized patients. N Engl J Med 352:969, 2005.
20. Piazza G, Rosenbaum EJ, Pendergast W, et al: Physician alerts to prevent symptomatic venous thromboembolism in hospitalized patients. Circulation 119:2196, 2009.

Epidemiology

21. Parasuraman S, Goldhaber SZ: Venous thromboembolism in children. Circulation 113:e12, 2006.
22. Naess IA, Christiansen SC, Romundstad P, et al: Incidence and mortality of venous thrombosis: A population-based study. J Thromb Haemost 5:692, 2007.
23. Cushman M, Tsai AW, White RH, et al: Deep vein thrombosis and pulmonary embolism in two cohorts: The longitudinal investigation of thromboembolism etiology. Am J Med 117:19, 2004.
24. Zee RY, Cook NR, Cheng S, et al: Polymorphism in the beta$_2$-adrenergic receptor and lipoprotein lipase genes as risk determinants for idiopathic venous thromboembolism: A multilocus, population-based, prospective genetic analysis. Circulation 113:2193, 2006.

25. Laporte S, Mismetti P, Decousus H, et al: Clinical predictors for fatal pulmonary embolism in 15,520 patients with venous thromboembolism: Findings from the Registro Informatizado de la Enfermedad TromboEmbolica venosa (RIETE) Registry. Circulation 117:1711, 2008.
26. Zhu T, Martinez I, Emmerich J: Venous thromboembolism: Risk factors for recurrence. Arterioscler Thromb Vasc Biol 29:298, 2009.
27. Goldhaber SZ, Tapson VF: A prospective registry of 5,451 patients with ultrasound-confirmed deep vein thrombosis. Am J Cardiol 93:259, 2004.
28. Sorensen HT, Horvath-Puho E, Pedersen L, et al: Venous thromboembolism and subsequent hospitalisation due to acute arterial cardiovascular events: A 20-year cohort study. Lancet 370:1773, 2007.
29. Ageno W, Becattini C, Brighton T, et al: Cardiovascular risk factors and venous thromboembolism: A meta-analysis. Circulation 117:93, 2008.
30. Borch KH, Braekkan SK, Mathiesen EB, et al: Abdominal obesity is essential for the risk of venous thromboembolism in the metabolic syndrome: The Tromsø study. J Thromb Haemost 7:739, 2009.
31. Rosengren A, Freden M, Hansson PO, et al: Psychosocial factors and venous thromboembolism: A long-term follow-up study of Swedish men. J Thromb Haemost 6:558, 2008.
32. Steffen LM, Folsom AR, Cushman M, et al: Greater fish, fruit, and vegetable intakes are related to lower incidence of venous thromboembolism: The Longitudinal Investigation of Thromboembolism Etiology. Circulation 115:188, 2007.
33. Stein PD, Beemath A, Olson RE: Obesity as a risk factor in venous thromboembolism. Am J Med 118:978, 2005.
34. Smeeth L, Cook C, Thomas S, et al: Risk of deep vein thrombosis and pulmonary embolism after acute infection in a community setting. Lancet 367:1075, 2006.
35. Stein PD, Beemath A, Meyers FA, et al: Incidence of venous thromboembolism in patients hospitalized with cancer. Am J Med 119:60, 2006.
36. Douketis JD, Gu C, Piccioli A, et al: The long-term risk of cancer in patients with a first episode of venous thromboembolism. J Thromb Haemost 7:546, 2009.
37. Marik PE, Plante LA: Venous thromboembolic disease and pregnancy. N Engl J Med 359:2025, 2008.
38. Blanco-Molina A, Trujillo-Santos J, Tirado R, et al: Venous thromboembolism in women using hormonal contraceptives. Findings from the RIETE Registry. Thromb Haemost 101:478, 2009.
39. Cushman M, Kuller LH, Prentice R, et al: Estrogen plus progestin and risk of venous thrombosis. JAMA 292:1573, 2004.
40. Rizkallah J, Man SF, Sin DD: Prevalence of pulmonary embolism in acute exacerbations of COPD: A systematic review and metaanalysis. Chest 135:786, 2009.
41. Mahmoodi BK, ten Kate MK, Waanders F, et al: High absolute risks and predictors of venous and arterial thromboembolic events in patients with nephrotic syndrome: Results from a large retrospective cohort study. Circulation 117:224, 2008.
42. Baccarelli A, Martinelli I, Pegoraro V, et al: Living near major traffic roads and risk of deep vein thrombosis. Circulation 119:3118, 2009.
43. Schreijer AJ, Cannegieter SC, Meijers JC, et al: Activation of coagulation system during air travel: A crossover study. Lancet 367:832, 2006.
44. Chandra D, Parisini E, Mozaffarian D: Travel and risk for venous thromboembolism. Ann Intern Med 151:1, 2009.
45. Rooden CJ, Tesselaar ME, Osanto S, et al: Deep vein thrombosis associated with central venous catheters—a review. J Thromb Haemost 3:2409, 2005.
46. Spencer FA, Gore JM, Lessard D, et al: Venous thromboembolism in the elderly. A community-based perspective. Thromb Haemost 100:780, 2008.

Pathophysiology

47. Segal JB, Brotman DJ, Necochea AJ, et al: Predictive value of factor V Leiden and prothrombin G20210A in adults with venous thromboembolism and in family members of those with a mutation: a systematic review. JAMA 301:2472, 2009.
48. Dalen JE: Should patients with venous thromboembolism be screened for thrombophilia? Am J Med 121:458, 2008.
49. Lim W, Crowther MA, Eikelboom JW: Management of antiphospholipid antibody syndrome: A systematic review. JAMA 295:1050, 2006.
50. Konstantinides S: Pulmonary embolism: Impact of right ventricular dysfunction. Curr Opin Cardiol 20:496, 2005.
51. Piazza G, Goldhaber SZ: The acutely decompensated right ventricle: Pathways for diagnosis and management. Chest 128:1836, 2005.
52. Kucher N, Goldhaber SZ: Management of massive pulmonary embolism. Circulation 112:e28, 2005.
53. Tapson VF: Acute pulmonary embolism. N Engl J Med 358:1037, 2008.

Diagnosis

54. Elliott CG, Goldhaber SZ, Jensen RL: Delays in diagnosis of deep vein thrombosis and pulmonary embolism. Chest 128:3372, 2005.
55. Kabrhel C, Camargo CA Jr, Goldhaber SZ: Clinical gestalt and the diagnosis of pulmonary embolism: Does experience matter? Chest 127:1627, 2005.
56. van Belle A, Buller HR, Huisman MV, et al: Effectiveness of managing suspected pulmonary embolism using an algorithm combining clinical probability, D-dimer testing, and computed tomography. JAMA 295:172, 2006.
57. Douma RA, Gibson NS, Gerdes VE, et al: Validity and clinical utility of the simplified Wells rule for assessing clinical probability for the exclusion of pulmonary embolism. Thromb Haemost 101:197, 2009.
58. Stein PD, Hull RD, Patel KC, et al: D-dimer for the exclusion of acute venous thrombosis and pulmonary embolism: A systematic review. Ann Intern Med 140:589, 2004.
59. Kearon C, Ginsberg JS, Douketis J, et al: An evaluation of D-dimer in the diagnosis of pulmonary embolism: A randomized trial. Ann Intern Med 144:812, 2006.
60. Vanni S, Polidori G, Vergara R, et al: Prognostic value of ECG among patients with acute pulmonary embolism and normal blood pressure. Am J Med 122:257, 2009.
61. Stein PD, Kayali F, Olson RE: Trends in the use of diagnostic imaging in patients hospitalized with acute pulmonary embolism. Am J Cardiol 93:1316, 2004.
62. Goldhaber SZ: Multislice computed tomography for pulmonary embolism—a technological marvel. N Engl J Med 352:1812, 2005.
63. Quiroz R, Kucher N, Zou KH, et al: Clinical validity of a negative computed tomography scan in patients with suspected pulmonary embolism: A systematic review. JAMA 293:2012, 2005.
64. Perrier A, Roy PM, Sanchez O, et al: Multidetector-row computed tomography in suspected pulmonary embolism. N Engl J Med 352:1760, 2005.
65. Hunsaker AR, Zou KH, Poh AC, et al: Routine pelvic and lower extremity CT venography in patients undergoing pulmonary CT angiography. AJR Am J Roentgenol 190:322, 2008.
66. Schoepf UJ, Goldhaber SZ, Costello P: Spiral computed tomography for acute pulmonary embolism. Circulation 109:2160, 2004.
67. Stein PD, Fowler SE, Goodman LR, et al: Multidetector computed tomography for acute pulmonary embolism. N Engl J Med 354:2317, 2006.
68. Stein PD, Chenevert TL, Fowler SE, et al. Gadolinium-enhanced magnetic resonance angiography for pulmonary embolism: a multicenter prospective study (PIOPED III). Ann Intern Med 152:434, 2010.
69. Schellong SM, Beyer J, Kakkar AK, et al: Ultrasound screening for asymptomatic deep vein thrombosis after major orthopaedic surgery: The VENUS study. J Thromb Haemost 5:1431, 2007.
70. Righini M, Le Gal G, Aujesky D, et al: Diagnosis of pulmonary embolism by multidetector CT alone or combined with venous ultrasonography of the leg: A randomised non-inferiority trial. Lancet 371:1343, 2008.

Management

71. Jimenez D, Uresandi F, Otero R, et al: Troponin-based risk stratification of patients with acute nonmassive pulmonary embolism: Systematic review and metaanalysis. Chest 136:974, 2009.
72. Donze J, Le Gal G, Fine MJ, et al: Prospective validation of the Pulmonary Embolism Severity Index. A clinical prognostic model for pulmonary embolism. Thromb Haemost 100:943, 2008.
73. Fremont B, Pacouret G, Jacobi D, et al: Prognostic value of echocardiographic right/left ventricular end-diastolic diameter ratio in patients with acute pulmonary embolism: Results from a monocenter registry of 1,416 patients. Chest 133:358, 2008.
74. Schoepf UJ, Kucher N, Kipfmueller F, et al: Right ventricular enlargement on chest computed tomography: A predictor of early death in acute pulmonary embolism. Circulation 110:3276, 2004.
75. Becattini C, Vedovati MC, Agnelli G: Prognostic value of troponins in acute pulmonary embolism: A meta-analysis. Circulation 116:427, 2007.
76. Scridon T, Scridon C, Skali H, et al: Prognostic significance of troponin elevation and right ventricular enlargement in acute pulmonary embolism. Am J Cardiol 96:303, 2005.
77. Aujesky D, Jimenez D, Mor MK, et al: Weekend versus weekday admission and mortality after acute pulmonary embolism. Circulation 119:962, 2009.
78. Aujesky D, Stone RA, Kim S, et al: Length of hospital stay and postdischarge mortality in patients with pulmonary embolism: A statewide perspective. Arch Intern Med 168:706, 2008.
79. Aujesky D, Mor MK, Geng M, et al: Predictors of early hospital readmission after acute pulmonary embolism. Arch Intern Med 169:287, 2009.
80. Konstantinides S: Clinical practice. Acute pulmonary embolism. N Engl J Med 359:2804, 2008.
81. Kearon C, Ginsberg JS, Julian JA, et al: Comparison of fixed-dose weight-adjusted unfractionated heparin and low-molecular-weight heparin for acute treatment of venous thromboembolism. JAMA 296:935, 2006.
82. Prandoni P, Carnovali M, Marchiori A: Subcutaneous adjusted-dose unfractionated heparin vs fixed-dose low-molecular-weight heparin in the initial treatment of venous thromboembolism. Arch Intern Med 164:1077, 2004.
83. Blossom DB, Kallen AJ, Patel PR, et al: Outbreak of adverse reactions associated with contaminated heparin. N Engl J Med 359:2674, 2008.
84. Kishimoto TK, Viswanathan K, Ganguly T, et al: Contaminated heparin associated with adverse clinical events and activation of the contact system. N Engl J Med 358:2457, 2008.
85. Hull RD: Treatment of pulmonary embolism: The use of low-molecular-weight heparin in the inpatient and outpatient settings. Thromb Haemost 99:502, 2008.
86. Lee AY, Levine MN, Baker RI, et al: Low-molecular-weight heparin versus a coumarin for the prevention of recurrent venous thromboembolism in patients with cancer. N Engl J Med 349:146, 2003.
87. Kucher N, Quiroz R, McKean S, et al: Extended enoxaparin monotherapy for acute symptomatic pulmonary embolism. Vasc Med 10:251, 2005.
88. Buller HR, Davidson BL, Decousus H, et al: Fondaparinux or enoxaparin for the initial treatment of symptomatic deep venous thrombosis: A randomized trial. Ann Intern Med 140:867, 2004.
89. Baroletti S, Labreche M, Niles M, et al: Prescription of fondaparinux in hospitalised patients. Thromb Haemost 101:1091, 2009.
90. Shetty R, Seddighzadeh A, Parasuraman S, et al: Once-daily fondaparinux monotherapy without warfarin for long-term treatment of venous thromboembolism. Thromb Haemost 98:1384, 2007.
91. Oliveira GB, Crespo EM, Becker RC, et al: Incidence and prognostic significance of thrombocytopenia in patients treated with prolonged heparin therapy. Arch Intern Med 168:94, 2008.
92. Baroletti S, Piovella C, Fanikos J, et al: Heparin-induced thrombocytopenia (HIT): Clinical and economic outcomes. Thromb Haemost 100:1130, 2008.
93. Arepally GM, Ortel TL: Clinical practice. Heparin-induced thrombocytopenia. N Engl J Med 355:809, 2006.
94. Di Nisio M, Middeldorp S, Buller HR: Direct thrombin inhibitors. N Engl J Med 353:1028, 2005.
95. Quiroz R, Gerhard-Herman M, Kosowsky JM, et al: Comparison of a single end point to determine optimal initial warfarin dosing (5 mg versus 10 mg) for venous thromboembolism. Am J Cardiol 98:535, 2006.
96. Poller L, Keown M, Ibrahim S, et al: A multicentre randomised assessment of the DAWN AC computer-assisted oral anticoagulant dosage program. Thromb Haemost 101:487, 2009.
97. Jowett S, Bryan S, Poller L, et al: The cost-effectiveness of computer-assisted anticoagulant dosage: Results from the European Action on Anticoagulation (EAA) multicentre study. J Thromb Haemost 7:1482, 2009.
98. Sconce E, Avery P, Wynne H, et al: Vitamin K supplementation can improve stability of anticoagulation for patients with unexplained variability in response to warfarin. Blood 109:2419, 2007.

99. Koo S, Kucher N, Nguyen PL, et al: The effect of excessive anticoagulation on mortality and morbidity in hospitalized patients with anticoagulant-related major hemorrhage. Arch Intern Med 164:1557, 2004.
100. Baker WL, Cios DA, Sander SD, et al: Meta-analysis to assess the quality of warfarin control in atrial fibrillation patients in the United States. J Manag Care Pharm 15:244, 2009.
101. van Walraven C, Jennings A, Oake N, et al: Effect of study setting on anticoagulation control: A systematic review and metaregression. Chest 129:1155, 2006.
102. Heneghan C, Alonso-Coello P, Garcia-Alamino JM, et al: Self-monitoring of oral anticoagulation: A systematic review and meta-analysis. Lancet 367:404, 2006.
103. Schwarz UI, Ritchie MD, Bradford Y, et al: Genetic determinants of response to warfarin during initial anticoagulation. N Engl J Med 358:999, 2008.
104. Wadelius M, Chen LY, Lindh JD, et al: The largest prospective warfarin-treated cohort supports genetic forecasting. Blood 113:784, 2009.
105. Eckman MH, Rosand J, Greenberg SM, et al: Cost-effectiveness of using pharmacogenetic information in warfarin dosing for patients with nonvalvular atrial fibrillation. Ann Intern Med 150:73, 2009.
106. Anderson JL, Horne BD, Stevens SM, et al: Randomized trial of genotype-guided versus standard warfarin dosing in patients initiating oral anticoagulation. Circulation 116:2563, 2007.
107. Rosand J, Eckman MH, Knudsen KA, et al: The effect of warfarin and intensity of anticoagulation on outcome of intracerebral hemorrhage. Arch Intern Med 164:880, 2004.
108. Dorfman DM, Goonan EM, Boutilier MK, et al: Point-of-care (POC) versus central laboratory instrumentation for monitoring oral anticoagulation. Vasc Med 10:23, 2005.
109. Eikelboom JE, Weitz JI: Dabigatran etexilate for prevention of venous thromboembolism. Thromb Haemost 101:2, 2009.
110. Kearon C, Kahn SR, Agnelli G, et al: Antithrombotic therapy for venous thromboembolic disease: American College of Chest Physicians Evidence-Based Clinical Practice Guidelines (8th Edition). Chest 133:454S, 2008.
111. Wagman LD, Baird MF, Bennett CL, et al: Venous thromboembolic disease. Clinical practice guidelines in oncology. J Natl Compr Canc Netw 4:838, 2006.
112. Lyman GH, Khorana AA, Falanga A, et al: American Society of Clinical Oncology guideline: Recommendations for venous thromboembolism prophylaxis and treatment in patients with cancer. J Clin Oncol 25:5490, 2007.
113. Goldhaber SZ: Optimal duration of anticoagulation after venous thromboembolism: Fixed and evidence-based, or flexible and personalized? Ann Intern Med 150:644, 2009.
114. Ridker PM: Long-term low-dose warfarin use is effective in the prevention of recurrent venous thromboembolism: Yes. J Thromb Haemost 2:1034, 2004.
115. Nijkeuter M, Sohne M, Tick LW, et al: The natural course of hemodynamically stable pulmonary embolism: Clinical outcome and risk factors in a large prospective cohort study. Chest 131:517, 2007.
116. Douketis JD, Gu CS, Schulman S, et al: The risk for fatal pulmonary embolism after discontinuing anticoagulant therapy for venous thromboembolism. Ann Intern Med 147:766, 2007.
117. Grifoni S, Vanni S, Magazzini S, et al: Association of persistent right ventricular dysfunction at hospital discharge after acute pulmonary embolism with recurrent thromboembolic events. Arch Intern Med 166:2151, 2006.
118. Christiansen SC, Cannegieter SC, Koster T, et al: Thrombophilia, clinical factors, and recurrent venous thrombotic events. JAMA 293:2352, 2005.
119. Cushman M, Glynn RJ, Goldhaber SZ, et al: Hormonal factors and risk of recurrent venous thrombosis: The prevention of recurrent venous thromboembolism trial. J Thromb Haemost 4:2199, 2006.
120. Kyrle PA, Minar E, Bialonczyk C, et al: The risk of recurrent venous thromboembolism in men and women. N Engl J Med 350:2558, 2004.
121. Eichinger S, Hron G, Bialonczyk C, et al: Overweight, obesity, and the risk of recurrent venous thromboembolism. Arch Intern Med 168:1678, 2008.
122. Eichinger S, Weltermann A, Minar E, et al: Symptomatic pulmonary embolism and the risk of recurrent venous thromboembolism. Arch Intern Med 164:92, 2004.
123. Eichinger S, Pecheniuk NM, Hron G, et al: High-density lipoprotein and the risk of recurrent venous thromboembolism. Circulation 115:1609, 2007.
124. Prandoni P, Prins MH, Lensing AW, et al: Residual thrombosis on ultrasonography to guide the duration of anticoagulation in patients with deep venous thrombosis: A randomized trial. Ann Intern Med 150:577, 2009.
125. Nijkeuter M, Hovens MM, Davidson BL, et al: Resolution of thromboemboli in patients with acute pulmonary embolism: A systematic review. Chest 129:192, 2006.
126. Shrivastava S, Ridker PM, Glynn RJ, et al: D-dimer, factor VIII coagulant activity, low-intensity warfarin and the risk of recurrent venous thromboembolism. J Thromb Haemost 4:1208, 2006.
127. Verhovsek M, Douketis JD, Yi Q, et al: Systematic review: D-dimer to predict recurrent disease after stopping anticoagulant therapy for unprovoked venous thromboembolism. Ann Intern Med 149:481, W494, 2008.
128. Bruinstroop E, Klok FA, Van De Ree MA, et al: Elevated D-dimer levels predict recurrence in patients with idiopathic venous thromboembolism: A meta-analysis. J Thromb Haemost 7:611, 2009.
129. The PREPIC Study Group: Eight-year follow-up of patients with permanent vena cava filters in the prevention of pulmonary embolism: The PREPIC (Prevention du Risque d'Embolie Pulmonaire par Interruption Cave) randomized study. Circulation 112:416, 2005.
130. Stein PD, Kayali F, Olson RE: Twenty-one-year trends in the use of inferior vena cava filters. Arch Intern Med 164:1541, 2004.
131. Jaff MR, Goldhaber SZ, Tapson VF: High utilization rate of vena cava filters in deep vein thrombosis. Thromb Haemost 93:1117, 2005.
132. Stein PD, Alnas M, Skaf E, et al: Outcome and complications of retrievable inferior vena cava filters. Am J Cardiol 94:1090, 2004.
133. Todd JL, Tapson VF: Thrombolytic therapy for acute pulmonary embolism: A critical appraisal. Chest 135:1321, 2009.
134. Geibel A, Olschewski M, Zehender M, et al: Possible gender-related differences in the risk-to-benefit ratio of thrombolysis for acute submassive pulmonary embolism. Am J Cardiol 99:103, 2007.
135. Ibrahim SA, Stone RA, Obrosky DS, et al: Thrombolytic therapy and mortality in patients with acute pulmonary embolism. Arch Intern Med 168:2183; discussion 2191, 2008.
136. Kucher N, Rossi E, De Rosa M, et al: Massive pulmonary embolism. Circulation 113:577, 2006.
137. Fiumara K, Kucher N, Fanikos J, et al: Predictors of major hemorrhage following fibrinolysis for acute pulmonary embolism. Am J Cardiol 97:127, 2006.
138. Kucher N: Catheter embolectomy for acute pulmonary embolism. Chest 132:657, 2007.
139. Margheri M, Vittori G, Vecchio S, et al: Early and long-term clinical results of AngioJet rheolytic thrombectomy in patients with acute pulmonary embolism. Am J Cardiol 101:252, 2008.
140. Eid-Lidt G, Gaspar J, Sandoval J, et al: Combined clot fragmentation and aspiration in patients with acute pulmonary embolism. Chest 134:54, 2008.
141. Kuo WT, van den Bosch MA, Hofmann LV, et al: Catheter-directed embolectomy, fragmentation, and thrombolysis for the treatment of massive pulmonary embolism after failure of systemic thrombolysis. Chest 134:250, 2008.
142. Sukhija R, Aronow WS, Lee J, et al: Association of right ventricular dysfunction with in-hospital mortality in patients with acute pulmonary embolism and reduction in mortality in patients with right ventricular dysfunction by pulmonary embolectomy. Am J Cardiol 95:695, 2005.
143. Meneveau N, Seronde MF, Blonde MC, et al: Management of unsuccessful thrombolysis in acute massive pulmonary embolism. Chest 129:1043, 2006.
144. Leacche M, Unic D, Goldhaber SZ, et al: Modern surgical treatment of massive pulmonary embolism: Results in 47 consecutive patients after rapid diagnosis and aggressive surgical approach. J Thorac Cardiovasc Surg 129:1018, 2005.
145. Bergan JJ, Schmid-Schonbein GW, Smith PD, et al: Chronic venous disease. N Engl J Med 355:488, 2006.
146. Stain M, Schonauer V, Minar E, et al: The post-thrombotic syndrome: Risk factors and impact on the course of thrombotic disease. J Thromb Haemost 3:2671, 2005.
147. McLaughlin VV, Archer SL, Badesch DB, et al: ACCF/AHA 2009 expert consensus document on pulmonary hypertension: A report of the American College of Cardiology Foundation Task Force on Expert Consensus Documents and the American Heart Association: Developed in collaboration with the American College of Chest Physicians, American Thoracic Society, Inc., and the Pulmonary Hypertension Association. Circulation 119:2250, 2009.
148. Hoeper MM, Mayer E, Simonneau G, et al: Chronic thromboembolic pulmonary hypertension. Circulation 113:2011, 2006.
149. Corsico AG, D'Armini AM, Cerveri I, et al: Long-term outcome after pulmonary endarterectomy. Am J Respir Crit Care Med 178:419, 2008.
150. Suntharalingam J, Treacy CM, Doughty NJ, et al: Long-term use of sildenafil in inoperable chronic thromboembolic pulmonary hypertension. Chest 134:229, 2008.
151. Jais X, D'Armini AM, Jansa P, et al: Bosentan for treatment of inoperable chronic thromboembolic pulmonary hypertension: BENEFiT (Bosentan Effects in iNopErable Forms of chronIc Thromboembolic pulmonary hypertension), a randomized, placebo-controlled trial. J Am Coll Cardiol 52:2127, 2008.

Prevention

152. Wein L, Wein S, Haas SJ, et al: Pharmacological venous thromboembolism prophylaxis in hospitalized medical patients: A meta-analysis of randomized controlled trials. Arch Intern Med 167:1476, 2007.
153. Nicolaides AN, Breddin HK, Carpenter P, et al: Thrombophilia and venous thromboembolism. International consensus statement. Guidelines according to scientific evidence. Int Angiol 24:1, 2005.
154. Lecumberri R, Marques M, Diaz-Navarlaz MT, et al: Maintained effectiveness of an electronic alert system to prevent venous thromboembolism among hospitalized patients. Thromb Haemost 100:699, 2008.
155. Amin A, Stemkowski S, Lin J, et al: Thromboprophylaxis rates in US medical centers: Success or failure? J Thromb Haemost 5:1610, 2007.
156. Streiff MB, Haut ER: The CMS ruling on venous thromboembolism after total knee or hip arthroplasty: Weighing risks and benefits. JAMA 301:1063, 2009.
157. Urbankova J, Quiroz R, Kucher N, et al: Intermittent pneumatic compression and deep vein thrombosis prevention. A meta-analysis in postoperative patients. Thromb Haemost 94:1181, 2005.
158. Nicolaides A, Goldhaber SZ, Maxwell GL, et al: Cost benefit of intermittent pneumatic compression for venous thromboembolism prophylaxis in general surgery. Int Angiol 27:500, 2008.
159. Dennis M, Sandercock PA, Reid J, et al: Effectiveness of thigh-length graduated compression stockings to reduce the risk of deep vein thrombosis after stroke (CLOTS trial 1): A multicentre, randomised controlled trial. Lancet 373:1958, 2009.
160. Turpie AG, Bauer KA, Caprini JA, et al: Fondaparinux combined with intermittent pneumatic compression vs. intermittent pneumatic compression alone for prevention of venous thromboembolism after abdominal surgery: A randomized, double-blind comparison. J Thromb Haemost 5:1854, 2007.
161. Glynn RJ, Ridker PM, Goldhaber SZ, et al: Effects of random allocation to vitamin E supplementation on the occurrence of venous thromboembolism: Report from the Women's Health Study. Circulation 116:1497, 2007.

CHAPTER 78 Pulmonary Hypertension

Stuart Rich

Normal Pulmonary Circulation

The lung has a unique double arterial blood supply from the pulmonary and bronchial arteries, as well as double venous drainage into the pulmonary and azygos veins.[1] Each pulmonary artery accompanies the appropriate-generation bronchus and divides with it down to the level of the respiratory bronchiole. The pulmonary arteries are classified as elastic or muscular. The elastic arteries are conducting vessels, highly distensible at low transmural pressure. As the arteries decrease in size, the number of elastic laminae decreases and smooth muscle increases. Eventually, in vessels between 100 and 500 μm, elastic tissue is lost from the media and the arteries become muscular. The intima of the pulmonary arteries consists of a single layer of endothelial cells and their basement membrane. The adventitia is composed of dense connective tissue in direct continuity with the peribronchial connective tissue sheath. The muscular arteries are 500 μm in diameter or smaller and are characterized by a muscular media bounded by internal and external elastic laminae. Arterioles are precapillary arteries smaller than 100 μm in outer diameter and composed solely of a thin intima and single elastic lamina. The alveolar capillaries are lined with a continuous layer of endothelium resting on a continuous basement membrane and focally connected to scattered pericytes located beneath the basement membrane. Within the respiratory units, the pulmonary arteries and arterioles are centrally located and give rise to precapillary arterioles, from which a network of capillaries radiates into the alveolar walls. The alveolar capillaries collect at the periphery of the acini and then drain into venules located in the interlobular and interlobar septa.

The bronchial circulation provides nutrition to the airways. The bronchial arteries ramify into a capillary network drained by bronchial veins; some empty into the pulmonary veins, and the remainder empty into the systemic venous bed. The bronchial circulation therefore constitutes a physiologic right-to-left shunt. Normally, blood flow through this system amounts to approximately 1% of the cardiac output; the resulting desaturation of left atrial blood is usually trivial. However, in some forms of pulmonary disease (e.g., severe bronchiectasis) and in the presence of many congenital cardiovascular malformations that cause cyanosis, blood flow through the bronchial circulation can increase to as much as 30% of left ventricular output and produce a significant right-to-left shunt.

The pulmonary circulation is characterized by high flow and by low pressure and low resistance (**Table 78-1**) The normal pulmonary vascular bed offers less than 10% of the resistance to flow offered by the systemic bed and can be approximated as the ratio of pressure drop (ΔP, in mm Hg) to mean flow (Q, in liters per minute). The ratio can be multiplied by 80 to express the results in dyne-sec · cm^{-5}, or expressed in mm Hg/liter/min, which is referred to as a Wood unit. The calculated pulmonary vascular resistance in normal adults is 67 ± 23 (standard deviation, SD) dyne-sec · cm^{-5}, or 1 Wood unit.

FETAL AND NEONATAL CIRCULATION. In the fetus, oxygenated blood enters the heart from the inferior vena cava and streams across the foramen ovale to the left atrium (see Chap. 65). Desaturated blood returns from the superior vena cava and into the right ventricle and pulmonary artery. Because the resistance of the pulmonary vascular bed in the collapsed fetal lung is extremely high, only 10% to 30% of the right ventricular output passes through the lungs, with the remainder being shunted across the ductus arteriosus to the descending aorta and then back to the placenta. An abrupt change in the pulmonary circulation occurs at birth. With the first breath, expansion of the lungs and the abrupt rise in the partial pressure of oxygen (P_{O_2}) of blood lead to a reversal of pulmonary arteriolar vasoconstriction and stretching and dilation of muscular pulmonary arteries and arterioles, with a marked drop in vascular resistance. This decreased resistance facilitates a large increase in pulmonary blood flow and raises left atrial volume and pressure. The latter closes the flap valve of the foramen ovale, and interatrial right-to-left shunting ordinarily ceases within the first hour of life. Normally, the ductus arteriosus closes over the next 10 hours as a result of contraction of the thick smooth muscle bundles within its wall in response to rising arterial oxygen tension and a change in the prostaglandin milieu. Following the initial dramatic fall in pulmonary vascular resistance at birth, a continuous decline occurs over the first few months of life, associated with thinning of the media of muscular pulmonary arteries and arterioles until the normal adult pattern is achieved.

AGING. In older adults, the main pulmonary artery becomes mildly dilated, and shallow atheromas may develop in the elastic pulmonary arteries. Mild medial thickening and eccentric intimal fibrosis may occur in the muscular pulmonary arteries; the capillaries become slightly thicker and the veins are frequently involved by intimal hyalinization, with mild luminal narrowing. Pulmonary artery pressure and pulmonary vascular resistance increase with advanced age. Changes in the pulmonary arteries are also affected by the reduced compliance of left ventricular filling with age that is reflected back in the pulmonary vascular bed.

EXERCISE. With moderate exercise, a large increase in pulmonary blood flow is normally accompanied by only a small increase in pulmonary artery pressure. Exercise results in an increase in left atrial pressure that is progressive with exercise intensity and accounts for most of the increase in observed pulmonary arterial pressure. This

TABLE 78-1 Hemodynamic Comparison of the Pulmonary and Systemic Circulations

	Pulmonary Circulation		*Systemic Circulation*	
PARAMETER	RANGE	MEAN	RANGE	MEAN
Arterial pressure, mm Hg	25/10	15	120/80	90
Capillary pressure, mm Hg	6-9	7	10-30	17
Venous pressure, mm Hg	1-4	2	0-10	6
Arterial M/D ratio, %*	3-7	5	15-25	20
Venous M/D ratio, %*	2-5	3	3-6	5
Vascular resistance, units	1-4	3	10-25	15
Blood flow, liter/min	4-6	5	4-6	5

*M/D ratio = ratio of the medial thickness to the external diameter of the vessel.

marked effect of downstream pressure on upstream pressure is unique to the lung circulation. Because of the high vascular compliance in the normal lung microcirculation, an increase in left atrial pressure that results from the increased flow will act to distend the small vessels, contributing to the fall in pulmonary vascular resistance during exercise.

ALTITUDE. Life at high altitudes is associated with pulmonary hypertension of variable severity, reflecting the range of susceptibilities of different persons to the pulmonary vasoconstrictive effect of chronic hypoxia. Altitude decreases the inspired P_{O_2} because of a decrease in barometric pressure. At sea level, P_{O_2} is on average 150 mm Hg. At high altitudes (3000 to 5500 m), P_{O_2} decreases to 80 to 100 mm Hg and, and at extreme altitudes (5500 to 8840 m), P_{O_2} decreases to 40 to 80 mm Hg. Corresponding alveolar P_{O_2} (P_{AO_2}) and arterial P_{O_2} (P_{aO_2}) depend on the hypoxic ventilatory response and associated respiratory alkalosis. Mild pulmonary hypertension in adults living at high altitudes occurs at rest and may increase substantially with exercise.[2] It is not immediately reversed by breathing of oxygen, does not seem to limit exercise capacity, and is rarely the cause of right ventricular failure. Severe pulmonary hypertension may occur with high-altitude pulmonary edema, subacute mountain sickness, and chronic mountain sickness. Transient right ventricular dysfunction has also been described with strenuous exercise at high altitudes.

Regulation of Pulmonary Vascular Tone and Blood Flow

ALVEOLAR OXYGENATION. Changes in alveolar oxygenation affect the small pulmonary arteries and arterioles by direct gaseous diffusion from the alveoli, respiratory bronchioles, and alveolar ducts in the pulmonary arterioles, even though the latter are upstream in relation to the alveoli. This fact, taken together with evidence for a reduction in pulmonary arterial blood volume during hypoxia, supports the view that the small pulmonary arteries and arterioles are the main sites of vasoconstriction and increased resistance in the pulmonary circulation during hypoxia. Although alveolar oxygen tension is a major physiologic determinant of pulmonary arteriolar tone, a reduction in oxygen tension in the mixed venous blood flowing through the small pulmonary arteries and arterioles may also contribute to pulmonary arterial vasoconstriction.[3]

The effect of oxygen on the pulmonary vasculature is the most distinctive characteristic by which it differs from the systemic vasculature. The hypoxic pulmonary vasoconstrictor response is an important adaptive mechanism in human physiology. Alveolar hypoxia results in local vasoconstriction so that blood flow is shunted away from hypoxic regions toward better ventilated areas of the lung, improving the ventilation-perfusion matching in the lung. Although the acute effects of this response are beneficial, chronic hypoxemia can result in sustained elevation of pulmonary artery pressure, vascular remodeling, and development of pulmonary arterial hypertension (PAH). The response of smooth muscle cells in the pulmonary arteries to hypoxia begins within seconds. Hypoxia causes pulmonary vascular smooth muscle membrane depolarization and inhibition of potassium currents (Kv 1.5 channels) as a result of changes in the membrane redox status. Increased calcium ion (Ca^{2+}) entry into the vascular smooth muscle cells via Ca^{2+} (L-type) channels also mediates hypoxic pulmonary vasoconstriction. Within the cell, Ca^{2+} can be mobilized from the sarcoplasmic reticulum and mitochondrial membrane, or the inner aspect of the cell membrane. Pulmonary vascular tone is also modulated by the balance between local kinase and phosphatase activities.

Whereas acute hypoxia causes reversible changes in vascular tone, chronic hypoxia induces structural remodeling and is mediated by a number of growth factors. The endothelial cell manifests marked changes in permeability, coagulant, inflammatory, and protein synthetic capabilities in response to chronic hypoxic exposure. Distinct smooth muscle cell populations with membrane-bound receptors sensitive to hypoxic activation engage specific intracellular signaling pathways, conferring unique hypoxic proliferative responses. Vascular endothelial growth factor (VEGF), an endothelial cell-specific mitogen, is upregulated during exposure to chronic hypoxia; this is thought to be a protective mechanism. Hypoxia-inducible factor-1α (HIF-1α) has been identified as a nuclear factor that is induced by hypoxia and bound to a site in the erythropoietin response element. HIF-1α represents a vital link between oxygen sensing, gene transcription, and the physiologic adaptation to chronic hypoxia in vivo. Expression of HIF-1α is tightly regulated by cellular oxygen tension. Acidosis increases pulmonary vascular resistance and acts synergistically with hypoxia. In contrast, an increase in arterial P_{CO_2} seems to exert no direct effect but rather operates by way of the induced increase in hydrogen ion concentration. Hypoxia and acidemia frequently coexist and their interaction, which is clinically important, follows a predictable pattern.

NITRIC OXIDE. Nitric oxide (NO) relaxes vascular smooth muscle by raising levels of cyclic guanosine monophosphate (cGMP).[4] Endothelial NO synthase is found in the vascular endothelium of the normal pulmonary vasculature, where it generates NO to regulate vascular tone. Release of NO occurs in response to a multitude of physiologic stimuli, including thrombin and shear stress. In addition to its direct hemodynamic effects, NO inhibits platelet activation and confers an important antithrombotic property on the endothelial surface. NO also inhibits the growth of vascular smooth muscle cells and is probably involved in vascular remodeling in response to injury. NO is also important in the signal transduction of angiogenesis in that VEGF receptor activation results in increased NO production.

ADRENERGIC CONTROL. The pulmonary vasculature expresses both alpha and beta adrenoreceptors, which help regulate pulmonary vascular tone by producing vasoconstriction or vasodilation, respectively. Alpha$_1$ adrenoreceptors in the pulmonary arteries have increased affinity and responsiveness to their agonists when compared with other vessels. The downstream signaling events in alpha$_1$-adrenergic stimulation are an increase in Ca^{2+} levels and activation of protein kinase, which mediate vascular contractile and proliferative responses. The increased sensitivity of alpha$_1$ adrenoreceptors to norepinephrine in the pulmonary arteries may facilitate local regulation of vascular tone in response to acute changes in oxygen concentrations, thereby adjusting regional perfusion. Excessive stimulation of alpha$_1$-adrenergic receptors produces smooth muscle contraction, proliferation, and growth.

Pathobiology of Pulmonary Arterial Hypertension

By definition, the precise cause of idiopathic pulmonary arterial hypertension (IPAH) is unknown, but it likely represents the clinical expression of PAH as the final common pathway from multiple biologic abnormalities in the pulmonary circulation.[5] Our understanding of the underlying pathobiology of pulmonary hypertension associated with clinical disease states has become increasingly complex as a multitude of genetic and molecular pathways have been identified.[6] Overall, it appears that varying degrees of thrombosis, vasoconstriction, vascular proliferation, and inflammation underlie chronic PAH. The initiating cell line remains unclear, but abnormalities in pulmonary endothelial cell (EC) function and pulmonary artery smooth muscle cells (PASMCs) may cause or contribute to the development of pulmonary hypertension in humans.[7] Disease progression is invariably accompanied by worsening of cellular function, which itself can further promote disease progression.

THROMBOSIS. The observation that chronic warfarin anticoagulation has been associated with a marked survival advantage in several longitudinal studies lends support to the important role of thrombosis in PAH.[8] Several lines of evidence point to the widespread development of in situ thrombosis of the small pulmonary arteries, with intraluminal thrombin deposition as an important causative feature of PAH. In studies of pulmonary vascular histopathology in IPAH, the prevalence rates of thrombotic lesions were more than 50%.[9] The promotion of PAH through the coagulation and fibrinolytic systems is likely a result of endothelial dysfunction. Thrombin appears to play a key role. Receptors for thrombin are present on ECs and PASMCs. Thrombin activation directly upregulates angiogenesis-related genes, including VEGF, VEGF receptors, tissue factor (TF), basic fibroblast growth factor (bFGF), and matrix metalloproteinase-2, all of which have been reported to be increased in PAH.[10,11] Thrombin indirectly upregulates the transcription of VEGF by inducing the production of reactive oxygen species (ROS) and the expression of the HIF-1α transcription factor. Thrombin also activates platelets.

There is increased expression of TF in the vasculature of patients with severe PAH. TF activation leads to rapid initiation of coagulation when a vessel is damaged and is involved in the migration and proliferation of PASMCs (**Fig. 78-1**). TF can induce angiogenesis by clotting-dependent mechanisms via thrombin generation and fibrin deposition.[12] Plasma levels of fibrinopeptide A, a byproduct and marker of fibrin generation, are elevated in PAH patients.

Abnormalities in platelet activation and function also occur in PAH. In addition to promoting thrombosis, platelet activation leads to the release of granules that contain mitogenic and vasoconstrictive substances, including VEGF, bFGF, platelet-derived growth factor (PDGF), and serotonin, which contribute to increased endothelial cell proliferation and migration.

VASOCONSTRICTION. The initial report of a patient with IPAH demonstrated a reversible fall in PA pressure in response to intravenous vasodilators. As a result, PAH has traditionally been thought of as a disease of inappropriate pulmonary vasoconstriction. However, clinical experiences from multiple registries and large referral centers have documented that reversible vasoconstriction plays an important role in less than 20% of patients with PAH.[13] Although it has not been possible to relate the presence of vasoreactivity specifically to the vascular changes noted on histology, one study reported a qualitative relationship in patients, showing that those with more advanced lesions had a reduced likelihood to respond to acute vasodilator testing.

An important concept in the pathobiology of PAH is that the disease develops in patients with an underlying genetic predisposition following exposure to specific stimuli, which serve as triggers. The finding of increased pulmonary vascular reactivity and vasoconstriction in patients with IPAH suggests that a vasoconstrictive tendency underlies the development of IPAH in predisposed individuals. Voltage-dependent and calcium-dependent potassium channels found throughout the pulmonary vascular bed (see Chap. 52) modulate pulmonary vascular tone. Inhibition of the voltage-regulated potassium channel by hypoxia or drugs can produce vasoconstriction and has been described in PASMCs harvested from patients with IPAH.[14] It has been suggested that abnormalities in the potassium channel of PASMCs are involved in the initiation or progression of pulmonary hypertension[15] (**Fig. 78-2**).

VASCULAR PROLIFERATION. A striking feature of the pulmonary vasculature in patients with PAH is intimal proliferation, which in some vessels causes complete vascular occlusion. Several growth factors have been implicated in the development of this type of vascular pathology. Enhanced growth factor release, activation, and intracellular signaling may lead to PASMC proliferation and migration, as well as extracellular matrix synthesis.[16] Even advanced lesions show evidence of in situ activity of ongoing synthesis of connective tissue proteins such as elastin, collagen, and fibronectin. In PAH, PASMCs have abnormalities that favor decreased apoptosis and enhanced proliferation. The impaired apoptosis appears to be multifactorial, related to abnormal mitochondrial hyperpolarization, activation of transcription factors such as HIF-1α[17] and the nuclear factor of activated T cells (NFAT),[18] and de novo expression of the antiapoptotic protein survivin.[19] The PASMCs in PAH also display excessive proliferation in response to transforming growth factor-β (TGF-β), which is exacerbated by impaired smooth muscle cell apoptosis.[20] Other processes,

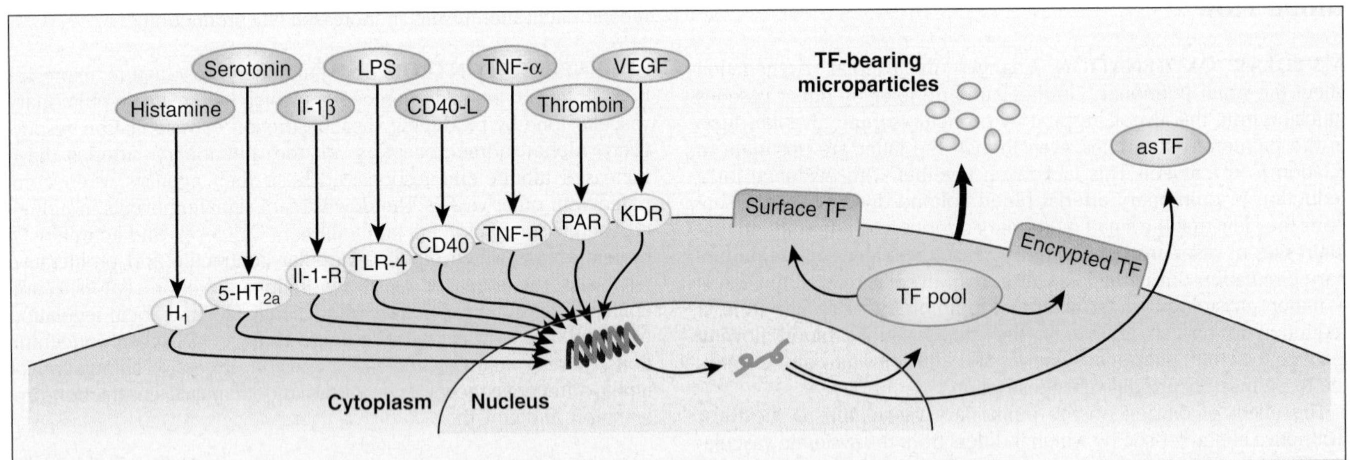

FIGURE 78-1 Molecular mechanisms of thrombosis-mediated remodeling. Induction of tissue factor (TF) is exemplified in an endothelial cell. Various mediators induce TF expression through activation of their receptors. Induction of TF primarily occurs at the transcriptional level, resulting in an increase in TF mRNA and, eventually, in TF protein expression. TF is distributed in three cellular pools as cytoplasmic TF, surface TF, and encrypted TF. Moreover, TF-containing microparticles are released from the cell. Alternative splicing results in a soluble secreted form of TF (asTF). CD40-L = CD40-ligand; H_1 = histamine H1 receptor; 5-HT_{2a} = 5-hydroxytryptamine 2a receptor; IL-1-R = interleukin-1 receptor; KDR = VEGF receptor 2; LPS = lipopolysaccharide; PAR = protease-activated receptor; TLR-4 = Toll-like receptor 4; TNF-R = tumor necrosis factor receptor. *(From Steffel J, Lüscher TF, Tanner FC: Tissue factor in cardiovascular diseases: Molecular mechanisms and clinical implications. Circulation 113:722, 2006.)*

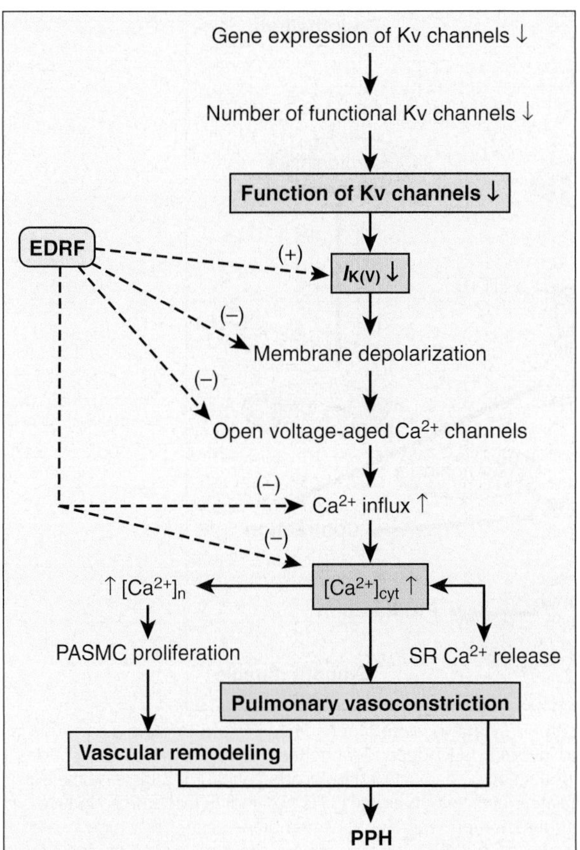

FIGURE 78-2 Molecular mechanisms of vasoconstriction-mediated remodeling. The process may be initiated by abnormal gene transcription and expression of Kv channels. Resultant reduction of Kv currents [$I_{K(V)}$] causes membrane depolarization and opens voltage-gated Ca^{2+} channels. Increased Ca^{2+} influx through sarcolemmal Ca^{2+} channels and Ca^{2+}-induced Ca^{2+} release from intracellular Ca^{2+} stores (mainly sarcoplasmic reticulum [SR]) raise cytoplasmic Ca^{2+} concentrations ($[Ca^{2+}]_{cyt}$), which triggers pulmonary vasoconstriction. An increase in $[Ca^{2+}]_{cyt}$ would also increase nuclear Ca^{2+} concentration ($[Ca^{2+}]_n$) and stimulate cell proliferation, which causes pulmonary vascular remodeling. Endothelium-derived relaxing factors (EDRFs) may participate in regulating Em and $[Ca^{2+}]_{cyt}$ through activation of K^+ (KCa and Kv) channels and/or inhibition of voltage-gated Ca^{2+} channels in PASMCs. (+) = increase (or enhance); (–) = decrease (or inhibit). *(From Yuan J, Aldinger A, Juhaszova M, et al: Dysfunctional voltage-gated K+ channels in pulmonary artery smooth muscle cells of patients with primary pulmonary hypertension. Circulation 98:1400, 1998.)*

such as mitochondrial and ion channel dysregulation, seem to convey a state of cellular resistance to apoptosis; this has recently emerged as a necessary event in the pathogenesis of pulmonary vascular remodeling.

Animal and human data point to a key role for serotonin in PAH (**Fig. 78-3**). Serotonin is an important constituent of platelet-dense granules and is released on activation. It is a vasoconstrictor that promotes smooth muscle cell hypertrophy and hyperplasia by exerting mitogenic effects on PASMCs.[21] Elevated plasma levels of serotonin and reduced platelet serotonin concentration have been described in IPAH patients. One series reported increased serotonin levels in patients with PAH associated with the use of fenfluramine and with connective tissue disease. Data indicate that the serotonin transporter (SERT) in the lung is a key determinant of pulmonary vessel remodeling because of its effects on PASMC growth.[22,23] The SERT is abundantly expressed in the lung and appears specific to PASMCs, because no similar effect has been reported with other SMC types. Mutations in the SERT and 5-hydroxytryptamine 2B receptor have now been reported in patients with IPAH.[24]

INFLAMMATION. The frequent association of PAH in well-defined inflammatory conditions, as well as the presence of PAH associated with connective tissue diseases (CTDs; see Chap. 89), indicate a role for vascular inflammation leading remodeling of the vessel in PAH[25,26] (**Fig. 78-4**). Macrophages and both T and B lymphocytes are present in the vascular lesions of IPAH and PAH related to CTD and human immunodeficiency virus (HIV; see Chap. 72). Inflammatory infiltrates have been identified in plexiform lesions in the lungs of patients with severe IPAH and mononuclear inflammatory cells surround vascular sites of plexiform growth in patients with scleroderma-related PAH. Autoantibodies from patients with CTD have been shown to induce upregulation of immunoactive molecules, such as intercellular adhesion molecule-1, endothelial leukocyte adhesion molecule-1, and major histocompatibility complex class II, on human pulmonary ECs. The nuclear factor of activated T-cells (NFAT) increases the transcription of multiple inflammatory mediators and activating T and B cells.[18] NFAT activation causes myocardial downregulation of Kv1.5, and NFATc2-activated circulating inflammatory cells are found in the blood and pulmonary arterial wall in PAH patients. Several interleukins and tumor necrosis factor-α are increased in patients with PAH,[27] and many of these cytokines are regulated by NFAT.

Inflammation has been observed in affected vessels in HIV patients with PAH, although development of severe PAH seems to be unrelated to the degree of immune deficiency. HIV patients with PAH also had significantly higher autoantibody levels than a matched HIV non-PAH control group. Similarly, the presence of circulating chemokines and cytokines, viral protein components (e.g., HIV-1 Nef), and increased expression of growth factors (e.g., VEGF, PDGF) in these patients are thought to contribute directly to further recruitment of inflammatory cells.[28] Many IPAH patients without immunodeficiency or other associated systemic diseases have evidence of autoimmunity and/or active inflammation. These include detectable levels of antinuclear antibodies, elevated serum levels of the proinflammatory cytokines interleukin-1 (IL-1) and IL-6, and increased pulmonary expression of PDGF or macrophage inflammatory protein-1. Clinically, there is also an association of IPAH with autoimmune thyroid disease

Cellular Pathology of Pulmonary Arterial Hypertension

Morphologic abnormalities in each cell line of the pulmonary vasculature have been described in PAH[29] (**Fig. 78-5**). Although endothelial dysfunction has been described in PAH, it is not known at what stage during the evolution of PAH that EC proliferation occurs. It has been proposed, however, that a somatic mutation rather than nonselective cell proliferation in response to injury accounts for the growth advantage of ECs in patients with IPAH. Heterogeneity in the PASMC and fibroblast populations also contributes to discordance between phenotype and function. Interconversion between cell types (fibroblast to smooth muscle cell, or endothelium to smooth muscle cell), in addition to neovascularization, may occur. PASMC hypertrophy and increased connective tissue and extracellular matrix are found in the large muscular and elastic arteries. In the subendothelial layer, increased thickness may be the result of recruitment and/or proliferation of smooth muscle-like cells. It is possible that precursor smooth muscle cells are in a continuous layer in the subendothelial layer along the entire pulmonary artery. These cells are similar to the pericytes responsible for the appearance of muscle in normally nonmuscular arteries and that contribute to intimal thickening in larger arteries. Alterations in the extracellular matrix secondary to proteolytic enzymes also play a role in the pathology of PAH. Matrix-degrading enzymes can release mitogenically active growth factors that stimulate PASMC proliferation. In addition, elastase and matrix metalloproteinases contribute to the upregulation of proliferation. Degradation of elastin has also been shown to stimulate upregulation of the glycoprotein fibronectin, which in turn stimulates smooth muscle cell migration.

The most common vascular changes in PAH are characterized as a hypertensive pulmonary arteriopathy, which is present in 85% of cases (**Table 78-2**). These changes involve medial hypertrophy of the arteries and arterioles, often in conjunction with other vascular changes. Isolated medial hypertrophy is uncommon and, when present, has

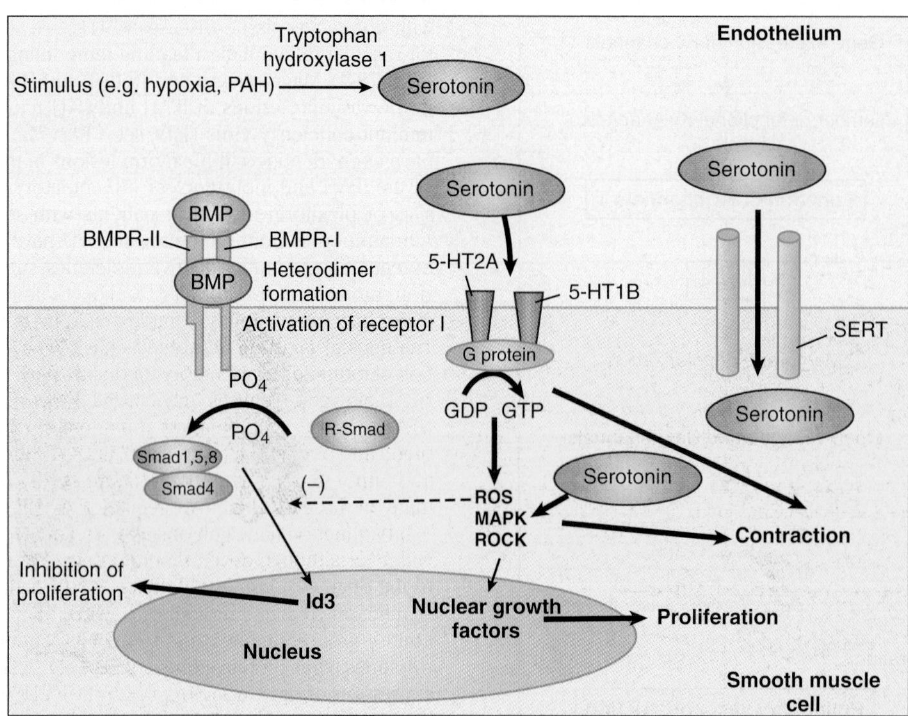

FIGURE 78-3 Molecular mechanisms of cellular proliferation–mediated remodeling. Serotonin synthesis via tryptophan hydroxylase 1 acts in a paracrine fashion on underlying PASMCs. Serotonin enters PASMC via SERT and signal transduction is initiated involving SERT-dependent generation of reactive oxygen species (ROS), rho kinase (ROCK), and mitogen-activated protein kinases (MAPK). This may contribute to contraction or, via nuclear translocation of pERK1/2, increase the expression of nuclear growth factors such as GATA 4, leading to proliferation. Serotonin may also stimulate 5-hydroxytryptamine (5-HT) 1A and 2B receptors to induce contraction and ROS, ROCK, and MAPK activation. Signaling by wild-type BMPRII involves heterodimerization with the transmembrane serine-threonine kinases type I BMPR-IA and BMPR-IB receptors at the cell membrane. On ligand binding, the constitutively active BMPR-II phosphorylates the type I receptor. Activated type I receptors phosphorylate the cytoplasmic signaling proteins known as receptor-mediated Smads (R-Smads) 1, 5, and 8. These complex with Smad4 and translocate to the nucleus, where they activate downstream target genes such as the inhibitors of DNA binding 3 (Ids), which inhibit proliferation. Serotonin may antagonize the antiproliferative BMPR-II/Smad 1, 5, 8 pathway, inhibit Id3 activation, and facilitate proliferation. (–) = inhibitory effect. *(From MacLean MR, Dempsie Y: Serotonin and pulmonary hypertension—from bench to bedside? Curr Opin Pharmacol 9:281, 2009.)*

been assumed to represent an early stage of the disease. The intimal proliferation may appear as concentric laminar intimal fibrosis, eccentric intimal fibrosis, or concentric nonlaminar intimal fibrosis. The frequency of these findings differs from case to case and within regions of the same lung in the same patient. In addition, plexiform and dilation lesions, as well as a necrotizing arteritis, may be seen throughout the lungs. The fundamental nature of the plexiform lesion remains a mystery. Morphologically, it represents a mass of disorganized vessels with proliferating ECs, PASMCs, myofibroblasts, and macrophages. Whether the plexiform lesion represents impaired proliferation or angiogenesis remains unclear (**Fig. 78-6**).

The other major pattern of vascular changes in PAH is that of a thrombotic pulmonary arteriopathy. Typical features include medial hypertrophy of the arteries and arterioles, with both eccentric and concentric nonlaminar intimal fibrosis. The presence of colander lesions, which represent recanalized thrombi, is also typical. These lesions are believed to arise as a result of primary in situ thrombosis of the small vascular arteries and not from recurrent pulmonary embolism. Many patients have characteristics of both patterns of arteriopathy in varying degrees. This suggests that the vascular changes from PAH occur across a spectrum and are likely influenced by genetic and environmental factors.

Role of Genetics in Pulmonary Arterial Hypertension

An important concept in the development of PAH is that the disease develops in patients with an underlying genetic predisposition following exposure to specific stimuli, which serve as triggers.[30] Predisposition to the development of pulmonary hypertension has been noted by the marked heterogeneity in responses of the pulmonary vasculature in various disease states. Examples include the considerable variability among individuals to vasoconstrictive stimuli such as hypoxia or acidosis, which can produce marked pulmonary hypertension in one person and be essentially without effect in another. Also, the severity of pulmonary hypertension and level of pulmonary vascular resistance vary considerably among individuals with congenital heart disease and comparably sized ventricular septal defects.

Using linkage analysis, the locus designated PPH-1 on chromosome 2q33 led to the discovery of the PPH-1 gene.[31] The bone morphogenetic protein receptor type II gene (*BMPR-II*) codes for a receptor member of the TGF-β family (**Fig. 78-7**). *BMPR-II* modulates vascular cell growth by activating the intracellular pathways of Smad and LIM kinase. The mutations ascribed to the locus interrupt the BMP-mediated signaling pathway, resulting in a predisposition to proliferation rather than apoptosis of cells in small pulmonary arteries.[32] These molecular studies have suggested that the target cells within the pulmonary arterial wall are sensitive to *BMPR-II* gene dosage and that the TGF-β pathway mediated through *BMPR-II* is critical for the maintenance and/or normal response to injury of the pulmonary vasculature. It is clear, however, that additional factors, environmental or genetic, are required in the pathogenesis of the disease.[33] Recent data have supported the hypothesis that the dominant genetic mechanism underlying PAH is haploinsufficiency for *BMPR-II*.[34] How defects in BMPR-II contribute to EC proliferation, PASMC hypertrophy, and fibroblast deposition in patients with PAH remains unclear. It is interesting to note that about one in four cases of IPAH actually have germline mutations in the gene encoding the *BMPR-II* receptor.[35] Patients with hereditary hemorrhagic telangiectasia and IPAH have been described and found to have mutations of the *ALK1* gene, also within the TGF-β superfamily.

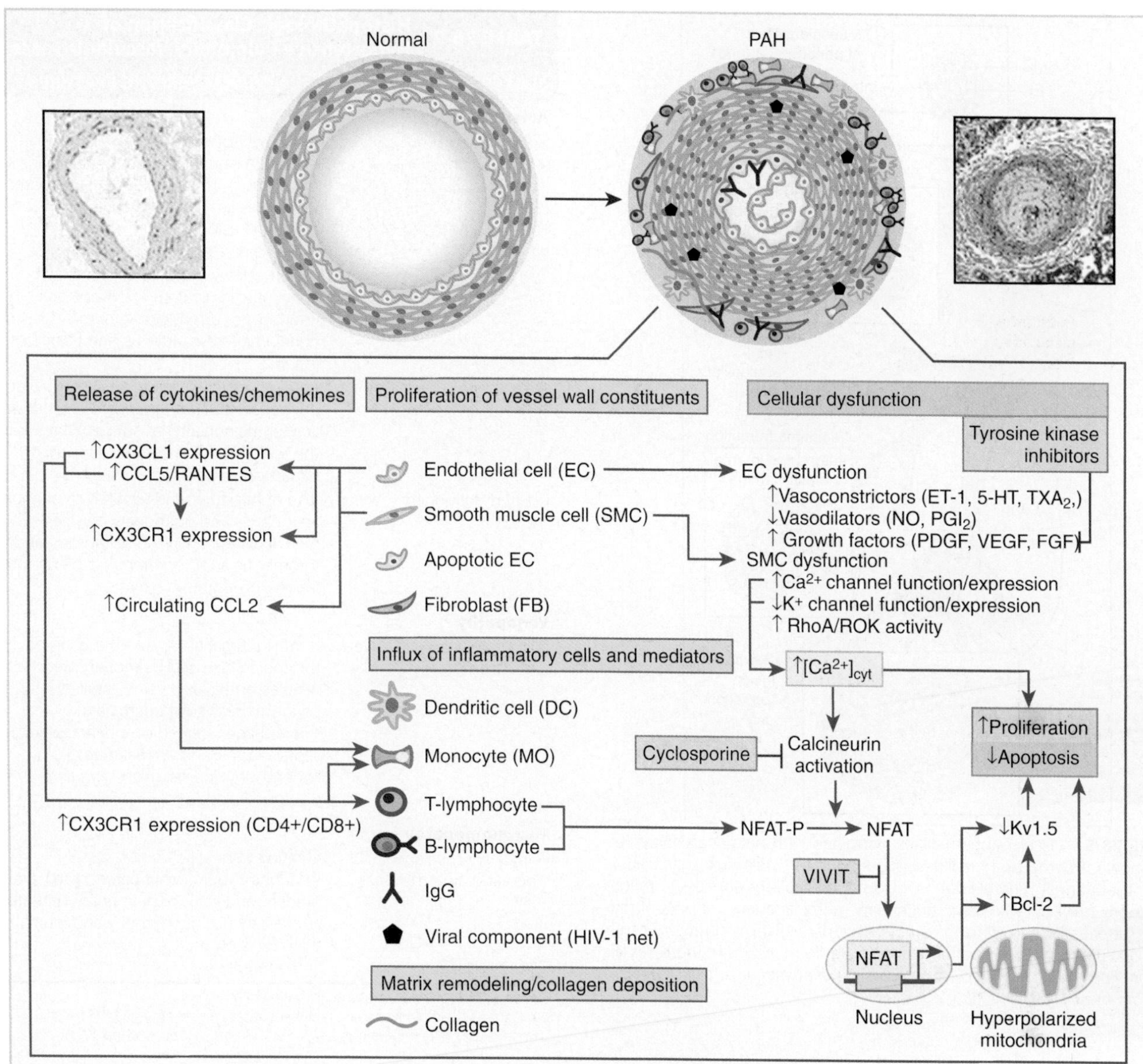

FIGURE 78-4 Molecular mechanisms of inflammation-mediated remodeling. This schematic features inflammatory mediators, cells, and mechanisms involved in pulmonary vascular remodeling as well as potential therapeutic targets. Release of cytokines and chemokines in remodeled vessels (e.g., plexiform lesions) or in the circulation, from activated ECs and smooth muscle cells (SMCs), mediate the influx of inflammatory cells (e.g., monocytes, T and B lymphocytes). Cellular dysfunction (particularly involving ECs and SMCs) contributes to the release of vasomotor and growth mediators, activation of transcriptional factors (e.g., nuclear factor of activated T lymphocytes [NFAT]), influx of calcium, and mitochondrial dysfunction. The net effect is a shift of balance in favor of cell proliferation and decreased apoptosis, leading to remodeling and narrowing of the pulmonary vascular lumen. Potential therapeutic target sites include inhibition of growth factors with tyrosine kinase inhibitors, calcineurin with cyclosporine, and prevention of NFAT activation with VIVIT polypeptide, a competitive peptide that inhibits the docking of NFAT to calcineurin. Specific mechanisms are detailed further in the text. bcl2 = B-cell lymphoma 2; CCL2 = chemokine (C-C motif) ligand 2; CCL5 = chemokine (C-C motif) ligand 5 or RANTES (**r**egulated upon **a**ctivation, **n**ormal ***T*** cell **e**xpressed and **s**ecreted); CX3CL1 = chemokine (C-X3-C motif) ligand 1 (fractalkine); CX3CR1 = chemokine (C-X3-C motif) receptor 1; DC = dendritic cells; FB = fibroblasts; FGF = fibroblast growth factor; 5-HT = serotonin; HIV-1 = human immunodeficiency virus 1; IgG = immunoglobulin G; MO = monocyte; PGI2 = prostacyclin; ROK = rho kinase. *(From Hassoun PM, Mouthon L, Barbera JA, et al: Inflammation, growth factors, and pulmonary vascular remodeling. J Am Coll Cardiol 54:S10, 2009.)*

Other genetic factors that have been associated with PAH suggest that polymorphisms in other genes could contribute to the development of PAH. The overexpression of SERT in pulmonary arteries and platelets from patients with PAH has been reported, with the increased activity of SERT responsible for the associated PASMC hyperplasia.[36] In addition, increased PASMC proliferation is related to SERT expression and activity in cultured PASMCs from patients with PAH. SERT is encoded by a single gene on chromosome 17q11.2, and a variant in the upstream promotor region of the SERT gene has been described. This polymorphism, with long (L) and short (S) forms, affects SERT expression and function, with the L allele inducing a greater rate of SERT gene transcription than the S allele. One study has shown that the L-allelic variant is found to be present in homozygous form in 65% of IPAH patients but in only 27% of control subjects.

Clinical Assessment of Patients with Suspected Pulmonary Hypertension

History

A careful and detailed history of the patient with suspected pulmonary hypertension is often revealing. Because the earliest symptoms in patients with pulmonary hypertension are manifest with exercise,

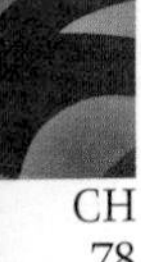

CH 78

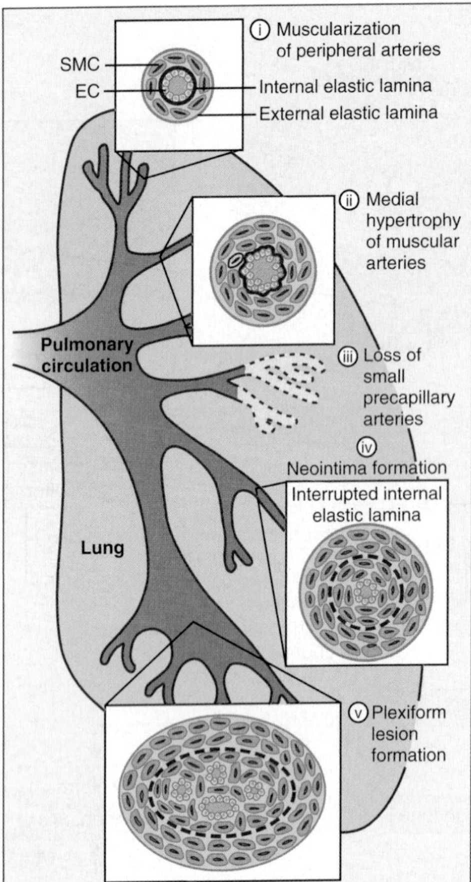

FIGURE 78-5 Vascular abnormalities associated with pulmonary hypertension. Shown are the abnormalities throughout the pulmonary circulation, including abnormal muscularization of distal precapillary arteries (i), medial hypertrophy (thickening) of large pulmonary muscular arteries (ii), loss of precapillary arteries (iii), neointima formation that is particularly occlusive in vessels 100 to 500 μM in size (iv), and formation of plexiform lesions in these vessels (v). *(From Rabinovitch M: Molecular pathogenesis of pulmonary arterial hypertension. J Clin Invest 118:2372, 2008.)*

TABLE 78-2 Histopathologic Classification of Hypertensive Pulmonary Vascular Disease

CLASSIFICATION	CHARACTERISTIC FEATURES
Arteriopathy	
Isolated medial hypertrophy*	Medial hypertrophy—increase of medial muscle in muscular arteries, muscularization of nonmuscularized arterioles; no appreciable intimal or luminal obstructive lesions; no plexiform lesions
Plexogenic	Plexiform and dilation lesions; medial hypertrophy; pulmonary eccentric or concentric laminar and nonlaminar arteriopathy, arteriopathy, intimal thickening; fibrinoid necrosis, arteritis, and thrombotic lesions
Thrombotic	Thrombi (fresh, organizing, or organized and pulmonary colander lesions); eccentric and concentric nonlaminar arteriopathy, intimal thickening, varying degrees of medial hypertrophy; no plexiform lesions
Isolated pulmonary arteritis	Active or healed arteritis, limited to pulmonary arteries; varying pulmonary degrees of medial hypertrophy, intimal fibrosis, and thrombotic arteritis lesions; no plexiform lesions; no systemic arteritis
Venopathy	
Pulmonary venoocclusive disease	Eccentric intimal fibrosis and recanalized thrombi in diseased pulmonary veins and venules; arterialized veins, capillary congestion, alveolar edema and siderophages, dilated lymphatics, pleural and septal edema, and arterial medial hypertrophy; intimal thickening and thrombotic lesions
Microangiopathy	
Pulmonary capillary hemangiomatosis	Infiltrating thin-walled blood vessels throughout pulmonary parenchyma, pleura, bronchi, and walls of pulmonary veins and arteries; medial hypertrophy and intimal thickening of muscular pulmonary arteries and arterioles

*Medial hypertrophy includes muscularization of arterioles.
From Pietra GG: Pathology of primary pulmonary hypertension. *In* Rubin LJ, Rich S (eds): Primary Pulmonary Hypertension. New York, Marcel Dekker, 1997, pp 19-61.

pulmonary hypertension can have an insidious onset. With the onset of right ventricular failure, lower extremity edema from venous congestion is characteristic. Angina is also common, likely reflecting reduced coronary blood flow to a markedly hypertrophied right ventricle.[37] As the cardiac output becomes fixed and eventually falls, patients may have episodes of syncope or near-syncope. Patients with pulmonary hypertension related to left ventricular diastolic dysfunction will characteristically have orthopnea and paroxysmal nocturnal dyspnea. Patients with underlying lung disease may also report episodes of coughing. Hemoptysis is relatively uncommon in patients with pulmonary hypertension and may be associated with underlying thromboembolism and pulmonary infarction. Some patients with advanced mitral stenosis also present with hemoptysis (see Chap. 66).

Physical Examination

Cardiovascular findings consistent with pulmonary hypertension and right ventricular pressure overload include a large *a* wave in the jugular venous pulse, low-volume carotid arterial pulse with a normal upstroke, left parasternal (right ventricular) heave, systolic pulsation produced by a dilated pulmonary artery in the second left interspace, ejection click and flow murmur in the same area, narrowly split second heart sound with a loud pulmonic component, and fourth heart sound of right ventricular origin. Late in the course, signs of right ventricular failure (e.g., hepatomegaly, peripheral edema, ascites) may be present. Patients with severe pulmonary hypertension may also have prominent *v* waves in the jugular venous pulse as a result of tricuspid regurgitation, third heart sound of right ventricular origin, a high-pitched early diastolic murmur of pulmonic regurgitation, and holosystolic murmur of tricuspid regurgitation. Tricuspid regurgitation is a reflection of right ventricular dilation. Cyanosis is a late finding and, unless the patient has associated lung disease, is usually attributable to a markedly reduced cardiac output, with systemic vasoconstriction and ventilation-perfusion mismatch in the lung. Uncommonly, the left laryngeal nerve becomes paralyzed as a consequence of compression by a dilated pulmonary artery (Ortner syndrome).

Diagnostic Tests

LABORATORY TESTS. The results of these studies (**Table 78-3**) are usually normal in patients with pulmonary hypertension. If chronic arterial oxygen desaturation exists, polycythemia should be present. Hypercoagulable states, abnormal platelet function, defects in fibrinolysis, and other abnormalities of coagulation are found in some patients with PAH. Brain natriuretic peptide (BNP) levels are elevated in patients with pulmonary hypertension and correlate with the pulmonary artery pressure.[38] Uric acid levels are elevated in patients with

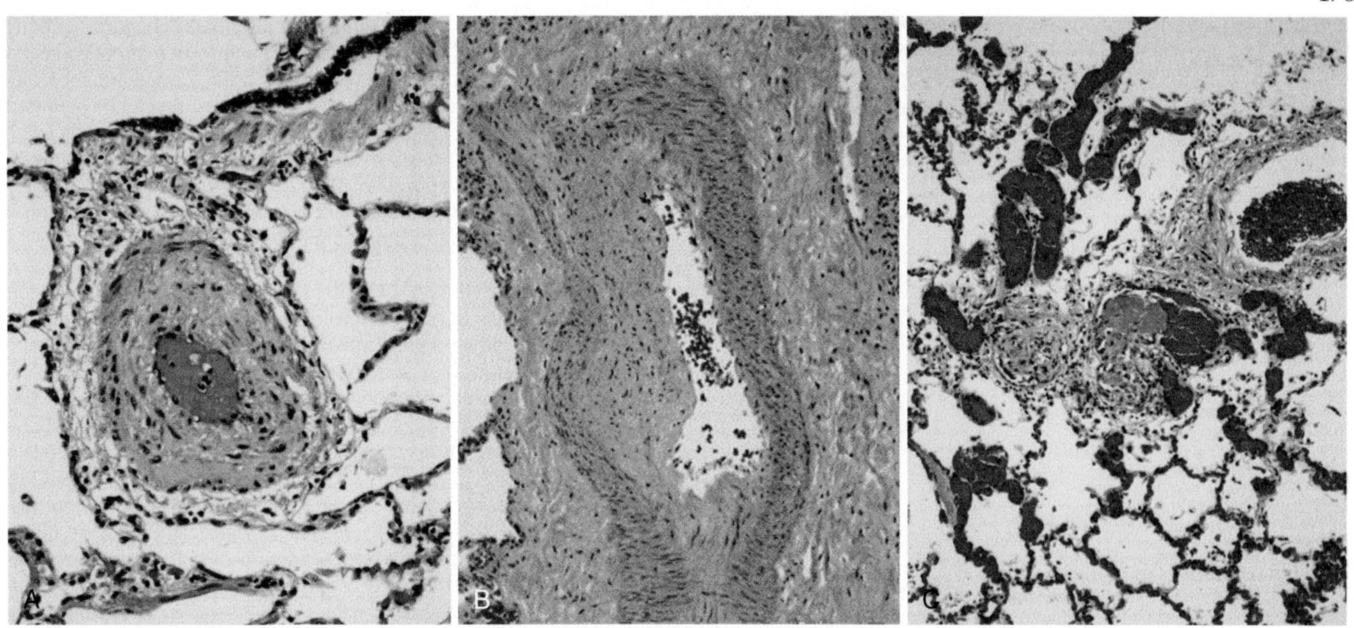

FIGURE 78-6 Photomicrographs of PA histologic lesions seen in cases of clinically unexplained pulmonary hypertension. **A,** Medical hypertrophy with intimal proliferation. The vascular lumen is markedly reduced, contributing to the elevated resistance. **B,** Eccentric intimal fibrosis. These are believed to be related to local thrombin deposition. **C,** Plexiform lesion demonstrating obstruction in the arterial lumen, aneurysmal dilation, and proliferation of anastomosing vascular channels. Hematoxolyn and eosin stains. **A** and **B,** magnification ×20; **C,** magnification ×4.

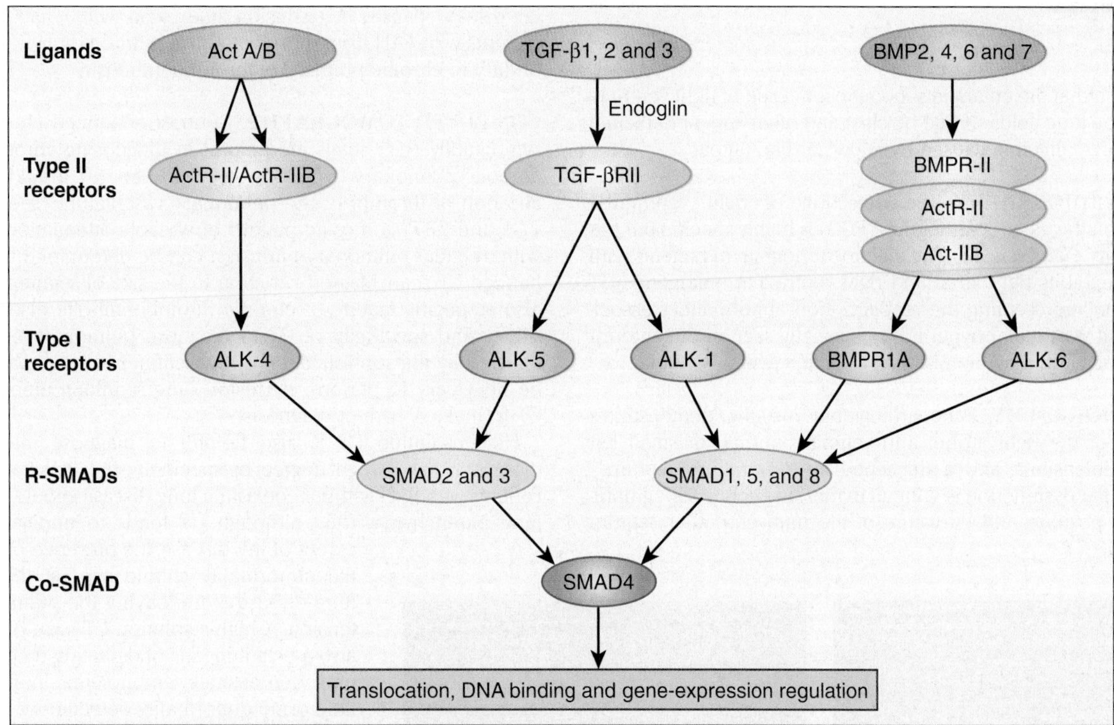

FIGURE 78-7 Transforming growth factor-β (TGF-β) signaling pathway. TGF ligands bind to a range of type II receptors to form complexes that interact with type I receptors. The receptors then form heterotetramers, which result in the phosphorylation and activation of receptor-regulated SMADs (R-SMADs) that subsequently form complexes with the common SMAD (Co-SMAD) SMAD4. This complex translocates to the nucleus, where it regulates gene transcription directly or indirectly. Endoglin is a coreceptor for both TGF-1 and TGF-3. Act = activin; ActR = activin receptor; ALK = activin-like kinase; TGF-R = TGF receptor. *(From Waite KA, Eng C: Developmental disorder to heritable cancer: It's all in the BMP/TGF family. Nat Rev Genet 4:763, 2003.)*

pulmonary hypertension and correlate with hemodynamics. Although the mechanism is uncertain, it may relate to overproduction and impaired uric acid excretion caused by the low cardiac output and tissue hypoxia. There is an increased incidence of thyroid disease in patients with PAH (see Chap. 86), which can mimic the symptoms of right ventricular failure.[39] Consequently, it is advised that thyroid function tests be monitored serially in all patients.

CHEST RADIOGRAPHY. A chest radiograph (see Chap. 16) shows enlargement of the main pulmonary artery and its major branches, with marked tapering of peripheral arteries. The right ventricle and atrium may also be enlarged. Dilation of the right ventricle gives the heart a globular appearance, but right ventricular hypertrophy or dilation is not easily discernible on a plain chest radiograph. Encroachment of the retrosternal air space on the lateral film may be a helpful

TABLE 78-3 Clues for Interpretation of Diagnostic Tests for Pulmonary Hypertension

TEST	NOTABLE FINDINGS
Chest x-ray	Enlargement of central pulmonary arteries reflects level of PA pressure and duration
Electrocardiography	Right axis deviation and precordial T wave abnormalities are early signs.
Pulmonary function tests	Elevated pulmonary artery pressure causes restrictive physiology.
Perfusion lung scan	Nonsegmental perfusion abnormalities can occur from severe pulmonary vascular disease.
Chest computed scan	Minor interstitial changes may reflect diffuse disease; mosaic tomography perfusion pattern indicates thromboembolism and/or left heart failure.
Echocardiography	Right ventricular enlargement will parallel the severity of the pulmonary hypertension.
Contrast echocardiography	Minor right to left shunting rarely produces hypoxemia.
Doppler echocardiography	This is too unreliable for following serial measurements to monitor therapy
Exercise testing	This is very helpful to assess the efficacy of therapy. Severe exercise-induced hypoxemia should cause consideration of a right-to-left shunt.

sign to confirm that the enlarged silhouette is a result of right ventricular dilation. The lung fields should be clear and often appear darkened from the relative oligemia caused by a low cardiac output.

ELECTROCARDIOGRAPHY. The detection of right ventricular hypertrophy on the electrocardiogram (ECG) is highly specific but has a low sensitivity (see Chap. 13). The electrocardiogram in patients with PAH usually exhibits right atrial and right ventricular enlargement. T wave inversion, representing the repolarization abnormalities associated with right ventricular hypertrophy, is usually seen in the anterior precordial leads and may be mistaken for anteroseptal ischemia.

ECHOCARDIOGRAPHY. Echocardiography usually demonstrates enlargement of the right atrium and ventricle, normal or small left ventricular dimensions, and a thickened interventricular septum.[40] Right ventricular dysfunction is difficult to measure echocardiographically, but the position and curvature of the intraventricular septum provide an indication of right ventricular afterload. Echocardiographic findings that portend a poor prognosis include pericardial effusion and a markedly diminished left ventricular cavity. Doppler echocardiographic estimates of right ventricular systolic pressures can be obtained by measuring the velocity of the tricuspid regurgitant jet and by using the Bernoulli formula (see Chap. 15). Although Doppler measurements correlate with right ventricular systolic pressure, they are relatively imprecise (±20 mm Hg) and are not a substitute for catheterization if a correct measurement of pulmonary pressure is needed.[41]

PULMONARY FUNCTION TESTS. Although pulmonary function in patients with PAH is often completely normal, reductions in lung volumes of 20% are common, making the differentiation from interstitial lung disease on the basis of pulmonary function tests (PFTs) difficult.[40] A significant obstructive pattern is not characteristic and should suggest obstructive airways disease. In patients with PAH, the diffusing lung capacity for carbon monoxide (DLCO) is reduced to approximately 60% to 80% of that predicted. The presence of mild to moderate arterial hypoxemia is caused by ventilation-perfusion mismatch and/or reduced mixed venous oxygen saturations resulting from low cardiac output. A severe reduction of both pulmonary arterial and systemic arterial oxygen saturations can be caused by right-to-left intracardiac or extracardiac shunts and/or intrapulmonary shunts. Consequently, PaO_2 and SaO_2 may vary markedly among patients with different constellations of associated abnormalities.

LUNG SCINTIGRAPHY. Patients with PAH may reveal a relatively normal perfusion pattern or diffuse, patchy perfusion abnormalities (**Fig. 78-8**). The latter is associated with a variety of pulmonary vascular disease causes. A perfusion lung scan will reliably distinguish patients with PAH from those who have pulmonary hypertension secondary to chronic pulmonary thromboembolism

COMPUTED TOMOGRAPHY. Contrast enhanced chest computed tomography (CT) scans are helpful in diagnosing chronic thromboembolic pulmonary hypertension (see Chap. 19). In addition to visualization of thrombi in the pulmonary vasculature (see Figs. 19-23C, 77-4, and 77-7), a mosaic pattern of variable attenuation compatible with irregular pulmonary perfusion can be determined in the nonenhanced CT scan. Marked variation in the size of segmental vessels is also a specific feature of chronic thromboembolic disease. The sensitivity and specificity of CT to diagnose pulmonary embolism are affected by the sophistication of the scanner. In some patients, it may be necessary to perform perfusion lung scanning along with chest CT to make a correct diagnosis.

High-resolution CT is also helpful to diagnose interstitial lung disease. It has a high degree of specificity, but its sensitivity is low. Patients with PAH without coexisting lung disease should have normal lung parenchyma. Thus, although CT tends to underrepresent the extent of the disease, the presence of any interstitial abnormality should suggest that interstitial lung disease is underlying the pulmonary hypertension. A high-resolution CT scan of the chest is also a useful means of detecting emphysema and may demonstrate emphysema in patients with little or no abnormality detected by PFTs.

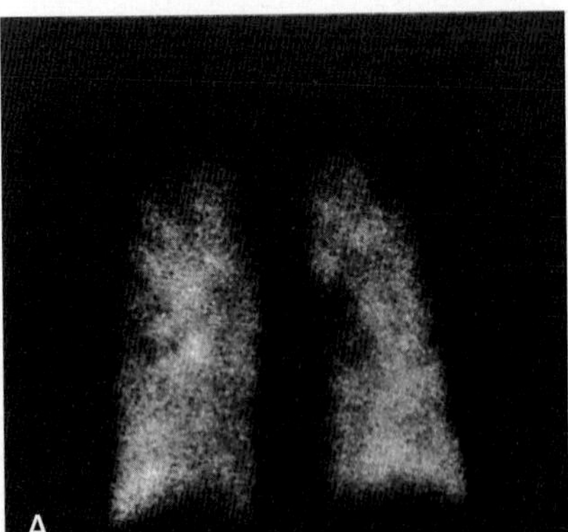

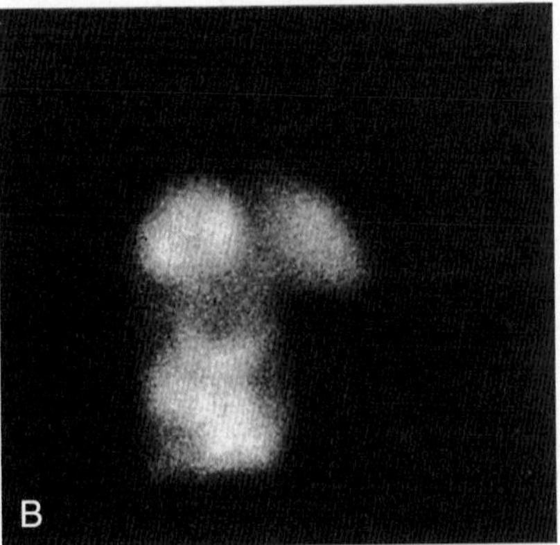

FIGURE 78-8 Perfusion lung scans in patients with pulmonary hypertension. **A,** Patient with IPAH. **B,** Patient with CTEPH. Both perfusion scans are abnormal. The scan in **A** shows a mottled distribution in a nonsegmental nonanatomic manner. The scan in **B** reveals lobar, segmental, and subsegmental defects, highly suggestive of an anatomic obstruction to pulmonary blood flow.

CARDIAC MAGNETIC RESONANCE IMAGING. Advances in magnetic resonance imaging technology (see Chap. 18) have led to the development of techniques for the assessment of hemodynamics in the pulmonary circulation and identification of right ventricular morphologic changes. Cardiovascular magnetic resonance (CMR) is now regarded as the reference standard for the assessment of right ventricular structure and function via the measurement of right ventricular volumes and ejection fraction, which makes CMR an attractive modality for serial follow-up in PAH management to determine treatment response.[42] One study that used CMR to assess the response to continuous intravenous epoprostenol in IPAH patients over 1 year showed a significant increase in right ventricular stroke volume and reduction in pulmonary vascular resistance.

EXERCISE TESTING. The use of a symptom-limited exercise test (see Chap. 14) can be very helpful in the evaluation of patients with pulmonary hypertension. The 6-minute walk test is commonly used in clinical trials as an endpoint for the efficacy of therapy in patients with pulmonary hypertension.[43] It has been correlated with workload, heart rate, oxygen saturation, and dyspnea response. Its drawbacks include the fact that anthropometric factors such as gait speed, age, weight, muscle mass, and length of stride can affect the test results. Treadmill testing using the Naughton-Balke protocol, which creates increases in work of 1-MET (metabolic equivalent) increments at 2-minute stages has also been used and compares with the 6-minute walk test in reflecting drug efficacy. Cardiopulmonary exercise testing using an upright bicycle and measurements of gas exchange have the potential to grade the severity of exercise limitation in patients with pulmonary hypertension noninvasively.[44]

CARDIAC CATHETERIZATION. In addition to confirming the diagnosis and allowing the exclusion of other causes, cardiac catheterization (see Chap. 20) also establishes the severity of disease and allows an assessment of prognosis. By definition, patients with PAH should have a low or normal pulmonary capillary wedge pressure. Because this is a critical measurement in distinguishing a patient with PAH from one with pulmonary venous hypertension, quality measures must be established in the catheterization laboratory to ensure that correct values are obtained.[45] The transducers must be carefully adjusted to reflect the height of the midchest of every patient. Pressures should never be determined by the electronically integrated mean pressure from the laboratory's computer, because these measurements ignore respiratory influences.[46] Instead, measurements of all pressures are properly made at end-expiration to avoid incorporating negative intrathoracic pressures. When a reproducible wedge pressure cannot be obtained, direct measurement of left ventricular end-diastolic pressure is advised. If the wedge pressure is increased, it should be correlated with left ventricular end-diastolic pressure and not attributed to a falsely elevated reading.

It can be difficult to pass a catheter into the pulmonary artery in patients with pulmonary hypertension because of the tricuspid regurgitation, dilated right atrium and ventricle, and low cardiac output. A specific flow-directed thermodilution balloon catheter has been developed for patients with pulmonary hypertension (American Edwards Laboratories, Irvine, Calif); it has an extra port for the placement of a 0.25-inch guidewire to provide better stiffness to the catheter, which greatly facilitates the procedure.

VASODILATOR TESTING. Several vasodilators are of value in the assessment of pulmonary vasoreactivity in patients with PAH (**Table 78-4**). All appear to have similar efficacy in identifying patients who are vasoreactive. Adenosine and epoprostenol are vasodilators at low doses but they possess potent inotropic properties which become manifest at higher doses, whereas NO has little effect on cardiac output at any dose. An increase in cardiac output with no change in pulmonary arterial pressure will result in a reduction in calculated pulmonary vascular resistance, and may be erroneously interpreted as a vasodilator response[45] (**Table 78-5**). Changes in pulmonary capillary wedge pressure can also have important influences on the

TABLE 78-4 Agents Used for Determination of Acute Pulmonary Vasoreactivity

AGENT	MODE OF ADMINISTRATION	DOSAGE	ADVANTAGES	DISADVANTAGES
Prostacyclin	Intravenous	2 ng/kg/min (stepwise increase every 10-15 min); maximum dose, 10 ng/kg/min	Affects PA pressure, cardiac output; can be used as chronic therapy	Systemic hypotension; dramatic side effects
Adenosine	Intravenous	50 μg/kg/min increased by 50 μg/kg/min every 2 min; maximum dose, 250 μg/kg/min	Affects PA pressure, cardiac output; rapid onset, rapid washout	Bradycardia
Nitric oxide	Inhaled	5-80 ppm for 10 min	Affects PA pressure alone; rapid onset, rapid washout	Rebound pulmonary hypertension in a few cases
Iloprost	Inhaled	2.5-5.0 μg/inhaled dose	Affects PA pressure selectively with minimal effects on cardiac output; can be used as chronic therapy	Potential dosing variabilities depending on investigator experience, inhalation device, and breathing pattern of patient

TABLE 78-5 Hemodynamic Assessment of Vasodilators in Pulmonary Hypertension

PARAMETER MEASURED	DESIRED ACUTE CHANGES	COMMENTS
Mean pulmonary artery pressure (PAP)	>10-mm Hg decrease; ideally, mean PAP < 30 mm Hg	Must not be associated with significant fall in systemic blood pressure
Pulmonary vascular resistance (PVR)	>33% decrease; ideally PVR < 6 units	Cardiac output unchanged or increased
Pulmonary capillary wedge pressure	No change	Increase in wedge pressure suggests pulmonary venoocclusive disease or coexisting left ventricular dysfunction
Cardiac output	Increase	Increase should be from increased stroke volume rather than increased heart rate
Heart rate	No significant change	Chronic increased heart rate will result in RV failure; watch for bradycardia if using high doses of diltiazem
Systemic arterial oxygen saturation	Increase if reduced on room air, little change if normal	Decrease in systemic arterial oxygen saturation suggests lung disease or right-to-left shunt; prohibits chronic use
Pulmonary artery (mixed venous) oxygen saturation	Increase; should parallel increase in cardiac output and reflect improved tissue oxygenation	

calculation of pulmonary vascular resistance. A rising capillary wedge pressure secondary to increased cardiac output may be the first sign of impending left ventricular failure and an adverse effect of a drug, whereas the calculated pulmonary vascular resistance may be lower and suggest a beneficial effect. The resting heart rate is a physiologic parameter of marked importance in patients with congestive heart failure, and treatments that cause an increased heart rate are likely to yield deleterious long-term results. Finally, the systemic arterial oxygen content should be evaluated in patients with pulmonary hypertension. Vasodilator drugs can result in vasodilation of blood vessels supplying poorly ventilated areas of the lung and can worsen hypoxemia. This effect is particularly noticeable in patients with underlying chronic lung disease.

CLASSIFICATION OF PULMONARY HYPERTENSION

Pulmonary hypertension, in its simplest sense, refers to any elevation in the pulmonary arterial pressure above normal. The presence of pulmonary hypertension may reflect a serious underlying pulmonary vascular disease or a manifestation of high cardiac output from thyrotoxicosis. Consequently, an accurate diagnosis of the cause of pulmonary hypertension in a patient is essential to establish an effective treatment plan. In addition, therapies that may be beneficial for patients with some types of pulmonary hypertension may be harmful for patients with other types.

The diagnosis of pulmonary hypertension relies on establishing an elevation in pulmonary artery pressure above normal. The upper limit of normal for pulmonary artery mean pressure is 19 mm Hg. However, this assumes that there are no abnormalities in downstream pressures of the left atrium or left ventricle, or an increased cardiac output. That is why a patient can have pulmonary hypertension from the standpoint of an elevated pulmonary artery pressure, but normal pulmonary vascular resistance. Parameters for normal pulmonary arterial systolic pressure derived by echocardiographic Doppler studies have suggested that the upper limit of normal of pulmonary arterial systolic pressure in the general population may be higher than previously appreciated.

In 1998, a new clinical classification for pulmonary hypertension was developed. This classification catalogued clinical conditions based on common causative features to serve as a guide in the clinical assessment and treatment of these patients (**Table 78-6**). Several modifications to this classification have since been proposed.[47] In addition, a functional classification, similar to the New York Heart Association (NYHA) functional classification for heart disease, has been developed to allow comparisons of patients with respect to the clinical severity of their symptoms. Because heart and lung diseases commonly coexist in these patients, a worsening functional class may not necessarily reflect worsening pulmonary hypertension.

PAH refers to pulmonary vascular disease originating from the arterioles that results in an elevation in pressure and vascular resistance and a normal pulmonary capillary wedge pressure. Although IPAH (formerly referred to as primary pulmonary hypertension, or PPH) is relatively rare, with an estimated incidence of 1 to 2/million, severe PAH associated with other conditions such as connective tissue CTDs and congenital heart defects is considerably more common. The Centers for Disease Control and Prevention has surveyed the number of hospitalizations of persons with pulmonary hypertension from any cause in the United States from 1980 to 2002 and found a dramatic increase since 1990, with 260,000 hospitalizations and 15,668 deaths reported annually since 2000.[48]

TABLE 78-6 Clinical Classification of Pulmonary Hypertension

Category 1: Pulmonary Arterial Hypertension

Key feature: Elevation in PAP with normal pulmonary capillary wedge pressure (PCWP)

Includes the following:

Idiopathic (IPAH)
- Sporadic
- Familial
- From exposure to drugs or toxins
- From exposure to HIV infection
- Persistent pulmonary hypertension of the newborn

Associated with other active conditions:
- Congenital systemic to pulmonary shunts
- Collagen vascular disease
- Portal hypertension

Pulmonary capillary hemangiomatosis (PCH)

Category 2: Pulmonary Venous Hypertension

Key feature: Elevation in PAP with elevation in PCWP

Includes the following:
- Left-sided atrial or ventricular heart disease
- Left-sided valvular heart disease
- Pulmonary venous obstruction
- Pulmonary venoocclusive disease (PVOD)

Category 3: Pulmonary Hypertension Associated with Hypoxemic Lung Disease

Key feature: Chronic hypoxia with mild elevation of PA pressure

Includes the following:
- Chronic obstructive lung disease
- Interstitial lung disease
- Sleep-disordered breathing
- Alveolar hypoventilation disorders
- Chronic exposure to high altitude
- Developmental abnormalities

Category 4: Pulmonary Hypertension Caused by Chronic Thromboembolic Disease

Key feature: Elevation of PAP with documentation of PA obstruction for >3 mo

Includes the following:
- Chronic pulmonary thromboembolism
- Nonthrombotic pulmonary embolism (tumor, foreign material)

Category 5: Pulmonary Hypertension from Conditions with Uncertain Mechanisms

Key feature: Elevation in PAP pressure in association with systemic disease where a causal relationship is possible but not clearly understood

Includes the following:
- Sarcoidosis
- Chronic anemias
- Schistosomiasis
- Histiocytosis X
- Lymphangiomatosis

Pulmonary Arterial Hypertension

IDIOPATHIC PULMONARY ARTERIAL HYPERTENSION. IPAH is the diagnosis given to patients with pulmonary hypertension of unexplained cause. However, the clinical features, usual age of onset, progression of the disease, and autopsy findings make IPAH a distinct clinical entity. There are sporadic and familial forms. The prevalence of familial PAH (FPAH) is uncertain, but it occurs in at least 6% of IPAH cases, and the incidence is likely higher. Many unique features are associated with the transmission and development of FPAH. The age of onset is variable and the low penetrance of the gene confers only about a 10% to 20% likelihood of development of the disease. Many individuals in families with PAH inherit the gene and have progeny in whom PAH never develops. Patients with FPAH have a similar female-to-male ratio, age of onset, and natural history of the disease as those with IPAH.

Documentation of FPAH can be difficult because remote common ancestry occurs in patients with PAH and skip generations caused by incomplete penetrance or by variable expression can mimic sporadic disease. Vertical transmission has been demonstrated in as many as five generations in one family and is indicative of a single autosomal dominant gene for PAH. Genetic anticipation has been described in FPAH since the early reports. Most cases of FPAH can be attributed to the mutation of *BMPR-2*. On clinical grounds, FPAH and IPAH appear identical.

Natural History and Symptoms

The most extensive study on the natural history of IPAH was reported from the National Institutes of Health (NIH) Registry on Primary Pulmonary Hypertension from 1981 to 1987. Of the patients, 63% were female, and the mean age was 36 ± 15 years (range, 1 to 81 years) at the time of diagnosis. The mean interval from the onset of symptoms to diagnosis was 2 years, and the most common initial symptoms were dyspnea (80%), fatigue (19%), and syncope or near-syncope (13%). No ethnic or racial differentiation was observed, with 12.3% of patients being black and 2.3% being Hispanic.

RIGHT VENTRICULAR FUNCTION. Right ventricular failure from pulmonary hypertension is a result of chronic pressure overload and associated volume overload, with the development of tricuspid regurgitation. The mechanism of right ventricular failure in patients with pulmonary hypertension is complex. The chronic pressure overload that induces right ventricular hypertrophy and reduced contractility has been shown to cause a reduction in coronary blood flow to the right ventricular myocardium, which can produce right ventricular ischemia acutely and chronically.[37] Such right ventricular dysfunction appears to be a result of a reduction in right ventricular coronary artery driving pressure. In animals, acute right ventricular failure secondary to right ventricular hypertension was overcome by increasing aortic pressure, which resulted in an increase in right ventricular coronary driving pressure.

LEFT VENTRICULAR FUNCTION. On occasion, patients with pulmonary hypertension have a reduced left ventricular ejection fraction and even regional wall motion abnormalities of the left ventricle. These findings had been attributed to mechanisms related to interventricular dependence, which suggests that in some way a dysfunctional right ventricle can lead to a dysfunctional left ventricle. More recently, extrinsic compression of the left main coronary artery by the pulmonary artery in patients with chronic pulmonary hypertension has been described and may be associated with classic angina-like symptoms. It is advisable to look for extrinsic compression of the left main coronary artery with coronary angiography in patients with long-standing pulmonary hypertension who have abnormal left ventricular function.

Clinical Course

The clinical course of patients with IPAH can be highly variable. The NIH registry demonstrated that the mean right atrial pressure, mean pulmonary artery pressure, and cardiac index were significantly related to mortality. The NYHA functional classification was also strongly related to survival. However, with the onset of overt right ventricular failure manifested by worsening symptoms and systemic venous congestion, patient survival is generally limited to approximately 6 months. The most common cause of death in patients with IPAH in the NIH registry was progressive right-sided heart failure. Sudden cardiac death was limited to patients who were in NYHA functional Class IV, suggesting that it is a manifestation of end-stage disease rather than a phenomenon that occurs early or unpredictably in the clinical course of the disease. The remainder of the patients died of other medical complications, such as pneumonia or bleeding, which suggests that patients with IPAH do not tolerate coexistent medical conditions well.

Management

With the current classification system, patients within a category of pulmonary hypertension are commonly treated alike. Differences in the efficacy and safety of therapies for pulmonary hypertension associated with other conditions are discussed later. However, the general principles surrounding the management of pulmonary hypertension patients are usually consistent.

LIFESTYLE CHANGES. The diagnosis of PAH does not necessarily imply total disability for the patient. However, marked increases in pulmonary artery have been documented to occur early in the onset of increased physical activity. For that reason, graded exercise activities, such as bicycle riding or swimming, in which patients can gradually increase their workload and easily limit the extent of their work, are thought to be safer than isometric activities. Isometric activities such as lifting weights or stair climbing can be associated with syncopal events and should be limited or avoided. One recent study has reported an improvement in exercise capacity in patients who underwent a training program that far exceeded the effects of vasodilator treatments.[49]

PREGNANCY. Pregnancy should be discussed with women of childbearing age. The physiologic changes that occur in pregnancy can potentially activate the disease and result in death of the mother and/or fetus. In addition to the increased circulating blood volume and oxygen consumption that will increase right ventricular work, circulating procoagulant factors and the risk of pulmonary embolism from deep vein thrombosis and amniotic fluid are serious concerns. Syncope and cardiac arrest have also been reported to occur during active labor and delivery, and a syndrome of postpartum circulatory collapse has been described. For these reasons, surgical sterilization should be given strong consideration by women with PAH or their husbands, and pregnancy should be strongly discouraged.

MEDICAL THERAPY. The mainstay of therapy has focused on the use of vasodilators. However, these patients suffer from right heart failure; thus, measures that have been shown to be effective for the treatment of heart failure are often used.

Digoxin

Animal studies of right ventricular systolic overload have shown that prior administration of digoxin helps prevent the reduction in contractility of the right ventricle. Clinically, digoxin can increase cardiac output by approximately 10% when given acutely to patients with right ventricular failure from pulmonary hypertension, which is similar to observations made in patients with left ventricular systolic failure. In addition, digoxin caused a reduction in circulating norepinephrine, which is markedly increased.

Diuretics

These drugs appear to be of marked benefit in symptom relief of patients with PAH. Their traditional role has been limited to patients manifesting right ventricular failure and systemic venous congestion. However, patients with advanced PAH can have increased left ventricular filling pressures that contribute to the symptoms of dyspnea and orthopnea, which can be relieved with diuretics. Diuretics may also serve to reduce right ventricular wall stress in patients with concomitant tricuspid regurgitation and volume overload. The fear that diuretics will induce systemic hypotension is unfounded, because the main factor limiting cardiac output is pulmonary vascular resistance and not pulmonary blood volume. Patients with severe venous congestion may require high doses of loop diuretics or the use of combined diuretics. In these cases, electrolyte levels need to be carefully monitored to avoid hyponatremia and hypokalemia. Elevated plasma aldosterone concentrations are associated with endothelial dysfunction, left ventricular hypertrophy, and cardiac death in left heart failure. Given the similarities between left and right heart failure in regard to activation of the renin-angiotensin-aldosterone system, it seems reasonable to use aldosterone antagonists in patients with PAH.

Supplemental Oxygen

Hypoxic pulmonary vasoconstriction can contribute to pulmonary vascular disease. Patients with PAH who exhibit resting hypoxemia or arterial oxygen desaturation with activity may benefit from supplemental oxygen because increased oxygen extraction occurs with fixed oxygen delivery. Patients with severe right-sided heart failure and resting hypoxemia resulting from markedly increased oxygen extraction at rest should be treated with continuous oxygen therapy to maintain their arterial oxygen saturation above 90%. Patients with hypoxemia caused by a right-to-left shunt may not improve their level of oxygenation to an appreciable degree with supplemental oxygen.

Anticoagulants

Oral anticoagulant therapy is widely recommended for patients with PAH, supported by the numerous studies implicating thrombin as contributing to disease progression.[50] A number of retrospective and prospective observational studies have shown a significant survival advantage in patients with PAH treated with warfarin. The current recommendation is to use warfarin in relatively low doses, as has been recommended for the prophylaxis of venous thromboembolism, with the international normalized ratio (INR) maintained at 2.0 to 3.0 times that of controls.

PRINCIPLES OF VASODILATOR DRUG TREATMENT OF PULMONARY ARTERIAL HYPERTENSION

- Establish a correct diagnosis. The symptoms of pulmonary hypertension attributable to PAH can be indistinguishable from pulmonary hypertension of other causes. In addition, treatments that may be helpful in PAH can often be harmful or dangerous in other conditions. For these reasons, it is essential that a correct diagnosis of the cause be made in every case. Lack of an obvious history should not be relied on as adequate, because patients with congenital heart disease may never have been told of a heart murmur, and patients with chronic thromboembolic pulmonary hypertension often have no antecedent history of pulmonary embolism. Given the poor survival of pulmonary hypertension of any cause, every patient should undergo thorough testing, including cardiac catheterization, prior to initiating therapy.

- Obtain baseline assessments of the disease. To determine whether a treatment of PAH is effective, it is important to evaluate the patient's response objectively. Regardless of which test or tests are used (e.g., exercise testing, catheterization), an adequate baseline assessment of the patient's disease must be obtained to monitor the patient's response to therapy.
- Test vasoreactivity. Because of the dramatic effect that calcium blockers have on improving survival in patients who are vasoreactive, patients should be tested at the time of diagnosis so that potentially reactive patients are not missed.
- Vasoreactive patients should undergo a trial of calcium channel blockers. Calcium blockers are the drugs of choice for those patients who demonstrate vasoreactivity at the time of testing. There is no evidence to suggest that these patients would have a similarly beneficial response with other therapies. Some patients who demonstrate reactivity may not respond to calcium blockers or may respond for only a limited period. It is essential that the drugs are used in the high doses that have been described to realize full benefit for the patient.

  Nonreactive patients should be offered other therapies. Currently, there are no comparative trials regarding the efficacy of the various approved therapies, so no specific treatment can or should be considered first-line treatment. However, foremost should be consideration of which treatment the physician believes will offer the patient the best chance for improved symptoms and long-term survival. This will often depend on personal opinion, because there are no long-term controlled trials of any therapies for pulmonary hypertension.
- Follow-up assessment of drug efficacy is essential. In all the clinical trials for pulmonary hypertension, the full treatment effect was reached within 1 month of the patient receiving the active drug at full dose. There are no data to suggest that patients who do not respond initially might respond over time with longer exposure. Thus, it is recommended that a repeat measure of drug efficacy be performed within 2 months of starting any new drug treatment.
- Treatments that are ineffective should be replaced. All approved therapies for PAH have inherent risks and are expensive. If a treatment is deemed ineffective by an assessment of efficacy, a different treatment should be substituted rather than added. Patients who clinically fail all treatments should be considered for lung transplantation.
- Benefits and risks of combination therapies are largely unknown. The use of these treatments in combination is becoming popular. However, the only randomized controlled trial of combination therapy demonstrating efficacy has been the addition of oral sildenafil to stable patients with PAH on intravenous epoprostenol.[51] Trials evaluating the combination of bosentan with epoprostenol and bosentan with tadalafil have failed to demonstrate increased efficacy.
- Repeated measures of efficacy should be adhered to. Evidence suggests that some therapies may lose efficacy over time. Thus, even in patients in whom it has been shown that drug therapy has been helpful initially, serial assessments of drug efficacy should be performed periodically to check for loss of efficacy over time.

VASODILATOR THERAPIES. All the approved therapies for pulmonary hypertension are considered to be pulmonary vasodilators. Current practice guidelines recommend that calcium channel blockers be used in vasoreactive patients, which is not an U.S. Food and Drug Administration (FDA)-approved use.[8] The approved vasodilators are recommended for patients who are shown to be nonresponsive to acute vasodilator testing. Regulatory approval has been based on the demonstration that they improve exercise tolerance over 12 to 16 weeks and is not based on a fall in pulmonary artery pressure. Although there is a presumption that they also lower pulmonary arterial pressure, the usual decrease in pulmonary artery pressure is less than 10%.

Calcium Channel Blockers

It has been reported that up to 20% of patients with IPAH are vasoreactive and will respond to high doses of calcium channel blockers, with a dramatic reduction in pulmonary artery pressure and pulmonary vascular resistance; on serial catheterization, this has been maintained for more than 20 years.[52] It appears essential that high doses (e.g., amlodipine, 20 to 30 mg/day; nifedipine, 180 to 240 mg/day; diltiazem, 720 to 960 mg/day) must be used to realize full benefit. When patients respond favorably, quality of life is restored, with improved functional class, and survival (94% at 5 years) is improved when compared with nonresponders and historical control subjects. This experience suggests that a select subset of patients with IPAH have the ability to have their pulmonary hypertension reversed and their quality of life and length of survival enhanced. It is unknown whether the response to calcium channel blockers identifies two subsets of patients with IPAH, different stages of IPAH, or a combination of both. However, patients who do not exhibit a dramatic hemodynamic response to calcium channel blockers do not appear to benefit from their long-term administration.

Prostacyclins

Prostacyclin is produced by vascular endothelial cells and has vasodilatory and antiproliferative activities. It is also a potent inhibitor of platelet aggregation. Abnormalities in prostacyclin production and metabolism have been described in PAH. Continuous intravenous infusion of epoprostenol (synthetic prostacyclin) has been shown in randomized clinical trials to improve symptoms related to IPAH, exercise tolerance, hemodynamics, and short-term survival.[53] It appears effective when given chronically, even if it does not seem effective acutely. Epoprostenol is administered through a central venous catheter that is surgically implanted and delivered by an ambulatory infusion system. The delivery system is complex and requires patients to learn the techniques of sterile drug preparation, operation of the pump, and care of the intravenous catheter. Most serious complications that have occurred with epoprostenol therapy have been attributable to the delivery system; these include catheter-related infections and temporary interruption of the infusion because of pump malfunction. The short half-life (6 minutes) of epoprostenol is believed to contribute to the hemodynamic collapse that has occurred when the infusion is abruptly interrupted. Side effects related to epoprostenol include flushing, headache, diarrhea, and a unique type of jaw discomfort that occurs with eating. In most patients, these symptoms are minimal and well tolerated. Chronic foot pain and a diffuse rash develop in some patients. To date, epoprostenol has been given to patients with PAH for more than 15 years with sustained effectiveness. In some patients (NYHA Class IV) who are critically ill, it serves as a bridge to lung transplantation by stabilizing the patient to a more favorable preoperative state. Patients who are less critically ill may do so well with epoprostenol therapy that the need to consider transplantation may be delayed, perhaps indefinitely.

The optimal dose of epoprostenol has never been determined, but doses between 25 and 40 ng/kg/min are typical. A high cardiac output state has been reported in a series of patients with IPAH receiving chronic epoprostenol therapy and is consistent with the drug having positive inotropic effects. The development of a chronic high-output state could have long-term detrimental effects on underlying cardiac function and should be avoided. The follow-up assessment of patients receiving intravenous epoprostenol is variable among medical centers, but it does appear important to determine the cardiac output response to therapy periodically to optimize dosing. The experience

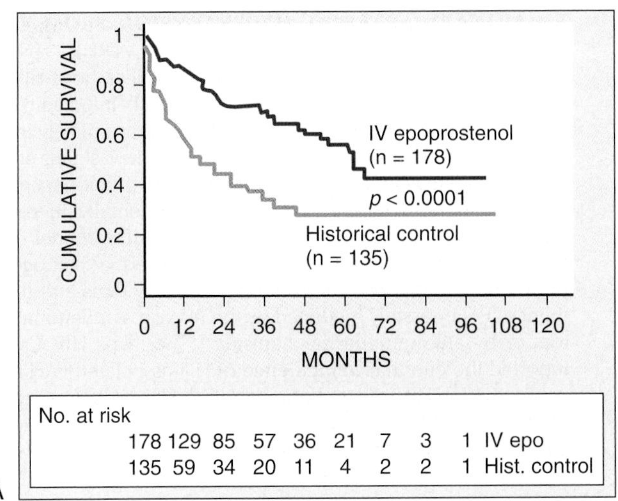

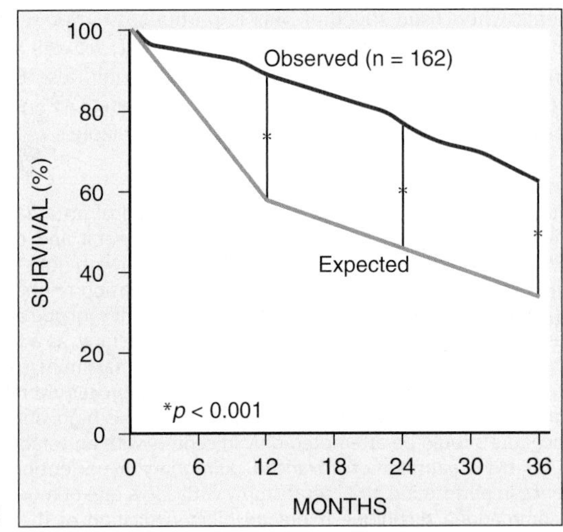

FIGURE 78-9 Kaplan-Meier survival estimates in patients with IPAH treated with epoprostenol therapy. **A,** Patient survival is compared with patients with IPAH matched for NYHA functional class who never received epoprostenol therapy. **B,** Patient survival compared with untreated patients with IPAH from the NIH registry survival prediction equation. The observed survival with epoprostenol therapy from both studies was remarkably similar and considerably better than what would have been expected. *(**A** from Sitbon O, Humbert M, Nunes H, et al: Long-term intravenous epoprostenol infusion in primary pulmonary hypertension. J Am Coll Cardiol 40:780, 2002; **B** from McLaughlin V, Shillington A, Rich S: Survival in primary pulmonary hypertension: The impact of epoprostenol therapy. Circulation 106:1477, 2002.)*

with epoprostenol in patients with IPAH for more than 10 years has been reported by two large centers (**Fig. 78-9**). Survival rates longer than 5 years were improved compared with survival in historical control subjects and the natural history predicted by the NIH Registry. Predictors of survival included NYHA functional class, exercise tolerance, and acute vasodilator responsiveness. Both studies provided important data for identifying patients who would do well over the long term, versus those in whom transplantation should be considered.

Treprostinil is a stable prostacyclin analogue that has pharmacologic actions similar to those of epoprostenol, but differs in that it is chemically stable at room temperature and has a longer half-life (4 hours). This allows it to be administered through continuous subcutaneous infusion, although infusion site pain is common. In a large, randomized clinical trial in patients with PAH, treprostinil was effective in reducing symptoms of dyspnea associated with exercise.[54] Treprostinil has also been approved for intravenous administration. The optimal dose of treprostinil has never been determined, but doses of 75 to 150 ng/kg/min are typical. Because there is no difference in bioavailability between the subcutaneous and intravenous routes, patients can be transitioned from one route of administration to the other without the need for adjusting the dosage. It has been reported that the use of intravenous treprostinil is associated with a higher incidence of gram-negative sepsis than intravenous epoprostenol.

A key element of the long-term efficacy of the parenteral prostacyclins appears to be related to the strategy of upward dose titration of the drug over time. It is important to increase the dose to tolerated side effects in patients who remain symptomatic because there is a direct relationship between the dose of drug and improvement in exercise testing and hemodynamics. Once an optimal dose has been achieved, the dose is kept constant thereafter. Patients who deteriorate after a long period of stability usually do not respond to further dose increases.

Iloprost, an analogue of prostacyclin, has been approved for use via inhalation. Because of the short half-life of iloprost, however, it requires frequent (up to 12/day) inhalations. Iloprost is given by 2.5- or 5.0-μg ampules via a dedicated nebulizer that limits the dose of drug that can be delivered. Beraprost is an orally active prostacyclin analogue that improved exercise capacity and symptoms over a 12-week period in a European trial. A similar trial conducted in the United States, however, showed similar efficacy at 12 weeks, only to document the loss of effectiveness over 1 year. This is the only randomized clinical trial to follow patients for a period of 1 year and underscores how initial improvements with therapies might not be sustained for longer periods. At present, beraprost is only approved for use in Japan.

Phosphodiesterase Type 5 Inhibitors

Inhibition of the phosphodiesterase type 5 (PDE5) enzyme produces pulmonary vasodilation by promoting an enhanced and sustained level of cGMP, an identical effect to that of inhaled NO. Sildenafil is a PDE5 inhibitor that has been shown to be a selective pulmonary vasodilator with similar efficacy to that of inhaled NO in lowering pulmonary artery pressure. Sildenafil has a preferential effect on the pulmonary circulation because of the high expression of the PDE5 isoform in the lung. Recent studies have also suggested that PDE5 inhibitors may improve cardiac function by direct effects on the myocardium.[55] In a large, randomized clinical trial sildenafil caused significant improvements in 6-minute walk distance and hemodynamics in patients with PAH.[56] The recommended dosage is 20 mg three times daily, but dosages as high as 80 mg three times daily have been used safely, and in some patients may be more effective. Side effects are generally mild and mainly related to vasodilation (headache, flushing, and nasal congestion). Tadalafil is a long-acting selective PDE5 inhibitor that has been recently approved for PAH.[57] In the pivotal clinical trial, it was similarly well tolerated and improved exercise tolerance and quality of life measures. The effective dose was 40 mg once daily.

Endothelin Receptor Blockers

Endothelin (ET)-1 exerts vasoconstrictor and mitogenic effects and is activated in PAH. Three endothelin receptor blockers have been approved for PAH. Although there have never been direct comparative trials, all three appear to have similar efficacy.[58] Bosentan, a nonselective ET receptor blocker, has produced an improvement in 6-minute walk distance after 16 weeks as compared with placebo in several clinical trials. It also has been shown to lengthen a composite endpoint of time to clinical worsening. The approved dosage of bosentan is 125 mg twice daily. Ambrisentan is an ET_A-selective endothelin receptor blocker that can be given once daily at a 5-mg dose, which can be increased to 10 mg if the drug is well tolerated. Sitaxsentan is an ET_A-selective endothelin receptor blocker that can be given once daily at a 100 mg dose. Sitaxsentan is currently approved only in the European Union, Canada, and Australia.

These drugs have similar side effects, which include peripheral edema. They also have a potential of causing liver toxicity requiring monthly monitoring of liver enzyme levels, and have interactions with warfarin that require careful monitoring of the INR and dose adjustments when used together. This is particularly important with sitaxsentan. Pregnancy monitoring (when indicated), as well as quarterly hematocrit testing, is also advised. Caution should also be used when they are coadministered with cyclosporine, strong CYP3A4 inhibitors (ketoconazole), or CYP2C19 inhibitors (omeprazole).

Surgical Therapy

Atrial Septostomy. The rationale for the creation of an atrial septostomy in patients with PAH is based on experimental and clinical observations suggesting that an intra-atrial defect allowing right-to-left shunting in the setting of severe pulmonary hypertension might be of benefit. Indications for the procedure include recurrent syncope and/or right ventricular failure despite maximum medical therapy, as a bridge to transplantation if deterioration occurs in the face of maximum medical therapy, or when no other option exists.[59] The rate of procedure-related mortality with atrial septostomy in patients with PAH is high, and thus the procedure should be attempted only in centers with an established record for the treatment of advanced pulmonary hypertension and experience in performing atrial septostomy with a low rate of morbidity. The recommended technique is graded balloon dilation of the fosse ovalis, which can be achieved in stages over several weeks in unstable patients. It should not be performed in a patient with impending death and severe right ventricular failure. Predictors of procedure-related failure or death include a mean right atrial pressure higher than 20 mm Hg, a pulmonary vascular resistance index higher than 55 units/m^2, or a predicted 1-year survival rate of less than 40%. The mechanisms responsible for the beneficial effects of atrial septostomy remain unclear. Possibilities include increased oxygen delivery at rest and/or with exercise, reduced right ventricular end-diastolic pressure or wall stress, improvement in right ventricular function, or relief of right ventricular ischemia.

Heart-Lung and Lung Transplantation. Heart-lung transplantation (see Chap. 31) has been performed successfully in patients with PAH since 1981. Currently, bilateral lung transplantation has become the procedure of choice, allowing the donor heart to be given to another patient.[60] Hemodynamic studies have shown an immediate reduction in pulmonary artery pressure and pulmonary vascular resistance associated with an improvement in right ventricular function. The 1-year survival rate is 70% to 75%, the 2-year survival rate is 55% to 60%, and the 5-year survival rate is between 40% to 45%. The major long-term complications in patients are the high incidence of bronchiolitis obliterans in the transplanted lungs, acute organ rejection, and opportunistic infection.

Transplantation should be reserved for patients with pulmonary hypertension that has progressed despite optimal medical management. It is generally accepted that patients should be considered for transplantation when they are in NYHA functional Class III or IV despite therapy with a parenteral prostacyclin. However, the recent adoption of a lung allocation score system for candidates has made it increasingly difficult for these patients to become transplanted. The scoring system was developed to reduce the mortality of patients on the waiting list, prioritize candidates on the basis of urgency, and avoid futile transplants. Because patients with pulmonary hypertension have a higher postoperative mortality than patients with lung disease, they receive a lower score. However, their long-term survival is comparable.

PULMONARY ARTERIAL HYPERTENSION FROM EXPOSURE TO ANOREXIGENS. Several anorexigens have been demonstrated to cause pulmonary hypertension in humans. The first observation was made in 1967, when an epidemic of PAH in Europe was associated with the use of aminorex, which has similarities to adrenaline and ephedrine in its chemical structure. The clinical features of pulmonary hypertension were identical to those attributed to IPAH. The association between the use of fenfluramine appetite suppressants and the development of PAH was established in a case-control study conducted in Europe in 1992 to 1994. Anorexigens such as amphetamines were also implicated. Ultimately, the marked increase in the number of cases of PAH and cardiac valvulopathy ascribed to the use of fenfluramine drugs in the United States led to their withdrawal in 1997. In most patients, the development of pulmonary hypertension was progressive, despite withdrawal of the anorexigen. In addition, many of the patients did not develop clinical symptoms of PAH for more than 5 years after their last ingestion. Animal models have suggested that the fenfluramines produce pulmonary hypertension via the SERT by allowing for serotonin to stimulate PASMC proliferation by some type of permissive effect.[61]

PULMONARY ARTERIAL HYPERTENSION FROM EXPOSURE TO HUMAN IMMUNODEFICIENCY VIRUS INFECTION. Although well documented, it remains unclear how HIV infection results in an increased incidence of PAH in HIV-infected patients (see Chap. 72). A direct pathogenic role of HIV seems unlikely inasmuch as no viral constituents have been detected in the vascular endothelium of these patients. On the other hand, reports of pulmonary arteriopathy with intimal proliferation in monkeys experimentally infected with the simian immunodeficiency virus and in a murine model of acquired immunodeficiency syndrome have suggested a pathogenetic link between infection with an immunodeficiency virus and the development of PAH, possibly mediated by the release of inflammatory mediators or by autoimmune mechanisms.[28] The Swiss HIV Cohort Study reported the cumulative incidence of HIV-associated PAH to be 1/200 patients in the HIV-infected population. PAH was diagnosed in patients in all stages of HIV infection; it was unrelated to the CD4 cell counts. The clinical and hemodynamic features of these patients were similar to those of patients with IPAH.

PERSISTENT PULMONARY HYPERTENSION OF THE NEWBORN. Three forms of persistent pulmonary hypertension of the newborn (PPHN) have been described. In the hypertrophic type, the muscular tissue of the pulmonary arteries is hypertrophied and extends peripherally to the acini, which causes narrowing of the arteries, an increase in pulmonary pressure, and a reduction in pulmonary blood flow. It is believed to be the result of sustained fetal hypertension from vasoconstriction caused by chronic fetal distress. In the hypoplastic type, the lungs and pulmonary arteries are underdeveloped, usually as the result of a congenital diaphragmatic hernia or prolonged leakage of amniotic fluid. The cross-sectional area of the pulmonary vascular bed is inadequate for normal neonatal pulmonary blood flow. In the reactive type, lung histology is presumably normal but vasoconstriction causes pulmonary hypertension. High levels of vasoconstrictive mediators such as thromboxane, norepinephrine, and leukotrienes may be responsible and may result from streptococcal infection or acute asphyxia at birth. Although PPHN can vary in severity, severe cases are life-threatening. It is commonly associated with severe hypoxemia and the need for mechanical ventilation. Right-to-left shunting at the level of the ductus arteriosus or foramen ovale is common. Inhaled nitric oxide has provided encouraging results through improvement in oxygenation in these patients. Intravenous epoprostenol has also been used and may even have effects additive to those of inhaled NO.

Alveolar capillary dysplasia is a very rare cause of pulmonary hypertension in neonates and is characterized by a developmental abnormality in the pulmonary vasculature. The antemortem diagnosis can be made only with open lung biopsy. Despite aggressive treatment with NO, epoprostenol, and even extracorporeal membrane oxygenation, survival in the setting of alveolar capillary dysplasia is rare.

PULMONARY ARTERIAL HYPERTENSION ASSOCIATED WITH CONGENITAL HEART DISEASE. Pulmonary hypertension can develop from any congenital heart defect that increases pulmonary blood flow (see Chap. 65).[62] If a congenital defect causes pulmonary hypertension from the time of birth, the small muscular arteries of the fetal lung may undergo delayed or only partial involution, with subsequent persistently high levels of pulmonary vascular resistance. This is especially true in lesions in which a left-to-right shunt enters the right ventricle or pulmonary artery directly (i.e., a post-tricuspid shunt, such as ventricular septal defect or patent ductus arteriosus). These patients experience a higher incidence of severe and irreversible pulmonary vascular damage than those in whom the shunt is proximal to the tricuspid valve (pretricuspid shunts, as in atrial septal defect and partial anomalous pulmonary venous drainage). An important feature of PAH in congenital heart disease is the right ventricular adaptive response to elevated pulmonary arterial pressure. When the onset is early in life, there is marked hypertrophy and preservation of a fetal-like phenotype. As a result, these patients can sustain an increased afterload for many years or decades as compared with patients in whom the pulmonary hypertension occurs later in life.

The vascular changes that occur in pulmonary hypertension associated with congenital heart disease are identical to those seen in IPAH. It is believed that ECs release mediators that induce PASMC growth in response to changes in pulmonary blood flow or pressure. Experimental data have suggested that medial hypertrophy can be converted to a neointimal pattern when pulmonary vascular injury is coupled with increased pulmonary blood flow. Early changes, characterized by hypertrophy of the media and intimal proliferation of the muscular pulmonary arteries and arterioles, are believed to be reversible. Advanced disease, characterized by the presence of concentric laminar fibrosis, with obliteration of many arterioles and small arteries, and plexiform lesions are considered irreversible.

Eisenmenger Syndrome

Eisenmenger syndrome refers to any anomalous circulatory communication that leads to obliterative pulmonary vascular disease. The long-term prognosis of patients with Eisenmenger syndrome is better than that of patients with IPAH, with survival reported to be 80% at 10 years, 77% at 15 years, and 42% at 25 years. A major distinction between Eisenmenger syndrome and other forms of PAH is the presence of cyanosis. Pulse oximetry at rest and with exercise is a useful way to monitor the progress of these patients and their response to therapy. Patients with bidirectional shunting may have normal resting pulse oximetry that will fall during exercise, reflecting shunt reversal. The magnitude of the fall may be helpful in deciding how to intervene. Patients with advanced pulmonary vascular disease will have hypoxemia at rest that worsens significantly with any level of exercise activity. Although this can have deleterious effects on organ function, these patients commonly have significant secondary erythrocytosis, which can effectively improve tissue oxygenation. Because erythrocytosis provides an important compensatory mechanism, patients should take supplemental iron to maintain their hematocrit. The use of anticoagulants is somewhat controversial, because these patients generally have thrombosis of the pulmonary vasculature but an increased risk of hemoptysis. It is recommended that warfarin anticoagulation be prescribed unless there is a history of bleeding.

All the approved vasodilators for PAH have been used in congenital heart disease to improve exercise tolerance, but the only randomized clinical trial conducted specifically in these patients (BREATHE-5) was with bosentan.[63] Intravenous epoprostenol therapy has also been reported to be effective, but the presence of an underlying right-to-left shunt presents a risk for systemic embolization from the indwelling venous catheter, which needs to be monitored closely.

PULMONARY ARTERIAL HYPERTENSION ASSOCIATED WITH CONNECTIVE TISSUE DISEASES. All the CTDs have been associated with the development of PAH, which is the leading cause of death in patients with scleroderma (see Chap. 89). Advanced pulmonary hypertension has also been described in patients with systemic lupus erythematosus, mixed CTDs, polymyositis, dermatomyositis, rheumatoid arthritis, and Sjögren syndrome. Patients with severe pulmonary hypertension usually have a pulmonary vasculature with histologic features that resemble those of IPAH, but coexisting interstitial fibrosis is extremely common and likely contributes to hypoxemia. Because CTDs may have an insidious onset and slowly progressive course, early recognition of the symptoms of pulmonary hypertension may be difficult. Dyspnea is the most common initial symptom. A reduced DLCO on pulmonary function tests has been shown to be predictive of the presence of pulmonary vascular disease. Scleroderma is associated with mild pulmonary hypertension in as many as one third of patients, which would make periodic screening with echocardiography in these patients reasonable.

The prognosis for patients with CTD in whom pulmonary hypertension develops is poor. Conventional therapy with digitalis, diuretics, and anticoagulation has been recommended to provide a clinical benefit similar to the practice in IPAH. Because hypoxemia is so common, patients should be tested with pulse oximetry during exercise, and supplemental oxygen used whenever indicated. All the approved therapies for PAH apply to the CTDs. The principles of drug selection and management for IPAH are similar, but their long-term efficacy is considerably less.[64] Patients with coexisting lung disease must be watched carefully for worsening oxygenation from the vasodilators.

PULMONARY ARTERIAL HYPERTENSION ASSOCIATED WITH PORTAL HYPERTENSION. Pulmonary abnormalities are commonly associated with the development of hepatic cirrhosis and include hepatopulmonary syndrome (HPS), and portopulmonary hypertension (POPH). HPS is characterized by vascular dilation that produces severe arterial hypoxemia from intrapulmonary shunting in the setting of normal hemodynamics. No proven medical therapy exists for HPS, except for supplemental oxygen.

POPH hypertension is progressive and is unrelated to the severity of hepatic dysfunction, with no reports of spontaneous resolution.[65] There is a strong association between portal hypertension and pulmonary hypertension, regardless of whether liver disease is present. The prevalence of pulmonary hypertension in patients with portal hypertension is estimated as 2% to 6%, with an estimated 5-year survival of 10% to 30%. Patients with POPH are similar to patients with PAH without cirrhosis, with the exception that they tend to have higher cardiac output and consequently lower systemic and pulmonary vascular resistance, which is characteristic of the cirrhotic state. Treatment of POPH generally follows the guidelines developed for treating patients with IPAH, but many of these drugs pose a risk of liver toxicity and should not be used. Although severe pulmonary hypertension is considered a contraindication to liver transplantation because of the risk of irreversible right-sided heart failure, successful liver transplantation has been reported in patients with mild pulmonary hypertension treated successfully with intravenous epoprostenol.

Pulmonary Capillary Hemangiomatosis

Pulmonary capillary hemangiomatosis (PCH) was first described in 1978 as a very rare cause of pulmonary hypertension. The typical chest radiographic appearance is a diffuse, bilateral, reticular nodular pattern associated with enlarged central pulmonary arteries. The most characteristic finding on high-resolution CT scan is diffuse bilateral thickening of the interlobular septa and small centrilobular, poorly circumscribed, nodular opacities. Diffuse ground-glass opacities have also been described. Histologic findings often include irregular small nodular foci of thin-walled capillary-sized vessels that diffusely invade the lung parenchyma, bronchiolar walls, and adventitia of large vessels.[66] These nodular lesions are often associated with alveolar hemorrhage. Most patients appear to be young adults and present with dyspnea and/or hemoptysis. A hereditary form with probable autosomal recessive transmission has been reported. It can be difficult to distinguish PCH from IPAH clinically. The clinical course of patients with this condition is usually one of progressive deterioration, leading to severe pulmonary hypertension, right-sided heart failure, and death. The only definitive treatment for these patients is lung transplantation.

Pulmonary Venous Hypertension

Patients with pulmonary venous hypertension have elevated pulmonary venous pressure (as reflected in the pulmonary capillary wedge pressure) as a consequence of left ventricular dysfunction (see Chap. 25), mitral and aortic valve disease (see Chap. 66), cardiomyopathy (see Chap. 68), cor triatriatum (see Chap. 65), and pericardial disease (see Chap. 75). Although mitral stenosis was the most common cause of this disorder decades ago, left ventricular diastolic dysfunction is the most common cause of pulmonary venous hypertension seen in the Western world today. It is presumed that the mechanism of both is similar. Specifically, a chronic elevation in the diastolic filling pressure of the left heart causes a backward transmission of the pressure to the pulmonary venous system, which appears to trigger vasoconstriction in the pulmonary arterial bed.

PATHOLOGY. Histologically, abnormal thickening of the pulmonary veins and formation of a neointima are seen. The latter can be extensive. There is medial hypertrophy and thickening of the neointima on the arterial side of the pulmonary circulation as well. Patients with chronic severe pulmonary venous hypertension may show distention of pulmonary capillaries, thickening and rupture of the basement membranes of endothelial cells, and transudation of erythrocytes through these ruptured membranes into the alveolar spaces, which contain fragments of disintegrating erythrocytes. Pulmonary hemosiderosis is commonly observed and may progress to extensive fibrosis. In the late stages of pulmonary venous hypertension, areas of hemorrhage may be scattered throughout the lungs, edema fluid, coagulum may collect in the alveolar spaces, and widespread organization and fibrosis of pulmonary alveoli may be present. Pulmonary lymphatics may become markedly distended and give the appearance of lymphangiectasis, particularly when the pulmonary venous pressure exceeds 30 mm Hg.

PATHOPHYSIOLOGY. Increased resistance to pulmonary venous drainage will force the PA pressure to increase. The severity of pulmonary hypertension depends, in part, on the contractility of the right ventricle. In the presence of a normal right ventricle, an increase in left atrial pressure initially results in a decrease in pulmonary vascular resistance and the pressure gradient across the lungs, reflecting distention of compliant small vessels, recruitment of additional vascular channels, or both. With further increases in left atrial pressure, PA pressure rises along with pulmonary venous pressure, so that at a constant pulmonary blood flow, the pressure gradient between the pulmonary artery and veins and pulmonary vascular resistance remains constant. When pulmonary venous pressure approaches or exceeds 25 mm Hg on a chronic basis, a disproportionate elevation in pulmonary artery pressure occurs, so that the pressure gradient between the pulmonary artery and veins rises while pulmonary blood flow remains constant or falls. This is indicative of an elevation in pulmonary vascular resistance caused in part by pulmonary arterial vasoconstriction. Some patients may have a genetic predisposition, allowing the chronically elevated pulmonary venous pressures to serve as a trigger for the development of structural changes similar to those found in IPAH. Marked reactive pulmonary hypertension with PA systolic pressures in excess of 80 mm Hg occurs in less than one third of patients whose pulmonary venous pressures are elevated more than 25 mm Hg, which suggests a broad spectrum of pulmonary vascular reactivity to chronic increases in pulmonary venous pressure. The molecular mechanisms involved in elevating pulmonary vascular resistance are unclear.

CLINICAL IMPLICATIONS. Pulmonary hypertension is a common and well-recognized complication of left ventricular systolic dysfunction and is an independent predictor of survival in these patients. Patients with a high pulmonary artery pressure and a low right ventricular ejection fraction have a sevenfold higher risk of death compared with heart failure patients with a normal pulmonary artery pressure and right ventricular ejection fraction. Treatment of pulmonary venous hypertension as caused by left ventricular systolic dysfunction should include traditional therapy for the underlying disease. Both epoprostenol and endothelin receptor antagonists have been studied in these patients and have been demonstrated to increase mortality or have no benefit, respectively. Recently, sildenafil has been used with some success.

Pulmonary venous hypertension related to left ventricular diastolic dysfunction, now referred to as heart failure with preserved ejection fraction (HFpEF), is less appreciated than that related to systolic dysfunction, and is commonly mistaken for IPAH (see Chap. 30). The features of pulmonary hypertension in patients with HFpEF have recently been characterized.[67] Patients tend to be older than IPAH patients and often have other conditions that may contribute to pulmonary hypertension, including obesity and obstructive sleep apnea. However, important and distinctive symptoms are orthopnea and paroxysmal nocturnal dyspnea, which is not a feature of PAH. Atrial fibrillation and absence of right axis deviation on the ECG should increase the suspicion for pulmonary venous hypertension. The chest x-ray will often show pulmonary vascular congestion, pleural effusions and, on occasion, pulmonary edema. A high-resolution chest CT scan can be particularly helpful because it will often reveal ground-glass opacities consistent with chronic pulmonary edema and a mosaic perfusion pattern. Left atrial enlargement on the echocardiogram also suggests pulmonary venous hypertension rather than PAH. Although echocardiographic techniques for the assessment of left ventricular diastolic function are advancing, heart catheterization is required to document left heart filling pressures in those with pulmonary hypertension. To make the diagnosis of PAH, the pulmonary capillary wedge pressure or left ventricular end-diastolic pressure must be less than 16 mm Hg. If an ideal wedge pressure tracing cannot be obtained, left ventricular end diastolic pressure should be directly measured. The reduction in diastolic filling time that occurs with an increased heart rate during exercise may further increase left heart filling pressures and, as a result, pulmonary artery (PA) pressures (**Fig. 78-10**).

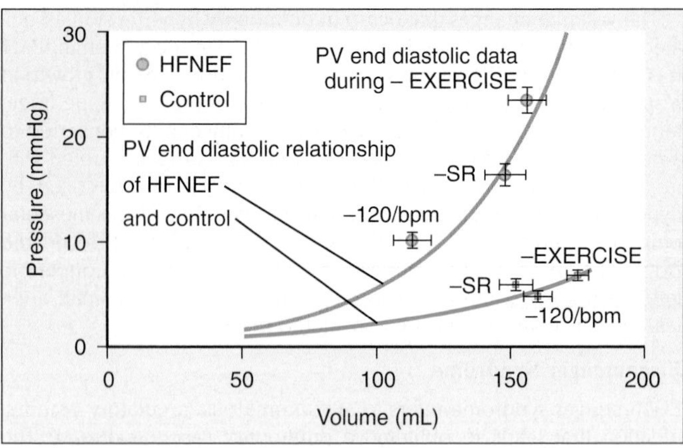

FIGURE 78-10 End-diastolic pressure-volume relationships from patients with heart failure with normal ejection fraction (HFNEF) and control subjects (arrows indicate curve for HFNEF and control subjects, respectively). Yellow circles indicate mean end-diastolic volume (EDV, with horizontal error bars indicating the standard error of the mean [SEM]) and pressure (with vertical error bars indicating SEM) during sinus rhythm (SR), during pacing with 120 bpm (beats/min), or during exercise of the HFNEF group. Blue squares indicate mean EDV and pressure (with vertical and horizontal error bars indicating SEM) of control subjects. The abnormal curve illustrates why patients with elevated left ventricular EDV or pulmonary wedge pressures experience such severe dyspnea with exercise, because any increase in stroke volume causes the pressure to rise. Conversely, a reduction in left ventricular filling pressure may relieve the symptoms of orthopnea and dyspnea and obscure the clinical picture of heart failure with a normal ejection fraction. *(From Westermann D, Kasner M, Steendijk P, et al: Role of left ventricular stiffness in heart failure with normal ejection fraction. Circulation 117:2051, 2008.)*

Two hemodynamic profiles have been described that are common in these patients. Some patients will have an elevation in pulmonary arterial pressure, with only a minimal increase in the transpulmonary gradient (mean PA pressure – pulmonary capillary wedge pressure), as a reflection of the passive increase in PA pressure necessary to overcome the increased downstream resistance. A preserved right ventricle must generate high systolic pressures to ensure adequate forward blood flow in these patients, and thus moderate degrees of pulmonary hypertension are not only characteristic but also favorable. Other patients will have reactive pulmonary vasoconstriction resulting in marked elevations in pulmonary arterial pressure beyond that which is necessary to maintain cardiac output. These patients are frequently distinguished by a marked elevation in PA diastolic pressure. This has been studied extensively in patients with mitral stenosis but is less well characterized in patients with left ventricular diastolic dysfunction.

TREATMENT. Treatment of HFpEF is difficult (see Chap. 30). The goal is to reduce or remove the elevated pulmonary venous resistance with medications such as nitrates, diuretics, and aggressive treatment of systemic hypertension. When successful, the pulmonary arterial pressure will also fall and the cardiac output will increase. Comorbid diseases such as obesity, diabetes, and obstructive sleep apnea must be addressed. Atrial fibrillation is not well tolerated in these patients and every attempt should be made to maintain sinus rhythm. Pulmonary vasodilators are not indicated, because their major hemodynamic effect is to raise cardiac output, and thus will predictably cause a worsening of pulmonary edema if the pulmonary venous obstruction is not being relieved. There are a number of reports of rapid deterioration and death when pulmonary vasodilators are used in the presence of pulmonary venous hypertension.

Pulmonary hypertension as a result of mitral stenosis has been well characterized, and tends to resolve with time after mitral valve repair or replacement[68] (see Chap. 66). The resolution is highly variable, and can occur immediately or over more than 1 year. Although pulmonary hypertension is associated with an increased operative risk, it should not interfere with appropriate treatment, regardless of severity. Pulmonary hypertension occasionally occurs in the setting of severe aortic stenosis, and portends a worse prognosis. Although severe pulmonary hypertension is an independent predictor of perioperative mortality, aortic valve replacement is associated with a reduction in pulmonary artery pressures and improvement in NYHA functional class. The prognosis of those with pulmonary hypertension and severe aortic stenosis who do not undergo surgery is poor, with a 20% survival after a median of 436 days.

Pulmonary Venoocclusive Disease

Pulmonary venoocclusive disease (PVOD) is a rare form of PAH. The histopathologic diagnosis is based on the presence of obstructive eccentric fibrous intimal pads in the pulmonary veins and venules. Arterialization of the pulmonary veins is often present and is associated with alveolar capillary congestion.[66] Other changes of chronic pulmonary hypertension, such as medial hypertrophy and muscularization of the arterioles with eccentric intimal fibrosis, may also be seen. The pulmonary venous obstruction explains the increased pulmonary capillary wedge pressure described in patients in the late stages of the disease and the increase in basilar bronchovascular markings noted on the chest radiograph. The chest CT scan may be helpful, revealing smooth interlobular septal thickening, ground-glass opacities, and a mosaic perfusion pattern. A perfusion lung scan showing multiple perfusion defects and a CT scan showing no evidence of pulmonary embolism are highly suggestive of the diagnosis. The treatment of PVOD is unsatisfactory.[69] Warfarin anticoagulation is essential. Anecdotal reports of success with calcium blockers or epoprostenol have been tempered by reports of these treatments producing fulminant pulmonary edema. Any therapy needs particularly close supervision, and early referral of the patient for lung transplantation should be considered.

Pulmonary Arterial Hypertension Associated with Hypoxic Lung Diseases

Diseases of the lung parenchyma associated with hypoxia are a common cause of mild pulmonary hypertension. Hypoxia induces muscularization of distal vessels and medial hypertrophy of more proximal arteries, as well as a loss of vessels, which is compounded by a loss of lung parenchyma in the setting of lung disease. Intimal thickening appears to be an early event that occurs in association with progressive air flow limitation. The development of plexiform lesions is not observed.

CHRONIC OBSTRUCTIVE PULMONARY DISEASE. Chronic obstructive pulmonary disease (COPD) refers to a heterogeneous group of diseases that share a common feature—the airways are narrowed, which results in an inability to exhale completely. Although there are numerous disorders that fall under the heading of COPD, the most common are emphysema and chronic bronchitis. Pulmonary hypertension in COPD has multiple causative factors, including pulmonary vasoconstriction caused by alveolar hypoxia, acidemia, and hypercarbia, compression of pulmonary vessels by the high lung volume, loss of small vessels in the vascular bed in regions of the emphysema and lung destruction, and increased cardiac output and blood viscosity from polycythemia secondary to hypoxia. Of these, hypoxia is the most important factor. Changes in airway resistance may augment pulmonary vascular resistance in patients with COPD by increasing the alveolar pressure. The effect of airway resistance on pulmonary artery pressure may be particularly important when ventilation increases (e.g., in cases of acute exacerbation of COPD). In patients with COPD, even small increases in flow that occur during mild exercise may increase pulmonary artery pressure significantly. Alveolar hypoxia is a potent pulmonary arterial constrictor that reduces perfusion with respect to ventilation in an attempt to restore Pa_{O_2}. There is also a positive correlation between the Pa_{CO_2} and PA pressure in COPD.

Clinically, patients with COPD present with dyspnea and signs of right heart failure, usually in the setting of marked hypoxemia. At cardiac catheterization, the level of the mean pulmonary arterial pressure is usually less than 30 mm Hg. The mean PA pressure typically seen in these patients is lower than the mean PA pressure in patients with IPAH who respond favorably to pulmonary vasodilator therapy. The fact that these patients are clinically failing may indicate that it is not the severity of the pulmonary hypertension but the degree of hypoxemia that is determining their clinical symptomatology. Because right ventricular failure occurs at this level of pulmonary hypertension, it is probable that the right ventricle in these patients is profoundly affected by the hypoxemia and behaves more like an ischemic right ventricle than a pressure-loaded right ventricle.

Although relatively mild, the level of the pulmonary arterial hypertension is predictive of prognosis in patients with COPD. Nonetheless, there has never been a clinical trial showing a beneficial effect of any pulmonary vasodilator in these patients. Concern over worsening ventilation-perfusion mismatch from vasodilators that has been demonstrated with acute testing is likely why these medications are not used. The only effective treatment for patients with COPD and pulmonary hypertension has been supplemental oxygen, with several studies showing an improvement in morbidity and mortality. Clinicians also need to follow the level of hemoglobin in these patients. Patients with hypoxemia should have reactive polycythemia as a fundamental biologic mechanism to compensate for their cardiopulmonary disease. A hemoglobin in the low-normal range, although well tolerated in patients with normal oxygenation, may not be tolerated in patients with hypoxemia and mild pulmonary hypertension

Patients who present with severe pulmonary hypertension should be evaluated for another disease process responsible for the high pulmonary arterial pressures before it is attributed to the COPD. However, there is a small subset of patients with COPD who do develop severe pulmonary arterial hypertension (mean PA pressure [PAP] > 45 mm Hg).[70] These patients have a distinctive pattern of cardiopulmonary abnormalities with mild to moderate airway obstruction, severe hypoxemia, hypocapnia, and a low DLCO. It is possible that the severe pulmonary hypertension is occurring in the presence of lung disease rather than as a result of the lung disease. Clinically, these patients have a hemodynamic profile more typical of PAH, with a marked increase in PA pressure, normal pulmonary capillary wedge pressures, and markedly elevated pulmonary vascular resistance. Pulmonary vasodilators have been associated with clinical worsening and should not be used.[71]

INTERSTITIAL LUNG DISEASES. Interstitial lung diseases (ILDs) represent various conditions that involve the alveolar walls, perialveolar tissue, and other contiguous supporting structures. Pulmonary hypertension in patients with ILD is often associated with obliteration of the pulmonary vascular bed by lung destruction and fibrosis.[72] The mechanism for pulmonary hypertension may be related to hypoxemia, a loss of effective pulmonary vasculature from lung destruction, and/or by indirectly triggering a pulmonary vasculopathy. Although ILD may be caused by environmental inhalant exposures, drugs, radiation, and recurring aspiration pneumonias, a large number of patients have ILD of unknown origin, the most common being idiopathic pulmonary fibrosis. ILD associated with CTD (e.g., scleroderma), represents an additional diagnostic challenge, because these patients may have only parenchymal disease, only vascular disease, or various stages of both.

The hemodynamic profile of patients with ILD and pulmonary hypertension is distinct from that of patients with IPAH. It is uncommon for the mean PA pressure ever to exceed 40 mm Hg in these patients, whereas it is unusual for the mean PA pressure to be less than 40 mm Hg in patients with IPAH. Consequently the combination of an abnormality consistent with interstitial lung disease on the chest CT scan and mild pulmonary hypertension should indicate the diagnosis of pulmonary hypertension associated with ILD and not IPAH (**Fig. 78-11**).

Most therapies for ILD have been directed toward halting progression or inducing regression of the interstitial disease process with immunosuppressive and anti-inflammatory agents. Overall, the results

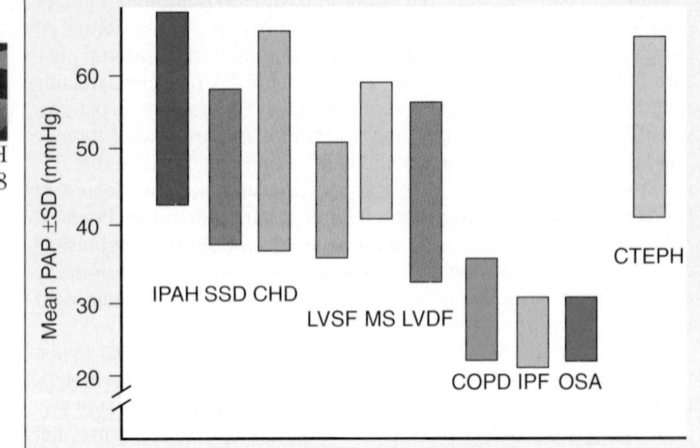

FIGURE 78-11 Mean PAP in patients with different causes of pulmonary hypertension (PH). The mean PAP ± 1 SDs (standard deviations) are shown from published series of patients with pulmonary hypertension from a variety of causes undergoing catheterization. From the graph, it would be difficult to determine the cause of the PH based on the mean PA pressure, with the exception of those with underlying lung disease. CHD = congenital heart disease; IPF = idiopathic pulmonary fibrosis; LVDF = left ventricular diastolic failure; LVSF = left ventricular systolic failure; MS = mitral stenosis; SSD = scleroderma spectrum of diseases.

of these trials have been disappointing, which makes the treatment of any associated pulmonary hypertension an attractive therapeutic target. Although vasodilator therapy has been available for decades, there are no randomized clinical trials showing benefit of these agents in ILD. Given the expense and morbidity associated with these therapies, we would caution against their anecdotal use in any patient until more definitive data support their chronic use. To date, lung transplantation is the only intervention proven to improve survival.

SLEEP-DISORDERED BREATHING. Observational studies have demonstrated a wide variation in the incidence of pulmonary hypertension as a complication of obstructive sleep apnea (OSA), with a wide range of severity (see Chap. 79). OSA is associated with repetitive nocturnal arterial oxygen desaturation and hypercapnia, large intrathoracic negative pressure swings, and acute increases in PA pressure. Mild pulmonary hypertension has been reported to occur in 20% to 40% of patients,[73] although the diagnosis of pulmonary hypertension in OSA is clouded by the frequent coexistence of systemic hypertension, obesity, and diastolic dysfunction. Right heart catheterization is usually necessary to make a clear diagnosis. Acute pulmonary hemodynamic changes during obstructive apneas have been well defined; however, the extent to which these translate into persistent daytime pulmonary hypertension remains less certain. Right ventricular failure from OSA is distinctly uncommon. Treatment with continuous positive airway pressure improves pulmonary hemodynamics in patients with OSA.

ALVEOLAR HYPOVENTILATION DISORDERS. Restrictive lung disease may result from neuromuscular diseases or other factors that affect chest wall expansion, including severe obesity. Chronic alveolar hypoventilation can lead to hypoxemia, hypercapnia, and acidosis and cause pulmonary hypertension. Thoracovertebral deformities that can result in chronic alveolar hypoventilation and pulmonary hypertension include idiopathic kyphoscoliosis, spinal tuberculosis, congenital spinal developmental abnormalities, spinal cord injury, ankylosing spondylitis, or other congenital and acquired muscular skeletal conditions, such as pectus excavatum. Pulmonary hypertension is related to the reduction of the vascular bed caused by hypoventilation and hypoxia. Usually, symptoms are slowly progressive. Hypoxemia can occur from both ventilation-perfusion mismatch and underlying atelectasis. In patients with advanced disease, intermittent positive pressure breathing and noninvasive ventilation have been used successfully, as well as supplemental oxygen in patients who are hypoxemic. The development of right-sided heart failure is an unusual manifestation of respiratory failure caused solely by respiratory muscle weakness from neuromuscular disease. It usually develops in response to hypoxic and hypercapnic stimuli in patients with chronic forms of these disorders.

Bilateral diaphragmatic paralysis as a result of phrenic nerve injury, which can be traumatic or secondary to an underlying motor neuron disease, is an uncommon and rarely recognized cause of pulmonary hypertension. It may occur after cardiac surgery, as a manifestation of Lyme disease, after radiation therapy, or as a manifestation of other neurologic disorders. When an affected patient is upright, ventilation may be normal or almost normal, but when the patient is supine, gas exchange deteriorates. The diagnosis may be suspected in a patient with supine breathlessness, disturbed sleep pattern, paradoxical motion of the abdomen on inspiration, and low vital capacity in the upright position. Patients with nontraumatic bilateral diaphragmatic paralysis may go unrecognized until they present with respiratory failure or pulmonary hypertension. The diagnosis can be made when the vital capacity is reduced by more than 40% of predicted and paradoxical motion of the hemidiaphragms is noted with fluoroscopy. Patients can also have unilateral paralysis of the diaphragm, which is more common but is associated with fewer symptoms and physiological abnormalities. The treatment should always be directed toward correcting the underlying chronic neuromuscular disease, if present, and addressing nocturnal hypoventilation with noninvasive ventilatory techniques.

Pulmonary Hypertension Caused by Chronic Thromboembolic Disease

Chronic thromboembolic pulmonary hypertension (CTEPH) is an underdiagnosed disorder (see Chap. 77).[74] Pulmonary embolism, either as a single episode or as recurrent events, is thought to be the typical initiating process, followed by progressive vascular remodeling and in situ propagation of the thrombus. However, more than half of patients with CTEPH may not have a history of clinically overt pulmonary embolism. Whereas the incidence was originally believed to be approximately 0.1% to 0.5% of patients who survive an acute pulmonary embolus, more recent data have suggested a higher incidence, as much as 5%. An identifiable hypercoagulable state is found in only a minority of patients. The lupus anticoagulant is present in 10% to 20% of patients with CTEPH whereas inherited deficiencies of protein C, protein S, and antithrombin III as a group can be identified in up to 5% of this population. Other risk factors for the development of chronic thromboembolic pulmonary hypertension have been identified, including chronic inflammatory disorders, myeloproliferative syndromes, presence of a ventriculoatrial shunt, and splenectomy.

Rather than having inherent fibrinolytic resolution of the thromboembolism with restoration of vascular patency, the thromboemboli in these patients fail to resolve adequately. They undergo organization and incomplete recanalization and become incorporated into the vascular wall. Usually, they are in the subsegmental, segmental, and lobar vessels, although it is believed that chronic thromboembolism tends to propagate in a retrograde manner, leading to slowly progressive vascular obstruction. The development of a pulmonary hypertensive arteriopathy, similar to that seen in patients with other forms of pulmonary hypertension, has been documented in nonobstructive lung regions as well as in vessels distal to partially or completely occluded proximal pulmonary arteries. These small-vessel changes therefore appear to be a significant contributor to the hemodynamic progression seen in some patients. The pathology of CTEPH has features that distinguish it from IPAH. The lesions are frequently more variable—that is, there are arterial pathways that appear relatively unaffected by vascular disease and others that typically show recanalized vascular thromboses.

PATIENT EVALUATION. CTEPH involving the proximal pulmonary arteries is a well-characterized entity. The slowly progressive nature of the course of CTEPH allows right ventricular hypertrophy to ensue, which compensates for the increased pulmonary vascular resistance. However, because of progressive thrombosis or vascular changes in the uninvolved vascular bed, the pulmonary hypertension becomes progressive and the patient manifests the clinical symptoms of dyspnea, fatigue, hypoxemia, and right-sided heart failure. Patients may present with progressive dyspnea on exertion and/or signs of right heart failure after a single or recurrent episode of overt pulmonary embolism. Some patients experience a reprieve between the acute event and clinical signs of CTEPH, which may last from a few months to many years. The findings on clinical examination of patients with CTEPH are similar to those of other patients with pulmonary hypertension, with the exception that these patients tend to have lower cardiac outputs than patients with IPAH, which is often reflected in the reduced carotid arterial pulse volume. On occasion, bruits can be heard over areas of the lung that represent vessels with partial occlusions, but they must be carefully listened for. Thrombophilia screening, including testing for antiphospholipid antibodies, lupus anticoagulant, and anticardiolipin antibodies, should be performed.

The perfusion lung scan has a high sensitivity for the detection of CTEPH and is an important reason why lung scans are recommended for all patients who present with pulmonary hypertension (see Fig. 78-8). However, the lung scan typically underestimates the severity of the central pulmonary arterial obstruction. Therefore, patients who present with one or more mismatched segmental or larger defects should undergo contrast-enhanced CT scanning[75] (see Chaps. 19 and 77; **Fig. 78-12**). The contrast-enhanced CT features of CTEPH include evidence of organized thrombus lining the pulmonary vessels in an eccentric or concentric fashion, enlargement of the right ventricle and central pulmonary arteries, variation in size of segmental arteries, bronchial artery collaterals, and parenchymal changes from pulmonary infarcts. Marked variation in the size of the segmental vessels is specific for CTEPH and is believed to represent involvement of the segmental vessels caused by thromboemboli. With nonenhanced CT, areas of increased attenuation that do not obscure the vessels and that have a ground-glass appearance have been characterized as a mosaic pattern corresponding to hypoperfusion of the lung. Although this pattern is consistent with CTEPH, it may also be seen in patients with cystic fibrosis and those with bronchiectasis, but is almost never seen in patients with IPAH.

Pulmonary angiography continues to be the standard for defining the pulmonary vascular anatomy and is performed in patients thought to be amenable to surgical intervention to determine the location and surgical accessibility of the thromboemboli and to rule out other diagnostic possibilities. Maturation and organization of clot results in vessel retraction and partial recanalization, resulting in several angiographic patterns suggestive of chronic thromboembolic disease–pouch defect, pulmonary webs or bands, intimal irregularities, abrupt narrowing of major pulmonary vessels, and obstruction of main, lobar, or segmental pulmonary arteries, frequently at their point of origin. Bronchial artery collaterals may be present. Because CTEPH is usually bilateral, the presence of unilateral central PA obstruction should prompt consideration of other diagnoses, such as pulmonary vascular tumors or extravascular compression from a lung carcinoma, hilar or mediastinal adenopathy, or mediastinal fibrosis.

Hemodynamically, these patients may be indistinguishable from patients with IPAH. However, it can be misleading to rely on the pulmonary capillary wedge pressure, because there is no way for the clinician to know whether the vessel that is used to obtain the wedge pressure tracing has distal thrombus. Thus, these patients need to have a direct measurement of left ventricular end-diastolic pressure when the diagnosis is made. Patients with CTEPH tend to have higher right atrial pressures and lower cardiac outputs than comparable patients with IPAH for the same level of PA pressure. Some patients will have a reactive component to their pulmonary hypertension believed to be attributable to pulmonary vasoconstriction in the vasculature that is uninvolved with pulmonary thromboemboli. One clinical dilemma is the patient with a documented solitary pulmonary embolism who develops pulmonary hypertension. Whether this represents coincidence, a cause and effect phenomenon, or a subset of genetically susceptible individuals may be impossible to resolve.

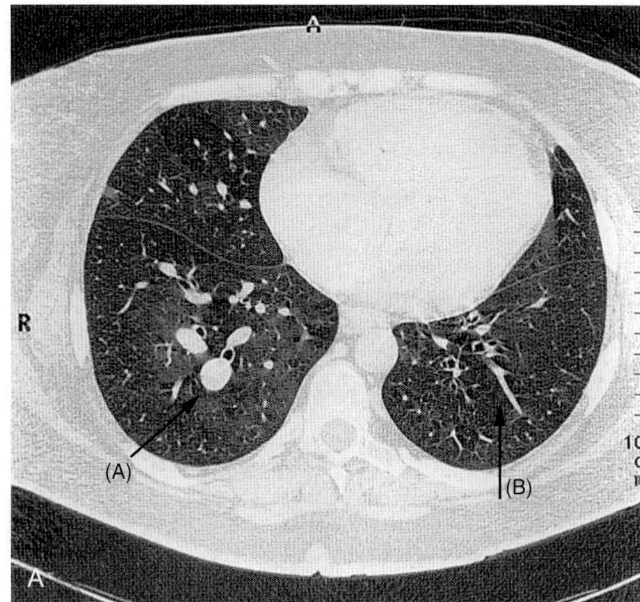

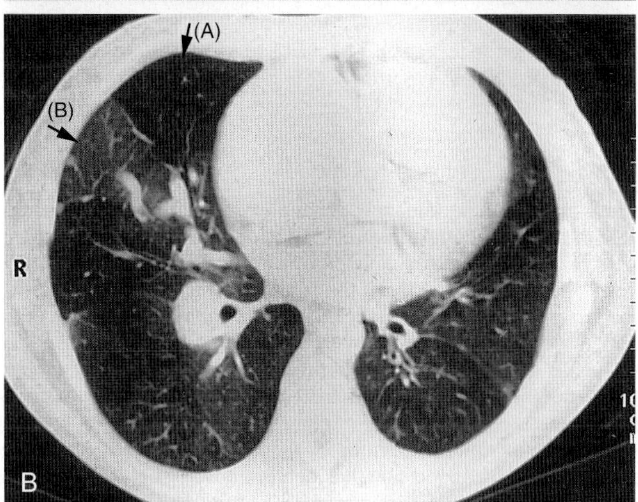

FIGURE 78-12 Chest CT scans in a patient with CTEPH. **A,** Helical scan with contrast medium enhancement of the pulmonary vasculature shows a marked disparity in vessel size between the involved vessels (A), which are enlarged from thrombus, and the uninvolved vessels (B). **B,** Noncontrast-enhanced high-resolution scan illustrates a marked mosaic pattern manifest by differences in density of regions of the lung parenchyma reflecting the perfused areas (B) and the nonperfused areas (A), also consistent with underlying thromboembolic disease.

TREATMENT. The natural history of CTEPH is poor and is related to the severity of the pulmonary hypertension. It is important to make the diagnostic distinction between patients with CTEPH and those with other forms of pulmonary hypertension because the treatments are so different. For the former group, a potentially curative therapy through pulmonary thromboendarterectomy (PTEA) is available (**Fig. 78-13**). In specialized centers, these patients can have a dramatic improvement in their symptoms, hemodynamics, and survival and is the treatment of choice. Because this disease is generally progressive, the hemodynamic indications for surgical intervention are an elevation of PA pressure and pulmonary vascular resistance for a period of more than 3 months, despite adequate anticoagulation. Operability is determined by the location and extent of proximal thromboemboli and should involve the main, lobar, or proximal segmental arteries. It

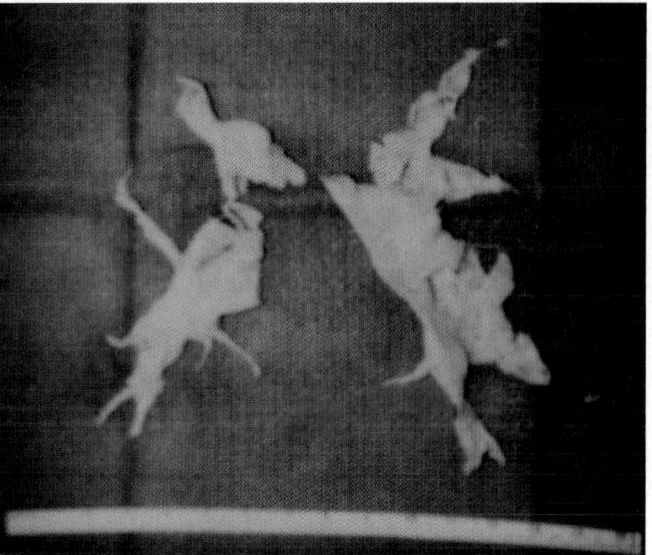

FIGURE 78-13 Specimen removed from a patient undergoing pulmonary thromboendarterectomy. The thrombus is highly organized and fibrous and represents a cast of the pulmonary circulation. Because the procedure is a true endarterectomy, the thrombosis can often be removed as a single unit. The more thrombus removed, the greater clinical improvement expected as a result of the surgery.

is also important to evaluate whether the amount of surgically accessible thrombus is compatible with a degree of hemodynamic impairment. Failure to reduce the pulmonary vascular resistance significantly with PTEA, usually a result of the small-vessel arteriopathy that may accompany this disease, is associated with a higher perioperative mortality rate and worse long-term outcome.

There is a close relationship between preoperative pulmonary vascular resistance and perioperative mortality. Right ventricular dysfunction is not considered a contraindication to surgery because right ventricular function has been noted to improve once the obstruction of the pulmonary blood flow has been removed. The operation is a true endarterectomy, requiring establishment of a dissection plane at the level of the media. The procedure is performed on cardiopulmonary bypass and usually requires periods of complete circulatory arrest to allow for a bloodless field and define an adequate dissection plane.

Postoperative management can be extremely challenging. Patients in whom a large volume of central thrombus is removed (see Fig. 78-13), associated with backbleeding from the distal vascular segments and an immediate fall in the PA pressure, usually have an extremely good postoperative course and long-term follow-up. Patients in whom small amounts of thrombus can be removed, the thrombus becomes fragmented at the time of PTEA, or there is no distal backbleeding from the segment where the thrombus was removed usually have a difficult postoperative course. In addition, lack of a significant fall in PA pressure or increase in cardiac output portends a difficult postoperative recovery. Much of the mortality risk appears to be related to severe right ventricular dysfunction, which actually initially worsens during the surgical procedure. Reperfusion injury, manifest by profound hypoxemia and pulmonary infiltrates corresponding to the segments where thrombus was removed, occurs in approximately 15% to 20% of patients and can be extensive. The only effective management of this complication is sustained assisted ventilation and oxygen supplementation. Survivors who have a good result, with a significant reduction in postoperative pulmonary vascular resistance at 48 hours, can expect to realize an improvement in functional class and exercise tolerance. Lifelong anticoagulation with a goal INR ratio of 2.5 to 3.5 is indicated postoperatively.

Some patients will have extensive disease that is inoperable or only partially amenable to surgical removal. The use of pulmonary vasodilators has been tested in anecdotal short-term studies with some success.[76] Both bosentan and sildenafil have been associated with an improvement in symptoms and exercise tolerance. It is assumed that the drugs affect the uninvolved pulmonary vasculature. Because there have been no prospective randomized trials of vasodilators in CTEPH, it remains unknown whether their use will translate into a clinically meaningful and sustained improvement in these patients. Nonetheless, in patients with inoperable CTEPH a clinical trial of pulmonary vasodilator therapy may be warranted, with the goal of improving the patient's symptomatology and quality of life.

Pulmonary Hypertension from Conditions with Uncertain Mechanisms

SICKLE CELL DISEASE. Cardiopulmonary complications are common in sickle cell disease. The cause of pulmonary hypertension, which has been reported in 20% to 32% of sickle cell disease patients, is multifactorial, with contributing factors that include hemolysis, impaired NO bioavailability, chronic hypoxemia, high cardiac output, thromboembolism, and parenchymal and vascular injury caused by sequestration of sickle erythrocytes, chronic liver disease, and asplenia.[77] In general, the hemodynamic profile of most patients with pulmonary hypertension in the setting of sickle cell disease is distinct from those with IPAH. It is characterized by a more modest elevation in PA pressure, an elevation in left heart filling pressures, and invariably a markedly elevated cardiac output. Left-sided heart disease, or pulmonary venous hypertension, is a contributing factor in most patients. Whether the pulmonary hypertension reduces survival or is simply a marker of more advanced sickle cell disease remains unclear. Intensification of sickle cell disease therapy, such as with hydroxyurea or exchange transfusions, should be the mainstay of treatment. There have been no controlled trials demonstrating benefit from pulmonary vasodilator therapy.

SCHISTOSOMIASIS. Although schistosomiasis is extremely rare in North America, hundreds of millions of people are affected worldwide, particularly in developing countries.[78] The development of pulmonary hypertension almost always occurs in the setting of hepatosplenic disease. Clinical features appear when ova embolize to the lungs, where they induce formation of delayed hypersensitivity granulomas. In addition, deposition of fibrous tissue may cause narrowing, thickening, and occlusion of the pulmonary arterioles. Histologically, focal changes related directly to the presence of schistosome ova may be located in the alveolar tissue or in the pulmonary arteries. However, classic changes typical of IPAH are also found, including plexiform lesions. The clinical symptoms and radiographic findings in these patients who develop pulmonary hypertension are not distinctive. In developing countries, this condition can be confused with IPAH.[79] The diagnosis of schistosomiasis-induced pulmonary hypertension is confirmed by finding the parasite ova in the urine or stool of persons with symptoms. However, the insidious onset of pulmonary vascular disease years after infection makes finding these parasite ova difficult. Active infections are treated with praziquantel, which kills the adult worms and stops further destruction of tissue by ova deposition. However, eradication of the infection does not seem to alter the progression of the pulmonary vascular disease.

SARCOIDOSIS. Sarcoidosis is a multisystemic granulomatous disease of unknown origin characterized by an enhanced cellular immune response at the sites of involvement. Although any organ can be involved, sarcoidosis most commonly affects the lungs and intrathoracic lymph nodes. The clinical manifestation and natural history of sarcoidosis vary greatly, but the lung is involved in more than 90% of patients. The most common presenting symptoms are cough and shortness of breath, which is of a progressive nature. As the disease progresses in the lung parenchyma, extensive interstitial fibrosis is the result. In addition, obstructive airway disease, fibrocystic disease, bronchiectasis, endobronchial granulomas, and lobar atelectasis are common consequences of lung involvement. Cardiac involvement from sarcoidosis appears to be more common than previously thought and may be present in up to one third of cases.[80] Consequently, patients presenting with dyspnea should undergo a thorough cardiac evaluation for the possibility of cardiac involvement. Noncaseating granulomas may infiltrate the myocardium and lead to the development of a restrictive cardiomyopathy (see Chap. 68). Patients with cardiac involvement from sarcoidosis also present with varying degrees of heart block, arrhythmias, and/or clinical features of biventricular diastolic heart failure. The prognosis of patients with cardiac involvement from sarcoidosis is variable but can be poor.

Pulmonary hypertension is usually the result of chronic severe fibrocystic sarcoidosis. Patients have chronic progressive dyspnea with effort, a chest radiograph demonstrating severe diffuse interstitial fibrotic lung disease, and pulmonary function test results that reflect severe restrictive physiology and marked hypoxemia. In these cases, the resulting pulmonary hypertension is usually mild to moderate and typical of patients presenting with restrictive lung disease of any cause. Management is generally focused on reversing any acute exacerbations of the lung disease and giving supplemental oxygen, when indicated. A subset of patients present with severe pulmonary hypertension thought to be caused by pulmonary vascular involvement, often in the setting of quiescent disease. It appears that these patients develop pulmonary vascular disease triggered in some way by the sarcoid disease process. The use of intravenous epoprostenol chronically may reverse the right-sided heart failure and improve hemodynamics, but will not affect the underlying fibrotic lung disease, and most patients will remain symptomatic and dyspneic.[81]

Future Perspectives

It has become apparent that the clinical manifestation of pulmonary hypertension is a final common pathway originating from diverse abnormalities in the pulmonary circulation associated with a number of risk factors. Animal models of pulmonary hypertension have illustrated how changes in specific molecular pathways can produce pulmonary hypertension, and how blocking these pathways can lead to reversal of advanced disease. Whether the reversal of the disease can be achieved in patients with therapy remains unknown, but to date has never been demonstrated. As the molecular pathways involved in pulmonary hypertension are becoming elucidated and understood, drugs that block these pathways will hold promise as future treatment. Although the presence of redundant pathways and multiple abnormalities will make clinical progress more challenging, clinical trials using growth factor inhibitors are being conducted. Many patients with long-standing pulmonary hypertension can function at a reasonable level as long as their right ventricular function remains intact. Novel therapies aimed at improving right ventricular adaptation to pulmonary hypertension with medications, or augmenting right ventricular function with medical devices, is another area that has great potential.

REFERENCES

Normal Pulmonary Circulation

1. Kasper M: Phenotypic characterization of pulmonary arteries in normal and diseased lung. Chest 128:547S, 2005.
2. Bartsch P, Gibbs JS: Effect of altitude on the heart and the lungs. Circulation 116:2191, 2007.
3. Weir EK, Lopez-Barneo J, Buckler KJ, Archer SL: Acute oxygen-sensing mechanisms. N Engl J Med 353:2042, 2005.
4. Ichinose F, Roberts JD Jr, Zapol WM: Inhaled nitric oxide: A selective pulmonary vasodilator: Current uses and therapeutic potential. Circulation 109:3106, 2004.

Pathobiology of Pulmonary Arterial Hypertension

5. Rabinovitch M: Molecular pathogenesis of pulmonary arterial hypertension. J Clin Invest 118:2372, 2008.
6. Morrell NW, Adnot S, Archer SL, et al: Cellular and molecular basis of pulmonary arterial hypertension. J Am Coll Cardiol 54:S20, 2009.
7. Budhiraja R, Tuder RM, Hassoun PM: Endothelial dysfunction in pulmonary hypertension. Circulation 109:159, 2004.
8. McLaughlin VV, Archer SL, Badesch DB, et al: ACCF/AHA 2009 expert consensus document on pulmonary hypertension. Circulation 119:2250, 2009.
9. Pietra GG, Capron F, Stewart S, et al: Pathologic assessment of vasculopathies in pulmonary hypertension. J Am Coll Cardiol 43:25S, 2004.
10. Gorlach A, BelAiba RS, Hess J, Kietzmann T: Thrombin activates the p21-activated kinase in pulmonary artery smooth muscle cells. Role in tissue factor expression. Thromb Haemost 93:1168, 2005.
11. Benisty JI, McLaughlin VV, Landzberg MJ, et al: Elevated basic fibroblast growth factor levels in patients with pulmonary arterial hypertension. Chest 126:1255, 2004.
12. White RJ, Meoli DF, Swarthout RF, et al: Plexiform-like lesions and increased tissue factor expression in a rat model of severe pulmonary arterial hypertension. Am J Physiol Lung Cell Mol Physiol 293:L583, 2007.
13. Barst RJ, McGoon M, Torbicki A, et al: Diagnosis and differential assessment of pulmonary arterial hypertension. J Am Coll Cardiol 43:40S, 2004.
14. Yu Y, Fantozzi I, Remillard CV, et al: Enhanced expression of transient receptor potential channels in idiopathic pulmonary arterial hypertension. Proc Natl Acad Sci USA 101:13861, 2004.
15. Hong Z, Smith AJ, Archer SL, et al: Pergolide is an inhibitor of voltage-gated potassium channels, including Kv1.5, and causes pulmonary vasoconstriction. Circulation 112:1494, 2005.
16. Humbert M, Morrell NW, Archer SL, et al: Cellular and molecular pathobiology of pulmonary arterial hypertension. J Am Coll Cardiol 43:13S, 2004.
17. Bonnet S, Michelakis ED, Porter CJ, et al: An abnormal mitochondrial-hypoxia inducible factor-1alpha-Kv channel pathway disrupts oxygen sensing and triggers pulmonary arterial hypertension in fawn hooded rats: Similarities to human pulmonary arterial hypertension. Circulation 113:2630, 2006.
18. Bonnet S, Rochefort G, Sutendra G, et al: The nuclear factor of activated T cells in pulmonary arterial hypertension can be therapeutically targeted. Proc Natl Acad Sci USA 104:11418, 2007.
19. McMurtry MS, Archer SL, Altieri DC, et al: Gene therapy targeting survivin selectively induces pulmonary vascular apoptosis and reverses pulmonary arterial hypertension. J Clin Invest 115:1479, 2005.
20. Richter A, Yeager ME, Zaiman A, et al: Impaired transforming growth factor-beta signaling in idiopathic pulmonary arterial hypertension. Am J Respir Crit Care Med 170:1340, 2004.
21. Marcos E, Fadel E, Sanchez O, et al: Serotonin-induced smooth muscle hyperplasia in various forms of human pulmonary hypertension. Circ Res 94:1263, 2004.
22. Eddahibi S, Guignabert C, Barlier-Mur AM, et al: Cross talk between endothelial and smooth muscle cells in pulmonary hypertension: Critical role for serotonin-induced smooth muscle hyperplasia. Circulation 113:1857, 2006.
23. de Caestecker M: Serotonin signaling in pulmonary hypertension. Circ Res 98:1229, 2006.
24. Machado RD, Koehler R, Glissmeyer E, et al: Genetic association of the serotonin transporter in pulmonary arterial hypertension. Am J Respir Crit Care Med 173:793, 2006.
25. Hassoun PM, Mouthon L, Barbera JA, et al: Inflammation, growth factors, and pulmonary vascular remodeling. J Am Coll Cardiol 54:S10, 2009.
26. Hamid R, Newman JH: Evidence for inflammatory signaling in idiopathic pulmonary artery hypertension: TRPC6 and nuclear factor-kappaB. Circulation 119:2297, 2009.
27. Csiszar A, Smith KE, Koller A, et al: Regulation of bone morphogenetic protein-2 expression in endothelial cells: Role of nuclear factor-kappaB activation by tumor necrosis factor-alpha, H_2O_2, and high intravascular pressure. Circulation 111:2364, 2005.
28. Marecki JC, Cool CD, Parr JE, et al: HIV-1 Nef is associated with complex pulmonary vascular lesions in SHIV-nef-infected macaques. Am J Respir Crit Care Med 174:437, 2006.
29. Tuder RM, Abman SH, Braun T, et al: Development and pathology of pulmonary hypertension. J Am Coll Cardiol 54:S3, 2009.
30. Newman JH, Trembath RC, Morse JA, et al: Genetic basis of pulmonary arterial hypertension. J Am Coll Cardiol 43:33S, 2004.
31. Cogan JD, Vnencak-Jones CL, Phillips JA 3rd, et al: Gross BMPR2 gene rearrangements constitute a new cause for primary pulmonary hypertension. Genet Med 7:169, 2005.
32. Teichert-Kuliszewska K, Kutryk MJ, Kuliszewski MA, et al: Bone morphogenetic protein receptor-2 signaling promotes pulmonary arterial endothelial cell survival: Implications for loss-of-function mutations in the pathogenesis of pulmonary hypertension. Circ Res 98:209, 2006.
33. Machado RD, James V, Southwood M, et al: Investigation of second genetic hits at the BMPR2 locus as a modulator of disease progression in familial pulmonary arterial hypertension. Circulation 111:607, 2005.
34. Machado RD, Aldred MA, James V, et al: Mutations of the TGF-beta type II receptor BMPR2 in pulmonary arterial hypertension. Hum Mutat 27:121, 2006.
35. Aldred MA, Vijayakrishnan J, James V, et al: BMPR2 gene rearrangements account for a significant proportion of mutations in familial and idiopathic pulmonary arterial hypertension. Hum Mutat 27:212, 2006.
36. Long L, MacLean MR, Jeffery TK, et al: Serotonin increases susceptibility to pulmonary hypertension in BMPR2-deficient mice. Circ Res 98:818, 2006.

Clinical Assessment of the Patient

37. van Wolferen SA, Marcus JT, Westerhof N, et al: Right coronary artery flow impairment in patients with pulmonary hypertension. Eur Heart J 29:120, 2008.
38. Souza R, Bogossian HB, Humbert M, et al: N-terminal-pro-brain natriuretic peptide as a haemodynamic marker in idiopathic pulmonary arterial hypertension. Eur Respir J 25:509, 2005.
39. Li JH, Safford RE, Aduen JF, et al: Pulmonary hypertension and thyroid disease. Chest 132:793, 2007.
40. McGoon M, Gutterman D, Steen V, et al: Screening, early detection, and diagnosis of pulmonary arterial hypertension: ACCP evidence-based clinical practice guidelines. Chest 126:14S, 2004.
41. Fisher MR, Forfia PR, Chamera E, et al: Accuracy of Doppler echocardiography in the hemodynamic assessment of pulmonary hypertension. Am J Respir Crit Care Med 179:615, 2009.
42. Benza R, Biederman R, Murali S, et al: Role of cardiac magnetic resonance imaging in the management of patients with pulmonary arterial hypertension. J Am Coll Cardiol 52:1683, 2008.
43. Salzman SH: The 6-min walk test: clinical and research role, technique, coding, and reimbursement. Chest 135:1345, 2009.
44. Oudiz RJ, Barst RJ, Hansen JE, et al: Cardiopulmonary exercise testing and six-minute walk correlations in pulmonary arterial hypertension. Am J Cardiol 97:123, 2006.
45. Ghofrani HA, Wilkins MW, Rich S: Uncertainties in the diagnosis and treatment of pulmonary arterial hypertension. Circulation 118:1195, 2008.
46. Halpern SD, Taichman DB: Misclassification of pulmonary hypertension due to reliance in pulmonary capillary wedge pressure rather than left ventricular end-diastolic pressure. Chest 136:37, 2009.

47. Simonneau G, Robbins IM, Beghetti M, et al: Updated clinical classification of pulmonary hypertension. J Am Coll Cardiol 54:S43, 2009.
48. Hyduk A, Croft J, Ayala C, et al: Pulmonary hypertension surveillance—United States, 1980-2002. MMRWR Surveill Summ 54:1, 2005.

Pulmonary Arterial Hypertension

49. Mereles D, Ehlken N, Kreuscher S, et al: Exercise and respiratory training improve exercise capacity and quality of life in patients with severe chronic pulmonary hypertension. Circulation 114:1482, 2006.
50. Johnson SR, Mehta S, Granton JT: Anticoagulation in pulmonary arterial hypertension: A qualitative systematic review. Eur Respir J 28:999, 2006.
51. Simonneau G, Rubin LJ, Galie N, et al: Addition of sildenafil to long-term intravenous epoprostenol therapy in patients with pulmonary arterial hypertension: A randomized trial. Ann Intern Med 149:521, 2008.
52. Sitbon O, Humbert M, Jais X, et al: Long-term response to calcium channel blockers in idiopathic pulmonary arterial hypertension. Circulation 111:3105, 2005.
53. Gomberg-Maitland M, Olschewski H: Prostacyclin therapies for the treatment of pulmonary arterial hypertension. Eur Respir J 31:891, 2008.
54. Lang I, Gomez-Sanchez M, Kneussl M, et al: Efficacy of long-term subcutaneous treprostinil sodium therapy in pulmonary hypertension. Chest 129:1636, 2006.
55. Nagendran J, Archer SL, Soliman D, et al: Phosphodiesterase type 5 is highly expressed in the hypertrophied human right ventricle, and acute inhibition of phosphodiesterase type 5 improves contractility. Circulation 116:238, 2007.
56. Galie N, Ghofrani HA, Torbicki A, et al: Sildenafil citrate therapy for pulmonary arterial hypertension. N Engl J Med 353:2148, 2005.
57. Galie N, Brundage BH, Ghofrani HA, et al: Tadalafil therapy for pulmonary arterial hypertension. Circulation 119:2894, 2009.
58. Dupuis J, Hoeper MM: Endothelin receptor antagonists in pulmonary arterial hypertension. Eur Respir J 31:407, 2008.
59. Kurzyna M, Dabrowski M, Bielecki D, et al: Atrial septostomy in treatment of end-stage right heart failure in patients with pulmonary hypertension. Chest 131:977, 2007.
60. Orens JB, Garrity ER Jr: General overview of lung transplantation and review of organ allocation. Proc Am Thorac Soc 6:13, 2009.
61. Dempsie Y, Morecroft I, Welsh DJ, et al: Converging evidence in support of the serotonin hypothesis of dexfenfluramine-induced pulmonary hypertension with novel transgenic mice. Circulation 117:2928, 2008.
62. Berger RMF: Pulmonary hypertension associated with congenital cardiac disease. Cardiol Young 19:311, 2009.
63. Galie N, Beghetti M, Gatzoulis MA, et al: Bosentan therapy in patients with Eisenmenger syndrome: A multicenter, double-blind, randomized, placebo-controlled study. Circulation 114:48, 2006.
64. Condliffe R, Kiely DG, Peacock AJ, et al: Connective tissue disease-associated pulmonary arterial hypertension in the modern treatment era. Am J Respir Crit Care Med 179:151, 2009.
65. Krowka MJ: Evolving dilemmas and management of portopulmonary hypertension. Semin Liver Dis 26:265, 2006.
66. Frazier AA, Franks TJ, Mohammed TL, et al: From the Archives of the AFIP: Pulmonary veno-occlusive disease and pulmonary capillary hemangiomatosis. Radiographics 27:867, 2007.

Pulmonary Venous Hypertension

67. Lam CS, Roger VL, Rodeheffer RJ, et al: Pulmonary hypertension in heart failure with preserved ejection fraction: A community-based study. J Am Coll Cardiol 53:1119, 2009.
68. Fawzy ME, Hassan W, Stefadouros M, et al: Prevalence and fate of severe pulmonary hypertension in 559 consecutive patients with severe rheumatic mitral stenosis undergoing mitral balloon valvotomy. J Heart Valve Dis 13:942, 2004.
69. Montani D, Price LC, Dorfmuller P, et al: Pulmonary veno-occlusive disease. Eur Respir J 33:189, 2009.

Pulmonary Arterial Hypertension Associated with Hypoxic Lung Disease

70. Chaouat A, Bugnet AS, Kadaoui N, et al: Severe pulmonary hypertension and chronic obstructive pulmonary disease. Am J Respir Crit Care Med 172:189, 2005.
71. Stolz D, Rasch H, Linka A, et al: A randomised, controlled trial of bosentan in severe COPD. Eur Respir J 32:619, 2008.
72. Behr J, Ryu JH: Pulmonary hypertension in interstitial lung disease. Eur Respir J 31:1357, 2008.
73. Atwood CW, McCrory D, Garcia JGN, et al: Pulmonary artery hypertension and sleep-disordered breathing: ACCP evidence-based clinical practice guidelines. Chest 126:72S, 2004.

Pulmonary Hypertension Caused by Chronic Thromboembolic Disease

74. Auger WR, Fedullo PF: Chronic thromboembolic pulmonary hypertension. Semin Respir Crit Care Med 30:471, 2009.
75. Coulden R: State-of-the-art imaging techniques in chronic thromboembolic pulmonary hypertension. Proc Am Thorac Soc 3:577, 2006.
76. Condliffe R, Kiely DG, Gibbs JS, et al: Improved outcomes in medically and surgically treated chronic thromboembolic pulmonary hypertension. Am J Respir Crit Care Med 177:1122, 2008.

Pulmonary Hypertension with Uncertain or Multifactorial Mechanisms

77. Machado RF, Gladwin MT: Chronic sickle cell lung disease: New insights into the diagnosis, pathogenesis and treatment of pulmonary hypertension. Br J Haematol 129:449, 2005.
78. Butrous G, Ghofrani HA, Grimminger F: Pulmonary vascular disease in the developing world. Circulation 118:1758, 2008.
79. Lapa M, Dias B, Jardim C, et al: Cardiopulmonary manifestations of hepatosplenic schistosomiasis. Circulation 119:1518, 2009.
80. Mehta D, Lubitz SA, Frankel Z, et al: Cardiac involvement in patients with sarcoidosis: Diagnostic and prognostic value of outpatient testing. Chest 133:1426, 2008.
81. Fisher KA, Serlin DM, Wilson KC, et al: Sarcoidosis-associated pulmonary hypertension: Outcome with long-term epoprostenol treatment. Chest 130:1481, 2006.

CHAPTER 79 Sleep Apnea and Cardiovascular Disease

Virend K. Somers

Normal Sleep Physiology

Sleep, which usually comprises up to one third of our lifetime, is a complex and dynamic physiologic process.[1] Rapid eye movement (REM) sleep makes up about 25% of a night of sleep. It is a tonic state punctuated by periods of phasic activity, during which autonomic and cardiac functions are erratic.[2] Thermoregulation is reduced, and sympathetic neural drive, heart rate, and blood pressure increase. Non–rapid eye movement (NREM) sleep comprises about 75% of sleep. During NREM sleep, in contrast to REM sleep, autonomic and cardiac regulation is stable. Sympathetic neural activity decreases and parasympathetic tone predominates, which decreases the arterial baroreceptor set point, heart rate, blood pressure, cardiac output, and systemic vascular resistance. Because of the predominance of parasympathetic neural tone, it is not unusual for healthy individuals to have sinus bradycardia, marked sinus arrhythmia, sinus pauses, or first-degree and type I second-degree atrioventricular block during sleep. Thus, the majority of sleep is quiescent with respect to cardiac function, with the exception being the dynamic changes of phasic REM sleep.

Sleep Disorders

The two principal sleep disorders with a recognized impact on cardiovascular function and disease are obstructive sleep apnea (OSA) and central sleep apnea (CSA).

Obstructive Sleep Apnea

DEFINITION AND PHYSIOLOGY. OSA is a sleep-related breathing disorder. Its principal feature is upper airway occlusion, which causes partial or complete cessation of air flow. This causes hypoxia and strenuous ventilatory efforts, followed by a transient arousal and restoration of airway patency and air flow. This sequence of events can recur hundreds of times nightly. In symptomatic individuals, the condition is called the obstructive sleep apnea syndrome.

An obstructive apnea is defined as the absence of air flow for at least 10 seconds in the presence of active ventilatory efforts, which are reflected by thoracoabdominal movements. An obstructive hypopnea is defined as a decrease of more than 50% in thoracoabdominal movements for at least 10 seconds associated with a decrease of more than 4% in oxygen saturation. The apnea-hypopnea index (AHI) is the average number of apneic and hypopneic events per hour of sleep, and it is the most common metric to describe the severity of OSA. OSA is present when the AHI is 5 or more and is considered severe when the AHI is 30 or more; however, these are essentially arbitrary thresholds created by expert consensus. In the context of cardiovascular disease and risk assessment,[3,4] low AHI thresholds are reasonable because clinically important cardiovascular outcomes are associated with an AHI as low as (and even lower than) 5 events/hour.[2]

The mechanisms of OSA relate to the structure and function of the pharyngeal musculature and the state of the central nervous system during sleep.[3,5] The patency of the upper airway is determined by pharyngeal dilator and abductor muscle tone competing against negative transmural pharyngeal pressures during inspiration. The supine position makes airway collapse more likely because of the posterior displacement of the tongue, soft palate, and mandible. People with micrognathia, retrognathia, tonsillar hypertrophy, macroglossia, and acromegaly are especially predisposed to OSA. Also, changes in central nervous system activity during sleep, particularly in REM sleep, decrease diaphragmatic activity (i.e., ventilatory drive) and pharyngeal muscle tone, which destabilizes the airway and favors airway collapse. Sedative-hypnotic medications or alcohol may compound these effects and increase the risk of obstructive apneas. Apneas terminate because of transient arousals to a lighter sleep stage, which are demonstrable with electroencephalographic recordings but may not result in subjective awakening or awareness. Chemoreceptors, which are activated by the hypoxemia and hypercapnia of apnea, elicit postapneic hyperventilation, also contributing to arousals.

PATHOPHYSIOLOGIC MECHANISMS LINKING OBSTRUCTIVE SLEEP APNEA TO CARDIOVASCULAR DISEASE. Individuals with OSA demonstrate an increased sensitivity of the peripheral chemoreceptors, which results in an increased ventilatory response to hypoxemia during sleep and wakefulness.[3] Activation of the chemoreceptors also stimulates sympathetic traffic to skeletal muscle vasculature, which results in peripheral vasoconstriction. During apneas, as hypoxemia worsens, peripheral sympathetic activity markedly increases and blood pressure acutely rises.[2] Severe oxygen desaturations may be associated with ventricular ectopy. In some individuals, peripheral sympathetic overactivity may be accompanied by cardiac parasympathetic activation, which results in peripheral vasoconstriction and bradycardia (i.e., the homeostatic "diving reflex" that simultaneously decreases myocardial oxygen demand and increases cerebral and cardiac perfusion).[2,3] Even during daytime wakefulness, individuals with OSA have persistently heightened sympathetic activity, partly because of tonic chemoreflex activation.

These mechanisms may be manifested clinically by a lack of the usual dip in nocturnal blood pressure, drug-resistant hypertension (see Chaps. 45 and 46), automatic tachycardias driven by sympathetic activity, and profound nocturnal bradycardias caused by cardiac vagal activity. Common nocturnal arrhythmias, such as marked sinus arrhythmia and second-degree atrioventricular block (Mobitz type I), are exacerbated, and higher degree conduction abnormalities, such as long sinus pauses and advanced atrioventricular block, may occur transiently (see Chaps. 36 and 39).[2-4] The chronically elevated sympathetic activity results in increased resting heart rates, decreased heart rate variability, and increased blood pressure variability. In conjunction with structural heart disease or heart failure, this may have prognostic implications.

The inspiratory efforts against a collapsed airway during an obstructive apnea generate marked negative intrathoracic pressures, which themselves cause acute cardiac structural and hemodynamic effects.[3,4,6]

Whereas normal inspiratory pressures are about −8 cm H_2O, individuals with OSA can generate intrathoracic pressures of −30 cm H_2O or lower. This increases venous return to the right side of the heart, produces ventricular interdependence, decreases left ventricular compliance and filling, and results in decreased cardiac output. Coupled with heightened peripheral sympathetic activity, these changes can directly increase cardiac afterload and detrimentally affect left ventricular systolic function. Acute diastolic dysfunction and increases in left atrial transmural pressure also occur, which may cause atrial or pulmonary vein stretch. This is evidenced by increased atrial volume, increases in atrial natriuretic peptide levels, and the common symptom of nocturia in individuals with OSA. The intrathoracic pressure fluctuations may cause chronic diastolic dysfunction and left atrial enlargement,[7] associated with OSA independently of obesity and hypertension. These changes, together with oscillations in sympathetic and parasympathetic tone, may promote the initiation of atrial fibrillation during sleep.[8] OSA also results in the release of important neurohumoral mediators of cardiac and vascular disease.[9] Individuals with OSA have increased production of the potent vasoconstrictor endothelin and impaired endothelial function, which affect vasomotion. OSA has also been associated with systemic inflammation, which may advance atherosclerosis. Perhaps through its effects on sympathetic activity or because of sleep deprivation, OSA may increase insulin resistance, which promotes cardiovascular risk through multiple pathways.[10] Last, OSA is associated with increased levels of leptin, a hormone secreted by fat cells that is also associated with cardiovascular events.[9]

OBSTRUCTIVE SLEEP APNEA AND CARDIOVASCULAR DISEASE ASSOCIATIONS AND OUTCOMES. The true prevalence of OSA in the population is unknown because most people with OSA have not undergone polysomnography and remain undiagnosed. Population-based studies estimate that 1 in 5 middle-aged Western adults with a body mass index (BMI) of 25 to 28 kg/m^2 have OSA, and 1 in 20 are symptomatic with the OSA syndrome. OSA is strongly associated with obesity, and there is a direct relationship between BMI and the AHI.[3] OSA is present in more than 40% of those with a BMI of 30 and is especially common in individuals with a BMI of 40. OSA is also associated with multiple metabolic abnormalities, including abdominal obesity, diabetes, and dyslipidemia, and it is highly prevalent in patients with the metabolic syndrome.[10] Given its putative roles in predisposing to and exacerbating insulin resistance,[9-11] OSA may conceivably contribute to the underlying pathophysiologic process of the metabolic syndrome.

OSA is highly prevalent in patients with cardiovascular disease (**Table 79-1**). Estimates of prevalence may differ geographically according to the BMI of patient populations. Many of these cardiovascular disease associations may occur because of the comorbidities of OSA, namely, obesity and its metabolic consequences, which together increase the risk of organic heart disease. However, observational studies have suggested that OSA itself may lead to incident cardiovascular disease. In a large population sample, the AHI correlated independently and directly with the development of hypertension during a period of 4 years.[3] OSA may also be a risk factor for new-onset atrial fibrillation. In 3542 people observed for an average of about 5 years after diagnostic polysomnography, non-elderly adults (younger than 65 years) with OSA (AHI = 5) were more likely than those without OSA to have incident atrial fibrillation (**Fig. 79-1**). The severity of nocturnal oxygen desaturation was associated with the magnitude of this risk independently of other atrial fibrillation risk factors, including obesity, hypertension, and heart failure.[12] OSA may be present in up to 50% of patients requiring cardioversion for atrial

TABLE 79-1 Estimated Prevalence of Obstructive Sleep Apnea in Patients with Cardiovascular Diseases

CARDIOVASCULAR DISEASE	PREVALENCE (%)
Hypertension	50
Coronary artery disease	33
Acute coronary syndrome	50
Myocardial infarction	50-60
Heart failure with systolic dysfunction	30-40
Acute stroke	50
Atrial fibrillation requiring cardioversion	50
Lone atrial fibrillation	33

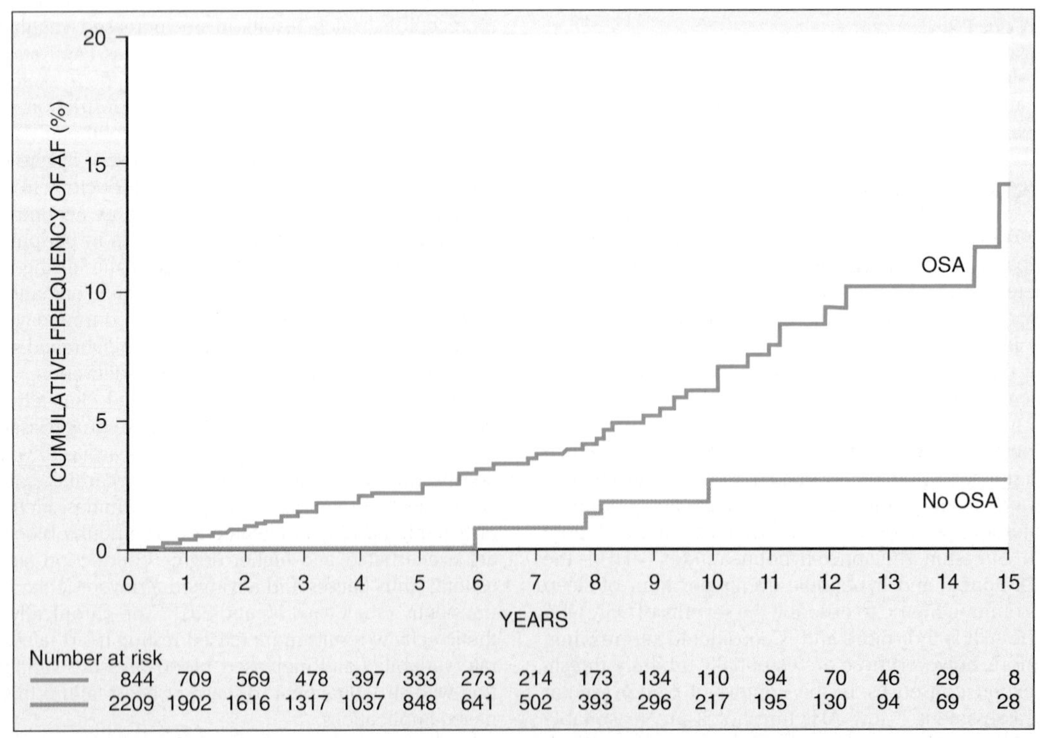

FIGURE 79-1 The cumulative frequency of new-onset atrial fibrillation (AF) in 3542 adults younger than 65 years, observed for an average of 4.6 years after diagnostic polysomnography. Individuals with OSA are shown with the blue line, and individuals without OSA are shown by the orange line. *(Modified from Gami AS, Hodge DO, Herges RM, et al: Obstructive sleep apnea, obesity, and the risk of incident atrial fibrillation. J Am Coll Cardiol 49:565, 2007.)*

fibrillation,[13] and untreated OSA may increase the likelihood of recurrence of atrial fibrillation after cardioversion.[3] There is emerging evidence implicating obstructive apnea in the pathophysiologic process and complications of hypertrophic cardiomyopathy.[14] Reliable evidence also exists for the direct effects of OSA in heart failure. Interventional studies of continuous positive airway pressure, which can effectively abolish obstructive apneas and hypopneas (see later), have shown increases in left ventricular ejection fraction.[4] OSA also can increase the risk of stroke, myocardial infarction, and death. In 1022 older adults observed for an average of about 3.5 years after diagnostic polysomnography, OSA (AHI = 5) was independently associated with a doubling of the risk of incident stroke or death.[15] In another 1651 men observed for an average of about 10 years, those with untreated severe OSA (AHI = 30) had a nearly threefold risk of death from stroke or myocardial infarction and a more than threefold risk of coronary revascularization or nonfatal myocardial infarction or stroke, independently of important comorbidities, compared with healthy men (**Fig. 79-2**).[16] Data from the Sleep Heart Health Study of more than 6000 subjects suggest that nocturnal desaturations of 4% or more are independently associated with cardiovascular disease.[17] A prospective cohort of 6441 men and women from the same study demonstrated that sleep disordered breathing was accompanied by an increase in all-cause mortality and coronary artery disease–related mortality in men aged 40 to 70 years (**Fig. 79-3**).[18] Finally, the unique nocturnal pathophysiology of OSA may be associated with an increased risk of nocturnal cardiac events. A retrospective study of 112 individuals who had undergone polysomnography and then had sudden cardiac death found that those with OSA had a peak in sudden cardiac death during the sleeping hours, which contrasted with the nadir of sudden cardiac death during this period in those without OSA and in the general population (**Fig. 79-4**).[19] In a related prospective study of patients admitted for myocardial infarction, patients with nocturnal onset of myocardial infarction had a much greater likelihood of having OSA (**Fig. 79-5**),[20] suggesting that OSA may have triggered the nocturnal myocardial infarction. Of patients with myocardial infarction onset between 12 AM and 6 AM, about 90% had OSA. Currently, however, available evidence does not definitively implicate OSA as an independent cause of cardiovascular events. **Figure 79-6** summarizes the pathophysiology of OSA, its possible intermediate cardiovascular disease mechanisms, and its cardiovascular disease associations and risks.

Central Sleep Apnea (Cheyne-Stokes Respirations)

DEFINITION AND PHYSIOLOGY. CSA refers to multiple forms of periodic breathing in which ventilation waxes and wanes, gradually alternating between hyperpnea and apnea. CSA may occur in infants and in people traveling to high altitudes. CSA, sometimes in the form of Cheyne-Stokes respirations, is also associated with heart failure (see Chaps. 25 to 27).[3,21]

CSA, like OSA, is considered a sleep-related breathing disorder, even though its characteristic ventilatory patterns can also present subtly during wakefulness. Its principal defect is an instability of ventilatory control, which results in oscillations in the arterial partial pressure of carbon dioxide ($Paco_2$) above and below the apneic threshold, producing periodic hyperpnea and apnea.[5] Ventilation is controlled by feedback loops that integrate information from multiple sources (e.g., central and peripheral chemoreceptors, intrapulmonary receptors, ventilatory muscle afferents) to limit fluctuations in $Paco_2$ and the arterial partial pressure of oxygen (Pao_2). Control of ventilation becomes unstable when a phase delay exists between the inputs (chemosensors) and responses (ventilatory muscles) in these feedback loops and also when the gain of these feedback loops is increased so that small inputs produce exaggerated responses.[5]

Patients with heart failure (see Chap. 25) have ventilatory instability and CSA because of their heightened chemosensitivity to $Paco_2$ (high loop gain) and long circulation time (phase delay). Increased chemosensitivity chronically decreases $Paco_2$ closer to the apneic threshold. Also, stimulation of pulmonary irritant mechanoreceptors by increased left ventricular filling pressures and pulmonary edema causes hyperventilation beyond what is necessary to normalize the $Paco_2$.[5] This hyperpnea leads to hypocapnia beyond the apneic threshold, and the central efferents to the ventilatory muscles become suppressed, resulting in apnea. In heart failure, this may be exacerbated by the prolonged lung to periphery circulation time, which is inversely proportional to cardiac output. During apnea, declining Pao_2 and rising $Paco_2$ ultimately initiate breathing, which may or may not be

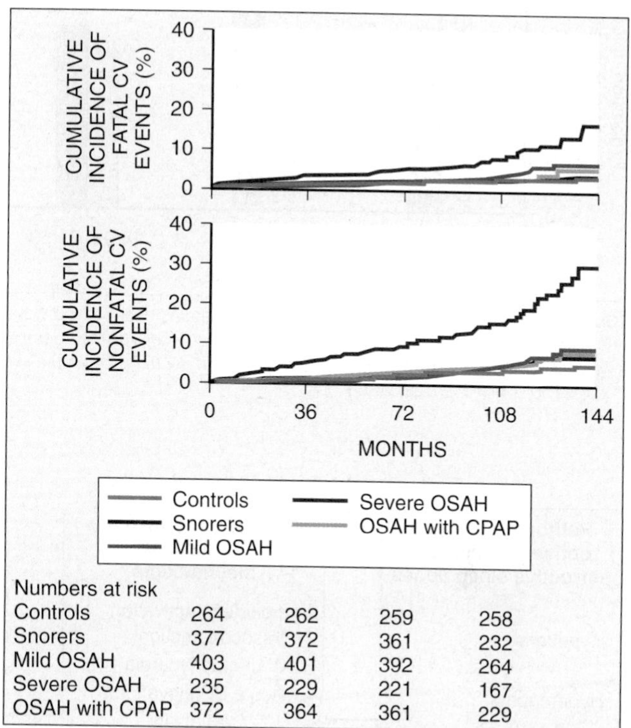

Numbers at risk				
Controls	264	262	259	258
Snorers	377	372	361	232
Mild OSAH	403	401	392	264
Severe OSAH	235	229	221	167
OSAH with CPAP	372	364	361	229

FIGURE 79-2 Cumulative frequency of fatal **(top)** and nonfatal **(bottom)** cardiovascular (CV) events in 1651 men observed for an average of 10.1 years. CPAP = continuous positive airway pressure; OSAH = obstructive sleep apnea–hypopnea syndrome. *(Modified from Marin JM, Carrizo SJ, Vicente E, et al: Long-term cardiovascular outcomes in men with obstructive sleep apnoea–hypopnoea with or without treatment with continuous positive airway pressure: An observational study. Lancet 365:1046, 2005.)*

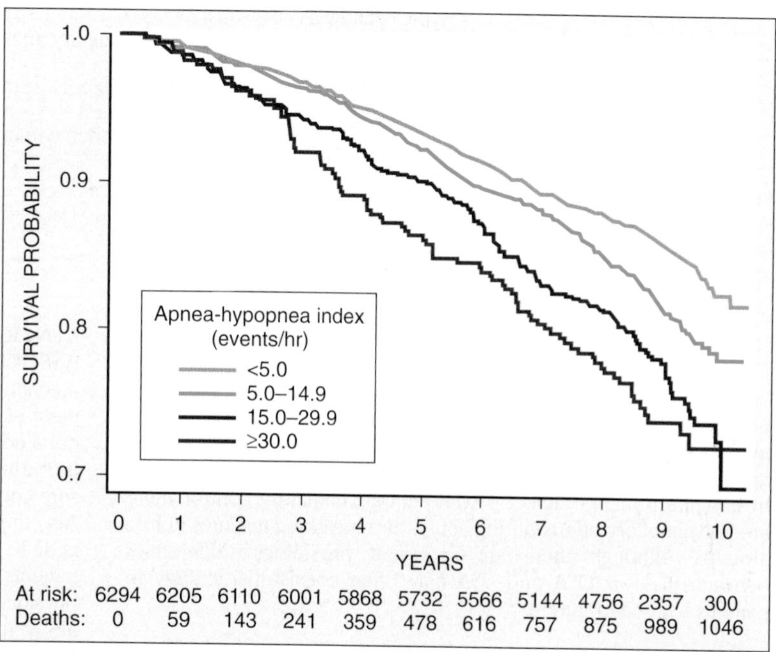

	0	1	2	3	4	5	6	7	8	9	10
At risk:	6294	6205	6110	6001	5868	5732	5566	5144	4756	2357	300
Deaths:	0	59	143	241	359	478	616	757	875	989	1046

FIGURE 79-3 Kaplan-Meier survival curves across categories of the apnea-hypopnea index. *(Modified from Punjabi NM, Caffo BS, Goodwin JL, et al: Sleep-disordered breathing and mortality: A prospective cohort study. PLoS Med 6:e1000132, 2009.)*

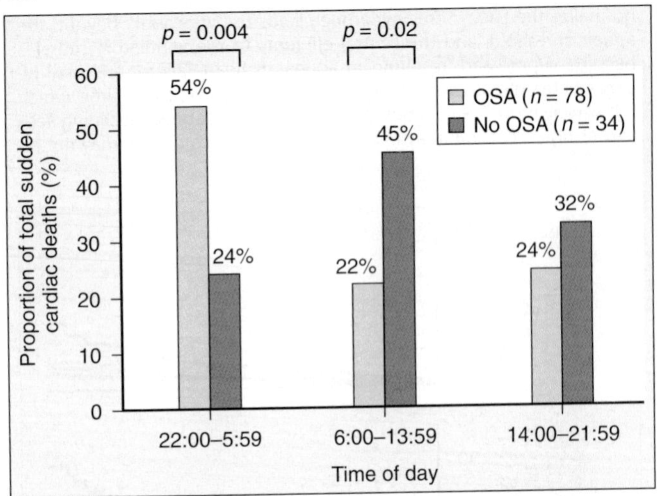

FIGURE 79-4 The day-night pattern of sudden cardiac death in individuals with and without polysomnogram-confirmed OSA. *(Modified from Gami AS, Howard DE, Olson EJ, et al: Day-night pattern of sudden death in obstructive sleep apnea. N Engl J Med 352:1206, 2005.)*

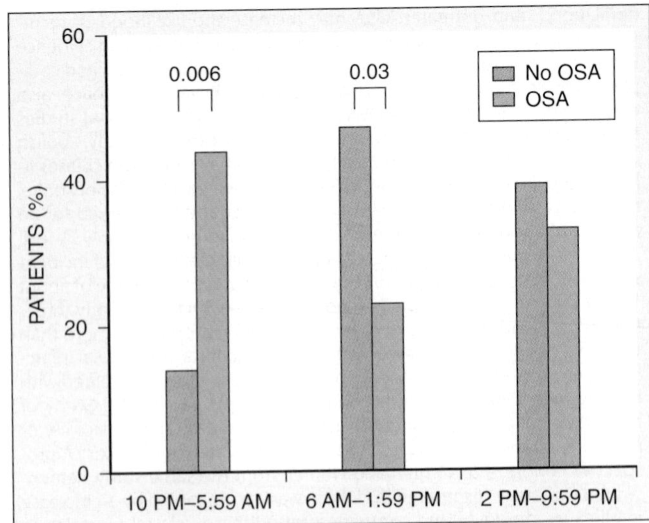

FIGURE 79-5 Day-night pattern of myocardial infarction based on three 8-hour time intervals in OSA (n = 64) and non-OSA (n = 28) patients. *(Reprinted with permission from Kuniyoshi FH, Garcia-Touchard A, Gami AS, et al: Day-night variation of acute myocardial infarction in obstructive sleep apnea. J Am Coll Cardiol 52:343, 2008.)*

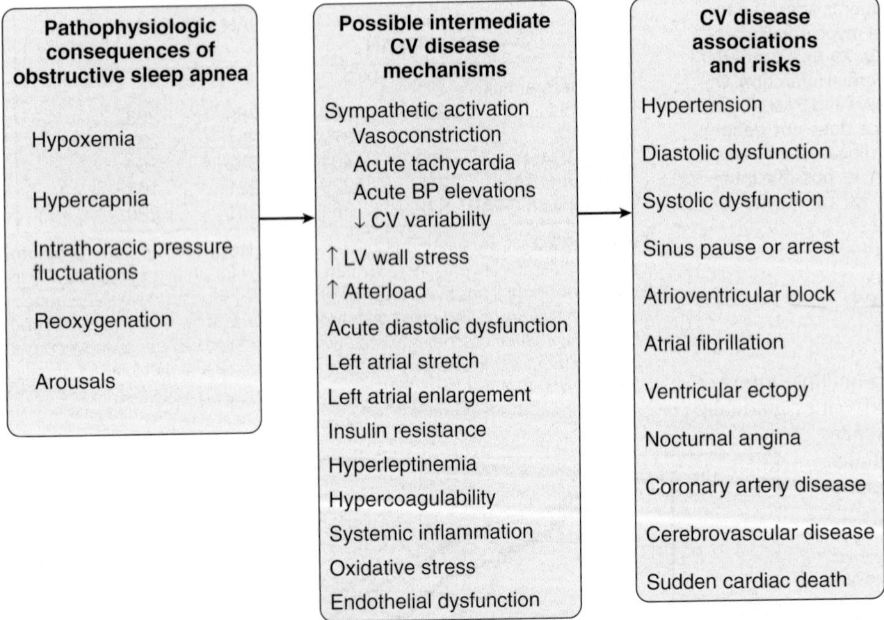

FIGURE 79-6 The pathophysiologic consequences of OSA may acutely and chronically elicit multiple intermediate cardiovascular (CV) disease mechanisms, which may promote the association of OSA with a number of cardiovascular conditions and diseases.

followed by an arousal. Arousals directly lead to hyperpnea and promote the periodic breathing of CSA because the same P_{CO_2} that was present during sleep is relatively hypercapnic for the awake state.

It is important to note the fundamental physiologic differences between OSA and CSA. In OSA, the principal defect is with pharyngeal muscle structure and function, ventilatory efforts continue during apnea, and arousals lead to airway patency and resumed breathing. In CSA, the principal defect is with central ventilatory control, there are no ventilatory efforts during apnea, and breathing resumes before arousals. Although there are important physiologic differences between the two, OSA and CSA may often coexist, particularly in patients with heart failure.[3,21]

PATHOPHYSIOLOGIC MECHANISMS LINKING CENTRAL SLEEP APNEA TO CARDIOVASCULAR DISEASE. CSA has important clinical implications for heart failure. Sleep deprivation and daytime somnolence may be especially problematic sequelae in heart failure patients who already have fatigue and functional limitations. The repetitive episodes of hypoxemia can have detrimental effects on myocardial oxygen supply, ventricular performance, and electrical stability. Individuals with CSA have heightened peripheral muscle sympathetic nerve activity and elevated levels of circulating catecholamines, which may be directly related to the severity of CSA.[3] Heart rate and blood pressure increase gradually with the rate of ventilation and peak with hyperpnea. The mechanisms of the elevated heart rate and blood pressure are not directly related to hypoxemia or sympathetic activity but instead are directly related to the periodic breathing itself and even manifested during periodic breathing in the awake state. Indeed, there is increasing evidence that daytime periodic breathing is itself associated with poor outcomes in heart failure patients.[22] Whereas CSA is associated with sleep fragmentation, cyclical hypoxemia, sympathetic overactivity, and periodicity of increased heart rate and blood pressure, its direct consequences for the cardiovascular system are unclear (see later).

CENTRAL SLEEP APNEA AND CARDIOVASCULAR DISEASE ASSOCIATIONS AND OUTCOMES. The prognostic role of CSA, the mechanisms by which it could increase cardiac risk, and the usefulness of targeting these mechanisms for intervention have been debated. CSA is associated with more severe forms of heart failure.[3,21] Individuals with CSA have elevated pulmonary capillary wedge pressure compared with patients with heart failure who do not have CSA. Also, the degree of hypocapnia in patients with CSA and heart failure is directly related to left ventricular filling pressures. However, not all patients with severe heart failure have CSA because the key pathophysiologic elements that cause unstable ventilatory control are not always present. The prevalence of CSA in patients with heart failure has been estimated at 30% to 40%.[23] Some small prospective studies assessing its prognostic value have suggested that the risk of cardiac transplantation and death are directly related to the severity of CSA, represented by the central apnea–hypopnea index.[24] It is possible that this is partly because of the associated increase in sympathetic activity, which is a known prognostic factor in heart failure. Also, patients with heart failure and CSA are more likely to have premature ventricular contractions, which may reflect ventricular electrical instability and a heightened risk of sudden cardiac death. This may not necessarily follow for patients with CSA but without heart failure. In a 10-year follow-up of 130 patients with stroke, OSA but not CSA was associated with an increased risk of early death.[25] However, large prospective systematic analyses of the relationship of CSA with significant heart failure outcomes or sudden cardiac death are lacking.[24]

Screening and Diagnosis of Sleep Disorders

History and Examination

After snoring, which is ubiquitous in people with OSA, the most common symptom of OSA is excessive daytime sleepiness, which is defined as falling asleep during daytime activities such as reading, conversing, eating, and driving. However, for unclear reasons, daytime somnolence may be less common in OSA patients with comorbid cardiovascular disease, such as heart failure. Another related but distinct symptom is tiredness on waking from sleep. An important symptom of OSA is witnessed nocturnal apnea, which is usually reported by the bed partner of the patient. Other symptoms may include nightly gasping or choking episodes, nighttime or morning headaches, morning dry mouth or sore throat, gastroesophageal acid reflux, and nocturia. Cognitive and memory difficulties as well as psychological and behavioral changes may be associated with severe OSA.[1]

The physical examination findings in people with OSA may be normal, but it is usually notable for an overweight or obese body habitus. However, about 40% of obese people do not have OSA (and about 30% of people with OSA are not obese). Increased neck circumference, particularly more than 17 inches, is more specific than the BMI for predicting OSA. Certain cranial features, such as a low soft palate, narrow oropharynx, large uvula, micrognathia, and retrognathia, also predispose to OSA.

Symptoms of CSA are not very specific, particularly in those with symptomatic heart failure. Snoring may not be present in individuals with CSA. Observations of the characteristic crescendo-decrescendo ventilatory pattern by a patient's bed partner may be helpful but may be difficult for them to identify. The physical examination is not specific for CSA beyond the findings of heart failure, although CSA is more common in male or lean heart failure patients.

Screening Tools for Obstructive Sleep Apnea

Even an expert's subjective prediction of OSA based on a patient's history and physical examination alone has a diagnostic accuracy of only about 50%. Multiple prediction models and questionnaires have been developed by researchers to assess the likelihood of OSA. Most agree that age, BMI, neck circumference, hypertension, loud and habitual snoring, and witnessed apneas are the most sensitive and specific characteristics of OSA. However, the predictive accuracy of any model is determined by the prevalence of OSA in the population in which it is applied. In patients with cardiovascular disease, in whom the prevalence of OSA is high, it is especially important to use variables with a high specificity for OSA, such as neck circumference and witnessed apneas. Overnight pulse oximetry has been used to screen for OSA; however, there are several limitations to its use, and more research is necessary to identify its appropriate role.[26]

Polysomnography

Polysomnography is the current gold standard test for the diagnosis of sleep disordered breathing, including OSA and CSA.[1] Traditionally, this is performed during a full night and, if indicated, repeated on another night to apply and to titrate continuous positive airway pressure (CPAP) therapy. Split-night studies, in which the diagnostic study occurs during the first half of the night and CPAP titration occurs during the second half of the night, are increasingly used as a more cost-effective diagnostic-therapeutic strategy. Polysomnography provides comprehensive information about sleep efficiency, sleep architecture, arousals and their causes, disordered breathing events, oscillations in oxygen saturation, and cardiac arrhythmias during specific sleep stages or events. Major limitations to obtaining polysomnography in the large population of patients with cardiovascular disease who probably have OSA or CSA are the cost and access to sleep centers. In fact, it has been estimated that more than 60% of U.S. adults with OSA are undiagnosed. In response to this, the use of portable sleep monitoring[26] for the evaluation of OSA has recently received approval for reimbursement, provided very specific monitoring criteria are met.[3]

Sleep Apnea Therapy

Obstructive Sleep Apnea

POSITIVE AIRWAY PRESSURE THERAPY. Positive airway pressure (PAP) therapy effectively splints open the airway, preventing its collapse and resultant apneas.[1] It is applied by naso-oral masks, nasal masks, or nasal pillows. A memory card records time of use for assessment of adherence. Continuous PAP is the principal therapy used. Autotitrating PAP machines and bilevel PAP machines are sometimes used for patients who do not tolerate standard continuous PAP.

A number of potential drawbacks of PAP therapy create obstacles to widespread acceptance by individual patients. These include claustrophobia, rhinitis or nasal congestion, nose bleeds, abrasions of the bridge of the nose, and air leaks because of poor fit of the device. Usually, these can be managed with conscientious attention to the patient's specific needs and regular follow-up.

Multiple cardiovascular benefits have been demonstrated with effective PAP therapy in individuals with OSA.[27] Nocturnal hypoxemia is relieved and sympathetic activity decreases, not only during sleep but also in daytime normoxic wakefulness. Similarly, PAP can promote decreases in blood pressure during sleep and daytime, particularly in patients with uncontrolled hypertension. PAP therapy is effective in relieving symptoms in some OSA patients with nocturnal myocardial ischemia or angina. In patients with heart failure and OSA, PAP causes direct improvements in left ventricular systolic function and, during several months of therapy, leads to increased left ventricular ejection fraction and improved functional status.[3,4] Long-term observational studies have suggested that OSA patients who use PAP are at decreased risk of major adverse cardiovascular events, such as myocardial infarction, coronary revascularization, stroke, and death.[16] Large randomized controlled trials assessing the effects of PAP on long-term cardiovascular outcomes have not been reported and it is unknown whether PAP will truly reduce cardiovascular events or death.[3,27] Current indications for CPAP therapy in patients with OSA are listed in **Table 79-2**.

OTHER THERAPIES. Treatment of obesity by lifestyle modification is effective in attenuating or curing OSA.[28] Pharmacologic therapy for OSA

TABLE 79-2 Indications for Continuous Positive Airway Pressure (CPAP) for Obstructive Sleep Apnea Treatment

Adults for whom surgery is a likely alternative to CPAP, with either
- An apnea-hypopnea index ≥15

or

- An apnea-hypopnea index ≥5 in a patient with symptoms (e.g., excessive daytime sleepiness, impaired cognition, mood disorders, insomnia), hypertension, ischemic heart disease, or history of stroke

Based on the Centers for Medicare and Medicaid Services, U.S. Department of Health and Human Services: Medicare Coverage Database, National Coverage, Continuous Positive Airway Pressure (CPAP) Therapy for Obstructive Sleep Apnea (OSA) (http://www.cms.hhs.gov/mcd).

is ineffective.[29] Mechanical devices other than PAP include oral appliances that maintain an anterior position of the tongue or the entire mandible.[30] These may be efficacious in patients with OSA that is mild or exclusive to the supine position. For patients with positional (supine) OSA, wearing a well-fitting shirt with a tennis ball sewn tightly to the midback should maintain a nonsupine sleep position, although there are insufficient data to prove its efficacy.

Surgical options exist for the treatment of OSA.[31] Bariatric surgery incidentally cures OSA in most morbidly obese patients; however, OSA returns if weight is regained. A number of surgeries that modify the oropharynx should be considered second-line therapies to weight loss and PAP. These are options for patients with specific craniofacial characteristics amenable to each specific approach. Tonsillectomy is more effective in children or thin adults. Tracheostomy, which was the first treatment ever effectively applied for OSA, is completely successful in abolishing obstructive apneas but should be reserved for patients with the motivation and support to maintain the apparatus.

Central Sleep Apnea

POSITIVE AIRWAY PRESSURE THERAPY. The rationale for use of positive-pressure ventilation in patients with CSA is based not on treatment of CSA per se but rather on treatment of heart failure. The same hemodynamic benefits of continuous PAP therapy shown in OSA patients have been reported in patients with heart failure and CSA, namely, decreased sympathetic activity, decreased ventricular afterload, and increased left ventricular ejection fraction.[32] Concomitant with these changes, the severity of CSA decreases. In the largest controlled trial performed to clarify the potential benefits of continuous PAP in this population, 258 patients with New York Heart Association Class II to IV heart failure and CSA were randomized to effective therapy with continuous PAP or no therapy.[33] The trial was stopped early, in part because of concerns about early divergence of transplantation-free survival favoring the control group, and no survival benefit was observed for the CPAP-treated group. A subsequent post hoc analysis proposed that survival may have been improved in those patients in whom CPAP effectively suppressed CSA, suggesting that alternative effective therapies may improve survival in these patients.[34] Adaptive pressure support servoventilation, another form of PAP, has been shown in short-term controlled trials to improve CSA. However, long-term outcome studies have not been reported.

OTHER THERAPIES. Low-flow oxygen supplementation may abolish CSA in some patients.[24] Two randomized placebo-controlled trials in heart failure patients have shown that nocturnal administration of low-flow oxygen by nasal cannula immediately improved the AHI, oxygen saturation, and sleep architecture and that 1 week of nocturnal oxygen supplementation improved functional capacity. A controlled study of 24 patients with heart failure has shown that implantation of a biventricular permanent pacemaker improves indices of CSA (both the AHI and minimum nocturnal oxygen saturation) and sleep quality after about 4 months.[35]

Small studies have shown improvements in CSA with the administration of theophylline; however, there are no large long-term studies assessing the safety of theophylline, a methylxanthine, in heart failure patients.[24,32] Another experimental intervention successful in directly abolishing CSA is the inhalation of a gas mixture that has a carbon dioxide tension as low as 1 to 3 mm Hg higher than ambient air. This resets the resting hypocapnic state of heart failure further from the apneic threshold.[24] The safety of delivery of carbon dioxide–enriched air to heart failure patients has not been assessed, and this is not applied clinically.

Future Perspectives

Whereas OSA has been implicated in cardiovascular disease generally and hypertension in particular, whether it is an independent risk factor for conditions such as myocardial infarction, stroke, and atrial fibrillation remains to be definitively established. More important, longitudinal controlled intervention trials are needed to ascertain whether treatment of OSA reduces cardiovascular events and mortality. In the meantime, treatment of patients with OSA and coexisting cardiovascular disease will need to be individualized on the basis of the overall clinical context.

Whether CSA is a marker of the severity of the underlying heart disease rather than a mediator of risk and whether it is a worthwhile target for intervention to improve cardiovascular prognosis also remain to be determined. In general, therapies that improve heart failure (e.g., angiotensin-converting enzyme inhibitors, biventricular pacing) also improve CSA. Pending further longitudinal controlled outcome studies, treatment directed specifically at CSA, such as oxygen or PAP, should probably be reserved for patients with severe daytime somnolence or symptoms attributable to nocturnal hypoxemia (angina or significant arrhythmias). Otherwise, optimization of heart failure management should remain the principal goal.

ACKNOWLEDGMENT

The author is grateful to Apoor Gami, MD, for contributions to the earlier edition of this chapter.

REFERENCES

Obstructive Sleep Apnea

1. Kryger MH, Roth T, Dement WC (eds): Principles and Practice of Sleep Medicine. 4th ed. Philadelphia, Elsevier Saunders, 2005.
2. Verrier RL, Josephson ME: Impact of sleep on arrhythmogenesis. Circ Arrhythmia Electrophysiol 2:450, 2009.
3. Somers VK, White DP, Amin R, et al: Sleep apnea and cardiovascular disease: An American Heart Association/American College of Cardiology Foundation Scientific Statement from the American Heart Association Council for High Blood Pressure Research Professional Education Committee, Council on Clinical Cardiology, Stroke Council, and Council on Cardiovascular Nursing. In collaboration with the National Heart, Lung, and Blood Institute National Center on Sleep Disorders Research (National Institutes of Health). Circulation 118:1080, 2008.
4. Bradley TD, Floras JS: Obstructive sleep apnoea and its cardiovascular consequences. Lancet 373:82, 2009.
5. White DP: Pathogenesis of obstructive and central sleep apnea. Am J Respir Crit Care Med 172:1363, 2005.
6. Shivalkar B, Van de Heyning C, Kerremans M, et al: Obstructive sleep apnea syndrome: More insights on structural and functional cardiac alterations, and the effects of treatment with continuous positive airway pressure. J Am Coll Cardiol 47:1433, 2006.
7. Otto ME, Belohlavek M, Romero-Corral A, et al: Comparison of cardiac structural and functional changes in obese otherwise healthy adults with versus without obstructive sleep apnea. Am J Cardiol 99:1298, 2007.
8. Gami AS, Friedman PA, Chung MK, et al: Therapy insight: Interactions between atrial fibrillation and obstructive sleep apnea. Nat Clin Pract Cardiovasc Med 2:145, 2005.
9. Wolk R, Gami AS, Garcia-Touchard A, Somers VK: Sleep and cardiovascular disease. Curr Probl Cardiol 30:625, 2005.
10. Svatikova A, Wolk R, Gami AS, et al: Interactions between obstructive sleep apnea and the metabolic syndrome. Curr Diab Rep 5:53, 2005.
11. McArdle N, Hillman D, Beilin L, Watts G: Metabolic risk factors for vascular disease in obstructive sleep apnea: A matched controlled study. Am J Respir Crit Care Med 175:190, 2007.
12. Gami AS, Hodge DO, Herges RM, et al: Obstructive sleep apnea, obesity, and the risk of incident atrial fibrillation. J Am Coll Cardiol 49:565, 2007.
13. Gami AS, Pressman G, Caples SM, et al: Association of atrial fibrillation and obstructive sleep apnea. Circulation 110:364, 2004.
14. Sengupta PP, Sorajja D, Eleid MF, et al: Hypertrophic obstructive cardiomyopathy and sleep-disordered breathing: An unfavorable combination. Nat Clin Pract Cardiovasc Med 6:14-15, 2009.
15. Yaggi HK, Concato J, Kernan WN, et al: Obstructive sleep apnea as a risk factor for stroke and death. N Engl J Med 353:2034, 2005.
16. Marin JM, Carrizo SJ, Vicente E, Agusti AG: Long-term cardiovascular outcomes in men with obstructive sleep apnoea-hypopnoea with or without treatment with continuous positive airway pressure: An observational study. Lancet 365:1046, 2005.
17. Punjabi NM, Newman AB, Young TB, et al: Sleep-disordered breathing and cardiovascular disease: An outcome-based definition of hypopneas. Am J Respir Crit Care Med 177:1150, 2008.
18. Punjabi NM, Caffo BS, Goodwin JL, et al: Sleep-disordered breathing and mortality: A prospective cohort study. PLoS Med 6:e1000132, 2009.
19. Gami AS, Howard DE, Olson EJ, Somers VK: Day-night pattern of sudden death in obstructive sleep apnea. N Engl J Med 352:1206, 2005.
20. Kuniyoshi FH, Garcia-Touchard A, Gami AS, et al: Day-night variation of acute myocardial infarction in obstructive sleep apnea. J Am Coll Cardiol 52:343, 2008.

Central Sleep Apnea

21. Caples SM, Somers VK: Influence of cardiac function and failure on sleep disordered breathing: Evidence for a causative role. J Appl Physiol 99:2433, 2005.
22. Brack T, Thuer I, Clarenbach CV, et al: Daytime Cheyne-Stokes respiration in ambulatory patients with severe congestive heart failure is associated with increased mortality. Chest 132:1463, 2007.
23. Oldenburg O, Lamp B, Faber L, et al: Sleep-disordered breathing in patients with symptomatic heart failure. A contemporary study of prevalence in and characteristics of 700 patients. Eur J Heart Fail 9:251, 2007.
24. Pepin JL, Chouri-Pontarollo N, Tamisier R, Levy P: Cheyne-Stokes respiration with central sleep apnoea in chronic heart failure: Proposals for a diagnostic and therapeutic strategy. Sleep Med Rev 10:33, 2006.
25. Sahlin C, Sandberg O, Gustafson Y, et al: Obstructive sleep apnea is a risk factor for death in patients with stroke: A 10-year follow-up. Arch Intern Med 168:297, 2008.

Screening and Diagnosis of Sleep Disorders

26. Littner MR: Portable monitoring in the diagnosis of the obstructive sleep apnea syndrome. Semin Respir Crit Care Med 26:56, 2005.

Sleep Apnea Therapy

27. Giles TL, Lasserson TJ, Smith BJ, et al: Continuous positive airways pressure for obstructive sleep apnoea in adults. Cochrane Database Syst Rev (1):CD001106, 2006.
28. Veasey SC, Guilleminault C, Strohl KP, et al: Medical therapy for obstructive sleep apnea: A review by the Medical Therapy for Obstructive Sleep Apnea Task Force of the Standards of Practice Committee of the American Academy of Sleep Medicine. Sleep 29:1036, 2006.
29. Smith I, Lasserson TJ, Wright J: Drug therapy for obstructive sleep apnoea in adults. Cochrane Database Syst Rev (2):CD003002, 2006.
30. Ng A, Gotsopoulos H, Darendeliler AM, Cistulli PA: Oral appliance therapy for obstructive sleep apnea. Treat Respir Med 4:409, 2005.
31. Sundaram S, Bridgman SA, Lim J, Lasserson TJ: Surgery for obstructive sleep apnoea. Cochrane Database Syst Rev (2):CD001004, 2005.
32. Javaheri S: Central sleep apnea in congestive heart failure: Prevalence, mechanisms, impact, and therapeutic options. Semin Respir Crit Care Med 26:44, 2005.
33. Bradley TD, Logan AG, Kimoff RJ, et al: Continuous positive airway pressure for central sleep apnea and heart failure. N Engl J Med 353:2025, 2005.
34. Arzt M, Floras JS, Logan AG, et al: Suppression of central sleep apnea by continuous positive airway pressure and transplant-free survival in heart failure: A post hoc analysis of the Canadian Continuous Positive Airway Pressure for Patients with Central Sleep Apnea and Heart Failure Trial (CANPAP). Circulation 115:3173, 2007.
35. Sinha AM, Skobel EC, Breithardt OA, et al: Cardiac resynchronization therapy improves central sleep apnea and Cheyne-Stokes respiration in patients with chronic heart failure. J Am Coll Cardiol 44:68, 2004.

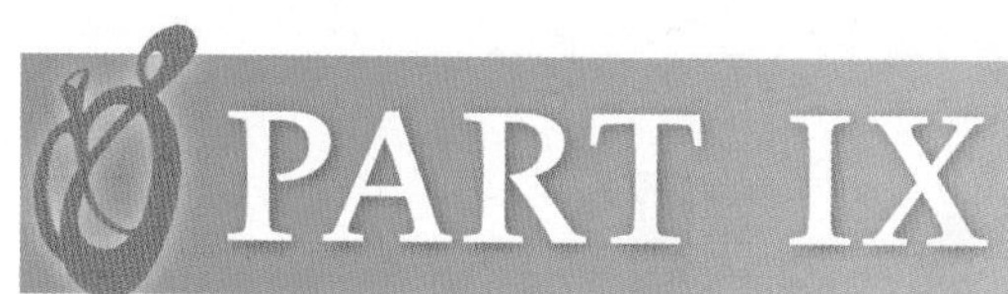

PART IX

CARDIOVASCULAR DISEASE IN SPECIAL POPULATIONS

CHAPTER 80 Cardiovascular Disease in the Elderly

Janice B. Schwartz and Douglas P. Zipes

Demographics and Epidemiology

The proportion of people aged 65 years and older in the United States is projected to increase from 12.4% (35 million) of the population in 2000 to 19.6% (71 million) in 2030 and to 82 million in 2050 (*www.cdc.gov*). The number of people older than 80 years is projected to double from 9.3 million in 2000 to 19.5 million in 2030 and to more than triple by 2050. Women represented 59% of persons older than 65 years in 2000 and are estimated to compose 56% of the older population in 2030 (**Fig. 80-1**). If current projections hold, there will be increases in the percentage of racial minorities (see Chap. 2). From 2000 to 2030, the proportion of persons aged ≥65 years who are members of racial minority groups (i.e., African American, American Indian–Alaska Native, Asian–Pacific Islander) is expected to increase from 11.3% to 16.5%, and the proportion of Hispanics is expected to increase from 5.6% to 10.9%. Almost half of people older than 65 years in the United States in 2000 had after-tax incomes at the poverty level (41% of 65- to 74-year-olds and 56% of those older than 75 years), and this trend is likely to continue.[1] Global trends are similar, with the worldwide population older than 65 years projected to increase to 973 million or 12% in 2030 and to make up about 20% of the population in 2050 (see Chap. 1). Increases will be greatest in undeveloped nations. Estimates are for twice as many women as men older than 80 years and three times as many women as men older than 90 years.

Cardiovascular disease is both the most frequent diagnosis and the leading cause of death in both men and women older than 65 years. Hypertension occurs in one half to two thirds of people older than 65 years, and heart failure is the most frequent hospital discharge diagnosis among older Americans. The profile of these common cardiovascular diseases in older patients differs from that in younger patients. Systolic but not diastolic blood pressure increases with aging, resulting in increased pulse pressure. Systolic hypertension becomes a stronger predictor of cardiovascular events, especially in women (see Chap. 81). Heart failure with preserved systolic function becomes more common at older ages and is more common in women. Coronary artery disease (CAD) is more likely to involve multiple vessels and the left main artery and is equally likely in women and men older than 65 years. Equal numbers of older men and women present with acute myocardial infarction (MI) until the age of 80 years, after which more women present. Non-ST rather than ST elevation MI accounts for two thirds of MI in older patients. More than 80% of all deaths attributable to cardiovascular disease occur in people older than 65 years, with approximately 60% of deaths in patients older than 75 years.

Importantly, cardiovascular disease in older people is not seen in isolation; 80% of older Americans have at least one chronic medical condition, and 50% have at least two. Arthritis affects about 60% of persons older than 65 years, cancer is present in 34%, and diabetes affects about 20% (**Fig. 80-2**). Also common are ear, nose, and throat problems and vision disorders and orthopedic problems. As U.S. adults live longer, the prevalence and incidence of dementia that impairs memory, decision-making capability, orientation to physical surroundings, and language also increase. The prevalence of dementia is estimated at 13% in community-dwelling white people older than 65 years and is higher in women than in men and African American and Hispanic populations.[2] By the age of 80 years, approximately 40% of people may be affected. Of Medicare beneficiaries with dementias, 60% have hypertension, 26% have CAD, 25% have had a stroke, 23% have diabetes, and 16% have heart failure.[2] Patients with dementia are three times more likely to be hospitalized and to remain in the hospital longer than are Medicare beneficiaries without dementias, such that about one quarter of all hospital patients aged 65 and older have dementia at any one time.[2]

The high morbidity and mortality from cardiovascular disease in the elderly warrant aggressive approaches to prevention and treatment that have been shown to be effective in older patients. Compelling data demonstrate reduced morbidity and mortality rates for the treatment of hypertension, heart failure, atrial fibrillation, acute coronary syndromes, CAD, stroke, diabetes, and lipid abnormalities in older patients 60 to 74 years of age, although data on minorities and women

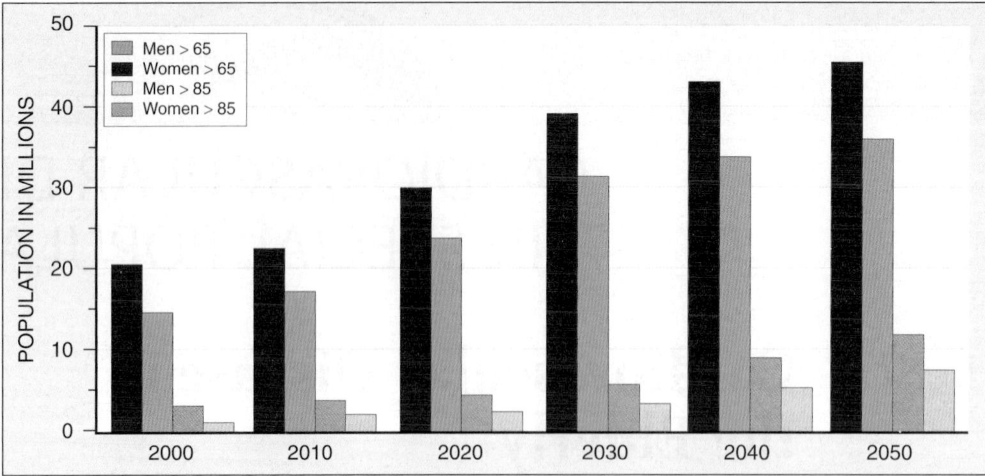

FIGURE 80-1 United States population estimates projected from 2000 until 2050. Dark pink bars represent numbers of women older than 65 years, and dark blue bars represent numbers of men older than 65 years; lighter pink bars represent numbers of women older than 85 years, and lighter blue bars represent numbers of men older than 85 years in millions of people. *(Source: U.S. Census Bureau.)*

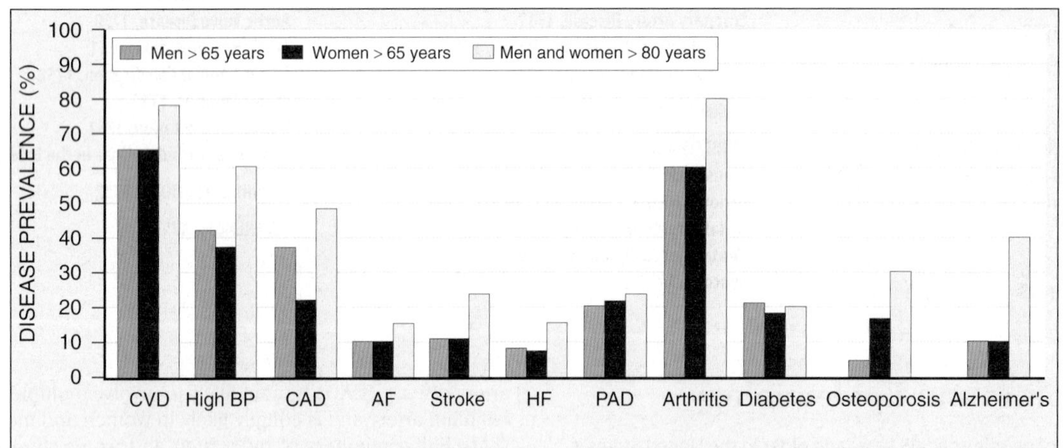

FIGURE 80-2 Prevalence of cardiovascular and other common chronic medical illnesses in older persons in the United States. Data are percentages. AF = atrial fibrillation; CAD = coronary artery disease; CVD = cardiovascular disease; HF = heart failure; high BP = hypertension (all forms); PAD = peripheral artery disease. Blue bars represent data for men older than 65 years, pink bars represent women older than 65 years, and yellow bars represent men and women older than 80 years.

are limited. Fewer trials of cardiovascular therapies have enrolled significant numbers of men or women older than 75 years, elderly patients with multisystem disease, or elderly patients with cognitive impairment, and none has addressed cardiovascular therapies in the nursing home population. When clinical trials enroll older patients, participants differ markedly from the majority of older patients. The projected increase in numbers of older people from previously understudied and undertreated groups presents both medical and economic challenges for cardiovascular disease treatment.

Pathophysiology

No universal definition of "elderly" or an accurate biomarker for aging exists. Whereas physiologic changes associated with aging do not appear at a specific age and do not proceed at the same pace in all individuals, most definitions of elderly are based on chronologic age. The World Health Organization uses 60 years of age to define elderly, whereas most U.S. classifications use the age of 65 years. Gerontologists subclassify older age groups into young old (60 to 74 years), old old (75 to 85 years), and very old (older than 85 years). Cardiovascular society statements have addressed differences in responses of patients younger than 65 years, those 65 to 74 years, and those 75 to 84 years separately from those of patients older than 85 years.[3,4] Clinicians often separate older patients into two subgroups, those 65 to 80 years of age and those older than 80 years, to highlight the frailty, reduced capacity (physical and mental), and presence of multiple disorders that are more common after 80 years of age.

Hallmarks of cardiovascular aging in humans include progressive increases in systolic blood pressure, pulse pressure, pulse wave velocity, and left ventricular mass and increased incidence of CAD and atrial fibrillation.[5-9] Reproducible age-related decreases are seen in rates of early left ventricular diastolic filling, maximal heart rates, maximal cardiac output, maximum aerobic capacity or maximal oxygen consumption ($\dot{V}O_2$max), exercise-induced augmentation of ejection fraction, reflex responses of heart rate, heart rate variability, and vasodilation in response to beta-adrenergic stimuli or endothelium-mediated vasodilator compounds.

Cellular, enzymatic, and molecular alterations in the arterial vessel wall include migration of activated vascular smooth muscle cells into the intima, with increased matrix production due to altered activity of matrix metalloproteinases, angiotensin II, transforming growth factor-β, intercellular cell adhesion molecules, and production of collagen and collagen cross-linking. There is also loss of elastic fibers, increases in fibronectin, and calcification. These processes lead to arterial dilation and increased intimal thickness, resulting in increased vascular stiffness. Increased arterial stiffness is manifested by increases in pulse wave velocity away from the heart and increased and earlier pulse wave reflections back toward the heart (often estimated as the aortic augmentation index). Typical arterial and radial waveforms from a young and older individual are shown in **Figure 80-3**. In both animal and human models of aging, endothelial cell production of nitric oxide (NO) decreases with age; there is decreased endothelial cell mass associated with increased cell senescence and apoptosis and increased NO consumption due to an age-dependent increase in vascular superoxide anion production. These changes contribute to reduced endothelial cell NO-mediated vasodilatory responses of the peripheral and coronary vasculature. Vascular responses to beta-adrenergic agonists and alpha-adrenergic blockade are also reduced with aging. In contrast, responses to non–endothelial cell–derived compounds such as nitrates and nitroprusside are preserved with aging but may vary by vascular bed or be altered by diseases such as hypertension and diabetes.

Changes in the extracellular matrix of the myocardium parallel those in the vasculature, with increased collagen, increased fibril diameter and collagen cross-linking, an increase in the ratio of type I to type III collagen, decreased elastin content, and an increase in fibronectin. There may also be a shift in the balance between matrix metalloproteinases and tissue inhibitors of matrix metalloproteinases that favors increased production of extracellular matrix. Fibroblast proliferation is induced by growth factors, in particular angiotensin, transforming growth factors, tumor necrosis factor-α, and platelet-derived growth factor. These changes are accompanied by cell loss and altered cellular function.[5] In the atria, decreased sinus node cells, decreased L-type calcium channels within sinus node cells, and extracellular matrix changes contribute to sinus node dysfunction and atrial fibrillation. Collagen, elastic tissue, and calcification changes in or near the central fibrous body and the atrioventricular (AV) node or proximal bundle branches contribute to conduction abnormalities and annular valvular calcification. In the ventricle, collagen deposition and extracellular matrix changes contribute to loss of cells, hypertrophy of myocytes with changes in myosin subforms, and altered myocardial calcium handling.[9] Changes in myocardial calcium handling include reduced or delayed inactivation of L-type transmembrane calcium current, decreased and delayed intracellular ionized calcium uptake by cardiac myocyte sarcoplasmic reticulum, and reduced and delayed outwardly directed potassium rectifier current activation. The result is prolongation of the membrane action potential and inward calcium current with prolongation of both contraction and relaxation.[5]

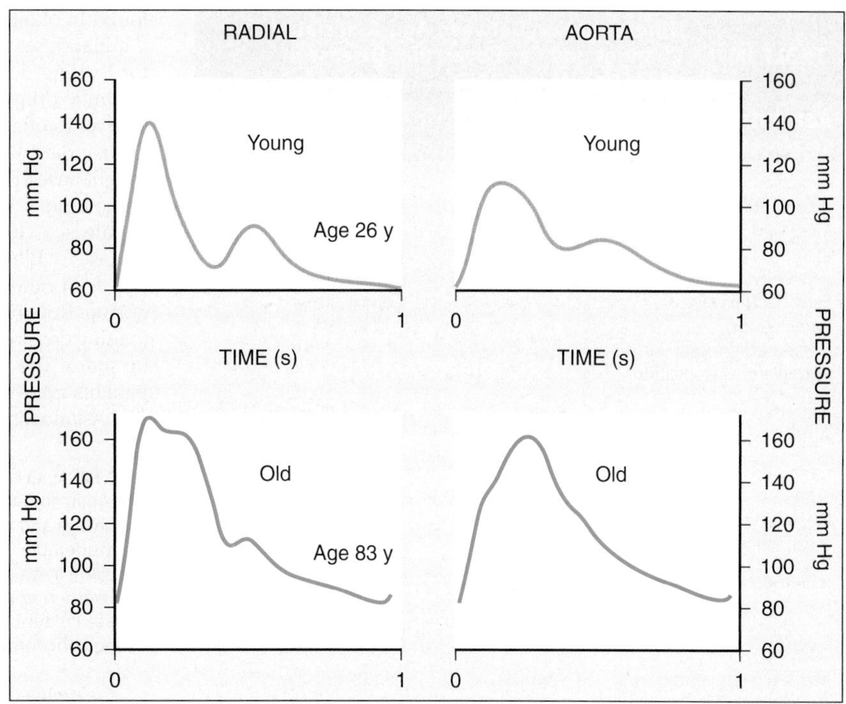

FIGURE 80-3 Directly measured arterial waveforms from a peripheral artery (radial) and calculated aortic pressure waves for a young man aged 26 years in the upper panels and his 83-year-old grandfather in the lower panels. *(Courtesy of Michael O'Rourke, MD, University of Sydney, Australia.)*

Age-related changes are also seen in the intravascular environment. Increases in fibrinogen, coagulation factors (V, VIII and IX, XIIa), and von Willebrand factor are seen without countering increases in anticoagulant factors (see Chap. 87). Platelet phospholipid content is altered and platelet activity is increased with increased binding of platelet-derived growth factor to the arterial wall in older individuals compared with younger individuals. Increased levels of plasminogen activator inhibitor (PAI-1) are seen with aging, especially during stress, resulting in impaired fibrinolysis. Circulating prothrombotic inflammatory cytokines, especially interleukin-6, also increase with age and may play a role in the pathogenesis of acute coronary syndromes. All these changes also potentiate development of atherosclerosis.[9]

Consistent changes in the autonomic nervous system accompany aging and influence cardiovascular function. For the beta-adrenergic system, age-related changes include decreased receptor numbers, altered G protein coupling, and altered G protein–mediated signal transduction. Age-related decreases in alpha-adrenergic platelet receptors and decreased alpha-adrenergic–mediated arterial vasoreactivity of forearm blood vessels occur, whereas alpha-adrenergic–mediated changes in human hand veins appear to be preserved. Dopaminergic receptor content and dopaminergic transporters decrease and cardiac contractile responses to dopaminergic stimulation may be blunted with aging. Decreased sensitivity and responses to parasympathetic stimulation are seen in cardiac and vascular tissues, whereas increased central nervous system effects are frequently seen in aging models. The combined age-related autonomic changes lead to decreased baroreflex function and responses to physiologic stressors with increased sensitivity to parasympathetic stimulation of the central nervous system.

Unifying hypotheses for age-related changes throughout the body include cumulative oxidative damage, inflammatory responses to cellular stress or infection, and programmed cell death. Some age-related cardiovascular changes can be partially if not totally reversed. Exercise improves endothelial function, measures of arterial stiffness, and baroreceptor function in older people. Calorie restriction slows aging and cardiac changes as well as increasing maximal life span in several small animal models. In humans, calorie restriction decreases weight, blood pressure, and risk factors for atherosclerosis and has improved indices of diastolic function in cross-sectional studies.[10,11] Medications such as angiotensin-converting enzyme (ACE) inhibitors, aldosterone antagonists, and beta blockers may influence the vascular and cardiac remodeling associated with hypertension, atherosclerosis, or heart failure.[9] Pilot studies suggest that combined exercise, stress management, and specialized diets that lower low-density lipoprotein (LDL) also increase telomerase activity and that cellular aging processes can be slowed.[12] Dietary antioxidant intake has been associated with slowing of age-related changes in the vasculature, but pharmacologic approaches with anti-inflammatory and antioxidant vitamin administration or omega-3 free fatty acids for either primary or secondary prevention have not been successful in humans.[13] Similarly, dehydroepiandrosterone has not been shown to have significant beneficial effects in older women or men. The most recent vitamin to be targeted for study is vitamin D. Decreased nutritional intake of vitamin D and sun exposure has resulted in vitamin D deficiency in high proportions of Americans, especially the elderly. A large study of vitamin D supplementation in older men and women to determine effects on cardiovascular events and cancer occurrence is under way. Other potential antiaging agents under investigation include those that directly target advanced glycation end products, inflammation, and collagen cross-links.

Age-related changes create a cardiovascular system faced with increased pulsatile load and one that is less able to increase output in response to stress. Age-related changes also limit maximal capacity and decrease reserve capacity, contributing to lower thresholds for symptoms in the presence of cardiovascular diseases that become more common with increasing age. **Table 80-1** summarizes age-related cardiovascular changes contrasted with cardiovascular disease.

Medication Therapy: Modifications for the Older Patient

Most of the therapeutic interventions for the elderly are pharmacologic, making appropriate drug selection and modification of dosing regimens for the older patient important (see Chap. 5).

TABLE 80-1 Differentiation Between Age-Associated Changes and Cardiovascular Disease in Older People

AGE-ASSOCIATED CHANGES	ORGAN	CARDIOVASCULAR DISEASE
Increased intimal thickness Arterial stiffening Increased pulse pressure Increased pulse wave velocity Early central wave reflections Decreased endothelium-mediated vasodilation	Vasculature	Systolic hypertension Coronary artery obstruction Peripheral artery disease Carotid artery obstruction
Increased left atrial size Atrial premature complexes	Atria	Atrial fibrillation
Decreased maximal heart rate Decreased heart rate variability	Sinus node	Sinus node dysfunction, sick sinus syndrome
Increased conduction time	Atrioventricular node	Type II block, third-degree block
Sclerosis, calcification	Valves	Stenosis, regurgitation
Increased left ventricular wall tension Prolonged myocardial contraction Prolonged early diastolic filling rate Decreased maximal cardiac output Right bundle branch block Ventricular premature complexes	Ventricle	Left ventricular hypertrophy Heart failure (with or without preserved systolic function) Ventricular tachycardia, fibrillation

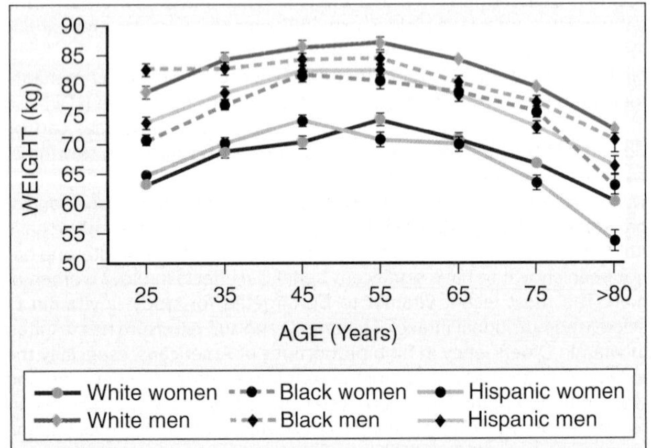

FIGURE 80-4 Mean weight in kilograms (±SE) by age, ethnicity/race, and sex/gender. *(Modified from Schwartz JB: The current state of knowledge on age, sex, and their interactions on clinical pharmacology. Clin Pharmacol Ther 82:87, 2007. Data source: NHANES: www.cdc.gov.)*

Loading Doses of Medications (see Chap. 10)

On average, body size decreases with aging and body composition changes, resulting in decreased total body water, intravascular volume, and muscle mass. Age-related changes are continuous but most pronounced after 75 to 80 years. Women, with the exception of African American women, tend to weigh less and to have smaller body and intravascular volumes and muscle mass than do men at all ages (**Fig. 80-4**). Higher serum concentrations of medications will be found in older patients, and especially older white and Asian women, if initial doses are the same as in younger patients. Weight adjustment for loading doses of the cardiovascular drugs digoxin, type I antiarrhythmic drugs, and type III antiarrhythmic drugs and for aminoglycoside antibiotics, chemotherapy regimens, and unfractionated heparin are standard. When fibrinolytic drugs have been administered without weight-based dosage adjustments, increased risk of intracranial hemorrhage results in patients with older age, smaller body weight, and female sex (in addition to hypertension and prior cerebrovascular disease).[14] Bleeding with low-molecular-weight heparins in combination with other lytic agents can be reduced by use of weight-based dosing. Routine dosage adjustments for weight should be made in loading doses of medications, especially those with a narrow therapeutic index. The result is usually a loading dose that is lower in older patients compared with younger patients and lowest in older white and Asian women.

Chronic Medication Administration

Renal Clearance (see Chap. 93)**.** Renal clearance by all routes (glomerular filtration, renal tubular reabsorption and secretion) decreases with age and is lower in women compared with men at all ages. There is considerable intersubject variability, but a general estimate is a 10% decline in glomerular filtration per decade, with 15% to 25% lower rates in women compared with men. The Cockcroft-Gault algorithm to estimate creatinine clearance includes age, sex, weight, and serum creatinine concentration as variables:

$$\text{Creatinine clearance} = (140 - \text{age[yr]} \times \text{weight[kg]})/(\text{creatinine} \times 72)$$
multiplied by 0.85 for women[15]

and highlights that significant decreases in renal elimination can be present in older patients in the presence of normal serum creatinine measurements. With elevations of serum creatinine, severe renal impairment is likely to be present. The Modification of Diet in Renal Disease (MDRD) algorithm incorporates serum creatinine (S_{Cr}), age, race, and sex as variables nonlinearly and may better estimate glomerular filtration rate (eGFR) in community-dwelling elderly and obese people and has been used in risk estimates.[16]

$$\text{eGFR}(\text{mL/min/m}^2) = 186.3^* \times S_{Cr}^{-1.154} \times \text{age}^{-0.203} \times \text{sex}\ (\times 0.742 \text{ if female}) \times \text{race}\ (\times 1.212 \text{ if African American})^{\dagger}$$

Online creatinine clearance and eGFR calculators are available at *http://www.kidney.org*.

The Cockcroft-Gault formula predicts a linear decrease with age that is steeper than the nonlinear decline predicted by the MDRD eGFR formula (**Fig. 80-5**). The result is underestimates with the Cockcroft-Gault formula and overestimates with the MDRD formula.[17] Most guidelines base dosage adjustments on estimated creatinine clearance (Cockcroft-Gault) to reduce excess dosing. The eGFR (MDRD) algorithm is used to classify renal status, risk of procedures, and renal complications and is reported routinely by most clinical laboratories. Both algorithms predict an "average" white woman older than 65 years to have stage 3 renal function (*http://www.kidney.org*) or moderate renal failure (see Fig. 80-5). Failure to adjust dosages of renally cleared narrow therapeutic index medications, such as thrombolytic agents, low-molecular-weight heparin, and glycoprotein (GP) IIb/IIIa inhibitors, has resulted in increased bleeding and intracerebral hemorrhages.[18-20]

Limitations of current methods to estimate renal clearance include lack of accuracy during hemodynamic instability or acute renal damage and reliance on creatinine measurements. Cystatin is a marker of renal clearance that reflects changes in renal function more rapidly and may reflect age-related changes without sex differences.[21-24] Estimates using cystatin differ from those with creatinine but appear to correlate with outcomes.[25] Incorporation of albuminuria in algorithms may also improve assessment of renal disease.

Even with limitations of current creatinine-based algorithms, routine estimation of creatinine clearance for dosages of renally cleared

*Note: use 175 if a standardized serum creatinine assay is used.
†For SI units: $\text{eGFR} = (3.1 \times S_{Cr}/88.4)^{-1.154} \times \text{age}^{-0.203} \times \text{sex} \times \text{race}$.

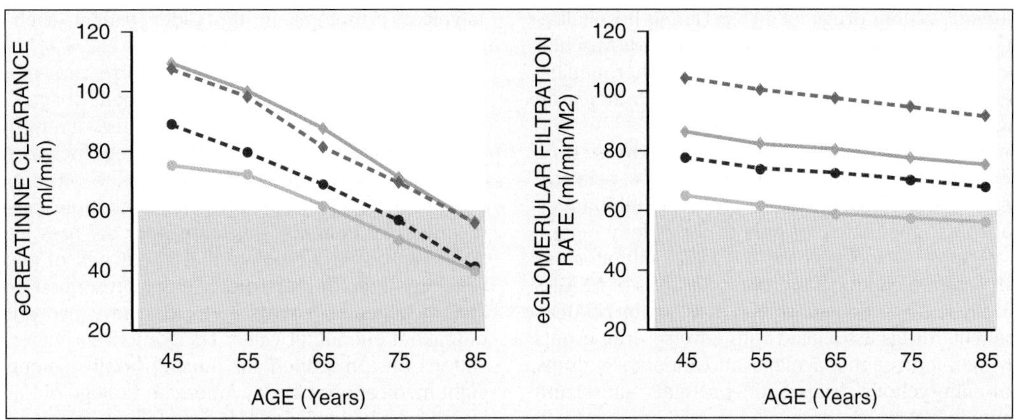

FIGURE 80-5 Estimates of creatinine clearance with the Cockcroft and Gault formula **(left panel)** and estimates of glomerular filtration rate with the MDRD simplified algorithm **(right panel)** for men and women aged 45 to 85 years. For calculations, mean weight and height by decade were obtained from U.S. survey data (NHANES, *http://www.cdc.gov*); serum creatinine is 1.0 mg/dL (average for older than 65 years in NHANES). Pink lines and circles represent estimates for women; blue lines and diamonds are estimates for men; lighter symbols are estimates for whites, and darker symbols represent estimates for African Americans. The shaded areas indicate GFR estimates of 30 to 59 mL/min/m^2 classified as stage 3 renal disease or moderate GFR decrease. Cockcroft and Gault estimates show a steeper decline with age. Both formulas estimate lower clearance in women compared with men and higher clearances in African Americans compared with whites (based on average height and weights and the same creatinine concentration). *(Modified from Schwartz JB: The current state of knowledge on age, sex, and their interactions on clinical pharmacology. Clin Pharmacol Ther 82:87, 2007.)*

medications and estimates of glomerular filtration for risk assessment before contrast agent administration, procedures, or surgery can guide efforts to reduce adverse effects and provides an opportunity for quality improvement. Consensus guidelines for oral dosing of renally excreted medications used frequently in the elderly may also be helpful.[26]

HEPATIC (AND INTESTINAL) CLEARANCE. No algorithms for estimation of age-related changes in hepatic and extrahepatic drug biotransformation have been validated clinically. In part, this is because hepatic and extrahepatic drug biotransformation processes may be influenced by more complex and heterogeneous factors that include both genetic and environmental influences, and enzymes can be both inhibited and induced (see Chap. 10).

Drugs metabolized by the conjugative reactions of glucuronidation (morphine, diazepam), sulfation (methyldopa), or acetylation (procainamide) do not appear to be affected by aging but show disease-related effects, may show frailty-related decreases, and show consistently lower clearance in women compared with men. Age-related changes are usually in phase I oxidative biotransformations by the membrane-bound cytochrome P-450 oxidative group of enzymes responsible for elimination of more than 50% of metabolized drugs.[27] Cardiovascular drugs showing age-related decreases in cytochrome P (CYP)–mediated clearance in research publications include alpha blockers (doxazosin, prazosin, terazosin), some beta blockers (metoprolol, propranolol, timolol), calcium channel blockers (dihydropyridines, diltiazem, verapamil), several HMG-CoA reductase inhibitors (fluvastatin and, in some studies, atorvastatin), and the benzodiazepine midazolam. Decreases in oxidative drug metabolism or clearance would suggest that lower amounts of drug per unit time (or day) should be given to older patients compared with younger patients, leading to the conventional dosing recommendation to "start low and go slow" for the older patient. Unfortunately, age-related changes have not been found in population studies of patients including women and patients receiving multiple medications.[28] Disease, environment, gender, and co-medications may have greater effects than age alone. Therefore, it is important to titrate to clinical effect if one starts with reduced dosages.

Attention has focused on genetic variation in explaining variability in drug metabolism, and allelic variants for many CYP enzymes have been described (see Chap. 10). Warfarin has polymorphisms of the CYP enzyme responsible for its metabolism (2C9) that are associated with lower warfarin requirements, and variants in the vitamin K epoxide reductase complex (VKORC) can either increase or decrease sensitivity to warfarin (see Fig. 80-e1 on website).[29] Increased age also increases sensitivity to warfarin, and estimates from different series suggest that age explains 40% of the variance in dosing; genetic variation of *VKORC1* can explain 25% of dosing variation, and variants of *CYP2C9* can explain 12% of dosing variation. Lower initial warfarin doses should be used in older patients and women (2 to 5 mg), and most often a loading dose is either not recommended or limited to 5 mg (see Chap. 87 and *www.ags.org*). Algorithms that incorporate age, race, sex, height and weight, and comedications in combination with other factors (including genetics) may help in estimating doses for individual patients. (see *www.warfarindosing.org*). With use of lower initial doses and multiple variable estimation algorithms in older patients, genotyping may not confer additional bleeding risk reduction, and the cost of genotyping for warfarin dosing estimation is not currently reimbursed by the Centers for Medicare and Medicaid Services.

Another drug with important genetic influences is clopidogrel. Clopidogrel is administered as a prodrug that requires metabolism by CYP2C19, and to a lesser extent CYP3A, for antiplatelet effects[29] (see Chap. 87). As with warfarin, age (in combination with body mass index and lipid levels) also contributes to platelet responses, and women tend to respond less well than men.[30]

ELIMINATION HALF-LIVES. In general, elimination half-lives of drugs increase with age, so the time between dosage adjustments needs to be increased in older patients before the full effect of a given dose can be assessed. Conversely, increased time is needed for complete drug elimination from the body and dissipation of drug effects.

Age-related changes in protein binding of drugs are not usually found. Changes in free drug concentrations due to the competition of drugs for binding sites can occur, but changes are predicted to be transitory. Clinically significant examples involve warfarin and changes in anticoagulation when additional drugs are added to warfarin therapy.

Table 80-2 summarizes general guidelines for drug dosing in older patients.

Adverse Drug Events and Drug Interactions

Adverse drug events are estimated to affect millions of people per year and account for up to 5% of total hospital admissions. A recent literature review found adverse drug event admission rates of 10.7% in elderly patients, with cardiovascular drugs accounting for about half of the admissions, nonsteroidal anti-inflammatory drugs (NSAIDs) for

20%, and central nervous system drugs for 14%.[31] During hospitalization, the odds ratio of severe adverse drug events with cardiovascular medications has been reported to be 2.4 times that of other medications. Heart failure, especially in women, is associated with increased risk of adverse drug reactions during hospitalization.[32]

The classes of drugs most commonly associated with adverse drug events in the elderly include diuretics, warfarin, NSAIDs, selective serotonin reuptake inhibitors, beta blockers, and ACE inhibitors.[33] Current pain management guidelines for pain in the elderly recommend NSAID and selective cyclooxygenase 2 (COX-2) inhibitor use only rarely and with extreme caution. Cardiovascular risks of NSAIDs in patients with CAD are less well delineated and may vary by NSAID.[34] In nursing home patients, drugs associated with adverse drug events are more frequently antibiotics, anticoagulants and antiplatelet drugs, atypical and typical antipsychotic drugs, antidepressants, antiseizure medications, or opioids.[35] Adverse drug effects may present with "atypical" symptoms in the older patient, such as mental status changes and impaired cognition.

TABLE 80-2 Guidelines for Medication Prescribing in Older Patients

In general, loading doses should be reduced. Weight (or body surface area) can be used to estimate loading dose requirements. Weight differences between the sexes are greatest for white people.

Use estimates of glomerular filtration to guide dosing of renally cleared medications and contrast agent administration. Reduce initial doses of metabolically or hepatically cleared drugs but titrate to effect.

Time between dosage adjustments and evaluation of dosing changes should be longer in older patients than in younger patients.

Routine use of strategies to avoid drug interactions is essential. Incorporation of reference materials, a team approach, and quality improvement efforts are effective strategies.

Knowledge of effects of noncardiac medications is critical.

Assessment of adherence and attention to factors contributing to nonadherence should be part of the prescribing process.

Physicians must be familiar with the patient's source of prescription medication coverage and provide education and assistance with obtaining critical medications.

Multidisciplinary approaches to monitoring of medication therapy may improve outcomes.

The strongest risk factor for adverse drug-related events is the number of drugs prescribed, independent of age. Chronic administration of four drugs is associated with a risk of adverse effects of 50% to 60%; administration of eight or nine drugs increases the risk to almost 100% (**Fig. 80-6**). Whereas the goal is to prescribe as few drugs as possible in the elderly, the presence of multiple diseases and multidrug regimens for common cardiovascular diseases often results in polypharmacy. Surveys estimate that about half of people older than 65 years use three or more medications prescribed on a daily basis, and 20% of patients 75 years and older have five drugs prescribed per outpatient encounter (*www.cdc.gov*). Even higher numbers of medications are prescribed for nursing home patients, averaging six to eight medications per day. American College of Cardiology/American Heart Association (ACC/AHA) guidelines for the pharmacologic treatment of patients after uncomplicated MI and for the management of chronic heart failure recommend use of more than three drugs (available at *ACC.org* or *heart.org*). Current regimens for treatment of the common disorders of diabetes and osteoporosis in the elderly similarly include two to four drugs. Strategies that minimize the chance of drug interactions and adverse drug effects are thus essential.

PHARMACOKINETIC INTERACTIONS. Pharmacokinetic interactions that alter the concentration of concomitantly administered medications are more likely if they are metabolized by or inhibit the same pathway. Tables 10-1 and 10-2 in Chapter 10 list examples of cardiovascular drugs by metabolic pathway with examples of inducers and inhibitors and interactions (also see *www.fda.gov/cder*). The most potent inhibitors of the cytochrome P-450 oxidative enzymes are amiodarone (all CYP isoforms) and dronedarone (CYP3A), the azole antifungal drugs itraconazole and ketoconazole (CYP3A), and protease inhibitors (CYP3A), followed by diltiazem (CYP3A) and erythromycin (CYP3A) (see *http://medicine.iupui.edu/clinpharm/ddis/table.asp*). Oral hypoglycemic agents are commonly prescribed drugs in the elderly, and coadministration of sulfonamide antibiotics with sulfonylureas can lead to hypoglycemia, in part because of CYP2C9 inhibition. Some drugs are administered as prodrugs and metabolized to active agents (cardiovascular examples include many ACE inhibitors and clopidogrel). Inhibition of the antiplatelet effects of clopidogrel has been reported with coadministration of atorvastatin that decreases clopidogrel activation by CYP3A, or proton pump inhibitors that inhibit CYP2C19-mediated clopidogrel activation.

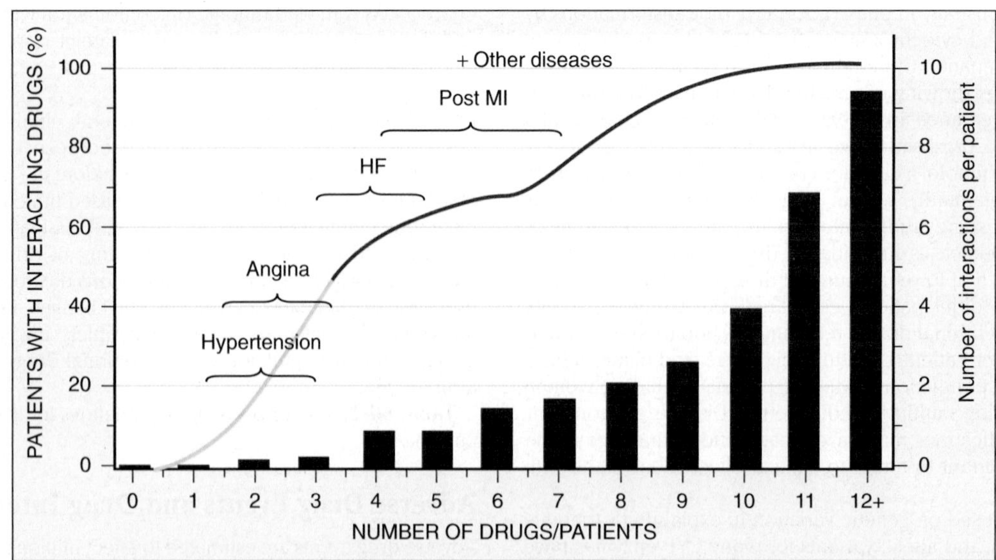

FIGURE 80-6 The relationship between the number of drugs consumed and drug interactions. Current guidelines for the pharmacologic management of patients with heart failure (HF) or myocardial infarction (post MI) place them at high risk for drug interactions. *(From Schwartz JB: Clinical Pharmacology, ACCSAP V, 2003. As modified from Nolan L, O'Malley K: The need for a more rational approach to drug prescribing for elderly people in nursing homes. Age Aging 18:52, 1989; and Denham MJ: Adverse drug reactions. Br Med Bull 46:53, 1990.)*

Inducibility of hepatic enzyme activity can lower concentrations of medications and lead to ineffective therapy. The antituberculous drug rifampin is the most potent inducer of CYP1A and CYP3A. With mandatory screening for tuberculosis, treatment with rifampin may be initiated. Dosages of coadministered drugs cleared by CYP1A and CYP3A may need to be increased during rifampin administration and decreased on discontinuation of rifampin. Markedly decreased cyclosporine levels and reduced clopidogrel inhibition of platelet aggregation during rifampin coadministration have been reported.[36] Other clinically relevant CYP inducers include carbamazepine (all CYPs); dexamethasone and phenytoin (CYP2C); caffeine, cigarette smoke, lansoprazole, omeprazole (CYP1A), and St. John's wort (CYP3A) (see *http://medicine.iupui.edu/clinpharm/ddis/table.asp*). Diet-drug and herb-drug interactions also occur.[37]

Despite the predictability of some interactions, many hospital admissions of elderly patients for drug toxicity involve administration of drugs known to interact.[38] Because of the multiplicity of potential interactions and release of new medications and discovery of new interactions, use of pharmacy or computerized and online tools that provide comprehensive up-to-date information and guidelines for avoidance of drug interactions is highly recommended. Available tools include the *Physicians' Desk Reference* (traditional, pocket, or online versions), *PDR Guide to Drug Interactions, Side Effects, and Indications* (traditional, computer version, or hand-held computer version available free of charge at *www.PDR.net*), Lexi-comp (software for smartphones, PDAs, and desktops), the *Medical Letter* and the *Medical Letter Drug Interactions Program* (computer based), Epocrates for the handheld computer or iPhone (available free of charge at *www.epocrates.com*), and online pharmacology texts or data bases (the Food and Drug Administration: *www.fda.gov/cder*, drug reactions section; *www.druginteractions.org* or *http://medicine.iupui.edu/flockhart*). Many individual hospitals, health care systems, and pharmacies provide internal reference sources.

Specialized clinics and use of specific algorithms or computer-based dosage programs to monitor oral anticoagulant therapy in outpatients have been shown to reduce bleeding-related complications. Other approaches that have been shown to reduce adverse drug reactions in older patients include involvement of pharmacy-trained individuals to assess the appropriateness of doses and medication counseling by multidisciplinary care team members. Algorithms have been developed for older patients to identify both medications that are potentially inappropriate and should be discontinued (STOPP criteria) and ones that appear indicated and should be initiated (START criteria).[39,40] A major limitation is the frequent lack of complete and readily accessible information on medication consumption and disease states in the older patient with multiple diseases and physicians. Integrated medical record and pharmacy information, interactive data bases, and computerized physician order entry with clinical decision support can reduce adverse drug events and improve medication therapy. Such systems, however, are not yet widely implemented. In contrast, mandated drug use review efforts appear ineffective.[41]

ADVERSE PHARMACODYNAMIC EFFECTS. Age-related changes in cardiovascular physiology and dynamics affect pharmacodynamics (see Table 80-1). Greater age-related nervous system sensitivity to parasympathetic stimulation may explain adverse effects such as urinary retention, constipation and fecal impaction, or worsened cognition in older patients who receive drugs with anticholinergic properties. Gastrointestinal transit time is generally increased in the elderly, and constipation is a frequent complaint of hospitalized elderly, less active elderly, and institutionalized elderly. Drug-induced constipation and bowel obstruction can occur in older patients receiving bile acid sequestrants, anticholinergic medications, opiates, and verapamil.

Pharmacodynamic drug interactions are more likely to occur between drugs acting on the same system. A classic example of additive effects that can produce hypotension and postural hypotension in the elderly is the coadministration of direct vasodilators or nitrates with alpha blockers, beta blockers, calcium channel blockers, ACE inhibitors, angiotensin receptor blockers (ARBs), diuretics, sildenafil, or tricyclic antidepressants. Other examples are bradycardia with combinations of amiodarone, beta-adrenergic blocking drugs, digoxin, diltiazem, or verapamil; and bleeding due to increased inhibition of platelet and clotting factors with combinations of aspirin, NSAIDs (including some COX-2–selective inhibitors), warfarin, or clopidogrel. Increased potassium concentrations due to combined administration of ACE inhibitors, ARBs, aldosterone and renin antagonists, and potassium-sparing diuretics in older patients are cited as causes of serious adverse drug reactions that are preventable.[35,42] Combinations of NSAIDs, including selective COX-2 inhibitors, with ACE inhibitors can also decrease potassium excretion with resultant hyperkalemia or can cause a decrease in renal function in the older patient. Combinations of drugs that produce QT interval prolongation can result in marked QT interval prolongation and torsades de pointes arrhythmias (see Chap. 39). Importantly, noncardiac drugs such as antibiotics (azithromycin, clarithromycin, erythromycin, gatifloxacin, gemifloxacin, moxifloxacin), antidepressants (amitriptyline, fluoxetine, lithium, venlafaxine), antipsychotics (haloperidol, risperidone), tamoxifen, and vardenafil used in the elderly may have additive effects with cardiovascular drugs such as the class IA, class IC, and class III antiarrhythmic drugs, isradipine, nicardipine, and ranolazine (see Chap. 37; online updated lists of medications that prolong the QT are available at *www.Qtdrugs.org*).

Examples of pharmacodynamic interactions with antagonistic effects include increased angina when beta agonists and theophylline are given to patients with CAD receiving beta blockers or nondihydropyridine calcium channel antagonists and loss of hypertension control when a drug such as fludrocortisone acetate is given for postural hypotension. Concern has also been raised about the ability of ibuprofen to block aspirin's binding to platelets and to diminish the cardioprotective effects of aspirin. The COX-2–selective NSAIDs rofecoxib and valdecoxib were removed from the market because of increased cardiovascular events, and other selective and nonselective NSAIDs are undergoing scrutiny.[34] Concern has also been raised with the weight gain and edema and possible increased incidence of heart failure with newer thiazolidinedione oral agents for the treatment of diabetes (rosiglitazone and pioglitazone).[43] Nicotinic acid raises high-density lipoprotein (HDL) concentration and reduces triglyceride levels but worsens insulin resistance and can exacerbate hyperglycemia in diabetics, as can beta blockers (with the exception of carvedilol) and thiazides. Selective estrogen receptor modulators and aromatase inhibitors can increase cholesterol and increase the risk of venous thromboembolic events, and serious cardiac events appear increased with some agents.[44] Familiarity with effects of noncardiac medications is necessary during pharmacotherapy of the elderly.

Inappropriate Prescribing in the Elderly

A number of lists of medications considered "inappropriate" for routine use in the elderly because of adverse effects or lack of efficacy have been compiled. The updated 2003 Beers criteria[45] can be accessed online (*archinte.ama-assn.org/cgi/reprint/163/22/2716.pdf*). Long-acting benzodiazepines, sedative and hypnotic agents, long-acting oral hypoglycemic agents, selected analgesics and NSAIDs, first-generation antihistamines, antiemetics, and gastrointestinal antispasmodics are usually considered inappropriate in the elderly. Amiodarone, clonidine, disopyramide, doxazosin, ethacrynic acid, guanethidine, and guanadrel have been classified as generally inappropriate in the elderly. More recent definitions of "inappropriate drug use" include failure to consider drug-disease interactions and failure to adjust drug dosages for age-related changes (i.e., digoxin at doses above 0.125 mg/day), drug duplication, drug-drug interactions, and duration of use. By use of these criteria, most drug use review studies concluded that inappropriate drug prescribing occurs in a significant fraction of older patients.[35,46] Resources such as the *Physicians' Desk Reference* may not contain geriatric prescribing information on older medications or present data on minimally effective doses established after drug marketing approval or in guidelines. Disturbingly, analyses suggest that inappropriate prescribing of medications to older patients

TABLE 80-3 Estimation of 4-Year Mortality in Community-Dwelling Elderly by Medical and Function Information

	Points
Age (year)	
60-64	1
65-69	2
70-74	3
75-79	4
80-84	5
>85	7
Male sex	2
Diabetes mellitus	1
Cancer	2
Lung disease	2
Heart failure	2
Body mass index <25	1
Current smoker	2
Assistance needed for	
Bathing	2
Managing finances	2
Difficulty	
Walking several blocks	2
Pushing or pulling heavy objects	1

→

Score	4-Year Mortality (%)
0	0-1
1	1
2	1.5
3	3.5
4	5
5	5-8
6	9
7	12-15
8	19-20
9	20-24
10	27-28
11	43-45
12	44-48
13	54-59
≥14	64-67

Modified from Lee S, Lindquist K, Segal M, Covinsky K: Development and validation of a prognostic index for 4-year mortality in older adults. JAMA 295:801, 2006.

in both the community and nursing homes has not decreased in recent years.[46-48]

Appropriate prescribing of medications is evolving to include consideration of discontinuing guideline-recommended medications in patients with life expectancy that may be too short to achieve long-term benefits or in whom concomitant diseases such as end-stage dementia result in therapeutic goals related primarily to quality of life. Estimation of life expectancy from both comorbid conditions and functional measures is gaining acceptance in determining appropriateness for screening for diseases, preventive strategies, and therapeutic decision making for older adults.[49-52] Recent models that estimate life expectancy use data likely to be available during routine clinical care or at the time of hospital discharge.[50,53] **Table 80-3** presents one model developed from a large and diverse sample of community-dwelling elderly in the United States. It identifies noncardiac factors that contribute significantly to overall mortality in the elderly. Another overall mortality prediction tool based on common laboratory tests plus age may also be useful in the hospital setting.[53] A logical approach to choosing appropriate medications, as well as other therapies, would incorporate consideration of remaining life expectancy, time until benefit, treatment targets, and goals of care for the individual older patient.

Adherence

Adherence with medications is commonly thought to be lower in older patients compared with younger patients. Contributing factors include the cost of medications; difficulty with understanding directions because of small print of written directions, hearing impairment, or impaired memory; inadequate instructions; complex dosing regimens; difficulties with packaging materials; and insufficient education of the patient, family, or caregiver on medication use. Of these, the most limiting are thought to be the cost of medications, poor education of the patient about medications, and cognitive impairment in elderly patients, especially those living alone. Use of HMG-CoA reductase inhibitors has been directly related to drug payment coverage and copayment requirements in Medicare recipients and in veterans.[54]

Physicians routinely overestimate the patient's adherence with medications. Assessment of adherence should be part of care, and issues related to potential contributors to medication nonadherence should be addressed by prescribing health care professionals. Unfortunately, there are few trials of interventions to improve medication adherence with resources usually available in clinical settings or that address adherence with multiple medication regimens. Strategies to improve adherence include programs for low-income seniors, visual or memory aids, medication-dispensing tools, use of geriatric-friendly packaging, assessment of cognitive status and the patient's understanding and inclusion of caregivers or family members in discussion about medications, and use of multidisciplinary teams or collaboration with pharmacists. Nonadherence is multifactorial, and it is likely that multiple strategies will need to be used.

Medicare D

January 1, 2006, marked the beginning of prescription drug coverage under the Medicare Prescription Drug and Modernization Act of 2003 in the United States. The Medicare D legislation created a complex plan involving government-contracted private industry coverage requiring individual enrollment. All plans include deductibles of $250 per year and partial payment of annual drug costs up to the estimated average annual drug expenditure for seniors of $2250 per year and then a gap in payment until costs exceed $3600 for all but low-income seniors (i.e., patients "dually eligible" for Medicaid and Medicare and those with incomes of 100% to 150% poverty levels). A multitude of plans are offered in regions that vary in benefits, co-pays, covered formulary medications, and tiers of medications with differing levels of co-pays within formularies. Physicians and pharmacists have had the task of educating a significant number of patients and families. Specific medications excluded from coverage by the law include those inappropriate for use in the elderly (such as barbiturates and benzodiazepines; see earlier) but also over-the-counter medications, vitamins, and products for symptomatic relief of colds or cough and medications not used for "medically accepted" indications. Information for physicians and patients on plans and formularies is available from many sources, including *www.Medicare.gov*, *www.MedicareToday.org*, *www.HLC.org*, *www.cms.hhs.gov*, *www.ama-assn.org*, and *www.accesstobenefits.org* or at 800-Medicare (800-633-4227).

The program created the potential for improving medication access, adherence, and therapy and has achieved some of these goals. Only about 10% of Medicare beneficiaries are currently without prescription coverage compared with 25% to 38% in preceding years, and a small but significant decrease in cost-related medication nonadherence has been documented.[55] Unfortunately, those in the poorest health or with multiple morbidities have not appeared to have improvements in cost-related medication nonadherence.

Current Controversies. Current controversies include the following: relative importance of factors influencing drug clearance rates (i.e., age, sex, genetics, environmental factors, disease state, comedications); relative importance of factors influencing drug responses in older patients (age, genetics, disease state, adherence, comedications); most efficacious approaches to decrease adverse medication events; role of electronic prescribing; optimization of medication alert system; and how to achieve universally available medical and medication information.

Vascular Disease

Hypertension (see Chaps. 45 and 46)

Prevalence and Incidence. Either diastolic (>90 mm Hg) or systolic (>140 mm Hg) hypertension occurs in one half to two thirds of people older than 65 years and in 75% of people older than 80 years.[56] The prevalence varies by race (or genetics) and is slightly higher in African Americans and Hispanics compared with non-Hispanic whites (see Chap. 2). The profile of hypertension is altered by aging, with systolic hypertension becoming more prevalent than diastolic hypertension. Systolic blood pressure rises with aging in both men and women but rises more steeply in women (see Chap. 81). After the age of 65 years, average systolic blood pressures are higher in women than in men. In contrast, diastolic blood pressure is relatively constant from 50 to 80 years of age, with average diastolic pressures higher in men than in women from the age of 50 to 80 years. "Isolated" systolic hypertension, without elevation of diastolic blood pressure, is present in about 8% of sexagenarians and more than 25% of the population older than 80 years. A large number of older people are unaware that they have hypertension. Even when it is recognized, hypertension is not controlled in many older patients, and older age is considered one of the strongest risk factors for resistant hypertension.[56,57]

TREATMENT. Relative risks for cardiovascular events associated with increasing blood pressure do not decline with older age, and absolute risk increases markedly in older patients, emphasizing the need for treatment of hypertension in the elderly.[56] Randomized placebo-controlled clinical trials of elderly patients during the past three decades have unequivocally demonstrated that treatment of diastolic or systolic hypertension confers cardiovascular benefits (see Table 80-e1 on website). Most of these studies used thiazide diuretics, beta blockers, or calcium channel blockers as first-line therapy with addition of secondary agents. ARBs were used in one study that showed only stroke benefits, and ACE inhibitors and ARBs have been used in comparative trials of newer drugs to older drugs that show stroke and cardiovascular benefits. Importantly, a recent trial enrolling the very old has demonstrated the safety and efficacy of carefully monitored treatment of systolic hypertension to a target of 150/80 mm Hg using indapamide with or without an ACE inhibitor in patients older than 80 years.[58] The participants were relatively "healthy" elderly (less than 12% had cardiovascular disease, only 7% had prior strokes or diabetes), and beneficial effects of treatment were seen within 1 year. In addition to reduced stroke, heart failure, and deaths from cardiovascular causes, overall mortality was also reduced. These findings counter prior meta-analysis and guideline concerns about risks of treatment of systolic hypertension in people older than 80 years but add to the controversy over the optimal target systolic blood pressure. Whereas other trials and American College of Cardiology clinical performance measures state a target of <140 mm Hg, many participants in the trials showing benefits did not achieve this goal.

There is no clear distinction in relative benefits between one pharmacologic agent or combination of agents and others for the treatment of uncomplicated hypertension in the elderly, although some data support varying benefit of agents on individual cardiovascular outcomes (see Table 80-e1 on website). Morbidity and mortality benefits of treatment of hypertension in the elderly have been seen with the five major antihypertensive classes—diuretics, beta blockers, calcium antagonists, ACE inhibitors, and angiotensin receptor antagonists.[59] Limited data show antihypertensive efficacy for a renin inhibitor, but longer term morbidity and mortality studies have not been completed. It appears that it is the control of both systolic and diastolic blood pressure that confers beneficial outcomes, that more than one medication has been administered to most trial participants, and that combination regimens are usually required to even approach blood pressure targets in older patients. The emphasis should be on diagnosis and treatment of hypertension rather than on the choice of initial individual therapeutic agents. Most guidelines and societies recommend basing the selection of combinations of pharmacologic agents on individual cardiovascular risk factors, concomitant diseases, side effect profiles, and ease of use.

The impact of common noncardiovascular conditions on both the efficacy and side effects of antihypertensive agents should be considered (**Table 80-4**). Arthritis is second in prevalence to cardiovascular disease in the elderly, and NSAIDs are among the most frequently consumed drugs (prescription and over-the-counter) in older people. In addition to the potential for cardiovascular ischemic events, adverse renal effects or hyperkalemia may occur when NSAIDs are given in combination with ACE inhibitors, ARBs, aldosterone, or renin antagonists. Loss of blood pressure control and heart failure have been precipitated by administration of nonselective NSAIDs as well as COX-2–selective NSAIDs. Age-related bone loss accelerates in older men and women and is the major contributing cause of osteoporosis. Osteoporosis in turn is a major risk factor for fractures in older people; the lifetime risk of osteoporotic fracture in Americans is estimated at 40% for women and 13% for men. Thiazides have been shown to preserve bone mineral density compared with placebo in randomized controlled trials and have been associated with higher bone mineral density and a reduction in risk of hip fractures in epidemiologic studies, providing a noncardiac treatment benefit in older patients.[60,61] Older patients for whom thiazide diuretics may not be a good choice include patients with urinary frequency problems (stress incontinence, urinary frequency with or without incontinence due to prostatic hypertrophy, overactive bladders, and patients needing assistance with toileting) because drugs that do not increase urinary frequency may have higher adherence.

Table 80-4 presents suggested antihypertensive regimens in older patients based on the presence of hypertension *and* concomitant conditions. Further data on frequent geriatric problems and medications to use or to avoid are available at *www.geriatricsatyourfingertips.com*. Education of the patient and caregiver should also be a component of care. A meta-analysis of randomized trials concluded that chronic disease self-management programs for older adults with hypertension produced clinically important benefits but could not identify key features of such programs.[62] A recent large randomized trial to improve blood pressure control in older male hypertensives found the best results with education of the patient on medication adherence, low-sodium diet, exercise, and the frequent need for more than one medication for blood pressure control, in combination with provider education and pharmacy alerts to providers regarding patients' responses to medications.[63]

ADDITIONAL CONSIDERATIONS IN THE OLDER PATIENT WITH HYPERTENSION. Both the Seventh Report of the Joint National Committee on Prevention, Detection, Evaluation, and Treatment of High Blood Pressure (JNC 7)[64] and the European Guidelines for the Management of Arterial Hypertension[65] recommend lower initial drug dosages and slower medication titration in older patients as well as the need to monitor for postural hypotension. A decrease in standing systolic blood pressure is estimated to be present in 15% of 70- to 74-year old community-dwelling men or women and in up to 30% of patients with systolic hypertension. Postural hypotension of >20 mm Hg or 20% of systolic pressure is a risk factor for falls and fractures that carry significant morbidity and mortality. Antihypertensive medications add to the risk of postural hypotension, as do many antiparkinson agents, antipsychotic agents, and tricyclic antidepressant drugs. The frailest and oldest of the elderly may reside in long-term care facilities. It is estimated that 30% to 70% are hypertensive and 30% have postural hypotension. Diuretic therapy appears to be effective in controlling systolic blood pressure in these patients and may also decrease postural hypotension. Postural blood pressure changes should be assessed (after ≥5 minutes supine, immediately after standing, and 2 minutes after standing) in older patients and volume depletion avoided.

TABLE 80-4 Considerations for Pharmacologic Therapy for Older Patients with Hypertension and Other Disorders

HYPERTENSION +	EFFICACY CONSIDERATIONS	TOXICITY OR ADVERSE EFFECT CONSIDERATIONS
Arthritis	—	ACE, ARB, aldosterone, and renin antagonist interactions with NSAIDs
Atrial fibrillation		Interactions with warfarin
Recurrent	ARB, ACE[*]	
Permanent	Beta blocker, calcium channel blocker (non-DHP)[*,†]	
Atrioventricular block	—	Beta blockers, non-DHP calcium channel blockers
Carotid disease or stroke	Calcium channel blocker,[†] ACE[*]	
Constipation	—	Verapamil
Coronary artery disease	Beta blocker[*,†] calcium channel blocker[*,†]	Nitrates and postural hypotension
Dementia	Clonidine[‡]	
Depression	—	SSRIs and hyponatremia
Diabetes	ACE,[*,†] ARB,[*,†] CCB (non-DHP) , beta blocker	Chlorpropamide and hyponatremia ACE or ARB + renin inhibitor and hyperkalemia
Glaucoma	Beta blocker	
Gout		Thiazide diuretics[*]
Heart failure	ACE,[*,†] ARB,[*,†] + loop diuretic,[*,†] beta blocker,[*,†] ± aldosterone antagonist[*,†,§]	Calcium channel blockers (possible)[*] ACE, ARB, aldosterone antagonist and hyperkalemia
Hyponatremia	—	Diuretic (especially with SSRI)
Incontinence	—	Diuretic
Metabolic syndrome	ACE,[*] ARB,[*] calcium channel blocker[*]	Beta blockers, diuretics
Myocardial infarction	Beta blocker,[*,†] ± ACE,[*,†] ± aldosterone antagonist[*]	ACE, ARB, aldosterone antagonist and hyperkalemia
Osteoporosis	Thiazides (beta blocker, ACE neutral or protect); potassium (K) phosphate (versus KCl)	Furosemide (bone loss)
Peripheral artery disease	Calcium channel blocker (DHP),[*,†] ACE + diuretics[‖]	Beta blocker (only if severe)
Postural hypotension	Thiazide[¶]	Alpha blocker, calcium channel blockers (DHP)
Prostatic hypertrophy	Alpha blocker[†]	
Pulmonary disease (asthma, COPD)		Beta blocker
Renal failure	ACE,[*,†] ARB,[*,†] ACE + ARB; loop diuretic[*,†]	Aldosterone antagonists (? renin inhibitors) and hyperkalemia
Ventricular arrhythmias	Beta blocker[†]	Thiazide, loop diuretics and hypokalemia

ACE = angiotensin-converting enzyme inhibitor; ARB = angiotensin receptor blocker; COPD = chronic obstructive pulmonary disease; NSAIDs = nonsteroidal anti-inflammatory drugs; DHP = dihydropyridine; SSRI = selective serotonin reuptake inhibitor.

*Recommendations for second-line agents usually added to thiazide diuretics from Chobanian AV, Bakris GL, Black HR, et al: The Seventh Report of the Joint National Committee on Prevention, Detection, Evaluation, and Treatment of High Blood Pressure. The JNC 7 Report. JAMA 289:2560, 2003.

†Mancia G, De Backer G, Dominiczak A, et al: 2007 Guidelines for the management of arterial hypertension. The Task Force for the management of arterial hypertension of the European Society of Hypertension (ESH) and of the European Society of Cardiology (ESC). Eur Heart J 28:1462, 2007.

‡Only available transdermal formulation for patients unable to swallow or who refuse oral medications.

§Systolic heart failure only.

‖Norgren L, Hiatt W, Dormandy J, et al: Inter-Society consensus for the management of peripheral arterial disease (TASC II). J Vasc Surg 45:S5A, 2007.

¶Nursing home patients.

Postprandial declines in both systolic and diastolic blood pressure occur in hospitalized, institutionalized, and community-dwelling elderly. The greatest decline occurs about 1 hour after eating, with blood pressure returning to fasting levels at 3 to 4 hours after eating. Vasoactive medications with rapid absorption and peaks should not be administered with meals.

New onset or worsening of hypertension occurs in 10% to 40% of cancer patients during administration of inhibitors of the vascular endothelial growth factor (VEGF) signaling pathway (bevacizumab, sunitinib, sorafenib) and has been associated with cardiac events and heart failure. Blood pressure should be controlled before administration of these drugs and monitored during VEGF therapy. If hypertension occurs, it should be promptly treated. Blood pressure has usually been controlled by oral antihypertensive therapy with ACE inhibitors, ARBs, beta blockers, diuretics, and occasionally nitrates. Verapamil and diltiazem are contraindicated in combination with VEGF inhibitors that are metabolized by CYP3A, and nifedipine may induce VEGF secretion and should be avoided. In cases of severe or persistent hypertension despite the initiation of antihypertensive treatment, temporary or permanent discontinuation of angiogenic inhibitors should be considered.[66]

Table 80-5 summarizes the approach to hypertension in older patients.

CURRENT CONTROVERSIES. Current controversies include the following: target blood pressures for systolic blood pressure in the very old (>80 years); lowest acceptable diastolic blood pressure during antihypertensive therapy; impact of differences in central versus peripheral blood pressure; initial therapy with single agents versus combination regimens; use of lifestyle modifications; impact of blood pressure treatment on development of dementia; safety and efficacy of aldosterone and renin inhibitors in the elderly; and role of aortic stiffness in predicting systolic blood pressure responses or as a target for systolic blood pressure–lowering agents.

Note: Updated JNC 8 recommendations will be published soon and are expected to address some of these controversies.

TABLE 80-5 Approach to Hypertension in Older Patients

Systolic as well as diastolic hypertension should be treated; current recommendations are based on brachial artery measurements:
- Diastolic target is <90 mm Hg.
- Systolic target is <140 mm Hg for most (<150 mm Hg for patients older than 80 years).

The focus should be on achieving blood pressure control, not initial therapy.

Multiple medications are usually required in older patients, and combinations should be based on concomitant diseases.

Drug dosing regimens should be adjusted for age and disease-related changes in drug metabolism and potential drug-drug interactions.

Patients should be monitored for adverse effects and drug interactions, especially
- Postural hypotension and postprandial hypotension
- Hypovolemia with diuretics
- Hyperkalemia with ACE inhibitors, ARBs, aldosterone, renin antagonists

Coronary Artery Disease (see Chaps. 49 and 57)

PREVALENCE AND INCIDENCE. Both the prevalence and severity of atherosclerotic CAD increase with age in men and women. Autopsy studies show that more than half of people older than 60 years have significant CAD, with increasing prevalence of left main or triple-vessel CAD with older age. By use of electrocardiographic evidence of MI, abnormal echocardiogram, carotid intimal thickness, and abnormal ankle-brachial index as measures of subclinical vascular disease in community-dwelling people older than 65 years, abnormalities were detected in 22% of women and 33% of men aged 65 to 70 years and 43% of women and 45% of men older than 85 years (see *http://www.chs-nhlbi.org/*). By 80 years of age, the frequency of symptomatic CAD is about 20% to 30% in both men and women. Because of the increasing proportion of women at older ages, however, there are more older women with angina presenting for care. These women have been less likely to receive evidence-based therapy for stable angina, aggressive therapy for acute coronary syndromes, or diagnostic evaluations.[67-70]

DIAGNOSIS

Estimation of Risk

Risk factors such as hypertension, total cholesterol level, and LDL-cholesterol concentration and tools such as those developed from the Framingham Study in younger populations may be less accurate in the very old or in women.[71,72] The Reynolds Risk Score may improve risk estimates in women up to age 80 years thought to be at intermediate risk (*http://www.reynoldsriskscore.org/*). Data suggest that HDL-cholesterol concentration, increased pulse pressure, and measures of arterial stiffness assume importance in risk assessment in older people. Chronic kidney disease (as defined by eGFR) has also been identified as a risk factor for cardiovascular disease and progression of cardiovascular disease, but it is not yet incorporated into risk models. Predictive models that incorporate both traditional risk factors (such as smoking, blood pressure, selected lipid levels, diabetes) and age-specific markers (such as pulse pressure, arterial stiffness, and possibly albuminuria with further adjustment for sex) may provide the best current estimates of cardiovascular risk in older people without known CAD.[73-75] In estimating risk of all-cause mortality, data from large populations including those undergoing angiography found that sex-specific risk scores combining complete blood count and basic metabolic profile components and age were highly predictive of mortality at 30 days, 1 year, and 5 years.[53] Such risk scores and estimates of life expectancy based on geriatric factors warrant use to assist in therapeutic decision making.

History

Anginal symptoms are more likely to be absent or ischemia silent in older patients compared with young patients. Symptoms are termed atypical because the description differs from the classic description of substernal pressure with exertion. Symptoms may primarily be dyspnea, shoulder or back pain, weakness, fatigue (in women), or epigastric discomfort and may be precipitated by concurrent illnesses. Some older patients describe symptoms with effort, but those with limited physical exertion may not report symptoms, and those with altered manifestations of pain due to concomitant diabetes or age-related changes may have symptoms at rest or during mental stress. Memory impairment may also limit the accuracy of the history. Lack of symptoms during evidence of myocardial ischemia on electrocardiography has been reported in 20% to 50% of patients 65 years or older.

Testing for Ischemia (see Chap. 53)

The prevalence of resting ST-T wave abnormalities on electrocardiography in older people results in a modest age-associated reduction in specificity of exercise electrocardiography (see Chap. 14). Treadmill exercise testing can provide prognostic information in patients able to exercise sufficiently and can also provide information about functional capacity and exercise tolerance. Exercise results can be enhanced by the use of modified protocols beginning with low-intensity exercise. Most series report slightly higher sensitivity (84%) and lower specificity (70%) in patients older than 75 years than in younger patients. Echocardiography and nuclear testing can overcome some of the limitations of electrocardiographic interpretation (see Chaps. 15 and 17). In older patients unable to exercise, pharmacologic agents such as dipyridamole and adenosine can be used with nuclear scintigraphy to assess myocardial perfusion at rest and after vasodilation; or agents such as dobutamine can be combined with echocardiography or other imaging techniques to assess ventricular function at rest and during increased myocardial demand.

The value of screening for asymptomatic CAD in the elderly is not known. The presence of coronary calcifications is high (**Fig. 80-7**), and neither the presence nor degree of coronary calcification has correlated with coronary flow decrease in the older population, and data are especially limited for women.[76-78] The high prevalence of hypertension, diabetes, obesity, and inactivity in the elderly, including those aged 65 to 75 years, would suggest that increased efforts to improve diet and

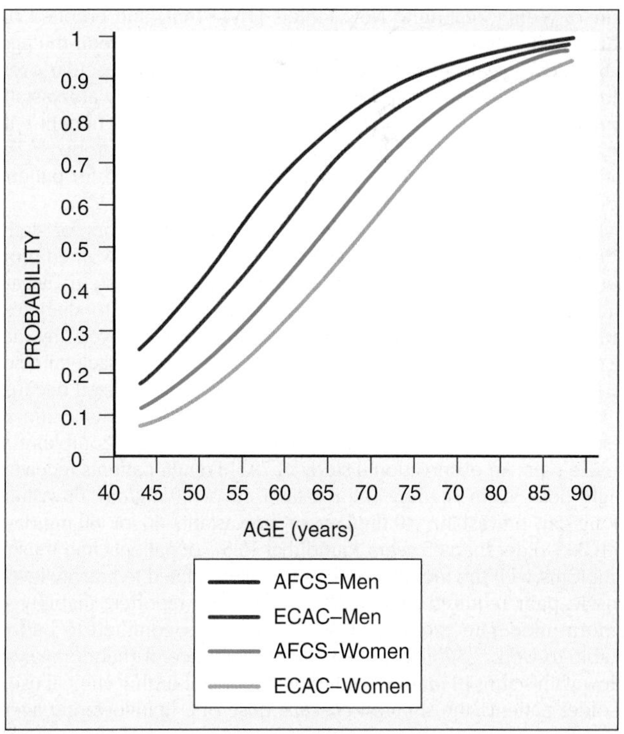

FIGURE 80-7 Predicted probability of presence of detectable coronary artery calcification among Amish Family Calcification Study (AFCS) and Epidemiology of Coronary Artery Calcification (ECAC; Lancaster County, Penn.) study participants. *(From Bielak LF, Yu PF, Ryan KA, et al. Differences in prevalence and severity of coronary artery calcification between two non-Hispanic white populations with diverse lifestyles. Atherosclerosis 196:888, 2008.)*

activity levels, smoking cessation, treatment of hypertension and diabetes, and optimization of renal function would be of greater benefit on overall morbidity and mortality than screening with vascular imaging studies in the asymptomatic elderly.

TREATMENT (see Chaps. 49 and 57)

Medical

Optimization of medical care warrants greater emphasis.[79] Optimal medical therapy for patients with stable coronary disease, including the elderly and diabetics with multivessel CAD, has recently been shown to produce results equivalent to those of percutaneous coronary intervention in reducing the risk of cardiovascular events.[80,81] Therapeutic goals and management goals for chronic stable angina are targeted at (1) symptom relief with nitrates, beta blockers, calcium antagonists, and partial free fatty acid inhibitors and (2) risk reduction and slowing of the progression of disease with control of hypertension and diabetes, weight control, lipid lowering (including triglycerides), exercise, and smoking cessation.[79] Aspirin at 75 to 162 mg/day is recommended, although benefits in women, especially older women, are not as clear as in men.[82] Secondary prevention efforts should be targeted at interventions conferring benefit within the anticipated life span of the patient. Lifestyle changes of smoking cessation, increased activity, and weight control provide improvements in a short time frame, whereas benefits of lipid lowering may take longer. Annual influenza vaccinations reduce cardiovascular events in older populations.

LIPID LOWERING IN THE ELDERLY (see Chaps. 47 and 49). Lipid lowering may not confer benefit until after 3 to 5 years of treatment on the basis of data from secondary prevention trials of HMG-CoA reductase inhibitors that enrolled significant numbers of older patients (summarized in Table 80-e2 on the website). These trials used 40 mg/day pravastatin, 20 to 40 mg/day simvastatin, or 1200 mg/day gemfibrozil (see Table 80-e2 on the website). Whereas increasingly lower LDL-cholesterol targets (<100 mg/dL) are recommended in CAD guidelines with higher doses of statins being used, the major trial on which these recommendations are based explicitly excluded CAD patients older than 75 years (Treating to New Targets [TNT] trial) and enrolled primarily white men.[79,83] Post hoc analyses of patients between the ages of 65 and 75 years showed reduced combined cardiovascular event endpoints (10.3% compared with 12.6%) with 80 mg/day atorvastatin compared with 10 mg/day atorvastatin but no mortality benefit with the higher dose for the elderly subgroup (or the entire group).[83] The optimal lipid target has not been definitively established for patients older than 75 years.

Dose considerations are important because risk factors for statin-induced myopathy include older age (>80 years and in women more than in men), smaller body frame, frailty, and multisystem disease (including chronic renal insufficiency, especially due to diabetes), and myopathy also increases with increasing dosages. Myopathy may be difficult to differentiate from other types of musculoskeletal disorders or pain in the older patient, or it may not be recognized because of cognitive impairment. Complaints may also be nonspecific or described as "flulike," with fatigue nearly as common a complaint as muscle pain. An observational study of 7924 French patients receiving "high"-dose statin therapy (atorvastatin 40 or 80 mg/day, fluvastatin 80 mg/day, pravastatin 40 mg/day, or simvastatin 40 or 80 mg/day), with 30% older than 65 years, found that 10.5% of patients had muscle symptoms, with the incidence of muscle pain related to activity levels. Muscle pain required analgesics in 39%, 38% reported inability to perform moderate exertion, and 4% were either confined to bed or unable to work.[84] Similarly, whereas the incidence of rhabdomyolysis is low with statins in randomized trials, it is higher during clinical use.[85] In older patients, the smallest *effective* dose of a lipid-lowering agent should be used and signs and symptoms monitored. Muscle strength testing may be helpful in evaluation of symptoms in older patients, including simple assessments of ability to rise from a chair or to climb stairs.

STATINS FOR PRIMARY PREVENTION (see Chap. 49). The elderly have not been the target of most primary prevention trials of lipid lowering. Older patients with hypertension and CAD risk factors have not had all-cause mortality benefits when they are studied as part of randomized trials of lipid lowering (see Table 80-e2 on website). Data on reductions in cardiovascular endpoints differ between studies, but in the largest that showed reduction in a composite cardiovascular endpoint (ASCOT-LLA), prespecified subgroups of women, diabetics, patients with metabolic syndrome, nonobese patients, and those with prior vascular diseases did not show coronary heart disease benefit. Aggressive lipid lowering as primary prevention should be reserved for elderly patients with longer life expectancy and should be accompanied by monitoring for adverse effects.

CURRENT CONTROVERSIES: LIPID-LOWERING STRATEGIES IN THE ELDERLY WITH OR AT RISK FOR CAD. Current controversies include the following: primary prevention with statins in the elderly, especially women; optimal targets for lipid lowering, especially in the very old and in nonwhites; frequency and management of statin-induced myalgias or myopathy in older patients; coronary heart disease and mortality and risk related to lipid subfractions (HDL-cholesterol versus LDL-cholesterol or apolipoprotein B).

Additional lipid-lowering agents are discussed in Chapter 47.

Special Considerations with Pharmacologic Treatment of the Elderly CAD Patient

See also Medication Therapy: Modifications for the Older Patient.

Marked vasodilation due to rapid absorption or higher peak effects of isosorbide dinitrates can exacerbate postural hypotension, so agents with smooth concentration versus time profiles such as mononitrates or transdermal formulations may be preferred for daily administration, although cost may be prohibitive. Beta blockers have not been shown to increase the occurrence of depression in randomized trials, but beta blockers that are not lipophilic (e.g., atenolol, nadolol) may produce fewer central nervous system effects. Calcium channel blockers, especially the dihydropyridines, can produce pedal edema more frequently in the older patient. Shorter acting formulations can produce or exacerbate postural hypotension and should be avoided. Verapamil can exacerbate constipation, especially in the inactive elderly. Both beta blockers and nondihydropyridine calcium channel blockers should be avoided in the presence of sick sinus node disease. Hormone replacement therapy is not indicated for either primary prevention of coronary heart disease or treatment of coronary heart disease.[86] Adverse effects of dizziness, constipation, nausea, asthenia, headache, dyspepsia, and abdominal pain with the piperazine derivative ranolazine are more common in elderly patients, and women may have less exercise benefit with ranolazine compared with men.[87] Individual antianginal agents are further discussed in Chapter 57.

Revascularization (see Chaps. 57 and 58)

Revascularization procedures in the elderly are increasing, with greater increases in the numbers of percutaneous coronary intervention (PCI) procedures than in coronary artery bypass grafting (CABG).[88] At least half of PCI procedures and CABG are performed in patients older than 65 years, with one third in patients older than 70 years. In randomized trials, patients aged 65 to 80 years have been reported to have higher early morbidity and mortality after CABG compared with PCI but greater angina relief and fewer repeated procedures after CABG. Stroke is more common after CABG than after PCI (1.7% versus 0.2%), and heart failure and pulmonary edema are more common after PCI (4.0% versus 1.3%). Five-year survival rates are above 80% for both procedures, but there is considerable selection bias in patients undergoing these procedures; women and minorities are underrepresented, and those at lowest and intermediate risk undergo the bulk of procedures.[88]

Information about elderly patients after revascularization as part of "routine" clinical care has emerged from clinical and administrative databases (**Fig. 80-8**). These patients tend to be older and to have more multivessel disease and comorbid conditions than those in randomized studies, and long-term survival rates are lower and complication rates are higher than in randomized trials. Early CABG mortality increases from below 2% in patients younger than 60 years to between

5% and 8% in patients older than 75 years, approaching 10% in patients older than 80 years. Elderly women are at highest risk, in part because of comorbid conditions. For patients older than 90 years, operative mortality has been reported as 11.8% in the Society of Thoracic Surgeons database.[89] An online risk calculator incorporating patient risk factors and risks for specific surgical procedures can be accessed at the Society of Thoracic Surgeons website. The Mayo Clinic Risk Score for PCI also appears to estimate in-hospital mortality risk for CABG.[90]

PCI. Registry data from 2000 found PCI in-hospital mortality risk of less than 1% in patients younger than 60 years that increased to 2% to 5% in patients older than 75 years and to more than 5% in patients older than 80 years. Data on PCI during 2004-2006 found similar in-hospital mortality rates (up to 1% for those up to 70 years of age, about 2% for 70- to 80-year-olds, and 3.2% for those older than 80 years).[90] These represent highly selected older patients, and risk estimates need to be adjusted before application to patients with differing characteristics.[90]

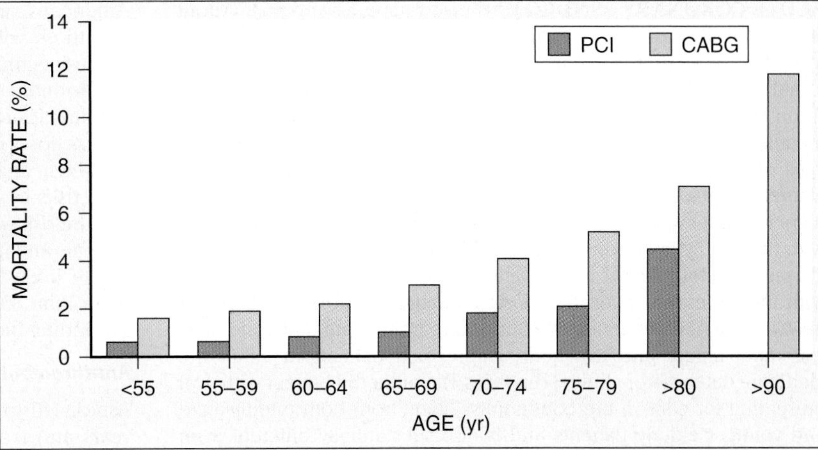

FIGURE 80-8 In-hospital mortality rates reported for revascularization procedures by age group. PCI = percutaneous coronary intervention of all types; CABG = coronary artery bypass graft surgery. *(Data are from the National Cardiovascular Revascularization Network as reported by Alexander K, Anstrom K, Muhlbaier L, et al: Outcomes of cardiac surgery in patients ≥80 years: Results from the National Cardiovascular Network. J Am Coll Cardiol 35:731, 2000; Batchelor W, Anstrom K, Muhlbaier L, et al: Contemporary outcome trends in the elderly undergoing percutaneous coronary interventions: Results in 7,472 octogenarians. National Cardiovascular Network Collaboration. J Am Coll Cardiol 36:723, 2000; and the Society of Thoracic Surgeons data base, Bridges C, Edwards F, Peterson E, et al: Cardiac surgery in nonagenarians and centenarians. J Am Coll Cardiol 197:347, 2003.)* Data were not available for PCI in patients older than 90 years. See text for further discussion of results for drug-eluting stents and newer surgical approaches.

PCI VERSUS CABG. One initial study of nearly 1700 patients older than 80 years (two- or three-vessel disease, excluding left main) found better in-hospital mortality and short-term survival for PCI versus CABG (3% versus 6%),[91] but survival was better after CABG for those surviving 6 months. The larger New York State database of more diverse patients older than 80 years (n = 5550) with multivessel disease (excluding left main) found risk-adjusted mortality and need for revascularization lower in patients treated with CABG (on-pump) compared with those who underwent PCI (bare metal stents).[92] Combined postmarketing registry and trial data compared bare metal stents and paclitaxel drug-eluting stents in patients older than 70 years.[93] Bare metal stents and drug-eluting stents had similar death, MI, and stent thrombosis rates, although repeated revascularization was more common with bare metal stents. A registry-based comparison of drug-eluting stents and CABG for multivessel disease (excluding left main, prior CABG, or recent MI) found that CABG had lower adjusted death rates and MI than drug-eluting stents, with clear advantages of CABG in those older than 80 years.[94] However, death or MI occurred in 16% to 17% of patients older than 80 years at 18-month follow-up.

PCI is associated with a slightly less than 1% risk of permanent stroke or coma, and CABG is associated with a 3% to 6% incidence of permanent stroke or coma in patients older than 75 years.[95] In the immediate postoperative period, longer durations of ventilatory support, greater need for inotropic support and intra-aortic balloon placement, and greater incidence of atrial fibrillation, bleeding, delirium, renal failure, perioperative infarction, and infection are seen in older patients compared with younger patients (see Chap. 84). The highest rate of complications is usually seen in older women and in patients undergoing emergency procedures. The length of disability and rehabilitation after procedures is also usually longer. Postoperative cognitive impairment in older patients detected with neuropsychological testing has been estimated at 25% to 50% after CABG. Randomized trials have reported both improved cognitive outcomes and no difference in cognitive outcomes of off-pump versus on-pump CABG.[96] Prerevascularization considerations in the older patients should address cognition and the potential need for in-home assistance after the procedure or extended care hospitalization. Postprocedure considerations should also include evaluation for depression (see later).

Comparison of Medical Therapy with Revascularization

(see Chap. 57)

A pivotal randomized study TIME[97] compared invasive (PCI or CABG) versus optimized medical therapy for CAD patients older than 75 years with angina refractory to therapy with at least two antianginal drugs (mean 2.5 ± 0.7) (see Table 80-e3 on website). Initial 6-month analyses favored revascularization, but the advantage was not present at 1 year. Revascularization presented an early risk of death and complications, and optimized medical therapy carried a chance of later events (hospitalization and revascularization), without a clear advantage of either strategy. Similarly, comparisons of revascularization with medical therapy in diabetics, including women and the elderly[81] (see Table 80-e3 on website), found no significant difference in outcomes between the approaches. Prompt revascularization decreased major cardiovascular events in CABG-treated patients compared with the medically treated but not in prompt PCI patients compared with medical treatment. Evolving data also suggest that PCI may not have fewer neurocognitive consequences.

Clinical Perspective

Age alone should not be the only criterion in considering revascularization procedures. There is a clear role for individualized risk assessment and respect for the patient's preference in the decision-making process. Short-term and long-term benefit should be considered in the context of anticipated life span and quality of life of the patient. Medical therapy has become more aggressive and compares favorably with revascularization in randomized trials of stable CAD patients older than 75 years, especially women. In contrast to the relatively low complication rates of revascularization in randomized trials of highly selected elderly patients, morbidity and mortality with revascularization in routine clinical care in patients older than 75 years are high. PCI is attractive in concept, but even drug-eluting stents may not confer the benefit of CABG in older patients with longer anticipated life spans. The possibility of disability or prolonged hospitalization after interventions and especially surgery must be considered and accurately conveyed to the patient and family. Death, recurrent angina, or MI may not be viewed as carrying the same negative impact as a disabling stroke by many older patients. For the patient unable to make decisions, involvement of family members or agents is key to decisions that reflect the wishes of the patient.

CURRENT ISSUES IN REVASCULARIZATION OF THE ELDERLY. Current issues include the following: appropriate selection criteria for specific therapies for octogenarians and nonagenarians; modifiable risk factors for revascularization mortality and morbidity in older patients; age-adjusted PCI and CABG protocol regimens; role of transradial approaches for PCI; benefits of on-pump versus off-pump CABG surgery (see Chap. 84); prevention of cognitive decline after revascularization procedures; and comparisons between modern medical therapy and revascularization.

ACUTE CORONARY SYNDROMES (see Chaps. 54 and 55). About 60% of hospital admissions for acute myocardial infarction (AMI) are in people older than 65 years, and approximately 85% of deaths due to AMI occur in this group.[98,99] With increasing age, the gender composition of patients presenting with AMI changes: from predominantly men in middle age, to equal numbers of men and women between the ages of 75 and 84 years, to the majority of patients with AMI being women at ages over 80 years (see Chap. 81). Mortality rates are usually higher in older women than in men with AMI, as are adverse outcomes with thrombolytics, fibrinolytics, and GP IIb/IIIa inhibitors. Mortality is at least threefold higher in the patient older than 85 years compared with the patient younger than 65 years. Patients enrolled in trials for treatment of AMI are generally younger, are more often male, and have less renal failure and less heart failure than patients in either the Medicare database or clinical registries. The older old patient with AMI presenting for care in the community differs from both middle-aged and younger elderly patients and is also substantially different from highly selected patients older than 65 years enrolled in randomized clinical trials.[3]

Diagnosis

Chest pain or discomfort is the most common complaint in patients up to the age of 75 years, but after the age of 80 years, complaints of diaphoresis increase and chest discomfort decreases (see Chap. 53). Altered mental status, confusion, and fatigue become common manifestations of MI in the oldest patients. Older patients may also present with sudden pulmonary edema or neurologic symptoms such as syncope or stroke. The electrocardiogram (ECG) is also more likely to be nondiagnostic (see Chap. 13). Nonspecific symptoms and nondiagnostic electrocardiographic findings lead to delays in diagnosis and implementation of therapy and highlight the importance of rapid laboratory testing for circulating markers of myocardial damage.

Treatment

Treatment decisions are often considered separately for ST elevation MI (STEMI) and non–ST elevation MI (NSTEMI) in the older patient analogous to other guidelines.[3,4,98,99] There is general agreement that eligible STEMI patients who receive reperfusion therapy (fibrinolytic therapy or PCI) have a lower risk of death, but few patients older than 75 years were enrolled in trials that serve as the basis for this recommendation. Lack of consensus on the best approach for reperfusion for acute MI in the elderly reflects the lack of data and the comorbidities and delayed presentation of older patients as well as the lack of widespread rapid access to high-volume PCI facilities and the higher incidence of serious adverse effects with pharmacologic reperfusion strategies. For NSTEMI, the debate centers on early versus delayed or selective risk-stratified invasive strategies after antiplatelet and antithrombin therapy and initiation of beta blockade and ACE inhibitors or ARBs in the presence of left ventricular dysfunction. It is unlikely that randomized trials will provide the answers to these questions in the very old patient, and registry data that include significant numbers of women and older patients with comorbidities serve an important role for this group. These data show that results in the community setting do not currently achieve the same results as reported in clinical trials.

REPERFUSION. Non–age-adjusted guidelines recommend reperfusion approaches in STEMI patients without contraindications if they present within 12 hours of symptom onset. PCI and fibrinolytic therapy have similar outcomes when they are delivered within 3 hours from symptom onset. In elderly patients who present in shock or are in a high-risk category or present later, PCI can offer better results.

Thrombolysis or Fibrinolysis (see Chap. 55)

For patients up to the age of 75 years, most trials show that fibrinolytic, antiplatelet, and antithrombin therapy is associated with a survival advantage compared with placebo that may be similar to or less than that seen in younger patients.[3,4,98-100] Bleeding and transfusion rates are higher in older patients, especially with improper dosing of antiplatelet and antithrombin agents.[98,99] Those at high risk for intracerebral hemorrhage include patients older than 75 years, women, African Americans, smaller patients (<65 kg for women and <80 kg for men), and those with prior stroke or systolic blood pressure >160 mm Hg. Fibrin-specific agents are also associated with increased stroke risk due to intracerebral hemorrhage in those older than 75 to 80 years. Coadministered low-molecular-weight or unfractionated heparin at excess doses contributes to the excess bleeding.[3] Dosage adjustments for weight and estimated renal clearance may decrease but not eliminate risks of bleeding in very old patients and in women. Cardiac rupture risk with thrombolysis is also increased in patients older than 70 years and in women (0.5% to 2%) and does not appear to be related to the intensity of anticoagulation. Risks of reperfusion in patients older than 85 years appear to differ from those in younger patients, supporting individualized clinical decisions.

Antithrombotic Agents

Aspirin (81 to 325 mg/day) reduces mortality in patients older than 70 years and is recommended for older patients with acute coronary syndromes of all types. Clopidogrel is added to aspirin in patients not considered for surgical revascularization, before PCI, or before discharge for medically treated patients. GP IIb/IIIa inhibitors in high-risk non–ST elevation acute coronary syndromes, especially if catheterization and PCI are planned, appear efficacious in patients older than 70 years, although net benefit may decline with increasing age. Bleeding risk including intracerebral hemorrhage is increased about twofold with GP IIb/IIIa inhibitors, rising to 7.2% for eptifibatide in patients older than 80 years.[3]

Antiplatelet and antithrombin agents have narrow therapeutic windows with dosing recommendations based on weight and renal function. More than 65% of patients older than 75 years with acute coronary syndromes receive an excess dose.[18,101] Women are more likely to receive excess GP IIb/IIIa doses than are men in both clinical practice and randomized trials, and about 25% of the bleeding risk in women is attributable to excess dosing.[20,102] These data highlight the need for adjustment of dosing of antithrombotic and antiplatelet agents for estimated renal clearance.

Invasive Strategies

In elderly patients with acute STEMI, primary angioplasty in experienced centers is associated with improved outcomes compared with thrombolytic strategies (see Chap. 55). This potential benefit, however, has not been seen in octogenarians.[103] Acute procedural success rates are somewhat lower in older patients and are associated with increased bleeding and increased risk for contrast-mediated renal dysfunction. Facilitated PCI is not endorsed for elderly patients secondary to increased bleeding risk.[4]

Antiplatelet therapy with clopidogrel (or prasugrel) has a routine role before PCI but should not be used in patients considered for CABG. Prasugrel has increased risk of fatal bleeding events compared with clopidogrel in patients older than 75 years with acute coronary syndromes and should not be used in older patients. Early versus delayed eptifibatide before angiography is not recommended.[104]

In-hospital mortality of patients older than 75 years is estimated to be fourfold to fivefold higher than in younger patients. For those older than 80 years, 2005 registry data for primary PCI for STEMI show in-hospital mortality as 16.6%. Two randomized trials have attempted to compare PCI with fibrinolysis in older patients with STEMI, and both were terminated prematurely because of inability to meet recruitment goals: the Senior PAMI[105] and the recently presented TRIANA trial.[106] It is clear that this question will not be answered in clinical trials. The published data suggest that benefits of invasive strategies relate primarily to later events and need for subsequent revascularization, except in older patients with cardiogenic shock due to left ventricular failure who have improved long-term survival with early invasive strategies.[107] There is growing evidence to support an invasive strategy that can be "delayed" for a period of hours to days to allow stabilization, initiation of pharmacologic therapy, and risk assessment. The Timing of Intervention in Acute Coronary Syndromes (TIMACS) trial[108] included patients older than 75 years and found no difference between early and delayed invasive strategies in low- to intermediate-risk patients (by GRACE score). For higher risk patients, early intervention reduced composite short-term cardiovascular endpoints. A recent randomized comparison of immediate invasive strategy with next working day invasive intervention in patients with NSTEMI using modern antiplatelet regimens found no difference in peak troponin levels between the two strategies in patients older or younger than 75 years.[109] Death rates were the same with both approaches. These data were published after the updated 2007 guidelines,[14] which stated that an initial conservative strategy (selected invasive) could be considered but favored rapid revascularization for older unstable angina/NSTEMI patients. The best strategy currently appears to be to initiate pharmacologic therapy and assess risk at the time of presentation, to consider urgent revascularization for older patients at highest risk and nonurgently for those at intermediate risk, and to be guided by symptoms and evolving clinical status for those at low risk. The patient's preferences should be considered in all scenarios.

For additional information on pharmacologic agents, see Chap. 55.

Current Perspective

Despite increased morbidity and mortality for older patients with CAD and acute coronary syndromes compared with younger patients, risk-adjusted AMI mortality in the United States has decreased from 1995-2006 in the Medicare population.[110] In analyses of community practice outcomes of five recommended therapies (early use of aspirin, beta blockers, heparin, GP IIb/IIIa inhibitors, and cardiac catheterization), in-hospital mortality declined as a function of the number of guideline-recommended therapies given in patients aged 75 years and older, with greater benefit with use of guideline-recommended therapies in older than in younger patients. With special attention to altered dosing for and sensitivity of older patients and close observation for adverse effects of intensive medical and interventional management in elderly subgroups with acute coronary syndromes, short-term morbidity can potentially be further reduced. In contrast to current trends for increased rates of cardiac catheterization and revascularization in lower risk MI patients, use of early invasive strategies should be redirected to high-risk patients, who may have greater benefit.

POST–MYOCARDIAL INFARCTION

Medications

Administration of aspirin, beta blockers, ACE inhibitors, or ARBs in patients with left ventricular dysfunction and lipid-lowering drugs for the post-MI patient is based on clinical trial data showing benefit in populations that have included elderly patients. With the caveat of adjustment of dosing for age and renal status, recommendations are the same as in younger patients (see Chap. 49 and earlier). In contrast, eplerenone did not show either cardiovascular mortality or all-cause mortality benefits for patients older than 65 years with heart failure after MI.[111] The addition of clopidogrel to aspirin after non–ST elevation MI has similar benefits in patients younger and older than 65 years, without significant data on patients older than 75 years.[112] Considerations that may be unique to the elderly patient after MI are the use of antidepressants and hormonal replacement therapy.

Depression affects 10% of community-dwelling older people (see Chap. 91). The prevalence of depression in patients after MI is estimated at 20% to 30% for major depression[113] and up to 50% for potentially significant symptoms of depression.[114] Studies show associations between depression and low perceived social support and increased cardiac morbidity and mortality in post-MI patients and in patients undergoing CABG. Individual trials of counseling interventions in patients with depression have not shown cardiac benefit, but meta-analyses suggest benefit. Trials of selective serotonin reuptake inhibitor (SSRI) antidepressant therapy in patients with depression after acute coronary syndromes or MI suggest benefits of SSRI use on either cardiac events and mortality (perhaps due to antiplatelet properties) or quality of life and overall function, especially in patients with a prior history of depression. Screening for depression can take the form of a simple two-question test followed by additional evaluation for patients with answers suggesting the presence of depression. Alternatively, the nine-item self-report Patient Health Questionnaire screening instrument can be used in literate patients, or the geriatric depression screen for older patients can be administered.[115] Increasing use of SSRI and mixed-mechanism antidepressants has led to recognition of hyponatremia with SSRIs and that SSRI antiplatelet effects can increase the risk of bleeding in combination with warfarin, low-molecular-weight heparin, or aspirin and in patients with hereditary platelet defects.[116] The first-generation SSRI fluoxetine confers increased risk of syncope in elderly patients.

Randomized trials comparing administration of hormone replacement therapy in the form of combined estrogen and progesterone or estrogen alone have shown overall lack of cardiovascular morbidity or mortality benefit and potential harm for both secondary and primary prevention in postmenopausal women (see Chap. 81).[117] Similar to estrogen, the selective estrogen modulator raloxifene lowered LDL-cholesterol and increased HDL-cholesterol but did not decrease coronary event rates and increased stroke rates and thromboembolism.[118] A comparison of raloxifene to tamoxifen for prevention of breast cancer in women found equivalent efficacy in invasive breast cancer reduction, equivalent risks for ischemic disease and stroke, and lower risk of thromboembolic events with raloxifene.[119] Neither estrogen nor estrogen plus progesterone, raloxifene, or tamoxifen can be recommended for cardiovascular disease prevention or treatment.

Rehabilitation Programs (see Chap. 50)

The feasibility of and improvement with intensive exercise interventions have been shown for the elderly, including the frail elderly, residing in the community as well as in the nursing home. The Cardiac Rehabilitation in Advanced Age (CR-AGE) trial compared hospital-based cardiac rehabilitation with home-based cardiac rehabilitation in cognitively intact patients from the ages of 46 to 86 years with recent MI.[120] Similar improvement in total work capacity and health-related quality of life was seen with home-based rehabilitation and hospital-based rehabilitation in all age groups without improvement in the control group. Improvement was somewhat smaller in the group older than 75 years. Benefits decreased over time after hospital rehabilitation but were maintained with home cardiac rehabilitation, and costs were lower in the home rehabilitation group.

Table 80-6 summarizes the approach to the older patient with CAD.

Carotid Artery Disease and Stroke (see Chap. 62)

Prevalence and Incidence. Stroke is the third leading cause of death and is the most common cause of major adult disability in the United States. The risk of stroke increases with age and doubles for each decade after the age of 55 years. Framingham data estimate the 10-year probability of stroke at 11% for men at the age of 65 years and 7% for women at the age of 65 years. At the age of 80 years, the probability increases to 22% and 24% for men and women, respectively. After the age of 85 years, women are at greater risk than are men. Carotid stenosis is responsible for about 15% to 25% of strokes and atrial fibrillation for about 15%. Whereas a transient ischemic attack (TIA) signals a high short-term risk of stroke, 70% of strokes are first events, stressing the importance of primary prevention and treatment of risk factors.[121] Modifiable risk factors for noncardioembolic ischemic stroke or TIA in the elderly are hypertension, diabetes, smoking and passive smoking, hyperlipidemia, lack of physical activity, inadequate treatment of atrial fibrillation, carotid artery disease, heart failure, estrogen administration to postmenopausal women, and sleep apnea (see Chap. 79). Nonmodifiable risk factors for stroke include age, sex (risk greater in men than in women), race/ethnicity (risk greater in African Americans compared with whites), and family history of stroke.

DIAGNOSIS

Transient Ischemic Attack

The traditional diagnosis of TIA—an episode of neurologic impairment lasting less than 24 hours attributable to focal ischemia in the brain or retina—was usually based on clinical history and was not associated with a new permanent neurologic deficit. Recently, high-resolution computed tomography (CT) and diffusion-weighted magnetic resonance imaging (MRI) studies have demonstrated that 15% to 50% of ischemic episodes with symptoms lasting less than 24 hours

TABLE 80-6 Approach to the Older Patient with Coronary Artery Disease

Optimization of medical care warrants greater emphasis.
- Exercise for all, weight loss for the overweight, and smoking cessation in smokers
- Control of hypertension and diabetes
- For relief of symptoms—beta blockers, nitrates, calcium channel blockers
- For prevention of complications—antiplatelet drugs and lipid lowering
- Pharmacologic treatments must incorporate age-related adjustments in dosing; consider altered reflex responses and drug interactions.

Morbidity and mortality from CAD and CAD treated medically or with revascularization increase with age, especially at ages older than 75 years, and there are no advantages of revascularization over optimal medical care for the older patient with stable or nondisabling CAD or who has a satisfactory quality of life.
- Decisions about medical therapy versus revascularization, or for PCI versus CABG, should be based on the role of CAD in the context of the individual older patient's overall health, lifestyle, projected life span, and preferences.

For acute coronary syndromes
- Older patients presenting with acute coronary syndromes in the community are substantially older, are more often women, and have more comorbidity than patients enrolled in randomized studies that are the basis for care guidelines, and clinical outcomes for the oldest patients are generally worse than trial results.
- ST elevation MI has a high mortality in the oldest patients.
- Immediate invasive strategies show the greatest benefit in higher risk patients.
- For patients at lower or intermediate risk, treatment choices should be based on consideration of patient and family preferences, quality of life issues, end-of-life preferences, sociocultural differences, and the experience and capabilities of the site of care.
- All treatment regimens must be adjusted for renal status and size.

Anticipated procedural complication rates should reflect the age and health status of the patient, not complication rates from randomized studies or younger patients.
- Recovery times will be prolonged from all procedures.
- Depression should be evaluated.

For patients older than 80 years, there are limited data.
- Recommendations are based on extrapolations from younger and less sick populations.
- Incremental benefits between therapies are small.
- Decisions between PCI and fibrinolytics or neither in patients older than 75 years should be individualized.

are associated with new cerebral infarction. These insights have led to tissue-based definitions of TIA and stroke. A recent American Heart Association–endorsed statement defines TIA as "a transient episode of neurological dysfunction caused by focal brain or retinal ischemia without evidence of acute infarction" and has no time limit for symptoms.[122] Ischemic stroke is defined as infarction of central nervous system tissue.

Scoring systems may help estimate short-term risk of stroke after a TIA. The ABCD^2 score (see Table 62-1) is calculated by **A**ge ≥60 years (1 point) and **B**lood pressure ≥140/90 mm Hg (1 point), **C**linical features (1 point for speech impairment without weakness, 2 points for unilateral weakness), **D**uration of TIA (≥60 minutes = 2 points and <60 minutes = 1 point), and **D**iabetes (1 point), with 2-day risk of stroke of 0% for scores of 0 or 1, 1.3% for 2 or 3, 4.1% for 4 or 5, and 8.1% for 6 or 7. High scores also appear to identify patients with moderate or severe carotid stenosis. The presence of a new infarct on brain imaging is also associated with an increased short-term risk of subsequent stroke, but it is unclear whether there is additive predictive value of MRI changes to scoring rules such as the ABCD^2.

Stroke

A lopsided face, weak arm, and garbled speech are the most common warning signs of stroke. The mnemonic FAST (face, arm, speech, time) can help identify patients with a potential stroke. Assessment should include a detailed neurologic examination with a stroke rating scale (see Chap. 62) and rapid triage to neuroimaging. Brain imaging guides selection of acute interventions. Non–contrast-enhanced CT is most commonly available, but MRI allows greater tissue definition.[123] Specialized or certified stroke centers are not universally available across the United States but provide the best opportunity for optimal care for older patients likely to have multiorgan disease and complex stroke types.[123]

TREATMENT

Acute Stroke Management[123,124]

Intravenous recombinant tissue plasminogen activator (rtPA) is the only medical therapy approved by the Food and Drug Administration proven to reduce effects of an ischemic stroke. Thrombolysis with rtPA is recommended for selected patients with ischemic stroke with a measurable neurologic deficit (see Chap. 62) in whom it can be administered within hours of stroke onset. Recent guidelines extend the time window for administration of rtPA to 3 to 4.5 hours after stroke onset. Because bleeding risk increases with age and with administration of rtPA at increasing times after onset of symptoms, the recommended time window for patients older than 80 years, however, remains within 3 hours of stroke onset.[125] A persistent systolic blood pressure >185 mm Hg or a diastolic blood pressure >110 mm Hg despite treatment is a contraindication to intravenous administration of rtPA. Other contraindications include recent trauma, surgery, MI, active bleeding, anticoagulation, low platelet levels, prior intracranial hemorrhage, and suggestion of subarachnoid hemorrhage. A major neurologic deficit denotes a poor prognosis, and a number of experts consider use of tPA in these patients. Subtypes of ischemic stroke are not thought to influence responses to rtPA. Symptomatic hemorrhagic transformation of the infarction after rtPA administration occurs in 5.2% of patients but can be reduced by proper selection of patients. Orolingual angioedema occurs in about 5% and is more common in patients taking ACE inhibitors and those with ischemia in the frontal cortex and insula. Intra-arterial thrombolysis is an option for selected patients with major stroke of <6 hours in duration who are not candidates for intravenous rtPA if they are at an experienced stroke center with immediate access to cerebral angiography and qualified interventionalists.

Data support administration of aspirin within 24 to 48 hours of stroke for most patients (not within 24 hours of intravenous rtPA) but not early anticoagulation with unfractionated or low-molecular-weight heparin or acute use of clopidogrel or GP IIb/IIIa receptor inhibitors outside the setting of clinical trials. Endovascular techniques and devices to extract thrombus are under evaluation. Current use should be limited to comprehensive stroke centers or clinical trials, as should use of combination pharmacologic regimens for reperfusion.

Blood pressure management in the setting of acute stroke remains controversial. Aggressive reduction in pressure is not generally recommended, but blood pressure control should precede any thrombolytic therapy. Randomized trials of blood pressure control in the acute stroke setting are ongoing and have passed the 1-year follow-up of data safety monitoring without termination, suggesting that judicious lowering of blood pressure does not have excessive risk. When hypertension is treated, intravenous and short-acting agents are recommended in consensus guidelines for initial therapy (labetalol or nicardipine, with nitropaste in ongoing trials). Poststroke management should include the early initiation of rehabilitation therapy, a swallow screening test for dysphagia, an active secondary stroke prevention program, and the proactive prevention of venous thrombi. Evaluation for depression is also strongly recommended.[126]

Prevention

Secondary and primary prevention is targeted at modifiable risk factors.[121] Evidence-based recommendations are for antiplatelet therapy in patients with prior stroke, TIA, or MI and anticoagulation in high-risk patients such as those with atrial fibrillation (see Chap. 39). Carotid artery interventions should be considered for patients with symptomatic disease or severe lesions.[127] Clinical trials with limited numbers of elderly and excluding the very elderly have also demonstrated that LDL-cholesterol reduction reduces the risk of stroke in

TABLE 80-9 Approach to the Older Patient with Peripheral Artery Disease

Treatment of cardiovascular risk factors and supervised walking-based exercise programs are first-line therapy.
Antiplatelet therapy with aspirin or clopidogrel is usually recommended.
Medications can improve symptoms (cilostazol > pentoxifylline); cilostazol should not be used in patients with heart failure.
Thorough examinations of the feet should be included in examinations.
Patients with decreased sensation or at risk for lesions should be referred to foot care specialists.
Revascularization options include PCI for iliac disease, but long-term efficacy requires surgical approaches at the femoropopliteal and infrapopliteal level.
Surgical morbidity and mortality increase with age, and postoperative recovery times can be prolonged. All are highest in the setting of surgery for critical ischemia or limb salvage.

and ginkgo biloba are less clear. Supplementation with folate, vitamin E, or omega-3 fatty acids is not recommended, nor is chelation therapy.[142]

Decreased sensation due to age, cognitive impairment, neuropathy or diabetes, increased risk of cutaneous damage from minor trauma with age, and decreased vision increase the chance of missing early signs of critical limb ischemia in older patients. The patient with PAD and the caregiver should be educated on limb hygiene, frequent examination, and early reporting of lesions, and health care professionals must inspect limbs as a routine part of clinical care. It appears that only about a quarter of patients with intermittent claudication will deteriorate significantly, although measured walking time does decrease progressively over time. Multidisciplinary care can help patients with critical limb ischemia avoid limb loss.

Revascularization can be performed by endovascular or surgical techniques for individuals with unacceptable responses to pharmacologic or lifestyle modifications, limiting disability, or critical limb ischemia. For acute limb ischemia, time to diagnosis and initiation of treatment is inversely related to successful outcome (see Chap. 61). Options include percutaneous catheter-directed thrombolytic therapy, percutaneous mechanical thrombus extraction with or without thrombolytic therapy, and surgical thrombectomy or bypass. Initial thrombolytic therapy is recommended for ischemia of ≤14 days' duration or graft occlusions, and initial surgical revascularization is recommended for those with ischemia of >14 days' duration or native arterial occlusions.[146] Interventional procedures have been most successful for disease of the iliac arteries. Guidelines address choices between surgical and catheter-based approaches as well as methods of catheter-based approaches that continue to evolve (see TransAtlantic Inter-Society consensus statements, Chaps. 61 and 63).[140,142,146] Decisions should be based on symptoms, responses to therapies, comorbid conditions, quality of life, and recognition of higher morbidity and longer surgical recovery times of older patients as well as the morbidity and mortality results of the operator.

Table 80-9 presents the general approach to the older patient with lower extremity PAD. Disease of the aorta is discussed in Chapter 60.

Current Controversies. Current controversies include the following: optimal pharmacologic therapies for PAD; role of prostaglandins and angiogenesis therapy; optimal endovascular techniques; and role of endovascular procedures versus surgical procedures.

Heart Failure (see Chaps. 25 to 30)

Heart failure has become primarily a disorder of the elderly. Heart failure contributes to at least 20% of hospital admissions of patients older than 65 years, with approximately three quarters of heart failure hospitalizations occurring in patients older than 65 years and more than 85% of heart failure deaths occurring in patients older than 65 years. Heart failure is self-reported by 0.1% of people at ages 18 to 39 years, by about 4% at ages 65 to 74 years, and by about 6% at ages 75 to 105 years. In the Cardiovascular Health Study of independent community-dwelling subjects aged 66 to 103 years, heart failure developed at a rate of 19.3/1000 patient-years. The incidence increased from 10.6/1000 person-years in participants 65 to 69 years of age to 42.5/1000 person-years in those older than 80 years.[147] Similar data have been reported among Medicare beneficiaries (**Fig. 80-10**). Asymptomatic left ventricular systolic dysfunction is estimated to occur in another 3% to 5% of the community, with higher prevalence at older ages. The incidence and prevalence of heart failure are higher in men than in women at all ages, and heart failure is more likely to result from CAD in men than in women. With more women alive at older ages, there are more older women than older men presenting for care for heart failure, and the etiology is less likely to be ischemic (see Chap. 81). Heart failure of any type is associated with a reduction in life span as well as decreased quality of life and recurrent hospitalizations.[148] Average 5-year mortality for heart failure patients with systolic dysfunction is approximately 50% and may be only slightly lower for heart failure patients with preserved systolic function (see Fig. 30-4).[149,150] Prognosis both for systolic heart failure and for heart failure with preserved ejection fraction is worse in patients older than 65 years, and the presence of preserved ejection fraction has less impact on survival than in younger patients. In community-based cohorts, overall survival after onset of heart failure has improved during the past two decades, but there has been less improvement among women and elderly patients with heart failure (**Fig. 80-11**).[151,152]

In contrast to middle-aged patients with heart failure, factors other than left ventricular systolic function contribute to heart failure in the elderly population. Heart failure in the presence of a normal or preserved ejection fraction may be seen in 40% to 80% of older patients with heart failure and is almost twice as frequent in women as in men.[149,153] A history of hypertension is often present, and increased circulating blood volume is present in a subset.[149,154] The pathophysiology is primarily attributed to left ventricular diastolic dysfunction (a leftward- and upward-shifted end-diastolic pressure-volume relationship); left ventricular diastolic chamber size is normal or reduced despite elevated filling pressures,

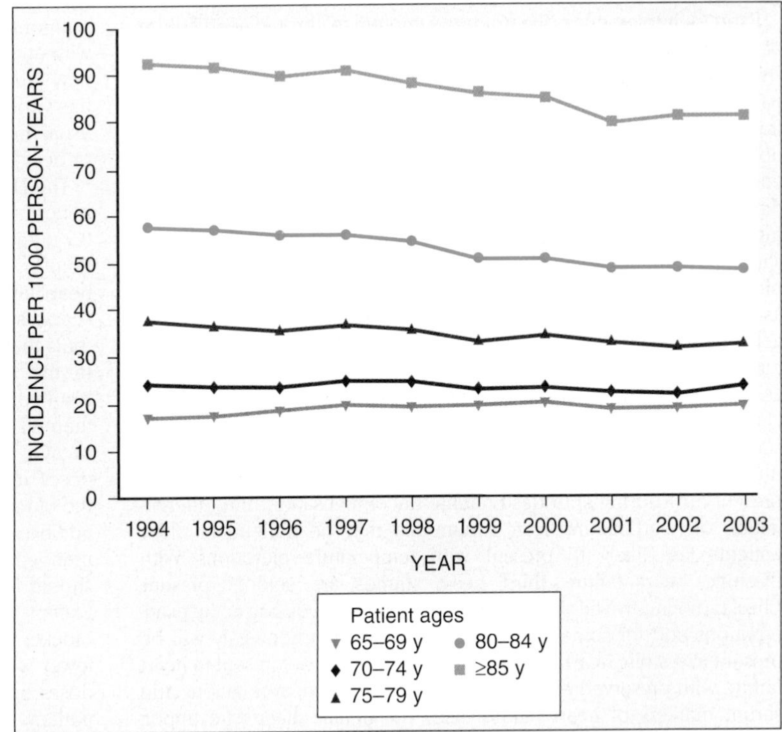

FIGURE 80-10 Incidence rates of heart failure by age in a nationally representative sample of nearly 3 million Medicare beneficiaries. The incidence of heart failure increases with increasing age within the Medicare population. *(From Curtis L, Whellan D, Hammill B, et al: Incidence and prevalence of heart failure in elderly persons, 1994-2003. Arch Intern Med 168:418, 2008.)*

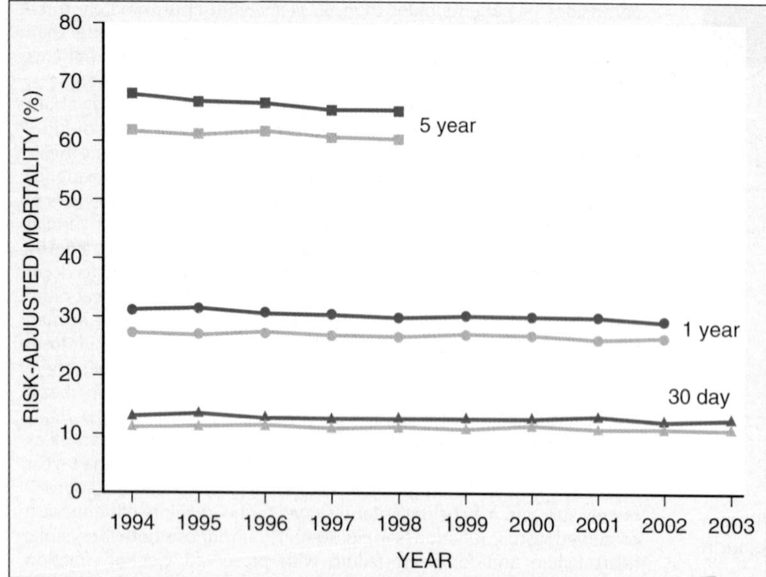

FIGURE 80-11 Risk-adjusted mortality after onset of heart failure by year of incidence and sex in a nationally representative sample of nearly 3 million Medicare beneficiaries. Mortality declined only slightly and was consistently lower for women. *(From Curtis L, Whellan D, Hammill B, et al: Incidence and prevalence of heart failure in elderly persons, 1994-2003. Arch Intern Med 168:418, 2008.)*

resulting in decreased stroke volume and cardiac output (see Fig. 30-10). Thus, some call the disorder diastolic heart failure. Endocardial biopsy specimens from heart failure patients without CAD show structural and functional differences in cardiomyocytes compared with cardiomyocytes from patients with abnormal ejection fraction (systolic heart failure).[155] Myocytes from patients with diastolic heart failure had increased diameter and higher myofibrillar density and developed greater passive force and had greater calcium sensitivity. Myocardial collagen volume fraction was equally elevated.

Exercise intolerance is the primary symptom in chronic heart failure of either systolic (see Chap. 28) or diastolic (see Chap. 30) etiology. Dyspnea and fatigue are prominent symptoms, but fatigue also accompanies many chronic illnesses and is part of the clinical syndrome of frailty in the elderly. Shortness of breath, orthopnea or development of nocturnal cough, and paroxysmal nocturnal dyspnea suggest the presence of heart failure. Less than half of patients with moderate or severe diastolic or systolic dysfunction as measured by Doppler echocardiography had recognized heart failure in a large community-based study.[156] Potential explanations for unrecognized heart failure in the older patient include the nonspecificity of complaints of fatigue, ascribing of symptoms to aging or comorbid conditions, reduction in activities to avoid symptoms, and memory impairment leading to poor historical information. Physical examination may not be as definitive as in younger individuals. Peripheral edema can be due to age-related changes in venous tone, decreased skin turgor, or prolonged sedentary states, and evaluation of volume status based on neck veins may be difficult in the older patient. Rales and a third heart sound may be present only during episodes of acute decompensation, and differentiation of heart failure from pneumonia may be difficult in older patients less likely to present with temperature elevations. With diastolic heart failure, third heart sounds are seldom present. Chest radiography will show pulmonary congestion during acute exacerbations and for some time after an episode; cardiomegaly will be present in systolic heart failure but may or may not be present in heart failure with preserved ejection fraction. Use of echocardiography and serum markers of heart failure takes on greater diagnostic importance.[155,157] Measurement of natriuretic peptides such as B-type natriuretic peptide (BNP) and N-terminal pro-BNP (NT-proBNP) can improve diagnostic accuracy of patients with dyspnea presenting for acute care and may be helpful in evaluating older patients with dyspnea and nonspecific symptoms or multiple comorbidities. Levels of natriuretic peptides increase with age and with renal decline, and are higher in women than in men, so interpretation requires consideration of these factors. For NT-proBNP, cutoffs for heart failure diagnosis are age specific, with an almost fourfold higher cutoff value for patients older than 75 years compared with those younger than 75 years. For BNP, a twofold higher cutoff value has been suggested for patients with eGFR less than 60 mL/min/1.73 m^2 (the eGFR for most white women older than 65 years; see earlier).

Most data from randomized double-blind studies of therapy for heart failure are from studies of younger middle-aged men with systolic dysfunction resulting from ischemic CAD and few major medical comorbidities. Notably, initial landmark studies of the treatment of systolic heart failure with the ACE inhibitor enalapril as well as hydralazine plus isosorbide excluded patients older than 75 or 80 years. More recent studies have included subsets of elderly (see Chaps. 27 and 28 and **Table 80-10**), and guidelines for the management of patients with chronic heart failure are based on the aggregate data[157-160] and are available at *www.acc.org*, *www.heart.org* or *www.onlinejcf.com*. Limited trial data are available to guide treatment of the older patient with heart failure and preserved or normal ejection fraction, and recent trials have not demonstrated survival benefits with ACE inhibitors or ARBs in these patients (see Table 80-10). Because the direct applicability of clinical trial findings and heart failure treatment guidelines to the majority of older heart failure patients is unknown and the limited data suggest that outcomes differ from trial results in younger systolic heart failure patients, it is important to consider care in the context of the individual patients and their goals, comorbid conditions, and estimated life expectancy.

HEART FAILURE WITH DECREASED SYSTOLIC FUNCTION (SYSTOLIC HEART FAILURE) (see Chap. 28). Pharmacologic therapy is targeted at control of systolic and diastolic hypertension (see earlier), use of diuretics to control pulmonary congestion and pulmonary edema, and control of ventricular response rate in patients with atrial fibrillation. Most systolic heart failure trials have tested the new therapy or intervention on a background of "usual therapy" that has varied over time. Earlier trials included digitalis and diuretics as usual therapy, but more recent usual therapy is an ACE inhibitor or ARB or beta blocker plus a diuretic, with lower rates of digoxin use.

The DIG trial analyses suggest that a morbidity and hospitalization benefit can accompany digoxin concentrations between 0.5 and 0.9 ng/mL, and the optimal use may be in those with atrial fibrillation.[161,162] Efficacy for ACE inhibitors in post-MI patients with systolic heart failure (SAVE, AIRE, TRACE) and ARBs in systolic heart failure (candesartan in the CHARM programs) has been demonstrated in trials that have included significant numbers of elderly patients.[163-168] In the carefully controlled and monitored setting, dose titration resulted in lower daily doses in older patients, especially those older than 80 years. Caution and close monitoring are necessary with use of ACE inhibitors or ARBs in the elderly, and in general, the "full doses" used in studies of younger patients should not be the target for the oldest patients. Combined use of ACE inhibitors and ARBs has no additive benefit, may have additive adverse effects, and is not recommended. Vasodilating beta blockers are usually considered and should be instituted at low doses during periods of clinical stability. Except for trials with non–U.S.-approved bucindolol, large beta blocker trials excluded patients older than 80 years and have enrolled fewer women than men. Trials with bisoprolol showed benefit at all doses, but doses titrated to tolerance were lower in the oldest enrolled patients with the greater medical comorbidities and in those with the most severe heart failure.[169] At least one trial of a vasodilating beta blocker not available in the United States (nebivolol, see Table 80-10) in exclusively elderly patients with heart failure has reported reduced combined endpoints of all-cause death or hospitalization for heart

Table 80-10 Investigations of Heart Failure Therapies in Elderly Patients

STUDY	PATIENTS	N (% WOMEN)	% >65 YEARS, MEDIAN AGE	DRUG (DOSE)	COMEDICATIONS	MAJOR RESULTS
SENIORS (randomized, placebo controlled) 2005	Heart failure (decreased EF in 64%; preserved EF in 36%)	2128 (37)	100% >70, 76	Nebivolol (10 mg/day)	Diuretic in 86%, ACE or ARB in 88%, aldosterone antagonist in 28%, digoxin in 39%	Overall advantage (low and preserved EF) Subgroups: survival advantage in <75 yr; no advantage in >75 yr
PEP-CHF (randomized, placebo controlled) 2006	Heart failure (preserved EF; hospitalized within 6 months)	850 (56)	100% >70, 76	Perindopril (4 mg/day) (+ diuretic)	Loop diuretics in 44%-47%, thiazide diuretics in 55%, beta blockers in 54%, digoxin in 12%, aldosterone antagonist in 10%	No survival benefit with intention-to-treat analyses but underpowered Reduced heart failure hospitalizations, but 30% not on assigned treatment at 1 yr Equal numbers in both groups taking ACE at end
OPTIMIZE-HF (registry and Medicare data) 2009	Decreased EF	7529 (45)	100%, 78 treated, 80 untreated	Beta blocker compared with no beta blocker	Diuretic in 83%, ACE or ARB in 62%-77%, aldosterone antagonist in 11%-18%, digoxin in 38%	Survival advantage for decreased EF
	Preserved EF	9712 (66)	100%, 80 treated, 81 untreated		Diuretic in 80%, ACE or ARB in 54%-65%, digoxin in 20%-23%, aldosterone antagonist in 7%-9%	No benefit in preserved EF group
I-PRESERVE (randomized, placebo controlled) 2008	Preserved EF	4128 (60)	100% >60, 72 35% >75	Irbesartan (300 mg/day)	Diuretic in 83%, beta blocker in 58%, ACE in 25%, aldosterone antagonist in 15%, digoxin in 13%	No benefit for death from any cause or hospitalization versus placebo

ACE = angiotensin-converting enzyme inhibitor; ARB = angiotensin receptor blocker; EF = ejection fraction.

SENIORS: Flather M, Shibata M, Coats A, et al: Randomized trial to determine the effect of nebivolol on mortality and cardiovascular hospital admission in elderly patients with heart failure (SENIORS). Eur Heart J 26:212, 2005. PEP-CHF: Cleland J, Tendera M, Adamus J, et al: The perindopril in elderly people with chronic heart failure (PEP-CHF) study. Eur Heart J 27:2338, 2006. OPTIMIZE-HF: Hernandez A, Hammill B, O'Connor C, et al: Findings from the OPTIMIZE-HF (Organized Program to Initiate Lifesaving Treatment in Hospitalized Patients with Heart Failure) Registry. Clinical effectiveness of beta-blockers in heart failure. J Am Coll Cardiol 53:184, 2009. I-PRESERVE: Massie B, Carson P, McMurray J, et al: Irbesartan in patients with heart failure and preserved ejection fraction. N Engl J Med 359:359, 2008.

failure, with nonsignificant differences in all-cause death.[170,171] U.S. Registry and Medicare data analyses of exclusively older patients support the conclusion that beta blocker use in clinical populations with heart failure diagnoses is associated with a survival advantage.[150] Ongoing studies are comparing individual beta blockers in elderly heart failure patients.

Studies of aldosterone antagonists have enrolled older patients, primarily white men. Benefit may be seen with these drugs used at lower doses in patients with severe heart failure, but increased use of spironolactone has been accompanied by increased incidence of hyperkalemia in older patients with heart failure, and close monitoring is necessary. Trial data on eplerenone are limited to heart failure in the post-MI setting in younger elderly with the suggestion of no benefit in those older than 65 years.[111] Caution is warranted for its use, especially without data for efficacy and known risks of hyperkalemia in patients with reduced renal clearance common in the elderly. Direct vasodilators such as hydralazine and nitrates have a limited role in older patients because of the increased likelihood of orthostatic hypotension.

Nonpharmacologic Strategies

Dietary sodium restriction is advised, and moderate physical activity should be encouraged if feasible. Supervised exercise training programs based on cardiac rehabilitation algorithms have shown modest benefit on all-cause mortality and hospitalization rates in middle-aged and younger elderly patients with systolic heart failure receiving optimal therapy by heart failure guidelines (age range, 51 to 68 years; 70% were men).[172] Perhaps more relevantly, self-reported health status was improved in the exercise group compared with placebo.[173] Exercise programs similar to those used in cardiac rehabilitation programs should be considered for older patients with systolic heart failure receiving optimal medical therapy to improve heart failure–related quality of life.

Cardiac resynchronization therapy (CRT) can decrease hospitalizations and reduce mortality in selected patients with prolonged cardiac repolarization or QRS intervals on the ECG and symptomatic systolic heart failure despite optimal medical therapy. Most trials excluded patients with atrial fibrillation. CRT trials to determine the efficacy of defibrillator implantation have not included significant numbers of elderly patients. Guidelines as well as clinical judgment dictate that such therapies be considered on an individual basis and when estimated longevity from all causes is long enough to confer benefit (see Chaps. 29 and 38). Revascularization therapies are considered in the setting of ischemia (see Chaps. 31, 32, and 57). The few highly selected patients older than 65 years who have received cardiac transplantation appear to have survival times similar to those of younger patients, with slightly more morbidity and mortality due to the surgical procedure but lower rates of rejection compared with younger patients (see Chap. 31).

HEART FAILURE WITH NORMAL OR PRESERVED LEFT VENTRICULAR EJECTION FRACTION (DIASTOLIC HEART FAILURE). Management is based on control of physiologic factors (blood pressure, heart rate, blood volume, and myocardial ischemia) that are known to exert important effects on ventricular relaxation and the treatment of diseases known to cause diastolic heart failure. Diuretics are effective in the presence of signs and symptoms of volume overload.[157,160] Circulating blood volume is a major determinant of ventricular filling pressure, and the use of diuretics may improve breathlessness in patients with diastolic heart failure (as well as in those with systolic heart failure), but overdiuresis must be avoided. ACE inhibitors and ARBs have been advocated on the basis of the potential for left ventricular regression and reduction of interstitial fibrosis and arterial stiffness. However, larger randomized trials of ACE inhibitors or ARBs for diastolic heart failure in the elderly have not found a survival or hospitalization benefit.[174,175] In these trials, an ACE inhibitor or ARB was added to baseline therapy with diuretics in three quarters of patients, beta blockers in more than half, calcium channel blockers in about one third, spironolactone in 10% to 15%, and digoxin in 15% to 28% (higher in earlier studies). Thus, ACE inhibitors and ARBs may help alleviate symptoms in individual patients, but they have not demonstrated the improved outcomes for diastolic heart failure that they have for systolic heart failure. Their use should be guided by symptomatic responses and the patient's tolerance.

Beta blockers and rate-slowing calcium channel blockers are often advocated on the premise that they decrease blood pressure and afterload and prolong the diastolic filling period. However, a comprehensive study of heart failure registry data linked to Medicare claims data incorporating a broad cohort of patients from all regions of the United States failed to find a survival benefit with the use of a variety of beta blockers in heart failure patients with preserved ejection fraction.[150] Nondihydropyridine calcium channel antagonists can improve measures of diastolic function during short-term use, but definitive data on outcomes with chronic administration for diastolic heart failure are not available. Digoxin was reported to yield symptomatic improvement and decreased hospitalizations (without mortality benefit) in the DIG study of patients with diastolic or systolic heart failure.[176] In analyses of the subset of patients with normal ejection fractions, no benefit of digoxin was detected in patients with mild to moderate heart failure who were in normal sinus rhythm and receiving diuretics and ACE inhibitors.[162] The risk-to-benefit ratio of digoxin in women with heart failure has also been questioned. Data are also lacking on nitrates, but some clinicians find them helpful in reducing orthopnea if they are given at bedtime.

The search for more effective therapies for diastolic heart failure is ongoing with investigations of the aldosterone antagonists spironolactone and eplerenone, the renin inhibitor aliskiren, endothelin receptor antagonists, statins, ion channel inhibitors ivabradine and ranolazine, and use of erythropoietin in patients with anemia. Studies of the collagen cross-link breaker alagebrium were terminated before enrollment was completed, and no other agents of this class are currently under study (*www.clinicaltrials.gov*).

ADDITIONAL CONSIDERATIONS FOR THE OLDER PATIENT WITH HEART FAILURE. Elderly patients with heart failure have the highest rehospitalization rate of all adult patient groups. Education and involvement of the patient, family members, and caregivers are key to the management of older patients with heart failure. Recognition of warning signs of worsening failure, understanding of medication regimens, diet adjustments, and regular moderate physical activity should be emphasized. Reliance cannot be placed on classic symptoms of heart failure, and weight should be measured daily with a mechanism for rapid communication of information and timely adjustment of diuretic dosages to prevent exacerbations of heart failure. Although diagnosis of heart failure may be improved by measurement of natriuretic peptides, a comparison of symptom-guided therapy with BNP-guided therapy did not improve overall clinical outcomes or quality of life in older patients and cannot be recommended as a routine monitoring strategy.[177] Multidisciplinary team approaches with patient contacts between office visits and more frequent contact during the transitional period after hospital discharge can be highly beneficial and reduce rehospitalization rates.[178,179] Use of primary care preventive strategies such as influenza vaccination can also reduce hospitalizations for heart failure in older people.[180] For very old patients or those with progressive symptoms of severe heart failure, goals of improving symptoms and quality of life and preventing acute exacerbations and hospitalization rather than prolongation of life become the emphasis. Palliative care programs may have special expertise in the management of symptoms such as dyspnea with opiates and in providing support for family and caregivers as well as for the patient with advanced heart failure.[181] See **Table 80-11** for the approach to the older patient with heart failure.

TABLE 80-11 Approach to the Older Patient with Heart Failure

Symptoms may be nonspecific in the older patient—suspect heart failure.
  Consider heart failure diagnosis in patients with fatigue, dyspnea, exercise intolerance, or low activity.
Diagnosis may be facilitated by use of echocardiography or serum markers of heart failure.
Heart failure may be present in the older patient with preserved systolic function (ejection fraction), especially in older women.
Aggressive treatment of hypertension or diabetes, when present, may improve heart failure outcomes.
Treat symptoms with a goal of improving quality of life and morbidity.
  Control blood pressure—systolic and diastolic.
  Treat ischemia.
  Control atrial fibrillation rate.
  Promote physical activity.
  Adjust medications for age- and disease-related changes in kinetics and dynamics.
Educate and involve patients, family members, or caregivers in management of heart failure.
  Monitor weight.
Consider use of multidisciplinary team approaches.

CURRENT CONTROVERSIES AND ISSUES IN HEART FAILURE IN THE ELDERLY. Current controversies include the following: blood pressure target for older patients with heart failure; efficacious treatment of diastolic heart failure; impact of exercise training on mortality; optimal use of case management teams for heart failure in the elderly; role of nutrition; role of renal dysfunction, anemia, or treatment with erythropoietin on outcomes; role of ultrafiltration; role of devices in patients older than 75 to 80 years or older patients with significant comorbid conditions; role of cross-link breaking agents to reduce ventricular stiffening; and role of testosterone in older men with heart failure.

Arrhythmias

Cell loss and collagen infiltration occur in the area of the sinus node, throughout the atria, the central fibrous body, and the cytoskeleton of the heart with increasing age. Changes are most marked in the area of the sinus node, with destruction of as many as 90% of cells by the age of 75 years. In the center of the sinus node, expression of the L-type calcium channel protein $Ca_v1.2$ responsible for the upstroke of the action potential and depolarization is also decreased with aging.[182] The correlation between pathology and sinus node function, however, is poor, and sinus node function is preserved in most elderly patients, although sinoatrial conduction is decreased. Collagen infiltration and fibrosis are of lesser magnitude in the area of the AV node and more marked in the left and right bundle branches. Conduction times through the AV node increase with aging, with the site of delay above the His bundle. Despite age-related collagen infiltration, His-Purkinje conduction times are not usually increased by aging alone.

Resting heart rate is not altered by age, but maximal heart rate and beat-to-beat variability in heart rate decrease with age because of decreases in sinus node responses to beta-adrenergic and parasympathetic stimulation (see Chap. 94). On the surface ECG, the PR interval increases and the R, S, and T wave amplitudes decrease. The QRS axis shifts leftward. This shift may reflect increased left ventricular mass or interstitial fibrosis of the anterior fascicular radiation. Right bundle branch block is found in 3% of healthy people older than 85 years and in up to 20% of centenarians and in 8% to 10% of older patients with heart disease, but it is not associated with cardiac morbidity or mortality. The presence of left bundle branch block increases with age and is more likely to be associated with cardiovascular disease.

Nonspecific intraventricular conduction delays become more frequent with increasing age and are usually related to underlying myocardial disease. Repolarization times throughout the myocardium increase with age, and surface ECG QT intervals increase.

Atrial ectopy has been found on electrocardiographic recordings in 10% of community-dwelling elderly without known cardiac disease and in up to 80% during 24-hour ambulatory electrocardiographic recordings. Brief episodes of atrial tachyarrhythmias are seen on 24-hour ambulatory ECGs in up to 50% of community-dwelling elderly. Premature ventricular complexes also increase in prevalence and frequency with age. Ventricular ectopic beats are seen on electrocardiography in 6% to 11% of elderly without known cardiovascular disease and in as many as 76% on 24-hour ambulatory electrocardiographic recordings. In the absence of cardiac disease, these age-related changes have not been associated with subsequent cardiovascular events (see Table 80-1).

Sinus Node Dysfunction

Bradycardia due to sinus node dysfunction or AV conduction disease is more common as age increases. The mean age of patients undergoing permanent pacemaker implantation is about 74 years, with 70% of new pacemaker recipients being older than 70 years. In the United States, 85% of pacemaker implantations are in patients older than 65 years, with up to 30% implanted in patients older than 80 years. The most common indication is for sinus node dysfunction.

Atrioventricular Conduction Disease

First-degree AV block is diagnosed in 6% to 10% of healthy elderly. Higher degree AV block is less common. Transient type II AV block occurs on 0.4% to 0.8% of 24-hour ambulatory ECGs of community-dwelling elderly and transient third-degree AV block in less than 0.2%. These arrhythmias usually represent advanced conduction system disease, requiring pacemaker implantation (see Chap. 39). Acquired AV block is the second most important indication for permanent pacemaker implantation.

Studies have compared outcomes with single-chamber versus dual-chamber pacing devices in older patients with sinus node dysfunction or AV node disease (see Chap. 38). The overall conclusion is that dual-chamber pacing does not provide a significant 2- to 6-year survival advantage or benefit with respect to cardiovascular death or stroke. For some patients, quality of life or heart failure symptoms may be improved or atrial fibrillation may be less common with atrial-based pacing, but procedural complication rates and reoperation rates before discharge are higher with dual-chamber pacemaker implantation.[183-185] For further discussion of pacing, see Chap. 38.

CURRENT CONTROVERSIES. Current controversies include the optimal pacing mode for individual patients with sinus and AV node disease and the role of resynchronization therapy in the elderly.

Atrial Arrhythmias

ATRIAL FIBRILLATION (see Chap. 39). Atrial fibrillation is seen on 24-hour ambulatory recordings in 10% of community-dwelling older patients. The incidence doubles with each decade beginning at the age of 60 years, so that by the age of 80 to 89 years, the incidence of atrial fibrillation is currently estimated to be 8% to 10%. Median age of patients with atrial fibrillation in the United States is about 75 years, with approximately 70% of patients with atrial fibrillation between the ages of 65 and 85 years. Atrial fibrillation is projected to increase, with a 2.5-fold increase in the prevalence during the next 50 years. Hospitalizations for atrial fibrillation have already increased.[186] Atrial fibrillation is rarely an isolated condition in the older patient. Hypertension, ischemic heart disease, heart failure, valvular disease, and diabetes are the most common conditions associated with atrial fibrillation, and thyroid disease should also be considered. The risk for stroke associated with atrial fibrillation combined with the high prevalence of other stroke risk factors mandates a focus on antithrombotic therapy (anticoagulation), management of associated conditions, and rate control to improve symptoms.

Currently, warfarin remains the first-line agent in the United States on the basis of long-term experience with its efficacy and adverse effects. Patients should be anticoagulated with warfarin in the absence of contraindications. The target international normalized ratio (INR) is 2 to 2.5 in older patients in whom close monitoring of INRs can be performed. Low fixed warfarin doses of 1 mg are not efficacious. Patients older than 75 years may require less than half the dose of middle-aged patients for equivalent anticoagulation. Warfarin dosing guidelines for the elderly recommend initiation of warfarin at the estimated maintenance dosage of warfarin, usually 2 to 5 mg daily, and it can be better estimated with algorithms that incorporate multiple clinical factors (*www.warfarindosing.org*). As discussed before, genotyping is not currently recommended or reimbursed for warfarin dosing estimation. Drug interaction information should be consulted whenever warfarin is being initiated or a drug is added to or deleted from a patient's medications. Chronic warfarin administration may contribute to osteoporosis. Vitamin K plays a role in bone metabolism, and oral anticoagulation with warfarin antagonizes vitamin K. In analyses of women receiving chronic oral anticoagulation compared with nonanticoagulated cohorts, increased risk of osteoporosis and higher rates of vertebral and rib fractures were associated with oral anticoagulation for more than 12 months.[187] Measures to prevent osteoporosis should accompany long-term anticoagulation with warfarin (calcium and vitamin D in most; bisphosphonates, calcitonin if needed).

In older patients who are unable to tolerate or who are not candidates for warfarin, aspirin combined with clopidogrel (75 mg/day) may reduce the risk of major vascular events, but as with warfarin, the risk of major hemorrhage is increased.[188] A large international trial of elderly patients with atrial fibrillation found the oral direct thrombin inhibitor dabigatran noninferior to warfarin for stroke prevention and to be associated with less bleeding at the lower (110 mg/day) of two doses but with a trend for increased risk of MI; the higher dose (150 mg/day) had lower stroke rates but increased bleeding and increased risk of MI.[189] Hepatotoxicity is stated to be less than that with the previously promising thrombin inhibitor ximelagatran. As experience with and access to dabigatran increase, current antithrombotic strategies may need to be reevaluated.

Randomized studies have found no significant difference in long-term outcome between rate control and rhythm control, even in the presence of heart failure, and it is the unusual older patient who requires rhythm control to provide symptom relief.[190-195] Agents effective in controlling heart rate include beta blockers, non-dihydropyridine calcium channel antagonists, amiodarone, and digoxin (for less active elderly). Dronedarone, an amiodarone-like drug without iodine moieties, has recently become available and is effective for control of heart rate and may improve cardiovascular outcomes with fewer adverse effects than with amiodarone.[196,197] Like amiodarone, it is a strong CYP3A inhibitor and increases digoxin, creatinine, and simvastatin levels. There are limited data on dose response or dose alterations for use in the elderly, and it should not be used in patients with systolic heart failure. Other recent data show that neither ARBs nor statins prevent recurrences of atrial fibrillation and that the beta blocker nebivolol improves atrial fibrillation outcomes in older patients.[171,198]

See **Table 80-12** for a summary of the approach to the older patient with atrial fibrillation.

CURRENT CONTROVERSIES. Current controversies include the following: optimal rate control; optimal use of dronedarone; best strategies to reduce bleeding risk with warfarin; estimating risk of complications of atrial fibrillation; role of self-monitoring of INR to improve warfarin therapy; and role and safety of dabigatran.

Ventricular Arrhythmias

Treatment of premature ventricular contractions with most type I antiarrhythmic agents either has been of no benefit or has decreased survival. If patients have symptoms, administration of a beta blocker may be helpful. Sustained ventricular tachycardia and ventricular fibrillation require treatment in patients of any age[199] (see Chap. 39).

TABLE 80-12 Approach to the Older Patient with Atrial Fibrillation

Atrial fibrillation is frequent in the elderly and confers a risk of stroke.
Routine examinations or electrocardiographic evaluations should be targeted toward detection of atrial fibrillation.
Thyroid disease and medical conditions should be controlled.
Anticoagulation with warfarin is the chief weapon against stroke.
- The potential for both greater benefit and fatal intracranial bleeding is present at ages older than 75 years, especially in women.
- Careful attention to anticoagulation monitoring is needed.
- Aspirin plus clopidogrel (75 mg/day) can reduce stroke risk in patients who are not candidates for warfarin or are warfarin intolerant, with overall bleeding risks similar to those with warfarin.
- Aspirin alone does not prevent stroke but increases bleeding risk.

Rate control produces equivalent benefits with lower costs and morbidity than attempts at rhythm control.
- Useful agents in the elderly include digoxin (rest control), beta blockers, nondihydropyridine calcium channel blockers, and amiodarone or dronedarone with dose adjustments for age, weight, and diseases.

Syncope

It is estimated that 40% of people older than 70 years fall at least once a year, and there is significant overlap between falls and syncope in older adults, with an estimated 30% of falls being due to syncope in the elderly. Syncope accounts for 1% to 3% of emergency department visits and as much as 6% of hospital admissions, and it is the sixth most common cause of hospitalization of patients older than 65 years. The cause of syncope often remains undetermined. The San Francisco Syncope Rule (high risk if any of the following are present: history of heart failure or hematocrit lower than 30%, abnormal ECG, shortness of breath, systolic blood pressure <90 mm Hg at presentation) or other more complex algorithms can help identify patients at high and low risk for short-term consequences and guide evaluations.[200] Dedicated syncope units and the rapid access multidisciplinary approach may also increase the diagnostic yield and reduce the need for hospitalization but are not widely available.[201] In a review of diagnostic testing in a series of older patients (mean age, 79 years) with syncope, the lowest likelihood of useful test results was found with electroencephalography, head CT scans, and cardiac enzyme tests.[59] Postural blood pressure recordings had the highest yield but were obtained uncommonly. In addition, carotid ultrasonography and tilt-table testing seldom identify the cause. A careful history and physical examination and use of a risk stratification algorithm can help identify patients likely to benefit from cardiac enzyme and heart rhythm monitoring.

Valvular Disease (see Chap. 66)

Age-related changes in the fibromuscular skeleton of the heart include myxomatous degeneration and collagen infiltration termed sclerosis. Another change is calcification of the aortic valve leaflets, aortic annulus, base of the semilunar cusps, and mitral annulus. The underlying processes involve lipid accumulation, inflammation, remodeling of the extracellular matrix, angiogenesis, and finally calcification.[202] Calcification progresses from the base of the cusps to the leaflets, eventually causing a reduction in leaflet motion and effective valve area without commissural fusion. Increasing calcification with progression to stenosis is now the most common cause of valvular stenoses in older patients, especially at the aortic position. Ischemic or hypertensive disease has become the most common cause of valvular regurgitation, especially at the mitral valve. Similarly, pulmonary regurgitation and tricuspid regurgitation in the elderly are usually secondary to pulmonary hypertension and dilation of the right ventricle resulting from left ventricular ischemia, heart failure, or pulmonary disease. Less common causes of mild to moderate mitral or aortic regurgitation are ruptured chordae, endocarditis, trauma, aortic dissection, and rheumatic heart disease.

Infective endocarditis is seen in about equal frequency in younger and older patients, but it is more likely to be associated with nosocomial infections with the use of intravascular catheters or devices, the presence of prosthetic implants, pacemaker leads, atheromas, or mitral annular calcification in older patients. Polymicrobial infections are uncommon in the elderly, and the most frequent pathogens are group D streptococci and enterococcus, *Staphylococcus epidermidis,* and viridans streptococci (see Chap. 67).

Treatment of symptomatic valvular disease relies on surgical approaches.[203] Surgery in older patients between 70 and 80 years of age is increasingly common, but experience with those older than 90 years is limited and carries a high surgical mortality rate.

Aortic Valve Disease

AORTIC STENOSIS. Sclerosis of the aortic valve is present in as many as 30% of the elderly, and the prevalence increases as age increases from 65 years to more than 85 years. Mild aortic stenosis is present in about 9% of people older than 65 years, moderate stenosis in 5%, and severe aortic stenosis in about 2%. Risk factors for progression from sclerosis to stenosis include a congenitally bicuspid valve, hypertension, hyperlipidemia, smoking, end-stage renal disease, and, in some series, diabetes, shorter stature, or male sex. No correlations have been found between C-reactive protein and calcification or rate of progression of stenosis. Intriguingly, telomere length has been reported to be shorter in older patients with critical calcific aortic valve stenosis compared with age-matched controls.

The pathophysiologic consequences of aortic stenosis are independent of cause and include left ventricular hypertrophy, elevated left ventricular diastolic pressures, and decreased stroke volume in patients of all ages. However, for any given degree of aortic stenosis, left ventricular hypertrophy and decreased left ventricular compliance are greater in patients older than 65 years compared with younger patients. Approximately 50% of patients with severe aortic stenosis will have significant CAD, further influencing left ventricular function, symptoms, and morbidity.

Diagnosis

Symptoms can be exertional angina, syncope, or heart failure and may be precipitated by atrial arrhythmias such as atrial fibrillation. Symptoms may be absent in inactive older patients, may be subtle, or may not be elicited from patients with memory impairment. Physical findings of calcific aortic valve stenosis in older patients differ from those seen with young patients with biscuspid aortic valves or rheumatic aortic stenosis and do not accurately reflect the degree of stenosis. The age-related arterial changes of decreased compliance and increased stiffness mask the carotid artery findings associated with aortic stenosis in younger individuals. The carotid artery upstroke and peak may appear normal, and carotid amplitude may be unaltered or increased even in the presence of severe calcific stenosis. The presence of decreased carotid upstroke and volume (in the absence of carotid disease) usually indicates severe stenosis. Aortic sclerosis and aortic stenosis both produce systolic ejection murmurs, but the murmur of aortic stenosis is late peaking (links to audio examples are found on the website). The volume of the murmur depends on flow as well as the pressure gradient and does not reflect the severity of stenosis. A murmur may be absent in low-output states, reflecting severe aortic valve obstruction. The murmur may also be high pitched and musical as opposed to harsh and low frequency, and the second heart sound may be preserved. Hypertension is common in the elderly, making left ventricular hypertrophy on electrocardiography or ventricular enlargement on chest radiography similarly of little diagnostic help. Thus, Doppler echocardiography has become the clinical standard for diagnosis of aortic stenosis in the elderly. In the patient with low cardiac output (low flow), maneuvers to increase output (exercise or inotropes such as dobutamine) are helpful in quantifying stenosis. Catheterization is less commonly used to make the diagnosis, but coronary angiography is usually performed to evaluate CAD in older patients before valvular interventions.

Management

Management of the older patient with aortic stenosis (**Table 80-13**) is similar to that of younger patients, with recognition of the increased likelihood of concomitant coronary disease and diseases of other organs (see Chap. 66).[203,204] Risk factors should be treated. Neither U.S.

TABLE 80-13 Approach to the Older Patient with Suspected Valvular Disease

Physical examination cannot reliably assess the severity of valvular lesions in most older patients.
Doppler echocardiography is the clinical standard for diagnosis and evaluation of the severity of valve lesions.
- Differentiates sclerosis from stenosis
- Can assist in monitoring progression of stenosis
- Quantitates regurgitation
- Assesses calcification of valves and supporting structures

Age is a predictor of worse outcomes for the natural history of valvular lesions as well as for surgical approaches.
Surgery is definitive therapy for valvular lesions. Age, coronary artery disease, additional diseases, projected life span, and desired lifestyle are factors in evaluation of surgical options.

nor European guidelines recommend routine antibiotic prophylaxis before dental, gastrointestinal (GI), or genitourinary (GU) procedures except in patients at high risk of infection, defined as those with implanted devices or grafts, prior endocarditis, and congenital heart disease.[203,204] The guidelines note the lack of multicenter randomized trial data on the effects of antibiotic prophylaxis and that it may be reasonable to use antibiotic prophylaxis in individual patients. The authors of this chapter might consider this to include older patients with frequent infections with recurrent sepsis, those receiving chemotherapeutic agents with a lowered white blood cell count, or patients within 60 days of implantation of cardiac devices or non-cardiac bioprostheses as examples of patients for whom antibiotic prophylaxis might be considered. In addition to careful clinical monitoring of symptoms, reevaluation with transthoracic echocardiography is currently recommended every 3 to 5 years for patients with mild stenosis, every 1 to 2 years for patients with moderate stenosis, and more frequently in those with severe stenosis.[203] Monitoring for iron deficiency anemia should also be performed because of the acquired coagulopathy and bleeding from intestinal angiodysplasia that is being increasingly recognized in older patients with aortic stenosis. Although valvular calcification processes have similarities to atherosclerotic processes, randomized double-blind placebo-controlled trials have failed to demonstrate slowing of progression of calcific aortic stenosis with lipid-lowering agents.[205-207] Evidence to support the use of ACE inhibitors or ARBs to slow calcification or the use of the selective aldosterone receptor antagonist eplerenone to slow progression of aortic stenosis does not exist. Treatment of symptomatic and severe aortic stenosis requires valve replacement.

Surgical morbidity and mortality relate to the severity and duration of aortic stenosis, degree of left ventricular hypertrophy, presence or absence of heart failure or CAD, comorbidities (especially renal), urgency and complexity of the procedure, and age of the patient. Combined valve replacement and CABG is associated with higher perioperative morbidity and mortality than is isolated valve replacement. Estimates of average operative mortality for older patients who have undergone valve replacement with or without CABG have been reported as 6% for high surgery volume centers and 13% in low surgery volume centers.[208] Operative mortality for aortic valve replacement in patients 80 years and older is estimated at 8% to 15%.[209] Perioperative renal failure, pulmonary insufficiency, stroke, late cognitive impairment, and late death rates are higher than in younger individuals. Postoperative hospitalization and rehabilitation times are also usually longer in older patients (see Chap. 84).

Minimally invasive and percutaneous approaches to the aortic valve are currently under investigation, but this technology is still evolving.[209,209a] Aortic balloon valvotomy is not a substitute for surgery because mortality after aortic valvuloplasty is similar to that in patients with severe symptomatic aortic stenosis who do not undergo surgery. Procedural morbidity and mortality are high (>10%), and initial improvement is followed by rapid restenosis and recurrence of symptoms within months in most series.[203,204] A limited role for valvotomy as a bridge to valve surgery in hemodynamically unstable patients (cardiogenic shock), in patients undergoing emergent noncardiac surgery, and in patients with severe comorbidities who are too ill to undergo cardiac surgery has been supported by some.[210]

Appropriate selection of patients for aortic valve replacement includes assessment of the burden of disease in addition to the valve disease, anticipated life span independent of valve disease, and symptom status. Surgical risk assessment tools that incorporate comorbidities and clinical status as well as individual and combined procedures in calculations may be helpful[211-213] (online tools are available at *www.sts.org or www.euroscore.org*; *http://www.sts.org/sections/stsnationaldatabase/riskcalculator/*, and *http://www.euroscore.org/calc.html*). Although not specifically developed for older patients, they incorporate the major risk factors of New York Heart Association functional class, diabetes, hypertension, renal insufficiency, and low ejection fraction that were identified in a European report on outcomes of valve surgery in octogenarians.[208,214] Combined procedures (CABG or multiple valves) also have almost twofold greater risk than single-valve surgeries in older patients. The more comorbidities and the frailer the patient, and the more complicated the procedure, the more likely that perioperative mortality and postoperative morbidity[214a] will outweigh the benefit (see Chap. 84).

Biologic tissue valves are frequently implanted in elderly patients on the basis of factors including avoidance of chronic anticoagulation, longer bioprosthesis durability with older age, and shorter anticipated life expectancy (see Chap. 66). Estimated structural failure rates of current bioprosthetic valves are about 1% per patient-year in patients older than 65 years.

Asymptomatic older patients with aortic stenosis and their families should be educated on signs and symptoms related to aortic stenosis and observed regularly for development of symptoms and by Doppler echocardiography for changes in aortic valve area. Sudden death in asymptomatic patients with aortic stenosis occurs, but the frequency in prospective studies using echocardiography is estimated at less than 1%, much lower than previous estimates of 3% to 5% in retrospective studies. Operative mortality in older patients exceeds either of these rates. Thus, asymptomatic older patients with severe aortic stenosis are not usually recommended for surgical interventions.[203,204]

CURRENT CONTROVERSIES. Current controversies include the following: role of pharmacotherapy or biologicals in prevention of or slowing of aortic valve calcification; management and frequency of monitoring of asymptomatic older patients with aortic stenosis; potential biomarkers of progression of stenosis; relative risks, benefits, and methods of minimally invasive and percutaneous aortic valve replacement; duration and type of antithrombotic therapy after surgical implantation of a biologic valve; and indications for early valve replacement in asymptomatic elderly patients with very severe aortic stenosis.

Aortic Regurgitation

The prevalence of aortic regurgitation also increases with age. Mild aortic regurgitation was detected by Doppler echocardiography in 13% of patients older than 80 years and moderate or severe regurgitation in 16% in one series.[215] Causes of aortic regurgitation in the older patient include primary valvular disease (myxomatous or infective) or aortic root disease and dilation secondary to hypertension or dissection. Most often, significant aortic regurgitation in older patients is seen in combination with aortic stenosis.

Older age is a predictor of worse outcome for the natural history of aortic regurgitation. The life span of older patients with chronic severe aortic regurgitation who did not undergo valve replacement in the presurgical era was estimated at 2 years after onset of heart failure. When infective aortic regurgitation occurs in the elderly, the clinical manifestations may be insidious and nonspecific and symptoms fewer than in younger patients (see Chap. 67). Central nervous system symptoms are common and may predict a less favorable clinical outcome. Patients who have acute heart failure and pulmonary congestion as the manifestation of aortic valve endocarditis have a mortality rate of 50% to 80%.

Aortic regurgitation can be diagnosed by the classic diastolic murmur on physical examination. The finding of a widened pulse pressure usually associated with aortic regurgitation in younger patients is of limited diagnostic value in the older patient because age-related changes in the vasculature usually produce a widened pulse pressure in older people. Doppler echocardiography is the usual method of quantitation of the regurgitation and assessment of ventricular function. Patients older than 75 years are more likely to develop symptoms or left ventricular dysfunction at earlier stages of left ventricular dilation, have more persistent ventricular dysfunction and heart failure symptoms after surgery, and have worse postoperative survival rates than younger patients.

Mitral Annular Calcification

Mitral annular calcification is a chronic degenerative process that is age related and is seen more commonly in women than in men and in people older than 70 years (see Fig. 16-21). An increased prevalence of mitral annular calcification is seen in patients with systemic hypertension, increased mitral valve stress, mitral valve prolapse, elevated left ventricular systolic pressure, aortic valve stenosis, chronic renal failure, secondary hyperparathyroidism, atrial fibrillation, and aortic atherosclerosis. Like aortic valve calcification, mitral annular calcification is associated with risk factors for the development of atherosclerosis. Mitral annular calcification may produce mitral stenosis, mitral regurgitation, atrial arrhythmias, and AV conduction delay and predispose to infective endocarditis. It is an independent risk factor for systemic embolism and stroke, with the risk of stroke directly related to the degree of mitral annular calcification. It has also been identified as an independent risk factor for cardiovascular death in some series.

Mitral Stenosis

Increasing numbers of older patients now present with symptomatic mitral stenosis. Symptoms are the same as in the younger patient and include exertional dyspnea, orthopnea, paroxysmal nocturnal dyspnea, and pulmonary edema or right-sided heart failure. Atrial fibrillation is more common in older patients. Physical findings of calcific mitral stenosis differ from those of rheumatic mitral stenosis, and neither a loud first heart sound nor opening snap is usually heard. The characteristic diastolic rumbling murmur is usually present. Quantification of stenosis is usually accomplished by Doppler echocardiography. Older patients are more likely to have heavy calcification and fibrosis of the valve leaflets and subvalvular fusion, making them less likely than younger patients to benefit from percutaneous valvotomy. The success rate of valvotomy in older patients is less than 50%; procedural mortality rates approach 3%, and there are higher complication rates including pericardial tamponade in 5% and thromboembolism in 3%. Selected older patients with favorable valve morphology may be candidates for percutaneous approaches, but long-term clinical improvement is considerably less and mortality is higher in older than in younger patients. Mitral valve surgery also carries higher risks in the older patient. In the older patient with concomitant medical problems or pulmonary hypertension at systemic levels, perioperative mortality for surgical mitral valve replacement may be as high as 10% to 20% compared with 6% for the average patient. Decisions must be individualized, but surgical valvular replacement is usually the procedure of choice for the older patient without severe pulmonary hypertension and with a longer projected life span discounting the mitral stenosis.

Mitral Regurgitation

Myxomatous degeneration and functional mitral regurgitation from left ventricular dysfunction after MI as causes of mitral regurgitation in the older patient are increasing (see Chap. 66). Rheumatic mitral disease is declining, and endocarditis etiology is unchanged. Mitral regurgitation may also be seen in the setting of left ventricular dilation due to heart failure.

Acute mitral regurgitation presents with heart failure and pulmonary edema, but this may also be the initial presentation for medical care of the older patient with chronic mitral regurgitation. Chronic mitral regurgitation may be asymptomatic, especially in the sedentary patient. In symptomatic patients, initial complaints are usually easy fatigability and decreasing exercise tolerance because of low forward cardiac output followed by dyspnea on exertion, orthopnea, paroxysmal nocturnal dyspnea, and dyspnea at rest as the left ventricle function fails. Right-sided heart failure may also occur. Findings on examination are not altered by age, and a holosystolic murmur is usually present along with displacement of the left ventricular apical impulse and third heart sound or early diastolic flow rumble. Comprehensive two-dimensional transthoracic echocardiography with Doppler study is recommended to evaluate left ventricular size and function, right ventricular and left atrial size, pulmonary artery pressure, and severity of mitral regurgitation. Transesophageal echocardiography is used when transthoracic echocardiography is suboptimal. Surgical options are based on symptoms, valvular anatomy, left ventricular function, atrial fibrillation, pulmonary hypertension, and extent of comorbid diseases.[203,204] Transesophageal echocardiography is recommended in the evaluation of surgical candidates to assess feasibility and to guide repair. Cardiac catheterization is used when there is a discrepancy between symptoms and noninvasive findings and to evaluate CAD. Medical treatment of chronic mitral regurgitation is age independent and includes therapy for heart failure and management of atrial fibrillation. Older age is a risk factor for hospital mortality with isolated mitral valve surgery. Elderly patients with mitral regurgitation have less successful surgical outcomes than do older patients with aortic stenosis. The average operative mortality for mitral valve replacement in the elderly exceeds 14% in the United States and is above 20% in low-volume centers.[208] Risks are reduced somewhat if mitral repair rather than mitral valve replacement is performed but increased with the need for combined CABG surgery for CAD that is often present in older patients. Mitral valve repair is preferred to mitral valve replacement when possible in the older patient, and repair rates now equal (or exceed) replacement rates. Series reporting mitral valve repair results (alone and with CABG) estimate early death rates in patients older than 70 years of 5%-9%.[216,217] Survival after combined mitral valve replacement and CABG at 5 years may be as low as 50%. When valve repair is not possible, mitral valve replacement is primarily performed with tissue valves in patients older than 65 years.[203,204] Although there is increasing evidence to support early intervention in patients with mitral valve regurgitation, the increased surgical risks related to age, common co-morbid conditions, and the likelihood of concomitant coronary artery disease necessitating a combined procedure with high morbidity and mortality in the older patient are the basis for the current AHA/ACC guideline recommendation that under most circumstances asymptomatic elderly patients or patients with mild symptoms should be treated medically.

Additional Considerations in the Elderly

Drug-induced valve disease is uncommon but was recently associated with chronic therapy with ergot-derived dopamine agonists such as pergolide (and cabergoline) in older patients with Parkinson disease. Fibroproliferative lesions produced valvular insufficiency or regurgitation that necessitated valve replacement in some patients and ultimately resulted in removal of pergolide from the U.S. market. Valvular fibrotic changes have not been seen with non–ergot dopamine agonists used for Parkinson disease. Papillary muscle rupture occurs in 1% to 3% of patients with acute MI and is primarily a disease of the elderly. Surgical treatment is recommended, and in this setting, the outcome of combined CABG plus mitral valve surgery is the same as or better than that of mitral valve repair alone.

Future Directions

Increasing emphasis is being placed on preventive strategies for cardiovascular disease in older patients and improving the quality of care by current therapies that were not designed for the elderly. A major limitation is the lack of understanding of the mechanisms underlying many age-related cardiovascular changes or diseases and the marked differences between older patients enrolled in clinical trials and the much larger population of older patients presenting for care. Increased investigation at both the basic level and the clinical level is needed to identify therapies that will benefit older patients based on both the pathophysiology of age-related cardiovascular disease and the frequent presence of comorbid diseases. Caring for patients near the end of their lives is different from caring for patients with longer life expectancies. Research and training will be needed to achieve coordinated care for the older patient that must consider both medical and social factors to provide optimal care.

REFERENCES

Demographics, Epidemiology, and Pathophysiology

1. U.S. Census Bureau: Income 2001 (http://www.census.gov/hhes/income). Accessed July 15, 2003.
2. 2009 Alzheimer's Disease Facts and Figures (www.alz.org).
3. Alexander K, Newby L, Cannon C, et al: Acute coronary care in the elderly, part I: Non–ST-segment elevation acute coronary syndromes: A scientific statement for healthcare professionals from the American Heart Association Council on Clinical Cardiology: In collaboration with the Society of Geriatric Cardiology. Circulation 115:2549, 2007.
4. Alexander K, Newby L, Armstrong P, et al: Acute coronary care in the elderly, part II: ST-segment-elevation myocardial infarction: A scientific statement for healthcare professionals from the American Heart Association Council on Clinical Cardiology: In collaboration with the Society of Geriatric Cardiology. Circulation 115:2570, 2007.
5. Lakatta E: Arterial and cardiac aging: Major shareholders in cardiovascular disease enterprises: Part III: Cellular and molecular clues to heart and arterial aging. Circulation 107:490, 2003.
6. Lakatta E: Arterial and cardiac aging: Major shareholders in cardiovascular disease enterprises: Part II: The aging heart in health: links to heart disease. Circulation 107:346, 2003.
7. Lakatta E, Levy D: Arterial and cardiac aging: Major shareholders in cardiovascular disease enterprises: Part I: Aging arteries: A "set up" for vascular disease. Circulation 107:139, 2003.
8. O'Rourke M, Hashimoto J: Mechanical factors in arterial aging: A clinical perspective. J Am Coll Cardiol 50:1, 2007.
9. Lakatta E, Wang M, Najjar S: Arterial aging and subclinical arterial disease are fundamentally intertwined at macroscopic and molecular levels. Med Clin North Am 93:583, 2009.
10. Fontana L, Meyer T, Klein S, Holloszy J: Long-term calorie restriction is highly effective in reducing the risk for atherosclerosis in humans. Proc Natl Acad Sci U S A 101:6659, 2004.
11. Meyer TE, Kovacs SJ, Ehsani AA, et al: Long-term caloric restriction ameliorates the decline in diastolic function in humans. J Am Coll Cardiol 47:398, 2006.
12. Ornish D, Lin J, Daubenmier J, et al: Increased telomerase activity and comprehensive lifestyle changes: A pilot study. Lancet Oncol 9:1048, 2008.
13. Honarbakhsh S, Schachter M: Vitamins and cardiovascular disease. Br J Nutr 101:1113, 2009.

Medication Therapy

14. Anderson J, Adams C, Antman E , et al: ACC/AHA 2007 guidelines for the management of patients with unstable angina/non ST-elevation myocardial infarction: Executive Summary: A report of the American College of Cardiology/American Heart Association Task Force on Practice Guidelines (Writing Committee to revise the 2001 guidelines for the management of patients with unstable angina/non ST-elevation myocardial infarction): Developed in collaboration with the American College of Emergency Physicians, the Society for Cardiovascular Angiography and Interventions, the Society of Thoracic Surgeons: Endorsed by the American Association of Cardiovascular and Pulmonary Rehabilitation and the Society for Academic Emergency Medicine. Circulation 116:803, 2007.
15. Cockcroft DW, Gault MH: Prediction of creatinine clearance from serum creatinine. Nephron 16:31, 1976.
16. Stevens L, Coresh J, Greene T, Levey A: Assessing kidney function—measured and estimated glomerular filtration rate. N Engl J Med 354:2473, 2006.
17. Pequignot R, Belmin J, Chauvelier S, et al: Renal function in older hospital patients is more accurately estimated using the Cockcroft-Gault formula than the Modification Diet in Renal Disease formula. J Am Geriatr Soc 57:1638, 2009.
18. Alexander K, Chen A, Roe M, et al: Excess dosing of antiplatelet and antithrombin agents in the treatment of non–ST-segment elevation acute coronary syndromes. JAMA 294:3108, 2005.
19. Lansky A, Pietras C, Costa R, et al: Gender differences in outcomes after primary angioplasty versus primary stenting with and without abciximab for acute myocardial infarction: Results of the Controlled Abciximab and Device Investigation to Lower Late Angioplasty Complications (CADILLAC) trial. Circulation 111:1611, 2005.
20. Kirtane A, Piazza G, Murphy S, et al: Correlates of bleeding events among moderate- to high-risk patients undergoing percutaneous coronary intervention and treated with eptifibatide. Observations from the PROTECT–TIMI-30 Trial. J Am Coll Cardiol 47:2374, 2006.
21. Shlipak M, Wassel Fyr C, Chertow G, et al: Cystatin C and mortality risk in the elderly: The health, aging, and body composition study. J Am Soc Nephrol 17:254, 2006.
22. Ognibene A, Mannucci E, Caldini A, et al: Cystatin C reference values and aging. Clin Biochem 39:658, 2006.
23. Wasen E, Isoaho R, Mattila K, et al: Estimation of glomerular filtration rate in the elderly: A comparison of creatinine-based formulae with serum cystatin C. J Intern Med 256:70, 2004.
24. Grubb A, Bjork J, Lindstrom V, et al: A cystatin-C based formula without anthropometric variables estimates glomerular filtration rate better than creatinine clearance using the Cockcroft-Gault formula. Scand J Clin Lab Invest 65:153, 2005.
25. Shlipak M, Katz R, Kestenbaum B, et al: Rate of kidney function decline in older adults: A comparison using creatinine and cystatin C. Am J Nephrol 30:171, 2009.
26. Hanlon J, Aspinall S, Semla T, et al: Consensus guidelines for oral dosing of primarily renally cleared medications in older adults. J Am Geriatr Soc 57:335, 2009.
27. Schwartz J: The current state of knowledge on age, sex, and their interactions on clinical pharmacology. Clin Pharmacol Ther 82:87, 2007.
28. Schwartz J, Abernethy D: Aging and medications: Past, present, future. Clin Pharmacol Ther 85:3, 2009.
29. Marin F, Gonzalez-Conejero R, Capanzano P, et al: Pharmacogenetics in cardiovascular antithrombotic therapy. J Am Col Cardiol 54:1041, 2009.
30. Shuldiner A, O'Connell J, Bliden K, et al: Association of cytochrome P450 2C19 genotype with the antiplatelet effect and clinical efficacy of clopidogrel therapy. JAMA 302:849, 2009.
31. Kongkaew C, Noyce P, Ashcroft D: Hospital admissions associated with adverse drug reactions: A systematic review of prospective observational studies. Ann Pharmacother 42:1017, 2008.
32. Catananti C, Liperoti R, Settanni S, et al: Heart failure and adverse drug reactions among hospitalized older adults. Clin Pharmacol Ther 86:307, 2009.
33. Cresswell K, Fernando B, McKinstry B, Sheikh A: Adverse drug events in the elderly. Br Med Bull 83:259, 2007.
34. Ray W, Varas-Lorenzo C, Chung C, et al: Cardiovascular risks of nonsteroidal antiinflammatory drugs in patients after hospitalization for serious coronary heart disease. Circ Cardiovasc Qual Outcomes 2:155, 2009.
35. Gurwitz J, Field T, Judge J, et al: The incidence of adverse drug events in two large academic long-term care facilities. Am J Med 118:251, 2005.
36. Lau WC, Waskell LA, Watkins PB, et al: Atorvastatin reduces the ability of clopidogrel to inhibit platelet aggregation: A new drug-drug interaction. Circulation 2002:32, 2003.
37. De Smet P: Herbal remedies. N Engl J Med 347:2046, 2002.
38. Juurlink D, Mamdani M, Kopp A, et al: Drug-drug interactions among elderly patients hospitalized for drug toxicity. JAMA 289:1652, 2003.
39. Barry P, Gallagher P, Ryan C, O'Mahony D: START (screening tool to alert doctors to the right treatment)—an evidence-based screening tool to detect prescribing omissions in elderly patients. Age Ageing 36:632, 2007.
40. Gallagher P, O'Mahony D: STOPP (Screening Tool of Older Persons' potentially inappropriate Prescriptions): Application to acutely ill elderly patients and comparison with Beers' criteria. Age Ageing 37:673, 2008.
41. Briesacher B, Limcangco R, Simoni-Wastila L, et al: Evaluation of nationally mandated drug use reviews to improve patient safety in nursing homes: A natural experiment. J Am Geriatr Soc 53:991, 2005.
42. Juurlink D, Mamdani M, Lee D, et al: Rates of hyperkalemia after publication of the Randomized Aldactone Evaluation Study. N Engl J Med 351:543, 2004.
43. McGuire D, Inzucchi S: New drugs for the treatment of diabetes mellitus. Circulation 117:440, 2008.
44. A comparison of letrozole and tamoxifen in postmenopausal women with early breast cancer. The Breast International Group (BIG) 1-98 Collaborative Group. N Engl J Med 353:2747, 2005.
45. Fick D, Cooper J, Wade W, et al: Updating the Beers criteria for potentially inappropriate medication use in older adults: Results of a US consensus panel of experts. Arch Intern Med 163:2716, 2003.
46. Simon S, Chan K, Soumerai S, et al: Potentially inappropriate medication use by elderly persons in U.S. Health Maintenance Organizations, 2000-2001. J Am Geriatr Soc 53:227, 2005.
47. Rochon P, Lane C, Bronskill S, et al: Potentially inappropriate prescribing in Canada relative to the US. Drugs Aging 21:939, 2004.
48. Curtis L, Ostbye T, Sendersky V, et al: Inappropriate prescribing for elderly Americans in a large outpatient population. Arch Intern Med 164:1621, 2004.
49. Lin O, Kozarek R, Schembre D, et al: Screening colonoscopy in very elderly patients. JAMA 295:2357, 2006.
50. Lee S, Lindquist K, Segal M, Covinsky K: Development and validation of a prognostic index for 4-year mortality in older adults. JAMA 295:801, 2006.
51. Walter L, Lewis C, Barton M: Screening for colorectal, breast, and cervical cancer in the elderly: A review of the evidence. Am J Med 118:1078, 2005.
52. O'Connor P: Adding value to evidence-based clinical guidelines. JAMA 294:741, 2005.
53. Horne B, May H, Muhlestein J, et al: Exceptional mortality prediction by risk scores from common laboratory tests. Am J Med 122:550, 2009.
54. Doshi JA, Zhu J, Lee BY, et al: Impact of a prescription copayment increase on lipid-lowering medication adherence in veterans. Circulation 119:390, 2009.
55. Madden J, Graves A, Zhang F, et al: Cost-related medication nonadherence and spending on basic needs following implementation of Medicare Part D. JAMA 299:1922, 2008.
56. Lloyd-Jones D, Evans J, Levy D: Hypertension in adults across the age spectrum. Current outcomes and control in the community. JAMA 294:466, 2005.

Hypertension

57. Calhoun D, Jones D, Textor S, et al: Resistant hypertension: Diagnosis, evaluation, and treatment. A scientific statement from the American Heart Association Professional Education Committee of the Council for High Blood Pressure Research. Hypertension 51:1403, 2008.
58. Beckett NS, Peters R, Fletcher AE, et al: Treatment of hypertension in patients 80 years of age or older. N Engl J Med 358:1887, 2008.
59. Mendu M, McAvay G, Lampert R, et al: Yield of diagnostic tests in evaluating syncopal episodes in older patients. Arch Intern Med 169:1299, 2009.
60. Lacroix A, Ott S, Ichikawa L, et al: Low-dose hydrochlorothiazide and preservation of bone mineral density in older adults. A randomized double-blind, placebo-controlled trial. Ann Intern Med 133:516, 2000.
61. Bolland M, Ames R, Horne A, et al: The effect of treatment with a thiazide diuretic for 4 years on bone density in normal postmenopausal women. Osteoporos Int 18:479, 2007.
62. Chodosh J, Morton S, Mojica W, et al: Meta-analysis: Chronic disease self-management programs for older adults. Ann Intern Med 143:427, 2005.
63. Roumie C, Elasy T, Greevy R, et al: Improving blood pressure control through provider education, provider alerts, and patient education. A cluster randomized trial. Ann Intern Med 145:165, 2006.
64. Chobanian AV, Bakris GL, Black HR, et al: The Seventh Report of the Joint National Committee on Prevention, Detection, Evaluation, and Treatment of High Blood Pressure. The JNC 7 Report. JAMA 289:2560, 2003.
65. Mancia G, De Backer G, Dominiczak A, et al: 2007 Guidelines for the management of arterial hypertension. The Task Force for the Management of Arterial Hypertension of the European Society of Hypertension (ESH) and of the European Society of Cardiology (ESC). Eur Heart J 28:1462, 2007.

66. Izzedine H, Ederhy S, Goldwasser F, et al: Management of hypertension in angiogenesis inhibitor-treated patients [review]. Ann Oncol 20:807, 2009.

Coronary Artery Disease

67. Daly C, Clemens F, Sendon JLL, et al: Gender differences in the management and clinical outcome of stable angina. Circulation 113:490, 2006.
68. Vaccarino V, Rathore S, Wenger N, et al: Sex and racial differences in the management of acute myocardial infarction, 1994 through 2002. N Engl J Med 353:671, 2005.
69. Anand S, Xie C, Mehta SR, et al: Differences in the management and prognosis of women and men who suffer from acute coronary syndromes. J Am Coll Cardiol 46:1845, 2005.
70. Blomkalns A, Chen A, Hochman J, et al: Gender disparities in the diagnosis and treatment of non–ST-segment elevation acute coronary syndromes: Large-scale observations from the CRUSADE (Can Rapid Risk Stratification of Unstable Angina Patients Suppress Adverse Outcomes With Early Implementation of the American College of Cardiology/American Heart Association Guidelines) National Quality Improvement Inititiative. J Am Coll Cardiol 45:832, 2005.
71. Psaty B, Anderson M, Kronmal R, et al: The association between lipid levels and the risks of incident myocardial infarction, stroke, and total mortality: The Cardiovascular Health Study. J Am Geriatr Soc 52:1639, 2004.
72. Stork S, Feelders R, van den Beld A, et al: Prediction of mortality risk in the elderly. Am J Med 119:519, 2006.
73. Mattace-Raso F, van der Cammen T, Hofman A, et al: Arterial stiffness and risk of coronary heart disease and stroke. The Rotterdam Study. Circulation 113:657, 2006.
74. Hansen T, Staessen J, Torp-Pederson C, et al: Prognostic value of aortic pulse wave velocity as index of arterial stiffness in the general population. Circulation 113:664, 2006.
75. Cao J, Biggs M, Barzilay J, et al: Cardiovascular and mortality risk prediction and stratification using urinary albumin excretion in older adults ages 68-102: The Cardiovascular Health Study. Atherosclerosis 197:806, 2008.
76. Mieres J, Shaw L, Arai A, et al: Role of noninvasive testing in the clinical evaluation of women with suspected coronary artery disease: Consensus statement from the Cardiac Imaging Committee, Council on Clinical Cardiology, and the Cardiovascular Imaging and Intervention Committee, Council on Cardiovascular Radiology and Intervention, American Heart Association. Circulation 111:682, 2005.
77. Redberg R: Coronary artery calcium: Should we rely on this surrogate marker? Circulation 113:336, 2006.
78. Bielak LF, Yu PF, Ryan KA, et al: Differences in prevalence and severity of coronary artery calcification between two non-Hispanic white populations with diverse lifestyles. Atherosclerosis 196:888, 2008.
79. Fraker TD Jr, Fihn SD, Gibbons RJ, et al: 2007 Chronic angina focused update of the ACC/AHA 2002 guidelines for the management of patients with chronic stable angina: A report of the American College of Cardiology/American Heart Association Task Force on Practice Guidelines Writing Group to develop the focused update of the 2002 Guidelines for the management of patients with chronic stable angina. Circulation 116:2762, 2007.
80. Boden W, O'Rourke R, Teo K, et al: Optimal medical therapy with or without PCI for stable coronary artery disease. N Engl J Med 356:1503, 2007.
81. The BARI 2D Study Group: A randomized trial of therapies for type 2 diabetes and coronary artery disease. N Engl J Med 360:2503, 2009.
82. Gasparyan A, Watson T, Lip G: The role of aspirin in cardiovascular prevention. J Am Coll Cardiol 51:1829, 2009.
83. LaRosa J, Grundy S, Waters D, et al: Intensive lipid lowering with atorvastatin in patients with stable coronary disease. N Engl J Med 352:1425, 2005.
84. Bruckert E, Hayem G, Dejager S, et al: Mild to moderate muscular symptoms with high-dosage statin therapy in hyperlipidemic patients—the PRIMO Study. Cardiovasc Drugs Ther 19:403, 2005.
85. Antons K, Williams C, Baker S, Phillips P: Clinical perspectives of statin-induced rhabdomyolysis. Am J Med 119:400, 2006.
86. Ouyang P, Michos E, Karas R: Hormone replacement therapy and the cardiovascular system: Lessons learned and unanswered questions. J Am Coll Cardiol 47:1741, 2006.
87. Chaitman B: Ranolazine for the treatment of chronic angina and potential use in other cardiovascular conditions. Circulation 113:2462, 2006.
88. Dunlay S, Rihal C, Sundt T, et al: Current trends in coronary revascularization. Curr Treat Options Cardiovasc Med 11:61, 2009.
89. Bridges C, Edwards F, Peterson E, et al: Cardiac surgery in nonagenarians and centenarians. J Am Coll Surg 197:347, 2003.
90. Singh M, Peterson E, Milford-Beland S, et al: Validation of the Mayo Clinic Risk Score for in-hospital mortality after percutaneous coronary interventions using the National Cardiovascular Data Registry. Circ Cardiovasc Interv 1:36, 2008.
91. Dacey L, Likosky D, Ryan T, et al: Long-term survival in octogenarians with multivessel coronary disease after surgery versus percutaneous intervention. Ann Thorac Surg 84:1904, 2007.
92. Hannan E, Racz M, Walford G, et al: Long-term outcomes of coronary-artery bypass grafting versus stent implantation. N Engl J Med. 325:2174, 2005.
93. Forman D, Cox D, Ellis S, et al: Long-term paclitaxel-eluting stent outcomes in elderly patients. Circ Cardiovasc Interv 2:178, 2009.
94. Hannan E, Wu C, Walford G, et al: Drug-eluting stents vs coronary artery bypass grafting in multivessel coronary disease. N Engl J Med 358:331, 2008.
95. King S, Smith S, Hirshfeld J, et al: 2007 Focused Update of the ACC/AHA/SCAI 2005 Guideline update for percutaneous coronary intervention: A report of the American College of Cardiology/American Heart Association Task Force on Practice Guidelines: 2007 Writing Group to review new evidence and update the ACC/AHA/SCAI 2005 Guideline Update for Percutaneous Coronary Intervention, Writing on behalf of the 2005 Writing Committee. Circulation 117:261, 2008.
96. Panesar S, Athanasious T, Nair S, et al: Early outcomes in the elderly: A meta-analysis of 4921 patients undergoing coronary artery bypass grafting—a comparison between off-pump and on-pump techniques. Heart 12:1808, 2006.
97. Pfisterer M, Buser P, Osswald S, et al: Outcome of elderly patients with chronic symptomatic coronary artery disease with an invasive vs. optimized medical treatment strategy: One-year results of the randomized TIME trial. JAMA 289:1117, 2003.
98. Antman E, Hand M, Armstrong P, et al: 2007 Focused Update of the ACC/AHA 2004 Guidelines for the Management of Patients With ST-Elevation Myocardial Infarction: A report of the American College of Cardiology/American Heart Association Task Force on Practice Guidelines: Developed in collaboration With the Canadian Cardiovascular Society endorsed by the American Academy of Family Physicians: 2007 Writing Group to Review New Evidence and Update the ACC/AHA 2004 Guidelines for the Management of Patients With ST-Elevation Myocardial Infarction, Writing on Behalf of the 2004 Writing Committee. Circulation 117:296, 2008.
99. Anderson J, Adams C, Antman E, et al: ACC/AHA 2007 guidelines for the management of patients with unstable angina/non–ST-elevation myocardial infarction: A report of the American College of Cardiology/American Heart Association Task Force on Practice Guidelines (Writing Committee to Revise the 2002 Guidelines for the Management of Patients With Unstable Angina/Non–ST-Elevation Myocardial Infarction) developed in collaboration with the American College of Emergency Physicians, the Society for Cardiovascular Angiography and Interventions, and the Society of Thoracic Surgeons endorsed by the American Association of Cardiovascular and Pulmonary Rehabilitation and the Society for Academic Emergency Medicine. J Am Coll Cardiol 50:e1, 2007.
100. Mehta R, Granger C, Alexander K, et al: Reperfusion strategies for acute myocardial infarction in the elderly. State of the art paper. J Am Coll Cardiol 45:471, 2005.
101. Alexander K, Roe M, Kulkarni S, et al: Evolution of cardiovascular care for elderly patients with non–ST-segment elevation acute coronary syndromes. Results from CRUSADE. J Am Coll Cardiol 46:1490, 2005.
102. Alexander K, Chen A, Newby L, et al: Sex differences in major bleeding with glycoprotein IIb/IIIa inhibitors: Results from CRUSADE. Circulation 114:1380, 2006.
103. Sixon S, Grines C, O'Neill W: The year in interventional cardiology. J Am Coll Cardiol 47:1689, 2006.
104. Giugliano RP, White JA, Bode C, et al: Early versus delayed, provisional eptifibatide in acute coronary syndromes. N Engl J Med 360:2176, 2009.
105. Grines C: Senior PAMI Trial. 2002.
106. Bardají A, Bueno H, Fernández-Ortiz A, et al: Type of treatment and short-term outcome in elderly patients with acute myocardial infarction admitted to hospitals with a primary coronary angioplasty facility. The TRIANA (TRatamiento del Infarto Agudo de miocardio eN Ancianos) Registry. Rev Esp Cardiol 58:351, 2005).
107. Hochman J, Sleeper L, Webb J, et al: Early revascularization and long-term survival in cardiogenic shock complicating acute myocardial infarction. JAMA 295:2511, 2006.
108. Mehta S, Granger C, Boden W, et al: Early versus delayed invasive intervention in acute coronary syndromes. N Engl J Med 360:2165, 2009.
109. Montalescot G, Cayla G, Collet JP, et al: Immediate vs. delayed intervention for acute coronary syndromes: A randomized clinical trial. JAMA 302:947, 2009.
110. Krumholz H, Wang Y, Chen J, et al: Reduction in acute myocardial infarction mortality in the United States. Risk-standardized mortality rates from 1995-2006. JAMA 302:767, 2009.
111. Pitt B, Remme W, Zannad F, et al: Eplerenone, a selective aldosterone blocker, in patients with left ventricular dysfunction after myocardial infarction. N Engl J Med 348:1309, 2003.
112. Sabatine M, Cannon C, Gibson C, et al: Addition of clopidogrel to aspirin and fibrinolytic therapy for myocardial infarction with ST-segment elevation. N Engl J Med 352:1179, 2005.
113. Thombs B, Bass E, Ford D, et al: Prevalence of depression in survivors of acute myocardial infarction. J Gen Intern Med 21:30, 2006.
114. Bush D, Ziegelstein R, Patel U, et al: Post–Myocardial Infarction Depression. Evidence Report/ Technology Assessment No. 123. (Prepared by the Johns Hopkins University Evidence-based Practice Center under Contract No. 290-02-0018). Rockville, Md, Agency for Healthcare Research and Quality, 2005. AHRQ publication No. 05-E018-2.
115. Whooley M: Depression and cardiovascular disease. JAMA 296:2874, 2006.
116. Serebruany VL: Selective serotonin reuptake inhibitors and increased bleeding risk: Are we missing something? Am J Med 119:113, 2006.
117. Hulley S, Grady D: Postmenopausal hormone treatment. JAMA 301:2493, 2009.
118. Barrett-Connor E, Mosca L, Collins et al: Effects of raloxifene on cardiovascular events and breast cancer in postmenopausal women. N Engl J Med 355:125, 2006.
119. Vogel V, Costantino J, Wickerham D, et al, National Surgical Adjuvant Breast and Bowel Project (NSABP): Effects of tamoxifen vs raloxifene on the risk of developing invasive breast cancer and other disease outcomes: The NSABP Study of Tamoxifen and Raloxifene (STAR) P-2 trial. JAMA 295:2727, 2006.
120. Marchionni N, Fattirolli F, Fumagalli S, et al: Improved exercise tolerance and quality of life with cardiac rehabilitation of older patients after myocardial infarction. Results of a randomized, controlled trial. Circulation 107:2201, 2003.

Carotid Artery Disease and Stroke

121. Goldstein L, Adams R, Alberts M, et al: Primary prevention of ischemic stroke: A guideline from the American Heart Association/American Stroke Association Stroke Council: Cosponsored by the Atherosclerotic Peripheral Vascular Disease Interdisciplinary Working Group; Cardiovascular Nursing Council; Clinical Cardiology Council; Nutrition, Physical Activity, and Metabolism Council; and the Quality of Care and Outcomes Research Interdisciplinary Working Group. Circulation 113:e873, 2006.
122. Easton J, Saver J, Albers G, et al: Definition and evaluation of transient ischemic attack: A Scientific Statement for healthcare professionals from the American Heart Association/ American Stroke Association Stroke Council, Council on Cardiovascular Surgery and Anesthesia; Council on Cardiovascular Radiology and Intervention; Council on Cardiovascular Nursing; and the Interdisciplinary Council on Peripheral Vascular Disease. The American Academy of Neurology affirms the value of this statement as an educational tool for neurologists. Stroke 40:2276, 2009.
123. Adams H, Del Zoppo G, Alberts M, et al: Guidelines for the Early Management of Adults With Ischemic Stroke: A guideline from the American Heart Association/American Stroke Association Stroke Council, Clinical Cardiology Council, Cardiovascular Radiology and Intervention Council and the Atherosclerotic Peripheral Vascular Disease and Quality of Care Outcomes in Research Interdisciplinary Working Groups. Stroke 38:1655, 2007.
124. Alberts M, Felberg R, Guterman L, Levine S: Atherosclerotic Peripheral Vascular Disease Symposium II. Stroke intervention: State of the art. Circulation 118:2845, 2008.

125. Del Zoppo G, Saver J, Jauch E, Adams H: Expansion of the time window for treatment of acute ischemic stroke with intravenous tissue plasminogen activator: A science advisory from the American Heart Association Stroke Council. Stroke 40:2945, 2009.
126. Bates B, Choi J, Duncan P, et al: Veterans Affairs/Department of Defense clinical practice guideline for the management of adult stroke rehabilitation care. Executive summary. Circulation 36:2049, 2005.
127. Sacco R, Adams R, Alberts M, et al: Guidelines for prevention of stroke in patients with ischemic stroke or transient ischemic attack. A statement for healthcare professionals from the American Heart Association/American Stroke Association Council on Stroke: Co-sponsored by the Council on Cardiovascular Radiology and Intervention: The American Academy of Nerurology affirms the value of this guideline. Circulation 113:e409, 2006.
128. ESPRIT Study Group: Aspirin plus dipyridamole versus aspirin alone after cerebral ischaemia of arterial origin (ESPRIT): Randomised controlled trial. Lancet 367:1665, 2006.
129. Adams R, Albers G, Alberts M, et al: Update to the AHA/ASA recommendations for the prevention of stroke in patients with stroke and transient ischemic attack. Stroke 39:1647, 2008.
130. CAPRIE Steering Committee: A randomised, blinded, trial of clopidogrel versus aspirin in patients at risk of ischaemic events (CAPRIE). Lancet 348:1329, 1996.
131. Sacco R, Diener H-C, Yusuf S, et al: Aspirin and extended-release dipyridamole versus clopidogrel for recurrent stroke. N Engl J Med 359:1238, 2008.
132. Mohr J, Thompson J, Lazar R, et al: A comparison of warfarin and aspirin for the prevention of recurrent ischemic stroke. N Engl J Med 345:1444, 2001.
133. Antiplatelet Trialists' Collaboration: Collaborative meta-analysis of randomised trials of antiplatelet therapy for prevention of death, myocardial infarction and stroke in high risk patients. BMJ 324:71, 2002.
134. Barnett H, Meldrum H, Eliasziw M: The appropriate use of carotid endarterectomy. CMAJ 166:1169, 2002.
135. Gurm HS, Yadav JS, Fayad P, et al: Long-term results of carotid stenting versus endarterectomy in high-risk patients. N Engl J Med 358:1572, 2008.
136. Mas J-L, Chatellier G, Beyssen B, et al: Endarterectomy vs. stenting in patients with symptomatic severe carotid stenosis. N Engl J Med 355:1660, 2006.
137. Hobson R, Howard V, Roubin G, et al: Carotid stenting is associated with increased complications in octogenarians: 30 day stroke and death rates in the CREST lead-in phase. J Vasc Surg 40:1106, 2004.
138. White C, Beckman J, Cambria R, et al, American Heart Association Writing Group 5: Atherosclerotic Peripheral Vascular Disease Symposium II. Controversies in carotid artery revascularization. Circulation 118:2852, 2008.
139. Massop D, Dave R, Metzger C, et al, SAPPHIRE Worldwide Investigators: Stenting and angioplasty with protection in patients at high-risk for endarterectomy: SAPPHIRE Worldwide Registry first 2,001 patients. Catheter Cardiovasc Interv 73:129, 2009.

Peripheral Arterial Disease

140. Hirsh A, Haskal Z, Hertzer N, et al: ACC/AHA 2005 Practice Guidelines for the management of patients with peripheral arterial disease (lower extremity, renal, mesenteric, and abdominal aortic): Executive Summary: A collaborative report from the American Association for Vascular Surgery/Society for Vascular Surgery, Society for Cardiovascular Angiography and Interventions, Society for Vascular Medicine and Biology, Society of Interventional Radiology, and the ACC/AHA Task Force on Practice Guidelines (Writing Committee to Develop Guidelines for the Management of Patients with Peripheral Arterial Disease). Circulation 113:1474, 2006.
141. Hankey G, Norman P, Eikelboom J: Medical treatment of peripheral artery disease. JAMA 295:547, 2006.
142. Norgren L, Hiatt W, Dormandy J, et al: Inter-Society Consensus for the Management of Peripheral Arterial Disease (TASC II). J Vasc Surg 45(Suppl 1):S5, 2007.
143. Berger JK, Krantz MJ, Kittelson J, Hiatt W: Aspirin for the prevention of cardiovascular events in patients with peripheral artery disease. A meta-analysis of randomized trials. JAMA 301:1909, 2009.
144. McDermott M, Criqui M: Aspirin and secondary prevention in peripheral artery disease. A perspective for the early 21st century. JAMA 301:1927, 2009.
145. The Warfarin Antiplatelet Vascular Evaluation Trial Investigators: Oral anticoagulant and antiplatelet therapy and peripheral arterial disease. N Engl J Med 357:217, 2007.
146. Gray B, Conte M, Dake M, et al: Atherosclerotic Peripheral Vascular Disease Symposium II. Lower extremity revascularization: State of the art. Circulation 118:2864, 2008.

Heart Failure

147. Gottdiener J, Arnold A, Aurigemma G, et al: Predictors of congestive heart failure in the elderly: The Cardiovascular Health Study. J Am Coll Cardiol 35:1628, 2000.
148. Solomon S, Anavekar N, Skali H, et al: Influence of ejection fraction on cardiovascular outcomes in a broad spectrum of heart failure patients. Circulation 112:3738, 2005.
149. Lee D, Gona P, Vasan R, et al: Relation of disease pathogenesis and risk factors to heart failure with preserved or reduced ejection fraction. Insights from the Framingham Heart Study of the National Heart, Lung, and Blood Institute. Circulation 119:3070, 2009.
150. Hernandez A, Hammill B, O'Connor C, et al: Clinical effectiveness of beta-blockers in heart failure. Findings from the OPTIMIZE-HF (Organized Program to Initiate Lifesaving Treatment in Hospitalized Patients with Heart Failure) Registry. J Am Coll Cardiol 53:184, 2009.
151. Roger VL, Weston S, Redfield M, et al: Trends in heart failure incidence and survival in a community-based population. JAMA 292:344, 2004.
152. Barker W, Mullooly J, Getchell W: Changing incidence and survival for heart failure in a well-defined older population, 1970-1974 and 1990-1994. Circulation 113:799, 2006.
153. Maeder M, Kaye D: Heart failure with normal left ventricular ejection fraction. J Am Coll Cardiol 53:905, 2009.
154. Maurer M, King D, Rumbarger E, et al: Left heart failure with a normal ejection fraction: Identification of different pathophysiologic mechanisms. J Card Fail 11:177, 2005.
155. van Heerebeek L, Borbely A, Niessen H, et al: Myocardial structure and function differ in systolic and diastolic heart failure. Circulation 113:1966, 2006.
156. Redfield M, Jacobsen S, Burnett J, et al: Burden of systolic and diastolic ventricular dysfunction in the community: Appreciating the scope of the heart failure epidemic. JAMA 289:194, 2003.
157. Jessup M, Abraham W, Casey D, et al: 2009 Focused update: ACCF/AHA guidelines for the diagnosis and management of heart failure in adults: A report of the American College of Cardiology Foundation/American Heart Association Task Force on Practice Guidelines. Circulation 119:1977, 2009.
158. Hunt S, Abraham W, Chin M, et al: ACC/AHA 2005 Guideline update for the diagnosis and management of chronic heart failure in the adult. Circulation 112:e154, 2005.
159. Adams K, Lindenfeld J, Arnold J, et al: Executive Summary: HFSA 2006 Comprehensive Heart Failure Practice Guideline. J Card Fail 12:10, 2006.
160. Dickstein K, Cohen-Solal A, Filippatos G, et al: ESC guidelines for the diagnosis and treatment of acute and chronic heart failure 2008: The Task Force for the diagnosis and treatment of acute and chronic heart failure 2008 of the European Society of Cardiology. Developed in collaboration with the Heart Failure Association of the ESC (HFA) and endorsed by the European Society of Intensive Care Medicine (ESICM). Eur J Heart Fail 10:933, 2008.
161. Ahmed A, Waagstein F, Pitt B, et al: Effectiveness of digoxin in reducing one-year mortality in chronic heart failure in the Digitalis Investigation Group trial. Am J Cardiol 103:82, 2009.
162. Ahmed A, Rich M, Fleg J, et al: Effects of digoxin on morbidity and mortality in diastolic heart failure: The ancillary digitalis investigation group trial. Circulation 114:397, 2006.
163. Garg R, Yusuf S: Overview of randomized trials of angiotensin converting enzyme inhibitors on mortality and morbidity in patients with heart failure. JAMA 273:1450, 1995.
164. Flather M, Yusuf S, Kober L, et al: Long-term ACE-inhibitor therapy in patients with heart failure or left-ventricular dysfunction: A systematic overview of data from individual patients. Lancet 355:1575, 2000.
165. Dahlöf B, Devereux RB, Kjeldsen SE, et al: Cardiovascular morbidity and mortality in the Losartan Intervention For Endpoint reduction in hypertension study (LIFE): A randomised trial against atenolol. Lancet 359:995, 2002.
166. Blood Pressure Lowering Treatment Trialists' Collaboration: Effects of different blood-pressure-lowering regimens on major cardiovascular events: Results of prospectively-designed overviews of randomised trials. Lancet 362:1527, 2003.
167. Blood Pressure Lowering Treatment Trialists' Collaboration: Effects of different blood pressure–lowering regimens on major cardiovascular events in individuals with and without diabetes mellitus: Results of prospectively designed overviews of randomized trials. Arch Intern Med 165:1410, 2005.
168. Cohen-Solal A, McMurray J, Swedberg K, et al: Benefits and safety of candesartan treatment in heart failure are independent of age: Insights from the Candesartan in Heart failure–Assessment of Reduction in Mortality and morbidity programme. Eur Heart J 29:3022, 2008.
169. Simon T, Mary-Krause M, Funck-Brentano C, et al: Bisoprolol dose-response relationship in patients with congestive heart failure: A subgroup analysis in the cardiac insufficiency bisoprolol study (CIBIS II). Eur Heart J 24:552, 2003.
170. Flather M, Shibata M, Coats A, et al: Randomized trial to determine the effect of nebivolol on mortality and cardiovascular hospital admission in elderly patients with heart failure (SENIORS). Eur Heart J 26:215, 2005.
171. Ghio S, Magrini G, Serio A, et al, SENIORS Investigators: Effects of nebivolol in elderly heart failure patients with or without systolic left ventricular dysfunction: Results of the SENIORS echocardiographic substudy. Eur Heart J 27:562, 2006.
172. O'Connor C, Whellan D, Lee K, et al: Efficacy and safety of exercise training in patients with chronic heart failure: HF-ACTION Randomized Controlled Trial. JAMA 301:1439, 2009.
173. Flynn K, Pina I, Whellan D, et al: Effects of exercise training on health status in patients with chronic heart failure: HF-ACTION Randomized Controlled Trial. JAMA 301:1451, 2009.
174. Yusuf S, Pfeffer M, Swedberg K, et al: Effects of candesartan in patients with chronic heart failure and preserved left-ventricular ejection fraction: The CHARM-Preserved trial. Lancet 362:777, 2003.
175. Cleland J, Tendera M, Adamus J, et al: The perindopril in elderly people with chronic heart failure (PEP-CHF) study. Eur Heart J 27:2338, 2006.
176. The Digoxin Investigators Group: The effect of digoxin on mortality and morbidity in patients with heart failure. N Engl J Med 336:525, 1997.
177. Pfisterer M, Buser P, Rickli H, et al: BNP-guided vs. symptom-guided heart failure therapy. The Trial of Intensified vs. Standard Medical Therapy in Elderly Patients with Congestive Heart Failure (TIME-CHF) Randomized Trial. JAMA 301:383, 2009.
178. Whellan D, Vic Hasselblad V, Peterson E, et al: Metaanalysis and review of heart failure disease management randomized controlled clinical trials. Am Heart J 149:722, 2005.
179. Sochalski J, Jaarsma T, Krumholz H, et al: What works in chronic care management: The case of heart failure. Health Aff (Millwood) 28:179, 2009.
180. Nichol K, Nordin J, Mullooly J, et al: Influenza vaccination and reduction in hospitalizations for cardiac disease and stroke among the elderly. N Engl J Med 348:1322, 2003.
181. Pantilat S, Steimle A: Palliative care for patients with heart failure. JAMA 291:2476, 2004.

Arrhythmias

182. Jones S, Boyett M, Lancaster M: Declining into failure. The age-dependent loss of the L-type calcium channel within the sinoatrial node. Circulation 115:1183, 2007.
183. Healey J, Toff W, Lamas G, et al: Cardiovascular outcomes with atrial-based pacing compared with ventricular pacing: Meta-analysis of randomized trials, using individual patient data. Circulation 114:11, 2006.
184. Kaszala K, Kalahasty G, Ellenbogen K: Cardiac pacing in the elderly. Am J Geriatr Cardiol 15:77, 2006.
185. Martinez C, Tzur A, Hrachian H, et al: Pacemakers and defibrillators: Recent and ongoing studies that impact the elderly. Am J Geriatr Cardiol 15:82, 2006.
186. Fuster V, Rydén L, Cannom D, et al: ACC/AHA/ESC 2006 Guidelines for the Management of Patients with Atrial Fibrillation: A report of the American College of Cardiology/American Heart Association Task Force on Practice Guidelines and the European Heart Society of Cardiology Committee for Practice Guidelines (Writing Committee to Revise the 2001 Guidelines for the Management of Patients with Atrial Fibrillation). J Am Coll Cardiol 48:e149, 2006.
187. Caraballo P, Heit J, Atkinson E, et al: Long-term use of oral anticoagulants and the risk of fracture. Arch Intern Med 159:1750, 1999.
188. The ACTIVE Investigators: Effect of clopidogrel added to aspirin in patients with atrial fibrillation. N Engl J Med 360:2066, 2009.
189. Connolly S, Ezekowitz M, Yusuf S, et al: Dabigatran versus warfarin in patients with atrial fibrillation. N Engl J Med 361:1139, 2009.

190. Wyse D, Waldo A, DiMarco J, et al: A comparison of rate control and rhythm control in patients with atrial fibrillation. N Engl J Med 347:1825, 2002.
191. Van Gelder I, Hagens V, Bosker H, et al: A comparison of rate control and rhythm control in patients with recurrent persistent atrial fibrillation. N Engl J Med 347:1834, 2002.
192. Carlsson J, Miketic S, Windeler J, et al: Randomized trial of rate-control versus rhythm-control in persistent atrial fibrillation: The strategies of treatment of atrial fibrillation (STAF) study. J Am Coll Cardiol 41:1690, 2003.
193. Opolski G, Torbicki A, Kosior D, et al: Rate control vs rhythm control in patients with nonvalvular persistent atrial fibrillation: The results of the Polish How to Treat Chronic Atrial Fibrillation (HOT CAFE) Study. Chest 126:476, 2004.
194. de Denus S, Sanoski C, Carlsson J, et al: Rate vs. rhythm control in patients with atrial fibrillation: A meta-analysis. Arch Intern Med 165:258, 2005.
195. Roy D, Talajic M, Nattel S, et al: Rhythm control versus rate control for atrial fibrillation and heart failure. N Engl J Med 358:2667, 2008.
196. Hohnloser S, Crijns H, van Eikels M, et al: Effect of dronedarone on cardiovascular events in atrial fibrillation. N Engl J Med 360:668, 2009.
197. Patel C, Yan G-X, Kowey P: Droneradone. Circulation 120:636, 2009.
198. The GISSI-AF Investigators: Valsartan for prevention of recurrent atrial fibrillation. N Engl J Med 360:1606, 2009.
199. Zipes DP, Camm AJ, Borggrefe M, et al: ACC/AHA/ESC 2006 guidelines for management of patients with ventricular arrhythmias and the prevention of sudden cardiac death—executive summary: A report of the American College of Cardiology/American Heart Association Task Force and the European Society of Cardiology Committee for Practice Guidelines (Writing Committee to Develop Guidelines for Management of Patients With Ventricular Arrhythmias and the Prevention of Sudden Cardiac Death). Circulation 114:e385, 2006.
200. Quinn J, McDermott D, Steiell I, et al: Prospective validation of the San Francisco syncope rule to predict patients with serious outcomes. Ann Emerg Med. 47:448, 2006.
201. Chen L, Benditt D, Shen W-K: Management of syncope in adults: An update. Mayo Clin Proc 83:1280, 2008.
202. Akat K, Borggrefe M, Kaden J: Aortic valve calcification: Basic science to clinical practice. Heart 95:616, 2009.
203. Bonow R, Carabello B, Cahatterjee K, et al: 2008 focused update incorporated into the ACC/AHA 2006 Guidelines for the Management of Patients With Valvular Heart Disease. A Report of the American College of Cardiology/American Heart Association Task Force on Practice Guidelines (Writing Committee to Develop Guidelines on Management of Patients With Valvular Heart Disease). J Am Coll Cardiol 52:e1, 2008.
204. Vahanian A, Baumgartner H, Bax J, et al: Guidelines on the management of valvular heart disease: The Task Force on the Management of Valvular Heart Disease of the European Society of Cardiology. Eur Heart J 28:230, 2007.
205. Cowell S, Newby D, Prescott R, et al: A randomized trial of intensive lipid-lowering therapy in calcific aortic stenosis. N Engl J Med 352:2389, 2005.
206. Rossebø A, Pedersen T, Boman K, et al: Intensive lipid lowering with simvastatin and ezetimibe in aortic stenosis. N Engl J Med 359:1343, 2008.
207. Chan KL, Teo K, Dumesnil JG, et al: Effect of lipid lowering with rosuvastatin on progression of aortic stenosis: Results of the Aortic Stenosis Progression Observation: Measuring Effects of Rosuvastatin (ASTRONOMER) Trial. Circulation 121:306, 2010.
208. Goodney P, O'Connor G, Wennberg D, Birkmeyer J: Do hospitals with low mortality rates in coronary artery bypass also perform well in valve replacement? Ann Thorac Surg 76:1131, 2003.
209. Rosengart T, Fedman T, Borger M, et al: Percutaneous and minimally invasive valve procedures. A scientific statement from the American Heart Association Council on Cardiovascular Surgery and Anesthesia, Council on Clinical Cardiology, Functional Genomics and Translational Biology Interdisciplinary Working Group, and Quality of Care and Outcomes Research Interdisciplinary Working Group. Circulation 117:1750, 2008.
209a. Leon MB, Smith CR, Mack M, et al: Transcatheter aortic-valve implantation for aortic stenosis in patients who cannot undergo surgery. N Engl J Med 363:1667, 2010.
210. Kauterman K, Michaels A, Ports T: Is there any indication for aortic valvuloplasty in the elderly? Am J Geriatr Cardiol 12:190, 2003.
211. Nashef S, Roques F, Hammill B, et al: Validation of European System for Cardiac Operative Risk Evaluation (EuroSCORE) in North American cardiac surgery. Eur J Cardiothorac Surg 22:101, 2002.
212. Shroyer A, Coombs L, Peterson E, et al: The Society of Thoracic Surgeons: 30-day operative mortality and morbidity risk models. Ann Thorac Surg 75:1856, 2003.
213. Ambler G, Omar R, Royston P, et al: Generic, simple risk stratification model for heart valve surgery. Circulation 112:224, 2005.
214. Bossone E, Di Bendetto G, Frigiola A, et al: Valve surgery in octogenarians: In-hospital and long-term outcomes. Can J Cardiol 23:223, 2006.
214a. Maillet JM, Sommeb D, Hennel E, et al: Frailty after aortic valve replacement (AVR) in octogenarians. Arch Gerontol Geriatrics 48:391, 2009.
215. Aronow W, Ahn C, Kronzon I: Comparison of echocardiographic abnormalities in African-American, Hispanic, and white men and women aged >60 years. Am J Cardiol 87:1131, 2001.
216. Lee R, Sundt TI, Moon M, et al: Mitral valve repair in the elderly: Operative risk for patients over 70 years of age is acceptable. J Cardiovasc Surg 44:157, 2003.
217. Chikwe J, Goldstone AB, Passage J, et al: A propensity score-adjusted retrospective comparison of early and mid-term results of mitral valve repair versus replacement in octogenarians. Eur Heart J. published ahead of print doi:10.1093/eurheartj/ehq331

CHAPTER 81 Cardiovascular Disease in Women

L. Kristin Newby and Pamela S. Douglas

Background

Throughout history, differences between men and women in health and in illness have fascinated researchers and clinicians alike. The Institute of Medicine's Committee on Understanding the Biology of Sex and Gender Differences defined *sex* as "the classification of living things, generally as male or female according to their reproductive organs and functions assigned by the chromosomal complement."[1] *Gender*, on the other hand, was defined as "a person's self-representation as male or female or how that person is responded to by social institutions on the basis of the individual's gender presentation." Women (XX) and men (XY) differ in their genetic complement by a single chromosome of the 46 that define the human species. The influence of this single chromosomal difference affects the mechanisms and expression of disease as well as the psychosocial and behavioral characteristics and environments of individuals, which may protect from or enhance susceptibility to cardiovascular disease. In this discussion of cardiovascular disease in women, both of these definitions help explain differences in the occurrence, presentation, or course of cardiovascular disease—and, in some cases, in treatment and response to therapy.

Scope of the Problem

Cardiovascular disease is the leading cause of death among women, regardless of race or ethnicity, accounting for approximately 455,000 deaths in the United States in 2005 and causing the deaths of 1 in 3 women; this amounts to more deaths from heart disease than from stroke, lung cancer, chronic obstructive lung disease, and breast cancer combined.[2] About half of these deaths (1 in 6) result from coronary heart disease. Estimates of the lifetime costs from coronary heart disease in a woman range from $0.77 million to $1.1 million, depending on the severity of coronary disease.[3] Encouragingly, between 1980 and 2002, age-adjusted mortality from heart disease decreased in both men (52%) and women (49%).[2] For coronary heart disease specifically, mortality rates fell in both men and women by 4.4% from 2000 to 2002.[2] Approximately 47% of this decrease was due to the influence of evidence-based medicine (post–myocardial infarction [MI] secondary prevention, initial treatment of acute coronary syndromes [ACS], heart failure treatment, revascularization for chronic angina, and use of antihypertensive and lipid-lowering therapy) and approximately 44% to a reduction in several risk factors (hypertension, cholesterol, smoking, and physical inactivity) in the general population.[4] However, although overall mortality among women decreased, mortality among young women (between 35 and 44 years of age) increased by 1.3% per year from 1997 to 2002.[5]

Whether there are fundamental differences between women and men in mortality after MI, or whether such observed differences reflect corresponding differences in baseline characteristics, has long been a topic of discussion. In addition to differences in patient-related factors, two studies suggest that mortality may differ among women and men according to the type of ACS at presentation. In an analysis of a population-based cohort (N = 78,254) from the American Heart Association's Get With the Guidelines, after adjustment for baseline confounders, mortality was similar among women and men (adjusted OR, 1.04; 95% CI, 0.99 to 1.10). Among patients with ST-segment elevation MI, however, women had significantly higher mortality even after adjustment for age and other comorbidities (adjusted OR, 1.12; 95% CI, 1.02 to 1.23).[6] Results were similar in a meta-analysis of 136,247 patients randomized in 11 ACS trials from 1993 to 2006. In this analysis, women with ST-segment elevation MI were at a higher 30-day mortality risk than men (adjusted OR, 1.15; 95% CI, 1.06 to 1.24), and women with non–ST-segment elevation MI (adjusted OR, 0.77; 95% CI, 0.63 to 0.95) and unstable angina (adjusted OR, 0.55; 95% CI, 0.43 to 0.70) were at a lower 30-day mortality risk than men.[7] In a subset in which angiographic data were available, these differences may have been explained by the extent of coronary disease. These conclusions warrant caution, given known selection bias in the use of angiography in women, as discussed in later sections. In general, however, these observations suggest that understanding of the differences between men and women in the development or progression of cardiovascular disease, factors associated with outcome, use of proven therapies, and response to therapy is paramount.

Prevention and management of cardiovascular disease in women begin with awareness of the problem. Despite estimates that a 40-year-old woman has a lifetime risk of cardiovascular disease of 32%,[8] only about 55% of women identified cardiovascular disease as their greatest health risk in a 2006 survey conducted by the American Heart Association (AHA).[9] Physician awareness of women's cardiovascular risks is also suboptimal. In one study, only 71.2% of surveyed internists and obstetrics and gynecology specialists responded correctly to all 13 questions assessing knowledge about cardiac risk factors.[10]

Experts in industrialized societies have long recognized that the first presentation with coronary heart disease occurs approximately 10 years later among women than among men, and most commonly after menopause. The worldwide INTERHEART study, a large study of more than 52,000 individuals with MI, first demonstrated that this approximate 8- to 10-year difference in age at onset holds widely around the world, across various socioeconomic, climatic, and cultural environments (see Chap. 1).[11] Although coronary artery disease in general is manifested earlier in less developed countries, the age gap in time of onset between men and women is universal (**Table 81-1**). Despite this delay in onset, mortality from coronary heart disease is increasing more rapidly among women than among men in both the developed and developing world.[12] Risk factors were similar in all regions of the world, although the strength of association of some risk factors with MI varied between women and men, as discussed later.[11] Another important observation that supports the critical role of risk awareness

TABLE 81-1 Comparison of Age at First Myocardial Infarction Among Women and Men Across Geographic Regions

REGION	MEDIAN AGE, WOMEN	MEDIAN AGE, MEN
Western Europe	68 (59-76)	61 (53-70)
Central and eastern Europe	68 (59-74)	59 (50-68)
North America	64 (52-75)	58 (49-68)
South America and Mexico	65 (56-73)	59 (50-68)
Australia and New Zealand	66 (59-74)	58 (50-67)
Middle East	57 (50-65)	50 (44-57)
Africa	56 (49-65)	52 (46-61)
South Asia	60 (50-66)	52 (45-60)
China and Hong Kong	67 (62-72)	60 (50-68)
Southeast Asia and Japan	63 (56-68)	55 (47-64)

Modified from Yusuf S, Hawken S, Ôunpuu S, et al: Effect of potentially modifiable risk factors associated with myocardial infarction in 52 countries (the INTERHEART study): Case-control study. Lancet 364:937, 2004.

is that younger, premenopausal women—not older women—carry a mortality excess compared with similarly aged men presenting with MI in the National Registry of Myocardial Infarction (NRMI).[13]

Experts have widely speculated that this age difference reflects premenopausal protection from the development of atherosclerotic coronary disease afforded by circulating estrogen, which is markedly reduced at menopause. Despite this plausible biologic explanation, replacement of estrogen after menopause does not prevent clinical cardiovascular events.[14-17] An excellent review by Ouyang and colleagues[18] provides a summary of hormonal influence on atherosclerotic vascular disease and the spectrum of observational and clinical trials research on postmenopausal hormone therapy.

Coronary Artery Disease Risk Factors and Risk Factor Modification (see Chaps. 1, 2, 44, and 49)

The classic risk factors for coronary atherosclerosis are commonly divided into those that are potentially modifiable to mitigate risk (diabetes, hypertension, hyperlipidemia, cigarette smoking, obesity, and sedentary lifestyle) and those that are not modifiable (age and family history). With a few exceptions, these factors have similar influence on cardiovascular risk in both sexes.

Unmodifiable Risk Factors

AGE (see Chap. 80). Age is one of the most powerful risk factors for the development of cardiovascular disease and accompanying clinical events. Although the prevalence of cardiovascular disease with increasing age varies modestly by sex (prior to the fifth decade of life, prevalence in men is greater than in women, but prevalence equalizes in the sixth decade and in subsequent decades becomes greater in women), the magnitude of the association of age with clinical cardiovascular events is similar among men and women.[2]

FAMILY HISTORY. Coronary heart disease and death from cardiovascular disease have a hereditary component.[19,20] In a few families, the predilection for coronary disease is monogenic, with transmission occurring in a mendelian pattern (see Chaps. 8 and 44). In contrast, the majority of coronary artery disease is complex, likely reflecting multiple genes, each contributing modestly to a predisposition to atherosclerosis and atherothrombotic clinical events. The current use of genome-wide association studies is shedding considerable light in this regard (see Chaps. 7, 8 and 44).[21]

Whether sex differences exist in the frequency of genetic polymorphisms that influence the occurrence of cardiovascular events remains an open question. The statistical association of gene variants with coronary disease differs in men and women, suggesting that different pathways may operate in the manifestation of cardiovascular disease between the sexes.[22] Two of 112 polymorphisms in 71 candidate genes associated with MI in women: stromelysin 1, a member of the matrix metalloproteinase family of enzymes that are believed to be involved in plaque rupture (RR, 4.7; 99% CI, 2.0 to 12.2), and (much less strongly) plasminogen activator inhibitor 1 (PAI-1). In contrast, in men, two different genes associate with MI: the gap junction protein connexin37 (RR, 1.7; 95% CI, 1.1 to 1.6) and p22 (phox), a component of the NAD(P)H redox system (RR, 0.7; 95% CI, 0.6 to 0.9). This apparent sex-related difference in the association of genetic polymorphisms with clinical disease phenotypes may be less related to the presence or absence of the genetic mutation itself than to the influences of sex on variation in the expression of various genes or the downstream responses to gene products.

Variations in sex hormones and their levels between men and women or other differences related to the presence or absence of Y chromosome genes, including but not limited to those that regulate cellular function, could influence these observed associations. Indeed, ex vivo male macrophages responded to androgens with augmentation of 27 atherosclerosis-associated genes, resulting in increased foam cell formation and enhanced lysosomal low-density lipoprotein (LDL) cholesterol degradation, whereas ex vivo female cells did not show a response in any of the 588 genes tested.[23] Such differences may explain observed differences in the pathophysiology of atherosclerosis, including plaque composition (more cellular and fibrous tissue in women),[24] endothelial function (estrogen-induced coronary vasodilation), and hemostasis (higher fibrinogen and factor VII levels in women).[25-27] Furthermore, the underlying inciting pathophysiologic change of atherothrombotic coronary events varies in women and men and may be influenced by both genetics and sex-based differences, including the effects of estrogen that influence gene expression and protein production or activity. For example, women are twice as likely to have plaque erosion (37% in women versus 18% in men), and men more frequently have plaque rupture as the underlying inciting event (82% in men versus 63% in women).[28] With the continued evolution of ribonucleic acid (RNA) microarray technology, metabolomics, and proteomic capabilities, it will become increasingly feasible to determine expression patterns of tens of thousands of genes and the presence and relative abundance of their protein and metabolite products simultaneously. Although only limited work has explored sex differences in gene expression, proteomics, or metabolomics, further work in these areas may provide important insights into development, diagnosis, and tailored treatment of cardiovascular disease in women and men.

Potentially Modifiable Risk Factors

HYPERTENSION (see Chaps. 45 and 46). Hypertension is an increasingly common risk factor among the U.S. population, with 65 million affected individuals in National Health and Nutrition Examination Surveys (NHANES) from 1999 to 2000.[29] Overall, more than 35 million women had hypertension, a 15% higher prevalence than that in men. The prevalence of hypertension increased with age in both sexes, but from 45 to 54 years of age, the escalation was greater among women than among men, the difference in prevalence reaching statistical significance at 75 years of age and older. In subjects younger than 35 years of age, hypertension was significantly more prevalent among men than among women.

In a meta-analysis of 61 prospective studies of hypertension involving more than 1 million previously healthy adults between 49 and 89 years of age, the association with ischemic heart disease risk was only slightly stronger in women than in men.[30] The slope of the association between ischemic heart disease mortality and blood pressure was fairly constant, arguing against a "threshold" systolic pressure below which disease risk is not further reduced. An analysis of men and women in the Framingham Heart Study supports this position by showing that the gradient of cardiovascular risk extended to high-normal and normal blood pressures in both sexes.[31]

Unfortunately, women remain one of the populations most likely to be undertreated when they have an established diagnosis of hypertension and, even more concerning, little progress has been made in improving rates of treatment and control during the past decade.

Whereas treatment and control rates in men increased by an absolute 9.8% and 15.3%, respectively, between the NHANE surveys spanning 1988 to 1994 and a follow-up survey from 1999 to 2000, the treatment and control rates in women were essentially unchanged (increases of only 1.9% and 0.5%, respectively).[32]

DIABETES AND THE METABOLIC SYNDROME (see Chaps. 44 and 64). The prevalence of diabetes in the United States is escalating rapidly. Between 2000 and 2001, it rose by 8.2%, and in the 11 years between 1990 and 2001, it rose by 61%; it is expected to double by 2050 across all age and sex groupings.[2] In 2006, women older than 20 years of age represented more than half (9.5 million) of the 17 million patients with known diabetes and accounted for 2.5 million of the estimated 6.4 million with undiagnosed diabetes.[2] Furthermore, of the 57 million people in the United States with prediabetes, defined as impaired glucose tolerance or a fasting blood glucose concentration of 110 to <126 mg/dL, women accounted for 23 million.[2] Cardiovascular disease is twice as common among women with diabetes as among those without, they are four times as likely to be hospitalized, and women have a higher risk for most clinical events and are less likely to be treated to HbA1c goal than men are.[2]

Metabolic syndrome relates closely to insulin resistance and comprises a constellation of at least three of the following risk factors: abdominal obesity, atherogenic lipid profile (excessive triglycerides or inadequate high-density lipoprotein [HDL] cholesterol), blood pressure of 130/85 mm Hg or higher, and fasting glucose concentration of 110 mg/dL or greater. At any given LDL-cholesterol level, metabolic syndrome increases the risk for coronary heart disease. Because of this, the National Cholesterol Education Program (NCEP) Adult Treatment Panel III considers metabolic syndrome a secondary target of risk reduction therapy.[33] After adjustment for age, metabolic syndrome appears to be highly prevalent in both sexes, with little difference in rates between women and men.[34]

HYPERLIPIDEMIA (see Chap. 47). According to summary statistics from the AHA, 47% of women older than 20 years of age have a total serum cholesterol level ≥200 mg/dL, and 31.7% have an LDL-cholesterol level ≥130 mg/dL—incidences similar to those in the general population.[2] More favorably, whereas 15.5% of Americans overall have an HDL level less than 40 mg/dL, only 6.7% of women are in this range.[2] The relative risk for coronary disease events associated with elevation of various lipid variables was determined in a nested case-control study from the Nurses' Health Study. Among 32,826 healthy women who provided blood samples at baseline, the multivariable adjusted relative risks (adjusted for high-sensitivity C-reactive protein [hs-CRP], homocysteine, and other traditional cardiac risk factors) for the highest quintiles of lipid variables were apolipoprotein B (RR, 4.1; 95% CI, 2 to 8.3), low levels of HDL (RR, 2.6; 95% CI, 1.4 to 5), LDL (RR, 3.1; 95% CI, 1.7 to 5.8), and triglycerides (RR, 1.9; 95% CI, 1.0 to 3.9).[35] Adverse changes in lipid profiles accompany menopause.[36] Perimenopausal triglyceride levels are the most erratic but follow roughly the same pattern of increase as total cholesterol and LDL cholesterol, which increase on average by an absolute 10% from levels at 6 months before menopause. Menopause influences HDL cholesterol less dramatically. HDL concentration declines gradually in the two years preceding menopause and then levels off after menopause. The postmenopausal increase in cardiovascular disease risk may result partly from these lipid alterations.

The 1988-1994 NHANES showed that serum cholesterol concentrations in U.S. adults were on a downward trend, but lipid profiles changed little between the 1988-1994 and 1999-2002 NHANES. In the follow-up survey, the prevalence of hypercholesterolemia was similar for men and women, and of all adults with high total cholesterol, only 35% were aware of their diagnosis, and rates were similar among men and women. Only 10.2% of dyslipidemic women were under treatment, compared with 12% overall, and among treated women, only 3.7% achieved a total cholesterol concentration of 5.2 mmol/liter compared with 5.4% overall.[37] As with hypertension, these findings highlight the need for a stronger commitment to prevention, treatment, and control of hypercholesterolemia, with an enhanced focus on women.

Lifestyle Risk Factors

In 2006, 60.5% of American women were overweight or obese, defined as a body mass index (BMI) greater than 25 kg/m^2.[2] The prevalence of obesity (BMI >30 kg/m^2) in women increased gradually but markedly, from 12.2% in 1991 to 20.8% in 2001.[38] The 2005-2006 NHANES identified 35.3% of women as obese.[39] Furthermore, as summarized in the 2009 AHA Heart Disease and Stroke Statistics,[2] in conjunction with the obesity epidemic, the National Center for Health Statistics reported in 2005 that 12% of women engaged in no moderate to vigorous leisure time physical activity, and a 2007 National Health Interview Survey found that 66.3% of women never engaged in vigorous physical activity and only 9.8% of women engaged in vigorous activity 5 days or more per week. Objective NHANES accelerometer data were even more sobering; only 3.2% of women 20 to 59 years of age and only 2.5% older than 60 years of age met recommendations for at least 30 minutes of moderate to vigorous physical activity at least 5 days per week.[40] Perhaps more concerning for the future of heart disease in women, 31.8% of girls in grades 9 through 12 had not engaged in moderate to vigorous physical activity in the preceding 7 days,[41] and in another study, 31% of white girls and 56% of black girls 16 to 17 years of age engaged in no leisure time physical activity at all.[42] In 2006, the estimated prevalence of cigarette smoking among women 18 years of age or older was 18.1%, and 10.7% of girls 12 to 17 years of age and 23.6% 18 years of age or older reported smoking in the past month.[2]

Global Assessment of Risk Factors for Coronary Heart Disease (see Chap. 44)

Primary findings of the large, case-control INTERHEART study provide some of the best data to date on the relation of clinical parameters to the risk of ischemic heart disease worldwide, including patterns of association of MI risk among women compared with men.[11] Overall, after adjustment, nine risk factors accounted for 90.4% of the population attributable risk for MI (94% of the population attributable risk among women and 90% among men). The risk factors were apolipoprotein B/apolipoprotein A-I ratio, cigarette smoking, hypertension, diabetes, abdominal obesity, psychosocial factors (an index based on combining parameter estimates for depression, stress at work or home, financial stress, one or more life events, and locus of control scores), fruit and vegetable intake, exercise, and alcohol intake.

Although the strength of association of most risk factors with MI was similar among women and men, the INTERHEART study confirmed a markedly stronger association of diabetes with MI among women (**Fig. 81-1**).[11] Psychosocial factors also tended to associate more strongly with increased risk among women, although the difference was less in magnitude. In addition, healthy lifestyle choices including regular exercise and modest alcohol consumption provided stronger protection among women than among men, and fruit and vegetable intake tended to more greatly benefit women. Although further work is necessary to define the underpinnings of these observations, they nonetheless have important implications for counseling and management of women to prevent the development of cardiovascular disease.

The Framingham Risk Score remains the most widely used and authoritative tool to estimate global, long-term coronary artery disease risk in women, as in men. However, it may underestimate risk, especially in younger women,[43] and alternative algorithms have been proposed. These include the Reynolds Risk Score, which adds hs-CRP, HbA1c, and family history, increasing the predictive value from a C-statistic of 0.75 to 0.80.[44] Still other data suggest that atherosclerosis imaging may have particular value in women; in the MESA study, 32% of low-risk women had measurable coronary artery calcification, and the likelihood of death was closely related to coronary artery calcification score.[45]

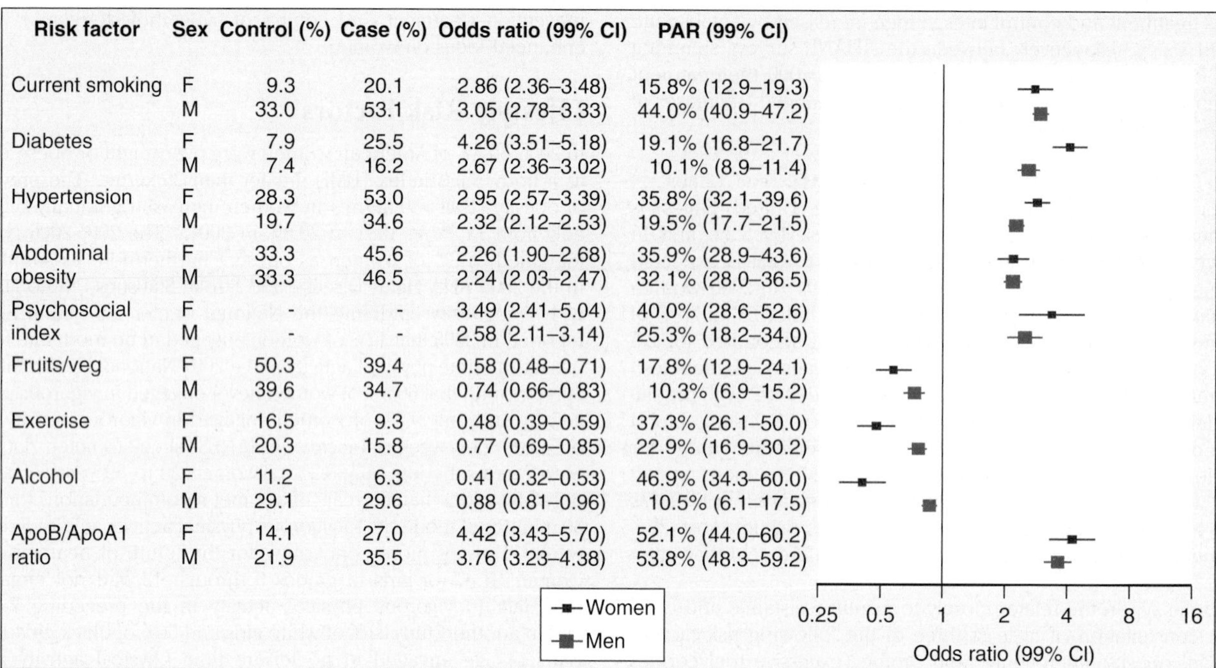

Risk factor	Sex	Control (%)	Case (%)	Odds ratio (99% CI)	PAR (99% CI)
Current smoking	F	9.3	20.1	2.86 (2.36–3.48)	15.8% (12.9–19.3)
	M	33.0	53.1	3.05 (2.78–3.33)	44.0% (40.9–47.2)
Diabetes	F	7.9	25.5	4.26 (3.51–5.18)	19.1% (16.8–21.7)
	M	7.4	16.2	2.67 (2.36–3.02)	10.1% (8.9–11.4)
Hypertension	F	28.3	53.0	2.95 (2.57–3.39)	35.8% (32.1–39.6)
	M	19.7	34.6	2.32 (2.12–2.53)	19.5% (17.7–21.5)
Abdominal obesity	F	33.3	45.6	2.26 (1.90–2.68)	35.9% (28.9–43.6)
	M	33.3	46.5	2.24 (2.03–2.47)	32.1% (28.0–36.5)
Psychosocial index	F	-	-	3.49 (2.41–5.04)	40.0% (28.6–52.6)
	M	-	-	2.58 (2.11–3.14)	25.3% (18.2–34.0)
Fruits/veg	F	50.3	39.4	0.58 (0.48–0.71)	17.8% (12.9–24.1)
	M	39.6	34.7	0.74 (0.66–0.83)	10.3% (6.9–15.2)
Exercise	F	16.5	9.3	0.48 (0.39–0.59)	37.3% (26.1–50.0)
	M	20.3	15.8	0.77 (0.69–0.85)	22.9% (16.9–30.2)
Alcohol	F	11.2	6.3	0.41 (0.32–0.53)	46.9% (34.3–60.0)
	M	29.1	29.6	0.88 (0.81–0.96)	10.5% (6.1–17.5)
ApoB/ApoA1 ratio	F	14.1	27.0	4.42 (3.43–5.70)	52.1% (44.0–60.2)
	M	21.9	35.5	3.76 (3.23–4.38)	53.8% (48.3–59.2)

FIGURE 81-1 Relative risks associated with various cardiac risk factors among men (M) and women (F) in the INTERHEART study. PAR = population attributable risk. *(From Yusuf S, Hawken S, Ôunpuu S, et al: Effect of potentially modifiable risk factors associated with myocardial infarction in 52 countries [the INTERHEART study]: Case-control study. Lancet 364:937, 2004.)*

Presentation with Acute Coronary Disease (see Chap. 53)

Symptoms commonly associated with MI in both sexes include chest pain, pressure, or squeezing; pain radiating to the neck, shoulder, back, arms, or jaw; palpitations; dyspnea; heartburn, nausea, vomiting, or abdominal pain; diaphoresis; and dizziness. Women may experience milder symptoms or describe them somewhat differently and may more frequently experience nonspecific prodromal symptoms, such as fatigue.[46] A study of 127 men and 90 women by Milner and colleagues[47] showed that among patients who presented to the emergency department with symptoms of coronary disease other than chest pain, there were several sex-related differences in symptoms. Dyspnea, nausea and vomiting, indigestion, fatigue, sweating, and arm or shoulder pain as presenting symptoms in the absence of chest pain were all more frequent among women than among men, but the Myocardial Infarction Triage and Intervention (MITI) Project investigators demonstrated that chest pain was present in almost all women (99.6%) and men (99%) who experienced a documented acute MI.[48] In addition to symptom differences, women with MI have more comorbidities, including hypertension, and present later in the course of symptoms and more frequently with high-risk clinical findings of heart failure and tachycardia.[49]

Women (4 million visits/year) are hospitalized more frequently than men (2.4 million visits/year) for the evaluation of chest pain,[2] but women who present with chest pain or even more clearly with ACS are more likely than men to have a noncardiac cause or other nonatherosclerotic causes, such as vasospasm.[50] The National Institutes of Health–sponsored Women's Ischemia Syndrome Evaluation (WISE) study confirmed a marked discordance between observed rates of obstructive coronary artery disease and the predicted probability of coronary disease (**Fig. 81-2**).[51] This discordance was pervasive across age groups, regardless of whether angina was classified as typical or atypical.

Imaging for Diagnosis and Prognosis

Compounding observations of differences in presentation and the discordance between predicted probability of disease and actual disease, there is a paucity of data regarding the best diagnostic strategy for assessment of women with chest pain to establish or to exclude a diagnosis of coronary artery disease. Thus, recommendations for the use of stress testing in women often derive from studies performed predominantly in men. Accuracy in the clinical setting is often confounded by the use of tests among women with low pretest probability, yielding multiple false-positive results. In one small study, however, the results of exercise stress testing according to the Duke Treadmill Score appeared as good for both diagnosis and prognosis in women as in men, with a higher negative predictive value in women.[52]

In general, recommendations for stress testing with imaging in women parallel those in men.[53] In a consensus statement from the AHA on imaging in women, Mieres and colleagues[54] summarized the available data on diagnostic stress testing and derived an algorithm to guide the use of exercise testing with or without cardiac imaging in women with chest pain. **Figure 81-3** demonstrates the algorithm for use in intermediate- or high-risk women with atypical or typical chest pain symptoms. Imaging in symptomatic women generally is recommended for those at intermediate or high risk for coronary artery disease. Both stress echocardiographic and stress gated myocardial single-photon emission computed tomographic nuclear imaging appear to perform similarly in women for diagnosis,[55] and both were given similar recommendations for stress testing in women in the AHA position statement.[54] Evidence suggests that the prognostic utility of either form of imaging with stress testing is similar (**Fig. 81-4**) and describes a gradient of risk that is similar in men and women.[55]

Evidence-Based Therapy in Women

WOMEN IN CLINICAL RESEARCH (see Chaps. 6 and 44). Randomized clinical trials with adequate power to demonstrate clinically meaningful differences between treatments, interventions, or management strategies should guide clinical practice. Assessment of treatment effect within a subgroup is usually underpowered and also fraught with the likelihood of type I error resulting from multiple comparisons. That said, consistency of findings across subgroups provides reassurance that the trial results are generalizable. Use of observational studies to assess treatment benefits and risks is complex and subject to multiple recognized and unrecognized biases, which may lead to erroneous conclusions. The story of hormone replacement therapy for primary and secondary prevention of cardiovascular events is an excellent example of the problems encountered in drawing inferences about treatment effects from nonrandomized cohorts. Multiple observational studies had shown dramatic reductions in coronary heart disease death or MI among users of hormone replacement therapy. However, a series of large randomized clinical trials later demonstrated that not only did hormone replacement therapy fail to reduce coronary heart disease events, but events actually increased in some cases among those randomly assigned to receive hormone therapy compared with those assigned to placebo treatment.[14-17]

Unfortunately, in a systematic review surveying the literature for all randomized controlled trials of MI from 1966 to 2000, Lee and colleagues[56] demonstrated that there was a marked discordance between the representation of women among MI patients and their representation in clinical trials (**Fig. 81-5**). Even in the most recent years of the survey, women sustained 45% of all MIs but represented only 27% of patients enrolled in randomized controlled trials of treatments for acute MI. Women were similarly underrepresented in the randomized controlled trials that formed the evidence base of support for the 2007 update of the AHA cardiovascular prevention guidelines for women.[57] These observations highlight that recruitment of women in proportion to their representation among patients with the cardiovascular disease of interest is paramount to support the application of the results of clinical trials to women. A 2007 "think tank" meeting of representatives from academia, industry, and regulatory agencies led to the suggestion of a number of strategies in four major areas to improve representation of women in the evidence base for the treatment of heart disease: improved clinical trial designs to optimize the study of women; appropriate incentives to conduct research in women; strategies to improve enrollment of women in clinical trials; and mandated reporting of results of clinical trials by sex.[58]

PRACTICE GUIDELINES TO CODIFY TREATMENT RECOMMENDATIONS. In general, American College of Cardiology/American Heart Association (ACC/AHA) guidelines for the management of ST-segment elevation and non–ST-segment elevation MI, as well as for chronic coronary disease, are silent or neutral on treatment by sex.[50,59-61] In addition to these "gender-neutral"

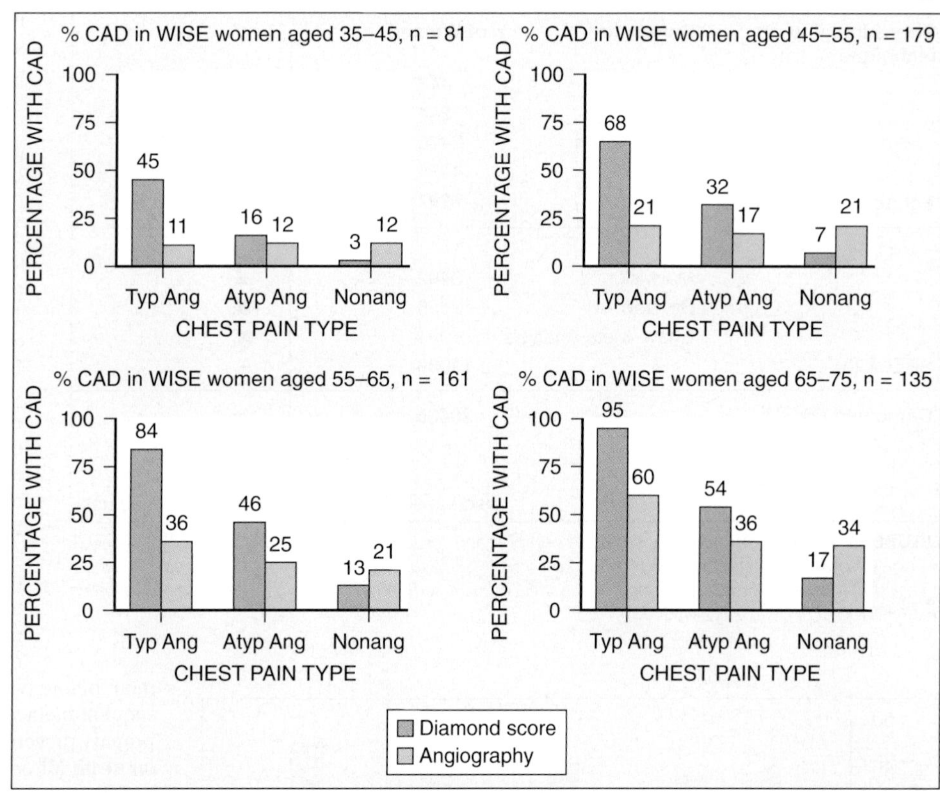

FIGURE 81-2 Observed rates of coronary artery disease (CAD) at angiography (yellow bars) compared with Diamond probability of CAD (purple bars). Atyp Ang = atypical angina; Nonang = nonanginal pain; Typ Ang = typical angina. *(From Shaw LJ, Bairey Merz CN, Pepine CJ, et al: Insights from the NHLBI-sponsored Women's Ischemia Syndrome Evaluation [WISE] Study. Part I: Gender differences in traditional and novel risk factors, symptom evaluation, and gender-optimized diagnostic strategies. J Am Coll Cardiol 47:4S, 2006.)*

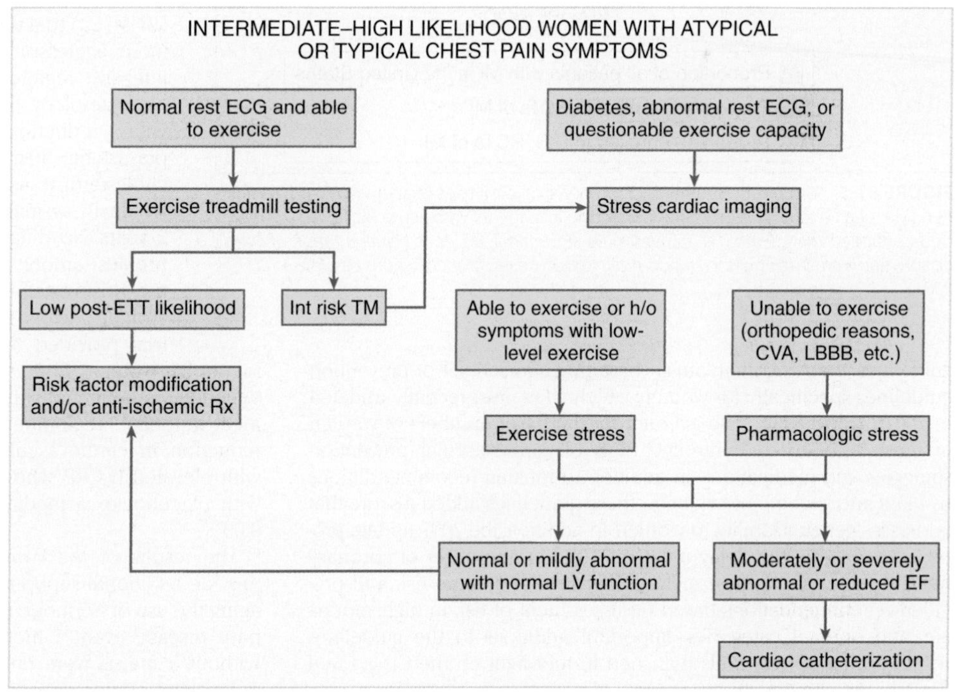

FIGURE 81-3 Algorithm for stress testing in women with moderate to high risk of coronary artery disease presenting with typical or atypical symptoms. CVA = cerebrovascular accident; ECG = electrocardiogram; EF = ejection fraction; ETT = exercise treadmill test; h/o = history of; LBBB = left bundle branch block; LV = left ventricular; TM = treadmill. *(From Mieres JH, Shaw LJ, Arai A, et al: Role of noninvasive testing in the clinical evaluation of women with suspected coronary artery disease: Consensus statement from the Cardiac Imaging Committee, Council of Clinical Cardiology, and the Cardiovascular Imaging and Intervention Committee, Council on Cardiovascular Radiology and Intervention, American Heart Association. Circulation 111:682, 2005.)*

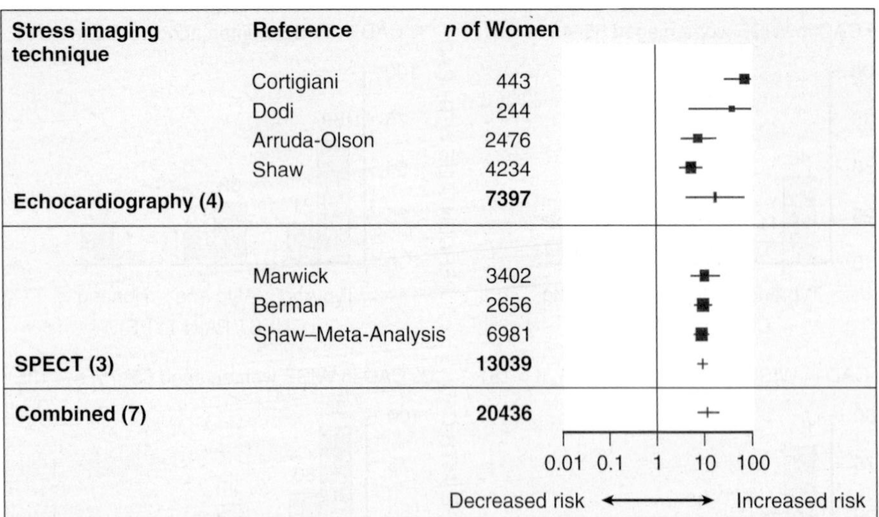

FIGURE 81-4 Prognostic utility of echocardiographic and nuclear stress imaging among women. SPECT = single-photon emission computed tomography. *(From Shaw LJ, Vasey C, Sawada S, et al: Impact of gender on risk stratification by exercise and dobutamine stress echocardiography: Long-term mortality in 4234 women and 6898 men. Eur Heart J 26:447, 2005.)*

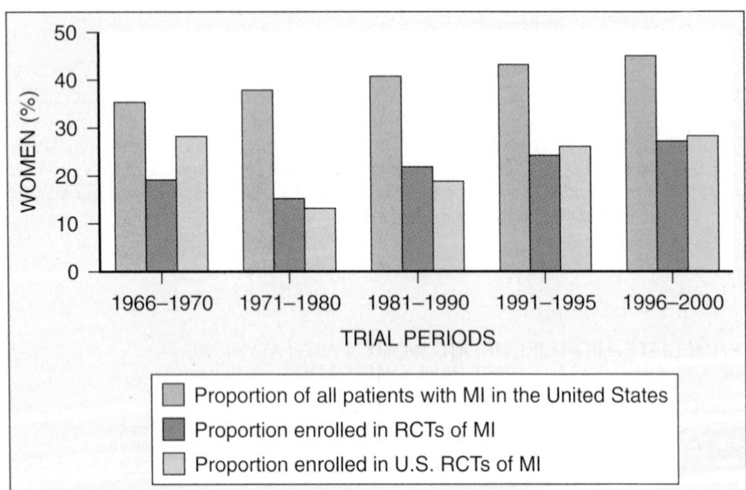

FIGURE 81-5 Underrepresentation of women in clinical trials of acute myocardial infarction (MI) relative to their representation among all patients with acute MI. RCTs = randomized controlled trials. *(From Lee PY, Alexander KP, Hammill BG, et al: Representation of elderly persons and women in published randomized trials of acute coronary syndromes. JAMA 286:708, 2001.)*

guidelines, the AHA maintains a broadly endorsed set of prevention guidelines specifically for women, which were most recently updated in 2007 (**Table 81-2**).[62] To account for the lower numbers of women in most randomized controlled trials of cardiovascular prevention strategies and medications, in addition to ranking recommendations by class and strength of evidence, these guidelines added a score that addresses generalizability to women. In addition, the 2007 update proposed managing the delay relative to men in the onset of coronary heart disease by emphasizing a perspective of lifetime risk and provided recommendations based on assessment of risk in high, moderate, and optimal categories. Important additions to the guidelines resulted from several trials that shed further light on the Class I and Class III recommendations.

The Women's Health Study randomized 39,876 healthy women older than 45 years to low-dose aspirin (100 mg on alternate days) or placebo and observed them for 10 years for first occurrence of death, nonfatal MI, or nonfatal stroke.[63] This trial provided important insights into the use of aspirin for primary prevention in women (see Chap. 44). Although the overall study showed a nonsignificant 9% reduction in the primary composite endpoint (RR, 0.91; 95% CI, 0.80 to 1.03), when the individual endpoints were examined, there was heterogeneity of effect. There was no effect of aspirin on the rate of nonfatal MI (RR, 1.02; 95% CI, 0.84 to 1.25) or cardiovascular death (RR, 0.95; 95% CI, 0.74 to 1.22), but aspirin reduced stroke risk by 17% overall (RR, 0.83; 95% CI, 0.69 to 0.99) and ischemic stroke by 24% (RR, 0.76; 95% CI, 0.63 to 0.93). Hemorrhagic stroke increased nonsignificantly (RR, 1.24; 95% CI, 0.82 to 1.87), but gastrointestinal bleeding requiring transfusion was significantly increased (RR, 1.40; 95% CI, 1.07 to 1.83). This study revealed significant age × treatment interactions for the effect of aspirin on the primary composite endpoint and the individual endpoint of nonfatal MI. Whereas the benefit of aspirin in reducing ischemic stroke was consistent across all age groups, only in those older than 65 years of age did aspirin significantly reduce the risk of nonfatal MI (RR, 0.66; 95% CI, 0.44 to 0.97). Thus, the use of aspirin in primary prevention requires a careful assessment of multiple potential risks and benefits of treatment before prescription in an individual woman. In a subsequent meta-analysis of all randomized trials of aspirin in primary prevention, aspirin reduced the rate of cardiovascular death, MI, or stroke by 12% (OR, 0.88; 95% CI, 0.79 to 0.99), largely because of a reduction in ischemic stroke (OR, 0.76; 95% CI, 0.63 to 0.93). There was no reduction in cardiovascular death or in MI alone, in contrast to men, in whom there was a 14% reduction in the composite of death, MI, or stroke, with a 32% reduction in MI but no reduction in ischemic stroke or cardiovascular death. Rates of bleeding were increased similarly in women and men.[64]

The Pravastatin or Atorvastatin Evaluation and Infection Trial–Thrombolysis In Myocardial Infarction 22 (PROVE IT-TIMI 22) trial demonstrated the safety and effectiveness of more aggressive lipid-lowering therapy with statins.[65] An intensive regimen of 80 mg of atorvastatin reduced LDL cholesterol by 51% to a median of 62 mg/dL, compared with a reduction of 22% to a median of 95 mg/dL in the pravastatin 40-mg arm. This greater reduction of LDL cholesterol translated into a 16% reduction in the hazard for death or major cardiac events at a mean follow-up of 2 years. No differences occurred in the safety or efficacy profiles among women and men. Even more recently, the Rosuvastatin to Prevent Vascular Events in Men and Women with Elevated C-Reactive Protein (JUPITER) trial provided firm evidence in primary prevention that for both women and men, treatment guided by hsCRP was beneficial among individuals whose cholesterol levels would not meet guideline recommendations for treatment. There was a 15% reduction in cardiovascular death, MI, and stroke among patients with elevated hsCRP who were treated with rosuvastatin compared with placebo for a median of 1.9 years (HR, 0.53; 95% CI, 0.40 to 0.69).[66]

The results of the Women's Health Initiative estrogen-only trial provide additional support for the Class III recommendation discouraging the use of hormone replacement therapy to prevent a first coronary disease event.[12] In this trial, 10,739 postmenopausal women without a uterus were randomized to placebo or 0.625 mg of oral conjugated equine estrogens daily. The trial was stopped early by its Data and Safety Monitoring Board in February 2004. At that point, there was no significant benefit of conjugated equine estrogens on the primary composite endpoint of death or nonfatal MI (RR, 0.91; 95% CI, 0.75 to 1.12), but the incidences of stroke (RR, 1.39; 95% CI, 1.10 to 1.77) and pulmonary embolus (RR, 1.34; 95% CI, 0.87 to 2.06) increased in the estrogen arm. Thus, it appears that no cardiovascular

TABLE 81-2 Recommendations from the 2007 American Heart Association Women's Evidence-Based Prevention Guidelines

CLINICAL AREA	RECOMMENDATIONS
Class I Recommendations	
Lifestyle interventions	Smoking cessation; avoid second-hand smoke
	30 minutes of moderate-intensity physical activity on most (preferably all) days of the week
	Cardiac rehabilitation/risk reduction program post-MI, post–coronary intervention, and if chronic angina
	Overall healthy eating pattern; limit saturated fat to <10% of calories, cholesterol to <300 mg/day; limit *trans* fatty acids
	Weight maintenance/reduction to BMI 18.5-24.9 kg/m^2 and waist circumference ≤35 inches
Major risk factor interventions	Encourage optimal BP <120/80 through lifestyle approaches
	Pharmacotherapy if BP <140/90 or lower if end-organ damage or diabetes
	Use thiazide diuretics unless absolute contraindication
	Optimal lipid targets: LDL <100 mg/dL, HDL <50 mg/dL, triglycerides <150 mg/dL, non–HDL cholesterol <130 mg/dL
	In high-risk women or elevated LDL, reduce intake of saturated fat to <7% of calories and cholesterol to <200 mg/day and reduce *trans* fatty acids
	Drug therapy for lipid abnormalities:
	High risk: initiate if LDL >100 mg/dL; statin therapy if high risk and LDL >100 mg/dL; niacin or fibrate if HDL is low or non–HDL cholesterol is high
	Intermediate risk: initiate if LDL >130 mg/dL; niacin or fibrate if HDL is low or non–HDL cholesterol is high
	Lifestyle approaches and pharmacotherapy to achieve near-normal (<7%) HbA1c in women with diabetes
Preventive drug regimens	Aspirin in high-risk women (75-162 mg daily) or clopidogrel if aspirin allergic or intolerant
	Beta blockers indefinitely post-MI unless contraindicated
	ACE inhibitors in high-risk women (post-MI, EF ≤40, or diabetes) unless contraindicated; ARBs in high-risk women who are intolerant of ACE inhibitors
Aldosterone blockade	Aldosterone blockade after MI if renal function and potassium are normal in women who are receiving therapeutic doses of ACE inhibitors and beta blockers who have EF ≤40 with symptomatic heart failure
Atrial fibrillation/stroke prevention	For chronic or paroxysmal atrial fibrillation, warfarin to INR 2.0-3.0 unless low risk
	Aspirin (325 mg daily) if contraindication to warfarin or at low risk for stroke (<1%/yr)
Class III Recommendations	
Hormone therapy	Do not start or continue estrogen plus progestin for primary or secondary prevention. Do not initiate or continue other forms of hormone therapy for prevention of cardiovascular disease pending results of ongoing trials.
Antioxidants	Do not use antioxidant supplements for cardiovascular disease prevention.
Folic acid	Do not use folic acid, with or without B_6 or B_{12} supplementation, for cardiovascular disease prevention.
Aspirin	Routine use of aspirin in women <65 years of age is not recommended for MI prevention.

ACE = angiotensin-converting enzyme; ARB = angiotensin receptor blocker; BMI = body mass index; BP = blood pressure; EF = ejection fraction; HbA1c = hemoglobin A1c; HDL = high-density lipoprotein; INR = international normalized ratio; LDL = low-density lipoprotein; MI = myocardial infarction.

Modified from Mosca L, Banka CL, Benjamin EJ, et al: American Heart Association evidence-based guidelines for cardiovascular disease prevention in women: 2007 update. J Am Coll Cardiol 49:1230, 2007.

benefits and potential harm result from postmenopausal administration of conjugated equine estrogens. Because of these and similar results of other studies of hormone replacement therapy, the U.S. Food and Drug Administration has placed a black box warning on the labeling of all estrogen-containing compounds.

Finally, several trials of vitamin supplementation revealed no benefit and potential harm and resulted in Class III recommendations in the 2007 update of the Women's Prevention Guidelines (see Table 81-2).

ACC/AHA STEMI and UA/NSTEMI ACS Guidelines

The ST-segment elevation MI (STEMI) guidelines are silent on sex-specific recommendations, providing completely sex-neutral treatment recommendations.[59] The unstable angina/non–ST-segment elevation MI (UA/NSTEMI) guidelines provide the following Class I summary recommendation regarding the treatment of women: "Women with UA/NSTEMI should be managed in a manner similar to men. Specifically, women, like men with UA/NSTEMI, should receive aspirin and clopidogrel. Indications for noninvasive and invasive testing are similar in women and men. (*Level of Evidence: B*)."[50] However, the literature suggests that subtle differences exist between the sexes and that these have relevance to the care of individual patients (see later discussion).

Invasive Management and Revascularization

A meta-analysis of trials of percutaneous coronary intervention (PCI) confirmed that women suffer vascular complications of their procedures more frequently than men do.[67] In addition, many studies of predominantly elective PCI demonstrated higher in-hospital mortality among women than among men. Late mortality was similar between the sexes. Findings were similar for the use of primary PCI to treat acute MI, showing higher in-hospital mortality but similar late mortality.

Three randomized controlled trials of early invasive strategies for the management of non–ST-segment elevation MI showed conflicting results with regard to treatment benefit in women.[68-70] Although differences in the frequency of use of bypass surgery and the early hazard discussed may have contributed to these observations, Glaser and colleagues[68] demonstrated a critical principle of the relationship of risk-to-treatment benefit that may be even more salient in explaining the results of these trials. For low-risk patients (as evidenced by normal troponin levels), treatment effect becomes neutral, whereas it is modest overall and substantial among high-risk patients with positive troponins. These observations held with use of either the TIMI risk score or the presence or absence of ST-segment shifts to define risk categories. More recently, in a meta-analysis of eight randomized trials enrolling 3075 women and 7075 men (**Fig. 81-6** and Fig. 56-16), O'Donoghue and colleagues[71] confirmed that women benefit significantly from an invasive management strategy if they are biomarker positive (OR for death, MI, or rehospitalization for ACS, 0.67; 95% CI, 0.50 to 0.88) but not when they are biomarker negative (OR, 0.94; 95% CI, 0.61 to 1.44). Men benefited substantially if they were biomarker positive (OR, 0.56, 95% CI, 0.46 to 0.67) and trended toward benefit even when biomarker negative (OR 0.72; 95% CI, 0.51 to 1.01).

For a summary of coronary artery bypass grafting in women, consult the ACC/AHA guidelines for coronary artery bypass graft surgery.[72] In general, women have a higher risk for perioperative morbidity and mortality, but in many studies, much of this difference is explained by presentation of women at older ages and with more severe coronary disease, risk factors, and left ventricular dysfunction. Even at younger ages, and after adjustment for body size and other risk factors, women

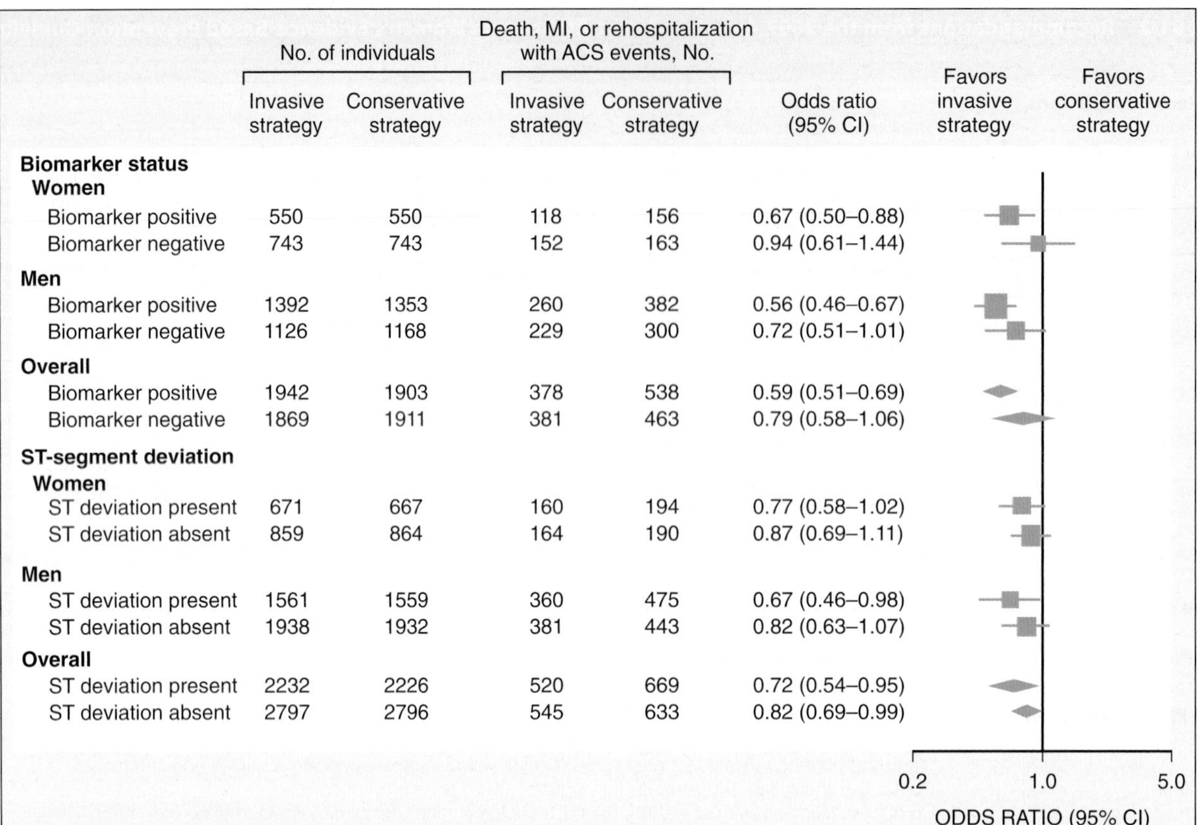

	No. of individuals		Death, MI, or rehospitalization with ACS events, No.			
	Invasive strategy	Conservative strategy	Invasive strategy	Conservative strategy	Odds ratio (95% CI)	Favors invasive strategy / Favors conservative strategy
Biomarker status						
Women						
Biomarker positive	550	550	118	156	0.67 (0.50–0.88)	
Biomarker negative	743	743	152	163	0.94 (0.61–1.44)	
Men						
Biomarker positive	1392	1353	260	382	0.56 (0.46–0.67)	
Biomarker negative	1126	1168	229	300	0.72 (0.51–1.01)	
Overall						
Biomarker positive	1942	1903	378	538	0.59 (0.51–0.69)	
Biomarker negative	1869	1911	381	463	0.79 (0.58–1.06)	
ST-segment deviation						
Women						
ST deviation present	671	667	160	194	0.77 (0.58–1.02)	
ST deviation absent	859	864	164	190	0.87 (0.69–1.11)	
Men						
ST deviation present	1561	1559	360	475	0.67 (0.46–0.98)	
ST deviation absent	1938	1932	381	443	0.82 (0.63–1.07)	
Overall						
ST deviation present	2232	2226	520	669	0.72 (0.54–0.95)	
ST deviation absent	2797	2796	545	633	0.82 (0.69–0.99)	

FIGURE 81-6 Death, MI, or rehospitalization with ACS for biomarker status and ST-segment deviation in trials of an invasive versus conservative treatment strategy in non–ST-segment elevation ACS, from a meta-analysis of several trials. Odds ratios were generated from random-effects models. Size of data markers is weighted on the basis of the inverse variance. The odds ratios and corresponding *P* values for the interaction terms for the efficacy of an invasive over a conservative strategy in biomarker-positive versus biomarker-negative patients were as follows: for all patients, OR for interaction, 0.79; *P* for interaction = 0.18; for women, OR for interaction, 0.75; *P* for interaction = 0.36; and for men, OR for interaction, 0.77; *P* for interaction = 0.09. The analogous data for patients with versus without ST-segment deviation were as follows: for all patients, OR for interaction, 0.83; *P* for interaction = 0.07; for women, OR for interaction, 0.87; *P* for interaction = 0.76; and for men, OR for interaction, 0.79; *P* for interaction = 0.07. VINO, VANQWISH, and ICTUS trials were excluded from the primary biomarker analysis because they enrolled only patients with elevated biomarkers, thus precluding the comparison of biomarker-positive and biomarker-negative subgroups. The meta-analysis ORs and 95% CIs for the efficacy of an invasive strategy versus conservative strategy if those three trials were also included were as follows: for all patients biomarker positive, OR, 0.72; 95% CI, 0.53-0.98; for all patients biomarker negative, OR, 0.79; 95% CI, 0.60-1.03; for biomarker-positive men, OR, 0.71; 95% CI, 0.49-1.01; for biomarker-negative men, OR, 0.72; 95% CI, 0.54-0.98; for biomarker-positive women, OR, 0.71; 95% CI, 0.56-0.91; and for biomarker-negative women, OR, 0.94; 95% CI, 0.61-1.44. *(From O'Donoghue M, Boden WE, Braunwald E, et al: Early invasive vs conservative treatment strategies in women and men with unstable angina and non–ST-segment elevation myocardial infarction: A meta-analysis. JAMA 300:71, 2008.)*

may be at slightly higher perioperative risk than men are.[73] Women have more postoperative depression than men but ultimately appear to recover similarly, although some reports suggest that quality of life may be rated lower in women than in men as far out as 1 year.[74-76] Long-term survival depends more on concomitant disease and risk factors, and after adjustment, it is similar in women and men. Thus, the guidelines recommend: "Coronary bypass surgery should therefore not be delayed or denied to women who have the appropriate indications for revascularization."[72]

Glycoprotein IIb/IIIa Inhibitors

A similar picture emerges with the small molecule glycoprotein IIb/IIIa inhibitors, with initial studies indicating heterogeneity of treatment effect by sex. Although men appeared to benefit from eptifibatide treatment, women had an increased rate of death or MI at 30 days in the Platelet Glycoprotein IIb/IIIa in Unstable Angina: Receptor Suppression Using Integrilin Therapy (PURSUIT) trial.[77] A subsequent meta-analysis of all small molecule glycoprotein IIb/IIIa inhibitor (eptifibatide or tirofiban) trials revealed similar results in aggregate.[78] However, once patients were stratified by risk with troponin results, it was clear that the treatment benefit extended to both men and women at high risk for adverse outcomes, and that adverse outcomes occurred mostly in low-risk individuals.

The recently completed Early Glycoprotein IIb/IIIa Inhibition in Non–ST-Segment Elevation Acute Coronary Syndrome (EARLY ACS) trial of early versus delayed provisional eptifibatide use among patients with non–ST-segment elevation ACS provides additional assurance of the safety of glycoprotein IIb/IIIa inhibitors among women who are at high risk at presentation.[79] Among patients who had at least two of the following—age ≥60 years, ST-segment shifts on the presenting electrocardiogram, or positive biomarkers of myocardial necrosis (84% of patients were troponin positive)—women and men had similar reductions in the primary endpoint of death, MI, recurrent ischemia requiring urgent revascularization, or thrombotic bailout at 96 hours (8% for men versus 7% for women; *P* for interaction, 0.949). Surprisingly, there was a trend toward a reduction in death or MI at 30 days among women (OR, 0.80; 95% CI, 0.64 to 1.004; $P = 0.052$) but not among men (OR, 0.94; 95% CI, 0.81 to 1.09). In aggregate, these results suggest that selected properly, women stand to benefit similarly from glycoprotein IIb/IIIa inhibition, but in situations in which treatment benefit is less certain (e.g., biomarker-negative patients), risks—particularly of bleeding—may predominate.

Bleeding with Antithrombotic Therapy

The differential treatment effects observed among women and men with the small molecule glycoprotein IIb/IIIa inhibitors and the relationship with risk for ischemic complications may be explained partly by the counterbalancing higher risk for complications of therapy, particularly bleeding. In a recent analysis from the Can Rapid Risk Stratification of Unstable Angina Patients Suppress Adverse Outcomes with Early Implementation of the ACC/AHA Guidelines (CRUSADE) registry, of patients receiving antithrombotic therapy with unfractionated heparin, enoxaparin, or a small molecule glycoprotein IIb/IIIa inhibitor, 42% received at least one initial dose outside of recommended dosing ranges.[80] Such overdosing associated with increased likelihood of bleeding that increased with the number of agents that were overdosed. Women were significantly more likely to be overdosed than were men, in part because of advanced age and associated renal impairment as well as lower body weight. Several studies have now shown that bleeding and the use of blood transfusions are associated with increased ischemic outcomes among patients with ACS[81-83]; thus, treatment of women at lower risk for adverse ischemic outcomes exposes them to both inherent bleeding risks of treatment and those associated with inappropriate dosing, to which they are more prone, that may offset or exceed any benefit of therapy. Careful attention, particularly to adjustments in dosing for body weight and estimated creatinine clearance, is critically important to ensure safe use of these therapies.

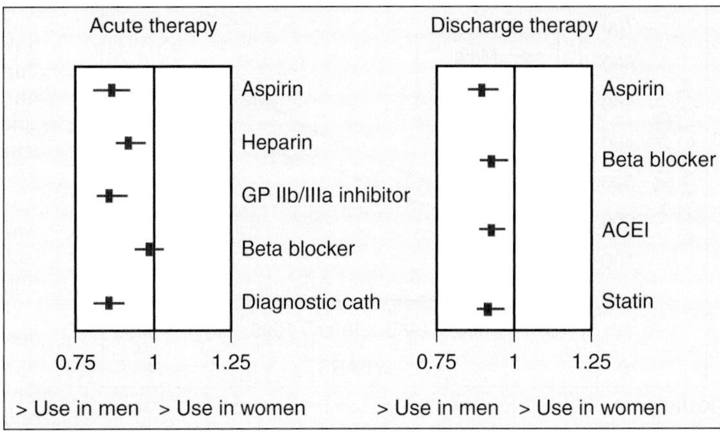

FIGURE 81-7 Use of guidelines-recommended therapies among women compared with men in the CRUSADE registry. ACEI = angiotensin-converting enzyme inhibitor; cath = cardiac catheterization; GP IIb/IIIa = glycoprotein IIb/IIIa. *(From Blomkalns AL, Chen AY, Hochman JS, et al; CRUSADE Investigators: Gender disparities in the diagnosis and treatment of non–ST-segment elevation acute coronary syndromes: Large-scale observations from the CRUSADE [Can Rapid Risk Stratification of Unstable Angina Patients Suppress Adverse Outcomes with Early Implementation of the American College of Cardiology/American Heart Association Guidelines] National Quality Improvement Initiative. J Am Coll Cardiol 45:832, 2005.)*

Sex Differences in Treatment

Despite abundant data in aggregate to support the use of existing evidence-based therapy similarly among women and men and sex-neutral practice guidelines for their use, undertreatment of women relative to men persists. In an analysis from the CRUSADE registry of patients with non–ST-segment elevation ACS, use of all therapies for acute management, including invasive management, and discharge management were suboptimal; but after adjustment for confounders, use of guidelines-recommended therapies and invasive management was lower in women than in men for all agents except beta-adrenergic receptor blockers (beta blockers) in the acute setting (**Fig. 81-7**).[84] These differences do not appear to be influenced by differences in objective measures of risk, such as troponin positivity or level of troponin elevation.[85] Among more than 345,000 patients with ST-segment elevation MI, the NRMI-1 investigators similarly observed lower rates of use of aspirin, beta blockers, and heparin in women compared with men and later administration of fibrinolytic therapy among women.[86] Using data from 78,254 patients in the Guidelines Applied in Practice data base, Jneid and colleagues[87] showed that in addition to lower use of guidelines-recommended medications, women had lower use of reperfusion therapy when eligible and also had longer times to either fibrinolytic therapy or primary PCI for ST-segment elevation MI. Equally important, women appear to have greater risk than men for nonadherence to long-term use of evidence-based medications in secondary prevention, particularly aspirin, statins, and angiotensin-converting enzyme (ACE) inhibitors.[88] Although the cause of these disparities in treatment and adherence is likely multifactorial, concerted efforts to correct them will be necessary for women to achieve the full potential of available therapies.

One important component of the strategy to improve adherence to cardiovascular disease guidelines is women's awareness of disease risk and physicians' awareness of guidelines and ability to correctly assess and assign risk level. Although the number of women who recognize cardiovascular disease as the leading cause of death among women has increased to 55% in a recent survey, in that same survey only 48% of women correctly identified the optimal level for blood pressure, 37% for HDL, 21% for LDL, and 31% for blood glucose concentration.[89] When present, though, individual awareness that one's level was not healthy did prompt initiation of steps to lower risk.

In a related study, 500 randomly selected physicians were surveyed about their awareness of and adherence to cardiovascular prevention guidelines.[90] Surprisingly, fewer than 1 in 5 physicians knew that more women than men die each year from cardiovascular disease. Using case studies, the investigators evaluated physicians' assessment of a patient's risk. Regardless of specialty, assignment of risk strongly associated with the recommendation for lifestyle or treatment interventions, but more women at calculated intermediate risk were perceived by physicians as being at low risk than occurred for intermediate-risk men. Thus, improved physician assessment of risk may be important in reducing undertreatment relative to guidelines recommendations.

Use of standardized treatment algorithms and participation in quality improvement programs may improve overall adherence to treatment guidelines and lessen sex-related undertreatment. The ACC's Guidelines Applied in Practice discharge tool is one such strategy that appears to be effective in increasing the use of guidelines-recommended therapies at discharge in both men and women.[91] Use of the tool may be associated with lower mortality among women at 1 year.

Cardiac Rehabilitation (see Chap. 50)

In a 2004 systematic review and meta-analysis of randomized controlled trials of exercised-based cardiac rehabilitation after MI that represented 48 trials since 1970, 21 included only men, 26 included both men and women, and 20% of all participants were women.[92] In aggregate, these trials showed a 20% reduction in total mortality and a 26% reduction in cardiac mortality among patients randomized to exercise-based cardiac rehabilitation compared with controls receiving usual care. Improvements in lipid levels and blood pressure and greater rates of smoking cessation were also found. Detailed analyses of men and women were not performed, but conclusions were general regarding the benefits of exercise-based cardiac rehabilitation after MI. In keeping with these findings, the ACC/AHA guidelines for the management of patients with ST-segment elevation MI provide a Class I recommendation for "cardiac rehabilitation/secondary prevention programs, when available … for patients with STEMI, particularly those with multiple modifiable risk factors and/or those moderate- to high-risk patients in whom supervised exercise training is warranted. (*Level of Evidence: C*)."[56] The guidelines for the management of patients with non–ST-segment elevation ACS recommend such programs especially for individuals who smoke.[50] Despite these recommendations, women are less likely than men to participate in cardiac rehabilitation after acute MI.[93]

Heart Failure (see Chaps. 26 to 30)

The prevalence of heart failure is increasing in both sexes. Although both the incidence and prevalence of heart failure are greater among

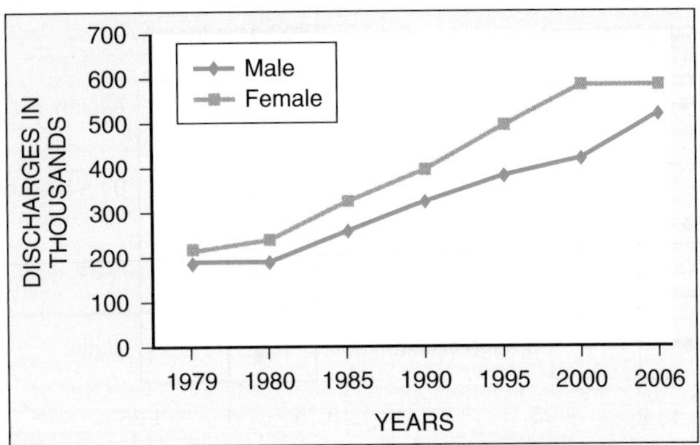

FIGURE 81-8 Trends in hospital discharges for heart failure from 1979 to 2006 by sex. *(From Lloyd-Jones D, Adams R, Carnethon M, et al: Heart disease and stroke statistics—2009 update: A report from the American Heart Association Statistics Committee and Stroke Statistics Subcommittee. Circulation 119:e21, 2009.)*

men than among women, the lifetime risk for development of heart failure among women and men at the age of 40 years is greater among women (1 in 6) than among men (1 in 9).[2] In 2004, women accounted for 57% of heart failure deaths, and heart failure continues to complicate acute MI more frequently in women than in men.[2] Although women accounted for more hospital discharges for heart failure each year than did men through 2000, that gap has narrowed through most recent estimates in 2006 (**Fig. 81-8**).[2]

The underlying pathophysiologic process of heart failure may be different in women and men. In the Medicare population, 80% of patients with heart failure and preserved systolic function are women (see Chap. 30).[94] Alcoholic cardiomyopathy occurs less frequently in women than in men, but this may be because of the lower prevalence of alcoholism among women; alcohol may actually be more toxic to the myocardium in women, with a lower total dose required to produce cardiomyopathy.[95] In a study of 105,388 patients admitted with acute decompensated heart failure, women accounted for 52% of cases but had preserved left ventricular function more frequently than men did (51% versus 28%).[96] Men and women had similar length of stay and adjusted in-hospital mortality; diuretic therapy was used similarly, but women received vasoactive agents less frequently. Although both sexes were undertreated with evidence-based oral therapies for heart failure, women were less likely than men to receive them. Additional data from the Acute Decompensated Heart Failure National Registry (ADHERE) indicate that approximately half of patients admitted for management of heart failure have preserved systolic function, and that these patients are more frequently women.[97] Reports from both the Mayo Clinic and the province of Ontario, Canada, reflect these findings of female prevalence among patients with heart failure with preserved left ventricular function.[98,99] Furthermore, these reports show an increasing prevalence of heart failure with preserved left ventricular function and indicate that its prognosis, which is similar to that of heart failure with systolic dysfunction, has remained essentially unchanged for more than a decade.

Because most evidence for the management of heart failure arises from trials in which left ventricular systolic dysfunction predominated or was a critical inclusion criterion and in which men predominated, assessment of the utility of these therapies in women is challenging—particularly when preserved systolic function is much more prominent among women with heart failure. The Candesartan in Heart Failure: Assessment of Reduction in Mortality and Morbidity (CHARM) clinical trials shed light on the treatment of both women and men with heart failure with preserved systolic function. In an aggregate analysis of CHARM trials, women more frequently had preserved systolic function (50%) than did men (35%). In these trials, despite generally lower use of evidence-based treatments for heart failure, women had lower adjusted mortality and the composite of death or heart failure hospitalization, regardless of cause of heart failure or left ventricular function. Benefit from treatment with candesartan, an angiotensin II receptor blocker, was identical in women and men.[100]

The current ACC/AHA heart failure guidelines recommend the following as a Class I recommendation: "Groups of patients including (a) high-risk ethnic minorities (e.g., blacks), (b) groups underrepresented in clinical trials, and (c) any groups believed to be underserved should, in the absence of specific evidence to direct otherwise, have clinical screening and therapy in a manner identical to that applied to the broader population. (*Level of Evidence: B*)."[101] In women, caution should be used in digoxin dosing, especially among elderly women with diminished renal function, and recognition of different side effect profiles, such as increased frequency of cough with ACE inhibitors, may be important.[101]

Implantable cardioverter-defibrillator (ICD) device implantation and cardiac resynchronization therapy are increasingly important components of the management of patients with heart failure and ischemic heart disease with left ventricular systolic dysfunction. The utility of and indication for ICD implantation and cardiac resynchronization therapy are reviewed in Chaps. 29 and 38. An excellent review on this topic by Goldberger and Lampert[102] is also available. Although multiple studies have provided evidence for use of these therapies, none of the studies, alone or in aggregate, have enrolled sufficient numbers of patients to allow meaningful conclusions about utility in women compared with men. Guidelines are therefore broadly inclusive and recommend use of ICD therapy for secondary prevention in all patients with "otherwise good clinical function and prognosis, for whom prolongation of survival is a goal."[101] As with the application of many therapies discussed previously, however, there is a substantial gap between men and women in the use of ICD therapy. In an analysis from the Guidelines Applied in Practice data base, only 35.4% of eligible patients received ICD therapy after MI. Relative to white men, both white women and black women were substantially less likely to receive an ICD (white women: OR, 0.62; 95% CI, 0.56 to 0.68; black women: OR, 0.56; 95% CI, 0.44 to 0.71).[103] Results were similar in older patients in the 2005 Centers for Medicare and Medicaid Services 5% sample data base. In this analysis of patients older than 65 years of age, men were more than three times as likely as women to receive an ICD when indicated for primary prevention (HR, 3.15; 95% CI, 2.86 to 3.47), but there was no reduction in mortality in the year after implantation among those who received an ICD.[104] For secondary prevention, men also more frequently received ICD therapy than women did (HR, 2.44; 95% CI, 2.30 to 2.59). In this setting, ICD therapy associated with 35% lower mortality among those who received an ICD.

Transplantation for the treatment of heart failure is used less frequently in women than in men. This is in part because of the older age of women with heart failure and differences in women's desires for transplantation.[105] According to AHA statistics, in the United States in 2004, 72.4% of transplant patients were men.[2] Among transplanted patients, 1-year survival rates were only slightly less among women (84.6%) compared with men (86.4%). This gap widened slightly at 3 years (76.1% versus 78.9%, respectively, in women and men) and at 5 years (68.5% versus 72.2%).

For a recent summary of heart failure etiology, diagnosis, and treatment in women, consult the excellent review by Hsich and Piña.[106]

Peripheral Arterial Disease (see Chap. 61)

Approximately 8 million Americans are believed to have lower extremity peripheral arterial disease, and their risk of death from cardiovascular disease is nearly sixfold greater than that of individuals without peripheral arterial disease.[2] As with coronary disease, the prevalence is slightly higher in men than in women.[107] Smoking and diabetes are the most potent risk factors for peripheral arterial disease. According to AHA 2009 summary statistics, only 10% of patients complain of classic intermittent claudication (ranging from 6/10,000 among men 30 to 44 years of age and 3/10,000 among women 30 to 44 years of age to 61/10,000 among men 65 to 74 years of age and 54/10,000 among women 65 to 74 years of age); 40% have no leg symptoms, and 50% have other atypical symptoms.[2] Particularly in elderly women, up to 66% may have no symptoms at all. For an in-depth summary of the epidemiology, diagnosis, and management of peripheral arterial disease, consult the 2005 AHA/ACC practice guidelines.[108] Recommendations for diagnosis and management generally are sex neutral. Interestingly, despite the higher cardiovascular risk among patients with peripheral vascular disease, use of aspirin for primary prevention among patients with ankle-brachial indices below 0.95 did not significantly improve outcomes compared with placebo in the 3350-patient Aspirin for Asymptomatic Atherosclerosis trial (results presented at the 2009 Scientific Sessions of the European Society of Cardiology, August 30, 2009), but the trial may have been underpowered considering the 12% reduction in primary prevention in the recent Antithrombotic Trialists' meta-analysis.[109]

The population prevalence of renal artery stenosis is not well established; but in older adults, it was determined in one study to be 8.4% and was more common in men (9.1%) than in women (5.5%).[110] About 90% of lesions are caused by atherosclerosis, but fibromuscular dysplasia is a particularly prevalent pathophysiologic finding in young women with hypertension and renal artery stenosis.[108] Guidelines for diagnosis and treatment are similar in women and in men.

Mesenteric arterial disease predominates in women; approximately two thirds of acute presentations are in elderly women (median age, 70 years), and 70% of chronic intestinal ischemia occurs in women.[108] Without treatment, acute intestinal ischemia is nearly always fatal. Surgical treatment to remove ischemic bowel and revascularize is given a Class I, B level of evidence recommendation in the guidelines for management of peripheral arterial disease.[108] Despite surgical treatment, mortality remains at approximately 70%. Percutaneous revascularization and surgical revascularization are recommended in the appropriate settings (see Chap. 63).[108] Abdominal aortic aneurysms caused by atherosclerotic disease are more prevalent in men than in women and are more prevalent in both sexes among older individuals and smokers.[108] Although treatment recommendations are sex neutral, screening of asymptomatic individuals is recommended in men but not in women because of the low number of abdominal aortic aneurysm–related deaths in women <75 years and the many competing health risks in older women.[111]

Future Perspectives

Cardiovascular disease is common among women, and as the population ages, the number of women living with coronary disease and its sequelae, such as heart failure, will only increase. In general, although underrepresentation of women in clinical trials persists, most existing treatments appear to be equally effective in women and men. Despite increasing awareness among physicians and women about cardiovascular disease risk, women are more likely to be undertreated and for some therapies are more susceptible to complications. Increased attention to careful selection of therapies according to risk and careful monitoring of dosing will be imperative to modulate the balance of benefit and risk in women. The growth in our understanding of genetic susceptibility to cardiovascular disease and rapid advances in genomic, proteomic, and metabolomic techniques promise to elucidate further the underpinnings of differences in disease pathophysiology in men and women that may ultimately lead to new therapies and perhaps the sex-specific application of new or existing therapies in the coming years.

REFERENCES

General and Risk Factors in Women

1. Wizemann TM, Pardue ML (eds): Institute of Medicine Committee on Understanding the Biology of Sex and Gender Differences. Exploring the Biological Contributions to Human Health. Does Sex Matter? Washington, DC, National Academy Press, 2001.
2. Lloyd-Jones D, Adams R, Carnethon M, et al: Heart disease and stroke statistics—2009 update: A report from the American Heart Association Statistics Committee and Stroke Statistics Subcommittee. Circulation 119:e21, 2009.
3. Shaw LJ, Merz CN, Pepine CJ, et al: The economic burden of angina in women with suspected ischemic heart disease: Results from the National Institutes of Health–National Heart, Lung and Blood Institute–sponsored Women's Ischemia Syndrome Evaluation. Circulation 114:894, 2006.
4. Ford ES, Ajani UA, Croft JB, et al: Explaining the decrease in U.S. deaths from coronary disease, 1980-2000. N Engl J Med 356:2388, 2007.
5. Ford ES, Capewell S: Coronary heart disease mortality among young adults in the U.S. from 1980 through 2002: Concealed leveling of mortality rates. J Am Coll Cardiol 50:2128, 2007.
6. Jneid H, Fonarow GC, Cannon CP, et al: Sex differences in medical care and early death after acute myocardial infarction. Circulation 118:2803, 2008.
7. Berger JS, Elliott L, Gallup D, et al: Sex differences in mortality following acute coronary syndromes. JAMA 302:874, 2009.
8. Lloyd-Jones DM, Larson MG, Beiser A, Levy D: Lifetime risk of developing coronary heart disease. Lancet 353:89, 1999.
9. Mosca L, Mochari H, Christian A, et al: National study of women's awareness, preventive action, and barriers to cardiovascular health. Circulation 113:525, 2006.
10. Barnhart J, Lewis V, Houghton JL, Charney P: Physician knowledge levels and barriers to coronary risk prevention in women: Survey results from the women and heart disease physician education initiative. Women's Health Issues 17:93, 2007.
11. Yusuf S, Hawken S, Ôunpuu S, et al: Effect of potentially modifiable risk factors associated with myocardial infarction in 52 countries (the INTERHEART study): Case-control study. Lancet 364:937, 2004.
12. Yusuf S, Reddy S, Ôunpuu S, Anand S: Global burden of cardiovascular diseases: Part I: General considerations, the epidemiologic transition, risk factors, and impact of urbanization. Circulation 104:2746, 2001.
13. Vaccarino V, Parsons L, Every NR, et al: Sex-based differences in early mortality after myocardial infarction. National Registry of Myocardial Infarction 2 Participants. N Engl J Med 341:217, 1999.

Hormone Therapy

14. Hulley S, Grady D, Bush T, et al: Randomized trial of estrogen plus progestin for secondary prevention of coronary heart disease in postmenopausal women. JAMA 280:605, 1998.
15. Grady D, Herrington D, Bittner V, et al: Cardiovascular disease outcomes during 6.8 years of hormone therapy: Heart and Estrogen/Progestin Replacement Study follow-up (HERS II) [erratum in JAMA 288:1064, 2002]. JAMA 288:49, 2002.
16. Manson JE, Hsia J, Johnson KC, et al: Estrogen plus progestin and the risk of coronary heart disease. N Engl J Med 349:523, 2003.
17. Women's Health Initiative Steering Committee: Effects of conjugated equine estrogen in postmenopausal women with hysterectomy: The Women's Health Initiative randomized controlled trial. JAMA 291:1701, 2004.
18. Ouyang P, Michos ED, Karas RH: Hormone replacement therapy and the cardiovascular system: Lessons learned and unanswered questions. J Am Coll Cardiol 47:1741, 2006.

Genetics

19. Zdravkovic S, Wienke A, Pedersen NL, et al: Heritability of death from coronary heart disease: A 36-year follow-up of 20 966 Swedish twins. J Intern Med 252:247, 2002.
20. Murabito JM, Pencina MJ, Nam BH, et al: Sibling cardiovascular disease as a risk factor for cardiovascular disease in middle-aged adults. JAMA 294:3117, 2005.
21. Paynter NP, Chasman DI, Pare G, et al: Association between a literature-based genetic risk score and cardiovascular events in women. JAMA 303:631, 2010.
22. Yamada Y, Izawa H, Ichihara S, et al: Prediction of the risk of myocardial infarction from polymorphisms in candidate genes. N Engl J Med 347:1916, 2002.

Mechanisms of Coronary Artery Disease in Women

23. Ng MKC, Quinn CM, McCrohon JA, et al: Androgens up-regulate atherosclerosis-related genes in macrophages from males but not females: Molecular insights into gender differences in atherosclerosis. J Am Coll Cardiol 42:1306, 2003.
24. Kramer MC, Rittersma SZ, de Winter RJ, et al: Relationship of thrombus healing to underlying plaque morphology in sudden coronary death. J Am Coll Cardiol 55:122, 2010.
25. English JL, Jacobs LO, Green G, et al: Effect of the menstrual cycle on endothelium dependent vasodilation of the brachial artery in normal young women. Am J Cardiol 82:256, 1998.
26. Sader MA, McCredie RJ, Griffiths KA, et al: Oestradiol improves arterial endothelial function in healthy men receiving testosterone. Clin Endocrinol (Oxf) 54:175, 2001.
27. Weksler B: Hemostasis and thrombosis. *In* Douglas PS (ed): Cardiovascular Health and Disease in Women. 2nd ed. Philadelphia, WB Saunders, 2002, pp 157-177.
28. Virmani R, Burke AP, Farb A, Kolodgie FD: Pathology of the vulnerable plaque. J Am Coll Cardiol 47(Suppl):C13, 2006.

Specific Risk Factors in Women

29. Fields LE, Burt VL, Cutler JA, et al: The burden of adult hypertension in the United States 1999 to 2000: A rising tide. Hypertension 44:398, 2004.
30. Prospective Studies Collaboration: Age-specific relevance of usual blood pressure to vascular mortality: A meta-analysis of individual data for one million adults in 61 prospective studies. Lancet 360:1903, 2002.
31. Vasan RS, Larson MG, Leip EP, et al: Impact of high-normal blood pressure on the risk of cardiovascular disease. N Engl J Med 345:1291, 2001.
32. Hajjar I, Kotchen TA: Trends in prevalence, awareness, treatment, and control of hypertension in the United States, 1988-2000. JAMA 290:199, 2003.
33. Expert Panel on Detection, Evaluation, and Treatment of High Blood Cholesterol in Adults: Executive Summary of the Third Report of the National Cholesterol Education Program (NCEP) Expert Panel on Detection, Evaluation, and Treatment of High Blood Cholesterol in Adults (Adult Treatment Panel III). JAMA 285:2486, 2001.
34. Ford ES, Giles WH, Dietz WH: Prevalence of the metabolic syndrome among US adults: Findings from the third National Health and Nutrition Examination Survey. JAMA 287:356, 2002.
35. Shai I, Rimm EB, Hankinson SE, et al: Multivariate assessment of lipid parameters as predictors of coronary heart disease among postmenopausal women: Potential implications for clinical guidelines. Circulation 110:2824, 2004.
36. Jensen J, Nilas L, Christiansen C: Influence of menopause on serum lipids and lipoproteins. Maturitas 12:321, 1990.
37. Ford ES, Mokdad AH, Giles WH, Mensah GA: Serum total cholesterol concentrations and awareness, treatment, and control of hypercholesterolemia among US adults: Findings from the National Health and Nutrition Examination Survey, 1999 to 2000. Circulation 107:2185, 2003.

38. Mokdad AH, Ford ES, Bowman BA, et al: Prevalence of obesity, diabetes, and obesity-related health risk factors, 2001. JAMA 289:76, 2003.
39. Ogden CL, Carroll MD, McDowell MA, Flegal KM: Obesity among adults in the United States: No statistically significant change since 2003-2004. NCHS Data Brief No 1. Hyattsville, Md, National Center for Health Statistics, 2007.
40. Troiano RP, Berrigan D, Dodd KW, et al: Physical activity in the United States measured by accelerometer. Med Sci Sports Exerc 40:181, 2008.
41. Eaton DK, Kann L, Kinchen S, et al; Centers for Disease Control and Prevention (CDC): Youth risk behavior surveillance: United States, 2007. MMWR Surveill Summ 57:1, 2008.
42. Kimm SY, Glynn NW, Kriska AM, et al. Decline in physical activity in black girls and white girls during adolescence. N Engl J Med 347:709, 2002.
43. Ford ES, Giles WH, Mokdad AH: The distribution of 10-year risk for coronary heart disease among US adults: Findings from the National Health and Nutrition Examination Survey III. J Am Coll Cardiol 43:1791, 2004.
44. Ridker PM, Buring JE, Rifai N, Cook NR: Development and validation of improved algorithms for the assessment of global cardiovascular risk in women: The Reynolds Risk Score. JAMA 297:611, 2007.
45. Lakoski SG, Greenland G, Wong ND, et al: Coronary artery calcium scores and risk for cardiovascular events in women classified as "low risk" based on Framingham Risk Score: The Multi-Ethnic Study of Atherosclerosis (MESA). Arch Intern Med 167:2437, 2007.
46. Kyker KA, Limacher MC: Gender differences in presentation and symptoms of coronary artery disease. Curr Womens Health Rep 2:115, 2002.
47. Milner KA, Funk M, Richards S, et al: Gender differences in symptom presentation associated with coronary heart disease. Am J Cardiol 84:396, 1999.
48. Kudenchuk PJ, Maynard C, Martin JS, et al: Comparison of presentation, treatment, and outcome of acute myocardial infarction in men versus women (The Myocardial Infarction Triage and Intervention Registry). Am J Cardiol 78:9, 1996.
49. McGuire DK, Newby LK, Biswas MS, Hochman JS: The elderly, women, and patients with diabetes mellitus. *In* Theroux P (ed): Acute Coronary Syndromes: A Companion to Braunwald's Heart Disease. Philadelphia, Elsevier Science, 2003, pp 553-573.
50. Braunwald E, Antman EM, Beasley JW, et al: ACC/AHA guidelines update for the management of patients with unstable angina and non–ST-segment elevation myocardial infarction. A report of the American College of Cardiology/American Heart Association Task Force on Practice Guidelines (Committee on the Management of Patients with Unstable Angina), 2002. Available at: http://www.acc.org/clinical/guidelines/unstable/unstable.pdf. Accessed June 30, 2006.
51. Shaw LJ, Bairey Merz CN, Pepine CJ, et al: Insights from the NHLBI-sponsored Women's Ischemia Syndrome Evaluation (WISE) Study. Part I: Gender differences in traditional and novel risk factors, symptom evaluation, and gender-optimized diagnostic strategies. J Am Coll Cardiol 47:4S, 2006.
52. Alexander KP, Shaw LJ, DeLong ER, et al: Value of exercise treadmill testing in women. J Am Coll Cardiol 32:1657, 1998.
53. Gibbons RJ, Balady GJ, Bricker JT, et al: ACC/AHA Guidelines update for exercise testing. A report of the American College of Cardiology/American Heart Association Task Force on Practice Guidelines (Committee on Exercise Testing), 2002. Available at: www.acc.org/clinical/guidelines/exercise/dirIndex.htm. Accessed July 16, 2006.
54. Mieres JH, Shaw LJ, Arai A, et al: Role of noninvasive testing in the clinical evaluation of women with suspected coronary artery disease: Consensus statement from the Cardiac Imaging Committee, Council of Clinical Cardiology, and the Cardiovascular Imaging and Intervention Committee, Council on Cardiovascular Radiology and Intervention, American Heart Association. Circulation 111:682, 2005.
55. Shaw LJ, Vasey C, Sawada S, et al: Impact of gender on risk stratification by exercise and dobutamine stress echocardiography: Long-term mortality in 4234 women and 6898 men. Eur Heart J 26:447, 2005.
56. Lee PY, Alexander KP, Hammill BG, et al: Representation of elderly persons and women in published randomized trials of acute coronary syndromes. JAMA 286:708, 2001.
57. Melloni C, Wang TY, Pieper KS, et al: Representation of women in randomized clinical trials of cardiovascular disease prevention [abstract]. J Am Coll Cardiol 51:A249, 2008.
58. Berger JS, Bairey-Merz CN, Redberg RF, Douglas PS: Improving the quality of care for women with cardiovascular disease: Report of a DCRI Think Tank, March 8 to 9, 2007. Am Heart J 156:816; 825.e1, 2008.

Evidence Base for Cardiovascular Therapy in Women

59. Antman EM, Anbe DT, Armstrong PW, et al: ACC/AHA guidelines for the management of patients with ST-elevation myocardial infarction. A report of the American College of Cardiology/American Heart Association Task Force on Practice Guidelines (Committee to Revise the 1999 Guidelines for the Management of Patients with Acute Myocardial Infarction. Circulation 110:e82, 2004.
60. Smith SC Jr, Allen J, Blair SN, et al: AHA/ACC guidelines for secondary prevention for patients with coronary and other atherosclerotic vascular disease: 2006 update. J Am Coll Cardiol 47:2130, 2006.
61. Gibbons RJ, Abrams J, Chatterjee K, et al: ACC/AHA guidelines update for the management of patients with chronic stable angina—summary article. A report of the American College of Cardiology/American Heart Association Task Force on Practice Guidelines (Committee on the Management of Patients with Chronic Stable Angina). Circulation 107:149, 2003.
62. Mosca L, Banka CL, Benjamin EJ, et al: American Heart Association evidence-based guidelines for cardiovascular disease prevention in women: 2007 update. J Am Coll Cardiol 49:1230, 2007.
63. Ridker PM, Cook NR, Lee I-M, et al: A randomized trial of low-dose aspirin in the primary prevention of cardiovascular disease in women. N Engl J Med 352:1293, 2005.
64. Berger JS, Roncaglioni MC, Avanzini F, et al: Aspirin for the primary prevention of cardiovascular events in women and men: A sex-specific meta-analysis of randomized controlled trials. JAMA 295:306, 2006.
65. Cannon CP, Braunwald E, McCabe CH, et al: Intensive versus moderate lipid lowering with statins after acute coronary syndromes [erratum in N Engl J Med 354:778, 2006]. N Engl J Med 350:1495, 2004.
66. Ridker PM, Danielson E, Fonseca FA, et al: Rosuvastatin to prevent vascular events in men and women with elevated C-reactive protein. N Engl J Med 359:2195, 2008.
67. Lansky AJ, Hochman JS, Ward PA, et al: Percutaneous coronary intervention and adjunctive pharmacotherapy in women: A statement for healthcare professionals from the American Heart Association. Circulation 111:940, 2005.
68. Glaser R, Herrmann HC, Murphy SA, et al: Benefit of an early invasive management strategy in women with acute coronary syndromes. JAMA 288:3124, 2002.
69. Lagerqvist B, Safstrom K, Stahle E, et al: Is early invasive treatment of unstable coronary artery disease equally effective for both women and men? FRISC II Study Group Investigators. J Am Coll Cardiol 38:41, 2001.
70. Clayton TC, Pocock SJ, Henderson RA, et al: Do men benefit more than women from an interventional strategy in patients with unstable angina or non–ST-elevation myocardial infarction? The impact of gender in the RITA 3 trial. Eur Heart J 25:1641, 2004.
71. O'Donoghue M, Boden WE, Braunwald E, et al: Early invasive versus conservative treatment strategies in women and men with unstable angina and non–ST-segment elevation myocardial infarction: A metaanalysis. JAMA 300:71, 2008.
72. Eagle KA, Guyton RA, Davidoff R, et al: ACC/AHA guideline update for coronary artery bypass graft surgery. A report of the American College of Cardiology/American Heart Association Task Force on Practice Guidelines (Committee to Update the 1999 Guidelines for Coronary Artery Bypass Graft Surgery), 2004. Available at: http://www.acc.org/clinical/guidelines/cabg/cabg.pdf. Accessed July 12, 2006.
73. Vaccarino V, Abramson JL, Veledar E, Weintraub WS: Sex differences in hospital mortality after coronary artery bypass surgery: Evidence for a higher mortality in younger women. Circulation 105:1176, 2002.
74. Vaccarino V, Lin ZQ, Kasl SV, et al: Sex differences in health status after coronary artery bypass surgery. Circulation 108:2642, 2003.
75. Keresztes PA, Merritt SL, Holm K, et al: The coronary artery bypass experience: Gender differences. Heart Lung 32:308, 2003.
76. Le Grande MR, Elliott PC, Murphy BM, et al: Health related quality of life trajectories and predictors following coronary artery bypass surgery. Health Qual Life Outcomes 4:49, 2006.
77. The PURSUIT Trial Investigators: Inhibition of platelet glycoprotein IIb/IIIa with eptifibatide in patients with acute coronary syndromes. Platelet Glycoprotein IIb/IIIa in Unstable Angina: Receptor Suppression Using Integrilin Therapy. N Engl J Med 339:436, 1998.
78. Boersma E, Harrington RA, Moliterno DJ, et al: Platelet glycoprotein IIb/IIIa inhibitors in acute coronary syndromes: A meta-analysis of all major randomised clinical trials [erratum in Lancet 359:2120, 2002]. Lancet 359:189, 2002.
79. Giugliano RP, White JA, Bode C, et al: Early versus delayed, provisional eptifibatide in acute coronary syndromes. N Engl J Med 360:2176, 2009.
80. Alexander KP, Chen AY, Roe MT, et al: Excess dosing of antiplatelet and antithrombin agents in the treatment of non–ST-segment elevation acute coronary syndromes. JAMA 294:3108, 2005.
81. Rao SV, Jollis JG, Harrington RA, et al: Relationship of blood transfusion and clinical outcomes in patients with acute coronary syndromes. JAMA 292:1555, 2004.
82. Rao SV, O'Grady K, Pieper KS, et al: Impact of bleeding severity on clinical outcomes among patients with acute coronary syndromes. Am J Cardiol 96:1200, 2005.
83. Yusuf S, Mehta SR, Chrolavicius S, et al: Comparison of fondaparinux and enoxaparin in acute coronary syndromes. N Engl J Med 354:1464, 2006.
84. Blomkalns AL, Chen AY, Hochman JS, et al: Gender disparities in the diagnosis and treatment of non–ST-segment elevation acute coronary syndromes: Large-scale observations from the CRUSADE (Can Rapid Risk Stratification of Unstable Angina Patients Suppress Adverse Outcomes with Early Implementation of the American College of Cardiology/American Heart Association Guidelines) National Quality Improvement Initiative. J Am Coll Cardiol 45:832, 2005.
85. Halim SA, Mulgund J, Chen AY, et al: Use of guidelines-recommended management and outcomes among women and men with low-level troponin elevation: Insights from CRUSADE. Circ Cardiovasc Qual Outcomes 2:199, 2009.
86. Vaccarino V, Rathore SS, Wenger NK, et al: Sex and racial differences in the management of acute myocardial infarction, 1994 through 2002. N Engl J Med 353:671, 2005.
87. Jneid H, Fonarow GC, Cannon CP, et al: Sex differences in medical care and early death after acute myocardial infarction. Circulation 118:2803, 2008.
88. Newby LK, Allen LaPointe NM, et al: Long-term adherence to evidence-based secondary prevention therapies in coronary artery disease. Circulation 113:203, 2006.
89. Mosca L, Mochari H, Christian A, et al: National study of women's awareness, preventive action, and barriers to cardiovascular health. Circulation 113:525, 2006.
90. Mosca L, Linfante AH, Benjamin EJ, et al: National study of physician awareness and adherence to cardiovascular disease prevention guidelines. Circulation 111:499, 2005.
91. Jani SM, Montoye C, Mehta R, et al: Sex differences in the application of evidence-based therapies for the treatment of acute myocardial infarction. Arch Intern Med 166:1164, 2006.
92. Taylor RS, Brown A, Ebrahim S, et al: Exercise-based rehabilitation for patients with coronary heart disease: Systematic review and meta-analysis of randomized controlled trials. Am J Med 116:682, 2004.
93. Witt BJ, Jacobsen SJ, Weston SA, et al: Cardiac rehabilitation after myocardial infarction in the community. J Am Coll Cardiol 44:988, 2004.

Heart Failure in Women

94. Masoudi FA, Havranek EP, Smith G, et al: Gender, age, and heart failure with preserved left ventricular systolic function. J Am Coll Cardiol 41:217, 2003.
95. Fernandez-Sola J, Nicolas-Arfelis JM: Gender differences in alcoholic cardiomyopathy. J Gend Specif Med 5:41, 2002.
96. Galvao M, Kalman J, DeMarco T, et al: Gender differences in in-hospital management and outcomes in patients with decompensated heart failure: Analysis from the Acute Decompensated Heart Failure National Registry (ADHERE). J Card Fail 12:100, 2006.
97. Yancy CW, Lopatin M, Stevenson LW, et al: Clinical presentation, management, and in-hospital outcomes of patients admitted with acute decompensated heart failure with preserved systolic function: A report from the Acute Decompensated Heart Failure National Registry (ADHERE) Database [erratum in J Am Coll Cardiol 47:1502, 2006]. J Am Coll Cardiol 47:76, 2006.

98. Owan TE, Hodge DO, Herges RM, et al: Trends in prevalence and outcome of heart failure with preserved ejection fraction. N Engl J Med 355:251, 2006.
99. Bhatia RS, Tu JV, Lee DS, et al: Outcome of heart failure with preserved ejection fraction in a population-based study. N Engl J Med 355:260, 2006.
100. O'Meara E, Clayton T, McEntegart MB, et al: Sex differences in clinical characteristics and prognosis in a broad spectrum of patients with heart failure: Results of the Candesartan in Heart failure: Assessment of Reduction in Mortality and morbidity (CHARM) program. Circulation 115:3111, 2007.
101. Hunt SA, Abraham WT, Chin MH, et al: ACC/AHA Guideline update for the diagnosis and management of chronic heart failure in the adult. A report of the American College of Cardiology/American Heart Association Task Force on Practice Guidelines (Writing Committee to Update the 2001 Guidelines for the Evaluation and Management of Heart Failure), 2005. Available at: http://www.acc.org/clinical/guidelines/failure//index.pdf. Accessed June 25, 2006.
102. Goldberger Z, Lampert R: Implantable cardioverter-defibrillators: Expanding indication and technologies. JAMA 295:809, 2006.
103. Hernandez AF, Fonarow GC, Liang L, et al: Sex and racial differences in the use of implantable cardioverter-defibrillators among patients hospitalized with heart failure. JAMA 298:1525, 2007.
104. Curtis LH, Al-Khatib SM, Shea AM, et al: Sex differences in the use of implantable cardioverter-defibrillators for primary and secondary prevention of sudden cardiac death. JAMA 298:1517, 2007.
105. Aaronson KD, Schwartz JS, Goin JE, et al: Sex differences in patient acceptance of cardiac transplant candidacy. Circulation 91:2753, 1995.
106. Hsich EM, Piña IL: Heart failure in women: A need for prospective data. J Am Coll Cardiol 54:491, 2009.

Peripheral Arterial Disease in Women

107. Criqui MH: Peripheral arterial disease—epidemiological aspects. Vasc Med 6(Suppl):3, 2001.
108. Hirsch AT, Haskal ZJ, Hertzer NR, et al: ACC/AHA 2005 guidelines for the management of patients with peripheral arterial disease (lower extremity, renal, mesenteric, and abdominal aortic): A collaborative report from the American Association for Vascular Surgery/Society for Vascular Surgery, Society for Cardiovascular Angiography and Interventions, Society for Vascular Medicine and Biology, Society of Interventional Radiology, and the ACC/AHA Task Force on Practice Guidelines (Writing Committee to Develop Guidelines for the Management of Patients with Peripheral Arterial Disease), 2005. Available at: http://www.acc.org/clinical/guidelines/pad/index.pdf. Accessed July 16, 2006.
109. Antithrombotic Trialists' Collaboration: Aspirin in the primary and secondary prevention of vascular disease: Collaborative meta-analysis of individual participant data from randomized trials. Lancet 373:1849, 2009.
110. Hansen KJ, Edwards MS, Craven TE, et al: Prevalence of renovascular disease in the elderly: A population-based study. J Vasc Surg 36:443, 2002.
111. U.S. Preventive Services Task Force: Screening for abdominal aortic aneurysm: Recommendation statement. Ann Intern Med 142:198, 2005.

CHAPTER 82 Pregnancy and Heart Disease

Carole A. Warnes

Approximately 2% of pregnancies involve maternal cardiovascular disease, and as such, this poses an increased risk to both mother and fetus. Most women with cardiovascular disease can have a pregnancy with proper care, but a careful pre-pregnancy evaluation is mandatory. Cardiac disease may sometimes be manifested for the first time in pregnancy because the hemodynamic changes may compromise a limited cardiac reserve.[1] Conversely, the symptoms and signs of a normal pregnancy may mimic the presence of cardiac disease. Lightheadedness, dizziness, shortness of breath, peripheral edema, and even syncope often occur in the course of a normal pregnancy, and for the unwary physician, cardiac disease may be suspected. An understanding of the normal cardiac examination of a pregnant patient is therefore important. For those physicians counseling patients with cardiac disease about the potential risks of a pregnancy, a comprehensive knowledge of the underlying defect as well as of the hemodynamic changes that pregnancy will impose is imperative.

With the declining incidence of rheumatic heart disease in Western countries, most maternal cardiac disease is now congenital in origin. Other cardiovascular problems seen include cardiomyopathies, both dilated and hypertrophic, and valvular disease, such as bicuspid aortic valve and mitral valve prolapse. Less common problems include pulmonary hypertension and, rarely, coronary artery disease. Prepregnancy counseling is important to give prospective mothers appropriate information about the advisability of pregnancy and to discuss the risks to her and the fetus. Such patients should be seen in a high-risk pregnancy unit and have a clinical examination, electrocardiogram, and chest radiograph. An echocardiogram facilitates a detailed evaluation of myocardial function, valvular disease, and pulmonary pressures. For patients with congenital heart disease, their perception of normal activity may be skewed, and an exercise test is helpful in delineating their true functional aerobic capacity. In general, patients who cannot achieve more than 70% of their predicted functional aerobic capacity are unlikely to tolerate a pregnancy safely. During this visit, it is important to take a careful family history to assess whether there is any congenital heart disease in the family. Genetic counseling may also be considered, if necessary. A careful discussion of the maternal and fetal risks should be made at the time of prepregnancy counseling, and if the mother is going to pursue a pregnancy, a strategy should be outlined regarding the frequency of follow-up by the cardiologist, and a plan should be put in place for labor and delivery.[2]

A multicenter Canadian study has suggested that maternal cardiac risk may be predicted by the use of a risk index.[3] Four predictors of maternal cardiac events are as follows: (1) prior cardiac event (e.g., heart failure, transient ischemic attack, or stroke before pregnancy) or arrhythmia; (2) baseline New York Heart Association (NYHA) class higher than Class II or cyanosis; (3) left-sided heart obstruction (mitral valve area smaller than 2 cm^2, aortic valve area less than 1.5 cm^2, or peak left ventricular outflow tract gradient more than 30 mm Hg by echocardiography); and (4) reduced systemic ventricular systolic function (ejection fraction less than 40%). Each of 599 pregnancies was assigned 1 point when each predictor was present. No pregnancy received more than 3 points. The estimated risk of a cardiac event in pregnancies with 0, 1, and more than 1 point was 5%, 27%, and 75%, respectively. It was concluded that those with a low cardiac risk of 0 could safely be delivered in a community hospital, but those at intermediate or high cardiac risk (risk score of 1 or more) should be delivered at a regional center.

During pregnancy, a multidisciplinary team approach is recommended, with close collaboration with the obstetrician so that the mode, timing, and location of delivery can be planned.[4] The management should be tailored to the specific needs of the patient. During pregnancy, fetal growth is monitored by the obstetric team, and for the woman with congenital heart disease, a fetal cardiac echocardiogram is offered at about 22 to 26 weeks of pregnancy to determine whether the baby has a congenital cardiac anomaly.

Hemodynamic Changes

During Pregnancy

The hemodynamic changes are profound and begin early in the first trimester. The plasma volume begins to increase in the sixth week of pregnancy and by the second trimester approaches 50% above baseline (**Fig. 82-1**). The plasma volume then tends to plateau until delivery. This increased plasma volume is followed by a slightly lesser rise in red cell mass, which results in the relative anemia of pregnancy. The heart rate begins to increase to about 20% above baseline to facilitate the increase in cardiac output (**Fig. 82-2**). Uterine blood flow increases with placental growth, and there is a fall in peripheral resistance. This decreased peripheral resistance may result in a slight fall in blood pressure, which also begins in the first trimester. The venous pressure in the lower extremities rises, which is why approximately 80% of healthy pregnant women develop pedal edema. The adaptive changes of a normal pregnancy result in an increase in cardiac output, which also begins in the first trimester and by the end of the second trimester approaches 30% to 50% above baseline.

These hemodynamic changes may cause problems for the mother with cardiac disease. The added volume load may obviously compromise a patient who has impaired ventricular function and limited cardiac reserve. Stenotic valvular lesions (e.g., aortic stenosis) are less well tolerated than regurgitant lesions because the decrease in peripheral resistance exaggerates the gradient across the aortic valve.

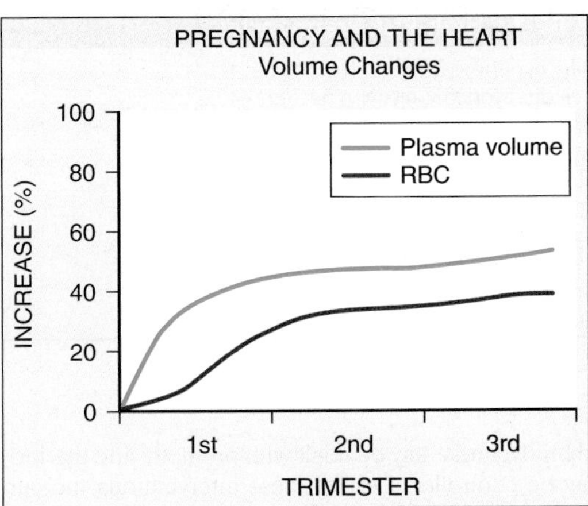

FIGURE 82-1 Plasma volume and red blood cell (RBC) increase during the trimesters of pregnancy. The plasma volume increases to approximately 50% above baseline by the second trimester and then virtually plateaus until delivery.

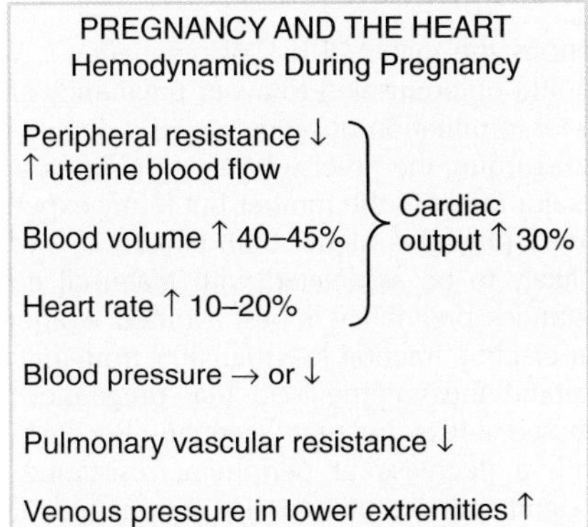

FIGURE 82-2 Hemodynamic changes during pregnancy relate to increased cardiac output and a fall in peripheral resistance. Blood pressure in most patients remains the same or falls slightly. Venous pressure in the legs increases, causing pedal edema in many patients.

Similarly, the tachycardia of pregnancy reduces the time for diastolic filling in a patient with mitral stenosis, with resultant increase in left atrial pressure. In contrast, with a lesion such as mitral regurgitation, the afterload reduction helps offset the volume load on the left ventricle that gestation imposes.

During Labor and Delivery

The hemodynamic changes during labor and delivery are abrupt. With each uterine contraction, up to 500 mL of blood is released into the circulation, prompting a rapid increase in cardiac output and blood pressure. The cardiac output is often 50% above baseline during the second stage of labor and may be even higher at the time of delivery. During a normal vaginal delivery, approximately 400 mL of blood is lost. In contrast, with a cesarean section, about 800 mL of blood is often lost and may pose a more significant hemodynamic burden to the parturient. After delivery of the baby, there is an abrupt increase in venous return, in part because of autotransfusion from the uterus but also because the baby no longer compresses the inferior vena cava. In addition, there continues to be autotransfusion of blood in the 24 to 72 hours after delivery, and this is when pulmonary edema may occur.

All these abrupt changes mandate that for the high-risk patient with cardiac disease, a multidisciplinary approach during labor and delivery is essential. The cardiologist and obstetrician should work with the anesthesiologist to determine the safest mode of delivery.

For most patients with cardiac disease, a vaginal delivery is feasible and preferable; a cesarean section is indicated only for obstetric reasons. Exceptions to this include the patient who is anticoagulated with warfarin because the baby is also anticoagulated, and vaginal delivery carries an increased risk to the fetus of intracranial hemorrhage. Cesarean section may also be considered in patients who have a dilated unstable aorta (e.g., Marfan syndrome), severe pulmonary hypertension, or a severe obstructive lesion such as aortic stenosis. High-risk patients should be delivered in a center where expertise is available to monitor the hemodynamic changes of labor and delivery and to intervene when necessary. If vaginal delivery is elected, fetal and maternal electrocardiographic monitoring should be performed. Delivery can be accomplished with the mother in the left lateral position so that the fetus does not compress the inferior vena cava, thereby maintaining venous return. The second stage should be assisted, if necessary (e.g., forceps or vacuum extraction), to avoid a long labor. Blood and volume loss should be replaced promptly. For those patients with tenuous hemodynamics, Swan-Ganz catheterization before active labor facilitates optimization of the hemodynamics and should be continued for at least 24 hours after delivery, when pulmonary edema commonly occurs.

Although there is no consensus regarding the administration of antibiotic prophylaxis at the time of delivery for patients with lesions vulnerable to infective endocarditis, many institutions routinely give antibiotics because of the documented bacteremia. This can occur even during an uncomplicated delivery.[5] Patients who are most vulnerable to the deleterious effects of endocarditis are those with cyanotic heart disease and prosthetic valves.[6]

Evaluation

Physical Examination (see Chap. 12)

Because of the altered hemodynamics during pregnancy, the physical examination findings of a healthy pregnant woman change and may mimic cardiac disease. The heart rate increases and the pulse volume is often bounding. By the middle of the second trimester, the jugular venous pressure may be elevated, with brisk descents, because of the volume overload and reduced peripheral resistance. The apical impulse is more prominent, and on auscultation, the first sound may appear loud. Commonly, there is an ejection systolic murmur at the left sternal edge, never more than grade 3/6 in intensity, which relates to increased flow through the left or right ventricular outflow tract. A third sound is very common. There should be no diastolic murmur. The second sound may also appear accentuated, and these combined auscultatory features may suggest an atrial septal defect or pulmonary hypertension. Continuous murmurs may also be heard, from either a cervical venous hum or a mammary souffle. Peripheral edema is common as pregnancy advances. If there is any concern that the physical examination suggests cardiac disease, transthoracic echocardiography should be performed. This facilitates the evaluation of ventricular size and function, valvular heart disease, and any potential shunts (e.g., atrial septal defect, ventricular septal defect) and the noninvasive assessment of pulmonary artery pressure.

Imaging (see Chaps. 15 to 19)

CHEST RADIOGRAPHY. A chest radiograph is not obtained routinely in any pregnant patient because of concern about radiation to the fetus, but it should be considered in any patient when there are concerns about her cardiac status and new onset of dyspnea or failure. The chest radiograph in a normal healthy patient may show slight prominence of the pulmonary artery, and as pregnancy advances, elevation of the diaphragm may suggest an increase in the cardiothoracic ratio.

TRANSTHORACIC ECHOCARDIOGRAPHY. This is the cornerstone of cardiac evaluation in pregnancy and facilitates differentiation of the features of cardiac disease from those of a normal pregnancy. It is used most frequently to determine the ventricular function, to assess the status of native and prosthetic valve disease, and, by use of the tricuspid regurgitant velocity, to assess pulmonary artery pressure. For those patients with congenital heart disease, a detailed assessment of any shunt and complex anatomy may be made.

During pregnancy, because of the increased cardiac output, the velocities across the left and right ventricular outflow tracts increase, which may mimic an increase in outflow tract gradient. Careful examination of the two-dimensional anatomic appearances will help differentiate this from a true valvular abnormality, and calculation of valve area will be helpful. Similarly, because of the increased stroke volume, any valvular regurgitation will appear to be accentuated. Serial echocardiograms may be particularly useful in a patient with a mechanical valve prosthesis who is vulnerable to thrombosis during pregnancy. The valve area calculation, in addition to pressure half-time determination, may be more helpful than a simple measurement of valve gradient; this may appear to be increased as pregnancy advances because the circulation becomes more hyperkinetic and cardiac output increases.

In patients with impaired ventricular function, particularly those with cardiomyopathy, echocardiography plays the most important role in assessing left ventricular function. In a normal pregnancy, the left ventricular end-diastolic measurement is increased, and there may be similar increases in right ventricular size as well as in the volumes of both atria. Measurement of ejection fraction is determined by changes in preload and afterload, and in the supine position, preload may be reduced because the fetus may compress the inferior vena cava.

TRANSESOPHAGEAL ECHOCARDIOGRAPHY. Transesophageal echocardiography is seldom performed during pregnancy but may be necessary to provide more detailed imaging of valvular disease, the presence or absence of a shunt, or intracardiac thrombus. In addition, it may be useful to determine the presence or absence of endocarditis to facilitate the detection of a valvular vegetation or perivalvular abscess. Transesophageal echocardiography can be performed safely, although careful monitoring of maternal oxygen saturation is necessary if midazolam is used for sedation. Antibiotic prophylaxis is unnecessary.

FETAL ECHOCARDIOGRAPHY. Excellent imaging of the fetal heart can usually be obtained by 20 weeks' gestation. The four-chamber view may be obtained in most pregnancies and should demonstrate two atrioventricular valves, the crux of the heart, and whether two ventricles of equal size are present. The patent foramen ovale should also be demonstrated. Typically, the heart should be smaller than one third of the size of the fetal thorax.

Management During Pregnancy

Medical Therapy

Patients who are otherwise healthy may require little or no specific treatment other than the usual obstetric recommendations and monitoring. Patients who are NYHA Class I or II may need to limit strenuous exercise and to have adequate rest, supplementation of iron and vitamins to minimize the anemia of pregnancy, low-salt diet if there is concern about ventricular dysfunction, and regular cardiac and obstetric evaluations, the frequency of which must be individualized. Patients who are NYHA Class III or IV may need hospital admission for bed rest and close monitoring and may require early delivery if there is maternal hemodynamic compromise.

Surgical Management

Cardiac surgery is seldom necessary during pregnancy and should be avoided whenever possible. There is a higher risk of fetal malformation and loss if cardiopulmonary bypass is performed in the first trimester; if it is performed in the last trimester, there is a higher likelihood of precipitating premature labor. The "optimal time" appears to be between 20 and 28 weeks of gestation, and the fetal outcome may be improved by use of normothermic rather than hypothermic extracorporeal circulation, higher pump flows, higher pressures (mean blood pressure of 60 mm Hg), and as short a bypass time as possible. Obstetric monitoring of the fetus during the procedure is recommended so that fetal bradycardia may be dealt with promptly and uterine contractions may be controlled. Despite these interventions, the current risk of fetal loss is still at least 10% and is probably higher when the cardiac surgery is emergent. Maternal functional class is an important predictive factor for maternal death. A multidisciplinary approach is preferable to optimize the outcome for both mother and baby.

TABLE 82-1 High-Risk Pregnancies

Pulmonary hypertension
Dilated cardiomyopathy, ejection fraction <40%
Symptomatic obstructive lesions
Aortic stenosis
Mitral stenosis
Pulmonary stenosis
Coarctation of the aorta
Marfan syndrome with aortic root >40 mm
Cyanotic lesions
Mechanical prosthetic valves

High-Risk Pregnancies

In some situations, the maternal risk of pregnancy is very high, and the patient should be counseled to avoid pregnancy and sometimes even to consider termination of pregnancy if it occurs (**Table 82-1**). No data exist regarding the precise level of pulmonary hypertension that poses a major threat to the mother, but in my experience, systolic pulmonary artery pressures higher than 60% to 70% of the systemic pressure are likely to be associated with maternal compromise; in these circumstances, pregnancy is best avoided. Women who have a left ventricular ejection fraction less than 40% from any cause are not likely to withstand the volume load that pregnancy imposes and should be advised not to become pregnant. Because pregnancy is associated with a decrease in peripheral resistance, symptomatic patients with significant stenotic cardiac lesions (see Table 82-1) are likely to deteriorate during a pregnancy. Patients with a dilated aortic root more than 40 mm are vulnerable to progressive aortic dilation, dissection, and rupture during pregnancy, particularly those patients with Marfan syndrome. This occurs not only because of the increased stroke volume but probably also because the gestational hormonal changes may be additive to the underlying histologic abnormality in the aortic media. Estrogen inhibits collagen and elastin synthesis in the aorta, and progesterone has been shown to accelerate the deposition of noncollagenous proteins in the aortas of rats.

Cardiovascular Diseases

Congenital Heart Disease (see Chap. 65)

Most maternal cardiac disease in Western societies is now congenital in origin. This relates to the enormous advances in congenital cardiac surgery during the last 50 years, so that most babies born with congenital heart disease, even with complex lesions, now survive to adulthood. Some patients will present for the first time in pregnancy with symptoms and learn that they have congenital heart disease. Other patients with repaired defects may encounter cardiac problems during pregnancy, the most common being heart failure and arrhythmias.[7] All patients, whether or not they have had cardiac repair, should have a detailed evaluation and appropriate counseling before pregnancy is considered.[8]

ATRIAL SEPTAL DEFECT. Secundum atrial septal defect is one of the most common congenital heart defects. Patients with even a large secundum atrial septal defect usually tolerate pregnancy without complication unless there is coexistent pulmonary hypertension or atrial fibrillation. The volume load on the right ventricle is usually well tolerated. Meticulous attention should be paid to the maternal leg veins, particularly during peridelivery, because deep venous thrombosis could precipitate a paradoxical embolus and stroke. Elective closure of an atrial septal defect by device or operative repair is preferable before pregnancy is contemplated.

VENTRICULAR SEPTAL DEFECT. Patients with small defects usually tolerate pregnancy without difficulty. In the setting of a large ventricular septal defect and pulmonary hypertension, patients should be counseled not to proceed with a pregnancy (see later discussion of Eisenmenger syndrome).

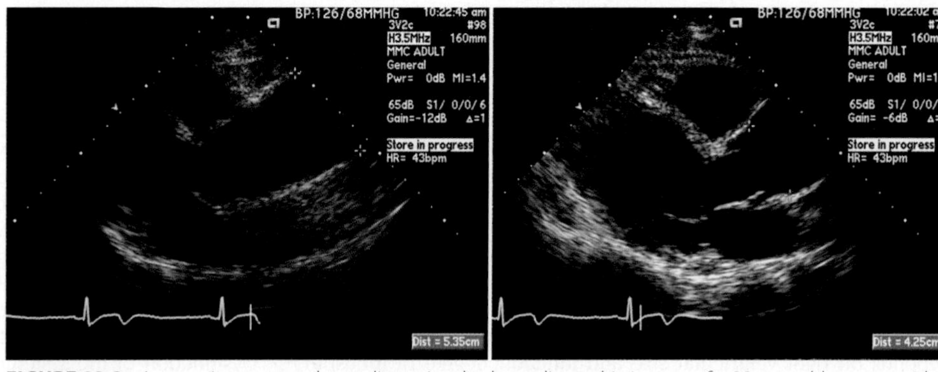

FIGURE 82-3 Long-axis parasternal two-dimensional echocardiographic images of a 30-year-old woman with a normal functioning bicuspid aortic valve. Her ascending aorta measures 4.25 cm at the sinotubular junction **(left)** and 5.35 cm at the mid ascending aorta **(right)**. An aortic root replacement (valve sparing) was recommended before pregnancy.

PATENT DUCTUS ARTERIOSUS. Small ducts with normal or near-normal pressures usually cause no hemodynamic perturbations during pregnancy. In the setting of a large shunt, the added volume load of pregnancy might precipitate left ventricular failure. Those with pulmonary hypertension should be counseled not to have a pregnancy.

CONGENITAL AORTIC STENOSIS. (see Chap. 66) Aortic stenosis in women of childbearing age usually occurs secondary to a bicuspid aortic valve. A detailed two-dimensional anatomic and Doppler echocardiographic assessment of the valve function should be performed before pregnancy is contemplated. In addition, there should be a careful examination of the entire thoracic aorta because bicuspid aortic valve is associated with an aortopathy, and even with a functionally normal valve, an aortic dilation or ascending aortic aneurysm may be present. Pregnancy is usually considered to be contraindicated if the aortic dimension is larger than 4.5 cm (**Fig. 82-3**).

Mild aortic stenosis is usually well tolerated, provided the patient has a normal exercise capacity and no symptoms.[9] Moderate stenosis is sometimes well tolerated, but the patient needs to be evaluated carefully before pregnancy. In the absence of symptoms, with a normal exercise test without ST-T wave changes, pregnancy with a compliant patient who is carefully managed is likely to be successful. Those with severe aortic stenosis (valve area smaller than 1 cm^2) or a mean gradient greater than 50 mm Hg should be counseled not to have a pregnancy. The decrease in peripheral resistance during pregnancy will exaggerate the aortic gradient and may precipitate symptoms. Patients may respond to bed rest and the administration of beta blockers, but an early delivery may be necessary. The risk to the mother of continuing the pregnancy versus delivery of a baby early by cesarean section needs to be balanced. Labor and delivery can be particularly problematic in such patients because of the abrupt hemodynamic changes, particularly the abrupt fall in afterload when the baby is delivered. Blood loss at the time of parturition can also precipitate maternal collapse. Epidural analgesia needs to be carefully and slowly administered, and spinal block should be avoided because of the potential for hypotension. Delivery may be facilitated by central venous pressure monitoring or the use of a Swan-Ganz catheter to maintain optimum hemodynamics. This should be continued for at least 24 hours after delivery.

Several small reports have reviewed percutaneous aortic balloon valvuloplasty during pregnancy; this can be accomplished, provided the valve anatomy is favorable and the procedure is performed by an experienced interventionalist.[10] Radiation exposure of the fetus can be minimized by lead screening of the mother's abdomen and pelvis. It should be performed in centers with extensive experience and surgical back-up and, if performed after 26 weeks of pregnancy, should have obstetric standby in case of premature labor.

COARCTATION OF THE AORTA. (see Chaps. 60 and 65) Women with coarctation may present for the first time during pregnancy because of systemic hypertension. A significant coarctation causes diminished flow to both the uterus and fetus, which may result in small-for-dates babies or even fetal loss. Therapeutic options include antihypertensive therapies, percutaneous balloon or stenting of the coarctation, or surgical intervention. Because of the associated aortopathy, the entire aorta is vulnerable to dilation, aneurysm, and dissection. When the presence of a coarctation is known, the entire aorta should be imaged at the time of pre-pregnancy counseling. Most women, however, will have a successful pregnancy with proper care.

PULMONARY STENOSIS. Pulmonary stenosis is usually well tolerated during pregnancy, particularly if the right ventricular pressure is less than 70% of systemic pressure and sinus rhythm is maintained. If necessary, balloon pulmonary valvuloplasty can be performed, with shielding of the fetus from radiation.

CYANOTIC HEART DISEASE. Cyanosis poses risks for both mother and fetus.[11] The decrease in peripheral resistance that accompanies pregnancy augments the right-to-left shunt and may exaggerate the maternal cyanosis. Because of the erythrocytosis that accompanies cyanosis and the propensity to thrombosis, women who develop venous thrombosis are at risk of paradoxical embolus and stroke. Maternal hypoxia imposes a pronounced handicap to fetal growth and survival. Presbitero and colleagues[12] have evaluated 44 women with 96 pregnancies (excluding patients with Eisenmenger syndrome) and confirmed earlier study findings that the degree of maternal cyanosis has a profound impact on fetal outcome. When the maternal oxygen saturation is less than 85%, the fetal outcome is poor, with only 2 of 17 pregnancies (12%) resulting in live-born infants (**Table 82-2**). Conversely, when the maternal oxygen saturation is 90% or higher, 92% of the pregnancies result in a live birth. Maternal cardiovascular complications occurred in 14 patients (32%). Eight patients had heart

TABLE 82-2 Fetal Outcome in Cyanotic Congenital Heart Disease and Its Relationship with Maternal Cyanosis

	NO. OF PREGNANCIES	NO. OF LIVE BIRTHS	PERCENTAGE BORN ALIVE
Hemoglobin, g/dL*			
≤16	28	20	71
17-19	40	18	45
≥20	26	2	8
Arterial oxygen saturation (%)†			
≤85	17	2	12
85-89	22	10	45
≥90	13	12	92

*Hemoglobin concentration unknown in two pregnancies.
†Arterial oxygen saturation unknown in 44 pregnancies.
From Presbitero P, Somerville J, Stone S, et al: Pregnancy in cyanotic congenital heart disease. Outcome of mother and fetus. Circulation 89:2673, 1994.

failure, and bacterial endocarditis occurred in two patients, both with palliated tetralogy of Fallot. Two patients had thrombotic complications, one pulmonary and one cerebral.

In addition to the degree of maternal cyanosis, right ventricular function must be assessed before pregnancy by echocardiography or magnetic resonance imaging. The type of maternal cardiac lesion present will also affect the propensity of the baby to inherit congenital cardiac disease. For those women with conotruncal abnormalities (tetralogy or pulmonary atresia), screening for 22q11 deletion is recommended because this has autosomal dominant transmission, and the offspring have a 50% chance of inheriting the genetic defect.[13]

EBSTEIN ANOMALY. The safety of a pregnancy in these patients depends on right ventricular size and function, degree of tricuspid regurgitation, and presence or absence of an atrial communication. The last is present in approximately 50% of patients, and if the patient is cyanotic at rest, the risk of pregnancy increases considerably. An atrial communication poses the added potential risk of a stroke from a paradoxical embolus, and meticulous attention should be paid to the mother's leg veins for the possibility of deep venous thrombosis. Atrial arrhythmias may not be well tolerated in pregnancy with this anomaly, and both atrial fibrillation and reentry tachycardia are common. Accessory bypass tracts causing preexcitation may precipitate rapid tachycardias, which add to the burden of a poorly functioning right ventricle.

CONGENITALLY CORRECTED TRANSPOSITION (L-TRANSPOSITION). Patients with this anomaly have atrioventricular discordance and ventriculoarterial discordance; thus, the systemic ventricle is the morphologic right ventricle. Patients may have a successful pregnancy as long as the ejection fraction of the systemic ventricle is preserved and there are no significant associated anomalies. The most common of these is systemic atrioventricular valve (tricuspid) regurgitation, which contributes to systemic ventricular dysfunction. Other lesions, such as ventricular septal defect, pulmonary stenosis, and complete heart block, may coexist and may compromise the ability to have a successful pregnancy.

Repaired Congenital Heart Disease (see Chap. 65)

Very few operations for congenital heart disease can be considered curative, and almost all patients have residua and sequelae that must be carefully evaluated at the time of pre-pregnancy counseling.

TETRALOGY OF FALLOT. Most women of childbearing age with tetralogy of Fallot will have had prior surgical repair and should be free of cyanosis. An occasional patient will be seen in adulthood who has not had prior surgery or may have been palliated with a surgically created shunt (e.g., Blalock-Taussig). In these cases, pregnancy may pose a risk, depending on the degree of cyanosis, as noted earlier. The fall in peripheral resistance augments the right-to-left shunt through the ventricular septal defect, causing worsening cyanosis, and this poses a risk for mother and fetus.

For those patients with prior definitive surgical repair, a careful assessment of any hemodynamic residua and sequelae should be undertaken before advice is given about the safety of a pregnancy. The clinical and echocardiographic evaluation should focus on the presence of lesions, such as residual pulmonary regurgitation, which is common after repair, and associated right ventricular dysfunction and tricuspid regurgitation. The volume load of pregnancy may not be well tolerated in these circumstances,[14,15] and superimposed atrial and even ventricular arrhythmias may add to the hemodynamic stresses. Additional volume lesions, such as ventricular septal defects and aortic regurgitation, as well as residual right ventricular outflow tract obstruction should be evaluated. For those women with a good surgical repair, good exercise capacity, and minimal residua, pregnancy may be well tolerated, provided they are properly managed.[15,16] Genetic counseling should be offered during pre-pregnancy counseling to look for 22q11 deletion. If there is no parental chromosomal abnormality and no family history of other congenital cardiac disease, the risk of the fetus having a congenital cardiac anomaly is approximately 5% to 6%, similar to the risk of inheritance of many congenital cardiac lesions.

TRANSPOSITION OF THE GREAT ARTERIES (D-TRANSPOSITION). All patients will have had surgery in childhood, commonly an atrial baffle procedure (Mustard or Senning operation), which leaves the morphologic right ventricle as the systemic pump. Function of the systemic ventricle should be assessed clinically and echocardiographically before pregnancy, as well as the degree of tricuspid (systemic) atrioventricular valve regurgitation and degree of baffle obstruction, the residual atrial septal defect, and the presence or absence of atrial arrhythmias, which are common complications. Dysfunction of the systemic ventricle may be a contraindication to pregnancy.

COARCTATION. The evaluation of the woman with repaired coarctation should include an assessment of the coarctation repair site to exclude residual or recurrent coarctation or aneurysm formation and an imaging study to assess the entire aorta to rule out dilation or aneurysm formation, which is most common in the ascending aorta. The aortic valve and left ventricular function should also be assessed. The outcome for both mother and baby is usually favorable. For patients with mild dilation of the aorta, vaginal delivery with a short second stage is reasonable, but if there is evidence of aortic instability, a cesarean section is preferable.

UNIVENTRICULAR HEART AND FONTAN OPERATIONS. These women have an increased risk of maternal complications, particularly atrial arrhythmias, which may cause profound hemodynamic deterioration. They are particularly vulnerable to thrombosis in the Fontan circuit because of the sluggish flow and prothrombotic state of pregnancy. Function of the single ventricle may deteriorate because of the volume load of pregnancy, and the risk of miscarriage also appears to be increased.

Pulmonary Hypertension (see Chap. 78)

Pulmonary hypertension, regardless of the cause, carries a high mortality when it is associated with pregnancy.[17] Causes include thromboembolic disease, anorexic drugs, valvular heart disease, and primary pulmonary hypertension. The most common cause in childbearing years, however, is secondary to a shunt in the setting of congenital heart disease (e.g., ventricular septal defect, patent ductus arteriosus, or atrial septal defect). When the pulmonary hypertension exceeds approximately 60% of systemic levels, pregnancy is more likely to be associated with complications. In the setting of severe pulmonary vascular disease (Eisenmenger syndrome, see Chap. 65), maternal mortality may approach 50%. The volume load of pregnancy may compromise the poorly functioning right ventricle and precipitate heart failure. The fall in peripheral resistance augments right-to-left shunting and may precipitate more cyanosis.

The time around labor and delivery is particularly dangerous, and the highest incidence of maternal death is during parturition and the puerperium. There may be an abrupt decrease in afterload as the baby is delivered, and hypovolemia from blood loss can cause hypoxia, syncope, and sudden death. Vagal responses to pain may also be life-threatening. Death may also occur from pulmonary embolism or in situ pulmonary infarction. In the largest retrospective review, Gleicher and associates[18] reported 44 documented cases of Eisenmenger syndrome with 70 pregnancies. Of these patients, 52% died in connection with a pregnancy, and 34% of vaginal deliveries resulted in maternal death. Three of four cesarean sections also resulted in maternal death; however, the numbers were small, and it is likely that those patients represented a higher risk cohort because they were the most hemodynamically unstable. Only 25.6% of pregnancies reached term, and more than half of the deliveries were premature. Perinatal mortality was 28.3% and was significantly associated with prematurity. Current recommendations are still that termination of pregnancy is the safer option, although in patients with pulmonary hypertension, this too may be a more complex procedure, and cardiac anesthesia is probably helpful in this regard. Low-dose subcutaneous heparin may be administered during bed rest, but there is no evidence that it improves maternal survival. The mode of delivery needs to be discussed carefully. If the vaginal route is selected, it should be performed in an intensive care unit. Epidural analgesia must be cautiously administered to minimize peripheral vasodilation. A prolonged second stage should be avoided. Meticulous attention should be paid to the peripheral venous system, and a thromboguard or compression pump may help prevent peripheral venous thrombosis. Cesarean section delivery is probably preferable[19] with cardiac anesthesia. In-hospital monitoring should be continued for at least 2 weeks after delivery.

No studies have suggested a more favorable outcome with the use of pulmonary vasodilators, although case reports have suggested a more successful maternal outcome. Nitric oxide can be administered through nasal cannula or facemask, and successful pregnancy has also been reported with intravenous epoprostenol. Sildenafil has also been used, but with all these agents, maternal death may still occur days or weeks after delivery.[20]

In summary, the mortality for patients with severe pulmonary hypertension and pregnancy is prohibitively high. Appropriate advice about contraception should be given to all patients. Estrogen-containing contraceptives are contraindicated in this setting.

Valvular Heart Disease (see Chap. 66)

Because of the declining incidence of rheumatic heart disease in Western countries, rheumatic heart disease is infrequent in North America but remains prevalent in developing countries. The most common problems encountered are bicuspid aortic stenosis (discussed previously) and mitral stenosis, which tends to worsen during pregnancy because of the increase in cardiac output coupled with the increase in heart rate; this shortens the diastolic filling time and exaggerates the mitral valve gradient. Any decrease in stroke volume causes a further reflex tachycardia, which contributes to an elevated left atrial pressure. The onset of atrial fibrillation may precipitate acute pulmonary edema. Patients should have a careful echocardiographic evaluation of their mitral valve gradient, valve area, and pulmonary pressures before proceeding with a pregnancy. Exercise echocardiography may also be helpful in delineating the hemodynamic response to effort in terms of mitral gradient and the presence or absence of pulmonary hypertension.

The cornerstone of therapy for the symptomatic patient is beta blockade. This slows the heart rate, prolongs the diastolic filling time, and can result in marked improvement in symptoms. Bed rest may also be helpful to slow the heart rate and to minimize cardiac demands. The judicious use of diuretics is appropriate if there is pulmonary edema. Anticoagulants should probably be given if the patient is on bed rest and should certainly be administered in the setting of atrial fibrillation. In unusual circumstances, when the mother is refractory to medical therapy, balloon valvuloplasty may be performed if the valve anatomy is favorable and there is no concomitant mitral regurgitation.[21,22] Rarer still, surgical valvotomy may be performed, with the caveats described earlier.

Mitral and aortic regurgitation are fairly well tolerated in pregnancy, provided the regurgitation is no more than moderate, the mother is symptom free before pregnancy, and ventricular function is well preserved. Closer monitoring during pregnancy is usually warranted, however, particularly for those with mitral regurgitation, because the left ventricle tends to dilate as pregnancy progresses, and this may exacerbate the degree of mitral regurgitation. Early delivery may be necessary if there is maternal hemodynamic compromise.

PROSTHETIC VALVES. Pregnancy for the woman with a prosthetic valve poses risks for mother and baby and has been called a "double jeopardy" situation.[23] The choice of a prosthetic valve for the woman of childbearing age involves a detailed discussion of the relative risks so that she can make an informed decision about whether to select a tissue or mechanical prosthesis. Tissue valves are less thrombogenic than mechanical valves and therefore are less problematic in pregnancy because they do not routinely involve the use of warfarin. The disadvantage is their tendency to degenerate after an average of 10 years, necessitating a reoperation, with its attendant risks and potential mortality. Mechanical prostheses, in contrast, have a greater longevity but require anticoagulation, and whichever anticoagulant strategy is chosen during pregnancy, there is a higher chance of fetal loss, placental hemorrhage, and prosthetic valve thrombosis. Thus, each type of valve has a risk-to-benefit ratio; the choices are reviewed here.

TISSUE PROSTHESES. The most common types of tissue valves used currently are porcine and pericardial valves. For patients in sinus rhythm, they confer the advantage that warfarin is not required, although many patients take a daily baby aspirin (81 mg). These valves are vulnerable to structural degeneration and calcification, which occurs more rapidly in younger patients. In addition, mitral prostheses tend to degenerate faster than those in the aortic position. There is some evidence that pregnancy may accelerate valve degeneration, and in some retrospective series, a second valve replacement was necessary in approximately one third of patients within 2 years of delivery. This is not universally accepted, however, and other large series have shown no difference in structural valve degeneration in young women who had a pregnancy versus those who did not.[24] Nonetheless, all tissue valves will degenerate, necessitating a second operation with an operative risk that is usually higher than the first. In some series, the mortality of a second valve replacement may be as high as 6%, and it must be recognized that if death occurs after the mother has had a successful pregnancy, the young child is left without a mother. Thus, at the time of counseling women of childbearing age about valve choice, the surgical results from the individual's institution should be reviewed. These may vary considerably on the basis of both surgical volume and expertise.

Homografts pose similar problems of structural deterioration and reoperation. The Ross operation, in which an autograft pulmonary valve is placed in the aortic position and a tissue prosthesis (usually porcine) is implanted in the pulmonary position, is associated with good outcomes during pregnancy when the hemodynamic indices are good. Nonetheless, the Ross procedure essentially exchanges one valvular problem for two, and ultimately the tissue pulmonary prosthesis as well as the aortic prosthesis must be replaced.

MECHANICAL PROSTHESES AND ANTICOAGULANT TREATMENT. The management of pregnancy when the mother has a mechanical valve prosthesis is controversial, and no universal consensus exists. There is no perfect strategy, and each modality is associated with some hazard for the mother or the fetus. Before any approach is adopted, it is crucial to explain the risks to the patient. During pregnancy, maternal blood is highly thrombogenic because there is an increased concentration of clotting factors and increased platelet adhesiveness combined with decreased fibrinolysis. These changes in clotting parameters make the risk of valve thrombosis and thromboembolism significant.

Unfractionated Heparin

Unfractionated heparin is a large molecule that does not cross the placenta and does not cause developmental abnormalities in the fetus. Laboratory control of activated partial thromboplastin time (aPTT) is difficult, however, in part because of the variation in response to standard doses and the wide variation in the reagents used to monitor doses. The aPTT ratio should be maintained at a level of at least 2, which corresponds to an anti–factor Xa (anti-Xa) level of more than 0.55 unit/mL in approximately 90% of patients.[25] Unfractionated heparin has been used subcutaneously and intravenously and is often begun in the first trimester, as soon as pregnancy is diagnosed, to minimize fetal exposure to warfarin at the critical time of fetal embryogenesis. It is usually continued until week 13 or 14 of pregnancy, when fetal embryogenesis is almost complete, and then warfarin is substituted. Some physicians continue heparin throughout pregnancy to avoid any fetal exposure to warfarin, but unfractionated heparin has been shown to be a poor anticoagulant in pregnancy. One large retrospective European study comparing different anticoagulation strategies has shown that most maternal complications (e.g., valve thrombosis, stroke, death) occur while mothers are taking heparin.[26] Most complications occur with mechanical mitral tilting disc prostheses, and this observation has been supported by many other studies, particularly with older generation prostheses.[27] One meta-analysis by Chan and colleagues[28] has shown that use of heparin early in the first trimester virtually eliminates the risk of fetal embryopathy but at the expense of maternal valve thrombosis, which occurred with a frequency of 9%. If unfractionated heparin is the selected treatment strategy, the midinterval aPTT should be at least twice that of the control, or an anti-Xa level of 0.35 to 0.7 unit/mL should be maintained.[25]

Low-Molecular-Weight Heparin

Low-molecular-weight heparin is an attractive alternative to unfractionated heparin because of its ease of use and superior bioavailability. Deaths have been reported with its use, however, usually associated with maternal valve thrombosis. The American College of Chest Physicians has suggested that it may be used and the anticoagulant effect carefully monitored by measuring the anti-Xa level. It is recommended that it be administered subcutaneously every 12 hours and the dose adjusted so that a 4-hour postinjection anti-Xa level is maintained at approximately 1.0 to 1.2 unit/mL, perhaps measured weekly.[25] The addition of low-dose aspirin, 75 to 162 mg/day, has also been recommended. There are no large prospective trials to confirm the usefulness of low-molecular-weight heparin in this setting, however, and reported studies are confined to small groups. Certainly, dosing based on weight alone has been shown to be inadequate to maintain most pregnant women in the therapeutic range as measured by anti-Xa activity,[29] and the pharmacokinetics changes throughout pregnancy. One retrospective study has reviewed published series between 1989 and 2004.[30] There were 74 women with 81 pregnancies, most of whom had mitral prostheses. Thromboemboli occurred in 10 of 81 pregnancies (12%), and all these patients had mitral prostheses. Low-molecular-weight heparin was used throughout in 60 pregnancies; in 21 pregnancies, it was used only in the first trimester and again at term. In 51 pregnancies, anti-Xa levels were monitored, and in 30 pregnancies, a fixed dose was used. All 10 patients with thromboemboli were receiving heparin throughout pregnancy, and 9 of them were on a fixed-dose regimen. This underscores the need for meticulous monitoring of anti-Xa levels, and Oran and associates[30] have recommended that the 4- to 6-hour postinjection level be maintained at 1 IU/mL. Thus, the use of low-molecular-weight heparin remains controversial, with no large prospective series and no evidence-based data to support which levels of anti-Xa should be maintained. It should be discontinued at least 24 hours before delivery if epidural analgesia is to be used because it has a prolonged effect and there is risk of spinal hematoma. Unfractionated heparin can be substituted peridelivery because it can be started and stopped abruptly. With all strategies, anticoagulants should be resumed as soon as possible after delivery.

Warfarin

Fetal exposure to warfarin in the first trimester may be associated with fetal embryopathy. In its mildest form, this may be only bone stippling (chondrodysplasia punctata); but in its most severe form, it may be manifested as nasal hypoplasia, optic atrophy, and mental retardation. The reported fetal risk of embryopathy varies widely but probably averages 6%. This risk is reduced by initiation of heparin before 6 weeks of pregnancy, but the disadvantage is an increased risk of maternal valve thrombosis. Warfarin also appears to increase the risk of fetal loss and spontaneous abortion.

The risk of fetal embryopathy may be dose related, and a study by Vitale and colleagues[31] has suggested that the risk is very low if the maternal warfarin dose is 5 mg or less. Thus, the anticoagulant approach for the woman with a mechanical valve needs to be individualized. For the woman with an older generation or tilting disc mitral prosthesis, particularly if she is in atrial fibrillation, the safer approach may be to treat her with warfarin for the first 34 to 35 weeks of pregnancy, particularly if her dose is less than 5 mg/day. This must be fully discussed with the patient before she becomes pregnant, not only for the medicolegal implications but so that all the risks and benefits are understood. For those patients at lesser risk, heparin therapy (with the provisos noted earlier) may be selected as soon as pregnancy is diagnosed, warfarin substituted at 13 to 14 weeks, and heparin restarted at approximately 35 weeks in anticipation of delivery.

Connective Tissue Disorders

The most common connective tissue disorder is the Marfan syndrome, a disorder of fibrillin that is inherited in an autosomal dominant pattern (see Chap. 60). Preconception counseling is essential to advise prospective parents about the risks of transmission to the offspring and the risks of cardiovascular complications for the mother. A careful clinical and echocardiographic cardiovascular evaluation should be performed. This would usually include magnetic resonance imaging or computed tomography assessment of the entire aorta to look for aortic dilation or dissection. Pregnancy is usually contraindicated if the ascending aorta is larger than 40 mm in diameter, although the exact dimension is still a matter of debate. It should be underscored to all women with Marfan syndrome that pregnancy is not uniformly safe, and aortic dilation and dissection may be unpredictable although more likely when the aorta is larger than 40 mm. One study has suggested that pregnancy is relatively safe up to a diameter of 45 mm.[32] Associated cardiovascular problems also need to be evaluated, including the presence or absence of aortic regurgitation and mitral valve prolapse with associated regurgitation. Many patients are receiving long-term treatment with beta-adrenergic blockers to slow the progression of aortic regurgitation. These should be continued during pregnancy if there is any aortic dilation. Periodic echocardiographic surveillance every 6 to 8 weeks is recommended to monitor the mother's aortic root size, with the interval dependent on the initial echocardiographic findings. Any chest pain should be promptly evaluated to rule out dissection. During labor and delivery, pushing should be avoided, with an assisted second stage if necessary.

Cardiomyopathies (see Chaps. 68 and 69)

DILATED CARDIOMYOPATHY. Patients with idiopathic dilated cardiomyopathy are usually counseled not to have a pregnancy if the ejection fraction is lower than 40%. Because angiotensin-converting enzyme (ACE) inhibitors are contraindicated in pregnancy, ventricular function must be assessed without this drug. Careful echocardiographic evaluation should be performed before pregnancy. Exercise testing may also be helpful because women with ejection fractions of 40% to 50% may not tolerate pregnancy well if they have a poor functional aerobic capacity. Symptomatic patients who proceed with a pregnancy may need hydralazine for afterload reduction, bed rest, and low-dose diuretics for heart failure. Early delivery may also be necessary.

PERIPARTUM CARDIOMYOPATHY. Peripartum cardiomyopathy (PPCM) is a dilated cardiomyopathy documented with echocardiographic left ventricular dysfunction occurring in the last month of pregnancy or within 5 months of delivery. Patients with a prior history of myocardial disease are excluded from this definition, although this makes the diagnosis challenging in many women who have had neither a chest radiograph nor an echocardiogram to confirm that they had previously normal ventricular function. The actual incidence is unknown, but it is probably approximately 1 in 3000. Risk factors include multiparity, being black, older maternal age, and preeclampsia. In a retrospective study of 123 women with PPCM,[33] a history of hypertension was obtained in 43% of patients, and twin pregnancies were reported in 13%. Consistent with earlier studies, most patients (75%) presented in the first month post partum, perhaps suggesting an autoimmune cause rather than the pregnancy's exacerbating a pre-existing cardiomyopathy. This theory is supported by the documentation of autoantibodies in some cases.

The treatment of PPCM is the same as for other forms of congestive heart failure, except that ACE inhibitors and angiotensin receptor blocking agents are contraindicated in pregnancy. Hydralazine, beta blockers, and digoxin have been used and are safe, and diuretics may decrease preload and improve symptoms.[34] Intracardiac thrombus and embolism are common, and consideration should be given to anticoagulation with unfractionated heparin in those with an ejection fraction lower than 35%.[35] Early fetal delivery may be necessary in women needing hospitalization for heart failure. Myocarditis is a causative factor in some cases, with a reported incidence between 8.8% and 78%. The role of endomyocardial biopsy is controversial, but it probably should be considered and performed by those with considerable experience. Immunosuppressive treatment should be given to those with proven myocarditis.

Normalization of ventricular function occurs in about 50% of patients and appears more likely if the ejection fraction is more than 30% at the time of diagnosis.[33] Most physicians counsel against a second pregnancy, even if the ventricular function does return to normal, because PPCM will recur in approximately 30% of cases. This may result in significant clinical deterioration and even death.[36]

HYPERTROPHIC CARDIOMYOPATHY. A wide spectrum of anatomic and hemodynamic abnormalities exist in hypertrophic cardiomyopathy, including left ventricular outflow tract obstruction, mitral regurgitation, arrhythmias, and diastolic dysfunction. Some patients are asymptomatic with minimal hemodynamic disturbance; others are profoundly limited, with marked hemodynamic perturbations. A careful personal history, review of family history, electrocardiography, exercise test, and transthoracic echocardiography should precede counseling about the advisability of a pregnancy. The prospective parents should be informed about the autosomal dominant inheritance pattern, which has variable penetrance. Currently, more than 200 genetic mutations have been identified, and genetic counseling and family screening are appropriate before pregnancy is contemplated.

Most women with hypertrophic cardiomyopathy tolerate pregnancy well. The decrease in afterload that might exacerbate the outflow gradient is largely offset by the maternal increase in plasma volume. Medications such as beta blockers, which alleviate the outflow tract obstruction, may be continued throughout pregnancy, but the dose may need to be increased. Patients who have significant symptoms before pregnancy (usually related to severe left ventricular outflow tract obstruction) may not do well and become hemodynamically unstable. Common symptoms include palpitation, angina, and breathlessness. In a retrospective study of 127 women with 271 pregnancies, 36 women (28.3%) reported cardiac symptoms but 90% were symptomatic before pregnancy.[37] Heart failure occurred postnatally in two women, but there were no maternal deaths. Arrhythmia-related deaths in pregnancy have been reported, however. Low-dose diuretics may be helpful to treat heart failure in pregnancy, but care must be taken not to volume deplete the patient and exacerbate the left ventricular outflow gradient. Meticulous attention should be paid to hemodynamics at the time of delivery. Epidural anesthesia and spinal block should be avoided in case of hypotension, and blood loss should be promptly replaced. The Valsalva maneuver should be avoided, and the second stage should be facilitated as necessary. Cesarean section is indicated for obstetric reasons only.

Coronary Artery Disease (see Chaps. 54 to 57)

Coronary artery disease is uncommon in women of childbearing age but may occur, particularly in the setting of diabetes and tobacco abuse. Acute myocardial infarction is rare, and when it occurs, pregnancy increases the maternal risk threefold to fourfold. The most common cause is coronary artery dissection,[38] and the most common site is in the left anterior descending coronary artery.[39] The treatment should be urgent coronary angiography, with a consideration of percutaneous coronary intervention and stenting. The vulnerability to coronary artery dissection during pregnancy may relate to the presence of hypertension and also to the changes in elastin and collagen synthesis incurred by the hormonal changes of pregnancy.

A U.S. population-based study[40] has reported 44 deaths related to acute myocardial infarction, for a case fatality rate of 5.1%. The odds of acute myocardial infarction were 30-fold higher for women aged 40 years and older than for women younger than 20 years. The odds were more than fivefold higher for black women aged 35 years and older. Thrombus may also occur without atherosclerotic disease, and atherosclerosis with or without intracoronary thrombus is found in some cases, presumably related to the clotting diathesis that occurs during pregnancy.

Hypertension (see Chaps. 45 and 46)

Hypertension in pregnancy is an important cause of maternal morbidity and mortality. The different types of hypertension seen in pregnancy are defined in **Table 82-3**.[41] Gestational hypertension is distinguished from preeclampsia by the lack of proteinuria. About 50% of patients will develop preeclampsia, however, so close monitoring is warranted. It develops in approximately 25% of patients with chronic hypertension. Preeclampsia is a much more worrisome development and tends to occur more commonly in primiparous women and those with twin pregnancies. They do not usually develop frank hypertension until the second half of gestation. The cause is not entirely clear but may relate to endothelial dysfunction causing abnormal remodeling of the placental spiral arteries. Hypertension is just one feature of the diffuse endothelial dysfunction, which is associated with vasospasm, reduced end-organ perfusion, and activation of the coagulation cascade.

Although antihypertensive medications are effective in treating chronic hypertension that has worsened during pregnancy, they are not effective in preventing preeclampsia. When preeclampsia develops, bed rest is usually initiated, with salt restriction and close monitoring, and magnesium sulfate is often administered in an effort to prevent eclamptic seizures and to prolong the pregnancy, thereby facilitating fetal maturity. Urgent delivery is usually necessary, however, after which the blood pressure usually normalizes rapidly.

The treatment of other types of hypertension in pregnancy involves bed rest, salt restriction, and antihypertensive medications. Beta blockers, particularly labetalol (see Cardiovascular Drug Therapy and **Table 82-4**), have been used with good effect, although there is a

TABLE 82-3 Classification of Hypertension in Pregnancy

Chronic hypertension	Hypertension (blood pressure ≥140 mm Hg systolic or ≥90 mm Hg diastolic) present before pregnancy or that is diagnosed before the 20th week of gestation
Gestational hypertension	New hypertension with a blood pressure of 140/90 mm Hg on two separate occasions, without proteinuria, arising de novo after the 20th week of pregnancy. Blood pressure normalizes by 12 weeks post partum.
Preeclampsia superimposed on chronic hypertension	Increased blood pressure above the patient's baseline, a change in proteinuria, or evidence of end-organ dysfunction
Preeclampsia-eclampsia	Proteinuria (>0.3 g during 24 hours or ++ in two urine samples) in addition to new hypertension. Edema is no longer included in the diagnosis because of poor specificity. When proteinuria is absent, suspect the disease when increased blood pressure is associated with headache, blurred vision, abdominal pain, low platelets, or abnormal liver enzymes.

From Gifford RW, August PA, Cunningham G, et al: Report of the National High Blood Pressure Education Program Working Group on High Blood Pressure in Pregnancy. Am J Obstet Gynecol 183:S1, 2000.

TABLE 82-4 Cardiovascular Drugs in Pregnancy

DRUG	POTENTIAL FETAL SIDE EFFECTS
Amiodarone	Goiter, hypothyroidism and hyperthyroidism, IUGR
Angiotensin-converting enzyme inhibitors	Contraindicated; IUGR, oligohydramnios, renal failure, abnormal bone ossification; FDA class X
Aspirin	Baby aspirin not harmful
Beta blockers	Relatively safe; IUGR, neonatal bradycardia, and hypoglycemia
Calcium channel blockers	Relatively safe; few data; concern regarding uterine tone at the time of delivery
Digoxin	Safe; no adverse effects
Flecainide	Relatively safe; limited data; used to treat fetal arrhythmias
Hydralazine	Safe; no major adverse effects
Lasix	Safe; caution regarding maternal hypovolemia and reduced placental blood flow
Lidocaine	Safe; high doses may cause neonatal central nervous system depression
Methyldopa	Safe; considered by some to be the drug of choice for hypertension in pregnancy
Procainamide	Relatively safe; limited data; has been used to treat fetal arrhythmias, no major fetal side effects
Propafenone	Limited data
Quinidine	Relatively safe; rarely associated with neonatal thrombocytopenia; minimal oxytocic effect
Warfarin	Fetal embryopathy, placental and fetal hemorrhage, central nervous system abnormalities; FDA class X

IUGR = intrauterine growth retardation.

long safety record with methyldopa, which has no adverse effect on mother or baby.

Coarctation of the aorta needs to be considered (**Fig. 82-4**).

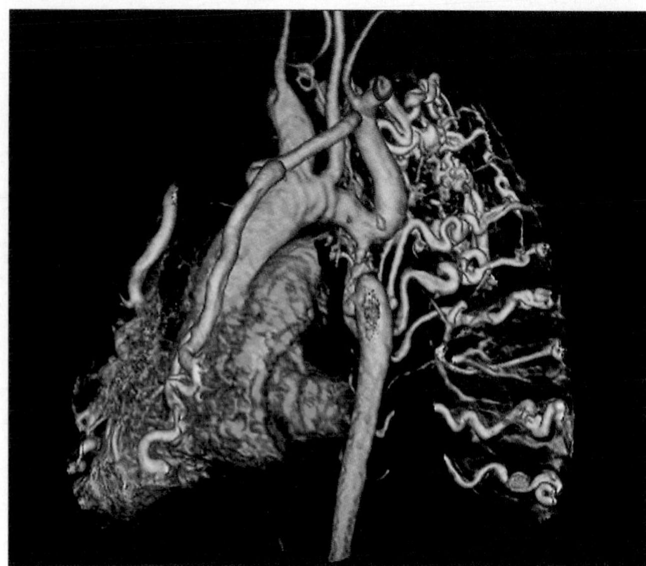

FIGURE 82-4 Magnetic resonance imaging scan of a 34-year-old with severe coarctation of the aorta (near interruption), with multiple and very large collateral vessels. She had had two prior pregnancies with preeclampsia and the coarctation had gone unnoticed.

Arrhythmias (see Chaps. 36 to 39)

Because of the physiologic changes of pregnancy, the heart may be more vulnerable to arrhythmias during this time. Potential contributing factors include the increase in preload, causing more myocardial irritability; increased heart rate, which may affect the refractory period; fluid and electrolyte shifts; and changes in catecholamine levels. Worsening of arrhythmias is not a consistent feature, however, and many women with a past history of tachycardia may not notice any change in the frequency of symptoms, and some even improve. The presenting symptom complex may be difficult to separate from the normal symptoms of pregnancy, including a sensation of fast heartbeat and skipped beats, which most commonly are supraventricular ectopics. The general approach should include taking a careful history, looking for any precipitating causes, and ruling out any concomitant medical problems (e.g., thyroid disease) by performing appropriate laboratory tests, such as complete blood count, electrolyte level measurement, and thyroid function determination. The clinical examination may help define whether the arrhythmia occurs in the setting of a normal heart or whether there is any underlying organic heart disease. If there is any doubt after the clinical examination, a transthoracic echocardiogram should be obtained. If the mother has no underlying cardiac disease, pharmacologic treatment should be administered if she is symptomatic or if the arrhythmia poses a risk to the mother or baby. In general, supraventricular and ventricular ectopic beats require no therapy. If there is underlying organic disease, the precipitating cause should be treated, if possible, and if this does not resolve, the arrhythmia medical therapy should be initiated.

The most common arrhythmia is atrial reentry tachycardia. Treatment of this type of arrhythmia is generally the same as for nonpregnant women, but with added concern about the effects of medications on the fetus (see Table 82-4). In general, the lowest dose necessary to treat the arrhythmia should be administered, and there should be a periodic evaluation of whether it is necessary to continue treatment. Atrial fibrillation is usually an indication that there is underlying structural heart disease. If the arrhythmia is unresponsive to medical therapy, electrical cardioversion may be performed and is not usually harmful to the fetus. Some have recommended that during elective cardioversion, fetal monitoring should be performed in case transient fetal bradycardia is present.

Premature ventricular complexes are common during pregnancy and usually require no treatment. Ventricular tachycardia is rare but may be a consequence of ischemic heart disease or cardiomyopathy. The treatment depends on the rate of tachycardia and the hemodynamic status of the mother. The choices of medications are listed in Table 82-4; electrical cardioversion should be performed if there is hemodynamic compromise.

Cardiovascular Drug Therapy (see Chap. 10)

When administration of cardiovascular drugs is being contemplated during pregnancy, the U.S. Food and Drug Administration (FDA) classification of these drugs must be considered. The reader is referred to more detailed information in this regard. Category X drugs are those for which fetal abnormalities have been demonstrated in animal or human studies, and the drug is contraindicated (e.g., warfarin). Almost all cardiovascular drugs are classified as category C, which means that animal studies have revealed adverse fetal effects, but there are no controlled data in women. A medication should be given only if the benefits outweigh the potential risk to the fetus. Important principles to be considered in using cardiovascular medications for pregnant women include the use of drugs with the longest safety record, the use of the lowest dose and shortest duration necessary, and in general the avoidance of a multidrug regimen, if possible. All these issues need to be reviewed carefully with the prospective mother at the time of pre-pregnancy counseling. A list of cardiovascular medications that might be considered in pregnancy is given in Table 82-4.

ASPIRIN. Aspirin crosses the placenta, and concern exists about its effect on fetal prostaglandins, which might cause closure of the fetal ductus arteriosus. Baby aspirin (81 mg), however, has been used safely in pregnancy without premature closure of the fetal duct. It may be useful adjunctive therapy when the mother has a mechanical valve prosthesis, and it can help prevent valve thrombosis.

AMIODARONE. Amiodarone and its iodine component cross the placenta and may cause neonatal goiter. The risks and benefits of its use, however, need to be balanced. If it has proved effective in controlling serious maternal arrhythmias, it may be safer for the mother to continue its use during pregnancy.

ANGIOTENSIN-CONVERTING ENZYME INHIBITORS. These are contraindicated in pregnancy because they are associated with abnormal renal development in the fetus as well as oligohydramnios and intrauterine growth retardation.

BETA-ADRENERGIC RECEPTOR BLOCKERS. These have been used extensively during pregnancy for treatment of arrhythmias, hypertrophic cardiomyopathy, and hypertension. They cross the placenta but are not teratogenic. Concern exists, however, particularly regarding fetal growth, because they have been demonstrated to cause fetal growth retardation. They may also be associated with neonatal bradycardia and hypoglycemia. More concern exists with regard to atenolol than some of the other beta-blocking agents. From a practical perspective, however, although the risk-to-benefit ratio needs to be considered, beta blockers have been used safely during pregnancy, although it is recommended that fetal growth be monitored more carefully.

CALCIUM CHANNEL BLOCKERS. These have been used to treat both arrhythmias and hypertension. There are limited data regarding their use. Most experience probably exists with verapamil, and no major adverse fetal effects have been recorded. Diltiazem and nifedipine have also been used, but studies are limited.

DIGOXIN. Digoxin has been used during pregnancy for many decades, and although it does cross the placenta, no adverse effects with its use have been reported.

DIURETICS. These agents, most commonly furosemide, may be used to treat congestive heart failure during pregnancy and sometimes are used for the treatment of hypertension. Aggressive use of diuretics, however, may cause reduction in placental blood flow and have a detrimental effect on fetal growth.

WARFARIN. Warfarin is usually contraindicated in the first trimester of pregnancy because it crosses the placenta and may cause fetal embryopathy. As noted earlier (see Mechanical Prostheses and Anticoagulant Treatment), however, there may be some high-risk situations in which the mother and physician determine that the safer approach is to continue warfarin therapy, particularly when the maternal dose is 5 mg or lower. Concern exists in the third trimester about labor and delivery because the immature fetal liver does not metabolize warfarin as rapidly as the mother's liver. After discontinuation of warfarin, reversal of anticoagulation occurs more rapidly in the mother, whereas reversal of anticoagulation in the fetus may take up to 1 week because of the immature fetal liver. Vaginal delivery when the fetus is anticoagulated is contraindicated because of the risk of fetal hemorrhage. Therefore, switching to an alternative anticoagulant such as heparin must be done well before labor is anticipated.

Contraception

For women with cardiac disease, appropriate contraceptive advice should be given before they become sexually active. This is particularly true for those with congenital heart disease, who, like other adolescents without heart disease, often become sexually active in their early teens. For some, pregnancy may pose a high risk of morbidity and even mortality. Patients need to be given detailed advice about various contraceptive methods and their effectiveness, and each patient should understand the relative risks and benefits of each modality.[42] The approach should be individualized, also bearing in mind the patient's likely compliance.[43]

BARRIER CONTRACEPTION. Male and female condoms help protect against sexually transmitted disease but must be used correctly and require some dexterity. Even when used appropriately, they have a recognized failure rate of approximately 15 pregnancies/100 woman-years of use. The decision to use a barrier method therefore depends on how critical it is for the woman to avoid pregnancy and on compliance and the ability to use a condom correctly.

INTRAUTERINE DEVICES. Intrauterine devices (IUDs) may be used in parous women, with failure rates of approximately 3 pregnancies/100 woman-years. Complications include infection and arrhythmia at the time of insertion. A vasovagal response occurring in a patient with idiopathic pulmonary arterial hypertension or secondary pulmonary hypertension, such as Eisenmenger syndrome, could be life-threatening, and many physicians therefore avoid use of an IUD in such patients. More recently developed IUDs are more effective than earlier devices in preventing pregnancy, particularly those that are loaded with progesterone, which suppresses endometrial activity and thickens cervical mucus.

Oral Contraceptives

Combination estrogen-progesterone oral preparations are very effective, with an extremely low failure rate, and for this reason, coupled with ease of use, are widely taken. For the woman with heart disease, however, concern exists because of increased risk of venous thromboembolism, atherosclerosis, hyperlipidemia, hypertension, and ischemic heart disease, particularly for those who are older than 40 years and for those who smoke. In addition, patients with congenital heart disease who have cyanosis, atrial fibrillation or flutter, mechanical prosthetic heart valves, or a Fontan circulation probably should avoid estrogen-containing preparations. Those with impaired ventricular function from any cause (probably an ejection fraction less than 40%) or with a history of any prior thromboembolic event should avoid estrogen.

Progesterone-only contraceptives are less reliable than combined preparations, with failure rates of 2 to 5 pregnancies/100 woman-years. The woman must take the pill at the same time every day for optimum efficacy, and this requires considerable motivation on the part of the patient. There is a paucity of data about adverse effects of progesterone agents on the cardiovascular system, but these are probably safe for most women with heart disease.

ALTERNATIVE COMBINED HORMONAL PREPARATIONS. Newer modalities include a vaginal ring, which is a once-monthly device that is removed after three weeks. A contraceptive patch containing estrogen and progesterone is also available as well as an injectable preparation, both of which have similar efficacy rates.

DEPOT PROGESTERONE. Injectable progesterone, given once every 3 months, is effective and is an attractive alternative for patients who may have problems with compliance with oral medications. Some patients find fluid retention and irregular menstruation to be problems, but cardiovascular contraindications are otherwise the same as those for progesterone.

ALTERNATIVE PROGESTERONE MODALITIES. Subdermal implants, which are inserted into the arm, are also available.

Tubal Sterilization

Tubal sterilization may be performed laparoscopically or through a laparotomy. For patients who have tenuous cardiac hemodynamics, there may be some risk of cardiac instability, and cardiac anesthesia may be preferable. This is particularly important, for example, in patients with primary or secondary pulmonary hypertension when general anesthesia may be hazardous and insufflation of the abdomen may elevate the diaphragm and contribute to unstable cardiorespiratory function. More recently, tubal sterilization has been accomplished with the use of an intrafallopian plug, which is inserted endoscopically.[44]

Future Perspectives

Appropriate pregnancy counseling for women with cardiac disease is problematic. Few physicians have expertise or training to manage such patients, particularly those women with congenital heart disease. Few evidence-based guidelines are available, and most published data involve isolated case reports or small cohort studies. Many questions remain unanswered. Although successful pregnancy is possible in many women with heart disease, does the volume load cause subtle long-term deterioration in ventricular function in those with limited cardiac reserve?[45] What is the ideal management strategy for women with mechanical valve prostheses? These continued uncertainties emphasize the need for multicenter research initiatives to answer prospectively the many questions that remain.

REFERENCES

General

1. Roos-Hesselink JW, Duvekot JJ, Thorne SA: Pregnancy in high risk cardiac conditions. Heart 95:680, 2009.
2. Connolly H, Warnes C: Pregnancy and contraception. *In* Gatzoulis MA, Webb GD, Daubeney PE (eds): Diagnosis and Management of Adult Congenital Heart Disease. Edinburgh, Churchill Livingstone, 2003, pp 135-177.
3. Siu SC, Sermer M, Colman JM, et al: Prospective multicenter study of pregnancy outcomes in women with heart disease. Circulation 104:515, 2001.
4. Thorne SA: Pregnancy in heart disease. Heart 90:450, 2004.
5. Elkayam U, Bitar F: Valvular heart disease and pregnancy part I: Native valves. J Am Coll Cardiol 46:223, 2005.

Congenital Heart Disease

6. Warnes CA, Williams RG, Bashore TM, et al: ACC/AHA 2008 Guidelines for the Management of Adults with Congenital Heart Disease: A report of the American College of Cardiology/American Heart Association Task Force on Practice Guidelines (writing committee to develop guidelines on the management of adults with congenital heart disease). Circulation 118:e714, 2008.
7. Drenthen W, Pieper PG, Roos-Hesselink JW, et al: Outcome of pregnancy in women with congenital heart disease: A literature review. J Am Coll Cardiol 49:2303, 2007.
8. Stout K: Pregnancy in women with congenital heart disease: The importance of evaluation and counselling [comment]. Heart 91:713, 2005.
9. Silversides CK, Colman JM, Sermer M, et al: Early and intermediate-term outcomes of pregnancy with congenital aortic stenosis. Am J Cardiol 91:1386, 2003.
10. Myerson SG, Mitchell AR, Ormerod OJ, Banning AP: What is the role of balloon dilatation for severe aortic stenosis during pregnancy? [see comment]. J Heart Valve Dis 14:147, 2005.
11. Warnes CA: Cyanotic congenital heart disease. *In* Oakley C, Warnes CA (eds): Heart Disease in Pregnancy. Malden, Mass, Blackwell, 2007, pp 43-58.
12. Presbitero P, Somerville J, Stone S, et al: Pregnancy in cyanotic congenital heart disease. Outcome of mother and fetus. Circulation 89:2673, 1994.
13. Beauchesne LM, Warnes CA, Connolly HM, et al: Prevalence and clinical manifestations of 22q11.2 microdeletion in adults with selected conotruncal anomalies [see comment]. J Am Coll Cardiol 45:595, 2005.
14. Khairy P, Ouyang DW, Fernandes SM, et al: Pregnancy outcomes in women with congenital heart disease. Circulation 113:517, 2006.
15. Meijer JM, Pieper PG, Drenthen W, et al: Pregnancy, fertility, and recurrence risk in corrected tetralogy of Fallot [see comment]. Heart 91:801, 2005.
16. Veldtman GR, Connolly HM, Grogan M, et al: Outcomes of pregnancy in women with tetralogy of Fallot [see comment]. J Am Coll Cardiol 44:174, 2004.
17. Warnes CA: Pregnancy and pulmonary hypertension. Int J Cardiol 97(Suppl 1):11, 2004.
18. Gleicher N, Midwall J, Hochberger D, Jaffin H: Eisenmenger's syndrome and pregnancy. Obstet Gynecol Surv 34:721, 1979.
19. Bonnin M, Mercier FJ, Sitbon O, et al: Severe pulmonary hypertension during pregnancy: Mode of delivery and anesthetic management of 15 consecutive cases [see comment]. Anesthesiology 102:1133; discussion 5A, 2005.
20. Lacassie HJ, Germain AM, Valdes G, et al: Management of Eisenmenger syndrome in pregnancy with sildenafil and L-arginine. Obstet Gynecol 103:1118, 2004.

Rheumatic and Acquired Valvular Heart Disease

21. Routray SN, Mishra TK, Swain S, et al: Balloon mitral valvuloplasty during pregnancy. Int J Gynaecol Obstet 85:18, 2004.
22. Aggarwal N, Suri V, Goyal A, et al: Closed mitral valvotomy in pregnancy and labor. Int J Gynaecol Obstet 88:118, 2005.
23. Elkayam U, Singh H, Irani A, Akhter MW: Anticoagulation in pregnant women with prosthetic heart valves. J Cardiovasc Pharmacol Ther 9:107, 2004.
24. Jamieson WR, Miller DC, Akins CW, et al: Pregnancy and bioprostheses: Influence on structural valve deterioration. Ann Thorac Surg 60:S282; discussion S287, 1995.
25. Bates SM, Greer IA, Hirsh J, Ginsberg JS: Use of antithrombotic agents during pregnancy: The Seventh ACCP Conference on Antithrombotic and Thrombolytic Therapy. Chest 126:627S, 2004.
26. Sbarouni E, Oakley CM: Outcome of pregnancy in women with valve prostheses. Br Heart J 71:196, 1994.
27. Elkayam U, Bitar F: Valvular heart disease and pregnancy: Part II: Prosthetic valves. J Am Coll Cardiol 46:403, 2005.
28. Chan WS, Anand S, Ginsberg JS: Anticoagulation of pregnant women with mechanical heart valves: A systematic review of the literature. Arch Intern Med 160:191, 2000.
29. Barbour LA, Oja JL, Schultz LK: A prospective trial that demonstrates that dalteparin requirements increase in pregnancy to maintain therapeutic levels of anticoagulation. Am J Obstet Gynecol 191:1024, 2004.
30. Oran B, Lee-Parritz A, Ansell J: Low molecular weight heparin for the prophylaxis of thromboembolism in women with prosthetic mechanical heart valves during pregnancy. Thromb Haemost 92:747, 2004.
31. Vitale N, De Feo M, De Santo LS, et al: Dose-dependent fetal complications of warfarin in pregnant women with mechanical heart valves [see comment]. J Am Coll Cardiol 33:1637, 1999.

Connective Tissue Disorders

32. Meijboom LJ, Vos FE, Timmermans J, et al: Pregnancy and aortic root growth in the Marfan syndrome: A prospective study [see comment]. Eur Heart J 26:914, 2005.

Cardiomyopathies

33. Elkayam U, Akhter MW, Singh H, et al: Pregnancy-associated cardiomyopathy: Clinical characteristics and a comparison between early and late presentation. Circulation 111:2050, 2005.
34. Sliwa K, Fett J, Elkayam U: Peripartum cardiomyopathy. Lancet 368:687, 2006.
35. Phillips SD, Warnes CA: Peripartum cardiomyopathy: Current therapeutic perspectives. Curr Treat Options Cardiovasc Med 6:481, 2004.
36. Sliwa K, Forster O, Zhanje F, et al: Outcome of subsequent pregnancy in patients with documented peripartum cardiomyopathy. Am J Cardiol 93:1441, 2004.
37. Thaman R, Varnava A, Hamid MS, et al: Pregnancy related complications in women with hypertrophic cardiomyopathy. Heart 89:752, 2003.

Coronary Artery Disease

38. Roth A, Elkayam U: Acute myocardial infarction associated with pregnancy. J Am Coll Cardiol 52:171, 2008.
39. Maeder M, Ammann P, Angehrn W, Rickli H: Idiopathic spontaneous coronary artery dissection: Incidence, diagnosis and treatment. Int J Cardiol 101:363, 2005.
40. James AH, Jamison MG, Biswas MS, et al: Acute myocardial infarction in pregnancy: A United States population-based study. Circulation 113:1564, 2006.

Hypertension

41. Gifford RW, August PA, Cunningham G, et al: Report of the National High Blood Pressure Education Program Working Group on High Blood Pressure in Pregnancy. Am J Obstet Gynecol 183:S1, 2000.

Contraception

42. Wald R, Colman J: Pregnancy and contraception. *In* Warnes C (ed): The AHA Clinical Series: Adult Congenital Heart Disease. Hoboken, NJ, Wiley-Blackwell, 2009, pp 237-259.
43. Thorne S, MacGregor A, Nelson-Piercy C: Risks of contraception and pregnancy in heart disease. Heart 92:1520, 2006.
44. Famuyide AO, Hopkins MR, El-Nashar SA, et al: Hysteroscopic sterilization in women with severe cardiac disease: Experience at a tertiary center. Mayo Clin Proc 83:431, 2008.
45. Guedes A, Mercier LA, Leduc L, et al: Impact of pregnancy on the systemic right ventricle after a Mustard operation for transposition of the great arteries. J Am Coll Cardiol 44:433, 2004.

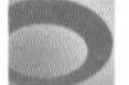

GUIDELINES Carole A. Warnes and Thomas H. Lee

Pregnancy and Heart Disease

Recommendations for the management of heart disease in pregnancy appear in various American College of Cardiology/American Heart Association (ACC/AHA) guidelines. These include guidelines on valvular heart disease,[1] atrial fibrillation,[2] and stroke.[3] The European Society of Cardiology also published guidelines on the management of valvular heart disease[4] as well as a position paper on use of anticoagulants in heart disease.[5]

ATRIAL FIBRILLATION

Atrial fibrillation is rare during pregnancy and is usually associated with another underlying cause, such as mitral stenosis, congenital heart disease, or hyperthyroidism. Diagnosis and treatment of the underlying condition causing the dysrhythmia are of utmost importance. Antithrombotic therapy is recommended for all pregnant women with atrial fibrillation.

The type of therapy should be chosen with regard to the stage of pregnancy (**Table 82G-1**).[2] The ventricular rate should be controlled with digoxin, calcium channel antagonist, or beta blocker. Direct-current cardioversion can be performed without fetal damage in women who become hemodynamically unstable because of atrial fibrillation. Administration of quinidine or procainamide is a reasonable approach for cardioversion in pregnant women with atrial fibrillation who are hemodynamically stable.

VALVULAR DISEASE

Many women with valvular heart disease can be successfully managed throughout pregnancy, labor, and delivery with conservative medical measures. Symptomatic or severe valvular lesions should be addressed and rectified before conception and pregnancy whenever possible. Drugs should be avoided when possible.[1]

Mitral Stenosis

Pregnant women with mild to moderate mitral stenosis can almost always be managed with judicious use of diuretics and beta blockade. A cardioselective beta blocker may prevent deleterious effects of epinephrine blockade on myometrial tissue. Women with severe mitral stenosis should be considered for percutaneous balloon mitral valvotomy before conception, if possible. Percutaneous balloon valvotomy is a reasonable option for women who develop severe symptoms during pregnancy.

Mitral Regurgitation

Mitral regurgitation can usually be managed medically with diuretics and vasodilator therapy. If surgery is required, repair is always preferred.

Aortic Stenosis

Pregnant women with mild obstruction and normal left ventricular systolic function can be managed conservatively throughout pregnancy. Those with moderate to severe obstruction or symptoms should be advised to delay conception until aortic stenosis can be corrected. Women with severe aortic stenosis who develop symptoms may require either early delivery of the baby or percutaneous aortic balloon valvotomy or surgery before delivery.

Aortic Regurgitation

Isolated aortic regurgitation can usually be managed with diuretics and vasodilator therapy when needed. Surgery during pregnancy should be contemplated only for control of refractory symptoms.

Endocarditis Prophylaxis

The guidelines do not recommend routine antibiotic prophylaxis in patients with valvular heart disease undergoing uncomplicated vaginal delivery or cesarean section unless infection is suspected. For high-risk patients, such as those with cyanotic heart disease, prosthetic heart valves, or a prior history of endocarditis, antibiotics are considered optional.[6]

SUPRAVENTRICULAR TACHYCARDIAS

Premature atrial beats, which are commonly observed during pregnancy, are generally benign and well tolerated. In patients with mild symptoms and structurally normal hearts, no treatment other than reassurance should be provided. Given that all commonly used antiarrhythmic drugs cross the placental barrier to some extent, antiarrhythmic drug therapy should be used only if symptoms are intolerable or if the tachycardia causes hemodynamic compromise (**Table 82G-2**).[7]

Catheter ablation should be recommended for women with symptomatic tachyarrhythmias before they contemplate pregnancy. Because of the potential problem of recurring tachyarrhythmias during pregnancy, the policy of withdrawing antiarrhythmic drugs and resuming them later can be recommended only as an alternative in selected cases. Catheter ablation is the procedure of choice for drug-refractory, poorly tolerated supraventricular tachycardia. If needed, it should be performed in the second trimester.

TABLE 82G-1 ACC/AHA Recommendations for Management of Atrial Fibrillation (AF) During Pregnancy

CLASS	INDICATION	LEVEL OF EVIDENCE
Class I (indicated)	Control the rate of ventricular response with digoxin, a beta blocker, or a calcium channel antagonist.	C
	Perform electrical cardioversion in patients who become hemodynamically unstable because of the dysrhythmia.	C
	Administer antithrombotic therapy (anticoagulant or aspirin) throughout pregnancy to all patients with AF (except those with lone AF).	C
Class IIb (weak supportive evidence)	Attempt pharmacologic cardioversion by administration of quinidine, procainamide, or sotalol in hemodynamically stable patients who develop AF during pregnancy.	C
	Administer heparin to patients with risk factors for thromboembolism during the first trimester and last month of pregnancy. Unfractionated heparin may be administered either by continuous intravenous infusion in a dose sufficient to prolong the activated partial thromboplastin time to 1.5 to 2 times the control (reference) value or by intermittent subcutaneous injection in a dose of 10,000 to 20,000 units every 12 hours, adjusted to prolong the midinterval (6 hours after injection) activated partial thromboplastin time to 1.5 times control. Limited data are available to support the subcutaneous administration of low-molecular-weight heparin for this indication.	C
	Administer an oral anticoagulant during the second trimester to patients at high thromboembolic risk.	C

TABLE 82G-2 ACC/AHA Recommendations for Treatment Strategies for Supraventricular Tachycardias During Pregnancy

INDICATION	CLASS I (INDICATED) [LEVEL OF EVIDENCE]	CLASS IIa (STRONG SUPPORTIVE EVIDENCE) [LEVEL OF EVIDENCE]	CLASS IIb (WEAK SUPPORTIVE EVIDENCE) [LEVEL OF EVIDENCE]	CLASS III (NOT INDICATED) [LEVEL OF EVIDENCE]
Acute conversion of PSVT	Vagal maneuver [C] Adenosine [C] Direct-current cardioversion [C]	Metoprolol,* propranolol* [C]	Verapamil [C]	
Prophylactic therapy	Digoxin [C] Metoprolol*	Propranolol* [B] Sotalol,* flecainide† [C]	Quinidine, propafenone,† verapamil [C] Procainamide [B] Catheter ablation [C]	Atenolol‡ [B] Amiodarone [C]

*Beta-blocking agents should not be taken in the first trimester, if possible.
†Consider atrioventricular node–blocking agents in conjunction with flecainide and propafenone for certain tachycardias.
‡Atenolol is categorized in class C (drug classification for use during pregnancy) by legal authorities in some European countries.
PSVT = paroxysmal supraventricular tachycardia.

STROKE

Pregnancy increases the risk for stroke and complicates the selection of acute and preventive treatments. Guidelines for acute treatment have not yet been established. Recommendations for stroke prevention in pregnant women made by the American Heart Association and American Stroke Association (AHA/ASA)[4] focus on anticoagulation and antiplatelet strategies (**Table 82G-3**), which are similar to those for management of valvular heart disease during pregnancy.

HYPERTENSION

The European Society of Hypertension and the European Society of Cardiology (ESH/ESC) issued guidelines in 2007 that address the management of hypertension in pregnancy (**Table 82G-4**).[8]

ANTICOAGULATION

The 2006 ACC/AHA guidelines on valvular heart disease emphasize the importance of pre-pregnancy counseling about anticoagulation strategies before pregnancy and the need for meticulous and frequent monitoring of anticoagulation once pregnancy occurs. The guidelines reflect the high complication rates in pregnant women with mechanical prosthetic heart valves managed with subcutaneous heparin and support the use of intravenous heparin during the first trimester. After the 36th week of pregnancy, transition from warfarin to heparin is recommended in anticipation of labor. There is no consensus on the ideal management strategy for women with mechanical prosthetic heart valves given the paucity of data regarding their comparative efficacy. A menu of options is proposed for anticoagulation strategies (**Table 82G-5**).

These strategies are complicated by the fact that low-molecular-weight heparin is not approved by the U.S. Food and Drug Administration (FDA) for use in any patient with a mechanical prosthetic heart valve, and the FDA has issued an advisory warning against the use of enoxaparin (Lovenox) in pregnant women with mechanical prosthetic heart valves. The guidelines note that some data indicate that low-molecular-weight heparin appears to be safe in nonpregnant patients with mechanical heart valves, but the expert panel could not recommend its use directly, given the status of FDA-approved indications. The ACC/AHA Guidelines for Adult Congenital Heart Disease emphasize that whichever anticoagulant

TABLE 82G-3 AHA/ASA Recommendations for Stroke Prevention During Pregnancy

CLASS	INDICATION	LEVEL OF EVIDENCE
Class IIb (weak supportive evidence)	For pregnant women with ischemic stroke or TIA and high-risk thromboembolic conditions, such as known coagulopathy or mechanical heart valves, the following options may be considered: adjusted-dose UFH throughout pregnancy, e.g., a subcutaneous dose every 12 hours with activated partial thromboplastin time monitoring; adjusted-dose LMWH with factor Xa monitoring throughout pregnancy; or UFH or LMWH until week 13, followed by warfarin until the middle of the third trimester, when UFH or LMWH is then reinstituted until delivery.	C
	Pregnant women with lower risk conditions may be considered for treatment with UFH or LMWH in the first trimester, followed by low-dose aspirin for the remainder of the pregnancy.	C

LMWH = low-molecular-weight heparin; TIA = transient ischemic attack; UFH = unfractionated heparin.

TABLE 82G-4 ESH/ESC Guidelines for the Management of Hypertension During Pregnancy

Nonpharmacologic treatment (including close supervision and restriction of activities) should be considered with SBP 140-149 mm Hg or DBP 90-95 mm Hg. In the presence of gestational hypertension (with or without proteinuria), drug treatment is indicated at blood pressure ≥140/90 mm Hg. SBP levels ≥170 or DBP >110 mm Hg should be considered an emergency requiring hospitalization.

In nonsevere hypertension, oral methyldopa, labetalol, calcium antagonists, and (less frequently) beta blockers are drugs of choice.

In preeclampsia with pulmonary edema, nitroglycerin is the drug of choice. Diuretic therapy is inappropriate because plasma volume is reduced.

As emergency, IV labetalol, oral methyldopa, and oral nifedipine are indicated; IV hydralazine is no longer the drug of choice because of excess perinatal adverse effects. IV infusion of sodium nitroprusside is useful in hypertensive crises, but prolonged administration should be avoided.

Calcium supplementation, fish oil, and low-dose aspirin are not recommended. However, low-dose aspirin may be used prophylactically in women with a history of early-onset preeclampsia.

DBP = diastolic blood pressure; IV = intravenous; SBP = systolic blood pressure.

TABLE 82G-5 ACC/AHA Recommendations for Anticoagulation Regimens in Pregnant Patients with Mechanical Prosthetic Valves

CLASS	INDICATION	LEVEL OF EVIDENCE
Class I (indicated)	Continuous therapeutic anticoagulation with frequent monitoring	B
	If warfarin is discontinued between weeks 6 and 12 of gestation, replace with continuous intravenous UFH, dose-adjusted UFH, or dose-adjusted subcutaneous LMWH.	C
	Up to 36 weeks of gestation, the therapeutic choice of continuous intravenous or dose-adjusted subcutaneous UFH, dose-adjusted LMWH, or warfarin should be discussed fully.	C
	If dose-adjusted LMWH is used, the LMWH should be administered twice daily subcutaneously to maintain the anti-Xa level between 0.7 and 1.2 unit/mL 4 hours after administration.	C
	If dose-adjusted UFH is used, the aPTT should be at least twice control.	C
	If warfarin is used, the INR goal should be 3.0 (range, 2.5 to 3.5).	C
	Warfarin should be discontinued starting 2 to 3 weeks before planned delivery and continuous intravenous UFH given instead.	C
Class IIa (strong supportive evidence)	It is reasonable to avoid warfarin between weeks 6 and 12 of gestation because of the high risk of fetal defects.	C
	It is reasonable to resume UFH 4 to 6 hours after delivery and begin oral warfarin in the absence of significant bleeding.	C
	It is reasonable to give low-dose aspirin (75 to 100 mg/day) in the second and third trimesters of pregnancy in addition to anticoagulation with warfarin or heparin.	C
Class III (not indicated)	LMWH should not be administered unless anti-Xa levels are monitored 4 to 6 hours after administration.	C
	Dipyridamole should not be used instead of aspirin as an alternative antiplatelet agent because of its harmful effects on the fetus.	B

aPTT = activated partial thromboplastin time; INR = international normalized ratio; LMWH = low-molecular-weight heparin; UFH = unfractionated heparin.

strategy is chosen, women with mechanical prosthetic heart valves should be cared for at tertiary care centers where a multidisciplinary team with expertise and training in the management of such patients is responsible for their care.[6]

REFERENCES

1. Bonow RO, Carabello BA, Chatterjee K, et al: ACC/AHA 2006 guidelines for the management of patients with valvular heart disease: A report of the American College of Cardiology/American Heart Association Task Force on Practice Guidelines (writing committee to revise the 1998 Guidelines for the Management of Patients With Valvular Heart Disease): Developed in collaboration with the Society of Cardiovascular Anesthesiologists: Endorsed by the Society for Cardiovascular Angiography and Interventions and the Society of Thoracic Surgeons [erratum appears in Circulation 115:e409, 2007]. Circulation 114:e84, 2006.
2. Fuster V, Ryden LE, Cannom DS, et al: ACC/AHA/ESC 2006 Guidelines for the Management of Patients with Atrial Fibrillation: A report of the American College of Cardiology/American Heart Association Task Force on Practice Guidelines and the European Society of Cardiology Committee for Practice Guidelines (Writing Committee to Revise the 2001 Guidelines for the Management of Patients With Atrial Fibrillation): Developed in collaboration with the European Heart Rhythm Association and the Heart Rhythm Society [erratum appears in Circulation 116:e138, 2007]. Circulation 114:e257, 2006.
3. Adams H, Adams R, Del Zoppo G, Goldstein LB: Guidelines for the early management of patients with ischemic stroke: 2005 guidelines update. A scientific statement from the Stroke Council of the American Heart Association/American Stroke Association [erratum appears in Stroke 36:1626, 2005]. Stroke 36:916, 2005.
4. Vahanian A, Baumgartner H, Bax J, et al: Guidelines on the management of valvular heart disease: The Task Force on the Management of Valvular Heart Disease of the European Society of Cardiology [see comment]. Eur Heart J 28:230, 2007.
5. De Caterina R, Husted S, Wallentin L, et al: Anticoagulants in heart disease: Current status and perspectives [see comment]. Eur Heart J 28:880, 2007.
6. Warnes CA, Williams RG, Bashore TM, et al: ACC/AHA 2008 Guidelines for the Management of Adults with Congenital Heart Disease: A report of the American College of Cardiology/American Heart Association Task Force on Practice Guidelines (writing committee to develop guidelines on the management of adults with congenital heart disease). Circulation 118:e714, 2008.
7. Blomstrom-Lundqvist C, Scheinman MM, Aliot EM, et al: ACC/AHA/ESC guidelines for the management of patients with supraventricular arrhythmias—executive summary. A report of the American College of Cardiology/American Heart Association Task Force on Practice Guidelines and the European Society of Cardiology Committee for Practice Guidelines (writing committee to develop guidelines for the management of patients with supraventricular arrhythmias) developed in collaboration with NASPE–Heart Rhythm Society. J Am Coll Cardiol 42:1493, 2003.
8. Mancia G, De Backer G, Dominiczak A, et al: 2007 Guidelines for the management of arterial hypertension: The Task Force for the Management of Arterial Hypertension of the European Society of Hypertension (ESH) and of the European Society of Cardiology (ESC). Eur Heart J 28:1462, 2007.

CHAPTER 83 Exercise and Sports Cardiology

Gary J. Balady and Philip A. Ades

The importance of exercise and sports were recognized by the ancient Greeks thousands of years ago, but an interesting paradox now exists. A large volume of evidence from epidemiologic observational studies, cohort studies, randomized controlled trials, and basic research, primarily conducted during the past four decades, demonstrates unequivocal evidence that exercise and physical activity confer health. The publication of the seminal 1996 Surgeon General's Report on Physical Activity and Health[1] moved the promotion of physical activity to the top of America's national public health agenda. Physical inactivity is now recognized as an independent risk factor for the development of cardiovascular disease (CVD)[2] (see Chap. 49). In the face of these events, however, only a small proportion of Americans engage in adequate physical activity. The Centers for Disease Control and Prevention has indicated that approximately 31% of adult Americans participate in recommended levels of physical activity, and almost 40% report no regular leisure time physical activity whatsoever.[3] Although the world benefits from advancements in technology that lead to increased productivity and improved quality of life, the price is paid in part by the generation of a sedentary society that spends much of its time in cars, at computer stations, and in front of televisions and video screens.

Medical professionals and public health and community leaders continue their unprecedented efforts to promote increased physical activity through venues that range from casual walks to participation in organized sports, and health care providers need to support these efforts for their patients in regard to optimizing the benefits of participation while minimizing the small but potential associated risks. This chapter presents these issues with an overview of the classifications of exercise and sports, data regarding the benefits of exercise and mechanisms by which these benefits occur, risks of exercise, exercise prescription, and screening and recommendations for participation in exercise and athletic competition with a particular emphasis on those with specific cardiovascular conditions.

Physical Activity, Exercise, and Sports

To understand the many issues regarding exercise and sports, and subsequently make important activity-related clinical decisions, a review of standard definitions[1] is essential. Physical activity refers to any activity in which skeletal muscle contraction and relaxation result in bodily movement and require energy. The intensity of physical activity can be described in terms of the energy required per unit of time for the performance of the activity. This variable can be quantified in absolute terms by measuring the oxygen uptake during the activity using respiratory gas analysis. It can also be estimated using standard regression equations as a multiple of resting energy expenditure (MET), where one MET is defined as the oxygen requirement in the resting awake individual (3.5 mL/kg of body weight/min). The intensity of a physical activity can also be defined in relative terms by expressing it as a proportion of the individual's maximal capacity (e.g., the percentage of maximal oxygen uptake or the percentage of maximum heart rate). Alternatively, activity intensity can be expressed as a measure of the force of muscle contraction required (in pounds or kilograms). When defining the amount of physical activity or exercise, an important interrelationship exists between the total dose of activity and the intensity at which the activity is performed. Dose refers to the total amount of energy expended in physical activity expressed in terms of kilocalories or MET-hours, whereas intensity reflects the rate of energy expenditure during such activity.

Exercise or exercise training is planned physical activity performed with the goal of improving or preserving physical fitness. Physical fitness is a set of attributes that enables an individual to perform physical activity. Physical fitness is best assessed by directly measuring peak or maximum oxygen uptake during a graded exercise test. Although this is not always practical, it is more commonly estimated from the peak MET level attained or reporting the peak work rate (e.g., speed and grade of a treadmill, watts on a stationary cycle) during graded exercise tests.[1]

Most types of exercise involve both endurance and resistance training, but one training type usually predominates (**Table 83-1**). The physiologic responses to exercise depend on the type of exercise performed. Endurance exercise, also referred to as aerobic, dynamic, or isotonic exercise, consists of activity involving high-repetition movements against low resistance. Regular endurance exercise is also referred to as endurance training, because it usually leads to an improved exercise capacity, thereby enabling the individual to exercise for a longer duration or at a higher work rate. Resistance exercise involves low-repetition movements against high resistance, in which muscle tension develops predominantly without much muscle shortening. Regular resistance training leads to increased strength and is also referred to as power or strength training. **Figure 83-1** demonstrates the classification of several types of sports as related to the peak static and dynamic components achieved during competition.[4] The classification does not take into account differences in environment (e.g., altitude, temperature, air quality) in which the sport is performed. Each of these variables can influence the physiologic responses during sports activity as well.

Finally, a distinction must be made between competitive and recreational sports, because the physiologic and emotional demands during training and performance may differ markedly.[5] Competitive athletes participate in an organized sport that places a high premium on athletic excellence and achievement, and requires systematic training and regular competition. These athletes characteristically extend themselves to high levels of effort for long periods of time,

TABLE 83-1 Exercise Prescription for Endurance and Resistance Training

Endurance Training		
Frequency	3-5 days/wk	***Modality****
		Aerobics
		Arm ergometry
		Cross country ski machines
		Combined arm-leg cycle
Intensity	55%-90% maximum HR *or* 40%-85% maximum Vo_2 or HRR	Elliptical machines
		Jogging, running
		Rowing
		Stair climber
		Swimming
		Walking
Duration:	20-60 min	
Resistance Training		
Frequency	2-3 days/wk	***All Major Muscle Groups***
		Arms and shoulders
		Biceps curl
Intensity	One to three sets of 8-15 RM for each muscle group	Tricepextension
		Overhead press
		Lateral raises
		Chest and back
		Bench press
		Lateral pull-downs, pull-ups
		Bent over, seated row
		Legs
		Leg extensions, curls, press
		Adductor, abductor

*Modalities listed are not all-inclusive.

HR = heart rate; maximum HR= 220 − age, or peak HR on exercise test; HRR = heart rate reserve = [(peak HR minus resting HR) × %] plus (resting HR); RM = maximum number of times a load can be lifted before fatigue; Vo_2 = measured oxygen uptake.

Modified from American College of Sports Medicine: ASCM's Guidelines for Exercise Testing and Prescription: 8th ed. Philadelphia, Lippincott Williams & Wilkins, 2009; and Fletcher GF, Balady GJ, Amsterdam EA, et al: Exercise standards for testing and training: A statement for health professionals from the American Heart Association. Circulation 104:1694, 2001.

often doing so regardless of other considerations. Recreational athletes engage in activities, on a regular or inconsistent basis, which do not require regular systematic training or the pursuit of excellence. Hence, they do not have the same pressure to excel as do competitive athletes.

Benefits of Exercise

Physical activity is associated with lower all-cause mortality rates in healthy individuals,[2,4,6,7] individuals with chronic diseases,[8] diabetic persons,[9] and older adults (see Chaps. 49 and 50).[10] Although studies of men and women have demonstrated that physical activity performed decades earlier without subsequent maintenance appears to have no long-term benefit, the risk for all-cause mortality decreases in inactive men and women who subsequently become more physically active.[2] Physical fitness can be more readily measured than physical activity. A consistent and graded relationship exists between peak exercise capacity attained during exercise testing and subsequent mortality in both men and women.[4,6] Regular exercise training in patients with coronary artery disease has demonstrated a reduction in mortality and cardiovascular events in meta-analyses[11] and in a recent large cross -sectional study,[12] but this benefit has not yet been conclusively demonstrated in any single, prospective, randomized trial. In the recently reported HF-ACTION trial, such training in patients with heart failure yielded modest significant reductions in the combined endpoint of all-cause mortality and hospitalizations after prespecified adjusted analysis.[13]

The specific mechanisms whereby physical activity reduces mortality and cardiovascular events are likely multifactorial, and extend beyond a reduction in cardiovascular risk factors, because beneficial effects have been shown on thrombosis, endothelial function, inflammation, and autonomic tone. The magnitude of blood pressure reduction attained with exercise is modest and, in mildly hypertensive persons, yields an effect that resembles that of pharmacologic monotherapy.[14] Physical activity and exercise induce several important and beneficial effects on glucose metabolism, including increased insulin sensitivity, decreased hepatic glucose production, preferential use of glucose over fatty acids by exercising muscle, and reduced obesity.[15] In addition, regular exercise may prevent the onset of diabetes mellitus.[16] Overweight and obesity are associated with significant increases in cardiovascular morbidity and mortality.[17] Exercise training appears to be an important component of weight loss programs, although most randomized controlled trials have shown only modest reductions in weight. Studies have suggested that physical activity and exercise help prevent obesity, maintain weight loss, and prevent weight regain after diet-induced weight loss.[18] The effects of exercise on lipid profiles demonstrate the greatest benefit on triglyceride levels, modest changes in high-density lipoprotein (HDL) levels, and little to no change in low-density lipoprotein (LDL) levels.[2] However, some data have suggested that exercise training reduces the concentration of atherogenic, small, dense LDL particles.[19] A unique study of monozygotic twins has shown that there is a strong genetic component to HDL levels that can be slightly but favorably modified by vigorous activity.[20]

Further evidence suggests that exercise training has beneficial effects on the fibrinolytic system, and many studies have reported an inverse relationship between physical activity or fitness and inflammatory markers.[21] Chronic exercise training appears to have an important and favorable influence on endothelial function in the peripheral arteries[22] as well as the coronary circulation.[23] This effect may depend in part on increased nitric oxide production, and yield a net reduction in oxidative stress[24] and an increase in endothelial progenitor cells.[25] Such improvements have been linked to a reduction in adverse cardiovascular events.[26] Finally, exercise training appears to modulate the balance between sympathetic and parasympathetic tone favorably, an effect associated with improvements in survival.[27]

Changes in the muscular, cardiovascular, and neurohumoral systems that result from exercise training lead to improvement in functional capacity and strength. These changes are referred to as the training effect, and they enable an individual to exercise to higher peak work rates with lower heart rates at each submaximal level of exercise. Aging is associated with a decline in maximal exercise capacity, and a longitudinal study has demonstrated that this decline accelerates with each successive decade of life.[28] Although regular exercise may attenuate this loss of exercise capacity at any age, it does not appear to prevent the progressively greater decline with advancing age.[28]

Risks of Exercise

Although there are many benefits to exercise, the risks during exercise and sports activities are low.[29] Most hazards involve the cardiovascular and musculoskeletal systems. These differ relative to the participant's age, sex, physical fitness, underlying cardiovascular and medical conditions, and the particular activity or sport. Accordingly, the cardiovascular risk-benefit ratio should be assessed for each individual for any given activity.

Age exerts a major influence on cardiovascular risk during exercise. Exercise-related death in persons older than 35 years of age usually results from atherosclerotic coronary artery disease, whereas genetic or congenital cardiac malformations are the predominant causes in younger individuals.[29] Although no centralized program requires mandatory reporting of sudden death in young athletes in the United States, the best available data come from the U.S. National Registry of Sudden Death in Athletes.[30] A recent comprehensive report from this registry has demonstrated that among 1866 sudden deaths in athletes younger than 40 years (mean, 19 years), 56% were deemed to be caused by a cardiovascular cause, at a rate of less than 100 cases/year and an incidence of 0.61/100,000 person-years. A prospective series of somewhat older Italian athletes (mean age, 26 years) who had undergone a national preparticipation screening program has reported the rate of sudden death to be 2.3/100,000 athletes/year, with a rate in men that is more than twice that in women.[31] The cardiovascular causes of sudden death in young athletes younger than 40 years of age are shown in **Table 83-2**, and a detailed report of sudden deaths per specific sport is provided in **Table 83-3**.

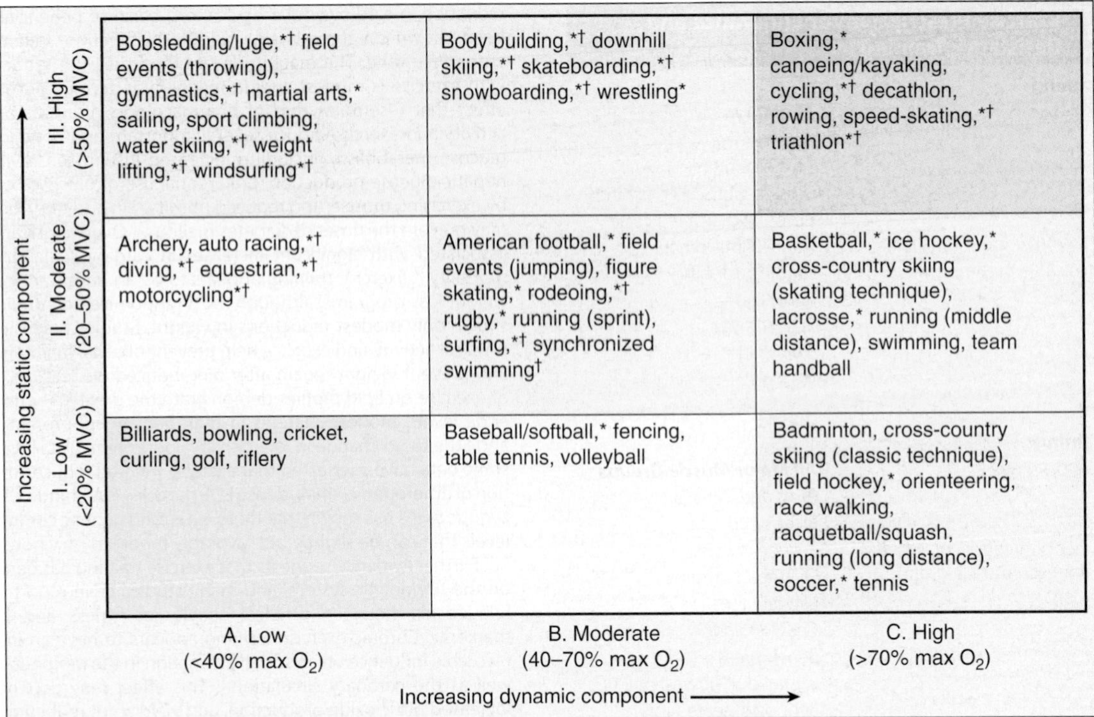

FIGURE 83-1 Classification of sports. This classification is based on peak static and dynamic components achieved during competition. The increasing dynamic component is related to the estimated percentage of maximal oxygen uptake (max O_2) achieved and results in an increasing cardiac output. The increasing static component is related to the estimated percentage of maximal voluntary contraction (MVC) attained and results in an increasing blood pressure. The lowest total cardiovascular demands are shown in green and the highest in red. Blue, yellow, and lavender depict low moderate, moderate, and high moderate total cardiovascular demands. *Danger of bodily collision. †Increased risk if syncope occurs. *(From Mitchell JH, Haskell W, Snell P, Van Camp SP: Task Force 8: Classification of sports. J Am Coll Cardiol 45:1364, 2005.)*

TABLE 83-2 Cardiovascular Causes of Sudden Death in Young Athletes ($N = 690$)

CAUSE	PROPORTION OF ALL CAUSES (%)
Hypertrophic cardiomyopathy	36
Coronary artery anomalies	17
Possible hypertrophic cardiomyopathy*	8
Myocarditis	6
Arrhythmogenic right ventricular cardiomyopathy	4
Ion channel disease	4
Mitral valve prolapse	3
Bridged left anterior descending coronary artery	3
Atherosclerotic coronary artery disease	3
Aortic rupture	3
Aortic stenosis	2
Dilated cardiomyopathy	2
Wolff-Parkinson-White syndrome	2
Other	5

*Findings suggestive but not diagnostic of hypertrophic cardiomyopathy.
Data from Maron BJ, Doerer JJ, Haas TS, et : Sudden death in young competitive athletes: Analysis of 1866 deaths in the United States, 1980-2006. Circulation 119:1085, 2009 (see Chap. 69).

The reported rates of exertionally related sudden death among middle-aged persons vary in part because of the method of data collection and reporting the type of activity involved, and the population studied. Prospectively collected data on men[32] and women[33] have demonstrated that the risk of sudden death during moderate to vigorous exertion is low. Among middle-aged men without known CVD in the Physicians' Health Study, the absolute risk during any episode of vigorous exertion was 1/1.51 million episodes of exertion,[32] whereas that reported in middle-aged women of the Nurses' Health Study during moderate to vigorous exertion was 1/36.5 million hours of exertion.[33] There is also evidence that heavy exertion may trigger an acute myocardial infarction; however, even less precise estimates are available for this occurrence in the general population. Importantly, these studies[32,33] and others clearly demonstrate that the risk of an adverse event increases transiently during the period of exertion, particularly in sedentary persons with occult or known coronary artery disease when performing an unaccustomed, vigorous physical activity. Conversely, the overall risk is significantly lower among those who engage in habitual moderate to vigorous physical activity and exercise.

Traumatic and musculoskeletal injuries during exercise and sports activities constitute an important and sometimes disabling risk of participation, but exceed the scope of this chapter. However, blunt, nonpenetrating chest blows may trigger ventricular fibrillation and sudden cardiac death. This condition is known as commotio cordis and causes approximately 3% of sudden deaths in young athletes in the United States.[30] It most commonly occurs in baseball, ice hockey, lacrosse, football, and martial arts, and is often the result of direct bodily contact from the ball or puck, or between players. Methods for preventing this devastating and often fatal event are discussed in detail elsewhere[34] (see Chap. 41).

Although the risks of each sport vary, long-distance marathon racing deserves special mention. Marathoning in the United States is becoming widely popular, particularly among middle-aged individuals. Of the 340 marathons that took place in 2007, there were 403,000 finishing times recorded. Approximately 69% of male marathoners and 55% of female marathoners are 35 years of age or older, and 6% of men and 3% of female are 60 years of age or older.[35] Studies have demonstrated that the risk of sudden cardiac death during marathon road racing is

TABLE 83-3 Demographics of Sudden Death in Young Athletes

SPORT	NO. (%)	AGE, yr	MALE, *N* (%)	FEMALE, *N* (%)	WHITE	BLACK	OTHER*	SURVIVORS, *N* (%)	TRAUMA INJURY	COMMOTIO CORDIS	CV DISEASES†
Football	565 (30)	17 ± 4	564 (99.8)	1 (0.2)	280	205	80	13 (2)	140 (25)	12 (2)	281 (50)
Basketball	405 (22)	17 ± 4	364 (90)	41 (10)	142	243	20	30 (7)	4 (1.0)	0	349 (86)
Soccer	115 (6)	16 ± 4	93 (81)	22 (19)	81	14	20	7 (6)	11 (10)	4 (4)	80 (70)
Baseball	111 (6)	16 ± 4	111 (100)	0	95	5	11	14 (13)	16 (14)	30 (27)	54 (49)
Motor vehicle racing‡	104 (6)	28 ± 8	103 (99)	1 (1)	102	0	2	0	97 (93)	0	5 (5)
Track and field	96 (5)	17 ± 4	74 (77)	22 (23)	62	22	12	3 (3)	25 (26)	0	61 (64)
Wrestling	69 (4)	22 ± 8	69 (100)	0	56	4	9	2 (3)	7 (10)	1 (1.4)	37 (54)
Boxing	56 (3)	25 ± 6	55 (98)	1 (2)	21	19	16	0	42 (75)	0	11 (1.8)
Swimming§	46 (2)	17 ± 4	30 (65)	16 (35)	43	1	2	1 (2)	0	0	35 (76)
Cross country	38 (2)	17 ± 4	29 (76)	9 (24)	30	6	2	2 (5)	0	0	29 (76)
Hockey	29 (1.5)	18 ± 5	29 (100)	0	28	1	0	3 (10)	4 (14)	7 (24)	11 (38)
Horse riding‖	27 (1.4)	27 ± 8	17 (63)	10 (37)	21	1	5	0	24 (89)	0	2 (7)
Softball	22 (1.2)	19 ± 6	6 (27)	16 (73)	19	0	3	2 (9)	3 (14)	1 (5)	12 (55)
Marathon	20 (1.1)	28 ± 7	15 (75)	5 (25)	16	0	4	3 (15)	0	0	13 (65)
Lacrosse	19 (1.0)	18 ± 2	19 (100)	0	18	1	0	2 (11)	1 (5)	8 (42)	9 (47)
Skiing¶	19 (1.0)	25 ± 8	14 (74)	5 (26)	19	0	0	0	15 (79)	0	1 (5)
Triathlon	17 (0.9)	32 ± 5	15 (88)	2 (12)	16	0	1	0	3 (18)	0	8 (47)
Rugby	16 (0.9)	21 ± 3	16 (100)	0	13	2	1	0	3 (19)	0	7 (44)
Martial arts	15 (0.8)	23 ± 7	14 (93)	1 (7)	12	3	0	0	5 (33)	2 (13)	2 (13)
Others**	14 (0.8)	26 ± 9	12 (86)	2 (14)	14	0	0	2 (14)	3 (21)	0	5 (36)
Rowing	11 (0.6)	22 ± 6	8 (73)	3 (27)	10	0	1	0	0	0	9 (82)
Cycling	10 (0.5)	29 ± 8	8 (80)	2 (20)	7	2	1	0	7 (70)	0	3 (30)
Tennis	10 (0.5)	19 ± 4	8 (80)	2 (20)	8	0	2	0	0	0	8 (80)
Volleyball	10 (0.5)	18 ± 5	1 (10)	9 (90)	5	3	2	1 (10)	0	0	10 (100)
Gymnastics	9 (0.5)	15 ± 3	5 (56)	4 (44)	6	0	3	0	4 (44)	0	3 (33)
Surfing	9 (0.5)	23 ± 8	9 (100)	0	7	0	2	0	2 (22)	0	1 (11)
Figure skating	2 (0.1)	24 ± 6	2 (100)	0	2	0	0	0	0	0	1 (50)
Golf	2 (0.1)	18 ± 0.7	2 (100)	0	2	0	0	0	0	0	2 (100)
Totals	1866	19 ± 6	1692	174	1135	532	199	85	416	65	1049

*Hispanic (*n* = 103); Asian (*n* = 20); Native American (*n* = 5); Pacific Islander (*n* = 5); Middle Eastern (*n* = 3); Indian (*n* = 1); Japanese (*n* = 1); mixed (*n* = 6); unknown (*n* = 55).
†Documented by autopsy and/or clinical findings.
‡Includes automobile (*n* = 63) and motorcycle (*n* = 41) racing.
§Swimming (*n* = 40); water polo (*n* = 6).
‖Jockey (*n* = 16); equestrian (*n* = 11).
¶Skiing (*n* = 12); snowboarding (*n* = 5); ski-jumping (*n* = 2).
** Skateboarding (*n* = 5); jai-alai (*n* = 4); field hockey (*n* = 2); bobsledding (*n* = 1); bowling (*n* = 1); riflery (*n* = 1).
From Maron BJ, Doerer JJ, Haas TS, et al: Sudden death in young competitive athletes: Analysis of 1866 deaths in the United States, 1980-2006. Circulation 119:1085, 2009.

approximately 0.8 to 1.1/100,000 race participants,[36,37] and that this risk appears to be decreasing relative to prior estimates, while the likelihood of survival is increasing. Improved survival may result from the greater availability of automated cardiac defibrillators at these events.[36] The risk of marathon racing among persons with recognized or occult CVD is not known, but it would be expected to be greater. Although marathon racing can lead to metabolic derangements, hyponatremia caused by overhydration recently has been recognized as an important and preventable risk.[38] Several studies have demonstrated structural and biochemical evidence of transient myocardial injury and systolic and diastolic dysfunction in the right and left ventricles. Some of these abnormalities may persist up to 1 month after a race,[39,39a] but the clinical significance of these findings is uncertain.

Exercise Prescription for Health and Fitness

Consensus papers and guidelines from the American Heart Association and the American College of Sports Medicine,[2,40,41] Institute of Medicine,[42] and U.S. Surgeon General[1] all recommend that adults exercise for 30 to 60 minutes at moderate-intensity levels (e.g., brisk walking) on most, if not all, days of the week, with the goal of achieving a weekly energy expenditure of at least 1000 kcal. This is considered the most basic exercise prescription. It is simple, effective, and based on scientific evidence. This recommendation has been further modified to specify that alternatively, vigorous-intensity aerobic physical activity should be performed for a minimum of 20 minutes on 3 days/

week, and that every adult should perform activities that maintain or increase muscular strength and endurance a minimum of 2 days/week.[40] The recommended daily physical activity can be accomplished in a single session or during multiple shorter intervals throughout the day. If exercise is of low intensity (e.g., slow walking), it should be performed more frequently and for longer duration.

Numerous exercise training studies have evaluated the frequency, intensity, and duration of the training sessions required to achieve physical fitness and muscular strength (see Table 83-1). Improvements in peak oxygen uptake of 15% to 30% are usually achieved for sedentary individuals using the regimen as outlined for endurance training. Intermittent activity at comparable exercise intensity and total duration can confer fitness benefits similar to those of continuous activity.[2] Details regarding the exercise prescription are provided elsewhere.[41]

The prescription for exercise training in persons with known CVD is presented in detail in Chap. 50. Issues regarding exercise and sports participation in those with specific cardiovascular conditions are discussed later in this chapter. Exercise tests should be performed on all cardiac patients who are about to begin an exercise training program, and should be repeated periodically or whenever the patient's condition warrants. Exercise intensity can be ascertained by an exercise test using the heart rate reserve method and peak heart rate (see Table 83-1). If angina or ischemic ST-segment depression occurs during the exercise test, the training heart rate should be a minimum of 10 beats/min below the heart rate at which the abnormality occurs. Modalities for training can be categorized by the specific muscle groups that are exercised, such as arms, legs, or both. In addition, different modalities emphasize predominantly endurance or resistance exercises (see Table 4.1.3 on website).

Screening

Concerted efforts to promote physical activity and exercise aim to increase levels of regular physical activity throughout the U.S. population, including the almost 25% of adult Americans who have some form of CVD. Although the benefits of exercise generally outweigh the risks, adequate screening and evaluation are important to identify and counsel persons with underlying CVD to minimize those risks before they begin exercising at vigorous levels (≥60% heart rate reserve or ≥77% peak heart rate; see Table 83-1). However, screening should not constitute an impediment to the widespread implementation of physical activity.

Screening can take place in many different settings and venues, such as the following: during office visits to the health care provider[40,41,43]; at health and fitness centers on enrollment or periodic guest use[44]; using self-screening tools from the American Heart Association and other organizations; and during preseason physical examinations for young athletes about to engage in a particular sport.[45,46] If underlying CVD is suspected or detected by any of these evaluations, then appropriate medical referral for further assessment is needed.

Medical Office Setting

Details regarding medical screening are provided elsewhere.[41,43,45,46] Abnormalities in any of the key elements of the history and physical examination, as shown in **Table 83-4**, should prompt further evaluation and testing. Using the American Heart Association risk classification scheme (**Table 83-5**), health care providers can assess whether vigorous exercise training can be permitted and what level of supervision and monitoring, if any, are needed.[47] Exercise testing is important in the risk stratification process for those deemed to be at greater risk of having underlying heart disease, particularly coronary artery disease, or those with diabetes. It also allows the establishment of appropriate and specific safety precautions, target exercise training heart rate, and initial levels of exercise training work rates.

Health and Fitness Facilities

The American Heart Association recommends that all facilities offering exercise equipment or services should conduct cardiovascular screening of all new members and/or prospective users.[44] The use of simple screening tools, such as the Physical Activity Readiness Questionnaire (PAR-Q), are recommended, with appropriate medical evaluation and follow-up as indicated.

TABLE 83-4 American Heart Association Consensus Panel Recommendations for Preparticipation Athletic Screening

Family History
1. Premature sudden cardiac death
2. Heart disease in surviving relatives < 50 yr
Personal History
3. Heart murmur
4. Systemic hypertension
5. Fatigue
6. Syncope, near-syncope
7. Excessive, unexplained exertional dyspnea
8. Exertional chest pain
Physical Examination
9. Heart murmur (supine/standing)
10. Femoral arterial pulses (to exclude coarctation of aorta)
11. Stigmata of Marfan syndrome
12. Brachial blood pressure measurement (sitting)

From Maron BJ, Douglas PS, Graham TP, et : Task Force 1: Preparticipation screening and diagnosis of cardiovascular disease in athletes. J Am Coll Cardiol 45:1322, 2005.

Athletes

Screening of competitive athletes prior to participation in organized sports is a particularly challenging issue, and is discussed in detail elsewhere.[43,45,46,48,49] There are approximately 10 to 15 million athletes in the United States. Although sudden cardiac death among these athletes is uncommon, it is nonetheless a tragic and potentially avoidable event. The risk for sudden death during exercise in young persons is much lower than in middle-aged adults because few young persons have advanced coronary artery disease, and because congenital and genetic cardiovascular problems that cause sudden cardiac death (e.g., hypertrophic cardiomyopathy, anomalous coronary arteries, congenital long-QT syndrome) are so rare (see Table 83-2). The estimated prevalence of these conditions in the young athletic population is 0.2%.[48] Mass screening of athletes can be particularly difficult, because individuals with these life-threatening conditions are often asymptomatic and their physical examination is generally unrevealing. In addition, the evaluation can be confounded by the normal physiologic changes in autonomic tone and in cardiac size and structure that occur with prolonged and intense training, known as the athlete's heart.[45] These changes are reflected in the electrocardiogram (ECG), which can appear abnormal in about 40% of elite athletes, and in the echocardiogram, which may demonstrate increased cardiac mass, chamber dimensions, and wall thickness. Chap. 69 discusses criteria for distinguishing hypertrophic cardiomyopathy from the athlete's heart.

Because no screening test or procedure will yield 100% sensitivity and specificity for the detection of a life-threatening cardiovascular abnormality or guarantee a zero-risk outcome, what more can be done to promote their detection and reduce the occurrence of adverse events? Although the specifics of screening remain controversial,[50] the American Heart Association does not recommend routine electrocardiography or echocardiography in the initial mass screening evaluation of young athletes because of their diagnostic and cost limitations when applied to this population.[46] However, these tests may be an important part of subsequent evaluations in the medical office setting, as clinically indicated. Those responsible for screening evaluations and supervision of athletes should be informed about the most common causes of sudden death in athletes (see Table 83-2). This will heighten their awareness of the signs and symptoms of associated cardiac conditions during the initial assessment and at any time during athletic participation. The initial medical history and physical should include

TABLE 83-5 American Heart Association Risk Classification for Exercise Training

Class A: Apparently healthy individuals.

This classification includes the following:

A1. Children, adolescents, men < 45 yr, and women < 55 yr who have no symptoms or known presence of heart disease or major coronary risk factors.
A2. Men ≥ 45 yr and women ≥55 yr who have no symptoms or known presence of heart disease and with less than two major cardiovascular risk factors.
A3. Men ≥ 45 yr and women ≥ 55 yr who have no symptoms or known presence of heart disease and with two or more major cardiovascular risk factors.

Activity guidelines: No restrictions other than basic guidelines

Supervision required: None

ECG and blood pressure monitoring: Not required

Note: It is suggested that persons classified as Class A2, and particularly Class A3, undergo a medical examination and possibly a medically supervised exercise test before engaging in vigorous exercise.

Class B: Presence of known, stable cardiovascular disease with low risk for complications with vigorous exercise, but slightly greater than for apparently healthy individuals.

This classification includes individuals with any of the following diagnoses:

1. Coronary artery disease (angina, myocardial infarction, coronary revascularization, abnormal exercise test, and abnormal coronary angiograms), whose condition is stable and who have the clinical characteristics outlined below
2. Valvular heart disease, excluding severe valvular stenosis or regurgitation with the clinical characteristics as outlined below
3. Congenital heart disease—risk stratification for patients with congenital heart disease should be guided by 36th Bethesda Conference recommendations[60]
4. Cardiomyopathy—ejection fraction ≤ 30%; includes stable patients with heart failure with clinical characteristics as outlined below; not hypertrophic cardiomyopathy or recent myocarditis
5. Exercise test abnormalities that do not meet any of the high-risk criteria outlined in class C, below

Clinical characteristics (must include all of the following):

1. NYHA Class I or II
2. Exercise capacity ≥ 6 METs
3. No evidence of "congestive" heart failure
4. No evidence of myocardial ischemia or angina at rest nor on the exercise test ≤ 6 METs
5. Appropriate rise in systolic blood pressure during exercise
6. Absence of sustained or nonsustained ventricular tachycardia at rest or with exercise
7. Ability to self-monitor intensity of activity satisfactorily

Activity guidelines: Activity should be individualized with exercise prescription provided by qualified individuals and approved by primary health care provider.

Supervision required: Medical supervision during initial prescription session is beneficial. Supervision by appropriate trained nonmedical personnel for other exercise sessions is recommended until the individual understands how to monitor his or her activity. Medical personnel should be trained and certified in Advanced Cardiac Life Support (ACLS). Nonmedical personnel should be trained and certified in basic life support, which includes cardiopulmonary resuscitation.

ECG and blood pressure monitoring: Useful during the early prescription phase of training, usually 6 to 12 sessions.

Class C: Those at moderate to high risk for cardiac complications during exercise and/or unable to self-regulate activity or to understand recommended activity level.

This classification includes individuals with any of the following diagnoses:

1. CAD with the clinical characteristics outlined below
2. Valvular heart disease—excluding severe valvular stenosis or regurgitation with the clinical characteristics as outlined below
3. Congenital heart disease—risk stratification for patients with congenital heart disease should be guided by 36th Bethesda Conference recommendations[60]
4. Cardiomyopathy—ejection fraction < 30%; includes stable patients with heart failure with clinical characteristics as outlined below; not hypertrophic cardiomyopathy or recent myocarditis
5. Complex ventricular arrhythmias not well controlled

Clinical characteristics (any of the following):

1. NYHA Class III or IV
2. Exercise test results:
   - Exercise capacity < 6 METs
   - Angina or ischemic ST depression at a workload < 6 METs
   - Fall in systolic blood pressure below resting levels during exercise
   - Nonsustained ventricular tachycardia with exercise
3. Previous episode of primary cardiac arrest (i.e., cardiac arrest that did not occur in the presence of an acute myocardial infarction or during a cardiac procedure)
4. A medical problem that the physician believes may be life-threatening

Activity guidelines: Activity should be individualized with exercise prescription provided by qualified individuals and approved by primary health care provider.

Supervision: Medical supervision during all exercise sessions until safety is established.

ECG and blood pressure monitoring: Continuous during exercise sessions until safety is established, usually 12 sessions or more.

Note: Class C patients who have successfully completed a series of supervised exercise sessions may be reclassified to Class B, providing that the safety of exercise at the prescribed intensity is satisfactorily established by appropriate medical personnel, and that the patient has demonstrated the ability to self-monitor.

Class D: Unstable disease with activity restriction. Exercise for conditioning purposes is not recommended.

This classification includes individuals with any of the following:

1. Unstable ischemia
2. Severe and symptomatic valvular stenosis or regurgitation
3. Congenital heart disease—criteria for risk that would prohibit exercise conditioning in patients with congenital heart disease should be guided by 36th Bethesda Conference recommendations[60]
4. Heart failure that is not compensated
5. Uncontrolled arrhythmias
6. Other medical conditions that could be aggravated by exercise

Activity guidelines: No activity is recommended for conditioning purposes. Attention should be directed to treating and restoring patient to Class C or better. Daily activities must be prescribed based on individual assessment by the patient's personal physician.

Modified from Fletcher GF, Balady GJ, Amsterdam EA, et : Exercise standards for testing and training: A statement for health professionals from the American Heart Association. Circulation 104:1694, 2001.

all the key elements as defined by the American Heart Association (see Table 83-4). Abnormal findings should prompt appropriate medical referral and further cardiovascular testing, as indicated. Finally, athletes and coaches should be advised that if the athlete develops chest discomfort, syncope or near-syncope, excessive dyspnea, palpitations, or other unusual symptoms during training or competition, they should report to medical personnel for an appropriate evaluation.

Exercise and Sports in Persons with Cardiovascular Disease

The presence of structural heart disease once signified the imposition of a sedentary lifestyle and an almost total avoidance of physical activity and competitive sports. There is now compelling evidence that regular exercise can reduce cardiovascular events and cardiovascular mortality in individuals with known coronary heart disease (CHD).[11,12] Furthermore, in the setting of other cardiovascular conditions, such as arterial hypertension, valvular heart disease, and chronic heart failure, regular exercise results in an increased functional capacity, improved quality of life, and improved cardiovascular risk factors.[13,51,52] Thus, after careful evaluation, most individuals with structural heart disease can safely participate in prescribed physical activity. Participation in competitive sports for individuals with structural heart disease depends on its type and severity, the type and intensity of the sport being pursued, and the level of risk or harm that could occur pursuant to participation.[5] Details regarding recommendations for participation have been presented in the 36th Bethesda Conference report.[53] Participation in competitive sports should be precluded only after a full cardiovascular examination and a knowledgeable assessment of potential harm from participation. In the heat of competition, however, individuals participating in competitive sports may not properly judge the significance of cardiac-related symptoms or if is prudent to terminate physical exertion.

Coronary Artery Disease

A large body of scientific evidence developed since the 1970s, primarily in cardiac rehabilitation programs, has shown that regular exercise reduces total and cardiovascular mortality in individuals with recently diagnosed CHD[11,12] (see Chap. 50). However, a relative paucity of data exists for competitive athletes with established CHD regarding the risk of athletic participation. The risk of competitive athletics likely increases to some degree in all patients with established CHD, and the risk of exercise-related events parallels the extent of disease, presence of left ventricular (LV) dysfunction, inducible ischemia, and electrical instability, along with the intensity of the competitive sport and intensity of effort.[54] Athletes with CHD diagnosed by any method should have their LV function assessed and undergo maximal exercise testing to assess exercise capacity, the presence of angina or inducible ischemia, and the presence of exercise-induced arrhythmias. In general, two levels of risk can be defined on the basis of testing.[54] First, mildly increased risk is predicted by the presence of preserved LV function at rest, normal exercise tolerance for age, absence of exercise-induced ischemia or complex ventricular arrhythmias, absence of hemodynamically significant coronary stenosis, and/or having undergone successful coronary revascularization. Second, substantially increased risk is identified by the presence of any of the following: impaired LV systolic function at rest (ejection fraction < 50%); evidence of exercise-induced myocardial ischemia or complex ventricular arrhythmias; and hemodynamically significant stenosis of a major coronary artery to 50% or more luminal narrowing if coronary angiography was performed. The 36th Bethesda Conference recommendations for participation in competitive sports have suggested that athletes in the mildly increased risk group can participate in low dynamic and low to moderate static competitive sports such as golf, bowling, diving, or motorcycling, but not in more strenuous competitive sports such as cycling, running, or basketball[54] (see Fig. 83-1). Athletes in the substantially increased risk category should generally be restricted to only the lowest intensity competitive sports. They should be reminded of the nature of prodromal symptoms and instructed to cease sports activity promptly should such symptoms appear.

Hypertension

Arterial hypertension is the most common cardiovascular condition observed in competitive athletes. Regular physical activity benefits individuals with systemic hypertension because it reduces blood pressure,[14] protects against stroke,[51] and protects against obesity-induced hypertension.[55] The presence of stage I hypertension in the absence of target organ damage, including left ventricular hypertrophy (LVH) on echocardiography, should not limit eligibility for any competitive sport, assuming that blood pressure has been adequately controlled with medication or lifestyle therapies. Athletes with more severe hypertension (stage 2), even without target organ damage such as LVH, should be restricted particularly from high static sports until blood pressure is controlled by lifestyle modification or drug therapy.[56] Hypertension per se has not been incriminated as a cause of sudden cardiac death in young competitive athletes; thus, the goal of treatment is to prevent target organ damage and long-term sequelae such as stroke or myocardial infarction.

Valvular Heart Disease

In general, patients with mild left-sided valvular regurgitation or stenosis who are asymptomatic with exercise testing, without other contraindications, can participate in regular physical activity and in essentially all competitive sports (see Chap. 66). In mitral stenosis, most patients with significant stenosis are sufficiently symptomatic, so that participation in competitive sports is not an issue. If atrial fibrillation and anticoagulation are present, the patient should not participate in sports with a risk for bodily contact. Individuals with mild to moderate mitral regurgitation who are in sinus rhythm, with normal LV size and function and normal pulmonary artery pressures, can participate in all competitive sports.[57] Patients with significant mitral regurgitation should be followed longitudinally with serial echocardiograms for changes in LV ejection fraction and end-systolic volume.[57] Individuals with severe mitral regurgitation and definite LV enlargement, pulmonary hypertension, or LV systolic dysfunction should not participate in any competitive sports.

Aortic stenosis can cause sudden death in young competitive athletes.[30] The severity of aortic stenosis is assessed by echocardiography or Doppler. It is important to note that most, but not all, episodes of exertional sudden death have occurred in individuals in whom aortic stenosis is severe. Because aortic stenosis is often progressive, follow-up should be longitudinal with serial echocardiography. Although athletes with mild aortic stenosis (valve area > 1.5 cm^2) can participate in exercise and competitive sports, those with asymptomatic, moderate aortic stenosis should engage only in lower-intensity sports and/or competition limited to sports with a moderate or low component of static or dynamic effort (see Fig. 83-1). Individuals with severe aortic stenosis or moderate stenosis with symptoms should not engage in any competitive sports and should also limit the intensity of regular exercise. Finally, the risk of exercise and competitive sports in patients with aortic insufficiency depends on its severity and clinical setting. For example, in the setting of a dilated proximal aorta, even with only mild regurgitation, only low-intensity exercise or sports can be recommended.[57] On the other hand, in the setting of mild or moderate aortic insufficiency, with normal or only mildly increased end-diastolic volume and a normal aorta, athletes can participate in all competitive sports. Finally, patients with severe aortic insufficiency and LV diastolic diameters larger than 67 mm, or mild to moderate insufficiency with symptoms, should not participate in any competitive sports.

Cardiomyopathy

Hypertrophic cardiomyopathy (see Chap. 69), myocarditis, and arrhythmogenic right ventricular dysplasia are known antecedents to sudden cardiac death in young athletes,[30] and thus are a contraindication to intense exercise and most competitive sports, with the possible exception of those of low intensity.[58] On the other hand, patients with stable New York Heart Association (NYHA) Class II or III chronic heart failure caused by ischemic cardiomyopathy or idiopathic dilated cardiomyopathy appear to be able to participate in supervised cardiac rehabilitation training programs safely, with transition to home programs without a substantially increased risk of cardiac death (see Chap. 50).[13] These programs have demonstrated clinical benefits, including an increased exercise capacity, improved quality of life, and possible survival benefit.[13] Individuals with NYHA Class II or III chronic heart failure and systolic LV dysfunction are generally too symptomatic to participate in high-intensity competitive sports.

Arrhythmias

A complaint of syncope or of palpitations occurring during physical exertion or sports participation mandates full evaluation. In particular, structural heart disease needs to be ruled out and the cause of these symptoms needs to be determined, if possible. These evaluations should include, but not be limited to, echocardiography, electrocardiography, exercise stress testing, and ambulatory monitoring. In the presence of structural heart disease, individuals with ventricular or supraventricular tachyarrhythmias should generally be excluded from intensive exercise or sports competition until definitive therapy can be accomplished.[59] In some cases, depending on the severity of the structural heart disease, if arrhythmias are controlled with medications or ablation, exercise and competition can be reconsidered. However, the presence of an intracardiac defibrillator to prevent sudden cardiac death has not been deemed to be an adequately tested therapy in a setting in which sudden cardiac death might otherwise be brought on by exercise.[59] Sinus bradycardia, sinus pause, and sinus arrest of less than 3 seconds are common in endurance-trained athletes and generally require no further evaluation or preclusion of exercise. When vasovagal syncope is diagnosed, despite its favorable prognosis, athletes with this condition should not participate in sports in which even a momentary loss of consciousness could be hazardous, such as automobile racing or downhill ski racing. For more details relating to the risk of specific arrhythmias, see the 36th Bethesda Conference report.[59]

Congenital Heart Disease

The most common congenital heart diseases that have been associated with untoward events during sports competition are hypertrophic cardiomyopathy (see Chap. 69), coronary artery anomalies, Marfan syndrome, and congenital aortic valve stenosis.[60] Other congenital lesions that are frequently associated with elevated pulmonary resistance also need to be considered (see Chap. 65). Hypertrophic cardiomyopathy is the most common underlying cause of sudden cardiac death during sports participation in young athletes and therefore is considered a disqualifying diagnosis for sports competition and intensive exercise.[30] Congenital coronary anomalies of wrong sinus origin, in which a coronary artery passes between great arteries, are the second most common cause of sudden death in young athletes.[30] As such, this diagnosis should result in exclusion from all participation in sports. Participation can be reconsidered after successful surgical correction in an athlete without ischemia or arrhythmias during maximal exercise testing. Coronary anomalies should be considered in athletes with exertional syncope, chest pain, or symptomatic ventricular arrhythmias and can be diagnosed by echocardiography, computed tomography, magnetic resonance imaging, or coronary arteriography.

Marfan syndrome is an autosomal dominant disorder of connective tissue, with an estimated prevalence of 1/5,000 to 10,000 (see Chaps. 8 and 60). Cardiac manifestations include progressive dilation of the aortic root or descending aorta, which predisposes to dissection and rupture, and mitral valve prolapse with associated mitral regurgitation. The risk for aortic rupture is usually linked to dilation of the proximal aorta to more than 50 mm, although even lesser levels of dilation increase risk. Athletes with aortic root dilations of more than 40 mm, moderate or worse mitral regurgitation, or a family history of dissection or sudden death in a relative with Marfan syndrome can only participate in low-intensity competitive sports (see Fig. 83-1). Weightlifting has been specifically linked with aortic dissection in athletes with cystic medial necrosis, and it should be considered relatively contraindicated in Marfan syndrome.[61]

Finally, a variety of congenital heart lesions linked to pulmonary hypertension present a risk during exercise and competitive sports.[60] In general, in the absence of other contraindications, if the pulmonary artery systolic pressure is less than 30 mm Hg, athletes can participate in all sports. If, however, the pulmonary systolic pressure is more than 30 mm Hg in the presence of an uncorrected intracardiac shunt, a full evaluation and individual exercise prescription are required for athletic participation. Patients with cyanotic congenital heart disease are generally too symptomatic to participate in intense exercise or competitive sports, although from a medical point of view, they should be precluded from participation. Variants of tetralogy of Fallot, atrial septal defects, ventricular septal defects, and Ebstein anomaly all require full evaluation on an individual basis before a decision can be made regarding athletic participation. The final decision should be based on the severity of the lesion, pulmonary pressure at rest and during exercise, and intensity of the sport being considered. In cases of mild or fully corrected lesions with normal pulmonary pressures, full participation can be considered. Details of these and other congenital conditions can be reviewed in the proceedings of the 36th Bethesda Conference report.[60]

Future Perspectives

As our society becomes more sedentary, and adverse health consequences such as obesity and diabetes increase, major and sustained efforts at physical activity promotion are needed. Whereas a broad approach requires concerted and multifaceted efforts that involve health policy makers, schools, worksites, insurers, the media, and others, health care providers have a primary responsibility to the individual. Medical education of physicians, nurses, and other health care providers needs to incorporate training in physical activity and exercise counseling, as well as screening for exercise- and sports-related risks. Health care providers need to evaluate the activity status of their patients routinely and promote the adoption of a physically active lifestyle. Accordingly, health care providers must be familiar with the physiologic demands of exercise and specific sports so that they may evaluate and mitigate risk appropriately, while not unduly proscribing participation.

Many of the recommendations made regarding screening and counseling individuals about their participation in exercise and sports are based on expert consensus. Because of the wide range and varied nature of the physiologic demands of sports and associated training, and the great variation in the presence and severity of underlying CVD and comorbidities of prospective participants, it is unlikely that there will ever be adequate scientific data to define individual risk precisely. However, the continued generation of carefully collected outcome data regarding adverse event rates during specific sports-related activities, and the underlying cause of those events, can fill many gaps in the available information and help further refine risk assessment. In the meantime, available guidelines need to be implemented by the medical community and those involved with athletic screening and training. Standardization of medical screening forms to contain key elements of the history and physical examination (see Table 83-4), and algorithms that outline steps for further evaluation, should be established for athletic screening at all levels of competition, from school to professional athletics. Finally, all those involved with directly supervising exercise and sports-related activities in any venue need to be facile with the prompt recognition of an adverse event, alerting of emergency medical systems, provision of cardiopulmonary resuscitation, and use of the automated external defibrillator (AED), where available. The American Heart Association and 36th Bethesda Conference Report[62] have outlined recommendations regarding the availability of AEDs at health and fitness facilities, sports arenas, and other venues of competitive athletic programs.

REFERENCES

Physical Activity, Benefits, and Risks of Exercise

1. U.S. Department of Health and Human Services: Physical Activity and Health: A Report of the Surgeon General. Atlanta, Centers for Disease Control and Prevention, 1996.
2. Thompson PD, Buchner D, Pina IL, et al: Exercise and physical activity in the prevention and treatment of atherosclerotic cardiovascular disease: A statement from the Council on Clinical Cardiology (Subcommittee on Exercise, Rehabilitation, and Prevention) and the Council on Nutrition, Physical Activity, and Metabolism (Subcommittee on Physical Activity). Circulation 107:3109, 2003.
3. Centers for Disease Control and Prevention: Exercise or Physical Activity, 2009 (http://www.cdc.gov/nchs/fastats/exercise.htm).
4. Kodama S, Saito K, Tanaka S, et al: Cardiorespiratory fitness as a quantitative predictor of all-cause mortality and cardiovascular events in healthy men and women: A meta-analysis. JAMA 301:2024, 2009.
5. Mitchell JH, Haskell W, Snell P, Van Camp SP: Task Force 8: Classification of sports. J Am Coll Cardiol 45:1364, 2005.
6. Gulati M, Pandey DK, Arnsdorf MF, et al: Exercise capacity and the risk of death in women: The St. James Women Take Heart Project. Circulation 108:1554, 2003.
7. Paffenbarger RS, Hyde RT, Wing A, et al: Physical activity, all-cause mortality, and longevity of college alumni. N Eng J Med 314:605-613, 1986.
8. Martinson BC, O'Connor PJ, Pronk NP: Physical inactivity and short-term all-cause mortality in adults with chronic disease. Arch Intern Med 161:1173, 2001.
9. Tanasescu M, Leitzmann MF, Rimm EB, et al: Physical activity in relation to cardiovascular disease and total mortality among men with type 2 diabetes. Circulation 107:2435, 2003.
10. Landi F, Cesari M, Lattanzio F, et al: Physical activity and mortality in frail, community-living, elderly patients. J Gerontol A Biol Sci Med Sci 59:833, 2004,
11. Taylor RS, Brown A, Ebrahim S, et al: Exercise-based rehabilitation for patients with coronary heart disease: Systematic review and meta-analysis of randomized controlled trials. Am J Med 116:682, 2004.
12. Suaya JA, Stason WB, Ades PA, et al: Cardiac rehabilitation and survival in older coronary patients. J Am Coll Cardiol 54:25, 2009.
13. O'Connor CM, Whellan DJ, Lee KL, et al: Efficacy and safety of exercise training in patients with chronic heart failure: HF-ACTION randomized controlled trial. JAMA 301:1439, 2009.
14. Whelton SP, Chin A, Xin X, et al: Effect of aerobic exercise on blood pressure: A meta-analysis of randomized, controlled trials. Ann IntERN Med 136:493, 2002.
15. Sigal RJ, Kenney GP, Wasserman DH, et al: Physical activity/exercise and type 2 diabetes: A consensus statement from the American Diabetes Association. Diabetes Care 29:1433, 2006.
16. Knowler WC, Barrett-Connor E, Fowler SE, et al: Reduction in the incidence of type 2 diabetes with lifestyle intervention or metformin. N Eng J Med 346:393, 2002.
17. Klein S, Burke LE, Bray GA, et al: Clinical implications of obesity with specific focus on cardiovascular disease. A statement for professionals from the American Heart Association Council on Nutrition, Physical Activity, and Metabolism. Circulation 110:2952, 2004.
18. Kumayika SK, Obarzanek E, Stettler J, et al: Population-based prevention of obesity: The need for comprehensive promotion of healthful eating, physical activity, and energy balance: A scientific statement from the American Heart Association. Circulation 118:428, 2008.
19. Slentz CA, Houmard JA, Johnson JL, et al: Inactivity, exercise training and detraining, and plasma lipoproteins. STRIDE: A randomized, controlled study of exercise intensity and amount. J Appl Physio 103:432, 2007.
20. Williams PT, Blanche PJ, Krauss RM: Behavioral versus genetic correlates of lipoproteins and adiposity in identical twins discordant for exercise. Circulation 112:350, 2005.
21. Kasapis C, Thompson PD: The effects of physical activity on C-reactive protein and inflammatory markers: A systematic review. J Am Coll Cardiol 45:1563, 2005.
22. Vona M, Codeluppi GM, Iannino T, et al: Effects of different types of exercise training followed by detraining on endothelium-dependent dilation in patients with recent myocardial infarction. Circulation 119:1601, 2009.
23. Hambrecht R, Wolf A, Geilen S, et al: Effect of exercise on coronary endothelial function in patients with coronary artery disease. N Eng J Med 342:454, 2000.
24. Adams V, Linke A, Krankel N, et al: Impact of regular physical activity on the NAD(P)H kinase and angiotensin receptor system in patients with coronary artery disease. Circulation 111:555, 2005.
25. Steiner S, Neissner A, Ziegler S, et al: Endurance training increases the number of endothelial progenitor cells in patients with cardiovascular risk and coronary disease. Atherosclerosis 181:305, 2005.
26. Halcox JP, Schenki WH, Zalos G, et al: Prognostic value of coronary vascular endothelial dysfunction. Circulation 106:653, 2002.
27. Adamson PB, Smith AL, Abraham WT, et al: Continuous autonomic assessment in patients with symptomatic heart failure: prognostic value of heart rate variability measured by implanted cardiac resynchronization device. Circulation 110:2389, 2004.
28. Fleg JL, Morrell CH, Bos AG, et al: Accelerated longitudinal decline of aerobic capacity in healthy older adults. Circulation 112:674, 2005.
29. Thompson PS, Franklin BA, Balady GJ, et al: Exercise and acute cardiovascular events: Placing the risks into perspective. A scientific statement from the American Heart Association. Circulation 115:2358, 2007.
30. Maron BJ, Doerer JJ, Haas TS, et al: Sudden death in young competitive athletes: Analysis of 1866 deaths in the United States, 1980-2006. Circulation 119:1085, 2009.
31. Corrado D, Hasso C, Rizzoli G, et al: Does sports activity enhance the risk of sudden death in adolescents and young adults? J Am Coll Cardiol 42:1959, 2003.
32. Albert CM, Mittleman MA, Chae CU, et al: Triggering of sudden death from cardiac causes by vigorous exertion. N Engl J Med 343:1355, 2000.
33. Whang W, Manson JE, Hu FB, et al: Physical exertion, exercise, and sudden cardiac death in women. JAMA 295:1399, 2006.
34. Maron BJ, Estes NAM, Link MA: Task Force 11: Commotio cordis Task Force 8: Classification of sports. J Am Coll Cardiol 45:1371, 2005.
35. MarathonGuide.com Staff: USA Marathoning: 2007 Overview (http://www.marathonguide.com/features/Articles/2007RecapOverview.cfm).
36. Roberts WO, Maron BJ: Evidence for decreasing occurrence of sudden cardiac death associated with the marathon. J Am Coll Cardiol 46:1373, 2005.
37. Redelmeier DA, Greenwald JA: Competing risks of mortality with marathons: Retrospective analysis. BMJ 335:1275, 2007.
38. Almond CSD, Shin AY, Fortescue EB, et al: Hyponatremia among runners in the Boston Marathon. N Engl J Med 352:1550, 2005.
39. Neilan TG, Yoerer DM, Douglas PS, et al: Persistent and reversible cardiac dysfunction among amateur marathon runners. Eur Heart J 27:1079, 2006.

39a. Saravia SG, Knebel F, Schroeckh S, et al: Cardiac troponin T release and inflammation demonstrated in marathon runners. Clin Lab 56:51, 2010.

Exercise Prescription and Screening

40. Haskell WL, Lee IM, Pate RR, et al: Physical activity and public health. Updated recommendation for adults from the American College of Sports Medicine and the American Heart Association. Circulation 116:1081, 2007.
41. American College of Sports Medicine: ASCM's Guidelines for Exercise Testing and Prescription. 8th ed. Philadelphia, Lippincott Williams & Wilkins, 2009.
42. Brooks GA, Butte NF, Rand WM, et al: Chronical of the Institute of Medicine physical activity recommendation: How a physical activity recommendation came to be among dietary recommendations. Am J Clin Nutr 79(Suppl):921S, 2004.
43. Maron B, Arujo C, Thompson P, et al: Recommendations for preparticipation screening and the assessment of cardiovascular disease in master athletes. Circulation 103:327, 2001.
44. Balady GJ, Chaitman B, Driscoll D, et al: American Heart Association/American College of Sports Medicine joint scientific statement: Recommendations for cardiovascular screening, staffing, and emergency policies at health/fitness facilities. Circulation 97:2283, 1998.
45. Maron BJ, Douglas PS, Graham TP, et al: Task Force 1: Preparticipation screening and diagnosis of cardiovascular disease in athletes. J Am Coll Cardiol 45:1322, 2005.
46. Maron BJ, Thompson PD, Ackerman MJ, et al: Recommendations and considerations related to preparticipation screening for cardiovascular abnormalities in competitive athletes: 2007 update: A scientific statement from the AHA. Circulation 115:1643, 2007.
47. Fletcher GF, Balady GJ, Amsterdam EA, et al: Exercise standards for testing and training: A statement for health professionals from the AHA. Circulation 104:1694, 2001.
48. Maron BJ, Zipes DP: Introduction: Eligibility recommendations for competitive athletes with cardiovascular abnormalities—general considerations. J Am Coll Cardiol 45:1318, 2005.
49. Maron BJ, Chaitman BR, Ackerman MJ, et al: Recommendations for physical activity and recreational sports participation for young patients with genetic cardiovascular diseases. Circulation 109:2807, 2004.
50. Thompson PD: Preparticipation screening of competitive athletes: Seeking simple solutions to a complex problem. Circulation 119:1072, 2009.

Exercise and Cardiovascular Disease

51. Ades PA: Cardiac rehabilitation and the secondary prevention of coronary heart disease. N Engl J Med 345:892, 2001.
52. Flynn KE, Piña IL, Whellan DJ, et al: Effects of exercise training on health status in patients with chronic heart failure: HF-ACTION randomized controlled trial. JAMA 301:1451, 2009.
53. Mitten MJ, Zipes DP: 36th Bethesda Conference: Eligibility recommendations for competitive athletes with cardiovascular abnormalities. J Am Coll Cardiol 45:1318, 2005.
54. Thompson PD, Balady GJ, Chaitman BR, et al: Task Force 6: Coronary artery disease. J Am Coll Cardiol 45:1348, 2005.
55. Lee CD, Folsom AR, Blair SN: Physical activity and stroke risk: A meta-analysis. Stroke 34:2475, 2003.
56. Kaplan NM, Gidding SS, Pickering TG, Wright JT Jr: Task Force 5: Systemic hypertension. J Am Coll Cardiol 45:1346, 2005.
57. Bonow RO, Cheitlin MD, Crawford MH, Douglas PS: Task Force 3: Valvular heart disease. J Am Coll Cardiol 45:1334, 2005.
58. Maron BJ, Ackerman MJ, Nishimura RA, et al: Task Force 4: HCM and other cardiomyopathies, mitral valve prolapse, myocarditis, and Marfan syndrome. J Am Coll Cardiol 45:1340, 2005.
59. Zipes DP, Ackerman MJ, Estes NA 3rd, et al: Task Force 7: Arrhythmias. J Am Coll Cardiol 45:1354, 2005.
60. Graham TP Jr, Driscoll DJ, Gersony WM, et al: Task Force 2: Congenital heart disease. J Am Coll Cardiol 45:1326, 2005.
61. Elefteriades JA, Hatzaras I, Tranquilli MA, et al: Weight lifting and rupture of silent aortic aneurysms [letter]. JAMA 290:2803, 2003.
62. Myerberg RJ, Estes NAM, Fontaine JM, et al: Task Force 10: Automated external defibrillators. J Am Coll Cardiol 45:1369, 2005.

CHAPTER 84 Medical Management of the Patient Undergoing Cardiac Surgery

Richard J. Gray and Dhun H. Sethna

Organization of the Program

Organization of the most successful programs, defined by low surgical mortality and morbidity, is generally characterized by larger surgical volume (and large per-surgeon volume), often with a single or small number of separate surgical practice groups under an enlightened surgical leadership. Application of goal-directed, multidisciplinary protocols and a quality improvement program have been shown to be associated with lower mortality after cardiac surgery. This decline may be less prominent in patients with diabetes, and focused quality improvement protocols are often required for this subset of patients.[1,2] The process of cardiac surgery has been shown to benefit from interventions to improve teamwork and communication, such as preoperative briefings, revised approach to structuring of operative teams to favor members who have gained familiarity with the operating surgeon, standardized communication practices, multidisciplinary grand rounds, and postoperative debriefings. Such forums may also be the venue to discuss ethical issues in cardiac surgery, such as refusal to operate on a noncompliant intravenous drug–abusing patient with recurrent prosthetic valve infections. Quality assurance is a must in any program; given the scope of the usual team, inclusion of nursing, anesthesia, cardiology, critical care, and others is important, with time spent reviewing data on surgical outcomes.

In a retrospective study using the Medicare Provider Analysis and Review file of 114,233 Medicare beneficiaries who survived coronary artery bypass graft (CABG) surgery without concomitant valve repair during a hospitalization for fiscal year 2005,[3] the mean cost of a hospitalization was $32,201 ± $23,059, and the mean length of stay was 9.9 ± 7.8 days. After adjustment for patient demographics and comorbid conditions, 13.6% of Medicare beneficiaries who were experiencing complications consumed significantly more hospital resources (incremental cost, $15,468) and had a longer length of stay (incremental stay, 5.3 days). In the Commonwealth of Virginia, the baseline cost of isolated CABG cases with no complications between 2004 and 2007 was $26,056.[4] Isolated atrial fibrillation (AF) was the most frequently cited complication and had the lowest additive cost ($2,574). Additive costs were greatest for prolonged ventilation ($40,704), renal failure ($49,128), mediastinitis ($62,773), and operative mortality ($49,242). The average hospital costs related to excessive postoperative hemorrhage in cardiac surgery are substantial. These observations suggest that the significant cost currently spent on treatment of complications of cardiac surgery can be better contained by redirecting resources to patient safety initiatives, such as evidence-based preoperative risk stratification, and perioperative best practices guidelines that have been shown to reduce selected complications.

Preoperative Risk Analysis

Advanced Age and Gender

Long-term survival of octogenarians submitted to a wide variety of cardiac operations is satisfactory despite substantial rates of early complications and deaths (see Chap. 80).[5] Most survivors are free from cardiac symptoms. Postoperative complications are stronger risk factors for hospital deaths and long-term survival than are preoperative comorbidities and procedural variables. Time spent on cardiopulmonary bypass (CPB) is associated with long-term survival.[6] Notwithstanding, with optimal perioperative patient management and patient selection, octogenarians can expect a long-term survival and quality of life similar to that of their younger colleagues after primary and redo cardiac surgery. Surviving octogenarians remain at home, function independently, and engage in regular leisure activities years after cardiac surgery.[7] Octogenarians undergoing aortic valve replacement (AVR) can experience a life expectancy similar to that of the general population based on actuarial curves, with more than half the patients surviving more than 6 years after their surgery.[8] More perioperative complications occur in patients older than 75 years who have low body mass index (BMI <23).[9] Off-pump CABG (OPCAB) using only arterial conduits confers an operative survival benefit leading to an enhanced long-term quality of life.[10] High operative mortality (13%) and postoperative complication (43%) rates are to be expected in nonagenarians.[11] However, select nonagenarians can also undergo elective CABG with a 95% 30-day survival; the main risk factor for death is emergency surgery. Physiologic indicators, social factors, and patient preferences should be integrated in the patient selection process, with more proactive intervention in symptomatic nonagenarian patients as it relates to earlier consideration of elective rather than emergency cardiac operations. Notwithstanding, complications result in prolonged average intensive care unit (ICU) stay (12 days; median, 5 days) and longer average hospital stay (17.5 days; median, 11 days).

In retrospective cohort studies of large data bases involving 15,000 to 54,425 patients undergoing CABG, early mortality was found to be significantly higher in women (see Chap. 81) after adjustment for confounding factors, including low body surface area.[12,13] This gender differential increases from top- to bottom-tier hospitals, suggesting that female patients could benefit from having CABG performed at tertiary care medical centers rather than at small community hospitals. On the other hand, a survey conducted between 1992 and 2002 of 3760 consecutive patients who underwent isolated CABG showed no differences in in-hospital mortality or 5-year survival between men and women.[14] Malignant ventricular arrhythmias, calcified aorta, and preoperative renal failure are poor prognostic signs in women. The benefit of open heart surgery at 2-year follow-up is equivalent in both genders in terms of quality of life as assessed by the 36-item short-form health survey questionnaire (SF-36), although women show lower baseline scores. Although women have more late strokes after valve replacement, they undergo fewer reoperations and have better overall long-term survival compared with men.[15]

Ethnicity and Race

In a survey conducted between 1997 and 2007 involving 12,874 consecutive CABG patients including 2033 (15.8%) blacks and 10,841 (84.2%) whites, survival at 3, 5, and 10 years for blacks was significantly lower than for whites (see Chap. 2).[16] Off-pump surgery did not narrow the disparity in outcomes between blacks and whites. In the Bypass Angioplasty Revascularization Investigation trial, clinical outcomes of black patients after coronary revascularization were worse than those of white patients in a clinical trial setting with similar treatment and access to care.[17] The differences in outcome between black and white patients were not completely attributable to the greater levels of comorbidity among black patients at study entry. Black patients were also less likely to be admitted at cardiac hospitals for coronary revascularization compared with general hospitals in the same area.[18]

Socioeconomic and IQ Status. Lower socioeconomic status is associated with a poorer early outcome after CABG and is independent of other recognized risk factors. Lower scores on measures of IQ at two time points have been shown to be associated with general cardiovascular morbidity and, particularly, total mortality, at a level of magnitude greater than several other established risk factors.[19]

Body Weight. Underweight is an independent predictor for early mortality, and morbid obesity is an independent predictor for late mortality after CABG.[20]

Case Volume. As a discriminator of quality of care and mortality, the use of hospital volumes of cardiac surgery, which may combine the experience of a wide range of individual surgeons, has been said to be "only slightly better than a coin flip."[21] There is considerable outcomes variability not explained by hospital volume, and low volume does not preclude excellent performance. Except for internal thoracic artery (ITA) use, care processes and morbidity rates are not associated with volume.[22] A retrospective cohort of 948,093 Medicare patients undergoing CABG with CPB in 870 U.S. hospitals from 1996 to 2001 showed considerable variation in adjusted mortality within the low-volume group (1% to 17%) as well as within the high-volume group (2% to 11%) so that the volume criterion alone was a poor discriminator of mortality (C-statistic = 0.51). Of the 660 low-volume hospitals, 253 (38%) had risk-adjusted mortality rates that were similar to or lower than the overall risk-adjusted mortality of some of the high-volume hospitals. Volume statistics of individual surgeons seem to be a better quality criterion of early mortality and postoperative complications. In a study of first-time isolated CABG operations, patients treated by low-volume surgeons (1 to 50 cases annually) had significantly higher mortality rates than those treated by medium-volume surgeons (51 to 100 cases annually; 7.0% versus 3.8%), high-volume surgeons (101 to 150 cases annually; 7.0% versus 2.7%), or very-high-volume surgeons (>151 cases annually; 7.0% versus 3.2%).[23] The adjusted odds ratio of hospital in-patient deaths declined with increasing surgeon volume. Hospital volume and surgeon volume effects on CABG outcomes are probably interdependent. High-volume hospitals invariably have some processes, infrastructure and personnel factors, or both that seem to produce not only better short-term outcomes but also better long-term outcomes.[24] Despite significant reduction in the volume of patients referred for surgical revascularization, risk profiles of patients undergoing isolated CABG in Washington State changed only modestly, and CABG mortality was not adversely affected and morbidity was reduced.[25] Thus, although minimal volume standards might be effective to improve quality to some extent, volume has limitations as a marker of quality because of its wide range of variance. In terms of case volume, for hospitals in the highest percentage OPCAB quartile, adjusted mortality and complication rates for patients having OPCAB were significantly lower than for the on-pump group; by contrast, for hospitals in the lowest percentage OPCAB quartile, mortality and complications were similar in off-pump and on-pump groups.[26] A surgeon performance index has been described that, with appropriate feedback, has been shown to improve performance of an individual surgeon with improvements in the range and mean of the overall performance of the surgical team.[27]

Surgical Technique. Conventional sternotomy with CPB is still the standard in most institutions (see Chap. 57). Alternative approaches should be used as tools within a decision-making algorithm driven by patient-related factors of coronary anatomy and comorbidity and the surgeon's experience, wherein thinking "better bypass" must override thinking "off pump." Beating-heart OPCAB has the potential to eliminate intraoperative global myocardial ischemia and to be an acceptable surgical option for patients after acute myocardial infarction (MI). It is associated with lower postoperative mortality and morbidity—the cytokine and chemokine production profile of the inflammatory response associated with CABG is largely similar with the off-pump and on-pump techniques in low-risk patients, but slightly higher concentrations of eotaxin, macrophage inflammatory protein 1ß, and interleukin (IL)-12 were found in the on-pump group.[28] Minimally invasive direct CABG (MIDCAB), conducted through a left thoracotomy, is limited to patients with amenable coronary anatomy.[29] Port-access CABG requires CPB with cardiac arrest but avoids sternotomy. OPCAB may be considered with a median sternotomy or with MIDCAB procedures.

Meta-analysis indicates that OPCAB appears to be as good as or superior to on-pump CABG in terms of reduced length of hospital stay and operative morbidity and mortality, including decreased need for intra-aortic balloon pump placement, rate of postoperative renal failure, hemorrhage-related reexploration, and stroke, especially in high-risk patients (see Chap. 57).[30] A very short preoperative course of erythropoietin administration is a safe and easy method to reduce the need for blood transfusions at OPCAB.[31] Although both OPCAB and on-pump CABG can be performed in high-risk patients with low short-term complications at 30-day follow-up,[32] a randomized trial by the Veterans Affairs study group showed the 1-year composite outcome to be higher for OPCAB than for on-pump CABG. The proportion of patients with fewer grafts completed than originally planned was higher with OPCAB than with on-pump CABG. Follow-up angiograms in 1371 patients who underwent 4093 grafts revealed that the overall rate of graft patency was lower in the OPCAB group than in the on-pump group. There were no treatment-based differences in neuropsychological outcomes or short-term use of major resources.[33] Risk factors for wound infection after OPCAB are comparable to those previously reported for conventional bypass grafting. In one study, diabetic patients had a comparative operative mortality and perioperative MI rate to that of nondiabetic patients.[34] However, they had an increased prevalence of postoperative acute renal insufficiency and infections. In patients with diabetes, the use of bilateral ITA conduits, even when they are harvested in a skeletonized fashion, is a risk factor. OPCAB is associated with favorable early outcomes in the elderly population, but these early benefits may not be maintained in the long term, and OPCAB shows trends toward worse long-term results. High-risk patients undergoing beating-heart myocardial revascularization with left ventricular (LV) assisted technique show reduced inflammatory response compared with patients treated with minimal extracorporeal circulation. Although the benefit of OPCAB increases as the relative use of the procedure at a hospital increases, OPCAB today can be safely implemented across numerous hospitals.

After risk adjustment, patients with critical left main stem stenosis or those with diffuse coronary artery disease (CAD) requiring endarterectomy can undergo OPCAB safely, with results comparable to those of on-pump CABG. Anatomic factors against OPCAB include target vessel size less than 1.25 mm, calcification, intramyocardial location of target vessels, and multiple stenoses. The risk of reduced graft patency also needs to be considered in choosing OPCAB as a tailored strategy in selected patients. Given that OPCAB can be performed safely, patients in the moderate- or high-risk range (i.e., elderly with multiple comorbidities or emergency patients operated on within the first 48 hours of acute MI) could preferentially be treated by use of OPCAB. Compared with men, women are a high-risk group and benefit from off-pump operation in terms of early mortality after CABG. Conversely, during follow-up, women have high adjusted risks of major cardiac and cerebral events after OPCAB.[35] Experienced OPCAB surgeons have a low risk of acute conversion to CPB. Acutely converted patients have a moderately increased risk of in-hospital death and serious complications that are difficult to quantify because conversion is infrequent and unpredictable.

Reoperation. Although hospital mortality for reoperative CABG is approaching that of primary CABG in many centers, it still remains a significant risk factor for operative mortality in contemporary practice. Aggressive risk-factor reduction (see Chap. 49) and complete arterial coronary revascularization at primary CABG should result in fewer coronary reoperations. In a study of elective redo CABG patients, minimal tissue dissection and target vessel revascularization without CPB did not add significant benefit with regard to perioperative morbidity and mortality. Routine use of preoperative multidetector computed tomography (CT) angiography to detect high-risk findings (see Chap. 19) has a strong association with adoption of preventive surgical strategies in high-risk patients undergoing redo cardiac surgery.[36]

Seasonal Variation. Hospital mortality and ICU stay after CABG have been shown to be increased during the winter season compared with the rest of the year.[37]

Baseline Laboratory Values

A lower preoperative hemoglobin level (13 g/dL for men and 12 g/dL for women) is an independent predictor of late mortality in patients undergoing CABG, whereas anemia is a risk factor for early and late mortality. In another analysis, preoperative hemoglobin level less than 10 g/dL was not a strong independent predictor of 30-day operative mortality or perioperative morbidity in multivariate models for on-pump CABG-only patients.[38] Preoperative anemia is also independently associated with acute kidney injury (AKI) after CABG. Moderate or severe anemia may be intertwined with other risk factors, such as serum creatinine concentration or heart failure, making risk assessment in complex patients difficult. Elevated preprocedural systemic markers of inflammation have been associated with adverse clinical outcomes after CABG. Higher preoperative white blood cell count has been independently associated with higher perioperative myocardial necrosis (creatine kinase MB isoenzyme [CK-MB] release) and 1-year mortality,[39] and it can have a significant impact on the risk for perioperative cerebrovascular accident and neuropsychological outcomes. However, reducing the perioperative inflammatory response with leukocyte filtration does not seem to be efficacious in improving short-term outcomes. High residual platelet reactivity as estimated by the PFA-100 point-of-care test independently correlates with a worse clinical outcome in patients undergoing CABG.[40] Poor preoperative glycemic control, as measured by an elevated hemoglobin A1c level, is associated with reduced in-hospital and lower long-term survival after CABG. For each unit increase in hemoglobin A1c, there is a significantly increased risk of perioperative MI and deep sternal wound infection.[41] Preoperative C-reactive protein (CRP) concentration greater than 1.0 mg/dL carries a higher risk of overall postoperative death, cardiac death, low cardiac output syndrome, and any cerebrovascular complication, with reduced overall long-term survival.[42] A CRP level greater than 10 mg/liter is a risk factor for early mortality, whereas a level greater than 5 mg/liter is a risk factor for late mortality.[43] Patients with high baseline CRP levels are also at higher risk of having postoperative AF after on-pump and off-pump surgery. Low basal free triiodothyronine (T_3) concentration has been shown to reliably predict the occurrence of postoperative AF in CABG patients (see Chap. 86).[44] Preoperative plasma B-type natriuretic peptide independently predicted in-hospital ventricular dysfunction, hospital stay, and up to 5-year all-cause mortality after primary CABG, but it does not predict the occurrence of postoperative AF.[45,46] The serum level of cardiac troponin I (cTnI) measured within 24 hours before elective CABG further identifies a subgroup of patients with higher risk for perioperative MI, low cardiac output syndrome, and high in-hospital mortality. Meta-analysis also shows an association between postoperative troponin release with mid- and short-term all-cause mortality after adult cardiac surgery.[47] Preoperative cTnI measurement before emergency CABG is a powerful and independent determinant of in-hospital mortality and major adverse cardiac events in acute coronary syndromes (see Chap. 56).[48]

Preoperative Drug Therapy

Preoperative aspirin taken within 5 days preceding CABG is associated with significantly lower in-hospital mortality without increased risk of reoperation for bleeding or need for blood transfusion. In patients who have had OPCAB, it does not increase bleeding-related complications, mortality rate, or other morbidities.

The risk versus benefit of preoperative administration of clopidogrel remains unresolved. On the basis of multivariable models, preoperative clopidogrel is an independent risk factor for increased transfusion requirements and prolonged ICU and hospital length of stay. Among in-hospital referral patients, preoperative clopidogrel administered within 5 days before CABG has been shown to increase early mortality and morbidity, and the risk of death is greatest when the drug is given within 48 hours of surgery.[49] Preoperative use of aspirin plus clopidogrel may be associated with an increased risk of infection after CABG. On the other hand, preoperative use of clopidogrel has also been shown not to be associated with increased major or life-threatening bleeding or need for surgical reexploration or higher risk of blood and blood product transfusion after CABG.[50] The ACUITY trial concluded that clopidogrel therapy in acute coronary syndrome in patients who underwent early CABG led to less ischemic events after surgery with no increased risk of bleeding.[51] A post hoc analysis of the CURE trial reported that patients who underwent early CABG after non–ST elevation acute coronary syndrome showed significant improvement in cardiovascular outcomes with preoperative clopidogrel therapy, with no significant increase in life-threatening postoperative bleeding.[52] It is recommended that surgery in patients receiving clopidogrel be performed with standard heparinization and antifibrinolytic strategies; platelets transfused before chest closure have a beneficial effect on hemostasis. Aprotinin may reduce bleeding and transfusion requirements of packed red blood cells, platelets, and total blood units in patients receiving clopidogrel who need urgent or elective CABG.[53] Recent use of clopidogrel before OPCAB is associated with greater risk for bleeding with similar mortality rate.[54] However, discontinuation of clopidogrel 3 days (72 hours) before the operation demonstrated a similar blood loss pattern compared with a control group.[55]

Preoperative enoxaparin given less than 12 hours before CABG is associated with lower postoperative hemoglobin values and higher rates of transfusion compared with preoperative continuous unfractionated heparin administration. Intraoperative heparin resistance may also be increased, requiring more heparin to maintain the desired activated clotting time, leading to higher heparin concentrations and lower antithrombin values compared with control patients. Patients with heparin-induced antibodies (heparin/PF4 antibodies) are more likely to develop thrombosis after cardiac surgery. Patients in whom antibodies are present before surgery show longer persistence of antibodies and increased incidence of thrombotic events over time and may be at risk for development of thrombosis, and therefore further exposure to heparin should be limited.

The multiple benefits of perioperative use of statins in cardiac surgery have been reviewed.[56] Preoperative statin therapy confers a protective benefit on postoperative outcomes in patients undergoing CABG regardless of inflammatory markers, with additional protection observed in patients with positive troponin T levels (see Chaps. 47 and 49). Myocardial damage is reduced, and both short- and long-term results can be improved.[57] Statin therapy in patients undergoing cardiac valve procedures has been associated with decreased postoperative morbidity and death,[58] even in the absence of CAD.[59] One large series (10,061 patients) failed to detect a protective effect of preoperative statin therapy on perioperative outcomes or long-term survival in patients undergoing isolated valve surgery. Valve patients undergoing concomitant CABG, however, appeared to receive a long-term survival benefit from statins.[60] The influence of preoperative statin therapy on postoperative AF has been reviewed,[61] with studies showing a higher or a lower incidence after elective CABG. Higher dose statins may offer the best preventive effect for AF as low-dose statins do not influence postoperative AF.

Preoperative angiotensin-converting enzyme inhibitors are associated with a reduced rate of AKI after on-pump CABG surgery.[62] Meta-analysis of 3323 patients from 50 randomized controlled trials shows that low-dose (1000 mg) corticosteroid prophylaxis given before CPB is as effective as higher doses in reducing the risk of AF and the duration of mechanical ventilation in adults undergoing cardiac surgery but with a higher incidence of postoperative hyperglycemia requiring insulin infusion.[63] The risk of all-cause infection is not increased. High-dose insulin therapy, titrated to maintain blood glucose concentrations below 180 mg/dL, has also been shown to blunt the early postoperative surge in inflammatory response to CPB as reflected by decreased levels of IL-6, IL-8, and tumor necrosis factor.[64]

Preoperative Medical Conditions

Pregnancy

Cardiac surgery during pregnancy is associated with increased maternal (8.6%) and fetal (18.6%) mortality rates. Poor functional class has been associated with a higher risk of maternal death, as is the use of vasoactive drugs, age, type of surgery, and reoperation. Maternal age older than 35 years, functional class, reoperation, emergency surgery, type of myocardial protection, and anoxic time can have adverse effects on fetal survival.

Cardiovascular Risk Factors (see Chap. 44)

CIGARETTE SMOKING. Smoking is a strong risk factor for the development of postoperative respiratory complications, which are twice as common in smokers (29.5%) as in nonsmokers (13.6%) and ex-smokers (14.7%). Patients who have stopped smoking for more than 6 months have complication rates similar to those who have never smoked. Even smoking cessation for more than 2 months can significantly reduce the rate of respiratory complications (57.1% versus 14.5%).

OBESITY. Despite the perception that obesity increases the risk of in-hospital and early (1 year) mortality and morbidity in CABG operations, the clinical outcomes of these patients are not so different from those of other patients when proper attention is given to detail. However, long-term survival may be reduced, and higher rates of AF, bleeding, reoperation, renal dysfunction, and gastrointestinal complications may occur. In addition, the relationship of BMI with post-CABG mortality and morbidity is U shaped, with the minimum risk located around a BMI of 30 kg/m^2, indicating that patients classified as overweight have the lowest risk, and those in the lower end of the obese range may not have seriously elevated risk.[65] BMI greater than 40 leads to significantly more complications, including a higher incidence of postoperative sternal wound infections, prolonged ventilation, and longer hospital stay.

DIABETES. The outcome in patients after cardiac surgery using CPB is negatively influenced by the presence of diabetes (see Chap. 64), with insulin-dependent type 2 diabetics showing a significantly higher rate of major postoperative complications including AKI, deep sternal wound infection, and prolonged postoperative stay compared with nondiabetics and those not taking insulin.[66] Patients with undiagnosed and insulin-treated diabetes have a higher risk of pulmonary complications in the perioperative course of CABG than do nondiabetic patients. These results may be explained if one considers the lung as another target organ of the diabetic disease. Although there may not be a higher risk of in-hospital mortality, longevity has been shown to be significantly reduced during a 5-year follow-up period. In-hospital resource use may be expected to be higher in diabetics; each 50 mg/dL blood glucose increase has been shown to be associated with longer postoperative days, higher hospitalization charges by $2824, and increased hospitalization cost by $1769. OPCAB in diabetic patients can significantly reduce postoperative morbidity and length of stay compared with coronary operation on CPB. The absence of diabetes-related target organ damage, specifically renal failure or peripheral vascular disease, is associated with long-term survival after CABG that is similar to or only slightly less than that of patients without diabetes. Diabetes does not affect the early postoperative and midterm results, including 1-year graft patency, in patients with multivessel disease undergoing total arterial vascularization and OPCAB.

METABOLIC SYNDROME. Postoperative stroke occurs in 4.7% of patients with metabolic syndrome and 2.1% of patients without metabolic syndrome, and postoperative AKI occurs in 3.8% of patients with metabolic syndrome and 1.1% of patients without metabolic syndrome, both of which are significantly high.[67]

PERIPHERAL VASCULAR DISEASE. Patients with peripheral vascular disease (see Chap. 61) undergoing CABG have better intermediate survival out to 3 years than do similar patients undergoing percutaneous coronary intervention. It is an independent risk factor for late mortality but not for early mortality.[68] OPCAB is safe in such patients with acceptable results and a reduced incidence of postoperative stroke. However, they are at higher risk for limb ischemia, impaired leg wound healing, and infection, especially after intra-aortic balloon counterpulsation therapy. About 10% of patients scheduled for CABG have associated unsuspected abdominal aortic aneurysm (see Chap. 60); whether this justifies routine preoperative echocardiographic screening remains undetermined. When calcification of the ascending aorta is detected on chest radiography, multidetector CT evaluation should be considered to map out the locations of calcium. Alternatively, intraoperative epiaortic ultrasound may be useful to avoid vascular disruption or stroke during cannulation or proximal anastomoses of bypass grafts. The most severe aortic calcification, known as porcelain aorta, may require OPCAB or an alternative approach to cannulation or proximal grafting.

Renal Dysfunction (see Chap. 93)

The RIFLE (R, renal risk; I, injury; F, failure; L, loss of kidney function; E, end-stage renal disease) classification or its recent modification, the Acute Kidney Injury Network definition and classification system, is becoming the standard for determination of postoperative AKI after cardiac surgery and is an independent risk factor for 90-day mortality.[69] In a small study of elderly cardiac surgery patients, serum cystatin C, a protease inhibitor, and plasma creatinine correlated equally in the detection of mild postoperative AKI as defined by the RIFLE criteria.[70] The Thakar scoring system for predicting the incidence of postoperative AKI requiring dialysis (AKI-D) allows the discrimination between patients with higher or lower risks of AKI-D.[71] Preoperative serum creatinine concentration between 1.47 and 2.25 mg/dL is an important predictor of worse in-hospital mortality, morbidity, and midterm survival after CABG, isolated valve surgery, and combined valve and CABG procedures. Mild elevation of preoperative creatinine level (1.3 to 2.0 mg/dL) can significantly increase the probability of perioperative mortality, low cardiac output, hemodialysis, and prolonged hospital stay. Total mortality in patients with lower calculated glomerular filtration rate (<71.1 mL $\cdot$ min^{-1} $\cdot$ 1.73 m^{-2}) is significantly increased, and its impact on these patients is evident at up to 15 years of follow-up. Mini-CPB is associated with a lower incidence of AKI compared with conventional CPB among patients undergoing CABG. Bilateral ITA grafting provides better long-term survival than single ITA grafting in patients with chronic kidney disease.[72]

Atrial Fibrillation

Preoperative AF is associated with an increased risk for perioperative mortality and morbidity, late mortality, and recurrent cardiovascular events in patients undergoing cardiac surgery.[73] The negative effect of AF might be more significant in patients with an ejection fraction greater than 40%. Both the EuroSCORE and, until recently, the Society of Thoracic Surgeons (STS) risk calculator do not include AF as a potential risk modifier; however, it should be identified as a variable to be investigated and incorporated into future risk calculators (see Chap. 40). Spontaneous cardioversion to sinus rhythm during surgery is transient in the majority of patients and is not associated with midterm survival benefit. Notwithstanding, if patients in AF require surgical revascularization, it is appropriate to consider performing a concomitant surgical ablation procedure. Preoperative values of atrial natriuretic peptide, angiotensin II, the sialylated carbohydrate antigen KL-6, hyaluronic acid, and pyridinoline cross-linked telopeptide of type I collagen in the blood have been proposed as new indices to predict the occurrence of AF after CABG.[74] Subclinical hypothyroidism appears to influence the development of transient postoperative AF after CABG. However, it is still unproven whether preoperative thyroxine replacement therapy might prevent this event.

Pulmonary Disease

Preoperative assessment of chronic obstructive pulmonary disease (COPD), currently reported to the STS data base by either clinical interview including medication and oxygen use or spirometric testing, may result in underestimation of risk.[75] COPD is associated with a higher mortality (7%) and higher incidence (50%) of postoperative respiratory complications, especially pneumonia, requiring prolonged ICU and hospital stay. Although not an independent predictor of increased early mortality and morbidity, it is a continuing detrimental risk factor for long-term survival. The subgroup of elderly patients (>75 years) with COPD who are receiving steroids have prohibitive postoperative mortality. A logistic risk model to predict the development of respiratory failure after valve surgery has been described,[76] as has also a simple score to identify patients with a strong likelihood of success in rapid weaning from mechanical ventilation.[77]

Neurologic Disease

The National Institutes of Health Stroke Scale and Mini-Mental State Examination scores can be used to predict both serious adverse neurologic outcome and deterioration of intellectual function in type I (clinically diagnosed stroke, transient ischemic attack, encephalopathy, or coma) or type II (deterioration of intellectual function) neurologic outcomes after CABG.[78] Preoperative stroke carries a higher risk for development of postoperative neurologic complications. An accepted rule of thumb is to wait 2 or 3 months after a stroke before placing a patient on CPB. Patients with remote cerebrovascular accident, even though they may have completely recovered, often exhibit signs of reactivation whereby some or all of the previous symptoms reappear, albeit in a milder form. Although the prognosis for recovery is good, several weeks are sometimes needed.

Carotid artery occlusive disease occurs in 1.5% to 6% of patients with CAD and may be associated with postoperative stroke. Although mandatory preoperative screening with bilateral duplex ultrasound of all patients is still done in some institutions, limiting this process to patients older than 65 years, those with a carotid bruit, or those with suspected or established cerebrovascular disease can reduce the screening load by nearly 40% with negligible impact on surgical management or neurologic outcomes. In those patients in whom critical, symptomatic carotid artery stenosis coexists at the time of scheduled CABG, a combined or staged CABG and carotid endarterectomy procedure can be done with excellent results. It still remains unclear whether a combined or staged technique shows superior outcomes over the other.

Patients with advanced parkinsonism require considerable nursing care after cardiac surgery, and their inability to generate a good cough effort requires aggressive respiratory care. ICU and hospital stay may be prolonged, and discharge to an extended care facility is often necessary. Abnormal peripheral vascular tone secondary to autonomic dysfunction, manifested in its extreme form as the Shy-Drager syndrome, can cause hemodynamic problems in the perioperative period. Although there is no absolute score from the Mini-Mental State Examination that provides a cutoff for declaring a patient inoperable, the indications for surgery in patients with Alzheimer disease who are severely disoriented, confused, and incapable of independent living should be strongly considered on an individual basis with a view against operation. Preoperative depression is an independent risk factor for postoperative mortality.

Hepatic Cirrhosis

Liver disease may be associated with complex multifactorial coagulopathies. Cardiac operation can be performed safely in patients with mild or moderately advanced hepatic cirrhosis with a 6% early mortality. Complication rates can be high at 39% for Pugh class A patients and 80% for Pugh class B and C on the basis of one study,[79] but rates may be lower for OPCAB in such patients.[80] Careful consideration of operative indications and methods is necessary in cirrhotic patients with low platelet counts or high MELD (the Model for End-Stage Liver Disease) scores. A high incidence of hospital morbidity is predicted in patients with platelet counts of less than $9.6 \times 10^4/\mu L$ or MELD scores exceeding 13.[81]

Connective Tissue Disease

CABG appears to be safe in patients with connective tissue diseases (see Chap. 89; rheumatoid arthritis and systemic lupus) with acceptable early results. Wound complications may be a problem, and the use of steroids or other immunomodulating agents is associated with increased postoperative complications. Chronic steroid therapy in general does not increase mortality or overall morbidity, but it may be associated with a greater chance for development of atrial arrhythmias or of requiring prolonged ventilation.

Human Immunodeficiency Virus Type 1

Although the incidence of active infectious endocarditis in patients with human immunodeficiency virus type 1 (HIV-1) has been reduced, noninfectious valvular disease and CAD are on the rise in such patients (see Chap. 72). Those patients requiring cardiac surgery show a high (22%) overall mortality with 58% actuarial 15-year survival and no blunting of the CD4 response induced by antiretrovirals.[82] The late causes of death are usually not AIDS related.

Hematology and Oncology

Whether cardiac surgery is justifiable in patients with malignant tumors is determined by the long-term outcome of the treated malignant neoplasm. Fatal progression of the tumor can occur if the time interval between the occurrence of the malignant neoplasm and cardiac surgery is short. Cardiac operations can be performed with acceptable mortality (4.1%) in patients with hematologic malignant neoplasms but with significant morbidity rates (50%), most often bleeding and infection.[83]

Antiphospholipid syndrome (APS) is a rare coagulation disorder associated with recurrent arterial and venous thrombotic events (see Chap. 87). The effects of surgery in APS have been reviewed.[84] Patients with APS undergoing cardiac surgery belong to a high-risk subgroup, and some patients with unexplained perioperative thromboembolic complications, such as graft occlusion, may turn out to have undiagnosed APS. Patients with glucose-6-phosphate dehydrogenase deficiency who are undergoing cardiac surgery may have a more complicated course with a longer ventilation time, more hypoxia, increased hemolysis, and a need for more blood transfusion. Because this difference may be caused by subnormal free radical deactivation, strategies that minimize bypass in general and free radicals specifically may be beneficial. Patients with glycoprotein IIIa allele $Pl^{A1/A2}$ genetic polymorphism (Pl^{A1} homozygotes) who undergo CABG show increased postoperative bleeding that is further accentuated by preoperative aspirin therapy.[85] Heart valve surgery and surgery for congenital heart diseases can be performed safely in patients with sickle cell disease or sickle cell trait with acceptable outcome and survival rates. Perioperative anemia from excessive hemodilution during CPB is a risk factor for major morbidity even in the absence of blood transfusions.

Preoperative Risk Calculation

On a background of increasingly complex preoperative profiles, outcomes after first CABG seem to have improved in routine clinical practice since the 1990s and compare well to those seen in clinical trials. Three mortality measures have traditionally been used to estimate perioperative outcomes: in-hospital, 30-day, and procedural (either in-hospital or 30-day) mortality. In the same population of patients, the in-hospital mortality is generally the lowest rate, whereas the procedural mortality rate is usually the highest. In addition, because complications occur more frequently than death, risk-adjusted major morbidity may differentially affect quality of care and enhance a surgical team's ability to assess their quality. A limitation of standard risk models is that risk associated with some preoperative variables can change significantly over time after surgery, and assessments that assume constant risk during the postoperative follow-up period may substantially overestimate or underestimate risk. Diabetes adds little incremental risk immediately after surgery, but the risk increases steadily and doubles at 9.5 years after surgery (see Chap. 64). Age, COPD, and urgent or emergent status also show risk, changing by 50% to 60% during a decade. Avoidance of CPB does not confer significant clinical advantages in all high-risk coronary patients; instead, there are particular subsets of patients for whom beating-heart surgery can be particularly indicated and others for whom on-pump revascularization seems a better solution (see Chap. 57). Off-pump surgery improves in-hospital outcome only in the subset of patients at highest risk. Off-pump patients have more early and late cardiac complications, whereas patients operated on-pump exhibit a higher incidence of postoperative systemic organ dysfunction. Adaptation of the operation to the individual patient is probably the best way to improve outcomes.

Two successful and widely used risk models are the EuroSCORE additive model, which also comes in a full logistic version, and the STS model. Notwithstanding, preoperative risk calculation remains an imperfect art. With use of the STS data base, models have been developed for postoperative mortality and composite endpoint and for postoperative morbidity, including stroke, renal failure, reoperation, prolonged ventilation, and sternal infection.[86] Severe diastolic dysfunction is a strong predictor of adverse outcome and mortality after on-pump CABG, and this high risk is not adequately predicted by EuroSCORE and the STS model. Measures of diastolic function should be included in routine preoperative risk assessment.[87] A preoperative echocardiographic wall motion score index is a surrogate measure of residual remote myocardial function and is a promising tool for better selection of patients to improve results after surgical ventricular restoration procedures for advanced ischemic heart failure.[88]

EuroSCORE. The EuroSCORE (**Table 84-1**) is the most rigorously evaluated scoring system in modern cardiac surgery. It has a significantly better discriminatory power to predict 30-day mortality than the STS risk algorithm for patients undergoing CABG. It has been used not only to estimate perioperative mortality risk but also to assess 3-month mortality, length of stay, and specific postoperative complications such as renal failure, sepsis or endocarditis, and respiratory failure in the whole context of cardiac surgery and to predict ICU cost and ICU stay of more than 2 days after open heart surgery. The additive EuroSCORE gives excellent discrimination that is as good as the logistic version of the model, but it greatly underestimates risk in high-risk patients compared with the logistic version. Recalibration of the logistic EuroSCORE in high-risk patients is needed because of its tendency to overestimate the mortality risk.[89] Internationally, the evidence is highly suggestive that the additive version generally overestimates mortality at lower scores (EuroSCORE 6) and underestimates mortality at higher values (EuroSCORE >13). The additive model is also less precise and exhibits a predictive distortion, which should be accounted for, particularly when it is employed at the individual patient level. The logistic EuroSCORE is more accurate at predicting mortality in simultaneous CABG and valve surgery as the additive EuroSCORE significantly underpredicts in this high-risk group. The logistic version should be used to predict mortality when possible. If this is not feasible, a modified additive score could be employed at the bedside. It may be necessary to validate the EuroSCORE when it is applied to new international populations. In addition, certain independent risk factors obtained in the standard logistic EuroSCORE may not be as important in a newly calibrated EuroSCORE based on current information. An example given is that of age. Whereas previous data would have suggested a significantly increased risk for an octogenarian undergoing isolated CABG, improvements in surgical technique and perioperative care have improved the outcomes associated with CABG in this elderly group. All of this has important implications when an individual surgeon's performance is analyzed in the current era, in which risk stratification may actually be different when a risk stratification model derived from obsolete data is used. A modified EuroSCORE with only five variables has been suggested.[90]

For valvular heart disease, the EuroSCORE has been used to predict not only in-hospital mortality, for which it was originally designed, but also long-term mortality in the whole context of heart valve surgery (see Chap. 66). Meta-analysis shows that the EuroSCORE has low discrimination ability for valve surgery, and it overpredicts risk.[91] Moreover, EuroSCORE risk stratification may be inferior to the STS model in patients undergoing AVR,[92] and it has been shown to be imprecise for prediction of perioperative mortality among octogenarian AVR patients, but it may be useful for predicting mortality during medium-term follow-up. The Northern New England Cardiovascular Disease Study Group risk model and the Providence Health System Cardiovascular Study Group risk model are additional commonly applied algorithms for valvular heart disease. Both allow similar assessment of prevalence and mortality, and a new unified model has been proposed.[93] A scoring system using blood tests and clinical risk factors to determine thromboembolic risk after heart valve replacement has been described and may be used to guide prosthesis choice and antithrombotic management.[94]

The "Normal" Postoperative Convalescence

The usual postoperative course is influenced by physiologic changes as a result of anesthesia, surgical trauma, and CPB, which make these

TABLE 84-1 The Additive EuroSCORE

RISK FACTOR	DEFINITION	SCORE
Patient-Related Factors		
Age	Per 5 years or part thereof (>60 yr)	1
Sex	Female	1
Chronic pulmonary disease	Long-term use of bronchodilators or steroids for lung disease	1
Extracardiac arteriopathy	Any one or more of the following: claudication; carotid occlusion or >50% stenosis; previous or planned intervention on the abdominal aorta, limb arteries, or carotid arteries	2
Neurologic dysfunction	Disease severely affecting ambulation or day-to-day functioning	2
Previous cardiac surgery	Requiring opening of the pericardium	3
Serum creatinine	>200 mmol/liter preoperatively	2
Active endocarditis	Patient still receiving antibiotic treatment for endocarditis at the time of surgery	3
Critical preoperative state	Any one or more of the following: ventricular tachycardia or fibrillation or aborted sudden death, preoperative cardiac massage, preoperative ventilation before arrival in the operating room, preoperative inotropic support, intra-aortic balloon counterpulsation, or preoperative acute renal failure (anuria or oliguria <10 mL/hr)	3
Cardiac-Related Factors		
Unstable angina	Rest angina requiring IV nitrates until arrival in the operating room	2
LV dysfunction	Moderate or LVEF 0.30-0.50	1
	Poor or LVEF <0.30	3
Recent myocardial infarct	<90 days	2
Pulmonary hypertension	Systolic PA pressure >60 mm Hg	2
Operation-Related Factors		
Emergency	Carried out on referral before the beginning of the next working day	2
Other than isolated CABG	Major cardiac procedure other than or in addition to CABG	2
Surgery on thoracic aorta	For disorder of ascending, arch, or descending aorta	3
Postinfarct septal rupture		4

EUROSCORE	PATIENTS	DIED (%)	OBSERVED	EXPECTED
0-2 (low risk)	4,529	36 (0.8)	(0.56-1.10)	(1.27-1.29)
3-5 (medium risk)	5,977	182 (3.0)	(2.62-3.51)	(2.90-2.94)
6 or greater (high risk)	4,293	480 (11.2)	(10.25-12.16)	(10.93-11.54)
Total	14,799	698 (4.7)	(4.37-5.06)	(4.72-4.95)

CABG = coronary artery bypass grafting; IV = intravenous; LV = left ventricular; LVEF = left ventricular ejection fraction; PA = pulmonary artery.

Modified from Nashef SA, Rogues F, Michel P, et al: European system for cardiac operative risk evaluation (EuroSCORE). Eur J Cardiothorac Surg 16:9, 1999.

patients unique from other hospitalized medical and surgical patients. The use of CPB and ischemia-reperfusion injury can be associated with a systemic inflammatory response syndrome. Significant activation of complement, platelets, neutrophils, monocytes and macrophages, coagulation, fibrinolysis, and kallikrein cascades results in elevated concentrations of tumor necrosis factor, CRP, IL-6, and IL-8 within the first few days after operation. This "whole-body inflammation" can lead to a "post-pump syndrome" that is clinically expressed as fever, leukocytosis, abnormal coagulation, hypoxemia (from neutrophil aggregation and lysis in pulmonary vasculature), increased pulmonary capillary permeability, renal dysfunction, and cognitive dysfunction. Preoperative treatment with statins is associated with lower biochemical parameters of systemic inflammatory response and myocardial damage after cardiac surgery with CPB.

Cardiovascular Convalescence

Sinus tachycardia of 100 to 120 beats/min may occur a few hours after surgery without apparent cause and should lead to assessment of adequacy of blood volume, low cardiac output syndrome, pericardial effusion or tamponade, infection (even without fever), and occult hyperthyroidism. Orthostatic hypotension can be a problem in some patients, persisting for up to 2 weeks or so after surgery. It may be associated with persistent sinus tachycardia with the heart rate relatively fixed at 100 to 120 beats/min. Investigation of intravascular volume status, liberalization of salt intake, and reevaluation of antihypertensive medications or diuretics that may have been ordered are indicated. Tightly fitting veno-occlusive stockings as well as instructions to the patient about slowly arising from lying or sitting positions are occasionally helpful.

Pulmonary Convalescence

Current practice is to extubate patients ideally within 4 to 6 hours after operation. Such rapid weaning or "fast tracking" should be encouraged in elective, hemodynamically stable patients with adequate gas exchange who have no evidence of heart failure, excessive bleeding, or neurologic complications. In one study, the 30-day mortality rate for fast tracked patients was 0.34%, mean intensive care time was 5 hours 52 minutes, mean time to extubation was 3 hours 10 minutes, mean readmission rate to intensive care was 0.34%, and mean hospital stay from day of operation (inclusive) was 5.7 days. This process increased throughput by 14.6% (compared with standard practices), allowing intensive care beds to be used by more than one patient each day, leading to significant cost savings by reducing the nursing ratio per patient. Immediate extubation after OPCAB appears to reduce the incidence of postoperative AF independent of comorbidities. Periextubation tachycardia should be controlled with intravenous esmolol.

Atelectasis is common. The usual suspects include general anesthesia; manual compression of the lung during operation; one-lung ventilation during minimally invasive surgery; apnea during CPB; and postoperative poor coughing or deep inspirations, gastric distention, interstitial lung water, and pleural effusions. Systematic literature reviews and a randomized study have failed to show that routine, prophylactic use of incentive spirometry, continuous positive airway pressure, or physical therapy lowers pulmonary morbidity in the usual patient, reflecting the low morbidity of most cases of postoperative atelectasis. However, preoperative inspiratory muscle training in high-risk patients may reduce the incidence of postoperative pulmonary complications. Pleural effusions occurring 2 to 3 weeks after surgery may represent a postpericardiotomy syndrome that occurs in 10% to 40% of patients; they, too, resolve spontaneously during a few months.

The incidence of pneumothorax after pleural and mediastinal drain removal is very low. The decision to obtain routine chest radiographs could be based on clinical judgment. Although the presence of an air leak is currently a contraindication to chest tube removal, a retrospective study of 6038 patients demonstrated that patients with air leaks can be safely discharged home with their chest tubes, which can then be safely removed even in the presence of a small pneumothorax if the patients are asymptomatic and have no subcutaneous emphysema after 14 days on a portable device at home and the pleural space deficit has not increased in size.[95]

Neurologic Convalescence

Ulnar and median nerve injury has been described after CABG in 1.9% to 18% of patients as a result of a fractured first rib after sternotomy, stretch or compression injury of the brachial plexus from sternal retraction, awkward arm positioning, or needle trauma at internal jugular puncture. In one small study, fracture of the first rib or of the costotransverse articulation as diagnosed by radionuclide bone scan was described in 15% of patients. Ulnar involvement follows the typical pattern of sensory distribution, generally numbness of the small finger and the medial portion of the ring finger in the affected limb. Median neuropathy results in motor weakness of the muscles of the hand and forearm, typically noted when the patient is unable to grasp a cup or eating cutlery. Resolution occurs in even the most serious cases, usually by 2 to 3 months. Numbness or tingling related to the leg incision wound has been reported in 61% of patients, of whom 37% improve within 3 months. However, up to 41% may have persistent numbness beyond 2 years. Incisional leg pain has been reported by 46% of patients, of whom 77% show improvement by 3 months and only 10% experience pain persisting beyond 2 years.

Neurologic dysfunction may occur in 32% of patients because of surgical trauma or ischemic neuropathy after the radial artery is removed as a conduit for CABG. There are no major neurologic hand complications in the presence of adequate collateral arterial blood supply. All reported neurologic complaints were associated with sensory conduction deceleration of no clinical significance in electromyographic investigations of median nerve sensory-motor and ulnar nerve motor conduction. Preoperative and postoperative radial nerve motor and sensory conduction records were statistically similar. The technique of radial artery harvesting does not seem to influence outcomes.

Visual symptoms are common and often consist of poor visual acuity, blurring, or scotoma. Many patients will describe prominent "floaters" that they had not experienced previously; others report seeing various spots and stripes. Because spontaneous recovery may take up to 6 months, it is ill-advised to change eyeglasses during this time in all but the most severely affected patients.

Postoperative Laboratory Values

Perioperative hematocrit levels are usually in the low 30s; even though the root cause of the usual postoperative anemia is related to hemodilution and blood loss, there may be features of anemia of "chronic disease." Platelet count <100,000 is common, but thrombocytopenia much below 50,000 should be investigated. Postoperative thrombotic thrombocytopenic purpura should be recognized as a possible pathophysiologic mechanism for unexplained postoperative thrombocytopenia, and treatment should be initiated once the diagnosis is established. Mild metabolic acidosis with serum bicarbonate levels of 18 to 26 mEq/liter and pH of 7.3 or above may occur and usually resolve with rewarming and improvement in cardiac output. Potassium levels can change rapidly and need regular and frequent surveillance and a replacement protocol. Calcium levels may often be depressed to 7.0 mg/dL or less because of hemodilution; this rarely requires treatment, but more profound lowering, especially in the presence of hypotension, should be treated. Phosphate levels should be routinely measured immediately after surgery and appropriate therapy instituted because significant hypophosphatemia is common (34.3%) and may be associated with considerable morbidity, including prolonged ventilation, increased cardioactive drug requirements, and prolonged hospital stay.[96] CPB is associated with increases in insulin consumption, and high catecholamine and cortisol levels exacerbate hyperglycemia; these changes are induced to a lesser degree by OPCAB. High serum glucose levels during and after CPB are independent risk factors for early death and morbidity in both diabetic and nondiabetic patients, but especially in diabetic women. An insulin nomogram or protocol is needed at least briefly to avoid diabetic ketoacidosis in diabetic patients and to improve leukocyte chemotaxis. Cardiac troponin T (cTnT) elevation is observed in nearly all subjects, with a median cTnT concentration of 1.08 ng/mL overall.[97] Direct predictors of postoperative cTnT values include preoperative MI; preoperative, intraoperative, or postoperative intra-aortic balloon pump; number of distal anastomoses; bypass time; and number of intraoperative defibrillations. Glomerular filtration rate, OPCAB, and use of warm cardioplegia are inversely associated with cTnT values. A linear association is seen between cTnT levels and length of stay and ventilator hours, and in an analysis adjusted for the STS risk model, cTnT remained independently prognostic for death, death or heart failure, death or need for vasopressors, and the composite of all three. In contrast to consensus-endorsed cTnT cut points for postoperative evaluation, a cTnT <1.60 ng/mL has a negative predictive value of 93% to 99% for exclusion of various post-CABG complications. Serum cTnI levels measured 24 hours after cardiac surgery predict short-, medium-, and long-term mortality and remain independently predictive when adjusted for all other potentially confounding variables. CABG is associated with a marked reduction in serum homocysteine and folate levels in the early postoperative period. This reduction is, at least in part, independent of hemodilution and may be caused by an altered homocysteine turnover because of an increased consumption of glutathione during and soon after CABG.

Perioperative Electrocardiographic Changes

Hemiblocks are the most common postoperative anomaly and are generally transient; many are gone within 48 hours and the majority by hospital discharge. There is dispute about the long-term significance, with some believing that they do not worsen prognosis. Conversely, left bundle branch block and nonspecific interventricular conduction delay, both seen less often, are associated with a worse long-term prognosis and may be associated with a significant risk of cardiac death in the first year after surgery. The appearance of new Q waves should raise the concern of an MI, but unmasking of previously evident Q waves of a remote inferior wall MI has been reported, as has disappearance of anterior Q waves. Atrioventricular (AV) block is a common complication of AVR. There is also a 23% incidence of postoperative complete AV block after mitral valve surgery, which may be the outcome of damage of the AV node artery.

Postoperative Drug Therapy

The use of antiplatelet therapy after CABG has been reviewed.[98] Clopidogrel (75 mg/day for 5 days) may not inhibit platelet aggregation in the first 5 postoperative days and therefore should not be used as a sole antiplatelet agent early after CABG.[99] However, there is also evidence that either clopidogrel plus aspirin or clopidogrel alone can maintain high graft patency in the early postoperative phase after CABG.[100] OPCAB patients can safely receive clopidogrel in the early postoperative period without increased risk for mediastinal hemorrhage when it is started 4 hours postoperatively, if the chest tube output is <100 mL/hr for 4 hours, and then daily. Clopidogrel therapy was independently associated with decreased symptom recurrence and reduced adverse cardiac events after OPCAB. Extending clopidogrel use beyond 30 days does not have a significant effect on defined endpoints. Early postoperative use of enoxaparin or unfractionated heparin is associated with a significant increase in reexploration for postoperative bleeding, often at a significantly delayed time after the initial surgery. Statin treatment initiated early after grafting improves long-term survival in patients with a single ITA graft but not in those with bilateral ITA grafts. Survival of statin-treated patients with single ITA grafts was similar to that of patients with bilateral ITA grafts. Calcium channel blockers may be associated with significantly reduced mortality after cardiac surgery, including CABG.

Hospital Course

Fast-track anesthesia routinely allows early (<24 hours) transfer out of the ICU. Virtually all patients are suitable for fast-track recovery. Patients with advanced age, high APACHE score, and reexploration are likely to have prolonged ICU stays (>3 days) with higher ICU mortality when renal, respiratory, or heart failure is present. Readmission to the ICU after fast-track anesthesia, although uncommon at 3.3%, is associated with a longer second ICU stay and significant mortality.[101] Forty-three percent of ICU readmissions occur within 24 hours of discharge and are commonly the result of pulmonary problems (47%), usually difficulty in clearing secretions, or arrhythmias (20%).

Although length of hospital stay will vary with the surgical procedure and many other factors, hospital discharge on the third to fifth postoperative day should be the goal for the patient having a straightforward CABG or valve procedure with CPB. Earlier discharge is possible in OPCAB patients; in one study, 55.8% of patients were discharged on the day after OPCAB with no deaths, but they had a high readmission rate of 12.7%. Early discharge is unusual in patients with diabetes, renal failure, or recent MI. Previous bypass, obesity, acute MI, and hypertension are associated with readmission. Prolonged ICU stay (>10 days) leads to high early mortality (33%), especially in patients who require dialysis, and quality of life is worse compared with the general population in both physical and mental aspects, but the difference is moderate. Discharge medications should include aspirin (81 to 325 mg), other antithrombotic drugs as dictated by a valve procedure or prior drug-eluting coronary stent, statins for those with CAD, oral analgesic such as acetaminophen with codeine, stool softener, beta blocker, and short-term use of any special agents used for arrhythmia management.

A nationwide inpatient sample of 8,398,554 discharges after CABG conducted between 1988 and 2005 showed that whereas median length of stay decreased from 11 to 8 days between 1988 and 2005 ($P < 0.0001$), there was a simultaneous increase in nonroutine discharges (patients discharged with continued health care needs) from 12% in 1988 to 45% in 2005 ($P < 0.0001$), primarily comprising home health care and long-term facility use. Multivariable regression models showed age, female gender, comorbidities, concurrent valve surgery, and surgery in lower volume hospitals to be associated with nonroutine discharge.[102] Thus, the significant shortening of length of stay during CABG may be counterbalanced by the increased requirement for additional expensive postoperative health care resources and services. Frailty is a newly recognized risk for postoperative complications and an independent predictor of in-hospital mortality, institutional discharge, and reduced midterm survival.[103]

Postoperative Morbidity

Cardiovascular Morbidity

HYPOTENSION AND LOW CARDIAC OUTPUT. Preoperative LV dysfunction is the most important determinant of postoperative low output. Additional determinants of low cardiac output include poor myocardial preservation with a long CPB pump run resulting in myocardial edema, loss of high-energy phosphates, and accumulation of oxygen free radicals; surgical technical mishap; and perioperative MI. Distinction between intrinsic cardiac dysfunction and pericardial tamponade is essential and can present challenges not seen in nonsurgical patients. Although equalized right atrial and pulmonary capillary wedge pressures may be the presenting situation in the surgical patient when both are low (8 to 10 mm Hg), clots can form in the pericardium, resulting in nonuniform cavity compression. A common area for such clots is around the right atrium at the site of venous cannulation. This can result, for instance, in compression of the right atrium with cervical vein distention with low cardiac filling pressures. Selective restriction of left atrial filling has also been observed in association with high right-sided filling pressures and low left atrial pressures. With intravenous fluid administration, pulmonary capillary wedge pressure should increase out of proportion to right atrial pressure (eventually exceeding the right atrial pressure by 5 mm Hg) in the absence of tamponade. The exception will be the patient with single-chamber (right atrial) compression by pericardial clot or even a lower pulmonary capillary wedge pressure caused by clot in the region of the left atrium. Transthoracic or transesophageal bedside echocardiography is useful to confirm normal LV contraction and the presence of pericardial blood. Technetium-tagged red blood cell nuclear studies with delayed imaging have proved useful in difficult cases. Many surgeons simply prefer taking the patient back for exploration if tamponade is suspected but cannot be confirmed. The diagnosis of postoperative diastolic dysfunction has been reviewed.[104]

Hemodynamic monitoring is essential in the management of postoperative low output syndromes; however, there are pitfalls, some unique to the cardiac surgical patient. The correlation of pulmonary capillary wedge pressure or pulmonary artery diastolic pressure with LV end-diastolic pressure has been questioned in the early hours after surgery because of altered ventricular compliance from hypothermia and myocardial edema and elevated pulmonary vascular resistance. Pulmonary ventilation using positive end-expiratory pressure in excess of the left atrial pressure will also invalidate this relationship. Directly measured diastolic systemic or pulmonary pressures can be falsely low because of underdamping of monitoring systems. Pulmonary capillary wedge pressures can appear spuriously low because of overwedging of the balloon device. Thermodilution output calculations can be inaccurate in the setting of severe tricuspid regurgitation. For these reasons, overall clinical assessment of the patient and the trend of hemodynamic performance are more important than any single measurement.

Management of hypotension or low output syndrome starts with ensuring adequate oxygenation and hematocrit and a check for acidosis. Filling pressures should then be optimized with intravenous volume to raise pulmonary capillary wedge pressure to 18 to 20 mm Hg, but this may need to be higher if there is LV hypertrophy or other cause of LV diastolic stiffness. There may be a blunted elevation of filling pressures with fluid administration in the vasodilated patient caused by sedation, fever, rewarming, or other factors. The heart rate may need to be adjusted with atrial or AV sequential pacing to a maximum of 90 to 100 beats/min. AV synchrony is vital to maintenance of cardiac function at this time.

Vasoactive Drugs. There is marked hospital variation in the use of vasoactive therapies in high-risk CABG patients in clinical practice. Hospital-level risk-adjusted rates of any inotrope use can vary from 35% to 100%, and vasodilator rates vary from 10% to 100%. If low output or hypotension persists, vasoactive drugs are needed and should be chosen on the basis of the framework shown in **Table 84-2**. Dobutamine is a good choice; because it does not release norepinephrine from endogenous stores (unlike dopamine), it may be useful when endogenous stores of norepinephrine are depleted, as in chronic heart failure. Epinephrine is generally reserved for unresponsiveness to dopamine or dobutamine; there is significant renal vascular constriction with epinephrine. Norepinephrine raises blood pressure with little effect on heart rate or tachyarrhythmias. It can also be used in conjunction with other agents, such as phentolamine (a weak alpha blocker and direct vascular smooth muscle relaxant) or dopamine, to blunt the intense alpha constricting effects, resulting in increases in blood pressure and vascular resistance with no change in heart rate, cardiac output, or filling pressures and with less renal vascular constriction. The "inodilators" amrinone and milrinone improve cardiac output by a reduction in vascular resistance and some increase in inotropy with little increase in heart rate. Unlike virtually all other vasoactive drugs, their relatively long duration of action must be kept in mind (<3 hours for amrinone; <2 hours for milrinone) during weaning to fully appreciate intrinsic cardiac performance. Levosimendan (12 μg/kg bolus, followed by an infusion of 0.2 μg/kg/min) started immediately after induction can significantly enhance primary weaning from CPB compared with placebo in patients undergoing three-vessel on-pump CABG. The need for additional inotropic or mechanical therapy is decreased.

Right Ventricular Failure. Acute right ventricular decompensation can lead to LV failure with catastrophic results. As with LV dysfunction, checking for oxygen saturation, optimizing heart rate and maintaining AV synchrony, correcting acidosis, and optimizing preload, afterload, and intrinsic ventricular performance are all important. Maintaining ventilator settings to avoid high peak inspiratory pressures will help reduce pulmonary vascular resistance. However, there are certain caveats. In the surgical patient, unlike the medical patient with right ventricular infarction, fluid administration can be useful to improve right ventricular function, but the limits of right atrial pressure elevation are less forgiving and can lead to rapid deterioration of LV function. Because the right-sided cardiac chambers are capacious, significant volume increase may occur with only modest increases in right atrial pressure, resulting in leftward shift of the intraventricular septum, thereby encroaching on LV filling. Inotropic agents that improve ventricular function but reduce pulmonary artery pressures are important, so dobutamine would be preferred to dopamine and epinephrine would be preferred to norepinephrine.

Phosphodiesterase inhibitors such as vardenafil may play a useful role, depending on systemic pressure (see Chap. 78).[105] They generally improve ventricular contractility and reduce pulmonary artery pressures and also may have positive lusitropic effects on diastolic relaxation. However, they may also lower blood pressure, which as a rule is the limiting factor in managing severe right-sided failure. This usually requires a combination of agents with careful titration of each. Prostaglandin E_1 given in smaller doses will have a selective effect on pulmonary vascular resistance with little systemic effects. The selective infusion of different drugs into the right side (intravenous vasodilator/inotrope) and left side (inotrope/constrictor into the left atrium), although attractive, has not been successful in the authors' experience because of the dominantly systemic effect of these agents, especially in the presence of poor cardiac function. Exceptions would be various inhaled agents such as nitric oxide, which because of its unique route of administration and short half-life results in a decrease in pulmonary resistance with little effect on systemic vascular resistance (SVR) and systemic blood pressure. Epoprostenol (prostacyclin, prostaglandin I_2) is a short-acting, selective pulmonary vasodilator that, when inhaled, will lower pulmonary afterload with little effect on systemic pressure. Iloprost, another prostacyclin analogue, lowers pulmonary vascular resistance for up to 2 hours with little effect on systemic pressures when it is given by aerosol.

Cardiac Arrest. MI is the predominant precipitating cause of cardiac arrest after CABG or AVR, and ventricular fibrillation or tachycardia is the most common mechanism. Despite aggressive resuscitation, outcome is poor (69% survival after respiratory arrest and 50% after cardiac arrest). Young patients with good LV function have a better probability of survival if they do not suffer a postoperative MI. Guidelines for resuscitation in cardiac arrest after cardiac surgery have been released by the EACTS Clinical Guidelines Committee.[106] Resternotomy at the bedside may be lifesaving. In an international survey from 53 countries, the incidence of cardiac arrest reported was 1.8%; emergency resternotomy after arrest, 0.5%; and emergency reinstitution of bypass, 0.2%.[107] Respondents indicated that they would perform three attempts at defibrillation for ventricular fibrillation without intervening external cardiac massage and for all arrests perform emergency resternotomy within 5 minutes if within 24 hours of the operation. Fifty percent of respondents would give epinephrine immediately, 58% would permit a nonsurgeon to perform an emergency resternotomy, and 76% would allow a surgeon's assistant and 30% an anesthesiologist to do this.

Mechanical Circulatory Support. The preoperative use of intra-aortic balloon pumping appears to shift high-risk patients undergoing CABG on pump and off pump into a lower risk category and is associated with comparable perioperative troponin leakage and short-term and long-term outcomes similar to those of low-risk patients not receiving intra-aortic balloon pumping. It can be placed preoperatively to stabilize the patient with high-risk ischemic heart disease, including those with recurring ischemia with precarious coronary anatomy, severe LV dysfunction, or mechanical complications of MI, such as ventricular septal rupture or acute mitral regurgitation. The postoperative indication is persistent low output or hypotension, despite safely tolerated dosages of inotropic drugs. As cardiac function improves in anticipation of balloon removal, drug support should be reduced and maintained at low levels.

Other devices can be used short term when maximal medical therapy and intra-aortic balloon counterpulsation are not sufficient, including extracorporeal membrane oxygenation and ventricular assist devices (see Chap. 32).

POSTOPERATIVE HYPERTENSION. Defined by a mean arterial pressure of 105 mm Hg, an increase of 20 mm Hg over baseline, or a systolic pressure above 140 mm Hg, postoperative hypertension is especially common and severe after valve surgery, particularly after relief of aortic stenosis. Patients who were hypertensive preoperatively and those receiving beta blockers preoperatively are also more prone to exhibit postoperative hypertension. Because it usually is manifested early (within 1 to 2 hours), the risk is that of arterial anastomosis disruption and mediastinal bleeding, myocardial ischemia caused by excessive afterload, and, if severe, the risk of stroke. Integrity of saphenous vein or ITA grafts may also be compromised.

Elevated serum catecholamines have been implicated as an etiologic factor, along with elevation of renin, angiotensin, vasopressin, and

TABLE 84-2 Hemodynamic Manipulation

BP	PCWP	CO	SVR	TREATMENT
↓	N or ↑	↓	↑	Inotrope
↓	N	N or ↑	↓	Alpha agent
↑	↑	↓	↑	Vasodilator

BP = blood pressure; CO = cardiac output; N = normal; PCWP = pulmonary capillary wedge pressure; SVR = systemic vascular resistance.

sympathetic activity. Although it is epinephrine levels that are most profoundly elevated in the first several hours after surgery, the norepinephrine levels remain elevated for several days. Further evidence of the central role played by norepinephrine is the observation that patients with postoperative hypertension have norepinephrine levels that are consistently elevated at twofold to sevenfold the upper limits of normal, whereas epinephrine levels are normal in some and only modestly elevated in others.

The hemodynamic picture is often that of normal or slightly reduced cardiac output and significant elevation of SVR. Consequently, a vasodilator, most commonly nitroglycerin, is used in this situation. Postoperative hypertension can also be seen in the setting of hyperdynamic cardiovascular function with sinus tachycardia, normal or elevated cardiac output, and normal or slightly elevated SVR. Esmolol or labetalol given as a continuous infusion is a common choice in this setting.

PERIOPERATIVE MYOCARDIAL INFARCTION. Common genetic variants in the 9p21 locus, previously known to be associated with MI in nonsurgical populations, are also associated with perioperative myocardial injury after CABG.[108] Acute ischemic injury of the myocardium is caused primarily by the limitations of myocardial protection during the procedure. Because coronary blood flow is absent during aortic cross-clamping for surgery with CABG, success depends directly on the ability to reduce myocardial oxygen requirements to a negligible level. The STS data base reports the national incidence of perioperative MI for 2005 to be 1.1%, based on the diagnostic criteria of CK-MB (or CK) at least five times the upper limits of normal at <24 hours postoperatively and one of the following if >24 hours: evolutionary ST-segment elevation, new Q waves in two or more contiguous leads or new left bundle branch block, or CK-MB (or CK) at least three times the upper limits of normal. The clinical risk factors appear to be older age and longer pump time as well as elevated LV end-diastolic pressure, unstable angina, and left main CAD.

The patient with perioperative MI usually emerges from the surgery with new Q waves that persist. "Pseudo" Q waves mimicking inferior wall MI may occur as a result of a marked left axis shift. The occurrence of perioperative MI seems to have an adverse impact on survival acutely, but there is disagreement about any impact on long-term survival, with some reporting reduced survival and others showing impact related only to enzyme level.

The mechanism of MI occurring days or weeks after the procedure is often bypass graft closure. The pattern of enzyme release, climbing to a peak a few hours after surgery rather than the more common immediate tapering, suggests a mechanism other than the expected enzyme release from inadequate myocardial preservation and other operative events. In one report, cTnI cutoff levels of 13 ng/mL identified patients at higher risk of hospital death (9.5% versus 0.7%) and were the only independent predictor but had no influence on mortality at 2 years' follow-up. In the case of CK-MB, a cutoff of >40 ng/mL was associated with higher perioperative mortality, but this association no longer persisted at 1 year. OPCAB appears to be associated with less release of cardiac enzymes but with no influence on survival at 1 year.

PERICARDIAL EFFUSION AND POSTCARDIOTOMY SYNDROME. Pericardial effusion occurs in 1.5% of patients, and symptoms are nonspecific. Several factors, mainly related to preoperative characteristics and type of operation, predispose patients to effusion. Echocardiography-guided pericardiocentesis is effective and safe in these patients.

Controversy still exists about the etiology of the postcardiotomy syndrome. Anti–heart antibodies, present in high titers in virtually all cases, have implicated an autoimmune response. Antibody to adenovirus or coxsackievirus B1 to B6 is present in 70% of affected patients, leading to the speculation that this is an immunologic reaction triggered by acute or latent virus infection. Signs and symptoms (**Table 84-3**) range from a low-grade fever, with or without white blood cell count elevation, to a profound illness with pericardial and pleuritic pain, myalgias, and lassitude with fever up to 104°F. A pericardial friction rub and often a pleural rub along with effusions are common. Elevated white cell count with a leftward shift and elevated sedimentation rate are also seen commonly. The electrocardiogram may show diffuse ST-segment elevation or can be entirely normal. The echocardiographic finding of a small pericardial effusion is also not specific.

TABLE 84-3 Typical Signs and Symptoms in Postpericardiotomy Syndrome Patients

SIGN OR SYMPTOM	NO. OF PATIENTS	INCIDENCE, %
Fever	45	100
Increased incisional pain	43	95
Pericardial or pleural rub	43	95
Malaise and weakness	31	69
Increased white blood cell count	38	84
Increased erythrocyte sedimentation rate	36	80
Pericardial or pleural fluid	30	67
Asymptomatic	2	4

Modified from Urschel HC, Razzuk MA, Gardner M: Coronary artery bypass occlusion secondary to postcardiotomy syndrome. Ann Thorac Surg 22:528, 1976.

The time of appearance can be as early as 1 week after surgery, but most cases appear 2 to 3 weeks after surgery and can appear for up to 2 months. The most serious consequences are pericardial constriction, bypass graft closure, and tamponade. Tamponade itself is uncommon. Therapy with oral prednisone 70 to 80 mg/day with tapering during 10 to 14 days is indicated. In the early phase of the presentation, inpatient treatment is appropriate unless the symptoms and involvement are very mild. Specifically, the systolic pressure should be above 100 mm Hg, the pulse pressure above 30 mm Hg, and the heart rate no higher than 110 beats/min. The patient should be examined frequently for evidence of increasing pulsus paradoxus or decreased urine output. Pericardial drainage is indicated when these parameters suggest tamponade (see Chap. 75), although, as noted, tamponade is uncommon. Pericardiocentesis poses special risks in patients with anteriorly placed coronary grafts. The fluid can be loculated, and catheter drainage should not be attempted unless there is echocardiographic evidence of fluid anteriorly or around the cardiac apex. For these reasons, pericardiocentesis should be done in the operating room or in an ICU setting, with use of echocardiographic guidance and only by experienced individuals. Special care is needed in skin preparation to avoid bacterial contamination. Fluid accumulation recurs with a reported incidence of 13% in a pediatric population to as high as 50% in adults in one report. A significant rate of early bypass graft occlusion as a consequence of postpericardiotomy syndrome has been reported with and without constriction and, along with the goal of symptomatic relief, is a reason for aggressive medical therapy.

CONSTRICTIVE PERICARDITIS. The diagnosis and management of postoperative constrictive pericarditis have been reviewed.[109] Constrictive pericarditis after open heart surgery may appear as early as 2 weeks or as late as several years after the procedure, the majority appearing between 3 and 12 months postoperatively. The presentation is similar to that of other causes of constriction (see Chap. 75), in which the hallmarks are distended neck veins, peripheral edema, ascites, and hepatosplenomegaly. Echocardiography is valuable in making the diagnosis (see Chap. 15), and definitive diagnosis by cardiac CT has also been reported (see Chap. 19). When constriction is suspected but cannot be confirmed by equalized diastolic pressures, rapid intravenous volume infusion may illustrate the true hemodynamic features. Most patients will require surgery, consisting of either localized or radical pericardiectomy, and the surgical results are generally favorable. Patients presenting within 2 months of surgery warrant a trial of medical therapy consisting of diuretics and steroids because of the high likelihood of a more inflammatory component with less fibrosis. The mechanisms proposed for constriction include the postpericardiotomy syndrome, the use of povidone-iodine pericardial irrigation, and the late effects of hemopericardium.

PERIOPERATIVE ARRHYTHMIAS

Atrial Fibrillation

The prevalence, risks, and management of perioperative AF have been reviewed.[110] The incidence of atrial tachyarrhythmias is 33% after CABG and 35% to 50% after valve-related procedures. AF is the most common arrhythmia, with an incidence of 20% to 40%, usually occurring between postoperative days 3 and 5. Age-related myocardial fibrosis is believed to be closely related to the occurrence of AF after

CABG. Independent predictors of AF include age older than 75 years, history of AF, diabetes, duration of CPB and crossclamp time, bicaval cannulation, inadequate protection of the atria during crossclamping, postoperative serum elevation of both epinephrine and norepinephrine, and postoperative high doses of nonsteroidal anti-inflammatory drugs. Meta-analysis of 14 studies (16,505 patients) has shown a slightly lower incidence of AF (19%) with OPCAB than with CABG with CPB (24%), including the elderly. Similar arrhythmias also occur in patients having noncardiac thoracic surgical procedures, but at reduced frequency. New-onset post-CABG AF is associated with increased long-term risk of mortality independent of the patient's preoperative severity. After control for a comprehensive array of risk factors associated with post-CABG adverse outcomes, risk of long-term mortality in patients who developed new-onset post-CABG AF after isolated CABG is 29% higher than in patients without it.[111]

No preventive strategies have been successful in eliminating the problem of postoperative AF, and the most successful approaches reduce the incidence by about half. Sotalol has been shown to be more effective than beta blockers in prevention but is a negative inotropic agent and can cause QT prolongation with polymorphic ventricular tachycardia including torsades de pointes. In a meta-analysis, beta blockers decreased the incidence of AF by approximately 40%. Amiodarone is effective when it is started preoperatively, intraoperatively, or postoperatively. Routine use of postoperative prophylactic intravenous bolus and subsequent 5 days of oral amiodarone therapy after CABG decrease the total cost of care.[112] Biatrial pacing has also shown efficacy when it is applied for the first 3 days postoperatively. Continuous monitoring of oxygen saturation and subsequent oxygen therapy for hypoxia have been shown to reduce the incidence of AF.

The management of AF after cardiac surgery has been reviewed.[113] Treatment of AF or atrial flutter begins with control of the heart rate (see Chap. 40) by use of intravenous metoprolol or esmolol, which has the advantage of rapid onset of action and 50% likelihood of conversion to sinus rhythm. Diltiazem affects rate control and cardioversion to a lesser extent and may be associated with hypotension or worsening heart failure. There is the possibility of complete AV block when intravenous beta blockers and calcium antagonists are combined, so that pacing wires should be in place and connected to a pacing device. Digoxin is not a first-line agent for prophylaxis, but it may be given intravenously in low daily doses (0.125 mg) to supplement beta blocker effects. Other approaches to acute pharmacologic conversion include procainamide, propafenone, ibutilide, and dofetilide. The last two agents are useful when negative inotropism is not tolerated or if bronchospasm is an issue with beta-blocking agents. Both prolong the QT interval and exhibit proarrhythmic properties and should be stopped as soon as cardioversion takes place.

Low-energy cardioversion with use of biatrial epicardial wires implanted during surgery is effective and safe in conscious patients. Overdrive atrial pacing is effective with use of temporary epicardial atrial pacing wires placed at surgery if the underlying rhythm is atrial flutter or paroxysmal atrial tachycardia. When the type of rhythm is not clear, an atrial electrogram can be helpful. Bipolar electrograms can be recorded by attaching one epicardial lead to each of the two arm leads of the electrocardiographic patient cable by an alligator clip. By recording standard lead I on the lead selector, a bipolar atrial electrogram is recorded. A unipolar recording can be performed by attaching the atrial lead to the precordial patient monitoring lead. If there is any sign of organized regular depolarization of the left atrium, a trial of overdrive pacing is indicated. Starting at a pacing rate of just under the atrial flutter rate with maximal stimulus output, the pacing rate is slowly increased by 10-beat increments until atrial entrainment occurs. Failure to correct the rhythm can be caused by a number of factors, including a broken pacemaker wire or loss of contact with the epicardial surface. If only one such wire is broken or available, unipolar pacing is possible with use of the functioning wire as a negative pole and an electrode patch close to the wire as the other electrode. The threshold for capture may rise above the level of output of commercially available pacing units (which is usually 20 mA), in which case repeated attempts after dosing with an antiarrhythmic agent may be successful. On occasion, atrial pacing will convert atrial flutter to AF. Because the ventricular response rate is often slower and more responsive to negative chronotropic agents, this is usually a preferred rhythm. Rapid atrial pacing that is unable to be converted to sinus rhythm may induce a level of higher grade AV blockade, resulting in a more controlled ventricular response rate despite persistent flutter. Heparin anticoagulation should be considered for the patient who has not converted in 24 hours and earlier if there is a history of atrial tachyarrhythmias before surgery. Cardioversion is reserved for patients exhibiting acute hemodynamic instability. It is desirable to have an anesthesiologist performing the sedation if possible. For elective cardioversion, anterior-posterior paddles are preferred, with the posterior paddle placed at the lower tip of the scapula. In one study of 640 consecutive CABG patients, amiodarone and early electrical cardioversion were more effective than non-amiodarone therapies for restoration of sinus rhythm. Hemodynamic compromise, systemic embolism, and anticoagulation-related complications, including pericardial tamponade, may complicate the management of AF.

Ventricular Arrhythmias. Ventricular ectopy including nonsustained ventricular tachycardia requiring at least a short course of therapy has been reported in up to 50% of patients, with high occurrence between postoperative days 3 and 5. Possible mechanisms include the previously mentioned elevation of circulating catecholamines, clinical or subclinical myocardial necrosis, and electrolyte abnormalities. Until more definitive data are available, it is prudent to individualize therapy on the basis of known or suspected risk factors, such as LV function and the patient's medical history. An initial approach is to use atrial pacing, which will often reduce the ectopy without resorting to drugs. For nonsustained ventricular tachycardia, magnesium and amiodarone are commonly used. For sustained ventricular tachycardia, overdrive pacing, cardioversion, or intravenous amiodarone is used.

Conduction Defects. Complete AV block, like lesser degrees of AV block, can be caused by incomplete washout of cardioplegia solution and antiarrhythmic drugs or their toxicity and is generally transient. Surgical transection of the node during AVR is a well-known complication and leads to permanent AV blockade. Improvement in preoperative complete heart block may occur in up to 29% of patients after successful AVR and can occur for up to 18 months after surgery. Factors weighing against recovery with the potential need for a permanent pacemaker include a heavily calcified AV node or aortic valve ring with extension into the septum, appearance of AV block hours or days after surgery, and, to a lesser extent, a significant preoperative conduction defect. In the absence of excessive calcification, optimism is warranted, and it may be realistic to wait for up to 10 days for recovery before implantation of a permanent pacemaker. Surgically placed epicardial pacemaker wires are commonly used and can be lifesaving. Paired placement on the right atrium and right ventricle enhances diagnostic capability and allows pacing of all modes of bradycardia and for overdrive pacing.

Postoperative Pulmonary Morbidity

Pulmonary complications after cardiac surgery have been reviewed in detail.[114] In a large, multicenter administrative data base of 51,351 patients who underwent CABG, the incidence of adult respiratory distress syndrome/pulmonary edema was 4.9%; pneumonia, 0.8%; and other respiratory complications, 3.0%. Clinical observations suggest a 7.5% incidence of pulmonary morbidity, with an associated 21% mortality, in cardiac surgery patients with use of CPB. Heart failure is a major cause of postoperative pulmonary morbidity, and preoperative LV systolic dysfunction has a greater correlation than reduced preoperative pulmonary function with postoperative respiratory failure. Observational and randomized studies, and one propensity analysis study from the STS data base, suggest that the incidence of pulmonary complications is lower in patients receiving OPCAB. Small studies of patients undergoing mini-sternotomy or anterior thoracotomy have not convincingly shown reductions in respiratory complications.

Data from the STS data base indicate that 6.0% of patients undergoing CABG by median sternotomy require mechanical ventilation for more than 48 hours, with higher incidence of 2-week hospital stay (6%) and higher mortality (11.3%) than in patients undergoing OPCAB, including patients with COPD. Factors that predispose to prolonged ventilation include low albumin, low cardiac output state, persistent postoperative bleeding, neurologic complications, acute renal failure, bloodstream infections, and intra-abdominal complications. Postoperative AF may lead to hemodynamic instability requiring reintubation.

Pneumonia. Pneumonia has been reported in 2% to 22% of cardiac surgery patients and may be associated with up to 27% mortality. Clinical presentation occurs, on average, 4 days after surgery and ranges from fever with productive cough to acute respiratory failure requiring prolonged ventilation. Silent aspiration leading to pneumonia occurs commonly in the elderly, especially those with neurologic or cognitive impairment. Other reported predisposing factors include use of H2 receptor blockers (which increase colonization of gastric fluid with gram-negative organisms, which are then microaspirated) or broad-spectrum antibiotics, presence of nasogastric tube (which facilitates microaspiration), reintubation, prolonged mechanical ventilation, and transfusion of four or more units of blood products. Diagnosis is difficult because of frequent concomitant atelectasis and pleural effusions, and hence a high index of suspicion is warranted. Gram-negative organisms are the most common, but gram-positive bacteria appearing in the sputum before surgery are often the culprits in pneumonia occurring within 3 days of CABG. Resistant strains are emerging. Ventilator-associated pneumonia occurs in 8% of patients after cardiac surgery, rising to 9% to 21% in those with respiratory failure and 44% when intubation is longer than 7 days. It has been suggested that the risk of pneumonia increases by 1% with each day of mechanical ventilation. Mortality of ventilator-associated pneumonia can be as high as 75% because of associated multiorgan failure.

Acute Respiratory Distress Syndrome. Acute respiratory distress syndrome (ARDS) is characterized by the presence of bilateral interstitial infiltrates on the chest radiograph, a pulmonary capillary wedge pressure of less than 18 mm Hg, and the presence of arterial hypoxemia leading to PaO_2/FiO_2 ratio less than 200. It occurs in less than 2% of patients undergoing CPB but is associated with mortality up to 80% because of associated multiorgan failure. It remains unclear whether off-pump or minimally invasive procedures reduce the occurrence of ARDS. The etiology of ARDS is multifactorial and includes pulmonary endothelial trauma caused by the whole-body inflammation on CPB, cessation of ventilation during CPB, translocation of enteric endotoxins secondary to intestinal hypoperfusion, and ischemia-reperfusion injury and hypothermia, with contributions from untoward reactions to protamine and transfusion products. Management is aimed at general multiorgan supportive care. Prevention of ventilator-associated pulmonary mechanotrauma through the use of small tidal volumes (6 mL/kg) has been shown to reduce mortality by 25%; the associated permissive hypercapnia is not detrimental. The use of heparin-coated circuits, hollow-fiber membrane oxygenators, or high-dose steroids to modulate the systemic inflammatory response has not been shown consistently to improve outcomes.

Postoperative Bleeding

Coagulopathy is common after CPB and is related to reductions in coagulation factors, fibrinolysis, inadequate reversal of heparinization, excessive protamine administration, other perioperative drugs, and defective platelet formation. It has been suggested that CPB-induced platelet aggregation may not be caused by factors released from the tubing or its coating but may be initiated by short bouts of high shear stress, and its continuation is critically dependent on adenosine diphosphate. Patients undergoing OPCAB show protection against activation of coagulation and fibrinolysis and against endothelial injury only during the intraoperative period; this is followed by the development of a prothrombotic pattern comparable to that of patients undergoing on-pump surgery lasting at least as late as 30 days after surgery. In addition, in patients undergoing OPCAB, the intraoperative administration of hetastarch increases the postoperative transfusion requirement and the volume of blood drained postoperatively. Hemodilution with low intraoperative hematocrit levels (<19%) has been shown not to contribute to postoperative bleeding. In contrast to standard coagulation testing (prothrombin time, fibrinogen level, D-dimer, and platelet count), platelet function as assessed by thromboelastography and whole-blood aggregometry may predict both bleeding and thrombosis after OPCAB.

Pharmacologic approaches and perioperative use of antithrombotic drugs (see Chap. 87) to reduce blood loss and transfusions in the perioperative period have been reviewed.[115] Meta-analysis has shown no significant difference in efficacy between the inexpensive lysine analogues, such as epsilon–aminocaproic acid or tranexamic acid, and more expensive serine protease inhibitors, such as high-dose aprotinin.

The specific use of aprotinin during cardiac surgery and its safety remain unresolved; cumulative evidence suggests that the risk associated with aprotinin may not be worth the hemostatic benefit. In a retrospective study of 1524 cardiac surgery patients at high risk for postoperative stroke, the administration of full-dose aprotinin but not half-dose aprotinin was associated with a lower incidence of stroke.[116] It has been proposed that the higher level of kallikrein inhibition obtained with full dosing may be required for end-organ protection. Another study concluded that its use is not associated with a change in mortality, MI, or renal failure risk but is associated with a reduced risk of stroke and a trend toward reduced incidence of AF.[117] The drug reduces perioperative bleeding during OPCAB. However, there is evidence showing an increased risk of death associated with aprotinin. A multicenter, blinded, randomized trial in high-risk cardiac surgery patients demonstrated a significantly higher occurrence of all-cause 30-day mortality with aprotinin compared with aminocaproic acid or tranexamic acid.[118] Analysis of electronic administrative records showed a 64% higher mortality on the day of CABG in patients who received aprotinin alone (n = 33,517) than in those who received aminocaproic acid alone (n = 44,682).[119] In another retrospective analysis of patients who underwent isolated CABG or combined CABG with valve operations, those who received aprotinin had a higher mortality rate and larger increases in serum creatinine levels than did patients who received aminocaproic acid or no antifibrinolytic agent.[120] On the other hand, there are studies indicating that full-dose aprotinin use is not associated with MI, neurologic dysfunction, renal insufficiency, or death after CABG or valve operations but does result in less postoperative bleeding and blood product transfusion and early extubation.[121] In another single-institution observational study involving 7836 consecutive patients (1998-2006), aprotinin was effective in reducing bleeding after cardiac surgery, was safe, and did not affect short- or medium-term survival.[122] The risk of hypersensitivity reactions is low (0.09%) after primary exposure to aprotinin. This risk after reexposure reaches a maximum between the 4th day and the 30th day after previous exposure and declines considerably after 6 months.

Desmopressin acetate (DDAVP) causes a 2- to 20-fold increase in plasma levels of factor VIII and von Willebrand factor and releases tissue plasminogen activator and prostacyclin from vascular endothelium. The drug may be useful in mild to moderate forms of hemophilia or von Willebrand disease, in uremic patients with platelet dysfunction, and in certain forms of postoperative platelet dysfunction based on specific testing.

Recombinant activated factor VII (rFVIIa) as rescue therapy in severe, uncontrollable hemorrhage after cardiac surgery is efficacious and safe and is not associated with adverse neurologic or cardiovascular effects. The median dose is 93 μg/kg, and 85% of patients need a single dose. In a registry cohort of 304 patients, the documented response rate to a single dose of rFVIIa was 84%, of which 23% experienced cessation of bleeding and 61% showed a reduction in bleeding. The percentage of patients alive at 28 days was 95% if bleeding ceased after rFVIIa, 86% if bleeding was reduced, and 60% if there was no response.[123]

Risk factors for surgical reexploration include advanced age, smaller BMI, nonelective cases, and five or more distal anastomoses. Preoperative aspirin and heparin are risk factors for the on-pump CABG group. Patients needing reexploration are at higher risk of complications if the time to reexploration is prolonged. Chest reexploration in the ICU for bleeding or tamponade after heart surgery can be a safe alternative to return to the operating room.

The main determinant of morbidity and mortality for patients requiring a surgical reexploration after cardiac operations is the amount of packed red blood cells transfused. Packed red blood cells must be used judiciously as perioperative packed red blood cell transfusion carries the potential for exposure to a variety of cellular and humoral antigens, disease transmission, and immunomodulation. A multidisciplinary approach to blood conservation has been proposed and can result in lower transfusion rates and equivalent patient outcomes. Transfusion is associated with reduced risk-adjusted 1-year survival after CABG, with the largest proportion of deaths occurring within 30 days. In a group of cardiac surgery patients, the risk of pneumonia increased by 5% per unit of red blood cells or platelets received, with higher risk for each day that the blood was stored. However, the administration of blood per se may not lead to increased postoperative infection. Point-of-care coagulation monitoring using thromboelastography has been shown to reduce postoperative transfusion requirements. Preoperative erythropoietin administered during weeks is associated with higher postoperative hemoglobin concentrations with modest reductions in transfusion requirements. Alternatively, intraoperative autologous heparinized blood removal before CPB in hemodynamically stable patients and retransfusion after CPB, intraoperative cell salvage, and autotransfusion of washed salvaged red blood cells also reduce need for transfusion. The mechanical cell salvage procedure reduces the red blood cell deformability and the cell 2,3-diphosphoglycerate content. Retransfusion of the processed blood by a cell-saving device does not further compromise the red blood cell function in patients undergoing cardiac surgery with CPB. Based on IL-6 and free hemoglobin washout, the quality of the processed blood remains constant even with multiple runs of the cell-saving device.

The volume remaining in the oxygenator and tubing set should be returned without cell processing or hemofiltration. Using the hard shell cardiotomy reservoir from the heart-lung machine, autotransfusion of the shed mediastinal blood can be continued hourly up to 18 hours after operation. By these methods, homologous red blood cell transfusion may be avoided in up to 98.6% of patients. However, cardiotomy suction and autotransfusion of mediastinal shed blood may contribute to the perioperative inflammatory response. Lipid particles in the size range of 10 to 60 μm in shed mediastinal blood with more than 300,000 particles per milliliter of blood can certainly contribute to microembolic complications.[124] Triglyceride profiles in these lipid particles and in adipose tissue are similar, suggesting that their origin is the mediastinum. Closed circuit extracorporeal circulation (CCECC) for CABG is associated with a significant reduction of red blood cell damage and activation of coagulation cascades similar to off-pump surgery compared with conventional CPB; in contrast, fibrinolysis markers and IL-6 were markedly increased in CCECC postoperatively. A substantially lower need for postoperative blood transfusions and a comparable hemorrhage-related reexploration rate suggest that OPCAB may avoid the morbidity and mortality associated with excessive postoperative blood loss. There is a tendency toward less activation of coagulation and fibrinolysis in low-risk patients during elective OPCAB compared with on-pump surgery.

Postoperative Renal Dysfunction

The development of AKI after cardiac surgery (see Chap. 93) is a devastating complication with high morbidity and up to 42% 30-day mortality.[125] Risk factors for the development of AKI include advanced age, diabetes, COPD, peripheral vascular disease, emergency operation, previous cardiac surgery, low preoperative hemoglobin level, high preoperative CRP level, perioperative MI, reexploration, and number of blood transfusions.[126] In the immediately postoperative period, neutrophil gelatinase–associated lipocalin and cystatin C correlate with and are independent predictors of duration and severity of AKI and duration of intensive care stay after adult cardiac surgery; however, the combination of both renal biomarkers does not add predictive value. The risk of adverse clinical events is not associated with ITA and saphenous vein graft failure, suggesting that factors other than graft failure account for the worse clinical outcomes, at least during the first year. In one study, three thresholds of AKI (>25%, >50%, and >75% decrease in estimated glomerular filtration rate within 1 week of surgery or need for postoperative dialysis) occurred in 24%, 7%, and 3% of the cohort, respectively. All three thresholds were independently associated with a more than fourfold increase in the odds of dying.[127] Early recovery of renal function is associated with improved long-term survival. Significant risk factors for death are complex procedures, gastrointestinal complications, long crossclamp time (>88 minutes), reexploration, advanced age (>75 years), elevated preoperative creatinine, postoperative pulmonary edema, sepsis, multiple organ failure, and hypotension. Although CPB is considered to be an important contributor to AKI, OPCAB improves only early mortality; long-term survival has been shown to be better in those revascularized on-pump, possibly because of more complete revascularization with CPB.

The use of various forms of renal replacement therapy after cardiac surgery (hemodialysis, hemofiltration, or combination) has been reviewed.[128] Patients with normal preoperative renal function can develop unexpected postoperative AKI requiring dialysis when they undergo urgent or emergent surgery or experience intraoperative technical complications requiring longer CPB and crossclamp times. Patients with even mild preoperative renal dysfunction commonly experience worsening of renal function even when the perioperative course is uncomplicated and often require dialysis in the hospital or after discharge. The decision to initiate dialysis in renal failure patients not on dialysis who develop further postoperative AKI can be difficult. Dialysis in such patients has been shown to reduce neurologic and gastrointestinal complications, to reduce major adverse events with lower length of stay, and probably to lower the rate of multiorgan failure. However, although in-hospital mortality may be relatively low, midterm mortality is increased compared with those who do not undergo dialysis. Preoperative renal failure patients on dialysis show a significant increase in hospital mortality, postoperative sepsis, and respiratory failure after cardiac surgery. The risk of dialysis dependence may be reduced with OPCAB. Patients who have undergone kidney transplantation show better survival than those on dialysis. Patients with serum creatinine concentration >2.0 mg/dL or dialysis dependence who have had an acute or recent MI and undergo CABG show an 8% to 10% hospital mortality and a higher risk of pulmonary complications and AF.

In patients with elevated preoperative serum creatinine, mannitol (25 g) or dopamine infusion at 3.0 to 4.5 μg/kg/min is often given intraoperatively; furosemide (20 to 100 mg) or hemofiltration should be considered during CPB. Sustained mild hypothermia does not improve renal outcomes. However, rewarming on CPB is associated with increased renal injury and should be avoided. *N*-Acetylcysteine is not beneficial in the prevention of renal dysfunction after cardiac surgery, and its routine use should be avoided. Likewise, there is no benefit of high-dose furosemide (Lasix) given postoperatively. Fenoldopam mesylate (0.08 μg/kg/min) infusion starting at the induction of anesthesia and continued for at least the next 24 hours may reduce the risk of acute renal failure in high-risk patients.[129] Maintaining high mean perfusion pressure (around 80 mm Hg), reducing pump time, and optimizing hemodynamics with pharmacologic or mechanical support are also beneficial. Infection control and renal protection must be stressed. Early and aggressive use of continuous venovenous hemofiltration postoperatively in patients with volume overload and high serum creatinine concentration is associated with better than expected survival. Off-pump surgery offers better early and late outcomes in patients with normal preoperative creatinine concentration. When the preoperative creatinine concentration is abnormal, the surgical strategy does not seem to have any influence.[130]

Postoperative Neurologic Morbidity

COGNITIVE DYSFUNCTION. Cognitive dysfunction after cardiac surgery has been reviewed.[131] It is a common short-term (33% to 83%) and long-term (20% to 60%) occurrence and may resolve after days to weeks or may remain as a permanent disorder, especially in terms of memory impairment. Often, longitudinal cognitive performance of patients with CABG shows a two-stage course with early improvement followed by later decline. Long-term cognitive deficit is predicted by early cognitive decline but not by ischemic brain lesions on magnetic resonance imaging (MRI). However, small studies indicate that prospective longitudinal neuropsychological performance of patients with CABG may be no different from that of comparable nonsurgical control subjects with CAD at 3 months or 1 year after baseline examination. This suggests that the generally reported cognitive decline during the early postoperative period after CABG may be transient and reversible. Subjective memory assessments have been correlated with objective performance on several memory tests.[132] Although subjective memory complaints are more common in patients with depression, they cannot be explained by depression alone. Baseline impairment before surgery in patients with CAD may also be higher than generally suspected. Pathologic findings point to a complex etiology involving the interplay of anesthesia effects, systemic inflammation, cerebral microemboli, and cerebral hypoperfusion with cerebral oxygen desaturation. Intraoperative hemodynamic instability, hypoxia, elevated preoperative creatinine, poor preoperative LV function, medications, postoperative infections, and intraoperative hyperglycemia in nondiabetic patients have been described as additional risk factors. Reduced preoperative endotoxin immunity has been proposed as a predictor of postoperative cognitive dysfunction in the elderly; a significant positive association between serum concentrations of S100B protein and neuropsychological function has been reported. Preoperative cerebral MRI may be used to predict the risk for cognitive dysfunction after CABG. Long-term cognitive function and MRI evidence of brain injury are similar after off-pump and on-pump CABG. OPCAB does not appear to consistently offer immunity from adverse neurocognitive outcomes, suggesting that the clinical decline may not be specific to the use of CPB but may also occur in patients with similar risk factors for cardiovascular and cerebrovascular disease.[133]

Cognitive dysfunction is clinically expressed as impairment of memory, concentration, language comprehension, and social integration and is usually evaluated with a battery of neuropsychological tests assessing the cognitive domains of attention, language, verbal and visual memory, visual construction, executive function, and psychomotor and motor speed. The clinical syndrome occurs more commonly in the elderly and those with low educational status, limited social support, diabetes, and severe noncoronary atherosclerotic disease. Women appear more likely to suffer injury to brain areas subserving visuospatial processing. The success of neuroprotective therapeutic interventions, including high-dose steroids, has been limited.

STROKE. Stroke and encephalopathy after cardiac surgery have been reviewed in detail.[134] Early stroke after CPB is independently associated with higher stroke-related death and is associated with increased need for skilled rehabilitation at discharge. Neuroprotective strategies aimed at reducing early postoperative stroke may have a positive impact on death and neurologic disability after CPB. Stroke after cardiac surgery is defined as any new permanent (manifest stroke) or temporary neurologic deficit or deterioration (transient ischemic attack or prolonged reversible ischemic neurologic deficit) and is confirmed by CT or MRI whenever possible. Brain MRI with diffusion-weighted imaging is the most sensitive and accurate neurologic imaging technique and is preferred to conventional MRI (T2 and FLAIR) because it can reveal significantly more lesions, especially in a "watershed" distribution. Stroke patients with hypoperfused brain tissue may be identified by comparing the mismatch between diffusion-weighted imaging and perfusion-weighted imaging. If diffusion-weighted imaging is not feasible, then head CT should be obtained.

The development of major stroke after CABG has been reported to be 1.5% to 5% in prospective studies and about 0.8% to 3.2% in retrospective analysis. When neurologic or psychometric analyses are performed before and after the operation, the occurrence of cerebral damage has varied from 15% to 40%. When more sensitive biochemical markers of brain cell damage are used, there is evidence of neurologic abnormality in more than 60% of patients. Clinically silent infarction may be far more frequent and could contribute to long-term cognitive dysfunction in patients after cardiac procedures. Serial measurement of serum S100B protein in the initial 12 hours after CPB has been used to predict early postoperative brain injury. Preoperative assessment of white matter disease by cerebral MRI may also help predict the patient's risk for development of cerebral injury. Use of a risk prediction model for stroke indicates that most strokes occur among patients at low or medium preoperative risk, suggesting that many of these strokes may be preventable.

Most strokes develop within the first 2 days after surgery and are up to two times more common in combined cardiac procedures or technically challenging operations. Multivariable analysis has identified 10 variables that were independent predictors of stroke: history of cerebrovascular disease, peripheral vascular disease, diabetes, hypertension, previous cardiac surgery, preoperative infection, urgent operation, CPB time more than 2 hours, need for intraoperative hemofiltration, and high transfusion requirement. The temperature at which CPB is performed is not a significant factor. Undergoing OPCAB reduces the incidence of perioperative stroke mainly by minimizing early strokes; however, the risk of delayed strokes is not different between patients undergoing on-pump and off-pump CABG.[135] Perioperative stroke confers significant mortality and morbidity. The 30-day mortality for stroke patients can be 10 times greater than that for those who do not suffer stroke. The greatest risk of death is noted within the first year after surgery. Five-year survival is lower among patients who had major functional limitations before discharge, among those who had hypoperfusion strokes, and among patients who were discharged to locations other than home or rehabilitation facilities. Patients with ascending aortic atherosclerosis, older age (>70 years), preoperative unstable angina, COPD, and carotid artery disease are at risk for late postoperative stroke (new strokes during 5-year follow-up) after CABG. Approximately 20% of patients with valve prostheses have a late embolic stroke within 15 years after valve replacement. Some risk factors, such as smoking, mitral mechanical prostheses, aortic tilting disc valves, and mitral valve surgery in the setting of LV dysfunction, are potentially modifiable.

ENCEPHALOPATHY. Encephalopathy, defined as diffuse brain injury, occurs in 8% to 32% of patients, depending on its manifestation, which can range from coma to confusion, agitation, and combativeness. Like stroke, it is associated with high mortality and prolonged length of hospital stay, with additional convalescence often required in a nursing home or assisted living facility. Psychotic symptoms are independently associated with prolonged ICU length of stay, multiorgan failure or shock, cardiac arrest, and higher in-hospital death after surgery. Important risk factors are advanced age, carotid bruits, hypertension, diabetes, and previous history of stroke. Perioperative hypothermia (<33°C), hypoxemia, low hematocrit, renal failure, increased serum sodium levels, infection, and stroke can be independent precipitating factors. Postoperative delirium is frequent after cardiac operations, especially in the elderly, and is associated with a higher mortality and readmissions, memory and concentration problems, and sleep disturbances. The Delirium Observation Screening (DOS) scale is a checklist developed for use before and after surgery to assess whether delirium has developed in patients.[136] The increased use of beating-heart surgery without CPB may lead to a lower occurrence of this complication.

REDUCING RISK OF POSTOPERATIVE STROKE AND ENCEPHALOPATHY. Evidence is accumulating that patients with perioperative encephalopathy and stroke have more pre-existing cerebrovascular disease than was recognized earlier, as evidenced by routine preoperative MRI scans. The main perioperative causes of neurologic dysfunction are microemboli caused by air, blood cell aggregates, calcium, or aortic atheroma associated with the pump oxygenator; the potential risk of air embolization during aortic cannulation; atheroembolism from the ascending aorta; and clots from the left ventricle. There is an independent, direct association between degree of hemodilution during CPB and risk of perioperative stroke, with each percentage decrease in hematocrit being associated with a 10% increase in the odds of suffering perioperative stroke. CT studies of the head suggest that a main mechanism of brain injury is cerebral embolization rather than cerebral hypoperfusion. Studies have also demonstrated a higher incidence of perioperative stroke (5%) in patients with abnormal preoperative regional cerebral perfusion, which is associated with older age, current tobacco use, and diabetes mellitus. The role of atheroembolism as a recognized complication of cardiac surgery has been reviewed by Djaiani.[137] Prophylactic cerebrovascular interventions and the selective use of aorta no-touch OPCAB can significantly reduce the incidence of perioperative stroke. Carbon dioxide field flooding can efficiently reduce air emboli released from incompletely deaired cardiac chambers and should be advocated for patients undergoing open heart surgery. AF after CABG has also been shown to be associated with the development of embolic postoperative stroke, usually occurring late (>7 days) after operation.

Although macroembolization is less common during modern cardiac surgery, microembolization remains a problem despite attention to routine precautions such as arterial filtration, reservoir filtration, filtration within the pump oxygenator, venting of the aorta, and (in the case of a diseased aorta) use of femoral cannulation, retrograde cardioplegia through the coronary sinus, bilateral ITA conduits, and insertion of proximal anastomoses on the carotid or innominate arteries. Transesophageal echocardiography, epiaortic scanning, and transcranial Doppler studies have documented embolic showers to the head during aortic crossclamping and unclamping. Superior neurologic outcomes are achieved by use of intra-aortic filters to capture particulate debris and avoidance of partial aortic clamping during OPCAB (no-touch technique). In one study of 700 consecutive patients, the incidence of stroke was significantly lower in the no-touch group.[138] Logistic regression has identified partial aortic clamping as the only independent predictor of stroke, influencing this risk 28-fold. Pulsatile flow, despite modest improvements in cerebral perfusion, does not seem to offer benefits in the incidence of stroke. Maintenance of high mean arterial pressure (80 to 100 mm Hg) on CPB does lead to fewer strokes than with lower mean pressure (50 to 60 mm Hg). The role of perioperative lidocaine for cerebral protection remains uncertain. Magnesium administration is safe and improves short-term postoperative neurologic function after cardiac surgery, particularly in preserving short-term memory and cortical control over brainstem functions.

Neuropathy. Phrenic nerve injury is a function of pericardial slush use and surgical dissection of the ITA. When no topical ice slush is used, an elevated left hemidiaphragm, manifested as the diaphragm's being two or more intercostal spaces higher than the opposite side, occurs in 2.5% of cases. This incidence is increased to 26% when topical ice slush is used and is further raised to 39% when the left ITA is dissected. The right phrenic nerve is at risk of injury in 4% of patients during high mobilization of the right ITA. Phrenic nerve injury can be prevented if the pericardiophrenic branch of the ITA is preserved. The hemidiaphragm remains elevated in 80% of patients at the end of 1 month and in 22% at the end of 1 year. Spontaneous recovery may be anticipated in two thirds of patients in whom the injury is identified postoperatively. High right ITA harvesting should be used with caution in patients with preoperative pulmonary dysfunction, in whom phrenic nerve injury would be poorly tolerated. Bilateral diaphragmatic paralysis has a prolonged time course of recovery.

Vocal cord palsy after adult cardiac surgery has been comprehensively reviewed.[139] The cumulative incidence is 1.1% (33 of 2980 patients). It may also be caused by injury of the recurrent laryngeal nerves by surgical dissection or nonsurgical mechanisms such as tracheal intubation and central venous catheterization. Other reported surgical mechanisms of injury are harvesting of ITA and topical cold cardioprotection. Bilateral nerve palsy has been lethal on at least one occasion.

The risk of perioperative optic neuropathy associated with cardiac surgery in which CPB is used is low (roughly 0.1%), but the outcomes can be devastating. Factors that lead to the condition remain unknown, although the presence of systemic vascular disease and both an absolute and relative drop in hemoglobin during the perioperative period seem to be important. Because this condition often causes profound permanent visual loss, it has been recommended that patients, particularly those with systemic vascular disease, be made aware of this potential complication when cardiac surgery with CPB is planned. In one study of neurologic complications after CABG, 17% had evidence of retinal infarction. Half were asymptomatic; others complained of visual disturbances such as reading difficulty or haziness in the peripheral vision. Despite the presence of definite pathologic changes, recovery of visual acuity can be expected. Cortical blindness can occur and may be missed during brief daily hospital visits with patients. One should be alerted when the patient appears to stare through rather than to focus on the objects of intended vision. When asked, the patient is unable to read or comprehend the content, often turning the reading material in various directions to help clarify confusion. Despite profound dysfunction, patients may not spontaneously mention such symptoms and occasionally may flatly deny their presence (Anton syndrome). CT or diffusion-weighted MRI may be useful in differentiating retinal from cortical causes of visual disturbances. The prognosis for symptomatic improvement is good, but detectable visual abnormalities often remain.

Neuropsychiatric Changes. Depression is common after surgery, especially in patients with the tendency preoperatively. It can start in the first week, worsens for 2 to 3 weeks, and usually resolves by 6 weeks. Clinically significant depression such as that which interferes with daily activity and postoperative recovery, not showing signs of improvement by 4 to 6 weeks, should be formally evaluated and treated, especially if it is present before surgery. Severe psychotic symptoms are seen in 2.1% of postoperative patients. Higher age, renal failure, dyspnea, heart failure, and LV hypertrophy are independent preoperative predisposing factors. Perioperative hypothermia (<33°C), hypoxemia, low hematocrit, renal failure, hypernatremia, infection, and stroke are independent precipitating factors. Psychotic symptoms have been shown to be independently associated with a prolonged length of stay in the ICU, multiorgan failure or shock, cardiopulmonary resuscitation, and in-hospital death after surgery.

Postoperative Gastrointestinal Morbidity

Abdominal organ morbidity after cardiac surgery has been thoughtfully reviewed by Hessel.[140] In his analysis of 37 reports between 1976 and 2004 covering more than 172,000 operations, the incidence of gastrointestinal complications averaged about 1.2% (range, 0.2% to 5.5%) and was associated with a high 33% average mortality (range, 13% to 87%), accounting for nearly 15% of all cardiac surgery deaths. In the STS data base for 1997 (*www.sts.org/doc/2986*), the incidence was 2.8% in 206,143 reported cases, which was about the same frequency as reoperation for bleeding, renal failure, and stroke and nearly two to three times more frequent than sternal infection, perioperative MI, acute respiratory failure, dialysis, and multiorgan failure. Gastrointestinal bleeding was the most common; mesenteric ischemia, pancreatitis, and cholecystitis were next in frequency; paralytic ileus, perforated peptic ulcer, hepatic failure, diverticular disease, pseudo-obstruction of the colon, small bowel obstruction, and multiorgan failure were less common. Intestinal infarction was invariably fatal, and high mortalities, averaging 70%, were associated with intestinal ischemia (which is usually of the nonocclusive type) and hepatic failure.

Damage to gastrointestinal organs can occur from hypoperfusion caused by vasoconstriction on CPB, atheroembolism, or perioperative hemodynamic instability leading to reduced mucosal blood flow with mucosal ischemia characterized by low mucosal pH. The systemic inflammatory response syndrome from endotoxemia, which can be initiated by splanchnic ischemia, has also been proposed as a mechanism. Complement activation on CPB, release of leukotriene B_4 and tumor necrosis factor, and plasmin formation result in damage to endothelial and mucosal cells and extracellular matrix as well as capillary leakage and microthrombi.

Identification of patients at higher risk for gastrointestinal morbidity and optimization of their perioperative hemodynamic management are the cornerstones for lowering of this complication. Prolonged postoperative mechanical ventilation longer than 24 hours is a risk factor; others include advanced age, low ejection fraction, perioperative inotropic or mechanical support, transfusions, arrhythmias, history of renal dysfunction, reoperation, emergency surgery, and poor New York Heart Association functional classification. Splanchnic blood flow may be improved with preoperative volume loading (1.5 mL/kg/hr of crystalloid or up to 600 mL of 6% hetastarch), phosphodiesterase inhibitors (milrinone), and selective gut decontamination (oral polymyxin, tobramycin, and amphotericin preoperatively for 3 days). Vasopressors should be avoided; the benefits of dopamine and dobutamine remain uncertain. The conduct of CPB may be of value; high flows, minimized circuits with low prime volumes, pulsatile flow, maintenance of hematocrit >25%, minimization of atheroembolization, and perioperative administration of aspirin have been shown to contribute to reduced gastrointestinal morbidity. Early diagnosis of bowel ischemia is difficult, although very high lactate levels, persistent metabolic acidosis, leukocytosis, and ileus may be clues. An aggressive approach including early use of colonoscopy, peritoneal lavage, and early interventional angiography with dilation or papaverine infusion and, occasionally, surgical intervention may be lifesaving.

Postoperative Wound Infection

The incidence of deep sternal wound infection appears to be decreasing, partly from the use of perioperative intravenous insulin.[141] Obesity is still the single most important risk factor for postoperative sternal dehiscence, with or without infection, after any type of cardiac operation. In a multivariate analysis, preoperative AF and an elevated CRP level were found to be significant predictors of mediastinitis in patients undergoing CABG.[142] Postoperative sternal wound complications after cardiac surgical procedures are classified as uninfected dehiscence (El Oakley class 1), superficial infections (El Oakley class 2A), and deep sternal wound infections (El Oakley class 2B). Recurrence rates of sternal infections remain high at nearly 20%. An algorithm for the management of poststernotomy complications has been proposed.[143] Prophylactic sternal reinforcement seems to prevent this complication by preventing nonunion or malunion, which can subsequently lead to deep sternal wound infections and mediastinitis. The current standard for sternotomy closure remains the method of wire cerclage. Bilateral ITA harvesting has carried a higher risk of sternal infection; skeletonization of both ITAs, in contrast to harvesting in a pedicled fashion, significantly reduces this risk.[144] There is no difference in the incidence of sternal dehiscence or superficial or deep sternal infection among diabetic patients receiving a single ITA or double skeletonized ITAs. Moreover, a study did not find tracheostomy to confer additional risk, suggesting that early tracheostomy may be considered in postoperative patients in respiratory failure.[145] Prophylactic antibiotics, usually cefazolin, are traditionally given at induction and a second dose before wound closure, with *Staphylococcus aureus* as the indicator microorganism. It has been shown that conventional doses do not provide targeted antimicrobial cefazolin plasma levels during the entire surgical procedure when CPB time exceeds 120 minutes. Patients with shorter bypass times and those undergoing profound hypothermic circulatory arrest are better protected, but the generally used protocol of prophylaxis is not optimal for all patients.

Leg wound complications are common, with an incidence of about 32% after traditional saphenous vein harvesting, with 65% of the patients requiring antibiotics. Single-dose cefazolin used as antibiotic prophylaxis in cardiac surgery is associated with a higher surgical site infection rate than a 24-hour, multiple-dose cefazolin regimen. Endoscopic saphenous vein harvesting of a short vein segment from the thigh results in less wound morbidity and better cosmetic results compared with open venous harvesting of a short vein segment from the calf. Prophylactic application of low-energy shock wave therapy may improve wound healing after vein harvesting for CABG. A retrospective analysis concluded that application of platelet-rich and platelet-poor plasma significantly reduced occurrences of chest wound infection, chest drainage, and leg wound drainage.[146] Radial artery infections secondary to catheterization for blood pressure monitoring are rare (0.2%) but potentially serious complications. Strict, systematic changing of arterial lines on a timely basis is warranted. A high suspicion index, aggressive surgical treatment of bacterial arteritis, and appropriate intravenous antibiotics are critical. Early surgical intervention is necessary in cases of infected radial artery pseudoaneurysms.

Postoperative Endocrine Abnormalities

Tight glucose control, defined as glucose concentration below 130 mg/dL for more than 50% of measurements, is mandatory after cardiac surgery and requires a standard protocol and metrics to track protocol performance. Reduced postoperative infections, especially mediastinitis, are experienced in diabetic patients and even in nondiabetic patients when intensive insulin therapy is used to keep blood glucose concentration below 110 mg/dL.

Diabetes insipidus after CABG has been ascribed to altered left atrial non-osmoreceptor function that provokes altered antidiuretic hormone activity during the period of asystole on CPB.[147] The euthyroid sick syndrome (non–thyroid illness syndrome) in CABG patients is considered to be a nonspecific response to stress. Reduction in serum total T_3 and free T_3 levels is associated with substantially elevated reversed T_3 levels, with values of thyroid-stimulating hormone, thyroxine, and free thyroxine remaining within normal limits. Off-pump surgery is associated with thyroid hormone changes similar to conventional surgical revascularization. It has been proposed that intravenous T_3 may have a potential role in the management of postoperative low cardiac output states (see Chap. 86).

REFERENCES

1. Stamou SC, Camp SL, Stiegel RM, et al: Quality improvement program decreases mortality after cardiac surgery. J Thorac Cardiovasc Surg 136:494, 2008.
2. Auerbach AD, Hilton JF, Maselli J, et al: Shop for quality or volume? Volume, quality, and outcomes of coronary artery bypass surgery. Ann Intern Med 150:696, 2009.
3. Brown PP, Kugelmass AD, Cohen DJ, et al: The frequency and cost of complications associated with coronary artery bypass grafting surgery: Results from the United States Medicare program. Ann Thorac Surg 85:1980, 2008.
4. Speir AM, Kasirajan V, Barnet SD, et al: Additive costs of postoperative complications for isolated coronary artery bypass grafting patients in Virginia. Ann Thorac Surg 88:40, 2009.

Preoperative Risk Analysis

5. Nissinen J, Wistbacka J-O, Loponen P, et al: Coronary artery bypass surgery in octogenarians: Long-term outcome can be better than expected. Ann Thorac Surg 89:1119, 2010.
6. Rohde SL, Baker RA, Tully PJ, et al: Preoperative and intraoperative factors associated with long-term survival in octogenarian cardiac surgery patients. Ann Thorac Surg 89:105, 2010.
7. Chaturvedi RK, Blaise M, Verdon J, et al: Cardiac surgery in octogenarians: Long-term survival, functional status, living arrangements, and leisure activities. Ann Thorac Surg 89:805, 2010.
8. Likosky DS, Sorensen MJ, Dacey LJ, et al: Long-term survival of the very elderly undergoing aortic valve surgery for valvular heart disease. Circulation 120(Suppl 1):S127, 2009.
9. Maurer MS, Luchsinger JA, Wellner R, et al: The effect of body mass index on complications of cardiac surgery in the oldest old. J Am Geriatr Soc 50:988, 2002.
10. Matsuura K, Kobayashi J, Tagusari O, et al: Off-pump coronary artery bypass grafting using only arterial grafts in elderly patients. Ann Thorac Surg 80:144, 2005.
11. Speziale G, Nasso G, Barattoni MC, et al: Operative and middle-term results of cardiac surgery in nonagenarians: A bridge toward routine practice. Circulation 121:208, 2010.
12. Guru V, Fremes SE, Tu JV, et al: Time-related mortality for women after coronary artery bypass graft surgery: A population-based study. J Thorac Cardiovasc Surg 127:1158, 2004.
13. Blankstein R, Ward RP, Arnsdorf M, et al: Female gender is an independent predictor of operative mortality after coronary artery bypass graft surgery. Circulation 112(Suppl I):I-323, 2005.
14. Ioannis K, Toumpoulis CE, Anagnostopoulos SK, et al: Assessment of independent predictors for long-term mortality between women and men after coronary artery bypass grafting: Are women different from men? J Thorac Cardiovasc Surg 131:343, 2006.
15. Kulik A, Lam B-K, Rubens FD, et al: Gender differences in the long-term outcomes after valve replacement surgery. Heart 95:318, 2009.
16. Cooper WA, Thourani VH, Guyton RA, et al: Racial disparity persists after on-pump and off-pump coronary artery bypass grafting surgery for coronary artery disease. Circulation 120(Suppl 1):S59, 2009.
17. Melsop K, Brooks MM, Boothroyd DB, et al: Effect of race on the clinical outcomes in the Bypass Angioplasty Revascularization Investigation trial. Circ Cardiovasc Qual Outcomes 12:186, 2009.
18. Nallamothu BK, Lu X, Vaughan-Sarrazin MS, et al: Coronary revascularization at specialty cardiac hospitals and peer general hospitals in black Medicare beneficiaries. Circ Cardiovasc Qual Outcomes 1:116, 2009.
19. Batty GD, Shipley MJ, Gale CR, et al: Does IQ predict total and cardiovascular disease mortality as strongly as other risk factors? Comparison of effect estimates using the Vietnam Experience Study. Heart 94:1541, 2008.
20. van Straten AHM, Bramer S, Soliman Hamad MA, et al: Effect of body mass index on early and late mortality after coronary artery bypass grafting. Ann Thorac Surg 89:30, 2010.
21. Karl F, Welke MJ, Barnett MS, et al: Limitations of hospital volume as a measure of quality of care for coronary artery bypass graft surgery. Ann Thorac Surg 80:2114, 2005.
22. Shahian DM, O'Brien SM, Normand SL, et al: Association of hospital coronary artery bypass volume with processes of care, mortality, morbidity, and the Society of Thoracic Surgeons composite quality score. Thorac Cardiovasc Surg 139:273, 2010.
23. Wen HC, Tang CH, Lin HC, et al: Association between surgeon and hospital volume in coronary artery bypass graft surgery outcomes: A population-based study. Ann Thorac Surg 81:835, 2006.
24. Lin HC, Xirasagar S, Tsao NW, et al: Volume-outcome relationships in coronary artery bypass graft surgery patients: 5-year major cardiovascular event outcomes. J Thorac Cardiovasc Surg 135:923, 2008.
25. Aldea GS, Mokadam NA, Melford R Jr, et al: Changing volumes, risk profiles, and outcomes of coronary artery bypass grafting and percutaneous coronary interventions. Ann Thorac Surg 87:1828, 2009.
26. Konety SH, Rosenthal GE, Vaughan-Sarrazin MS: Surgical volume and outcomes of off-pump coronary artery bypass graft surgery: Does it matter? J Thorac Cardiovasc Surg 137:1116, 2009.
27. Hartrumpf M, Claus T, Erb M, et al: Surgeon performance index: Tool for assessment of individual surgical quality in total quality management. Eur J Cardiothorac Surg 35:751, 2009.
28. Castellheim A, Hoel TN, Videm V, et al: Biomarker profile in off-pump and on-pump coronary artery bypass grafting surgery in low-risk patients. Ann Thorac Surg 85:1994, 2008.
29. Biancari F , Rimpiläinen R: Meta-analysis of randomised trials comparing the effectiveness of miniaturised versus conventional cardiopulmonary bypass in adult cardiac surgery. Heart 95:964, 2009.
30. Abu-Omar Y, Taggart DP: The present status of off-pump coronary artery bypass grafting. Eur J Cardiothorac Surg 36:312, 2009.
31. Weltert L, D'Alessandro S, Nardella S, et al: Preoperative very short-term, high-dose erythropoietin administration diminishes blood transfusion rate in off-pump coronary artery bypass: A randomized blind controlled study. J Thorac Cardiovasc Surg 139:621, 2010.
32. Molle CH, Perko MJ, Lund JT, et al: No major differences in 30-day outcomes in high-risk patients randomized to off-pump versus on-pump coronary bypass surgery: The Best Bypass Surgery Trial. Circulation 121:498, 2010.
33. Shroyer AL, Grover FL, Hattler B, et al: On-pump versus off-pump coronary artery bypass surgery. N Engl J Med 361:1827, 2009.
34. Marcheix B, Vanden Eynden F, Demers P, et al: Influence of diabetes mellitus on long-term survival in systematic off-pump coronary artery bypass surgery. Ann Thorac Surg 86:1181, 2008.
35. Fu SP, Zheng Z, Yuan X, et al: Impact of off-pump techniques on sex differences in early and late outcomes after isolated coronary artery bypass grafts. Ann Thorac Surg 87:1090, 2009.
36. Kamdar AR, Meadows TA, Roselli EE, et al: Multidetector computed tomographic angiography in planning of reoperative cardiothoracic surgery. Ann Thorac Surg 85:1239, 2008.
37. Shuhaiber JH, Goldsmith K, Nashef SA: The influence of seasonal variation on cardiac surgery: A time-related clinical outcome predictor. J Thorac Cardiovasc Surg 136:894, 2008.
38. Bell ML, Grunwald GK, Baltz JH, et al: Does preoperative hemoglobin independently predict short-term outcomes after coronary artery bypass graft surgery? Ann Thorac Surg 86:1415, 2008.
39. Newall N, Grayson AD, Oo AY, et al: Preoperative white blood cell count is independently associated with higher perioperative cardiac enzyme release and increased 1-year mortality after coronary artery bypass grafting. Ann Thorac Surg 81:583, 2006.

40. Bevilacqua S, Alkodami A, Volpi E, et al: Risk stratification after coronary artery bypass surgery by a point-of-care test of platelet function. Ann Thorac Surg 87:496, 2009.
41. Halkos ME, Puskas JD, Lattouf OM, et al: Elevated preoperative hemoglobin A1c level is predictive of adverse events after coronary artery bypass surgery. J Thorac Cardiovasc Surg 136:631, 2008.
42. Kangasniemi OP, Biancari F, Luukkonen F, et al: Preoperative C-reactive protein is predictive of long-term outcome after coronary artery bypass surgery. Eur J Cardiothorac Surg 29:983, 2006.
43. van Straten AHM, Soliman Hamad MA, van Zundert AJ, et al: Preoperative C-reactive protein levels to predict early and late mortalities after coronary artery bypass surgery: Eight years of follow-up. J Thorac Cardiovasc Surg 138:954, 2009.
44. Cerillo AG, Bevilacqua S, Storti S, et al: Free triiodothyronine: A novel predictor of postoperative atrial fibrillation. Eur J Cardiothorac Surg 24:487, 2003.
45. Fox AA, Shernan SS, Collard CD, et al: Preoperative B-type natriuretic peptide is an independent predictor of ventricular dysfunction and mortality after primary coronary artery bypass grafting. J Thorac Cardiovasc Surg 136:452, 2008.
46. Tavakol M, Hassan KZ, Abdula RK, et al: Utility of brain natriuretic peptide as a predictor of atrial fibrillation after cardiac operations. Ann Thorac Surg 88:802, 2009.
47. Lurati Buse GA, Koller MT, Grapow M, et al: The prognostic value of troponin release after adult cardiac surgery: A meta-analysis. Eur J Cardiothorac Surg 37:399, 2010.

Preoperative Laboratory Values and Drug Treatment

48. Thielmann M, Massoudy P, Neuhauser M, et al: Prognostic value of preoperative cardiac troponin I in patients undergoing emergency coronary artery bypass surgery with non ST-elevation or ST-elevation acute coronary syndromes. Circulation 114(Suppl I):I-448, 2006.
49. Herman CR, Buth KJ, Kent BA, et al: Clopidogrel increases blood transfusion and hemorrhagic complications in patients undergoing cardiac surgery. Ann Thorac Surg 89:397, 2010.
50. Karabulut H, Toraman F, Evrenkaya S, et al: Clopidogrel does not increase bleeding and allogenic blood transfusion in coronary artery surgery. Eur J Cardiothorac Surg 25:419, 2004.
51. Ebrahimi R, Dyke C, Mehran R, et al: Outcomes following pre-operative clopidogrel administration in patients with acute coronary syndromes undergoing coronary artery bypass surgery: The ACUITY (Acute Catheterization and Urgent Intervention Triage strategy) Trial. J Am Coll Cardiol 53:1965, 2009.
52. Fox KA, Mehta SR, Peters R, et al: Benefits and risks of the combination of clopidogrel and aspirin in patients undergoing surgical revascularization for non–ST-elevation acute coronary syndrome: The Clopidogrel in Unstable angina to prevent Recurrent ischemic Events (CURE) Trial. Circulation 110:1202, 2004.
53. Lindvall G, Sartipy I, van der Linden J: Aprotinin reduces bleeding and blood product use in patients treated with clopidogrel before coronary artery bypass grafting. Ann Thorac Surg 80:922, 2005.
54. Vaccarino GN, Thierer J, Albertal M, et al: Impact of preoperative clopidogrel in off pump coronary artery bypass surgery: A propensity score analysis. J Thorac Cardiovasc Surg 137:309, 2009.
55. Maltais S, Perrault LP, Do QB: Effect of clopidogrel on bleeding and transfusions after off-pump coronary artery bypass graft surgery: Impact of discontinuation prior to surgery. Eur J Cardiothorac Surg 34:127, 2008.
56. Paraskevas KI: Applications of statins in cardiothoracic surgery: More than just lipid-lowering. Eur J Cardiothorac Surg 33:377, 2008.
57. Mannacio VA, Iorio D, de Amicis V, et al: Effect of rosuvastatin pretreatment on myocardial damage after coronary surgery: A randomized trial. J Thorac Cardiovasc Surg 136:1541, 2009.
58. Fedoruk LM, Wang H, Conaway MR, et al: Statin therapy improves outcomes after valvular heart surgery. Ann Thorac Surg 85:1521, 2008.
59. Tabata M, Khalpey Z, Cohn LH, et al: Effect of preoperative statins in patients without coronary artery disease who undergo cardiac surgery. J Thorac Cardiovasc Surg 136:1510, 2009.
60. Borger MA, Seeburger J, Walther T, et al: Effect of preoperative statin therapy on patients undergoing isolated and combined valvular heart surgery. Ann Thorac Surg 89:773, 2010.
61. Liakopoulos OJ, Choi Y-H, Kuhn EW, et al: Statins for prevention of atrial fibrillation after cardiac surgery: A systematic literature review. J Thorac Cardiovasc Surg 138:678, 2009.
62. Benedetto U, Sciarretta S, Roscitano A, et al: Preoperative angiotensin-converting enzyme inhibitors and acute kidney injury after coronary artery bypass grafting. Ann Thorac Surg 86:1160, 2008.
63. Ho KM, Tan JA: Benefits and risks of corticosteroid prophylaxis in adult cardiac surgery: A dose-response meta-analysis. Circulation 119:1853, 2009.
64. Albacker T, Carvalho G, Schricker T, et al: High-dose insulin therapy attenuates systemic inflammatory response in coronary artery bypass grafting patients. Ann Thorac Surg 86:20, 2008.

Preoperative Medical Conditions

65. Wagner BD, Grunwald GK, Rumsfeld J, et al: Relationship of body mass index with outcomes after coronary artery bypass graft surgery. Ann Thorac Surg 84:10, 2007.
66. Alserius T, Hammar N, Nordqvist T, et al: Improved survival after coronary artery bypass grafting has not influenced the mortality disadvantage in patients with diabetes mellitus. J Thorac Cardiovasc Surg 138:1115, 2009.
67. Kajimoto K, Miyauchi K, Kasai T, et al: Metabolic syndrome is an independent risk factor for stroke and acute renal failure after coronary artery bypass grafting. J Thorac Cardiovasc Surg 137:658, 2009.
68. van Straten AHM, Firanescu C, Soliman Hamad MA, et al: Peripheral vascular disease as a predictor of survival after coronary artery bypass grafting: Comparison with a matched general population. Ann Thorac Surg 89:414, 2010.
69. Haase M, Bellomo R, Matalanis G, et al: A comparison of the RIFLE and Acute Kidney Injury Network classifications for cardiac surgery–associated acute kidney injury: A prospective cohort study. Thorac Cardiovasc Surg 138:1370, 2009.
70. Ristikankare A, Pöyhiä R, Kuitunen A, et al: Serum cystatin C in elderly cardiac surgery patients. Ann Thorac Surg 89:689, 2010.
71. Heise D, Sundermann D, Braeuer A, et al: Validation of a clinical score to determine the risk of acute renal failure after cardiac surgery. Eur J Cardiothorac Surg 37:710, 2010.
72. Kinoshita T, Asai T, Murakami Y, et al: Efficacy of bilateral internal thoracic artery grafting in patients with chronic kidney disease. Ann Thorac Surg 89:1106, 2010.
73. Ad N, Barnett SD, Haan CK, et al: Does preoperative atrial fibrillation increase the risk for mortality and morbidity after coronary artery bypass grafting? J Thorac Cardiovasc Surg 137:901, 2009.
74. Sezai A, Hata M, Niino T, et al: Study of the factors related to atrial fibrillation after coronary artery bypass grafting: A search for a marker to predict the occurrence of atrial fibrillation before surgical intervention. J Thorac Cardiovasc Surg 137:895, 2009.
75. Ad N, Henry L, Halpin L, et al: The use of spirometry testing prior to cardiac surgery may impact the Society of Thoracic Surgeons risk prediction score: A prospective study in a cohort of patients at high risk for chronic lung disease. J Thorac Cardiovasc Surg 139:686, 2010.
76. Filsoufi F, Rahmanian PB, Castillo JG, et al: Logistic risk model predicting postoperative respiratory failure in patients undergoing valve surgery. Eur J Cardiothorac Surg 34:953, 2008.
77. Trouillet J-L, Combes A, Vaissier E, et al: Prolonged mechanical ventilation after cardiac surgery: Outcome and predictors. J Thorac Cardiovasc Surg 138:948, 2009.
78. Nussmeier NA, Miao Y, Roach GW, et al: Predictive value of the National Institutes of Health Stroke Scale and the Mini-Mental State Examination for neurologic outcome after coronary artery bypass graft surgery. J Thorac Cardiovasc Surg 139:901, 2010.
79. Lin CH, Lin FY, Wang SS, et al: Cardiac surgery in patients with liver cirrhosis. Ann Thorac Surg 79:1551, 2005.
80. Hayashida N, Shoujima T, Teshima H, et al: Clinical outcome after cardiac operations in patients with cirrhosis. Ann Thorac Surg 77:500, 2004.
81. Morisaki A, Hosono M, Sasaki Y, et al: Risk factor analysis in patients with liver cirrhosis undergoing cardiovascular operations. Ann Thorac Surg 89:811, 2010.
82. Mestres CA, Chuquiure JE, Claramonte X, et al: Long-term results after cardiac surgery in patients infected with the human immunodeficiency virus type-1 (HIV-1). Eur J Cardiothorac Surg 23:1007, 2003.
83. Fecher AM, Birdas TJ, Haybron D, et al: Cardiac operations in patients with hematologic malignancies. Eur J Cardiothorac Surg 25:537, 2004.
84. Gorki H, Malinovski V, Stanbridge RDL: The antiphospholipid syndrome and heart valve surgery. Eur J Cardiothorac Surg 33:168, 2008.
85. Morawski W, Sanak M, Cisowski M, et al: Prediction of the excessive perioperative bleeding in patients undergoing coronary artery bypass grafting: Role of aspirin and platelet glycoprotein IIIa polymorphism. J Thorac Cardiovasc Surg 130:791, 2005.

Preoperative Risk Calculation

86. Laurie A, Shroyer W, Coombs LP, et al: The society of thoracic surgeons: 30-day operative mortality and morbidity risk models. Ann Thorac Surg 75:1856, 2003.
87. Merello L, Riesle E, Alburquerque J, et al: Risk scores do not predict high mortality after coronary artery bypass surgery in the presence of diastolic dysfunction. Ann Thorac Surg 85:1247, 2008.
88. Klein P, Holman ER, Versteegh MIM, et al: Wall motion score index predicts mortality and functional result after surgical ventricular restoration for advanced ischemic heart failure. Eur J Cardiothorac Surg 35:847, 2009.
89. Ranucci M, Castelvecchio S, Menicanti L, et al: An adjusted EuroSCORE model for high-risk cardiac patients. Eur J Cardiothorac Surg 36:791, 2009.
90. Ranucci M, Castelvecchio S, Menicanti L, et al: Accuracy, calibration and clinical performance of the EuroSCORE: Can we reduce the number of variables? Eur J Cardiothorac Surg 37:724, 2010.
91. Parolari A, Pesce LL, Trezzi M, et al: EuroSCORE performance in valve surgery: A meta-analysis. Ann Thorac Surg 89:787, 2010.
92. Wendt D, Osswald BR, Kayser K, et al: Society of Thoracic Surgeons Score is superior to the EuroSCORE determining mortality in high risk patients undergoing isolated aortic valve replacement. Ann Thorac Surg 88:468, 2009.
93. Jin R, Grunkemeier GL, Starr AS, et al: Validation and refinement of mortality risk models for heart valve surgery. Ann Thorac Surg 80:471, 2005.
94. Butchart EG, Ionescu A, Payne N, et al: A new scoring system to determine thromboembolic risk after heart valve replacement. Circulation 108(Suppl II):II-68, 2003.

The "Normal" Postoperative Convalescence

95. Cerfolio RJ, Minnich DJ, Bryant AS: The removal of chest tubes despite an air leak or a pneumothorax. Ann Thorac Surg 87:1690, 2009.
96. Cohen J, Kogan A, Sahar G, et al: Hypophosphatemia following open heart surgery: Incidence and consequences. Eur J Cardiothorac Surg 26:306, 2004.
97. Mohammed AA, Agnihotri AK, van Kimmenade RRJ, et al: Prospective, comprehensive assessment of cardiac troponin T testing after coronary artery bypass graft surgery. Circulation 120:843, 2009.
98. Zimmermann N, Gams E, Hohlfeld T: Aspirin in coronary artery bypass surgery: New aspects of and alternatives for an old antithrombotic agent. Eur J Cardiothorac Surg 34:93, 2008.
99. Lim E, Cornelissen J, Routledge T, et al: Clopidogrel did not inhibit platelet function early after coronary bypass surgery: A prospective randomized trial. J Thorac Cardiovasc Surg 128:432, 2004.
100. Gao C, Ren C, Li D, et al: Clopidogrel and aspirin versus clopidogrel alone on graft patency after coronary artery bypass grafting. Ann Thorac Surg 88:59, 2009.
101. Kogan A, Cohen J, Raanani E, et al: Readmission to the intensive care unit after "fast-track" cardiac surgery: Risk factors and outcomes. Ann Thorac Surg 76:503, 2003.
102. Swaminathan M, Phillips-Bute BG, Patel UD, et al: Increasing healthcare resource utilization after coronary artery bypass graft surgery in the United States. Circ Cardiovasc Qual Outcomes 2:305, 2009.
103. Lee DH, Buth KJ, Martin B-J, et al: Frail patients are at increased risk for mortality and prolonged institutional care after cardiac surgery. Circulation 121:973, 2010.

Postoperative Morbidity

104. Alsaddique AA: Recognition of diastolic heart failure in the postoperative heart. Eur J Cardiothorac Surg 34:1141, 2008.
105. Jing Z-C, Jiang X, Wu BX, et al: Vardenafil treatment for patients with pulmonary arterial hypertension: A multicentre, open-label study. Heart 95:1531, 2009.
106. Dunning J, Fabbri A, Kolh PH, et al: Guideline for resuscitation in cardiac arrest after cardiac surgery. Eur J Cardiothorac Surg 36:3, 2009.

107. Adam Z, Adam S, Everngam RL, et al: Resuscitation after cardiac surgery: Results of an international survey. Eur J Cardiothorac Surg 36:29, 2009.
108. Liu K-Y, Muehlschlegel JD, Perry TE, et al: Common genetic variants on chromosome 9p21 predict perioperative myocardial injury after coronary artery bypass graft surgery. J Thorac Cardiovasc Surg 139:483, 2010.
109. Schwefer M, Aschenbach R, Heidemann J, et al: Constrictive pericarditis, still a diagnostic challenge: Comprehensive review of clinical management. Eur J Cardiothorac Surg 36:502, 2009.
110. Kaireviciute D, Aidietis A, Lip GY: Atrial fibrillation following cardiac surgery: Clinical features and preventative strategies. Eur Heart J 30:410, 2009.
111. Filardo G, Hamilton C, Hebeler RF Jr, et al: New-onset postoperative atrial fibrillation after isolated coronary artery bypass graft surgery and long-term survival. Circ Cardiovasc Qual Outcomes 2:164, 2009.
112. Zebis LR, Christensen TD, Kristiansen IR, et al: Amiodarone cost effectiveness in preventing atrial fibrillation after coronary artery bypass graft surgery. Ann Thorac Surg 85:28, 2008.
113. Rho RW: The management of atrial fibrillation after cardiac surgery. Heart 95:422, 2009.
114. Weissman C: Pulmonary complications after cardiac surgery. Semin Cardiothorac Vasc Anesth 8:185, 2004.
115. Dunning J, Versteegh M, Fabbri A, et al: Guideline on antiplatelet and anticoagulation management in cardiac surgery. Eur J Cardiothorac Surg 34:73, 2008.
116. Frumento RJ, O'Malley CM, Bennett-Guerrero E, et al: Stroke after cardiac surgery: A retrospective analysis of the effect of aprotinin dosing regimens. Ann Thorac Surg 75:479, 2003.
117. Sedrakyan A, Treasure T, Elefteriades JA: Effect of aprotinin on clinical outcomes in coronary artery bypass graft surgery: A systematic review and meta-analysis of randomized clinical trials. J Thorac Cardiovasc Surg 128:442, 2004.
118. Fergusson DA, Hébert PC, Mazer CD, et al: A Comparison of aprotinin and lysine analogues in high-risk cardiac surgery. N Engl J Med 358:2319, 2008.
119. Schneeweiss S, Seeger JD, Landon J, et al: Aprotinin during coronary-artery bypass grafting and risk of death. N Engl J Med 358:771, 2008.
120. Shaw AD, Stafford-Smith M, White WD, et al: The effect of aprotinin on outcome after coronary-artery bypass grafting. N Engl J Med 358:784, 2008.
121. Later AFL, Maas JJ, Engbers FHM, et al: Tranexamic acid and aprotinin in low- and intermediate-risk cardiac surgery: A non-sponsored, double-blind, randomised, placebo-controlled trial. Eur J Cardiothorac Surg 36:322, 2009.
122. Pagano D, Howell NJ, Freemantle N, et al: Bleeding in cardiac surgery: The use of aprotinin does not affect survival. J Thorac Cardiovasc Surg 135:495, 2008.
123. Dunkley C, Phillips L, McCall P, et al: Recombinant activated factor VII in cardiac surgery: Experience from the Australian and New Zealand Haemostasis Registry. Ann Thorac Surg 85:836, 2008.
124. Eyjolfsson A, Scicluna S, Johnsson P, et al: Characterization of lipid particles in shed mediastinal blood. Ann Thorac Surg 85:978, 2008.
125. Mehta R, Hafley GE, Gibson CM, et al: Influence of preoperative renal dysfunction on one-year bypass graft patency and two-year outcomes in patients undergoing coronary artery bypass surgery. J Thorac Cardiovasc Surg 136:1149, 2009.
126. van Straten AHM, Soliman Hamad MA, van Zundert AAAJ, et al: Risk factors for deterioration of renal function after coronary artery bypass grafting. Eur J Cardiothorac Surg 37:106, 2010.
127. Karkouti K, Wijeysundera DN, Yau TM, et al: Acute kidney injury after cardiac surgery: Focus on modifiable risk factors. Circulation 119:495, 2009.
128. Elahi M, Asopa A, Pflueger A, et al: Acute kidney injury following cardiac surgery: Impact of early versus late haemofiltration on morbidity and mortality. Eur J Cardiothorac Surg 35:854, 2009.
129. Ranucci M, Soro G, Barzaghi N, et al: Fenoldopam prophylaxis of postoperative acute renal failure in high-risk cardiac surgery patients. Ann Thorac Surg 78:1332, 2004.
130. Di Mauro M, Gagliardi M, Iacò AL, et al: Does off-pump coronary surgery reduce postoperative acute renal failure? The importance of preoperative renal function. Ann Thorac Surg 84:1496, 2007.
131. Gao L, Taha R, Gauvin D, et al: Postoperative cognitive dysfunction after cardiac surgery. Chest 128:3664, 2005.
132. McKhann GM, Selnes OA, Grega MA, et al: Subjective memory symptoms in surgical and nonsurgical coronary artery patients: 6-year follow-up. Ann Thorac Surg 87:27, 2009.
133. Selnes OA, Grega MA, Bailey MM, et al: Do management strategies for coronary artery disease influence 6-year cognitive outcomes? Ann Thorac Surg 88:445, 2009.
134. McKhann GM, Grega MA, Borowicz LM Jr, et al: Stroke and encephalopathy after cardiac surgery: An update. Stroke 37:562, 2006.
135. Nishiyama K, Horiguchi M, Shizuta S, et al: Temporal pattern of strokes after on-pump and off-pump coronary artery bypass graft surgery. Ann Thorac Surg 87:1839, 2009.
136. Koster S, Oosterveld FCJ, Hensens AG, et al: Delirium after cardiac surgery and predictive validity of a risk checklist. Ann Thorac Surg 86:1883, 2008.
137. Djaiani GN: Aortic arch atheroma: Stroke reduction in cardiac surgical patients. Semin Cardiothorac Vasc Anesth 10:143, 2006.
138. Lev-Ran O, Braunstein R, Sharony R, et al: No-touch aorta off-pump coronary surgery: The effect on stroke. J Thorac Cardiovasc Surg 129:307, 2005.
139. Dimarakis I, Protopapas AD: Vocal cord palsy as a complication of adult cardiac surgery: Surgical correlations and analysis. Eur J Cardiothorac Surg 26:773, 2004.
140. Hessel EA II: Abdominal organ injury after cardiac surgery. Semin Cardiothorac Vasc Anesth 8:243, 2004.
141. Matros E, Aranki SF, Bayer LR, et al: Reduction in incidence of deep sternal wound infections: Random or real? J Thorac Cardiovasc Surg 139:680, 2010.
142. Elenbaas TW, Soliman Hamad MA, Schönberger JP, et al: Preoperative atrial fibrillation and elevated C-reactive protein levels as predictors of mediastinitis after coronary artery bypass grafting. Ann Thorac Surg 89:704, 2010.
143. Doyle AJ, Large SR, Murphy F: Sternal wound dehiscence after internal mammary artery harvesting. Logical management. Part 2. Interact Cardiovasc Thorac Surg 4:511, 2005.
144. De Paulis R, de Notaris S, Scaffa R, et al: The effect of bilateral internal thoracic artery harvesting on superficial and deep sternal infection: The role of skeletonization. J Thorac Cardiovasc Surg 129:536, 2005.
145. Parwis B, Rahmanian DH, Adams JG, et al: Tracheostomy is not a risk factor for deep sternal wound infection after cardiac surgery. Ann Thorac Surg 84:1984, 2007.
146. Khalafi RS, Bradford DW, Wilson MG: Topical application of autologous blood products during surgical closure following a coronary artery bypass graft. Eur J Cardiothorac Surg 34:360, 2008.
147. Kuan P, Messenger JC, Ellestad MH: Transient central diabetes insipidus after aortocoronary bypass operations. Am J Cardiol 52:1181, 1983.

CHAPTER 85 Anesthesia and Noncardiac Surgery in Patients with Heart Disease

Lee A. Fleisher and Joshua Beckman

Cardiovascular morbidity and mortality represent a special concern in the patient with known (or risk factors for) cardiovascular disease who undergoes noncardiac surgery. The costs of perioperative myocardial injury add substantially to total health care expenditures, with an average increased length of stay of 6.8 days for patients with perioperative myocardial ischemic injury. Perioperative cardiovascular complications not only affect the immediate period, but also may influence outcome over subsequent years. The evidence base for managing patients with cardiovascular disease peri–noncardiac surgery has grown in recent decades, beginning with identification of those at greatest risk and progressing to recent randomized trials to identify strategies to reduce perioperative cardiovascular complications. Guidelines provide information for the management of high-risk patients and disseminate best practices. This chapter attempts to distill this information, incorporating the available guidelines from the American College of Cardiology (ACC)/American Heart Association (AHA) and from the European Society of Cardiology (ESC) while acknowledging that these guidelines undergo constant evolution.[1,2]

Assessment of Risk

The identification of perioperative cardiac risk has been studied for three decades, and much of the work has focused on the development of clinical risk indices. The most recent index was developed in a study of 4315 patients 50 years of age or older undergoing elective major noncardiac procedures in a tertiary-care teaching hospital. Six independent predictors of complications were identified and included in a revised cardiac risk index (RCRI): high-risk type of surgery, history of ischemic heart disease, history of congestive heart failure, history of cerebrovascular disease, preoperative treatment with insulin, and preoperative serum creatinine higher than 2 mg/dL, with increasing cardiac complication rates noted with an increasing number of risk factors. Patients can be stratified into low, intermediate, and high cardiovascular risk on the basis of having zero, one or two, or three or more RCRI risk factors, respectively. The RCRI has become the standard tool for assessing the probability of perioperative cardiac risk in a given individual, and directs the decision to perform cardiovascular testing and implement perioperative management protocols. The RCRI has been validated in vascular surgery populations and predicts long-term outcome and quality of life, although one group has advocated inclusion of age as a risk factor. The RCRI is discussed throughout the rest of this chapter.

Ischemic Heart Disease

A patient may be evaluated by those in a number of health care systems before undergoing noncardiac surgery; he or she may be seen by a primary caregiver or a cardiologist. However, many patients are only evaluated immediately before surgery by the surgeon or anesthesiologist. The stress of noncardiac surgery may raise heart rate (HR) preoperatively, which associates with a high incidence of symptomatic and asymptomatic myocardial ischemia. Therefore, the preoperative clinical evaluation of the patient may identify stable or unstable coronary artery disease (CAD). Patients with acute coronary syndromes, such as unstable angina or decompensated heart failure of ischemic origin, have a high risk of developing further decompensation or myocardial necrosis and of death during the perioperative period. Such patients clearly warrant further evaluation and medical stabilization. If the noncardiac surgery is truly emergent, there are several older case series using intra-aortic balloon bump counterpulsation to provide short-term myocardial protection beyond maximal medical therapy, although this measure is rarely used today.

If the patient does not have unstable symptoms, the identification of known or symptomatic stable CAD or risk factors for CAD can guide further diagnostic evaluation or changes in perioperative management. In determining the extent of the preoperative evaluation, it is important not to perform testing unless the results will affect perioperative management. These management changes include cancellation of surgery for prohibitive risk compared with benefit, delay of surgery for further medical management, coronary interventions before surgery, use of an intensive care unit, and changes in monitoring. As discussed later, the potential benefit of preoperative coronary revascularization has been questioned, often limiting the need for extensive testing.

The patient with stable angina represents a continuum from mild angina with extreme exertion to dyspnea with angina after walking up a few stairs. The patient who only manifests angina after strenuous exercise often does not demonstrate signs of left ventricular dysfunction and generally can be stabilized with adequate medical therapy, particularly treatment with aspirin, beta-adrenergic blocking agents (beta blockers), and statins (see Chaps. 49 and 57). In contrast, a patient with dyspnea on mild exertion would be at high risk for developing perioperative ventricular dysfunction, myocardial ischemia, and possible myocardial infarction (MI). Such patients have a high probability of having extensive CAD, and additional monitoring or cardiovascular testing should be considered (see Chap. 17), depending on the surgical procedure, institutional factors, and prior evaluation.

Traditionally, coronary risk assessment for noncardiac surgery in patients with a prior MI was based on the time interval between the MI and surgery. Multiple studies have demonstrated an increased incidence of reinfarction after noncardiac surgery if the prior MI was within 6 months of the operation. Improvements in perioperative care have shortened this time interval, but its relative importance is less relevant in the current era of thrombolytics, angioplasty, and routine coronary risk stratification after an acute MI. Although some patients with a recent MI may continue to have myocardium at risk for subsequent ischemia and infarction, most patients in the United States will have had their critical coronary stenosis evaluated and revascularized or will be on maximal medical therapy. The AHA/ACC Task Force on Perioperative Evaluation of the Cardiac Patient Undergoing Noncardiac Surgery has suggested that the highest risk cohort is made up of patients within 30 days of MI, during which plaque and myocardial healing occur. After that period, risk stratification is based on the presentation of disease (i.e., those with active ischemia are at highest risk).

Hypertension

In the 1970s, a series of case studies changed the prevailing concept that antihypertensive agents should be discontinued before surgery. The reports suggested that poorly controlled hypertension was associated with untoward hemodynamic responses, and that antihypertensive agents should be continued perioperatively. However, several large prospective studies did not establish mild to moderate hypertension as an independent predictor of postoperative cardiac complications such as cardiac death, postoperative MI, heart failure, or arrhythmias. The approach to the patient with hypertension therefore mostly relies on management strategies from the nonsurgical literature.

A hypertensive crisis in the postoperative period, defined as a diastolic blood pressure (BP) higher than 120 mm Hg and clinical evidence of impending or actual end organ damage, poses a definite risk of MI and cerebrovascular accident (see Chap. 45). Diagnostic criteria include papilledema or other evidence of increased intracranial pressure, myocardial ischemia, or acute renal failure. Several precipitants of hypertensive crises have been identified, including preeclampsia or eclampsia, pheochromocytomas, abrupt clonidine withdrawal before surgery, use of chronic monoamine oxidase inhibitors with or without sympathomimetic drugs in combination, and inadvertent discontinuation of antihypertensive therapy.

Chronic hypertension may predispose patients to perioperative myocardial ischemia because CAD is more prevalent in these patients. Recent clinical trials have yielded mixed conclusions regarding the relevance of hypertension to perioperative outcomes. A retrospective evaluation of 2462 patients undergoing vascular surgery has shown that adding hypertension to a risk prediction model improved its prognostic ability.[3] In contrast, in the Perioperative Ischemic Evaluation (POISE) trial of beta-adrenergic blockade, chronic hypertension was present in 62% of the 8351 subjects, yet was not a predictor of postoperative stroke or death.[4] Thus, hypertensive patients with known peripheral and coronary vascular disease should have preoperative BP levels monitored and controlled.

Whether patients with mild to moderate hypertension should be considered at greater risk for perioperative myocardial ischemia remains uncertain. Surgery generally need not be postponed or canceled in the otherwise uncomplicated patient with mild to moderate hypertension. Antihypertensive medications should be continued perioperatively, and BP should be maintained near preoperative levels to reduce the risk of myocardial ischemia. In patients with more severe hypertension, such as diastolic BP higher than 110 mm Hg, the potential benefits of delaying surgery to optimize antihypertensive medications should be weighed against the risk of delaying the surgical procedure. With rapid-acting intravenous agents, BP can usually be controlled within several hours. Weksler and colleagues studied 989 chronically treated hypertensive patients who presented for noncardiac surgery with diastolic BP between 110 and 130 mm Hg and with no previous MI, unstable or severe angina pectoris, renal failure, pregnancy-induced hypertension, left ventricular hypertrophy, previous coronary revascularization, aortic stenosis, preoperative dysrhythmias, conduction defects, or stroke. The control group had their surgery postponed and remained in the hospital for BP control, and the study patients received 10 mg of nifedipine, delivered intranasally.[1] No statistically significant differences in postoperative complications were observed, suggesting that this subset of patients without significant cardiovascular comorbidities can proceed with surgery despite elevated BP on the day of surgery.

Heart Failure

Heart failure associates with perioperative cardiac morbidity after noncardiac surgery in almost all studies. Goldman and colleagues have identified a third heart sound or signs of heart failure as portending the highest perioperative risks. For patients who present for noncardiac surgery with signs or symptoms of heart failure, its underpinnings require characterization.[1] The preoperative evaluation should aim to identify the underlying coronary, myocardial, and/or valvular heart disease and assess the severity of systolic and diastolic dysfunction. Hammill and associates[5] have evaluated short-term outcomes in patients with heart failure, CAD, or neither who underwent major noncardiac surgery, using Medicare Claims data. Older patients with heart failure who undergo major surgical procedures have substantially higher risks of operative mortality and hospital readmission than other patients, including those with coronary disease, admitted for the same procedures. Treatment of decompensated hypertrophic cardiomyopathy is different than treatment for dilated cardiomyopathy (see Chap. 69), and thus the preoperative evaluation can influence perioperative management; in particular, this assessment may influence perioperative fluid and vasopressor management. Ischemic cardiomyopathy is of greatest concern because the patient has a substantial risk for developing further ischemia, leading to myocardial necrosis and potentially a downward spiral. A pulmonary artery catheter or transesophageal echocardiography may be helpful for such patients.

Obstructed hypertrophic cardiomyopathy was formerly regarded as a high-risk condition associated with high perioperative morbidity. A retrospective review of perioperative care in 35 patients, however, has suggested that the risk of general anesthesia and major noncardiac surgery is low in such patients. This study did suggest relative contraindication of spinal anesthesia in view of the sensitivity of cardiac output to preload in this condition. Haering and coworkers have studied 77 patients with asymmetrical septal hypertrophy who were retrospectively identified from a large database.[1] Of these patients, 40% had one or more adverse perioperative cardiac events, including one patient who had an MI and ventricular tachycardia that required emergent cardioversion. Most of the events were perioperative congestive heart failure, and no perioperative deaths occurred. Unlike in the original cohort of patients, the type of anesthesia was not an independent risk factor. Important independent risk factors for adverse outcomes (as seen generally) included major surgery and increasing duration of surgery.

Valvular Heart Disease

Aortic stenosis places a patient at increased risk, with those with critical stenosis associated with the highest risk of cardiac decompensation in patients undergoing elective noncardiac surgery (see Chap. 66). Kertai has reported a substantially higher rate of perioperative complications in patients with severe aortic stenosis, compared with patients with moderate aortic stenosis—31% (5/16) versus 11% (10/92).[1,6] The presence of any of the classic triad of angina, syncope, and heart failure in a patient with aortic stenosis should prompt further evaluation and potential interventions, usually valve replacement. Many patients with severe or critical aortic stenosis are asymptomatic.

Preoperative patients with aortic systolic murmurs warrant a careful history and physical examination, and often further evaluation. Several recent case series of patients with critical aortic stenosis have demonstrated that when necessary, noncardiac surgery can be performed with acceptable risk. For the most part, these series have included patients with few or no symptoms but a valve area smaller than 0.5 cm^2. Aortic valvuloplasty is an alternative option for some patients. Although the long-term outcome of patients who undergo aortic balloon valvuloplasty is generally poor, primarily because of restenosis, this procedure can provide temporary benefit surrounding noncardiac surgery in patients who cannot undergo valve replacement in the short term. The considerable procedure-related morbidity and mortality risk must be carefully considered before recommending this strategy to lower the risk of noncardiac surgery.

Mitral valve disease tends to cause less risk of perioperative complications than aortic stenosis, although occult mitral stenosis from rheumatic heart disease is still encountered on occasion and can lead to severe left heart failure in the presence of tachycardia (e.g., uncontrolled atrial fibrillation) and/or volume loading. In contrast to aortic valvuloplasty, mitral valve balloon valvuloplasty often yields short-term and long-term benefit, especially in younger patients with predominant mitral stenosis but without severe mitral valve leaflet thickening or significant subvalvular fibrosis and calcification.

In the perioperative patient with a functioning prosthetic heart valve, antibiotic prophylaxis and anticoagulation are major issues. All patients with prosthetic valves who undergo procedures that can cause transient bacteremia should receive prophylaxis (see Chap. 67). In patients with prosthetic valves, the risk of increased bleeding during a procedure while receiving antithrombotic therapy must be weighed against the increased risk of a thromboembolism caused by stopping the therapy. The common practice for patients undergoing noncardiac surgery with a mechanical prosthetic valve in place is cessation of oral anticoagulants 3 days before surgery (see Chap. 66). This allows the international normalized ratio (INR) to fall to less than 1.5 times normal; oral anticoagulants can then be resumed on postoperative day 1. An alternative approach in patients at high risk for thromboembolism is conversion to heparin during the perioperative period, which can then be discontinued 4 to 6 hours before surgery and resumed shortly thereafter. The use of low-molecular-weight heparins (LMWHs) in preoperative warfarin anticoagulation bridging was investigated in a multicenter, single-arm cohort study[7] of 224 high-risk patients (prosthetic valves, atrial fibrillation, and a major risk factor). Warfarin was held for 5 days; LMWHs were given 3 days preoperatively and at least 4 days postoperatively. The overall rate of thromboembolism was 3.6%, and the overall rate of cardioembolism was 0.9%. Major bleeding was seen in 6.7% of subjects, although only 8 of 15 episodes occurred during LMWH administration. LMWHs are cost-effective because of reduction in hospital admission duration, but two studies have shown a residual anticoagulation effect in as many as two thirds of patients.[8,9]

Many current prosthetic valves have a lower risk of valve thrombosis than the older ball-in-cage valves, so the risk of heparin may outweigh the benefit in the perioperative setting. According to the AHA/ACC guidelines, heparin can usually be reserved for high-risk patients. High risk is defined by the presence of a mechanical mitral or tricuspid valve or mechanical aortic valve and of risk factors (e.g., atrial fibrillation, previous thromboembolism, hypercoagulable condition, older generation mechanical valves, ejection fraction less than 30%, or more than one mechanical valve).[10] Subcutaneous LMWHs or unfractionated heparin offers an alternative outpatient approach but receives a tentative recommendation. Discussion between the surgeon and cardiologist regarding the optimal perioperative management is critical.

Congenital Heart Disease in Adults

Congenital heart disease afflicts 500,000 to 1 million U.S. adults (see Chap. 65). The nature of the underlying anatomy and any anatomic correction affect the perioperative plan and incidence of complications, which include infection, bleeding, hypoxemia, hypotension, and paradoxical embolization. A major concern in the patient with congenital heart disease is the presence of pulmonary hypertension and Eisenmenger syndrome. Regional anesthesia traditionally has been avoided in these patients because of the potential for sympathetic blockade and worsening of the right to left shunt. However, a review of the published literature incorporating 103 cases has found that overall perioperative mortality is 14%; patients receiving regional anesthesia had a mortality of 5%, whereas those receiving general anesthesia had a mortality of 18%.[6] The authors concluded that most deaths probably occurred as a result of the surgical procedure and disease, and not from anesthesia. Although perioperative and peripartum mortalities were high, many anesthetic agents and techniques had been used with success. Patients with congenital heart disease are at risk for infective endocarditis and should receive antibiotic prophylaxis. This recent review discusses the anesthetic management of these patients in detail.

Arrhythmias

Cardiac arrhythmias are common in the perioperative period, particularly in older patients or in patients undergoing thoracic surgery (see Chaps. 36 to 41). Predisposing factors include prior arrhythmias, underlying heart disease, hypertension, perioperative pain (e.g., hip fracture), severe anxiety, and other situations that heighten adrenergic tone. A prospective study of 4181 patients aged 50 years or older found supraventricular arrhythmia in 2% of patients during surgery and in 6.1% of patients after surgery. Perioperative atrial fibrillation raises several concerns, including an incidence of stroke (see Chap. 40). Winkel and colleagues[11] evaluated 317 patients undergoing major vascular surgery without atrial fibrillation to determine the incidence of new-onset atrial fibrillation and its association with adverse cardiovascular outcomes. They reported an incidence of 4.7% and a more than sixfold increase in cardiovascular death, MI, unstable angina, and stroke in the first 30 days, and a fourfold increase over the next 12 months. Early treatment to restore sinus rhythm or to control the ventricular response and initiate anticoagulation is therefore indicated. Prophylactic intravenous diltiazem in randomized, placebo-controlled trials in high-risk thoracic surgery has reduced the incidence of clinically significant atrial arrhythmias.[1] Balser and associates have studied 64 cases of postoperative supraventricular tachyarrhythmia. After adenosine administration, patients who remained in supraventricular tachyarrhythmia were prospectively randomized to receive intravenous diltiazem or intravenous esmolol for ventricular rate control; it was reported that intravenous esmolol produces a more rapid (2-hour) conversion to sinus rhythm than does intravenous diltiazem.[1] **Figure 85-1** presents an algorithm for atrial fibrillation management.

Although ventricular arrhythmias were originally identified as a risk factor for perioperative morbidity, recent studies have not confirmed this finding. O'Kelly studied a consecutive sample of 230 male patients with known CAD or at high risk of CAD who were undergoing major noncardiac surgical procedures.[1] Preoperative arrhythmias associated with intraoperative and postoperative arrhythmias, but nonfatal MI and cardiac death were not substantially more frequent in those with prior perioperative arrhythmias. Amar and coworkers[12] studied 412 patients undergoing major thoracic surgery and determined that the incidence of nonsustained ventricular tachycardia is 15% but is not associated with poor outcome. Despite this finding, the presence of an arrhythmia in the preoperative setting should provoke a search for underlying cardiopulmonary disease, ongoing myocardial ischemia or infarction, drug toxicity, or metabolic derangements.

Conduction abnormalities can increase perioperative risk and may require the placement of a temporary or permanent pacemaker. On the other hand, patients with intraventricular conduction delays, even in the presence of a left or right bundle branch block, and with no history of advanced heart block or symptoms, rarely progress to complete heart block perioperatively. The availability of transthoracic pacing units has decreased the need for temporary transvenous pacemakers.

CH 85

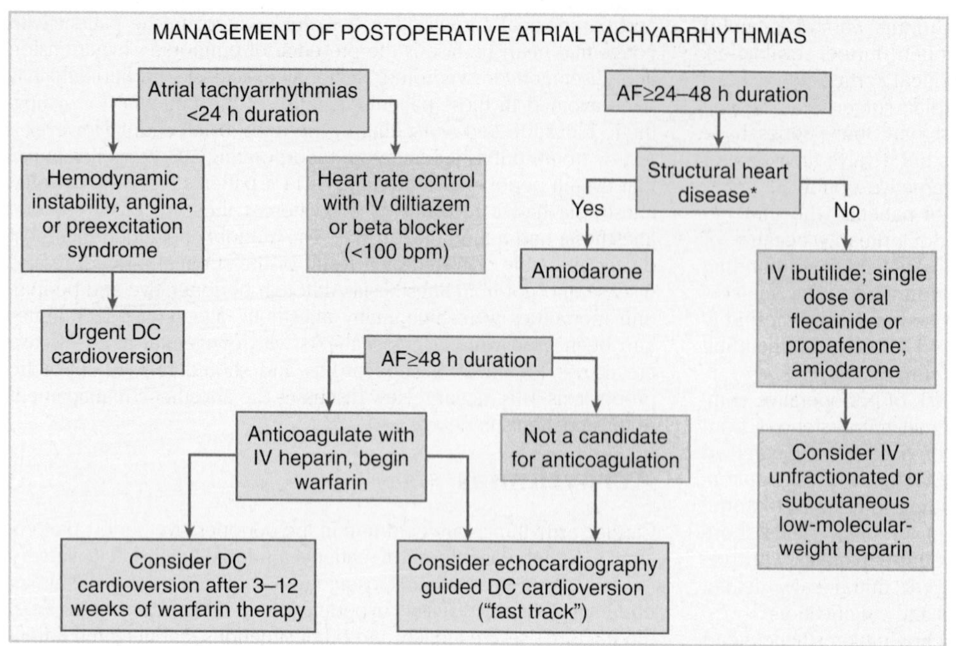

FIGURE 85-1 Proposed algorithm for the treatment of postoperative atrial tachyarrhythmias. AF = atrial fibrillation or flutter; bpm = beats/min; DC = direct current. *Structural heart disease is defined as the presence of one of the following: left ventricular hypertrophy with wall thickness > 1.4 cm, mitral valve disease, coronary artery disease, or heart failure. *(From Amar D: Perioperative atrial tachyarrhythmias. Anesthesiology 97:1618, 2002.)*

number of blocks that could be walked or flights of stairs that could be climbed. Several scales based on activities of daily living have been proposed to assess exercise tolerance. Current guidelines advocate one such scale (the Duke Activity Scale Index; see Chaps. 50 and 83).

The type of surgical procedure itself has a significant impact on perioperative risks and the amount of preparation required to perform anesthesia safely. For surgical procedures not associated with significant stress or a high incidence of perioperative myocardial ischemia or morbidity, the costs of the evaluation often exceed any benefits from the information gained by preoperative assessment. For example, outpatient procedures cause little morbidity and mortality; in such patients, perioperative management is rarely changed by cardiovascular status unless the patient demonstrates unstable angina or overt congestive heart failure. In fact, 30-day mortality after outpatient surgery may actually be lower than expected if the patients did not have surgery. In contrast, open surgery for vascular disease entails a high risk of morbidity and ischemic potential (see Chap. 61). Intra-abdominal, thoracic, and orthopedic procedures entail intermediate risk (**Table 85-3**). Endovascular procedures fall into this intermediate-risk category on the basis of their perioperative morbidity and mortality, although long-term survival appears similar to that in patients who undergo open procedures.

In addition to the risk of the surgical procedure itself, risk also correlates with the surgical volume in a given center. Several studies have demonstrated differential mortality rates in cancer and vascular surgeries, with higher mortality seen in low-volume centers, although recent studies have demonstrated that low-volume centers may also have low mortality rates if proper care systems are in place. Therefore, surgical mortality rates may be institution specific, which may influence the decision to perform further perioperative evaluations and interventions.

The AHA/ACC guidelines[1] presented their recommendations in algorithmic form as a framework for determining which patients are candidates for cardiac testing (see Fig. 85-2). Given the availability of the evidence, the Writing Committee chose to include the level of the recommendations and strength of evidence for each of the pathways:

- Step 1: The consultant should determine the urgency of noncardiac surgery. In many cases, patient-specific or surgery-specific factors dictate an obvious strategy (e.g., emergent surgery) that may not allow for further cardiac assessment or treatment.
- Step 2: Does the patient have an active cardiac condition? In patients being considered for elective noncardiac surgery, the presence of unstable coronary disease, decompensated heart failure, or severe arrhythmia or valvular heart disease usually leads to cancellation or delay of surgery until the cardiac problem has been clarified and treated appropriately. Examples of unstable coronary syndromes include previous MI with evidence of important ischemic risk by clinical symptoms or noninvasive study, unstable or severe angina, and new or poorly controlled ischemia-mediated heart failure. Depending on the results of tests or interventions and the risk of delaying surgery, it may be appropriate to proceed to the planned surgery with maximal medical therapy.
- Step 3: Is the patient undergoing low-risk surgery? Interventions based on cardiovascular testing in stable patients would rarely result in a change in management, and it would be appropriate to proceed with the planned surgical procedure.

Diagnostic and Nondiagnostic Testing

Decision to Undergo Diagnostic Testing

The ACC/AHA[1] and ESC[2] guidelines have both proposed algorithms based on the available evidence and incorporating class of recommendations and level of evidence in each step (**Fig. 85-2**). The current algorithms use a stepwise bayesian strategy that relies on assessment of clinical markers, prior coronary evaluation and treatment, functional capacity, and surgery-specific risk (see later). Successful use of the algorithms requires an appreciation for different levels of risk attributable to certain clinical circumstances, levels of functional capacity, and types of surgery, and for how the information from any diagnostic testing will influence perioperative management.

A number of studies have attempted to identify clinical risk markers for perioperative cardiovascular morbidity and mortality. As noted, patients with unstable coronary syndromes and severe valvular disease have active cardiac conditions. Patients with known stable CAD have intermediate risk. Other clinical risk factors in the RCRI make up the remainder of the intermediate risk predictors (e.g., history of congestive heart failure, history of cerebrovascular disease, preoperative treatment with insulin, preoperative serum creatinine level > 2 mg/dL). Cardiovascular disease has clinical risk markers, each associated with variable levels of perioperative risk, which have been classified as low-risk factors. The classification of perioperative clinical risk markers for assessing the need for further testing is shown in **Table 85-1**.

As described with regard to anginal pattern, exercise tolerance is one of the strongest determinants of perioperative risk and the need for invasive monitoring (see Chap. 14). In one study of outpatients referred for evaluation before major noncardiac procedures,[1] patients were asked to estimate the number of blocks they could walk and how many flights of stairs they could climb without experiencing cardiac symptoms (**Table 85-2**). Patients who could not walk four blocks and could not climb two flights of stairs were considered to have poor exercise tolerance, and had twice as many perioperative cardiovascular complications as those with better functional status. The likelihood of a serious complication occurring was inversely related to the

- Step 4: Does the patient have moderate functional capacity without symptoms? In highly functional asymptomatic patients, management will rarely change on the basis of results of any further cardiovascular testing, and it is therefore appropriate to proceed with the planned surgery. If the patient has poor functional capacity, is symptomatic, or has unknown functional capacity, the presence of clinical risk factors will determine the need for further evaluation. If the patient has no clinical risk factors, it is appropriate to proceed with the planned surgery, and no further change in management is indicated.

If the patient has one or two clinical risk factors, it is reasonable to proceed with the planned surgery (with heart rate control) or to consider testing if it will change management. In patients with three or more clinical risk factors, if the patient is undergoing vascular surgery, it has been suggested that testing should only be considered if it will change management. In nonvascular surgery in which the perioperative morbidity related to the procedure ranges from 1% to 5% (intermediate-risk surgery), there are insufficient data to determine the best strategy—proceeding with the planned surgery with tight heart rate control with beta blockade, or further cardiovascular testing if it will change management.

Falcone and coworkers performed a small randomized trial of 99 patients undergoing elective vascular surgery.[1] Patients at low or intermediate clinical risk were randomized to testing or no testing, with no difference in perioperative or long-term outcome. The vast majority of these patients were highly functional and placed on perioperative beta blocker therapy, suggesting that exercise capacity can help determine the need for further diagnostic testing preoperatively.

Poldermans and colleagues[13] randomized 770 intermediate-risk patients to cardiac stress testing ($N = 386$) or no testing. Those with extensive stress-induced ischemia were considered for revascularization, with the choice of procedure at the discretion of the primary physician. HR was tightly controlled with beta blockers in all patients. Patients assigned to no testing had similar incidences of cardiac death or MI at 30 days after surgery, as did those assigned to testing (1.8% versus 2.3%; odds ratio [OR], 0.78; 95% confidence interval [CI], 0.28 to 2.1; $P = 0.62$). Regardless of allocated strategy, patients with a HR less than 65 beats/min had lower risk than the remaining patients (1.3% versus 5.2%; OR, 0.24; 95% CI, 0.09 to 0.66; $P < 0.003$). The authors suggested that testing is not required in patients at intermediate risk if HR is controlled; however, we believe that testing may still be indicated if the results will change management.

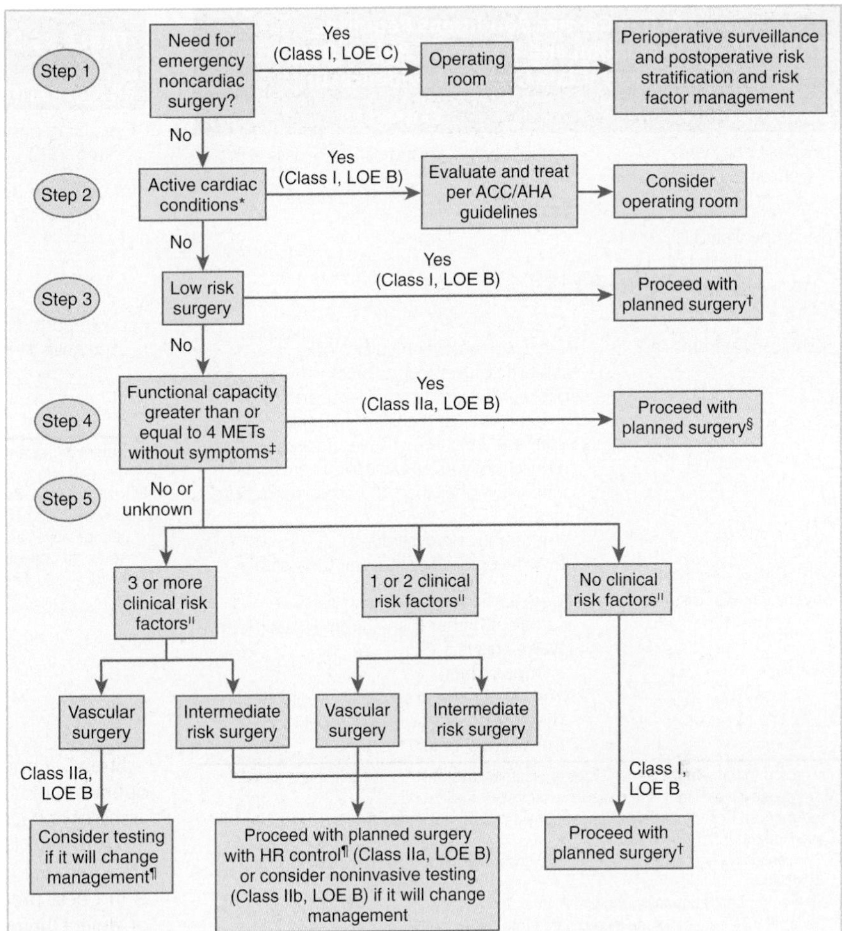

FIGURE 85-2 American College of Cardiology/American Heart Association (ACC/AHA) Task Force on Perioperative Evaluation of Cardiac Patients Undergoing Noncardiac Surgery proposed algorithm for decisions regarding the need for further evaluation. This represents one of a number of such algorithms in the literature. This incorporates the class of recommendation for each step and level of evidence (LOE). *See Table 85-1 for active cardiac conditions. †See Class III recommendations in Section 5.2.3. Noninvasive Stress Testing in the guidelines. ‡See Table 85-2 for estimated MET level equivalent. §Noninvasive testing may be considered before surgery in specific patients with risk factors if it will change management. ||Clinical risk factors include ischemic heart disease, compensated or prior heart failure, diabetes mellitus, renal insufficiency, and cerebrovascular disease. ¶Consider perioperative beta blockade (see Table 11 in the source article listed below for populations in which this has been shown to reduce cardiac morbidity/mortality. MET = metabolic equivalent. *(From Fleisher LA, Beckman JA, Brown KA, et al: 2009 ACCF/AHA focused update on perioperative beta blockade incorporated into the ACC/AHA 2007 guidelines on perioperative cardiovascular evaluation and care for noncardiac surgery: A report of the American College of Cardiology Foundation/American Heart Association Task Force on Practice Guidelines. Circulation 120:e169, 2009.)*

Tests to Improve Identification and Definition of Cardiovascular Disease

Several noninvasive diagnostic methods can evaluate the extent of CAD before noncardiac surgery. The exercise electrocardiogram has traditionally evaluated individuals for the presence of CAD, but as noted, patients with excellent exercise tolerance in daily life will rarely benefit from further testing. Patients with poor exercise capacity, in contrast, may not achieve adequate HR and BP for diagnostic purposes on electrocardiographic stress tests. Such patients often require concomitant imaging.

A substantial number of high-risk patients either cannot exercise or have contraindications to exercise (e.g., patients with claudication or an abdominal aortic aneurysm undergoing vascular surgery, both of which have a high rate of perioperative cardiac morbidity). Pharmacologic stress testing therefore has become popular, particularly as a preoperative test in vascular surgery patients. Several studies have shown that the presence of a redistribution defect on dipyridamole or adenosine thallium or sestamibi imaging in patients undergoing peripheral vascular surgery predicts postoperative cardiac events (see Chap. 17). Pharmacologic stress imaging is best used in patients at moderate clinical risk. Several strategies may increase the predictive value of such tests. The redistribution defect can be quantitated, with larger areas of defect associating with increased risk. Additionally, both increased lung uptake and left ventricular cavity dilation indicate ventricular dysfunction with ischemia. It has been shown that the delineation of low-risk and high-risk thallium scans (larger area of defect, increased lung uptake, and left ventricular cavity dilation) markedly improve the test's predictive value; patients with high-risk thallium scans have particularly increased risk for perioperative morbidity and long-term mortality.

TABLE 85-1 Active Cardiac Conditions Requiring Evaluation and Treatment Before Noncardiac Surgery (Class I, level of evidence: B)

CONDITION	EXAMPLES
Unstable coronary syndromes	Unstable or severe angina* (CCS class III or IV)† Recent MI‡
Decompensated HF (NYHA functional class IV; worsening or new-onset HF)	
Significant arrhythmias	High-grade atrioventricular block Mobitz II atrioventricular block Third-degree atrioventricular heart block Symptomatic ventricular arrhythmias Supraventricular arrhythmias (including atrial fibrillation) with uncontrolled ventricular rate (HR higher than 100 beats per minute at rest) Symptomatic bradycardia Newly recognized ventricular tachycardia
Severe valvular disease	Severe aortic stenosis (mean pressure gradient higher than 40 mm Hg, aortic valve area less than 1 cm^2, or symptomatic) Symptomatic mitral stenosis (progressive dyspnea on exertion, exertional presyncope, or HF)

*According to Campeau L: Letter: grading of angina pectoris. Circulation 54:522, 1976.
†May include "stable" angina in patients who are unusually sedentary.
‡The American College of Cardiology National Cardiovascular Data Registry defines recent MI as >7 days but ≤1 month (within 30 days).
CCS = Canadian Cardiovascular Society; HF = heart failure; NYHA = New York Heart Association.
From Fleisher LA, Beckman JA, Brown KA, et al: 2009 ACCF/AHA focused update on perioperative beta blockade incorporated into the ACC/AHA 2007 guidelines on perioperative cardiovascular evaluation and care for noncardiac surgery: A report of the American College of Cardiology Foundation/American Heart Association Task Force on Practice Guidelines. Circulation 120:e169, 2009.

TABLE 85-2 Estimated Energy Requirements for Various Activities

NO. OF METS	QUESTION: CAN YOU ...
1	Take care of yourself? Eat, dress, or use the toilet? Walk indoors around the house? Walk a block or two on level ground at 2 to 3 mph (3.2-4.8 kph)?
4	Do light work around the house like dusting or washing dishes? Climb a flight of stairs or walk up a hill? Walk on level ground at 4 mph (6.4 kph)? Run a short distance? Do heavy work around the house, like scrubbing floors or lifting or moving heavy furniture? Participate in moderate recreational activities like golf, bowling, dancing, doubles tennis, or throwing a baseball or football?
>10	Participate in strenuous sports like swimming, singles tennis, football, basketball, or skiing?

kph = km/hr; MET = metabolic equivalent; mph = miles/hr.
Modified from Fleisher LA, Beckman JA, Brown KA, et al: 2009 ACCF/AHA focused update on perioperative beta blockade incorporated into the ACC/AHA 2007 guidelines on perioperative cardiovascular evaluation and care for noncardiac surgery: A report of the American College of Cardiology Foundation/American Heart Association Task Force on Practice Guidelines. Circulation 120:e169, 2009.

TABLE 85-3 Cardiac Risk Stratification for Noncardiac Surgical Procedures*

RISK STRATIFICATION	EXAMPLES OF PROCEDURES
Vascular (reported cardiac risk often >5%)	Aortic and other major vascular surgery Peripheral vascular surgery
Intermediate (reported cardiac risk generally = 1%-5%)	Intraperitoneal and intrathoracic surgery Carotid endarterectomy Head and neck surgery Orthopedic surgery Prostate surgery
Low (reported cardiac risk generally <1%)†	Endoscopic procedures Superficial procedure Cataract surgery Breast surgery Ambulatory surgery

*Combined incidence of cardiac death and nonfatal MI.
†These procedures generally do not require further preoperative cardiac testing.
From Fleisher LA, Beckman JA, Brown KA, et al: 2009 ACCF/AHA focused update on perioperative beta blockade incorporated into the ACC/AHA 2007 guidelines on perioperative cardiovascular evaluation and care for noncardiac surgery: A report of the American College of Cardiology Foundation/American Heart Association Task Force on Practice Guidelines. Circulation 120:e169, 2009.

Stress echocardiography has also been widely used as a preoperative test (see Chap. 15). One advantage of this test is that it assesses myocardial ischemia dynamically in response to increased inotropy and HR, such as may occur during the perioperative period. The presence of new wall motion abnormalities that occur at low HR is the best predictor of increased perioperative risk, with large areas of defect being of secondary importance. Boersma and colleagues have assessed the value of dobutamine stress echocardiography with respect to the extent of wall motion abnormalities and the ability of preoperative beta blocker treatment to attenuate risk in patients undergoing major aortic surgery.[1] They assigned one point for each of the following characteristics: age older than 70 years, current angina, MI, congestive heart failure, prior cerebrovascular disease, diabetes mellitus, and renal failure. As the total number of clinical risk factors increases, perioperative cardiac event rates also increase.

So, which diagnostic test should be used for preoperative risk assessment? Several groups have published meta-analyses examining the various preoperative diagnostic tests. Good predictive values for ambulatory electrocardiogram monitoring, radionuclide angiography, dipyridamole thallium imaging, and dobutamine stress echocardiography have been demonstrated. Shaw and associates have also demonstrated excellent predictive values for dipyridamole thallium imaging and dobutamine stress echocardiography.[1] Beattie and coworkers have performed a meta-analysis of 25 stress echocardiography studies and 50 thallium imaging studies.[1] The likelihood ratio for stress echocardiography was more indicative of a postoperative cardiac event than that for thallium imaging (likelihood ratio, 4.09; 95% CI, 3.21 to 6.56, versus likelihood ratio, 1.83; 95% CI, 1.59 to 2.10; $P < 0.001$). The difference was attributable to fewer false-negative stress echocardiograms. A moderate to large perfusion defect by either test predicted postoperative MI and death. An important determinant with respect to the choice of preoperative testing is the expertise at the local institution. Another factor is whether assessment of valve function or myocardial thickness is of interest, where echocardiography may be preferred. Stress nuclear imaging may have slightly higher sensitivity, but stress echocardiography may be less likely to yield false–positive results. The role in preoperative risk assessment of newer imaging modalities for preoperative assessment using magnetic resonance imaging, multislice computed tomography, coronary calcium scores, and positron emission tomography is rapidly evolving.

(>24-hour) elevation of cTnI. The authors suggested that these two patterns represent two distinct pathophysiologies—acute coronary occlusion for early morbidity and prolonged myocardial ischemia for late events. Mohler and coworkers[19] evaluated cTn-I and CK-MB in 784 high-risk vascular surgery patients on the day of surgery and at 24, 72, and 120 hours postoperatively. They reported a sensitivity of 51% and a specificity of 91% for the defined cardiovascular event, using a receiver operating characteristic (ROC)–defined cut point for CK-MB of 3.1 ng/mL.

Recently, brain natriuretic peptide (BNP) has been studied in the perioperative period. Mahla and colleagues[20] measured preoperative and postoperative N-terminal pro-BNP (NT-proBNP) in 218 vascular surgery patients. Using ROC analysis-defined cut points, patients with elevated NT-proBNP had an almost 20-fold in-hospital and fivefold long-term risk of cardiac events. Goei and associates[21] have evaluated the predictive capacity of preoperative levels of NT-proBNP in 356 vascular surgery patients; they found that BNP elevations are associated with adverse 30-day cardiovascular events in subjects with normal renal function but not in those with severe renal impairment. In a meta-analysis of seven prospective observational studies, BNP or NT-proBNP above the ROC-determined optimal threshold was associated with marked increases in 30-day and intermediate-term cardiac death, nonfatal MI, and major adverse cardiac events.[22] A subsequent meta-analysis demonstrated that preoperative BNP measurement independently predicts perioperative cardiovascular events in studies that only considered the outcomes of death, cardiovascular death, or MI (OR, 44.2; 95% CI, 7.6 to 257.0; I(2) = 51.6%) and studies that included other outcomes (OR, 14.7; 95% CI, 5.7 to 38.2; I(2) = 62.2%); the P value for interaction was 0.28.[23]

Traditionally, PMIs were associated with a 30% to 50% short-term mortality, but recent series have reported a fatality rate of perioperative MIs of less than 20%. Whether these shifts in timing relate to reductions or better detection of hypotension-related subendocardial ischemia, or a change in the timing of true plaque rupture events, remains unclear. Studies from the 1980s suggested a peak incidence of the second and third postoperative days. Badner and coworkers, using troponin I as a marker for MI, have suggested that the immediate and first postoperative days show the highest incidence, as confirmed in other studies.[1] The finding that postanesthetic care unit hypotension best predicted troponin release suggests a hemodynamic rather than plaque rupture event. Thus, the change likely relates to more robust surveillance methods, not a fundamental shift in how or when myocardial ischemia or infarct occur.

Increasing evidence associates a perioperative MI or biomarker elevation with worse long-term outcome. Lopez-Jimenez and colleagues found that abnormal troponin T levels were associated with an increased incidence of cardiovascular complications within 6 months of surgery.[1] Kim and associates studied perioperative troponin I levels in 229 patients having aortic or infrainguinal vascular surgery or lower extremity amputation.[1] Twenty-eight patients (12%) had postoperative troponin I levels higher than 1.5 ng/mL, which was associated with a sixfold increased risk of 6-month mortality and a 27-fold increased risk of MI. Furthermore, they observed a relationship between troponin I concentration and mortality. Landesberg and coworkers demonstrated that postoperative CK-MB and troponin, even at low cutoff levels, are independent and complementary predictors of long-term mortality after major vascular surgery.[1] Mahla and colleagues[20] also demonstrated that elevations in BNP levels are associated with a fivefold long-term risk of cardiac events. The appropriate use of screening biomarkers in current preoperative risk assessment algorithms remains unstudied.

Reducing Cardiac Risk of Noncardiac Surgery

Surgical Revascularization

Coronary revascularization has been suggested as a means of reducing perioperative risk surrounding noncardiac surgery. Retrospective evidence indicates that prior successful preoperative revascularization may decrease postoperative cardiac risk two- to four-fold in patients undergoing elective vascular surgery. The strongest evidence comes from the Coronary Artery Surgery Study (CASS) Registry, which enrolled patients from 1978 to 1981.[1] The operative mortality for patients with CABG before noncardiac surgery was 0.9% but was significantly higher (2.4%) in patients without prior CABG. However, a 1.4% mortality rate was associated with the CABG procedure itself. Eagle and associates have reported a long-term analysis of patients entered into CASS and assigned to medical or surgical therapy for CAD for more than 10 years who subsequently underwent 3368 noncardiac operations in the years following assignment of coronary treatment.[1] Intermediate-risk surgery such as abdominal, thoracic, or carotid endarterectomy associated with a combined morbidity and mortality of 1% to 5%, with a small but substantial improvement in outcome in patients who had undergone prior revascularization. The most improvement in outcome occurred in patients undergoing major vascular surgery, such as abdominal or lower extremity revascularization. This observational study did not randomize patients, however, and was undertaken in the 1970s and 1980s, before significant advances in medical, surgical, and percutaneous coronary strategies.

Several cohort studies have examined the benefit of percutaneous coronary intervention (PCI) before noncardiac surgery. Posner and colleagues used an administrative data set of patients who underwent PCI and noncardiac surgery in Washington State.[1] They matched patients with coronary disease undergoing noncardiac surgery with and without prior PCI and looked at cardiac complications. In this nonrandomized design, they noted a significantly lower rate of 30-day cardiac complications in patients who underwent PCI at least 90 days before the noncardiac surgery. PCI within 90 days of noncardiac surgery did not improve outcome. The advent of drug-eluting stents requiring prolonged antiplatelet therapy may promote operative bleeding complications or increase subacute stent thrombosis if antiplatelet treatment stops perioperatively (see Chap. 58).

Several randomized trials have addressed the value of both CABG and PCI in a subset of patients. McFalls and colleagues[24] reported the results of a multicenter randomized trial in the Veterans Affairs Health System in which patients with documented CAD on coronary angiography, excluding those with left main disease or severely depressed ejection fraction (<20%), were randomized before elective major vascular surgery to CABG (59%) or PCI (41%) versus routine medical therapy. At 2.7 years after randomization, mortality in the revascularization group was not significantly different (22%) compared with the no-revascularization group (23%). Within 30 days after the vascular operation, a postoperative MI, defined by elevated troponin levels, occurred in 12% of the revascularization group and 14% of the no-revascularization group ($P = 0.37$). The authors suggested that coronary revascularization is not indicated in patients with stable CAD, and further support the lack of efficacy of PCI or CABG for single- or double-vessel disease before noncardiac surgery. In a reanalysis of the data, the completeness of the revascularization affects the rate of perioperative MI, with CABG being more effective than PCI.

Poldermans and associates[25] have evaluated the role of coronary artery revascularization in 101 vascular surgery patients with three or more Lee index risk factors and extensive stress-induced ischemia, on a background of beta blocker therapy. Coronary angiography showed two-vessel disease in 12 patients (24%), three-vessel disease in 33 patients (67%), and left main disease in 4 patients (8%). Revascularization improved neither 30-day nor 1-year outcome ($P > 0.2$ for both). Long-term benefit was only shown in those with corrected left main disease.[26] Most recently, Garcia and coworkers[27] analyzed randomized and nonrandomized patients who had preoperative coronary angiography, and unprotected left main CAD was present in 4.6% of patients who underwent coronary angiography before vascular surgery; this was the only subset of patients showing a benefit with preoperative coronary artery revascularization.

As described earlier, Poldermans and colleagues[13] randomized vascular patients at intermediate risk to testing and interventions or no testing, and found no difference in 30-day cardiac events with beta blocker therapy provided to all subjects. Monaco and associates[28] studied 208 patients at moderate clinical risk who were undergoing major vascular surgery and were randomly allocated to a selective strategy group, in whom coronary angiography was performed based on the results of noninvasive tests, or to a systematic strategy group, who systematically underwent preoperative coronary angiography. The strategy of routine coronary angiography had no effect on short-term outcome, but positively affected long-term outcome of peripheral arterial disease surgical patients at medium to high risk.

One issue in interpreting the results is that the length of time between coronary revascularization and noncardiac surgery most likely affects its protective effect and potential risks. Back and coworkers[29] have studied 425 consecutive patients undergoing 481 elective major vascular operations at an academic Veterans Affairs Medical Center. Coronary revascularization was classified as recent (CABG, <1 year; percutaneous transluminal coronary angioplasty [PTCA], <6 months) in 35 cases, as prior (CABG, 1 to 5 years; PTCA, 6 months to 2 years) in 45 cases, and as remote (CABG, >5 years; PTCA, >2 years) in 48 cases. Outcomes in patients with previous PTCAs were similar to those after CABG. Significant differences in adverse cardiac events and mortality were found between patients with CABG done within 5 years or PTCA within 2 years (6.3% and 1.3%, respectively), individuals with remote revascularization (10.4% and 6.3%, respectively), and nonrevascularized patients stratified at high risk (13.3% and 3.3%, respectively) or intermediate or low risk (2.8% and 0.9%, respectively). The authors concluded that previous coronary revascularization (CABG, >5 years; PTCA, >2 years) provides only modest protection against adverse cardiac events and mortality following major arterial reconstruction.

Coronary Stenting and Noncardiac Surgery

PCI using coronary stenting poses several special issues. Kaluza and colleagues reported the outcome in 40 patients who underwent prophylactic coronary stent placement less than six weeks before major noncardiac surgery requiring general anesthesia.[1] They reported 7 MIs, 11 major bleeding episodes, and 8 deaths. All of the deaths and MIs, as well as 8 of the 11 bleeding episodes, occurred in patients who underwent surgery fewer than 14 days after stenting. Four patients died after undergoing surgery 1 day after stenting. Wilson and associates reported on 207 patients who underwent noncardiac surgery within 2 months of stent placement.[1] Eight patients died or suffered an MI, and all of those were among the 168 patients undergoing surgery 6 weeks after stent placement. Vincenzi and coworkers studied 103 patients and reported that the risk of a perioperative cardiac event was 2.11-fold greater in patients with recent stents (<35 days before surgery) as compared with PCI more than 90 days before surgery.[1] The importance of delaying surgery was reported, even though the investigators either continued antiplatelet drug therapy or only briefly interrupted it; heparin was administered to all patients. Leibowitz and colleagues studied 216 consecutive patients who had PCI within 3 months of noncardiac surgery (112 had PTCA and 94 had stenting).[1] A total of 26 patients (12%) died, 13 in the stent group (14%) and 13 in the PTCA group (11%)—a nonsignificant difference. The incidence of acute MI and death within 6 months did not differ significantly (7% and 14% in the stent group and 6% and 11% in the PTCA group, respectively). Many more events occurred in the two groups when noncardiac surgery was performed within 2 weeks of PCI. On the basis of the accumulating data, elective noncardiac surgery after PCI, with or without stent placement, should be delayed for 4 to 6 weeks.

Drug-eluting stents may represent an even greater problem during the perioperative period. Emerging data from a series of recent analyses in the nonoperative setting and several perioperative case reports suggest that the risk of thrombosis continues for at least one year after insertion (see Chap. 58).[1] Several reports have suggested that drug-eluting stents may represent an additional risk over a prolonged period (up to 12 months), particularly if antiplatelet agents are discontinued. Schouten and colleagues[30] retrospectively evaluated 192 patients who underwent noncardiac surgery and had a successful PCI because of unstable CAD within 2 years of the procedure. Drug-eluting stents accounted for 52% of the stents placed. Of the 192 patients, 30 underwent surgery prior to the recommended discontinuation of dual antiplatelet therapy for the particular stent (30 days for bare metal stents and up to 6 months for sirolimus-eluting stents). In patients in whom antiplatelet therapy was stopped before the required time for clopidogrel use (early surgery group), the incidence of death or nonfatal MI was 30.7%, compared with 0% in patients who continued antiplatelet therapy. The elevated risk of stent thrombosis and cardiovascular events, however, seems to abate over time. Godet and associates[31] investigated the risk of postoperative adverse cardiovascular events at a mean of 14 months after drug-eluting stent placement in 96 consecutive patients, noting a 2% in-stent thrombosis rate. More recently, Anwaruddin and coworkers[32] determined the risk of postoperative complications in 481 patients with drug-eluting stent placement an average of 1.1 years prior to the operation. They reported a 9% risk of death, nonfatal MI, or stent thrombosis by 30 days. A 2007 science advisory from the AHA, ACC, Society for Cardiovascular Angiography and Interventions, American College of Surgeons, and American Dental Association stressed the importance of 12 months of dual antiplatelet therapy after placement of a drug-eluting stent.[1] This advisory also recommended postponing elective surgery for 1 year and, if surgery cannot be deferred, considering the continuation of aspirin during the perioperative period in high-risk patients with drug-eluting stents. In patients with illness requiring more timely surgery, strategies for bridging the cessation of antiplatelet therapy until the procedure include the use of intravenous eptifibatide and tirofiban, but these have not been tested in adequate numbers to permit recommendation.

Pharmacologic Interventions

BETA-ADRENERGIC BLOCKING AGENTS. Beta blockers (**Table 85-4**) are the best-studied medical treatment, and guidelines for their use in the perioperative period have been published recently. Mangano and colleagues administered atenolol or placebo, beginning on the morning of surgery and continuing for 7 days postoperatively, in a cohort of 200 patients with known coronary disease or risk factors for CAD who were undergoing high-risk noncardiac surgery.[1] They demonstrated a marked reduction in the incidence of perioperative myocardial ischemia, although no differences in the rates of perioperative MI. Survival improved markedly at 6 months in the atenolol group and continued for at least 2 years. The authors speculated that the lower incidence of myocardial ischemia resulted from less plaque destabilization, with a resultant reduction in subsequent MI or death in the 6 months after noncardiac surgery. Issues of randomization and uneven distribution of risk factors and treatment at baseline and on discharge with beta blockers may account for the findings, at least in part. However, Poldermans and associates have studied the perioperative use of bisoprolol versus routine care in elective major vascular surgery in the Dutch Echocardiographic Cardiac Risk Evaluation Applying Stress Echo (DECREASE) trial.[1] This medication was started at least 7 days preoperatively, titrated to achieve a resting HR less than 60 beats/min, and continued postoperatively for 30 days. The study was confined to patients with at least one clinical marker of cardiac risk (prior MI, diabetes, angina pectoris, heart failure, age older than 70 years, or poor functional status), and evidence of inducible myocardial ischemia on a preoperative dobutamine stress echocardiogram. Patients with extensive regional wall abnormalities (large zones of myocardial ischemia) were excluded. Bisoprolol reduced perioperative MI or cardiac death by almost 80% in this high-risk population. Because of the selection criteria, the efficacy of bisoprolol in the highest risk group—those who would be considered for coronary revascularization or modification or cancellation of the surgical procedure—cannot be determined from this trial. The event rate in the placebo group (almost 40%) suggests, however, that all but the highest risk patients were enrolled in the trial.

Boersma and coworkers have reevaluated the value of dobutamine stress echocardiography with respect to the extent of wall motion abnormalities and the use of beta blockers during surgery for the entire cohort of patients screened for the DECREASE trial.[1] They assigned one point for each of the following characteristics: age older

TABLE 85-4 Beta-Adrenergic Blocking Agents

STUDY	NO. OF PATIENTS IN STUDY	BETA BLOCKER REGIMEN	PATIENT RISK GROUP	SURGICAL PROCEDURE	DURATION OF BETA BLOCKADE	WERE BETA BLOCKERS FULLY TITRATED?	WERE BETA BLOCKERS OF BENEFIT?
MSCPI	200	Atenolol, 50-100 mg	Known CAD or at risk for CAD with ≥ two risk factors	Vascular, abdominal, orthopedic, neurosurgery	Duration of hospitalization	No	Yes, at 6-8 mo
DECREASE I	112	Bisoprolol, varying doses	≥ One or more RCRI risk factor and positive DBA stress echo	Major vascular surgery	1 wk before until 30 days after surgery	Yes, to heart rate of 60 beats/min	Yes, 90% reduction in MI and death
MaVS	496	Metoprolol, single dose	ASA class 1-3	Major vascular surgery	2 hr before until 5 days after surgery	No. Metoprolol dosed by patient weight.	No; more intraoperative treatment requiring bradycardia in metoprolol arm
DIPOM	921	Metoprolol succinate, two doses	Diabetic patients; <10% had history of CAD	Intermediate risk surgery	1 day before until a maximum of 8 days after surgery (mean 4.6 days)	Two doses; 100 mg/day or 50 mg/day if heart rate = 55-65 beats/min	No benefit or harm
POISE	8351	Metoprolol succinate	History of CAD, PVD, stroke, CHF, undergoing vascular surgery, or ≥ three or more RCRI risk factors	Noncardiac surgery (major vascular surgery 36%, intraperitoneal 21%, orthopedic 21%)	2-4 hr before surgery to 30 days after surgery	No, dose limitation for low heart rate	Yes and no; reduction in CV death, NFMI, NF cardiac arrest; increase in mortality and stroke
DECREASE IV	1066	Bisoprolol	Intermediate risk (risk estimate, 1%-6% MI or death)	General, urologic, orthopedic, ENT surgery	Within 30 days of surgery until 30 days after	Yes, to target heart rate 50-70 beats/min	Yes, 66% reduction in NFMI and cardiac death

DBA = dobutamine; ENT = ear, nose, and throat; NFMI = nonfatal MI.
Modified from Chopra V, Eagle KA: Perioperative beta-blockers for cardiac risk reduction: Time for clarity. JAMA 303:551, 2010.

than 70 years, current angina, MI, congestive heart failure, prior cerebrovascular event, diabetes mellitus, and renal failure. As the total number of clinical risk factors increased, perioperative cardiac event rates also increased. When the risk of death or MI was stratified by perioperative beta blocker usage, there was no significant improvement in those without any of the prior risk factors. In those with a risk factor score between 1 and 3, which represented more than half of all patients, the rate of cardiac events fell from 3% to 0.9% by effective beta blockade. Most importantly, in those with fewer than three risk factors, comprising 70% of the population, beta blocker therapy was effective in reducing cardiac events in those with new wall motion abnormalities in one to four segments (33% versus 2.8%), having a smaller effect in those without new wall motion abnormalities (5.8% versus 2%). Beta blockers were not protective in those patients with new wall motion abnormalities in more than five segments. This group with risk factors and extensive wall motion abnormalities on preoperative stress echo may be the group to consider for prophylactic coronary revascularization. Dunkelgrun and colleagues[33] investigated the role of beta blockade in intermediate-risk noncardiac surgery patients (defined as a predicted risk of cardiac event of 1% to 6%) in an open-label randomized trial. Bisoprolol, titrated to a heart rate of 50 to 70 beats/min preoperatively and maintained during the hospitalization, reduced the rate of perioperative cardiac death and nonfatal MI from 66% to 2.1%.

The trial data supporting the use of beta blockers are not uniformly positive. Brady and associates randomized 103 patients without previous MI who had infrarenal vascular surgery to oral metoprolol or placebo from admission until 7 days after surgery.[1] Perioperative beta blockade with metoprolol did not seem to reduce 30-day cardiovascular events, but it was underpowered to do so. The study did show that metoprolol reduced the time from surgery to discharge. Lindenauer and colleagues[34] retrospectively reviewed the records of 782,969 patients and determined who received beta blocker treatment during the first 2 hospital days. The relationship between perioperative beta blocker treatment and the risk of death varied directly with cardiac risk; among the 580,665 patients with an RCRI score of 0 or 1, treatment was associated with no benefit and possible harm, whereas among the patients with an RCRI score of 2, 3, or 4 or higher, the adjusted odds ratios for death in the hospital were 0.88 (95% CI, 0.80 to 0.98), 0.71 (95% CI, 0.63 to 0.80), and 0.58 (95% CI, 0.50 to 0.67), respectively.

A study of 497 vascular surgery patients randomized to a fixed dose of metoprolol versus placebo demonstrated no difference in perioperative outcome. A trial of metoprolol in diabetic patients without known coronary disease undergoing a diverse group of surgical procedures was unable to demonstrate any difference in perioperative outcomes.[1] In the POISE trial, Devereaux and colleagues randomized 8351 high-risk patients undergoing noncardiac surgery to metoprolol succinate 200 mg daily, or matching placebo.[4] The long-acting metoprolol was first administered at 100 mg 2 to 4 hours before surgery, within 6 hours after surgery, and then at 200 mg daily thereafter. Active treatment with a beta blocker reduced the composite of cardiovascular death, nonfatal MI, and nonfatal cardiac arrest at 30 days after randomization by 1.1%, but increased mortality by 0.8% and stroke by 0.5%. Why was this variance seen? One prominent difference among these trials is the use of titration. In the clinical trials showing reductions in events, beta blockers were titrated to ensure appropriate effect, whereas in the trials in which beta blockers did not improve outcomes or instead worsened them, titration was limited or absent. The timing of medication administration is another possible cause; preoperative titration associated with better outcomes than administration at or just after surgery.

In 2009, an update to the ACC/AHA guidelines on perioperative beta blockade modified previous recommendations based on recent evidence.[1] The continuation of beta blockers in patients undergoing surgery who are receiving beta blockers remains a Class I recommendation. No other Class I recommendations are stated. The use of beta

TABLE 85-5 Recommendations for Perioperative Beta Blocker Therapy

Class I

1. Beta blockers should be continued in patients undergoing surgery who are receiving beta blockers for treatment of conditions with ACCF/AHA Class I guideline indications for the drugs (level of evidence: C).

Class IIa

1. Beta blockers titrated to heart rate and blood pressure are probably recommended for patients undergoing vascular surgery who are at high cardiac risk because of coronary artery disease or the finding of cardiac ischemia on preoperative testing (level of evidence: B).
2. Beta blockers titrated to heart rate and blood pressure are reasonable for patients in whom preoperative assessment for vascular surgery identifies high cardiac risk, as defined by the presence of more than one clinical risk factor* (level of evidence: C).
3. Beta blockers titrated to heart rate and blood pressure are reasonable for patients in whom preoperative assessment identifies coronary artery disease or high cardiac risk, as defined by the presence of more than one clinical risk factor,* who are undergoing intermediate-risk surgery (level of evidence: B).

Class IIb

1. The usefulness of beta blockers is uncertain for patients who are undergoing intermediate-risk procedures or vascular surgery in whom preoperative assessment identifies a single clinical risk factor in the absence of coronary artery disease* (level of evidence: C).
2. The usefulness of beta blockers is uncertain in patients undergoing vascular surgery with no clinical risk factors who are not currently taking beta blockers (level of evidence: B).

Class III

1. Beta blockers should not be given to patients undergoing surgery who have absolute contraindications to beta blockade (level of evidence: C).
2. Routine administration of high-dose beta blockers in the absence of dose titration is not useful and may be harmful to patients not currently taking beta blockers who are undergoing noncardiac surgery (level of evidence: B).

*Clinical risk factors include history of ischemic heart disease, history of compensated or prior heart failure, history of cerebrovascular disease, diabetes mellitus, and renal insufficiency (defined in the Revised Cardiac Risk Index as a preoperative serum creatinine of 2 mg/dL).

From Fleischmann KE: Perioperative focused update. J Am Coll Cardiol 54:2102, 2009.

blockers titrated to heart rate and blood pressure are all Class IIa recommendations for the following: (1) patients undergoing vascular surgery who are at high cardiac risk because of CAD; (2) the finding of cardiac ischemia on preoperative testing in patients for whom preoperative assessment for vascular surgery identified high cardiac risk, as defined by the presence of more than one RCRI clinical risk factor; and (3) for patients in whom preoperative assessment identified CAD or high cardiac risk, as defined by the presence of more than one clinical risk factor, who are undergoing intermediate-risk surgery. A new Class III recommendation is that the routine administration of high-dose beta blockers in the absence of dose titration is not useful, and may be harmful to patients not currently taking beta blockers who are undergoing noncardiac surgery (**Table 85-5**).

Several pragmatic considerations pertain to the use of perioperative beta blockers in those not currently taking these agents. Several authors have recently demonstrated that most patients presenting for noncardiac surgery, and even for vascular surgery, have not been started on beta blockers.[1] One concern of anesthesiologists is related to the acute administration of beta-blocking agents on the morning of surgery. The combined effect of acute HR decrease and the induction of anesthesia in a patient who had previously been beta blocker–naïve has anecdotally been associated with marked bradycardia and hypotension. Treatment of these events may lead to wide swings in HR and BP and less HR control than desired. Thus, the approach to the use of beta blockers depends on the preoperative status, type of surgery, cardiac risk factors, and any results of cardiac stress testing. Ideally, beta blocker therapy should be initiated more than seven days in advance,[35] and longer-acting agents such as atenolol or bisoprolol should be used. Analyzing a large data base, Redelmeier and associates have demonstrated improved perioperative survival in patients given atenolol as compared with metoprolol.[1] If the patient is undergoing nonvascular surgery or vascular surgery and has indications for beta blocker therapy independent of surgery, but is not currently taking beta blockers, then initiation of beta blockers several days preoperatively by the internist, cardiologist, or other primary care provider is appropriate to ensure a stable beta blocker level on the day of surgery. If several days of beta blocker therapy cannot be achieved, the potential risks of new-onset beta blocker therapy during induction of general, epidural, or spinal anesthesia may outweigh the benefits of beginning drug therapy the morning of surgery. Because the study by Mangano and coworkers did not demonstrate any difference in in-hospital outcome, and the approach of Raby and colleagues demonstrated similar efficacy with respect to perioperative ischemia,[1] we suggest inducing general anesthesia or providing regional anesthesia before starting beta blocker therapy. If the induction is associated with tachycardia, then administration of esmolol is appropriate. After adequate anesthesia and analgesia are achieved, HR should be controlled and maintained below 70 beats/min. Feringa and coworkers[16] have demonstrated that higher doses of beta blockers and tight HR control are associated with reduced perioperative myocardial ischemia and troponin T release and with improved long-term outcome in vascular surgery patients.

STATIN THERAPY. In addition to their cholesterol-lowering properties, statins have anti-inflammatory and plaque-stabilizing properties (see Chap. 47). Given the potential mechanisms of perioperative MIs, statins could have theoretical benefits. Poldermans and colleagues performed a case-control study of 2816 patients who underwent major vascular surgery from 1991 to 2000. Statin therapy was significantly less common in patients experiencing a postoperative MI compared with controls (8% versus 25%; $P < 0.001$).[1] The adjusted odds ratio for perioperative mortality among statin users as compared with nonusers was 0.22 (95% CI, 0.10 to 0.47). Lindenauer and associates used administrative data to study a cohort of 780,591 patients; 77,082 patients (9.9%) received lipid-lowering therapy perioperatively, and 23,100 (2.96%) died during hospitalization.[1] Using multivariate modeling and propensity matching, the number needed to treat to prevent a postoperative death was 85 (95% CI, 77 to 98) and varied from 186 among patients at lowest risk to 30 among those with an RCRI score of 4 or more. Durazzo and colleagues randomized 100 patients to receive 20 mg atorvastatin or placebo once a day for 45 days.[1] The incidence of cardiac events was more than three times higher with placebo (26%) compared with atorvastatin (8%; $P < 0.031$). Patients given atorvastatin exhibited a significant decrease in the rate of cardiac events, compared with the placebo group, within 6 months after vascular surgery ($P < 0.018$). In DECREASE IV, Dunkelgrun and coworkers[33] used a 2 × 2 factorial design to evaluate high-dose fluvastatin and beta blockade in intermediate-risk patients. Nonsignificant reductions in cardiovascular death and MI were noted. Accumulating evidence suggests that statin therapy should continue during the perioperative period, and consideration should be given for starting statin therapy in high-risk patients, particularly those who meet the National Cholesterol Education Program's Adult Treatment Panel III's recommendations, because it could be argued that the patient should have been on a statin already.

NITROGLYCERIN. Only two randomized trials have evaluated the potential protective effect of prophylactic nitroglycerin for reducing perioperative cardiac complications after noncardiac surgery. In a small study by Coriat and colleagues in patients undergoing carotid endarterectomy, high-dose (1 μg/kg/min) nitroglycerin was more effective than low-dose (0.5 μg/kg/min) nitroglycerin in reducing the incidence of myocardial ischemia, but MI did not occur in either group.[1] The anesthetic used in this study was an oxygen-pancuronium-fentanyl method, and therefore inhalational agents were not administered. Dodds and associates have studied nitroglycerin versus placebo using a balanced anesthetic technique and reported no difference in the rates of myocardial ischemia or infarction.[1] Taken together, the evidence suggests that prophylactic nitroglycerin does not reduce the incidence of perioperative cardiac morbidity, although neither trial was powered to detect a modest benefit of nitroglycerin. Because prophylactic nitroglycerin has considerable hemodynamic effects and is not known to prevent MI or cardiac death, it would seem prudent to avoid the prophylactic use of nitroglycerin, although there are clear indications for its use once myocardial ischemia develops.

Nonpharmacologic Interventions

TEMPERATURE. Frank and coworkers completed a randomized trial of regional versus general anesthesia for lower extremity vascular bypass procedures and noted an association between hypothermia (temperature < 35°C) and myocardial ischemia.[1] They subsequently performed a trial in 300 high-risk patients undergoing a diverse group of intermediate-risk and high-risk procedures, randomizing patients to maintenance of normothermia or routine care. They observed a significantly reduced incidence of perioperative cardiac morbidity and mortality within 24 hours of surgery in the group that was kept normothermic.

ELECTROCARDIOGRAPHIC, HEMODYNAMIC, AND ECHOCARDIOGRAPHIC MONITORING. A number of studies have demonstrated the predictive value of correlating perioperative ST-segment changes and major cardiac events (see earlier). Furthermore, the duration of cumulative or continuous perioperative ST changes strongly predicts poor outcomes. ST-segment monitoring therefore has become a standard during the intraoperative and ICU periods for high-risk patients. Patients at low to moderate risk may also develop ST-segment changes, but these changes may not reflect true myocardial ischemia, as suggested in a recent series.[1]

The time of greatest risk of a postoperative cardiac event may be when the patient is on the ward and unmonitored. ST-segment telemetry monitors have not been tested to any large degree in the perioperative period. The issue of whether early treatment of prolonged ST-segment changes leads to improved outcomes remains unresolved. Until such studies are completed, the efficacy of such monitors remains debatable.

Much controversy surrounds the value of pulmonary artery catheterization for noncardiac surgery. Several small randomized trials did not demonstrate a significant reduction in major cardiac morbidity and mortality in patients undergoing aortic surgery. A large-scale cohort study by Polanczyk and colleagues, in which patients who had pulmonary catheters placed were matched to those who did not, that used a propensity score also failed to demonstrate any significant benefit.[1] An increased incidence of congestive heart failure and untoward noncardiac outcomes in the pulmonary artery catheter group were observed. A total of 1994 patients were randomized to goal-directed therapy guided by a pulmonary catheter, with standard care without the use of a pulmonary catheter for patients undergoing urgent or elective major surgery. No difference in survival occurred, but there was a higher rate of pulmonary embolism in the catheter group compared with the standard-care group. Therefore, current evidence does not support the routine use of pulmonary artery catheterization for high-risk patients undergoing major noncardiac surgery. Further work will be required to understand whether these results can be generalized to the high-risk vascular surgical population and to determine the benefits of pulmonary artery catheters in specific clinical situations.

Transesophageal echocardiography (TEE) represents another means of assessing intraoperative cardiac function (see Chap. 15). It is an extremely sensitive, noninvasive tool to monitor intraoperative wall motion abnormalities and fluid status. In patients undergoing aortic cross clamping, TEE proved to have a significantly better sensitivity for detecting intraoperative ischemia than electrocardiographic monitoring. For noncardiac surgery, a study of TEE, two-lead electrocardiography, and 12-lead electrocardiography demonstrated minimal additive value of TEE over two-lead electrocardiography. Although TEE for the routine monitoring of intraoperative ischemia in noncardiac surgery may have minimal additive value over ST-segment recording for predicting patients who will sustain perioperative morbidity, TEE monitoring may be valuable to guide treatment in patients with unstable hemodynamics for whom filling status and/or myocardial function are uncertain.

TRANSFUSION THRESHOLD. Much controversy surrounds the optimal hemoglobin level at which to transfuse high-risk noncardiac surgical patients. No randomized trials have evaluated the optimal transfusion threshold, although there is a great deal of anecdotal evidence. Several small cohort studies have shown that hematocrits in the 27% to 29% range represent the point below which the incidence of myocardial ischemia and potentially MI increases. A large-scale trial of transfusion triggers in the ICU did not document increased morbidity and mortality with a transfusion threshold of hemoglobin less than 7 g/dL, but there were trends toward increased morbidity in the subset of patients with ischemic heart disease.[1] The evidence suggests that patients with known ischemic heart disease that has not been revascularized should be maintained perioperatively with a hemoglobin level higher than 9 g/dL.

REFERENCES

Assessment of Risk

1. Fleisher LA, Beckman JA, Brown KA, et al: 2009 ACCF/AHA focused update on perioperative beta blockade incorporated into the ACC/AHA 2007 guidelines on perioperative cardiovascular evaluation and care for noncardiac surgery: A report of the American College of Cardiology Foundation/American Heart Association Task Force on Practice Guidelines. Circulation 120:e169, 2009.
2. Poldermans D, Bax JJ, Boersma E, et al: Guidelines for pre-operative cardiac risk assessment and perioperative cardiac management in non-cardiac surgery: The Task Force for Preoperative Cardiac Risk Assessment and Perioperative Cardiac Management in Non-cardiac Surgery of the European Society of Cardiology (ESC) and endorsed by the European Society of Anaesthesiology (ESA). Eur Heart J 30:2769, 2009.
3. Welten GM, Schouten O, van Domburg RT, et al: The influence of aging on the prognostic value of the revised cardiac risk index for postoperative cardiac complications in vascular surgery patients. Eur J Vasc Endovasc Surg 34:632, 2007.
4. Devereaux PJ, Yang H, Yusuf S, et al: Effects of extended-release metoprolol succinate in patients undergoing non-cardiac surgery (POISE trial): A randomised controlled trial. Lancet 371:1839, 2008.

Congenital and Valvular Heart Disease

5. Hammill BG, Curtis LH, Bennett-Guerrero E, et al: Impact of heart failure on patients undergoing major noncardiac surgery. Anesthesiology 108:559, 2008.
6. Cannesson M, Earing MG, Collange V, Kersten JR: Anesthesia for noncardiac surgery in adults with congenital heart disease. Anesthesiology 111:432, 2009.
7. Kovacs MJ, Kearon C, Rodger M, et al: Single-arm study of bridging therapy with low-molecular-weight heparin for patients at risk of arterial embolism who require temporary interruption of warfarin. Circulation 110:1658, 2004.
8. O'Donnell MJ, Kearon C, Johnson J, et al: Brief communication: Preoperative anticoagulant activity after bridging low-molecular-weight heparin for temporary interruption of warfarin. Ann Intern Med 146:184, 2007.
9. Douketis JD, Woods K, Foster GA, Crowther MA: Bridging anticoagulation with low-molecular-weight heparin after interruption of warfarin therapy is associated with a residual anticoagulant effect prior to surgery. Thromb Haemost 94:528, 2005.
10. Bonow RO, Carabello BA, Chatterjee K, et al: 2008 Focused update incorporated into the ACC/AHA 2006 guidelines for the management of patients with valvular heart disease: A report of the American College of Cardiology/American Heart Association Task Force on Practice Guidelines (Writing Committee to Revise the 1998 Guidelines for the Management of Patients With Valvular Heart Disease): Endorsed by the Society of Cardiovascular Anesthesiologists, Society for Cardiovascular Angiography and Interventions, and Society of Thoracic Surgeons. Circulation 118:e523, 2008.

Arrhythmias

11. Winkel TA, Schouten O, Hoeks SE, et al: Prognosis of transient new-onset atrial fibrillation during vascular surgery. Eur J Vasc Endovasc Surg 38:683, 2009.
12. Amar D, Zhang H, Roistacher N: The incidence and outcome of ventricular arrhythmias after noncardiac thoracic surgery. Anesth Analg 95:537, 2002.

Diagnostic Testing

13. Poldermans D, Bax JJ, Schouten O, et al: Should major vascular surgery be delayed because of preoperative cardiac testing in intermediate-risk patients receiving beta-blocker therapy with tight heart rate control? J Am Coll Cardiol 48:964, 2006.

Anesthesia and Postoperative Management

14. Rodgers A, Walker N, Schug S, et al: Reduction of postoperative mortality and morbidity with epidural or spinal anaesthesia: Results from overview of randomised trials. BMJ 321:1493, 2000.
15. Bhananker SM, Posner KL, Cheney FW, et al: Injury and liability associated with monitored anesthesia care: A closed claims analysis. Anesthesiology 104:228, 2006.
16. Feringa HH, Bax JJ, Boersma E, et al: High-dose beta-blockers and tight heart rate control reduce myocardial ischemia and troponin T release in vascular surgery patients. Circulation 114:I344, 2006.
17. Landesberg G, Beattie WS, Mosseri M, et al: Perioperative myocardial infarction. Circulation 119:2936, 2009.

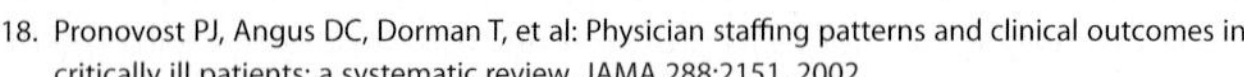

18. Pronovost PJ, Angus DC, Dorman T, et al: Physician staffing patterns and clinical outcomes in critically ill patients: a systematic review. JAMA 288:2151, 2002.
19. Mohler ER 3rd, Mantha S, Miller AB, et al: Should troponin and creatinine kinase be routinely measured after vascular surgery? Vasc Med 12:175, 2007.

Reducing Cardiac Risks

20. Mahla E, Baumann A, Rehak P, et al: N-terminal pro-brain natriuretic peptide identifies patients at high risk for adverse cardiac outcome after vascular surgery. Anesthesiology 106:1088, 2007.
21. Goei D, Schouten O, Boersma E, et al: Influence of renal function on the usefulness of N-terminal pro-B-type natriuretic peptide as a prognostic cardiac risk marker in patients undergoing noncardiac vascular surgery. Am J Cardiol 101:122, 2008.
22. Rodseth RN, Padayachee L, Biccard BM: A meta-analysis of the utility of pre-operative brain natriuretic peptide in predicting early and intermediate-term mortality and major adverse cardiac events in vascular surgical patients. Anaesthesia 63:1226, 2008.
23. Karthikeyan G, Moncur RA, Levine O, et al: Is a pre-operative brain natriuretic peptide or N-terminal pro-B-type natriuretic peptide measurement an independent predictor of adverse cardiovascular outcomes within 30 days of noncardiac surgery? A systematic review and meta-analysis of observational studies. J Am Coll Cardiol 54:1599, 2009.
24. McFalls EO, Ward HB, Moritz TE, et al: Coronary-artery revascularization before elective major vascular surgery. N Engl J Med 351:2795, 2004.
25. Poldermans D, Schouten O, Vidakovic R, et al: A clinical randomized trial to evaluate the safety of a noninvasive approach in high-risk patients undergoing major vascular surgery: The DECREASE-V Pilot Study. J Am Coll Cardiol 49:1763, 2007.
26. Schouten O, van Kuijk JP, Flu WJ, et al: Long-term outcome of prophylactic coronary revascularization in cardiac high-risk patients undergoing major vascular surgery (from the randomized DECREASE-V Pilot Study). Am J Cardiol 103:897, 2009.
27. Garcia S, Moritz TE, Ward HB, et al: Usefulness of revascularization of patients with multivessel coronary artery disease before elective vascular surgery for abdominal aortic and peripheral occlusive disease. Am J Cardiol 102:809, 2008.
28. Monaco M, Stassano P, Di Tommaso L, et al: Systematic strategy of prophylactic coronary angiography improves long-term outcome after major vascular surgery in medium- to high-risk patients: A prospective, randomized study. J Am Coll Cardiol 54:989, 2009.
29. Back MR, Leo F, Cuthbertson D, et al: Long-term survival after vascular surgery: specific influence of cardiac factors and implications for preoperative evaluation. J Vasc Surg 40:752, 2004.
30. Feringa HH, Elhendy A, Karagiannis SE, et al: Improving risk assessment with cardiac testing in peripheral arterial disease. Am J Med 120:531, 2007.
31. Godet G, Le Manach Y, Lesache F, et al: Drug-eluting stent thrombosis in patients undergoing non-cardiac surgery: is it always a problem? Br J Anaesth 100:472, 2008.
32. Anwaruddin S, Askari AT, Saudye H, et al: Characterization of post-operative risk associated with prior drug-eluting stent use. JACC Cardiovasc Interv 2:542, 2009.
33. Dunkelgrun M, Boersma E, Schouten O, et al: Bisoprolol and fluvastatin for the reduction of perioperative cardiac mortality and myocardial infarction in intermediate-risk patients undergoing noncardiovascular surgery: A randomized controlled trial (DECREASE-IV). Ann Surg 249:921, 2009.
34. Lindenauer PK, Pekow P, Wang K, et al: Perioperative beta-blocker therapy and mortality after major noncardiac surgery. N Engl J Med 353:349, 2005.
35. Chopra V, Eagle KA: Perioperative beta-blockers for cardiac risk reduction: Time for clarity. JAMA 303:551, 2010.

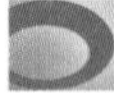

GUIDELINES Lee A. Fleisher and Joshua Beckman

Reducing Cardiac Risk with Noncardiac Surgery

Currently, specialty societies have published two sets of guidelines on perioperative cardiovascular evaluation and management for noncardiac surgery. An American College of Cardiology/American Heart Association (ACC/AHA) task force published guidelines in 1996, and updated them in 2009.[1] The Task Force for Preoperative Cardiac Risk Assessment and Perioperative Cardiac Management in Non-cardiac Surgery of the European Society of Cardiology (ESC), and endorsed by the European Society of Anaesthesiology (ESA), published guidelines in 2009.[2] The two sets of guidelines are similar and use a sequential algorithmic approach to testing, but differ in how they rate the evidence on beta-adrenergic receptor blocking agents (beta blockers). For details of the European guidelines, see additional content on the website.

The ACC/AHA guidelines emphasize the importance of a directed history and physical examination, including assessment of functional capacity and the revised cardiac risk index (RCRI) or Lee index risk factors. Risk factors include age older than 70 years, prior myocardial infarction, angina, congestive heart failure, prior cerebrovascular event, diabetes mellitus, and renal insufficiency. Clinicians should give attention to noncardiac comorbid conditions as well as cardiac issues. The ACC/AHA guidelines do not endorse any single risk prediction decision aid, but instead recommend a stepwise algorithm to identify patients most appropriate for noninvasive testing for further risk stratification (see Fig. 85-2). Each step includes the class of recommendation and the level of evidence.

ANCILLARY TESTING

ACC/AHA recommendations for the use of tests in patients undergoing noncardiac surgery are summarized in **Table 85G-1**. In the ACC/AHA guidelines, the routine 12-lead electrocardiogram (ECG) is recommended for patients undergoing vascular surgery or with at least one RCRI clinical risk factor. They recommend restraint in the use of ECGs for asymptomatic patients undergoing low-risk procedures. Routine use of echocardiography to assess left ventricular (LV) function is discouraged unless patients have worsening heart failure or dyspnea of unknown cause. Similarly, routine use of exercise or pharmacologic stress testing in asymptomatic patients without evidence of coronary artery disease is considered a Class III indication (not supported by evidence).

The ACC/AHA recommendations for the use of coronary revascularization (**Table 85G-2**) aim to improve the patient's long-term cardiovascular prognosis and minimize the risk of an acute complication during the procedure. In general, the same indications determine whether a nonsurgical patient warrants coronary angiography in the preoperative setting. For patients who require percutaneous revascularization, a strategy using balloon angioplasty alone or in conjunction with a bare metal stent is recommended because of the mandate for 12 months of dual antiplatelet therapy after drug-eluting stent deployment.[3] The ESC guidelines recommended that percutaneous coronary intervention (PCI) or coronary artery bypass grafting (CABG) be performed according to the applicable guidelines for management in stable angina pectoris. **Table 85G-3** lists the recommendations regarding timing of noncardiac surgery after coronary revascularization, particularly PCI. Both the ACC/AHA and ESC guidelines propose algorithms regarding the optimal management of surgery based on previous PCI (**Fig. 85G-1**; see website).[2]

RISK REDUCTION INTERVENTIONS

The ACC/AHA guidelines emphasize that "It is almost never appropriate to recommend coronary bypass surgery or other invasive interventions such as coronary angioplasty in an effort to reduce the risk of noncardiac surgery when they would not otherwise be indicated." Thus, they give more attention to medical therapies and monitoring interventions for higher-risk patients.

In 2009, ACC/AHA published a focused update on the perioperative use of beta blockers that responded to new data from clinical trials.[4] The updated guidelines support the use of beta blockers in various patient subgroups (**Fig. 85G-2**), especially patients with coronary heart disease or at high cardiac risk who are undergoing vascular surgery; those who are taking a beta blocker to treat angina, hypertension, or symptomatic arrhythmias; and those with other ACC/AHA Class I guideline recommendations. The guidelines are somewhat less supportive of beta blocker use in other populations, for whom the ideal target populations, doses, and routes of administration have yet to be delineated. The answers to practical questions, such as how, when, and how long to continue perioperative beta blocker therapy, also remain uncertain. The guidelines are uniform in the recommendation of dose titration to heart rate and blood pressure. A large clinical trial has shown that administration of oral, long-acting beta blockers initiated at the time of surgery in the absence of dose titration results in increased total mortality and stroke.[5] This strategy received a Class III (not supported by the evidence and may be harmful) recommendation. The ESC guidelines are more supportive of perioperative beta blockers; they are recommended for patients who have known ischemic heart disease (IHD) or myocardial ischemia according to preoperative stress testing, and for patients scheduled for high-risk surgery.

TABLE 85G-1 Recommendations for Noninvasive Stress Testing Before Noncardiac Surgery

Class I

1. Patients with active cardiac conditions in whom noncardiac surgery is planned should be evaluated and treated per ACC/AHA guidelines* before noncardiac surgery (level of evidence: B).

Class IIa

1. Noninvasive stress testing of patients with three or more clinical risk factors and poor functional capacity (less than 4 METs) who require vascular surgery† is reasonable if it will change management (level of evidence: B).

Class IIb

1. Noninvasive stress testing may be considered for patients with at least one or two clinical risk factors and poor functional capacity (less than 4 metabolic equivalents [METs]) who require intermediate risk or vascular surgery if it will change management (level of evidence: B).

Class III

1. Noninvasive testing is not useful for patients with no clinical risk factors undergoing intermediate-risk noncardiac surgery (level of evidence: C).
2. Noninvasive testing is not useful for patients undergoing low-risk noncardiac surgery (level of evidence: C).

*See Fleisher and colleagues[1] for the following references: ACC/AHA/ESC Guidelines for the Management of Patients With Atrial Fibrillation,[108] ACC/AHA/ACP Guidelines for the Management of Patients with Chronic Stable Angina,[188] ACC/AHA 2005 Guideline Update for the Diagnosis and Management of Chronic Heart Failure in the Adult,[189] ACC/AHA Guidelines for the Management of Patients with ST-Elevation Myocardial Infarction,[49] ACC/AHA/ESC Guidelines for the Management of Patients With Supraventricular Arryhthmias,[190] ACC/AHA 2002 Guideline Update for the Management of Patients With Unstable Angina and Non-ST-Segment Elevation Myocardial Infarction[187] ACC/AHA 2006 Guidelines for the Management of Patients With Valvular Heart Disease,[102] and ACC/AHA/ESC Guidelines for the Management of Patients With Ventricular Arrhythmias and the Prevention of Sudden Cardiac Death.[191]

†Vascular surgery is defined by emergency aortic and other major vascular surgery and peripheral vascular surgery.

From Fleisher LA, Beckman JA, Brown KA, et al: 2009 ACCF/AHA focused update on perioperative beta blockade incorporated into the ACC/AHA 2007 guidelines on perioperative cardiovascular evaluation and care for noncardiac surgery. J Am Coll Cardiol 54:e13, 2009.

TABLE 85G-2 Preoperative Coronary Revascularization with CABG or Percutaneous Coronary Intervention

Class I*

1. Coronary revascularization before noncardiac surgery is useful in patients with stable angina who have significant left main coronary artery stenosis (level of evidence: A).
2. Coronary revascularization before noncardiac surgery is useful in patients with stable angina who have three-vessel disease (survival benefit is greater when LV ejection fraction [EF] is less than 0.50; level of evidence: A).
3. Coronary revascularization before noncardiac surgery is useful in patients with stable angina who have two-vessel disease with significant proximal left anterior descending artery stenosis and either EF less than 0.50 or demonstrable ischemia on noninvasive testing (level of evidence: A).
4. Coronary revascularization before noncardiac surgery is recommended for patients with high-risk unstable angina or non–ST-segment elevation myocardial infarction (MI; level of evidence: A).
5. Coronary revascularization before noncardiac surgery is recommended for patients with acute ST-elevation MI (level of evidence: A).

Class IIa

1. In patients in whom coronary revascularization with PCI is appropriate for mitigation of cardiac symptoms and who need elective noncardiac surgery in the subsequent 12 months, a strategy of balloon angioplasty or bare metal stent placement followed by 4 to 6 weeks of dual antiplatelet therapy is probably indicated (level of evidence: B).
2. In patients who have received drug-eluting coronary stents and who must undergo urgent surgical procedures that mandate the discontinuation of thienopyridine therapy, it is reasonable to continue aspirin if at all possible and restart the thienopyridine as soon as possible (level of evidence: C).

Class IIb

1. The usefulness of preoperative coronary revascularization is not well established in high-risk ischemic patients (e.g., abnormal dobutamine stress echocardiogram, with at least five segments of wall motion abnormalities; level of evidence: C).
2. The usefulness of preoperative coronary revascularization is not well established for low-risk ischemic patients with an abnormal dobutamine stress echocardiogram (segments 1 to 4; level of evidence: B).

Class III

1. It is not recommended that routine prophylactic coronary revascularization be performed in patients with stable coronary artery disease (CAD) before noncardiac surgery (level of evidence: B).
2. Elective noncardiac surgery is not recommended within 4 to 6 weeks of bare metal coronary stent implantation or within 12 months of drug-eluting coronary stent implantation in patients for whom thienopyridine therapy, or aspirin and thienopyridine therapy, will need to be discontinued perioperatively (level of evidence: B).
3. Elective noncardiac surgery is not recommended within 4 weeks of coronary revascularization with balloon angioplasty (level of evidence: B).

*All Class I indications are consistent with the ACC/AHA 2004 Guideline Update for Coronary Artery Bypass Graft Surgery. (Eagle KA, Guyton RA, Davidoff R, et al: ACC/AHA 2004 guideline update for coronary artery bypass graft surgery: A report of the American College of Cardiology/American Heart Association Task Force on Practice Guidelines [Committee to Update the 1999 Guidelines for Coronary Artery Bypass Graft Surgery]. Circulation 110:e340-437, 2004).

From Fleisher LA, Beckman JA, Brown KA, et al: 2009 ACCF/AHA focused update on perioperative beta blockade incorporated into the ACC/AHA 2007 guidelines on perioperative cardiovascular evaluation and care for noncardiac surgery. J Am Coll Cardiol 54:e13, 2009.

CH 85

TABLE 85G-3 Recommendations on Timing of Noncardiac Surgery in Cardiac-Stable or Asymptomatic Patients with Prior Revascularization

RECOMMENDATIONS	CLASS OF RECOMMENDATION	LEVEL OF EVIDENCE
It is recommended that patients with previous CABG in the last 5 years be sent for noncardiac surgery without further delay.	I	C
It is recommended that noncardiac surgery be performed in patients with recent bare metal stent implantation after a minimum of 6 weeks and optimally 3 months following the intervention.	I	B
It is recommended that noncardiac surgery be performed in patients with recent drug-eluting stent implantation no sooner than 12 months following the intervention.	I	B
Consideration should be given to postponing noncardiac surgery in patients with recent balloon angioplasty until at least 2 weeks following the intervention.	IIa	B

From Poldermans D, Bax JJ, Boersma E, et al: Guidelines for pre-operative cardiac risk assessment and perioperative cardiac management in non-cardiac surgery: The Task Force for Preoperative Cardiac Risk Assessment and Perioperative Cardiac Management in Non-cardiac Surgery of the European Society of Cardiology (ESC) and endorsed by the European Society of Anaesthesiology (ESA). Eur Heart J 30:2769-812, 2009.

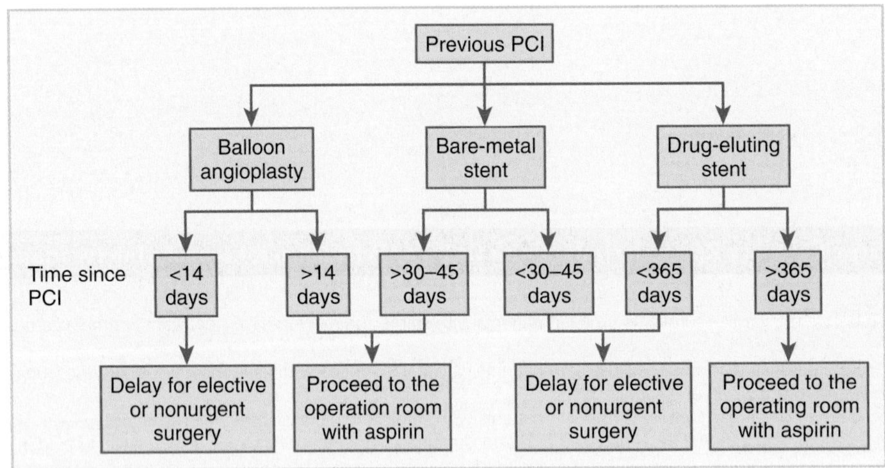

FIGURE 85G-1 Proposed approach to the management of patients with previous PCI requiring noncardiac surgery. *(From Fleisher LA, Beckman JA, Brown KA, et al: 2009 ACCF/AHA focused update on perioperative beta blockade incorporated into the ACC/AHA 2007 guidelines on perioperative cardiovascular evaluation and care for noncardiac surgery. J Am Coll Cardiol 54:e13, 2009.)*

Similar to the ACC/AHA guidelines, continuation of beta blockers is recommended for patients previously treated with beta blockers because of IHD, arrhythmias, or hypertension (see website).

Intraoperative nitroglycerin is supported for patients with acute ischemic syndromes who must undergo urgent noncardiac procedures. The ACC/AHA guidelines warn that prophylactic use of nitroglycerin must take into account the anesthetic plan and patient's hemodynamics, and must recognize the risk of vasodilation and hypovolemia during anesthesia and surgery. The ACC/AHA task force did not find sufficient evidence to balance risks and benefits of intra-aortic balloon counterpulsation for patients with myocardial ischemic syndromes or routine use of transesophageal echocardiography.

The ACC/AHA guidelines acknowledge that the use of a pulmonary artery catheter (PAC) may be reasonable for patients at risk for major hemodynamic disturbances easily detected by a PAC. However, because incorrect interpretation of data from a PAC may cause harm, the decision must be based on three parameters—patient disease, surgical procedure (i.e., intraoperative and postoperative fluid shifts), and practice setting (experience in PAC use and interpretation of results). ST-segment monitoring to detect perioperative ischemia in patients with coronary heart disease can be useful, but the guidelines acknowledge that no studies have shown that this intervention directs therapy that improves outcome.

According to the ACC/AHA guidelines, perioperative surveillance for acute coronary syndromes using routine electrocardiography and cardiac serum biomarkers is unnecessary for clinically low-risk patients undergoing low-risk procedures. In patients with high or intermediate clinical risk with known or suspected coronary artery disease who are undergoing high- or intermediate-risk procedures, the guidelines recommend performance of electrocardiography at baseline, immediately after the surgical procedure, and daily on the first 2 days after surgery. The guidelines support cardiac troponin measurements for detection of myocardial injury in patients with evidence of myocardial ischemia, but not their routine measurement.

2007 Perioperative guideline recommendations	2009 Perioperative focused update recommendations	Comments
	Class I	
1. Beta blockers should be continued in patients undergoing surgery who are receiving beta blockers to treat angina, symptomatic arrhythmias, hypertension, or other ACC/AHA Class I guideline indications. *(Level of Evidence: C)*	1. Beta blockers should be continued in patients undergoing surgery who are receiving beta blockers for treatment of conditions with ACCF/AHA Class I guideline indications for the drugs. *(Level of Evidence: C)*	2007 recommendation remains current in 2009 update with revised wording.
2. Beta blockers should be given to patients undergoing vascular surgery who are at high cardiac risk owing to the finding of ischemia on preoperative testing. *(Level of Evidence: B)*		Deleted/combined recommendation (class of recommendation changed from I to IIa for patients with cardiac ischemia on preoperative testing).
	Class IIa	
1. Beta blockers are probably recommended for patients undergoing vascular surgery in whom preoperative assessment indentifies coronary heart disease. *(Level of Evidence: B)*	1. Beta blockers titrated to heart rate and blood pressure are probably recommended for patients undergoing vascular surgery who are at high cardiac risk owing to coronary artery disease or the finding of cardiac ischemia on preoperative testing. *(Level of Evidence: B)*	Modified/combined recommendation (wording revised and class of recommendation changed from I to IIa for patients with cardiac ischemia on preoperative testing).
2. Beta blockers are probably recommended for patients in whom preoperative assessment for vascular surgery identifies high cardiac risk, as defined by the presence of more than 1 clinical risk factor.* *(Level of Evidence: B)*	2. Beta blockers titrated to heart rate and blood pressure are reasonable for patients in whom preoperative assessment for vascular surgery identifies high cardiac risk, as defined by the presence of more than 1 clinical risk factor.* *(Level of Evidence: C)*	Modified recommendation (level of evidence changed from B to C).
3. Beta blockers are probably recommended for patients in whom preoperative assessment identifies coronary heart disease or high cardiac risk, as defined by the presence of more than 1 clinical risk factor,* who are undergoing intermediate-risk or vascular surgery. *(Level of Evidence: B)*	3. Beta blockers titrated to heart rate and blood pressure are reasonable for patients in whom preoperative assessment identifies coronary artery disease or high cardiac risk, as defined by the presence of more than 1 clinical risk factor,* who are undergoing intermediate-risk surgery. *(Level of Evidence: B)*	2007 recommendation remains current in 2009 update with revised wording.
	Class IIb	
1. The usefulness of beta blockers is uncertain for patients who are undergoing either intermediate-risk procedures or vascular surgery, in whom preoperative assessment identifies a single clinical risk factor.* *(Level of Evidence: C)*	1. The usefulness of beta blockers is uncertain for patients who are undergoing either intermediate-risk procedures or vascular surgery in whom preoperative assessment identifies a single clinical risk factor in the absence of coronary artery disease.* *(Level of Evidence: C)*	2007 recommendation remains current in 2009 update with revised wording.
2. The usefulness of beta blockers is uncertain in patients undergoing vascular surgery with no clinical risk factors who are not currently taking beta blockers. *(Level of Evidence: B)*	2. The usefulness of beta blockers is uncertain for patients undergoing vascular surgery with no clinical risk factors* who are not currently taking beta blockers. *(Level of Evidence: B)*	2007 recommendation remains current in 2009 update.
	Class III	
1. Beta blockers should not be given to patients undergoing surgery who have absolute contraindications to beta blockade. *(Level of Evidence: B)*	1. Beta blockers should not be given to patients undergoing surgery who have absolute contraindications to beta blockade. *(Level of Evidence: C)*	2007 recommendation remains current in 2009 update.
	2. Routine administration of high-dose beta blockers in the absence of dose titration is not useful and may be harmful to patients not currently taking beta blockers who are undergoing noncardiac surgery. *(Level of Evidence: B)*	New recommendation

* Clinical risk factors include history of ischemic heart disease, history of compensated or prior heart failure, history of cerebrovascular disease, diabetes mellitus, and renal insufficiency (defined in the Revised Cardiac Risk Index as a preoperative serum creatinine of >2 mg/dL). ACC indicates American College of Cardiology; and AHA, American Heart Association.

FIGURE 85G-2 ACC/AHA recommendations for use of perioperative beta blockers. *(From Fleischmann KE, Beckman JA, Buller CE, et al: 2009 ACCF/AHA focused update on perioperative beta blockade. J Am Coll Cardiol 54:2102, 2009.)*

REFERENCES

1. Fleisher LA, Beckman JA, Brown KA, et al: 2009 ACCF/AHA focused update on perioperative beta blockade incorporated into the ACC/AHA 2007 guidelines on perioperative cardiovascular evaluation and care for noncardiac surgery. J Am Coll Cardiol 54:e13, 2009.
2. Poldermans D, Bax JJ, Boersma E, et al: Guidelines for pre-operative cardiac risk assessment and perioperative cardiac management in non-cardiac surgery: The Task Force for Preoperative Cardiac Risk Assessment and Perioperative Cardiac Management in Non-cardiac Surgery of the European Society of Cardiology (ESC) and endorsed by the European Society of Anaesthesiology (ESA). Eur Heart J 30:2769, 2009.
3. Grines CL, Bonow RO, Casey DE Jr, et al: Prevention of premature discontinuation of dual antiplatelet therapy in patients with coronary artery stents: A science advisory from the American Heart Association, American College of Cardiology, Society for Cardiovascular Angiography and Interventions, American College of Surgeons, and American Dental Association, with representation from the American College of Physicians. J Am Coll Cardiol 49:734, 2007.
4. Fleischmann KE, Beckman JA, Buller CE, et al: 2009 ACCF/AHA focused update on perioperative beta blockade. J Am Coll Cardiol 54:2102, 2009.
5. Devereaux PJ, Yang H, Yusuf S, et al: Effects of extended-release metoprolol succinate in patients undergoing non-cardiac surgery (POISE trial): A randomised controlled trial. Lancet 371:1839, 2008.

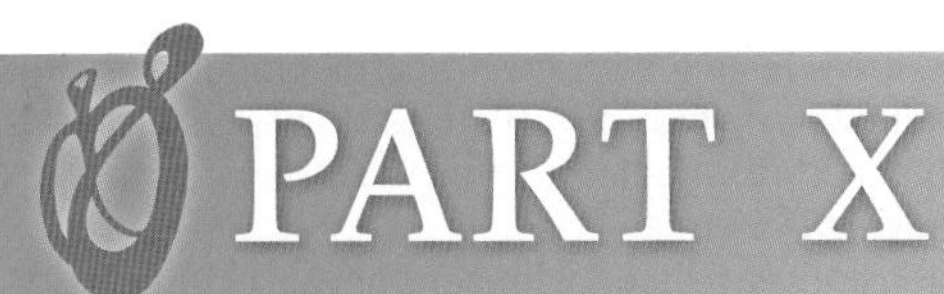

PART X

CARDIOVASCULAR DISEASE AND DISORDERS OF OTHER ORGANS

CHAPTER 86 Endocrine Disorders and Cardiovascular Disease

Irwin Klein

Medical science has few areas in which basic science investigation is linked more closely to clinical observations and therapy than in cardiovascular endocrinology. As our understanding of the cellular and molecular effects of various hormones has evolved, we can better understand the clinical manifestations that arise from excess hormone secretion and glandular failure, leading to hormone deficiency states. More than 200 years ago, English physician Caleb Hillier Parry described a woman with goiter and palpitations whose "each systole shook the whole thorax." He was the first to suggest a connection between diseases of the heart and enlargement of the thyroid gland. The cardiovascular abnormalities associated with pathologic changes of endocrine glands were recognized before the identification of the specific hormones produced by these glands. This chapter reviews the spectrum of cardiac disease states that arise from changes in specific endocrine function. This approach allows us to explore the cellular mechanisms whereby various hormones can alter the cardiovascular system through actions on cardiac myocytes, vascular smooth muscle cells, and other target cells and tissues.

Pituitary Gland

The pituitary gland consists of two distinct anatomic portions. The anterior pituitary, or adenohypophysis, contains six different cell types; five of these produce polypeptide or glycoprotein hormones, and the sixth is classically referred to as being composed of nonsecretory chromophobic cells. Of these cell types, the somatotropic cells, which secrete human growth hormone (hGH), and the corticotropic cells, which produce adrenocorticotropic hormone (ACTH), can contribute to cardiac disease. The posterior pituitary, or neurohypophysis, is the anatomic location for the nerve terminals that secrete vasopressin (antidiuretic hormone) or oxytocin.

Growth Hormone

In adults, excessive growth hormone secretion before the fusion of bony epiphysis leads to gigantism, whereas increased secretion of hGH after maturation of the long bones leads to acromegaly. Growth hormone exerts its cellular effects through two major pathways. The first is by hormone binding to specific growth hormone receptors on target cells. These receptors have been identified in the heart, skeletal muscle, fat, liver, and kidneys, as well as in many additional cell types throughout fetal development.[1] The second growth-promoting effect of hGH results from stimulation of synthesis of insulin-like growth factor type 1 (IGF-1). This protein is produced primarily in the liver, but other cell types can produce IGF-1 under the influence of hGH.

Shortly after the identification of the IGF family, it was proposed that most actions of growth hormone are mediated through this second messenger. Clinical disease activity of patients with growth hormone excess (acromegaly) correlates better with serum levels of IGF-1 than with hGH levels. The ability to promote glucose uptake and cellular protein synthesis gave rise to the term *insulin-like*. IGF-1 binds to its cognate IGF-1 receptor, localized on almost all cell types. Transgenic experiments have demonstrated that the presence of IGF-1 receptors on cell types is closely linked to the ability of those cells to divide. Studies in which the IGF-1 receptor was overexpressed in cardiac myocytes reportedly produced an increased myocyte number and mitotic rate, and enhanced the replication of postdifferentiated myocytes. The harnessing of this action potentially could benefit genetic manipulation and repair of the diseased myocardium.

Infusion of hGH or IGF-1 acutely changes hemodynamics. The acute increases in cardiac contractility and cardiac output may be caused, at least in part, by a decrease in systemic vascular resistance and cardiac afterload.[2] Short-term administration of hGH and IGF-1 does not increase blood pressure, implying that the increase in cardiac output results from changes in systemic vascular resistance.[3,4]

Cardiovascular Manifestations of Acromegaly

Acromegaly is a relatively uncommon condition (approximately 900 new cases each year in the United States). Acromegaly and pituitary-dependent human gigantism are associated with markedly increased morbidity and mortality, primarily from cardiovascular disease. Untreated acromegaly, identified by its characteristic clinical signs and symptoms and by increased hGH secretion, markedly shortens life expectancy, with less than 20% of patients surviving beyond 60 years. Multiple studies have implicated increased neoplasia arising from the gastrointestinal tract, colon polyps, colon cancer, and pulmonary disease in this increased mortality.[5] However, cardiovascular and cerebrovascular changes, including hypertension, cardiomegaly, congestive heart failure, and cerebral vascular accidents, are the major events that limit survival.[6]

The cardiovascular and hemodynamic effects of acromegaly vary considerably depending on age, severity of disease, and disease duration.[7] Patients diagnosed with less than 5 years of disease activity had no significant change in systolic or diastolic blood pressure, but echocardiographic determination of left ventricular mass index increased almost 35% and cardiac index increased 24%.[8] Measures of systolic function, including stroke index, increased significantly, and systemic vascular resistance rose by 20%. Left ventricular diastolic function was normal.[6] These studies contrast with reports that longer duration of acromegaly produces left ventricular dysfunction and cardiomyopathy. In untreated acromegaly, global left ventricular diastolic dysfunction accompanies cardiac hypertrophy. Regional myocardial systolic strain abnormalities, identified by Doppler imaging, reversed with treatment.[9]

Known cardiac disease risk factors—including hypertension, insulin resistance, diabetes mellitus, and hyperlipidemia—frequently occur in patients with acromegaly. Although initial reports suggested that accelerated atherosclerosis caused impairment of cardiac function in long-standing acromegaly, a postmortem study revealed significant coronary artery disease in only 11% of patients dying from disease-related causes. Angiography shows normal or dilated coronary arteries in most cases. Nuclear stress testing is positive in less than 25% of patients, indicating that atherosclerosis and ischemic heart disease are unlikely to account for the marked degrees of biventricular cardiac hypertrophy, cardiac failure, and cardiovascular mortality. A rather specific functional and histologic myocyte change appears to arise from prolonged excess serum levels of hGH and IGF-1.[8] As many as two thirds of acromegaly patients have echocardiographic criteria for left ventricular hypertrophy (LVH).[6,7] Right ventricular mass also increases in acromegaly, indicating a more generalized process beyond systemic hypertension.[9] Asymmetrical septal hypertrophy, initially thought to be common in patients with acromegaly, is an unusual finding. Acromegaly increases the prevalence of aortic and mitral valve disease, which persists despite disease cure.[10] Progressive mitral valve regurgitation and left ventricular strain occur in patients with uncontrolled acromegaly.[11] Acromegaly patients may present with dilation of the aortic root and/or defects of the cardiac conduction system.[7,12]

Histologic evaluation of acromegaly cardiac tissue reveals an increase in myocyte size (hypertrophy) without an increase in cell number. Acromegaly produces interstitial fibrosis and infiltration of a variety of inflammatory cells, including mononuclear cells consistent with myocarditis.[6] The absence of cell necrosis in the presence of an inflammatory reaction has raised the question of whether some of these histologic findings can be accounted for by IGF-1–promoted programmed cell death (apoptosis).

Functional changes accompany pathologic involvement of the heart in acromegaly.[8,9] Although approximately 10% of newly diagnosed patients have signs and symptoms of cardiac compromise, this percentage increases markedly with disease duration.[11-13] Some studies have reported a low incidence of overt left ventricular failure, suggesting that supervening factors, including hypertension, type 2 diabetes, and hyperlipidemia, are necessary to impair function. In acromegaly, LVH and congestive heart failure can occur in long-standing disease without hypertension, indicating that high levels of growth hormone and/or IGF-1 can produce cardiac myopathic changes per se. Successful therapy reverses many, if not all, of these findings.[14,15]

Abnormalities on the electrocardiogram (ECG), including left axis deviation, septal Q waves, ST-T wave depression, abnormal QT dispersion, and conduction system defects, occur in up to 50% of acromegaly patients. A variety of dysrhythmias can occur, including atrial and ventricular ectopic beats, sick sinus syndrome, and supraventricular and ventricular tachycardias.[6] Fourfold increases in complex ventricular arrhythmias and late potentials observed in a signal-averaged ECG, thought to be predictors of ventricular irritability, were also more common in active acromegaly when compared with treated patients.[12] In contrast, exercise stress testing with electrocardiographic monitoring did not show inducible rhythm disturbances or evidence of ischemia, suggesting that left ventricular rhythm disturbances are not related to any underlying ischemia.

Secondary hypertension associated with acromegaly occurs in 20% to 40% of patients.[5-7] Given the overall high prevalence rate of hypertension in the adult population and the insidious onset of acromegaly, determining whether hypertension is secondary or merely coincidental is difficult. Improvement with therapy, however, suggests that they are related.[15] Although observational studies of survival in acromegaly initially suggested that hypertension was not an independent risk factor for mortality, a survey of patients dying of the disease found that mean blood pressures were higher than in those who survived.[5] The mechanism underlying hypertension in acromegaly is not clearly understood. Newly diagnosed patients with short-duration disease had systolic and diastolic blood pressures no different from those in age- and sex-matched controls, whereas the cardiac index was significantly increased. In long-standing acromegaly patients, the arterial intimal thickness is increased, and these changes respond to hGH lowering.[2]

Growth hormone administration promotes sodium retention and volume expansion, and appears to have a potent antinatriuretic effect independent of any effect on aldosterone.[3,16] Studies of the renin-angiotensin-aldosterone system have shown a failure to inhibit renin release optimally by volume expansion. Angiotensin II inhibitors cause a paradoxical increase in blood pressure in patients with acromegaly. The role of hyperinsulinemia in the hypertension of acromegaly has been questioned. Increased serum insulin can contribute to urinary sodium retention, impairment of endothelial-dependent vasodilation, and increased sympathetic activity.

DIAGNOSIS. In 99% of cases, acromegaly arises from benign adenomas of the anterior pituitary gland.[5,15] At diagnosis, most of these neoplasms are classified as macroadenomas (>10 mm), and patients have clinical evidence of disease for longer than 10 years. The diagnosis can be confirmed by demonstrating a serum growth hormone level higher than 5 ng/dL and a serum IGF-1 level higher than 300 mIU/mL, measured 1 hour after a 100-g glucose load. In most patients, fasting growth hormone levels are higher than 10 ng/mL. Tumor localization can be established by magnetic resonance imaging (MRI) dedicated to the pituitary gland. Rarely, growth hormone–releasing hormone (GH-RH) can be secreted, causing diffuse hyperplasia of the pituitary. Such changes must prompt consideration of a neoplastic lesion residing in other parts (ectopic) of the endocrine system.

THERAPY. Transsphenoidal surgery with resection of the adenoma is the procedure of choice for initial management. If hGH and/or IGF-1 levels remain elevated, radiotherapy in older patients or dopamine or somatostatin receptor agonists in younger patients can restore normal serum growth hormone and IGF-1 levels. Octreotide acetate is a pharmacologic analogue to somatostatin and is effective in the vast majority of patients to lower hGH to less than 5 ng/mL. Primary therapy might involve lowering IGF-1 levels and shrinking tumor size in selected cases.[15,17] The cardiovascular complications of acromegaly, including hypertension, LVH, and left ventricular dysfunction, improve with treatment, and survival is significantly better in patients achieving disease remission.[7,11] Pegvisomant, a growth hormone receptor antagonist, can normalize IGF-1 levels in long-term therapy and may play a role in somatostatin-resistant patients.[14]

Adrenal Gland

Adrenocorticotropic Hormone and Cortisol

The adrenocorticotropic cells in the anterior pituitary synthesize a large protein (pro-opiomelanocortin), which is then processed within the corticotropic cell into a family of smaller proteins that include alpha-melanocyte–stimulating hormone, beta-endorphin, and ACTH. ACTH, in turn, binds to specific cells within the adrenal gland. The adrenal gland anatomically consists of two major segments, the cortex and medulla.

The cortex zona glomerulosa produces aldosterone and the zona fasciculata produces primarily cortisol and some androgenic steroids. The zona reticularis also produces cortisol and androgens. ACTH regulates the synthesis of cortisol in the zona fasciculata and reticularis. The zona glomerulosa shows much less ACTH responsiveness and responds primarily to angiotensin II by increased aldosterone secretion.

Cushing Disease

Excess cortisol secretion and its attendant clinical disease states can arise from excess pituitary release of ACTH (Cushing disease) or through the adenomatous or rarely malignant neoplastic process arising in the adrenal gland itself (Cushing syndrome). Well-characterized conditions of adrenal glucocorticoid and mineralocorticoid excess appear to result from the excessively high levels of (ectopic) ACTH produced by small cell carcinoma of the lung, carcinoid tumors, pancreatic islet cell tumors, medullary thyroid cancer, and other adenocarcinomas and hematologic malignancies.

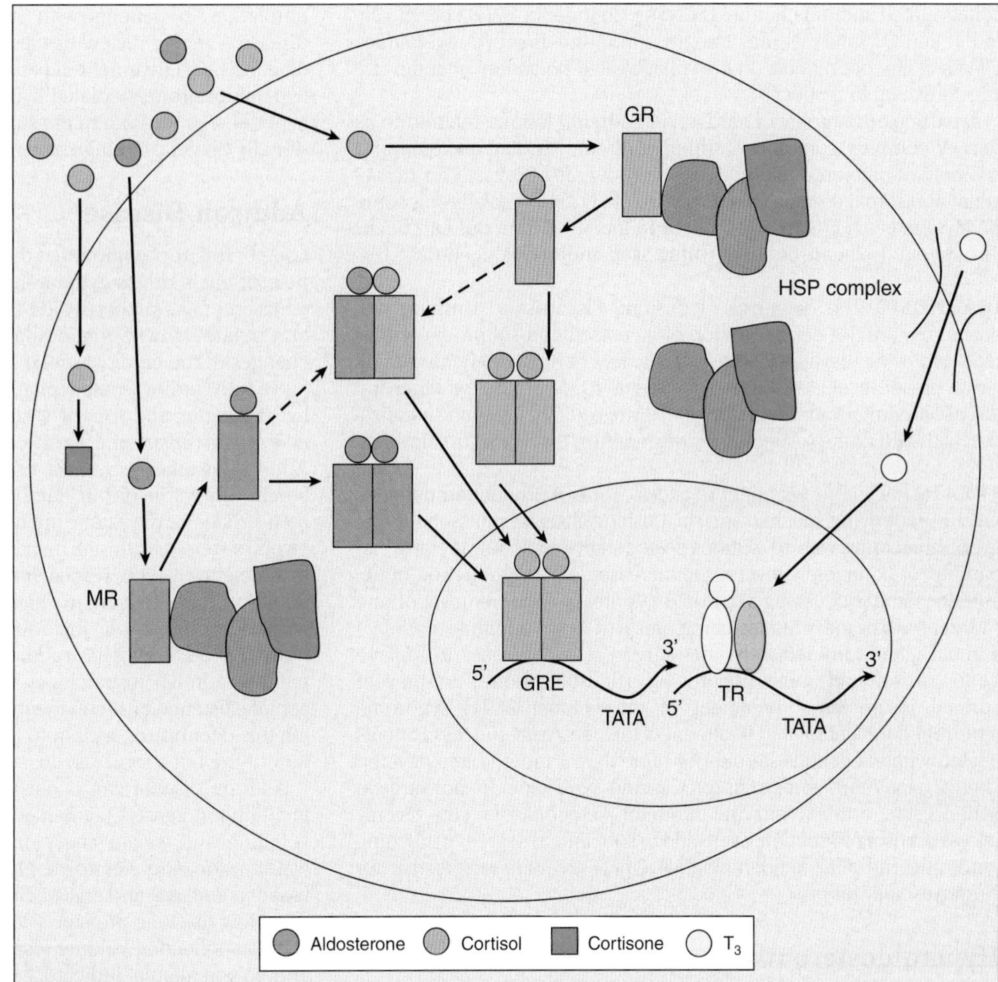

FIGURE 86-1 Schematic representation of a generalized nuclear hormone receptor mechanism of action. The mineralocorticoid receptor (MR) has similar affinities for aldosterone and cortisol. Circulating levels of cortisol are 100 to 1000 times greater than that of aldosterone. In MR-responsive cells, the enzyme 11-beta-hydroxysteroid dehydrogenase metabolizes cortisol to cortisone, thereby allowing aldosterone to bind to MR. MR and the glucocorticoid receptor (GR) are cytoplasmic receptors that after binding ligand, translocate to the nucleus and bind to glucocorticoid response elements (GREs) in the promoter regions of responsive genes. T_3 is transported into the cell via specific membrane proteins and binds to thyroid hormone receptors (TRs), which are bound to TREs in the promoter regions of T_3-responsive genes. HSP = heat shock protein; TATA = TATA box promoter region. *(Courtesy of Dr. S. Danzi.)*

Cortisol, a member of the glucocorticoid family of steroid hormones, binds to monomeric receptors located within the cytoplasm of many cell types (**Fig. 86-1**). The unliganded glucocorticoid receptors are bound to heat shock protein complexes. After binding cortisol, the receptors dissociate from these complexes, homodimerize or occasionally heterodimerize, translocate to the nucleus, and function as transcription factors. Several cardiac genes contain glucocorticoid response elements in their promoter regions that confer glucocorticoid responsiveness.[18] These genes include those that encode the voltage-gated potassium channel, as well as protein kinases, which serve to phosphorylate and regulate voltage-gated sodium channels. This expression may be chamber-specific and play a role in the developing fetal heart.[19]

The cardiac effects of glucocorticoid excess in Cushing disease rise from the effects of glucocorticoids on the heart, liver, skeletal muscle, and fat tissue.[18-20] Accelerated atherosclerosis can result from abnormal glucose metabolism with hyperglycemia and hyperinsulinemia, hypertension, and altered clotting and platelet function. The mechanism for cortisol-mediated hypertension is multifactorial. In contrast to aldosterone-induced hypertension, the central administration of glucocorticoids lowers blood pressure.[21] Thus, cortisol-mediated hypertension appears not to result from activation of the mineralocorticoid receptor. In addition, antagonism of glucocorticoid effects via its cytosolic receptor can block cortisol-induced elevations of glucose and insulin levels, but not those related to blood pressure.[22,23] Interestingly, one study has suggested that inhibition of sodium retention is also insufficient to block the cortisol-mediated rise in blood pressure, pointing to the changes in vascular reactivity, systemic vascular resistance, and nitric oxide–mediated vasodilation as candidates for the hypertensive effect.[18]

The rise in serum glucose levels and the development of insulin resistance may activate proinflammatory cytokines such as tumor necrosis factor-α and interleukin-6 (IL-6), which may underlie the accelerated atherosclerosis of insulin resistance found in other endocrine disease states.[22] Thus, although typically acting as an anti-inflammatory hormone, cortisol excess can promote inflammation and accelerate atherosclerosis by producing insulin resistance, changes in corticosteroid binding protein, and regulation of proinflammatory cytokines.[24] The centripetal obesity characteristic of glucocorticoid excess resembles that seen in the insulin resistance syndromes. Excess androgen production resulting from increased ACTH stimulation of the adrenal cortex may also accelerate atherosclerosis in men and women.

The increased cardiovascular morbidity and mortality of Cushing syndrome can in large part be explained by cerebrovascular disease, peripheral vascular disease, coronary artery disease with myocardial infarction, and chronic congestive heart failure.[20,23] All expected changes in the setting of accelerated atherosclerosis result from hypertension and hyperlipidemia. Studies of left ventricular structure and function have shown hypertrophy and impaired contractility in 40% of patients.[25] Cushing syndrome can present as dilated cardiomyopathy.[26] In addition, the marked muscle weakness resulting from corticosteroid-induced skeletal myopathy contributes to impaired exercise tolerance.

Patients with Cushing disease can exhibit a variety of electrocardiographic changes. The duration of the P-R interval appears to correlate inversely with adrenal cortisol production rates. The mechanism underlying this may relate to the expression or regulation of the voltage-gated sodium channel (SCN5A). Changes in ECGs, specifically in P-R and QT intervals, may also arise from the direct (nongenomic) effects of glucocorticoids on the voltage-gated potassium channel (Kv 1.5) in excitable tissues.[18,20]

A particular complex of cardiac and adrenal lesions, referred to as Carney complex, combines Cushing syndrome, cardiac myxoma, and a variety of pigmented dermal lesions (not café-au-lait).[27] This monogenic autosomal dominant trait maps to the Q2 region of chromosome 17. Myxomas most commonly occur in the left atrium but can occur throughout the heart, occur at young ages, and be multicentric.

DIAGNOSIS. The diagnosis of Cushing disease and Cushing syndrome require the demonstration of increased cortisol production as reflected by an elevated 24-hour, urinary-free cortisol or nocturnal salivary cortisol level.[24] ACTH measurements to determine whether the disease is pituitary, adrenal, or ectopically based, and anatomic localization with MRI of the suspected lesions, confirm the laboratory findings.

TREATMENT. The treatment of excess cortisol production depends on the underlying mechanisms. In Cushing disease, transsphenoidal hypophysectomy with or without postoperative radiation therapy can partially or completely reverse the increased ACTH production of the anterior pituitary. Cushing syndrome requires surgical removal of one (adrenal adenoma, adrenal carcinoma) or both (multiple nodular) adrenal glands. Immediately after surgery, it is necessary to replace both cortisol and mineralocorticoid (fludrocortisone) to prevent adrenal insufficiency. Treatment of the ectopic ACTH syndrome requires identification and treatment of the neoplastic process. Patients treated with exogenous steroids for more than 1 month often develop clinical signs and symptoms of Cushing syndrome. In nonsurgical patients, the adrenal enzyme inhibitor ketoconazole can reverse excess cortisol production. Even mild or subclinical degrees of Cushing syndrome (adrenal incidentaloma) appear to increase the risk for cardiovascular disease.

Hyperaldosteronism

Aldosterone production by the zona glomerulosa is under the control of the renin-angiotensin system. Renin secretion responds primarily to changes in intravascular volume. Aldosterone synthesis and secretion is primarily regulated by angiotensin II, which binds to the angiotensin II type I receptor on the cells of the zona glomerulosa.[28]

The mechanism of action of aldosterone on target tissues resembles that reported for glucocorticoids (see Fig. 86-1). Aldosterone enters cells and binds to the mineralocorticoid receptor, which then translocates to the nucleus and promotes the expression of aldosterone-responsive genes. In addition to kidney cells, in which mineralocorticoid receptors control sodium transport, in vitro studies have demonstrated these receptors in rat cardiac myocytes; they respond to mineralocorticoid stimulation with an increase in protein synthesis. Whether these changes correspond to any relevant in vivo cardiac effects is unclear, but aldosterone may augment the development of cardiac hypertrophy in hypertension.[29]

The aldosterone antagonists spironolactone and eplerenone compete for receptor binding in the cytosol (see Fig. 86-1). They are the most recent class of compounds approved for the treatment of heart failure.[30] Recent studies have defined a role for these agents after acute myocardial infarction and for the treatment of left ventricular dysfunction, heart failure, and hypertension.[31,32]

Although the major cause of increased serum aldosterone levels is in the physiologic response to the activation of the renin-angiotensin system, there are well-recognized aldosterone-producing benign adrenal adenomas (Conn syndrome). Primary hyperaldosteronism augments sodium retention, causes hypertension, increases renal loss of magnesium and potassium, decreases arterial compliance with a rise in systemic vascular resistance and resulting vascular damage, and alters the sympathetic and parasympathetic neural regulation. Many of the changes in the heart and cardiovascular system in hyperaldosteronism result from the associated hypertension.[32] A recent report has linked primary aldosteronism to the development of atrial fibrillation in patients with hypertension but no structural heart disease. A recent review has discussed the approach to the detection, diagnosis, and treatment of patients with primary aldosteronism.[33] The hyperaldosterone-mediated hypokalemia and much of the associated hypertension respond to the surgical removal of a unilateral (or occasionally bilateral) benign adrenal adenoma(s).[34]

Addison Disease

Long before recognition that the glands situated just above the upper pole of each kidney (suprarenal) synthesize and secrete glucocorticoids and mineralocorticoids, Thomas Addison described the association of atrophy with loss of function of these structures, with marked changes in the cardiovascular system. The hypovolemia, hypotension, and acute cardiovascular collapse resulting from renal sodium wasting, hyperkalemia, and loss of vascular tone are the hallmarks of acute addisonian crisis, one of the most severe endocrine emergencies. Adrenal insufficiency most commonly arises from bilateral loss of adrenal function on an autoimmune basis, as a result of infection, hemorrhage, or metastatic malignancy—or in selected cases, of inborn errors of steroid hormone metabolism.[35] In contrast, secondary adrenal insufficiency, which results from pituitary-dependent loss of ACTH secretion, leads to a fall in glucocorticoid production while mineralocorticoid production, including aldosterone, remains at relatively normal levels. Studies have addressed the issue of relative hypothalamic-pituitary-adrenal insufficiency in acutely ill patients.[36] Although the actual existence of such an entity and diagnostic criteria for establishing this occurrence remain to be validated, it has reopened the question of the need for stress-dose cortisol treatment of critical illness.

Addison disease can occur at any age. The noncardiac symptoms, including increased pigmentation, abdominal pain with nausea and vomiting, and weight loss, can be chronic, whereas the tachycardia, hypotension, and electrolyte abnormalities herald impending cardiovascular collapse and crisis.[35] Blood pressure measurements uniformly show low diastolic pressure (<60 mm Hg), with significant orthostatic changes reflecting volume loss. Laboratory findings of hyponatremia and hyperkalemia indicate loss of aldosterone production (renin levels are high). Hyperkalemia can alter the ECG, producing low-amplitude P waves and peaked T waves.[36] Newly diagnosed untreated patients with Addison disease have reduced left ventricular, end-systolic, and end-diastolic dimensions compared with controls. Cardiac atrophy is an unusual condition; it is seen in malnutrition caused by anorexia, in astronauts after prolonged space flight, in populations with sodium-deficient diets, and characteristically with Addison disease (teardrop heart; **Fig. 86-2**). This atrophy reflects a response to decreases in cardiac workload, because restoration of normal plasma volume with mineralocorticoid and glucocorticoid replacement increases ventricular mass.

DIAGNOSIS. Acute adrenal insufficiency characteristically occurs in the setting of acute stress, infection, or trauma in a patient with chronic autoimmune adrenal insufficiency, or in children with congenital abnormalities of cortisol metabolism. It can also occur from bilateral adrenal hemorrhage in patients with severe systemic infection or diffuse intravascular coagulation.[35] Secondary adrenal insufficiency can occur in the setting of hypopituitarism, which is usually chronic, but acute changes caused by pituitary hemorrhage (apoplexy) or pituitary inflammation (lymphocytic hypophysitis) can occur. Patients treated with long-term suppressive doses of corticosteroids (>10 mg of prednisone for more than 1 month) can develop acute adrenal insufficiency if treatment is precipitously stopped.

The diagnosis is established when, in the morning or during severe stress, cortisol levels are low (<8 mg/dL) and fail to rise above 20 μg/dL 30 minutes after an intravenous (IV) injection of 0.25 mg of cosyntropin. Diagnosis in the setting of acute illness may be more difficult, and a low (<10 μg/dL) morning serum level of cortisol may suffice to suggest impaired control of secretion.[36]

TREATMENT. Management of acute addisonian crisis needs to address three major issues. The first is adequate hydrocortisone

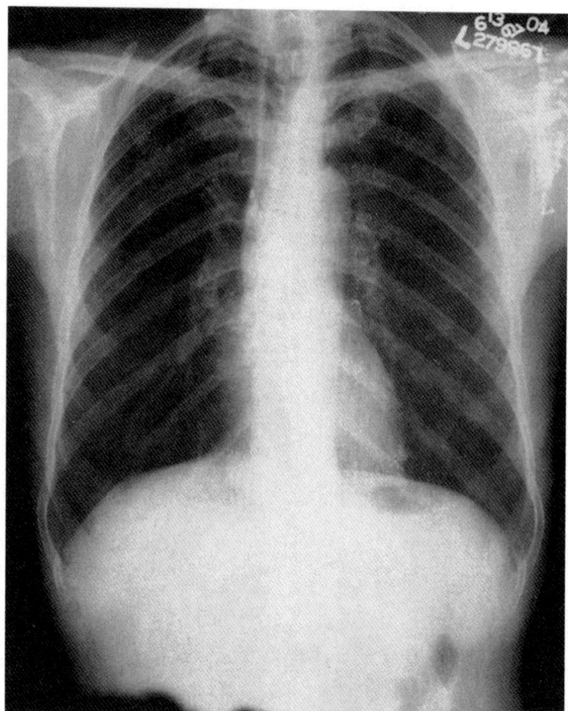

FIGURE 86-2 Routine chest radiograph of a patient with Addison disease related to tuberculosis. In addition to the small cardiac silhouette, there are calcified lymph nodes in the hilum of the right lung. *(Courtesy of Dr. J. B. Naidich.)*

replacement—100 mg given as an initial IV bolus, then 100 mg every 8 hours for the first 24 hours, tapering the dose for the next 72 to 96 hours. The second is the restoration of intravascular fluid deficit using large volumes of normal saline with 5% dextrose. The third is identifying and treating any underlying precipitating cause, including infection, acute cardiac or cerebral ischemia, or intra-abdominal emergency. Chronic treatment is oral corticosteroid and mineralocorticoid (fludrocortisone, 0.1 mg/day) replacement, but these patients are at increased risk for all-cause and cardiovascular mortality.[37]

Parathyroid Disease

Diseases of the parathyroid glands can produce cardiovascular disease and alter cardiac function by two mechanisms. The first is changes in the secretion of parathyroid hormone (PTH), a protein hormone, which affects the heart, vascular smooth muscle cells, and endothelial cells. The second mechanism is changes in serum calcium levels. Serum ionized calcium regulates the synthesis and secretion of PTH by an exquisitely sensitive negative feedback mechanism.[38]

PTH can bind to its receptor and alter the spontaneous beating rate of neonatal cardiac myocytes through an increase in intracellular cyclic adenosine monophosphate (cAMP). PTH can also alter calcium influx and cardiac contractility in adult cardiac myocytes and relaxation of vascular smooth muscle cells. In addition to PTH, a structurally related parathyroid hormone–related peptide (PTHrP) is synthesized and secreted in a variety of tissues, including cardiac myocytes. PTHrP can bind to the PTH receptor on cardiac cells and stimulate cAMP accumulation and contractile activity, as well as regulate L-type calcium currents. Thus, the direct effects of increased serum levels of PTHrP on the heart and systemic vasculature can accompany paraneoplastic syndromes characterized by hypercalcemia.[38]

Hyperparathyroidism

Classic primary hyperparathyroidism producing hypercalcemia most often results from the adenomatous enlargement of one of the four parathyroid glands. The cardiovascular actions of hypercalcemia include the following: an increase in cardiac contractility; shortening of the ventricular action potential duration, primarily through changes in phase 2; and blunting of the T wave and changes in the ST segment, occasionally suggesting cardiac ischemia.[39] The Q-T interval is shortened and occasionally accompanied by decreases in the P-R interval. Treatment with digitalis glycosides appears to increase sensitivity of the heart to hypercalcemia.

Hypercalcemia has been linked to pathologic changes in the heart, including the myocardial interstitium, conducting system, and calcific deposits in the valve cusps and annuli. Although initially observed in fairly long-standing and severe hypercalcemia, so-called metastatic calcifications can also occur in secondary parathyroid disease arising from chronic renal failure, in which the serum calcium–phosphorus product constant is exceeded. Whereas left ventricular systolic function is generally maintained in primary hyperparathyroidism, severe or chronic disease may impair diastolic function. Changes in left ventricular structure and function do not appear to improve by 1 year after successful parathyroid surgery.[39]

A simultaneous increase in serum immunoreactive PTH (best represented by the intact PTH assay), with an elevation of the serum calcium level, establishes the diagnosis of primary hyperparathyroidism. Other causes include hypercalcemia of malignancy with an increased level of PTHrP or arising from direct bony metastasis, or neoplastic (lymphoma) or non-neoplastic (sarcoidosis) disease leading to an increase in synthesis and release of 1,25-dihydroxyvitamin D_3. Treatment for hyperparathyroidism is the surgical removal of the parathyroid adenoma.

Hypocalcemia

Low serum levels of total and ionized calcium directly alter myocyte function. Hypocalcemia prolongs phase 2 of the action potential duration and the Q-T interval. Severe hypocalcemia can impair cardiac contractility and gives rise to a diffuse musculoskeletal syndrome, including tetany and rhabdomyolysis. Primary hypoparathyroidism is rare and can be seen after surgical removal of the parathyroid glands, in the setting of polyglandular dysfunction syndromes, as the result of glandular agenesis (DiGeorge) syndrome, and in the rare heritable disorder pseudohypoparathyroidism.

The most common cause of low serum calcium levels is chronic renal failure and high PTH levels. In such patients, the effects of chronically high levels of PTH (secondary hyperparathyroidism) on the heart and cardiovascular system predominate.[38] The ability of PTH to stimulate G protein–coupled receptors may impair myocyte contractility and contribute to the LVH commonly observed in patients with chronic renal failure. Cinacalcet, a recently approved calcimimetic agent, can treat the secondary hyperparathyroidism associated with chronic renal failure. A trial to assess its effectiveness on cardiovascular events is ongoing.[40]

Vitamin D

Recent evidence has suggested that lower levels of vitamin D (<30 ng/mL of 25-hydroxyvitamin D) are associated with increased all-cause and cardiovascular morbidity.[41] In postmenopausal women, increased vitamin D intake reduces the relative risk of developing cancer. Although low levels of vitamin D occur in chronic renal disease and heart failure, it is too soon to draw conclusions regarding vitamin D supplementation to prevent cardiac disease.[42]

Thyroid Gland

The thyroid gland and heart share a close relationship, arising in embryology. In ontogeny, the thyroid and heart anlage migrate together. The close physiologic relationship is affirmed by predictable changes in cardiovascular function across the entire range of thyroid disease states; cardiovascular manifestations are some of the most common and characteristic findings of hyperthyroidism. The diagnosis and management of thyroid hormone–mediated cardiac disease states require understanding of the cellular mechanisms of thyroid hormone on the heart and vascular smooth muscle cells.[43]

Cellular Mechanisms of Thyroid Hormone Action on the Heart

Under the regulation of thyroid-stimulating hormone (thyrotropin, TSH), the thyroid gland has the unique property of concentrating iodide and, through a series of enzymatic steps, synthesizes predominantly tetraiodothyronine (T_4, 85%) and a smaller percentage of triiodothyronine (T_3, 15%; **Fig. 86-3**). The major source of T_3 synthesis is by conversion by 5′-monodeiodination, primarily in the liver and skeletal muscle and in the kidneys. Studies have confirmed T_3 as the active form of thyroid hormone that accounts for the vast majority of biologic effects, including stimulation of tissue thermogenesis, alterations in the expression of various cellular proteins, and actions on the heart and vascular smooth muscle cells.[44,45] Serum-free T_3, in turn, is taken up by transport proteins (**Fig. 86-4**). Most data indicate that the cardiac myocyte cannot metabolize T_4 to T_3. Therefore, despite the presence of the relevant enzymes, all the observed nuclear actions and changes in gene expression result from changes in blood levels of T_3. As reported for the steroid and retinoic acid families of receptor proteins, the thyroid hormone receptors (TRs) bind as homodimers or heterodimers to the thyroid hormone response elements (TREs) in a promoter region of specific genes. Binding to the promoter regions can activate or repress gene expression.[46]

Thyroid hormone transcriptionally regulates many cardiac proteins (**Table 86-1**). These include structural and regulatory proteins, cardiac membrane ion channels, and cell surface receptors, thus providing a molecular mechanism to explain many of the diverse effects of thyroid hormone on the heart. The first reported and best studied to date have been the myosin heavy chain isoforms (alpha and beta). The human ventricle expresses primarily beta myosin, and there are limited alterations in isoform expression accompanying thyroid disease states. Changes in myosin heavy chain isoform expression occur in the human atria in various

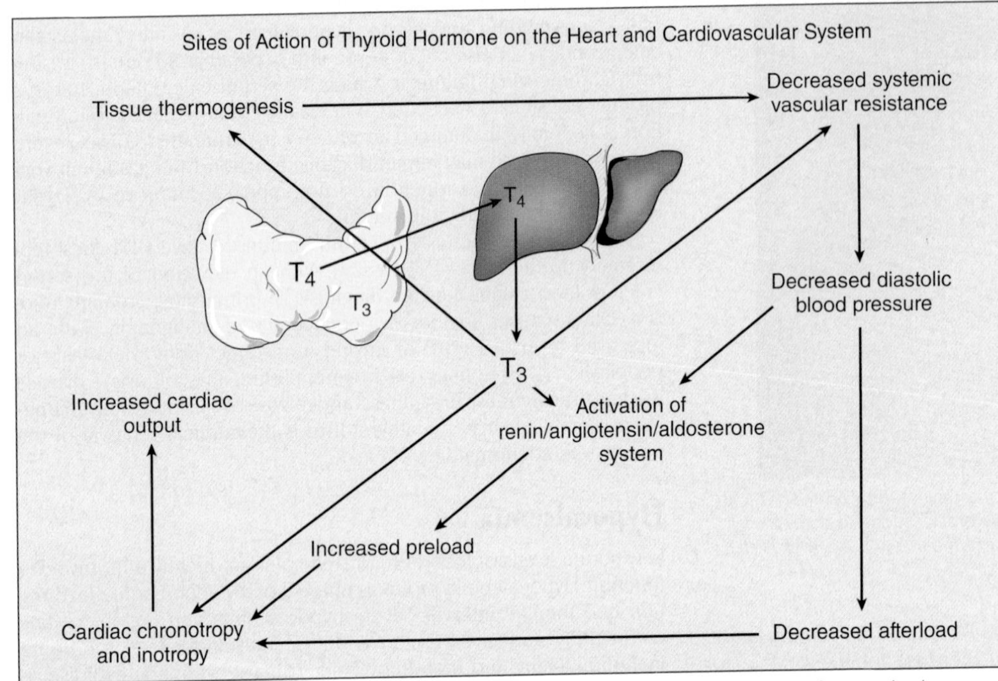

FIGURE 86-3 Schematic representation of thyroid hormone metabolism and the effects of T_3 on the heart and systemic vasculature.

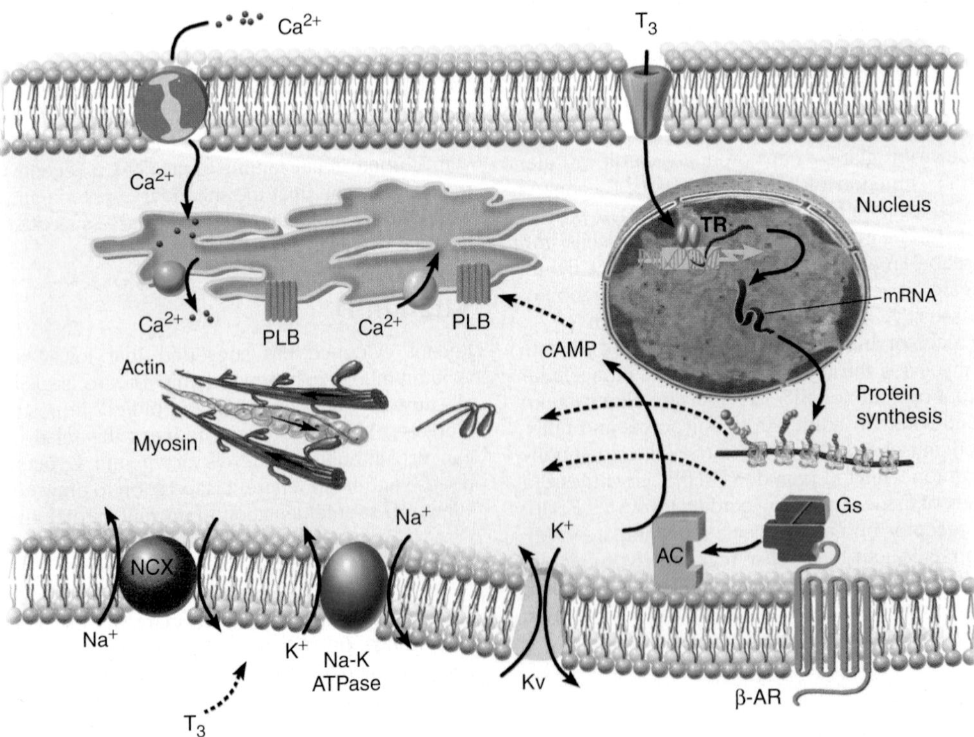

FIGURE 86-4 T_3 enters the cell via specific membrane transporters and binds to nuclear T_3 receptors. The complex binds to thyroid hormone response elements and regulates transcription of specific genes. Non-nuclear T_3 actions on channels for Na^+, K^+, and Ca^{2+} ions are indicated. AC = adenylyl cyclase; ATPase = adenosine triphosphatase; β-AR = beta-adrenergic receptor; Gs = guanine nucleotide binding protein subunit; Kv = voltage-gated potassium channel; mRNA = messenger RNA; NCX = sodium calcium exchanger; PLB = phospholamban; TR = T_3 receptor protein.

TABLE 86-1 Thyroid Hormone Regulation of Cardiac Gene Expression

Positively Regulated
Alpha-myosin heavy chain
Sarcoplasmic reticulum Ca^{2+}-ATPase
Na^+, K^+-ATPase
Voltage-gated potassium channels (Kv 1.5, Kv 4.2, Kv 4.3)
Atrial and brain natriuretic peptide
Malic enzyme
Beta-adrenergic receptor
Guanine nucleotide-binding protein G_s
Adenine nucleotide transporter 1
Negatively Regulated
Beta-myosin heavy chain
Phospholamban
Na^+, Ca^{2+} exchanger
Thyroid hormone receptor $alpha_1$
Adenylyl cyclase (AC) types V, VI
Guanine nucleotide-binding protein G_i
Monocarboxylate transporters 8 and 10

ATPase = adenosine triphosphatase.

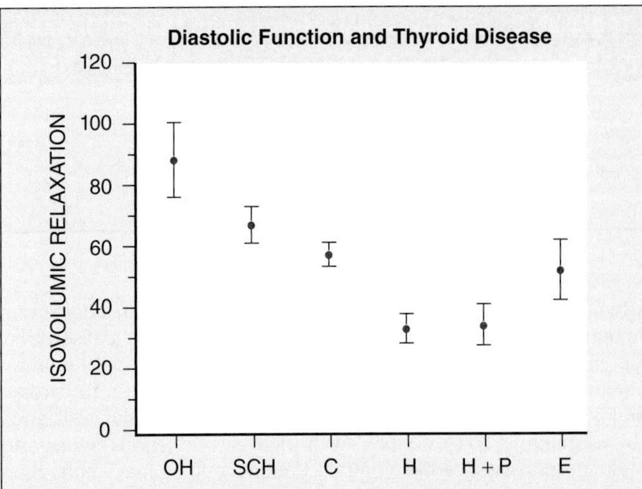

FIGURE 86-5 Diastolic function, as measured by the isovolumic relaxation time, varies over the entire range of thyroid disease, including overt hypothyroidism (OH), subclinical hypothyroidism (SCH), control (C), hyperthyroidism (H), hyperthyroidism after beta-adrenergic blockade (H + P), and hyperthyroidism after treatment to restore normal thyroid function (E).

diseases, including congestive heart failure, and whether these changes are thyroid hormone–mediated remains to be determined.[47]

Sarcoendoplasmic reticulum Ca^{2+}-ATPase (SERCA) is an important ion pump that determines the magnitude of myocyte calcium cycling (see Chap. 24). The reuptake of calcium into the sarcoendoplasmic reticulum early in diastole in part determines the rate at which the left ventricle relaxes (isovolumetric relaxation time [IVRT]).[43] The activity of SERCA2 in turn is regulated by the polymeric protein phospholamban, with its ability to inhibit SERCA activity further modified by the level of phosphorylation of the individual phospholamban monomers.[48] Inotropic agents that enhance cardiac contractility through increases in myocyte cAMP do so by stimulating the phosphorylation of phospholamban. Thyroid hormone inhibits the expression of phospholamban and increases phospholamban phosphorylation.[49] Genetically engineered animals deficient in phospholamban do not increase cardiac contractility further after exposure to excess thyroid hormone.[48] These data indicate that thyroid hormone exerts most of its direct effects on cardiac contractility by regulating calcium cycling through the SERCA-phospholamban system transcriptionally and post-transcriptionally. This molecular mechanism can explain why diastolic function varies inversely across the entire spectrum of thyroid disease states, including even mild subclinical hypothyroidism (**Fig. 86-5**).[50,51] In addition, beta-adrenergic blockade of the heart in hyperthyroidism does not decrease the rapid diastolic relaxation, further dissociating the thyroid hormone from the adrenergic effects of thyrotoxicosis.

Changes in other myocyte genes, including Na^+,K^+-ATPase, account for the increase in basal oxygen consumption of the experimental hyperthyroid heart and explain the decrease in digitalis sensitivity of hyperthyroid patients. Studies have shown that thyroid hormone can regulate the genetic expression of its own nuclear receptors and plasma membrane transport proteins (MCT8 and 10) within the cardiac myocyte (see Table 86-1).

In addition to the well-characterized nuclear effects of thyroid hormone, some cardiac responses to thyroid hormone appear to be mediated through nongenomic mechanisms,[52] as suggested by their relatively rapid onset of action—faster than can be accounted for by changes in gene expression and protein synthesis—and failure to be affected by inhibitors of gene transcription. The significance of these diverse actions remains to be established, but may explain the ability of acute T_3 treatment to alter cardiovascular hemodynamics. They may alter the functional properties of membrane ion channels and pumps, including the sodium channel and inward rectifying potassium current (I_K).

Thyroid Function Testing

A number of sensitive and specific laboratory tests can establish a diagnosis of thyroid disease with a high degree of precision. The serum TSH level is the most widely used and sensitive measure for the diagnosis of hypothyroidism and hyperthyroidism.[53] Serum TSH levels uniformly increase (>5 mIU/mL) in patients with primary hypothyroidism and, conversely, because of the normal feedback of excess levels of T_4 (and T_3) on the pituitary synthesis and secretion of TSH, the levels are low in hyperthyroidism (<0.1 mIU/mL). Measures of free T_4 can be useful when coexistent hepatic, nutritional, or genetic disease may alter thyroxine-binding globulin content. Autoimmune thyroid disease (Hashimoto and Graves) can be further diagnosed by the use of serologic measures of antithyroid antibodies, most specifically antithyroid peroxidase (anti-TPO) or antithyroglobulin antibodies.

Thyroid Hormone–Catecholamine Interaction

Early observations of the heart in hyperthyroidism emphasized the similarity to that of hyperadrenergic states, and moreover proposed enhanced sensitivity to catecholamines in this setting. This postulate formed the basis for the test described by Emil Goetsch in 1918, in which hyperthyroidism could be diagnosed by demonstrating a marked cardioacceleration and blood pressure response to small subcutaneous doses of epinephrine. Hyperthyroid subjects have decreased circulating catecholamine concentrations, despite the appearance of increased adrenergic signs and symptoms. Increased $beta_1$-adrenergic receptors on cardiac myocytes observed in experimental hyperthyroidism provide a mechanism for enhanced catecholamine sensitivity. A carefully controlled study of nonhuman primates, however, found no increase in sensitivity of the heart or cardiovascular system to catecholamines in experimental hyperthyroidism.[54] Accompanying the increased levels of $beta_1$-adrenergic receptors and guanosine triphosphate–binding proteins, thyroid hormone decreases the expression of cardiac-specific adenylyl cyclase catalytic subunit isoforms (V, VI), and thereby maintains the cellular response to beta-adrenergic agonists within normal limits.[55]

Hemodynamic Alterations in Thyroid Disease

Changes in myocardial contractility and hemodynamics occur across the entire spectrum of thyroid disease (**Table 86-2**; see Fig. 86-5). Multiple studies, including those in experimental animals, as well as invasive and noninvasive measurements in patients, have indicated that T_3 regulates cardiac inotropy and chronotropy through both direct and indirect mechanisms.[56-59] T_3 acts on tissues throughout the body to increase tissue thermogenesis (see Fig. 86-3). Direct effects on vascular smooth muscle cells decrease systemic vascular resistance of the arterioles of the peripheral circulation. A decrease in mean

TABLE 86-2 Cardiovascular Changes with Thyroid Disease

PARAMETER	NORMAL	HYPERTHYROID	HYPOTHYROID
Systemic vascular resistance (dyne-cm · sec^{-5})	1500-1700	700-1200	2100-2700
Heart rate (beats/min)	72-84	88-130	60-80
Cardiac output (liter/min)	5.8	>7.0	<4.5
Blood volume (% of normal)	100	105.5	84.5

arterial pressure and activation of the renin-angiotensin-aldosterone system occurs, as does an increase in renal sodium reabsorption. The increase in plasma volume, coupled with an increase in erythropoietin, leads to an increase in blood volume and a rise in cardiac preload. Thus, a combination of lower systemic vascular resistance (by as much as 50%), coupled with increases in venous return and preload, increases cardiac output. Cardiac output may more than double in hyperthyroidism and, conversely, may decrease by as much as 30% to 40% in hypothyroidism. Studies using positron emission tomography (PET) measurements of acetate metabolism have demonstrated that the marked increase in cardiac output in hyperthyroidism causes no change in energy efficiency.[60]

T_3 appears to reduce systemic vascular resistance by direct effects on vascular smooth muscle cells and through changes in the vascular endothelium potentially involving the synthesis and secretion of nitric oxide.[56] T_3 can produce vasodilation within hours after administration to patients undergoing coronary artery bypass grafting (CABG) and to patients with chronic congestive heart failure.[47,59] Arterial compliance also falls in hyperthyroidism, and may explain why mean arterial and diastolic pressures are low and peak systolic pressures increase.[57] Thus, the combination of increased cardiac output and decreased arterial compliance, which may be more pronounced in older patients with some degree of arterial vascular disease, leads to systolic hypertension in up to 30% of patients. In hypothyroidism, systemic vascular resistance may increase as much as 30%. Mean arterial pressure rises, with up to 20% of patients having diastolic hypertension. Even mild hypothyroidism may decrease endothelial-derived relaxing factors.[61] The diastolic hypertension of hypothyroidism is frequently associated with a low renin level and a decrease in hepatic synthesis of renin substrate. This leads to a characteristically low level of salt sensitivity, again reinforcing the importance of an increase in systemic vascular resistance underlying the mechanism for diastolic hypertension.

Hyperthyroidism

Cardiovascular symptoms are an integral and often the predominant clinical presentation of patients with hyperthyroidism. Most patients experience palpitations resulting from increases in the rate and force of cardiac contractility. The increase in heart rate results from a decrease in parasympathetic stimulation and an increase in sympathetic tone. Heart rates higher than 90 beats/min at rest and during sleep commonly occur, the normal diurnal variation in heart rate is blunted, and the increase during exercise is exaggerated. Many hyperthyroid patients experience exercise intolerance and exertional dyspnea, caused in part by skeletal and respiratory muscle weakness.[62,63] In the setting of a low vascular resistance and increased preload, cardiac functional reserve is compromised and cannot rise further to accommodate the demands of submaximal or maximal exercise.

A subset of thyrotoxic patients can experience angina-like chest pain. In older patients with known or suspected coronary artery disease, the increase in cardiac work associated with the increase in cardiac output and cardiac contractility of hyperthyroidism can produce myocardial ischemia, which can respond to beta-adrenergic blocking agents (beta blockers) or the restoration of a euthyroid state. Rare patients, usually younger women, experience a syndrome of chest pain at rest associated with ischemic electrocardiographic changes. Cardiac catheterization has demonstrated that most of these patients have angiographically normal coronary arteries, but coronary vasospasm similar to that found in variant angina can occur. Myocardial infarction rarely develops, and these patients appear to respond to calcium channel blockers or nitroglycerin.[43] Recent reports have documented cerebrovascular ischemic symptoms in young, primarily Asian women with Graves disease. This syndrome, Moyamoya disease, is characterized by anatomic occlusion of the terminal portions of internal carotid arteries. Treatment of hyperthyroidism can prevent further cerebral ischemic symptoms and reinforces the importance of routine thyroid function tests, including TSH, in patients who present with cardiac or cerebral vascular ischemic symptoms.

Hyperthyroidism is associated with a substantial degree of pulmonary hypertension (pulmonary artery systolic pressure > 75 mm Hg), which is reversible after treatment of Graves disease.[64] This observation implies that although systemic vascular resistance is decreased with thyrotoxicosis, pulmonary vascular resistance is not. Evaluation for thyroid disease with measurement of the serum TSH level may benefit all patients with unexplained pulmonary hypertension.[57]

ATRIAL FIBRILLATION. The most common rhythm disturbance in patients with hyperthyroidism is sinus tachycardia,[43] but its clinical impact is overshadowed by patients with atrial fibrillation resulting from thyrotoxicosis (see Chap. 40). The prevalence of atrial fibrillation and the less common forms of supraventricular tachycardia in this disease ranges from 2% to 20%.[65,66] When compared with a control population with normal thyroid function and a 2.3% prevalence of atrial fibrillation, the prevalence of atrial fibrillation in overt hyperthyroidism was 13.8%. In a study of more than 13,000 hyperthyroid patients, the prevalence for atrial fibrillation was less than 2%, perhaps because of earlier recognition and disease treatment.[65] When that same group of patients was analyzed for age distribution, prevalence increased stepwise in each decade, peaking at approximately 15% in patients older than 70 years. This study confirms that atrial fibrillation caused by hyperthyroidism is more common with advancing age. In a study of unselected patients presenting with atrial fibrillation, less than 1% of cases was caused by overt hyperthyroidism. Thus, the yield of abnormal thyroid function testing, including a low serum TSH level, appears to be low in patients with new-onset atrial fibrillation. However, the ability to restore thyrotoxic patients to a euthyroid state and sinus rhythm justifies TSH testing in most patients with recent onset of otherwise unexplained atrial fibrillation or other supraventricular arrhythmias.

Treatment of atrial fibrillation in the setting of hyperthyroidism includes beta-adrenergic blockade using a $beta_1$ selective or nonselective agent to control the ventricular response (**Table 86-3**). This symptomatic measure can be accomplished rapidly, whereas treatments leading to restoration of the euthyroid state require more time. Digitalis has been used to control the ventricular response in hyperthyroidism-associated atrial fibrillation, but because of the increased rate of digitalis clearance, decreased sensitivity of the drug action resulting from high cellular levels of Na^+,K^+-ATPase, and decreased parasympathetic tone, patients usually require higher doses of this medication. Anticoagulation in patients with hyperthyroidism and atrial fibrillation is controversial.[43,67] The potential for systemic or cerebral embolization must be weighed against the risk of bleeding and complications. Whether hyperthyroid patients are at increased risk for systemic embolization per se is not totally resolved.[68] In a retrospective study of patients with hyperthyroidism, age rather than atrial fibrillation was the main risk factor for embolization. Retrospective analysis of large series of patients has not demonstrated a prevalence of thromboembolic

TABLE 86-3 Beta-Adrenergic Receptor Blockade in the Treatment of Hyperthyroidism*

DRUG	DOSAGE	FREQUENCY	CONSIDERATIONS
Propranolol	10-40 mg	tid or qid	Nonselective β-AR blockade; longest experience
Atenolol	25-100 mg	bid	Relative $beta_1$ selectivity; increased patient compliance
Metoprolol	25-50 mg	qid	Relative $beta_1$ selectivity
Nadolol	40-160 mg	qd	Nonselective β-AR blockade; once daily; least experience to date
Esmolol	IV pump, 50-100 μg/kg/min		In ICU setting of severe hyperthyroidism or storm

*Each of these drugs has been approved for the treatment of cardiovascular diseases, but to date none has been approved for the treatment of hyperthyroidism.
β-AR = beta-adrenergic receptor; ICU = intensive care unit.

events greater than the reported risk of major bleeding from warfarin treatment. Thus, in younger patients with hyperthyroidism and atrial fibrillation in the absence of other heart disease, hypertension, or other independent risk factors for embolization, the benefits of anticoagulation have not been proven and might be outweighed by the risk. Aspirin provides an alternative for lowering the risk for embolic events in younger individuals and can be used safely.

Successful treatment of hyperthyroidism with radioiodine or antithyroid drugs and restoration of normal serum levels of T_4 and T_3 are associated with reversion to sinus rhythm in two thirds of patients within 2 to 3 months.[65] In older patients or in the setting of atrial fibrillation of longer duration, the rate of reversion to sinus rhythm is lower and electrical or pharmacologic cardioversion therefore should be attempted, but only after the patient has been rendered euthyroid. Most patients (90%) can be restored to sinus rhythm by electrical cardioversion or pharmacologic measures, and many will remain in sinus rhythm for up to 5 years or more. In a regimen that added disopyramide, 300 mg/day, for 3 months after successful cardioversion, patients were more likely to remain in sinus rhythm than those not treated.[67]

HEART FAILURE IN THYROID DISEASE. The cardiovascular alterations in hyperthyroidism include increased resting cardiac output and enhanced cardiac contractility (**Fig. 86-6**; see Table 86-2). Nevertheless, a minority of patients presents with symptoms, including dyspnea on exertion, orthopnea, and paroxysmal nocturnal dyspnea, as well as signs demonstrating peripheral edema, elevated jugular venous pressure, or an S_3 indicative of heart failure. This complex of findings, coupled with a failure to increase the LV ejection fraction with exercise, has suggested a hyperthyroid cardiomyopathy. The term often used in this setting, *high-output failure*, is not appropriate, because although resting cardiac output is as much as two to three times normal, the exercise intolerance does not appear to be a result of cardiac failure, but rather of skeletal muscle weakness[43,63] and perhaps associated pulmonary hypertension.[64] High-output states, however, can increase renal sodium reabsorption, expand plasma volume, and cause development of peripheral edema, pleural effusions, and venous hypertension. Whereas systemic vascular resistance falls with hyperthyroidism, the pulmonary vascular bed is not similarly affected and, as a result of the increase in output to the pulmonary circulation, there is an increase in pulmonary artery pressures.[57] This results in a rise in mean venous pressure, jugular venous hypertension, hepatic congestion, and peripheral edema of the type associated with primary pulmonary hypertension or right heart failure.

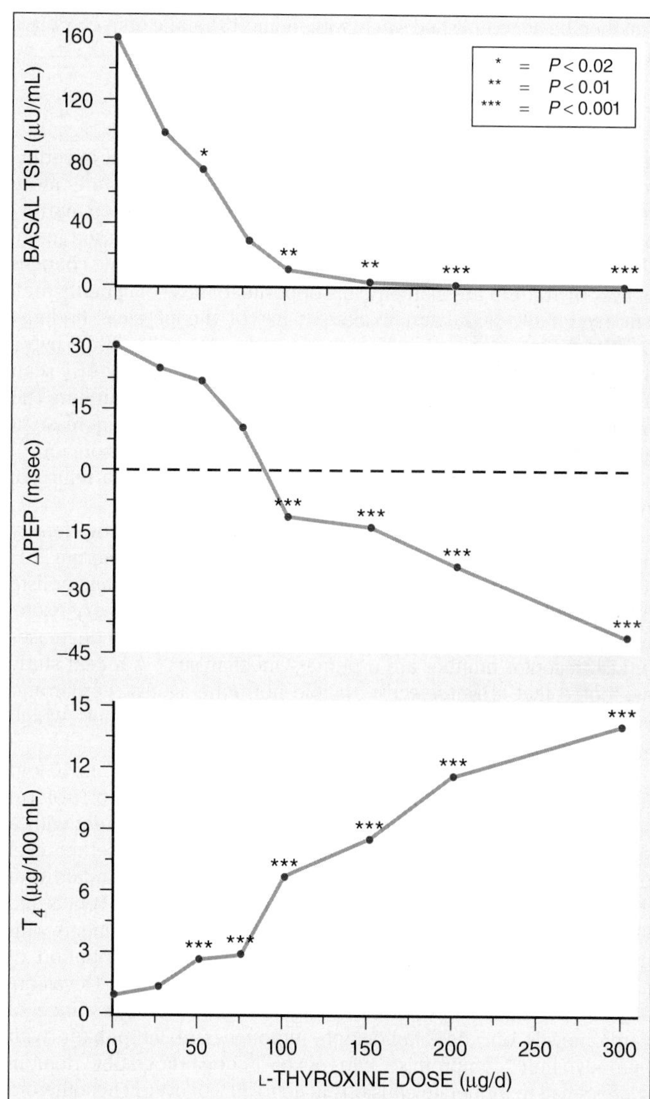

FIGURE 86-6 Response to stepwise L-thyroxine sodium treatment of hypothyroid patients as assessed by serum TSH and T_4 levels and by improvement in left ventricular contractility as measured noninvasively by the change in the pre-ejection period (PEP). *(From Crowley WF Jr, Ridgway EC, Bough EW, et al: Noninvasive evaluation of cardiac function in hypothyroidism. Response to gradual thyroxine replacement. N Engl J Med 296:1, 1977.)*

Patients with long-standing hyperthyroidism and marked sinus tachycardia or atrial fibrillation can develop low cardiac output, impaired cardiac contractility with a low ejection fraction, an S_3, and pulmonary congestion, all consistent with congestive heart failure.[43] Review of such cases suggests that impairment in left ventricular function results from prolonged high heart rate and the development of rate-related heart failure. When the left ventricle becomes dilated, mitral regurgitation may also develop (see Chap. 66). Recognition of this entity is important because treatment aimed at slowing heart rate or controlling the ventricular response in atrial fibrillation appears to improve left ventricular function, even before initiation of antithyroid therapy. Because these patients are critically ill, they should be managed in an intensive care unit setting. Some patients with hyperthyroidism, similar to the overall congestive heart failure population, do not tolerate initiation of beta blockers in full doses. Treatment can be started with lower doses of short-acting beta blockers in conjunction with classic forms of treatment of acute congestive heart failure, including diuresis.

The increase in rate-pressure product and oxygen consumption that results from hyperthyroidism can impair cardiac function in older patients with known or suspected ischemic, hypertensive, or valvular heart disease. It is important to recognize hyperthyroidism in older patients promptly, because they are at higher risk of cardiovascular and cerebral vascular events before[69] and subsequent to treatment.[70]

TREATMENT. Treatment of patients with thyrotoxic cardiac disease should include a beta-adrenergic antagonist to lower the heart rate to 10% or 15% above normal. This causes the tachycardia-mediated component of ventricular dysfunction to improve, whereas the direct inotropic effects of thyroid hormone will persist (see Table 86-3 and Fig. 86-4).[43] The rapid onset of action and improvement in many of the signs and symptoms of hyperthyroidism indicate that most patients with overt symptoms should receive beta blockers. Definitive therapy can then be accomplished safely with iodine-131 alone or in combination with an antithyroid drug.

Hypothyroidism

In contrast to the dramatic clinical signs and symptoms of hyperthyroidism, the cardiovascular findings of hypothyroidism are more subtle.[71] Mild degrees of bradycardia, diastolic hypertension, narrow pulse pressure and relatively quiet precordium, and decreased intensity of the apical impulse are all characteristic. Hemodynamic changes of hypothyroidism are diametrically opposite to those of hyperthyroidism (see Table 86-2) and explain many of the physical findings. Despite the decrease in cardiac output and contractility of the hypothyroid myocardium, studies of myocardial metabolism by PET scan have shown energy inefficiency of the hypothyroid myocardium. The oxygen cost of work increases primarily as a result of the increase in afterload.[72] Treatment of hypothyroid patients with the restoration of a euthyroid state resolves these changes in parallel with a return of systemic vascular resistance to lower levels.

Hypothyroidism also produces increases in total and low-density lipoprotein (LDL) cholesterol in proportion to the rise in serum TSH levels.[73] Although thyroid hormone can alter cholesterol metabolism through multiple mechanisms, including a decrease in biliary excretion, it appears that changes in LDL metabolism caused by decreases in LDL receptor number are a primary mechanism.[74] A recent study has noted that a liver-selective thyroid hormone agonist, eprotirome, can further lower cholesterol levels in statin-treated patients, which supports this concept.[75]

The serum creatine kinase (CK) level is elevated by 50% to 10-fold in up to 30% of patients with hypothyroidism. Analysis of isoform specificity indicates that more than 96% is CK-MM, consistent with a skeletal muscle origin of increased enzyme release.[74] The serum level of creatine kinase in hypothyroidism after initiation of standard oral thyroid hormone replacement declines slowly over weeks. Pericardial effusions can occur consistent with the observation that patients with hypothyroidism have an increase in the volume of distribution of albumin and a decrease in lymphatic clearance function. Occasionally, the pericardial effusions are large, causing the appearance of cardiomegaly on chest radiograph. Although rare, tamponade with hemodynamic compromise can occur. Echocardiography demonstrates small to moderate effusions in up to 30% of overtly hypothyroid patients, which resolve over a period of weeks to months after initiation of thyroid hormone replacement.[71]

As a result of changes in ion channel expression, the ECG in hypothyroidism is characterized by sinus bradycardia, low voltage, and prolongation of the action potential duration and QT interval. The latter predisposes patients to ventricular arrhythmias, and some patients with acquired torsade de pointes have improved or completely resolved with thyroid hormone replacement.[43]

Increases in risk factors for atherosclerosis, including hypercholesterolemia, hypertension, and elevated levels of homocysteine, may elevate the risk for atherosclerosis and coronary and systemic vascular disease in patients with hypothyroidism (see Chaps. 44 and 47).[73,74] One study has reported increases in abdominal aortic atherosclerosis in older female patients with even mild hypothyroidism.[76] Whether patients with hypothyroidism have an increase in coronary artery disease is an important clinical issue. One report has suggested increased cardiovascular morbidity and mortality with untreated subclinical hypothyroidism,[77] and that increases in carotid intimal medial thickness resolve with thyroid hormone replacement.[78] Noninvasive studies, including nuclear scans, have demonstrated abnormalities in perfusion suggestive of myocardial ischemia, but these defects appear to resolve with thyroid hormone treatment.

In patients younger than 50 years of age with no history of heart disease, it is possible to initiate full replacement doses of L-thyroxine (100 to 150 μg/day) without concern for untoward cardiac effects. In patients older than 50 years of age with known or suspected coronary artery disease, the issue is more complicated.

In patients with known coronary artery disease and coexistent hypothyroidism, three major issues need to be addressed. The first is whether coronary artery revascularization is required before initiating thyroid hormone replacement. If patients are not candidates for percutaneous intervention, CABG can be accomplished in patients with unstable angina, left main coronary artery disease, or three-vessel disease with impaired left ventricular function, even in the setting of overt hypothyroidism. Rarely, a patient has sufficiently profound hypothyroidism to prolong bleeding times and partial thromboplastin times, requiring preoperative supplementation of clotting factors. Thyroid hormone replacement can be delayed until the postoperative period, when it can be administered in full doses parenterally or orally.[43]

The second issue is in patients with known stable cardiac disease, in whom cardiac revascularization is not clinically indicated. Treatment of such patients should begin with low doses (12.5 μg) of L-thyroxine and increased stepwise (12.5 to 25 μg) every 6 to 8 weeks until the serum TSH level is normal. Thyroid hormone replacement in this setting and its ability to lower systemic vascular resistance and decrease afterload, as well as improve myocardial efficiency, can actually decrease clinical signs of myocardial ischemia. Beta blockers are an ideal concomitant therapy to control heart rate.

The third important issue involves patients who, although potentially at risk for coronary artery disease, exhibit no clinical signs or symptoms. In this group, thyroid hormone replacement can be started at low doses, generally in the range of 25 to 50 μg/day, and increased by 25 μg every 6 to 8 weeks until the serum TSH level is normal. If signs or symptoms of ischemic heart disease develop, the same recommendations apply as to patients with known underlying heart disease.

In all patients, thyroid hormone replacement should be sufficient to restore the serum TSH level to normal and the patients are clinically euthyroid. The concept that these patients benefit from maintenance of mild hypothyroidism is not supported by the known effects of thyroid hormone on the heart and cardiovascular system.[43,71,72] Thyroid hormone replacement should be accomplished by purified preparations of levothyroxine sodium. Preparations containing T_4 with T_3 (thyroid extract) or the existing purified preparations of T_3 do not offer benefit. The short half-life of T_3 and the inability to maintain serum levels within the normal range in patients so treated can add to cardiac risk.[78] An interesting issue is whether some patients with statin-induced myopathy have underlying thyroid disease as a contributing factor. The myopathy or myalgia symptoms of both conditions are similar (**Table 86-4**), and thyroid function testing with TSH should be part of the evaluation of these patients.[74]

DIAGNOSIS. Hashimoto disease, post–radioiodine therapy for Graves disease, and iodine deficiency (in parts of the world where that remains a public health problem) are the leading causes of hypothyroidism and produce diagnostic elevation in serum TSH levels.[53] Thus, the finding of an elevated TSH level is sufficient to establish the diagnosis and form the basis for treatment. In routine practice, additional testing with a serum T_4 and T_3 resin uptake is confirmatory. The prevalence of hypothyroidism is estimated at 3% to 4% for overt disease and 7% to 10% for the milder forms of disease, and increases with advancing age. TSH screening can therefore be advised for all adults, particularly patients with hypertension, hypercholesterolemia, hypertriglyceridemia, coronary or peripheral vascular disease, and unexplained pericardial or pleural effusions and for various musculoskeletal syndromes or statin-associated myopathy.[43,74]

contractile function.[43] A recent study of T_3 treatment of humans with NYHA Class III or IV heart failure has shown similar results.[93]

Children and adults undergoing cardiac surgery with cardiopulmonary bypass demonstrate a predictable fall in serum T_3 levels in the perioperative period.[94] Although treatment strategies using acute administration of intravenous T_3 to adults after CABG have shown an improvement in cardiac output and a fall in systemic vascular resistance, there was no alteration in overall mortality. In this group of patients, atrial fibrillation decreased by as much as 50% when compared with age-matched controls.[95] Pediatric cardiac patients, especially those undergoing surgery in the neonatal period, demonstrate an even greater decline in serum T_3 levels that can last longer. The low postoperative T_3 level identifies patients at increased risk for morbidity and mortality.[96] A prospective randomized study has shown that especially in neonates, the degree of therapeutic intervention and the need for postoperative inotropic agents is decreased by the administration of T_3 in doses sufficient to restore serum T_3 levels to normal.[97]

In patients with chronic congestive heart failure, the fall in serum T_3 levels correlates with the severity of heart failure as assessed by NYHA classification.[47,93] Up to 30% of patients with heart failure have a low serum T_3 level, which occurs in patients treated with amiodarone and in those who are not. In view of the deleterious effects of hypothyroidism on the myocardium, T_3 replacement may provide benefit. Human studies using a novel form of T_3 that can restore serum T_3 levels to normal and avoid the peaks and valleys of drug levels currently associated with existing drug preparations are needed to answer this question.

Pheochromocytoma

Pheochromocytomas (see Chaps. 45 and 94) are primarily benign tumors arising from neuroectodermal chromaffin cells usually within the adrenal medulla and abdomen, but they may arise anywhere within the plexus of sympathetic adrenergic nerves. Although the prevalence is probably less than 1/2000 cases of diastolic hypertension, the importance of pheochromocytoma derives from the dramatic mode in which symptoms can present. Autopsy studies have shown that in 75% of patients, the diagnosis was not clinically suspected and, in more than 50% of patients, it contributed to mortality.[98]

Most pheochromocytomas are 1 cm or larger, the vast majority arise as a unilateral adrenal lesion, and extra-adrenal tumors are more common in children.[99] Although most tumors are sporadic, approximately 10% are familial, and the latter are more often bilateral or occur in an extra-adrenal location. When pheochromocytoma coexists with medullary thyroid carcinoma or occasionally with hyperparathyroidism, it is designated as multiple endocrine neoplasia (MEN) syndrome type 2. These patients have a mutation in the RET proto-oncogene. In patients with MEN 2B, pheochromocytomas coexist with medullary thyroid cancer and mucosal neuromas frequently seen on the lips and tongue. In patients with neurofibromatosis, pheochromocytoma may be present in up to 1% of patients; in von Hippel–Lindau disease, pheochromocytoma develops in association with cerebellar or retinal angiomas and may have specific gene expression indicating a propensity for malignancy.[100]

Pheochromocytoma presents clinically with headache, palpitations, excessive sweating, tremulousness, chest pain, weight loss, and a variety of other constitutional complaints. Hypertension may be episodic but is usually constant, and is paradoxically associated with orthostatic hypotension on arising in the morning. The paroxysmal attacks and classic symptoms result from episodic excess catecholamine secretion.[98]

The first onset of hypertension caused by pheochromocytoma can be at the time of elective surgical intervention for an unrelated condition. As a result of norepinephrine release, with an increase in systemic vascular resistance, cardiac output is minimally (if at all) increased, despite increases in heart rate. The ECG can show LVH as well as the presence of inverted T waves, suggesting left ventricular strain. Although ventricular and atrial ectopy and episodes of supraventricular tachycardia can occur, there is little to distinguish the LVH from that of essential hypertension.[98]

Impaired left ventricular function and cardiomyopathy have occurred in patients with pheochromocytoma. The mechanism underlying this is complex and includes the following: increased left ventricular work and LVH from associated hypertension; potential adverse effects of excess catecholamines on myocyte structure and contractility; and changes in coronary arteries, including thickening of the media, presumably potentially impairing blood flow to the myocardium. Histologic evidence of myocarditis is present postmortem in patients with previously diagnosed or undiagnosed disease.[98] The possibility of catecholamine-stimulated tachycardia in turn mediating left ventricular dysfunction should be addressed, because treatments designed to slow heart rate may improve left ventricular function.

The release of catecholamines from pheochromocytomas involves diffusion out of chromaffin cells, as well as release of storage vessels, accounting for the demonstration of chromogranin A in the circulation. The primary catecholamine released is norepinephrine, but epinephrine can also increase. Demonstration of elevated serum dopamine levels implies malignant transformation, which in turn suggests that the tumor may arise in an extra-adrenal site and have certain gene expression profiles.[100] Rarely, pheochromocytoma can arise within the heart, presumably from chromaffin cells, which are part of the adrenergic autonomic paraganglia.[101]

DIAGNOSIS. Diagnosis is established by demonstrating an increase in norepinephrine or epinephrine or its metabolites in serum or blood. Quantitative 24-hour urinary metanephrine levels are the most reliable screening procedures, and plasma catecholamine levels, when determined under proper conditions, are also fairly sensitive.[101,102] Provocative tests aim to increase plasma catecholamine levels in patients with episodic disease; in contrast, the clonidine suppression test is safe and suppresses plasma norepinephrine levels by more than 50% in essential hypertensive patients, but not in those with pheochromocytoma.[99] Imaging modalities include MRI, which has a high degree of specificity, and computed tomography (CT), which has a high degree of sensitivity because adrenal lesions are large enough to be detected. Further studies with isotopic precursors of catecholamine biosynthesis, including ^{131}I-metaiodobenzylguanidine (MIBG), can confirm that anatomic lesions are producing catecholamines.

TREATMENT. Definitive treatment of pheochromocytoma requires removal of the lesion. Accurate preoperative localization reduces operative mortality and eliminates the need for exploratory laparotomy. Endoscopic procedures are now standard.[103] Preoperative pharmacologic management includes 7 to 14 days of alpha-adrenergic blockade, usually with prazosin or phenoxybenzamine. Beta blocker therapy is contraindicated before establishing sufficient alpha blockade. If supraventricular arrhythmias or unremitting tachycardia is present, beta$_1$-selective agents such as atenolol are preferred.[102] Operative intervention requires constant blood pressure monitoring and intravenous phentolamine or sodium nitroprusside may be required to treat episodic hypertension.[98] Postoperative management includes the use of large volumes of crystalloid-containing fluids to maintain blood volume and prevent hypotension. Glucose may be necessary to replace depleted liver glycogen stores. Success of surgery can be determined by effective blood pressure and symptomatic improvement, but also with measurement of urinary catecholamines 4 weeks after the procedure. In patients who are not candidates for surgical treatment, metyrosine can decrease catecholamine synthesis and improve most cardiovascular signs and symptoms.

Future Perspectives

The recognition that a variety of naturally occurring hormones have such profound effects on the heart and cardiovascular system suggests that these actions can be captured to treat a variety of cardiovascular diseases. The ability of thyroid hormone to lower cholesterol levels,[75] enhance cardiac contractility (especially diastolic function) via novel transcription-based mechanisms,[104] and at the same time lower systemic vascular resistance provides a platform for developing novel therapies. Similarly, the ability of vasoactive intestinal peptide to lower pulmonary artery pressure opens the possibility of treating patients with pulmonary hypertension from many different causes.

REFERENCES

(For references to the older literature, please consult the 8th edition of *Braunwald's Heart Disease*, Chap. 81.)

Acromegaly

1. Lu C, Schwartzbauer G, Sperling MA, et al: Demonstration of direct effects of growth hormone on neonatal cardiomyocytes. J Biol Chem 276:22892, 2001.
2. Napoli R, Guardasole V, Angelini V, et al: Acute effects of growth hormone on vascular function in human subjects. J Clin Endocrinol Metab 88:2817, 2003.
3. Colao A, Vitale G, Pivonello R, et al: The heart: An end-organ of GH action. Eur J Endocrinol 151(Suppl):S93, 2004.
4. Brevetti G, Marzullo P, Silvestro A, et al: Early vascular alterations in acromegaly. J Clin Endocrinol Metab 87:3174, 2002.
5. Mestron A, Webb SM, Astorga R, et al: Epidemiology, clinical characteristics, outcome, morbidity and mortality in acromegaly based on the Spanish Acromegaly Registry (Registro Espanol de Acromegalia, REA). Eur J Endocrinol 151:439, 2004.
6. Clayton RN: Cardiovascular function in acromegaly. Endocr Rev 24:272, 2003.
7. Bruch C, Herrmann B, Schmermund A, et al: Impact of disease activity on left ventricular performance in patients with acromegaly. Am Heart J 144:538, 2002.
8. Colao A, Spinelli L, Cuocolo A, et al: Cardiovascular consequences of early-onset growth hormone excess. J Clin Endocrinol Metab 87:3097, 2002.
9. Di Bello V, Bogazzi F, Di Cori A, et al: Myocardial systolic strain abnormalities in patients with acromegaly: A prospective color Doppler imaging study. J Endocrinol Invest 29:544, 2006.
10. Colao A, Spinelli L, Marzullo P, et al: High prevalence of cardiac valve disease in acromegaly: An observational, analytical, case-control study. J Clin Endocrinol Metab 88:3196, 2003.
11. van der Klaauw AA, Bax JJ, Roelfsema F, et al: Uncontrolled acromegaly is associated with progressive mitral valvular regurgitation. Growth Horm IGF Res 16:101, 2006.
12. Herrmann BL, Bruch C, Saller B, et al: Acromegaly: Evidence for a direct relation between disease activity and cardiac dysfunction in patients without ventricular hypertrophy. Clin Endocrinol (Oxf) 56:595, 2002.
13. Damjanovics SS, Neskovic AN, Petakov MS, et al: High output heart failure in patients with newly diagnosed acromegaly. Am J Med 112:610, 2002.
14. Trainer PJ, Drake WM, Katznelson L, et al: Treatment of acromegaly with the growth hormone-receptor antagonist pegvisomant. N Engl J Med 342:1171, 2000.
15. Clemmons DR, Chihara K, Freda PU, et al: Optimizing control of acromegaly: Integrating a growth hormone receptor antagonist into the treatment algorithm. J Clin Endocrinol Metab 88:4759, 2003.
16. Fazio S, Cittadini A, Biondi B, et al: Cardiovascular effects of short-term growth hormone hypersecretion. J Clin Endocrinol Metab 85:179, 2000.
17. Colao A, Pivonello R, Auriemma RS, et al: Predictors of tumor shrinkage after primary therapy with somatostatin analogues in acromegaly: A prospective study in 99 patients. J Clin Endocrinol Metab 91:2112, 2006.

Adrenal Cortex

18. Whitworth JA, Mangos GJ, Kelly JJ: Cushing, cortisol, and cardiovascular disease. Hypertension 36:912, 2000.
19. Wintour EM: Cortisol as a growth hormone for the fetal heart. Endocrinology 147:3641, 2006.
20. Colao A, Pivonello R, Spiezia S, et al: Persistence of increased cardiovascular risk in patients with Cushing disease after five years of successful cure. J Clin Endocrinol Metab 84:2664, 1999.
21. Maron BA, Leopold JA: Mineralocorticoid receptor antagonists and endothelial function. Curr Opin Investig Drugs 9:963, 2008.
22. Fernandez-Real J, Ricard W: Insulin resistance and chronic cardiovascular inflammatory syndrome. Endocr Rev 24:278, 2003.
23. Suzuki T, Shibata H, Ando T, et al: Risk factors associated with persistent postoperative hypertension in Cushing syndrome. Endocr Res 26:791, 2000.
24. Dekker MJ, Koper JW, van Aken MO, et al: Salivary cortisol is related to atherosclerosis of carotid arteries. J Clin Endocrinol Metab 93:3741, 2008.
25. Muiesan ML, Lupia M, Salvetti M, et al: Left ventricular structural and functional characteristics in Cushing syndrome. J Am Coll Cardiol 41:2275, 2003.
26. Marazuela M, Aguilar-Torres R, Benedicto A, et al: Dilated cardiomyopathy as a presenting feature of Cushing syndrome. Int J Cardiol 88:331, 2003.
27. Bertherat J: Carney complex (CNC). Orphanet J Rare Dis 6:21, 2006.
28. Carey RM, Siragy HM: Newly recognized components of the renin-angiotensin system: Potential roles in cardiovascular and renal regulation. Endocr Rev 24:261, 2003.
29. Young MJ, Funder JW: Mineralocorticoid receptors and pathophysiological roles for aldosterone in the cardiovascular system. J Hypertens 20:1465, 2002.
30. Szucs TD, Holm MV, Schwenkglenks M, et al: Cost-effectiveness of eplerenone in patients with left ventricular dysfunction after myocardial infarction—an analysis of the Ephesus Study from a Swiss perspective. Cardiovasc Drugs Ther 20:193, 2006.
31. Verma A, Solomon SD: Optimizing care of heart failure after acute MI with an aldosterone receptor antagonist. Curr Heart Fail Rep 4:183, 2007.
32. Matsumura K, Fujii K, Oniki H, et al: Role of aldosterone in left ventricular hypertrophy in hypertension. Am J Hypertens 19:13, 2006.
33. Watson T, Karthikeyan VJ, Lip GYH, Beevers DG: Atrial fibrillation in primary aldosteronism. J Renin Angiotensin Aldosterone Syst 10:190, 2009.
34. Funder JW, Carey RM, Fardella C: Case detection, diagnosis, and treatment of patients with primary aldosteronism: An endocrine society clinical practice guideline. J Clin Endocrinol Metab 93:3266, 2008.
35. Espinosa G, Santos E, Cervera R, et al: Adrenal involvement in the antiphospholipid syndrome: Clinical and immunologic characteristics of 86 patients. Medicine (Baltimore) 82:106, 2003.
36. Cooper MS, Stewart PM: Corticosteroid insufficiency in acutely ill patients. N Engl J Med 348:727, 2003.
37. Bergthorsdottir R, Leonsson-Zachrisson M, Oden A, Johannsson G: Premature mortality in patients with Addison's disease: A population-based study. J Clin Endocrinol Metab 91:4849, 2006.

Parathyroid Disease

38. Stefenelli T, Abela C, Frank H, et al: Cardiac abnormalities in patients with primary hyperparathyroidism: Implications for follow-up. J Clin Endocrinol Metab 82:106, 1997.
39. Birgander M, Bondeson A-G, Bondeson L, et al: Cardiac structure and function before and after parathyroidectomy in patients with asymptomatic primary hyperparathyroidism. Endocrinologist 19:154, 2009.
40. Floege J, Raggi P, Block GA, et al: Study design and subject baseline characteristics in the ADVANCE Study: Effects of cinacalcet on vascular calcification in haemodialysis patients. Nephrol Dial Transplant 25:1916, 2010.

Vitamin D

41. Holick MF: Vitamin D deficiency. New Engl J Med 357:266, 2007.
42. Vanga SR, Good M, Howard PA, Vacek JL: Role of vitamin D in cardiovascular health. Am J Cardiol 106:798, 2010.

Thyroid Disease

43. Klein I, Danzi S: Thyroid disease and the heart. Circulation 116:1725, 2007.
44. Gereben B, Zavacki AM, Ribich S, et al: Cellular and molecular basis of deiodinase-regulated thyroid hormone signaling. Endocr Rev 29:898, 2008.
45. Bassett JH, Harvey CB, Williams GR: Mechanisms of thyroid hormone receptor–specific nuclear and extra nuclear actions. Mol Cell Endocrinol 213:1, 2003.
46. Danzi S, Dubon P, Klein I: Effect of serum triiodothyronine on regulation of cardiac gene expression: Role of histone acetylation. Am J Physiol Heart Circ Physiol 289:H1506, 2005.
47. Danzi S, Klein I: Changes in thyroid hormone metabolism and gene expression in the failing heart: Therapeutic implications. *In* Iervasi G, Pingitore A (eds): Thyroid and Heart Failure: From Pathophysiology to Clinics. Milan, Italy, Springer-Verlag, 2009, pp 97-108.
48. Carr AN, Kranias EG: Thyroid hormone regulation of calcium cycling proteins. Thyroid 12:453, 2002.
49. Ojamaa K, Kenessey A, Klein I: Thyroid hormone regulation of phospholamban phosphorylation in the rat heart. Endocrinology 141:2139, 2000.
50. Biondi B, Klein I: Hypothyroidism as a risk factor for hypothyroidism. Endocrine 24:1, 2004.
51. Virtanen VK, Saha HH, Groundstroem KW, et al: Thyroid hormone substitution therapy rapidly enhances left-ventricular diastolic function in hypothyroid patients. Cardiology 96:59, 2001.
52. Davis PJ, Davis FB, Lin HY, et al: Translational implications of nongenomic actions of thyroid hormone initiated at its integrin receptor. Am J Physiol Endocrinol Metab 297:E1238, 2009.
53. Demers LM, Spencer CA: Laboratory medicine practice guidelines, laboratory support for the diagnosis and monitoring of thyroid disease. Thyroid 13:3, 2003.
54. Hoit BD, Khoury SF, Shao Y, et al: Effects of thyroid hormone on cardiac beta-adrenergic responsiveness in conscious baboons. Circulation 96:592, 1997.
55. Ojamaa K, Klein I, Sabet A, et al: Changes in adenylyl cyclase isoforms as a mechanism for thyroid hormone modulation of cardiac beta-adrenergic receptor responsiveness. Metabolism 49:275, 2000.
56. Park KW, Kai HB, Ojamaa K, et al: The direct vasomotor effect of thyroid hormones on rat skeletal muscle resistance arteries. Anesth Analg 85:734, 1997.
57. Danzi S, Klein I: Thyroid hormone and blood pressure regulation. Curr Hypertens Rep 5:513, 2003.
58. Biondi B, Palmieri EA, Lombardi G, et al: Effects of thyroid hormone on cardiac function: The relative importance of heart rate, loading conditions, and myocardial contractility in the regulation of cardiac performance in human hyperthyroidism. J Clin Endocrinol Metab 87:968, 2002.
59. Schmidt B, Martin N, Georgens AC, et al: Nongenomic cardiovascular effects of triiodothyronine in euthyroid male volunteers. J Clin Endocrinol Metab 87:1681, 2002.
60. Bengel FM, Lehnert J, Ibrahim T, et al: Cardiac oxidative metabolism, function, and metabolic performance in mild hyperthyroidism: A noninvasive study using positron emission tomography and magnetic resonance imaging. Thyroid 13:471, 2003.
61. Taddei S, Caraccio N, Virdis A, et al: Impaired endothelium-dependent vasodilatation in subclinical hypothyroidism: Beneficial effect of levothyroxine therapy. J Clin Endocrinol Metab 88:3731, 2003.
62. Kahaly GJ, Kampmann C, Mohr-Kahaly S: Cardiovascular hemodynamics and exercise tolerance in thyroid disease. Thyroid 12:473, 2002.
63. Im SH, Oh CW, Kwon OK, et al: Moyamoya disease associated with Graves' disease: Special considerations regarding clinical significance and management. J Neurosurg 102:1013, 2005.
64. Marvisi M, Zambrelli P, Brianti M: Pulmonary hypertension is frequent in hyperthyroidism and normalizes after therapy. Eur J Intern Med 17:267, 2006.
65. Shimizu T, Koide S, Noh JY, et al: Hyperthyroidism and the management of atrial fibrillation. Thyroid 12:489, 2002.
66. Auer J, Scheibner P, Mische T, et al: Subclinical hyperthyroidism as a risk factor for atrial fibrillation. Am Heart J 142:838, 2001.
67. Nakazawa H, Lythall DA, Noh J, et al: Is there a place for the late cardioversion of atrial fibrillation? A long-term follow-up study of patients with post-thyrotoxic atrial fibrillation. Eur Heart J 21:327, 2000.
68. Fuster V, Ryden LE, Asinger RW, et al: ACC/AHA/ESC guidelines for the management of patients with atrial fibrillation. J Am Coll Cardiol 38:1266, 2001.
69. Franklyn JA, Maisonneuve P, Sheppard MC, et al: Mortality after the treatment of hyperthyroidism with radioactive iodine. N Engl J Med 338:712, 1998.
70. Flynn RW, MacDonald TM, Jung RT, et al: Some cardiovascular diseases occur with increased frequency in patients treated for hyperthyroidism or hypothyroidism. J Clin Endocrinol Metab 91:2159, 2006.
71. Klein I: The cardiovascular system in hypothyroidism. *In* Braverman LE, Utiger RD (eds): Werner & Ingbar's The Thyroid: A Fundamental and Clinical Text. 9th ed. Philadelphia, Lippincott Williams & Wilkins, 2005, pp 774-780.

72. Bengel FM, Nekolla SC, Ibrahim T, et al: Effect of thyroid hormones on cardiac function, geometry, and oxidative metabolism assessed noninvasively by positron emission tomography and magnetic resonance imaging. J Clin Endocrinol Metab 85:1822, 2000.
73. Cappola AR, Ladenson PW: Hypothyroidism and atherosclerosis. J Clin Endocrinol Metab 88:2438, 2003.
74. Rush J, Danzi S, Klein I: Role of thyroid disease in the development of statin-induced myopathy. Endocrinologist 16:279, 2006.
75. Ladenson PW, Kristensen JD, Ridgway EC, et al: Use of the thyroid hormone analogue eprotirome in statin-treated dyslipidemia. N Engl J Med 362:906, 2010.
76. Hak AE, Pols HAP, Visser TJ, et al: Subclinical hypothyroidism is an independent risk factor for atherosclerosis and myocardial infarction in elderly women: The Rotterdam Study. Ann Intern Med 132:270, 2000.
77. Walsh JP, Bremmer AP, Bulsara MK, et al: Subclinical thyroid dysfunction as a risk factor for cardiovascular disease. Arch Intern Med 165:2467, 2005.
78. Kim SD, Kim SH, Park KS, et al: Regression of the increased common carotid artery-intima media thickness in subclinical hypothyroidism after thyroid hormone replacement. Endocr J 56:753, 2009.
79. Rodondi N, Bauer DC, Cappola AR: Subclinical thyroid dysfunction, cardiac function, and the risk of heart failure. The Cardiovascular Health study. J Am Coll Cardiol 52:1152, 2008.
80. Rodondi N, den Elzen WPJ, Bauer DC, et al: Subclinical hypothyroidism and the risk of coronary heart disease and mortality. JAMA 304:1365, 2010.
81. Biondi B, Cooper DS: The clinical significance of subclinical thyroid dysfunction. Endocr Rev 29:76, 2008.
82. Razvi SS, Pearce SH: Treatment of subclinical hypothyroidism and cardiovascular morbidity and mortality—analysis of the United Kingdom General Practitioner Research Database. Abstract, International Thyroid Congress, 2010.
83. Sawin CT: Subclinical hyperthyroidism and atrial fibrillation. Thyroid 12:501, 2002.
84. Cappola AR, Fried LP, Arnold AM, et al: Thyroid status, cardiovascular risk, and mortality in older adults. JAMA 295:1033, 2006.
85. Parle, JV, Maisonneuve P, Sheppard MC, et al: Prediction of all-cause and cardiovascular mortality in elderly people from one low serum thyrotropin result: A 10-year cohort study. Lancet 358:861, 2001.
86. Mitchell AL, Pearce SH: How should we treat patients with low serum thyrotropin concentrations? Clin Endocrinol (Oxf) Epub Sept 10, 2009.

Amiodarone

87. Cohen-Lehman J, Dahl P, Danzi S, Klein I: Effects of amiodarone on thyroid function. Nat Rev Endocrinol 6:34, 2010.
88. Multaq (Dronedarone): Briefing Document: Advisory Committee Meeting of the Cardiovascular and Renal Drugs Division of the US Food and Drug Administration, March 18, 2009 (http://www.fda.gov/downloads/AdvisoryCommittees/CommitteesMeetingMaterials/Drugs/CardiovascularandRenalDrugsAdvisoryCommittee/UCM134981.pdf).
89. Bogazzi F, Bartalena L, Cosci C, et al: Treatment of type II amiodarone-induced thyrotoxicosis by either iopanoic acid or glucocorticoids: A prospective, randomized study. J Clin Endocrinol Metab 88:1999, 2003.
90. Yiu KH, Jim MH, Siu CW, et al: Amiodarone-induced thyrotoxicosis is associated with a nearly threefold increased risk for major adverse cardiovascular events that must be identified and treated. J Clin Endocrinol Metab 94:109, 2009.
91. Williams M, Lo Gerfo P: Thyroidectomy using local anesthesia in critically ill patients with amiodarone-induced thyrotoxicosis: A review and description of the technique. Thyroid 12:523, 2002.

Changes in Thyroid Hormone Metabolism in Cardiac Disease

92. Iervasi G, Pingitore A, Landi P, et al: Low-T_3 syndrome: A strong prognostic predictor of death in patients with heart disease. Circulation 107:708, 2003.
93. Pingitore A, Galli E, Barison A, et al: Acute effects of triiodothyronine (T_3) replacement therapy in patients with chronic heart failure and low-T3 syndrome: A randomized, placebo-controlled study. J Clin Endocrinol Metab 93:1351, 2008.
94. Portman MA, Fearneyhough C, Ning W, et al: Triiodothyronine repletion in infants during cardiopulmonary bypass for congenital heart disease. J Thorac Cardiovasc Surg 120:604, 2000.
95. Klemperer JD, Klein I, Ojamaa K, et al: Triiodothyronine therapy lowers the incidence of atrial fibrillation after cardiac operations. Ann Thorac Surg 61:1323, 1996.
96. Portman MA, Slee A, Olson AK, et al: Triiodothyronine supplementation in infants and children undergoing cardiopulmonary bypass (TRICC): A multicenter placebo-controlled randomized trial: Age analysis. Circulation 122(suppl 1):S224, 2010.
97. Chowdhury D, Parnell V, Ojamaa, K, et al: Usefulness of triiodothyronine (T_3) treatment after surgery for complex congenital heart disease in infants and children. Am J Cardiol 84:1107, 1999.

Pheochromocytoma

98. Bravo EL: Pheochromocytoma. Cardiol Rev 10:44, 2002.
99. Manger WM, Gifford RW: Pheochromocytoma. J Clin Hypertens (Greenwich) 4:62, 2002.
100. Brouwers FM, Elkahloun AG, Munson PJ, et al: Gene expression profiling of benign and malignant pheochromocytoma. Ann N Y Acad Sci 1073:541, 2006.
101. Lenders JW, Pacak K, Eisenhofer G: New advances in the biochemical diagnosis of pheochromocytoma: Moving beyond catecholamines. Ann N Y Acad Sci 970:29, 2002.
102. Schiff RL, Welsh GA: Perioperative evaluation and management of the patient with endocrine dysfunction. Med Clin North Am 87:175, 2003.
103. Eigelberger MS, Duh QY: Pheochromocytoma. Curr Treat Options Oncol 2:321, 2001.
104. Danzi S, Klein I: Thyroid hormone treatment to mend a broken heart. J Clin Endocrinol Metab 93:1172, 2008.

CHAPTER 87 Hemostasis, Thrombosis, Fibrinolysis, and Cardiovascular Disease

Jeffrey I. Weitz

Hemostasis preserves vascular integrity by balancing the physiologic processes that maintain blood fluidity under normal circumstances and prevent excessive bleeding after vascular injury. Preservation of blood fluidity depends on an intact vascular endothelium and a complex series of regulatory pathways that maintain platelets in a quiescent state and keep the coagulation system in check. In contrast, arrest of bleeding requires rapid formation of hemostatic plugs at sites of vascular injury to prevent exsanguination. Perturbation of hemostasis can lead to thrombosis, which can occur in arteries or veins and is a major cause of morbidity and mortality. Arterial thrombosis is the most common cause of acute coronary syndromes, ischemic stroke, and limb gangrene, whereas thrombosis in the deep veins of the leg leads to the postphlebitic syndrome and to pulmonary embolism, which can be fatal.

Most arterial thrombi form on top of disrupted atherosclerotic plaques, because plaque rupture exposes thrombogenic material in the plaque core to the blood. This material then triggers platelet aggregation and fibrin formation, which results in the generation of a platelet-rich thrombus that temporarily or permanently occludes blood flow.[1,2] Temporary occlusion of blood flow in coronary arteries may trigger unstable angina, whereas persistent obstruction causes myocardial infarction. The same processes can occur in the cerebral circulation, where temporary arterial occlusion may manifest as a transient ischemic attack and permanent occlusion can lead to a stroke.

In contrast to arterial thrombi, venous thrombi rarely form at sites of obvious vascular disruption.[2] Although they can develop after surgical trauma to veins, or secondary to indwelling venous catheters, they usually originate in the valve cusps of the deep veins of the calf or in the muscular sinuses, where there is stasis. Sluggish blood flow in these veins reduces the oxygen supply to the avascular valve cusps. Hypoxemia induces endothelial cells lining the valve cusps to express adhesion molecules, which tether tissue factor–bearing leukocytes and microparticles onto their surface. Tissue factor–bearing leukocytes and microparticles adhere to these activated cells and induce coagulation. Impaired blood flow exacerbates local thrombus formation by reducing clearance of activated clotting factors. Calf vein thrombi that extend into the proximal veins of the leg can dislodge and travel to the lungs to produce pulmonary embolism.

Arterial and venous thrombi contain platelets and fibrin, but the proportions differ. Arterial thrombi are rich in platelets because of the high shear in the injured arteries. In contrast, venous thrombi, which form under low shear conditions, contain relatively few platelets and consist mostly of fibrin and trapped red cells.[2] Because of the predominance of platelets, arterial thrombi appear white, whereas venous thrombi appear red, reflecting the trapped red cells.

The antithrombotic drugs used for prevention and treatment of thrombosis target components of thrombi, and include antiplatelet drugs, which inhibit platelets; anticoagulants, which attenuate coagulation; and fibrinolytic agents, which induce fibrin degradation (**Fig. 87-1**). With the predominance of platelets in arterial thrombi, strategies to inhibit or treat arterial thrombosis focus mainly on antiplatelet agents,[2] although in the acute setting, strategies often include anticoagulants and fibrinolytic agents. When arterial thrombi are occlusive and rapid restoration of blood flow is required, mechanical and pharmacologic methods enable thrombus extraction, compression, or degradation. Although rarely used for this indication, anticoagulants can also prevent recurrent ischemic events after acute myocardial infarction. Anticoagulants are the mainstay for prevention and treatment of venous thromboembolism because fibrin is the predominant component of venous thrombi. Antiplatelet drugs are less effective than anticoagulants because of the limited platelet content of venous thrombi. Selected patients with venous thromboembolism benefit from fibrinolytic therapy[3]—for example, patients with massive or submassive pulmonary embolism—achieve more rapid restoration of pulmonary blood flow with systemic or catheter-directed fibrinolytic therapy than with anticoagulant therapy alone (see Chap. 77). Selected patients with extensive deep vein thrombosis in the iliac and/or femoral veins also may have a better outcome with catheter-directed fibrinolytic therapy and/or mechanical thrombus extraction in addition to anticoagulants.

Building on a review of hemostasis and thrombosis that highlights the processes involved in platelet activation and aggregation, blood coagulation, and fibrinolysis, this chapter focuses on antiplatelet, anticoagulant, and fibrinolytic drugs in common use. It also provides a brief overview of new antithrombotic drugs in advanced stages of development.

Hemostatic System

The major components of the hemostatic system are the vascular endothelium, platelets, and the coagulation and fibrinolytic systems.

Vascular Endothelium

A monolayer of endothelial cells lines the intimal surface of the circulatory tree and separates the blood from the prothrombotic subendothelial components of the vessel wall. As such, the vascular endothelium (see Chap. 43) encompasses about 10^{13} cells and covers a vast surface area. Rather than serving as a static barrier, the healthy vascular endothelium is a dynamic organ that actively regulates hemostasis by inhibiting platelets, suppressing coagulation, and promoting fibrinolysis.[1,2]

PLATELET INHIBITION. Endothelial cells synthesize prostacyclin and nitric oxide and release them into the blood. These agents not

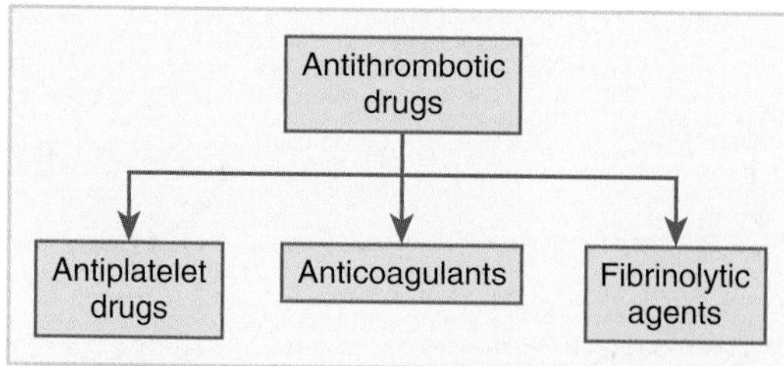

FIGURE 87-1 Classification of antithrombotic drugs.

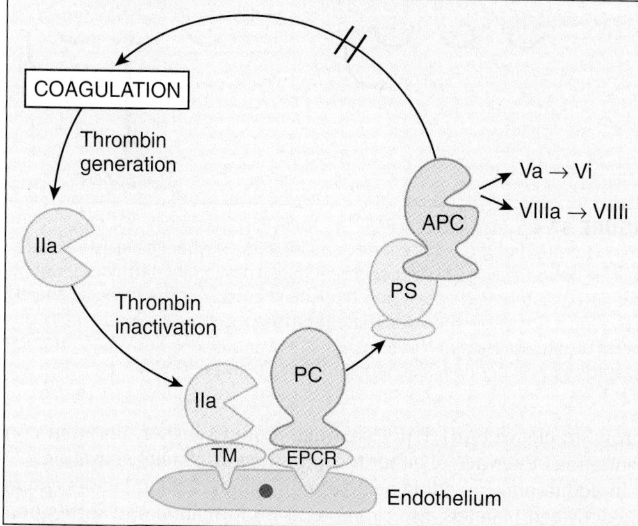

FIGURE 87-2 Protein C pathway. Activation of coagulation triggers thrombin (IIa) generation. Excess thrombin binds to thrombomodulin (TM) on the endothelial cell surface. Once bound, the substrate specificity of thrombin alters such that it no longer acts as a procoagulant, but becomes a potent activator of protein C (PC). EPCR binds protein C and presents it to thrombomodulin-bound thrombin for activation. Activated protein C (APC), together with its cofactor, protein S (PS), binds to the activated platelet surface and proteolytically degrades factors Va and VIIIa into inactive fragments (Vi and VIIIi). Degradation of these activated cofactors inhibits thrombin generation (double bar).

only serve as potent vasodilators, but also inhibit platelet activation and subsequent aggregation by stimulating adenylate cyclase and increasing intracellular levels of cyclic adenosine monophosphate (cAMP). In addition, endothelial cells express CD39 on their surface, a membrane-associated ecto adenosine diphosphatase (ADPase). By degrading ADP, a platelet agonist, CD39 attenuates platelet activation.[4]

ANTICOAGULANT ACTIVITY. Intact endothelial cells play an essential part in the regulation of thrombin generation through various mechanisms. Endothelial cells produce heparan sulfate proteoglycans, which bind circulating antithrombin and accelerate the rate at which it inhibits thrombin and other coagulation enzymes.[5] Tissue factor pathway inhibitor (TFPI), a naturally occurring inhibitor of coagulation, binds heparan sulfate on the endothelial cell surface.[6] Administration of heparin or low-molecular-weight heparin (LMWH) displaces glycosaminoglycan-bound TFPI from the vascular endothelium, and released TFPI may contribute to the antithrombotic activity of these drugs.[7] Endothelial cells express thrombomodulin and endothelial cell protein C receptor (EPCR) on their surface.[8]

Thrombomodulin binds thrombin and alters this enzyme's substrate specificity so that it no longer acts as a procoagulant, but becomes a potent activator of protein C (**Fig. 87-2**). Activated protein C serves as an anticoagulant by degrading and inactivating activated factors V and VIII (factor Va and VIIIa, respectively), key cofactors involved in thrombin generation. EPCR on the endothelial cell surface enhances this pathway by binding protein C and presenting it to the thrombin–thrombomodulin complex for activation.[9]

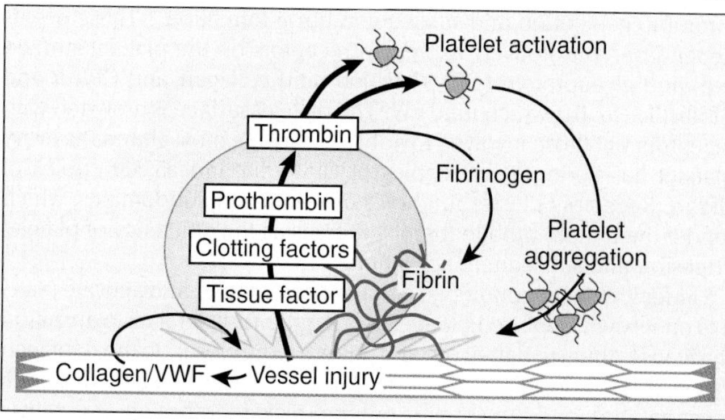

FIGURE 87-3 Central role of thrombin in thrombogenesis. Vascular injury simultaneously triggers platelet adhesion and activation, as well as activation of the coagulation system. Platelet activation is initiated by exposure of subendothelial collagen and vWF, onto which platelets adhere. Adherent platelets become activated and release ADP and thromboxane A_2, platelet agonists that activate ambient platelets and recruit them to the site of injury. Coagulation, which is triggered by tissue factor exposed at the site of injury, results in thrombin generation. Thrombin not only converts fibrinogen to fibrin, but also serves as a potent platelet agonist. When platelets are activated, glycoprotein IIb/IIIa on their surface undergoes a conformational change that endows it with the capacity to ligate fibrinogen and mediate platelet aggregation. Fibrin strands then weave the platelet aggregates together to form a platelet-fibrin thrombus (see Fig. 56-3).

FIBRINOLYTIC ACTIVITY. The vascular endothelium promotes fibrinolysis by synthesizing and releasing tissue and urokinase plasminogen activator (t-PA and u-PA, respectively), which initiate fibrinolysis by converting plasminogen to plasmin.[10] Endothelial cells in most vascular beds synthesize t-PA constitutively. In contrast, perturbed endothelial cells produce u-PA in the settings of inflammation and wound repair.

Endothelial cells also produce type 1 plasminogen activator inhibitor (PAI-1), the major regulator of t-PA and u-PA. Therefore, net fibrinolytic activity depends on the dynamic balance between the release of plasminogen activators and PAI-1. Fibrinolysis localizes to the endothelial cell surface because these cells express annexin II, a coreceptor for plasminogen and t-PA that promotes their interaction. Therefore, healthy vessels actively resist thrombosis and help maintain platelets in a quiescent state.[10]

Platelets

Platelets are anucleate particles released into the circulation after fragmentation of bone marrow megakaryocytes. Because they are anucleate, platelets have limited capacity to synthesize proteins. Thrombopoietin, a glycoprotein synthesized in the liver and kidneys, regulates megakaryocytic proliferation and maturation as well as platelet production.[11] Once they enter the circulation, platelets have a life span of 7 to 10 days.

Damage to the intimal lining of the vessel exposes the underlying subendothelial matrix. Platelets home to sites of vascular disruption and adhere to the exposed matrix proteins. Adherent platelets undergo activation and not only release substances that recruit additional platelets to the site of injury, but also promote thrombin generation and subsequent fibrin formation (**Fig. 87-3**). A potent platelet agonist, thrombin amplifies platelet recruitment and activation. Activated platelets then aggregate to form a plug that seals the leak in the vasculature. Understanding the steps in these highly integrated processes helps pinpoint the sites of action of the antiplatelet drugs and rationalizes the usefulness of anticoagulants for the treatment of arterial thrombosis and venous thrombosis.

ADHESION. Platelets adhere to exposed collagen and von Willebrand factor (vWF) and form a monolayer that supports and promotes thrombin generation and subsequent fibrin formation.[12] These events depend on constitutively expressed receptors on the platelet surface, $\alpha_2\beta_1$ and glycoprotein (GP) VI, which bind collagen, and GPIbα and GPIIb/IIIa ($\alpha_{IIb}\beta_3$), which bind vWF. The platelet surface is crowded with receptors, but those involved in adhesion are the most abundant: every platelet has about 80,000 copies of GPIIb/IIIa and 25,000 copies of GPIbα. Receptors cluster in cholesterol-enriched subdomains, which render them more mobile, thereby increasing the efficiency of platelet adhesion and subsequent activation.[13]

Under low shear conditions, collagen can capture and activate platelets on its own. Captured platelets undergo cytoskeletal reorganization that causes them to flatten out and adhere more closely to the damaged vessel wall. Under high shear conditions, however, collagen and vWF must act in concert to support optimal platelet adhesion and activation. vWF synthesized by endothelial cells and megakaryocytes assembles into multimers that range from 550 to over 10,000 kDa.[14] When released from storage in the Weibel-Palade bodies of endothelial cells or the alpha granules of platelets, most of the vWF enters the circulation, but the vWF released from the abluminal surface of endothelial cells accumulates in the subendothelial matrix, where it binds collagen via its A3 domain. This surface-immobilized vWF can simultaneously bind platelets via its A1 domain. In contrast, circulating vWF does not react with unstimulated platelets. This difference in reactivity likely reflects vWF conformation; circulating vWF is in a coiled conformation that prevents access of its platelet-binding domain to vWF receptors on the platelet surface, whereas immobilized vWF assumes an elongated shape that exposes the A1 domain. In their extended conformation, large vWF multimers act as the molecular glue that tethers platelets to the damaged vessel wall with sufficient strength to withstand higher shear forces. Large vWF multimers provide additional binding sites for collagen, and heighten platelet adhesion because platelets have more vWF receptors than collagen receptors.[15] Adhesion to collagen or vWF results in platelet activation, the next step in platelet plug formation.

ACTIVATION. Adhesion to collagen and vWF initiates signaling pathways that result in platelet activation. These pathways induce cyclooxygenase-1 (COX-1)–dependent synthesis and release of thromboxane A_2, and trigger the release of ADP from storage granules. Thromboxane A_2 is a potent vasoconstrictor and, like ADP, locally activates ambient platelets and recruits them to the site of injury. This process results in expansion of the platelet plug. To activate platelets, thromboxane A_2 and ADP must bind to their respective receptors on the platelet membrane. The thromboxane receptor (TP) is a G protein–coupled receptor that is found on platelets and on the endothelium, which explains why thromboxane A_2 induces vasoconstriction as well as platelet activation.[16] ADP interacts with a family of G protein–coupled receptors on the platelet membrane.[17,18] Most important of these is $P2Y_{12}$, which is the target of the thienopyridines, but $P2Y_1$ also contributes to ADP-induced platelet activation, and maximal ADP-induced platelet activation requires activation of both receptors. A third ADP receptor, $P2X_1$, is an ATP-gated calcium channel. Platelet storage granules contain ATP and ADP; ATP released during the platelet activation process may contribute to the platelet recruitment process in a $P2X_1$-dependent fashion.

Although TP and the various ADP receptors signal through different pathways, they all increase the intracellular calcium concentration in platelets. This in turn induces shape change via cytoskeletal rearrangement, granule mobilization and release, and subsequent platelet aggregation. Activated platelets promote coagulation by expressing phosphatidyl serine on their surface, an anionic phospholipid that supports assembly of coagulation factor complexes. Once assembled, these clotting factor complexes trigger a burst of thrombin generation and subsequent fibrin formation. In addition to converting fibrinogen to fibrin, thrombin amplifies platelet recruitment and activation and promotes expansion of the platelet plug. Thrombin binds to protease-activated receptors types 1 and 4 (PAR1 and PAR4, respectively) on the platelet surface and cleaves their extended amino termini (**Fig. 87-4**), thereby generating new amino termini that serve as tethered ligands that bind and activate the receptors.[17,19] Whereas low concentrations of

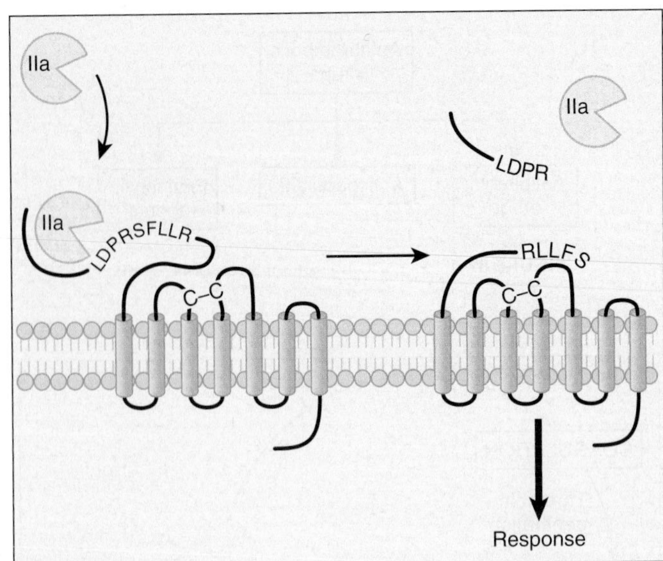

FIGURE 87-4 Activation of PAR1 by thrombin. Thrombin (IIa) binds to the amino terminus of the extracellular domain of PAR1, where it cleaves a specific peptide bond. Cleavage of this bond generates a new amino-terminus sequence that acts as a tethered ligand and binds to the body of the receptor, thereby activating it. Thrombin then dissociates from the receptor. Analogues of the first five or six amino acids of the tethered ligand sequences, known as thrombin receptor agonist peptides, can independently activate PAR1.

thrombin cleave PAR1, PAR4 cleavage requires higher thrombin concentrations. Cleavage of either receptor triggers platelet activation.

In addition to providing a surface on which clotting factors assemble, activated platelets also promote fibrin formation and subsequent stabilization by releasing factor V, factor XI, fibrinogen, and factor XIII. Thus, there is coordinated activation of platelets and coagulation, and the fibrin network that results from thrombin action helps anchor the platelet aggregates at the site of injury. Activated platelets also release adhesive proteins, such as vWF, thrombospondin, and fibronectin, which may augment platelet adhesion at sites of injury, as well as growth factors, such as platelet-derived growth factor (PDGF) and transforming growth factor-β (TGF-β), which promote wound healing. Platelet aggregation is the final step in the formation of the platelet plug.

AGGREGATION. Platelet aggregation links platelets to each other to form clumps. GPIIb/IIIa mediates these platelet-to-platelet linkages. On nonactivated platelets, GPIIb/IIIa exhibits minimal affinity for its ligands. On platelet activation, GPIIb/IIIa undergoes a conformational transformation, which reflects transmission of inside-out signals from its cytoplasmic domain to its extracellular domain.[15] This transformation enhances the affinity of GPIIb/IIIa for its ligands, fibrinogen, and under high shear conditions, vWF. Arg-Gly-Asp (RGD) sequences located on fibrinogen and vWF, as well as a platelet-binding Lys-Gly-Asp (KGD) sequence on fibrinogen, mediate their interaction with GPIIb/IIIa. When subjected to high shear, circulating vWF elongates and exposes its platelet-binding domain, which enables its interaction with the conformationally activated GPIIb/IIIa.[14] Divalent fibrinogen and multivalent vWF molecules serve as bridges and bind adjacent platelets together. Once bound to GPIIb/IIIa, fibrinogen and vWF induce outside-inside signals that augment platelet activation and result in the activation of additional GPIIb/IIIa receptors, creating a positive feedback loop. Because GPIIb/IIIa acts as the final effector in platelet aggregation, it is a logical target for potent antiplatelet drugs. Fibrin, the ultimate product of the coagulation system, tethers the platelet aggregates together and anchors them to the site of injury.

Coagulation

Coagulation results in the generation of thrombin, which converts soluble fibrinogen to fibrin. Coagulation occurs through the action of discrete enzyme complexes, which are composed of a vitamin K–dependent enzyme and a nonenzyme cofactor, and assemble on anionic phospholipid membranes in a calcium-dependent fashion. Each enzyme complex activates a vitamin K–dependent substrate that becomes the enzyme component of the subsequent complex (**Fig. 87-5**). Together, these complexes generate a small amount of thrombin that amplifies its own generation by activating the nonenzyme cofactors and platelets, which then provide an anionic surface on which the complexes assemble. The three enzyme complexes involved in thrombin generation are extrinsic tenase, intrinsic tenase, and prothrombinase. Although extrinsic tenase initiates the system under most circumstances, the contact system also plays a role in some situations.

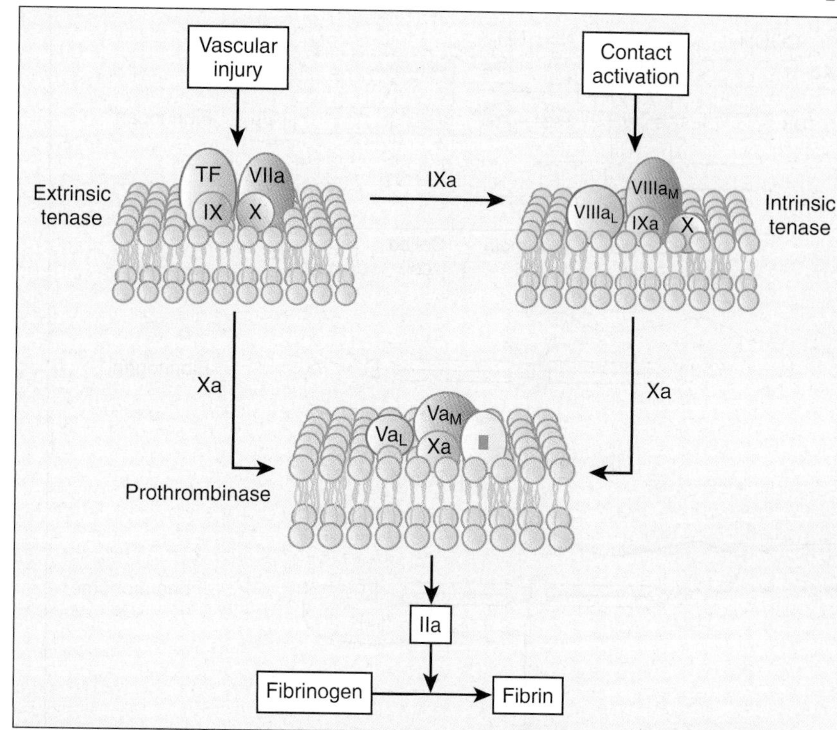

FIGURE 87-5 Coagulation system. Coagulation occurs through the action of discrete enzyme complexes, which are composed of a vitamin K–dependent enzyme and a nonenzyme cofactor. These complexes assemble on anionic phospholipid membranes in a calcium-dependent fashion. Vascular injury exposes tissue factor (TF), which binds factor VIIa to form extrinsic tenase. Extrinsic tenase activates factors IX and X. Factor IXa binds to factor VIIIa to form intrinsic tenase, which activates factor X. Factor Xa binds to factor Va to form prothrombinase, which converts prothrombin (II) to thrombin (IIa). Thrombin then converts soluble fibrinogen into insoluble fibrin.

EXTRINSIC TENASE. This complex forms on exposure of tissue factor–expressing cells to the blood. Tissue factor exposure occurs after atherosclerotic plaque rupture because the core of the plaque is rich in cells that express tissue factor. Denuding injury to the vessel wall also exposes tissue factor constitutively expressed by subendothelial fibroblasts and smooth muscle cells. In addition to cells in the vessel wall, circulating monocytes and monocyte-derived microparticles (small membrane fragments) also provide a source of tissue factor.[20] When tissue factor–bearing monocytes or microparticles bind to platelets or other leukocytes and their plasma membranes fuse, tissue factor transfer occurs. By binding to adhesion molecules expressed on activated endothelial cells or to P-selectin on activated platelets, these tissue factor–bearing cells or microparticles can initiate or augment coagulation.[21] This phenomenon likely explains how venous thrombi develop in the absence of obvious vessel wall injury.[2]

Tissue factor is an integral membrane protein that serves as a receptor for factor VIIa. The blood contains trace amounts of factor VIIa, which has negligible activity in the absence of tissue factor.[22] With tissue factor exposure on anionic cell surfaces, factor VIIa binds in a calcium-dependent fashion to form the extrinsic tenase complex, which is a potent activator of factors IX and X. Once activated, factors IXa and Xa serve as the enzyme components of intrinsic tenase and prothrombinase, respectively.

INTRINSIC TENASE. Factor IXa binds to factor VIIIa on anionic cell surfaces to form the intrinsic tenase complex. Factor VIII circulates in blood in complex with vWF. Thrombin cleaves factor VIII and releases it from vWF, converting it to its activated form. Activated platelets express binding sites for factor VIIIa. Once bound, factor VIIIa binds factor IXa in a calcium-dependent fashion to form the intrinsic tenase complex, which then activates factor X. The reduction in catalytic efficiency of factor IXa–mediated activation of factor X that occurs with deletion of individual components of the intrinsic tenase complex highlights their importance. Absence of the membrane or factor VIIIa almost completely abolishes enzymatic activity, and the catalytic efficiency of the complete complex is 10^9-fold greater than that of factor IXa alone. Because intrinsic tenase activates factor X at a rate 50- to 100-fold faster than extrinsic tenase, it plays a critical role in the amplification of factor Xa and subsequent thrombin generation.

PROTHROMBINASE. Factor Xa binds to factor Va, its activated cofactor, on anionic phospholipid membrane surfaces to form the prothrombinase complex. Activated platelets release factor V from their alpha granules, and this platelet-derived factor V may be more important in hemostasis than its plasma counterpart. Whereas plasma factor V requires thrombin activation to exert its cofactor activity, the partially activated factor V released from platelets already exhibits substantial cofactor activity. Activated platelets express specific factor Va binding sites on their surface, and bound factor Va serves as a receptor for factor Xa. The catalytic efficiency of factor Xa activation of prothrombin increases by 10^9-fold when factor Xa is incorporated into the prothrombinase complex. Prothrombin binds to the prothrombinase complex, where it undergoes conversion to thrombin in a reaction that releases prothrombin fragment 1.2 (F1.2). Plasma levels of F1.2, therefore, provide a marker of prothrombin activation.

FIBRIN FORMATION. The final effector in coagulation is thrombin. Thrombin converts soluble fibrinogen into insoluble fibrin. Fibrinogen is a dimeric molecule, each half of which is composed of three polypeptide chains—the Aα, Bβ, and γ chains. Numerous disulfide bonds covalently link the chains together and join the two halves of the fibrinogen molecule (**Fig. 87-6**). Electron micrographic studies of fibrinogen reveal a trinodular structure, with a central E domain flanked by two D domains. Crystal structures show symmetry of design with the central E domain, which contains the amino termini of the fibrinogen chains joined to the lateral D domains by coiled coil regions.

Fibrinogen, the most abundant plasma protein involved in coagulation, circulates in an inactive form. Thrombin binds to the amino termini of the Aα and Bβ chains of fibrinogen, where it cleaves specific peptide bonds to release fibrinopeptide A and fibrinopeptide B and generates fibrin monomer (see Fig. 87-6). Because they are products of thrombin action on fibrinogen, plasma levels of these fibrinopeptides provide an index of thrombin activity. Fibrinopeptide release creates new amino termini that extend as knobs from the E domain of one fibrin monomer and insert into preformed holes in the D domains of other fibrin monomers. This creates long strands known as protofibrils, consisting of fibrin monomers noncovalently linked together in a half-staggered overlapping fashion.

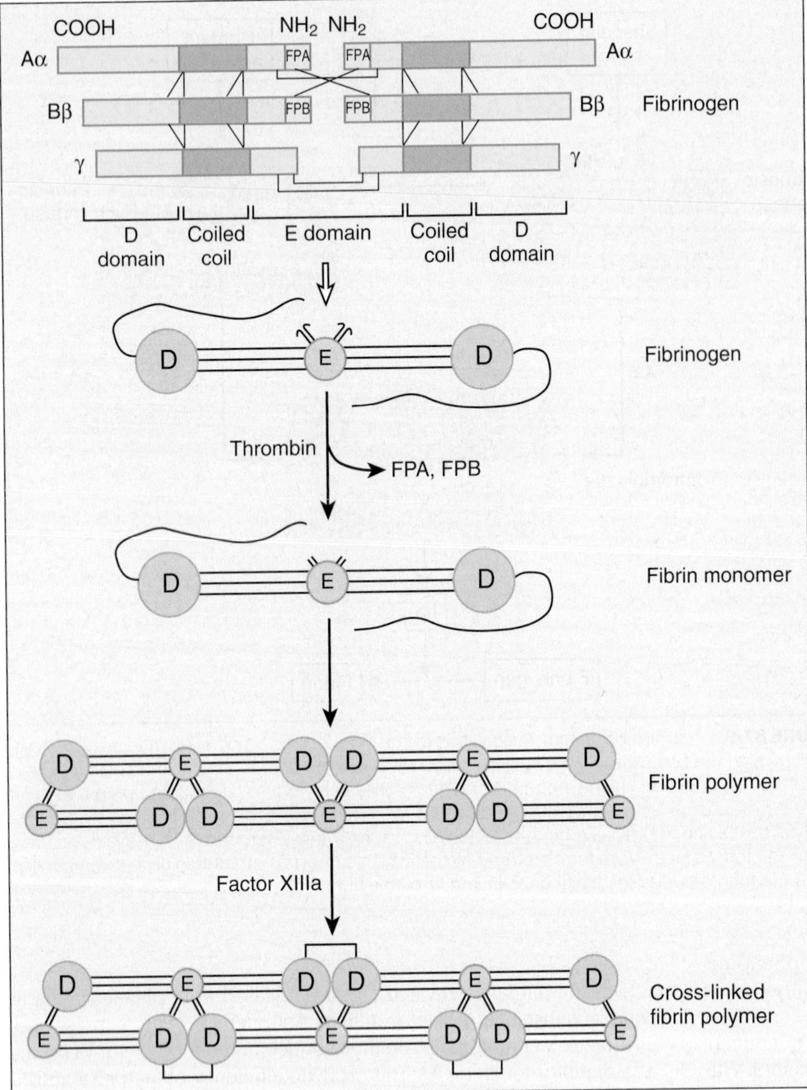

FIGURE 87-6 Fibrinogen structure and conversion of fibrinogen to fibrin. A chimeric molecule, each half of fibrinogen is composed of three polypeptide chains—the Aα, Bβ, and γ chains. Numerous disulfide bonds (lines) covalently link the chains together and join the two halves of the fibrinogen molecule to yield a trinodular structure with a central E domain linked via the coiled coil regions to two lateral D domains. To convert fibrinogen to fibrin, thrombin cleaves specific peptide bonds at the amino (NH_2) termini of the Aα and Bβ chains of fibrinogen to release fibrinopeptide A (FPA) and fibrinopeptide B (FPB), thereby generating fibrin monomer. Fibrin monomers polymerize to generate protofibrils arranged in a half-staggered overlapping fashion. By covalently cross-linking α and γ chains of adjacent fibrin monomers, factor XIIIa stabilizes the fibrin network and renders it resistant to degradation.

Noncovalently linked fibrin protofibrils are unstable. By covalently cross-linking alpha and gamma chains of adjacent fibrin monomers, factor XIIIa stabilizes the fibrin in a calcium-dependent fashion and renders it relatively resistant to degradation. Factor XIII circulates in blood as a heterodimer consisting of two A and two B subunits. The active site and calcium binding site of factor XIII are localized to the A subunit. Platelets contain large amounts of factor XIII in their cytoplasm, but platelet-derived factor XIII consists only of A subunits. Both plasma and platelet factor XIII are activated by thrombin.

CONTACT PATHWAY. Current thinking is that tissue factor exposure represents the sole pathway for activation of coagulation and that the contact system, which includes factor XII, prekallikrein, and high-molecular-weight kininogen, is unimportant for hemostasis because patients deficient in these factors do not have bleeding problems. The physiologic role of factor XI is more difficult to assess because the plasma level of factor XI does not predict the propensity for bleeding. Although the capacity of thrombin to feed back and activate platelet-bound factor XI may explain this phenomenon, platelet-derived factor XI may be more important for hemostasis than circulating factor XI.

The contact pathway cannot be ignored, however, because coronary catheters and other blood-contacting medical devices, such as stents or mechanical valves, likely trigger clotting through this mechanism.[23] Factor XII bound to the surface of catheters or devices undergoes a conformational change that results in its activation. Factor XIIa converts prekallikrein to kallikrein in a reaction accelerated by high-molecular-weight kininogen, and factor XIIa and kallikrein then feed back to activate additional factor XII. Factor XIIa propagates coagulation by activating factor XI (**Fig. 87-7**).

In addition to its role in device-related thrombosis, the contact pathway may also contribute to arterial thrombosis. RNA released from damaged cells in atherosclerotic plaques activates factor XII, and mice given RNA-degrading enzymes exhibit attenuated thrombosis at sites of arterial injury. Polyphosphates released from activated platelets also activate factor XII, and may provide another stimulus for contact pathway activation. Mice deficient in factor XI or XII form small unstable thrombi at sites of arterial damage, suggesting that factors XI and XII contribute to thrombogenesis.[24] It is unknown whether the same is true in humans. Patients with unstable angina have increased plasma levels of factor XIa,[25] but it is unclear whether this reflects activation by factor XIIa or thrombin. Although the contribution of the contact pathway to thrombin generation remains uncertain, the final product of coagulation is fibrin. Hemostasis depends on the dynamic balance between the formation of fibrin and its degradation. The fibrinolytic system mediates fibrin breakdown.

Fibrinolytic System

Fibrinolysis is initiated when plasminogen activators convert plasminogen to plasmin, which then degrades fibrin into soluble fragments (**Fig. 87-8**). Blood contains two immunologically and functionally distinct plasminogen activators, t-PA and u-PA. t-PA mediates intravascular fibrin degradation, whereas u-PA binds to a specific u-PA receptor (u-PAR) on the surface of cells, where it activates cell-bound plasminogen.[10] Consequently, pericellular proteolysis during cell migration and tissue remodeling and repair are the major functions of u-PA.

Regulation of fibrinolysis occurs at two levels. PAI-1 and, to a lesser extent, PAI-2, inhibit the plasminogen activators, whereas alpha$_2$-antiplasmin inhibits plasmin. Endothelial cells synthesize PAI-1, which inhibits both t-PA and u-PA, whereas monocytes and the placenta synthesize PAI-2, which specifically inhibits u-PA.[10] Thrombin-activated fibrinolysis inhibitor (TAFI) also modulates fibrinolysis and provides a link between fibrinolysis and coagulation.[26] Thrombosis can occur if there is impaired activation of the fibrinolytic system, whereas excessive activation leads to bleeding. Therefore, a review of the mechanisms of action of t-PA, u-PA, and TAFI is worthwhile.

MECHANISM OF ACTION OF TISSUE PLASMINOGEN ACTIVATOR. t-PA, a serine protease, contains five discrete domains—a fibronectin-like finger domain, an epidermal growth factor (EGF) domain, two kringle domains, and a protease domain. Synthesized as a single-chain polypeptide, plasmin readily converts t-PA into a two-chain form. Single- and two-chain forms of t-PA convert plasminogen to plasmin. Native Glu-plasminogen is a single-chain polypeptide with

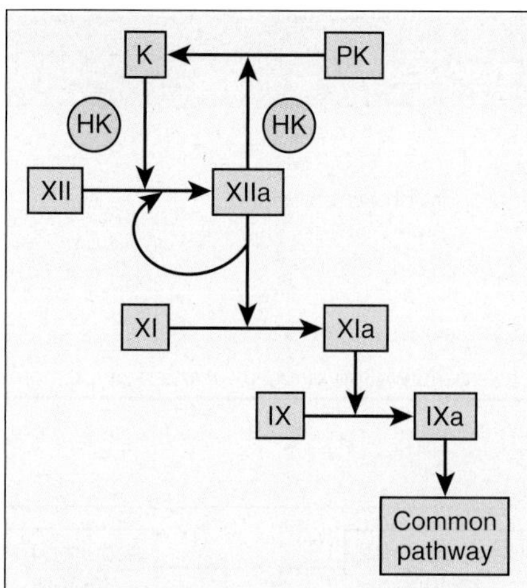

FIGURE 87-7 Contact system. Factor XII (fXII) is activated by contact with negatively charged surfaces. XIIa converts prekallikrein (PK) to kallikrein (K) and can feed back to activate more XII. Similarly, XIIa also can feed back to amplify its own generation. About 75% of circulating PK is bound to high-molecular-weight kininogen (HK), which localizes it to anionic surfaces and promotes PK activation. XIIa propagates clotting by activating XI, which then activates IX. The resultant IXa assembles into the intrinsic tenase complex, which activates X to initiate the common pathway of coagulation.

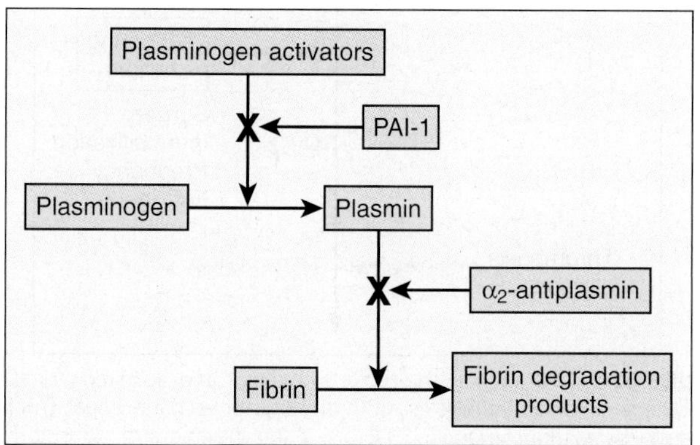

FIGURE 87-8 Fibrinolytic system and its regulation. Plasminogen activators convert plasminogen to plasmin. Plasmin then degrades fibrin into soluble fibrin degradation products. The system is regulated at two levels. Type 1 plasminogen activator inhibitor (PAI-1) regulates the plasminogen activators, whereas alpha$_2$-antiplasmin serves as the major inhibitor of plasmin.

a Glu residue at its amino-terminus. Plasmin cleavage at the amino terminus generates Lys-plasminogen, a truncated form with a Lys residue at its new amino terminus. t-PA cleaves a single peptide bond to convert single-chain Glu- or Lys-plasminogen into two-chain plasmin, composed of a heavy chain containing five kringle domains and a light chain containing the catalytic domain. Because its open conformation exposes the t-PA cleavage site, Lys-plasminogen is a better substrate than Glu-plasminogen, which assumes a circular conformation that renders this bond less accessible.

t-PA has little enzymatic activity in the absence of fibrin, but its activity increases by at least three orders of magnitude when fibrin is present.[10] This increase in activity reflects the capacity of fibrin to serve as a template that binds t-PA and plasminogen and promotes their interaction. t-PA binds to fibrin via its finger and second kringle domains, whereas plasminogen binds fibrin via its kringle domains. Kringle domains are looplike structures that bind Lys residues on fibrin. As fibrin undergoes degradation, more Lys residues are exposed, which provide additional binding sites for t-PA and plasminogen. Consequently, degraded fibrin stimulates t-PA activation of plasminogen more than intact fibrin.

Alpha$_2$-antiplasmin rapidly inhibits circulating plasmin by docking to its first kringle domain and then inhibiting the active site.[10] Because plasmin binds to fibrin via its kringle domains, plasmin generated on the fibrin surface resists inhibition by alpha$_2$-antiplasmin. This phenomenon endows fibrin-bound plasmin with the capacity to degrade fibrin. Factor XIIIa cross-links small amounts of alpha$_2$-antiplasmin onto fibrin, which prevents premature fibrinolysis.

Like fibrin, annexin II on endothelial cells binds t-PA and plasminogen and promotes their interaction. Cell-surface gangliosides and alpha-enolase also may bind plasminogen and promote its activation by altering its conformation into the more readily activated open form. Plasminogen binds to endothelial cells via its kringle domains. Lipoprotein(a), which also possesses kringle domains, impairs cell-based fibrinolysis by competing with plasminogen for cell-surface binding. This phenomenon may explain the association between elevated levels of lipoprotein(a) and atherothrombosis.[27]

MECHANISM OF ACTION OF UROKINASE PLASMINOGEN ACTIVATOR. Synthesized as a single-chain polypeptide, single-chain u-PA (scu-PA) has minimal enzymatic activity. Plasmin readily converts scu-PA into a two-chain form that is enzymatically active and capable of binding u-PAR on cell surfaces. Further cleavage at the amino terminus of two-chain u-PA yields a truncated, lower molecular weight form that lacks the u-PAR binding domain.[10]

Two-chain forms of u-PA readily convert plasminogen to plasmin in the absence or presence of fibrin. In contrast, scu-PA does not activate plasminogen in the absence of fibrin, but it can activate fibrin-bound plasminogen, because plasminogen adopts a more open and readily activatable conformation when immobilized on fibrin. Like the higher molecular weight form of two-chain u-PA, scu-PA binds to cell surface u-PAR, where plasmin can activate it. Many tumor cells elaborate u-PA and express u-PAR on their surface. Plasmin generated on these cells endows them with the capacity for metastasis.[28]

MECHANISM OF ACTION OF THROMBIN-ACTIVATED FIBRINOLYSIS INHIBITOR. TAFI, a procarboxypeptidase B–like molecule synthesized in the liver, circulates in blood in a latent form where thrombin bound to thrombomodulin can activate it. Unless bound to thrombomodulin, thrombin activates TAFI inefficiently.[26] TAFI attenuates fibrinolysis by cleaving Lys residues from the carboxy termini of chains of degrading fibrin, thereby removing binding sites for plasminogen, plasmin, and t-PA. TAFI links fibrinolysis to coagulation because the thrombin-thrombomodulin complex not only activates TAFI, which attenuates fibrinolysis, but also activates protein C, which mutes thrombin generation.

TAFI has a short half-life in plasma because the enzyme is unstable.[26] Genetic polymorphisms can result in synthesis of more stable forms of TAFI. Persistent attenuation of fibrinolysis by these variant forms of TAFI may render patients susceptible to thrombosis.

Thrombosis

A physiologic host defense mechanism, hemostasis focuses on arrest of bleeding by forming hemostatic plugs composed of platelets and fibrin at sites of vessel injury. In contrast, thrombosis reflects a pathologic process associated with intravascular thrombi that fill the lumens of arteries or veins.

Arterial Thrombosis

Most arterial thrombi occur on top of disrupted atherosclerotic plaques (see Chap. 43). Coronary plaques with a thin fibrous cap and a lipid-rich core are most prone to disruption.[1,2] Rupture of the fibrous cap exposes thrombogenic material in the lipid-rich core to the blood and triggers platelet activation and thrombin generation. The extent of plaque disruption and the content of thrombogenic material in the plaque determine the consequences of the event, but host factors also contribute. Breakdown of regulatory mechanisms that limit platelet activation and inhibit coagulation can augment thrombosis at sites of plaque disruption.

Decreased production of nitric oxide and prostacyclin by diseased endothelial cells can trigger vasoconstriction and platelet activation.[29]

TABLE 87-1 Classification of Hypercoagulable States

HEREDITARY	MIXED	ACQUIRED
Loss of Function		
Antithrombin deficiency	Hyperhomocysteinemia	Advanced age
Protein C deficiency		Previous venous thromboembolism
Protein S Deficiency		Surgery
Gain of Function		Immobilization
Factor V Leiden		Obesity
Prothrombin gene mutation		Cancer
Elevated factor VIII, IX, or XI levels		Pregnancy, puerperium; drug-induced—L-asparaginase, hormone therapy

Proinflammatory cytokines lower thrombomodulin expression by endothelial cells, which promotes thrombin generation, and stimulate PAI-1 expression, which inhibits fibrinolysis.[30]

Products of blood coagulation contribute to atherogenesis, as well as to its complications. Microscopic erosions in the vessel wall trigger the formation of tiny platelet-rich thrombi. Activated platelets release PDGF and TGF-β, which promote a fibrotic response.[31] Thrombin generated at the site of injury not only activates platelets and converts fibrinogen to fibrin, but also activates PAR-1 on smooth muscle cells and induces their proliferation, migration, and elaboration of extracellular matrix. Microthrombi incorporation into plaques promotes their growth, and decreased endothelial cell production of heparan sulfate, which normally limits smooth muscle proliferation, contributes to plaque expansion. The multiple links between atherosclerosis and thrombosis have prompted the term *atherothrombosis*.

Venous Thrombosis

The causes of venous thrombosis (see Chap. 77) include those associated with hypercoagulability, which can be genetic or acquired, and the mainly acquired risk factors, such as advanced age, obesity, or cancer, which are associated with immobility (**Table 87-1**). Inherited hypercoagulable states and these acquired risk factors combine to establish the intrinsic risk of thrombosis for each individual. Superimposed triggering factors, such as surgery, pregnancy, or hormonal therapy, modify this risk, and thrombosis occurs when the combination of genetic, acquired, and triggering forces exceed a critical threshold (**Fig. 87-9**).

Some acquired or triggering factors entail a higher risk than others. For example, major orthopedic surgery, neurosurgery, multiple trauma, and metastatic cancer (particularly adenocarcinoma) associate with the highest risk, whereas prolonged bed rest, antiphospholipid antibodies, and the puerperium are associated with an intermediate risk, and pregnancy, obesity, long-distance travel, or the use of oral contraceptives or hormonal replacement therapy are mild risk factors. Up to 50% of patients who present with venous thromboembolism before 45 years of age have inherited hypercoagulable disorders—so-called thrombophilia—particularly those whose events occurred in the absence of risk factors or with minimal provocation, such as after minor trauma or a long-haul flight or with estrogen use. The following sections describe the inherited and acquired hypercoagulable states.

Hypercoagulable States

INHERITED HYPERCOAGULABLE STATES. Inherited hypercoagulable states fall into two categories. Some are associated with gain of function in procoagulant pathways (e.g., factor V Leiden, the prothrombin gene mutation, and increased levels of procoagulant proteins); others are associated with loss of function of endogenous anticoagulant proteins (e.g., deficiencies of antithrombin, protein C, and protein S). Although all these inherited hypercoagulable disorders increase the risk of venous thromboembolism, only increased levels of procoagulant proteins are clearly associated with an increased risk of arterial thrombosis.

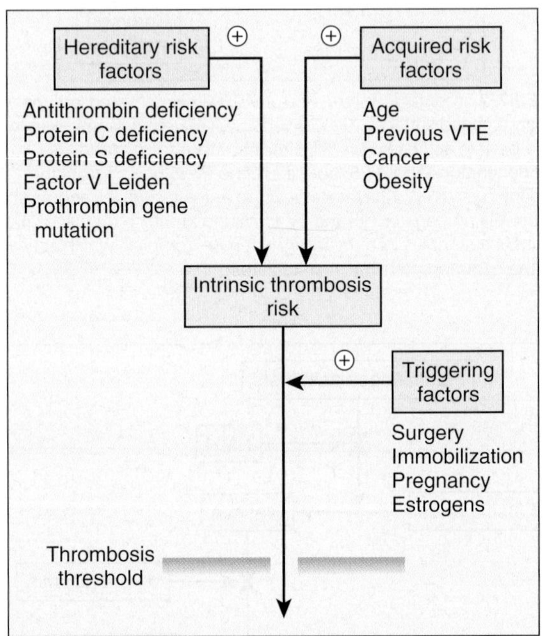

FIGURE 87-9 Thrombosis threshold. Hereditary and acquired risk factors combine to create an intrinsic risk of thrombosis for each individual. This risk is increased by extrinsic triggering factors. If the intrinsic and extrinsic forces exceed a critical threshold where thrombin generation overwhelms protective mechanisms, thrombosis occurs. VTE = venous thromboembolism.

Factor V Leiden

Factor V Leiden mutation, present in about 5% of whites, is the most common inherited thrombophilia. Because of a founder effect, the mutation is less common in Hispanics and blacks and rare in Asians. Caused by a point mutation in the factor V gene, the defect results in the synthesis of a factor V molecule with a Gln residue in place of an Arg residue at position 506, one of three sites at which activated protein C cleaves factor Va to inactivate it. Consequently, activated factor V Leiden resists rapid proteolysis and persists 10-fold longer in the presence of activated protein C than its wild-type counterpart. Inherited in an autosomal dominant fashion, individuals heterozygous for the factor V Leiden mutation have a fivefold increase in the risk of venous thromboembolism; those homozygous for the mutation have a higher risk. However, the absolute risk of venous thrombosis is low with factor V Leiden, and with an annual risk of 0.1% to 0.3%, subjects with this disorder have a lifetime risk of thrombosis of only 5% to 10%.

An activated protein C resistance assay establishes the diagnosis of factor V Leiden in most cases. This assay involves calculation of the ratio of the activated partial thromboplastin time (aPTT) measured after activated protein C addition, divided by that determined prior to its addition. Use of factor V–deficient plasma increases the specificity of the test. If the clotting assay result is equivocal, genetic testing using a polymerase chain reaction (PCR)–based assay confirms the diagnosis.

Prothrombin Gene Mutation

The second most common thrombophilic disorder, the prothrombin gene mutation, reflects a G to A nucleotide transition at position 20210 in the 3′-untranslated region of the prothrombin gene. This mutation causes elevated levels of prothrombin, which enhance thrombin generation and may limit factor Va inactivation by activated protein C. The exact mechanism whereby the G20210A mutation increases prothrombin levels remains controversial. Enhanced protein synthesis may result from more efficient 3′-end formation, increased messenger RNA stability, increased translation efficiency, or some combination of these mechanisms.

The prevalence of the prothrombin gene mutation is about 3% in whites and lower in Asians and blacks. The mutation increases the risk of venous thrombosis to a similar extent as factor V Leiden. Laboratory diagnosis depends on genetic screening after PCR amplification of the 3′-untranslated region of the prothrombin gene. Although heterozygotes have 30% higher levels of prothrombin than noncarriers, the wide range of prothrombin levels in healthy individuals precludes the use of this phenotype for carrier identification.

Elevated Levels of Procoagulant Proteins

Elevated levels of factor VIII and other coagulation factors, including fibrinogen and factors IX and XI, appear to be independent risk factors for venous thrombosis. Increased levels of factor VIII also have been associated with up to a threefold increase in the risk of myocardial infarction.[32] Although the molecular bases for the high levels of these coagulation factors have yet to be identified, genetic mechanisms likely contribute because these quantitative abnormalities have high hereditability.

Antithrombin Deficiency

Synthesized in the liver, antithrombin regulates coagulation by forming a 1:1 covalent complex with thrombin, factor Xa, or other activated clotting factors. Heparan sulfate or heparin accelerates the rate of antithrombin interaction with its target proteases. Inherited antithrombin deficiency is rare, occurring in about 1/2000 people, and can be caused by decreased synthesis of a normal protein or synthesis of a dysfunctional protein. A parallel reduction in the levels of antithrombin antigen and activity identifies deficiencies caused by decreased synthesis, whereas decreased antithrombin activity in the face of normal antigen levels identifies dysfunctional forms of antithrombin. A measurement of antithrombin activity, with or without added heparin, identifies variants with impaired heparin-binding capacity.

Acquired antithrombin deficiency results from decreased synthesis, increased consumption, or enhanced clearance. Decreased synthesis can occur in patients with severe hepatic disease, particularly cirrhosis, or in those given L-asparaginase. Increased activation of coagulation can result in antithrombin consumption in disorders such as extensive thrombosis, disseminated intravascular coagulation, severe sepsis, disseminated malignancy, or prolonged extracorporeal circulation. Heparin treatment also can reduce antithrombin levels up to 20% by enhancing its clearance. Severe antithrombin deficiency can occur in some patients with nephrotic syndrome caused by loss of protein in the urine.

Protein C Deficiency

Thrombin initiates the protein C pathway when it binds thrombomodulin on the endothelial cell surface (see Fig. 87-2). Thrombin bound to thrombomodulin activates protein C about 1000-fold more efficiently than free thrombin.[8] EPCR augments this process 20-fold by binding protein C and presenting it to the thrombin-thrombomodulin complex for activation.[9] Activated protein C then dissociates from the activation complex and decreases thrombin generation by inactivating factors Va and VIIIa on the activated platelet surface. For efficient inactivation of these factors, activated protein C must bind to protein S, its cofactor.

There are inherited and acquired forms of protein C deficiency. About 1 in 200 adults has heterozygous protein C deficiency inherited in an autosomal dominant fashion, but most have no history of thrombosis.[8] The variable phenotypic expression of hereditary protein C deficiency suggests the existence of other, yet unrecognized, modifying factors. In contrast to antithrombin deficiency, in which the homozygous state is embryonic lethal, homozygous or doubly heterozygous protein C deficiency can occur. Newborns with these disorders often present with purpura fulminans characterized by widespread thrombosis.

Inherited protein C deficiency can result from decreased synthesis of normal protein or synthesis of dysfunctional forms of protein C. Identification of the type of deficiency requires simultaneous measurement of protein C antigen and activity; reduced synthesis of a normal protein results in a parallel reduction in protein C antigen and activity, whereas synthesis of a dysfunctional protein results in normal antigen and reduced activity.

Acquired protein C deficiency can be caused by decreased synthesis or increased consumption. Decreased synthesis can occur in patients with liver disease or in those given warfarin. Protein C consumption can occur with severe sepsis, with disseminated intravascular coagulation, and after surgery. Whereas antithrombin levels can be low in patients with nephrotic syndrome, protein C levels are normal or elevated in such patients.

Protein S Deficiency

Protein S serves as a cofactor for activated protein C (see Fig. 87-3). In addition, protein S may directly inhibit prothrombin activation because of its capacity to bind factor Va or Xa, components of the prothrombinase complex. The importance of the direct anticoagulant activity of protein S is uncertain.

In the circulation, about 60% of total protein S is bound to C4b-binding protein, a complement component; only the remaining free 40% is functionally active. Diagnosis of protein S deficiency requires measurement of the free and bound forms of protein S. Inherited protein S deficiency can result from reduced synthesis of the protein or synthesis of a dysfunctional protein. Acquired protein S deficiency can be caused by decreased synthesis, increased consumption, loss, or shift of free protein S to the bound form. Decreased synthesis can occur in patients with severe liver disease or in those given warfarin or L-asparaginase. Increased consumption of protein S occurs in patients with acute thrombosis or disseminated intravascular coagulation. Patients with nephrotic syndrome can excrete free protein S in their urine, causing decreased protein S activity. Total protein S levels in these patients are often normal because the levels of C4b-binding protein increase, shifting more protein S to the bound form. C4b-binding protein levels also increase in pregnancy and with the use of oral contraceptives. This shifts more protein S to the bound form and lowers the levels of free protein S and protein S activity. The consequences of this phenomenon are uncertain.

Other Hereditary Disorders

A polymorphism in the gene that encodes EPCR is associated with venous thrombosis. Linked to EPCR shedding and high levels of soluble EPCR, this polymorphism reduces endothelial EPCR, and soluble EPCR competes with its endothelial cell counterpart for protein C binding.[33]

A polymorphism in factor XIII that results in more rapid activation by thrombin is associated with a reduced risk of thrombosis.[34] Unexpectedly, in some case-control studies, this polymorphism was associated with a small reduction in the risk of myocardial infarction. The mechanism responsible for this protection is unclear.

ACQUIRED HYPERCOAGULABLE STATES. These states include surgery and immobilization, advanced age, obesity, cancer, pregnancy and estrogen therapy (oral contraception or hormone replacement therapy), prior history of venous thromboembolism, antiphospholipid antibody syndrome, and hyperhomocysteinemia (see Table 87-1). These conditions can occur in isolation or in conjunction with hereditary hypercoagulable states.

Surgery and Immobilization

Surgery can directly damage veins, and immobilization after surgery leads to stasis in the deep veins of the leg. The risk of venous thromboembolism in surgical patients depends on patient age, type of surgery, and presence of active cancer. Patients older than 65 years of age are at greater risk; high-risk types of surgery include major orthopedic procedures, neurosurgery, or extensive abdominal or pelvic surgery, especially for cancer. Because the risk of venous thromboembolism increases up to 20-fold in these patients, they require vigorous thromboprophylaxis until they are fully mobile.

Hospitalization and nursing home confinement account for about 60% of cases of venous thromboembolism, again reflecting the impact of immobilization. Hospitalization for medical illness accounts for a similar proportion of cases as hospitalization for surgery, highlighting the need for thromboprophylaxis in medical patients and in surgical patients.

Advanced Age

Predominantly a disease of older age, venous thromboembolism in those younger than 50 years of age has an incidence of 1/10,000 and increases about 10-fold/decade thereafter. Men have an overall age-adjusted incidence rate about 1.2-fold higher than that in women. Although incidence rates are higher in women during their reproductive years, men have higher incidence rates after 45 years of age. There are many potential reasons for the increase in the incidence of venous thromboembolism with advanced age, including decreased mobility, intercurrent diseases, and a vascular endothelium that is less resistant to thrombosis. Levels of procoagulant proteins also increase with age.

Obesity

The risk of venous thromboembolism increases about 1.2-fold for every 10-kg/m^2 increase in body mass index, but the basis for the association between obesity and venous thromboembolism is unclear. Obesity leads to immobility; in addition, adipose tissue, particularly visceral fat, expresses proinflammatory cytokines and adipokines, which may promote coagulation by increasing levels of procoagulant proteins or may impair fibrinolysis by elevating PAI-1 levels. With the growing epidemic of obesity, the incidence of venous thromboembolism may increase.

Cancer

About 20% of patients with venous thromboembolism have cancer (see Chap. 90).[35] Cancer patients who develop venous thromboembolism have reduced survival compared with those without venous thromboembolism. Patients with brain tumors and advanced ovarian or prostate cancer have particularly high rates of venous thromboembolism. Treatment with chemotherapy, hormonal therapy, and biologic agents (e.g., erythropoietin and antiangiogenic drugs) further increases the risk, as do central venous catheters and surgery for cancer.

The pathogenesis of thrombosis in cancer patients is multifactorial in origin and represents a complex interplay between the tumor, patient characteristics, and hemostatic system.[35] Many types of tumor cells express tissue factor or other procoagulants that can initiate coagulation. In addition to its role in coagulation, tissue factor also acts as a signaling molecule that promotes tumor proliferation and spread.[36]

Patient characteristics that contribute to venous thromboembolism include immobility and venous stasis secondary to extrinsic compression of major veins by tumor. Surgical procedures, central venous catheters, and chemotherapy can injure vessel walls. In addition, tamoxifen and selective estrogen receptor modulators (SERMs) induce an acquired hypercoagulable state by reducing the levels of natural anticoagulant proteins.

A proportion of patients who present with unprovoked venous thromboembolism have occult cancer. This observation has prompted some experts to recommend extensive screening for cancer in such patients, but potential harm—including procedure-related morbidity, the psychological impact of false-positive tests, and the cost of screening—offsets any benefits of this approach. Small studies comparing extensive cancer screening with no screening in patients with unprovoked venous thromboembolism have not demonstrated a reduction in cancer-related mortality with screening. Therefore, unless there are symptoms suggestive of underlying cancer, only age-appropriate screening for breast, cervical, colon, and possibly prostate cancer is indicated, because screening for these cancers may reduce mortality.

Pregnancy

Pregnant women have a five- to sixfold higher risk of venous thromboembolism than age-matched nonpregnant women (see Chap. 82). Venous thromboembolism occurs in about 1 in 1000 pregnancies, and about 1 in 1000 women develop venous thromboembolism in the postpartum period. Venous thromboembolism is the leading cause of maternal morbidity and mortality. Patient-related factors influence the risk of venous thromboembolism in pregnancy and the puerperium. These include age older than 35 years, body mass index higher than 29, cesarean delivery, thrombophilia, and personal or family history of venous thromboembolism. Ovarian hyperstimulation and multiparity also are risk factors.

More than 90% of deep vein thrombi in pregnancy occur in the left leg, because the enlarged uterus compresses the left iliac vein by exerting pressure on the overlying right iliac and ovarian arteries. Hypercoagulability occurs in pregnancy because of the combination of venous stasis and changes in the blood. Uterine enlargement reduces venous blood flow from the lower extremities. This is not the only mechanism responsible for venous stasis, however, because blood flow from the lower extremities begins to decrease by the end of the first trimester, likely reflecting hormonally induced venous dilation. Systemic factors also contribute to hypercoagulability. Thus, the levels of procoagulant proteins, such as factor VIII, fibrinogen, and vWF, increase in the third trimester of pregnancy. Coincidentally, there is suppression of natural anticoagulant pathways. The net effect of these changes is enhanced thrombin generation, as evidenced by elevated levels of F1.2 and thrombin-antithrombin complexes.

About half of the episodes of venous thromboembolism in pregnancy occur in women with thrombophilia. The risk of venous thromboembolism in women with thrombophilic defects depends on the type of abnormality and the presence of other risk factors. The risk appears to be highest in women with antithrombin, protein C, or protein S deficiency, and lower in those with factor V Leiden or the prothrombin gene mutation. In general, the daily risk of venous thromboembolism in these women is higher in the postpartum period than during pregnancy. The risk during pregnancy is similar in all three trimesters. Therefore, women needing thromboprophylaxis require treatment throughout pregnancy and for at least 6 weeks postpartum.

Sex Hormone Therapy

Oral contraceptives, estrogen replacement therapy, and SERMs all associate with an increased risk of venous thrombosis (see Chap. 81). The relatively high risk of venous thromboembolism associated with first-generation oral contraceptives prompted the development of low-dose formulations. Currently available low-estrogen combination oral contraceptives contain 20 to 50 μg of ethinylestradiol and one of several different progestins. Even these low-dose combination contraceptives are associated with a three- to fourfold increased risk of venous thromboembolism compared with nonusers. In absolute terms, this translates to an incidence of 3 to 4/10,000 compared with 5 to 10/100,000 in nonusers of reproductive age.

Whereas smoking increases the risk of myocardial infarction and stroke in women taking oral contraceptives, it is unclear whether smoking affects the risk of venous thromboembolism. Obesity, however, affects the risk of arterial and venous thrombosis. The risk of venous thromboembolism is highest during the first year of oral contraceptive use and persists only for the duration of use.

Case-control studies have suggested a 20- to 30-fold higher risk of venous thromboembolism in women with inherited thrombophilia who use oral contraceptives compared with nonusers with thrombophilia or users without these defects. Despite the increased risk, there is no need for routine screening for thrombophilia in young women considering oral contraceptive use. Based on the incidence and case fatality rate of thrombotic events, estimates have suggested that screening 400,000 women would detect 20,000 factor V Leiden carriers and that prevention of a single death would necessitate withholding oral contraceptives in all these women. Even larger numbers of women with less prevalent thrombophilic defects would require screening. Based on these considerations, routine screening is not recommended.

Evidence has mounted that hormonal replacement therapy with conjugated equine estrogen, with or without a progestin, increases the risk of myocardial infarction, ischemic stroke, and venous thromboembolism. Consequently, the use of hormone replacement therapy has markedly decreased. SERMs, such as tamoxifen, are estrogen-like compounds that serve as an estrogen antagonist in the breast but as estrogen agonists in other tissues, such as bone and the uterus. Like estrogens, tamoxifen increases the risk of venous thromboembolism three- to fourfold. The risk is higher in postmenopausal women, particularly those receiving systemic combination chemotherapy. Aromatase inhibitors are replacing tamoxifen for the treatment of estrogen receptor–positive breast cancer. These newer agents are associated with a lower risk of venous thromboembolism than tamoxifen. Raloxifene, a SERM used to prevent osteoporosis, increases the risk of venous thromboembolism threefold compared with placebo, which contraindicates raloxifene for the prevention of osteoporosis in women with a history of venous thromboembolism.

History of Prior Venous Thromboembolism

A history of previous venous thromboembolism places patients at risk for recurrence. When anticoagulation treatment stops, patients with unprovoked venous thromboembolism have a risk of recurrence of about 10% at 1 year and 30% at 5 years. This risk appears to be independent of whether or not there is an underlying thrombophilic defect, such as factor V Leiden or the prothrombin gene mutation.

The risk of recurrent venous thromboembolism is lower in patients whose incident event occurred in association with a transient risk factor, such as major surgery or prolonged immobilization. These patients have a risk of recurrence of about 4% at 1 year and 10% at 5 years. Patients whose venous thromboembolism occurred on the background of minor risk factors, such as oral contraceptive use or a long-haul flight, likely have an intermediate risk of recurrence. Patients at the highest risk for recurrence are those with inherited deficiencies of antithrombin, protein C, or protein S, antiphospholipid antibody syndrome, or advanced malignancy, or those homozygous for factor V Leiden or the prothrombin gene mutation. Their risk of recurrence is likely to be 15% at 1 year and up to 50% at 5 years.

Antiphospholipid Antibody Syndrome (see Chap. 89)

A heterogeneous group of autoantibodies directed against proteins that bind phospholipid, antiphospholipid antibodies can be categorized into those that prolong phospholipid-dependent coagulation assays, so-called lupus anticoagulants (LAs) or anticardiolipin antibodies (ACLs), which target cardiolipin. A subset of ACLs recognizes other phospholipid-bound proteins, particularly beta$_2$-glycoprotein I.

Patients with thrombosis in association with a persistent LA and/or ACL antibody have antiphospholipid syndrome. Primary antiphospholipid syndrome occurs in isolation, whereas secondary forms are associated with autoimmune disorders, such as systemic lupus erythematosus or other connective tissue diseases. Thrombosis in these patients can be arterial, venous, or placental. Arterial thrombosis can manifest as a transient ischemic attack, stroke, or myocardial infarction. In addition to deep vein thrombosis and pulmonary embolism, sagittal sinus thrombosis also can occur. Placental thrombosis is likely the root cause of the pregnancy-related complications that characterize antiphospholipid syndrome. These complications include fetal loss before 10 weeks' gestation and unexplained fetal death after 10 weeks' gestation. Intrauterine growth retardation, pre-eclampsia, and eclampsia also can occur. Treatment with aspirin and/or LMWH during pregnancy may reduce the risk of these complications in women with documented thrombophilic defects.

Laboratory diagnosis of antiphospholipid syndrome requires the presence of an LA or ACL antibody on tests done at least 6 weeks apart. Diagnosis of a LA requires a battery of phospholipid-dependent clotting tests, whereas immunoassays detect ACL antibodies. Only antibodies of medium to high titer and of the IgG or IgM subclass are associated with thrombosis. About 3% to 10% of healthy individuals have ACL antibodies. Such antibodies also occur with certain infections, such as mycobacterial pneumonia, malaria, or parasitic disorders, and after exposure to some medications. Often, these antibodies are of low titer and are transient. About 30% to 50% of patients with systemic lupus erythematosus or other connective tissue disorders have ACL antibodies, and 10% to 20% have an LA.

The mechanism whereby antiphospholipid antibodies trigger thrombosis is unclear. These antibodies directly activate endothelial cells in culture and induce the expression of adhesion molecules that can tether tissue factor-bearing leukocytes or microparticles onto their surface. ACL antibodies also interfere with the protein C pathway, inhibit antithrombin catalysis by endothelial heparan sulfate, and impair fibrinolysis. The importance of these mechanisms in humans remains unclear.

Hyperhomocysteinemia

Homocysteine is an intermediate sulfur-containing amino acid that serves as a methyl group donor during the metabolism of methionine, an essential amino acid derived from the diet. The interconversion of methionine and homocysteine depends on the availability of 5-methyltetrahydrofolate, a methyl group donor; vitamin B_{12} and folate, cofactors in the interconversion; and the enzyme methionine synthase. Increased levels of homocysteine can result from increased production or reduced metabolism. Severe hyperhomocysteinemia and cystinuria, which are rare, usually result from deficiency of cystathionine in beta-synthetase. Mild to moderate hyperhomocysteinemia is more common, and can be caused by genetic mutations in methylenetetrahydrofolate reductase (MTHFR) when they are accompanied by nutritional deficiency of folate, vitamin B_{12}, or vitamin B_6. Common polymorphisms in MTHFR, C677T and A1298C, are associated with reduced enzymatic activity and increased thermolability, which increase the requirement for nutritional cofactors. Hyperhomocysteinemia also can be associated with certain drugs, such as methotrexate, theophylline, cyclosporine, and most anticonvulsants, as well as some chronic diseases, such as end-stage renal disease, severe hepatic dysfunction, and hypothyroidism.

A fasting serum homocysteine level higher than 15 mmol/liter is considered elevated. Although elevated levels once were a common finding, routine fortification of flour in North America with folic acid has resulted in lower homocysteine levels in the general population. Elevated serum levels of homocysteine may be associated with an increased risk of myocardial infarction, stroke, and peripheral arterial disease, as well as venous thromboembolism.

Although administration of folate, along with vitamin B_{12} and vitamin B_6, reduces levels of homocysteine, randomized trials have shown that such therapy does not lower the risk of recurrent cardiovascular events in patients with coronary artery disease or stroke, nor does it lower the risk of recurrent venous thromboembolism (see Chap. 49). Based on these negative trials and the declining incidence of hyperhomocysteinemia, enthusiasm for screening for hyperhomocysteinemia has declined.

Treatment of Thrombosis

Antiplatelet Drugs

The commonly used antiplatelet drugs include aspirin, thienopyridines (e.g., ticlopidine, clopidogrel, prasugrel), dipyridamole, and GPIIb/IIIa antagonists, with distinct sites of action (see Fig. 87-9).

ASPIRIN. The most widely used antiplatelet agent worldwide is aspirin. As an inexpensive and effective drug, aspirin serves as the foundation of most antiplatelet strategies.

Mechanism of Action

Aspirin produces its antithrombotic effect by irreversibly acetylating and inhibiting platelet COX-1 (**Fig. 87-10**), a critical enzyme in the biosynthesis of thromboxane A_2. At high doses (about 1 g/day), aspirin also inhibits COX-2, an inducible COX isoform found in

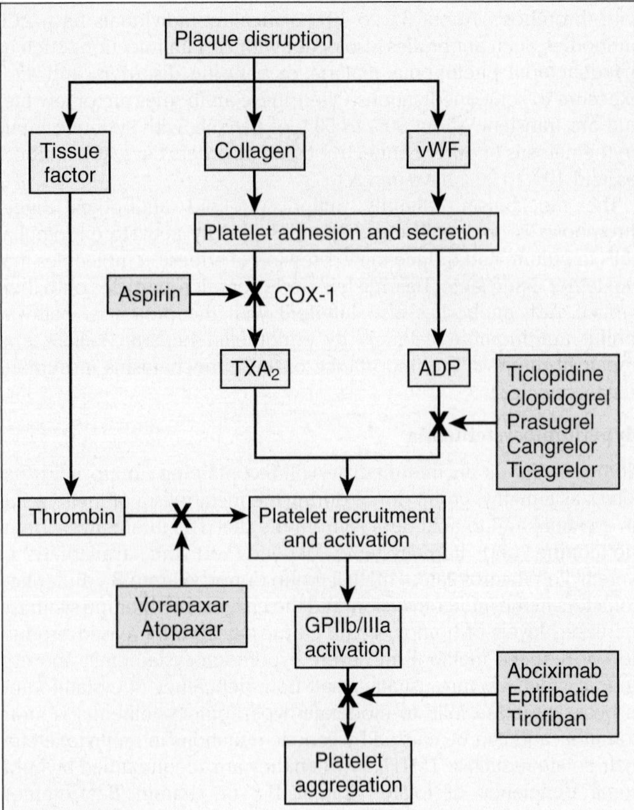

FIGURE 87-10 Sites of action of antiplatelet drugs. Aspirin inhibits thromboxane A_2 (TXA_2) synthesis by irreversibly acetylating COX-1. Reduced TXA_2 release attenuates platelet activation and recruitment to the site of vascular injury. Ticlopidine, clopidogrel, and prasugrel irreversibly block $P2Y_{12}$, a key ADP receptor on the platelet surface; cangrelor and ticagrelor are reversible inhibitors of $P2Y_{12}$. Abciximab, eptifibatide, and tirofiban inhibit the final common pathway of platelet aggregation by blocking fibrinogen and vWF binding to activated GPIIb/IIIa. Vorapaxar and atopaxar inhibit thrombin-mediated platelet activation by targeting PAR1, the major thrombin receptor on platelets.

endothelial cells and inflammatory cells.[37] In endothelial cells, COX-2 initiates the synthesis of prostacyclin, a potent vasodilator and inhibitor of platelet activation, which antagonizes the effects of thromboxane A_2.

Indications

Aspirin is widely used for the secondary prevention of cardiovascular events in patients with coronary artery disease, cerebrovascular disease, or peripheral vascular disease (see Chaps. 55-57 and 61). Compared with placebo, aspirin produces a 25% reduction in the risk of cardiovascular death, myocardial infarction, or stroke in these patients.[37] Aspirin also is used for primary prevention in patients whose estimated annual risk of myocardial infarction is in excess of 1%, a point at which benefits are likely to outweigh harms.[38] This includes patients older than 40 years, with two or more major risk factors for cardiovascular disease, or those older than 50 years, with one or more such risk factors. Aspirin is equally effective in men and women. In men, aspirin mainly reduces the risk of myocardial infarction, whereas in women, aspirin lowers the risk of stroke.

Dosage

Usually administered at doses of 75 to 325 mg once daily, there is no evidence that higher dose aspirin is more effective than lower doses, and some meta-analyses have suggested reduced efficacy with higher doses.[37] Because the side effects of aspirin depend on dose, daily aspirin doses of 75 to 150 mg are recommended for most indications. When rapid platelet inhibition is required, the initial dose of aspirin should be at least 160 mg.

Side Effects

Most common side effects are gastrointestinal and range from dyspepsia to erosive gastritis or peptic ulcers with bleeding and perforation.[37] Use of enteric-coated or buffered aspirin in place of plain aspirin does not eliminate the risk of gastrointestinal side effects. The risk of major bleeding with aspirin is 1% to 3% per year.[37] With concomitant use of aspirin and anticoagulants such as warfarin, the risk of bleeding increases. When combined with warfarin, use of low-dose aspirin (75 to 100 mg daily) is best. Eradication of *Helicobacter pylori* infection and administration of proton pump inhibitors may reduce the risk of aspirin-induced gastrointestinal bleeding in patients with peptic ulcer disease.

Patients with a history of aspirin allergy characterized by bronchospasm should not be given aspirin. This problem occurs in about 0.3% of the general population but is more common in patients with chronic urticaria or asthma, particularly those with coexisting nasal polyps or chronic rhinitis.[39] Aspirin overdose is associated with hepatic and renal toxicity.

Aspirin Resistance

The term *aspirin resistance* is used to describe clinical and laboratory phenomena.[40] A diagnosis of clinical aspirin resistance, defined as the failure of aspirin to protect patients from ischemic vascular events, can only be made after such an event occurs. This retrospective diagnosis provides no opportunity to modify therapy. Furthermore, it is unrealistic to expect aspirin, which selectively blocks thromboxane A_2–induced platelet activation, to prevent all vascular events.

Aspirin resistance also has been described biochemically as failure of the drug to produce its expected inhibitory effects on tests of platelet function, such as thromboxane A_2 synthesis or arachidonic acid–induced platelet aggregation.[37] However, the tests of platelet function used for the diagnosis of biochemical aspirin resistance have not been standardized.[37,40] Furthermore, no definitive evidence shows that these tests identify patients at risk of recurrent vascular events, or that resistance can be reversed either by giving higher doses of aspirin or by adding other antiplatelet drugs. Until such information is available, testing for aspirin resistance remains a research tool.

THIENOPYRIDINES. The thienopyridines include ticlopidine, clopidogrel, and prasugrel—drugs that target $P2Y_{12}$, a key ADP receptor on platelets. Prasugrel is the newest addition to the thienopyridine class.

Mechanism of action

The thienopyridines selectively inhibit ADP-induced platelet aggregation by irreversibly blocking P2Y12 (see Fig. 87-10). Ticlopidine and clopidogrel, are prodrugs that require metabolism by the hepatic cytochrome P-450 (CYP450) enzyme system to be activated. Consequently, when given in usual doses, ticlopidine and clopidogrel have a delayed onset of action. Although prasugrel also is a prodrug that requires metabolic activation, its onset of action is more rapid than ticlopidine or clopidogrel, and it produces greater and more predictable inhibition of ADP-induced platelet aggregation.[41] These characteristics reflect the rapid and complete absorption of prasugrel from the gut and its more efficient activation pathways. Whereas all the absorbed prasugrel undergoes activation, only 15% of absorbed clopidogrel undergoes metabolic activation, with the remainder inactivated by esterases.

The active metabolites of all of the thienopyridines bind irreversibly to the receptor $P2Y_{12}$. Consequently, these drugs have prolonged action—a problem if patients require urgent surgery. Such patients have increased risk for bleeding, which necessitates stopping the thienopyridine at least 5 days prior to the procedure.

Indications

Like aspirin, ticlopidine is more effective than placebo at reducing the risk of cardiovascular death, myocardial infarction, and stroke in patients with atherosclerotic disease.[42] Because of its delayed onset of action, ticlopidine is not recommended for patients with acute myocardial infarction. Ticlopidine is used little because of the risk of myelosuppression and because of the greater potency and better safety profile of newer drugs.[42]

When compared with aspirin in patients with recent ischemic stroke, myocardial infarction, or peripheral arterial disease, clopidogrel reduced the risk of cardiovascular death, myocardial infarction, and stroke by 8.7%. Therefore, clopidogrel is more effective than aspirin, but at greater cost. The combination of clopidogrel and aspirin capitalizes on their capability to block complementary pathways of platelet activation. For example, this combination is recommended for at least 4 weeks after implantation of a bare-metal stent in a coronary artery and for at least 1 year in those with a drug-eluting stent.[42] Recent concerns about late in-stent thrombosis with drug-eluting stents have led some experts to recommend long-term use of clopidogrel plus aspirin for this indication (see Chap. 58).[43,44]

The combination of clopidogrel and aspirin also is effective in patients with unstable angina (see Chap. 56). In 12,562 such patients, the risk of cardiovascular death, myocardial infarction, or stroke was 9.3% in those randomized to the combination of clopidogrel and aspirin, and 11.4% in those given aspirin alone. This 20% relative risk reduction with combination therapy was highly statistically significant, but combining clopidogrel with aspirin increases the risk of major bleeding to about 2% per year—a risk that persists even with a daily aspirin dose of 100 mg or less.[45] Therefore, clopidogrel plus aspirin use should be restricted to situations in which there is clear evidence of benefit. For example, this combination has not proven to be superior to clopidogrel alone in patients with acute ischemic stroke[46] or to aspirin alone for primary prevention in those at risk for cardiovascular events.[47]

Prasugrel was compared with clopidogrel in 13,608 patients with acute coronary syndromes who were scheduled to undergo a percutaneous coronary intervention (PCI).[48] The incidence of the primary efficacy endpoint, a composite of cardiovascular death, myocardial infarction, and stroke, was significantly lower with prasugrel than with clopidogrel (9.9% and 12.1%, respectively), mainly reflecting a reduction in the incidence of nonfatal myocardial infarction. The incidence of stent thrombosis also was significantly lower with prasugrel than with clopidogrel (1.1% and 2.4%, respectively). These advantages, however, were at the expense of significantly higher rates of fatal bleeding (0.4% and 0.1%, respectively) and life-threatening bleeding (1.4% and 0.9%, respectively) with prasugrel. Because patients older than 75 years of age and those with a history of prior stroke or transient ischemic attack have a particularly high risk of bleeding, prasugrel should generally be avoided in older patients, and the drug is contraindicated in those with a history of cerebrovascular disease. Caution is required if prasugrel is used for patients weighing less than 60 kg or those with renal impairment.

Dosage. Ticlopidine is given twice daily at a dose of 250 mg. The more potent clopidogrel is given once daily at a dose of 75 mg.[42] Because its onset of action is delayed for several days, loading doses of clopidogrel are given when rapid ADP receptor blockade is desired (see Chap. 58). After a loading dose of 60 mg, prasugrel is given once daily at a dose of 10 mg. Patients older than 75 years of age or weighing less than 60 kg may do better with a daily prasugrel dose of 5 mg.[49]

Side Effects. The most common side effects of ticlopidine are gastrointestinal. More serious are the hematologic side effects, which include neutropenia, thrombocytopenia, and thrombotic thrombocytopenic purpura. These side effects usually occur within the first few months of starting treatment. Therefore, blood counts must be carefully monitored when initiating therapy with ticlopidine. Gastrointestinal and hematologic side effects are rare with clopidogrel[42] and prasugrel.[49]

Thienopyridine Resistance. The capacity of clopidogrel to inhibit ADP-induced platelet aggregation varies among subjects.[50] This variability reflects, at least in part, genetic polymorphisms in the CYP isoenzymes involved in the metabolic activation of clopidogrel. The most important of these is *CYP2C19*.[51,52] Clopidogrel-treated patients with the loss-of-function *CYP2C19*2* allele exhibit reduced platelet inhibition compared with those with the wild-type *CYP2C19*1* allele, and experience a higher rate of cardiovascular events.[53,54] This is important because estimates suggest that up to 25% of whites, 30% of blacks, and 50% of Asians carry the loss-of-function allele, which would render them resistant to clopidogrel. Even patients with reduced-function CYP2C19*3, *4, or *5* alleles may derive less benefit from clopidogrel than those with the full-function *CYP2C19*1* allele. Concomitant administration of clopidogrel and proton pump inhibitors, which are inhibitors of *CYP2C19*, produces a small reduction in the inhibitory effects of clopidogrel on ADP-induced platelet aggregation. This interaction does not appear to increase the risk of cardiovascular events.[55]

In contrast to their effect on the metabolic activation of clopidogrel, *CYP2C19* polymorphisms appear to be less important determinants of the activation of prasugrel. There was no association between the loss-of-function allele and decreased platelet inhibition or increased rate of cardiovascular events with prasugrel.[56,57]

Although *CYP3A4* also contributes to the metabolic activation of clopidogrel, polymorphisms in this enzyme do not appear to influence clopidogrel responsiveness. However, a small study in patients undergoing PCI has revealed that atorvastatin, a competitive inhibitor of *CYP3A4*, reduces the inhibitory effect of clopidogrel on ADP-induced platelet aggregation. This finding was not confirmed in a subsequent study.[58] The impact of this interaction on clinical outcomes is unknown. Clopidogrel-treated patients with polymorphisms in *ABCB1* may exhibit reduced drug absorption, which may render them at higher risk for cardiovascular events.

The observation that genetic polymorphisms affecting clopidogrel absorption or metabolism influence clinical outcomes raises the possibilities that pharmacogenetic profiling may help identify clopidogrel resistant patients, and that point-of-care assessment of the extent of clopidogrel-induced platelet inhibition may help detect patients at higher risk for subsequent cardiovascular events.[59] It is unknown whether administration of higher doses of clopidogrel to such patients will overcome this resistance. Instead, prasugrel or newer $P2Y_{12}$ inhibitors may be better choices for these patients. For an update on recent experience with newer P2Y12 antagonists, including ticagrelor, see below and Chaps. 55 and 56.

DIPYRIDAMOLE. A relatively weak antiplatelet agent on its own,[37] an extended-release formulation of dipyridamole combined with low-dose aspirin, a preparation marketed as Aggrenox, is used for the prevention of stroke in patients with transient ischemic attacks.

Mechanism of Action

By inhibiting phosphodiesterase, dipyridamole blocks the breakdown of cAMP. Increased levels of cAMP reduce intracellular calcium and inhibit platelet activation. Dipyridamole also blocks the uptake of adenosine by platelets and other cells. With more extracellular adenosine, there is a further increase in local cAMP levels because the platelet adenosine A_2 receptor and adenylate cyclase are coupled (**Fig. 87-11**).

Dosage. Aggrenox is given twice daily. Each capsule contains 200 mg of extended-release dipyridamole and 25 mg of aspirin.[37]

Side Effects. Because dipyridamole has vasodilatory effects, caution is necessary in patients with coronary artery disease. Gastrointestinal

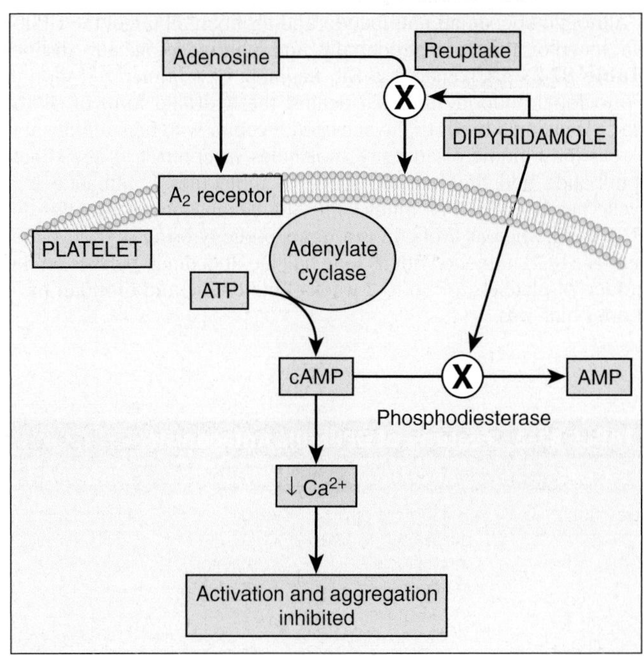

FIGURE 87-11 Mechanism of action of dipyridamole. Dipyridamole increases levels of cAMP in platelets by blocking the reuptake of adenosine, thereby increasing the concentration of adenosine available to bind to the A2 receptor, and by inhibiting phosphodiesterase-mediated cAMP degradation. By promoting calcium uptake, cAMP reduces intracellular levels of calcium. This, in turn, inhibits platelet activation and aggregation.

complaints, headache, facial flushing, dizziness, and hypotension also can occur. These symptoms often subside with continued use of the drug.

INDICATIONS. Dipyridamole plus aspirin was compared with aspirin or dipyridamole alone, or with placebo, in patients with an ischemic stroke or transient ischemic attack (see Chap. 62). The combination reduced the risk of stroke by 22.1% compared with aspirin and by 24.4% compared with dipyridamole. A second trial compared dipyridamole plus aspirin with aspirin alone for secondary prevention in patients with ischemic stroke. Vascular death, stroke, or myocardial infarction occurred in 13% of patients given combination therapy and in 16% of those treated with aspirin alone.[60] Although the combination of dipyridamole plus aspirin compares favorably with aspirin, the combination is not superior to clopidogrel. In a large randomized trial that compared dipyridamole plus aspirin with clopidogrel for secondary prevention in patients with ischemic stroke,[61] recurrent stroke event rates were similar (9.0% and 8.8%, respectively), as were the rates of vascular death, stroke, and myocardial infarction (13.1% in both treatment arms). However, there was a trend for more hemorrhagic strokes with dipyridamole plus aspirin than with clopidogrel (0.8% and 0.4%, respectively) and more major bleeding (4.1% and 3.8%, respectively).

Although Aggrenox can replace aspirin for stroke prevention, because of the vasodilatory effects of dipyridamole and the paucity of data supporting the usefulness of this drug in patients with symptomatic coronary artery disease, Aggrenox should be avoided in such patients. Clopidogrel is a better choice for patients with coronary artery disease.

GPIIb/IIIa RECEPTOR ANTAGONISTS. As a class, parenteral GPIIb/IIIa receptor antagonists have an established niche in patients with acute coronary syndromes. The three agents in this class are abciximab, eptifibatide, and tirofiban.

Mechanism of Action

A member of the integrin family of adhesion receptors, GPIIb/IIIa is expressed on the surface of platelets and megakaryocytes. With about 80,000 copies per platelet, GPIIb/IIIa is the most abundant receptor.[15] Consisting of a noncovalently linked heterodimer, GPIIb/IIIa is inactive on resting platelets. With platelet activation, inside-outside signal transduction pathways trigger conformational activation of the receptor. Once activated, GPIIb/IIIa binds fibrinogen and, under high shear conditions, vWF. Once bound, fibrinogen and vWF bridge adjacent platelets together to induce platelet aggregation.

Although abciximab, eptifibatide, and tirofiban all target the GPIIb/IIIa receptor, they are structurally and pharmacologically distinct (**Table 87-2**). Abciximab is a Fab fragment of a humanized murine monoclonal antibody directed against the activated form of GPIIb/IIIa.[62] Abciximab binds to the activated receptor with high affinity and blocks the binding of adhesive molecules. In contrast to abciximab, eptifibatide and tirofiban are synthetic molecules. Eptifibatide is a cyclic heptapeptide that binds GPIIb/IIIa because it incorporates the KGD motif, whereas tirofiban is a nonpeptidic tyrosine derivative that acts as a RGD mimetic. With its long half-life, abciximab persists on the surface of platelets for up to 2 weeks. Eptifibatide and tirofiban have shorter half-lives.

TABLE 87-2 Features of GPIIb/IIIa Antagonists

FEATURE	ABCIXIMAB	EPTIFIBATIDE	TIROFIBAN
Description	Fab fragment of humanized mouse monoclonal antibody	Cyclical KGD-containing heptapeptide	Nonpeptidic RGD mimetic
Specific for GPIIb/IIIa	No	Yes	Yes
Plasma half-life	Short (min)	Long (2.5 hr)	Long (2.0 hr)
Platelet-bound half-life	Long (days)	Short (sec)	Short (sec)
Renal clearance	No	Yes	Yes

In addition to targeting the GPIIb/IIIa receptor, abciximab (but not eptifibatide or tirofiban) also inhibits the closely related $\alpha_v\beta_3$ receptor, which binds vitronectin, and $\alpha_M\beta_2$, a leukocyte integrin. Inhibition of $\alpha_v\beta_3$ and $\alpha_M\beta_2$ may endow abciximab with anti-inflammatory and/or antiproliferative properties that extend beyond platelet inhibition.[62]

DOSAGE. All the GPIIb/IIIa antagonists are given as an intravenous bolus followed by an infusion. Because of their renal clearance, eptifibatide and tirofiban doses require reduction in patients with renal insufficiency.[62]

SIDE EFFECTS. In addition to bleeding, thrombocytopenia is the most serious complication. Antibodies directed against neoantigens on GPIIb/IIIa that are exposed on antagonist binding[63] cause thrombocytopenia, which is immune-mediated. With abciximab, thrombocytopenia occurs in up to 5% of patients and is severe in about 1% of these individuals. Thrombocytopenia is less common with the other two agents, occurring in about 1% of patients.

INDICATIONS. Abciximab and eptifibatide are used in patients undergoing PCI, particularly those with acute myocardial infarction, whereas tirofiban and eptifibatide are used for high-risk patients with unstable angina (see Chaps. 55, 56, and 58).[64,65]

NEWER ANTIPLATELET AGENTS. New agents in advanced stages of development include cangrelor and ticagrelor, direct-acting reversible $P2Y_{12}$ antagonists, and vorapaxar and atopaxar, orally active inhibitors of PAR-1, the major thrombin receptor on platelets (see Fig. 87-10). Cangrelor is an adenosine analogue that binds reversibly to $P2Y_{12}$ and inhibits its activity. The drug has a half-life of 3 to 6 minutes and is given intravenously as a bolus followed by an infusion. When stopped, platelet function recovers within 60 minutes. Recent trials comparing cangrelor with placebo during PCI or comparing cangrelor with clopidogrel after such procedures revealed little or no advantage of cangrelor.[66,67] Consequently, identification of a role for cangrelor requires additional studies.

Ticagrelor is an orally active, reversible inhibitor of $P2Y_{12}$. The drug is given twice daily and not only has a more rapid onset and offset of action than clopidogrel, but also produces greater and more predictable inhibition of ADP-induced platelet aggregation. When compared with clopidogrel in patients with acute coronary syndromes,[68] ticagrelor produced a greater reduction in the primary efficacy endpoint, a composite of cardiovascular death, myocardial infarction, and stroke at 1 year, than clopidogrel (9.8% and 11.7%, respectively; $P = 0.001$). This difference reflected a significant reduction in cardiovascular death (4.0% and 5.1%, respectively; $P = 0.001$) and myocardial infarction (5.8% and 6.9%, respectively; $P = 0.005$) with ticagrelor relative to clopidogrel. Rates of stroke were similar with ticagrelor and clopidogrel (1.5% and 1.3%, respectively) and there was no difference in rates of major bleeding. When minor bleeding was added to the major bleeding results, however, ticagrelor showed an increase relative to clopidogrel (16.1% and 14.6%, respectively; $P = 0.008$). Ticagrelor also was superior to clopidogrel in patients with acute coronary syndrome who underwent PCI or cardiac surgery. Although not yet licensed, in one study, ticagrelor demonstrated a reduction in cardiovascular death compared with clopidogrel in patients with acute coronary syndromes (see Chaps. 55 and 56).

Vorapaxar, an orally active inhibitor of the thrombin receptor PAR-1,[69] is under investigation as an adjunct to aspirin or aspirin plus clopidogrel. Two large phase III trials are underway. Atopaxar, a second oral PAR-1 antagonist, also is in development.[70]

Anticoagulants

There are parenteral and oral anticoagulants. Currently available parenteral anticoagulants include heparin, LMWH and fondaparinux, a synthetic pentasaccharide. The only available oral anticoagulants in the United States are vitamin K antagonists; of these, warfarin is the agent most often used in North America.

Dabigatran etexilate, an oral thrombin inhibitor, and rivaroxaban, an oral factor Xa inhibitor, are available in Europe and Canada for short-term thromboprophylaxis after elective hip or knee replacement surgery.[71]

TABLE 87-3 Comparison of the Features of Heparin, Low-Molecular-Weight Heparin, and Fondaparinux

FEATURE	HEPARIN	LMWH	FONDAPARINUX
Source	Biologic	Biologic	Synthetic
Molecular weight	15,000	5000	1728
Target	Xa and IIa	Xa and IIa	Xa
Bioavailability (%)	30	90	100
Half-life (hr)	1	4	17
Renal excretion	No	Yes	Yes
Antidote	Complete	Partial	No
HIT	<5%	<1%	Never

PARENTERAL ANTICOAGULANTS

HEPARIN. A sulfated polysaccharide, heparin is isolated from mammalian tissues rich in mast cells (**Table 87-3**). Most commercial heparin is derived from porcine intestinal mucosa and is a polymer of alternating D-glucuronic acid and *N*-acetyl-D-glucosamine residues.[72]

Mechanism of Action

Heparin acts as an anticoagulant by activating antithrombin (previously known as antithrombin III) and accelerating the rate at which it inhibits clotting enzymes, particularly thrombin and factor Xa.[72] Antithrombin, the obligatory plasma cofactor for heparin, is a member of the serine protease inhibitor (serpin) superfamily. Synthesized in the liver and circulating in plasma at a concentration of 2.6 ± 0.4 μM, antithrombin acts as a suicide substrate for its target enzymes.

To activate antithrombin, heparin binds to the serpin via a unique pentasaccharide sequence found on one third of the chains of commercial heparin (**Fig. 87-12**). Heparin chains lacking this pentasaccharide sequence have little or no anticoagulant activity.[72] Once bound to antithrombin, heparin induces a conformational change in the reactive center loop of antithrombin that renders it more readily accessible to its target proteases. This conformational change enhances the rate at which antithrombin inhibits factor Xa by at least two orders of magnitude, but has little effect on the rate of thrombin inhibition by antithrombin. To catalyze thrombin inhibition, heparin serves as a template that binds antithrombin and thrombin simultaneously. Formation of this ternary complex brings the enzyme in close apposition to the inhibitor, thereby promoting the formation of a stable covalent thrombin-antithrombin complex.

Only pentasaccharide-containing heparin chains composed of at least 18 saccharide units, which correspond to a molecular weight of 5400, are long enough to bridge thrombin and antithrombin together.[72] With a mean molecular weight of 15,000 (range, 5000 to 30,000), almost all the chains of unfractionated heparin are long enough to provide this bridging function. Consequently, by definition, heparin has equal capacity to promote the inhibition of thrombin and factor Xa by antithrombin, and has an anti-factor Xa–to–anti-factor IIa (thrombin) ratio of 1:1. Heparin causes the release of TFPI from the endothelium. A factor Xa–dependent inhibitor of tissue factor–bound factor VIIa,[6] TFPI may contribute to the antithrombotic activity of heparin. Longer heparin chains induce the release of more TFPI than shorter chains.

Pharmacology of Heparin

Heparin requires parenteral administration; it usually is administered subcutaneously or by continuous intravenous infusion. The intravenous route is most often used for therapeutic purposes. If given subcutaneously for the treatment of thrombosis, the dose must be high enough to overcome the limited bioavailability associated with this method of delivery.[72]

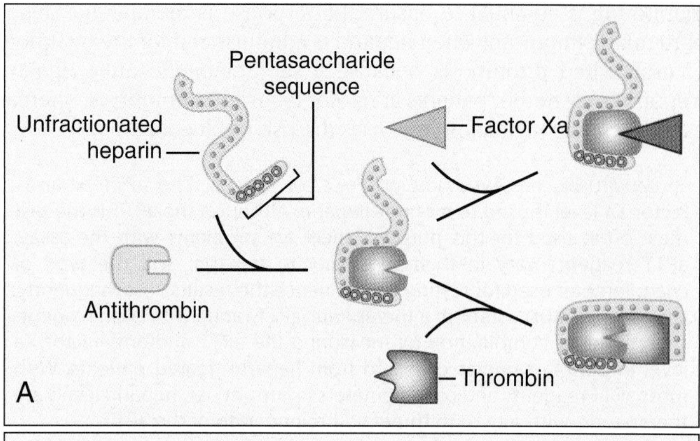

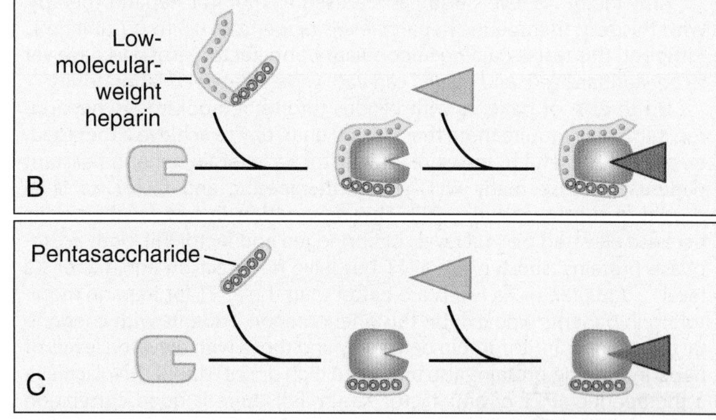

FIGURE 87-12 Mechanism of action of heparin, LMWH, and fondaparinux, a synthetic pentasaccharide. **A,** Heparin binds to antithrombin via its pentasaccharide sequence. This induces a conformational change in the reactive center loop of antithrombin that accelerates its interaction with factor Xa. To potentiate thrombin inhibition, heparin must simultaneously bind to antithrombin and thrombin. Only heparin chains composed of at least 18 saccharide units, which corresponds to a molecular weight of 5400, are of sufficient length to perform this bridging function. With a mean molecular weight of 15,000, all the heparin chains are long enough to do this. **B,** LMWH has greater capacity to potentiate factor Xa inhibition by antithrombin than thrombin because, with a mean molecular weight of 4500 to 5000, at least half of the LMWH chains are too short to bridge antithrombin to thrombin. **C,** The pentasaccharide only accelerates factor Xa inhibition by antithrombin because the pentasaccharide is too short to bridge antithrombin to thrombin.

In the circulation, heparin binds to the endothelium and to plasma proteins other than antithrombin. Heparin binding to endothelial cells explains its dose-dependent clearance. At low doses, the half-life of heparin is short because it rapidly binds to the endothelium. With higher doses of heparin, the half-life is longer, because heparin clearance is slower once the endothelium is saturated. Clearance is mainly extrarenal; heparin binds to macrophages, which internalize and depolymerize the long heparin chains and secrete shorter chains back into the circulation. Because of its dose-dependent clearance mechanism, the plasma half-life of heparin ranges from 30 to 60 minutes with bolus intravenous doses of 25 and 100 U/kg, respectively.[72]

Once heparin enters the circulation, it binds to plasma proteins other than antithrombin—a phenomenon that reduces the anticoagulant activity of heparin. Some of the heparin-binding proteins found in plasma are acute-phase reactants whose levels are elevated in ill patients. Activated platelets or endothelial cells release other proteins that can bind heparin, such as large multimers of vWF. Activated platelets also release platelet factor 4 (PF4), a highly cationic protein that binds heparin with high affinity. The large amounts of PF4 associated with platelet-rich arterial thrombi can neutralize the anticoagulant activity of heparin. This phenomenon may attenuate heparin's capacity to suppress thrombus growth.

Because the levels of heparin-binding proteins in plasma vary from person to person, the anticoagulant response to fixed or weight-adjusted doses of heparin is unpredictable. Consequently, coagulation monitoring is essential to ensure the response is therapeutic. This is particularly important when heparin is administered for the treatment of established thrombosis because a subtherapeutic anticoagulant response may render patients at risk for recurrent thrombosis, whereas excessive anticoagulation increases the risk of bleeding.[72]

Monitoring the Anticoagulant Effect of Heparin. The aPTT or anti–factor Xa level is used to monitor heparin. Although the aPTT is the test most often used for this purpose, there are problems with the assay; aPTT reagents vary in their sensitivity to heparin, and the type of coagulometer used for testing can influence the results.[72] Consequently, laboratories must establish a therapeutic aPTT range with each reagent-coagulometer combination by measuring the aPTT and anti–factor Xa level in plasma samples collected from heparin-treated patients. With most aPTT reagents and coagulometers in current use, heparin levels are therapeutic, with a two- to threefold prolongation of the aPTT.

Anti–factor Xa levels also can be used to monitor heparin therapy. With this test, therapeutic heparin levels range from 0.3 to 0.7 units/mL. Although this test is gaining in popularity, anti–factor Xa assays have yet to be standardized, and results can vary widely between laboratories.

Up to 25% of patients with venous thromboembolism are heparin-resistant; they require more than 35,000 units/day to achieve a therapeutic aPTT. It is useful to measure anti–factor Xa levels in heparin-resistant patients because many will have a therapeutic anti–factor Xa level despite a subtherapeutic aPTT. This dissociation in test results occurs because elevated plasma levels of fibrinogen and factor VIII, both acute-phase proteins, shorten the aPTT but have no effect on anti–factor Xa levels.[72] Anti–factor Xa levels are better than the aPTT for heparin monitoring in patients who exhibit this phenomenon. Patients with congenital or acquired antithrombin deficiency and those with elevated levels of heparin-binding proteins also may need high doses of heparin to achieve a therapeutic aPTT or anti–factor Xa level. If there is good correlation between the aPTT and the anti–factor Xa level, either test can be used for monitoring heparin therapy.

Dosage. For prophylaxis, heparin is usually given in fixed doses of 5000 units subcutaneously two or three times daily. With these low doses, coagulation monitoring is unnecessary.[73] In contrast, monitoring is essential when the drug is given in therapeutic doses. Fixed-dose or weight-based heparin nomograms are used to standardize heparin dosing and to shorten the time required to achieve a therapeutic anticoagulant response. At least two heparin nomograms have been validated in patients with venous thromboembolism, and both reduce the time required to achieve a therapeutic aPTT. Weight-adjusted heparin nomograms also have been evaluated in patients with acute coronary syndromes. After an intravenous heparin bolus of 5000 units, or 70 units/kg, a heparin infusion rate of 12 to 15 units/kg/hour is usually administered.[72] In contrast, weight-adjusted heparin nomograms for patients with venous thromboembolism use an initial bolus of 5000 units, or 80 units/kg, followed by an infusion of 18 units/kg/hour. Thus, achievement of a therapeutic aPTT requires higher doses of heparin in patients with venous thromboembolism than in those with acute coronary syndromes. This may reflect differences in the thrombus burden. Heparin binds to fibrin, and the fibrin content of extensive deep vein thrombi is more than that of small coronary thrombi.

Heparin manufacturers in North America measure heparin potency in USP units, with a unit defined as the concentration of heparin that prevents 1 mL of citrated sheep plasma from clotting for 1 hour after calcium addition. In contrast, manufacturers in Europe measure heparin potency with anti–factor Xa assays using an international heparin standard for comparison. Because of problems with heparin contamination with oversulfated chondroitin sulfate,[74] which the USP assay system does not detect, North American heparin manufacturers now use the anti–factor Xa assay to measure heparin potency. Use of international units in place of USP units results in a 10% to 15% reduction in heparin dose. This change is unlikely to affect patient care because heparin has been dosed this way in Europe for many years. Furthermore, heparin monitoring ensures a therapeutic anticoagulant response in high-risk situations, such as cardiopulmonary bypass surgery or PCI.

Limitations of Heparin

Heparin has pharmacokinetic and biophysical limitations (**Table 87-4**). The pharmacokinetic limitations reflect heparin's propensity to bind in a pentasaccharide-independent fashion to cells and plasma proteins. Heparin binding to endothelial cells explains its dose-dependent clearance, whereas binding to plasma proteins results in a variable anticoagulant response and can lead to heparin resistance.

TABLE 87-4 Pharmacokinetic and Biophysical Limitations of Heparin

LIMITATION	MECHANISM
Poor bioavailability	Limited absorption of long heparin chains
Dose-dependent clearance	Binds to endothelial cells
Variable anticoagulant response	Binds to plasma proteins; levels vary from patient to patient
Reduced activity in the vicinity of platelet-rich thrombi	Neutralized by platelet factor 4 released from activated platelets
Limited activity against factor Xa incorporated into the prothrombinase complex and thrombin bound to fibrin	Reduced capacity of heparin-antithrombin complex to inhibit factor Xa bound to activated platelets and thrombin bound to fibrin

The biophysical limitations of heparin reflect the inability of the heparin-antithrombin complex to inhibit factor Xa when it is incorporated into the prothrombinase complex that converts prothrombin to thrombin, and to inhibit thrombin bound to fibrin.[72] Consequently, factor Xa bound to activated platelets within platelet-rich thrombi can generate thrombin, even in the face of heparin. Thrombin bound to fibrin is protected from inhibition by the heparin-antithrombin complex. Clot-associated thrombin can then trigger thrombus growth by locally activating platelets and amplifying its own generation through feedback activation of factors V, VIII, and XI. Heparin neutralization by the high concentrations of PF4 released from activated platelets within the platelet-rich thrombus further compounds this problem.

Side Effects

The most common side effect of heparin is bleeding. Other complications include thrombocytopenia, osteoporosis, and elevated levels of transaminases.

BLEEDING. The risk of heparin-induced bleeding increases with higher heparin doses. Concomitant administration of drugs that affect hemostasis, such as antiplatelet or fibrinolytic agents, increases the risk of bleeding, as does recent surgery or trauma.[75] Protamine sulfate will neutralize heparin in patients with serious bleeding. A mixture of basic polypeptides isolated from salmon sperm, protamine sulfate binds heparin with high affinity to form protamine-heparin complexes that undergo renal clearance. Typically, 1 mg of intravenous protamine sulfate neutralizes 100 units of heparin. Anaphylactoid reactions to protamine sulfate can occur, but administration by slow intravenous infusion reduces the risk of these problems.[72]

THROMBOCYTOPENIA. Heparin-induced thrombocytopenia (HIT) is an antibody-mediated process triggered by antibodies against neoantigens on PF4 that are exposed when heparin binds to this protein.[76] These antibodies, which usually are of the IgG subtype, bind simultaneously to the heparin-PF4 complex and to platelet Fc receptors. Such binding activates the platelets and generates platelet microparticles. Circulating microparticles are procoagulant because they express anionic phospholipids on their surface and can bind clotting factors, thereby promoting thrombin generation.

Typically, HIT occurs 5 to 14 days after initiation of heparin therapy, but can manifest earlier if the patient has received heparin within the past 3 months (**Table 87-5**). It is rare for the platelet count to fall below 100,000/μL in patients with HIT, and even a 50% decrease in the platelet count from the pretreatment value should raise the suspicion of HIT in those receiving heparin. HIT is more common in surgical patients than in medical patients and, like many autoimmune disorders, occurs more frequently in women than in men.[77]

HIT can be associated with arterial or venous thrombosis. Venous thrombosis, which manifests as deep vein thrombosis and/or pulmonary embolism, is more common than arterial thrombosis. Arterial thrombosis can manifest as ischemic stroke or acute myocardial

TABLE 87-5 Features of Heparin-Induced Thrombocytopenia

FEATURE	DETAILS
Thrombocytopenia	Platelet count of 100,000/μL or less or decrease in platelet count of 50% or more from baseline
Timing	Platelet count falls 5-10 days after starting heparin
Type of heparin	More common with unfractionated heparin than with LMWH
Type of patient	More common in surgical patients than medical patients; more common in women than in men
Thrombosis	Venous thrombosis more common than arterial thrombosis

TABLE 87-6 Management of Heparin-Induced Thrombocytopenia

- Stop all heparin.
- Give an alternative anticoagulant, such as lepirudin, argatroban, bivalirudin, or fondaparinux.
- Do not give platelet transfusions.
- Do not give warfarin until the platelet count returns to baseline levels; if warfarin was administered, give vitamin K to restore INR to normal.
- Evaluate for thrombosis, particularly deep vein thrombosis.

infarction. Rarely, platelet-rich thrombi in the distal aorta or iliac arteries can cause critical limb ischemia.[76,77]

The diagnosis of HIT is established with enzyme-linked assays to detect antibodies against heparin-PF4 complexes or with platelet activation assays. Enzyme-linked assays are sensitive, but can be positive in the absence of any clinical evidence of HIT.[78] The most specific diagnostic test is the serotonin release assay. This test involves quantification of serotonin release after exposure of washed platelets loaded with labeled serotonin to patient serum in the absence or presence of varying concentrations of heparin. If the patient serum contains HIT antibody, heparin addition induces platelet activation and subsequent serotonin release.

To manage HIT, heparin should be stopped in patients with suspected or documented HIT, and an alternative anticoagulant should be administered to prevent or treat thrombosis (**Table 87-6**).[79] The agents most often used for this indication are parenteral direct thrombin inhibitors, such as lepirudin, argatroban, or bivalirudin, or factor Xa inhibitors, such as fondaparinux.

Patients with HIT, particularly those with associated thrombosis, often have evidence of increased thrombin generation that can lead to consumption of protein C. If these patients receive warfarin without a concomitant parenteral anticoagulant, the further decrease in protein C levels induced by the vitamin K antagonist can trigger skin necrosis.[80] To avoid this problem, patients with HIT require treatment with a direct thrombin inhibitor or fondaparinux until the platelet count returns to normal levels. At this point, low-dose warfarin therapy can be introduced and the thrombin inhibitor can be discontinued when the anticoagulant response to warfarin has been therapeutic for at least 2 days.[76-79]

OSTEOPOROSIS. Treatment with therapeutic doses of heparin for longer than 1 month can cause a reduction in bone density. This occurs in up to 30% of patients given long-term heparin therapy,[72] and symptomatic vertebral fractures occur in 2% to 3% of these individuals.

Studies in vitro and in laboratory animals have provided insights into the pathogenesis of heparin-induced osteoporosis. These investigations suggest that heparin causes bone resorption by decreasing bone formation and enhancing bone resorption. Thus, heparin affects the activity of osteoclasts and osteoblasts.[72]

ELEVATED LEVELS OF TRANSAMINASES. Therapeutic doses of heparin frequently cause modest elevations in the serum levels of hepatic transaminases, without a concomitant increase in the level of bilirubin. The levels of transaminases rapidly return to normal when the drug is stopped. The mechanism responsible for this phenomenon is unknown.

TABLE 87-7 Advantages of Low-Molecular-Weight Heparin and Fondaparinux over Heparin

ADVANTAGE	CONSEQUENCE
Better bioavailability and longer half-life after subcutaneous injection	Can be given subcutaneously once or twice daily for both prophylaxis and treatment
Dose-independent clearance	Simplified dosing
Predictable anticoagulant response	Coagulation monitoring unnecessary for most patients
Lower risk of heparin-induced thrombocytopenia	Safer than heparin for short- or long-term administration
Lower risk of osteoporosis	Safer than heparin for long-term administration

LOW-MOLECULAR-WEIGHT HEPARIN. Consisting of smaller fragments of heparin, LMWH is prepared from unfractionated heparin by controlled enzymatic or chemical depolymerization. The mean molecular weight of LMWH is about 5000, one third the mean molecular weight of unfractionated heparin.[72] Because of its advantages over heparin (**Table 87-7**), LMWH has replaced heparin for many indications.

Mechanism of Action

Like heparin, LMWH exerts its anticoagulant activity by activating antithrombin. With a mean molecular weight of about 5000, which corresponds to about 17 saccharide units, at least half of the pentasaccharide-containing chains of LMWH are too short to bridge thrombin to antithrombin (see Fig. 87-12). These chains retain the capacity to accelerate factor Xa inhibition by antithrombin, because this activity largely results from the conformational changes in antithrombin evoked by pentasaccharide binding. Consequently, LMWH catalyzes factor Xa inhibition by antithrombin more than thrombin inhibition.[72] Depending on their unique molecular weight distributions, LMWH preparations have anti–factor Xa–to–anti–factor IIa ratios ranging from 2:1 to 4:1 (see Table 87-3).

Pharmacology of Low-Molecular-Weight Heparin

Although usually given subcutaneously, LMWH can be administered intravenously if a rapid anticoagulant response is needed. LMWH has pharmacokinetic advantages over heparin. These advantages arise because the shorter heparin chains bind less avidly to endothelial cells, macrophages, and heparin-binding plasma proteins.[72] Reduced binding to endothelial cells and macrophages eliminates the rapid, dose-dependent, and saturable mechanism of clearance that is a characteristic of unfractionated heparin. Instead, the clearance of LMWH is dose-independent and its plasma half-life is longer. Based on the measurement of anti–factor Xa levels, LMWH has a plasma half-life of about 4 hours. Because of its renal clearance, LMWH can accumulate in patients with renal insufficiency.

LMWH exhibits about 90% bioavailability after subcutaneous injection.[72] Because LMWH binds less avidly than heparin to heparin-binding proteins in plasma, LMWH produces a more predictable dose response, and resistance to LMWH is rare. With a longer half-life and more predictable anticoagulant response, LMWH can be given subcutaneously once or twice daily without coagulation monitoring, even when the drug is given in treatment doses. These properties render LMWH more convenient than unfractionated heparin. Capitalizing on this feature, studies in patients with venous thromboembolism have shown that home treatment with LMWH is as effective and safe as in-hospital treatment with continuous intravenous infusions of heparin. Outpatient treatment with LMWH streamlines care, reduces health care costs, and increases patient satisfaction.

Low-Molecular-Weight Heparin Monitoring. In most patients, LMWH does not require coagulation monitoring. If monitoring is necessary, the anti–factor Xa level is measured, because most LMWH preparations have little effect on the aPTT. Therapeutic anti–factor Xa levels with LMWH range from 0.5 to 1.2 units/mL when measured 3 to 4 hours after drug administration. With prophylactic doses of LMWH, peak anti–factor Xa levels of 0.2 to 0.5 units/mL are desirable.[72]

Situations that may require LMWH monitoring include renal insufficiency and obesity. LMWH monitoring in patients with a creatinine clearance of 50 mL/min or less is advisable to ensure that there is no drug accumulation. Although weight-adjusted LMWH dosing appears to produce therapeutic anti–factor Xa levels in overweight patients, this approach has not been well studied in those with morbid obesity. It may also be advisable to monitor the anticoagulant activity of LMWH during pregnancy because dose requirements can change, particularly in the third trimester. Monitoring also should be considered in high-risk settings, such as in patients with mechanical heart valves who are given LMWH for the prevention of valve thrombosis.

Dosage. The doses of LMWH recommended for prophylaxis or treatment vary depending on the preparation. For prophylaxis, once-daily subcutaneous doses of 4000 to 5000 units are often used, whereas doses of 2500 to 3000 units are given when the drug is administered twice daily. For treatment of venous thromboembolism, a dose of 150 to 200 units/kg is given if the drug is administered once daily. If a twice-daily regimen is used, a dose of 100 units/kg is given. In patients with unstable angina, LMWH is given subcutaneously on a twice-daily basis at a dose of 100 to 120 units/kg. The dose is reduced in patients with renal impairment.

Side Effects. The major complication of LMWH is bleeding. Meta-analyses have suggested that the risk of major bleeding may be lower with LMWH than with unfractionated heparin.[81] HIT and osteoporosis are less common with LMWH than with unfractionated heparin.[76-78]

Bleeding. The risk of bleeding with LMWH increases when antiplatelet or fibrinolytic drugs are given concomitantly. Recent surgery, trauma, or underlying hemostatic defects also increase the risk of bleeding with LMWH.[75]

Although protamine sulfate serves as an antidote for LMWH, it incompletely neutralizes the anticoagulant activity of LMWH because it only binds the longer chains.[72] Because longer chains are responsible for the catalysis of thrombin inhibition by antithrombin, protamine sulfate completely reverses the anti–factor IIa activity of LMWH. In contrast, protamine sulfate only partially reverses the anti–factor Xa activity of LMWH because the shorter pentasaccharide-containing chains of LMWH do not bind protamine sulfate. Consequently, continuous intravenous unfractionated heparin may be safer than subcutaneous LMWH for patients at high risk for bleeding.

Thrombocytopenia. The risk of HIT is about fivefold lower with LMWH than with heparin.[76-78] LMWH binds less avidly to platelets and causes less PF4 release. Furthermore, with lower affinity for PF4 than heparin, LMWH is less likely to induce the conformational changes in PF4 that trigger the formation of HIT antibodies. LMWH should not be used to treat HIT patients because most HIT antibodies exhibit cross-reactivity with LMWH. This in vitro cross-reactivity is not simply a laboratory phenomenon; there are case reports of thrombosis in HIT patients treated with LMWH.

Osteoporosis. The risk of osteoporosis is lower with long-term LMWH than with heparin.[72] For extended treatment, therefore, LMWH is a better choice than heparin because of the lower risk of osteoporosis and HIT.

FONDAPARINUX. A synthetic analogue of the antithrombin-binding pentasaccharide sequence, fondaparinux differs from LMWH in several ways (see Table 87-3). Fondaparinux is licensed for thromboprophylaxis in medical, general surgical, or high-risk orthopedic patients and as an alternative to heparin or LMWH for the initial treatment of patients with established venous thromboembolism. The drug is not yet licensed in the United States as an alternative to heparin or LMWH in patients with acute coronary syndromes.

Mechanism of action

As a synthetic analogue of the antithrombin-binding pentasaccharide sequence found in heparin and LMWH, fondaparinux has a molecular weight of 1728. Fondaparinux binds only to antithrombin (see Fig. 87-12) and is too short to bridge thrombin to antithrombin. Consequently, fondaparinux catalyzes factor Xa inhibition by antithrombin and does not enhance the rate of thrombin inhibition.[72]

Pharmacology of Fondaparinux. Fondaparinux exhibits complete bioavailability after subcutaneous injection. With no binding to endothelial cells or plasma proteins, the clearance of fondaparinux is dose-independent and its plasma half-life is 17 hours. The drug is given subcutaneously once daily. Because of its renal clearance, fondaparinux is contraindicated in patients with a creatinine clearance less than 30 mL/min, and it should be used with caution in those with a creatinine clearance less than 50 mL/min.[72]

Fondaparinux produces a predictable anticoagulant response after administration in fixed doses because it does not bind to plasma proteins. It is given at a dose of 2.5 mg once daily for prevention of venous thromboembolism. For initial treatment of established venous thromboembolism, fondaparinux is given at a dose of 7.5 mg once daily. The dose can be reduced to 5 mg once daily for those weighing less than 50 kg and increased to 10 mg for those weighing more than 100 kg. When given in these doses, fondaparinux is as effective as heparin or LMWH for the initial treatment of patients with deep vein thrombosis or pulmonary embolism, and produces similar rates of bleeding.[82]

Fondaparinux is used at a dose of 2.5 mg once daily in patients with acute coronary syndromes. When this prophylactic dose of fondaparinux was compared with treatment doses of enoxaparin in patients with non–ST-segment elevation acute coronary syndromes, there was no difference in the rate of cardiovascular death, myocardial infarction, or stroke at 9 days.[83] In one study, however, the rate of major bleeding, was 50% lower with fondaparinux than with enoxaparin, a difference that likely reflects that the dose of fondaparinux was lower than that of enoxaparin. In acute coronary syndrome patients who require PCI, there is a risk of catheter thrombosis with fondaparinux unless adjunctive heparin is given.[84]

Side Effects. Although fondaparinux can induce the formation of HIT antibodies, HIT does not occur.[85] This apparent paradox reflects the fact that induction of HIT requires heparin chains of sufficient length to bind multiple PF4 molecules. Fondaparinux is too short to do this. In contrast to LMWH, there is no cross-reactivity of fondaparinux with HIT antibodies. Consequently, fondaparinux appears to be effective for the treatment of HIT,[86,87] although large clinical trials supporting its use are lacking.

The major side effect of fondaparinux is bleeding, and it has no antidote. Protamine sulfate has no effect on the anticoagulant activity of fondaparinux because it fails to bind to the drug. Recombinant activated factor VII reverses the anticoagulant effects of fondaparinux in volunteers,[72] but it is unknown whether this agent controls fondaparinux-induced bleeding.

PARENTERAL DIRECT THROMBIN INHIBITORS

Heparin and LMWH indirectly inhibit thrombin because they require antithrombin to exert their anticoagulant activity. In contrast, direct thrombin inhibitors do not require a plasma cofactor; instead, they bind directly to thrombin and block its interaction with its substrates. Approved parenteral direct thrombin inhibitors include lepirudin, argatroban, and bivalirudin (**Table 87-8**). Lepirudin and argatroban are licensed for the treatment of patients with HIT, whereas bivalirudin is approved as an alternative to heparin in patients undergoing PCI, including those with HIT.

LEPIRUDIN. A recombinant form of hirudin, lepirudin is a bivalent direct thrombin inhibitor that interacts with the active site of thrombin and exosite 1, the substrate binding site.[72] For rapid anticoagulation, lepirudin is given by continuous intravenous infusion, but the drug can

TABLE 87-8 Comparison of the Properties of Hirudin, Bivalirudin, and Argatroban

PARAMETER	HIRUDIN	BIVALIRUDIN	ARGATROBAN
Molecular mass	7000	1980	527
Site(s) of interaction with thrombin	Active site and exosite 1	Active site and exosite 1	Active site
Renal clearance	Yes	No	No
Hepatic metabolism	No	No	Yes
Plasma half-life (min)	60	25	45

be given subcutaneously for thromboprophylaxis. Lepirudin has a plasma half-life of 60 minutes after intravenous infusion and is cleared by the kidneys. Consequently, lepirudin accumulates in patients with renal insufficiency. A high proportion of lepirudin-treated patients develop antibodies against the drug. Although these antibodies rarely cause problems, in a small subset of patients they can delay lepirudin clearance and enhance its anticoagulant activity; some of these patients experience serious bleeding.

Lepirudin is usually monitored using the aPTT, and the dose is adjusted to maintain an aPTT that is 1.5 to 2.5 times the control. The aPTT is not an ideal test for monitoring lepirudin therapy because the clotting time plateaus with higher drug concentrations. Although the ecarin clotting time provides a better index of lepirudin dose than the aPTT, the ecarin clotting time has yet to be standardized and the test is not available in all coagulation laboratories.

ARGATROBAN. Argatroban, a univalent inhibitor that targets the active site of thrombin, is metabolized in the liver.[72] Consequently, it must be used with caution in patients with hepatic insufficiency. Because it is not cleared by the kidneys, argatroban is safer than lepirudin for HIT patients with renal impairment.

Argatroban is administered by continuous intravenous infusion and has a plasma half-life of about 45 minutes. The aPTT is used to monitor its anticoagulant effect, and the dose is adjusted to achieve an aPTT 1.5 to 3 times the baseline value, but not to exceed 100 seconds. Argatroban also prolongs the international normalized ratio (INR), a feature that can complicate the transitioning of patients to warfarin. This problem can be circumvented by using the levels of factor X to monitor warfarin in place of the INR. Alternatively, argatroban can be stopped for 2 to 3 hours before INR determination.

BIVALIRUDIN. A synthetic 20–amino acid analogue of hirudin, bivalirudin is a divalent thrombin inhibitor.[72] Thus, the N-terminal portion of bivalirudin interacts with the active site of thrombin, whereas its C-terminal tail binds to exosite 1, the substrate-binding domain on thrombin. Bivalirudin has a plasma half-life of 25 minutes, the shortest half-life of all the parenteral direct thrombin inhibitors. Bivalirudin is degraded by peptidases and is partially excreted via the kidneys. When given in high doses in the cardiac catheterization laboratory, the anticoagulant activity of bivalirudin is monitored using the activated clotting time. With lower doses, its activity can be assessed using the aPTT.

Studies comparing bivalirudin with heparin have suggested that bivalirudin produces less bleeding. This feature, plus its short half-life, renders bivalirudin an attractive alternative to heparin in patients undergoing PCI. Bivalirudin also has been used successfully in HIT patients who require PCI.[72]

ORAL ANTICOAGULANTS

Vitamin K antagonists were identified more than 60 years ago during investigations into the cause of hemorrhagic disease in cattle. Characterized by decreased prothrombin levels, this disorder occurs after ingestion of hay containing spoiled sweet clover. Hydroxycoumarin, which was isolated from bacterial contaminants in the hay, interferes with vitamin K metabolism, thereby causing a syndrome similar to vitamin K deficiency. This compound spawned the development of other vitamin K antagonists, including warfarin.

WARFARIN. A water-soluble vitamin K antagonist initially developed as a rodenticide, warfarin is the coumarin derivative most often prescribed in North America. Like other vitamin K antagonists, warfarin interferes with the synthesis of the vitamin K–dependent clotting proteins, which include prothrombin (factor II) and factors VII, IX, and X. Warfarin also impairs synthesis of the vitamin K–dependent anticoagulant proteins C and S.[88]

Mechanism of Action

All the vitamin K–dependent clotting factors possess glutamic acid residues at their N termini. A post-translational modification adds a

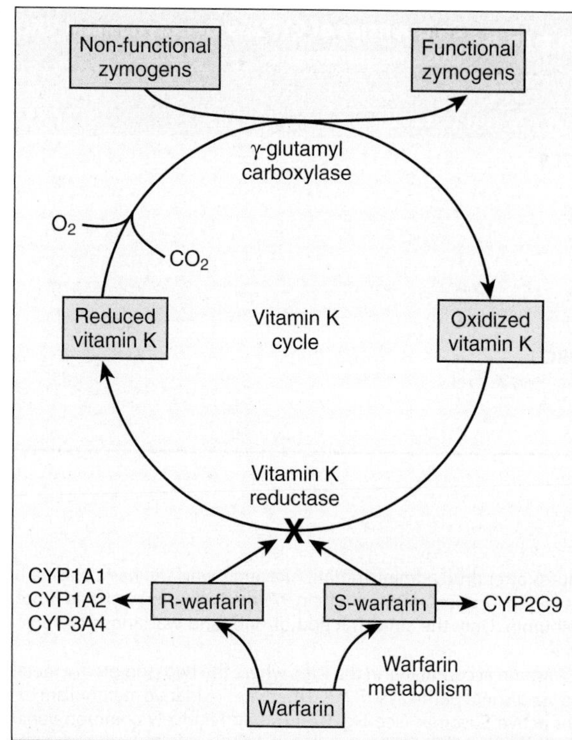

FIGURE 87-13 Mechanism of action of warfarin. A racemic mixture of S and R enantiomers, S-warfarin is most active. By blocking vitamin K epoxide reductase, warfarin inhibits the conversion of oxidized vitamin K into its reduced form. This inhibits vitamin K–dependent γ-carboxylation of factors II, VII, IX, and X, because reduced vitamin K serves as a cofactor for a γ-glutamyl carboxylase that catalyzes the γ-carboxylation process, thereby converting prozymogens to zymogens capable of binding calcium and interacting with anionic phospholipid surfaces. S-warfarin is metabolized by *CYP2C9*. Common genetic polymorphisms in this enzyme can influence warfarin metabolism. Polymorphisms in the C1 subunit of vitamin K reductase (VKORC1) also can affect the susceptibility of the enzyme to warfarin-induced inhibition, thereby influencing warfarin dosage requirements.

carboxyl group to the γ carbon of these residues to generate γ-carboxyglutamic acid. This modification is essential for expression of the activity of these clotting factors because it permits their calcium-dependent binding to anionic phospholipid surfaces.[88] The γ-carboxylation process is catalyzed by a vitamin K–dependent carboxylase. Thus, vitamin K from the diet is reduced to vitamin K hydroquinone by vitamin K reductase (**Fig. 87-13**). Vitamin K hydroquinone serves as a cofactor for the carboxylase enzyme, which in the presence of carbon dioxide, replaces the hydrogen on the γ carbon of glutamic acid residues with a carboxyl group. During this process, vitamin K hydroquinone is oxidized to vitamin K epoxide, which is then reduced to vitamin K by vitamin K epoxide reductase (VKOR).

Warfarin inhibits VKOR, thereby blocking the γ-carboxylation process. This results in the synthesis of vitamin K–dependent clotting proteins that are only partially γ-carboxylated.[88] Warfarin acts as an anticoagulant because these partially γ-carboxylated proteins have reduced or absent biologic activity. The onset of action of warfarin is delayed until the newly synthesized clotting factors with reduced activity gradually replace their fully active counterparts.

The antithrombotic effect of warfarin depends on a reduction in the functional levels of factor X and prothrombin, clotting factors that have half-lives of 24 and 72 hours, respectively.[88] Because of the delay in achieving an antithrombotic effect, initial treatment with warfarin is supported by concomitant administration of a rapidly acting parenteral anticoagulant, such as heparin, LMWH, or fondaparinux, in patients with established thrombosis or at high risk for thrombosis.

PHARMACOLOGY OF WARFARIN. Warfarin is a racemic mixture of R and S isomers. Warfarin is rapidly and almost completely absorbed from the gastrointestinal tract. Levels of warfarin in the blood peak about 90

TABLE 87-9 Frequencies of CYP2C9 Genotypes and VKORC1 Haplotypes in Different Populations and Their Effect on Warfarin Dose Requirements

	Frequency %			
GENOTYPE/HAPLOTYPE	WHITES	BLACKS	ASIANS	DOSE REDUCTION COMPARED WITH WILD TYPE
CYP2C9				
*1/*1	70	90	95	—
*1/*2	17	2	0	22
*1/*3	9	3	4	34
*2/*2	2	0	0	43
*2/*3	1	0	0	53
*3/*3	0	0	1	76
VKORC 1				
Non-A, non-A	37	82	7	—
Non-A/A	45	12	30	26
A/A	18	6	63	50

minutes after drug administration.[88] Racemic warfarin has a plasma half-life of 36 to 42 hours, and more than 97% of circulating warfarin is bound to albumin. Only the small fraction of unbound warfarin is biologically active.

Warfarin accumulates in the liver, where the two isomers are metabolized via distinct pathways. *CYP2C9* mediates oxidative metabolism of the more active S isomer (see Fig. 87-12). Two relatively common variants, *CYP2C9*2* and *CYP2C9*3*, encode an enzyme with reduced activity. Patients with these variants require lower maintenance doses of warfarin. Approximately 25% of whites have at least one variant allele of *CYP2C9*2* or *CYP2C9*3*, whereas these variant alleles are less common in blacks and Asians (**Table 87-9**). Heterozygosity for *CYP2C9*2* or *CYP2C9*3* decreases the warfarin dose requirement by 20% to 30% relative to that required in subjects with the wild-type *CYP2C9*1/*1* alleles, whereas homozygosity for the *CYP2C9*2* or *CYP2C9*3* allele reduces the warfarin dose requirement by 50% to 70%. Consistent with their decreased warfarin dose requirement, subjects with at least one *CYP2C9* variant allele are at increased risk for bleeding. Compared with individuals with no variant alleles, the relative risks for warfarin-associated bleeding in *CYP2C9*2* or *CYP2C9*3* carriers are 1.91 and 1.77, respectively.[89,90]

Polymorphisms in *VKORC1* also can influence the anticoagulant response to warfarin.[90-94] Several genetic variations of *VKORC1* are in strong linkage disequilibrium and have been designated as non-A haplotypes. *VKORC1* variants are more prevalent than variants of *CYP2C9*. Asians have the highest prevalence of *VKORC1* variants, followed by whites and blacks (see Table 87-9). Polymorphisms in *VKORC1* likely explain 30% of the variability in warfarin dose requirements. Compared with *VKORC1* non-A, non-A homozygotes, the warfarin dose requirement decreases by 25% and 50% in A/A heterozygotes and homozygotes, respectively. These findings prompted the U.S. Food and Drug Administration (FDA) to amend the prescribing information for warfarin to indicate that lower initiation doses should be considered for patients with *CYP2C9* and *VKORC1* genetic variants. In addition to genotype data, other pertinent patient information has been incorporated into warfarin dosing algorithms. Although such algorithms help predict suitable warfarin doses, it remains unclear whether better dose identification improves patient outcome in terms of reducing hemorrhagic complications or recurrent thrombotic events.

In addition to genetic factors, diet, drugs, and various disease states influence the anticoagulant effect of warfarin. Fluctuations in dietary vitamin K intake affect the activity of warfarin. A wide variety of drugs can alter absorption, clearance, or metabolism of warfarin.[88] Because of the variability in the anticoagulant response to warfarin, coagulation monitoring is essential to ensure a therapeutic response.

Monitoring

Warfarin therapy is most often monitored using the prothrombin time, a test sensitive to reductions in the levels of prothrombin, factor VII, and factor X. The test involves the addition of thromboplastin, a reagent that contains tissue factor, phospholipid, and calcium, to citrated plasma and determining the time to clot formation. Thromboplastins vary in their sensitivity to reductions in the levels of the vitamin K–dependent clotting factors. Consequently, less sensitive thromboplastins will trigger the administration of higher doses of warfarin to achieve a target prothrombin time. This is problematic, because higher doses of warfarin increase the risk of bleeding.

The INR was developed to circumvent many of the problems associated with the prothrombin time. To calculate the INR, the patient's prothrombin time is divided by the mean normal prothrombin time, and this ratio is then multiplied by the international sensitivity index (ISI), an index of the sensitivity of the thromboplastin used for prothrombin time determination to reductions in the levels of the vitamin K–dependent clotting factors. Highly sensitive thromboplastins have an ISI of 1.0. Most current thromboplastins have ISI values that range from 1.0 to 1.4.[88]

Although the INR has helped standardize anticoagulant practice, problems persist. The precision of INR determination varies depending on reagent-coagulometer combinations, leading to variability in the INR results. Also complicating INR determination is unreliable reporting of the ISI by thromboplastin manufacturers. Furthermore, every laboratory must establish the mean normal prothrombin time with each new batch of thromboplastin reagent. To accomplish this, the prothrombin time must be measured in fresh plasma samples from at least 20 healthy volunteers using the same coagulometer used for patient samples.

For most indications, warfarin is administered in doses that produce a target INR of 2.0 to 3.0. An exception is patients with high-risk mechanical heart valves, for whom a target INR of 2.5 to 3.5 is recommended.[88] Studies in atrial fibrillation have demonstrated an increased risk of cardioembolic stroke when the INR falls below 1.7, and an increase in bleeding with INR values above 4.5.[95] These findings highlight the narrow therapeutic window of vitamin K antagonists. In support of this concept, a study in patients receiving long-term warfarin therapy for unprovoked venous thromboembolism has demonstrated a higher rate of recurrent venous thromboembolism with a target INR of 1.5 to 1.9 compared with a target INR of 2.0 to 3.0.[88]

Dosing

Warfarin is usually started at a dose of 5 to 10 mg. Lower doses are used for patients with *CYP2C9* or *VKORC1* polymorphisms that affect the pharmacodynamics or pharmacokinetics of warfarin and render patients more sensitive to the drug. The dose is then titrated to achieve the desired target INR.[88] Because of its delayed onset of action, patients with established thrombosis or those at high risk for thrombosis are given concomitant treatment with a rapidly acting parenteral anticoagulant, such as heparin, LMWH, or fondaparinux. Initial prolongation of the INR reflects a reduction in the functional levels of factor VII. Consequently, concomitant treatment with the parenteral anticoagulant should be continued until the INR has been therapeutic for at least 2 consecutive days. A minimum 5-day course of parenteral anticoagulation is recommended to ensure that the levels of prothrombin have fallen into the therapeutic range with warfarin.[72]

Because warfarin has a narrow therapeutic window, frequent coagulation monitoring is essential to ensure that the anticoagulant response is therapeutic. Even patients with stable warfarin dose requirements should have their INR determined every 3 to 4 weeks. More frequent monitoring is necessary with the introduction of new medications, because many drugs enhance or reduce the anticoagulant effects of warfarin.

Side Effects

Like all anticoagulants, the major side effect of warfarin is bleeding; a rare complication is skin necrosis. Warfarin crosses the placenta and can cause fetal abnormalities, so it should not be used during pregnancy.[88]

BLEEDING. At least half of bleeding complications with warfarin occur when the INR exceeds the therapeutic range. Bleeding complications may be mild, such as epistaxis or hematuria, or more severe, such as retroperitoneal or gastrointestinal bleeding. Life-threatening intracranial bleeding also can occur.[75]

To minimize the risk of bleeding, the INR should be maintained in the therapeutic range. In asymptomatic patients whose INR is between 3.5 and 4.5, warfarin should be withheld until the INR returns to the therapeutic range. If the INR is over 4.5, a therapeutic INR can be achieved more rapidly by administration of low doses of sublingual vitamin K.[96] A vitamin K dose of 1 mg usually is adequate for patients with an INR between 4.9 and 9, whereas 2 to 3 mg can be used for those with an INR higher than 9. Higher doses of vitamin K can be administered if more rapid reversal of the INR is required, or if the INR is excessively high. Although vitamin K administration results in a more rapid reduction in the INR, there is no evidence that it reduces the risk of hemorrhage.[96]

Patients with serious bleeding need additional treatment. These patients should be given 10 mg of vitamin K by slow intravenous infusion. Additional vitamin K should be given until the INR is in the normal range. Treatment with vitamin K should be supplemented with fresh-frozen plasma as a source of vitamin K–dependent clotting proteins. For life-threatening bleeds, or if patients cannot tolerate the volume load, prothrombin complex concentrates can be used.[88]

Warfarin-treated patients who experience bleeding when their INR is in the therapeutic range require investigation into the cause of the bleeding. Those with gastrointestinal bleeding often have underlying peptic ulcer disease or a tumor. Similarly, investigation of hematuria or uterine bleeding in patients with a therapeutic INR may unmask a tumor of the genitourinary tract.

SKIN NECROSIS. A rare complication of warfarin, skin necrosis usually occurs 2 to 5 days after initiation of therapy. Well-demarcated erythematous lesions form on the thighs, buttocks, breasts, or toes. Typically, the center of the lesion becomes progressively necrotic. Examination of skin biopsies taken from the borders of these lesions reveals thrombi in the microvasculature.

Warfarin-induced skin necrosis occurs in patients with congenital or acquired deficiencies of protein C or protein S.[88] Initiation of warfarin therapy in these patients produces a precipitous fall in plasma levels of proteins C or S, thereby eliminating this important anticoagulant pathway before warfarin exerts an antithrombotic effect through lowering of the functional levels of factor X and prothrombin. The resultant procoagulant state triggers thrombosis, but the reason that the thrombosis localizes to the microvasculature of fatty tissues is unclear.

Treatment involves discontinuation of warfarin and reversal with vitamin K, if needed. An alternative anticoagulant, such as heparin or LMWH, should be given to patients with thrombosis. Protein C concentrates or recombinant activated protein C may accelerate healing of the skin lesions in protein C deficient patients; fresh-frozen plasma may be of value for those with protein S deficiency. Occasionally, skin grafting is necessary when there is extensive skin loss.

Because of the potential for skin necrosis, patients with known protein C or protein S deficiency require overlapping treatment with a parenteral anticoagulant when initiating warfarin therapy. Warfarin should be started in low doses in these patients, and the parenteral anticoagulant should be continued until the INR is therapeutic for at least 2 to 3 consecutive days.

Pregnancy

Warfarin crosses the placenta and can cause fetal abnormalities or bleeding. The fetal abnormalities include a characteristic embryopathy, which consists of nasal hypoplasia and stippled epiphyses. The risk of embryopathy is highest with warfarin administration in the first trimester of pregnancy.[97] Central nervous system abnormalities also can occur with warfarin exposure at any time during pregnancy. Finally, maternal administration of warfarin produces an anticoagulant effect in the fetus that can cause bleeding. This is of particular concern at delivery, when trauma to the head during passage through the birth canal can lead to intracranial bleeding. Because of these potential problems, warfarin is contraindicated in pregnancy, particularly in the first and third trimesters (see Chaps. 66 and 82). Instead, heparin, LMWH, or fondaparinux can be given during pregnancy for prevention or treatment of thrombosis. Warfarin does not pass into breast milk, and thus is safe for nursing mothers.

Special Problems

Patients with an LA or those who need urgent or elective surgery present special challenges. Although observational studies have suggested that patients with thrombosis complicating APL require higher-intensity warfarin regimens to prevent recurrent thromboembolic events, two randomized trials have demonstrated that targeting an INR of 2.0 to 3.0 is as effective as higher-intensity treatment and produces less bleeding.[98] Monitoring warfarin therapy can prove difficult in patients with APL if the LA prolongs the baseline INR. Warfarin can be dosed based on measurements of factor X levels in such patients.

If patients receiving long-term warfarin treatment require an elective invasive procedure, warfarin can be stopped 5 days prior to the procedure to allow the INR to return to normal levels. Those at high risk for recurrent thrombosis can be bridged with once- or twice-daily subcutaneous injections of LMWH when the INR falls below 2.0. The last dose of LMWH should be given 12 to 24 hours prior to the procedure, depending on whether LMWH is administered twice or once daily, respectively. After the procedure, warfarin can be restarted.

NEW ORAL ANTICOAGULANTS

New oral anticoagulants that target thrombin or factor Xa are under development.[99-102] These drugs have a rapid onset of action and have half-lives that permit once- or twice-daily administration. Designed to produce a predictable level of anticoagulation, these new oral agents are given in fixed doses without routine coagulation monitoring. Therefore, these drugs are more convenient to administer than warfarin.

Dabigatran etexilate, an oral thrombin inhibitor, and rivaroxaban, an oral factor Xa inhibitor, are licensed in Europe and Canada for short-term thromboprophylaxis after elective hip or knee replacement surgery, and in the United States for atrial fibrillation. Phase III trials with apixaban, another oral factor Xa inhibitor, also have been completed in patients undergoing major orthopedic surgery (**Table 87-10**).

The recently reported RE-LY trial[101] shows the promise of these new agents for long-term indications. This trial compared two different dose regimens of dabigatran etexilate (110 or 150 mg twice daily) with warfarin (dose-adjusted to achieve an INR between 2.0 and 3.0) for stroke prevention in 18,113 patients with nonvalvular atrial fibrillation. The annual rates of the primary efficacy outcome, stroke or systemic embolism, were 1.7% with warfarin, 1.5% with the lower dose dabigatran regimen, and 1.1% with the higher-dose regimen. Thus, the lower-dose dabigatran regimen was noninferior to warfarin, whereas the higher-dose regimen was superior. Annual rates of major bleeding were 3.4% with warfarin, compared with 2.7% and 3.1% with the lower-dose and higher-dose dabigatran regimens, respectively. Thus, the lower-dose dabigatran regimen was associated with less major bleeding than warfarin, whereas the rate of major bleeding with the higher-dose regimen was not significantly different from that with warfarin. Rates of intracerebral bleeding were significantly lower with both doses of dabigatran than with warfarin, as were rates of life-threatening bleeding. There was no evidence of hepatotoxicity with dabigatran.

TABLE 87-10 Comparison of Features of New Oral Anticoagulants in Advanced Stages of Development

FEATURE	RIVAROXABAN	APIXABAN	DABIGATRAN ETEXILATE
Target	Xa	Xa	IIa
Molecular weight	436	460	628
Prodrug	No	No	Yes
Bioavailability (%)	80	50	6
Time to peak (hr)	3	3	2
Half-life (hr)	9	9-14	12-17
Renal excretion (%)	65	25	80
Antidote	None	None	None

Unmonitored dabigatran etexilate (150 mg twice daily) was compared with warfarin for treatment of venous thromboembolism in the RE-COVER trial.[102] The primary efficacy outcome, recurrent venous thromboembolism and related deaths, occurred in 2.4% of patients randomized to dabigatran and in 2.1% of those given warfarin. Major bleeding episodes occurred in 1.5% of patients randomized to dabigatran and in 1.9% of those assigned to warfarin. Therefore, dabigatran appears to be as effective and safe as warfarin for the treatment of venous thromboembolism. The promising results of these trials indicate that replacements for warfarin will soon be available.

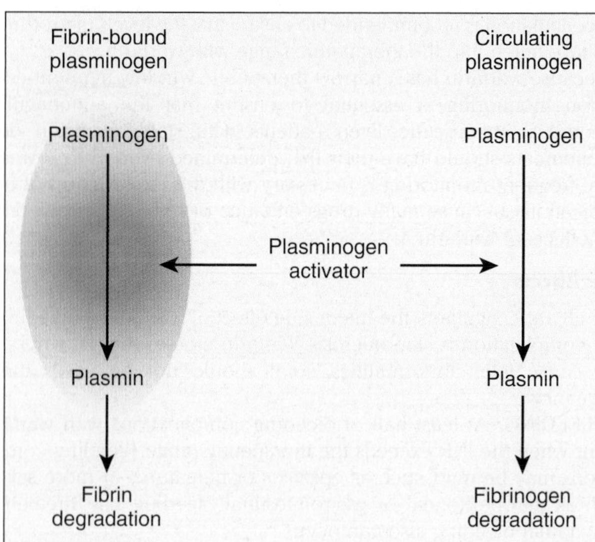

FIGURE 87-14 Consequences of activation of fibrin-bound or circulating plasminogen. The fibrin specificity of plasminogen activators reflects their capacity to distinguish between fibrin-bound and circulating plasminogen, which depends on their affinity for fibrin. Plasminogen activators with high affinity for fibrin preferentially activate fibrin-bound plasminogen. This results in the generation of plasmin on the fibrin surface. Fibrin-bound plasmin, which is protected from inactivation by alpha$_2$-antiplasmin, degrades fibrin to yield soluble fibrin degradation products. In contrast, plasminogen activators with little or no affinity for fibrin do not distinguish between fibrin-bound and circulating plasminogen. Activation of circulating plasminogen results in systemic plasminemia and subsequent degradation of fibrinogen and other clotting factors.

Fibrinolytic Drugs

Used to degrade thrombi, fibrinolytic drugs (see Chap. 55) can be administered systemically or delivered via catheters directly into the substance of the thrombus. Currently approved fibrinolytic agents include streptokinase, acylated plasminogen streptokinase activator complex (anistreplase), urokinase, recombinant tissue plasminogen activator (rt-PA; also known as alteplase or activase), and two recombinant derivatives of rt-PA, tenecteplase and reteplase. All these agents act by converting the proenzyme, plasminogen, to plasmin, the active enzyme.[10] There are two pools of plasminogen: circulating plasminogen and fibrin-bound plasminogen (**Fig. 87-14**). Plasminogen activators that preferentially activate fibrin-bound plasminogen are fibrin-specific. In contrast, nonspecific plasminogen activators do not discriminate between fibrin-bound and circulating plasminogen.[103] Activation of circulating plasminogen results in the generation of unopposed plasmin that can trigger the systemic lytic state. Alteplase and its derivatives are fibrin-specific plasminogen activators, whereas streptokinase, anistreplase, and urokinase are nonspecific agents.

STREPTOKINASE. Unlike other plasminogen activators, streptokinase is not an enzyme and does not directly convert plasminogen to plasmin. Instead, it forms a 1:1 stoichiometric complex with plasminogen, thus inducing a conformational change in plasminogen that exposes its active site (**Fig. 87-15**). This conformationally altered plasminogen then converts additional plasminogen molecules to plasmin.[10] Streptokinase has no affinity for fibrin, and the streptokinase-plasminogen complex activates free and fibrin-bound plasminogen. Activation of circulating plasminogen generates sufficient amounts of plasmin to overwhelm alpha$_2$-antiplasmin. Unopposed plasmin not only degrades fibrin in the occlusive thrombus, but also induces a systemic lytic state.[103]

When given systemically to patients with acute myocardial infarction, streptokinase reduces mortality. For this indication, the drug is usually given as an intravenous infusion of 1.5 million units over 30 to 60 minutes. Patients who receive streptokinase can develop antibodies against it, as can patients with prior streptococcal injection. These antibodies can reduce the effectiveness of streptokinase.

Allergic reactions occur in about 5% of patients treated with streptokinase. These may manifest as a rash, fever, chills, and rigors; rarely, anaphylactic reactions can occur. Transient hypotension is common with streptokinase and likely reflects plasmin-mediated release of bradykinin. The hypotension usually responds to leg elevation and administration of intravenous fluids and low doses of vasopressors, such as dopamine or norepinephrine.

ANISTREPLASE. To generate this drug, streptokinase is mixed with equimolar amounts of Lys-plasminogen, a plasmin-cleaved form of plasminogen with a Lys residue at its N terminal. The active site of Lys-plasminogen exposed on combination with streptokinase is blocked with an anisoyl group. After intravenous infusion, the anisoyl group is slowly removed by deacylation, giving the complex a half-life of about 100 minutes. This allows drug administration via a single bolus infusion. Although it is more convenient to administer, anistreplase offers few mechanistic advantages over streptokinase. Like streptokinase, anistreplase does not distinguish between fibrin-bound and circulating plasminogen. Consequently, anistreplase produces a systemic lytic state. Similarly, allergic reactions and hypotension are just as frequent with anistreplase as they are with streptokinase.[104]

When anistreplase was compared with alteplase in patients with acute myocardial infarction, reperfusion was obtained more rapidly with alteplase than with anistreplase.[104] Improved reperfusion was associated with a trend toward better clinical outcomes and reduced mortality with alteplase. These results and the high cost of anistreplase have dampened enthusiasm for its use.

UROKINASE. Derived from cultured fetal kidney cells, urokinase is a two-chain serine protease with a molecular weight of 34,000.[105] Urokinase directly converts plasminogen to plasmin. Unlike streptokinase, urokinase is not immunogenic, and allergic reactions are rare. Urokinase produces a systemic lytic state because it does not discriminate between fibrin-bound and circulating plasminogen.[103] Despite many years of use, systemic urokinase has never been evaluated for coronary fibrinolysis; instead, it is used for catheter-directed lysis of thrombi in the deep veins or in coronary or peripheral arteries.

ALTEPLASE. A recombinant form of single-chain t-PA, alteplase has a molecular weight of 68,000. Plasmin rapidly converts alteplase into its two-chain form. The interaction of alteplase with fibrin is mediated by the finger domain and, to a lesser extent, by the second kringle domain (**Fig. 87-16**).[10] The affinity of alteplase for fibrin is considerably higher than that for fibrinogen. Consequently, the catalytic efficiency of plasminogen activation by alteplase is two to three orders of magnitude higher in the presence of fibrin than in the presence of fibrinogen.[103]

Although alteplase preferentially activates plasminogen in the presence of fibrin, alteplase is not as fibrin-selective as was first predicted. Its

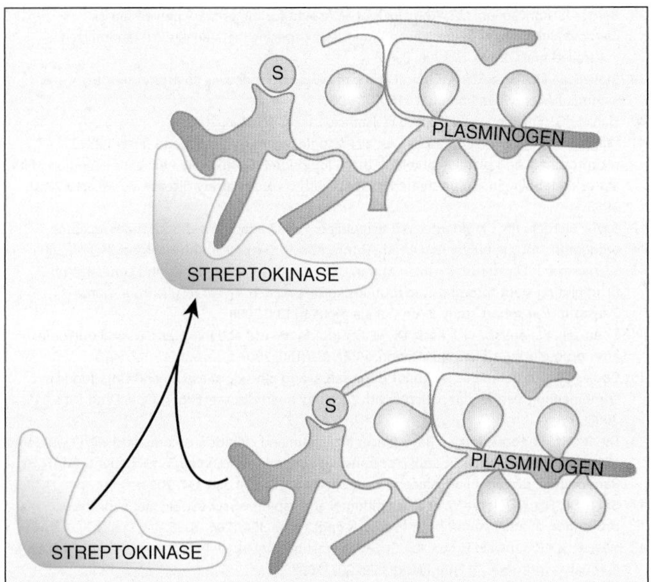

FIGURE 87-15 Mechanism of action of streptokinase. Streptokinase binds to plasminogen and induces a conformational change in plasminogen that exposes its active site. The streptokinase-plasmin(ogen) complex then serves as the activator of additional plasminogen molecules.

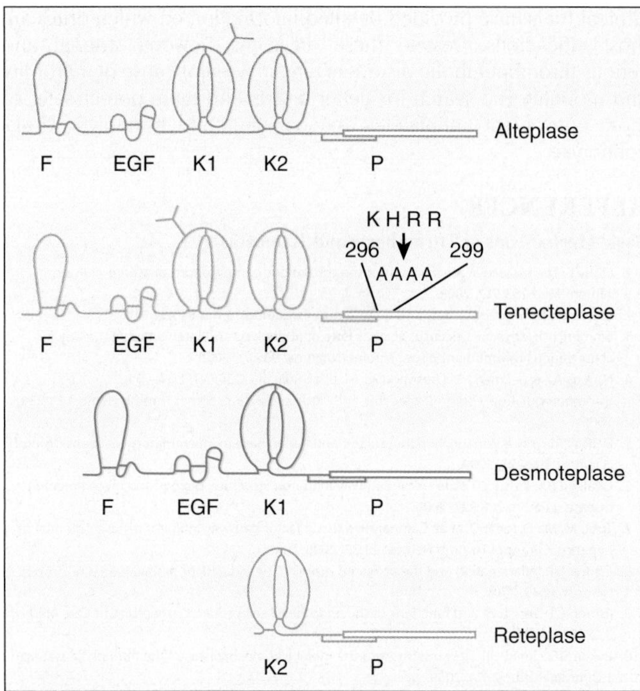

FIGURE 87-16 Domain structures of alteplase, tenecteplase, desmoteplase, and reteplase (see Fig. 55-14). The finger (F), epidermal growth factor (EGF), first and second kringles (K1 and K2, respectively), and protease (P) domains are illustrated. The glycosylation site (Y) on K1 has been repositioned in tenecteplase to endow it with a longer half-life. In addition, a tetra-alanine substitution in the protease domain renders tenecteplase resistant to PAI-1 inhibition. Desmoteplase differs from alteplase and tenecteplase in that it lacks a K2 domain. Reteplase is a truncated variant that lacks the F, EGF, and K1 domains.

fibrin specificity is limited because like fibrin, (DD)E, the major soluble degradation product of cross-linked fibrin, binds alteplase and plasminogen with high affinity. Consequently, (DD)E is as potent as fibrin as a stimulator of plasminogen activation by alteplase. Whereas plasmin generated on the fibrin surface results in thrombolysis, plasmin generated on the surface of circulating (DD)E degrades fibrinogen. Fibrinogenolysis results in the accumulation of fragment X, a high-molecular-weight clottable fibrinogen degradation product. Incorporation of fragment X into hemostatic plugs formed at sites of vascular injury renders them susceptible to lysis.[106] This phenomenon may contribute to alteplase-induced bleeding.

A trial comparing alteplase with streptokinase for the treatment of patients with acute myocardial infarction demonstrated significantly lower mortality with alteplase than with streptokinase, although the absolute difference was small.[106a] Patients younger than 75 years of age with anterior myocardial infarction who presented less than 6 hours after symptom onset derived the greatest benefit from alteplase. For treatment of acute myocardial infarction or acute ischemic stroke, alteplase is given as an intravenous infusion over 60 to 90 minutes. The total dose of alteplase usually ranges from 90 to 100 mg. Allergic reactions and hypotension are rare, and alteplase is not immunogenic.

Tenecteplase. A genetically engineered variant of t-PA, tenecteplase was designed to have a longer half-life than t-PA and to be resistant to inactivation by PAI-1.[107] To prolong its half-life, a new glycosylation site was added to the first kringle domain (see Fig. 87-16). Because addition of this extra carbohydrate side chain reduced fibrin affinity, the existing glycosylation site on the first kringle domain was removed. To render the molecule resistant to inhibition by PAI-1, a tetra-alanine substitution was introduced at residues 296-299 in the protease domain, the region responsible for the interaction of t-PA with PAI-1.

Tenecteplase is more fibrin-specific than t-PA. Although both agents bind to fibrin with similar affinity, the affinity of tenecteplase for (DD)E is significantly lower than that of t-PA.[107] Consequently, (DD)E does not stimulate systemic plasminogen activation by tenecteplase to the same extent as t-PA. As a result, tenecteplase produces less fibrinogenolysis than t-PA.

For coronary fibrinolysis, tenecteplase is given as a single intravenous bolus. In a large phase III trial that enrolled more than 16,000 patients, the 30-day mortality rate with single-bolus tenecteplase was similar to that with accelerated dose t-PA. Although rates of intracranial hemorrhage also were similar with both treatments, patients given tenecteplase had fewer noncerebral bleeds and a reduced need for blood transfusions compared with those treated with t-PA.[107] The improved safety profile of tenecteplase likely reflects its enhanced fibrin specificity.

Reteplase. A recombinant t-PA derivative, reteplase is a single-chain variant that lacks the finger, epidermal growth factor, and first kringle domains (see Fig. 87-16). This truncated derivative has a molecular weight of 39,000. Reteplase binds fibrin more weakly than t-PA because it lacks the finger domain. Because it is produced in *Escherichia coli*, reteplase is not glycosylated; this endows it with a plasma half-life longer than that of t-PA. Consequently, reteplase is given as two intravenous boluses separated by 30 minutes. Clinical trials have demonstrated that reteplase is at least as effective as streptokinase for treatment of acute myocardial infarction,[108] but is not superior to t-PA.

Newer Fibrinolytic Agents. Newer fibrinolytic agents include desmoteplase (see Fig. 87-16), a recombinant form of the full-length plasminogen activator isolated from the saliva of the vampire bat,[109] and alfimeprase, a truncated form of fibrolase, an enzyme isolated from the venom of the southern copperhead snake.[110] Clinical studies with these agents have proven disappointing. Desmoteplase, which is more fibrin-specific than t-PA, was investigated for the treatment of acute ischemic stroke.[111] Patients presenting 3 to 9 hours after symptom onset were randomized to one of two doses of desmoteplase or to placebo. Overall response rates were low, and were no different with desmoteplase than with placebo. Mortality was higher in the desmoteplase arms.

Alfimeprase is a metalloproteinase that degrades fibrin and fibrinogen in a plasmin-independent fashion.[110] In the circulation, alfimeprase is inhibited by alpha$_2$-macroglobulin, so it must be delivered via a catheter directly into the thrombus. Despite promising phase III results,[112] studies of alfimeprase for the treatment of peripheral arterial occlusion or for restoration of flow in blocked central venous catheters were stopped because of lack of efficacy. The disappointing results with desmoteplase and alfimeprase highlight the challenges of introducing new fibrinolytic drugs.

Conclusions and Future Directions

Thrombosis in the arteries or veins reflects a complex interplay among the vessel wall, platelets, coagulation system, and fibrinolytic pathways. Activation of coagulation also triggers inflammatory pathways that may contribute to thrombogenesis. A better understanding of the biochemistry of platelet aggregation and blood coagulation and advances in structure-based drug design have identified new targets and resulted in the development of novel antithrombotic drugs. Well-designed clinical trials have provided detailed information on which drugs are most efficacious. Despite these advances, however, arterial and venous thromboembolic disorders remain a major cause of morbidity and mortality. The search for better targets and more potent, safer, or more convenient antiplatelet, anticoagulant, and fibrinolytic drugs continues.

REFERENCES

Basic Mechanisms of Thrombosis and Hemostasis

1. Libby P: The molecular mechanisms of the thrombotic complications of atherosclerosis. J Intern Med 263:517, 2008.
2. Mackman N: Triggers, targets and treatments of thrombosis. Nature 451:914, 2008.
3. Emmerich J, Meyer G, Decousus H, et al: Role of fibrinolysis and interventional therapy for acute venous thromboembolism. Thromb Haemost 96:251, 2006.
4. Marcus AJ, Broekman MJ, Drosopoulos JH, et al: Role of CD39 (NTPDase-1) in thromboregulation, cerebroprotection, and cardioprotection. Semin Thromb Hemost 31:234, 2005.
5. Li JP, Vlodavsky I: Heparin, heparan sulfate and heparanase in inflammatory reactions. Thromb Haemost 102:823, 2009.
6. Lwaleed BA, Bass PS: Tissue factor pathway inhibitor: Structure, biology and involvement in disease. J Pathol 208:327, 2006.
7. Tobu M, Ma Q, Iqbal O, et al: Comparative tissue factor pathway inhibitor release potential of heparins. Clin Appl Thromb Hemost 11:37, 2005.
8. Esmon CT: Inflammation and the activated protein C anticoagulant pathway. Semin Thromb Hemost 32:49, 2006.
9. Esmon CT: Structure and functions of the endothelial cell protein C receptor. Crit Care Med 32:S298, 2004.
10. Rijken DC, Lijnen HR: New insights into the molecular mechanisms of the fibrinolytic system. J Thromb Haemost 7:4, 2009.
11. Kaushansky K: The molecular mechanisms that control thrombopoiesis. J Clin Invest 115:3339, 2005.
12. Watson SP: Platelet activation by extracellular matrix proteins in haemostasis and thrombosis. Curr Pharm Des 15:1358, 2009.
13. López JA, del Conde I, Shrimpton CN: Receptors, rafts, and microvesicles in thrombosis and inflammation. J Thromb Haemost 3:1737, 2005.
14. Turner NA, Nolasco L, Ruggeri ZM, Moake JL: Endothelial cell ADAMTS-13 and VWF: Production, release, and VWF string cleavage. Blood 114:5102, 2009.
15. Sadler JE: von Willebrand factor assembly and secretion. J Thromb Haemost 7(Suppl 1):24, 2009.
16. Nakahata NL: Thromboxane A2: Physiology/pathophysiology, cellular signal transduction and pharmacology. Pharmacol Ther 118:18, 2008.
17. Smyth SS, Woulfe DS, Weitz JI, et al: G-protein-coupled receptors as signaling targets for antiplatelet therapy. Arterioscler Thromb Vasc Biol 29:449, 2009.
18. Cattaneo M: Platelet P2 receptors: Old and new targets for antithrombotic drugs. Expert Rev Cardiovasc Ther 5:45, 2007.
19. McEachron TA, Pawlinski R, Richards KL, et al: Protease-activated receptors mediate cross-talk between coagulation and fibrinolysis. Blood Aug. 24, 2010 [Epub ahead of print].
20. Butenas S, Orfeo T, Mann KG: Tissue factor in coagulation: Which? Where? When? Arterioscler Thromb Vasc Biol 29:1989, 2009.
21. Blann A, Shantsila E, Shantsila A: Microparticles and arterial disease. Semin Thromb Hemost 35:488, 2009.
22. Morrissey J, Mackman N: Tissue factor and factor VIIa: Understanding the molecular mechanism. Thromb Res 122(Suppl 1):S1, 2008.
23. Vogler EA, Siedecki CA: Contact activation of blood-plasma coagulation. Biomaterials 30:1857, 2009.
24. Müller F, Renné T: Novel roles for factor XII-driven plasma contact activation system. Curr Opin Hematol 15:516, 2008.
25. Butenas S, Undas A, Gissel MT, et al: Factor XIa and tissue factor activity in patients with coronary artery disease. Thromb Haemost 99:142, 2008.
26. Marx PF, Verkleij CJ, Seron MV, Meijers JC: Recent developments in thrombin-activatable fibrinolysis inhibitor research. Mini Rev Med Chem 9:1165, 2009.
27. Tziomalos K, Athyros VG, Wierzbicki AS, Mikhailidis DP: Lipoprotein a: Where are we now? Curr Opin Cardiol 24:351, 2009.
28. McMahon B, Kwaan HC: The plasminogen activator system and cancer. Pathophysiol Haemost Thromb 36:184, 2008.
29. Tang EH, Vanhoutte PM: Prostanoids and reactive oxygen species: Team players in endothelium-dependent contractions. Pharmacol Ther 122:140, 2009.
30. Zhang C: The role of inflammatory cytokines in endothelial dysfunction. Basic Res Cardiol 103:398, 2008.
31. Jennings LK: Role of platelets in atherothrombosis. Am J Cardiol 103:4A, 2009.
32. Bank I, Libourel EJ, Middeldorp S, et al: Elevated levels of FVIII:C within families are associated with an increased risk for venous and arterial thrombosis. J Thromb Haemost 1:79, 2005.
33. Saposnik B, Reny JL, Gaussem P, et al: A haplotype of the EPCR gene is associated with increased plasma levels of sEPCR and is a candidate risk factor for thrombosis. Blood 103:1311, 2004.
34. Kobbervig C, Williams E: FXIII polymorphisms, fibrin clot structure and thrombotic risk. Biophys Chem 112:223, 2004.
35. Falanga A, Marchetti M: Venous thromboembolism in the hematologic malignancies. J Clin Oncol 27:4848, 2009.
36. Kasthuri RS, Taubman MB, Mackman N: Role of tissue factor in cancer. J Clin Oncol 27:4834, 2009.

Antiplatelet Agents

37. Patrono C, Baigent C, Hirsh J, et al: Antiplatelet drugs: American College of Chest Physicians Evidence-Based Clinical Practice Guidelines (8th Edition). Chest 133:199S, 2008.
38. Berger JS, Roncaglioni MC, Avanzini F, et al: Aspirin for the primary prevention of cardiovascular events in women and men: A sex-specific meta-analysis of randomized controlled trials. JAMA 295:306, 2006.
39. Stevenson DD, Szczeklik A: Clinical and pathologic perspectives on aspirin sensitivity and asthma. J Allergy Clin Immunol 118:773, 2006.
40. Hankey GJ, Eikelboom JW: Aspirin resistance. Lancet 367:606, 2006.
41. Wallentin L, Varenhorst C, James S, et al: Prasugrel achieves greater and faster P2Y12 receptor-mediated platelet inhibition than clopidogrel due to more efficient generation of its active metabolite in aspirin-treated patients with coronary artery disease. Eur Heart J 29:21, 2008.
42. Savi P, Herbert JM: Clopidogrel and ticlopidine: P2Y12 adenosine diphosphate-receptor antagonists for the prevention of atherothrombosis. Semin Thromb Haemost 31:174, 2005.
43. Wenaweser P, Daemen J, Zwahlen M, van Domburg R, et al: Incidence and correlates of drug-eluting stent thrombosis in routine clinical practice: 4-year results from a large 2-institutional cohort study. J Am Coll Cardiol 52:1134, 2008.
44. Eisenstein EL, Anstrom KJ, Kong DF, et al: Clopidogrel use and long-term clinical outcomes after drug-eluting stent implantation. JAMA 297:159, 2007.
45. Cooke GE, Goldschmidt-Clermont PJ: The safety and efficacy of aspirin and clopidogrel as a combination treatment in patients with coronary heart disease. Expert Opin Drug Saf 5:815, 2006.
46. Diener HC, Bogousslavsky J, Brass LM, et al: Aspirin and clopidogrel compared with clopidogrel alone after recent ischemic stroke or transient ischemic attack in high-risk patients (MATCH): Randomised, double-blind, placebo-controlled trial. Lancet 364:331, 2004.
47. Bhatt DL, Fox KA, Hacke W, et al: Clopidogrel and aspirin versus aspirin alone for the prevention of atherothrombotic events. N Engl J Med 354:1706, 2006.
48. Wiviott SD, Braunwald E, McCabe CH, et al: Prasugrel versus clopidogrel in patients with acute coronary syndromes. N Engl J Med 357:2001, 2007.
49. Tantry US, Bliden KP, Gurbel PA: Prasugrel. Expert Opin Invest Drugs 15:1627, 2006.
50. Nguyen TA, Diodati JG, Pharand C: Resistance to clopidogrel: A review of the evidence. J Am Coll Cardiol 45:1157, 2005.
51. Hulot JS, Bura A, Villard E, et al: Cytochrome P450 2C19 loss-of-function polymorphism is a major determinant of clopidogrel responsiveness in healthy subjects. Blood 108:2244, 2006.
52. Angiolillo DJ, Fernandez-Ortiz A, Bernardo E, et al: Contribution of gene sequence variations of the hepatic cytochrome P450 3A4 enzyme to variability in individual responsiveness to clopidogrel. Arterioscler. Thromb. Vasc. Biol 26:1895, 2006.
53. Simon T, Verstuyft C, Mary-Krause M, et al: Genetic determinants of response to clopidogrel and cardiovascular events. N Engl J Med 360:363, 2009.
54. Mega JL, Close SL, Wiviott SD, et al: Cytochrome P-450 polymorphisms and response to clopidogrel. N Engl J Med 360:354, 2009.
55. O'Donoghue ML, Braunwald E, Antman EM, et al: Pharmacodynamic effect and clinical efficacy of clopidogrel and prasugrel with or without a proton-pump inhibitor: An analysis of two randomized trials. Lancet 374:989, 2009.
56. Varenhorst C, James S, Erlinge D, et al: Genetic variation of CYP2C19 affects both pharmacokinetic and pharmacodymamic responses to clopidogrel but not prasugrel in aspirin-treated patients with coronary artery disease. Eur Heart J 30:1744, 2009.
57. Mega JL, Close SL, Wiviott SD, et al: Cytochrome P450 genetic polymorphisms and the response to prasugrel: Relationship to pharmacokinetic, pharmacodynamic, and clinical outcomes. Circulation 119:2553, 2009.
58. Malmstrom RE, Ostergren J, Jorgensen L, Hjemdahl P, et al: Influence of statin treatment on platelet inhibition by clopidogrel—a randomized comparison of rosuvastatin, atorvastatin and simvastatin co-treatment. J Intern Med 266:457, 2009.
59. Michelson AD: Platelet function testing in cardiovascular diseases. Circulation 119:e489, 2004.
60. ESPRIT Study Group; Halkes PH, van Gijn J, Kappelle LJ, et al: Aspirin plus dipyridamole versus aspirin alone after cerebral ischaemia of arterial origin (ESPRIT): Randomised controlled trial. Lancet 367:1665, 2006.
61. Diener HC, Sacco RL, Yusuf S, Cotton D, et al: Effects of aspirin plus extended-release dipyridamole versus clopidogrel and telmisartan on disability and cognitive function after recurrent stroke in patients with ischemic stroke in the Prevention Regimen for Effectively Avoiding Second Strokes (PRoFESS) trial: A double-blind, active and placebo-controlled study. Lancet Neurol 7:875, 2008.
62. Rossi ML, Zavalloni D: Inhibitors of platelets glycoprotein IIb/IIIa (GPIIb/IIIa) receptor: Rationale for their use in clinical cardiology. Mini Rev Med Chem 4:703, 2004.
63. Aster RH: Immune thrombocytopenia caused by glycoprotein IIb/IIIa inhibitors. Chest 127:53S, 2005.
64. Harrington RA, Becker RC, Cannon CP, Gutterman D, et al: Antithrombotic therapy for non-ST-segment elevation acute coronary syndromes: American College of Chest Physicians Evidence-Based Clinical Practice Guidelines (8th Edition). Chest 133:670S, 2008.
65. Goodman SG, Menon V, Cannon CP, Steg G, et al: Acute ST-segment elevation myocardial infarction: American College of Chest Physicians Evidence-Based Clinical Practice Guidelines (8th Edition). Chest 133:708S, 2008.
66. Bhatt DL, Lincoff MA, Gibson CM, et al: Intravenous platelet blockade with cangrelor during PCI. N Engl J Med 361:2330, 2009.
67. Harrington RA, Stone GW, McNulty S, et al: Platelet inhibition with cangrelor in patients undergoing PCI. N Engl J Med 361:2318, 2009.
68. Wallentin L, Becker RC, Budaj A, Cannon CP, et al: Ticagrelor versus clopidogrel in patients with acute coronary syndromes. N Engl J Med 361:1045, 2009.
69. Oestreich J: SCH-530348, a thrombin receptor (PAR-1) antagonist for the prevention and treatment of atherothrombosis. Curr Opin Invest Drugs 10:988, 2009.
70. Serebruany VL, Kogushi M, Dastros-Pitei D, Flather M, et al: The in-vitro effects of E5555, a protease-activated receptor (PAR)-1 antagonist, on platelet biomarkers in healthy volunteers and patients with coronary artery disease. Thromb Haemost 102:111, 2009.

Anticoagulants

71. Gross PL, Weitz JI: New antithrombotic drugs. Clin Pharmacol Ther 86:139, 2009.
72. Hirsh J, Bauer KA, Donati MB, Gould M, et al: Parenteral anticoagulants: American College of Chest Physicians Evidence-Based Clinical Practice Guidelines (8th Edition). Chest 133:141S, 2008.

73. Geerts WH, Bergqvist D, Pineo, GF, et al: Prevention of venous thromboembolism: American College of Chest Physicians Evidence-Based Clinical Practice Guidelines (8th Edition). Chest 133:381S, 2008.
74. Blossom DB, Kallen AJ, Patel PR, et al: Outbreak of adverse reactions assocated with contaminated heparin. N Engl J Med 359:2674, 2008.
75. Schulman S, Beyth RJ, Kearon C, Levine MN: Hemorrhagic complications of anticoagulant and thrombolytic treatment: American College of Chest Physicians Evidence-based Clinical Practice Guidelines (8th Edition). Chest 133:257S, 2008.
76. Shantsila E, Lip GY, Chong BH: Heparin-induced thrombocytopenia. A contemporary clinical approach to diagnosis and management. Chest 135:1651, 2009.
77. Greinacher A: Heparin-induced thrombocytopenia. J Thromb Haemost 7(Suppl 1):9, 2009.
78. Warkentin TE, Linkins LA: Immunoassays are not created equal. J Thromb Haemost 7:1256, 2009.
79. Hirsh J, Heddle N, Kelton JG: Treatment of heparin-induced thrombocytopenia: A critical review. Arch Intern Med 164:361, 2004.
80. Srinivasan AF, Rice L, Bartholomew JR, et al: Warfarin-induced skin necrosis and venous limb gangrene in the setting of heparin-induced thrombocytopenia. Arch Intern Med 164:66, 2004.
81. Quinlan DJ, McQuillan A, Eikelboom JW: Low-molecular-weight heparin compared with intravenous unfractionated heparin for treatment of pulmonary embolism: A meta-analysis of randomized, controlled trials. Ann Intern Med 140:175, 2004.
82. Buller HR, Davidson BL, Decousus H, et al: Fondaparinux or enoxaparin for the initial treatment of symptomatic deep venous thrombosis: A randomized trial. Ann Intern Med 140:867, 2004.
83. Fifth Organization to Assess Strategies in Acute Ischemic Syndromes Investigators: Comparison of fondaparinux and enoxaparin in acute coronary syndromes. N Engl J Med 354:1464, 2006.
84. Yusuf S, Mehta SR, Chrolavicius S, et al: Effects of fondaparinux on mortality and reinfarction in patients with acute ST-segment elevation myocardial infarction: The OASIS-6 randomized trial. JAMA 295:1519, 2006.
85. Warkentin TE, Cook RJ, Marder VJ, et al: Anti-platelet factor 4/heparin antibodies in orthopedic surgery patients receiving antithrombotic prophylaxis with fondaparinux or enoxaparin. Blood 106:3791, 2005.
86. Kuo KH, Kovacs MJ: Fondaparinux: A potential new therapy for HIT. Hematology 10:271, 2005.
87. Grouzi E, Kyriakou E, Panagou I, Spilliotopoulou I: Fondaparinux for the treatment of acute heparin-induced thrombocytopenia: A single-center experience. Clin Appl Thromb Hemost 16:663, 2010.
88. Ansell J, Hirsh J, Hylek E, Jacobson A, et al: Pharmacology and management of the vitamin K antagonists: American College of Chest Physicians Evidence-Based Clinical Practice Guidelines (8th Edition). Chest 133:160S, 2008.
89. Sanderson S, Emery J, Higgins J: CYP2C9 gene variants; drug dose and bleeding risk in warfarin-treated patients: A HUGEnet™ systematic review and meta-analysis. Genet Med 7:97, 2005.
90. Sconce EA, Khan TI, Wynne HA, et al: The impact of CYP2C9 and VKORC1 genetic polymorphism and patient characteristics on warfarin dose requirements: Proposal for a new dosing regimen. Blood 106:2329, 2005.
91. Wadelius M, Chen LY, Eriksson N, et al: Association of warfarin dose with genes involved in its action and metabolism. Hum Genet 121:23, 2007.
92. McClain M, Palomaki GE, Piper M, et al: A rapid-ACCE review of CYP2C9 and VKORC1 alleles testing to inform warfarin dosing in adults at elevated risk for thrombotic events and to avoid serious bleeding. Genet Med 10:89, 2008.
93. Rieder MJ, Reiner AP, Gage BF: Effects of VKORC1 haplotypes on the transcriptional regulation and warfarin dose. N Engl J Med 352:2285, 2005.
94. International Warfarin Pharmacogenetics Consortium: Estimation of the warfarin dose with clinical and pharmacogenetic data. N Engl J Med 360:753, 2009.
95. Singer DE, Albers GW, Dalen JE, Fang MC, et al: Antithrombotic therapy in atrial fibrillation: American College of Chest Physicians Evidence-Based Clinical Practice Guidelines (8th Edition). Chest 133:546S, 2008.
96. Crowther MA, Ageno W, Garcia D, et al: Oral vitamin K versus placebo to correct excessive anticoagulation in patients receiving warfarin: A randomized trial. Ann Intern Med 150:293, 2009.
97. Bates SM, Greer IA, Pabinger I, Sofaer S, et al: Venous thromboembolism, thrombophilia, antithrombotic therapy, and pregnancy: American College of Chest Physicians Evidence-Based Clinical Practice Guidelines (8th Edition). Chest 133:844S, 2008.
98. Finazzi G, Marchioli R, Brancaccio V, et al: A randomized clinical trial of high-intensity warfarin vs. conventional antithrombotic therapy for the prevention of recurrent thrombosis in patients with the antiphospholipid syndrome (WAPS). J Thromb Haemost 3:848, 2005.
99. Bates SM, Weitz JI: The status of new anticoagulants. Br J Haematol 134:3, 2006.
100. Gross PL, Weitz JI: New antithrombotic drugs. Clin Pharmacol Ther 86:139, 2009.
101. Connolly SJ, Ezekowitz MD, Yusuf S, et al: Dabigatran versus warfarin in patients with atrial fibrillation. N Engl J Med 361:1139, 2009.
102. Schulman S, Kearon C, Kakkar AK, Mismetti P, et al: Dabigatran versus warfarin in the treatment of acute venous thromboembolism. N Engl J Med 361:2342, 2009.

Fibrinolytic Drugs

103. Longstaff C, William S, Thelwell C: Fibrin binding and the regulation of plasminogen activators during thrombolytic therapy. Cardiovasc Hematol Agents Med Chem 6:212, 2008.
104. Bell WR Jr: Evaluation of thrombolytic agents. Drugs 54:11, 1997.
105. Vincenza Carriero M, Franco P, Vocca I, Alfano D, et al: Structure, function and antagonists of urokinase-type plasminogen activators. Front Biosci 14:3782, 2009.
106. Schaefer AV, Leslie BA, Rischke JA, et al: Incorporation of fragment X into fibrin clots renders them more susceptible to lysis by plasmin. Biochemistry 45:4257, 2006.
106a. The Gusto Investigators: An international randomized trial comparing four thrombolytic strategies for acute myocardial infarction. N Engl J Med 329:673, 1993.
107. Melandri G, Vagnarelli F, Calabrese D, Semprini F, et al: Review of tenecteplase (TNKase) in the treatment of acute myocardial infarction. Vasc Health Risk Manag 5:249, 2009.
108. Simpson D, Siddiqui MA, Scott LJ, Hilleman DE: Spotlight on reteplase in thrombotic occlusive disorders. BioDrugs 21:65, 2007.
109. Paciaroni M, Medeiros E, Bogousslavsky J. Desmoteplase: Expert Opin Biol Ther 9:773, 2009.
110. Deitcher SR, Funk WD, Buchanan J, et al: Alfimeprase: A novel recombinant direct-acting fibrinolytic. Expert Opin Biol Ther 6:1361, 2006.
111. Hacke W, Furlan AJ, Al-Rawi Y, Davalos A, et al: Intravenous desmoteplase in patients with acute ischaemic stroke selected by MRI perfusion-diffusion weighted imaging or perfusion CT (DIAS-2): A prospective, randomized, double-blind, placebo-controlled study. Lancet Neurol 8:141, 2009.
112. Moll S, Kenyon P, Bertolli L, De Maio J, et al: Phase II trial of alfimeprase, a novel-acting fibrin degradation agent, for occluded central venous access devices. J Clin Oncol 24:3056, 2006.

CHAPTER 88 Rheumatic Fever

B. Soma Raju and Zoltan G. Turi

Rheumatic fever (RF) is an autoimmune disorder that remains incompletely characterized with regard to its basic elements—cause, pathophysiology, diagnosis, and treatment—despite evidence of its existence dating to at least the 1600s. The classic understanding that the disease is a post–suppurative streptococcal pharyngitis cascade, leading variably to arthritis, chorea, dermal manifestations, and, most important, carditis, has largely withstood challenge. Immunologic studies have confirmed the presence of epitopes on the bacterial surface that mimic cardiac myosin as well as antigens found in valve, skin, joint, and brain tissue that account for the immunologic cross-reactive attack characteristic of RF. No single diagnostic tool or laboratory test exists for RF. Hence, the diagnosis depends on a composite of clinical criteria.

The sequelae of only one manifestation, carditis, account for most of the morbidity and essentially all of the mortality associated with RF. As a cause of heart disease in adults, RF has declined dramatically in industrialized nations but remains a major source of morbidity and mortality in developing countries and in some selected aboriginal populations in wealthy nations. The primary consequences of RF, rheumatic mitral and aortic valve disease in adults, are also declining worldwide but remain a major burden on the limited health care resources of the countries where the disease is most prevalent (see Chap. 1). The diagnostic and treatment algorithms for RF are still largely based on descriptive series and expert opinion panels. Because failure to diagnose RF and to institute secondary prophylaxis results in rheumatic heart disease (RHD), increasing attention is being focused on improving sensitivity of diagnosis in areas where the disease is endemic.

Epidemiology

Streptococcus pyogenes is responsible for diseases ranging from pharyngitis to glomerulonephritis, necrotizing fasciitis, and toxic shock syndrome. Suppurative pharyngitis is the only clearly established prequel to RF. In 2005, 15.6 million people were estimated to have RF or RHD on the basis of traditional clinical measures that may represent substantial underestimation.[1] The majority of these cases are from sub-Saharan Africa and south central Asia, which along with indigenous populations in Australia and New Zealand represent the world's highest prevalence.

Given a causal association between group A beta-hemolytic streptococci (GABHS) and RF, their epidemiology is also linked. Whereas most pharyngitis (80%) is viral in etiology, GABHS is isolated in up to 75% of cases from children with symptoms of severe bacterial pharyngitis.[2] Antistreptolysin O titers more than 200 Todd units are found in up to 50% of asymptomatic children 6 to 15 years old, the prime age group for RF. This reflects the frequent occurrence of pharyngitis in this age group (estimated to be once yearly), approximately 15% to 20% of which is caused by GABHS.[3] Recurrence is most common in adolescents and young adults and is uncommon beyond the age of 34 years. Data from the early antibiotic era suggest that 0.3% to 3% of those with untreated GABHS pharyngitis develop RF. Although there is no clear gender predisposition, postpubertal chorea and the development of mitral stenosis are more common in females. GABHS is present in 10% to 30% of asymptomatic individuals in the prime RF age groups in the United States, but it is higher in many countries. A history of pharyngitis has been reported in approximately two thirds of RF cases. Carriers (patients with positive throat cultures without clinical history or rise in antibody titers) do not appear predisposed to RF. The possibility that RF may follow nonpharyngeal streptococcal infection, in particular pyoderma, continues to be explored.

Decline in Rheumatic Fever. The decline in RF began before the antibiotic era. Explanations include improvement in environmental factors, decrease in rheumatogenicity of streptococcal strains, and improved specificity in diagnosis. The last was largely due to the introduction of the Jones criteria, before which children with minor manifestations such as isolated arthralgias were frequently assigned a diagnosis of RF. The decrease in mortality from acute carditis in the preantibiotic era suggests that the virulence of rheumatogenic strains decreased as well. **Figure 88-1** demonstrates the dramatic decline in mortality associated with RF in the United States in the past century along with milestones in diagnosis and management. Whereas the incidence of RF in industrialized states is now estimated to be less than 1/100,000 people, it is 100-fold higher in endemic areas.[4] RHD occurs in up to 3% of children in some developing nations.[1] Socioeconomic, epidemiologic, cultural, and other factors influence applicability of some of the standard RF algorithms in these countries. As a cause of valvular disease seen at autopsy or surgery, RHD has declined exponentially since the 1920s, when 39.5% of New England cardiac admissions were related to RHD; it now accounts for less than 0.5% of primary discharge diagnoses in the United States. In contrast, rates remain comparable to those of the 1950s in the poorest nations as well as in isolated subpopulations such as the aboriginal people of Austrailia. Crowding, inadequate medical facilities, lack of antibiotics for primary therapy and secondary prevention, and lack of medical personnel have sustained the prevalence of RF and RHD. There is a trend in some developing nations toward declining frequency, in part because of better availability of basic care, sometimes associated with over-the-counter dispensing of antibiotics.

The outbreaks of RF in the United States in the 1980s prompted extensive investigation of the disease in an industrialized nation. RF occurred in areas without the risk factors attributed to susceptible populations, and some evidence suggests an association with the reappearance of rheumatogenic strains of *S. pyogenes*.[5] The diagnosis remains rare in industrialized countries, accounting for approximately 0.1% of pediatric hospitalizations in the United States, with geographic clusters and some evidence of ethnic susceptibility, in particular Asians and Pacific Islanders.

Pathobiology

The classic triad of agent, host, and environment plays a major role in the pathogenesis of RF. GABHS has more than 130 subtypes defined by M-protein surface molecules.[3] Some of these appear to be rheumatogenic, typically mucoid strains that adhere well to pharyngeal tissue and have antiphagocytic properties that allow persistence of bacteria in tissues for up to 2 weeks, until specific antibodies are created. M protein, *N*-acetylglucosamine, and several other epitopes mimic myocardium (myosin and tropomyosin), heart valves (laminin),

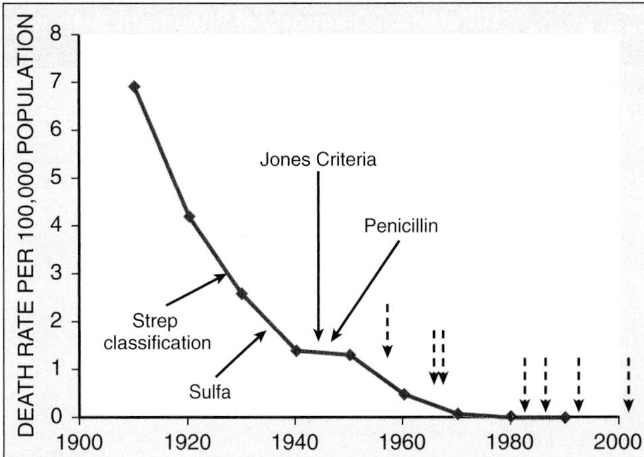

FIGURE 88-1 Decline in mortality from rheumatic fever in the United States during the 20th century. Note that the decline began well before the availability of penicillin. Dashed arrows mark the multiple modifications or revisions of the Jones criteria or World Health Organization expert opinion reviews and recommendations. *(Modified from Gordis L: The virtual disappearance of rheumatic fever in the United States: Lessons in the rise and fall of disease. T. Duckett Jones memorial lecture. Circulation 72:1155, 1985.)*

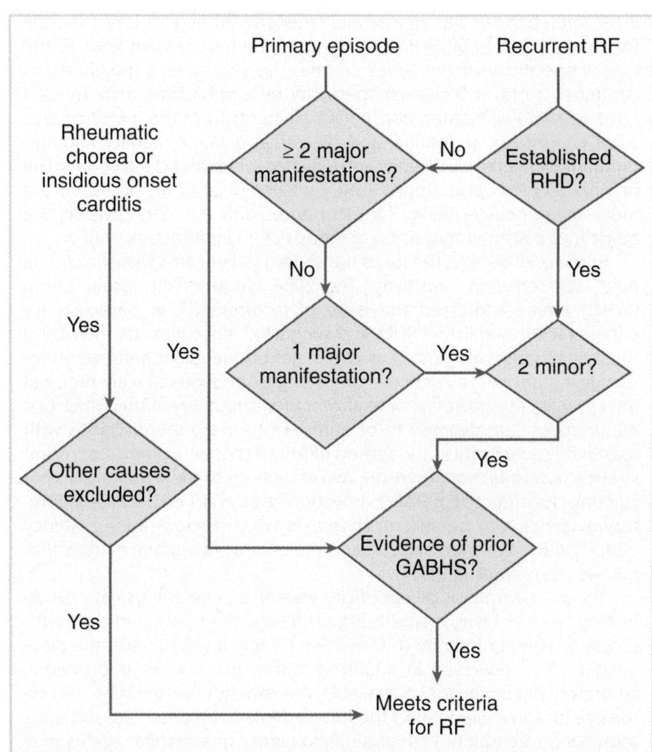

FIGURE 88-2 Algorithm for diagnosis of acute rheumatic fever, incorporating the 1992 revision of the Jones criteria and the World Health Organization (WHO) expert consultation report (2002-2003). The WHO modifications incorporated in the flow chart are more sensitive and less specific than those incorporated in the American Heart Association criteria. GABHS = group A beta-hemolytic streptococci; RF = rheumatic fever; RHD = rheumatic heart disease.

synovia (vimentin), skin (keratin), and subthalamic and caudate nuclei in the brain (lysogangliosides).[6] Superantigenic activity triggered by M-protein fragments as well as streptococcal toxins have also been implicated in autoimmune reactivity mediated by B cells and T cells. T cells activated against myosin and bacterial epitopes react to valve tissue with as yet incompletely defined host factors that may enhance the inflammatory response in heart valves. Considerable heterogeneity exists in the epitopes associated with RF in different geographic areas as well as in the genes that encode M proteins, in particular the chromosomal *emm* sequence types that have been associated with GABHS pharyngitis and RF. Other properties of GABHS, such as production of serum opacity factor, differentiate strains associated with RF from those associated with glomerulonephritis. Patients who develop RF appear to manifest a hyperimmune response to GABHS, the level of which appears to correlate with the severity of RF manifestations. The decline in incidence of RF has paralleled the decrease in rheumatogenic M-protein strains isolated from the throats of children with pharyngitis, whereas conversely, the reappearance of RF in the United States has been associated with an increase in strains known to be rheumatogenic.[5] Unfortunately, strains that vary from those classically associated with rheumatogenicity continue to be isolated, confounding development of a widely applicable vaccine; there is evidence that GABHS may have evolved to prevent clearance by the immune system.

The risk for development of RF after GABHS pharyngitis is associated with genetic susceptibility and is also much higher in those with prior RF, in whom risk is as high as 50%. This provides a strong mandate for long-term secondary antibiotic prophylaxis. The evidence that hosts are genetically predisposed to RF is significant, with varying human leukocyte antigen (HLA) class II alleles and tumor necrosis factor-α as well as other genetic markers identified in populations known to be susceptible.[7] The issue of susceptibility is confounded by markers that either may reflect genetic susceptibility or may be expressed as a consequence of repeated exposure to group A streptococci.[8] In particular, a B-cell alloantigen, D8/17, appears to be both sensitive and specific in some endemic areas for screening of patients with RF as well as patients with prior RF in first-degree relatives.

Finally, environmental elements correlate strongly with development of RF. Where epidemic pharyngitis has been documented, such as in military barracks before antibiotic availability, approximately 3% developed RF. With the element of overcrowding removed, during the same period, the RF rate was approximately one tenth as common. It has been hypothesized that there is increased virulence associated with rapid transmission across multiple hosts.

Pathology

In patients dying of rheumatic carditis, autopsy examination has demonstrated verrucous vegetations on the valve leaflets, along with extensive inflammation and edema.[9] In the exudative phase, during the first few weeks after the onset of RF, fibrinoid degeneration of collagen is noted. Inflammation is seen in left ventricular (LV) endocardium, with lymphocytic, macrophage, and, in a minority of cases, plasma cell, polymorphonuclear leukocyte, eosinophil, and mast cell infiltration. In the proliferative phase, 1 to 6 months after the onset of RF, Aschoff bodies, granulomatous lesions pathognomonic for rheumatic carditis, are seen and can be found in valve tissue as well as in endocardium, myocardium, and pericardium. Although Aschoff bodies can be demonstrated as early as the second week of onset of RF, they may be present chronically without evidence of carditis. Rheumatic arthritis is manifested by edema, lymphocytic and polymorphonuclear infiltration, and fibrinoid lesions that resolve. In patients with chorea, inflammatory changes have been noted in the cerebral cortex, cerebellum, and basal ganglia.

Diagnosis

Jones Criteria (Fig. 88-2)

Before the initial 1944 Jones criteria, RF diagnosis was based on a wide, inconsistent range of nonspecific symptoms, including minor arthralgias, fevers, and abdominal pain. Because RF was a major cause of mortality, the criteria were designed to address the need for accurate diagnosis to allow assessment of disease incidence and treatment outcomes. Thus, specificity was emphasized over sensitivity, which remained the prevailing focus of multiple revisions. The major criteria—carditis, polyarthritis, chorea, erythema marginatum, and subcutaneous nodules—have been unchanged since the first revision in 1956. Minor criteria include the clinical findings of arthralgia and fever and elevated acute-phase reactants. Evidence of a prior group A streptococcal infection was incorporated in 1965 as an *essential* criterion. Although it is not specific for an acute attack of GABHS pharyngitis, the requirement adds to the overall specificity of the Jones criteria. The subsequent modifications continued to favor increased specificity by emphasizing arthritis over arthralgia and eliminated nonspecific elements from the minor criteria, such as epistaxis, abdominal and precordial pain, pulmonary findings, prolonged PR interval, anemia, and elevated white blood cell counts. The original revisions also emphasized evidence of prior RF, based on the much greater susceptibility for recurrence. With the 1992 revision, the guidelines placed emphasis on diagnosis of an *initial* attack of RF.

In the past decade, the focus has shifted to concerns that the criteria now lack sufficient sensitivity. The 2004 World Health Organization (WHO) report addressed the issue of recurrent RF, in particular for patients with established RHD, and suggested algorithms for increasing the overall sensitivity.[3] Whereas two major or one major and two minor manifestations plus evidence of preceding GABHS infection are required for a primary episode of RF or recurrent RF without established RHD, two minor criteria are deemed to be sufficient to make the diagnosis with reasonable specificity in the setting of RHD if there is evidence of recent streptococcal infection. There are two exceptions to the requirement that evidence for antecedent GABHS infection be established because laboratory evidence may be absent: chorea, in which there is a long latency period before symptoms occur; and the chronic low-grade carditis that follows many cases of RF.

The prior emphasis on specificity warned against the use of a single finding, such as fever, monarthritis, arthralgia, or elevation of the erythrocyte sedimentation rate or C-reactive protein level, to make the diagnosis of RF.[10] However, in countries where the disease is prevalent, laboratory data may not be available, the patient's presentation may be too late for some elements of the Jones criteria to be observed, and over-the-counter treatment with anti-inflammatory or antibiotic agents may obscure elements of the criteria. In this setting, clinical findings such as monarthritis or polyarthralgias are used by practitioners to make a diagnosis of "probable rheumatic fever" in vulnerable age groups when a number of minor manifestations are present, in particular if there is evidence of antecedent GABHS infection. The importance of such a controversial "probable" category is the suspicion raised for possible subsequent development of carditis, with the benefits of serial follow-up examinations and, in particular, the administration of chronic secondary antibiotic prophylaxis.

A number of clinical conditions mimic RF, including some associated with GABHS infections (**Table 88-1**).[11] Special considerations apply if a first attack of RF occurs in adulthood. In this setting, arthritis dominates, with a lower incidence of carditis; the other major manifestations are rare. Although the Jones criteria may be met, they become less specific, and other causes need to be excluded.

Carditis

Approximately 40% to 60% of RF episodes result in RHD,[4,11] with progression dependent on the severity of carditis, recurrences of RF, and availability of and compliance with secondary prophylaxis. Carditis typically is manifested as valvulitis, classically detected by the presence of mitral regurgitation (MR) or, less commonly, aortic regurgitation (AR). It can be responsible for acute and chronic myocardial dysfunction and acute, although not chronic, pericardial disease. Neither myocarditis nor pericarditis appears to occur in the absence of valvulitis, and if evidence of valvular involvement is not present, nonrheumatic causes must be considered. Whereas carditis typically is manifested in children as MR, with AR seen in approximately 20% to 40%, mitral stenosis is the most frequent clinically important valvular lesion in adults. Rheumatic tricuspid stenosis is less common and isolated rheumatic aortic stenosis is rare.

The severity of LV dysfunction appears to correlate with the extent of valvulitis rather than myocardial injury. A clinical syndrome suggesting rheumatic myocarditis is not associated with the troponin level elevation seen in viral myocarditides. When severe heart failure does occur in RF, both echocardiographic data and postmortem pathology findings point to altered myocardial mechanics caused by valvular regurgitation rather than by myocarditis. Traditionally, the diagnosis has been made on the basis of auscultation of MR or, less commonly, AR in the setting of heart failure, with cardiomegaly in the most severe cases. Severe MR is most commonly associated with the worst prognosis, acute and sometimes refractory and fatal heart failure.[12] This subgroup is most likely to develop significant chronic RHD, with an incidence as high as 90%. There is a linear relationship between the severity of MR during the first episode of RF and subsequent RHD.

Because valvulitis can be transient, serial evaluation is appropriate. In a significant percentage of patients, the carditis is subclinical,

TABLE 88-1 Differential Diagnosis of Rheumatic Arthritis, Carditis, and Chorea

Arthritis
- Infectious
  - Staphylococcal, gonococcal
  - Endocarditis
  - Lyme disease
  - Mycobacterial, fungal
  - Viral
- Reactive
  - Poststreptococcal
  - Enteric infection
  - Reiter syndrome
  - Inflammatory bowel
- Connective tissue disease
  - Rheumatoid arthritis
  - Systemic lupus
  - Systemic vasculitis
- Miscellaneous
  - Gout
  - Leukemia, lymphoma
  - Sarcoidosis
  - Cancer
  - Familial Mediterranean fever
  - Henoch-Schönlein purpura
  - Mucocutaneous disorders
  - "Growth pains" in children
  - Serum sickness

Carditis
- Murmur
  - Physiologic murmur
  - Mitral valve prolapse
  - Bicuspid aortic valve
  - Anemia
  - Straight back syndrome
- Congenital heart disease
  - Ventricular septal defect
  - Subvalvular aortic stenosis
  - Primum atrial septal defect
- Viral myocarditis
- Endocarditis
- Pericarditis

Chorea
- Familial chorea—Huntington
- Hormone induced
  - Oral contraceptives
  - Pregnancy
- Drug induced
  - Anticonvulsants
  - Antidepressants
  - Metoclopramide
  - Phenothiazines
- Connective tissue
  - Systemic lupus
  - Periarteritis
- Lyme disease
- Wilson disease
- Atypical seizures
- Hyperthyroidism
- Hypoparathyroidism
- Tourette syndrome
- PANDAS

PANDAS = ***p***ediatric ***a***utoimmune ***n***europsychiatric ***d***isorders ***a***ssociated with ***s***treptococcal infection.

Modified from Pinals RS: Polyarthritis and fever. N Engl J Med 330:769, 1994; Kothari SS: Active rheumatic carditis. *In* Narula J, Virman R, Srinath Reddy K, Tandon R (eds): Rheumatic Fever. Washington, DC, American Registry of Pathology, Armed Forces Institute of Pathology, 1999, p 265; and Swedo SE: Sydenham's chorea: A model for childhood autoimmune neuropsychiatric disorders. JAMA 272:1788, 1994.

setting the stage for scarring of the mitral or aortic valve apparatus with manifestations occurring years or decades later. Although valvulitis does account for the majority of myocardial dysfunction, there is a characteristic regional wall motion abnormality in the inferobasal segment adjacent to the mitral valve. The inflammatory process typically involves the leaflets and often extends into the submitral apparatus. Because pericarditis alone is not diagnostic of rheumatic carditis, detection of an associated valvular lesion is important. Pericardial involvement may result in effusion, but large effusions, chronic constriction, and tamponade are rare. Tachycardia and various arrhythmias are nonspecific. The use of endomyocardial biopsy or radionuclide tracers for detection of inflammation has not been of additional diagnostic benefit.

Recurrent episodes of RF result in a very high incidence of carditis. The diagnosis of recurrent or "mimetic" carditis has traditionally been based on new cardiac murmurs, pericarditis, and an increase in cardiac silhouette size. The greater environmental exposure to infections in a population already susceptible to RF makes exclusion of endocarditis in patients with fever and heart murmurs especially important, particularly when other major Jones criteria are absent.

Physical Examination. There are a number of hallmarks of acute carditis on physical examination during an initial episode of RF. There may be a prominent LV impulse secondary to cardiac enlargement but not as localized as with chronic MR. Because of recent onset, there is usually at most only mild LV dilation. Sinus tachycardia is common, but atrial fibrillation is rare. The first heart sound may vary in intensity from normal to diminished because of MR, prolonged PR interval, or both. The second heart sound is normally or widely or variably split, depending on degree of the MR. The pulmonary component of the second sound is accentuated with the presence of pulmonary hypertension in severe MR. Whereas the aortic second sound is classically diminished in chronic AR, it is usually normal in RF because mobility of the aortic valve is not affected early. A third heart sound is common, but not specific for severity of MR, because children frequently have an S_3 without associated disease.

The soft, blowing, high-pitched pansystolic murmur of MR is a hallmark of carditis in RF, best heard at the apex and selectively transmitted to the axilla and back; the latter suggests severe MR. A non-pansystolic murmur may occur when MR is mild, although it retains its high-frequency, soft, blowing character, distinguishing it from physiologic murmurs. The apical diastolic murmur of Carey Coombs is often related to the severity of MR but is also associated with flow disturbances caused by mitral valve deformity secondary to valvulitis, in addition to the increased flow in diastole. Unlike the late diastolic accentuation seen with mitral stenosis, this murmur is typically mid-diastolic. When the aortic valve is involved, there is an early decrescendo diastolic murmur best heard along the base and left sternal border. AR in the absence of MR is uncommon. A murmur of functional tricuspid regurgitation may occur in the setting of severe heart failure, pulmonary hypertension, and right ventricular dilation, with associated neck vein distention and other hallmarks of tricuspid insufficiency. It has been suggested that echocardiography may be helpful in settings such as concomitant pericarditis, in which auscultation may be difficult. However, MR is usually moderate or severe when pericarditis is secondary to RF and the murmur is often detectable, despite a friction rub, which may be intermittent.

Echocardiography. Increasing attention has been paid to echocardiography as a more sensitive tool than auscultation to detect carditis and RHD. Studies in developing countries have suggested that the increased sensitivity provided by ultrasound may be as high as 10-fold.[1] Defining echocardiographic Doppler findings that are specific for rheumatic valvulitis in the absence of auscultatable murmurs is a subject of controversy, as is the use of echocardiography alone to justify a diagnosis of carditis for this major Jones criterion.[10] MR is the most common echocardiographic finding. Mitral valve thickening or concomitant AR is seen with moderate frequency in the period after RF.[13] Several sets of echocardiographic criteria have been developed to differentiate pathologic from functional MR, including posterior direction, length and velocity of the mitral jet, holosystolic flow, significant turbulence, and MR seen in orthogonal planes. Consensus recommendations for diagnosis of MR secondary to RHD include a regurgitant jet >1 cm in length seen in at least two planes and a mosaic pattern with peak velocity >2.5 m/sec persistent throughout systole.[3] Specificity can be increased by the addition of morphologic valve features consistent with rheumatic deformities, such as valvular or subvalvular thickening or restricted leaflet mobility. Nodular lesions are seen in roughly 25%. Use of morphologic abnormalities consistent with RHD combined with concomitant regurgitation (without the Doppler features described before) results in up to a fourfold increase in sensitivity compared with use of Doppler criteria alone.[14]

Echocardiography is useful to confirm findings on auscultation, to exclude nonrheumatic causes, and to sequentially follow up valvular insufficiency, cardiac chamber size, pulmonary hypertension, valve thickening, and LV systolic function (see Chaps. 15 and 66). Importantly, in patients without clinical findings for carditis, an important minority of those with arthritis and, in particular, chorea manifest echocardiographic abnormalities. An additional argument for the routine use of echocardiography is a reduction in the false-positive rate. The latter is substantial when only auscultation and other clinical criteria are used for diagnosis of valvulitis.[1]

It has been argued that diagnosis of carditis on the basis of echocardiography without physical examination findings ("echocarditis") results in overdiagnosis. In particular, MR may be detected by echocardiography in other febrile illnesses. Longitudinal studies of such patients will shed light on the long-term implications of "silent carditis." There is modest evidence that these patients may have a milder course, but study design issues make this uncertain.[15] Whereas WHO consensus criteria do not accept echocardiographic findings alone for the major Jones criterion of carditis, the controversy has led some workers in endemic areas to establish independent criteria that do. The potential benefits of long-term antibiotic prophylaxis and serial cardiac evaluation in these patients need to be weighed against cost and logistics; relatively less expensive echocardiographic equipment may tip the balance.

Arthritis

Polyarthritis is the earliest and most frequent manifestation of RF, occurring in up to 75% of those with acute symptoms. It is typically migratory, very painful, and limited to the major joints of the arms and legs. Arthritis occurs within 2 to 3 weeks after onset of RF and is the only clinically apparent manifestation in one third to one half of patients. The arthritis is self-limited, with symptoms and findings varying from minor arthralgias to severe arthritis with erythema, warmth, and swelling. Joint aspiration may reveal moderate leukocytosis. Commonly, tenderness is out of proportion to other findings. During the migratory phase, multiple joints can be involved in different phases of inception and resolution. Inflammation in individual joints lasts 1 to 2 weeks, and the polyarthritis as a whole resolves in 1 month or less. Chronic sequelae and disability do not appear to occur, with the rare exception of Jaccoud arthropathy, an unusual periarticular fibrosis that is not specific for RF. The arthritis phase frequently overlaps the onset of carditis, and the two manifestations appear to be inversely related in severity—patients with severe arthritis appear to have less severe manifestations of carditis, and vice versa. Considerable debate has taken place over the differing patterns of joint manifestations in industrialized and developing countries and whether arthralgias or single-joint arthritis should be made a major criterion in areas where the diagnosis may otherwise be missed, largely because of late presentation. In general, because it resolves completely, the long-term importance of the arthritis of RF is that it draws attention to the presence of carditis, which may otherwise be missed in asymptomatic individuals.

A number of conditions resemble the migratory polyarthritis of RF (see Table 88-1). In general, failure to respond to salicylates suggests nonrheumatic etiology. If salicylates (or nonsteroidals) are given early, they may blunt the full appearance of the syndrome, resulting in monoarthritis. Other forms of infectious arthritis including Lyme disease, other autoimmune disorders, and acute leukemia can present with polyarthritis, ironically including a serum sickness syndrome induced by penicillin. Bacterial endocarditis with joint involvement is especially important to consider. Because the peak antistreptolysin O titer typically occurs at the same time as the onset of rheumatic arthritis, joint inflammation in the absence of an elevated antistreptolysin O titer is unlikely to be related to RF.

A major consideration in the differential diagnosis is poststreptococcal reactive arthritis (PSRA). It occurs early after streptococcal pharyngitis without other manifestations of RF, may affect the small joints of the upper extremities, is much less responsive to salicylates, and has longer duration. There is substantial commonality between RF and PSRA, including evidence of similar genetic susceptibility. A formula based on laboratory data, clinical course, and response to anti-inflammatory agents helps differentiate this entity from RF.[16] The consensus has been that these patients should be monitored for the development of RHD, and secondary prophylaxis is recommended for children. However, serial echocardiography in adults with PSRA has not demonstrated increased development of RHD compared with matched controls.[17]

Chorea

Sydenham chorea is manifested as involuntary irregular movements, fibrillation of the tongue, characteristic spooning with external rotation of the hands, and abolition of the movements with sleep. It occurs as the sole manifestation of RF in 20% of patients and in conjunction with arthritis in 30%. Concomitant subclinical carditis detected by echocardiography appears to be as high as 70%.[18] Chorea is a uniquely delayed manifestation of RF, with a wide range in reported incidence between 5% and 35%, latency of 1 to 7 months, and choreiform manifestations that may last for months and occasionally years. Importantly, there is a substantial risk of subsequent RHD in these patients, found in one study to be more than 50%.[19] Attention has focused on psychological manifestations of the disease, including short- and long-term emotional lability, obsessive-compulsive behavior, attention deficit/hyperactivity disorder, and other central nervous system manifestations such as seizures and chronic migraine. These too appear to be immunologically mediated, with evidence of antibodies to brain tissue. Although neurologic deficits typically resolve within 2 years, residual psychiatric disturbances occur in a small but significant number of patients in the subsequent decades. Recurrences are common. Because of the late manifestation of chorea, laboratory evidence of prior streptococcal infection is far less common than with carditis or arthritis. Thus, consideration of the differential diagnosis is particularly relevant; this includes epilepsy, connective tissue diseases, other choreas, primary psychiatric disorders, Lyme disease, and toxic reactions to various drugs including oral contraceptives. The diagnosis is made on clinical grounds, as neuroimaging has not been diagnostic. A syndrome of pediatric autoimmune neuropsychiatric disorders associated with streptococcal infections (PANDAS), in a fashion similar to poststreptococcal reactive arthritis, has a temporal relationship to GABHS infection but is not associated with other features of RF. Immunologic cross-reactivity between basal ganglia and GABHS epitopes has been hypothesized, but the evidence base is incomplete and the diagnostic and therapeutic management algorithms used for patients with Sydenham chorea, including secondary antibiotic prophylaxis, are not recommended.[2]

Cutaneous Manifestations

Both major cutaneous criteria of RF occur in less than 10% of cases, and neither is specific for RF. Subcutaneous nodules are usually seen concomitant with moderate to severe rheumatic carditis, occur several weeks after onset of cardiac findings, consist of firm nodules found over major joints and bone prominences, are asymptomatic and sometimes evanescent, and typically resolve within a few weeks to 2 months. They can be seen with other autoimmune disorders. Erythema marginatum typically also occurs in conjunction with carditis, with a milder course, but it may last for months or years. It tends to occur early in the course of RF and localizes over the trunk or proximal extremities. It resembles the cutaneous findings associated with juvenile rheumatoid arthritis and Lyme disease and is seen in settings that include sepsis and drug reactions.

Laboratory Findings

There is no specific laboratory test for RF. Erythrocyte sedimentation rate and C-reactive protein are reliable markers for the severity of the autoimmune response and inflammatory activity, and the time course generally correlates with activity of the disease, although masking may be induced by anti-inflammatory agents. Because of the late onset of chorea, the acute-phase reactants, like the anti-GABHS titers, are frequently no longer elevated at presentation. The electrocardiographic findings of RF include sinus arrhythmias, with tachycardia related to fever, pericarditis, or myocarditis; bradycardia occurs in a minority. First-degree but occasionally second- or third-degree AV block occurs in 30% or more of patients but is not specific for valvular involvement or carditis. Heart block is secondary to inflammation of peri–atrioventricular nodal tissues and possibly increased vagal tone; lesions in or around the His bundle have been demonstrated. There is no correlation with prognosis or subsequent valvular manifestations. The QT interval is frequently prolonged, and QT dispersion has been reported to correlate with acute rheumatic carditis. There have been rare episodes of torsades de pointes and sudden death.

In general, the most important test in the diagnostic algorithm relates to detection of GABHS.[2] A positive throat culture is of limited value because many individuals are carriers; conversely, a negative culture may be secondary to elimination of GABHS from the pharynx because of immune response or antibiotics. The rapid streptococcal antigen detection test (RADT) is highly specific but less sensitive. Immunoassays that are both sensitive and specific have not been widely adopted.

Because only a minority of pharyngitis is secondary to GABHS, and because GABHS is present in a significant number of patients in a carrier state, the decision to treat with antibiotics is ultimately based on the clinical manifestations of pharyngitis and perceived risk, including the age of the patient and prevalence of RF in the community. A clinical spectrum that suggests bacterial infection, including lymphadenopathy, fever, headache, severe throat symptoms, and tonsillar-pharyngeal swelling or exudate in the absence of viral upper respiratory symptoms, makes the clinical diagnosis relatively specific. The highest sensitivity and specificity and the least antibiotic overuse appear to be associated with treatment of patients with acute pharyngitis who have a positive RADT result or negative RADT result but positive subsequent throat culture. In adults, in regions where RF risk is low, empiric treatment without positive throat culture or RADT is generally unnecessary and associated with substantial overtreatment. In general, use of the formal criteria for diagnosis and treatment of GABHS pharyngitis has led to undertreatment in developing countries; the opposite is true in industrialized nations, where thousands need to be treated with antibiotics to prevent one case of RF.

Baseline antibody levels exhibit substantial age and geographic variability, with high levels during the peak ages of vulnerability to RF. In contrast, *rising* streptococcal antibody titers, including antistreptolysin O, anti-deoxyribonuclease B, antihyaluronidase, and streptozyme, are more specific although variably affected by non-GABHS infections. Up to 20% of patients developing RF may have negative antistreptolysin O titers. The time course of antibody level increase is within 1 month of onset of streptococcal pharyngitis and plateaus for 3 to 6 months, after which a decline is seen, with levels elevated from the patient's baseline that typically last 1 year or less. A variety of increasingly sophisticated laboratory tests, many not available in areas where RF is endemic, are specific for a host of other rheumatic disorders that can be differentiated from RF and its sequelae.

Treatment

The sine qua non of treatment is acute antimicrobial therapy to eliminate GABHS from the pharynx and subsequent continuous antibiotics for secondary prevention (**Table 88-2**). Primary prevention, with effective antibiotic treatment starting less than 10 days after the onset of pharyngitis, largely eliminates risk of RF and is the most cost-effective approach. Once the RF is manifested, the treatment algorithm varies, depending on manifestations of major criteria (**Fig. 88-3**). The course of RF covers a spectrum from mild, resolving without treatment, to severe and recurrent with consequent end-stage RHD. Long-term monitoring is warranted, even if symptoms resolve early, because approximately half of carditis patients develop RHD.[4,11] The first line of symptomatic therapy has traditionally been anti-inflammatory agents, ranging from salicylates to steroids, although the course of the disease is not influenced by anti-inflammatory therapy.[20] Evidence for bed rest is from the preantibiotic era, and many practitioners now treat RF patients on an outpatient basis, except for those presenting with carditis, for whom bed rest, at a minimum during the symptomatic stage, is empirically applied.

TABLE 88-2 Antibiotic Therapy for Acute Rheumatic Fever and Long-Term Prophylaxis

Initial Treatment of Group A Beta-Hemolytic Streptococcal Pharyngitis (Adult Dosages)					
ANTIBIOTIC	DOSE	FREQUENCY	DURATION	COMMENTS	CLASS
Benzathine penicillin G	1.2 million units IM	One time	Acutely only	↓ Compliance issues↑ Pain	I
Penicillin V	500 mg PO	Twice daily	10 days		I
Amoxicillin	1000 mg PO	Daily	10 days		I
Penicillin Allergic					
Narrow-spectrum cephalosporins*	Varies by drug	Varies by drug	10 days	Avoid if history of anaphylaxis secondary to penicillin	I
Clindamycin*,†	300 mg PO	Twice daily	10 days		IIa
Azithromycin*,‡	500 mg PO day 1 250 mg PO days 2-5	Daily	5 days		IIa
Clarithromycin*,‡	250 mg PO	Twice daily	10 days		IIa
Secondary Prophylaxis Regimen for Patients with Documented RF (Adult Dosages)§					
ANTIBIOTIC	DOSE	FREQUENCY		COMMENTS	CLASS
Benzathine penicillin G	1.2 million units IM	Every 3 to 4 weeks¶		↓ Compliance issues ↑ Pain	I
Penicillin V	250 mg PO	Twice daily			I
Erythromycin*,‡	250 mg PO	Twice daily			I
Sulfadiazine*	1 g PO	Daily			I
Sulfisoxazole*	1 g PO	Daily			IIa

*Alternative for penicillin-allergic patients. Erythromycin for secondary prophylaxis is an alternative for patients allergic to both penicillin and sulfa.

†Dosage is empiric. For severe pharyngitis, doses up to 1.2 g daily in two to four divided doses.

‡Some areas have a high rate of macrolide-resistant group A streptococci. In addition, erythromycin toxicity, including gastrointestinal intolerance and long-QT syndrome, limits its use.

§Duration of therapy ranges from 5 years to life-long (see text). For patients with poststreptococcal reactive arthritis, recommended duration is 1 year in nonendemic areas, 5 years where RF is prevalent if no evidence of carditis appears.

¶In endemic areas, benzathine penicillin every 3 weeks should be considered to maintain optimal drug levels (Class I indication). In nonendemic areas, benzathine penicillin is given every 3 weeks if RF recurs on the regimen of every 4 weeks (Class I).

Modified from Gerber MA, Baltimore RS, Eaton CB, et al: Prevention of rheumatic fever and diagnosis and treatment of acute streptococcal pharyngitis. A scientific statement from the American Heart Association Rheumatic Fever, Endocarditis, and Kawasaki Disease Committee. Circulation 119:1541, 2009; and Rheumatic fever and rheumatic heart disease. World Health Organ Tech Rep Ser 923:1, 2004.

Prevention Strategies

PRIMARY PREVENTION. Effective eradication of GABHS from the pharynx defines the role of primary prevention. Patients with apparent bacterial pharyngitis and positive test results for GABHS should be treated as early as possible in the suppurative phase. The differential diagnosis, in addition to viral infection, includes non-GABHS and gonococcal pharyngitis. Penicillin is uniformly effective for GABHS if it is taken orally for a full 10-day course or if intramuscular benzathine penicillin is administered because penicillin-resistant GABHS has not been demonstrated. The particular advantage of intramuscular benzathine penicillin G is that it avoids compliance issues. Oral cephalosporins, indicated for penicillin-allergic patients, have been used in shorter than 10-day courses with high compliance, with bacterial elimination and clinical response that may be superior to penicillin treatment, but the evidence base is insufficient to recommend this regimen for treatment in endemic areas. Aggressive antibiotic therapy for primary prevention is essential in areas where RF is prevalent and may represent the best hope for decreasing the overall health care burden of RHD.[21] In contrast, in populations where RF is rare, antibiotic use results in modest therapeutic benefit, and the risk-to-benefit ratio has been called into question.

SECONDARY PREVENTION. The method of choice for prevention of RF recurrence is continuous administration of benzathine penicillin G every 4 weeks. Because of low penicillin levels during the fourth week, 3-week intervals should be considered in endemic areas or for patients at high risk. Those with documented RF should have continuous secondary prevention as soon as the primary GABHS treatment regimen has been completed. An oral regimen should be reserved primarily for patients deemed to be at low risk for recurrent RF or those allergic to penicillin or otherwise intolerant of intramuscular therapy. The duration of therapy depends on the patient's age, known RHD, time since last episode of RF, number of episodes, family history, occupational exposure, and environmental factors, such as living in endemic areas.[3] The Class I recommendations are 5 years or until the age of 21 years (whichever is longer) in the absence of carditis, 10 years or until the age of 21 years for patients with mild or apparently healed carditis, and 10 years or until the age of 40 years for patients who develop RHD.[2] Patients at high risk for repeated episodes of RF, such as those at significant risk of recurrent exposure to GABHS infection, should be considered for life-long antibiotic prophylaxis. Confounding factors have been reluctance of rural practitioners to administer parenteral antibiotics for fear of allergic reactions and, for similar reasons, regulations prohibiting parenteral administration in hospitals in some developing countries. The actual risk of anaphylaxis, estimated to be 0.2%, is less in children younger than 12 years.

Therapeutic Modalities

CARDITIS. Salicylates and nonsteroidals have no specific role in rheumatic carditis, with the exception of treatment of concomitant pericarditis. Acute carditis has generally been treated with steroids even though a meta-analysis of eight randomized controlled trials failed to demonstrate superiority of steroids, immunoglobulins, or salicylates over placebo in the progression of RHD.[20] Nevertheless, in the setting of severe, potentially life-threatening heart failure, steroid administration is widespread. Withdrawal of steroids or salicylates can result in rebound or relapse. Treatment of cardiac manifestations otherwise follows established guidelines, including management of congestive heart failure and severe valvular regurgitation, although special attention should be paid to use of digitalis because these patients are sensitive to development of heart block.

Unless valvular regurgitation and severe congestive heart failure are refractory to drug therapy, valve surgery is avoided whenever possible during RF. Surgical morbidity and mortality have been significant, and failed repair leading to valve replacement has been frequent. However, when surgery is necessary, LV function generally improves significantly, consistent with valve regurgitation rather than myocardial dysfunction being the primary mechanism leading to heart failure.

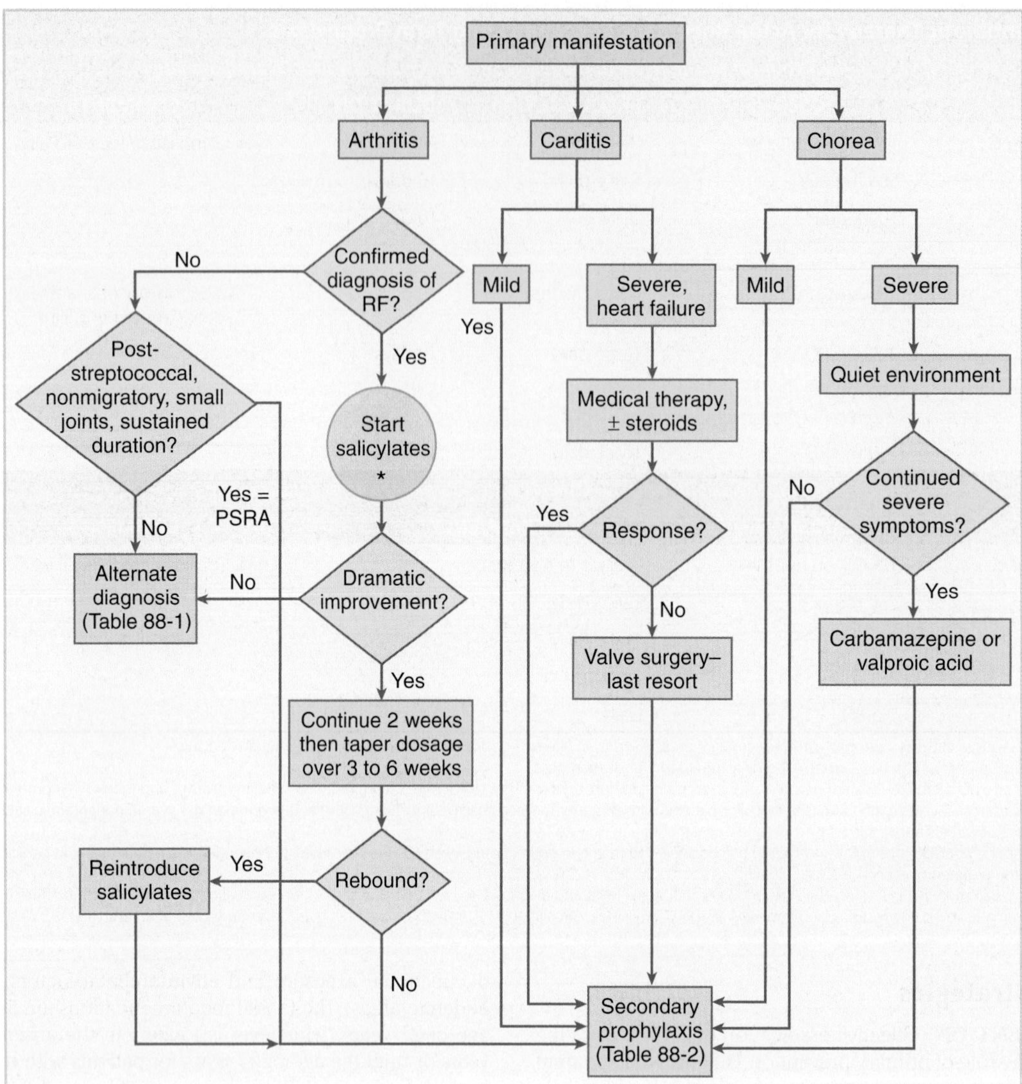

FIGURE 88-3 Algorithm for management of rheumatic fever and its primary manifestations. *Salicylates are also indicated for fever and arthralgia, but there is no evidence of effectiveness for carditis or chorea. PSRA = poststreptococcal reactive arthritis; RF = rheumatic fever. *(Modified from Thatai D, Turi ZG: Current guidelines for the treatment of patients with rheumatic fever. Drugs 57:545, 1999.)*

Arthritis. Salicylates are the first line of therapy for migratory polyarthritis because of their highly effective analgesic, anti-inflammatory, and antipyretic properties. Nonsteroidals are effective alternatives. Aspirin (up to 100 mg/kg/day in four or more divided doses) is both therapeutic and diagnostic; failure of the pain to resolve within 24 hours suggests alternative causes of arthritis. Although salicylate levels can be followed (15 to 30 mg/dL is the therapeutic range), these data are usually not available in endemic areas; instead, patients are monitored for tinnitus and gastrointestinal toxicity. Early administration does have the potential to mask the evolving clinical picture (e.g., arthritis when medication is given for arthralgias). Steroids are typically not used because they offer no therapeutic advantage and may mask the presence of other illnesses causing arthritis, such as lupus, or exacerbate other causes, such as infectious arthritis.

Chorea. Traditional treatment has included sedation and empiric use of antiseizure or antipsychotic medications. Small series have studied corticosteroids, along with plasmapheresis and intravenous immunoglobulins, to assess their influence on the severity and time course of symptoms. The duration of symptoms does appear to be shortened with treatment. However, the evidence base is not conclusive, some of the interventions are potentially toxic, and, pending larger studies, a conservative approach to a largely self-limited disorder has been deemed appropriate. For patients with refractory symptoms, there is modest evidence favoring use of carbamazepine or valproic acid. Because of the high incidence of carditis,[18] whether clinical or subclinical, and potential progression to RHD, these patients require long-term antibiotic therapy.

Future Directions

A universal streptococcal vaccine has been elusive, partly because of the number and variability of antigenic stimulants, making the use of a vaccine that identifies specific epitopes ineffective. A simple and inexpensive screening test for identification of patients and populations genetically susceptible to RF has not been developed, nor is there a readily available, universally applicable, and inexpensive screening test for GABHS antibodies. Given the relatively modest cost of secondary prophylaxis and the prohibitive expense associated with RHD in developing countries where RF remains endemic, systematic longitudinal studies of more sensitive diagnostic tools, in particular portable echocardiography, have been an important research focus in the past decade.[1] RF still receives <0.4% of research funds aimed at the so-called neglected diseases. Competition for limited health care resources, with a growing prevalence of ischemic heart disease in developing countries (see Chap. 1), has limited the financing of potentially highly cost-effective preventive health care programs.

REFERENCES

Epidemiology

1. Marijon E, Ou P, Celermajer DS, et al: Prevalence of rheumatic heart disease detected by echocardiographic screening. N Engl J Med 357:470, 2007.

2. Gerber MA, Baltimore RS, Eaton CB, et al: Prevention of rheumatic fever and diagnosis and treatment of acute Streptococcal pharyngitis: A scientific statement from the American Heart Association Rheumatic Fever, Endocarditis, and Kawasaki Disease Committee. Circulation 119:1541, 2009.
3. Rheumatic fever and rheumatic heart disease. World Health Organ Tech Rep Ser 923:1, 2004.
4. Carapetis JR, Steer AC, Mulholland EK, et al: The global burden of group A streptococcal diseases. Lancet Infect Dis 5:685, 2005.
5. Shulman ST, Stollerman G, Beall B, et al: Temporal changes in streptococcal M protein types and the near-disappearance of acute rheumatic fever in the United States. Clin Infect Dis 42:441, 2006.

Pathobiology and Pathology

6. Martins TB, Veasy LG, Hill HR: Antibody responses to group A streptococcal infections in acute rheumatic fever. Pediatr Infect Dis J 25:832, 2006.
7. Guilherme L, Kalil J: Rheumatic fever: From innate to acquired immune response. Ann N Y Acad Sci 1107:426, 2007.
8. Bryant PA, Robins-Browne R, Carapetis JR, et al: Some of the people, some of the time: Susceptibility to acute rheumatic fever. Circulation 119:742, 2009.
9. Virmani R, Farb A, Burke AP, Narula J: Pathology of acute rheumatic carditis. *In* Narula J, Virmani R, Reddy KS, Tandon R (eds): Rheumatic Fever. Washington, DC, American Registry of Pathology, 1999, pp 217-234.

Diagnosis

10. Ferrieri P: Proceedings of the Jones Criteria workshop. Circulation 106:2521, 2002.
11. Lee JL, Naguwa SM, Cheema GS, et al: Acute rheumatic fever and its consequences: A persistent threat to developing nations in the 21st century. Autoimmun Rev 9:117, 2009.
12. Kamblock J, N'Guyen L, Pagis B, et al: Acute severe mitral regurgitation during first attacks of rheumatic fever: Clinical spectrum, mechanisms and prognostic factors. J Heart Valve Dis 14:440, 2005.
13. Caldas AM, Terreri MT, Moises VA, et al: The case for utilizing more strict quantitative Doppler echocardiographic criterions for diagnosis of subclinical rheumatic carditis. Cardiol Young 17:42, 2007.
14. Marijon E, Celermajer DS, Tafflet M, et al: Rheumatic heart disease screening by echocardiography: The inadequacy of World Health Organization criteria for optimizing the diagnosis of subclinical disease. Circulation 120:663, 2009.
15. Tubridy-Clark M, Carapetis JR: Subclinical carditis in rheumatic fever: A systematic review. Int J Cardiol 119:54, 2007.
16. Barash J, Mashiach E, Navon-Elkan P, et al: Differentiation of post-streptococcal reactive arthritis from acute rheumatic fever. J Pediatr 153:696, 2008.
17. van Bemmel JM, Delgado V, Holman ER, et al: No increased risk of valvular heart disease in adult poststreptococcal reactive arthritis. Arthritis Rheum 60:987, 2009.
18. Demiroren K, Yavuz H, Cam L, et al: Sydenham's chorea: A clinical follow-up of 65 patients. J Child Neurol 22:550, 2007.
19. Carapetis JR, McDonald M, Wilson NJ: Acute rheumatic fever. Lancet 366:155, 2005.

Treatment

20. Cilliers AM, Manyemba J, Saloojee H: Anti-inflammatory treatment for carditis in acute rheumatic fever. Cochrane Database Syst Rev (2):CD003176, 2003.
21. Karthikeyan G, Mayosi BM: Is primary prevention of rheumatic fever the missing link in the control of rheumatic heart disease in Africa? Circulation 120:709, 2009.

CHAPTER 89 Rheumatic Diseases and the Cardiovascular System

Alexandra Villa-Forte and Brian F. Mandell

Systemic rheumatologic disorders may involve the cardiovascular system directly or indirectly. Patients often seek medical attention because of constitutional symptoms, musculoskeletal pain, fever, peripheral or visceral ischemia, or organ failure without apparent involvement of the cardiovascular system. Involvement of the heart and vessels can range from clinically silent to catastrophic. Alternatively, the cardiovascular specialist may first recognize that cardiovascular symptoms may have a primary immunologic basis. Examples include patients who present with claudication, ischemic heart disease, or aortic aneurysms caused by arteritis, and patients with systemic lupus erythematosus (SLE) who develop acute myocarditis, pericarditis, or valvular dysfunction. Patients with several systemic inflammatory diseases have a documented elevated risk for coronary and cerebrovascular events in the absence of excessive traditional cardiovascular risk factors.

Vasculitis

Discrimination among the various forms of vasculitis begins with the concept of primary (immune dysregulation, without a known trigger) versus secondary. Secondary vasculitis is associated with another condition (e.g., drug allergy, viral hepatitis, bacterial endocarditis) or with rheumatic disease. Secondary vasculitis requires treatment of the underlying disease or removal of the causative agent. Misclassification could lead to inappropriate use of immunosuppressive therapy, with adverse or lethal consequences. Examples include vasculitis secondary to sepsis, particularly endocarditis, drug toxicity, and poisonings, malignancies, cardiac myxomas, and multifocal emboli from large-vessel aneurysms (**Table 89-1**). These conditions can mimic vasculitis or cause multifocal ischemia or infarction, with accompanying vasculitis.

The greatest certainty in the diagnosis of primary vasculitis is in the setting of classic clinical and laboratory patterns with supportive histopathology—for example, a 70-year-old woman with new-onset severe headache, temporal region pain, hip and shoulder girdle stiffness, visual aberration (amaurosis or blindness), and a high erythrocyte sedimentation rate (ESR). This picture would be so compatible with giant cell arteritis that empiric therapy could be started without biopsy evidence of the diagnosis, but a positive biopsy would remove any doubt and would be useful if the response to steroids is delayed. Unfortunately, many patients with vasculitis do not present with such recognizable features. Instead, one may have to depend on combinations of less typical clues. A patient with ischemic digits, active urinary sediment, and peripheral neuropathy is likely to have vasculitis, especially if mimics have already been ruled out. The presence of a purpuric rash, particularly if it is palpable (**Fig. 89-1**), furthers the probability of a small-vessel vasculitis but will not exclude a secondary cause, such as a malignancy or hepatitis C–associated vasculitis.

Approach to Proving the Diagnosis of Vasculitis

Definitive diagnosis depends on documenting lesions in affected tissue. The greatest success in achieving a tissue diagnosis comes from a biopsy of abnormal or symptomatic sites. In patients with proven vasculitis, the yield from biopsies of clinically normal sites (i.e., blind biopsy) is considerably less than 20%. Therefore, a biopsy of apparently normal tissue is not recommended. Biopsies of abnormal organs provide diagnostically useful information in about 65% of cases. Needle biopsies are small and often do not contain affected tissue; uniform involvement of vessels in affected viscera is uncommon.

A biopsy may not be practical in certain circumstances, such as systemic illness with symptoms of intestinal ischemia, carotidynia, or findings of unequal pulses or blood pressures. Because biopsy of large vessels is usually impractical, angiography may be helpful. In this setting, vascular stenoses and/or aneurysms that cannot be explained by atherosclerosis or infection may provide sufficient circumstantial evidence to proceed with treatment for primary vasculitis.

Forms of Vasculitis Relevant to Cardiologists and Cardiovascular Surgeons

TAKAYASU ARTERITIS

Takayasu arteritis (TA) is an idiopathic large-vessel vasculitis of young adults that affects the aorta and its major branches.

EPIDEMIOLOGY. Women are affected about 10 times more often than men. The median age at onset is 25 years. Best known in Asia, TA can occur worldwide and can affect individuals of all races and ethnicities. The prevalence of TA is estimated as 2.6/1,000,000 persons in the United States and 1.26/1,000,000 in northern Europe.[1] An autopsy series from Japan noted features of TA in 1 in every 3000 autopsies.[2]

PATHOGENESIS. The cause of TA is unknown. Acute lesions contain mononuclear cell infiltrates that appear to have entered the vessel wall through the vasa vasorum and subsequently migrate to the arterial intima. These cells are predominantly macrophages and T cells (gamma-delta, cytotoxic, and natural killer). The presence of various cytokines, including interleukin-6 (IL-6) and tumor necrosis factor (TNF) in these granulomatous lesions has prompted various therapeutic approaches using cytokine-targeted biologic agents.[3]

TABLE 89-1 Diseases That Can Mimic Primary Systemic Vasculitis

Sepsis, especially endocarditis
Drug toxicity, poisoning
  Cocaine
  Amphetamines
  Ephedra
  Phenylpropanolamine
Coagulopathy
  Anticardiolipin antibody syndrome
  Disseminated intravascular coagulation
Malignancy (solid organ or liquid tumors)
Cardiac myxoma
Multifocal emboli from large-vessel aneurysms (cholesterol, mycotic)
Ehlers-Danlos syndrome (vascular ectatic type)
Fibromuscular dysplasia

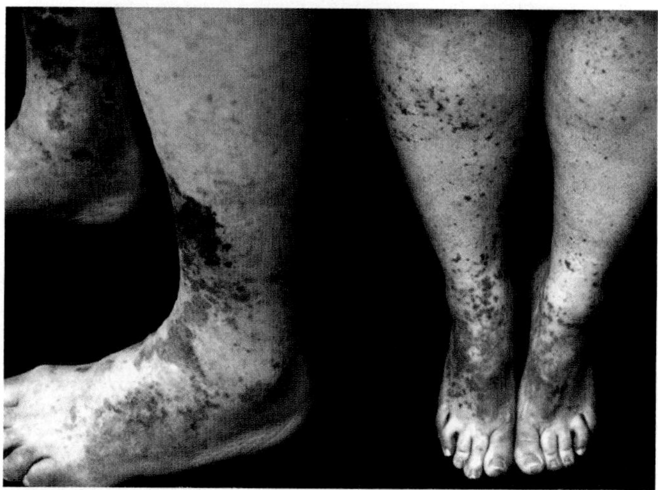

FIGURE 89-1 Palpable purpura. Vascular inflammation at the level of capillaries and venules leads to exudation of formed elements and the color and texture of lesions noted in these patients. The person on the right is a young woman with Henoch-Schönlein vasculitis or purpura (HSP). The older man on the left has a similar lesion, but in this case, it was associated with hepatitis C, acquired in the course of transfusions for heart surgery. HCV infection led to cryoglobulinemia and secondary vasculitis. The treatment for each patient is different. The patient with HSP, who does not have extracutaneous disease, only requires reassurance and monitoring for her usually self-limiting problem, whereas the patient with HCV and vasculitis requires antiviral therapy.

CLINICAL FEATURES. In TA, arterial stenoses occur three to four times more often than aneurysms. Claudication (>60% upper versus 30% lower extremities) is the most common complaint and bruits (approximately 80%), blood pressure, or pulse asymmetries (60 to 80%) are the most common findings. Aneurysms are most common and clinically most significant in the aortic root, where they can lead to valvular regurgitation (**Fig. 89-2A**, left; see Fig. 89-2B). Hypertension results most often from renal artery stenosis, but can also be associated with suprarenal aortic stenosis or a chronically damaged, rigid aorta. Cardiac, renal, and central nervous system (CNS) vascular complications cause most severe morbidity and mortality. Estimates of mortality range from a low of approximately 3% to approximately 35% at 5-year follow-up.[1,4]

Symptoms of claudication, Raynaud phenomenon, ischemia, or the finding of hypertension, especially in young patients, necessitate examination for asymmetry of extremity pulses, blood pressure, and bruits. Increasing extremity or visceral ischemia, malaise, myalgias, arthralgias, night sweats, and fever may indicate active disease. Occurrence of such symptoms in the setting of an elevated ESR indicates active disease. Many patients still experience progressive disease[1,4] but do not have any constitutional or new vascular symptoms, and as many as 50% may have normal ESRs. Active disease in these patients is suggested by the following:

1. New vascular abnormalities on sequential angiographic studies despite suspected remission.
2. Presence of inflammatory changes in bypass biopsy specimens from patients in whom surgery was performed because of critical flow abnormalities in the setting of clinically quiescent disease.[1,4]

Determining disease activity in TA is a major challenge because of poor correlation among clinical, laboratory, radiologic, and histologic data. Studies using refinements in magnetic resonance imaging (MRI)[5] may enable the clinician to detect qualitative abnormalities in the vessel wall that imply inflammatory change. ^{18}F-fluorodeoxyglucose–positron emission tomography (FDG-PET) has been evaluated in the assessment of disease activity; preliminary results were encouraging, showing high sensitivity and specificity for the presence of inflammation.[6] However, the clinical usefulness of this test remains uncertain, and its correlation with disease activity has been questioned.[7] The value of FDG-PET may be limited by the presence of atherosclerotic disease and other conditions that could lead to false-positive results. Prospective studies with large numbers of patients to define the operating characteristics of PET clearly are necessary.

Cardiac sequelae of TA result more often from aortic regurgitation and inadequately treated hypertension than from arteritis affecting the coronary vessels.[1,4] Indirect evidence from echocardiography suggests that left ventricular systolic dysfunction caused by myocarditis may affect approximately 18% of patients.[8] When coronary artery vasculitis is detected (less than 5%), it is most frequent in the ostial regions. More distal involvement may also occur, and both types of lesions may affect the same patient. These observations underscore the importance of considering vasculitis in the differential diagnosis of young patients with ischemic symptoms.

DIFFERENTIAL DIAGNOSIS. Certain congenital diseases cause abnormalities of arterial extracellular matrix and aortic regurgitation (e.g., Marfan syndrome, Ehlers-Danlos syndrome). However, these conditions do not cause stenotic lesions in large vessels, the most common feature of TA. Inborn genetic errors that affect arterial matrix do not cause systemic symptoms, abnormal acute-phase reactants, anemia, or thrombocytosis, which may accompany large-vessel vasculitis. The young female predominance of TA distinguishes it from patients with typical atherosclerosis, a disease much more likely to affect the lower extremity large vessels than the arms, and the abdominal aorta more than the aortic root. Infectious causes of large-vessel aneurysms (e.g., bacterial, syphilitic, mycobacterial, fungal) must be considered in both sexes and all age groups, but are not usually associated with vascular stenoses affecting the arch vessels. Other autoimmune diseases may be complicated by large-vessel vasculitis, but they are discerned by their associated characteristics (e.g., SLE, Cogan syndrome, Behçet disease, spondyloarthropathies) and age predilections (e.g., Kawasaki disease in younger individuals or giant-cell arteritis in older adults). Sarcoidosis can closely mimic TA. Making the correct diagnosis depends on finding other characteristic features of sarcoidosis (e.g., proliferative synovitis, skin lesions, Bell's palsy, adenopathy). There are no specific diagnostic tests for TA. The diagnosis depends on clinical features in conjunction with vascular imaging abnormalities. In patients who undergo vascular surgery, histopathologic abnormalities may support the diagnosis, but the surgeon must recognize the need to send tissue for this purpose.

TREATMENT. Almost all patients with TA improve when treated with high doses of a corticosteroid (e.g., prednisone, 1 mg/kg/day); relapses are common with tapering of corticosteroid therapy. Corticosteroid-resistant or relapsing patients may respond to the addition to daily therapy of cyclophosphamide (approximately 2 mg/kg) or weekly therapy with methotrexate (approximately 20 mg).[1,4,9] Approximately 40% of patients who receive a cytotoxic agent and corticosteroids will achieve remission but, over time, about half these patients will also relapse, leading to the need for chronic immunosuppressive therapy

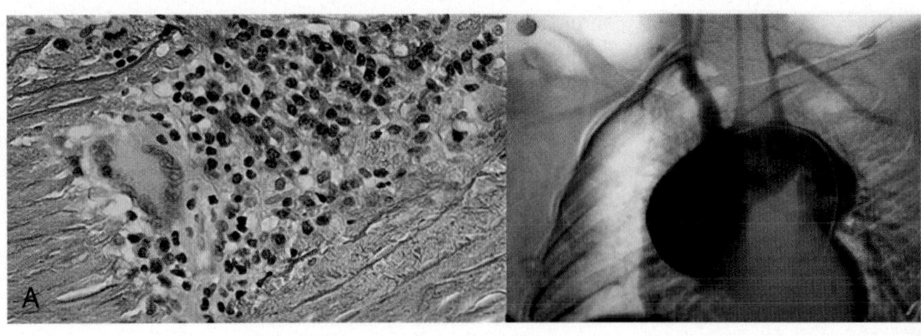

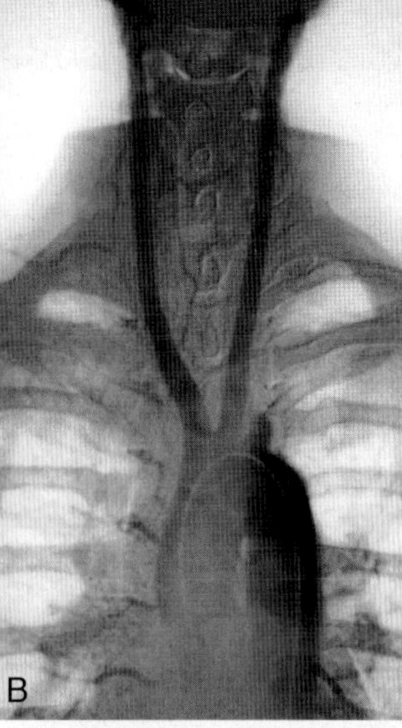

FIGURE 89-2 Takayasu disease. **A,** Takayasu arteritis. Granulomatous inflammation and medial destruction (left) has led to marked aortic root dilation (right) in a 17-year-old female high school student who developed symptoms of congestive heart failure and exertional angina. She also had diffuse narrowing of the left common carotid artery and irregular dilation of the innominate artery. (Hematoxylin-eosin stain; magnification ×40.) **B,** Occlusion of both subclavian arteries led to leg pressures being the only reliable measure of central aortic pressure.

in many patients. Such unsatisfactory results have led to ongoing studies that seek to take advantage of new insights into pathogenesis. Preliminary studies have shown that treatment designed to block TNF may dramatically improve most patients (14 of 15) with TA who have relapsed during tapering of steroid therapy.[10,11]

A discussion of pharmacologic therapy for TA only addresses one important aspect of care. Other important issues include treatment of the anatomic effects of vascular lesions; fibrotic stenosis and thrombosed vessels will not respond to corticosteroids. Patients with TA may have signs of clinical deterioration caused by fixed critical stenoses or aneurysms. Hypertension affects approximately 40% to 90% of patients.[1,4] In Asia, India, and Mexico, TA is one of the most common causes of hypertension in adolescents and young adults. One of the most common traps in clinical management relates to not knowing whether blood pressure recordings in an extremity represent aortic root pressure. Because more than 90% of patients have stenotic lesions, and the most common site of stenosis is the subclavian and innominate arteries, blood pressure in one or both arms may underestimate pressure in the aorta. Elevated aortic root pressure, when unrecognized and untreated, enhances the risks of hypertensive complications. Intravascular pressure recordings during angiographic procedures can address this issue. The importance of knowing the distribution and severity of all vascular lesions cannot be overemphasized. In the setting of renal insufficiency, the potential of contrast agents to cause further renal impairment may limit exploring the extent of all potential vascular lesions. However, in the absence of contraindications, patients should have the entire aorta and its primary branches included in vascular imaging studies. MR angiography does not affect the opportunity to measure intravascular pressures, but may suffice to delineate vascular lesions without resorting to catheter-guided angiography.

Whenever feasible, anatomic correction of clinically significant lesions should be considered, especially in the setting of renal artery stenosis and hypertension. In about 20% of patients, aortic root involvement may lead to valvular insufficiency, angina, and congestive heart failure (see Fig. 89-2).[1,4] Severe or progressive changes may require aortic surgery, with or without valve replacement. Because of the high prevalence of subclavian and carotid stenoses in TA, severe symptomatic stenoses of these vessels should be treated by grafts that originate from the aortic root and not from an arch vessel to another arch vessel. The latter may be followed by loss of the graft because of new stenosis in an initially spared subclavian or carotid artery. Conversely, a graft from the ascending aorta is a safer long-term conduit because the ascending aorta in TA essentially never becomes stenotic. Mesenteric and celiac artery stenoses are usually asymptomatic and only rarely require surgery. Angioplasty and intravascular stents have met with restenosis far more often than bypass, which is preferred whenever feasible. It is always best to operate on patients who are in remission; however, judgment of disease activity in TA may be difficult. Consequently, all bypass surgeries should include vascular biopsy specimens for histopathologic evaluation. Findings from surgical specimens may help guide the need for postoperative immunosuppressive treatment. Even high-flow grafts can occlude spontaneously soon after surgery, often for unclear reasons.

The care of patients with TA requires a team approach that includes clinicians familiar with the proper use of immunosuppressive therapies, vascular imaging and intervention specialists and, in the setting of critical stenoses or aneurysms, cardiovascular surgeons. For most patients, medical and surgical therapies provide important palliation.

GIANT CELL ARTERITIS OF OLDER ADULTS

Giant cell arteritis (GCA) and Takayasu arteritis are the principal diseases associated with sterile granulomatous inflammation of large and medium-sized vessels.

EPIDEMIOLOGY. In the United States, GCA affects approximately 18/100,000 population older than 50 years of age (mean, 74 years of age). GCA is more common in northern latitudes. In Iceland and Denmark, the prevalence is 27 and 21/100,000, respectively, in the group older than 50 years of age. Although females predominate (2 to 3:1), this sex difference is less striking than in TA (6 to 10:1). The demographic characteristics of GCA are the same as for patients with polymyalgia rheumatica (PMR), and 30% to 50% of patients with GCA concurrently have features of PMR.[12]

PATHOGENESIS. The cause of GCA remains unknown; the inflammatory lesion begins in the adventitia. The vasa vasorum furnish the conduit for the mononuclear cells (dendritic cells, macrophages, and Th1-type lymphocytes) that mediate vascular injury. Dendritic cells participate in the process by presenting to lymphocytes the putative antigen that is believed to promote the development of GCA. The finding of clonality of approximately 4% of T lymphocytes without clonality of peripheral blood lymphocytes in the vessel wall supports this conjecture. Vascular lesions initially overexpress proinflammatory cytokines such as IL-1, IL-6, TNF, and interferon-γ (IFN-γ). Intermediate

TABLE 89-2 Clinical Profile of Giant Cell Arteritis

ABNORMALITY	FREQUENCY (%)
Atypical headache	60-90
Tender temporal artery	40-70
Systemic symptoms not attributable to other diseases	20-50
Fever	20-50
Polymyalgia rheumatica	30-50
Acute visual abnormalities	12-40
Transient ischemic attack or stroke	5-10
Claudication	
Jaw	30-70
Extremity	5-15
Aortic aneurysm	15-20
Dramatic response to corticosteroid therapy	~100
Positive temporal artery biopsy	~50-80

lesions harbor mediators of matrix destruction (e.g., metalloproteinases, reactive oxygen and nitrogen species). In later stages, growth factors such as platelet-derived growth factor (PDGF) and fibroblast growth factor (FGF) participate in stimulating myointimal proliferation, leading to vessel stenosis.

CLINICAL FEATURES. The most characteristic features of GCA are new onset of atypical and often severe headaches, scalp and temporal artery tenderness, acute visual loss, polymyalgia rheumatica, and pain in the muscles of mastication (**Table 89-2**). Concurrence of such abnormalities with an increase in the ESR supports a clinical diagnosis of GCA and mandates treatment, even without proof of diagnosis from a temporal artery biopsy. The diagnosis is doubtful if dramatic improvement does not occur within 24 to 72 hours. The yield of positive temporal artery biopsies in patients clinically diagnosed with GCA is about 50% to 80%, depending on the clinical pattern of disease. Patients with a high ESR who have presented to an ophthalmologist with symptoms of new-onset atypical headache and visual loss are more likely to have a positive biopsy than patients who present with symptoms of vague limb girdle pain, chronic headache, and malaise, or patients with predominant aortitis.

GCA may produce clinically apparent aortitis in at least 15% of cases and involve the primary branches of the aorta, especially the subclavian arteries, in a similar number of individuals.[12,13] Postmortem studies have suggested that large-vessel involvement is far more common than clinically appreciated. Consequently, some patients with GCA may present with features that resemble those of TA. Among older adults with inflammatory large-vessel disease, the same considerations and precautions must be applied in GCA as in patients with TA—the need to identify an extremity that provides a reliable blood pressure equivalent to aortic root pressure and follow-up to include careful observation for new bruits, pulse, and blood pressure asymmetry. Patients with GCA are more than 17 times more likely than age-matched controls to have thoracic aortic aneurysms, and about 2.5 times more likely than age-matched controls to have abdominal aortic aneurysms. Half of patients with thoracic aortic aneurysms die as a result of those lesions. Because aneurysms were found in the course of routine care or at postmortem, these may be conservative estimates. The finding of large-vessel disease, including aortic aneurysms, in older adults with GCA should not be assumed to be caused by atherosclerosis. It is not surprising that about half of patients with GCA have objective features of cardiac disease. Myocardial infarction (MI) caused by GCA is rare or rarely appreciated; histopathologic findings in coronary arteries are infrequently sought in the group of patients whose mean age is 74 years.

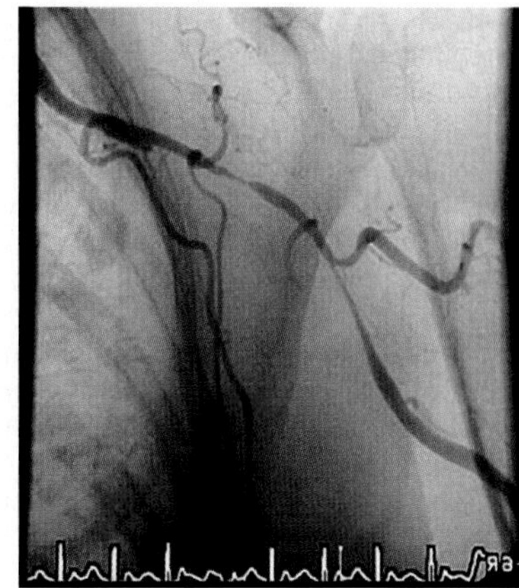

FIGURE 89-3 Giant cell arteritis. Here, Takayasu-like lesions involving the subclavian and axillary arteries are shown.

DIFFERENTIAL DIAGNOSIS. Mimics of GCA include other vasculitides that may cause musculoskeletal pain, headache, visual aberrations, fever, and malaise. Although these include Wegener granulomatosis, microscopic polyangiitis, and others, it is relatively simple to exclude these based on the presence of more characteristic features of those illnesses (e.g., upper and/or lower airway disease and features of small-vessel vasculitis). Rarely, the GCA phenotype may be part of a paraneoplastic process. If polymyalgia rheumatica is the most compelling symptom of GCA, the differential then also includes polymyositis and proximal-onset rheumatoid arthritis. No precise serologic test exists for GCA. Diagnosis is based on a clinically compatible presentation, concurrent elevated acute-phase reactants (more than 80% of cases), a positive temporal artery biopsy (50% to 80% of cases) or angiographic abnormalities of large vessels (**Fig. 89-3**) compatible with GCA.

TREATMENT. Corticosteroid treatment continues to be the most effective therapy for GCA. Prednisone (≈0.7 to 1 mg/kg/day) will reduce symptoms within 1 to 2 days and often eliminate symptoms within 1 week. Approximately 2 to 4 weeks after clinical and laboratory measurement, particularly of the ESR, normalized tapering of corticosteroids can begin. Unfortunately, the ESR does not always normalize, even with disease control, so it should not be relied on as the only measure of disease activity. Occasional patients may either not achieve complete remission or not tolerate weaning of corticosteroid therapy. Cytotoxic and other immunosuppressive agents, including anti-TNF agents, have not proved efficacious in controlled comparative trials.[14,15] Two retrospective studies have demonstrated that the use of low-dose aspirin reduces cranial ischemic events (blindness and stroke) three- to fourfold compared with patients who had not received such therapy; in the absence of contraindications, all patients with GCA should receive low-dose aspirin.[16,17]

IDIOPATHIC AORTITIS

Aortitis can occur in TA and GCA, Behçet disease, and Cogan syndrome, and in children as a complication of Kawasaki disease. Occasionally, it is an unanticipated finding in patients undergoing surgery for aortic valve regurgitation, aneurysm resection, or coarctation.[18] Little is known about the frequency and clinical characteristics of idiopathic aortitis. Aortitis in the context of retroperitoneal fibrosis is a separate topic that will not be discussed in this chapter.

EPIDEMIOLOGY. A 20-year review of pathologic specimens from consecutive aortic surgeries at the Cleveland Clinic Foundation has revealed that 52 of 1204 specimens (4.3%) showed findings of idiopathic aortitis. Of patients with idiopathic aortitis, 67% were women.[18]

PATHOGENESIS. Unless the patient with idiopathic aortitis had a past history of GCA or TA, the mechanisms of disease remain unexplored.

CLINICAL FEATURES. In our series, 96% of patients with idiopathic aortitis had findings limited to the thoracic aorta. These data resemble those from large postmortem series in which aortas were examined in spite of the absence of overt aortic disease during life. In 69% of cases, idiopathic aortitis was not related to a current or past history of systemic disease. However, in 31% (16 of 52), aortitis was associated with a past history of GCA, TA, SLE, Wegener granulomatosis, or various other disorders.

DIFFERENTIAL DIAGNOSIS. Patients with idiopathic aortitis vary in age from childhood to the very elderly. Consequently, differential diagnosis should consider Kawasaki disease, TA, GCA, SLE, sarcoidosis, Cogan syndrome, Behçet disease, spondyloarthropathies, rheumatoid arthritis, rheumatic fever, and aortitis caused by infectious agents (e.g., tuberculosis, syphilis, mycoses, bacteria). Symptoms or findings of these diseases may immediately allow prioritization of diagnostic choices. However, some processes may be clinically silent, and ancillary laboratory studies (e.g., rapid plasma reagin [RPR], antinuclear antibody [ANA], skin tests such as purified protein derivative [PPD]), cultures, and special stains of surgical specimens may aid diagnosis. The diagnosis of idiopathic aortitis requires ruling out all causes of aortitis that may have specific therapies.

TREATMENT. In our experience with 36 patients, followed for a mean period of 42 months and analyzed retrospectively, new aneurysms were identified in 6 of 25 patients not treated with corticosteroids and in 0 of 11 patients treated postoperatively with corticosteroids. Although this observation could suggest that such therapy is warranted, there were marked variations of dose and duration of therapy that led to uncertainty about corticosteroid efficacy. Because only 17% of all patients subsequently developed new aneurysms over 3.5 years, we do not believe that all such patients require medical treatment.[18] These observations suggest isolated inflammatory disease of the aortic root in most patients. Treatment should depend on documentation of ongoing inflammatory disease. We approach this by history and physical examination, laboratory evaluation (complete blood count [CBC], ESR, C-reactive protein [CRP]), and imaging studies (MRI or MR angiography of the entire aorta and its primary branches). These tests should not be done in the immediate postoperative period. Because new lesions may occur over time, patients with idiopathic aortitis identified at the time of surgery should be periodically evaluated for recurrence. If disease definitely recurs, treatment should be pursued as recommended for TA and GCA. Although proof of the effectiveness of this approach is lacking, it can be defended based on the similarities of these conditions and demonstrated efficacy in GCA and TA.

KAWASAKI DISEASE

Kawasaki disease (KD) is an acute febrile systemic illness of childhood. It is the principal cause of acquired heart disease in children in Japan and the United States.

EPIDEMIOLOGY. KD occurs primarily in children younger than 4 or 5 years of age. Peak incidence is in children younger than 2 years of age. Boys are affected 1.5 times more often than girls. KD almost never occurs beyond 8 years of age (mean age in Japan is 12 months and, in the United States, 2.8 years of age). Although all racial groups can be affected, Asian children have the highest incidence of KD (50 to 200/100,000 children younger than 5 years of age versus 6 to 15/100,000 in the United States). Asian Americans have a higher incidence of KD than black Americans, in whom the incidence exceeds that of white Americans.[19] Although siblings of patients with KD are infrequently affected, KD does affect siblings more often than the general age-matched population (2.1% versus 0.19%). When siblings are affected, symptoms often occur shortly after their family member becomes ill. This raises questions about an infectious cause in the setting of an immunologic predisposition.[19-22]

PATHOGENESIS. Fever, rash, conjunctivitis, adenopathy, and geographic clustering suggest an infectious cause, but no agent has yet been identified. The essential absence of disease in neonates invites speculation about protection from maternal antibodies, and the rarity of KD in adults suggests protection through acquired immunity.[21,22]

The acute phase of illness is characterized by immunoinflammatory activation. This includes high levels of acute-phase reactants, leukocytosis with a left shift, lymphocytosis with a predominance of polyclonal B cells, and thrombocytosis that frequently reaches 1,000,000/mm^3. Blood T lymphocytes, including $CD4^+$ and $CD8^+$ cells, increase in number and show signs of activation. In spite of these observations, children with acute KD are often transiently anergic. Increased blood levels of a broad range of cytokines and soluble forms of endothelial cell adhesion molecules indicate immune activation. Cytokine-mediated endothelial cell activation and cytotoxic factors to endothelial cells may play an important early role in pathogenesis. Tissue specimens reveal vasculitis with endothelial cell edema, necrosis, desquamation, and a changing profile of leukocytes in the vessel wall—first, neutrophils and later, macrophages and T lymphocytes. After months, the inflammatory infiltrate diminishes and, as it fades, myointimal proliferation may produce stenoses or wall weakening resulting in coronary aneurysm formation. Either situation sets the stage for subsequent thrombosis.[21,22]

TABLE 89-3 Definition of Kawasaki Disease

Fever ≥ 5 days, without other explanation, plus at least four of the following:
1. Bilateral conjunctival injection
2. Mucous membrane changes—injected or fissured lips; injected pharynx or strawberry tongue
3. Extremity abnormality—erythema of palms, soles, edema of hands, feet, or generalized or peripheral desquamation (hands, feet)
4. Rash (polymorphous)
5. Cervical lymphadenopathy (usually a single node > 1.5 cm)

Associated manifestations
- Irritability
- Sterile pyuria, meatitis
- Perineal erythema and desquamation
- Arthralgias, arthritis
- Abdominal pain, diarrhea
- Aseptic meningitis
- Hepatitis
- Obstructive jaundice
- Hydrops of gallbladder
- Uveitis
- Sensorineural hearing loss
- Cardiovascular changes

80% cases < 4 years; rare, >8 years.
CDC = Centers for Disease Control and Prevention.
Modified from Barron K: Kawasaki disease: Etiology, pathogenesis and treatment. Cleve Clin J Med 69(Suppl 2):69, 2002.

CLINICAL FEATURES. The most prominent features of KD are included in the case definition guidelines of the Centers for Disease Control and Prevention (**Table 89-3**). These guidelines lack any specific serologic diagnostic test. The illness is usually self-limiting, within 4 to 8 weeks, and mortality is 2%.

Cardiac abnormalities include pericardial effusions (approximately 30%), myocarditis, mitral regurgitation (approximately 30%), aortitis and aortic regurgitation (infrequent), congestive heart failure, and atrial and ventricular arrhythmias.[21,22] Electrocardiographic findings include decreased R wave voltage, ST-segment depression, and low-amplitude or inverted T waves. Slowed atrioventricular conduction can occur. In untreated patients or patients treated with aspirin alone, coronary artery aneurysms occur in 20% to 25% of cases within 2 weeks and are associated with a mortality rate of approximately 2%. Early diagnosis and treatment with aspirin and intravenous immune globulin (IVIG) have reduced the death rate to well below 1% and the prevalence of coronary artery aneurysms to approximately 5%. Deaths usually result from acute coronary artery thrombosis in aneurysms that form following vasculitis. Noninvasive techniques disclose coronary artery aneurysms in approximately 20% of patients, compared with

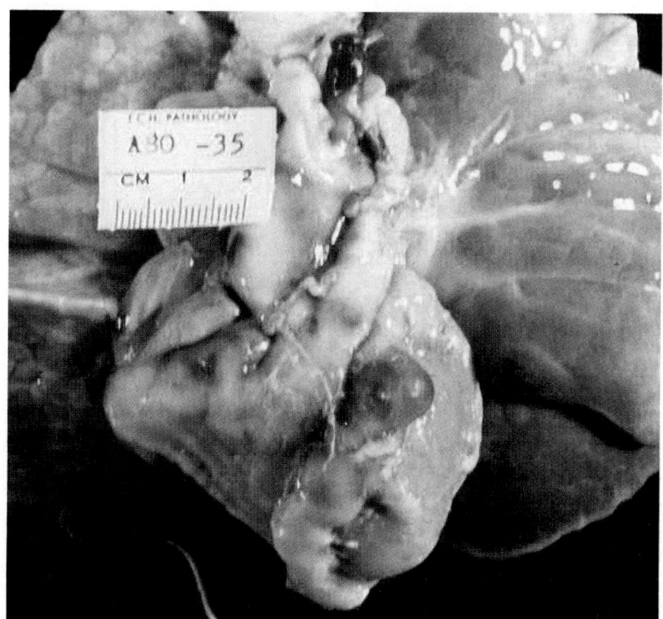

FIGURE 89-4 Giant coronary artery aneurysms caused by Kawasaki disease. Note the bulbous protrusion from the left anterior descending coronary artery. *(Courtesy of Dr. Karyl Barron.)*

60% shown by angiography. Aneurysms usually appear 1 to 4 weeks after onset of fever. New aneurysms seldom form after 6 weeks. Aneurysms are more common in the proximal than distal coronary arteries. Giant aneurysms (larger than 8 mm; **Fig. 89-4**) are the most likely to thrombose later and occlude, leading to infarction and even sudden death; endothelial abnormalities and intimal proliferation in smaller lesions (<4 mm) may lead to cardiac ischemia as well. About half of all small aneurysms will undergo angiographic regression within 1 to 2 years. Giant aneurysms rarely regress. MI may result from thrombus formation in aneurysms or severe stenoses and occurs most commonly in the first year after illness, but may occur years later.[19]

Postmortem studies have also demonstrated vasculitis of the aorta and of the celiac, carotid, subclavian, and pulmonary arteries. Rare case reports of gut vasculitis in KD exist. Gastrointestinal (GI) morbidity may depend more on small-vessel than large-vessel disease.

DIFFERENTIAL DIAGNOSIS. Given the resemblance of KD to infectious diseases, competing diagnoses include bacterial, spirochetal (e.g., leptospirosis), rickettsial (e.g., Rocky Mountain spotted fever), and viral illnesses. Drug reactions, poisonings, juvenile rheumatoid arthritis, SLE, other vasculitides, and malignancies, especially lymphomas and leukemias, may also share aspects of KD.

TREATMENT. Before the use of high dosages of aspirin and IVIG, coronary artery aneurysms were relatively common. The current standard of care consists of 2 g/kg of IVIG as a single infusion. Treatment provided within the first 10 days of illness shows efficacy most convincingly. Aspirin (80 to 100 mg/kg/day until the patient is afebrile) has both anti-inflammatory and antithrombotic effects. After fever subsides, the dose of aspirin is reduced (3 to 5 mg/kg/day) to achieve primarily antiplatelet effects. This treatment should continue until the platelet count and other inflammatory markers return to normal (about 8 weeks). Long-term, low-dose aspirin is recommended for children with echocardiographically demonstrated aneurysms, although controlled studies have not proved the efficacy of such therapy. A small subset of KD patients resists conventional therapy and is prone to aneurysm formation and long-term disease sequelae. The use of corticosteroids in this group and other patients remains controversial. The increased frequency of coronary artery aneurysms in an early report of corticosteroid-treated patients has not been seen by others.[21]

Recommendations for long-term follow-up by the American Heart Association include consideration of anticoagulation therapy in children with multiple giant aneurysms and known obstructive lesions, and evaluation by stress testing during adolescence. Severe coronary artery lesions have been treated by bypass, but if disease is widespread and bypass not possible, transplantation should be considered.[19] Coronary artery bypass procedures have been reserved for patients with severe obstructive lesions, such as those involving the main left coronary artery (LCA) or at least two of three major coronary arteries. Internal thoracic artery grafts appear to fare better than saphenous vein grafts. Data on percutaneous interventions, including those using drug-eluting stents, are limited.

Vasculitis of Small or Medium-Sized Vessels That May Affect the Cardiovascular System

Churg-Strauss Syndrome

Churg-Strauss syndrome (CSS; allergic angiitis and granulomatosis) is a very rare syndrome that typically includes a history of asthma; eosinophilia; pulmonary infiltrates; upper airway inflammation; and variable renal, neurologic, cutaneous, and cardiac involvement. Histopathologic observations from involved lesions reveal eosinophilic granulomatous infiltrates and vasculitis.

EPIDEMIOLOGY. The most generous estimates of incidence of CSS are 2.4 cases/1,000,000 persons annually. Those affected may be children or adults, with the peak group being 35 to 50 years of age and with no sex bias.[23]

PATHOGENESIS. The cause of CSS remains unknown. Nonetheless, authorities have recommended withdrawal of any newly introduced drugs or treatments (e.g., desensitization), and avoidance of new environmental stimuli (e.g., farm, workplace, if relevant to the medical history). A role for leukotriene antagonists, as used in the treatment of asthma, in precipitating CSS is the subject of controversy. Most would agree that if such an agent were introduced just before the emergence of CSS, it should be discontinued.

The granulomatous nature of CSS lesions suggests an involvement of Th1 lymphocytes and macrophages, although antineutrophil cytoplasmic antibody (ANCA), if relevant, and eosinophils argue for a role of Th2-biased lymphocytes. The latter produce IL-5, a cytokine that increases eosinophil production and release from the bone marrow.

CLINICAL FEATURES. By definition, the diagnosis of CSS requires a past or present history of atopy, usually asthma. Systemic symptoms are present in 70% to 100% of cases from different series. Chest imaging reveals infiltrates, usually multifocal, in 30% to 75%. Much less often, pulmonary nodules may be seen, as in Wegener granulomatosis (WG). In CSS, nodules seldom cavitate, a finding that is common in WG. Cardiac disease in CSS is the most common cause of death. It is reported in 15% to 55% of cases and may include pericarditis, myocarditis, and coronary arteritis. Congestive heart failure occurs in 15% to 30% of cases. Mesenteric ischemia (≈5%) contributes significantly to morbidity and mortality, and may cause frank blood per rectum, melena, or bowel perforation. Many more patients have abdominal pain (30% to 60%) for which the ultimate cause is suspected to be CSS. The small intestine and colon are the sites more often affected. Peripheral neurologic abnormalities (sensory and/or motor) affect more than two thirds of patients. Approximately 50% of patients have musculoskeletal symptoms and rashes, and renal disease (glomerulonephritis) affects at least one third.

DIFFERENTIAL DIAGNOSIS. CSS may be confused with WG. Patients who suffer from WG do not have an unusually high frequency of allergies, asthma, and striking eosinophilia, but some patients with WG have a more modest peripheral eosinophilia (≈10%).

Other considerations in the differential diagnosis include parasitic infections, especially helminths (e.g., larvae and adults of hookworm, ascaris, trichinella, strongyloides, filaria, flukes) that may produce chronic eosinophilia by stimulating IL-5 in affected organs. Because helminths may migrate through the lungs, infiltrates and bronchospasm may result, producing a picture of eosinophilic pneumonia and asthma. Idiopathic hypereosinophilic syndrome (HES) is a diagnosis to be considered only after exclusion of all other causes of eosinophilia. In some cases, HES is part of a leukoproliferative syndrome and may be associated with splenomegaly, cytogenetic abnormalities, myelofibrosis, myelodysplasia, anemia, and abnormal red blood cell forms. The absence of vasculitis and asthma distinguishes HES from CSS. HES has particular interest for cardiologists because of the risks of cardiac fibrosis, ventricular apical necrosis, valvular dysfunction, and intraventricular thrombus formation. Myocarditis and cardiac fibrosis may lead to a restrictive cardiomyopathy.

TREATMENT. Corticosteroids (usually prednisone, 1 mg/kg/day orally) usually produce dramatic improvement. In patients with critical organ system involvement (heart, brain, kidneys, gut), it may be prudent to provide pulse IV therapy (methylprednisolone, 1 g/day) for 1 to 3 days. Although recommended, this regimen has never been the subject of controlled clinical trials. Patients who are critically ill should also receive a second agent (usually cyclophosphamide). Cyclophosphamide is used daily in a dose of 2 mg/kg, assuming normal renal function. In the presence of renal impairment, the dose must be proportionately reduced to avoid severe bone marrow suppression. Long-term cyclophosphamide therapy carries many risks, and cyclophosphamide is now used to induce remission. Then, after 3 to 6 months, if remission continues, cyclophosphamide is switched to maintenance therapy with daily azathioprine or weekly methotrexate.

Polyarteritis Nodosa

Polyarteritis nodosa (PAN) is a nongranulomatous disease of only medium-sized arteries. The older PAN literature has been a source of confusion. Those series included patients with both PAN and microscopic polyangiitis (MPA), a disease that can have features of PAN but is defined by the presence of small-vessel vasculitis (capillaries, venules, and arterioles). Today, cases of nongranulomatous vasculitis with glomerulonephritis (renal capillaritis) and pulmonary infiltrates (alveolitis or capillaritis) would be considered MPA and not PAN, according to the Chapel Hill Consensus Conference (CHCC) on Nomenclature. The guidelines also stress that PAN and MPA are not mediated by immune complex and are not secondary forms of vasculitis, although hepatitis B and C can produce similar syndromes.

EPIDEMIOLOGY. Because not all researchers strictly adhere to the CHCC guidelines, it is difficult to know the incidence of PAN. Even liberal application of these guidelines indicates that PAN is a rare disease, with an annual incidence of less than 1/100,000. Some include vasculitis caused by hepatitis, mediated by immune complexes and cryoglobulins, in this figure. Men and women are equally affected. PAN may affect people of any age, but the incidence peaks between 40 and 60 years of age.

PATHOGENESIS. When one properly excludes cases associated with hepatitis, the cause of medium-sized vessel vasculitis compatible with PAN is unknown. The histopathology of lesions varies and often evolves over time, at first having a predominance of neutrophils and later, of mononuclear cells. Granulomas and increased numbers of eosinophils are not present. Necrotizing changes may follow, with weakening of the vessel wall and aneurysm formation (**Fig. 89-5**) or myointimal proliferation, causing stenosis and occlusion.

CLINICAL FEATURES. Systemic symptoms occur in at least half of patients in different series. Any organ system can be involved. However, if one adheres to CHCC guidelines, several features should not be included because they reflect microvascular (capillary or venule) disease—palpable purpura, pulmonary infiltrates, or hemorrhage and glomerulonephritis. In contrast, these findings occur in MPA.

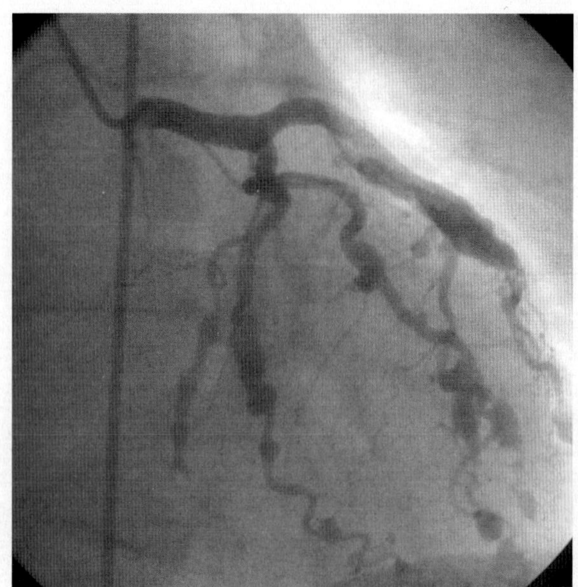

FIGURE 89-5 Coronary artery aneurysms caused by PAN.

PAN would more typically include deep skin inflammatory changes that may produce painful nodules (similar to erythema nodosum) or progress to infarction and gangrene (30% to 50%), neuropathy (especially mononeuritis multiplex, 20% to 50%), renal infarction and insufficiency (≈10% to 30%), hypertension (approximately 30%), segmental pulmonary infarctions (<40%), and cardiac disease (10% to 30%—congestive failure, angina, infarction, pericarditis). Although musculoskeletal symptoms occur in over 50% of all PAN patients, they are not a helpful differential diagnostic feature. As noted for CSS, markers of poor prognosis include ischemia or infarction of critical organs (brain, gut, kidneys, and heart). Although clinically apparent heart disease may only affect less than one third of cases, postmortem examination may reveal medium-sized vessel vasculitis or consequences of hypertension (left ventricular hypertrophy, congestive heart failure) in up to 75%.

DIFFERENTIAL DIAGNOSIS. It is important to reemphasize that certain infections may cause inflammation of medium-sized vessels. All patients with clinical findings that resemble those of PAN should be tested for hepatitis B and C. A PAN-like presentation is usually associated with hepatitis B virus (HBV) and cryoglobulinemia, whereas an MPA-like presentation occurs more frequently in association with hepatitis C virus (HCV) infection and cryoglobulinemia. Rarely, infection with human immunodeficiency virus (HIV) may present in this fashion. In immunocompromised hosts, cytomegalovirus (CMV) should also be sought as a possible cause of small and medium-sized vessel disease. The PAN-MPA–like spectrum obligates a search for bacterial and fungal infections as causes of endocarditis or endovascular vegetations. Use and abuse of vasoactive drugs (e.g., cocaine, amphetamines, ephedrine) should also be considered (see Chap. 73). PAN is not associated with ANCA. No serologic diagnostic tests exist for PAN; the diagnosis depends on biopsy or angiographic proof of medium-sized vessel inflammation (**Fig. 89-6**), but the angiograms are not specific for PAN.

TREATMENT. The guidelines for treatment are the same as those for CSS. Not all patients with PAN require the addition of a cytotoxic agent (cyclophosphamide, methotrexate, or azathioprine) to the corticosteroid. In the setting of critical organ disease, however, one should not hesitate to use these agents.

Other primary vasculitides such as hypersensitivity vasculitis, Henoch-Schönlein purpura, and WG may all have cardiac consequences. However, because vasculitis-mediated heart disease is infrequent in these disorders, they will not be addressed further here. The principles of treatment resemble those noted for CSS and PAN, except that WG therapy always requires the addition of a cytotoxic agent. Although primary cardiac involvement from vasculitis is not common in WG, accelerated atherosclerosis may occur in these patients, compared with controls that are matched for age, sex, and conventional risk factors.[24,25]

Systemic Rheumatologic Disorders

Rheumatoid Arthritis

Rheumatoid arthritis (RA) is the most common form of chronic inflammatory polyarthritis. Approximately 70% of patients have rheumatoid factor (RF). The presence of RF does not confirm the diagnosis of RA, because some healthy persons and those with other diseases, including chronic viral hepatitis and bacterial endocarditis, may also have RF. Use of the anticyclic citrullinated peptide (anti-CCP) test, adds some specificity to the serologic diagnosis; it is not detected in RF-positive patients with hepatitis C. Similar to RF, anti-CCP in a patient with RA marks more aggressive disease. Systemic complications of RA include pericarditis, pleuritis, vasculitis, interstitial lung disease, atherosclerotic cardiovascular disease, and Sjögren and Felty syndromes. Patients with RA also have a slightly increased prevalence of lymphoma, an important consideration when estimating the risk of drug-induced lymphoproliferative disease in patients with RA.

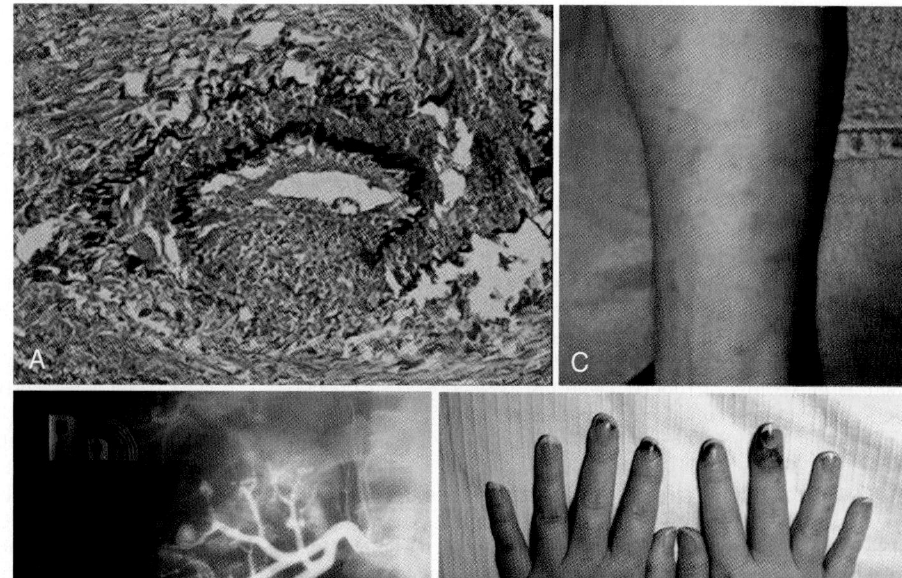

FIGURE 89-6 In PAN, the likelihood of having adequate collateral circulation to maintain tissue viability following vasoocclusion is less than that seen in other vasculitides. **A,** Section of a muscular artery showing destruction of the internal elastic lamina (from 5 to 8 o'clock), as well as intimal thickening and stenosis. **B,** Although aneurysms may be visually more striking on angiography, renovascular occlusive lesions may contribute to high-renin hypertension and renal failure. **C,** Palpable subcutaneous nodules on the patient's forearms that were painful. **D,** Infarcts on the fingers caused by severe digital artery involvement. **A,** Hematoxylin-eosin stain; magnification ×20.

EPIDEMIOLOGY. RA affects approximately 1% to 3% of the population. The disease affects those of all ages, but is most frequently diagnosed in women (>2:1) during their third to fifth decades of life.

PATHOGENESIS. The cause of RA is unknown. There is a genetic predisposition, but this is seemingly polygenic. There may be an infectious trigger, but no agent has been identified. An abnormal and persistent T-cell response triggers macrophage activation. TNF, IL-1, and other cytokines sustain the chronic inflammatory response, which includes angiogenesis, proliferation of synovial tissue, and bone remodeling. The dramatic efficacy of specific anti-TNF and anti–B-cell therapies suggest a dominant role for these targets in the pathogenesis of the disease.

CLINICAL FEATURES. RA is a chronic symmetrical polyarthritis that affects small and large joints, especially the metacarpophalangeal joints and wrists, sparing the lumbar and thoracic spine and distal interphalangeal joints. It affects the pericardium in approximately 40% of patients, as indicated by echocardiographic and necropsy studies (see Chap. 75). Chronic, asymptomatic effusive pericardial disease is far more common than acute pericarditis.[26] Asymptomatic pericardial abnormalities were commonly observed by echocardiography in the era before current aggressive approaches to treatment of the disease. The electrocardiogram (ECG) is usually normal in patients with chronic pericardial disease, but may show characteristic changes in acute pericarditis. Coexistent small pleural effusions are common and may reflect rheumatoid serositis or hemodynamic effects of the pericarditis. Pericardial calcification can occur, mimicking tuberculous pericarditis, but this is rare.

Limited data describe the nature of pericardial fluid in RA. Fluid is frequently blood-tinged, with leukocyte counts ranging from scant to more than 30,000/mm^3, generally with a neutrophil predominance. The glucose level in the pericardial fluid may be low when compared with serum glucose levels, similar to markedly depressed glucose levels reported in rheumatoid pleural effusions. The presence of rheumatoid factor in the fluid does not confirm the diagnosis of RA pericarditis. Constrictive pericarditis can occur and must be distinguished from restrictive cardiomyopathy, a rare complication of secondary amyloidosis in patients with longstanding RA.

Treatment of clinical pericarditis includes the use of nonsteroidal anti-inflammatory drugs (NSAIDs), intensified systemic immunosuppressive therapy, pericardial steroid injections, or pericardiocentesis if hemodynamic compromise occurs. If systemic therapy is ineffective or already at an intense level, patients with recurrent pericardial effusions may require a pericardial window. There are no data on colchicine therapy in RA pericarditis. The current use of aggressive medical therapy early in the course of rheumatoid disease may decrease the frequency of extra-articular complications of RA, including pericardial involvement.

RA does not usually cause clinically apparent myocarditis, but congestive heart failure probably occurs with increased prevalence. Secondary amyloidosis is rare in rheumatoid disease, but can cause cardiomyopathy and atrioventricular block. Focal cardiac involvement with rheumatoid nodules can occur and may be associated with conduction block. All levels of block have been described and, once established, may not respond to anti-inflammatory or immunosuppressive therapies.

Autopsy studies have indicated frequent involvement of the cardiac valves and aorta, but valve abnormalities in RA rarely cause clinical problems. Slowly progressive granulomatous valvulitis may be difficult, if not impossible, to distinguish from disease unrelated to RA. A rapidly progressive aortic valvulitis, advancing to the need for valve replacement caused by regurgitation for less than 5 years, has been described. Rheumatoid aortitis, with involvement of the aortic valve, has been reported, but aortitis is not frequently recognized antemortem. Pulmonary hypertension (PHtn) may result from rheumatoid lung disease.

Patients with RA have an increased incidence of coronary artery disease (CAD), which may be masked by limited physical activity because of joint disease. Hence, special consideration should be given to the patient with RA about to undergo major noncardiac surgery. Although currently unsupported by adequate evidence, it is reasonable to consider longstanding RA as an intermediate risk factor in assessing preoperative risk, similar to patients with renal insufficiency in the American Heart Association (AHA) guidelines. Coronary arteritis is a rarely reported complication of RA.

DIFFERENTIAL DIAGNOSIS. Rheumatoid arthritis, in the absence of characteristic radiographic erosive changes, remains a diagnosis of exclusion. Other conditions that can cause a symmetrical small and large joint polyarthritis include chronic hepatitis B and C, SLE, several vasculitides, and crystal-induced arthropathies. Early or acute RA can also be confused with bacterial endocarditis and other infections, such as parvovirus or rubella. Lyme disease (*Borrelia* sp. infection), which can cause cardiac conduction disease, produces an oligoarticular large joint arthritis that does not mimic RA.

TREATMENT. Current treatment regimens for the treatment of RA emphasize aggressive disease-modifying therapy as soon as the diagnosis is made. Combination therapy with agents such as methotrexate, sulfasalazine, leflunomide, hydroxychloroquine, and low-dose prednisone is frequently used. NSAIDs are not a mainstay of therapy because of the following: (1) they have not been shown to alter the course of RA; (2) they can increase risk of GI bleeding; and (3) chronic use of cyclooxygenase 1 (COX-1) or COX-2 inhibitors can cause renal dysfunction and hypertension.

Antagonists of TNF are extremely effective agents, although cost and the unknown long-term effects of therapy are of concern in their use. The increased use of effective therapy may be associated with a decreased incidence of extra-articular complications of RA. The use of high-dose infliximab in patients with severe CHF and RA has raised a concern over increased cardiac morbidity and mortality.[27] The data available do not clearly preclude the use of anti-TNF agents in patients with mild and controlled CHF, but warrant increased vigilance.

HLA-B27–Associated Spondyloarthropathies

The RF-negative spondyloarthropathies include ankylosing spondylitis, psoriatic arthritis, inflammatory bowel disease–associated arthritis, and postinfectious reactive arthritis.

EPIDEMIOLOGY. The vast majority of white patients with ankylosing spondylitis and many patients with other spondyloarthropathies have the HLA-B27 gene; however, most who carry this gene do not have spondyloarthritis, and gene typing should not be a routine diagnostic test. Patients with spondyloarthropathy share several features that distinguish them from rheumatoid arthritis. Although females do suffer from these disorders, ankylosing spondylitis and reactive arthritis are male-dominant diseases. The spondyloarthropathies are less common than RA.

PATHOGENESIS. The spondyloarthropathies have been historically grouped together because of some shared clinical characteristics and the disproportionate presence of the B27 antigen. Studies with transgenic rats expressing the human B27 antigen have shown that these animals, when raised in a non–germ-free environment, exhibit inflammation of skin, spine, and other tissues similar to that seen in human patients. These observations support a role for B27 in the pathogenesis of the inflammation. The B27 gene may permit an abnormal immune response to gut or mucosal bacterial antigens, which cross-react with tissue antigens present in joints, skin, and other tissues. The abnormal response includes the breakdown of tolerance to unknown self-antigens and the perpetuation of localized inflammation, a conjecture that lacks confirmation. Not all patients with spondyloarthropathies have the B27 antigen; either there are alternative pathogenic mechanisms, or the current ability to define the HLA-B locus at a molecular rather than serological level limits our full understanding of its pathogenetic role.

CLINICAL FEATURES. Unlike rheumatoid arthritis, the entire spine, not just the cervical region, may be involved. Sacroiliac joint involvement is frequent, and may be the only musculoskeletal manifestation. Large peripheral joints are commonly involved, but unlike in RA, involvement tends to be asymmetrical. There frequently is inflammation of the tendons, ligaments, or joint capsules at the point of attachment to bone (enthesis; thus, the term *enthesitis*). Diffuse tendon sheath involvement may produce sausage digits (not seen in RA). In the United States, 90% of white patients with ankylosing spondylitis and approximately 60% of patients with inflammatory bowel disease–related spondylitis have the HLA-B27 gene. The carriage rate of HLA-B27 in healthy U.S. whites is approximately 10%. It is much lower in blacks and Asians. Presence of the gene predisposes to anterior uveitis and perhaps cardiac conduction disease and proximal aortitis. Thus, patients with psoriatic arthritis, enteropathic arthritis, and reactive arthritis, as well as ankylosing spondylitis, are predisposed to these complications. Patients may express extraskeletal B27-associated complications without overt rheumatic disease.

Pericarditis, although reported, is not characteristic of the spondyloarthropathies. CAD occurs at an increased rate in psoriasis and psoriatic arthritis, but it has not been well studied in other disorders. Diastolic dysfunction may occur in patients who have HLA-B27 but rarely has clinical significance. Cardiac conduction disease can complicate ankylosing spondylitis and other B27-associated disorders. Up to one third of patients with ankylosing spondylitis develop conduction disease. Atrioventricular (AV) conduction block may initially be intermittent, but tends to progress. Conduction disease is more common in male patients, and as many as 20% of men with permanent pacemakers carry the HLA-B27 gene. Conduction disease may be the only abnormality associated with the HLA-B27 gene. Electrophysiologic studies have indicated that the level of block is usually at the AV node and is not fascicular.[28] Atrial fibrillation may occur more commonly than expected in patients with the HLA-B27 gene.

Aortic root disease has been reported in up to 100% of ankylosing spondylitis patients who also had aortic valve involvement in an autopsy series.[29] Characteristic findings include thickening of the aortic root, with subsequent dilation. Aortic cusp nodularity with proximal thickening comprises the subaortic hump, which was found in 74% of 44 selected patients with ankylosing spondylitis[30] using transesophageal echocardiography. In this study, aortic regurgitation developed in 50% of patients, and 20% of patients developed congestive heart failure, underwent valve replacement, had a stroke, or died, as compared with only 3% of age- and sex-matched volunteers. The aortic lesions progressed in 24% of patients and resolved in an additional 20% over an approximately 2-year follow-up. The severity of aortic root disease was associated with the patient's age and duration of spondylitis. Dilation and stiffening of the aortic root may contribute to the aortic regurgitation. Hence, the regurgitant murmur, as in syphilitic aortitis, may be best heard along the right sternal border. However, an electrocardiographic and transthoracic echocardiographic study of 100 Swiss men with ankylosing spondylitis of more than 15 years' duration has shown no significant increase in valvular or conduction disease.[30]

DIFFERENTIAL DIAGNOSIS. The B27-associated spondyloarthropathies are characterized by inflammation of the spine, with morning stiffness of the involved areas. Unlike RA, the peripheral arthritis is usually asymmetrical, with frequent involvement of large joints. The specific spondyloarthropathies are clinically distinguished by their associated extra-articular features (e.g., psoriasis, balanitis, urethritis, oral and/or genital ulcers). Psoriatic arthritis may be present, and severe, in the absence of significant cutaneous psoriasis. Cardiac involvement seems linked more to the presence of the HLA-B27 gene than to any specific rheumatic disorder.

TREATMENT. For years, the spondyloarthropathies have been treated symptomatically, with marginal success, with NSAIDs and physical therapy. Modification of the disease course has not been well documented with such therapy. The disease-modifying drugs used successfully in patients with RA (methotrexate, sulfasalazine) have minimal efficacy in relieving the symptoms and findings of spinal inflammation, although they often successfully relieve peripheral arthritis. The B27 extra-articular manifestations are treated, as needed, with corticosteroids (uveitis) or surgery (aortic regurgitation, aortitis). Anti-TNF agents (etanercept, infliximab, adalimumab) have demonstrated impressive clinical efficacy in treating the symptoms of spondylitis; whether they will be beneficial for treating or preventing cardiovascular manifestations is currently unknown. As noted, the use of these agents in patients with heart failure warrants vigilance.

Systemic Lupus Erythematosus

SLE is a systemic autoimmune disease characterized by the presence of immune complexes, autoantibodies, and ANAs in the setting of a constellation of clinical features, which may include serositis, arthritis, glomerulonephritis, CNS dysfunction, hemolytic anemia, thrombocytopenia, and leukopenia. More than 20% of patients with SLE have antiphospholipid antibodies (APLAs) that predispose to arterial and venous thrombosis, pulmonary hypertension, valvular dysfunction, or miscarriage (see Chap. 87).

EPIDEMIOLOGY. SLE is more common in women and can occur at any age. Both idiopathic and drug-induced SLE have cardiac manifestations. Reversible drug-induced SLE is well recognized following treatment with various cardiac medications, including procainamide, hydralazine, and quinidine.

PATHOGENESIS. Over 95% of patients with SLE have a positive ANA; however, even high titers of ANA are not diagnostic of SLE. Anti–double-stranded DNA is more specific for SLE but is present in only 50% to 70% of patients with idiopathic SLE, often in those with glomerulonephritis. SLE is an autoantibody and immune complex disorder, with immunoglobulin and complement deposition in involved organs, including the heart. The serologic findings may be detectable years before clinical disease manifests. However, the view of SLE as only an immune complex disorder is an oversimplification. Some animal models of SLE have been associated with retroviral infections, but there are no consistently demonstrable viral agents in humans with SLE. Studies of twins have suggested a role for genetic factors, and recent data support the involvement of IFN-α in SLE pathogenesis.

CLINICAL FEATURES. Pericarditis is the most commonly recognized cardiac problem in SLE (see Chap. 75).[31] Imaging and autopsy series have demonstrated pericardial involvement in more than 60% of patients, although clinically significant pericarditis occurs in less than 30%. Unexplained chest pain is common in patients with SLE, but is more likely caused by manifestations other than pericarditis. Pericarditis may occur as the initial manifestation of SLE, appear at any point during the disease course, or occur as a complication of chronic renal disease. Pericardial fluid has generally demonstrated a neutrophil predominance, elevated protein level, and low or normal glucose concentration. Complement levels in pericardial fluid tend to be low, but this is not a characteristic unique to SLE. The fluid is indistinguishable from that obtained from patients with bacterial pericarditis, and infection must therefore be excluded. Pericardial tamponade may (rarely) occur at any point in the course of SLE, including the initial presentation. When effusions occur in the setting of chronic renal failure, it is difficult to distinguish uremic from SLE pericarditis. Pericarditis, as well as tamponade, can occur with drug-induced lupus. Constrictive pericarditis, presumably as a sequela of SLE pericarditis, can occur.

Coronary arteritis, resulting in ischemic syndromes, occurs rarely in patients with SLE. The distinction between atherosclerotic CAD, which is far more common, and coronary arteritis has been inferred from sequential angiographic studies that show more rapid changes in luminal images with arteritis than those characteristic of CAD.

Additional causes of acute coronary syndromes in SLE include thrombosis, often related to the presence of APLAs and, very rarely, embolism from nonbacterial vegetative endocarditis (Libman-Sacks). APLAs are associated in some echocardiographic studies with valve thickening and nonbacterial endocarditis. Antiendothelial cell antibodies may accelerate atherogenesis (see Fig. 15-62). The presence of APLAs independently predicted CAD in a subset analysis of the Helsinki heart study. The rare patient with coronary arteritis should be treated with high-dose corticosteroids, and patients with thrombotic disease related to APLAs should receive long-term anticoagulation. Aspirin is probably not sufficient as an anticoagulant, although therapeutic trial evidence is lacking in patients with APLAs. Thrombocytopenia is common in patients with APLAs, and may complicate therapeutic decisions.

Myocardial dysfunction in SLE is usually multifactorial and may result from immunologic injury, ischemia, valvular disease, or coexistent problems such as hypertension. Acute myocarditis is infrequent, but can be the initial presentation of SLE. Patients with peripheral skeletal myositis are reportedly at increased risk for myocarditis. Measurement of troponin I may help in the assessment of cardiac involvement, but the MB fraction of creatine kinase (CK) may be significantly elevated in the presence of skeletal myositis, even in the absence of myocarditis. Noninvasive studies have demonstrated abnormal systolic and diastolic function in patients with active SLE. These changes often reverse with control of disease activity. Acute or chronic congestive heart failure caused by SLE, in the absence of other contributing factors, is not common. Endomyocardial biopsy of the patient with cardiomyopathy and suspected SLE will not likely provide a specific diagnosis of SLE. The biopsy generally reveals patches of myocardial fibrosis, sparse interstitial mononuclear cell infiltrates, and occasional myocyte necrosis with immune complex deposition, even in areas devoid of inflammatory changes. Unexplained acute left ventricular (LV) failure in a patient with active SLE warrants a trial of corticosteroid therapy. Hydroxychloroquine-induced cardiomyopathy should be considered in patients on this drug.

Tachyarrhythmias can occur in patients with SLE with pericarditis. Sinus tachycardia may be the earliest manifestation of myocarditis. Abnormal heart rate variability may be caused by autonomic dysfunction or occult myocarditis. Unexplained sinus tachycardia, which resolves with treatment of SLE, can occur in the presence of active SLE, even when evidence of cardiac dysfunction is absent. Occult pulmonary embolism should be considered as a cause of tachycardia in patients with SLE, especially in the presence of APLAs. Abnormal myocardial single-photon emission computed tomography (SPECT) scans have been noted, even in some patients with a normal resting echocardiogram.[32]

Conduction disease is not expected in adults with SLE, but infants born to mothers with SLE, and some other systemic autoimmune diseases, have an increased incidence of congenital complete AV block. The pathogenic mechanism is the transmission of maternal anti-Ro and anti-La antibodies in utero, causing myocardial inflammation and fibrosis of the conduction system.[33] The risk for developing complete AV block in infants born to mothers carrying this antibody is low. However, women with systemic autoimmune diseases known to be associated with this antibody should be screened for its presence prior to pregnancy. If present, the fetus should be followed throughout pregnancy with ultrasound studies to detect fetal conduction abnormality or hydrops. AV block usually appears early in pregnancy and is almost always irreversible. If recognized early, dexamethasone may reverse fetal myocarditis in utero. Data to support this intervention are limited.

Valvular pathology in SLE is common. Recognized 50 years ago as noninfectious vegetations (Libman-Sacks endocarditis), transesophageal studies have shown valvular abnormalities in over 50% of patients with SLE.[34] Valvular thickening is the most common echocardiographic finding, followed by vegetations and valvular insufficiency. The vegetations generally localize on the atrial side of the mitral valve and the arterial side of the aortic valve and are usually nonmobile. Over time, the lesions may resolve or worsen; fibrosis may cause retraction of the valve, causing regurgitation. Less commonly, the vegetations on the valve may occlude the orifice, causing stenosis. Valvulitis (**Fig. 89-7**), with valve fenestrations and rapidly progressing dysfunction, can occur. The nonbacterial vegetations rarely embolize

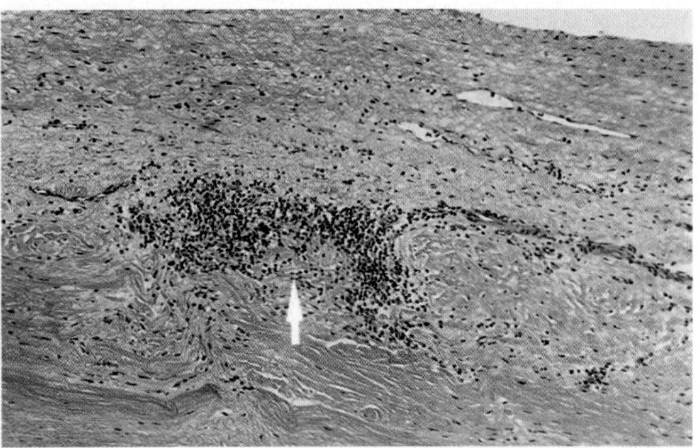

FIGURE 89-7 Valvulitis in SLE. Patients with SLE can develop valve dysfunction caused by bland vegetations (Libman-Sacks endocarditis), valve-associated thrombosis, and rarely true valvulitis. This photomicrograph illustrates aortic valve valvulitis that was discovered at the time of surgery for aortitis and aortic insufficiency (×400). The white arrow indicates a cluster of infiltrating leukocytes.

and cause stroke syndromes. Several studies have demonstrated an increased prevalence of cardiac valve dysfunction in the presence of APLA, with or without SLE. Because vegetations may occur in APLA-negative patients with SLE, multiple mechanisms may affect heart valve damage in SLE patients. Because of the high prevalence of valvular abnormalities in patients with SLE, it has been suggested that antibiotic prophylaxis for endocarditis be considered for all patients with SLE before high-risk procedures are carried out. Adequate studies do not exist to provide evidence for this proposal. There are reports of mitral and aortic valve replacement in patients with SLE.[35] Valve repair has also been described.[36] Recurrence of valve disease, particularly thrombosis, may affect prosthetic valves.

Pulmonary artery hypertension is common in SLE.[37] Clinically significant pulmonary hypertension is less common. Causes of the development of pulmonary hypertension include thromboembolic disease associated with APLAs, intimal proliferation of the pulmonary artery and, very rarely, arteritis of the pulmonary vessels. Successful heart-lung transplantation has been reported in a patient with SLE and progressive pulmonary hypertension. Aortitis with associated valvular insufficiency can occur rarely in SLE.[38]

DIFFERENTIAL DIAGNOSIS. Among the most common features of SLE are ANAs (>95%), arthralgias and arthritis (60% to 90%), constitutional symptoms (50% to 75%), rash (50% to 80%), Raynaud vasospasm (30% to 60%), and glomerulonephritis (30% to 75%). Characteristic features that enhance diagnostic likelihood include butterfly rash, sun-sensitive skin eruptions, discoid skin lesions, cytopenias (especially thrombocytopenia and leukopenia), antibodies to double-stranded DNA and Sm (anti-Smith), hypocomplementemia, and characteristic findings on biopsies of involved sites. Diseases that can be confused with SLE include dermatomyositis, infections, particularly endocarditis, lymphomas, thrombotic thrombocytopenic purpura, immune thrombocytopenic purpura, Still disease, and sarcoidosis. The pattern of cardiac involvement in SLE is not diagnostic.

TREATMENT. There is no single treatment for SLE. The specific manifestations are managed on an individual basis. Life-threatening organ involvement is controlled by high-dose corticosteroids, often with the addition of cyclophosphamide, azathioprine, or mycophenolate. Patients with mild pericarditis without threat of hemodynamic compromise are generally treated with a short course of NSAID therapy, unless there is a contraindication, such as renal insufficiency. Corticosteroids are used for more severe disease. There are no data on colchicine for the treatment of lupoid pericarditis. If prompt response to steroid therapy does not occur, large sterile pericardial effusions, particularly those accompanied by fever and/or hemodynamic compromise, are best treated with drainage and, if recurrent, consideration of a pericardial window. Arteritis and myocarditis are treated with high-dose corticosteroids, with or without adjunctive cyclophosphamide or azathioprine. Corticosteroid therapy may be tried for acute valvulitis; the indications for surgery are the same as for other causes of valvular dysfunction.

Antiphospholipid Antibody Syndrome

APLA syndrome (APLAS; see Chap. 87) is defined as the presence of either APLA or a lupus anticoagulant and a history of otherwise unexplained recurrent venous or arterial thrombosis, or frequent second- or third-trimester miscarriages. Thrombocytopenia, hemolytic anemia, and livedo reticularis are commonly present. APLAs are common (10% to 30%) in SLE, although not all these patients will exhibit the clinical syndrome. Low to moderate levels of APLA can also accompany a number of infectious and other autoimmune diseases, usually without clinical consequence. In the absence of an underlying systemic disease, APLAS is termed *primary*. The presence of APLA or a lupus anticoagulant, in the absence of sequelae, does not routinely warrant therapy.

EPIDEMIOLOGY. The true prevalence of the antiphospholipid antibody syndrome is unknown. The demonstration of a lupus anticoagulant or APLAs alone does not define the clinical syndrome, which requires a coincident clinical thrombotic or embolic event(s).

PATHOGENESIS. (see Chap. 87)

CLINICAL FEATURES. Venous thromboembolic disease is the most common manifestation and usually occurs in the legs and lungs (see Chap. 77). Arterial thrombosis often causes stroke, but can occur in a wide range of locations. Primary APLAS is not associated with pericarditis, myocarditis, or conduction disease. Cardiac manifestations include thrombotic CAD, intracardiac thrombi, and nonbacterial endocarditis.[39] Heart valve abnormalities occur in approximately 30% of patients with primary APLAS and include leaflet thickening, thrombotic masses extending from the valve ring or leaflets, or vegetations. The mitral valve is affected more frequently than the aortic valve and regurgitation is far more common than stenosis (**Fig. 89-8**). Most valvular involvement is clinically silent. The first manifestation of valvular involvement with APLAS may be a thromboembolic event, such as stroke. The incidence of superimposed bacterial endocarditis is not known. Treatment of clinically significant valvular or intracardiac thrombotic masses is high-dose anticoagulation with heparin and then chronic warfarin,[40] with or without the addition of aspirin. Management of heparin dosing, in the setting of a lupus anticoagulant, which prolongs the baseline partial thromboplastin time (PTT), may require consultation with the coagulation laboratory[41] and use of special assays. Vegetations may resolve with anticoagulation therapy over several months,[42] but may also resolve spontaneously. Patients with APLAS have elevated risk for MI and reocclusion following coronary intervention or bypass grafting. Aggressive prophylactic anticoagulation should be used perioperatively in patients with APLAS and previous thrombosis. Pulmonary hypertension can occur in patients with APLAS secondary to chronic thromboembolic disease, or pulmonary arteriolar intimal proliferation.

DIFFERENTIAL DIAGNOSIS. The differential diagnosis of APLAS includes SLE, thrombocytopenic purpura (TTP), idiopathic thrombocytopenic purpura (ITP), and occult neoplasia. SLE can involve the heart, as discussed earlier. TTP can cause myocardial ischemia, but not valvular disease; occult neoplasia is associated with nonbacterial thrombotic endocarditis.

TREATMENT. The primary therapy of APLAS is anticoagulation, generally to a level similar to that for patients with prosthetic valves. Preliminary studies have supported aspirin treatment for arterial disease, although many clinicians prefer to use warfarin, and prospective trials have indicated that an international normalized ratio (INR) of approximately 2.0 to 2.5 is sufficient (older, retrospective studies

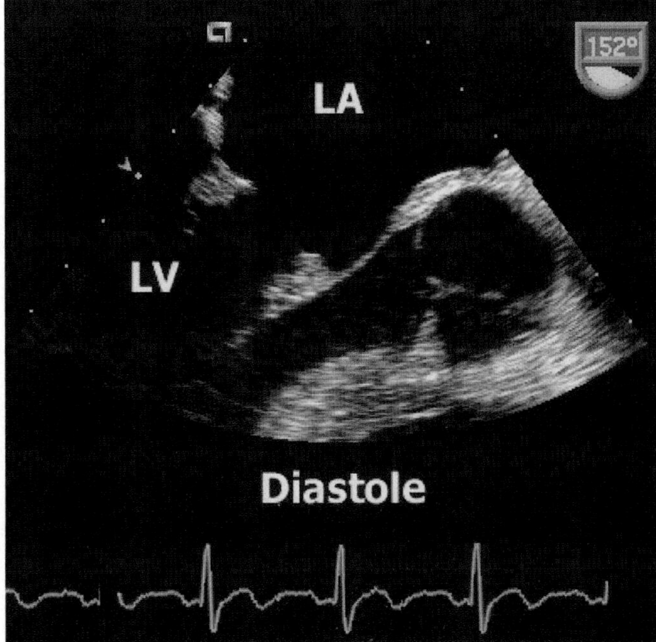

A

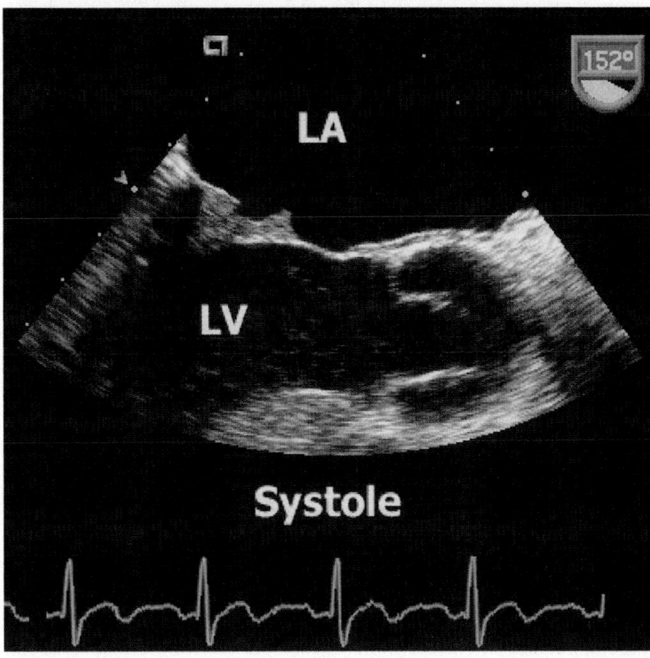

B

FIGURE 89-8 A, B, Transesophageal echocardiogram demonstrating large masses representing sterile vegetations in a 41-year-old male with a previous history of deep venous thrombosis, symptoms of dyspnea on exertion, and a holosystolic apical murmur. A transthoracic echocardiogram demonstrated severe mitral regurgitation. The presence of opposing lesions on both the anterior (right) and posterior (left) leaflets of the mitral valve, also known as kissing vegetations, is characteristic of the anticardiolipin antibody syndrome. *(Courtesy of Dr. Mario Garcia, Cleveland Clinic, Cleveland.)*

had suggested a target INR of 3.0) for venous thrombosis. Monitoring the anticoagulation level can be difficult in the presence of a prolonged PTT, but use of weight-based algorithms or low-molecular-weight heparin while waiting for a full warfarin effect makes this easier. There are no long-term controlled studies on the effect of chronic anticoagulation and valve disease. Valve replacement can be successful in these patients; the indications for surgery are the same as for other patients. The need for lifelong anticoagulation in these patients may influence the choice of valve. Patients with baseline prolonged PT or INR because of the presence of lupus anticoagulant may require that warfarin therapy be monitored by the activity levels of factors II and X.

Scleroderma

Scleroderma (progressive systemic sclerosis [PSS]; CREST syndrome) and its variants are characterized by microvascular occlusive disease with vasospasm and intimal proliferation in conjunction with various patterns of cutaneous and parenchymal fibrosis. Although early lesions are inflammatory, the most obvious clinical manifestations result from enhanced fibrosis.

EPIDEMIOLOGY. Scleroderma is a rare disease. An increased prevalence occurs in certain populations, such as the Choctaw Native Americans. The average onset occurs between 45 and 65 years of age. Children are infrequently affected. Among younger individuals, there is a female bias (approximately 7:1 versus 3:1 for entire scleroderma cohorts).

PATHOGENESIS. The cause of scleroderma is unknown. An increased frequency of autoimmune disorders and autoantibodies in relatives of patients suggests the importance of genetic factors. Nonetheless, scleroderma affects both members of twin pairs extremely rarely, indicating that if inheritance plays a role, it is complex, almost certainly polygenic, and perhaps influenced by environmental factors. The latter view is supported by the association of scleroderma-like conditions with exposure to tainted oils (e.g., rapeseed oil) and drugs (e.g., certain preparations of L-tryptophan).

The earliest lesions are mononuclear infiltrates, primarily T lymphocytes, surrounding small arteries. Endothelial injury and vascular leak probably accounts for the edema seen in the early stages of scleroderma in some patients. Immunocyte and endothelial cell activation yields release of cytokines (e.g., transforming growth factor-β, PDGF, IL-4), stimulating an increase in fibroblast production of extracellular matrix macromolecules, especially types I and III collagen and glycosaminoglycans. Over 90% of patients are ANA-positive in both PSS and the more limited CREST (***c***alcinosis, ***R***aynaud phenomenon, ***e***sophageal dysmotility, ***s***clerodactyly, ***t***elangiectasia) variant.

CLINICAL FEATURES. Raynaud phenomenon usually precedes skin hardening and ultimately occurs in more than 90% of patients, supporting the initial and critical role of vascular dysfunction. Common features among patients with limited CREST or generalized PSS are arthralgias (more than 90%), esophageal dysmotility (more than 80%), telangiectasias (90% with CREST, approximately 60% with generalized disease) and pulmonary fibrosis (35% of CREST, 70% generalized). Renal crisis[43] is 20-fold more common in generalized disease than in CREST (20% versus 1%). Calcinosis may occur in both subtypes, but is twice as common in the CREST variant (40% versus 20%). Generalized PSS is distinguished by proximal cutaneous fibrosis. Thus, the term *limited* is not meant to indicate the absence of risk of visceral disease, but only refers to the distribution of skin involvement. The pattern of visceral involvement differs somewhat between CREST and PSS.

Pericardial involvement is common in PSS, and includes fibrinous pericarditis in up to 70% of patients at autopsy (see Chap. 75).[44] Echocardiography demonstrates small pericardial effusions in less than 40% of patients. Acute pericarditis syndromes, including large effusions, occasionally occur. Pericarditis with effusions may require corticosteroid therapy, but there is concern over the risk of inducing scleroderma renal crisis with the use of corticosteroids.

Necropsy and endomyocardial biopsies have demonstrated the presence of patchy fibrosis, occasionally with contraction band necrosis. These findings may result from intermittent intense ischemia produced by microvascular occlusion, perhaps caused by vasospasm. The epicardial coronary arteries are generally angiographically normal. However, approximately 80% of PSS and 65% of CREST patients have fixed perfusion defects on scintigraphic imaging. MIs can occur in PSS patients who have angiographically normal coronary arteries. Ventricular conduction abnormalities are common and, along with a septal pseudoinfarct pattern, correlate with reduced myocardial function with exercise. Abnormalities can be found throughout the conduction system, and more than 60% of patients have ventricular ectopy. Patients with scleroderma, especially those with a history of palpitations or syncope, are prone to sudden death.[45] The risk of sudden death is further increased in patients with coexistent skeletal myositis. Primary valvular disease is not common. Renal crisis[43] may be associated with minimal or extreme hypertension, rapidly rising creatinine level, microangiopathy, thrombocytopenia, and left ventricular failure. Treatment is with angiotensin-converting enzyme (ACE) inhibitors, and other antihypertensive medications, if needed—not with corticosteroids. The goal is rapid control of the blood pressure in the low-normal range.

Pulmonary hypertension occurs in limited scleroderma and PSS and is a major clinical problem (see Chap. 78). This complication may result from intrinsic pulmonary artery disease or from interstitial fibrosis.[46] Patients with CREST, as well as PSS, should undergo periodic echocardiography to screen for asymptomatic pulmonary hypertension.

DIFFERENTIAL DIAGNOSIS. Initially, before skin hardening occurs, SLE, RA, or severe primary Raynaud disease can be confused with scleroderma. Buerger disease does not lead to thick tight skin and is more often seen in male smokers, but can cause Raynaud phenomenon and digital necrosis (see Chap. 61). Cryoglobulinemia and its primary causes (hepatitis, malignancy, other systemic autoimmune diseases) should be excluded in patients who present with principally vascular symptoms and ischemic lesions. Eosinophilic fasciitis, carcinoid syndrome, nephrogenic sclerosis associated with gadolinium exposure, and several paraneoplastic syndromes can, rarely, also cause some diagnostic confusion. In time, the emergence of features typical of scleroderma usually enables clarification of diagnosis.

TREATMENT. At present, there is no proven effective treatment to limit the progression of PSS. A controlled trial has suggested that cyclophosphamide may slightly slow the progression of pulmonary involvement in some patients. Treatment of Raynaud vasospasm is symptomatic. Gastric reflux is often severe and can be improved by avoiding food and liquid intake before reclining, not assuming a fully horizontal position (wedged pillows for beds or raising the head of the bed), and by aggressive antacid regimens with proton pump inhibitors. Renal crisis usually responds to aggressive control of blood pressure; ACE inhibitors are the initial agents of choice, and the need for renal replacement therapy may be temporary. A few complications (e.g., myositis, alveolitis, pericarditis) may respond to corticosteroids, but steroid use increases the risk for renal crisis. Conduction disease and arrhythmias are treated as they would be in the absence of PSS. Pulmonary hypertension may respond to vasodilator therapy with endothelin antagonists or prostanoids.

Polymyositis and Dermatomyositis

Weakness of proximal more than distal skeletal muscles characterizes polymyositis (PM) and dermatomyositis. The CK level is usually elevated. Respiratory muscles can be clinically involved. Both conditions can be associated with fever, interstitial lung disease, and sometimes myalgias. Other visceral organ involvement is uncommon in adults. Dermatomyositis has characteristic skin lesions, which include extensor surface and extensor tendon erythema; Gottron papules overlying the knuckles, elbows, and knees; edema of the eyelids; and a photosensitive diffuse papular eruption with scaling. Dermatomyositis may be a paraneoplastic syndrome in patients older than 40 years of age.

EPIDEMIOLOGY. The incidence of inflammatory myositis is about 2 to 10 new cases/1,000,000 population annually. People of all races and ethnicities may develop PM or dermatomyositis. There is a female dominance of 2.5:1. In children, there is less sex bias (1:1), but when myositis coexists with other autoimmune diseases (e.g., SLE, scleroderma—overlap syndromes), the bias is enhanced (10:1 females). When myositis coexists with malignancy in the adult population (mean age, 60 years), it is not sex-biased. Inflammatory myositis can affect patients of all ages. Juvenile dermatomyositis has no association with malignancy, but may be associated with arteritis, which can cause bowel ischemia.

PATHOGENESIS. The cause of these disorders is unknown. Involved muscles are infiltrated with lymphocytes, and the lymphocyte subsets and histopathologic pattern of inflammation differ between the two disorders. PM is characterized by endomysial mononuclear cell infiltration, although in dermatomyositis there is a greater amount of perivascular inflammation and perifascicular atrophy is seen. Autoantibodies are demonstrable, and certain antibody profiles may be associated with specific clinical patterns of presentation of PM and response to therapy; currently, however, these autoantibodies cannot be used to dictate therapeutic decisions.

CLINICAL FEATURES. Both diseases affect skeletal muscle, but can also affect the heart. Pericarditis is not common but can occur when polymyositis occurs as part of an overlap syndrome with other autoimmune diseases, such as SLE or PSS. Localized or generalized myocardial dysfunction is common by echocardiographic assessment, but infrequently causes clinical heart failure. The cardiomyopathy may be steroid-responsive. Corticosteroid myopathy, a complication of treatment that can mimic PM, although with a normal CK level, generally affects skeletal but not respiratory or cardiac muscle. PM and dermatomyositis frequently affect the conduction system. In an electrocardiographic study of 77 patients, 23% had conduction block,[47] which can occur in the absence of cardiomyopathy. Pulmonary hypertension can occur, but is usually related to interstitial lung disease. Acute alveolitis can at times mimic acute heart failure. Acute dysphagia caused by muscle dysfunction can predispose to aspiration.

DIFFERENTIAL DIAGNOSIS. PM causes a chronically elevated CK level and/or proximal weakness. Statin therapy can cause myopathy, and occasionally an elevated CK level, and thus can mimic PM. Myalgias are more common than in PM, and weakness less common in statin-associated myopathy. Other drugs (e.g., colchicine, hydroxychloroquine, azidothymidine [AZT]) can also induce elevations in the CK level, and drug-induced myopathy should always be considered before proceeding with diagnostic tests for PM (e.g., electromyography, biopsy). Hypothyroidism can mimic PM. Inclusion body myositis causes an elevated CK level, but usually is more indolent than PM and frequently also involves the distal muscles. The distinction is important, because it is less responsive to therapy. Polymyalgia rheumatica is not associated with an increase in muscle enzyme levels or weakness, but causes proximal muscle stiffness and pain. Dermatomyositis is recognized by one of several characteristic rashes, although SLE can mimic the rash in some patients.

TREATMENT. There are no controlled trials to guide treatment decisions. Nonetheless, initial therapy of inflammatory myositis when an underlying malignancy is not identified includes high doses of daily oral corticosteroids. In severe disease—that is, in the setting of dysphagia or myocarditis—a pulse regimen of several grams of methylprednisolone is often prescribed. Many clinicians frequently use a second agent (e.g., methotrexate, azathioprine, cyclosporine, tacrolimus) along with corticosteroids from the outset or if the patient demonstrates a chronic requirement for high-dose corticosteroid therapy. Long-term immunosuppressive therapy is frequently required. Refractory cases may respond to the addition of monthly high-dose IVIG therapy (~2 g/kg).

Sarcoidosis

Sarcoidosis is a granulomatous inflammatory disease of unknown cause that primarily affects the lung parenchyma, but can cause

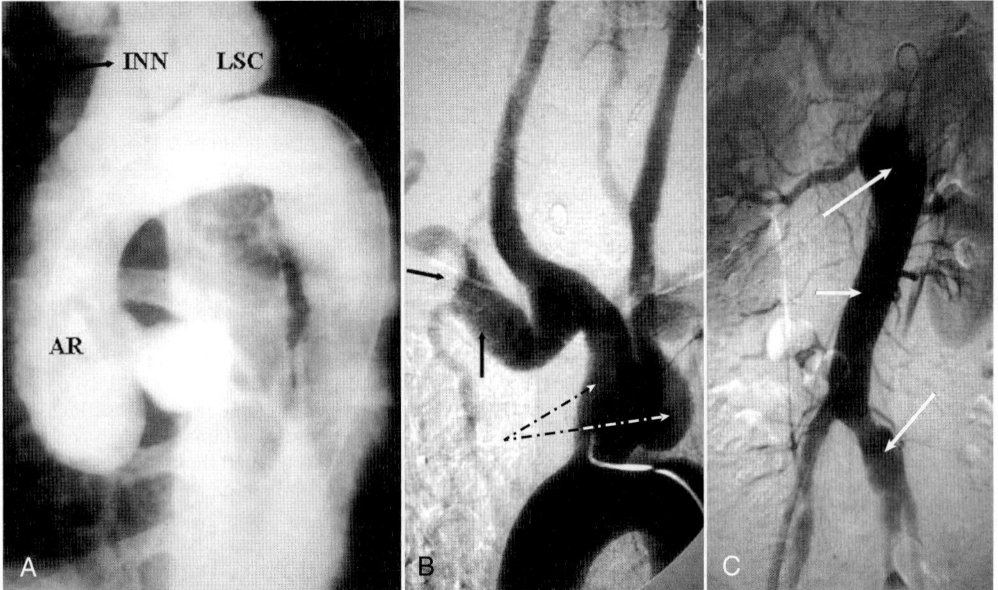

FIGURE 89-9 Sarcoid vasculitis shown in this aortogram from a 20-year-old black man who presented with chronic polyarthritis, uveitis, Bell's palsy, and upper extremity claudication. The angiogram shows aneurysmal dilation of the innominate and proximal subclavian arteries (dashed arrows), the entire aortic root (AR; **A**), occlusion of both subclavian vessels (arrows) associated with arm claudication **(B),** and stenosis of the iliac vessels **(C).** Note how sarcoid vasculitis can mimic TA. However, TA is associated with stenoses three to four times more often than aneurysms. Therefore, this angiographic picture should raise the differential diagnosis of TA. INN = innominate artery; LSC = left subclavian artery.

adenopathy, arthropathy, myositis, fever, renal, CNS, liver, skin, eye, aortitis, and cardiac disease.

EPIDEMIOLOGY. Sarcoidosis can affect men and women of all ages; peak incidence is in the second to fourth decade. The prevalence varies with the degree of vigilance applied to screening and susceptibility of populations. Consequently, in Sweden, the prevalence is 64/100,000, although in the United States it has variably been reported as 10 to 40/100,000. The manifestations of the disease are seemingly different in different populations. Scandinavians seem more predisposed to acute sarcoid (Löfgren syndrome). There is a preponderance of cases with cardiac involvement reported from Japan. Blacks and Hispanics seem more prone to severe multisystem disease.

PATHOGENESIS. The cause of sarcoidosis is unknown. A multicenter U.S. study has found limited evidence to support an environmental or occupational exposure cause. In contrast, studies have linked infectious agents, including mycobacterial and propionibacterial organisms, with sarcoidosis. Evidence of polyclonal B-cell activation in the blood and several reports of transmission of sarcoidosis to recipients of organs donated by patients with sarcoidosis have also supported the presence of a transmissible agent, despite the generally successful use of immunosuppressive therapy. There is evidence for a genetic predisposition to sarcoidosis, including familial clustering and shared HLA haplotypes in different populations. Some data link TNF to the pathogenesis of sarcoidosis—hence, the use of anti-TNF therapies for severe manifestations. Scarring from granulomatous inflammation may result in a focus for arrhythmia.

CLINICAL FEATURES. Pericarditis has been described and necropsy studies have documented cardiac involvement in 27% of patients. Clinically significant pericarditis is uncommon. The granulomatous infiltrative disease of the myocardium is often asymptomatic, but can cause arrhythmias, conduction disease and, rarely, otherwise unexplained congestive heart failure (see Chap. 70). Granulomatous infiltration may be patchy, with a predilection toward involvement of the left ventricle, particularly the upper septal area. This distribution influences the likelihood of obtaining a diagnostic right-sided endomyocardial biopsy. MRI with gadolinium may be helpful in determining and the need for and duration of immunosuppressive therapy, but this approach has not been proven in any formal trial (see Chap. 18 and Fig. 18-13). Sarcoid-dilated cardiomyopathy may be difficult to distinguish from idiopathic cardiomyopathy or occasionally from giant cell myocarditis. Conduction disease is more common than pump dysfunction in patients with sarcoidosis.[48] Biopsy may help distinguish sarcoidosis from idiopathic or giant cell myocarditis, but the diagnostic yield of endomyocardial biopsy is low.[49] Active sarcoidosis is generally believed to be steroid-responsive. However, myocardial involvement with sarcoid can result in large patches of fibrotic scar that may be arrhythmogenic and not responsive to steroids.

Pulmonary artery hypertension and cor pulmonale can occur in sarcoidosis, generally as a result of pulmonary fibrosis. Systemic vasculitis is an uncommon complication of sarcoidosis. Its prevalence remains unknown. Sarcoid vasculitis can affect small- to large-caliber vessels, including the aorta. The latter presentation can be easily confused with Takayasu arteritis (**Fig. 89-9**). Black patients appear predisposed to developing large-vessel involvement.

DIFFERENTIAL DIAGNOSIS. Clinically, there are many mimics of systemic sarcoidosis, including chronic viral hepatitis, granulomatous hepatitis, SLE, Still disease, lymphoma, HIV infection, fungal infections, and Sjögren syndrome. When tissue specimens are available, special stain and culture assays should be performed to seek fungal and mycobacterial infection. The ACE level should not be relied on as a diagnostic test. Cardiac sarcoidosis is usually diagnosed by the presence of otherwise unexplained cardiomyopathy or conduction disease in the presence of documented pulmonary or hepatic sarcoidosis. Patients thought to have arrhythmogenic right ventricular dysplasia have a high (15%) prevalence of probable sarcoidosis on biopsy.

TREATMENT. Although corticosteroid therapy may be palliative for all forms of sarcoidosis, including vasculitis, relapses of the disease are common and may preclude total withdrawal of treatment. Myocardial involvement is generally treated with long-term therapy, and frequently steroid-sparing therapies such as methotrexate are added empirically. Morbidity from disease and treatment is common. There are no controlled trials of therapeutic interventions in cardiac sarcoidosis, and specifically there is no evidence to guide the duration of therapy. The serum ACE level is an imperfect guide to therapy.

Because ventricular arrhythmias may result from scarring, they may not respond to anti-inflammatory therapies and may require an implantable device.

Cardiovascular Risk in Rheumatic Diseases

Systemic rheumatic diseases have been associated with increased cardiovascular (CV) morbidity and mortality and a high prevalence of subclinical atherosclerosis. These chronic inflammatory diseases may share some pathogenic pathways with atherosclerosis, a disease that shares inflammatory mechanisms.

Patients with RA have an increased mortality rate as compared with the general population,[50] mostly attributable to cardiovascular disease (CVD), with a relative risk of at least 2 compared with age-matched normal controls. The risk remains similar after adjusting for known and potential CV risk factors.[51,52] Coronary artery atherosclerosis, as detected by the presence of calcification on cardiac computed tomography (CT) of the coronary arteries (see Chap. 19), appears more severe and prevalent in patients with RA present for more than 10 years than in those with early RA (<5 years) and control subjects.[53] Subclinical atherosclerosis detected as an increase in the intima-media thickness of the carotid artery was also higher in patients with RA than in controls.[54] Excess CV morbidity, with increased prevalence of MI and congestive heart failure, and a higher event fatality, also occurs in RA. The cause of increased atherosclerosis in patients with RA is not known and cannot be explained solely by traditional CV risk factors. Epidemiologic studies have not shown a strikingly higher prevalence of traditional CV risk factors in patients with RA, and corticosteroid use does not explain the increased risk, although dyslipidemia may precede the development of clinical RA. RA may be associated with proatherogenic lipid profiles such as low total and high-density lipoprotein (HDL) cholesterol and high triglyceride levels, a pattern that is associated with a more atherogenic low-density lipoprotein particle.[55] HDL in patients with RA may not exert antioxidant activity and thus may not be protective.[56] Inflammation may contribute to the increased CVD in RA. Elevated systemic levels of proinflammatory cytokines as seen in RA may promote the development of atherosclerosis. Patients with more severe and active RA, advanced joint damage, extra-articular disease, and rheumatoid factor positivity appear to have a higher risk of CV mortality.[57-59] Other confounding risk factors in patients with RA include use of selective or nonselective NSAIDs, underusage of aspirin, and use of corticosteroids, which may accelerate atherosclerosis. The observation that psoriasis and psoriatic arthritis also increase CVD and the possibility that anti-inflammatory therapies may reduce CVD risk strengthen the argument that systemic inflammation (or its mediators) exacerbates atherosclerotic CVD.

The use of disease-modifying agents may reduce risk for heart failure hospitalization in RA patients.[60] Despite the known proatherogenic effects of corticosteroids, they may actually decrease the risk for CV complications in RA by decreasing inflammation. Given the limited interventional data, aggressive prevention and treatment of traditional risk factors and suppression of systemic inflammation in RA are reasonable goals.

Premature MI in patients with SLE, observed in 1976 by Urowitz and colleagues, still occurs.[61] Patients with SLE have significantly increased morbidity and mortality from CVD. The incidence of CAD in SLE patients has been estimated to be 50-fold higher than in age- and sex-matched controls without SLE. In several studies, CVD led the causes of death in patients with SLE.[62-64]

MI may be the initial manifestation of CAD in young patients with SLE. The prevalence of subclinical CAD is high, as determined by scintigraphy, cardiac CT, and autopsy studies. Evidence is increasing that traditional CV risk factors do not fully account for the increased rate of atherosclerosis in these patients, and the disease appears to be an independent risk factor. Atherosclerosis in SLE has been associated with longer duration of disease and less aggressive immunosuppressive therapy.[65] Dyslipidemia with raised triglyceride and lipoprotein(a) levels and nonprotective forms of HDL have been described in patients with SLE.[66] Treatment of SLE patients should include close monitoring and aggressive management of traditional risk factors for CVD.

Many studies have evaluated the risk of CVD in hyperuricemic patients, and a small number of studies have suggested an association between clinical gout and CVD. Data from two large prospective studies have suggested an independent association of gout with CVD and mortality.[67,68] Individuals with gout have a higher risk of death from all causes. Among men without preexisting CAD, the increased mortality risk is primarily caused by an elevated risk of CV death. The mechanism for excess risk of CV death is not clear. Although a cause-and-effect relationship between gout and cardiovascular disease cannot be determined from current data, patients with gout should have aggressive management of CV risk factors. The components of the metabolic syndrome are extremely common in patients with gout.[69] Animal and a few human studies have demonstrated a direct role for hyperuricemia in causing hypertension.

Nonsteroidal Anti-Inflammatory Drugs and the Risk of Cardiovascular Disease

There has been great interest in the CV effect of nonselective NSAIDs and selective COX-2 inhibitors. Published data have supported either a detrimental or salubrious effect on CV events. Initially, attention was given to the selective COX-2 inhibitors after rofecoxib was shown to increase the risk of major coronary events.[70] Epidemiologic studies have raised concern over the use of NSAIDs and have suggested that these drugs may increase CVD by increasing systolic blood pressure, exacerbating congestive heart failure, antagonizing the beneficial effect of aspirin, or promoting thrombosis.[71] Despite anti-inflammatory and (generally reversible) antiplatelet effects, the nonselective NSAIDs do not seem to protect against MI. Instead, one large-population, case-control study has shown an increased risk of MI with the use of rofecoxib, diclofenac, and ibuprofen, even when adjusted for many potential confounders.[72] Another large population-based, matched, case-control study has found that traditional NSAIDs and COX-2 inhibitors are associated with an increased risk of first MI of approximately 40%.[73] A major potential confounder in nonrandomized studies is related to the study populations. Many patients may have an increased baseline risk of CVD and, without appropriate control data, even randomized trials are difficult to interpret. In addition, the timing of exposure of patients to the drugs, in relation to the cardiac event, is often unclear.

In contrast, the use of naproxen is associated with reduced rates of CVD events in patients with RA, and a meta-analysis of observational studies has suggested a modest CVD protective association with naproxen.[74] In a relatively small cohort of patients with early inflammatory polyarthritis, NSAID use was not associated with increased risk of all-cause mortality or CV mortality. Patients who were exposed to NSAIDs tended to have a lower risk of dying than patients who did not receive NSAIDs. This relationship was particularly strong for CV mortality, and ever being exposed to NSAIDs was associated with a 2.5-fold reduction in the risk of CV death. Control of inflammation may result in a beneficial effect on the CV system, although the anti-inflammatory efficacy of these drugs in the doses used is arguable. The study did not show any further CVD benefit from increasing duration of NSAID exposure. Despite the lack of evidence of a true cardioprotective effect of NSAIDs, this study suggested that NSAID use alone does not explain the increased risk of CVD in patients with arthritis.[75]

Despite the concerns from observational and a few prospective trials, the absolute risk of an NSAID inducing a cardiovascular event in a given patient seems to be low, and the benefits of pain reduction must be taken into consideration. Nonetheless, when using NSAIDS, their tendency to increase blood pressure and water retention, cause renal insufficiency, and induce gastropathy and enteritis must always be taken into consideration.

Acknowledgment

We gratefully acknowledge the contributions of Dr. Gary S. Hoffman to an earlier version of this chapter, and to our understanding of the vasculitic disorders.

REFERENCES

Takayasu Arteritis

1. Kerr GS, Hallahan CW, Giordano J, et al: Takayasu's arteritis. Ann Intern Med 120:919, 1994.
2. Hashimoto Y, Tanaka M, Hata A, et al: Four years follow-up study in patients with Takayasu arteritis and severe aortic regurgitation; assessment by echocardiography. Int J Cardiol 54(Suppl):173, 1997.
3. Seko Y, Sato O, Takagi A, et al: Restricted usage of T-cell receptor V alpha-V beta genes in infiltrating cells in aortic tissue of patients with Takayasu's arteritis. Circulation 93:1788, 1996.
4. Maksimowicz-McKinnon K, Clark TM, Hoffman GS: Takayasu's arteritis: Limitations of therapy and guarded prognosis in an American cohort. Arthritis Rheum 56:1000, 2007.
5. Tso E, Flamm SD, White RD, et al: Takayasu's arteritis: Utility of magnetic resonance imaging in diagnosis and treatment. Arthritis Rheum 46:1634, 2002.
6. Webb M, Chambers A, Al-Nahhas A, et al: The role of F-FDG PET in characterizing disease activity in Takayasu arteritis. Eur J Nucl Med Mol Imaging 31:627, 2004.
7. Arnaud L, Haroche J, Malek Z, et al: Is ^{18}F-Fluorodeoxyglucose positron emission tomography scanning a reliable way to assess disease activity in Takayasu arteritis? Arthritis Rheum 60:1193, 2009.
8. Pfizenmaier DH, Al Atawi FO, Castillo K, et al: Predictor of left ventricular dysfunction in patients with Takayasu's arteritis or giant cell aortitis. Clin Exp Rheumatol 22(Suppl 36):S41, 2004.
9. Hoffman GS, Leavitt RY, Kerr GS, et al: Treatment of Takayasu's with methotrexate. Arthritis Rheum 37:578, 1994.
10. Hoffman GS, Merkel PA, Brasington RD, et al: Anti-tumor necrosis factor therapy in patients with difficult to treat Takayasu arteritis. Arthritis Rheum 50:2296, 2004.
11. Molloy ES, Langford CA, Clark TM, et al: Anti-tumour necrosis factor therapy in patients with refractory Takayasu arteritis: long-term follow-up. Ann Rheum Dis 67:1567, 2008.

Giant Cell Arteritis

12. Weyand CM, Goronzy JJ: Medium and large vessel vasculitis. N Engl J Med 349:160, 2003.
13. Evans JM, O'Fallon WM, Hunder GG: Increased incidence of aortic aneurysm and dissection in giant cell (temporal) arteritis. Ann Intern Med 122:502, 1995.
14. Hoffman GS, Cid MC, Rendt-Zagar KE, et al: Infliximab-GCA Study Group: Infliximab for maintenance of glucocorticosteroid-induced remission of giant cell arteritis: a randomized trial. Ann Intern Med 146:621, 2007.
15. Hoffman GS, Cid MC, Hellmann DB, et al: A multicenter, randomized, double-blind, placebo-controlled trial of adjuvant methotrexate treatment for giant cell arteritis. Arthritis Rheum 46:1309, 2002.
16. Nesher GN, Berkun Y, Mates M, et al: Low-dose aspirin and prevention of cranial ischemic complications in GCA. Arthritis Rheum 50:1332, 2004.
17. Lee MS, Smith SD, Galor A, Hoffman GS: Antiplatelet and anticoagulant therapy in patients with giant cell arteritis. Arthritis Rheum 54:3306, 2006.

Idiopathic Aortitis

18. Rojo-Leyva F, Ratliff N, Cosgrove DM, Hoffman GS: Study of 52 patients with idiopathic aortitis from a cohort of 1,204 surgical cases. Arthritis Rheum 43:901, 2000.

Kawasaki Disease

19. Newburger JW, Takahashi M, Gerber MA, et al: Diagnosis, treatment, and long-term management of Kawasaki disease: A statement for health professionals from the Committee on Rheumatic Fever, Endocarditis and Kawasaki Disease, Council on Cardiovascular Disease in the Young, American Heart Association. Circulation 110:2747, 2004.
20. Davis RL, Waller PL, Mueller BA, et al: Kawasaki syndrome in Washington state: Race-specific incidence rates and residential proximity to water. Arch Pediatr Adolesc Med 149:66, 1995.
21. Barron K: Kawasaki disease: Etiology, pathogenesis and treatment. Cleve Clin J Med 69(Suppl 2): 69, 2002.
22. Barron KS: Kawasaki disease. *In* Hoffman GS, Weyand CM (eds): Inflammatory Disease of Blood Vessels. New York, Marcel Dekker, 2002, pp 305-319.

Churg-Strauss Syndrome and Polyarteritis Nodosa

23. Watts RA, Scott DG, Lane SE: Epidemiology of Wegener's granulomatosis, microscopic polyangiitis, and Churg-Strauss syndrome. Cleve Clin J Med 69 (Suppl 2):SII84, 2002
24. deLeeuw K, Sanders J-S, Stegeman C, et al: Accelerated atherosclerosis in patients with Wegener's granulomatosis. Ann Rheum Dis 64:753, 2005.
25. Faurschou M, Mellemkjaer L, Sorensen IJ, et al: Increased morbidity from ischemic heart disease in patients with Wegener's granulomatosis. Arthritis Rheum 60:1187, 2009.

Rheumatoid Arthritis

26. Kitas G, Banks MJ, Bacon PB: Cardiac involvement in rheumatoid disease. Clin Med 1:18, 2001.
27. Sarzi-Puttini P, Atzeni F, Shoenfeld Y, Ferraccioli G: TNF-alpha, rheumatoid arthritis, and heart failure: A rheumatological dilemma. Autoimmun Rev 4:153, 2005.

HLA-B27–Associated Spondyloarthropathies

28. Bergfeldt L: HLA-B27–associated cardiac disease. Ann Intern Med 127:621, 1997.
29. Roldan CA, Chavez J, Wiest PW, et al: Aortic root disease associated with ankylosing spondylitis. J Am Coll Cardiol 32:1397, 1998.
30. Brunner F, Kunz A, Weber U, Kissling R: Ankylosing spondylitis and heart abnormalities: Do cardiac conduction disorders, valve regurgitation and diastolic dysfunction occur more often in male patients with diagnosed ankylosing spondylitis for over 15 years than in the normal population? Clin Rheumatol 25:24, 2005.

Systemic Lupus Erythematosus

31. Moder KG, Miller TD, Tazelaar HD: Cardiac involvement in systemic lupus erythematosus. Mayo Clin Proc 74:275, 1999.
32. Laganà B, Schillaci O, Tubani L, et al: Lupus carditis: Evaluation with technetium-99m MIBI myocardial SPECT and heart rate variability. Angiology 50:143, 1999.
33. Finkelstein Y, Adler Y, Harel L, et al: Anti-Ro (SSA) and anti-La (SSB) antibodies and complete congenital heart block. Ann Intern Med 148:204, 1997.
34. Roldan CA, Shively BK, Crawford MH: An echocardiographic study of valvular heart disease associated with systemic lupus erythematosus. N Engl J Med 335:1424, 1996.
35. Fluture A, Chaudhari S, Frishman WH: Valvular heart disease and systemic lupus erythematosus: Therapeutic implications. Heart Dis 5:349, 2003.
36. Perez-Villa F, Font J, Azqueta M, et al: Severe valvular regurgitation and antiphospholipid antibodies in systemic lupus erythematosus: A prospective, long-term follow-up study. Arthritis Rheum 53:460, 2005.
37. Johnson SR, Gladman DD, Urowitz MB, et al: Pulmonary hypertension in systemic lupus. Lupus 13:506, 2004.
38. Ohara N, Myiata T, Kurata A, et al: Ten years' experience of aortic aneurysm associated with systemic lupus erythematosus. Eur J Vasc Endovasc Surg 19:288, 2000.

Antiphospholipid Antibody Syndrome

39. Hojnik M, George J, Ziporen L, Shoenfeld Y: Heart valve involvement (Libman- Sacks endocarditis) in the antiphospholipid syndrome. Circulation 92:1579, 1996.
40. Lim W, Crowther MA, Eikelboom JW: Management of antiphospholipid antibody syndrome: A systematic review. JAMA 295:1050, 2006.
41. Bartholomew J: Dosing of heparin in the presence of a lupus anticoagulant. J Clin Rheumatol 4:307, 1998.
42. Agirbasli MA, Hansen DE, Byrde BF: Resolution of vegetations with anticoagulation after myocardial infarction in primary antiphospholipid syndrome. Echocardiography 10:877, 1997.

Scleroderma

43. Rhew EY, Barr WG: Scleroderma renal crisis: New insights and developments. Curr Rheumatol Rep 6:129, 2004.
44. Byers RJ, Marshall DAS, Freemont AJ: Pericardial involvement in systemic sclerosis. Ann Rheum Dis 45:393, 1997.
45. Kahan A, Coghlan G, McLaughlin V: Cardiac complications of systemic sclerosis. Rheumatology 48(Suppl 3):iii45, 2009.
46. Chang B, Schachna L, White B, et al: Natural history of mild-moderate pulmonary hypertension and the risk factors for severe pulmonary hypertension in scleroderma. J Rheumatol 33:269, 2006.

Polymyositis and Dermatomyositis

47. Stern R, Godblold J, Chess Q, Kagen L: ECG abnormalities in polymyositis. Arch Intern Med 144:2185, 1984.

Sarcoidosis

48. Kim Jessica SD, Hudson MA, Donnino R, et al: Cardiac sarcoidosis. Am Heart J 157:9, 2009.
49. Uemura A, Morimoto SI, Hiramissu S, et al: Histological diagnostic rate of cardiac sarcoidosis: Evaluation of endomyocardial biopsies. Am Heart J 138:299, 1999.
50. Avina-Zubieta JA, Choi HK, Sadatsafavi M, et al: Risk of cardiovascular mortality in patients with rheumatoid arthritis: A meta-analysis of observational studies. Arthritis Rheum 59:1690, 2008.
51. del Rincon ID, Williams K, Stern MP, et al: High incidence of cardiovascular events in a rheumatoid arthritis cohort not explained by traditional cardiac risk factors. Arthritis Rheum 44:2737, 2001.
52. Solomon DH, Karlson EW, Rimm EB, et al: Cardiovascular morbidity and mortality in women diagnosed with rheumatoid arthritis. Circulation 11:1307, 2003.
53. Chung CP, Oeser A, Raggi P, et al: Increased coronary-artery atherosclerosis in rheumatoid arthritis. Arthritis Rheum 52:3045, 2005.
54. Salmon JE, Roman MJ: Subclinical atherosclerosis in rheumatoid arthritis and systemic lupus erythematosus. Am J Med 121:S3, 2008.
55. Nurmohamed MT: Atherogenic lipid profiles and its management in patients with rheumatoid arthritis. Vasc Health Risk Manag 3:845, 2007.
56. Nurmohamed MT, Dijkmans BAC: Dyslipidemia, statins and rheumatoid arthritis. Ann Rheum Dis 68:453, 2009.
57. Gabriel SE, Crowson CS, Maradit-Kremers H, et al: Survival in rheumatoid arthritis: A population-based analysis of trends over 40 years. Arthritis Rheum 48:54, 2003.
58. Navarro-Cano G, del Rincon I, Pogosian S, et al: Association of mortality with disease severity in rheumatoid arthritis, independent of comorbodity. Arthritis Rheum 48:2425, 2003.
59. Gonzalez A, Icen M, Maradit-Kramers H, et al: Mortality trends in rheumatoid arthritis: The role of rheumatoid factor. J Rheumatol 35:1009, 2008.
60. Bernatsky S, Hudson M, Suissa S: Anti-rheumatic drug use and risk of hospitalization for congestive heart failure in rheumatoid arthritis. Rheumatology 44:677, 2005.
61. Urowitz, MB, Bookman AA, Koehler BE, et al: The bimodal mortality pattern of systemic lupus erythematosus. Am J Med 60:221, 1976.
62. Manzi S, Meilahn EN, Rairie JE, et al: Age-specific incidence rates of myocardial infarction and angina in women with systemic lupus erythematosus: Comparison with the Framingham study. Am J Epidemiol 145:408, 1997.
63. Asanuma Y, Oeser A, Shintani AK, et al: Premature coronary artery atherosclerosis in systemic lupus erythematosus. N Engl J Med 349:2407, 2003.
64. Roman MJ, Shanker BA, Davis A, et al: Prevalence and correlates of accelerated atherosclerosis in systemic lupus erythematosus. N Engl J Med 349:2399, 2003.
65. Roman MJ , Crow MK, Lockshin MD, et al: Rate and determinants of progression of atherosclerosis in systemic lupus erythematosus. Arthritis Rheum 56:3412, 2007.
66. Magadmi ME, Ahmad X, Tuskie W et al: Hyperinsulinemia, Insulin resistance and circulating oxidized low density lipoprotein in women with systemic lupus erythematosus. J Rheumol 33:50, 2006.
67. Krishnan E, Baker JF, Furst DE, et al: Gout and the risk of acute myocardial infarction. Arthritis Rheum 54:2688, 2006.

68. Choi HK, Curhan G: Independent impact of gout on mortality and risk for coronary artery disease. Circulation 116:894, 2007.
69. Feig DI, Kang DH, Johnson RJ: Uric acid and cardiovascular risk. N Engl J Med 359:1811, 2008.
70. Bresalier RS, Sandler RS, Quan H, et al: Cardiovascular events associated with rofecoxib in a colorectal adenoma chemoprevention trial. N Engl J Med 352:1092, 2005.
71. Scott PA, Kingsley GH, Scott DL: Non-steroidal anti-inflammatory drugs and cardiac failure: Meta-analyses of observational studies and randomised controlled trials. Eur J Heart Fail 10:1102, 2008.
72. Hippisley-Cox J, Coupland C: Risk of myocardial infarction in patients taking cyclo-oxygenase-2 inhibitors or conventional non-steroidal anti-inflammatory drugs: Population based nested case-control analysis. BMJ 330:1366, 2005.
73. Helin-Salmivaara A, Virtanen A, Vesalainen R, et al: NSAID use and the risk of hospitalization for first myocardial infarction in the general population: A nationwide case-control study from Finland. Eur Heart J 27:1657, 2006.
74. Watson DJ, Rhodes T, Cai B, Guess HA. Lower risk of thromboembolic cardiovascular events with naproxen among patients with rheumatoid arthritis. Arch Intern Med 162:1105, 2002.
75. Goodson NJ, Brookhart AM, Symmons DPM, et al: Non-steroidal anti-inflammatory drug use does not appear to be associated with increased cardiovascular mortality in patients with inflammatory polyarthritis: results from a primary care based inception cohort of patients. Ann Rheum Dis 68:367, 2009.

CHAPTER 90 The Cancer Patient and Cardiovascular Disease

Thomas Force and Ming Hui Chen

Patients with cancer frequently develop complications in the cardiovascular system. These complications can occur as a result of locally invasive disease or distant spread. Pericardial effusions with tamponade and superior vena cava syndrome are relatively common manifestations of advanced cancers. The cardiovascular system can also be affected by indirect complications, most notably hyperviscosity syndromes, resulting from myeloproliferative disorders or leukemias. Finally, several of the therapies used to treat cancer, including radiation, traditional chemotherapeutics, and so-called targeted therapeutics aimed at factors that are causal or that promote cancer growth and metastasis, can also be toxic to the heart and cardiovascular system. Because cardiovascular disease and cancer are common diseases and share common risk factors, they often coexist in patients. It has become increasingly clear that optimal care of oncology patients by cardiologists and oncologists requires an understanding of both disciplines.

Direct Complications of Neoplasia

Cardiac Tumors

Primary tumors of the heart are uncommon and are usually benign (see Chap. 74). Briefly, the classes of primary tumors that involve the heart include myxomas (which account for 25% to 50% of all primary cardiac tumors), papillary fibroelastomas (10%), rhabdomyomas (of which approximately 50% occur in association with tuberous sclerosis), and lipomas and hemangiomas (5% to 10%).[1] Malignant tumors are usually sarcomas (angiosarcoma being most common) or lymphomas, although primary lymphomas of the heart occur much less frequently than secondary involvement.

In contrast, direct extension of tumors, hematogenous spread, and retrograde lymphatic extension to the heart are common.[2] Based on autopsy studies, involvement of the heart or pericardium occurs in 10% to 12% of all patients with malignant neoplasms. Tumors most likely to involve the heart are primary lung tumors (36% of all patients with cardiac involvement). The grouping of lymphoma, leukemia, and Kaposi sarcoma accounts for 20%, breast cancer for 7%, and esophageal cancer for 6%. Most of these involve the heart by direct extension or regional lymphatic invasion. Metastases to the myocardium are much less common and are often caused by hematogenous spread of melanomas or lymphomas (see Figs. 18-18 and 72-4). From 46% to 71% of patients with melanoma have metastases to the myocardium or pericardium. Although a relatively rare cancer, mesotheliomas commonly invade the pericardium (74% of patients) or myocardium (25% of patients). Patients with myocardial metastases of any origin often present with sudden onset of arrhythmia or, more rarely, conduction abnormalities.

Pericardial Involvement (see Chap. 75)

PERICARDIAL EFFUSION. The differential diagnosis of a pericardial effusion in a patient with a known malignant neoplasm includes malignant effusion, radiation-induced or drug-induced pericarditis, idiopathic pericarditis, infectious (including tuberculosis, fungal, or bacterial), and iatrogenic secondary to procedures. In one series, approximately 40% of patients with cancer and a pericardial effusion were found to have either radiation-induced (10%) or idiopathic (32%) effusions,[2] although other series have reported even higher rates.[3] Drug-induced pericarditis is typically seen after high-dose anthracycline or cyclophosphamide therapy (see later, Cardiovascular Complications of Cancer Therapeutic Agents).

CARDIAC TAMPONADE. Approximately one third of patients with pericardial involvement will present with impaired cardiac function, and cardiac compression can progress to tamponade, demanding immediate drainage. Patients' symptoms include chest pain, fever, dyspnea, cough, and peripheral edema. Tamponade without two or more signs of an inflammatory process (typical pain, friction rub, fever, diffuse ST-segment elevation) is more likely to be malignant (2.9-fold increase in risk).[3] Findings on physical examination, electrocardiography, and chest radiography are typically similar to those of pericardial effusions due to any cause. Echocardiography demonstrates the effusion, which is usually large, although it does not have to be if the fluid has accumulated quickly. However, tamponade can occur with loculated effusions, and in these cases, typical echocardiographic signs may be absent.

The acute treatment of tamponade includes careful fluid replacement as a temporizing measure if the patient is believed to be volume depleted and hemodynamic status is compromised.[3] Echocardiography-guided pericardiocentesis is required. Fluid should be sent for a full battery of diagnostic tests because, as noted, the cause is commonly noncancerous, even in patients with known cancer. If the effusion is malignant, cytologic examination of the pericardial fluid is positive in approximately 85% of patients.

Although no randomized clinical trials of various strategies have been done, the risk of recurrence of the effusion appears to be reduced by extended catheter drainage (3 ± 2 days; 11.5% recurrence) as opposed to simple pericardiocentesis (36% recurrence).[4] Recurrence of pericardial effusion can often be treated with repeated pericardiocentesis with extended catheter drainage. Some have used intrapericardial instillation of chemotherapeutic agents or sclerosing agents, but it is not clear that this approach is more effective than extended catheter drainage. On occasion, percutaneous balloon pericardiotomy or pericardiectomy may be required, but patients with malignant effusions have such a poor prognosis (median survival of

135 days in one series of 275 patients) that invasive procedures should be avoided, if possible. Therapy is directed at the underlying tumor.

CONSTRICTIVE PERICARDITIS. Constrictive or effusive-constrictive pericarditis is a late complication of chest irradiation that may be becoming more common because of the longer survival of patients with breast cancer and Hodgkin disease who typically receive chest irradiation. In a retrospective study of 635 patients with Hodgkin disease, 44 patients developed delayed pericarditis, and pericardiectomy was required in 12.[5] This study included patients who had received mantle irradiation with and without subcarinal block, and rates are lower when blocking is used (see later). The median range for time between radiation therapy and pericardiectomy is 7 to 13 years.[6] In a series of 163 patients undergoing pericardiectomy for constrictive pericarditis of various causes, prior irradiation significantly adversely affected both perioperative mortality (21.4% versus 2.7% for postradiation versus idiopathic constrictive pericarditis) and long-term survival.[3,6] Reasons for this include mediastinal fibrosis from the radiation, which limits the amount of pericardium that can be removed, increasing the risk of residual constriction. In addition, a restrictive myopathy that can follow chest irradiation and can accompany constrictive pericarditis adds significant morbidity and mortality. Patients may have underlying myocardial fibrosis and should be evaluated for this before consideration of pericardiectomy because exclusion of these patients reduces perioperative mortality.[3]

Superior Vena Cava Obstruction

Superior vena cava syndrome (SVCS) occurs when obstruction of the thin-walled superior vena cava (SVC) interrupts venous return of blood to the right atrium from the head, upper extremities, and thorax. The SVC is encircled by lymph nodes that drain from the right thoracic cavity and the lower left thorax (**Fig. 90-1**; see Fig. 16-7). SVCS often is manifested with slowly progressive symptoms worsening during weeks and recruitment of collateral circulation through several venous systems, including the azygos and internal mammary. When symptoms occur abruptly, SVCS can constitute a medical emergency.[7]

SYMPTOMS. Obstruction of the SVC can be caused by malignant or benign disease. Clinically, patients report the progressive development of shortness of breath (60%), facial swelling (50%), cough (24%), arm swelling (18%), chest pain (15%), and dysphagia (9%) as well as distorted vision, hoarseness, nausea, headache, and syncope. Physical findings include venous distention over the neck (66%) and chest wall (54%), facial edema (46%), plethora (19%), and cyanosis (19%). Symptoms may be exacerbated by lying in a supine position or bending forward. Patients with this syndrome may develop life-threatening complications, such as laryngeal or cerebral edema.

CAUSATIVE FACTORS. Seventy-five percent to 85% of cases of SVCS result from neoplasia (**Table 90-1**), with lung cancer

TABLE 90-1 Malignant Neoplasms Associated with Superior Vena Cava Syndrome in Adults*

NEOPLASTIC DIAGNOSIS	PERCENTAGE OF SVCS	DISEASE-ASSOCIATED SVCS (%)
Lung cancer, stage 3B or 4	48-81	
Small cell lung cancer		15-45
Squamous cell cancer		20-25
Adenocarcinoma		5-25
Large cell carcinoma		4-30
Lymphoma	2-21	
Diffuse large cell lymphoma		64
Lymphoblastic lymphoma		33
Breast cancer	11	

*Includes lung cancer, lymphomas, and metastases from other solid tumors; 75% to 85% of patients with SVCS have neoplastic disease.

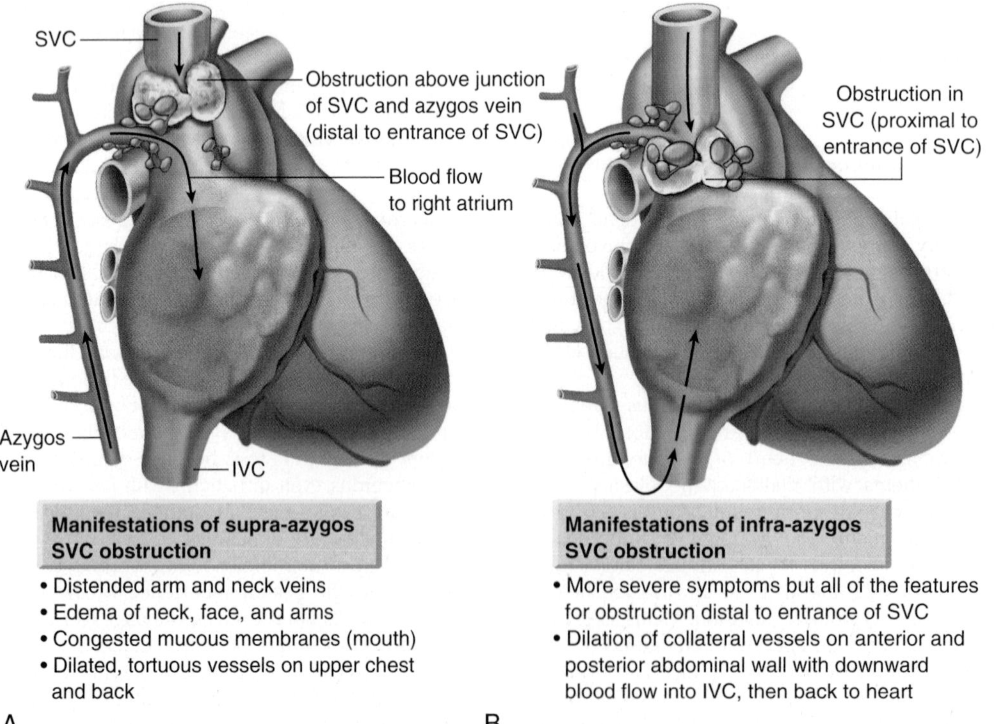

FIGURE 90-1 Anatomy of superior vena cava (SVC) syndrome. Lymph nodes may obstruct blood return above the entrance of the azygos vein **(A)**, resulting in edema of the face, neck, and arms and distended veins in the neck and arms and over the upper chest. Obstruction below the return of the azygos vein **(B)** results in retrograde flow through the azygos through collateral veins to the inferior vena cava (IVC), with all the symptoms and signs in **A** plus dilation of the veins over the abdomen as well. *(Modified from Skatin AT [ed]: Atlas of Diagnostic Oncology. 3rd ed. Philadelphia, Elsevier Science, 2003.)*

accounting for most cases.[7] Of patients with lung cancer, 2% to 5% develop SVCS. However, 10% to 20% of patients with small cell lung cancer (SCLC), which constitutes only 20% of lung cancers, develop SVCS, accounting for almost 40% of patients with SVCS and lung cancer. Of patients with lung cancer–associated SVCS, 80% have right-sided primary lesions.

Lymphoma is the second most common cause of neoplasia-associated SVCS, occurring in 2% to 21% of SVCS patients. Similar to patients with lung cancer, only 1% to 5% of patients with lymphoma develop SVCS (21% of lymphoblastic lymphomas and 7% of diffuse large cell lymphomas). Of patients with primary mediastinal B-cell lymphoma with sclerosis, 57% developed SVCS. Although Hodgkin lymphoma often involves the mediastinum, SVCS rarely develops. Thymoma and germ cell tumors are other primary mediastinal malignant neoplasms that occasionally cause SVCS. The most common metastatic disease that causes SVCS is breast cancer, accounting for 11% of SVCS cases.

DIFFERENTIAL DIAGNOSIS. Benign causes of SVC obstruction not associated with neoplasia result from mediastinal fibrosis caused by radiotherapy or histoplasmosis, tuberculosis, collagen-vascular disease, arteriovenous shunts, or SVC thrombosis as a complication of central venous catheters, pacemaker leads, peritoneovenous shunts, Swan-Ganz catheters, or hyperalimentation catheters. Pacemakers and implantable cardioverter-defibrillators result in up to 30% of local venous thrombosis, in some cases associated with infection; however, SVC obstruction is uncommon and relates to acute or previous lead infection or retention of a severed lead.[8] Other benign causes include granulomas, congenital anomalies, and mediastinal fibrosis from histoplasmosis.

DIAGNOSTIC PROCEDURES. In a patient with characteristic symptoms of SVC obstruction, physical evaluation is usually informative and raises a high level of suspicion. In patients with SVCS caused by neoplasia, 60% lack a prior history of cancer. A mass is generally present on the chest radiograph, with superior mediastinal widening and often pleural effusions. Computed tomography (CT) provides critical additional information. Contrast-enhanced CT can document the presence of obstruction and establish the level, extent, and therapeutic options by mapping collateral and patent vasculature to aid interventional access and to document any pulmonary emboli. Increased use of imaging in patients with cancer has identified many asymptomatic patients with impending SVC obstruction, allowing early radiation therapy to prevent or to delay obstruction. The CT scan can illustrate the strategic relationship of growing tumor masses or the development of nonocclusive, early intraluminal thrombus. Cardiac magnetic resonance imaging (CMR) can also perform this role effectively.

The causes of SVCS include intraluminal, mural, and extraluminal obstruction. Intraluminal causes include bland and neoplastic thrombus as well as direct tumor extension. Bland thrombus is usually associated with intravenous lines or infected pacemaker leads, although it is an uncommon cause of complete occlusion. A paraneoplastic bland thrombus can also occur, and tumor vascularization can be used to differentiate a bland from a neoplastic thrombus. Mural causes include strictures resulting from radiation therapy. Extraluminal causes are usually direct compression by bronchogenic tumors or malignant lymphadenopathy and represent the most common causes detected by imaging.

Because the underlying cause will guide any therapeutic recommendations, obtaining tissue samples to define the cause is essential. Sputum cytology can establish the diagnosis in almost half of patients. Biopsy of enlarged lymph nodes, when present, is frequently a relatively noninvasive method to obtain reliable tissue diagnosis. Thoracentesis can establish the diagnosis of malignancy in 70% of patients with pleural effusions. A diagnosis is made in most of the remaining cases with bronchoscopy, including brushing, washing, and biopsy samples. A marrow biopsy may be diagnostic of lymphoma or SCLC. If the diagnosis remains obscure, percutaneous transthoracic CT-guided fine-needle biopsy is a safe and effective method of diagnosis. When other methods have been unsuccessful, mediastinoscopy has a high diagnostic yield but a somewhat higher risk of complications (5%).

MANAGEMENT. During medical evaluation and before institution of specific therapy, oxygen is administered to reduce the cardiac output and venous pressure; head elevation, diuretics, and a low-salt diet are used to reduce edema. Dehydration increases the risk of further thrombosis, however. In patients with SVCS caused by malignant tumors, radiotherapy and chemotherapy are the most common first-line treatment options. Steroids can, in some cases, decrease inflammation or tumor-associated obstruction but may obscure the diagnosis of lymphoma.

Increasingly, endovascular stenting is proving to provide more rapid and longer lasting relief of the obstruction (see Chap. 63).[9] Stent insertion has a high percentage of technical success, with rapid relief of symptoms. Adjuvant radiation therapy and chemotherapy can be used. Anticoagulation has not been proven to provide benefit in patients with neoplasia-associated SVCS and may interfere with diagnostic biopsies and interventions. Surgical treatment involves the insertion of a bypass graft between the left innominate or jugular vein and the right atrial appendage, with use of an autologous or Dacron graft. However, this operation is very invasive and difficult. In the chronic situation devoid of vascular interventions, patients may develop a network of chest wall and azygos-hemiazygos collateral vessels that effectively restore venous return to the right side of the heart.

Oncologic treatment of SVCS focuses on determining as rapidly as possible the histologic type of the primary lesion so that curative therapy for lymphomas, germ cell tumors, and even SCLC can be instituted or so that palliation for advanced non-SCLCs and other metastatic solid tumors can be provided. The prognosis of patients who present with SVCS depends greatly on the prognosis of the underlying neoplasm. Combination chemotherapy with or without radiation therapy relieves SVCS symptoms within 1 to 2 weeks in patients with newly diagnosed SCLC and lymphoma.

Valvular Heart Disease

Cardiac valves can be involved directly by primary or metastatic tumor, by bacterial or candidal infections, with nonbacterial thrombotic endocarditis, by trauma from semipermanent catheters inserted to facilitate treatment, and as a late effect of radiation therapy (see later, Complications of Radiation Therapy).

Nonbacterial thrombotic endocarditis can be seen in autoimmune disorders and can also complicate the course of various malignant neoplasms, most commonly adenocarcinomas from the gastrointestinal tract and lung.[10] Morbidity and mortality mainly result from systemic embolism. In one study of 200 nonselected ambulatory patients with solid tumors evaluated for evidence of thromboembolic events and for plasma D-dimer levels, 38 patients had cardiac valvular vegetations. The valves affected were mitral (19), aortic (18), and tricuspid (1). Primary lesions were lymphoma (10), lung (9), and pancreatic (3). Thromboembolism to extremities was diagnosed in 4 patients, cerebrovascular accidents were diagnosed in 2, and 4 patients had silent segmental left ventricular (LV) wall motion abnormalities on echocardiography. Nine of 38 patients (24%) with vegetations developed thromboembolism. D-Dimer levels were increased in 19 of 21 patients (90%) with thromboembolism.[10] Treatment of cancer-related nonbacterial thrombotic endocarditis remains difficult.

Ischemic Heart Disease

Given the similar risk factors for certain cancers and coronary artery disease (CAD), especially smoking, particulate matter air pollution, and age, patients will commonly have both diseases. Furthermore, as discussed in detail later, several cancer therapies can be toxic to the cardiovascular system, producing unstable angina, myocardial infarction (MI), and heart failure (HF). Depending on the type and level of aggressiveness of the chosen cancer therapeutic approach and the risk factor profile of the patient, it is reasonable to consider a baseline evaluation for the presence and severity of CAD or LV dysfunction before initiation of the therapy, even in the absence of symptoms or objective signs of disease. Although there are no firm guidelines that address this issue, patients who will receive agents known to induce unstable angina or MI (see later) should probably undergo stress and imaging studies to screen for CAD before treatment.

Arrhythmias

Arrhythmias in cancer patients are caused most commonly by coexisting abnormalities rather than by the cancer itself. Thus, although arrhythmia-inducing metastases to the myocardium or pericardium certainly occur, more commonly arrhythmias will be caused by hypoxemia (as a result of extensive carcinomas of the lung, metastases to the lung, or pulmonary infection), electrolyte imbalances, cardiotoxic radiation and cancer therapeutics, or comorbidities such as chronic obstructive pulmonary disease. Resuscitation of patients with end-stage cancer is often attempted, but the chance of survival is low. In one series, 0 of 171 patients in whom cardiac arrest was anticipated because of worsening metabolic status survived to discharge. In contrast, 22% survived in whom the arrest was not anticipated.[11] These findings highlight the need for careful attention to end-of-life decisions with end-stage patients, thereby avoiding painful and costly interventions that are usually futile.

Indirect Cardiovascular Complications of Neoplasia

Hyperviscosity

Hyperviscosity can result from a number of causes, including erythrocytosis (from polycythemia vera); thrombocytosis, which can be reactive or secondary to a myeloproliferative disorder (essential thrombocytosis); leukocytosis, occasionally seen in acute leukemias; and an increase in plasma protein levels (seen with multiple myeloma and Waldenström macroglobulinemia). For further information on the cardiovascular complications of hyperviscosity and its treatment, see Chap. 90 Online Supplement on the website.

Cardiovascular Complications of Cancer Therapeutic Agents

Drug development in cancer therapeutics has changed more dramatically in the last decade than in any other era. In this section, the cardiovascular toxicity of traditional chemotherapeutic agents and of the newer targeted therapeutic agents are discussed (see Chap. 73).

Traditional Chemotherapeutic Agents

ANTHRACYCLINES. The anthracyclines currently approved in the United States, doxorubicin (Adriamycin), daunorubicin (Cerubidine), epirubicin (Ellence), and idarubicin (Idamycin PFS), are key components of many chemotherapeutic regimens, having demonstrated efficacy in lymphomas and many solid tumors, including breast and SCLC.[12] This class of agents is clearly the most cardiotoxic to date (**Table 90-2**; see Table 73-7), acutely producing arrhythmias, LV dysfunction, and pericarditis and chronically producing LV dysfunction and HF. The toxicity is strongly dose related. Initial retrospective analyses have suggested that the incidence of HF is 2.2% overall and 7.5% in patients receiving a cumulative dose of 550 mg/m^2. However, more recent studies have suggested that the incidence is higher than this.[13] The incidence rises significantly for cumulative doses above 400 to 450 mg/m^2 for doxorubicin. Consequently, for most tumors, oncologists typically limit the dose to 450 to 500 mg/m^2.[12] If patients develop anthracycline cardiomyopathy, it is often within the first year of completing therapy, with a median of 5 to 9 months. However, the cardiomyopathy may be progressive during years.

Risk factors for cardiotoxicity, in addition to doses above 450 mg/m^2, include advanced age, history of cardiac disease, and prior mediastinal irradiation (**Fig. 90-2**). Predictors of cardiotoxicity based on assessment of LV function include a baseline LV ejection fraction (LVEF) less than 50% or a decline in LVEF of more than 10% on treatment to a level less than 50%. Diastolic dysfunction may be the first abnormality noted. Children may be particularly susceptible to anthracycline cardiotoxicity; in one series, 5% developed HF at 15 years of follow-up, and the incidence increased to 10% for cumulative doses of 550 mg/m^2.[14] In addition to dose and mediastinal irradiation, age at diagnosis and female gender are predictors for adverse outcomes in children. Unlike in adults, HF may appear years after treatment has been stopped and may be progressive.[15]

Endomyocardial biopsy is the most sensitive method to detect anthracycline cardiotoxicity, with typical findings being cytosolic vacuolization, lysis of myofibrils, and cellular swelling, findings more typical of a necrotic form of cell death. However, abnormalities on electron microscopy have not been shown to correlate highly with risk for development of HF and are often present in patients at cumulative doses well below those associated with an increased risk of HF. Given the technical nature of the procedure and inherent risks, this is not a practical way to detect or to observe patients with anthracycline cardiotoxicity, and serial determination of LV function, although insensitive, is the currently accepted method.

The cellular mechanisms leading to anthracycline cardiotoxicity remain unclear but are believed, in part, to involve oxidant stress leading to iron oxidation and generation of free radicals that damage cell and organelle membranes through peroxidation of lipids.[16] The oxidized iron hypothesis has led to the use of dexrazoxane (Zinecard), a chelator of intracellular iron. Although the compound does reduce the incidence of cardiotoxicity, concerns were raised in one trial that it might also reduce efficacy of the anthracycline.[17] This was not seen in a later meta-analysis, however, and the drug is approved in the United States. American Society of Clinical Oncology recommendations have suggested that the use of dexrazoxane be limited to patients who have received more than 300 mg/m^2 of doxorubicin or the equivalent.

Other strategies have been used to limit anthracycline cardiotoxicity, including the use of epirubicin, a stereoisomer of doxorubicin. This agent has less cardiotoxicity than doxorubicin at comparable doses, and 900 to 1000 mg/m^2 of epirubicin produces cardiotoxicity comparable to 450 to 500 mg/m^2 of doxorubicin. However, efficacy of the two agents appears to be comparable at equivalent doses. Patients should have a baseline determination of LV function before initiation of anthracycline therapy and should be monitored periodically after that, especially when the cumulative dose rises above 300 to 350 mg/m^2 for doxorubicin or above the comparable doses for the other anthracyclines. The criteria noted earlier concerning risk factors, baseline LV function, and deterioration of LV function, in combination with dosage consideration, can be used to risk stratify patients for the development of HF. Routine use of troponin measurements is not highly predictive except in patients receiving high-dose chemotherapy (for treatment of aggressive malignant neoplasms). In those patients, an elevated troponin I level predicted those going on to develop LV dysfunction with high sensitivity albeit low predictive accuracy. A negative troponin I strongly predicted patients whose LV function would not deteriorate.[18] A recent report has suggested that prophylactic angiotensin-converting enzyme inhibitor therapy in patients with elevated troponin I levels can prevent progression to HF. Earlier studies of anthracycline cardiotoxicity have suggested a high mortality rate, but with more modern approaches to the management of patients with HF, the prognosis is better (see Fig. 90-2).

TAXANES. The taxanes paclitaxel (Taxol) and docetaxel (Taxotere) disrupt microtubular networks as their mechanism of antitumor activity and are effective in breast cancer. Used alone, they have relatively little cardiotoxicity (see Table 90-2). In one large study, cardiac toxicity occurred in 14% of patients, but 76% of these events were asymptomatic bradycardia. Heart block can also occur. However, when paclitaxel is combined with doxorubicin, cardiotoxicity is increased, and 18% of patients developed HF in one trial. This was found to be secondary to retardation of metabolism of the doxorubicin. When paclitaxel was administered 30 minutes after doxorubicin and the

TABLE 90-2 Clinical Syndromes of Cardiotoxicity

PARAMETER	FREQUENCY	COMMENTS
Left Ventricular Dysfunction–Heart Failure		
Chemotherapeutics		
Anthracyclines		
Doxorubicin	+++	Highly dose dependent
Epirubicin	+	Risk factors include age (old and young), prior mediastinal XRT, history of heart disease, decreased EF, drop in EF on drug therapy, female gender (for children), and other agents (especially trastuzumab)
Idarubicin	++	Risk decreased by liposomal encapsulation or dexrazoxane
Alkylating agents		
Cyclophosphamide	+++	Primarily seen with high-dose "conditioning" regimens
Ifosfamide	+++	Risk factors are prior mediastinal XRT or anthracycline drug therapy Also can have myocarditis, pericarditis, myocardial necrosis
Taxanes		
Paclitaxel	+	Also employed in paclitaxel-eluting stent
Docetaxel	+/++	
Proteasome inhibitor		
Bortezomib	+/++	Moderately high rates of HF seen in trials (5%), but rates only minimally higher than in patients receiving dexamethasone
Targeted Therapeutics		
Monoclonal antibodies		
Trastuzumab	++	Not common as single agent Increased risk with anthracyclines, paclitaxel, cyclophosphamide
Pertuzumab	+/++	Targets HER2 Rates of LV dysfunction as high as ~25% in one series
Bevacizumab	+/++	Targets VEGF-A (ligand for VEGFRs) and serves as a trap, not allowing VEGF-A to interact with receptor HF can be seen in setting of severe hypertension, which occurs in 10%-25% of patients, depending on dose; anthracyclines may increase HF risk
Tyrosine kinase inhibitors		
Imatinib, nilotinib	+	Can cause severe fluid retention with peripheral edema, pleural and pericardial effusion not secondary to LV dysfunction
Dasatinib	++	Same as above re fluid retention
Sunitinib	+++	LV dysfunction common; hypertension likely plays role
Ischemic Syndromes		
Fluorouracil, capecitabine	++	ACS; patients with CAD at increased risk Recurs with rechallenge; multiple mechanisms proposed; etiology remains unknown
Cisplatin, carboplatin	+	ACS caused by vasospasm or vascular injury Hypertension common; thromboembolism more common (see below)
Interferon-α	+	Risk of ischemia increased in patients with CAD; hypertension common
Paclitaxel	+	Myocardial ischemia in 1%-5%; serious ischemic cardiac events not common
Docetaxel	+	Limited data but rate probably ~1%
Bevacizumab	++	Arterial thrombotic events not common but occurred in 8.5% of patients >65 yr
Vinca alkaloids	+	~1% risk of cardiac events; ischemia possibly caused by coronary spasm
Sorafenib	+ – ++	~2.5% risk of ACS
Erlotinib	+ – ++	Limited data but rate ~2%
Hypertension		
Cisplatin	++++	
Bevacizumab	++++	Extremely common with all anti-VEGF therapeutics to date
Sunitinib	++++	Intrinsic in mechanism of action of these agents
Sorafenib	++++	
Venous Thrombosis		
Cisplatin	+++	DVT or PE in 8.5%; most occur early in treatment; additional risk factors for DVT are often present
Thalidomide	++++	Uncommon with monotherapy but risk rises with concurrent chemotherapy
Lenalidomide	+++	See comments re thalidomide
Erlotinib	++	Rate with erlotinib plus gemcitabine ~2% over that seen with gemcitabine alone

Relative frequency of the cardiotoxicity is scored as follows: + = ≤1%; ++ = 1% to 5%; +++ = 6% to 10%; ++++ = >10%.
ACS = acute coronary syndromes; CAD = coronary artery disease; DVT = deep venous thrombosis; EF = ejection fraction; HF = heart failure; LV = left ventricular; PE = pulmonary embolism; VEGF = vascular endothelial cell growth factor; VEGFR = vascular endothelial cell growth factor receptor; XRT = radiation therapy.
Modified from Yeh ET, Bickford CL: Cardiovascular complications of cancer therapy: Incidence, pathogenesis, diagnosis, and management. J Am Coll Cardiol 53:2231, 2009.

doxorubicin dose was kept to 360 mg/m^2, the decline in LVEF was greater than that with the combination of doxorubicin plus cyclophosphamide, although the rates of HF were low and not statistically different between the groups.[19] Docetaxel does not retard metabolism of doxorubicin and appears to lead to only a minimal increase in HF.

ALKYLATING AGENTS AND ANTIMETABOLITES. These classes of agents generally have low incidences of cardiotoxicity (see Table 90-2). Cyclophosphamide (Cytoxan) is relatively well tolerated when it is used at conventional doses, but in patients receiving conditioning regimens before autologous stem cell transplantation, which use high-dose cyclophosphamide, acute cardiotoxicity can occur.[20] As opposed to the total cumulative dosage for anthracyclines, dosage of an individual course of treatment is more predictive for cyclophosphamide. Risk factors include prior anthracycline therapy or mediastinal irradiation and possibly prior imatinib therapy.[21] Clinically, patients may present with HF, myocarditis, or pericarditis. In one series of 17 consecutive patients receiving induction therapy, none of whom devel-

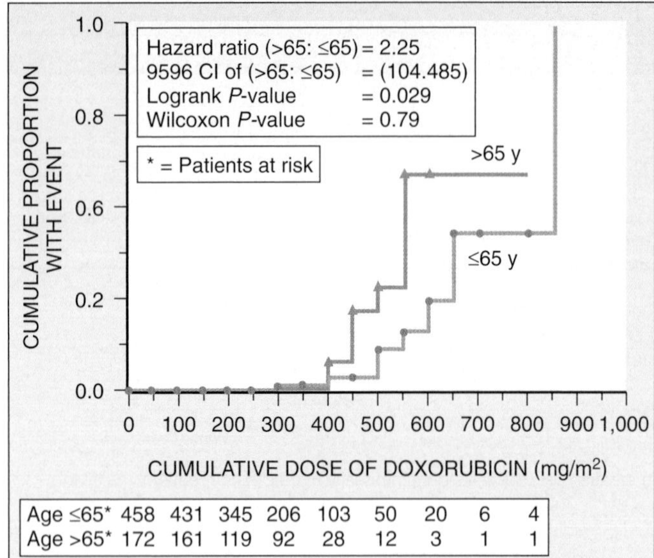

FIGURE 90-2 Risk of doxorubicin-associated congestive heart failure by patient age. This graphically depicts the cumulative doxorubicin dose at the onset of doxorubicin-associated congestive heart failure in 630 patients according to patient age older or younger than 65 years. *(Redrawn from Swain SM, Whaley FS, Ewer MS: Congestive heart failure in patients treated with doxorubicin: A retrospective analysis of three trials. Cancer 97:2869, 2003.)*

oped HF, LV dilation by CMR was evident from the onset.[20] Mechanisms underlying the toxicity are believed to be injury of both endothelial cells and myocytes, and a picture of hemorrhagic myocardial necrosis can emerge. Those who survive the acute phase typically do not have residual LV dysfunction. High-dose ifosfamide (Ifex) induced HF in 17% of patients.[22]

Cisplatin (Platinol)–based regimens are the cornerstone of therapy for testicular germ cell cancer, the most common malignant neoplasm in men aged 20 to 40 years; 80% of those with disseminated nonseminoma achieve long-term survival. Thus, in addition to short-term toxicity, long-term toxicity is a concern in this group. Cisplatin is notable for causing hypertension, which is sometimes severe. Acute chest pain syndromes, including MI, have also been reported, possibly related to coronary spasm. Because cisplatin is often used in combination with bleomycin, an agent that can induce Raynaud phenomenon in approximately one third of patients, long-term vascular toxicity is particularly a concern. Indeed, after a median 10-year follow-up of patients treated with platinum-based regimens (cisplatin or carboplatin [Paraplatin]) versus radiation therapy, 6.7% of patients after chemotherapy and 10% of patients after irradiation suffered a cardiac event, for a relative risk of 2.4- to 2.8-fold compared with patients treated with surgery only. Changes in the ratio of carotid intima-media thickness were detected as early as 10 weeks after a course of cisplatin-based chemotherapy. The morbidity data have led to calls for more conservative approaches to patients at low risk for cancer recurrence.

Fluorouracil (Adrucil) is used in the treatment of many solid tumors, and regimens based on this agent are the mainstay for treatment of colorectal cancer. Fluorouracil can cause acute ischemic syndromes ranging from angina to MI, and this can occur in patients without CAD (approximately 1% of patients), although it is more common in patients with pre-existing disease (4% to 5%). Overall, rates range from 0.55% to 8%, although more sensitive methods of detecting possible subclinical ischemia (ambulatory electrocardiographic monitoring) find much higher rates. Discontinuation of treatment and standard antianginal therapies usually lead to resolution of symptoms, but ischemia often recurs if therapy is reinitiated. An alternative agent, capecitabine (Xeloda), is metabolized to fluorouracil, preferentially in tumor cells, suggesting that it may have less cardiotoxicity. However, one retrospective review (that excluded patients with "significant" cardiac disease) has found an incidence of 6.5% major cardiac events for the combination, including angina (4.6%), MI, ventricular tachycardia, and sudden death.[21] Vasospasm is believed to be the mechanism triggering ischemia, although thromboembolic events are also increased. It is not clear at this point whether prophylactic nitrates prevent ischemic events. Capecitabine monotherapy appears to have a lower incidence of cardiac toxicity compared with fluorouracil monotherapy.

OTHER CHEMOTHERAPEUTIC AGENTS

Tamoxifen

Tamoxifen (Nolvadex) is widely used in the treatment of breast cancer. On the basis of largely experimental data, it had been proposed to have cardioprotective effects. However, in a large trial of 13,388 patients, in women both with and without CAD, tamoxifen therapy did not reduce or increase the incidence of fatal MI, nonfatal MI, unstable angina, or severe angina.[23] Concerns have been raised, however, that stroke risk might be increased somewhat.

Proteasome Inhibitors

Bortezomib (Velcade) is an inhibitor of the proteasome system responsible for degrading improperly folded proteins and proteins that are no longer needed in the cell. The drug is approved for use in patients with multiple myeloma. The concept behind its use is that malignant cells have altered proteins regulating the cell cycle, leading to more rapid cell division and increased accumulation of damaged proteins as a result. Therefore, the continued health of the malignant cell, as opposed to normal cells, may be more dependent on degradation of the damaged proteins. In support of this concept, proteasome inhibitors are more toxic to proliferating malignant cells in culture than to normal cells. Targets include activation of endoplasmic reticulum stress pathways leading to activation of proapoptotic factors and inactivation of survival factors. Cardiomyocytes have an active proteasome system, raising concerns that inhibitors may be cardiotoxic. However, in the phase III trials of bortezomib, HF was reported in 5% of patients but was also reported in 4% of patients in the dexamethasone arm of the trial.[24]

Additional Agents

A discussion of the cardiotoxicity of additional agents, including cytokines (interleukin-2, aldesleukin [Proleukin], and denileukin diftitox) and interferons, histone deacetylase inhibitors (trichostatin A and suberoylanilide hydroxamic acid), topoisomerase inhibitors (etoposide and teniposide), purine analogues (pentostatin and cladribine), all-*trans*-retinoic acid, arsenic trioxide, and thalidomide and lenalidomide, can be found in the Chap. 90 Online Supplement on the website.

Targeted Therapeutics

The treatment of a number of malignant neoplasms has changed radically during the past few years with the advent of so-called targeted therapies. As opposed to traditional chemotherapeutics, which target basic cellular processes present in most cells, these therapies target factors that are specifically dysregulated in cancerous cells. It was hoped that this approach would reduce toxicities typical of standard chemotherapeutics (e.g., alopecia, gastrointestinal toxicity, myelotoxicity) and at the same time be more effective at treating the cancer. In some situations, this has been the case, but concerns about cardiotoxicity have surfaced for some agents.[25,26]

Most of the targeted cancer therapeutics inhibit the activity of tyrosine kinases (**Table 90-3**).[27] Tyrosine kinases (TKs) attach phosphate groups to tyrosine residues of other proteins, thereby changing the activity, subcellular localization, or rate of degradation of the protein. In the normal cell, these wild-type (i.e., normal) tyrosine kinases play many roles in regulating basic cellular functions. However, in leukemias and cancers, the gene encoding the causal (or contributory) TK is amplified (leading to overexpression) or mutated, leading to a constitutively activated state that drives proliferation of the cancerous

TABLE 90-3 Kinase Inhibitors in Cancer, Their Targets, and Representative Malignant Neoplasms

AGENT (TRADE NAME)	Targets: PRIMARY	Targets: OTHER	REPRESENTATIVE MALIGNANT NEOPLASMS
Tyrosine Kinase Inhibitors			
FDA Approved			
Imatinib (Gleevec)	Bcr-Abl	Abl, c-Kit, PDGFRs, DDR1, Cdc2	CML, Ph+ ALL, CMML, HES, GIST
Nilotinib (Tasigna)	Bcr-Abl and most IRMs	Abl, c-Kit, PDGFRs	Imatinib-resistant CML, ALL, GIST
Dasatinib (Sprycel)	Bcr-Abl and most IRMs	Abl, c-Kit, PDGFRs, DDR1, SFKs, EphB4	Imatinib-resistant CML, ALL, GIST
Sunitinib (Sutent)	VEGFRs	*PDGFRs, c-Kit, CSF-1R, FLT3, RET	RCC, GIST
Sorafenib (Nexavar)	VEGFRs	†PDGFRs, c-Kit, FLT3, Raf-1/B-Raf	RCC, hepatocellular carcinoma
Lapatinib (Tykerb)	EGFR (ERBB1), HER2 (ERBB2)	NI	HER2+ breast cancer, ovarian cancer, gliomas, NSCLC
Gefitinib (Iressa)	EGFR	NI	NSCLC, gliomas
Erlotinib (Tarceva)	EGFR	NI	NSCLC, pancreatic cancer, gliomas
Temsirolimus (Torisel)	mTOR	NI	RCC
Everolimus (Afinitor)	mTOR	NI	RCC
Sirolimus (Rapamune)	mTOR	NI	RCC
Projected			
Bosutinib	Bcr-Abl and several IRMs	Abl, SFKs, DDR1, EphB4	Imatinib-resistant CML
Lestaurtinib	JAK2, FLT3	TrkA/B/C	MPD (PCV, ET, IMF), AML
Pazopanib	VEGFR, PDGFR, c-Kit	NK	RCC
Vandetanib	VEGFR, EGFR	NK	NSCLC
Cediranib	VEGFR	NK	Colorectal cancer
Alvocidib	CDK	NK	CLL
Enzastaurin	PKCβ	NK	Diffuse large B-cell lymphoma
Deforolimus	mTOR	NK	RCC, metastatic sarcomas
Monoclonal Antibodies			
Trastuzumab (Herceptin)	HER2/ErbB2	NI	Breast
Pertuzumab (Omnitarg)	HER2/ErbB2	NI	Breast
Bevacizumab (Avastin)	VEGF-A	NI	Colon, renal cell, NSCLC, other

*≥50 targets.
†≥15 targets.
ALL = acute lymphoblastic leukemia; AML = acute myeloid leukemia; CDK = cyclin-dependent kinase; CLL = chronic lymphocytic leukemia; CML = chronic myeloid leukemia; CMML = chronic myelomonocytic leukemia; EGFR = epidermal growth factor receptor; EphB4 = ephrin receptor tyrosine kinase B4; ET = essential thrombocytosis; FDA = Food and Drug Administration; FLT3 = FMS-like tyrosine kinase 3; GIST = gastrointestinal stromal tumors; HES = hypereosinophilic syndrome; IMF = idiopathic myelofibrosis; IRMs = imatinib-resistant Abl mutants; JAK2 = Janus kinase 2; MPDs = myeloproliferative disorders; mTOR = mammalian target of rapamycin; NI = none identified; NK = not known; NSCLC = non–small cell lung cancer; PCV = polycythemia vera; PDGFR = platelet-derived growth factor receptor; Ph+ ALL = Philadelphia chromosome–positive acute lymphocytic leukemia; PKCβ = protein kinase C β; RCC = renal cell carcinoma; RET = rearranged during transfection; SFKs = SRC family kinases; VEGF = vascular endothelial cell growth factor; VEGFR = vascular endothelial cell growth factor receptor.
From Cheng H, Force T: Molecular mechanisms of cardiovascular toxicity of targeted cancer therapeutics. Circ Res 106:21, 2010.

clonal cells or blocks their normal death (see Table 90-3).[27] Inhibition of these kinases could then retard cell proliferation or induce cell death. Cardiotoxicity arises when the normal kinase, which is often present in cardiomyocytes and is also inhibited by the agent, plays a central role in maintenance of cardiomyocyte homeostasis. In some cases, cardiotoxicity of these drugs may be predictable, but usually it is not. This is because the targeted kinase is typically not known to provide an important function in the heart or because of off-target effects (i.e., inhibition of TKs other than those the drug was designed to target). Most tyrosine kinase inhibitors (TKIs) compete with ATP for binding to a pocket in the kinase that is moderately well conserved across many TKs. There are approximately 500 protein kinases in the human genome, of which approximately 90 are TKs. Although these drugs are typically designed to target two to five kinases, in truth it is unusual for this class of drugs to inhibit fewer than 10 kinases, and some in use inhibit 30 or more kinases. Furthermore, there may be several additional TKs that are inhibited and many additional serine or threonine kinases (the other major family) that are inhibited, and these will generally not be known to the oncologist or cardiologist caring for the patient. Therefore, if patients present with HF after initiation of therapy, the possibilities of off-target effects accounting for toxicity versus HF from other causes must be considered.

DRUGS AND THEIR TARGETS. Table 90-3 lists approved TKIs, several others that are well along in development, and the monoclonal antibodies most relevant to the heart. The first molecularly targeted therapies, trastuzumab (Herceptin) and imatinib (Gleevec), illustrate the two general classes of these agents—humanized monoclonal antibodies targeting growth factor receptors on the surface of the cancer cell (trastuzumab) and small molecule inhibitors of receptors or of intracellular pathways regulating growth of the cancer cells (imatinib) (**Fig. 90-3**). All generic names for monoclonal antibodies end in -mab, and all small molecule inhibitors end in -nib.

HER2 Receptor and Its Antagonists: Trastuzumab, Lapatinib, and Pertuzumab

The growth factor receptor HER2 (human epidermal growth factor receptor 2) is amplified in 15% to 30% of breast cancers, and HER2-positive cancers carry a worse prognosis. This amplification, and the resulting overexpression (up to 100-fold) and activation of HER2, both enhances cell cycle progression (and thus proliferation) and inhibits apoptosis of the cancer cells. Trastuzumab is a humanized monoclonal antibody that binds to and inhibits the activity of the HER2 receptor.[25] Treatment with trastuzumab improves survival in patients with metastatic disease and, when used in the adjuvant setting after surgery, reduces recurrences of the cancer.

Trastuzumab is well tolerated as far as its side effect profile. However, it can induce HF in a percentage of patients. The original trials with trastuzumab indicated that 3% to 7% of patients developed LV dysfunction, and this incidence was increased to 27% by concomitant use of doxorubicin (with 16% being New York Heart Association [NYHA] Class III or IV).[25] This is in comparison to rates of 8% total and 3% NYHA Class III or IV HF with anthracyclines plus cyclophosphamide. When trastuzumab was used with paclitaxel, 13% of patients developed cardiotoxicity versus only 1% with paclitaxel alone.

More recently, trastuzumab cardiotoxicity has been analyzed in three key trials in breast cancer patients that assessed efficacy of the agent in the adjuvant setting. In one trial, patients who underwent surgery plus adjuvant or neoadjuvant chemotherapy or radiotherapy were randomized to receive trastuzumab or simply observation. At 1 year of follow-up, 7.1%

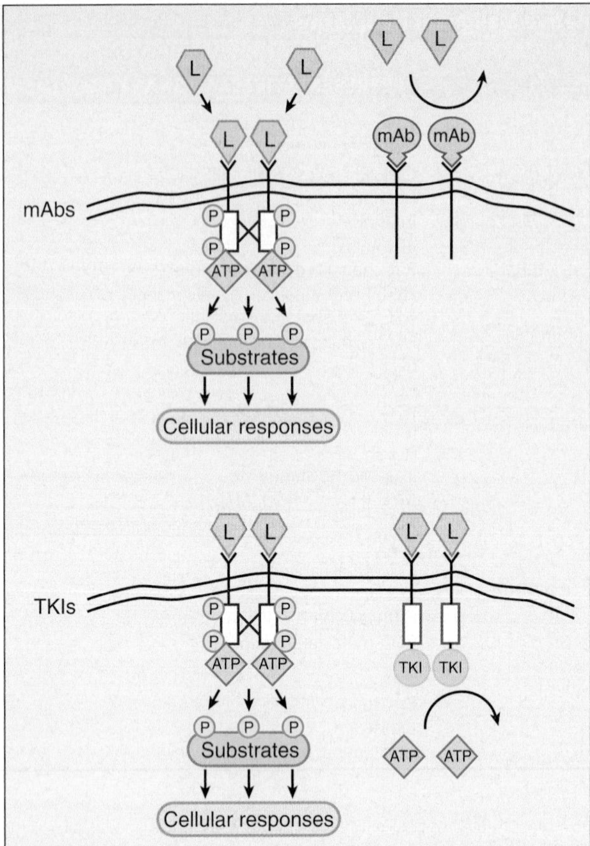

FIGURE 90-3 Mechanisms of action of monoclonal antibodies (mAbs) versus small molecule tyrosine kinase inhibitors (TKIs). Ligand (L) binding to receptor tyrosine kinases leads to receptor dimerization, cross-phosphorylation (purple lines and P), and activation of the intracellular tyrosine kinase domain. Substrates are then phosphorylated, leading to cellular responses. Monoclonal antibodies **(top)** interfere with ligand binding to receptor or receptor dimerization and cross-phosphorylation, blocking activation of the receptor tyrosine kinases.[17] TKIs **(bottom)** do not prevent ligand binding or dimerization. By preventing adenosine triphosphate (ATP) from binding to the kinase domain, they block cross-phosphorylation of receptors and phosphorylation of substrates. *(From Chen MH, Kerkelä R, Force T: Mechanisms of cardiac dysfunction associated with tyrosine kinase inhibitor cancer therapeutics. Circulation 118:86, 2008.)*

of patients in the trastuzumab arm versus 2.2% in the observation arm had significant declines in LVEF, and only 1.7% in the trastuzumab arm versus 0% in the observation arm developed symptomatic HF. These figures represent short-term risks for trastuzumab in otherwise healthy patients with no cardiac morbidities and normal LV function who had received moderate doses of adjuvant chemotherapy and no mediastinal irradiation.

The other two studies, which also excluded patients with a cardiac history and low ejection fraction or a decline in ejection fraction on doxorubicin-cyclophosphamide therapy, examined patients treated with more aggressive regimens. Follow-up was for a mean of 27 months. In this trial, 8.7% of patients in the trastuzumab arm versus 1.6% in the no-trastuzumab arm developed symptomatic HF. Furthermore, 2.2% to 4.1% developed severe HF on trastuzumab versus 0.2% to 0.8% on placebo. The lower rates in these later three trials, compared with earlier studies, reflect not only enrollment of more highly selected patients but also administration of doxorubicin and trastuzumab sequentially rather than concurrently. Even given the lower rates, overall approximately 20% of patients were withdrawn from this trial for cardiac reasons.[28] The more recent trials largely enrolled node-positive patients. However, it is possible that clinical practice will move toward treatment of node-negative patients, for whom the prognostic significance of HER2 positivity is only modest. It will be important to analyze risk-benefit in node-negative patients, in whom even the relatively low rates of HF may outweigh benefits.

MECHANISMS OF TRASTUZUMAB CARDIOTOXICITY. That trastuzumab was cardiotoxic is not altogether surprising because mice in which the HER2 gene (designated ErbB2 in mice) was knocked out developed a dilated cardiomyopathy.[29] Thus, the ErbB2 receptor, at least in mice, appears to serve a "maintenance" function in cardiomyocytes. Furthermore, cardiomyocytes isolated from the knockout hearts were more susceptible to anthracycline toxicity, consistent with the concept that inhibition of HER2 in patients may have amplified the severity of doxorubicin toxicity by preventing repair. Consistent with this, neuregulin, the endogenous ligand for HER2, can decrease anthracycline cardiotoxicity.[16] Cellular mechanisms of the toxicity of ErbB2 inhibition remain a matter of debate.[30] That the story is more complex is underscored by the reported very low rates of LV dysfunction (1.4%) and HF (0.2%) in a review of trials with lapatinib, the TKI that targets HER2.[30] In contrast, the monoclonal antibody pertuzumab, which interferes with dimerization of HER2 with the HER3 receptor, has induced LV dysfunction (defined as a decline in ejection fraction of ≥10%) in as many as 27% of patients.[31] This highlights the point that not all HER2 antagonists appear to be equivalent in inducing LV dysfunction, with lapatinib being the apparent outlier. This apparent difference could be due to the different mechanisms of action of the TKIs versus monoclonal antibodies or to distinct differences in trial design.[30]

NATURAL HISTORY OF TRASTUZUMAB TOXICITY. Debate continues about the degree to which trastuzumab cardiotoxicity is reversible. Clearly, ultrastructural abnormalities on biopsy appear to be minimal, and patients respond well to standard HF regimens.[32] Some can continue on treatment without recurrence of HF. In follow-up in one of the adjuvant trials, of 27 patients with trastuzumab-induced HF (trastuzumab given after anthracycline plus cyclophosphamide, with or without paclitaxel), only one patient was persistently symptomatic.[28] Furthermore, overall LV function at more than 6 months of follow-up improved for the group versus on-treatment values. However, LV function remained depressed compared with baseline in 17 of 24 patients. Longer term follow-up is required to evaluate this issue fully.

Bcr-Abl and Imatinib

The first targeted small molecule kinase inhibitor to be used successfully in malignant neoplasms was imatinib. This agent inhibits the activity of the fusion protein Bcr-Abl, which arises from the chromosomal translocation that creates the Philadelphia chromosome and is the causal factor in approximately 90% of cases of chronic myeloid leukemia and some cases of B-cell acute lymphoblastic leukemia.[27] This translocation creates a constitutively active protein kinase that drives proliferation and inhibits apoptosis in bone marrow stem cells, leading to the leukemias. Imatinib has revolutionized the treatment of chronic myeloid leukemia, and now 90% of patients are alive 5 years after diagnosis with a disease that was uniformly fatal before the development of imatinib. Imatinib was the first TKI to be associated with HF, although the overall incidence is low.[21,25]

Dasatinib and nilotinib are more potent Bcr-Abl inhibitors, with dasatinib being decidedly less selective than the others. HF is uncommon with imatinib and nilotinib, but HF or LV dysfunction can occur in as many as 4% of patients receiving dasatinib.[21] Furthermore, the median duration of treatment in this trial was only 6 months. However, patients need to be on treatment for life because chronic myeloid leukemia recurs when the drug is stopped. Patients were excluded from the trial if they had abnormal cardiac function, again highlighting the fact that patients in clinical trials may not reflect the population of patients as a whole that will be receiving the drug. Nilotinib also prolongs the QT interval by 15 to 30 milliseconds.

Epidermal Growth Factor Receptor Antagonists

Epidermal growth factor receptor (EGFR) antagonists are in fairly widespread use for a number of solid tumors, although their efficacy has been generally modest. These agents are either monoclonal antibodies (e.g., cetuximab [Erbitux], panitumumab) or small molecule inhibitors (gefitinib [Iressa] or erlotinib [Tarceva]). In contrast to inhibition of HER2, cardiotoxicity with EGFR inhibitors seems to be quite rare. Thus, other causes of HF should be aggressively sought in patients receiving these agents presenting with HF. However, acute MI has been reported with erlotinib (2.3% risk versus 1.2% in patients receiving gemcitabine). Erlotinib is also associated with venous thromboembolism, with rates varying from ~4% to 10%.[21]

Vascular Endothelial Growth Factor and Vascular Endothelial Growth Factor Receptor Antagonists

There is great interest in drug development for agents targeting the vascular supply of tumors. Because vascular endothelial cell growth factor (VEGF) and two of its receptors, VEGFR1 and VEGFR2, are key regulators of angiogenesis and are overexpressed in many solid tumors, they represent prime candidates.[33] The monoclonal antibody bevacizumab (Avastin) targets VEGF-A and, combined with chemotherapy, enhanced survival in metastatic colorectal cancer and metastatic, nonsquamous, non-SCLC,[33] leading many to suggest that "antivascular" therapies may soon be incorporated into many regimens for solid tumors. Sunitinib and sorafenib are TKIs that also target VEGFRs, and many others are in development. Sunitinib and sorafenib are part of a recent trend toward targeting of multiple kinases involved in cancer progression. Although this makes sense for treatment of cancers, multitargeted TKIs raise additional concerns about cardiotoxicity. Hypertension is very common with all three of these VEGF/VEGFR antagonists and can be severe in 8% to 20% of patients. Thus, hypertension appears to be a class effect related to VEGFR inhibition.

All three agents are associated with HF; bevacizumab and sorafenib appear to be less problematic than sunitinib. Rates of HF with bevacizumab monotherapy are low but rise when patients have received prior anthracyclines or irradiation. In one case series of sunitinib-treated patients, 8% developed NYHA Class III or IV HF and an additional 10% suffered asymptomatic but significant declines in ejection fraction.[34]

On the basis of a meta-analysis of five trials, concerns have also been raised about the approximately twofold increase in arterial (but not venous) thromboembolic events with bevacizumab.[35] Age and prior thromboembolic events were risk factors. In patients older than 65 years, 8.5% developed arterial thromboembolic events versus 2.9% for the chemotherapy-alone arm. Stroke risk was increased approximately fourfold (1.9% versus 0.5%).

Sorafenib is also associated with acute coronary syndromes; in one study, the rate was 2.9% for patients receiving sorafenib compared with 0.4% in the placebo arm (*www.univgraph.com/bayer/inserts/nexavar.pdf*; Bayer Pharmaceuticals, Inc., 2006).

There are no guidelines at present concerning screening evaluations and follow-up of patients who will receive VEGF/VEGFR-targeted therapeutics. Until more data are available, a baseline evaluation of LV function should be considered for patients who will receive sunitinib if there are significant risk factors. Patients receiving therapy, especially those with cardiac disease, should be observed closely, and obviously, strict attention should be paid to hypertension management for all of the VEGF/VEGFR therapeutics.

Vascular Disrupting Agents

Another class of agents, the so-called vascular disrupting agents, target endothelial cells. A phase I trial of one such agent, ZD6126, which targets the tubulin network of the endothelial cell, was complicated by pulmonary thromboembolism, asymptomatic creatine kinase MB release, and declines in LVEF. An additional clinical trial of this agent, which appears to target normal as well as tumor vasculature, found an 11% incidence of cardiac events.

Histone Deacetylase Inhibitors

This relatively new class of agents negatively regulates cell proliferation by preventing the removal of acetyl moieties by histone deacetylases. Vorinostat has been approved for use in cutaneous T-cell lymphoma, but several additional trials are ongoing for this and other histone deacetylase inhibitors. In one trial, pulmonary embolism was noted in 5.4% of patients (*http://www.cancer.gov/cancertopics/druginfo/fda-vorinostat*). It is not clear if this is an on-target or off-target effect of the drug, nor is the mechanism known.

CONCERNS ABOUT DRUGS IN DEVELOPMENT. There are literally hundreds of agents in development, but one area of significant concern is inhibition of multiple factors along the phosphoinositide 3-kinase (PI3K)/Akt pathway. Indeed, the most active drug development in cancer is probably directed at the many components that make up this pathway. This pathway is very notable in that all of the major factors in it have been found to be mutated or amplified in a wide range of cancers, making this pathway an ideal target in cancer therapy.[36] Furthermore, it is believed that effective cancer therapy will require targeting of multiple components of the pathway.[36] Whereas this is undoubtedly true from a cancer perspective, with the central role played by the PI3K/Akt pathway in cardiomyocyte survival in the setting of stress, concerns about aggressive targeting of this pathway are obvious. In spite of that, several agents are currently in clinical trials.[36] This PI3K/Akt pathway, more than any other, epitomizes the similarity between cancer signaling and survival signaling in cardiomyocytes.

Complications of Radiation Therapy

Cardiovascular disease is one of the leading causes of mortality in long-term cancer survivors treated with mediastinal irradiation. Patients with lymphomas and breast, lung, and esophageal cancers frequently receive high doses of radiation to the heart and vasculature. Late cardiovascular effects range from valvular heart disease to premature CAD, stroke, cardiomyopathy, HF, constrictive pericarditis, and complete heart block.[37] Similar to anthracycline cardiomyopathy, radiation-induced cardiovascular dysfunction is progressive with time after radiation therapy, with cardiac events typically occurring 10 to 20 years after radiation therapy.[38] In approaching cardiac complications in patients exposed to chest radiation, however, it is important to recognize that the distribution of disease is defined by the geometry of the radiation portal. In other words, it predominantly involves cardiac structures that happen to fall within the portal while leaving nonirradiated adjacent structures relatively intact, hence occasionally producing atypical clinical presentations.[38]

PATHOPHYSIOLOGY. Radiation is believed to cause endothelial dysfunction of the microvasculature leading to thrombosis and small-vessel disease. Furthermore, irradiation of larger vessels included in the field, such as the proximal coronary arteries, results in intimal hyperplasia, eventually leading to premature atherosclerosis and coronary stenosis.[39] Irradiation of the myocardium leads to progressive fibrosis resulting in diastolic dysfunction and finally restrictive cardiomyopathy in long-term survivors.[40]

Much of our understanding of late cardiac effects of radiation therapy comes from the study of Hodgkin lymphoma, in which therapy entails a relatively stereotyped radiation portal and generally good longer term survival. Furthermore, many long-term Hodgkin lymphoma survivors receive radiation therapy alone, separating the contribution of radiation therapy from the additive effects of chemotherapy on the heart.[5,41]

STROKE AND TRANSIENT ISCHEMIC ATTACKS. Long-term cancer survivors who have received head and neck irradiation have a twofold to threefold increased risk of stroke and transient ischemic attacks.[42,43] At 25 years after treatment, the cumulative risk for ischemic cerebral events (cerebrovascular accident, transient ischemic attack) approaches 6% to 7%.[42,43] Importantly, peripheral vascular complications of radiation therapy may also include arterial stenoses and occlusions of any vessels in the radiation fields. Depending on the type of cancer, the subclavian, internal mammary, and coronary arteries also may have been irradiated.

CORONARY ARTERY DISEASE. Premature cardiovascular disease accounts for 25% of non–primary cancer–related deaths in long-term survivors of mantle irradiation.[44] Risk of cardiovascular disease increases with time elapsed since exposure to radiation. Radiation-associated relative risk of ischemia, sudden death, or HF is 2.9% at 10 years and increases with time since exposure to 24.7% at 25 years.[45] Nineteen years after exposure to radiation therapy, standardized incidence ratios for CAD in Hodgkin lymphoma survivors are 3.6 times greater than those in an age- and gender-matched population.[46] Importantly, radiation-associated coronary disease may be difficult to diagnose because many patients do not experience anginal "warning" symptoms after mediastinal irradiation, apparently reflecting irradiation of sensory nerves in the chest.[38] Therefore, a high index of suspicion along with an understanding of cardiovascular risk for CAD is important in the care of this population. The combination of radiation therapy with anthracycline exposure and the presence of traditional cardiac risk factors further increase the risk of cardiovascular disease in long-term survivors.[46,47]

Valvular Heart Disease. As previously discussed, chest irradiation also increases risk for clinically significant valvular disease, especially involving the aortic valve. Sixty percent of Hodgkin lymphoma survivors treated with high-dose radiation therapy have moderate to severe valvular dysfunction 20 years after treatment.[44] Patients who have received <30 Gy of radiation are less likely to have significant valve disease.[40] Anthracycline chemotherapy also further increases the risk of valve disease and HF after mediastinal radiation therapy.[37,46] Therefore, routine periodic screening for valve disease in patients treated with radiation has been recommended because many patients who are asymptomatic have been found to have subclinical valvular disease.[48]

Cardiomyopathy. Patients who have received radiation therapy are at risk for development of diastolic dysfunction, restrictive cardiomyopathy, and subsequent HF. Systolic dysfunction is relatively infrequent with radiation therapy alone, occurring in >10% of patients.[40,44] Childhood survivors of radiation therapy demonstrate a complex of decreased LV mass, decreased chamber size, and decreased wall thickness.[49] Diastolic dysfunction was also common in adult long-term survivors and associated with worsened event-free survival.[37] Furthermore, significant decrease in peak oxygen uptake to <20 mL/kg/m^2, values that are graded as severely reduced in typical HF populations, may be seen in 30% of childhood survivors of Hodgkin lymphoma.[40]

Conduction Block. Bundle branch block and even complete heart block requiring pacemaker placement may occur, presumably reflecting radiation-induced fibrosis of the conduction system.

Breast cancer survivors may also be at risk for radiation-associated cardiovascular disease, including MI[21,50]; however, late cardiac effects in this population may vary according to the dose, the laterality of the radiation field (left versus right breast), and the era in which the patient was treated.[51] With improved radiation technique, cardiovascular disease deaths declined from 13% to 5.5% in patients treated before 1980 versus those treated after 1985.[52] Survivors treated with older radiation techniques have a higher risk for fatal cardiovascular disease than do patients treated more recently. In contrast, survivors treated with modern techniques of radiation therapy have not shown an increase in cardiovascular disease after 10 to 15 years compared with those who received no breast irradiation.[52] However, longer follow-up is necessary to confirm the lack of increased cardiovascular risk in those treated with modern radiation therapy protocols.

MONITORING. Subclinical cardiovascular disease is common in long-term cancer survivors.[44] Noninvasive cardiac imaging is important in the long-term follow-up of cancer survivors.[38] Echocardiography with tissue Doppler imaging is important for detection of systolic and diastolic dysfunction and for assessment of valvular and pericardial disease. Stress testing, with or without imaging, should be considered in long-term survivors of mediastinal irradiation. Recommendations for cardiac assessment of children and adults are available.[21,48,53]

PREVENTION. Alterations in radiation treatment technique, such as reductions in dose-volume, field size, and cardiac shielding, have decreased cardiac irradiation.[53] Additional approaches to reduce cardiac irradiation at time of therapy include deep inspiratory breath-holding that decreases the amount of myocardium in the field without altering irradiation of the breast.[54-56] These techniques have been validated in clinical trials and are beginning to be implemented in radiation treatment protocols (*www.ClinicalTrials.gov*). Beyond improvements in radiation delivery, however, treatment of modifiable cardiac risk factors in long-term survivors remains central to the reduction of overall cardiovascular risk.[46,48]

Management of Heart Failure Induced by Cancer Therapeutic Agents

At present, the guidelines of the Heart Failure Society of America and the American Heart Association/American College of Cardiology (AHA/ACC) do not contain specific recommendations for treatment of patients with what is presumed to be cancer therapeutic–induced HF. However, it is probably most reasonable at this time to approach the patient as one would any patient with newly diagnosed HF, as discussed in Chap. 28. In this regard, it is critical to exclude other potential causes of HF before assuming that chemotherapy has caused the HF. Several of the agents discussed earlier, including trastuzumab and sunitinib, appear to have some degree of reversibility of LV dysfunction with aggressive treatment with angiotensin-converting enzyme inhibitors and beta blockers. In many cases, patients need to continue the cancer treatment, and a number of anecdotal case reports have suggested that patients whose LV dysfunction largely resolves after withdrawal of the agent and institution of an HF regimen may be safely rechallenged with the agent, although continuing the HF regimen. Clearly, however, at this point there is insufficient evidence to conclude whether this approach is generally safe, so no clear recommendations can be made, and any rechallenge should be undertaken with great caution.

Future Perspectives

Many more targets exist for drug development for leukemias and solid tumors. Given the intense interest in this area by the pharmaceutical industry, inhibitors will likely become available at some point. Clinicians will be faced with a host of novel therapeutics and the prospect of trying to predict which will have adverse effects on the cardiovascular system. The key for the future will be to develop better strategies to identify targets to be avoided, thereby limiting cardiotoxicity. When the target cannot be avoided (i.e., when it is causal), the goal will be to develop prophylactic therapies to prevent or to minimize cardiotoxicity in high-risk patients. When that fails, we need to develop effective approaches to the management of patients with cardiotoxicity so that progression of HF can be prevented and patients can continue on what is often lifesaving treatment. In this endeavor, oncologists and cardiologists must collaborate.

REFERENCES

Direct and Indirect Complications of Neoplasia

1. Luna A, Ribes R, Caro P, et al: Evaluation of cardiac tumors with magnetic resonance imaging. Eur Radiol 15:1446, 2005.
2. Chiles C, Woodard PK, Gutierrez FR, Link KM: Metastatic involvement of the heart and pericardium: CT and MRI imaging. Radiographics 21:439, 2001.
3. Maisch B, Seferovic PM, Ristic AD, et al: Guidelines on the diagnosis and management of pericardial diseases. Eur Heart J 25:587, 2004.
4. Tsang TS, Barnes ME, Gersh BJ: Outcomes of clinically significant idiopathic pericardial effusion requiring intervention. Am J Cardiol 91:704, 2002.
5. Lee PJ, Mallik R: Cardiovascular effects of radiation therapy. Cardiol Rev 13:80, 2005.
6. Bertog SC, Thambidorai SK, Prarakh K, et al: Constrictive pericarditis: Etiology and cause-specific survival after pericardiectomy. J Am Coll Cardiol 43:1445, 2004.
7. Wudel LJ, Nesbitt JC: Superior vena cava syndrome. Curr Treat Options Oncol 2:77, 2001.
8. Teo N, Sabharwal T, Rowland E, et al: Treatment of superior vena cava obstruction secondary to pacemaker wires with balloon venoplasty and insertion of metallic stents. Eur Heart J 23:1465, 2002.
9. Rowell NP, Gleeson FV: Steroids, radiotherapy, chemotherapy and stents for superior vena cava obstruction in carcinoma of the bronchus: A systematic review. Clin Oncol 14:338, 2002.
10. Edoute Y, Haim N, Rinkevich D, et al: Cardiac valvular vegetations in cancer patients: A prospective echocardiographic study of 200 patients. Am J Med 102:252, 1997.
11. Ewer MS, Kish SK, Martin CG, et al: Characteristics of cardiac arrest in cancer patients as a predictor of survival after cardiopulmonary resuscitation. Cancer 92:1905, 2001.

Cardiovascular Complications of Cancer Therapeutic Agents

12. Ng R, Better N, Green MD: Anticancer agents and cardiotoxicity. Semin Oncol 33:2, 2006.
13. Swain SM, Whaley FS, Ewer MS: Congestive heart failure in patients treated with doxorubicin: A retrospective analysis of three trials. Cancer 97:2869, 2003.
14. Kremer LC, van Dalen EC, Offringa M, et al: Anthracycline-induced clinical heart failure in a cohort of 607 children: Long-term follow-up study. J Clin Oncol 19:191, 2001.
15. Lipshultz SE, Lipsitz SR, Sallan SE, et al: Chronic progressive cardiac dysfunction years after doxorubicin therapy for childhood acute lymphoblastic leukemia. J Clin Oncol 23:2629, 2005.
16. Peng X, Chen B, Lim CC, Sawyer DB: The cardiotoxicity of anthracycline chemotherapeutics. Mol Interv 5:163, 2005.
17. Swain SM, Whaley FS, Gerber MC, et al: Cardioprotection with dexrazoxane for doxorubicin-containing therapy in advanced breast cancer. J Clin Oncol 15:1318, 1997.
18. Cardinale D, Sandri MT, Colombo A, et al: Prognostic value of troponin I in cardiac risk stratification of cancer patients undergoing high-dose chemotherapy. Circulation 109:2749, 2004.

19. Biganzoli L, Cufer T, Bruning P, et al: Doxorubicin-paclitaxel: A safe regimen in terms of cardiac toxicity in metastatic breast carcinoma patients. Results from a European Organization for Research and Treatment of Cancer multicenter trial. Cancer 97:40, 2003.
20. Kuittinen T, Husso-Saastamoinen M, Sipola P, et al: Very acute cardiac toxicity during BEAC chemotherapy in non-Hodgkin's lymphoma patients undergoing autologous stem cell transplantation. Bone Marrow Transplant 36:1077, 2005.
21. Yeh ET, Bickford CL: Cardiovascular complications of cancer therapy: Incidence, pathogenesis, diagnosis, and management. J Am Coll Cardiol 53:2231, 2009.
22. Pai VB, Nahata MC: Cardiotoxicity of chemotherapeutic agents: Incidence, treatment and prevention. Drug Safety 22:263, 2000.
23. Reis SE, Costantino JP, Wickerham DL, et al: Cardiovascular effects of tamoxifen in women with and without heart disease: Breast cancer prevention trial. National Surgical Adjuvant Breast and Bowel Project Breast Cancer Prevention Trial Investigators. J Natl Cancer Inst 93:16, 2001.
24. Richardson PG, Sonneveld P, Schuster MW, et al: Bortezomib or high-dose dexamethasone for relapsed multiple myeloma. N Engl J Med 352:2487, 2005.
25. Chen MH, Kerkela R, Force T: Mechanisms of cardiac dysfunction associated with tyrosine kinase inhibitor cancer therapeutics. Circulation 118:84, 2008.
26. Force T, Krause DS, Van Etten RA: Molecular mechanisms of cardiotoxicity of tyrosine kinase inhibition. Nat Rev Cancer 7:332, 2007.
27. Krause DS, Van Etten RA: Tyrosine kinases as targets for cancer therapy. N Engl J Med 353:172, 2005.
28. Tan-Chiu E, Yothers G, Romond E, et al: Assessment of cardiac dysfunction in a randomized trial comparing doxorubicin and cyclophosphamide followed by paclitaxel, with or without trastuzumab as adjuvant therapy in node-positive, human epidermal growth factor receptor 2–overexpressing breast cancer: NSABP B-31. J Clin Oncol 23:7811, 2005.
29. Crone SA, Zhao YY, Fan L, et al: ErbB2 is essential in the prevention of dilated cardiomyopathy. Nat Med 8:459, 2002.
30. De Keulenaer GW, Doggen K, Lemmens K: The vulnerability of the heart as a pluricellular paracrine organ: Lessons from unexpected triggers of heart failure in targeted ErbB2 anticancer therapy. Circ Res 106:35, 2010.
31. Agus DB, Sweeney CJ, Morris MJ, et al: Efficacy and safety of single-agent pertuzumab (rhuMAb 2C4), a human epidermal growth factor receptor dimerization inhibitor, in castration-resistant prostate cancer after progression from taxane-based therapy. J Clin Oncol 25:675, 2007.
32. Ewer MS, Vooletich MT, Durand JB, et al: Reversibility of trastuzumab-related cardiotoxicity: New insights based on clinical course and response to medical treatment. J Clin Oncol 23:7820, 2005.
33. Morabito A, De Maio E, Di Maio M, et al: Tyrosine kinase inhibitors of vascular endothelial growth factor receptors in clinical trials: Current status and future directions. Oncologist 11:753, 2006.
34. Chu T, Rupnick MA, Kerkela R, et al: Cardiotoxicity associated with the tyrosine kinase inhibitor sunitinib. Lancet 270:2011, 2007.
35. Scappaticci FA, Skillings JR, Holden SN, et al: Arterial thromboembolic events in patients with metastatic carcinoma treated with chemotherapy and bevacizumab. J Natl Cancer Inst 99:1232, 2007.
36. Yuan TL, Cantley LC: PI3K pathway alterations in cancer: Variations on a theme. Oncogene 27:5497, 2008.

Cardiovascular Complications of Radiation Therapy

37. Heidenreich PA, Kapoor JR: Radiation induced heart disease: Systemic disorders in heart disease. Heart 95:252, 2009.
38. Chen MH, Diller L: Cardiovascular disease in cancer survivors: From bench to bedside. Circ Res 2010; in press.
39. Fajardo LF: The pathology of ionizing radiation as defined by morphologic patterns. Acta Oncol 44:13, 2005.
40. Adams MJ, Lipsitz SR, Colan SD, et al: Cardiovascular status in long-term survivors of Hodgkin's disease treated with chest radiotherapy. J Clin Oncol 22:3139, 2004.
41. Hull MC, Morris CG, Pepine CJ, Mendenhall NP: Valvular dysfunction and carotid, subclavian, and coronary artery disease in survivors of Hodgkin lymphoma treated with radiation therapy. JAMA 290:2831, 2003.
42. De Bruin ML, Dorresteijn LD, van't Veer MB, et al: Increased risk of stroke and transient ischemic attack in 5-year survivors of Hodgkin lymphoma. J Natl Cancer Inst 101:928, 2009.
43. Bowers DC, Liu Y, Leisenring W, et al: Late-occurring stroke among long-term survivors of childhood leukemia and brain tumors: A report from the Childhood Cancer Survivor Study. J Clin Oncol 24:5277, 2006.
44. Heidenreich PA, Hancock SL, Lee BK, et al: Asymptomatic cardiac disease following mediastinal irradiation. J Am Coll Cardiol 42:743, 2003.
45. Glanzmann C, Kaufmann P, Jenni R, et al: Cardiac risk after mediastinal irradiation for Hodgkin's disease. Radiother Oncol 46:51, 1998.
46. Aleman BM, van den Belt-Dusebout AW, De Bruin ML, et al: Late cardiotoxicity after treatment for Hodgkin lymphoma. Blood 109:1878, 2007.
47. Swerdlow AJ, Higgins CD, Smith P, et al: Myocardial infarction mortality risk after treatment for Hodgkin disease: A collaborative British cohort study. J Natl Cancer Inst 99:206, 2007.
48. Shankar SM, Marina N, Hudson MM, et al: Monitoring for cardiovascular disease in survivors of childhood cancer: Report from the Cardiovascular Disease Task Force of the Children's Oncology Group. Pediatrics 121:e387, 2008.
49. Adams MJ, Lipshultz SE: Pathophysiology of anthracycline- and radiation-associated cardiomyopathies: Implications for screening and prevention. Pediatr Blood Cancer 44:600, 2005.
50. Carver JR, Shapiro CL, Ng A, et al: American Society of Clinical Oncology clinical evidence review on the ongoing care of adult cancer survivors: Cardiac and pulmonary late effects. J Clin Oncol 25:3991, 2007.
51. Early Breast Cancer Trialists' Collaborative Group: Favourable and unfavourable effects on long-term survival of radiotherapy for early breast cancer: An overview of the randomised trials. Lancet 355:1757, 2000.
52. Giordano SH, Kuo YF, Freeman JL, et al: Risk of cardiac death after adjuvant radiotherapy for breast cancer. J Natl Cancer Inst 97:419, 2005.
53. Ng D, Constine LS, Deming RL, et al: American College of Radiology ACR Appropriateness Criteria. Follow-up of Hodgkin's Lymphoma. Available at: http:www/acr.org/SecondaryMainMenuCategories/quality_safety/app_criteria/pdf/ExpertPanelonRadiationOncologyHodgkinsWorkGroup/FollowUpofHodgkinsDiseaseDoc2.aspx.
54. Chen MH, Chuang ML, Bornstein BA, et al: Impact of respiratory maneuvers on cardiac volume within left-breast radiation portals. Circulation 96:3269, 1997.
55. Lu HM, Cash E, Chen MH, et al: Reduction of cardiac volume in left-breast treatment fields by respiratory maneuvers: A CT study. Int J Radiat Oncol Biol Phys 47:895, 2000.
56. Korreman SS, Pedersen AN, Aarup LR, et al: Reduction of cardiac and pulmonary complication probabilities after breathing adapted radiotherapy for breast cancer. Int J Radiat Oncol Biol Phys 65:1375, 2006.

CHAPTER 91 Psychiatric and Behavioral Aspects of Cardiovascular Disease

Viola Vaccarino and J. Douglas Bremner

Stress, Emotions, and Cardiovascular Disease: General Considerations

The cardiovascular system has long been considered vulnerable to the effects of psychological factors, and popular wisdom holds stress and emotions as important risk factors for cardiovascular disease (CVD). There are ample physiologic and experimental data to substantiate this belief and to support a link between a number of psychosocial factors and cardiovascular risk.

The stress response, an adaptive physiologic mechanism that allows the organism to counteract potentially damaging stimuli, results in stimulation of the sympathoadrenal system and the hypothalamus-pituitary-adrenal axis with release of cortisol and norepinephrine. Activation of the stress system is physiologically useful to counteract the stressor. However, repeated or excessive activation due to psychological stress is believed to be damaging because of adverse effects of neuroendocrine activation on hemodynamics, metabolism, and immune function.[1] For the cardiovascular system, psychological factors have been implicated both as triggers of acute coronary events and as promoters of the atherosclerotic process. Potential underlying biologic mechanisms are numerous and include repeated or sustained increase in blood pressure and heart rate, effects on insulin resistance and other metabolic abnormalities, enhanced platelet activity, endothelial dysfunction, increased systemic vascular resistance, autonomic dysfunction, ventricular arrhythmias, plaque instability, and disruption of coronary flow dynamics.[2] Furthermore, inflammation and immune function are emerging as key intermediary factors of the stress response in many biologic systems.[3]

From Animal Models to Human Populations

Research in nonhuman primates has provided some of the strongest experimental evidence of the adverse cardiovascular effects of chronic stress. Spanning many decades, these studies have demonstrated that chronic psychosocial stress causes endothelial damage and accelerated atherosclerosis; they have also indicated that males and females may be affected differently. Cynomolgus monkeys under social stress develop endothelial injury, and this effect is blocked by propranolol, the beta-adrenergic receptor antagonist, indicating that it is mediated by norepinephrine. Among males, dominant individuals develop more extensive atherosclerosis than subordinates do when housed in recurrently reorganized (unstable) social groups. By contrast, it is the subordinate females who develop more atherosclerosis, rather than the dominants.[4] Subordinate females are more likely than dominant ones to have visceral obesity and to have behavioral and physiologic characteristics consistent with a stressed state.

In humans, the adverse effects of experimentally induced stress on the cardiovascular system are well documented (described later; see Mental Stress); yet, the effects of naturally occurring stressors on cardiovascular function and CVD risk have been more difficult to demonstrate. One problem is the definition of exposure. Under the general term of *psychosocial stress*, investigators have included interrelated but different elements, encompassing a variety of environmental exposures (from traumatic events to job or family difficulties to minor everyday hassles) as well as individuals' responses or emotional states, such as depression and anxiety. Another problem is the lack of standardized measures to consistently define and to quantify type and severity of psychological stress. As discussed in this chapter, the most robust evidence to date implicates low socioeconomic status, work stress, caregiving stress, social isolation, and depression as risk factors for CVD. In addition to manifest disease, many of these factors have been associated with subclinical markers of atherosclerosis. Findings related to other psychosocial and psychiatric factors, such as other forms of chronic stress, anxiety, and anger or hostility, have been less consistent.

Psychological and Psychiatric Conditions in the Cardiac Patient

Recognition of psychological and psychiatric factors is important in the management of the cardiac patient not only because many of these conditions are prevalent and have been linked to adverse cardiovascular outcomes but also because they are related to health behaviors and lifestyle risk factors that have prognostic significance. These include factors such as lower adherence to treatment recommendations, lower physical activity, unhealthy diet, and tobacco smoking. However, psychological and psychiatric conditions are less likely than traditional CVD risk factors to be recognized and managed in current cardiology practice. This is because of complexities in definition and assessment, as mentioned before, but also because many symptoms of psychological distress are easily confused with physical disease, for example, fatigue, weight loss, poor appetite, or trouble sleeping.

Current recommendations call for cardiologists to be more proactive in addressing this important domain of patient care.[5,6] The goals of this chapter, therefore, are to review key epidemiologic and pathophysiologic evidence linking psychological factors to CVD and to discuss their management in the current practice of cardiology. For clarity, we classify psychological and psychiatric conditions into general categories of acute stressful events, chronic stressors, emotional factors (including affective disorders), and personality traits.

Acute Stress

Stressful and Emotional Triggers of Acute Ischemia (see Chaps. 54 and 56)

A key pathophysiologic event underlying acute cardiac ischemia is the disruption of a vulnerable atherosclerotic plaque because of plaque rupture or plaque erosion with superimposed thrombus formation. However, plaque disruption does not always result in an acute coronary syndrome. It is hypothesized that stressful, emotional episodes act as triggers of acute coronary events by causing pathophysiologic derangements that are necessary for an ischemic event to occur in susceptible individuals. These pathophysiologic effects, discussed later, include hemodynamic responses to cardiovascular activation, coronary vasoconstriction, inflammation, and prothrombotic effects (**Fig. 91-1**).[2]

Many studies, albeit not all, have demonstrated an increase in hospital admissions for acute coronary syndromes after emotionally stressful events, such as natural and industrial disasters, terrorist attacks, and sporting events.[2] During the 1994 Northridge earthquake in the Los Angeles area, there was a 35% increase in hospital admissions for acute myocardial infarction in the week after the earthquake compared with the week before. On the basis of coroners' records, sudden cardiac death increased from an average of 4.6 events per day in the week before the earthquake to 24 events on the day of the earthquake and then fell to 2.7 per day in the next 6 days. Only three of these cases were associated with unusual physical exertion. An analysis of all deaths in Los Angeles County confirmed these data and showed that coronary deaths tended to be clustered around the epicenter of the earthquake; by contrast, there was no increase in noncoronary deaths.[7] Studies of the 1995 Hanshin-Awaji earthquake in Japan showed similar results. However, the 1989 Loma Prieta earthquake in the San Francisco Bay Area was not associated with an increase in coronary events. One explanation may be the timing of the earthquakes. Both the Northridge and Hanshin-Awaji quakes occurred in winter and early in the morning, when there is a greater susceptibility to acute coronary syndromes, whereas the Loma Prieta earthquake struck on an October afternoon.

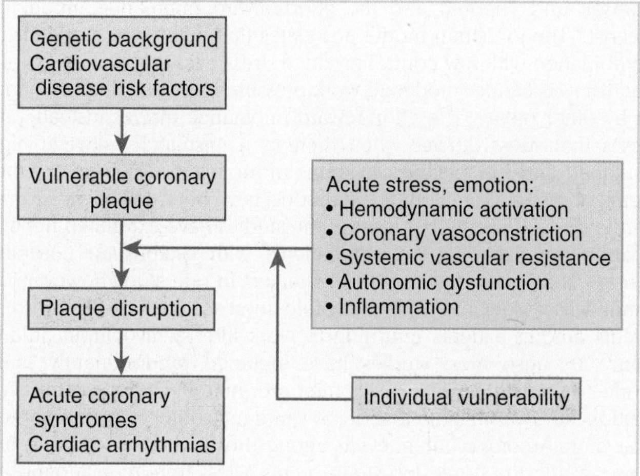

FIGURE 91-1 Potential mechanisms underlying the acute triggering of adverse cardiac events by psychological factors.

War and terrorist attacks have also been associated with an increase in acute coronary events, but again, results are mixed. During the initial phases of the Gulf War in the Tel Aviv area in 1991, there was an increase in the incidence of acute myocardial infarction and sudden death. By contrast, the World Trade Center terrorist attack in New York City on September 11, 2001, was not linked to an increase in cardiac death or admissions to acute coronary care in New York City immediately after the attack. It is possible that this event, which was observed by most New Yorkers through news reports on television, did not cause acute stress to the same extent as an incident that poses a direct threat to personal safety. However, the incidence of cardiovascular ailments diagnosed by physicians increased by more than 50% in the next 3 years, therefore suggesting a more chronic impact of the attack rather than an acute triggering effect. In addition, after the attack, ventricular arrhythmias increased by more than twofold among patients with implantable cardioverter-defibrillators (ICDs), but this increase did not occur until 3 days after the event and persisted in the next 30 days.[8] These data again suggest that subacute stress may have played a role.

A limitation of these studies is the lack of information on the circumstances surrounding cardiac events, making it difficult to rule out alternative explanations. Apart from emotional stress, cardiac events could be triggered by concomitant factors, for example, vigorous physical exertion (such as running away) or heavy eating and drinking. In this respect, studies of individual emotional triggers, in which patients are asked about their experiences before symptom onset, provide more information. On the other hand, self-reports of patients may be affected by recall bias.

Among individual emotional triggers, acute anger has been studied most extensively.[2] In the Determinants of Myocardial Infarction Onset study, 2.4% of patients reported being very angry or furious in the 2 hours before acute myocardial infarction. In comparison with a matched control period 24 hours earlier, the odds of acute myocardial infarction after acute anger were increased fourfold, and the risk of anger triggering was particularly high in subjects of lower socioeconomic status. The Stockholm Heart Epidemiology Program (SHEEP) study and other studies found similar results, but the incidence of an acute anger episode before symptom onset varies substantially in all these reports, from 1% to 17%, depending on the definition of the anger episode.

In addition to anger, episodes of acute stress or emotions have been reported as triggers of CVD events. Acute work-related stress has been linked to myocardial infarction. In the SHEEP study, patients reporting a sudden, short-term increase in workload, such as a high-pressure deadline, exhibited a sixfold increase in the odds of myocardial infarction during the next 24 hours in comparison with the period between 24 and 48 hours before the infarction.[9] Exposure to heavy traffic has also been associated with increased risk of myocardial infarction.[10] The time the subjects spend in cars or public transportation is directly related to the risk; in addition to stress, however, pollution and noise may contribute to this effect. Stressful life events have been linked to acute myocardial stunning in susceptible individuals with severe, reversible left ventricular dysfunction.[11] These patients, almost all women, also show exaggerated sympathetic nervous system stimulation as indicated by markedly elevated plasma catecholamine levels. Finally, episodes of depression and sadness have also been linked to the triggering of acute myocardial ischemia. Such episodes appear to be common (18%) in the 2 hours before onset of cardiac symptoms[12] and are associated with substantially increased odds of acute coronary syndromes, between 2.5 and 5 (depending on the severity of depression), compared with a control period for each patient.

Mental Stress

A useful method of assessing the effects of stress and emotion on cardiac function is to measure transient ischemic responses to a standardized psychological stress challenge in the laboratory, or "mental stress test," using mental arithmetic, color naming, public speeches, and similar tasks. Mental stress–induced myocardial ischemia is analogous to exercise stress ischemia, except that the stimulus is psychological rather than physical.[13]

Mental stress ischemia has been studied with a variety of imaging techniques and a range of stressful stimuli.[14] This literature indicates that mental stress ischemia can be induced in one third to two thirds of coronary heart disease patients. It is typically painless and occurs at lower levels of oxygen demand than ischemia due to physical exertion. In addition, mental stress ischemia is generally not related to the severity of coronary artery disease, suggesting that it is not simply a reflection of coronary disease severity. Patients may develop ischemia with mental stress but not with exercise or pharmacologic stress,[15] although results vary. Ischemic responses are induced not only by severe emotional stress but also by milder challenges similar to those that might be encountered in everyday life. In fact, mental stress–induced (but not exercise-induced) myocardial ischemia correlates with ischemia measured in daily life ambulatory monitoring. Thus, mental stress testing could potentially provide a means for the identification of patients vulnerable to myocardial ischemia in everyday life.

In addition to ischemia, mental stress may affect the electrical properties of the heart; a mental stress task in coronary heart disease patients with defibrillators was associated with an increase in T wave alternans and with lower heart rates than with exercise.[16] Mental stress was also associated with a decrease in heart rate variability.[17]

All the results published to date have indicated that mental stress–induced ischemia is a predictor of poor prognosis. Several patient series followed from 1 to 5 years have found substantial increases, between 70% and threefold, in cardiovascular events, revascularization procedures, and death comparing coronary patients with mental stress ischemia with those without, independent of coronary disease severity and CVD risk factors.[13,14] Although the samples of patients followed up longitudinally to date are relatively small, current evidence indicates that myocardial ischemic responses to standardized mental stress are prognostically important at least as much as exercise-induced ischemia.

Potential Mechanisms of Acute Stress

The mechanisms behind emotional triggering of cardiac events are likely to be multiple and may include hemodynamic changes, such as increases in blood pressure, heart rate, systemic vascular resistance, and coronary artery vasoconstriction.[2,13,14] It is clear, however, that different hemodynamic responses underlie ischemia triggered by psychological stress compared with exercise stress. Myocardial ischemic responses to mental stress occur at a lower rate-pressure product than does exercise-induced ischemia in the same patients, although the hemodynamic response tends to be larger than in patients who do not become ischemic. Both people with and without pre-existing coronary heart disease who develop mental stress ischemia show an increase in systemic vascular resistance, suggesting that a rise in afterload caused by peripheral vasoconstriction may play a role in ischemia induced by psychological stress. By contrast, systemic vascular resistance is decreased by exercise. These effects may be secondary to a centrally mediated neurogenic peripheral vasoconstriction; in fact, plasma catecholamines increase rapidly with mental stress and correlate with hemodynamic changes.[18]

Abnormal coronary artery vasomotor response is also observed during mental stress. Patients with atherosclerosis may undergo a paradoxical constriction during mental stress, particularly at points of stenosis, which may reduce myocardial blood flow and thus result in ischemia. This vasomotor response correlates with the endothelium-dependent response to an infusion of acetylcholine, suggesting coronary endothelial dysfunction as a mechanism. The degree of constriction may not, however, be sufficient to explain the decrease in coronary flow during mental stress, which can be reversed by alpha-adrenergic blockade through intracoronary administration of phentolamine; in the absence of epicardial coronary artery constriction, this suggests sympathetically mediated coronary microvascular dysfunction.[13,14,18] Thus, both coronary endothelial dysfunction and vasomotor abnormalities in the coronary microvasculature appear to play a role in myocardial ischemia triggered by psychological stress.

Autonomic dysfunction is another likely process underlying the acute effects of stress on the heart. Both sympathetic activation and parasympathetic withdrawal can stimulate arrhythmias and lower the threshold for ventricular fibrillation. Heart rate variability, a measure of the beat-to-beat changes in heart rate as the heart responds to internal and external stimuli, is an accepted noninvasive measure of overall cardiac autonomic function. Reduced heart rate variability predicts coronary heart disease incidence in population studies as well as mortality, particularly sudden death, in patients after acute myocardial infarction.[19] Heart rate variability is reduced by acute mental stress in the laboratory and was found to be reduced during major disasters, such as earthquakes and terrorist attacks, in studies of patients who were undergoing ambulatory electrocardiographic monitoring at the time of the event.[2]

Inflammation and immunity are increasingly recognized as key factors in mediation of cellular responses to acute psychological stress. Norepinephrine-dependent adrenergic stimulation due to stress activates the transcription factor nuclear factor κB in circulating monocytes, resulting in initiation of the inflammation cascade.[3] Thus, psychosocial stress stimulates mononuclear cell activation and subsequent immune and inflammatory response, which may result in myocardial ischemia.

On the basis of current evidence, therefore, psychological stress induces physiologic responses that could trigger cardiac ischemia or sudden death. However, it is likely that this risk affects only a subset of vulnerable individuals. In one study, patients who reported emotional triggers of their acute coronary syndrome had more prolonged systolic blood pressure responses and enhanced platelet activation in response to a laboratory stressful challenge compared with the non-trigger group.[20] Therefore, some patients may be particularly susceptible to physiologic responses to emotional stimuli and therefore be at higher risk of unfavorable cardiovascular consequences due to stress. If such patients could be identified in advance, specific procedures could be put in place to minimize their exposure to emotional triggers as well as to reduce their risks associated with such exposure.

Chronic Stress

Work Stress

The belief that work-related stress may be harmful to the heart is highly rooted in popular wisdom; thus, work stress has been extensively studied for its potential adverse cardiovascular effects. Two dominant models of work stress include the job strain model developed by Karasek and Theorell and the effort-reward imbalance model by Siegrist.[5] The job strain model postulates that high work demands in combination with low control produce stress because workers in low-control jobs cannot moderate work pressure by organizing their time or by other means. The effort-reward imbalance model, instead, proposes that stress derives when there is a mismatch between high workload and low payback in terms of money, job security, or other forms of recognition. Both these models have been linked to adverse cardiovascular events, but most of the studies have examined initially healthy populations.[21] Among patients with established coronary disease, studies are few and results mixed. In one study, however, job strain was associated with a twofold increase in risk of recurrent events among patients returning to work after a myocardial infarction.[22] Because most studies have included predominantly male worker populations, data on women are limited. There is some suggestion, however, that the role of job strain may differ between women and men. Among women, even among those who are working full time outside the home, job strain seems a less important prognostic factor than for men, whereas stress in other life domains, such as family and social relations, may be more important.[23]

Low Socioeconomic Status

Socioeconomic status is generally defined by interrelated factors such as occupational status, economic resources, education, and social class. The existence of a social gradient in health and disease has long been recognized.[24] Beginning many decades ago, the Whitehall study of British civil servants reported that even among people who are not poor, there is a social gradient in mortality and morbidity, including CVD, from the bottom to the top of society. Such results have been confirmed in many other contexts including the United States. Low socioeconomic status is accompanied by poorer health habits and higher frequencies of standard CVD risk factors, such as hypertension, obesity, smoking, and unhealthy diet, which, however, only partially account for the CVD gradient due to social class. Many adverse psychosocial characteristics are also related to socioeconomic status. These include financial hardship, poorer housing, neighborhood status, social discrimination and isolation, depression, and adverse working conditions. Thus, low socioeconomic status can be viewed as a composite of chronic stressors that may result in adverse behavioral and physiologic consequences.

Hypothalamic-pituitary-adrenal axis and autonomic dysfunction is observed as socioeconomic status levels decline and may increase the risk for central obesity and metabolic risk factors. The Whitehall II study, for example, described a close relationship between lower social position and increased prevalence of metabolic syndrome, an association that was minimally affected by differences in health behaviors.[25,26] Disturbances in neuroendocrine and cardiac autonomic activity, compatible with activation of the neuroendocrine stress axes, were also noted in subjects with metabolic syndrome and subjects of lower socioeconomic status. Notably, psychosocial factors (socioeconomic status and job-related stress) explained a large portion of the association between adrenal or autonomic disturbances and metabolic syndrome.

Marital and Caregiving Stress

Whereas work stress has been primarily studied among men, marital stress and caregiving stress have been primarily studied among women. In the Stockholm Female Coronary Risk Study, women who underwent a myocardial infarction and reported marital stress had an almost threefold higher risk of recurrent cardiac events than did women with less marital stress after adjustment for other risk factors.[23] Marital stress has also been linked to atherosclerosis progression in women[27]; thus, it appears to be an important risk factor for women. Overall, however, few studies are available on this dimension of chronic stress, and data on sex differences in the response to this stressor are also needed.

Caregiving for an ill family member is common, particularly among women, can be quite stressful, and has been associated with CVD risk and mortality.[5,28] In the Nurses' Health Study, caregiving for an ill or disabled spouse was associated with nearly double increased risk of coronary events after adjustment for other risk factors. Similarly, in the Caregiver Health Effects Study, caregiving was associated with a 63% higher adjusted mortality risk. The adverse effects of caregiving, however, apply only to caregivers who report strain; caregivers not experiencing strain do not have elevated mortality rates. Looking at potential mechanisms, the San Diego Caregiver Study showed that distressed caregivers had an increased likelihood of developing hypertension during the follow-up than controls; they also had higher levels of D-dimer (a circulating procoagulant factor), more sleep disruption, and higher levels of plasma inflammatory cytokines.[28]

Early Life Stress

Psychological trauma, particularly if it occurs early in life, such as childhood maltreatment, is an emerging risk factor for CVD. Its effects may be in part mediated by symptoms of depression, which is associated with trauma exposure. Anda and colleagues, in a series of studies, showed that early adverse life experiences are associated with dramatic increases in anxiety, substance abuse, obesity, and smoking and predict incident coronary heart disease in adulthood independent of these factors.[29] Having 7 or more (of 10) adverse childhood events was associated with an adjusted 3.6-fold increased risk of coronary heart disease. A large proportion of early adverse experiences include childhood sexual or physical abuse, which is common particularly among girls; such history is found in about 20% of women.

A recent meta-analysis confirmed a link between childhood maltreatment and a number of medical outcomes in adulthood, including CVD.[30] Despite heterogeneity of effects across studies, the association is seen both when abuse is measured by self-report and when it is measured objectively. Many potential behavioral, emotional, and biologic explanations may underlie this relationship. Recently, a prospective study linked childhood maltreatment to adult inflammation.[31] Maltreated children showed a significant and graded increase in the risk of having elevated C-reactive protein and other markers of inflammation 20 years later, which persisted after accounting for co-occurring early life risks and health behaviors. This study provides evidence for a long-term effect of early life stress on physical health.

Social Isolation and Lack of Support

Both the size and the quality of a person's social contacts have been related to CVD and total mortality. Social relationships may improve health in a variety of ways, including provision of instrumental and emotional support and encouragement toward a healthy lifestyle and health care seeking. Emotional support may also buffer the adverse effects of psychological stressors. Reverse causation is also possible, however, because individuals who are diseased or otherwise at risk may be less socially engaged.

Despite scientific interest in this construct, there is little theoretical integration on its meaning and little consensus on measurement and mechanisms. Although a number of population studies have shown elevated risk of CVD associated with social isolation or lack of support, results are not consistent, perhaps reflecting variations in measurements and definitions.[21] The effects appear more robust in prognostic studies of patients with coronary heart disease. Factors such as living alone, lacking a confidant, being socially isolated, and perceiving low support have been linked to increased mortality in cardiac populations; in general, the association persisted after adjustment for lifestyle behaviors and disease severity.[21] Thus, instrumental and emotional aspects of social contacts may be particularly beneficial for high-risk individuals such as cardiac patients.

General Stress

Relatively few studies have examined the relationship between nonspecific perceived daily life stress and the onset or exacerbation of CVD. In general, these studies are limited in their measurement of stress and have yielded conflicting results in terms of effect size, sex differences, and other subgroup analyses. For example, the Copenhagen City Heart Study found a relative risk of 2.6 for incident ischemic heart disease comparing high stress versus low stress in men younger than 55 years but no association in women and older men.[32] The largest study addressing this question was the INTERHEART, a large international case-control study of risk factors for myocardial infarction.[33] This study included brief assessments of depression, locus of control, perceived stress at home or work, financial stress, and adverse life events. High general stress at home or work was significantly associated with myocardial infarction, with an odds ratio of 1.55, adjusted for geographic region, age, sex, and smoking. This estimate was similar across regions, ethnic groups, and sex. Permanent general stress, representing the highest severity level of the general stress classification, had an odds ratio of 2.17 for myocardial infarction. The study also evaluated a composite score of psychosocial risk factors and found that in terms of both odds ratio and population attributable risk, the risk associated with psychosocial factors was comparable to that of standard CVD risk factors.[34]

Emotional Factors and Psychiatric Diagnoses

Depression and anxiety differ from other psychological factors considered in this chapter because they are psychiatric disorders and as such amenable to drug treatment or other types of clinical management. Most of the evidence linking these factors to CVD risk, however, has involved the measurement of symptom scales rather than psychiatric diagnoses. In this group, depression has received particular attention and has shown the most robust results for a relationship with CVD.

Depression

Depression is a highly prevalent condition and growing global problem. By 2030, depression is projected to be the second leading cause of disability worldwide (after HIV infection and AIDS) and the number one cause of disability in high-income countries.[35] Depression is three times more common among cardiac patients than among controls, and 15% to 30% of cardiac patients have significant depression. This prevalence is higher in women than in men; among myocardial infarction patients, the prevalence of depression is particularly high, about 40%, among younger women (<60 years old).[36]

Depression as a risk factor varies from mild (subclinical) depressive symptoms to a clinical diagnosis of major depression. As defined by the *Diagnostic and Statistical Manual of Mental Disorders,* fourth edition, major depression is characterized by depressed mood or anhedonia (inability to experience pleasure from normally pleasurable life activities) for at least 2 weeks accompanied by significant functional impairment and additional somatic or cognitive symptoms.

Many meta-analyses of observational studies have provided evidence for an association between clinical depression (or depressive symptoms) and CVD risk, both among individuals initially free of heart disease[37] and in a variety of populations of heart disease patients, including patients with acute coronary syndromes,[37,38] congestive heart failure,[39] stable coronary heart disease,[40] and post–coronary bypass surgery.[37] However, individual studies have produced significantly heterogeneous risk estimates and have varied in their ability to adjust for potential confounding factors such as smoking, physical inactivity, and severity of coronary heart disease. Among individuals initially free of heart disease, a recent meta-analysis reported a pooled unadjusted relative risk for future coronary events of 1.81 (95% confidence interval, 1.53-2.15) comparing depressed with nondepressed persons.[37] Among coronary heart disease patients, the pooled relative risk for recurrent events or mortality was similar, 1.80 (95% confidence interval, 1.50-2.15). However, adjustment for disease severity attenuated the association in coronary heart disease patients by almost 50%, suggesting possible reverse causation (severe coronary heart disease leading to depression).

Most epidemiologic studies of depression as a risk factor for CVD have examined depressive symptoms rather than major depression. Those that did consider major depression tended to find larger risk estimates than those assessing symptom scales, although many were limited in their adjustment for potential confounding factors.[37,40] There is evidence for a gradient of risk linking level of depressive symptoms to likelihood of adverse cardiac events, beginning at relatively low levels of depressive symptoms.

Many potential mechanisms have been postulated for the relationship between depression and CVD.[41] Depression is associated with other cardiovascular risk factors including smoking, sedentary lifestyle, obesity, diabetes, and hypertension, but many studies have shown an independent effect of depression on cardiac outcomes after adjustment for these factors. In heart disease patients, depression is also associated with severity of functional impairment. If functional limitations translate into a decrement in physical activity or self-care, this could accelerate progression of coronary heart disease. In addition, depressed patients show lower adherence to medication regimens, lifestyle risk factor modification, and cardiac rehabilitation. Thus, depression may affect cardiac outcomes through behavioral mechanisms involving healthy lifestyle, delay in seeking treatment, and nonadherence to secondary prevention.[42]

Depression is characterized by an overactivity of the hypothalamic-pituitary-adrenal axis and the sympathoadrenal system that resembles the neuroendocrine response to stress, with increased, or prolonged, release of cortisol and norepinephrine and disruption of normal circadian patterns. These abnormalities may lead to repeated or sustained elevations in blood pressure, heart rate, and plasma glucose concentration and insulin resistance and dyslipidemia.[43]

Depressed individuals also show reduced parasympathetic flow, which contributes to autonomic nervous system dysregulation in depression.[43] Heart rate variability, a noninvasive measure of cardiac autonomic function, is lower in depressed patients. Other indications of autonomic dysfunction in depressed cardiac patients include increased heart rate response to orthostatic challenge, abnormal heart rate response to premature ventricular contractions, and abnormal ventricular repolarization. All these factors are predictors of mortality in cardiac patients.

Enhanced platelet activity in depression has also been proposed as a potential link between depression and cardiac events, but data are limited and results mixed.[44] Other postulated mechanisms involve endothelial dysfunction and inflammation. Psychological stress has been related to impaired endothelial function both in primates and in humans; these findings have been extended to depression.[45] Many studies have shown an association between depression and elevated levels of acute-phase proteins, such as C-reactive protein, and inflammatory cytokines, such as interleukin-6, in subjects with and without CVD. However, results in CVD patients are somewhat inconsistent, and to date there is no evidence that inflammation is a mechanism in the link between depression and cardiovascular outcomes.[46]

Finally, growing evidence suggests that depression and CVD may be different phenotypic expressions of the same genetic substrates.[47] Genetic pleiotropy, however, does not eliminate other causal possibilities, for example, the fact that certain genes cause depression and depression, in turn, causes or complicates CVD.

Despite the important comorbidity between depression and physical illness, less than half of depressed medical patients are recognized by their physicians.[48] During an admission for acute myocardial infarction, less than 15% of patients with depression are identified.[49] One reason for this may be uncertainty about whether depression treatment will improve outcomes and thus whether systematic depression screening is warranted in cardiac patients.[50] Indeed, studies to date have not proved that treatment of depression can improve cardiovascular outcomes. Investigation in this area has been limited, however. Furthermore, depression remains an important illness in and of itself that deserves proper evaluation and treatment. In addition to prognosis, depression substantially affects the quality of life of cardiac patients and is one of the strongest predictors of nonadherence with medical treatment regimens.[51] By recognizing and treating depression, we can improve patients' overall well-being and their adherence to medical treatments and healthy lifestyle behaviors.

Anxiety

Anxiety, like depression, includes a large spectrum of conditions, from psychiatric diagnoses amenable to clinical treatment to subthreshold symptoms that are common in the general population. As for depression, most studies examining the relationship between anxiety and coronary heart disease have considered anxiety symptom scales rather than a clinical diagnosis of anxiety disorder. A systematic review of both etiologic and prognostic studies found highly inconsistent results.[21] About half of the studies failed to find an association between anxiety and CVD risk, both in initially healthy populations and among patients with established coronary heart disease. As with other psychosocial factors, these inconsistencies may be due to differences in the measurement of anxiety and the fact that symptom scales may not discriminate among anxiety disorders that may differ in their biologic substrate and therefore their relationship with CVD. For example, phobic anxiety, rather than other forms of anxiety, has shown more consistent associations with CVD risk, particularly sudden death, in population studies. There is emerging evidence that another anxiety disorder, post-traumatic stress disorder, may increase CVD risk, but studies to date are few and methodologically limited.[52]

Other Psychosocial Characteristics and Personality Traits

Anger and Hostility

Anger and hostility have been intensively studied for their relation with CVD. Despite being different constructs, anger and hostility are often used interchangeably, and their interconnection is poorly defined. Hostility is one of the dimensions of type A personality that was believed, in early research, to be a risk factor for CVD, a relationship not supported by later investigation. Hostility is a personality/cognitive trait characterized by a negative attitude toward others. Anger is an emotional state characterized by feelings ranging from mild irritation to intense fury or rage toward others. A recent meta-analysis found substantial heterogeneity of results, with half to two thirds of the studies failing to find a significant association between anger or hostility and CVD risk.[53] The summary combined estimate for anger and hostility indicated a modest but significant 19% increase in coronary heart disease incidence in initially healthy populations and a 24% increase in recurrent coronary heart disease events in patients with preexisting coronary heart disease. However, studies of higher quality tended to show smaller and nonsignificant effects. The risk associated with anger or hostility appears to be more marked in men and is in large part explained by behavioral factors such as smoking and physical activity.[53]

Type D Personality

Type D (or "distressed") personality, first introduced in 1995 by Denollet and colleagues, is a personality type that combines negative affectivity and social inhibition.[54] It describes individuals who tend to experience negative emotions (dysphoria, tension, worry) and at the same time are inhibited in their expression of emotions, thoughts, and behaviors in a social context. These investigators were able to link this construct to adverse cardiovascular outcomes and total death in a number of studies of CVD patients. Because type D personality is related to other psychosocial characteristics (hostility, anger, depression, and social isolation), its interconnection with and independence from these other factors need more evaluation. However, this personality type seems to be a predictor even after depression and other psychosocial stressors are accounted for. These authors propose that it is the combination of these two traits (negative affect and social inhibition) that is damaging, rather than either one alone.

Psychiatric Care of the Cardiac Patient

Psychotherapy for Depression

In many cases, life events contribute to the development of symptoms of depression and anxiety. Early life stress plays an important role in the development of depression for many people. Relationships and stress in the workplace are also important contributors, and often these factors combine. Dysfunctional relationships or jobs can also contribute to depression. In many cases, medication alone may not suffice for the treatment of depression; psychotherapy plus medication is often better than taking medication alone.

Psychotherapy helps people with depression understand the behaviors, emotions, and ideas that contribute to depression, regain a sense of control and pleasure in life, and learn coping skills. Psychodynamic therapy is based on the assumption that a person is depressed because of unresolved, generally unconscious conflicts, often stemming from childhood. Interpersonal therapy focuses on the behaviors and interactions a depressed patient has with family and friends. The primary goal of this therapy is to improve communication skills and increase self-esteem during a short time. Cognitive-behavioral therapy involves examination of thought patterns that can be negative and self-defeating and going over the basis of such thoughts and how they contribute to emotions. Psychotherapy has been shown to be as effective for depression as medications, and some people, especially with early life stress issues, may not respond to medication without psychotherapy.

Because of the increased risk of mortality in cardiac patients with depression, it was assumed that successful treatment of depression would reduce this risk. The ENRICHD (Enhancing Recover in Coronary Heart Disease Patients) trial, however, did not find such a beneficial effect of cognitive-behavioral therapy for cardiac outcomes[55]; however, the improvement in depression in comparison to placebo was modest.

Other types of therapy have been shown to be useful for depression and anxiety. These include interpersonal therapy, stress management, and stress reduction. In addition, yoga, meditation, and mindfulness-based stress reduction training can be useful.

Antidepressant Medications

Antidepressant medications are another proven method for the treatment of depression. Antidepressants act on the serotonin and norepinephrine systems as well as other neurotransmitter systems in the brain. Drugs that increase brain levels of serotonin and norepinephrine have been shown to be effective treatment of depression and anxiety. Antidepressants typically bind to proteins called transporters that are responsible for taking the neurotransmitter back up into the neuron after it has been released into the synapse, the space between neurons. Drugs that block uptake of the transmitter by the transporter result in an increase in neurotransmitter in the synapse, which accounts for at least part of the reason that these drugs work. Many of the antidepressant drugs block the serotonin transporter, the norepinephrine transporter, or a combination of the two. The original drugs, the tricyclics, had a more general effect on blockage of neurotransmitter uptake.

TRICYCLIC ANTIDEPRESSANTS. The first medication found to work for the treatment of depression was discovered by accident. The tricyclic drug imipramine (Tofranil) was developed in the 1940s for the treatment of tuberculosis. It was noticed that a number of the depressed patients on the tuberculosis wards were getting better in terms of their depression (if not tuberculosis). This led psychiatrists in France, and later the United States, to try this drug for patients hospitalized for depression, demonstrating its usefulness. This was the birth of the tricyclic medications.

Tricyclics, in addition to imipramine, include doxepin (Sinequan), amoxapine (Asendin), and amitriptyline (Elavil). Tricyclics increase norepinephrine and serotonin levels in the synapse. The most common side effects of the tricyclics are the anticholinergic side effects, which include dry mouth, constipation, memory problems, confusion, blurred vision, sexual dysfunction, and decreased urination. Specific cardiac effects include heart arrhythmias and hypotension. Tricyclics have properties like quinidine, leading to an increase in the PR interval, a prolongation of QRS duration and QT interval, and a flattening of the T wave on the electrocardiogram (see Chap. 36). These effects are usually not of clinical significance. However, tricyclics should be avoided in patients with preexisting cardiac conduction defects, congestive heart failure, or recent myocardial infarction. Prolongation of the QT interval beyond 0.44 second is associated with an increased risk of malignant ventricular arrhythmias (torsades de pointes; see Chap. 39).

The anticholinergic side effects of the tricyclics are especially troublesome for the elderly because they are more susceptible to the memory impairment and orthostatic hypotension that can be associated with these medications. For this reason, it is recommended that the tricyclics amitriptyline and doxepin not be prescribed to the elderly.

Tricyclic medications have been associated with an increased risk of malignant ventricular arrhythmias and sudden cardiac death[56] (see Chap. 41). For patients who suffer a cardiac event while being treated with a tricyclic, abrupt withdrawal from the tricyclic medication can be associated with an increased risk of arrhythmias. Therefore, these medications should be tapered slowly. If prolongation of the QT interval or development of hypotension in patients treated with a tricyclic becomes a problem, tricyclics should be slowly tapered and patients treated with a selective serotonin reuptake inhibitor, venlafaxine, or bupropion (see later). These medications are preferred in patients with new onset of depression after an acute myocardial infarction.

NOREPINEPHRINE REUPTAKE INHIBITORS. Antidepressant medications designed specifically to block reuptake of norepinephrine into the synapse are called norepinephrine reuptake inhibitors (NRIs). Medications in this group include desipramine (Norpramin) and nortriptyline (Aventyl, Pamelor). They have a more favorable profile in terms of anticholinergic side effects and effects on the heart and blood pressure than the tricyclics.

MONOAMINE OXIDASE INHIBITORS. Drugs that block the monoamine oxidase inhibitor enzyme (MAOI drugs) and therefore boost the monoamines (serotonin, norepinephrine) include phenelzine (Nardil) and tranylcypromine (Parnate). They have a more favorable cardiovascular profile than the tricyclics, with little or no effect on cardiac conduction, although they can be associated with orthostatic hypotension and weight gain. They can cause a "wine and cheese reaction" of potentially life-threatening elevations of blood pressure if taken with foods that are high in tyramine content, including wine, cheese, chocolate, and beer. Medications that can precipitate hypertensive reactions if a patient is also taking an MAOI include those with sympathomimetic effects (e.g., amphetamines, ephedrine, cocaine). MAOIs should also not be taken together with meperidine (Demerol). Because of the risk of hypertensive crises, the MAOIs are not recommended for use in cardiac patients and indeed they are no longer commonly prescribed in general.

ANTIDEPRESSANTS WITH NOVEL MECHANISMS OF ACTION. Some drugs act on various neurotransmitter systems or in general are poorly understood in terms of mechanism of action. These include bupropion (Wellbutrin), which primarily acts on dopamine systems and is used for both depression and smoking cessation under the brand name Zyban. Side effects include weight loss and restlessness as well as possible increases in blood pressure. High doses of bupropion can rarely cause seizures. A randomized controlled trial of bupropion versus placebo for the treatment of depression in patients hospitalized after cardiovascular events did not find an increase in mortality or cardiovascular events with bupropion.[57]

Drugs with mixed actions are trazodone (Desyrel) and maprotiline (Ludiomil). These medications have lesser degrees of anticholinergic side effects and effects on the heart and blood pressure than other antidepressant medications do. Trazodone can rarely cause priapism (extended painful erection that requires emergency treatment), however.

Nefazodone (Serzone) has both serotonin reuptake inhibition and postsynaptic serotonin receptor blockade properties. It blocks the reuptake of serotonin into the neuron and also blocks a receptor for serotonin on the neuron on the receiving end. It therefore has a chemically unique mode of action. Nefazodone has been associated with several cases of fatal liver failure. It also has been shown to have teratogenic effects in animal studies and is therefore contraindicated for use in pregnancy. Other side effects include dry mouth, nausea, headache, and upset stomach. Nefazodone has mild effects on the alpha-adrenergic receptor, which means that it can cause mild orthostatic hypotension. Given that alternative antidepressants that do not cause liver failure are just as effective, nefazodone should not be used except as a last resort in the cardiac patient.

Mirtazapine (Remeron) is a tetracyclic antidepressant that has actions on a number of different receptor systems. It blocks presynaptic noradrenergic alpha$_2$ receptors with associated enhancement of norepinephrine release. Mirtazapine also increases serotonin release. Side effects include sweating and shivering, tiredness, strange dreams, dyslipidemia, weight gain, upset stomach, anxiety, and agitation. It can be associated with mild orthostatic hypotension and anticholinergic side effects. It has not been shown to have effects on the heart's electrical properties. In the Myocardial Infarction and Depression-Intervention Trial (MIND-IT), 91 post–myocardial infarction patients with depression were randomly assigned to 8 weeks of mirtazapine or placebo. There was no difference in cardiovascular events between the two groups. Mirtazapine was associated with an increase in fatigue and appetite changes.

SELECTIVE SEROTONIN REUPTAKE INHIBITORS. As the tricyclics went off patent, a new generation of drugs, the selective serotonin reuptake inhibitors (SSRIs), were developed. These medications more specifically act on the serotonin transporter and therefore have a side effect profile different from that of the older tricyclic medications, specifically fewer anticholinergic and cardiac effects, which makes them the antidepressant medications of choice in the population of cardiac patients.

SSRI medications include fluoxetine (Prozac, Sarafem), paroxetine (Paxil), fluvoxamine (Luvox), citalopram (Celexa), escitalopram (Lexapro), and sertraline (Zoloft). They act by blocking the transporter that brings the serotonin back from the synapse into the neuron, effectively increasing the levels of serotonin in the synapse. Fluoxetine, paroxetine, sertraline, and other SSRIs are free of anticholinergic side effects and have no known effects on blood pressure and the heart.

The SSRI medications have not been shown to have greater efficacy than the older tricyclics in the treatment of depression, although a larger number of patients drop out of treatment while receiving tricyclics because of side effects. For example, the Danish Study Group found that the older tricyclic medication clomipramine worked better for severe depression than did paroxetine, although it had more side effects. In general, SSRIs, like the older tricyclics, have only modest efficacy over placebo. A review from 15 years ago showed that more than 80% of the improvement with fluoxetine was accounted for by a placebo effect. A more recent meta-analysis from data submitted to the Food and Drug Administration (FDA) also showed that 80% of the improvement with antidepressants comes from the placebo response.[58] Patients with mild or moderate depression do not have clinically meaningful responses to antidepressants, whereas those with severe depression do.[59]

The primary advantage of SSRIs in the cardiac patient is lesser risk of cardiovascular and anticholinergic side effects. Side effects of SSRIs include nausea, diarrhea, headache, insomnia, and agitation. One of the most troubling side effects of the SSRIs is sexual dysfunction, which includes loss of libido, delayed ejaculation, and erectile dysfunction. Antidepressants without sexual dysfunction side effects can be given instead of an SSRI in these cases, including bupropion, mirtazapine, and trazodone, drugs not in the SSRI class.

SSRI treatment, especially fluoxetine, is also associated with an increase in risk of bleeding.[60] For the cardiac patient taking an aspirin or other antiplatelet or anticoagulation treatment, this can be an important issue; therefore, potential bleeding risks should be carefully evaluated.

SSRIs stopped suddenly can result in a potent withdrawal syndrome, including agitation, nervousness, and sometimes suicidal thoughts. SSRIs can cause akathisia and other extrapyramidal side effects, like the antipsychotics. Akathisia includes feelings of restlessness, pacing, and internal stiffness, which subjectively are very uncomfortable. However, these symptoms are not common and are treatable with benzodiazepines or low doses of propranolol.

A more troubling problem is the potential for suicidality associated with SSRIs. Several recent meta-analyses have shown an increase in suicidal attempts in adults taking SSRIs, and the FDA recently added a warning that SSRI antidepressants may increase the risk of suicidal thoughts or suicide. Studies, however, have shown no difference between SSRIs and the older tricyclic antidepressants in suicide risk, suggesting that *all* antidepressant medications may carry an increased risk of suicide.

Short-term trials of SSRIs have found them to be safe and effective for cardiac patients.[55,61] For instance, in the Sertraline Antidepressant Heart Attack Randomized Trial (SADHART), 369 patients hospitalized for a myocardial infarction or unstable angina with the diagnosis of depression were randomly assigned to receive sertraline at a flexible dose or placebo for 24 weeks. There was no difference in cardiovascular parameters (ejection fraction, QT interval, premature ventricular contractions), cardiovascular events, or death between the two groups. Treatment responders, however, appeared to have better cardiac outcomes than nonresponders. The Canadian Cardiac Randomized Evaluation of Antidepressant and Psychotherapy Efficacy (CREATE) trial found 12 weeks of treatment with the SSRI citalopram to be more efficacious than placebo for the treatment of depression and not to be associated with an increased risk for cardiovascular events.[62] Other studies have not shown differences in cardiovascular outcomes after short-term treatment with fluoxetine in comparison to placebo.[55]

Several cohort studies, however, have shown increased cardiac risk with longer term use of SSRIs. For example, the Nurses' Health Study, which looked at more than 60,000 women without a history of heart disease, found that women taking antidepressants were three times as likely as women not taking antidepressants to have a sudden cardiac death, even after adjustment for severity of depression and risk factors for heart disease.[63] Furthermore, there was an equal risk for SSRIs and other antidepressants outside of the SSRI class. However, sudden cardiac death in healthy women is fairly rare, and in this study, only 46 of 100,000 women taking an SSRI had a sudden cardiac death. The Women's Ischemia Syndrome Evaluation (WISE) study compared women with and without antidepressant and anxiolytic therapy.[64] Antidepressant use was associated with a doubling of risk for cardiovascular events and death. Although anxiolytic use alone was not associated with an increased risk, women who were taking both antidepressants and anxiolytics had a fourfold or greater risk of cardiovascular events and mortality.

SEROTONIN AND NOREPINEPHRINE DUAL REUPTAKE INHIBITORS. The latest group of antidepressants has dual reuptake inhibition for serotonin and norepinephrine (SNRIs) and includes venlafaxine (Effexor) and duloxetine (Cymbalta). In general, these drugs have shown better treatment response for depression than SSRIs and tricyclics. When multiple studies were combined, with treatment response defined as a 50% reduction in symptoms of depression, venlafaxine had a success rate of 74% that was significantly better than that of SSRIs (a 61% success rate) and tricyclics (a 58% success rate).

Both venlafaxine and duloxetine can cause dizziness, constipation, dry mouth, headache, and changes in sleep or more rarely a serotonin syndrome, with restlessness, shivering, and sweating. Venlafaxine has been associated with a dose-dependent increase in blood pressure, which is of particular concern for cardiac patients, especially those with pre-existing hypertension. Although not well studied, there is a good possibility that duloxetine has similar effects. Venlafaxine seems to carry the greatest risk of suicidality among all of the antidepressants, with a threefold increased risk of attempted or completed suicides.

Mood-Stabilizing Agents

Mood-stabilizing agents are used conventionally in the treatment of epilepsy, but they may have efficacy in the stabilization of mood in patients with psychiatric disorders, especially patients with bipolar disorder. Bipolar disorder (formerly known as manic-depressive disorder) is a condition that affects more than 2 million Americans. People who have this illness tend to experience extreme mood swings along with other specific symptoms and behaviors.

It is not known how mood-stabilizing drugs work for bipolar disorder, but many of them modulate function of the excitatory amino acid glutamate, a brain neurotransmitter that plays a critical role in memory and has been implicated in both epilepsy and mood and anxiety disorders. Mood-stabilizing agents include valproic acid (Valproate), carbamazepine (Tegretol), topiramate (Topamax), lamotrigine (Lamictal), phenytoin (Dilantin), and neurontin (Gabapentin). These are commonly used in clinical practice, often in combination with SSRI medications. Valproate can cause a potentially fatal liver failure, although this is very rare. Side effects of carbamazepine include ataxia, diplopia, and sedation, which are dose related. It can also cause neutropenia and hyponatremia, and in rare cases it is associated with aplastic anemia or life-threatening hepatic toxicity. Carbamazepine has quinidine-like effects on cardiac conduction, similar to the tricyclics, and should be used with caution in cardiac patients. It has interactions with numerous other medications and can affect blood levels of other medications. Lamotrigine in rare cases can cause Stevens-Johnson syndrome, a potentially lethal disease. Lithium (Eskalith, Lithobid, Lithonate) is a primary mineral that has been shown to stabilize the mood of patients with bipolar disorder. Dose-dependent side effects include diarrhea, increased thirst, nausea, trembling, rash, and fatigue. Dose adjustments can eliminate these symptoms. In rare cases, lithium can unmask or exacerbate a sinus node arrhythmia.

Electroconvulsive Therapy

Electroconvulsive therapy (ECT) is used as a last resort for the treatment of depression in patients who have had multiple failed trials of psychotherapy and medication. ECT has an 80% response rate, which is a better response rate than for medications, and contrary to popular belief, it is a safe procedure. ECT causes profound hemodynamic changes, including bradycardia (up to frank asystole, which may last for a few seconds), followed by tachycardia and hypertension. These effects, however, are transient and typically resolve within 20 minutes. Possible complications include persistent hypertension, arrhythmias, asystole lasting more than 5 seconds, chest pain, ischemia, and heart failure. Older age and pre-existing CVD, including hypertension, coronary artery disease, congestive heart failure, aortic stenosis, implanted cardiac devices, and atrial fibrillation, have been associated with increased complication rates. However, most complications remain minor and transient, and most patients can safely complete treatment.[65]

There are no absolute contraindications to ECT. However, the procedure should be delayed in patients who are hemodynamically unstable or have new-onset or uncontrolled hypertension. In patients with stable coronary heart disease and controlled hypertension, medications can be continued through the morning of the procedure. In patients with an implanted pacemaker, the pacemaker should be tested before and after ECT; the magnet should be placed at the patient's bedside in the event that electrical interference leads to pacemaker inhibition and bradycardia. ECT appears safe in patients with an ICD. Detection mode of the ICD should be turned off during ECT, and continuous electrocardiographic monitoring should be performed, with resuscitative equipment by the patient's bedside in the event that external defibrillation is necessary.[65]

Antipsychotics

The typical antipsychotic medications block the dopamine D_2 receptor in the brain, which is thought to be involved in the symptoms of psychosis. Probably more important, antipsychotics (previously known as major tranquilizers) are very sedating, which leads to their use in patients who have agitated behavior.

The antipsychotic drugs developed for schizophrenia are also used as an adjunct to antidepressants for treatment-resistant depression. Some studies, however, have shown an increased risk of death when antipsychotics are used in the elderly. Therefore, they should be used with caution in this population.

The first generation of antipsychotic medications included chlorpromazine (Thorazine), haloperidol (Haldol), thioridazine (Mellaril), and perphenazine (Trilafon). These medications can be associated with troubling extrapyramidal side effects, including twitching, jerking movements, and lip smacking. They also can cause orthostatic hypotension and have anticholinergic side effects and therefore may interfere with memory in the elderly, especially the low-potency antipsychotics thioridazine and chlorpromazine. Typical antipsychotics have mild effects on cardiac conduction, to a lesser degree than tricyclics and greater in the low-potency antipsychotics. High doses of haloperidol have been associated with rare cases of ventricular arrhythmia (torsades de pointes) when given to the agitated, delirious patient.

The second generation of antipsychotic medications, atypical antipsychotics, act by blocking a wide range of different dopamine receptors in addition to other receptors like the serotonin receptors. It is thought that this is the reason they are not associated with risks of extrapyramidal side effects similar to those with the older antipsychotic medications. The first atypical to be produced, clozapine (Clozaril), is associated in rare cases with agranulocytosis, which can be fatal. For this reason, patients taking clozapine have to have their blood counts tested on a regular basis. Clozapine is also associated with anticholinergic side effects and orthostatic hypotension and is not ideal for the cardiac patient. Other atypicals include olanzapine (Zyprexa), risperidone (Risperdal), and quetiapine (Seroquel). These medications have fewer neurologic side effects, although they are not without their own problems. They can interfere with glucose metabolism, increasing the tendency to development of type 2 diabetes.[66] They can also increase lipids and cause weight gain. All of these side effects are particularly adverse for patients with coronary heart disease. Increased diabetes has been seen with olanzapine and clozapine, with less risk with risperidone. There are conflicting results for quetiapine.

Anxiolytic Medications

BENZODIAZEPINE MEDICATIONS. In the 1960s, benzodiazepines displaced barbiturates as the most commonly used treatment of insomnia and became commonly used in patients with anxiety and depression. They were originally marketed as having less potential for dependence and abuse, although this did not bear out over time. Benzodiazepines act on a receptor in the brain called the gamma-aminobutyric acid (GABA)–benzodiazepine receptor complex. This is the same complex to which alcohol and the inhibitory transmitter GABA bind, although benzodiazepines have their own binding site. Like alcohol, they act by increasing a general inhibition on neurons in the brain that results in a calming effect.

Benzodiazepines most commonly prescribed today include alprazolam (Xanax), which is mainly used for anxiety attacks and panic disorder; clonazepam (Klonopin), which is used for epilepsy; and temazepam (Restoril). Triazolam (Halcion) is a very short acting benzodiazepine that was formerly widely prescribed, but it can cause patients to wake up in the night. It also has been associated with a number of negative psychiatric side effects, including violence and aggression thought to be related to disinhibition, especially in the elderly, for which it dropped out of favor.

Other benzodiazepine medications that are longer acting and that are still sometimes used in the treatment of insomnia include oxazepam (Serax), lorazepam (Ativan), chlordiazepoxide (Librium), clorazepate (Tranxene), halazepam (Paxipam), prazepam (Centrax), quazepam (Doral), estazolam (Prosom), diazepam (Valium), and flurazepam (Dalmane). Differences in the individual benzodiazepines are related to the time of onset of action and duration of effect.

Benzodiazepines have not been shown to be better in terms of inducing sleep than other drugs such as diphenhydramine and promethazine. They decrease the average time it takes to fall asleep by just 4 minutes. However, individuals taking benzodiazepines report that they *feel* like they fall asleep faster than they actually do. On average, benzodiazepines increase the user's sleep time by about 1 hour per night.

The side effects from benzodiazepines during the day can cause serious problems. Compared with placebo, individuals taking benzodiazepines had 80% more daytime drowsiness, dizziness, and lightheadedness. Other side effects are problems the next day with memory and increased motor vehicle accidents. Use of benzodiazepine medications is associated with a 60% increase in road traffic accidents. This increased risk is not seen with other psychotropics, including antidepressants. Risk is increased further with concurrent alcohol use and in older age.

The long-acting benzodiazepines can cause significant mental impairment the next day in older patients and are associated with a 50% increase in hip fracture because older people who take them do not have full motor skills back the following day, and this increases the risk of falls. Oxazepam has the least effect on memory and as a result is recommended as the best benzodiazepine for use as a sleeping pill, although it should be used for less than 4 weeks. Long-term use is not recommended for all medications for insomnia.

The primary concern in the cardiac patient using benzodiazepines is a potential risk of respiratory suppression. For this reason, benzodiazepines with shorter half-lives should be preferred to those with longer half-lives in cardiac patients. In patients with cardiac disease and associated pulmonary impairment, these medications should be used with caution.

NONBENZODIAZEPINE "Z-DRUG" MEDICATIONS. The newer generation of insomnia medications, zaleplon (Sonata), zolpidem (Ambien), eszopiclone (Lunesta), and zopiclone (Imovane), or Z drugs, act on specific subsets of the GABA receptor. They are commonly called nonbenzodiazepine medications, but the name is misleading because they bind to the same GABA-benzodiazepine receptor complex in the brain as benzodiazepines and alcohol do. The difference is that they bind to a different part of the same receptor complex. They have been marketed as having less dependency and fewer side effects than the older generation of benzodiazepine medications, and some argue that these drugs have less potential for abuse than the benzodiazepines do. However, studies have not shown them to be more effective or safe than the benzodiazepines, and no difference between the different Z drugs for safety or efficacy has been established. As for benzodiazepines, general side effects for all of these medications include memory impairment, drowsiness, headache, dizziness, nausea, and nervousness. An increased risk of road traffic accidents was also seen with zopiclone. Zaleplon has a much shorter half-life (1 hour) than zolpidem (2.5 hours) and eszopiclone (6 hours) and is therefore promoted as being associated with less drowsiness the next day.

A side effect that has been seen in some patients taking zolpidem is sleepwalking. Zolpidem increases slow-wave sleep, which has been associated with sleepwalking. Cases have been reported of people getting out of bed after taking zolpidem, driving, and getting into car accidents, with no memory of what happened. Patients taking zolpidem should not drink any alcohol, as that can increase the risk of having a dangerous sleepwalking accident.

ANTIHISTAMINES. Drugs developed for the treatment of allergies were found to have sedative properties that are useful for insomnia, and versions for this purpose are available both by prescription and over-the-counter. The most commonly prescribed antihistamine for insomnia is hydroxyzine (Atarax, Vistaril). Over-the-counter diphenhydramine (Benadryl, Simply Sleep, Tylenol PM, Excedrin PM, and their "store brand" counterparts) is often used as a sleep aid and is effective for many people. These medications are relatively free of potential for addiction or abuse. Side effects are less common than for benzodiazepines or Z drugs and include dry mouth, urinary retention, and more rarely confusion, nightmares, nervousness, and irritability.

MEDICATIONS WITH OTHER ACTIONS. Ramelteon (Rozerem) is a melatonin receptor agonist that is used for insomnia. Melatonin is a hormone involved in the sleep-wake cycle. Side effects include headache, drowsiness, fatigue, nausea, dizziness, and more rarely diarrhea and depression. Advantages of this medication are the absence of abuse potential and the lack of withdrawal symptoms.

Buspirone (BuSpar), an agonist of the serotonin 1A receptor, is relatively free of next-day drowsiness and memory impairment or the potential for dependence or abuse. Buspirone is efficacious in the treatment of anxiety and is preferable to the benzodiazepines for the treatment of the cardiac patient as it lacks respiratory suppressive effects. Side effects are minimal and include nausea, headache, and lightheadedness. There are no known adverse cardiac effects.

Anxiolytic medications, when used alone, have not been shown to be associated with increased mortality or cardiovascular events in cardiac patients. However, as mentioned before, when used in combination with antidepressants, they have been associated with a fourfold or greater increase in cardiovascular events and mortality in an observational study.[64] Although treatment of anxiety has not been shown to decrease cardiovascular mortality, it does lead to an improvement in wellness and quality of life, which is an important consideration in cardiac patients with anxiety.[67]

Alternative Medicines, Herbs, and Supplements

There are some natural remedies that have been recommended for depression and anxiety (see Chap. 51).

ST. JOHN'S WORT. St. John's wort (*Hypericum perforatum*) is a popular medication for the over-the-counter treatment of mild depression; 12% of Americans report using it at least once a year. St. John's wort has action similar to that of antidepressants, including monoamine oxidase inhibition, serotonin reuptake inhibition, and actions on sigma receptors. St. John's wort has been shown to be better than placebo in some earlier controlled studies and as effective as tricyclic antidepressants in the treatment of depression. However, most of these earlier studies were poorly controlled and did not use standard definitions of depression, making it difficult to draw conclusions about the efficacy of St. John's wort.

A large placebo-controlled randomized trial using appropriate methodology in patients with severe cases of major depression showed no difference between St. John's wort and placebo. However, a direct head-to-head comparison of St. John's wort with the SSRI paroxetine showed that it was better in reducing symptoms of depression in patients with severe major depression; 71% of St. John's wort–treated patients had a 50% reduction in symptoms compared with 60% of those taking paroxetine. In this study, headache was the only side effect with St. John's wort that was more common than with placebo.

A second study funded by the National Institutes of Health and performed by the Hypericum Depression Trial Study Group (HDTSG) showed that St. John's wort was not more effective than placebo but not worse than an antidepressant comparison. In fact, the placebo effect did best; it was effective in 32% of patients compared with 25% for sertraline and 24% for St. John's wort. However, patients taking St. John's wort experienced fewer side effects than did those who took the antidepressant. St. John's wort caused an increase in swelling, frequent urination, and sexual dysfunction; sertraline caused diarrhea, nausea, sexual dysfunction, forgetfulness, frequent urination, and sweating.

Critics of these studies said that selection of only patients with severe depression obscured the potential benefits for patients with mild depression. One recent meta-analysis of patients with severe depression did not show consistent effects for St. John's wort. There was about a 15% increase in efficacy over placebo for severe depression. Another meta-analysis of St. John's wort for both major and minor depression was consistent with greater efficacy, about a 60% increase over placebo. Finally, a recent Cochrane review noted substantial heterogeneity of results across trials but nonetheless concluded that on the basis of the available evidence, the *Hypericum* extracts are 28% superior to placebo in patients with major depression, are similarly effective as standard antidepressants, and have fewer side effects than standard antidepressants.[68]

St. John's wort can interact with a number of medications, including digoxin, theophylline, protease inhibitors, and cyclosporine.

SAMe. *S*-Adenosylmethionine (SAMe), a molecule found in all human cells, is also promoted as a supplement for the treatment of depression. It plays a role in methylation reactions, including gene expression, maintenance of cell membranes, and neurotransmitter synthesis. Administration of SAMe has been shown to increase levels of serotonin in the brain. A meta-analysis from Italy that pooled data from several small studies concluded that SAMe was better than placebo and equivalent to tricyclic antidepressants in efficacy with fewer side effects. However, there was considerable variability in the studies conducted. Studies have also not had adequate long-term follow-up to determine long-term benefits of SAMe for depression, although it does not appear that SAMe has potential long-term toxicity.

KAVA. Kava (or kava-kava) is an extract of the roots of the Polynesian plant *Piper methysticum* used in the South Pacific for its sedative, aphrodisiac, and stimulatory effects. Active compounds include the kava pyrones, which may have effects on the brain. Some controlled trials have shown that kava reduces anxiety in patients with anxiety disorders. Side effects of kava, however, are not insignificant and include dizziness, dry mouth, gastric disturbance, diarrhea, drowsiness, depression, and more rarely liver failure, which has caused it to be banned in some countries. Because of the real risk of liver failure, kava is not recommended for the treatment of mood disorders.

OMEGA-3 FATTY ACIDS. Low dietary intake and low serum or red blood cell levels of omega-3 fatty acids are associated with depression in patients with and without coronary heart disease and with an increased risk for cardiac mortality. Two omega-3 fatty acids, eicosapentaenoic acid and docosahexaenoic acid, are found in high concentrations at neuronal synapses in the human brain and are essential for neuronal functioning. In depressed psychiatric patients who were otherwise medically healthy, some studies have indicated that supplementation with omega-3 fatty acids dramatically improves the efficacy of antidepressants; however, few controlled studies have been conducted. A study in patients with stable coronary heart disease and depression, however, showed no improvement in depression after 10 weeks of treatment with omega-3 fatty acids plus sertraline versus a placebo plus sertraline.[69]

VITAMINS. Vitamin E, because of its antioxidant properties, was initially thought to have beneficial effects on the inflammatory processes related to plaque formation in the brains of patients with Alzheimer disease. Trials, however, have not found that vitamin E is beneficial for cognition. Both vitamin E and vitamin A have been associated with increased risk of CVD in several large placebo-controlled trials, contrary to initial theories that they would have the opposite effect.

The use of B vitamins has also been advocated as a way to improve cognition and depression because high plasma levels of the amino acid homocysteine have been associated with Alzheimer disease and depression. Because homocysteine is involved in vitamin B pathways, it was thought that lowering homocysteine with vitamin B therapy would lead to an improvement in cognition and depression. In one study, 276 healthy persons older than 65 years with elevated homocysteine concentrations were given folate and vitamins B_{12} and B_6 or a placebo. Neither folate nor vitamin B supplementation resulted in an improvement in scores of cognition after 2 years.[70]

VALERIAN. Valerian is an extract of the valerian root *(Valeriana officinalis)* and is widely prescribed in Europe for the treatment of insomnia. Valerian is available as a supplement in the United States. In an early study, 166 volunteers were given a valerian-containing commercial product or placebo. After three doses, valerian was associated with a significant decrease in the time it takes to fall asleep and improvement in sleep quality. This study did not measure, however, how well the blinding worked, which is important because valerian has a strong and distinctive smell.

An uncontrolled study of 54 subjects showed a reduction in heart rate, blood pressure, and subjective distress to a stressful task after receiving valerian. This study suggests that valerian may have sedative properties. Valerian does not have major side effects and is probably safe in cardiac patients. However, few data are available to prove its efficacy.

Exercise

A number of studies, dating from the mid-1990s to more recently, show that cardiovascular and resistance or weight training improves depression. These effects may be related in part to an increased growth in brain cells. Regular exercise has favorable effects on the immune system as well, which may promote health, especially in stressed or depressed individuals.

A study of 12,028 randomly selected individuals aged 20 to 79 years showed that increasing physical activity was associated with a 70% reduction in self-reported stress as well as a decrease in life dissatisfaction. Even 2 to 4 hours of walking per week was associated with significant gains. Another study of a group of employees showed reductions in stress levels and depression and improvements in feelings of health and vitality after a 24-week program of aerobic exercise compared with a control group. A 1985 study looked at 43 patients with depression; about half were treated for the condition with antidepressants. Patients were randomized to receive 9 weeks of exercise training (aerobic for 1 hour, three times a week, at 50% to 70% maximum aerobic capacity) or occupational therapy. Exercise was associated with a statistically significant greater decrease in depressive symptoms. In another study, 86 patients with depression who were treated with antidepressants but did not have a therapeutic response were randomized to exercise or health education classes. Exercise involved weight bearing for 45 minutes twice a week for 10 weeks. More patients treated with exercise had an improvement in depression, as defined by a 30% lower Hamilton Depression Scale score; 55% got better with exercise versus 33% without, a difference that was statistically significant. In another study, 156 patients with major depression older than 50 years were randomly assigned to aerobic exercise, antidepressants (sertraline), or a combination of the two for 16 weeks. All patients showed an improvement in symptoms of depression with an essentially identical response between the groups, suggesting that the effect of exercise is at least as large as that of antidepressant medications.

A study found that a half-hour a day of exercise 6 days a week is an effective exercise "dose" to improve the mood of people who have mild to moderate depression, whereas a lower dose is comparable to placebo effect. The study compared two exercise regimens in depressed patients and found that whereas the group that performed 80 minutes of exercise a week received little or no mental health benefit (30% reduction in depressive symptoms versus 29% reduction in the control group), the 3-hour-a-week group had a substantial (47%) reduction in depressive symptoms.[71] Therefore, aerobic exercise at a dose consistent with public health recommendations for CVD prevention is also an effective treatment of mild to moderate depression. Exercise may also complement the effects of antidepressant medication in depressed patients who do not have a complete response to medication.

Treatment Approaches to the Cardiac Patient with Depression and Anxiety

Even though treatment of depression or anxiety has not been shown to improve cardiovascular outcomes in the cardiac patient, it is still necessary to evaluate and to manage these problems to promote the patient's wellness and quality of life as well as to improve patients' ability to adhere to treatments and lifestyle recommendations.

In many cases in which the cardiac patient reports symptoms of depression or anxiety, the cardiologist can address the problem without the need for an immediate referral to a psychiatrist. Many patients complaining of "anxiety" may actually have worry about their cardiac condition. In this situation, education about the cardiac condition, listening to the patient's concerns, and allowing patients to ventilate their worries may go a long way to relieving distress. The next step is to determine if the patient is having thoughts of taking his or her own life or is having severe impairment in functioning that would necessitate referral to a psychiatrist.

A referral to a psychologist or social worker for psychotherapy or counseling may be useful for cardiac patients with symptoms of depression or anxiety. In addition, these patients may benefit from training in stress reduction and stress management techniques, such as yoga, meditation, or mindfulness-based stress reduction classes. The cardiologist may also start a trial of medication. Benzodiazepines can be used short term but should be limited to less than 2 weeks to reduce the risk for development of dependence. They can be useful, however, in the period before antidepressants start working. An alternative for the treatment of anxiety that does not have the risk of dependence or respiratory suppression is buspirone. Antidepressants useful in the cardiac patient include SSRIs (paroxetine, fluoxetine, sertraline, and others), mirtazapine, and bupropion. Patients who fail to respond to these medications may respond to venlafaxine or duloxetine, with careful monitoring of blood pressure. Healthy lifestyle, especially physical activity, should always be recommended, tailored to patients' functional capabilities, to decrease depression and to improve well-being.

REFERENCES

Stress, Emotions, and Cardiovascular Disease: General Considerations

1. McEwen BS: Central effects of stress hormones in health and disease: Understanding the protective and damaging effects of stress and stress mediators. Eur J Pharmacol 583:174, 2008.
2. Steptoe A, Brydon L: Emotional triggering of cardiac events. Neurosci Biobehav Rev 33:63, 2009.
3. Bierhaus A, Wolf J, Andrassy M, et al: A mechanism converting psychosocial stress into mononuclear cell activation. Proc Natl Acad Sci U S A 100:1920, 2003.
4. Kaplan JR, Chen H, Manuck SB: The relationship between social status and atherosclerosis in male and female monkeys as revealed by meta-analysis. Am J Primatol 71:732, 2009.
5. Rozanski A, Blumenthal JA, Davidson KW, et al: The epidemiology, pathophysiology, and management of psychosocial risk factors in cardiac practice: The emerging field of behavioral cardiology. J Am Coll Cardiol 45:637, 2005.
6. Lichtman JH, Bigger JT Jr, Blumenthal JA, et al: Depression and coronary heart disease: Recommendations for screening, referral, and treatment: A science advisory from the American Heart Association Prevention Committee of the Council on Cardiovascular Nursing, Council on Clinical Cardiology, Council on Epidemiology and Prevention, and Interdisciplinary Council on Quality of Care and Outcomes Research: Endorsed by the American Psychiatric Association. Circulation 118:1768, 2008.

Acute Stress

7. Kloner RA: Natural and unnatural triggers of myocardial infarction. Prog Cardiovasc Dis 48:285, 2006.
8. Steinberg JS, Arshad A, Kowalski M, et al: Increased incidence of life-threatening ventricular arrhythmias in implantable defibrillator patients after the World Trade Center attack. J Am Coll Cardiol 44:1261, 2004.
9. Moller J, Theorell T, de Faire U, et al: Work related stressful life events and the risk of myocardial infarction. Case-control and case-crossover analyses within the Stockholm heart epidemiology programme (SHEEP). J Epidemiol Community Health 59:23, 2005.
10. Peters A, von Klot S, Heier M, et al: Exposure to traffic and the onset of myocardial infarction. N Engl J Med 351:1721, 2004.
11. Wittstein IS, Thiemann DR, Lima JAC, et al: Neurohumoral features of myocardial stunning due to sudden emotional stress. N Engl J Med 352:539, 2005.
12. Steptoe A, Strike PC, Perkins-Porras L, et al: Acute depressed mood as a trigger of acute coronary syndromes. Biol Psychiatry 60:837, 2006.
13. Holmes SD, Krantz DS, Rogers H, et al: Mental stress and coronary artery disease: A multidisciplinary guide. Prog Cardiovasc Dis 49:106, 2006.
14. Strike PC, Steptoe A: Systematic review of mental stress-induced myocardial ischaemia. Eur Heart J 24:690, 2003.
15. Ramachandruni S, Fillingim RB, McGorray SP, et al: Mental stress provokes ischemia in coronary artery disease subjects without exercise- or adenosine-induced ischemia. J Am Coll Cardiol 47:987, 2006.
16. Kop WJ, Krantz DS, Nearing BD, et al: Effects of acute mental stress and exercise on T-wave alternans in patients with implantable cardioverter defibrillators and controls. Circulation 109:1864, 2004.
17. Hamer M, Steptoe A: Association between physical fitness, parasympathetic control, and proinflammatory responses to mental stress. Psychosom Med 69:660, 2007.
18. Soufer R, Jain H, Yoon AJ: Heart-brain interactions in mental stress–induced myocardial ischemia. Curr Cardiol Rep 11:133, 2009.
19. Thayer JF, Lane RD: The role of vagal function in the risk for cardiovascular disease and mortality. Biol Psychol 74:224, 2007.
20. Strike PC, Magid K, Whitehead DL, et al: Pathophysiological processes underlying emotional triggering of acute cardiac events. Proc Natl Acad Sci U S A 103:4322, 2006.
21. Kuper H, Marmot M, Hemingway H: Systematic review of prospective cohort studies of psychosocial factors in the etiology and prognosis of coronary heart disease. Semin Vasc Med 2:267, 2002.

Chronic Stress

22. Aboa-Eboule C, Brisson C, Maunsell E, et al: Job strain and risk of acute recurrent coronary heart disease events. JAMA 298:1652, 2007.
23. Orth-Gomer K: Psychosocial and behavioral aspects of cardiovascular disease prevention in men and women. Curr Opin Psychiatry 20:147, 2007.
24. Siegrist J, Marmot M: Health inequalities and the psychosocial environment—two scientific challenges. Soc Sci Med 58:1463, 2004.
25. Brunner EJ, Hemingway H, Walker BR, et al: Adrenocortical, autonomic, and inflammatory causes of the metabolic syndrome: Nested case-control study. Circulation 106:2659, 2002.
26. Hemingway H, Shipley M, Brunner E, et al: Does autonomic function link social position to coronary risk? The Whitehall II study. Circulation 111:3071, 2005.
27. Wang HX, Leineweber C, Kirkeeide R, et al: Psychosocial stress and atherosclerosis: Family and work stress accelerate progression of coronary disease in women. The Stockholm Female Coronary Angiography Study. J Intern Med 261:245, 2007.

28. Dimsdale JE: Psychological stress and cardiovascular disease. J Am Coll Cardiol 51:1237, 2008.
29. Dong M, Giles WH, Felitti VJ, et al: Insights into causal pathways for ischemic heart disease: Adverse childhood experiences study. Circulation 110:1761, 2004.
30. Wegman HL, Stetler C: A meta-analytic review of the effects of childhood abuse on medical outcomes in adulthood. Psychosom Med 71:805, 2009.
31. Danese A, Pariante CM, Caspi A, et al: Childhood maltreatment predicts adult inflammation in a life-course study. Proc Natl Acad Sci U S A 104:1319, 2007.
32. Nielsen NR, Kristensen TS, Schnohr P, Gronbaek M: Perceived stress and cause-specific mortality among men and women: Results from a prospective cohort study. Am J Epidemiol 168:481; discussion 492, 2008.
33. Rosengren A, Hawken S, Ounpuu S, et al: Association of psychosocial risk factors with risk of acute myocardial infarction in 11 119 cases and 13 648 controls from 52 countries (the INTERHEART study): Case-control study. Lancet 364:953, 2004.
34. Yusuf S, Hawken S, Ounpuu S, et al: Effect of potentially modifiable risk factors associated with myocardial infarction in 52 countries (the INTERHEART study): Case-control study. Lancet 364:937, 2004.

Emotional Factors and Psychiatric Diagnoses

35. Mathers CD, Loncar D: Projections of global mortality and burden of disease from 2002 to 2030. PLoS Med 3:e442, 2006.
36. Mallik S, Spertus JA, Reid KJ, et al: Depressive symptoms after acute myocardial infarction: Evidence for highest rates in younger women. Arch Intern Med 166:876, 2006.
37. Nicholson A, Kuper H, Hemingway H: Depression as an aetiologic and prognostic factor in coronary heart disease: A meta-analysis of 6362 events among 146 538 participants in 54 observational studies. Eur Heart J 27:2763, 2006.
38. van Melle JP, de Jonge P, Spijkerman TA, et al: Prognostic association of depression following myocardial infarction with mortality and cardiovascular events: A meta-analysis. Psychosom Med 66:814, 2004.
39. Rutledge T, Reis VA, Linke SE, et al: Depression in heart failure: A meta-analytic review of prevalence, intervention effects, and associations with clinical outcomes. J Am Coll Cardiol 48:1527, 2006.
40. Barth J, Schumacher M, Herrmann-Lingen C: Depression as a risk factor for mortality in patients with coronary heart disease: A meta-analysis. Psychosom Med 66:802, 2004.
41. Skala JA, Freedland KE, Carney RM: Coronary heart disease and depression: A review of recent mechanistic research. Can J Psychiatry 51:738, 2006.
42. Whooley MA, de Jonge P, Vittinghoff E, et al: Depressive symptoms, health behaviors, and risk of cardiovascular events in patients with coronary heart disease. JAMA 300:2379, 2008.
43. Carney RM, Freedland KE, Veith RC: Depression, the autonomic nervous system, and coronary heart disease. Psychosom Med 67:S29, 2005.
44. von Kanel R: Platelet hyperactivity in clinical depression and the beneficial effect of antidepressant drug treatment: How strong is the evidence? Acta Psychiatr Scand 110:163, 2004.
45. Sherwood A, Hinderliter AL, Watkins LL, et al: Impaired endothelial function in coronary heart disease patients with depressive symptomatology. J Am Coll Cardiol 46:656, 2005.
46. Vaccarino V, Johnson BD, Sheps DS, et al: Depression, inflammation, and incident cardiovascular disease in women with suspected coronary ischemia: The National Heart, Lung, and Blood Institute–sponsored WISE study. J Am Coll Cardiol 50:2044, 2007.
47. de Geus EJ: Genetic pleiotropy in depression and coronary artery disease. Psychosom Med 68:185, 2006.
48. Cepoiu M, McCusker J, Cole MG, et al: Recognition of depression by non-psychiatric physicians: A systematic literature review and meta-analysis. J Gen Intern Med 23:25, 2008.
49. Huffman JC, Smith FA, Blais MA, et al: Recognition and treatment of depression and anxiety in patients with acute myocardial infarction. Am J Cardiol 98:319, 2006.
50. Thombs BD, de Jonge P, Coyne JC, et al: Depression screening and patient outcomes in cardiovascular care: A systematic review. JAMA 300:2161, 2008.
51. Rieckmann N, Gerin W, Kronish IM, et al: Course of depressive symptoms and medication adherence after acute coronary syndromes: An electronic medication monitoring study. J Am Coll Cardiol 48:2218, 2006.
52. Qureshi S, Pyne J, Magruder K, et al: The link between post-traumatic stress disorder and physical comorbidities: A systematic review. Psychiatr Q 80:87, 2009.

Other Psychosocial Characteristics and Personality Traits

53. Chida Y, Steptoe A: The association of anger and hostility with future coronary heart disease: A meta-analytic review of prospective evidence. J Am Coll Cardiol 53:936, 2009.
54. Kupper N, Denollet J: Type D personality as a prognostic factor in heart disease: Assessment and mediating mechanisms. J Pers Assess 89:265, 2007.

Psychiatric Care of the Cardiac Patient

55. Shimbo D, Davidson KW, Haas DC, et al: Negative impact of depression on outcomes in patients with coronary artery disease: Mechanisms, treatment considerations, and future directions. J Thromb Haemost 3:897, 2005.
56. Sala M, Coppa F, Cappucciati C, et al: Antidepressants: Their effects on cardiac channels, QT prolongation and torsades de pointes. Curr Opin Investig Drugs 7:256, 2006.
57. Rigotti NA, Thorndike AN, Regan S, et al: Bupropion for smokers hospitalized with acute cardiovascular disease. Am J Med 119:1080, 2006.
58. Kirsch I, Deacon BJ, Huedo-Medina TB, et al: Initial severity and antidepressant benefits: A meta-analysis of data submitted to the Food and Drug Administration. PLoS Med 5:e45, 2008.
59. Fournier JC, DeRubeis RJ, Hollon SD, et al: Antidepressant drug effects and depression severity: A patient-level meta-analysis. JAMA 303:47, 2010.
60. Ziegelstein RC, Parakh K, Sakhuja A, Bhat U: Platelet function in patients with major depression. Intern Med J 39:38, 2009.
61. Carney RM, Freedland KE: Depression in patients with coronary heart disease. Am J Med 121:S20, 2008.
62. Lesperance F, Frasure-Smith N, Koszycki D, et al: Effects of citalopram and interpersonal psychotherapy on depression in patients with coronary artery disease. JAMA 297:367, 2007.
63. Whang W, Kubzansky LD, Kawachi I, et al: Depression and risk of sudden cardiac death and coronary heart disease in women: Results from the Nurses' Health Study. J Am Coll Cardiol 53:950, 2009.
64. Krantz DS, Whittaker KS, Francis JL, et al: Psychotropic medication use and risk of adverse cardiovascular events in women with suspected coronary artery disease: Outcomes from the Women's Ischemia Syndrome Evaluation (WISE) study. Heart 95:1901, 2009.
65. Tess AV, Smetana GW: Medical evaluation of patients undergoing electroconvulsive therapy. N Engl J Med 360:1437, 2009.
66. Newcomer JW: Abnormalities of glucose metabolism associated with atypical antipsychotic drugs. J Clin Psychiatry 18:36, 2004.
67. Janeway DDO: An integrated approach to the diagnosis and treatment of anxiety within the practice of cardiology. Cardiol Rev 17:36, 2009.

Alternative Medicines, Herbs, and Supplements

68. Linde K, Berner MM, Kriston L: St John's wort for major depression. Cochrane Database Syst Rev (4):CD000448, 2008.
69. Carney RM, Freedland KE, Rubin EH, et al: Omega-3 augmentation of sertraline in treatment of depression in patients with coronary heart disease: A randomized controlled trial. JAMA 302:1651, 2009.
70. McMahon JA, Green TJ, Skeaff CM, et al: A controlled trial of homocysteine lowering and cognitive performance. N Engl J Med 354:2764, 2006.
71. Dunn AL, Trivedi MH, Kampert JB, et al: Exercise treatment for depression: Efficacy and dose response. Am J Prev Med 28:1, 2005.

CHAPTER 92 Neurologic Disorders and Cardiovascular Disease

William J. Groh and Douglas P. Zipes

Cardiac disease occurring secondary to an underlying neurologic disorder is related either to a direct involvement of the heart or is caused by induced neurohormonal abnormalities that act on the heart. In several neurologic disorders, the cardiovascular manifestations are responsible for a greater risk of morbidity and mortality than the neurologic manifestations. This chapter will review those neurologic disorders associated with important cardiovascular sequelae.

Muscular Dystrophies

The muscular dystrophies are a diffuse group of heritable disorders in which direct involvement of cardiac muscle is present to a variable degree. The muscular dystrophies that manifest cardiovascular involvement can be classified into the following:

1. Duchenne and Becker muscular dystrophies
2. Myotonic dystrophies
3. Emery-Dreifuss muscular dystrophies and associated disorders
4. Limb-girdle muscular dystrophies
5. Facioscapulohumeral muscular dystrophy

Duchenne and Becker Muscular Dystrophies

GENETICS. Both Duchenne and Becker muscular dystrophy are X-linked recessive disorders in which the genetic locus has been identified as an abnormality in the dystrophin gene. The dystrophin protein and dystrophin-associated glycoproteins provide a structural link between the myocyte cytoskeleton and extracellular matrix functioning to link contractile proteins to the cell membrane. Dystrophin messenger RNA is expressed predominantly in skeletal, cardiac, and smooth muscle with lower levels in the brain. Absence of dystrophin can lead to membrane fragility, resulting in myofibril necrosis and eventual loss of muscle fibers, with fibrotic replacement. Abnormalities in dystrophin and in dystrophin-associated glycoproteins underlie the degeneration of cardiac and skeletal muscle in several inherited myopathies, including X-linked dilated cardiomyopathy. Beyond the inherited disorders, the loss of dystrophin plays a role in myocyte failure in other cardiomyopathies, including sporadic idiopathic, viral myocarditis, and those associated with coronary artery disease. In Duchenne muscular dystrophy, dystrophin is almost absent whereas in Becker muscular dystrophy, dystrophin is present but reduced in size or amount. This leads to the characteristic rapidly progressive skeletal muscle disease in Duchenne and the more benign course in Becker muscular dystrophy. The heart as a muscle is involved in both disorders. Specific dystrophin gene mutations are associated with a higher prevalence of cardiomyopathy.[1]

CLINICAL PRESENTATION. Duchenne muscular dystrophy is the most common inherited neuromuscular disorder, with an incidence of 1/3,500 live male births. Patients typically become symptomatic before the age of 5 years, presenting with skeletal muscle weakness that progresses if untreated so that the boy becomes wheelchair-bound before the age of 13 years (**Fig. 92-1**). Historically, death occurs commonly by age 25 years, primarily from respiratory dysfunction and, less commonly, from heart failure. A multidisciplinary treatment approach including steroids, cardiac therapy, and ventilatory support has lengthened survival. Becker muscular dystrophy is less common, with an incidence of 1/33,000 live male births, has a more variable presentation of skeletal muscle weakness (see Fig. 92-1), and has a better prognosis, with most patients surviving to age 40 to 50 years.

In both Duchenne and Becker muscular dystrophies, elevated serum creatine kinase activity is observed, over 10- and fivefold normal values, respectively.

CARDIOVASCULAR MANIFESTATIONS. Most patients with Duchenne muscular dystrophy develop a cardiomyopathy, but symptoms can be masked by severe skeletal muscle weakness. Preclinical cardiac involvement is present in 25% by age 6, with the onset of clinically apparent cardiomyopathy after age 10 years common. Up to 90% of Duchenne muscular dystrophy patients 18 years of age or older have a dilated cardiomyopathy by echocardiography. Predilection for involvement in the inferobasal and lateral left ventricle has been observed (**Fig. 92-2**). As with the skeletal muscle weakness, cardiac involvement in Becker muscular dystrophy is more variable than in Duchenne muscular dystrophy, ranging from none or subclinical to severe cardiomyopathy requiring transplantation. Cardiac involvement in Becker muscular dystrophy is independent of the severity of skeletal muscle involvement, with some but not all investigators observing increased likelihood of cardiovascular disease in older patients. More than 50% of patients with subclinical or benign skeletal muscle disease were noted to have cardiac involvement if carefully evaluated. Progression in the severity of cardiac involvement is common. Cardiomyopathy can initially involve only the right ventricle.

Thoracic deformities and a high diaphragm can alter the cardiovascular examination in Duchenne muscular dystrophy. A reduction in the anterior-posterior chest dimension is commonly responsible for a systolic impulse displaced to the left sternal border, a grade 1-3/6 short midsystolic murmur in the second left interspace, and a loud pulmonary component of the second heart sound. In Duchenne and Becker muscular dystrophies, mitral regurgitation is commonly observed. The presence of mitral regurgitation is related to posterior papillary muscle dysfunction in Duchenne muscular dystrophy and to mitral annular dilation in Becker muscular dystrophy.

Female carriers of Duchenne and Becker muscular dystrophies are at increased risk of dilated cardiomyopathy.

Electrocardiography

In most patients with Duchenne muscular dystrophy, the electrocardiogram (ECG) is abnormal (see Chap. 13). The classically described electrocardiographic pattern shows distinctive tall R waves and increased R/S amplitude in V_1 and deep narrow Q waves in the left precordial leads, possibly related to the posterolateral left ventricular involvement (**Fig. 92-3**). Other common findings include a short PR interval and right ventricular hypertrophy. There does not appear to be an association between the presence of a dilated cardiomyopathy and electrocardiographic abnormalities.[2] In patients with Becker muscular dystrophy, electrocardiographic abnormalities are present in up to 75%. These include tall R waves and increased R/S amplitude in V_1, akin to that seen in Duchenne muscular dystrophy, but can also show frequent incomplete right bundle branch block. This may be related to early involvement of the right ventricle. In patients with congestive heart failure, left bundle branch block is common.

Echocardiography

Diastolic dysfunction and regional wall motion abnormalities as observed by echocardiography (see Chap. 15) can precede the global systolic dysfunction in Duchenne and Becker muscular dystrophies. Regional abnormalities in the posterobasal and lateral wall typically occur earlier than in other areas (see Fig. 92-2). A process akin to left ventricular noncompaction can be observed, possibly resulting from compensatory mechanisms in response to the failing dystrophic myocardium. Mitral regurgitation can result from dystrophic changes in the posterior leaflet papillary muscles.

Arrhythmias

In Duchenne muscular dystrophy, persistent or labile sinus tachycardia is the most common arrhythmia recognized (see Chap. 39). Atrial arrhythmias, including atrial fibrillation and atrial flutter, occur primarily as a preterminal rhythm. Abnormalities in atrioventricular conduction have been observed, with both short and prolonged PR intervals recognized. Ventricular arrhythmias occur on monitoring in 30%, primarily ventricular premature beats. Complex ventricular arrhythmias have been reported, more commonly in patients with severe skeletal muscle disease. Sudden

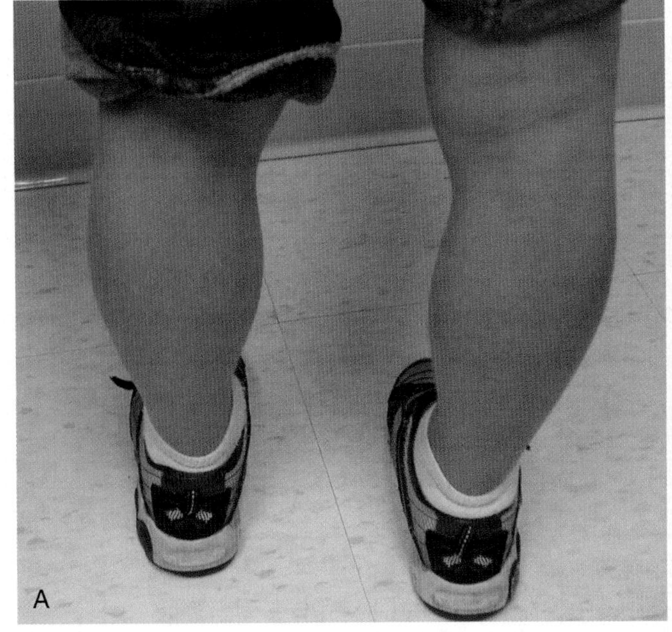

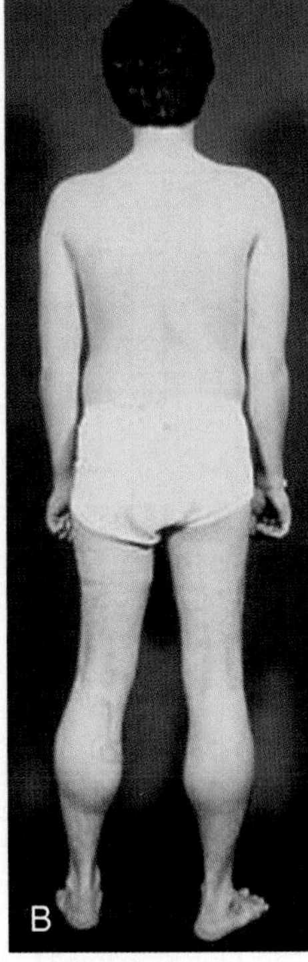

FIGURE 92-1 **A,** Calf pseudohypertrophy in an 8-year-old boy with Duchenne muscular dystrophy. **B,** Becker muscular dystrophy in a 24-year-old man. There is dystrophy of the shoulder girdle and calf pseudohypertrophy. *(**A** courtesy of Dr. Laurence E. Walsh; **B** courtesy of Dr. Robert M. Pascuzzi.)*

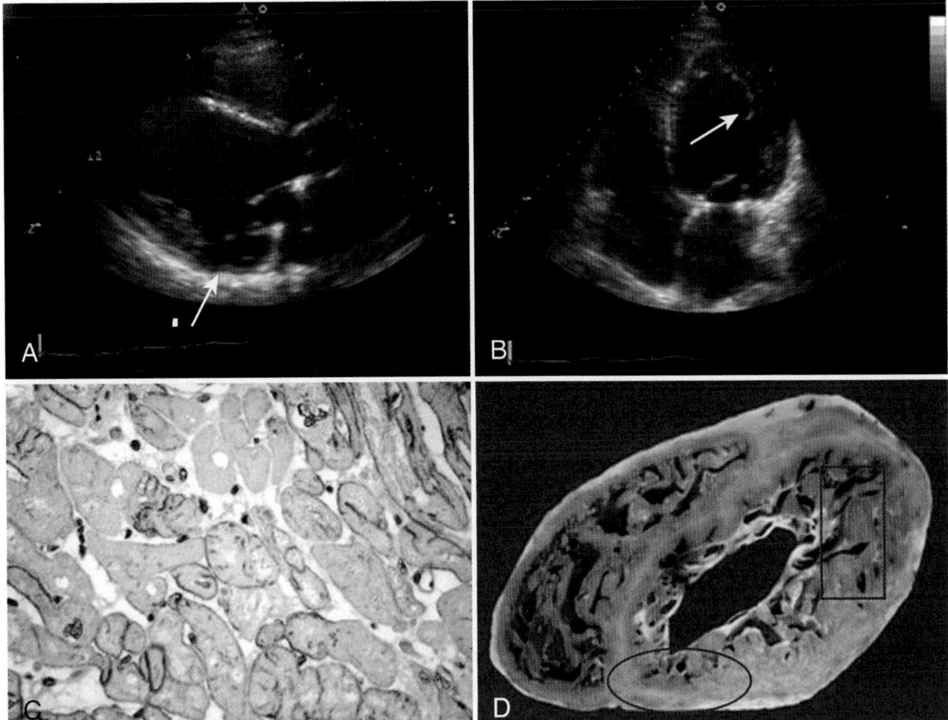

FIGURE 92-2 Cardiac involvement in a 32-year-old man with Becker muscular dystrophy. **A, B,** Transthoracic echocardiogram showing localized thinning and noncompaction in the inferobasal (A, arrow) and apicolateral left ventricle (B, arrow). **C,** Myocardial biopsy showing discontinuous and absent staining consistent with Becker muscular dystrophy. **D,** Explanted heart obtained at transplantation correlating with the echocardiogram with involvement in the inferobasal (oval) and apicolateral left ventricle (rectangle). (**C** stained for dystrophin antibody.) *(From Rapezzi C, Leone O, Biagini E, et al: Echocardiographic clues to diagnosis of dystrophin-related dilated cardiomyopathy. Heart 93:10, 2007.)*

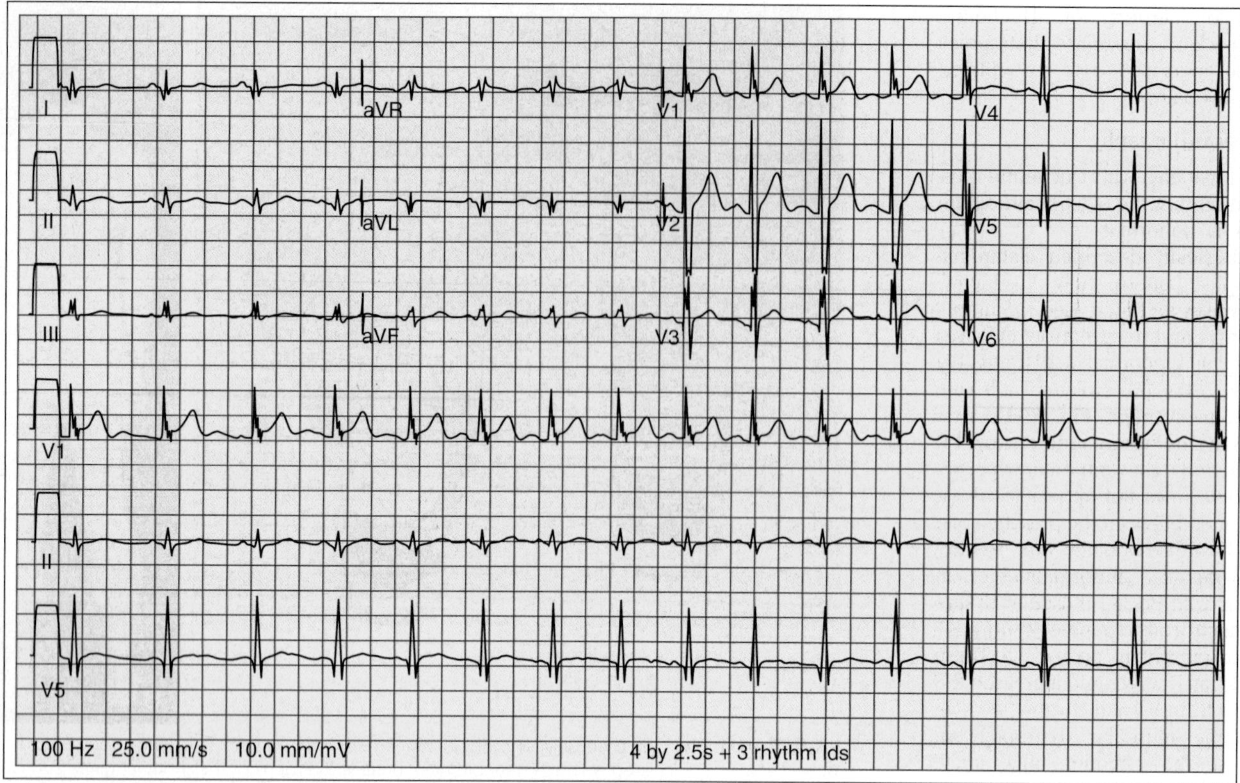

A

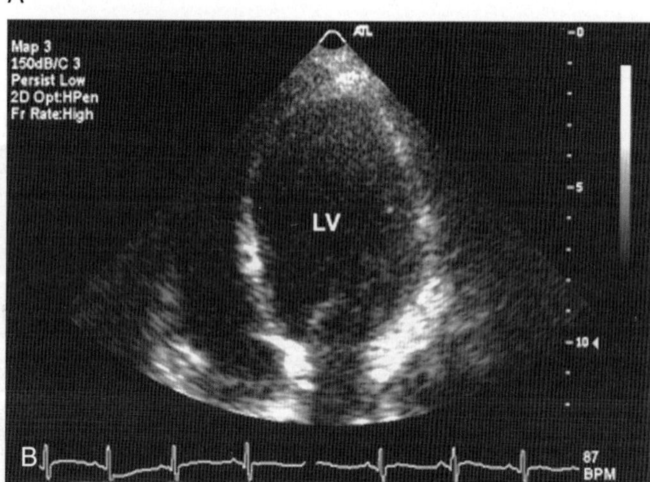

FIGURE 92-3 Dilated cardiomyopathy in a 19-year-old man with Duchenne muscular dystrophy. **A,** ECG showing a QRS complex that is typical of Duchenne dystrophy, with tall R waves in V_1 and deep narrow Q waves in leads I and aVL. **B,** Two-dimensional echocardiogram (parasternal four chamber) showing a dilated, thinned left ventricle (LV).

death occurs in Duchenne muscular dystrophy, typically in patients with end stage muscular disease. Whether the sudden death is caused by arrhythmias is unclear. Several follow-up studies have shown a correlation between sudden death and the presence of complex ventricular arrhythmias. The presence of ventricular arrhythmias was not a predictor for all-cause mortality.

Arrhythmia manifestations in Becker muscular dystrophy typically relates to the severity of the associated structural cardiomyopathy. Distal conduction system disease with complete heart block and bundle branch reentry ventricular tachycardia has been observed.

TREATMENT AND PROGNOSIS. Duchenne muscular dystrophy is a progressive disorder, with death from a respiratory or cardiac cause. Steroids and steroid derivatives are effective in delaying skeletal muscle disease progression and appear also to decrease the progression of the dilated cardiomyopathy.[3] Gene replacement therapy holds future promise. A primary cardiac cause of death occurs in 25% of patients but appears to be playing an increasingly significant role because of delayed mortality with improved respiratory support. There is an equal distribution of cardiac death from heart failure and sudden death. Annual imaging for assessment of left ventricular function should be initiated in patients at approximately 10 years of age. Angiotensin-converting enzyme (ACE) inhibitors and beta blockers can improve left ventricular function in patients treated early.[1,4] Whether these heart failure therapies improve long-term outcomes is unclear.

In patients with Becker muscular dystrophy, an improvement in left ventricular function is also observed after treatment with ACE inhibitors and beta blockers.[1] Screening left ventricular imaging should occur as in Duchenne muscular dystrophy. Female carriers of Duchenne and Becker muscular dystrophies do not develop a cardiomyopathy during childhood and screening can be delayed until later in

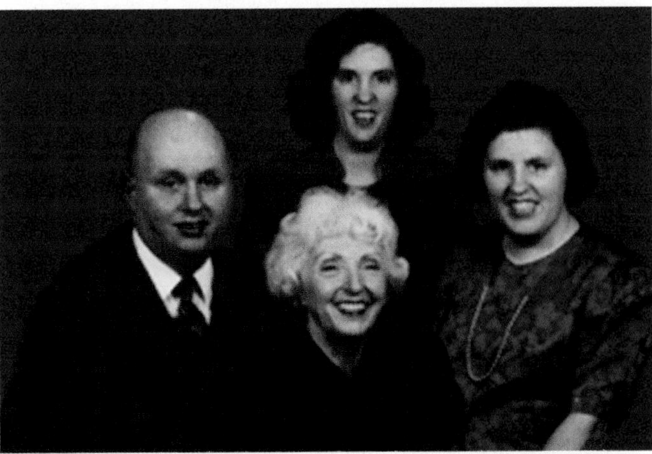

FIGURE 92-4 Myotonic muscular dystrophy in three siblings. The mother (front) is unaffected. Premature balding (left) and characteristic thin facies (rear) are demonstrated.

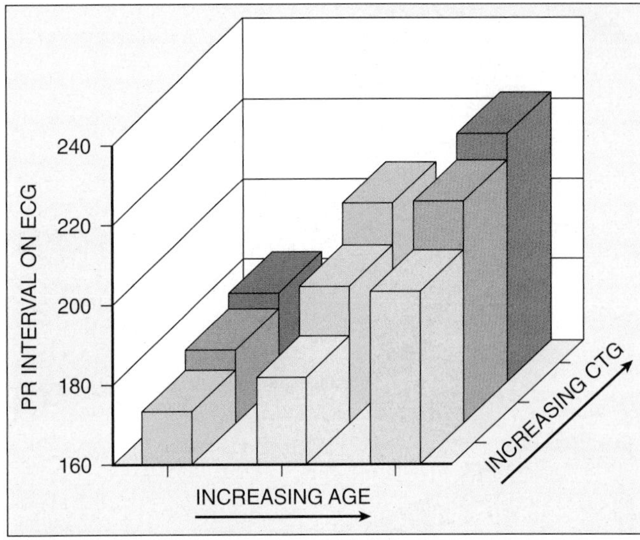

FIGURE 92-5 Relationship between the PR interval on the ECG and age and CTG repeat sequence expansion in 342 patients with myotonic dystrophy type 1. There is a direct relationship between age and CTG repeat sequence expansion and the severity of cardiac conduction disease as quantified by the PR interval. The relationship suggests that cardiac involvement in myotonic dystrophy type 1 is a time-dependent degenerative process, with the rate of progression modulated by the extent of CTG repeat expansion. *(From Groh WJ, Lowe MR, Zipes DP: Severity of cardiac conduction involvement and arrhythmias in myotonic dystrophy type 1 correlates with age and CTG repeat length. J Cardiovasc Electrophysiol 13:444, 2002.)*

adolescence. Whether carriers benefit from afterload reduction therapy is unknown but would seem reasonable based on shared mechanisms. Once heart failure is established, conventional therapy is indicated. Cardiac transplantation has been reported.

Myotonic Dystrophies

Genetics. The myotonic dystrophies are autosomal dominant inherited disorders characterized by reflex and percussion myotonia, weakness and atrophy of distal skeletal muscles, and systemic manifestations including endocrine abnormalities, cataracts, cognitive impairment, and cardiac involvement (**Fig. 92-4**). Two distinct genetic mutations are known to be responsible for the myotonic dystrophies and are reflected in an updated disease classification. In myotonic dystrophy type 1, the gene mutation is an amplified and unstable trinucleotide, cytosine-thymine-guanine (CTG) repeat found on chromosome 19q13.3. Whereas unaffected patients have 5 to 37 copies of the repeat, patients with myotonic dystrophy have 50 to several thousand repeats. A direct correlation exists between an increasing number of CTG repeats and earlier age of onset and increasing severity of neuromuscular involvement. Cardiac involvement, including conduction disease and arrhythmias, also correlates with the length of repeat expansion (**Fig. 92-5**). It is typical for the CTG repeat to expand as it is passed from parents to their offspring, giving the characteristic worsening clinical manifestations in subsequent generations that is termed *anticipation*.

Myotonic dystrophy type 2, also called proximal myotonic myopathy, has generally less severe skeletal muscle and cardiac involvement than type 1.[5] There is no congenital presentation or cognitive impairment in myotonic dystrophy type 2, typically the most severely involved subsets of the type 1 patients. The genetic mutation responsible for myotonic dystrophy type 2 is a large and unstable tetranucleotide repeat expansion, cytosine-CTG, found on chromosome 3q21. Intergenerational contraction of the repeat expansion has been reported and there is no apparent relationship between the degree of expansion and clinical severity.

The molecular mechanism whereby both myotonic dystrophies exert their similar phenotypic presentations is by the toxic effects of the large mutant RNA expansion on nuclear RNA binding proteins.[6]

CLINICAL PRESENTATION. The myotonic dystrophies are the most common inherited neuromuscular disorders in patients presenting as adults. Until recently, studies have not genetically differentiated myotonic dystrophy types 1 and 2, and therefore the clinical characteristics described are likely for a mixed group. Type 1 is significantly more common than type 2, except possibly in certain areas of northern Europe. The global incidence of myotonic dystrophy type 1 has been estimated to be 1/8000, although it is higher in certain populations, such as French Canadians, and lower to nonexistent in other populations, such as African blacks. The age at onset of symptoms and diagnosis averages 20 to 25 years. Common early manifestations are weakness in the muscles of the face, neck, and distal extremities. On examination, myotonia (delayed muscle relaxation) can be demonstrated in the grip, thenar muscle group, and tongue (**Fig. 92-6**). Diagnosis when the patient is asymptomatic is possible using electromyography and genetic testing. In general, cardiac symptoms occur after the onset of skeletal muscle weakness but can be the initial manifestation of the disease.

Myotonic dystrophy type 2 also manifests with myotonia, muscle weakness, cataracts, and endocrine abnormalities, as in type 1. Age at symptom onset is typically older in myotonic dystrophy type 2.

CARDIOVASCULAR MANIFESTATIONS. Cardiac pathology in the myotonic dystrophies primarily involves degeneration, fibrosis, and fatty infiltration of the specialized conduction tissue, including the sinus node, atrioventricular node, and His-Purkinje system. Degenerative changes are observed in working atrial and ventricular tissue but only rarely progress to a symptomatic dilated cardiomyopathy (**Fig. 92-7**). It is not clear whether there are differences in the cardiac pathology observed between myotonic dystrophy types 1 and 2. The primary cardiac manifestations of the myotonic dystrophies are arrhythmias.

ELECTROCARDIOGRAPHY. Most adult patients with myotonic dystrophy type 1 have electrocardiographic abnormalities. In a large, unselected middle-aged myotonic population followed in a U.S. neuromuscular clinic setting, 65% of patients had an abnormal ECG.[7] Abnormalities included first-degree atrioventricular block in 42%, right bundle branch block in 3%, left bundle branch block in 4%, and nonspecific intraventricular conduction delay in 12%. Q waves not associated with a known myocardial infarction are common. Electrocardiographic abnormalities progress as the patient ages (**Fig. 92-8**).

Electrocardiographic abnormalities are less common in myotonic dystrophy type 2, occurring in approximately 20% of middle-aged patients.

ECHOCARDIOGRAPHY. Left ventricular systolic and diastolic dysfunction, left ventricular hypertrophy, mitral valve prolapse, regional

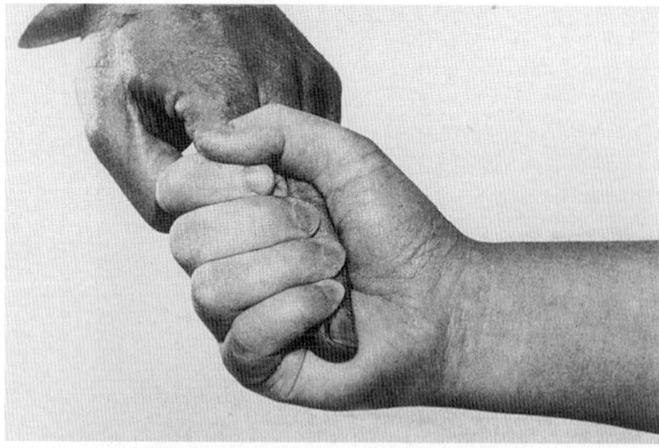

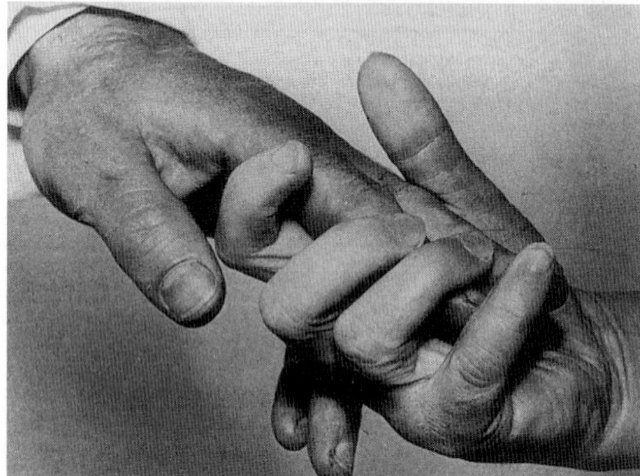

FIGURE 92-6 Grip myotonia in myotonic muscular dystrophy. This patient had an inability to release (bottom) after exerting grip (top). *(From Engel AG, Franzini-Armstrong C [eds]: Myology: Basic and Clinical. 2nd ed. vol. II. New York, McGraw Hill, 1994.)*

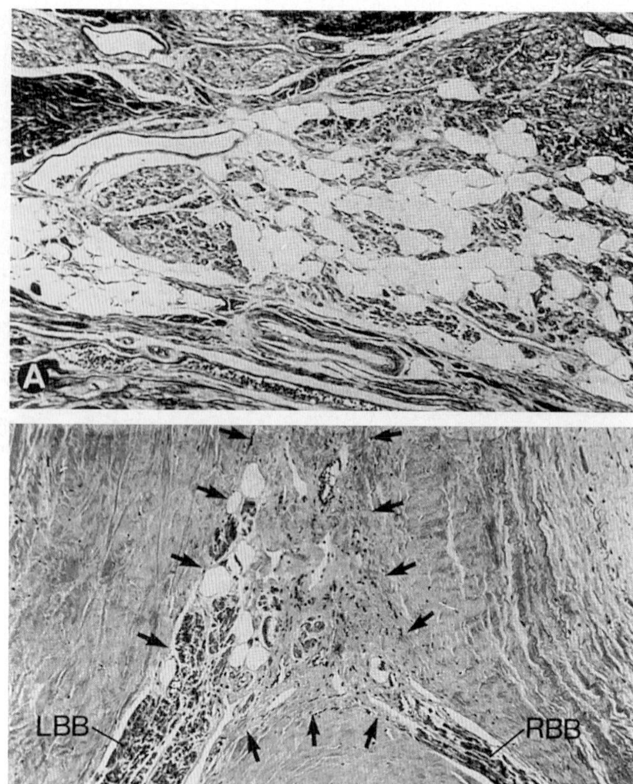

FIGURE 92-7 Histopathology of the atrioventricular bundle in myotonic dystrophy. **A,** Fatty infiltration in a 57-year-old man. **B,** Focal replacement fibrosis and atrophy in a 48-year-old woman. Arrows demarcate expected size and shape of the branching atrioventricular bundle. (**A,** Masson trichrome stain, ×90; **B,** hematoxylin-eosin stain, ×90). LBB = left bundle branch; RBB = right bundle branch. *(From Nguyen HH, Wolfe JT III, Holmes DR Jr, Edwards WD: Pathology of the cardiac conduction system in myotonic dystrophy: A study of 12 cases. J Am Coll Cardiol 11:662, 1988.)*

wall motion abnormalities, and left atrial dilation have been reported in myotonic dystrophy type 1 patients with moderate prevalence rates, as observed by echocardiography (see Chap. 15).[8] However, the prevalence of clinical heart failure is significantly lower, estimated at 2%. Left ventricular hypertrophy and ventricular dilation have been reported in myotonic dystrophy type 2.

Arrhythmias

Patients with myotonic dystrophy type 1 demonstrate a wide range of arrhythmias. With a cardiac electrophysiologic study, the most commonly found abnormality is a prolonged His-ventricular (H-V) interval. Conduction system disease can progress to symptomatic atrioventricular block and necessitate pacemaker implantation. The prevalence of permanent cardiac pacing in patients with myotonic dystrophy type 1 varies widely among studies based on referral patterns and the indications used for implantation. Updated practice guidelines have recognized that asymptomatic conduction abnormalities in neuromuscular diseases such as myotonic dystrophy may warrant special consideration for pacing.

Atrial arrhythmias, primarily atrial fibrillation and atrial flutter, are the most common arrhythmias observed.[7] Ventricular tachycardia can occur. Myotonic dystrophy type 1 patients are at risk of ventricular tachycardia because of reentry in the diseased distal conduction system, as characterized by bundle branch reentry and interfascicular reentry tachycardia (**Fig. 92-9**). Therapy with right bundle branch or fascicular radiofrequency ablation can be curative.

The incidence of sudden death in patients with myotonic dystrophy type 1 is substantial and thought to be caused by primarily arrhythmias. In a prospective registry of 406 myotonic dystrophy type 1 patients from the United States, one third of deaths were sudden, presumably caused by arrhythmias.[7] Sudden death was secondary only to respiratory failure as a cause of death. The mechanisms leading to sudden death in myotonic dystrophy type 1 are not clear. Distal conduction disease producing atrioventricular block can result in the lack of an appropriate escape rhythm and asystole or bradycardia-mediated ventricular fibrillation. Sudden death can occur in myotonic dystrophy type 1, despite previous permanent cardiac pacing, implicating the role of ventricular arrhythmias. Whether a nonarrhythmic cause of sudden death plays a role remains uncertain.

Arrhythmias and sudden death have been reported in myotonic dystrophy type 2 but seem to be rarer than in type 1.[9]

TREATMENT AND PROGNOSIS. Because cardiac manifestations can occur in myotonic dystrophy types 1 and 2, diagnostic evaluation and appropriate therapy should be done for both. However, cardiac management in patients with the myotonic dystrophies is not well established. An echocardiogram can determine whether structural abnormalities are present. In the unusual patient with a dilated cardiomyopathy, standard therapy, including ACE inhibitors and beta blockers, has improved symptoms. Patients presenting with symptoms indicative of arrhythmias, such as syncope and palpitations, should undergo an evaluation, often including a cardiac electrophysiologic study, to determine a cause. Annual ECGs and 24-hour ambulatory monitoring have been recommended for asymptomatic patients. Significant or progressive electrocardiographic abnormalities, despite a lack of symptoms, can be an indication for prophylactic pacing or further diagnostic testing. The presence of significant electrocardiographic conduction

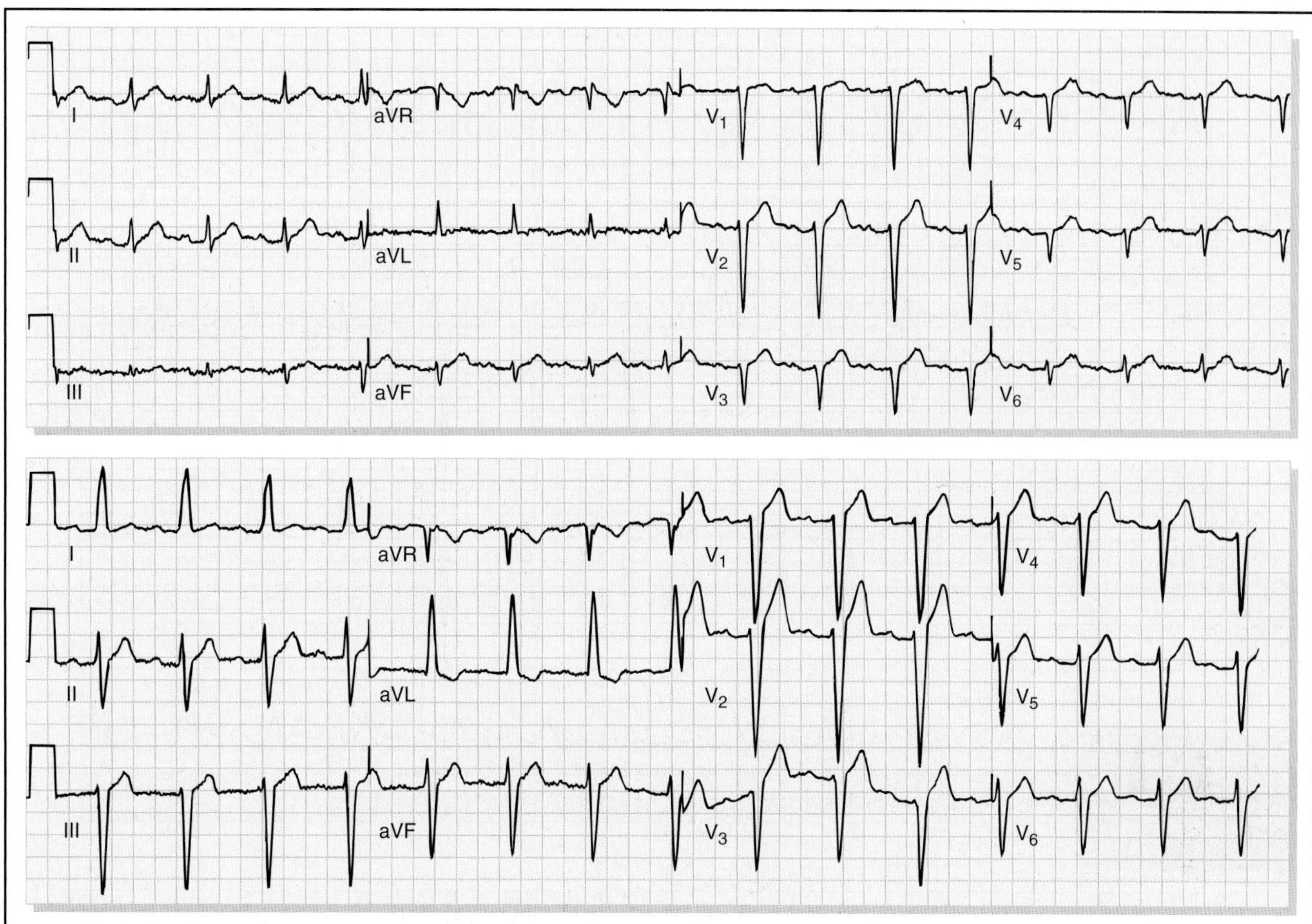

FIGURE 92-8 ECGs obtained 1 year apart in a 36-year-old man with myotonic dystrophy (the top set is older). Note the abnormal Q waves in the precordial leads. An increasing PR interval and QRS duration are observed, consistent with increasing severity of conduction disease.

abnormalities and clinical atrial arrhythmias have been determined to be independent risk factors for sudden death.[7] Whether permanent pacemakers protect against sudden death is unclear, and whether implantable cardioverter-defibrillators (ICDs) would be a more appropriate prophylactic therapy in the myotonic dystrophy patient is untested. Certain families may be more prone to arrhythmia manifestations of myotonic dystrophy. Anesthesia in patients with myotonic dystrophy can increase the risk of atrioventricular block and other arrhythmias. Careful monitoring during the perioperative period, with a low threshold for prophylactic temporary pacing, is recommended.

In patients presenting with wide complex tachycardia, a cardiac electrophysiologic study with particular evaluation for bundle branch reentry tachycardia should be carried out. ICDs are being increasingly used in myotonic dystrophy patients.

The course of neuromuscular abnormalities in the myotonic dystrophies is variable. Death from respiratory dysfunction can occur in advanced skeletal muscle disease. Other patients may be only minimally limited by weakness, up to 60 to70 years of age. Sudden death can reduce survival in patients with the myotonic dystrophies, including those minimally symptomatic from a neuromuscular status. Which evaluation and interventions are appropriate and the degree of effectiveness needed to decrease the risk of sudden death are unclear.

Emery-Dreifuss Muscular Dystrophy and Associated Disorders

Genetics and Cardiac Pathology. Emery-Dreifuss muscular dystrophy is a rare familial disorder in which skeletal muscle symptoms are often mild, but with cardiac involvement that is common and life-threatening. The disease is typically inherited in an X-linked recessive fashion but there is heterogeneity, in that families have been reported that fit an X-linked dominant, autosomal dominant, and autosomal recessive inheritance pattern. The gene responsible for the X-linked Emery-Dreifuss muscular dystrophy, *STA*, encodes a nuclear membrane protein termed *emerin*. The lack of emerin in skeletal and cardiac muscle is responsible for the disease phenotype. Mutations in genes found on chromosome 1 encoding two other nuclear membrane proteins, lamins A and C, have been identified as being responsible for a variety of other disorders, with a phenotypic expression related to X-linked Emery-Dreifuss muscular dystrophy. These disorders include autosomal dominant and recessive Emery-Dreifuss muscular dystrophy, autosomal dominant dilated cardiomyopathy with conduction disease, autosomal dominant limb-girdle muscular dystrophy with conduction disease, and lipodystrophy with associated cardiac abnormalities.[10]

Nuclear membrane proteins, such as emerin and lamins A and C, provide structural support for the nucleus and interact with the cell's cytoskeletal proteins. Mutations in the tail regions of lamins A and C are responsible for most cases of autosomal dominant Emery-Dreifuss muscular dystrophy, with a phenotype of cardiac and skeletal muscle involvement. Mutations in the rod domain of the lamin A/C gene primarily cause isolated cardiac disease, including dilated cardiomyopathy, conduction system degeneration, and atrial and ventricular arrhythmias.

Clinical Presentation. Emery-Dreifuss muscular dystrophy is characterized by a triad of the following: (1) early contractures of the elbow, Achilles tendon, and posterior cervical muscles; (2) slowly progressing muscle weakness and atrophy, primarily in humeroperoneal muscles; and (3) cardiac involvement (**Fig. 92-10**). The disorder has been labeled benign X-linked muscular dystrophy to differentiate the slowly progressive muscular weakness from that of Duchenne muscular dystrophy. A definitive diagnosis can be made in

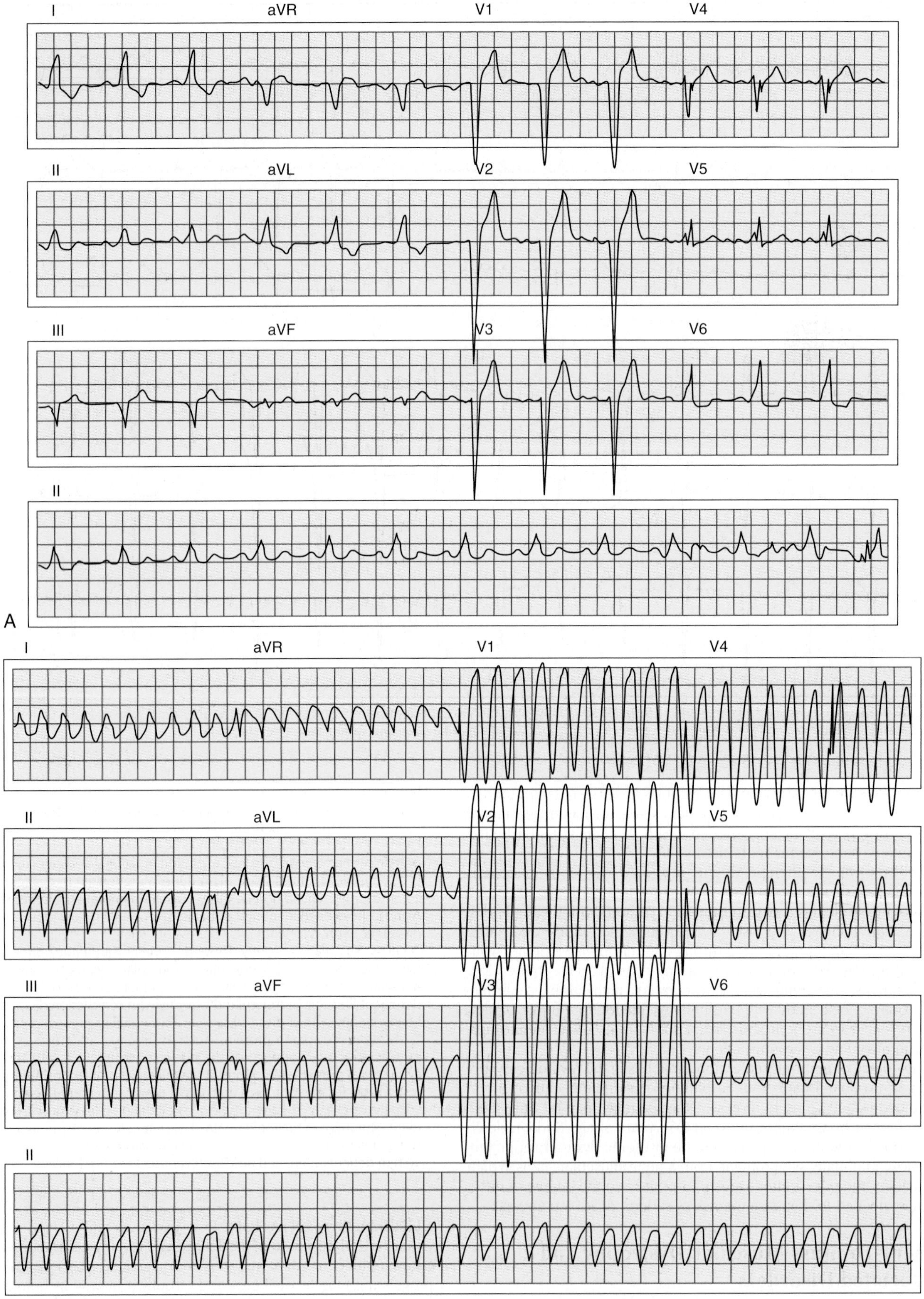

I aVR V1 V4

II aVL V2 V5

III aVF V3 V6

II

A

I aVR V1 V4

II aVL V2 V5

III aVF V3 V6

II

B

FIGURE 92-9 Bundle branch reentry tachycardia in a 34-year-old woman with myotonic dystrophy type 1 presenting with a symptomatic (recurrent syncope) wide-complex tachycardia. **A,** ECG showing sinus rhythm and a QRS complex with left bundle branch block. **B,** ECG showing a rapid monomorphic tachycardia easily inducible at electrophysiologic study, with left bundle morphology.

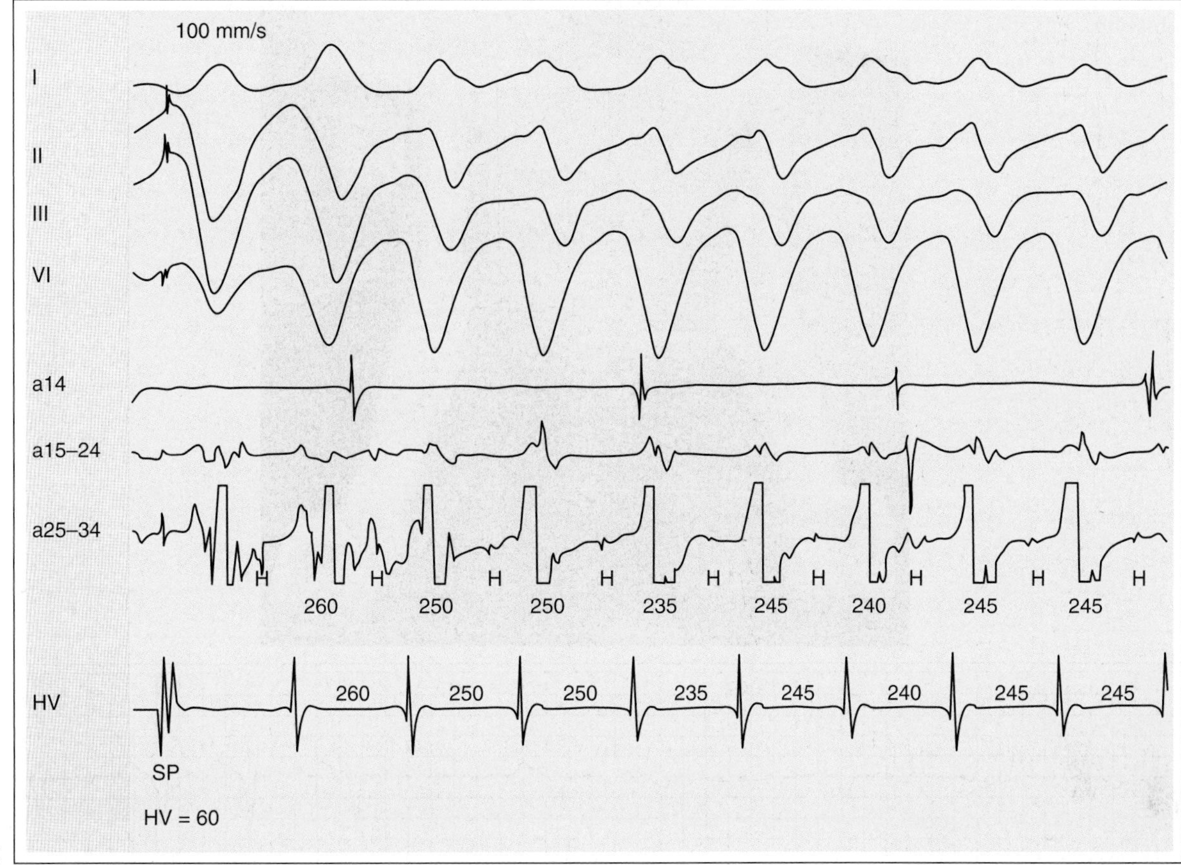

FIGURE 92-9, cont'd C, Recordings during electrophysiologic study, including the surface ECG (leads I, II, III, V1) and intracardiac ECGs. A monomorphic ventricular tachycardia is induced with atrial-ventricular (A-V) dissociation and His association consistent with bundle branch reentry tachycardia. H = His recording; HRA = high right atrium; HV = RV; RV = right ventricle; a14 = HRA; a15-24 = His proximal; a25-34 = His distal.

Emery-Dreifuss muscular dystrophy with genetic testing and anti–emerin antibody staining in skeletal muscle biopsy.

In the autosomal dominant and recessive inheritance of Emery-Dreifuss muscular dystrophy, a more variable phenotypic expression and penetrance are typically observed.

A mutation in the lamin A/C gene is also responsible for an autosomal dominant inherited familial partial lipodystrophy, characterized by marked loss of subcutaneous fat, diabetes, hypertriglyceridemia, and cardiac abnormalities.

CARDIOVASCULAR MANIFESTATIONS. Arrhythmias and dilated cardiomyopathy are the major manifestations of cardiac disease in Emery-Dreifuss muscular dystrophy and associated disorders. In X-linked recessive Emery-Dreifuss muscular dystrophy, abnormalities in impulse generation and conduction are exceedingly frequent. ECGs are generally abnormal by age 20 to 30 years, commonly showing first-degree atrioventricular block. The atria appear to be involved earlier than the ventricles, with atrial fibrillation and atrial flutter or, more typically, permanent atrial standstill and junctional bradycardia observed. Abnormalities in impulse generation or conduction are present in the ECG of virtually all patients by age 35 to 40 years and pacing is often required. Ventricular arrhythmias, including sustained ventricular tachycardia and ventricular fibrillation, have been reported. Invasive cardiac electrophysiologic study data are limited in this rare condition. Mild prolongation of the H-V interval and atrial, atrioventricular nodal, and ventricular refractory periods have been observed. Sudden, presumably cardiac, death before age 50 years is common. The incidence of sudden death may decrease with prophylactic pacing.

A nonrandomized study has shown frequent appropriate therapies for ventricular arrhythmias in patients with conduction disease who received prophylactic ICDs.[11] Female carriers of X-linked recessive Emery-Dreifuss muscular dystrophy do not develop skeletal muscle disease but late cardiac disease, including conduction abnormalities and sudden death, can occur. Although arrhythmia disease is the most common presentation of cardiac involvement in X-linked recessive Emery-Dreifuss muscular dystrophy, a dilated cardiomyopathy can rarely develop. The dilated cardiomyopathy is more common in patients in whom survival has been improved with pacemaker implantation. Both autopsy and endomyocardial biopsies have shown abnormal cardiac fibrosis.

An X-linked dominant Emery-Dreifuss muscular dystrophy with incomplete and age-dependent penetrance has been reported.[12] In the families observed, skeletal muscle involvement was absent or mild and the primary cardiac manifestations were atrial fibrillation, heart block, and sudden death. Women were affected later in life than men.

Patients with disorders caused by lamin A and C mutations typically present at age 20 to 40 years with cardiac conduction disease, atrial fibrillation, and dilated cardiomyopathy. Skeletal muscle disease is typically subclinical or absent. Progression of a cardiomyopathy to an extent that heart transplantation is required has been observed. Sudden death in patients with a dilated cardiomyopathy is common. Pacing is often required for symptomatic heart block.

TREATMENT AND PROGNOSIS. Affected patients should be monitored for the development of electrocardiographic conduction abnormalities and other arrhythmias. Atrioventricular block can occur with anesthesia. In X-linked recessive Emery-Dreifuss muscular dystrophy, permanent pacing is recommended once conduction disease is evident, and can be lifesaving. Sudden death, even in patients with pacemakers, can occur. Prophylactic placement of an ICD has been advocated for patients with disorders caused by lamin A and C

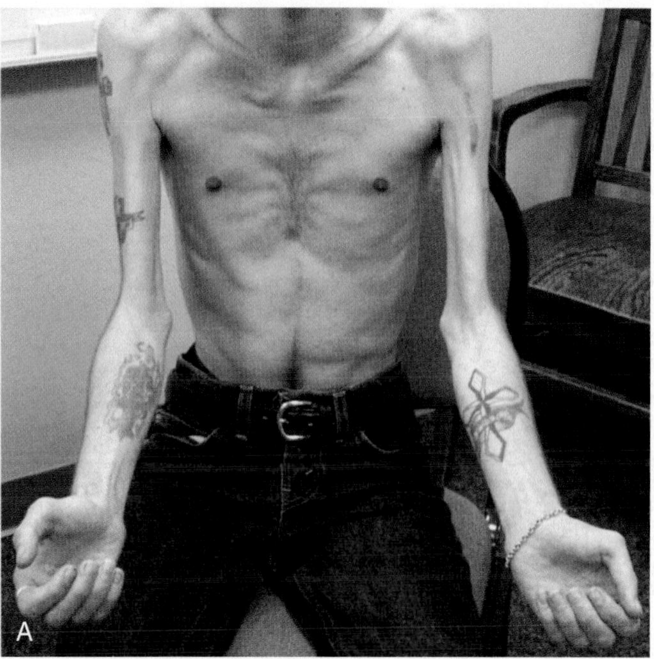

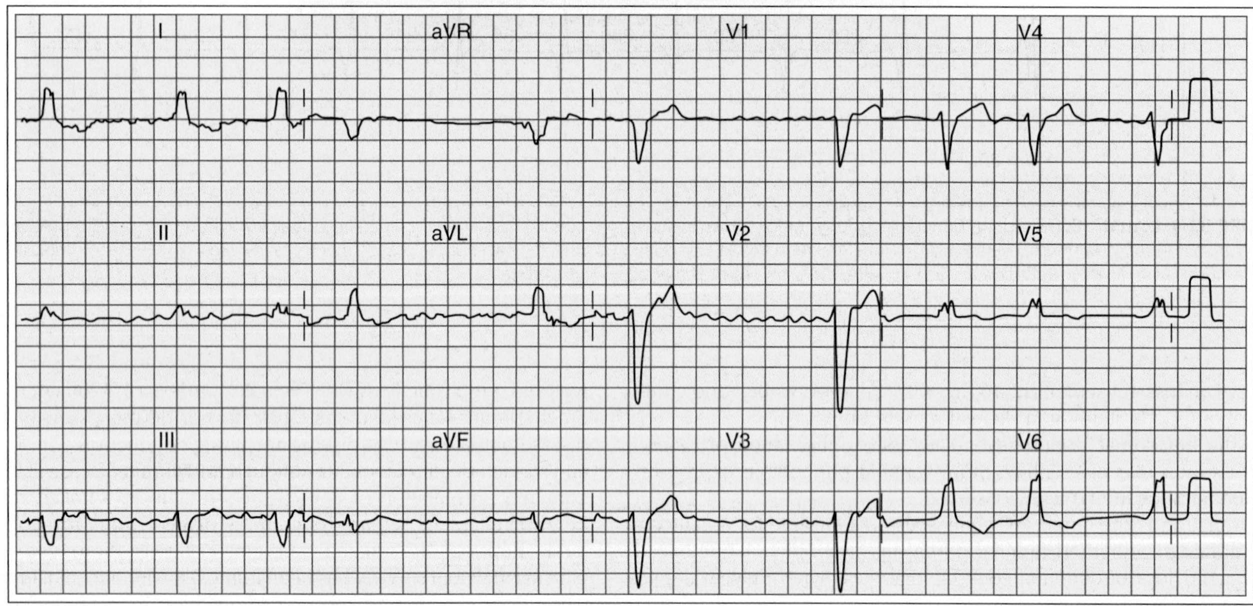

FIGURE 92-10 Emery-Dreifuss muscular dystrophy in a 28-year-old man presenting with syncope. **A,** Contractures of the elbow and atrophy in the humeroperoneal muscles. **B,** ECG at patient presentation showing atrial fibrillation with slow ventricular rate and a QRS complex with left bundle branch block. *(Courtesy of Dr. Robert M. Pascuzzi.)*

mutations if significant electrocardiographic conduction disease is present and pacing is being considered.[11] Whether prophylactic ICDs should be considered only for a certain subgroups of patients or in all patients with Emery-Dreifuss muscular dystrophy and associated disorders, with significant conduction disease or cardiomyopathy, is not clear. History, examination, and cardiac imaging for evaluation of left ventricular function are appropriate for all patients with Emery-Dreifuss muscular dystrophy and associated disorders. Patients with left ventricular dysfunction should benefit from appropriate pharmacologic therapy. Patients appear to benefit from heart transplantation. Female carriers of X-linked recessive Emery-Dreifuss muscular dystrophy develop conduction disease and electrocardiographic monitoring on a routine basis is appropriate.

Limb-Girdle Muscular Dystrophies

GENETICS. The limb-girdle muscular dystrophies constitutes a group of disorders with a limb–pelvic girdle distribution of weakness, but with otherwise heterogeneous inheritance and genetic cause.[13] Inheritance is most commonly autosomal recessive (limb-girdle muscular dystrophy type 2) but sporadic and autosomal dominant (limb-girdle muscular dystrophy type 1) inheritance is also observed. A genetically based nomenclature (e.g., 1A, 1B, 2A) was introduced to categorize an increasing number of recognized disorders. The genes involved encode dystrophin-associated glycoproteins, sarcomeric proteins, nuclear membrane proteins, and cellular enzymes.

CLINICAL PRESENTATION. The onset of muscle weakness is variable but usually occurs before 30 years of age. The recessive disorders tend to cause earlier and more severe weakness than the dominant disorders. Creatine kinase levels are typically moderately elevated. Patients commonly present with complaints of difficulty with walking or running secondary to pelvic girdle involvement. As the disease progresses, involvement of the shoulder muscles and then more distal muscles occurs, with sparing of facial involvement. Slow progression to severe disability and death can occur.

CARDIOVASCULAR MANIFESTATIONS. As with many of the features of the limb-girdle muscular dystrophies, there is heterogeneity observed in the presence and degree of cardiac involvement.

Limb-girdle muscular dystrophies types 2C to F are autosomal recessive disorders caused by mutations in a subunit of the sarcoglycan complex. Patients with sarcoglycanopathies commonly manifest a dilated cardiomyopathy. ECGs show similar abnormalities as in Duchenne and Becker muscular dystrophies, including an increased R wave in V_1 and lateral Q waves. Using electrocardiographic or echocardiographic evaluations, cardiac abnormalities are detected in up to 80% of patients with a smaller proportion symptomatic. A severe cardiomyopathy, including presentation with heart failure in childhood, can occur. Sudden death associated with the cardiomyopathy has been reported. Mechanisms whereby sarcoglycan abnormalities lead to a dilated cardiomyopathy may include a direct myopathic effect exacerbated by vascular spasm and ischemia, increasing cellular dysfunction, and death.[14]

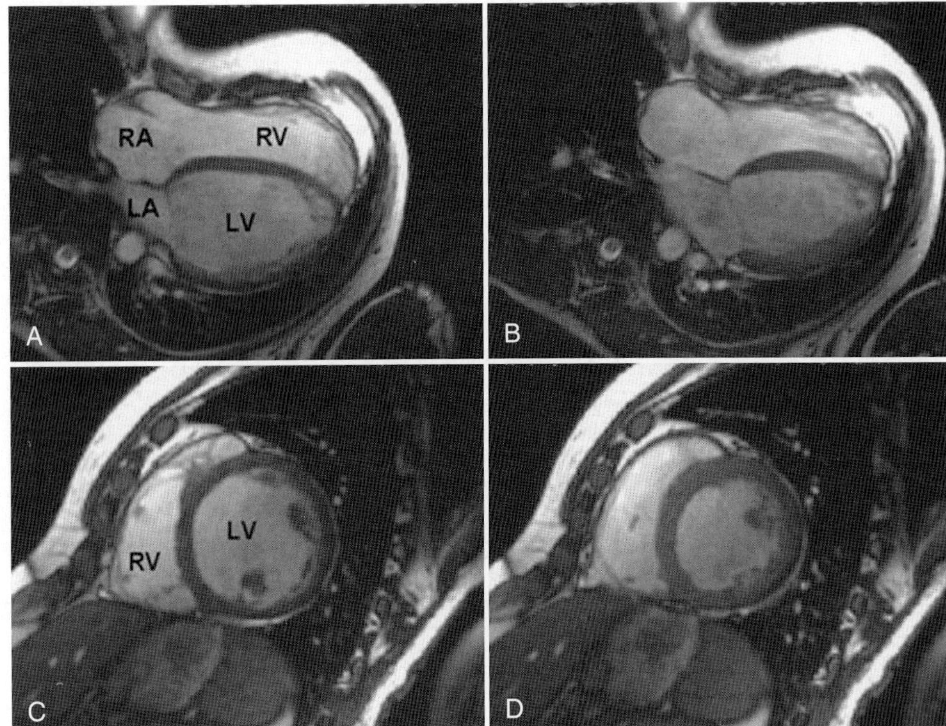

FIGURE 92-11 Cardiac involvement in a 33-year-old man with limb-girdle muscular dystrophy type 2I demonstrated by magnetic resonance imaging. Four-chamber view in diastole **(A)** and systole **(B)**; midventricular short axis in diastole **(C)** and systole **(D)**. The images demonstrate enlarged left and right ventricles, with moderately impaired left ventricular function (calculated ejection fraction = 39%). RA = right atrium; RV = right ventricle; LA = left atrium; LV = left ventricle. *(From Gaul C, Deschauer M, Tempelmann C, et al: Cardiac involvement in limb-girdle muscular dystrophy 2I: Conventional cardiac diagnostic and cardiovascular magnetic resonance. J Neurol 253:1317, 2006.)*

Limb-girdle muscular dystrophy type 2I is an autosomal recessive disorder caused by a mutation in the fukutin-related protein gene located on chromosome 19. The mutation is also responsible for a form of congenital muscular dystrophy. The gene abnormality affects glycosylation of a dystrophin-associated glycoprotein. The age at disease onset and severity of skeletal muscle involvement in limb-girdle muscular dystrophy type 2I is variable, with some patients symptomatic in childhood but, more typically, symptoms developing between age 20 and 40 years. Similar to the sarcoglycanopathies, a high proportion of patients with limb-girdle muscular dystrophy type 2I develop a dilated cardiomyopathy (**Fig. 92-11**).[15] In one series, almost all patients had evidence of cardiac involvement by age 60 years. About 50% of all patients had heart failure symptoms and some were being considered for cardiac transplantation. In limb-girdle muscular dystrophy type 2I, conduction disease did not occur separately from the structural cardiac involvement.

Autosomal dominant limb-girdle muscular dystrophy type 1B is caused by mutations in the gene encoding lamins A and C, similar to that observed in Emery-Dreifuss muscular dystrophy. It is not surprising that the clinical phenotype is also similar to that of Emery-Dreifuss muscular dystrophy, with mild skeletal muscle symptoms and more severe cardiac involvement, primarily arrhythmias. Affected patients develop atrioventricular block by early middle age, often necessitating pacing. Sudden death, thought to be cardiac, is common, including in those in whom pacing was previously instituted. A dilated cardiomyopathy can occur.

TREATMENT AND PROGNOSIS. Because of the heterogeneous nature of limb-girdle muscular dystrophy, specific recommendations for routine cardiac evaluation and therapy are based on the genetic classification. Genetic testing can determine those with limb-girdle types 2C to F, 2I, or 1B, who are at the highest risk for cardiac involvement. In these patients (and their families), cardiac evaluation for arrhythmias and ventricular dysfunction should be done. Patients with dilated cardiomyopathies respond to standard heart failure therapy.[15] Prophylactic placement of an ICD instead of a pacemaker has been recommended in those with lamin A and C mutations after conduction disease is observed.[11]

Facioscapulohumeral Muscular Dystrophy

GENETICS. Facioscapulohumeral muscular dystrophy is the third most common muscular dystrophy after Duchenne and myotonic dystrophy, with a prevalence of 1/20,000 persons. It is an autosomal dominant disorder in which the genetic locus has been mapped to chromosome 4q35. Genetic heterogeneity has been reported. The diagnosis can be confirmed by a 4q35 EcoRI allele size of 38 kb or smaller. This repeat region, known as D4Z4, is responsible for binding to a regulatory protein complex that suppresses transcription of adjacent genes. The lack of an appropriate number of D4Z4 repeats results in an overexpression of 4q35 genes and is proposed as the mechanism leading to the facioscapulohumeral muscular dystrophy phenotype. The exact genes that are overexpressed and their protein products are not clear.

CLINICAL PRESENTATION. Muscle weakness tends to follow a slowly progressive but variable course, presenting with facial and/or shoulder girdle muscle weakness and progressing to involve the pelvic musculature. Major disability affecting walking eventually occurs in 20% of patients.

CARDIOVASCULAR MANIFESTATIONS. Cardiac involvement in facioscapulohumeral muscular dystrophy is reported but does not constitute as much of a problem in prevalence or severity as in other muscular dystrophies. In some series, no evidence of cardiac abnormalities were found. Other series have reported a propensity toward arrhythmias, primarily atrial in origin, with atrioventricular conduction abnormalities less common.[16]

TREATMENT AND PROGNOSIS. Because significant clinical cardiac involvement is rare in facioscapulohumeral muscular dystrophy, specific monitoring or treatment recommendations are not well defined. Annual ECGs have been recommended.

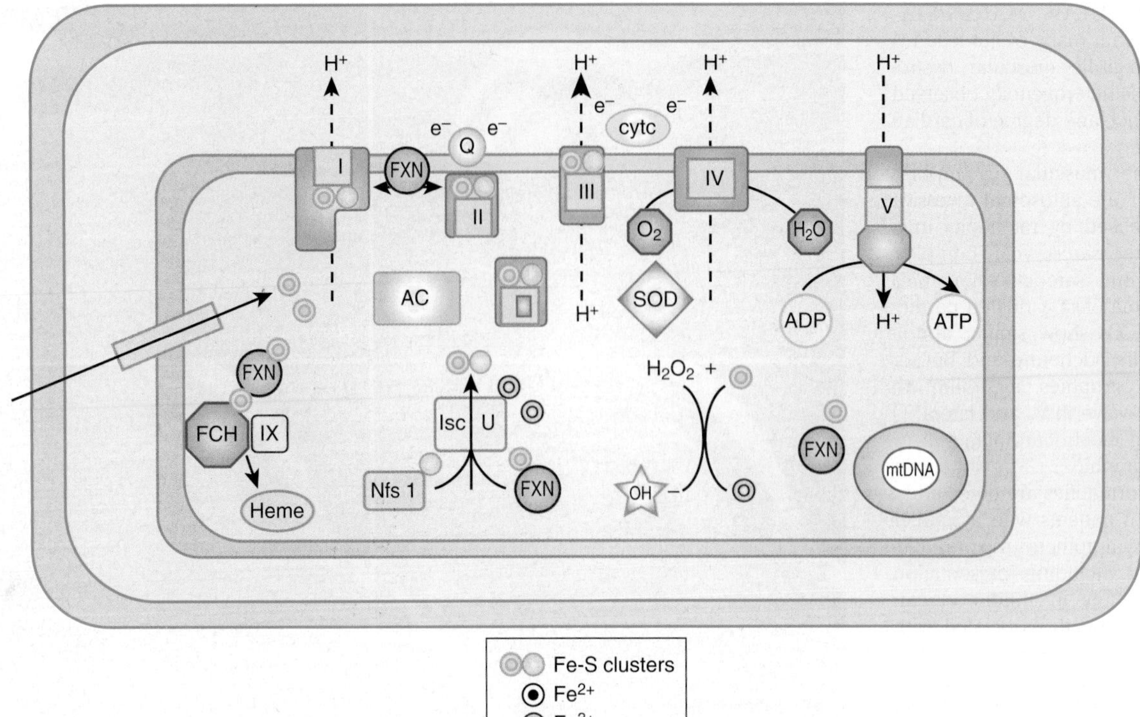

FIGURE 92-12 Postulated functions of frataxin (FXN). 1. Frataxin is a general iron chaperone, providing Fe^{2+} to ferrochelatase (FCH) for heme biosynthesis, mitochondrial iron-sulfur (Fe-S) clusters biogenesis, and maintenance of the mitochondrial aconitase (AC) Fe-S cluster. 2. Frataxin may have a direct interaction with respiratory chain complexes (I-V). 3. Frataxin prevents oxidative stress and protects mitochondrial proteins and mitochondrial DNA (mtDNA) from free Fe^{2+}. It prevents the Fenton reaction by converting Fe^{2+} to Fe^{3+} and thus prevents hydroxyl radical formation. ADP = adenosine diphosphate; ATP = adenosine triphosphate; cytc = cytochrome C; e^- = electron; Q = coenzyme Q (ubiquinone); SOD = superoxide dismutase. *(From Pandolfo M: Friedreich ataxia. Arch Neurol 65:1296, 2008.)*

Friedreich Ataxia

Genetics. Friedreich ataxia is an autosomal recessive, spinocerebellar, degenerative disease characterized clinically by ataxia of the limbs and trunk, dysarthria, loss of deep tendon reflexes, sensory abnormalities, skeletal deformities, diabetes mellitus, and cardiac involvement.[17] The disease is linked to chromosome 9, with the gene mutation affecting the encoding of a 210–amino acid protein, frataxin. Frataxin is a mitochondrial protein important in iron homeostasis and respiratory function (**Fig. 92-12**). Messenger RNA for frataxin is highly expressed in the heart. The mutation responsible for Friedreich ataxia is an amplified trinucleotide (guanine-adenine-adenine [GAA]) repeat found in the first intron of the gene encoding frataxin. Whereas normal patients have fewer than 33 repeats, patients with Friedreich ataxia have 66 to 1500 GAA repeats. In 95% of patients, both alleles of the gene have the expanded repeat. In 5% of patients, a point mutation occurs on one allele in association with an expanded repeat on the other. The GAA repeat disrupts transcription, severely decreasing frataxin synthesis. The decrease in frataxin leads to mitochondrial dysfunction, poor cellular response to oxidative stress, and apoptosis. Endomyocardial biopsies in patients with Friedreich ataxia have shown deficient function in mitochondrial respiratory complex subunits and in aconitase, an iron-sulfur enzyme involved in iron homeostasis. Abnormal cardiac bioenergetics appear to result from the abnormalities in respiratory function and iron handling. As the GAA triplet size increases, an earlier age of symptom onset, increasing severity of neurologic symptoms, and worsening left ventricular hypertrophy by echocardiography are observed.

CLINICAL PRESENTATION. Friedreich ataxia is the most common inherited spinocerebellar degenerative disease, with a prevalence of 1/50,000. Neurologic symptoms usually manifest around puberty and almost always before the age of 25 years. Progressive loss of neuromuscular function, with the patient wheelchair-bound 10 to 20 years after symptom onset, is the norm. Neurologic symptoms precede cardiac symptoms in most but not all cases.

CARDIOVASCULAR MANIFESTATIONS. Friedreich ataxia is generally associated with a concentric hypertrophic cardiomyopathy (**Fig. 92-13**). Less commonly, asymmetric septal hypertrophy is observed (see Chap. 69). The presence of a left ventricular outflow gradient associated with the septal hypertrophy has been reported. Presentation with a dilated cardiomyopathy is rarer but can occur (**Fig. 92-14**). The dilated cardiomyopathy appears to occur as a progressive transition from a hypertrophic cardiomyopathy. The prevalence of hypertrophy varies among studies but increases in prevalence with a younger age at diagnosis and with increasing GAA trinucleotide repeat length. Up to 95% of neurologically symptomatic patients have abnormalities on electrocardiographic and echocardiographic evaluation. Findings are primarily consistent with ventricular hypertrophy. Left ventricular hypertrophy is not always present on ECGs despite echocardiographic evidence. Widespread T wave inversions are common (**Fig. 92-15**). Patients with left ventricular hypertrophy without systolic dysfunction typically have no cardiac symptoms.

Arrhythmias occur in Friedreich ataxia but are less common than what might be expected considering the high incidence of cardiac hypertrophy. Atrial arrhythmias, including atrial fibrillation and flutter, are associated with the progression to a dilated cardiomyopathy. Ventricular tachycardia, again in the setting of a dilated cardiomyopathy, has been observed. The hypertrophic cardiomyopathy of Friedreich ataxia is not associated with serious ventricular arrhythmias as observed in the other types of heritable hypertrophic cardiomyopathies. Myocardial fiber disarray is not commonly seen in the hypertrophic cardiomyopathy of Friedreich ataxia. Sudden death has been reported but a mechanism has not been well characterized.

Endomyocardial biopsies in Friedreich ataxia have demonstrated myocyte hypertrophy and interstitial fibrosis. Histopathologic examination has revealed myocyte hypertrophy and degeneration, interstitial fibrosis, active muscle necrosis, bizarre pleomorphic nuclei, and periodic acid-Schiff–positive deposition in large and small coronary arteries. Degeneration and fibrosis in cardiac nerves and ganglia and in the conduction system have also been observed. Deposition of calcium salts and iron has been reported.

TREATMENT AND PROGNOSIS. Idebenone, a free radical scavenger, modestly decreases left ventricular hypertrophy and mass in Friedreich ataxia patients.[18] Patients with a greater degree of hypertrophy respond best. It is not clear if idebenone improves left ventricular systolic function. Whether the modest improvement in cardiac imaging parameters with idebenone also leads to any alteration in the clinical cardiovascular course has not been tested. Idebenone does not appear to improve neurologic outcomes.

In most patients with Friedreich ataxia, progressive neurologic dysfunction is the norm, with death from respiratory failure or infection in the fourth or fifth decade. Cardiac death occurs primarily in those developing a dilated cardiomyopathy. These patients tend to do poorly with rapid progression to end-stage congestive heart failure. It is unclear whether pharmacologic or ICD therapy improves outcomes in Friedreich ataxia and dilated cardiomyopathy.

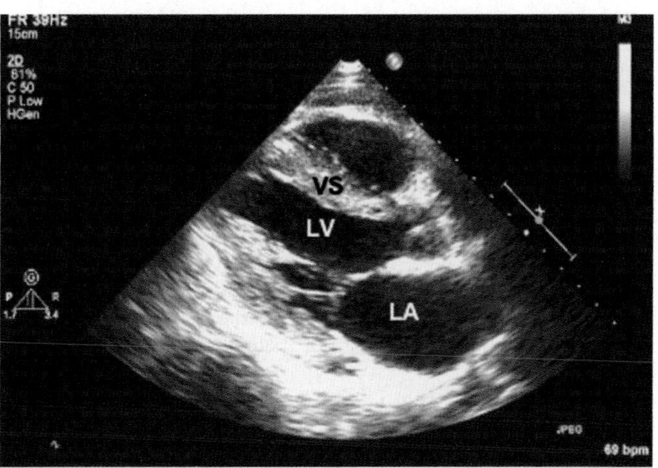

FIGURE 92-13 Hypertrophic cardiomyopathy in a 28-year-old man with Friedreich ataxia. This two-dimensional echocardiogram (parasternal two chamber) shows a thickened ventricular septum (VS) and a dilated left atrium (LA). LV = left ventricle.

Less Common Neuromuscular Diseases Associated with Cardiac Manifestations

Periodic Paralyses

Genetics. The primary periodic paralyses are rare, nondystrophic, autosomal dominant disorders that result from abnormalities in ion channel genes.[19] They can be classified into hypokalemic, hyperkalemic, and normokalemic periodic paralyses, with several subclassifications in each. In addition, acquired hypokalemic periodic paralysis may complicate thyrotoxicosis, especially in men of Asian descent.

Hypokalemic periodic paralysis is characterized by episodic attacks of weakness in association with decreased serum potassium levels. Penetrance is almost complete in males and approximately 50% in females. Most hypokalemic periodic paralysis have mapped to chromosome 1q31-32, with mutations occurring in the alpha$_1$ subunit of the dihydropyridine-sensitive calcium channel. The disease is genetically heterogeneous, with a mutation at chromosome 17q23 causing abnormalities in the alpha subunit of the skeletal muscle sodium channel (*SCN4A*).

Hyperkalemic periodic paralysis also manifests with episodic weakness but with symptoms worsening with potassium supplementation. Complete penetrance is observed. Potassium levels are usually high but may be normal during an attack. Hyperkalemic periodic paralysis is caused primarily by mutations in the alpha subunit of *SCN4A* found at chromosome 17q23. Multiple different mutations in this gene have been reported that result in a potassium-sensitive failure of inactivation (gain of function) in the sodium channel. Hyperkalemic periodic paralysis is genetically heterogeneous, with most affected individuals having an *SCN4A* mutation but with other loci also identified.

Andersen-Tawil syndrome is a distinct periodic paralysis associated with characteristic dysmorphic physical features, an abnormal QT-U wave pattern, and ventricular arrhythmias (**Fig. 92-16**).[20] The periodic paralysis can be hypo-, hyper-, or normokalemic. Phenotypic variability and incomplete penetrance is observed, making the diagnosis in a family difficult. Approximately two thirds of Andersen-Tawil syndrome patients link to chromosome 17q23, with the mutations responsible occurring in the *KCNJ2* gene encoding the inward rectifier potassium protein, Kir2.1. The result of the mutation is a loss of function in the inward rectifier potassium channel, I_{Kir}, affecting terminal repolarization of the cardiac action potential. The genetic cause of Andersen-Tawil syndrome in the other third of patients remains unknown. Andersen-Tawil syndrome has been given a long-QT syndrome 7 nomenclature.

CLINICAL PRESENTATION. The primary manifestation of all the periodic paralyses is episodic weakness. Attacks of weakness tend to be more severe and of longer duration with hypokalemic periodic

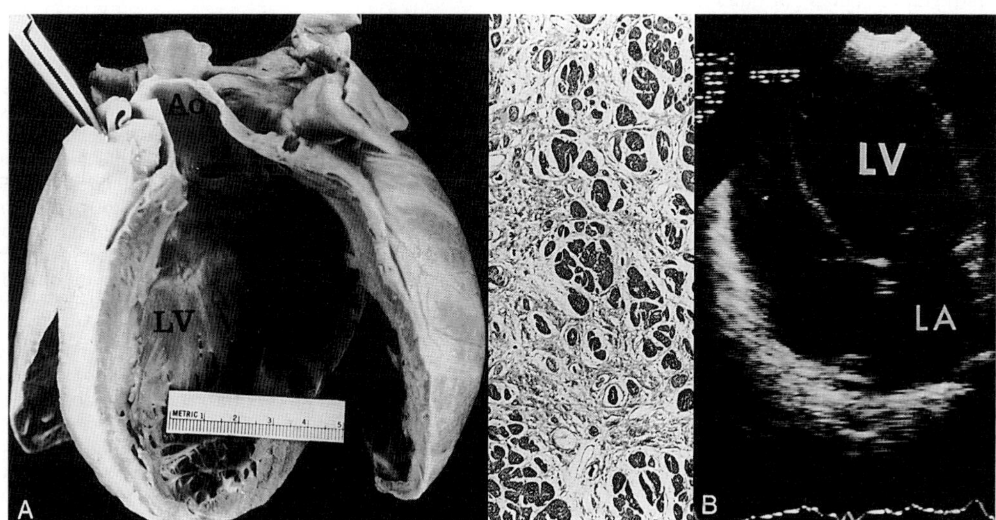

FIGURE 92-14 **A,** Gross and histologic specimens from a 17-year-old boy with Friedreich ataxia whose echocardiogram progressed from normal at age 13 years to a minimally dilated, hypocontractile left ventricle (LV) 3 to 4 years later. The gross specimen shows a mildly dilated LV with normal wall thickness; the walls were flabby. The microscopic section from the left ventricular free wall **(middle panel)** shows marked connective tissue replacement. Although specifically sought, small-vessel coronary artery disease was not identified. **B,** Two-dimensional echocardiogram (apical window) showing the mildly dilated, thin-walled LV. LA = left atrium. ***(A, B,*** *From Child JS, Perloff JK, Bach PM, et al: Cardiac involvement in Friedreich ataxia. J Am Coll Cardiol 7:1370, 1986.)*

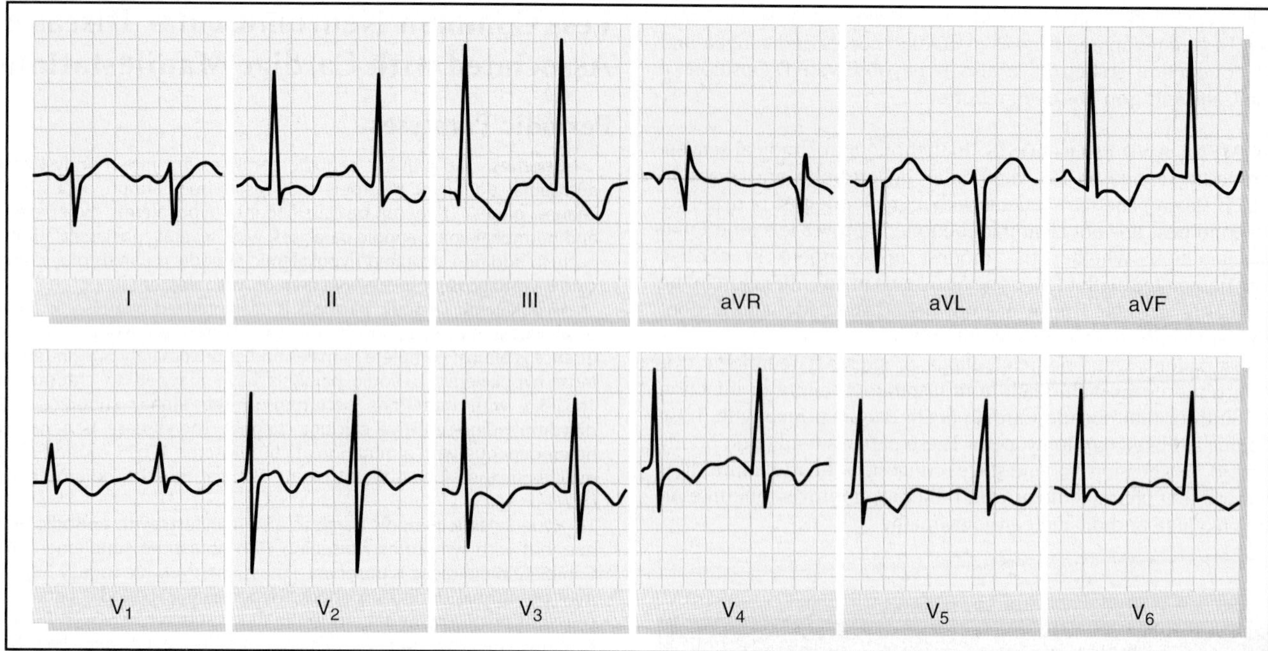

FIGURE 92-15 ECG from a 34-year-old man with Friedreich ataxia. Widespread ST and T changes are observed. *(Courtesy of Dr. Charles Fisch, Indiana University School of Medicine, Indianapolis.)*

paralysis than with hyperkalemic periodic paralysis. In all the periodic paralyses, cold, exercise, and rest after exercise can trigger an attack. Ingestion of carbohydrates can trigger an attack in hypokalemic periodic paralysis but may ameliorate an attack in hyperkalemic periodic paralysis.

CARDIOVASCULAR MANIFESTATIONS. The periodic paralyses are associated with ventricular arrhythmias. Arrhythmias occur primarily in hyperkalemic periodic paralysis and Andersen-Tawil syndrome. Bidirectional ventricular tachycardia has been observed independently of digitalis intoxication. The episodes of bidirectional ventricular tachycardia are independent of attacks of muscle weakness, do not correlate with serum potassium levels, and can convert to sinus rhythm with exercise. Ventricular ectopy is common.

A prolonged QT interval can be observed. In some reports, the prolonged QT interval is episodic and associated with weakness, hypokalemia, or antiarrhythmia therapy. In other cases, a prolonged QT interval can be constant. Andersen-Tawil syndrome is associated with a modest prolongation in the QT interval but more specifically a prolonged and prominent U wave. Ventricular arrhythmias, including premature ventricular contractions, ventricular bigeminy, and nonsustained polymorphic ventricular tachycardia, primarily bidirectional tachycardia, is commonly observed in Andersen-Tawil syndrome. Cardiac conduction abnormalities, atypical of long-QT syndromes, have been observed in Andersen-Tawil syndrome. Torsades de pointes is observed in Andersen-Tawil syndrome but is less common than in the other long-QT syndromes. A family with Andersen-Tawil syndrome and a dilated cardiomyopathy, with an unknown interrelationship, has been reported.

Syncope, cardiac arrest, and sudden death have been reported in the periodic paralyses, most prominently in the Andersen-Tawil syndrome. The factors that portend an increased risk of life-threatening arrhythmias are not clear.

TREATMENT AND PROGNOSIS. The episodes of weakness typically respond to measures that normalize potassium levels. Weakness in hyperkalemic periodic paralysis can respond to mexiletine. Weakness in hypokalemic periodic paralysis can respond to acetazolamide. Treatment of electrolytes usually does not improve arrhythmias or, if it does, only transiently. Improvement in symptomatic nonsustained ventricular tachycardia associated with a prolonged QT interval has been reported with beta blocker therapy. Class 1A antiarrhythmic agents can worsen muscle weakness and exacerbate arrhythmias associated with a prolonged QT interval. Bidirectional ventricular tachycardia, not associated with a prolonged QT interval, may not respond to beta blocker therapy. Amiodarone has been observed to decrease episodes of polymorphic ventricular tachycardia in Andersen-Tawil syndrome. ICDs have been used for patients with Andersen-Tawil syndrome.

Mitochondrial Disorders

GENETICS. The mitochondrial disorders are a heterogeneous group of diseases resulting from abnormalities in mitochondrial DNA and respiratory chain function.[21] The number of distinct disorders is extensive. Mitochondrial DNA is inherited maternally and most of these disorders are thus transmitted from mother to children of both genders. Some of the disorders occur sporadically or are inherited in an autosomal fashion. Disease severity can vary between patients and family members because both mutant and normal mitochondrial DNA can be present in tissue in a variable proportion. It is not surprising, based on the important metabolic function of mitochondria, that these disorders manifest with systemic pathology. Tissue with a high respiratory workload such as the brain, skeletal muscle, and cardiac muscle are especially affected.

Mitochondrial disorders that have cardiac manifestations present as several clinical phenotypes, including the following: chronic progressive external ophthalmoplegia, which includes the Kearns-Sayre syndrome; *m*yoclonus *e*pilepsy with *r*ed *r*agged *f*ibers (MERRF); *m*itochondrial myopathy, *e*ncephalopathy, *l*actic *a*cidosis, and *s*trokelike episodes, abbreviated MELAS; and Leber hereditary optic neuropathy. Other, rarer mitochondrial point mutation disorders present primarily with cardiac manifestations, typically a hypertrophic or dilated cardiomyopathy. Chronic progressive external ophthalmoplegia is primarily a sporadic disease, whereas the others are maternally inherited.

CLINICAL PRESENTATION. Kearns-Sayre syndrome is characterized by the clinical triad of progressive external ophthalmoplegia, pigmentary retinopathy, and atrioventricular block. Diabetes, deafness, and ataxia can also be associated. Clinical features of MERRF include myoclonus, seizures, ataxia, dementia, and skeletal muscle weakness. MELAS is the most common of the maternally inherited mitochondrial disorders and is characterized by encephalopathy, subacute strokelike events, migraine-like headaches, recurrent emesis, extremity weakness, and short stature. Leber hereditary optic neuropathy manifests as a severe, subacute, painless loss of central vision, predominantly affecting young men.

CARDIOVASCULAR MANIFESTATIONS. In chronic progressive external ophthalmoplegia, most commonly in the Kearns-Sayre syndrome, cardiac involvement manifests primarily as conduction abnormalities. A

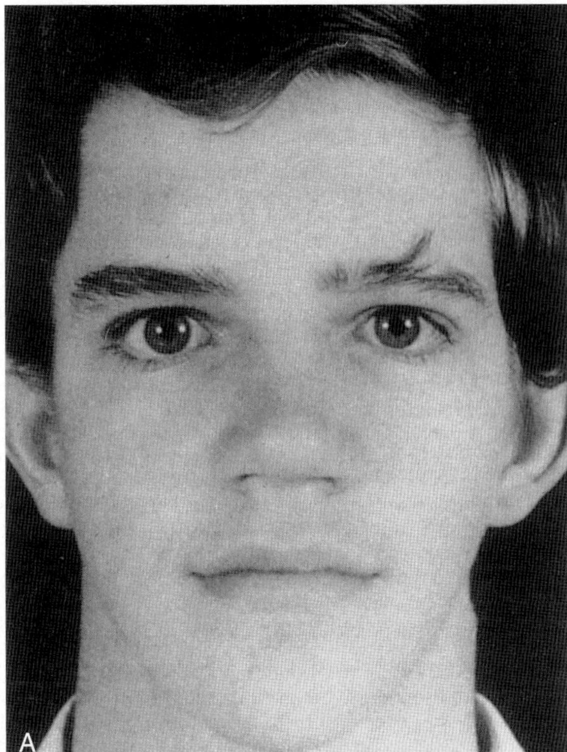

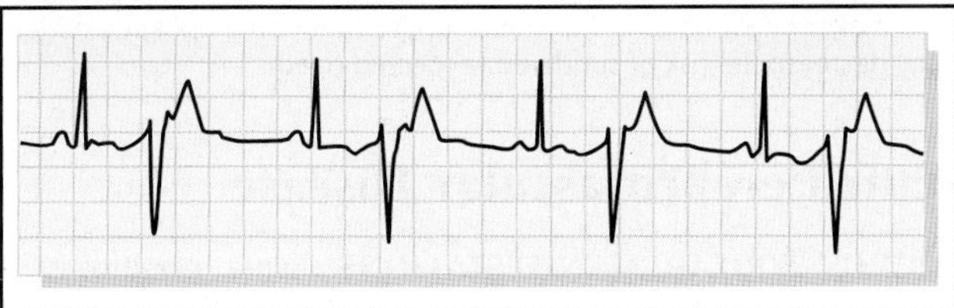

FIGURE 92-16 Andersen-Tawil syndrome in a 22-year-old man. **A,** Characteristic low-set ears and hypoplastic mandible. **B,** Electrocardiographic recording revealing ventricular bigeminy. *(From Tawil R, Ptacek LJ, Pavlakis SG, et al: Andersen's syndrome: Potassium-sensitive periodic paralysis, ventricular ectopy, and dysmorphic features. Ann Neurol 35:326, 1994.)*

dilated cardiomyopathy has been reported. In the Kearns-Sayre syndrome, atrioventricular block is observed, usually presenting after eye involvement. The H-V interval is prolonged, consistent with distal conduction disease. Permanent pacing is often required by age 20. An increased prevalence of electrocardiographic preexcitation has also been reported.

Leber hereditary optic neuropathy can be associated with a short PR interval on the ECG and preexcitation. Supraventricular tachycardia has been reported.

In MERRF and MELAS, cardiac involvement manifesting as hypertrophic (symmetrical or asymmetrical) or dilated cardiomyopathy is observed. Other disorders caused by mitochondrial point mutations can present with a similar cardiac phenotype. Patients can present with chest pain with electrocardiographic abnormalities and myocardial perfusion defects. Whether the dilated cardiomyopathy represents a progression from the hypertrophic cardiomyopathy or a separate syndrome is not clear. The dilated cardiomyopathy can result in heart failure and death. MELAS is also associated with an increased risk of preexcitation and Wolff-Parkinson-White syndrome.[22]

Treatment and Prognosis. In Kearns-Sayre syndrome, the implantation of a pacemaker has been advocated when significant or progressive conduction disease is evident, including in asymptomatic patients. The degree of conduction disease that warrants prophylactic pacing is not clear. In Leber hereditary optic neuropathy, a baseline ECG is prudent. In the other mitochondrial disorders, an understanding of the potential for cardiac involvement is necessary. Screening echocardiography has been recommended. Whether other specific screening evaluations are warranted in these disorders is uncertain. Therapy directed at improvement in the respiratory chain defects—for example, with coenzyme Q10—have not been uniformly demonstrated to be of benefit.

Spinal Muscular Atrophy

Genetics and Clinical Presentation. Spinal muscular atrophy is a lower motor neuron disorder presenting as progressive, symmetrical proximal muscular weakness.[23] Spinal muscular atrophy is the leading hereditary cause of infant death. The disorder is inherited in an autosomal recessive fashion or is sporadic. Spinal muscular atrophy is classified clinically by the age at symptom onset and disease severity into type I (Werdnig-Hoffman disease), type II (intermediate form), type III (Kugelberg-Welander disease), and type IV (adult onset).

Spinal muscular atrophy links to chromosome 5q13. Mutations or deletions in the telomeric *SMN* (survival of motor neuron) gene occur in more than 98% of patients. The loss of functional SMN protein results in premature neuronal cell death.

Cardiovascular Manifestations. Cardiac involvement in spinal muscular atrophy includes coexisting complex congenital heart disease, cardiomyopathy, and arrhythmias. Congenital heart disease has been associated with types I and III spinal muscular atrophy. The most common abnormality is atrial septal defect, with other abnormalities reported. In spinal muscular atrophy type III, a dilated cardiomyopathy can occur, with endomyocardial biopsies demonstrating fibrosis. Progression leading to a fatal outcome has been reported. Arrhythmia abnormalities, including atrial standstill, atrial fibrillation, atrial flutter, and atrioventricular block, appear to be the most common cardiac manifestation in these diseases. Permanent pacing for atrial standstill and atrioventricular block has been reported.

Treatment and Prognosis. In spinal muscular atrophy type I, severe skeletal muscle involvement with respiratory failure can limit the life span to a significant degree, so that treatment of associated cardiac abnormalities is often not indicated. In spinal muscular atrophy type III, awareness of the potential for associated cardiac abnormalities is necessary. Permanent pacing may be required. Directed therapy to improve functional SMN protein holds future promise.

Desmin-Related Myopathy

Genetics and Clinical Presentation. Desmin-related myofibrillar myopathy is a rare inherited skeletal muscle dystrophic disorder associated with a cardiomyopathy in more than 50% of affected patients. The disorder is inherited in an autosomal dominant fashion or is sporadic. Desmin mutations are the cause of 1% to 2% of cases of familial dilated cardiomyopathy.[24] Desmin is a cytoskeletal protein that functions as the chief intermediate filament providing support to contracting skeletal and cardiac muscle. Mutations in the desmin gene lead to the inability for the protein to form functioning intermediate filaments. Some mutations cause a cardiomyopathy without an apparent skeletal myopathy.

Patients typically present in their late 20s, with distal weakness that progresses proximally. Difficulty with ambulation and, in severe cases, with respiration, can occur. Creatine kinase levels are mildly elevated in some patients. Muscle biopsy is diagnostic, showing desmin and other myofibrillar protein deposition with immunostaining. Genetic testing is available.

Cardiovascular Manifestations. The cardiomyopathy associated with the desmin-related myopathies can occur before or after the diagnosis of a skeletal myopathy. The cardiac involvement observed typically consists of conduction system dysfunction prior to the onset of a dilated or restrictive cardiomyopathy. Syncope, with the need for pacemaker implantation, has been described. Both sudden and heart failure–related deaths can occur. Sudden death can occur despite pacemaker implantation.

Treatment and Prognosis. The desmin-related myopathies should be considered in the differential diagnosis of individuals or families presenting with skeletal and cardiac myopathies. Monitoring for the development of cardiac conduction and structural disease is indicated in affected families. Prophylactic pacemakers or ICDs should be considered for those patients with significant conduction disease, as in other neuromuscular disorders. Heart failure therapy for appropriate patients is indicated.

Guillain-Barré Syndrome

Clinical Presentation. Guillain-Barré syndrome is an acute inflammatory demyelinating neuropathy characterized by peripheral, cranial, and autonomic nerve dysfunction.[25] It is the most common acquired demyelinating neuropathy, with an annual incidence of 1 to 2/100,000 population. Men are more commonly affected than women. In two thirds of affected patients, an acute viral or bacterial illness, typically respiratory or gastrointestinal, precedes the onset of neurologic symptoms by up to 6 weeks. The disorder typically presents with pain, paresthesias, and

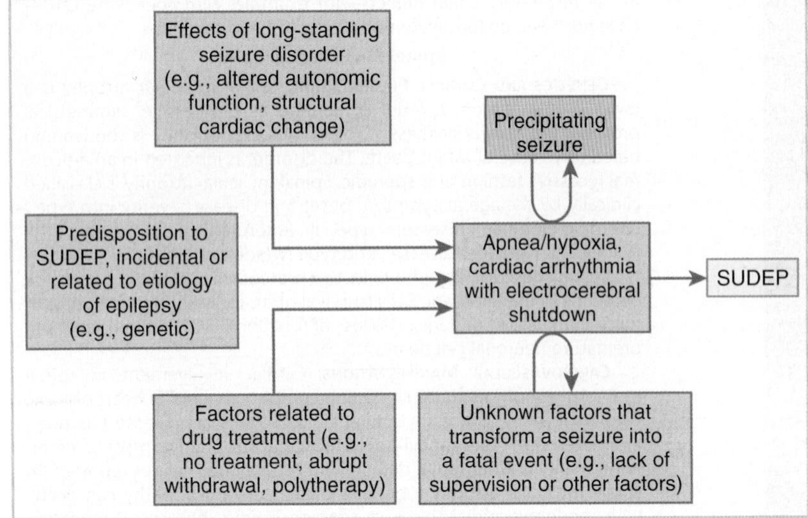

FIGURE 92-17 Interaction between proposed risk factors and triggers for sudden unexpected death in epilepsy. *(From Tomson T, Nashef L, Ryvlin P: Sudden unexpected death in epilepsy: Current knowledge and future directions. Lancet Neurol 7:1021, 2008.)*

symmetrical limb weakness that progresses proximally and can involve cranial and respiratory muscles. Approximately 25% of patients require assisted ventilation.

Cardiovascular Manifestations. Nonambulatory patients are at increased risk for deep venous thrombosis and pulmonary emboli. Cardiac involvement in Guillain-Barré syndrome is related to accompanying autonomic nervous system dysfunction that manifests as hypertension, orthostatic hypotension, resting sinus tachycardia, loss of heart rate variability, electrocardiographic ST-segment abnormalities and both bradycardia and tachycardias. Significant autonomic nervous system dysfunction occurs in about 20% of patients with Guillain-Barré syndrome, primarily in severe cases.[25] Microneurographic recordings have shown increased sympathetic outflow during the acute illness, which normalizes with recovery.

Life-threatening arrhythmias are common in severe cases of Guillain-Barré syndrome, primarily those requiring assisted ventilation. Arrhythmias observed include asystole, symptomatic bradycardia, rapid atrial fibrillation, and ventricular tachycardia or fibrillation. Deaths caused by arrhythmias can occur. Asystole has been commonly associated with tracheal suctioning.

Treatment and Prognosis. Supportive care should include deep venous thrombosis prophylaxis in nonambulatory patients. Early plasmapheresis or intravenous immunoglobulin can improve recovery. In severely affected patients, especially those requiring assisted ventilation, cardiac rhythm monitoring is mandatory. If serious bradycardia or asystole is observed, temporary or permanent pacing can improve survival. Atropine or isoproterenol during tracheal suctioning can be of benefit. The mortality rate in patients hospitalized with Guillain-Barré syndrome is as high as 15%. In patients who recover from Guillain-Barré syndrome, autonomic function also recovers and long-term arrhythmia risk has not been observed.

Myasthenia Gravis

Clinical Presentation. Myasthenia gravis is a disorder of neuromuscular transmission resulting from the production of antibody targeted against the nicotinic acetylcholine receptor. The primary symptom, fluctuating weakness, usually begins with the eye and facial muscles and later can involve the large muscles of the limbs. Patients can present at any age, typically at a younger age in women and an older age in men. Myasthenia gravis is usually associated with hyperplasia or a benign or malignant tumor (thymoma) of the thymus gland. The prevalence of myasthenia gravis is 50 to 125 cases/1,000,000.

Cardiovascular Manifestations. A myocarditis can occur in patients with myasthenia gravis, especially in those with thymoma.[26] Up to 16% of patients with myasthenia gravis have cardiac manifestations not explained by another cause. Presentation with arrhythmia symptoms, including atrial fibrillation, atrioventricular block, asystole, ventricular tachycardia, sudden death, or heart failure is typical. Autopsy findings are consistent with myocarditis.

Treatment and Prognosis. Myasthenia gravis is treated with anticholinesterase and immunosuppressive agents. Thymectomy is often indicated. Anticholinesterase agents may slow heart rate and cause hypotension. Whether immunosuppressive agents or thymectomy improve associated cardiac disease is unknown. Case reports have described patients developing rapidly progressive and fatal heart failure within weeks after thymoma resection, with histology showing giant cell myocarditis.

EPILEPSY

Cardiovascular Manifestations. Epilepsy is a complex brain disorder characterized by chronic seizures. Patients with epilepsy are at an increased risk of sudden death of unknown cause. Sudden unexpected death in epilepsy (SUDEP) is responsible for 2% to 17% of deaths, with an incidence ranging from 0.1 to 9.3/1,000 patient-years, depending on the population studied.[27] The underlying mechanisms leading to sudden death in epilepsy are not clear but may involve apnea, excessive respiratory secretions, acute pulmonary edema, or arrhythmias (**Fig. 92-17**). Most witnessed sudden deaths occur at or in proximity to the time of a seizure. Severe bradycardia with sinus arrest has been documented in a small number of monitored patients during seizures. Whether bradycardia has a role in epileptic patients undergoing sudden death is not clear.

Observational studies have assessed risk factors for sudden unexpected death in epilepsy. These include a high seizure frequency, long duration of epilepsy, poor compliance with antiepileptic drug therapy, and the need for polytherapy to control seizures.

Treatment and Prognosis. A primary arrhythmia disorder needs to be considered in the differential diagnosis of epilepsy. Patients with poorly controlled epilepsy should be aggressively evaluated and treated. Patients with ictal-associated bradycardia have undergone permanent pacemaker implantation. Nighttime supervision of the epileptic patient may decrease the risk of sudden unexpected death.

Acute Cerebrovascular Disease

CARDIOVASCULAR MANIFESTATIONS. Acute cerebrovascular diseases, including subarachnoid hemorrhage, other stroke syndromes, and head injury, can be associated with severe cardiac manifestations.[28] The mechanism whereby cardiac abnormalities occur with brain injury is related to autonomic nervous system dysfunction, with increased sympathetic and parasympathetic output. Excessive myocardial catecholamine release is primarily responsible for the observed cardiac pathology. Hypothalamic stimulation can reproduce the electrocardiographic changes observed in acute cerebrovascular disease. Electrocardiographic changes associated with hypothalamic stimulation or blood in the subarachnoid space can be diminished with spinal cord transection, stellate ganglion blockade, vagolytics, and adrenergic blockers.

Electrocardiographic abnormalities are observed in approximately 70% of patients with subarachnoid hemorrhage. Abnormalities, including ST-segment elevation and depression, T wave inversion, and pathologic Q waves are observed. Peaked inverted T waves and a prolonged QT interval can occur in a significant proportion of patients with abnormal ECGs (**Fig. 92-18**). Hypokalemia can be seen in patients with subarachnoid hemorrhage and can increase the likelihood of QT interval prolongation. Other stroke syndromes are often associated with abnormal ECGs but whether these are related to the stroke syndrome or to underlying intrinsic cardiac disease is often difficult to discern. A prolonged QT interval is more common in subarachnoid hemorrhage than other stroke syndromes. Closed head trauma can cause electrocardiographic abnormalities similar to those of subarachnoid hemorrhage, including a prolonged QT interval.

Myocardial damage, with liberation of enzymes and subendocardial hemorrhage or fibrosis at autopsy, can occur in the setting of acute cerebral disease.[28,29] The term *neurogenic stunned myocardium* is used to describe the reversible syndrome. The process can present with selective apical involvement, a takotsubo cardiomyopathy (see Chap. 68). Cardiac troponin I level elevation and echocardiographic evidence of left ventricular dysfunction is present in a significant proportion of patients with subarachnoid hemorrhage. Patients with poorer

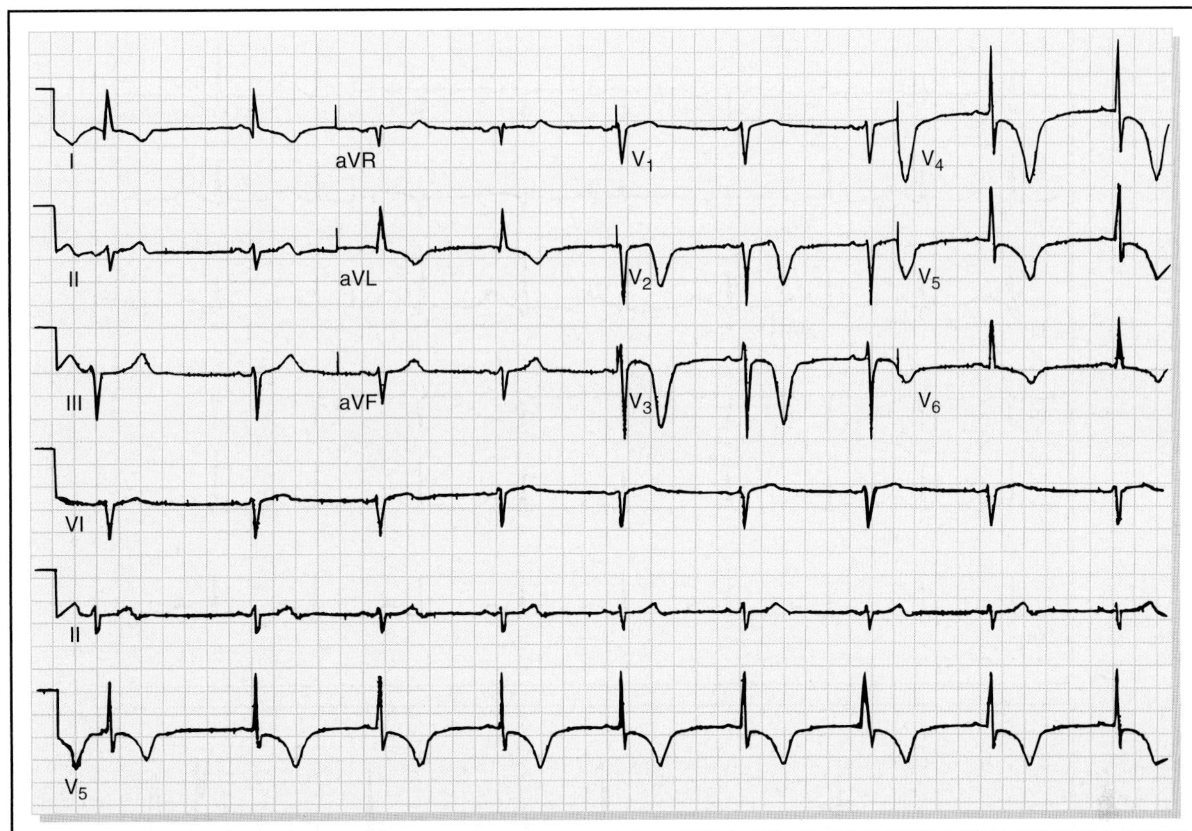

FIGURE 92-18 ECG from a patient with cerebral hemorrhage. Deep and symmetrical T wave inversions are observed. *(Courtesy of Dr. Charles Fisch, Indiana University School of Medicine, Indianapolis.)*

neurologic status at admission are more likely to have an increased peak troponin level. Women are at higher risk of myocardial necrosis.

Pulmonary edema may accompany the acute neurologic insult. The edema can have both a cardiogenic component, related to systemic hypertension and left ventricular dysfunction, and a neurogenic (pulmonary capillary leak) component.

Life-threatening arrhythmias can occur in the setting of acute cerebrovascular disease. Ventricular tachycardia or fibrillation has been observed in patients with subarachnoid hemorrhage and head trauma. A torsades de pointes–type ventricular tachycardia can occur (**Fig. 92-19**). This is often observed in the setting of a prolonged QT interval and hypokalemia. Stroke syndromes, other than subarachnoid hemorrhage, appear to be only rarely associated with serious ventricular tachycardias. Atrial arrhythmias, including atrial fibrillation and regular supraventricular tachycardia, have been observed. Atrial fibrillation is most common in patients presenting with an acute thromboembolic stroke. Separating an effect from the cause can be difficult. Bradycardias, including sinoatrial block, sinus arrest, and atrioventricular block, occur in up to 10% of patients with subarachnoid hemorrhage.

TREATMENT AND PROGNOSIS. Beta-adrenergic blockers appear to be effective for decreasing myocardial damage and controlling supraventricular and ventricular arrhythmias associated with subarachnoid hemorrhage and head trauma. Beta-adrenergic blockers increase the likelihood of bradycardia and cannot be used in patients with hypotension requiring vasopressors. Life-threatening arrhythmias occur primarily in the first day following a neurologic event. Continuous electrocardiographic monitoring during this period is indicated. Careful monitoring of potassium levels, especially in patients with subarachnoid hemorrhage, is warranted. Refractory ventricular arrhythmias have been controlled effectively with stellate ganglion blockade. Electrocardiographic abnormalities reflect unfavorable intracranial factors but do not appear to portend a poor cardiovascular outcome. The magnitude of peak troponin level elevation is predictive for adverse patient outcomes, including severe disability at hospital discharge and death.[28] Other than the mortality occurring secondary to acute arrhythmias, the myocardial necrosis does not appear to play a major factor affecting outcome.

Head injury (e.g., blunt trauma, gunshot wound) and cerebrovascular accidents are the leading causes of brain death in patients being considered as heart donors. These donors can manifest electrocardiographic abnormalities, hemodynamic instability, and myocardial dysfunction related primarily to adrenergic storm and not to intrinsic cardiac disease. Experimental studies on whether contractile performance recovers with transplantation are still controversial. Optimization of volume status and inotropic support, with careful echocardiographic evaluation and possibly left heart catheterization, can allow the use of some donor hearts that would otherwise have been rejected.

Future Perspectives

The molecular mechanisms responsible for cardiac involvement in the neurologic diseases are increasingly better understood. Patients with dystrophic muscular diseases will continue to have their quality and quantity of life improved by supportive clinical care. A prolonged life span will result in a greater proportion of patients manifesting symptoms related to cardiac involvement. Cardiologists and electrophysiologists will be increasingly consulted about the management of these patients. Controversies regarding the appropriate use of pharmacotherapy and device therapy to manage cardiac manifestations in the neurologic diseases will be addressed further with patient series and nonrandomized trials. Gene therapy continues to hold future promise.

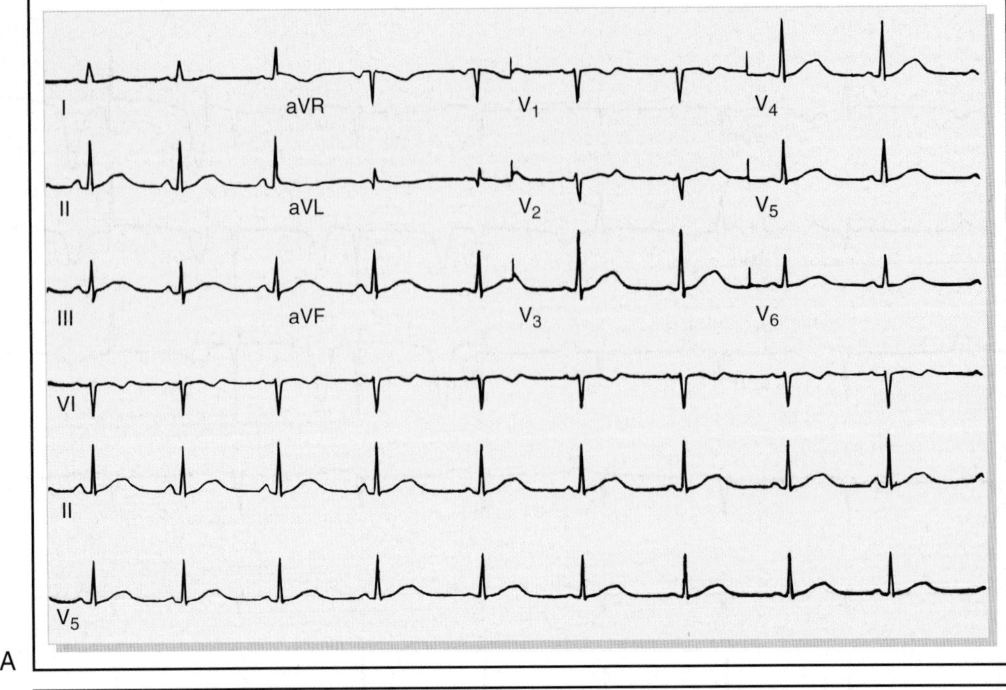

A

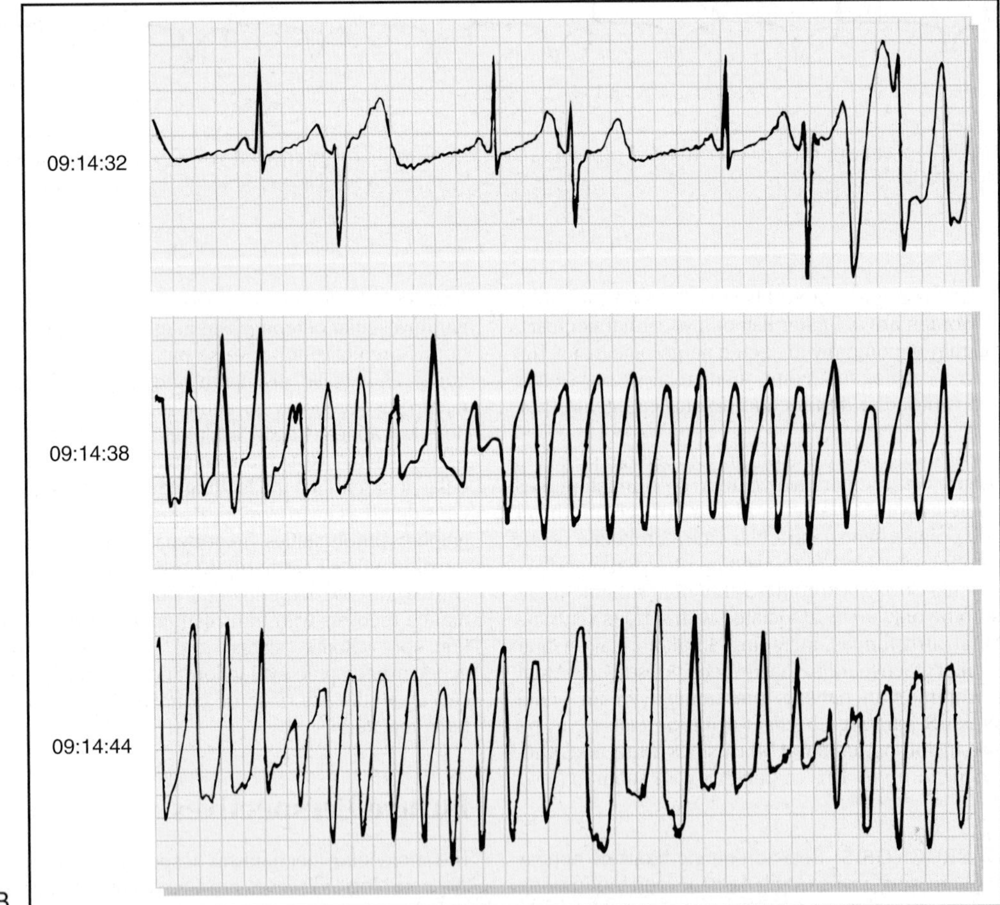

B

FIGURE 92-19 49-year-old patient with cerebral hemorrhage. **A,** ECG recorded within 3 hours of admission and 4 hours after onset of symptoms. QT interval prolongation is observed. **B,** Electrocardiographic monitoring 6 hours after admission. Ventricular bigeminy precedes the onset of polymorphic ventricular tachycardia. Cardioversion was required. The patient was subsequently treated with a beta-adrenergic blocker without further ventricular tachycardia.

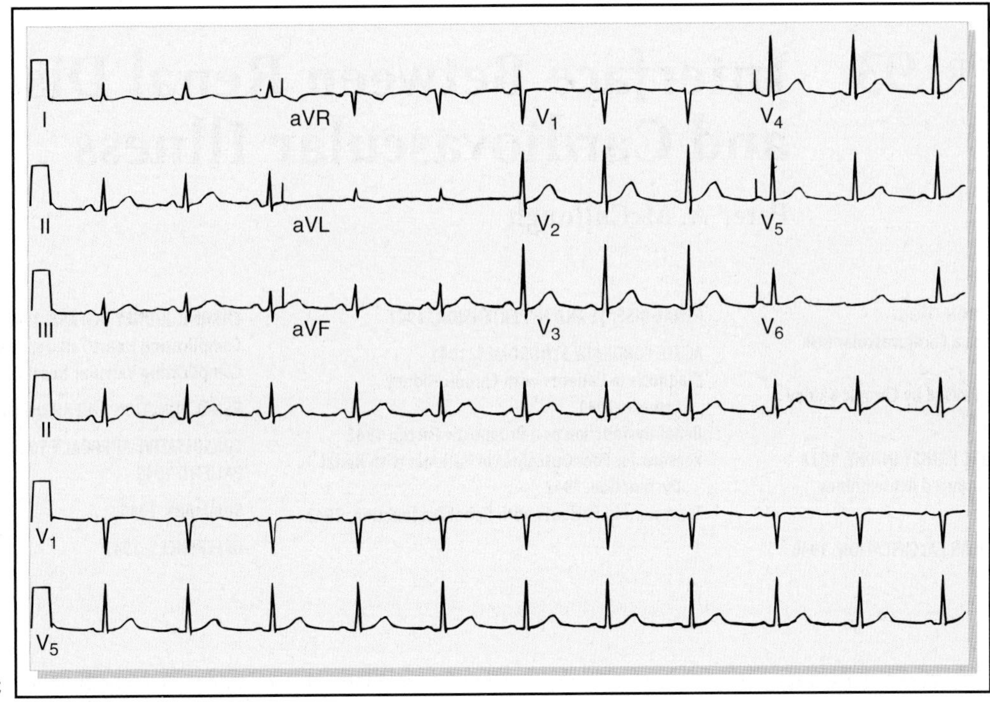

FIGURE 92-19, cont'd C, ECG obtained 2 weeks after admission. The QT interval has normalized.

REFERENCES

Duchenne and Becker Muscular Dystrophies

1. Jefferies JL, Eidem BW, Belmont JW, et al: Genetic predictors and remodeling of dilated cardiomyopathy in muscular dystrophy. Circulation 112:2799, 2005.
2. Thrush PT, Allen HD, Viollet L, et al: Re-examination of the electrocardiogram in boys with Duchenne muscular dystrophy and correlation with its dilated cardiomyopathy. Am J Cardiol 103:262, 2009.
3. Manzur AY, Kuntzer T, Pike M, et al: Glucocorticoid corticosteroids for Duchenne muscular dystrophy. Cochrane Database System Rev (1):CD003725, 2008.
4. Duboc D, Meune C, Lerebours G, et al: Effect of perindopril on the onset and progression of left ventricular dysfunction in Duchenne muscular dystrophy. J Am Coll Cardiol 45:855, 2005.

Myotonic Dystrophies

5. Meola G, Moxley RT: Myotonic dystrophy type 2 and related myotonic disorders. J Neurol 251:1173, 2004.
6. Day JW, Ranum LP: RNA pathogenesis of the myotonic dystrophies. Neuromusc Disord 15:5, 2005.
7. Groh WJ, Lowe MR, Chandan S, et al: Electrocardiographic abnormalities and risk of sudden death in myotonic dystrophy type 1. N Engl J Med 358:2688, 2008.
8. Bhakta D, Lowe MR, Groh WJ: Prevalence of structural cardiac abnormalities in patients with myotonic dystrophy type I. Am Heart J 147:224, 2004.
9. Schoser BG, Ricker K, Schneider-Gold C, et al: Sudden cardiac death in myotonic dystrophy type 2. Neurology 63:2402, 2004.

Emery-Dreifuss Muscular Dystrophy and Associated Disorders

10. Worman HJ, Bonne G: "Laminopathies": A wide spectrum of human diseases. Exper Cell Res 313:2121, 2007.
11. Meune C, Van Berlo JH, Anselme F, et al: Primary prevention of sudden death in patients with lamin A/C gene mutations. N Engl J Med 354:209, 2006.
12. Sakata K, Shimizu M, Ino H, et al: High incidence of sudden cardiac death with conduction disturbances and atrial cardiomyopathy caused by a nonsense mutation in the STA gene. Circulation 111:3352, 2005.

Limb-girdle Muscular Dystrophies

13. Guglieri M, Straub V, Bushby K, et al: Limb-girdle muscular dystrophies. Curr Opin Neurol 21:576, 2008.
14. Wheeler MT, Allikian MJ, Heydemann A, et al: Smooth muscle cell-extrinsic vascular spasm arises from cardiomyocyte degeneration in sarcoglycan-deficient cardiomyopathy. J Clin Invest 113:668, 2004.
15. Poppe M, Bourke J, Eagle M, et al: Cardiac and respiratory failure in limb-girdle muscular dystrophy 2I. Ann Neurol 56:738, 2004.

Facioscapulohumeral Muscular Dystrophy

16. Trevisan CP, Pastorello E, Armani M, et al: Facioscapulohumeral muscular dystrophy and occurrence of heart arrhythmia. Eur Neurol 56:1, 2006.

Friedreich Ataxia

17. Pandolfo M: Friedreich ataxia. Arch Neurol 65:1296, 2008.
18. Ribai P, Pousset F, Tanguy ML, et al: Neurological, cardiological, and oculomotor progression in 104 patients with Friedreich ataxia during long-term follow-up. Arch Neurol 64:558, 2007.

Less Common Neuromuscular Diseases Associated with Cardiac Manifestations

19. Finsterer J: Primary periodic paralyses. Acta Neurol Scand 117:145, 2008.
20. Yoon G, Oberoi S, Tristani-Firouzi M, et al: Andersen-Tawil syndrome: Prospective cohort analysis and expansion of the phenotype. Am J Med Genet 140:312, 2006.
21. DiMauro S: Mitochondrial myopathies. Curr Opin Rheum 18:636, 2006.
22. Sproule DM, Kaufmann P, Engelstad K, et al: Wolff-Parkinson-White syndrome in patients with MELAS. Arch Neurol 64:1625, 2007.
23. Lunn MR, Wang CH: Spinal muscular atrophy. Lancet 371:2120, 2008.
24. Taylor MR, Slavov D, Ku L, et al: Prevalence of desmin mutations in dilated cardiomyopathy. Circulation 115:1244, 2007.
25. Hughes RA, Cornblath DR: Guillain-Barré syndrome. Lancet 366:1653, 2005.
26. Joudinaud TM, Fadel E, Thomas-de-Montpreville V, et al: Fatal giant cell myocarditis after thymoma resection in myasthenia gravis. J Thor Cardiovasc Surg 131:494, 2006.
27. Tomson T, Nashef L, Ryvlin P: Sudden unexpected death in epilepsy: Current knowledge and future directions. Lancet Neurol 7:1021, 2008.

Acute Cerebrovascular Disease

28. Naidech AM, Kreiter KT, Janjua N, et al: Cardiac troponin elevation, cardiovascular morbidity, and outcome after subarachnoid hemorrhage. Circulation 112:2851, 2005.
29. Tung P, Kopelnik A, Banki N, et al: Predictors of neurocardiogenic injury after subarachnoid hemorrhage. Stroke 35:548, 2004.

CHAPTER 93 Interface Between Renal Disease and Cardiovascular Illness

Peter A. McCullough

Cardiorenal Intersection

Hemodynamic and regulatory functions inextricably link the heart and kidneys. In a normal 70-kg man, each kidney weighs about 130 to 170 g and receives blood flow of 400 mL/min/100 g, which is approximately 20% to 25% of the cardiac output, allowing the needed flow to maintain glomerular filtration by approximately 1 million nephrons (**Fig. 93-1**). This flow exceeds by severalfold the blood flow through most other organs on a weight basis. Although the oxygen extraction is low, the kidneys account for about 8% of the total oxygen consumption of the body. The kidney has a central role in electrolyte balance, volume, and blood pressure regulation. Communication between these two organs occurs at multiple levels, including the sympathetic nervous system, the renin-angiotensin-aldosterone system (RAAS), antidiuretic hormone, endothelin, and the natriuretic peptides (**Fig. 93-2**). In addition, the kidneys produce active hormones, including 1,25-dihydroxyvitamin D and erythropoietin (EPO), which have cardiovascular sites of action. With the understanding of these systems has come the development of key diagnostic and therapeutic targets in cardiovascular medicine.

The obesity pandemic in developed countries is a central driver of secondary epidemics of type 2 diabetes (DM) and hypertension (HTN), often leading to combined chronic kidney disease (CKD) and cardiovascular disease (CVD).[1] Among those who have DM for 25 years or longer, the prevalence of diabetic nephropathy in types 1 and 2 DM is 57% and 48%, respectively.[2] Approximately 50% of all cases of end-stage renal disease (ESRD) are caused by diabetic nephropathy. With the aging of the general population and cardiovascular care shifting toward the older population, an understanding of why decreasing levels of renal function act as a major adverse prognostic factor after a variety of cardiac events is imperative. Considerable evidence has shown that CKD accelerates atherosclerosis, myocardial disease, and valvular disease and promotes an array of cardiac arrhythmias that can lead to sudden death.[3]

Chronic Kidney Disease as a Cardiovascular Risk State

Chronic kidney disease is defined through a range of estimated glomerular filtration rate (eGFR) values by the National Kidney Foundation Kidney Disease Outcomes Quality Initiative (KDOQI).[4] A common definition for CKD stipulates an eGFR of less than 60 mL/min/1.73 m^2 or the presence of kidney damage (**Fig. 93-3**). Although with normative aging (age 20 to 80 years), the eGFR declines from about 130 to 60 mL/min/1.73 m^2, a variety of pathobiologic processes appear to begin when the eGFR drops below 60 mL/min/1.73 m^2. Most studies of cardiovascular outcomes have found that a critical cut point for the development of contrast-induced acute kidney injury (CI-AKI), restenosis after percutaneous coronary intervention (PCI), recurrent myocardial infarction (MI), diastolic or systolic heart failure (HF), arrhythmias, and cardiovascular death is an eGFR of 60 mL/min/1.73 m^2—which roughly corresponds to a serum creatinine (Cr) level higher than 1.5 mg/dL in the general population (**Fig. 93-4**).[4-8] Because Cr is a crude indicator of renal function and often underestimates renal dysfunction in women and older adults, calculated measures of eGFR or creatinine clearance (CrCl) using the Cockcroft-Gault equation or the modification of diet in renal disease equation are superior methods for the assessment of renal function. The four-variable modification of diet in renal disease equation for eGFR is the preferred method because it does not rely on body weight. The equation is given by the following:

$$\text{eGFR} = 186.3 \times (\text{serum Cr}^{-1.154}) \times (\text{age}^{-0.203})$$

Calculated values are multiplied by 0.742 for women and by 1.21 for blacks. Another blood test reflecting renal filtration function is cystatin C.[9] Cystatin C is a nonglycosylated protein with low molecular mass (13-kDa) produced by all nucleated cells. Its low molecular mass and high isoelectric point allow it to be filtered freely by the glomerular membrane and 100% reabsorbed by the proximal tubule. The serum concentration of cystatin C correlates with renal filtration, and because of a stable production rate, it provides a more accurate marker of renal filtration function than the serum Cr level. Serum levels of cystatin C do not depend on weight and height, muscle mass, age, or sex making it less variable than the Cr level. Furthermore, measurements can be made and interpreted from a single random sample, with reference values of 0.54 to 1.21 mg/liter (median, 0.85 mg/liter; range, 0.42 to 1.39 mg/liter).

In addition, microalbuminuria at any level of eGFR indicates CKD and may reflect endothelial dysfunction in glomerular capillaries caused by the metabolic syndrome, DM, or HTN (see Chaps. 45 and 64). Microalbuminuria can be defined as a random urine albumin-to-Cr ratio (ACR) of 30 to 300 mg/g. An ACR higher than 300 mg/g is considered gross proteinuria. The random, spot urine ACR is the office test for microalbuminuria recommended as part of the cardiovascular risk assessment done by cardiologists and other specialists. Microalbuminuria as an independent CVD risk factor for diabetics and those without DM is discussed in Chap. 64. The Seventh Report of the Joint National Committee on Prevention, Detection, Evaluation, and Treatment of High Blood Pressure (JNC 7) has recognized CKD as an independent cardiovascular risk state,[10] which has many vascular and metabolic abnormalities (see later; **Fig. 93-5**).[11]

Implications of Anemia Caused by Chronic Kidney Disease

There is increasing recognition of the associations between the blood hemoglobin (Hb) level, CKD, and CVD. The most common cut point for the definition of anemia by the World Health Organization is a Hb level lower than 13 g/dL in men and lower than 12 g/dL in women. Approximately 9% of the general adult population meets the definition of anemia at these levels. In general, anemia caused by CKD is present in 20% of patients with stable coronary disease and 30% to 60% of patients with HF. Hence, anemia is a common and easily identifiable potential diagnostic and therapeutic target.[12,13]

Anemia contributes to multiple adverse outcomes, in part because of decreased tissue oxygen delivery and uptake.[13] The cause of anemia in patients with CKD can be multifactorial, with a central component being a relative deficiency of EPO as well as an increase in hepcidin produced by the liver, resulting in attenuated maturation of hemangioblasts combined with an iron reuptake defect. In response to oxygen tension, the kidneys produce 90% of plasma EPO levels and maintain a range between 10 and 30 IU/mL; however, during anemic periods, these levels may exceed 100 IU/mL. Patients with CKD and HF appear to have a relative EPO deficiency, with an inappropriately low EPO level for the measured blood Hb level. In the setting of CKD and HF, there are increased levels of tumor necrosis factor-α, interleukin-1 (IL-1) and interleukin-6 (IL-6), endothelin, matrix metalloproteinases, and other inflammation-related proteins produced by many organs. These factors can reduce directly red cell production at the level of the bone marrow and aggravate the anemia. Of 29 large prospective studies of HF, 28 found anemia to predict mortality independently.[14] On average, in those patients with HF, for each 1-g/dL decrement in Hb, there is a 13% increase in risk for all-cause mortality. In addition, patients with anemia and CKD will more likely progress to ESRD irrespective of their baseline level of renal function. As Hb drops over time, there is a graded increase in HF hospitalizations and death. Conversely, those patients who have had a rise in Hb—whether as a result of improved nutrition, reduced neurohormonal factors, or other unknown factors—enjoy a significant reduction in endpoints over the next several years. This improvement has been associated with a significant reduction in left ventricular mass index, suggesting a favorable change in left ventricular remodeling.[15] The observational data suggest that changes in Hb, either up or down, are associated with clinical consequences. Hence, there is a rationale for therapeutic intervention on the Hb level to change the natural history of cardiorenal disease.

In addition to the effect on Hb levels, the pleiotropic effects of erythrocyte-stimulating proteins (ESPs) include positive effects on coronary endothelium, resulting in an increase in coronary flow reserve. This effect may be mediated through the activation of endothelial nitric oxide synthase via protein kinase B phosphorylation and by preventing endothelial cell apoptosis. These proteins may also enhance myocardial repair in patients with myocardial injury. This could minimize the progression of left ventricular dysfunction by recruiting vascular progenitor cells, which can become functional myocardial cells, thereby increasing the contractile function of the injured ventricle. The molecular targets for ESPs include receptors expressed on cardiac myocytes, endothelial cells, and endothelial progenitor cells, in addition to hematopoietic stem cells.

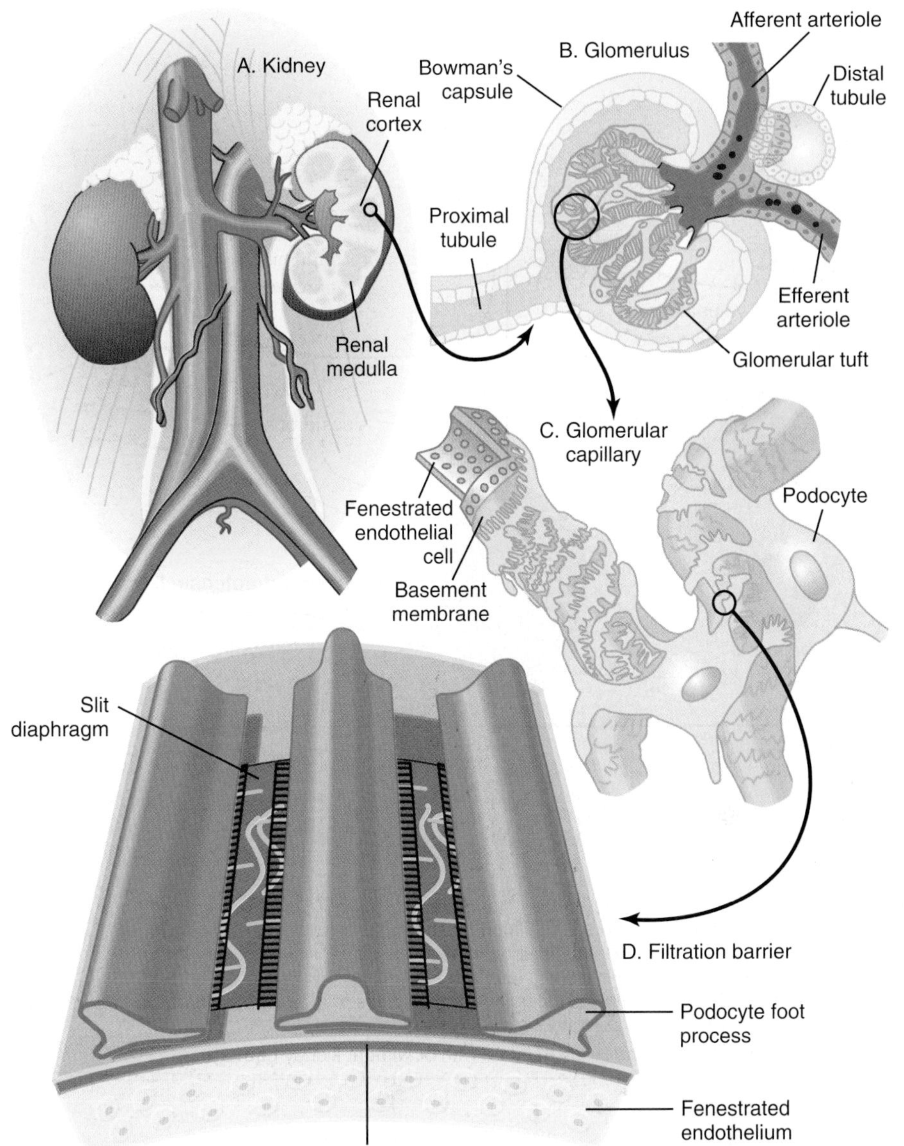

FIGURE 93-1 Normal structure of the glomerular vasculature. **A,** Each kidney contains about 1 million glomeruli in the renal cortex. **B,** Afferent arteriole entering Bowman's capsule and branching into several capillaries that form the glomerular tuft. The walls of the capillaries constitute the actual filter. The plasma filtrate (primary urine) is directed to the proximal tubule, whereas the unfiltered blood returns to the circulation through the efferent arteriole. **C,** The filtration barrier of the capillary wall contains an innermost fenestrated endothelium, the glomerular basement membrane, and a layer of interdigitating podocyte foot processes. **D,** Cross section through the glomerular capillary depicts the fenestrated endothelial layer and the glomerular basement membrane, with overlying podocyte foot processes. An ultrathin slit diaphragm spans the filtration slit between the foot processes, slightly above the basement membrane. To show the slit diaphragm, the foot processes are drawn smaller than actual scale. *(Modified from Tryggvason K, Patrakka J, Wartiovaara J: Hereditary proteinuria syndromes and mechanisms of proteinuria. N Engl J Med 354:1387, 2006.)*

Treatment of anemia with exogenous ESPs (EPO and darbepoetin alfa) in CKD has been disappointing in reducing morbidity, particularly that of cardiovascular origin, and in improving survival and quality of

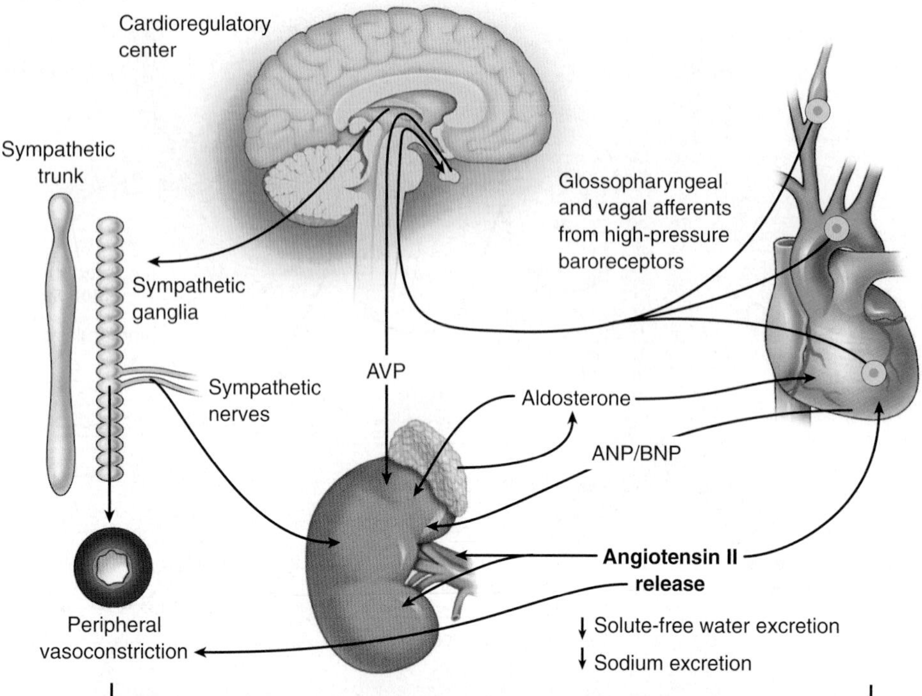

FIGURE 93-2 Major neurohumoral communication systems between the heart and kidney. ANP = A-type natriuretic peptide; AVP = arginine vasopressin; BNP = B-type natriuretic peptide. *(Modified from Schrier RW, Abraham WT: Hormones and hemodynamics in heart failure. N Engl J Med 341:577, 1999.) (see Fig. 45-10)*

Criteria

1. Kidney damage for ≥ 3 months, as defined by structural or functional abnormalities of the kidney, with or without decreased GFR, manifest by *either:*
   - Pathological abnormalities; or
   - Markers of kidney damage, including abnormalities in the composition of the blood or urine, or abnormalities in imaging tests
2. eGFR <60 mL/min/1.73m^2 for ≥ 3 months, with or without kidney damage

Markers of kidney damage	Findings indicating kidney damage
Proteinuria	Albumin-to-creatinine ratio >30 mg/g
Urine sediment abnormalities	Cellular casts, coarse granular casts, fat
Imaging tests	Abnormalities in kidney size Asymmetry in kidney size or function Irregularities in shape (cysts, scars, mass lesions) Stones Hydronephrosis and other abnormalities of the urinary tract Arterial stenosis and other vascular lesions
Abnormalities in blood or urine composition	Nephrotic syndrome Tubular syndromes (renal tubular acidosis, potassium secretory defects, renal glycosuria, renal phosphaturia, Fanconi's syndrome)

FIGURE 93-3 Diagnostic criteria for chronic kidney disease and kidney damage.

life. Darbepoetin alfa (Aranesp) is a genetically engineered form of EPO designed to have a longer half-life, making once-monthly injections an attractive treatment option.[13] Increasing the Hb level from below 10 to 12 g/dL has been linked to favorable changes in biomarkers, such as left ventricular remodeling, improved ejection fraction, improved functional classification, and higher levels of peak oxygen consumption with exercise testing. These biomarkers may not reflect clinical outcomes, because treatment with EPO and supplemental iron, which is needed in approximately 70% of patients, can cause three problems: (1) increased platelet activity, thrombin generation, and resultant increased risk of thrombosis; (2) increased endothelin levels and increased asymmetrical dimethylarginine, which theoretically reduces nitric oxide availability, and results in HTN; and (3) worsened measures of oxidative stress. Three randomized trials in CKD have indicated that treatment with ESPs to a higher hemoglobin results in higher CVD events. The Cardiovascular Risk Reduction by Early Anemic Treatment with Epoetin beta in Chronic Kidney Disease Patients (CREATE) trial randomized 603 patients to treatment with EPO to a target of 13.0 to 15.0 g/dL versus 10.5 to 11.5 g/dL for 2.5 years, and found higher rates of CVD and progression to ESRD in the 13.0 to 15.0 g/dL group.[16] The Correction of Hemoglobin and Outcomes in Renal Insufficiency (CHOIR) trial randomized 1432 patients with CKD and treated with EPO to a target of 13.5 versus 11.3 g/dL.[17] The composite endpoint, a combination of mortality and cardiovascular outcomes (stroke, MI, hospitalization because of HF), occurred in 125 events in the 13.5-g/dL arm and 97 events in the 11.3-g/dL arm (P = 0.03). A placebo-controlled trial on this issue is critical because it appears that treatment to higher hemoglobin targets results in worsened CVD outcomes. The Trial to Reduce Cardiovascular Events with Aranesp Therapy (TREAT), a multicenter, double-blind, placebo-controlled randomized trial, was specifically designed to determine whether patients with CKD (eGFR = 20 to 60 mL/min/1.73 m^2), type 2 DM, and anemia (Hb < 11 g/dL) would experience a reduction in the risk of the composite endpoint of death or cardiovascular morbidity (nonfatal MI, hospitalization for myocardial ischemia, HF, or stroke) when treated with darbepoetin alfa to raise the Hb level to 13 g/dL. This study did not show a reduction in the risk of cardiovascular or renal events or death, but showed an excess of stroke in the darbepoetin alfa group.[18] Until there is clear evidence that the partial correction of anemia has favorable outcomes in CVD, this form of treatment is not recommended for the primary purpose of improving the natural history of CVD.

Contrast-Induced Acute Kidney Injury

Contrast-induced acute kidney injury has been defined as a composite rise in the serum Cr level of more than 25% or 0.5 mg/dL, or an increase of 50% (or 0.3 mg/dL) or more from baseline, with a reduction in urine output to less than 0.5 mL/kg/hour for 6 hours after intravascular administration of iodinated contrast (see Chap. 20).[19] The frequency of CI-AKI is approximately 13% in nondiabetics and 20% in diabetics undergoing PCI (see Chap. 58). It is critical to understand that the risk of CI-AKI is related in a curvilinear fashion to the eGFR (**Fig. 93-6**).[20] Fortunately, in patients undergoing PCI, cases of CI-AKI leading to dialysis are rare (0.5% to 2.0%). When this does occur, it portends a catastrophic outcome, including a 36% in-hospital mortality rate and a 2-year survival of only 19%.[21] Although not always attributed to CI-AKI, transient rises in the Cr level relate directly to longer intensive care unit and hospital ward stays (3 and 4 more days, respectively) after bypass surgery. Even transient rises in the Cr level translate to differences in mortality after PCI (**Fig. 93-7**).[22]

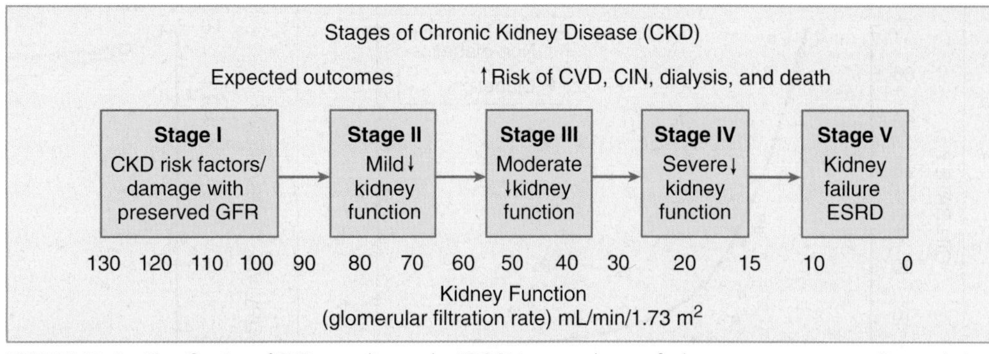

FIGURE 93-4 Classification of CKD according to the KDOQI. Increased rates of adverse events are generally seen below an eGFR of 60 mL/min/1.73 m^2. CIN = contrast-induced nephropathy. *(From McCullough PA, Sandberg KR: Epidemiology of contrast-induced nephropathy. Rev Cardiovasc Med 4[Suppl 5]: S3, 2003.)*

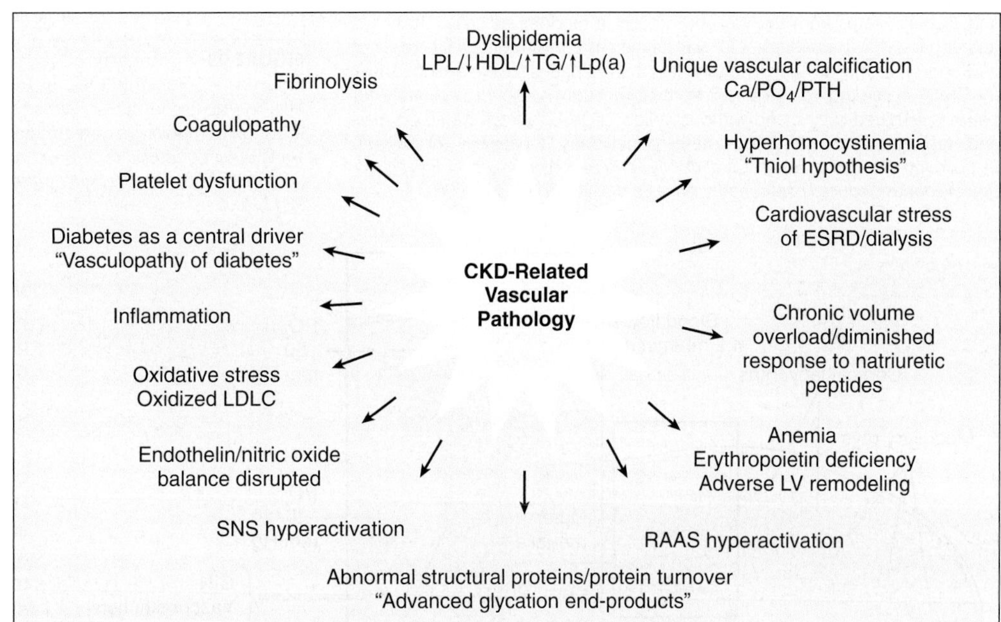

FIGURE 93-5 Pathobiology of the CKD state and its effects on the cardiovascular system. Lp(a) = lipoprotein(a); LPL = lipoprotein lipase; LV = left ventricle; NO = nitric oxide; SNS = sympathetic nervous system. *(Modified from McCullough PA: Why is chronic kidney disease the "spoiler" for cardiovascular outcomes? J Am Coll Cardiol 41:725, 2003.)*

Three core elements contribute to the pathophysiology of CI-AKI: (1) direct toxicity of iodinated contrast material to nephrons; (2) microshowers of atheroemboli to the kidneys; and (3) contrast material- and atheroemboli-induced intrarenal vasoconstriction. Furthermore, as renal function declines, a host of chronic perturbations occur in hemostasis, lipids, endothelial function, protein metabolism, calcium-phosphorus balance, and oxidative stress.[23] Direct toxicity to nephrons with iodinated contrast media appears to be related to the ionic strength and osmolality of the contrast media.[24] Microshowers of cholesterol emboli occur in about 50% of PCIs when a guiding catheter is passed through the aorta.[25] Most of these showers are clinically silent. In approximately 1% of high-risk cases, however, an acute cholesterol emboli syndrome can develop, manifested by acute renal failure, mesenteric ischemia, decreased microcirculation to the extremities and, in some cases, embolic stroke. Because acute renal failure occurs after coronary artery bypass surgery with almost the same risk predictors as in procedures involving contrast media, atheroembolism represents a common pathogenic feature of both causes of renal failure.[26] Intrarenal vasoconstriction as a pathologic vascular response to contrast medium and perhaps as an organ response to cholesterol emboli is a final hypoxic-ischemic injury to the kidney in PCI. Hypoxia triggers activation of neurohumoral systems and results in further reduction in renal blood flow. When contrast agents are given to animals, there is transient vasodilation caused by nitric oxide release from endothelial cells followed by sustained vascular smooth muscle cell constriction.[27-29] But when there is vascular disease, endothelial dysfunction, and a reduction in the overall number of nephron units, contrast agents evoke longer periods of renal vasoconstriction and have a prolonged transit time in the kidney in the vascular and urinary spaces. Thus, there is extravasation of iodinated contrast molecules from the renal tubules into the vascular peritubular space, causing additional vasoconstriction and cellular injury (**Fig. 93-8**). The most important predictor of CI-AKI is underlying renal dysfunction. The remnant nephron theory postulates that after sufficient chronic kidney damage has occurred and the eGFR is reduced to less than 60 mL/min/1.73 m^2, the remaining nephrons are vulnerable. Residual nephrons have increased oxygen demands and are more susceptible to ischemic and oxidative injury. Emerging blood and urine biomarkers become elevated before the rise in the serum Cr level, including neutrophil–gelatinase-associated lipocalin (siderocalin), kidney injury molecule-1, interleukin-18 (IL-18), liver fatty acid binding protein, a variety of tubular enzymes, and cystatin C (see earlier). The clinical use of such markers for CI-AKI is expected in the future.[30]

Prevention of Contrast-Induced Acute Kidney Injury (see Chap. 20)

A prevention strategy for CI-AKI should be used for patients with preexisting CKD (baseline eGFR < 60 mL/min/1.73 m^2), and in particular,

CH 93

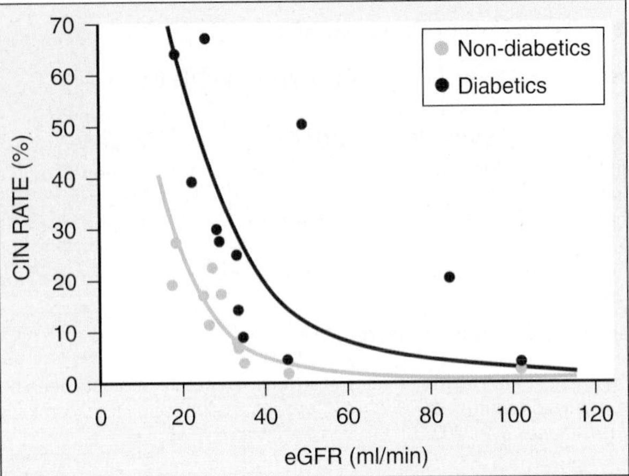

FIGURE 93-6 Rates of contrast-induced acute kidney injury (CI-AKI) by eGFR and diabetic status from the placebo groups of randomized trials. The fitted function is a drawn quadratic. CIN was defined as a serum Cr level increase of 25% and/or 0.5 mg/dL. Trials including less than 25 patients were excluded. Risk for CI-AKI according to the baseline renal function is shown separately for patients with (red circles) and without (yellow circles) diabetes, based on trials and registries that presented these populations separately. *(Data from McCullough PA, Adam A, Becker CR, et al; CIN Consensus Working Panel: Risk prediction of contrast-induced nephropathy. Am J Cardiol 98[Suppl 1]:27, 2006.)*

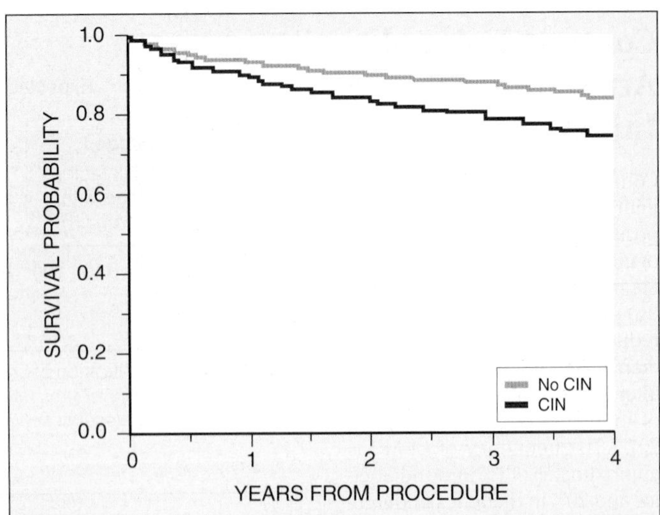

FIGURE 93-7 Mortality in 7230 patients with and without CKD and contrast-induced nephropathy (CIN), or CI-AKI, after PCI. CIN is defined as ≥25% or ≥0.5-mg/dL rise in the Cr level at 48 hours after PCI. Patients with STEMI and those on hemodialysis were excluded. *(Modified from Dangas G, Iakovou I, Nikolsky E, et al: Contrast-induced nephropathy after percutaneous coronary interventions in relation to chronic kidney disease and hemodynamic variables. Am J Cardiol 95:13, 2005.)*

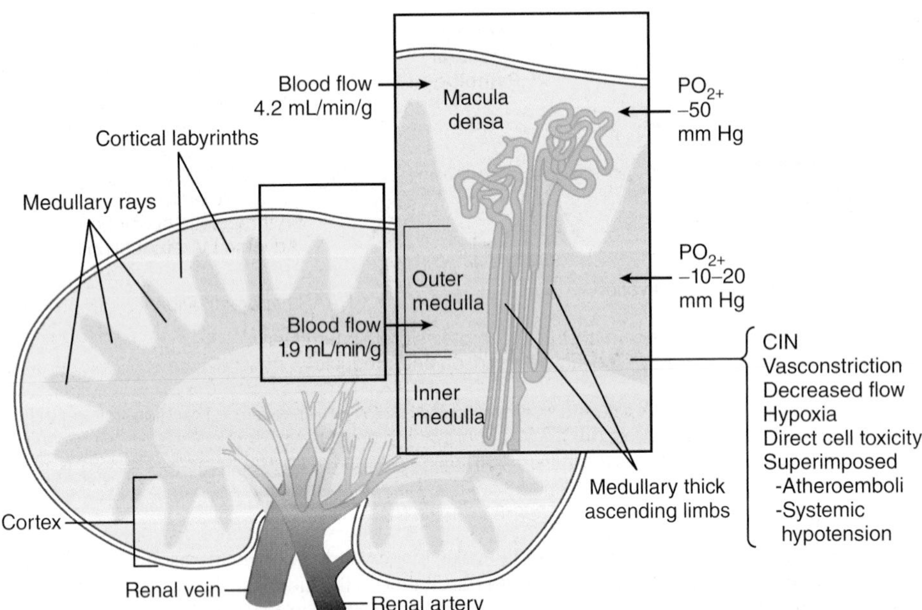

FIGURE 93-8 Pathophysiology of CI-AKI demonstrating, in the presence of a reduced nephron mass, that the remaining nephrons are vulnerable to injury. Iodinated contrast, after causing a brief (minutes) period of vasodilation, causes sustained (hours to days) intrarenal vasoconstriction and ischemic injury. The ischemic injury sets off a cascade of events, largely driven by oxidative injury, causing death of renal tubular cells. If a sufficient mass of nephron units is affected, a recognizable rise in the serum Cr level will occur. *(Modified from McCullough PA: Contrast-induced acute kidney injury. J Am Coll Cardiol 51:1419, 2008.)*

those with CKD and DM. The presence of CKD, DM, and other risk factors including hemodynamic instability, use of intra-aortic balloon counterpulsation, HF, older age, hyperglycemia, and anemia in the same patient can produce a predicted probability of CI-AKI more than 50% (**Fig. 93-9**).[31] Thus, CI-AKI must be discussed in detail during the informed consent process of high-risk patients before the use of intravascular iodinated contrast. Four basic concepts apply to CI-AKI prevention: (1) hydration and volume expansion; (2) choice and quantity of contrast material; (3) pre-, intra-, and postprocedural end-organ protection with pharmacotherapy; and (4) postprocedural monitoring and expectant care.

Hydration with intravenous normal saline or isotonic sodium bicarbonate is reasonable, starting 3 to 12 hours before the procedure at a rate of 1.5 mL/kg/hr or more.[32,33] Those at risk should receive at least 300 to 500 mL of intravenous hydration before administration of the contrast material. If there are particular concerns regarding volume overload or HF in individuals in whom clinical assessment of volume status is difficult, a right-heart catheterization may aid management during and after the procedure. The postprocedure hydration target is a urine output of 150 mL/hr. If patients have a diuresis of more than 150 mL/hr, their extra losses should be replaced with more intravenous fluid. In general, this strategy calls for hydration orders of normal saline or sodium bicarbonate at 150 mL/hr for at least 6 hours after the procedure. Achieving adequate urine flow rates may reduce the rate of CI-AKI by 50%.

Head-to-head randomized trials of iodinated contrast agents have demonstrated the lowest rates of CI-AKI with nonionic, iso-osmolar iodixanol, particularly in those with CKD and DM. A meta-analysis included 16 prospective, double-blind, randomized controlled trials that compared iodixanol with low-osmolar contrast media (LOCM) in adult patients undergoing angiographic examinations and reported Cr values at baseline and following CM administration.[34] The pooled data demonstrated a reduced risk of CI-AKI (≥0.5 mg/dL rise at 72 hours) with iodixanol (overall odds ratio [OR] = 0.39; 95% confidence interval [CI], 0.23 to 0.66; P = 0.0004). A 2009 tabular meta-analysis restricted to trials of iodixanol and nonionic LOCM found an overall nonsignificant trend in favor of iodixanol; however, the impact on the subset with CKD and DM could not be evaluated (**Fig. 93-10**).[35] These data support the hypothesis that iodixanol (290 mOsm/kg) is less nephrotoxic than LOCM agents with osmolality ranging from 600 to 800 mOsm/kg; however, this finding applies only to those who have both CKD and DM.

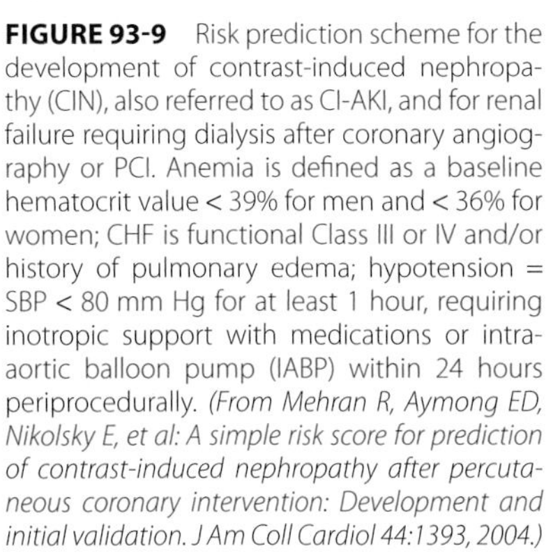

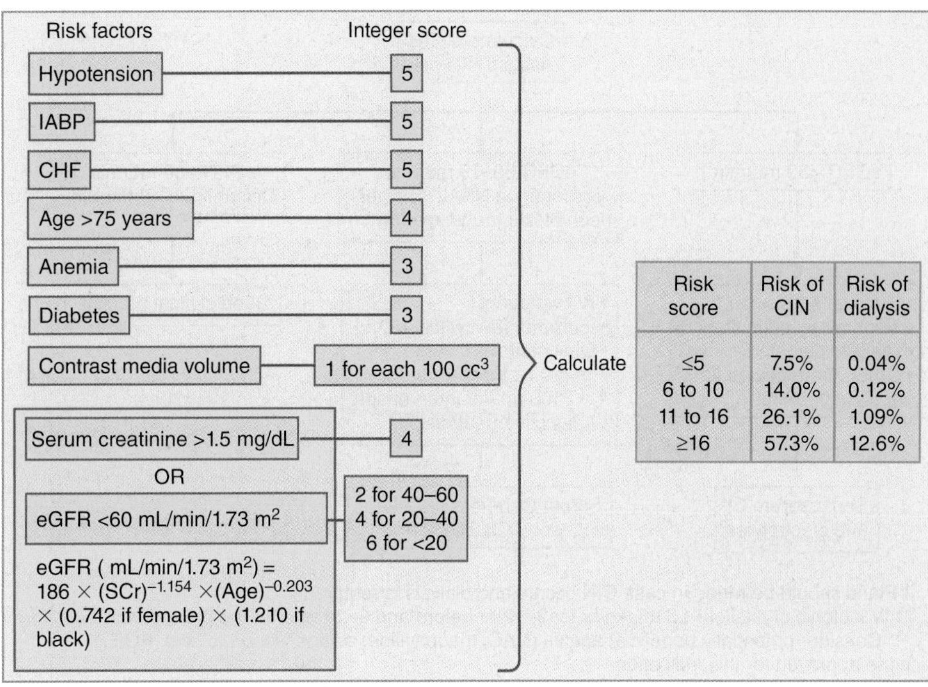

FIGURE 93-9 Risk prediction scheme for the development of contrast-induced nephropathy (CIN), also referred to as CI-AKI, and for renal failure requiring dialysis after coronary angiography or PCI. Anemia is defined as a baseline hematocrit value < 39% for men and < 36% for women; CHF is functional Class III or IV and/or history of pulmonary edema; hypotension = SBP < 80 mm Hg for at least 1 hour, requiring inotropic support with medications or intra-aortic balloon pump (IABP) within 24 hours periprocedurally. *(From Mehran R, Aymong ED, Nikolsky E, et al: A simple risk score for prediction of contrast-induced nephropathy after percutaneous coronary intervention: Development and initial validation. J Am Coll Cardiol 44:1393, 2004.)*

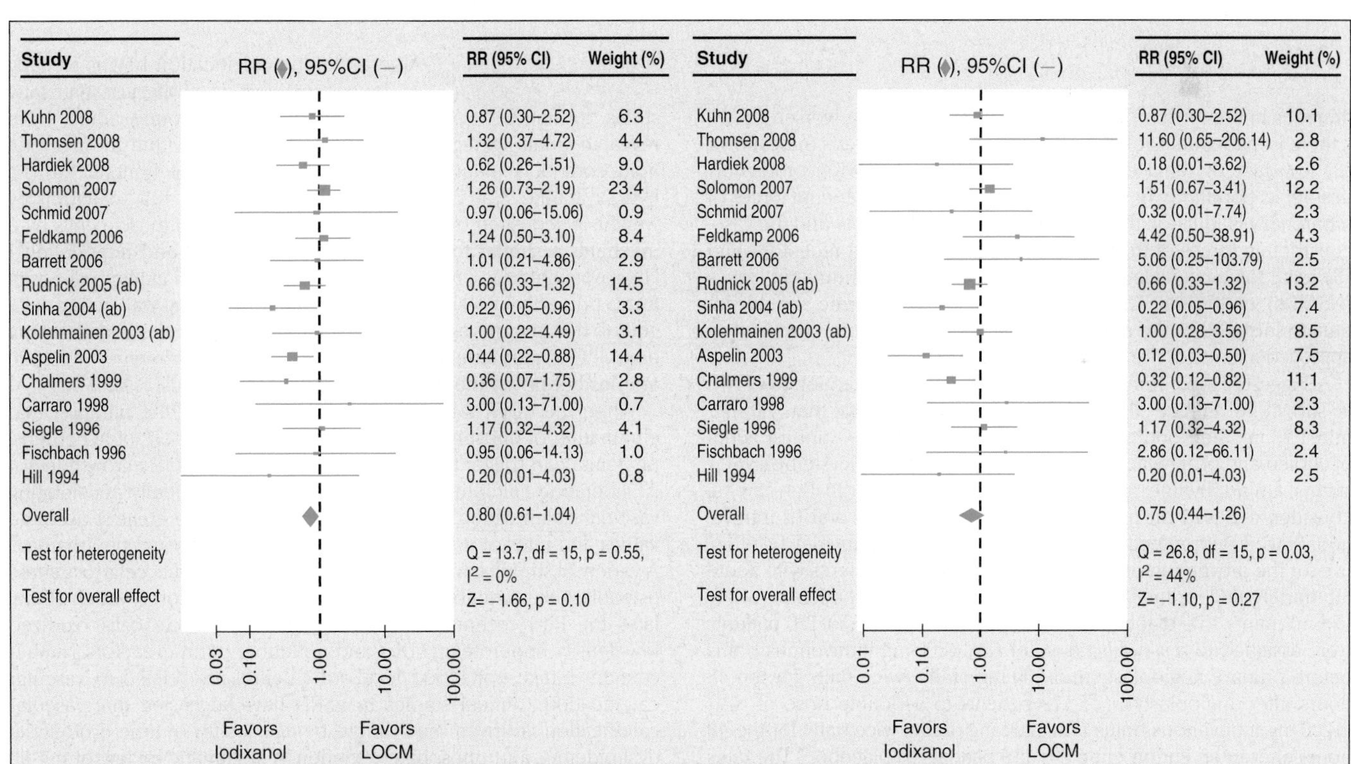

FIGURE 93-10 Incidence of CI-AKI from a 2009 meta-analysis of trials comparing iso-osmolar iodixanol with all nonionic low-osmolar agents, demonstrating an overall trend in favor of a treatment effect with iodixanol (not statistically significant). **Left and right panels,** Results for ≥25% and ≥0.5-mg/dL rise in serum Cr level, respectively. *(From Heinrich MC, Häberle L, Müller V, et al: Nephrotoxicity of iso-osmolar iodixanol compared with nonionic low-osmolar contrast media: Meta-analysis of randomized controlled trials. Radiology 250:68, 2009.)*

The American College of Cardiology/American Heart Association (ACC/AHA) guidelines for the management of acute coronary syndrome (ACS) recommends iodixanol for patients with CKD at risk for CI-AKI undergoing urgent angiography.[36] Although it is desirable to limit contrast to the smallest volume possible in any setting, there is disagreement about a safe contrast limit. The lower the eGFR, the smaller the amount of contrast material needed to cause CI-AKI. In general, contrast medium should be limited to less than 30 mL for a diagnostic and less than 100 mL for an interventional procedure. If staged procedures are planned, it is advantageous to have more than 10 days between the first and second contrast exposures if contrast nephropathy has occurred with the first procedure.

More than 40 randomized trials have tested various adjunctive strategies for the prevention of CI-AKI.[37] Most of these trials were small, underpowered, and did not find the preventive strategy under investigation superior to placebo. These trials permit several conclusions: (1)

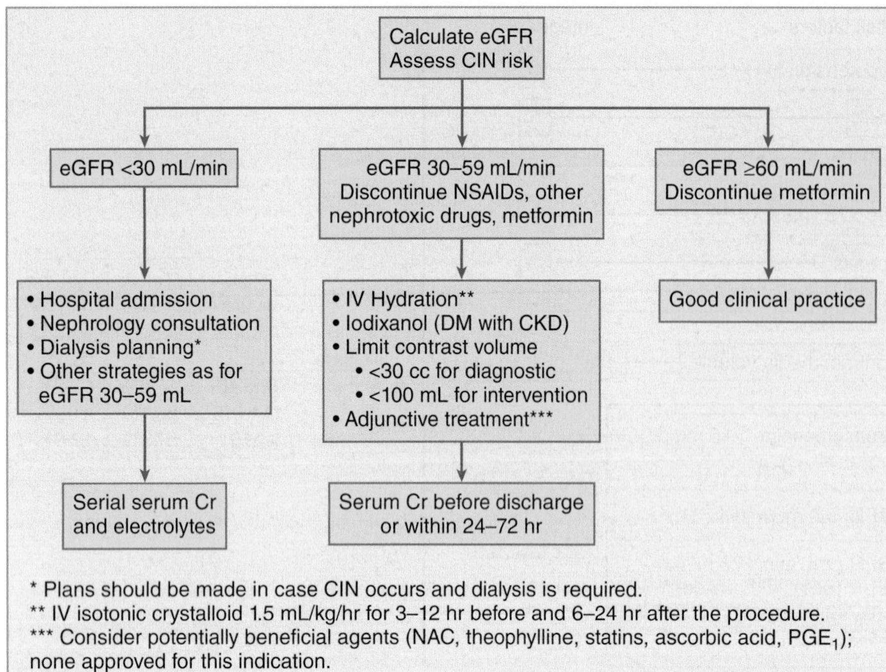

FIGURE 93-11 Algorithm for the management of patients receiving iodinated contrast media. PGE_1 = prostaglandin E_1. *(Modified from McCullough PA: Contrast-induced acute kidney injury. J Am Coll Cardiol 51:1419, 2008.)*

diuretics in the form of loop diuretics or mannitol can worsen CI-AKI if there is inadequate volume replacement for the diuresis that follows; (2) low-dose or renal dose dopamine does not provide protection, despite its popularity in practice, given the counterbalancing forces of intrarenal vasodilation through the dopamine-1 receptor and the vasoconstricting forces of the dopamine-2, alpha, and beta receptors; and (3) renal toxic agents including nonsteroidal antiinflammatory drugs (NSAIDs), metformin, aminoglycosides, and cyclosporine should not be administered in the periprocedural period. There are currently no approved agents for the prevention of CI-AKI.

A suggested algorithm for risk stratification and prevention of CI-AKI is shown in **Figure 93-11**. When the eGFR is less than 60 mL/min/1.73 m^2, then optimal hydration, iodixanol as the contrast agent of choice, and prophylactic agents—including *N*-acetylcysteine (NAC), statins, aminophylline, ascorbic acid, and prostaglandin E_1—can be considered. Based on many small randomized trials, oral or intravenous NAC, a cytoprotective agent against oxidative injury, may be effective for the prevention of CI-AKI.[37] A trial of NAC in patients with acute MI undergoing primary angioplasty assigned 354 patients (eGFR, ~78 mL/min; ~15% diabetics) to one of three groups: (1) 116 patients were assigned to a standard dose of NAC (600-mg intravenous bolus before primary angioplasty and 600 mg orally twice daily for the 48 hours after angioplasty); (2) 119 patients to a double dose of NAC (1200-mg intravenous bolus and 1200 mg orally twice daily for the 48 hours after intervention); and (3) 119 patients to placebo.[38] The rates of CI-AKI (>25% rise in the Cr level from baseline) were 39 (33%) in controls, 17 (15%) for standard-dose NAC, and 10 (8%) for double-dose NAC ($P < 0.001$). Overall in-hospital mortality was as follows: 13 (11%) in the control group died, 5 (4%) in the standard-dose NAC group, and 3 (3%) in the high-dose NAC group ($P = 0.02$). The rate for the composite endpoint of death, acute renal failure requiring temporary renal replacement therapy, or the need for mechanical ventilation was 21 (18%), 8 (7%), and 6 (5%) in the three groups, respectively ($P = 0.002$). Most operators believe—given the seriousness of CI-AKI, the relative safety of the strategies used, and the evolution of clinical trials shaping our practice—that the combination of hydration, use of iodixanol, and use of prophylactic NAC is a reasonable three-pronged approach to minimize CI-AKI and the risk of acute renal failure requiring dialysis.

Postprocedural monitoring is critical in the current era of short hospital stays and outpatient procedures. In general, high-risk patients in the hospital should have hydration started 12 hours before the procedure and continued for at least 6 hours afterward. A serum Cr level should be measured 24 hours after the procedure. For outpatients, particularly those with eGFR less than 60 mL/min/1.73 m^2, either an overnight stay or discharge to home with 48-hour follow-up and Cr level measurement is advised. Individuals in whom severe CI-AKI develops have an increased Cr level greater than 0.5 mg/dL in the first 24 hours after the procedure.[39] Thus, for those who do not have this degree of Cr level elevation and an otherwise uneventful course, discharge to home may be considered. For those with eGFR lower than 30 mL/min/1.73 m^2, the possibility of dialysis should be discussed with the patient; preprocedure nephrology consultation is advised for possible pre- and postprocedure hemofiltration and dialysis management.

Acceleration of Vascular Calcification

Atherosclerotic calcification begins as early as the second decade of life, just after fatty streak formation.[40] Coronary artery lesions of young adults have revealed small aggregates of crystalline calcium within the necrotic lipid core of a plaque.[40] Calcium phosphate—the mineral form is hydroxyapatite, $Ca_5(PO_4)_3(OH)$—which contains 40% calcium by weight, is deposited by modulated vascular smooth muscle cells by a mechanism similar to that found in osteogenesis and remodeling.[41] Hydroxyapatite, the predominant crystalline form in calcium deposits, forms primarily in vesicles that pinch off from arterial wall cells, analogous to how matrix vesicles pinch off from chondrocytes in developing bone.[41] Coronary artery calcification (CAC) occurs in atherosclerotic arteries but not in the normal vessel wall (see Chaps. 19 and 43).

When the eGFR falls below 60 mL/min/1.73 m^2, the filtration and elimination of phosphorus are reduced. Subtle degrees of hyperphosphatemia can trigger the increased release of fibroblast growth factor 23, liberating calcium stores from bone and potentially accelerating vascular calcification. Patients with ESRD have the greatest absolute values and rates of accumulation of CAC of any patient population.[42] A variety of stimuli can induce vascular smooth muscle cells to assume osteoblast-like functions in vitro, including phosphorus, which stimulates the Pit-1 receptor on vascular smooth muscle cells, oxidized low-density lipoprotein (LDL), and a number of other factors. Neither calcium intake nor blood levels of calcium are related to vascular calcification. Clinical studies in ESRD have suggested that vascular calcification is driven much more by age, length of time on dialysis, dyslipidemia, and phosphate retention. A systematic review of the literature in CKD and ESRD ($N = 2919$) found 31 studies that were split on finding or not finding the significance of serum Ca, serum phosphate (PO_4), calcium-phosphate product, parathyroid hormone (PTH), or treatments for Ca-PO_4 balance, including phosphate binders, calcium, and vitamin D analogues, in relation to CAC.[43] When taken into consideration, the lipid profiles (primarily reduced high-density lipoprotein cholesterol [HDL-C], elevated triglyceride [TG], elevated LDL-C, and elevated total cholesterol levels) were the most predictive factors of CAC in ESRD.

There have been 10 randomized trials (N = 2612) of therapies aimed to attenuate CAC measured by electron beam, helical, and multislice computed tomography (CT) (see Chap. 19).[44] Therapies included the following: statins, n = 1113; placebo, n = 829; and antihypertensives, n = 201. In patients with CKD (N = 477), treatments included low-phosphorus diet (n = 29), sevelamer phosphate binder (n = 229), and calcium-based phosphate binders (n = 219). The overall mean weighted annualized CAC progression was 17.2% ± 6.7%. Patients with CVD and CKD had rates of 16.9% ± 5.2% and 18.4% ± 11.1%, respectively (P < 0.0001). Progression rates ranged among classes of therapy from 13.5% to 19.3% and 14.2% to 24.1%. In contrast, the rate of CAC progression in patients assigned to placebo was 13.5%. Thus, despite earlier enthusiasm about statins, calcium restriction in ESRD, and sevelamer, it appears that no management approach influences the steady progression of arterial calcification.

Sevelamer was also tested in the Dialysis Clinical Outcomes Revisited (DCOR) trial.[45] This 3-year trial involving more than 2100 patients found no difference in mortality and morbidity for those receiving sevelamer hydrochloride versus those using calcium-based phosphate binders (9% relative risk reduction with sevelamer; P = 0.30). There have been two large outcomes trials testing statins in ESRD. The 4D Trial (Deutsche Diabetes Dialyse Studie) randomized 1255 type 2 DM patients with new ESRD to atorvastatin 20 mg daily or placebo for a median of 4 years.[46] The statin was effective in reducing the median serum LDL-C by 42% throughout the study period. The primary endpoint, however, defined as the composite of cardiac death, nonfatal MI, and fatal or nonfatal stroke, was only reduced by 8% with atorvastatin (P = 0.37). The AURORA Trial (A Study to Evaluate the Use of Rosuvastatin in Subjects on Regular Hemodialysis: An Assessment of Survival and Cardiovascular Events) randomized 2776 hemodialysis patients 50 to 80 years of age to rosuvastatin 10 mg daily or placebo over 4 years.[47] The mean reduction in LDL-C was 43% in patients receiving rosuvastatin, from a baseline level of 100 mg/dL. The combined primary endpoints of death from cardiovascular causes, nonfatal MI, or nonfatal stroke were similar (9.2 and 9.5 events/100 patient-years, respectively; hazard ratio, 0.96; P = 0.59). Rosuvastatin had no effect on individual components of the primary endpoint. There was also no significant effect on all-cause mortality (13.5 versus 14.0 events/100 patient-years; hazard ratio, 0.96; P = 0.51). It appears from DCOR, 4D, and AURORA that avoidance of calcium-based phosphate binders or LDL-C reduction in ESRD does not affect cardiovascular events or mortality. Explanations for this lack of effect include the following: advanced calcific atherosclerosis that is not influenced by reductions in LDL-C; nonischemic cardiovascular mechanisms unaffected by lipid status in terminal events in ESRD (e.g., pump failure, non-ischemic arrhythmias); and competing non-cardiovascular causes of mortality (e.g., sepsis, venous thromboembolism). Thus, as of this writing, using statins or any particular phosphate binder in patients with ESRD cannot be expected to influence CAC or clinical outcomes. There have been no trials testing the degree of phosphate lowering or control of PTH on CAC progression and CVD events.

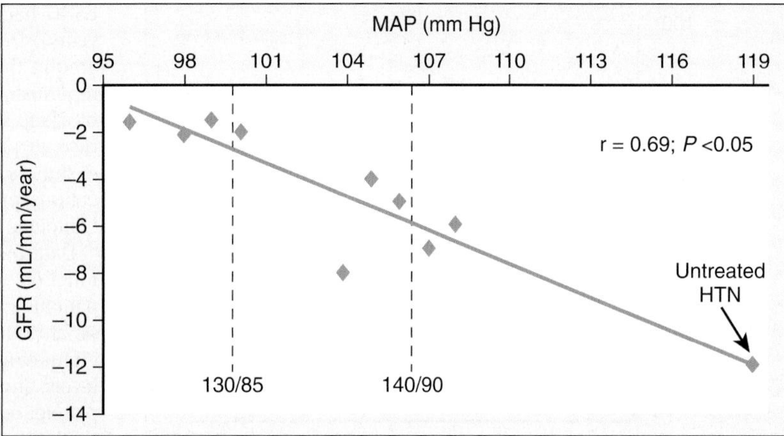

FIGURE 93-12 Influence of SBP on the rate of decline in renal function. MAP = mean arterial pressure. *(Modified from Bakris GL, Williams M, Dworkin L, et al: Preserving renal function in adults with hypertension and diabetes: A consensus approach. National Kidney Foundation Hypertension and Diabetes Executive Committees Working Group. Am J Kidney Dis 36:646, 2003.)*

Renal Disease and Hypertension

The kidney is a central regulator of blood pressure and controls intraglomerular pressure through autoregulation. Glomerular injury activates a variety of pathways that increase systemic blood pressure. This effect sets up a vicious circle of more glomerular and tubulointerstitial injury and worsened HTN (see Chap. 45). A cornerstone of management of combined CKD and CVD is strict blood pressure control (**Fig. 93-12**). An optimal blood pressure can be defined as less than 120/80 mm Hg (with systolic blood pressure [SBP] being the more important target), and most patients with CKD and HTN require three or more antihypertensive agents to achieve a goal blood pressure lower than 130/80 mm Hg.[11] The key lifestyle issues with CKD and HTN include dietary changes with sodium restriction, weight reduction to a target body mass index lower than 25 kg/m^2, and exercise for 60 minutes/day most days of the week. Pharmacologic therapy aims for strict blood pressure control with an agent that antagonizes the RAAS, often in combination with a thiazide-type diuretic. ONTARGET (ONgoing Telmisartan Alone and in combination with Ramipril Global Endpoint Trial) randomized 25,620 participants with DM or known vascular disease to ramipril 10 mg orally every day (n = 8,576), telmisartan 80 mg every day (n = 8,542), or a combination of the two (n = 8,502) over 4.7 years.[48] The secondary renal outcome, dialysis or doubling of the serum Cr level, was similar with telmisartan (2.21%) and ramipril (2.03%) and more frequent with combination therapy (2.49%; P = 0.038). The eGFR decreased least with ramipril compared with telmisartan (−2.82 ± 17.2 versus −4.12 ± 17.4 mL/min/1.73 m^2; P < 0.0001) or combination therapy (−6.11 ± 17.9 mL/min/1.73 m^2; P < 0.0001). Thus, unless a patient has systolic HF and meets the criteria for prior angiotensin-converting enzyme inhibitor (ACEI) + angiotensin receptor blocker (ARB) trials, patients with DM and CVD should be treated with an ACEI or an ARB, but not both. Dihydropyridine calcium channel blockers alone should also be avoided because of the relative afferent arteriolar dilation, which increases intraglomerular pressure and worsens glomerular injury. Special diagnostic consideration should be given to the possibility of underlying bilateral renal artery stenosis from the clinical clues of poorly controlled blood pressure on more than three agents, abdominal bruits, smoking history, peripheral arterial disease, and a marked change in the serum Cr level with the administration of an ACEI or ARB.[49] Although renal artery stenosis accounts for less than 3% of ESRD cases, it represents a potentially treatable condition[50] (see Chaps. 45 and 63).

Acute Coronary Syndromes

Diagnosis in Patients with Chronic Kidney Disease

Patients with CKD have shown a higher burden of silent ischemia, which clusters with serious arrhythmias, HF, and other cardiac events. Hemodialysis patients bear considerable hemodynamic stress three times weekly during dialysis sessions. Several studies have demonstrated a relationship between ST-segment depression and release of cardiac biomarkers (primarily troponin) before or during dialysis and poor long-term survival.[51] From a practical perspective, it is important to realize that patients with CKD presenting to the hospital with chest discomfort represent a high-risk group, having a 40% cardiac event rate at 30 days.[52] In making the diagnosis of acute MI (AMI) in patients with CKD or ESRD, troponin I is the preferred biomarker on the basis of its kinetic profile in patients with renal impairment.[53] The skeletal myopathy of CKD can elevate creatine kinase, myoglobin, and some troponin T assay results, making these tests less desirable. In addition to an elevated biomarker of cardiac injury, supporting evidence of the

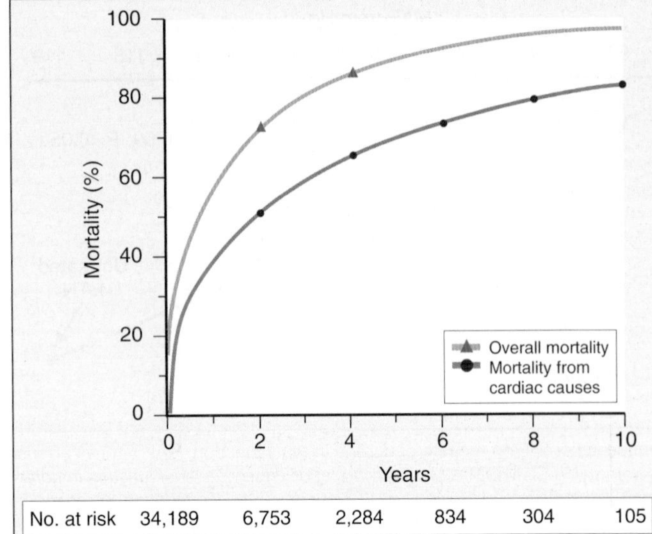

FIGURE 93-13 Cumulative mortality after myocardial infarction in patients with end-stage renal disease from the U.S. Renal Data System. *(Modified from Herzog CA, Ma JZ, Collins AJ: Poor long-term survival after acute myocardial infarction among patients on long-term dialysis. N Engl J Med 339:799, 1998.)*

diagnosis of AMI could be characteristic chest pain, electrocardiographic changes (ST-segment elevation or depression, new Q waves), or the identification of a culprit lesion on angiography. Because of the high event rate and prevalence of CVD in patients with CKD, it is advisable to consider admission to the hospital when the presenting symptom is chest discomfort and the eGFR is lower than 60 mL/min/1.73 m^2 or the patient has ESRD and is receiving dialysis.[54]

Renal Dysfunction as a Prognostic Factor

In the last several decades, considerable advances have been made in the diagnosis and treatment of ACS in the general population (see Chaps. 55 and 56). These advances include early paramedic response and defibrillation, coronary care units, and pharmacotherapy, including antiplatelet agents, antithrombotics, beta-adrenergic receptor blocking agents (beta blockers), ACEIs, and intravenous thrombolytic agents. Primary angioplasty for ST-segment elevation MI (STEMI) has become a well-accepted mode of treatment. These advances, however, have not been tested in patients with CKD or ESRD, primarily because these patients have generally been excluded from randomized treatment trials. Retrospective studies of patients in coronary care units have identified renal dysfunction as the most significant prognostic factor for long-term mortality when adjusting for other clinical factors, including age, sex, and comorbidities.[55] In addition, retrospective studies of patients with AMI consistently identify renal dysfunction as an independent predictor of death, with a greater impact on mortality than baseline demographics or therapies received.[55] Patients with ESRD have the highest mortality after AMI of any large chronic disease population (**Fig. 93-13**).[56]

Reasons for Poor Outcomes in Patients with Renal Dysfunction

Four reasons may underlie poor cardiovascular outcomes in patients with renal dysfunction after an ACS: (1) excess comorbidities associated with CKD and ESRD, in particular DM and HF; (2) therapeutic nihilism; (3) toxicity of therapies; and (4) special biologic and pathophysiologic factors in renal dysfunction that worsen outcomes.[55] In one study by Beattie and coworkers, the comorbidities of patients with STEMI and CKD (mean Cr = 2.7 mg/dL) included older age (mean, 70.2 years), DM (38.1%), and prior HF (23.2%).[6] Those with ESRD had similar rates of comorbidities, including age (mean, 64.9 years), DM (40.4%), and prior HF (31.7%). This study found that among the CKD and ESRD groups, there are lower rates of use of reperfusion therapy (thrombolysis or primary angioplasty) and beta blockers, suggesting some contribution to poor outcomes from underuse of proven therapies (therapeutic nihilism). Patients with renal dysfunction may present later in their course, have more contraindications, or have other aspects about their presentations that prompt clinicians to use fewer therapies or take a more conservative approach.

Data on the toxicity of treatments for an ACS related to renal dysfunction are often unavailable, primarily because of exclusion of patients with CKD from these trials. The primary defects in thrombosis attributable to uremia are excess thrombin generation, increased circulating thrombin-antithrombin complexes, lower antithrombin III levels, increased plasminogen activation inhibitor, and decreased platelet aggregation. Decreased platelet aggregation is further related to the following: (1) reductions in the dense granule content of adenosine triphosphate, serotonin, and von Willebrand factor; (2) diminished thromboxane A2 generation in response to thrombin; and (3) diminished availability and function of glycoprotein IIb/IIIa. In the balance, patients with CKD and ESRD, when untreated, are more susceptible to atherothrombosis; however, after receiving any form of antiplatelet or antithrombotic therapy, these patients are more prone to bleeding complications.[57] In patients with renal dysfunction, the best measure of bleeding risk is the bleeding time. Unfortunately, the bleeding time is not a practical test for the ACS patient; consequently, clinicians cannot readily assess the a priori bleeding risk for any given CKD or ESRD patient. It is unlikely that bleeding complications alone account for the large differences seen in mortality between CKD and ESRD and those with preserved renal function with AMI.

The final and most important reason why patients with CKD and ESRD have poor outcomes after an ACS is the enhanced vascular pathobiology induced by the chronic renal failure state.[55] The processes that contribute to accelerated atherosclerosis include a dyslipidemia characterized by decreased function of lipoprotein lipase and decreased HDL-C and elevated TG and LDL levels. Levels of homocysteine and other thiols rise when the eGFR drops below 60 mL/min/1.73 m^2, enhancing the oxidation of LDL-C and progression of atherosclerotic lesions.[23] Renal dysfunction is a systemic inflammatory state, associated with higher rates of plaque rupture and incident CVD events. Finally, chronic hyperactivation of the sympathetic nervous system and an imbalance between endothelin, a powerful vasoconstrictor, and nitric oxide, a local paracrine vasodilator, may worsen HTN and may augment intravascular wall stress, which could further contribute to incident CVD events.

Treatment in Patients with Renal Dysfunction

Clinicians must confront ACS in high-risk populations with CKD and ESRD with little evidence on which to base treatment decisions (see Chaps. 55 and 56). Therapies that benefit the general population often yield enhanced benefit in patients with CKD and ESRD. A favorable risk-benefit ratio has now been demonstrated for aspirin, beta blockers, ACEIs, ARBs, aldosterone receptor antagonists, and statins.[58] Therapies that require dose adjustment on the basis of CrCl include low-molecular-weight heparins, bivalirudin, and glycoprotein IIb/IIIa antagonists (**Table 93-1**). Given that the major inputs for bleeding risks include older age, low body weight, and renal dysfunction, Table 93-1 also lists agents that are approved in a weight-adjusted dose form and gives the currently recommended dose adjustments for commonly used antiplatelet and antithrombotic agents.[57] Greater use of such therapies, despite the heightened risk for complications, may attenuate the excess mortality reported in the CKD and ESRD populations. There have been no randomized trials of PCI or bypass surgery in patients with CKD or ESRD. In the Bypass Angioplasty Revascularization Investigation (BARI) trial, however, whether PCI or surgery was used in the management of multivessel coronary disease, CKD and DM associated with worsened long-term survival (**Fig. 93-14**).[8] Further research is needed into the particular pathogenic mechanisms in the renal failure

TABLE 93-1 Recommended Dose Adjustment of Conventional Antithrombotics Used for Acute Coronary Syndromes*

ANTITHROMBOTIC AGENT	eGFR (mL/min/1.73 m^2) (CrCl in mL/min) 60-90	30-60	<30	DIALYSIS-DEPENDENT
Aspirin	No adjustment needed	No adjustment needed	No adjustment needed	No adjustment needed
Clopidogrel	No adjustment needed	No adjustment needed	No adjustment needed	No adjustment needed
Ticlopidine	No adjustment needed	No adjustment needed	No adjustment needed	No adjustment needed
Heparin	No guidelines	No guidelines	No guidelines	No guidelines
LMWH	No guidelines	No guidelines	Reduce dose by 30%; factor Xa monitoring advocated	No guidelines
Lepirudin	No guidelines	CrCl = 45-60 mL/min or SrCr = 1.6-2 mg/dL—reduce bolus to 0.2 mg/kg IV + decrease infusion rate by 50% (0.075 mg/kg/hr IV) CrCl = 30-44 mL/min or SrCr = 2.1-3 mg/dL—reduce bolus to 0.2 mg/kg IV + decrease standard initial infusion rate by 70% (0.045 mg/kg/hr IV)	CrCl = 15-29 mL/min or SrCr = 3.1-6 mg/dL—reduce bolus to 0.2 mg/kg IV + decrease infusion rate by 85% (0.0225 mg/kg/hr IV) CrCl < 15 mL/min or SrCr > 6 mg/dL—reduce bolus to 0.2 mg/kg IV; no infusion	Reduce bolus dose to 0.2 mg/kg IV; no infusion
Bivalirudin	No guidelines	Reduce infusion dose by 20%	Reduce infusion dose by 60%	Reduce infusion dose by 90%
Argatroban	No dose adjustment	No dose adjustment	No dose adjustment	
Abciximab	No guidelines Monitoring advocated	No guidelines Monitoring advocated	No guidelines Monitoring advocated	No guidelines; monitoring advocated
Eptifibatide	No guidelines	SrCr = 2-4 mg/dL—135 mg/kg IV bolus + 0.5 mg/kg/min IV infusion	SrCr > 4.0 mg/dL; contraindicated	No clinical data; in vitro data demonstrate clearance
Tirofiban	No dose adjustment	No dose adjustment	0.2 mg/kg/min IV for 30 min, followed by 0.05 mg/kg/min IV	No clinical data; in vitro data demonstrate clearance

*In patients with CKD and ESRD.
LMWH = low-molecular-weight heparin; SrCr = serum creatinine.
Modified from Sica D: The implications of renal impairment among patients undergoing percutaneous coronary intervention. J Invasive Cardiol 14(Suppl B):30B, 2002.

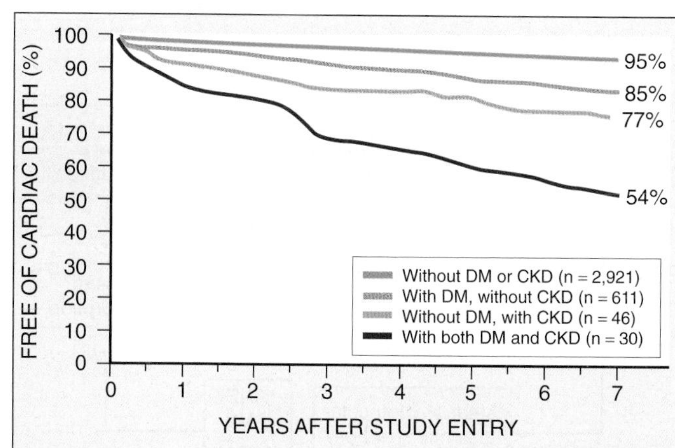

FIGURE 93-14 Freedom from cardiovascular death after angioplasty or bypass surgery in the BARI trial and registry (*N* = 3608). *(Modified from Szczech LA, Best PJ, Crowley E, et al: Outcomes of patients with chronic renal insufficiency in the Bypass Angioplasty Revascularization Investigation. Circulation 105:2253, 2002.)*

state that promote plaque rupture, accelerate atherosclerosis, lead to ACS complications, and promote the development of HF and arrhythmias.

Chronic Kidney Disease

Complicating Heart Failure

The diagnosis of HF with concomitant renal failure presents a particular challenge. Patients with CKD, and in particular ESRD, frequently have three key mechanical contributors to HF—pressure overload (related to HTN), volume overload, and cardiomyopathy. Approximately 20% of patients approaching hemodialysis have a diagnosis of HF.[59] It is unclear how much of this diagnosis results from chronic volume overload from renal failure or from impaired systolic or diastolic function. Notably, CKD influences the levels of BNP, a diagnostic blood test for HF. In general, when the eGFR is lower than 60 mL/min/1.73 m^2, a higher BNP cut point of 200 pg/mL should be used in the diagnosis of HF.[60] CKD (eGFR < 60 mL/min/1.73 m^2), when present in patients with HF, independently predicts poor outcomes.[61] Estimated and actual GFRs clearly can be reduced by decreased renal blood flow related to low cardiac output. However, multiple studies of patients with classes II and III HF who do not have a low cardiac output state have shown decreased survival in a graded fashion related to renal impairment.

The combination of HF and CKD presents a challenge to cardiologists with respect to proven treatment options. ACEIs, if tolerated (or ARBs if ACEIs are not tolerated) beta blockers, aldosterone antagonists, and loop diuretics are all acceptable combination therapies (see Chap. 28).[62] Caveats in the use of ACEIs and ARBs are the marked elevation in the serum Cr level and acute renal failure, which are more likely to occur when the patient is volume-depleted or in the presence of occult bilateral renal artery stenosis or its equivalent (e.g., unilateral renal artery stenosis present in a renal transplant recipient).[63] When initiating therapy to block the RAAS, it is advisable to have the SBP stable and greater than 90 mm Hg, euvolemia, and a drug regimen without concurrent renal toxic agents. Clinicians should realize that CKD patients enjoy an improved survival and reduced rates of ESRD on ACEIs or ARBs, even though the serum Cr level is chronically elevated on these agents because of reduced intraglomerular pressure. Discontinuation of ACEIs or ARBs because of moderate asymptomatic rises in the Cr level is a common management error. In general, an attempt should be made to use ACEIs or ARBs in patients down to an eGFR of 15 mL/min/1.73 m^2. Below this level, case reports suggest a high rate

TABLE 93-2 Recommended Dose Adjustment of Selected Medical Therapy for Hypertension, Dyslipidemia, Heart Failure, and Arrhythmias*

AGENT USED	ELIMINATION ROUTE	eGFR (mL/min/1.73 m^2) (CrCl in mL/min) 90-60	60-30	<30	DIALYSIS-DEPENDENT
Central Adrenergic Blockers					
Clonidine	Renal				↓ Dose 50%
Methyldopa	Renal	qid	qid	↓ tid	↓ bid or qd
Angiotensin-Converting Enzyme Inhibitors					
Captopril	Renal				↓ Dose 50%
Enalapril	Hepatic			↓ Dose 25%	↓ Dose 50%
Lisinopril	Renal			↓ Dose 25%	↓ Dose 50%
Ramipril	Renal, GI			↓ Dose 75%	↓ Dose 75%
Benazepril	Renal			↓ Dose 25%	↓ Dose 75%
Inotropic Agents					
Digoxin	Renal, nonrenal		↓ Dose 50%	↓ Dose 50%	↓ Dose 75%; change to qod
Milrinone	Renal		↓ Dose 25%	↓ Dose 50%	↓ Dose 75%
Antiarrhythmics					
Disopyramide	Renal, hepatic	bid	bid	↓ qd	↓ qod
Flecainide	Renal, hepatic				↓ Dose 25%-50%
Mexiletine	Renal, hepatic				↓ Dose 50%-75%
Procainamide	Renal, hepatic	qid	↓ tid	↓ bid	↓ bid or qd
Dofetilide	Renal, nonrenal		↓ Dose 50%	↓ Dose 75%	Contraindicated
Beta Blockers					
Atenolol	Renal			↓ Dose 50%	↓ Dose 75%; ↓ qod
Sotalol	Renal			↓ Dose 50%	↓ Dose 75%
Others					
Verapamil	Hepatic				↓ Dose 50%-75%
Hydralazine	Hepatic	qid	↓ tid	↓ tid	↓ bid
Gemfibrozil	Renal			↓ Dose 50%	↓ Dose 75%
Fenofibrate	Renal				Contraindicated
Nicotinic acid	Renal, hepatic			↓ Dose 25%	↓ Dose 25%

*In patients with CKD and ESRD.
GI = gastrointestinal.

of hyperkalemia and the concern of accelerating the course to ESRD and dialysis.

The management of the patient who is already receiving dialysis and has HF requires particular care. In general, proven HF therapies, provided they are tolerated, should be used along with regular and ad hoc dialysis as needed to control volume overload. In a randomized trial, carvedilol did provide additional benefit in this scenario.[64] In addition, a retrospective analysis has supported the use of ACEIs in patients with ESRD admitted with HF.[65] Finally, the acute management of decompensated HF in patients with impaired eGFR poses a particularly difficult challenge.[66] In fact, an elevated Cr level is the single most common reason for using positive inotropes or inodilators in hospitalized patients with HF.[67] There are no published reports of dobutamine leading to long-term favorable outcomes and, in the short term, it increases arrhythmias and mortality. Similarly, milrinone has not been shown to reduce mortality, causes arrhythmias, and must be dose-adjusted when the eGFR drops below 45 mL/min/1.73 m^2 (**Table 93-2**). Another option is the use of intravenous BNP (nesiritide), which causes primarily venodilation and natriuresis.[68] Completed studies with nesiritide have evaluated the CKD subgroups and found benefit in CKD equal to that in those with preserved renal function, although the overall effect is modestly better than that with intravenous nitroglycerin.[69] Patients with advanced HF have reduced renal blood flow, decreased glomerular filtration rate, enhanced proximal reabsorption of water, and an overall reduced capacity of the nephron to excrete water (**Fig. 93-15**). Furthermore, reduced effective arterial blood volume is a stimulus for antidiuretic hormone release, which plays a dominant role in worsening water retention. The clinical signs of this cardiorenal syndrome are an elevation in the serum Cr and blood urea nitrogen levels, hyponatremia, volume retention, and excessive thirst.

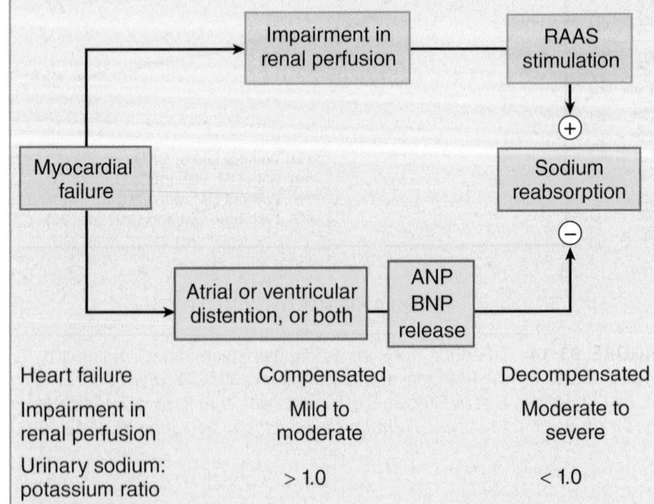

FIGURE 93-15 Pathophysiologic processes in combined heart and kidney failure. ANP = A-type natriuretic peptide; BNP = B-type natriuretic peptide. *(From Weber KT: Aldosterone in congestive heart failure. N Engl J Med 345:1689, 2001.)*

Treatment efforts should be aimed at improving left ventricular systolic function, often in the hospital setting, with the intravenous therapies mentioned earlier (see Chap. 28). Small trials using continuous venovenous ultrafiltration have demonstrated short-term reductions in symptoms, shorter hospital stays, and reductions in rehospitalizations.[70] Until larger trials confirm longer-term benefits in hospitalization and mortality, ultrafiltration can be considered a last-line approach for the patient with refractory cardiorenal failure.

In summary, CKD and HF present a particularly challenging scenario for clinicians and patients. Frequent monitoring and the combined use of renal and cardioprotective strategies are critical. Future research is needed to confirm anemia correction and ultrafiltration as additional strategies in patients who have cardiorenal syndrome. Dialysis patients, despite having volume reduction with mechanical fluid removal, should have medical therapy with ACEIs or ARBs, beta blockers, and additional agents for blood pressure control if needed.

Complicating Valvular Heart Disease

Impaired renal function has been linked to mitral annular calcification and aortic sclerosis (see Chap. 66). Advanced thickening of the cardiac valves and calcification can accompany ESRD.[71] Approximately 80% of patients with ESRD have the murmur of aortic sclerosis. Neither of these lesions usually progresses to the point where studies beyond echocardiography are needed. Bacterial endocarditis may develop in patients with ESRD who have temporary dialysis access catheters.[72] Endocarditis with common pathogens, including *Staphylococcus*, *Streptococcus*, and *Enterococcus* spp., in the aortic or mitral position, is associated with a mortality rate higher than 50% in this setting (see Chap. 67). It becomes difficult to treat given the continued need for dialysis access and the delay in surgical placement of permanent arteriovenous shunts or fistulas. Unfortunately, surgical mortality associated with valve replacement in ESRD related to endocarditis is high. In the setting of ESRD, when valve surgery is carried out for endocarditis or other causes of valve failure, there has been no difference in survival among those who received tissue or mechanical valve prostheses. Thus, tissue valves are a reasonable choice given the complicating issue of chronic anticoagulation and bleeding with dialysis vascular access.

Renal Function and Arrhythmias

Uremia, hyperkalemia, acidosis, and disorders of calcium-phosphate balance have all been linked to higher rates of atrial and ventricular arrhythmias.[73] Given a concurrent substrate of left ventricular hypertrophy, left ventricular dilation, HF, and valvular disease, it is not surprising that higher rates of almost all arrhythmias have been reported in CKD, including bradyarrhythmias and heart block. Caveats for practical management include dose adjustment for many antiarrhythmic medications, including digoxin, sotalol, and procainamide (see Table 93-2). Of concern, CKD, and ESRD in particular, may cause elevated defibrillation thresholds and failure of implantable cardioverter-defibrillators (ICDs).[74] Until this association is better understood, patients receiving ICDs should have frequent surveillance and consideration for noninvasive programmed stimulation for appropriate antitachycardia and defibrillation therapy. Considering the high rates of sudden death in patients with ESRD, clinical trials of prophylactic ICDs in this population are under consideration.

Consultative Approach to the Hemodialysis Patient

The prevalence of angiographically significant coronary artery disease (CAD) ranges from 25% in young, nondiabetic hemodialysis patients to 85% in older ESRD patients with long-standing DM.[75,76] Cardiac death in dialysis patients younger than age 45 years is approximately 100-fold greater than that in the general population. The prevalence and severity of CAD among patients with ESRD is daunting in terms of occurrence and extent of poor outcomes. Medicare beneficiaries with CKD prior to the initiation of dialysis are 60% more likely to have a billing claim submitted for the diagnosis of CVD and 70% more likely to have a claim submitted for atherosclerotic heart disease.[77] Of those receiving dialysis, a substantial proportion, perhaps the most of them, have established CAD. In diabetic renal transplant candidates, 30% will have one or more coronary artery lesions with more than 75% stenosis. When comparing the patients who undergo evaluation for CAD, those with ESRD have substantially more numerous and severe coronary artery lesions, as well as more severe left ventricular dysfunction.[76]

The patient with incipient ESRD who has been placed on dialysis can be considered to be the highest cardiovascular risk patient in medicine, with expected rates of CVD death that are many times higher than that expected for a non-ESRD patient, even those with a burden of several cardiovascular risk factors. ESRD is more than a cardiovascular risk equivalent, warranting meticulous efforts to achieve goals mandated by guidelines (**Table 93-3**).

Despite the use of multiple medications, most published series of ESRD patients from clinical trials or registries have indicated that the mean systolic blood pressure is approximately 155 mm Hg. Indeed, 80% of ESRD patients have HTN, but only 30% achieve adequate control.[78] Long-term cardiorenal protection involves two important concepts—blood pressure control to a much lower target (SBP < 130 mm Hg), and use of an agent that blocks the RAAS, such as an

TABLE 93-3 Therapeutic Opportunities to Improve Cardiovascular Care in Patients with Chronic Kidney Disease

THERAPEUTIC OPPORTUNITY	RATIONALE
Weight loss, weight maintenance at BMI < 25 kg/m²	Improve dysmetabolic syndrome and diabetes
Low sodium intake	Reduce blood pressure Make blood pressure more responsive to medications Reduce volume retention between dialysis sessions
Aspirin 81 mg qd or clopidogrel 75 mg orally qd if aspirin-intolerant	Primary prevention of AMI and stroke
Lipid control (e.g., diet, statin, fibrates, niacin) ▪ LDLC < 70 mg/dL ▪ Non–HDL-C < 100 mg/dL ▪ Apo B < 80 mg/dL	Possible prevention of AMI, stroke, and CVD death in CKD Possible reduction in progression of CKD No proven impact on outcomes in ESRD
Blood pressure control to target SBP < 130 mm Hg (optimal, ~120 mm Hg) ▪ RAAS blocking agents (ACE or ARB) ▪ Beta-blocking agents ▪ Diuretics ▪ Calcium channel blockers ▪ Other add-on agents	Primary prevention of AMI, stroke, heart failure, and CVD death Preserve residual urine volume in peritoneal dialysis patients Reduce LVH Treat subclinical cardiac ischemia
Blood glucose control in diabetes (target HbA1C, 7.0%)	Reduction in risk of AMI, stroke, and CVD death Reduction in worsened nephropathy, retinopathy
Treatment of anemia (target < 12 g/dL and/or lowest ESP or iron doses) ▪ ESPs ▪ Iron	Improve symptoms of anemia Improve quality of life Possible reduction in LVH Unproven impact on AMI, stroke, HF, and CVD death
Treatment of CKD mineral and bone disorder (targets for ESRD: PO_4 = 3.5-5.5 mg/dL; iPTH = 150-300 pg/mL; Ca × PO_4 product < 55) ▪ Phosphate binders ▪ Calcitriol, vitamin D analogues	Reduce the risk of soft tissue calcification Reduce risk of symptomatic hyper- or hypocalcemia Possible reduction in all-cause mortality Unproven impact on skeletal fractures, bone pain, AMI, stroke, HF, and CVD death

BMI = body mass index; ESP = erythrocyte-stimulating protein; HbA1C = hemoglobin A1C; non-HDL-C = non-HDL cholesterol.

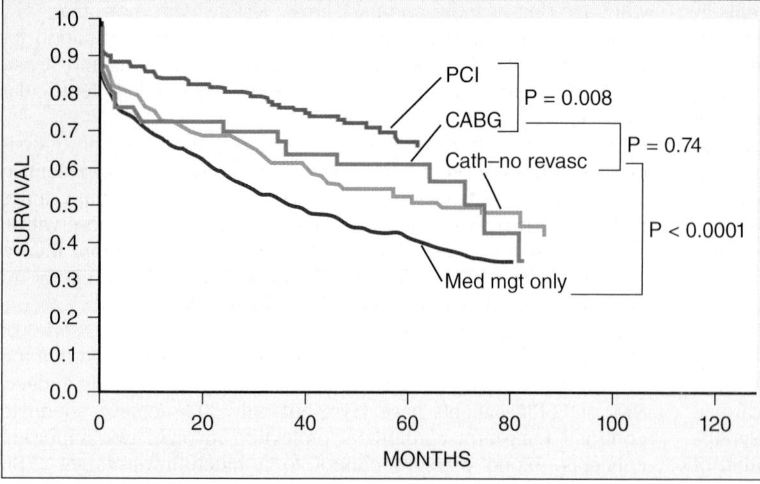

FIGURE 93-16 Long-term survival according to CAD management strategy in patients with CrCl < 60 mL/min or ESRD on dialysis. *(From Keeley EC, Kadakia R, Soman S, et al: Analysis of long-term survival after revascularization in patients with chronic kidney disease presenting with acute coronary syndromes. Am J Cardiol 92:509, 2003.)*

ACEI or ARB as the base of therapy. How can an ACEI or ARB be effective in a patient with ESRD, particularly one who is anephric? The RAAS appears to have considerable redundancy and is able to maintain its function, if not increase its overall level of activity, without participation by the kidneys.[79] Hence, this hyperactivation of the RAAS is a target for therapy in ESRD because ACEIs and ARBs have been demonstrated to reduce left ventricular hypertrophy (LVH) and possibly improve survival in ESRD.[80] A small trial has demonstrated that ramipril is related to preservation of residual urine output in those receiving peritoneal dialysis, which is a consistently favorable management issue in ESRD.[81] A retrospective study has found that although only approximately 20% of patients with ESRD and CAD receive ACEI, those who are given these agents after CAD events have improved all-cause mortality over the next 5 years.[82] The common difficulty with ACEIs or ARBs is worsened hyperkalemia in patients with ESRD. As tolerated, the clinician should consider adjusting the dialytic regimen to improve potassium removal. From all sources of evidence to date, patients with ESRD appear to benefit from ACEI or ARB therapy, provided the serum potassium level and blood pressure can be adequately controlled.

With an ACEI or ARB as a base of therapy, the antihypertensive regimen can be further modified according to blood pressure–lowering efficacy and CAD event reduction. Beta blockers can be used as antihypertensive and anti-ischemic agents.[83] In those with HF, beta blockers improve left ventricular ejection fraction and reduce rates of hospitalization, sudden death, and all-cause mortality.[84,85] Large relative risk reductions in all-cause mortality have been reported for patients who receive beta blockers with ESRD after CAD events.

After inclusion of an ACEI or ARB and beta blockers in the ESRD blood pressure regimen, the remaining choices should be based on ease of management, compliance, and lack of adverse effects. The goal is to create a blood pressure environment for the cardiovascular system in which the mean SBP—on 24-hour monitoring, for example—is at least lower than 130 mm Hg. Guidelines for non-ESRD patients state that the optimal systolic blood pressure should be approximately 120 mm Hg.[11] The difficult task in the ESRD patient is to achieve these goals without having hypotension during dialysis sessions. Given the high rates of severe CAD in ESRD, hypotension during dialysis can worsen clinical and subclinical ischemia recognized as chest discomfort, shortness of breath, ST-segment depression on electrocardiography, and elevations of cardiac troponin on blood testing.[86]

The National Kidney Foundation guidelines support LDL-C reduction, in most cases with a statin, in patients with CKD despite the lack of risk reductions in CVD events observed to date in clinical trials such as 4-D and AURORA.[87,88] In addition, agents that reduce non–HDL-C, including nicotinic acid and fibrates, can be used according to the National Cholesterol Education Project Adult Treatment Panel III (NCEP-ATP-III) guidelines.[89]

In ESRD with DM, blood glucose control to a target glycohemoglobin level lower than 7 mg/dL can be expected to reduce rates of microvascular (retinopathy) and, to a lesser extent, clinically important atherosclerotic disease elsewhere (AMI, stroke, CVD death).[90] Similarly, smoking cessation is recommended for patients with ESRD.[91] The effect of aspirin on renal endpoints is unknown; however, given its CVD protective effect, it is recommended for adult patients with ESRD.[92] For those who are aspirin-intolerant, general cardiology guidelines recommend the use of clopidogrel, although there are no published studies of clopidogrel on cardiovascular outcomes in ESRD.

Several analyses have suggested that ESRD patients with CAD who receive conservative medical management fare the worst of all groups (**Fig. 93-16**).[92-95] Thus, the first step after stress imaging in an ESRD patient with symptomatic CAD is to make an attempt at angiography and revascularization. Usually, multivessel CAD is found, so the next question is, what is the optimal approach—multivessel PCI or coronary artery bypass grafting (CABG)? It is widely accepted that patients with ESRD undergoing mechanical coronary revascularization procedures are at increased risk for adverse events, including death. Dialysis-dependent patients undergoing CABG face a 4.4 times greater risk of in-hospital death, a 3.1 times greater risk of mediastinitis, and a 2.6 times greater risk of stroke compared with those patients undergoing CABG who were not on dialysis.[96] Although newer surgical techniques have been successful in high-risk patients with renal failure, the long-term results, compared with traditional surgical and percutaneous techniques, are not yet known. In general, despite this significant up-front risk of surgery, the literature suggests the superiority of CABG compared with PCI in patients with ESRD. In single-vessel CAD and multivessel CAD without good bypass targets, recent trends have suggested that PCI with stenting is a favorable approach for patients with ESRD. Drug-eluting stents have reduced restenosis rates in this population and may tip the risk-benefit scale in favor of PCI.[97]

In summary, patients with ESRD have more than coronary artery disease risk-equivalent status in their baseline CAD risk assessment. An aggressive approach to medical management for CAD is warranted, even in the case of subclinical CAD. A low threshold for diagnostic testing should apply to ESRD patients (**Fig. 93-17**). When significant CAD is found, ESRD patients appear to benefit from revascularization compared with conservative medical management and, if clinically reasonable, should be given that opportunity for improved survival and reduction in future cardiac events.

Summary

Recognition that patients with CKD have an elevated CVD risk has increased over the last decade. Frequent clinical scenarios in which renal function influences care include CI-AKI, ACS, HF, valvular disease, and arrhythmias. Results from retrospective studies and clinical trial

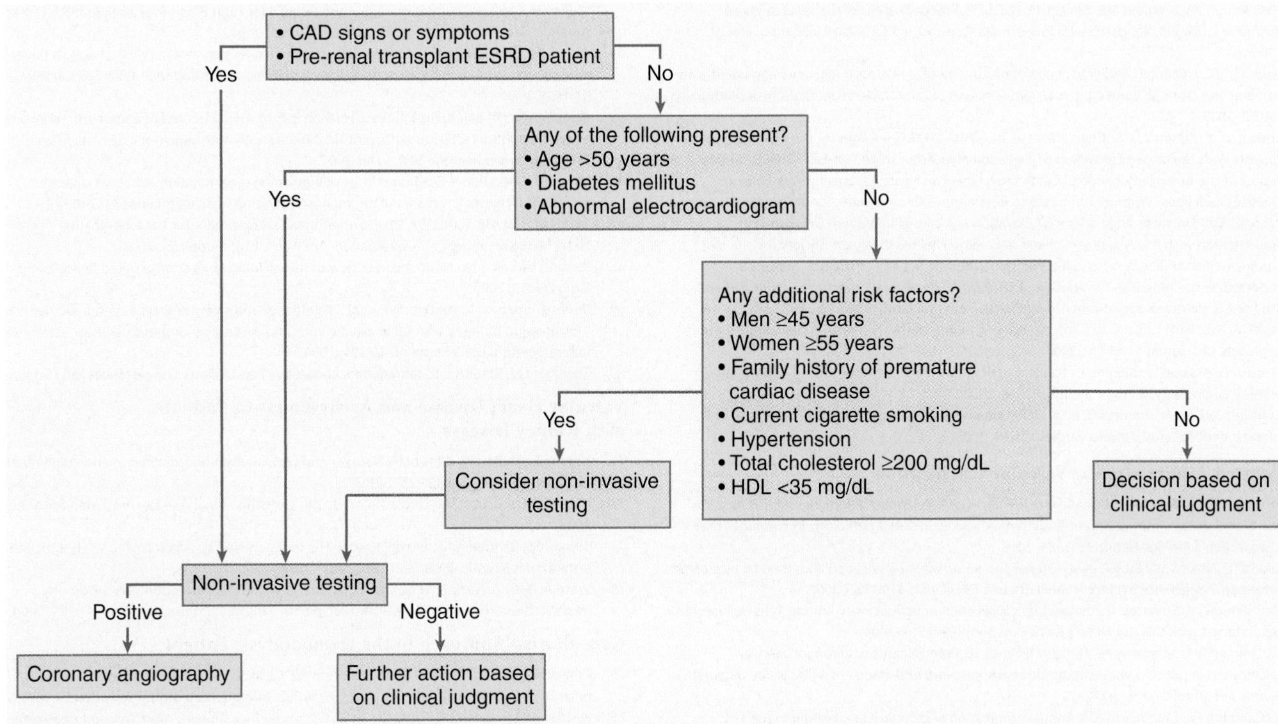

FIGURE 93-17 Approach to the ESRD patient with CAD or being considered for renal transplantation. HDL = high-density lipoprotein cholesterol. *(Modified from McCullough PA: Evaluation and treatment of coronary artery disease in patients with end-stage renal disease. Kidney Int Suppl [95]:S51, 2005.)*

subgroups form the basis of current recommendations, given the lack of prospective randomized trials of CKD and ESRD. Further study of the adverse metabolic milieu of CKD is likely to lead to generalizable diagnostic and therapeutic targets for the future management of renal patients with cardiovascular illness.

REFERENCES

Epidemiology and Outcomes

1. Lewis CE, Jacobs DR Jr, McCreath H, et al: Weight gain continues in the 1990s: 10-year trends in weight and overweight from the CARDIA study. Am J Epidemiol 151:1172, 2000.
2. Bakris GL, Williams M, Dworkin L, et al: Preserving renal function in adults with hypertension and diabetes: A consensus approach. National Kidney Foundation Hypertension and Diabetes Executive Committees Working Group. Am J Kidney Dis 36:646, 2000.
3. McCullough PA: Cardiorenal risk: An important clinical intersection. Rev Cardiovasc Med 3:71, 2002.
4. National Kidney Foundation: Clinical practice guidelines for chronic kidney disease: Evaluation, classification, and stratification. Am J Kidney Dis 2(Suppl 1):S46, 2002.
5. McCullough PA, Soman SS, Shah SS, et al: Risks associated with renal dysfunction in patients in the coronary care unit. J Am Coll Cardiol 36:679, 2000.
6. Beattie JN, Soman SS, Sandberg KR, et al: Determinants of mortality after myocardial infarction in patients with advanced renal dysfunction. Am J Kidney Dis 37:1191, 2001.
7. Chertow GM, Lazarus JM, Christiansen CL, et al: Preoperative renal risk stratification. Circulation 95:878, 1997.
8. Szczech LA, Best PJ, Crowley E, et al: Outcomes of patients with chronic renal insufficiency in the Bypass Angioplasty Revascularization Investigation. Circulation 105:2253, 2002.
9. Filler G, Bokenkamp A, Hofmann W, et al: Cystatin C as a marker of GFR–history, indications, and future research. Clin Biochem 38:1, 2005.
10. Sarnak MJ, Levey AS, Schoolwerth AC, et al: Kidney disease as a risk factor for development of cardiovascular disease: A statement from the American Heart Association Councils on Kidney in Cardiovascular Disease, High Blood Pressure Research, Clinical Cardiology, and Epidemiology and Prevention. Circulation 108:2154, 2003.
11. Chobanian AV, Bakris GL, Black HR, et al: The Seventh Report of the Joint National Committee on Prevention, Detection, Evaluation, and Treatment of High Blood Pressure: The JNC 7 report. JAMA 289:2560, 2003.

Anemia and Chronic Kidney Disease

12. NKF-DOQI clinical practice guidelines for the treatment of anemia of chronic renal failure. National Kidney Foundation-Dialysis Outcomes Quality Initiative. Am J Kidney Dis 30(Suppl 3):S192, 1997.
13. McCullough PA, Lepor NE: The deadly triangle of anemia, renal insufficiency, and cardiovascular disease: Implications for prognosis and treatment. Rev Cardiovasc Med 6:1, 2005.
14. Silverberg DS, Wexler D, Iaina A: The role of anemia in the progression of congestive heart failure. Is there a place for erythropoietin and intravenous iron? J Nephrol 17:749, 2004.
15. Anand I, McMurray JJ, Whitmore J, et al: Anemia and its relationship to clinical outcome in heart failure. Circulation 110:149, 2004.
16. Drüeke TB, Locatelli F, Clyne N, et al: Normalization of hemoglobin level in patients with chronic kidney disease and anemia. N Engl J Med 355:2071, 2006.
17. Singh A, Reddan D: Correction of Hemoglobin and Outcomes in Renal Insufficiency (CHOIR) trial. Presented at the National Kidney Foundation 2006 Spring Clinical Meeting, Chicago, April 19-23, 2006.
18. Pfeffer MA, Burdmann EA, Chen CY, et al: A trial of darbepoetin alfa in type 2 diabetes and chronic kidney disease. N Engl J Med 361:2019, 2009.

Percutaneous Coronary Interventions and Contrast-Induced Acute Kidney Injury

19. McCullough P: Outcomes of contrast-induced nephropathy: Experience in patients undergoing cardiovascular intervention. Catheter Cardiovasc Interv 67:335, 2006.
20. McCullough PA, Manley HJ: Prediction and prevention of contrast nephropathy. J Interv Cardiol 14:547, 2001.
21. Pannu N, Wiebe N, Tonelli M, Alberta Kidney Disease Network: Prophylaxis strategies for contrast-induced nephropathy. JAMA 295:2765, 2006.
22. Rihal CS, Textor SC, Grill DE, et al: Incidence and prognostic importance of acute renal failure after percutaneous coronary intervention. Circulation 105:2259, 2002.
23. Yerkey MW, Kernis SJ, Franklin BA, et al: Renal dysfunction and acceleration of coronary disease. Heart 90:961, 2004.
24. Andersen KJ, Christensen EI, Vik H: Effects of iodinated x-ray contrast media on renal epithelial cells in culture. Invest Radiol 29:955, 1994.
25. Keeley EC, Grines CL: Scraping of aortic debris by coronary guiding catheters: A prospective evaluation of 1,000 cases. J Am Coll Cardiol 32:1861, 1998.
26. Wijeysundera DN, Karkouti K, Beattie WS, et al: Improving the identification of patients at risk of postoperative renal failure after cardiac surgery. Anesthesiology 104:65, 2006.
27. Denton KM, Shweta A, Anderson WP: Preglomerular and postglomerular resistance responses to different levels of sympathetic activation by hypoxia. J Am Soc Nephrol 13:27, 2002.
28. Uder M, Humke U, Pahl M, et al: Nonionic contrast media iohexol and iomeprol decrease renal arterial tone: Comparative studies on human and porcine isolated vascular segments. Invest Radiol 37:440, 2002.
29. Rauch D, Drescher P, Pereira FJ, et al: Comparison of iodinated contrast media-induced renal vasoconstriction in human, rabbit, dog, and pig arteries. Invest Radiol 32:315, 1997.
30. Endre ZH: Acute kidney injury: Definitions and new paradigms. Adv Chronic Kidney Dis 15:213, 2008.
31. Mehran R, Aymong ED, Nikolsky E, et al: A simple risk score for prediction of contrast-induced nephropathy after percutaneous coronary intervention: Development and initial validation. J Am Coll Cardiol 44:1393, 2004.
32. McCullough PA: Contrast-induced acute kidney injury. J Am Coll Cardiol 51:1419, 2008.
33. Stevens MA, McCullough PA, Tobin KJ, et al: A prospective randomized trial of prevention measures in patients at high risk for contrast nephropathy: Results of the P.R.I.N.C.E. Study. Prevention of Radiocontrast-Induced Nephropathy Clinical Evaluation. J Am Coll Cardiol 33:403, 1999.

34. McCullough PA, Bertrand ME, Brinker JA, Stacul F: A meta-analysis of the renal safety of isosmolar iodixanol compared with low-osmolar contrast media. J Am Coll Cardiol 48:692, 2006.
35. Heinrich MC, Häberle L, Müller V, et al: Nephrotoxicity of iso-osmolar iodixanol compared with nonionic low-osmolar contrast media: Meta-analysis of randomized controlled trials. Radiology 250:68, 2009.
36. Anderson JL, Adams CD, Antman EM, et al: ACC/AHA 2007 Guidelines for the Management of Patients With Unstable Angina/Non-ST-Elevation Myocardial Infarction-Executive Summary: A Report of the American College of Cardiology/American Heart Association Task Force on Practice Guidelines (Writing Committee to Revise the 2002 Guidelines for the Management of Patients With Unstable Angina/Non-ST-Elevation Myocardial Infarction) Developed in Collaboration with the American College of Emergency Physicians, the Society for Cardiovascular Angiography and Interventions, and the Society of Thoracic Surgeons: Endorsed by the American Association of Cardiovascular and Pulmonary Rehabilitation and the Society for Academic Emergency Medicine. J Am Coll Cardiol 50:652, 2007.
37. Tepel M, Aspelin P, Lameire N: Contrast-induced nephropathy: A clinical and evidence-based approach. Circulation 113:1799, 2006.
38. Marenzi G, Assanelli E, Marana I, et al: N-acetylcysteine and contrast-induced nephropathy in primary angioplasty. N Engl J Med 354:2773, 2006.
39. Guitterez N, Diaz A, Timmis GC, et al: Determinants of serum creatinine trajectory in acute contrast nephropathy. J Interv Cardiol 15:349, 2002.

Accelerated Atherosclerotic Vascular Calcification

40. McCullough PA, Agrawal V, Danielewicz E, Abela GS: Accelerated atherosclerotic calcification and Monckeberg's sclerosis: A continuum of advanced vascular pathology in chronic kidney disease. Clin J Am Soc Nephrol 3:1585, 2008.
41. Aikawa E, Aikawa M, Libby P, et al: Arterial and aortic valve calcification abolished by elastolytic cathepsin S deficiency in chronic renal disease. Circulation 119:1785, 2009.
42. McCullough PA, Soman S: Cardiovascular calcification in patients with chronic renal failure: Are we on target with this risk factor? Kidney Int Suppl (90):S18, 2004.
43. McCullough PA, Sandberg KR, DumLer F, Yanez JE: Determinants of coronary vascular calcification in patients with chronic kidney disease and end-stage renal disease: A systematic review. J Nephrol 17:205, 2004.
44. McCullough PA, Chinnaiyan KM: Annual progression of coronary calcification in trials of preventive therapies. Arch Int Med 169:2064, 2009.
45. Suki WN, Zabaneh R, Cangiano JL, et al: Effects of sevelamer and calcium-based phosphate binders on mortality in hemodialysis patients. Kidney Int 72:1130, 2007.
46. Wanner C, Krane V, Marz W, et al: Atorvastatin in patients with type 2 diabetes mellitus undergoing hemodialysis. N Engl J Med 353:238, 2005.
47. Fellström BC, Jardine AG, Schmieder RE, et al: Rosuvastatin and cardiovascular events in patients undergoing hemodialysis. N Engl J Med 360:1395, 2009.

Renal Disease and Hypertension

48. Mann JF, Schmieder RE, McQueen M, et al: Renal outcomes with telmisartan, ramipril, or both, in people at high vascular risk (the ONTARGET study): A multicentre, randomised, double-blind, controlled trial. Lancet 372:547, 2008.
49. Cohen MG, Pascua JA, Garcia-Ben M, et al: A simple prediction rule for significant renal artery stenosis in patients undergoing cardiac catheterization. Am Heart J 150:1204, 2005.
50. Fatica RA, Port FK, Young EW: Incidence trends and mortality in end-stage renal disease attributed to renovascular disease in the United States. Am J Kidney Dis 37:1184, 2001.

Ischemic Heart Diseases in Patients with Impaired Renal Function

51. Freda BJ, Tang WH, Van Lente F, et al: Cardiac troponins in renal insufficiency: Review and clinical implications. J Am Coll Cardiol 40:2065, 2002.
52. McCullough PA, Nowak RM, Foreback C, et al: Emergency evaluation of chest pain in patients with advanced kidney disease. Arch Intern Med 162:2464, 2002.
53. McCullough PA, Nowak RM, Foreback C, et al: Performance of multiple cardiac biomarkers measured in the emergency department in patients with chronic kidney disease and chest pain. Acad Emerg Med 9:1389, 2002.
54. McCullough PA: Acute coronary syndromes in patients with renal failure. Curr Cardiol Rep 5:266, 2003.
55. McCullough PA: Why is chronic kidney disease the "spoiler" for cardiovascular outcomes? J Am Coll Cardiol 41:725, 2003.
56. Herzog CA, Ma JZ, Collins AJ: Poor long-term survival after acute myocardial infarction among patients on long-term dialysis. N Engl J Med 339:799, 1998.
57. Sica D: The implications of renal impairment among patients undergoing percutaneous coronary intervention. J Invasive Cardiol 14(Suppl B):30B, 2002.
58. McCullough PA: Evaluation and treatment of coronary artery disease in patients with end-stage renal disease. Kidney Int Suppl (95):S51, 2005.

Heart Failure in Patients with Kidney Disease

59. Schreiber BD: Congestive heart failure in patients with chronic kidney disease and on dialysis. Am J Med Sci 325:179, 2003.
60. McCullough PA, Duc P, OmLand T, et al: B-type natriuretic peptide and renal function in the diagnosis of heart failure: An analysis from the Breathing Not Properly Multinational Study. Am J Kidney Dis 41:571, 2003.
61. Al-Ahmad A, Rand WM, Manjunath G, et al: Reduced kidney function and anemia as risk factors for mortality in patients with left ventricular dysfunction. J Am Coll Cardiol 38:955, 2001.
62. Shlipak MG: Pharmacotherapy for heart failure in patients with renal insufficiency. Ann Intern Med 138:917, 2003.
63. Schoolwerth AC, Sica DA, Ballermann BJ, et al: Renal considerations in angiotensin converting enzyme inhibitor therapy: A statement for healthcare professionals from the Council on the Kidney in Cardiovascular Disease and the Council for High Blood Pressure Research of the American Heart Association. Circulation 104:1985, 2001.
64. Cice G, Ferrara L, D'Andrea A, et al: Carvedilol increases two-year survival in dialysis patients with dilated cardiomyopathy: A prospective, placebo-controlled trial. J Am Coll Cardiol 41:1438, 2003.
65. McCullough PA, Sandberg KR, Yee J, Hudson MP: Mortality benefit of angiotensin-converting enzyme inhibitors after cardiac events in patients with end-stage renal disease. J Renin Angiotensin Aldosterone Syst 3:188, 2002.
66. Smith GL, Vaccarino V, Kosiborod M, et al: Worsening renal function: What is a clinically meaningful change in creatinine during hospitalization with heart failure? J Card Fail 9:13, 2003.
67. Jain P, Massie BM, Gattis WA, et al: Current medical treatment for the exacerbation of chronic heart failure resulting in hospitalization. Am Heart J 145(Suppl):S3, 2003.
68. Keating GM, Goa KL: Nesiritide: A review of its use in acute decompensated heart failure. Drugs 63:47, 2003.
69. Butler J, Emerson C, Peacock WF, et al: The efficacy and safety of B-type natriuretic peptide (nesiritide) in patients with renal insufficiency and acutely decompensated congestive heart failure. Nephrol Dial Transplant 19:391, 2004.
70. Thorsgard M, Bart BA: Ultrafiltration for congestive heart failure. Congest Heart Fail 15:136, 2009.

Valvular Heart Disease and Arrhythmias in Patients with Kidney Disease

71. Umana E, Ahmed W, Alpert MA: Valvular and perivalvular abnormalities in end-stage renal disease. Am J Med Sci 325:237, 2003.
72. Manian FA: Vascular and cardiac infections in end-stage renal disease. Am J Med Sci 325:243, 2003.
73. Soman SS, Sandberg KR, Borzak S, et al: The independent association of renal dysfunction and arrhythmias in critically ill patients. Chest 122:669, 2002.
74. Wase A, Basit A, Nazir R, et al: Impact of chronic kidney disease upon survival among implantable cardioverter-defibrillator recipients. J Interv Card Electrophysiol 11:199, 2004.

Consultative Approach to the Hemodialysis Patient

75. Centers for Disease Control and Prevention (CDC): Incidence of end-stage renal disease among persons with diabetes–United States, 1990-2002. MMWR Morb Mortal Wkly Rep 54:1097, 2005.
76. Reddan DN, Szczech LA, Tuttle RH, et al: Chronic kidney disease, mortality, and treatment strategies among patients with clinically significant coronary artery disease. J Am Soc Nephrol 14:2373, 2003.
77. Szczech LA, Reddan DN, Owen WF, et al: Differential survival following coronary revascularization procedures among patients with renal insufficiency. Kidney Int 60:292, 2001.
78. Agarwal R, Nissenson AR, Batlle D, et al: Prevalence, treatment, and control of hypertension in chronic hemodialysis patients in the United States. Am J 115:291, 2003.
79. Vlahakos DV, Hahalis G, Vassilakos P, et al: Relationship between left ventricular hypertrophy and plasma renin activity in chronic hemodialysis patients. J Am Soc Nephrol 8:1764, 1997.
80. Hampl H, Sternberg C, Berweck S, et al: Regression of left ventricular hypertrophy in hemodialysis patients is possible. Clin Nephrol 58(Suppl 1):S73, 2002.
81. Li PK, Chow KM, Wong TY, et al: Effects of an angiotensin-converting enzyme inhibitor on residual renal function in patients receiving peritoneal dialysis. A randomized, controlled study. Ann Intern Med 139:105, 2003.
82. McCullough PA: Opportunities for improvement in the cardiovascular care of patients with end-stage renal disease. Adv Chronic Kidney Dis 11:294, 2004.
83. Bakris GL: Role for beta-blockers in the management of diabetic kidney disease. Am J Hypertens 16(Pt 2):7S, 2003.
84. Cice G, Ferrara L, D'Andrea A, et al: Carvedilol increases two-year survival in dialysis patients with dilated cardiomyopathy: A prospective, placebo-controlled trial. J Am Coll Cardiol 41:1438, 2003.
85. McCullough PA, Sandberg KR, Borzak S, et al: Benefits of aspirin and beta-blockade after myocardial infarction in patients with chronic kidney disease. Am Heart J 144:226, 2002.
86. Porter GA, Norton TL, Lindsley J, et al: Relationship between elevated serum troponin values in end-stage renal disease patients and abnormal isotopic cardiac scans following stress. Ren Fail 25:55, 2003.
87. Buemi M, Senatore M, Corica F, et al: Statins and progressive renal disease. Med Res Rev 22:76, 2002.
88. National Kidney Foundation: K/DOQI Clinical Practice Guidelines For Managing Dyslipidemias in Chronic Kidney Disease. Executive Summary. New York, National Kidney Foundation, 2003.
89. Grundy SM, Cleeman JI, Merz CN, et al: Implications of recent clinical trials for the National Cholesterol Education Program Adult Treatment Panel III guidelines. Circulation 110:227, 2004.
90. American Diabetes Association: Standards of medical care for patients with diabetes mellitus. Diabetes Care 26(Suppl 1):S33, 2003.
91. Biesenbach G, Zazgornik J: Influence of smoking on the survival rate of diabetic patients requiring hemodialysis. Diabetes Care 19:625, 1996.
92. Winchester JF: Therapeutic uses of aspirin in renal diseases. Am J Kidney Dis 28(Suppl 1):S20, 1996.
93. Keeley EC, McCullough PA: Coronary revascularization in patients with coronary artery disease and chronic kidney disease. Adv Chronic Kidney Dis 11:254, 2004.
94. Reddan DN, Szczech LA, Tuttle RH, et al: Chronic kidney disease, mortality, and treatment strategies among patients with clinically significant coronary artery disease. J Am Soc Nephrol 14:2373, 2003.
95. Keeley EC, Kadakia R, Soman S, et al: Analysis of long-term survival after revascularization in patients with chronic kidney disease presenting with acute coronary syndromes. Am J Cardiol 92:509, 2003.
96. Opsahl JA, Husebye DG, Helseth HK, et al: Coronary artery bypass surgery in patients on maintenance dialysis: Long-term survival. Am J Kidney Dis 12:271, 1988.
97. Mishkel GJ, Varghese JJ, Moore AL, et al: Short- and long-term clinical outcomes of coronary drug-eluting stent recipients presenting with chronic renal disease. J Invasive Cardiol 19:331, 2007.

CHAPTER 94 Cardiovascular Manifestations of Autonomic Disorders

Virend K. Somers*

Cardiovascular function is closely linked and responsive to numerous endogenous and exogenous factors. This interplay is mediated through rapid and often subtle neurohormonal changes. One of the most important mechanisms whereby rapid circulatory control is achieved is the autonomic nervous system, which modulates cardiac function through direct effects on the heart and vascular tone.

Overview of Neural Circulatory Control

The autonomic nervous system can be subdivided into sympathetic, parasympathetic, and enteric components. The principal cardiovascular influences are mediated through the sympathetic and parasympathetic systems. The interplay between these two systems and their relative balance help determine cardiovascular responses under a variety of conditions. These responses usually take the form of changes in blood pressure or heart rate. The physiology whereby blood pressure and heart rate react to autonomic modulation is important to understanding how disorders of the autonomic nervous system can affect cardiovascular function.[1]

Baroreceptors

Autonomic responses, capillary shift mechanisms, hormonal responses, and kidney and fluid balance mechanisms all interact to maintain blood pressure control. Of these, the autonomic nervous system offers the most rapid response system. Neural circulatory regulation occurs via increased contractility of the heart or vasoconstriction of the arterial or venous circulations in response to information received from baroreceptors. This afferent information is synthesized and integrated, and appropriate responses are generated, in the vasomotor center of the brain.

The reflexes by which blood pressure is maintained are collectively known as the baroreflex, which includes arterial baroreceptors (also known as the high pressure receptors) and cardiopulmonary receptors (the low pressure receptors). Under normal physiologic circumstances, sympathetic activity is inhibited and parasympathetic activity predominates.

Arterial Baroreceptors. Arterial baroreceptors, which are the most sensitive, are located in the carotid sinuses, aortic arch, and at the origin of the right subclavian artery. The carotid sinus baroreceptors are innervated by the glossopharyngeal nerve (CN IX), and the aortic arch baroreceptors are innervated by the vagus nerve (CN X). Baroreceptors are stretch-dependent mechanoreceptors that sense changes in pressure, transmitting via afferents to the nucleus tractus solitarius (NTS) in the brainstem. When distended, the baroreceptors are activated and generate action potentials increasing in frequency in correlation to the amount of stretch. Thus, spike frequency is used as a surrogate measure of blood pressure at the level of the NTS, with higher frequency correlating with higher blood pressure.

The arterial baroreceptors are tonically active under normal circumstances at a mean arterial pressure (MAP) above 70 mm Hg, which is termed the *baroreceptor set point*. With MAPs below the set point, baroreceptors become essentially silent. However, the set point may vary with persistent blood pressure changes, such as in chronic hypertension, in which the set point is increased, or in chronic hypotension, in which it is decreased (see Chap. 45). The set point may vary, depending on other endogenous factors and disease states.

Integration of baroreceptor afferent signals is achieved at the level of the NTS. The NTS sends inhibitory fibers to the vasomotor center, which regulates the sympathetic nervous system, and excitatory fibers to vagal nuclei that regulate the parasympathetic system. Activation of the NTS (associated with increased action potential frequency from arterial baroreceptors) stimulates parasympathetic outflow while an inactive nucleus induces sympathetic activation and parasympathetic inhibition. Sympathetic activation leads to increased cardiac contractility, increased heart rate, venoconstriction, and arterial vasoconstriction, ultimately leading to increased blood pressure via elevation of total peripheral resistance and cardiac output. Parasympathetic activation leads to a decrease in heart rate and a minor decrease in contractility, resulting in a decrease in blood pressure.

Coupling of sympathetic inhibition with parasympathetic activation allows the baroreflex to maximize blood pressure reduction. Conversely, sympathetic activation with parasympathetic inhibition allows for an increase in blood pressure.

Cardiopulmonary Baroreceptors

Although the arterial baroreceptors are the most sensitive receptors, low-pressure receptors in the heart and venae cavae termed *cardiopulmonary receptors* also play a role in blood pressure modulation. They primarily respond to changes in volume but also to chemical stimuli. They project via vagal afferents to the NTS and via spinal sympathetic afferents to the spinal cord. Stimulation results in vasodilation and inhibition of vasopressin release. Furthermore, a stretch stimulus depresses renal sympathetic nerve activity[2] and has been shown to play a role in modulating renin release, resulting in diuresis and natriuresis,[3] thus regulating whole-body fluid volume to maintain blood pressure homeostasis.[1]

*The author is grateful to Drs. Rose Marie Robertson, David Robertson, and Suraj Kapa for contributions to the prior editions of this chapter.

Heart Rate Modulation

Modulation of heart rate is another means whereby the autonomic nervous system maintains normal blood pressure and exerts control over the cardiovascular system. Increases in heart rate are achieved through increases in contractile frequency via sympathetic activation. This is in part mediated through the arterial baroreflex. The cardiopulmonary receptors have only limited direct influence on heart rate control.

Under normal circumstances, at rest, the intrinsic sinus nodal rate is 95 to 110 beats/min, but efferent parasympathetic input via the vagus nerve suppresses the sinus nodal rate to 60 to 70 beats/min. During rest, there is little sympathetic efferent input and a low concentration of catecholamines. This changes with any movement away from the resting state, as with physical exertion, when sympathetic activity increases and parasympathetic activity decreases. On termination of exertion, the recovery of resting heart rate is again largely governed by parasympathetic dominance.

Although cardiac automaticity is intrinsic to pacemaker activity (see Chap. 35), the autonomic nervous system plays a primary role under normal conditions in defining heart rate and rhythm. The parasympathetic influence is achieved via acetylcholine release from the vagus nerve, which increases conductance of potassium across the cell membrane. In addition, acetylcholine inhibits the hyperpolarization-activated pacemaker current. This effect is quickly dispersed because of the high acetylcholinesterase concentration around the sinus node. The sympathetic influence is achieved by release of epinephrine and norepinephrine, which causes cAMP-mediated phosphorylation of membrane proteins and a resultant increase in the inward calcium current, resulting in accelerated slow diastolic depolarization. Also, other endogenous factors, such as nitric oxide, influence channel function and further modulate autonomic control of heart rate.

Breathing and Chemoreflexes

The chemoreflexes are modulators of sympathetic activation and play an important role in cardiovascular autonomic tone. The chemoreceptors are most simply divided into their central and peripheral components. The peripheral chemoreceptors are located in the carotid bodies and respond to hypoxemia, whereas the central chemoreceptors are in the brainstem and respond mostly to hypercapnia. Hypoxemia or hypercapnia results in hyperventilation and vascular sympathetic activation. Inhibitory influences on the chemoreflex drive are seen with stretch of the pulmonary afferents and with activation of the baroreflex, both of which have a greater influence on peripheral rather than central chemoreflexes.[4,5]

In numerous clinical conditions there is a substantial role of the chemoreflexes in the modulation of neural circulatory control. One is sleep apnea (see Chap. 79), in which the sympathetic vasoconstrictor response to hypoxia is potentiated because of elimination of the inhibitory influence on the chemoreflexes by stretch of the pulmonary afferents.[5] Another is hypertension, in which the ventilatory response to hypoxemia is increased and there is also an increase in sympathetic tone. This may be caused in part by impaired baroreflex sensitivity in hypertensive patients, but also by an increased chemoreflex drive. The tornic chemoreflex drive in obstructive sleep apnea patients can be reversed by the use of 100% oxygen, with which reductions in heart rate, blood pressure, and sympathetic outflow are seen. Administering 100% oxygen to patients with borderline hypertension and to spontaneously hypertensive rats also reduces not only ventilation but vasoconstrictor tone.

Diving Reflex. Under circumstances of prolonged apnea, a unique state of simultaneous increased parasympathetic drive to the heart and increased sympathetic drive to the vasculature occurs (**Fig. 94-1**). This is seen in diving mammals and sometimes in humans during prolonged submersion in water. In response to hypoxia, the body usually seeks to increase ventilation and blood flow to end-organs to maintain tissue oxygenation. However, in response to prolonged hypoxia in the absence of breathing, the body no longer experiences replenishment of oxygen stores and the normal homeostatic mechanisms alter so as to maintain oxygen delivery to organs vital to life—the brain and heart. This is achieved by decreasing oxygen delivery to much of the rest of the body via increased sympathetic vasoconstriction. This increased sympathetic outflow, however, does not constrict the cerebral vasculature because cerebral vascular tone is under autoregulatory control. Furthermore, myocardial oxygen demand is decreased because of bradycardia caused by an increase in parasympathetic tone. Thus, it is possible for individuals under exceptional circumstances to survive for prolonged periods of up to 5 minutes or more under anoxic conditions.

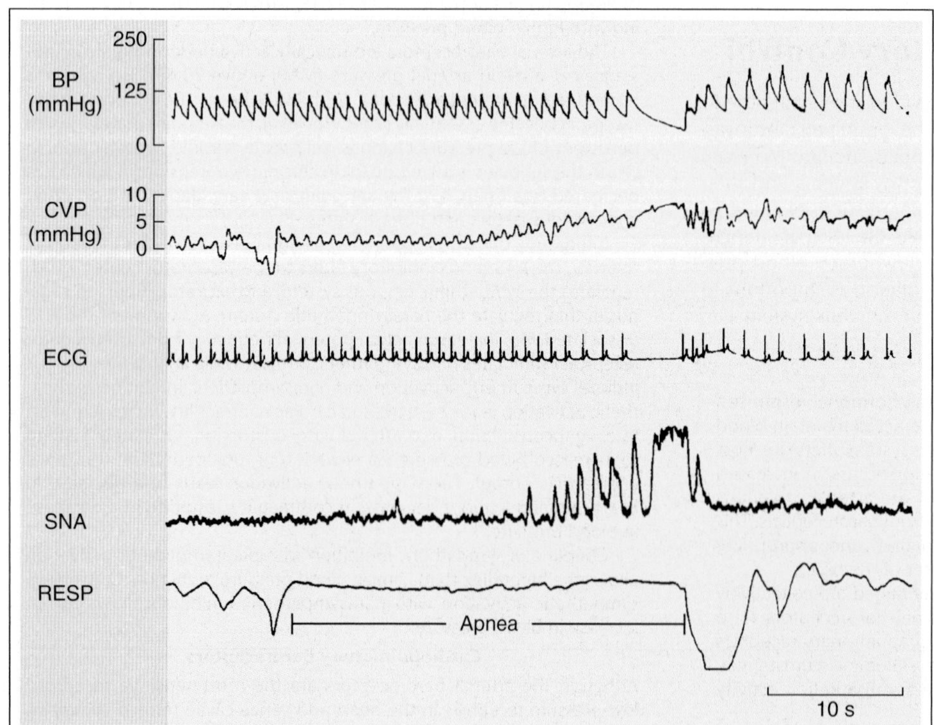

FIGURE 94-1 Components of the diving reflex. Shown are recordings of intra-arterial BP, central venous pressure (CVP), electrocardiogram (ECG), sympathetic nerve activity (SNA), and respiration (RESP) during apnea lasting 30 seconds. SNA is reflected by frequency and amplitude of bursts. Toward the end of the apneic period increases in BP, CVP, and SNA are noted, in addition to progressive bradycardia with eventual complete heart block. Furthermore, O_2 saturation fell to 92%. With release of apnea, electrocardiographic and SNA changes resolve, with some temporarily continued elevation in BP. *(From Somers VK, Dyken ME, Mark AL, Abboud FM: Parasympathetic hyperresponsiveness and bradyarrhythmias during apnoea in hypertension. Clin Auton Res 2:171, 1992.)*

Autonomic Testing

Testing of autonomic function may occur at the bedside or via sophisticated instrumentation and long-term studies. Experimental evidence for an association between lethal arrhythmias and increased sympathetic or reduced vagal activity has spurred development of several quantitative markers of autonomic activity. Generally, the two easiest and most economical means of studying the interplay between autonomic and cardiac function are via orthostatics and the Valsalva maneuver, although both are nonspecific. When a patient presents with syncope, a cost-effective means of exploring a neurocardiogenic cause is with a tilt-table test (see Chaps. 36 and 42). Furthermore, studies of baroreflex sensitivity, heart rate variability, heart rate recovery, and chemoreflexes have been shown to help in direct assessment of autonomic dysfunction. Finally, blood levels of norepinephrine and its metabolites may assist in discriminating between different types of dysautonomias.

Orthostatics

Orthostatic hypotension is defined as a decrease of more than 20 mm Hg in systolic pressure or a decrease of more than 10 mm Hg in diastolic pressure after rising to a standing position from a supine position. Blood pressure and heart rate measurement should be done once symptoms develop or after 3 minutes have passed after rising to the standing position. If the patient is unable to stand, then orthostatics may be done after the patient has risen to a sitting position, with the feet dangling over the edge of the bed. Orthostatic hypotension is an inability of the cardiopulmonary system to maintain sufficient blood pressure and adequate cerebral perfusion against gravity. Generally, on rising from a supine position, an average person may lose about 700 mL of blood from the thorax. This results in decreased stroke volume, as well as a decreased systolic pressure and increased diastolic pressure. Compensation occurs via an increase in heart rate and slight peripheral vasoconstriction. Individuals intolerant of orthostasis may get venous pooling secondary to decreased muscle and vascular tone and develop a decreased circulating blood volume in response to standing. When testing orthostatics, it is important to note that a significant decrease in blood pressure without a corresponding rise in heart rate suggests abnormal autonomic innervation to the heart and may represent an underlying neuropathy, chronotropic incompetence or drug therapy, such as beta blockade, that blunts the heart rate response.

Valsalva Maneuver

The Valsalva maneuver becomes useful for testing patients at the bedside when done in conjunction with continuous electrocardiographic monitoring. During monitoring, the patient will blow continuously into a closed system for 12 seconds at 40 mm Hg and the fastest heart rate during the maneuver is divided by the slowest heart rate immediately afterward. A quotient of less than 1.4 is suggestive of autonomic impairment. However, this is nonspecific. For example, patients with congestive heart failure are less able to restrict blood return to the right atrium and do not exhibit the typical hemodynamic response.[1] Recovery of BP after the Valsalva may provide a useful measure of adrenergic vasoconstrictor reserve (see later).

Other Tests of Autonomic Function

BAROREFLEX SENSITIVITY. Baroreflex sensitivity is a measure of parasympathetic input to the sinus node. Testing baroreflex control of heart rate involves measuring the reflex increase in R-R interval in response to an increase in blood pressure. The increase in blood pressure has historically been achieved by the use of an alpha-adrenergic agonist, most often phenylephrine. Intravenous injection of a bolus of phenylephrine induces a 20- to 30-mm Hg increase in systolic pressure. Generally, a linear relationship exists between the increase in the R-R interval and increase in systolic pressure. The slope is used to quantify the sensitivity of the arterial baroreflex; it is typically steep in healthy individuals but decreases with advancing age and flattens even more with severe cardiovascular disease, such as hypertension or heart failure.

As a measure of autonomic function, baroreflex sensitivity decreases (i.e., shows a flatter slope) with sympathetic dominance and increases (i.e., shows a steeper slope) with parasympathetic dominance. In the search for noninvasive ways to measure baroreflex sensitivity, various devices and maneuvers have been used. The FINAPRES (from finger arterial pressure) device is one such example and has been used in the Autonomic Tone and Reflexes After Myocardial Infarction (ATRAMI) study. Spontaneous increases and decreases in blood pressure, as well as associated RR changes, have been used to determine the spontaneous baroreflex. Furthermore, spectral techniques used to analyze the relationship between beat to beat oscillations of blood pressure (BP) and R-R intervals are being studied as possible alternatives to the more invasive method of phenylephrine infusion.

Generally, autonomic testing evaluates the baroreflex by measuring heart rate changes in response to increases and decreases in BP. However, the baroreflex regulates BP by changing not only heart rate (vagal component) but also peripheral resistance (adrenergic component). A potentially useful nuance in baroreflex testing has been the differentiation between adrenergic and vagal baroreflex sensitivity.[6] Adrenergic baroreflex sensitivity relates the BP recovery time to the preceding BP decrease induced by the Valsalva maneuver, in a sense measuring the sympathetic vasoconstrictor response to hypotension. This may provide a helpful index for evaluating and following patients with adrenergic failure.

CHEMOREFLEXES. Studies of chemoreflex function are one way of determining the dominant respiratory response, as well as the breathing–heart rate–blood pressure interactions, in certain diseases. As noted, the hypercapnic response is mediated mainly by central chemoreceptors, whereas the hypoxemic response is mediated by peripheral chemoreceptors.

HEART RATE VARIABILITY. Heart rate variability has become a commonly used but difficult to interpret means of studying the interplay between the autonomic nervous system and cardiovascular function. The phenomenon being measured in heart rate variability is that of the oscillation in the interval between consecutive heartbeats, as well as the variance of heart rates. Thus, heart rate variability studies the oscillation of heart rate and R-R intervals.

The actual measurement of heart rate variability has been achieved via multiple different modalities, most notably using time domain and frequency domain methods. It is usually calculated by analyzing the time series of beat to beat intervals from electrocardiographic or arterial pressure tracings. A simple example of time domain measurement of heart rate variability is calculation of the standard deviation of beat to beat intervals. The time domain graph of a value shows how the signal varies over time. The frequency domain graph, however, shows how much of a signal lies within given frequency bands over a range of frequencies. It involves the use of mathematical transforms, such as the Fourier transform, to decompose a function into an infinite or finite number of frequencies. Spectral density analysis is the most common frequency domain method used and involves measurement of how the power of a signal or time series is distributed at any particular frequency.

A common frequency domain method involves application of the discrete Fourier transform to the beat to beat interval time series. The frequency bands of most interest in humans are the high-frequency (HF) band, low-frequency (LF) band, very low frequency (VLF) band, and the ultralow-frequency (ULF) band, each of which has its own physiologic correlate. The HF band lies between 0.15 and 0.4 Hz and is driven by respiration, appearing to derive mainly from vagal activity. The LF band, which lies between 0.04 and 0.15 Hz, appears to derive from vagal and sympathetic activity and is believed to reflect delay in the baroreceptor loop. The VLF band lies between 0.0033 and 0.04 Hz and has been attributed to physical activity. Finally, the ULF band lies between 0 and 0.0033 Hz and is associated with day-night variation.

Other means of calculating heart rate variability include phase domain measurement and other nonlinear dynamic methods. The information provided by each measuring method, however, is complementary and ought to be taken together to define and understand the characteristics of heart rate variability in a given disorder.

The usefulness of heart rate variability as a measure of autonomic function and as a predictor of mortality has been suggested by a number of studies. In the 1970s, Wolf and colleagues showed a higher risk of postinfarction mortality with reduced heart rate variability, and Ewing and associates developed simple bedside tests to use short-term R-R differences as a means of detecting autonomic neuropathy in diabetics. In the late 1980s, heart rate variability was shown to be an independent predictor of post–myocardial infarction mortality. More recently, altered heart rate variability has been associated with other pathologic conditions such as hypertension, hemorrhagic shock,[7] and septic shock.[8] Heart rate variability has been accepted via international consensus as an independent predictor of mortality after myocardial infarction and as an early warning sign for diabetic neuropathy.

Heart rate turbulence, thought to be a reflection of baroreflex sensitivity, may also provide prognostically useful information. Abnormal heart rate turbulence has been linked to total mortality and sudden death in patients after myocardial infarction and patients with heart failure.[9]

HEART RATE RECOVERY. During exercise, heart rate rises, initially secondary to a reduction in vagal tone and then because of increased sympathetic activity. After exercise, parasympathetic reactivation and reduced sympathetic activity contribute to the recovery of resting heart rate. The rate at which the heart rate returns to baseline, measured over the first minute after exercise, is termed the *heart rate recovery*. A delayed heart rate recovery is a marker of decreased vagal activity, which has been shown to be an independent risk factor for sudden cardiac death.[10]

TILT-TABLE TESTING. Tilt-table testing is often conducted in patients presenting with a history of syncope to diagnose possible dysautonomic causes of syncope (see Chap. 42). The test is considered positive if the patient experiences symptoms associated with a blood pressure drop or an arrhythmia. These abnormalities are suggestive of dysfunction of the autonomic system. Normally, blood pressure will compensate via an increase in heart rate and constriction of blood vessels in the legs. In some patients, fainting or syncope could be associated with a precipitous drop in blood pressure (vasodepressor syncope) or pulse rate (cardioinhibitory syncope), or a mixed response, thus requiring continuous monitoring of both.

ORTHOSTATIC HYPOTENSION. Orthostatic hypotension (not the same as orthostatic intolerance; see later) is secondary to neurogenic and non-neurogenic conditions.[11] Neurogenic causes are addressed later (see Autonomic Dysregulation). Non-neurogenic causes include hypovolemia, cardiac dysfunction, and medications (including those used to treat hypertension, myocardial ischemia, depression, psychosis, and Alzheimer and Parkinson disease). It is especially prevalent in older adults, in whom the consequences of the predisposing factors noted can be magnified. Orthostatic hypotension and tachycardia may also occur after prolonged bed rest or after exposure to microgravity, such as in space flight. In some patients, orthostatic hypotension may be accompanied by fatigue, cognitive dysfunction, and emotional difficulties, as well as by gait abnormalities and falls.[12,13] Symptoms can be debilitating and confine patients to bed; the consequent physical deconditioning may worsen the overall problem. Longitudinal studies have suggested that orthostatic hypotension can increase the risk of stroke, myocardial ischemia, and mortality. The therapeutic goal is to attenuate or eliminate symptoms, rather than restore normotension. Pharmacologic therapy is often suboptimal and should be combined with interventions such as compression of venous capacitance beds, use of physical countermaneuvers, and intermittent water bolus treatment. Treatment can be difficult and development of supine hypertension should be minimized, especially in patients with diabetes, heart failure, or cardiac ischemia.

Autonomic Dysregulation

Dysautonomias refer to any dysfunction of the autonomic nervous system, whether central, peripheral, or secondary to other disease processes. In general, the most common dysautonomias are those affecting the sympathetic system. However, the parasympathetic system and conditions of increased parasympathetic tone, such as during sleep or with endurance training, are also important to understand because they can have significant implications for cardiovascular health.

The sympathetic dysautonomias are the most common and may be characterized by disorders of release, function, or reuptake of the main sympathetic chemical messenger, norepinephrine. Furthermore, local blood flow and clearance of norepinephrine from the circulation can manifest as a dysautonomia. The sympathetic dysautonomias can be generally divided into two groups—those associated with decreased function, in which orthostasis often occurs, and those associated with increased outflow, in which hypertension and/or tachycardia may be present.

Primary Chronic Autonomic Failure

Orthostatic intolerance is a key manifestation of neurocirculatory failure. It often serves as the presenting symptom. However, not all orthostatic hypotension is symptomatic of neurocirculatory failure. Most cases of orthostatic hypotension result from blood loss, volume depletion, or a prolonged bedridden state. Only rarely does it result from true autonomic failure.

Chronic autonomic failure is distinguishable from acute-onset autonomic dysfunction syndromes by its progressive nature and prognosis. Generally, chronic autonomic failure can be subdivided into secondary and primary failure, with secondary failure being far more common. In cases of secondary failure, the cause is usually clear and treatment involves therapy for the underlying disorder. However, when autonomic failure dominates the clinical presentation and a clear cause is not apparent, this is termed *primary chronic autonomic failure*.[1]

Primary autonomic failure may be subdivided into three major syndromes—pure autonomic failure, multisystem atrophy, and Parkinson disease. Major overlap among these three syndromes exists, and treatment differs between them.

PURE AUTONOMIC FAILURE. Pure autonomic failure involves orthostatic hypotension in the absence of symptoms or signs of central neurodegeneration. Thus, the dysfunction occurs at the level of peripheral neurons and not in the central nervous system. The functional error lies in available levels of norepinephrine, which are low when supine and rise minimally with standing.[1] Orthostatic hypotension and an inadequate chronotropic response to standing and the Valsalva maneuver are therefore evident. No direct effect on longevity occurs in these patients.

MULTISYSTEM ATROPHY. Multisystem atrophy includes autonomic failure with signs and symptoms of progressive central neurodegeneration. It is generally divided into Parkinsonian, cerebellar, and mixed forms. Patients develop symptoms in the sixth or seventh decade of life, exhibiting sympathetic and parasympathetic dysfunction.[1] In addition to orthostatic hypotension, findings may include impotence, loss of sweating, abnormal pupillary responses, reduced intraocular pressure, sleep apnea, and urinary incontinence. In some patients, orthostatic angina, which is actually exacerbated by the use of nitroglycerin, may occur. The angina appears to be caused by severe orthostatic hypotension and resultant inadequate coronary perfusion. Furthermore, urine production is greater in these patients during the night, leaving patients more hypovolemic in the morning and exaggerating symptoms further.

Orthostatic changes in this disease may be striking, with as much as a 100-mm Hg fall in systolic pressure on standing and a minimal rise in heart rate. Because of the progressive nature and the chronicity, patients may tolerate this precipitous drop in blood pressure relatively well. Patients often exhibit hypertension when supine, suggesting an inappropriate level of circulating catecholamines. In fact, plasma levels of catecholamines and their metabolites are preserved but not appropriately elevated on standing.

Lifespan in multisystem atrophy is diminished, and patients live on average 9 years from diagnosis. Movement abnormalities are centrally mediated and do not often respond to pharmacologic intervention. Furthermore, respiratory compromise can occur progressively, with development of nocturnal stridor that may require continuous positive airway pressure.[1]

PARKINSON DISEASE WITH AUTONOMIC FAILURE. This entity is similar in clinical appearance to multisystem atrophy with parkinsonian features. The most common cause is diffuse disease of autonomic centers in the brain, resulting in autonomic dysfunction similar to that described earlier, affecting organs diffusely.

DIAGNOSIS AND THERAPY. Distinguishing pure autonomic failure from multisystem atrophy and from Parkinson disease with autonomic failure tends to be easier than distinguishing between the latter two. Magnetic resonance imaging (MRI) of the brain in pure autonomic failure will not reveal any central nervous system abnormalities, whereas in the other two it will demonstrate central lesions. Differentiating between multisystem atrophy and Parkinson disease is important, because the prognosis in multisystem atrophy is much worse. It has been suggested that levodopa-carbidopa can be used to distinguish patients with Parkinson disease, but this drug can worsen orthostatic hypotension and there have been reports of patients diagnosed with multisystem atrophy showing some improvement with therapy.

Neuroimaging techniques have been used to distinguish the three types of autonomic failure. Cardiac sympathetic nerves take up ^{123}I-metaiodobenzylguanidine (^{123}I-MIBG) and 6-(^{18}F) fluorodopamine, postganglionic adrenergic markers that radiolabel vesicles in the sympathetic nerve terminals, thus allowing for visualization of cardiac innervation. In patients with multisystem atrophy, normal uptake and hence intact cardiac sympathetic innervation are noted. However, patients with Parkinson disease or pure autonomic failure show no detectable activity in the myocardium on emission scans, consistent with loss of sympathetic innervation of the heart. Thus, even though Parkinson disease with autonomic failure may demonstrate central lesions, there is a suggestion of an additional postganglionic lesion in these patients, which is distinct from the isolated preganglionic lesion of multisystem atrophy (MSA).

The recently updated consensus statement for the diagnosis of MSA reflects the advances and challenges in this field.[14] Preliminary results of an ongoing prospective study comparing patients with MSA to those with Parkinson disease have shown that autonomic defects are more strikingly abnormal in MSA versus those in Parkinson disease.[15] These differences were sustained and greater at 1-year follow-up, suggesting a more rapid progression of dysautonomia in multisystem atrophy than in Parkinson disease. These findings further support the concept that the primary lesion in multisystem atrophy is preganglionic and in Parkinson disease is ganglionic and postganglionic.

Therapy depends on changes in lifestyle in addition to pharmacologic therapy. Ingestion of carbohydrates can lower blood pressure, and a meal before bedtime may be helpful in reducing nighttime supine hypertension. This depressor effect can be difficult for patients after meals during the day, so caffeine ingestion or use of somatostatin in the case of severe blood pressure decreases can be used to attenuate the hemodynamic response to food. Furthermore, water intake can help increase blood pressure. Physical maneuvers that cause compression of the lower extremities have also been noted to help patients symptomatically.[1]

Pharmacologically, the two main areas of intervention include volume expansion and pressor administration. Use of fludrocortisone and adding sodium to the diet can help with volume expansion. The use of pressor agents should be considered in the context of the postganglionic or preganglionic nature of the different diseases. In patients with sympathetic cardiac denervation (i.e., pure autonomic failure or Parkinson disease with autonomic failure), midorine (an alpha-adrenoreceptor agonist) or L-threo-3,4-dihydroxyphenylserine (a norepinephrine precursor converted by parenchymal cells) may be useful. However, patients with MSA in whom sympathetic innervation is intact may benefit from use of a sympathomimetic amine or alpha$_2$-adrenoreceptor blocker. Also, ma-huang or yohimbine may be useful because it induces release of norepinephrine from the sympathetic nerve terminal, but could cause acute hypertension if used improperly.[1]

Secondary Autonomic Failure

More commonly, autonomic failure occurs in the context of some other disease process and treatment of the underlying process may or may not relieve the autonomic dysfunction. The most common cause of secondary autonomic failure is diabetes (see Chap. 64). Diabetic neuropathy is a well-known, long-term complication and all nerves may be affected, both somatic and autonomic. Cardiovascular complications secondary to dysfunction of autonomic control have been described in patients with and without orthostatic hypotension. Heart rate variability and baroreflex testing[16] may help in the detection of diabetic autonomic neuropathy. Nerve conduction abnormalities may not be the only component of autonomic dysfunction in diabetes. Relationships between vascular stiffness and dysfunction of the baroreflex have also been noted. Furthermore, some studies have suggested that the primary dysfunction may be in defective activation of central parasympathetic pathways. Thus, there appear to be afferent and efferent, as well as sympathetic and parasympathetic, components to the autonomic dysregulation associated with diabetes.

Glucose and blood pressure control may protect against neuropathic and microvascular complications and improve autonomic function. A recent study has evaluated the effects of prior intensive versus conventional insulin therapy on the prevalence of cardiac autonomic neuropathy in former subjects of the Diabetic Control and Complications Trial (DCCT).[17] DCCT autonomic measures (R-R variation with paced breathing, Valsalva ratio, postural blood pressure changes, and autonomic symptoms) were repeated in 1226 subjects, studied 13 to 14 years after the end of the DCCT. Although the prevalence of cardiac autonomic neuropathy was higher in both groups after 13 to 14 years, the incidence was much lower (odds ratio [OR], 0.69; 95% confidence interval [CI], 0.51 to 0.96) in the former intensive group versus the conventional group, suggesting that the benefits of intensive insulin therapy in reducing risk of autonomic neuropathy may be sustained for many years.[17]

Amyloidosis can also result in secondary autonomic failure[18] (see Chap. 68). A recent retrospective study of 65 patients who had biopsy-proven amyloidosis and also had autonomic function testing suggested that patients with peripheral neuropathy of unknown origin should undergo autonomic testing, even in the absence of symptoms of autonomic failure.[19] Early recognition of autonomic failure in those patients may lead to earlier diagnosis of underlying amyloidosis, and hence earlier treatment.

Other common causes of secondary autonomic failure include renal failure[20] (see Chap. 93), paraneoplastic syndromes, and vitamin B_{12} deficiency. If antibodies against components of the autonomic nervous system are present in the absence of clinically apparent neoplasm, further assessment for neoplasm should be made, given that clinical improvement can be achieved following treatment.[21] HIV infection can cause autonomic dysfunction independent of effects on cardiac function (see Chap. 72), as can heavy metal intoxication, particularly with copper, lead, mercury, or thallium.

AUTOIMMUNE AUTONOMIC FAILURE. Severe autonomic failure can result from autoimmune damage to neurons. Disease progression is variable and ranges from days to years. Because of the variable time of presentation, it may be difficult to separate autoimmune autonomic failure from other types of autonomic dysfunction. In addition to orthostatic hypotension, bowel and bladder dysfunction may occur. Plasma catecholamine levels are usually low and rise minimally with standing. Some reports have shown the beneficial effect of intravenous gamma globulin in treatment. One case report has also suggested a role for plasma exchange pheresis in treatment.[22]

In addition to autoimmune autonomic failure, autonomic dysfunction may be seen as a complication in severe cases of Guillain-Barré syndrome. In these patients, treatment is often supportive and orthostatic intolerance may be the only symptom. Furthermore, autonomic function may completely return with general motor function. Orthostatic intolerance may also occur as a sequela of prolonged bed rest in these patients.[1]

CONGENITAL AUTONOMIC FAILURE. The first autonomic disorder associated with a defined genetic abnormality was dopamine beta-hydroxylase deficiency. Dopamine beta-hydroxylase converts dopamine to norepinephrine in vesicles in noradrenergic neurons. Thus, this is a disorder of sympathetic noradrenergic function. As a result of the norepinephrine deficiency, patients cannot mount a vasoconstrictor response to upright posture and have marked orthostatic hypotension with a blunted rise in heart rate.[1] Also, they have excess quantities of dopamine, which is released in place of norepinephrine, resulting in increased urinary sodium excretion, ptosis, nasal stuffiness, joint hyperextensibility, and retrograde ejaculation in men. Dihydroxyphenylserine has been used with some benefit to restore norepinephrine levels because these patients have normal levels of dopa decarboxylase.[23]

Orthostatic Intolerance

Orthostatic intolerance (see Chap. 42) is an entity distinct from orthostatic hypotension and is only occasionally characterized by the rapid development of orthostatic hypotension. Generally, symptoms are seen in young women who report visual changes, poor concentration while standing, fatigue while standing, tremor, and often syncope. Several diseases are associated with orthostatic intolerance. These range from problems of localized excess noradrenergic stimulation to abnormalities of the baroreflex response. However, there is considerable overlap in terms of diagnosis, especially among postural

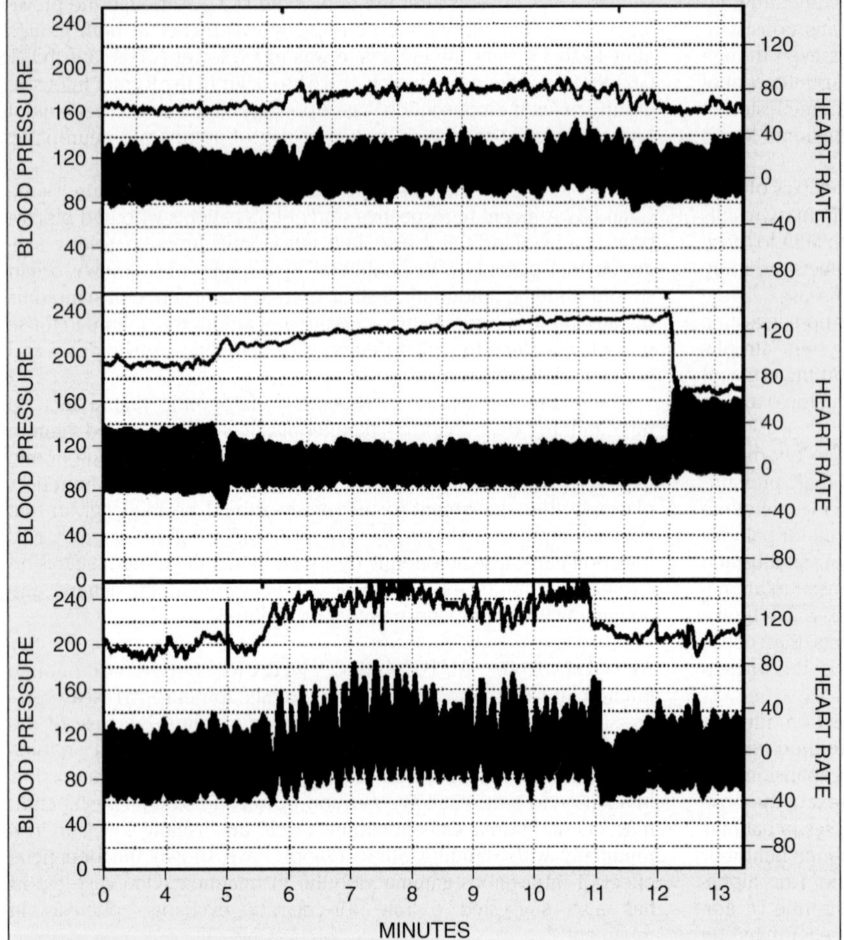

FIGURE 94-2 Examples of BP and heart rate recordings from a normal subject **(top panel),** a patient with neuropathic POTS **(middle panel),** and a patient with hyperadrenergic POTS **(bottom panel).** Note the modest reduction in BP in neuropathic POTS. Hyperadrenergic POTS is associated with prominent BP oscillations, an orthostatic increment in systolic BP, and a prominent norepinephrine response to head-up tilt. *(From Low PA, Sandroni P, Joyner M, Shen W-K: Postural tachycardia syndrome. J Cardiovasc Electrophysiol 20:352, 2009.)*

tachycardia syndrome, neurally mediated syncope, and chronic fatigue syndrome, which often coexist in patients presenting with orthostatic intolerance.

Postural Tachycardia Syndrome

Postural orthostatic tachycardia syndrome (POTS) presents primarily with orthostatic symptoms, tachycardia, and the absence of significant hypotension.[24] Symptoms of orthostatic intolerance include those elicited by brain hypoperfusion and by sympathetic excitation.[25] POTS affects females in a 5:1 ratio over males, and most patients are between 20 to 40 years of age. POTS is heterogenous in mechanisms, as well as in presentation. Major mechanisms are denervation (neuropathic POTS), deconditioning, and a hyperadrenergic state (**Fig. 94-2**). Each of these three major mechanisms is exacerbated by hypovolemia.

Diagnostic criteria for postural orthostatic tachycardia syndrome are controversial and may be based on several criteria, including the following:

- Orthostatic tachycardia greater than 30 beats/min, usually to 120 beats/min or higher
- Transient systolic blood pressure decrease of more than 20 mm Hg, with recovery within the first minute of tilt
- Standing plasma norepinephrine level higher than 600 pg/mL
- Severe orthostatic symptoms

Although patients with POTS often have increased anxiety and somatic hypervigilance, the excessive tachycardia during orthostatic stress is not secondary to anxiety, but is a physiologic response that helps maintain arterial pressure during venous pooling.[26] POTS patients also demonstrate excessive tachycardia during exercise. Recent data have suggested that the tachycardia during exercise in POTS is not secondary to abnormal baroreflex regulation of heart rate.[27] Treatment of POTS[25] includes increasing intravascular volume with high levels of salt and fluids, supplemented by compression garments. Pharmacologic interventions include low-dose beta blockers, and low dose vasoconstrictors such as midodrine and fludrocortisone. A recent, randomized, crossover acute drug trial has compared low-dose (20-mg) propranolol to placebo and found that propranolol reduces supine and standing heart rates and improves symptoms at 2 hours after dosing.[28] In a comparison between the low-dose and a higher (80-mg) dose propranolol, the higher dose had a great effect on attenuating standing heart rate and orthostatic tachycardia, but the lower dose elicited a greater improvement in symptoms at 2 hours after dosing. The therapeutic importance of exercise training and improved physical conditioning is becoming increasingly apparent as an important strategy for the deconditioned patient.

Neurally Mediated Syncope

Neurally mediated syncope, also known as *neurocardiogenic syncope*, is characterized by periodic syncopal episodes with normal autonomic function between episodes (**Fig. 94-3**; see Chap. 42). Patients frequently have vasovagal-like fainting and a reduction in vascular sympathetic activity during the syncopal episode. Several variants of neurally mediated syncope are discussed later in this chapter.

The mechanisms underlying neurally mediated syncope remain controversial but are presumed to be secondary to decreased venous return to the heart resulting from increased peripheral venous pooling of blood, which results in cardiac hypercontractility. One study has documented the complete disappearance of peroneal sympathetic nerve recordings during syncopal episodes in these patients. The hypercontractile response activates cardiac mechanoreceptors, resulting in a paradoxical reflex bradycardia and decreased systemic vascular resistance, despite the already decreased venous return, eliciting the characteristic presyncopal symptoms of weakness, light-headedness, feelings of warmth or cold, and ultimate brief loss of consciousness. This reflex bradycardia and hypotension are similar to those evoked by the Bezold-Jarisch reflex. In the absence of any underlying cardiovascular, neurologic, or other disease, isolated vasovagal syncope may represent a variation of normal; because spontaneous syncope may affect up to 50% of everyone, subjects are generally normotensive with otherwise normal blood pressure regulation,[29] and long-term prognosis is usually excellent,[30] aside from sequelae of any falls that may occur with a syncopal event.

Potential cardiac causes of syncope must be considered before this diagnosis of exclusion can be made. However, even then, diagnosis can be difficult. Situational syncope must be excluded, as well as phobia syndromes or other organic causes. Tilt-table testing has good specificity but uncertain sensitivity in diagnosis and is not always reproducible. Implantable loop recorders, which store 45 minutes of retrospective electrocardiographic data, may also be used and can be activated by patients after each syncopal event. However, the cost is high and the diagnostic benefit remains undefined.

Typically, treatment in these patients is conservative and involves education, particularly in determining potential predisposing factors and recognizing prodromal symptoms when they occur. Increasing fluid and salt intake may also help in avoiding the development of syncope. Pharmacologic therapy includes beta blockers, which presumably work via inhibition of mechanoreceptor activation; fludrocortisone, which expands central fluid volume via retention of sodium; and vasoconstrictors and selective serotonin reuptake inhibitors, which may have a role in regulating sympathetic nervous system activity. Although cardiac pacing addresses the bradycardia, it is incompletely effective because it does not compensate for the vasodepressor component.

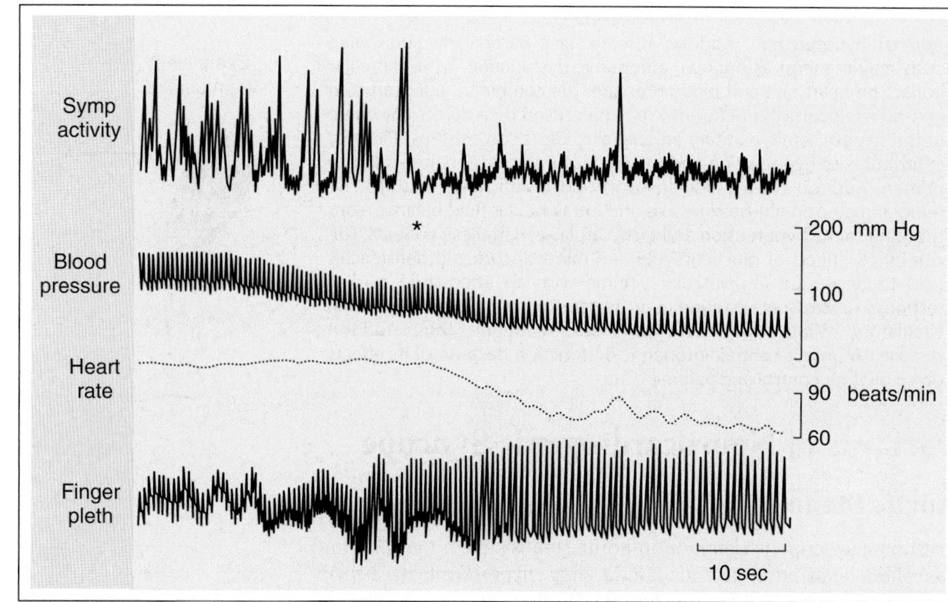

FIGURE 94-3 Recordings of sympathetic nerve activity and blood pressure before and during vasovagal syncope. Note the simultaneous reductions in sympathetic nerve activity, heart rate, and blood pressure associated with the episode of syncope (*). Pleth = plethysmography; symp = sympathetic. *(From Wallin BG, Sundlof G: Sympathetic outflow to muscles during vasovagal syncope. J Auton Nerv Syst 6:287, 1982.)*

Chronic Fatigue Syndrome

Chronic fatigue syndrome is characterized by new, unexplained fatigue that lasts for at least 6 months, is unrelieved by rest, and has no clear cause. The etiology of this syndrome is unclear. Some studies have suggested that dysautonomia may be common in patients with chronic fatigue syndrome. On the basis of tilt-table testing, more than 60% of patients with chronic fatigue show abnormal blood pressure or heart rate responses, with sudden hypotension or severe bradycardia or tachycardia, along with decreased consciousness. Syncopal episodes in these patients are usually associated with a decrease in sympathetic outflow in the absence of ventricular hypovolemia or hypercontractility.

Chronic fatigue patients have not been shown to benefit from treatment with fludrocortisone and high salt intake, unlike most patients suffering from orthostatic intolerance secondary to sympathetic neurocirculatory failure. Thus, the exact mechanism of orthostatic intolerance in these patients is unclear. Alternative treatments may include midorine or beta-adrenoreceptor blockers. Whether relief of any dysautonomic symptoms in these patients may relieve the symptoms of fatigue is unclear. Because these patients are often physically inactive, an exercise conditioning program implemented to improve well-being may help alleviate symptoms.

Baroreflex Failure

Causes of baroreflex failure most often include surgery, radiation therapy, and cerebrovascular accidents. Failure results from damage to afferent neuronal input (via the vagus and glossopharyngeal nerves) or from damage to brainstem nuclei or interneurons.[1] As a result, there is a loss of response to arterial baroreceptor stimulation.

These patients often present acutely with significant pheochromocytoma-like pressor crises associated with palpitations, diaphoresis, and severe headaches. Patients may present after surgical intervention, trauma, or stroke. Blood pressure is labile and may rise to extremely high levels. Some studies have shown that 9% to 30% of patients exhibit hypertension consistent with baroreflex failure after carotid endarterectomy.[1] Patients with unilateral involvement may show almost complete failure as well. The right carotid baroreflex may be more effective than the left carotid, suggesting a difference in clinical outcome depending on which carotid artery is affected.

The clinical presentation can vary over time, and acute episodes during waking hours may mimic a pheochromocytoma; severe hypotension and bradycardia may occur during sleep. Heart rate and blood pressure change together (concomitant rises or falls in both). Furthermore, there is little or no orthostatic hypotension initially, but it may appear later with prolonged standing. Apneic episodes may occur because of loss of neural afferents from carotid chemoreceptors.

Loss of the baroreflex buffering mechanism results in prolonged and exaggerated responses to a variety of tests, such as the cold pressor test. Plasma and urinary norepinephrine levels may be high, with plasma levels in the 1000- to 3000-pg/mL range. Minor stimuli can result in pressor crises, even after successful initial treatment in these patients, and long-term therapy may be necessary. Diagnostically, patients may show a depressor response to a small dose of clonidine but no heart rate response to depressor or pressor infusions, even though heart rate will change with sedation or cortical stimuli.[1]

Initial therapy over the first 72 hours can include nitroprusside and clonidine. Chronically, patients may continue to have labile hypertension and tachycardia alternating with hypotension and bradycardia. This may be effectively treated with clonidine and methyldopa. During periods of excess cortical stimulation (e.g., stress, anxiety), low-dose benzodiazepines and clonidine may help relieve symptoms.[1]

Carotid Sinus Hypersensitivity

Carotid sinus hypersensitivity is defined as a ventricular pause longer than 3 seconds and/or a fall in systolic BP of more than 50 mm Hg with carotid sinus massage.[30] Carotid sinus syndrome refers to the association of carotid sinus hypersensitivity with spontaneous syncope. Carotid sinus massage should be avoided in patients with prior transient ischemic attacks (TIAs), stroke within 3 months, or carotid bruits, unless Doppler studies exclude significant carotid artery disease. Cardiac pacing has been considered as a therapeutic option, although a recent randomized, double-blind, placebo-controlled crossover trial has shown no benefit of dual-chamber pacing[31] (see Chap. 38).

Norepinephrine Transporter Deficiency

In norepinephrine transporter deficiency, there is a deficiency of the membrane norepinephrine transporter. As a result, there is a more than 98% reduction in reuptake of norepinephrine at the sympathetic nerve ending. This results in elevated levels of norepinephrine at the synapse and resultant tachycardia, especially on standing, when norepinephrine delivery is increased, despite the already elevated synaptic concentration.

Addison Disease

Adrenal hypofunction, Addison disease, and particularly addisonian crisis may manifest as a global autonomic dysfunction, with particular impact on heart rate and blood pressure. The combined glucocorticoid and mineralocorticoid deficiency may be caused by a defect anywhere in the hypothalamic-pituitary-adrenal axis. Glucocorticoid insufficiency contributes to hypotension and may reduce myocardial contractility. In primary Addison disease, mineralocorticoid insufficiency disturbs the renin-angiotensin-aldosterone axis and intravascular fluid balance, contributing to the hypotension and tachycardia seen in these patients. The combined effects of glucocorticoid and mineralocorticoid deficiencies lead to decreased intravascular volume with an attenuated cardiac response to stressors, resulting in orthostatic hypotension and eventual circulatory collapse without appropriate treatment. Thus, Addison disease can mimic central autonomic dysfunction because of its effects on circulatory control and volume status.

Variants of Neurocardiogenic Syncope

Aortic Stenosis

Exertional syncope is common in aortic stenosis (see Chap. 66) and has often been attributed to carotid sinus hypersensitivity, arrhythmias, or left ventricular failure (**Fig. 94-4**). The normal compensatory response to exercise involves a rise in blood pressure and heart rate resulting from an increase in cardiac output, peripheral vasoconstriction in inactive muscles, and vasodilation in active muscles. The onset of near-syncope in patients with aortic stenosis has been associated with a large reduction in blood pressure and cardiac output to resting levels in the absence of appropriate reflex vasoconstriction. Patients with aortic stenosis and a history of exertional syncope develop paradoxical forearm vasodilation during leg exercise. This muscular vasodilation is presumed to be caused by activation of mechanosensitive vagal afferents in response to an outflow obstruction–associated increase in left ventricular end-diastolic pressure. The net effect of this process is a reflex vasodilation. However, the vasodilator response is not accompanied by bradycardia, suggesting that the syncopal response to exertion in aortic stenosis is primarily vasodepressor rather than cardioinhibitory in nature.

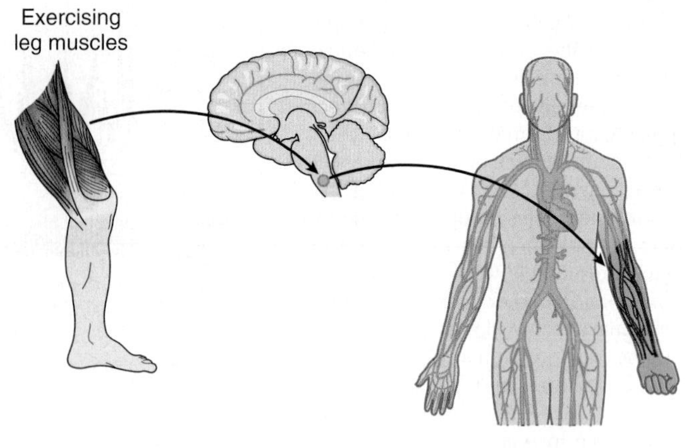

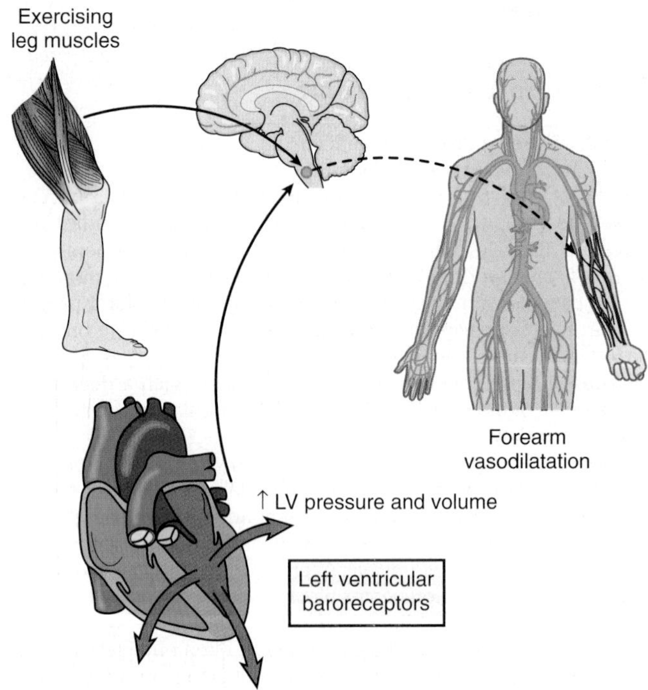

FIGURE 94-4 Syncope in severe aortic stenosis. The schematic shows how afferent impulses from exercising leg muscles relayed to the brainstem normally elicit reflex vasoconstriction in the nonexercising forearm. However, in patients with severe aortic stenosis, increased left ventricular pressure and volume during exercise inhibits and even reverses forearm vasoconstriction by inducing sympathetic withdrawal during exercise. This sympathetic withdrawal has the potential to result in exertional syncope. *(Modified from Mark AL: The Bezold-Jarisch reflex revisited: Clinical implications of inhibitory reflexes originating in the heart. J Am Coll Cardiol 1:90, 1983.)*

Renal Failure and Hemodialysis

Acute hypotension is a common complication of hemodialysis, although the precise cause is poorly defined (**Fig. 94-5**; see Chap. 93). Presumably, the mechanism may be similar to that in hypotension associated with acute hemorrhage, in which there is paradoxical sympathetic withdrawal, vasodilation, and bradycardia. This appears to result from activation of cardiac vagal afferents caused by tachycardia and decreased ventricular filling. Hypotension-prone hemodialysis patients have an initial tachycardia, sympathetic activation, and vasoconstriction, followed by profound hypotension caused by paradoxical bradycardia, vasodilation, and sympathetic inhibition. This is different from patients not prone to hypotension who exhibit progressive rises in heart rate and sympathetic activity during dialysis. Furthermore, there is a clear difference in cardiac adaptation to changes in fluid volume, with hypotension-prone patients exhibiting a progressive reduction to near-obliteration of left ventricular end-systolic dimensions, whereas there is little change in hypotension-resistant patients. This suggests that the mechanism whereby hypotension develops in hypotension-prone hemodialysis patients may be via excessive myocardial contraction around an empty chamber, resulting in activation of ventricular mechanoreceptors and consequent cardiac inhibition. The differential diagnosis of hypotension during dialysis should also include simple hypovolemia, pericardial effusion with development of tamponade as cardiac filling pressures decrease, and cardiac ischemia.

Right Coronary Thrombolysis

Patients with right coronary artery occlusion following intracoronary thrombolytic therapy and resultant reperfusion exhibit a greater incidence of bradycardia and hypotension (≈80%) than patients with left coronary occlusion (≈14%; see Chap. 58). This perceived difference may be caused in part by the preferential distribution of inhibitory cardiac receptors in the inferoposterior wall of the ventricle. Activation of the inhibitory reflex may be caused by sudden improvement in contractile force of the previously akinetic segment of myocardium, resulting in activation of mechanosensitive vagal afferents, or by the release of free radicals and other metabolic products, resulting in activation of chemosensitive vagal afferents.

Inferior Wall Myocardial Infarction

As noted, there is a preferential localization of inhibitory cardiac receptors in the inferoposterior wall of the left ventricle. With infarction, there would be an expected reflex tachycardia, and this is often the case in patients who suffer from an anterior wall infarction. However, patients suffering from an inferior wall infarction (see Chap. 55) may have a relatively increased incidence of bradycardia and hypotension. During Prinzmetal angina, spasm of vessels supplying the inferior wall more often results in bradycardia when compared with spasm of those vessels supplying the anterior wall, which more often results in tachycardia. This reflex activation of cardiac inhibitory signals also appears to result in inhibition of renal sympathetic activity, further potentiating neurogenic hypotension.

Reflex reduction in cardiac afterload and heart rate may be beneficial in the context of myocardial infarction caused by a decrease in myocardial oxygen demand. Thus, low-grade activation of the cardiac inhibitory reflex may conceivably contribute to the more favorable prognosis associated with inferior wall myocardial infarction.

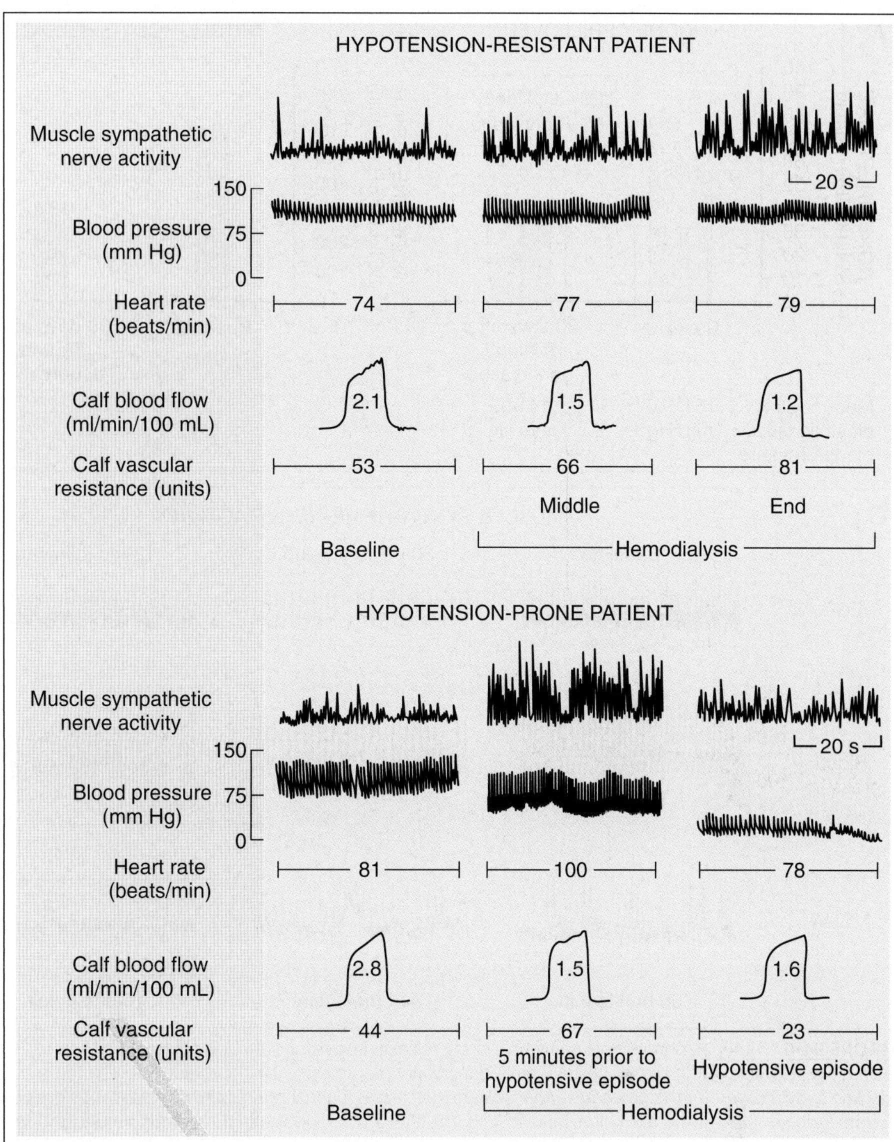

FIGURE 94-5 Mechanisms of hypotension during hemodialysis. **Top,** Measurements in a patient resistant to dialysis-induced hypotension. **Bottom,** Measurements in a patient prone to hypotension during dialysis. In a hypotension-resistant patient, hemodialysis induces a gradual increase in sympathetic activity and accompanying fall in calf blood flow and increased vascular resistance. This vasoconstriction works in concert with increased heart rate to maintain blood pressure. However, in a hypotension-prone patient, hemodialysis initially induces sympathetic activation that is qualitatively similar to that in the hypotension-resistant patient. However, further hemodialysis causes a marked fall in BP, with an associated reduction in sympathetic nerve activity, heart rate, and vascular resistance. This is likely caused by activation of ventricular mechanoreceptors because of volume depletion in the setting of tachycardia and increased contractility, resulting in a relative bradycardia and sympathetic inhibition with vasodilation and consequent profound hypotension. *(From Converse RL, Jacobsen TN, Jost CMT, et al: Paradoxical withdrawal of reflex vasoconstriction as a cause of hemodialysis-induced hypotension. J Clin Invest 90:1657, 1992.)*

Hypertrophic Obstructive Cardiomyopathy

Syncope in hypertrophic obstructive cardiomyopathy (HCM) is associated with a high risk of sudden death (see Chap. 69). In these patients, sudden death has generally been associated with a tendency to develop malignant arrhythmias. However, patients with HCM also demonstrate syncope during sinus rhythm and an abnormal blood pressure response to exercise, suggesting that activation of left ventricular baroreceptors may cause the associated hypotension and hemodynamic collapse. The predisposition to hypotension and bradycardia in these patients appears to result from activation of left ventricular mechanoreceptors. Studies with tilt-table testing in these patients resulted in hypotension in a significant number of patients with a prior history of syncope. Head-up tilt was paired with echocardiography, which revealed reduced cavity sizes and increased fractional shortening with head-up tilt, consistent with conditions that would be favorable to activation of left ventricular mechanoreceptors. This suggests that the cause of syncope in patients with HCM may not just be malignant arrhythmias but may also occur because of inappropriate activation of inhibitory left ventricular mechanoreceptors in response to vigorous ventricular contraction or reduced ventricular cavity size.

Blood Phobia

Many people suffer from blood or injury phobia and experience syncope or presyncope in response to these visual stimuli. Syncope in these patients has been thought to be largely neurogenic and anticipatory in origin because of the high correlation with situational stressors. It has been suggested that patients suffering from syncope secondary to blood or injury phobia actually have an underlying predisposition toward neurocardiogenic syncope. Patients with a history of blood phobia syncope have been shown to have a higher rate of tilt-induced syncope than controls. These findings suggest that fainting in response to blood or injury may be caused by dysfunction in neural circulatory control and has an associated organic origin. It has been proposed that this dysfunction may secondarily lead to the phobia because of repeated syncopal events.

Disorders of Increased Sympathetic Outflow

Increased sympathetic outflow may occur in a number of diseases, either as a primary event contributing to development of the disease or as secondary to the underlying disease. For example, many patients

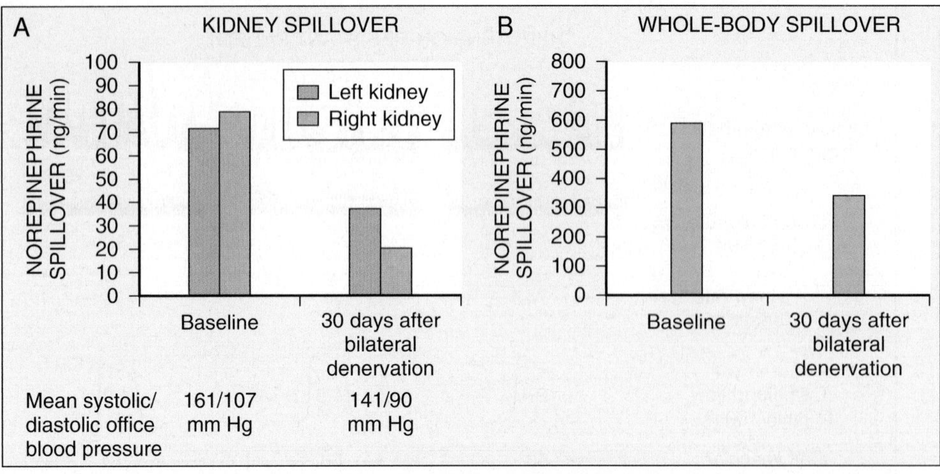

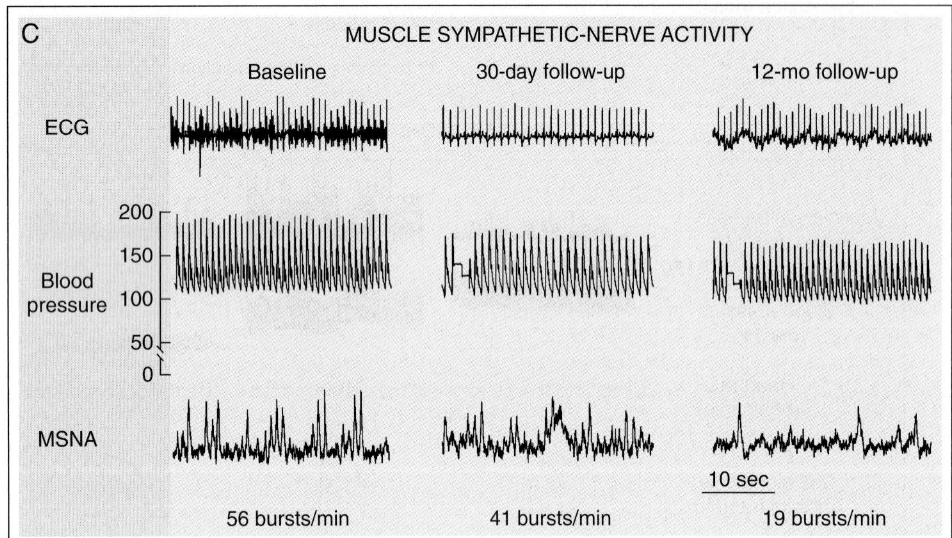

FIGURE 94-6 Norepinephrine renal and whole-body spillover and results of microneurography before and after renal nerve ablation. **A,** Results of bilateral renal denervation, as assessed by the radiotracer dilution method, at baseline and 30 days after the procedure. After ablation, decreases in renal norepinephrine spillover were observed in both kidneys (48% in the left kidney and 75% in the right kidney), indicating substantial modulation of renal sympathetic efferent-nerve activity after the procedure. Simultaneously, a marked reduction in whole-body sympathetic nerve activity was apparent, with a decrease in whole-body norepinephrine spillover of 42% **(B). C,** Reduction in muscle sympathetic nerve activity (MSNA), as assessed in the peroneal nerve on microneurography, after bilateral renal nerve ablation, which highlights the possibility that inhibition of afferent renal nerve activity may contribute to a reduction in central sympathetic drive. *(From Schlaich MP, Sobotka PA, Krum H, et al: Renal sympathetic-nerve ablation for uncontrolled hypertension. N Engl J Med 361:932, 2009.)*

with essential hypertension have chronic sympathetic activation, which may precede the development of sustained hypertension (see Chap. 40). Patients with panic disorder exhibit acute episodes that evoke sympathetic neuronal and adrenomedullary activation, with precipitation of coronary artery spasm. In heart failure patients, chronic elevation in sympathetic tone is noted, as is seen in patients with obstructive sleep apnea, in whom associated hypoxia and hypercapnia during nocturnal apneas may elicit further increases in sympathetic outflow.

Sympathetic activation increases with age, even in the absence of disease,[32] and can contribute to the age-related increased risk of hypertension.[33] Although women have lower muscle sympathetic activity than men, their age-related rise in sympathetic drive is greater, so the difference in sympathetic activation between men and women is attenuated by menopause.

Neurogenic Essential Hypertension

Patients with early essential hypertension (see Chap. 45) may have a hyperdynamic circulation driven by increased efferent sympathetic nerve firing to skeletal muscle and elevated levels of norepinephrine in the heart and kidneys. High sympathetic outflow may be secondary to one or more of the following: impaired baroreflex gain, increased chemoreflex gain, insulin resistance, and/or genetic factors. Sympathetic activation stimulates the heart, elevating cardiac output, causing neurally mediated vasoconstriction, and augmenting renin secretion and tubular reabsorption of sodium, increasing total body fluid volume. In the long term, secondary end-organ and vascular changes may sustain established hypertension, even in the absence of overt sympathetic activation and tachycardia.

Recent studies have suggested that catheter-based radiofrequency ablation of renal nerves (efferent sympathetic and afferent sensory) bilaterally in patients with resistant hypertension may elicit significant and sustained (up to 12 months postprocedure) reductions in systolic and diastolic pressure.[34] In a recent case study, bilateral renal sympathetic nerve ablation was accompanied by marked falls in renal sympathetic activity, decrease of renin activity by 50%, reduced whole-body norepinephrine spillover, increased baroreflex gain, and decrease in BP.[35] At 12 months postprocedure, BP remained significantly lower, microneurography showed reduced sympathetic activity, and cardiac MRI showed a decrease in left ventricular mass (**Fig. 94-6**).

Panic Disorder

Cardiovascular events during a panic episode may be triggered by increased sympathetic outflow (see Chap. 91). Although the true risk is unknown, it seems that there may be some increased ischemic heart disease in patients with a history of panic disorder. During a panic attack, sympathetic nerve firing increases, as does adrenomedullary secretion of epinephrine. Patients who describe angina pectoris–like symptoms during a panic attack may or may not have electrocardiographic changes consistent with myocardial ischemia. It has been suggested that some patients may experience angina-like attacks secondary to coronary artery spasm.

Coronary Artery Disease

Sympathetic activity is increased in unstable angina and after a myocardial infarction[32] (see Chap. 54). The heightened sympathetic drive may persist for 6 to 9 months and may be implicated in subsequent cardiovascular morbidity and mortality.

Congestive Heart Failure

The failing heart becomes partly sympathetically denervated (**Fig. 94-7**; see Chap. 27). Thus, historically, adrenergic agonists were used to treat these patients, although this turned out to be more dangerous than helpful. In fact, beta blocker use in these patients contributed to long-term improvement rather than worsening of heart failure. The reason for this may be partially because although there is low myocardial tissue concentration of norepinephrine, cardiac norepinephrine spillover is increased to levels associated with near-maximal aerobic exercise. Heart failure patients may also exhibit baroreflex and chemoreflex dysfunction and disrupted heart rate variability and ventilatory control. In patients

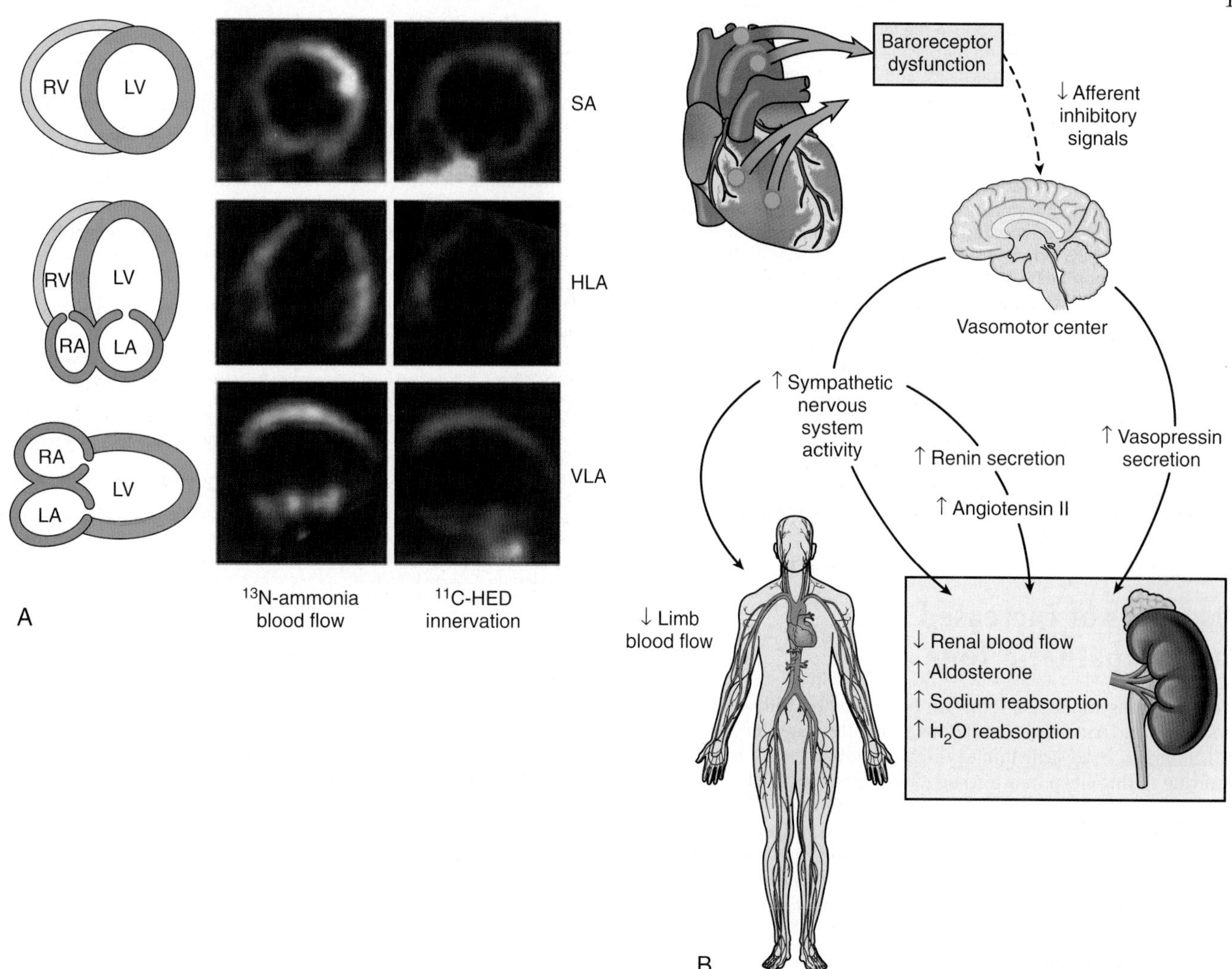

FIGURE 94-7 **A,** Autonomic denervation of the failing heart. Positron emission tomography images obtained from patients with congestive heart failure (CHF) demonstrate that there is partial denervation of the left ventricle in these patients. The images above demonstrate the short-axis (SA), horizontal long-axis (HLA), and vertical long-axis (VLA) views of the heart. Ammonia uptake is seen to be relatively homogeneous, which is consistent with intact myocardial perfusion. C-11 hydroxyephedrine (C-HED) uptake marks innervation of the heart and, in patients with heart failure, there is reduced retention that appears to be relatively heterogeneous, suggesting partial denervation of the left ventricle. A known association exists between the extent of denervation and clinical outcome, with higher degrees of denervation associated with increased mortality. Denervation of the heart may affect cardiac and vascular control secondary to defective afferent autonomic input from mechanoreceptors in the left ventricle. **B,** Increased sympathetic activity in CHF. Baroreceptor dysfunction may partly account for the increased sympathetic activity seen in patients with congestive heart failure. Baroreceptor function is impaired in heart failure, in part because of partial sympathetic denervation of the heart. Thus, inhibitory input from cardiac mechanoreceptors is decreased, despite increased intracardiac volumes. Typically, stimulation of these mechanoreceptors via increased stretch will result in vasodilation and depression of renal sympathetic nerve activity. However, because of partial denervation, there is a lack of appropriate inhibition of the sympathetic nervous system, leading to excess sympathetic activity to the kidney, worsening fluid retention, and to peripheral blood vessels, potentiating vasoconstriction. Therefore, partial denervation of cardiac mechanoreceptors may result in a neural circulatory profile mimicking that seen in hypovolemia and may, in part, explain the sympathetic activation and fluid retention seen in heart failure. *(**A,** from Schwaiger M, Bengal F: Atlas of Heart Diseases: Nuclear Cardiology. In Dilsizian V, Narula J, Braunwald E [series eds]: Current Medicine LLC, Philadelphia, PA, 2006; **B,** modified from Nohria A, Cusco J, Creager M: Atlas of Heart Diseases: Heart Failure. In Colucci WS, Braunwald E [series eds]: Current Medicine LLC, Philadelphia, PA, 2004.)*

with dilated cardiomyopathy, the presence of sleep apnea may further increase cardiac sympathetic activation,[36] perhaps because of heightened central chemosensitivity.[37] Increased cardiac sympathetic activation, altered baroreflex gain, chemoreflex dysfunction, blunted heart rate variability, and disordered breathing control have been associated with poorer long-term outcomes. It has been proposed that development of heart failure and increase in sympathetic outflow may occur in conjunction with and feed off one another to affect cardiac status further adversely. Although cardiac transplantation may improve some of the autonomic disturbances seen in heart failure, residual autonomic dysfunction may persist.

Obstructive Sleep Apnea

An increase in sympathetic outflow occurs during both sleep and waking hours in patients with obstructive sleep apnea (OSA; see Chap. 79). This is in part caused by the hypoxemia and hypercapnia during apneic episodes. During waking hours, the increased sympathetic outflow may be related to increased tonic chemoreflex sensitivity. Most OSA patients are also obese, and the interaction between obesity and OSA in increasing sympathetic activity awaits further clarification. Continuous positive airway pressure treatment during sleep appears to attenuate sympathetic outflow, even during daytime wakefulness.

Pheochromocytoma

Pheochromocytoma is a rare catecholamine-secreting tumor derived from the chromaffin cells of the adrenal gland or the paraganglion chromaffin tissue of the sympathetic nervous system (see Chaps. 45 and 86). Most commonly, these tumors arise from the adrenal glands, but it is also possible to develop extra-adrenal pheochromocytomas in the sympathetic ganglia anywhere from the brain to the bladder. Because of the increased secretion of catecholamines, there is excess sympathetic drive, resulting in life-threatening hypertension or cardiac arrhythmias. The excess secretion is associated with lack of normal innervation to the adrenal medulla. The exact mechanism of secretion is not completely clear, although it may be caused by direct pressure or changes in tumor blood flow. Pheochromocytomas may also be sporadic or familial, with primarily norepinephrine secretion in the former and epinephrine in the latter. Diagnosis requires testing for plasma metanephrine, which has a higher sensitivity and lower specificity, and 24-hour urine collection for total catecholamines, vanillylmandelic acid, and metanephrines, which have a higher specificity and lower sensitivity. Computed tomography (CT) of the abdomen and pelvis is the typical imaging modality used but is neither the most sensitive nor the most specific, particularly for adrenal tumors smaller than 1 cm. MRI has almost 100% sensitivity for detection of adrenal pheochromocytomas. When the clinical suspicion is high because of positive laboratory test results but imaging reveals no source, a scan with ^{131}I-MIBG may be useful. Definitive treatment is via surgical resection with appropriate alpha and beta blockade preoperatively.

Sleep-Associated Disorders

In general, parasympathetic tone increases during non–rapid eye movement (REM) sleep. This is associated with a fall in heart rate during sleep. However, REM sleep, which is predominant in the later hours of sleep, just before waking, may be associated with significant sympathetic activation.[38] This may be relevant to nocturnal angina associated with REM and to the predominance of cardiac events during the early waking hours following sleep. Although parasympathetic activity largely dominates sleep, the increase in sympathetic outflow during REM sleep, when dreams are most likely to occur, may conceivably contribute to tachycardia and cardiac ischemia.

Disorders of Increased Parasympathetic Tone

Increased parasympathetic tone can be associated with a number of physiologic and pathologic conditions, including weight loss and spinal cord trauma.[39] Bradyarrhythmias, such as Mobitz type I heart block occurring during sleep, may also be caused by abrupt but physiologic increases in parasympathetic tone during REM sleep[38] (see Chap. 39). Also, the decrease in resting heart rate seen in well-conditioned athletes may be associated with an elevated parasympathetic outflow at rest. However, in general, pathologic disorders of sympathetic outflow are more common than those of parasympathetic tone.

Sinus Arrhythmia

Under normal circumstances, the heart is under parasympathetic dominance. Variations from the resting state occur with each breath because of the influence of breathing on the flow of sympathetic and vagal activity to the sinoatrial node.[40] With inhalation, vagus nerve activity is inhibited and heart rate begins to increase. With exhalation, this process reverses. This variation of heart rate with breathing is normal and is a sign of cardiac health. Absence of heart rate change with inspiration suggests cardiac disease and disturbed or diseased neural circulatory control (see Chap. 39).

Future Perspectives

Dysautonomias and other autonomic disorders can be debilitating and are often difficult to treat. Challenges in diagnosing and treating autonomic disorders include the ubiquitous nature of the autonomic nervous system, difficulties in differentiating autonomic symptoms from those caused by emotional or psychological disorders, relative paucity of quantitative measurements of autonomic dysfunction, and difficulties in accessing and modulating autonomic neural control. For example, evaluating cardiac sympathetic innervation requires expensive imaging techniques or invasive measures of cardiac norepinephrine spillover, and cardiac vagal activation is usually extrapolated from measures of heart rate control.

Technologies for inexpensive, noninvasive, and accurate measures of human autonomic tone are sorely needed to advance diagnosis and modulate therapeutic interventions. Improvements in information technology and rapid signal acquisition and processing are already forming the foundation for acutely responsive software and hardware, which can sense hemodynamic changes and respond in quick but measured fashion (e.g., could be enabled by an artificial baroreflex[41] or implanted cardiac[42] or vascular assist device). These could mimic autonomic function by modulating blood pressure via pharmacologic intervention (infusion of vasoactive agents) or triggering physical maneuvers, as needed.

Recent insights into the role of autonomic innervation of the heart and great vessels and the usefulness of ablation in treating tachyarrythmias have also renewed interest in cardiac ganglia and their role in potentiating or inhibiting cardiac electrical instability. As methods develop for accessing these ganglia safely in humans, it is likely that therapeutic innovations will emerge that are based on perturbing or inhibiting their structure and function.

REFERENCES

Neural Circulatory Control

1. Robertson RH, Robertson D: Cardiovascular manifestations of autonomic disorders. *In* Zipes DP, Libby P, Bonow R, Braunwald E (eds): Braunwald's Heart Disease: A Textbook of Cardiovascular Disease, 7th edition. Philadelphia, WB Saunders, 2004, pp 2173-2184.
2. Ditting T, Hilgers KF, Scrogin KE, et al: Influence of short-term versus long-term cardiopulmonary receptor stimulation on renal and preganglionic adrenal sympathetic nerve activity in rats. Basic Res Cardiol 101:223, 2006.
3. DiBona GF: Physiology in perspective: The wisdom of the body: Neural control of the kidney. Am J Physiol Regul Integr Comp Physiol 289:R633, 2005.
4. Spicuzza L, Porta C, Bramanti A, et al: Interaction between central-peripheral chemoreflexes and cerebro-cardiovascular control. Clin Auton Res 15:373, 2005.
5. Caples SM, Gami A, Somers VK: Obstructive sleep apnea. Ann Intern Med 142:187, 2005.
6. Schrezenmaier C, Singer W, Swift NM, et al: Adrenergic and vagal baroreflex sensitivity in autonomic failure. Arch Neurol 64:381, 2007.

Autonomic Testing

7. Cooke WH, Convertino VA: Heart rate variability and spontaneous baroreflex sequences: Implications for autonomic monitoring during hemorrhage. J Trauma Inj Infect Crit Care 58:798, 2005.
8. Soriano F, Nogueira A, Cappi S, et al: Heart dysfunction and heart rate variability prognoses in sepsis. Crit Care 8:P75, 2005.
9. Cygankiewicz I, Wojciech Z, Vazquez R, et al: Heart rate turbulence predicts all-cause mortality and sudden death in congestive heart failure patients. Heart Rhythm 5:1095, 2008.
10. Tiukinhoy S: Heart rate profile during exercise as a predictor of sudden death. J Cardiopul Rehab 25:387, 2005.

Orthostatic Hypotension

11. Maule S, Papotti G, Naso D, et al: Orthostatic hypotension: Evaluation and treatment. Cardiovasc Hematol Disord Drug Targets 7:63, 2007.
12. Low PA, Singer W: Management of neurogenic orthostatic hypotension: An update. Lancet Neurol 7:451, 2008.
13. Mosnaim AD, Abiola R, Wolf ME, Perlmuter LC: Etiology and risk factors for developing orthostatic hypotension. Am J Ther 17:86, 2010.

Autonomic Dysregulation

14. Gilman S, Wenning GK, Low PA, et al: Second consensus statement on the diagnosis of multisystem atrophy. Neurology 71:670, 2008.
15. Lipp A, Sandroni P, Ahlskog E, et al: Prospective differentiation of multisystem atrophy from Parkinson disease, with and without autonomic failure. Arch Neurol 66:742, 2009.
16. Skrapari I, Tentolouris N, Katsilambros N: Baroreflex function: Determinants in health subjects and disturbances in diabetes, obesity and metabolic syndrome. Curr Diabetes Rev 2:329, 2006.
17. Pop-Busui R, Low PA, Waberski BH, et al: Effects of prior intensive insulin therapy on cardiac autonomic nervous system function in type 1 diabetes mellitus: The Diabetes Control and Complications Trial/Epidemiology of Diabetes Interventions and Complications Study. Circulation 119:2886, 2009.
18. Ito T, Sakakibara R, Yamamoto T, et al: Urinary dysfunction and autonomic control in amyloid neuropathy. Clin Auton Res 16:66, 2006.
19. Wang AK, Fealey RD, Gehrking TL, Low PA: Patterns of neuropathy and autonomic failure in patients with amyloidosis. Mayo Clin Proc 83:1226, 2008.
20. Koomans HA, Blankestijn PJ, Joles JA: Sympathetic hyperactivity in chronic renal failure: A wake-up call. J Am Soc Nephrol 15:524, 2004.
21. Low PA: Autonomic neuropathies. Curr Opin Neurol 15:605, 2002.
22. Schroeder C, Vernino S, Birkenfeld AL, et al: Plasma exchange for primary autoimmune autonomic failure. N Engl J Med 353:1585, 2005.
23. Vincent S, Robertson D: The broader view: Catecholamine abnormalities. Clin Auton Res 12(Suppl):I44, 2002.
24. Low PA, Sandroni P, Joyner MJ, Shen W-K: Postural tachycardia syndrome. *In* Low PA, Benarroch EE (eds): Clinical Autonomic Disorders. 3rd ed. Philadelphia, Lippincott Williams & Wilkins, 2008, pp 515-533.
25. Low PA, Sandroni P, Joyner M, Shen WK: Postural tachycardia syndrome (POTS). J Cardiovasc Electrophysiol 20:352, 2009.
26. Masuki S, Eisenach JH, Johnson CP, et al: Excessive heart rate response to orthostatic stress in postural tachycardia syndrome is not caused by anxiety. J Appl Physiol 102:896, 2007.
27. Masuki S, Eisenach JH, Schrage WG, et al: Arterial baroreflex control of heart rate during exercise in postural tachycardia syndrome. J Appl Physiol 103:1136, 2007.
28. Raj SR, Black BK, Biaggioni I, et al: Propranolol decreased tachycardia and improves symptoms in the postural tachycardia syndrome—less is more. Circulation 120:725, 2009.
29. Alboni P, Brignole M, Degli Uberti EC: Is vasovagal syncope a disease? Europace 9:83, 2007.
30. Moya A, Sutton R, Ammirati F, et al: Guidelines for the diagnosis and management of syncope (version 2009). The task force for the diagnosis and management of syncope of the European Society of Cardiology (ESC). Developed in collaboration with the European Heart Rhythm

Association (EHRA), Heart Failure Association (HFA), and Heart Rhythm Society (HRS). Eur Heart J 30:2631, 2009.

31. Parry SW, Steen N, Tynan M, et al: Pacing in elderly recurrent fallers with carotid sinus hypersensitivity: A randomised, double-blind, placebo controlled crossover trial. Heart 95:405, 2009.

Disorders of Increased Sympathetic Outflow

32. Charkoudian N, Rabbitts JA: Sympathetic neural mechanisms in human cardiovascular health and disease. Mayo Clin Proc 84:822, 2009.
33. Narkiewicz K, Phillips BG, Kato M, et al: Gender-selective interactions between aging, blood pressure, and sympathetic nerve activity. Hypertension 45:522, 2005.
34. Krum H, Schlaich M, Whitbourn R, et al: Catheter-based renal sympathetic denervation for resistant hypertension: A multi-centre safety and proof-of-principle cohort study. Lancet 373:1275, 2009.
35. Schlaich MP, Sobotka PA, Krum H, et al: Renal sympathetic-nerve ablation for uncontrolled hypertension. N Engl J Med 361:932, 2009.
36. Nanjo S, Yamashiro Y, Fujimoto S, et al: Evaluation of sympathetic activity by ^{123}I-metaiodobenzylguanidine myocardial scintigraphy in dilated cardiomyopathy patients with sleep breathing disorder. Circ J 73:686, 2009.
37. Mequro K, Toyama T, Adachi H, et al: Assessment of central chemosensitivity and cardiac sympathetic nerve activity using I-123 MIBG imaging in central sleep apnea syndrome in patients with dilated cardiomyopathy. Ann Nucl Med 21:73, 2007.
38. Verrier RL, Josephson ME: Impact of sleep on arrhythmogenesis. Circ Arrhythmia Electrophysiol 2:450, 2009.

Disorders of Increased Parasympathetic Tone

39. Gondim FAA, Lopes ACA, Oliveira GR, et al: Cardiovascular control after spinal cord injury. Curr Vasc Pharmacol 2:71, 2004.
40. Grossman P, Wilhelm, FH, Spoerle M: Respiratory sinus arrhythmia, cardiac vagal control, and daily activity. Am J Physiol Heart Circ Physiol 287:H728, 2004.

Future Perspectives

41. Yamasaki F, Ushida T, Yokoyama T, et al: Artificial baroreflex: Clinical application of a bionic baroreflex system. Circulation 113:634, 2006.
42. Birks EJ, Tansley PD, Hardy J, et al: Left ventricular assist device and drug therapy for the reversal of heart failure. New Engl J Med 355:1873, 2006.

DISCLOSURE INDEX

The following contributors have indicated that they have a relationship that, in the context of their participation in the writing of a chapter for the ninth edition of *Braunwald's Heart Disease,* could be perceived by some people as a real or apparent conflict of interest, but do not consider that it has influenced the writing of their chapter. Codes for the disclosure information (institution[s] and nature of relationship[s]) are provided below.

Relationship Codes

A—Stock options or bond holdings in a for-profit corporation or self-directed pension plan
B—Research grants
C—Employment (full or part-time)
D—Ownership or partnership
E—Consulting fees or other remuneration received by the contributor or immediate family
F—Nonremunerative positions, such as board member, trustee, or public spokesperson
G—Receipt of royalties
H—"Speaker's bureau"

Institution and Company Codes

001—Abbott Laboratories
002—Abiomed
003—ACC & ABIM
004—Accumetrics
005—Acorn Cardiovascular
006—Actelion Pharmaceuticals
007—Active Biotic
008—Adolor
009—AGA Medical
010—Alexion Pharmaceuticals
011—Alnylam
012—Alteon
013—American Board of Vascular Medicine
014—American College of Nutrition
015—American Heart Association
016—Amgen
017—Amorcyte Inc.
018—Anexon
019—Angiodynamics
020—Apnex
021—Apotex
022—Aptus Endosystems, Inc.
023—ARCA
024—Arena
025—Armgo Pharma
026—Arstasis
027—Astellas
028—AstraZeneca, Inc.
029—AtheroGenics, Inc.
030—Atlas Venture Advisors, Inc.
031—Automedics
032—Avanir
033—Aventis
034—Baker Brothers Advisors LLC
035—Barr-Teva Litigation
036—BASS Medical
037—Bayer Healthcare
038—Bayer Italy
039—Beckman-Coulter
040—Berkeley Heart Labs
041—BG Medicine
042—BGB-New York
043—Biomarin Pharmaceuticals
044—Bioscience Webster
045—Biosite, Inc.
046—Biotronik
047—Blackwell Publishing
048—Bluhm Cardiovascular Institute
049—BMS
050—BMS-Sanofi
051—Boeringer Ingelheim
052—Boston Scientific Corporation
053—Boston Scientific Inc.
054—Bracco
055—Brahms
056—Bristol Meyers Squibb, Co.
057—Bristol Meyers Squibb, Co. & BMS-Sanofi
058—Cardiac Concepts Inc.
059—Cardiac Dimensions
060—Cardio DX
061—CardioDynamics
062—Cardiokine Inc.
063—CardioMems Inc.
064—CDC
065—Centocor
066—Certification Board of Cardiovascular Computed Tomography
067—CHF Solutions
068—Circ HF
069—Circulation
070—Clinical Data Inc.
071—Cook Medical Inc.
072—Cordis Corporation
073—Corthera
074—Critical Diagnostics
075—Cryocor
076—Current Protocols in Human Genetics
077—CV Therapeutics, Inc.
078—Cytokinetics, Inc.
079—Dade Behring
080—Daiichi Sankyo
081—DebioPharm
082—Dime
083—Drugs for the Heart
084—Duke University
085—E Z EM
086—Edwards Lifesciences
087—Eisai
088—Eli Lilly and Company
089—Elsevier
090—Emisphere
091—Encysive
092—Endologix, Inc.
093—ErreKappa Terapeutici
094—European Union
095—F. Hoffmann–La Roche Ltd.
096—FoldRx
097—Forest Labs
098—GE Healthcare
099—Gene Ox
100—Genentech
101—Genzyme
102—Geron
103—Gilead Sciences
104—Glaxo SmithKline
105—Griffin & Schwartz Scientific Services
106—GSK
107—Guidant Corporation
108—Heart Ware
109—I3DNL
110—IBM
111—Intekrin Therapeutics
112—Interleukin Genetics
113—Int'l Life Sciences Health & Environmental Sciences Institue
114—Inverness Medical Inc.
115—ISIS
116—Johnson & Johnson
117—Kowa Research Institute
118—LabCorp
119—Laboratory of Molecular Medicine/ HPCGG
120—Lantheus Medical Imaging
121—Lippincott
122—LPath
123—Lung RX

124—Mallinckrodt
125—MAP Pharmaceuticals
126—Massachusetts Medical Society, Mayo Press
127—Mayo Health Solutions and Industry Partners
128—Medicines Company
129—Medicure
130—Medscape
131—Medtronic Vascular
132—Medtronic, Inc.
133—Merck & Co., Inc.
134—Merck-Schering Plough Corp.
135—Merck Cardiovascular Scientific
136—MG Medicine
137—Millennium Pharmaceuticals
138—Mitsubishi-Tanabe Pharma
139—Molecular Insight Pharmaceuticals
140—Myogen
141—Nanosphere
142—National Heart, Lung and Blood Institute
143—NCME
144—Nektar Therapeutics
145—Neurological Technologies
146—NIH
147—NIH/Agency for Healthcare Research and Quality
148—Nitromed
149—NormOxys
150—Northpoint Domain
151—NovaCardia
152—Novartis, Inc.
153—Ortho-Clinical Diagnostics
154—Otsuka Pharmaceuticals
155—PeriCor Therapeutics
156—Pfizer, Inc.
157—PGxHealth
158—Philips Medical
159—Physical logic
160—Pixel Velocity
161—Preventicum
162—Prime
163—Private companies
164—Proctor and Gamble
165—Protein Design Labs
166—Regado
167—Regeneron
168—Reliant Pharmaceuticals
169—Resmed Foundation
170—Respironics
171—Roche Diagnostics
172—SAB
173—Sanofi-Aventis
174—Sapphire Therapeutics, Inc.
175—Schering
176—Schering Plough Corp.
177—Sciele, Inc.
178—Scios, Inc.
179—Select research
180—Servier France
181—Shionogi
182—Siemens
183—Siemens Medical Solutions
184–Sigma Tau
185—Society of Cardiac Angiography and Interventions
186—Society of cardiovascular computed tomography
187—Society of Chest Pain Centers
188—Solvay Pharmaceuticals
189—Sorin Medical
190—Springer
191—St. Jude Medical
192—Stereotaxis
193—T2 BioSystems
194—T2cure
195—Takeda
196—Terumo Heart, Inc.
197—Tethys
198—Thoratec
199—Toshiba
200—Translational Research in Oncology
201—TriVascular Inc.,
202—United Health
203—United Therapeutics, Inc.
204—University of California
205—UpToDate (Wolters-Kluwer)
206—VA
207—Vanderbilt/Genaissance
208—Vascular Biogenics
209—Vascular Disease foundation
210—Vasculitis Foundation
211—Ventracor Inc.
212—Vertex
213—Viacor
214—Vifor
215—Visen Scientific
216—Vitae Pharamceutical
217—W.L. Gore & Associates, Inc.
218—Wyeth
219—Xceed Molecular Scientific Advisory Board
220—Xoma
221—Zoll

Contributors

Ackerman, Michael J. F-052, F-132, F-157, F-191, G-157
Ades, Philip A. B-146
Antman, Elliott M. B-080, B-088, B-173, F-015
Bhatt, Deepak L. B-028, B-056, B-087, B-128, B-173
Boden, William E. B-001, E-001, E-103, E-117, E-173, H-001, H-056, H-103, H-173
Bonow, Robert O. E-086
Bremner, James Douglas B-146, B-206
Cannon, Christopher A-031, B-004, B-028, B-104, B-111, B-133, B-195, E-011, E-057, E-152
Canty, John M. Jr. B-146, B-206, C-206
Chaitman, Bernard B-098
Creager, Marc B-146, E-101, E-134, E-149, F-013, F-209, G-089, G-190
Dilsizian, Vasken A-098, A-139, B-098, E-027, E-098, E-120, E-139
Douglas, Pamela S. B-002, B-016, B-086, B-125, B-142, B-147, B-213, C-084, E-060, E-200
Emanuel, Linda B-146, B-147, G-089
Felker, Michael B-016, B-041, B-078, B-116, B-142, B-171, E-016, E-041, E-078, E-102, E-171
Filippatos, Gerasimos B-073, B-094, B-114, B-141, B-171, B-184, B-214
Fisher, Stacy D. H-006
Force, Thomas H-133, H-134
Gaziano, Michael John B-016, E-037
Gheorghiade, Mihai E-001, E-027, E-028, E-037, E-073, E-078, E-081, E-093, E-104, E-116, E-132, E-133, E-152, E-154, E-155, E-165, E-173, E-184, E-188
Goldberger, Ary L. B-146, G-089
Goldhaber, Samuel Z. B-049, B-051, B-087, B-116, E-130, B-173, E-049, E-051, E-087, E-173
Gray, Andrew T. C-204
Greenberg, Barry A-122, B-146, E-045, E-077, E-103, E-132, H-103, H-133, H-152, H-173
Groh, William J. E-088
Hayes, David L. E-046, E-052, E-132, E-191, E-189, E-160, G-047
Jaffer, Farouc A-215, E-215
Jessup, Mariell B-108, F-015, E-053
Kaplan, Norman M. H-051, H-097, G-015, G-121
Krumholz, Harian M. B-147, E-202, F-003
Lange, Richard Allen B-146
Lipshultz B-142, B-146, B-152, B-156, B-171
Mann, Douglas L. A-062, B-142, E-005, E-104, E-132, F-025, G-089
Maron, Barry B-132, E-099
McGuire, Darren K. E-080, E-095, E-138, E-197
McManus, Bruce B-027, B-156
Mehra, Mandeep R. B-142, B-146, E-102, E-104, E-116, E-132, E-191
Miller, John M. E-052, E-132, E-191, E-192
Mirvis, David G-089, G-205
Morady, Fred E-107, E-132, E-191
Mueller, Paul S. E-053, E-126, G-126
Myerburg, Robert J. E-051, E-104, E-142, E-168, E-173, H-052, H-098, H-173, H-191
Newby, Kristin L. B-049, B-104, B-133, B-166, B-176, E-028, E-104, E-181, F-187
O'Gara, Patrick E-120, B-146
Oh, Jae K. B-146, B-199, G-121
Olgin, Jeffrey B-044, B-053, B-132, B-191, B-221
Opie, Lionel G-083, G-089
Otto, Catherine M. G-089, G-205
Redfield, Margaret M. B-130, B-146, B-218, E-068, E-152
Ridker, Paul M. B-016, B-028, B-146, E-101, E-208, G-028, G-079, G-182
Roden, Dan B-146, C-023, C-027, C-032, C-080, C-135, C-156, C-173, C-216, G-070
Rubart-von der Lohe, Michael B-146
Sabatine, Marc S. B-028, B-055, B-056, B-080, B-153, B-173, B-176, F-056, F-080, F-173, H-088
Sanchez, Luis A. E-022, E-071, E-092, E-201, E-217, E-131

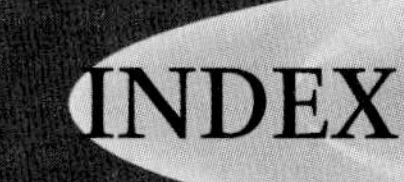

INDEX

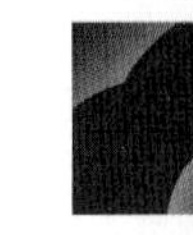

INDEX

INDEX

D

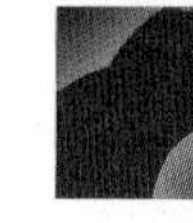

INDEX

INDEX

N

INDEX

S

W

X

Y

Z